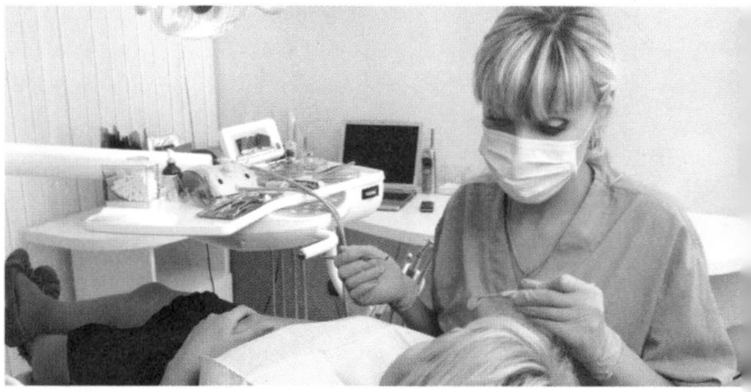

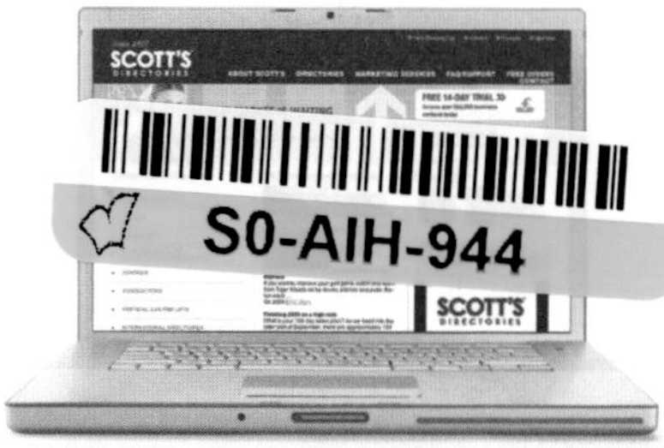

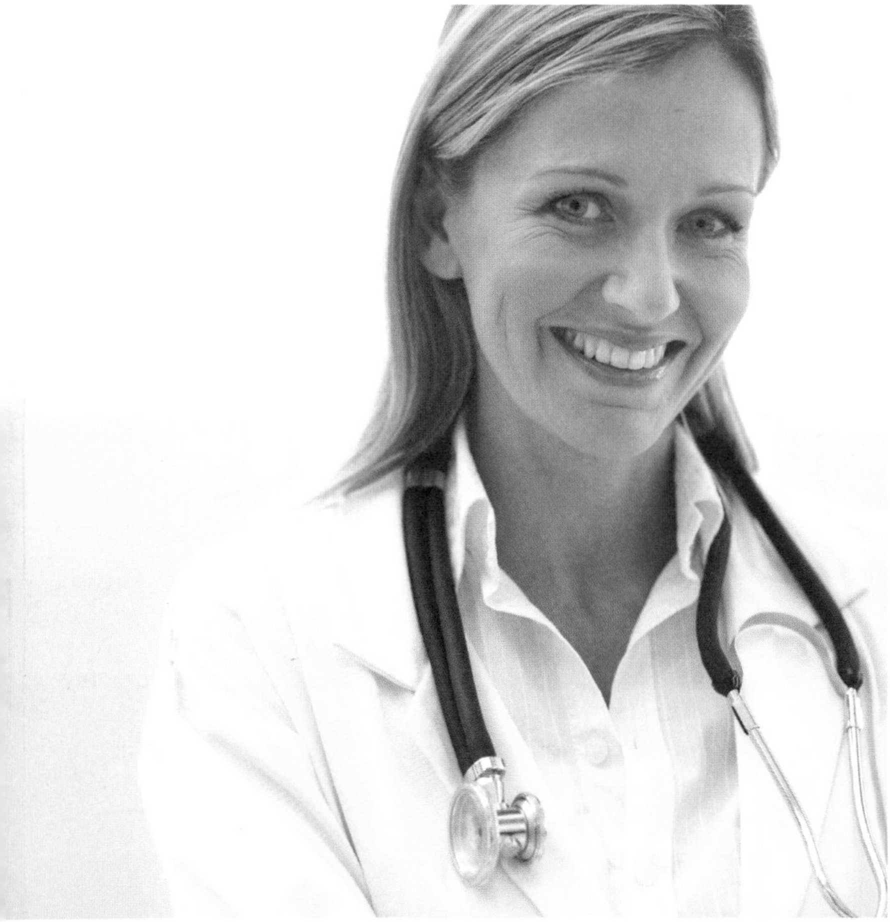

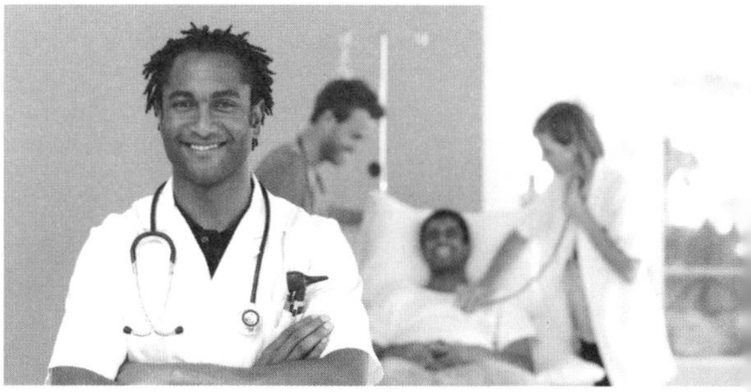

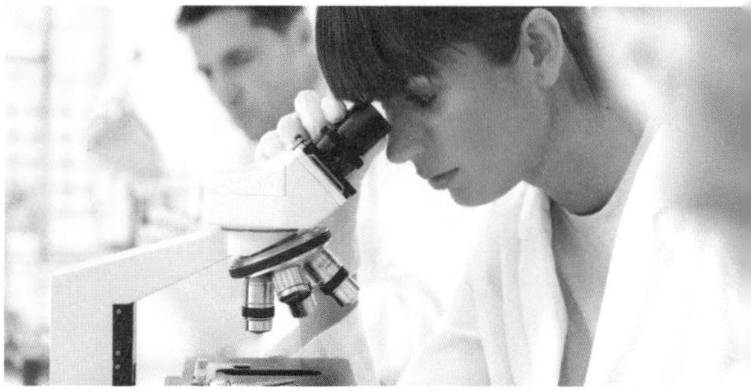

59th Edition

CANADIAN MEDICAL DIRECTORY

Published by Scott's Directories
BIG Directories Limited Partnership
In association with the Canadian Medical Association
80 Valleybrook Dr., Toronto, Ontario M3B 2S9
Email: medical@scottsdirectories.com

Group Publisher
Paul Stuckey

Director, Data Services
Cindy Gardiner

Editor
Christopher Rajan
Tel.: (416) 442-5600 X3529 Fax: (416) 510-5128

Assistant Editor
Asha Bajaj

Senior Technical Editor
Dave de Jong

Technical Editor
Jenna Jozic

Customer Service Desk
Tel: (416) 442-2122 Fax: (416) 442-2191

Medical Data Research Department
Manager, Mila Marvida

Medical Research Clerks:
Babes Andal, Sheila Marbella, Jean Soriano, Silva Telian

Canadian Cataloguing in Publication Data

The National Library of Canada has catalogued this publication as follows:

Canadian Medical Directory

1st (1955)
ISSN 0068-9203
ISBN-13: 978-1-55257-236-8
1. Physicians—Canada—Directories. 2. Surgeons—Canada—Directories.

R713.01C3 610.69'52'02571C75-034334-6

IMPORTANT NOTICE

TABLE OF CONTENTS

SECTION ONE

SECTION TWO

SECTION THREE

SECTION FOUR

SECTION FIVE

SECTION SIX

SECTION SEVEN

NOTE FROM THE EDITOR

Welcome to the 59th edition of the *Canadian Medical Directory!*

Scott's Directories will soon offer you an easy-to-use web service dedicated to connecting you to the most highly qualified physicians in the country - each of them willing to serve as a Medical Expert. Comprised of nearly **4,700 Medical Experts** across hundreds of Specialties and Subspecialties, our network of medical experts can:

- Testify in a court of law
- Comment on TV, radio and print
- Write medical-legal reports
- Manage clinical trials for pharmaceutical companies . . . and more!

For more detailed information on Canadian hospitals such as administrative and medical personnel; bed size and breakdown; annual budgets and much more, refer to the annual **Directory of Canadian Healthcare Personnel**. This companion edition also contains detailed information on Long Term Care facilities and Medical Clinics and Laboratories from across the country. The directory is available in print and Online.

We acknowledge the participation of the Canadian Medical Association which provides the annual Year in Review section. CMA's participation is limited to providing the annual Year in Review featuring medical news and does not include the sharing of any membership information due to privacy limitations.

The use of personal information in Canadian commercial activities is protected by federal legislation under the Personal Information Protection and Electronic Documents Act (PIPEDA). The Act is not applicable to business contact information which includes business addresses, telephone numbers and fax numbers. When no business address is available, we will confirm the individual's home address and contact information via questionnaire or by telephone. The Canadian Medical Directory intends to continue treating personal information with the same care and concern we have demonstrated in the past. We will respect and protect the privacy of individuals listed in our publications according to the law.

The cooperation of physicians in returning their annual verification forms promptly and fully completed is greatly appreciated — this is THE single most important source for ensuring accuracy in the directory. The Royal College, Provincial Registrars, The College of Family Physicians of Canada, Medical Associations, Health Departments and our own research department are thanked for their continued contributions, without which we could not produce such a comprehensive directory.

The *Canadian Medical Directory* makes every effort to ensure the completeness and accuracy of each edition. However, occasional errors are unavoidable with an undertaking of this size. The onus is on the directory user to confirm doctor fax numbers and email addresses before sending out mass market campaigns. In the event that errors appear, the directory's sole responsibility will be to correct the errors in future editions. Notification of inaccuracies should be sent to: The Editor, Canadian Medical Directory, 80 Valleybrook Dr, Toronto, ON M3B 2S9.

Medical interns and residents are not listed in the directory. This omission is due to the mobility of these physicians, making it difficult to list them accurately. Canadian physicians practising abroad and retired physicians are not listed in the directory.

The directory accepts no responsibility for the improper use of a medical name found in the directory to write a prescription: the final authority of a license to practise medicine rests with the Registrars in each of the provinces and territories.

Verification forms, emails, or other pertinent information regarding listings must be received before April 30th, 2014 for inclusion in the next edition of the directory.

Thank you for using the *Canadian Medical Directory!*

Christopher Rajan

Christopher Rajan, Editor
June 2013

PLEASE NOTE

- **that over 30% of doctors approved their own listings between September 1, 2012, and April 15, 2013.**
- **that changes of address, etc., occurring thereafter have not been incorporated.**
- **and that in the next year 100,000+ changes will be made in the Directory records.**
- **annual editions of the Directory are necessary to provide an up-to-date reference source.**

The preparation of the next edition of the Directory will be simplified if doctors will advise the Canadian Medical Directory, 80 Valleybrook Dr, Toronto, Ontario, Canada M3B 2S9 of all changes of address.

All doctors who can be contacted will be given the opportunity to revise their listings for the next edition.

The publishers of the Canadian Medical Directory make every effort to ensure accuracy, but they do not hold themselves responsible for any consequences that may arise from errors or omissions.

USER'S GUIDE

Please note that over 30% of the listings were compiled or approved by the doctors themselves during a eight month period. However, some doctors may have changed address, etc., outside of that time frame.

The Directory contains seven sections:

- Section One – Biographical listings of physicians, followed by the Index of Languages Spoken
- Section Two – General Practitioners and Family Medicine physicians by geographical location
- Section Three – Certified Specialists by geographic location
- Section Four – Hospitals & Health Centres in Canada and Index
- Section Five – Resource section, including medical associations and universities
- Section Six – Canadian Health Care Associations
- Section Seven – The 2012 Year in Review and the Canadian Medical Hall of Fame

SECTION ONE — PHYSICIANS IN CANADA

In the white pages will be found biographical listings, in alphabetical order, for qualified doctors known to be in Canada at the time of publication, with the exception of those doctors who graduated from Canadian medical schools in 2012. New medical graduates' names are located at the end of Section Five. Interns, hospital residents and retired doctors are excluded from the directory.

The following information is given, when applicable, for each doctor: surname, given name and initials; office address (if in private practice); university and year of graduation; medical degrees, specialist certifications (area of practice); hospital, university appointments; office telephone number, fax number, email address and languages spoken (when indicated).

The alphabetical listing of physicians is arranged as follows:

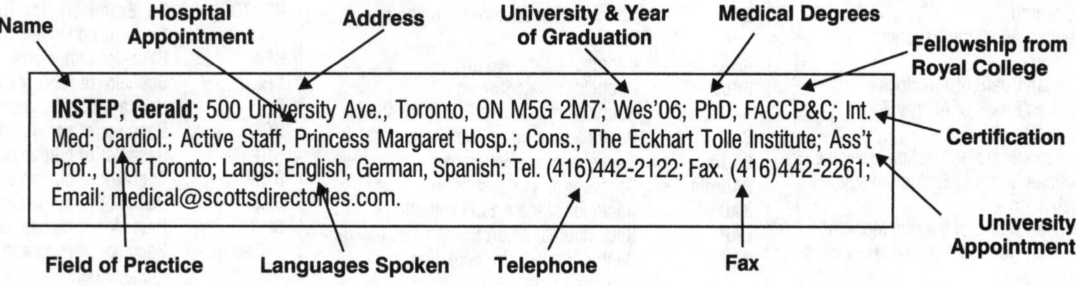

SECTION TWO — PHYSICIANS BY GEOGRAPHIC LOCATION

This Section includes General Practitioners and Family Medicine physicians listed alphabetically by region. Interns, hospital residents and retired doctors are excluded from this list.

SECTION THREE — PHYSICIANS BY CERTIFIED SPECIALTY

This Section includes Certified Specialists listed by specialty and geographic location.

SECTION FOUR — HOSPITALS & HEALTH CENTRES IN CANADA

This Section includes all Canadian Hospitals & Health Centres and an Index.

SECTION FIVE — RESOURCE SECTION

This Section includes the 2012 graduates in medicine from Canadian universities, excluded from the alphabetical and geographic sections, along with information about Medical Associations, Health Departments and Universities.

SECTION SIX — CANADIAN HEALTHCARE ASSOCIATIONS

This section contains listings of numerous Canadian Healthcare Associations arranged alphabetically by association name.

SECTION SEVEN — 2012 YEAR IN REVIEW / CANADIAN MEDICAL HALL OF FAME

This Section includes the 2012 Year in Review, which is a summary of major medical news items from the *Canadian Medical Association Journal*, and the Canadian Medical Hall of Fame, which highlights and honours physicians, researchers and healthcare builders who have made significant contributions to healthcare in Canada.

ABBREVIATIONS

UNIVERSITIES

Canadian universities are abbreviated as follows (other universities are shown in full):

Alb	Alberta
Cal	Calgary
Dal	Dalhousie
Lav	Laval
Man	Manitoba
McG	McGill
McM	McMaster
Mem	Memorial
Mon	Montreal
NOSM	Northern Ontario School of Medicine
Ott	Ottawa
Qns	Queens
Sask	Saskatchewan
Sher	Sherbrooke
Tor	Toronto
UBC	British Columbia
Wes	Western Ontario

DEGREES

Certificates, Degrees, Diplomas, Fellowships, and Titles are abbreviated as follows:

AA	Associate in arts
AACP	Assoc. American College of Physicians
AACS	Assoc. American College of Surgeons
AACT	American Academy Clin. Toxicology
AAD	American Academy of Dermatology
AAFP & RS	American Academy Facial, Plastic & Reconstructive Surgery
AAPCC	American Assoc. of Psychiatric Clinics for Children
AAPN	American Academy Psychiatry & Neurology
ABA	American Board of Anesthesia
ABAI	American Board of Allergy & Immunology
ABAvM	American Board of Aviation Medicine
ABEM	American Board of Endocrinology & Metabolism
ABIM	American Board of Internal Medicine
ABIMC	American Board of Internal Medicine & Cardiology
ABMH	American Board of Medical Hypnosis
ABMM	American Board of Medical Management
ABMO	American Board of Medical Oncology
ABMT	American Board of Medical Toxicology
ABNM	American Board of Nuclear Medicine
ABNS	American Board of Neurosurgery
ABOG	American Board of Obstetrics & Gynecology
ABOM	American Board of Occupational Medicine
ABPMR	American Board of Physical Med. and Rehab.
ABQAURP	American Board of Quality Assurance & Utilization Review Physicians
ABREI	American Board of Reproductive Endocrinology & Infertility
ABRM	American Board of Respiratory Medicine
ABS	American Board of Surgery
ABTS	American Board of Thoracic Surgery
ACLS	Advanced Cardiac Life Support
ACPE	American College of Physician Executives
AFCCP	Assoc. Fellow Coll. Chest Physicians
AFOM	Assoc. Faculty Occupational Medicine
AICS	Assoc. Intern. College of Surgeons
AIUM	American Inst. of Ultra Sound Medicine
AM	Associate in music
AMA	American Medical Association
AMCAA	Assoc. Member, Canadian Acad. Allergy
AMCGP	Assoc. Member, College of General Practice of Canada
AMLFC	Assoc. Medecin Langue Francais du Canada
AMO	Assist. Medical Officer
APA	American Psychiatric Assoc.
ARIC	Assoc., Royal Institute of Chemistry
ARSH	Associate of the Royal Society of Health
ARSM	Affiliate, Royal Society of Medicine
AS	Associate in science
ASAM	American Society of Addiction Medicine
ASFPS	American Society of Facial Plastic Surgery
ASH	American Society of Hemotology
ATLS	Advanced Trauma Life Support
BA	Bachelor of arts
BAA	Baccalauréat en administration des affaires
BAA	Bachelor of applied arts
BAcc	Bachelor of accounting
BACS	Bachelor of arts in community studies
BAD	Baccalauréat en art dramatique
BAdm	Bachelor of administration
BAdmin	Bachelor of administration
BAO	Bachelor of the Art of Obstetrics
BAP	Baccalauréat en architecture de paysage
BARA	Bachelor of arts in recreation administration
BArch	Bachelor of architecture
BArtsSc	Bachelor of arts and science
BAS	Bachelor of administrative studies
BASc	Bachelor of applied science
BAV	Baccalauréat en arts visuels
BBA	Bachelor of business administration
BBE	Bachelor of business economics
BBM	Bachelor of business management
BCB	Bachelor of computing and business
BCEd	Bachelor of Christian education
BChir	Bachelor of Chirurgie
BCIS	Bachelor of computer information systems
BCL	Bachelor of canon law
BCL	Bachelor of civil law
BCLS	Basic Cardiac Life Support
BComm	Bachelor of commerce
BCompSc	Bachelor of computer science
BCR	Bachelor of community rehabilitation
BCS	Bachelor of Christian studies
BCS	Bachelor of computer science
BCSc	Bachelor of computer science
BDes	Bachelor of design
BDesign	Bachelor of design
BDI	Baccalauréat en design industriel
BDSc	Bachelor of dental science
BE	Bachelor of science in engineering
BEAD	Bachelor of education after degree
BEd	Bachelor of education
BED	Bachelor of environmental design
BEDS	Bachelor of environmental design studies
BEd(Voc)	Bachelor of vocational education
BEng	Bachelor of engineering
BEngCS	Bachelor of engineering and computer systems
BEngMgt	Bachelor of engineering and management
BEngSoc	Bachelor of engineering and society
BEP	Baccalauréat en éducation physique
BEPS	Baccalauréat en éducation physique et santé
BES	Bachelor of environmental studies
BESc	Bachelor of engineering science
BESTCO	Bd. Examiners Sex Therapy & Counselling Ontario
BFA	Bachelor of fine arts
BFS	Bachelor of food science
BG	Baccalauréat en génie
BGS	Bachelor of general studies
BHE	Bachelor of human ecology
BHEc	Bachelor of human ecology
BHJ	Bachelor of human justice
BHK	Bachelor of human kinetics
BHRM	Bachelor of hotel and resort management
BHSc	Bachelor of health sciences
BHSc(OT)	Bachelor of health sciences in occupational therapy
BHSc(PT)	Bachelor of health sciences in physiotherapy
BHum	Bachelor of humanities
BIA	Baccalauréat en informatique appliquée
BIB	Bachelor of international business
BID	Bachelor of industrial design
BID	Bachelor of interior design
BIng	Baccalauréat en ingénierie
BIS	Bachelor of independent studies
BIS	Bachelor of information systems
BISW	Bachelor of Indian social work
BISys	Bachelor of information systems
BJ	Bachelor of journalism
BKin	Bachelor of kinesiology
BL	Baccalauréat en loisir
BLA	Bachelor of landscape architecture
BLIM	Board of Life Insurance Medicine
BLT	Bachelor of laboratory technology
BM	Bachelor of music
BMA	Bachelor of musical arts
BMath	Bachelor of mathematics
BMedSc	Bachelor of medical science
BMgt	Bachelor of management
BMLS	Bachelor of medical laboratory science
BMLSc	Bachelor of medical laboratory science
BMR(OT)	Bachelor of medical rehabilitation (occupational therapy)
BMR(PT)	Bachelor of medical rehabilitation (physical therapy)
BMS	Bachelor of maritime studies
BMSc	Bachelor of medical science
BMT	Bachelor of music therapy
BMus	Bachelor of music

BMusA	Bachelor of musical arts
BMusEd	Bachelor of music education
BMus(MusEd)	Bachelor of music (music education)
BMusTh	Bachelor of music therapy
BN	Bachelor of nursing
BOM	Bachelor of office management
BOR	Bachelor of outdoor recreation
BOT	Bachelor of occupational therapy
BPA	Bachelor of professional arts
BPA	Bachelor of public administration
BPAS	Bachelor of physical activity studies
BPE	Bachelor of physical education
BPh	Bachelor of philosophy
BPharm	Bachelor of Pharmacy
BPHE	Bachelor of physical and health education
BPhEd	Bachelor of physical education
BPR	Bachelor of public relations
BPs	Baccalauréat en psychologie
BPT	Bachelor of physical therapy
BRec	Bachelor of recreation
BRLS	Bachelor of recreation and leisure studies
BRM	Bachelor of recreation management
BRS	Bachelor of recreation studies
BSA	Bachelor of science in agriculture
BSc	Bachelor of science
BSc(Agr)	Bachelor of science in agriculture
BSc(AgrEng)	Bachelor of science in agricultural engineering
BSc(Arch)	Bachelor of science in architecture
BSc(CS)	Bachelor of science in computer science
BSc(Eng)	Bachelor of science in engineering
BSc(Env)	Bachelor of science in environmental sciences
BSc(Ergo)	Baccalauréat ès sciences en ergothérapie
BSc(FSc)	Bachelor of science in food science
BSc(HE)	Bachelor of science in health education
BSc(HEc)	Bachelor of science in home economics
BSc(Med)	Bachelor of science in medicine
BSc(N)	Bachelor of science in nursing
BSc(NRC)	Bachelor of science (natural resource conservation)
BSc(Nutr)	Bachelor of science in nutrition
BSc(NutrSc)	Bachelor of science in nutritional science
BSc(OT)	Bachelor of science in occupational therapy
BSc(Pharm)	Bachelor of science in pharmacy
BSc(PT)	Bachelor of science in physical therapy
BScA	Baccalauréat ès sciences appliquèes
BScD	Bachelor of science in dentistry
BScDA	Bachelor of science in data analysis
BScE	Bachelor of science in engineering
BScF	Bachelor of science in forestry
BScFE	Bachelor of science in forest engineering
BScG	Baccalauréat ès sciences en génie
BScHE	Bachelor of science in human ecology
BScInf	Baccalauréat en sciences infirmières
BScKin	Bachelor of science in kinesiology
BScMH	Bachelor of science in mental health
BScN	Bachelor of science in nursing
BScOT	Bachelor of science in occupational therapy
BScPhm	Bachelor of science in pharmacy
BScPN	Bachelor of science in psychiatric nursing
BScPT	Bachelor of science in physiotherapy
BScSoc	Baccalauréat ès sciences sociales
BServSoc	Baccalauréat en service social
BSF	Bachelor of science in forestry
BSL	Bachelor of science in language
BSM	Bachelor of sports management
BSN	Bachelor of science in nursing
BSN	Bachelor of science in nutrition
BSocSc	Bachelor of social sciences
BSP	Bachelor of science in pharmacy
BSPE	Bachelor of science in physical education
BSpecEd	Bachelor of special education
BSS	Baccalauréat en service social
BSW	Bachelor of social work
BT	Bachelor of technology
BTech	Bachelor of technology
BTh	Bachelor of theology
BTHM	Bachelor of tourism and hospitality management
BTM	Bachelor of technology management
BTrad	Baccalaurèat en traduction
BTS	Baccalauréat en travail social
BV/TE	Bachelor of vocational/technical education
BVocEd	Bachelor of vocational education
CABEM	Certificant, American Board of Emergency Medicine
CABS	Certificant, American Board of Surgery
CAFC	Certificant, Acupuncture Foundation of Canada
CASAM	Certificant, American Society of Addiction Medicine
CBLIE	Certificant, Board of Life Insurance Examiners
CCAMA	Certificant, Canadian Academy of Medical Acupuncture
CCBOM	Certificant, Canadian Board of Occupational Medicine
CCFP	Certificate, College of Family Physicians
CCFP(EM)	Certificant, College of Family Physicians, Emergency Medicine
CCMG	Canadian College of Med. Geneticists
CGP	Certified Group Psychotherapist
CGPP	Certificant in General Practice Psychotherapy
CHA	Certificate, Hospital Administration
ChB	Bachelor of Chirurgie
CHE	Certified Health Executive
CIH	Certificate in Industrial Hygiene
CM	Master of surgery
CMHA	Certificate, Mental Health Assoc.
COSCH	Certificant, Ontario Society of Clinical Hypnosis
CPA	Canadian Psychiatric Association
CPH	Certificate in Public Health
CRS	Colon Rectal Surgery
CSCC	Certificate Society of Clinical Chemists
CST	Certificate Health in the Workplace
CTM&H	Certificate Tropical Medicine & Hygiene
DA	Diploma in Anesthesia
DAAPM	Diploma, American Academy of Pain Management
DABA	Diploma, American Board of Anesthesia
DABA & CI	Diploma, American Board of Allergy & Clinical Immunology
DABCC	Diploma, American Board of Clinical Chemists
DABD	Diploma, American Board of Dermatology
DABDS	Diploma, American Board of Dermatology and Syphilology
DABEM	Diploma, American Board of Emergency Medicine
DABFP	Diploma, American Board of Family Practice
DABIM	Diploma, American Board of Internal Medicine
DABN	Diploma, American Board of Neurology
DABNS	Diploma, American Board of Neurosurgery
DABOG	Diploma, American Board of Obstetrics and Gynecology
DABOph	Diploma, American Board of Ophthalmology
DABOS	Diploma, American Board of Orthopedic Surgery
DABOtol	Diploma, American Board of Otolaryngology
DABPath	Diploma, American Board of Pathology
DABPath & MA	Diploma, American Board of Pathology and Morbid Anatomy
DABPathAnat	Diploma, American Board of Pathological Anatomy
DABPed	Diploma, American Board of Pediatrics
DABPH	Diploma, American Board of Public Health
DABPM	Diploma, American Board of Physical Medicine
DABPMR	Diploma, American Board of Physical Med. and Rehab.
DABPN	Diploma, American Board of Psychiatry and Neurology
DABPrevMed	Diploma, American Board, Preventive Medicine
DABPS	Diploma, American Board of Plastic Surgery
DABR	Diploma, American Board of Radiology
DABS	Diploma, American Board of Surgery
DABTR	Diploma, American Board of Therap. Radiology
DABTS	Diploma, American Board of Thoracic Surgery
DABU	Diploma, American Board of Urology
DACR	Diploma, American College of Radiology
DAIP	Diploma, American Inst. of Psychoanalysis
DAvMed	Diploma, Aviation Medicine
DC	Docteur en chiropratique
DCH	Diploma, Child Health
DCL	Doctor of canon law
DCL	Doctor of civil law
DCMT	Diploma in Clin. Med. of Tropics
DCNP	Diploma in Clin. Neuropsychology
DCP	Diploma Clinical Pathology
DDAM	Diploma, Direction & Admin. Med.
DDC	Doctorat en droit canonique
DDR	Diploma, Diagnostic Radiology
DDS	Doctor of dental surgery
DECH	Diploma, Epidemiology & Community Health
DESS	Diplôme d'études supérieures specialisées
DGS	Diploma, General Surgery
DHA	Diploma, Hospital Administration
DHMSA	Diploma in the History of Medicine, Society of Apothecaries
DHOM	Diploma, Hospital Organization & Management
DIFA	Diploma, International Fertility Assoc.
DIH	Diploma, Industrial Health
DIMOH	Diploma Industrial Medicine & Occupational Health
Dip. Bact.	Diploma in Bacteriology
DJur	Doctor of jurisprudence
DLIM	Diploma in Life Ins. Medicine
DLO	Diploma, Laryngology and Otology
DMA	Doctor of musical arts
DMD	Doctor of dental medicine
DMI	Doctor of ministry
DMin	Doctor of ministry
DMJ	Diploma, Medical Jurisprudence
DMO	District Medical Officer
DMRD	Diploma in Medicine, Radio-Diagnostic
DMRE	Diploma, Medical Radiology and Electrology
DMRT	Diploma, Medical Radiotherapy
DMus	Doctor of music
DMV	Doctorat en médicine vétérinaire

DO	Diploma, Ophthalmology
DO	Doctor of Osteopathy
DOH&S	Diploma, Occupational Health & Safety
DOMFS	Diploma, Oral & Maxillofacial Surgery
DOMS	Diploma, Ophth. Med. and Surgery
DPH	Diploma, Public Health
DPharm	Doctor of pharmacy
DPM	Diploma, Psychological Medicine
DPs	Doctorat en psychologie
DR	Diploma, Radiology
DRACR	Diploma of Royal Australasian College of Radiologists
DRCOG	Diploma, Royal College of Obstetricians and Gynecologists
DS	Diploma in Surgery
DSc	Doctor of Science
DSSc	Diploma, Sanitary Science
DST	Diploma, Santé du Travail
DSW	Doctor of social work
DTCD	Diploma, Tuberculous and Chest Diseases
DTD	Diploma in Tuberculous Diseases
DTH	Diploma, Tropical Hygiene
DTh	Doctor of theology
DTM	Diploma, Tropical Medicine
DTM&H	Diploma, Tropical Medicine & Hygiene
DTPH	Diploma, Tropical Public Health
DU	Diploma, Urology
DV	Diploma, Venereology (Liverpool)
DVM	Doctor of veterinary medicine
DVSc	Doctor of veterinary science
EdD	Doctor of education
EMBA	Executive master of business administration
FAAA	Fellow, American Academy of Allergy
FAAAS	Fellow, American Assoc. for Advancement of Science
FAACIA	Fellow, American Assoc. of Clinical Immunology & Allergy
FAAD	Fellow, American Academy of Dermatology
FAAFP	Fellow, American Academy of Family Practice
FAAMD	Fellow, American Assoc. on Mental Deficiency
FAAN&OS	Fellow, American Academy of Neurological & Orthopedic Surgeons
FAAO	Fellow, American Academy of Ophthalmology
FAAOO	Fellow, American Academy of Ophthalmology and Otolaryngology
FAAOS	Fellow, American Academy of Orthopedic Surgeons
FAAP/FASIP	Fellow, American Academy of Pediatrics
FAAST	Fellow, American Academy of Surgery of Trauma
FAATS	Fellow, American Academy of Thoracic Surgeons
FABAS	Fellow, American Bd. of Abdominal Surg.
FABAT	Fellow, American Board Allergy & Immunology
FABMB	Fellow, American Bd. of Med. Genetics
FABMLAMSC	Fellow, American Board Medical Legal Analysis in Medicine & Surgery
FABPrevM	Fellow, American Board of Preventive Medicine
FACA	Fellow, American College of Allergists
FACA	Fellow, American College of Anesthesia
FACB	Fellow, American College of Biochemistry
FACC	Fellow, American College of Cardiology
FACCP	Fellow, American College Clin. Pharmacology
FACCP&C	Fellow, American College of Clin. Pharm. & Chemotherapy
FACD	Fellow, American College of Dermatology
FACE	Fellow, American College of Endocrinology
FACEP	Fellow, American College of Emergency Physicians
FACFP	Fellow, American College of Forensic Psychiatry
FACG	Fellow, American College of Gastroenterology
FACGE	Fellow, American College of Gastrointestinal Endoscopy
FACHA	Fellow, American College of Hospital Administration
FACLM	Fellow, American College of Legal Medicine
FACN	Fellow, American College of Nutrition
FACNM	Fellow, American College Nuclear Medicine
FACO	Fellow, American College of Otolaryngology
FACOCCP	Fellow, American College of Occupational Physicians
FACOG	Fellow, American College of Obstetrics & Gynecologists
FACOM	Fellow, Australian College of Occupational Med.
FACON	Fellow, American College of Neuropsychopharmacology
FACP	Fellow, American College of Physicians
FACP&RM	Fellow, American College of Physical & Rehab. Medicine
FACPath	Fellow, American College of Pathology
FACPh	Fellow, American College of Phlebology
FACPsyA	Fellow, American College Psychiatry (Psychoanalysis)
FACPT	Fellow, American College of Physical Therapy
FACR	Fellow, American College of Radiology
FACS	Fellow, American College of Surgeons
FACSM	Fellow, American College of Sports Medicine
FACTM	Fellow, American College of Tropical Medicine
FAFC	Fellow, Acupuncture Fdn. of Canada
FAGS	Fellow, American Geriatric Society
FAHACCS	Fellow, American Heart Association, Council of Cardiovascular Surgery
FAIM	Fellow, Academy of Internal Medicine
FAMWA	Fellow, American Medical Writers' Assoc.
FANZCP	Fellow, Australian & New Zealand College of Psychiatrists
FAOMA	Fellow, American Occupational Medical Association
FAPA	Fellow, American Pediatric Assn.
FAPA	Fellow, American Psychiatric Association
FAPHA	Fellow, American Public Health Assn.
FAPM	Fellow, Academy of Psychosomatic Medicine
FARA	Fellow, American Rheumatism Association
FASAS	Fellow, American Society of Abdominal Surgeons
FASCH	Fellow, American Soc. Clin. Hypnosis
FASCP	Fellow, American Society of Clinical Pathologists
FASCRS	Fellow, American Society of Colon & Rectal Surgeons
FASEA	Fellow, Assoc. of Surgeons of East Africa
FASHA	Fellow, American Surgery of Hand Assoc.
FASHNS	Fellow, American Society of Head & Neck Surgery
FAsMA	Fellow, Aerospace Medical Association
FASOO	Fellow, American Society of Ophthalmologists and Otolaryngologists
FASPS	Fellow, American Society of Plastic & Reconstructive Surgeons
FBLIM	Fellow, Bd. of Life Insurance Medicine
FBPsS	Fellow, British Psychological Society
FCAMA	Fellow, Canadian Academy of Medical Acupuncture
FCAP	Fellow, College of American Pathologists
FCCAHA	Fellow, Clinical Cardiology, American Health Assoc.
FCCMG	Fellow, Canadian College Med. Genetics
FCCP	Fellow of the College of Chest Physicians
FCFP	Fellow, College of Family Physicians Canada
FCIFPS	Fellow, Canadian Inst. of Facial Plastic Surgery
FCPS	Fellow, Canadian Pediatric Society
FCSAIC	Fellow, Canadian Society of Allergy & Clinical Immunology
FCSCC	Fellow, Canadian Society of Clinical Chemists
FCSE	Fellow, Canadian Soc. Electroencephalographers
FESC	Fellow, European Society of Cardiology
FFARACS	Fellow, Fac. of Anesthesia, Royal Australian College of Surgeons
FFARCS	Fellow, Fac. of Anesthesia, Royal College of Surgeons (Eng.)
FFCM	Fellow, Faculty of Community Medicine
FFMG	Fellow, Family Medicine in Geriatrics
FFR	Fellow, Faculty of Radiology
FHCS	Fellow, Hungarian College of Surgeons
FHKAM	Fellow, Hong Kong Academy of Medicine
FIAA	Fellow, International Assn. Allergists
FIAC	Fellow, International Academy of Cytology
FIACS	Fellow, International Academy Cosmetic Surgery
FICA	Fellow, International College of Anesthetists
FICA(An)	Fellow, International College of Anatomists
FICA(Ang)	Fellow, International College of Angiology
FICP	Fellow, International College of Pediatricians
FICPM	Fellow, International College of Physical Medicine
FICPSM	Fellow, International College of Psychosomatic Medicine
FICS	Fellow, International College of Surgery
FIGA	Fellow, International Geriatric Association
FIGS	Fellow, International Gastroenterologist's Society
FIMA	Fellow, Industrial Medical Association
FIPA	Fellow, International Psychiatric Association
FISH	Fellow, International Soc. Hematology
FMH	Federation of the Swiss Physicians
FNGS	Fellow, National Gastroenterologists Soc.
FRACOG	Fellow of the Royal Australian College of Obstetricians and Gynecologists
FRACP	Fellow, Royal Australasian College of Physicians
FRACR	Fellow, Royal Australasian College of Radiologists
FRACS	Fellow, Royal Australasian College of Surgeons
FRAI	Fellow, Royal Anthropological Institute
FRAM	Fellow, Royal Academy of Medicine
FRANZCP	Fellow, Royal Australian & New Zealand College of Psychiatrists

FRCGP	Fellow, Royal College of General Practice
FRCM	Fellow, Royal College of Medicine
FRCOG	Fellow, Royal College of Obstetrics & Gyn.
FRCP	Fellow, Royal College of Physicians
FRCPA	Fellow, Royal College of Pathologists Australia
FRCPath	Fellow, Royal College of Pathology
FRCPC	Fellow, Royal College of Physicians Canada
FRCR	Fellow, Royal College of Radiology
FRCS	Fellow, Royal College of Surgeons
FRCSC	Fellow, Royal College of Surgeons Canada
FRFPS	Fellow, Royal Faculty of Physicians and Surgeons
FRIC	Fellow, Royal Institute of Chemistry
FRIPHH	Fellow, Royal Institute, Public Health & Hygiene
FRS	Fellow of the Royal Society
FRSA	Fellow, Royal Society of Arts
FRSC	Fellow, Royal Society of Canada
FRSH	Fellow, Royal Soc. of Health
FRSM	Fellow, Royal Society of Medicine
FRSTM	Fellow, Royal Soc. Trop. Med. (Lond.)
FSAM	Fellow Society of Adolescent Medicine
FSCEH	Fellow, Society for Clinical & Experimental Hypnosis
FSIH	Fellow, Society of Industrial Hygiene
FSOGC	Fellow, Society of Obst. & Gyn. Canada
FWACS	Fellow of the West African College of Surgeons
IMBA	International master of business administration
JCHMT	Joint Committee for Higher Medical Training
JSD	Doctor in the science of law
LABIM	Licentiate, American Board of International Medicine
LABO	Licentiate, American Board of Ophthalmology
LABP	Licentiate, American Board of Pediatrics
LABR	Licentiate, American Board of Radiology
LAH	Licentiate Apothecaries Hall, Dublin
LCL	Licentiate in canon law
LDC	Licence en droit canonique
LGMCUK	Lic. Gen. Med. Council of the United Kingdom
LICA	Licentiate, International College of Anesthetists
LLB	Bachelor of laws
LLD	Doctor of laws
LLL	Licentiate of laws
LLM	Master of laws
LM	Licentiate in Midwifery
LMCC	Licentiate of the Medical Council of Canada
LMCFP	Life Memb., College of Family Physicians
LMRSH	Licentiate Member of the Royal Society of Health
LMSSA	Licentiate in Medicine and Surgery Society of Apothecaries
LMus	Licentiate in music
LPh	Licentiate in philosophy
LPs	Licentiate in psychiatry
LRCP	Licentiate, Royal College of Physicians
LRCS	Licentiate, Royal College of Surgeons
LRFPS	Licent. of Royal Faculty of Physicians & Surgeons
LTh	Licentiate in theology
MA	Master of arts
MA(CL)	Master of arts in canon law
MA(DC)	Maîtrise ès arts en droit canonique
MA(Ed)	Master of Arts in Education
MA(Miss)	Master of arts in missiology
MA(PastSt)	Master of arts in pastoral studies
MA(ScPast)	Maîtrise ès arts en sciences pastorales
MA(Th)	Master of arts in theology
MAAGP	Member, American Academy of General Practice
MAAP	Member, American Assoc. of Physicians
MABIM	Member, American Board of Internal Medicine
MABR	Member, American Board of Radiologists
MAC	Master of art conservation
MAcc	Master of accounting
MACHA	Member, American College of Hospital Administration
MAdEd	Master of adult education
MAdmin	Master of administration
MADTR	Maîtrise en aménagement du territoire et développement
MAEd	Master of arts in education
MAES	Master of applied environmental studies
MAg	Master of agriculture
MAgr	Master of agriculture
MAHE	Master of arts in human ecology
MAIS	Member Assoc. Industrial Surgeons
MAL	Master of arts, liberal studies
MANZCP	Member, Australian & New Zealand College of Psychiatry
MAO	Master, Art of Obstetrics
MAP	Maîtrise en administration publique
MAPs	Maîtrise ès arts en psychologie
MAqua	Master of aquaculture
MArch	Master of architecture
MARS	Member Assoc. Railway Surgeons
MAS	Master of applied statistics
MAS	Master of archival studies
MASA	Master of advanced studies in architecture
MASc	Master of applied science
MASCP&T	Member, American Society for Clinical Pharmacology & Therapeutics
MAT	Master of arts in teaching
MATh	Master of arts in theology
MB, BS	Bachelor of Medicine, Bachelor of Surgery
MBA	Master of business administration
MBSI	Maîtrise en bibliothéconomie et sciences de l'information
MC	Master of counselling
MCA	Master of criminology (applied)
MCAA	Member Canadian Acad. Allergy
MCE	Master of continuing education
MCEd	Master of continuing education
MCFP	Member College of Family Physicians
MCFP(EM)	Member College of Family Physicians (Emergency Medicine)
MChOrth	Master of Orthopedic Surgery
MCID	Master of clinical dentistry
MClSc	Master of clinical science
MCL	Master of civil law
MClSc	Master of Clinical Science
MCNS	Member, Congress of Neurological Surgeons
MCompSc	Master of computer science
MCP	Master of city planning
MCPS	Member of the College of Physicians & Surgeons
MCS	Master of communication studies
MCS	Master of computer science
MCSc	Master of computer science
MD	Doctor of medicine
MDC	Maîtrise en droit canonique
MDE	Master of development economics
MDE	Master of distance education
MDEs	Master of design
MDI	Master of divinity
MDiv	Master of divinity
MEc	Master of economics
MEd	Master of education
MEDes	Master of environmental design
MEDS	Master of environmental design studies
MEE	Maîtrise en études de l'environnement
MEng	Master of engineering
MEngSc	Master of engineering science
MEnv	Maîtrise en environnement
MEnvSc	Master of environmental science
MES	Master, environmental studies
MESc	Master of engineering science
MF	Master of forestry
MFA	Master of fine arts
MFC	Master of forest conservation
MFE	Master of forest engineering
MFisc	Maîtrise en fiscalité
MFOM	Member Faculty of Occupational Medicine
MFPHM	Member Faculty of Public Health Medicine
MG	Maîtrise en génie
MGP	Maîtrise en gestion de projet
MGSS	Maîtrise en gestion des services de santé
MHA	Master of health administration
MHA	Master, hospital administration
MHE	Master of human ecology
MHK	Master of human kinetics
MHPEd	Master of Health Professions Education
MHSA	Master of health services administration
MHSc	Master of health sciences
MI	Maîtrise en informatique
MIAASM	Member, International Academy of Aviation & Space Medicine
MIMA	Member, Industrial Medical Assoc.
MIng	Maîtrise en ingénierie
MIR	Master of industrial relations
MJ	Master of journalism
MKin	Master of kinesiology
MLA	Master of landscape architecture
MLandArch	Master of landscape architecture
MLE	Master of linguistics and exegesis
MLIS	Master of library and information studies
MMath	Master of mathematics
MMedEd	Master of Medical Education
MMFT	Master of marriage and family therapy
MMin	Master of ministry
MMM	Master of marine management
MMS	Master of management studies
MMS	Master of museum studies
MMSA	Member, Medical Specialists' Assoc.
MMSBC	Master, Medical Science in Biomedical Communication
MMus	Master of music
MN	Master of nursing
MNRM	Master of natural resources management
MOA	Maîtrise en orthophonie et audiologie
MOH	Master, Occupational Health
MPA	Master of public administration
MPAS	Master of physical activity studies
MPE	Master of physical education
MPH	Master of public health
MPharm	Master of pharmacy and pharmaceutical sciences
MPhil	Master of philosophy
MPL	Master of planning
MPM	Master of pest management
MPM	Master of public management
MProfpast	Maîtrise professionnelle en pastorale
MPs	Maîtrise en psychologie
MPT	Masters program in physical therapy
MRACP*	Memb., Royal Australasian College of Physicians
MRACR*	Member, Royal Australasian College of Radiologists

MRCGP	Member, Royal College of General Practice
MRCOG	Member, Royal College of Obstetricians and Gynecologists
MRCPath	Member, Royal College of Pathologists
MRCPsy	Member, Royal College of Psychiatrists
MRCS	Member, Royal College of Surgeons
MRE	Master of religious education
MRel	Master of religion
MRM	Master of resources management
MROCC	Medical Review Officer Certificate, Canada
MRSH	Member, Royal Society of Health
MS	Master of surgery
MSc	Master of science
MSc(EdPsych)	Master of science in educational psychology
MSc(Eng)	Master of science in engineering
MSc(Pharm)	Master of science in pharmacy
MScA	Master of science, applied
MScE	Master of science in engineering
MScF	Master of science in forestry
MScFE	Master of science in forest engineering
MScHE	Master of science in human ecology
MScN	Master of science in nursing
MScPl	Master of science in planning
MScS	Maîtrise ès sciences de la santé
MServSoc	Maîtrise en service social
MSL	Licentiate in medieval studies
MSL	Master of studies in law
MSLP	Master of speech languages pathology
MSN	Master of science in nursing
MSS	Maîtrise en service social
MSW	Master of social work
MTech	Maîtrise en technologie des systèmes
MTh	Master of theology
MThP	Maîtrise en théologie pastorale
MTM	Master in the teaching of mathematics
MTS	Master of theological studies
MTSC	Master of theological studies in counselling
MUP	Master urban planning
MUrb	Maîtrise en urbanisme
MURP	Master of urban and rural planning
MusBac	Bachelor of music
MusDoc	Doctor of music
MusM	Master of music
MV/TEd	Master of vocational/technical education
MVA	Master of visual arts
MVetSc	Master of veterinary science
MWS	Master of women's studies
OD	Doctor of optometry
P&OT	Phys. & Occup. Therapy
PCN(Fr.)	Physics, Chemistry & Natural Science France
PharmD	Doctor of pharmacy
PhD	Doctor of philosophy
PhD(CL)	Doctor of philosophy in canon law
PhD(DC)	Doctorat en philosophie, en droit canonique
PhD(Th)	Doctor of philosophy in theology
PhilM	Master of philosophy
SAGES	Society American Gastrointestinal Endoscopic Surgery
SJD	Doctor of juridical science
SM	Science Maître
SMO	Senior Medical Officer
STM	Master of sacred theology
TDD	Tuberculosis Diseases, Diploma
ThD	Doctor of theology
ThM	Master of theology

* Australasian = Australia & New Zealand

APPOINTMENTS

A.C.P.	Accredited Clinical Polysomnographer
Assoc.	Associate
Ass't.	Assistant
Att'd.	Attending
Chmn.	Chairman
Clin.	Clinical
C.F.M.C.	Canadian Forces Medical Council
C.F.M.S.	Canadian Forces Medical Service
C.M.P.A.	Canadian Medical Protective Assn.
C.N.R.	Canadian National Railway
Comm.	Commission
Cons.	Consultant
C.O.	Commanding Officer
Court.	Courtesy
C.P.R.	Canadian Pacific Railway
C.P.S.O.	College of Physicians & Surgeons of Ontario
Dem.	Demonstrator
Dir.	Director
Dist.	District
D.M.S.	Director of Medical Services
D.O.T.	Department of Transport
D.V.A.	Department of Veterans Affairs
Ed.	Edinburgh
Emer.	Emeritus
Extn.	External
Fell.	Fellow
Fr.	France
Gen.	General
Germ.	Germany
Govt.	Government
Hon.	Honourary
Hosp.	Hospital
Hung.	Hungary
Ins.	Insurance
Inst.	Institute
Instr.	Instructor
Ire.	Ireland
It.	Italy
Jr.	Junior
Lect.	Lecturer
Lith.	Lithuania
Mil.	Military
M.L.A.	Member, Legislative Assembly
M.O.H.	Medical Officer of Health
Mun.	Municipal
M.P.	Member of Parliament
M.P.P.	Member of Provincial Parliament
Neth.	Netherlands
N.I.P.	Not in Practice
O.H.I.P.	Ontario Health Insurance Plan
O.P.D.	Outpatient Dept.
P.G.	Postgraduate
Phys.	Physician
Pres.	President
Prof.	Professor
Prov.	Provincial
Q.C.	Queen's Counsel
Q.H.P.	Queen's Honourary Physician
Q.H.S.	Queen's Honourary Surgeon
San.	Sanitorium
S.Africa	South Africa
Sec.	Secretary
Serv.	Service
Scot.	Scotland
Spec.	Specialist
Sr.	Senior
S.M.O.	Senior Medical Officer
S.T.D.	Sexually Transmitted Disease
Supt.	Superintendent
Switz.	Switzerland
T.T.C.	Toronto Transit Commission
Twp.	Township
U.	University
Vis.	Visiting
Vol.	Voluntary
W.C.B.	Workers' Compensation Board
W.H.O.	World Health Organization
W.M.A.	World Medical Association

DECORATIONS AND MEDALS

A.F.C.	Air Force Cross
B.E.M.	British Empire Medal
C.B.	Companion, Order of Bath
C.B.E.	Commander, Order of British Empire
C.C.	Companion, Order of Canada
C.D.	Canadian Forces Decoration
C.H.	Companion of Honour
C.M.	Member, Order of Canada
C.M.G.	Companion, Order of St. Michael and St. George
C.M.M.	Commander of the Order of Military Merit
C.St.J.	Commander, Venerable Order of St. John of Jerusalem
D.C.M.	Distinguished Conduct Medal
D.F.C.	Distinguished Flying Cross
D.F.M.	Distinguished Flying Medal
D.S.C.	Distinguished Service Cross
D.S.O.	Distinguished Service Order
D.U.	Honorary Doctorate
E.D.	Efficiency Decoration
G.B.E.	Knight Grand Cross, Order of British Empire
G.C.	George Cross
G.C.V.O.	Knight Grand Cross, Royal Victoria Order
G.M.	George Medal
K.B.E.	Knight Commander of British Empire
K.C.B.	Knight Commander, Order of Bath
K.St.J.	Knight Venerable, Order of St. John of Jerusalem
M.B.E.	Member, Order of British Empire
M.C.	Military Cross
M.M.	Military Medal
M.M.M.	Member Military Merit
O.B.E.	Officer, Order of British Empire
O.C.	Officer, Order of Canada
O.M.	Order of Merit
O.M.M.	Officer of the Order of Military Merit
O.Ont.	Order of Ontario
O.St.J.	Officer, Venerable Order of St. John of Jerusalem
S.B.St.J.	Serving Brother, Venerable Order of St. John of Jerusalem
S.O.M.	Saskatchewan Order of Merit
T.D.	Territorial Decoration
V.C.	Victoria Cross
V.D.	Volunteer Decoration

CERTIFICATION

The specialties and subspecialties recognized by The Royal College of Physicians and Surgeons of Canada (RCPSC) are shown below. Certification by the Province of Quebec is distinguished by the addition of the recognized abbreviation, e.g., IntMed(P.Q.) — certified in internal medicine by the CPMQ. If a doctor is certified in different specialties, the provincial certification is shown first. A Royal College Specialty Certificate shall be understood to mean that the Certificant has met the Royal College credentials standards (including an acceptable medical qualification), has satisfactorily completed a defined period of specialty residency education in a program recognized by the Royal College, has provided the College with a document confirming the satisfactory completion of residency education and has been successful at the specialty examinations.

RCPSC specialty certificates and certificates of special competence:

MEDICINE

Anesthesia
Cardiology[1]
Clinical Immunology & Allergy[1]
Community Medicine
Dermatology
Diagnostic Radiology
Emergency Medicine
Endocrinology & Metabolism[1]
Gastroenterology[1]
Geriatric Medicine[1]
Hematology[1]
Infectious Diseases[1]
Internal Medicine
Medical Genetics
Medical Oncology[1]
Nephrology[1]
Neurology
Nuclear Medicine
Occupational Medicine
Pediatrics
Physical Medicine & Rehabilitation
Psychiatry
Radiation Oncology
Respirology[1]
Rheumatology[1]

LABORATORY MEDICINE

Anatomical Pathology
General Pathology
Hematological Pathology
Medical Biochemistry
Medical Microbiology
Neuropathology

SURGERY

Cardiac Surgery
General Surgery
Neurosurgery
Obstetrics & Gynecology
Ophthalmology
Orthopedic Surgery
Otolaryngology
Pediatric General Surgery[1]
Plastic Surgery
Thoracic Surgery
Urology
Vascular Surgery[1]

[1]Subspecialty recognized by a certificate of special competence

The RCPSC accredits the following subspecialty residency programs but does not offer examinations for the certification of individuals completing these programs: clinical pharmacology, clinician investigator program, colorectal surgery, critical care medicine, general surgical oncology, gynecologic oncology, gynecologic reproductive endocrinology and infertility, maternal-fetal medicine, neonatal-perinatal medicine, neuroradiology, pediatric radiology.

POLICY REGARDING PUBLICATION OF RCPSC QUALIFICATIONS

The Fellowship designations of The Royal College of Physicians and Surgeons of Canada are:

DIVISION OF MEDICINE (including laboratory specialties)
FRCPC — Fellow of The Royal College of Physicians of Canada

DIVISION OF SURGERY
FRCSC — Fellow of The Royal College of Surgeons of Canada

Only Fellows in good standing may use the Fellowship designations.

CMA CODE OF ETHICS

This Code has been prepared by the Canadian Medical Association as an ethical guide for Canadian physicians, including residents, and medical students. Its focus is the core activities of medicine – such as health promotion, advocacy, disease prevention, diagnosis, treatment, rehabilitation, palliation, education and research. It is based on the fundamental principles and values of medical ethics, especially compassion, beneficence, non-maleficence, respect for persons, justice and accountability. The Code, together with CMA policies on specific topics, constitutes a compilation of guidelines that can provide a common ethical framework for Canadian physicians.

Physicians should be aware of the legal and regulatory requirements that govern medical practice in their jurisdictions.

Physicians may experience tension between different ethical principles, between ethical and legal or regulatory requirements, or between their own ethical convictions and the demands of other parties. Training in ethical analysis and decision-making during undergraduate, postgraduate and continuing medical education is recommended for physicians to develop their knowledge, skills and attitudes needed to deal with these conflicts. Consultation with colleagues, regulatory authorities, ethicists, ethics committees or others who have relevant expertise is also recommended.

FUNDAMENTAL RESPONSIBILITIES

1. Consider first the well-being of the patient.
2. Practise the profession of medicine in a manner that treats the patient with dignity and as a person worthy of respect.
3. Provide for appropriate care for your patient, even when cure is no longer possible, including physical comfort and spiritual and psychosocial support.
4. Consider the well-being of society in matters affecting health.
5. Practise the art and science of medicine competently, with integrity and without impairment.
6. Engage in lifelong learning to maintain and improve your professional knowledge, skills and attitudes.
7. Resist any influence or interference that could undermine your professional integrity.
8. Contribute to the development of the medical profession, whether through clinical practice, research, teaching, administration or advocating on behalf of the profession or the public.
9. Refuse to participate in or support practices that violate basic human rights.
10. Promote and maintain your own health and well-being.

RESPONSIBILITIES TO THE PATIENT

General Responsibilities

11. Recognize and disclose conflicts of interest that arise in the course of your professional duties and activities, and resolve them in the best interest of patients.
12. Inform your patient when your personal values would influence the recommendation or practice of any medical procedure that the patient needs or wants.
13. Do not exploit patients for personal advantage.
14. Take all reasonable steps to prevent harm to patients; should harm occur, disclose it to the patient.
15. Recognize your limitations and, when indicated, recommend or seek additional opinions and services.
16. In determining professional fees to patients for non-insured services, consider both the nature of the service provided and the ability of the patient to pay, and be prepared to discuss the fee with the patient.

Initiating and Dissolving a Patient—Physician Relationship

17. In providing medical service, do not discriminate against any patient on such grounds as age, gender, marital status, medical condition, national or ethnic origin, physical or mental disability, political affiliation, race, religion, sexual orientation, or socioeconomic status. This does not abrogate the physician's right to refuse to accept a patient for legitimate reasons.
18. Provide whatever appropriate assistance you can to any person with an urgent need for medical care.
19. Having accepted professional responsibility for a patient, continue to provide services until they are no longer required or wanted; until another suitable physician has assumed responsibility for the patient; or until the patient has been given reasonable notice that you intend to terminate the relationship.
20. Limit treatment of yourself or members of your immediate family to minor or emergency services and only when another physician is not readily available; there should be no fee for such treatment.

Communication, Decision Making and Consent

21. Provide your patients with the information they need to make informed decisions about their medical care, and answer their questions to the best of your ability.

22. Make every reasonable effort to communicate with your patients in such a way that information exchanged is understood.

23. Recommend only those diagnostic and therapeutic services that you consider to be beneficial to your patient or to others. If a service is recommended for the benefit of others, as for example in matters of public health, inform your patient of this fact and proceed only with explicit informed consent or where required by law.

24. Respect the right of a competent patient to accept or reject any medical care recommended.

25. Recognize the need to balance the developing competency of minors and the role of families in medical decision-making. Respect the autonomy of those minors who are authorized to consent to treatment.

26. Respect your patient's reasonable request for a second opinion from a physician of the patient's choice.

27. Ascertain wherever possible and recognize your patient's wishes about the initiation, continuation or cessation of life-sustaining treatment.

28. Respect the intentions of an incompetent patient as they were expressed (e.g., through a valid advance directive or proxy designation) before the patient became incompetent.

29. When the intentions of an incompetent patient are unknown and when no formal mechanism for making treatment decisions is in place, render such treatment as you believe to be in accordance with the patient's values or, if these are unknown, the patient's best interests.

30. Be considerate of the patient's family and significant others and cooperate with them in the patient's interest.

Privacy and Confidentiality

31. Protect the personal health information of your patients.

32. Provide information reasonable in the circumstances to patients about the reasons for the collection, use and disclosure of their personal health information.

33. Be aware of your patient's rights with respect to the collection, use, disclosure and access to their personal health information; ensure that such information is recorded accurately.

34. Avoid public discussions or comments about patients that could reasonably be seen as revealing confidential or identifying information.

35. Disclose your patients' personal health information to third parties only with their consent, or as provided for by law, such as when the maintenance of confidentiality would result in a significant risk of substantial harm to others or, in the case of incompetent patients, to the patients themselves. In such cases take all reasonable steps to inform the patients that the usual requirements for confidentiality will be breached.

36. When acting on behalf of a third party, take reasonable steps to ensure that the patient understands the nature and extent of your responsibility to the third party.

37. Upon a patient's request, provide the patient or a third party with a copy of his or her medical record, unless there is a compelling reason to believe that information contained in the record will result in substantial harm to the patient or others.

Research

38. Ensure that any research in which you participate is evaluated both scientifically and ethically and is approved by a research ethics board that meets current standards of practice.

39. Inform the potential research subject, or proxy, about the purpose of the study, its source of funding, the nature and relative probability of harms and benefits, and the nature of your participation including any compensation.

40. Before proceeding with the study, obtain the informed consent of the subject, or proxy, and advise prospective subjects that they have the right to decline or withdraw from the study at any time, without prejudice to their ongoing care.

RESPONSIBILITIES TO SOCIETY

41. Recognize that community, society and the environment are important factors in the health of individual patients.

42. Recognize the profession's responsibility to society in matters relating to public health, health education, environmental protection, legislation affecting the health or well-being of the community and the need for testimony at judicial proceedings.

43. Recognize the responsibility of physicians to promote equitable access to health care resources.

44. Use health care resources prudently.

45. Recognize a responsibility to give generally held opinions of the profession when interpreting scientific knowledge to the public; when presenting an opinion that is contrary to the generally held opinion of the profession, so indicate.

RESPONSIBILITIES TO THE PROFESSION

46. Recognize that the self-regulation of the profession is a privilege and that each physician has a continuing responsibility to merit this privilege and to support its institutions.

47. Be willing to teach and learn from medical students, residents, other colleagues and other health professionals.

48. Avoid impugning the reputation of colleagues for personal motives; however, report to the appropriate authority any unprofessional conduct by colleagues.

49. Be willing to participate in peer review of other physicians and to undergo review by your peers. Enter into associations, contracts and agreements only if you can maintain your professional integrity and safeguard the interests of your patients.

50. Avoid promoting, as a member of the medical profession, any service (except your own) or product for personal gain.

51. Do not keep secret from colleagues the diagnostic or therapeutic agents and procedures that you employ.

52. Collaborate with other physicians and health professionals in the care of patients and the functioning and improvement of health services. Treat your colleagues with dignity and as persons worthy of respect.

RESPONSIBILITIES TO ONESELF

53. Seek help from colleagues and appropriately qualified professionals for personal problems that might adversely affect your service to patients, society or the profession.

54. Protect and enhance your own health and well-being by identifying those stress factors in your professional and personal lives that can be managed by developing and practising appropriate coping strategies.

SECTION 1 — PHYSICIANS IN CANADA

AAD, Imad; Ctr Hosp Rouyn-Noranda, 4e 9e rue, Rouyn-Noranda QC J9X 2B2; (Lebanon)'93; Staff, Centre Hospitalier Rouyn-Noranda; (819)764-5131

AALAMIAN, Armand; GMF Côté-des-Neiges, 500-5700 ch Cote-des-Neiges, Montreal QC H3T 2A8; McG'88; CCFP; FCFP; (514)731-8531; Fax. (514)731-0536; armand.aalamian@mcgill.ca.

AARON, Lorne E; Service d'Urologie Rive-Sud, 304-3234 boul Taschereau, Greenfield Park QC J4V 2H3; McG'91; FRCSC; Urol. Staff, Hôpital Anna-Laberge; (450)671-2945; Fax. (450)671-8045.

AARON, Shawn D; The Ottawa Hosp-Gen Campus, L1267-501 Smyth Rd, Ottawa ON K1H 8L6; McG'90; FRCPC; IntMed; Critical Care Medicine; Respir. Staff, The Ottawa Hospital - General Campus; Prof, University of Ottawa; Langs: Bilingual(English/French); (613)737-8899 x74729; Fax. (613)739-6807.

AARON, Stephen L; Heritage Med Research Centre, 562-107 University Campus NW, Edmonton AB T6G 2S2; Alb'77; ABIM; FRCPC; IntMed; Rheum. Ac Staff, University of Alberta Hospital; Prof, University of Alberta; (780)407-6762; Fax. (780)407-6055; stephen.aaron@ualberta.ca.

AARONS, Gilbert H; 305-1017 Wilson Ave, North York ON M3K 1Z1; (Jamaica)'67; (416)638-2484; Fax. (416)638-3141.

AARTS, Mary-Anne W; 304-840 Coxwell Ave, Toronto ON M4C 5T2; Qns'98; FRCSC; GenSurg (Minimal Invasive Surgery); Critical Care Medicine. Staff Surg, Toronto East General Hospital Inc; Asst Prof, University of Toronto; (416)461-8363

AASHEIM, Lise H; Peterborough Clinic FHT, 203-26 Hospital Dr, Peterborough ON K9J 7C3; Tor'94; CCFP; (705)740-6873; Fax. (705)740-6858; laasheim@ptboclinic.com.

AASMAN, Edward J; Rocky Med Clinic, PO Box 99 Stn Main, Rocky-Mtn-Hse AB T4T 1A1; Alb'95; CCFP; (403)845-3315; Fax. (403)845-2177.

AAZAMI, Pejman; The Doctor's Office, 406-2299 Dundas St W, Toronto ON M6R 1X7; Tor'97; CCFP; (416)535-3511

ABADI, Babak; CAMH Pace Clinic, 1326-80 Workman Way, Toronto ON M6J 1H4; UBC'93; FRCPC; Psy (Geriatric Psychiatry). Staff, Centre for Addiction & Mental Health (CAMH) - Russell Street Site; Staff, Centre for Addiction & Mental Health Pace Clinic; Langs: Farsi; (416)535-8501 x2722; Fax. (416)535-1296.

ABADIE, Pascale; Hop Riviere-des-Prairies, 7070 boul Perras, Montreal QC H1E 1A4; Caen (France)'93; Staff, Hôpital Riviere des Prairies; (514)323-7260 x4564

ABADIE, Simon; Ctr Hosp Affilie-St-Sacrement, 1050 ch Sainte-Foy, Quebec QC G1S 4L8; Laval'06; CCFP; CCFP(E.M.); Staff, Centre Hospitalier Affilié Universitaire de Québec - Hôpital du St-Sacrement; (418)682-7511

ABADIR, Amir; Postgrad Med Education, 602-500 University Ave, Toronto ON M5G 1V7; Qns'06; FRCPC; IntMed; Gastroent.

ABADIR, Sylvia; Hop Ste-Justine, 3175 ch Cote-Sainte-Catherine, Montreal QC H3T 1C5; Toulouse III (France)'07; (514)345-4931

ABADIR, Wadid W K; 305-2347 Kennedy Rd, Scarborough ON M1T 3T8; Alexandria (Egypt)'85; FRCPC; Derm. Staff, Sunnybrook Health Sciences Centre; (416)297-8800; Fax. (416)297-6502.

ABARA, O Emmanuel; 9755 Bathurst St, Richmond Hill ON L4C 3X5; Ibadan (Nigeria)'76; FRCSC; Urol (Endoscopy Urology). Staff, Mackenzie Richmond Hill Hospital; Staff, Kirkland & District Hospital; Staff, Sensenbrenner Hospital; (905)883-3666; Fax. (905)883-0080.

ABASKHAROUN, Ramy R D; The Ottawa Hosp-Civic Campus, Gl A194-1053 Carling Ave, Ottawa ON K1Y 4E9; McG'01; FRCPC; IntMed; Gastroent. Staff, The Ottawa Hospital - Civic Campus; (613)798-5555 x18941; Fax. (613)798-5068.

ABAWI, Shakker; Bronte Med Group, 78 Jones St, Oakville ON L6L 6C5; Tor'80; Ac Staff, Halton Healthcare Services Corporation - Oakville Site; (905)827-9865; Fax. (905)827-3583.

ABAWI, Walid; Rudd Clinic, 123 Edward St, Toronto ON M5G 1E2; Cal'90; FRCSC; GenSurg. (416)597-0997; Fax. (416)597-2912.

ABAYA-COMENDADOR, Albina; Mackenzie Richmond Hill Hosp, 10 Trench St, Richmond Hill ON L4C 4Z3; Manila (Philippines)'74; FRCPC; Psy. Consultant, Mackenzie Richmond Hill Hospital; (905)832-1406 x2205; Fax. (905)832-1952.

ABAZID, Nizar R; Health Sciences Centre, 820 Sherbrook St, Winnipeg MB R3A 1R9; Damascus (Syria)'96; Staff, Health Sciences Centre.

ABBA, Zaheera; Cachet Family Physicians, 2-9255 Woodbine Ave, Markham ON L6C 1Y9; Pretoria (South Africa)'98; CCFP; (905)887-2222

ABBAS, Fadwa; CSSS du Nord de Lanaudière, 1000 boul Sainte-Anne, St-Charles-Brromee QC J6E 6J2; (Lebanon)'94; Staff, Centre Hospitalier Régional de Lanaudière; (450)759-8222

ABBAS, Harith A; Banting Institute, 302-100 College St, Toronto ON M5G 1L5; Baghdad (Iraq)'97; FRCSC; OrthSurg.

ABBAS, Mohammad A; CSSS Du Haut Saint-Maurice, 885 boul Ducharme, La Tuque QC G9X 3C1; Aleppo (Syria)'00; (819)523-4581 x2011; Fax. (819)523-6819.

ABBAS, Tahir; Saskatoon Cancer Centre, 20 Campus Dr, Saskatoon SK S7N 4H4; (306)655-2710; Fax. (306)655-0633.

ABBAS, Wassan; 2 Caprice Crt, Hamilton ON L9C 2N5; (Other Foreign)'96.

ABBASI, Khawar M; 3043 Sixth Line, Oakville ON L6H 7C5; Punjab (Pakistan)'92; CCFP; Staff, New Best Care Medical Centre; (905)897-9000; Fax. (905)879-1818; kabbasi@sasktel.net.

ABBASI, Marjan; Misericordia Community Hosp, 16940 87 Ave NW, Edmonton AB T5R 4H5; (Iran)'96; CCFP; Staff, Covenant Health - Misericordia Community Hospital; (780)735-2362; Fax. (780)735-2533.

ABBASI, Qamar A; Western Mem Reg Hosp, PO Box 2005 Stn Main 1 Brookfield Ave, Corner Brook NL A2H 6J7; Santo Domingo (Dominican Republic)'84; Staff, Western Memorial Regional Hospital; (709)637-5601

ABBASI DEZFOULY, Nader; 5790 Mullen Way NW PO Box 36555 Mactaggart RPO, Edmonton AB T6R 0S0; Tehran (Iran)'97; FRCPC; OccupMed. Staff, University of Alberta Hospital.

ABBASIAN, Ali; Cape Breton Healthcare Complex, 1482 George St, Sydney NS B1P 1P3; Tehran (Iran)'91; FRCPC; DiagRad. Staff, Cape Breton Healthcare Complex; (902)567-8000

ABBASS, Allan A; Abbie J Lane Mem Bldg, 8203-5909 Veterans Memorial La, Halifax NS B3H 2E2; Dal'87; BSc; FRC; FRCPC; Psy (Brief Psychotherapy). Staff Psy, Queen Elizabeth II Health Sciences Centre - Victoria General Site; Dir Education, Dalhousie University; (902)473-2514; Fax. (902)473-4545; allan.abbass@dal.ca.

ABBASS, Syed Akbar; St Joseph's Health Centre, 30 The Queensway, Toronto ON M6R 1B5; Wes'02; FRCPC; Anes. Staff, St Joseph's Health Centre; (416)530-6000

ABBASS, Syed Ashgar; The Cleveland Clinic, Box 818 3000-181 Bay St, Toronto ON M5J 2T3; Wes'02; FRCPC; Anes. Staff, Humber River Regional Hospital - Finch Avenue Site; Staff, Lakeview Surgery Centre; Staff, Greene Stone Clinic Toronto; Staff, Albany Medical Clinic; Staff, Cottrelle Gastroenterology Centre; (416)507-6600; sabbass@cheo.on.ca.

ABBEY, Bruce V; 4-21 College Ave W, Guelph ON N1G 1R7; Tor'71; DABD; Langs: French; (519)654-2200; Fax. (519)654-9105; chevalvolantlibre@yahoo.com.

ABBEY, Mark D; 2768 Broadway W PO Box 74611 Rpo Kitsilano, Vancouver BC V6K 4P4; UBC'88; CCFP; (604)875-1137

ABBEY, Susan E; Dept of Psy, 11C 1114-585 University Ave, Toronto ON M5G 2N2; Tor'81; BSc; FRCPC; Psy (Transplant Psychiatry). Dir Med Psy, Toronto General Hospital - UHN; (416)340-4447; susan.abbey@uhn.on.ca.

ABBI, Arun K; Foothills Med Centre, C231-1403 29 St NW, Calgary AB T2N 2T9; Alb'90; FRCPC; EmergMed. Staff, Foothills Medical Centre; (403)816-1848

ABBOTT, Beverly J; Medical Serv Solutions Inc, 114 Empire Ave, St. John's NL A1C 3G2; Mem'80; CCFP; (709)738-1919

ABBOTT, Burton B; 2300 McPhillips St, Winnipeg MB R2V 3M3; Sask'98; BSc; BMR(PT); CCFP; FRCPC; Staff, Seven Oaks General Hospital; Staff, St Boniface General Hospital; Asst Prof EmergMed/Lecturer Physical Therapy, University of Manitoba; (204)632-3113

ABBOTT, David F; 117-1350 Burrard St, Vancouver BC V6Z 0C2; (United Kingdom)'67; Staff, Mackenzie & District Hospital & Health Centre; (250)997-7892; david.abbott@northernhealth.ca.

ABBOTT, Laura L; Waterford Family Health Centre, 23 Main St, Waterford ON N0E 1Y0; Tor'92; CCFP; FCFP; (519)443-6694; Fax. (519)443-6829.

ABBOTT, Lesleigh S; The Hosp for Sick Children, 555 University Ave, Toronto ON M5G 1X8; Ott'07; FRCPC; Peds (Hematological Oncology). Staff, The Hospital For Sick Children; (416)813-7742

ABBOTT, Michael M; 65 Park Lane Circle, North York ON M3C 2N4; Tor'51; FACP; FACC; FCCP; FAHA; FRCPC; IntMed (Cardiology). Staff, Mount Sinai Hospital; Staff, North York General Hospital - Branson Division; (416)222-8800; Fax. (416)222-5246.

ABBOTT, William E; St Paul's Hosp, 1081 Burrard St, Vancouver BC V6Z 1Y6; McM'75; FRCPC; Anes. Staff, Providence Health Care - St Paul's Hospital; (604)682-2344

ABBOUD, Fayez; CSSSG-Hop de Gatineau, CP 2000 Succ Bureau-Chef 909 boul de la Verendrye O, Gatineau QC J8P 7H2; Paris (France)'80; ac Staff, Hôpital de Gatineau; Prof, McGill University; Langs: Arabic; English; (819)561-8100

ABBOUD, Jeffrey; Carling-Broadview Med Bldg, 306-770 Broadview Ave, Ottawa ON K2A 3Z3; Ott'87; Staff, Carleton Place & District Memorial Hospital; (613)321-8328

ABBOUD, Olivier; Hop du Sacre-Coeur de Mtl, 5400 boul Gouin O, Montreal QC H4J 1C5; Mon'07; Otol. Staff, Hôpital du Sacre-Coeur de Montréal; (514)338-2222

ABBOUD, Rana; Seneca Sports Centre, G2652-1750 Finch Ave E, North York ON M2J 2X5; Man'05; CCFP; Staff, St George's Medical Centre; Staff The Seneca Health Centre, Seneca College; (416)491-5050

ABBOUD, Samir; Centre Med Notre-Dame, 1515 rue Notre-Dame, Lachine QC H8S 2E4; Montpellier (France)'71; FRCSC; Otol (P.Q.). (514)637-1138

ABBU, Ganesan P; Dr C W Wiebe Med Centre, 385 Main St, Winkler MB R6W 1J2; Natal (South Africa)'87; MB ChB; CCFP; FCFP; (204)325-4312

ABBUD, Saad L; St Lawrence Med Clinic, PO Box 772 36 Ottawa St, Morrisburg ON K0C 1X0; Baghdad (Iraq)'79; MSc; MB ChB; CCFP; (613)543-2963

ABCARIUS, Fredericka N; Mount Sinai Hosp Centre, 5690 boul Cavendish, Cote Saint-Luc QC H4W 1S7; McG'91; CCFP; FCFP; Staff, Mount Sinai Hospital Center; Staff, McGill University Health Centre - Montreal Chest Institute; (514)369-2222 x2200; Fax. (514)369-6187.

ABD EL MESIH, Sameh A B M N; Hamiota Health Centre, 177 Birch Ave E, Hamiota MB R0M 0T0.

ABD HALIM, Siti R; Health Sciences Centre, 300 Prince Philip Dr, St. John's NL A1B 3V6; Staff, Health Sciences Centre.

ABDALIAN, Rupert S; 2038 Victoria Park Ave, North York ON M1R 1V2; McG'03; FRCPC; IntMed; Gastroent. Staff, North York General Hospital; (416)447-7000; Fax. (416)447-7072.

ABDALLA, Abdallah H; 9711 101 Ave, Fort St. John BC V1J 6S1; Tanta (Egypt)'78; Staff, Fort St John Hospital & Health Centre; (250)262-5282

ABDALLA, Anwer; Millbourne Mall Med Centre, 115 Millbourne Shopp Ctr NW, Edmonton AB T6K 3L6; (Libya)'01; MB BCh; CCFP; (587)521-2022; Fax. (587)521-2023.

ABDALLA, Mohamed A A; Tillsonburg Dist Mem Hosp, 167 Rolph St, Tillsonburg ON N4G 3Y9; Nairobi (Kenya)'00; Staff, Tillsonburg District Memorial Hospital; (519)842-3611; Fax. (519)842-6733.

ABDALLA, Mohamed E; 204-535 Belmont Ave W, Kitchener ON N2M 5E9; Ain Shams (Egypt)'79; MB ChB; CCFP; (519)571-3295; Fax. (519)571-8378.

ABDALLA, Shaza E E; Carman Commun Health Centre, PO Box 1570, Carman MB R0G 0J0; CCFP.

ABDALLAH, Amel; Fort William Family Hlth Team, 117 McKellar St S, Thunder Bay ON P7E 1H5; Tunis (Tunisia)'92; CCFP; Staff, Anishnawbe Mushkiki Health Centre; Langs: French; Arabic; (807)626-1257; Fax. (807)622-2541.

ABDALLAH, Omar E M; North Walkerville Med Centre, 110-2425 Tecumseh Rd E, Windsor ON N8W 1E6; Cairo (Egypt)'75; Otol (Head & Neck Surgery). (519)252-9196; Fax. (519)252-0375.

ABDEEN, Aboosaly Z; 104 Main St PO Box 507 Stn Main, Stephenville NL A2N 3B4; Colombo (Sri Lanka)'61; MRCS; Dip Ortho(Lond.); DABOph; FRCS; FRCSC; Ophth (Surgical & Medical Ophthalmology). Consultant, Sir Thomas Roddick Hospital; (709)643-5217; Fax. (709)643-3041.

ABDEEN, Nishard; CSSSG Hop de Hull, 116 boul Lionel-Emond, Gatineau QC J8Y 1W7; McG'88; FRCPC; DiagRad. Staff, Hull Hospital; (819)595-6000; Fax. (819)595-6076.

ABDEL-BAKI, Amal; CHUM-Hôp Notre-Dame, 1560 rue Sherbrooke E, Montreal QC H2L 4M1; Laval'96; MSc; FRCPC; Psy (Early Intervention Psychosis). Staff, Centre Hospitalier l'Université de Montréal (CHUM) - Hôpital Notre-Dame; Prof clin agrégé, Universite de Montreal; Langs: English; (514)890-8242; amalbaki@hotmail.com.

ABDEL-BARR, Sara J; Business Bldg, 510-1200 Burrard St, Vancouver BC V6Z 2C7; UBC'89; Vis Staff, Providence Health Care - St Paul's Hospital; (604)681-9022

ABDEL-BARY, Mona A M; 8A-1390 Major Mackenzie Dr E, Richmond Hill ON L4S 0A1; Ain Shams (Egypt)'80; MB BS; CCFP; Langs: Arabic; (905)884-7711

ABDEL-FATTAH, Mohamed M; 201-2030 Marine Dr, North Vancouver BC V7P 1V7; Cairo (Egypt)'76; MB ChB; MHA; FRCPC; Psy (Psychosomatic Medicine). Staff, Lions Gate Hospital; Langs: Arabic; (604)770-4211

ABDEL-GALIL, Ramzy; CFB Edmonton, PO Box 10500 Stn Forces, Edmonton AB T5J 4J5; Wes'07; CCFP; (780)973-4011

ABDEL HADI, Farid M; 16-1615 Dundas St E, Whitby ON L1N 2L1; Cairo (Egypt)'89; MHSc(Bioethics); FRCSC; ObstGyn (Infertility). Staff, Lakeridge Health - Oshawa Site; Locum Tenens, Northumberland Hills Hospital; Locum Tenens, Ross Memorial Hospital; Asst Prof ObstGyn, Queen's University; Langs: Russian; Arabic; (905)245-0711; Fax. (905)245-0522; obclinic@rogers.com.

ABDEL-HAFEZ, Mohammed S; Harvest Hills Med Clinic, 715-500 Country Hills Blvd NE, Calgary AB T3K 4Y7; (Egypt)'92; MB ChB; CCFP; (403)226-8647

ABDEL-HAMID, M Nabile; 2F-905 Victoria Ave E, Thunder Bay ON P7C 1B3; Cairo (Egypt)'68; LRCPS(Glas); DGS; FRCS(Ed); FRCS(Glas); FRCSC; Otol (Head & Neck Surgery). Ac Staff, Thunder Bay Regional Health Sciences Centre; (807)623-5678; Fax. (807)622-1586.

ABDEL-KADER, Mahmoud A K; 3410 28 Ave, Vernon BC V1T 1W9; Cairo (Egypt)'78; MB ChB; MRCPsy(UK); FRCPC; Psy. Consultant Psy, Vernon Jubilee Hospital; (250)542-3475; Fax. (250)542-0954.

ABDEL-KERIEM, Mohamed A; Peter Lougheed Centre, 3722-3500 26 Ave NE, Calgary AB T1Y 6J4; Alexandria (Egypt)'75; MB ChB; MRCPsy(UK); FRCPC; Psy (General Psychiatry). Consultant Forensic Psy, Peter Lougheed Centre; Clin Assoc Prof Psy, University of Calgary; Langs: Arabic; (403)297-7701; Fax. (403)297-7790; mohamed.abdel-keriem@calgaryhealthregion.ca.

ABDEL-MALAK, Maher N M; Halton Healthcare Serv Corp, 327 Reynolds St, Oakville ON L6J 3L7; Cairo (Egypt)'80; CCFP; Staff, Halton Healthcare Services Corporation - Oakville Site; (905)845-2571

ABDEL-MALAK, Mamdouh Z; 410-101 Syndicate Ave N, Thunder Bay ON P7C 3V4; Cairo (Egypt)'82; FRCSC; Urol. Staff Urol, Thunder Bay Regional Health Sciences Centre; Assoc Prof, North West Medical School; Langs: Arabic; (807)623-8896; Fax. (807)623-1533.

ABDEL MALAK, Nagy M; North Hamilton Commun Hlth Ctr, 438 Hughson St N, Hamilton ON L8L 4N5; Asiyut (Egypt)'82; MB ChB; CCFP; Staff, Burlington Walk-In Clinic; Staff, Derry Medical Clinic; (905)523-6611

ABDEL MALEK, Gihan F K; Thames Valley FHT-W London FH, 2F-785 Wonderland Rd S, London ON N6K 1M6; Cairo (Egypt)'83; CCFP; Staff, Strathroy Middlesex General Hospital - Middlesex Hospital Alliance; (519)641-6712; Fax. (519)641-6189.

ABDEL-MALEK, Maximous Y M; Lisgar Woods Med Centre, B2-6970 Lisgar Dr, Mississauga ON L5N 8C8; Asyut (Egypt)'78; LMCC; CCFP; FCFP; Langs: Arabic; (905)824-4441; Fax. (905)824-4431.

ABDEL MALEK, Mira G K; 2670 County Rd 43 PO Box 1119, Kemptville ON K0G 1J0; Ain Shams (Egypt)'00; CCFP; Staff, Strandherd Crossing Medical Centre; (613)258-4131; Fax. (613)258-2799.

ABDEL-MALEK, Nada; Gates of Maple Family Practice, 201-955 Major Mackenzie Dr W, Maple ON L6A 4P9; Ott'10; CCFP; (905)417-7899

ABDEL MALEK, Wafik F; 2-310 Guelph St, Georgetown ON L7G 4B1; Alexandria (Egypt)'82; CCFP; Staff, South Georgetown Medical Clinic; (905)877-2220

ABDEL-MALIK GHALI, Rafik R; 205-477 King St, Welland ON L3B 3K4; Cairo (Egypt)'83; MB ChB; FRCSC; GenSurg. Staff, Niagara Health System - Welland Hospital Site; (905)732-6660; Fax. (905)732-6669.

ABDEL MEGUID, Abdel M K; Streetsville Glen Med Centre, 1-7955 Financial Dr, Brampton ON L6Y 0J8; Cairo (Egypt)'69; MB BCh; Langs: Arabic; (905)455-8877; Fax. (905)455-8867.

ABDEL-MESIH, Amal; St Joseph's Healthcare, 50 Charlton Ave E, Hamilton ON L8N 4A6; McM'06; FRCPC; AnatPath. Staff Path & Molecular Med, St Joseph's Healthcare - Charlton Campus; (905)522-1155; Fax. (905)521-6192.

ABDEL-QADIR, Husam-Eldin M; Univ Hlth Network-Toronto Western Hosp, EW5 559-399 Bathurst St, Toronto ON M5T 2S8; Tor'07; FRCPC; IntMed. Staff, Toronto Western Hospital - University Health Network; Langs: Arabic; (416)603-5815; Fax. (416)603-5398.

ABDEL-RAZEK, Khaled H; Orillia Med/Dental Centre, 200-16 O'Brien St, Orillia ON L3V 5S2; Ain Shams (Egypt)'86; FRCSC; ObstGyn. Staff ObstGyn, Orillia Soldiers' Memorial Hospital; (705)325-3111; Fax. (705)325-1089.

ABDEL-SALAM, Hama S I; Espanola & Area Family Hlth Team, 801 McKinnon Dr, Espanola ON P5E 1T2; Dundee (Scotland)'79; MB ChB; CCFP; FCFP; Ac Staff, Anson General Hospital; Langs: Arabic; French; (705)258-4156; Fax. (705)258-4159.

ABDEL SALAM, Suzan Y; LMC Endocrinology Centres, 306-5 Quarry Ridge Rd, Barrie ON L4M 7G1; Punjab (Pakistan)'86; FRCPC; IntMed (Endocrinology). (705)737-0830; Fax. (705)737-0679.

ABDEL SAMAD, Nizar; The Moncton Hosp, 135 av MacBeath, Moncton NB E1C 6Z8; Beirut (Lebanon)'98; Staff, The Moncton Hospital; (506)857-5111

ABDEL-SAYED, Farid I; 105-195 boul Greber, Gatineau QC J8T 3R1; Cairo (Egypt)'61; MB ChB; AB; (819)243-0010; Fax. (819)243-0088.

ABDEL SHAHID, Raafat A A; Pollard's Point Med Clinic, GD, Pollards Point NL A0K 4B0; University of Cairo (Egypt)'86; MB BCh.

ABDELATY, Amr Nour E; Colchester East Hants Hlth Ctr, 600 Abenaki Rd, Truro NS B2N 5A1; Ain Shams University (Egypt)'94; MB BCh; Staff, Colchester East Hants Health Centre.

ABDELBARY, Hesham A M M; Mount Sinai Hosp, 600 University Ave, Toronto ON M5G 1X5; McM'03; FRCSC; OrthSurg. Staff, Mount Sinai Hospital; (416)596-4200

ABDELGADER, Abdelgalel; Windsor Health Centre, 101-700 Tecumseh Rd E, Windsor ON N8X 4T2; Libya (Libya)'93; FRCPC; IntMed; Rheum. Staff, Windsor Regional Hospital - Metropolitan Site; Staff, Hôtel-Dieu Grace Hospital; Langs: Arabic; (519)258-5335

ABDELGADIR, Ibrahim M; St Martha's Reg Hosp, 25 Bay St, Antigonish NS B2G 2G5; Garyounis (Libya)'98; FRCPC; IntMed; Gastroent. Staff, St Martha's Regional Hospital; (902)863-4500

ABDELHALEEM, Mohamed M M S; The Hosp for Sick Children, 3691-555 University Ave, Toronto ON M5G 1X8; Zagazig (Egypt)'86; MB ChB; MSc; PhD; FRCPC; HemPath. Head Div of HemPath, The Hospital For Sick Children; Asst Prof Med, University of Toronto; Langs: Arabic; (416)813-6434; Fax. (416)813-6257; mohamed.abdelhaleem@sickkids.ca.

ABDELHALIM-AMDISS, Fatima; Ctr Hosp Pierre-Janet, 20 rue Pharand Gatineau, Gatineau QC J9A 1K7; Mohamad V (Morocco)'81; Staff, Centre Hospitalier Pierre-Janet; Prof, University of Ottawa; (819)771-7761

ABDELHUSSEIN, Hussein S; Plains Med Centre, 141 Plains Rd W, Burlington ON L7T 1G1; Baghdad (Iraq)'02; MB ChB; CCFP; (905)218-6444; Fax. (905)521-2775.

ABDELLATIF, Dalia M A; East Edmonton Health Centre, 7910 112 Ave NW, Edmonton AB T5B 0C2; CCFP; (780)757-4220

ABDELMALAK, Ehab M T; Apple Wellness Center, 229 1 St SW, Airdrie AB T4B 3L8; Ain Shams (Egypt)'95; (403)948-3342

ABDELMALEK, Ihab; Tyne Valley Medical Centre, PO Box 145, 6905 Rte 12, Tyne Valley PE C0B 2C0; (Egypt)'94; (902)831-5800; Fax. (902)831-5828.

ABDELMALLEK, Irini A A; Kenderdine Med Clinic, 110-1804 McOrmond Dr, Saskatoon SK S7S 0A6; (306)934-6606; Fax. (306)955-3180.

ABDELMOTTAL, Essam A Y; Providence Care-Mental Health, PO Box 603 Stn Main 752 King St W, Kingston ON K7L 4X3; Benha (Egypt)'94; Staff, Providence Care - Mental Health Services; Asst Prof, Queen's University; Langs: Arabic; (613)546-1101; Fax. (613)548-5580.

ABDELNOUR, Dona; Clinique Med Riviere-des-Prair, CP 149, Montreal QC H1E 0A1; Mon'02; CCFP; (514)494-6973

ABDELNOUR, Miriam; St Mary's Hospital Centre, 3830 av Lacombe, Montreal QC H3T 1M5; Mon'03; CCFP; Staff, St Mary's Hospital Centre; (514)345-3511 x3453

ABDELRAZEK, Nermean M; 210-1920 Ellesmere Rd, Scarborough ON M1H 2V6; Tennessee(TN) (USA)'97; FRCSC; ObstGyn. (416)289-2287; Fax. (416)289-1555.

ABDELSALAM, Ghanim I; 20-1901 Weston Rd, York ON M9N 3P5; Khartoum (Sudan)'81; MB BS; MSc; CCFP; Langs: Arabic; (416)241-7770; Fax. (416)241-5480.

ABDELSALAM, Mahmoud; The Moncton Hosp, 135 MacBeath Ave, Moncton NB E1C 6Z8; Cairo (Egypt)'90; Staff, The Moncton Hospital; (506)857-5111

ABDELSAYED, Nagy S I; Kenderdine Med Clinic, 110-1804 McOrmond Dr, Saskatoon SK S7S 0A6; (306)934-6606; Fax. (306)955-3180.

ABDELSHAHEED, Nabegh N; City Centre Med Clinic, 201-3420 Hurontario St, Mississauga ON L5B 4A9; Cairo (Egypt)'74; FRCPC; MedBiochem. Staff, Trillium Health Centre - Mississauga; (905)848-0045; Fax. (905)848-0047.

ABDESSAMAD, Hasan; PO Box 93666 Nelson Park, Vancouver BC V6E 4L7; Beirut (Lebanon)'03; FRCSC; ObstGyn. Langs: Arabic.

ABDOLLAH, Azad; Kingston Gen Hosp, 76 Stuart St, Kingston ON K7L 2V7; Qns'86; FRCPC; Neur. Staff, Kingston General Hospital; (613)549-6666 x3232

ABDOLLAH, Hoshiar; Kingston Gen Hosp, FAPC3-76 Stuart St, Kingston ON K7L 2V7; Baghdad (Iraq)'72; MB ChB; ABIM; ABCD; FRCPC; Cardiol (Clinical Electro Physiology). Ac Staff, Kingston General Hospital; Prof Dept of Med, Queen's University; Langs: Kurdish; (613)549-6666 x3380; Fax. (613)548-1387; abdollah@kgh.kari.net.

ABDOULRAMAN, Hamed; 206-145 15th St W, North Vancouver BC V7M 1R9; RCS (Ireland)'82; MB ChB; LRCP; LRCS; MRCPsy(UK); BAO; FRCPC; Psy (Child & Adolescent Psychiatry). Staff, Lions Gate Hospital; Langs: English; French; (604)980-0811; Fax. (604)980-9811.

ABDUELMULA, Kamal A A; 205-505 Queen St, Spruce Grove AB T7X 2V2; (780)962-2001; Fax. (780)962-8176.

ABDUKADR, Almuez A K; Access Med Centre, 13718 113A St NW, Edmonton AB T5X 4H7; Al-Fateh (Libya)'01; (780)456-3067

ABDUL HADI, Deema S O; Brampton Medical Plex, 10-27 Ruth Ave, Brampton ON L6Z 4R2; (Ireland)'04; CCFP; (905)495-5888; Fax. (905)495-5822.

ABDUL-HADI, Ibada; Ctr Hosp Affilie-St-Sacrement, 1050 ch Sainte-Foy, Quebec QC G1S 4L8; Laval'03; Staff, Centre Hospitalier Affilié Universitaire de Québec - Hôpital du St-Sacrement; (418)682-7511

ABDUL HADI, Reem S O; Saskatoon Community Clinic, 455 2nd Ave N, Saskatoon SK S7K 2C2; (Ireland)'06; CCFP; (306)652-0300; Fax. (306)664-4120.

ABDUL HAMEED, Saleema; Belle River Med Clinic, PO Box 990 190 Chisholm St, Belle River ON N0R 1A0; Kerala (India)'85; BSc; MB BS; CCFP; (519)728-4495; Fax. (519)728-3895.

ABDUL KADIR, Najeeb A; Cumberland Reg Hlth Care Ctr, 19428 Highway 2, Amherst NS B4H 1N6; Baghdad (Iraq)'82; MB ChB; DGS; FRCS(Glasg.); Staff, Cumberland Regional Health Care Center; (902)667-3361; abidalkader@yahoo.com.

ABDUL-RAHMAN, Ibrahim; Oshawa Med Centre, 675 King St E, Oshawa ON L1H 1G4; Basra (Iraq)'94; MB ChB; LMCC; CCFP; Langs: Arabic; (905)448-9443; Fax. (905)448-1942.

ABDUL RAZAK, Albiruni R; Univ Hlth Network-Princess M, WS33 5-610 University Ave, Toronto ON M5G 2M9; (Ireland)'00; Staff, Princess Margaret Hospital - University Health Network; (416)946-4501

ABDUL-RAZZAK, Amane; Halton Healtcare Serv-Oakville, 327 Reynolds St, Oakville ON L6J 3L7; McM'07; CCFP; Staff, Halton Healthcare Services Corporation - Oakville Site; (905)845-2571

ABDUL WAHAB, Muzafar G; Postgrad Med Education, MDCL 3101A-1280 Main St W, Hamilton ON L8S 4K1; Madurai Kamaraj (India)'93.

ABDULALI, Mufaddal; Unimedico Family Practice, 110-955 Major Mackenzie Dr, Vaughan ON L6A 4P9; Saba University (Netherlands Antilles)'08; (289)553-3300

ABDULHADI, Mohamed H; Broad Med Specialists, 2275 Broad St, Regina SK S4P 1Y7; Benghazi (Libya)'77; MB BS; ABIM; FACP; FRCPC; IntMed; Nephrol. Langs: Arabic; (306)757-2477; Fax. (306)790-1059; abdulhadi@sasktel.net.

ABDULHAFID, Adel H; Barrhead Healthcare Centre, 18-4815 51 Ave, Barrhead AB T7N 1M1; Al Fateh (Libya)'91; Staff, Barrhead Healthcare Centre; (780)674-2221

ABDULHAMEED, Abdulnasser N; Musquodoboit-Harbour Med Clini, 7907 Highway 7, Musquodoboit-Harbr NS B0J 2L0; Baghdad (Iraq)'95; MB ChB; abdulhameed@mun.ca.

ABDULHUSEIN, Abbas G; 5-3098 Falconbridge Hwy, Garson ON P3L 1P5; Cardiff (Wales)'78; MB ChB; Lecturer Clinical Sciences Faculty, Northern Ontario School of Medicine-Laurentian University; Langs: Gujarati; (705)693-4200; Fax. (705)693-2666.

ABDULHUSEIN, Mustafa H; Doctors-R-Us, 12-205 Van Kirk Dr, Brampton ON L7A 3V4; Carribean (Montserrat)'97; CRCP; DABFP; Langs: Gujarati; Hindi; Punjabi; Urdu; (905)495-2254; Fax. (905)495-5350; doctors.r.us@gmail.com.

ABDULHUSSEIN, Rahim; 1-1127 Markham Rd, Scarborough ON M1H 2Y5; Tor'09; CCFP; (416)264-4446; Fax. (416)264-4456.

ABDULHUSSEIN, Salam N; Burin Peninsula Health Care Ct, PO Box 340, Burin NL A0E 1E0; Baghdad (Iraq)'94; MB ChB; Staff, Burin Peninsula Health Care Centre; (709)891-1040

ABDULJALIL, Nabil; Kingston Gen Hosp, 76 Stuart St, Kingston ON K7L 2V7; Al-Fateh (Libya)'99; CCFP; Staff, Kingston General Hospital; (613)549-6666

ABDULKAREEM, Ali Ihsan; Bonavista Peninsula Health Ctr, Postal Service 1 Hospital Rd, Bonavista NL A0C 1B0; Al-Mustansiriyah (Iraq)'92; MB ChB; Staff, Bonavista Peninsula Health Centre; (709)468-7881

ABDULKARIM, Bassam S; MUHC-Montreal Gen Hosp, 1650 av Cedar, Montreal QC H3G 1A4; Aix-Marseille (France)'97; FRCPC; MedOncol (Radiation Oncology). Staff, McGill University Health Centre - Montreal General Campus; (514)934-1934

ABDULKARIM, Emad H; Southbank Med Centre, 3-2430 Bank St, Ottawa ON K1V 0T7; Mosul (Iraq)'88; (613)736-6946; Fax. (613)736-6948.

ABDULKARIM, Soran S; Rouge Valley HS-Centenary, 2867 Ellesmere Rd, Scarborough ON M1E 4B9; Univ of Al-Mustansiriyah (Iraq)'96; FRCPC; AnatPath. Staff, Rouge Valley Health System - Centenary Health Centre Site; Staff, Rouge Valley Health System - Ajax & Pickering Health Centre Site; (416)284-8131

ABDULKHALIQ, Anas; Waterford Hosp, 306 Waterford Bridge Rd, St. John's NL A1E 4J8; U of Al-Mustansiriyah (Iraq)'02; MB ChB; CCFP; Staff, Waterford Hospital; (709)777-3300

ABDULKHALIQ, Taha; Dr William H Newhook Comm HC, PO Box 449, Whitbourne NL A0B 3K0; Baghdad (Iraq)'86; MB ChB; CCFP; Staff, Dr William H Newhook Health Centre; (709)873-2330; abdulkhaliq@mun.ca.

ABDULLA, Agiela M K; Prairie North Health Centre, 4806 50th St, Lloydminster SK S9V 0M9; IntMed. (306)820-5997; Fax. (306)820-5978.

ABDULLA, Alnoor; 2902-583 Beach Cres, Vancouver BC V6Z 3E6; UBC'75; FACP; FACC; FCCP; ABIM; ABCD; FRCP; LMCC; FRCPC; IntMed (Cardiology); Cardiol. Langs: Gujarati; Urdu; Swahili; (604)377-9929; abdulla@cardiaccare.ca.

ABDULLA, Alykhan S; The Kingsway Health Centre, PO Box 819 Stn Main 1F-5542 Ann St, Manotick ON K4M 1A7; Cal'92; Dip SportMed; LMCC; BSc; FCFP; DTMed; AAFPhys; CCFP; FCFP; Med Dir, The Kingsway Health Centre; Med Dir, The Kingsway Travel Clinic; Med Dir, The Healthy Performer; Langs: Gujarati; Kacchi; (613)692-5433; Fax. (613)692-5435.

ABDULLA, Ramzan H; 1821 Rose St, Regina SK S4P 1Z7; Makerere (Uganda)'71; MB ChB; ABIM; FCCP; FRCPC; IntMed; Respir. Staff, Regina General Hospital; Head Med/Sec Head Respiratory, Regina Qu'Appelle Health Region; Clin Prof Med, University of Saskatchewan; (306)525-2270; Fax. (306)359-1068.

ABDULLA, Safwat S A; James Paton Mem Hosp, 125 Trans Canada Hwy, Gander NL A1V 1P7; Al Fateh (Libya)'91; MB BCh; Staff, James Paton Memorial Hospital; (709)256-2500

ABDULLAH, Ali R; Meridian Clinic, 3-4402 37 St, Stony Plain AB T7Z 2A9; (Iraq)'92; (780)963-7800

ABDULLAH, Amid K; Calgary Lab Services, 9-3535 Research Rd NW, Calgary AB T2L 2K8; Baghdad (Iraq)'84; FRCPC; GenPath. Staff, Calgary Laboratory Services; Langs: Arabic; Kurdish; Farsi; (403)770-3670; Fax. (403)770-3292.

ABDULLAH, Nadine; Univ Hlth Network-Toronto Western Hosp, EW8 417-399 Bathurst St, Toronto ON M5T 2S8; Tor'98; LMCC; BSc; FRCP; MD; MEd; FRCPC; IntMed. Staff, Toronto Western Hospital - University Health Network; (416)603-6467

ABDULLAH, Rukhsana A; Trillium Hlth Ctr-Mississauga, 100 Queensway W, Mississauga ON L5B 1B8; Karachi (Pakistan)'90; FRCPC; Peds. Staff, Trillium Health Centre - Mississauga; (905)848-7580

ABDULLAH, Ubaidullah; Alberta Hosp Edmonton, PO Box 307 Stn Main, Edmonton AB T5J 2J7; Staff, Alberta Hospital Edmonton; Staff, Alberta Mental Health Board; (780)342-5439; Fax. (780)342-5233.

ABDULMAJID AL HAMAMI, Ihsan; Malvern Med Centre, 100-1333 Neilson Rd, Toronto ON M1B 4Y9; Alexandria (Egypt)'79; MB ChB; PhD; CCFP; FCFP; (416)291-7719; Fax. (416)787-3775.

ABDULNOUR, Elias M; CHUM-Hop St-Luc, 1058 rue Saint-Denis, Montreal QC H2X 3J4; St. Joseph (Lebanon)'75; FRCSC; GenSurg; Cardiovasc&ThorSurg. Staff, Centre Hospitalier l'Université De Montréal (CHUM) - Hôpital Saint-luc; (514)890-8000

ABDULRAHMAN, Abdulqadir M; Bluewater Health-Norman Site, 89 Norman St, Sarnia ON N7T 6S3; (Somalia)'90; FRCPC; Anes. Staff, Bluewater Health - Mitton Site; Staff, Rouge Valley Health System - Centenary Health Centre Site; Staff, Rouge Valley Health System - Ajax & Pickering Health Centre Site; Staff, Bluewater Health - Norman Site; (519)464-4400; Fax. (519)464-4501.

ABDULRAHMAN ALANSARI, Nabeel M M; 465 University Ave PO Box 21120 Rpo University, Charlottetown PE C1A 9H6; Volgograd (Russia (Federation))'84.

ABDULREHMAN, Abdulhamid S; 200 St Anne's Rd, Winnipeg MB R2M 3A1; Bristol (England)'73; DRCOG; LMCC; Ac Staff, Victoria General Hospital; Staff, Concordia General Hospital; Staff, St Boniface General Hospital; (204)255-3998

ABDULSAMAD, Atef A M; Lessard Med Clinic, 6633 177 St NW, Edmonton AB T5T 4K3; Al-Fateh (Libya)'00; ABIM; FRCPC; IntMed;CCFP; Attending Academic Staff, University of Alberta; Langs: Arabic; (780)757-7999; Fax. (780)757-7991.

ABDURAHMAN, Adel; Sault Area Hosp, 750 Great Northern Rd, Sault Ste. Marie ON P6B 0A8; Ott'04; GenSurg. Staff, Sault Area Hospital - Sault Ste Marie; Staff, Temiskaming Hospital; (705)759-3434

ABDURRAHMAN, Murtala B; Baywood Med Centre, 202-95 Bayly St W, Ajax ON L1S 7K8; Ibadan (Nigeria)'67; MB BS; MD; FRCPC; Peds (Nephrology). Staff Peds, Rouge Valley Health System - Ajax & Pickering Health Centre Site; (905)683-7593; Fax. (905)683-7669; pediatricgroup@sympatico.ca.

ABDURRAHMAN, Zainab B; PG Med Educ McMaster Univ, MDCL 3101A-1280 Main St W, Hamilton ON L8S 4K1; Tor'07; FRCPC; Peds; ClinImmunol&Allergy.

ABED, Abeer K E; 3461 Cook St, Victoria BC V8X 1B3; Zagazig (Egypt)'91; MB BCh; CCFP; (250)386-6161

ABED, Mohammed M; Cornwall Prof Bldg, 416-2125 11th Ave, Regina SK S4P 3X3; Tehran (Iran)'62; FAB; FRCSC; ObstGyn (Ultrasound). Obstetrics & Gynecology, Pasqua Hospital; Ac Staff, Regina General Hospital; Physician, Regina Health District; Clin Prof, University of Saskatchewan; Langs: Farsi; (306)352-7800; Fax. (306)757-3694; dr.abed@accesscomm.ca.

ABEDI, Syed T H; Scarborough Hosp-Birchmount, 3030 Birchmount Rd, Scarborough ON M1W 3W3; Osmania (India)'75; MB BS; MSc; FCAP; FRCPC; AnatPath (Hematology Pathology). Staff, The Scarborough Hospital - Birchmount Campus; Consultant Pathologist, Canadian Medical Laboratories; Langs: Persian; Urdu; (416)495-2701; Fax. (416)495-2477.

ABEDPOUR DARDASHTI, Marzieh; Centre Med Brunswick, 955 boul Saint-Jean, Pointe-Claire QC H9R 5K3; CCFP; (514)426-6677

ABEJ, Esmail; Health Sciences Centre, GC425-820 Sherbrook St, Winnipeg MB R3A 1R9; Al Fateh (Libya)'00; CCFP; Staff, Health Sciences Centre; Langs: Arabic; (204)787-4930; eaabej@hotmail.com.

ABEL, James G; St Paul's Hosp, B492-1081 Burrard St, Vancouver BC V6Z 1Y6; Tor'83; BSc; MSc; FRCSC; GenSurg (Cardiovascular Surgery); Cardiovasc&ThorSurg. Staff Surg, Providence Health Care - St Paul's Hospital; Staff Surg, Vancouver General Hospital - Centennial Pavillion; Clin Assoc Prof Surg, University of British Columbia; (604)806-8503; Fax. (604)806-9453; jabel@providencehealth.bc.ca.

ABEL, Julie; CHUS-Hop Fleurimont, 3001 12e av N, Sherbrooke QC J1H 5N4; Sher'95; FRCPC; IntMed. Staff, Centre Hospitalier Universitaire de Sherbrooke-Hopital Fleurimont; (819)346-1110 x14948; Fax. (819)820-6406.

ABEL, Katherine J M; LA Medical Clinic, 30-5201 50 St, Leduc AB T9E 6T4; Alb'02; BSc; CCFP; Staff, Leduc Community Hospital; Staff, Covenant Health - Grey Nuns Community Hospital; (780)986-9600; Fax. (780)986-9732.

ABEL, Rachel D; Health Park, 206-45 Weatherbee Rd, Sydney NS B1M 0A1; Punjab (Pakistan)'89; MB BS; CCFP; (902)270-3340; Fax. (902)270-3339.

ABEL, Selwyn L; 401-3101 Bloor St W, Etobicoke ON M8X 2W2; Witwatersrand (South Africa)'73; FRCSC; Ophth (Cataract Surgery). Staff, St Joseph's Health Centre; (416)239-1968; Fax. (416)233-4763.

ABEL, Sylvain; Ctr Hosp du Centre la Mauricie, 50 119e rue, Shawinigan-Sud QC G9P 5K1; Laval'93; FRCSC; GenSurg. General Surgery, Centre Hospitalier du Centre la Mauricie; (819)536-7500; Fax. (819)536-7611.

ABELA, Anthony; Clinique Med de l'Est Inc, 100-30 boul Saint-Joseph E, Montreal QC H2T 1G9; Beyrouth (Lebanon)'69; CSPQ; FRCSC; Otol (Pediatric Otolaryngology). ac Membre, Hôpital Ste-Justine; adj Prof Surg, Universite de Montreal; Langs: Arabic; English; (514)845-4240; Fax. (514)845-5493.

ABELE, Jonathan T; Hys Med Centre, 202-11010 101 St NW, Edmonton AB T5H 4B9; Wes'99; FRCPC; DiagRad; NuclearMed. Staff, University of Alberta Hospital; (780)428-1121

ABELL, Margaret E; Abell Med Clinic, PO Box 70 134 First St, Wawanesa MB R0K 2G0; Leeds (England)'63; MB ChB(Leeds,UK); (204)824-2327; Fax. (204)824-2361; abellmedclinic@shaw.ca.

ABELL, Nicholas A; Hanover Med Associates, 118 7th Ave, Hanover ON N4N 2G9; Man'99; CCFP; FRCPC; (519)364-2820

ABELL, William R; Rosser Avenue Med Clinic, 841 Rosser Ave, Brandon MB R7A 0L1; Leeds (England)'64; MRCS; LRCP; DObstRCOG; Ac Staff, Glenboro Health District Hospital; Ac Staff, Baldur Health Centre; Chief/Medical Staff, Wawanesa & District Memorial Health Centre; University of Manitoba.

ABELLS, Yoel B; Forest Hill Family Health Cent, 491 Eglinton Ave W, Toronto ON M5N 1A8; McM'84; CCFP; FCFP; Staff, Mount Sinai Hospital; Staff, Humber River Regional Hospital - Keele Street Site; (416)782-6111

ABELSETH, David P; PO Box 266 Stn Postal Box Ctr, Red Deer AB T4N 5E8; Cal'82; FRCPC; Psy (Child & Adolescent Psychiatry). Staff, Red Deer Regional Hospital Centre; Consultant, Alberta Mental Health Board; (403)314-1100; Fax. (403)314-1178; abelseth@telusplanet.net.

ABELSETH, Gregory A; Gulf Canada Square, 335-401 9 Ave SW, Calgary AB T2P 3C5; Cal'88; BEng; FRCSC; OrthSurg (General Orthopedics). Ac Staff, Rockyview General Hospital; Ac Staff, Peter Lougheed Centre; Clin Assoc Prof Orth, University of Calgary; (403)221-4322; Fax. (403)221-4387; gregory.abelseth@calgaryhealthregion.ca.

ABELSOHN, Alan R; 205-1466 Bathurst St, Toronto ON M5R 3S3; Cape Town (South Africa)'74; MB ChB; CCFP; FCFP; Langs: Afrikaans; (416)483-8111; Fax. (416)483-8182; alan.abelsohn@utoronto.ca.

ABELSON, William H; Victoria Med Bldg, 512-1669 Victoria St, Prince George BC V2L 2L5; Tor'80; FRCPC; Peds; InfectDis. Staff, University Hospital of Northern British Columbia; (250)563-4550; Fax. (250)563-4045.

ABENHAIM, Haim A; H325-5790 ch Cote-des-Neiges, Montreal QC H3S 1Y9; McG'01; FRCS; MPH; FRCSC; ObstGyn (Maternal Fetal Medicine). Staff/Dir Perinatal Research, Sir Mortimer B Davis Jewish General; (514)340-8222 x5488; Fax. (514)340-7941.

ABENHEIMER, Martin S M; 97 Bentinck St, Sydney NS B1P 1G3; Glasgow (Scotland)'75; FRCPC; Peds. Chief Peds, Cape Breton Healthcare Complex; (902)562-8501; Fax. (902)562-8255.

ABERGEL, Heidi A; Clinique Med Mondiale, 1-5598 ch de la Cote-des-Neige, Montreal QC H3T 1Y8; McG'00; CCFP; (514)733-9899

ABERMAN, Arnold; 585 University Ave, Toronto ON M5G 2N2; McG'67; FRCPC; IntMed (Respirology). Staff, Toronto General Hospital - UHN; (416)821-1321; arnie.aberman@utoronto.ca.

ABERMAN, Arnold B; CLSC Seigneurie de Beauharnois, 142 rue Saint-Laurent, Beauharnois QC J6N 1V9; McG'74; (450)429-6455; Fax. (450)429-1119.

ABESAMIS, Gregorio R; Royal Alexandra Hosp, 10240 Kingsway Ave NW, Edmonton AB T5H 3V9; (Philippines)'83; Staff, Royal Alexandra Hospital; (780)735-4111

ABEYSEKERA, Rathnayake M M S; Cumberland Reg Hlth Care Ctr, 19428 Highway 2, Amherst NS B4H 1N6; Ceylon (Sri Lanka)'76; MB BS; DA(Eng.); FRCA(UK); Staff, Sackville Memorial Hospital; Staff, Cumberland Regional Health Care Center; (902)667-3361; Fax. (902)667-6031.

ABEYSINGHE, Chitralekha R; Ashgrove Med Bldg, 101-6633 Highway 7, Markham ON L3P 7P2; Colombo (Sri Lanka)'92; MB BS; CCFP; Langs: Sinhalese; Tamil; (905)471-6621

ABEYSINGHE, Nilanga M; Near North Med Clinic, 202-66 Josephine St, North Bay ON P1B 0A7; Colombo (Sri Lanka)'02; CCFP; (705)474-2106; Fax. (705)474-6613.

ABI DAOUD, Marie; Calgary Lab Services, 3535 Research Rd NW, Calgary AB T2L 2K8; Dal'04; FRCPC; AnatPath. Staff, Calgary Laboratory Services; (403)770-3569; Fax. (403)770-3788.

ABI-JAOUDE, Elia; Univ Hlth Network-Toronto Western Hosp, 3W 402-399 Bathurst St, Toronto ON M5T 2S8; Man'04; FRCPC; Psy. Fellow, Toronto Western Hospital - University Health Network; (416)603-2581; Fax. (416)603-5180.

ABI RAAD, Camille; CSSS de Trois-Rivieres, 1991 boul du Carmel, Trois-Rivieres QC G8Z 3R9; (Lebanon)'93; Staff, CSSS de Trois-Rivières; (819)697-3333

ABID, Simona; Halton HC Serv Corp-Oakville, 327 Reynolds St, Oakville ON L6J 3L7; Timisoara (Romania)'93; FRCPC; IntMed; GeriatricMed. Staff, Halton Healthcare Services Corporation - Oakville Site; (905)845-2571

ABIDI, Rabbiya N; Castlemore Health Centre, 3-65 Braydon Blvd, Brampton ON L6P 2S4; Peshawar (Pakistan)'97; CCFP; (905)794-7649; Fax. (905)794-7650.

ABIDI, Sabina; IWK Health Centre, PO Box 9700 Rpo CSC 5850-5980 University Ave, Halifax NS B3K 6R8; Dal'00; FRCPC; Psy. Staff, IWK Health Centre; (902)470-8888

ABIDI, Shuayb M; Pacific Place Mall, 999 36 St SE, Calgary AB T2A 7X6; Kabul (Afghanistan)'88; CCFP; (403)387-3300

ABIDULLAH, Mohammad; Westman Reg Laboratory, L 108A-150 McTavish Ave E, Brandon MB R7A 7H8; Peshawar (Pakistan)'95; FRCPC; AnatPath. (204)578-4480

ABIKHZER, Gad S; SMBD Jewish Gen Hosp, 3755 ch Cote-Sainte-Catherine, Montreal QC H3T 1E2; McG'06; MDCM; NuclearMed. Staff, Sir Mortimer B Davis Jewish General; (514)340-8222

ABIKHZER, Myriam; 350-5950 ch de la Cote-des-Nei, Montreal QC H3S 1Z6; McG'04; CCFP; (514)733-0987; Fax. (514)733-7704.

ABIKHZER, Victor; 350-5950 Ch de la Cote-des-Nei, Montreal QC H3S 1Z6; Strasbourg (France)'76; Staff, Centre Hospitalier l'Université de Montréal (CHUM) - Hôpital Notre-Dame; Staff, Sir Mortimer B Davis Jewish General; Langs: Hebrew; Arabic; English; (514)733-9192; Fax. (514)733-7704.

ABIKHZER, Yael; 350-5950 ch Cote-des-Neiges, Montreal QC H3S 1Z6; McG'08; CCFP; (514)733-0987; Fax. (514)733-7704.

ABINADER, Naji; 393 boul Marcotte, Roberval QC G8H 1Z5; St. Joseph (Lebanon)'81; FRCSC; OrthSurg. Staff, Hotel-Dieu de Roberval; (418)275-2935

ABISCOTT, Joshua; Access Med Centre, 6-3098 Carling Ave, Nepean ON K2B 7K2; Ott'97; CCFP; (613)596-9840; Fax. (613)596-0496.

ABISH, Sharon B; MUHC-Montreal Children's Hosp, B335-2300 rue Tupper, Montreal QC H3H 1P3; McG'83; FRCPC; Peds (Pediatric Hematology Oncology); MedOncol (P.Q.); Hem (P.Q.). Staff, McGill University Health Centre - Montreal Children's Hospital; McGill University; (514)412-4445; sharon.abish@muhc.mcgill.ca.

ABLA, Oussama A; The Hosp For Sick Children, 555 University Ave, Toronto ON M5G 1X8; Genoa (Italy)'89; Staff, The Hospital For Sick Children; Langs: Arabic; Italian; Spanish; (416)813-7879; Fax. (416)813-5327.

ABLEMAN, Darryl J; Able-Care Med Clinic, 56-2991 Lougheed Hwy, Coquitlam BC V3B 6J6; Witwatersrand (South Africa)'84; Staff, Royal Columbian Hospital; Staff, Eagle Ridge Hospital & Health Care Centre; (604)945-7819; Fax. (604)945-2884.

ABLETT, David P J; Rockyview Gen Hosp, 7007 14 St SW, Calgary AB T2V 1P9; Leeds (England)'74; MB ChB; FRCPC; Anes (Chronic Pain). Staff, Rockyview General Hospital; (403)943-3410; Fax. (403)943-3360.

ABOELNAZAR, Saber A; University of Alberta Hosp, 8440 112 St NW, Edmonton AB T6G 2B7; Alexandria (Egypt)'84; FRCSC; CardSurg. Staff, University of Alberta Hospital; (780)407-8822

ABOELNOUR, Mustafa S; All Well Primary Care, 4217 23 Ave NW, Edmonton AB T6L 5Z8; Al Fateh (Libya)'96; CCFP; (780)462-0442; Fax. (780)462-0577.

ABOGUDDAH, Ayman A; Neil Prof Bldg, 201-2550 12th Ave, Regina SK S4P 3X1; Baghdad (Iraq)'82; ABIM; FACC; FRCPC; IntMed (Echocardiography); Cardiol. Dir Echo Lab, Regina General Hospital; Assoc Prof, University of Saskatchewan; Langs: Arabic; (306)359-7885; Fax. (306)359-2656.

ABOLARIN, Mofoluwaso A; Wellpoint Health, 103-240 Midpark Way SE, Calgary AB T2X 1N4; (Nigeria)'87; MB BS; FRCSEd(Scot); CCFP; Med Dir, Canadian Back Institute; Langs: Yoruba; (403)201-9600; Fax. (403)201-9610.

ABONOWARA, Abdulgani A M; Niagara HS-St Catharines, 142 Queenston St, St. Catharines ON L2R 7C6; Al-Fateh (Libya)'98; FRCPC; IntMed; Cardiol. Staff, Niagara Health System - St Catharines General Site.

ABOO, Aboobaker; Kilborn Med Centre, 100-1385 Bank St, Ottawa ON K1H 8N4; Craiova (Romania)'81; Langs: Portuguese; Romanian; French; Spanish; Italian; (613)523-4874; Fax. (613)523-7440.

ABOO, Ismail Y; Grey Bruce HS-Owen Sound, PO Box 1800 Stn Main 1800 8th St E, Owen Sound ON N4K 6M9; Karachi (Pakistan)'87; MB BS; Staff MedOncol & Hematologist, Grey Bruce Health Services - Owen Sound; Langs: Urdu; Hindi; Gujarati; (519)376-2121

ABOOBAKER, Suleman; Central Mall Medical Clinic, 3691 Tecumseh Rd E, Windsor ON N8W 1H8; Medunsa (South Africa)'97; (519)948-0011; Fax. (519)948-0338.

ABOOD, Muhanned F; Percy E Moore Hosp, PO Box 190, Hodgson MB R0C 1N0; Staff, Percy E Moore Hospital; (204)372-8444

ABOOD, Saifee; 9623 66 AVE NW, Edmonton AB T6E 0M2; (Iraq)'94; (780)434-0102

ABORAWI, Abdelbasat; Chinook Paediatric Clinic, 951 19 St S, Lethbridge AB T1J 3H5; Al-Arab (Libya)'94; (403)320-7825; Fax. (403)320-8613.

ABOSH, Dory B; St Michael's Hosp, 30 Bond St, Toronto ON M5B 1W8; Man'98; FRCPC; IntMed. Staff, St Michael's Hospital; (416)864-5431

ABOU ABDO, Mirna; CLSC d'Aylmer, 425 rue Leguerrier, Gatineau QC J9H 6N8; Mon'03; Staff, Hull Hospital; Langs: Arabic; English; (819)684-2251

ABOU CHACRA, Zahi; Group Health Westmount Square, 550-1 Westmount Sq, Montreal QC H3Z 2P9; McG'05; FRCSC; Otol. (514)934-2334

ABOU-GAREEB, Iman; Cambie Plaza Med Clinic, 180-11700 Cambie Rd, Richmond BC V6X 1L5; Alexandria (Egypt)'82; MHSc(Epidemiol); MB BCh; CCFP; Clin Asst Prof Family Med, University of British Columbia; Langs: Arabic; (604)270-9833; Fax. (604)270-8127.

ABOU-KHAMIS, Rami; Burntwood Reg Health Authority, 867 Thompson Dr S, Thompson MB R8N 1Z4; Staff, Northern Health Thompson Regional Office; (204)788-6375

ABOU MOURAD, Yasser; Gordon & Leslie Diamond HCC, 10F-2775 Laurel St, Vancouver BC V5Z 1M9; Sofia (Bulgaria)'96; FRCPC; IntMed. Sr Hematologist, BC Cancer Agency Vancouver Centre; Asst Prof Med, University of British Columbia; Langs: Bulgarian; Arabic; (604)875-4863; Fax. (604)875-4763.

ABOU-NASSAR, Awni; South Common Med Centre, 3-2110 Burnhamthorpe Rd W, Mississauga ON L5L 5Z5; Jerusalem (Israel)'86; Langs: Arabic; Hebrew; (905)820-3209; Fax. (905)820-2576.

ABOU-NASSAR, Karim E; CSSSG-Hop de Gatineau, CP 2000 Succ Bureau-Chef 909 boul de la Verendrye O, Gatineau QC J8P 7H2; Ott'03; FRCPC; IntMed; Hem. Staff, Hôpital de Gatineau; (819)966-6100; Fax. (819)966-6289.

ABOU SAID, Edith; Appletree Med Centre, 2573 Baseline Rd, Ottawa ON K2H 7B3; (Hungary)'93; CCFP; Langs: Arabic; Hungarian; Bilingual(English/French); (613)721-8630; Fax. (613)721-8643.

ABOU-SEIDO, Maher K M; Springdale Prof Bldg, 503-2250 Bovaird Dr E, Brampton ON L6R 0W3; (Kuwait)'86; BSc; MB ChB; FRCOG; FRCSC; ObstGyn. Obstetrics & Gynecology, William Osler Health System - Brampton Civic Hospital; Langs: Arabic; (905)595-4960; Fax. (905)595-4965; maher2001@hotmail.com.

ABOUALI, Jihad A K; Mount Sinai Hosp, 476-600 University Ave, Toronto ON M5G 1X5; McM'07; OrthSurg. Staff, Mount Sinai Hospital; (416)596-4200

ABOUBZOU, Nour-Eddine; CSSS des Aurores Boreales, CP 6000 Succ Bureau-Chef 679 2e rue E, La Sarre QC J9Z 2X7; Bucharest (Romania)'89; Gen Practice, Centre Hospitalier La Sarre; (819)333-2311

ABOUELNASR, Wahid A; East Toronto Health Centre, 1496 Danforth Ave, Toronto ON M4J 1N4; Ein Shams (Egypt)'81; FRCPC; Psy. Staff, Ontario Shores Centre for Mental Health Sciences; (416)778-1496

ABOUHAMRA, Musbah M; Lloyd Women's Clinic, 3308 50 Ave, Lloydminster AB T9V 0V6; Jamahiriya (Libya)'88; MB ChB; FRCSC; ObstGyn. (780)875-8755; Fax. (780)875-5868.

ABOUHASSAN, Tyceer; Jackson Park Med Centre, 201-2475 McDougall St, Windsor ON N8X 3N9; Ott'05; BSc; BA; BEd; MBA; FRCPC; IntMed (Diabetes); Endocrin&Metab. Assoc Prof, Schulich School of Medicine & Dentistry; (519)915-6432; Fax. (519)915-6083.

ABOUJAMRA, Jamal; Pape Med Centre, 1018 Pape Ave, Toronto ON M4K 3V9; Damascus (Syria)'82; CCFP; Langs: Arabic; (416)469-6668; Fax. (416)429-0022.

ABOULISAYEN, Abdullah M; 201-630 Tecumseh Rd E, Windsor ON N8X 4W2; Al-Fateh (Libya)'86; MD; FRCPC; IntMed (Cardiology). (519)258-4900; Fax. (519)258-4901.

ABOUNA, Samir; Matheson Centre, 15-801 Matheson Blvd W, Mississauga ON L5V 2N6; Baghdad (Iraq)'78; MD; MB ChB; CCFP; Langs: Assyrian; Arabic; (905)890-5600; Fax. (905)890-5633; dr_abouna@hotmail.com.

ABOUNAJA, Mohamed A; Rouge Valley-Centenary HC, 2867 Ellesmere Rd, Scarborough ON M1E 4B9; Al-Fateh (Libya)'00; CCFP; Staff, Rouge Valley Health System - Centenary Health Centre Site; (416)797-6577; Fax. (416)281-7438.

ABOURBIH, Jacques; Northern Ontario School of Med, 935 Ramsey Lake Rd, Sudbury ON P3E 2C6; McG'73; FRCSC; Urol. Ac Staff, Health Sciences North-Laurentian Site; Ac Staff, Health Sciences North-St Joseph's Health Centre; Ac Staff, Health Sciences North - Memorial Site; (705)673-8455; Fax. (705)673-8676.

ABOURJAILI, Radwan; Centre medical de Cowansville, 101-370 rue de la Riviere, Cowansville QC J2K 1N3; Sher'87; FRCSC; Otol (Allergy & Respirology). ac Membre, Hôpital Brome-Missisquoi-Perkins; (450)263-0774; Fax. (450)263-6457.

ABOUSSAFY, Andre; CSSS de la Matapedia, 135 av Gaetan-Archambault, Amqui QC G5J 2K5; Laval'86; Staff, CSSS de la Matapedia; (418)629-2211

ABOUSSOUAN, Francis; Cabinet Dr Francis Aboussouan, 34 av Glencoe, Outremont QC H3T 1P9; Mon'82; ac Staff, Centre Hospitalier l'Université de Montréal (CHUM) - Hôtel-Dieu; (514)345-9794; Fax. (514)738-8293.

ABRAHAM, Alan; Langley Health Services, 22051 Fraser Hwy, Langley BC V3A 4H4; Cal'99; FRCPC; Anes. Staff, Langley Memorial Hospital; (604)534-4121

ABRAHAM, Cherrie Z; SMBD Jewish Gen Hosp, E110-3755 ch Cote-Sainte-Cathe, Montreal QC H3T 1E2; Dal'94; FRCSC; GenSurg; VascSurg. Staff, Sir Mortimer B Davis Jewish General; (514)340-8222 x3324

ABRAHAM, Christopher I; Kingston Gen Hosp, 76 Stuart St, Kingston ON K7L 2V7; UBC'96; FRCPC; DiagRad. Staff, Kingston General Hospital; (613)548-2301

ABRAHAM, E George; 115 Maclean Pl, Welland ON L3B 5X9; Bombay (India)'72; MB BS; MRCP(UK); FACC; FRCPC; IntMed (Cardiology). Consultant, Niagara Health System - Welland Hospital Site; Consultant, Niagara Health System - Port Colborne General Site; (905)788-0960; Fax. (905)788-9278.

ABRAHAM, Edward P; Saint John Reg Hosp, PO Box 2100 Stn Main 400 University Ave, Saint John NB E2L 4L2; Dal'82; FRCSC; OrthSurg. Staff, Saint John Regional Hospital; (506)648-7971; Fax. (506)648-7973; abred@reg2.health.nb.ca.

ABRAHAM, Gary C; 101-157 Queen St E, Brampton ON L6W 3X4; Tor'90; BSc(Kinesiol); Staff, William Osler Health System - Brampton Civic Hospital; (905)453-1340; Fax. (905)453-5493.

ABRAHAM, Gebrehiwot; Addiction & Mental Hlth-Queen, 1001 Queen St W, Toronto ON M6J 1H4; Addis Ababa (Ethiopia)'75; FRCPC; Psy. Staff, Centre for Addiction & Mental Health (CAMH) - Queen Site; (416)535-8501 x2254; Fax. (416)583-1334.

ABRAHAM, Hany G; Alpha Care Clinic, 2-310 Guelph St, Georgetown ON L7G 4B1; Ain Shams (Egypt)'87; CCFP; (905)877-2220; Fax. (905)877-5554.

ABRAHAM, J Mathew; Broad Street Clinic, 2210 Broad St, Regina SK S4P 4V6; (Other Foreign)'04; (306)781-8080; Fax. (306)781-5644.

ABRAHAM, Jacob; Pine Med Clinic, 5110 5th Ave, Whitehorse YT Y1A 1L4; (India)'82; MB BS; CCFP; (867)668-4353; mail2jacs@yahoo.ca.

ABRAHAM, Jessica; 2050-11300 Tuscany Blvd NW PO BOX 27066, Calgary AB T3L 2V0; Cal'98; FRCSC; GenSurg.

ABRAHAM, Marilyn; Advanced Walk-In Med Clinic, 111-21 Queensway W, Mississauga ON L5B 1B6; Tor'98; MPH; FRCPC; Peds. Staff, The Hospital For Sick Children; (905)897-0788

ABRAHAM, Robert J; Queen Elizabeth II HSC-Halifax, 3316-1796 Summer St, Halifax NS B3H 3A7; Dal'87; FRCPC; DiagRad (Vascular & Interventional Radiology). Staff, Queen Elizabeth II Health Sciences Centre - Halifax Infirmary Site; Ac Staff, Queen Elizabeth II Health Sciences Centre - Victoria General Site; Dalhousie University; (902)473-3666; Fax. (902)473-5323.

ABRAHAM, Ronnie P; 109-15388 24 Ave, Surrey BC V4A 2J2; Witwatersrand (South Africa)'08; (604)531-4131

ABRAHAM, Suma R; Colchester East Hants Hlth Ctr, 600 Abenaki Rd, Truro NS B2N 5A1; RCS (Ireland)'74; Staff, St Martha's Regional Hospital; Staff, Colchester East Hants Health Centre; (902)893-4321

ABRAHAM, T Easo; The Rudd Clinic, 825-123 Edward St, Toronto ON M5G 1E2; Madras (India)'66; MB; BSc; FRCSC; GenSurg. (416)597-0997; Fax. (416)597-2912.

ABRAHAM, Thoppil M; 30A East Main St, Welland ON L3B 3W3; Kerala (India)'70; MB BS; FRCPC; Psy. Physician Psy, Abraham & Singi Healthcare Network Inc; Langs: Malayalam; Hindi; Tamil; (905)735-6530; Fax. (905)735-6713; doetma@aol.com.

ABRAHAMIAN, Dikran J; Waypoint Centre for Mental H C, 500 Church St, Penetanguishene ON L9M 1G3; Yerevan (Armenia (Republic))'80; Staff, Waypoint Centre for Mental Health Care; Langs: Armenian; Arabic; French; (705)549-4474

ABRAHAMS, Heather R; SMBD Jewish Gen Hosp, 3755 ch Cote-Sainte-Catherine, Montreal QC H3T 1E2; McG'94; CCFP; Staff, Sir Mortimer B Davis Jewish General; (514)340-8253; Fax. (514)340-8298.

ABRAHAMS, Ismail; 7-13665 96 Ave, Surrey BC V3V 1Z1; Cape Town (South Africa)'57; MB BCh; MD; LRCP; FACOG; FRCOG; MRCS; FRCSC; ObstGyn (Infertility). (604)588-8381; Fax. (604)588-8312.

ABRAHAMS, Pauline E; 77 Victoria Park Ave, Scarborough ON M4E 3S2; Edinburgh (Scotland)'78; MB ChB; CCFP; Staff, Mount Sinai Hospital; (416)694-8254; Fax. (416)694-9983.

ABRAHAMS, Ronald R; Hycroft Med Bldg, 115-3195 Granville St, Vancouver BC V6H 3K2; Qns'77; CCFP; FCFP; Med Dir Perinatal Addictions, BC Women's Hospital & Health Centre; Clin Prof Family Pract, University of British Columbia; (604)732-0525

ABRAHAMS, Ruth S; 21561 Old Yale Rd, Langley BC V3A 4M9; Tor'87; MD; BSc; FACOG; FRCSC; ObstGyn. (604)534-4441; Fax. (604)534-4491; DRRSA@telus.net.

ABRAHAMS, Zuheir; 7-13665 96 Ave, Surrey BC V3V 1Z1; UBC'00; FRCPC; IntMed. (604)588-8381

ABRAHAMSE, Cornelis J; 377 Reid St, Peterborough ON K9H 4G4; Ott'75; (705)740-1078; Fax. (705)740-1048.

ABRAHAMSON, Carrie N; 300 3 St S, Lethbridge AB T1J 1Y9; (South Africa)'04; MB ChB; CCFP; (403)394-2002; Fax. (403)394-2066.

ABRAHAMSON, John L A; Toronto East Gen Hosp Inc, 825 Coxwell Ave, Toronto ON M4C 3E7; Ott'88; MSc; FRCPC; IntMed; Rheum. Staff, Toronto East General Hospital Inc; (416)469-6252

ABRAHAMSON, Simon D; St Michael's Hosp, SW1 026-30 Bond St, Toronto ON M5B 1W8; Cape Town (South Africa)'80; FRCPC; Anes. Staff, St Michael's Hospital; (416)864-5071; Fax. (416)864-6014.

ABRAHIM, Ken S I; 8-8123 Lundy's Lane, Niagara Falls ON L2H 1H3; Our Lady of Fatima Univ (Other Foreign)'99; CCFP; (289)296-4712; Fax. (289)296-3545.

ABRAHIM, Mohammed; Halton HCS Corp-Milton, 7030 Derry Rd E, Milton ON L9T 7H6; Ain Shams (Egypt)'00; CCFP; Staff, Halton Healthcare Services Corporation - Milton District Hospital; Staff, Niagara Health System - Welland Hospital Site; (905)876-7606; Fax. (905)876-7000.

ABRAM, Nancy L; 43 Victoria Terr, Grimsby ON L3M 2E9; McM'89; DC; CCFP; Clinical Asst Prof, McMaster University; (905)563-5315

ABRAMENKO, Heather M; 95 Spring St PO Box 310, Almonte ON K0A 1A0; UBC'85; BScN; (613)256-5656; Fax. (613)256-5445.

ABRAMOVITCH, Allan; Scarborough North Med Arts, 306-4040 Finch Ave E, Scarborough ON M1S 4V5; McG'76; FRCSC; Urol (Male Infertility). Langs: English; French; (416)754-1017; Fax. (416)754-4994.

ABRAMS, H Joel; 301-2797 Bathurst St, North York ON M6B 4B9; Tor'71; Staff, North York General Hospital; Staff, Mount Sinai Hospital; Staff, Baycrest Centre for Geriatric Care; (416)787-1297; Fax. (416)781-9580.

ABRAMS, Howard B; Univ Hlth Network-Toronto Gen, EN14 216-200 Elizabeth St, Toronto ON M5G 2C4; McM'81; BSc(Eng); FRCPC; IntMed. Div Head Gen IntMed, Toronto General Hospital - UHN; Div Head Gen IntMed, Mount Sinai Hospital; Assoc Prof Med, University of Toronto; (416)340-4195; Fax. (416)595-5826; howard.abrams@uhn.on.ca.

ABRAMS, Jason A; Medcan Health Mgmt Inc, 1500-150 York St, Toronto ON M5H 3S5; Wes'07; CCFP; (416)350-5900

ABRAMS, Jonathan C; Mount Sinai Fam Hlth Team, 4F-60 Murray St Box 13, Toronto ON M5T 3L9; Tor'99; MPH; CCFP; Staff, Mount Sinai Hospital; Staff, Temmy Latner Centre for Palliative Care; (416)586-4800 x6833; Fax. (416)586-4804; j.abrams@tlcpc.org.

ABRAMS, Karen M; Univ Hlth Network-Toronto Gen, 8EN-200 Elizabeth St, Toronto ON M5G 2C4; Tor'88; FRCPC; Psy (Women's Mental Health). Ac Staff, Toronto General Hospital - UHN; (416)340-4825; Fax. (416)340-4198; karen.abrams@utoronto.ca.

ABRAMS, Mitchell W; Cambridge Mem Hosp, 700 Coronation Blvd, Cambridge ON N1R 3G2; Dal'02; FRCPC; DiagRad. Staff, Cambridge Memorial Hospital; (519)621-2330

ABRAMSON, Beth L; 6 039QC-30 Bond St, Toronto ON M5B 1W8; Tor'91; MSc; FRCPC; IntMed (Cardiac Consultation); Cardiol. Dir Prevention & Rehab Centre/Assoc Prof Med, St Michael's Hospital; (416)864-5968; Fax. (416)864-5974.

ABRAMSON, Harry; Bathurst Med Centre, 205-4256 Bathurst St, North York ON M3H 5Y8; Tor'54; FRCPC; IntMed. Staff, North York General Hospital - Branson Division; (416)635-0148; Fax. (416)635-0120.

ABRAMSON, Norman; First Med Place, 202-170 Queensway W, Mississauga ON L5B 3A8; McM'77; (905)275-0023; Fax. (905)275-4001.

ABRAMSON, Sydney L; Applegrove Med Clinic, 135 Applegrove St, Sudbury ON P3C 1N2; McM'81; CCFP; Staff, The Oaks Centre; Langs: Bilingual(English/French); (705)673-3111

ABRIEL, David L; Fishermen's Mem Hosp, PO Box 1180, Lunenburg NS B0J 2C0; Dal'81; Staff, Fishermen's Memorial Hospital; Staff, South Shore Regional Hospital; Med Officer of Hlth, City of Mahone Bay; (902)624-7362; Fax. (902)527-5403.

ABRIEL KEREN, Avital; Dept of Respiratory Medicine, 585 University Ave, Toronto ON M5G 2C4; Technion-Israel Institute of Technology (Israel)'03.

ABROL, Kaajal; LIfe Quest Ctre Reproductive M, 18F-655 Bay St, Toronto ON M5G 2K4; McM'05; FRCSC; ObstGyn (Gynecological Reproductive Endocrinology). Staff, True North Imaging; (416)217-3971

ABROUS, Fariza; CSSS du Rocher Perce, CP 3300 451 rue Monseigneur Ross E, Chandler QC G0C 1K0; Tizi-Ouzou (Algeria)'95; Staff, Centre Hospitalier de Chandler; (418)689-2261 x2718; Fax. (418)689-4620.

ABSI, Farid; CSSS de Trois-Rivieres, 1991 boul Du Carmel, Trois-Rivieres QC G8Z 3R9; Alexandria (Egypt)'81; FRCPC; IntMed. Staff, CSSS de Trois-Rivières; Langs: Arabic; English; (819)697-3333

ABTAHI, Forough; Pitt Street Med Centre, 1335 Pitt St, Cornwall ON K6J 3T7; Tehran (Iran)'70; Affil Staff, Cornwall Community Hospital - Second Street Site; Affil Staff, Cornwall Community Hospital; Langs: Persian; French; (613)932-6163

ABTAHI, Maryam; The Ottawa Hosp-Gen Campus, 501 Smyth Rd, Ottawa ON K1H 8L6; Iran University of Medical Sciences (Iran)'00.

ABU-ABED, Mohamed I; William Osler HC-Brampton, 2100 Bovaird Dr E, Brampton ON L6R 3J7; McM'09; CCFP; Staff, William Osler Health System - Brampton Civic Hospital; (905)494-2120

ABU-ABED, Suzan; Kingston Gen Hosp, D2 8 216-76 Stuart St, Kingston ON K7L 2V7; Tor'06; FRCPC; AnatPath. Staff, Kingston General Hospital; (613)549-6666

ABU AISH, Mohammed; Fraser Children's & Fam Clinic, 6447 Fraser St, Vancouver BC V5W 3A6; Jeddah (Saudi Arabia)'98; MB BCh; FRCPC; Peds. Staff, BC Children's Hospital; (604)324-8262

ABU-ALMAALI, Abeer; Dr A A Wilkinson Mem Hlth Ctre, PO Box 70, Old Perlican NL A0A 3G0; Baghdad (Iraq)'97; MB ChB; CCFP; Staff, Dr A A Wilkinson Memorial Health Centre; (709)587-2200

ABU-ASSI, Rammy; The Hosp for Sick Children, 555 University Ave, Toronto ON M5G 1X8; University of Adelaide (Australia)'96; Clin Fellow Gastroent, The Hospital For Sick Children; (416)813-6185

ABU-BAKARE, Asiru; Port Arthur Health Centre Inc, 194 Court St N, Thunder Bay ON P7A 4V7; Tor'70; ABIM; FACP; FACE; DTMH(Liverpool); FRCPC; IntMed; Endocrin&Metab. Staff, Thunder Bay Regional Health Sciences Centre Port-Arthur; Staff, St Joseph's Care Group - St Joseph's Hospital; Langs: Edo; (807)346-1000; Fax. (807)346-6206; Abubakar@tbaytel.net.

ABU DIEH, Anwar H M; Kanata Prof Centre, 209-99 Kakulu Rd, Kanata ON K2L 3C8; Crimean (Ukraine)'97; MD; CCFP; Langs: Arabic; Russian; (613)592-4222; Fax. (613)592-2224.

ABU-HAKIMA, Maysan; Osteoporosis Centre, 2F-1820 Richmond Rd SW, Calgary AB T2T 5C7; Cal'87; BSc(Hon); FRCPC; IntMed (Osteoporosis). Assoc Physician, Grace Osteoporosis Centre; Clinical Asst Prof Med, University of Calgary; Langs: Arabic; French; (403)955-8130; Fax. (403)955-8634.

ABU HALEEQA, Khaled E M E; Bldg A 2-800 Southdown Rd, Mississauga ON L5J 2Y4; RCS (Ireland)'98; (905)822-2020

ABU KUWAIK, Ghassan Z K; 302-600 Sherbourne St, Toronto ON M4X 1W4; Himachal Pradesh University (India)'93; FRCPC; Peds (Developmental Pediatrics). Staff, The Hospital For Sick Children; (416)929-1919; Fax. (416)929-1959.

ABU-LABAN, Riyad B; Vancouver Gen Hosp, 855 12th Ave W, Vancouver BC V5Z 1M9; Alb'84; MHSc; FRCPC; EmergMed (AIDS/HIV). Att Physician EmergMed/Associate Research Dir, Vancouver General Hospital - Centennial Pavillion; Clinical Asst Prof, University of British Columbia; (604)875-4700; Fax. (604)875-4872; abulaban@interchange.ubc.ca.

ABU RAFEA, Basim F A; IWK Health Centre, PO Box 9700 Rpo CSC 2141-5980 University Ave, Halifax NS B3K 6R8; Riyadh (Saudi Arabia)'95; MB BS; FRCSC; ObstGyn. Staff, IWK Health Centre; (902)470-7098; Fax. (902)425-1125.

ABU-RASHED, Kamal A; Windsor River Walk-In Clinic, 500 Wyandotte St E, Windsor ON N9A 3H9; St Christopher Iba Mar Diop College (Other Foreign)'05; Staff, Hôtel-Dieu Grace Hospital; (519)254-2999; Fax. (519)254-4999.

ABU-SA'DA, Omar S D; Sturgeon Community Hosp, 25-201 Boudreau Rd, St. Albert AB T8N 6C4; (Jordan)'95; FRCPC; Peds (Neonatal & Perinatal Medicine). Staff, Sturgeon Community Hospital; (780)418-7325; Fax. (780)418-7393.

ABU SETTEH, Nihad M A; Mavis Wellness, 7-5025 Heatherleigh Ave, Mississauga ON L5V 2Y7; Dubai (United Arab Emirates)'94; CCFP; (905)501-9115

ABU SHAHMA, Mohamed S; 10-5233 Stanley Ave, Niagara Falls ON L2E 7C2; Al Fateh (Libya)'97; CCFP; (289)296-7757; Fax. (289)296-8856.

ABU SHARAR, Ziad; Children's & Women's HC of BC, 4480 Oak St, Vancouver BC V6H 3V4; Minsk (Belarus)'95; Staff, BC Children's Hospital; (604)875-2121

ABU SHULLAIH, Zaki Omar; Cape Breton Healthcare Complex, 1482 George St, Sydney NS B1P 1P3; Romania (Romania)'98; Staff, Cape Breton Healthcare Complex; (902)567-8092; Fax. (902)567-7905.

ABU-WASEL, Bassam; Queen Elizabeth II HSC, 6 302-1278 Tower Rd, Halifax NS B3H 2Y9; Universita Degli Studi di Catania (Other Foreign)'01; Staff, Queen Elizabeth II Health Sciences Centre - Victoria General Site; (902)473-2700

ABU-ZAHRA, Hakam T; Windsor Reg Cancer Centre, 2220 Kildare Rd, Windsor ON N8W 2X3; Cairo (Egypt)'61; MB ChB; FRCPC; IntMed; Hem. Ac Staff, Windsor Regional Hospital - Metropolitan Site; Ac Staff, Windsor Regional Hospital - Windsor Regional Cancer Centre; (519)253-3191 x58519; hakam_abuzahra@wrh.on.ca.

ABUALROSS, Hani S; Addiction & Mental Hlth-Clarke, 250 College St, Toronto ON M5T 1R8; Abdul Aziz (Saudi Arabia)'96; Clin Fellow, Centre for Addiction & Mental Health (CAMH) - College Street Site; (416)535-8501

ABUD, Lely; 413 Main St PO Box 170, Mahone Bay NS B0J 2E0; Taubate (Brazil)'91; CCFP; (902)624-8373; Fax. (902)624-1524.

ABUDERBALA, Najat M; 6633 177 ST NW, Edmonton AB T5T 4K3; (780)757-7999; Fax. (780)757-7991.

ABUELALAA, Enas; Halton Family Centre, 2951 Walker's Line, Burlington ON L7M 4Y1; (Egypt)'90; CCFP; (905)336-3437

ABUFAYED, Mohamed A; Access Med Centre, 13718 113A St NW, Edmonton AB T5X 4H7; Al-Fateh (Libya)'92; MB ChB; CCFP; Langs: Arabic; (780)456-3067

ABUFAYYAH, Mohammed; Univ Hlth Network-Toronto Western Hosp, 1 412EW-399 Bathurst St, Toronto ON M5T 2S8; Abdul Aziz (Saudi Arabia)'99; FRCPC; IntMed; Rheum. Staff, Toronto Western Hospital - University Health Network; (416)603-5905; Fax. (416)603-9387.

ABUGHADUMA, Read M A; 104-200 Consillium Place, Scarborough ON M1H 3E4; Tripoli (Libya)'94; FRCSC; OrthSurg (Joint Replacement). Staff, The Scarborough Hospital - General Campus; Langs: Arabic; (416)479-8686

ABUGHAMJA, Tareq S M; 1169 Bloor St W, Toronto ON M6H 1M9; Al Fateh (Libya)'01; MB BCh; CCFP; Langs: Arabic.

ABUHAMED, Kusai; 12620A 132 Ave NW, Edmonton AB T5L 3P9; (Libya)'06; (780)990-1820

ABUHAMED, Louai; 3236 82 St, Edmonton AB T6K 3Y3; (780)761-3335

ABUHELALA, Ahmed M; 15121 121 St NW, Edmonton AB T5X 3C8; (Libya)'01; MB ChB; Langs: Arabic; (780)472-7171; Fax. (780)478-9179; abuhelala@gmail.com.

ABUHJAR, Abdussalam K; Regina Med Centre, 100-2550 12th Ave, Regina SK S4P 3X1; Garyounis (Libya)'94; Urol. (306)566-4120; Fax. (306)566-4150.

ABUJAZIA, Abdurrezagh F; Dr C W Wiebe Med Centre, 385 Main St, Winkler MB R6W 1J2; Al Fateh (Libya)'96; FRCSC; GenSurg.

ABUJRAD, Hussein A; 1995 Merivale Rd, Ottawa ON K2G 3K2; Al Fateh (Libya)'00; Endocrin&Metab; IntMed. Staff, The Ottawa Hospital - Riverside Campus; (613)482-0118; Fax. (613)680-6420.

ABUKHADIR, Sofian; Country Hills Village, 220-5149 Country Hills Blvd NW, Calgary AB T3A 5K8; (403)241-8848; Fax. (403)241-8849.

ABULAEHA, Rida M A; James Paton Mem Hosp, 125 Trans Canada Hwy, Gander NL A1V 1P7; Locum Tenens, James Paton Memorial Hospital; (709)256-2500

ABULBIDA, Tarik A; Fogo Island Health Centre, PO Box 9, Fogo NL A0G 2B0; Al Fateh (Libya)'00; MB BCh; Staff, Fogo Island Health Centre; (709)266-2221

ABULOMRAIN, Ghalib A I; Strait of Belle Isle Health Ce, PO Box 59, Flowers Cove NL A0K 2N0; Garyounis (Libya)'02; MB ChB; Staff, Strait of Belle Isle Health Centre; (709)456-2401

ABUMEESS, Ahmed A R; Dr William Newhook Comm HC, GD, Whitbourne NL A0B 3K0; Al Fateh (Libya)'04; CCFP; Staff, Dr William H Newhook Health Centre; (709)759-2300; abumeess@mun.ca.

ABUNAJI, Mohamed A; Sunnybrook Health Sciences Ctr, M1600-2075 Bayview Ave, Toronto ON M4N 3M5; Al Fateh (Libya)'97; FRCPC; Neur. Staff, Sunnybrook Health Sciences Centre; Staff, The Scarborough Hospital - Birchmount Campus; (416)480-4475

ABUNASSAR, Joseph G; Postgrad Med Education, 2044-451 Smyth Rd, Ottawa ON K1H 8M5; Ott'08; IntMed.

ABUNASSAR, Ramzi Y; Smyth Med Centre, 324-1929 Russell Rd, Ottawa ON K1G 4G3; Ott'73; FRCPC; IntMed (Gastroenterology). Ac Staff, The Ottawa Hospital - General Campus; Ac Staff IntMed/Gastroenterol, The Ottawa Hospital - Riverside Campus; Langs: Arabic; Hebrew; (613)737-7726; Fax. (613)737-2856.

ABUSHAWISH, Ghassan; Alexandra Hosp, 29 Noxon St, Ingersoll ON N5C 1B8; Tichreen (Syria)'94; CCFP; Staff, Alexandra Hospital; (519)485-1700; Fax. (519)681-5657.

ABUSWIDER, Samer A; The Ottawa Hosp-Gen Campus, W3301-501 Smyth Rd, Ottawa ON K1H 8L6; Al Fateh (Libya)'98; Clin Fellow Ophth, The Ottawa Hospital - General Campus; (613)737-8575

ABUZEID, Wael; Postgrad Med Education, 602-500 University Ave, Toronto ON M5G 1V7; Ott'08; FRCPC; IntMed. (416)978-6976

ABUZGAYA, Fathi H; Ajax Med Arts Bldg, 207-601 Harwood Ave S, Ajax ON L1S 2J5; Garyunis (Libya)'82; FRCSC; OrthSurg (Joint Replacement). Staff, Rouge Valley Health System - Ajax & Pickering Health Centre Site; (905)686-0882; Fax. (905)686-7940.

ACAR, Behram; Saint John Reg Hosp, PO Box 2100 Stn Main 400 University Ave, Saint John NB E2L 4L2; Dokuz Eylul (Turkey)'91; Staff, Saint John Regional Hospital; (506)648-6000

ACCARDO, Marco A; Pine Seven Med Centre, 205-4600 Highway 7, Woodbridge ON L4L 4Y7; Tor'83; BSc; (905)850-7788; Fax. (905)850-7790.

ACEVEDO MENDEZ, Francisco E; Summerhill Med Clinic, 207-130 Conception Bay Hwy, Conception Bay S NL A1W 3A6; Cali (Colombia)'01; (709)834-2039

ACEVEDO MENDEZ, Luis A; Humber Med Clinic, PO Box 670, Bay Roberts NL A0A 1G0; Cali (Colombia)'02; Staff, Western Memorial Regional Hospital; Langs: Spanish; (709)786-7144

ACHARYA, Anish P; The Alex Seniors Commun Hlth, 630 9 Ave SE, Calgary AB T2G 4V9; Cal'00; CCFP; (403)920-0011

ACHARYA, Chhaya V; Bluewater Health-Norman Site, 89 Norman St, Sarnia ON N7T 6S3; Baroda (India)'92; FRCPC; AnatPath. Staff Lab Services, Bluewater Health - Norman Site; Staff, Bluewater Health - Mitton Site; (519)464-4400 x5486; Fax. (519)383-7274.

ACHARYA, Hernish J; 10942 124 St NW, Edmonton AB T5M 0H5; Alb'07; FRCPC; PhysMed&Rehab. Staff, University of Alberta Hospital; (780)447-4924

ACHARYA, Meenaxi S; Bay L'Argent Med Clinic, PO Box 40, Bay l'Argent NL A0E 1B0; Gujarat (India)'73; MB BS; AB; DABPM; FRCPC; PhysMed&Rehab (Chronic Pain). Langs: Hindi; Gujarati; (709)461-2308

ACHARYA, Sanjay V; Queensway-Carleton Hosp, 3045 Baseline Rd, Ottawa ON K2H 8P4; Mem'92; FRCPC; Anes. Staff, Queensway Carleton Hospital; Staff, The Ottawa Hospital - Civic Campus; (613)721-2000

ACHARYA, Surendra D P; Bay L'Argent Med Clinic, PO Box 40, Bay L'Argent NL A0E 1B0; Bangalore (India)'70; MB BS; (709)461-2308; Fax. (709)461-2415.

ACHARYA, Virbala C; The Ottawa Hosp-Gen Campus, 501 Smyth Rd, Ottawa ON K1H 8L6; Bombay (India)'67; MB BS; FCAP; FRCPC; AnatPath (Gynecological Pathology). Ac Staff, The Ottawa Hospital - General Campus; Asst Prof Health Sciences Centre, University of Ottawa; Langs: Gujarati; (613)737-8833; vacharya@ottawahospital.on.ca.

ACHARYYA, Partha; William Osler HC-Brampton, 2100 Bovaird Dr E, Brampton ON L6R 3J7; Calcutta (India)'78; FRCPC; Psy. Staff, William Osler Health System - Brampton Civic Hospital; (905)494-2120; Fax. (905)494-6710.

ACHEBE, Ifeoma F; Johnstone Crossing Comm Hlth C, 300 Jordan Pkwy, Red Deer AB T4P 0G8; (Nigeria)'96; (403)356-6424

ACHEN, Blaine M; University of Alberta Hosp, 8440 112 St NW, Edmonton AB T6G 2B7; Alb'99; FRCPC; Anes. Staff, University of Alberta Hospital; (780)407-8861

ACHENBACH, Jillian M; Public Gardens Med Clinic, 200-5675 Spring Garden Rd, Halifax NS B3H 1H1; Dal'08; CCFP; (902)425-5440; Fax. (902)482-6019.

ACHESON, Donald K; PO Box 331 Stn Main, St Stephen NB E3L 2X2; Dal'83; (506)466-3878

ACHESON, Todd M; BC Cancer Agency, 13750 96 Ave, Surrey BC V3V 1Z2; (Montserrat)'07; Staff, BC Cancer Agency Fraser Valley Centre; (604)581-2211

ACHIAM, Cimi; Royal Columbian Hosp, 330 Columbia St E, New Westminster BC V3L 3W7; Wes'06; FRCPC; EmergMed. Staff, Royal Columbian Hospital; (604)365-5130

ACHIM, Catherine; CHUQ-Ctr Hosp Univ Laval, 2705 boul Laurier, Quebec QC G1V 4G2; Laval'05; FRCSC; Ophth. Staff, Centre Hospitalier Universitaire de Quebec-CHUL; (418)525-4444

ACHIM, Michel; Villa Medica, 225 Sherbrooke E, Montreal QC H2X 1C9; Mon'82; Staff, Institut de Réadaptation Gingras-Lindsay de Montréal; (514)288-8201; Fax. (514)288-6370; jnolet@ssss.gouv.qc.ca.

ACHIR, Sanaa; Clinique Force Medic, 200-1021 rue Jean-Talon E, Montreal QC H2R 1V6; Rabat (Morocco)'03; (514)787-1818

ACHIUME, J Kirkwood; 115 Christopher Dr, Cambridge ON N1R 4S1; Tor'67; (519)740-2444; Fax. (519)740-3405.

ACHIUME, Patricia M; North Bay Reg Health Centre, 50 College Dr, North Bay ON P1B 0A4; Tor'66; FRCPC; Psy (Acute Adult Psychiatry). Staff Acute In-Patient Psy Unit, North Bay Regional Health Centre - Regional Mental Health; Psychiatrist, Muskoka-Parry Sound Community Mental Health Service; (705)474-1200 x2154; Fax. (705)495-7890; pachiume@nembc.on.ca.

ACHKAR, Madeleine; CLSC Ruisseau Papineau, 1665 rue Du Couvent, Laval QC H7W 3A8; Ain Shams (Egypt)'77; Langs: English; Arabic; (450)687-5690; Fax. (450)687-5998.

ACHONG, Eamon H; Haney Health Associates, 22338 Selkirk Ave, Maple Ridge BC V2X 2X5; McG'60; Psy (Psychotherapy). Consultant, Ridge Meadows Hospital & Health Care Centre; (604)477-7202

ACHONG, Michael R; Medical Arts Bldg, 501-1 Young St, Hamilton ON L8N 1T8; Edinburgh (Scotland)'70; MB ChB; BSc(Pharm); FRCPC; IntMed (Infectious Diseases). Ac Staff Med, St Joseph's Healthcare - Charlton Campus; Clin Assoc Prof, McMaster University; (905)528-0430; Fax. (905)528-0432.

ACHTEM, Benjamin; 3021B Pandosy St, Kelowna BC V1Y 1W3; UBC'00; FRCSC; Otol (Head & Neck Surgery). Staff, Fort St John Hospital & Health Centre; Staff, Kelowna General Hospital; (250)763-3322; Fax. (250)763-3328.

ACHTYMICHUK, Audrey; Nose Hill Med Clinic, 137-1829 Ranchlands Blvd NW, Calgary AB T3G 2A7; Sask'85; CCFP; (403)239-8888; Fax. (403)241-1506.

ACHTYMICHUK, Gerald W; 201-20 Hobson St, Cambridge ON N1S 2M6; Cal'82; Staff, Cambridge Memorial Hospital; House Physician, Queen's Square Terrace; (519)621-2560

ACHYUTHAN, Geeta; Regina Med Centre, 103-2550 12th Ave, Regina SK S4P 3X1; Sask'84; Ac Staff, Pasqua Hospital; Ac Staff, Regina Health District; University of Saskatchewan; Langs: Malayalam; (306)566-4100; Fax. (306)566-4115; gachyuthan@sasktel.net.

ACKAOUI, Alexandre; Centre de Sante de Rigaud, 1 rue Hotel-de-Ville, Rigaud QC J0P 1P0; Mon'88; (450)451-5336; Fax. (450)451-5214; ackaoui.berube@sympatico.ca.

ACKAOUI, Elias G; Centre Med Hochelaga, 9080 rue Hochelaga, Montreal QC H1L 2N9; Alexandria (Egypt)'71; (514)353-8742; Fax. (514)353-2351.

ACKER, Amy E; Hotel-Dieu Hosp, Brock3-166 Brock St, Kingston ON K7L 5G2; Dal'03; FRCPC; Peds. Staff, Hotel-Dieu Hospital; (613)544-3400; Fax. (613)544-3559.

ACKER, John C; 17 Beach Dr, Rothesay NB E2E 4X3; Dal'65; BSc; FRCS; OrthSurg (Sports Medicine). Consultant MSK Clinical Skills, Saint John Regional Hospital; Staff, St Joseph's Hospital; Teacher, Dalhousie University; (506)849-8212; Fax. (506)849-9157.

ACKER, John J; Scarborough North Med Arts, 301-4040 Finch Ave E, Scarborough ON M1S 4V5; Wes'77; FRCPC; IntMed; Rheum. Ac Staff, The Scarborough Hospital - Birchmount Campus; (416)298-0111; Fax. (416)298-1574.

ACKERMAN, Ida; Sunnybrook Odette Cancer Ctre, T2 156-2075 Bayview Ave, Toronto ON M4N 3M5; Tor'75; FRCPC; RadOncol (Gynecologic Oncology). Staff, Sunnybrook Health Sciences Centre; (416)480-6165; Fax. (416)480-6002; ida.ackerman@sunnybrook.ca.

ACKERMAN, Margaret J; Hamilton HS-General Site, 237 Barton St E, Hamilton ON L8L 2X2; McM'78; DAB; FRCPC; EmergMed. Staff Emerg, Hamilton Health Sciences Centre - Hamilton General Hospital; Clin Assoc Prof Emerg Med, McMaster University; (905)527-0271 x46368; Fax. (905)527-1941; mackerma@mcmaster.ca.

ACKERMAN, Thomas E; Hys Medical Centre, 11010 101 St NW, Edmonton AB T5H 4B9; Man'87; FRCPC; DiagRad. Staff, University of Alberta Hospital; (780)426-1121; Fax. (780)425-5979.

ACKERMANN, Carel W; 200-300 Columbia St, Kamloops BC V2C 6L1; Stellenbosch (South Africa)'88; MB ChB; FRCSC; OrthSurg (Adult Reconstructive Surgery). Staff, Royal Inland Hospital; Langs: Afrikaans; (250)374-1448; Fax. (250)374-2663; callieaIetta@yahoo.com.

ACKERMANN, Frank P; East Kootenay Reg Hosp, 13 24th Ave N, Cranbrook BC V1C 3H9; Tor'95; CCFP; CCFP(E.M.); FCFP; Staff, East Kootenay Regional Hospital; (250)426-5281

ACKERMANN, Michael J M; St Mary's Med Clinic, PO Box 297, Sherbrooke NS B0J 3C0; Dal'88; BSc; Med Dir Family Med, St Mary's Memorial Hospital; Preceptor Undergrad Family Med, Dalhousie University; Langs: Chinese; French; German; (902)522-2275; Fax. (902)522-2556.

ACKERMANN, Wendy C; Associated Medical Clinica, PO Box 510 10017 101 Ave, Lac La Biche AB T0A 2C0; (780)623-4421; Fax. (780)623-1920.

ACKLAND, Susan; St Paul's Hosp, B512-1081 Burrard St, Vancouver BC V6Z 1Y6; UBC'81; Staff, Providence Health Care - St Paul's Hospital; (604)806-8060

ACKLAND-SNOW, Julia C; Misericordia Community Hosp, 16940 87 Ave NW, Edmonton AB T5R 4H5; Cal'98; FRCPC; Peds. Staff, Covenant Health - Misericordia Community Hospital; (780)735-2731; Fax. (780)735-2794.

ACOB, Constante A; Visiting Spec Clinic Work Safe, 6951 Westminster Hwy, Vancouver BC V6B 5L5; Far Eastern (Philippines)'64; MD; FRCPC; PhysMed&Rehab. (604)214-6700

ACOTT, Philip D; IWK Health Centre, PO Box 9700 Rpo Csc 5850 University Ave, Halifax NS B3K 6R8; Dal'86; FRCPC; Peds. Staff, IWK Health Centre; (902)470-8195; Fax. (902)470-8900.

ACRE, Yael; 660-5025 rue Sherbrooke O, Montreal QC H4A 1S9; McG'01; CCFP; Physician, St Andrew's Nursing Home; Langs: Spanish; French; (514)932-6122; yaelacre@yahoo.com.

ACRES, John C; 5668 South St PO Box 1150 Stn Central, Halifax NS B3J 2Y2; Dal'70; FRCPC; IntMed (Occupational Medicine); Respir. Med Advisor, Worker's Compensation Board of NS; (902)695-5348; john.acres@wcb.gov.ns.ca.

ACSAI, Megan S; Maple Leaf Clinic, 601-14 College St, Toronto ON M5G 1K2; Wes'07; CCFP.

ACTON, David C; Valley Reg Hosp, 150 Exhibition St, Kentville NS B4N 5E3; Dublin (Ireland)'78; MB ChB; BAO; FRCR; FRCPC; DiagRad. Ac Staff, Valley Regional Hospital; Ac Staff, Western Kings Memorial Health Centre; Lecturer Med, Dalhousie University; (902)678-7381 x2702; Fax. (902)678-0098.

ACTON, Gillian R; 701 Highway 97 S, Vernon BC V1B 3W4; Alb'82; FRCPC; Psy. Staff, Alberta Hospital Edmonton; (250)938-1209

ACTON, Lise-Marie; 105-75 Dyrgas Gate, Canmore AB T1W 0A6; Ott'10; CCFP.

ACTON, Saskia E; Gaia Collaborative Medicine, 101-75 Dyrgas Gate, Canmore AB T1W 0A6; UBC'90; CCFP; (403)675-4242; Fax. (403)675-4243.

AD-DAB'BAGH, Yasser; Children's Hosp Eastern Ontari, 317-1385 Bank St, Ottawa ON K1H 8N4; Riyadh (Saudi Arabia)'93; MB BS(Dublin); CCST; LMCC; FRC; DPM; DPsy; Dip; FRCPC; Psy (Developmental Disability). Langs: Arabic.

ADACHI, Jonathan D Rick; Charlton Med Centre, 501-25 Charlton Ave E, Hamilton ON L8N 1Y2; McM'79; BSc; FRCPC; IntMed (Osteoporosis); Rheum. Ac Staff, St Joseph's Healthcare - Charlton Campus; Prof, McMaster University; (905)529-1317; Fax. (905)521-1297.

ADAIR, John D; Northmount Med Centre, 502-145 13th St E, North Vancouver BC V7L 2L4; UBC'81; (604)988-4744; Fax. (604)988-4725.

ADAM, Abbas F Y; 15 Allan Dr, Bolton ON L7E 2B5; University of Al-Mustansiriyah (Iraq)'02; MB BS; CCFP; (905)951-1234

ADAM, Christian; Southside Medical Clinic, 202-640 Prospect St, Fredericton NB E3B 9M7; Cape Town (South Africa)'81; MB ChB; FACOG; FRCSC; ObstGyn. Staff, Dr Everett Chalmers Regional Hospital; Staff, Oromocto Public Hospital; Langs: French; (506)459-2803

ADAM, Christina M; St Joseph's Healthcare, 50 Charlton Ave E, Hamilton ON L8N 4A6; McM'00; FRCPC; Psy. Staff, St Joseph's Healthcare - Charlton Campus; (905)521-1155

ADAM, Christopher J E; Legacy Sport Med Clinic, 14-160 Meadowood Dr, Winnipeg MB R2M 5L6; Man'99; CCFP; FCFP; (204)667-1560

ADAM, David N; G02-95 Bayly St W, Ajax ON L1S 7K8; Tor'02; FRCPC; Derm. (905)427-3996

ADAM, Derek L; Spall Med Clinic, 150-1940 Harvey Ave, Kelowna BC V1Y 8J8; Alb'97; CCFP; FCFP; (250)860-9909; Fax. (250)860-9906.

ADAM, Fhameeda; CSSS de la Vallée de l'Or, 725 6e rue, Val-d'Or QC J9P 3Y1; Laval'10; CCFP; Staff, Centre Hospitalier de Val d'Or; (819)825-5858

ADAM, Genevieve; Hop Brome-Missisquoi-Perkins, 950 rue Principale, Cowansville QC J2K 1K3; Mon'06; Staff, Hôpital Brome-Missisquoi-Perkins; (450)266-4342; Fax. (450)263-8669.

ADAM, George A; North York Gen Hosp, 4001 Leslie St, North York ON M2K 1E1; Tor'74; CCFP; FCFP; Ac Staff Emerg & Family Pract, North York General Hospital; Assoc Staff Emerg & Family Pract, The Scarborough Hospital - General Campus; Ac Staff, Humber River Regional Hospital - Finch Avenue Site; (416)756-6002; Fax. (416)756-6793; adam8353@rogers.com.

ADAM, Germain; Centre Hosp Honore-Mercier, 2750 boul Laframboise, Saint-Hyacinthe QC J2S 4Y8; Mon'70; FRCPC; Psy (Pediatric Psychiatry). Chef Pedo-Psy Services, Centre Hospitalier Honore-Mercier; (450)771-3222; Fax. (450)771-3273; germain.adam@csss16.gouv.qc.ca.

ADAM, John E; Parkdale Med Tower, 308-1081 Carling Ave, Ottawa ON K1Y 4G2; Qns'61; MHA; FAAD; FRCPC; Derm. Staff Consultant Div of Derm, The Ottawa Hospital - Civic Campus; Clin Prof Div of Derm, University of Ottawa; (613)722-8532; Fax. (613)722-8727.

ADAM, Josee; Clarence-Rockland Fam Hlth Team, 2741 Chamberland St, Rockland ON K4K 0B4; Ott'03; CCFP; Langs: Bilingual(English/French); (613)446-7677

ADAM, Larry J; Tsawwassen Med Clinic, 201-1077 56 St, Delta BC V4L 2A2; Sask'79; (604)943-1131; Fax. (604)943-2617.

ADAM, Paul; Rosedale Med Centre, 411-600 Sherbourne St, Toronto ON M4X 1W4; Tor'72; AB; ABIM; DABD; FRCPC; IntMed; Derm. Ac Staff/Head Derm, St Michael's Hospital; Asst Prof, University of Toronto; (416)922-3417; Fax. (416)961-0383.

ADAM, Robert A; 553 1re rue O, Amos QC J9T 2M9; Laval'65; FRCSC; OrthSurg (Trauma). Assoc Member, CH Hôtel-Dieu d'Amos; Consultant, Centre Hospitalier de Val d'Or; (819)732-6066; Fax. (819)732-6066; radam@cableamos.com.

ADAM, Robert S; St Joseph's Health Centre, 30 The Queensway, Toronto ON M6R 1B5; Tor'05; FRCSC; Ophth. Staff, St Joseph's Health Centre; (416)530-6565; Fax. (416)530-6291.

ADAM, Rogelia F R; Markham College Med Clinic, 200-474 College St, Toronto ON M6G 1A4; San Marcos (Peru)'76; (416)975-1598; Fax. (416)975-9668.

ADAM, Suleman V; Broadview Med Clinic, PO Box 39, Broadview SK S0G 0K0; RCS (Ireland)'71; LRCP; LRCS; LM; (306)696-2266; Fax. (306)696-2676.

ADAM, Trudy J; The Richmond Hosp, 7000 Westminster Hwy, Richmond BC V6X 1A2; Cal'06; FRCPC; Psy. Staff, Richmond Hospital; (604)339-8331

ADAM-SDROLIAS, Heather; Victoria Gen Hosp, 2340 Pembina Hwy, Winnipeg MB R3T 2E8; CCFP; Staff, Victoria General Hospital; (204)269-3570

ADAMIAK, Anna; Southlake Reg Health Centre, 596 Davis Dr, Newmarket ON L3Y 2P9; Wes'05; FRCPC; AnatPath. Staff, Southlake Regional Health Centre; (905)895-4521

ADAMIAK, Eugene J; Mayfair Place, 215-6707 Elbow Dr SW, Calgary AB T2V 0E4; Sydney (Australia)'72; ABIM; FRCPC; IntMed (Respirology). Ac Staff, Foothills Medical Centre; Ac Staff, Rockyview General Hospital; (403)255-4833; Fax. (403)255-4912.

ADAMIS, Jon M; 852 119 St SW, Edmonton AB T6W 0J1; Alb'01; FRCSC; Otol. (780)438-1884; Fax. (780)988-2609.

ADAMKO, Darryl J; Royal University Hosp, 103 Hospital Dr, Saskatoon SK S7N 0W8; Sask'93; FRCPC; Peds (Pediatric Respirology); Respir. Staff, Royal University Hospital; (306)966-8158

ADAMO, Ciro A; Bluewater Imaging, 100-2010 Eglinton Ave W, Toronto ON M6E 2K3; Sask'86; FRCPC; DiagRad. (416)781-2050

ADAMO, George; 945 rue Saint-Jean, Roberval QC G8H 2H3; Aleppo (Syria)'88; FRCSC; Urol. (418)275-3122

ADAMO, Niam; Grand Park Medical, 208-719 Central Parkway W, Mississauga ON L5B 4L1; Mosul (Iraq)'97; MB ChB; CCFP; Langs: Arabic; Spanish; (905)270-3636; Fax. (905)270-8881.

ADAMOWSKI, Susan; Carrefour Vanier Med Centre, 305-150 Montreal Rd, Vanier ON K1L 8H2; Ott'76; BSc; MSc; (613)744-4978; Fax. (613)744-2151.

ADAMS, Amanda J; Markham Med Centre, 214-6633 Highway 7, Markham ON L3P 7P2; McM'96; BSc; MSc; CCFP; FCFP; (905)294-2290; Fax. (905)294-0029.

ADAMS, Barrett R; Smyth Paediatric Group, 220-1929 Russell Rd, Ottawa ON K1G 4G3; Ott'59; Peds (Consultant & Primary Care). Emeritus Staff, Children's Hospital of Eastern Ontario (CHEO); Clin Assoc Prof, University of Ottawa; (613)737-7707; Fax. (613)737-4867.

ADAMS, Beverly L; Foothills Med Centre, AW259B-1403 29 St NW, Calgary AB T2N 2T9; Sask'87; FRCPC; Psy. Staff, Foothills Medical Centre; (403)944-1296; Fax. (403)944-2165.

ADAMS, Brendan D; 17-152 MacLaurin Dr, Calgary AB T3Z 3S4; Cal'81; CCFP; (403)269-5323; Fax. (403)264-5362.

ADAMS, Cherie-Lee; Hamilton HSC-McMaster Site, PO Bpx 2000 Stn Lcd 1 1200 Main St W, Hamilton ON L8N 3Z5; Dal'08; Staff, Hamilton Health Sciences Centre - McMaster Children's Hospital; (905)521-2100

ADAMS, David; Medecine Familiale Montclair, 207-15 boul Montclair, Gatineau QC J8Y 2E2; Sher'88; (819)772-2003; Fax. (819)772-4080.

ADAMS, David O; Meadowlark Health Centre, 184 Meadowlark Shopping Ctr NW, Edmonton AB T5R 5W9; Wes'69; FRCSC; GenSurg (Breast Cancer). Site Leader Surg, Covenant Health - Misericordia Community Hospital; Clinical Asst Prof Surg, University of Alberta; (780)484-1122; Fax. (780)489-4121.

ADAMS, Dermot A A; 302-3001 Tutt St, Kelowna BC V1Y 2H4; LRCS (Ireland)'83; MB ChB; FRCPC; Neur. Staff, Kelowna General Hospital; (250)979-1634; Fax. (250)979-1639.

ADAMS, Erin R M; 520 Nicola St, Kamloops BC V2C 2R1; UBC'05; FRCSC; ObstGyn. (250)374-4456

ADAMS, Fatin M H; 2940 17 Ave SW, Calgary AB T3E 0A9; Baghdad (Iraq)'85; FRCPC; IntMed; Gastroent. Clin Prof/Staff, Rockyview General Hospital; (403)244-4844; Fax. (403)244-2268.

ADAMS, Gerald S; Kingston Gen Hosp, 76 Stuart St, Kingston ON K7L 2V7; Mem'80; FRCPC; IntMed (Angioplasty); Cardiol. Dir Cardiovasc Lab & Staff, Kingston General Hospital; Dir Cardiovasc Lab & Staff, Hotel-Dieu Hospital; Asst Prof Med, Queen's University; (613)548-1383; Fax. (613)548-2400; adamsg@kgh.kari.net.

ADAMS, Gheorghita C; Royal University Hosp, EH 119-103 Hospital Dr, Saskatoon SK S7N 0W8; (Romania)'97; FRCPC; Psy. Staff, Royal University Hospital; (306)966-8230

ADAMS, Grenfell B; Health Sciences Centre, 300 Prince Philip Dr, St. John's NL A1B 3V6; McG'64; MD; FRCPC; IntMed (Hematology). Staff, Health Sciences Centre; Prof Med, Memorial University Of Newfoundland; (709)777-6545

ADAMS, Helika D; 2018 Hwy 224 PO Box 315, Shubenacadie NS B0N 2H0; Dal'79; (902)758-3340

ADAMS, Hilary; 321-11245 Valley Ridge Dr NW, Calgary AB T3B 5V4; Cal'87; CCFP; (403)282-3806; Fax. (403)284-5601.

ADAMS, Howard F; Windsor Health Centre, 103-700 Tecumseh Rd E, Windsor ON N8X 4T2; Wes'74; DAB; FRCSC; PlasSurg (Reconstructive Surgery). Staff, Windsor Regional Hospital - Metropolitan Site; Staff, Hôtel-Dieu Grace Hospital; Staff, Essex County Regional Burn Unit; (519)258-1415; Fax. (519)258-7454; adamsh@mnsi.net.

ADAMS, J H; Dartmouth Med Centre, 310-46 Portland St, Dartmouth NS B2Y 1H4; Mem'74; (902)465-4531; Fax. (902)464-4906.

ADAMS, James R; Athabascan Place, 215-80 Chippewa Rd, Sherwood Park AB T8A 4W6; Alb'83; (780)464-1179; Fax. (780)467-3100; jamesradams@shaw.ca.

ADAMS, Jennifer H; South Nepean Satellite CHC, 201-4100 Strandherd Dr, Nepean ON K2J 0V2; McM'06; CCFP; (613)288-2820; Fax. (613)288-3690.

ADAMS, Jeremy; Univ Hlth Network-Toronto Western Hosp, NE 470-399 Bathurst St, Toronto ON M5T 2S8; Tor'08; IntMed. Staff, Toronto Western Hospital - University Health Network; (416)603-5818

ADAMS, John M; Dr John Adams Family Prac Inc, PO Box 1106 131 Vermillion Ave, Princeton BC V0X 1W0; Liverpool (England)'63; MRC(UK); DLO; DCH; CCFP; Staff, Princeton General Hospital; (250)295-6331; Fax. (250)295-6379; jadams@cablerocket.com.

ADAMS, John R; Centre for Movement Disorders, 2780 Bur Oak Ave, Markham ON L6B 1C9; Qns'98; BSc(Hon)Life Science; MSc; FRCPC; Neur (Movement Disorders). Consultant, Markham Stouffville Hospital; (905)472-7082; Fax. (905)472-6270.

ADAMS, Julian F; Niagara Med Prof Centre, PO Box 10 1882 Highway 55, Virgil ON L0S 1T0; Belfast (Ireland)'66; BAO; BCh; Chief Med Staff, Niagara Health System - Niagara-on-the-Lake Hospital Site; (905)468-3275; Fax. (905)468-7960; jadams@niagara.com.

ADAMS, Karen; CHUQ-Ctr Hosp Univ Laval, H.1365-2705 boul Laurier, Quebec QC G1V 4G2; Laval'04; FRCPC; IntMed; Rheum. Staff, Centre Hospitalier Universitaire de Quebec-CHUL; (418)525-4444

ADAMS, Kenneth W; Advanced Med Therapeutics Clin, 509-1200 Sheppard Ave E, North York ON M2K 2S5; Wes'81; (416)633-3905; Fax. (416)633-3907.

ADAMS, Lenley S; Queen Elizabeth Hosp, PO Box 6600 Stn Central, Charlottetown PE C1A 8T5; Dal'91; FRCPC; IntMed. Staff, Queen Elizabeth Hospital; (902)894-2111

ADAMS, Leona; St Paul's Hosp, 1081 Burrard St, Vancouver BC V6Z 1Y6; UBC'02; FRCPC; Psy. Staff, Providence Health Care - St Paul's Hospital; (604)682-2344 x69423

ADAMS, Leyland M; Royal Alexandra Hosp, 6408-10240 Kingsway NW, Edmonton AB T5H 3V9; McG'68; FRCPC; Psy. Ac Staff, Royal Alexandra Hospital; (780)735-4567; Fax. (780)735-4797.

ADAMS, Lorna; Southlake Reg Health Centre, 596 Davis Dr, Newmarket ON L3Y 2P9; McM'85; CCFP; Staff, Southlake Regional Health Centre; (905)895-4521

ADAMS, Lorne W; Plaza Med Clinic, 12 Gleneyre St, St. John's NL A1A 2M7; Dal'74; (709)722-9000

ADAMS, Marc; Polyclinique Med Pierre LeGard, 300-1000 montee des Pionniers, Terrebonne QC J6V 1S8; Mon'97; CCFP; Staff, Centre Hospitalier Pierre le Gardeur; (450)657-5799

ADAMS, Mark P; Inst of Commun & Family Psy, 4333 ch Cote-Sainte-Catherine, Montreal QC H3T 1E4; Sher'71; FRCPC; Psy (Consultation-Liaison). Ac Staff, Sir Mortimer B Davis Jewish General; adj Prof, McGill University; (514)340-8210

ADAMS, Martha E; 35 Rumsey Rd, Toronto ON M4G 1N7; Tor'82; FRCPC; Psy. (416)425-6095; Fax. (416)425-2444.

ADAMS, Michael W H; St Joseph's Health Centre, 710 Victoria Ave E, Thunder Bay ON P7C 5P7; Tor'69; Court Staff, Thunder Bay Regional Health Sciences Centre; (807)624-3400; Fax. (807)624-3522.

ADAMS, Mohamed M; 100-410 Baseline Rd PO BOX 3560 Stn Main, Sherwood Park AB T8H 2T4; Cairo (Egypt)'69; LRCP; MRCS(Eng); (780)464-2004

ADAMS, Mohamed N Z; Broad Street Clinic, 2210 Broad St, Regina SK S4P 4V6; Bombay (India)'77; MB BS; Langs: Afrikaans; (306)781-8080

ADAMS, Moustafa A A; Medical & Foot Clinic, 2544 Guardian Rd NW, Edmonton AB T5T 1K8; Cairo (Egypt)'79; MB ChB; Langs: Arabic; (780)444-2252; drmadams@telus.net.

ADAMS, Nigel J; Ultima Med Services, 300-4440 Stark St, Richmond BC V7B 1A1; London (England)'75; MB BS; MRCS; LRCP; CCFP; (604)270-1370; Fax. (604)270-3306.

ADAMS, Paul C; London HSC-University Hosp, PO Box 5339 Stn B 339 Windermere Rd, London ON N6A 5A5; Qns'80; ABIM; AB; FRCPC; IntMed. Ac Staff, London Health Sciences Centre - University Hospital; Prof, University of Western Ontario; (519)685-8500 x35375; Fax. (519)663-3549; padams@uwo.ca.

ADAMS, Rachael E; West Carleton Family Hlth Team, PO Box 218 119 Langstaff Dr, Carp ON K0A 1L0; Qns'08; CCFP; (613)839-3271; Fax. (613)839-3273.

ADAMS, Rebecca A; 735 4th Ave PO Box 1000, Hope BC V0X 1L0; UBC'07; CCFP; (604)869-5648

ADAMS, Richard M; Medical Assoc Of Port Perry, 462 Paxton St, Port Perry ON L9L 1L9; Tor'98; CCFP; Staff, Lakeridge Health - Port Perry Site; (905)985-8425

ADAMS, Robert F; Glengarry Mem Hosp, 20260 County Rd #43, Alexandria ON K0C 1A0; St. George's (Grenada)'88; AB; CCFP; Staff, Glengarry Memorial Hospital; (613)525-3929; Fax. (613)525-5072.

ADAMS, Robert; Professional Arts Bldg, 504-100 Arden St, Moncton NB E1C 4B7; Sher'97; FRCSC; Neursurg (Surgical Oncology). Langs: Bilingual(English/French); (506)857-5376; Fax. (506)857-5378.

ADAMS, Stephen G; Royal University Hosp, 103 Hospital Dr, Saskatoon SK S7N 0W8; Sask'04; BSc; FRCPC; Psy. Staff, Royal University Hospital; (306)966-8226; Fax. (306)966-8232; stephen.adams@saskatoonhealthregion.ca.

ADAMS, Stewart P A; Market Mall Prof Bldg, 206-4935 40 Ave NW, Calgary AB T3A 2N1; Sask'86; FRCPC; Derm. Staff, Foothills Medical Centre; Clin Assoc Prof, University of Calgary; (403)284-4222; Fax. (403)284-5272.

ADAMS, Susan; North Bay Reg Health Centre, PO Box 2500 50 College Dr, North Bay ON P1B 0A4; Southampton (England)'84; MRCPsy; FRCPC; Psy. Staff, North Bay Regional Health Centre - Regional Mental Health; Asst Prof, University of Western Ontario; (705)474-1200 x7808; Fax. (705)472-1694.

ADAMS JR., Winston E; Radiology Associates Of Regina, 6-2727 Parliament Ave, Regina SK S4S 6X5; Dublin (Ireland)'84; MB ChB; FRCPC; DiagRad. Staff, Radiology Associates of Regina; (306)352-7653; Fax. (306)522-4311.

ADAMSON, Charles R; 3024 Bridge St PO Box 170, South Mountain ON K0E 1W0; Ott'77; CCFP; FCFP; Ac Staff, Winchester District Memorial Hospital; (613)989-2205; Fax. (613)989-2207; adamson@magma.ca.

ADAMSON, Henry; Dr Henry Adamson Med Clinic, 5780 Southwood Dr, Halifax NS B3H 4P4; Dundee (Scotland)'76; FRCPC; Anes. Staff, Dartmouth General Hospital; (902)229-9160

ADAMSON, Margaret E M; 312-3024 Hurontario St, Mississauga ON L5B 4M4; Tor'75; Ac Staff Family Pract, Trillium Health Centre - Mississauga; (905)848-1711; Fax. (905)848-1714.

ADAMSON, Maureen E; 601-22259 48 Ave PO Box 12025 Rpo Murrayville, Langley BC V3A 9J5; Ott'86; CCFP; FCFP; Vis Consultant Palliative Care, Langley Memorial Hospital; Vis Consultant Palliative Care, Peace Arch Hospital; (604)514-6144

ADAMSON, Peter A; Renaissance Plaza, M110-150 Bloor St W, Toronto ON M5S 2X9; Tor'72; ABFPS; FACS(Otol); BSc(Hon); ABOtol; FRCSC; Otol (Facial Plastic Surgery). Consultant Surgeon, North York General Hospital; Prof/Head Div of Facial Plastic & Reconstructive Surg Dept of Otol Head & Neck Surg, Toronto General Hospital - UHN; (416)323-3900; Fax. (416)323-1344; paa@dradamson.com.

ADAMSON, Sandra C; Muskoka Algonquin Healthcare, 75 Ann St, Bracebridge ON P1L 2E4; NOSM'09; CCFP; Staff, South Muskoka Memorial Hospital - Muskoka Algonquin Healthcare; (705)645-4400

ADAMUS, Allison T K; West Hill Med Clinic, 1A-2995 2nd Ave W, Prince Albert SK S6V 5V5; Sask'08; CCFP; Coord Residency Training, University of Saskatchewan; (306)765-8500; Fax. (306)765-8501.

ADANLAWO, Adewumi M; Alpen Med Clinic, 346 Railway St W, Cochrane AB T4C 2E2; FRCSC; ObstGyn. (403)851-0091

ADATIA, Almas M; Family Walk-In Medical Clinic, 3018 Don Mills Rd, North York ON M2J 3C1; Makerere (Uganda)'72; MB ChB; Assoc Staff, Mount Sinai Hospital; (416)494-7599; Fax. (416)494-8149.

ADATIA, Feisal A; 200-5340 1 St SW, Calgary AB T2H 0C8; Tor'03; FRCSC; Ophth. (403)286-6802; Fax. (403)286-6819.

ADATIA, Ian T K; University of Alberta Hosp, 4C1 19-8440 112 St NW, Edmonton AB T6G 2B7; Bristol (England)'80; FRCPC; Peds (General Pathology); Cardiol. Staff, Stollery Children's Hospital; (780)407-8361; Fax. (780)407-3954.

ADATIA, Sadruddin; Royal Oak Med Clinic, 192-8888 Country Hills Blvd NW, Calgary AB T3G 5T4; Makerere (Uganda)'68; MB ChB; DObstRCOG; CCFP; (403)239-3660; Fax. (403)239-4001.

ADCOCK, Lesley; Univ Hlth Network-Toronto Western Hosp, 2W 404-399 Bathurst St, Toronto ON M5T 2S8; Dal'97; BSc; CCFP; FCFP; Staff, Toronto General Hospital - UHN; Staff Family Health Centre, Toronto Western Hospital - University Health Network; (416)603-5888; Fax. (416)603-5448.

ADDAE, Gina A O; 90A Isabella St, Toronto ON M4Y 1N4; (Ghana)'81; MB ChB; FRCPC; Psy. (416)929-7729

ADDAI, Stephen A; City Plaza Specialist Clinic, 3-330 Central Ave N, Swift Current SK S9H 0L4; (Ghana)'90; MRCP(UK); MB ChB; DPH(Cambridge); (306)778-3988; Fax. (306)778-3989.

ADDERLEY, Robert J; Children's & Women's HC of BC, 2L5-4480 Oak St, Vancouver BC V6H 3V4; UBC'76; FRCPC; Peds (Pediatric Intensive Care). Pediatrics, BC Children's Hospital; Clin Prof Peds, University of British Columbia; (604)875-2729; Fax. (604)875-2728.

ADDETIA, Karima; MUHC-Royal Victoria Hosp, M4.76-687 av des Pins O, Montreal QC H3A 1A1; Mem'01; FRCPC; IntMed; Cardiol. Staff, McGill University Health Centre - Royal Victoria Hospital; (514)289-2300

ADDINGTON, Donald E; Foothills Med Centre, 1403 29 St NW, Calgary AB T2N 2T9; London (England)'72; MB BS; MRCPsy; FRCPC; Psy (Schizophrenia). Staff Psy, Foothills Medical Centre; (403)944-4548

ADDISON, Anthony M; 110 Queen's Plate Dr, Etobicoke ON M9W 0B4; London (England)'63; MB BS; MRCS; LRCP; FRCOG; FRCSC; ObstGyn. Consultant, St Michael's Hospital; Staff, William Osler Health System - Etobicoke General Hospital; (416)741-6057; Fax. (416)741-6058.

ADDISON, Cynthia A; The Medical Clinic Associates, 4794A Joyce Ave, Powell River BC V8A 3B6; Cal'86; (604)485-6261; Fax. (604)485-2820.

ADDISON, Kirsten; Fort William Family Hlth Team, 117 McKellar St S, Thunder Bay ON P7E 1H5; Ott'04; CCFP; (807)626-1223

ADDISON, Mark J W; Cottage Med Clinic, PO Box 2140 300 Miette St, Jasper AB T0E 1E0; Cape Town (South Africa)'81; DA(SA); Chief Med Staff, Seton Jasper Healthcare Centre; (780)852-4885; Fax. (780)852-2199.

ADDLEMAN, Benjamin; Alexandra Comm Health Centre, 101-1318 Centre St NE, Calgary AB T2E 2R7; Dal'01; CCFP; (403)266-2622; Fax. (403)266-2692.

ADDLEMAN, David; Victoria Health Centre, 65 Brunswick St, Fredericton NB E3B 1G5; McG'70; FRCPC; Psy. Staff Psy, Dr Everett Chalmers Regional Hospital; Clin Instructor, Dalhousie University; (506)444-3636; Fax. (506)444-2247.

ADDLEMAN-FRANKEL, Sarah; The Ottawa Hosp-Civic Campus, 1053 Carling Ave, Ottawa ON K1Y 4E9; McG'07; MDCM; CCFP; CCFP(E.M.); Staff, The Ottawa Hospital - Civic Campus; (613)722-7000

ADDO, Sylvia M; BC Public Service Agency, 201-3200 Shelbourne St, Victoria BC V8W 9V1; FRCPC; OccupMed. (250)952-4228

ADDURI, V Rao; Medical Arts Bldg, 703-233 Kennedy St, Winnipeg MB R3C 3J5; Andhra (India)'64; MSc(Ortho); FRCSC; OrthSurg. Orthopedic Surgery, Concordia General Hospital; Ac Staff, Victoria General Hospital; (204)943-2559; Fax. (204)943-4275.

ADE-CONDE, Adetunji J; Chatham-Kent Hlth Alliance, PO Box 2030 Stn Main 80 Grand Ave W, Chatham ON N7M 5L9; Lagos (Nigeria)'96; Staff, Chatham-Kent Health Alliance; (519)352-6400

ADEAGBO, Bamidele A; Office of the Chief Med Examin, 4070 Bowness Rd NW, Calgary AB T3B 3R7; (403)297-8123

ADEAGBO, Francis; Labrador Health Centre, PO Box 7000 Stn C 227 Hamilton River Rd, Happy-Valley-Goose NL A0P 1C0; Staff, Labrador Health Centre; (709)897-2000

ADEBAYO, Adeleye A M; Blue Spruce Med Centre, 16729 100 St NW, Edmonton AB T5X 3Z9; (Nigeria)'92; DPH; CCFP; (780)457-1351; dalemi42@hotmail.com.

ADEBAYO, Ayodele L; Primecare Health, 120-109 Quarry Park Blvd SE, Calgary AB T2C 5E7; (403)930-7111; Fax. (403)930-7114.

ADEBAYO, Francis O; 5002 51 St PO Box 326, St Paul AB T0A 3A0; (780)645-3666; Fax. (780)645-3688.

ADEBISI, Omoniyi Y; Tower Clinic, 5520 50th Ave, Wetaskiwin AB T9A 0T3; (Nigeria)'92; CCFP; (780)352-9700; Fax. (780)352-9739.

ADEBISI, Timothy A; Three Hills Med Clinic, PO Box 1818 779 2nd St, Three Hills AB T0M 2A0; (Nigeria)'91; MB BS; FRCS; MRCGPract; CCFP; (403)443-5522; Fax. (403)443-5497; boyeadebisi@hotmail.com.

ADEBOWALE, Akinade O; Sault Area Hosp, 750 Great Northern Rd, Sault Ste Marie ON P6B 0A8; Ibadan (Nigeria)'04; Staff, Sault Area Hospital - Sault Ste Marie; (705)759-3434; adebowalea@sah.on.ca.

ADEDIPE, Olusola A; Regina Qu'Appelle HR-Regina, 122-1440 14th Ave, Regina SK S4P 0W5; Locum Tenens, Regina General Hospital; (306)781-7229; Fax. (306)352-0499.

ADEDIRAN, T Peter; IWK Health Centre, PO Box 9700 Rpo CSC 5980 University Ave, Halifax NS B3K 6R8; Lagos (Other Foreign)'97; MB BS; Staff, IWK Health Centre; (902)470-8888

ADEFOLARIN, Oluremi A; Yorkton Mental Health Centre, 270 Bradbrooke Dr, Yorkton SK S3N 2K6; Ibadan (Nigeria)'95; MRCPsy(UK); MB BS; FRCPC; Psy. Psychiatrist, Yorkton Mental Health & Addiction Centre; (306)786-0558; Fax. (306)786-0556; oluremi.adefolarin@shr.sk.ca.

ADEGBITE, A Manna; Queensway-Carleton Hosp, 3045 Baseline Rd, Ottawa ON K2H 8P4; Lagos (Nigeria)'94; MB BS; FRCPC; Peds. Staff Ped, Queensway Carleton Hospital; (613)721-2000

ADEGBITE, Andrew B O; Sudbury Med Centre, 312-65 Larch St, Sudbury ON P3E 1B8; Ibadan (Nigeria)'76; FRCSC; Neursurg. Ac Staff, Health Sciences North-St Joseph's Health Centre; (705)673-3130; Fax. (705)673-7296.

ADEGBOYEGA-CONDE, Omotola; Chatham-Kent Health Alliance, PO Box 2030 Stn Main 80 Grand Ave W, Chatham ON N7M 5L9; Lagos (Nigeria)'98; Staff, Chatham-Kent Health Alliance; (519)351-6144

ADEGBULU, Adekunle K; 504-3 Stonegate Rd NW, Airdrie AB T4B 0N2; Ilorin (Nigeria)'88; MB BS; MCFP; CCFP; (403)945-8216; Fax. (403)945-8276.

ADEKEYE, Olufemi A; Primecare Health Inc, 120-109 Quarry Park Blvd SE, Calgary AB T2C 5E7; (Nigeria)'94; CCFP; (403)930-7111

ADEKOYA, David A; Windsor Reg Hosp-Metropolitan, 1995 Lens Ave, Windsor ON N8W 1L9; New York (USA)'96; CCFP; CCFP(E. M.); Staff, Windsor Regional Hospital - Metropolitan Site; (519)254-5577

ADEL, Anoushirvan; Peterborough Reg HC-Hospital, 1 Hospital Dr, Peterborough ON K9J 7C6; (Iran)'86; ABPN; BSc; FRCPC; Psy (Geriatric Psychiatry). Staff, Peterborough Regional Health Centre - Hospital Drive; (705)876-5028

ADELASOYE, Oluremi F; 15 Williams St N, Lindsay ON K9V 3Z8; (Nigeria)'94; FRCSC; ObstGyn. Staff, Aberdeen Regional Hospital; (705)324-7117; Fax. (705)324-4884; radelasoye@gmail.com.

ADELMAN, Karin A E; North Kingston Comm Health Ctr, 400 Elliott Ave, Kingston ON K7K 6M9; University of Massachusetts (USA)'82; CCFP; (613)542-2949

ADELSON, Edward I; 501-5885 ch Cote-des-Neiges, Montreal QC H3S 2T2; Qns'62; BSc; FACC; CSPQ; FRCPC; IntMed (Aerobic Sports Medicine & Cardiology); Cardiol (P.Q.). Assoc Staff, Sir Mortimer B Davis Jewish General; McGill University; Langs: Yiddish; French; (514)738-8897; Fax. (514)738-1061.

ADELSTEIN, Mitchell; North York Gen Hosp, 1NE 126-4001 Leslie St, North York ON M2K 1E1; Boston (USA)'01; Staff, North York General Hospital; (416)756-6165

ADELSTEIN, Raquel; 206-815 College St, Toronto ON M6G 1C9; Tor'98; CCFP; Staff, Sunnybrook Health Sciences Centre; (416)923-5500; Fax. (416)923-2249.

ADELUGBA, Olajide O; Regional Psychiatric Centre, PO Box 9243 Stn Main 2520 Central Ave, Saskatoon SK S7K 3X5; Ibadan (Nigeria)'85; Staff, Regional Psychiatric Centre - Prairies; (306)975-5411; Fax. (306)875-6024.

ADEM, Doris; Polyclinique Med Fabreville, 380 boul Cure-Labelle, Laval QC H7P 5L3; Laval'75; (450)628-5800; Fax. (450)628-0217.

ADEMIDUN, Aderotimi O; 203-210 Dundas St E, Belleville ON K8N 5G8; Ibadan (Nigeria)'85; FRCSC; ObstGyn. (613)966-2586

ADENUGA, Olugbenga A; 207-44 Mapleton Rd, Moncton NB E1C 7W8; Ibadan (Nigeria)'95; MD; MMed; DipHIV; CCFP; Staff Faculty, Dalhousie University; (506)382-2183

ADENWALA, Tasneem; Goodfellow Prof Bldg, 205-170 McEwan Dr E, Bolton ON L7E 4C8; Bombay (India)'93; CCFP; Physician, Tuscany Medical Centre; Physician, Markham Road Medical Centre; Langs: Hindi; Marathi; Gujarati; Urdu; (905)857-5368; Fax. (905)857-5364.

ADERIBIGBE, Taiwo A A; Victoria Med Centre, 502-304 Victoria Ave N, Hamilton ON L8L 5G4; Ibadan (Nigeria)'91; CCFP; (905)522-8906

ADERINTO, Rasheedah A; Dr Hugh Twomey Health Ctre, PO Box 250 25 Twomey Dr, Botwood NL A0H 1E0; Obafemi Awolowo (Nigeria)'94; MB ChB; CCFP; Physician, Dr Hugh Twomey Health Care Centre; (709)257-2874; Fax. (709)257-4687.

ADESANYA, Arinola O; Oncology Clinic, 150 Sherway Dr, Etobicoke ON M9C 1A5; Ibadan (Nigeria)'76; MB BS; FRCPC; HemPath (Hematological Oncology); IntMed. Consultant Hematologist & Internist, Trillium Health Centre - Mississauga; (416)521-4110; Fax. (416)521-4122.

ADESANYA, Augustine T; Medical Office, C-640 Ross Ave E, Timmins ON P4N 0A2; Ibadan (Nigeria)'75; MB BS; FRCPC; IntMed. Staff, Anson General Hospital; Staff, Lady Minto Hospital Cochrane; Staff, Bingham Memorial Hospital; Staff, Sensenbrenner Hospital; (705)268-9788; Fax. (705)268-2077.

ADETOLA, Ejibunmi; 490 Main St PO Box 726, Winchester ON K0C 2K0; Ogun State (Nigeria)'91; FRCSC; ObstGyn;CCFP; Staff ObstGyn, Winchester District Memorial Hospital; (613)774-9990; Fax. (613)774-9991.

ADETOLA, Motunrayo J; 600-1400 Carling Ave, Ottawa ON K1Z 7L8; Ago-Iwoye (Nigeria)'90; MCFP(SA); CCFP; Staff Emerg, St Francis Memorial Hospital; Asst Prof, University of Ottawa; Langs: Yoruba; (613)820-3694; Fax. (613)820-3695.

ADEWALE, Adesegun A; 1710B 20 St PO Box 309, Didsbury AB T0M 0W0; Lagos (Nigeria)'98; CCFP; (403)335-8895; Fax. (403)335-8867.

ADEWALE, Oluwayemisi O; 103-1800 Market St SE, Airdrie AB T4A 0K9; (Nigeria)'99; (403)980-9929; Fax. (403)980-9925.

ADEWUMI, Adegboyega A; Moose Jaw Union Hosp, 455 Fairford St E, Moose Jaw SK S6H 1H3; FRCPC; Psy. Staff, Moose Jaw Union Hospital; (306)691-6461; Fax. (306)691-6462.

ADEY, Christopher K; CML Healthcare, 120-2462 Howard Ave, Windsor ON N8X 3V6; Mem'77; BSc; BMedSci; AB; FRCPC; DiagRad. (519)255-1265; Fax. (519)256-0265.

ADEY, Frances M; 101-284 Helmcken Rd, Victoria BC V9B 1T2; Manchester (England)'66; MB BCh; (250)474-7715

ADEY, Tanis L; St Clare's Mercy Hosp, W3-154 LeMarchant Rd, St. John's NL A1C 5B8; Mem'91; FRCPC; Psy. Staff Start Clinic, St Clare's Mercy Hospital; Asst Prof, Memorial University Of Newfoundland; (709)777-5111

ADEYEYE, Adeola; 205-599 Main St, Hampton NB E5N 6C2; Obafemi (Other Foreign)'00; MD; MPA; CCFP; Lecturer, Dalhousie University; (506)832-0576; Fax. (506)638-1426.

ADEYI, Oyedele A; Univ Hlth Network-Toronto Gen, 11F 206-200 Elizabeth St, Toronto ON M5G 2C4; Ibadan (Nigeria)'87; FRCPC; AnatPath. Staff Path, Toronto General Hospital - UHN; (416)340-3136

ADHAM, Tamer M H; Queen Elizabeth II Hosp, 10409 98 St, Grande Prairie AB T8V 2E8; Staff, Queen Elizabeth II Hospital; (780)538-7100

ADHIKARI, Neill; Sunnybrook Hlth Sciences Ctre, D1 08-2075 Bayview Ave, Toronto ON M4N 3M5; McG'95; FRCPC; IntMed (Critical Care Medicine); Respir. Staff, Sunnybrook Health Sciences Centre; (416)480-4522

ADIB AZAD, Hamid; East Calgary Health Centre, 4715 8 Ave SE, Calgary AB T2A 3N4; (Germany)'99; CCFP; (403)955-1400

ADIBFAR, Ali; Elements, 195 Avenue Rd, Toronto ON M5R 2J3; Richmond(VA) (USA)'98; DDS; MD; FRCSC; PlasSurg (Cosmetic Surgery). Dir PlasSurg, Oak Ridge Medical Center; Dir PlasSurg, Elements Wellness & Medispa; Langs: Bilingual(English/French); (416)929-6609; Fax. (416)929-0736.

ADIE, Mohammad A; Windsor Reg Hosp-Metropolitan, 1995 Lens Ave, Windsor ON N8W 1L9; Aleppo (Syria)'92; FRCPC; Peds (Neonatology). Staff Neonatologist, Windsor Regional Hospital - Metropolitan Site; (519)254-6741; Fax. (519)255-1735; mohammad_adie@wrh.on.ca.

ADIL, Aliya; Brooklin Med Centre, 1A-5959 Anderson St, Whitby ON L1M 2E9; (Pakistan)'89; MB BS; CCFP; Langs: Urdu; (905)655-3321; Fax. (905)655-4848.

ADILI, Anthony; St Joseph's Healthcare, 8F-50 Charlton Ave E, Hamilton ON L8N 4A6; McM'97; FRCSC; OrthSurg. Staff, St Joseph's Healthcare - Charlton Campus; (905)521-6062

ADILMAN, Stephen M; Royal Jubilee Hosp, 1952 Bay St, Victoria BC V8R 1J8; UBC'90; Staff, Royal Jubilee Hospital; (250)370-8000

ADISESH, Linganatha A; Saint John Reg Hosp, PO Box 2100 Stn Main 400 University Ave, Saint John NB E2L 4L2; Liverpool (England)'86; Staff, Saint John Regional Hospital; (506)648-6000

ADJAHOTO, Etsé; Centre Sante Comm-St Joseph's, 1-280 Victoria St, Dalhousie NB E8C 2R6; (Benin)'87; Staff, Centre de santé Communitaire - St-Joseph; (506)684-7000

ADJAMI, Adele; Clinique Med Saint-Henri, 3966 rue Notre-Dame O, Montreal QC H4C 1R1; St. Joseph (Lebanon)'70; (514)935-4330; Fax. (514)935-4292.

ADJAOUD, Amelie; Clinique Sante Jacques-Cartier, 200-1815 rue King O, Sherbrooke QC J1J 2E3; Sher'99; (819)565-7446; Fax. (819)565-7780.

ADJEMIAN, Raffi A; Clinique Mistissini, 395 boul Mistissini, Mistissini QC G0W 1C0; McG'96; FRCPC; EmergMed;CCFP; Staff, McGill University Health Centre - Royal Victoria Hospital; (418)923-9919

ADKINS, L John; Orillia Soldiers' Mem Hosp, 170 Colborne St W, Orillia ON L3V 2Z3; Tor'87; FRCPC; DiagRad. Staff Radiol, Orillia Soldiers' Memorial Hospital; (705)327-9130

ADL GOLCHIN, Oveis; The Pas Health Complex Inc, PO Box 240 Stn Main 67 1st St W, The Pas MB R9A 1K4; (Other Foreign)'94; Staff, St. Anthony General Hospital; Langs: Farsi; (204)623-3334; Fax. (204)623-2088; oadl@normanrha.mb.ca.

ADLAM, Anita; PO Box 426 Stn Main, Terrace BC V8G 4B1; Orange Free State (South Africa)'90; MB ChB; MMed(Ped); FRCPC; Peds. Staff, Mills Memorial Hospital; Staff, Sleeping Beauty Medical Clinic; Langs: Afrikaans; (250)638-4089; Fax. (250)615-5418; anita.adlam@northernhealth.ca.

ADLE, Mansour; 710-4060 rue Sainte-Catherine, Westmount QC H3Z 2Z3; Teheran (Iran)'72; LMCC; CSPQ; GenSurg (P.Q.) (Liposuction). gén Chirurgien, Centre Hospitalier de LaSalle; gén Chirurgien, CSSS de Dorval-Lachine-Lasalle; Langs: Spanish; Farsi; Turkish; French; (514)935-6555; Fax. (514)935-8686; mansour.adle@sympatico.ca.

ADLEMAN, Neil L; 305-101 Queensway W, Mississauga ON L5B 2P7; Man'78; FRCPC; Peds; Cardiol. (905)273-4055

ADLER, Adam J; Scarborough Hosp-Birchmount, 3030 Birchmount Rd, Scarborough ON M1W 3W3; Tor'99; FRCPC; EmergMed. Staff, The Scarborough Hospital - Birchmount Campus; (416)495-2550

ADLER, Reva N; Bridgepoint Health Centre, 14 St Matthews Rd, Toronto ON M4M 2B5; State Univ(New York) (USA)'83; FRCPC; IntMed; GeriatricMed. Staff, Bridgepoint Health Centre; (416)461-8252

ADLER, Ruth I; New Vision Family Health Team, 421 Greenbrook Dr, Kitchener ON N2M 4K1; Sheffield (England)'80; Ad Staff Privil, St Mary's General Hospital; Ad Staff Privil, Grand River Hospital - Kitchener/Waterloo Health Centre; (519)578-3510; Fax. (519)578-6040.

ADLER NEVO, Gili W; Sunnybrook Hlth Sciences Ctre, FG 22-2075 Bayview Ave, Toronto ON M4N 3M5; Tel Aviv (Israel)'98; Staff, Sunnybrook Health Sciences Centre; (416)480-6833

ADLINGTON, Jay B; Grey Bruce HS-Owen Sound, PO Box 1800 Stn Main 7102-1800 8th St E, Owen Sound ON N4K 6M9; Wes'01; FRCSC; OrthSurg. Staff, Grey Bruce Health Services - Owen Sound; (519)376-2663; Fax. (519)376-4163.

ADNAMS, Bruce; Cowichan Med Centre, 3106 Gibbins Rd, Duncan BC V9L 1E8; Cape Town (South Africa)'79; MB ChB; MMed(Otol); FRCS(Ed); Staff, Kootenay Boundary Regional Hospital; (250)746-7711

ADNO, Brian; Albany Med Clinic, 807 Broadview Ave, Toronto ON M4K 2P8; Witwatersrand (South Africa)'80; Assoc Staff, Toronto East General Hospital Inc; Att Staff, Chester Village for the Aged; (416)461-9471; Fax. (416)461-2710.

ADOLPH, Allyson J; 1022 20 St S, Lethbridge AB T1K 2C9; Sask'96; FRCSC; ObstGyn (Laparoscopy). (403)381-4410; Fax. (403)381-4402.

ADOLPHE, Sarah; Hop Marie Clarac, 3530 boul Gouin E, Montreal-Nord QC H1H 1B7; Mon'04; Staff, Hopital Marie Clarac; (514)321-8800

ADOR-DIONISIO, Jorge B; Grey Bruce HS-Owen Sound, PO Box 1800 Stn Main 1800 8th St E, Owen Sound ON N4K 6M9; U of the East (Philippines)'73; FRCPC; DiagRad. Chief Dept of Diag Imaging, Grey Bruce Health Services - Owen Sound; (519)376-2121 x2201; Fax. (519)376-0423.

ADOUBALI, Abdurahman; Miramichi Reg Hosp, 500 Water St, Miramichi NB E1V 3G5; Al-Fateh (Libya)'92; Staff, Miramichi Regional Hospital; (506)623-3000

ADREWI, Hosen S; 10-5233 Stanley Ave, Niagara Falls ON L2E 7C2; Al Fateh (Libya)'00; CCFP; Staff, Roblin & District Health Centre; (289)296-7757

ADRIAN, Carl H D; Foothills Med Centre, 1403 29 St NW, Calgary AB T2N 2T9; Cal'00; FRCPC; Psy. Staff, Foothills Medical Centre; (403)944-1567; Fax. (403)944-2838.

ADRIAN, Mark D; Vancouver Spine Clinic, 6F-818 10th Ave W, Vancouver BC V5Z 1M9; Man'93; FRCPC; PhysMed&Rehab. (604)742-9940

ADRIANO, Alvin; Oasis Med Centre, 405-9650 Harvest Hills Blvd, Calgary AB T3K 0B3; CCFP; (403)954-2775; Fax. (403)984-2767.

ADRIEN, Alix; Dir de la Sante Publique-Mtl, 1301 rue Sherbrooke E, Montreal QC H2L 1M3; McG'79; FRCPC; CommunMed. Staff, McGill University Health Centre - Montreal General Campus; (514)528-2400 x3681; Fax. (514)528-2452.

ADU-POKU, Yaw; 165 Foster Ave, Belleville ON K8N 3P8; (Ghana)'74; FRCSC; ObstGyn. (613)969-2278

ADVANI, Andrew; St Michael's Health Centre, 6 151-61 Queen St E, Toronto ON M5C 2T2; Edinburgh (United Kingdom)'96; (416)864-6060; Fax. (416)867-3696.

ADVENT, Donald A; Royal Court Med Centre, 301-1 Quarry Ridge Rd, Barrie ON L4M 7G1; Ott'77; (705)726-2991; Fax. (705)726-1069; don.advent@rogers.com.

ADWEDAA, Ebenezer O; Cypress Reg Health Centre, 2004 Saskatchewan Dr, Swift Current SK S9H 5M8; (306)778-9400; Fax. (306)778-9431.

ADZICH, Kim P; Rimbey Med Clinic, PO Box 650, Rimbey AB T0C 2J0; Alb'81; DTMH; Ac Staff, Rimbey Hospital & Care Centre; (403)843-2256; Fax. (403)843-2255.

AEDY, Lawrence J; 103-26 Hiscott St, St Catharines ON L2R 1C6; McM'76; FRCSC; Ophth. (905)687-8844; Fax. (905)687-8844.

AERY, Navrup; Norway House Health Services, PO Box 1060, Norway House MB R0B 1B0; (Other Foreign)'03.

AETA, Hany A M M; Orleans Urgent Care Clinic, 100-1220 Place D'Orleans Dr, Orleans ON K1C 7K3; Cairo (Egypt)'80; Staff Emerg, The Ottawa Hospital - General Campus; Staff Emerg, The Ottawa Hospital - Civic Campus; Physician Family Med, Kent Family Medical Centre; Teach Staff Emergency Dept, University of Ottawa; Langs: Arabic; (613)841-5389; Fax. (613)841-5393.

AFADAPA-IPAYE, Morenike A; Guelph Med Place 1, 204-83 Dawson Rd, Guelph ON N1H 1B1; (Nigeria)'88; FRCPC; Peds. (519)780-1700

AFFIFI, Rasheed A E; Shouldice Hosp, 7750 Bayview Ave, Thornhill ON L3T 4A3; Alexandria (Egypt)'55; MB ChB; FRCSC; GenSurg. Staff, Shouldice Hospital; Langs: Arabic; French; (905)889-1125; Fax. (905)889-4216.

AFFLECK, Andrew W; 197 Chercover Dr, Thunder Bay ON P7G 1A6; Qns'83; CCFP; CCFP(E.M.); Ac Staff Emerg Service, Thunder Bay Regional Health Sciences Centre; (807)767-6729; Fax. (807)767-6729.

AFFLECK, Rita M; Cochrane Family Health Team, PO Box 2050 233 8th St, Cochrane ON P0L 1C0; McG'86; CCFP; (705)272-4331; Fax. (705)272-2638.

AFFOO, Clifford L; Carmen Vanderwater Med Centre, PO Box 790 Stn Main 33-180 Parsons Rd, Alliston ON L9R 1V9; London (England)'78; MB BS; MRCS; LRCP; CCFP; Ac Staff, Stevenson Memorial Hospital; Med Consultant, Honda of Canada Mfg.; (705)435-6225; Fax. (705)435-6062.

AFIF, Waqqas; MUHC-Royal Victoria Hosp, 2.28-687 av des Pins O, Montreal QC H3A 1A1; McG'03; FRCPC; IntMed; Gastroent. Staff, McGill University Health Centre - Royal Victoria Hospital; (514)843-1616

AFIFI, Tarek J; Winnipeg Clinic, 425 St Mary Ave, Winnipeg MB R3C 0N2; Man'04; FRCPC; Derm.

AFILALO, Jonathan; SMBD-Jewish Gen Hosp, 3755 ch Cote-Sainte-Catherine, Montreal QC H3T 1E2; McG'04; FRCPC; IntMed; Cardiol. Staff, Sir Mortimer B Davis Jewish General; (514)340-8222 x59; Fax. (514)340-7534.

AFILALO, Marc; SMBD Jewish Gen Hosp, 3755 ch Cote-Sainte-Catherine, Montreal QC H3T 1E2; Mon'79; MCFP(EM); FACEP; LMCC; FRC; FRCPC; EmergMed. Dir Emerg Dept, Sir Mortimer B Davis Jewish General; assoc Prof, McGill University; (514)340-8222 x5568; Fax. (514)340-7519; marc.afilalo@mcgill.ca.

AFOLABI, Oluwatola; Univ Hlth Network-Toronto Western Hosp, 4F-399 Bathurst St, Toronto ON M5T 2S8; Tor'07; FRCSC; PlasSurg. Staff, Toronto Western Hospital - University Health Network; (416)603-2581; Fax. (416)603-5553.

AFOLABI, Oyewale A; Moose Jaw Union Hosp, 455 Fairford St E, Moose Jaw SK S6H 1H3; Staff, Moose Jaw Union Hospital.

AFSAR, Afsaneh; 302-3025 Hurontario St, Mississauga ON L5A 2H1; Tor'90; Court Staff Family Pract, Trillium Health Centre - Mississauga; Court Staff Family Pract, The Credit Valley Hospital; (905)279-6661; Fax. (905)279-0319.

AFSHAR, Kourosh; Children's & Women's HC of BC, ACB KO 134-4480 Oak St, Vancouver BC V6H 3V4; Tehran (Iran)'91; FRCSC; Urol. Urology, BC Children's Hospital; (604)875-2734

AFSHAR, Maryam; The Credit Valley Hosp, 2200 Eglinton Ave W, Mississauga ON L5M 2N1; Ankara (Turkey)'91; Staff, The Credit Valley Hospital; (905)813-2200

AFSHAR-GHOTLI, Zohreh; Thunder Bay Reg HSC-T-Bay, 980 Oliver Rd, Thunder Bay ON P7B 6V4; Tehran (Iran)'94; FRCPC; AnatPath. Staff, Thunder Bay Regional Health Sciences Centre; (807)684-6000

AFSHARI-AZAD, Nahid; The Ottawa Hosp-Civic Campus, 1053 Carling Ave, Ottawa ON K1Y 4E9; Ott'83; FRCPC; IntMed; GeriatricMed. Dir Geriatric Assessment Unit, The Ottawa Hospital - Civic Campus; Dir Equity Diversity & Gender/Asst Prof, University of Ottawa; Langs: Persian; (613)761-4195; Fax. (613)761-5334; nazad@ottawahospital.on.ca.

AFTAB, Huma; Royal University Hosp, 103 Hospital Dr, Saskatoon SK S7N 0W8; Peshawar (India)'99; FRCPC; Psy. Staff, Royal University Hospital; (306)655-1000

AFZAL, Ayesha N; Langley Mem Hosp, 22051 Fraser Hwy, Langley BC V3A 4H4; Rawalpindi (Pakistan)'95; MB BS; Staff, Langley Memorial Hospital; (604)534-4370

AFZAL, Samina; IWK Health Centre, PO Box 9700 Rpo CSC 5850-5980 University Ave, Halifax NS B3K 6R8; Punjab (Pakistan)'88; Staff, IWK Health Centre; (902)470-8229; Fax. (902)470-7975.

AG BAZET, Albaka; Clinique Med Adoncour, 505 rue Adoncour, Longueuil QC J4G 2M6; Mon'05; CCFP; (450)646-4445

AGAIBI, Samuel M; Queen Elizabeth II HSC, 1796 Summer St, Halifax NS B3H 2Y9; Punjab University (India)'88; MB BS; Staff, Queen Elizabeth II Health Sciences Centre - Victoria General Site; (902)473-4153; Fax. (902)473-6293.

AGANABA, Tari L; Dawson Creek & Dist Hosp, 11100 13 St, Dawson Creek BC V1G 3W8; Ibadan (Nigeria)'76; MB BS; Staff, Dawson Creek & District Hospital; (250)784-7361

AGAPITOS, Peter J; Riverside Prof Centre, 209-1919 Riverside Dr, Ottawa ON K1H 1A2; Ott'82; FRCSC; Ophth. Staff, The Ottawa Hospital - Civic Campus; Staff, The Ottawa Hospital - General Campus; Asst Prof Ophth, University of Ottawa; (613)236-9929; Fax. (613)236-6801.

AGARWAL, Anil; 103-77 Westmount Rd, Guelph ON N1H 5J1; New Delhi (India)'80; MB BS; DMRD; FRCPC; IntMed. Staff, Guelph General Hospital; Langs: Hindi; (519)822-7347

AGARWAL, Parul; Youthdale Treatment Centre, 227 Victoria St, Toronto ON M5B 1T8; New Delhi (India)'96; FRCPC; Psy. (416)363-3751; Fax. (416)363-7945.

AGARWAL, Ragini; McMaster Family Practice, A-690 Main St W, Hamilton ON L8S 1A4; London (England)'92; CCFP; FCFP; (905)521-5015; Fax. (905)521-5010.

AGARWAL, Sanjay; 200-300 Main St N, Brampton ON L6V 4H6; Tor'94; CCFP; CCFP(E.M.); Staff, William Osler Health System - Brampton Civic Hospital; (905)451-1806; Fax. (905)451-8272.

AGARWAL, Shashi; Credit Valley Prof Bldg, 306-2300 Eglinton Ave W, Mississauga ON L5M 2V8; Bhopal (India)'77; (905)828-1027; Fax. (905)828-1509.

AGARWAL, Vikas; Mountain Med Walk-In Clinic, 880 Upper Wentworth St, Hamilton ON L9A 5H2; Wes'04; CCFP; Staff, Mountain Medical Walk-In Clinic; (905)575-0808

AGARWALA, Ravi; Niagara HS-St Catherines, 142 Queenston St, St. Catharines ON L2R 7C6; Ott'94; FRCPC; IntMed (Respirology). Staff, Niagara Health System - St Catharines General Site; Staff Pulmonary & Critical Care Division, University of Rochester(NY); Langs: Spanish; French; (905)684-7271

AGARWALA, Vinod K; The Ottawa Hosp-Gen Campus, 501 Smyth Rd Box 502, Ottawa ON K1H 8L6; Lucknow (India)'61; FRCSC; OrthSurg. Staff, The Ottawa Hospital - General Campus; Staff, The Ottawa Hospital - Riverside Campus; (613)235-9930; Fax. (613)235-2538.

AGATE, William A; The Health Centre Of Maple, 1-2810 Major Mackenzie Dr, Maple ON L6A 3L2; Tor'83; CCFP; CCFP(E.M.); Ac Staff, Mackenzie Richmond Hill Hospital; (905)832-3838 x1; Fax. (905)832-9097.

AGBAHOVE, Onome T; Abbotsford Reg Hosp & Cancer C, 32900 Marshall Rd, Abbotsford BC V2S 0C2; Ibadan (Nigeria)'92; Staff, Abbotsford Regional Hospital & Cancer Centre; (604)851-4700

AGBAYANI, Regina N; Albion-Kipling Med Centre, 206-1525 Albion Rd, Etobicoke ON M9V 5G5; (Philippines)'82; CCFP; Staff, William Osler Health System - Etobicoke General Hospital; (416)744-7890; Fax. (416)744-8106.

AGBAYEWA, M Oluwafemi; Burnaby Hosp, 3935 Kincaid St, Burnaby BC V5G 2X6; Ibadan (Nigeria)'74; MB BS; MRCPsy(Lond); FRCPC; Psy (Administrative Psychiatry). Consultant Geriatric Psy, Burnaby Hospital; Consultant Geriatric Psy, Government of Territory of Yukon; Clin Prof, University of British Columbia; Langs: Yoruba; (604)453-1923; agbayewa@interchange.ubc.ca.

AGBI, Adejumoke A; Dr Charles S Curtis Mem Hosp, 178-200 West St, St Anthony NL A0K 4S0; Ogun State (Nigeria)'03; MB ChB; Staff, Charles S Curtis Memorial Hospital; (709)454-3333

AGBI, Charles B; The Ottawa Hosp-Civic Campus, C2212-1053 Carling Ave, Ottawa ON K1Y 4E9; Ibadan (Nigeria)'77; FRCS(Ed); FRCSC; Neursurg. Staff, The Ottawa Hospital - Civic Campus; (613)761-5383; Fax. (613)761-4504.

AGBODO, Johnson C L; Penticton Reg Hosp, 550 Carmi Ave, Penticton BC V2A 3G6; Minsk (Belarus)'90; Staff, Penticton Regional Hospital; (250)492-9041

AGBOOLA, Julius A; 304-1950 Algonquin Ave, North Bay ON P1B 4Z2; Obafemi Awolowo (Nigeria)'88; FRCSC; ObstGyn. Staff, North Bay Regional Health Centre - Regional Mental Health; (705)840-9000; Fax. (705)840-9007.

AGBOOLA, Olaniyi B; Yarmouth Reg Hosp, 60 Vancouver St, Yarmouth NS B5A 2P5; Zaria (Nigeria)'87; FRCSC; ObstGyn. Staff, Yarmouth Regional Hospital; (902)742-3541

AGBOOLA, Olusegun O; 302-168 Charlotte St, Ottawa ON K1N 8K6; Ibadan (Nigeria)'71; MB BS; AB(T); FWACS; FRCPC; RadOncol (Lung Cancer). Staff RadOncol, The Ottawa Hospital - General Campus; Staff RadOncol, Ottawa Regional Cancer Centre; Assoc Prof, University of Ottawa; (613)789-4385

AGELLON, John D; St Joseph's Health Centre, 30 The Queensway, Toronto ON M6R 1B5; Tor'00; FRCPC; Anes. Staff, St Joseph's Health Centre; (416)530-6000

AGERANIOTI-BELANGER, Stacey; Hôpital Ste-Justine, 2123-3175 ch Cote-Sainte-Cathe, Montreal QC H3T 1C5; Alb'93; FRCPC; Peds. Staff, Hôpital Ste-Justine; Langs: Greek; Bilingual(French/English); (514)345-4931 x7727; stacey_ageranioti_belanger@hotmail.com.

AGES, Deena E; The Doctor's Office, 3089 Dufferin St, North York ON M6A 2S7; Tor'90; Langs: Hebrew; (416)256-9642; Fax. (416)256-9638.

AGGARWAL, Aaron N; Etherington Hall, 102 Stuart St, Kingston ON K7L 2V6; Alb'04; BSc; FRCPC; IntMed; Respir. Staff IntMed, Kingston General Hospital; (613)548-2342; Fax. (613)549-1459.

AGGARWAL, Anita; William Osler HC-Brampton, 2100 Bovaird Dr E, Brampton ON L6R 3J7; Tor'01; CCFP; CCFP(E.M.); Staff, Trillium Health Centre - Mississauga; Staff, William Osler Health System - Brampton Civic Hospital; (905)494-2120

AGGARWAL, Anita; 270 Riddell St, Woodstock ON N4S 6N6; Gulbarga University (India)'02; Staff, Woodstock General Hospital; (519)421-4211

AGGARWAL, Anjali; 304-855 Broadview Ave, Toronto ON M4K 3Z1; Qns'03; FRCSC; ObstGyn.

AGGARWAL, Dhiraj; Ontario Mental Hlth Services, 200-311 McArthur Ave, Vanier ON K1L 8M3; Ott'03; FRCPC; Psy. (613)738-6990

AGGARWAL, Jagan N; Coral Spring Medical, 5070 68 St NE, Calgary AB T3J 4J1; National(Wales) (United Kingdom)'66; Staff, Covenant Health - Our Lady of the Rosary Hospital; (403)568-0171; Fax. (403)568-0157.

AGGARWAL, Naresh K; Finclea Med Centre, 204-490 Bramalea Rd, Brampton ON L6Y 0G1; Himachal Pradesh (India)'78; MB BS; CCFP; FCFP; Langs: Hindi; Punjabi; (905)792-6500; Fax. (905)792-6853.

AGGARWAL, Neera; Kemptville Dist Hosp, PO Box 2007 2675 Concession Rd, Kemptville ON K0G 1J0; Punjabi (India)'94; CCFP; Staff, Kemptville District Hospital; Staff, Strandherd Crossing Medical Centre; (613)258-0100; Fax. (613)258-6171.

AGGARWAL, Rakesh M; Niagara H System-Welland Site, 65 Third St, Welland ON L3B 4W6; Liverpool (England)'77; MB ChB; MRC(UK); DMRD; FRCR; FRCPC; DiagRad (Diagnostic & Therapeutic Radiology). Staff, Niagara Health System - Welland Hospital Site; Staff, Niagara Health System - Port Colborne General Site; (905)732-6111 x3276; Fax. (905)732-9537.

AGGARWAL, Ram K; 19-6175 Hwy 7, Woodbridge ON L4H 0P6; Wisconsin (USA)'94; FRCPC; IntMed (Critical Care Medicine). Staff Med Critical Care & Cardiology, William Osler Health System - Etobicoke General Hospital; Staff, William Osler Health Centre; Langs: Punjabi; Hindi; (905)850-3091; raggarwal@rogers.com.

AGGARWAL, Ravinder K; 234A Colborne St W, Orillia ON L3V 2Z6; Tor'87; CCFP; FCFP; Staff Family Pract, Orillia Soldiers' Memorial Hospital; (705)325-2487; Fax. (705)325-1906.

AGGARWAL, Rohit; 4103 Wolfe Point Way, Ottawa ON K1V 1P3; Ott'09; CCFP; Staff, Pembroke Regional Hospital Inc.

AGGARWAL, Sandeep G; Bridgeland Med Bldg, 1F-803A 1 Ave NE, Calgary AB T2E 7C5; Tor'89; FRCPC; IntMed (Cardiac Rehabilitation); Cardiol. Staff, Foothills Medical Centre; Staff, Rockyview General Hospital; Staff, Peter Lougheed Centre; Staff, South Health Campus; University of Calgary; (403)571-8607; Fax. (403)237-8601.

AGGARWAL, Sandeep K; Oakmed Family Health Team, 110-231 Oak Park Blvd, Oakville ON L6H 7S8; Wes'06; BSc; CCFP; Staff, Village of Erin Meadows LTC; (905)901-5111; Fax. (905)901-5122.

AGGARWAL, Sanjay; GMF Cote-des-Neiges, 500-5700 ch Cote-des-Neiges, Montreal QC H3T 2A8; Qns'02; BSc; CCFP; (514)731-8531; Fax. (514)731-0563.

AGGARWAL, Seema; South Windor Med Centre, 2-3840 Howard Ave, Windsor ON N9E 3N9; (India)'95; MB BS; CCFP; Staff, Windsor Regional Hospital - Metropolitan Site; (519)969-3744; Fax. (519)969-4478.

AGGARWAL, Shilpa; Medical Clinic, 701 Oxford St E, London ON N5Y 4T7; Wes'98; CCFP; FCFP; (519)660-5799

AGHA, Amer; Clinique Med le Plein Ciel, 475 boul de la Cote-Vertu, Saint-Laurent QC H4L 1X7; Bucharest (Romania)'82; (514)337-3171; Fax. (514)337-5023.

AGHA KHANI, Yahya; South Health Campus, 480047-4448 Front St SE, Calgary AB T3M 1M4; Isfahan (Iran)'91; FRCPC; Neur. Staff, South Health Campus; (403)956-3444; Fax. (403)956-3494.

AGHAJAFARI, Fariba; Sunridge Family Med Teaching C, 2685 36 St NE, Calgary AB T1Y 5S3; Shahid Beheshti (Iran)'92; MSc; CCFP; Staff, Sunridge Family Medicine Teaching Centre; (403)943-5000; fariba_aghajafari@yahoo.com.

AGHANAJAFI, Effat; 3436 Broadway W, Vancouver BC V6R 2B3; Tehran (Iran)'88; CCFP; (604)732-8808

AGHARAZII, Mohsen; CHUQ-Hotel-Dieu de Quebec, 11 Cote Du Palais, Quebec QC G1R 2J6; Laval'94; CSPQ; LMCC; MRCP; FRCPC; IntMed (Hypertension Nephrology); Nephrol. Staff, Centre Hospitalier Universitaire de Québec (CHUQ) - Siege Social; adj Prof, Université Laval; Langs: Farsi; (418)691-5464; Fax. (418)691-5757; mohsen.agharazii@crhdq.ulaval.ca.

AGHAZAMAN KASHANI, Soudabeh; Lakeshore Village Walk-In Med, 2885 Lake Shore Blvd W, Etobicoke ON M8V 1J1; Tehran (Iran)'81; CCFP; Staff, Southdown Medical Centre; (416)259-5100; Fax. (416)259-6958.

AGID, Ofer; Addiction & Mental Hlth-Clarke, 250 College St, Toronto ON M5T 1R8; Hebrew (Israel)'94; Staff, Centre for Addiction & Mental Health (CAMH) - College Street Site; (416)535-8501

AGID, Ronit F; Univ Hlth Network-Toronto Western Hosp, 3MW 425-399 Bathurst St, Toronto ON M5T 2S8; Hebrew (Israel)'95; FRCPC; DiagRad (Neuro Radiology). Staff, Toronto Western Hospital - University Health Network; (416)603-5800

AGIER, Jean-Maurice; CSSS Couer-de-l'Ile, 7345 rue Garnier, Montreal QC H2E 2A1; Lyon (France)'78; (514)495-6767 x6065

AGIREB, Ahmed E A; Fogo Island Health Centre, PO Box 9, Fogo NL A0G 2B0; Al-Fateh (Libya)'02; MB BCh; Staff, Fogo Island Health Centre; (709)266-2221

AGNAOU, Hocine; 230-383 boul du Seminaire N, St-Jean-sur-Richel QC J3B 8C5; (Algeria)'96; FRCPC; Psy. (450)346-2222 x8472

AGNEW, Shane R; Kelowna Gastroent Associates, 564 Leon Ave, Kelowna BC V1Y 6J6; Wes'89; FRCPC; IntMed; Gastroent. Medical Staff, Kelowna General Hospital; (250)763-6433; Fax. (250)763-3818.

AGO, C Tetteh; Nova Scotia Cancer Centre, 5820 University Ave, Halifax NS B3H 1V7; Accra (Ghana)'74; MB ChB; DMRT; DAB; FRCR; FRCPC; RadOncol. Staff, Cape Breton Healthcare Complex; Head RadOncol/Asst Prof, Dalhousie University; (902)473-2030; Fax. (902)473-1273.

AGOHA, Victor K; Wal-Mart Canada, 1212 37 St SW, Calgary AB T3C 1S3; (Nigeria)'85; MB BS; CCFP; Staff, Peter Lougheed Centre; (403)451-5788; Fax. (403)451-5789.

AGOPSOWICZ, Barbara H; Dominion Med Centre, 2383 111 St NW, Edmonton AB T6J 5E5; Wroclaw (Poland)'81; Vis Staff Privil, University of Alberta Hospital; Langs: Polish; Ukrainian; (780)436-0020; Fax. (780)436-0603.

AGOSTINO, Holly; Dept of Adolescent Medicine, 1040 av Atwater, Montreal QC H3Z 1X3; McG'07; MDCM; FRCPC; Peds (Adolescent Medicine). (514)412-4481

AGOSTON, Hanga; Connor House Family Practice, 240 Pinnacle St, Belleville ON K8N 3A6; Wes'10; CCFP; (613)968-9840

AGOUES, Isabelle; Clinique Med Blainville, 519 boul du Curé-Labelle, Blainville QC J7C 2H6; Mon'93; (450)430-1274

AGOUMI, Younes; CHUM-Hop Notre-Dame, 1560 rue Sherbrooke E, Montreal QC H2L 4M1; Sher'03; FRCSC; Ophth. Staff, Centre Hospitalier l'Université de Montréal (CHUM) - Hôpital Notre-Dame; (514)890-8000

AGRANOVICH, Alexander L; BC Cancer Agency-Fraser Valley, 13750 96 Ave, Surrey BC V3V 1Z2; St Petersburg (Russia (Federation))'75; FRCPC; RadOncol (Central Nerous System Oncology). Ac Staff, BC Cancer Agency Fraser Valley Centre; Ac Staff, Surrey Memorial Hospital; Clin Assoc Prof Surg, University of British Columbia; Langs: Russian; (604)930-4036; Fax. (604)930-4065; aagranov@bccancer.bc.ca.

AGRANOVICH, Natalie V; Riverview Hosp, 2601 Lougheed Hwy, Coquitlam BC V3C 4J2; Leningrad (Russia (Federation))'75; Staff, BC Mental Health & Addiction Service; (604)524-7655; Fax. (604)543-0231.

AGRAWAL, Anita; Royal University Hosp, 4562-103 Hospital Dr, Saskatoon SK S7N 0W8; Ranchi (India)'93; FRCSC; ObstGyn. Staff, Royal University Hospital; (306)966-8693; Fax. (306)966-8040.

AGRAWAL, Sacha; East Region Mental Hlth Serv, 2757 King St E, Hamilton ON L8G 5E4; Tor'02; FRCPC; Psy. (905)573-4801

AGRAWAL, Sumit K; London HSC-University Hosp, PO Box 5339 Stn B B1 333-339 Windermere Rd, London ON N6A 5A5; Wes'01; FRCSC; Otol. Staff, London Health Sciences Centre - University Hospital; (519)663-3568; Fax. (519)663-3916.

AGUANNO, Jonathan J; Dundurn Med Group, 160 Dundurn St S, Hamilton ON L8P 4K3; Tor'96; CCFP; (905)528-5480; Fax. (905)389-1107.

AGUAYO, Pablo V; 203-1670 Dufferin St, Toronto ON M6H 3M2; (Chile)'99; CCFP; (416)652-7667

AGUILAR, Eslier G; Villa Nova Med Clinic, 119-120 Conception Bay Hwy, Conception-Bay-S NL A1W 3A6; Havana (Cuba)'93; CCFP; Staff, Cape Breton Healthcare Complex; (709)834-2131; Fax. (709)834-3101.

AGUILAR, Karenina; 204-119 Memorial Ave, Orillia ON L3V 5X1; Wes'10; CCFP; (705)323-9800

AGUILAR, Rodolfo P; Hope Medical Clinic, 4B-408 Main St, Stonewall MB R0C 2Z0.

AGUILAR RIVERA, Omar D J; St Clair Corporate Centre, 112-265 Front St N, Sarnia ON N7T 7X1; (Mexico)'85; FRCPC; Psy. Staff, Bluewater Health - Mitton Site; (519)344-6519

AGULNIK, David B; St Paul's Hosp, 1081 Burrard St, Vancouver BC V6Z 1Y6; Ott'95; BSc; CCFP; CCFP(E.M.); Staff, Providence Health Care - St Paul's Hospital; (604)682-2344

AGULNIK, Jason S; SMBD Jewish Gen Hosp, G.203-3755 ch Cote-Sainte-Cath, Montreal QC H3T 1E2; McG'97; FRCPC; IntMed; Respir. Staff, Sir Mortimer B Davis Jewish General; (514)340-8222 x3763; Fax. (514)340-7555.

AGWAZE, Agatha E; Good Health Med Centre, 1212 37 St SW, Calgary AB T3C 1S3; (Nigeria)'94; (403)451-5788; Fax. (403)451-5789.

AGWAZE, Monday M; 4-4710 50 St PO Box 1210, Stettler AB T0C 2L0; (Nigeria)'93; MB BS; MMed(FamMed); CCFP; (403)742-3441; Fax. (403)742-3299.

AH-LAN, Christopher; CSSS du Sud de Lanaudière, 911 rue Montee des Pionniers, Terrebonne QC J6V 2H2; McG'04; FRCPC; IntMed; MedOncol; Hem. Staff, Centre Hospitalier Pierre le Gardeur; (450)654-7525 x32131

AH-LAN, Khim C; 5975 boul Payer, Saint-Hubert QC J3Y 6W6; Bordeaux (France)'78; Langs: English; French; (450)656-8221; Fax. (450)656-0515.

AH NOW, Walter; 933 Liverpool Rd, Pickering ON L1W 1S7; Cape Town (South Africa)'63; MB ChB; BSc; CCFP; FCFP; Court Staff, Rouge Valley Health System - Centenary Health Centre Site; Court Staff, Rouge Valley Health System - Ajax & Pickering Health Centre Site; (905)839-1133

AH-SUE, Michael J; Clinique Med Urgence Brossard, 7601 boul Taschereau, Brossard QC J4Y 1A2; Dublin (Ireland)'69; FRCSC; ObstGyn. (450)462-0863

AH-SUE, Sheri L; Addiction & Mental Hlth-Queen, 1001 Queen St W, Toronto ON M6J 1H4; RCS (Ireland)'05; CCFP; Staff, Centre for Addiction & Mental Health (CAMH) - Queen Site; (416)535-8501; sheriahsue@yahoo.com.

AHAD, Victor A; Ctr Hosp de Verdun, 4000 boul Lasalle, Verdun QC H4G 2A3; Ein Shams (Egypt)'56; Nephrol (P.Q.); IntMed (P.Q.). Assoc Member Med, Centre Hospitalier de Verdun; Langs: Arabic; English; (514)362-1000; v.abdelahad@videotron.ca.

AHAMAD, Keith R; 265 Cordova St E, Vancouver BC V6A 4S7; UBC'10; (604)880-8073

AHAMED, Karim S; Sturgeon Community Hosp, 201 Boudreau Rd, St. Albert AB T8N 6C4; UBC'02; FRCPC; DiagRad. Staff, Sturgeon Community Hospital; (780)418-8219

AHAMED, Zahra S; 240-919 Centre St NW, Calgary AB T2E 2P6; UBC'05; CCFP.

AHEE, Richard E M; Peterborough Clinic FHT, 26 Hospital Dr, Peterborough ON K9J 7C3; Qns'82; CCFP; Staff, Peterborough Regional Health Centre - Hospital Drive; (705)740-6848; Fax. (705)740-6847.

AHEER, Mukhtiar S; South Georgetown Clinic, 333 Mountainview Rd S, Georgetown ON L7G 6E8; '09; CCFP; (905)873-2308

AHERN, Stephane P; Hop Maisonneuve-Rosemont, 5415 boul de l'Assomption, Montreal QC H1T 2M4; Sher'00; FRCPC; IntMed; Critical Care Medicine (P.Q.). Staff, Hopital Maisonneuve-Rosemont; (514)252-3400 x5793

AHLAN, Jennifer C M; Centre Regional du Diabete, 1515 boul Chomedey, Laval QC H7V 3Y7; Sher'06; FRCPC; IntMed (P.Q.); Endocrin&Metab. Staff, Hopital de la Cite de la santé; (450)978-8607

AHLGREN, Paul D; Medical Arts Bldg, 1001-1538 rue Sherbrooke O, Montreal QC H3G 1L5; Qns'78; ABIM; FRCPC; IntMed; MedOncol. Staff, St Mary's Hospital Centre; Staff, McGill University Health Centre - Montreal General Campus; Internal Med, Hôpital Santa Cabrini Ospedale; adj Prof, McGill University; Langs: French; (514)933-2778; info@villemariemed.com.

AHLIJAH, William K; 100-2550 12th Ave, Regina SK S4P 3X1; Nigeria (Nigeria)'64; DPM; MPhil(Psy.); (306)566-4140; Fax. (306)566-4150.

AHLUWALIA, Ajit K; Malton Med Arts Bldg, 209-3530 Derry Rd E, Mississauga ON L4T 4E3; Maulana Ajad (India)'73; MB BS; Staff, William Osler Health System - Etobicoke General Hospital; (905)677-1919; Fax. (905)677-1919.

AHLUWALIA, Amar K; Carlton Med Centre, 20-595 Carlton St, St Catharines ON L2M 4Y2; Delhi (India)'54; MB BS; MS; Langs: Hindi; Punjabi; (905)682-8161; Fax. (905)687-9400.

AHLUWALIA, Mohinderjit S; Malton Med Arts Bldg, 212-3530 Derry Rd E, Mississauga ON L4T 4E3; Glasgow (Scotland)'71; Ac Staff, William Osler Health System - Etobicoke General Hospital; Langs: Punjabi; (905)673-6037; Fax. (905)673-6038.

AHLUWALIA, Nalin K; Halton HCS Corp-Oakville, 327 Reynolds St, Oakville ON L6J 3L7; Dal'89; CCFP; CCFP(E.M.); Staff, Halton Healthcare Services Corporation - Oakville Site; (905)338-4618

AHLUWALIA, Rajpal S; Western Medical Institute, 101-1020 Lorimer Blvd, Winnipeg MB R3P 1C7; Manchester (England)'79; MB ChB; ATLS; (204)452-2220

AHLUWALIA, Ravjit S; Fowler Kennedy Sports Med Clin, 3M Centre-1151 Richmond St, London ON N6A 3K7; Ott'09; CCFP; (519)661-3011; Fax. (519)661-3379.

AHLUWALIA, Simran; Child & Parent Resource Inst, 600 Sanatorium Rd, London ON N6H 3W7; Punjabi (India)'96; FRCPC; Psy. Staff, Child & Parent Resource Institute; (519)858-2774

AHLUWALIA, Usha; Malton Med Arts Bldg, 212-3530 Derry Rd E, Mississauga ON L4T 4E3; Delhi (India)'77; (905)673-6037; Fax. (905)673-6038.

AHLUWALIA, Vandana; Finchgate Med Centre, 227-40 Finchgate Blvd, Brampton ON L6T 3J1; Tor'89; FRCPC; IntMed; Rheum. Court Staff, Headwaters Health Care Centre - Orangeville Site; Ac Staff, William Osler Health System - Brampton Civic Hospital; Langs: Hindi; Punjabi; Urdu; (905)799-1850 x21; Fax. (905)799-8040.

AHMAD, Afzaal; 1521 6th Ave W, Prince Albert SK S6V 5K1.

AHMAD, Afzal; Trillium Hlth Ctr-Mississauga, 100 Queensway W, Mississauga ON L5B 1B8; RCS (Ireland)'68; FRCPC; DiagRad. Staff, Trillium Health Centre - Mississauga; (905)848-7614; Fax. (905)848-7676.

AHMAD, Aijaz; Medicine Hat Reg Hosp, 666 5 St SW, Medicine Hat AB T1A 4H6; (Pakistan)'79; MB BS; Staff, Medicine Hat Regional Hospital; Clinical Asst Prof, University of Calgary; Langs: Urdu; Hindi; Punjabi; (403)528-2911; Fax. (403)526-5818.

AHMAD, Amer R; 59 Payzant Dr PO Box 2408, Windsor NS B0N 2T0; Dal'89; Staff, Hants Community Hospital; Med Examiner, Hants County; (902)798-8260

AHMAD, Asma R; Queen Elizabeth II HSC, 1276 South Park St, Halifax NS B3H 2Y9; Punjab (Pakistan)'60; MB BS; ABPath; FRCPC; AnatPath. Gen Pathol, Queen Elizabeth II Health Sciences Centre - Victoria General Site; Assoc Prof, Dalhousie University; (902)473-7471; Fax. (902)473-1049; asma.raza@cdha.nshealth.ca.

AHMAD, Belal; London Reg Cancer Centre, 790 Commissioners Rd E, London ON N6A 4L6; Qns'02; FRCPC; RadOncol. (519)685-8500; Fax. (519)685-8627.

AHMAD, Chaudhary E; Dr H Bliss Murphy Cancer Ctre, 300 Prince Philip Dr, St. John's NL A1B 3V6; Quaid-E-Azam (Pakistan)'87; MB BS; FRCPC; IntMed; MedOncol. Staff, Dr H Bliss Murphy Cancer Centre; (709)777-6934

AHMAD, Dildar; London Cardiac Institute, 302-256 Pall Mall St, London ON N6A 5P6; RCS (Ireland)'62; FRCP(Ire); FCCP; FRCPC; IntMed (Respirology). Emeritus Prof Med, University of Western Ontario; (519)645-0146; Fax. (519)645-1584.

AHMAD, Ejaz; Four Season Medical Clinic, 562 Ellice Ave, Winnipeg MB R3B 3C6; Punjab (Pakistan)'85; MB BS; CCFP; Staff, Selkirk Mental Health Centre; Langs: Urdu; Hindi; Punjabi; Bilingual(English/French).

AHMAD, Fuad; North Park Med Centre, 2355 Keele St, North York ON M6M 4A2; Peshawar (India)'91; CCFP; (416)244-4377; Fax. (416)244-1004.

AHMAD, Ghias; 309-741 Broadview Ave, Toronto ON M4K 3Y3; Lahore (India)'60; FRCPC; IntMed. (416)925-7011; Fax. (416)925-7323.

AHMAD, Iftikhar; 4713 48 AVE SS 3, St Paul AB T0A 3A3; (Pakistan)'90; (780)645-3331; Fax. (780)645-1702.

AHMAD, Imran; Hop Maisonneuve-Rosemont, 5415 boul de l'Assomption, Montreal QC H1T 2M4; Karachi (Pakistan)'92; MB BS; Staff, Hopital Maisonneuve-Rosemont; (514)252-3404

AHMAD, Ishtiaq; James Paton Mem Hosp, 125 Trans Canada Hwy, Gander NL A1V 1P7; Multan (Pakistan)'90; Staff, James Paton Memorial Hospital; (709)256-2500

AHMAD, Jamil; The Plastic Surgery Clinic, 1421 Hurontario St, Mississauga ON L5G 3H5; RCS (Ireland)'05; MD; FRCSC; PlasSurg. Staff, Women's College Hospital; Staff, Toronto Western Hospital - University Health Network; (905)278-7077; Fax. (905)275-1582; drahmad@theplasticsurgeryclinic.com.

AHMAD, Kamran; St Michael's Hosp, 6 050-30 Bond St, Toronto ON M5B 1W8; Tor'98; FRCPC; IntMed; Cardiol. Staff/Lecturer ElectroPhysiol, St Michael's Hospital; (416)360-4000

AHMAD, Khalil; Western Mem Reg Hosp, PO Box 2005 Stn Main 1 Brookfield Ave, Corner Brook NL A2H 6J7; Rawalpindi (Pakistan)'86; Staff, Western Memorial Regional Hospital; (709)637-5000

AHMAD, Khalil; Community Mental Health Centre, 1420-99 Wyse Rd, Dartmouth NS B3A 4S5; Karachi (Pakistan)'63; MB BS; DPM; Consultant Psy, IWK Health Centre; Lecturer, Dalhousie University; (902)469-8170; Fax. (902)461-0939.

AHMAD, Khawaja M N; Ironwood Med Clinic, 3100-11666 Steveston Hwy, Richmond BC V7A 5J3; Punjab (Pakistan)'83; MB BS; (604)448-9595

AHMAD, Marium F; Rouge Valley HS-Ajax/Pickering, 580 Harwood Ave S, Ajax ON L1S 2J4; McM'08; CCFP; Staff, Rouge Valley Health System - Ajax & Pickering Health Centre Site; Staff, Scarborough Centre for Healthy Communities; Staff, Scarborough Centre for Healthy Communities; (905)683-2320; Fax. (905)428-5231.

AHMAD, Mayraj; William Osler HC-Brampton, N2916-2100 Bovaird Dr E, Brampton ON L6R 3J7; Tor'00; FRCPC; IntMed; Cardiol. Staff, William Osler Health System - Brampton Civic Hospital; (905)494-6221

AHMAD, Mohamad; London HSC-Victoria Hosp, PO Box 5010 Stn B 800 Commissioners Rd E, London ON N6A 5W9; Wes'97; Anes. Staff, London Health Sciences Centre - Victoria Campus; (519)685-8500

AHMAD, Nazir; Saskatoon Cancer Centre, 20 Campus Dr, Saskatoon SK S7N 4H4; Staff, Saskatoon Cancer Centre; (306)655-2710; Fax. (306)655-0633.

AHMAD, Omar; Royal Columbian Hosp, 330 Columbia St E, New Westminster BC V3L 3W7; Ott'00; FRCPC; EmergMed; Critical Care Medicine. Staff, Royal Columbian Hospital; (604)520-4253

AHMAD, Rubeena M; Boyle McCauley Health Centre, 10628 96 St NW, Edmonton AB T5H 2J2; Man'94; BPE; CCFP; FCFP; (780)422-7333; Fax. (780)422-7343.

AHMAD, Rukshanda; Public Health Agency of Canada, PL 6809A-785 Carling Ave, Ottawa ON K1S 5H4; Nawabshah (Pakistan)'91; (613)948-2863; Fax. (613)960-0944.

AHMAD, S Zareen; Rebecca McDonald Centre, 2F-60 Murray St, Toronto ON M5T 3L9; Dal'01; FRCPC; IntMed; Rheum. Staff, Sunnybrook Health Sciences Centre; Langs: French; (416)586-4800 x8247

AHMAD, Saima W; Maryvale Adolesc & Family Serv, 3640 Wells St, Windsor ON N9C 1T9; Lahore (India)'95; FRCPC; Psy. (519)258-0484; Fax. (519)258-0488.

AHMAD, Semina; Etobicoke Urgent Care Centre, 10-25 Woodbine Downs Blvd, Etobicoke ON M9W 6N5; University of Sint Eustatius (Other Foreign)'06; (416)741-2273

AHMAD, Shahabuddin; Battleford's Med Centre, 1121 103rd St, North Battleford SK S9A 1K5; Dacca (Bangladesh)'61; (306)445-9459; Fax. (306)445-9450.

AHMAD, Suffia N; Southwood Med Centre, 3F-2385 Pembina Hwy, Winnipeg MB R3T 2H4; Man'95; BSc; CCFP; (204)988-1590; Fax. (204)988-1595; sufahmad@yahoo.ca.

AHMAD, Tahani M T K; The Hosp for Sick Children, 555 University Ave, Toronto ON M5G 1X8; (Jordan)'04; Fellow, The Hospital For Sick Children; (416)813-6025

AHMAD, Zafar D; Trillium Hlth Ctre-Mississauga, 100 Queensway W, Mississauga ON L5B 1B8; Tor'00; CCFP; CCFP(E.M.); Staff, Trillium Health Centre - Mississauga; (905)848-7100

AHMAD KHAN, Faiz; MUHC-Montreal Chest Institute, 3650 rue Saint-Urbain, Montreal QC H2X 2P4; McG'05; Respir; IntMed. Staff, McGill University Health Centre - Montreal Chest Institute; (514)934-1934

AHMADI, Hazhir; Lions Gate Hosp, 231 15th St E, North Vancouver BC V7L 2L7; UBC'91; FRCPC; Anes. Staff, Lions Gate Hospital; (604)984-5709; Fax. (604)984-5729.

AHMADI TORSHIZI, Ali; Health Sciences Centre, GA 252-820 Sherbrook St, Winnipeg MB R3A 1R9; FRCPC; IntMed. Staff, Health Sciences Centre; (204)290-0839

AHMADI TORSHIZI, Omid; Health Centre Med Clinic, PO Box 298 218 Caron St, St Jean Baptiste MB R0G 2B0; CCFP.

AHMADINEJAD, Saeed; Good Samaritan Senior's Clinic, 9534 87 St NW, Edmonton AB T6C 3J1; (Iran)'93; CCFP; Langs: Farsi; (780)440-8274; Fax. (780)469-6495.

AHMADO, Hend O I; Toronto Ctre Adv Reprod Tech, 2F-150 Bloor St W, Toronto ON M5S 2X9; Aziz (Saudi Arabia)'90; (416)972-0110

AHMAN, Frank W; Abbotsford Reg Hosp & Cancer C, 32900 Marshall Rd, Abbotsford BC V2S 0C2; Wes'76; FRCSC; ObstGyn (Colposcopy). Obstetrics & Gynecology, Abbotsford Regional Hospital & Cancer Centre; Clinical Asst Prof, University of British Columbia; (604)851-4767

AHMARANI, Christian; Clinique ORL & Facial PlasSurg, 5775 boul Leger, Montreal-Nord QC H1G 1K7; Mon'86; FRCSC; Otol (Facial Plastic Surgery). Staff, Centre Hospitalier l'Université de Montréal (CHUM) - Hôtel-Dieu; Prés assem Otol, Hopital Maisonneuve-Rosemont; Clin Prof Otol Maxillo Facial & Facial Plastic Surg, Universite de Montreal; Langs: Bilingual(French/English); (514)327-4040; Fax. (514)327-9001; lesorldemontrealnord@bellnet.ca.

AHMED, Abdelaziz A E; Jackson Park Health Centre, 150-2475 McDougall St, Windsor ON N8X 3N9; Khartoum (Sudan)'83; MRCP(UK); FRCPC; IntMed. Consultant IntMed, Hôtel-Dieu Grace Hospital; Aj Prof, University of Western Ontario; Langs: Arabic; (519)252-9861 x4; Fax. (519)252-7787.

AHMED, Abul B M; St George Med Centre, 16-585 Ontario St, Milton ON L9T 2N2; Dhaka (Bangladesh)'65; MB BS; DPM(Lond); MRCPsy(Eng); FRSM(Lond); FRCPC; Psy (Adult Psychiatry). Langs: Bengali; Urdu; Hindi; (905)369-0605; Fax. (905)369-0615.

AHMED, Adekunle G; Brockville Mental Health Ctre, PO Box 1050 Stn Main 1804 Highway 2 E, Brockville ON K6V 5W7; Zaria (Nigeria)'86; MB; BSc; MRCPsy(UK); FRCPC; Psy. Staff, Royal Ottawa Mental Health Centre - Royal Ottawa Health Care Group; Staff, Brockville Mental Health Centre - Royal Ottawa Health Care Group; Staff, Centre for Rational & Cognitive Therapies; (613)345-1461; Fax. (613)345-7276.

AHMED, Ahmed A A; Kanata Children's Clinic, 9B-7 Kakulu Rd, Ottawa ON K2L 2L4; (Jordan)'97; FRCPC; Peds. Staff, QHC Belleville General; (613)271-1110; Fax. (613)271-1114.

AHMED, Ayesha A; Saskatoon Nephrology Group, 434-230 Avenue R S, Saskatoon SK S7M 2Z1; Sask'97; FRCPC; IntMed; Nephrol. Clinical Asst Prof Med, University of Saskatchewan; (306)934-3300; Fax. (306)934-3355.

AHMED, Bashir; Montreal Road Med Centre, 398 Montreal Rd, Ottawa ON K1K 0V4; All India Inst (India)'82; MB BS; Langs: Persian; Urdu; Hindi; (613)244-2005; Fax. (613)244-2004.

AHMED, Bedri U; Rouge Valley-Ajax & Pickering, 580 Harwood Ave S, Ajax ON L1S 2J4; '94; CCFP; Staff, Rouge Valley Health System - Ajax & Pickering Health Centre Site; Staff, Morningside Medical Centre; Staff, Milner Medical Centre; (905)683-2320

AHMED, Diana R; Brant Comm HS-Brantford Gen, 200 Terrace Hill St, Brantford ON N3R 1G9; McM'98; BSc; CCFP; FCFP; Court Staff, The Brant Community Healthcare System - Brantford General Hospital Site; Court Staff Privileges FamMed, St Joseph's Healthcare - Charlton Campus; Langs: Russian; (519)752-7871; ahmed@nhchc.ca.

AHMED, Ghalib; Ottewell Med Clinic, 6138 90 Ave NW, Edmonton AB T6B 0P2; Qns'96; CCFP; (780)468-6409; Fax. (780)469-1261; ghalib_ahmed@hotmail.com.

AHMED, Ghazanfar; 5662 Main St, Niagara Falls ON L2G 5Z4; American University of the Caribbean (St Maarten)'02; (905)356-3562

AHMED, Hala M A; Semma Medical Clinic, 15160 Fraser Hwy, Surrey BC V3R 3P1; Cairo (Egypt)'96; MB ChB; CCFP; Langs: Arabic; (604)855-6661

AHMED, Imran; Sherwood Park Medicentre, 9-101 Bremner Dr, Sherwood Park AB T8H 0M5; (Pakistan)'93; (780)467-4717; Fax. (780)467-9316.

AHMED, Iqbal H; Richmond Health Science Ctre, 560-6091 Gilbert Rd, Richmond BC V7C 5L9; Manchester (England)'77; MB ChB; MSc; MRC(UK); FCCP; MPH(Johns Hopkins); FRCPC; Respir (Asthma); IntMed. Staff Respirologist, Richmond Hospital; (604)214-0600; Fax. (604)214-0602.

AHMED, Iqbal K; Credit Valley Eye Centre, 1-3200 Erin Mills Pky, Mississauga ON L5L 1W8; Tor'95; Ophth (Anterior Segment). Staff, The Credit Valley Hospital; Clinical Asst Prof, University of Utah(USA); Staff, Credit Valley Eye Care; (905)820-6789; Fax. (905)820-0111; ike.ahmed@utoronto.ca.

AHMED, Iram F; Niagara Falls Comm Health Cent, PO Box 123, Niagara Falls ON L2E 6S8; Florida (USA)'01; BSc; MD; Langs: Urdu; Gujarati; (905)356-4222; Fax. (905)356-5676.

AHMED, Ishtiaq; Bowmanville Prof Bldg, 302-222 King St E, Bowmanville ON L1C 1P6; Tor'05; CCFP; Staff, Lakeridge Health - Bowmanville Site; Staff, Rouge River Medical Centre; (905)697-8847; Fax. (905)697-7745.

AHMED, Itrat; Dr Everett Chalmers Reg Hosp, PO Box 9000 Stn A 700 Priestman St, Fredericton NB E3B 5N5; Punjab (India)'86; FRCPC; AnatPath. Staff, Dr Everett Chalmers Regional Hospital; (506)452-5400

AHMED, Maheen; Ottawa Children's Clinic, 402-1105 Carling Ave, Ottawa ON K1Y 4G5; Aga Khan (Pakistan)'00; FRCPC; Peds; Nephrol. Staff, Children's Hospital of Eastern Ontario (CHEO); (613)728-5437

AHMED, Matin A; 981 Hollingsworth Bend NW, Edmonton AB T6R 3G7; (Pakistan)'82; MB; BSc; Staff, Royal Alexandra Hospital; (780)438-9365

AHMED, Moheddin M B A; Jasper Avenue Med Centre, 11464 Jasper Ave NW, Edmonton AB T5K 0M1; (Libya)'03; Staff, Northern Lights Regional Health Centre; (780)756-5262; Fax. (780)756-9211; oya.clinic@yahoo.ca.

AHMED, Muhammad E; The Ottawa Hosp-Civic Campus, 1053 Carling Ave, Ottawa ON K1Y 4E9; Punjab (Pakistan)'00; Fellow Radiol, The Ottawa Hospital - Civic Campus; (613)798-5555

AHMED, Munir; Melita Health Centre, PO Box 459 147 Summit St, Melita MB R0M 1L0; (Other Foreign)'94; (204)522-8353

AHMED, Nadeem A; Thunder Bay Reg HSC-T-Bay, 980 Oliver Rd, Thunder Bay ON P7B 6V4; Ott'93; FRCPC; IntMed;CCFP; Gastroent. Staff, Thunder Bay Regional Health Sciences Centre; (807)684-6000

AHMED, Nafeesa Q; Al Shiffa Med Clinic, 219 Mccraney St W, Oakville ON L6H 1H8; (Pakistan)'68; MB BS; MD; Court Staff Privil, Trillium Health Centre - Mississauga; Langs: Urdu; Arabic; Hindi; (905)338-1920

AHMED, Najma A; St Michael's Hosp, QW 3073-30 Bond St, Toronto ON M5B 1W8; McG'92; BSc(Hon); FRCSC; GenSurg (Endocrinology Surgery); Critical Care Medicine. Staff, St Michael's Hospital; Langs: Urdu; (416)864-5481; Fax. (416)864-3083; ahmedn@smh.toronto.on.ca.

AHMED, Najma N; MUHC-Montreal Children's Hosp, D562-2300 rue Tupper, Montreal QC H3H 1P3; Tor'95; FRCPC; Peds (Pediatric Gastroenterology). Staff Ped Gastroenterol, McGill University Health Centre - Montreal Children's Hospital; Asst Prof Peds, McGill University; Langs: Bilingual(French/English); (514)412-4474; Fax. (514)412-4392.

AHMED, Najneen; Miramichi Reg Hosp, 500 Water St, Miramichi NB E1V 3G5; Dhaka (Bangladesh)'96; Staff, Miramichi Regional Hospital; (506)623-3150

AHMED, Naseer; Cancercare Manitoba, 675 McDermot Ave, Winnipeg MB R3E 0V9; Karachi (Pakistan)'81; MB BS; FRCPC; RadOncol. (204)787-4183; Fax. (204)786-0194; naseer.ahmed@cancercare.mb.ca.

AHMED, Osama S E; Saskatoon Cancer Centre, 20 Campus Dr, Saskatoon SK S7N 4H4; Staff, Saskatoon Cancer Centre; (306)655-2662; Fax. (306)655-2210.

AHMED, Rabia A; Royal Alexandra Hosp, 324-10240 Kingsway NW, Edmonton AB T5H 3V9; Sask'00; ABIM; ABIM(InfectDis); FRCPC; IntMed; InfectDis. Staff, Royal Alexandra Hospital; (780)944-8690

AHMED, Rahel; Whitehorse Med Services Ltd, 406 Lambert St, Whitehorse YT Y1A 1Z7; Tor'01; BSc; CCFP; CCFP(E.M.); Staff, Whitehorse Medical Services Ltd; (867)393-6600; Fax. (867)393-6601.

AHMED, S Nizamuddin; University of Alberta Hosp, 2E3. 12WCM-8440 112 St NW, Edmonton AB T6G 2B7; Karachi (Pakistan)'92; DABCN; DABN; FRCPC; Neur (Epilepsy). Staff, University of Alberta Hospital; Dir Clinical Neurophysiology Lab & Ass't Prof, University of Alberta; Langs: Urdu; (780)407-1010; Fax. (780)407-1325.

AHMED, Sabera; Halton Family Health Centre, 2951 Walker's Line, Burlington ON L7M 4Y1; Dhaka (Bangladesh)'96; CCFP; (905)336-3437; Fax. (905)336-9632.

AHMED, Sabrina; Clinique Med Urgence Brossard, 7601 boul Taschereau, Brossard QC J4Y 1A2; Qns'02; CCFP; (450)462-0863

AHMED, Sadaf K; Halton Family Health Centre, 2952 Walker's Line, Burlington ON L7M 4Y1; London (England)'99; CCFP; (905)592-3950

AHMED, Salah O; Horner Med Clinic, 202-440 Browns Line, Etobicoke ON M8W 3T9; Zagazig (Egypt)'82; MB ChB; CCFP; Staff, Mississauga Urgent Care; (416)259-0300

AHMED, Salim; Miramichi Reg Hosp, 500 Water St, Miramichi NB E1V 3G5; Dhaka (Bangladesh)'89; Staff, Miramichi Regional Hospital; (506)623-3000

AHMED, Samar M S; Univ Hlth Network-Toronto Gen, 200 Elizabeth St, Toronto ON M5G 2C4; Jeddah (Saudi Arabia)'01; Staff, Toronto General Hospital - UHN.

AHMED, Sana A; St Michael's Hosp, 30 Bond St, Toronto ON M5B 1W8; Sask'06; FRCPC; Anes. Staff, St Michael's Hospital; (416)360-4000

AHMED, Sarwat M; Appletree Clinic, 2573 Baseline Rd, Ottawa ON K2H 7B3; Ott'79; CCFP; FCFP; (613)721-8630

AHMED, Shabbeer; Queen Elizabeth II HSC, 417-1276 South Park St, Halifax NS B3H 2Y9; Rajasthan (India)'73; Staff, Queen Elizabeth II Health Sciences Centre - Victoria General Site.

AHMED, Shafqat M; Trillium Cardiovascular Assoc, 608-89 Queensway W, Mississauga ON L5B 2V2; McG'90; FRCSC; CardSurg; Cardiovasc&ThorSurg (P.Q.). (905)848-7513; Fax. (905)848-7515.

AHMED, Shaheeda M; Sunnybrook Hlth Sciences Ctre, E222-2075 Bayview Ave, Toronto ON M4N 3M5; McG'96; FRCPC; IntMed; Cardiol. Staff, Sunnybrook Health Sciences Centre; (416)480-6043; Fax. (416)480-6715.

AHMED, Shaheen; 6602 Main St, Vancouver BC V5X 3H2; Dhaka (Bangladesh)'97; (604)558-1803

AHMED, Shahid; Saskatoon Cancer Centre, 20 Campus Dr, Saskatoon SK S7N 4H4; Karachi (Pakistan)'95; FACP; FRCPC; IntMed; MedOncol. Staff, Saskatoon Cancer Centre; Clin Assoc Prof Med, Royal University Hospital; Prof Med, University of Saskatchewan; Langs: Urdu; (306)655-2710; shahid.ahmed@saskcancer.ca.

AHMED, Shahida; Cancercare Manitoba, 675 McDermot Ave, Winnipeg MB R3E 0V9; Karachi (Pakistan)'81; MB BS; FRCPC; RadOncol. (204)787-1152; Fax. (204)786-0194; shahida.ahmed@cancercare.mb.ca.

AHMED, Shajan; London HSC-Victoria Hosp, PO Box 5010 Stn B E1 102-800 Commissioners Rd E, London ON N6A 5W9; Xavier Univ School of Medicine (Aruba)'08; CCFP; Staff, London Health Sciences Centre - Victoria Campus; (519)685-8500

AHMED, Shakeela R; North Bay Pediatric Group, 400 McKeown Ave, North Bay ON P1B 0B2; Karachi (Pakistan)'88; MB BS; FRCPC; Peds. Staff, North Bay Regional Health Centre - Regional Mental Health; (705)495-8135; Fax. (705)495-8132.

AHMED, Shehla; Burntwood Commun Hlth Resource, 50 Selkirk Ave, Thompson MB R8N 0M7.

AHMED, Sheikh N; BC Cancer Agency, 32900 Marshall Rd, Abbotsford BC V2S 0C2; Punjab (Pakistan)'88; MB BS; FRCPC; RadOncol. Staff, Abbotsford Regional Hospital & Cancer Centre; Langs: Urdu; Punjabi; (604)851-4743; Fax. (604)851-4726.

AHMED, Sofia B; Foothills Med Centre, C210-1403 29 St NW, Calgary AB T2N 2T9; Tor'99; FRCPC; IntMed; Nephrol. Staff, Foothills Medical Centre; (403)944-2745; Fax. (403)944-2876.

AHMED, Somaiah; 140 Rolling Hills Dr, Orangeville ON L9W 4X8; McM'07; CCFP; Staff, Headwaters Health Care Centre - Orangeville Site; (519)941-7575; Fax. (519)941-7060.

AHMED, Syed A; Niagara H System-G Niagara, PO Box 1018 Stn Main 5546 Portage Rd, Niagara Falls ON L2E 6X2; Karachi (Pakistan)'62; MB BS; DPM(Dublin & Lond); FRCPC; Psy (General Adult Psychiatry). Ac Staff, Niagara Health System - Greater Niagara General Site; (905)358-0171 x3810

AHMED, Syed K S; 674 Barclay Rd, London ON N6K 1K3; NOSM'10; CCFP.

AHMED, Syed S; Miramichi Reg Hosp, 500 Water St, Miramichi NB E1V 3G5; Dhaka (Bangladesh)'88; CCFP; Staff, Miramichi Regional Hospital; (506)623-3451

AHMED, Syed T; 103-426 Talbot St, St Thomas ON N5P 1B9; Srinagar (India)'87; MB BS; FRCP(UK); FRCPC; Peds. Consultant Ped, London Health Sciences Centre - Children's Hospital; Consultant Peds, Children's Hospital of Eastern Ontario (CHEO); Consultant Peds, St Thomas Elgin General Hospital; Aj Prof Dept of Peds, University of Western Ontario; Langs: Urdu; Hindi; Arabic; (519)637-8074; Fax. (519)637-2646; humtar@yahoo.com.

AHMED, Syed Z; Thunder Bay Reg HSC-T-Bay, 980 Oliver Rd, Thunder Bay ON P7B 6V4; Karachi (Pakistan)'00; FRCPC; IntMed; Critical Care Medicine. Staff, Thunder Bay Regional Health Sciences Centre; (807)684-6000

AHMED, Tahira S; Medical Bldg, 242-600 Tecumseh Rd E, Windsor ON N8X 4X9; Khyber (Pakistan)'70; Langs: Urdu; Arabic; (519)252-6400

AHMED, Uzma; Meadowvale Prof Centre, 206-6855 Meadowvale Town Ctre, Mississauga ON L5N 2Y1; Pakistan (Pakistan)'89; MB BS; FRCPC; Peds (Emergency Medicine). Staff, The Credit Valley Hospital; Langs: Urdu; (905)819-8370; Fax. (905)819-8785.

AHMED, Youmna; Markham Stouffville Hosp, PO Box 1800 Stn Main 381 Church St, Markham ON L3P 7P3; Lahore (Pakistan)'01; Staff, Markham Stouffville Hospital; Resd Supvr Family Practice, University of Toronto; (905)472-7000; Fax. (905)472-7621; ysaqqib200@yahoo.ca.

AHMED-BENTLEY, Jasmine; Dynacare Kasper Med Lab, 200-10150 102 St NW, Edmonton AB T5J 5E2; Alb'00; FRCPC; MedMicrobiol. (780)447-8449; Fax. (780)452-8488.

AHMER, Abubaker A; 104-510 Ingersoll Ave, Woodstock ON N4S 4X9; Al-Fateh (Libya)'90; MB ChB; FRCSC; OrthSurg. Staff, Woodstock General Hospital; Langs: Arabic; (519)536-7843

AHMET, Alexandra H; Children's Hosp Eastern Ont, 401 Smyth Rd, Ottawa ON K1H 8L1; McM'00; FRCPC; Peds (Pediatric Endocrinology); Endocrin&Metab. Endocrinologist Peds, Children's Hospital of Eastern Ontario (CHEO); Asst Prof, University of Ottawa; Langs: French; (613)737-7600; aahmet@cheo.on.ca.

AHMODU, Olorunfemi S; Community Mental Health Servic, 350 Cheadle St W, Swift Current SK S9H 4G3; (306)778-5280; Fax. (306)773-9890.

AHN, Henry; St Michael's Orthopaedic, 800-55 Queen St E, Toronto ON M5C 1R6; Tor'99; FRCSC; OrthSurg (Trauma). Staff, St Michael's Hospital; (416)864-6005

AHN, Richard A; St Joseph's Health Centre, 30 The Queensway, Toronto ON M6R 1B5; Qns'04; FRCPC; Anes. Staff, St Joseph's Health Centre; (416)530-6000

AHOOJA, Vineeta; Rouge Valley Cardiology, 406-1371 Neilson Rd, Scarborough ON M1B 4Z8; West Indies (Jamaica)'99; (416)281-9499; Fax. (416)283-5705.

AHRONHEIM, Gerald A; Hillside Pediatric Clinic, 65 av Hillside, Westmount QC H3Z 1W1; Michigan (USA)'66; BS; MD; ABPeds; MedMicrobiol (P.Q.); Peds (P.Q.) (Pediatric Infectious Diseases). assoc Staff, McGill University Health Centre - Montreal Children's Hospital; Clin Asst Prof, McGill University; Langs: Bilingual(French/English); (514)931-2524; Fax. (514)931-2625.

AHRONHEIM, Sara R; MUHC-Royal Victoria Hosp, 687 av des Pins O, Montreal QC H3A 1A1; McG'07; MDCM; Staff, McGill University Health Centre - Royal Victoria Hospital; (514)934-1934

AHSAN, Muhammad R; St Michael's Hosp, BW 8F-30 Bond St, Toronto ON M5B 1W8; Karachi (Pakistan)'94; FRCSC; CardSurg. Staff, St Michael's Hospital; (416)864-5110

AHSAN, Sania; The Hosp for Sick Children, 555 University Ave, Toronto ON M5G 1X8; Dhaka (Bangladesh)'94; Fellow, The Hospital For Sick Children; (416)813-6025

AHSANUDDIN, Arshad N; Health Sciences Centre, MS559Q-820 Sherbrook St, Winnipeg MB R3A 1R9; Staff, Health Sciences Centre; (204)774-6511

AHUJA, Amit R; 100-3001 Gordon Ave, Coquitlam BC V3C 2K7; UBC'04; FRCPC; DiagRad. (604)941-7611

AHUJA, Jan; Orleans Urgent Care Clinic, 100-1220 Place D'Orleans Dr, Orleans ON K1C 7K3; Tor'74; FACEP; FRCPC; EmergMed. Assoc Prof EmergMed, University of Ottawa; (613)841-5389; Fax. (613)841-5393.

AHUJA, Nina; 536 Concession St, Hamilton ON L8V 1A6; McM'98; BSc(Hons); FRCSC; Ophth (Comprehensive Ophthalmology). Staff, St Joseph's Healthcare - Charlton Campus; Clin Assoc Prof Surg, McMaster University; (905)575-7050; Fax. (905)297-7597.

AHWENG, Andrew G C; Brandon Clinic, 620 Dennis St, Brandon MB R7A 5E7; Staff, Northern Health Thompson Regional Office.

AICHER, Joseph; Saint John Reg Hosp, PO Box 2100 Stn Main 400 University Ave, Saint John NB E2L 4L2; McM'98; MPH; MCP; FRCPC; Psy (Community Mental Health). Staff, Saint John Regional Hospital; Langs: French; (506)648-6000; joseph.aicher@gnb.ca.

AIDOO, Rosemond; Portage Med FHT-Morrison St Si, 103-6453 Morrison St, Niagara Falls ON L2E 7H1; (Ghana)'85; CCFP; Staff, Niagara Health System - Greater Niagara General Site; Staff, Niagara Health System - St Catharines General Site; Staff, Niagara Health System - Ontario Street Site; (905)357-6636; Fax. (905)356-7100.

AIELLO, Marie-Jose; Clin Externe de Psychiatrie, 200-2924 boul Taschereau, Greenfield Park QC J4V 2G8; Mon'76; FRCPC; Psy (Adolescent Psychiatry). Psychiatrist, Hopital Charles LeMoyne; Langs: Italian; English; (450)466-5000 x6119

AIELLO, Michael J; 5303 Canotek Rd, Ottawa ON K1J 9M1; Ott'08; CCFP; (613)746-6223; Fax. (613)746-6018.

AIKEN, Amanda M; Hys Med Centre, 510-11010 101 St NW, Edmonton AB T5H 4B9; Man'07; FRCSC; ObstGyn. (780)414-0782; Fax. (780)414-0784.

AIKEN, Caroline L M; McMaster University, 1280 Main St W, Hamilton ON L8S 4K1; Wes'95; CCFP; Fellow Sports & Exercise Med, McMaster University.

AIKEN, Jonathan; 270-1641 Hillside Ave, Victoria BC V8T 5G1; UBC'05; CCFP; (250)592-8783; Fax. (250)592-3897.

AIKEN, Paula A; Lougheed Med Clinic, 145-9855 Austin Rd, Burnaby BC V3J 1N4; UBC'88; (604)421-2555; Fax. (604)421-1554.

AIKEN, Trevor C; Riverside Med Clinic, 304-1101 Dewdney Ave, Trail BC V1R 4T1; Edinburgh (Scotland)'89; MB ChB; CCFP; (250)368-5656

AIKIN, Kenneth A; Centre Med Ormstown, RR 4 24 rue Gale, Ormstown QC J0S 1K0; McG'74; FACS; CAB; FRCSC; GenSurg. ac Staff, Barrie Memorial Hospital; ac Staff, Centre Hospitalier Régional du Suroît; Conférencier Surg, McGill University; (450)829-2331; Fax. (450)829-3636.

AIKMAN, Peter J; Nova Scotia Rehab Centre, 1341 Summer St, Halifax NS B3H 4K4; Qns'98; CCFP; Staff, Nova Scotia Rehabilitation Centre; (902)473-5232; Fax. (902)473-3204.

AILANE, Tassadit; CSSS du Lac-des-Deux-Montagnes, 520 boul Arthur-Sauve, Saint-Eustache QC J7R 5B1; Algiers (Algeria)'88; FRCPC; Anes. Staff, Hôpital de Saint-Eustache; (450)473-6811

AILON, Jonathan I; Univ Hlth Network-Toronto Gen, 200 Elizabeth St, Toronto ON M5G 2C4; McG'09; Staff, Toronto General Hospital - UHN; (416)340-3111

AILSBY, Ronald L; Regina Qu'Appelle Hr-Pasqua, 6-4101 Dewdney Ave, Regina SK S4T 1A5; Sask'69; MSc(Surg.); FACS; FRCSC; OrthSurg. Staff, Pasqua Hospital; Asst Prof Clin Surg, University of Saskatchewan; (306)766-7016; Fax. (306)766-7025; ron@dragonflyllama.com.

AINA, Judy; Medicentre Lasalle, 208-1500 av Dollard, LaSalle QC H8N 1T5; Mon'93; (514)366-5732; Fax. (514)366-2474.

AINA, Rima; The Ottawa Hosp-Civic Campus, 1053 Carling Ave, Ottawa ON K1Y 4E9; Sher'96; FRCPC; DiagRad. Staff, The Ottawa Hospital - Civic Campus; (613)798-5555 x15078

AINAMO, Jyri S; PO Box 289, Kingston NS B0P 1R0; Dal'87; Ac Staff, Soldiers Memorial Hospital; (902)765-2268; Fax. (902)765-2268.

AINMELK, Youssef; CHUS-Hop Fleurimont, 3001 12e av N, Sherbrooke QC J1H 5N4; Damascus (Syria)'65; DAB; FRCSC; ObstGyn (Fertility). ac Staff, Centre Hospitalier Universitaire de Sherbrooke-Hopital Fleurimont; Consultant, Centre Hospitalier Universitaire de Sherbrooke-Hôpital Hôtel-Dieu; Prof, Universite de Sherbrooke; Langs: Arabic; English; (819)346-1110 x13056; Fax. (819)820-6434; youssef.ainmelk@usherbrook.ca.

AINSLIE, Martha D; Health Sciences Centre, 820 Sherbrook St, Winnipeg MB R3A 1R9; Qns'87; FRCPC; IntMed; Critical Care Medicine; Respir. Staff, Health Sciences Centre; (204)774-8511

AINSLIE, Scott A; 3107 35 Ave, Vernon BC V1T 2T2; Cal'03; FRCSC; GenSurg. (250)545-6443

AINSLIE, William H; Niagara H System-G Niagara, PO Box 1018 Stn Main 5546 Portage Rd, Niagara Falls ON L2E 6X2; Tor'54; DAB; FACS; FRCSC; GenSurg (Administration). Staff Surg Asst, Niagara Health System - Greater Niagara General Site; (905)358-0171 x2007; Fax. (905)358-8435; wainslie@niagarahealth.on.ca.

AINSWORTH, Craig D; Hamilton HS-General Site, NW 8N 01-237 Barton St E, Hamilton ON L8L 2X2; Wes'05; FRCPC; IntMed; Critical Care Medicine; Cardiol. Staff, Hamilton Health Sciences Centre - Hamilton General Hospital; (905)527-0271

AINSWORTH, Erin A E; 203-2825 Clearbrook Rd, Abbotsford BC V2T 6S3; Cal'10; CCFP; (604)852-1567

AINSWORTH, Geoffrey; Medical Bldg, 1503-805 Broadway W, Vancouver BC V5Z 1K1; Leeds (England)'70; MB ChB; FRCPC; Psy. Liaison, BC Children's Hospital; (604)879-1503

AINSWORTH, Kelly E; The Hosp for Sick Children, 555 University Ave, Toronto ON M5G 1X8; McM'07; DiagRad. Staff, The Hospital For Sick Children; (416)813-6025; Fax. (416)813-7163.

AINSWORTH, Leslie A; 506-168 Charlotte St, Ottawa ON K1N 8K6; McM'79; (613)789-1133

AINSWORTH, Peter; London HSC-Victoria Hosp, PO Box 5010 Stn B E3 013A-800 Commissioners Rd E, London ON N6A 5W9; National (Ireland)'78; PhD; FRCPC; MedBiochem (Molecular Genetics Diagnostics). Staff, London Health Sciences Centre - Victoria Campus; Aj Prof Biochem, University of Western Ontario; (519)685-8122; ainswort@uwo.ca.

AIRD, Mary M; PO Box 1260, Mayerthorpe AB T0E 1N0; National (Ireland)'81; MB ChB; BAO; (780)786-2412; Fax. (780)786-2249.

AIRD, Natalie J; 102-1757 Beaufort Ave, Comox BC V9M 1R8; Sask'98; FRCPC; Peds. (250)339-5254; Fax. (250)339-5236; dr.aird@shaw.ca.

AIRIA, Parisa; Reflex Med Clinic, 1-3470 Laird Rd, Mississauga ON L5L 5Y4; Tehran (Iran)'02; CCFP; (905)820-6000; Fax. (905)820-6090.

AIRIR, Abdelhafid; 405-4045 Rae St, Regina SK S4S 6Y8; (306)585-3560

AIT BENTALEB, Lahcen; Centre Med Brunswick, 305-955 rue Saint-Jean, Pointe-Claire QC H9R 5K3; Hassan II (Morocco)'85; FRCPC; Psy. Staff, Centre Hospitalier l'Université de Montréal (CHUM) - Hôpital Notre-Dame; Staff, Hopital Louis-H Lafontaine; (514)459-3192

AIT HAMOUDA, Karima; CHUM-Hop Notre-Dame, 1560 rue Sherbrooke E, Montreal QC H2L 4M1; Oran (Algeria)'96; CCFP; Staff, Centre Hospitalier l'Université de Montréal (CHUM) - Hôpital Notre-Dame; (514)890-8000

AITCHISON, Juliann M; Shuswap Family Practice, 102-571 6 St NE, Salmon Arm BC V1E 1R6; Tor'92; CCFP; FCFP; (250)832-2151; Fax. (250)832-3669.

AITCHISON, Katherine J; Edmonton Mental Health Clinic, 9942 108 St NW, Edmonton AB T5K 2J5; (England)'90; (780)342-7764

AITKEN, A Stewart; Royal Victoria Hosp, 201 Georgian Dr, Barrie ON L4M 6M2; Tor'92; FRCPC; IntMed; Critical Care Medicine. Staff, Royal Victoria Regional Health Centre; (705)728-9802

AITKEN, George S; The North Surrey Med Bldg, 302-9656 King George Blvd, Surrey BC V3T 2V5; Glasgow (Scotland)'68; MB ChB; FRCSC; OrthSurg (Musculoskeletal Injury). (604)588-6467; Fax. (604)581-2691; gsaitken@telus.net.

AITKEN, Susan E; Nose Hill Med Clinic, 137-1829 Ranchlands Blvd NW, Calgary AB T3G 2A7; Alb'75; FRCPC; Peds. (403)239-8888; Fax. (403)241-1506.

AIZENMAN, Allan I; A238-101 Tunney Pasture Drivew, Ottawa ON K1A 0K9; Alb'69; (613)941-3198

AJABOR, Kenneth U; Hamiota District Hlth Ctre, 177 Birch Ave, Hamiota MB R0M 0T0; Staff, Hamiota District Health Centre; (204)764-2412; kajabor@arha.ca.

AJAMIAN, Faria; The Allin Clinic, 10155 120 St NW, Edmonton AB T5K 2A2; (Iran)'91; Clinical Asst Prof, University of Alberta; Staff, Stollery Children's Hospital; Staff, Covenant Health - Misericordia Community Hospital; Staff, University of Alberta Hospital; Langs: Persian; Farsi; (780)482-7551; Fax. (780)488-2056.

AJANI, Olufemi A; Alberta Children Hosp, 2888 Shaganappi Trail NW, Calgary AB T3B 6A8; Ife (Nigeria)'88; FRCSC; Neursurg. Staff, Alberta Children's Hospital; (403)955-5041; Fax. (403)955-7634.

AJAO, Olarenwaju O; Burntwood Reg Health Authority, 50 Selkirk Ave, Thompson MB R8N 0M7; CCFP; Staff, Thompson General Hospital; Staff, Burntwood Regional Health Authority; (204)778-1731

AJAYI, Abayomi; 124-217 Terrace Hill St, Brantford ON N3R 1G8; Ilorin (Nigeria)'92; FRCPC; IntMed. (519)757-1110; Fax. (519)757-1146.

AJAYI, Raphael O; Murals Clinic, 105-22314 Fraser Hwy, Langley BC V3A 8M6; CCFP; (604)532-9944

AJAYI-OBE, J Oluwagbenga; London Diagnostic Centre, 481 London Rd, Sarnia ON N7T 4X3; Ibadan (Nigeria)'94; MB BS; DOHS; CCFP; Physician, Bluewater Health - Norman Site; Langs: Fanti; Ghanaian; Nigerian; Pidgin; Yoruba; (519)336-6019; Fax. (519)336-7136; gbenga.ajayi-obe@ontariomd.ca.

AJEGBO, Obiora N; Border City Clinic, 2707 50 Ave, Lloydminster SK S9V 2A8; (306)825-4427; Fax. (306)825-2028.

AJIBOYE, P Ayodele; Central Nfld Reg Health Centre, 50 Union St, Grnd-Falls-Windsor NL A2A 2E1; North Carolina (USA)'79; Staff, Central Newfoundland Regional Health Centre; (709)489-8198

AJISAFE, Olaniyi F; Safecare Med Services, 205-2780 Jane St, North York ON M3N 2J2; Ibadan (Nigeria)'84; CCFP; Langs: Yoruba; (416)740-7233; Fax. (416)744-7233.

AJISEBUTU, Tewogbola S; Airport Health Centre, 113-2985 Drew Rd, Mississauga ON L4T 0A4; Ibadan (Nigeria)'81; CCFP; (905)677-0658; Fax. (905)677-0659.

AJMO, Ian; Centre Hosp Honore-Mercier, 2750 boul Laframboise, Saint-Hyacinthe QC J2S 4Y8; Mon'04; Staff, Centre Hospitalier Honore-Mercier; (450)771-3333

AJOGWU, Chamberlain; Shellbrook Primary Hlth Care C, Box 1030 206 2nd Ave W, Shellbrook SK S0J 2E0; (306)747-2552; Fax. (306)747-2141.

AJUEZE, Peter C; Northeast Mental Health Centre, 680 Kirkwood Dr, Sudbury ON P3E 1X3; Benin (Nigeria)'03; (705)675-5900

AKABUTU, John J; College Plaza 3, 408-8215 112 St NW, Edmonton AB T6G 2C8; Dal'67; Att Staff, University of Alberta Hospital; Med Dir, Alberta Cord Blood Bank; Pres, Canadian Cord Blood Registry; Emeritus Prof PedHem, University of Alberta; (780)492-2397; Fax. (780)492-8704; john.akabutu@ualberta.ca.

AKAGAMI, Ryojo; 8109-2775 Laurel St, Vancouver BC V5Z 1M9; Tor'93; FRCS; MD; BSc; MHSc; FRCSC; Neursurg (Skull Base Surgery). Neurosurgery, BC Children's Hospital; Staff, Vancouver General Hospital - Centennial Pavillion; Staff, BC Cancer Agency Vancouver Centre; Langs: Japanese; (604)875-5734; Fax. (604)269-3734.

AKAI, Peter S; 12224 41 Ave NW, Edmonton AB T6J 0V7; Wes'83; ABIM; PhD; FRCPC; IntMed (Opiate Addiction); InfectDis. Consultant InfectDis, Covenant Health - Misericordia Community Hospital; (780)951-9398; akai@shaw.ca.

AKANAYEVA, Alnura; Peter Lougheed Centre, 3500 26 Ave NE, Calgary AB T1Y 6J4; Staff, Peter Lougheed Centre; (403)943-2801

AKBAR, Shafiq F; 124 Street Med Group, 10839 124 St NW, Edmonton AB T5M 0H4; Karachi (Pakistan)'87; MB BS; MD; ABIM; FRCPC; IntMed (Rheumatology); Rheum. Langs: Urdu; Punjabi; Hindi; (780)758-1111; Fax. (780)758-1118.

AKBAR, Zaubaria; 101-13805 104 Ave, Surrey BC V3T 1W7; Rawalpindi Medical College (Pakistan)'96; MB BS; Langs: Hindi; Punjabi; Urdu; (604)594-2714

AKBAR-ZADEH, Ali; Royal Columbian Hosp, 330 Columbia St E, New Westminster BC V3L 3W7; Kerman (Iran)'99; CCFP; Staff, Royal Columbian Hospital; (604)520-4253

AKBARALI, Nurjehan; Ellesmere Health Care Centre, 1-2060 Ellesmere Rd, Scarborough ON M1H 2V6; Punjab (Pakistan)'75; MB BS; MHSc; CCFP; FCFP; Ac Staff, Rouge Valley Health System - Centenary Health Centre Site; Lecturer, University of Toronto; (416)439-2273; Fax. (416)439-2244.

AKBARALY, Tasnime; Hop Charles Lemoyne, 3120 boul Taschereau, Greenfield Park QC J4V 2H1; Laval'01; Staff, Hopital Charles LeMoyne; (450)466-5000

AKBARI, Ayub; The Ottawa Hosp-Riverside, 5 25-1967 Riverside Dr, Ottawa ON K1H 7W9; Karachi (Pakistan)'88; FRCPC; IntMed; Nephrol. Staff, The Ottawa Hospital - General Campus; Staff, The Ottawa Hospital - Civic Campus; Staff, The Ottawa Hospital - Riverside Campus; (613)738-8400 x82537; Fax. (613)738-8337; aakbari@ottawahospital.on.ca.

AKBARI, Majid; Lions Gate Hosp, 231 15th St E, North Vancouver BC V7L 2L7; Mashhad (Iran)'92; FRCPC; AnatPath., Lions Gate Hospital; (604)984-5762

AKBARI-NASAB, Ardalan; Humber River Reg Hosp-Finch, 2111 Finch Ave W, North York ON M3N 1N1; Saba (Netherlands Antilles)'06; Staff, Humber River Regional Hospital - Finch Avenue Site; (416)744-2500

AKBARINEJAD MOOSAVI, Seyed M; Hôpital régional Chaleur, 1750 Sunset Dr, Bathurst NB E2A 4L7; Tehran (Iran)'88; Staff, Hopital Regional Chaleur; (506)545-6543

AKCAKIR, Berna; Family Med Associates, 500-267 O'Connor St, Ottawa ON K2P 1V3; Tor'94; MHSc; CCFP; FCFP; Langs: Turkish; (613)231-6849; Fax. (613)232-4818.

AKEF, Reza; Lakeridge Health-Oshawa Site, 1 Hospital Crt, Oshawa ON L1G 2B9; Shaheed Beheshti University (Iran)'01; CCFP; Staff, Lakeridge Health - Oshawa Site; (905)576-8711

AKENA, Charles; Lakewood Med Centre, 30 Lakewood Blvd, Winnipeg MB R2J 2M6; (204)257-3395

AKHAVEIN, Katayoon; Lions Gate Maternity Clinic, 3F-231 15th St E, North Vancouver BC V7L 2L7; Tehran (Iran)'92; CCFP; Staff, Peace Arch Hospital; (604)985-6408

AKHLAGHI-KAKROUDI, Fatereh; Willowdale Med Clinic, 6023 Yonge St, North York ON M2M 3W2; Tehran (Iran)'94; CCFP; (416)916-2733; Fax. (416)916-2315.

AKHRAS, Ronald; Centre Med L'Acadie, 101A-9825 boul de l'Acadie, Montreal QC H4N 2W2; St. Joseph (Lebanon)'84; CCFP; Langs: Spanish; English; Arabic; (514)336-6655; Fax. (514)336-6659.

AKHTAR, Hammad; Watrous Med Clinic, PO Box 1059, Watrous SK S0K 4T0; CCFP; (306)946-2075; Fax. (306)946-2072.

AKHTAR, Javed; Dr Charles A Janeway Child HC, 300 Prince Philip Dr, St. John's NL A1B 3V6; Peshawar (Pakistan)'79; MB BS; FRCSC; GenSurg; PedGenSurg. Staff, Janeway Children's Health & Rehabilitation Centre; (709)777-4964

AKHTAR, Jawed; 202-315 22nd St E, Saskatoon SK S7K 0G6; McG'88; FRCPC; IntMed (Echocardiography); Cardiol. Staff, Royal University Hospital; Staff, Saskatoon City Hospital; Staff, St Paul's Hospital (Grey Nuns) of Saskatoon; Staff Cardiol, University of Saskatchewan; (306)374-3278; Fax. (306)373-5247; fax_in@mac.com.

AKHTAR, Muhammad; University Hosp of Northern BC, 1475 Edmonton St, Prince George BC V2M 1S2; Rawalpindi (Pakistan)'89; MD; Staff, University Hospital of Northern British Columbia; (250)565-2000

AKHTAR, Nadeem; Regional Mental HC-London, PO Box 5532 Stn B 850 Highbury Ave, London ON N6A 4H1; London (England)'03; Staff, Regional Mental Health Care-St Joseph's Health Care; (519)455-5110

AKHTAR, Sabrina N; Univ Hlth Network-Toronto Western Hosp, 2W428-399 Bathurst St, Toronto ON M5T 2S8; Wes'07; CCFP; Staff, The Hospital For Sick Children; Staff, Toronto Western Hospital - University Health Network; (416)603-5888 x3147; Fax. (416)603-6228.

AKHTAR, Saima S; London HSC-Victoria Hosp, PO Box 5010 Stn B 800 Commissioners Rd E, London ON N6A 5W9; Dal'91; FRCSC; ObstGyn. Staff, St Joseph's Hospital - St Joseph's Health Care; Staff, London Health Sciences Centre - Victoria Campus; (519)685-8002; Fax. (519)685-8071.

AKHTAR, Shazia; Medmart Med Centre, 68 Centennial Pky N, Hamilton ON L8E 1H6; Lahore (Pakistan)'98; CCFP; (905)560-5800

AKHTAR, Yasmeen J; Dr Charles A Janeway Child HC, 300 Prince Philip Dr, St. John's NL A1B 3V6; (Pakistan)'80; FRCPC; Peds. Staff, Janeway Children's Health & Rehabilitation Centre; (709)777-6300

AKHTARI, Shahrzad; A202-11685 Yonge St, Richmond Hill ON L4E 0K7; (Iran)'96; MD; CCFP; Langs: Farsi; (905)884-6500; Fax. (905)884-6100; drshahrzad.akhtari@gmail.com.

AKIERMAN, Albert R; Peter Lougheed Centre, 3500 26 Ave NE, Calgary AB T1Y 6J4; (Jamaica)'76; MB BS; FRCPC; Peds. Dir Div of Neonatol, Peter Lougheed Centre; Staff Neonatol, Foothills Medical Centre; Consultant, Alberta Children's Hospital; Assoc Prof, University of Calgary; (403)943-4892; Fax. (403)943-2565.

AKIL, Philippe; Ctr Hosp Rouyn-Noranda, 4 9e rue, Rouyn-Noranda QC J9X 2B2; Staff, Centre Hospitalier Rouyn-Noranda; (819)764-5131

AKIN, Suzan S; Regina Qu'Appelle HR-Regina, 1440 14th Ave, Regina SK S4P 0W5; Sask'04; FRCPC; Anes. Staff, Regina General Hospital; (306)766-4444

AKINBIYI, Amos A; Gardiner Park Medical Clinic, 358 University Park Dr, Regina SK S4V 0Y8; Ibadan (Nigeria)'80; MB BS; LRCP(Lond); MRCS(Eng); FRCOG; FRCSC; ObstGyn (Gynecologic Oncology). Vis Consultant, Weyburn General Hospital; Staff ObstGyn, Regina General Hospital; Asst Prof, University of Saskatchewan; Langs: Yoruba; (306)569-1522

AKINBIYI, Oluwatosin A; 101-9815 97 St, Grande Prairie AB T8V 8B9; Sask'05; FRCSC; OrthSurg. Staff, Queen Elizabeth II Hospital; (780)402-7181

AKINBIYI, Tolulola T A A; William Jackman Mem Hosp, 410 Booth Ave, Labrador City NL A2V 2K1; Staff, Captain William Jackman Memorial Hospital; (709)944-6960; Fax. (709)944-6690.

AKINBOLUE, Oladele S; Halton HSC-Oakville Site, 327 Reynolds St, Oakville ON L6J 3L7; Ibadan (Nigeria)'84; MB BS; FRCPC; Anes. Staff, Halton Healthcare Services Corporation - Oakville Site; (905)338-4647

AKINCIOGLU, Cigdem; London HSC-University Hosp, PO Box 5339 Stn B C3 209-339 Windermere Rd, London ON N6A 5A5; Gazi (Turkey)'96; FRCPC; NuclearMed. Staff, London Health Sciences Centre - Victoria Campus; Staff, London Health Sciences Centre - University Hospital; (519)663-3528; Fax. (519)663-3860.

AKINDELE, Florence O; St Paul Women's Clinic, PO Box 680 4918 50 Ave, St Paul AB T0A 3A0; Ile-Ife (Nigeria)'91; FCOG(SA); FWACS; MB ChB; MPH(Wits); Langs: Yoruba; (780)645-1719 x2211; Fax. (780)645-1707.

AKINDELE, Olufunmi O; Mount Sinai Hosp, 775-600 University Ave, Toronto ON M5G 1X5; Ibadan (Nigeria)'88; MB BS; DCH; Staff, The Hospital For Sick Children; Staff, Mount Sinai Hospital; (416)586-4800 x5558; Fax. (416)586-8745.

AKINFEMIWA, Omotayo B; Humber River Reg Hosp-Church, 200 Church St, Toronto ON M9N 1N8; (Nigeria)'80; CCFP; Staff, Humber River Regional Hospital - Church Street Site; (416)249-8111; Fax. (416)243-4547.

AKINFOLARIN, Josephine; Hop Reg d'Edmundston, 275 Hebert Blvd, Edmundston NB E3V 4E4; Sofia (Bulgaria)'91; Staff, Hôpital regional d'Edmundston; (506)739-2200

AKINGBOLA, Olurotimi A; Dundas Med Centre, 305-220 Dundas St W, Whitby ON L1N 8M7; Ibadan (Nigeria)'86; MRC(UK); FRCSC; ObstGyn. Consultant ObstGyn, Lakeridge Health - Oshawa Site; Clin Lecturer ObstGyn, Queen's University; (905)668-5560; Fax. (905)668-5561.

AKINJISE, Idowu C; Tamarack Health Centre, 109-9616 Franklin Ave, Fort McMurray AB T9H 2J9; (Nigeria)'88; CCFP; Langs: Yoruba; (780)790-0366; Fax. (780)743-0323; iakinjise@wbpcm.ca.

AKINLAJA, Adeola B; Cape Breton Healthcare Complex, 1482 George St, Sydney NS B1P 1P3; Ibadan (Nigeria)'99; MB BS; Staff, Cape Breton Healthcare Complex; (902)567-8000

AKINLAJA, Ayodeji O; Cape Breton Healthcare Complex, 1482 George St, Sydney NS B1P 1P3; Ogun State (Nigeria)'97; Staff, Cape Breton Healthcare Complex; (902)567-8000

AKINLOSOTU, Adewale A; Hotel-Dieu Grace Hosp, 1030 Ouellette Ave, Windsor ON N9A 1E1; Obafemi Awolowo (Nigeria)'93; FRCPC; Psy. Staff, Hôtel-Dieu Grace Hospital; Staff, Windsor Regional Hospital - Tayfour Site; (519)973-4411

AKINLOYE, Olayiwola O; Quance East Medical Clinic, 49-2223 Victoria Ave E, Regina SK S4N 6E4; Staff, Wynyard Community Health Centre; Staff, Northgate Medical Centre; (306)522-2278; Fax. (306)522-2281.

AKINLOYE, Olusegun; Saint John Reg Hosp, PO Box 2100 Stn Main 400 University Ave, Saint John NB E2L 4L2; Ibadan (Nigeria)'98; Staff, Saint John Regional Hospital; (506)648-6000

AKINMOKUN, Adebusola; The Moncton Hosp, 135 MacBeath Ave, Moncton NB E1C 6Z8; Ibadan (Nigeria)'99; FRCPC; Psy. Staff, The Moncton Hospital; (506)857-5520

AKINNAWONU, Anthony; Yorkton Mental Health Centre, 270 Bradbrooke Dr, Yorkton SK S3N 2K6; Staff, Yorkton Mental Health & Addiction Centre; (306)786-0558; Fax. (306)786-0556; anthony.akinnawonu@shr.sk.ca.

AKINSETE, Folajimi; Estevan Med Clinic, 110-1175 Nicholson Rd, Estevan SK S4A 2S7; (306)634-2661; Fax. (306)634-8821.

AKINSOLA, Oluwatosin A; Cape Breton Healthcare Complex, 1482 George St, Sydney NS B1P 1P3; Obafemi Awolowo College (Other Foreign)'97; FRCPC; Psy. Staff, Cape Breton Healthcare Complex; (902)849-4413

AKINSOLA, Sunday A; Dr G B Cross Mem Hosp, 67 Manitoba Dr, Clarenville NL A5A 1K3; Kiev Medical Institute (Ukraine)'81; Staff, The Dr G B Cross Memorial Hospital; (709)466-3411

AKINSOOTO, Victor S; Hamilton HS-McMaster Site, PO Box 2000 Stn Lcd 1 1200 Main St W, Hamilton ON L8N 3Z5; Ilorin (Nigeria)'91; FRCSC; ObstGyn (Gynecological Reproductive Endocrinology). Staff, Hamilton Health Sciences Centre - McMaster University Medical Centre; Staff, Hamilton Health Sciences Centre - McMaster Children's Hospital; (905)521-2100; Fax. (905)562-3708.

AKINTAN, Abosede; Georgian Bay Gen Hosp, 25 Jeffery St, Penetanguishene ON L9M 1K6; American University of Antigua (Other Foreign)'08; Staff, Georgian Bay General Hospital - Penetanguishene; (705)534-7913

AKINTAN, Olabode O; Hamilton HS-McMaster Site, PO Box 2000 Stn Lcd 1 1200 Main St W, Hamilton ON L8N 3Z5; University of Jos (Other Foreign)'96; FRCPC; Psy. Staff, Hamilton Health Sciences Centre - McMaster University Medical Centre; (905)521-2100; Fax. (905)521-7938.

AKINTOLA, D Raphael; Queen Elizabeth II Hosp, 10409 98 St, Grande Prairie AB T8V 2E8; Ilorin (Nigeria)'92; MB BS; CCFP; CCFP(E.M.); Staff, Queen Elizabeth II Hospital; (780)538-7100; Fax. (780)539-7846.

AKINTOLA, Olalekan M; Brandon Clinic Med Corp, 620 Dennis St, Brandon MB R7A 5E7; Ibadan (Nigeria)'95; MRCOG; FRCSC; ObstGyn. (204)728-4440; Fax. (204)726-1765.

AKINYELE, Adegboyega A; 31 Saint Marie St, Collingwood ON L9Y 3J9; Ibadan (Nigeria)'76; MB BS; FRCS(Glas); FACS; FRCSC; GenSurg. Consultant, Collingwood General & Marine Hospital; Consultant, Grey Bruce Health Services - Meaford Site; (705)444-5695; Fax. (705)444-6043; dakinyele@sympatico.ca.

AKIYAMA, Tomoyuki; The Hosp for Sick Children, 555 University Ave, Toronto ON M5G 1X8; Okayama (Japan)'95; Staff, The Hospital For Sick Children; (416)813-6332

AKKOR, Sueda; Business Bldg, 503-1200 Burrard St, Vancouver BC V6Z 2C7; Istanbul (Turkey)'81; FRCSC; Ophth (General Ophthalmic Surgery). Ac Staff Ophth, Vancouver General Hospital - Centennial Pavillion; Clin Assoc Prof, University of British Columbia; Langs: Turkish; (604)609-2022; Fax. (604)609-2019.

AKLADIOS, Hala N; Medica One, 1275 Rymal Rd E, Hamilton ON L8W 3N1; Tanta (Egypt)'83; CCFP; (905)387-0005

AKLILU, Fasika; Grey Nuns Commun Hosp, 1100 Youville Drive West NW, Edmonton AB T6L 5X8; Alb'05; CCFP; CCFP(E.M.); Staff, Covenant Health - Grey Nuns Community Hospital; (780)735-7000

AKOT, Mawien M; Northgate Med Centre, 2711 Avonhurst Dr, Regina SK S4R 3J3; Alexandria (Egypt)'96; MB ChB; Staff, Northgate Medical Centre; (306)543-4566; Fax. (306)543-4441.

AKOTOYE, Christian K; Humber Valley Med Centre, 4-2630 Kipling Ave, Etobicoke ON M9V 4B9; (Ghana)'81; CCFP; FCFP; Staff, William Osler Health System - Etobicoke General Hospital; (416)744-2756; Fax. (416)744-2756.

AKOURY, Hani A G; St Joseph Health Centre, SB WW301-30 The Queensway, Toronto ON M6R 1B5; Alexandria (Egypt)'73; MB ChB; DAB; FRCSC; ObstGyn (Maternal Fetal Medicine). Staff, St Joseph's Health Centre; (416)530-6373; Fax. (416)530-6377.

AKPAN, Udeme E; Moose Jaw Union Hosp, 455 Fairford St E, Moose Jaw SK S6H 1H3; Staff, Moose Jaw Union Hospital; (306)691-6464; Fax. (306)691-6461.

AKRA, Mohamed A M; Cancercare Manitoba, ON3258-675 McDermot Ave, Winnipeg MB R3E 0V9; Benghazi (Libya)'93; MB ChB; FRCPC; RadOncol.

AKRIGG, Marian R; Fairmont Med Bldg, 1112-750 Broadway W, Vancouver BC V5Z 1J1; UBC'72; FRCPC; Derm. Vis Specialist, Dawson Creek & District Hospital; Vis Specialist, Fort St John Hospital & Health Centre; Consultant, Vancouver General Hospital - Centennial Pavillion; (604)879-9023

AKRIOTIS, Van J; 34-462 Birchmount Rd, Scarborough ON M1K 1N8; Wes'86; CCFP; (416)698-9988; Fax. (416)698-1055.

AKSOY, Davut E; 168 Garrison Rd, Fort Erie ON L2A 1M4; Wes'89; (905)994-9494

AKTAS, Murat; Windsor Med Centre, 3-130 Ouellette Place, Windsor ON N8X 1L9; Wes'90; (519)971-2901; Fax. (519)971-2902.

AKTER, Nazma; Eastwood Med Clinic, 7919 118 Ave NW, Edmonton AB T5B 0R5; (Bangladesh)'02; MB BS; MD; Langs: Bengali; (780)756-3666; Fax. (780)756-2598.

AKULA, Hari P; Grand Valley Med Clinic, 21 Main St N, Orangeville ON L9W 5S6; Karnataka (India)'02; CCFP; (519)928-5666; Fax. (519)928-3260.

AKYUREKLI, Deniz; 250 10th St E, Owen Sound ON N4K 1S5; Ott'93; FRCSC; Otol. Staff, Grey Bruce Health Services - Owen Sound; (519)371-5769; Fax. (519)371-8708.

AL-AAMA, Tareef Y A; St Joseph's HC-Parkwood Hosp, A280-801 Commissioners Rd E, London ON N6C 5J1; Jeddah (Saudi Arabia)'00; FRCPC; IntMed; GeriatricMed. Staff, Parkwood Hospital - St Joseph's Health Care; (519)685-4000

AL ABDULMOHSIN, Mohammed A H; Postgrad Med Education, MDCL 3101A-1280 Main St W, Hamilton ON L8S 4K1; Bahrain (Saudi Arabia)'03; GenSurg.

AL-ADRA, David P; University of Alberta Hosp, 8440 112 St NW, Edmonton AB T6G 2B7; Alb'07; Staff, University of Alberta Hospital; (780)407-8822

AL-AGHA, Osama M; Regina Qu'Appelle HR-Pasqua, 4101 Dewdney Ave, Regina SK S4T 1A5; (Yemen)'00; FRCPC; AnatPath (Surgical Pathology-Cytopath). Staff Path, Pasqua Hospital; Langs: Arabic; (306)766-2434; Fax. (306)766-2752.

AL-AGHA, Rany B; Royal Alexandra Hosp, 323-10240 Kingsway NW, Edmonton AB T5H 3V9; National U. (Ireland)'00; Staff, Royal Alexandra Hospital; (780)944-1440

AL-ALI, Kaes A S; Port Hope Med Centre, 209-249 Ontario St, Port Hope ON L1A 3Y9; Baghdad (Iraq)'97; FRCSC; GenSurg. (905)885-8949; Fax. (905)885-0716.

AL-AMODI, Hussein A O; Eastwood Med Clinic, 7919 118 Ave NW, Edmonton AB T5B 0R5; (Yemen)'07; (780)756-3666

AL-AMRI, Ahmed S A; Saint John Reg Hosp, PO Box 2100 Stn Main 400 University Ave, Saint John NB E2L 4L2; Jeddah (Saudi Arabia)'99; FRCPC; Neur. Staff, Saint John Regional Hospital; (506)648-6000

AL ANEE, Bassam I M; Family Practice Clinic, 84 Memorial Ave, Grnd-Falls-Windsor NL A2A 1R9; (709)489-6688

AL-AQEEL, Aqeel I M; 86 Kent St N, Simcoe ON N3Y 3S4; Riyadh (Saudi Arabia)'89; MD; FRCSC; GenSurg (Minimal Invasive Surgery). Staff, Norfolk General Hospital; Langs: Arabic; (519)426-8800; Fax. (519)426-5700.

AL-ARABI, Ayman M A; MCI The Doctor's Office, 595 Bay St, Toronto ON M5G 2C2; Riyadh (Saudi Arabia)'94; CCFP; (416)598-1703

AL-AREIBI, Arif R A; London HSC-Victoria Hosp, PO Box 5010 Stn B D2 315-800 Commissioners Rd E, London ON N6A 5W9; Al-Arab (Libya)'91; FRCPC; Anes. Staff, London Health Sciences Centre - Victoria Campus; (519)685-8500; arif.al-areibi@lhsc.on.ca.

AL-ATASSI, Talal; Lakeridge Health-Oshawa Site, 1 Hospital Crt, Oshawa ON L1G 2B9; McG'09; Staff, Lakeridge Health - Oshawa Site; (905)576-8711

AL-AWAD, Essa H; Peter Lougheed Ctr/Calgary GH, 35B-3500 26 Ave NE, Calgary AB T1Y 6J4; (Syria)'94; MB BS; Staff, Peter Lougheed Centre; (403)943-4892; Fax. (403)943-2565.

AL AWAMY, Mohammed B H; Univ Hlth Network-Toronto Western Hosp, 399 Bathurst St, Toronto ON M5T 2S8; Dammam (Saudi Arabia)'06; FRCPC; IntMed (Gastroenterology). Fellow Gastroent, Toronto Western Hospital - University Health Network; (416)603-5724

AL-BAAJ, Tholfkar M H; Strait of Belle Isle Hlth Care, PO Box 59, Flowers Cove NL A0K 2N0; University of Al-Mustansiriyah (Iraq)'00; MB ChB; Staff, Strait of Belle Isle Health Centre; (709)456-2401

AL-BADOOSH, Auday M A; Terrenceville Medical Clinic, PO Box 119, Terrenceville NL A0E 2X0; Al-Nahrain (Iraq)'99; MB ChB; Locum Tenens, Burin Peninsula Health Care Centre.

AL-BAKKAL, Sahar; Montreal Road Med Centre, 398 Montreal Rd, Ottawa ON K1K 0V4; Damascus (Syria)'90; Peds (Attention Deficit Hyperactivity Disorder). (613)244-2005; Fax. (613)244-2001.

AL-BATTRAN, Mazin H M; Grand River Hosp-KW Hlth Ctre, PO Box 9056 Stn C 835 King St W, Kitchener ON N2G 1G3; Baghdad (Iraq)'99; MB ChB; FRCPC; Psy (Consultant Liaison Psychiatry). Consultant Liaison Psy, Grand River Hospital - Kitchener/Waterloo Health Centre; (519)749-4300; Fax. (519)749-4289.

AL-BEER, Ali; Kent Place Mall, 207-189 Kent St, Lindsay ON K9V 5G6; Baghdad (Iraq)'92; FRCSC; OrthSurg. (705)328-0222; Fax. (705)328-1333.

AL-BEGAMY, Youssef S; Moose Jaw Union Hosp, 455 Fairford St E, Moose Jaw SK S6H 1H3; CCFP; Staff, Moose Jaw Union Hospital; (306)684-2204

AL BESHIR, Mohammad S A; Charles S Curtis Mem Hosp, 178-200 West St, St Anthony NL A0K 4S0; Dammam (Saudi Arabia)'06; FRCPC; IntMed; Gastroent. Staff, Charles S Curtis Memorial Hospital; (519)646-6000 x64312; Fax. (519)646-6130.

AL-BREIKI, Danah H M S; The Ottawa Hosp-Gen Campus, 501 Smyth Rd, Ottawa ON K1H 8L6; Dammam (Saudi Arabia)'03; Ophth. Staff, The Ottawa Hospital - General Campus; (613)715-8524

AL-BUSAIDI, Mujahid; Sunnybrook Hlth Sciences Ctre, D108-2075 Bayview Ave, Toronto ON M4N 3M5; Oman (Saudi Arabia)'04; FRCPC; IntMed; Critical Care Medicine. Staff, Sunnybrook Health Sciences Centre; (416)480-5291; Fax. (416)480-4999.

AL-CHADDAD, Elias; CSSS de Jonquiere, CP 1200 Stn Pdf Jonquiere 2230 rue de l'Hopital, Jonquiere QC G7X 7X2; Beirut (Lebanon)'69; LMCC; GenSurg (P.Q.) (Endoscopy). Staff, Centre Hospitalier Jonquiere; Langs: Arabic; English; (418)695-7700; Fax. (418)695-7715.

AL-DABBAGH, Haider M; 5-5035 Hurontario St, Mississauga ON L4Z 3X7; Baghdad (Iraq)'88; MB ChB; CCFP; Langs: Arabic; Hindi; (905)275-4895; Fax. (905)275-5472.

AL-DABBAGH, Muroog; North York Gen Hosp-Branson, 3W EDC-555 Finch Ave W, North York ON M2R 1N5; Iraq (Iraq)'86; FRCPC; Peds. Staff, North York General Hospital; Staff, North York General Hospital - Branson Division; (416)635-2575

AL-DANDAN, Sadeq W A; Vancouver Gen Hosp, 3410-899 12th Ave W, Vancouver BC V5Z 1M9; Dammam (Saudi Arabia)'01; NeurPath; AnatPath. Staff, Vancouver General Hospital - Centennial Pavillion; (604)875-4111

AL-DARAZI, Youness; Welland Paediatric Associates, 390 Lincoln St, Welland ON L3B 4N4; Beirut (Lebanon)'95; FRCPC; Peds (Infectious Diseases). Asst Prof, Hamilton Health Sciences Centre - McMaster University Medical Centre; Staff, Niagara Health System - Welland Hospital Site; (905)788-1915; Fax. (905)788-1779.

AL DARWISH, Mahdi E A; 375 South St, Goderich ON N7A 3M7; Karachi (Pakistan)'99; Psy. (519)667-6667; Fax. (519)667-6564.

AL-DHAHER, Firas F; 431 King St, Petrolia ON N0N 1R0; Wes'05; CCFP; Langs: Arabic; (519)852-2500; Fax. (519)882-4321.

AL-DHAMIN, Ammar S S; Queen Elizabeth II HSC-Halifax, 4443-1796 Summer St, Halifax NS B3H 3A7; Baghdad (Iraq)'95; MB ChB; Staff, Queen Elizabeth II Health Sciences Centre - Halifax Infirmary Site; (902)473-8773

AL-DOURI, Faten M; William Osler HC-Brampton, 2100 Bovaird Dr E, Brampton ON L6R 3J7; Saddam (Iraq)'97; FRCPC; DiagRad. Staff, William Osler Health System - Brampton Civic Hospital; (905)494-2120; Fax. (905)494-6614.

AL ESSAWI, Turki H M; Health Sciences Centre, AD203-820 Sherbrook St, Winnipeg MB R3A 1R9; King Saud University (Saudi Arabia)'99; FRCSC; Urol. Staff, Health Sciences Centre; (204)774-8511

AL FARAJ, Noura J B; Alberta Med Association, 12230 106 Ave NW, Edmonton AB T5N 3Z1; Dammam (Saudi Arabia)'03; FRCPC; Psy. (780)732-3366

AL FARIS, Jamila A H; The Ottawa Hosp-Gen Campus, C2433-501 Smyth Rd, Ottawa ON K1H 8L6; Dammam (Saudi Arabia)'87; Staff Med Oncol Cancer Centre, The Ottawa Hospital - General Campus; (613)798-5555

AL-FARRA, Bassel; South Walkerville Med Centre, 115-2224 Walker Rd, Windsor ON N8W 5L7; Aleppo (Syria)'81; FRCSC; Urol (Impotence & Neurological Urology). Ac Staff, Windsor Regional Hospital - Metropolitan Site; Ac Staff, Hôtel-Dieu Grace Hospital; Langs: Arabic; (519)254-9906; Fax. (519)254-8301; balfarra@hotmail.com.

AL-FEELI, Aziz K; Parkland Med Associates, 205-505 Queen St, Spruce Grove AB T7X 2V2; Leicester (England)'96; FRCPC; PhysMed&Rehab. (780)962-2001; Fax. (780)453-8176.

AL-GASIM, Abeer A M; 1169 Bloor St W, Toronto ON M6H 1M9; (Saudi Arabia)'01; CCFP; Langs: Arabic; (647)427-3574; Fax. (647)427-3590.

AL-GHAITHI, Ibrahim S M; Alberta Children's Hosp, 2888 Shaganappi Trail NW, Calgary AB T3B 6A8; Oman (Saudi Arabia)'01; FRCPC; Peds. Staff, Alberta Children's Hospital; (403)955-2293; Fax. (403)955-3065.

AL-GHAMDI, Hamed S A; Pleasantview Prof Bldg, 407-11044 51 Ave NW, Edmonton AB T6H 5B4; Jeddah (Saudi Arabia)'01; FRCPC; IntMed; Cardiol. Staff, Foothills Medical Centre.

AL-GHAMDI, Khalid H S; Plaza II Mall, 604-8600 Franklin Ave, Fort McMurray AB T9H 4G8; Jeddah (Saudi Arabia)'04; FRCPC; IntMed (Respirology). Staff, University of Alberta Hospital; Staff, Northern Lights Regional Health Centre; (780)750-0725

AL-GHAMDI, Mohammed; Queen Elizabeth II Hosp, 10409 98 St, Grande Prairie AB T8V 2E8; Jeddah (Saudi Arabia)'94; FRCSC; OrthSurg. Staff, Queen Elizabeth II Hospital; (780)882-0602; Fax. (780)532-3236.

AL-GHAMDI, Mohammad S; University of Alberta Hosp, 8440 112 St NW, Edmonton AB T6G 2B7; Jeddah (Saudi Arabia)'02; Psy. Staff, University of Alberta Hospital; (780)833-1514

AL GHANIM, Nayef S A; Univ Hlth Network-Toronto Western Hosp, MP10 306-399 Bathurst St, Toronto ON M5T 2S8; Bahrain (Saudi Arabia)'01; FRCPC; Rheum; IntMed. Fellow, Toronto Western Hospital - University Health Network; (416)603-5800

AL-GHOUL, Ahmed R; Seema Eye Care Centre, 110-1016 68 Ave SW, Calgary AB T2V 4J2; Sask'01; FRCSC; Ophth (Corneal Transplantation). Clin Lecturer, University of Calgary; (403)253-5300; Fax. (403)253-8608; office@seemaeye.com.

AL HABEEB, Ayman S; Univ Hlth Network-Toronto Gen, 200 Elizabeth St, Toronto ON M5G 2C4; Riyadh (Saudi Arabia)'99; FRCPC; AnatPath. Staff, Toronto General Hospital - UHN; (416)340-3543; Fax. (416)340-5517.

AL-HABIB, Saed S; 101-1614 Dundas St E, Whitby ON L1N 8Y8; Riyadh (Saudi Arabia)'96; Staff, The Scarborough Hospital - General Campus; Langs: Arabic; Fax. (905)438-9001.

AL-HADDAD, Sahar F H; St Michael's Hosp, CCW2 091-30 Bond St, Toronto ON M5B 1W8; Baghdad (Iraq)'90; FRCPC; AnatPath (Gastrointestinal Pathology)., St Michael's Hospital; (416)864-5851; Fax. (416)864-5648.

AL HADDAD, Wael J T; Postgrad Med Education, MDCL 3101A-1280 Main St W, Hamilton ON L8S 4K1; (Jordan)'98; Teach Staff, McMaster University.

AL HADI, Mouafak; Mindemoya Med Clinic, PO Box 150 2120B Highway 551, Mindemoya ON P0P 1S0; Ott'06; CCFP; Langs: Czech; Arabic; (705)377-5371

AL-HALIMI, Maha; Fredericton Med Clinic, 301A-1015 Regent St, Fredericton NB E3B 6H5; Dubai (Saudi Arabia)'06; CCFP; Staff, Dr Everett Chalmers Regional Hospital; (506)447-4470; Fax. (506)447-4066.

AL-HAMID, Sameer M; MedEmerg Inc, 9-6400 Millcreek Dr, Mississauga ON L5N 3E7; Dammam (Saudi Arabia)'93; (905)858-1368

AL HARBI, Faiz M F; Arnprior & District Mem Hosp, WW 18-350 John St N, Arnprior ON K7S 2P6; Riyadh (Saudi Arabia)'03; Staff, Arnprior & District Memorial Hospital; (613)623-3166

AL-HARBI, Hatem H J A; Hamilton HS-McMaster Site, PO Box 2000 Stn Lcd 1 1200 Main St W, Hamilton ON L8N 3Z5; Jeddah (Saudi Arabia)'98; Staff, Hamilton Health Sciences Centre - McMaster University Medical Centre; (905)521-2100

AL-HARBI, Khalid E A; Hamilton HS-McMaster Site, PO Box 2000 Stn Lcd 1 HSC 4E4-1200 Main St W, Hamilton ON L8N 3Z5; King Abdul Aziz University (Saudi Arabia)'88; FRCSC; GenSurg; PedGenSurg. Staff, Hamilton Health Sciences Centre - McMaster University Medical Centre; Langs: Arabic; (519)521-2100

AL HARBI, Mousa A R; Dartmouth Gen Hosp, 325 Pleasant St, Dartmouth NS B2Y 4G8; Dammam (Saudi Arabia)'05; MB BS; FRCPC; IntMed. Staff, Dartmouth General Hospital; (902)465-8300

AL HARBI, Nasser S T; The Hosp for Sick Children, 555 University Ave, Toronto ON M5G 1X8; Riyadh (Saudi Arabia)'02; Clin Fellow Peds, The Hospital For Sick Children; (416)813-1500

AL-HARBI, Othman R A; Ontario Endoscopy Clinic, 302-1315 Finch Ave W, North York ON M3J 2G6; King Saud University (Saudi Arabia)'99; Gastroent; IntMed. (416)634-0001

AL HARITHY, Ru'aa S K A; Sunnybrook Hlth Sciences Ctre, 2075 Bayview Ave, Toronto ON M4N 3M5; Riyadh (Saudi Arabia)'02; FRCPC; Derm. Staff, Sunnybrook Health Sciences Centre; Staff, Women's College Hospital; (416)480-6100

AL HASHMI, Amal; MUHC-Montreal Neurology Inst, 144-3801 rue University, Montreal QC H3A 2B4; Oman (Saudi Arabia)'01; Neur. Staff, McGill University Health Centre - Montreal Neurological Hospital; (514)398-6644

AL-HASHMI, Hani; Tom Baker Cancer Centre, 1331 29 St NW, Calgary AB T2N 4N2; McM'03; FRCPC; IntMed; MedOncol; Hem. Staff, Tom Baker Cancer Centre; (403)521-3038

AL-HASHMI, Ibrahim M M; 5A-5230 Dundas St W, Etobicoke ON M9B 1A8; Riyadh (Saudi Arabia)'86; MB BS; FRCPC; Peds (Pediatric Hematology). Staff, St Joseph's Health Centre; Staff, Guelph General Hospital; Langs: Arabic; (416)234-5442; Fax. (416)234-1483.

AL HAYEK, Ali I K; Regina Qu'Appelle HR-Regina, 122-1440 14th Ave, Regina SK S4P 0W5; King Faisal University (Saudi Arabia)'98; FRCSC; Neursurg. Staff, Regina General Hospital; (306)781-7229; Fax. (306)352-0499.

AL-HAYKI, Maryam M A; 7-5875 Rochdale Blvd, Regina SK S4X 2P9; (Bahrain)'93; (306)502-5031; Fax. (306)205-6108.

AL-HEJILY, Wesam A S; Foothills Med Centre, 1403 29 St NW, Calgary AB T2N 2T9; King Abdul Aziz University (Saudi Arabia)'03; FRCPC; IntMed; Cardiol. Staff, Foothills Medical Centre; (403)944-1110; Fax. (403)944-1592.

AL-HELLAWI, Ali Z D; 214-1448 Lawrence Ave E, North York ON M4A 2V6; Baghdad (Iraq)'88; FRCPC; IntMed. Staff, Humber River Regional Hospital - Finch Avenue Site; (647)344-5990

AL-HERTANI, Walla; MUHC-Montreal Gen Hosp, 2300 rue Tupper, Montreal QC H3H 1P3; Dal'05; FRCPC; MedGenetics. Staff, McGill University Health Centre - Montreal Children's Hospital; (514)726-9726

AL-HESAYEN, Abdurrahman O S; St Michael's Hosp, QW6 036-30 Bond St, Toronto ON M5B 1W8; Riyadh (Saudi Arabia)'91; FRCPC; IntMed (Heart Failure); Cardiol. Staff Cardiol/Prof Med, St Michael's Hospital; Langs: Arabic; (416)864-5952; al_hesayen@smh.ca.

AL-HOUSSAN, Walid; Sunrise Med Centre, 1460 Merivale Rd, Nepean ON K2E 5P2; (Syria)'86; CCFP; (613)727-7473; Fax. (613)727-2754.

AL-HOWARY, Ala A; IWK Health Centre, PO Box 9700 Rpo CSC 5850-5980 University Ave, Halifax NS B3K 6R8; Al-Mustansiriya U (Iraq)'02; MB ChB; BAO; Staff, IWK Health Centre; (902)470-8888

AL-HUMAYYD, Saad S; Fitzgerald Bldg, 112-150 College St, Toronto ON M5S 3E2; Riyadh (Saudi Arabia)'03; DiagRad. (416)978-6801

AL-HUSARI, Muhanad A J; Niagara H System-Welland Site, 65 Third St, Welland ON L3B 4W6; Baghdad (Iraq)'92; CCFP; Staff, Niagara Health System - Welland Hospital Site; (905)732-6111

AL HUSSEIN, Mosaad A; Univ Hlth Network-Toronto Western Hosp, EW5F 470-399 Bathurst St, Toronto ON M5T 2S8; Riyadh (Saudi Arabia)'07; IntMed. Fellow, Toronto Western Hospital - University Health Network.

AL-IZZI, Saif S A L; Eastwood Med Clinic, 7919 118 Ave NW, Edmonton AB T5B 0R5; (Other Foreign)'08; (780)756-3666; Fax. (780)756-2598.

AL JAHASH, Ibrahim M A; 11408 Jasper Ave NW, Edmonton AB T5K 0M1; (780)488-4242; Fax. (780)488-4141.

AL-JANABI, Hasan; Bluewater Health-Norman Site, 89 Norman St, Sarnia ON N7T 6S3; Saba (Netherlands Antilles)'04; Staff, Bluewater Health - Norman Site; (519)464-4400

AL-JARRAH, Dirgham; Niagara H System-G Niagara, 5546 Portage Rd, Niagara Falls ON L2E 6X2; (Iraq)'76; CCFP; Staff, Niagara Health System - Greater Niagara General Site; (905)358-0171

AL JAWAD, Mohammed S; London HSC-Victoria Hosp, E3 640-800 Commissioners Rd E, London ON N6A 5W9; Dammam (Saudi Arabia)'06; IntMed.

AL-JAWADI, Omar; 113-2922 Glen Dr PO Box 52569 Rpo Coquitlam Ctr, New Westminster BC V3B 7J4; Mosul (Iraq)'85; MB ChB; MSc; CCFP; (604)496-5182

AL-JAZRAWI, Nadir; CPM Pain Clinic, 9-6400 Millcreek Dr, Mississauga ON L5N 3E7; Baghdad (Iraq)'97; MB ChB; CCFP; (905)288-1045

AL-JEFFRI, Abdulla; The Hosp for Sick Children, 555 University Ave, Toronto ON M5G 1X8; King Faisal (Saudi Arabia)'86; Staff, The Hospital For Sick Children; (416)813-1500

AL-KAABI, Atheer; Health Sciences Centre, GF543-820 Sherbrook St, Winnipeg MB R3A 1R9; Alb'04; FRCPC; Neur. Staff, Health Sciences Centre; (204)774-8511

AL-KADHALY, Mothafar; Thompson Gen Hosp, 871 Thompson Dr S, Thompson MB R8N 0C8; Staff, Thompson General Hospital; (204)677-2381

AL KANDARI, Salem; The Ottawa Hosp-Gen Campus, 3301-501 Smyth Rd, Ottawa ON K1H 8L6; Dublin (Ireland)'02; Ophth. Staff, The Ottawa Hospital - General Campus; (613)798-5555

AL-KARAIN, Mohammad Y M; Professional Arts Bldg, 221-100 Arden St, Moncton NB E1C 4B7; (Jordan)'94; FRCPC; IntMed; Gastroent. Staff, The Moncton Hospital; Lecturer, Dalhousie University; (506)386-7131; Fax. (506)386-8074.

AL KARMI, Rani N I; 114-500 Kings Rd, Sydney NS B1S 1B1; Irkutsk State Medical University (Russia (Federation))'95; FRCSC; Ophth. Staff, Cape Breton Healthcare Complex; (902)270-3882; Fax. (902)270-3879.

AL-KASSEM, Anas; 223 West Street Upper, Simcoe ON N3Y 1S9; Damascus (Syria)'97; FRCSC; GenSurg. Staff, Ross Memorial Hospital; (226)440-3055

AL KATHEERI, Ali M A; London HSC-University Hosp, PO Box 5339 Stn B ALL 139-339 Windermere Rd, London ON N6A 5A5; Mecca (Saudi Arabia)'02; FRCPC; IntMed; Nephrol. Fellow Nephrol, London Health Sciences Centre - University Hospital; (519)685-8500

AL-KATIB, Fatih M W; Acadia Med Centre, 3310 8th St E, Saskatoon SK S7H 5M3; London (England)'63; MB BS; LRCP; MRCS; Staff, Saskatoon District Health Board; Staff Privil, Heartland Health Region; Coroner, Province of Saskatchewan; Langs: Turkish; Arabic; French; (306)373-6000; Fax. (306)477-5000; fatih.al-katib@gov.sk.ca.

AL-KAYSSI, Nabil M; Hermitage Medicentre, 12747 50 St NW, Edmonton AB T5A 4L8; Al-Mustansyriha (Iraq)'84; MSc; MB ChB; CCFP; Staff Pt-Time, Sturgeon Community Hospital; Staff Pt-Time, Devon General Hospital; Staff Pt-Time, Westlock Healthcare Centre; Langs: Arabic; (780)473-2102; Fax. (780)478-9061.

AL KHAROUF, Esam J; IWK Health Centre, PO Box 9700 Rpo CSC 5980 University Ave, Halifax NS B3K 6R8; Homs (Syria)'05; MD; Staff, IWK Health Centre; (902)470-8731

AL-KHATIB, Dina; 1066 Sycamore Ave, Bathurst NB E2A 4T8; (Jordan)'96; CCFP; (506)543-6991

AL-KHAYYAT, Shadi S M; Scarborough Hosp-Birchmount, 3030 Birchmount Rd, Scarborough ON M1W 3W3; Jeddah (Saudi Arabia)'01; FRCPC; IntMed; MedOncol. Staff, The Scarborough Hospital - Birchmount Campus; (416)495-3600; Fax. (416)667-6620.

AL-KHAZRAJI, Wassan S K; Bonavista Peninsula Health Ctr, Postal Service 1 Hospital Rd, Bonavista NL A0C 1B0; Locum Tenens, Bonavista Peninsula Health Centre.

AL KHDAIR, Darar A; Hamilton HSC- Hamilton Gen, C3 11A-237 Barton St E, Hamilton ON L8L 2X2; (Kuwait)'04; FRCPC; IntMed; Cardiol. Staff, Hamilton Health Sciences Centre - Hamilton General Hospital; (905)521-2631; Fax. (905)296-0086.

AL-KUDMANI, Basheer S B; Sunnybrook Hlth Sciences Ctre, 2075 Bayview Ave, Toronto ON M4N 3M5; Kign Saud University (Saudi Arabia)'99; Staff, Sunnybrook Health Sciences Centre; (416)480-6100

AL-KURTASS, Suhaib; Misericordia Community Hosp, 16940 87 Ave NW, Edmonton AB T5R 4H5; (Saudi Arabia)'97; Staff, Covenant Health - Misericordia Community Hospital; Langs: Arabic; (780)735-2255

AL LAWATI, Hatim A A H; Postgrad Med Education, 2F-500 University Ave, Toronto ON M5G 1V7; Oman (Saudi Arabia)'02; FRCPC; IntMed; Cardiol.

AL-MAANI, Amal S S; The Hosp for Sick Children, 555 University Ave, Toronto ON M5G 1X8; Sultan Qaboos University (Saudi Arabia)'01; FRCPC; Peds; InfectDis. Staff, The Hospital For Sick Children; (416)813-6230

AL-MAGHRABY, Hatim Q I; Univ Hlth Network-Toronto Western Hosp, 600 University Ave, Toronto ON M5G 1X5; Jeddah (Saudi Arabia)'00; FRCPC; AnatPath. Staff, Mount Sinai Hospital; (416)586-4800; Fax. (416)586-8481.

AL-MAHMUDI, Maha; BC Cancer Agency-Vanc Isl Ctr, 2410 Lee Ave, Victoria BC V8R 6V5; Al-Fateh University (Libya)'99; MB BCh; Staff, BC Cancer Agency Vancouver Island Centre; (250)519-5500

AL MAINI, Mustafa H A; 301-294 Main St, Toronto ON M4C 4X5; Sultan Qaboos University (Oman)'97; ABIM; FACRheum; FAAAI; FRFPS; ClinImmunol&Allergy; Rheum; IntMed (Adult Rheumatology). Langs: Arabic; (416)693-3030; almaini@acir.ca.

AL-MANAHI, Rasha N A; Eastside Collaborative Practic, 688A East River Rd, New Glasgow NS B2H 3S1; Baghdad (Iraq)'02; MB ChB; Langs: Arabic; (902)752-3632; Fax. (902)755-5532.

AL MANDIL, Majid; CSSS du Suroît, 150 rue Saint-Thomas, Salaber-de-Valleyf QC J6T 6C1; Riyadh (Saudi Arabia)'98; FRCSC; Urol. Staff, Centre Hospitalier Régional du Suroît; (450)371-9920

AL-MANE, Faisal M; 104-527 Admiral St, Woodstock ON N4S 5B2; RCS (Ireland)'91; FRCPC; IntMed. (519)421-3323; Fax. (519)421-3933.

AL MASOUDI, Faisal K H; GP Med Clinic, 12225 99 ST, Grande Prairie AB T8V 6X9; (780)533-4444; Fax. (780)533-4443.

AL-MEJAL, Zahra; The Hosp for Sick Children, 555 University Ave, Toronto ON M5G 1X8; Bahrain (Saudi Arabia)'02; Clin Fellow Psy, The Hospital For Sick Children; (416)813-1500

AL MOHRI, Huda A G; 100 International Blvd, Etobicoke ON M9W 6J6; Oman (Saudi Arabia)'99; FRCPC; IntMed; MedMicrobiol; InfectDis. (416)675-4530

AL MOSYAB, Nemer; University of Toronto, 2F-500 University Ave, Toronto ON M5G 1V7; Dammam (Saudi Arabia)'05; Psy.

AL-MUDAFFER, Mudaffer A; 203-3030 Lincoln Ave, New Westminster BC V3B 6B4; Al-Mustansiriyah (Iraq)'90; MB ChB; Peds. (604)942-1119

AL-MULLA HUMMADI, Yasmin K A; Dr Walter Templeman Hlth Ctr, PO Box 580, Bell Island NL A0A 4H0; Baghdad (Iraq)'98; MB ChB; Staff, Dr Walter Templeman Health Centre; (709)488-2821

AL-NAAMI, Ghassan; Morrison Centre, 202-9914 Morrison St, Fort McMurray AB T9H 4A4; (Jordan)'96; MB BS; (780)799-4616; Fax. (780)799-4914.

AL NABBOT, Salah E E; Dr Charles L LeGrow Hlth Ctr, PO Box 250 1 Grand Bay Rd, Port-aux-Basques NL A0M 1C0; Staff, Rufus Guinchard Health Centre; (709)695-2175

AL-NAIMI, Amal; The Hosp for Sick Children, 555 University Ave, Toronto ON M5G 1X8; Dammam (Saudi Arabia)'02; Clin Fellow Respirol, The Hospital For Sick Children; (416)813-1500

AL-NAKHLI, Mohammed; Quinte Health CC-Belleville Si, 265 Dundas St E, Belleville ON K8N 5A9; Jeddah (Saudi Arabia)'97; FRCPC; Psy. Staff, QHC Belleville General; (613)969-7400

AL-NASSAR, Rafid S; 69 Abercrombie Rd, New Glasgow NS B2H 1K4; Al-Mustansiriyah (Iraq) MB ChB; Staff, Aberdeen Regional Hospital; (902)755-3000; Fax. (902)752-1611.

AL-ODHAYB, Sami; Scarborough Gen Med Bldg, BC 12-3000 Lawrence Ave E, Scarborough ON M1P 2V1; King Saud University (Saudi Arabia)'00; Clin Fellow Ophth, The Scarborough Hospital - General Campus; (416)289-4000

AL-OTIBI, Merdas H F; London HSC-University Hosp, PO Box 5339 Stn B 339 Windermere Rd, London ON N6A 5A5; Riyadh (Saudi Arabia)'99; Neursurg. Fellow NeuroSurg, London Health Sciences Centre - University Hospital; (519)663-3982

AL-QADHI, Firas A L N; Guelph Gen Hosp, 115 Delhi St, Guelph ON N1E 4J4; Baghdad (Iraq)'97; FRCPC; Anes. Staff, Guelph General Hospital; (519)837-6440

AL QARSHOUBI, Issa S M; Ontario Endoscopy Clinic, 302-1315 Finch Ave W, North York ON M3J 2G6; Oman (Saudi Arabia)'01; FRCPC; IntMed; Gastroent. Staff, St Michael's Hospital; (416)634-0001; Fax. (416)634-0002.

AL QASEER, Ziad N F; 21 McGivern St PO Box 1300, Walkerton ON N0G 2V0; Baghdad (Iraq)'91; MB ChB; CCFP; (519)507-1021; Fax. (519)370-2513.

AL-QOOFI, Faisal T Y; Calgary Heart Centre, 403-3280 Hospital Dr NW, Calgary AB T2N 4Z6; King Saud (Saudi Arabia)'98; FRCPC; IntMed; Cardiol. Staff, Foothills Medical Centre; (403)521-2227

AL-QUTUB, Salma T A; Fitzgerald Bldg, 113-150 College St, Toronto ON M5S 3E2; King Abdul Aziz University (Saudi Arabia)'92; (416)978-6801

AL RAISI, Marwan S D; Children Hosp of Eastern Ont, 401 Smyth Rd, Ottawa ON K1H 8L1; Sultan Qaboos University (Saudi Arabia)'01; PedEmergMed; EmergMed. Staff, Children's Hospital of Eastern Ontario (CHEO); (613)737-7600

AL RAWAHI, Ghada N; BC Women's Hosp & Health Ctre, 2G27-4500 Oak St, Vancouver BC V6H 3N1; Oman (Saudi Arabia)'99; FRCPC; MedMicrobiol. Fellow, BC Women's Hospital & Health Centre; (604)875-2424

AL-REJJAL, Rafat; 1045 Sycamore Ave, Bathurst NB E2A 4M9; (Jordan)'94.

AL-RIKABI, Anwar; CSSS de Beauce-Etchemin, 1515 17e rue, Saint-Georges QC G5Y 4T8; Baghdad (Iraq)'97; Staff, Centre Hospitalier Beauce-Etchemin; (418)228-2031 x7231

AL-RUJAIB, Mashael K K; The Ottawa Hosp-Gen Campus, 1466-501 Smyth Rd, Ottawa ON K1H 8L6; Dammam (Saudi Arabia)'97; FRCPC; DiagRad. Staff, The Ottawa Hospital - General Campus; (613)737-8899

AL-RUJAIB, Turky; Women's Hosp, WR 120-735 Notre Dame Ave, Winnipeg MB R3E 0L8; King Faisal (Saudi Arabia)'92; GynOnco; ObstGyn.

AL-SAADON, Khalid; Cornwall Community Hosp, PO Box 100 Stn Main 113-840 McConnell Ave, Cornwall ON K6H 5S5; Kuwait (Kuwait)'84; FRCPC; IntMed. Internal Med, Cornwall Community Hospital; (613)933-1214

AL SAATI, Basem; Kingston Gen Hosp, 76 Stuart St, Kingston ON K7L 2V7; Damascus (Syria)'85; Staff, Kingston General Hospital; Staff, Hotel-Dieu Hospital; (613)549-6666; Fax. (613)548-1368.

AL-SABBAGH, Ahmad; Credit Valley Med Arts Centre, 507-2000 Credit Valley Rd, Mississauga ON L5M 4N4; Damascus (Syria)'80; FRCPC; IntMed (Respirology). (905)232-5900

AL SABEH, Nayla; CSSS de la Haute-Yamaska, 205 boul Leclerc O, Granby QC J2G 1T7; Aleppo (Syria)'82; CSPQ; AnatPath. Chief Dept of AnatPath, Centre Hospitalier de Granby; (450)372-5491 x2212; josee.senecal@rrsss16.gouv.qc.ca.

AL-SADKHAN, Haydar K M; Bluewater Health-Norman Site, 89 Norman St, Sarnia ON N7T 6S3; Baghdad (Iraq)'90; FRCPC; Anes. Staff, Bluewater Health - Norman Site; (519)464-4400; Fax. (519)336-8780.

AL-SAFAR, Anmar S; Dr A A Wilkinson Mem Hlth Ctre, PO Box 70 Main St, Old Perlican NL A0A 3G0; Baghdad (Iraq)'91; MB ChB; Staff, Dr A A Wilkinson Memorial Health Centre; (709)587-2200

AL-SAFFAR, Hussain A A; Univ Hlth Network-Princess M, 610 University Ave, Toronto ON M5G 2M9; Dammam (Saudi Arabia)'04; Otol. Staff, Princess Margaret Hospital - University Health Network; (416)946-2149

AL-SAHAN, Mohammad; Timmins & District Hosp, 700 Ross Ave E, Timmins ON P4N 8P2; Riyadh (Saudi Arabia)'98; OrthSurg. Staff, Timmins & District Hospital; (705)267-2131

AL SAIED, Mohamed; Family Practice & Walk-In Clin, 815 College St, Toronto ON M6G 1C9; Al-Fateh (Libya)'97; MB ChB; FRCSC; OrthSurg;CCFP; (416)533-1145

AL-SAIGH, Basil B; Finch Weston Med Clinic, C1-3492 Weston Rd, North York ON M9M 2W1; Saba (Netherlands Antilles)'05; (416)509-0909

AL-SALEH, Ayman M O; Hamilton HS-General Site, NW 8N 01-237 Barton St E, Hamilton ON L8L 2X2; Riyadh (Saudi Arabia)'04; FRCPC; IntMed. Staff, Hamilton Health Sciences Centre - Hamilton General Hospital; (905)521-2100

AL SALEH, Hani Q A M; The Hosp for Sick Children, 555 University Ave, Toronto ON M5G 1X8; (Kuwait)'06; FRCPC; Peds. Staff, The Hospital For Sick Children; (416)813-6248

AL SALIH, Hala; Harbourside Family Health Ctre, 243 Harbour Dr, Summerside PE C1N 5R1; (902)432-2600

AL-SAMAK, Sofian M A; PO Box 619, Vulcan AB T0L 2B0; Mosul (Iraq)'97; MB ChB; CCFP; CCFP(E.M.); (403)485-2216; Fax. (403)485-2218.

AL SAWAFI, Yaqoub A R; Univ Hlth Network-Toronto Gen, 9N 955-200 Elizabeth St, Toronto ON M5G 2C4; Sultan Qaboos (Saudi Arabia)'99; GenSurg (Thoracic Surgery). Clin Fellow Gen Surg, Toronto General Hospital - UHN; (416)340-3120

AL SAWI, Mohamed A M; 21 Queensway Rd, Mississauga ON L5B 1B6; Ain Shams (Egypt)'87; FRCPC; IntMed; Nephrol.

AL-SELAHI, Eiman M S A; London HSC-South St, 375 South St, London ON N6A 4G5; Arabian Gulf University (Saudi Arabia)'03; Peds. Staff Clinical Allergy & Immunology, London Health Sciences Centre - South Street; (519)685-8167

AL SHAAR, Wasan; 751 Victoria St S, Kitchener ON N2M 5N4; Baghdad (Iraq)'98; CCFP.

AL SHABANAH, Hasan A H; Hamilton HS-McMaster Site, PO Box 2000 Stn Lcd 1 3A-1200 Main St W, Hamilton ON L8N 3Z5; Riyadh (Saudi Arabia)'97; Staff, Hamilton Health Sciences Centre - McMaster University Medical Centre; (905)521-2100

AL-SHAIBANI, Wifaq; Alberta Children's Hosp, 2888 Shaganappi Trail NW, Calgary AB T3B 6A8; Cal'06; FRCPC; Peds. Staff, Alberta Children's Hospital; (403)955-2200

AL SHAIBI, Maha A N; Univ Hlth Network-Princess M, 3 130-610 University Ave, Toronto ON M5G 2M9; Sultan Qaboos (Saudi Arabia)'00; GenSurg. Staff, Princess Margaret Hospital - University Health Network; (416)946-6583

AL-SHAKARJI, Nather N; Acton Med & Urgent Care, 10 Eastern Ave, Acton ON L7J 0A5; Baghdad (Iraq)'91; CCFP; Staff, Halton Healthcare Services Corporation - Milton District Hospital; Langs: Arabic; (519)853-4449; Fax. (519)853-5242; nalshakarji@rogers.com.

AL-SHAMAM, Ali O; Western Mem Reg Hosp, PO Box 2005 Stn Main 1 Brookfield Ave, Corner Brook NL A2H 6J7; Staff, Western Memorial Regional Hospital; (709)637-5000

AL-SHAMI, Eman; 113-385 Silver Star Blvd, Scarborough ON M1V 0E3; Baghdad (Iraq)'85; MB ChB; Staff, Yarmouth Regional Hospital.

AL-SHAMI, Mohamad-Rakan; 101-60 Alpine Pl, St. Albert AB T8N 3Y2.

AL-SHAMMAA, Ameer K A; James Paton Mem Hosp, 125 Trans Canada Hwy, Gander NL A1V 1P7; Baghdad (Iraq)'94; MB BS; Staff, James Paton Memorial Hospital; (709)256-2500

AL-SHAMSI, Humaid O; Juravinski Cancer Center, 699 Concession St, Hamilton ON L8V 5C2; FRCPC; IntMed; MedOncol. (905)387-9711

AL SHAMSI, Mohamed S M; Children's Hosp of Eastern Ont, 401 Smyth Rd, Ottawa ON K1H 8L1; Oman (Saudi Arabia)'99; EmergMed. Staff, Children's Hospital of Eastern Ontario (CHEO); (613)737-7600

AL SHAREEF, Basem H M; Sunnybrook Hlth Sciences Ctre, H1 86-2075 Bayview Ave, Toronto ON M4N 3M5; Umm Al Qura (Saudi Arabia)'02; GenSurg. Staff, Sunnybrook Health Sciences Centre; (416)480-5850

AL-SHARIEF, Alaa; Upper River Valley Hosp, 11300 130 Rte, Waterville NB E7P 0A4; Aden (Yemen)'98; CCFP; Staff, Upper River Valley Hospital - Waterville; (506)375-5900

AL-SHARIEF, Khaled; Gibson Health Clinic, PO Box 9000 Stn A, Fredericton NB E3B 5N5; Yemen (United Arab Emirates)'95; MB BS; CCFP; (506)447-4220; khaled.al-sharief@rvh.nb.ca.

AL-SHAYJI, Ayman F; Saint John Reg Hosp, PO Box 2100 Stn Main 400 University Ave, Saint John NB E2L 4L2; Dublin (Ireland)'92; MB ChB; FRCSC; Neursurg. Staff, Saint John Regional Hospital; Assoc Prof, Dalhousie University; (506)648-6650; Fax. (506)648-6649.

AL SHELLEH, Sameeha; Univ Hlth Network-Toronto Gen, 8N 840-200 Elizabeth St, Toronto ON M5G 2C4; (Jordan)'02; Clin Fellow Nephrol, Toronto General Hospital - UHN; (416)340-3303

AL-SHIBANI, Abdelmagid S M; Parkland Med Associates, 205-505 Queen St, Spruce Grove AB T7X 2V2; Al-Fateh (Libya)'99; (780)962-2001; Fax. (780)962-8176.

AL-SIBANI, Nasser K M; University of Alberta Hosp, 8440 112 St NW, Edmonton AB T6G 2B7; FRCPC; Psy. Staff, University of Alberta Hospital; (780)407-8822

AL SUWAIH, Addnan R; White Bay Central Health Centr, PO Box 70 63 Cloud Dr, Roddickton NL A0K 4P0; Staff, White Bay Central Health Centre; (709)457-2215

AL-TARSHI, Muna T A; Univ Hlth Network-Princess M, 610 University Ave, Toronto ON M5G 2M9; Oman (Saudi Arabia)'99; Hem; IntMed. Clin Fellow Haematology, Princess Margaret Hospital - University Health Network; (416)946-6541

AL-TATARI, Hossam M; 210-2224 Walker Rd, Windsor ON N8W 5L7; Debrecen (Hungary)'94; Langs: Arabic; (519)255-9991; Fax. (519)255-7086.

AL-TIKRITI, Bakir Y D; Family Medical Clinic, PO Box 1195 490 Main St, Lewisporte NL A0G 3A0; Locum Tenens, Brookfield Bonnews Health Care Centre; Staff, Green Bay Community Health Centre.

AL-TOURAH, Abdulwahab J; Surrey Mem Hosp, 13750 96 Ave, Surrey BC V3V 1Z2; Dublin (Ireland)'96; MB BCh; BAO; FRCPC; IntMed; MedOncol. Staff, Surrey Memorial Hospital; Langs: Arabic; (604)930-2098

AL-TUKMACHI, Ahmad M S; Grey Bruce HS-Markdale, PO Box 406 55 Isla St, Markdale ON N0C 1H0; Kufa (Iraq)'90; MB ChB; Staff, Grey Bruce Health Services - Markdale; (519)986-3040

AL-TURBAK, Haytham; University of Ottawa, 2044-451 Smyth Rd, Ottawa ON K1H 8M5; Riyadh (Saudi Arabia)'02; FRCPC; IntMed. Teach Staff, University of Ottawa.

AL-WARD, Harith H A; Westney Heights Med Centre, 2-15 Westney Rd N, Ajax ON L1T 1P4; Baghdad (Iraq)'90; CCFP; (905)428-8055

AL WASSIA, Haydi; Foothills Med Centre, 1403 29 St NW, Calgary AB T2N 2T9; Jeddah (Saudi Arabia)'00; FRCPC; Peds (Neonatal & Perinatal Medicine). Staff, Foothills Medical Centre; (403)944-4638

AL-YOUSIF, Bahn H H; Claresholm Med Centre, PO Box 2050, Claresholm AB T0L 0T0; (Other Foreign)'96; (403)625-4484; Fax. (403)625-3969.

AL ZAIN, Khalid A H; 3-800 College St, Bathurst NB E2A 2T6; Jeddah (Saudi Arabia)'83; IntMed. (506)545-3681; Fax. (506)545-1079.

ALA, Brigitte D; 1568 Ouellette Ave, Windsor ON N8X 1K7; Wes'91; FRCPC; DiagRad. Staff Radiol, Hôtel-Dieu Grace Hospital; (519)256-4914; Fax. (519)973-9556; bala@hdgh.org.

ALAARAJI, Yassir; 204-22112 52 Ave, Langley BC V2Y 2M6; (Ireland)'87; (604)533-1140

ALABASTER, Charlotte; Bowmont Med Clinic, 6535 Bowness Rd NW, Calgary AB T3B 0E8; London (England)'82; MB BS; DRCOG; LMCC; CCFP; Staff Maternity Privil, Foothills Medical Centre; Langs: German; Spanish; (403)247-9797; Fax. (403)247-0014; stewartworden@hotmail.com.

ALABBAS, Abdullah E; University of Alberta Hosp, 2B2.42 WMC-8440 112 St NW, Edmonton AB T6G 2B7; Bahrain (Saudi Arabia)'00; FRCPC; Peds; Nephrol. Staff, University of Alberta Hospital; (780)407-8822

ALADETOYINBO, Adenike; Saint John Reg Hosp, PO Box 2100 Stn Main 400 University Ave, Saint John NB E2L 4L2; Ilorin (Nigeria)'98; Staff Peds, Saint John Regional Hospital; (506)648-6000

ALADETOYINBO, Kehinde; Saint John Reg Hosp, PO Box 2100 Stn Main 400 University Ave, Saint John NB E2L 4L2; Ilorin (Nigeria)'97; Staff, Saint John Regional Hospital; (506)648-6000

ALADI, Flora O; 48-6060 Memorial Dr NE, Calgary AB T2A 5Z5; (403)272-8130; Fax. (403)248-1535.

ALAGBE, Sylvie; Hopital Regional Chaleur, 1750 Sunset Dr, Bathurst NB E2A 4L7; Staff, Hopital Regional Chaleur; (506)544-3000

ALAGHBAND-RAD, Javad; IWK Health Centre, PO Box 9700 Rpo Csc 5850-5980 University Ave, Halifax NS B3K 6R8; Tehran (Iran)'89; MD; Staff, IWK Health Centre; Assoc Prof Psy, Dalhousie University; Langs: Farsi; Persian; (902)470-6300; Fax. (902)470-7062; rad@dal.ca.

ALAGIAKRISHNAN, Kannayiram; Clinical Sciences Bldg, B139-152 University Campus NW, Edmonton AB T6G 2G3; Tamil Nadu (India)'83; FRCPC; IntMed; GeriatricMed. (780)407-6947; Fax. (780)407-2006.

ALAGIC, Emer; 204-217 Terrace Hill St, Brantford ON N3R 1G8; Sarajevo (Bosnia-Herzegovina)'88; CCFP; (519)750-1331

ALAILY, Hana; Hop Fleury, 2180 rue Fleury E, Montreal QC H2B 1K3; Mon'89; Staff, Centre Hospitalier Fleury; (514)324-2000

ALAIN, Guylaine; Clinique Med de l'Outaouais, 25 ch de la Savane, Gatineau QC J8T 8A4; Laval'88; AB; FRCPC; Derm. Langs: English; (819)561-6611

ALAIN, Isabelle; Clin Perinatalitie Trois-Rivie, 100-4900 boul des Forges, Trois-Rivieres QC G8Y 1X1; Sher'01; Médecin Family Med, Clinique de Perinatalite de Trois-Rivieres; Langs: Bilingual(French/English); (819)373-2303; Fax. (819)373-0765.

ALAIN, Jean; CP 2000 Succ Bureau-Chef, Gatineau QC J8P 7H2; Laval'78; MRCP(Exp.Med.); CSPQ; MSc; FRCPC; MedBiochem. Chief Dept of Biochem, Hôpital de Gatineau; Consultant-Med Biochem, Pontiac Hospital Centre; Consultant, Centre Hospitalier de Val d'Or; Langs: Bilingual(French/English); Esperanto; (819)966-6100 x8349; jean.alain@ssss.gouv.qc.ca.

ALAIN, Jimmy; Dermatology du Quebec-Metro, 2880 ch des Quatre-Bourgeois, Quebec QC G1V 4X7; Laval'96; FRCPC; Derm. (418)650-3555; Fax. (418)650-1260.

ALAIN, Michel; Clinique Med Havre Sante, 521 boul Du Havre, Salaber-de-Valleyf QC J6S 4Z5; Mon'74; assoc Staff, Centre Hospitalier Régional du Suroît; (450)371-6444; Fax. (450)371-5315.

ALAIN, Pierre; CHUQ-St-Francois d'Assise, 10 rue de l'Espinay, Quebec QC G1L 3L5; Laval'76; CSPQ; FRCPC; Cardiol. Ac Staff, Centre Hospitalier Universitaire De Québec - Pavillon De St-françois-d'assise; (418)525-4303

ALAKIJA, Pauline; Dynalife DX, 200-10150 102 St NW, Edmonton AB T5J 5E2; UBC'90; MSc; FRCPC; AnatPath (Cardiovascular Pathology). (780)451-3702; pauline.alakija@albertahealthservices.ca.

ALAKKAD, Husni A O; Fitzgerald Bldg, 121-150 College St, Toronto ON M5S 3E2; Dammam (Saudi Arabia)'05; FRCPC; Anes. (416)946-0608

ALAKLABI, Mohammed; Univ of Alberta Hosp, 2D4.34-8440 112 St NW, Edmonton AB T6G 2B7; Staff, University of Alberta Hospital; (780)407-1959; Fax. (780)407-3672.

ALALLAM, A Aboubaker; Port Arthur Health Centre Inc, 194 Court St N, Thunder Bay ON P7A 4V7; Al Fateh (Libya)'00; FRCPC; IntMed; Gastroent. (807)346-1000; Fax. (807)346-6206.

ALAM, Ahsan; MUHC-Royal Victoria Hosp, R2.38-687 av des Pins O, Montreal QC H3A 1A1; McG'01; FRCPC; IntMed; Nephrol. Staff, McGill University Health Centre - Royal Victoria Hospital; (514)934-1934 x34672

ALAM, Huma A; London Intercommunity Hlth Ctr, 659 Dundas St, London ON N5W 2Z1; Punjab (Pakistan)'88; CCFP; Staff, London Intercommunity Health Centre - Dundas Street; (519)660-0874 x272

ALAM, M Mumtaz; 611 Wonderland Rd N, London ON N6H 4V6; (Other Foreign)'91; CCFP; (519)471-6686; Fax. (519)471-2801.

ALAM, Mahmood; Queen Elizabeth II HSC, 2269-1796 Summer St, Halifax NS B3H 3A7; Punjab University (India)'94; MB BS; Staff, Queen Elizabeth II Health Sciences Centre - Halifax Infirmary Site; (902)473-3808; Fax. (902)473-4448.

ALAM, Mohammad N; MUHC-Royal Victoria Hosp, 687 av des Pins O, Montreal QC H3A 1A1; Alb'03; CCFP; CCFP(E.M.); Staff, McGill University Health Centre - Royal Victoria Hospital; Staff, McGill University Health Centre - Montreal General Campus; (514)934-1934

ALAM, Mohammad S; Nanton Med Clinic, PO Box 940 2214 20 St, Nanton AB T0L 1R0; (Pakistan)'89; LMCC; MD; (403)646-2218; Fax. (403)646-3046.

ALAM, M. Shafiqul; Thompson Gen Hosp, 871 Thompson Dr, Thompson MB R8N 0C8; Dhaka (Bangladesh)'00; MB BS; MD; CCFP; Staff Emerg, Thompson General Hospital; (204)677-2381; Fax. (204)778-1413.

ALAM, Mohammed S; Dundas Med Clinic, 101-160 Dundas St E, Mississauga ON L5A 1W4; Dhaka (Bangladesh)'86; MB BS; CCFP; (905)273-3777; Fax. (905)277-9882; alamhm@hotmail.com.

ALAM, Muhammad F; Dr Charles A Janeway Child HC, 300 Prince Philip Dr, St. John's NL A1B 3V6; Karachi (Pakistan)'90; MB BS; DABPN; FRCPC; Neur (Pediatric Neurology). Staff Neurol, Janeway Children's Health & Rehabilitation Centre; Clinical Asst Prof Peds, Memorial University Of Newfoundland; Langs: Urdu; (709)777-4324; Fax. (709)777-4361.

ALAM, Muhammad M; 611 Wonderland Rd N, London ON N6H 4V6; Lahore (Pakistan)'91; (519)471-6686; Fax. (519)471-2801.

ALAM, Nadia; Halton HCS Corp-Georgetown, 1 Princess Anne Dr, Georgetown ON L7G 2B8; Dal'06; CCFP; Staff, Halton Healthcare Services Corporation - Georgetown Hospital; (905)873-0111

ALAM, Tasriqul M; 220-279 Wharncliffe Rd N, London ON N6H 2C2; Dhaka (Bangladesh)'82; MB BS; CCFP; Physician, Oxford Medical Walk-In Clinic; Langs: Bengali; Hindi; Urdu; (519)936-9900; Fax. (519)936-9894.

ALAM, Zeenat Y; Windsor Reg Cancer Centre, 2220 Kildare Rd, Windsor ON N8W 2X3; Dacca (Bangladesh)'72; MRC(UK); FRCPC; IntMed (Medical Oncology). Ac Staff Med, Hôtel-Dieu Grace Hospital; Ac Staff, Windsor Regional Hospital - Metropolitan Site; Langs: Bengali; Urdu; Hindi; (519)253-5253; Fax. (519)253-6494.

ALAME-ASSI, Saada; 204-1789 Mountain Rd, Moncton NB E1G 5C4; Beirut (Lebanon)'99; MD; (506)382-8880; Fax. (506)860-2760; saalame@serha.ca.

ALAMEEL, Turki A S; Ziedler Ledcor Centre, 2 39-130 University Campus NW, Edmonton AB T6G 2X8; Riyadh (Saudi Arabia)'04; FRCPC; IntMed; Gastroent. (780)492-8243; Fax. (780)492-1455.

ALAMELDIN, Mona; MUHC-Montreal Gen Hosp, 1650 av Cedar, Montreal QC H3G 1A4; Alexandria (Egypt)'91; AnatPath (P.Q.). Staff, Sir Mortimer B Davis Jewish General; Staff, McGill University Health Centre - Montreal General Campus; (514)934-1934

ALAMELHUDA, Elsayed E; Family Practice & Walk-In Clin, 2-3020 Dougall Ave, Windsor ON N9E 1S4; Cluj (Romania)'79; CCFP; Langs: Arabic; German; Romanian; (519)967-8867; Fax. (519)967-8859; elsayed53@hotmail.com.

ALAMI, Ghassan; CSSS de Saint-Jerome, 290 rue de Montigny, Saint-Jerome QC J7Z 5T3; McG'03; FRCSC; OrthSurg. Staff, Hôtel-Dieu de Saint-Jérôme; (450)431-8201

ALAMI, Ziad; Clinique Med le Plein-Ciel, 475 boul de la Cote-Vertu, Saint-Laurent QC H4L 1X7; Tours (France)'70; Otol (P.Q.). (514)337-3171

ALANAZI, Haitham A S; Univ of Ottawa Heart Institute, 40 Ruskin St, Ottawa ON K1Y 4W7; Riyadh (Saudi Arabia)'02; Cardiol; IntMed. Staff, University of Ottawa Heart Institute; (613)761-5000

ALANDEJANI, Talal; St Paul's Hosp, 1081 Burrard St, Vancouver BC V6Z 1Y6; Jeddah (Saudi Arabia)'03; Otol (Head & Neck Surgery). Staff, Providence Health Care - St Paul's Hospital; (604)682-2344

ALANEN, Kenneth W; Bow River Prof Centre, 242-4411 16 Ave NW, Calgary AB T3B 0M3; Wes'94; FRCPC; AnatPath; Derm. (403)457-1900

ALANJARI, Abdulmohsen K A A; Mount Sinai Hosp, 600 University Ave, Toronto ON M5G 1X5; (Kuwait)'02; ObstGyn (Maternal Fetal Medicine). Staff, Mount Sinai Hospital; (416)586-4800

ALANSARI, Nabeel M; 465 University Ave PO Box 21120, Charlottetown PE C1A 9H6; (Other Foreign)'84; Staff, Aberdeen Regional Hospital; (902)314-4035

ALANT, Jacob D V; Foothills Med Centre, 1403 29 St NW, Calgary AB T2N 2T9; Pretoria (South Africa)'97; FRCSC; Neursurg. Staff, Foothills Medical Centre; (403)944-4496

ALARAB, May A G; 8 816-700 University Ave, Toronto ON M5G 1Z5; Baghdad (Iraq)'89; MB ChB; MSc; MRCOG; MRCP; Staff/Asst Prof, Mount Sinai Hospital; Staff/Asst Prof, University of Toronto; Langs: Arabic; (416)586-8428; Fax. (416)586-8387.

ALARAKHIA, Mohamed; Centre for Family Medicine, 623-1187 Fisher-Hallman Rd, Kitchener ON N2E 4H9; Wes'08; CCFP; (519)570-3008; Fax. (519)570-0043.

ALARAPE, Akadri A; All Well Primary Care Centre, 2835 Millwoods Rd NW, Edmonton AB T6K 4A9; (Nigeria)'87; (780)450-4550; Fax. (780)461-1985.

ALARIE, Hughette; 380 rue Germain, Trois-Rivieres QC G8W 1J4; Laval'77; Med Consultant Family Planning Cllinic & Private Office, CSSS de Trois-Rivières; Langs: Bilingual(French/English); (819)376-1133; Fax. (819)372-6879.

ALARIE, Isabelle; CHUS-Hop Fleurimont, 3001 12e av N, Sherbrooke QC J1H 5N4; Laval'95; FRCPC; MedMicrobiol. Staff, Centre Hospitalier Universitaire de Sherbrooke-Hopital Fleurimont; (819)346-1110

ALARIE, Marie-Claude; CSSS de Trois-Rivieres, 155 rue Toupin, Trois-Rivieres QC G8T 3Z8; Laval'99; CCFP; Staff, Centre de santé Cloutier-du-Rivage; (819)370-2108; Fax. (819)370-2010.

ALARIE, Pierre; 4173 rue Berri, Montreal QC H2L 4H4; Mon'68; Member GenMed, Centre Hospitalier l'Université De Montréal (CHUM) - Hôpital Saint-luc; Clinical Asst Prof, Universite de Montreal; (514)875-0051; Fax. (514)875-1191.

ALARIE, Rejean; Centre Medical Fusey, 101-200 rue Fusey, Trois-Rivieres QC G8T 2V8; Laval'67; Physician, Le Trifluvien; (819)376-3669; Fax. (819)374-3041.

ALARY, Michel; Ctr Hosp Affilie-St-Sacrement, 1050 ch Sainte-Foy, Quebec QC G1S 4L8; Sher'74; MSc; PhD; Consultant, Centre Hospitalier Affilié Universitaire de Québec - Hôpital du St-Sacrement; Teach Staff, Université Laval; Langs: English; (418)682-7387; Fax. (418)682-7949; malary@uresp.ulaval.ca.

ALAS LOPEZ, Juan P; 64 Main St PO Box 1019, Springhill NS B0M 1X0; (El Salvador)'85; CCFP; (902)597-3829; Fax. (902)597-3066.

ALASAAD, Hani G M; LMC Diabetes and Endocrinology, 5-306 Quarry Rd, Barrie ON L4M 7G1; King Saud University (Saudi Arabia)'89; (705)737-0830; Fax. (705)737-0679.

ALASSAF, Hossam A M; The Ottawa Hosp-Gen Campus, 501 Smyth Rd, Ottawa ON K1H 8L6; Qassim (Saudi Arabia)'08.

ALATISHE, Moses A; 101 Cameron St, Moncton NB E1C 5Y7; Leningrad (Russia (Federation))'70; FRSM; FRCPC; Psy (Child & Adolescent Psychiatry). Consultant Psy, Shepody Healing Centre & Community Mental Hlth Initiative; Langs: Russian; Yoruba; (506)859-4495; Fax. (506)859-4431.

ALATISHE, Yuri; St Joseph's Mountain H Service, PO Box 585 Stn Lcd 1 100 5th St W, Hamilton ON L8N 3K7; Ross University (Other Foreign)'06; FRCPC; Psy. Staff, St Joseph's Healthcare Hamilton - West 5th Campus; (905)388-2511; Fax. (905)575-6038.

ALATRASH, Akrem K M; Jasper Avenue Med Centre, 11464 Jasper Ave, Edmonton AB T5K 0M1; (Libya)'02; MB BCh; (780)756-9212; Fax. (780)756-9211.

ALAVI, Afsaneh; 210-1077 North Service Rd, Mississauga ON L4Y 1A6; Kerman (Iran)'90; FRCPC; Derm. Staff, Women's College Hospital; (905)273-9009; Fax. (905)273-6409.

ALAVI, Shazia; Grandview Med Centre, 167 Hespeler Rd, Cambridge ON N1R 3H7; Punjab (Pakistan)'97; CCFP; (519)623-4200

ALAVIAN GHAVANINI, Ahmad; London HSC-University Hosp, PO Box 5339 Stn B C7 119A-339 Windermere Rd, London ON N6A 5A5; Shiraz (Iran)'98; FRCPC; Neur. Staff, London Health Sciences Centre - University Hospital; (519)685-8300

ALAWADHI, Maryam A Z E; Postgrad Med Education, 451 Smyth Rd, Ottawa ON K1H 8M5; (Kuwait)'02; (613)737-8010; Fax. (613)737-8115.

ALAWIYE, Alaba A; PO Box 120, Bassano AB T0J 0B0; CCFP; (403)641-6130; Fax. (403)641-6134.

ALAWSI, Maysarah; Iroquois Ridge Medical Centre, B5-360 Dundas St E, Oakville ON L6H 6Z9; Al Fateh (Libya)'04; CCFP; (905)257-8777; Fax. (905)257-0437.

ALAWSI, Sarwah A A A; Central Nfld Reg Health Centre, 50 Union St, Grnd-Falls-Windsor NL A2A 2E1; Staff, Central Newfoundland Regional Health Centre; (709)292-2500

ALAZHARI, Khalid E A; Rouge Valley HS-Ajax/Pickering, 580 Harwood Ave S, Ajax ON L1S 2J4; Al Fateh (Libya)'00; CCFP; CCFP(E.M.); Leamington District Memorial Hospital; Staff, Rouge Valley Health System - Ajax & Pickering Health Centre Site; (905)683-2320

ALAZRAGH, Waled A; 210-282 Linwell Rd, St. Catharines ON L2N 6N5; Al Fateh (Libya)'99; CCFP; (905)984-8944; Fax. (905)984-4477.

ALBADINE, Roula; CHUM-Hop St-Luc, 1058 rue Saint-Denis, Montreal QC H2X 3J4; Damascus (Syria)'93; Staff, Centre Hospitalier l'Université De Montréal (CHUM) - Hôpital Saint-luc; (514)890-0000 x36218

ALBAK, Russell E; Assiniboine Clinic, 633 Lodge Ave, Winnipeg MB R3J 0S9; Man'84; CCFP; FCFP; Lecturer Family Med, University of Manitoba; (204)958-6707; Fax. (204)888-1750.

ALBAYRAM, Mehmet S; Alberta Children's Hosp, 2888 Shaganappi Trail NW, Calgary AB T3B 6A8; Staff, Alberta Children's Hospital; (403)955-7985; Fax. (403)955-7656.

ALBERS, Jan-Martin; Dr Bernstein Health & Diet Cli, PO Box 342 Stn 1st Can Place 77 Adelaine St W, Toronto ON M5X 1E1; Qns'91; CCFP; FCFP; Langs: Dutch; German; (416)869-3118; Fax. (416)362-2728.

ALBERSHEIM, Susan G; Children's & Women's HC of BC, 1R47-4480 Oak St, Vancouver BC V6H 3V4; Man'77; DAA; FRCPC; Peds (Neonatal & Perinatal Medicine). Staff Newborn Serv, BC Children's Hospital; Clin Prof, University of British Columbia; (604)875-2135; Fax. (604)875-3106.

ALBERT, Alexandra; CHUQ-Ctr Hosp Univ Laval, 2705 boul Laurier, Quebec QC G1V 4G2; Laval'06; FRCPC; IntMed; Rheum. Staff, Centre Hospitalier Universitaire de Quebec-CHUL; (418)525-4444

ALBERT, Andrew; Burk's Falls Health Centre, PO Box 860 150 Huston St RR 1, Burks Falls ON P0A 1C0; Ott'82; CCFP; FCFP; Staff, Huntsville District Memorial Hospital - Muskoka Algonquin Healthcare; Lecturer, University of Ottawa; (705)382-2900 x253; Fax. (705)382-3473.

ALBERT, Clifford; Centre Medical du College, 1500 av Atwater, Montreal QC H3Z 1X5; McG'95; LMCC; MDCM; FASLMS; CCFP; Staff EmergMed, CSSS du Coeur de l'Isle Hôpital Jean-Talon; Med Dir, Canadian Institute For Laser Surgery; Langs: Bilingual(English/French); (514)937-9070; Fax. (514)937-2564.

ALBERT, Darren L; Eye Health MD, 440-8000 boul Decarie, Montreal QC H4P 2S4; McG'89; Ophth (Cataract). Staff, Sir Mortimer B Davis Jewish General; Staff, Hôpital Anna-Laberge; adj Prof, McGill University; Langs: French; (514)340-3937; Fax. (514)340-2729.

ALBERT, Diane; Agence de la SSS du Bas-St-Lau, 288 rue Pierre-Saindon, Rimouski QC G5L 9A8; Sher'06; CCFP; Langs: Bilingual(French/English); (418)727-4562

ALBERT, Emilie; Clin de Gynecology du Haut Ric, 630 boul du Seminaire N, St-Jean-sur-Richel QC J3B 7X6; McG'05; FRCSC; ObstGyn. (450)348-1171

ALBERT, Francois; CSSS du Haut Saint-Maurice, 885 boul Ducharme, La Tuque QC G9X 3C1; Staff, Centre Hospitalier Saint-Joseph de la Turque; (819)523-4581

ALBERT, Frederick L; 248 King St W PO Box 1269, Prescott ON K0E 1T0; (Jamaica)'67; Assoc Staff, Brockville General Hospital - Charles Street; Assoc Prof Family Med, Providence Continuing Care Centre (PCCC) - St Vincent de Paul Hospital; Langs: Bilingual(English/French); (613)925-3216; Fax. (613)925-3387.

ALBERT, Gabriella; Hôpital Laval, 2725 ch Sainte-Foy, Quebec QC G1V 4G5; Tirgu Mures (Romania)'98; Staff, Hôpital Laval; (418)656-8711 x5143

ALBERT, Gilles R; Clinique Med Payer, 5975 boul Payer, Saint-Hubert QC J3Y 6W6; Mon'74; FRCPC; Peds. Langs: Bilingual(French/English); (450)656-8221; Fax. (450)656-0515.

ALBERT, Guy; Hop du Sacre-Coeur de Mtl, 5400 boul Gouin O, Montreal QC H4J 1C5; Mon'67; MedMicrobiol. Ac Staff, Hôpital du Sacre-Coeur de Montréal; (514)338-2050; Fax. (514)338-2909.

ALBERT, Jacques; The Moncton Hosp, 135 MacBeath Ave, Moncton NB E1C 6Z8; Sher'99; CCFP; CCFP(E.M.); Staff, The Moncton Hospital; (506)857-5353

ALBERT, Jean-Francois; CSSS de Trois-Rivieres, 1991 boul du Carmel, Trois-Rivieres QC G8Z 3R9; Mon'88; LMCC; CSPQ; Anes (Intensive Care). Staff, CSSS de Trois-Rivières; Langs: English; (819)697-3333 x69856; jfalbert@mac.com.

ALBERT, Jean-Marie; CSSS du Nord de Lanaudière, 1000 boul Sainte-Anne, St-Charles-Brromee QC J6E 6J2; Mon'63; FRCPC; Psy (General Psychiatry). Staff, Centre Hospitalier l'Université de Montréal (CHUM) - Hôpital Notre-Dame; Staff, Centre Hospitalier Régional de Lanaudière; Staff, Hopital Louis-H Lafontaine; Commissioner, Commission on Social Affairs; adj Prof, Universite de Montreal; (450)759-8222; Fax. (450)759-0011.

ALBERT, Lori J; 1E 424-399 Bathurst St, Toronto ON M5T 2S8; Tor'88; FRCPC; IntMed; Rheum. Staff, Toronto Western Hospital - University Health Network; (416)603-6484; Fax. (416)603-4348; lori.albert@uhn.ca.

ALBERT, Maha A; 202-5293 Highway 7, Markham ON L3P 7M7; Ain Shams (Egypt)'80; MB ChB; DCH(Ire); Staff, Markham Stouffville Hospital; (905)472-9493; Fax. (905)472-1880.

ALBERT, Martin; Hop du Sacre-Coeur de Mtl, 5400 boul Gouin O, Montreal QC H4J 1C5; Mon'96; FRCPC; IntMed; Critical Care Medicine (P.Q.). Staff Intensive Care, Hôpital du Sacre-Coeur de Montréal; Universite de Montreal; Langs: Bilingual(English/French); (514)338-2050; m.albert@umontreal.ca.

ALBERT, Michel; 980 Oliver Rd, Thunder Bay ON P7B 6V4; Ott'04; CCFP; CCFP(E.M.); Staff, Thunder Bay Regional Health Sciences Centre; Langs: French; (807)684-6100

ALBERT, Michelle S; Courtice Health Centre, 2F-1450 Highway 2, Courtice ON L1E 3C3; Tor'88; BSc; CCFP; FCFP; Ac Staff, Lakeridge Health - Bowmanville Site; (905)721-4946; Fax. (905)721-6170.

ALBERT, Natalie; CHUQ-Ctr Hosp Univ Laval, 2705 boul Laurier, Quebec QC G1V 4G2; Laval'96; CSPQ; FRCPC; Anes (Regional Anesthesia). Staff, Centre Hospitalier Universitaire de Quebec-CHUL; Langs: Bilingual(English/French); (418)656-4141; natt.albert@sympatico.ca.

ALBERT, Paul; Dr Georges-L Dumont Reg Hosp, 330 av Universite, Moncton NB E1C 2Z3; Sher'99; CCFP; CCFP(E.M.); Staff, Dr Georges-L-Dumont University Hospital Centre; (506)862-4113

ALBERT, Shelley E; Sunnybrook Hlth Sciences Ctre, A224-2075 Bayview Ave, Toronto ON M4N 3M5; Tor'85; FRCPC; IntMed (Hypertension); Nephrol. Staff, Sunnybrook Health Sciences Centre; Staff, North York General Hospital; (416)480-6950; Fax. (416)480-4571.

ALBERT-DAIGLE, Luce; 160 rue Principale, Saint-Jacques NB E7B 1W4; Sher'93; CCFP; Staff, Hôpital regional d'Edmundston; Langs: Bilingual(French/English); (506)739-7708; Fax. (506)739-5839.

ALBERTON, Bruno G; Clinique Med Centre-Ville, 5-167 rue de la Reine, Gaspe QC G4X 2W6; UBC'85; CCFP; (418)368-1811; Fax. (418)368-2616.

ALBERTS, Hendrik; Welland McMaster Family Hlth Team, 555 Prince Charles Dr, Welland ON L3C 6B5; Pretoria (South Africa)'92; MB ChB; LMCC; CCFP; Langs: Afrikaans; Zulu; (905)734-9699

ALBERTS, Martin J A; Moose Jaw Union Hosp, 455 Fairford St E, Moose Jaw SK S6H 1H3; Pretoria (South Africa)'04; MB ChB; CCFP; Staff, Moose Jaw Union Hospital; (306)694-0200; Fax. (306)694-0282.

ALBERTS, Melissa; Welland McMaster Family Hlth Team, 555 Prince Charles Dr, Welland ON L3C 6B5; Pretoria (South Africa)'95; MB ChB; CCFP; (905)734-9699

ALBERTYN, Albert R; Nipawin Med Group, PO Box 2135, Nipawin SK S0E 1E0; Pretoria (South Africa) MB ChB; Langs: Afrikaans; Dutch; (306)862-4626; Fax. (306)862-3522.

ALBIANI, David A; UBC Eye Care Centre, 2550 Willow St, Vancouver BC V5Z 3N9; Qns'02; FRCSC; Ophth. (604)875-4656

ALBIN-COOK, Krystyna A; 2-452 Rathburn Rd, Etobicoke ON M9C 3S8; Warsaw (Poland)'71; Court Staff, Trillium Health Centre - West Toronto; Med Dir, Queensway Health Centre; Langs: Polish; French; (416)621-2323; Fax. (416)621-2321.

ALBIR, Yousra Y; Placentia Health Centre, PO Box 480 1 Corrigan Pl, Placentia NL A0B 2Y0; Baghdad (Iraq)'08; MB ChB; Locum Tenens, Placentia Health Centre; (709)227-2061

ALBISTON, Brigit J; South Shore Reg Hosp, 90 Glen Allan Dr, Bridgewater NS B4V 3S6; UBC'05; GenPath. Staff, South Shore Regional Hospital; (902)527-5068; Fax. (902)543-1562.

ALBORG, Frances J; Woodstock Med Clinic, 8-110 Chapel St, Woodstock NB E7M 1H1; Wayne State(MI) (USA)'78; CCFP; (506)328-3154; Fax. (506)328-8400.

ALBRBAR, Mohamed J H; Access Med Centre, 13718 113A St NW, Edmonton AB T5X 4H7; Al Fateh (Libya)'00; CCFP; Langs: Arabic; (780)456-3067; Fax. (780)478-6384; spadina3580@yahoo.com.

ALBRECHT, Ana-Ruth; New Westminster Med Centre, 102-600 Royal Ave, New Westminster BC V3M 1J3; UBC'72; Assoc Staff, Royal Columbian Hospital; (604)522-1648; Fax. (604)522-1650.

ALBRECHT, Craig; 1145 Concession Rd, Cambridge ON N3H 4L5; Wes'00; CCFP; Hd FamilyMed, Grand Bend Community Health Centre - Hensall Site; (519)653-1470

ALBRECHT, Gaylord D; Guelph Family Health Team, 83 Dawson Rd, Guelph ON N1H 1B1; McM'07; CCFP; (519)766-1360

ALBRECHT, John E; New Westminster Med Centre, 101-600 Royal Ave, New Westminster BC V3M 1J3; UBC'71; Assoc Staff, Royal Columbian Hospital; (604)526-4277; Fax. (604)521-3644.

ALBRECHT, Kelly D; ISIS Women's Health Clinic, 144-1402 8 Ave NW, Calgary AB T2N 1B9; Cal'06; FRCSC; ObstGyn. (403)289-8996; Fax. (403)289-8956.

ALBRECHT, Lorne E; Guildford Med Dental Centre, 20-15300 105 Ave, Surrey BC V3R 6A7; Alb'85; FRCPC; Derm. Asst Prof, University of British Columbia; (604)585-1110; Fax. (604)585-1170; lalbrecht@primus.ca.

ALBRECHT, Steffen; MUHC-Montreal Children's Hosp, D. 469-2300 rue Tupper, Montreal QC H3H 1P3; Sher'85; CSPQ; NeurPath; AnatPath. Staff, McGill University Health Centre - Montreal Children's Hospital; (514)412-4495; Fax. (514)412-4258.

ALBRITTON, William L; University of Saskatchewan, 6B61-107 Wiggins Rd, Saskatoon SK S7N 5E5; Birmingham (USA)'70; PhD; FRCPC; Peds. Dean Faculty of Med/Prof, University of Saskatchewan; (306)966-6655; Fax. (306)966-4298; dean.medicine@usask.ca.

ALBUQUERQUE, Joy M; 900-150 Bloor St W, Toronto ON M5S 3C1; Man'89; FRCPC; Psy. (416)340-2954; Fax. (416)340-2860.

ALBUQUERQUE, Sandra; 207-8120 Beddington Blvd NW, Calgary AB T3K 2A8; (India)'94; CCFP; (403)275-4611

ALBUS, Wayne W; 109-13278 Tecumseh Rd E, Windsor ON N8N 3T6; Wes'86; CCFP; (519)735-8310; Fax. (519)735-6073.

ALCAIDINHO, Duarte; Polyclinique St-Jerome, 304-200 rue Durand, Saint-Jerome QC J7Z 7E2; Mon'79; Urol. Staff, Hôtel-Dieu de Saint-Jérôme; (450)436-7173; Fax. (450)436-7617.

ALCARAZ-LIMCANGCO, Yolanda; Centennial Ctre for Mental Hea, PO Box 1000, Ponoka AB T4J 1R8; (Philippines)'90; CCFP; (403)783-7810

ALCHALABI, Karam R A; Burin Peninsula Hlth Care Ctr, PO Box 340, Burin NL A0E 1E0; (Iraq)'96; Staff, Grand Bank Health Centre; (709)891-1040

ALCINDOR, Antony; 205-529 rue Jarry E, Montreal QC H2P 1V4; Port-au-Prince (Haiti)'58; CSPQ; GenPath. Langs: Creole; English; (514)272-5341; jacda@sympatico.ca.

ALCINDOR, Jean Joseph Thierry; MUHC-Montreal Gen Hosp, A7 130-1650 av Cedar, Montreal QC H3G 1A4; Université d'État d'Haïti (Haiti)'91; ABIM; MedOncol (P.Q.); Hem (P.Q.). Staff, McGill University Health Centre - Montreal General Campus; Langs: Bilingual(English/French); Creole; Spanish; (514)934-1934 x43118; Fax. (514)934-8379; thierry.alcindor@muhc.mcgill.ca.

ALCINDOR, M C Michele; Clinique Med Colombus, 204-1140 rue Jean-Talon E, Montreal QC H2R 1V9; Seville (Spain)'73; Ac Staff, Hôpital du Sacre-Coeur de Montréal; (514)270-2141; Fax. (514)270-6920.

ALCOCK, Carl J; Henley Gardens Clinic, 4B-1089 Kingston Rd, Scarborough ON M1N 4E4; Mem'75; (416)690-7200; Fax. (416)690-7679.

ALDA, Martin; Abbie J Lane Mem Bldg, 3088-5909 Veterans Memorial La, Halifax NS B3H 2E2; Karlova (Czech Republic)'82; FRCPC; Psy. (902)473-2585; Fax. (902)473-4877.

ALDANDASHI, Samer; Royal Alexandra Hosp, 10240 Kingsway NW, Edmonton AB T5H 3V9; (Syria)'95; MD; Staff Psy, Royal Alexandra Hospital; Langs: Arabic; (780)735-4567; Fax. (780)735-4797.

ALDAOUD, Abdullah M A; Addiction & Mental Hlth-ARF, 33 Russell St, Toronto ON M5S 2S1; Riyadh (Saudi Arabia)'01; Staff, Centre for Addiction & Mental Health (CAMH) - Russell Street Site; (416)535-8501

ALDEA, Michael S; Campbellton Reg Hosp, PO Box 880 Stn Main 189 Lily Lake Rd, Campbellton NB E3N 3H3; Manila (Philippines)'94; Staff, Hôpital Régional Campbellton; (506)789-5000

ALDERDICE, Catherine A; St Joseph's Health Care, 100 Westmount Rd, Guelph ON N1H 5H8; Mem'76; FRCPC; Rheum. Staff, St Joseph's Health Centre; (519)824-6000 x4330; Fax. (519)767-3431; calderdice@gghorg.ca.

ALDIS, Ann E; MUHC-Montreal Gen Hosp, D5371-1650 av Cedar, Montreal QC H3G 1A4; Wes'76; DiagRad. Staff Radiol, McGill University Health Centre - Montreal General Campus; (514)934-1934 x48003; Fax. (514)934-8263.

ALDIS, Hugh W; Peterborough Reg HC-Hospital, 1 Hospital Dr, Peterborough ON K9J 7C6; Wes'74; DABR; DiagRad. Staff, St Francis Memorial Hospital; Staff, Peterborough Regional Health Centre - Rogers St Site; Ac Staff Radiol, Peterborough Regional Health Centre - Hospital Drive; (705)876-5039; Fax. (705)743-1713.

ALDRIDGE, Christopher; Family Pract & Chronic Pain Mg, 202-688 Coxwell Ave, Toronto ON M4C 3B7; Tor'02; CCFP; (416)463-4632; Fax. (416)463-4639.

ALDRIDGE, David J; Cape Breton Hlthcare Complex, 1482 George St, Sydney NS B1P 1P3; London (England)'69; MB BS; BSc(Hons); MRCPsy; FRCPC; Psy (Child & Adolescent Psychiatry). Att Staff Child & Adolesc Mental Health Serv, Cape Breton Healthcare Complex; Consultant Child & Adolescent Psy, Cape Breton District Health Authority; (902)567-7731; Fax. (902)567-7918; aldridged@cbdha.nshealth.ca.

ALDRIDGE, E Jane; Sheddon Avenue Med Assoc, 308-331 Sheddon Ave, Oakville ON L6J 1X8; McM'85; BSc(Hon); CCFP; FCFP; Assoc Staff, Halton Healthcare Services Corporation - Oakville Site; (905)845-8771; Fax. (905)845-8379.

ALDRIDGE, Leonard L; Fanning Extended Care Centre, 722 16 Ave NE, Calgary AB T2E 6V7; Alb'69; Ac Staff, Calgary Aux Hospital(Carewest) District 7; Asst Prof Div of Family Med, University of Calgary; (403)230-6900; laldridge@ucalgary.ca.

ALDRIDGE, Lisa; 253-99 Fifth Ave, Ottawa ON K1S 5P5; Mem'03; CCFP.

ALEEM, Abdul; 101-1617 Baker St, Cranbrook BC V1C 1B4; Punjab (Pakistan)'65; MB BS; LRCP; MRCS; FRCSC; GenSurg. Staff, East Kootenay Regional Hospital; (250)489-3044; Fax. (250)489-2878.

ALEEM, Nadia; Addiction & Mental Hlth-Clarke, 250 College St, Toronto ON M5T 1R8; UBC'01; Psy. Staff, Centre for Addiction & Mental Health (CAMH) - College Street Site; (416)979-6819; Fax. (416)979-6853.

ALEGADO, Eli; 4119 Bathurst St, North York ON M3H 3P4; Philippines (Philippines)'82; FRCPC; IntMed. (647)349-1270; Fax. (647)349-1271.

ALEGRE, Hugo T; 94 Laughton Ave, Toronto ON M6N 2W9; Tor'73; (416)656-4847

ALEKER, Junaid; 5035 51 St PO Box 1076 Stn Main, Whitecourt AB T7S 1P9; (South Africa)'04; (780)778-2224

ALEKSANDROVA, Iryna G; North York Gen Hosp, 4001 Leslie St, North York ON M2K 1E1; Doneck (Ukraine)'98; FRCPC; Anes. Staff, North York General Hospital; (416)756-6520

ALEKSIC, Slavica; Centre médicale Centrale, 4-135 rue Saint-Antoine N, Granby QC J2G 5G7; Mon'93; Staff, Centre Hospitalier de Granby; (450)372-5401; Fax. (450)372-4174.

ALEKSIEJUK, Janusz; Niagara H System-Welland Site, 65 Third St, Welland ON L3B 4W6; Bialystok (Poland)'79; Staff, Niagara Health System - Welland Hospital Site; Langs: Polish; (905)732-6111

ALEKSIEJUK, Zofia K; 1558 Haig Blvd, Mississauga ON L5E 2N3; Bialystok (Poland)'79; FRCPC; Psy. Asst Prof, University of Ottawa; (905)271-8777

ALEM, Atalay E; Whitby Mental Health Centre, 700 Gordon St, Whitby ON L1N 5S9; Addis Ababa (Ethiopia)'83; Acad Staff Visitor, Ontario Shores Centre for Mental Health Sciences; (905)668-5881

ALEMAYEHU, Efrem; 202-1011 Dufferin St, Toronto ON M6H 4B5; Addis Ababa (Ethiopia)'76; BSc(PublicHealth); MSc; Langs: Amharic; Tigrigna; (416)539-9002; Fax. (416)539-0309.

ALENEZI, Osamah H S S; Infectious Diseases Clinic, 201-1200 Burrard St, Vancouver BC V6Z 2C7; (Kuwait)'00; FRCPC; IntMed. (604)642-6429

ALESSANDRINI, Renato S; Oshawa Clinic, 117 King St E, Oshawa ON L1H 1B9; Wes'89; FRCPC; IntMed; Cardiol. Staff, Lakeridge Health - Oshawa Site; (905)723-8551 x5438; Fax. (905)721-4961.

ALEWAN, Salem; Carbonear General Hosp, 86 Highroad S, Carbonear NL A1Y 1A4; Al Fateh (Libya)'03; MB BCh; CCFP; Locum Tenens, Carbonear General Hospital; (709)945-5111; alewan@mun.ca.

ALEX, Erica S; 2-7398 Edmonds St, Burnaby BC V3N 1A8; (Other Foreign)'98; CCFP; (604)522-1711

ALEXANDER, Abraham S; BC Cancer Agency-Vanc Isl Ctr, 2410 Lee Ave, Victoria BC V8R 6V5; Alb'00; FRCPC; RadOncol. Staff, BC Cancer Agency Vancouver Island Centre; (250)519-5500

ALEXANDER, Alexander M; 200-1840 Eglinton Ave W, Toronto ON M6E 2J4; Mem'87; (416)789-6100; Fax. (416)789-3735.

ALEXANDER, Cherupushpam; St Joseph's Health Centre, 30 The Queensway, Toronto ON M6R 1B5; Kerala (India)'78; MB BS; FRCPC; GenPath. Staff Path, St Joseph's Health Centre; (416)530-6000 x4623

ALEXANDER, David I; Queen Elizabeth II HSC-Halifax, 4863-1796 Summer St, Halifax NS B3H 3A7; Dal'74; FRCSC; OrthSurg (Spine). Staff, Queen Elizabeth II Health Sciences Centre - Halifax Infirmary Site; Staff, Queen Elizabeth II Health Sciences Centre - Victoria General Site; (902)473-4092; Fax. (902)473-2054.

ALEXANDER, David J; 306-100 Colborne St W, Orillia ON L3V 2Y9; Qns'85; FRCPC; IntMed; Respir. Med Dir Sleep Lab, Orillia Soldiers' Memorial Hospital; (705)327-6652; Fax. (705)327-6693.

ALEXANDER, Kimberly A; Springdale Prof Bldg, 503-2250 Bovaird Dr E, Brampton ON L6R 0W3; McM'01; FRCSC; ObstGyn. Staff, William Osler Health System - Brampton Civic Hospital; (905)595-4960

ALEXANDER, Kunniparampil N; William Osler HC-Brampton, 2100 Bovaird Dr E, Brampton ON L6R 3J7; Kerala (India)'74; FRCPC; AnatPath. Staff, William Osler Health System - Brampton Civic Hospital; (905)494-2120 x58722; Fax. (905)494-6622.

ALEXANDER, Mary E; Trafalgar Prof Centre, 312-1235 Trafalgar Rd, Oakville ON L6H 3P1; (Jamaica)'81; MB BS; CGPA; CCFP; FCFP; (905)842-1510; Fax. (905)844-3811.

ALEXANDER, Michael A J; Shouldice Hosp, 7750 Bayview Ave, Thornhill ON L3T 4A3; Lagos (Nigeria)'69; MB BS; FACS; FRCSC; GenSurg (Herniology). Chief Surgeon/Chief Staff, Shouldice Hospital; Court Staff Surgeon, St Michael's Hospital; Aj Lecturer Surg, University of Toronto; (905)889-1125; Fax. (905)889-4216; postoffice@shouldice.com.

ALEXANDER, Michael; Allied Health Centre, 102-5673 North St, Niagara Falls ON L2G 1J4; Manchester (England)'78; MB ChB; FCCP; FACP; FRCP; FRCPC; IntMed (Sleep Medicine); ClinImmunol&Allergy. Staff Physician, Niagara Health System - Greater Niagara General Site; Asst Prof, McMaster University; Aj Prof, Brock University; (905)374-1405; Fax. (905)374-1428; doc911@cogeco.ca.

ALEXANDER, Michelle L; Markham Family Health Team, 1-122 Cornell Park Ave, Markham ON L6B 1B6; Tor'93; CCFP; (905)471-9999; Fax. (905)471-3627; malexander@msh.on.ca.

ALEXANDER, Pradeep J; 48-2140 North Park Dr, Brampton ON L6S 0C9; Tor'99; FRCSC; OrthSurg (Foot & Ankle Surgery). Ac Staff, William Osler Health System - Brampton Civic Hospital; Lecturer, University of Toronto; (905)793-7787

ALEXANDER, Robert; Edmonton Clinic Health Academy, 4 557-11405 87 Ave NW, Edmonton AB T6G 1C9; Wes'99; FRCPC; Peds (Pediatric Nephrology); Nephrol. Staff, University of Alberta Hospital; Staff, Edmonton Clinic Health Academy; (780)248-5560; Fax. (780)248-5627.

ALEXANDER, Sarah W; The Hosp for Sick Children, 555 University Ave, Toronto ON M5G 1X8; Harvard (USA)'94; Staff, The Hospital For Sick Children; (416)813-7654; Fax. (416)813-5327.

ALEXANDER, Timothy W; University of Alberta Hosp, 8440 112 St NW, Edmonton AB T6G 2B7; Newcastle-Upon-Tyne (England)'82; FRCR; FRCPC; DiagRad. Ac Staff Radiol, University of Alberta Hospital; Clin Assoc Prof, University of Alberta; (780)407-6907; Fax. (780)407-6176.

ALEXANDER, Wendy J; 40 Grove Ave, Rothesay NB E2E 5K6; Mem'90; FRCPC; Peds (Respirology). (506)849-0099; Fax. (506)849-8877; wendyalexander@nb.aibn.com.

ALEXANDER-WILLIAMS, Karen A; Lawrence-Victoria Park Med Ctr, 1715 Lawrence Ave E, Scarborough ON M1R 2X7; Dal'89; (416)701-1650

ALEXIADIS, Alexandros; The Richmond Hosp, SPCU-7000 Westminster Hwy, Richmond BC V6X 1A2; Dal'92; Staff, Richmond Hospital; (604)278-9711 x4127

ALEXIADIS, Maria; Mayflower Medical Clinic, 204-998 Parkland Dr, Halifax NS B3M 0A6; Dal'88; BSc(Biology); Staff GP in Psy, Early Psychosis Program; Langs: Greek; (902)835-1628; Fax. (902)835-1151.

ALEXIEVA, Nedalina K; Lakeridge Health-Oshawa Site, 1 Hospital Crt, Oshawa ON L1G 2B9; Varna (Bulgaria)'93; CCFP; Staff, Lakeridge Health - Oshawa Site; (905)576-8711

ALEXIS, Mercy E; Islington Med Clinic, 1000-1243 Islington Ave, Etobicoke ON M8X 1Y9; Amsterdam (Netherlands)'71; DAB; FRCPC; Derm. Court Staff, Trillium Health Centre - Mississauga; Court Staff, Women's College Hospital; (416)231-0100

ALEXIS, Michele L; 2135 Pitt St, Cornwall ON K6K 1A1; Ott'85; Assoc Staff, Cornwall Community Hospital; Assoc Staff, Cornwall Community Hospital - Second Street Site; (613)936-2511; Fax. (613)936-2098.

ALEXOPOULOS, Karen N; Dr KN Alexopoulos Med Prof, 208-55 Wyndham St N, Guelph ON N1H 7T8; Wes'93; CCFP; FCFP; Court Staff Privil, Guelph General Hospital; (519)837-2283; Fax. (519)767-2262.

ALEXOPOULOU, Iakovina; Hamilton HS-McMaster Site, PO Box 2000 Stn Lcd 1 2N19-1200 Main St W, Hamilton ON L8N 3Z5; Athens (Greece)'74; FRCPC; AnatPath (Renal Pathology). Dir AnatPath/Dep Chief Dept of LabMed, Hamilton Health Sciences Centre - McMaster University Medical Centre; Staff, St Joseph's Healthcare - Charlton Campus; Prof Path & Molecular Med, McMaster University; Langs: Greek; (905)521-2100 x76317; alexopou@mcmaster.ca.

ALEXOV, Lubomir; 301-1920 Ellesmere Rd, Scarborough ON M1H 2V6; Guadalajara (Mexico)'85; BSc; Staff, Rouge Valley Health System - Centenary Health Centre Site; Langs: Spanish; Bulgarian; (416)438-1987; Fax. (416)438-0448.

ALEXY, Julius; Selkirk Mental Health Centre, PO Box 9600 Stn Main 825 Manitoba Ave, Selkirk MB R1A 2B5; Komensky (Slovakia)'77; IntMed(Czech); Staff Physician, Selkirk Mental Health Centre; Lecturer, University of Manitoba; Langs: Slovak; German; Hungarian; (204)482-1661 x661; Fax. (204)482-6390.

ALEYASEEN, Maryam; Baywood Med Centre, 402-95 Bayly St W, Ajax ON L1S 7K8; Tor'98; FRCSC; GenSurg. Staff, Rouge Valley Health System - Ajax & Pickering Health Centre Site; (905)686-8679

ALEYASSINE, Hassan; MUHC-Montreal Gen Hosp, 1650 av Cedar, Montreal QC H3G 1A4; Lausanne (Switzerland)'62; CSPQ; FRCPC; MedBiochem (Endocrinology). Staff, McGill University Health Centre - Montreal General Campus; assoc Prof Med, McGill University; (514)934-1934 x42780

ALEYKINA, Natalya O; 12 West St, Corner Brook NL A2H 2Y8; Zaporizhzhya (Ukraine)'00; MD; CCFP; Staff, Western Memorial Regional Hospital; (709)637-5000; Fax. (709)634-5577; aleykina@gmail.com.

ALFALAH, Ibrahim M; 309-505 Main St, Airdrie AB T4B 3K3; Al-Fateh (Libya)'96; MB ChB; CCFP; (403)945-0770

ALFAYADH, Ridhab A B R; Niagara HS-Greater Niagara Gen, 5546 Portage Rd, Niagara Falls ON L2E 6X2; Baghdad (Iraq)'93; CCFP; CCFP(E.M.); Staff, Niagara Health System - Greater Niagara General Site; (905)378-4647

ALFIERI, Joanne; MUHC-Montreal Gen Hosp, D5.400-1650 av Cedar, Montreal QC H3G 1A4; McG'04; FRCPC; RadOncol. Staff, McGill University Health Centre - Montreal General Campus; (514)934-8040; Fax. (514)934-8425.

ALFLLOUSE, Atya; Royal Alexandra Hosp, 10240 Kingsway NW, Edmonton AB T5H 3V9; (Libya)'94; FRCSC; Neursurg. Staff, Royal Alexandra Hospital; (780)491-0036

ALFRED, Premini C P; Malvern Med Arts Bldg, 100-1333 Neilson Rd, Scarborough ON M1B 4Y9; Jaffna (Sri Lanka)'84; CCFP; FCFP; (416)291-7719; Fax. (416)287-3775.

ALGARIANI, Tarek G M; Lessard Med Clinic, 6633 177 ST NW, Edmonton AB T5T 4K3; (780)757-7999; Fax. (780)757-7991.

ALGER, Sheryl; Kootenay Lake Hosp, 410-3 View St, Nelson BC V1L 2V1; McM'03; FRCSC; ObstGyn. Staff, Kootenay Lake General Hospital; (250)352-1122; Fax. (250)352-1183; sheryl.alger@interiorhealth.ca.

ALGHALYINI, Baraa M K; 199-3044 Bloor St W, Etobicoke ON M8X 2Y8; Riyadh (Saudi Arabia)'99; CCFP.

ALGHAMDI, Hassan U; Queen Elizabeth II HSC, 1276 South Park St, Halifax NS B3H 2Y9; Abha (Saudi Arabia)'04; MB BS; Staff, Queen Elizabeth II Health Sciences Centre - Victoria General Site; (902)473-2700

ALGHAMDI, Khalid H S; London HSC-University Hosp, PO Box 5339 Stn Main B2 194-339 Windermere Rd, London ON N6A 5A5; King Abdul Aziz University (Saudi Arabia)'03; Staff, London Health Sciences Centre - University Hospital; (519)685-8300

ALGHAMDI, Mohammad S; Child Psychiatry Associates, 407-11044 51 Ave NW, Edmonton AB T6H 5B4; Jeddah (Saudi Arabia)'02; FRCPC; Psy (Child & Adolescent Psychiatry). (780)438-6181; Fax. (780)437-3499.

ALGHAMDI, Mohammed; The Hosp for Sick Children, 555 University Ave, Toronto ON M5G 1X8; Riyadh (Saudi Arabia)'00; Cardiol; Peds. Staff, The Hospital For Sick Children; (416)813-7467

ALGIE, Robert I; Nelson Med Prof Corp, 301 Victoria Ave, Fort Frances ON P9A 2C1; Qns'80; CCFP; FCFP; Staff, La Verendrye Hospital - Riverside Health Care Facility; Liaison, Occupational Health & Safety; (807)274-3287; Fax. (807)274-7882.

ALGIRD, Almunder R R; Hamilton HS-General Site, 237 Barton St E, Hamilton ON L8L 2X2; Al-Fateh (Libya)'99; FRCSC; Neursurg. Staff, Hamilton Health Sciences Centre - Hamilton General Hospital; (905)527-4322; Fax. (905)521-0578.

ALGOM, David; Greenbank Med Centre, 105-139 Greenbank Rd, Nepean ON K2H 9A5; Hebrew (Israel)'64; FRCPC; ClinImmunol&Allergy (Allergic Respiratory Syndrome). Clin Assoc Prof Med, University of Ottawa; Langs: Hebrew; French; Russian; Bulgarian; (613)828-8611; Fax. (613)733-0505.

ALGU, Kemchand; Synergy Wellness Centre, 221-501 Bethel Dr, Sherwood Park AB T8H 0N2; Natal (South Africa)'79; MB ChB; CCFP; Assoc Staff, Alberta Mental Health Board-Ponoka Site; (780)464-0123; kemalgu@hotmail.com.

ALGUACIL-GARCIA, Antonio; Sudbury Reg Hosp-SJHC, 700 Paris St, Sudbury ON P3E 3B5; Madrid (Spain)'69; AnatPath. Staff, Health Sciences North-St Joseph's Health Centre; (705)523-7100 x1642

ALGUNDI, Abdullah A Y; Fox Creek Med Clinic, PO BOX 640 600 3 St, Fox Creek AB T0H 1P0; (780)662-3010; Fax. (780)622-4169.

ALGUWAIHES, Abdullah M A; Main Health Clinic, 301-294 Main St, Toronto ON M4C 4X5; Riyadh (Saudi Arabia)'02; FRCPC; IntMed; Endocrin&Metab. (416)693-3030; Fax. (416)693-3033.

ALHADDAD, Mohamed O; 309-505 Main St SW, Airdrie AB T4B 3K3; (403)945-0770; Fax. (403)945-8997.

ALHAJ IMHMED, Hasan A M; 17719 98A Ave NW, Edmonton AB T5T 5W8; (Libya) MB BCh; (780)481-5555; Fax. (780)487-5666.

ALHARBI, Abdulrahman M F; Red Deer Reg Hosp Centre, 3942 50A Ave, Red Deer AB T4N 4E7; Jeddah (Saudi Arabia)'00; FRCPC; IntMed; Cardiol. Staff, Red Deer Regional Hospital Centre; (780)735-6833

ALHARBI, Fawaz S D; Mount Sinai Hosp, 600 University Ave, Toronto ON M5G 1X5; Riyadh (Saudi Arabia)'03; FRCPC; DiagRad. Staff, Mount Sinai Hospital; (416)596-4200

ALHEIT, Berthold; Victoria Hosp, PO Box 3000 Stn Main 1200 24th St W, Prince Albert SK S6V 5T4; Staff, Victoria Hospital; (306)765-6200; Fax. (306)756-6224.

ALHERBISH, Aws J A; Grey Nuns Community Hosp & HC, 1100 Youville Drive West NW, Edmonton AB T6L 5X8; (Saudi Arabia)'06; IntMed. Staff, Covenant Health - Grey Nuns Community Hospital; (780)735-7000

ALHOZALI, Hanadi; Univ of Western Ontario, M106-1151 Richmond St, London ON N6A 5C1; Jeddah (Saudi Arabia)'02; FRCPC; IntMed; Nephrol. Teach Staff, University of Western Ontario.

ALHUJAIRI, Mohammed; Palliser Health Authority, 666 5 St SW, Medicine Hat AB T1A 4H6; King Faisal University (Saudi Arabia)'00; FRCPC; Anes. (403)529-8998

ALHULAIMI, Naji M A; University of Alberta Hosp, 2C2WCM-8440 112 St NW, Edmonton AB T6G 2B7; King Faisal (Saudi Arabia)'94; FRCPC; IntMed; Cardiol. Staff Mazankowski Alberta Heart Institute, University of Alberta Hospital; Langs: Arabic; (780)407-3990; Fax. (780)407-6452.

ALHUSAYEN, Ra'ed O S; Sunnybrook Hlth Sciences Ctre, M1 700-2075 Bayview Ave, Toronto ON M4N 3M5; Riyadh (Saudi Arabia)'01; FRCPC; Derm. Fellow, Sunnybrook Health Sciences Centre; (416)480-6100

ALI, Abdalla M; Children's Hosp, 840 Sherbrook St, Winnipeg MB R3A 1S1; FRCPC; Peds.

ALI, Abdulhafid O; East Tower, 201-1615 Dundas St E, Whitby ON L1N 2L1; Tripoli (Libya)'80; MB ChB; FRCSC; OrthSurg (Arthroscopy). (905)404-9055

ALI, Abdullah; McMaster University, MDCL 3113-1200 Main St W, Hamilton ON L8N 3Z5; (Kuwait)'01; FRCSC; GenSurg (Pediatric General Surgery). Teach Staff, McMaster University.

ALI, Adib S; North Hamilton Comm Health Ctr, 438 Hughson St N, Hamilton ON L8L 4N5; McM'08; CCFP; (905)523-6611; Fax. (905)523-8735.

ALI, Alaa H; Horizon Square Med Centre, 3508 32 AVE NE, Calgary AB T1Y 6J2; (403)291-5599; Fax. (403)250-6730.

ALI, Amjad; Northgate Medi Clinic, 489 Albert St N, Regina SK S4R 3C3; St George's (Grenada)'93; (306)924-4727; Fax. (306)924-4729.

ALI, Amna; Parkland Med Associates, 205-505 Queen St, Spruce Grove AB T7X 2V2; (South Africa)'92; (780)962-2001; Fax. (780)962-8176.

ALI, Asim; The Hosp for Sick Children, 555 University Ave, Toronto ON M5G 1X8; Tor'99; FRCSC; Ophth. Staff, The Hospital For Sick Children; Langs: Urdu; (416)813-7190; asim.ali@sickkids.ca.

ALI, Asma; Hamilton Reg Cancer Centre, 699 Concession St, Hamilton ON L8V 5C2; Riyadh (Saudi Arabia)'99; MedOncol; IntMed. Staff, Hamilton Regional Cancer Centre; (905)387-9711; Fax. (905)575-6326.

ALI, Asser A A; Arnprior Family Hlth Team, 157-346 John St N, Arnprior ON K7S 2P6; Alexandria (Egypt)'05; CCFP; (613)623-8966; Fax. (613)623-0143.

ALI, Azra; North York Gen Hosp, 4001 Leslie St, North York ON M2K 1E1; Mem'97; CCFP; CCFP(E.M.); Staff, North York General Hospital; (416)756-6000

ALI, Durya; Bowmanville Prof Bldg, 302-222 King St E, Bowmanville ON L1C 1P6; Karachi (Pakistan)'97; CCFP; Staff, Lakeridge Health - Bowmanville Site; Langs: Urdu; (905)697-8282; Fax. (905)697-7745.

ALI, Ebtihal A; Women's Hosp, WS012-735 Notre Dame Ave, Winnipeg MB R3E 0L8.

ALI, Fadhil S; Deerfoot Meadows Med Clinic, 7979 11 St SE, Calgary AB T2H 0B8; (Iraq)'89; CCFP; Langs: Arabic; (403)251-2690; Fax. (403)251-2695.

ALI, Fahim H; Med Associates of Port Perry, 462 Paxton St, Port Perry ON L9L 1L9; Qns'01; CCFP; Staff Anes, Lakeridge Health - Port Perry Site; Staff Anes, Ross Memorial Hospital; Langs: Hindi; Urdu; (905)985-2895; Fax. (905)985-3464.

ALI, Faizal H; 476 Palmerston Blvd, Toronto ON M6G 2P1; Man'88; BSc(Med); FRCPC; Psy (Psychoanalysis). Staff Pt-Time Psy, Centre for Addiction & Mental Health (CAMH) - Queen Site; (416)588-8681; Fax. (416)583-1263; f.ali@utoronto.ca.

ALI, Fareed A; Ophtalmic Consultant Center, 1880 Sismet Rd, Mississauga ON L4W 1W9; Tor'92; FRCSC; Ophth. Physician, Ophtalmic Consultant Centres Inc; (905)212-9482 x232; Fax. (905)212-1012.

ALI, Farzan; 300A-18 Kensington Rd, Brampton ON L6T 4S5; Man'05; FRCSC; GenSurg. Staff, Hamilton Health Sciences Centre - Hamilton General Hospital; (905)497-8844; Fax. (905)801-9911.

ALI, Fatima; 102-16703 82 St NW, Edmonton AB T5Z 0H5; (Pakistan)'03; (780)457-7142; Fax. (780)457-7152.

ALI, Ghassan H; Grand Bank Community Hlth Ctre, PO Box 310, Grand Bank NL A0E 1W0; Mosul (Iraq)'94; MB ChB; Staff, Grand Bank Health Centre; (709)832-2500

ALI, Habeeb T; Alpen Med Clinic, 346 Railway St W, Cochrane AB T4C 2E2; (Nigeria)'92; (403)851-0091; Fax. (403)851-9958.

ALI, Haider; Humber River Reg Hosp-Finch, 2111 Finch Ave W, North York ON M3N 1N1; Baghdad (Iraq)'95; CCFP; Staff, Humber River Regional Hospital - Finch Avenue Site; (416)744-2500

ALI, Hira; Sherwood Park Medicentre, 101 Bremner Dr, Sherwood Park AB T8H 0M5; (780)467-4717

ALI, Humaira H; Old Quebec Street Mall, 208-55 Wyndham St N, Guelph ON N1H 7T8; Peshawar (Pakistan)'93; CCFP; (519)837-2283; Fax. (519)767-2262.

ALI, Idris M; Queen Elizabeth II HSC-Halifax, 2265-1796 Summer St, Halifax NS B3H 3A7; Garyunis (Libya)'79; FRC; FRCSC; GenSurg (Cardiac Surgery); Cardiovasc&ThorSurg. Staff Cardiovasc Surg, Queen Elizabeth II Health Sciences Centre - Victoria General Site; Staff, Queen Elizabeth II Health Sciences Centre - Halifax Infirmary Site; Prof Surg, Dalhousie University; (902)473-2116; Fax. (902)473-4448; idris.ali@dal.ca.

ALI, Iftikhar; Univ of Ottawa Heart Institute, 40 Ruskin St, Ottawa ON K1Y 4W7; Punjab (India)'92; Staff, University of Ottawa Heart Institute.

ALI, Imtiaz S; Foothills Med Centre, C831-1403 29 St NW, Calgary AB T2N 2T9; Dal'88; BSc(Hons); FRCSC; GenSurg (Cardio & Thoracic Surgery); CardiothorSurg. Staff, Foothills Medical Centre; (403)944-1090; Fax. (403)944-2906; imtiaz.ali@dal.ca.

ALI, Jameel; 402-55 Queen St E, Toronto ON M5C 1R6; Man'66; FACS; MMed(Ed.); FRCSC; GenSurg. Staff, St Michael's Hospital; Dir Postgrad Education Dept of Surg, University of Toronto; (416)864-6019; Fax. (416)864-6008; ali@smh.toronto.on.ca.

ALI, Javed E; 465 George St, Sydney NS B1P 1K5; Karachi (Pakistan)'78; FRCPC; Psy. Staff, Cape Breton Healthcare Complex; (902)539-6300

ALI, Karim F; Niagara H System-Ontario St, 155 Ontario St, St. Catharines ON L2R 5K3; Staff, Niagara Health System - Ontario Street Site; (905)378-4647

ALI, Karima M; The Doctor's Office, B-4701 130 Ave SE, Calgary AB T2Z 4J2; (Ireland)'98; BSc; MB BCh; BAO; LRCP; LMCC; CCFP; Langs: Gujarati; French; Urdu; (403)232-1000; Fax. (403)257-6353.

ALI, Kevin; Royal Victoria Reg Hlth Ctr, 201 Georgian Dr, Barrie ON L4N 1G4; (Other Foreign)'08; CCFP; Staff, Royal Victoria Regional Health Centre; (705)728-9802

ALI, Khaled; The Hosp for Sick Children, 602-555 University Ave, Toronto ON M5G 1X8; (Ireland)'06; Peds.

ALI, Khan; Rockyview Gen Hosp, 7007 14 St SW, Calgary AB T2V 1P9; RCS (Ireland)'93; FRCPC; IntMed. Staff, Rockyview General Hospital; (403)943-3000

ALI, Liaqat; Royal Victoria Hosp, 201 Georgian Dr, Barrie ON L4M 6M2; Punjab (Pakistan)'75; MB BS; DPM; MRCPsy; FRCPC; Psy (General Adult Psychiatry). Staff, Royal Victoria Regional Health Centre; Langs: Persian; Urdu; Hindi; (705)728-9802 x4452; Fax. (705)739-5631.

ALI, M Ben; Manitoba Clinic, 790 Sherbrook St, Winnipeg MB R3A 1M3; (Jamaica)'80; MB BS; BSc; FRCSC; PlasSurg. Assoc Staff, Seven Oaks General Hospital; (204)774-6541; Fax. (204)775-6373.

ALI, Iqbal; Surrey Mem Hosp, 13750 96 Ave, Surrey BC V3V 1Z2; Karnatak (India)'63; FCCP; FRCPC; IntMed. Staff, Surrey Memorial Hospital; Langs: Hindi; Urdu; (604)581-2211

ALI, Madi M M; Hamilton HS-McMaster Site, PO Box 2000 Stn Lcd 1 248-1200 Main St W, Hamilton ON L8N 3Z5; Al-Arab (Libya)'93; FRCPC; Anes; Critical Care Medicine. Staff, Hamilton Health Sciences Centre - McMaster University Medical Centre; (905)521-2100

ALI, Maqsood; Millwoods Medicentre, 6426 28 Ave NW, Edmonton AB T6L 6N3; (Pakistan)'88; Staff, Covenant Health - Misericordia Community Hospital; (780)462-3491; Fax. (780)461-2650.

ALI, Massud A A; Regina Internal Med Specialist, 1821 Rose St, Regina SK S4P 1Z7; Al Arab (Libya)'99; FRCPC; IntMed; Gastroent. (306)525-2405

ALI, Michael; Courtice Health Centre, 3F-1450 Highway 2, Courtice ON L1E 3C3; (Guyana)'94; CCFP; (905)721-6154; Fax. (905)721-6190.

ALI, Mohamed J; Mackenzie Richmond Hill Hosp, 10 Trench St, Richmond Hill ON L4C 4Z3; Ott'82; FRCPC; Anes (Anesthesia & Critical Care). Staff, Mackenzie Richmond Hill Hospital; (905)883-2110

ALI, Mohamed; 163 First Ave, Welland ON L3C 1Y5; Mem'76; BSc; Med Dir, Woodlands of Sunset; (905)735-6693; Fax. (905)735-0188.

ALI, Molud A; Deloraine Medical Clinic, PO Box 429, Deloraine MB R0M 0M0.

ALI, Muhammad; The Hosp for Sick Children, 555 University Ave, Toronto ON M5G 1X8; Balochistan (Pakistan)'98; Staff, The Hospital For Sick Children; (416)813-7742

ALI, Nabeel; MUHC-Royal Victoria Hosp, C7.68-687 av des Pins O, Montreal QC H3A 1A1; Mon'00; FRCPC; Peds (Neonatology). Staff Neonatologist, McGill University Health Centre - Royal Victoria Hospital; Langs: German; Bengali; (514)934-1934 x34876; Fax. (514)843-1741; nabeel.ali@mcgill.ca.

ALI, Naheed S; St Michael's Hosp, 30 Bond St, Toronto ON M5B 1W8; Punjab (Pakistan)'78; FRCPC; IntMed (Acute Coronary Care); Cardiol. Staff, St Michael's Hospital; (416)360-4000

ALI, Naved A; 101-1001 Broadway Ave W, Vancouver BC V6H 4E4; Alb'87; CCFP; Staff, BC Mental Health & Addiction Service; Staff, Sleeping Sotones Addiction Day Program; Staff, Physician Health Program of BC; (604)822-7121

ALI, Parveen S; 9820 101 Ave, Fort St. John BC V1J 2B2; Sir Salimullah (Bangladesh)'98; (250)787-1123

ALI, Pervez; Centric Health Atria 1, W300-2255 Sheppard Ave E, North York ON M2J 4Y1; McM'90; BSc; DAB; FRCSC; OrthSurg (Hip & Knee Reconstruction). Ac Staff, The Scarborough Hospital - General Campus; Ac Staff, The Scarborough Hospital - Birchmount Campus; Langs: Hindi; Urdu; (416)495-9902; Fax. (416)445-8692.

ALI, Rafaqat; The Malone Med Clinic, 4955 41 Ave, Drayton Valley AB T7A 1V4; (India)'85; (780)542-3366; Fax. (780)542-6207.

ALI, Rizwan; Family Med Clinic, 120-15277 Castledowns Rd NW, Edmonton AB T5X 3N5; (780)457-5511; Fax. (780)456-4004.

ALI, S Kaiser; Saskatoon Cancer Centre, 20 Campus Dr, Saskatoon SK S7N 4H4; Dacca (Bangladesh)'80; FAAP; MB BS; FRCPC; Peds (Pediatric Hematology Oncology). Staff, Saskatoon Cancer Centre; Leader Ped Oncology Program, Saskatchewan Cancer Agency; Head Div of Ped HemOncol/Clin Prof Pediatrics & Oncology, University of Saskatchewan; (306)655-2742; Fax. (306)655-2639; kaiser.ali@saskcancer.ca.

ALI, S Nasir; 168 Essex St, Sarnia ON N7T 4R9; Karachi (Pakistan)'81; MRC(UK); MRC(Dublin); FRCPC; IntMed (Cardiology). Med Dir Medicine Prog, Bluewater Health - Mitton Site; Ac Staff, Bluewater Health - Norman Site; (519)337-7535; Fax. (519)337-7536.

ALI, Salah-Eddin; Brampton Med Plex, 10-27 Ruth Ave, Brampton ON L6Z 4R2; Debrecen (Hungary)'93; CCFP; (905)495-5888; Fax. (905)495-5822.

ALI, Samana; Royal Alexandra Hosp, 5027-10240 Kingsway NW, Edmonton AB T5H 3V9; Karachi (Pakistan)'96; Staff, Royal Alexandra Hospital; (780)735-4647

ALI, Samia H A; Kingston Gen Hosp, 76 Stuart St, Kingston ON K7L 2V7; Khartoum (Sudan)'99; FRCPC; Anes. (613)548-7827

ALI, Samina; Edmonton Clinic Health Academy, 3 512-11405 87 Ave NW, Edmonton AB T6G 1C9; McG'96; FRCPC; Peds; PedEmergMed. Staff, University of Alberta Hospital; Staff, Edmonton Clinic Health Academy; (780)248-5575; Fax. (780)248-5626.

ALI, Syed A; 2727 2nd Ave W, Prince Albert SK S6V 5E5; Karachi (Pakistan)'94; ABIM; FRCPC; IntMed. Staff Internist, Yorkton Regional Health Centre; Staff, Prince Albert Parkland Health Region; (306)764-2870; Fax. (306)764-2873.

ALI, Syed A; Lymburm Med Centre, 7526 178 St NW, Edmonton AB T5T 2Y5; Decca (Bangladesh)'54; DCP(Lond); MRC; FRCP; Langs: Bengali; Urdu; Hindi; (780)481-2076; Fax. (780)481-1380.

ALI, Syed T; London HSC-University Hosp, PO Box 5339 Stn B 339 Windermere Rd, London ON N6A 5A5; Karachi (Pakistan)'03; GenSurg. Staff, London Health Sciences Centre - University Hospital; (519)685-8500

ALI, Syed Z; Cape Breton Hlthcare Complex, 1482 George St, Sydney NS B1P 1P3; Karachi (Pakistan)'98; Staff, Cape Breton Healthcare Complex; (902)567-8000

ALI, Taghreed H; Burin Peninsula Health Care Ct, PO Box 340, Burin NL A0E 1E0; Baghdad (Iraq)'95; MB BS; CCFP; Staff, Burin Peninsula Health Care Centre; (709)891-1040

ALI, Tahmeena T; 101A-2099 152 St, Surrey BC V4A 4N7; Man'00; BSc; CCFP; (604)538-5770

ALI, Tehmina K; Altona Clinic, PO Box 999, Altona MB R0G 0B0.

ALI, Vasima; Finch East Med Centre, 201-3850 Finch Ave E, Scarborough ON M1T 3T6; Jawahar Lal (India)'70; Ac Staff, The Scarborough Hospital - Birchmount Campus; Assoc Staff, North York General Hospital; Langs: Urdu; (416)298-2988; Fax. (416)298-3140.

ALI, Yaser M A; 4 The Market Place, East York ON M4C 5M1; Kuwait (Kuwait)'99; MSc; ABIM; MD; CDD; FRCPC; IntMed; ClinImmunol&Allergy; Rheum. Langs: Arabic; (416)690-1357; yaser.ali@utoronto.ca.

ALI, Yasmin; Eagle Ridge Med Clinic, 102-1173 The High St, Coquitlam BC V3B 0B1; Karachi (Pakistan)'83; MB BS; CCFP; FCFP; Med Staff, Royal Columbian Hospital; Med Staff, Eagle Ridge Hospital & Health Care Centre; Langs: Urdu; Hindi; Gujarati; (604)945-0032; Fax. (604)945-4739.

ALI AL-KAZELY, Luay H; Plains Med Center, 141 Plains Rd W, Burlington ON L7T 1G1; Baghdad (Iraq)'01; MB ChB; CCFP; (905)218-6444; Fax. (905)521-2775.

ALI MAJID, Nadia; Able-Care Med Clinic, 56-2991 Lougheed Hwy, New Westminster BC V3B 6J6; (Iraq)'95; (604)945-7819; Fax. (604)945-2884.

ALI NEJAD, Shahrokh; Virden Med Clinic, PO Box 730 455 Frame St, Virden MB R0M 2C0; (204)748-1345; Fax. (204)748-1640.

ALI-RIDHA, Nihad H; Lakeridge Hlth Corp-Oshawa, 1 Hospital Crt, Oshawa ON L1G 2B9; Baghdad (Iraq)'73; MB ChB; ABPath; FRCPC; AnatPath (Forensic Pathology). Staff LabMed, Lakeridge Health - Oshawa Site; Langs: Turkish; Arabic; (905)576-8711 x4277; Fax. (905)721-4757; naliridha@lakeridgehealth.on.ca.

ALIABADI, Hossein; Grand Manan Hosp, 196 Route 776, Grand Manan NB E5G 1A3; Mashhad (Iran)'92; Staff, Grand Manan Hospital; (506)662-4060

ALIBHAI, Haneef N; MD Cosmetic & Laser Clinic, 107-2051 McCallum Rd, Abbotsford BC V2S 3N5; McG'93; BSc; CCFP; FCFP; Clin Instructor Med, University of British Columbia; (604)557-7777; Fax. (604)557-7778; doctor@mdcosmetic.ca.

ALIBHAI, Karim N; Surgicorp Inc, 205-3017 66 St NW, Edmonton AB T6K 4B2; Alb'94; FRCSC; GenSurg; VascSurg. (780)461-6012; Fax. (780)461-5442.

ALIBHAI, Malyha; Victoria East Medical Clinic, 2068 Prince of Wales Dr, Regina SK S4V 3A6; (Other Foreign)'10; CCFP; (306)789-4677; Fax. (306)789-3422.

ALIBHAI, Nasimbanu S; Northgate Med Centre, 2711 Avonhurst Dr, Regina SK S4R 3J3; Man'80; (306)543-4566; Fax. (306)543-4441.

ALIBHAI, Shabbir M H; Univ Hlth Network-Toronto Gen, EN14 214-200 Elizabeth St, Toronto ON M5G 2C4; Tor'93; MSc; FRCPC; IntMed; GeriatricMed. Staff Physician, Mount Sinai Hospital; Consultant, Toronto Rehabilitation Institute - University Centre; Staff Physician, Toronto General Hospital - UHN; Langs: Gujarati.

ALIDINA, Diamond F H; 6B-1450 Kingston Rd, Pickering ON L1V 1C1; Makerere (Uganda)'71; Court Staff, Lakeridge Health - Oshawa Site; Ac Staff, Rouge Valley Health System - Ajax & Pickering Health Centre Site; (905)831-8333; Fax. (905)831-8858.

ALIDINA, Parviz D F; Pickering Urgent Care Practice, 6B-1450 Kingston Rd, Pickering ON L1V 1C1; Makerere (Uganda)'71; MB ChB; Court Staff, Lakeridge Health - Oshawa Site; Assoc Staff, Rouge Valley Health System - Ajax & Pickering Health Centre Site; (905)831-8333; Fax. (905)831-8858.

ALIDINA, Zahra; Pickering Medicenter, 6B-1450 Kingston Rd, Pickering ON L1V 1C1; Wes'01; CCFP; (905)831-8333; Fax. (905)831-8858.

ALIJA, Agron; South Western Med Centre, 813 Richmond St, London ON N6A 3H6; Pristina (Serbia)'98; CCFP; (519)433-4330; Fax. (519)433-4332.

ALIKHAN, Neetan; Markham Stoufville Urgent Care, 100-110 Copper Creek Dr, Markham ON L6B 0P9; Wes'99; CCFP; CCFP(E.M.); (905)472-8911; Fax. (905)472-6081.

ALIKHAN, Qasim R; West Ottawa Sleep Centre, 303-770 Broadview Ave, Ottawa ON K2A 3Z3; Wes'97; FRCPC; IntMed (Sleep Medicine); Respir. (613)722-9900; Fax. (613)722-9100.

ALIKHAN, Riyaaz; William Osler HC-Brampton, 2100 Bovaird Dr E, Brampton ON L6R 3J7; Ott'03; CCFP; CCFP(E.M.); Staff, William Osler Health System - Brampton Civic Hospital; (905)494-2120

ALIKHANI, Katayoun; South Health Campus, 480009-4448 Front St SE, Calgary AB T3M 1M4; Tehran (Iran)'92; Staff, Foothills Medical Centre; (403)956-2461; Fax. (403)956-2992.

ALIKOUZEHGARAN, Maryam; Alberta Hosp Edmonton, PO Box 307 Stn Main, Edmonton AB T5J 2J7; Tehran (Iran)'90; FRCPC; Psy. Staff, Alberta Hospital Edmonton; Staff, Edmonton Mental Health Clinic; (780)472-5457; Fax. (780)472-5411.

ALIMA, Limor H; Meadowlark Prof Bldg, 302-8702 Meadowlark Rd NW, Edmonton AB T5R 5W5; McM'93; CCFP; (780)487-5333; Fax. (780)487-3045.

ALIMENTI, Ariane; BC Women's Hosp & Health Ctre, E 600B-4500 Oak St, Vancouver BC V6H 3N1; Brussels (Belgium)'85; Clinical Asst Prof, BC Women's Hospital & Health Centre; Langs: Bilingual(French/English); Italian; Spanish; (604)875-2212; Fax. (604)875-3063; aalimenti@cw.bc.ca.

ALIMORADI, Ima; St Paul's Hosp, 9B-1081 Burrard St, Vancouver BC V6Z 1Y6; Tehran (Iran)'99; FRCPC; IntMed; GeriatricMed. Staff, Providence Health Care - St Paul's Hospital; (604)806-8029

ALIPIO, Al D S; 403-849 Upper Wentworth S, Hamilton ON L9A 5H4; Santo Tomas (Philippines)'01; CCFP; (905)388-5996

ALIPOUR MILAJERDI, Shahryar; Barrie Memorial Hosp, 28 rue Gale, Ormstown QC J0S 1K0; Tehran (Iran)'95; CCFP; CCFP(E.M.); Staff, Barrie Memorial Hospital; (450)829-2321

ALISHARAN, Robert M; Surrey Med Arts Bldg, 103-13710 94A Ave, Surrey BC V3V 1N1; West Indies (Jamaica)'72; MB BS; DCH; FRCPC; Peds. Consultant Peds, Surrey Memorial Hospital; (604)583-7070; Fax. (604)582-5536.

ALITER, Hashem F; Queen Elizabeth II HSC-Halifax, 2006-1796 Summer St, Halifax NS B3H 3A7; Ufa (Russia (Federation))'98; MD; Staff, Queen Elizabeth II Health Sciences Centre - Halifax Infirmary Site; (902)473-7890; Fax. (902)473-7149.

ALIU, Teuta; Lincoln Med Centre, 4413 Ontario St, Beamsville ON L0R 1B5; University of Pristina (Kosovo)'98; CCFP; Att Physician, West Lincoln Memorial Hospital; (905)563-1212; Fax. (905)563-4404.

ALIU-BERISHA, Shpresa; Stone Church, 1475 Upper Ottawa St, Hamilton ON L8W 3J6; Pristina (Serbia)'98; CCFP; (905)575-1300

ALIZADEH-EBADI, Mahmoud; 401-7900 Hurontario St, Brampton ON L6Y 0P6; Tabriz University (Other Foreign)'93; FRCSC; Ophth. (905)456-9500; Fax. (905)456-9508.

ALIZADEH-KHIAVI, Kamel; 409 8 Ave NE, Calgary AB T2E 0R3; Wes'97; CCFP; Langs: Turkish; Azeri; Farsi; (403)276-8711

ALIZADEHFAR, Reza; MUHC-Montreal Gen Hosp, 2300 rue Tupper, Montreal QC H3H 1P3; Mon'98; ClinImmunol&Allergy; Peds. Staff, McGill University Health Centre - Montreal Children's Hospital; (514)412-4400 x24470; reza.alizadehfar@muhc.mcgill.ca.

ALIZADEHRANJBAR, Keysun; Hys Centre, 350-11010 101 St NW, Edmonton AB T5H 4B9; (Iran)'95; Staff, Royal Alexandra Hospital; (780)428-3246; Fax. (780)425-0487.

ALJADA, Ibrahim S; Health Sciences Centre, 820 Sherbrook St, Winnipeg MB R3A 1R9; Amman (Jordan)'93; MB BS; FRCPC; AnatPath (Cytopath). Asst Prof Path, Health Sciences Centre; Asst Prof Family Med, University of Manitoba; (204)787-2036; ialjada@hsc.mb.ca.

ALJADI, Alhadi A M; 11408 Jasper Ave, Edmonton AB T5K 0M1; (Libya)'00; CCFP; (780)488-4242

ALJAFARI, AlHassan K; Corydon Medical Clinic, 894 Corydon Ave, Winnipeg MB R3M 0Y4; Al-Fateh(Libya) (Libya)'98; CCFP; Staff, Gimli Community Health Centre (Johnson Memorial Hospital).

ALJEHANI, Yasser; Queen Elizabeth II HSC, 8 845-1276 South Park St, Halifax NS B3H 2Y9; Dammam (Saudi Arabia)'02; MD; Staff, Queen Elizabeth II Health Sciences Centre - Victoria General Site; (902)473-7015; Fax. (902)473-4442.

ALKENBRACK, J Douglas; Richmond Med Centre, 307 Bridge St W, Napanee ON K7R 2G3; Qns'70; Att Staff, Lennox & Addington County General Hospital; Med Dir, J M Parral Home for the Aged; Coroner, Province of Ontario; (613)354-1779; Fax. (613)354-6992.

ALKHALAF, Sarah G A; 2-12287 Tenth Line, Stouffville ON L4A 0Y1; Basra (Iraq)'95; CCFP; (905)642-7008; Fax. (905)642-7009.

ALKHATER, Reem A A; The Hosp for Sick Children, RCH 6526-555 University Ave, Toronto ON M5G 1X8; Dammam (Saudi Arabia)'00; FRCPC; Neur.

ALKHERAYF, Fahad A E; The Ottawa Hosp-Civic Campus, C2R-1053 Carling Ave, Ottawa ON K1Y 4E9; Riyadh (Saudi Arabia)'01; FRCSC; Neursurg. Staff, The Ottawa Hospital - Civic Campus; (613)797-1239

ALKON MINTSOPOULOS, Sultana; Rouge Valley-Centenary HC, 2867 Ellesmere Rd, Scarborough ON M1E 4B9; Uzbekistan (Russia (Federation))'90; Staff, Rouge Valley Health System - Centenary Health Centre Site; (416)284-4894

ALKUDMANI, Amer S B; Univ Hlth Network-Toronto Western Hosp, 399 Bathurst St, Toronto ON M5T 2S8; Riyadh (Saudi Arabia)'00; FRCSC; PlasSurg. Staff, Toronto Western Hospital - University Health Network; (416)603-5790

ALLABY, Cheryl L; Hamilton HS-Juravinski Site, 711 Concession St, Hamilton ON L8V 1C3; McM'93; BSc(PT); CCFP; FCFP; Staff, Hamilton Health Sciences Centre-Juravinski Site; (905)521-2100

ALLABY, Leslie; 84 Dufferin Ave, Saint John NB E2K 2T8; Mem'85; (506)634-7374; Fax. (506)634-7378.

ALLADIN, Lenny C; Complexe Sante Reine-Elizabeth, 549-2100 av De Marlowe, Montreal QC H4A 3L5; McG'78; BSc; pers Médecin, St Mary's Hospital Centre; McGill University; Langs: English; French; (514)484-8331; Fax. (514)484-1223.

ALLADINA, Salima J A; Foothills Med Centre, 1403 29 St NW, Calgary AB T2N 2T9; UBC'08; CCFP; CCFP(E.M.); Staff, Foothills Medical Centre; (403)944-1110

ALLAIN, Dominic; Edmonton Clinic Health Academy, 11405 87 Ave NW, Edmonton AB T6G 1C9; Dal'03; FRCPC; Peds; PedEmergMed. Staff, University of Alberta Hospital; Staff, Edmonton Clinic Health Academy; (780)248-5575; Fax. (780)248-5626.

ALLAIN, Melanie; Health Centre, 33 rue Main, Rexton NB E4W 0E5; Sher'10; CCFP.

ALLAIN, Suzanne M; Lakehead Psychiatric Hosp, PO Box 2930 Stn P 580 Algoma St N, Thunder Bay ON P7B 5G4; Tor'88; FRCPC; Psy. Psychiatrist, Lakehead Psychiatric Hospital - St. Joseph's Care Group; Reg Dir Psy West, Northern Ontario School of Medicine-Laurentian University; (807)343-4300; Fax. (807)343-4361; allains@tbh.net.

ALLAIRE, Andre; CSSS du Nord de Lanaudière, 1000 boul Sainte-Anne, St-Charles-Brromee QC J6E 6J2; Mon'86; CSPQ; FRCPC; AnatPath. Staff AnatPath, Centre Hospitalier Régional de Lanaudière; Langs: English; (450)759-8222 x2933; andre.allaire.chrdl@ssss.gouv.qc.ca.

ALLAIRE, Catherine; BC Women's Hosp & Health Ctre, F2-4500 Oak St, Vancouver BC V6H 3N1; McG'90; FRCSC; ObstGyn (Infertility). Staff, BC Women's Hospital & Health Centre; Ac Staff, Vancouver General Hospital - Centennial Pavillion; Clin Instructor, University of British Columbia; (604)875-2534

ALLAIRE, Denis; Polyclinique St-Jerome, 305-200 rue Durand, Saint-Jerome QC J7Z 7E2; Mon'71; LMCC; AB; FRCS; Otol. Ac Member, Hôtel-Dieu de Saint-Jérôme; Langs: Bilingual(French/English); (450)565-9898; Fax. (450)565-2702.

ALLAIRE, Guy; CHUM-Hop Notre-Dame, 1560 rue Sherbrooke E, Montreal QC H2L 4M1; Mon'81; CSPQ; FRCPC; AnatPath (Hepatic Pathology). Anatomical Pathology, Centre Hospitalier l'Université de Montréal (CHUM) - Hôpital Notre-Dame; assoc Prof, Universite de Montreal; (514)890-8000 x27024; guy.allaire.chum@ssss.gouv.qc.ca.

ALLAIRE, Jasmine; Children's & Women's HC of BC, 4480 Oak St, Vancouver BC V6H 3N1; McG'07; MDCM; FRCPC; Peds. Staff, BC Women's Hospital & Health Centre; (604)875-2045

ALLAIRE, Sandra L; 150-4311 12 St NE, Calgary AB T2E 4P9; Sask'77; (403)517-6121; Fax. (403)205-8042.

ALLAIRE, Suzanne; Centre d'Urgence St-Laurent, 200-1605 boul Marcel-Laurin, Saint-Laurent QC H4R 0B7; Laval'79; LMCC; (514)747-2555; Fax. (514)747-7624.

ALLAN, Bruce B; Centre For Women Bonavista Sq, 707-12100 Macleod Trail SE, Calgary AB T2J 7G9; Cal'93; FRCSC; ObstGyn. Staff Physician, Rockyview General Hospital; Clinical Asst Prof, University of Calgary; (403)271-2550; Fax. (403)271-4546.

ALLAN, David; The Ottawa Hosp-Gen Campus, 7209-501 Smyth Rd, Ottawa ON K1H 8L6; Qns'97; FRCPC; IntMed; Hem. Staff, The Ottawa Hospital - General Campus; Langs: English; French; (613)737-8899 x71281; Fax. (613)737-8861; daallan@ottawahospital.on.ca.

ALLAN, Donald R; Health Sciences Centre, GE445 B-820 Sherbrook St, Winnipeg MB R3A 1R9; Man'85; FRCPC; IntMed; Nephrol. Staff, Health Sciences Centre; Asst Prof, University of Manitoba; (204)787-3583; Fax. (204)787-3326.

ALLAN, G Michael; North Edmonton Health Centre, 14007 50 St NW, Edmonton AB T5A 5E4; UBC'96; CCFP; FCFP; (780)342-4038; Fax. (780)342-4192.

ALLAN, James P; CSSS du Suroît, 150 rue Saint-Thomas, Salaber-de-Valleyf QC J6T 6C1; Mon'96; FRCPC; MedMicrobiol; InfectDis (P.Q.). Staff, Centre Hospitalier Régional du Suroît; (450)371-9920 x2561

ALLAN, John C; Saint John Reg Hosp, PO Box 2100 Stn Main 400 University Ave, Saint John NB E2L 4L2; Dal'88; FRCPC; DiagRad. Staff, Saint John Regional Hospital; (506)648-6923; Fax. (506)648-6925.

ALLAN, Margaret C; Hinton Med Clinic, 102 Allen Cove, Hinton AB T7V 2A6; Mem'78; BSc; CCFP; Staff, Hinton Healthcare Centre; (780)865-3338; clinic@hintonmedical.com.

ALLAN, Mark A; Medical Clinic 14 Wing, PO Box 5000, Greenwood NS B0P 1N0; Mem'84; (902)765-1494 x1408; Fax. (902)765-1534; allan.ma@forces.gc.ca.

ALLAN, Melissa; Sudbury Reg Hosp-Laurentian, 41 Ramsey Lake Rd, Sudbury ON P3E 5J1; Wes'99; CCFP; CCFP(E.M.); Staff, Health Sciences North-Laurentian Site; (705)523-7300; mallan@gov.nu.ca.

ALLAN, Patricia L; 203-220 Main St, Antigonish NS B2G 2C2; Mem'82; Staff, St Martha's Regional Hospital; (902)863-4070; Fax. (902)863-2575.

ALLAN, Rebecca J; Humber River Reg Hosp-Church, 200 Church St, Toronto ON M9N 1N8; Wes'01; FRCPC; IntMed; Cardiol. Staff, Humber River Regional Hospital - Church Street Site; (416)249-8111

ALLAN, Scott M; 77 Victoria Park Ave, Scarborough ON M4E 3S2; Tor'80; CCFP; Dir FM Residency Prog, The Scarborough Hospital - General Campus; (416)694-8254

ALLAN, Sharon J; BC Cancer Agency-Vanc Isl Ctr, 2410 Lee Ave, Victoria BC V8R 6V5; Alb'79; ABIM; AB; FRCPC; IntMed; MedOncol. Chief MedOncol, BC Cancer Agency Vancouver Island Centre; (250)519-5570

ALLANACH, R William; 123 ch Cap-Brule, Boudreau-Ouest NB E4P 6J2; Dal'68; Assoc Staff, The Moncton Hospital; Assoc Staff, Dr Georges-L-Dumont University Hospital Centre; (506)532-6946; Fax. (506)532-1569.

ALLANACH, William W; Professional Arts Bldg, 621-100 Arden St, Moncton NB E1C 4B7; Dal'97; FRCSC; OrthSurg. Staff, The Moncton Hospital; (506)877-1112; Fax. (506)877-1117.

ALLARD, Andre; Direction de la Sante Publique, 1000 rue Labelle, Saint-Jerome QC J7Z 5N6; Mon'75; Public Health & Preventive Med; CommunMed (P.Q.). Community Med, Hôtel-Dieu de Saint-Jérôme; Langs: Bilingual(English/French); (450)436-8622 x3209; Fax. (450)436-1761; andre_allard@ssss.gouv.qc.ca.

ALLARD, Andree; CSSS de Vaudreuil-Soulanges, 11 ch de la Cite-des-Jeunes, Saint-Polycarpe QC J0P 1X0; Mon'94; (450)265-3771; Fax. (450)265-3556; andree_allard@rrsss16.gouv.qc.ca.

ALLARD, Catherine; CHUS-Hop Fleurimont, 3001 12e av N, Sherbrooke QC J1H 5N4; Mon'03; FRCPC; MedMicrobiol; InfectDis (P.Q.). Staff, Centre Hospitalier Universitaire de Sherbrooke-Hopital Fleurimont; (819)346-1110 x14321

ALLARD, Christian; 114-475 boul Talbot, Chicoutimi QC G7H 4A3; Sher'83; FRCPC; IntMed (Pneumology); Respir. Staff, Complexe hospitalier de la Sagamie; Clin Prof, Universite de Sherbrooke; Clin Prof, Universite de Montreal; (418)549-5987; Fax. (418)549-9948; c.allardmd@videotron.ca.

ALLARD, Denis; Polyclinique St-Jerome, 304-200 rue Durand, Saint-Jerome QC J7Z 7E2; Mon'83; FRCSC; Urol (Urological Oncology). Staff, Hôtel-Dieu de Saint-Jérôme; Langs: Bilingual(French/English); (450)436-7173; Fax. (450)436-3420.

ALLARD, Denis G; Public Health Services, 81 Albert St, Moncton NB E1C 1B3; McG'73; MSc(Epidem); FRCPC; CommunMed (Infectious Diseases); Public Health & Preventive Med. Dep Chief MOH, Moncton Health Region; Dep Chief MOH, Vitalité Health Network Public Health Office Moncton; Langs: English; (506)856-2401; Fax. (506)869-6122.

ALLARD, Francine; Centre de Sante Publique, 2400 av D'Estimauville, Quebec QC G1E 7G9; Mon'72; Staff, Centre Hospitalier Universitaire de Quebec-CHUL; (418)666-7000 x436; Fax. (418)666-2776; francine.allard@ssss.gouv.qc.ca.

ALLARD, Gaston; Clin Med St Felix de Valois, 610 ch Joliette RR 1, St-Felix-de-Valois QC J0K 2M0; Mon'75; Langs: English; (450)889-5577; Fax. (450)889-4239.

ALLARD, Genevieve; CSSS Maria-Chapdelaine, 2000 boul du Sacre-Coeur, Dolbeau-Mistassini QC G8L 2R5; Mon'05; Staff, Centre Maria-Chapdelaine - CH de Dolbeau-Mistassini; (418)276-1234

ALLARD, Jacinthe; Clin Med St Felix de Valois, 610 ch Joliette RR 1, St-Felix-de-Valois QC J0K 2M0; Mon'82; (450)889-5577; Fax. (450)889-4239.

ALLARD, Jacques; Hop Santa Cabrini Ospedale, 5655 rue Saint-Zotique E, Montreal QC H1T 1P7; Laval'72; CSPQ; Anes (P.Q.). Anesthesiste, Hôpital Santa Cabrini Ospedale; (514)252-6582

ALLARD, Jacques; Inst U Geriatrie Sherbrooke, 1036 rue Belvedere S, Sherbrooke QC J1H 4C4; Sher'71; CCFP; FCFP; ac Membre CMDP, CSSS Institut universitaire de gériatrie de Sherbrooke; Prof Dept of Research, Universite de Sherbrooke; (819)780-2220

ALLARD, Jean B; Clinique Med Ste-Colette, 11520 boul Sainte-Colette, Montreal-Nord QC H1G 6J3; Mon'73; (514)323-0430; Fax. (514)328-9643.

ALLARD, Jean-Pascale; CSSS de Chicoutimi, 305 rue Saint-Valier, Chicoutimi QC G7H 5H6; Mon'01; FRCSC; OrthSurg. Staff, Complexe hospitalier de la Sagamie; (418)541-1000

ALLARD, Joffre C; CSSS de Rimouski-Neigette, CP 3150 Succ A 150 av Rouleau, Rimouski QC G5L 5T1; Mon'80; FRCPC; MedOncol; Hem; IntMed (P.Q.). Ac Staff Hem, Hôpital Regional Rimouski; Langs: Bilingual(French/English); (418)724-3000 x8478; Fax. (418)724-8613.

ALLARD, Johane; 9N 973-585 University Ave, Toronto ON M5G 2N2; Mon'81; ABIM; FRCPC; IntMed; Gastroent. Staff, Toronto General Hospital - UHN; Langs: English; French; (416)340-5159; Fax. (416)348-0065; johane.allard@uhn.on.ca.

ALLARD, Magali; CSSS du Nord de Lanaudière, 1000 boul Sainte-Anne, St-Charles-Brromee QC J6E 6J2; Mon'03; FRCPC; Psy. Staff, Centre Hospitalier Régional de Lanaudière; (450)834-5407

ALLARD, Manon; Centre Med Hillside, 65 av Hillside, Westmount QC H3Z 1W1; Mon'82; FRCPC; Peds. Assoc Member, McGill University Health Centre - Montreal Children's Hospital; McGill University; Langs: Bilingual(French/English); (514)931-2524; Fax. (514)931-2625.

ALLARD, Manon; CHUQ-St-Francois D'Assise, 10 rue de l'Espinay, Quebec QC G1L 3L5; Laval'05; CCFP; CCFP(E.M.); Staff, Centre Hospitalier Universitaire De Québec - Pavillon De St-françois-d'assise; (418)525-4388

ALLARD, Marc L; Osler Cardiology Associates, 200-3 Conestoga Dr, Brampton ON L6Z 4N5; Tor'01; FRCPC; IntMed; Cardiol. Staff Cardiol, William Osler Health System - Brampton Civic Hospital; (905)453-5023; Fax. (905)452-1052.

ALLARD, Marc; Clinique Med Berger, 116-1000 ch Sainte-Foy, Quebec QC G1S 2L6; Laval'91; MSc(Physiol.); LMCC; BSc(Biol.); Staff Geriatrics, Jeffery Hale Hospital-Saint Brigid's; (418)688-1385; Fax. (418)689-3249; marc_allard@ssss.gouv.qc.ca.

ALLARD, Marc-Andre; GMF Centre medical AJC, 110 rue Saint-Jean, Drummondville QC J2B 7T1; Sher'03; (819)477-1800

ALLARD, Mariannick; CSSS Haut-Richelieu-Rouville, 920 boul du Seminaire N, St-Jean-sur-Richel QC J3A 1B7; Sher'07; CCFP; CCFP(E.M.); Staff, Hôpital du Haut-Richelieu; (450)359-5000

ALLARD, Marie-Eve; CSSS de Saint-Jerome, 290 rue de Montigny, Saint-Jerome QC J7Z 5T3; Mon'01; FRCSC; ObstGyn. Staff, Hôtel-Dieu de Saint-Jérôme; (450)431-8200

ALLARD, Marie-Frederique A; CSSS de l'Energie-Ste-Therese, 1705 av Georges, Shawinigan QC G9N 2N1; Sher'94; FRCPC; Psy. Psychiatre, CH du Centre-de-la-Mauricie (Ste-Thérèse de Shawinigan); (819)536-7575 x4276; marie-frederique_allard@ssss.gouv.qc.ca.

ALLARD, Marie-Josee; 105-140 rue Champlain, Dieppe NB E1A 1N8; Laval'98; FRCSC; Otol. Consultant, Dr Georges-L-Dumont University Hospital Centre; Staff, The Moncton Hospital; (506)854-6273; Fax. (506)854-5945.

ALLARD, Melanie; CHUQ-St-Francois d'Assise, 10 rue de l'Espinay, Quebec QC G1L 3L5; Laval'00; CCFP; Staff Emerg, Centre Hospitalier Universitaire De Québec - Pavillon De St-françois-d'assise; Physician, Clinique Medicine Giffard; (418)525-4444

ALLARD, Michael F; UBC Hospital, G105-2211 Wesbrook Mall, Vancouver BC V6T 2B5; UBC'81; FRCPC; AnatPath (Clinical). Ac Staff Research Lab, Providence Health Care - St Paul's Hospital; Staff, UBC Hospital - Koerner Pavillion; Assoc Prof/Dept Head & School Dir Pathology & Laboratory Med, University of British Columbia; (604)822-7102

ALLARD, Michel; CSST Laurentides, 85 rue de Martigny O, Saint-Jerome QC J7Y 3R8; Mon'66; GenSurg. Staff, Hôpital du Sacre-Coeur de Montréal; (450)431-4000 x4013

ALLARD, Myriam; Clin Med St Felix de Valois, 610 ch Joliette RR 1, St-Felix-de-Valois QC J0K 2M0; Laval'10; CCFP; (450)889-5577

ALLARD, Nathalie; CSSS du Nord de Lanaudière, 1000 boul Sainte-Anne, St-Charles-Brromee QC J6E 6J2; Mon'89; Staff, Centre Hospitalier Régional de Lanaudière; (450)759-8222

ALLARD, Nathalie; Ctr de Med Familiale de Granby, 48 rue Denison E, Granby QC J2G 4C6; Sher'97; CCFP; (450)372-3996; Fax. (450)372-0430.

ALLARD, Nicole; Clinique Med Soleil, 64 1re Av O, Amos QC J9T 1T8; Sher'77; (819)732-8341; Fax. (819)732-1642.

ALLARD, Paul; Clin Med St Felix de Valois, 610 Ch Joliette RR 1, St-Felix-de-Valois QC J0K 2M0; Mon'76; Staff, Centre Hospitalier Régional de Lanaudière; (450)889-5577; Fax. (450)889-4239.

ALLARD, Pierre; Bruyere Continuing Centre, 43 Bruyere St, Ottawa ON K1N 5C8; Laval'71; MSc; PhD(Epidemiol); FRCPC; CommunMed (Palliative Care); Public Health & Preventive Med. Staff, The Ottawa Hospital - General Campus; (613)562-6262

ALLARD, Rene V; Kingston Gen Hosp, 76 Stuart St, Kingston ON K7L 2V7; Tor'01; FRCPC; Anes. Staff, Kingston General Hospital; (613)549-6666; Fax. (613)548-6019.

ALLARD, Robert; Dir de la Sante Publique-Mtl, 1301 rue Sherbrooke E, Montreal QC H2L 1M3; McG'74; FRCPC; CommunMed (Public Health). Staff Public Health Unit, McGill University Health Centre - Montreal General Campus; Clin Teacher, McGill University; (514)528-2400 x3689; Fax. (514)528-2452; rallard@santepub-mtl.qc.ca.

ALLARD, Rollande; Direction de la Sante Publique, 1255 rue Beauregard, Longueuil QC J4K 2M3; Laval'85; BSc(Biochem); Médecin, Agence de santé et des services sociaux de la Montérégie; Langs: English; (450)928-6777 x5552; Fax. (450)928-3760; r.allard@rrsss16.gouv.qc.ca.

ALLARD, Stephanie; CLSC La Region-Sherbrookoise, 1200 rue King E, Sherbrooke QC J1G 1E4; Sher'07; CCFP; (819)780-2222

ALLARD, Suzanne; I R D P Q-Site Francois-Charon, 525 boul Wilfrid-Hamel, Quebec QC G1M 2S8; Laval'80; Médecin Physical Readaptation, Institut de Readaption & Deficience Physique de Quebec; (418)529-9141 x6313; Fax. (418)529-3289; suzanne.allard@irdpq.qc.ca.

ALLARD, Sylvain; Clin de Med Familiale Saguenay, 220-874 boul de l'Universite E, Chicoutimi QC G7H 6B9; Laval'81; Staff, Complexe hospitalier de la Sagamie; (418)545-2998; Fax. (418)545-4782.

ALLARD, Sylvie; CHSLD Cartierville, 12235 rue Grenet, Montreal QC H4J 2N9; Mon'84; Clin Teach Staff Family Med, Hôpital du Sacre-Coeur de Montréal; (514)337-7300

ALLARD, Valere; CSSS de la Baie-des-Chaleurs, RR 2 419 boul Perron, Maria QC G0C 1Y0; Laval'89; FRCSC; GenSurg. Staff, CSSS de la Baie-des-Chaleurs; (418)759-3443

ALLARD, Yves; CSSS Drummond-Hop Sainte-Croix, 570 rue Heriot, Drummondville QC J2B 1C1; Laval'85; LMCC; FRCPC; IntMed (Oncology). ac Staff, Hôpital Sainte-croix; (819)478-6464; Fax. (819)478-6414.

ALLARD-DANSEREAU, Claire; Hôpital Ste-Justine, 3175 ch Cote-Sainte-Catherine, Montreal QC H3T 1C5; Sher'73; FRCPC; Peds (Child Abuse). Ac Member Peds, Hôpital Ste-Justine; Teach Staff, Universite de Montreal; (514)345-4866; Fax. (514)345-4869.

ALLARD-PIGEON, Marjorie; Clin Perinatalitie Trois-Rivie, 100-4900 boul des Forges, Trois-Rivieres QC G8Y 1X1; Laval'09; CCFP; (819)373-2303

ALLARD RIOPEL, Miriame; Centre Med Laval, 1110 boul Vanier, Laval QC H7C 2R8; Mon'08; (450)661-2521

ALLARD-WASAJJA, Kathleen A; CLSC de Limoilou, 1405 ch de la Canardiere, Quebec QC G1J 0A7; Laval'00; Médecin, CLSC de Limoilou; Langs: English; (418)529-2572; Fax. (418)648-9201; kathleen.allard-wasajja@csssuc.qc.ca.

ALLARDYCE, D Bruce; Crestwood Medical Dental, 311-6051 Gilbert Rd, Richmond BC V7C 3V3; UBC'62; FACS; FRCSC; GenSurg (Gastrointestinal Surgery). Ac Staff Surg, Richmond Hospital; Assoc Prof Emeritus, University of British Columbia; (604)244-0085; Fax. (604)244-0086; bdyce@shaw.ca.

ALLARDYCE, Pamela J; 104-3040 Tutt St, Kelowna BC V1Y 2H5; UBC'93; BSc; CCFP; (250)763-6922

ALLART, Annemarie; Univ of Ottawa Hlth Services, 300-100 Marie Curie Pvt, Ottawa ON K1N 1A2; (Grenada)'99; (613)564-3950; Fax. (613)564-6627.

ALLARY, Catherine; CHUS-Hop Hotel-Dieu, 580 rue Bowen S, Sherbrooke QC J1G 2E8; Nice (France)'82; Psy (P.Q.). Ac Staff, Centre Hospitalier Universitaire de Sherbrooke-Hôpital Hôtel-Dieu; Universite de Sherbrooke; (819)346-1110 x25545; Fax. (819)829-6284; catherineallary@hotmail.com.

ALLAYE-CHAN, Louise T; 6681 Victoria Dr, Vancouver BC V5P 3Y2; UBC'92; (604)321-8712

ALLAZZAM, Abdulmohsen; Kelowna Gen Hosp, 2268 Pandosy St, Kelowna BC V1Y 1T2; Riyadh (Saudi Arabia)'01; MB BS; FRCSC; PlasSurg. Staff, Kelowna General Hospital; (250)862-4000

ALLDRED, John Byron; 328 Worthington St W, North Bay ON P1B 3B6; Tor'75; CCFP; (705)472-3660; Fax. (705)472-4144.

ALLED, Jalal A; Advanced Walk-In Med Clinic, 111-21 Queensway W, Mississauga ON L5B 1B6; Al-Fateh (Libya)'87; FRCPC; IntMed. (905)897-9228

ALLEGA, Rossano L; 201-980 Queenston Rd, Stoney Creek ON L8G 1B9; McM'79; CCFP; FCFP; Staff, St Joseph's Healthcare - Charlton Campus; (905)664-2130; Fax. (905)664-3744.

ALLEGRETTO, Michael W; Univ of Alberta Hosp-SCC/WCM, 1E4WCM-8440 112 St NW, Edmonton AB T6G 2B7; Alb'96; FRCSC; Otol. Staff, University of Alberta Hospital; (780)407-8356; Fax. (780)407-6434.

ALLEGRO, Sabrina; Humber River Reg Hosp-Church, 200 Church St, Toronto ON M9N 1N8; McM'05; FRCPC; IntMed; MedOncol. Staff, Humber River Regional Hospital - Church Street Site; (416)243-4505; Fax. (416)243-4580.

ALLEGRUCCI, Philippe; Clinique Med 3000 Inc, 3000 rue Belanger, Montreal QC H1Y 1A9; Mon'87; BSc; (514)376-7702; Fax. (514)376-2639.

ALLEN, Alexander C; IWK Health Centre, PO Box 9700 Rpo CSC 5980 University Ave, Halifax NS B3K 6R8; McG'59; FAAP; DABPed; FRCPC; Peds (Neonatal & Perinatal Medicine). Staff Perinatal Med Div of Neonatol, IWK Health Centre; Prof, Dalhousie University; (902)470-6681; Fax. (902)470-6469; alexander.allen@dal.ca.

ALLEN, Christine G; Valley Med Imaging, 102-32475 Simon Ave, Abbotsford BC V2T 5E3; Alb'02; FRCPC; DiagRad. (604)226-5372

ALLEN, Christopher J; St Joseph's Healthcare, 50 Charlton Ave E, Hamilton ON L8N 4A6; Oxford (England)'74; BMus; BCh; MRC(UK); FRCPC; Respir. Ac Staff Reg Chest & Allergy Unit, St Joseph's Healthcare - Charlton Campus; Clin Assoc Prof Med, McMaster University; (905)522-1155 x33154; Fax. (905)521-6183; allencj@mcmaster.ca.

ALLEN, Christopher T B; Queen Elizabeth II HSC, 525-1276 South Park St, Halifax NS B3H 2Y9; London (England)'70; MB BS; FFARCS; FRCPC; Anes (Critical Care Medicine). Asst Prof, Queen Elizabeth II Health Sciences Centre - Victoria General Site; (902)473-1393

ALLEN, Christyne; CHUQ-Ctr Hosp Univ Laval, B0027-2705 boul Laurier, Quebec QC G1V 4G2; Sher'95; FRCPC; IntMed; Endocrin (P.Q.); Endocrin&Metab. Staff, Centre Hospitalier Universitaire de Quebec-CHUL; (418)654-2169; Fax. (418)654-2792.

ALLEN, David M; Manitoulin Hlth Centre, 11 Meredith St, Little Current ON P0P 1K0; Tor'80; CCFP; CCFP(E.M.); FCFP; Staff, West Nipissing General Hospital.

ALLEN, Diane; CSSS Les Eskers de l'Abitibi, 622 4e rue O, Amos QC J9T 2S2; Sher'93; FRCSC; ObstGyn. Staff, CH Hôtel-Dieu d'Amos; (819)732-3341; Fax. (819)732-6449.

ALLEN, Donna B; St Paul Family Health Organiza, 4F-99 Wayne Gretzky Pky, Brantford ON N3S 6T6; McM'99; BSc(Hons); CCFP; Ac Staff, The Brant Community Healthcare System - Brantford General Hospital Site; (519)756-6400; Fax. (519)756-7343.

ALLEN, Douglas L; Queen Elizabeth II HSC-Halifax, 1796 Summer St, Halifax NS B3H 3A7; Dal'75; FACEP; MCFP(EM); FCFP; Staff, Queen Elizabeth II Health Sciences Centre - Halifax Infirmary Site; Staff Emerg Dept, Queen Elizabeth II Health Sciences Centre - Victoria General Site; Lecturer, Dalhousie University; (902)473-2020

ALLEN, Edward C; 6-11 King St W, Toronto ON M5H 4C7; Tor'68; CCFP; FCFP; (416)864-0460; Fax. (416)864-1546.

ALLEN, Genevieve; Dr Everett Chalmers Reg Hosp, PO Box 9000 Stn A, Fredericton NB E3B 5N5; CCFP; Staff, Dr Everett Chalmers Regional Hospital; (506)447-4444

ALLEN, Gillian B; 206-726 Bloor St W, Toronto ON M6G 4A1; Tor'69; Langs: German; French; Italian; (416)516-5244

ALLEN, Jennifer M; Radiology Consultants Assoc, 120A-6707 Elbow Dr SW, Calgary AB T2V 0E3; Sask'91; FRCPC; DiagRad. (403)777-3003; Fax. (403)777-3008.

ALLEN, Joel; Westgrove Clinic, 203-505 Queen St, Spruce Grove AB T7X 2V2; Cape Town (South Africa)'85; FRCPC; IntMed. Asst Prof, University of Alberta; (780)960-1440; Fax. (780)960-1404.

ALLEN, John E; Dr CW Wiebe Med Centre, 385 Main St, Winkler MB R6W 1J2; Witwatersrand (South Africa)'80; MB ChB; Langs: Afrikaans; (204)325-4312; Fax. (204)325-4594.

ALLEN, Joseph A; Rouge Valley-Centenary HC, 2867 Ellesmere Rd, Scarborough ON M1E 4B9; Queen's (Ireland)'71; Staff, Rouge Valley Health System - Centenary Health Centre Site; (416)284-8131; Fax. (416)281-7323.

ALLEN, Judith M; 200-460 Nanaimo St, Vancouver BC V5L 4W3; Tor'85; FRCPC; Psy. Staff, UBC Hospital - Koerner Pavillion; Clin Instructor, University of British Columbia; (604)873-0103

ALLEN, Julie K; Wortley Village Med Centre, 215-190 Wortley Rd, London ON N6C 4Y7; Wes'88; CCFP; Assoc Staff Family Med, London Health Sciences Centre - Victoria Campus; Physician, Wortley Village Medical Centre; (519)438-7666; Fax. (519)438-5020.

ALLEN, Katherine P; 204-274 Dundas St E, Belleville ON K8N 1E6; Qns'79; CCFP; FCFP; Assoc Staff, QHC Belleville General; (613)969-7743; Fax. (613)969-7744.

ALLEN, Larry H; St Joseph's Health Care, PO Box 5777 Stn B 268 Grosvenor St, London ON N6A 4V2; Dublin (Ireland)'79; MB ChB; FRCSC; Ophth (Lacrimal). Staff Ivey Eye Inst, St Joseph's Hospital - St Joseph's Health Care; Asst Prof, University of Western Ontario; (519)646-6366; Fax. (519)646-6248; larry.allen@sjhc.london.on.ca.

ALLEN, Lauren A; Royal University Hosp, 103 Hospital Dr, Saskatoon SK S7N 0W8; Sask'02; FRCSC; OrthSurg (Pediatric Orthopedic Surgery). Staff, Royal University Hospital; (306)966-2783; Fax. (306)966-8573.

ALLEN, Lisa M; Hydro Place Bldg, 8 713-700 University Ave, Toronto ON M5G 1Z5; Wes'92; FRCSC; ObstGyn (Pediatric & Adolescent Gynecology). Assoc Staff, Toronto General Hospital - UHN; Head Gynecology, Mount Sinai Hospital; Head, The Hospital For Sick Children; (416)586-3162; Fax. (416)586-8287.

ALLEN, Maureen A; PO Box 1772 Stn Main, Antigonish NS B2G 2M5; Mem'89; CCFP; CCFP(E.M.); Staff, Health Sciences Centre.

ALLEN, Michael J; Dalhousie University, C106-5849 University Ave, Halifax NS B3H 4H7; Dal'75; Dir Special Projects, Dalhousie University; (902)494-2173; Fax. (902)494-1479.

ALLEN, Murray W; 01 M28-190 Melrose Ave, Ottawa ON K1Y 4E9; Ott'84; FACS(PlasSurg); FRCSC; PlasSurg (Head & Neck Surgery). Asst Prof, University of Ottawa; (613)798-5555 x12061; Fax. (613)761-4982.

ALLEN, Philippe; Queen Elizabeth II HSC, 818-1276 South Park St, Halifax NS B3H 2Y9; Tor'07; GenSurg. Staff, Queen Elizabeth II Health Sciences Centre - Victoria General Site; (902)473-2700

ALLEN, Raymond B; Piedmont Walk-In Clinic, 10-550 University Dr W, Lethbridge AB T1J 4T3; West Virginia(WV) (USA)'88; CCFP; (403)380-2024

ALLEN, Richard E; 410-4800 Leslie St, North York ON M2J 2K9; Tor'90; CCFP; CCFP(E.M.); FCFP; Ac Staff, North York General Hospital; Ac Staff, North York General Hospital - Branson Division; (416)497-9900; Fax. (416)497-6992.

ALLEN, Stephen M; The Group Health Centre, 240 Mcnabb St, Sault Ste. Marie ON P6B 1Y5; Dal'90; FACS; FRCSC; GenSurg. Ac Staff Surg, Sault Area Hospital - Sault Ste Marie; (705)759-1234

ALLEN, Susan J; 152-759 Hyde Park Rd, London ON N6H 3S2; Wes'82; FRCPC; IntMed (Psychotherapy); Psy. (519)679-3330; Fax. (519)963-0980.

ALLEN, Tara; The Credit Valley Hosp, 2200 Eglinton Ave W, Mississauga ON L5M 2N1; Wes'02; FRCPC; Peds (Neonatal & Perinatal Medicine); Respir. Staff, The Credit Valley Hospital; (416)271-4512

ALLEN, Timothy V; Academic Family Medicine, 2630 Skymark Ave, Mississauga ON L4W 5A4; Tor'70; MCFP(EM); FRCPC; EmergMed. ac Staff, Centre Hospitalier Universitaire de Quebec-CHUL; Staff, Merrickville District Community Health Centre; Prof Emerg Med, Université Laval; Langs: English; French; (905)629-0900; Fax. (905)629-0893.

ALLEN, Upton D; The Hosp For Sick Children, 555 University Ave, Toronto ON M5G 1X8; West Indies (Grenada)'81; MB BS; FAAP; FRCPC; Peds; InfectDis. Staff, The Hospital For Sick Children; (416)813-8129; upton.allen@sickkids.ca.

ALLEN, Vanessa G; Ontario Public Health Lab, 81 Resources Rd, Etobicoke ON M9P 3T1; McG'02; FRCPC; IntMed; MedMicrobiol; InfectDis. Staff, Mount Sinai Hospital; (416)235-5806; Fax. (416)235-6063.

ALLEN, Victoria M; PO Box 9700 Rpo CSC, Halifax NS B3K 6R8; Dal'93; BSc; MSc; FRCSC; ObstGyn (Maternal Fetal Medicine). Staff, IWK Health Centre; Assoc Prof ObstGyn Comm Health & Epidemiology, Dalhousie University; (902)470-6602; Fax. (902)425-1125; victoria.allen@dal.ca.

ALLEN BRADSHAW, Barbra Y; Vernon Jubilee Hosp, 2101 33 St, Vernon BC V1T 5L2; Alb'05; FRCPC; AnatPath. Staff, Vernon Jubilee Hospital; (250)558-4115

ALLEN DEMERS, Catherine; CSSS Becancour-Nicolet-Yamaska, 216 rue Principale, Fortierville QC G0S 1J0; Sher'03; (819)287-4442

ALLEVATO, Pat A; Windsor Reg Hosp-Metropolitan, 1995 Lens Ave, Windsor ON N8W 1L9; Tor'80; AB(CytoPath); FRCPC; AnatPath; GenPath. Ac Staff, Windsor Regional Hospital - Metropolitan Site; Ac Staff, Leamington District Memorial Hospital; Staff Gen. Path., Medical Laboratories of Windsor; (519)254-1661 x52445; Fax. (519)254-6861.

ALLEYNE, Julia M Klich; Women's College Hosp, 10F-76 Grenville St, Toronto ON M5S 1B2; McM'87; FACSM; BHSc; Dip SportMed; MD; CCFP; Ac Staff, Women's College Hospital; (416)323-6478; Fax. (416)323-6487; julia.alleyne@utoronto.ca.

ALLIBHAI, Sophia; West Hill Community Services, 3545 Kingston Rd, Scarborough ON M1M 1R6; Ott'93; CCFP; (416)284-5931

ALLIDINA, Diamond A; 77 Maclaren St, Ottawa ON K2P 0K5; Durham (England)'72; FRCPC; Psy. (613)232-6745; Fax. (613)739-7949.

ALLIN, Jeffrey C; Belleville Family Med Centre, 50-470 Dundas St E, Belleville ON K8N 1G1; Qns'79; (613)966-4045; Fax. (613)966-0072.

ALLIN, R Bruce; City of Kawartha Lakes FHT, 205 Francis St E, Fenelon Falls ON K0M 1N0; Qns'72; Med Staff, Ross Memorial Hospital; (705)887-1308; Fax. (705)887-4874.

ALLIN, Robert C; Medical Assoc Of Port Perry, 462 Paxton St, Port Perry ON L9L 1L9; Tor'65; CCFP; Ac Staff, Lakeridge Health - Port Perry Site; Coroner, Region of durham; Asst Prof Family & Commun Med, University of Toronto; (905)985-2895 x5412; Fax. (905)985-8931; r.allin@sympatico.ca.

ALLIN, Warren D; Credit Valley Eye Care, 3200 Erin Mills Pkwy, Mississauga ON L5L 1W8; Tor'63; FRCSC; Ophth (Cosmetic Surgery). Court Staff, The Credit Valley Hospital; Court Staff, Trillium Health Centre - Mississauga; Staff, William Osler Health System - Brampton Civic Hospital; Staff, Credit Valley Eye Care; Coroner, Province of Ontario; (905)451-4560; Fax. (905)459-5085.

ALLISON, David J; Eastern Hlth Comm Service, 760 Topsail Rd, Mount Pearl NL A1N 3J5; Qns'76; MD; FRCPC; CommunMed (Communicable Diseases & Environmental Health); Public Health & Preventive Med. Med Officer of Hlth, Eastern Health Corporate Office; Clin Assoc Prof Div of Community Health, Memorial University Of Newfoundland; (709)752-4192; Fax. (709)752-4989.

ALLISON, Francois; CLSC du Marigot, 250 boul Cartier O, Laval QC H7N 5S5; Laval'86; Universite de Montreal; (450)668-1803

ALLISON, James M; 205-285 Aurora Cres, Kelowna BC V1X 7N6; Trinity Coll. (Ireland)'78; MB ChB; BAO; Assoc Staff, Kelowna General Hospital; (250)765-4117; Fax. (250)765-9015.

ALLISON, Patrick J; South Hlth & Life Managment Ct, 2-2120 Regent St, Sudbury ON P3E 3Z9; Ott'04; FRCSC; OrthSurg. (705)522-9101; Fax. (705)522-5744.

ALLISON, Roy C; Port Arthur Health Centre Inc, 194 Court St N, Thunder Bay ON P7A 4V7; Belfast (Ireland)'73; Court Staff, Thunder Bay Regional Health Sciences Centre Port-Arthur; Ac Staff, St Joseph's Care Group - St Joseph's Hospital; (807)346-1000; Fax. (807)346-6206.

ALLISON, Sandra J; Western Regional Health, 20 7th St, Brandon MB R7A 6M8; Man'07; FRCPC; Public Health & Preventive Med;CCFP.

ALLISON, Simon M; Medical Arts Clinic, 30-650 Terminal Ave S, Nanaimo BC V9R 5E2; Liverpool (England)'01; MB ChB; CCFP; (250)753-3431

ALLODI, Federico A; Consent & Capacity Board of On, 151 Bloor St W, Toronto ON M5S 2T5; Madrid (Spain)'57; MRCPsy(UK); DPsy; FRCPC; Psy. Langs: Spanish; Italian; French; (416)327-4142; Fax. (416)327-4207.

ALLOO, Javed A; Nymark Med Centre, 4839 Leslie St, North York ON M2J 2K8; Qns'99; CCFP; Staff, The Scarborough Hospital - Birchmount Campus; (416)498-3600

ALLOUL, Sophie; CSSS de Laval, 1755 boul Rene-Laennec, Laval QC H7M 3L9; Mon'04; Peds. Staff, Hopital de la Cite de la santé; (514)345-4931

ALLY, Muhammad S C; Brooks Medical Clinic, 219B 3 St W, Brooks AB T1R 0S3; (403)362-3040; Fax. (403)362-0102.

ALMADANI, Mahmud H M; Lakeridge Hlth Corp-Oshawa, 1 Hospital Crt, Oshawa ON L1G 2B9; Al-Fateh (Libya),Al Fateh University (Libya)'90; FRCPC; Peds (Neonatology). Staff, Lakeridge Health - Oshawa Site; (905)576-8711 x4559

ALMADEN-CAMACHO, Emily A; 1050 91 St SW, Edmonton AB T6X 0P2; (Philippines)'95; CCFP; (780)463-7050

ALMAGOR, Doron; 711-1849 Yonge St, Toronto ON M4S 1Y2; Tor'90; FRCPC; Psy (Attention Deficit Hyperactivity Disorder). Staff, Toronto Western Hospital - University Health Network; Staff, Centre for Addiction & Mental Health (CAMH) - College Street Site; Langs: Hebrew; (416)304-1779; Fax. (416)304-0257; doron.almagor@gmail.com.

ALMAKKI, Nazar E M; 403-2863 Ellesmere Rd, Scarborough ON M1E 5E9; Khartoum (Sudan)'99; FRCPC; IntMed (Respirology). Staff, Rouge Valley Health System - Centenary Health Centre Site; (416)792-0836

ALMALKI, Youssef; Bluewater Health-Norman Site, 89 Norman St, Sarnia ON N7T 6S3; Wes'04; DiagRad. Staff, Bluewater Health - Mitton Site; Staff, Bluewater Health - Norman Site; (519)464-4400

ALMALKY, Ammar; Russell Med Clinic, PO Box 549, Russell MB R0J 1W0; (Other Foreign)'94; (204)773-2146

ALMAN, Benjamin A; The Hosp For Sick Children S107-555 University Ave, Toronto ON M5G 1X8; Philadelphia (USA)'86; FRCSC; OrthSurg. Staff, The Hospital For Sick Children; (416)813-7980; Fax. (416)813-6414; benjamin.alman@sickkids.ca.

ALMANFUD, Abdullah A A; Belmont Prof Bldg, 208-564 Belmont Ave W, Kitchener ON N2M 5N6; Al Fateh University (Libya)'99; (519)576-3099

ALMARZOUKI, Hani Z M; University of Alberta Hosp, 1E4. 29-8440 112 St NW, Edmonton AB T6G 2B7; Jeddah (Saudi Arabia)'07; Otol. Staff, University of Alberta Hospital; (780)407-8397; Fax. (780)407-3885.

ALMAS, Leilani T; Park Avenue Med Centre, 5F-4634 Park Ave, Terrace BC V8G 1V7; UBC'78; FRCSC; ObstGyn. (250)615-5051; Fax. (250)615-5054.

ALMAS, Naveed; Chilliwack Gen Hosp, 45600 Menholm Rd, Chilliwack BC V2P 1P7; Peshawar (Pakistan)'91; MB BS; Staff, Chilliwack General Hospital; (604)702-2885

ALMASI, Behzad; 304-622 College St, Toronto ON M6G 1B6; Saba University (Netherlands Antilles)'05; CCFP; (647)343-4687

ALMASI, Julie; Club Tiny Tots, 3550-6900 boul Decarie, Cote Saint-Luc QC H3X 2T8; Mon'06; CCFP; Langs: Bilingual(French/English); (514)342-9911; Fax. (514)342-2911.

ALMEKHLAFI, Mohammed A G; Foothills Medical Centre, 1149-1403 29 St NW, Calgary AB T2N 2T9; Jeddah (Saudi Arabia)'03; Neur. Staff, Foothills Medical Centre; (403)944-8671

ALMGRAHI, Abdulaziz; Royal University Hosp, 103 Hospital Dr, Saskatoon SK S7N 0W8; Benghazi (Libya)'93; FRCPC; NuclearMed. Staff, Royal University Hospital; (306)655-1797; Fax. (306)622-1742.

ALMIGHAIRBI, Adel M S; Hammonds Plains Medical Clinic, 2120 Hammonds Plains Rd, Hammonds Plains NS B4B 1P3; Al Fateh (Libya)'99; MB BCh; CCFP; Gen Physician, Fogo Island Health Centre; (902)832-9233; Fax. (902)832-7409.

ALMISKI, Muhamed S A F; Health Sciences Centre, 820 Sherbrook St, Winnipeg MB R3A 1R9; Staff, Health Sciences Centre; (204)774-8511

ALMOGBEL, Osama A; Univ of Toronto, 602-500 Unviersity Ave, Toronto ON M5G 1V7; Riyadh (Saudi Arabia)'06; IntMed.

ALMOHAMMEDI, Faisal; Sunnybrook Health Sciences Ctr, M1 700-2075 Bayview Ave, Toronto ON M4N 3M5; Jeddah (Saudi Arabia)'01; FRCPC; AnatPath; Derm. Staff Dermatology Clinic, Sunnybrook Health Sciences Centre; (416)480-4905

ALMOND, Christopher J; Lloydminster Hosp, 3820 43 Ave, Lloydminster SK S9V 1Y5; Sask'08; CCFP; CCFP(E.M.); Staff, Lloydminster Hospital; (306)820-6000

ALMOND, Richard G; Fort William Clinic, 117 Mckellar St S, Thunder Bay ON P7E 1H5; Wes'76; CCFP; FCFP; Ac Staff, Thunder Bay Regional Health Sciences Centre; Sec Chair/Prog Dir Family Med, Northern Ontario School of Medicine-Laurentian University; (807)626-1234; Fax. (807)623-2705.

ALMUTAIRI, Fawaz Q R; Univ of Ottawa Heart Institute, 40 Ruskin St, Ottawa ON K1Y 4W7; King Saud U (Saudi Arabia)'02; Cardiol; IntMed. Staff Cardiac Surg ICU, University of Ottawa Heart Institute; (613)761-4379

ALMUTAWA, Mohammad; University of Alberta Hosp, 2C2 WMC-8440 112 St NW, Edmonton AB T6G 2B7; Aberdeen (Scotland)'04; FRCPC; IntMed (Cardiology). Staff, University of Alberta Hospital; (780)407-6826; Fax. (780)407-6452.

ALNAJI, Fuad S; Children's Hosp Eastern Ont, 401 Smyth Rd, Ottawa ON K1H 8L1; Bahrain (Saudi Arabia)'00; FRCPC; Peds; Critical Care Medicine. Staff, Children's Hospital of Eastern Ontario (CHEO); (613)737-7600

ALNAJJAR, Abdulsalam; Univ of Ottawa, 2044-451 Smyth Rd, Ottawa ON K1H 8M5; Bahrain (Saudi Arabia)'95; IntMed. Teach Staff, University of Ottawa.

ALNAQBI, Khalid; Univ Hlth Network-Toronto Western Hosp, 1F-399 Bathurst St, Toronto ON M5T 2S8; Abu Dhabi (United Arab Emirates)'02; FRCPC; IntMed; Rheum. Staff, Toronto Western Hospital - University Health Network; (416)603-5869; Fax. (416)603-4348.

ALNASSAR, Mu'taz M A; Hamilton HSC-McMaster Site, O Box 2000 Stn Lcd 1 1200 Main St W, Hamilton ON L8N 3Z5; (Jordan)'98; Staff, Hamilton Health Sciences Centre - McMaster Children's Hospital; (905)521-2100

ALNHISI, Khaled M A; Grantham Med Clinic, 400 Scott St, St Catharines ON L2M 3W4; Al-Fateh (Libya)'99; CCFP; Langs: Arabic; (905)937-0000

ALO, Nadin; Tuscany Med Centre, 105-9100 Jane St, Vaughan ON L4K 0A4; Al-Mustansiriyah (Iraq)'01; MB ChB; CCFP; (905)760-1140; Fax. (905)760-5587.

ALOBAID, Abdulhakeem M S; The Ottawa Hosp-Civic Campus, 1053 Carling Ave, Ottawa ON K1Y 4E9; Riyadh (Saudi Arabia)'99; FRCSC; GenSurg. Staff, The Ottawa Hospital - Civic Campus; (613)737-8899

ALOMAR, Abdulaziz Z M; Fowler Kennedy Sport Med Clin, 3M-1151 Richmond St, London ON N6A 3K7; Riyadh (Saudi Arabia)'00; FRCSC; OrthSurg. Staff, Fowler Kennedy Sport Medicine Clinic; (519)661-3011

ALOMARI, Mohammad G; Windsor Reg Hosp-Metropolitan, 1995 Lens Ave, Windsor ON N8W 1L9; (Jordan)'92; FRCPC; AnatPath. Staff, Windsor Regional Hospital - Metropolitan Site; (519)254-5577

ALONSO, Erik J; Royal Alexandra Hosp, 541CSC-10240 Kingsway NW, Edmonton AB T5H 3V9; (Ireland)'06; MB BCh; BAO; CCFP; CCFP(E.M.); Staff, Royal Alexandra Hospital; (780)735-4449; Fax. (780)735-4916.

ALONSO, Wilfred J; Stadium Med Centre, 21-1941 Uxbridge Dr NW, Calgary AB T2N 2V2; CCFP; (403)248-8807; Fax. (403)248-8897.

ALONSO ESTEVE, Angela; Univ Hlth Network-Toronto Gen, 12EN 228-200 Elizabeth St, Toronto ON M5G 2C4; Universidad de la Laguna (Philippines)'01; Clin Fellow Nephrol, Toronto General Hospital - UHN; (416)340-3514; Fax. (416)340-4226.

ALONZO-PROULX, Isabel; CSSS Haut-Richelieu-Rouville, 920 boul du Seminaire N, St-Jean-sur-Richel QC J3A 1B7; Sher'02; Staff, Hôpital du Haut-Richelieu; (450)359-5000

ALOS, Nathalie; Hôpital Ste-Justine, 3175 ch Cote-Sainte-Catherine, Montreal QC H3T 1C5; Bordeaux (France)'91; Prof, Hôpital Ste-Justine; Langs: Bilingual(English/French); (514)345-4735; Fax. (514)345-4988; nathalie.alos@recherche-ste-justine.qc.ca.

ALOTAIBI, Majed; Clinique Ocularis, 100-4210 rue Sainte-Catherine, Westmount QC H3Z 1P4; Riyadh (Saudi Arabia)'02; MB BS; Ophth. (514)285-8808; Fax. (514)285-9191.

ALOTAIBI, Noor H A; Queen Elizabeth II HSC, 2035-1276 South Park St, Halifax NS B3H 2Y9; Umm Al Qura (Saudi Arabia)'04; MB BS; Ophth. Staff, Queen Elizabeth II Health Sciences Centre - Victoria General Site; (902)473-2700

ALOUDAT, Sarah I M; Kingston Gen Hosp, 76 Stuart St, Kingston ON K7L 2V7; (Jordan)'02; FRCPC; IntMed; Nephrol. Staff, Kingston General Hospital; (613)549-6666

ALOWAMI, Salem O S; St Joseph's Healthcare, L 222 6-50 Charlton Ave E, Hamilton ON L8N 4A6; Al-Arab (Libya)'89; FACP; FRCPC; AnatPath (Dermatological Pathology). Staff, St Joseph's Healthcare - Charlton Campus; Langs: Arabic; (905)522-1155; alowami@hotmail.com.

ALOYSIUS, Jeyaranee; Bayers Lake Med Clinic, 210 Chain Lake Dr, Halifax NS B3S 1C5; Jaffna (Sri Lanka)'84; DLO; MB BS; LMCC; CCFP; Physician, Bayers Lake Medical Clinic; Langs: Sinhalese; Tamil; (902)407-4012; Fax. (902)407-4013; jeyaloy@yahoo.com.

ALPER, Deborah; 605-5885 ch de la Cote-des-Nei, Montreal QC H3S 2T2; McG'92; MD; BSc; MSc; CCFP; Clin Asst Family Med, Sir Mortimer B Davis Jewish General; Lecturer Pt-Time Family Med, McGill University; Langs: French; (514)733-3389; Fax. (514)564-7789.

ALPER, Jennifer; SMBD Jewish Gen Hosp, 3755 ch Cote-Sainte-Catherine, Montreal QC H3T 1E2; McG'07; CCFP; CCFP(E.M.); Staff, Sir Mortimer B Davis Jewish General; (514)340-8222; Fax. (514)340-7510.

ALPERT, Brian; The Jacobs Pain Centre, 102-8920 Woodbine Ave, Markham ON L3R 9W9; Tor'82; FRCSC; OrthSurg. (905)305-9484; Fax. (905)305-7381.

ALPERT, Lesley C; SMBD Jewish Gen Hosp, 3755 ch Cote-Sainte-Catherine, Montreal QC H3T 1E2; Tufts(Boston) (USA)'79; PhD; CSPQ; GenPath (P.Q.) (Breast Pathology). Staff, Sir Mortimer B Davis Jewish General; Prof Path, McGill University; (514)340-8222 x4197; Fax. (514)340-8102.

ALPHIN, Mohamed T; 4-3295 Dunmore Rd SE, Medicine Hat AB T1B 3R2; Aleppo (Syria)'75; FRCSC; Urol (Pediatric Urology). Ac Staff Adult & Ped Urol, Medicine Hat Regional Hospital; Langs: Arabic; (403)528-2912; Fax. (403)529-9491; talalalphin@hotmail.com.

ALPORT, Edward C; Regina Qu'Appelle HR-Pasqua, 4101 Dewdney Ave, Regina SK S4T 1A5; Alb'76; DABPath; FRCPC; GenPath. Dir LabMed, Pasqua Hospital; Med Dir, Canadian Blood Service-Regina Centre; Clinical Asst Prof Path, University of Saskatchewan; (306)766-2244; edward.alport@rqhealth.ca.

ALQAHTANI, Abdulrahman; Univ of Ottawa Heart Institute, 40 Ruskin St, Ottawa ON K1Y 4W7; Otago (New Zealand)'06; IntMed. Staff, University of Ottawa Heart Institute; (613)761-5000

ALQAHTANI, Saleh A; 707A-5010 43 St, Red Deer AB T4N 6H2; Jeddah (Saudi Arabia)'98; FRCPC; IntMed; Gastroent. Staff, Foothills Medical Centre; (403)612-8585

ALQDAH, Maen A A; The Moncton Hosp, 135 MacBeath Ave, Moncton NB E1C 6Z8; (Jordan)'99; AB(Respirol Critical Care Med; FRCPC; IntMed (Critical Care Medicine); Respir. Staff, The Moncton Hospital; (506)857-5700; Fax. (506)857-5548.

ALQURASHI, Waleed D A; Children's Hosp Eastern Ont, 401 Smyth Rd, Ottawa ON K1H 8L1; Dammam (Saudi Arabia)'02; FRCPC; Peds; PedEmergMed. Staff, Children's Hospital of Eastern Ontario (CHEO); (613)737-7600; Fax. (613)738-4885.

ALQUTUB, Adel N H; London HSC-Children's Hosp, PO Box 5010 E1 317-800 Commissioners Rd E, London ON N6A 4G5; Riyadh (Saudi Arabia)'93; Gastroent; IntMed. Staff, London Health Sciences Centre - Children's Hospital; (519)667-6843; adel.alqutub@lhsc.on.ca.

ALRAJHI, Abdulaziz A M; The Ottawa Hosp-Civic Campus, 1053 Carling Ave, Ottawa ON K1Y 4E9; Riyadh (Saudi Arabia)'00; FRCPC; EmergMed. Staff, The Ottawa Hospital - Civic Campus; (613)737-8136; Fax. (613)739-6647.

ALRAJHI, Yaser A M; Univ of Alberta Hosp, 1E4.29-8440 112 St NW, Edmonton AB T6G 2B7; King Abdul Aziz University (Saudi Arabia)'00; Otol (Head & Neck Surgery). Staff, University of Alberta Hospital; (780)407-8397; Fax. (780)407-3558.

ALRAYES, Zeyad; Dartmouth Fam Focus Med Clinic, 201-240 Baker Dr, Dartmouth NS B2W 6L4; (Other Foreign)'02; (902)462-2038; Fax. (902)462-2015.

ALREZAQ, Abdalla; 144-146 West St, St Anthony NL A0K 4S0; Baghdad (Iraq)'99; MB; CCFP; Staff, Charles S Curtis Memorial Hospital; (709)454-3333

ALSADEN, Mohamed-Rida A; Windsor Reg Hosp-Metropolitan, 1995 Lens Ave, Windsor ON N8W 1L9; Baghdad (Iraq)'88; FRCPC; Anes. Staff, Windsor Regional Hospital - Metropolitan Site; Langs: Arabic; (519)254-5577

ALSADOON, Abdulaziz A Y; Hotel-Dieu Grace Hosp, 1030 Ouellette Ave, Windsor ON N9A 1E1; Dammam (Saudi Arabia)'05; FRCPC; EmergMed. Staff, Hôtel-Dieu Grace Hospital; (519)873-4444

ALSAFFAR, Heytham K; 302-168 Charlotte St, Ottawa ON K1N 8K6; RCS (Ireland)'79; MB ChB; BAO; LRCPS; Staff, The Ottawa Hospital - General Campus; Staff, The Ottawa Hospital - Civic Campus; Staff, Ottawa Regional Cancer Centre; Langs: Arabic; (613)789-4385; alsaffar2@hotmail.com.

ALSAGHIR, Abdullah; Campbellton Reg Hosp, PO Box 880 Stn Main 189 Lily Lake Rd, Campbellton NB E3N 3H3; Riyadh (Saudi Arabia)'94; Staff, Hôpital Régional Campbellton; (506)789-5000

ALSAHLI, Mazen; 309-531 Davis Dr, Newmarket ON L3Y 6P5; Aleppo University (Syria)'95; Staff, Southlake Regional Health Centre; (905)898-6100; Fax. (905)898-6105.

ALSARRAF, Adel; Humber River Reg Hosp-Church, 200 Church St, Toronto ON M9N 1N8; RCS (Ireland)'99; FRCPC; IntMed. Staff, Humber River Regional Hospital - Church Street Site; (416)243-4103

ALSEFAOU, Abdualla O A; Grand River Hosp-KW Hlth Ctre, PO Box 9056 Stn C 835 King St W, Kitchener ON N2G 1G3; Al-Fateh (Libya)'92; FRCPC; Anes. Staff, Grand River Hospital - Kitchener/Waterloo Health Centre; (519)749-4300

ALSEHLI, Riyadh N M; University of Alberta Hosp, 8440 112 St NW, Edmonton AB T6G 2B7; Riyadh (Saudi Arabia)'03; FRCPC; IntMed; Nephrol. Staff, University of Alberta Hospital; (780)407-8822

ALSENOSY, Nafa; St Mary's Hosp Centre, 3830 av Lacombe, Montreal QC H3T 1M5; Al Fateh (Libya)'97; FRCPC; Anes. Staff, St Mary's Hospital Centre; (514)345-3511 x3344

ALSERAYE, Faisal M; Regina Qu'Appelle HR-Regina, 1440 14th Ave, Regina SK S4P 0W5; Riyadh (Saudi Arabia)'99; FRCPC; HemPath. Staff, Regina General Hospital; (306)766-4444

ALSHAHABI, Qussay J L; Charles S Curtis Mem Hosp, 178-200 West Ave, St Anthony NL A0K 4S0; Baghdad (Iraq)'93; MB ChB; CCFP; Staff, Charles S Curtis Memorial Hospital; (709)454-3333

ALSHAHRANI, Ali M G; Univ of Ottawa Heart Institute, 40 Ruskin St, Ottawa ON K1Y 4W7; King Saud University (Saudi Arabia)'06; IntMed. Clin Fellow Cardiol, University of Ottawa Heart Institute; (613)761-5000

ALSHAIKHI, Abdullah Y; Carpe Diem Surgical Center, 5270 rue Bellechasse, Montreal QC H1T 2A9; Dammam (Saudi Arabia)'97; FRCSC; GenSurg; PlasSurg. (514)257-1860

ALSHAKMAN, Khalad; Hamilton HS-McMaster Site, PO Box 2000 Stn Lcd 1 1200 Main St W, Hamilton ON L8N 3Z5; Al Fateh (Libya)'96; FRCSC; OrthSurg. Staff Ortho Surg, Hamilton Health Sciences Centre - McMaster University Medical Centre; (905)521-2100

ALSHAMI, Haider A A; Brandon Reg Health Centre, 150 McTavish Ave E, Brandon MB R7A 2B3; (Other Foreign)'92; Gen Practice, Brandon Regional Health Centre; (204)726-1122

ALSHANKITI, Osamah H K; Clinical Sciences Bldg, 8 120-152 University Campus NW, Edmonton AB T6G 2G3; Riyadh (Saudi Arabia)'03; FRCPC; Anes. (780)407-8861; Fax. (780)407-3200.

ALSHARAF, Zuhair M A; Sunnybrook Hlth Sciences Ctre, C753-2075 Bayview Ave, Toronto ON M4N 3M5; Riyadh (Saudi Arabia)'99; Staff, Sunnybrook Health Sciences Centre; (416)480-4037

ALSHARIF, Jamal A H; 421 Shepherdson Rd, New Liskeard ON P0J 1P0; Benghazi (Libya)'96; FRCSC; GenSurg. (705)647-1088

ALSHAYA, Osama S I; McMaster University, MDCL 3101A-1280 Main St W, Hamilton ON L8S 4K1; Riyadh (Saudi Arabia)'04; OrthSurg.

ALSHEHHI, Maryam H A D; PG Med Educ McMaster Univ, MDCL 3101A-1280 Main St W, Hamilton ON L8S 4K1; Bahrain (Saudi Arabia)'02; FRCPC; IntMed.

ALSHGAGI, Husameddin A; Caernarvon Med Clinic, 11812 145 Ave NW, Edmonton AB T5X 2E3; (780)705-5005; Fax. (780)705-5215.

ALSHIGAGI, Emadalden A; Falher Med Clinic, PO Box 720 309 Main St, Falher AB T0H 1M0; (780)837-2275; Fax. (780)837-2630.

ALSHRIF, Moustfha A; U of Regina Hlth Centre, 225-3737 Wascana Pky, Regina SK S4S 0A2; Al Arab Medical University (Saudi Arabia)'99; FRCSC; OrthSurg. (306)337-3340; Fax. (306)337-3192.

ALSOMALI, Faisal M; St Boniface Hosp, A8023-409 Tache Ave, Winnipeg MB R2H 2A6; Dammam (Saudi Arabia)'00; FRCPC; Peds. Staff, St Boniface General Hospital; (204)233-8563

ALSUWAIDAN, Mohammad; Univ Hlth Network-Toronto Western Hosp, 9MP 325-399 Bathurst St, Toronto ON M5T 2S8; (Kuwait)'03; FRCPC; Psy. Staff, Toronto Western Hospital - University Health Network; (416)603-5800

ALTABBAA, Ghazwan; Rockyview Gen Hosp, 7007 14 St SW, Calgary AB T2V 1P9; Damascus (Syria)'90; FRCPC; IntMed; Nephrol. Staff, Rockyview General Hospital; (403)943-3111

ALTAF, Fawaz M N S; St Joseph's Healthcare, 50 Charlton Ave E, Hamilton ON L8N 4A6; Jeddah (Saudi Arabia)'98; FRCSC; CardSurg; ThorSurg. Staff, St Joseph's Healthcare - Charlton Campus; (905)522-1155

ALTAMIRANO DIAZ, Luis A; London HSC-Victoria Hosp, PO Box 5010 Stn B B1 146-800 Commissioners Rd E, London ON N6A 5W9; Cochabamba (Bolivia)'98; Staff, London Health Sciences Centre - Victoria Campus; (519)685-6060

ALTAS, Melanie J; 306-301 Columbia St E, New Westminster BC V3L 3W5; UBC'02; FRCSC; ObstGyn. (604)759-0241

ALTAWEEL, Alawi A M; Univ Hlth Network-Toronto Gen, 200 Elizabeth St, Toronto ON M5G 2C4; King Saud University (Saudi Arabia)'99; Staff, Toronto General Hospital - UHN; (416)340-3111

ALTAWEEL, Ziyad E K; Dr G B Cross Mem Hosp, 67 MAnitoba Dr, Clarenville NL A5A 1K3; Baghdad (Iraq)'04; MB ChB; Staff, The Dr G B Cross Memorial Hospital; (709)466-3411; ziyad.altaweel@easternhealth.ca.

ALTAYEB, Samee A; 11035 Groat Rd NW, Edmonton AB T5M 3J9; (780)705-4090; Fax. (780)705-4394.

ALTEEN, Caroline A S H; Wedgewood Med Centre, 12 Gleneyre St, St. John's NL A1A 2M7; Mem'83; (709)579-2606

ALTEEN, Lawrence W; Dept of Health Commun Services, PO Box 8700 Stn A 57 Margaret's Place, St. John's NL A1B 4J6; Mem'82; Dir Physician Services, Health & Community Services; (709)729-3531; Fax. (709)729-5238; larryalteen@gov.nl.ca.

ALTENKIRK, Gary B; Doc'N Talk Clinic, 68 Robie St, Truro NS B2N 1L2; Dal'96; CCFP; CCFP(E.M.); (902)843-7770; Fax. (902)895-3015.

ALTER, David A; 109-311 Commercial St, Milton ON L9T 3Z9; Tor'90; FRCPC; IntMed; Cardiol. Staff, St Michael's Hospital.

ALTER, Howard M; 435-131 Bloor St W, Toronto ON M5S 1R1; Tor'79; DPsy; FRCPC; Psy (Counselling). Staff Pt-Time, Centre for Addiction & Mental Health (CAMH) - College Street Site; (416)963-9985; Fax. (416)963-4430.

ALTER, Larry S; 132 The Queensway S, Keswick ON L4P 1Z7; Tor'86; BSc(Hon.); CCFP; FCFP; Ac Staff Family Med, Southlake Regional Health Centre; (905)989-2388; Fax. (905)989-0898.

ALTERESCU, Alexandre; North York Med Arts Bldg, 240-1333 Sheppard Ave E, North York ON M2J 1V1; Lausanne (Switzerland)'67; DU(McG.); DAB(Sexology); Staff, North York General Hospital; Langs: English; French; Italian; Romanian; (416)493-2666; Fax. (416)493-5116; malterescu@rogers.com.

ALTITANCHY, Hadeel; Dr G B Cross Mem Hosp, 67 Manitoba Dr, Clarenville NL A5A 1K3; Staff, The Dr G B Cross Memorial Hospital; (709)425-0863

ALTMAN, Alon; Health Sciences Centre, 820 Sherbrook St, Winnipeg MB R3A 1R9; UBC'04; FRCSC; ObstGyn (Gynecologic Oncology). Staff, Health Sciences Centre; (204)774-8511

ALTMAN, David L; Forest Hill Family Health Cent, 200-491 Eglinton Ave W, Toronto ON M5N 1A8; McM'05; LLB; LLM; MBA; CCFP; Staff Privilege, Mount Sinai Hospital; Lecturer, University of Toronto; (416)782-6111

ALTMAN, Gary N; St Boniface Gen Hosp, 409 Tache Ave, Winnipeg MB R2H 2A6; Man'83; FRCPC; Psy (Child Psychiatry). Staff, St Boniface General Hospital; (204)237-2690; Fax. (204)233-8051.

ALTMAN, Robert D; SMBD Jewish Gen Hosp, 3755 ch Cote-Sainte-Catherine, Montreal QC H3T 1E2; Mon'07; FRCPC; Neur. Staff, Sir Mortimer B Davis Jewish General; (514)340-8222

ALTMAN, Siemion; 5542 Sunshine Coast Hwy PO Box 949, Sechelt BC V0N 3A0; Katowice (Poland)'69; FRCPC; Psy. Consultant, Sunshine Coast Mental Health Services; University of British Columbia; (604)885-6101; Fax. (604)885-5842.

ALTMAN, Yevgeni; Langley Mem Hosp, 22051 Fraser Hwy, Langley BC V3A 4H4; UBC'90; CCFP; CCFP(E.M.); Staff, Langley Memorial Hospital; (604)534-4121

ALTMANN, Karolina; 404-450 Central Ave, London ON N6B 2E5; (Slovakia)'96; Langs: Slovak; Czech; (519)204-5761; Fax. (519)204-6817.

ALTMEYER, Ronald C; CFB Edmonton, PO Box 10500 Stn Forces, Edmonton AB T5J 4J5; Ott'09; BSc; CCFP; Physician, CFB Health Services Centre; (780)973-4011; Fax. (780)973-1635.

ALTO, Lauri E C; Manitoba Clinic, 790 Sherbrook St, Winnipeg MB R3A 1M3; Man'84; FRCPC; Peds. Assoc Staff, St Boniface General Hospital; (204)774-6541; Fax. (204)783-7163.

ALTOKHAIS, Tariq I S; Hamilton HS-McMaste Site, PO Box 2000 Stn Lcd 1 1200 Main St W, Hamilton ON L8N 3Z5; King Saud University (Saudi Arabia)'02; Clin Fellow Pediatric GenSurg, Hamilton Health Sciences Centre - McMaster Children's Hospital; (905)521-2100

ALTOMARE, Filiberto; 801-61 Queen St E, Toronto ON M5C 2T2; Tor'91; BSc; DAB; FRCSC; Ophth. Staff, Mount Sinai Hospital; Staff, Princess Margaret Hospital - University Health Network; Staff, St Michael's Hospital; (416)867-3708; Fax. (416)867-7482.

ALTON, Bryan J; Medical Arts Bldg, 700-1 Young St, Hamilton ON L8N 1T8; Wes'85; CCFP; FCFP; Ac Staff, St Joseph's Healthcare - Charlton Campus; Court Staff, Hamilton Health Sciences Centre - McMaster University Medical Centre; Clinical Asst Prof Family Med, McMaster University; (289)396-5105; Fax. (289)396-5683.

ALTON, Susan H; Whitehorse Med Services Ltd, 406 Lambert St, Whitehorse YT Y1A 1Z7; Alb'87; CCFP; Staff, Whitehorse Medical Services Ltd; (867)393-6600; Fax. (867)393-6601.

ALTURKISTANI, Majed; Dr Georges-L Dumont Reg Hosp, 330 av Universite, Moncton NB E1C 2Z3; Makkah (Saudi Arabia)'03; FRCPC; Anes. Staff, Dr Georges-L-Dumont University Hospital Centre; (506)862-4000

ALVAREZ, A Nanette; Peter Lougheed Centre, 3500 26 Ave NE, Calgary AB T1Y 6J4; Qns'81; FRCPC; IntMed (Adult Congenital Heart Disease); Cardiol. Staff Cardiol, Peter Lougheed Centre; Staff, Calgary Regional Health Authority; Assoc Prof, University of Calgary; Langs: Spanish; French; (403)943-4920; Fax. (403)250-9539.

ALVAREZ, Carlos A; Aberdeen Hosp, 835 East River Rd, New Glasgow NS B2H 3S6; (Mexico)'71; FRCSC; GenSurg (Laparoscopic Surgery). Staff, Aberdeen Regional Hospital; Langs: Spanish; (902)752-7600

ALVAREZ, Christine M; Children's & Women's HC of BC, A203-4480 Oak St, Vancouver BC V6H 3V4; UBC'93; BSc; MSc(Surg); FRCSC; OrthSurg (Pediatric Orthopedic Surgery). Staff, BC Children's Hospital; Asst Prof Med, University of British Columbia; (604)875-2178; Fax. (604)875-2275.

ALVAREZ, Elizabeth; 179 James St S, Hamilton ON L8P 3A3; Toledo (USA)'02; CCFP; (905)529-9779

ALVAREZ, Fernando; Hôpital Ste-Justine, 3175 ch Cote-Sainte-Catherine, Montreal QC H3T 1C5; Buenos Aires (Argentina)'74; Dir Peds, Hôpital Ste-Justine; Prof, Universite de Montreal; Langs: Spanish; French; (514)345-4626; Fax. (514)345-4999; fernando.alvarez@umontreal.ca.

ALVAREZ, Fresnel J; Ctr de Sante Vallee-Gatineau, 309 boul Desjardins, Maniwaki QC J9E 2E7; Laval'10; CCFP; Staff, CSSS de la Vallée de la Gatineau; (819)449-2300

ALVAREZ, George F; Rockyview Gen Hosp, 7007 14 St SW, Calgary AB T2V 1P9; Man'96; FRCPC; IntMed (Intensive Care). Staff, Rockyview General Hospital; (403)943-8781

ALVAREZ, Gonzalo G; The Ottawa Hosp-Gen Campus, L1243-501 Smyth Rd, Ottawa ON K1H 8L6; Ott'99; FRCPC; IntMed; Respir. Staff, The Ottawa Hospital - General Campus; Langs: Spanish; French; (613)737-8899 x79294

ALVAREZ, Isabel F; Markham Family Health Team, 1-122 Cornell Park Ave, Markham ON L6B 1B6; Wes'83; CCFP; FCFP; Ac Staff Family Med, Markham Stouffville Hospital; (905)471-9999; ialvarez@msh.on.ca.

ALVAREZ- HIGUERA, Andrea D; Homewood Health Centre, 150 Delhi St, Guelph ON N1E 6K9; Nueva Granada (Colombia)'99; FRCPC; Psy. Staff, Homewood Health Centre; (519)824-1010

ALVAREZ BERNAL, Cesar E; CSSS Pierre Boucher, 1333 boul Jacques-Cartier E, Longueuil QC J4M 2A5; Havana (Cuba)'85; Spécialiste Psy, Centre Hospitalier Pierre Boucher; Langs: Spanish; (450)468-8111

ALVARO, Ruben E; Women's Hosp, WR004-735 Notre Dame Ave, Winnipeg MB R3E 0L8; University of Rosario (Argentina)'81; Staff Neonatol, Health Sciences Centre; Med Dir Neonatol, St Boniface General Hospital; Assoc Prof Peds, University of Manitoba; Langs: Spanish; (204)787-4953; Fax. (204)787-1587.

ALVES, Cristina; The Hosp for Sick Children, 555 University Ave, Toronto ON M5G 1X8; Coimbra (Portugal)'96; Staff, The Hospital For Sick Children; (416)813-6686

ALVI, Fozia S; Doctors Plus Med Centre, 310-505 Main St SW, Airdrie AB T4B 3K3; (Pakistan)'97; CCFP; (403)945-0770

ALVI, Mansour I; Athlete's Care, 5095 Yonge St, North York ON M2N 6Z4; McM'04; FRCSC; OrthSurg. Staff, Mount Sinai Hospital; (416)479-8685

ALVI, Ruby M; Trillium Summerville Fam Med U, 700-101 Queensway W, Mississauga ON L5B 2P7; Tor'95; MHSc; CCFP; Physician, Trillium Health Centre - Mississauga; (905)272-9900; Fax. (905)272-9977.

ALWASAIDI, Turki A M; The Ottawa Hosp-Gen Campus, L2248-501 Smyth Rd, Ottawa ON K1H 8L6; Jeddah (Saudi Arabia)'01; Hem; IntMed. (613)737-8899; Fax. (613)739-6956.

ALWAYN, Ian P J; Queen Elizabeth II HSC, 6S 291-1276 South Park St, Halifax NS B3H 2Y9; Leiden (Netherlands)'94; MD; Staff, Queen Elizabeth II Health Sciences Centre - Victoria General Site; (902)473-6193; Fax. (902)473-6640.

ALWIN, David M; Ctr Hosp Anna-Laberge, 200 boul Brisebois, Chateauguay QC J6K 4W8; Yale (USA)'85; FRCPC; IntMed. Staff IntMed, Hôpital Anna-Laberge; Staff, St Mary's Hospital Centre; (450)699-2425; Fax. (450)699-2510; alwin@sympatico.ca.

ALY, Hazem M; Saint John Reg Hosp, PO Box 2100 Stn Main 400 University Ave, Saint John NB E2L 4L2; Staff, Saint John Regional Hospital; (506)648-6000

ALY, Hoda M M; 200-20 Wynford Dr, North York ON M3C 1J4; Ain Shams (Egypt)'03; CCFP; (416)444-6161; Fax. (416)444-5849.

ALY, Nahla Y S; Tiny Tots Med Centre, 6900 boul Decare, Cote Saint-Luc QC H3X 2T8; Cairo (Egypt)'82; CCFP; (514)342-9911

ALYAMI, Fahad; Dartmouth Gen Hosp, 325 Pleasant St, Dartmouth NS B2Y 4G8; Riyadh (Saudi Arabia)'05; MB BS; Staff, Dartmouth General Hospital; (902)465-8300

ALYOUSIF, Mohammad A S; Addiction & Mental Hlth-Clarke, 620-250 College St, Toronto ON M5T 1R8; Riyadh (Saudi Arabia)'01; Clin Fellow Psy, Centre for Addiction & Mental Health (CAMH) - College Street Site.

ALZABEN, Faten; London HSC-South Street Site, PO Box 5375 Stn B 5058-375 South St, London ON N6A 4G5; Jeddah (Saudi Arabia)'00; FRCPC; Psy. Fellow, London Health Sciences Centre - South Street; (519)685-8500

ALZRIGHE, Mohamed; 101-58 Tacoma Dr, Dartmouth NS B2W 3E5; Al-Fateh (Libya)'98; MB ChB; CCFP; (902)466-1531; Fax. (902)466-1352.

AMAD, Hani; Yonge-Eglinton Med Centre, LL07-2401 Yonge St, Toronto ON M4P 3H1; Alb'02; FRCPC; IntMed; Cardiol. Staff, Southlake Regional Health Centre; Staff, William Osler Health System - Etobicoke General Hospital; Staff, William Osler Health System - Brampton Civic Hospital; (647)345-5590

AMADALA, S; Foothills Med Centre, 1403 29 St NW, Calgary AB T2N 2T9; Nairobi (Kenya)'84; MB ChB; MRCPsy; DPM; DipAeroMed; FRCP; FRCPC; Psy (Addiction Psychiatry). Staff, Foothills Medical Centre; Langs: Kiswahili; Swahili; (403)944-1296; stephen.amadala@calgaryhealthregion.ca.

AMADEO, Ryan J J; Health Sciences Centre, GH6-820 Sherbrook St, Winnipeg MB R3A 1R9; Man'98; FRCPC; Anes. Staff, Health Sciences Centre; (204)774-6511

AMADU, Adam A; Thompson Gen Hosp, 871 Thompson Dr, Thompson MB R8N 0C8; Crimea (Ukraine)'92; CCFP; CCFP(E.M.); Staff, Thompson General Hospital; (204)677-2381

AMAHZOUNE, Mohamed; 309 boul Desjardins, Maniwaki QC J9E 2E7; (Morocco)'97; (819)449-4690

AMALADOSS, Antony S J; Integrated Psychiatric Service, 306-672 Brant St, Burlington ON L7R 2H4; Madras (India)'76; Langs: Tamil; (905)637-2586 x13

AMALADOSS, Noel R; Joseph Brant Mem Hosp, 1230 Northshore Blvd, Burlington ON L7S 1W7; Stellenbosch (South Africa)'04; Psy. Staff, Joseph Brant Memorial Hospital; (905)632-3737

AMAMOO, Adwoa B; Appletree Med Group, 15-1 Rossland Rd W, Ajax ON L1Z 1Z2; Mem'08; CCFP; (647)722-2370; Fax. (416)367-4301.

AMAN, Ijaz; Royal Alexandra Hosp, 10240 Kingsway NW, Edmonton AB T5H 3V9; Punjab (India)'88; Staff, Royal Alexandra Hospital; (780)735-4670

AMAND, Herve; CSSS du Nord de Lanaudière, 1000 boul Sainte-Anne, St-Charles-Brromee QC J6E 6J2; Louvain (Belgium)'89; Staff, Centre Hospitalier Régional de Lanaudière; (450)759-8222 x2004; Fax. (450)759-8152.

AMANI, Hossein; Toronto Rehab Univer Centre, 550 University Ave, Toronto ON M5G 2A2; Tor'92; FRCPC; PhysMed&Rehab (Pain Medicine). Clin Instructor, University of Toronto; Langs: Farsi; (416)597-3422

AMANI, Neda; 474 Elgin St, Ottawa ON K2P 2J6; Tor'98; BSc; Langs: Farsi; French; (613)825-7701; Fax. (613)825-1299.

AMANIE, John O; Cross Cancer Institute, 11560 University Ave NW, Edmonton AB T6G 1Z2; Sask'98; FRCPC; RadOncol. Staff, Cross Cancer Institute; (780)432-8518

AMANKWAH, Kofi S; Mackenzie Richmond Hill Hosp, 10 Trench St, Richmond Hill ON L4C 4Z3; Alb'67; CAB(Maternal&FetalMed.); FRCSC; ObstGyn (Perinatal). Staff, Mackenzie Richmond Hill Hospital; (905)883-1212

AMANKWAH, Yaa Obesebea; The Ottawa Hosp-Riverside, 7F-1967 Riverside Dr, Ottawa ON K1H 7W9; (Ghana)'98; MB ChB; FRCSC; ObstGyn (Menopause). Staff, The Ottawa Hospital - General Campus; Staff, The Ottawa Hospital - Riverside Campus; Asst Prof, University of Ottawa; (613)738-8400; Fax. (613)738-8524.

AMANKWE, Isaac O; Hilltop Med Clinic, 140-15321 16th Ave, Surrey BC V4A 1R6; (Other Foreign)'93; CCFP; (604)531-5575

AMANN, Eric W; Rosedale Med Centre, 310-600 Sherbourne St, Toronto ON M4X 1W4; Man'61; Langs: German; (416)463-1123; Fax. (416)463-5223; amann_eric@on.aibn.com.

AMANN, Justin H; London X-Ray Associates, 104-450 Central Ave, London ON N6B 2E8; Wes'94; FRCPC; DiagRad. Staff, St Joseph's Hospital - St Joseph's Health Care; (519)672-5270

AMANULLAH, Shabbir; Hillsborough Hsp & Special CC, PO Box 1929 Stn Central 115 Murchison Lane, Charlottetown PE C1A 7N5; Mysore (India)'94; FRCPC; Psy. Staff, Hillsborough Hospital & Special Care Centre; (902)368-5400

AMANULLAH, Syed F; 707A-5010 43 St, Red Deer AB T4N 6H2; (Pakistan)'87; (403)314-0355; Fax. (403)314-0499.

AMAR, Charles; Cite Sante St-Laurent, 1-1077 rue Decarie, Saint-Laurent QC H4L 3M8; Mon'88; Staff, Centre Hospitalier l'Université de Montréal (CHUM) - Hôtel-Dieu; Staff, CSSS du Coeur de l'Isle Hôpital Jean-Talon; (514)747-5556; Fax. (514)747-5557.

AMAR, Jack N; Pacific Gastroenterology Assoc, 770-1190 Hornby St, Vancouver BC V6Z 2K5; Tor'77; ABIM; FRCP; FRCPC; IntMed; Gastroent. Ac Staff, Providence Health Care - St Paul's Hospital; Asst Prof, University of British Columbia; (604)688-6332 x221; Fax. (604)689-2004; jackamar@shaw.ca.

AMAR, Maxime; Centre Affilie Universitaire, 3F-880 rue Pere-Marquette, Quebec QC G1S 2A4; Laval'89; assoc Membre, Centre Hospitalier Affilié Universitaire de Québec - Hôpital du St-Sacrement; Infectious Diseases, CSSS de la Vieille-Capitale; Langs: Italian; English; French; Spanish; (418)681-8787 x3857; Fax. (418)687-9694; maxime.amar@fmed.ulaval.ca.

AMAR, Simon; MUHC-Montreal Gen Hosp, 1650 av Cedar, Montreal QC H3G 1A4; McG'02; FRCPC; Psy. Staff, McGill University Health Centre - Montreal General Campus; (514)934-1934 x44758

AMAR, Yannick G; CSSS du Lac-des-Deux-Montagnes, 520 boul Arthur-Sauve, St-Eustache QC J7R 5B1; McG'98; FRCSC; Otol. Staff, Hôpital de Saint-Eustache; (450)473-6811

AMARAKONE, Inoka D; Ridgeview Med Centre, 212-1240 Railway Ave, Canmore AB T1W 1P4; (United Kingdom)'00; MB ChB; (403)609-8333

AMARAKONE, Samudrika H G; Southbank Med Centre, 3-2430 Bank St, Ottawa ON K1V 0T7; Peradeniya (Sri Lanka)'76; MB BS; CCFP; (613)736-6946; Fax. (613)736-6948.

AMARAL, Andre C K; Sunnybrook Hlth Sciences Ctre, D108-2075 Bayview Ave, Toronto ON M4N 3M5; Sao Paolo (Brazil)'98; Staff, Sunnybrook Health Sciences Centre; (416)480-6100

AMARAL, Joao G P V; The Hosp For Sick Children, 555 University Ave, Toronto ON M5G 1X8; Parana (Brazil)'97; Staff, The Hospital For Sick Children; (416)813-7654 x1652; joao.amaral@sickkids.ca.

AMARASEKERA, D Vimal S; One Step Med Centre, 1A-3585 Lawrence Ave E, Scarborough ON M1G 1P4; (Sri Lanka)'78; CCFP; (416)431-0736; Fax. (416)431-0648.

AMARASEKERA, Sukeshini; 8-700 Markham Rd, Scarborough ON M1H 2A7; Ceylon (Sri Lanka)'82; MB BS; FAAP; Peds. Staff Ped, Crescent Town Health Centre; Langs: Sinhalese; (416)264-3443; Fax. (416)264-3446.

AMARATUNGA, Kanchana R; PG Medical Education Office, MDCL 3101A-1280 Main St, Hamilton ON L8S 4K1; McM'08; IntMed.

AMARATUNGA, Ruwan T; The Ottawa Hosp-Gen Campus, 510 Smyth Rd Box 210, Ottawa ON K1H 8L6; Wes'08; IntMed. Staff, The Ottawa Hospital - General Campus; (613)722-7000

AMARIEI, I Camelia; Eagle Ridge Hosp & Hlth CC, 475 Guildford Way, New Westminster BC V3H 3W9; Iasi (Romania)'91; Staff, Eagle Ridge Hospital & Health Care Centre; (604)461-2022

AMARIYEN, Dawi H M; Univ of Toronto, 2F-500 University Ave, Toronto ON M5G 1V7; Benghazi (Libya)'98.

AMARO, Justine L; Th Ottawa Hosp-Gen Campus, 501 Smyth Rd, Ottawa ON K1H 8L6; Cal'01; CCFP; CCFP(E.M.); Staff, The Ottawa Hospital - General Campus; Langs: Bilingual(English/French); (613)722-7000

AMATO, Dominick J; 438-600 University Ave, Toronto ON M5G 1X5; Michigan (USA)'67; FRCPC; Hem (Clinical Hematology). Staff Physician, Mount Sinai Hospital; Assoc Prof Med, University of Toronto; (416)586-4800 x5189; Fax. (416)586-4677; damato@mtsinai.on.ca.

AMATO, Victor; Royal Alex Place, 225-10106 111 Ave NW, Edmonton AB T5G 0B4; Cape Town (South Africa)'65; CCFP; Ac Staff, Covenant Health - Misericordia Community Hospital; Court Staff, Covenant Health - Edmonton General Continuing Care Centre; (780)428-7751

AMATTO, Michael J; West Village Mall, 160 Columbia Blvd W, Lethbridge AB T1K 4J4; Alb'95; (403)381-7000; Fax. (403)381-8250.

AMBA, Sudhir; Wellington Med Arts Bldg, 202-121 Wellington St W, Barrie ON L4N 1L2; Delhi (India)'76; DABIM; ABIM(Rheum); FRCPC; IntMed (Rheumatology). Staff, Royal Victoria Regional Health Centre; (705)722-5333

AMBALAVANAR, Elancheliyan; Rouge Valley-Centenary HC, 2867 Ellesmere Rd, Scarborough ON M1E 4B9; Sri Jayewardenepura (Sri Lanka)'01; CCFP; Staff, Rouge Valley Health System - Centenary Health Centre Site; Langs: Tamil; (416)281-7270

AMBERG, Stephane J; CSSSG-Hop de Hull, 116 boul Lionel-Emond, Gatineau QC J8Y 1W7; Ott'03; FRCPC; Anes. Staff, Hull Hospital; (819)595-6000

AMBIS, Christopher J; Health Sciences Bldg, 310-15 Mountain Ave S, Stoney Creek ON L8G 2V6; McM'00; CCFP; (905)664-3730; Fax. (905)664-9921.

AMBIS, Robert J S; Health Sciences Bldg, 310-15 Mountain Ave S, Stoney Creek ON L8G 2V6; Ott'66; Asst Prof, McMaster University; (905)664-3730; Fax. (905)664-9921.

AMBLER, Kimberley L S; Gordon & Leslie Diamond HC, 10F-2775 Laurel St, Vancouver BC V5Z 1M9; Dal'06; FRCPC; IntMed; Hem. (604)875-4863

AMBREEN, Shazia; Stevenson Mem Hosp, PO Box 4000 Stn Main 200 Fletcher Cres, Alliston ON L9R 1W7; Karachi (Pakistan)'98; CCFP; Staff, Stevenson Memorial Hospital; (705)435-6281

AMBROSANO, Lorella; Plaza 2 Shopping Ctr, 609-8600 Franklin Ave, Fort McMurray AB T9H 4G8; (South Africa)'87; (780)743-0630; Fax. (780)791-7539.

AMBROSE, Devon J; 305-400 Tache Ave, Winnipeg MB R2H 3C3; Man'06; FRCSC; ObstGyn.

AMBROSE, Laura E; Surrey Prenatal Clinic, 9655 137 St, Surrey BC V3T 4G8; UBC'10; CCFP; (778)395-0085

AMBROZIC, Laura K; Lonsdale Med Dental Bldg, 108-1940 Lonsdale Ave, North Vancouver BC V7M 2K2; Qns'99; CCFP; (604)987-3347

AMBULGEKAR, Shivaji M; Murals Medical Clinic, 105-22314 Fraser Hwy, Langley BC V3A 8M6; Marathwuda (India)'73; MB BS; MRC(UK); CCFP; Staff, Langley Memorial Hospital; (604)532-9944; shivambulgekar@shaw.ca.

AMDEMICHAEL, Esiahas; Waterloo Sports Med Centre, 5-65 University Ave E, Waterloo ON N2J 2V9; Tor'90; FRCPC; CCFP; AnatPath (Dermatological Pathology); Derm. Asst Prof Med, Northern Ontario School of Medicine; (519)342-1307; esiahas@gmail.com.

AMDURSKY, David; Kildare Family Med Associates, 8-7005 ch Kildare, Cote Saint-Luc QC H4W 1C1; McG'76; CCFP; (514)489-5785; Fax. (514)489-5786.

AMED, Shazhan; BC Women's Hosp & Health Ctre, 4500 Oak St, Vancouver BC V6H 3N1; Cal'01; FRCPC; Peds; Endocrin&Metab. Staff, BC Women's Hospital & Health Centre; (604)875-2345 x4803

AMEDE, Kebede H; The Brandon Clinic, 620 Dennis St, Brandon MB R7A 5E7; Addis Ababa (Ethiopia)'84; LMCC; Staff, Rossburn Health Centre; Staff, Brandon Regional Health Centre; Langs: Amharic; (204)728-4440; Fax. (204)726-1765.

AMEEN, Rukhsana; 981 Hollingsworth Bend NW, Edmonton AB T6R 3G7; (Pakistan)'82; Staff, Royal Alexandra Hospital; (780)438-9365

AMEEN, Sakeenah; A8-1390 Major Mackenzie E, Richmond Hill ON L4S 0A1; Mahatma Gandhi Missions Med College (India)'01; CCFP; (905)884-7711

AMEIS, Arthur; 502-333 Wilson Ave, North York ON M3H 1T2; Tor'75; DABPM; FAAPMR; FRCPC; PhysMed&Rehab (Pain Management). Assoc Staff, North York General Hospital - Branson Division; Consultant, Multi-Disciplinary Assessment Centre; (416)388-3111

AMEIS, Stephanie; The Hosp for Sick Children, 555 University Ave, Toronto ON M5G 1X8; McM'04; FRCPC; Psy. Staff Psy, The Hospital For Sick Children; (416)813-6600

AMELI, F Michael; 605-55 Queen St E, Toronto ON M5C 1R6; Birmingham (England)'63; MB ChB; LRCP; FRCS(E); FACS; FRCSC; VascSurg (General Surgery). Chief Div of VascSurg/Assoc Prof Med, St Michael's Hospital; (416)864-5143; Fax. (416)864-5160.

AMENDY, Ulrich; Alberta Children's Hosp, 2888 Shaganappi Trail NW, Calgary AB T3B 6A8; (Germany)'92; Staff, Alberta Children's Hospital; (403)955-7985; Fax. (403)955-7656.

AMER, Amal A M M; Seaway Valley Comm Hlth Ctre, 353 Pitt St, Cornwall ON K6J 3R1; Alexandria (Egypt)'96; CCFP; (613)936-0306; Fax. (613)936-0521.

AMER, Emad E; Credit Valley Prof Bldg, 511-2300 Eglinton Ave W, Mississauga ON L5M 2V8; Cairo (Egypt)'63; MRCP(Lond); FCCP; FACP; IntMed (Respirology). Staff Div of Respirol, The Credit Valley Hospital; Staff Ontario Immigration & WSIB Roster, Worker's Safety & Insurance Board; Langs: Arabic; (905)820-7999; Fax. (905)820-7991.

AMER, Rebecca K; St Joseph's Healthcare, 50 Charlton Ave E, Hamilton ON L8N 4A6; McM'04; FRCPC; IntMed; Respir. Staff, St Joseph's Healthcare - Charlton Campus; Langs: Bilingual(English/French); (905)522-1155 x33714

AMER, Tehmina; 455 Trafalgar Rd, Oakville ON L6J 3H8; Punjab (India)'88; (905)338-9594

AMES, Christina M; SMBD Jewish Gen Hosp, 3755 ch Cote-Sainte-Catherine, Montreal QC H3T 1E2; UBC'08; CCFP; CCFP(E.M.); Staff, Sir Mortimer B Davis Jewish General; (514)340-8222

AMES, Janet E; 511-1669 Victoria St, Prince George BC V2L 2L5; McM'83; Dip SportMed; CCFP; FCFP; Staff, University Hospital of Northern British Columbia; (250)596-2454

AMES, Robert P E; Goodfelow Med Centre, 203-170 McEwan Dr E, Bolton ON L7E 4C8; Tor'91; Court Staff, Humber River Regional Hospital - Finch Avenue Site; (905)951-1575; Fax. (905)951-1786.

AMHALHAL, Ismeil M A; Sault Area Hosp, 750 Great Northern Rd, Sault Ste. Marie ON P6B 0A8; Benghazi (Libya)'97; FRCPC; IntMed; Cardiol. Staff, Sault Area Hospital - Sault Ste Marie; (705)759-3434

AMID, Ali; Children Hosp of Eastern Ont, 401 Smyth Rd, Ottawa ON K1H 8L1; Tehran (Iran)'02; Peds. Staff, Children's Hospital of Eastern Ontario (CHEO).

AMIEN, Bashrat A; Devon Gen Hosp, 101 Erie St S, Devon AB T9G 1A6; (South Africa)'03; MB ChB; Staff, Devon General Hospital; (780)987-4322; Fax. (780)987-4333; bashamien@gmail.com.

AMIES, David R; Moose Jaw Union Hosp, 455 Fairford St E, Moose Jaw SK S6H 1H3; Witwatersrand (South Africa)'52; MB ChB; FACP; FRCPC; IntMed (Hyperbaric Medicine). Dir Diagnostic Labs, Moose Jaw Union Hospital; (306)694-0200; drussellamies@sasktel.net.

AMIGO, Pablo Hernán; Grey Nuns Community Hosp & HC, STN 43-1100 Youville Drive Wes, Edmonton AB T6L 5X8; (Argentina)'93; MD; Att Physician Pallative Care Unit, Covenant Health - Grey Nuns Community Hospital; Clinical Asst Prof Div of Palliative Care Dept of Oncol, University of Alberta; Langs: Spanish; (780)735-7044; Fax. (780)735-7700; pablo.amigo@albertahealthservices.ca.

AMIMI, Myriam N; 1-677 Great Northern Rd, Sault Ste. Marie ON P6B 5A1; Ott'92; FRCSC; ObstGyn. Staff ObstGyn, Sault Area Hospital - Sault Ste Marie; Langs: English; French; (705)942-5151; Fax. (705)942-7421.

AMIN, Bita; Worker's Compensation Board, 333 Broadway, Winnipeg MB R3C 4W3; (Other Foreign)'00; Staff, Workers' Comp Board of MB; (204)954-4339

AMIN, Devendra H; Stonebridge Medical Clinic, 2-303 Stonebridge Rd, Saskatoon SK S7T 0G3; St. Andrews (Scotland)'65; MB ChB; (306)382-6666; Fax. (306)382-6686.

AMIN, Faizan Z; PG Medical Education Office, MDCL 3101A-1280 Main St W, Hamilton ON L8S 4K1; McM'10.

AMIN, Harish J; Alberta Children's Hosp, C4 615-2888 Shaganappi Tr NW, Calgary AB T3B 6A8; London (England)'81; MRC(UK); FAAP; FRCPC; Peds (Neonatology). Staff, Alberta Children's Hospital; Asst Prof, University of Calgary; (403)955-7251; Fax. (403)955-3045.

AMIN, Hussein M N; Lewisporte Med Clinic, PO Box 1195 1207 Main St, Lewisporte NL A0G 3A0; Baghdad (Iraq)'03; MB BS; CCFP; Staff, Green Bay Community Health Centre; Gen Physician, Connaigre Peninsula Community Health Centre; (709)535-8617; Fax. (709)535-0172; hussein.amin@easternhealth.ca.

AMIN, Jayshree; Cobourg Med Centre, 5-1060 Burnham St, Cobourg ON K9A 5V9; McG'79; Ac Staff, Northumberland Hills Hospital; (905)373-8333; Fax. (905)373-9333.

AMIN, Leena; William Osler HC-Etobicoke, 101 Humber College Blvd, Etobicoke ON M9V 1R8; Wes'08; FRCPC; IntMed. Staff, William Osler Health System - Etobicoke General Hospital; (416)494-2120

AMIN, Nalin K; St Joseph's Healthcare, 50 Charlton Ave E, Hamilton ON L8N 4A6; Man'00; BSc; FRCSC; GenSurg. Staff, St Joseph's Healthcare - Charlton Campus; (905)522-1155

AMIN, Parsa F; 224-40 Finchgate Blvd, Brampton ON L6T 3J1; Wes'06; CCFP; Langs: Urdu; (905)451-6959

AMIN, Prakash A; 3601-1499 Pender St W, Vancouver BC V6G 0A7; Indore (India)'70; MB BS; Vis Staff, Vancouver General Hospital - Centennial Pavillion; (604)434-7414

AMIN, Reham; William Osler HC-Brampton Civi, 2100 Bovaird Dr E, Brampton ON L6R 3J7; Dal'02; FRCPC; IntMed; Critical Care Medicine. Staff, William Osler Health System - Brampton Civic Hospital; (905)494-2120 x50554

AMIN, Shabbir F; Walk-In Med Clinic, 9368 Southfort Dr, Fort Saskatchewan AB T8L 0C5; Bombay (India)'66; MB BS; CCFP; Staff, Fort Saskatchewan Health Centre; Langs: Urdu; Hindi; Gujarati; (780)997-0177; Fax. (780)992-2065; walkinclinic@shaw.ca.

AMIN, Shaista; 2-310 Guelph St, Georgetown ON L7G 4B1; Karachi (Pakistan)'83; CCFP; Staff, Halton Healthcare Services Corporation - Georgetown Hospital; Physician, Winston Churchill Medical Centre; (289)428-1014; Fax. (905)877-5554.

AMIN, Sheikh N U; Recreation Athletic & Wellness, 3359 Mississauga Rd N, Mississauga ON L5L 1C6; Saba University School of Medicine (Netherlands Antilles)'07; CCFP; (905)820-9292; Fax. (905)820-9250.

AMIN, Shilpa; ONE Fertility Clinic, 3210 Harvester Rd, Burlington ON L7N 3T1; Man'96; BSc; FRCSC; ObstGyn (Reproductive Endocrinology & Infertility). Staff, Hamilton Health Sciences Centre - McMaster Children's Hospital; Asst Prof, McMaster University; Langs: Hindi; (905)634-4440; Fax. (905)639-3810; aminsh@mcmaster.ca.

AMIN, Smita; Sheppard Med Bldg, 304/305-701 Sheppard Ave E, North York ON M2K 2Z3; McG'87; FRCPC; IntMed; Derm. Langs: English; French; (416)590-9918; Fax. (416)590-9842; smita.amin@utoronto.ca.

AMIN, Surendra; Univ of Waterloo Health Servic, 200 University Ave W, Waterloo ON N2L 3G1; Glasgow (Scotland)'67; MB ChB; FRCS(Glas); CCFP; Physician, University Of Waterloo; (519)888-4567

AMIN, Sushma; Pelham Group Health Centre, 104-245 Pelham Rd, St Catharines ON L2S 1X8; McG'84; DABOT; FRCSC; Otol. Consultant, Niagara Health System - Greater Niagara General Site; Ac Staff, Niagara Health System - St Catharines General Site; Staff, Hôtel Dieu Shaver Health & Rehabilitation Centre; (905)641-0677; Fax. (905)641-0520.

AMIN, Zahir S; Sheldon Chumir Urgent CC, 1213 4th St SW, Calgary AB T2R 0X7; (Australia)'04; CCFP; (403)955-6011

AMIN HASHEM, Mohamed; Ctr Hosp Affilie-Enfant-Jesus, 1401 18e rue, Quebec QC G1J 1Z4; (Egypt)'93; Staff, Centre Hospitalier Affilié Universitaire de Québec - Hôpital De L'Enfant Jésus; (418)649-5700; Fax. (418)649-5856; m2amin@hotmail.com.

AMINAZADEH, Nasser; 2175 Sheppard Ave E, North York ON M2J 1W8; Tehran (Iran)'97; FRCSC; GenSurg. Staff, St Joseph's Healthcare - Charlton Campus; (416)492-7700; Fax. (416)492-5776.

AMINBAKHSH, Amin; 201-245 Columbia St E, New Westminster BC V3L 3W4; Tehran (Iran)'90; FRCPC; IntMed; Cardiol. (604)522-8667

AMINI, Zarlasht; Queensway Carleton Hosp, 3045 Baseline Rd, Ottawa ON K2H 8P4; Staff, Queensway Carleton Hospital; (613)828-3122

AMIOT, Louis-Philippe; Hop Maisonneuve-Rosemont, 5415 boul de l'Assomption, Montreal QC H1T 2M4; Mon'95; MSc; FRCSC; OrthSurg (Spine). Staff, Hopital Maisonneuve-Rosemont; Langs: English; (514)252-3400; Fax. (514)252-3506.

AMIR, Eitan; Univ Hlth Network-Princess M, 5 214-610 University Ave, Toronto ON M5G 2M9; Manchester (England)'03; PhD; Staff MedOncol, Princess Margaret Hospital - University Health Network; Langs: Hebrew; (416)946-4501 x5181; Fax. (416)946-4563.

AMIR, Igal M; A335-SMBD Jewish Gen Hosp, 3755 ch Cote-Sainte-Catherine, Montreal QC H3T 1E2; McG'91; CSPQ; FRCPC; Anes. Staff, Sir Mortimer B Davis Jewish General; (514)340-8222 x5701

AMIR, Mohammad F; St George Med Clinic, 16-585 Ontario St S, Milton ON L9T 2N2; Peshawar (Pakistan)'00; (905)693-9500; Fax. (905)693-8600.

AMIRALI, Evangelia-Lila; MUHC-Montreal Children's Hosp, D580-2300 rue Tupper, Montreal QC H3H 1P3; Athens (Greece)'86; FRCPC; Psy (Child Psychiatry). Staff, McGill University Health Centre - Montreal Children's Hospital; Langs: French; Greek; (514)412-4400 x22169; lila.amirali@mcgill.ca.

AMIRAULT, J David; Queen Elizabeth II HSC-Halifax, 4857-1796 Summer St, Halifax NS B3H 3A7; Dal'76; BSc; FRCSC; OrthSurg. Staff, Queen Elizabeth II Health Sciences Centre - Halifax Infirmary Site; Staff, Queen Elizabeth II Health Sciences Centre - Victoria General Site; Assoc Prof, Dalhousie University; (902)473-7108; Fax. (902)473-4580; david.amirault@cdha.nshealth.ca.

AMIRJANI, Nasim; Synergy Wellness Centre, 129-501 Bethel Dr, Sherwood Park AB T8H 0N2; Iran University (Iran)'98; FRCPC; PhysMed&Rehab. Staff, Glenrose Rehabilitation Hospital; (780)416-8747; Fax. (780)449-5461.

AMIRKHALKHALI, Baharak; IWK Health Centre, PO Box 9700 Rpo CSC, Halifax NS B3K 6R8; Dal'00; FRCSC; ObstGyn. Staff, IWK Health Centre; (902)470-6788; Fax. (902)470-8640.

AMISS, John D; Medical-Dental Bldg, 309-1120 Yates St, Victoria BC V8V 3M9; McG'67; FRCPC; Derm. Consultant, Vancouver Island Health Authority; Clin Instructor Derm, University of British Columbia; (250)384-4887; Fax. (250)384-4799.

AMISSAH-ARTHUR, Justice B; Burin Peninsula Hlth Care Ctr, PO Box 340, Burin NL A0E 1E0; (Ghana)'78; MB ChB; Staff, Burin Peninsula Health Care Centre; (709)891-1040

AMIT, Minoli N; St Martha's Doctor's Offices, 103-23 Bay St, Antigonish NS B2G 2G7; Dal'77; FRCPC; Peds. Staff, St Martha's Regional Hospital; (902)867-1417; Fax. (902)863-1186; m. amit@ns.sympatico.ca.

AMJAD, Afsari B; Royal Ottawa Hlth Care Group, 1145 Carling Ave, Ottawa ON K1Z 7K4; Osmania (India)'70; FRCPC; Psy (General Psychiatry). Staff Psy, Royal Ottawa Mental Health Centre - Royal Ottawa Health Care Group; Asst Prof, University of Ottawa; Langs: Hindi; Punjabi; Urdu; Telugu; (613)722-6521 x6918; Fax. (613)761-3602.

AMJAD, Asim; Allan Blair Cancer Centre, 300-4101 Dewdney Ave, Regina SK S4T 7T1; Staff, Saskatoon Cancer Centre; (306)766-2213; Fax. (306)766-2688.

AMJAD, Asma; 1595 Merivale Rd, Ottawa ON K2G 3K2; Ott'98; CCFP; (613)224-2800; Fax. (613)224-2804.

AMJAD, Saima; Glen Huron Med Centre, 4-1 Glen Hawthorne Blvd, Mississauga ON L5R 0C2; Punjab (Pakistan)'99; CCFP; Langs: Urdu; Punjabi; (905)366-0505; Fax. (905)366-0506.

AMJADI, Kayvan; The Ottawa Hosp-Civic Campus, 1053 Carling Ave, Ottawa ON K1Y 4E9; Qns'99; FRCPC; IntMed (Interventional Pulmonary Medicine); Respir. Staff Interventional Pulmonary, La Verendrye Hospital - Riverside Health Care Facility; Staff, The Ottawa Hospital - Civic Campus; (613)798-5555 x18139

AMLANI, Salima; St Joseph's Healthcare, 50 Charlton Ave E, Hamilton ON L8N 4A6; McM'05; FRCPC; IntMed; Respir. Staff, St Joseph's Healthcare - Charlton Campus; Staff, The Juravinski Cancer Centre; (905)522-1155

AMLANI, Shoaib; William Osler HC-Brampton, 2100 Bovaird Dr E, Brampton ON L6R 3J7; Tor'99; FRCPC; IntMed (Interventional Cardiology); Cardiol. Staff, William Osler Health System - Brampton Civic Hospital; (905)494-2120; Fax. (905)494-6717.

AMMAD, Mahjabeen; 10A-30 Eglinton Ave W, Mississauga ON L5R 3E7; Punjab (India)'86; CCFP; (905)712-2288

AMMANN, Walter; Royal Columbian Hosp, 330 Columbia St E, New Westminster BC V3L 3W7; Man'77; FRCPC; DiagRad; NuclearMed. Staff Nuclear Med, Royal Columbian Hospital; Staff Nuclear Med, Burnaby Hospital; (604)520-4436

AMMAR, Ahmed; CSSS de la Baie-des-Chaleurs, RR 2 419 boul Perron, Maria QC G0C 1Y0; (Tunisia)'96; Staff, CSSS de la Baie-des-Chaleurs; (418)759-1336

AMMARA, Yasmina; CHUM-Hop Notre-Dame, 1560 rue Sherbrooke E, Montreal QC H2L 4M1; Mon'89; Staff, Centre Hospitalier l'Université de Montréal (CHUM) - Hôpital Notre-Dame; Clin Prof Family Med, Universite de Montreal; (514)890-8000

AMOAH-GYAMPOH, Maxwell; Women's Hosp, 735 Notre Dame Ave, Winnipeg MB R3E 0L8; Legon (Ghana)'72; LMCC; Staff, Health Sciences Centre.

AMOG-KERR, Lea M; 120-115 Christopher Dr, Cambridge ON N1R 4S1; U. of The East (Philippines)'64; Ac Staff, Cambridge Memorial Hospital; Langs: Tagalog; (519)622-1210; Fax. (519)622-5322.

AMOLINS, Roland E; Oakville Health Centre, 208-1060 Speers Rd, Oakville ON L6L 2X4; Qns'77; CCFP; Ac Staff Family Med, Halton Healthcare Services Corporation - Oakville Site; Physician, Goodrich Landing Gear & Procor Ltd.; Langs: Estonian; French; (905)842-3735; Fax. (905)842-8001.

AMOO, Kazeem O; Capt William Jackman Mem Hosp, 410 Booth St, Labrador City NL A2V 2K1; (Other Foreign)'94; Locum Tenens, Captain William Jackman Memorial Hospital; (709)944-2632; Fax. (709)944-4155.

AMOODI, Hosam A M; Dartmouth ENT Associates, 35 Baker Dr, Dartmouth NS B2W 0H3; Jeddah (Saudi Arabia)'03; Otol (Head & Neck Surgery). (902)435-8588; Fax. (902)435-8695.

AMOOZEGAR, Farnaz; South Health Campus, 480043-4448 Front St SE, Calgary AB T3M 1M4; Cal'03; FRCPC; Neur (Headache). Staff Neurol, Foothills Medical Centre; Asst Prof, University of Calgary; Langs: Farsi; (403)956-2462; Fax. (403)952-2992.

AMPOFO, Theophilus; West Eglinton Med Centre, 200-2010 Eglinton Ave W, Toronto ON M6E 2K3; McG'71; Langs: Akan; (416)787-2322

AMRA, Suleman; CSSS du Sud de Lanaudière, 911 montee des Pionniers, Terrebonne QC J6V 2H2; Natal (South Africa)'67; MRC(UK); FACP; FRCPC; IntMed (Hepatology); Gastroent. Staff, Centre Hospitalier Pierre le Gardeur; (450)654-7525 x21300

AMRANI, Laila; CSSS de Trois-Rivieres, 1991 boul du Carmel, Trois-Rivieres QC G8Z 3R9; Casablanca (Morocco)'94; Staff, CSSS de Trois-Rivières; (819)697-3333

AMRE, Ramila D; 213-3775 rue University, Montreal QC H3A 2B4; Shivaji (India)'97; FRCPC; AnatPath. (514)398-7192

AMROLIA, Dinyar H; 8-5320 8 Ave SE, Calgary AB T2A 3P5; Vikram (India)'61; MB BS; LRCP; MRCS(Eng); FRCS(Eng); Langs: Gujarati; Hindi; Urdu; (403)273-4604

AMSELLEM, Maurice; Clin Med Henri-Bourassa, 3231 boul Henri-Bourassa E, Montreal-Nord QC H1H 1H2; Toulouse (France)'66; Staff, Centre Hospitalier Fleury; Langs: Spanish; Arabic; English; (514)323-2434; Fax. (514)323-1655.

AMSELLEM-ABECASSIS, Lydie; CLSC St-Andre-Avellin, 14 rue Saint-Andre, St-Andre-Avellin QC J0V 1W0; Paris (France)'94; (819)983-7341

AMSON, Bradley J; 230-1555 McKenzie Ave, Victoria BC V8N 1A4; Sask'83; FRCSC; GenSurg (Bariatric Surgery). Staff, Royal Jubilee Hospital; Staff, Victoria General Hospital; (250)220-8929

AMSTER, Solomon L; 206-13278 Tecumseh Rd E, Windsor ON N8N 3T6; St Maarten (Netherlands Antilles)'06; (519)735-1490; Fax. (519)735-6236.

AMSTUTZ, Ilona L; The Medical Clinic, 10011 96 St, Fort St. John BC V1J 3P3; Lublin (Poland)'95; Preceptor, Fort St John Family Med Residency Program; Langs: Polish; (250)785-6677; Fax. (250)787-0109.

AMSTUTZ, Nancy; CSSS de Trois-Rivieres, 155 rue Toupin, Trois-Rivieres QC G8T 3Z8; Mon'01; Staff, Centre de santé Cloutier-du-Rivage; (819)370-2221 x3311; Fax. (819)370-2401.

AMU-DARKO, Kofi; Maple Creek Primary Care Clini, PO Box 517 36A Pacific Ave, Maple Creek SK S0N 1N0; (Ghana)'89; CCFP; (306)662-2829

AMUNDSEN, Susan; PO Box 30232 Rpo Saanich Centr, Victoria BC V8X 5E1; Alb'04; CCFP.

AMUNDSON, Heather J; Ramblewood Med Clinic, 202-14 Ramblewood Dr, Wasaga Beach ON L9Z 0C4; Ott'87; CCFP; FCFP; (705)422-1888; Fax. (705)422-1078.

AMURAWAIYE, Emmanuel O; 2B-201 King St W, Oshawa ON L1J 2J5; Ibadan (Nigeria)'79; FRCSC; GenSurg (Critical Care/Trauma). Staff, Lakeridge Health - Oshawa Site; Assoc Prof, Queen's University; (905)576-1936; Fax. (905)576-2406.

AMUSAN, Isaac O; 5002 51 St PO Box 326, St Paul AB T0A 3A0; (Nigeria)'82; MB ChB; (780)645-3666; Fax. (780)645-3688.

AMY, Robert J P M; Trafalgar Prof Centre, 304-1235 Trafalgar Rd, Oakville ON L6H 3P1; Alb'72; FAAO; BSc; FRCSC; Ophth. Ac Staff Ophth, Halton Healthcare Services Corporation - Oakville Site; Court Staff, Joseph Brant Memorial Hospital; (905)842-3555; Fax. (905)849-6990.

AMYOT, Arthur; Hop du Sacre-Coeur de Mtl, 5400 boul Gouin O, Montreal QC H4J 1C5; Mon'64; Psy (Consultation). Membre Geriatric Psy, Hôpital du Sacre-Coeur de Montréal; Prof Psy, Universite de Montreal; (514)338-3563; Fax. (514)338-4359.

AMYOT, Diane; CLSC Drummond, 350 rue Saint-Jean, Drummondville QC J2B 5L4; Mon'85; (819)474-2572; damyot@9bit.qc.ca.

AMYOT, Isabelle; College des Medecins du Quebec, 2170 boul Rene-Levesque O, Montreal QC H3H 2T8; Mon'81; ABPeds; MBA; FRCPC; Peds. Langs: Bilingual(French/English); (514)933-4441; Fax. (514)933-2291.

AMYOT, Karyne; Ctr Hosp Anna-Laberge, 200 boul Brisebois, Chateauguay QC J6K 4W8; Sher'97; Staff, Hôpital Anna-Laberge; (450)699-2425

AMYOT, Luce; Polyclinique Med Fabreville, 380 boul Cure-Labelle, Laval QC H7P 5L3; Mon'82; Langs: English; (450)628-5800 x304; Fax. (450)628-0217.

AMYOT, Luce S; CSSS Pierre Boucher, 1333 boul Jacques-Cartier E, Longueuil QC J4M 2A5; Mon'88; Staff, Centre Hospitalier Pierre Boucher; (450)468-6223

AMYOT, Marc-Andre; CSSS du Nord de Lanaudière, 1000 boul Sainte-Anne, St-Charles-Brromee QC J6E 6J2; Sher'90; Staff, Centre Hospitalier Régional de Lanaudière; (450)759-8222; maamyot@videotron.ca.

AMYOT, Marcel A; Institut de L'Oeil de Montreal, 2300 boul Marce-Laurin, Saint-Laurent QC H4R 1J9; Mon'58; Ophth (Cataract). Staff, CSSS de Dorval-Lachine-Lasalle; Clin Prof, Universite de Montreal; Langs: Bilingual(French/English); (514)745-4445; Fax. (514)745-4636; mamyot2012@gmail.com.

AMYOT, Marie-Claudel; Polyclinique Pierre-Le-Gardeur, 1000 montee des Pionniers, Terrebonne QC J6V 2H2; Mon'00; CCFP; Staff, Centre Hospitalier Pierre le Gardeur; (450)657-1313

AMYOT, Robert; Hop du Sacre-Coeur de Mtl, 5400 boul Gouin O, Montreal QC H4J 1C5; Mon'92; CSPQ; FRCPC; IntMed (Echocardiography); Cardiol. Staff, Hôpital du Sacre-Coeur de Montréal; (514)338-2200; Fax. (514)338-2381.

AMYOT, Robert; CHUM-Hotel-Dieu, 3840 rue Saint-Urbain, Montreal QC H2W 1T8; Mon'68; Respir (P.Q.). Chef, Centre Hospitalier l'Université de Montréal (CHUM) - Hôtel-Dieu; (514)890-8170; Fax. (514)890-8179.

AMYOT, Shawn R; Royal Trust Bldg, 401-116 Albert St, Ottawa ON K1P 5G3; Ott'09; CCFP; (613)216-3932; Fax. (613)216-3930.

AMYOT, Sylvain L; CSSS de Saint-Jerome, 290 rue de Montigny, Saint-Jerome QC J7Z 5T3; Mon'95; Critical Care Medicine (P.Q.); IntMed. Staff, Hôtel-Dieu de Saint-Jérôme; (450)432-8208

AN, Pamela H; Harbourfront Medical, 4-8 York St, Toronto ON M5J 2Y2; McM'09; CCFP; (416)366-2273; Fax. (416)366-5665.

AN, Tianyou; CHUM-Hop Notre-Dame, 1560 rue Sherbrooke E, Montreal QC H2L 4M1; McG'05; Anes. Staff, Centre Hospitalier l'Université de Montréal (CHUM) - Hôpital Notre-Dame; (514)890-8000

ANAGNOSTOPOULOS, Nikolaos; Bayview-Finch Med Clinic, 301-3292 Bayview Ave, North York ON M2M 4J5; Tor'99; BScPharm; CCFP; Staff, North York General Hospital; (416)733-9991

ANAGNOSTOU, Evdokia; Holland Bloorview Kids Rehab, 150 Kilgour Rd, Toronto ON M4G 1R8; McG'98; FRCPC; Neur. Staff, Holland Bloorview Kids Rehabilitation Hospital; (416)425-6220; Fax. (416)753-6046.

ANAMARIA, Isabelle; CSSS du Rocher Percé, CP 3300 451 rue Mgr Ross E, Chandler QC G0C 1K0; Mon'92; Staff, Centre Hospitalier de Chandler; (418)689-2261

ANAN, Ghadeer; Dr Everett Chalmers Reg Hosp, PO Box 9000 Stn A 700 Priestman St, Fredericton NB E3B 5N5; Riyadh (Saudi Arabia)'97; FRCPC; MedOncol; IntMed. Staff, Dr Everett Chalmers Regional Hospital; (506)452-5199; Fax. (506)452-5233.

ANAND, Anju; St Michael's Hosp, 6045-30 Bond St, Toronto ON M5B 1W8; Tor'03; FRCPC; IntMed; Respir. Staff, St Michael's Hospital; (416)864-6060 x6026

ANAND, Jagdish R; Sunridge Prof Centre, 505-2675 36 St NE, Calgary AB T1Y 6H6; Guru Nanak (India)'82; FRCS(Ed); FRANZCO; FRCSC; Ophth. (403)452-6384

ANAND, Navin; Credit Valley Med Arts Centre, 309-2000 Credit Valley Rd, Mississauga ON L5M 4N4; Tor'88; FRCPC; IntMed; Gastroent. Staff, The Credit Valley Hospital; (905)607-9848; Fax. (905)607-9849.

ANAND, Neeru; Medical Clinic, 106-7445 120 St, Delta BC V4C 0B3; Rajasthan (India)'83; MB BS; CCFP; Staff, Yarmouth Regional Hospital; Langs: Hindi; Punjabi; Urdu; (604)503-0490

ANAND, Nitasha; 401-100 Colborne St W, Orillia ON L3V 2Y9; Qns'05; FRCPC; IntMed; Gastroent. Staff, Orillia Soldiers' Memorial Hospital; (705)326-2443; Fax. (705)326-2444.

ANAND, Pamela; Heart of Ottawa Medical Centre, 270 Elgin St, Ottawa ON K2P 1M2; McG'07; MDCM; CCFP; Assoc Physician, Kingston General Hospital; Asst Prof, Queen's University; Langs: Bilingual(French/English); (613)230-8885; Fax. (613)230-3666.

ANAND, Parvesh; Maitland Valley Family Hlth Team, 180 Cambria Rd N, Goderich ON N7A 4N8; Lucknow (India)'64; MB BS; FRCS(Ed); FRCSC; GenSurg (Consultation). Ac Staff, Clinton Public Hospital - Huron Perth Healthcare Alliance; Ac Staff, South Bruce Grey Health Centre - Kincardine Site; Ac Staff, Alexandra Marine & General Hospital; (519)524-6060

ANAND, Sanjiv; 203-123 Champlain St, Dieppe NB E1A 1N5; Laval'92; CCFP; Staff, Dr Georges-L-Dumont University Hospital Centre; Med Dir, Spencer Memorial Nursing Home; Langs: Bilingual(French/English); (506)863-0015; Fax. (506)858-9969.

ANAND, Sarah-Jane; 3809 Sunset St, Burnaby BC V5G 1T4; UBC'02; FRCSC; ObstGyn. Consultant, Burnaby Hospital; (604)565-9447

ANAND, Sondekere K; Windsor Reg Hosp-Metropolitan, 1995 Lens Ave, Windsor ON N8W 1L9; Nehru (India)'76; DA(UK); FFARCS(Ire); Staff, Windsor Regional Hospital - Metropolitan Site; (519)254-1661 x52201

ANAND, Sonia S; McMaster University, MDCL 3204-1280 Main St W, Hamilton ON L8S 4K1; McM'92; PhD(Epid.); FRCPC; IntMed (Vascular Medicine). Staff, Hamilton Health Sciences Centre - Hamilton General Hospital; Prof Med, McMaster University; (905)525-9140 x21523; Fax. (905)528-2814.

ANAND, Sumeet M; 3304-3000 Lawrence Ave E, Scarborough ON M1P 2V1; McM'04; FRCPC; Otol. (416)438-6292; Fax. (416)438-6405.

ANAND, Sundaram; North York Endoscopy Centre, 4646 Dufferin St, North York ON M3H 5S4; Agra (India)'53; MB BS; MPH(Johns Hopkins); FRCS; FACS; FRCSC; GenSurg (Colon & Rectal Surgery). Staff Surg, North York Endoscopy Centre; Langs: Hindi; (416)222-6160; Fax. (416)222-9604; rangoon@sympatico.ca.

ANAND, Vijay; University of Alberta Hosp, 8440 112 St NW, Edmonton AB T6G 2B7; Man'05; FRCPC; Peds; Critical Care Medicine. Staff, University of Alberta Hospital; (780)407-8822

ANANDAKRISHNAN, Canagasund; The Medical Centre, 7 Pinsent Dr, Grnd-Falls-Wi NL A2A 2S8; Ceylon (Sri Lanka)'69; MB BS; MRCP(UK); FRCPC; Derm. Staff, Central Newfoundland Regional Health Centre; Clinical Asst Prof Med, Memorial University Of Newfoundland; (709)489-1200; Fax. (709)489-6724.

ANANTH, Shobana; Markham-Stouffville Hosp, PO Box 1800 Stn Main 381 Church St, Markham ON L3P 7P3; Mem'97; CCFP; CCFP(E.M.); FCFP; Staff, Markham Stouffville Hospital; (905)472-7111

ANANTHAN, Jean P; Heart Lake Med Centre, 204-10425 Kennedy Rd, Brampton ON L6Z 0A4; Tor'81; BSc; CCFP; FCFP; (905)846-3777; Fax. (905)846-4498.

ANANTHAN, Yasotha D; William Osler HC-Etobicoke, 101 Humber College Blvd, Etobicoke ON M9V 1R8; (Aruba)'07; Staff, William Osler Health System - Etobicoke General Hospital; (416)494-2120

ANASHARA, Fouad H; Westwood Med Clinic, 3320 Portage Ave, Winnipeg MB R3K 0Z1; (Other Foreign)'09; CCFP; CCFP(E.M.); (204)832-1363

ANASPURE, Rahul S; St Joseph's Healthcare, 50 Charlton Ave E, Hamilton ON L8N 4A6; Pune University (India)'99; Clin Fellow DiagRad, St Joseph's Healthcare - Charlton Campus; (905)522-1155

ANASTAKIS, Dimitrios J; Univ Hlth Network-Toronto Western Hosp, EW2-399 Bathurst St, Toronto ON M5T 2S8; Tor'88; FACS; FICS; FRCSC; PlasSurg (Peripheral Nerve Surgery). Staff, Toronto Western Hospital - University Health Network; Prof Surg, University of Toronto; Langs: Bilingual(English/French); (416)603-5790; Fax. (416)603-6189.

ANASTASIADES, Lefkos; Winnipeg Clinic, 425 St Mary Ave, Winnipeg MB R3C 0N2; Athens (Greece)'74; FACP; FRCPC; IntMed (Cardiology). Consultant Privil, The Salvation Army Grace Hospital; Lecturer, University of Manitoba; Langs: Greek; (204)957-3270

ANASTASIO, Romulo F; A5-1575 Upper Ottawa St, Hamilton ON L8W 3E2; Santo Tomas (Philippines)'72; Court Staff, St Joseph's Healthcare - Charlton Campus; Court Staff, West Haldimand General Hospital; Ac Staff, Hamilton Health Sciences Centre - Hamilton General Hospital; Langs: Tagalog; (905)578-5776; Fax. (905)578-5779.

ANASTASSIADES, Tassos P; Queen's Univ-Etherington Hall, 2050-94 Stuart St, Kingston ON K7L 2V6; McG'62; MSc; PhD; FRCPC; IntMed (Rheumatology). Att Staff, Kingston General Hospital; Att Staff, Hotel-Dieu Hospital; Consultant, Providence Care - St Mary's of the Lake Hospital Site; Prof Med, Queen's University; (613)533-2971

ANAWATI, Alexandre G; Health Sciences North-Laurenti, 41 Ramsey Lake Rd, Sudbury ON P3E 6J1; NOSM'09; CCFP; CCFP(E.M.); Staff, Health Sciences North-Laurentian Site; Staff, West Nipissing General Hospital; (705)523-7100

ANAWATI, Jean I; G2-172 Ethel St, Sturgeon Falls ON P2B 1V9; Wes'73; Staff, West Nipissing General Hospital; Staff, North Bay Regional Health Centre - Regional Mental Health; Asst Prof Family Med, Northern Ontario School of Medicine; Asst Prof Family Med, University of Ottawa; Langs: Bilingual(English/French); Arabic; Italian; French; (705)753-0860; Fax. (705)753-0361.

ANAWATI, Michelle L; Univ of Ottawa Health Services, 204-2339 Ogilvie Rd, Ottawa ON K1J 8M6; Ott'10; CCFP; (613)842-7960

ANCA, Nicoleta I; Foothills Med Centre, 1403 29 St NW, Calgary AB T2N 2T9; Timisoara (Romania)'02; FRCPC; DiagRad. Staff, Foothills Medical Centre; (403)944-1110

ANCHALA, Krishnapriya; McMaster University, 1280 Main St W, Hamilton ON L8S 4K1; Kansas (USA)'98; Staff Peds, Hamilton Health Sciences Centre - McMaster University Medical Centre; (905)521-2100

ANCTIL, Audrey; GMF Montee de la Baie, 3942 ch Oka, St-Joseph-du-Lac QC J0N 1M0; Sher'10; CCFP; (450)473-7225

ANCTIL, Chantal; CSSS de Vaudreuil-Soulanges, 490 boul Harwood, Vaudreuil-Dorion QC J7V 7H4; Mon'92; LMCC; CCFP; FCFP; Staff, CSSS de Vaudreuil-Soulanges; Langs: Bilingual(French/English); (450)455-6171; Fax. (450)455-6145; chantal_anctil@rrsss16.gouv.qc.ca.

ANCTIL, Jean-Louis; Ctr Hosp Affilie-St-Sacrement, 1050 ch Sainte-Foy, Quebec QC G1S 4L8; Laval'72; Ophth. Consultant, Centre Hospitalier Universitaire De Québec - Pavillon De St-françois-d'assise; Ac Staff, Centre Hospitalier Affilié Universitaire de Québec - Hôpital du St-Sacrement; Consultant, Centre Hospitalier Affilié Universitaire de Québec - Hôpital De L'Enfant Jésus; Université Laval; (418)682-7680; Fax. (418)682-7534.

ANCTIL, Marylene; 210-1900 boul des Recollets, Trois-Rivieres QC G8Z 4K4; Laval'96; Langs: Bilingual(French/English); (819)376-0300; Fax. (819)373-7189.

ANCTIL, Mylene; CSSS Pierre Boucher, 1333 boul Jacques-Cartier E, Longueuil QC J4M 2A5; Sher'99; FRCPC; Psy. Staff, Centre Hospitalier Pierre Boucher; (450)468-8401

ANCTIL, Pierre-Yves; CSSS Les Eskers de l'Abitibi, 622 4e rue O, Amos QC J9T 2S2; Laval'02; FRCPC; Anes. Staff, CH Hôtel-Dieu d'Amos; (819)732-3341

ANCTIL, Suzanne; Clin Pedia des Mille-Iles, 203-233 rue Turgeon, Sainte-Therese QC J7E 3J8; Mon'00; CSPQ; Peds. Staff, Hôpital de Saint-Eustache; Langs: English; (450)434-8006

ANDARY, Leesha Y; 7875 Riverside Dr E, Windsor ON N8S 1E1; Tor'82; (519)974-4122; Fax. (519)974-0890.

ANDELFINGER, Gregor U; Hôpital Ste-Justine, 3175 ch Cote-Sainte-Catherine, Montreal QC H3T 1C5; Ulm (Germany)'92; FRCPC; Cardiol. Staff, Hôpital Ste-Justine; (514)345-4931

ANDERMANN, Anne; St Mary's Hosp Centre, 3830 av Lacombe, Montreal QC H3T 1M5; McG'02; FRCPC; CommunMed;CCFP; Public Health & Preventive Med. Staff, St Mary's Hospital Centre; (514)345-3511

ANDERMANN, Lisa F S; Mount Sinai Hosp, 600 University Ave, Toronto ON M5G 1X5; McG'96; FRCPC; Psy. Staff, Mount Sinai Hospital; (416)586-4800 x4514; Fax. (416)586-8654; landermann@mtsinai.on.ca.

ANDERS, Benjamin; 203-474 Columbia St, Kamloops BC V2C 2T5; UBC'76; CCFP; Assoc Staff Family Med, Royal Inland Hospital; (250)372-2422; Fax. (250)372-2399.

ANDERS, Karl H; South Health Campus, 4448 Front St SE, Calgary AB T3M 1M4; Man'82; Staff, Foothills Medical Centre; (403)956-1359

ANDERSEN, Joel E A; 1935 Paris St, Sudbury ON P3E 3C6; Qns'75; MSc; CCBOM; CCFP; Staff Physician, Occupational Health Clinic for Ontario Workers/Sudbury; (705)522-8718; Fax. (705)522-9562.

ANDERSEN, John C; Glenrose Rehab Hosp, 10230 111 Ave NW, Edmonton AB T5G 0B7; Cal'98; FRCPC; Peds (Pediatric Rehabilitation). Staff, Glenrose Rehabilitation Hospital; Asst Prof, University of Alberta; (780)735-7999; Fax. (780)735-7907.

ANDERSEN, Lee K; Royal Victoria Hosp, 201 Georgian Dr, Barrie ON L4M 6M2; Wes'02; CCFP; Staff, Royal Victoria Regional Health Centre; (705)728-9040

ANDERSEN, Michelle; Hop Reg D'Edmundston, 275 Hebert Blvd, Edmundston NB E3V 4E4; New South Wales (Australia)'00; Staff, Hôpital regional d'Edmundston; (506)273-7135

ANDERSEN-KAY, Michelle L; 729 Devonshire Ave, Woodstock ON N4S 5R3; Qns'97; CCFP; CCFP(E.M.); Staff, Woodstock General Hospital; (519)533-1444; Fax. (519)533-0499.

ANDERSON, A Robert; Cowichan Med Centre, 3106 Gibbins Rd, Duncan BC V9L 1E8; Cal'82; FRCSC; OrthSurg (Sports Medicine). Staff, Cowichan District Hospital; (250)746-7711; Fax. (250)746-8809; aranderson1951@gmail.com.

ANDERSON, Adarine; Nokomis Health Care Centre, PO Box 98, Nokomis SK S0G 3R0; Otago (New Zealand)'69; MB ChB; MRCP(Lond.); Staff, Nokomis Health Care Centre; (306)528-2114; Fax. (306)528-4655.

ANDERSON, Alvin J; 307-4195 Dundas St W, Etobicoke ON M8X 1Y4; Wes'52; FRCSC; GenSurg.

ANDERSON, Annette; 11300 130 Rte, Waterville NB E7P 0A4; UBC'92; MCPS; Staff, Upper River Valley Hospital - Waterville; Langs: German; (506)375-5900; dr.annette.anderson@horizonnb.ca.

ANDERSON, Barbara A; Mediclinic, 101-3333 8th St E, Saskatoon SK S7H 4K1; Sask'84; (306)955-1530; Fax. (306)955-8811.

ANDERSON, Barry J; Nelson Med Prof Corp, 301 Victoria Ave, Fort Frances ON P9A 2C1; Man'75; FACS; FRCSC; GenSurg (Endocrinology Surgery). Ac Staff, La Verendrye Hospital - Riverside Health Care Facility; Northern Ontario School of Medicine; (807)274-3287; Fax. (807)274-7882; bjanderson1@vianet.ca.

ANDERSON, Brent R; Seven Oaks Gen Hosp, 2DS12-2300 McPhillips St, Winnipeg MB R2V 3M3; Man'96; BSc; FRCSC; GenSurg (Breast Cancer). Staff Surg, Seven Oaks General Hospital; Staff, Boundary Trails Health Centre; Teach Staff, University of Manitoba; (204)632-7133

ANDERSON, Brian A; St Boniface Gen Hosp, C5014-409 Tache Ave, Winnipeg MB R2H 2A6; Sask'74; FRCPC; Neur (Adult Neurology). Staff, St Boniface General Hospital; (204)237-2222; Fax. (204)237-1461.

ANDERSON, Bruce M; PO Box 97, Cowley AB T0K 0P0; Alb'71; (403)628-2210

ANDERSON, Cameron M; Psychiatry-Health Centre, 715 12th Ave W, Vancouver BC V5Z 1M9; UBC'06; Psy. (604)875-5720

ANDERSON, Carmel R; Kelowna Dermatology Inc, 201-436 Cedar Ave, Kelowna BC V1Y 4X3; Sask'89; FRCPC; Derm (Medical Consultant). Consultant, Kelowna General Hospital; (250)860-4818

ANDERSON, Carol P; 8193-2775 Laurel St, Vancouver BC V5Z 1M9; UBC'87; (604)875-4809; Fax. (604)875-5652.

ANDERSON, Carolyn K; 201-20434 64 Ave, Langley BC V2Y 1N4; UBC'94; FRCS(Hons); FRCSC; Ophth (Cataract). Staff, Langley Memorial Hospital; (604)530-6838; Fax. (604)530-5292; dr.carolyn@andersoneyesurgery.com.

ANDERSON, Charles C; Tantallon Family Practice, 202-5110 St Margarets Bay Rd, Upper Tantallon NS B3Z 1E2; Dal'83; (902)826-2744; Fax. (902)826-2887; ca@ns.sympatico.ca.

ANDERSON, Cheryl D; 304-888 8th Ave W, Vancouver BC V5Z 3Y1; Washington (USA)'83; BA; BSc; MD; MHSc; Clin Assoc Prof School of Population & Public Health, University of British Columbia; (604)874-0261

ANDERSON, D Richard; Rockyview Gen Hosp, 7007 14 St SW, Calgary AB T2V 1P9; Alb'69; Staff, Rockyview General Hospital; Ac Medical Staff, Viewpoint Medical Assessment Services Ltd; Ac Staff, Calgary Regional Health Authority; (403)252-5702; Fax. (403)252-5953.

ANDERSON, Daphne L; Calgary Sports Therapy, 500-1060 7 St SW, Calgary AB T2R 0C4; Tor'96; CCFP; CCFP(E.M.); Physician, Calgary Sports Therapy; (403)237-0121; Fax. (403)237-0120.

ANDERSON, David A; Kelowna Gen Hosp, 2268 Pandosy St, Kelowna BC V1Y 1T2; Cal'86; FRCPC; DiagRad. Staff, Kelowna General Hospital; (250)862-4454; Fax. (250)862-4456.

ANDERSON, David K; Surrey Mem Hosp, 13750 96 Ave, Surrey BC V3V 1Z2; UBC'69; Assoc Staff, Surrey Memorial Hospital; (604)455-1008; Fax. (604)455-1009.

ANDERSON, David M; 8-715 Coronation Blvd, Cambridge ON N1R 7R1; Ott'65; FRCSC; Ophth (Cataract Surgery). Ac Staff, Cambridge Memorial Hospital; Court Staff, Grand River Hospital - Kitchener/Waterloo Health Centre; Court Staff, St Mary's General Hospital; (519)623-6250; Fax. (519)622-2990; eyedocda@rogers.com.

ANDERSON, David M; 101-15451 Russell Ave, White Rock BC V4B 2R5; Alb'71; Ac Staff, Peace Arch Hospital; (604)531-5595; Fax. (604)531-9818.

ANDERSON, David R; Queen Elizabeth II HSC, 442-1276 South Park St, Halifax NS B3H 2Y9; Dal'83; FRCPC; IntMed; Hem. Ac Staff Med, Queen Elizabeth II Health Sciences Centre - Victoria General Site; Head/Prof Med, Dalhousie University; (902)473-8562; Fax. (902)473-4600; david.anderson@dal.ca.

ANDERSON, Dawn L; Ville Marie Med Clinic, 1000-1538 rue Sherbrooke O, Montreal QC H3G 1L5; Man'88; BSc(Med); FRCSC; GenSurg (Surgical Oncology). Staff, St Mary's Hospital Centre; Asst Prof Surg, McGill University; Langs: English; French; (514)933-2778; Fax. (514)933-9635.

ANDERSON, Donald W; 4F-2775 Laurel St, Vancouver BC V5Z 1M9; Alb'78; FRCSC; Otol. Vis Staff, Providence Health Care - St Paul's Hospital; (604)945-0711

ANDERSON, Donella; Penticton Reg Hosp, 550 Carmi Ave, Penticton BC V2A 3G6; McM'92; CCFP; FCFP; Staff, Penticton Regional Hospital; (250)492-9032

ANDERSON, Donna M; 258-2025 Corydon Ave, Winnipeg MB R3P 0N5; Sask'74; FRCPC; Psy. (204)489-9680; Fax. (204)489-9680.

ANDERSON, Douglas J; Comox Med Clinic, 100-1695 Comox Ave, Comox BC V9M 3M1; UBC'92; CCFP; FCFP; (250)339-2266

ANDERSON, Douglas M; 203-30 Crystalridge Dr, Okotoks AB T1S 2C3; Cal'86; CCFP; FCFP; (403)995-0010; Fax. (403)995-0051.

ANDERSON, Duncan P; St Paul's Hosp, 1081 Burrard St, Vancouver BC V6Z 1Y6; McG'67; BSc; FRCSC; Ophth (Neuro Ophthalmology). Staff Ophth, Providence Health Care - St Paul's Hospital; Consultant Ophth, Vancouver General Hospital - Centennial Pavillion; Emeritus Associate Prof Ophth, University of British Columbia; Langs: English; French; (604)806-8168; Fax. (604)806-8058.

ANDERSON, E James; Main St PO Box 70, Lucan ON N0M 2J0; Wes'65; (519)227-4288

ANDERSON, Erin; St Boniface Gen Hosp, M1049-409 Tache Ave, Winnipeg MB R2H 2A6; Man'06; FRCPC; Psy. Staff, St Boniface General Hospital; (204)233-8563

ANDERSON, Geoffrey M; Dept of HPME-U of T, 400-155 College St, Toronto ON M5T 3M6; Ott'77; Teach Staff, University of Toronto; (416)946-3770; Fax. (416)978-7350.

ANDERSON, Glenn P J; White Rock Med Clinic, 101-15451 Russell Ave, White Rock BC V4B 2R5; Alb'72; CCFP; FCFP; Ac Staff, Peace Arch Hospital; (604)531-5595; Fax. (604)531-9818; glennlorna@shaw.ca.

ANDERSON, Gordon S; Wainwright Clinic, 501 10 St, Wainwright AB T9W 1R5; (South Africa)'87; (780)842-3341; dranders@telusplanet.net.

ANDERSON, Heather D; Burnaby Hosp, 3935 Kincaid St, Burnaby BC V5G 2X6; Alb'03; FRCPC; IntMed. Staff, Burnaby Hospital; (604)434-4211

ANDERSON, Helen L; BC Cancer Agency-Vanc Isl Ctr, 2410 Lee Ave, Victoria BC V8R 6V5; Auckland (New Zealand)'90; MB ChB; FRCPC; IntMed. Staff, BC Cancer Agency Vancouver Island Centre; (250)519-5572

ANDERSON, Ian A; Anaesthesia Associates, 100 Piccadilly St, London ON N6A 1R8; Aberdeen (Scotland)'69; MB ChB; DAB; Anes. Consultant, London Health Sciences Centre - University Hospital; University of Western Ontario; (519)672-2130

ANDERSON, Ian B; Foothills Med Centre, 1403 29 St NW, Calgary AB T2N 2T9; McG'78; FRCSC; GenSurg (Trauma Surgery); Critical Care Medicine. Staff, Foothills Medical Centre; Clinical Asst Prof Surg, University of Calgary; (403)944-4262; Fax. (403)944-4262.

ANDERSON, Ian H; Saint John Reg Hosp, PO Box 2100 Stn Main 400 University Ave, Saint John NB E2L 4L2; Dal'73; FRCPC; DiagRad. Ac Staff, St Joseph's Hospital; Diagnostic-Radiology, Saint John Regional Hospital; Asst Prof, Dalhousie University; (506)648-6923; Fax. (506)648-6925.

ANDERSON, James G; Medical-Surgical Eye Bldg, 879 Shefford Rd, Gloucester ON K1J 8H9; Ott'75; Staff, The Ottawa Hospital - Riverside Campus; Clin Preceptor, University of Ottawa; (613)746-7172; Fax. (613)746-9608.

ANDERSON, Jarrod R; Misericordia Community Hosp, 16940 87 Ave NW, Edmonton AB T5R 4H5; Alb'06; CCFP; CCFP(E.M.); Staff, Covenant Health - Misericordia Community Hospital; (780)735-2819

ANDERSON, Jennifer A; St Michael's Hosp, CC 8 129-30 Bond St, Toronto ON M5B 1W8; Tor'87; MSc; FRCSC; Otol (Head & Neck Surgery). Chief Otol/Head & Neck Surg/Med Dir Voice Disorders Clinic, St Michael's Hospital; (416)864-5278; Fax. (416)864-5367.

ANDERSON, Jennifer E; West Coast Family Med Clinic, 1300-6660 Sooke Rd Box 880, Sooke BC V9Z 1H4; Cal'77; BSc; MHSc; Clinical Asst Prof Family Med, University of British Columbia; (250)642-4233

ANDERSON, John F; Ctre Addiction Research of BC, PO Box 1700 Stn CSC, Victoria BC V8W 2Y2; McM'77; Physician, British Columbia Ministry Of Health; (250)472-5623; john.anderson@gov.bc.ca.

ANDERSON, Josdalyne; SCOHS-Elisabeth Bruyere Hosp, 3JB 375-43 Bruyere St, Ottawa ON K1N 5C8; Ott'09; CCFP; Staff, SCO Health Service - Élisabeth Bruyère Hospital; (613)562-6335

ANDERSON, Juanita M; 108-585 16th St, West Vancouver BC V7V 3R8; UBC'83; Staff, Lions Gate Hospital; Clin Instructor, University of British Columbia; (604)922-1122; Fax. (604)922-6535.

ANDERSON, Julie A; Summit Med Clinic, 4-1380 Summit Dr, Kamloops BC V2C 1T8; UBC'89; CCFP; Staff, Royal Inland Hospital; (250)374-9800; Fax. (250)374-9876.

ANDERSON, K Eric; Dartmouth Gen Hosp, 325 Pleasant St, Dartmouth NS B2Y 4G8; Dal'99; FRCSC; OrthSurg. Staff, Dartmouth General Hospital; (902)465-8300

ANDERSON, Karen E; Halifax Prof Center, 425-5991 Spring Garden Rd, Halifax NS B3H 1Y6; Dal'85; (902)422-6220; Fax. (902)422-6988.

ANDERSON, Keith H; Parkdale Med Tower, 702-1081 Carling Ave, Ottawa ON K1Y 4G2; Ott'70; DPsy; FRCPC; Psy. Staff, The Ottawa Hospital - Civic Campus; (613)725-2284; Fax. (613)725-9161.

ANDERSON, Keith J; Foothills Med Centre, C222B-1403 29 St NW, Calgary AB T2N 2T9; Staff, Foothills Medical Centre; (403)944-4309; Fax. (403)270-2268.

ANDERSON, Kelly B; Glenrose Rehab Hosp, 10230 111 Ave NW, Edmonton AB T5G 0B7; Cal'80; FRCPC; Peds. Staff, Glenrose Rehabilitation Hospital; Ac Staff, University of Alberta Hospital; (780)735-7999

ANDERSON, Kenneth E; Queensway Prof Centre, 109-190 Sherway Dr, Etobicoke ON M9C 5N2; Tor'79; (416)621-7333; Fax. (416)621-9054.

ANDERSON, Kenneth; Health Sciences Centre, 300 Prince Philip Dr, St. John's NL A1B 3V6; Dal'65; FACS; PlasSurg. Staff, Health Sciences Centre; (709)777-6300

ANDERSON, Kent S; Rockyview Gen Hosp, 7007 14 St SW, Calgary AB T2V 1P9; Alb'80; FRCPC; Psy (Geriatric Psychiatry). Med Dir Consultation Liason, Rockyview General Hospital; Clin Lecturer, University of Calgary; (403)943-3503; Fax. (403)212-1230.

ANDERSON, Kerry A; Paterson Med Centre, RR 1 Stn Main 45 Wolseley St, Kenora ON P9N 3W7; Man'04; CCFP; (807)468-3021

ANDERSON, Kim; Institut de Cardiologie de Mtl, 5000 Belanger St, Montreal QC H1T 1C8; Mon'07; IntMed. Staff, Institut de Cardiologie de Montréal; (514)376-3330

ANDERSON, Lucyna J; Kanata Prof Centre, 203-99 Kakulu Rd, Kanata ON K2L 3C8; Bialystok (Poland)'87; FRCSC; ObstGyn. Staff, Queensway Carleton Hospital; Langs: Polish; (613)592-8200; Fax. (613)592-0936.

ANDERSON, M Catherine; Upper Grand Family Health Team, LL-205 Queen St E, Fergus ON N1M 1T2; Qns'89; BSc; CCFP; FCFP; Staff, Groves Memorial Community Hospital; Clin Assoc Prof Family Med, McMaster University; Langs: Spanish; French; (519)787-1200; Fax. (519)787-1803.

ANDERSON, Manfred E; 95 King St W, Mississauga ON L5B 1H1; Tor'82; Staff, Trillium Health Centre - Mississauga; (905)848-2284; Fax. (905)896-7475.

ANDERSON, Mary C; Waterloo Walk In Clinic, 13-170 University Ave W, Waterloo ON N2L 3E9; Liverpool (England)'69; MB ChB; DA; (519)725-1514; Fax. (519)725-5137.

ANDERSON, Mary Lynn; Peterborough Clinic, 301-26 Hospital Dr, Peterborough ON K9J 7C3; Tor'73; CGPP; Court Staff Psy Dept, Peterborough Regional Health Centre - Hospital Drive; (705)743-2040 x368

ANDERSON, Michael; Royal Court Med Centre, 202-1 Quarry Ridge Rd, Barrie ON L4M 7G1; Qns'94; GenSurg (Surgical Oncology). Staff, Cancer Care Ontario - Provincial Office; Lecturer Surg, University of Toronto; (705)721-0040; Fax. (705)721-0575; michael.anderson@cancercare.con.ca.

ANDERSON, Nancy J; PO Box 247, Bella Coola BC V0T 1C0; Cal'80; BSc; CCFP; FCFP; Fam Med, Bella Coola General Hospital; Clin Instructor, University of British Columbia; (250)982-2150; nananderson@hotmail.com.

ANDERSON, P Paul A; Perth-Smiths Falls Dist Hosp, 33 Drummond St W, Perth ON K7H 2K1; Stellenbosch (South Africa)'77; FRCSC; OrthSurg (Spine Surgery). Staff, Perth & Smiths Falls District Hospital - Perth Site (Great War Memorial Site); Langs: Afrikaans; Dutch; (613)267-7020

ANDERSON, Patricia C; Panorama Village Med Clinic, 103-15157 56 Ave, Surrey BC V3S 9A5; Cal'96; BSc; MSc; (604)574-0481

ANDERSON, Peter A M; IWK Health Centre, PO Box 9700 Rpo CSC, Halifax NS B3K 6R8; Dal'82; FRCSC; Urol (Pediatric Urology). Div Head Urol, IWK Health Centre; Staff Urol, Queen Elizabeth II Health Sciences Centre - Victoria General Site; Prof Urol, Dalhousie University; (902)470-8861; Fax. (902)470-8267; maureen.macdonald@iwk.nshealth.ca.

ANDERSON, Peter J; Whitehorse Med Services Ltd, 406 Lambert St, Whitehorse YT Y1A 1Z7; UBC'82; Ac Staff, Whitehorse General Hospital; Staff, Whitehorse Medical Services Ltd; (867)393-6600; Fax. (867)393-6601; wmsl@klondiker.com.

ANDERSON, Peter L; 87 Adelaide St N, Lindsay ON K9V 4L4; McM'79; CCFP; FCFP; Staff, Ross Memorial Hospital; (705)324-6763; Fax. (705)328-1816.

ANDERSON, Peter R; East Wellington Family Hlth Team, 1-6 Thompson Cres, Erin ON N0B 1T0; McM'10; CCFP; (519)833-9396

ANDERSON, Raymond C; Comber Med Centre, PO Box 38 6405 Main St, Comber ON N0P 1J0; Wes'73; BSc; Court Staff, Windsor Regional Hospital - Metropolitan Site; Court Staff, Leamington District Memorial Hospital; (519)687-2333

ANDERSON, Reynald; CSSS Pierre Boucher, 1333 boul Jacques-Cartier E, Longueuil QC J4M 2A5; Sher'90; CSPQ; FRCPC; Anes. Staff, Centre Hospitalier Pierre Boucher; (450)468-8111

ANDERSON, Robert B; 401-1338 Broadway W, Vancouver BC V6H 1H2; Qns'90; BSc; MRCS; FRCSC; ObstGyn. Staff, Providence Health Care - St Paul's Hospital; Clinical Asst Prof Med, University of British Columbia; (604)736-0424; Fax. (604)736-5403.

ANDERSON, Robert J; Sudbury Reg Hosp-Laurentian, 41 Ramsey Lake Rd, Sudbury ON P3E 5J1; McM'00; FRCPC; Anes; Critical Care Medicine. Staff, Health Sciences North-Laurentian Site; Staff, Health Sciences North-St Joseph's Health Centre; Prog Dir Family Practice Anes, Northern Ontario School of Medicine; (705)523-7100

ANDERSON, Ronald A; Alberta Children's Hosp, 2888 Shaganappi Trail NW, Calgary AB T3B 6A8; McG'83; MDCM; FRCPC; Peds (Hematological Oncology). Staff, Alberta Children's Hospital; Assoc Prof Oncology & Peds, University of Calgary; (403)955-7203; ronald.anderson@albertahealthservices.ca.

ANDERSON, Ronald R; 234-20 Perron St, St. Albert AB T8N 1E4; Alb'81; CCFP; Clin Lecturer Med, University of Alberta; (780)418-3730; Fax. (780)419-3705.

ANDERSON, Ryan A; 278-2025 Corydon Ave, Winnipeg MB R3P 0N5; Man'03; FRCPC; Psy.

ANDERSON, S Lance; 1014 20th St S, Lethbridge AB T1K 2C9; UBC'03; BScPT; FRCSC; OrthSurg (Adult Hip & Knee Reconstruction). (403)942-4361

ANDERSON, Scott B; London HSC-South St, PO Box 5375 Stn B 800 Commissioners Rd E, London ON N6A 4G5; Wes'91; FRCPC; EmergMed; Critical Care Medicine. Staff Critical Care, St Joseph's Hospital - St Joseph's Health Care; Staff, London Health Sciences Centre - South Street; Asst Prof, University of Western Ontario; Langs: English; French; (519)667-6538; Fax. (519)667-6769.

ANDERSON, Shelley D; St Boniface Gen Hosp, M5-409 Tache Ave, Winnipeg MB R2H 2A6; Man'94; FRCPC; Psy. Staff Geriatric Psy, St Boniface General Hospital; Asst Prof Psy, University of Manitoba; (204)235-3285; Fax. (204)237-6264.

ANDERSON, Stephanie G; Health and Counselling Service, MBC 0164-8888 University Dr, Burnaby BC V5A 1S6; Alb'04; CCFP.

ANDERSON, Stephen D; 8193-2775 Laurel St, Vancouver BC V5Z 1M9; UBC'84; FRCPC; Psy (Consultant Liaison Psychiatry). Ac Staff, Vancouver General Hospital - Centennial Pavillion; Asst Prof, University of British Columbia; (604)875-4809; Fax. (604)875-5652.

ANDERSON, Terry D; St Anthony's X-Ray Clinic, 102-582 Goldstream Ave, Victoria BC V9B 2W7; Alb'71; FRCPC; DiagRad. (250)478-8812

ANDERSON, Thomas H; Scarborough Prof Centre, 311-1371 Neilson Rd, Scarborough ON M1B 4Z8; Tor'81; FRCSC; GenSurg; ThorSurg. (416)282-5557; Fax. (416)282-3930.

ANDERSON, Todd J; Foothills Med Centre, 1403 29 St NW, Calgary AB T2N 2T9; Cal'85; FRCPC; IntMed (General Cardiology); Cardiol. Staff, Foothills Medical Centre; Prof Med, Scholar of the Alberta Heritage Fdn. for Medical Research; Dept Head Cardiac Sciences, University of Calgary; (403)944-1033; todd.anderson@calgaryhealthregion.ca.

ANDERSON, Tyler J; Grey Nuns Community Hosp & HC, 1100 Youville Drive West NW, Edmonton AB T6L 5X8; Alb'02; CCFP; CCFP(E.M.); Staff, Covenant Health - Grey Nuns Community Hospital; (780)735-7000

ANDERSON, Vance E; 206-124 Main St, St George NB E5C 3S3; Dal'04; CCFP; (506)755-9024; Fax. (506)755-3440; vealg@hotmail.com.

ANDERSON, William D; Thunder Bay Reg HSC-T-Bay, 980 Oliver Rd, Thunder Bay ON P7B 6V4; Alb'97; BSc; FRCPC; IntMed (Pulmonary Medicine); Critical Care Medicine; Respir. Staff, Thunder Bay Regional Health Sciences Centre; (807)684-6000

ANDERSON, William W; Royal Alexandra Hosp, 1046 14. 1-10240 Kingsway NW, Edmonton AB T5H 3V9; Alb'80; FRCPC; DiagRad. Staff, Royal Alexandra Hospital; Clin Instructor, University of Alberta; (780)735-4327; Fax. (780)735-5794.

ANDERSON DECOTEAU, Marcia; Salvation Army Grace Gen Hosp, 300 Booth Dr, Winnipeg MB R3J 3M7; Man'02; FRCPC; IntMed. Staff, The Salvation Army Grace Hospital; (204)837-0391

ANDERSON-HILL, Kimberly; 225-501 Bethel Dr, Sherwood Park AB T8H 0N2; Alb'03; CCFP; (780)467-4343

ANDERSON PENNO, Ellen E; 209-8555 Scurfield Dr NW, Calgary AB T3L 1Z6; Minnesota (USA)'92; MD; FRCSC; Ophth. (403)247-1477; Fax. (403)247-9774.

ANDERSONS, Maris; 901-790 Bay St Box 34, Toronto ON M5G 1N8; Dal'72; CSAM; FASAM; CCFP; FCFP; Ac Staff Fam & CommunMed, St Michael's Hospital; Staff Consultant, Sunnybrook Health Sciences Centre; Consultant, Ministry Of Transportation; Langs: Latvian; (416)967-4788; Fax. (416)967-6623; marandersons@rogers.com.

ANDERSSON, Paul O; H2 Medical Centre, 7020 4 St NW, Calgary AB T2K 1C4; Alb'89; CCFP; (403)730-7663; Fax. (403)730-4466.

ANDERTON, Adrian G; Cranston Family Healthcare, 1020-356 Cranston Rd SE, Calgary AB T3M 0S9; (South Africa)'01; MB ChB; (587)353-5835; Fax. (587)353-5836.

ANDOLFATTO, Gary; Lions Gate Hosp, 231 15th St E, North Vancouver BC V7L 2L7; UBC'90; CCFP; CCFP(E.M.); FCFP; Staff, Lions Gate Hospital; (604)984-5799; Fax. (604)984-5828.

ANDONATOS, Stella; Maimonides Geriatric Centre, 5795 av Caldwell, Cote Saint-Luc QC H4W 1W3; McG'93; Langs: English; French; Greek; (514)483-2121

ANDONIAN, Sero; MUHC-Royal Victoria Hosp, S6.92-687 av des Pins O, Montreal QC H3A 1A1; McG'02; FRCSC; Urol. Staff, McGill University Health Centre - Royal Victoria Hospital; (514)843-2865; Fax. (514)843-1552.

ANDONOV, Igor; Campbellton Reg Hosp, PO Box 880 Stn Main 189 Lily Lake Rd, Campbellton NB E3N 3H3; (Macedonia)'96; Staff, Hôpital Régional Campbellton; (506)789-5000

ANDRADE, Danielle M D; Univ Hlth Network-Toronto Western Hosp, 5W 445-399 Bathurst St, Toronto ON M5T 2S8; Parana (Brazil)'95; Staff, Toronto Western Hospital - University Health Network; (416)603-5927; Fax. (416)603-5768.

ANDRADE, Jason; Institut de Cardiologie de Mtl, 5000 rue Belanger, Montreal QC H1T 1C8; Ott'04; FRCPC; IntMed; Cardiol. Staff, Institut de Cardiologie de Montréal; (514)376-3330

ANDRADE, Jennifer M; UWO Student Health Services, 11UCC-1151 Richmond St, London ON N6A 3K7; Wes'92; CCFP; FCFP; Physician Studen Health Services, University of Western Ontario; (519)661-3030

ANDRADE, William N; Newmarket Med Place, 305-712 Davis Dr, Newmarket ON L3Y 8C3; Tor'00; FRCSC; PlasSurg. Lecturer, University of Toronto; (905)898-2519; Fax. (905)898-7239.

ANDRAOS, Noel H; 25 rue Saint-Francois, Gatineau QC J9A 1B1; Cairo (Egypt)'65; CCFP; (819)776-5584

ANDRAWIS, Mamdouh N R; 89 Dundas St W, Napanee ON K7R 1Z7; Alexandria (Egypt)'88; CCFP; (613)354-3960; Fax. (613)354-8077.

ANDRE, Barnave; Polyclinique Med Pierre Le Gar, 300-1000 montee des Pionniers, Terrebonne QC J6V 1S8; Mon'02; CCFP; Staff, Centre Hospitalier Pierre le Gardeur; (450)657-1313

ANDRE, J Kurt; 10-10 Headdon Gate, Richmond Hill ON L4C 8A3; Wes'83; FAAP; FRCPC; Peds (Nephrology). (905)770-5661; Fax. (905)770-3381.

ANDRE, Liliane; Centre Med & Prof de Dorval, 667 ch Bord-Du-Lac Lakeshore, Dorval QC H9S 2B7; Mon'91; Staff, Hôpital de Saint-Eustache; (514)633-1510; Fax. (514)633-8299.

ANDREA, Glenn C; Dalhousie Health Services, PO Box 15000 Lcd 2 6230 Coburg Rd, Halifax NS B3H 4R2; Dal'90; (902)494-2171; Fax. (902)494-2727.

ANDREAE, Martin E; 4539 Marine Ave, Powell River BC V8A 2K5; Pretoria (South Africa)'09; MB ChB; (604)485-4713

ANDREAS, Cecile L; FW Green Med Clinic, 1629 Baker St, Cranbrook BC V1C 1B4; Stellenbosch (South Africa)'91; MB ChB; Staff, East Kootenay Regional Hospital; Langs: Afrikaans; (250)426-6601; Fax. (250)417-4601.

ANDREAS, Gregory S; FW Green Med Clinic, 1629 Baker St, Cranbrook BC V1C 1B4; Stellenbosch (South Africa)'91; MB ChB; BPharm; (250)426-6601

ANDREIUK, John R; PO Box 199, Fairview AB T0H 1L0; Alb'76; CCFP; FCFP; (780)835-4255; Fax. (780)835-5009.

ANDRENYI, Veronica; Queen Elizabeth Health Centre, 2100 av de Marlowe, Montreal QC H4A 3L5; Tirgu Mures (Romania)'59; FRCPC; DiagRad. Staff, McGill University Health Centre - Montreal General Campus; Langs: Hungarian; French; (514)485-5013

ANDREOU, Charalambos; Surrey Med Arts Bldg, 302-13798 94A Ave, Surrey BC V3V 1N1; Alb'87; Urol (Oncology). Staff, Surrey Memorial Hospital; Langs: Greek; (604)583-1789; Fax. (604)583-1792; andreou@telus.net.

ANDREOU, E Roseann; Toronto East Gen Hosp Inc, 825 Coxwell Ave, Toronto ON M4C 3E7; Wes'01; BSc; MSc; FRCPC; IntMed; Hem. Staff, Toronto East General Hospital Inc; Langs: Greek; (416)469-6410; randr@tegh.on.ca.

ANDRES, Cedric; CHUM-Hop Notre-Dame, 1560 rue Sherbrooke E, Montreal QC H2L 4M1; Sher'01; FRCPC; Psy. Staff, Centre Hospitalier l'Université de Montréal (CHUM) - Hôpital Notre-Dame; (514)890-8000

ANDRES, Deirdre E; City Centre Fam Physicians, 100-514 Queen St, Saskatoon SK S7K 0M5; Sask'76; CCFP; Court Staff, Saskatoon City Hospital; Staff Family Med, Royal University Hospital; Clinical Asst Prof Family Med, University of Saskatchewan; (306)244-3016; Fax. (306)244-4737.

ANDRES, Mario R; 202-800 Bathurst St, Toronto ON M5R 3M8; Manila (Philippines)'64; MD; FRCPC; IntMed (Cardiology). Langs: Tagalog; (416)535-4602; Fax. (416)532-6649.

ANDRES, Salvador J; Acadia Med Centre, 3310 8th St E, Saskatoon SK S7H 5M3; Santo Tomas (Philippines)'70; Staff, Saskatoon City Hospital; Staff, St Paul's Hospital (Grey Nuns) of Saskatoon; Staff, Royal University Hospital; Staff, St John's Ambulance; Clin Lecturer, University of Saskatchewan; Langs: Spanish; Tagalog; (306)373-6000; Fax. (306)477-5000.

ANDREW, Christopher G; St Boniface Gen Hosp, Z3043-409 Tache Ave, Winnipeg MB R2H 2A6; Man'98; BSc; FRCSC; GenSurg (Laparoscopic Surgery). Staff, St Boniface General Hospital; Staff, Concordia General Hospital; Staff, Victoria General Hospital; Asst Prof, University of Manitoba; Langs: Spanish; (204)235-3375; Fax. (204)237-3429; candrew@sbgh.mb.ca.

ANDREW, Deborah K; Capilano Centre, 302-9945 50 St NW, Edmonton AB T6A 0L4; UBC'85; CCFP; (780)490-5543

ANDREW, Donald M; 140C Hampton Rd, Rothesay NB E2E 2R1; Dal'84; CCFP; Staff, Saint John Regional Hospital; (506)849-0222

ANDREW, Gail H; Glenrose Rehab Hosp, 10230 111 Ave NW, Edmonton AB T5G 0B7; McG'71; FRCPC; Peds (Developmental Pediatrics). Staff, Glenrose Rehabilitation Hospital; Staff, University of Alberta Hospital; Clin Asst Peds, University of Alberta; (780)735-7963; Fax. (780)735-7907.

ANDREW, George C; Hys Med Centre, 11010 101 St NW, Edmonton AB T5H 4B9; Aberdeen (England)'69; MB ChB; DRCOG; DMRD; FRCR; FRCPC; DiagRad. (780)428-1121; Fax. (780)425-5979.

ANDREW, Hugh G; Manitoba Health, 3015-300 Carlton St, Winnipeg MB R3B 3M9; Man'66; DPsy; FRCPC; Psy (Administrative Psychiatry). Sr Staff Psy, Selkirk Mental Health Centre; Chief Provincial Psy, Manitoba Health; Asst Prof, University of Manitoba; (204)788-6677; Fax. (204)945-3105; hugh.andrew@gov.mb.ca.

ANDREW, John I; Tillsonburg Fam Physicians, 4-594 Broadway St, Tillsonburg ON N4G 5K9; Wes'77; CCFP; Staff, Tillsonburg District Memorial Hospital; (519)842-3636; Fax. (519)842-9522.

ANDREW, John; Royal Jubilee Hosp, 1952 Bay St, Victoria BC V8R 1J8; Tor'04; FRCPC; DiagRad; NuclearMed. Staff, Royal Jubilee Hospital; (250)370-8000

ANDREW, Melissa H; Providence Care-Mental Health, PO Box 603 Stn Main 752 King St W, Kingston ON K7L 4X3; Wes'93; FRCPC; Psy. Staff, Providence Care - Mental Health Services; (613)546-1101

ANDREW, Melissa K; Veteran's Memorial Bldg, 1314-5955 Veterans Memorial Ln, Halifax NS B3H 2E1; Dal'01; FRCPC; IntMed; GeriatricMed. (902)473-4995; Fax. (902)473-7133.

ANDREW, Philip J; 202-140 Oxford St E, London ON N6A 5R9; Alb'69; FRCPC; Cardiol; IntMed. (519)601-7005; Fax. (519)601-8009.

ANDREW, Rodney F; 1081 Burrard St. St. Paul's Hospital, Vancouver BC V6Z 1Y6; London (England)'62; MB BS; MRCS; CCFP; FCFP; Dir Med Education, Providence Health Care - St Paul's Hospital; Clin Prof, University of British Columbia; (604)682-2344 x62969; randrew@providencehealth.bc.ca.

ANDREWS, Catriona H; London Reg Cancer Centre, 790 Commissioners Rd E, London ON N6A 4L6; Man'89; (519)685-8600

ANDREWS, Christopher D; Plaza 33, PO Box 23122 Rpo Plaza 33, Kelowna BC V1X 7K7; UBC'93; CCFP; CCFP(E.M.); (250)765-5500

ANDREWS, Christopher N; GI Clinic, UCMC2-3330 Hospital Dr NW, Calgary AB T2N 4N1; McM'99; FRCPC; IntMed; Gastroent. Staff, Health Research Innovation Centre; (403)210-9325; Fax. (403)210-9340.

ANDREWS, Christopher W; Alberta Children's Hosp, 2888 Shaganappi Trail NW, Calgary AB T3B 6A8; Alb'06; FRCPC; Peds. Staff, Alberta Children's Hospital; (403)955-7211

ANDREWS, Kathee; Balance for Life Women's Healt, 201-157 Main St, Unionville ON L3R 2G8; Mem'85; BSc; BMedSci; Dir Womens Health, Balance for Life Women's Health; Consultant, Medisys Health Corporation; (905)477-7775; Fax. (905)477-3775; info@balanceforlifewomenshealth.com.

ANDREWS, David M H; 404-6389 Coburg Rd, Halifax NS B3H 2A5; Dal'69; FRCSC; Ophth. Ac Staff, IWK Health Centre; Ac Staff, Queen Elizabeth II Health Sciences Centre - Victoria General Site; Consultant, Dartmouth General Hospital; (902)420-9036; Fax. (902)492-0306; grand.oaks@ns.sympatico.ca.

ANDREWS, Debra; Glenrose Rehab Hosp, 121-10230 111 Ave NW, Edmonton AB T5G 0B7; Harvard (USA)'79; FAAP; MRCP; ABPeds; BSc; MD; FRCPC; Peds (Developmental Pediatrics). Staff, Glenrose Rehabilitation Hospital; Staff, University of Alberta Hospital; Assoc Prof Peds, University of Alberta; (780)735-7921; Fax. (780)735-7907.

ANDREWS, Eleanor J; 214 Med Place, 24-9909 102 St, Grande Prairie AB T8V 2V4; UBC'73; BSc; CCFP; FCFP; Chief Continuing Care, Queen Elizabeth II Hospital; (780)830-4101; Fax. (780)539-5544.

ANDREWS, Gordon T; UBC Hospital, 2211 Wesbrook Mall, Vancouver BC V6T 2B5; Sask'95; FRCPC; DiagRad. Staff, UBC Hospital - Koerner Pavillion; (604)822-7080

ANDREWS, James S; Saint John Reg Hosp, PO Box 2100 Stn Main 400 University Ave, Saint John NB E2L 4L2; Wes'04; FRCSC; ObstGyn (Maternal Fetal Medicine). Staff, Saint John Regional Hospital; (506)648-6000

ANDREWS, John E; 304 Mcintyre St E, North Bay ON P1B 1C8; London (England)'69; MB BS; LRCP; MRCS; FRCPC; IntMed. Ac Staff, North Bay Regional Health Centre - Regional Mental Health; (705)476-1430; Fax. (705)476-1431.

ANDREWS, Lorraine D; VCMHS-Hamber House, 233 15th Ave W, Vancouver BC V5Y 1Y1; UBC'89; BSc; FRCPC; Psy (Child & Adolescent Psychiatry). (604)876-9276; Fax. (604)873-4012.

ANDREWS, Wayne L; Dr Charles A Janeway Child HC, 3J312-300 Prince Philip Dr, St. John's NL A1B 3V6; Dal'73; FRCPC; Peds. Staff, Janeway Children's Health & Rehabilitation Centre; (709)777-4622

ANDREWS ALEXANDER, Amy L E; Canadian Forces Base, PO Box 1000 Stn Main 31 Canadian Forces Hosp, Borden ON L0M 1C0; McM'06; CCFP; (705)424-1200; Fax. (705)423-2088.

ANDRIAMAMPIONONA, Francis A; Inst U Geriatrie de Montreal, 4565 ch Queen Mary, Montreal QC H3W 1W5; Staff, Institut Universitaire de Gériatrie de Montréal; (514)340-3515

ANDRIASHEK, Diana M; Glenrose Rehab Hosp, 10230 111 Ave NW, Edmonton AB T5G 0B7; Alb'75; Staff, Glenrose Rehabilitation Hospital; (780)735-7913; Fax. (780)735-8200.

ANDRIGHETTI, Santina; Oakville Med Arts Bldg, 15-358 Reynolds St, Oakville ON L6J 3L9; McM'92; FRCSC; ObstGyn. Staff, Halton Healthcare Services Corporation - Oakville Site; (905)815-8885; Fax. (905)815-8560.

ANDRIUK, Debora; 133 rue Larouche, Cowansville QC J2K 1T2; Mon'92; Staff Geriatric Med & Psychogeriatric Prog, CSSS la Pommeraie; Langs: English; (450)263-3242 x2210; Fax. (450)263-8159.

ANDRONOWSKI, Adam K; Northeastern On Reg Cancer Ctr, 41 Ramsey Lake Rd, Sudbury ON P3E 5J1; Lodz (Poland)'84; FRCPC; RadOncol. Staff, Northeastern Ontario Regional Cancer Centre; Langs: Polish; (705)522-6237 x2451

ANDRUCHOW, Angela A; Mill Creek Family Medicine, 101-1912 Enterprise Way, Kelowna BC V1Y 9S9; Alb'98; BSc; CCFP; Staff, Kelowna General Hospital; (250)868-0700; Fax. (250)868-3003.

ANDRUCHOW, James E; Foothills Med Centre, 1403 29 St NW, Calgary AB T2N 2T9; McG'07; MDCM; FRCPC; EmergMed. Staff, Foothills Medical Centre; Fax. (403)944-1110.

ANDRUCHOW, Jennifer L; St Thomas Surgical Clinic, 4 St Joseph St, St. Albert AB T8N 0B5; Alb'98; FRCSC; GenSurg. Langs: Ukrainian; (780)459-6633; Fax. (780)459-6609.

ANDRUCHOW, Marshall F; Justik Med Clinic, 8225 105 St NW, Edmonton AB T6E 4H2; Alb'70; Assoc Staff, Covenant Health - Edmonton General Continuing Care Centre; (780)432-0211; Fax. (780)439-9349.

ANDRUCSON, Victor M; 240-255 Newport Rd, Port Moody BC V3H 5H1; Sask'61; Dir Diagnostic Imaging, Royal Columbian Hospital; Locum Tenens, Eagle Ridge Hospital & Health Care Centre; (778)839-2274; vma@shaw.ca.

ANDRUKO, Brent I; Trillium Hlth Ctr-Mississauga, 100 Queensway W, Mississauga ON L5B 1B8; Wes'89; Staff, Trillium Health Centre - Mississauga; (905)848-7100

ANDRUS, Paul G L; 72 King St W, Stoney Creek ON L8G 1H8; Qns'93; (905)662-9128; Fax. (905)662-4100.

ANDRUSKI, Benjamin; 201-303 9 Ave SW, High River AB T1V 0H2; Cal'10; CCFP; Staff, Foothills Medical Centre; (403)652-2929; Fax. (403)652-1510.

ANEES, Farah; Chatham Kent Commun Hlth Ctre, 150 Richmond St, Chatham ON N7M 1N9; Karachi (Pakistan)'00; (519)397-5455

ANEES, Iram; Health Sciences Centre, 300 Prince Philip Dr, St. John's NL A1B 3V6; Fatima Jinnah (Pakistan)'95; MB BS; FRCPC; IntMed; Nephrol. Staff IntMed, Health Sciences Centre; (709)777-8877

ANEES, Muhammad; 1271 100th St, North Battleford SK S9A 0V6; Staff, Battlefords Union Hospital; (306)445-6096; Fax. (306)445-6097.

ANEJA, Ambika; St Joseph's Health Centre, 30 The Queensway, Toronto ON M6R 1B5; Tor'04; ObstGyn. Staff, Sunnybrook Health Sciences Centre; Staff, St Joseph's Health Centre; (416)530-6000

ANELLO, Francesco A; 401 Laurel St, Cambridge ON N3H 3Y7; Wes'82; BSc(HonGenetics); CCFP; Staff, Grand River Hospital - Kitchener/Waterloo Health Centre; Langs: Italian; (519)653-3731; Fax. (519)653-3736.

ANG, Chrizette T; Advanced Walk-In Med Clinic, 111-21 Queensway W, Mississauga ON L5B 1B6; Alb'98; (905)897-0788

ANG, Lee-Cyn; London HSC-University Hosp, PO Box 5339 Stn B 339 Windermere Rd, London ON N6A 5A5; (Singapore)'74; MB BS; FRCPath(UK)AnatPat; LMCC; FRCPC; NeurPath. Staff, London Health Sciences Centre - University Hospital; Prof Path, University of Western Ontario; Langs: Cantonese; Chinese; Mandarin; (519)685-8500 x32289; Fax. (519)663-2930.

ANG, Miriam; Sunnybrook Hlth Sciences Ctre, 2075 Bayview Ave, Toronto ON M4N 3M5; Wes'07; ObstGyn. Staff, Sunnybrook Health Sciences Centre; (416)480-6100

ANG, Vivienne; 553 St Clair Ave W, Toronto ON M6C 1A3; Tor'89; (416)652-3307; Fax. (416)652-3413.

ANGARAN, Paul A; St Michael's Hosp, 6 050-30 Bond St, Toronto ON M5B 1W8; Tor'04; FRCPC; IntMed; Cardiol. Staff, St Michael's Hospital; (416)864-5104; Fax. (416)864-5849.

ANGEL, Aubie; Massey College U of Toronto, 4 Devonshire Pl, Toronto ON M5S 2E1; Man'59; BSc(Med.); MSc; FRCPC; IntMed (Diabetes). Consultant, Toronto General Hospital - UHN; Langs: Bilingual(English/French); (416)506-1597; aubie.angel@utoronto.ca.

ANGEL, Jonathan B; The Ottawa Hosp-Gen Campus, G12-501 Smyth Rd, Ottawa ON K1H 8L6; Tor'88; BSc; FRCPC; IntMed (Infectious Diseases-HIV/AIDS); InfectDis. Staff, The Ottawa Hospital - General Campus; Assoc Prof Med, University of Ottawa; (613)737-8442

ANGEL, Melissa S; Western Mem Reg Hosp, PO Box 2005 1 Brookfield Ave, Corner Brook NL A2H 6J7; Mem'07; CCFP; CCFP(E.M.); Locum Tenens, Western Memorial Regional Hospital; (709)637-5000

ANGEL, Michael J; William Osler HC-Brampton Civi, 2100 Bovaird Ave E, Brampton ON L6R 3J7; Tor'00; FRCP; PhD; MSc; BSc; FRCPC; Neur (Neuromuscular Diseases). Assoc Staff/Lecturer Dept of Med Division of Neurology, Toronto General Hospital - UHN; Staff, Baycrest Centre for Geriatric Care; Staff, William Osler Health System - Brampton Civic Hospital; (905)494-2120 x50554; Fax. (905)494-6481; mike.angel@utoronto.ca.

ANGEL, Steven F; Royal University Hosp, 103 Hospital Dr, Saskatoon SK S7N 0W8; Sask'95; LMCC; FRCPC; GenPath. Ac Staff, Royal University Hospital; (306)655-2940; Fax. (306)665-2223; s_f_angel@hotmail.com.

ANGELES, Hilda A N; East Calgary Health Centre, 4715 8 Ave SE, Calgary AB T2A 3N4; FRCPC; Peds. (403)955-1077; Fax. (403)955-1076.

ANGELES, M Carmen; Chatham-Kent Health Alliance, PO Box 2030 Stn Main 80 Grand Ave W, Chatham ON N7M 5L9; UST (Philippines)'95; FRCPC; Anes. Staff, Chatham-Kent Health Alliance; (519)352-6400

ANGELES, Ronald M; Regina Qu'Appelle HR-Pasqua, 4101 Dewdney Ave, Regina SK S4T 1A5; UST Manila (Philippines)'99; FRCPC; AnatPath. Anatomical Pathology, Pasqua Hospital; (306)766-2159; Fax. (306)766-2752.

ANGELINI, Mark P; Medical Clinic Bldg, 102-89 Humber College Blvd, Etobicoke ON M9V 4B8; Tor'01; BSc(Hons); FRCSC; OrthSurg (Hip & Knee Arthroplasty). Staff OrthSurg, William Osler Health System - Etobicoke General Hospital; Langs: Italian; (647)438-7195; Fax. (647)438-7277.

ANGELINI, Paola; The Hosp for Sick Children, 555 University Ave, Toronto ON M5G 1X8; Turin (Italy)'98; Staff HemOncol, The Hospital For Sick Children; (416)813-7500

ANGELOVA, Jordanka; PO Box 60153 Rpo U Of Alberta, Edmonton AB T6G 2S4; Alb'02; BSc(Pharm); CCFP; Langs: Bulgarian; Spanish; Portuguese; (780)438-2306

ANGELSKI, Carla L; Edmonton Clinic Health Academy, 3 512-11405 87 Ave NW, Edmonton AB T6G 1C9; Sask'05; FRCPC; Peds; PedEmergMed. Staff, Edmonton Clinic Health Academy; (780)248-5575; Fax. (780)248-5625.

ANGERS, Daniel; 538 rue Commerciale, La Tuque QC G9X 3A8; Laval'77; (819)523-4459

ANGERS, Magalie; CHUS-Hop Hotel-Dieu, 580 rue Bowen S, Sherbrooke QC J1G 2E8; Sher'06; OrthSurg. Staff, Centre Hospitalier Universitaire de Sherbrooke-Hôpital Hôtel-Dieu; (819)346-1110

ANGERS, Michele; CHUQ-Ctr Hosp Univ Laval, D 1211-2705 boul Laurier, Quebec QC G1V 4G2; Laval'05; FRCSC; OrthSurg. Staff, Centre Hospitalier Universitaire de Quebec-CHUL; (418)656-4444

ANGERS, Suzanne; Queen Elizabeth Urgent Care, 2111 av Northcliffe, Montreal QC H4A 3K6; Mon'82; (514)481-4343

ANGERS, Yves; Clinique d'Orthopedie de Levis, 6620 rue Saint-Georges, Levis QC G6V 4H1; Laval'79; FRCSC; OrthSurg. Ac Staff, Hôtel-Dieu de Lévis; (418)837-8251; Fax. (418)837-2033.

ANGILLETTA, Bruno; Norfinch Med Centre, 106-2100 Finch Ave W, North York ON M3N 2Z9; Genova (Italy)'83; Staff, Humber River Regional Hospital - Finch Avenue Site; (416)739-7600; Fax. (416)739-7601.

ANGL, Mohinder K; Courtice Health Centre, 1450 Highway 2, Courtice ON L1E 3C3; Punjab (India)'74; MB BS; Langs: Hindi; Punjabi; Urdu; (905)721-4069

ANGLE, James D; 200-2984 Boul Taschereau, Greenfield Park QC J4V 2G9; McG'84; FRCPC; IntMed; Rheum. Staff, Hopital Charles LeMoyne; Langs: English; French; (450)465-9789; Fax. (450)672-4578.

ANGLE, Michael R; MUHC-Montreal Neurology Inst, 539-3801 rue University, Montreal QC H3A 2B4; McG'76; CSPQ; Anes (P.Q.); IntMed. Staff, McGill University Health Centre - Montreal Neurological Hospital; Staff, McGill University Health Centre - Royal Victoria Hospital; (514)398-1922; Fax. (514)398-1352.

ANGLE, Pamela J; Sunnybrook Hlth Sciences Ctre, 2075 Bayview Ave, Toronto ON M4N 3M5; Harvard(Boston) (USA)'88; FRCPC; Anes. Staff, Sunnybrook Health Sciences Centre; (416)480-6100

ANGLIN, Peter J; Stronach Reg Cancer Centre, 596 Davis Dr, Newmarket ON L3Y 2P9; Qns'86; FRCPC; IntMed (Clinical Hematology); MedOncol; Hem. Staff, Southlake Regional Health Centre; Staff, Stronach Regional Cancer Centre; Instructor, University of Toronto; (905)895-4521 x6091; Fax. (905)952-3053.

ANGLIN, Rebecca E S; 4W8 H-1280 Main St W, Hamilton ON L8S 4K1; McM'05; FRCPC; Psy. Staff Mountain Health Services, St Joseph's Healthcare Hamilton - West 5th Campus; (905)521-2100

ANGUS, Donald R; Foothills Med Centre, 1403 29 St NW, Calgary AB T2N 2T9; Alb'71; FRCPC; Psy. Dir Psy Assessment Serv, Foothills Medical Centre; Clin Assoc Prof, University of Calgary; (403)944-1291; Fax. (403)944-2838; donald.angus@albertahealthservices.ca.

ANGUS, Eric E; PO Box 670, Lions Bay BC V0N 2E0; UBC'91; CCFP; CCFP(E.M.); Staff, Squamish General Hospital / Hilltop House; (604)626-7375

ANGUS, Karen E; Health Sciences Centre, 2420-300 Prince Philip Dr, St. John's NL A1B 3V6; Dal'06; CCFP; CCFP(E.M.); Staff, Health Sciences Centre; (709)777-6300

ANGUS, Robert J; St Joseph's Gen Hosp, 2137 Comox Ave, Comox BC V9M 1P2; McM'90; MASc; Staff, St Joseph's General Hospital; (250)339-1457

ANGYALFI, Steve J; Tom Baker Cancer Centre, 1331 29 St NW, Calgary AB T2N 4N2; Alb'82; FRCPC; RadOncol. Staff Oncol, Tom Baker Cancer Centre; Med Consultant Ped Oncol, Alberta Children's Hospital; Med Consultant, Foothills Medical Centre; Clin Assoc Prof Oncol, University of Calgary; Langs: Hungarian; (403)521-3095; Fax. (403)283-1651; stevea@cancerboard.ab.ca.

ANIAGU, Charles A; Bow Island Med Clinic, PO Box 990 502 1st St W, Bow Island AB T0K 0G0; Staff, Bow Island Health Centre; (403)545-2244; Fax. (403)545-2099.

ANID, Gabriel A; Thompson Gen Hosp, 871 Thompson Dr, Thompson MB R8N 0C8; Southampton (England)'83; FRCS; Consultant, Thompson General Hospital; (204)677-2381; Fax. (204)677-2389; ganid@BRHA.mb.ca.

ANIDJAR, Maurice; MUHC-Royal Victoria Hosp, 687 av des Pins O, Montreal QC H3A 1A1; Paris (France)'92; Staff, McGill University Health Centre - Royal Victoria Hospital; (514)934-1934 x34808; Fax. (514)843-1552.

ANIFOWOSHE, Akeem B; 40-1770 Albion Rd, Etobicoke ON M9V 1C2; University of Illinois (USA)'00; CCFP; (416)748-5678

ANIKI, Yahaya Y; Holistic Med Clinic, 603-8600 Franklin Ave, Fort McMurray AB T9H 4G8; Vinnitsa (Ukraine)'91; (780)750-1600; Fax. (780)750-1660.

ANIOL, Michael J; M Aniol Med Prof Corp, B1-1276 Lasalle Blvd, Sudbury ON P3A 1Y8; Tor'91; CCFP; FCFP; Asst Prof Med, Laurentian University; Asst Prof Med, Northern Ontario School of Medicine-Lakehead University; (705)525-2171; Fax. (705)525-2173.

ANIOL, Wojciech; Red Lake Med Group, PO Box 311, Red Lake ON P0V 2M0; Wes'76; Ac Staff, Red Lake Margaret Cochenour Memorial Hospital; Langs: Polish; (807)727-3378; Fax. (807)727-3122; vaniol@redlakehospital.ca.

ANIS, Hanaa N; Family Practice Clinic, 84 Memorial Ave, Grnd-Falls-Windsor NL A2A 1R9; Cairo (Egypt)'87; MB BCh; (709)489-6688

ANJEMA, Christopher; Dr Chris Anjema Med Prof Corp, 735 St Clair St, Chatham ON N7M 5J7; Wes'99; MEd; FRCSC; Ophth (Comprehensive Ophthalmology). Staff, Anjema Eye Institute; Aj Prof, Emory University; (519)380-0008; Fax. (519)354-9982.

ANJILVEL, George M; Columbia Drive Med Clinic, PO Box 1180, Marystown NL A0E 2M0; Madras (India)'54; MB BS; FRCSC; GenSurg. Att Staff Surg, Burin Peninsula Health Care Centre; (709)279-3696

ANJORIN, Adeyemi G; South Shore Reg Hosp, 90 Glen Allan Dr, Bridgewater NS B4V 3S6; Ilorin (Nigeria)'00; MB BS; Staff, South Shore Regional Hospital; (902)543-5400; Fax. (902)543-5400.

ANJUM, Mahraz; The Juravinski Cancer Centre, 699 Concession St, Hamilton ON L8V 5C2; Pradesh (India)'93; FRCPC; IntMed. (905)387-9711

ANKENBAUER, Martin R; Castlegar Med Associates, 1008 Columbia Ave, Castlegar BC V1N 1H2; Wuerzburg (Germany)'86; Langs: German; (250)365-2161; Fax. (250)365-2171.

ANKER, Chad H; South Urgent Care Center, 31 Sunpark Plaza SE, Calgary AB T2X 3W5; Alb'94; CCFP; Staff, Rockyview General Hospital; Med Staff, Foothills Medical Centre; (403)943-9476

ANNAKKAGE, Rannulu D; Stonewall & Dist Health Ctre, 589 3rd Ave S, Stonewall MB R0C 2Z0; Auckland (New Zealand)'99; Staff, Stonewall & District Health Centre; (204)467-5514

ANNAMALA, Ganesan; Sunnybrook Hlth Sciences Ctre, MG 183-2075 Bayview Ave, Toronto ON M4N 3M5; Belfast (Ireland)'93; Staff, Sunnybrook Health Sciences Centre; Langs: Malay; Tamil; (416)480-6100

ANNAMALAI, Sivakumar; 167 Townsend St, Sydney NS B1L 1E1; Tamil Nadu University (Sri Lanka)'93; MB BS; (902)270-3170; Fax. (902)270-3165.

ANNAN, Alastair W J; Enderby Community Hlth Ctre, PO Box 580 707 3 Ave, Enderby BC V0E 1V0; Pretoria (South Africa)'76; MB ChB; DA(SA); Langs: Dutch; (250)838-2450

ANNANDALE, Francois C; Cadillac Fairview Tower 2, 960-321 6 Ave SW, Calgary AB T2P 3H3; Pretoria (South Africa)'91; MB ChB; CCFP.

ANNAVUKADAVU, Abdul S; Chinook Reg Hosp, 960 19 St S, Lethbridge AB T1J 1W5; Staff, Chinook Regional Hospital; (403)388-6022; Fax. (403)388-6619.

ANNAWI, Hane A; North East Med Centre, 7210 144 Ave NW, Edmonton AB T5C 2R7; (Libya)'03; CCFP; (780)478-2995; Fax. (780)472-0215.

ANNEN, A Albert; 200-240 Wharncliffe Rd N, London ON N6H 4P2; Wes'77; CCFP; FCFP; Ad Staff, London Health Sciences Centre - University Hospital; Ac Staff, St Joseph's Hospital - St Joseph's Health Care; Ac Staff, Mount Hope Centre Long Term Care; Clinical Asst Prof Family Med, University of Western Ontario; (519)850-9199; Fax. (519)850-9399; aannen@uwo.ca.

ANNIS, Robert V; 101-586 Argus Rd, Oakville ON L6J 3J3; Tor'65; Staff, Halton Healthcare Services Corporation - Oakville Site; (905)842-2410; Fax. (905)842-7376.

ANNIS, Robert W K; 185 Inkerman St E, Listowel ON N4W 2N1; Tor'88; CCFP; Listowel Memorial Hospital - Listowel Wingham Hospitals Alliance; (519)291-4200

ANNISETTE, Garth K M; 410 Giles Blvd E, Windsor ON N9A 4C6; (Jamaica)'78; MB BS; BSc; FRCSC; OrthSurg. Staff, Hôtel-Dieu Grace Hospital; Staff, Windsor Regional Hospital - Metropolitan Site; (519)256-3626; Fax. (519)254-3849.

ANOSIKE, Jide E; Postmaster Med Clinic, 1-2520 Postmaster Dr, Oakville ON L6M 0N2; Ilorin (Nigeria)'89; MB BS; CCFP; (905)825-5999

ANOZIE, Amaraegbulam; 202-300 Merganser Dr W, Chestermere AB T1X 1L6; Nigeria (Nigeria)'82; CCFP; (403)235-3343; Fax. (403)248-3720.

ANQUIST, K Warren; 201-32310 South Fraser Way, Abbotsford BC V2T 1X1; Alb'86; FRCPC; Peds. Staff, Abbotsford Regional Hospital & Cancer Centre; Asst Prof, University of British Columbia; (604)853-8674; Fax. (604)853-8028.

ANRAKU, Masaki; Univ Hlth Network-Toronto Gen, 9N 947-200 Elizabeth St, Toronto ON M5G 2C4; Kagoshima (Japan)'96; Clin Fellow Thoracic Surg, Toronto General Hospital - UHN; (416)340-4798

ANSALDO, Carlos M; Hop du Sacre-Coeur de Mtl, 5400 boul Gouin O, Montreal QC H4J 1C5; Buenos Aires (Argentina)'93; Staff, Hôpital du Sacre-Coeur de Montréal; (514)338-2222 x2425

ANSAR, Roomana; 66 Eveline St, Selkirk MB R1A 1K6.

ANSARI, A Hashsham; One Stop Medical Centre, 3585 Lawrence Ave E, Scarborough ON M1G 1P4; Karachi (Pakistan)'95; CCFP; Langs: Punjabi; Urdu; Hindi; (416)431-0736; Fax. (416)431-0648.

ANSARI, Khalid; Grey Nuns Comm Hosp & HC, 4017-1100 Youville Drive West, Edmonton AB T6L 5X8; Alb'99; FRCSC; Otol (Facial Plastic Surgery). Staff, Covenant Health - Grey Nuns Community Hospital; Asst Prof, University of Alberta Hospital; (780)735-7254; Fax. (780)735-7537.

ANSARI, Muhammad Z; Health Sciences Centre, 820 Sherbrook St, Winnipeg MB R3A 1R9; Staff, Health Sciences Centre; (204)774-8511

ANSARI, Saira; Scarborough Hosp-General Div, 3050 Lawrence Ave E, Scarborough ON M1P 2V5; Bhopal (India)'81; MB BS; FRCPC; AnatPath. Staff Path, The Scarborough Hospital - General Campus; Langs: Urdu; Hindi; (416)438-2911 x6450

ANSARI, Shoaib R; Cape Breton Healthcare Complex, 1482 George St, Sydney NS B1P 1P3; Rawalpindi (Pakistan)'98; Staff, Cape Breton Healthcare Complex; (902)567-8592

ANSARI, Zeba I; Oakville Health Centre, 208-1060 Speers Rd, Oakville ON L6L 2X4; Aligarh (India)'81; FAAP; FRCPC; Peds. Att Staff Peds, Halton Healthcare Services Corporation - Oakville Site; (905)339-0008; Fax. (905)842-8001.

ANSARI, Ziaul B; Community Med Clinic, 5108 50 Ave, Wetaskiwin AB T9A 0S6; Karachi (Pakistan)'64; FRCS; Langs: Urdu; (780)352-2511; Fax. (780)352-7599.

ANSARIAN, Mohammad B; Misericordia Community Hosp, 16940 87 Ave NW, Edmonton AB T5R 4H5; (Iran)'78; Staff, Covenant Health - Misericordia Community Hospital; (780)735-2731; Fax. (780)735-2794.

ANSELL, Chantal D; Student Hlth & Counselling Ser, 1 Campus Dr, Saskatoon SK S7N 5A3; Sask'99; CCFP; Langs: French; (306)966-5768; Fax. (306)966-5786.

ANSELL, Richard J; Southridge Med Clinic, 300B Village Lane, Okotoks AB T1S 1Z6; Pretoria (South Africa)'84; MB ChB; Physician Emerg, Okotoks Health & Wellness Centre; Langs: Afrikaans; (403)938-7707; dransell@telus.net.

ANSELM, Anjali H; 96 Roncesvalles Ave, Toronto ON M6R 2K8; Ott'03; BSc; FRCPC; IntMed; Cardiol. Staff, St Joseph's Health Centre; (647)748-4897; ansela@stjoe.on.ca.

ANSELMO, Mark A; Alberta Children's Hosp, 2888 Shaganappi Trail NW, Calgary AB T3B 6A8; Alb'97; FRCPC; Respir; Peds. Staff, Alberta Children's Hospital; (403)955-7502; Fax. (403)955-7059.

ANSLEY, David M; Vancouver Gen Hosp, 2449-855 12th Ave W, Vancouver BC V5Z 1M9; Sask'81; FRCPC; Anes. Staff, Vancouver General Hospital - Centennial Pavillion; (604)875-4304

ANSON, Shelagh; Children's & Women's HC of BC, 1R47-4480 Oak St, Vancouver BC V6H 3V4; Dal'99; FRCPC; Peds. Staff, BC Children's Hospital; (604)875-2135

ANSTEAD, Keith S; Regina Qu'Appelle HR-Pasqua, 4101 Dewdney Ave, Regina SK S4T 1A5; London (England)'71; Staff, Pasqua Hospital; (306)766-2222

ANSTEE, Grizel C; The Ottawa Hosp-Gen Campus, 501 Smyth Rd, Ottawa ON K1H 8L6; Ott'81; CCFP; Clin Associate, The Ottawa Hospital - General Campus; (613)737-8158; Fax. (613)737-8861.

ANSTETT, Robert J; LL-920 King St W, Kitchener ON N2G 1G4; Wes'81; FRCSC; ObstGyn. Ac Staff, Grand River Hospital - Kitchener/Waterloo Health Centre; (519)745-2116; Fax. (519)745-3884.

ANTAKI, Aline; Clinique Ped La Courte Echelle, 86 boul Brien, Repentigny QC J6A 5K7; Mon'95; Peds. Staff Ped & Neonatal, Centre Hospitalier Pierre le Gardeur; Langs: Bilingual(French/English); (450)657-1705; Fax. (450)657-1800.

ANTAKI, Roland; CHUM-Hop St-Luc, 1058 rue Saint-Denis, Montreal QC H2X 3J4; University of Aleppo (Syria)'02; FRCSC; ObstGyn (Gynecological Reproductive Endocrinology). Staff, Centre Hospitalier l'Université De Montréal (CHUM) - Hôpital Saint-luc; (514)890-8000

ANTAO, Viola; Women's College Hosp, 76 Grenville St, Toronto ON M5S 1B2; Tor'99; MHSc; CCFP; Staff, Women's College Hospital; Asst Prof Family Comm Med, University of Toronto; (416)323-6060

ANTAR, Ramy; The Ottawa Hosp-Gen Campus, LM10-501 Smyth Rd, Ottawa ON K1H 8L6; Alexandria (Egypt)'04; IntMed. Staff, The Ottawa Hospital - General Campus; (613)798-5555

ANTEBI, Elie; Ctr Hosp Anna-Laberge, 200 boul Brisebois, Chateauguay QC J6K 4W8; Laval'04; FRCSC; Urol. Staff, Hôpital Anna-Laberge; (450)699-2425

ANTEL, Jack P; MUHC-Montreal Neurology Inst, 3801 rue University, Montreal QC H3A 2B4; Man'69; FRCPC; Neur. Ac Staff, McGill University Health Centre - Montreal Neurological Hospital; Prof Neurol & Neuro Surg, McGill University; (514)398-8550; jack.antel@mcgill.ca.

ANTHES, David L; Ridgeway Clinic, 1001 Ridgeway St E, Thunder Bay ON P7E 5H8; Tor'95; BASc; Pres, Physician Housecall Services; Pres, MedEng Computer Billing Systems; Teach Staff Biology, Lakehead University / Library; (807)622-0601; Fax. (807)623-0470.

ANTHES, Margaret L; Thunder Bay Reg HSC-T-Bay, 980 Oliver Rd, Thunder Bay ON P7B 6V4; Wes'91; FRCPC; RadOncol. Ac Staff, Thunder Bay Regional Health Sciences Centre; Clin Assoc Prof Med, Northern Ontario School of Medicine; (807)684-7211; Fax. (807)684-5801; anthesm@tbh.net.

ANTHIREYA-KAKANI, Sophia; Alexandra Medical Centre, 29 Noxon St, Ingersoll ON N5C 3V6; CCFP; (519)485-9617; Fax. (519)485-9620.

ANTHONISEN, Nicholas R; Respiratory Unit, RS315-810 Sherbrook St, Winnipeg MB R3A 1R8; Harvard(MA) (USA)'58; PhD(McG); FRCPC; MedScient(Med) (Respiratory Disease). Staff, Health Sciences Centre; Consultant, St Boniface General Hospital; Prof Med, University of Manitoba; (204)787-2562

ANTHONY, Francis R; 540 St. George Blvd, Moncton NB E1E 2B5; Agra (India)'62; LRCP; MRCS; FRCS(Lond); FRCSC; Urol. Staff, Dr Georges-L-Dumont University Hospital Centre; (506)857-0640; Fax. (506)382-1932.

ANTHONY, John S; Scarborough Prof Centre, 314-1371 Neilson Rd, Scarborough ON M1B 4Z8; Tor'72; FCCP; MASc; FRCPC; IntMed (Respirology). Staff, Rouge Valley Health System - Centenary Health Centre Site; (416)282-9112; Fax. (416)282-4282.

ANTHONY, Robert G; Langley Health Services, 22051 Fraser Hwy, Langley BC V3A 4H4; Qns'75; FACEP; FRCPC; EmergMed.

ANTHONY, Rozario; The Moncton Hosp, 135 MacBeath Ave, Moncton NB E1C 6Z8; Bangalore (India)'92; Staff, The Moncton Hospital; (506)857-5111

ANTMAN, Neil S; Trillium Hlth Ctr-Mississauga, 100 Queensway W, Mississauga ON L5B 1B8; Haifa (Israel)'89; FRCPC; IntMed; Critical Care Medicine; Respir. Dir ICU/Head, Trillium Health Centre - West Toronto; Staff, Trillium Health Centre - Mississauga; (905)848-7663; nantman@thc.on.ca.

ANTOCHI, Ruxandra M; The Ottawa Hosp-Gen Campus, 501 Smyth Rd, Ottawa ON K1H 8L6; Wes'98; FRCPC; Psy. Staff, The Ottawa Hospital - General Campus; (613)737-8010; Fax. (613)737-8115.

ANTOINE, Louis B; 969 Queen St E, Sault Ste. Marie ON P6A 2C2; (Haiti)'76; Staff, Sault Area Hospital - Sault Ste Marie.

ANTOLINEZ-URIBE, Edgar; 17 Wellington St N, Woodstock ON N4S 6P1; (Colombia)'92; FRCSC; ObstGyn (Maternal Fetal Medicine). Staff, St Joseph's Hospital - St Joseph's Health Care; Staff, Woodstock General Hospital; (519)290-5000

ANTON, Andrew R; Foothills Med Centre, 1403 29 St NW, Calgary AB T2N 2T9; Cal'92; FRCPC; EmergMed. Staff, Foothills Medical Centre; (403)538-7635; Fax. (403)944-2419.

ANTON, Annepa; Atlantic Medical Centre, 1054 McPhillips St, Winnipeg MB R2X 2K9; (Other Foreign)'09.

ANTON, Hubert A; Pacific Rehab Medicine, 140-943 Broadway W, Vancouver BC V5Z 4E1; Cal'78; BSc; FRCPC; PhysMed&Rehab., G F Strong Rehabilitation Centre; Ac Staff, Vancouver General Hospital - Centennial Pavillion; (604)733-2222; Fax. (604)733-2202; hubert.anton@vch.ca.

ANTON, Natalie R; 3A3.19-8440 112 St NW, Edmonton AB T6G 2B7; Cal'94; FRCPC; Peds; Critical Care Medicine. Staff, University of Alberta Hospital; (780)407-1673; Fax. (780)407-3214; natalie.anton@albertahealthservices.ca.

ANTONE, N Irwin; Meno-Ya_Win Health Centre, 71 Seventh Ave, Sioux Lookout ON P8T 1H6; Wes'76; CCFP; FCFP; Staff, Sioux Lookout Meno-Ya-Win Health Centre; (807)737-3030

ANTONENKO, Alexander; 5-4646 Dufferin St, North York ON M3H 5S4; Crimean State Medical University (Other Foreign)'95; CCFP; Langs: Russian; (416)222-6160; Fax. (416)222-9604.

ANTONENKO, Natalie E; Selkirk Mental Health Centre, PO Box 9600 Stn Main 825 Manitoba Ave, Selkirk MB R1A 2B5; UBC'90; BSc(Zool); Staff, Selkirk Mental Health Centre; Langs: Spanish; French; (204)482-3810

ANTONESCU, Serban M; Hop Santa Cabrini Ospedale, 5655 rue Saint-Zotique E, Montreal QC H1T 1P7; Bucharest (Romania)'85; Staff, Hôpital Santa Cabrini Ospedale; (514)252-6000 x6546

ANTONIADES, Marc; Clinique d'Orthopedie, 4370 Cote Rosemont, Trois-Rivieres QC G8Y 0A5; Sher'83; OrthSurg (P.Q.). Staff, Centre Hospitalier Regional de Trois-Rivieres; (819)374-5111; Fax. (819)374-8719.

ANTONIADIS, Gregory A; North Huron FHT-Wingham, PO Box 609 285 Catherine St, Wingham ON N0G 2W0; Ott'89; CCFP; Staff, Wingham & District Hospital - Listowel Wingham Hospitals Alliance; (519)357-2500; Fax. (519)357-1816.

ANTONIAK, Gregory P; Facial Surgery & Cosmetic Ctre, 308-1919 Riverside Dr, Ottawa ON K1H 1A2; Wes'82; FRCSC; Otol (Cosmetic Surgery). Ac Staff, The Ottawa Hospital - Riverside Campus; Ac Staff, Children's Hospital of Eastern Ontario (CHEO); Surgeon -In-Chief, The Facial Surgery & Cosmetic Centre of Ottawa Inc; (613)521-3223; Fax. (613)521-6017; mailbox@face.ca.

ANTONIOLLI, Lisa; CF Health Sevices Centre, PO Box 10500 Stn Forces, Edmonton AB T5J 4J5; Alb'96; CCFP; (780)973-1651; Fax. (780)973-1651.

ANTONIOU, Andreas; London HSC-University Hosp, PO Box 5339 Stn B 339 Windermere Rd, London ON N6A 5A5; Tor'05; FRCPC; Anes. Staff Anes & Periop Med, London Health Sciences Centre - University Hospital; (519)663-3283

ANTONIOU, John; SMBD Jewish Gen Hosp, E 003-3755 ch Cote-Sainte-Cath, Montreal QC H3T 1E2; McG'91; FRCSC; OrthSurg (Joint Arthroplasty). Staff, Sir Mortimer B Davis Jewish General; Langs: French; Greek; (514)340-8222 x4615; Fax. (514)340-7595.

ANTONISSEN, Ludovieus; Ear Falls Family Health Team, PO Box 250 25 Spruce St, Ear Falls ON P0V 1T0; Man'82; (807)222-3728

ANTONIUK, Craig D; 9368 Southfort Dr, Fort Saskatchewan AB T8L 0C5; Alb'01; CCFP; (780)997-0177

ANTONIUK, Karen M; 326 Wilson St E, Ancaster ON L9G 2C2; McM'93; CCFP; FCFP; Assoc Staff, Hamilton Health Sciences Centre - McMaster University Medical Centre; (905)648-0770; Fax. (905)648-0777.

ANTONIUK, Mark J; 4010 50 St NW, Edmonton AB T6L 5N3; Alb'89; CCFP; Staff Family Med, Covenant Health - Grey Nuns Community Hospital; (780)450-5646; Fax. (780)462-4406.

ANTONSEN, John E; 205-1990 Fort St, Victoria BC V8R 6V4; UBC'89; FRCPC; IntMed; Nephrol. (250)595-2511; Fax. (250)595-8503.

ANTONY, Saju; 105-9181 Main St, Chilliwack BC V2P 4M9; Punjab (India)'84; MB BS; MRCPsy(Lond); DPM(Ire); FRCP; FRCPC; Psy (General Adult Psychiatry). Consultant Psy, Chilliwack General Hospital; Physician, Mental Health Centre; Langs: Malayalam; Hindi; (604)792-1888; Fax. (604)792-1129.

ANTONY, Savarimuthiusosai; 24179 Highway 7 PO Box 41, Sheet Harbour NS B0J 3B0; Colombo (Sri Lanka)'84; MB BS; (902)885-5602

ANTONYSHYN, Oleh M; Sunnybrook Hlth Sciences Ctre, M520-2075 Bayview Ave, Toronto ON M4N 3M5; Tor'80; DrMedCh; FRCS; FRCSC; PlasSurg (Cosmetic Surgery). Head Craniofacial Prog/Consultant PlasSurg, Sunnybrook Health Sciences Centre; Prof PlasSurg, University of Toronto; Langs: Ukrainian; (416)480-4868; Fax. (416)480-6800.

ANTOWAN, Samir M; Iroquois Ridge Med Centre B5-360 Dundas St E, Oakville ON L6H 6Z9; Saddam College of Medicine (Iraq)'94; CCFP; (905)257-8777; Fax. (905)257-0437.

ANTRIM, Anne A; Children's & Women's HC of BC, 1R47-4480 Oak St, Vancouver BC V6H 3V4; UBC'86; BSc; FRCPC; Peds. Ac Staff, BC Children's Hospital; (604)875-2345

ANTTILA, Lisa K; Dominion Centre, 47 Marion St, Winnipeg MB R2H 0S8; Man'05; FRCSC; ObstGyn.

ANTUNES, Marcia O; Royal Alexandra Hosp, 5027-10240 Kingsway NW, Edmonton AB T5H 3V9; (Brazil)'89; Staff, Royal Alexandra Hospital; (780)735-4670; Fax. (780)735-4072.

ANTUNES, Paulo R M; Ctre de sante Comm de l'Estrie, 6-841 Sydney St, Cornwall ON K6H 3J7; Guadalajara (Mexico)'03; CCFP; (613)937-2683

ANTUNES, Rui L; Cornwall Comm Hosp-McConnell, PO Box 100 Stn Main 840 McConnell Ave, Cornwall ON K6H 5S5; Coimbra (Portugal)'61; FRCSC; GenSurg. Staff, Cornwall Community Hospital; Langs: Portuguese; English; (613)938-4240 x2217; rl.antunes@sympatico.ca.

ANVARI, Linda; Emerald Business Centre, 5-20 Kingsbridge Garden Cir, Mississauga ON L5R 3K7; Cape Town (South Africa)'01; MB ChB; CCFP; Physician, University of Lethbridge; (905)507-1111; Fax. (905)890-7102; anvari@uleth.ca.

ANVARI, Mehran; St Joseph's Healthcare, 50 Charlton Ave E, Hamilton ON L8N 4A6; Newcastle (England)'83; FRCSC; GenSurg (Laparoscopic Gastrointestinal Surgery). Ac Staff, St Joseph's Healthcare - Charlton Campus; Court Staff, Hamilton Health Sciences Centre - McMaster University Medical Centre; Prof Surg, McMaster University; Langs: Farsi; (905)522-2951; Fax. (905)521-6113.

ANWAR, Mariam; Campbellton Reg Hosp, PO Box 880 189 Lilly Lake Rd, Campbellton NB E3N 3H3; Aga Khan (Other Foreign)'04; Staff, Hôpital Régional Campbellton; (506)789-5000

ANWAR, Muhammad A Q; Health Sciences Centre, 300 Prince Philip Dr, St. John's NL A1B 3V6; Punjab (India)'94; FRCPC; IntMed (Respirology). Locum Tenens, James Paton Memorial Hospital; Locum Tenens, Charles S Curtis Memorial Hospital; Staff Respiratory Med, Health Sciences Centre; Staff, The Dr G B Cross Memorial Hospital; (709)737-6300

ANWAR, Muhammad M; 260 Sherbrooke St, New Westminster BC V3L 3M2; Multan (Pakistan)'95; MB BS; FRCPC; Psy. Staff, Royal Columbian Hospital; (604)777-8386

ANWAR, Shahgul; Health Sciences Centre, 300 Prince Philip Dr, St. John's NL A1B 3V6; Rawalpindi Medical College (Pakistan)'97; MB BS; Staff, Health Sciences Centre; (709)777-6648

ANWAR, Syed S; Dynacare Kasper Med Lab, 200-10150 102 St NW, Edmonton AB T5J 5E2; Karachi (Pakistan)'91; MB BS; FRCPC; AnatPath. (780)451-3702

ANWAR MASIH, Tahreem S; 23-1285 Elgin Mills Rd, Richmond Hill ON L4S 0B5; Peshawar (India)'93; CCFP; (289)637-1727; Fax. (289)637-1728.

ANWEILER, Laura L; 370 Select Dr PO Box 168, Kingston ON K7M 8T4; Wes'90; CCFP; FCFP; (613)536-3006

ANYA MENGUE, Pierre; CSSS des Collines, RR 2 101 ch Burnside, Wakefield QC J0X 3G0; (819)459-1112 x2411

ANYADIKE, Ignatius O; St Boniface Clinic, 343 Tache Ave, Winnipeg MB R2H 2A5; Jerusalem (Israel)'68; DABPed; FAAP; FRCPC; Peds (Neonatology). Staff, Health Sciences Centre; Staff Peds, St Boniface General Hospital; Lecturer Peds, University of Manitoba; (204)925-9550; Fax. (204)231-4567.

ANYAEGBUNA, Okechukwu; Saint John Reg Hosp, PO Box 2100 Stn Main 400 University Ave, Saint John NB E2L 4L2; (Nigeria)'99; Staff, Saint John Regional Hospital; (506)648-6000

ANYALEBECHI, Obinna; CBI Health, 100 Signal Rd, Fort McMurray AB T9H 5A3; (Nigeria)'95; MB BCh; Staff, Northern Lights Regional Health Centre; (780)715-3800

ANYANWU, Leonard U; Saskatoon Community Clinic, 455 2nd Ave N, Saskatoon SK S7K 2C2; Ibadan (Nigeria)'94; (306)652-0300; Fax. (306)664-4120.

ANZARUT, Alexander D; 201-2763 Beverly St, Duncan BC V9L 6X2; UBC'00; FRCSC; PlasSurg. (250)597-3390

ANZARUT, Andre R; 1148 7th Ave W, Vancouver BC V6H 1B4; Paris (France)'63; DCH(Eng); FRCPC; FRCPC; Neur; Peds (Dementia). Emeritus Clin Prof Med, University of British Columbia; Langs: French; Hebrew; Spanish; (604)732-8887; Fax. (604)732-9427.

ANZARUT, Jody E; Cook Medical Bldg, 326-1175 Cook St, Victoria BC V8V 4A1; UBC'00; CCFP; (250)386-2449

AOKI, Fred Y; Basic Medical Science Bldg, 510-745 Bannatyne Ave, Winnipeg MB R3E 0J9; Man'66; ABIM; FRCPC; IntMed (Clinical Pharmacology). Asst Physician, Health Sciences Centre; Consultant, St Boniface General Hospital; Internal Medicine, WRHA - Deer Lodge Centre; Prof Med Microbiol Pharmacol & Therapeutics, University of Manitoba; (204)789-3625; Fax. (204)789-3926; aokify@cc.umanitoba.ca.

AOTA, Eriko; Fairmont Med Bldg, 1317-750 Broadway W, Vancouver BC V5Z 1J3; UBC'94; CCFP; FCFP; Langs: Japanese; (604)876-0711; Fax. (604)876-0770.

AOUADI, Adila; 675 ch de Saint-Jean, La Prairie QC J5R 2L2; Mohammed V Sioussi (Morocco)'06; (450)444-2002

AOUIDA, Mohamed; Hop Reg D'Edmunston, 275 Hébert Blvd, Edmundston NB E3V 4E4; (Tunisia)'04; Staff, Hôpital regional d'Edmundston; (506)739-2200

AOUINATI, Sophia; Hop Maisonneuve-Rosemont, 5415 boul de l'Assomption, Montreal QC H1T 2M4; Mon'06; CCFP; Staff, Hopital Maisonneuve-Rosemont; (514)252-3400

AOUN, Lawrence; Hotel-Dieu Grace Hosp, 1030 Ouellette Ave, Windsor ON N9A 1E1; Tor'08; CCFP; Staff, Hôtel-Dieu Grace Hospital; (519)973-4411

APANTAKU, Olubukola J; 160-6900 Taylor Dr, Red Deer AB T4P 1K4; University of Ibadan (Nigeria)'97; FRCSC; ObstGyn. (403)342-2234; Fax. (403)342-2655.

APANTAKU, Olushola M; Medical & Dental Bldg, 101-3939 50A Ave, Red Deer AB T4N 4E6; (Nigeria)'99; MB BS; CCFP; (403)348-8100

APANTAKU-OLAJIDE, Babatunde; Saint John Reg Hosp, PO Box 2100 Stn Main 400 University Ave, Saint John NB E2L 4L2; Ilorin (Nigeria)'99; Staff, Saint John Regional Hospital; (506)648-6000

APARICIO, Carlos; CSSS de la Haute-Gaspésie, 50 rue du Belvedere, Ste-Anne-des-Monts QC G4V 1X4; Granada (Spain)'56; DiagRad (P.Q.). Staff, Centre Hospitalier des Monts; (418)763-2261

APARICIO, Catriona L; BC Cancer Agency-Vancouver CC, 600 10th Ave W, Vancouver BC V5Z 4E6; Oxford (United Kingdom)'89; Staff GP Palliative Care, BC Cancer Agency Vancouver Centre; (604)877-6000; Fax. (604)872-4596.

APEL, Maryana; 420-1011 Glenmore Trail SW, Calgary AB T2V 4R6; Odessa (Ukraine)'83; FRCPC; PhysMed&Rehab (Electrodiagnosis). Consultant Neurosciences, Foothills Medical Centre; Consultant Neurosciences, Rockyview General Hospital; Clinical Asst Prof, University of Calgary; (403)319-0400; Fax. (403)319-0401; drapel@arkzone.com.

APOSTLE, Kelly L; Fraser Orthopaedic Institute, 403-233 Nelson's Cres, New Westminster BC V3L 0E4; Wes'05; FRCSC; OrthSurg. (604)525-6885

APOSTLE, Nicole A; St Paul's Hosp, 1081 Burrard St, Vancouver BC V6Z 1Y6; Wes'06; CCFP; Staff, Providence Health Care - St Paul's Hospital; (604)682-2344

APOSTLE, Peter D; East Street Med Arts Centre, 202-170 East St, Sault Ste. Marie ON P6A 3C6; Wes'78; (705)759-3777; Fax. (705)949-1908.

APOSTOL, Georgeta; Royal Alexandra Hosp, 10240 Kingsway NW, Edmonton AB T5H 3V9; Iuliu Hatieganu University (Other Foreign)'96; Peds. Staff, Royal Alexandra Hospital; (780)735-4605; Fax. (780)735-4071.

APOSTOL, Tony A; 102-111 Waterloo St, London ON N6B 2M4; Tor'77; FRCSC; OrthSurg. (519)433-4857; Fax. (519)433-2516.

APOSTOLIDES, Constantine; 1202-5955 Veterans Memorial La, Halifax NS B3H 2E1; Dal'99; BSc(Biology); CCFP; Ac Staff, Capital Health Centre; Asst Prof Med, Dalhousie University; Langs: Greek; (902)473-2493; Fax. (902)473-7336; capostol@dal.ca.

APPAVOO, Lalitha L; Mayfair Place Med Centre, 303-6707 Elbow Dr SW, Calgary AB T2V 0E5; Sask'94; BSc; FRCPC; Psy. (403)571-2480; Fax. (403)571-2499.

APPAVOO, Samuel D; Maitland Valley Family Hlth Team, 180 Cambria Rd N, Goderich ON N7A 4N8; McM'89; CCFP; CCFP(E.M.); FCFP; Ac Staff, Alexandra Marine & General Hospital; Aj Prof, University of Western Ontario; (519)524-6060; Fax. (519)524-5225.

APPAVOO, Shushiela; Hys Med Centre, 202-11010 101 St NW, Edmonton AB T5H 4B9; Sask'89; FRCPC; DiagRad. (780)426-1121; Fax. (780)425-5979.

APPAVOO, Siva; 92 Erb St E, Waterloo ON N2J 1L9; Bombay (India)'76; FRCPC; Psy. (519)880-9878; Fax. (519)886-8545.

APPEL, Karen A; Northern Medical Unit, T150-770 Bannatyne Ave, Winnipeg MB R3E 0W3; Man'06; CCFP; (204)789-3711

APPELBY, Mark E; Uptown Health Centre, 243 Eglinton Ave W, Toronto ON M4R 1B1; Tor'98; CCFP; (416)489-2106

APPELL, William A; Medical Office, 202-840 Coxwell Ave, Toronto ON M4C 5T2; Tor'76; FRCPC; Gastroent; IntMed. Ac Staff, Toronto East General Hospital Inc; (416)690-6762; Fax. (416)690-6775.

APPELT, Gregory; Kelowna Respiratory Clinic, 302-3975 Lakeshore Rd, Kelowna BC V1W 1V3; Man'00; FRCPC; Peds; ClinImmunol&Allergy. (778)477-5806; Fax. (778)477-5808.

APPELTAUER, Luis C; Clinique Med Diamant, 355-1575 boul Henri-Bourassa O, Montreal QC H3M 3A9; (Uruguay)'66; Langs: Spanish; French; (514)744-9881; Fax. (514)744-1262.

APPENDINO, Juan P; Children's Hosp, AE308-840 Sherbrook St, Winnipeg MB R3A 1S1; Cordoba (Argentina)'00.

APPLEBY, James P; 1624 7th Ave, Prince George BC V2L 3P6; UBC'82; GenSurg (Endocrinology). Ac Staff, University Hospital of Northern British Columbia; Clin Associate, University of British Columbia; (250)561-2700; Fax. (250)561-2794.

APPLEBY, Kenneth J; 4349 Hastings St, Burnaby BC V5C 2J8; Qns'81; Staff, Burnaby Hospital; (604)299-4388; Fax. (604)299-1405.

APPLEBY, Michael B; Mission View Medical, 210-616 K L O Rd, Kelowna BC V1Y 4X4; Qns'85; Staff, Kelowna General Hospital; (250)763-7112; Fax. (250)763-8935.

APPLEGARTH, Christine W L; Broadway-Burrard Med Clinic, 1816 Broadway W, Vancouver BC V6J 1Y9; UBC'00; Langs: Cantonese; (604)736-1888; Fax. (604)736-5544.

APPLEGARTH, Oliver; UBC-Dept of Anes, 2N 2449-910 10th Ave W, Vancouver BC V5Z 1M9; UBC'00; FRCPC; Anes. (604)875-4304

APPLETON, Alison E; Peninsula FHT-Lions Head, 24 Moore St, Lions Head ON N0H 1W0; Tor'05; CCFP; (519)793-3445; alisonorganek@hotmail.com.

APPLETON, Brent E; 403-301 Columbia St E, New Westminster BC V3L 3W5; Ott'95; (604)526-2140

APPLETON, Darryl E; Appleton Sleep Clinic, 685 Finch Ave W, North York ON M2R 1P2; Tor'04; FRCPC; Psy (Sleep Medicine). (416)635-0909; Fax. (416)635-0300.

APPLETON, Erin E; Chinook Reg Hosp, 960 19 St S, Lethbridge AB T1J 1W5; McM'05; CCFP; Staff, Chinook Regional Hospital; (403)388-6111

APPLETON, Geoffrey M; Park Avenue Med Centre, 3F-4634 Park Ave, Terrace BC V8G 1V7; Edinburgh (Scotland)'70; MB ChB; Staff, Mills Memorial Hospital; Med Dir, Northern Health Authority; (250)615-5030; Fax. (250)615-5035.

APPLEYARD, Craig E; 552 Raglan St S, Renfrew ON K7V 1R8; Tor'73; CCFP; FCFP; Staff Consultant, Renfrew Victoria Hospital; (613)432-3240; Fax. (613)432-9567; drappleyard@bellnet.ca.

APPOO, Jehangir J; Foothills Med Centre, 1403 29 St NW, Calgary AB T2N 2T9; McG'97; FRCSC; CardSurg. Staff, Foothills Medical Centre; (403)944-2515; Fax. (403)944-2906.

APPS, David A; Central Park Med Clinic, 301-3965 Kingsway, Burnaby BC V5H 1Y8; McM'75; BSc; CCFP; FCFP; Ac Staff, Burnaby Hospital; (604)439-9333; Fax. (604)439-9572.

APPS, Robert C; L16-15 Elizabeth St, Orangeville ON L9W 3X3; Tor'66; FRCPC; IntMed. Staff, Headwaters Health Care Centre - Orangeville Site; (519)940-0211; Fax. (519)940-0610.

APRAMIAN, David A; Burk's Falls Health Centre, 150 Huston St RR 1 Box 550, Burks Falls ON P0A 1C0; McM'79; BSc; CCFP; FCFP; Court Staff Privil, Huntsville District Memorial Hospital - Muskoka Algonquin Healthcare; (705)382-2900; Fax. (705)382-3473.

APRIASZ, Izabela; St Joseph's Healthcare, 50 Charlton Ave E, Hamilton ON L8N 4A6; Krakow (Poland)'06; Staff, St Joseph's Healthcare - Charlton Campus; (905)522-1155

APRIKIAN, Armen-Garo; MUHC-Montreal Gen Hosp, L8 309-1650 av Cedar, Montreal QC H3G 1A4; Sher'85; FRCSC; Urol (Urological Oncology). Staff, McGill University Health Centre - Montreal General Campus; Asst Prof Surg, McGill University; (514)934-8295; Fax. (514)934-8297.

APRIL, Andre M; CSSS de Gatineau, 125 boul Lionel-Emond, Gatineau QC J8Y 5S8; Laval'90; Langs: English; (819)770-1880 x217; Fax. (819)770-8624.

APRIL, Claude; Clinique Med Pierre-Bertrand, 212-303 boul Pierre-Bertrand, Quebec QC G1M 3L7; Laval'79; Gen Practice, CSSS de Quebec-Sud; (418)683-2724; Fax. (418)683-8861; claude.april@orlo.ulaval.ca.

APRIL, Guy; Clinique Med Duberger, 2810 boul Pere-Lelievre, Quebec QC G1P 2Y1; Laval'81; LMCC; (418)688-8414; Fax. (418)688-4273.

APRIL, Nicole; Inst Nat'l de Sante Publique, 5F-945 av Wolfe, Quebec QC G1V 5B3; Laval'77; FRCPC; CommunMed (Public Health & Preventive Medicine). (418)650-5115 x5505; Fax. (418)654-3210; nicole.april@inspq.qc.ca.

APTEKAR, Nafisa J; The Medical Place, 201-178 John St, Brampton ON L6W 2A4; Nagpur (India)'79; MD; CCFP; Langs: Hindi; Gujarati; (905)456-2888; Fax. (905)456-2868.

APULLAN, Francisco J; CSSS du Nord de Lanaudière, 1000 boul Sainte-Anne, St-Charles-Brromee QC J6E 6J2; Cordoba (Argentina)'97; Staff, Centre Hospitalier Régional de Lanaudière; (450)759-8222

AQUINO, Emmanuel P B; The Nova Scotia Hosp, PO Box 1004 Stn Main 300 Pleasant St, Dartmouth NS B2Y 3Z9; Manila (Philippines)'68; MD; FACFP; Ac Staff, The Nova Scotia Hospital; Staff, The East Coast Forensic Psychiatry Hospital; Lecturer, Dalhousie University; Langs: Tagalog; (902)464-3336; Fax. (902)464-6079; emmanuel.aquino@cdha.nshealth.ca.

AQUINO, John M; 208-20 York Mills Rd, North York ON M2P 2C2; Tor'91; CCFP; FCFP; (416)512-6366

AQUINO JR, Jose; The Ottawa Hosp-Civic Campus, 1053 Carling Ave, Ottawa ON K1Y 4E9; Dal'87; FRCPC; DiagRad (Interventional Radiology). Staff Rad, The Ottawa Hospital - Civic Campus; Asst Prof, University of Ottawa; (613)761-5476; Fax. (613)761-5268.

AQUINO-PARSONS, Christina; BC Cancer Agency-Vancouver CC, 600 10th Ave W, Vancouver BC V5Z 4E6; McG'83; FRCPC; RadOncol. Staff, BC Cancer Agency Vancouver Centre; (604)877-6000; Fax. (604)708-2000; cparsons@bccancer.bc.ca.

AR-RUSHDI, Muna; 6 Cedar St PO Box 1311, Greenwood NS B0P 1N0; Washington(DC) (USA)'90; MD; CCFP; Staff, Labrador Health Centre; (709)896-6900; Fax. (709)896-6969.

ARA, Shamim; Hamilton HS-Henderson Site, 711 Concession St, Hamilton ON L8V 1C3; Chittagong (Bangladesh)'85; FRCPC; AnatPath. Staff, Hamilton Health Sciences Centre-Juravinski Site; (905)521-2100

ARAB-O'BRIEN, Donna M; St Joseph's Health Centre, 306SE-30 The Queensway, Toronto ON M6R 1B5; Dal'88; BSc; FRCPC; IntMed; Endocrin&Metab. Staff Endocrin, St Joseph's Health Centre; Langs: Arabic; (416)530-6466; Fax. (416)530-6510.

ARABI, Nezhat; AIM North Health Group, 302-235 North Centre Rd, London ON N5X 4E7; Iran University of Medical Sciences (Iran)'86; Staff, London Intercommunity Health Centre - Dundas Street; (519)645-2444

ARADI, Abdussalam M M; 221-501 Bethel Dr, Sherwood Park AB T8H 0N2; (780)464-0123; Fax. (780)449-1062.

ARAFA, Neema A; Main Square Med Centre, 2575 Danforth Ave, Toronto ON M4C 1L5; Alexandria (Egypt)'74; MB ChB; Langs: Arabic; (416)694-0500; Fax. (416)694-9767.

ARAGHI, Golbarg; Innova Medical, 115-1650 Elgin Mills Rd E, Richmond Hill ON L4S 0B2; McG'02; CCFP; Langs: Bilingual(French/English); (905)884-8846

ARAGOLA, Sanjay; St Boniface Gen Hosp, 409 Tache Ave, Winnipeg MB R2H 2A6; Bangalore (India)'95; FRCPC; Anes. Staff, St Boniface General Hospital; (204)233-8563

ARAGON, Jose V; Ctre Hosp de Lasalle, 8585 Tsse Champlain, LaSalle QC H8P 1C1; Cauca (Spain)'94; FRCPC; Anes. Anesthesiste, Centre Hospitalier de LaSalle; (514)362-8000

ARAGONES, Rafael; Clin Ext Psych Sainte-Therese, 2F-55 rue Saint-Joseph, Sainte-Therese QC J7E 4Y5; (Mexico)'76; Psy (P.Q.). Staff, Hôtel-Dieu de Saint-Jérôme; (450)430-3702; Fax. (450)430-6648.

ARAKELIAN, Jean; Clinique Med Cartier, 1100-1851 rue Sherbrooke E, Montreal QC H2K 4L5; St. Joseph (Lebanon)'71; Gastroent (P.Q.). ac Staff, Centre Hospitalier l'Université de Montréal (CHUM) - Hôpital Notre-Dame; (514)524-3569; Fax. (514)526-4594.

ARAKI, Michael T; Surrey Mem Hosp, 13750 96 Ave, Surrey BC V3V 1Z2; UBC'86; Assoc Staff Privil, Surrey Memorial Hospital; (604)588-3367; Fax. (604)585-5644.

ARAM, Omid; CSSS de la Haute-Gaspésie, 50 rue du Belvedere, Ste-Anne-des-Monts QC G4V 1X4; Mashhad (Iran)'00; (418)763-2261; Fax. (418)763-1827.

ARANEDA, M Carolina; Health Sciences Centre, 820 Sherbrook St, Winnipeg MB R3A 1R9; Man'89; Staff, Health Sciences Centre; (204)774-6511

ARANGO, Miguel F; London HSC-University Hosp, PO Box 5339 Stn B 339 Windermere Rd, London ON N6A 5A5; Spain (Spain)'93; FRCPC; Anes. Staff Anes & Perioperative Med, London Health Sciences Centre - University Hospital; (519)663-3022

ARANI, Arash M; Argus Med Centre, 300-581 Argus Rd, Oakville ON L6J 3J4; McM'98; BSc(BioChem.); CCFP; (905)338-9900; Fax. (905)338-9904.

ARARA, Mohammed E; Eriksdale Med Clinic, PO Box 130, Eriksdale MB R0C 0W0; Al-Fateh(Libya) (Libya)'98.

ARARAT, Alpay T; St Joseph Health Centre, 30 The Queensway, Toronto ON M6R 1B5; Wes'06; FRCPC; Anes. Staff, St Joseph's Health Centre; (416)530-6000

ARAS, Ziya; Burin Peninsula Hlth Care Ctr, PO Box 340, Burin NL A0E 1E0; (Turkey)'81; Staff, Burin Peninsula Health Care Centre; (709)891-1040

ARASU, Mala; Alberta Children's Hosp, 2888 Shaganappi Trail NW, Calgary AB T3B 6A8; Qns'03; FRCPC; Peds. Staff, Alberta Children's Hospital; (403)955-7211

ARATA, Martin; CSSS de la Region de Thetford, 1717 rue Notre-Dame E, Thetford Mines QC G6G 2V4; Laval'91; Staff, Hopital du CSS de la Region de Thetford; (418)338-7711; Fax. (418)338-7794.

ARAUJO, Adilson A M; 5-5030 Tenth Line W, Mississauga ON L5M 7Z5; Wes'94; Langs: Portuguese; (905)607-0700; Fax. (905)607-0779.

ARAVINDAKSHAN, Kenatingal S; Carbonear Gen Hosp, 86 Highroad South, Carbonear NL A1Y 1A4; Mysore (India)'78; MB BS; MRCP; DCH; Staff, Carbonear General Hospital; (709)945-5111

ARBEAU, Ryan P; London HSC-Victoria Hosp, PO Box 5010 Stn B ET-800 Commissioners Rd E, London ON N6A 5W9; Dal'08; Staff, London Health Sciences Centre - Victoria Campus.

ARBELAEZ CORREA, Luz J; 201-1801 Bowen Rd, Nanaimo BC V9S 1H1; Javier Pontifical (Colombia)'92; FRCSC; ObstGyn. (250)755-1763

ARBER, John W; Queens Student Hlth Ontario, 146 Stuart St, Kingston ON K7L 3N6; Qns'71; ABEM; CCFP; Locum Tenens, QHC Trenton Memorial; (613)533-6000; Fax. (613)533-6740.

ARBESS, Gordon A; Arbess Med Prof Corp, 410 Sherbourne St, Toronto ON M4X 1K2; Qns'96; CCFP; Staff Physician, St Michael's Hospital; Langs: Bilingual(English/French); (416)867-3728; Fax. (416)867-3726; g.arbess@utoronto.ca.

ARBIC, Diane; Hotel-Dieu de Levis, 143 rue Wolfe, Levis QC G6V 3Z1; Mon'86; Staff, Hôtel-Dieu de Lévis; (418)835-7121; Fax. (418)834-3009.

ARBILLAGA, Hector O; Solaire Bldg, 302-888 4 Ave SW, Calgary AB T2P 0V2; (Argentina)'90; Langs: Spanish; (403)265-7117; Fax. (403)351-1756; rheumatologyclinic@telus.net.

ARBITMAN, Ruben; 401-3500 Dufferin St, North York ON M3K 1N2; Univeristy of Valle (Colombia)'59; FRCPC; Psy (General Psychiatry). Langs: Spanish; (416)631-8100; Fax. (416)631-8144; indi@on.aibn.com.

ARBITMAN, Stella L; Thornhill Med Centre, 18 Centre St, Thornhill ON L4J 1E9; Tor'92; CCFP; Staff, Mackenzie Richmond Hill Hospital; Langs: English; French; Spanish; (905)889-3634; Fax. (905)889-3986.

ARBOLEDA-FLOREZ, Julio E; Quinte Health CC-Belleville Si, 265 Dundas St E, Belleville ON K8N 5A9; Nacional University (Colombia)'64; DPsy; DAB; FACFP; APA; FRSM; DFAPA; FRCPC; Psy (Forensic Psychiatry). Chief Psy, Providence Care - Mental Health Services; Chief Dept of Psy, Kingston General Hospital; Chief Dept of Psy, Hotel-Dieu Hospital; Dep Chief Psy, QHC Belleville General; Teach Staff, Queen's University; Langs: Spanish; Portuguese; French; Italian; (613)969-7400; julio.arboleda-florez@queensu.ca.

ARBOUR, Christiane; CHUM-Hop Notre-Dame, F1133-1560 rue Sherbrooke E, Montreal QC H2L 4M1; Laval'78; Staff, Centre Hospitalier l'Université de Montréal (CHUM) - Hôpital Notre-Dame; (514)890-8003

ARBOUR, Claude; CHUS-Hop Hotel-Dieu, 580 rue Bowen S, Sherbrooke QC J1G 2E8; Sher'84; FRCPC; Psy. Chief Inpatient Service, Centre Hospitalier Universitaire de Sherbrooke-Hôpital Hôtel-Dieu; assoc Prof, Universite de Sherbrooke; (819)346-1110 x26542; Fax. (819)820-6420.

ARBOUR, Jean-Daniel; CHUM-Hop Notre-Dame, 1560 rue Sherbrooke E, Montreal QC H2L 4M1; Mon'89; FRCSC; Ophth. Staff, Centre Hospitalier l'Université de Montréal (CHUM) - Hôpital Notre-Dame; dép Chef Ophth, Universite de Montreal; (514)890-8000 x27103; Fax. (514)849-5115.

ARBOUR, Jean-Francois; CSSS de Trois-Rivieres, 1991 boul Du Carmel, Trois-Rivieres QC G8Z 3R9; Mon'86; FRCPC; Neur; Electroenceph (P.Q.). Staff, CSSS de Trois-Rivières; (819)378-9700

ARBOUR, Laura T; Victoria Gen Hosp, 1 Hospital Way, Victoria BC V8Z 6R5; McM'91; FRCPC; Peds (Medical Genetics). Staff, Victoria General Hospital; Staff Teacher, University of British Columbia; (250)727-4420

ARBOUR, Maurice H; CHUM-Hotel-Dieu, 3840 rue Saint-Urbain, Montreal QC H2W 1T8; Mon'72; Staff, Centre Hospitalier l'Université de Montréal (CHUM) - Hôtel-Dieu; Universite de Montreal; (514)890-8000; mmterrault@videotron.ca.

ARBOUR, Rejean; Clinimedspa, 100-800 boul Leduc, Brossard QC J4Y 0K7; Sher'96; FRCSC; GenSurg. (450)676-3444; Fax. (450)676-0044.

ARBOUR-LEVERT, Melanie; CSSS de Laval, 1755 boul Rene-Laennec, Laval QC H7M 3L9; Sher'05; FRCSC; ObstGyn; GynOnco. Staff, Hopital de la Cite de la santé; (450)668-1010

ARCADI, Sonia; Care Point Medical Ctr, 140-555 Sixth St, New Westminster BC V3L 5H1; UBC'89; (604)523-1166; Fax. (604)523-1722.

ARCAND, Andre; 101-1251 boul Saint-Joseph E, Montreal QC H2J 1L9; Laval'71; Med Advisor Occu Med, St Mary's Hospital Centre; Med Consultant, Centre Hospitalier l'Université de Montréal (CHUM) - Hôtel-Dieu; Med Consultant, Centre Hospitalier l'Université de Montréal (CHUM) - Hôpital Notre-Dame; Med Dir, Goodyear Canada Valleyfield & Med. Advisor, Concordia University; (514)521-1223; Fax. (514)521-1413.

ARCAND, Andrew S; Markham Stouffville Hosp, PO Box 1800 Stn Main 381 Church St, Markham ON L3P 7P3; Qns'97; CCFP; CCFP(E.M.); Staff, Markham Stouffville Hospital; (905)472-7111

ARCAND, Genevieve; CHUM-Hop Notre-Dame, 1560 rue Sherbrooke E, Montreal QC H2L 4M1; Mon'00; CSPQ; Anes. Staff, Centre Hospitalier l'Université de Montréal (CHUM) - Hôpital Notre-Dame; (514)890-8000 x26876

ARCAND, Jennifer L; Renfrew Med Group, 510 Raglan St N, Renfrew ON K7V 1P5; Ott'10; CCFP.

ARCAND, Lyne; Inst Nat'l de Sante Publique Q, 100-190 boul Cremazie E, Montreal QC H2P 1E2; Sher'81; Consultant DSC, Hopital de la Cite de la santé; (514)864-1600 x3511; lyne_arcand@ssss.gouv.qc.ca.

ARCAND, Marcel; Inst U Geriatrie Sherbrooke, 1036 rue Belvedere S, Sherbrooke QC J1H 4C4; Sher'73; MSc(Pharm); CCFP; FCFP; Chef méd gén, CSSS Institut universitaire de gériatrie de Sherbrooke; Prof Family Med, Universite de Sherbrooke; Langs: Bilingual(English/French); (819)821-1150 x45088; Fax. (819)829-7153.

ARCAND, Pierre H; Hôpital Ste-Justine, 3175 ch Cote-Sainte-Catherine, Montreal QC H3T 1C5; Ott'74; ABOtol; CSPQ; FRCSC; Otol (Pediatric Otolaryngology). Clinical Asst Prof Otol Services, Hôpital Ste-Justine; (514)345-4931 x5627; Fax. (514)345-4791; pierre-arcand@ssss.gouv.qc.ca.

ARCAND, Robert; Hop Charles Lemoyne, 3120 boul Taschereau, Greenfield Park QC J4V 2H1; Sher'88; CSPQ; GenPath (P.Q.). Staff, Hopital Charles LeMoyne; (450)466-5000 x2366; robert.arcand@rrsss16.gouv.qc.ca.

ARCAND, Yves; CSSS de Memphremagog, 50 rue Saint-Patrice E, Magog QC J1X 3X3; Laval'75; Staff, Centre Hospitalier et CLSC de Memphremagog; (819)843-3381 x2314

ARCAND-BOSSE, Jean-Francois; Polyclinique de Trois-Rivieres, 365-1900 boul des Recollets, Trois-Rivieres QC G8Z 4K4; Laval'99; Nephrol; IntMed. Staff Nephrol, CSSS de Trois-Rivières; Langs: English; (819)373-1202; Fax. (819)693-1845.

ARCEGA, Rossana V; Oak Bay Med Centre, 159-2515 90 Ave SW, Calgary AB T2V 0L8; Cal'99; CCFP; (403)281-2020; Fax. (403)281-7785.

ARCELIN, Andre; 1155 boul Saint-Joseph E, Montreal QC H2J 1L3; Seville (Spain)'69; (514)490-0648; Fax. (514)490-0648.

ARCELIN, Katia; Hop Jean-Talon, 1385 rue Jean-Talon E, Montreal QC H2E 1S6; Iberoamericana (Mexico)'00; CCFP; Staff, CSSS du Coeur de l'Isle Hôpital Jean-Talon; (514)495-6767

ARCHAMBAULT, Andre; CHUM-St-Luc, 1058 rue Saint-Denis, Montreal QC H2X 3J4; Mon'82; CSPQ; FRCPC; Anes. Staff, Centre Hospitalier l'Université De Montréal (CHUM) - Hôpital Saint-luc; (514)890-8000 x36581

ARCHAMBAULT, Claude; Clinique Med Fabreville, 208-380 boul Curé-Labelle, Laval QC H7P 5L3; Mon'78; Assoc Staff, CSSS du Coeur de l'Isle Hôpital Jean-Talon; (450)628-5800 x319; Fax. (450)628-6621.

ARCHAMBAULT, Claude R; Coop Sante Aylmer, 67 rue du Couvent, Gatineau QC J9H 6A2; Laval'82; Ac Staff, Hull Hospital; (819)684-5336; Fax. (819)684-1240.

ARCHAMBAULT, Claudine; CLSC Suzor-Cote-Victoriaville, 100 rue de l'Ermitage, Victoriaville QC G6P 9N2; Sher'78; (819)758-7281; claudine_archambault@ssss.gouv.qc.ca.

ARCHAMBAULT, Denis; Clinique Med St-Francois, 201-8495 rue Adrien, Laval QC H7A 1J9; Laval'82; Consultant Med Staff, Hôtel-Dieu de Saint-Jérôme; (450)665-1702; Fax. (450)665-0240.

ARCHAMBAULT, Dominique; Ctr Hosp Anna-Laberge, 200 boul Brisebois, Chateauguay QC J6K 4W8; Mon'89; CCFP; Staff, Hôpital Anna-Laberge; (450)699-2425; Fax. (450)699-2525.

ARCHAMBAULT, Genevieve; CHSLD Drapeau-Deschambault, 100 rue du Chanoine-Lionel-Gro, Sainte-Therese QC J7E 5E1; Sher'98; Gen Practice, CSSS de Thérèse de Blainville; (450)437-4267

ARCHAMBAULT, Jean; CHUQ-Hotel-Dieu de Quebec, 11 Cote du Palais, Quebec QC G1R 2J6; Mon'04; FRCPC; RadOncol. Staff, Centre Hospitalier Universitaire de Québec (CHUQ) - Siege Social; (418)525-4444

ARCHAMBAULT, Julie; Polyclinique Med Pierre Le Gar, 300-1000 Montee des Pionniers, Terrebonne QC J6V 1S8; Sher'02; (450)589-5778

ARCHAMBAULT, Line; Hotel-Dieu du Sacre-Coeur, 1 av Du Sacre-Coeur, Quebec QC G1N 2W1; Laval'85; FRCPC; Psy. Staff, Hotel-Dieu du Sacre-Coeur de Jesus de Quebec; (418)529-6851

ARCHAMBAULT, Lisa M J; Consultation Pediatrique, 1801 av Dollard, Lasalle QC H8N 1T9; Dal'87; Peds. Langs: English; French; Spanish; (514)364-5223; Fax. (514)364-5221.

ARCHAMBAULT, Luc L P; Polyclinique Med Concorde, 300 boul de la Concorde E, Laval QC H7G 2E6; Mon'63; FRCPC; Neur; Electroenceph (P.Q.). ac Staff, Hopital de la Cite de la santé; (450)667-5310; Fax. (450)667-5248.

ARCHAMBAULT, Louise; CSSS de Laval, 1755 boul Rene-Laennec, Laval QC H7M 3L9; Mon'77; CSPQ; FRCPC; Anes. Staff, Hopital de la Cite de la santé; (450)668-1010; Fax. (450)629-1957.

ARCHAMBAULT, Martin; Clinique Med Monteuil, 200-4650 rue des Laurentides, Laval QC H7K 2J4; Sher'93; Staff, Hopital de la Cite de la santé; (450)628-8717; maiger@videotron.ca.

ARCHAMBAULT, Maryse; Ctr Hosp Affilie-Enfant-Jesus, 1401 18e rue, Quebec QC G1J 1Z4; Ott'99; CCFP; Staff, Centre Hospitalier Affilié Universitaire de Québec - Hôpital De L'Enfant Jésus; Langs: Spanish; English; (418)649-0252; amaryse@hotmail.com.

ARCHAMBAULT, Nicole; 8-216 av de la Cathédrale, Rimouski QC G5L 5J2; Mon'80; (418)722-6438

ARCHAMBAULT, Patrice; 240-315 boul Brunswick, Pointe-Claire QC H9R 5M7; McG'82; DAB; FRCSC; Ophth (Cataract Surgery). Asst Staff, Sir Mortimer B Davis Jewish General; ac Membre, Lakeshore General Hospital - Pointe Claire; adj Staff Ophth, McGill University Health Centre - Montreal General Campus; assoc Prof, McGill University; Langs: Bilingual(English/French); (514)694-2010; Fax. (514)694-0772.

ARCHAMBAULT, Patrick; Hotel-Dieu de Levis, 143 rue Wolfe, Levis QC G6V 3Z1; Laval'00; FRCPC; EmergMed; Critical Care Medicine (P.Q.). Staff, Hôtel-Dieu de Lévis; (418)835-7121 x3905

ARCHAMBAULT, Pierre; CSSS de Trois-Rivieres, 1991 boul du Carmel, Trois-Rivieres QC G8Z 3R9; Laval'91; Staff, CSSS de Trois-Rivières; (819)697-3333

ARCHAMBAULT, Robert; CSSSG-Hop de Gatineau, 909 boul de la Verendyre O, Gatineau QC J8P 7H2; Mon'78; FRCPC; RadOncol. Staff, Hôpital de Gatineau; (819)561-8100

ARCHAMBAULT, Stéphanie; CHUM-Hop St-Luc, 1058 rue Saint-Denis, Montreal QC H2X 3J4; Sher'07; CCFP; Staff, Centre Hospitalier l'Université De Montréal (CHUM) - Hôpital Saint-luc; (514)890-8000

ARCHAMBAULT-GRENIER, Marie-Anne; CSSS du Sud de Lanaudière, 911 montee des Pionniers, Terrebonne QC J6V 2H2; Mon'03; FRCPC; IntMed; MedOncol; Hem. Staff, Centre Hospitalier Pierre le Gardeur; (514)787-8814

ARCHAMBAULT-LEGER, Stephanie; Asclepios Med Clinic, 2-750 Taylor Creek Dr, Orleans ON K1C 1T1; McG'07; MDCM; CCFP; Langs: Bilingual(French/English); (613)830-8388; Fax. (613)830-8588.

ARCHDEKIN, Murray W; Chemainus Med Clinic, 9892 Explanade St RR1, Chemainus BC V0R 1K1; Cal'91; CCFP; FCFP; (250)246-3261; Fax. (250)246-9144.

ARCHER, Brian; 7 Cambridge Ave, Quispamsis NB E2E 4W7; Qns'88; FRCPC; DiagRad. Staff, Saint John Regional Hospital; Lecturer Med, Dalhousie University; (506)868-1096

ARCHER, David D; Kenderdine Med Clinic, 110-1804 McOrmond Dr, Saskatoon SK S7S 0A6; Sask'04; BSc; CCFP; Clin Lecturer, University of Saskatchewan; (306)934-6606; Fax. (306)955-3180.

ARCHER, David P; Foothills Med Centre, C229-1403 29 St NW, Calgary AB T2N 2T9; McG'75; CSPQ; FRCPC; Anes. Ac Staff Anes, Foothills Medical Centre; (403)944-2439; Fax. (403)944-2425.

ARCHER, Derek C; Credit Valley Imaging Assoc, G02-2300 Eglinton Ave W, Mississauga ON L5M 2V8; Tor'86; FRCPC; DiagRad. (905)828-0653

ARCHER, Jessie; CLSC Villeray, 1425 rue Jarry E, Montreal QC H2E 1A7; (Haiti)'79; (514)376-4141

ARCHER, John W; Simon Fraser Health Region, 600-22470 Dewdney Trunk Rd, Maple Ridge BC V2X 5Z6; Sheffield (England)'74; MB ChB; FRCPC; Peds. Head Pediatrics, Ridge Meadows Hospital & Health Care Centre; (604)466-5118; Fax. (604)476-1850.

ARCHER, Robert A; Huronia Med Centre, PO Box 790 Stn Main 200-240 Old Penetang Rd, Midland ON L4R 4P4; Qns'78; CCFP; Georgian Bay General Hospital - Midland; (705)526-8351; Fax. (705)526-0239.

ARCHER, Stephen; Kingston Gen Hosp, 76 Stuart St, Kingston ON K7L 2V7; Qns'81; FRCPC; IntMed. Staff, Kingston General Hospital; Dept Head Med, Queen's University; (613)549-6666

ARCHIBALD, Alison L; Cape Breton Healthcare Complex, 124. 1-1482 George St, Sydney NS B1P 1P3; Dal'07; GenSurg. Staff, Cape Breton Healthcare Complex; (902)567-6155; Fax. (902)567-3627.

ARCHIBALD, Christopher; 2354 LCDC Bldg-Tunney's Pastur, AL0602B-100 Eglantine Driveway, Ottawa ON K1A 0K9; McG'85; FRCPC; CommunMed. Staff Surveillance & Risk Assessment Div, Health Canada; Langs: English; French; (613)941-3155; Fax. (613)946-8695; chris.archibald@phac-aspc.gc.ca.

ARCHIBALD, Curtis W; 315-5595 Fenwick St, Halifax NS B3H 4M2; Dal'06; Ophth. (902)405-8477; Fax. (902)405-8479.

ARCHIBALD, Gregory C; 8512-5909 Veterans Memorial La, Halifax NS B3H 2E2; Mem'80; DrMedCh; CCFP; FCFP; Prof Med, Dalhousie University; (902)473-4624; Fax. (902)473-4760; greg.archibald@dal.ca.

ARCHIBALD, J David; Aberdeen Prof Centre, 825 East River Rd, New Glasgow NS B2H 3S6; Dal'70; FRCSC; Ophth (Medical & Surgery). Staff, Sutherland-Harris Memorial Hospital; Staff, Aberdeen Regional Hospital; (902)755-6460; Fax. (902)755-6663.

ARCHIBALD, J Fredric; Hydrostone Med Centre, 5521 Duffus St, Halifax NS B3K 2M5; Dal'75; CCFP; (902)482-2683; Fax. (902)453-5264; hydromed@eastlink.ca.

ARCHIBALD, James S; Hys Med Centre, 206-11010 101 St NW, Edmonton AB T5H 4B9; Edinburgh (Scotland)'71; MB ChB; BSc(MedSci); FCCP; FRCP(Ed); FRCPC; IntMed (Respirology). Clin Assoc Prof, University of Alberta; (780)424-2273; Fax. (780)425-9569.

ARCHIBALD, Jason D; St Joseph's Healthcare, 50 Charlton Ave E, Hamilton ON L8N 4A6; Dal'01; FRCSC; Otol. Staff, St Joseph's Healthcare - Charlton Campus; (905)522-1155

ARCHIBALD, John M; 558 Charlotte St, Sydney NS B1P 1E7; Dal'74; (902)539-7666; Fax. (902)567-1097.

ARCHIBALD, Jonathan M; Brookdale Family Clinic, 304 Bellevue St, Peterborough ON K9H 5G1; Dal'95; BSc; CCFP; Langs: Bilingual(English/French); (705)743-7100; Fax. (705)743-7104.

ARCHIBALD, Lise; Ctr Readaptation Ubald-Villene, 2525 ch de la Canardiere, Quebec QC G1J 2G3; Laval'75; Prog Dir, Centre de Readaptation Ubold Villeneuve; Langs: English; (418)663-5008; Fax. (418)687-3585.

ARCHIBALD, Marilyn; Region of Hamilton-Wentworth, 1447 Upper Ottawa St, Hamilton ON L8W 3J6; London (England)'76; MB BS; Staff Social & Public Health Services, City of Hamilton-Wentworth; (905)546-3274

ARCHIBALD, S B Wallace; 110 Craig St PO Box 69 Stn Main, Russell ON K4R 1C7; Dal'89; BSc; MD; CCFP; FCFP; Staff, Winchester District Memorial Hospital; Assoc Prof, University of Ottawa; (613)445-5333; Fax. (613)445-3659; wally.archibald@ontariomd.ca.

ARCHIBALD, Shauna M; Living Well Integrative Health, 2176 Windsor St, Halifax NS B3K 5B6; Dal'02; BSc(Hon); CCFP; Lecturer FamMed, Dalhousie University; (902)406-1500; Fax. (902)406-1501.

ARCHIBALD, Stuart D; St Joseph's Healthcare, 50 Charlton Ave E, Hamilton ON L8N 4A6; Tor'72; FRCSC; GenSurg (Medical Oncology). Ac Staff Head & Neck Surg, St Joseph's Healthcare - Charlton Campus; Assoc Prof Surg/Assoc Prof Hamilton Cancer Clinic, McMaster University; (905)522-3029; Fax. (905)521-6121.

ARCHIBALD, Susy R; Aldershot Family Health Org, 501 Plains Rd E, Burlington ON L7T 2E2; McM'89; BSc; CCFP; FCFP; (905)681-9200; Fax. (905)681-9404.

ARCHIE, Suzanne M; Cleghorn Program, 703-25 Charlton Ave E, Hamilton ON L8N 1Y2; McM'87; FRCPC; Psy (Psychotic Disorders). Staff, St Joseph's Healthcare - Charlton Campus; McMaster University; (905)540-6586; Fax. (905)525-2805.

ARCIA-BRAVO, Edgard A; Spingbank Med Centre, 311-460 Springbank Dr, London ON N6J 0A8; Nat'l (Nicaragua)'86; MD; Physician, Wortley Village Medical Centre; Langs: Spanish; (519)850-3335; Fax. (519)850-8788; info@santamarthamedical.com.

ARCIERI-PIERSANTI, Vincenzo; Peterborough Reg HC-Hospital, 1 Hospital Dr, Peterborough ON K9J 7C6; Dal'78; AB; CCFP; CCFP(E.M.); Staff, Peterborough Regional Health Centre - Hospital Drive; Fam Med, Peterborough Regional Health Centre - Rogers St Site; (705)876-5157

ARCISZEWSKA, Halszka T; St Joseph's Mountain H Service, PO Box 585 Stn Lcd 1 100 5th St W, Hamilton ON L8N 3K7; Warsaw (Poland)'59; FRCPC; Psy. Staff, St Joseph's Healthcare Hamilton - West 5th Campus; Asst Prof Psy, McMaster University; (905)388-2511 x4423; Fax. (905)575-6049.

ARCOUET, Celine; CLSC Grande-Vallee, 71 boul St-Francois-Xavier E, Grande-Vallee QC G0E 1K0; Mon'94; (418)393-2001; Fax. (418)393-2767.

ARDELL, Dale M R; Victoria Square Med Clinic, PO Box 5700 Stn Main 207-2345 10th Ave W, Prince Albert SK S6V 7V6; Sask'79; BSc; CCFP; Chief GenPract/Staff Fam Med, Victoria Hospital; (306)763-8888; Fax. (306)763-9038.

ARDELL, Robert A; Supermed Family Practice, 591 15 St E, Prince Albert SK S6V 1G3; Sask'86; CCFP; (306)763-4808; Fax. (306)764-0802; supermedadmin@sasktel.net.

ARDESHIRI, Farnaz; 200-5799 Yonge St, North York ON M2M 3V3; Tehran (Iran)'89; FRCPC; Peds. Staff, Mackenzie Richmond Hill Hospital; Langs: Farsi; (416)222-1020

ARDILA-ROMERO, Jesus A; Ctr Hosp de Lasalle, 8585 Tsse Champlain, LaSalle QC H8P 1C1; (Venezuela)'84; FRCPC; Peds (Neonatal & Perinatal Medicine). Staff Peds, Centre Hospitalier de LaSalle; Staff Peds, St Mary's Hospital Centre; Langs: Spanish; (514)362-8000

ARDILOUZE, Jean-Luc; CHUS-Hop Fleurimont, 3001 12e av N, Sherbrooke QC J1H 5N4; Limoges (France)'78; Endocrin&Metab (P.Q.) (Diabetology). Staff Endocrin, Centre Hospitalier Universitaire de Sherbrooke-Hopital Fleurimont; assoc Prof, Universite de Sherbrooke; (819)346-1110; Fax. (819)820-6420.

AREF, Karim G; Rouge Valley-Ajax & Pickering, 580 Harwood Ave S, Ajax ON L1S 2J4; Alexandria (Egypt)'91; FRCPC; Peds. Staff, Rouge Valley Health System - Ajax & Pickering Health Centre Site; (905)683-2320

AREL, Luc; CSSS du Nord de Lanaudière, 1000 boul Sainte-Anne, St-Charles-Brromee QC J6E 6J2; Mon'81; CSPQ; Anes. Staff, Centre Hospitalier Régional de Lanaudière; (450)759-8222 x2960; larel@videotron.ca.

AREL, Roxanne; St Mary's Hosp Centre, 3830 av Lacombe, Montreal QC H3T 1M5; McG'04; CCFP; Staff, St Mary's Hospital Centre; (514)345-3511; Fax. (514)734-2602.

ARELLANO, Luis-Ramiro J; Children's Hosp of Western Ont, 800 Commissioners Rd E, London ON N6C 2V5; Wes'84; MSc; FRCPC; Anes (Cardiac Anesthesia). Staff, Children's Hospital of Western Ontario; (519)685-8500

ARENA, Orazio; St Mary's Hosp Centre, 3830 av Lacombe, Montreal QC H3T 1M5; Catania (Italy)'97; FRCSC; GenSurg. Staff, St Mary's Hospital Centre; (514)345-3511

ARENAS, Patricia M; Casselman Med Centre PO Box 380, Casselman ON K0A 1M0; Ott'73; Langs: French; (613)764-5440; Fax. (613)764-9974.

ARENDSE, Regan E; Rheumatology Associates of SK, 103-39 23rd St E, Saskatoon SK S7K 0H6; (306)244-2277; Fax. (306)244-6755.

ARENSON, Anna M; Sunnybrook Hlth Sciences Ctre, 2075 Bayview Ave, Toronto ON M4N 3M5; Man'76; FRCPC; DiagRad. Staff, Sunnybrook Health Sciences Centre; (416)480-4360 x5733

ARENT, Robin; Edmonton Clinic Health Academy, 11405 87 Ave NW, Edmonton AB T6G 1C9; Buffalo(NY) (USA)'94; BSc; Staff, University of Alberta Hospital; Staff, Edmonton Clinic Health Academy; (780)248-5575; Fax. (780)248-5625.

ARES, Chantal; SMBD Jewish Gen Hosp, 3755 ch Cote-Sainte-Catherine, Montreal QC H3T 1E2; Alb'03; FRCSC; Ophth. Staff, Sir Mortimer B Davis Jewish General; (514)340-8280; Fax. (514)340-8215.

ARES, Francois; Centre de Sante Saint-Philippe, 5 rue Saint-Philippe, Windsor QC J1S 1C9; Sher'90; Staff, Carrefour de Sante et Services Sociaux-Pavillon St-Louis; (819)845-5005; Fax. (819)845-5010.

ARES, Isabelle; 63 rue Girouard, Victoriaville QC G6P 5T3; Laval'92; FRCPC; Psy. Staff, Hotel-Dieu d'Arthabaska; (819)260-3363; Fax. (819)260-3373.

AREVALO CENTENO, Ruben D; CSSS Drummond-Hop Sainte-Croix, 570 rue Heriot, Drummondville QC J2B 1C1; (Venezuela)'91; Staff, Hôpital Sainte-croix; (819)478-6464

ARFAI, Esmail K; 649 Sheppard Ave W, North York ON M3H 2S4; Tabriz (Iran)'63; DPM; MRCPsy; FRCPC; Psy (General Psychiatry). Langs: Azeri; Farsi; (416)630-0610; Fax. (416)398-5712.

ARFALI, Erfan; Brant Community HC-Brantford, 200 Terrace Hill St, Brantford ON N3R 1G9; Mosul (Iraq)'93; CCFP; CCFP(E.M.); Staff, The Brant Community Healthcare System - Brantford General Hospital Site; Langs: Kurdish; Arabic; (204)239-2243

ARGALS, Ivars J; Associate Clinic, 5215 49 Ave, Wetaskiwin AB T9A 0R1; Tor'75; CCFP; FCFP; Ac Staff, Wetaskiwin Hospital & Care Centre; (780)352-7157; Fax. (780)352-2273.

ARGATOFF, Larry H; Valley Med Laboratories, 105-537 Leon Ave, Kelowna BC V1Y 6J5; UBC'88; FRCPC; GenPath. (250)763-4813; Fax. (250)862-2843.

ARGENT, Nicholas B; 3105A-1600 Scott St, Ottawa ON K1A 0K9; Bristol (England)'85; MB ChB(Hons); FACP; MRCP(UK); MD; FRCPC; IntMed; Nephrol. Med Reviewer Therapeutic Products Directorate, Health Canada; (613)952-8115; Fax. (613)952-9656; nicholas_argent@hc-sc.gc.ca.

ARGENTIN, Stefania; CHUM-Hotel-Dieu, 3840 rue Saint-Urbain, Montreal QC H2W 1T8; McG'94; CSPQ; FRCPC; IntMed; Cardiol. Staff, Centre Hospitalier l'Université de Montréal (CHUM) - Hôtel-Dieu; (514)890-8174

ARGOUARCH, Sylvie J; Royal Jubilee Hosp, 1952 Bay St, Victoria BC V8R 1J8; Brest (France)'82; FRCPC; Psy (Geriatric Psychiatry). Staff Seniors Outpatient Clinic, Royal Jubilee Hospital; Physician, Vancouver Island Health Authority; Langs: English; French; (250)370-8111 x13440; Fax. (250)370-8814.

ARGOUIN, Isabelle; CSSS Pierre Boucher, 1333 boul Jacques-Cartier E, Longueuil QC J4M 2A5; Laval'98; Staff, Centre Hospitalier Pierre Boucher; (450)468-8111

ARGUE, Donald R; Brockville Mental Health Centr, 1804 Hwy 2 E, Brockville ON K6V 5W7; Qns'73; Staff, Brockville General Hospital - Charles Street; Staff, Providence Continuing Care Centre (PCCC) - St Vincent de Paul Hospital; Staff, Brockville Mental Health Centre - Royal Ottawa Health Care Group; (613)345-1461

ARGUIN, Denis A; CSSS de Rouyn-Noranda, 1 9e rue, Rouyn-Noranda QC J9X 2A9; Sher'77; Médecin, CSSS de Rouyn-Noranda; Prof Family Med, Universite de Sherbrooke; Langs: English; (819)764-5131 x45038; Fax. (819)762-0230.

ARGUIN, Frederic; Ctr Hosp Anna-Laberge, 200 boul Brisebois, Chateauguay QC J6K 4W8; Mon'08; CCFP; Staff, Hôpital Anna-Laberge; (450)699-2425

ARHAM, Muhammad N; Windermere Med Clinic, 204-32450 Simon Ave, Abbotsford BC V2T 5R3; (Other Foreign)'99; (604)859-6774

ARHANCHIAGUE, Eneko R; North York Gen Hosp, 4001 Leslie St, North York ON M2K 1E1; Ott'08; FRCPC; IntMed. Staff, North York General Hospital; (416)756-6000

ARIANA, Anahita; Century Group Inc, 5150 Cordova Bay Rd, Victoria BC V8Y 2K6; Illinois (USA)'02; CCFP; CCFP(E.M.); (705)368-6798

ARIANO, David M; Grey Nuns Community Hosp & HC, 1100 Youville Drive West NW, Edmonton AB T6L 5X8; Alb'95; CCFP; CCFP(E.M.); Staff, Covenant Health - Grey Nuns Community Hospital; (780)735-7000; Fax. (780)735-4698.

ARIF, Abu S M; Warden Family Practice & Walk-, 3502 Danforth Ave, Scarborough ON M1L 1E1; Chittagong (Bangladesh)'90; CCFP; (647)984-6172

ARIF, Beenish; Niagara H System-Welland Site, 65 Third St, Welland ON L3B 4W6; (Pakistan)'03; MB BS; CCFP; Staff, Niagara Health System - Welland Hospital Site; (905)378-4647

ARIF, Muhammad; Tillsonburg Dist Mem Hosp, 167 Rolph St, Tillsonburg ON N4G 3Y9; Karachi (Pakistan)'90; Staff, Tillsonburg District Memorial Hospital; (519)842-3611

ARIF, Saroosh; 150 Sherway Dr, Etobicoke ON M9C 1A5; Karachi (Pakistan)'90; FRCPC; IntMed. Staff, Trillium Health Centre - Mississauga; (416)521-4110; Fax. (416)521-4122.

ARIF, Stephen G; Chisel Peak Med Clinic, PO Box 2769 417 10th Ave, Invermere BC V0A 1K0; Ott'86; BA; CCFP; FCFP; Staff, Invermere & District Hospital; (250)341-6900; Fax. (250)341-3226.

ARIHAN, Oguz; Clinique Urgence Rive-Sud, 3200 boul Taschereau, Longueuil QC J4V 2H3; Ankara (Turkey)'54; (450)672-7658

ARIKAN, Yasemin; Keary Med Centre, 203-245 Columbia St E, New Westminster BC V3L 3W4; Cal'93; FRCPC; IntMed (Infectious Diseases). Med Staff Assoc, Royal Columbian Hospital; Med Staff Assoc, Eagle Ridge Hospital & Health Care Centre; Clin Assoc Prof Community IntMed & Assoc InfectDis, University of British Columbia; Langs: English; French; Turkish; (604)525-9666; Fax. (604)525-2173; id.neph@gmail.com.

ARIS, Fadi; Lakeshore Gen Hosp, 160 rue Stillview, Pointe-Claire QC H9R 2Y2; McG'05; DiagRad. Staff, Lakeshore General Hospital - Pointe Claire; (514)630-2108

ARIS-JILWAN, Nahla M; CHUM Hop Notre-Dame, 1560 rue Sherbrooke E, Montreal QC H2L 4M1; Angers (France)'72; Endocrin&Metab (P.Q.); IntMed. ac Staff, Centre Hospitalier l'Université de Montréal (CHUM) - Hôpital Notre-Dame; adj Prof, Universite de Montreal; Langs: Arabic; English; (514)890-8000 x26594; Fax. (514)412-7767; nahla.aris-jilwan.chum@ssss.gouv.qc.ca.

ARJANE, Georges; Ctr Hosp de Verdun, 4000 boul Lasalle, Verdun QC H4G 2A3; Beirut (Lebanon)'65; MedOncol; HemPath; Hem (P.Q.). Staff, Centre Hospitalier de Verdun; Langs: Arabic; English; (514)362-1000 x2609; Fax. (514)765-7306.

ARJANE, Mylene; Clinique Psyche, 400-400 av Laurier O, Montreal QC H2V 2K7; Mon'01; FRCPC; Psy. (514)279-4141

ARJANE, Philippe; Service d'Urologie Rive-Sud, 3234 boul Taschereau, Greenfield Park QC J4V 2H3; Sher'94; FRCSC; Urol (Laparoscopic Urology). Staff, Centre Hospitalier l'Université De Montréal (CHUM) - Hôpital Saint-luc; (450)671-2945; parjane@hotmail.com.

ARKILANDER, Adrianna; Guelph Gen Hosp, 115 Delhi St, Guelph ON N1E 4J4; McM'02; CCFP; CCFP(E.M.); Staff, Guelph General Hospital; (519)822-5350

ARKURAN, Cigdem; Richmond Health Science Ctre, 201-6091 Gilbert Rd, Richmond BC V7C 5L9; UBC'95; FRCSC; ObstGyn. Staff, Richmond Hospital; Staff, Delta Hospital; Langs: Turkish; (604)244-7657; Fax. (604)244-7917.

ARLEN, Dianne J; St Joseph's Healthcare, 50 Charlton Ave E, Hamilton ON L8N 4A6; McM'89; BSc; FRCPC; IntMed (Transplantation); Nephrol. Ac Staff, St Joseph's Healthcare - Charlton Campus; Assoc Prof Med, McMaster University; (905)522-4941 x34055; Fax. (905)521-6088; arlend@mcmaster.ca.

ARLETTE, John P; 202-636 45 St SW, Calgary AB T3C 2G2; Cal'76; FRCPC; Derm (Mohs Micrographic Surgery). Staff, Foothills Medical Centre; Asst Prof, University of Calgary; (403)216-4685; Fax. (403)216-4689; drjohn@johnarlette.com.

ARMAND, Genevieve; CLSC Arthur Buies, 430 rue Labelle, Saint-Jerome QC J7Z 5L3; Mon'81; (450)431-2221 x25571; Fax. (450)431-6538.

ARMAND, Jean-Claude; Douglas Mental Hlth Univ Inst, 6875 boul Lasalle, Verdun QC H4H 1R3; (Haiti)'71; Staff, Douglas Mental Health University Institute; Staff, Centre d'Accueil Louis Riel; Langs: Creole; English; (514)761-6131

ARMANI, Antonio Alvi; 340-10 Bay St, Toronto ON M5J 2R8; Tor'85; Langs: Italian; (416)363-6655; Fax. (416)363-1589; antonio@alviarmani.com.

ARMANIOUS, Finley; Vernon Jubilee Hosp, 2101 32 St, Vernon BC V1T 5L2; Cairo (Egypt)'50; FRCPC; IntMed. Staff, Vernon Jubilee Hospital; (250)545-2211 x1347

ARMANIOUS, Shadia; Lakeshore Gen Hosp, 160 av Stillview, Pointe-Claire QC H9R 2Y2; Cairo (Egypt)'64; FRCPC; DiagRad. Staff, Lakeshore General Hospital - Pointe Claire; (514)630-2225 x1333

ARMAS ENRIQUEZ, Ana T; Agassiz Med Centre, 130-30 Stephen St, Morden MB R6M 2G3; Havana (Cuba)'00; CCFP; (204)822-4474; Fax. (204)822-6886.

ARMITAGE, Kathleen J; 12-456 Vodden St E, Brampton ON L6S 5Y7; Wes'66; FRCPC; PhysMed&Rehab (Orthopedic Medicine). (905)455-4088; Fax. (905)455-9706.

ARMITAGE, Michael E; Dr Everett Chalmers Reg Hosp, PO Box 9000 Stn A, Fredericton NB E3B 5N5; Dal'85; CCFP; FCFP; Ac Staff, Dr Everett Chalmers Regional Hospital; (506)458-5100

ARMOGAM, Preianathan; Port McNeill Med Clinic, PO Box 14 2161 McNeill Rd, Port McNeill BC V0N 2R0; Witwatersrand (South Africa)'98; CCFP; (250)956-3377

ARMOGAN, E D; 769 Southdale Rd E, London ON N6E 3B9; Wes'90; CCFP; FCFP; (519)668-6074; Fax. (519)681-2753.

ARMOGAN, Narendra; Ophtalmic Consultant Centrs In, 1880 Sismet Rd, Mississauga ON L4W 1W9; Wes'93; FRCSC; Ophth (Vitreo Retinal Surgery). Staff Vitreo Retinal Surg, St Joseph's Health Centre; Physician, Ophtalmic Consultant Centres Inc; (905)212-9482; Fax. (905)212-1012; info@retinamd.ca.

ARMOUR, Christine M; 20 Barrie St, Kingston ON K7L 3J6; Qns'01; FRCPC; GeriatricMed. (613)533-6310

ARMOUR, Edouard F H; Tecumseh Commun Hlth Care Ctre, 13390 Lanoue St, Windsor ON N8N 5E1; West Indies (Jamaica)'61; MB BS; DABPed; FAAP; FRCPC; Peds. Hon Staff, Windsor Regional Hospital - Metropolitan Site; (519)979-5260; Fax. (519)979-8085.

ARMOUR, Paul W; 555 George St N, Peterborough ON K9H 3S1; Wes'72; (705)743-0030; Fax. (705)743-0047.

ARMOUR, Pauline D; Homewood Health Centre, 150 Delhi St, Guelph ON N1E 6K9; McM'77; CCFP; Staff, Homewood Health Centre; (519)824-1010 x2344; Fax. (519)767-3536.

ARMSON, B Anthony; G2141-5850/5980 University Ave PO Box 9700, Halifax NS B3K 6R8; Dal'81; BSc; MSc; AB; FRCSC; ObstGyn (Maternal Fetal Medicine). Ac Staff, IWK Health Centre; Staff Consultant, Queen Elizabeth II Health Sciences Centre - Victoria General Site; Head ObstGyn/Prof, Dalhousie University; (902)470-6460; Fax. (902)425-1125; anthony.armson@iwk.nshealth.ca.

ARMSON, Heather A; Sunridge Family Med Teaching C, 2685 36 St NE, Calgary AB T1Y 5S3; Cal'83; CCFP; FCFP; Asst Prof, University of Calgary; (403)943-5000; Fax. (403)476-8784; armson@ucalgary.ca.

ARMSTRONG, Ankelly L M; Med Associates of Port Perry, 462 Paxton St, Port Perry ON L9L 1L9; McM'06; CCFP; Staff Privil Family Med & Obst, Lakeridge Health - Port Perry Site; (905)985-2895; Fax. (905)985-9719.

ARMSTRONG, Barry D; PO Box 29165 RPO McIntyre Cent, Thunder Bay ON P7B 6P9; Cal'79; BSc; ATLS; ACLS; FRCSC; GenSurg (Trauma Surgery). Surgeon, Thunder Bay Regional Health Sciences Centre; Langs: English; French; (807)343-4748

ARMSTRONG, Brent J; Salvation Army Grace Gen Hosp, 300 Booth Dr, Winnipeg MB R3J 3M7; Man'83; FRCPC; Psy. Staff, The Salvation Army Grace Hospital; (204)837-0451; Fax. (204)885-3064.

ARMSTRONG, Bryan M; Haliburton Family Med Centre, PO Box 870 7217 Gelert Rd, Haliburton ON K0M 1S0; Tor'94; CCFP; (705)457-1212

ARMSTRONG, C Paul; Associate Clinic, 320-401 9 Ave SW, Calgary AB T2P 3C5; Cal'77; BSc(Hon); FRCS; FRCSC; GenSurg. Staff, Tom Baker Cancer Centre; Physician, Alberta Health Services; Clin Lecturer, University of Calgary; (403)221-4489; Fax. (403)221-4420.

ARMSTRONG, Christopher; London HSC-Victoria Hosp, PO Box 5010 Stn B 800 Commissioners Rd E, London ON N6A 5W9; Ott'93; FRCPC; AnatPath. Staff Path, London Health Sciences Centre - Victoria Campus; (519)685-8500

ARMSTRONG, David; McMaster University Med Centre, HSC 4W8F-1280 Main St W, Hamilton ON L8S 4K1; Cambridge (England)'77; MB ChB; MA; FRCP(UK); FRCPC; IntMed (Functional Bowel Disorder); Gastroent. Court Staff, St Joseph's Healthcare - Charlton Campus; Assoc Prof, McMaster University; Langs: German; French; (905)521-2100 x76404; Fax. (905)521-4958; armstro@mcmaster.ca.

ARMSTRONG, Derek C; 555 University Ave, Toronto ON M5G 1X8; West Indies (Jamaica)'76; MB BS; FRCPC; DiagRad (Pediatric Neuro Radiology). Ac Staff Radiol, The Hospital For Sick Children; (416)813-6035; Fax. (416)813-5471; derek.armstrong@sickkids.ca.

ARMSTRONG, Donald R; 102-73 Delhi St, Guelph ON N1E 6L9; Qns'82; FRCSC; OrthSurg. Staff, Guelph General Hospital; (519)763-7433; Fax. (519)763-6271.

ARMSTRONG, Duncan S; 513 King St, Bridgewater NS B4V 1B3; Dal'78; (902)543-1199

ARMSTRONG, Fraser W; Meadowlark Health Centre, 180 Meadowlark Shopping Ctr NW, Edmonton AB T5R 5W9; Cal'88; CCFP; FCFP; Ac Staff, Covenant Health - Misericordia Community Hospital; (780)484-7574; Fax. (780)486-4142.

ARMSTRONG, Gavin A; University of Alberta Hosp, 8440 112 St NW, Edmonton AB T6G 2B7; Staff, University of Alberta Hospital; (780)407-6907; Fax. (780)407-3853.

ARMSTRONG, Glen L E O; PO Box 449, High Prairie AB T0G 1E0; Alb'10; (780)523-4501; Fax. (780)523-4800.

ARMSTRONG, Harvey A; 184 Bayview Heights Dr, East York ON M4G 2Y9; Tor'64; DPsy; DCPsy; FRCPC; Psy (Child & Adolescent Psychiatry). (416)921-7688; Fax. (416)921-0747.

ARMSTRONG, Ian G; 11700 Sarcee Trail NW PO Box 80044 Rpo Beacon Hill, Calgary AB T3R 0B2; Alb'10; CCFP.

ARMSTRONG, Irene E; Toronto Public Health, 8F-277 Victoria St, Toronto ON M5B 1W2; Tor'98; FRCPC; CommunMed;CCFP; Staff, Toronto East General Hospital Inc.

ARMSTRONG, J Bradford; Hinton Med Clinic, 102 Allen Cove, Hinton AB T7V 2A6; Cal'78; BSc; CCFP; FCFP; Chief of Med Staff, Hinton Healthcare Centre; (780)865-3338; Fax. (780)865-2024; clinic@hintonmedical.com.

ARMSTRONG, J Neil G; 6604 Capilano Cres, Edmonton AB T6A 3R7; Cal'81; FRCPC; Anes. Staff, Foothills Medical Centre; Dept Head Anes, University Of Calgary; (403)944-4701

ARMSTRONG, J Gregory; 204-119 Memorial Ave, Orillia ON L3V 5X1; Tor'99; BSc; CCFP; Assoc Staff, Orillia Soldiers' Memorial Hospital; (705)323-9800; Fax. (705)323-9601.

ARMSTRONG, Janice P; Humber River Reg Hosp-Church, 200 Church St, Toronto ON M9N 1N8; Tor'80; Staff, Humber River Regional Hospital - Church Street Site.

ARMSTRONG, Jennifer M; 3364 Carling Ave, Nepean ON K2H 5A8; Tor'77; DAB(EnvironmentalMed); (613)721-9800; Fax. (613)721-9314; admin@oehc.ca.

ARMSTRONG, John; Tonquin Med Clinic, PO Box 189, Tofino BC V0R 2Z0; Ott'85; Clin Instructor, University of British Columbia; (250)725-3282; Fax. (250)725-3215.

ARMSTRONG, Judith-Anne; Peterborough Clinic FHT, 203-26 Hospital Dr, Peterborough ON K9J 7C3; Ott'81; CCFP; FCFP; Staff, Peterborough Regional Health Centre - Hospital Drive; (705)740-6875; Fax. (705)740-6858; jarmstrong@ptboclinic.com.

ARMSTRONG, Karen L; Timmins Family Health Team, 1-681 Algonquin Blvd E, Timmins ON P4N 8S6; McM'95; BASc; CCFP; FCFP; Asst Prof, Northern Ontario School of Medicine; Asst Prof, Laurentian University; Asst Prof, Lakehead University / Library; (705)267-5600; Fax. (705)268-3900.

ARMSTRONG, Kathryn G W; Royal Victoria Hosp, 201 Georgian Dr, Barrie ON L4M 6M2; Ott'05; FRCPC; EmergMed. Staff, Royal Victoria Regional Health Centre; (705)728-9802

ARMSTRONG, Kenneth T; 5400 Portage Rd, Niagara Falls ON L2G 5X7; McM'80; BSc(Physiol); DOHS; (905)358-3434

ARMSTRONG, Kevin P J; St Joseph's Health Care, PO Box 5777 Stn B 268 Grosvenor St, London ON N6A 4V2; Dal'91; FRCPC; Anes. Staff, St Joseph's Hospital - St Joseph's Health Care; (519)646-6000 x64219

ARMSTRONG, Kristy A; 710 Granville St PO Box 18479, Vancouver BC V6Z 0B3; Ott'10; CCFP; (778)988-4287

ARMSTRONG, Linlea; BC Women's Hosp & Health Ctre, C234-4500 Oak St, Vancouver BC V6H 3N1; UBC'98; FRCPC; MedGenetics. Staff, BC Women's Hospital & Health Centre; (604)875-2157

ARMSTRONG, N Jean; Ridgeview Med Clinic, 1240 Railway Ave, Canmore AB T1W 1P4; Alb'80; Dept Head Anes, University of Calgary; (403)609-8333; Fax. (403)609-3666.

ARMSTRONG, P Mark D; Ermineskin Med Clinic, 301-2377 111 St NW, Edmonton AB T6J 5E5; Qns'84; BSc; CCFP; FCFP; Staff, Covenant Health - Grey Nuns Community Hospital; (780)436-8731; Fax. (780)434-8732.

ARMSTRONG, Paidrig M J; St Joseph's Health Care, PO Box 5777 Stn B 268 Grosvenor St, London ON N6A 4V2; Dal'91; FRCPC; Anes. Staff, St Joseph's Hospital - St Joseph's Health Care; (519)646-6000

ARMSTRONG, Paul D; Timmins Family Health Team, 1-681 Algonquin Blvd E, Timmins ON P4N 8S6; McM'95; CCFP; FCFP; (705)267-5600; Fax. (705)268-3900.

ARMSTRONG, Paul W; Li Ka Shing Centre, 2 132-8308 114 St NW, Edmonton AB T6G 2E1; Qns'66; FACC; FRCPC; Cardiol. Staff, University of Alberta Hospital; Prof Med, University of Alberta; (780)492-0591; Fax. (780)492-9486; paul.armstrong@ualberta.ca.

ARMSTRONG, R Douglas; 206-672 Brant St, Burlington ON L7R 2H3; Wes'81; FRCSC; OrthSurg. Assoc Staff, Joseph Brant Memorial Hospital; Assoc Staff, Halton Healthcare Services Corporation - Oakville Site; (905)333-3311

ARMSTRONG, Robert D; 4-640 Hyde Park Rd, London ON N6H 3S1; Qns'77; CCFP; FCFP; (519)641-3627; Fax. (519)641-3628; robert.armstrong@sympatico.ca.

ARMSTRONG, Sarah A; London HSC-University Hosp, PO Box 5339 Stn B 339 Windermere Rd, London ON N6A 5A5; Wes'07; EmergMed. Staff, London Health Sciences Centre - University Hospital; (519)685-8500

ARMSTRONG, Sarah A; Child & Parent Resource Inst, 600 Sanatorium Rd, London ON N6H 3W7; New York (USA)'04; Staff, Child & Parent Resource Institute; (519)858-2774

ARMSTRONG, Sean W; Seven Oaks Gen Hosp, 2300 McPhillips St, Winnipeg MB R2V 3M3; Man'97; FRCPC; IntMed; Nephrol. Staff, Seven Oaks General Hospital; (204)632-7133

ARMSTRONG, Susan A; North York Gen Hosp, 4001 Leslie St, North York ON M2K 1E1; Tor'00; FRCPC; DiagRad. Staff, North York General Hospital; (416)756-6000

ARMSTRONG, Taylor C; The George Hull Centre, 3F-600 The East Mall, Etobicoke ON M9B 4B1; Tor'05; FRCPC; Psy.

ARMSTRONG, Thomas M; Huronia Urgent Care Clinic, 480 Huronia Rd, Barrie ON L4N 6M2; Tor'75; Ac Staff, Royal Victoria Regional Health Centre; (705)792-0933; tom.armstrong2@sympatico.ca.

ARMSTRONG, W Douglas; Meadowlark Health Centre, 180 Meadowlark Shopping Ctr NW, Edmonton AB T5R 5W9; Man'60; BSc; MSc; PhD(Immunol); Staff Consultant, Covenant Health - Misericordia Community Hospital; Clinical Asst Prof Family Med, University of Alberta; (780)484-7574; Fax. (780)481-2055; wda1@telus.net.

ARNAOUT, Amel; The Ottawa Hosp-Riverside, 4F-1967 Riverside Dr, Ottawa ON K1H 7W9; Dal'00; FRCPC; IntMed; Endocrin&Metab. Staff, The Ottawa Hospital - Riverside Campus; (613)738-8400 x8333

ARNAOUT, Angel; The Ottawa Hosp-Gen Campus, CW 1604-501 Smyth Rd, Ottawa ON K1H 8L6; Dal'99; FRCSC; GenSurg. Staff, The Ottawa Hospital - General Campus; (613)798-5555; Fax. (613)737-8371.

ARNASON, Jo Ann V; Lansdowne Professional Ctr II, 347-3066 Shelbourne St, Victoria BC V8R 6T9; Man'84; Staff, Victoria General Hospital; (250)598-0678

ARNASON, Stephen K; Dr Everett Chalmers Hosp, PO Box 9000 Stn A, Fredericton NB E3B 5N5; Dal'99; BSc; ABR; FRCPC; DiagRad (Vascular & Interventional Radiology). Staff, Dr Everett Chalmers Regional Hospital; (506)452-5130; dr.stephen.arnason@rvh.nb.ca.

ARNASON, Terra G; Royal Victoria Hosp, 3654-103 Hospital Dr, Saskatoon SK S7N 0W8; Alb'01; FRCPC; IntMed; Endocrin&Metab. Staff, Royal University Hospital; (306)966-7911; Fax. (306)966-7926.

ARNAUDON, Daniel H J; 322 Silverthorn Ave, Toronto ON M6N 3K6; Tor'84; Staff, St Joseph's Health Centre; (416)656-8777; Fax. (416)656-5489.

ARNDT, Susanne E; Regina Med Centre, 103-2550 12th Ave, Regina SK S4P 3X1; Sask'84; CCFP; FCFP; Staff Womens Health, Regina General Hospital; Clinical Asst Prof Family Med, University of Saskatchewan; (306)566-4100; Fax. (306)566-4115.

ARNDT, Talitha A T; Davisville Fam Practice, 600-1881 Yonge St, Toronto ON M4S 3C4; Tor'91; BScH; CCFP; FCFP; Ac Staff, Toronto General Hospital - UHN; Ac Staff, Mount Sinai Hospital; Court Staff, Women's College Hospital; (416)932-3172; Fax. (416)440-0238.

ARNEJA, Amarjit S; Rehabilitation Centre, 800 Sherbrook St, Winnipeg MB R3A 1M4; Rajasthan (India)'69; MB BS; FRCPC; PhysMed&Rehab (Geriatric Medicine). Dir Amputation Prog Day Hospital, Health Sciences Centre; Ac Staff Rehab Centre, St Boniface General Hospital; Assoc Prof, University of Manitoba; (204)787-2270; Fax. (204)787-1476; aarneja@hsc.mb.ca.

ARNEJA, Jagmit; St Boniface Clinic, 343 Tache Ave, Winnipeg MB R2H 2A5; Vikram (India)'68; FRCSC; ObstGyn. Ac Staff, Victoria General Hospital; Staff, Health Sciences Centre; (204)233-8537

ARNEJA, Jugpal S; BC Children's Hosp, PO Box 150 A237-4480 Oak St, Vancouver BC V6H 3V4; Man'99; FRCSC; PlasSurg. Staff, BC Children's Hospital; (604)875-2794

ARNETT, Gordon D; Orthopaedic Consultants, 10972 124 St NW, Edmonton AB T5M 0H8; Alb'70; FRCSC; OrthSurg (Arthroplasty). Ac Staff, Royal Alexandra Hospital; Ac Staff, Covenant Health - Misericordia Community Hospital; Ac Staff, Leduc Community Hospital; Staff, Covenant Health - Grey Nuns Community Hospital; Clin Assoc Prof Surg, University of Alberta; (780)453-6999; Fax. (780)451-1437.

ARNOLD, Andrew M; The Juravinski Cancer Centre, 699 Concession St, Hamilton ON L8V 5C2; London (England)'72; MB BS; MRCS; LRCP; MRC; FRCPC; IntMed (Medical Oncology). Staff, St Joseph's Healthcare - Charlton Campus; Staff MedOncol, Hamilton Health Sciences Centre-Juravinski Site; Head Dept of MedOncol, Hamilton Regional Cancer Centre; Prof Med, McMaster University; (905)387-9495 x64602; Fax. (905)575-6326.

ARNOLD, Angela J; Regina Qu'Appelle HR-Regina, 1440 14th Ave, Regina SK S4P 0W5; (Other Foreign)'08; CCFP; CCFP(E.M.); Staff, Regina General Hospital; (306)766-4213; Fax. (306)766-4357.

ARNOLD, Barbra J; STI Clinic, 655 12th Ave W, Vancouver BC V5Z 4R4; Alb'96; CCFP; (604)707-5600

ARNOLD, Cynthia E; 120 Vidal St N, Sarnia ON N7T 5X5; Wes'83; CCFP; CCFP(E.M.); FCFP; (519)332-8822; Fax. (519)332-8208.

ARNOLD, David H; R W Large Mem Hosp, 88 Waglisla St, Denny Island BC V0T 1Z0; Tor'79; CCFP; Staff/Med Dir, R W Large Memorial Hospital; (250)957-2332; Fax. (250)657-2360; david_arnold@rwlmh.ca.

ARNOLD, David W; Dr David Arnold Inc, 3407 32 Ave, Vernon BC V1T 2M9; UBC'82; CCFP; Clin Assoc Prof, University of British Columbia; (250)545-4422

ARNOLD, Donald M; McMaster University, HSC 3V50-1280 Main St W, Hamilton ON L8S 4K1; McG'97; MSc; FRCPC; IntMed; Hem. Staff, Hamilton Health Sciences Centre - McMaster University Medical Centre; Asst Prof Hematology, McMaster University; (905)521-2100 x76305; Fax. (905)521-4971.

ARNOLD, Douglas J; 326-119 Pine St S, Timmins ON P4N 2K3; Tor'89; CCFP; FCFP; Staff, Timmins & District Hospital; (705)267-2373

ARNOLD, Douglas L; MUHC-Montreal Neurology Inst, 3801 rue University, Montreal QC H3A 2B4; Cornell (USA)'76; MD; FRCPC; Neur (Magnetic Resonance Imaging). Att Staff Neurol, McGill University Health Centre - Montreal Neurological Hospital; Prof, McGill University; (514)398-8185; Fax. (514)398-2975; doug@mrs.mni.mcgill.ca.

ARNOLD, Florence P; Saskatoon Cancer Centre, 20 Campus Dr, Saskatoon SK S7N 4H4; UP Manila(Philippines) (Philippines)'91; MD; ABIM; ABMO; AB(Hem); Staff, Saskatoon Cancer Centre; Clinical Asst Prof, University of Saskatchewan; (306)655-2710; Fax. (306)655-2639.

ARNOLD, George M; Markham Stouffville Health Cen, 406-379 Church St, Markham ON L6B 0T1; Tor'86; FRCSC; ObstGyn. Chief ObstGyn, Markham Stouffville Hospital; (905)472-4553; Fax. (905)472-1877.

ARNOLD, Ian; Melrose Family Health Team, 210 Melrose Ave, Ottawa ON K1Y 4K7; Cal'79; CCFP; (613)761-4334; Fax. (613)761-4200; ian.arnoldmd@rogers.com.

ARNOLD, Ian M F; Occupational Hlth Prog-McGill, 627 Kochar Dr, Ottawa ON K2C 4H2; Qns'68; DOHS(McM); MSc(McG); FAB; CSPQ; FCBOM; FRCPC; GenSurg (P.Q.); OccupMed. Chair Workforce Advisory Committee, Mental Health Commission of Canada; Consultant Environment, Health & Safety Commission; Prof Med, McGill University; Langs: English; French; (613)228-3054; imfarnold@ca.inter.net.

ARNOLD, J Malcolm O; London HSC-University Hosp, PO Box 5339 Stn B C6124D-339 Windermere Rd, London ON N6A 5A5; Queen's (Ireland)'76; BSc; MB; MD; FRCP; FESC; FRCPC; IntMed (Heart Failure). Staff, London Health Sciences Centre - University Hospital; Chair, Canadian Heart Failure Network; Prof Med, University of Western Ontario; (519)663-3496

ARNOLD, Karen P; Downtown Commun Hlth Clinic, 569 Powell St, Vancouver BC V6A 1G8; Dal'85; CCFP; Staff, BC Mental Health & Addiction Service; Staff, Downtown Community Health Clinic; (604)255-3151

ARNOLD, Kenneth L; Port Arthur Health Centre, 194 Court St N, Thunder Bay ON P7A 4V7; Queen's (Ireland)'71; Staff, Thunder Bay Regional Health Sciences Centre Port-Arthur; Staff, St Joseph's Care Group - St Joseph's Hospital; (807)346-1000; Fax. (807)346-6206.

ARNOLD, Laura; 32 Merritt Rd, Toronto ON M4B 3K5; UBC'02; CCFP; larnold@bizinfogroup.ca

ARNOLD, M Renee; Lower Outaouis Family Hlth Tea, 206-1062 Ghislain St, Hawkesbury ON K6A 3B2; Sher'81; CCFP; FCFP; Staff, Hawkesbury & District General Hospital; Langs: Bilingual(French/English); (613)632-7061; Fax. (613)632-1736.

ARNOLD, Pamela J; Regina Qu'Appelle HR-Regina, 1440 14th Ave, Regina SK S4P 0W5; CCFP; Staff, Regina General Hospital; (306)766-4444

ARNOLD, Paul A; Daly Grove Shopping Centre, 4217 23 Ave NW, Edmonton AB T6L 5Z8; Andrews (Scotland)'69; (780)462-0442; Fax. (780)462-0577.

ARNOLD, Paul D; The Hosp for Sick Children, 555 University Ave, Toronto ON M5G 1X8; Tor'96; FRCPC; Psy. Staff, The Hospital For Sick Children; (416)813-7654

ARNOLD, Paul F; Univ Hlth Network-Toronto Gen, 200 Elizabeth St, Toronto ON M5G 2C4; Mem'80; MCFP(EM); Staff, Toronto General Hospital - UHN; (416)340-3856

ARNOLD, Robert C; Hillside Med Centre, 360 2nd Ave, Campbell River BC V9W 3T9; UBC'85; CCFP; Staff, Campbell River & District General Hospital; (250)287-7708; Fax. (250)287-3086.

ARNOLD, Robin A V; Scarborough Hosp-General Div, 3050 Lawrence Ave E, Scarborough ON M1P 2V5; Tor'56; Staff, The Scarborough Hospital - General Campus; (416)438-2911

ARNOLD, Rosemary J; 101-475 Park St, Kitchener ON N2G 4V5; Liverpool (England)'67; (519)579-4150; Fax. (519)579-2665.

ARNOLD, Stephen; CSSS des Iles, 430 ch Principal, Cap-aux-Meules QC G4T 1R9; UBC'88; CCFP; Staff, Hôpital de l'Archipel; Langs: Bilingual(English/French); (418)986-2121; Fax. (418)986-7010.

ARNOLD, Todd W; Surrey Mem Hosp, 13750 96 Ave, Surrey BC V3V 1Z2; Man'86; CCFP; Staff, Surrey Memorial Hospital; (604)581-2211

ARNOT, Alison; 1123AS-3359 Mississauga Rd, Mississauga ON L5L 1C6; Ott'81; BSc(Bio); CCFP; CCFP(E.M.); Ac Staff, The Credit Valley Hospital; Associate, University of Toronto; Langs: Bilingual(English/French); (905)828-5255; Fax. (905)828-3852.

ARNOT, James B; 333 Broadway, Winnipeg MB R3C 4W3; Edinburgh (Scotland)'55; MB ChB; FRCS(Ed); FRCSC; OrthSurg. Consultant OrthSurg, Workers' Comp Board of MB; (204)954-4339

ARNOTT, Alec H; Kent Place, 103-33774 Marshall Rd, Abbotsford BC V2S 1L1; Glasgow (Scotland)'77; BSc; MB ChB; FFARCSI; LMCC; (604)853-5424; Fax. (604)853-6879.

ARNOTT, Gail L; Mission Hills Med Clinic, 220-32530 Lougheed Hwy, Mission BC V2V 1A5; Glasgow (Scotland)'79; MB ChB; (604)826-7751

ARNOTT, James H; Scarborough Prof Centre, 406-1371 Neilson Rd, Scarborough ON M1B 4Z8; Tor'61; FRCPC; IntMed (Endocrinology). Court Staff, St Michael's Hospital; Ac Staff, Rouge Valley Health System - Centenary Health Centre Site; (416)281-9499; Fax. (416)283-5705.

ARNOTT, Peter C; McGregor Med Centre, 561 Machray Ave, Winnipeg MB R2W 1B1; Cape Town (South Africa)'79; MB ChB; BSc(Hons)(UK); MCFP; Staff, Stonewall & District Health Centre; parnott@ahwc.ca.

ARNTFIELD, Robert T; London HSC-Victoria Hosp, PO Box 5010 Stn B 800 Commissioners Rd E, London ON N6A 5W9; Wes'04; FRCPC; EmergMed (Critical Care Medicine). Staff, London Health Sciences Centre - Victoria Campus; (519)685-8500

ARNTFIELD, Shannon L; London HSC-Victoria Hosp, PO Box 5010 Stn B B2 430-800 Commissioners Rd, London ON N6A 5W9; Wes'04; FRCSC; ObstGyn. Staff, London Health Sciences Centre - Victoria Campus; (519)646-6098; Fax. (519)646-6180.

ARNTSEN, Helen M; Northside Med Group, 210-1465 Salisbury Ave, Port Coquitlam BC V3B 6J3; UBC'87; BScPharm; Physician Palliative, Crossroads Hospice; (604)941-8277; Fax. (604)941-5622.

AROCKIASAMY, Vincent S; University Hosp of Northern BC, 1475 Edmonton St, Prince George BC V2M 1S2; Bangalore (India)'85; FRCPC; Peds. Staff, University Hospital of Northern British Columbia; (250)565-2000; Fax. (250)565-2343.

AROICHANE, Maryam; 301-9600 Cameron St, Burnaby BC V3J 7N3; Mon'86; FRCSC; Ophth (Pediatric Ophthalmology). (604)563-3415

AROJOJOYE, Oyebode; 205-2790 Gladwin Rd, Abbotsford BC V2T 4S7; Lagos (Nigeria)'89; MB BS; MRCPsy(UK); LMCC; FRCPC; Psy. Staff, Lions Gate Hospital; (604)855-6571; droarojojoye@telus.net.

ARON, Margaret; Queen Elizabeth II HSC, 1276 South Park St, Halifax NS B3H 2Y9; McG'07; MDCM; Otol. Staff, Queen Elizabeth II Health Sciences Centre - Victoria General Site; (902)473-7015; Fax. (902)473-4442.

ARONNILAKKARA, Priya P; 2444 Hurontario St, Mississauga ON L5B 2V1; (India)'00; CCFP; (905)566-1414; pprasad_a@yahoo.ca.

ARONSHTAM, Grygory; Com El Med Bldg, 305-2620 Commercial Dr, Vancouver BC V5N 4C4; Moscow (Russia (Federation))'80; CCFP; Langs: Russian; Hebrew; (604)872-8577

ARONSON, Howard L; Chinook Reg Hosp, 960 19 St S, Lethbridge AB T1J 1W5; McG'79; CCFP; CCFP(E.M.); Staff, Chinook Regional Hospital; (403)388-6304

ARONSON, Ronnie; LMC Diabetes & Endo Centre, 107-1929 Bayview Ave, Toronto ON M4G 3E8; Tor'90; ABIM; FACE; FRCPC; IntMed (Diabetology); Endocrin&Metab. Exec Dir, LMC Diabetes & Endocrinology Centres-Eglinton; Langs: Hebrew; (416)645-2929; Fax. (416)645-2930; ronnie.aronson@lmc.ca.

ARONSON, Samuel A; SMBD Jewish Gen Hosp, 3755 ch Cote-Sainte-Catherine, Montreal QC H3T 1E2; Albany (USA)'68; FRCSC; Urol. Staff, Sir Mortimer B Davis Jewish General; (514)340-8222

ARONYK, Keith E; University of Alberta Hosp, 2D1.02WCM-8440 112 St NW, Edmonton AB T6G 2B7; Alb'77; FRCS; FRCSC; Neursurg (Pediatric Neuro Surgery). Div Dir NeuroSurg/Chief Ped/GenSurg, University of Alberta Hospital; Staff, Children's Health Centre; Assoc Prof Surg, University of Alberta; (780)407-6870; Fax. (780)407-7293; keith.aronyk@ualbertahealthservices.ca.

ARORA, Amritpal S; 202-7315 Edmonds St, Burnaby BC V3N 1A7; UBC'06; CCFP; (604)526-2401

ARORA, Gagan; Cumberland Reg Health Centre, 19428 Highway 2, Amherst NS B4H 1N6; Bangalore (India)'85; Staff, Cumberland Regional Health Care Center; (902)667-3361

ARORA, Harpreet S; Grandview Med Ctr Fam Hlth Team, 167 Hespeler Rd, Cambridge ON N1R 3H7; Medical University of the Americas (Saint Kitts-Nevis)'02; (519)623-4200; Fax. (519)623-2546.

ARORA, Monil; Medreach Med Centre, 1642 Merivale Rd, Ottawa ON K2G 4A1; Haryana (India)'97; CCFP.

ARORA, Nawaz; Dr Aurora's Clinic, 353 St Paul Ave, Brantford ON N3R 4N3; Bombay (India)'93; MB BS; CCFP; Langs: Punjabi; Hindi; (519)309-0066; Fax. (519)309-0068.

ARORA, Rajeev K; Castlemore Family Med Centre, 2-9960 Airport Rd, Brampton ON L6S 0C5; Ott'96; BSc; CCFP; (905)799-2273; Fax. (905)799-2467.

ARORA, Rakesh C; I H Asper Clinical Research In, CR3012-369 Tache Ave, Winnipeg MB R2H 2A6; Tor'96; FACS; BA; PhD; FRCSC; CardSurg; Critical Care Medicine. Staff Cardiac Surg/Intensivist, St Boniface General Hospital; Asst Prof, University of Manitoba; (204)258-1031; Fax. (204)231-4624; rarora.sbgh@me.com.

ARORA, Roopa D; 867 Upper Paradise Rd, Hamilton ON L9C 5R3; Qns'93; CCFP; Assoc Staff, Hamilton Health Sciences Centre - Hamilton General Hospital; (905)574-2500; roopa_arora@yahoo.com.

ARORA, Sarvsheel; Sunshine Med Clinic, 309-150 Montreal Rd, Ottawa ON K1L 8H2; Haryana (India)'91; CCFP; (613)695-9001

ARORA, Shefali D; Grandview Med Ctre Fam Hlth Team, 167 Hespeler Rd, Cambridge ON N1R 3H7; Medical University of the Americas (Saint Kitts-Nevis)'03; (519)623-4200

ARORA, Steven K; Hamilton HS-McMaster Site, PO Box 2000 Stn Lcd 1 3A53-1200 Main St W, Hamilton ON L8N 3Z5; McM'99; FRCPC; Peds; Nephrol. Staff, Hamilton Health Sciences Centre - McMaster University Medical Centre; (905)521-2100; Fax. (905)308-7548.

ARORA, Sunder S; Smyth Med Centre, 300-1929 Russell Rd, Ottawa ON K1G 4G3; Guru Nanak Dev (India)'77; DABPN; DPsy; FRCPC; Psy (Adult & Child Psychiatry). Court Staff, Children's Hospital of Eastern Ontario (CHEO); Consultant, Royal Ottawa Mental Health Centre - Royal Ottawa Health Care Group; Asst Prof, University of Ottawa; Langs: Hindi; Punjabi; Urdu; (613)739-7051; Fax. (613)739-7051; sarora101@hotmail.com.

ARORA, Vineet I; 867 Upper Paradise Rd, Hamilton ON L9C 5R3; McM'89; DAB; FRCSC; Ophth (Vitreo Retinal Surgery). Staff, St Joseph's Healthcare - Charlton Campus; Staff, Hamilton Health Sciences Centre - McMaster University Medical Centre; (905)574-2500; Fax. (905)574-9000.

ARPIN, Jacinthe; Centre Hosp Honore-Mercier, 2750 boul Laframboise, Saint-Hyacinthe QC J2S 4Y8; Sher'99; FRCPC; Psy. Staff, Centre Hospitalier Honore-Mercier; (450)771-3222

ARPIN, Marie-Helene; Centre Hosp Honore-Mercier, 2750 boul Laframboise, Saint-Hyacinthe QC J2S 4Y8; Mon'06; FRCSC; ObstGyn. Staff, Centre Hospitalier Honore-Mercier; (450)771-3333

ARPIN, Yves; Clinique Fam De St-Hyacinthe, 2955 boul Laframboise, Saint-Hyacinthe QC J2S 4Z3; Mon'74; (450)774-2428; Fax. (450)774-8986.

ARPS, Gina M; Associate Med Clinic, 203-10030 106 St, Westlock AB T7P 2K4; Alb'01; CCFP; (780)349-3341; Fax. (780)349-6686.

ARRAF, John; Foothills Med Centre, 1403 29 St NW, Calgary AB T2N 2T9; Sask'91; FRCPC; Anes. Staff, Foothills Medical Centre; (403)944-1110; Fax. (403)944-2425.

ARRAZAGHI, Abdelwahab A; 207-1920 Ellesmere Rd, Scarborough ON M1H 2V6; Al-Fateh (Libya)'92; MB ChB; DABIM; FRCPC; IntMed; Cardiol. Langs: Arabic; Spanish; (416)438-8667; Fax. (416)438-6358.

ARREDONDO, Jorge L; Hamilton HS-McMaster Site, PO Box 2000 Stn Lcd 1 1200 Main St W, Hamilton ON L8N 3Z5; Valle (Colombia)'86; FRCPC; AnatPath. Staff, Hamilton Health Sciences Centre - McMaster University Medical Centre; Teach Staff, McMaster University; (905)521-2100

ARREZAGHI, Mohamed; St Norbert Med Centre, 3554 Pembina Hwy, Winnipeg MB R3V 1A7; Al-Fateh (Libya)'95; Staff, Bethesda Hospital Steinbach; (204)433-7263; marrezaghi@sehealth.mb.ca.

ARRIETA, Maria-Jesus; Lakeshore Gen Hosp, 160 av Stillview, Pointe-Claire QC H9R 2Y2; McG'87; FRCPC; IntMed; MedMicrobiol; InfectDis. Staff, Lakeshore General Hospital - Pointe Claire; (514)630-2225

ARROWSMITH, Sarah C; 574 Princess St, Kingston ON K7L 1C9; Qns'06; CCFP; (613)767-6056

ARROYO, Jacky; CSSS du Nord de Lanaudière, 1000 boul Sainte-Anne, St-Charles-Brromee QC J6E 6J2; Laval'89; FRCPC; EmergMed. Staff, Centre Hospitalier Régional de Lanaudière; (450)759-8222 x2820; Fax. (450)759-2994.

ARRUDA, Horacio; Ministere de la Sante, 1075 ch Sainte-Foy, Quebec QC G1S 2M1; Sher'83; FRCPC; Public Health & Preventive Med; CommunMed (P.Q.). Clin Teach Staff Social & Preventive Med, Universite de Montreal; Langs: Portuguese; English; (418)266-6720; Fax. (418)266-6708; horacio.arruda@msss.gouv.qc.ca.

ARRUDA, Wilma G; 39-1925 Bowen Rd, Nanaimo BC V9S 1H1; UBC'93; BSc; BEd; FRCPC; Peds. Med Dir Child Youth & Family Prog, Vancouver Island Health Authority; (250)755-7945

ARRUJ, Nasim; 613A-8600 Franklin Ave, Fort McMurray AB T9H 4G8; (780)748-2974; Fax. (780)748-2978.

ARSENAULT, Andre M; Hop Jean-Talon, 1385 rue Jean-Talon E, Montreal QC H2E 1S6; Mon'67; NuclearMed (P.Q.). Consultant, Hôpital du Haut-Richelieu; Staff, CSSS du Coeur de l'Isle Hôpital Jean-Talon; Staff Public Health, Hopital Charles LeMoyne; Assoc Prof Rad, Universite de Montreal; Langs: Spanish; Bilingual(French/English); (514)495-6767 x6421; Fax. (514)495-6738; andre.arsenaultcdi@ssss.gouv.qc.ca.

ARSENAULT, Caroline; Clinique Med Pierre-Boucher, 1615 boul Jacques-Cartier E, Longueuil QC J4M 2X1; Mon'97; Langs: English; (450)468-6223; Fax. (450)468-5041.

ARSENAULT, Chantal; 203-140 Champlain St, Dieppe NB E1A 1N8; Laval'88; CCFP; FCFP; Staff FamMed, Dr Georges-L-Dumont University Hospital Centre; Clin Prof Psy, Universite de Sherbrooke; (506)856-5926; Fax. (506)855-2324.

ARSENAULT, Claude; CSSS Pierre Boucher, 1333 boul Jacques-Cartier E, Longueuil QC J4M 2A5; Mon'81; Staff, Centre Hospitalier Pierre Boucher; (450)468-8111

ARSENAULT, Francois; CSSS de la Haute-Yamaska, 205 boul Leclerc O, Granby QC J2G 1T7; Laval'95; LMCC; OrthSurg. Staff, Centre Hospitalier de Granby; (450)372-5491

ARSENAULT, Francois; CSSS de Chicoutimi, 305 rue Saint-Vallier, Chicoutimi QC G7H 5H6; Mon'88; Staff, Complexe hospitalier de la Sagamie; (418)541-1010

ARSENAULT, Frederic; Hotel-Dieu de Levis, 143 rue Wolfe, Levis QC G6V 3Z1; Laval'07; PlasSurg. Staff, Hôtel-Dieu de Lévis; (418)835-7121

ARSENAULT, Gillian R; Maple Ridge Public Health Unit, 400-22470 Dewdney Trunk Rd, Maple Ridge BC V2X 5Z6; UBC'76; BSc; MHSc; FRCPC; CommunMed (Public Health). (604)476-7076

ARSENAULT, Guylaine; CHUS-Hop Hotel-Dieu, 580 rue Bowen S, Sherbrooke QC J1G 2E8; Sher'03; FRCPC; IntMed; Rheum. Staff, Centre Hospitalier Universitaire de Sherbrooke-Hôpital Hôtel-Dieu; (819)346-1110; Fax. (819)564-5265.

ARSENAULT, Isabelle; CSSS de Saint-Jerome, 290 rue de Montigny, Saint-Jerome QC J7Z 5T3; Mon'99; Respir; IntMed. Staff, Hôtel-Dieu de Saint-Jérôme; (450)431-8200

ARSENAULT, Isabelle; UMF Charles Lemoyne, 201-299 Boul Sir-Wilfrid-Lauri, Saint-Lambert QC J4R 2L1; Mon'84; CCFP; FCFP; Langs: Bilingual(French/English); (450)466-5630; Fax. (450)466-5631.

ARSENAULT, Jean-Pierre; CSSS de Rivière-de-Loup, 75 rue Saint-Henri, Riviere-du-Loup QC G5R 2A4; Mon'01; FRCSC; GenSurg. Staff, Centre Hospitalier Regional du Grand-Portage; (418)868-1000

ARSENAULT, Lorne J A; CSSS des Iles, 430 ch Principal, Cap-aux-Meules QC G4T 1R9; Laval'60; FRCSC; GenSurg. Staff, Hôpital de l'Archipel; (418)986-2121; Fax. (418)986-6845.

ARSENAULT, Lyne; Centre Med Ruby, 101-361 Main St E, Hawkesbury ON K6A 1A8; Mon'95; CCFP; Langs: English; (613)632-0605; Fax. (613)632-7073.

ARSENAULT, Marc-Yvon; Maternity & Gynecology Centre, 1811 av Dollard, Lasalle QC H8N 1T9; Mon'92; FRCSC; ObstGyn. (514)364-3700; Fax. (514)364-9866; drarsenault@gynecolasalle.com.

ARSENAULT, Marie; Hôpital Laval, 2725 ch Sainte-Foy, Quebec QC G1V 4G5; Laval'89; CSPQ; FRCPC; IntMed; Cardiol (P.Q.). Staff, Hôpital Laval; (418)656-8711

ARSENAULT, Marie-Andree; Clinique Med Nepisiguit, 950 av Picot, Bathurst NB E2A 4Z9; Laval'07; CCFP; (506)546-1018; Fax. (506)545-7723.

ARSENAULT, Marie-Claude; CSSS de Chicoutimi, CP 263 305 rue Saint-Vallier, Chicoutimi QC G7H 5H6; Sher'04; CCFP; Staff, Complexe hospitalier de la Sagamie; (418)541-1079

ARSENAULT, Marie-Eve; CSSS de Trois-Rivieres, 1991 boul du Carmel, Trois-Rivieres QC G8Z 3R9; Sher'00; FRCPC; Neur. Staff, CSSS de Trois-Rivières; Langs: Bilingual(French/English); (819)378-9700

ARSENAULT, Marie-Eve; MD Centropolis, 227-655 Prom du Centropolis, Laval QC H7T 0A3; Mon'00; Staff, Hopital de la Cite de la santé; (514)739-5646

ARSENAULT, Marie-Josee; Hotel-Dieu de Sorel, 400 av de l'Hotel-Dieu, Sorel-Tracy QC J3P 1N5; Mon'93; CCFP; Fam Med, Hôtel-Dieu de Sorel; (450)746-6000

ARSENAULT, Melanie; Rexton Health Clinic, 33 rue Main, Rexton NB E4W 0E5; Sher'02; CCFP; Staff Family Med, Hôpital Stella-Maris-de-Kent; (506)523-2972; Fax. (506)523-2971.

ARSENAULT, Michael A; Hôpital Ste-Justine, 3175 ch Cote-Sainte-Catherine, Montreal QC H3T 1C5; Ott'92; FRCPC; Peds (Emergency Pediatrics). Ped Emerg, Hôpital Ste-Justine; Clinical Asst Prof, Universite de Montreal; Langs: Italian; (514)345-4932 x6276; Fax. (514)345-2358; michael.arsenault@umontreal.ca.

ARSENAULT, Mylene; Jewish Rehabilitation Hosp, 3205 Place Alton-Goldbloom, Laval QC H7V 1R2; McG'01; CCFP; Staff, Jewish Rehabilitation Hospital; Langs: English; (450)688-9550

ARSENAULT, Pierre; Clinique Med de Stoke, 202 Route 216, Stoke QC J0B 3G0; Mon'90; DSc; CCFP; Staff, Centre Hospitalier Universitaire de Sherbrooke-Hopital Fleurimont; (819)543-0511; Fax. (819)543-0515; pierre.arsenault@usherbrooke.ca.

ARSENAULT, Sarto; Clin de Chirurgie Orthopedique, 150-10445 av 1Re, Saint-Georges QC G5Y 6X8; Laval'72; OrthSurg. Langs: Bilingual(French/English); (418)228-2899; Fax. (418)228-2875; sarto.arsenault@cgocable.ca.

ARSENAULT, Sylvain; Groupe Med de Trois-Rivieres, 225-1900 boul Des Recollets, Trois-Rivieres QC G8Z 4K4; Sher'89; CCFP; (819)375-6666

ARSENAULT, Theodore; Drummond Med Bldg, 722-1414 rue Drummond, Montreal QC H3G 1W1; Laval'60; Derm. Associate Derm, McGill University Health Centre - Royal Victoria Hospital; adj Prof, McGill University; (514)849-8472

ARSENAULT, William E; 201 Humber Ave, Labrador City NL A2V 2Y3; Mem'75; CCFP; FCFP; Staff, Captain William Jackman Memorial Hospital; (709)944-2600; Fax. (709)944-3093.

ARSENAULT-SAMSON, Nadine; Harbourside Family Health Ctre, 243 Harbour Dr, Summerside PE C1N 5R1; Laval'03; CCFP; Staff, Prince County Hospital; Langs: Bilingual(French/English); (902)432-2600; Fax. (902)432-2610; nparsenault@ihis.org.

ARSENEAU, Christian; CSSS de Trois-Rivieres, 1991 boul du Carmel, Trois-Rivieres QC G8Z 3R9; Sher'00; FRCPC; DiagRad. Staff, CSSS de Trois-Rivières; (819)697-3333

ARSENEAU, Fernand G; PO Box 986 Stn Main, Moncton NB E1C 8P2; Mon'86; Dip SportMed; LMCC; Staff, Dr Georges-L-Dumont University Hospital Centre; Langs: English; (506)383-4339; Fax. (506)854-6574; fernanda@nbnet.nb.ca.

ARSENEAU, Jean-Louis; CSSS de Memphremagog, 50 rue Saint-Patrice E, Magog QC J1X 3X3; Laval'67; Staff, Centre Hospitalier et CLSC de Memphremagog; (819)843-3381

ARSENEAU, Jean-Pierre; Clinique Med Nepisiguit, 950 av Picot, Bathurst NB E2A 4Z9; Sher'92; LMCC; CCFP; (506)546-6696; Fax. (506)545-7723; cmni@nbnet.nb.ca.

ARSENEAU, Jocelyne; Lyman Duff Med Sciences Bldg, 3775 rue University, Montreal QC H3A 2B4; Laval'74; CSPQ; FRCPC; AnatPath. Assoc Prof Path & ObstGyn, McGill University Health Centre - Royal Victoria Hospital; (514)398-7192 x488; Fax. (514)398-2440.

ARSENEAU, Richard R; St Paul's Hosp, 1081 Burrard St, Vancouver BC V6Z 1Y6; Tor'87; FRCPC; IntMed. Assoc Staff, Providence Health Care - St Paul's Hospital; (604)682-2344 x62554; Fax. (604)806-8338.

ARSENEAULT, Daniel; Centre Med Christ-Roi, 102-40 rte du President-Kenned, Levis QC G6V 6C4; Mon'85; Staff, Hôtel-Dieu de Lévis; (418)833-4977; Fax. (418)833-9557.

ARSENEAULT, Denis; 8641 av Chaumont, Anjou QC H1K 1N4; Mon'76; (514)352-2482; Fax. (514)351-6866.

ARSENEAULT, Tania; Dr Georges-L Dumont Reg Hosp, 330 av Universite, Moncton NB E1C 2Z3; Sher'04; CCFP; CCFP(E.M.); Staff, Dr Georges-L-Dumont University Hospital Centre; (506)862-4000

ARSHAT, Daoud J D; 906 Brant St, Burlington ON L7R 2J5; (Iraq)'98; CCFP; (905)637-5885

ARSHINOFF, Steve; York-Finch Eye Associates, 316-2115 Finch Ave W, North York ON M3N 2V6; Baylor(TX) (USA)'75; FRCS; FRCSC; Ophth (Cataract Anterior Segment & Refractive Surgery). Staff Ophth, Humber River Regional Hospital - Finch Avenue Site; Clinical Asst Prof, McMaster University; Lecturer, University of Toronto; (416)745-6969; Fax. (416)745-6724; ifix2is@sympatico.ca.

ARSIRADAM, Neethia M; Victoria Hosp, PO Box 3000 Stn Main 1200 24th St W, Prince Albert SK S6V 5T4; Natal (South Africa)'88; MB ChB; FRCPC; Anes. Staff, Victoria Hospital; (306)765-6267

ARTAUD, Laurence; CHUM-Hop Notre-Dame, 1560 rue Sherbrooke E, Montreal QC H2L 4M1; Mon'98; FRCPC; Psy. Staff, Centre Hospitalier l'Université de Montréal (CHUM) - Hôpital Notre-Dame; (514)890-8242

ARTEAU, Annie; CHUQ-Hotel-Dieu de Quebec, 11 Cote du Palais, Quebec QC G1R 2J6; Laval'07; OrthSurg. Staff, Centre Hospitalier Universitaire de Québec (CHUQ) - Siege Social; (418)525-4444

ARTEAU-GAUTHIER, Isabelle; CSSS de l'Energie-Ste-Therese, 1705 av Georges, Shawinigan QC G9N 2N1; Sher'06; FRCSC; Otol. Staff, CH du Centre-de-la-Mauricie (Ste-Thérèse de Shawinigan); (819)536-7500; isabelle_arteau-gauthier@ssss.gouv.qc.ca.

ARTEAU-GAUTHIER, Myreille; ASSS Lanaudiere, 245 rue du Cure-Majeau, Joliette QC J6E 8S8; Laval'78; Staff, Centre Hospitalier Régional de Lanaudière; (450)759-1157 x4441

ARTHO, Giovanni P; MUHC-Montreal Gen Hosp, D5.989-1650 av Cedar, Montreal QC H3G 1A4; Bern (Switzerland)'90; Staff, McGill University Health Centre - Montreal General Campus; (514)934-1934 x43351; Fax. (514)934-8263.

ARTHUR, Brian W; Hotel-Dieu Hosp, 224A-166 Brock St, Kingston ON K7L 5G2; Qns'80; FRCSC; Ophth. Staff, Hotel-Dieu Hospital; (613)544-3400 x3100

ARTHUR, Frederick E; 975 Willow Ave, London ON N6E 1P4; Wes'88; CCFP; CCFP(E.M.); Staff Emerg Physician, Chatham-Kent Health Alliance - Sydenham Hospital Campus; (519)681-4982; Fax. (519)681-6634.

ARTHUR, Jane; Regina Qu'Appelle HR-Regina, 1440 14th Ave, Regina SK S4P 0W5; Witwatersrand (South Africa)'89; MB ChB; BSc; MSc; Staff, Regina General Hospital; (306)766-4444; Fax. (306)585-3593.

ARTHUR, John S; Richmond Health Science Ctre, 310-6091 Gilbert Rd, Richmond BC V7C 5L9; Cal'73; FRCSC; OrthSurg (Hip & Knee Arthroplasty). Staff, Delta Hospital; Staff, Richmond Hospital; (604)273-6148; Fax. (604)273-3421.

ARTHUR, Laverne S; Morton Comm Healthcare Ctre, PO Box 832 1-150 Strickland Rd, Lakefield ON K0L 2H0; McM'04; BA; BEd; CCFP; (705)652-6800; Fax. (705)652-8373.

ARTHUR, Marion F; Collingwood Health Centre, 200-186 Erie St, Collingwood ON L9Y 4T3; Wes'82; BSc; Staff, Collingwood General & Marine Hospital; Staff, Collingwood Health Centre; (705)444-7687; Fax. (705)444-1108.

ARTHUR, Rebecca H; Ctr for Fertility & Reproducti, 7F-250 Dundas St W, Toronto ON M5T 2Z5; McM'02; FRCSC; ObstGyn. (416)586-4748; Fax. (416)586-4686.

ARTHUR, Simon G; Foothills Prof Bldg, 350-1620 29 St NW, Calgary AB T2N 4L7; Cal'91; BSc; CCFP; (403)282-1245; Fax. (403)282-9545.

ARTHUR, Thomas D; Nisga'a Valley Hlth Authority, PO Box 234, Aiyansh BC V0J 1A0; McG'73; CCFP; (250)633-5000

ARTHURS, Bryan P; MUHC-Montreal Gen Hosp, L4.112-1650 av Cedar, Montreal QC H3G 1A4; Wes'79; FRCSC; Ophth (Oculo Plastic Surgery). Att Staff Ophth, McGill University Health Centre - Montreal General Campus; Assoc Prof Ophth, McGill University; Langs: English; French; (514)934-8055; Fax. (514)934-8223.

ARTHURS, James R; Northwestern Health Unit, RR 1 Stn Main 21 Wolsley St, Kenora ON P9N 3W7; Seattle (USA)'68; (807)468-3147; Fax. (807)468-4970.

ARTHURS, Michael J; North Bay Reg Health Centre, 50 College Dr, North Bay ON P1B 0A4; McM'79; Staff, North Bay Regional Health Centre - Regional Mental Health; (705)474-8600

ARTINIAN, Berdj; Halton HCS Corp-Oakville, 327 Reynolds St, Oakville ON L6J 3L7; Ain Shams (Egypt)'65; FRCPC; GenPath. Staff, Halton Healthcare Services Corporation - Oakville Site; (905)338-4675; bartinian@haltonhealthcare.on.ca.

ARTS, Rudolf J; Atrium Prof Bldg, 304-190 Cundles Rd E SS 103, Barrie ON L4M 4S5; Nijmegen (Netherlands)'75; MD; FRCPC; Neur (Clinical Neurophysiology). Staff, Royal Victoria Regional Health Centre; Langs: Dutch; (705)721-1060; Fax. (705)721-2442.

ARULCHELVAM, Pradeepan; Family Health Centre, 1125 Markham Rd, Scarborough ON M1H 2Y5; Colombo (Sri Lanka)'93; MB BS; CCFP; Lecturer, University of Toronto; Langs: Tamil; Sinhalese; Bilingual(English/French).

ARUMUGAM, Bhavani; North Burlington Med Centre, 18-1960 Appleby Line, Burlington ON L7L 0B7; Chennai (India)'92; MD; CCFP; Langs: Tamil; Malay; (905)319-2000; Fax. (905)319-6292.

ARUN-PRAKASH, M Venugopal; Regional Mental HC-St Thomas, PO Box 2004 Stn Main, St Thomas ON N5P 3V9; Mysore (India)'76; MB BS; MRCPsy; FRCPC; Psy (Forensic Psychiatry). Consultant Psych, Regional Mental Health Care-St Joseph's Health Care; (519)631-8510; Fax. (519)472-7585.

ARUNASALAM, Kiritharan; Headwaters Specialist Clinic, 125-150 Rolling Hills Dr, Orangeville ON L9W 4X8; (Grenada)'01; FRCPC; IntMed. Staff, Headwaters Health Care Centre - Orangeville Site; Langs: Tamil; (519)938-5596; Fax. (519)938-5597.

ARUNDELL, Geoffrey W; Lions Gate Hosp, 231 15th St E, North Vancouver BC V7L 2L7; UBC'66; FRCPC; Anes. Assoc Staff, Lions Gate Hospital; (604)988-3131

ARVANITIS, Jennifer M; Mount Sinai Hosp, 600 University Ave, Toronto ON M5G 1X5; Wes'93; CCFP; FCFP; Staff, Mount Sinai Hospital; (416)596-4200

ARVINTE, Andrei A; Niagara H System-St Catharine, PO Box 3018 Stn Main 142 Queenston St, St Catharines ON L2R 7C6; Bucharest (Romania)'90; FRCPC; DiagRad. Staff, Niagara Health System - St Catharines General Site; (905)684-7271

ARVINTE, Galina; 2-403 Ontario St, St. Catharines ON L2N 1L5; Kiev (Ukraine)'88; CCFP; Staff, Niagara Health System - Welland Hospital Site; (905)984-8766; Fax. (905)984-8242.

ARVISAIS, Nadine; Centre de Sante du Plateau, 103-195 rue de l'Atmosphere, Gatineau QC J9A 0A3; Ott'06; CCFP; (819)777-7270

ARWINI, Ahmed A S; Thunder Bay Reg HSC-T-Bay, 1713-980 Oliver Rd, Thunder Bay ON P7B 6V4; Al-Fateh (Libya)'93; FRCSI; FRCP; FRCPC; AnatPath (General Surgery). Staff, Thunder Bay Regional Health Sciences Centre; (807)684-6593; a.arwini@dr.com.

ARWINI, Mohamed A S; Southwest Medi-Centre, 500-1 Springs Dr, Swift Current SK S9H 3X6; Al-Fateh (Libya)'89; MB ChB; FRCSC; Urol. (306)773-4681; Fax. (306)778-3449.

ARYA, A Neil; The Centre for Family Medicine, 10B Victoria St S, Kitchener ON N2G 1C5; Qns'90; CCFP; FCFP; Staff, Grand River Hospital - Kitchener/Waterloo Health Centre; Staff, St Mary's General Hospital; Langs: Spanish; Hindi; French; (519)783-0021; Fax. (519)783-0031; neilarya@hotmail.com.

ARYA, Amit; Earlsbridge Plaza, 6-10 Earlsbridge Blvd, Brampton ON L7A 3P1; UBC'03; BSc; CCFP; Langs: Hindi; Punjabi; Urdu; (905)840-4776

ARYA, Naveen; 1-2125 Wyecroft Rd, Oakville ON L6L 5L7; Wes'98; FRCPC; IntMed (Therapeutic Endoscopy); Gastroent. Staff, Halton Healthcare Services Corporation - Oakville Site; (905)849-0688; Fax. (905)849-1596.

ARYA, Neehar; Sturgeon Community Hosp, 201 Boudreau Rd, St. Albert AB T8N 6C4; London (England)'95; MB BS; Staff, Sturgeon Community Hospital; (780)418-7361

ARZOLA VILLALOBOS, Gracian C; Mount Sinai Hosp, 1514-600 University Ave, Toronto ON M5G 1X5; (Chile)'96; Staff, Mount Sinai Hospital; (416)586-5270

ARZOUMANIAN, Yervant; Brockville Gen Hosp, 75 Charles St, Brockville ON K6V 1S8; McG'96; FRCPC; DiagRad. Staff, Brockville General Hospital - Charles Street; (613)345-5645

ASA, Sylvia L; Univ Hlth Network-Toronto Gen, 11F-200 Elizabeth St, Toronto ON M5G 2C4; Tor'77; FCAP; PhD; FRCPC; AnatPath (Endocrinology Pathology). Chief Pathologist, Toronto General Hospital - UHN; Langs: English; French; (416)340-4802; Fax. (416)340-5517.

ASADY, M Anwar; Trillium Hlth Ctr-Mississauga, 100 Queensway W, Mississauga ON L5B 1B8; Peshawar (Pakistan)'88; DCH; MRCP; Staff, Trillium Health Centre - Mississauga; Langs: Farsi; Urdu; (905)848-7100; aasady@thc.on.ca.

ASAI, Yuka; MUHC-Royal Victoria Hosp, A4.17-687 av des Pins O, Montreal QC H3A 1A1; Sask'05; FRCPC; Derm (P.Q.). Staff, McGill University Health Centre - Royal Victoria Hospital; (514)934-1934 x31550

ASANO, Tracey K; Centennary HC-The Court, 401-2863 Ellesmere Rd, Scarborough ON M1E 5E9; Tor'92; FRCSC; GenSurg. Staff, Rouge Valley Health System - Centenary Health Centre Site; (416)286-9729; Fax. (416)286-9175.

ASARIA, Jamil; 186 St George St, Toronto ON M5R 2N3; Tor'04; FRCSC; Otol (Head & Neck Surgery). (416)479-4244

ASARO, Rosalinda; 27-1077 North Service Rd, Mississauga ON L4Y 1A6; Tor'96; BSc; CCFP; (905)949-1700; Fax. (905)949-8625.

ASAYESH, Khalil; Peel Med Arts Bldg, 307-145 Queen St E, Brampton ON L6W 3P8; Tehran (Iran)'54; MD; FRCPC; Psy (Affective Disorders). Staff, William Osler Health System - Brampton Civic Hospital; Langs: Farsi; (905)450-8811; Fax. (905)450-8810.

ASBELL, Irwin J; 410-2333 Dundas St W Box 25, Toronto ON M6R 3A6; Tor'84; BSc; MSc; CCFP; (416)537-7000; Fax. (416)537-0132.

ASCAH, John G; 109-3265 Westwood Dr, Prince George BC V2N 1S4; Wes'81; FRCPC; Anes (Intensive Care). Staff, University Hospital of Northern British Columbia; (250)301-8270

ASCAH, Kathryn J; Univ of Ottawa Heart Institute, H1220-40 Ruskin St, Ottawa ON K1Y 4W7; Tor'77; ABC; FRCPC; IntMed (Echography Cardiac); Cardiol. Staff, University of Ottawa Heart Institute; Dir Stress Lab Ottawa Heart Inst, The Ottawa Hospital - Civic Campus; Assoc Prof Med, University of Ottawa; (613)761-4688; Fax. (613)761-4929; kascah@ottawaheart.ca.

ASCH, Murray R; Lakeridge Hlth Corp-Oshawa, 1 Hospital Crt, Oshawa ON L1G 2B9; Wes'83; FRCPC; DiagRad (Body Imaging). Staff, Lakeridge Health - Oshawa Site; Staff, The Hospital For Sick Children; (905)576-8711 x3497; Fax. (905)721-4770.

ASCHE, Gerd; 21393 Lakeview Cres RR 3, Hope BC V0X 1L1; Bonn (Germany)'51; AB; CCFP; Med Examiner, Civil Aviation Canada; Langs: German; Italian; (604)869-2043; Fax. (604)869-2053; gerdasch@uniserve.com.

ASCHE-QUINT, Ursula; 21393 Lakeview Cres, Hope BC V0X 1L1; Bonn (Germany)'54; CCFP; Fam Med, Fraser Canyon Hospital; Court Staff, Chilliwack General Hospital; ursula.asche-quint@fraserhealth.ca.

ASCHER, Ilana S; Shops on Steeles Med Centre, 206-2900 Steeles Ave E, Thornhill ON L3T 4X1; Ross U (USA)'07; (905)881-6667

ASCURRA DE ORTIZ, Ana Maria; Capital Dist Mental Hlth Prog, 300 Pleasant St, Dartmouth NS B2Y 3S3; San Marcos (Peru)'84; CCFP; (902)464-3111; Fax. (902)464-6519.

ASDAGHI, Negar; UBC Hospital, S169-2211 Wesbrook Mall, Vancouver BC V6T 2B5; Shahid Beheshti University (Israel)'02; FRCPC; Neur. Staff, UBC Hospital - Koerner Pavillion; (604)822-1789

ASEFA, Victor K K; Victoria Hosp, PO Box 3000 Stn Main 1200 24th St W, Prince Albert SK S6V 5T4; Staff, Victoria Hospital; (306)981-1324

ASEFI, Shirin; 9206 Yonge St, Richmond Hill ON L4C 7A2; Isfahan (Iran)'97; CCFP; (905)709-7716

ASEKOMHE, Ikhimhaigie F; Northgate Med Centre, 4-980 Central Park Dr, Brampton ON L6S 3L7; Ile-Ife (Nigeria)'91; CCFP; (905)458-4771

ASEM, Kevin D; Fowler Kennedy Sports Med Clin, 3M-1151 Richmond St, London ON N6A 3K7; Ott'08; CCFP; (519)661-3011

ASENJO, Juan F; MUHC-Montreal Gen Hosp, D10.152-1650 av Cedar, Montreal QC H3G 1A4; (Chile)'85; FRCPC; Anes. Staff, McGill University Health Centre - Montreal General Campus; (514)934-1934 x4261

ASFAHA, Samuel; Calgary Heart Centre, 3280 Hospital Dr NW, Calgary AB T2N 4Z6; Cal'03; FRCPC; IntMed; Gastroent. Staff, Foothills Medical Centre; Physician, Health Research Innovation Centre; (403)592-5025

ASFOUR, Nabil; 21st Medical Clinic, 502-402 21 St E, Saskatoon SK S7K 0C3; (306)956-3444; Fax. (306)956-3577.

ASGAR, Anita W; Institut de Cardiologie de Mtl, 5000 rue Belanger, Montreal QC H1T 1C8; Mem'99; FRCPC; IntMed; Cardiol. Staff, Institut de Cardiologie de Montréal; (514)376-3330

ASGARALI, Saied; Pickering Med Centre, 214-1885 Glenanna Rd, Pickering ON L1V 6R6; (Jamaica)'85; MB BS; FRCS(UK); FRCSC; Otol. Att Staff, Rouge Valley Health System - Ajax & Pickering Health Centre Site; (905)831-0505; Fax. (905)831-6503.

ASGARI, Nilfoofar; Prairie North Health Centre, 4806 50 St, Lloydminster SK S9V 0M9; (306)820-5997; Fax. (306)820-5978.

ASH, Judith M; Medvue Medical Imaging, 210-123 Edward St, Toronto ON M5G 1E2; Tor'69; DAB; DMRD; FRCPC; DiagRad; NuclearMed. Sr Staff Rad & Div of Nuclear Med, The Hospital For Sick Children; (416)593-5458; Fax. (416)593-4118; judith.ash@sickkids.ca.

ASH, Leslie C; Quinte HC Corp-Belleville Gen, 265 Dundas St E, Belleville ON K8N 5A9; Tor'63; FRCPC; Psy (Child Psychiatry). Ac Staff, QHC Belleville General; Aj Asst Prof of Family Med, Queen's University; (613)969-7400 x2232

ASH, Marla R; North York Family Health Team, 702-240 Duncan Mill Rd, North York ON M3B 3S6; Tor'94; CCFP; Ac Staff, North York General Hospital; (416)494-7435; Fax. (416)494-4819.

ASHAM-YOUSSEF, Amal A; Brittany Glen Med Centre, 102-5602 Tenth Line W, Mississauga ON L5M 7L9; Alexandria (Egypt)'90; CCFP; (905)858-9393

ASHAMALLA, Alison K; South Riverside Comm Hlth Ctre, 955 Queen St E, Toronto ON M4M 3P3; Tor'05; CCFP; (416)461-2493; Fax. (416)461-8245.

ASHAMALLA, Shady; Sunnybrook Hlth Sciences Ctre, T2015-2075 Bayview Ave, Toronto ON M4N 3M5; Tor'05; FRCSC; GenSurg. Staff, Sunnybrook Health Sciences Centre; (416)480-4027

ASHATER, Elsharif M M; Thunder Bay Reg HSC, 980 Oliver Rd, Thunder Bay ON P7B 6V4; Sirt (Libya)'00; FRCPC; IntMed; Rheum. Staff, Thunder Bay Regional Health Sciences Centre; Langs: Arabic; (807)684-6027

ASHBOURNE, John F; Peterborough Reg HC-Hospital, 1 Hospital Dr, Peterborough ON K9J 7C6; Cal'79; FRCPC; EmergMed. Staff, Peterborough Regional Health Centre - Hospital Drive; (705)876-5022

ASHBURY, Edwin L; Kingston Gen Hosp, 76 Stuart St, Kingston ON K7L 2V7; Qns'78; BA; FRCPC; Anes (Pediatric Anesthesia). Staff Anes, Kingston General Hospital; Staff Anes, Hotel-Dieu Hospital; Assoc Prof Anes & Peds, Queen's University; (613)548-7827; Fax. (613)548-1375.

ASHBY, David; Dept of Veteran's Affairs, PO Box 7700 Stn Central, Charlottetown PE C1A 8M9; McG'71; AB; FACS; FRCSC; GenSurg (Thoracic Surgery). Staff, Veterans Affairs Canada; Langs: Bilingual(French/English); (902)566-8888

ASHBY, Peter; Univ Hlth Network-Toronto Western Hosp, 4FP-399 Bathurst St, Toronto ON M5T 2S8; Queen's University (United Kingdom)'60; MB ChB; MD; FRCP(Ed); FAAN; MRCP(Lond); FRCPC; Neur (Neuromuscular Diseases). Staff EMG Lab, Toronto Western Hospital - University Health Network; Staff EMG Lab, The Credit Valley Hospital; Prof, University of Toronto; (416)603-5922; Fax. (416)603-7096.

ASHE, Gerald P; 70 Charles St, Brockville ON K6V 1T3; Ott'76; CCFP; FCFP; (613)345-1458; Fax. (613)345-5296.

ASHE, Kassem A; St Mary's Gen Hosp, 911 Queens Blvd, Kitchener ON N2M 1B2; Wes'84; CardSurg; VascSurg; GenSurg. Staff, St Mary's General Hospital; Langs: Arabic; (519)744-3311

ASHENHURST, Michael E; 344-933 17 Ave SW, Calgary AB T2T 5R6; Sask'85; FRCSC; Ophth (Oculo Plastic Surgery). Staff, Peter Lougheed Centre; Staff, Rockyview General Hospital; Staff, Alberta Children's Hospital; (403)245-3171; Fax. (403)245-4205.

ASHER, Ayesha; Wellpoint Health, 103-240 Midpark Way SE, Calgary AB T2X 1N4; CCFP; (403)256-8213; Fax. (403)254-8795.

ASHFAQ, Bushra; Northern Medical Unit, T162-770 Bannatyne Ave, Winnipeg MB R3E 0W3; CCFP.

ASHFAQ, Sirajuddin; Aberdeen Hosp, 835 East River Rd, New Glasgow NS B2H 3S6; Osmania (India)'61; MB BS; IntMed; GenPath. Staff, Aberdeen Regional Hospital; (902)752-7600; Fax. (902)752-1931.

ASHFIELD, James E; Saint John Reg Hosp, PO Box 2100 Stn Main 400 University Ave, Saint John NB E2L 4L2; Dal'97; FRCSC; Urol. Staff, Saint John Regional Hospital; (506)648-7790; Fax. (506)648-6894.

ASHFIELD, Jane G; 2-10 King George Crt, Saint John NB E2K 0H5; Dal'97; CCFP; (506)634-8706; Fax. (506)634-6654.

ASHFORTH, Robert A; University of Alberta Hosp, 8440 112 St NW, Edmonton AB T6G 2B7; Alb'82; DABR; FRCPC; DiagRad (Neuro Radiology). Staff Radiol, University of Alberta Hospital; Asst Prof, University of Alberta; (780)407-1210; Fax. (780)407-1202.

ASHIKIAN, Haig; Spratt Med Centre, 1-4188 Spratt Rd, Gloucester ON K1V 0Z6; Mon'90; CCFP; FCFP; Physician, Riverside South Family Health Organization; Langs: French; Spanish; Armenian; (613)822-0171; Fax. (613)822-1838; drhaigashikian@gmail.com.

ASHKAR, Laila K; Vancouver Breast Centre, 505-750 Broadway W, Vancouver BC V5Z 1H4; Jeddah (Saudi Arabia)'94; MB BS; FRCPC; DiagRad. Staff, BC Women's Hospital & Health Centre; (604)879-4177

ASHLEY, Jason B; Sudbury Reg Hosp-Laurentian, 41 Ramsey Lake Rd, Sudbury ON P3E 5J1; Wes'03; FRCPC; DiagRad. Staff, Health Sciences North-Laurentian Site; (705)522-2200

ASHLEY, Jeffrey M; Rexdale Med Centre, 2-123 Rexdale Blvd, Etobicoke ON M9W 1P1; Wes'88; Staff, William Osler Health System - Etobicoke General Hospital; (416)743-5853; Fax. (416)743-1358.

ASHOK, Dhandapani; London HSC-Victoria Hosp, PO Box 5010 Stn B 800 Commissioners Rd E, London ON N6A 5W9; Madras (India)'92; Staff, London Health Sciences Centre - Victoria Campus; (519)685-8500; Fax. (519)685-8127.

ASHRAF, Muhammad; Lloydminster Hosp, 3820 43 Ave, Lloydminster SK S9V 1Y5; Locum Tenens, Lloydminster Hospital; (306)820-6000

ASHRAF, Nazia; Phoenix Med Centre, 106-2155 10th Ave, Prince George BC V2M 5J6; (Other Foreign)'98; CCFP; (250)981-2367

ASHRAFI, Ahmad S; Surrey Med Arts Bldg, 214-13710 94A Ave, Surrey BC V3V 1N1; Ott'97; BSc; FRCSC; GenSurg (Critical Care Medicine); ThorSurg. Staff, Surrey Memorial Hospital; Langs: Persian; Urdu; Pashtu; Dari; German; Hindi; (604)588-5634

ASHTEKAR, Vijaykumar V; Mental Health Clinic, 350 Cheadle St W, Swift Current SK S9H 4G3; Poona (India)'73; MB BS; MRCPsy(U.K.); Chief Psychiatrist, Cypress Regional Hospital; Langs: Hindi; Marathi; (306)778-5250; Fax. (306)778-5408; vijay.ashtekar@cypressrha.ca.

ASHTON, Brian D; Sunnyside Mall, 302-1595 Bedford Hwy, Bedford NS B4A 3Y4; Dal'94; BSc; CCFP; FCFP; (902)835-3361

ASHTON, Deirdre A; Ermineskin Med Clinic, 301-2377 111 St NW, Edmonton AB T6J 5E5; London (England)'74; MB BS; MRCS; LRCP; (780)436-8731; Fax. (780)434-8732.

ASHTON, Martin; South Indian Lake Nursing Stn, GD, South Indian Lake MB R0B 1N0; Man'84; Staff, South Indian Lake Nursing Station; (204)374-2013

ASHTON, Russell W; Two Rivers FHT-Healthlink, 10B-350 Conestoga Blvd, Cambridge ON N1R 7L7; Qns'93; CCFP; FCFP; Chief Commun & Family Med, Cambridge Memorial Hospital; (519)740-5010

ASHTON, Thomas H; 577 Carmi Ave, Penticton BC V2A 3G7; UBC'67; FACC; FRCPC; IntMed (Cardiology). Staff, Penticton Regional Hospital; (250)493-1080; Fax. (250)492-7342; ashtonoffice@hotmail.com.

ASHUR, Mohamed S A; Hôpital régional Chaleur, 1750 Sunset Dr, Bathurst NB E2A 4L7; Al-Fateh (Libya)'85; FRCPC; Peds. Staff, Hopital Regional Chaleur; (506)544-2252; Fax. (506)544-2037; mashur@reg6.health.nb.ca.

ASHWELL, Stephen P; 1025 103 Ave, Dawson Creek BC V1G 2G6; UBC'87; CCFP; Staff, Dawson Creek & District Hospital; (250)782-1186; Fax. (250)782-9447.

ASHWORTH, Allison B; London Reg Cancer Centre, 790 Commissioners Rd E, London ON N6A 4L6; Alb'05; FRCPC; RadOncol.

ASHWORTH, Nigel L; Glenrose Rehab Hosp, 10230 111 Ave NW, Edmonton AB T5G 0B7; Leicester (England)'89; MB ChB; MSc(Ep.); FRCPC; PhysMed&Rehab (Clinical Neurophysiology). Staff, Glenrose Rehabilitation Hospital; Prof, University of Alberta; (780)735-8210; Fax. (780)735-6018; nigel.ashworth@albertahealthservices.ca.

ASIF, Anjum; 103-611 Holly Ave, Milton ON L9T 0K4; Karachi (Pakistan)'88; CCFP; (905)878-0086; Fax. (905)878-1562.

ASIF, Nusrat; Pacific Place Mall, 958-999 36 St NE, Calgary AB T2A 7X6; CCFP; (403)387-3300; Fax. (403)387-3305.

ASIM, Hammad; 305B-45 Weatherbee Rd, Mira Road NS B1M 0A1; Punjab (Pakistan)'87; MB BS; BSc; Assoc Staff, Cape Breton Healthcare Complex; (902)567-2270; Fax. (902)567-2272.

ASIM, Muhammad; The Hosp for Sick Children, 555 University Ave, Toronto ON M5G 1X8; Punjab (Pakistan)'00; Clin Fellow Peds, The Hospital For Sick Children; (416)813-8013

ASIRWATHAM, Ramesh I; Hope Med Centre, 3208A Eglinton Ave E, Scarborough ON M1J 2H6; Ceylon (Sri Lanka)'92; MB BS; CCFP; (416)267-6700; Fax. (416)267-0189.

ASKALAN, Rand A; 555 University Ave, Toronto ON M5G 1X8; Tor'01; FRCPC; Neur (Pediatric Neurology). Staff, The Hospital For Sick Children; Langs: Other language; (416)813-6659; Fax. (416)813-6334; rand.askalan@sickkids.ca.

ASKAR, Majdi R; All Well Primary Care Centre, 4217 23 Ave, Edmonton AB T6L 5Z8; Al-Fateh (Libya)'96; MB ChB; (780)462-0442; oska1118@hotmail.com.

ASKAR, Wanda M K; James Paton Mem Hosp, 125 Trans Canada Hwy, Gander NL A1V 1P7; Baghdad (Iraq)'06; MB ChB; Staff, James Paton Memorial Hospital; (709)256-2500

ASKARI, Sussan; Nova Scotia Rehab Centre, 285-1341 Summer St, Halifax NS B3H 4K4; Shiraz (Iran)'92; MD; Staff, Nova Scotia Rehabilitation Centre; (902)473-1238; Fax. (902)473-3204.

ASKARIFAR, Rasool; Beausejour Primary Health Ctre, PO Box 11208, Beausejour MB R0E 0C0; Man'10.

ASKEW, Gordon R; Hys Med Ctre, 11010 101 St NW, Edmonton AB T5H 4B9; Man'78; FRCPC; DiagRad (Radiology). Staff, Royal Alexandra Hospital; (780)426-1121

ASKIN, W Joseph; Ctre for Sleep & Human Perform, 106-51 Sunpark Dr SE, Calgary AB T2X 3V4; Cal'89; CCFP; FCFP; (403)254-6663; Fax. (403)254-6693.

ASLAHI, Ramona; St Michael's Hosp, 30 Bond St, Toronto ON M5B 1W8; Tehran (Iran)'00; FRCPC; IntMed; Nephrol. Staff, St Michael's Hospital; (416)864-6060

ASLAM, Muhammad R; Prairie North Specialist Clini, 107-4910 50 St, Lloydminster SK S9V 1Y5; Karachi (Pakistan)'91; (306)820-2599; Fax. (306)825-4774.

ASLAM, Nadeem; LMC Endocrinology Centres, 106-1929 Bayview Ave, Toronto ON M4G 3E8; Lahore (Pakistan)'91.

ASLAM, Zeeshan; Dr Everett Chalmers Reg Hosp, PO Box 9000 Stn A, Fredericton NB E3B 5N5; Peshawar (Pakistan)'94; MD; ABIM; ABIM(CriticalCare); FCCP; Med Dir ICU, Dr Everett Chalmers Regional Hospital; (506)452-5925; Fax. (506)447-4081.

ASLANIAN, Pierre; CHUM-Hop St-Luc, 1058 rue Saint-Denis, Montreal QC H2X 3J4; Mon'90; FRCPC; IntMed; Critical Care Medicine (P.Q.). Staff, Centre Hospitalier l'Université De Montréal (CHUM) - Hôpital Saint-luc; (514)890-8000

ASMAL, Mohammed Z D; Medcare Jane Finch, 3869 Jane St, North York ON M3N 2K1; (South Africa)'91; MB ChB; CCFP; (416)636-7077; Fax. (416)635-0562.

ASMIS, Timothy R; The Ottawa Hosp-Gen Campus, 501 Smyth Rd, Ottawa ON K1H 8L6; Ott'01; BSc; FRCPC; IntMed; MedOncol. Staff, The Ottawa Hospital - General Campus; (613)737-7700

ASNER, Sandra A H; The Hosp for Sick Children, 555 University Ave, Toronto ON M5G 1X8; Geneva (Switzerland)'02; Clin Fellow Ped, The Hospital For Sick Children; (416)813-1500

ASNONG, Veronique; Clinique Medi-Soleil, 383 boul du Seminaire N, St-Jean-sur-Richel QC J3B 8C5; Mon'10; CCFP; (450)349-5555

ASPE AYER, Diana M; Fanning Centre, 722 16 Ave NE, Calgary AB T2E 6V7; (Mexico)'91; CCFP; (403)230-6945; Fax. (403)230-6955.

ASPE LUCERO, Carlos; Allan Blair Cancer Centre, 4101 Dewdney Ave, Regina SK S4T 7T1; Locum Tenens, Regina General Hospital; (306)766-2213; Fax. (306)766-2777.

ASPIN, Derek G; Queen Square Doctors FHT, 201-366 Main St N, Brampton ON L6V 1P8; Guy's Hosp. (England)'70; Staff, William Osler Health System - Brampton Civic Hospital; (905)455-1455; Fax. (905)455-1331.

ASPIN, John D; IWK Health Centre, PO Box 9700 Rpo CSC, Halifax NS B3K 6R8; (England)'69; Staff, IWK Health Centre; (902)491-2361; john.aspin@iwk.nshealth.ca.

ASPINALL, Alexander I; South Health Campus, 7E GI-4448 Front St SE, Calgary AB T3M 1M4; Cal'99; FRCPC; IntMed (Hepatology); Gastroent. (403)956-3804

ASPINALL, Hugh; Avalon Med Clinic, 19851 Willoughby Dr, Langley BC V2Y 1A7; UBC'71; Staff, Langley Memorial Hospital; (604)534-9284; Fax. (604)534-1463.

ASPIROT, Ann; Hôpital Ste-Justine, 3175 ch Cote-Sainte-Catherine, Montreal QC H3T 1C5; Mon'00; FRCSC; GenSurg; PedGenSurg. Staff, Hôpital Ste-Justine; (514)345-4879

ASPLER, Aviva L; 100-8250 boul Decarie, Montreal QC H4P 2P5; McG'98; CCFP; (514)731-7717; Fax. (514)731-2228; aviva1@videotron.ca.

ASPY, William J; Kingston Family Health Team, 200-2437 Princess St, Kingston ON K7M 3G1; Qns'04; CCFP; (613)549-2255; waspy@kfhn.net.

ASQUITH, Philip R; Victoria Med Bldg, 513-1669 Victoria St, Prince George BC V2L 2L5; Alb'75; CCFP; Staff, University Hospital of Northern British Columbia; Chair of Economics, Society of General Practitioners of British Columbia; (250)563-9311; Fax. (250)563-7017.

ASRAT, Getnet A; Perth Med Clinic, 14 Isabella St, Perth ON K7H 2W6; (Ethiopia)'87; MHSc; CCFP; Langs: Amharic; (613)267-2820; Fax. (613)267-5706.

ASSAAD, Dalal M; Sunnybrook Hlth Sciences Ctre, M1 720-2075 Bayview Ave, Toronto ON M4N 3M5; Alexandria (Egypt)'71; FRCPC; AnatPath; Derm. Staff, Sunnybrook Health Sciences Centre; Langs: Arabic; (416)480-4908

ASSAAD, David M; Scarborough Eye Associates, 2941 Lawrence Ave E, Scarborough ON M1P 2V6; Tor'00; BSc; FRCSC; Ophth (Retina). Staff, St Michael's Hospital; (416)438-6000

ASSAAD, Hoda M A; 108-1309 Dawson Rd, Lorette MB R0A 0Y0; (Other Foreign)'88; CCFP.

ASSAAD, Ihab G R; The Credit Valley Hosp, 2200 Eglinton Ave W, Mississauga ON L5M 2N1; Cairo (Egypt)'88; FRCPC; Anes. Staff, The Credit Valley Hospital; (905)813-2200

ASSAD, Christopher J; 2-4300 Upper Middle Rd, Burlington ON L7M 4P6; Wes'92; BSc; FRCSC; PlasSurg (Breast Surgery). Assoc Staff, Halton Healthcare Services Corporation - Milton District Hospital; Staff, Halton Healthcare Services Corporation - Oakville Site; (905)315-9994; Fax. (905)315-9998.

ASSAD, P Paul; Clinique Med de Buckingham, 200-620 av de Buckingham, Gatineau QC J8L 2H5; Ott'73; EmergMed. (819)986-6006

ASSAD, Samir R G; Vaughan Comm Health Centre, 121-9401 Jane St, Maple ON L6A 4H7; Cairo (Egypt)'91; MB ChB; CCFP; Langs: Arabic; (905)303-2192; Fax. (905)303-7196.

ASSAF, Adel A; MUHC-Montreal Gen Hosp, D5 137-1650 av Cedar, Montreal QC H3G 1A4; Laval'87; BSc; MSc; FRCPC; DiagRad (Musculoskeletal). assoc Prof, McGill University Health Centre - Montreal General Campus; CEO, Westmount Square Medical Imaging; Langs: English; (514)934-8003; Fax. (514)934-8263; adelassaf@videotron.ca.

ASSAF, Christian; Ctr Hosp de Verdun, 4000 boul Lasalle, Verdun QC H4G 2A3; Mon'01; CCFP; Staff, Centre Hospitalier de Verdun; (514)765-7325

ASSAL, Michel; Clin Med Metro St-Michel, 7281 boul Shaughnessy, Montreal QC H2A 1J6; Mon'82; Staff, Centre Hospitalier Pierre Boucher; Physician, Union Carbide & Bio-Recherche & Staff, CLSC Rosemont; (514)374-0991; Fax. (514)374-0991.

ASSALIAN, Alfred; CSSS Pierre Boucher, 1333 boul Jacques-Cartier Est, Longueuil QC J4M 2A5; Mon'88; DAB; FRCSC; Ophth (Glaucoma). Staff, Centre Hospitalier Pierre Boucher; Staff, Centre Hospitalier l'Université de Montréal (CHUM) - Hôpital Notre-Dame; Langs: English; French; (450)468-8111

ASSALIAN, Pierre; MUHC-Montreal Gen Hosp, 1650 av Cedar, Montreal QC H3G 1A4; Cairo (Egypt)'68; Psy (P.Q.) (Depression). Staff Psy, McGill University Health Centre - Montreal General Campus; assoc Prof, McGill University; Langs: English; French; (514)934-1934 x42051; Fax. (514)934-8237; pierre.assalian@muhc.mcgill.ca.

ASSALY, Thomas R; Cornwall Comm Hosp-McConnell, PO Box 100 Stn Main 840 McConnell Ave, Cornwall ON K6H 5S5; McG'87; FRCPC; DiagRad. Staff, Cornwall Community Hospital; (613)938-4089; Fax. (613)938-4066.

ASSAYAG, Deborah; MUHC-Montreal Chest Institute, 3650 rue Saint-Urbain, Montreal QC H2X 2P4; McG'07; MDCM; Respir; IntMed. Staff, McGill University Health Centre - Montreal Chest Institute; (514)934-5201

ASSAYAG, Jacob G; Hop Jean-Talon, 1385 rue Jean-Talon E, Montreal QC H2E 1S6; Bruxelles (Belgium)'81; Staff, CSSS du Coeur de l'Isle Hôpital Jean-Talon; (514)495-6767

ASSAYAG, Y Raphael; Groupe Sante Physimed, 121-6363 rte Transcanadienne, Saint-Laurent QC H4T 1Z9; McG'06; MDCM; CCFP; (514)747-8888

ASSEDOU, Aaron; Hop du Sacre-Coeur de Mtl, 5400 boul Gouin O, Montreal QC H4J 1C5; Mon'08; CCFP; CCFP(E.M.); Staff, Hôpital du Sacre-Coeur de Montréal; (514)338-2000

ASSEF, Richard; Hop Santa Cabrini Ospedale, 5655 rue Saint-Zotique E, Montreal QC H1T 1P7; Dakar (Senegal)'87; CCFP; Staff, Hôpital Santa Cabrini Ospedale; (514)252-6000

ASSELAH, Jamil; MUHC-Montreal Gen Hosp, 1650 av Cedar, Montreal QC H3G 1A4; (Algeria)'00; Staff, McGill University Health Centre - Montreal General Campus; (514)934-1934

ASSELIN, Anne; Clin de Radiology de Granby, 66 rue Court, Granby QC J2G 4Y5; Sher'89; DiagRad. Staff, Centre Hospitalier de Granby; (450)378-0167

ASSELIN, Anne-Marie; CSSS de Trois-Rivieres, 1991 boul Du Carmel, Trois-Rivieres QC G8Z 3R9; Sher'93; CSPQ; FRCPC; Anes. Staff, CSSS de Trois-Rivières; (819)697-3333

ASSELIN, Clement; Clin d'Orthopedie Clement Asse, 306-176 av Rouleau, Rimouski QC G5L 8W1; Sher'86; LMCC; FRCSC; OrthSurg. Orthopedic Surgery, Hôpital Regional Rimouski; Langs: Bilingual(French/English); (418)721-2277; Fax. (418)721-2277.

ASSELIN, Fannie; CSSS de Trois-Rivieres, 155 rue Toupin, Trois-Rivieres QC G8T 3Z8; Mon'05; Staff, Centre de santé Cloutier-du-Rivage; (819)370-2100

ASSELIN, Francine; Centre Prof Belanger, 3871 rue Belanger, Montreal QC H1X 3M7; Laval'81; (514)722-1166; Fax. (514)722-1108.

ASSELIN, Guylaine; Hop Maisonneuve-Rosemont, 5415 boul de l'Assomption, Montreal QC H1T 2M4; Mon'88; FRCSC; ObstGyn (Pediatric Gynecology). Staff, Hopital Maisonneuve-Rosemont; (514)252-3400 x3820

ASSELIN, Johanne; CSSS du Nord de Lanaudière, 1000 boul Sainte-Anne, St-Charles-Brromee QC J6E 6J2; Mon'91; Staff, Centre Hospitalier Régional de Lanaudière; (450)759-8222

ASSELIN, Leandre; Hop Jeffrey Hale, 1250 ch Sainte-Foy, Quebec QC G1S 2M6; Laval'88; Staff, Jeffery Hale Hospital-Saint Brigid's; (418)683-4471; Fax. (418)683-8980.

ASSELIN, Marc-A; Clinique Med 3000 Inc, 3000 rue Belanger, Montreal QC H1Y 1A9; Sher'70; ac Staff, Hôpital Santa Cabrini Ospedale; (514)376-7702; Fax. (514)376-2639.

ASSELIN, Marcel; 604-3000 boul Notre-Dame, Laval QC H7V 4B8; Mon'71; (450)686-1986; Fax. (450)687-3720.

ASSELIN, Michel; CLSC de Matawinie, 485 rue Dupuis RR 2, Chertsey QC J0K 3K0; Mon'81; (450)882-2488; Fax. (450)882-9072.

ASSELIN, Yves; Clinique D'Ophth de Montmagny, 87 av de la Fabrique, Montmagny QC G5V 2J3; Sher'83; FRCSC; Ophth. Staff, CSSS de Montmagny-L'Islet; (418)248-2221; Fax. (418)248-3241.

ASSELSTINE, Robert C; Kingsway Health Centre, PO Box 819 Stn Main 5542 Ann St, Manotick ON K4M 1A7; Ott'68; (613)692-5433

ASSEMI, Ardavan; Walkley Med Centre, 1852 Bank St, Ottawa ON K1V 7Z8; Dal'98; BSc; CCFP; Langs: Farsi; French; (613)526-5200; Fax. (613)719-7807; a.assemi@rogers.com.

ASSEMI, Manutchehr; Strandherd Crossing Med Ctre, 305-3161 Strandherd Dr, Nepean ON K2J 5N1; Tehran (Iran)'60; FAAP; FRCPC; Peds (Neonatology). Langs: French; Farsi; Arabic; (613)823-5245

ASSI, Hazem; The Moncton Hosp, 135 MacBeath Ave, Moncton NB E1C 6Z8; Beirut (Lebanon)'98; MD; Staff, The Moncton Hospital; Langs: Arabic; Bilingual(French/English); (506)870-2920; Fax. (506)870-2922.

ASSI, Hussein; 5-1116 Mountain Rd, Moncton NB E1C 2T3; Bruxelles (Belgium)'83; Staff, The Moncton Hospital; (506)382-0690

ASSIMAKOPOULOS, Peter; E104-SMBD Jewish Gen Hosp, 3755 ch Cote-Sainte-Catherine, Montreal QC H3T 1E2; McG'93; FRCPC; IntMed; Endocrin (P.Q.); Endocrin&Metab. Staff, Sir Mortimer B Davis Jewish General; McGill University; Langs: Greek; (514)340-7550; Fax. (514)340-7529.

ASSKAR, Ramzi R; Red River Med Centre, 139 Carmen Ave, Winnipeg MB R2L 0E5; Al-Fateh (Libya)'96; CCFP.

ASSOULINE, Sarit; SMBD Jewish Gen Hosp, 3755 ch Cote-Sainte-Catherine, Montreal QC H3T 1E2; McG'97; BSc; MSc; FRCPC; IntMed (Leukemia & Lymphoma); Hem. Staff, Lakeshore General Hospital - Pointe Claire; Staff, Sir Mortimer B Davis Jewish General; assoc Prof Med/assoc Prof Oncol, McGill University; Langs: Bilingual(English/French); (514)340-8207; Fax. (514)340-8733.

ASSOULINE, Tony; Ctr Hosp de Lasalle, 8585 Tsse Champlain, LaSalle QC H8P 1C1; Grenoble (France)'90; CCFP; Staff, Centre Hospitalier de LaSalle; Langs: Bilingual(English/French); (514)362-8000; tonyassouline@hotmail.com.

ASSURAS, George N; Health Sciences Centre, GF431-820 Sherbrook St, Winnipeg MB R3A 1R9; Tor'84; FRCSC; GenSurg (Trauma). Ac Staff, Health Sciences Centre; Asst Prof, University of Manitoba; Langs: Greek; (204)787-3125; Fax. (204)787-4851.

ASSURAS, John W; London Reg Cancer Centre, 790 Commissioners Rd E, London ON N6A 4L6; Wes'85; Staff, London Regional Cancer Center; (519)685-8650; Fax. (519)685-8736.

ASTAWAN, Leanne; 120-121 Charles St W, Kitchener ON N2G 1H6; (Indonesia)'89; CCFP; (519)578-4230

ASTI, Melina; Niagara H System-St Catherine, PO Box 3018 Stn Main 142 Queenston St, St Catharines ON L2R 7C6; Milano (Italy)'97; FRCPC; Psy. Staff, Niagara Health System - St Catharines General Site; (905)378-4647 x46441; Fax. (905)397-1904.

ASTLE, William F; Alberta Children's Hosp, 2888 Shaganappi Trail NW, Calgary AB T3B 6A8; Cal'79; DAB; FRCSC; Ophth (Pediatric Ophthalmology & Strabismus). Staff Ophth, Alberta Children's Hospital; Prof, University of Calgary; (403)955-7940; Fax. (403)955-7672.

ASTORGA, Maria Fe V; Royal Alexandra Hosp, 6F 6408-10240 Kingsway NW, Edmonton AB T5H 3V9; UST Manila (Philippines)'92; FRCPC; Psy. Staff, Royal Alexandra Hospital; (780)735-4567; Fax. (780)735-4797.

ASTREIN, Alexey; Langley Mem Hosp, 22051 Fraser Hwy, Langley BC V3A 4H4; Novgorod (Russia (Federation))'84; Staff, Langley Memorial Hospital; (604)534-4121

ASTROPE, Valerie J; St Joseph's Gen Hosp, 2137 Comox Ave, Comox BC V9M 1P2; UBC'99; FRCPC; DiagRad. Staff, St Joseph's General Hospital; (250)339-1423

ASWALD, Jorg M; Springbank Med Centre, 210-460 Springbank Dr, London ON N6J 0A8; Munster (Germany),'07; MD; MSc; FRCPC; IntMed. (519)641-2102; Fax. (519)641-2103; drjorgaswald@sympatico.ca.

ASZTALOS, Elizabeth D V; Sunnybrook Hlth Sciences Ctre, M4 230-2075 Bayview Ave, Toronto ON M4N 3M5; Tor'84; FRCPC; Peds (Neonatology). Staff, Sunnybrook Health Sciences Centre; Staff, Women's College Hospital; (416)480-6100; elizabeth.asztalos@sunnybrook.ca.

ATACK, D Barry; Newmarket Med Place, 310-712 Davis Dr, Newmarket ON L3Y 8C3; Wes'82; FRCSC; ObstGyn. Staff Gyn, Alexandra Hospital; Staff Gyn, Tillsonburg District Memorial Hospital; Staff ObstGyn, Stratford General Hospital - Huron Perth Healthcare Alliance; (905)967-1249

ATACK, David M; 5795 Martin St N PO Box 1375, Almonte ON K0A 1A0; Ott'72; FRCPC; Neur (Nerve Conduction Studies). Consultant, Almonte General Hospital; Consultant, Carleton Place & District Memorial Hospital; Consultant, Arnprior & District Memorial Hospital; Consultant, The Ottawa Hospital - Civic Campus; (613)256-0219; Fax. (613)256-1308; satack@sympatico.ca.

ATAELLAHI, Mobin; Charlotte County Hosp, 4 Garden St, St Stephen NB E3L 2L9; (Other Foreign)'99; Staff, Charlotte County Hospital; (506)465-4485

ATALLA, Maher G Y; Conestoga Med Centre, 26-380 Bovaird Dr E, Brampton ON L6Z 2S8; Ain Shams (Egypt)'91; MB ChB; CCFP; Langs: Arabic; (905)840-3900; Fax. (905)840-3912; maheratalla@yahoo.ca.

ATALLA, Niveen; Selkirk Med Centre, 353 Eveline St, Selkirk MB R1A 1N1; (Other Foreign)'94.

ATALLA, Soheir; Centre Medical Mira, 1560 boul de Rome, Brossard QC J4W 3A1; Cairo (Egypt)'74; BSc; Langs: Arabic; French; (450)466-1880; Fax. (450)466-4884.

ATALLAH, Joseph; University of Alberta Hosp, 4C2.32-8440 112 St NW, Edmonton AB T6G 2B7; McG'01; MSc; MDCM; FRCPC; Peds (Pediatric Cardiology); Cardiol. Staff, University of Alberta Hospital; (780)407-3963; Fax. (780)407-3954.

ATAMNA, Chahinez; Ctr Hosp Chauveau, 11999 rue de l'Hopital, Quebec QC G2A 2T7; (Algeria)'90; Gen Practice, Centre Hospitalier Chauveau; (418)842-3651; Fax. (418)842-8931.

ATAPATTU, Vidura I; North Bay Reg Health Centre, 50 College Dr, North Bay ON P1B 5A4; Doneck Medical University (Other Foreign)'98; CCFP; (705)474-8600

ATCHA, Farida; William Osler HC-Brampton, 2100 Bovaird Dr E, Brampton ON L6R 3J7; Santo Domingo (Dominican Republic)'98; CCFP; Staff, William Osler Health System - Brampton Civic Hospital; (905)494-2120; Fax. (905)494-2120.

ATCHISON, Amy; 326-1175 Cook St, Victoria BC V8V 4A1; Sask'06; CCFP; (250)386-2449

ATCHISON, Katherine E; 210-4320 50 Ave, Red Deer AB T4N 3Z6; Sask'92; CCFP; FCFP; (403)346-5833; Fax. (403)346-5832.

ATEER, Khaled A; 15345 97 St NW, Edmonton AB T5X 5V3; (Libya)'01; MB BCh; Langs: Arabic; (780)457-6060; Fax. (780)457-6111.

ATEYAH, Wameed; Schomberg Med Centre, 12-17250 Highway 27, Schomberg ON L0G 1T0; Baghdad (Iraq)'94; CCFP; (905)939-4600

ATHAIDE, Gregory O; Whitby Med Arts Centre, 16-1615 Dundas St E, Whitby ON L1N 2L1; McM'04; FRCSC; ObstGyn. Staff, Lakeridge Health - Oshawa Site; (905)231-1555; Fax. (905)576-1234.

ATHAIDE, Sylvia B; 495-5 Fairview Mall Dr, North York ON M2J 2Z1; Punjab (Pakistan)'69; BSc(Microbiol); MB BS; Staff, North York General Hospital; Physician WSIB Assessment, Sunnybrook Health Sciences Centre; Staff N E L Assesment, Workers' Comp Board of ON; Physician, Medical Council of Canada Examination Board; Langs: Urdu; Concani; (416)496-0305; Fax. (416)496-3392.

ATHALE, Uma H; McMaster University, HSC 3N27-1280 Main St W, Hamilton ON L8S 4K1; Bombay (India)'84; FRCPC; Peds (Pediatric Hematology Oncology). Fellow, Hamilton Health Sciences Centre - McMaster University Medical Centre; Assoc Prof, McMaster University; (905)521-2100 x73428

ATHAR, Humera; Off Site Adolescent Clinic, 3640 Wells St, Windsor ON N9C 1T9; Punjab (Pakistan)'94; Staff, Hôtel-Dieu Grace Hospital; Staff, Windsor Regional Hospital - Metropolitan Site; Staff, Windsor Regional Hospital - Tayfour Site; (519)258-0484; Fax. (519)258-0488; hatgarmd@yahoo.com.

ATHAR, Saira; Fredericton Med Clinic, 509-1015 Regent St, Fredericton NB E3B 6H5; Dal'03; BSc; CCFP; (506)472-7141; Fax. (506)472-7503.

ATHAYDE, Jitendra I; The Credit Valley Hosp, 2200 Eglinton Ave W, Mississauga ON L5M 2N1; Bangalore (India)'86; FRCPC; Anes. Staff, The Credit Valley Hospital; (905)813-2220

ATHERSTONE, Juliet A; Vancouver Gen Hosp, 855 12th Ave W, Vancouver BC V5Z 1M9; UBC'03; FRCPC; Anes. Staff, Vancouver General Hospital - Centennial Pavillion; (604)875-4111

ATHERSTONE, Michael J; 1811 Crescent Rd, Victoria BC V8S 2G7; UBC'07; Anes. (778)265-1981

ATHERTON, Francis; Dept of Health and Wellness, PO Box 488 Stn Central, Halifax NS B3J 2R8; Leeds (England)'82; MB ChB; (902)424-2358; Fax. (902)424-4716.

ATHERTON, William; Holly Street Endoscopy Clinic, 301-40 Holly St, Toronto ON M4S 3C3; Alb'69; FRCSC; GenSurg (Colonoscopy); VascSurg. Staff Surg, Rudd Clinic; (416)486-8088; Fax. (416)486-7888.

ATHEY, Robert A; Streetsville Med Centre, 8-5425 Creditview Rd, Mississauga ON L5V 2P3; Tor'89; Ac Staff, The Credit Valley Hospital; (905)826-1164; Fax. (905)826-1214; robathey@rogers.com.

ATHREYA, Sriharsha; St Joseph's Healthcare, T0112-50 Charlton Ave E, Hamilton ON L8N 4A6; Mysore (India)'96; Staff, St Joseph's Healthcare - Charlton Campus; (905)522-1155

ATHWAL, Bali; Health Gate Medical, 13446 108 Ave, Surrey BC V3T 2K1; Qns'96; (604)583-6364

ATHWAL, George G S; St Joseph's Health Care, PO Box 5777 Stn B DO 205-268 Grosvenor St, London ON N6A 4V2; UBC'98; FRCSC; OrthSurg. Staff, London Health Sciences Centre - Victoria Campus; Staff, London Health Sciences Centre - University Hospital; Staff Hand & Upper Limb Centre, St Joseph's Hospital - St Joseph's Health Care; Staff, London Health Sciences Centre - South Street; (519)646-6081

ATIA, John N A; Amherst Family Health Clinic, 800-158 Robert Angus Dr, Amherst NS B4H 4R7; Cairo (Egypt)'89; MB BCh; (902)667-3330; Fax. (902)661-3411.

ATIF, Rabia; Healthsense, 2983 Westoak Trail Blvd, Oakville ON L6M 5E4; (Other Foreign)'01; CCFP.

ATIN, Mark D; The Endoscopy Clinic, 230-340 College St, Toronto ON M5T 3A9; Tor'83; BSc; FRCPC; IntMed (Gastroenterology). Staff Consultant, Toronto Western Hospital - University Health Network; (416)964-3457; Fax. (416)964-9241; drmarkd@bellnet.ca.

ATIYABI, Haleh; Medistat Med Familiale, 4965 rue Saint-Pierre, Pierrefonds QC H9H 5M9; Tehran (Iran)'97; CCFP; (514)624-4774

ATIYAH, Abdulrazzak O; New Waterford Consol Hosp, 716 King St, New Waterford NS B1H 3Z5; Dal'93; BSc; FRCSC; PlasSurg. Staff, New Waterford Consolidated Hospital; Staff, Cape Breton Healthcare Complex; Langs: Arabic; (902)862-7212; Fax. (902)862-9411; atiyah@eastlink.ca.

ATKINS, Barbara R; Penticton Health Care Centre, 740 Carmi Ave, Penticton BC V2A 8P9; UBC'86; (250)770-3434

ATKINS, Edward J; Eye Care Centre, 701 Queen St, Saskatoon SK S7K 0M7; McM'03; BScN; FRCPC; Neur (Neuro Ophthalmology). (306)655-8000; Fax. (306)655-8119; edward.atkins@usask.ca.

ATKINS, Harold L; The Ottawa Hosp-Gen Campus, 501 Smyth Rd, Ottawa ON K1H 8L6; Ott'83; FRCPC; IntMed (Bone Marrow Transplant). Staff, The Ottawa Hospital - General Campus; Assoc Prof, University of Ottawa; (613)737-7700 x70341; hatkins@toh.on.ca.

ATKINS, James A; MedEmerg Inc, 9-6400 Millcreek Dr, Mississauga ON L5N 3E7; UBC'81; CCFP; CCFP(E.M.); FCFP; Langs: Bilingual(English/French); (905)858-1368; jatkins@telus.net.

ATKINS, Kenneth W; 3 Geneva St, St Catharines ON L2R 4M2; Qns'99; (905)323-9765; Fax. (905)685-3247.

ATKINS, Mark H; 1625 Fort St PO Box 5639, Victoria BC V8R 4S6; UBC'97; FRCPC; Psy. (250)507-5930

ATKINSON, Adelle R; The Hosp For Sick Children, 555 University Ave, Toronto ON M5G 1X8; McM'94; BSc; FRCPC; Peds (Bone Marrow Transplant); ClinImmunol&Allergy. Staff Immunology & Bone Marrow Transplant, The Hospital For Sick Children; (416)813-8626; Fax. (416)813-8638.

ATKINSON, Anthony R; Medical Arts Bldg, 302-42 Glen Allan Dr, Bridgewater NS B4V 3N2; London (England)'75; FCCP; FRC; MA; FRCPC; IntMed (Respirology). Internal Med, South Shore Regional Hospital; Consultant, Fishermen's Memorial Hospital; Consultant, Queens General Hospital; Ac Staff, Nova Scotia Cancer Center; (902)543-8121; Fax. (902)543-6028; anthony.atkinson@cdha.nshealth.ca.

ATKINSON, Bradley C; PO Box 187, Sheet Harbour NS B0J 3B0; (Wales)'91; MB ChB; Med Pres, Eastern Shore Memorial Hospital; (902)885-2298; Fax. (902)885-3210.

ATKINSON, Carla M; 104-5 Richard Way SW, Calgary AB T3E 7M8; Cal'85; FRCPC; Psy (Anxiety Disorder). Staff, Alberta Children's Hospital; (403)240-1188

ATKINSON, Carolyn R; Canadian Med Protective Assoc, PO Box 8225 Stn T 875 Carling Ave, Ottawa ON K1G 3H7; McM'96; CCFP; Staff, Canadian Medical Protective Association; (613)725-2000; carolyn.atkinson@cha.nshealth.ca.

ATKINSON, Celia N; Toronto East Gen Hosp Inc, 825 Coxwell Ave, Toronto ON M4C 3E7; Tor'04; BSc; MSc; PhD; FRCPC; Peds. Staff, Toronto East General Hospital Inc; Staff, The Hospital For Sick Children; (416)461-8272; Fax. (416)469-6618.

ATKINSON, Christina M; Medicine in Motion Med Centre, 5-121 Ilsley Ave, Dartmouth NS B3B 1S4; Dal'95; CCFP; Staff, Medicine in Motion Medical Centre; (902)468-2774; Fax. (902)468-1359.

ATKINSON, David I; Children's After Hours Clinic, 101 Fanshawe Park Rd E, London ON N5X 3V9; Wes'65; AB; FRCPC; Peds (Clinical Immunology & Allergy). Staff, St Thomas Elgin General Hospital; (519)850-3800

ATKINSON, Donald H; Orillia Soldiers Mem Hosp, 170 Colborne St W, Orillia ON L3V 2Z3; Wes'76; BSc; CCFP; Staff, Orillia Soldiers' Memorial Hospital; (705)325-2201 x3480; dhatkinson@osmh.on.ca.

ATKINSON, Elaine L; 204-282 Linwell Rd, St. Catharines ON L2N 6N5; Ott'91; BSc; CCFP; FCFP; Court Staff, Niagara Health System - Ontario Street Site; Court Staff, Niagara Health System - St Catharines General Site; Clinical Asst Prof, McMaster University; (905)937-8888; Fax. (905)937-7889.

ATKINSON, Jeffrey D; MUHC-Montreal Children's Hosp, C1137-2300 rue Tupper, Montreal QC H3H 1P3; Tor'94; FRCSC; Neursurg (Pediatric Neuro Surgery). Staff, McGill University Health Centre - Montreal Children's Hospital; (514)412-4400 x25224; jeffrey.atkinson@muhc.mcgill.ca.

ATKINSON, Joan M; 33 Church St S, Ajax ON L1S 6A6; Tor'59; Staff, Rouge Valley Health System - Ajax & Pickering Health Centre Site; (905)683-0200; Fax. (905)683-0636; jmatkinson45@yahoo.ca.

ATKINSON, Kathryn J; Business Bldg, 510-1200 Burrard St, Vancouver BC V6Z 2C7; UBC'88; CCFP; (604)687-3387; Fax. (604)687-2015.

ATKINSON, Kenneth A; Columbia Med Bldg, 410-301 Columbia St E, New Westminster BC V3L 3W5; Ott'92; BSc; FRCPC; IntMed; Gastroent. Staff, Royal Columbian Hospital; Staff, Eagle Ridge Hospital & Health Care Centre; Langs: English; French; (604)525-0155; Fax. (604)525-1699; drkatkinson@public.medi.net.

ATKINSON, Martin H; 2025 Palermo Way SW, Calgary AB T2V 5J6; Alb'64; MSc(ClinMed); FACP; FRCPC; IntMed; Rheum. (403)281-7122; Fax. (403)281-7124.

ATKINSON, Mary L; Thunder Bay District Hlth Unit, 999 Balmoral St, Thunder Bay ON P7B 6E7; Ott'74; CCFP; FCFP; Staff, Thunder Bay Regional Health Sciences Centre; Staff, Nipigon District Memorial Hospital; (807)625-5940; matkinson@ndmh.ca.

ATKINSON, Paul R; Saint John Reg Hosp, PO Box 2100 Stn Main 400 University Ave, Saint John NB E2L 4L2; Belfast (Ireland)'95; Staff, Saint John Regional Hospital; (506)648-6000

ATKINSON, Susan M; Dalhousie Fam Med Mumford Clin, 0265-6960 Mumford Rd, Halifax NS B3L 4P1; Dal'90; BSc(Hons)(Psychol); CCFP; FCFP; Staff, Queen Elizabeth II Health Sciences Centre - Victoria General Site; Court Staff, IWK Health Centre; Clin Instructor, Dalhousie University; (902)473-4700; satkinso@dal.ca.

ATKINSON, Victoria E; The Richmond Hosp, 7000 Westminster Hwy, Richmond BC V6X 1A2; Tor'01; FRCPC; Peds. Staff, Richmond Hospital; (604)244-5183

ATKISON, Paul R; London HSC-Victoria Hosp, PO Box 5010 Stn B B1 160-800 Commissioners Rd E, London ON N6A 5W9; Cal'84; MSc; PhD; FRCPC; Peds (Diabetology). Dir Peds Transplant Program, London Health Sciences Centre - Victoria Campus; Assoc Prof Peds, University of Western Ontario; (519)685-8354; Fax. (519)685-8105; paul.atkison@lhsc.on.ca.

ATLAS, Henri; 100-100 ch Rockland, Mont-Royal QC H3P 2V9; Louvain (Belgium)'61; FRCSC; GenSurg (Trauma). Court Staff, Hôpital du Sacre-Coeur de Montréal; Langs: English; (514)331-4322; Fax. (514)331-8683.

ATLAS, Jason T; 250 Lawrence Ave, Toronto ON M5M 1B2; Wes'99; FRCSC; Otol. Staff, Cambridge Memorial Hospital; (416)787-4333

ATMURI, Nagasree; 104-389 Connell St, Woodstock NB E7M 5G5; Man'03; CCFP; Staff, Upper River Valley Hospital - Waterville.

ATOE, Dennis E; Chatham-Kent Family Health Team, 30 McNaughton Ave, Wallaceburg ON N8A 1R9; St. George's (Grenada)'91; BSc; MD; CCFP; FCFP; Staff, Chatham-Kent Health Alliance - Sydenham Hospital Campus; Aj Prof, University of Western Ontario; (519)627-1497; Fax. (519)627-1071.

ATOUI, Rony; Sudbury Reg Hosp-Mem Site, 131-865 Regent St, Sudbury ON P3E 3Y9; McG'03; FRCSC; CardSurg. Staff, Sudbury Regional Hospital Pharmacy-Memorial Site; (705)671-5353; Fax. (705)671-5352.

ATRENS-SHARKO, Maureen; Kelowna Gen Hosp, 2268 Pandosy St, Kelowna BC V1Y 1T2; Alb'88; BSc; CCFP; CCFP(E.M.); Staff, Kelowna General Hospital; (250)862-4000

ATRI, Mostafa; NCSB 1C-569, 585 University Ave, Toronto ON M5G 2N2; Tehran (Iran)'76; FRCPC; DiagRad. Staff, Mount Sinai Hospital; Staff, Toronto Western Hospital - University Health Network; Staff, Princess Margaret Hospital - University Health Network; Staff, Toronto General Hospital - UHN; Staff, Sunnybrook Health Sciences Centre; (416)340-4800 x3372

ATRIE, Damon; Hamilton HS-General Site, 251-237 Barton St E, Hamilton ON L8L 2X2; McM'09; Staff, Hamilton Health Sciences Centre - Hamilton General Hospital; (905)527-4322

ATTA, Imran; Clinicare Walk In Clinic, 844 Wonderland Rd S, London ON N6K 2V8; Multan (Pakistan)'84; CCFP; (519)471-1801; Fax. (519)471-1800.

ATTABIB, Najmedden A; Saint John Reg Hosp, PO Box 2100 Stn Main 400 University Ave, Saint John NB E2L 4L2; Al-Fateh (Libya)'94; FRCSC; Neursurg (Spine Surgery). Staff, Saint John Regional Hospital; Asst Prof, Dalhousie University; (506)648-6650; Fax. (506)648-6649.

ATTALLA, Amany A Y; Two Rivers FHT-Hespeler Med Cl, B12-350 Conestoga Blvd, Cambridge ON N1R 7L7; Cairo (Egypt)'85; MB ChB; CCFP; FCFP; Staff, Cambridge Memorial Hospital; Langs: Arabic; French; (519)629-4615; amyadel@hotmail.com.

ATTALLA, Hani F; Kirillos Walk-In Clinic, 13B-2458 Dundas St W, Mississauga ON L5K 1R8; Alexandria (Egypt)'79; CCFP; (905)822-2364; Fax. (905)822-0367.

ATTALLA, Mireille G; Dixie Road Med Associates, 2200 Dixie Rd, Mississauga ON L4Y 1Z4; Ain Shams (Egypt)'93; CCFP; (905)279-1700

ATTALLA, Mona S G; 1B-7955 Financial Dr, Brampton ON L6Y 0J8; Alexandria (Egypt)'89; CCFP; (905)455-8877

ATTALLAH, Gabriel N; 187 Queenston St, St Catharines ON L2R 3A3; Man'95; CCFP; (905)688-5125

ATTARD, Jo-Anne P; Saint John Reg Hosp, PO Box 2100 Stn Main 400 University Ave, Saint John NB E2L 4L2; Cal'99; BSc; FRCSC; GenSurg (Colon & Rectal Surgery). Staff, Saint John Regional Hospital; Asst Prof Surg, Dalhousie University; (506)649-2613; Fax. (506)648-7925.

ATTARIWALA, Rajpaul; AIM Medical Imaging, 1371 Broadway W, Vancouver BC V6H 1G9; Cal'98; FRCPC; DiagRad; NuclearMed. Staff, Providence Health Care - St Paul's Hospital.

ATTERSLEY, Edward M; North York Med Clinic, 303-2175 Sheppard Ave E, North York ON M2J 1W8; Tor'67; Ac Staff, North York General Hospital; Court Staff Privil, The Scarborough Hospital - General Campus; (416)492-7700; Fax. (416)492-5776; atter@rogers.com.

ATTIA, Amine N; Credit River Med Clinic, A02-6085 Creditview Rd, Mississauga ON L5V 2A8; Ain Shams (Egypt)'78; CCFP; Langs: Arabic; (905)826-6095; Fax. (905)826-9219.

ATTIA, Elham B; 5-3955 Erin Centre Blvd, Mississauga ON L5M 0H1; Assiut (Egypt)'94; CCFP; (905)607-4007

ATTIA, Tammy; 4-1230 Alward St, Prince George BC V2M 7B1; Dal'01; MCFP; CCFP; (250)564-8513; Fax. (250)564-8526; tattia01@hotmail.com.

ATTIA-ALLA, Ayman; Campbellton Reg Hosp, PO Box 880 189 Lily Lake Rd, Campbellton NB E3N 3H3; Ain Shams (Egypt)'92; Staff, Hôpital Régional Campbellton; (506)789-5000

ATTIA-GALAND, Samia; Ctr Hosp Pierre-Janet, 20 rue Pharand, Gatineau QC J9A 1K7; Paris (France)'74; FRCPC; Psy (P.Q.). Staff Psy, Centre Hospitalier Pierre-Janet; Assoc Prof Psy, University of Ottawa; Assoc Prof Psy, Universite de Montreal; Langs: Arabic; English; (819)771-7761 x8066; Fax. (819)776-8048.

ATTIE, Catherine; U of Ottawa Health Services, 300-100 Marie Curie Pvt, Ottawa ON K1N 6N5; Mon'91; ObstGyn. Staff, The Ottawa Hospital - General Campus; (613)564-3950; Fax. (613)564-0046.

ATTIE, Nabil; Clinique Medicale Viau, 4750 rue Jarry E, Saint-Leonard QC H1R 1X8; St. Joseph (Lebanon)'71; FRCPC; Rheum. Langs: Arabic; (514)326-7203; Fax. (514)326-3656.

ATTIG, Ezzedine; CSSS de Rivière-du-Loup, 75 rue Saint-Henri, Riviere-du-Loup QC G5R 2A4; (Belgium)'82; MSc; MD; CSPQ; FRCPC; Neur (Neuro Physiology). Staff, Centre Hospitalier Regional du Grand-Portage; Langs: Arabic; Belgian; English; (418)868-1010; Fax. (418)868-1059; eattig@bellnet.ca.

ATTIGNON, Ablavi S H N; GMF Coop Sante Aylmer, 67 rue du Couvent, Gatineau QC J9H 6A2; (819)687-5397

ATTISHA, Reneen F; Hamilton Care Medical & Dental, 11-969 Upper Ottawa St, Hamilton ON L8T 4V9; Baghdad (Iraq)'93; (289)755-3296; Fax. (289)755-3297.

ATTON, A Lance; Hotel-Dieu Grace Hosp, 1030 Ouellette Ave, Windsor ON N9A 1E1; Sask'87; Ac Staff Emerg, Hôtel-Dieu Grace Hospital; Ac Staff Emerg, Windsor Regional Hospital - Metropolitan Site; Physician, Canadian Armed Forces; (519)973-4401

ATTUAH, Kwame; Advanced Walk-In Med Clinic, 111-21 Queensway Blvd W, Mississauga ON L5B 1B6; (Ghana)'75; MB ChB; FRCSC; ObstGyn. Staff, Niagara Health System - Douglas Memorial Hospital Site; Staff, Niagara Health System - Welland Hospital Site; Staff, Niagara Health System - Port Colborne General Site; (905)897-0788

ATTWELL, A David; Jubilee Centre, 1823 Fort St, Victoria BC V8R 1J6; UBC'92; BSc; Ac Staff, Vancouver Island Health Authority; Ac Staff, Aberdeen Hospital; (250)592-6226; Fax. (250)592-2248.

ATTWELL, Andrew J; BC Cancer Agency-Vanc Isl Ctr, 2410 Lee Ave, Victoria BC V8R 6V5; McG'98; FRCPC; IntMed; MedOncol. Staff, BC Cancer Agency Vancouver Island Centre; (250)519-5571; Fax. (250)519-5590.

ATTWELL, Kristen A; 2587 Penrhyn St, Victoria BC V8N 1G4; UBC'98; FRCPC; Neur. (250)380-2545

ATTWOOD, David G; Royal Ottawa Hlth Care Group, 3F-1145 Carling Ave, Ottawa ON K1Z 7K4; Mem'94; FRCPC; Psy (Intensive Care). Staff, Royal Ottawa Mental Health Centre - Royal Ottawa Health Care Group; (613)722-6521

ATTWOOD, Zachary P; Bay St George Medical Clinic, 127 Montana Dr, Stephenville NL A2N 2T4; Mem'10; CCFP.

ATTYE, Aly; Clinique Med le Plein-Ciel, 475 boul de la Cote-Vertu, Saint-Laurent QC H4L 1X7; Dakar (Mauritius)'84; FRCPC; Peds. Staff, Centre Hospitalier Pierre le Gardeur; Staff Neonatol, Hôpital du Sacre-Coeur de Montréal; (514)337-3171; Fax. (514)337-6023.

ATWAL, Gulshandeep S; Southlake Reg Health Centre, 596 Davis Dr, Newmarket ON L3Y 2P9; St Petersburg (Russia (Federation))'00; FRCPC; IntMed. Staff, Southlake Regional Health Centre; (905)895-4521 x4521; gulshanatwal@gmail.com.

ATWAL, Jasdeep; Assiniboine Clinic, 633 Lodge Ave, Winnipeg MB R3J 0S9; Man'00; CCFP.

ATWAL, Kanwaldip S; Bathurst Walk-In Clinic, 101-4430 Bathurst St, North York ON M3H 3S3; Man'95; BSc(Hons); CCFP; CCFP(E.M.); Ac Staff, Toronto Western Hospital - University Health Network; Ac Staff, Toronto General Hospital - UHN; (416)633-3629; Fax. (416)633-3624.

ATWAL, Rajinder K; Bathurst Walk-In Clinic, 101-4430 Bathurst St, North York ON M3H 3S3; Cal'94; CCFP; Langs: Punjabi; (416)633-3629; Fax. (416)633-3624.

ATWAL, Sanita; 1 Field Ambulance Clinic, PO Box 10500 Stn Forces, Edmonton AB T5J 4J5; Alb'98; FRCSC; GenSurg (Sports Medicine). Langs: English; French; (780)973-4011

ATWOOD, Jennifer A; Fort William Clinic, 117 McKellar St S, Thunder Bay ON P7E 1H5; Ott'02; CCFP; Staff, Thunder Bay Regional Health Sciences Centre; Langs: Bilingual(English/French); (807)626-1256

ATWOOD, Lenisa J; Hotel-Dieu Grace Hosp, 1030 Ouellette Ave, Windsor ON N9A 1E1; Qns'98; CCFP; CCFP(E.M.); Staff, Hôtel-Dieu Grace Hospital; (519)973-4411

ATZEMA, Clare L; Sunnybrook Hlth Sciences Ctre, C753-2075 Bayview Ave, Toronto ON M4N 3M5; UBC'00; FRCPC; EmergMed. Staff, Sunnybrook Health Sciences Centre; (416)480-4037; Fax. (416)480-4704.

AU, Ambrose S S; Cornerstone Family Med Centre, 106-100 Strowger Blvd, Brockville ON K6V 5J9; Wes'95; BSc; MSc; CCFP; FCFP; Assoc Staff, Brockville General Hospital - Charles Street; Assoc Staff, Providence Continuing Care Centre (PCCC) - St Vincent de Paul Hospital; Physician, 3M Canada Company; Physician Occup Med, Invista Canada; Langs: Cantonese; (613)498-0444; Fax. (613)498-4850; ambroseaumd@gmail.com.

AU, Anita G; Wetaskiwin Lung Laboratory, 5217A 50 St, Wetaskiwin AB T9A 3B8; Alb'07; FRCPC; IntMed. (780)352-7085; Fax. (780)352-7870.

AU, Bryan L; St Michael's Hosp, 30 Bond St, Toronto ON M5B 1W8; Tor'97; FRCPC; EmergMed. Staff, St Michael's Hospital; (416)864-5095; Fax. (416)864-5341.

AU, Calvin L; UBC-Dept of Anes, JPP2 2449-910 10th Ave W, Vancouver BC V5Z 1M9; Ott'94; FRCPC; Anes. Head Vascular Anes, Vancouver General Hospital - Centennial Pavillion; Clinical Asst Prof, University of British Columbia; (604)875-4304

AU, Chi-Cheong; Haig Clinic, 601 6 Ave S, Lethbridge AB T1J 0Z2; (Taiwan)'61; FRCPC; IntMed (Hematology). Hematology, Chinook Regional Hospital; (403)328-6641; Fax. (403)328-6118.

AU, Daniel T S; 820 Dundas St W, Toronto ON M6J 1V3; Shanghai (China (Republic))'60; (416)603-9853; Fax. (416)603-9853.

AU, Dick; Misericordia Community Hosp, 16940 87 Ave NW, Edmonton AB T5R 4H5; Alb'91; FRCPC; IntMed. Staff, Covenant Health - Misericordia Community Hospital; (780)735-2611; Fax. (780)735-2930.

AU, Heather-Jane; Cross Cancer Institute, 11560 University Ave NW, Edmonton AB T6G 1Z2; Alb'91; FRCPC; IntMed (Breast Cancer); MedOncol. Staff, Cross Cancer Institute; Asst Prof, University of Alberta; Langs: French; (780)432-8762; Fax. (780)432-8888; heathera@cancerboard.ab.ca.

AU, Hosanna C M; The Hosp for Sick Children, 555 University Ave, Toronto ON M5G 1X8; Tor'01; FRCPC; Peds. Staff, The Hospital For Sick Children; (416)813-6275

AU, How Hoong; Scarborough Prof Centre, 411-1371 Neilson Rd, Scarborough ON M1B 4Z8; London (England)'72; MB BS; FACS; ABS; FRCSC; GenSurg; VascSurg. Staff, Rouge Valley Health System - Centenary Health Centre Site; Langs: Cantonese; (416)282-8391; Fax. (416)282-7406.

AU, Jana B; Health Sciences Centre, 300 Prince Philip Dr, St. John's NL A1B 3V6; Mem'07; CCFP; Staff, Health Sciences Centre; (709)737-6300

AU, Keegan P; 342 Pennywell Rd, St. John's NL A1E 1V9; Mem'03; FRCSC; OrthSurg. Staff, Health Sciences Centre; (709)726-4179

AU, Lillian L C; Dominion Health Centre, 2383 111 St NW, Edmonton AB T6J 5E5; Alb'95; BSc; CCFP; FCFP; (780)436-0020; Fax. (780)436-0603.

AU, Nicholas H; Children's & Women's HC of BC, 2K53-4480 Oak St, Vancouver BC V6H 3V4; UBC'02; FRCPC; HemPath. Staff, BC Children's Hospital; (604)875-2549

AU, Raymond; Richmond Mental Health Team, 200-6061 No. 3 Rd, Richmond BC V6Y 2B2; Alb'98; FRCPC; Psy. Psychiatrist, Richmond Hospital; Clin Instructor, University of British Columbia; (604)273-9121; raymond_t_au@yahoo.com.

AU, Selena S; South Health Campus, 260160-4448 Front St SE, Calgary AB T3M 1M4; UBC'07; FRCPC; IntMed; Critical Care Medicine. (403)956-2401; Fax. (403)956-2995.

AU, Sheila; St Paul's Hosp, 547-1081 Burrard St, Vancouver BC V6Z 1Y6; Ott'94; FRCPC; Peds; Derm. Ac Staff, Providence Health Care - St Paul's Hospital; Consultant Staff, BC Children's Hospital; Consultant staff, Vancouver General Hospital - Centennial Pavillion; (604)806-8735

AU, Stephanie Y P; 118-13798 94A St, Surrey BC V3V 1N1; UBC'06; FRCPC; IntMed; Cardiol. Staff, Foothills Medical Centre; (604)588-8100

AU, Susan J L; 2F-11 King St W Box 6, Toronto ON M5H 4C7; Wes'80; BSc; Court Staff, St Michael's Hospital; Court Staff, Women's College Hospital; (416)864-0727; Fax. (416)864-9742.

AU, W Frederick; NCSB 1C-571, 585 University Ave, Toronto ON M5G 2N2; (Hong Kong)'72; MB BS; ABR; FRCPC; DiagRad. Staff, Toronto General Hospital - UHN; (416)340-3372

AU-YEUNG, Elizabeth J; Toronto East Gen Hosp Inc, 825 Coxwell Ave, Toronto ON M4C 3E7; Wes'04; FRCPC; Anes. Staff, Toronto East General Hospital Inc; (416)461-8272

AUBE, Anne; Beamsville Med Ctr Fam Hlth Team, PO Box 430 4279 Hixon St, Beamsville ON L0R 1B0; Ott'07; CCFP; Staff, West Lincoln Memorial Hospital; Langs: Bilingual(English/French); (905)563-5315

AUBE, Denise; Inst Nat'l de Sante Publique, 5/F-945 av Wolfe, Quebec QC G1V 5B3; Laval'75; FRCPC; CommunMed. Ac Staff, Centre Hospitalier Universitaire de Quebec-CHUL; Teach Staff Social Preventive Med & Commun Med, Université Laval; Langs: English; (418)650-5115 x5603; Fax. (418)654-3210; denise.aube@inspq.qc.ca.

AUBE, Francois; CSSS du Sud de Lanaudière, 911 monte des Pionniers, Terrebonne QC J6V 2H2; Sher'06; DiagRad (P.Q.). Staff, Centre Hospitalier Pierre le Gardeur; (450)654-7525; Fax. (450)470-2640.

AUBE, Gilles; Clinique Medicale du Faubourg, 145-1160 boul Saint-Joseph, Gatineau QC J8Z 1T3; Laval'80; CCFP; ac Staff, Hull Hospital; (819)595-3296; Fax. (819)595-0486.

AUBE, Katherine; Clinique Med Mascouche, 100-1025 Montee Masson, Mascouche QC J7K 2L9; Sher'96; (450)474-6000; Fax. (450)474-6666.

AUBE, Marie-Helene; Centre Hosp Honore-Mercier, 2750 boul Laframboise, Saint-Hyacinthe QC J2S 4Y8; Mon'01; FRCSC; ObstGyn. Staff, Centre Hospitalier Honore-Mercier; (450)771-3333

AUBE, Michel; MUHC-Montreal Neurology Inst, 3801 rue University, Montreal QC H3A 2B4; Mon'69; FRCPC; Neur (Headache); Electroenceph (P.Q.). Associate Neurol, McGill University Health Centre - Montreal Neurological Hospital; Assoc Prof Neurol & NeurSurg, McGill University; Langs: English; (514)398-1911; Fax. (514)398-2745; michelaube@hotmail.com.

AUBE-MAURICE, Joanne; Agence de SSS du Bas-St-Lauren, 288 rue Pierre-Saindon, Rimouski QC G5L 9A8; Laval'06; FRCPC; Public Health & Preventive Med. (418)724-8184

AUBERTIN, Gudrun; Victoria Gen Hosp, 1 Hospital Way, Victoria BC V8Z 6R5; UBC'03; FRCPC; MedGenetics. Staff, Victoria General Hospital; (250)727-4212

AUBIN, Alain; Clinique Med St-Alphonse, 911 Rte 343 RR 1, St-Alphonse-Rodrig QC J0K 1W0; Mon'77; (450)883-2239; Fax. (450)883-3502.

AUBIN, Benoit; CHUM-Hop St-Luc, 1058 rue Saint-Denis, Montreal QC H2X 3J4; Mon'84; DiagRad. Staff, Centre Hospitalier l'Université De Montréal (CHUM) - Hôpital Saint-luc; Universite de Montreal; (514)890-8000 x36400

AUBIN, Christian; CSSS Pierre Boucher, 1333 boul Jacques-Cartier E, Longueuil QC J4M 2A5; Mon'89; CSPQ; Anes. Staff, Centre Hospitalier Pierre Boucher; (450)468-8111; Fax. (450)468-8240.

AUBIN, Dominique; CSSS Haut-Richelieu-Rouville, 920 boul Du Seminaire N, St-Jean-Sur-Richel QC J3A 1B7; Mon'91; ObstGyn. Staff Gynecology Clinic, Hôpital du Haut-Richelieu; Langs: English; (450)348-1171; Fax. (450)348-1172.

AUBIN, Donald; 930 rue Jacques-Cartier E, Chicoutimi QC G7H 7K9; Laval'86; Staff Emerg, CHSLD-CLSC Cleophas-Claveau; (418)545-4980 x309; Fax. (418)549-9710; donald.aubin@ssss.gouv.qc.ca.

AUBIN, Emmanuelle; CLSC Mercier-Est-Anjou, 9503 rue Sherbrooke E, Montreal QC H1L 6P2; Mon'09; CCFP; (514)356-2572

AUBIN, Fanny; 5-1968 boul Portobello, Orleans ON K4A 4E7; Sher'00; FRCSC; ObstGyn. Staff, Montfort Hospital; (613)837-7033; Fax. (613)837-5781.

AUBIN, Francine; CHUM-Hop Notre-Dame, 1560 rue Sherbrooke E, Montreal QC H2L 4M1; Mon'02; FRCPC; IntMed; MedOncol; Hem. Staff, Centre Hospitalier l'Université de Montréal (CHUM) - Hôpital Notre-Dame; (514)890-8000

AUBIN, Francois; Ctr Hosp Affilie-Enfant-Jesus, 1401 18e rue, Quebec QC G1J 1Z4; Laval'88; Staff, Centre Hospitalier Affilié Universitaire de Québec - Hôpital du St-Sacrement; Staff, Centre Hospitalier Affilié Universitaire de Québec - Hôpital De L'Enfant Jésus; (418)649-0252; francoisaubin57@hotmail.com.

AUBIN, Genevieve; Clinique Ped des Mille-Iles, 203-233 rue Turgeon, Sainte-Therese QC J7E 3J8; Sher'94; Peds. Staff, Hôpital de Saint-Eustache; Langs: Bilingual(French/English); (450)434-8006; ginogene@videotron.ca.

AUBIN, Linda; Polyclinique St-Eustache, 75 rue Grignon, St-Eustache QC J7P 4J2; Sher'84; CCFP; (450)473-6882; Fax. (450)473-1916.

AUBIN, Lydia; Centre Med Saint-Francois, 200-2125 boul Lemire, Drummondville QC J2B 8N8; Sher'06; CCFP; (819)477-6793

AUBIN, M Susan L; Riverside Prof Centre, 410-1919 Riverside Dr, Ottawa ON K1H 1A2; Qns'92; BScChemEng; FRCSC; ObstGyn (Colposcopy). Ac Staff, The Ottawa Hospital - Riverside Campus; Ac Staff, The Ottawa Hospital - Civic Campus; Asst Prof Fac of Med, University of Ottawa; Langs: German; (613)733-4411; Fax. (613)733-3990.

AUBIN, Marie; Clinique Med Monteuil, 200-4650 boul des Laurentides, Laval QC H7K 2J4; Mon'84; (450)628-8717; Fax. (450)628-5305.

AUBIN, Marie-Josee; Hop Maisonneuve-Rosemont, 5415 boul de l'Assomption, Montreal QC H1T 2M4; McG'93; FRCSC; Ophth. Staff, Hopital Maisonneuve-Rosemont; (514)252-3400 x1733; Fax. (514)252-3905.

AUBIN, Mario; CSSS Les Eskers de l'Abitibi, 622 4e rue O, Amos QC J9T 2S2; Mon'02; FRCSC; OrthSurg. Staff, CH Hôtel-Dieu d'Amos; (819)732-3341

AUBIN, Michele; UMF Laval, 2690 ch des Quatre-Bourgeois, Quebec QC G1V 0B7; Laval'80; MSc(Epidemiol.); PhD(Epidemiol); CCFP; FCFP; Staff Family Med & Research, Institut Universitaire Cardiologie & Pneumologie de Quebec; Prof, Université Laval; Langs: English; (418)656-4795; Fax. (418)656-4503.

AUBIN, Patrice; Ctr Hosp Trois-Riv-St-Joseph, 731 rue Sainte-Julie, Trois-Rivieres QC G9A 1Y1; Mon'95; CSPQ; FRCPC; Anes. Staff, Centre Hospitalier Regional de Trois-Rivieres; (819)697-3333

AUBIN, Philippe; Les Toubibs de la Baie, RR 2 427 boul Perron, Maria QC G0C 1Y0; Mon'91; CCFP; FCFP; Staff, CSSS de la Baie-des-Chaleurs; Langs: Bilingual(French/English); (418)759-5223; toubibs@globetrotter.net.

AUBIN, Raymond F; Orleans Urgent Care Clinic, 1220 Place D'Orleans Dr, Orleans ON K1C 7K3; Ott'75; MCFP(EM); (613)841-5389

AUBIN, Richard; 200-8 Place du Commerce, Verdun QC H3E 1N3; Laval'78; Langs: English; Spanish; (514)798-2228; Fax. (514)787-1929; aubin.r@videotron.ca.

AUBIN, Stephane; CSSS Haut-Richelieu-Rouville, 920 boul Du Seminaire N, St-Jean-Sur-Richel QC J3A 1B7; Mon'85; Staff, Hôpital du Haut-Richelieu; (450)359-5176; Fax. (450)359-5145.

AUBIN, Sylvie; Hop Jeffery Hale, 1250 ch Sainte-Foy, Quebec QC G1S 2M6; Laval'96; Staff, Jeffery Hale Hospital-Saint Brigid's; (418)683-4471

AUBIN, Yvan; 2041 rue de Lauzanne, Val-David QC J0T 2N0; Mon'67; FACOG; DAB; ObstGyn. assoc Membre, CSSS de la Vallée de la Gatineau; (819)326-5643

AUBREE, Nicolas; CSSS du Nord de Lanaudière, 1000 boul Sainte-Anne, St-Charles-Brromee QC J6E 6J2; Mon'96; FRCSC; GenSurg (Vascular Surgery). Staff, Centre Hospitalier Régional de Lanaudière; (450)759-8222

AUBREY, Michael E; Dixon Med Centre, 307-531 Davis Dr, Newmarket ON L3Y 6P5; McG'81; FRCPC; IntMed; Rheum. Ac Staff, Southlake Regional Health Centre; (905)853-1843; Fax. (905)853-1863.

AUBREY-BASSLER, Christine M; Family Medicine Clinic, 17-141 Torbay Rd, St. John's NL A1A 2H1; Mem'00; CCFP.

AUBREY-BASSLER, F Kris; Health Sciences Centre, 1772-300 Prince Philip Dr, St. John's NL A1B 3V6; Ott'01; MSc; CCFP; CCFP(E.M.); Staff, Health Sciences Centre; Langs: English; French; (709)777-8373; Fax. (709)777-6118; krisaubrey@canada.com.

AUBRY, Jean R; 1209 Cassells St, North Bay ON P1B 4B8; Ott'75; CAFCI; CCFP; Langs: English; French; (705)840-1212; Fax. (705)840-6903.

AUBRY, Joan; 204-1919 Riverside Dr, Ottawa ON K1H 1A2; McG'88; ObstGyn. (613)260-2684

AUBRY, Mark J; 220-214 boul de la Cite-des-Je, Gatineau QC J8Y 6S8; Ott'78; (819)772-9111

AUBRY, Martine; 102-39 rue Laurier E, Victoriaville QC G6P 6P6; Sher'95; FRCSC; ObstGyn. Langs: English; (819)357-4073; Fax. (819)357-4075.

AUBRY, Sylvain; Clinique Med Soleil, 64 1re Av O, Amos QC J9T 1T8; Mon'80; Staff, CH Hôtel-Dieu d'Amos; (819)732-8341; Fax. (819)732-1642.

AUBUT, Jocelyn; Clinique Globale, 7494 rue Saint-Denis, Montreal QC H2R 2E4; Mon'74; Psy (Biomedical Ethics). Dir gén, Institut Philippe-Pinel de Montreal; Clin Assoc Prof Med, Universite de Montreal; (514)648-8461

AUBUT, Luc; Polyclinique Med de Terrebonne, 201-901 boul des Seigneurs, Terrebonne QC J6W 1T8; Mon'82; (450)471-1117

AUBUT, Nicolas; Dermatogy Centre of Quebec, 105-2880 ch Quatre-Bourgeois, Quebec QC G1V 4X7; Mon'06; FRCPC; Derm (P.Q.). (418)650-3555; Fax. (418)650-1260.

AUBUT, Stephanie; CP 1321, Saint-Quentin NB E8A 1A2; Laval'08; CCFP.

AUCAMP, Marius H; Sterling Centre, 301-3210 25th Ave, Vernon BC V1T 1P1; Stellenbosch (South Africa)'06; MB ChB; Langs: Afrikaans; (306)752-4595; Fax. (306)752-4594.

AUCHINACHIE, Keith T; Medical Arts Bldg, 353 St Paul Ave, Brantford ON N3R 4N3; Aberdeen (Scotland)'70; DRCOG; MRCGPract; Staff, The Brant Community Healthcare System - Brantford General Hospital Site; (519)756-0331; Fax. (519)756-0332.

AUCLAIR, Francois; The Ottawa Hosp-Civic Campus, 1053 Carling Ave, Ottawa ON K1Y 4E9; Sher'79; FRCPC; IntMed. Staff, The Ottawa Hospital - Civic Campus; (613)761-4155; Fax. (613)761-5340; fauclair@ottawahospital.on.ca.

AUCLAIR, Genevieve; Inuulitsivik Health Centre, GD, Povungnituq QC J0M 1P0; Laval'05; CCFP; Staff, Inuulitsivik Health Centre; (819)988-2957

AUCLAIR, Nathalie; Sheldon Chumir Health Ctre, 1213 4 St SW, Calgary AB T2R 0X7; Mon'89; CCFP; FCFP; (403)955-6501

AUCOIN, Andre; 139 Victoria St, Edmundston NB E3V 2H7; Laval'88; LMCC; GenSurg (Digestive Endoscopy). Langs: English; (506)739-7175; Fax. (506)739-8400; 22ucoin@health.nb.ca.

AUCOIN, Colette; Dr Georges-L Dumont Reg Hosp, 330 av Universite, Moncton NB E1C 2Z3; Laval'98; LMCC; FRCPC; Psy (Adult General Psychiatry). Staff, Dr Georges-L-Dumont University Hospital Centre; Langs: Bilingual(French/English); (506)862-4177; Fax. (506)862-4325.

AUCOIN, J Claude; Cheticamp Med Clinic, PO Box 220, Cheticamp NS B0E 1H0; Dal'68; Pres Med Staff, Sacred Heart Hospital; Langs: Bilingual(English/French); (902)224-3110; Fax. (902)224-1905; molly.224@hotmail.ca.

AUCOIN, Jean-Sebastien; CSSS de Trois-Rivieres, 1991 boul du Carmel, Trois-Rivieres QC G8Z 3R9; McG'06; MDCM; MedOncol; Hem; IntMed. Staff, CSSS de Trois-Rivières; (819)697-3333

AUCOIN, Marc; Hôpital de Tracadie-Sheila, CP 3180 Stn Main 400 rue des Hospitalieres, Tracadie-Sheila NB E1X 1G5; Sher'08; CCFP; Staff, Hôpital de Tracadie-Sheila; (506)394-3000

AUCOIN, Marcel D; Cheticamp Med Clinic, PO Box 220, Cheticamp NS B0E 1H0; Sher'94; CCFP; FCFP; Fam Med, Sacred Heart Hospital; Langs: Bilingual(English/French); (902)224-3110; Fax. (902)224-1905.

AUCOIN, Maryse; CHUQ-Ctr Hosp Univ Laval, 2705 boul Laurier, Quebec QC G1V 4G2; Laval'99; CSPQ; Anes. Staff, Centre Hospitalier Universitaire de Quebec-CHUL; (418)525-4444

AUCOIN, Michael W; 1107 37 St SW, Calgary AB T3C 1S5; Dal'08; CCFP; (403)246-7788; Fax. (403)242-8850.

AUCOIN, Nathalie; CSSS de Laval, 1755 boul Rene-Laennec, Laval QC H7M 3L9; Mon'90; FRCPC; IntMed; MedOncol; Hem. Staff, Hopital de la Cite de la santé; (450)668-1010; Fax. (450)975-5044.

AUCOIN, Richard J; Radiology Associates Inc, 1122 Scenic Dr S, Lethbridge AB T1K 7E5; Dal'82; FRCPC; DiagRad; NuclearMed. Staff Radiol & Chief, Chinook Regional Hospital; (403)328-1122; Fax. (403)328-1218.

AUCOIN, Sylvie; The Moncton Hosp, 135 MacBeath Ave, Moncton NB E1C 6Z8; Ott'05; FRCPC; Anes. Staff, The Moncton Hospital; (506)857-5111

AUCOIN SAVOIE, Isabelle; Dr Geroges-L dumont Reg Hosp, 330 av Universite, Moncton NB E1C 2Z3; Sher'06; FRCSC; Ophth. Staff, Dr Georges-L-Dumont University Hospital Centre; (506)862-4000

AUDAIN, Colin V; Queen Elizabeth II HSC, 1276 South Park St, Halifax NS B3H 2Y9; Dal'02; FRCPC; Anes. Staff, Queen Elizabeth II Health Sciences Centre - Victoria General Site; (902)473-7736; Fax. (902)423-9495.

AUDCENT, Tobey A M; Children's Hosp Eastern Ont, 401 Smyth Rd, Ottawa ON K1H 8L1; McM'03; FRCPC; Peds. Staff, Children's Hospital of Eastern Ontario (CHEO); (613)737-7600

AUDELIN, Marie-Chantal; Hôpital Laval, 2725 ch Sainte-Foy, Quebec QC G1V 4G5; Mon'98; FRCPC; Cardiol. Staff, Hôpital Laval; (450)656-8711

AUDET, Alexandra; CSSS de la Matapedia, 135 rue de l'Hopital, Amqui QC G5J 2K5; Sher'10; CCFP; Staff, CSSS de la Matapedia; (418)629-2211

AUDET, Catherine; CSSS de Saint-Jerome, 290 rue de Montigny, Saint-Jerome QC J7Z 5T3; Sher'03; FRCPC; Peds. Pediatrics, Hôtel-Dieu de Saint-Jérôme; (450)431-8200

AUDET, Daniel; Clinique Fam Lac-Saint-Charles, 1514 rue Jacques-Bedard, Quebec QC G3G 3C1; Laval'81; (418)849-7171; Fax. (418)849-7613.

AUDET, Denis; 110-4850 boul Henri-Bourassa, Quebec QC G1H 3A7; Laval'72; Ac Staff, Centre Hospitalier Universitaire De Québec - Pavillon De St-françois-d'assise; (418)661-6959; Fax. (418)661-1016.

AUDET, Helene; Groupe Med de Trois-Rivieres, 225-1900 boul des Recollets, Trois-Rivieres QC G8Z 4K4; Mon'86; (819)373-4551

AUDET, Helene; Centre De L'Osteoporose, 100-1200 av de Germain-des-Pre, Quebec QC G1V 3M7; Laval'87; Langs: English; (418)650-2671; Fax. (418)650-3916.

AUDET, Jean; CHUQ-Hotel-Dieu de Quebec, 11 Cote Du Palais, Quebec QC G1R 2J6; Laval'75; CSPQ; Cardiol (P.Q.). Staff, Centre Hospitalier Universitaire de Québec (CHUQ) - Siege Social; (418)691-5151; Fax. (418)691-5415.

AUDET, Jean-Francois; Clinique d'Urologie Berger, 416-1000 ch Sainte-Foy, Quebec QC G1S 2L6; Laval'97; FRCSC; Urol (Laparoscopic Urology). Staff Urol, Centre Hospitalier Universitaire de Québec (CHUQ) - Siege Social; Université Laval; Langs: English; (418)266-2876; Fax. (418)266-2879; jf_audet@hotmail.com.

AUDET, Josee; CSSS de Beauce-Etchemin, 1515 17e rue, Saint-Georges QC G5Y 4T8; Laval'07; CCFP; Fam Med, Centre Hospitalier Beauce-Etchemin; (418)228-2031; Fax. (418)227-3825.

AUDET, Lyne; Riley Park Health Centre, 182-1402 8 Ave NW, Calgary AB T2N 1B9; Mon'87; CCFP; FCFP; Langs: English; (403)289-4312; Fax. (403)289-4377.

AUDET, Marc; 1-170 av de l'Eglise, Dolbeau-Mistassini QC G8L 4W6; Laval'77; Staff, Centre Maria-Chapdelaine - CH de Dolbeau-Mistassini; (418)276-4260; Fax. (418)276-6092.

AUDET, Marie-Christine; CSSS Maria-Chapdelaine, 2000 boul du Sacre-Coeur, Dolbeau-Mistassini QC G8L 2R5; Laval'06; CCFP; Staff, Centre Maria-Chapdelaine - CH de Dolbeau-Mistassini; (418)276-1234; Fax. (418)276-4355.

AUDET, Marie-Claude; Centre Racine Sainte-Foy, 102-2880 ch des Quatre-Bourgeo, Quebec QC G1V 4X7; Laval'76; Ac Staff, Centre Hospitalier Universitaire de Quebec-CHUL; (418)657-6363

AUDET, Marie-Eve; Ctr Hosp Affilie-Enfant-Jesus, 1401 18e rue, Quebec QC G1J 1Z4; Laval'02; FRCPC; DiagRad. Staff, Centre Hospitalier Affilié Universitaire de Québec - Hôpital De L'Enfant Jésus; (418)649-5782

AUDET, Marie-Josee; 1463 av Dobell, Quebec QC G1T 2L4; Laval'83; Psy. Member Teaching Committee in Med, Centre Hospitalier Affilié Universitaire de Québec - Hôpital du St-Sacrement; Member Res Committee in Psy, Université Laval; (418)650-2260; Fax. (418)650-0629.

AUDET, Maryse; CSSS de la région de Thetford, 1717 rue Notre-Dame E, Thetford Mines QC G6G 2V4; Laval'06; IntMed. Staff, Hopital du CSS de la Region de Thetford; (418)338-7777

AUDET, Nathalie; 110-2880 ch des Quatre-Bourgeo, Quebec QC G1V 4X7; McG'96; FRCS; ABOtol; FRCSC; Otol (Head & Neck Surgery). Clin Prof Otol & Ophth, Université Laval; Langs: Bilingual(English/French); (418)653-8717; Fax. (418)653-7199; nathalieaudet@hotmail.com.

AUDET, Nathalie; Centre Medical de l'Hetriere, 201-3520 rue de l'Hetriere, St-Augustin-D-Desm QC G3A 0B4; Mon'93; Staff, Centre d'hebergement Saint-Augustin; (418)651-3933; Fax. (418)651-0256.

AUDET, Neil; 12-8 45e Av, Lachine QC H8T 2L7; Mon'74; (514)634-3388

AUDET, Nicole; CSSS de Laval, 1755 boul Rene-Laennec, Laval QC H7M 3L9; Sher'80; MA; CCFP; FCFP; Staff, Hopital de la Cite de la santé; Asst Med Dir, Merck Frosst; Prof Family Med, Universite de Montreal; (450)668-1010

AUDET, Pascale; CHUM-Hop St-Luc, 1058 rue Saint-Denis, Montreal QC H2X 3J4; Mon'94; FRCPC; DiagRad. Staff, Centre Hospitalier l'Université De Montréal (CHUM) - Hôpital Saint-luc; (514)890-8350

AUDET, Patrice; CSSS de la Haute-Yamaska, 205 boul Leclerc O, Granby QC J2G 1T7; Sher'90; DiagRad. Staff, Centre Hospitalier de Granby; (450)372-5491; Fax. (450)372-7197.

AUDET, Richard; CSSS de la Baie-des-Chaleurs, RR 2 419 boul Perron, Maria QC G0C 1Y0; Laval'91; FRCPC; IntMed (Cardiology). Ac Member, CSSS de la Baie-des-Chaleurs; Assoc Member, Centre Hospitalier de Chandler; Langs: Bilingual(French/English); (418)759-3443; Fax. (418)759-5177.

AUDET, Sarah; CSSS de Lac-Saint Jean-Est, CP 1300 Succ Bureau-Chef 300 boul Champlain S, Alma QC G8B 5W3; Sher'07; CCFP; CCFP(E.M.); Staff, CSSS de Lac-Saint Jean-Est; (418)669-2000

AUDET, Sylvie; Hotel-Dieu de Roberval, 450 rue Brassard, Roberval QC G8H 1B9; Mon'84; Staff, Hotel-Dieu de Roberval; (418)275-0110

AUDET, William M; 17 Central Ave E, Brockville ON K6V 1W5; Ott'80; Staff, Brockville General Hospital - Charles Street; Staff, Providence Health Care - St Vincent's Hospital-Brock Fahrni Site; Staff, Brockville Mental Health Centre - Royal Ottawa Health Care Group; (613)342-6272; Fax. (613)342-8266; waudet@bcmhs.bc.ca.

AUDET-LAPOINTE, Pierre; Dir de la Sante Publique, 1301 rue Sherbrooke E, Montreal QC H2L 1M3; Mon'60; ABOG; ObstGyn (Gynecologic Oncology). Prof, Universite de Montreal; Langs: English; (514)528-2400 x3481; Fax. (514)527-1943; paudet@santepub-mtl.qc.ca.

AUDETTE, Myriam; GMF de Mascouche, 100-880 montee Masson, Mascouche QC J7K 2L7; Sher'90; Médecin, Centre Hospitalier Pierre le Gardeur; Langs: English; (450)474-2493; Fax. (450)966-0156.

AUDI, Nevine; Montfort Hosp, 713 Montreal Rd, Ottawa ON K1K 0T2; Alexandria (Egypt)'92; CCFP; CCFP(E.M.); Staff, Montfort Hospital; Langs: Arabic; French; (613)746-4621; n.audi@rogers.com.

AUDIBERT, Francois M; Hôpital Ste-Justine, 3175 ch Cote-Sainte-Catherine, Montreal QC H3T 1C5; Paris VII (France)'95; Staff, Hôpital Ste-Justine; Prof ObstGyn, Universite de Montreal; (514)345-7768; Fax. (514)345-4648.

AUDY, Daniel; Hop Maisonneuve-Rosemont, 5415 boul de l'Assomption, Montreal QC H1T 2M4; Laval'86; LMCC; CSPQ; FRCPC; Anes (Alternative Medicine). Staff Anes, Hopital Maisonneuve-Rosemont; Clin Staff Anes, Universite de Montreal; Langs: Bilingual(French/English); (514)252-3426; Fax. (514)252-3542.

AUDY, Marie; Centre Med Donnacona, 420 Route 138, Donnacona QC G3M 1C2; Laval'77; ac Membre, Centre Hospitalier Universitaire De Québec - Pavillon De St-françois-d'assise; Langs: English; Spanish; (418)285-1122; Fax. (418)285-0006; marie.audy@ssss.gouv.qc.ca.

AUER, Joseph M; Central Med Bldg, 202-1105 Carling Ave, Ottawa ON K1Y 4G5; Ott'73; Assoc Staff, The Ottawa Hospital - Riverside Campus; (613)722-0898

AUER, Rebecca A C; The Ottawa Hosp-Gen Campus, CCW 1617-501 Smyth Rd, Ottawa ON K1H 8L6; Qns'00; FRCSC; GenSurg. Staff, The Ottawa Hospital - General Campus; (613)737-8899

AUER, Roland N; Hôpital Ste-Justine, 3175 ch Cote-Sainte-Catherine, Montreal QC H3T 1C5; Alb'77; PhD(Sweden); FRCPC; NeurPath. Staff, Hôpital Ste-Justine; (514)345-4931 x4360; Fax. (514)345-4819.

AUER-GRZESIAK, Iwona A; Foothills Med Centre, 1403 29 St NW, Calgary AB T2N 2T9; Cal'90; FRCPC; AnatPath (Hematology Pathology). Staff, Foothills Medical Centre; Med Dir, Flow Cytometry Lab.; Langs: Polish; (403)944-8225; Fax. (403)270-4135.

AUERSPERG, Edward V; Simon Fraser Health Region, 600-22470 Dewdney Trunk Rd, Maple Ridge BC V2X 5Z6; UBC'83; FRCPC; IntMed. (604)467-5333; Fax. (604)467-1403.

AUFFREY, Jean-Marie; 201-387 Main St, Shediac NB E4P 2B5; McG'74; CCFP; FCFP; Ac Staff, Dr Georges-L-Dumont University Hospital Centre; (506)532-5780; Fax. (506)532-3296.

AUFRICHT, Margaret L P; Crowfoot Village Fam Practice, 210-600 Crowfoot Cres NW, Calgary AB T3G 0B4; Cal'84; CCFP; FCFP; Staff, Foothills Medical Centre; (403)239-9733; Fax. (403)241-8112.

AUGER, Alain; Clinique Med Bromont, C101-82 boul de Bromont, Bromont QC J2L 2K3; Mon'95; Staff, Hôpital Brome-Missisquoi-Perkins; (450)534-5474; Fax. (450)534-1725.

AUGER, Caroline; Clinique Med Familiale, 2185 boul de Tadoussac, Chicoutimi QC G7G 4X2; Mon'96; Staff, Complexe hospitalier de la Sagamie; (418)698-2414; Fax. (418)698-2413.

AUGER, Claire E; RC10-575 rue Saint-Amable, Quebec QC G1R 5R4; Laval'77; Member, Tribunal Administratif du Quebec; (418)643-3418; Fax. (418)643-0022; claire.auger@taq.gouv.qc.ca.

AUGER, Danielle; Direction de la Sante Publique, 2.03-201 boul Cremazie E, Montreal QC H2M 1L2; Laval'85; Staff, Ministry of Health & Social Services-Quebec; (514)864-2755; Fax. (514)864-2778; danielle.auger@msss.gouv.qc.ca.

AUGER, Dominique; Omniclinique de l'Outaouais, 202-28 boul du Mont-Bleu, Gatineau QC J8Z 1J1; Ott'93; CCFP; FCFP; Staff, Montfort Hospital; Staff, Centre Regional de Readoptation La Ressourse; Langs: Bilingual(French/English); (819)777-2111

AUGER, Dominique; CHUM-Hotel-Dieu, 3840 rue Saint-Urbain, Montreal QC H2W 1T8; Mon'03; FRCPC; IntMed; Cardiol. Staff, Centre Hospitalier l'Université de Montréal (CHUM) - Hôtel-Dieu; (514)890-8000

AUGER, Edouard; Clinique TSO du CHUQ, 184 rue Racine, Quebec QC G2B 1E3; Mon'93; FRCPC; Psy (Anxiety Disorder). Staff, Institut Universitaire Sante; Langs: Bilingual(English/French); (418)657-3696; Fax. (418)657-3697; edouard_auger@ssss.gouv.qc.ca.

AUGER, Eric; CSSS du Lac-des-Deux-Montagnes, 520 boul Arthur-Sauve, St-Eustache QC J7R 5B1; Laval'98; CSPQ; FRCPC; Anes. Staff, Hôpital de Saint-Eustache; (450)473-6811

AUGER, Francois; Ctr Hosp Affilie-Enfant-Jesus, 1401 18e rue, Quebec QC G1J 1Z4; Laval'77; FRCPC; MedMicrobiol (Infectiology). Staff, Centre Hospitalier Affilié Universitaire de Québec - Hôpital De L'Enfant Jésus; Dir Burn Research Lab, Centre Hospitalier Affilié Universitaire de Québec - Hôpital du St-Sacrement; Prof Surg, Université Laval; Langs: English; Spanish; (418)990-8255 x1662; Fax. (418)990-8242; francois.auger@chg.ulaval.ca.

AUGER, Francois; Clinique Med Neufchatel, 101-2425 boul Bastien, Quebec QC G2B 1B3; Laval'84; (418)843-3771; Fax. (418)843-3865.

AUGER, Gilles; CSSS de Saint-Jerome, 290 rue de Montigny, Saint-Jerome QC J7Z 5T3; Mon'82; Staff, Hôtel-Dieu de Saint-Jérôme; (450)431-8200

AUGER, Isabelle; CHUQ-Ctr Hosp Univ Laval, 2705 boul Laurier, Quebec QC G1V 4G2; Laval'00; FRCPC; Derm. Staff, Centre Hospitalier Universitaire de Quebec-CHUL; (418)654-2160

AUGER, Jean-Marie; UMF Laval, 2690 ch des Quatre-Bourgeois, Quebec QC G1V 0B7; Laval'81; LMCC; Staff, Hôpital Laval; Prof, Université Laval; Langs: Bilingual(French/English); (418)656-4795; Fax. (418)656-4503; jean-marie.auger@ssss.gouv.qc.ca.

AUGER, Julie R; Timmins & Dist Hosp, 700 Ross Ave E, Timmins ON P4N 8P2; Ott'95; CCFP; FCFP; Med Dir LTC, Timmins & District Hospital; Langs: English; French; (705)264-3099; Fax. (705)264-3099.

AUGER, Julien; CSSS de Saint-Jerome, 290 rue de Montigny, Saint-Jerome QC J7Z 5T3; Mon'10; CCFP; Staff, Hôtel-Dieu de Saint-Jérôme; (450)431-8200

AUGER, Louis; Clinique Med Grand-Boulevard, 200-353 boul des Bois-Francs S, Victoriaville QC G6P 4T2; Mon'93; Langs: Bilingual(French/English); (819)751-3006; Fax. (819)751-6625.

AUGER, Louise T; MUHC-Montreal Children's Hosp, B260-2300 rue Tupper, Montreal QC H3H 1P3; Baylor(TX) (USA)'80; FAAP; MD; PhD; FRCPC; Peds. Staff Peds, McGill University Health Centre - Montreal Children's Hospital; Assoc Prof Peds, McGill University; Langs: Bilingual(English/French); (514)412-4400 x22893; Fax. (514)412-4255.

AUGER, Manon; McGill University Health Centr, 3775 rue University, Montreal QC H3A 2B4; McG'86; CSPQ; FRCPC; AnatPath (Cytopath). Staff, McGill University Health Centre - Royal Victoria Hospital; Assoc Prof Path, McGill University; Langs: English; French; (514)398-7192 x495; Fax. (514)398-7446.

AUGER, Marc; Reseau de Sante du Temiscouata, 45 rue Du Foyer S RR 1, Riviere-Bleue QC G0L 2B0; Laval'77; Staff, Centre Hospitalier Regional du Grand-Portage; (418)893-5549; Fax. (418)893-1084.

AUGER, Marie-Claude; Centre Med Ruby, 101-361 Main St E, Hawkesbury ON K6A 1A8; Sher'06; CCFP; (613)632-0605; Fax. (613)632-7073.

AUGER, Martin; CSSS de Montmagny-L'Islet, 350 boul Tache O RR 1, Montmagny QC G5V 3R8; Laval'84; Staff, CSSS de Montmagny-L'Islet.

AUGER, Michel; Hotel-Dieu d'Arthabaska, 5 rue des Hospitalieres, Victoriaville QC G6P 6N2; Mon'62; Urol. Dir Tech Services, Hotel-Dieu d'Arthabaska; (819)357-2030

AUGER, Nathalie; Inst Nat'l de Sante Publique, 100-190 boul Crémazie E, Montreal QC H2P 1E2; UBC'97; FRCPC; CommunMed. Teach Staff Social & Prevetive Med, Universite de Montreal; Langs: Bilingual(French/English); (514)864-1600 x3717; Fax. (514)864-1616; nathalie.auger@inspq.qc.ca.

AUGER, Pascale; Centre Med Fontainebleau, 102-10 boul des Chateaux, Blainville QC J7B 1Z5; Mon'99; Staff, Hopital de la Cite de la santé; (450)419-8811

AUGER, Pierre L; Centre de Sante Publique, 2400 av D'Estimauville, Quebec QC G1E 7G9; Laval'67; MSc; CSPQ; FRCPC; Hem (P.Q.) (Environmental Health); OccupMed. ac Staff, Centre Hospitalier Universitaire de Quebec-CHUL; Langs: Bilingual(French/English); (418)666-7000 x321; Fax. (418)666-2776; pierre.auger@ssss.gouv.qc.ca.

AUGER, Pierre; Clin de Cardiologie de Levis, 600-4975 boul de la Rive-Sud, Levis QC G6V 4Z5; Laval'62; CSPQ; Cardiol (P.Q.); IntMed. ac Staff Med & Cardiol, Hôtel-Dieu de Lévis; Dir méd, Desjardins Financial Security; Langs: English; French; (418)833-5750; Fax. (418)833-5837; pierre.auger@dsf.ca.

AUGER, Pierre; Ctr Hosp Fleury, 2180 rue Fleury E, Montreal QC H2B 1K3; Mon'67; FRCPC; MedMicrobiol. Staff, Centre Hospitalier Fleury; Med Microbiol, Institut de Cardiologie de Montréal; Universite de Montreal; (514)383-5063; pierre.auger@umontreal.ca.

AUGER, Renee; Ctr Hosp Affilie-Enfant-Jesus, 1401 18e rue, Quebec QC G1J 1Z4; Laval'87; FRCPC; DiagRad. Diagnostic-Radiology, Centre Hospitalier Affilié Universitaire de Québec - Hôpital De L'Enfant Jésus; Langs: English; (418)649-5782; Fax. (418)649-5903.

AUGER, Veronique; Alder Med Clinic, 277 Evergreen Rd, Campbell River BC V9W 5Y4; UBC'01; CCFP; Langs: Bilingual(English/French); (250)287-7441; Fax. (250)287-4384.

AUGER-DUFOUR, Alexis; CSSS de Montmagny-L'Islet, 350 boul Tache O RR 1, Montmagny QC G5V 3R8; Laval'98; FRCPC; Psy. Staff, CSSS de Montmagny-L'Islet; (418)248-0630; Fax. (418)248-8472.

AUGER-DUFOUR, Etienne; Ctr Hosp Affilie-Enfant-Jesus, 1401 18e rue, Quebec QC G1J 1Z4; Laval'05; FRCSC; GenSurg (P.Q.). Staff, Centre Hospitalier Affilié Universitaire de Québec - Hôpital De L'Enfant Jésus; (418)649-0252

AUGLA, Salman H; Carbonear Gen Hosp, 86 Highroad South, Carbonear NL A1Y 1A4; Baghdad (Iraq)'89; Staff, Carbonear General Hospital; (709)945-5111

AUGUSTE, Ulrick; Tunney's Pasture, 100 Eglantine Drwy, Ottawa ON K1A 0K9; Port-au-Prince (Haiti)'82; Staff Surveillance Risk Assessment Division, Public Health Agency of Canada; Staff Surveillance Risk Assessment Division, Centre Communicable Diseases & Infection Control; (613)960-0829; Fax. (613)946-8695; ulrick.auguste@phac.aspc.gc.ca.

AUGUSTIN, Charles E; Hôpital Laval, 2725 ch Sainte-Foy, Quebec QC G1V 4G5; Montpellier (France)'71; CSPQ; Cardiol (P.Q.). Cardiology, Hôpital Laval; (418)656-8711

AUGUSTIN, Jean; 400B-2555 St. Joseph Blvd, Orleans ON K1C 1S6; (Haiti)'62; FRCPC; Psy. Staff, Montfort Hospital; Staff, Cornwall Community Hospital - Second Street Site; Staff, Cornwall Community Hospital; (613)837-8316; Fax. (613)837-2820.

AUGUSTINE, Anita; Living Hope Centre, 8-1224 Strachan Rd SE, Medicine Hat AB T1B 4R2; (India)'90; CCFP; (403)548-2500

AUJLA, Prince S S; Medical Bldg, 205-250 Harding Blvd W, Richmond Hill ON L4C 9M7; Tor'00; FRCPC; IntMed; Nephrol. Staff, Mackenzie Richmond Hill Hospital; Langs: Punjabi.

AUJLA, Ramandeep S; Primary Urgent Care Clinic, F1-7070 McLaughlin Rd, Mississauga ON L5W 1W7; (Ireland)'06; CCFP; (905)795-2873; Fax. (905)795-9114.

AUL, B Ritu; North York Gen Hosp, 3SE-4001 Leslie St, North York ON M2K 1E1; Qns'05; FRCPC; MedGenetics. Staff Medical Genetics, North York General Hospital; (416)756-6000

AUL, Madhurima; University of Calgary, 370-2500 University Dr NW, Calgary AB T2N 1N4; Cal'90; CCFP; FCFP; Teach Staff, University Of Calgary; (403)210-9355

AUL, Sewa S; Sudbury Reg Hosp-Laurentian, 41 Ramsey Lake Rd, Sudbury ON P3E 5J1; Shivaji (India)'73; MB BS; FCCP; FACC; FICS; Cardiovasc&ThorSurg; GenSurg. Chief Cardiovascular Dept, Health Sciences North - Memorial Site; Ac Staff, Health Sciences North-St Joseph's Health Centre; Ac Staff, Health Sciences North-Laurentian Site; (705)671-5252

AULAKH, Jasdeep S; Peace Arch Hosp, 15521 Russell Ave, White Rock BC V4B 2R4; Guru Nanak Dev (India)'92, Staff, Peace Arch Hospital; (604)541-7171

AULAKH, Lakyntiew P S; Sudbury Reg Hosp-Kirkwood, 680 Kirkwood Dr, Sudbury ON P3E 1X3; Assam (India)'91; Gen Practice, Health Sciences North-Kirkwood Site; Langs: Hindi; Punjabi; (705)675-5900; Fax. (705)671-3031; laulakh@hrsrh.on.ca.

AULAKH, Paramjit S; 101-8181 120A St, Surrey BC V3W 3P2; Punjab (India)'79; Staff, Surrey Memorial Hospital; Langs: Hindi; Punjabi; (604)599-6909; Fax. (604)599-4192.

AULD, Ian J; Canadian Sport Medicine, 2424 University Dr NW, Calgary AB T2N 3Y9; UBC'99; (403)289-8959; Fax. (403)284-9139.

AULD, Lindsay K; 214-11 Hidden Creek Dr NW, Calgary AB T3A 6K6; Tor'04; CCFP; (403)248-2273

AULD, Michael E; Grey Nuns Community Hosp & HC, 1100 Youville Drive West NW, Edmonton AB T6L 5X8; Alb'89; FRCPC; Anes. Staff, Covenant Health - Grey Nuns Community Hospital; (780)735-7020

AUM, Eull N; Shouldice Hosp, 7750 Bayview Ave, Thornhill ON L3T 4A3; (South Korea)'45; FRCPC; Anes. Staff, Shouldice Hospital; Langs: Japanese; Korean; (905)889-1125; Fax. (905)889-4216.

AUMAIS, Christian; Clinique Med Boisbriand, 877 boul de la Grande-Allee, Boisbriand QC J7G 1W6; Mon'82; (450)437-4600; Fax. (450)437-7038.

AUMAIS, Guy L; Hop Maisonneuve-Rosemont, 5415 boul de l'Assomption, Montreal QC H1T 2M4; Mon'76; Gastroent. Staff, Hopital Maisonneuve-Rosemont; Universite de Montreal; Langs: Bilingual(French/English); (514)252-3400

AUMEERALLY, Farouk L; Ctr Hosp Restigouche Inc, PO Box 10 Stn Main, Campbellton NB E3N 3G2; RCS (Ireland)'65; Psychiatrist, Centre Hospitalier Restigouche; (506)789-7000; Fax. (506)789-7065.

AUMOND, Francois; Hotel-Dieu de Levis, 143 rue Wolfe, Levis QC G6V 3Z1; Mon'97; CCFP; Staff, Hôtel-Dieu de Lévis; (418)835-7121; francoisaumond@ssss.gouv.qc.ca.

AUMOND, Ginette; CSSS d'Antoine-Labelle-l'Annon, 1525 rue l'Annonciation N, Riviere-Rouge QC J0T 1T0; Mon'84; Staff, Centre de L'Annonciation; Langs: Bilingual(French/English); (819)275-2118 x3124

AUMOND BEAUPRÉ, Tommy; CSSS du Lac-Temiscamingue, 22 rue Notre-Dame N, Ville-Marie QC J9V 1W8; Mon'06; Staff, CSSS du Témiscamingue; (819)622-2773; Fax. (819)629-3257.

AUMONT, Marie-France; Ctr Hosp Laurentien, 234 rue Saint-Vincent, Ste-Agathe-Des-Mts QC J8C 2B8; Sher'97; Fam Med, Centre Hospitalier Laurentien; (819)324-4000; Fax. (819)324-4010.

AUNG, Stephanie; 107-301 Columbia St E, New Westminster BC V3L 3W5; (Other Foreign)'09; (604)522-7363

AUNG, Steven K H; Dr Steven K H Aung's Med Clin, 9904 106 St NW, Edmonton AB T5K 1C4; Rangoon (Burma)'73; MB BS; PhD; FAAFP; FAB; Staff Consultant, University of Alberta Hospital; Staff Consultant, Royal Alexandra Hospital; Staff Consultant, Covenant Health - Misericordia Community Hospital; Member Executive Committee, Alberta Health & Wellness/Health Canada; Clin Prof Med Family Med School of Med & Dentistry/Aj Prof Pharmacy Rehab, University of Alberta; Langs: Chinese; Burmese; (780)426-2760; Fax. (780)424-8520; draung@aung.com.

AURET, Marnel; Wildrose Med Centre, PO Box 3955 4607 50 AVE, Olds AB T4H 1W1; (South Africa)'06; (403)556-7130; Fax. (403)556-1944.

AURON, Samuel; 202A-1685 Main St W, Hamilton ON L8S 1G5; (Mexico)'71; FRCPC; Psy. Staff Psy, Hamilton Health Sciences Centre - McMaster University Medical Centre; Asst Prof, McMaster University; Langs: Spanish; (905)527-7990

AUSFORD, Allen E G; Meadowlark Health Centre, 180 Meadowlark Shopping Ctr Nw, Edmonton AB T5R 5W9; Alb'79; CCFP; FCFP; Ac Staff Family Pract, Covenant Health - Misericordia Community Hospital; Instructor, Wilderness Medicine; (780)484-7574

AUSTEN, Daran L; Gulf Canada Square, 320-401 9 Ave SW, Calgary AB T2P 3C5; Cal'95; FRCSC; GenSurg. (403)221-4489; Fax. (403)221-4420.

AUSTGARDEN, Douglas A; Royal Victoria Hosp, 201 Georgian Dr, Barrie ON L4M 6M2; UBC'95; FRCPC; EmergMed (Critical Care Medicine). Staff, Royal Victoria Regional Health Centre; (705)728-9090 x4444

AUSTIN, David E; Markham Stouffville Hosp, PO Box 1800 Stn Main 381 Church St, Markham ON L3P 7P3; Tor'80; FRCPC; EmergMed. Chief Med Staff, Markham Stouffville Hospital; (905)472-7000 x6128; Fax. (905)472-7026; daustin@msh.on.ca.

AUSTIN, Heather A; Harbourside Family Health Ctre, 243 Harbour Dr, Summerside PE C1N 5R1; Dal'08; CCFP; (902)432-2600; Fax. (902)432-2610.

AUSTIN, Marc R; Bluewater Health-Norman Site, 89 Norman St, Sarnia ON N7T 6S3; McM'99; CCFP; Staff, Bluewater Health - Norman Site; (519)464-4400

AUSTIN, Monica L; Old Quebec Street Mall, 208-55 Wyndham St N, Guelph ON N1H 7T8; McM'85; CCFP; FCFP; Staff, Guelph General Hospital; (519)837-2283; Fax. (519)767-2262.

AUSTIN, Nancy E; The Richmond Hosp, 7000 Westminster Hwy, Richmond BC V6X 1A2; Tor'95; CCFP; CCFP(E.M.); Staff, Richmond Hospital; (604)244-5585

AUSTIN, Stephen J; Dr G B Cross Mem Hosp, 67 Manitoba Dr, Clarenville NL A5A 1K3; London (England)'81; MB BS; MRCP; Staff, The Dr G B Cross Memorial Hospital; (709)466-3411

AUSTIN, Tanya; 100-1695 Comox Ave, Comox BC V9M 3M1; Mem'79; CCFP; FCFP; (250)339-2266

AUSTIN, Thomas M; Cowichan Dist Hosp, 3045 Gibbins Rd, Duncan BC V9L 1E5; Cal'86; OrthSurg. Staff, Cowichan District Hospital; (250)746-4141

AUSTIN, Thomas W; London HSC-Victoria Hosp, PO Box 5010 Stn B 800 Commissioners Rd E, London ON N6A 5W9; Wes'65; FRCPC; IntMed (Infectious & Sexually Transmitted Diseases). Staff, London Health Sciences Centre - Victoria Campus; (519)685-8500

AUSTRUP, Mona L; Niagara H System-St Catharines, PO Box 3018 Stn Main 142 Queenston St, St Catharines ON L2R 7C6; Tor'92; FRCPC; Anes. Staff, Niagara Health System - St Catharines General Site; (905)684-7271 x45561

AUTHIER, Alain; CSSS de la Vallée de l'Or, 725 6e rue, Val-d'Or QC J9P 3Y1; Mon'95; Staff, Centre Hospitalier de Val d'Or; (819)825-5858

AUTHIER, Louis; Hop Charles LeMoyne, 3120 boul Taschereau, Greenfield Park QC J4V 2H1; Mon'65; CSPQ; Anes. Staff, Hopital Charles LeMoyne; (450)466-5000 x2680

AUTHIER, Louise; Pavillon Rosemont, 5689 boul Rosemont, Montreal QC H1T 2H1; Mon'73; CCFP; FCFP; Staff, Hopital Maisonneuve-Rosemont; Prog Dir Dept de Medecine, Universite de Montreal; (514)252-3814; Fax. (514)252-3854.

AUTMIZGUINE, Julie; Hôpital Ste-Justine, 3175 ch Cote-Sainte-Catherine, Montreal QC H3T 1C5; Sher'06; FRCPC; Peds; InfectDis. Staff, Hôpital Ste-Justine; (514)345-4931

AUYEUNG, Anthony; 34 Madison Ave, Toronto ON M5R 2S1; Tor'91; BSc; MSc; FACOG; FRCSC; ObstGyn (Reproductive Endocrinology & Infertility). (416)260-2004; Fax. (416)260-2794.

AUYEUNG, Grace C Y; Alexander Prof Bldg, 210-849 Alexander Crt, Peterborough ON K9J 7H8; Ott'89; CCFP; FCFP; Assoc Staff, Peterborough Regional Health Centre - Hospital Drive; Fam Med, Peterborough Regional Health Centre - Rogers St Site; (705)876-1066; Fax. (705)876-8763.

AVANESSIAN, Ardashes; Royal Inland Hosp, 311 Columbia St, Kamloops BC V2C 2T1; Shaheed Beheshti (Iran)'87; FRCPC; IntMed. Staff, Royal Inland Hospital; (250)314-2734

AVDIC, Sanja; St Joseph's Health Centre, 30 The Queensway, Toronto ON M6R 1B5; Belgrade (Serbia)'82; FRCPC; Peds (Neonatal & Perinatal Medicine). Head Neonatology, St Joseph's Health Centre; Langs: Croatian; Serbian; (416)530-6625

AVENANT, Christiaan R J; Cowichan Dist Hosp, 3045 Gibbins Rd, Duncan BC V9L 1E5; Stellenbosch (South Africa)'85; MB ChB; DA(SA); Staff, Cowichan District Hospital; (250)715-0430; Fax. (250)715-0430; cavenant@shaw.ca.

AVENDANO ALVAREZ, Monica; West Park Healthcare Centre, 82 Buttonwood Ave, Toronto ON M6M 2J5; (Chile)'63; FRCPC; IntMed (Tuberculosis). Internal Med, West Park Healthcare Centre; Staff, St Michael's Hospital; Langs: Spanish; (416)243-3631; Fax. (416)243-3696.

AVERBACK, Paul; 306-9900 boul Cavendish, Saint-Laurent QC H4M 2V2; Man'75; DAB; (514)426-8012; Fax. (514)426-8012.

AVERY, Bradley C; Family Practice Unit, 102-402 Hanson St, Whitehorse YT Y1A 1Y8; Alb'94; CCFP; Staff, Whitehorse General Hospital; (867)667-6421

AVERY, Chandra M; Dartmouth Gen Hosp, 325 Pleasant St, Dartmouth NS B2Y 4G8; Saba (Netherlands Antilles)'05; CCFP; CCFP(E.M.); Staff, Dartmouth General Hospital; (902)465-8300

AVERY, Granger R; Port McNeill Med Clinic, PO Box 14, Port Mcneill BC V0N 2R0; London (England)'70; MRCS; LRCP; (250)956-3377; Fax. (250)956-3299.

AVERY, Lisa S; Women's Hosp, WR120-735 Notre Dame Ave, Winnipeg MB R3E 0L8; Man'01; FRCSC; ObstGyn. Staff, Thompson General Hospital.

AVERY, Patricia K; 64 Alagash Dr, Sault Ste. Marie ON P6A 5K6; Tor'84; Ac Staff, Sault Area Hospital - Sault Ste Marie.

AVERY, Roger A; Health Sciences Centre, 300 Prince Philip Dr, St. John's NL A1B 3V6; Mem'97; FRCSC; Neursurg. Staff, Health Sciences Centre; (709)777-6300

AVERY, Ross A; Bridge Link Medical Clinic, 1186 Richards St, Richards Landing ON P0R 1J0; Wes'96; CCFP; (705)246-2477

AVERY, Susan M; Shea Heights Comm Health Ctre, PO Box 13122 Stn A 57B Linegar Ave, St. John's NL A1B 4A4; Mem'09; CCFP; (709)752-4301

AVILA, Maria L; The Hosp for Sick Children, 555 University Ave, Toronto ON M5G 1X8; Tucuman (Argentina)'02; Staff HemOncol, The Hospital For Sick Children; (416)813-7500

AVILA-CASADO, Maria del Carmen; Univ Hlth Network-Toronto Gen, 11E 226-200 Elizabeth St, Toronto ON M5G 2C4; (Mexico)'85; Staff, Toronto General Hospital - UHN; (416)340-3283

AVILA FLORES, Francisco; Brandon Reg Health Centre, 150 McTavish Ave E, Brandon MB R7A 2B3; FRCPC; DiagRad. Staff, Brandon Regional Health Centre; (204)578-4000

AVILA INSAMBERGTH, Arsenio J; Sunnybrook Hlth Sciences Ctre, M606-2075 Bayview Ave, Toronto ON M4N 3M5; Zulia (Venezuela)'77; FAMCCP; DABPainMed; FRCPC; Anes (Critical Care Medicine). Asst Prof Anes, Sunnybrook Health Sciences Centre; Asst Prof Anes, Health Sciences North-Laurentian Site; Asst Prof Anes, University of Toronto; Asst Prof Anes, University of Ottawa; Asst Prof Anes, Northern Ontario School of Medicine; Langs: Spanish; (416)480-6100 x4864; arsenio.avila@sunnybrook.ca.

AVILES, Alberto J; Blue Water Surgical Centre, 106-704 Mara St, Point Edward ON N7V 1X4; Chicago (USA)'99; (519)336-1555; Fax. (519)336-2193.

AVINA-ZUBIETA, Juan A; Arthritis Research Centre, 1F-5591 No. 3 Rd, Richmond BC V6X 2C7; Guadalajara (Mexico)'90; (604)207-4004

AVINASHI, Ramesh K; Kensington Med Clinic, 6548 Hastings St, Burnaby BC V5B 1S2; Aligarh (India)'70; MRCS; LRCP; CCFP; (604)299-9769

AVINASHI, Sanja; Aquarius Medical Clinic, 202-179 Davie St, Vancouver BC V5Z 2Y1; Sask'05; CCFP.

AVINASHI, Vishal; Children's & Women's HC of BC, K4 200-4480 Oak St, Vancouver BC V6H 3V4; Sask'05; FRCPC; Peds; Gastroent. Staff, BC Children's Hospital; (604)875-2332

AVINOAM-DAR, Galit; Women's College Hosp, 842-76 Grenville St, Toronto ON M5S 1B2; The Hebrew University (Israel)'98; Clin Fellow Derm, Women's College Hospital; (416)323-7732; Fax. (416)323-6306.

AVIS, Simon P; Province of Nfld & Labrador, PO Box 8700 Stn A, St. John's NL A1B 3V6; Mem'79; FRCPC; GenPath; AnatPath. Chief Forensic Path, Health Sciences Centre; Chief Med Examiner, Province of Newfoundland & Labrador; Chair Clinical Disciplines Lab Med/Prof, Memorial University Of Newfoundland; (709)777-6402; ocme@gov.nf.ca.

AVITAL, Ofer A; Clinique Med de l'Est Inc, 100-30 boul Saint-Joseph E, Montreal QC H2T 1G9; McG'95; (514)845-4240

AVITZUR, Yaron; The Hosp for Sick Children, 555 University Ave, Toronto ON M5G 1X8; Tel-Aviv (Israel)'95; Staff, The Hospital For Sick Children; (416)813-7733; Fax. (416)813-4972; yaron.avitzur@sickkids.ca.

AVIV, Richard I; Sunnybrook Hlth Sciences Ctre, 2075 Bayview Ave, Toronto ON M4N 3M5; Cape Town (South Africa)'93; FRCPC; DiagRad (Neuro Radiology). Staff, Sunnybrook Health Sciences Centre; (416)480-6100

AVRAM, Darrell R; 525-2550 15th Ave, Regina SK S4P 1A5; Sask'83; AB; FRCSC; Ophth (Oculo Plastic Surgery). Court Staff, Regina General Hospital; Ac Staff, Pasqua Hospital; Clinical Asst Prof Ophth, University of Saskatchewan; (306)522-4545; Fax. (306)347-3080.

AVRAM, Ronen; Hamilton HS-General Site, 703-237 Barton St E, Hamilton ON L8L 2X2; Wes'99; BSc; MSc; FRCSC; PlasSurg (Breast Reconstruction). Staff, Hamilton Health Sciences Centre - Juravinski Cancer Centre; Staff, Hamilton Health Sciences Centre - Hamilton General Hospital; (905)527-4322; Fax. (905)521-4825.

AVRAM, Victoria R A; Hamilton HS-Henderson Site, 10 70-711 Concession St, Hamilton ON L8V 1C3; McM'01; FRCSC; OrthSurg. Staff, Hamilton Health Sciences Centre-Juravinski Site; (905)389-4411; Fax. (905)381-7028.

AVRAMENKO, Victor W; Crystal Ridge Family Med Clin, 4-55 Wheatland Trail, Strathmore AB T1P 1R7; Alb'83; CCFP; Med Advisor, Viper Medical Services; Med Advisor, MD Rockyview EMS; (403)934-5911; Fax. (403)934-6672; vwamd1@efirehose.net.

AVRUCH, Leonard I; The Ottawa Hosp-Gen Campus, 501 Smyth Rd, Ottawa ON K1H 8L6; Tor'81; FRCPC; DiagRad. Staff Radiol, The Ottawa Hospital - General Campus; Asst Prof, University of Ottawa; (613)737-8624; Fax. (613)737-8538.

AW, Brian J; Medical Clinic, A8-1390 Major MacKenzie Dr E, Richmond Hill ON L4S 0A1; Tor'92; CCFP; Langs: Bilingual(English/French); (905)884-7711

AW, James J; Medcan Health Mgmt Inc, 1500-150 York St, Toronto ON M5H 3S5; Ott'91; DOHS; Chief Advisor, Scotiabank; Med Dir, Medcan Health Management Inc; (416)350-4880; Fax. (416)350-5981; jamesaw@medcan.com.

AWAD, A George; Humber River Reg Hosp-Keele, 2175 Keele St, Toronto ON M6M 3Z4; Cairo (Egypt)'57; PhD; Psy (Psycho Pharmacology). Chief Psy/Dir Physician, Humber River Regional Hospital - Keele Street Site; (416)658-2008; Fax. (416)658-2015.

AWAD, Awad I; 2-420 North Service Rd E, Oakville ON L6H 5R2; Cairo (Egypt)'72; FRCPC; Psy. (905)338-3331; Fax. (905)338-2923.

AWAD, Ayman T R A; Woodview Med Centre, 3236 Weston Rd, North York ON M9M 2T8; CCFP; (416)745-0600

AWAD, Imad T; Sunnybrook Health Sciences Ctr, M3 200-2075 Bayview Ave, Toronto ON M4N 3M5; Baghdad (Iraq)'89; Staff, Sunnybrook Health Sciences Centre; Langs: Arabic; (416)480-4864

AWAD, Jaklin A J; Winnipeg Clinic, 425 St Mary Ave, Winnipeg MB R3C 0N2; Assiut (Egypt)'82; CCFP.

AWAD, Lucy; Woodview Med Centre, 3236 Weston Rd, North York ON M9M 2T8; Ain Shams (Egypt)'92; MB ChB; CCFP; (416)745-0600; Fax. (416)745-0607.

AWAD, Nagy S H; James Paton Mem Hosp, 125 Trans Canada Hwy, Gander NL A1V 1P7; Cairo (Egypt)'98; MB BCh; Staff, James Paton Memorial Hospital; (709)256-2500

AWAD, Rita T S; Western Memorial Reg Hosp, PO Box 2005 1 Brookfield Dr, Corner Brook NL A2H 6J7; Alexandria (Egypt)'89; MB BCh; Staff, Western Memorial Regional Hospital; (709)637-5000

AWAD, S Michael; 1C-6315 Horn St, Red Deer AB T4N 6H5; Ein Shams (Egypt)'76; MB ChB; MRC; LMCC; FRCSC; ObstGyn (Infertility). Staff, Foothills Medical Centre; (403)347-2650

AWAD, Saadeldin M A; Chatham-Kent Health Alliance, PO Box 2030 Stn Main 80 Grand Ave W, Chatham ON N7M 5L9; Alexandria (Egypt)'72; FRCPC; AnatPath. Med Dir Lab/Hd AnatPath, Chatham-Kent Health Alliance; Aj Prof Path, University of Western Ontario; (519)352-6400; Fax. (519)437-6140.

AWAD, Stephanie; Clinique Med de l'Ouest, 103-4475 rue Bannantyne, Verdun QC H4G 1E2; Mon'07; CCFP; (514)765-3600; Fax. (514)765-9625.

AWAD-EL-KARIEM, Sawsan M; Moose Jaw Union Hosp, 455 Fairford St E, Moose Jaw SK S6H 1H3; Khartoum (Sudan)'78; MB BS; MRCPsy(UK); Staff, Moose Jaw Union Hospital; Langs: Arabic; (306)691-6464

AWADALLA, Alaa; 47 Marion St, Winnipeg MB R2H 0S8; Tanta (Egypt)'84; MB ChB; FRCOG; FRCSC; ObstGyn (Laparoscopic Surgery). Staff, Victoria General Hospital; Staff Women's Hosp, Health Sciences Centre; Staff, St Boniface General Hospital.

AWADDE ALLA GHATTAS, Suzan; Eglinton Churchill Med Centre, C3-2901 Eglinton Ave W, Mississauga ON L5M 6J3; Tanta (Egypt)'94; CCFP; Langs: Arabic; (905)608-1173; Fax. (905)608-1176.

AWAKAN, Babatunde A; 1-6601 48 Ave, Camrose AB T4V 3G8; (Nigeria)'95; MB BS; CCFP; Langs: Yoruba; (780)672-2425; Fax. (780)608-5897.

AWALT, Erin J; Lockview Med Clinic, 159 Cobequid Rd, Lower Sackville NS B4C 2N1; Dal'05; CCFP; (902)832-2311; Fax. (902)832-2312.

AWAN, Raza A; Synergy Sports Med & Rehab, 235 Wallace Ave, Toronto ON M6H 1V5; Tor'95; FRCPC; PhysMed&Rehab (Neuro Physiology). (416)703-3525

AWAN, Saeed-Ur-Rehman; Royal University Hosp, 103 Hospital Dr, Saskatoon SK S7N 0W8; Peshawar (Pakistan)'86; FRFPS; MB BS; FRCSC; GenSurg; PedGenSurg. Staff, Royal University Hospital; (306)966-8141; Fax. (306)966-7542; saeed1991@yahoo.ca.

AWAN, Tariq M; Northland Med Clinic, 101-4600 Crowchild Trail NW, Calgary AB T3A 2L6; Punjab (Pakistan)'89; MB BS; CCFP; Preceptor Examiner, Foothills Medical Centre; Preceptor Medical School, University of Calgary; Langs: Urdu; Punjabi; (403)286-3700; Fax. (403)286-3744.

AWDE, J Douglas; 210-101 Cherryhill Blvd, London ON N6H 4S4; Wes'90; Chief Dentistry Dept, London Health Sciences Centre - Victoria Campus; (519)672-5260; Fax. (519)672-5456.

AWDE, Murray G; 303-240 Wharncliffe Rd N, London ON N6H 4P2; Wes'73; CCFP; FCFP; Aj Prof Family Med, University of Western Ontario; (519)435-1230; Fax. (519)439-3636.

AWERBUCK, Bernard; LL4-1525 Albion Rd, Etobicoke ON M9V 5G5; Tor'54; DMRD; DiagRad. (416)741-5661; Fax. (416)741-6417.

AWERBUCK, Jonathan A; Addiction & Mental Hlth-Queen, 301-1001 Queen St W, Toronto ON M6J 1H4; Tor'93; CCFP; Staff, Centre for Addiction & Mental Health (CAMH) - Queen Site; (416)535-8501 x2663; Fax. (416)583-1266.

AWOSIKA, Ebi; Primecare Health, 120-109 Quarry Park Blvd SE, Calgary AB T2C 5E7; (403)930-7111; Fax. (403)930-7114.

AWOSIKA, Olukayode O; 120-109 Quarry Park Blvd SE, Calgary AB T2C 3G3; (403)930-7111

AWUKU, Mark A; Windsor Health Centre, 204-630 Tecumseh Rd E, Windsor ON N8X 4W2; (Ghana)'75; FRCPC; Peds (Consultant Pediatrics). Staff, Hôtel-Dieu Grace Hospital; Staff, Windsor Regional Hospital - Metropolitan Site; Assoc Prof Peds, Schulich School of Medicine & Dentistry; Assoc Dean Windsor Prog Faculty & Government Affairs, University of Western Ontario; (519)252-6464; Fax. (519)252-9303; mawuku@uwo.ca.

AWWAD, Bahaa E D H; Sault Area Hosp, 750 Great Northern Rd, Sault Ste. Marie ON P6B 0A8;Cairo (Egypt)'76; MB BCh; ObstGyn. Staff, Sault Area Hospital - Sault Ste Marie; (705)759-3720

AXELROD, Terry S; Sunnybrook Hlth Sciences Ctre, MG301-2075 Bayview Ave, Toronto ON M4N 3M5; Tor'81; FRCSC; OrthSurg (Hand Surgery). Staff, Sunnybrook Health Sciences Centre; (416)480-6769; Fax. (416)480-5886.

AXLER, Auby H; 201-1118 Homer St, Vancouver BC V6B 6L5; Alb'93; BSc; FRCPC; Psy (Psychotherapy). Staff Mood Disorder Clinic, UBC Hospital - Koerner Pavillion; Psychiatrist In-Cardiac Clinic, Vancouver General Hospital - Centennial Pavillion; Assoc Dir Training Psychotherapy/Assoc Clin Prof, University of British Columbia; (604)662-4776; Fax. (604)662-4772.

AXLER, Jeffrey L; Pine Seven Med Centre, 225-4600 Highway 7, Woodbridge ON L4L 4Y7; Tor'77; FRCPC; IntMed; Gastroent. Staff, William Osler Health System - Etobicoke General Hospital; Staff, Mount Sinai Hospital; Associate Research, Toronto Digestive Disease Associates.

AXLER, John T; Albany Med Clinic, 807 Broadview Ave, Toronto ON M4K 2P8; Tor'68; CCFP; FCFP; Staff G P Unit, Toronto East General Hospital Inc; (416)461-9471; Fax. (416)461-2710.

AXLER, Theodore; Royal Bank Plaza Med Centre, PO Box 134 LR8-200 Bay St, Toronto ON M5J 2J3; Qns'72; (416)368-6787; Fax. (416)368-7632.

AYAD, Hani I; Deerfoot Meadows Med Clinic, 7979 11 St SE, Calgary AB T2H 0B8; Cairo(Egypt) (Egypt)'95; (403)251-2690

AYAD, Misaa M S; Wilson Med Centre, 130 Wilson St, Hamilton ON L8R 1E2; Al-Fateh (Libya)'88; FRCPC; Peds. Staff, Hamilton Health Sciences Centre; Langs: Arabic; (905)526-6250

AYAD, Tareck; CHUM-Hop Notre-Dame, 1560 rue Sherbrooke E, Montreal QC H2L 4M1; Sher'00; FRCSC; Otol. Staff, Centre Hospitalier l'Université de Montréal (CHUM) - Hôpital Notre-Dame; (514)890-8000 x27201; tareck.ayad@mail.mcgill.ca.

AYALA AREVALO, M Angelica; CLSC Ste-Therese de Blainville, 2F-55 rue Saint-Joseph, Sainte-Therese QC J7E 4Y5; Mon'93; Psy (P.Q.) (Consultation-Liaison). Staff, Hôtel-Dieu de Saint-Jérôme; Langs: Spanish; (450)430-3702

AYALA-BUSTAMANTE, Everick N; Westmount Square Med Centre, C201-1 car Westmount, Westmount QC H3Z 2P9; Lima (Peru)'01; FRCPC; DiagRad. (514)939-9764

AYALA PAREDES, Felix A; CHUS-Hop Fleurimont, 3001 12e Av N, Sherbrooke QC J1H 5N4; La Plata (Argentina)'92; Staff, Centre Hospitalier Universitaire de Sherbrooke-Hopital Fleurimont; Langs: English; Spanish; (819)346-1110 x74947; Fax. (819)820-6897; felix.ayala-paredes@usherbrooke.ca.

AYANBADEJO, Benjamin O; Old Quebec Street Mall, 218-55 Wyndham St N, Guelph ON N1H 7T8; Ibadan (Nigeria)'76; MB BS; MRCOG; FRCSC; ObstGyn. Consultant, North Wellington Health Care - Louise Marshall Hospital; Consultant, Groves Memorial Community Hospital; Staff, Guelph General Hospital; (519)837-1848; Fax. (519)837-2363.

AYANBADEJO, Clement; Queen Elizabeth Hosp, PO Box 6600 Stn Central, Charlottetown PE C1A 8T5; (Other Foreign)'00; CCFP; Staff, Queen Elizabeth Hospital; (902)894-2111

AYANRINO, Femi B; Queen Elizabeth II Hospital, 10409 98 St, Grande Prairie AB T8V 2E8; (Nigeria)'92; MB BS; Staff, Queen Elizabeth II Hospital; (780)538-7173; Fax. (780)538-7277.

AYAS, Najib; St Paul's Hosp, 224-1081 Burrard St, Vancouver BC V6Z 1Y6; Alb'92; FRCPC; IntMed; Respir. Staff, Providence Health Care - St Paul's Hospital; (604)806-9420

AYAS, Raouf R; Centre Prof Belanger, 205-3871 rue Belanger, Montreal QC H1X 3M7; Ein Shams (Egypt)'69; CSPQ; FRCPC; Cardiol. Ac Staff, Hopital de la Cite de la santé; (514)727-6353; raouf@pharmaciegabriel.com.

AYAS, Timmy; Carnat Centre, 300-2580 32 St NE, Calgary AB T1Y 7M8; Cal'03; FRCPC; Psy;CCFP; (403)944-9800; Fax. (403)944-9850.

AYE, Lwin M; Dynacare Kasper Med Labs, 200-10150 102 St NW, Edmonton AB T5J 5E2; (Burma)'90; MB BS; ABPath; Clinical Asst Prof Path & LabMed, University of Alberta; (780)451-3702; Fax. (780)454-2845; mlwinaye@cha.ab.ca.

AYE, Tim M; St Mary's Gen Hosp, 911 Queens Blvd, Kitchener ON N2M 1B2; Tor'91; FRCPC; Anes. Staff, St Mary's General Hospital; (519)744-3311

AYENI, Olawale O; 303-132 Parkdale Ave S, Hamilton ON L8K 3P3; Ife Medical School (Other Foreign)'92; CCFP; (905)549-8863; Fax. (905)549-4706.

AYENI, Olubimpe; York Prof Bldg, 679 Davis Dr, Newmarket ON L3Y 5G8; Ott'06; FRCSC; PlasSurg. (905)853-6644; Fax. (905)853-1898.

AYENI, Olufemi R; Hamilton HS-McMaster Site, PO Box 2000 Stn Lcd 1 4E17-1200 Main St W, Hamilton ON L8N 3Z5; Ott'02; FRCSC; OrthSurg. Staff, Hamilton Health Sciences Centre - McMaster University Medical Centre; Langs: Yoruba; (905)521-2100

AYENI, R Oluwafemi; 3-105 Progress Cres, Kapuskasing ON P5N 3J4; Lagos (Nigeria)'71; MB BS; MSc(McGill); FACS; FWACS; FRCSC; GenSurg. Staff, Sensenbrenner Hospital; Asst Prof, Northern Ontario School of Medicine-Laurentian University; Langs: Yoruba; (705)335-4355; Fax. (705)335-3809.

AYERS, Christopher N; Symons Valley Firstcare, 214-11 Hidden Creek Dr NW, Calgary AB T3A 6K6; Man'96; CCFP; Langs: English; French; (403)248-2273

AYERS, Ian B; Vulcan Medical Clinic, PO Box 419, Vulcan AB T0L 2B0; McM'08; CCFP; Staff, Foothills Medical Centre; (403)485-2216

AYESHA, Qanta; The Scarborough Hosp-General, 3050 Lawrence Ave E, Scarborough ON M1P 2V5; Lahore (Pakistan)'95; CCFP; Staff, The Scarborough Hospital - General Campus; (416)438-2911

AYIBIOWU, Ogunroti; Wentworth Limeridge Med Ctre, 307-849 Upper Wentworth St, Hamilton ON L9A 5H4; Ibadan (Nigeria)'91; MB BS; CCFP; Langs: Yoruba; (905)383-8951; Fax. (905)383-8965; roteone@yahoo.com.

AYLETT, Alan A A; Near North Med Clinic, 202-66 Josephine St, North Bay ON P1B 0A7; Wes'74; BSc(Hons); Staff, North Bay Regional Health Centre - Regional Mental Health; (705)474-1441; Fax. (705)474-1137.

AYLING, Geraldine Z; Penticton Reg Hosp, 550 Carmi Ave, Penticton BC V2A 3G6; London (England)'96; MB BS; Staff, Penticton Regional Hospital; (250)492-9004

AYLING, Grant R; Westcoast Family Practice Ctre, 3F-2775 Laurel St, Vancouver BC V5Z 1M9; Otago (New Zealand)'76; MB ChB; Ac Staff, Vancouver General Hospital - Centennial Pavillion; (604)875-5691

AYLLON UGARTE, Jose; Hop Charles Lemoyne, 3120 boul Taschereau, Greenfield Park QC J4V 2H1; Lima (Peru)'93; Staff, Hopital Charles LeMoyne; Langs: Spanish; English; (450)466-5650; Fax. (450)466-5066.

AYLMER, Anne P; Dartmouth Gen Hosp, 325 Pleasant St, Dartmouth NS B2Y 4G8; Glasgow (Scotland)'75; FRCPC; Anes. Staff, Dartmouth General Hospital; (902)441-4613

AYLMER, David A; Colchester East Hants Hlth Ctr, 600 Abenaki Rd, Truro NS B2N 5A1; Glasgow (Scotland)'75; FFARCS(Ire); FRCPC; Anes. Staff, Colchester East Hants Health Centre; (902)893-4321

AYLWARD, Bedford Z; Dawson Creek Med Clinic, 816 103 Ave, Dawson Creek BC V1G 2G1; Dal'57; Staff, Dawson Creek & District Hospital; (250)782-5271; Fax. (250)782-6360.

AYLWARD, Darroch L; 207-10134 97 Ave, Grande Prairie AB T8V 7X6; Alb'85; AAFP; LMCC; (780)882-7797; Fax. (780)882-6617.

AYMONG, Eve D; St Paul's Hosp, 474A-1081 Burrard St, Vancouver BC V6Z 1Y6; Tor'93; MSc; FRCPC; IntMed (Interventional Cardiology); Cardiol. Staff Cardiol, Providence Health Care - St Paul's Hospital; Staff Cardiol, Vancouver General Hospital - Centennial Pavillion; Teach Staff, University of British Columbia; (604)682-2344

AYOADE, Gbade A; 110 Queens Plate Dr, Etobicoke ON M9W 0B4; Ibadan (Nigeria)'78; MB BS; MRCOG; FICS; FRCSC; ObstGyn. Langs: Yoruba.

AYODELE, Kayode I; Springdale Prof Bldg, 512-2250 Bovaird Dr E, Brampton ON L6R 0W3; Ibadan (Nigeria)'75; MB BS; MRC; MMed(Sci.); FRCSC; ObstGyn. Staff ObstGyn, The Scarborough Hospital - General Campus; (905)451-9486

AYOTTE, Charles; Hop Maisonneuve-Rosemont, 5415 boul de l'Assomption, Montreal QC H1T 2M4; Laval'95; Neur (Electroencephalography). Staff, Centre Hospitalier l'Université De Montréal (CHUM) - Hôpital Saint-luc; Staff, Hopital Maisonneuve-Rosemont; (514)252-3528; Fax. (514)252-3529; c_ayo70@hotmail.com.

AYOTTE, Evans C; Clinique Med Manseau, 584 boul Manseau, Joliette QC J6E 3E4; Sher'90; Staff, Centre Hospitalier Régional de Lanaudière; Langs: English; (450)753-9234; Fax. (450)755-1157.

AYOTTE, Louise; Agence Sante Montreal, 3725 rue Saint-Denis, Montreal QC H2X 3L9; Mon'76; Staff, Centre Hospitalier Universitaire de Sherbrooke-Hôpital Hôtel-Dieu; (514)286-6500 x6942

AYOTTE, Nancy; CSSS de Trois-Rivieres, 155 rue Toupin, Trois-Rivieres QC G8T 3Z8; Laval'99; Staff, Centre de santé Cloutier-du-Rivage; (819)370-2108

AYOTTE, Normand J; Clinique de Gynecologie, 304-1785 av Saint-Marc, Shawinigan QC G9N 2H6; Laval'71; FRCSC; ObstGyn (Clinical Research). ac Staff, CH du Centre-de-la-Mauricie (Ste-Thérèse de Shawinigan); Université Laval; Langs: Spanish; English; (819)536-2591; Fax. (819)536-5115.

AYOUB, Christian; Institut de Cardiologie de Mtl, 5000 rue Belanger, Montreal QC H1T 1C8; Laval'01; CSPQ; FRCPC; Anes. Staff, Institut de Cardiologie de Montréal; (514)376-3330 x3732

AYOUB, Haifa H; Guysborough Med Clinic, PO Box 260, Guysborough NS B0H 1N0; Mosul (Iraq)'84; MB ChB; Staff, Guysborough Memorial Hospital; (902)533-4040; Fax. (902)533-2040.

AYOUB, Jean-Pierre M; CHUM-Hop Notre-Dame, 1560 rue Sherbrooke E, Montreal QC H2L 4M1; McG'91; FRCP; LMCC; FRCPC; IntMed; MedOncol. Staff, Centre Hospitalier l'Université de Montréal (CHUM) - Hôpital Notre-Dame; Langs: French; Spanish; (514)890-8000 x27015; jean-pierre.ayoub.chum@ssss.gouv.qc.ca.

AYOUB, Joseph I; CHUM-Hop Notre-Dame, 1560 rue Sherbrooke E, Montreal QC H2L 4M1; Alexandria (Egypt)'61; FRCPC; Hem (P.Q.); MedOncol; HemPath. Staff Teacher, Centre Hospitalier l'Université de Montréal (CHUM) - Hôpital Notre-Dame; Aj Prof MedOncol, McGill University; Dir Program Oncol, Universite de Montreal; (514)890-8000 x25381

AYOUB, Patricia; Hop Maisonneuve-Rosemont, 5415 boul de l'Assomption, Montreal QC H1T 2M4; Sher'00; CCFP; Staff, Hopital Maisonneuve-Rosemont; (514)252-3400

AYOUB, Paul; Ctr Hosp De Verdun, 4000 boul Lasalle, Verdun QC H4G 2A3; Laval'99; FRCPC; IntMed; Nephrol. Staff, Centre Hospitalier de Verdun; (514)362-1000 x2141

AYOUB, Paul; CSSS-Hopital De Hull, 116 boul Lionel-Emond, Gatineau QC J8Y 1W7; Kharkov State (Ukraine)'92; Staff, Hull Hospital; (819)966-6200; Fax. (819)966-6306.

AYOW, Michael K; Humber River Reg Hosp-Church, 200 Church St, Toronto ON M9N 1N8; Alb'90; CCFP; CCFP(E.M.); FCFP; Staff, Humber River Regional Hospital - Church Street Site; (416)249-8111

AYROUD, Yasmine; The Ottawa Hosp-Gen Campus, 501 Smyth Rd, Ottawa ON K1H 8L6; Mon'79; CSPQ; FRCPC; AnatPath. Staff, The Ottawa Hospital - General Campus; (613)737-8899 x72013

AYTOUR, Ibrahim M; Sunridge Prof Centre, 2675 36 St NE, Calgary AB T1Y 6H6; (403)291-3315; Fax. (403)291-9308.

AYUB, Nasir; Athabasca Health Authority, PO Box 124, Black Lake SK S0J 0H0; Amritsar (India)'89; (306)439-2200; Fax. (306)439-2210.

AYUEN, Kim L; Sunnybrook Hlth Sciences Ctre, HG39-2075 Bayview Ave, Toronto ON M4N 3M5; McG'07; MDCM; CCFP; Staff, Sunnybrook Health Sciences Centre; Langs: Bilingual(English/French); (416)480-6100

AYYOBI, Amir; Sturgeon Community Hosp, 201 Boudreau Rd, St. Albert AB T8N 6C4; Cal'05; Staff, Sturgeon Community Hospital; Staff, University of Alberta Hospital; (780)418-8200

AZABI, Tareq O; 101-112 Queenston St, St Catharines ON L2R 2Z4; Al-Fateh (Libya)'90; MB ChB; FRCSC; GenSurg. Staff, Niagara Health System - St Catharines General Site; (905)685-0821

AZAD, Aristotle; Burris Clinic, 300-275 Lansdowne St, Kamloops BC V2C 6J3; UBC'81; PhD; FRCSC; GenSurg; VascSurg. Dir Vascular Lab, Royal Inland Hospital; (250)377-3331; Fax. (250)377-3783.

AZAD, Jason K; 206-13278 Tecumseh Rd E, Windsor ON N8N 3T6; Man'97; CCFP; (519)735-1946; Fax. (519)735-6236.

AZADEH, Minoo; Univ Hlth Network-Toronto Western Hosp, 399 Bathurst St, Toronto ON M5T 2S8; Tabriz (Iran)'95; FRCSC; Ophth. Staff, Toronto Western Hospital - University Health Network; (416)603-2581

AZADIAN, Abbas G; 7560 Bayview Ave, Thornhill ON L3T 2S1; Tor'95; FRCPC; Psy (Psychological Trauma). Langs: Farsi; (905)731-1133; Fax. (905)731-6752.

AZAGHDANI, Abdulhamid M; Carbonear Gen Hosp, 86 Highroad S, Carbonear NL A1Y 1A4; Al-Fateh University (Libya)'93; MB BCh; Staff, Carbonear General Hospital; (709)945-5111

AZAM, Adeel; 104-266 4 St SW, Medicine Hat AB T1A 4E5; Peshawar (Pakistan)'91; MB BS; ABIM; FRCPC; IntMed. Dir Diabetes Education Centre & ICU/CCU, Medicine Hat Regional Hospital; Clinical Asst Prof Med, University of Calgary; Langs: Urdu; (403)580-8288; Fax. (403)580-8233.

AZAM, Afshan; Malvern Med Centre, 100-1333 Neilson Rd, Scarborough ON M1B 4Y9; (416)291-7719

AZAM, Almas L; Oasis Med Centre, 486 Advance Blvd, Tecumseh ON N8N 0B8; Punjab (Pakistan)'95; CCFP; (519)727-3338

AZANCOT, Linda; CLSC Ahuntsic, 1165 boul Henri-Bourassa E, Montreal QC H2C 3K2; Mon'97; Langs: English; (514)384-2000 x8411; Fax. (514)381-0814; lindaazancot.csssamn@ssss.gouv.qc.ca.

AZAR, Rani M; CHUM-Hop Notre-Dame, 1560 rue Sherbrooke E, Montreal QC H2L 4M1; Beirut (Lebanon)'88; FRCPC; IntMed. Staff, Centre Hospitalier l'Université de Montréal (CHUM) - Hôpital Notre-Dame; (514)890-8000

AZARBAR, Sayena; Hop Jean-Talon, 1385 rue Jean Talon E, Montreal QC H2E 1S6; Mon'07; IntMed. Staff, CSSS du Coeur de l'Isle Hôpital Jean-Talon; (514)495-6767

AZER, Eman A M; Alpha-One Med Centre, 12-1891 Rathburn Rd E, Mississauga ON L4W 3Z3; Assiut (Egypt)'84; MB ChB; CCFP; (905)212-9955

AZER, Nivin F T; Agassiz Medical Centre, 130-30 Stephen St, Morden MB R6M 2G3; CCFP; (204)822-4474

AZER, Nivine N Z; Wheat City Medical Clinic, C1-1711 Kirkcaldy Dr, Brandon MB R7A 0B9.

AZER, Raed; 3304 Landry Ave, New Waterford NS B1H 1L5; Alexandria (Egypt)'84; MB ChB; LMCC; CCFP; FCFP; Staff, Cape Breton District Health Authority; Staff Chief, New Waterford Consolidated Hospital; Assoc Physician, Cancer Center & Palliative Care Services; Langs: Arabic; French; (902)862-8100; Fax. (902)862-9405; azerr@cbdha.nshealth.ca.

AZER, Salwa; 305-2347 Kennedy Rd, Scarborough ON M1T 3T8; Tor'86; CCFP; (416)297-8800; Fax. (416)297-6502.

AZER, Sameh C; Fort Saskatchewan Med Clinic, 9421 94 Ave, Fort Saskatchewan AB T8L 1N6; Alexandria (Egypt)'80; Staff, Fort Saskatchewan Health Centre; Staff Obst/Gynecol, Lamont Health Care Centre; Langs: English; French; (780)998-2231; Fax. (780)998-4399.

AZHARUDDIN, Mohammed; Hamilton HS-Hamilton Gen Site, 237 Barton St E, Hamilton ON L8L 2X2; Pradesh (India)'85; IntMed. Staff, Hamilton Health Sciences Centre - Hamilton General Hospital; (905)527-4322; Fax. (905)527-1941.

AZHARUDDIN, Tahera; Windsor Family Health Team, 245-2475 McDougall St, Windsor ON N8X 3N9; Dr NTR University of Health Sciences (Other Foreign)'00; CCFP; (519)250-5656

AZHER, Tanweer; St Clare's Mercy Hosp, 154 LeMarchant Rd, St. John's NL A1C 5B8; Punjab (Pakistan)'86; MB BS; MRCP(Ire); Staff, St Clare's Mercy Hospital; Clin Asst Prof, Memorial University Of Newfoundland; (709)777-5769; azher82@hotmail.com.

AZHER, Zaira; East End Med Centre, 2 Mount Cashel Rd, St. John's NL A1A 1X7; Bahawalpur (Pakistan)'97; MB BS; CCFP; (709)453-1450

AZI, Adaku M; Bowmanville Med Bldg, 302-222 King St E, Bowmanville ON L1C 1P6; (Nigeria)'00; CCFP; Staff, Lakeridge Health - Bowmanville Site; (905)697-8847; Fax. (905)697-7745.

AZIEZ, Abdelaâziz; Centre de Sante Valcartier, CP 1000 Bdp Succ Forces, Courcelette QC G0A 4Z0; CCFP; (418)844-5000

AZIM, Abdul; Queen Elizabeth II HSC-Halifax, 6896-1796 Summer St, Halifax NS B3H 3A7; Chittagong (Bangladesh)'83; Staff, Queen Elizabeth II Health Sciences Centre - Halifax Infirmary Site; (902)473-4153; Fax. (902)473-6293.

AZIM, Hassan F A; 620-100 Park Royal S, West Vancouver BC V7T 1A2; Cairo (Egypt)'55; MB ChB; FAPA; FRCPC; Psy (Family Therapy). (604)925-2441; Fax. (604)913-0316.

AZIZ, Abdul; Chinook Paediatric Clinic, 951 19 St S, Lethbridge AB T1J 3H5; Peshawar (Pakistan)'83; Langs: Hindi; Punjabi; Persian; Urdu; (403)320-7518

AZIZ, Ahmed T; G R Baker Mem Hosp, 543 Front St, Quesnel BC V2J 2K7; Baghdad (Iraq)'87; MB ChB; FRCPC; IntMed. Internal Medicine, G R Baker Memorial Hospital; Langs: Arabic; (250)992-0636; ahmed1806@yahoo.com.

AZIZ, Alnoor; Crescent Town Health Centre, 4 The Market Place, Toronto ON M4C 5M1; Tor'81; Staff Teacher Pt-Time Family Med, St Michael's Hospital; (416)690-3412; Fax. (416)691-2543.

AZIZ, Anis; Doctors Bldg, 335-955 Queen St E, Sault Ste. Marie ON P6A 2C3; Mon'04; FRCSC; Urol. Staff, Sault Area Hospital - Sault Ste Marie; Langs: Bilingual(French/English); (705)254-4364; Fax. (705)759-9355.

AZIZ, Aziz N N; Roblin District Health Centre, PO Box 940 15 Hospital St, Roblin MB R0L 1P0; Staff, Roblin & District Health Centre; (204)937-2142

AZIZ, Dalal A; 218-400 Bronte St S, Milton ON L9T 0H7; Beirut (Lebanon)'97; BSc; MD; FRCSC; GenSurg (Surgical Oncology). Staff Gen Surg, Halton Healthcare Services Corporation - Milton District Hospital; Langs: French; Arabic; (905)878-6635; Fax. (905)878-8111.

AZIZ, Khalid; Royal Alexandra Hosp, 5027 DTC-10240 Kingsway NW, Edmonton AB T5H 3V9; London (England)'81; MB BS; MRCGPract(UK); DRCOG; BA; FRCPC; Peds (Neonatal & Perinatal Medicine). Staff Neonatologist, Royal Alexandra Hospital; Assoc Prof Peds, University of Alberta; (780)735-4670; Fax. (780)735-4072.

AZIZ, Mariam; Halton Geriatric Mental Health, 5230 South Service Rd, Burlington ON L7L 5K2; McM'05; Psy. (905)681-8233; Fax. (905)681-8628.

AZIZ, Mohammed A G A; 201-293 Freshwater Rd, St. John's NL A1B 1B7; Baghdad (Iraq)'96; MB ChB; CCFP; Staff, Dr Walter Templeman Health Centre; (709)488-2821; Fax. (709)488-2600; mohammed.aziz@easternhealth.ca.

AZIZ, Nevine A; Crescent Town Health Centre, 4 The Market Place, Toronto ON M4C 5M1; Ott'81; Staff, The Scarborough Hospital - General Campus; (416)690-3412; Fax. (416)691-2543.

AZIZ, S Yasmin; Sound Care Med Centre, 560-1145 Hunt Club Rd, Ottawa ON K1V 0Y3; Ott'90; ObstGyn. Clin Asst, The Ottawa Hospital - General Campus; Langs: Punjabi; English; (613)738-2378

AZIZ, Sahar; Montebello Med Clinic, 249 Waverley Rd, Dartmouth NS B2X 2C5; Ain Shams (Egypt)'87; MB BCh; CCFP; (902)406-4444; Fax. (902)406-4447.

AZIZ, Samir B; Joseph Brant Mem Hosp, 1230 North Shore Blvd E, Burlington ON L7S 1W7; Baghdad (Iraq)'93; MB ChB; CCFP; CCFP(E.M.); Staff, Joseph Brant Memorial Hospital; (905)336-4116

AZIZ, Shiraz F; Ackroyd Med Clinic, 105-8056 King George Blvd, Surrey BC V3W 5B5; Makerere (Uganda)'71; MB BS; LRCP; MRCS; Langs: Kacchi; Hindi; Gujarati; Swahili; (604)593-5499; Fax. (604)593-5498.

AZIZ, Tariq; Hamilton HS-Henderson Site, 711 Concession St, Hamilton ON L8V 1C3; Karachi (Pakistan)'89; FRCPC; GenPath. Staff, Hamilton Health Sciences Centre-Juravinski Site; (905)521-2100

AZIZ, Zared A; St Joseph's Health Centre, 30 The Queensway, Toronto ON M6R 1B5; Ott'01; BSc; FRCPC; GenPath. Staff, St Joseph's Health Centre; (416)530-6285

AZIZ-FEW, Carolyn F; PO Box 78006 Rpo Callingwood, Edmonton AB T5T 6A1.

AZIZA, Jonathan; Scarborough Hosp-General Div, 3050 Lawrence Ave E, Scarborough ON M1P 2V5; Tor'83; FRCPC; DiagRad. Staff Radiol, The Scarborough Hospital - General Campus; (416)431-8107; Fax. (416)431-8141.

AZMAYESH-FARD, Arash; 117 Edenstone Pl NW, Calgary AB T3A 3Z3; Alb'98; FRCPC; Anes. Staff, Peter Lougheed Centre; (403)620-8193; Fax. (403)284-2061.

AZOUBEL, Gustavo A P; Scarborough Hosp-General Div, 3050 Lawrence Ave E, Scarborough ON M1P 2V5; Pernambuco (Portugal)'01; VascSurg; GenSurg. Staff, The Scarborough Hospital - General Campus; (416)483-2911

AZOUZ, E Michel; Westmount Square Med Imaging, C210-1 Car Westmount, Westmount QC H3Z 2P9; Alexandria (Egypt)'68; DABR; FRCPC; DiagRad (Pediatric Radiology). Langs: Arabic; (514)939-9764; Fax. (514)939-9363; michelazouz@yahoo.com.

AZRAN, Danielle; SMBD Jewish Gen Hosp, 3755 ch Cote-Sainte-Catherine, Montreal QC H3T 1E2; Mon'91; Staff, Sir Mortimer B Davis Jewish General; McGill University; (514)340-8222 x4974

AZUELOS, Alan; SMBD Jewish Gen Hosp, 3755 ch Cote-Sainte-Catherine, Montreal QC H3T 1E2; Ott'97; CCFP; CCFP(E.M.); Staff, Sir Mortimer B Davis Jewish General; (514)340-8222

AZUELOS, Elisabeth; Hop du Sacre-Coeur de Mtl, 5400 boul Gouin O, Montreal QC H4J 1C5; Mon'91; Staff, Hôpital du Sacre-Coeur de Montréal; Staff, Hopital de la Cite de la santé; (514)338-2050; Fax. (514)338-3228.

AZUELOS, Ilan; MUHC-Montreal Chest Institute, 3650 rue Saint-Urbain, Montreal QC H2X 2P4; McG'07; MDCM; FRCPC; IntMed; Respir. Staff, McGill University Health Centre - Montreal Chest Institute; (514)466-3481

AZUH, Victor I; Pillette Village Walk-In Clini, 100-4900 Wyandotte St E, Windsor ON N8Y 1H7; Lagos (Nigeria)'79; MB BS; MRCOG; (519)974-8682; Fax. (519)974-8836; victor_az@hotmail.com.

AZZAM, Hussam M; Thompson Gen Hosp, 871 Thompson Dr, Thompson MB R8N 0C8; FRCSC; ObstGyn. Staff, Thompson General Hospital; (204)677-2381

AZZAM, Joseph E; Avenue Med Centre, 221 Brant Ave, Brantford ON N3T 3J3; Tor'05; FRCSC; ObstGyn. (519)753-8666; Fax. (519)753-6880.

AZZAM, Khalid M; Hamilton HS-General Site, 626-237 Barton St E, Hamilton ON L8L 2X2; Rajasthan (India)'95; Staff, Hamilton Health Sciences Centre - Hamilton General Hospital; (905)527-4322 x45149; Fax. (905)523-8352.

AZZAM, Lina; Thompson Gen Hosp, 871 Thompson Drive, Thompson MB R8N 0C8; FRCSC; ObstGyn. Staff, Thompson General Hospital; (204)677-2381

AZZARI, Fabian A; CSSS de Rimouski-Neigette, CP 3150 Succ A 150 av Rouleau, Rimouski QC G5L 5T1; (Argentina)'93; Staff, Hôpital Regional Rimouski; (418)724-3000

AZZARIA, Samir; La Maison Michel Sarrazin, 2101 ch Saint-Louis, Quebec QC G1T 1P5; Laval'97; CCFP; Staff, Maison Michel Sarrazin; Langs: Spanish; (418)688-0878; Fax. (418)681-8636.

AZZI, Fadi-Boutros; Hawkesbury Dist Gen Hosp, 1111 Ghislain St, Hawkesbury ON K6A 3G5; Sher'02; CCFP; Staff, Hawkesbury & District General Hospital; Langs: Arabic; French; (613)632-1111

AZZI, Melhem; Ctre Hosp de Verdun, 4000 boul Lasalle, Verdun QC H4G 2A3; St. Joseph (Lebanon)'84; AB(Surg.); FRCSC; GenSurg (Endoscopy). Staff, Centre Hospitalier de Verdun; (514)362-1000

AZZI, Wadih B; PO Box 4010, Barrhead AB T7N 1A1; Sher'03; CCFP; azzi@ualberta.ca.

AZZIE, Georges R; The Hosp for Sick Children, RCH 1505-555 University Ave, Toronto ON M5G 1X8; Tor'86; FRCSC; GenSurg; PedGenSurg. Staff, The Hospital For Sick Children; (416)813-7654 x2413; georges.azzie@sickkids.ca.

AZZOPARDI, Mark J A; Port Hope Med Centre, 202-249 Ontario St, Port Hope ON L1A 3Y9; Tor'87; (905)885-6712; Fax. (905)885-7695.

AZZOPARDI, Peter; SGH Medical Mall, 407-3030 Lawrence Ave E, Scarborough ON M1P 2T7; Tor'85; FRCPC; Peds. Staff, The Scarborough Hospital - Birchmount Campus; Staff, The Scarborough Hospital - General Campus; (416)431-5292

AZZOUZI, Khalid; CSSSG-Hop de Gatineau, 909 boul de la Verendrye O, Gatineau QC J8P 7H2; Lille (France)'97; MedOncol (P.Q.); Hem (P.Q.). Staff, Hôpital de Gatineau; Langs: Bilingual(French/English); (819)561-8100

AZZUMEEA, Fahad M I; PG Medical Education Office, 500 University Ave, Toronto ON M5G 1V7; Riyadh (Saudi Arabia)'99; DiagRad.

BAARD, Johann; Nipawin Med Group, PO Box 2135, Nipawin SK S0E 1E0; (306)862-4626; Fax. (306)862-3522.

BAARS, Cornelius M; Orleans Urgent Care Clinic, 100-1220 Place D'Orleans Dr, Orleans ON K1C 7K3; McG'64; DECH; CCFP; FCFP; (613)841-4920

BAASCH, Erik J; Hilltop Med Clinic, 140-15321 16 Ave, Surrey BC V4A 1R6; Witwatersrand (South Africa)'87; MB ChB; CCFP; (604)531-5575; Fax. (604)535-0126.

BAASS, Alexis; MUHC-Royal Victoria Hosp, C6.88-687 av des Pins O, Montreal QC H3A 1A1; Mon'05; FRCPC; MedBiochem. Staff, McGill University Health Centre - Royal Victoria Hospital; (514)934-1934 x36790; Fax. (514)834-1499.

BAASS, Patricia C; 100-240 Wharncliffe Rd N, London ON N6H 4P2; Tor'00; CCFP; Langs: Bilingual(English/French); (519)685-3210

BAATH, Jasbir S; Sandalwood Med Centre, 5-2945 Sandalwood Pky E, Brampton ON L6R 3J6; Guru Nanak (India)'75; MB BS; FRCPC; IntMed; GeriatricMed. (905)463-1337

BAATH, Kulrajbir; Holly Street Endoscopy Clinic, 301-40 Holly St, Toronto ON M4S 3C3; Sask'06; FRCPC; IntMed; Gastroent. Teach Staff, McMaster University; (416)486-8088

BABA, Carolyn M; 403-3735 Casorso Rd, Kelowna BC V1W 5G1; UBC'85; Peds. (250)861-6200

BABAKIFARD, Katayoun; Hôpital Laval, 2725 ch Sainte-Foy, Quebec QC G1V 4G5; (Other Foreign)'92; CCFP; Staff, Hôpital Laval; (418)656-4550

BABAKISSA, Corentin; CHUS-Hop Fleurimont, 3001 12e Av N, Sherbrooke QC J1H 5N4; (France)'91; Gastroent (P.Q.). Staff, Centre Hospitalier Universitaire de Sherbrooke-Hopital Fleurimont; (819)346-1110; corentin.babakissa@usherbrooke.ca.

BABAPULLE, Mohan N; Medical Bldg, 404-18 Pine St, Kitchener ON N2H 5Z8; McG'98; FRCPC; IntMed; Cardiol. (519)576-8240; Fax. (519)576-8291.

BABBAGE, Christopher A; Sherbrook Centre, 4F-260 Sherbrooke St, New Westminster BC V3L 3M2; UBC'93; FRCPC; Psy.

BABCOCK, Courtney A; 1624 Seventh Ave, Prince George BC V2L 3P6; UBC'06; GenSurg. Staff, University Hospital of Northern British Columbia; (250)561-2700

BABCOCK, Lea J; Couchiching Family Health Team, 201B-119 Memorial St, Orillia ON L3V 5X1; Wes'93; CCFP; Staff, Orillia Soldiers' Memorial Hospital; (705)326-9334; Fax. (705)325-9498.

BABEN, Christo; Cambridge Mem Hosp, 700 Coronation Blvd, Cambridge ON N1R 3G2; Stellenbosch (South Africa)'80; MB ChB; CCFP; Staff, Cambridge Memorial Hospital; Langs: Afrikaans; (519)621-2333; Fax. (519)740-4921.

BABENSEE, Susan E; Kootenay-Boundary Reg Hosp, 1200 Hospital Bench, Trail BC V1R 4M1; Tor'87; FRCPC; DiagRad; NuclearMed. Dir Med Imaging, Kootenay Boundary Regional Hospital; (250)364-3416; Fax. (250)364-3435.

BABEY, Kenneth; Mount Forest Fam Health Team, 525 Dublin St SS 3, Mount Forest ON N0G 2L3; McM'76; Staff All Sites, North Wellington Health Care - Louise Marshall Hospital; (519)323-0255; Fax. (519)323-2113.

BABIAK, Taras; 201-15 Toronto St, Toronto ON M5C 2E3; Tor'76; ABNPath; ABPath; BA; MD; FRCPC; NeurPath (Chronic Psychiatric Disorders); Psy. Staff Consultant Psy, Centre for Addiction & Mental Health (CAMH) - College Street Site; Physician, IRIS Group & Memb., Toronto Psychoanalytic Institute; Langs: Ukrainian; Russian; (416)966-0835; Fax. (416)966-0837; alimacb@globalserve.net.

BABIC, Bojana; 201-15 Mountain Ave S, Stoney Creek ON L8G 2V6; McM'01; FRCPC; Peds; Endocrin&Metab. (905)664-9992

BABICK, Terry R; 201-952 Main St, Winnipeg MB R2W 3P4; Man'76; (204)589-7386; Fax. (204)589-7387.

BABIN, Antoine; Clinique Med St-Louis, 220-3165 ch Saint-Louis, Quebec QC G1W 4R4; Laval'72; (418)653-1970; antoine_babin@yahoo.com.

BABIN, Charles E; Centre Med de Huntingdon, RR 3 72A rue Chateauguay, Huntingdon QC J0S 1H0; Ott'60; Langs: English; French; (450)264-6101; Fax. (450)264-6101.

BABIN, Guillaume; Inst Univ Cardiol & Pneumologi, 2725 ch Sainte-Foy, Quebec QC G1V 4G5; Laval'08; FRCPC; IntMed. (418)656-4813

BABIN, Jacinthe; CSSS Haut-Richelieu-Rouville, 920 boul du Seminaire N, St-Jean-sur-Richel QC J3A 1B7; Laval'99; FRCPC; IntMed; Nephrol. Staff, Hôpital du Haut-Richelieu; Langs: Bilingual(French/English); (418)691-5151

BABIN, Lise M; 105-185 av Acadie, Dieppe NB E1A 1G6; Laval'94; CCFP; (506)862-4182; Fax. (506)862-4179.

BABIN, Martina; 2372 Highway 206 PO Box 3000, Arichat NS B0E 1A0; Laval'10; CCFP; (902)226-1674; Fax. (902)226-9312.

BABIN, Sandra; Clin d'Endocrinologie de l'Out, 3E-520 boul de l'Hopital, Gatineau QC J8V 2P5; Mon'90; FRCPC; IntMed; Endocrin&Metab; Endocrin (P.Q.). Langs: English; (819)369-5111; Fax. (819)771-7839.

BABINEAU, Gaetan; Coop Sante Aylmer, 67 rue du Couvent, Gatineau QC J9H 6A2; Mon'87; Staff, Centre Hospitalier Gatineau Mémorial; (819)684-1234

BABINEAU, Veronique; Clin de Gyn et D'Obsterique, 2235 7e av, Trois-Rivieres QC G8Z 3E2; McG'06; MDCM; FRCSC; ObstGyn. (819)379-5353

BABINS, Eric M; Southland Sport Med, 2000 Southland Dr SW, Calgary AB T2V 4S4; Cal'88; Dip SportMed; CCFP; FCFP; Clin Assoc Prof, University of Calgary; Langs: French; (403)251-9535; Fax. (403)252-9021; hockeymd@shaw.ca.

BABIUK, Danielle; 103-2489 Bloor St W, Toronto ON M6S 1R6; Sher'83; Staff, St Joseph's Health Centre.

BABIUK, Olga; Clinique Med du Plateau, 300-195 rue de l'Atmosphere, Gatineau QC J9A 0A3; Mon'84; (819)776-0001

BABKIS, Andrey Y; Meadow Lake Associate Clinic, PO Box 1510 218 Centre St, Meadow Lake SK S9X 1Z1; (306)236-5661; Fax. (306)236-4355.

BABLAD, Guru S; Forest Hill Family Health Cent, 302-491 Eglinton Ave W, Toronto ON M5N 1A8; Bombay (India)'60; DMRD; DABR; FRCPC; DiagRad. (416)640-1103; Fax. (416)640-1106.

BABLITZ, Harvey A; Whitecourt Med Clinic, PO Box 1076 Stn Main 5102 50 St, Whitecourt AB T7S 1P9; Alb'75; (780)778-2224; Fax. (780)778-2127.

BABOOLAL, Ranjit T; West Arthur Place, 707-1265 Arthur St E, Thunder Bay ON P7E 6E7; National Ireland (Ireland)'80; MB ChB; FAAP; MRC; FRCPC; Peds (Neonatology). (807)622-6366

BABST, Hans Van N; Nanaimo Reg Gen Hosp, 1200 Dufferin Cres, Nanaimo BC V9S 2B7; Witwatersrand (South Africa)'87; MB BCh; FRCPC; Anes. Staff, Nanaimo Regional General Hospital; (250)755-7605

BABUIN, Peter P E; Caledonian Med Clinic, 340 Campbell St, Nanaimo BC V9R 3G7; UBC'69; (250)753-3202; Fax. (250)753-1039.

BABURAM, Ashokchand; Bonnyville Healthcare Centre, PO Box 1008 Stn Main 5001 Lakeshore Dr, Bonnyville AB T9N 2J7; Mangalore (India)'93; Staff, Bonnyville Healthcare Centre; Consultant OrthSurg, Cold Lake Healthcare Centre; (780)826-8264; Fax. (780)826-6531.

BABWAH, Jesse P; Sunnybrook Hlth Sciences Ctre, 2075 Bayview Ave, Toronto ON M4N 3M5; Spartan St Lucia (Other Foreign)'06; Staff, Sunnybrook Health Sciences Centre; (416)480-4600

BABY, Benjamin J; Grove Medical Centre, 401-21183 88 Ave, Langley BC V1M 2G5; Newcastle-Upon-Tyne (England)'01; MB BS; CCFP; (604)882-1250

BABY, Marie-Claire; Hotel-Dieu de Levis, 143 rue Wolfe, Levis QC G6V 3Z1; Laval'98; CCFP; CCFP(E.M.); Staff, Hôtel-Dieu de Lévis; (418)835-7122 x6178; Fax. (418)835-7143.

BABY, Miriam T; 1915 17 St PO Box 180 Stn Main, Coaldale AB T1M 1M3; (South Africa)'03; (403)345-3072; Fax. (403)345-2141.

BABYN, Paul S; Royal University Hosp, 1566-103 Hospital Dr, Saskatoon SK S7N 0W8; McG'82; MDCM; FRCPC; DiagRad (Pediatrics). Staff, Royal University Hospital; Dept Head Med Imaging, University of Saskatchewan; (306)655-2379; Fax. (306)655-2370; paul.babyn@saskatoonhealthregion.ca.

BACANI, Julinor T; University of Alberta Hosp, 5B2.04-8440 112 St NW, Edmonton AB T6G 2B7; UBC'99; FRCPC; AnatPath. Staff, University of Alberta Hospital; (780)407-3419; Fax. (780)407-3009.

BACCHUS, Catherine M; Foothills Med Centre, 1403 29 St NW, Calgary AB T2N 2T9; Tor'85; MSc; FRCPC; IntMed. Staff, Foothills Medical Centre; Vice Chair Strategic Planning Dept of Med, University of Calgary; (403)944-3324; Fax. (403)944-1095; maria.bacchus@albertahealthservices.ca.

BACCHUS, Farzana R; Hamilton HS-General Site, 1 270-237 Barton St E, Hamilton ON L8L 2X2; McM'07; FRCPC; IntMed; Hem. Staff, Hamilton Health Sciences Centre - Hamilton General Hospital.

BACCHUS, Rahman; Dr R Bacchus Medical Prof Corp, 102-1106 Ouellette Ave, Windsor ON N9A 1C9; West Indies (Jamaica)'72; FRCPC; IntMed; Gastroent. Ac Staff, Hôtel-Dieu Grace Hospital; Court Staff, Windsor Regional Hospital - Metropolitan Site; Aj Prof, University of Western Ontario; (519)254-4511; Fax. (519)254-7226.

BACH, David B; London HSC-University Hosp, PO Box 5339 Stn B 339 Windermere Rd, London ON N6A 5A5; McG'80; FRCPC; DiagRad (Body Computed Tomography). Staff Radiologist, London Health Sciences Centre - University Hospital; Hon Treas, Canadian Medical Association; Emeritus Prof, University of Western Ontario; (519)663-3221; Fax. (519)663-8803.

BACH, Paul S; St Paul's Hosp, 1081 Burrard St, Vancouver BC V6Z 1Y6; Cal'88; FRCPC; Anes. Staff, Providence Health Care - St Paul's Hospital; (604)682-2344

BACHAND, Andre; Hop du Sacre-Coeur de Mtl, 5400 boul Gouin O, Montreal QC H4J 1C5; Mon'61; MedOncol (P.Q.); Hem (P.Q.). Staff, Hôpital du Sacre-Coeur de Montréal; (514)338-2150

BACHAND, Francois; BC Cancer Ctre-Southern Interi, 399 Royal Ave, Kelowna BC V1Y 5L3; Sher'04; FRCPC; RadOncol. Staff, BC Cancer Agency Sindi Ahluwalia Hawkins Centre for the Southern Interior; (250)712-3900

BACHAND, Gilles; Clinique Med Plateau Marquette, 200-731 rue Galt O, Sherbrooke QC J1H 1Z1; Sher'78; LMCC; (819)564-8662; Fax. (819)564-1294.

BACHAND, Isabelle; CSSS du Suroît, 150 rue Saint-Thomas, Salaber-de-Valleyf QC J6T 6C1; Sher'93; CSPQ; FRCPC; MedBiochem. Staff, Centre Hospitalier Régional du Suroît; (450)371-9920; Fax. (450)371-5275.

BACHAND, Jacques; Clinique Med Plateau Marquette, 200-731 rue Galt O, Sherbrooke QC J1H 1Z1; Sher'75; Staff, Centre Hospitalier Universitaire de Sherbrooke-Hôpital Hôtel-Dieu; (819)564-8662; Fax. (819)564-1294.

BACHAND, Marie-Pier; CHUS-Hop Hotel-Dieu, 580 rue Bowen S, Sherbrooke QC J1G 2E8; Sher'07; FRCPC; IntMed; Gastroent. Staff, Centre Hospitalier Universitaire de Sherbrooke-Hôpital Hôtel-Dieu; (819)346-1110

BACHAND, Monique; Clinique Medicale GMF-1851, 1100-1851 rue Sherbrooke E, Montreal QC H2K 4L5; Mon'76; Langs: English; (514)526-3351; Fax. (514)526-4594.

BACHAND, Stephane; Clinique Dr Stephane Bachand, 306-176 Av Rouleau, Rimouski QC G5L 8W1; Sher'86; FRCSC; OrthSurg (P.Q.) (Arthroplasty). Staff, Hôpital Regional Rimouski; Langs: Bilingual(French/English); (418)724-2818; Fax. (418)723-4550.

BACHER, Janice K; Davisville Family Practice, 1881 Yonge St, Toronto ON M4S 3C4; Tor'10; CCFP; (416)932-3172

BACHER, Larry; Malvern Med Arts Bldg, 100-1333 Neilson Rd, Scarborough ON M1B 4Y9; Tor'81; CCFP; FCFP; Staff, The Scarborough Hospital - General Campus; Staff, Rouge Valley Health System - Centenary Health Centre Site; (416)291-7719; Fax. (416)287-3775.

BACHER, Thomas S; Malvern Med Centre, 100-1333 Neilson Rd, Scarborough ON M1B 4Y9; Tor'75; Staff, The Scarborough Hospital - General Campus; (416)291-7719; Fax. (416)287-3775.

BACHER, Yves; MUHC-Royal Victoria Hosp, M812-687 av des Pins O, Montreal QC H3A 1A1; Mon'81; FRCPC; IntMed; GeriatricMed. Staff, McGill University Health Centre - Royal Victoria Hospital; (514)934-1934 x36972; Fax. (514)843-1400; yves.bacher@muhc.mcgill.ca.

BACHEYIE, Godfrey S; Windsor Reg Hosp-Metropolitan, ME1260-1995 Lens Ave, Windsor ON N8W 1L9; Accra (Ghana)'73; MB ChB; FAAP; FRCPC; Peds (Neonatology). Dir Neonatology, Windsor Regional Hospital - Metropolitan Site; Aj Prof Psychology, University Of Windsor; Clinical Asst Prof Peds, University of Western Ontario; (519)255-2379; Fax. (519)255-1735; godfrey_bacheyie@wrh.on.ca.

BACHIR, Ayda; CSSS Bordeaux-Cartierville-St-, 555 boul Gouin O, Montreal QC H3L 1K5; Mon'76; Gen Practice, Pavillon Notre-Dame de la Merci; (514)331-3020

BACHLER, Markus A; 1485 Merklin St, White Rock BC V4B 4C4; UBC'99; FRCPC; Anes. Staff, Lions Gate Hospital; (604)961-4070

BACHYNSKY, Theodore J; 135-5325 Cordova Bay Rd, Victoria BC V8Y 2L3; Dal'92; BSc; CCFP; Staff, Victoria General Hospital; Staff, Royal Jubilee Hospital; (250)385-6115

BACILY, Mervat A; Markham Prof Centre, 203-2265 Pembina Hwy, Winnipeg MB R3T 5J3; (Egypt)'86; CCFP; Physician, Greencrest Pembina Clinic; Langs: Arabic; (204)261-9881; mervatadly@hotmail.com.

BACIOWSKI, Chris K; 21 Morbank Dr, Scarborough ON M1V 2M1; Bialystok Acad. of Med. (Poland)'65; Staff, The Scarborough Hospital - General Campus; (416)292-5760; Fax. (416)292-9350.

BACKLER, John H; 100-4999 rue Sainte-Catherine, Westmount QC H3Z 1T3; Montpellier (France)'75; CCFP; Assoc Physician, Sir Mortimer B Davis Jewish General; Teach Staff Family Med, McGill University; Langs: French; (514)485-8226

BACKLIN, Samuel A; Rockyview Gen Hosp, 7007 14 St SW, Calgary AB T2V 1P9; Tor'82; CCFP; CCFP(E.M.); Staff, Rockyview General Hospital; (403)943-3449; Fax. (403)242-9104.

BACKMAN, Steven B; MUHC-Royal Victoria Hosp, 687 av des Pins O, Montreal QC H3A 1A1; McG'88; CSPQ; FRCPC; Anes. Dir Anes, McGill University Health Centre - Royal Victoria Hospital; Head Dept of Anes & Assoc Prof, McGill University; (514)934-1934 x36123; Fax. (514)843-1698; steven.backman@muhc.mcgill.ca.

BACKO-SHANNON, Mirjana; Oakmed Family Health Team, 110-231 Oak Park Blvd, Oakville ON L6H 7S8; Qns'00; BSc; CCFP; Staff, Halton Healthcare Services Corporation - Oakville Site; (905)901-5111; Fax. (905)901-5122.

BACKSTEIN, David J; Mount Sinai Hosp, 476D-600 University Ave, Toronto ON M5G 1X5; Tor'93; FRCSC; OrthSurg (Hip & Knee Arthroplasty). Assoc Prof, Mount Sinai Hospital; (416)586-8457; Fax. (416)586-8678.

BACKSTEIN, Robert S; Plastic Surgery Centre, 400-4256 Bathurst St, North York ON M3H 5Y8; Tor'94; FRCSC; PlasSurg. Staff, Toronto Dermatology Centre; (416)633-0001; Fax. (416)633-0002.

BACKUS, Richard D H; Rebalance MD, 104-3551 Blanshard St, Victoria BC V8Z 0B9; Alb'72; BSc; Dip SportMed; MD; DHMSA; Assoc Staff, Victoria General Hospital; Assoc Staff, Royal Jubilee Hospital; Asst Prof, University of Victoria; (250)940-4444

BACKWAY, Karen L; 205-751 Victoria St S, Kitchener ON N2M 5N4; Tor'99; FRCPC; Peds. (519)885-9153

BACON, Mark J; Lasalle Community Health Care, 2125 Front Rd, Windsor ON N9J 2C1; Wes'95; CCFP; (519)734-1234; Fax. (519)734-8674.

BACOPULOS, Sarah A; 106-3305 Harvester Rd, Burlington ON L7N 3N2; Wes'04; FRCSC; GenSurg. (905)333-6245; Fax. (905)333-6266.

BACSKAI, Istvan S; 356B Woodroffe Ave, Ottawa ON K2A 3V6; Pecs (Hungary)'81; Langs: Hungarian; (613)729-8278; Fax. (613)729-8359.

BADALATO, Heather A; Homewood Health Centre, 150 Delhi St, Guelph ON N1E 6K9; McM'06; CCFP; Staff, Homewood Health Centre; (519)824-1010

BADALI, Mary A; Sunnybrook Hlth Sciences Ctre, C753-2075 Bayview Ave, Toronto ON M4N 3M5; Tor'81; CCFP; CCFP(E.M.); Ac Staff, Sunnybrook Health Sciences Centre; (416)480-4037; Fax. (416)480-4704.

BADAWI, Abdelrahman K; Hamilton HS-McMaster Site, PO Box 2000 Stn Lcd 1, Hamilton ON L8N 3Z5; Al Fateh (Libya)'00; FRCSC; OrthSurg. Staff, Hamilton Health Sciences Centre - McMaster Children's Hospital.

BADAWI, Arieg Z E; Kelso Lake Med Centre, 205-330 Bronte St S, Milton ON L9T 7X1; Khartoum (Sudan)'01; CCFP; (905)876-1011; Fax. (905)876-3401.

BADAWI, Mohammad; Wetaskiwin Hosp & Care Centre, 4509-6910 47 St, Wetaskiwin AB T9A 3N3; (Syria)'94; FRCSC; ObstGyn (Prenatal Care). Staff, Wetaskiwin Hospital & Care Centre; (780)361-4360; Fax. (780)352-0300.

BADAWI, Osama K; Queenston Med & Dental Centre, 201-631 Queenston Rd, Hamilton ON L8K 6R5; Ein Shams (Egypt)'82; Assoc Staff Family Med, Hamilton Health Sciences Centre-Juravinski Site; (905)560-8645; Fax. (905)560-8647.

BADAWY, Mohamed; Ctr Hosp de Lasalle, 8585 Tsse Champlain, LaSalle QC H8P 1C1; Mon'07; FRCPC; Anes. Staff, Centre Hospitalier de LaSalle; (514)362-8000

BADCOCK, Beverley S; Ross Mem Hosp, 10 Angeline St N, Lindsay ON K9V 4M8; Mem'84; FRCPC; Anes. Staff, Ross Memorial Hospital; (705)324-6111 x4228; Fax. (705)328-6121.

BADDAR, Faisal; Pembroke Reg Hosp, 705 MacKay St, Pembroke ON K8A 1G8; McG'09; CCFP; Staff, Pembroke Regional Hospital Inc; (613)735-2811

BADENHORST, Bartholomeus L; Protea Med Clinic, 1-4440 44 Ave NE, Calgary AB T1Y 4W5; Orange Free State (South Africa)'95; MB ChB; CCFP; (403)285-8010

BADENHORST, Charl J; Fort St John Mental Health, 230-9900 100 Ave, Fort St. John BC V1J 5S7; Orange Free State (South Africa)'82; MB ChB; MMedSci; BSc(Hons); Physician, Fort St John Mental Health & Addiction Services; Asst Prof Commun Health, University of British Columbia; (250)793-2780; Fax. (250)262-4010; charl.badenhorst@northernhealth.ca.

BADENHORST, Este; Protea Med Clinic, 1-4440 44 Ave NE, Calgary AB T1Y 4W5; (South Africa)'02; (403)285-8010; estebadenhorst@yahoo.ca.

BADENHORST, Frederik J; Selkirk Medical Centre, 353 Eveline St, Selkirk MB R1A 1N1; (Other Foreign)'82; MB ChB; Langs: Afrikaans.

BADENHORST, Johannes G; Bayside Med Centre, 3 Beck Blvd, Penetanguishene ON L9M 1B9; Pretoria (South Africa)'91; DA(SA); CCFP; Staff, Georgian Bay General Hospital - Midland; Langs: Afrikaans; (705)549-3939; Fax. (705)549-0029.

BADENHORST, Josias S; 125-47 Clearview Market Way, Red Deer AB T4P 0M9; Stellenbosch (South Africa)'88; MB ChB; Langs: Afrikaans; (403)356-0222; Fax. (403)356-0223.

BADENHORST, Karen A; Protea Med Clinic, 1-4440 44 Ave NE, Calgary AB T1Y 4W5; Orange Free State (South Africa)'94; MB ChB; LMCC; CCFP; Langs: Afrikaans; (403)285-8010; Fax. (403)285-8801.

BADENHORST, Lynette; Riverview Health Centre, 455-1 Morley Ave, Winnipeg MB R3L 2P4; Stellenbosch (South Africa)'84; MB ChB; Ac Staff Behaviour Management Prog, Riverview Health Centre; Ac Staff, Winnipeg Regional Health Authority; Langs: Afrikaans.

BADENHORST, Stefanus M; Protea Med Centre, 1-4440 44 Ave NE, Calgary AB T1Y 4W5; (South Africa)'99; (403)285-8010; Fax. (403)285-8801.

BADER, Erin L; 604-11010 101 St NW, Edmonton AB T5H 4B9; Cal'04; FRCSC; ObstGyn. Staff General ObstGyn, Royal Alexandra Hospital; Staff Gen ObstGyn, Northeast Community Health Centre; (780)421-4728; Fax. (780)426-6698.

BADER, Jean-Francois; Queen Elizabeth Hosp, PO Box 6600 Stn Central, Charlottetown PE C1A 8T5; Sher'94; CCFP; CCFP(E.M.); FCFP; Staff, Queen Elizabeth Hospital; (902)894-0130

BADER, Mazen; Hamilton HS-Henderson Site, 508-711 Concession St, Hamilton ON L8V 1C3; Istanbul (Turkey)'96; MPH; FRCPC; IntMed; InfectDis. Staff, Hamilton Health Sciences Centre-Juravinski Site; (905)389-4411

BADER, Russell T; North York Gen Hosp, 4001 Leslie St, North York ON M2K 1E1; Ben-Gurion (Israel)'08; FRCPC; IntMed. Staff, North York General Hospital; (416)756-6000

BADESCU, Felicia; CSSS de la Vallée de l'Or, 725 6e rue, Val-d'Or QC J9P 3Y1; Bucarest (Romania)'88; Psy (P.Q.). Staff, Centre Hospitalier de Val d'Or; (819)825-6711

BADHAN, Harry S; Finchgate Med Centre, 105-40 Finchgate Blvd, Brampton ON L6T 3J1; Guru Nanak (India)'78; Staff, William Osler Health System - Brampton Civic Hospital; Langs: Punjabi; Hindi; Urdu; (905)791-8330; Fax. (905)791-8330.

BADHESHA, Jagdeep S; DB08A-7556 Falconridge Blvd NE, Calgary AB T3J 0C9; (India)'99; MD; LMCC; CCFP; Langs: Punjabi; Urdu; Hindi; (403)475-2500; Fax. (403)475-2504.

BADI, Entisar M; 200-10083 Keele St, Vaughan ON L6A 3Y8; Al-Fateh (Libya)'89; ObstGyn. Staff, Grey Bruce Health Services - Owen Sound; Langs: Arabic; (905)879-0506

BADI, Fathi A; Fishermen's Mem Hosp, PO Box 1180 14 High St, Lunenburg NS B0J 2C0; University of Al Fateh (Libya)'02; MB BCh; Staff, Fishermen's Memorial Hospital; (902)789-2526; dr. badi@yahoo.ca.

BADII, Maziar; 208-888 8th Ave W, Vancouver BC V5Z 3Y1; UBC'95; MHSc; FRCPC; IntMed (Spine); Rheum. Staff, Vancouver General Hospital - Centennial Pavillion; Dir Injury & Disability Prev, Occupational Hlth & Safety Agency for Healthcare; Teach Staff Rheum, University of British Columbia; Langs: Persian; (604)731-3125

BADIR, Badir Francis; Hop Santa Cabrini Ospedale, 5655 rue Saint-Zotique E, Montreal QC H1T 1P7; Ain Shams (Egypt)'87; MB ChB; MSc; ABIM; FRCPC; IntMed (Cardiology). Staff, Hôpital Santa Cabrini Ospedale; Langs: Bilingual(French/English); (514)252-6444

BADLEY, Bernard W D; 5890 Chain Rock Dr, Halifax NS B3H 1A1; London (England)'57; FRCP; IntMed (Gastroenterology). Consultant, Canadian Forces Health Services Centre (Atlantic); Med Dir Colon Cancer Prevention Prog, Cancer Care Manitoba; (902)423-1922; badley@eastlink.ca.

BADLISSI, Dalal; CSSS du Nord de Lanaudière, 1000 boul Sainte-Anne, St-Charles-Brromee QC J6E 6J2; Aleppo (Syria)'79; MPH; FRCPC; CommunMed (P.Q.); Public Health & Preventive Med. Staff, Centre Hospitalier Régional de Lanaudière; Public Health, Regie Regional de Lanaudiere; Langs: Arabic; Bilingual(French/English); (450)759-1157 x4426; Fax. (450)759-5149; dalal_badlissi@ssss.gouv.qc.ca.

BADMOS, Oluleke S; Toronto East Gen Hosp Inc, 825 Coxwell Ave, Toronto ON M4C 3E7; Ibadan (Nigeria)'85; MB BS; FRCS; FRCOG; FRCSC; ObstGyn. Staff, Toronto East General Hospital Inc; Lecturer ObstGyn, University of Toronto; (416)469-6333

BADNER, Neal; Kelowna Gen Hosp, 2268 Pandosy St, Kelowna BC V1Y 1T2; Qns'84; FRCPC; Anes. Staff, Kelowna General Hospital; (250)862-4003

BADOE, Kwame E; Trellis Mental Hlth & Dev Serv, 147 Delhi St, Guelph ON N1E 4J3; (Ghana)'76; MB ChB; FRCPC; Psy (General Adult Psychiatry). Consultant Privil, St Joseph's Hospital - St Joseph's Health Care; Consultant Psy, Guelph General Hospital; Langs: Nzima; Twi; (519)821-2060 x218; Fax. (519)821-5452; kbadoe@trellis.on.ca.

BADOWSKI, Deborah; Halton HSC Corp-Oakville, 327 Reynolds St, Oakville ON L6J 3L7; Tor'80; Staff, Halton Healthcare Services Corporation - Oakville Site; (905)338-4647

BADRA, Riad; Clinique Externe Pedopsy, 2924 boul Taschereau, Longueuil QC J4V 2G8; Lyon I (France)'76; (450)466-5496 x6169

BADRA QUIRION, Karine; St Paul's Hosp, 1081 Burrard St, Vancouver BC V6Z 1Y6; Sher'09; CCFP; Staff, Providence Health Care - St Paul's Hospital; Langs: Bilingual(English/French); (604)682-2344

BADRA VERDU, Mariano; CHUS-Hop Fleurimont, 3001 12e av N, Sherbrooke QC J1H 5N4; Staff, Centre Hospitalier Universitaire de Sherbrooke-Hopital Fleurimont; (819)346-1110 x14326

BADRAN, Haitham; CSSS de Saint-Jerome, 290 de Montigny, Saint-Jerome QC J7Z 5T3; McG'07; MDCM; FRCSC; PlasSurg. Staff, Hôtel-Dieu de Saint-Jérôme; (450)432-2777

BADRO, Emile; 7715 boul Newman, LaSalle QC H8N 1X7; Beirut (Lebanon)'72; FRCSC; GenSurg. assoc Staff, Hôpital Ste-Justine; (514)992-4404

BAECHLER, Marion G; 201-348 Muskoka Rd 3 N, Huntsville ON P1H 1H8; McM'91; CCFP; FCFP; (705)789-6137; Fax. (705)789-6175.

BAER, Carolyn E H; The Moncton Hosp, 135 MacBeath Ave, Moncton NB E1C 6Z8; Ott'87; FRCPC; IntMed. Staff Internist, The Moncton Hospital; Asst Prof, Dalhousie University; Clinical Asst Prof, Memorial University Of Newfoundland; Langs: English; French; (506)857-5111

BAER, Philip A; Malvern Med Arts Bldg, 305-1333 Neilson Rd, Scarborough ON M1B 4Y9; McG'80; ABIM; FACRheum; FRCPC; IntMed (Osteoporosis); Rheum. Ed in Chief CRAJ, Canadian Rheumatology Association; Med Consultant, Empire Insurance Group Inc; Med Dir, Transamerica Life Canada Inc; Med Dir, Canadian Premier Life; Chair Section of Rheumatology, Ontario Medical Association; Langs: French; (416)286-7686; Fax. (416)286-8413.

BAER, Susan; BC Women's Hosp & HC, 4500 Oak St, Vancouver BC V6H 3N1; UBC'98; FRCPC; Psy (Child & Adolescent Psychiatry). Staff Psy, BC Women's Hospital & Health Centre; Clin Instructor, University of British Columbia; (604)875-2345 x7396; Fax. (604)875-2099.

BAERG, Kerry J; Alder Med Centre, 277 Evergreen Rd, Campbell River BC V9W 5Y4; Tor'88; (250)287-7441; Fax. (250)287-4384.

BAERG, Krista L; Royal University Hosp, 103 Hospital Dr, Saskatoon SK S7N 0W8; Sask'98; FRCPC; Peds. Staff, Royal University Hospital; Asst Prof, University of Saskatchewan; (306)966-8911; Fax. (306)966-8640.

BAERG HALL, Elizabeth A; Langara Student Health, 100 49th Ave W, Vancouver BC V5Y 2Z6; McM'88; FRCPC; Psy. Staff, BC Women's Hospital & Health Centre; Clinical Asst Prof, University of British Columbia; Staff Student Health Centre, Langara College; (604)323-5256

BAERGEN, James G; 212-1240 Railway Ave, Canmore AB T1W 1P4; Cal'07; CCFP; (403)609-8333

BAERGEN, Kathleen G; 201-5651 Riverbend Rd NW, Edmonton AB T6H 5K4; Alb'87; CCFP; (780)438-8844; Fax. (780)436-9511.

BAERLOCHER, Mark; Georgian Radiology Consultants, 115-121 Wellington St W, Barrie ON L4N 1L2; Tor'05; FRCPC; DiagRad. (705)726-4531

BAETA, Basil R; 204-86 Angeline St S, Lindsay ON K9V 6C5; McG'74; BSc; FACS; FRCSC; GenSurg. Staff, Ross Memorial Hospital; (705)324-6159; Fax. (705)324-7091; basilbaeta@gmail.com.

BAETZ, Marilyn D A; Royal University Hosp, EH119-103 Hospital Dr, Saskatoon SK S7N 0W8; Sask'93; FRCPC; Psy. Staff, Royal University Hospital; Staff, Saskatoon Health Region; Dept Head Psy, University of Saskatchewan; (306)966-8223; Fax. (306)966-8761; m.baetz@usask.ca.

BAETZ, Tara D; Kingston Reg Cancer Centre, 25 King St W, Kingston ON K7L 5P9; Ott'95; BSc(Biol.); FRCPC; IntMed; MedOncol. Dir Experimental Therapeutics, Queen's University; (613)544-2630 x4503

BAFUNDI, Peter; The Doctor's Office, 3089 Dufferin St, North York ON M6A 2S7; Tor'94; BSc; CCFP; (416)256-9642; Fax. (416)256-9638.

BAGAI, Akshay; St Michael's Hosp, 30 Bond St, Toronto ON M5B 1W8; Tor'03; FRCPC; IntMed; Cardiol. Staff, St Michael's Hospital; (416)917-9497

BAGDAN, Barry M; Oceanview Women's Clinic, 101-1757 Beaufort Ave, Comox BC V9M 1R8; Alb'86; BMedSci; FRCSC; ObstGyn (Laparoscopic Surgery). Clinical Asst Prof, University of British Columbia; (250)339-3114; Fax. (250)339-4186.

BAGDAN, Bonnie L; Highwood Health Center, PO Box 5695 Stn Main 121 4th Ave W, High River AB T1V 1M7; Cal'94; CCFP; (403)652-7999; Fax. (403)652-7997.

BAGERIA, Charanjit S; 3348 Keele St, North York ON M3J 1L5; Tor'94; CCFP; Langs: Punjabi; (416)398-2505; Fax. (647)342-8478.

BAGG, Stephen D; St Mary's of the Lake Hosp, PO Box 3600 Stn Main, Kingston ON K7L 5A2; Qns'86; MSc; FRCPC; PhysMed&Rehab (Electrodiagnosis). Att Staff PhysMed&Rehab, Providence Care - St Mary's of the Lake Hospital Site; Att Staff, Kingston General Hospital; Att Staff, Hotel-Dieu Hospital; Dept Head Physical Med & Rehab, Queen's University; (613)544-4210; Fax. (613)544-4614; baggs@providencecare.ca.

BAGGA, Amit; 203-1106 Ouellette Ave, Windsor ON N9A 1C9; Wes'95; FRCPC; IntMed; Nephrol. Ac Staff Nephrol & IntMed, Hôtel-Dieu Grace Hospital; Cons Staff Nephrol, Windsor Regional Hospital - Metropolitan Site; Langs: Hindi; (519)255-2260; Fax. (519)946-9979; amitbagga108@gmail.com.

BAGGIO, Daniel; CSSS du Suroît, 150 rue Saint-Thomas, Salaber-de-Valleyf QC J6T 6C1; Mon'94; FRCPC; IntMed. Staff, Centre Hospitalier Régional du Suroît; (450)371-9920; Fax. (450)371-7454.

BAGGLEY, Anne M; 2948 Baseline Rd, Ottawa ON K2H 8T5; Tor'05; CCFP; Staff, Hawkesbury & District General Hospital; Langs: Bilingual(English/French); (613)482-0118

BAGGOO, Alan K; 213-145 15 St W, North Vancouver BC V7M 1R9; UBC'93; FRCSC; OrthSurg. Staff, Lions Gate Hospital; (604)980-0535; Fax. (604)988-0536.

BAGGOO, Darlene; Fairmont Med Bldg, 1317-750 Broadway W, Vancouver BC V5Z 1J3; UBC'92; CCFP; (604)876-0711; Fax. (604)876-0770.

BAGGS, Douglas K; Health Sciences Centre, 300 Prince Philip Dr, St. John's NL A1B 3V6; Mem'86; FRCPC; EmergMed. Clin Chief Emerg Trauma Prog, Health Sciences Centre; Asst Prof Med, Memorial University Of Newfoundland; (709)777-6335; hcc. bagd@hccsj.nf.ca.

BAGHAEE, Jalal; Parrsboro & Area Prof Centre, 76 Jenks Ave, Parrsboro NS B0M 1S0; (Iran)'94; MD; (902)254-3760; Fax. (902)254-3617.

BAGHBANNAZARY, Maryam; Vancouver Gen Hosp, 6A-855 12th Ave W, Vancouver BC V5Z 1M9; Alb'96; CCFP; Staff, Vancouver General Hospital - Centennial Pavillion; Langs: Farsi; (604)875-4073

BAGHDADLIAN, Hovsep; 406-4800 Sheppard Ave E, North York ON M2J 2K9; McG'82; ABIM; CSPQ; FRCPC; IntMed; MedMicrobiol; InfectDis. Staff, North York General Hospital; Staff, The Scarborough Hospital - General Campus; Langs: Armenian; French; (416)913-7224; Fax. (416)913-6286.

BAGHERI, Aghdas; 1206-180 Bloor St W, Toronto ON M5S 2V6; Tehran (Iran)'65; FRCPC; Psy. Sr Staff Psy, Centre for Addiction & Mental Health (CAMH) - Queen Site; (416)923-1640

BAGHIRZADA, Leyla B; Foothills Med Centre, 1403 29 St NW, Calgary AB T2N 2T9; (Azerbaijan)'98; FRCPC; Anes. Staff, Foothills Medical Centre; (403)944-1110

BAGLI, Darius J; The Hosp For Sick Children M292-555 University Ave, Toronto ON M5G 1X8; McG'84; FRCSC; Urol (Pediatric Urology). Staff Urol/Assoc Scientist Research Inst/Consultant Telemedicine, The Hospital For Sick Children; (416)813-6465 x8192; Fax. (416)813-6461; darius.bagli@sickkids.ca.

BAGNALL, Eric G; CFB Kingston, PO Box 17000 Stn Forces, Kingston ON K7K 7B4; Qns'83; (613)542-2813; Fax. (613)542-5486.

BAGNELL, Alexa L; IWK Health Centre, PO Box 9700 Rpo CSC 5850-5980 University Ave, Halifax NS B3K 6R8; Dal'97; FRCPC; Psy (Child & Adolescent Psychiatry). Staff, IWK Health Centre; Asst Prof, Dalhousie University; (902)470-8375; Fax. (902)470-8937.

BAGNELL, P Scott; Urology Consultants, 620-5991 Spring Garden Rd, Halifax NS B3H 1Y6; Dal'97; FRCSC; Urol. (902)425-3940; Fax. (902)422-0033.

BAGOVICH, Maria A; Rebecca McDonald Arthritis, 60 Murray St, Toronto ON M5T 3L9; McM'08; FRCPC; IntMed. (416)927-2027

BAGRY, Hema S; St Boniface Gen Hosp, L2035-409 Tache Ave, Winnipeg MB R2H 2A6; Bombay (India)'97; FRCPC; Anes. Staff, St Boniface General Hospital; (204)233-8563

BAGSHAW, Sean M; University of Alberta Hosp, 3C1.12-8440 112 St NW, Edmonton AB T6G 2B7; Cal'00; FRCPC; IntMed; Critical Care Medicine. Staff, University of Alberta Hospital; (780)407-6755

BAGUIO, Arnell; Southlake Reg Health Centre, 596 Davis Dr, Newmarket ON L3Y 2P9; Cebu (Philippines)'00; CCFP; Staff, Southlake Regional Health Centre; (905)895-4521

BAGUR, Rodrigo H; CHUQ-Hotel-Dieu de Quebec, 11 Cote du Palais, Quebec QC G1R 2J6; Staff, Centre Hospitalier Universitaire de Québec (CHUQ) - Siege Social; (418)691-5750

BAH, Abdoulaye; Clinique Millenia, CP 62 Succ Pl-Desjardins 303-4 Complexe Desjardins, Montreal QC H5B 1B2; Dakar (Senegal)'80; (514)287-2683; Fax. (514)287-1129.

BAH, Chaikou; 333-1804 boul Le Corbusier, Laval QC H7S 2N3; Sher'84; FRCSC; OrthSurg (Spine Surgery). Staff, CSSS du Coeur de l'Isle Hôpital Jean-Talon; Langs: English; French; (450)688-4451

BAHADUR, Randy; Grand River Hosp-KW Hlth Ctre, PO Box 9056 Stn C 835 King St W, Kitchener ON N2G 1G3; (Trinidad & Tobago)'08; CCFP; Staff, Grand River Hospital - Kitchener/Waterloo Health Centre; (519)749-4300

BAHAL, Maglin N; King West Village Med Centre, 201-626 King St W, Toronto ON M5V 1M7; Kasturba Medical College (India)'02; CCFP; (416)703-1313; Fax. (416)703-1310.

BAHARY, Jean-Paul; CHUM-Hop Notre-Dame, 1560 rue Sherbrooke E, Montreal QC H2L 4M1; Mon'86; FRCPC; RadOncol (Neuro Oncology). Staff, Centre Hospitalier l'Université de Montréal (CHUM) - Hôpital Notre-Dame; Prof, Universite de Montreal; (514)890-8254

BAHASADRI, Mohammad; Medical Clinic Bldg, 203-89 Humber College Blvd, Etobicoke ON M9V 4B8; (Iran)'92; FACS; MD; FRCSC; GenSurg (Advanced Laparoscopic Surgery). Staff GenSurg, William Osler Health System - Etobicoke General Hospital; Langs: Persian; Farsi; (416)913-6457

BAHL, Gaurav S; BC Cancer Agency-Abbotsford Ct, 32900 Marshall Rd, Abbotsford BC V2S 0C2; Nagpur (India)'02; FRCPC; RadOncol. (604)851-4742

BAHL, Mala; Grand River Hosp-KW Hlth Ctre, PO Box 9056 Stn C 835 King St W, Kitchener ON N2G 1G3; Jefferson(PA) (USA)'97; FRCPC; IntMed; MedOncol. Staff, Grand River Hospital - Kitchener/Waterloo Health Centre; (519)749-4380

BAHLER, Brad R; 101-190 Pelican Pl, Sylvan Lake AB T4S 1K2; Alb'02; CCFP; (403)887-2224; Fax. (403)887-2261.

BAHLIS, Nizar J; Foothills Med Centre, 681-1403 29 St NW, Calgary AB T2N 2T9; (Lebanon)'95; Staff, Foothills Medical Centre; (403)944-1564; Fax. (403)944-2102.

BAHMUTAN, Ana S; Health Sense Medical, 8-2983 Westoak Trails Blvd, Oakville ON L6M 5E4; CCFP; (905)901-1217

BAHORIC, Boris; SMBD Jewish Gen Hosp, 3755 ch Cote-Sainte-Catherine, Montreal QC H3T 1E2; Rijeka (Croatia)'85; FRCPC; RadOncol (Gynecologic Oncology). Staff RadOncol, McGill University Health Centre - Montreal General Campus; Staff, Sir Mortimer B Davis Jewish General; adj Prof, McGill University; Langs: Italian; Croatian; Bilingual(French/English); (514)340-8288; Fax. (514)340-7548; bbahoric@roc.jgh.mcgill.ca.

BAHRA, Parminder S; Brantford Urgent Care, 40 Shellington Pl, Brantford ON N3S 0C5; Tor'90; BSc; MSc; CCFP; CCFP(E.M.); Physician Emerg, The Brant Community Healthcare System - Brantford General Hospital Site; Ac Staff, Toronto East General Hospital Inc; (519)753-9581

BAHRAMI, Tahmoures; Atlantic Medical Centre, 1054 McPhillips St, Winnipeg MB R2X 2K9; Chittagong (Bangladesh)'96; CCFP.

BAHRAMI-ESFERJANI, Azar; 308-101 Queensway W, Mississauga ON L5B 2P7; Tehran (Iran)'97; FRCPC; IntMed; Rheum. (905)272-7200; Fax. (905)272-4500.

BAHREY, Lisa A L; Univ Hlth Network-Toronto Gen, 200 Elizabeth St, Toronto ON M5G 2C4; McM'95; FRCPC; Anes. Staff, Toronto General Hospital - UHN; (416)340-5164

BAHRGARD NIKOO, Mohammad J; St Mary's Gen Hosp, 911 Queens Blvd, Kitchener ON N2M 1B2; Guilan University (Iran)'01; FRCPC; IntMed; Critical Care Medicine. Staff, London Health Sciences Centre - University Hospital; Staff, Health Sciences North-Laurentian Site; Staff, St Mary's General Hospital; (519)749-6428; Fax. (519)749-6426.

BAHSALI, Georges I; CSSS de Laval, 1755 boul Rene-Laennec, Laval QC H7M 3L9; St. Joseph (Lebanon)'84; ABIM; LMCC; FRCPC; IntMed (Diabetes); Endocrin (P.Q.); Endocrin&Metab. Staff, Hopital de la Cite de la santé; Langs: Bilingual(French/English); (450)668-1010; Fax. (450)975-5052.

BAHSOUN, Rabih; CSSS d'Antoine-Labelle-Mt Laur, RR 1 2561 ch de la Lievre S, Mont-Laurier QC J9L 3G3; (Lebanon)'02; Staff, CSSS d'Antoine-Labelle; (819)623-1234

BAI, Helen H K; 210-6855 Meadowvale Town Centr, Mississauga ON L5N 2Y1; McG'84; FRCPC; Peds (Consultant Pediatrics). Ac Staff, The Credit Valley Hospital; (905)826-8993; Fax. (905)826-0520.

BAIBERGENOVA, Akerke T; Sunnybrook Hlth Sciences Ctre, M1-2075 Bayview Ave, Toronto ON M4N 3M5; (Kazakhstan)'93; MPH; PhD(Clin Epidemiol); Derm. Staff, Sunnybrook Health Sciences Centre; Asst Prof, University of Toronto; Langs: Russian; (416)480-4908

BAICHE, Nadia; Ctr Hosp Fleury, 2180 rue Fleury E, Montreal QC H2B 1K3; Mon'02; Staff, Centre Hospitalier Fleury; (514)384-2000

BAICI, Wayne C V; Addiction & Mental Hlth-Clarke, 533-250 College St, Toronto ON M5T 1R8; McM'06; FRCPC; Psy. (416)535-8501

BAIDWAN, Jatinder S; Medical Affairs, 2101 Richmond Ave, Victoria BC V8R 4R7; London (England)'94; MB BS; CCFP; Langs: Hindi; Punjabi; Urdu; (250)519-7700 x13802

BAIDWAN, Saminder K; Deer Lodge Centre Inc, 2109 Portage Ave, Winnipeg MB R3J 0L3; Punjab (India)'67; MB BS; MD; Ac Staff, WRHA - Deer Lodge Centre; (204)837-1301

BAIER, Paul A; Joseph Brant Mem Hosp, 1230 North Shore Blvd E, Burlington ON L7S 1W7; Wes'00; FRCPC; Anes. Anesthetist, Joseph Brant Memorial Hospital; (905)632-3730

BAIER, R John; Health Sciences Centre, CE408-820 Sherbrook St, Winnipeg MB R3A 1R9; Man'81; BSc; Peds (Neonatal & Perinatal Medicine). Staff, Health Sciences Centre.

BAIG, Kashif M; The Ottawa Hosp-Gen Campus, W6281-501 Smyth Rd, Ottawa ON K1H 8L6; McG'02; MBA; FRCPC; Ophth (Cornea). Staff, The Ottawa Hospital - General Campus; Langs: Bilingual(English/French); (613)737-8629; Fax. (613)739-6876.

BAIG, M Naseer; Trillium Hlth Ctr-Mississauga, 100 Queensway W, Mississauga ON L5B 1B8; Wes'94; BSc; FRCPC; Anes. Staff Anes, Trillium Health Centre - Mississauga; Langs: Urdu; (905)848-7100 x7628

BAIG, Mirza M W; London HSC-Victoria Hosp, 800 Commissioners Rd, London ON N6A 5W9; Allama Iqbal (Pakistan)'08; CCFP; CCFP(E.M.); Staff, London Health Sciences Centre - Victoria Campus; (519)667-6538; Fax. (519)667-6769.

BAIGRIE, Ronald S; Sudbury Med Centre, 200C-65 Larch St, Sudbury ON P3E 1B8; Tor'69; FACC; FRCPC; Cardiol (Adult Cardiology). Court Staff, Health Sciences North - Memorial Site; (705)674-5030; Fax. (705)671-3147; rsb@meetyourheart.com.

BAIKIE, Hilary A; 202-595 Columbia St W, Kamloops BC V2C 1K7; Mem'06; FRCSC; ObstGyn. (250)434-4762

BAIL, Monte H; 302-110 Eglinton Ave W, Toronto ON M4R 1A3; Mount Sinai (USA)'80; FRCPC; Psy (Medico Legal Assessments). Psychiatrist, West Park Healthcare Centre; (416)482-3530

BAILEY, Allan L; Westgrove Clinic, 201-505 Queen St, Spruce Grove AB T7X 2V2; Alb'88; CCFP; Staff Gen Practice, Covenant Health - Misericordia Community Hospital; Site Med Dir, Westview Health Centre; Associate Clinical Professor/Investigator Clinical Trials Bio Quest Research, University of Alberta; (780)962-9888; Fax. (780)960-5298.

BAILEY, Anthony J; Centre for Complex Disorders, A3 121 938-28 Ave W, Vancouver BC V5Z 4H4; London (England)'82; MB ChB; Teach Staff, University of British Columbia; (604)875-2000 x4729

BAILEY, Benoit; Hôpital Ste-Justine, 3175 ch Cote-Sainte-Catherine, Montreal QC H3T 1C5; Mon'90; MSc; FRCPC; Peds (Emergency Pediatrics). Staff Emerg Services & Section of Pharmacol & Toxicology, Hôpital Ste-Justine; Clinical Asst Prof Peds, Universite de Montreal; (514)345-4931 x6276; Fax. (514)345-4823; benoit.bailey@umontreal.ca.

BAILEY, Christopher; London HSC-Victoria Hosp, E4-800 Commissioners Rd E, London ON N6A 5W9; McM'96; MSc(Surg); FRCSC; OrthSurg (Spine Surgery). Staff, London Health Sciences Centre - Victoria Campus; (519)685-8500 x55358

BAILEY, Christopher J; 1-150 Strickland Rd, Lakefield ON K0L 2H0; Qns'82; BSc; Ac Staff, Peterborough Regional Health Centre - Rogers St Site; (705)652-6405

BAILEY, Darrin L; Cedars Prof Park, 2915 66 St NW, Edmonton AB T6K 4C1; Alb'99; BSc; PhD; FRCPC; Psy. Clin Staff Psy, Covenant Health - Grey Nuns Community Hospital; (780)450-9451; Fax. (780)461-6190.

BAILEY, Denis J; Univ Hlth Network-Toronto Gen, 11E 409-200 Elizabeth St, Toronto ON M5G 2C4; Tor'76; FRCPC; AnatPath. Staff, Princess Margaret Hospital - University Health Network; (416)340-3853

BAILEY, Gillian F; First Nations & Inuit Health A, 1525-1505 Barrington St, Halifax NS B3J 3K5; Bristol (England)'80; MRCGPract; DRCOG; Reg Physician Advisor, First Nations & Inuit Health Branch Atlantic; Langs: French; (902)426-6776; Fax. (902)426-8675; gillian.bailey@hc-sc.gc.ca.

BAILEY, Gordon R; Red Deer Med Centre, 108-3947 50A Ave, Red Deer AB T4N 6V7; Tor'72; BSc; FRCPC; IntMed (Atherosclerosis Prevention). Dir, The Bailey Clinic; (403)343-8972; Fax. (403)343-1919; gordon.bailey@thebaileyclinic.com.

BAILEY, Jason M; Winchester Dist Mem Hosp, 566 Louise St, Winchester ON K0C 2K0; Ott'05; CCFP; Staff, Winchester District Memorial Hospital; (613)774-2420

BAILEY, Jason P; St Joseph's Hlth Centre, 100 Westmount Rd, Guelph ON N1H 5H8; Dal'96; CCFP; FCFP; Staff, St Joseph's Health Centre; (519)824-2620; jbailey@gghorg.ca.

BAILEY, Jennifer L; 419-5920 1A St SW, Calgary AB T2H 0G3; Alb'05; FRCPC; IntMed; Gastroent. (403)452-1646

BAILEY, Jillian C; Highlands Health Network, 140 Rolling Hills Dr, Orangeville ON L9W 4X8; McM'05; CCFP; Staff, Headwaters Health Care Centre - Orangeville Site; (519)941-7575; Fax. (519)941-7060.

BAILEY, Joseph; Wellington Med Arts Bldg, 206-121 Wellington St W, Barrie ON L4N 1L2; Tor'85; Staff, Royal Victoria Regional Health Centre; (705)722-6707; Fax. (705)722-6724.

BAILEY, Karen A; Hamilton HS-McMaster Site, PO Box 2000 Stn Lcd 1 1200 Main St W, Hamilton ON L8N 3Z5; McM'98; FRCSC; GenSurg; PedGenSurg. Staff, Hamilton Health Sciences Centre - McMaster University Medical Centre; (905)521-2100

BAILEY, Karen J; 37 2 Ave SE, High River AB T1V 1G4; Alb'82; BSc; MD; FRCSC; ObstGyn;CCFP; Staff ObstGyn, High River General Hospital; (403)652-4505; Fax. (403)652-4724; kbaileymd99@shaw.ca.

BAILEY, Katherine M; Children's & Women's HC of BC, B321-4480 Oak St, Vancouver BC V6H 3V4; UBC'98; FRCPC; Anes. Staff, BC Children's Hospital; (604)875-2345 x2711

BAILEY, Kathryn A; Thamesview Family Health Team, 465 Grand Avenue W, Chatham ON N7L 1C5; Tor'84; BSc(Genetics); MD; MSc; CCFP; FCFP; Instructor FamMed, University of Western Ontario; (519)352-3210; Fax. (519)352-2176; kathryn.anne.bailey@gmail.com.

BAILEY, Luc; CSSS de Saint-Jerome, 290 rue de Montigny, Saint-Jerome QC J7Z 5T3; Mon'92; InfectDis (P.Q.); MedMicrobiol. Staff, Hôtel-Dieu de Saint-Jérôme; (450)432-2777; Fax. (450)431-8206.

BAILEY, Mark N; Orillia Soldiers Mem Hosp, 170 Colborne St W, Orillia ON L3V 2Z3; Ott'06; FRCPC; IntMed; Critical Care Medicine. Staff, Orillia Soldiers' Memorial Hospital; (705)259-0377; Fax. (705)259-3070.

BAILEY, Michelle J A; Alberta Children's Hosp, 2888 Shaganappi Trail NW, Calgary AB T3B 6A8; Cal'95; BSc; MSc(McGill); FRCPC; Peds. Staff, Alberta Children's Hospital; (403)955-3015

BAILEY, Robert F; St Mary's Hosp Centre, B207-3830 av Lacombe, Montreal QC H3T 1M5; Cal'73; FRCPC; IntMed; GeriatricMed. Staff Geriatric Med, St Mary's Hospital Centre; adj Prof Med, McGill University; Langs: English; French; (514)345-3511 x3453; Fax. (514)734-2663; robertbailey@videotron.ca.

BAILEY, Robert J; Hys Med Centre, 310-11010 101 St NW, Edmonton AB T5H 4B9; Ott'68; ABIM; FRCPC; IntMed (Gastroenterology). Med Dir, Northern Health Services Network; Clin Prof, University of Alberta; (780)421-1029; Fax. (780)425-5533; rjbailey@ualberta.ca.

BAILEY, Stewart; London HSC-Victoria Hosp, 4F-800 Commissioners Rd E, London ON N6A 5W9; Wes'68; FRCSC; OrthSurg. Staff, London Health Sciences Centre - Victoria Campus; (519)685-8055; Fax. (519)685-8059.

BAILEY, Thomas M; Westwind Med Clinic, 107-755 Goldstream Ave, Victoria BC V9B 0H9; UBC'76; CCFP; FCFP; Clinical Asst Prof, University of British Columbia; (250)478-1764; Fax. (250)478-1300.

BAILEY VERA, Dennis; CHUQ-Ctr Hosp Univ Laval, 2705 boul Laurier, Quebec QC G1V 4G2; Valparaiso (Chile)'96; Peds (P.Q.). Staff, Centre Hospitalier Universitaire de Quebec-CHUL; (418)656-4141

BAILLARGEON, Claude; CSSS de la Minganie, CP 190 1035 Prom des Anciens, Havre-Saint-Pierre QC G0G 1P0; Laval'91; Staff, CSSS de la Minganie; (418)538-2212

BAILLARGEON, David; CSSS de Laval, 1755 boul Rene-Laennec, Laval QC H7M 3L9; McG'98; FRCSC; OrthSurg (Knee & Shoulder). Staff, Hopital de la Cite de la santé; Langs: English; (450)668-1010

BAILLARGEON, Jean-Daniel; CHUS-Hop Hotel-Dieu, 580 rue Bowen S, Sherbrooke QC J1G 2E8; Mon'91; FRCPC; IntMed; Gastroent. Staff, Centre Hospitalier Universitaire de Sherbrooke-Hôpital Hôtel-Dieu; (819)346-1110 x23553; Fax. (819)820-6420; gastro-med@usherbrooke.ca.

BAILLARGEON, Jean-Martin; CHUM-Hop St-Luc, 1058 rue Saint-Denis, Montreal QC H2X 3J4; Laval'92; FRCPC; DiagRad. Staff, Centre Hospitalier l'Université De Montréal (CHUM) - Hôpital Saint-luc; Universite de Montreal; Langs: English; French; (514)890-8000 x36400

BAILLARGEON, Jean-Patrice; CHUS-Hop Fleurimont, 3001 12e Av N, Sherbrooke QC J1H 5N4; Mon'94; FRCPC; IntMed; Endocrin (P.Q.); Endocrin&Metab. Staff, Centre Hospitalier Universitaire de Sherbrooke-Hopital Fleurimont; (819)564-5241

BAILLARGEON, Joanne; Clinique Psyche, 400 av Laurier O, Montreal QC H2V 2K7; Mon'78; Psy. Staff, Institut Universitaire de Gériatrie de Montréal; (514)279-4141

BAILLARGEON, Lucie; UMF Laurier, 2875 boul Laurier, Quebec QC G1V 2M2; Laval'78; MSc(Epidemiol); Ac Staff Family Med, Centre Hospitalier Universitaire de Quebec-CHUL; (418)654-2701; Fax. (418)654-2138; lucie.baillargeon@crchul.ulaval.ca.

BAILLARGEON, Martine; Dir de la Sante Publique-Mtl, 1301 rue Sherbrooke E, Montreal QC H2L 1M3; Mon'78; FRCSC; PlasSurg; OccupMed (P.Q.). (514)528-2400

BAILLARGEON, Michel; Ctr Hosp Affilie-St-Sacrement, 1050 ch Sainte-Foy, Quebec QC G1S 4L8; Laval'68; FRCPC; IntMed (Diabetology); Endocrin&Metab (P.Q.). Chef Endocrin Service, Centre Hospitalier Affilié Universitaire de Québec - Hôpital du St-Sacrement; (418)652-7511; Fax. (418)688-8441.

BAILLARGEON, Robert; Hop Charles Lemoyne, 3120 boul Taschereau, Greenfield Park QC J4V 2H1; Mon'74; CSPQ; Anes. Staff Anes, Hopital Charles LeMoyne; (450)466-5000 x2680

BAILLARGEON-GAGNE, Sara; Centre Hosp Honore-Mercier, 2750 boul Laframboise, Saint-Hyacinthe QC J2S 4Y8; Mon'07; Urol. Staff, Centre Hospitalier Honore-Mercier; (514)287-7593

BAILLIE, Cory S; Manitoba Clinic, 790 Sherbrook St, Winnipeg MB R3A 1M3; Sask'94; ABIM; FRCPC; IntMed; Rheum. (204)788-5505

BAILLIE, Frank G H; Hamilton HS-General Site, 614-237 Barton St E, Hamilton ON L8L 2X2; Glasgow (Scotland)'72; MB ChB; FRCSC; GenSurg (Trauma). Staff, Hamilton Health Sciences Centre - Hamilton General Hospital; Assoc Prof, McMaster University; Langs: German; (905)527-0271 x44237; Fax. (905)577-9966; baillie@hhsc.ca.

BAILLIE, Hector M; Medical Centre, 24-1515 Dufferin Cres, Nanaimo BC V9S 2B8; Glasgow (Scotland)'81; MSc; MB ChB; FRCPC; IntMed. Staff General Internist, Nanaimo Regional General Hospital; (250)753-2446; Fax. (250)753-9686.

BAILLIE, Jane I; Burlington Prof Centre, 309-3155 Harvester Rd, Burlington ON L7N 3V2; McM'01; FRCSC; ObstGyn. (289)337-1663

BAILLIE, Mark S M; 105-2231 Louie Dr, Kelowna BC V4T 3K3; Witwatersrand (South Africa)'88; MB BCh; LMCC; CCFP.

BAILLIE, Nigel M; Haldimand War Mem Hosp, 206 John St, Dunnville ON N1A 2P7; London (England)'63; MB BS; DABA; FACA; Anes (Chronic Pain). Staff, Haldimand War Memorial Hospital; Ac Staff, Hamilton Health Sciences Centre - Hamilton General Hospital; Hon Staff, Hamilton Health Sciences Centre - McMaster University Medical Centre; Clin Assoc Prof, Hamilton Health Sciences Centre - McMaster Children's Hospital; (905)774-7431 x1324

BAILLIU, Leslie-Ann; SCOHS-Elisabeth Bruyere Hosp, 43 Bruyere St, Ottawa ON K1N 5C8; Ott'99; CCFP; Staff, SCO Health Service - Élisabeth Bruyère Hospital; Staff, Montfort Hospital; (613)562-6262

BAILLOD, Alanna B; Royal University Hosp, 113 EH-103 Hospital Dr, Saskatoon SK S7N 0W8; Sask'08; Staff, Royal University Hospital; (306)655-1000

BAILLOT, Richard; Hôpital Laval, 2725 ch Sainte-Foy, Quebec QC G1V 4G5; Mon'75; FRCSC; GenSurg; Cardiovasc&ThorSurg. Staff, Hôpital Laval; (418)656-4717; Fax. (418)656-4707.

BAILLY, Gregory G; Urology Consultants, 620-5991 Spring Garden Rd, Halifax NS B3H 1Y6; Dal'97; FRCSC; Urol (Incontinence). Prog Dir Dept of Urology/Asst Prof, Dalhousie University; (902)425-3940; Fax. (902)422-0033.

BAILON-POUJOL, Julie; CSSS de Laval, 1755 boul Rene-Laennec, Laval QC H7M 3L9; Mon'06; FRCPC; Peds. Staff, Hopital de la Cite de la santé; (450)668-1010

BAILY, Mark I; 208-341 Main St N, Brampton ON L6X 3C7; McG'78; Staff Family Pract, Toronto East General Hospital Inc; Staff, The Scarborough Hospital - Birchmount Campus; (905)451-7241; Fax. (905)451-9282.

BAIMEL, Evelyne; 302-1835 Yonge St, Toronto ON M4S 1X8; McG'79; CCFP; FCFP; Court Staff, Mount Sinai Hospital; Court Staff, Women's College Hospital; (416)487-0347; Fax. (416)481-6949.

BAIMEL, Melanie S; 302-1835 Yonge St, Toronto ON M4S 1X8; McM'08; CCFP; CCFP(E.M.); (416)487-0347

BAIN, Caroline E C; Deer Valley Family Med Centre, 101-83 Deerpoint Rd SE, Calgary AB T2J 6W5; Qns'92; CCFP; (403)271-5124; Fax. (403)225-1276; baince@telus.net.

BAIN, Douglas J G; Toronto East Gen Hosp Inc, 825 Coxwell Ave, Toronto ON M4C 3E7; Wes'88; FRCPC; IntMed; Respir. Staff The Respiratory Centre, Toronto East General Hospital Inc; (416)469-7777; Fax. (416)469-7717.

BAIN, James B; Campbellford Mem Hosp, PO Box 1027 146 Oliver Rd, Campbellford ON K0L 1L0; Man'96; BSc; MSc; DAvMed; PhD; CCFP; Staff, Campbellford Memorial Hospital; (705)653-1140

BAIN, James R; McMaster University HSC, PO Box 2000 Stn Lcd 1 4E16-1200 Main St W, Hamilton ON L8N 3Z5; Wes'84; FRCSC; PlasSurg (Hand Surgery). Chief Plastic Surg, Hamilton Health Sciences Centre - McMaster University Medical Centre; Assoc Chair Research, McMaster University; (905)521-2100 x73222; Fax. (905)521-9992; bainj@hhsc.ca.

BAIN, Jerald; 404-960 Lawrence Ave W, North York ON M6A 3B5; Wes'65; BSc(Pharm); MSc; FRCPC; IntMed (Reproductive Medicine); Endocrin&Metab. Langs: Yiddish; (416)783-4436; j.bain@utoronto.ca.

BAIN, John; Northfield Med Centre, 206-99 Northfield Dr E, Waterloo ON N2K 3P9; Glasgow (Scotland)'55; MB ChB; (519)744-2592

BAIN, Vincent G; Zeidler Ledcor Centre, 1 55-130 University Campus NW, Edmonton AB T6G 2X8; Alb'81; FACP; FRCPC; IntMed (Hepatology); Gastroent. Ac Staff, University of Alberta Hospital; Dir Liver Unit/Prof Med & Med, University of Alberta; (780)492-8128; Fax. (780)492-8130.

BAIN-ATOE, Gemma H; 182 Richmond St, Chatham ON N7M 1P2; St George (Grenada)'94; MD; BSc; FRCPC; IntMed. (519)380-0202; Fax. (519)380-9850.

BAINBRIDGE, Daniel T; London HSC-University Hosp, PO Box 5339 Stn B 339 Windermere Rd, London ON N6A 5A5; Sask'95; FRCPC; Anes. Staff, London Health Sciences Centre - University Hospital; (519)685-8500

BAINBRIDGE, J Andrew; Associate Med Clinic, PO Box 1076 Stn Main 5035 51 St, Whitecourt AB T7S 1P9; Liverpool (England)'76; MB ChB; LMCC; (780)778-2224; Fax. (780)778-2127; katahdin@telusplanet.net.

BAINBRIDGE, Monica T; London Reg Cancer Centre, 790 Commissioners Rd E, London ON N6A 4L6; Sask'95; BSc(Hons); CCFP; FCFP; (519)685-8640

BAINBRIDGE, Terry C; Kelowna Gen Hosp, 2268 Pandosy St, Kelowna BC V1Y 1T2; UBC'87; FRCPC; AnatPath (Oncology Surgical Pathology). Staff, Kelowna General Hospital; Fax. (250)980-6602.

BAINE, Sherri D; 503-1110 Sheppard Ave E, North York ON M2K 2W2; McM'94; BSc(Hons); FRCPC; Peds. (416)226-4294; Fax. (416)226-1928.

BAINES, Alexandra S; Royal Ottawa Hlth Care Group, 1145 Carling Ave, Ottawa ON K1Z 7K4; Qns'05; FRCPC; Psy. Staff, Royal Ottawa Mental Health Centre - Royal Ottawa Health Care Group; (613)722-6521

BAINEY, Kevin R; University of Alberta Hosp, 8440 112 St NW, Edmonton AB T6G 2B7; Alb'02; FRCPC; IntMed; Cardiol. Staff, University of Alberta Hospital; (780)407-2176; kbainey@ualberta.ca.

BAINS, Jason D; 101-12827 76 Ave, Surrey BC V3W 2V3; Alb'08; CCFP; Langs: Punjabi; (604)590-0443

BAINS, Paramjot; Health Sciences Centre, 300 Prince Philip Dr, St. John's NL A1B 3V6; Staff, Health Sciences Centre; (709)737-6300

BAINS, Perminder S; Gordon & Leslie Diamond Ctre, 9F-2775 Laurel St, Vancouver BC V5Z 1M9; UBC'08; IntMed. (604)875-4111

BAINS, Puneet; 207-126 15 St E, North Vancouver BC V7L 2P9; St George's Univ (Other Foreign)'05; FRCPC; IntMed; MedOncol. Langs: Punjabi; (604)988-4899

BAINS, Rajdeep; 6-875 Main St E, Milton ON L9T 0J4; Rajah Muthiah Medical College (India)'97; CCFP; (905)875-0955; Fax. (905)636-8620.

BAINS, Ravinder; Lake of the Woods Dist Hosp, 21 Sylvan St RR 1 Stn Main, Kenora ON P9N 3W7; Man'01; FRCPC; Psy. Staff, Lake of the Woods District Hospital; (807)468-9861

BAINS, Rick A B S; 5-320 Dundas St, London ON N6B 3R8; Man'87; Ophth (Refractive Cataract Surgery)., University of Western Ontario; (519)963-0911; rbains0209@rogers.com.

BAIR, F Douglas; 2125 Wyecroft Rd, Oakville ON L6L 5L7; Wes'97; MD; FRCPC; IntMed (Therapeutic Endoscopy); Gastroent. Staff, Halton Healthcare Services Corporation - Oakville Site; (905)338-0626; Fax. (905)338-0384.

BAIRAGI, Niranjan; 6-10030 12th Ave, North Battleford SK S9A 3A4; (306)446-0588

BAIRAGI, Ranjana; North Battleford Medical Clini, 102-11427 Railway Ave, North Battleford SK S9A 3G8; (306)445-4415; Fax. (306)445-5145.

BAIRAM, Aida; CHUQ-Ctr Hosp Univ Laval, 2705 boul Laurier, Quebec QC G1V 4G2; Aleppo (Syria),Nancy (France)'89; PhD; Peds (P.Q.). Staff Research, Centre Hospitalier Universitaire de Quebec-CHUL; Université Laval; Langs: Arabic; (418)656-4141; aida.bairam@crsfa.ulaval.ca.

BAIRATI, Isabelle; CHUQ-Hotel-Dieu de Quebec, 11 Cote Du Palais, Quebec QC G1R 2J6; Besancon (France)'89; PhD(Epidemiol); CommunMed (P.Q.). Staff Public Health, Centre Hospitalier Universitaire de Québec (CHUQ) - Siege Social; Asst Prof Cancerology Research Centre, Université Laval; (418)525-4444 x15569; Fax. (418)691-2470; isabelle.bairati@chuq.qc.ca.

BAIRD, Andrew C; The Medical Arts Centre, 103-650 South Terminal Ave, Nanaimo BC V9R 5E2; Edinburgh (Scotland)'70; MB ChB; DObstRCOG; CCFP; Staff, Nanaimo Regional General Hospital; (250)753-3431; Fax. (250)754-6897.

BAIRD, David F; Collingwood Gen & Marine Hosp, 459 Hume St, Collingwood ON L9Y 1W9; (Ireland)'06; CCFP; Staff, Collingwood General & Marine Hospital; (705)445-2550

BAIRD, Douglas A; Toronto East Gen Hosp Inc, 825 Coxwell Ave, Toronto ON M4C 3E7; Tor'61; Anes. Staff, Toronto East General Hospital Inc; (416)469-6588 x6219; Fax. (416)469-6874.

BAIRD, J Burke; Hamilton HSC-McMaster Site, PO Box 2000 Stn Lcd 1 3N10-1200 Main St W, Hamilton ON L8N 3Z5; Wes'94; BSc; FRCPC; Peds. Staff, Hamilton Health Sciences Centre - McMaster University Medical Centre; (905)521-2100

BAIRD, Jennifer E; Regina Qu'Appelle HR-Regina, 1440 14th Ave, Regina SK S4P 0W5; McG'94; FRCSC; GenSurg (Critical Care Medicine). Staff, Regina General Hospital; (306)766-6925; Fax. (306)766-6920.

BAIRD, Judy L; 1475 Upper Ottawa St, Hamilton ON L8W 3J6; Wes'93; CCFP; FCFP; (905)575-1300

BAIRD, Kevin J; University of Calgary, MSC 370-2500 University Dr NW, Calgary AB T2N 1N4; Cal'05; FRCPC; Psy. (403)210-9355

BAIRD, Lawson D; 2190 York Ave, Vancouver BC V6K 1C3; McG'79; Ac Staff, Providence Health Care - St Paul's Hospital; (604)733-9110; Fax. (604)733-9149.

BAIRD, Michael G; Hotel-Dieu Hosp, 166 Brock St, Kingston ON K7L 5G2; Ott'70; FACC; FAHA; FRCPC; Cardiol (Clinical Cardiology). Staff, Hotel-Dieu Hospital; Staff, Kingston General Hospital; Queen's University; (613)544-3400 x2250; Fax. (613)544-7250; bairdm@hdh.kari.net.

BAIRD, Nicole; SMBD-Jewish Gen Hosp, 3755 ch Cote-Sainte-Catherine, Montreal QC H3T 1E2; McG'80; Staff, Sir Mortimer B Davis Jewish General; (514)340-8222; Fax. (514)340-7931.

BAIRD, Robert; MUHC-Montreal Children's Hosp, C812-2300 rue Tupper, Montreal QC H3H 1P3; McG'02; FRCSC; GenSurg; PedGenSurg. Staff, McGill University Health Centre - Montreal Children's Hospital; (514)412-4400 x22869; Fax. (514)412-4289.

BAIRD, Rosemary D; Integrated Wellness Med Centre, 2-4655 Central Blvd, Burnaby BC V5H 3P2; UBC'85; BSc; (604)582-8820; Fax. (604)582-2103.

BAIRD, Wycliffe H; High Point Med Centre, 303-3461 Dixie Rd, Mississauga ON L4Y 3X4; Dal'72; (905)625-0889

BAISE, Taryn; Yellowbird Family Clinic, 3380 Gateway Blvd NW, Edmonton AB T6J 6V1; Witwatersrand (South Africa)'83; MB ChB; (780)434-2893; Fax. (780)435-1057.

BAITZ, Brian; Doctor's Office, 491 Lawrence Ave W, North York ON M5M 1C7; Cape Town (South Africa)'81; MB ChB; MMed(Rad.D.); FRCPC; DiagRad. (416)781-9375

BAITZ, Thomas; Mcconnell Med Centre, 113-820 McConnell Ave, Cornwall ON K6H 4M4; Alb'61; FRCPC; IntMed (Cardiology). Ac Staff, Cornwall Community Hospital - Second Street Site; Ac Staff, Cornwall Community Hospital; (613)933-1214; Fax. (613)933-4523.

BAJAJ, Girish; Hamilton HSC-McMaster Site, PO Box 2000 Stn Lcd 1 1200 Main St W, Hamilton ON L8N 3Z5; Delhi (India)'00; FRCPC; IntMed. Staff, Hamilton Health Sciences Centre - McMaster Children's Hospital; (905)521-2100

BAJAJ, Harminder P S; Healthplex Med Centre, 100-150 West Dr, Brampton ON L6T 4P9; (905)454-7410; Fax. (905)454-3220.

BAJAJ, Harpreet S; LMC Endocrinology Centre, 238-2130 North Park Dr, Brampton ON L6S 0C9; New Delhi (India)'01; MB BS; ABIM; Langs: Punjabi; Hindi; Urdu; Spanish; (905)595-0560; Fax. (905)595-0562.

BAJAJ, Parvesh; Access Med Clinic, 6-3098 Carling Ave, Nepean ON K2B 7K2; Delhi (India)'69; MB BS; LMCC; Vis Staff Privil, Queensway Carleton Hospital; Physician, Medex Nursing Home; Physician, Carlingview Manor Nursing Home; Langs: Hindi; Punjabi; Urdu; (613)721-0978; Fax. (613)596-0496.

BAJAJ, Renu; Auburn Centre, 901-570 University Ave E, Waterloo ON N2K 4P2; Wes'87; CCFP; CCFP(E.M.); Staff, St Mary's General Hospital; Staff, Grand River Hospital - Kitchener/Waterloo Health Centre; Langs: Punjabi; (519)578-6099

BAJAJ, Sangeeta; Brampton Med Bldg, 314-40 Finchgate Blvd, Brampton ON L6T 3J1; McG'93; FRCPC; IntMed; Rheum. Court Staff, Headwaters Health Care Centre - Orangeville Site; Staff, William Osler Health System - Brampton Civic Hospital; Langs: French; Hindi; (905)799-1850; Fax. (905)799-8040.

BAJELAN, Adnan; 116 Heron Ave, Summerside PE C1N 5R9; Baghdad (Iraq)'84; MB ChB; CCFP; Staff, A M Guy Memorial Health Centre; Langs: Arabic; Kurdish; (902)859-3929; Fax. (902)859-3922; abajelan@yahoo.com.

BAJNO, Lydia M; The Hosp for Sick Children, 555 University Ave, Toronto ON M5G 1X8; Man'04; FRCPC; DiagRad. Staff, The Hospital For Sick Children; (416)813-1500

BAJRAMOVIC, Fersada B; Riverside Prof Centre, 211-1919 Riverside Dr, Ottawa ON K1H 1A2; Sarajevo (Bosnia-Herzegovina)'70; MD; Physician, Ottawa Vein & Cosmetic Medical Clinic; (613)737-5675; Fax. (613)233-2540; hfbajramovic@hotmail.com.

BAJRAMOVIC, Hifzija H; The Ottawa Hosp-Gen Campus, 501 Smyth Rd, Ottawa ON K1H 8L6; Sarajevo (Bosnia-Herzegovina)'64; FRCPC; Psy (Cognitive Therapy). Ad Staff Privil, Royal Ottawa Mental Health Centre - Royal Ottawa Health Care Group; Dir Cognitive & Behavior Therapy Clinic & Staff, The Ottawa Hospital - General Campus; Asst Prof, University of Ottawa; Langs: Macedonian; Croatian; Serbian; (613)737-8010; Fax. (613)737-8115.

BAJURNY, Gary; 911 Yonge St PO Box 340, Walkerton ON N0G 2V0; Ott'67; Gen Practice, South Bruce Grey Health Centre - Walkerton Site; Med Dir, Bruce Lea Haven Nursing Home; (519)881-0564; Fax. (519)881-0565.

BAJWA, Amarjit K; Valley Med Imaging, 102-32475 Simon Ave, Abbotsford BC V2T 5E3; Punjabi (India)'87; MB BS; FRCPC; DiagRad. (604)859-8998

BAJWA, Amarjit S; 205-45625 Hodgins Ave, Chilliwack BC V2P 1P2; Guru Nanak (India)'88; MB BS; Staff OrthSurg, Chilliwack General Hospital; (604)795-4704

BAJWA, Gurjit; William Osler HC-Etobicoke, 101 Humber College Blvd, Etobicoke ON M9V 1R8; Tor'96; Staff, William Osler Health System - Etobicoke General Hospital; Langs: Punjabi; Hindi; (416)747-3400

BAJWA, Harjeet; Campbellton Reg Hosp, PO Box 880 Stn Main 189 Lily Lake Rd, Campbellton NB E3N 3H3; Guru-Nanak (India)'75; MB BS; Chief Radiol Diagnostic Imaging, Hôpital Régional Campbellton; Chief Radiol Diagnostic Imaging, Vitality Health Network; (506)789-5000; Fax. (506)789-5396.

BAJWA, Riffet R; Kozlov Shopping Centre, 242-400 Bayfield St, Barrie ON L4M 5A1; Punjab (Pakistan)'69; MB BS; DPM(Lond); MRCPsy(UK); Staff, Royal Victoria Regional Health Centre; (705)726-0411; Fax. (705)726-0455.

BAJWA, Sameena A; Evergreen Med Center, 205-4851 Westwinds Dr NE, Calgary AB T3J 4L4; Lahore (Pakistan)'99; MB BS; LMCC; DObst; CCFP; Langs: Punjabi; Urdu; Hindi; Arabic; (403)580-2008; Fax. (403)580-2009.

BAJZAK, Krisztina I; Health Sciences Centre, 2J557-300 Prince Philip Dr, St. John's NL A1B 3V6; Mem'93; MSc; FACOG; FRCSC; ObstGyn (Minimal Invasive Surgery). Staff, Health Sciences Centre; Asst Prof, Memorial University Of Newfoundland; (709)777-8935; Fax. (709)777-7455.

BAK, Adrian W; Kelowna Gastroent Associates, 564 Leon Ave, Kelowna BC V1Y 6J6; Ott'92; ABIM; FRCPC; IntMed; Gastroent. Med Staff, Kelowna General Hospital; (250)763-6433; Fax. (250)763-3818.

BAK, David M; Health & Wellness Centre, 125-589 South Pelham Rd, Welland ON L3C 3C7; Wes'92; Staff, Niagara Health System - Welland Hospital Site; (905)788-1500; Fax. (905)788-1510.

BAK, Malgorzata A; Delhi Community Health Centre, 105 Main St, Delhi ON N4B 2L8; Wroclaw Academy of Medicine (Poland)'85; Langs: Polish; (519)582-2323; Fax. (519)582-1513.

BAKALA, Cameron D; 204-3330 Richter St, Kelowna BC V1W 4V5; UBC'88; FRCSC; Otol (Facial Plastic Surgery). Staff, Kelowna General Hospital; (250)868-8056; cdbakala@silk.net.

BAKALEM-LOULI, Radia; Polyclinique Med Fabreville, 380 boul Cure-Labelle, Laval QC H7P 5L3; (Algeria)'93; CCFP; (450)628-5800; Fax. (450)628-0217.

BAKARE, Stephanee O; Clinique Brunswick, 200-955 boul Saint-Jean, Pointe-Claire QC H9R 5K3; McG'05; FRCSC; ObstGyn. (514)313-3414

BAKBAK, Asaad I; 117 King St E, Oshawa ON L1H 1B9; Tripoli (Libya)'84; MB ChB; FACC; FRSC; FRCPC; IntMed; Cardiol. Ac Staff, Lakeridge Health - Oshawa Site; Court Staff, Rouge Valley Health System - Centenary Health Centre Site; (905)721-4903; Fax. (905)723-3794; dr_bakbak@hotmail.com.

BAKDOUNES, Mhd Khldoun; St Mary's Hosp Centre, 3830 av Lacombe, Montreal QC H3T 1M5; Damascus (Syria)'94; FRCPC; AnatPath. Staff, St Mary's Hospital Centre; (514)345-3511 x3732

BAKER, Alison D; Avenue Med Centre, 1-221 Brant Ave, Brantford ON N3T 3J2; Tor'01; CCFP; (519)753-8666; Fax. (519)753-6880.

BAKER, Andrew D; 2100 Bovaird Dr E, Brampton ON L6R 3J7; Qns'97; FRCPC; IntMed (General Medicine); GeriatricMed. Staff, William Osler Health System - Brampton Civic Hospital; (905)494-6586; andrew.baker@williamoslerhs.ca.

BAKER, Andrew J; St Michael's Hosp, 30 Bond St, Toronto ON M5B 1W8; Tor'85; FRCPC; Anes (Critical Care/Trauma). Med Dir Trauma & Neurosurg, St Michael's Hospital; (416)864-5559

BAKER, Blair; The Royal Victoria Hosp, 201 Georgian Dr, Barrie ON L4M 6M2; (Ireland)'08; CCFP; Staff, Royal Victoria Regional Health Centre; (705)728-9090; b.baker@utoronto.ca.

BAKER, Brian; 308-1100 Sheppard Ave E, North York ON M2K 2W1; Cape Town (South Africa)'74; MB ChB; FRCPC; Psy (Cardiovascular Psychiatry). Assoc Staff, Toronto General Hospital - UHN; (416)222-5286; Fax. (416)446-0849; brian.bker@utoronto.ca.

BAKER, Chad F; 400-10924 107 Ave NW, Edmonton AB T5H 0X5; Alb'03; FRCSC; Ophth. (780)448-1801

BAKER, Chandran J; Health Sciences Ctr Gen Hosp, 700 William Ave, Winnipeg MB R3E 0Z3; Man'83; FRCPC; Anes. Staff, Health Sciences Centre; (204)774-6511

BAKER, Darrell Kurt; 340 Lock St W, Dunnville ON N1A 1V5; Tor'81; FACS; FRCSC; GenSurg. General Surgery, Haldimand War Memorial Hospital; (905)774-7533; Fax. (905)774-7534; dkbaker@sympatico.ca.

BAKER, Denis; CSSS de Montmagny-l'Islet, 430 rue Jean-Leclerc, St-Jean-Port-Joli QC G0R 3G0; Laval'90; CCFP; FCFP; Fam Med, CSSS de Montmagny-l'Islet; (418)598-3355; Fax. (418)598-9800.

BAKER, Eric C; Raymond Med Clinic, 20 Church Ave, Raymond AB T0K 2S0; UBC'07; CCFP; (403)752-3337

BAKER, Gary T; Carbonear Gen Hosp, 86 Highroad South, Carbonear NL A1Y 1A4; Mem'77; Carbonear General Hospital; (709)945-5260; gary.baker@easternhealth.ca.

BAKER, Gordon A; 309-500 Sheppard Ave E, North York ON M2N 6H7; Tor'58; Psy. (416)218-0529

BAKER, James E; St Michael's Hosp, 30 Bond St, Toronto ON M5B 1W8; Qns'95; FRCPC; Anes. Staff, St Michael's Hospital; (416)360-4000

BAKER, Jane L; Allin Clinic, 10155 120 St NW, Edmonton AB T5K 2A2; (United Kingdom)'04; CCFP; (780)482-7551

BAKER, Janet D; Riverside South Med Centre, 3-665 Earl Armstrong Rd, Gloucester ON K1V 2G2; Dal'95; BSc(Hons); CCFP; (613)822-0411

BAKER, Jason B; 110-200 St Clair Ave W, Toronto ON M4V 1R1; Wes'95; CCFP; CCFP(E.M.); FCFP; Staff, Toronto General Hospital - UHN; Physician, Hazelton Place Retirement Centre; Physician, Upper Canada College; (416)928-9343; Fax. (416)928-9368; jbaker@ucc.on.ca.

BAKER, Jay W; 46 Adam St, Cambridge ON N3C 2K3; Tor'74; CCFP; FCFP; Staff, Cambridge Memorial Hospital; Ethics Committee; Med Dir, St Luke's Home for the Aged; (519)658-0040; jay.baker@sickkids.ca.

BAKER, Jeffrey P; St Michael's Hosp, CW16F 050-30 Bond St, Toronto ON M5B 1W8; Tor'73; FRCPC; IntMed (Endoscopy); Gastroent. Staff, St Michael's Hospital; (416)864-5909; Fax. (416)864-5995; bakerj@smh.ca.

BAKER, Jillian M; St Michael's Hosp Pediatric Cl, 2F-61 Queen St E, Toronto ON M5C 2T2; Cal'99; FRCPC; Peds (Pediatric Hematology Oncology). Staff, The Hospital For Sick Children; (416)867-3655; Fax. (416)867-3736.

BAKER, Katarzyna; East Calgary Health Centre, 4715 8 Ave SE, Calgary AB T2A 3N4; (Poland)'08; CCFP; (403)455-1400

BAKER, Kevin R; The Ottawa Hosp-Civic Campus, D4-1053 Carling Ave, Ottawa ON K1Y 4E9; Qns'84; FRCSC; ObstGyn (Endoscopic Surgery). Head Section of Urogynecology & Reconstructive Pelvic Surg, The Ottawa Hospital - Civic Campus; Assoc Prof, University of Ottawa; Langs: French; (613)761-4522; Fax. (613)761-4915; kbaker@ottawahospital.on.ca.

BAKER, Laura L; Burnaby Hosp, 3935 Kincaid St, Burnaby BC V5G 2X6; Qns'80; FRCPC; Anes. Ac Staff, Burnaby Hospital; (604)434-4211; Fax. (604)412-6313.

BAKER, Laurie-Ann; Foothills Med Centre, C231-1403 29 St NW, Calgary AB T2N 2T9; McM'00; CCFP; CCFP(E.M.); Staff, Foothills Medical Centre; Staff Emerg Med, Calgary Health Region; Dir Off Service & Undergraduate Educ/Clerkship, University of Calgary; (403)944-1635

BAKER, Lawrence; Agincourt Prof Centre, 302-2330 Kennedy Rd, Scarborough ON M1T 0A2; Tor'74; Physician, Trench Electric Ltd; (416)298-1303; Fax. (416)298-4872.

BAKER, Leslie A; Student Health Services, 11-1151 Richmond St, London ON N6A 3K7; Wes'90; Staff University Community Centre, The University Of Western Ontario.

BAKER, Linda M; Rosthern Med Clinic, PO Box 1089, Rosthern SK S0K 3R0; Sask'76; Clin Lecturer, University of Saskatchewan; (306)232-4894; Fax. (306)232-4970.

BAKER, Michael A; Univ Hlth Network-Toronto Gen, 14EB 227-200 Elizabeth St, Toronto ON M5G 2C4; Tor'66; FACP; MD; FRCPC; Hem; IntMed. Staff, Toronto General Hospital - UHN; (416)340-5300; michael.baker@uhn.on.ca.

BAKER, Milton F; 218-3930 Shelbourne St, Victoria BC V8P 5P6; Alb'70; BSc; ABIM; FRCPC; IntMed (Fibromyalgia). Pres, SSPS of British Columbia; Clin Assoc Prof, University of British Columbia; (250)721-3353; Fax. (250)721-4730.

BAKER, Norma A; Rouge Valley-Ajax & Pickering, 580 Harwood Ave S, Ajax ON L1S 2J4; Tor'87; BSc(Hons.); Ac Staff, Rouge Valley Health System - Ajax & Pickering Health Centre Site; (905)683-2320 x3200; Fax. (905)428-5231.

BAKER, Patricia M; Health Sciences Centre, MS4-820 Sherbrook St, Winnipeg MB R3A 1R9; Man'91; FRCPC; AnatPath. Staff, Health Sciences Centre; Assoc Prof, University of Manitoba; pmbaker@hsc.mb.ca.

BAKER, Paul F; Royal Columbian Hosp, 330 Columbia St E, New Westminster BC V3L 3W7; UBC'80; FRCPC; Anes. Ac Staff Anes, Royal Columbian Hospital; (604)520-4602; Fax. (604)520-4899.

BAKER, Philip N; Health Sciences Centre, 2J2.01-132 University Campus N, Edmonton AB T6G 2R7; Nottingham (England)'85; BS; BMedSci; FRCOG; FRCSC; ObstGyn (Maternal Fetal Medicine). (780)492-9728; Fax. (780)492-7303.

BAKER, Raymond P; 303-4180 Lougheed Hwy, Burnaby BC V5C 6A7; Wes'75; BSc; FASAM; CCFP; FCFP; (604)718-6929

BAKER, Robert A; Steveston Med Group, 204-3811 Chatham St, Richmond BC V7E 2Z4; Man'73; Vis Staff Family Pract, Vancouver General Hospital - Centennial Pavillion; Staff, Richmond Hospital; Clin Instructor Family Pract, University of British Columbia; (604)277-7166; Fax. (604)277-3811.

BAKER, Robert S; Headwaters Health Care Centre, 100 Rolling Hills Dr, Orangeville ON L9W 4X9; Tor'60; FRCPC; Anes. Staff, Headwaters Health Care Centre - Orangeville Site; (519)941-2410; Fax. (519)942-0483.

BAKER, Sandra E; 2606 Pandosy St, Kelowna BC V1Y 1V6; Cal'96; MSc; BSc; FRCPC; IntMed; Cardiol. Staff Cardiol, Kelowna General Hospital; (250)762-9211; Fax. (250)762-8337; cardiologyclinic@shaw.ca.

BAKER, Sharon L; London HSC-University Hosp, PO Box 5339 Stn B 399 Windermere Rd, London ON N6A 5A5; Wes'84; Staff, London Health Sciences Centre - University Hospital; (519)685-8500

BAKER, Stephen M; 302-1625 Oak Bay Ave, Victoria BC V8R 1B1; Man'86; DAB; FRCSC; Ophth (Ophthalmic Plastic & Reconstructive Surgery). stephen.baker@dal.ca.

BAKER, Stephen R; 310-4800 Leslie St, North York ON M2J 2K9; McM'95; BSc; FAAP; FRCPC; Peds. Staff, North York General Hospital; Staff Pt-Time Emerg, The Hospital For Sick Children; (416)492-5888; Fax. (416)492-6569.

BAKER, Steven K; McMaster University HSC, PO Box 2000 Stn Lcd 1 2H22-1200 Main St W, Hamilton ON L8N 3Z5; McM'00; BA; BEd; MSc; CSCN; FRCPC; PhysMed&Rehab (Neuromuscular Diseases). Assoc Prof, McMaster University; (905)521-2100 x76946; Fax. (905)577-8380.

BAKER, Wayne K; 150-17475 56 Ave, Surrey BC V3S 2X6; UBC'86; CCFP; Ac Staff, Peace Arch Hospital; Staff, Surrey Memorial Hospital; (604)576-7701

BAKEZADEH, Farhad; 204-580 Main St, Saint John NB E2K 1J5; Mashhad (Iran)'89; MD; Staff, Saint John Regional Hospital; Langs: Persian; Farsi; (506)634-2197; Fax. (506)634-8209.

BAKHET, Maged M S; 204-9656 King George Blvd, Surrey BC V3T 2V5; Assiut (Egypt)'84; MB ChB; MRC; FRCSC; ObstGyn. (604)634-0500

BAKHSHI KAHNAMOUEI, Manijeh; 412-1100 Sheppard Ave E, North York ON M2K 2W1; (Iran)'98; CCFP; (647)748-7887

BAKHT, M Murad; William Osler HC-Brampton, 2100 Bovaird Dr E, Brampton ON L6R 3J7; Dhaka (Bangladesh)'73; MB BS; DCH; FRCPC; Psy (Child & Adolescent Psychiatry). Staff, Joseph Brant Memorial Hospital; Staff, William Osler Health System - Brampton Civic Hospital; Langs: Bengali; (905)494-2120 x50619

BAKISH, David; Ottawa Psychopharmacology Clin, 328-1929 Russell Rd, Ottawa ON K1G 4G3; Strasbourg (France)'80; BSc; FRCPC; Psy (Psycho Pharmacology). Dir, Ottawa Psychopharmaceo Clinic; Langs: English; French; (613)737-5454 x221; Fax. (613)737-0440; dbakish@opctrials.com.

BAKKEN, Maureen P; 500-80 Donlevy Ave, Red Deer AB T4R 2Y8; Alb'76; Ac Staff, Red Deer Regional Hospital Centre; (403)343-8484

BAKKER, Willemien G; Dixie Road Med Associates, 2200 Dixie Rd, Mississauga ON L4Y 1Z4; Qns'76; CCFP; FCFP; Staff, Trillium Health Centre - Mississauga; (905)279-1700; Fax. (905)897-9167.

BAKKER, Gerald J J; Medical Office, 233 Fourth Ave, Sudbury ON P3B 4C3; Qns'84; BSc; MSc; Staff, Health Sciences North - Memorial Site; (705)524-9152; Fax. (705)524-5723.

BAKKER, Jacqueline I; Central Alberta Prof Centre, 171-5201 43 St, Red Deer AB T4N 1C7; Cal'96; FRCPC; Neur (Multiple Sclerosis). Staff, Red Deer Regional Hospital Centre; (403)343-7731; Fax. (403)343-7856.

BAKKER, Scott R; 204-45625 Hodgins Ave, Chilliwack BC V2P 1P2; Wes'06; CCFP; (604)792-1908

BAKONYI, Judit; Vancouver Gen Hosp, C321-855 12th Ave W, Vancouver BC V5Z 1M9; Budapest (Hungary)'86; CCFP; Staff, Vancouver General Hospital - Centennial Pavillion; (604)875-4111

BAKOTA, Martin; 215 Charlotte St, Saint John NB E2L 2K1; Dal'95; CCFP; (506)634-1787; Fax. (506)649-5130; mbakota@nbnet.nb.ca.

BAKOWSKY, Volodko S; Nova Scotia Rehab Centre, 245-1341 Summer St, Halifax NS B3H 4K4; Qns'94; FRCPC; IntMed; Rheum. Staff, Nova Scotia Rehabilitation Centre; Staff, Queen Elizabeth II Health Sciences Centre - Halifax Infirmary Site; Assoc Prof, Dalhousie University; (902)473-3818; Fax. (902)473-7019; volodko.bakowsky@cdha.nshealth.ca.

BAKRI, A Majid; Mayo Gen Hosp, PO Box 238, Mayo YT Y0B 1M0; Moscow (Russia (Federation))'78; Staff, Mayo General Hospital; Staff, Mayo Health Centre; Fax. (867)996-2018.

BAKSH, Anton D; Children's Hosp Eastern Ont, 401 Smyth Rd, Ottawa ON K1H 8L1; Mem'97; FRCPC; Psy. Staff, Children's Hospital of Eastern Ontario (CHEO); (613)737-7600 x3413

BAKSH, Arlene D; Peace Arch Hosp, 15521 Russell Ave, White Rock BC V4B 2R4; UBC'95; FRCPC; Psy. Staff, Peace Arch Hospital; (604)538-4240; Fax. (604)538-8500.

BAKSHI, Amitabh; Courtenay Med Associates, 201-1350 England Ave, Courtenay BC V9N 8X6; Ravi Shankar (India)'96; MB BS; CCFP; (250)334-4411

BAKSHI, Darshan R; Radiology Consultants Assoc, 120-6707 Elbow Dr SW, Calgary AB T2V 0E3; (India)'96; Staff, Peter Lougheed Centre; (403)777-3003; Fax. (403)777-3008.

BAKSHI, Neeja; Royal Alexandra Hosp, 323 CSC-10240 Kingsway NW, Edmonton AB T5H 3V9; Staff, Royal Alexandra Hospital; (780)735-4111

BAKSHI, Nupura K; Mount Sinai Hosp, 600 University Ave, Toronto ON M5G 1X5; Tor'04; FRCSC; Ophth. Staff, Mount Sinai Hospital; (416)586-4800

BAKSHI, Shameet N; Addiction & Mental Hlth-Clarke, 250 College St, Toronto ON M5T 1R8; Wes'04; FRCPC; Psy. Staff, Centre for Addiction & Mental Health (CAMH) - College Street Site; (416)535-8501

BAKSHI, Tuhin K; Associate Clinic, 5215 49 Ave, Wetaskiwin AB T9A 0R1; Patna (India)'76; MB BS; CASM; Dip SportMed; CCFP; FCFP; Med Staff, Wetaskiwin Hospital & Care Centre; Med Examiner, Gov't of Alberta; Ac Staff, David Thompson Reg Health Centre; Clinical Asst Prof Family Med, University of Alberta; Langs: Bengali; Hindi; (780)352-7157; Fax. (780)352-2273; tkbakshi@telusplanet.net.

BAL, Sharon; B7A-350 Conestoga Blvd, Cambridge ON N1R 7L7; Tor'02; BSc; CCFP; Staff, Cambridge Memorial Hospital; (519)620-4533

BAL, Simerpreet S; Health Sciences Centre, GF535-820 Sherbrook St, Winnipeg MB R3A 1R9; Staff, Health Sciences Centre; (204)774-8511

BALA, Anand; Town Centre Prof Bldg, 214-6203 28 Ave NW, Edmonton AB T6L 6K3; Cal'95; FRCPC; IntMed; Gastroent. Staff, Covenant Health - Grey Nuns Community Hospital; Clinical Asst Prof, University of Alberta; (780)485-5515; Fax. (780)485-5516.

BALAA, Fady K; The Ottawa Hosp-Civic Campus, 305CPC-1053 Carling Ave, Ottawa ON K1Y 4E9; Wes'00; FRCSC; GenSurg (Hepatopancreatobiliary Surgery). Staff/Asst Prof Surg, The Ottawa Hospital - Civic Campus; Langs: Arabic; (613)761-5015; fbalaa@toh.on.ca.

BALABAN, Kayli; Mount Sinai Hosp, 9F-600 University Ave, Toronto ON M5G 1X5; Tor'04; FRCPC; Psy. Staff, Mount Sinai Hospital; (416)586-4800

BALABAN, Mihai; Lakeshore Gen Hosp, 160 av Stillview, Pointe-Claire QC H9R 2Y2; Bucarest (Romania)'64; CSPQ; Anes (P.Q.). Staff, Lakeshore General Hospital - Pointe Claire; (514)630-2225 x2699

BALACHANDRA, Bhamini; Alberta Hosp Edmonton, PO Box 307 Stn Main, Edmonton AB T5J 2J7; Peradeniya (Sri Lanka)'71; MB BS; FRCPC; Psy (Adult Psychiatry). Staff, Alberta Hospital Edmonton; Langs: Tamil; Sinhalese; (780)342-5439; Fax. (780)342-5233.

BALACHANDRA, Brinda; Royal Alexandra Hosp, DTC 50002-10240 Kingsway NW, Edmonton AB T5H 3V9; Man'00; FRCPC; AnatPath. Staff, Royal Alexandra Hospital; (780)735-5281; Fax. (780)735-4715; brinda.balachandra@albertahealthservices.ca.

BALACHANDRA, Krishna; Alberta Hosp Edmonton, PO Box 307 Stn Main 17480 Fort Rd, Edmonton AB T5J 2J7; Man'99; FRCPC; Psy. Staff, Alberta Hospital Edmonton; (780)342-5473; Fax. (780)342-5411.

BALACHANDRA, Thambirajah; Office of Chief Med Examiner, 210-1 Wesley Ave, Winnipeg MB R3C 4C6; (Sri Lanka)'71; MB BS; ABPath; FCAP; FRCPC; AnatPath (Forensic Pathology). Assoc Staff, Concordia General Hospital; Consultant, Health Sciences Centre; Ac Staff, St Boniface General Hospital; Chief Med Examiner, Province of MB; Head Forensic Sciences/Assoc Prof, University of Manitoba; Langs: Tamil; Sinhalese; (204)945-2088; thambirajah.balachandra@gov.mb.ca.

BALACHANDRA, Vasthare K; 116 Mitton St S, Sarnia ON N7T 3C4; Mysore (India)'63; MB BS; DABS; DABTS; FACS; FRCSC; GenSurg. Ac Staff, Bluewater Health - Mitton Site; General Surgery, Bluewater Health - Charlotte Eleanor Englehart Hospital; Ac Staff, Bluewater Health - Norman Site; (519)336-4615

BALAGEORGE, Dimitrios; Manitoba Clinic, 790 Sherbrook St, Winnipeg MB R3A 1M3; Man'89; FRCSC; OrthSurg. (204)774-6541; Fax. (204)774-5623.

BALAISIS, Elise M J; Clinical Tenant Support Team, 211 Gore Ave, Vancouver BC V6A 0B6; Ott'08; CCFP; Langs: Bilingual(English/French); (604)660-8848

BALAKRISHNA, Rangappa; Hilltop Med Clinic, 140-15321 16th Ave, Surrey BC V4A 1R6; Bangalore (India)'71; DA(Lond); CCFP; Staff, Peace Arch Hospital; (604)531-5575

BALAKRISHNAN, Kanapathi P; Nipawin Med Group, PO Box 2135, Nipawin SK S0E 1E0; (Sri Lanka)'71; MB BS; LRCP; CCFP; FCFP; (306)862-4626; Fax. (306)862-3522.

BALAKRISHNAN, Leela G; Millwoods Medicentre, 6426 28 Ave NW, Edmonton AB T6L 6N3; Madras (India)'75; MB BS; (780)462-3491; Fax. (780)461-2650.

BALAKRISHNAN, Pradeep; Homewood Health Centre, 150 Guelph St, Guelph ON N1E 6K9; Mysore (India)'80; MB BS; MRCPsy(Lond); LMCC; FRCPC; Psy (Adult General Psychiatry). Staff, Homewood Health Centre; Langs: Malayalam; (519)824-1010

BALAKRISHNAN, Sadhana L; WestOak Med Clinic, 2495 Old Bronte Rd, Oakville ON L6M 4J2; London (England)'06; FRCPC; Peds. (905)582-7533; Fax. (905)582-0766.

BALAKUMAR, Mahadeva; Delta Hosp, 5800 Mountain View Blvd, Delta BC V4K 3V6; Colombo (Sri Lanka)'81; MB BS; Staff, Delta Hospital; (604)943-1121

BALASINGAM, Sivadevi; Taylor Street Med Clinic, 3020 Taylor St E, Saskatoon SK S7H 4J2; (Other Foreign)'80; (306)374-8082; Fax. (306)374-0047.

BALASINGAM, Vijayabalan; Clinique Med McDermot, 37 av Donegani, Pointe-Claire QC H9R 2V7; McG'96; FRCSC; Neursurg (Brain Tumors). Chef, Hopital Maisonneuve-Rosemont; adj Prof, Universite de Montreal; Langs: English; (514)697-1410; Fax. (514)697-1411.

BALASINGHAM, Prabaharan; Miramichi Reg Hosp, 500 Water St, Miramichi NB E1V 3G5; Jaffna (Sri Lanka)'93; Staff, Miramichi Regional Hospital; (506)623-3327

BALASKA, Yasmina; Bradley Med Centre, 595 Bradley Ave, London ON N6E 3Z8; (Algeria)'88; CCFP; (519)681-6112

BALASUBRAMANIAM, Balaji; Chatham-Kent Hlth Alliance, PO Box 2030 Stn Main 80 Grand Ave W, Chatham ON N7M 5L9; Manipal (India)'95; Staff, Chatham-Kent Health Alliance; (519)352-6400

BALASUNDARAM, Manjula; Chatham Kent Family Health Team, 20 Emma St, Chatham ON N7L 5K5; (England)'94; (519)354-2172; mbalasundaram@ckha.on.ca.

BALASURIYA, Rajiv; 100-1 Belton Blvd, St Catharines ON L2T 3Y4; (Other Foreign)'08; (905)688-6460

BALATON, John L; Foothills Med Centre, 1403 29 St NW, Calgary AB T2N 2T9; Sask'85; FRCPC; Anes. Staff, Foothills Medical Centre; (403)944-1430; john.balaton@crha-health.ab.ca.

BALATON, Joseph M; Sutherland Family Med Clinic, 1108 Central Ave, Saskatoon SK S7N 2H1; Sask'81; CCFP; FCFP; (306)374-9121; Fax. (306)374-9744.

BALATON, Julianna E K; Sutherland Family Med Clinic, 1108 Central Ave, Saskatoon SK S7N 2H1; Sask'83; CCFP; FCFP; Langs: Hungarian; (306)374-9114; Fax. (306)374-9117.

BALAZSI, A Gordon; Centre Med Rene Laennec, 201-1100 av Beaumont, Mont-Royal QC H3P 3H5; McG'78; FRCSC; Ophth (Cataract Surgery). Staff Ophth, McGill University Health Centre - Royal Victoria Hospital; assoc Prof, McGill University; Langs: English; French; Hungarian; (514)738-6666; Fax. (514)738-1769.

BALBUL, Alfred; 5492 ch Queen-Mary, Montreal QC H3X 1V6; McG'82; DAB; FRCPC; Derm. Staff, McGill University Health Centre - Montreal General Campus; adj Prof Med, McGill University; (514)282-8815; Fax. (514)849-5833.

BALCAR, Petr; Royal Columbian Hosp, 330 Columbia St E, New Westminster BC V3L 3W7; Qns'04; FRCPC; EmergMed. Staff, Royal Columbian Hospital; (604)520-4253

BALCEWICZ, Malgorzata; The Oncology Group, 5F-2100 Bovaird Dr E, Brampton ON L6R 3J7; Pomeranian (Poland)'88; FRCPC; IntMed (Medical Oncology). Staff, William Osler Health System - Brampton Civic Hospital; Staff, The Oncology Group; (905)494-6542; Fax. (905)494-6416; malgorzata.balcewicz@williamoslerhs.ca.

BALCHA, Berhanu; 202-1385 Sargent Ave, Winnipeg MB R3E 3P8; Semmelweis (Hungary)'81; MD; LMCC; Staff, WRHA - Deer Lodge Centre; Staff, The Salvation Army Grace Hospital; Langs: Oromo; Amharic; Hungarian; (204)956-0988; Fax. (204)943-9954; drbalcha@netscape.net.

BALCHAND, Kamlesh; HE1 419-60 White Squirrel Way, Toronto ON M6J 1H4; Tor'01; FRCPC; Psy (Addiction Psychiatry). Staff, Centre for Addiction & Mental Health (CAMH) - Queen Site; (416)535-8501

BALDASSARE, Ronald D; 1571 Sutherland Ave, Kelowna BC V1Y 5Y7; McG'89; AB; FRCSC; Ophth (Cornea/External Disease). Div Head Ophth, Kelowna General Hospital; (250)979-2010; Fax. (250)979-2080; rbaldassare@shaw.ca.

BALDAUF, Christian G; Grey Bruce HS-Owen Sound, PO Box 1800 Stn Main 1800 8th St E, Owen Sound ON N4K 6M9; Ott'98; FRCPC; DiagRad. Staff, Grey Bruce Health Services - Owen Sound; (519)376-2121 x2297; Fax. (519)372-3954.

BALDELLI, Angela M; Medical Arts Bldg, 621-750 Spadina Cres E, Saskatoon SK S7K 3H3; Wes'90; FRCPC; IntMed (Infectious Diseases). Clin Assoc Prof Med, University of Saskatchewan; (306)651-2830; Fax. (306)651-2836; baldelli.associates@sasktel.net.

BALDELLI, Robert J; Kensington Med Clinic, 6548 Hastings St, Burnaby BC V5B 1S2; Cal'93; CCFP; (604)299-9769

BALDERSON, Jeffrey O; Sioux Lookout First Nation Hlt, PO Box 4000 Stn Main, Sioux Lookout ON P8T 1K2; Qns'92; MA; CCFP; FCFP; (807)737-5160

BALDERSON, Kenneth E; CCW 17033-30 Bond St, Toronto ON M5B 1W8; McG'90; FRCPC; Psy. Staff, St Michael's Hospital; (416)864-3082; Fax. (416)864-3091; baldersonk@smh.ca.

BALDERSTON, Janet I; 2634 South Parkside Dr, Lethbridge AB T1K 0C4; Dal'02; FRCSC; Otol. (403)524-3681; Fax. (403)524-3669.

BALDINI, Gabriele; MUHC-Montreal Gen Hosp, 1650 av Cedar, Montreal QC H3G 1A4; (Italy)'03; Staff, McGill University Health Centre - Montreal General Campus; (514)934-1934

BALDISERA, Tara; 5-2120 Regent St, Sudbury ON P3E 3Z9; Ott'06; BComm; CCFP; Asst Prof/Med Dir CME, Northern Ontario School of Medicine; (705)222-3737

BALDO, Allain; Ottawa Cardiovascular Centre, 502-1355 Bank St, Ottawa ON K1H 8K7; McG'97; FRCPC; IntMed. (613)738-1584

BALDOCK, Robert L; Langley Airport, 4A-5333 216 St, Langley BC V2Y 2N3; UBC'74; (604)488-4917; Fax. (604)576-5675.

BALDONADO, Narciso; Northern Lights Health Region, 7 Hospital St, Fort McMurray AB T9H 1P2; (Philippines)'82; Staff, Northern Lights Regional Health Centre; (780)791-6161; Fax. (780)748-2913.

BALDRY, Craig D; SMBD Jewish Gen Hosp, 335A-3755 ch Cote-Ste-Catherin, Montreal QC H3T 1E2; McG'95; CSPQ; FRCPC; Anes; Critical Care Medicine (P.Q.). Staff, Sir Mortimer B Davis Jewish General; Langs: Bilingual(French/English); (514)340-8222 x5701; Fax. (514)340-8108; craig_baldry@yahoo.com.

BALDWIN, Caroline L; St Paul's Hosp, 10D-1081 Burrard St, Vancouver BC V6Z 1Y6; UBC'08; CCFP; Staff, Providence Health Care - St Paul's Hospital; (604)682-2344

BALDWIN, Clark; London Intercommunity Hlth Ctr, 659 Dundas St, London ON N5W 2Z1; Tor'97; CCFP; Physician, London Intercommunity Health Centre - Dundas Street; Physician Consultant, Health Zone Nurse Practitioner Led Clinic; (519)660-0874; Fax. (519)642-1532.

BALDWIN, Gregory A; Kensington Med Clinic, 6548 Hastings St, Burnaby BC V5B 1S2; Ott'81; FRCPC; Peds (Pediatric Emergency Medicine). (604)299-9769; Fax. (604)299-9772.

BALDWIN, Joan F D; Wascana Rehab Centre, 2180 23rd Ave, Regina SK S4S 0A5; Sask'76; CCFP; FCFP; Staff, Wascana Rehabilitation Centre; (306)766-5781; Fax. (306)766-5359; joanbaldwin@hotmail.com.

BALDWIN, Katherine L; Children's Hosp Eastern Ont, 401 Smyth Rd, Ottawa ON K1H 8L1; Ott'05; FRCPC; Peds. Staff, Children's Hospital of Eastern Ontario (CHEO); (613)737-7600

BALDWIN, William E; SGH Medical Mall, 501-3030 Lawrence Ave E, Scarborough ON M1P 2T7; Tor'62; FRCSC; Urol. Staff, The Scarborough Hospital - General Campus; Court Staff, Toronto East General Hospital Inc; (416)438-6787; Fax. (416)438-2863; william.baldwin@sympatico.ca.

BALDZHIYSKI, Nikolay; Hôpital régional Chaleur, 1750 Sunset Dr, Bathurst NB E2A 4L7; Plovdiv (Bulgaria)'80; LMCC; Staff, Hopital Regional Chaleur; Langs: Bulgarian; Russian; Bilingual(French/English); (506)544-3000; Fax. (506)544-2326; nbaldzhiysky@reg6.health.nb.ca.

BALE, Michael; Chelsea House Fam Med Group, 33623 Wildwood Dr, Abbotsford BC V2S 1S2; London (England)'71; MB BS; PhD; BPharm(Hons); Ac Staff, Abbotsford Regional Hospital & Cancer Centre; (604)853-4100; Fax. (604)853-2626.

BALEC, Raymond J; Norwest Commun Health Centre, 525 Simpson St, Thunder Bay ON P7C 3J6; Man'08; CCFP; (807)622-8235

BALFOUR, Clive H; The Medical Arts Centre, 30-650 Terminal Ave, Nanaimo BC V9R 5E2; Cape Town (South Africa)'76; MB ChB; (250)753-3431; Fax. (250)734-6897.

BALFOUR, Jennifer; Helmcken Pediatric Associates, 212-284 Helmcken Rd, Victoria BC V9B 1T2; Alb'94; FRCPC; Peds. Staff, Victoria General Hospital; (250)881-7347

BALFOUR, Nicholas J B; Plaza 33, PO Box 23122 Rpo Plaza 33, Kelowna BC V1X 7K7; UBC'93; CCFP; CCFP(E.M.); FCFP; Staff, Kelowna General Hospital; (250)765-5500

BALFOUR, Shana C; 169 rue Botsford, Moncton NB E1C 4X4; Sher'03; FRCPC; Nephrol; IntMed. Langs: Bilingual(French/English); (506)857-3020; Fax. (506)855-2847.

BALG, Frederic; CHUS-Hop Fleurimont, 3001 12e Av N, Sherbrooke QC J1H 5N4; Sher'98; FRCSC; OrthSurg. Staff, Centre Hospitalier Universitaire de Sherbrooke-Hopital Fleurimont; (819)346-1110 x14233; frederic.balg@usherbrooke.ca.

BALHAJ, Abdelaati A; Stonewall & Dist Health Ctr, 589 3rd Ave S, Stonewall MB R0C 2Z0; (Other Foreign)'96; Staff, Stonewall & District Health Centre; (204)467-5514

BALHARRY, Richard C; Canmore MediSpa & Laser Ctre, 901B Main St, Canmore AB T1W 2B4; Andrews (Scotland)'69; MB ChB; Chief Medical Staff, Canmore General Hospital; Court Staff, Covenant Health - Banff Mineral Springs Hospital; (403)678-5511; Fax. (403)678-2727; balharry@medispa.com.

BALHOUS, Wassim; Ctr Sante Commun Hamilton/Niag, 810 Main St E, Welland ON L3B 3Y4; Ferrara (Italy)'90; CCFP; (905)734-1141

BALI, Amardeep K; AIM Health Group, 458 Central Ave, London ON N6B 2E5; (Mexico)'06; (519)432-1521

BALI, Neena; Royal Ottawa Hlth Care Group, 1145 Carling Ave, Ottawa ON K1Z 7K4; Dar-es-Salaam (Tanzania)'76; FRCPC; Psy (Adult Psychiatry). Staff, Royal Ottawa Mental Health Centre - Royal Ottawa Health Care Group; (613)722-6521 x6615; Fax. (613)798-2988.

BALICKI, Danuta M; Pavillon Masson, 3850 rue Saint-Urbain, Montreal QC H2W 1T7; Mon'87; FRCPC; IntMed; MedOncol; Hem. Staff, Centre Hospitalier l'Université de Montréal (CHUM) - Hôtel-Dieu; (514)890-8000 x15518; Fax. (514)412-7207.

BALINSON, Alex P; AIM Health Group, 100-19 Allstate Pkwy, Markham ON L3R 5A4; Wes'72; Ac Staff Family Med, St Joseph's Healthcare - Charlton Campus; (905)475-3353; abalinson@cogeco.ca.

BALISKI, Christopher R; 203-3040 Tutt St, Kelowna BC V1Y 2H5; Sask'95; BSc; FRCSC; GenSurg (Surgical Oncology). (250)763-2226

BALKI, Mrinalini S; Mount Sinai Hosp, 600 University Ave, Toronto ON M5G 1X5; Nagpur (India)'94; Staff, Mount Sinai Hospital; (416)586-5270

BALKISSOON, Eric J; Humber River Reg Hosp-Finch, 2111 Finch Ave W, North York ON M3N 1N1; Madras (India)'62; FRCPC; Anes. Ac Staff, Humber River Regional Hospital - Finch Avenue Site; Court Staff, The Scarborough Hospital - Birchmount Campus; (416)747-3835; Fax. (416)747-3773.

BALKISSOON, Mahadeo; 3225 Lawrence Ave E, Scarborough ON M1H 3C2; Tor'65; Staff, Rouge Valley Health System - Centenary Health Centre Site; Staff, The Scarborough Hospital - General Campus; (416)431-9577; Fax. (416)431-3904.

BALKO, George V; St Boniface Clinic, 343 Tache Ave, Winnipeg MB R2H 2A5; Man'90; CCFP; FCFP; (204)233-8537

BALKO, Justin P; 5201 50 St, Leduc AB T9E 6T4; Cal'08; CCFP; (780)986-9600; Fax. (780)986-9732.

BALKWILL, Susan L; BC Cancer Agency-Fraser Valley, 13750 96 Ave, Surrey BC V3V 1Z2; Cal'94; FRCPC; RadOncol. Staff, BC Cancer Agency Fraser Valley Centre; (604)930-4036; Fax. (604)930-4065.

BALL, Adrianne M M; 300-690 Dorval Dr, Oakville ON L6K 3W7; Qns'94; FRCPC; IntMed; Nephrol. (905)849-4567

BALL, Allison L; Tom Baker Cancer Centre, 1331 29 St NW, Calgary AB T2N 4N2; Cal'06; FRCSC; ObstGyn. Staff, Tom Baker Cancer Centre; (403)521-3721; Fax. (403)521-3573.

BALL, Arlene E; Bow River Prof Centre, 313-4411 16 Ave NW, Calgary AB T3B 0M3; Mem'87; FRCSC; Ophth. Ac Staff Ophth, Foothills Medical Centre; Consultant Privil Ophth, Rockyview General Hospital; Clin Lecturer Surg, University of Calgary; (403)286-3335; Fax. (403)286-3316.

BALL, Chad G; Foothills Med Centre, 1403 29 St NW, Calgary AB T2N 2T9; Tor'02; FRCSC; GenSurg. Staff, Foothills Medical Centre; (403)944-1110; Fax. (403)944-8799.

BALL, Daniel G; North Bay Reg Health Centre, 50 College St, North Bay ON P1B 0A4; Tor'68; FRCPC; DiagRad. Staff Radiol., North Bay Regional Health Centre - Regional Mental Health; (705)474-8600 x4023; Fax. (705)495-2787.

BALL, Fred; St Boniface Clinic, 343 Tache Ave, Winnipeg MB R2H 2A5; Man'05; CCFP; (204)925-9550

BALL, Ian C; Wellington Med Arts Bldg, 114-121 Wellington St W, Barrie ON L4N 1L2; Ott'79; FRCPC; DiagRad. Diagnostic Imaging, Royal Victoria Regional Health Centre; (705)726-4531

BALL, Ian M; Kingston Gen Hosp, 76 Stuart St, Kingston ON K7L 2V7; Wes'02; FRCPC; EmergMed (Critical Care Medicine). Staff, Kingston General Hospital; (613)549-6666 x4485

BALL, Mary Kate; 3403 32 Ave, Vernon BC V1T 2M9; UBC'03; FRCSC; OrthSurg. (250)545-2488

BALL, Nigel J; Vancouver Gen Hosp, 1250-855 12th Ave W, Vancouver BC V5Z 1M9; London (England)'84; MB BS; FRCPC; AnatPath (Dermatological Pathology). Staff, Vancouver General Hospital - Centennial Pavillion; Clin Assoc Prof Path, University of British Columbia; (604)875-4577

BALL, Warren T; The Peterborough Clinic, 327 Charlotte St, Peterborough ON K9J 0B2; Wes'02; FRCPC; IntMed; Cardiol. (705)775-0145

BALLA, Agneta; St Joseph Family Med Clinic, 402-2555 St Joseph Blvd, Orleans ON K1C 1S6; McG'08; CCFP; (613)830-1298; Fax. (613)841-6550.

BALLAGH, Robert H; Georgian Prof Centre, 203-125 Bell Farm Rd, Barrie ON L4M 6L2; Wes'88; FRCSC; Otol. (705)726-6966; Fax. (705)725-7330.

BALLANCE, D Lee-Ann; 3F-528 Wentworth St, Nanaimo BC V9R 3E4; Mem'97; BSc; MSc; FRCPC; Psy. Consultant Liaison Psy, West Coast General Hospital; (250)739-5868

BALLANTINE, Jane E; Richmond Square Med Centre, 70-3915 51 St SW, Calgary AB T3E 6N1; Queen's (Ireland)'85; (403)229-2273; Fax. (403)246-9688.

BALLANTYNE, Patricia K; 637 Wellington St, London ON N6A 3R8; Wes'81; CCFP; (519)672-6805

BALLANTYNE, Robert H; 530 Columbian St W, Waterloo ON N2T 0B1; Tor'69; BSc; CCFP; FCFP; (519)880-8444

BALLARD, Andrew M; 102-107 Edward St, St Thomas ON N5P 1Y8; Wes'86; CCFP; FCFP; Ac Staff, St Thomas Elgin General Hospital; (519)633-3221; Fax. (519)633-3225; aballard@uwo.ca.

BALLARD, Betty L H; Courtice Health Centre, 2F-1450 Highway 2, Courtice ON L1E 3C3; Dal'74; BSc; (905)723-8551 x5257; Fax. (905)721-6172.

BALLARD, James H; 415-645 Fort St, Victoria BC V8W 1G2; Wes'64; LMCC; Staff, Vancouver Island Health Authority; Member, Victoria Med. Society; Preceptor, University of British Columbia; Langs: English; (250)380-7033; Fax. (250)380-2644; jbmd@shaw.ca.

BALLARD, Tonya G; Cambridge Ctr for Hlth & Welln, B4D-350 Conestoga Blvd, Cambridge ON N1R 7L7; McM'04; FRCPC; PhysMed&Rehab. (519)624-5999

BALLAUF, Frank P; Vernon Jubilee Hosp, 2101 32 St, Vernon BC V1T 5L2; UBC'87; CCFP; CCFP(E.M.); Staff, Vernon Jubilee Hospital; (250)558-1200 x1401; Fax. (250)558-7830.

BALLEGEER, Trevor; Early Psychosis Prevention, 505-180 King St, Winnipeg MB R3B 3P7; Man'97; FRCPC; Psy.

BALLEM, Penny J D; 3695 10th Ave W, Vancouver BC V6R 2G2; UBC'78; FRCPC; Hem. Langs: Bilingual(English/French).

BALLEN, Jenifer L; St Boniface Gen Hosp, 409 Tache Ave, Winnipeg MB R2H 2A6; Sask'02; FRCPC; Anes. Staff, St Boniface General Hospital; (204)233-8563

BALLERMANN, Barbara J; Clinical Sciences Bldg, 13103CSB-11350 83 Ave, Edmonton AB T6G 2P4; Cal'76; MD; FRCPC; IntMed (Nephrology). Medical Staff, University of Alberta Hospital; Prof Med/Chair Dept of Med, University of Alberta; Langs: German; (780)248-1639; Fax. (780)248-1637.

BALLERMANN, Charlotte A; Capital City Women's Centre, 196-17010 90 Ave NW, Edmonton AB T5T 1L6; Alb'04; BSc(Biochem); FRCSC; ObstGyn. Att Physician, Covenant Health - Misericordia Community Hospital; Clin Lecturer ObstGyn, University of Alberta; (780)439-2007; Fax. (780)439-3080.

BALLINGER, Lisa M; 543 Eglinton Ave E, Toronto ON M4P 1N7; Tor'85; Staff Family Pract & Emerg Dept, Toronto East General Hospital Inc; (416)487-9454

BALLIVY, Olivier; Hop Charles Lemoyne, 3120 boul Taschereau, Greenfield Park QC J4V 2H1; Mon'97; FRCPC; RadOncol. Staff, Hopital Charles LeMoyne; (450)466-5650

BALLON, Bruce C; Addiction & Mental Hlth-ARF, 3108-33 Russell St, Toronto ON M5S 2S1; Man'93; BSc; FRCPC; Psy (Addiction Psychiatry). Clin Head Youth Addiction Services, Centre for Addiction & Mental Health (CAMH) - Russell Street Site; (416)535-8501 x4466; Fax. (416)595-6399.

BALLON, Lawrence L; 161 Admiral Rd, Toronto ON M5R 2L7; Ott'66; DPsy; FRCPC; Psy (Mindfulness-Based Stress Reduction). (416)961-6720; Fax. (416)923-2304; lawrence@centreformindfulness.com.

BALLOU, Stephen G; Bruyere Academic Fam Hlth Team, 75 Bruyere St, Ottawa ON K1N 5C7; McG'80; CCFP; FCFP; Asst Prof Family Med, University of Ottawa; (613)241-3344

BALLOUK, Fayez; Western Mem Reg Hosp, PO Box 2005 Stn Main 1 Brookfield Ave, Corner Brook NL A2H 6J7; Aleppo Univ (Syria)'82; Staff, Western Memorial Regional Hospital; (709)637-5000

BALLY, Gerry A; 125 Sussex Dr PO Box 500 New Delhi Stn A, Ottawa ON K1N 8T7; Ott'83; CCFP; Physician, Citizenship & Immigration Canada; Langs: English; French; (613)941-8336; Fax. (613)941-2179; gbally@magma.ca.

BALLYK, Catherine J; Brant Community HC-Brantford, 200 Terrace Hill St, Brantford ON N3R 1G9; Mem'81; FRCPC; PhysMed&Rehab. Staff, The Brant Community Healthcare System - Brantford General Hospital Site; (519)752-7871 x5822; Fax. (519)750-9972.

BALLYK, Peter D; St Joseph's Health Centre, 30 The Queensway, Toronto ON M6R 1B5; Tor'99; FRCPC; DiagRad. Staff, St Joseph's Health Centre; (416)530-6001

BALMACEDA, Rufino B; 1145 Carling Ave, Ottawa ON K1Z 7K4; UERMMMC (Philippines)'72; DrMedCh; BSc; FRCPC; Psy (Forensic Psychiatry). Staff Psychiatrist Integrated Forensic Program, Royal Ottawa Mental Health Centre - Royal Ottawa Health Care Group; Staff Psychiatrist, St Lawrence Correctional & Treatment Cente-Secure Treatment Unit; Asst Prof, University of Ottawa; Langs: Tagalog; (613)722-6521 x6365; Fax. (613)798-2992; rufino.balmaceda@theroyal.ca.

BALMAIN, Sean; Mount Sinai Hosp, 600 University Ave, Toronto ON M5G 1X5; Glasgow (Scotland)'97; Staff, Mount Sinai Hospital; (416)596-4200

BALOG, Stephanie A; 1780 Broadway W PO Box 14074, Vancouver BC V6J 0B9; Wes'10; CCFP; (778)989-9442

BALOGH, Alexander G; Tom Baker Cancer Centre, 1331 29 St NW, Calgary AB T2N 4N2; Qns'93; BSc; MSc; FRCPC; RadOncol (Genito Urinary Oncology). Staff, Tom Baker Cancer Centre; Att Staff, Foothills Medical Centre; Dir RadOncol Residency Prog & Clin Ass't Prof, University of Calgary; Langs: Hungarian; (403)521-3095; Fax. (403)283-1651; alexbalo@cancerboard.ab.ca.

BALOGH, Arpad; The Group Health Centre, 240 Mcnabb St, Sault Ste. Marie ON P6B 1Y5; Tor'72; Ac Staff Family Med, Sault Area Hospital - Sault Ste Marie; Med Dir, Algoma Steel Inc; (705)759-1234 x2290

BALOGH, Judith M; Odette Cancer Centre, T2 152-2075 Bayview Ave, Toronto ON M4N 3M5; Tor'81; FRCPC; RadOncol (Head & Neck). Staff, Sunnybrook Health Sciences Centre; (416)480-4951; Fax. (416)480-6002.

BALOGH, Louis; Newmarket Med Place, 301-712 Davis Dr, Newmarket ON L3Y 8C3; Wes'72; ABPeds; FRCPC; Peds. Vice Pres Reg Cardiac and Cancer Programs, Southlake Regional Health Centre; (905)898-5438; Fax. (905)898-6529; lbalogh@southlakeregional.org; Semi-Retired.

BALON, Jeffrey W; 1538 Stittsville Main St PO Box 959 Stn Main, Stittsville ON K2S 1B1; McM'92; BSc; DC; CCFP; (613)836-1711; Fax. (613)836-1712.

BALOUCH, Hamid M; 1030 1 Ave PO Box 209, Beaverlodge AB T0H 0C0; (Pakistan)'98; (780)354-8993; Fax. (780)354-8181.

BALOUN, Daniela; The Two Hundred, 306-200 St Clair Ave W, Toronto ON M4V 1R1; Prague (Czech Republic)'72; Langs: Czech; (416)920-1766; Fax. (416)920-2116.

BALSDON, Jeffrey L; 105-107 Edward St, St Thomas ON N5P 1Y8; Wes'89; (519)631-2610

BALSDON, Lewis A; 105-107 Edward St, St Thomas ON N5P 1Y8; Wes'62; (519)631-2610

BALSER, Eric F; Brooks & Balser Med Inc, PO Box 1599 452 Main St, Middleton NS B0S 1P0; Dal'97; BSc; CCFP; Ac Staff, Soldiers Memorial Hospital; Asst Prof, Dalhousie University; (902)825-2101; Fax. (902)825-6973.

BALSYS, Aras J; 219-1920 Weston Rd, York ON M9N 1W4; Tor'68; ABIM; FRCPC; IntMed (Critical Care Medicine). Langs: Lithuanian; (416)244-5565; Fax. (416)244-5566; abalsys@sympatico.ca.

BALTAZAR, Carmen; Institut de Cardiologie de Mtl, 5000 rue Belanger, Montreal QC H1T 1C8; Mon'00; CCFP; Staff EmergMed, Institut de Cardiologie de Montréal; Clin Staff, Universite de Montreal; (514)376-3330

BALTER, Meyer S; Mount Sinai Hosp, 6 207-600 University Ave, Toronto ON M5G 1X5; McG'81; ABIM; FACP; FCCP; FRCPC; IntMed (Respiratory Disease); Respir. Ac Staff, Mount Sinai Hospital; Assoc Staff, Toronto General Hospital - UHN; Prof Med, University of Toronto; (416)586-4800 x4663; Fax. (416)586-4736; mbalter@mtsinai.on.ca.

BALTHAZARD, Carole; Centre de Sante Sutton, GD 33 rue Principale S, Sutton QC J0E 2K0; Mon'94; Chef Geriatrie-readaptation, Hôpital Brome-Missisquoi-Perkins; (450)538-3983; Fax. (450)538-3983; cbalthazard@aol.com.

BALTZAN, Marcel A; Mount Sinai Hosp Centre, 5690 boul Cavendish, Cote Saint-Luc QC H4W 1S7; McG'91; FRCPC; IntMed (Sleep Disorders); Respir. Consultant, Mount Sinai Hospital Center; Langs: English; French; (514)369-2222; Fax. (514)369-0282.

BALTZAN, Richard B; Baltzan Associate Med Clinic, 204-321A 21st St E, Saskatoon SK S7K 0C1; McG'59; FACP; FRCPC; IntMed (Nephrology). Assoc Staff, St Paul's Hospital (Grey Nuns) of Saskatoon; Assoc Staff, Royal University Hospital; (306)653-1855; Fax. (306)653-0442; baltzanmedclinic@sasktel.net.

BALTZER, Franziska; Adolescent Medicine, W 120-1040 av Atwater, Westmount QC H3Z 1X3; Berne (Switzerland)'78; MD; Peds (P.Q.) (Adolescent Medicine). Dir Adolesc Med & Gynecol Prog, McGill University Health Centre - Montreal Children's Hospital; assoc Prof, McGill University; Langs: German; English; (514)412-4481; Fax. (514)412-4319; franziska.baltzer@muhc.mcgill.ca.

BALUYUT, Crystal A; Addiction & Mental Hlth-Clarke, 709-250 College St, Toronto ON M5T 1R8; Tor'02; FRCPC; Psy. Staff, Centre for Addiction & Mental Health (CAMH) - College Street Site; (416)535-8501

BALYK, Robert A; Strathcona Med Dental Bldg, 200-8225 105 St NW, Edmonton AB T6E 4H2; Man'83; FRCSC; OrthSurg (Sports Medicine). Staff, University of Alberta Hospital; Staff, Covenant Health - Grey Nuns Community Hospital; Dir, Northern Alberta Shoulder Program; (780)439-5858; Fax. (780)433-1344.

BALYS, Richard; 10-294 Cobequid Rd, Lower Sackville NS B4C 4C5; Ott'01; FRCSC; Otol. Lecturer, Dalhousie University; Langs: Bilingual(English/French); (902)435-8589; Fax. (902)435-8695; balysent@gmail.com.

BALZUN, Margaret A; Signal Hill Centre, 200-5986 Signal Hill Ctr SW, Calgary AB T3H 3P8; Cal'85; CCFP; FCFP; Staff, Rockyview General Hospital; (403)240-2660; Fax. (403)242-8390.

BAMBACE, Nadia; Inst de Readaptation de Mtl, 6300 av deDarlington, Montreal QC H3S 2J4; Mon'05; FRCPC; IntMed; Hem. Staff, Institut de Réadaptation Gingras-Lindsay de Montréal; (514)340-2085

BAMBAO, M Clarissa; Sunnyside Med Arts Centre, 407-27 Roncesvalles Ave, Toronto ON M6R 3B2; Qns'03; FRCSC; ObstGyn. (416)537-5289; Fax. (416)537-3698.

BAMBER, Karen E; B201-20641 Logan Ave, Langley BC V3A 7R3; UBC'89; FRCPC; Peds. (604)534-2900; Fax. (604)533-2905.

BAMBONYE, Miriam E; St Mary's Hosp Centre, 3830 av Lacombe, Montreal QC H3T 1M5; Mon'04; DiagRad. Staff, St Mary's Hospital Centre; (514)345-3511

BAMDADIAN, Farshid; CSSS Pierre Boucher, 1333 boul Jacques-Cartier E, Longueuil QC J4M 2A5; Tehran (Iran)'96; OrthSurg. Staff, Centre Hospitalier Pierre Boucher; (450)468-6223

BAMFORD, Diane F; 502-168 Charlotte St, Ottawa ON K1N 8K6; Ott'90; CCFP; FCFP; Langs: Bilingual(English/French); (613)563-0320; Fax. (613)563-2211.

BAMFORD, J D Russell; River Valley Med Clinic, 106 Lambert St, Whitehorse YT Y1A 1Z2; Dublin (Ireland)'79; MB ChB; BAO; CCFP; Physician Emerg, Whitehorse General Hospital; Vis Consultant, Haines Junction Health Centre; Langs: English; French; (867)667-6491; Fax. (867)633-3804.

BAMFORTH, Fiona; University of Alberta Hosp, 8440 112 St NW, Edmonton AB T6G 2B7; London (England)'76; MB BS; FRCPC; MedBiochem. Prof/Chair Lab Med & Path, University of Alberta Hospital; (780)407-7379; Fax. (780)407-8599.

BAMFORTH, J Stephen G; University of Alberta Hosp, 8 53MSB-8440 112 St NW, Edmonton AB T6G 2B7; London (England)'75; MRC(UK); DAB; FRCPC; MedGenetics (Pediatrics). Dir Clin Genetics Sect, University of Alberta Hospital; Assoc Prof Dept of Med Genetics, University of Alberta; (780)407-7327; Fax. (780)407-6845.

BAMGBADE, Olumuyiwa A; University Hosp of Northern BC, 1475 Edmonton St, Prince George BC V2M 1S2; Staff, University Hospital of Northern British Columbia; (250)565-2000

BAMI, Harmeet K; William Osler HC-Brampton, 1423-2100 Bovaird Dr E, Brampton ON L6R 3J7; Delhi (India)'87; FRCPC; Psy. Staff, William Osler Health System - Brampton Civic Hospital; Langs: Punjabi; Hindi; Urdu; (905)494-6695

BANACH, Ryan L; Norfinch Med Centre, 301-2100 Finch Ave W, North York ON M3N 2Z9; McM'08; CCFP; (416)739-8700

BANACH, Theodore M; Prana Medical Clinic, 208 Regent Ave W, Winnipeg MB R3C 1R2; Man'73.

BANACK, Alan D; 506-1200 Bay St, Toronto ON M5R 2A5; Tor'68; Court Staff, Mount Sinai Hospital; (416)920-9139; Fax. (416)920-5273; albanack@hotmail.com.

BANAGE, Christine L N; HSC-Div of Internal Med, 3330 Hospital Dr NW, Calgary AB T2N 4N1; Lusaka (Zambia)'89; MB ChB; Clin Assoc Prof, University of Calgary; (403)220-6882; Fax. (403)283-6151.

BANANDA SHAMBU, Sunil; Millbourne Road Med Clinic, 131 Millbourne Road East NW, Edmonton AB T6K 1P6; (Other Foreign)'97; (780)462-4229; Fax. (780)462-3315.

BANASCH, Jan L; Grey Nuns Community Hosp & HC, 1100 Youville Drive West NW, Edmonton AB T6L 5X8; Nottingham (England)'84; BMedSci; FRCPC; Psy (Psychosis). Staff, Covenant Health - Grey Nuns Community Hospital; Consultant Psy, Alberta Mental Health Services; Clin Prof, University of Alberta; (780)342-7783; Fax. (780)425-9317; jan.banasch@albertahealthservices.ca.

BANCE, Manohar L; Queen Elizabeth II HSC, DB3184-1276 South Park St, Halifax NS B3H 2Y9; Manchester (England)'85; BSc; MSc; FRCSC; Otol (Neuro Otolaryngology). Staff, Queen Elizabeth II Health Sciences Centre - Victoria General Site; (902)473-5975; Fax. (902)473-4345.

BANDALI, Ashraf M; Conestoga Med Centre, 26-380 Bovaird Dr E, Brampton ON L6Z 2S8; Makerere (Uganda)'72; MB ChB; Langs: Gujarati; (905)791-2230; Fax. (905)840-3912.

BANDER, Marek S; Digby Gen Hosp, PO Box 820, Digby NS B0V 1A0; Lublin (Poland)'66; Staff, Digby General Hospital; (902)245-4447; Fax. (902)245-2144.

BANDEY, Karl; C-59 Lorne Ave E, Stratford ON N5A 6S4; Wes'89; Ac Staff, Stratford General Hospital - Huron Perth Healthcare Alliance; (519)271-1731; Fax. (519)271-3124.

BANDI, Edith; St Mary's Hosp Centre, 3830 Lacombe Ave, Montreal QC H3T 1M5; Freiburg (Germany)'86; CSPQ; Anes (P.Q.) (Obstetrics Anesthesia). Staff, St Mary's Hospital Centre; Langs: German; Romanian; French; (514)345-3511 x3344; Fax. (514)734-2683.

BANDIERA, Glen W; St Michael's Hosp, 30 Bond St, Toronto ON M5B 1W8; McM'93; FRCPC; EmergMed (Trauma). Ac Staff Emerg, St Michael's Hospital; Assoc Dean PGME, University of Toronto; (416)864-5095; Fax. (416)864-5341.

BANDRAUK, Natalie A; Health Sciences Centre, 300 Prince Philip Dr, St. John's NL A1B 3V6; McG'93; FRCPC; IntMed; Critical Care Medicine. Staff Critical Care Offices, Health Sciences Centre; (709)777-6300

BANDS, Colin J; Peter Lougheed Centre, 3500 26 Ave NE, Calgary AB T1Y 6J4; Stellenbosch (South Africa)'83; MB ChB; DA(SA); FRCPC; Anes; Critical Care Medicine. Staff, Peter Lougheed Centre; Staff, Foothills Medical Centre; Asst Prof, University of Calgary; (403)943-4315; Fax. (403)291-1491; bandsc@cadvision.com.

BANDYAYERA, Etienne; 204-350 St. George St, Moncton NB E1C 1X1; Burundi (South Africa)'90; CCFP; Staff, The Moncton Hospital; (506)853-5125; Fax. (506)853-0494.

BANDYOPADHYAY, Subrata; Univ Hlth Network-Princess M, 16F-610 University Ave, Toronto ON M5G 2M9; Calcutta (India)'88; LMCC; AB; CCFP; Staff, Princess Margaret Hospital - University Health Network; (416)946-2000

BANE, Anita L; Hamilton HS-Henderson Site, 711 Concession St, Hamilton ON L8V 1C3; Galway (Ireland)'95; Staff, Hamilton Health Sciences Centre-Juravinski Site; (905)827-4322 x42063

BANERJEE, Avik U; 558 Belmont Ave W, Kitchener ON N2M 5E3; Tor'00; BSc; FRCSC; Otol (Facial Plastic Surgery). Langs: Bengali; (519)896-0949; Fax. (519)896-0957.

BANERJEE, Devi; MUHC-Montreal Gen Hosp, A6 170-1650 av Cedar, Montreal QC H3G 1A4; McG'99; BSc; MDCM; FRCPC; IntMed; ClinImmunol&Allergy. Staff, McGill University Health Centre - Montreal General Campus; Langs: Bilingual(English/French); (514)934-1934 x42531; Fax. (514)934-8570.

BANERJEE, Diponkar; BC Cancer Agency, 3225H-600 10th Ave W, Vancouver BC V5Z 4E6; Makerere University (Uganda)'71; PhD(Immunol); MB ChB; FRCPC; AnatPath (Lymphoma). Staff, BC Cancer Agency Vancouver Centre; Exec Med Dir, PHSA Laboratories; Teach Staff Lab Med & Path, University of British Columbia; (604)877-6074

BANERJEE, Lopita; Wise Elephant Family Hlth Team, 247 Main St N, Brampton ON L6X 1N3; Tor'00; CCFP; (905)459-4385; Fax. (905)459-6373; lbanerjee@ahealingplace.ca.

BANERJEE, P Joy; Guelph Gen Hosp, 115 Delhi St, Guelph ON N1E 4J4; Tor'97; FRCPC; DiagRad. Staff, Guelph General Hospital; (519)837-6440

BANERJEE, Prasenjit; Halton HSC Corp-Oakville, 327 Reynolds St, Oakville ON L6J 3L7; Wes'01; CCFP; CCFP(E.M.); Staff, Halton Healthcare Services Corporation - Oakville Site; (905)845-2571

BANERJEE, Susitna T; Koffler Student Services Centr, 2F-214 College St, Toronto ON M5T 2Z9; Ott'08; CCFP; (416)978-8030; Fax. (416)971-2089.

BANERJEE, Tamalina S; Royal University Hosp, 2841-103 Hospital Dr, Saskatoon SK S7N 0W8; Dublin (Ireland)'04; FRCPC; GenPath. Staff, Royal University Hospital; (306)655-2156; Fax. (306)655-2223.

BANERJEE, Tapas; Port Hope Med Centre, 203-249 Ontario St, Port Hope ON L1A 3Y9; Tor'81; Staff, Northumberland Hills Hospital; (905)885-1881

BANERJI, Anna; Immigrant Health & ID clinic, 2F-61 Queen St E, Toronto ON M5C 2T2; Tor'89; DTMH; MPH; FRCPC; Peds (Public Health); InfectDis. Staff Consul Pediatrics, St Michael's Hospital; Staff, St Joseph's Health Centre; Langs: Bengali; (416)867-3655; Fax. (416)867-3736.

BANERJI, Kunal; Workers' Comp Board, PO BOX 2415 9912 107 St NW, Edmonton AB T5K 1G5; Man'99; CCFP; Staff, Covenant Health - Misericordia Community Hospital; (780)498-3971

BANERJI, Shantanu; CancerCare Manitoba, ON2068-675 McDermot Ave, Winnipeg MB R3E 0V9; Man'02; FRCPC; IntMed; MedOncol.

BANERJI, Versha; CancerCare Manitoba, ON2020-675 McDermot Ave, Winnipeg MB R3E 0V9; Man'02; FRCPC; IntMed; Hem.

BANET, Joan; CSSS de Temiscouata, CP 310 58 rue de l'Eglise, Notre-Dame-du-Lac QC G0L 1X0; Gen Practice, Centre Hospitalier Notre-Dame-du-Lac; (418)899-6751; Fax. (418)899-2809.

BANFILL, Suzanne; Clinique Med de Coaticook, 206-18 rue du Manege, Coaticook QC J1A 3B3; Sher'00; CCFP; Staff, Centre Hospitalier de Coaticook; (819)849-4808; Fax. (819)849-7400.

BANGEE, Misbah; 210-5 Brockley Dr, Scarborough ON M1P 3J2; misbah1968@gmail.com.

BANH, Tu Van; Kingston Family Health Team, 500A Gardiners Rd, Kingston ON K7M 7W9; Dal'03; CCFP; (613)389-5974

BANH, Van-Ty; CHSLD Lucille-Teasdale, 3095 rue Sherbrooke E, Montreal QC H1W 1B2; Saigon (Vietnam)'71; Gen Practice, CHSLD Lucille-Teasdale; (514)523-1173

BANIC, Zlatko; Dr Everett Chalmers Reg Hosp, PO Box 9000 Stn A, Fredericton NB E3B 5N5; Novi Sad (Serbia)'81; Staff, Dr Everett Chalmers Regional Hospital; (506)452-5400

BANIHANI, Rudaina I H; Holland Bloorview Kids Rehab, 10 Kilgour, Toronto ON M4G 1R8; (Jordan)'00; Staff, Holland Bloorview Kids Rehabilitation Hospital; (416)813-7424

BANIHASHEMI, Ben; Univ of Ottawa Heart Institute, 40 Ruskin St, Ottawa ON K1Y 4W7; Ott'07; IntMed. (613)761-5000

BANIHASHEMI, Sayed B; Lakeridge Hlth Corp-Oshawa, 1 Hospital Crt, Oshawa ON L1G 2B9; Isfahan (Iran)'97; FRCPC; RadOncol (Gynecologic Oncology). Staff, Lakeridge Health - Oshawa Site; (905)576-8711 x4595

BANIJAMALI, Hamid S; Bridgeland Med Bldg, 207-803 1 Ave NE, Calgary AB T2E 7C5; Cal'95; FRCPC; IntMed; Cardiol. Staff, Peter Lougheed Centre; Staff, Foothills Medical Centre; Clin Assoc Prof Med & Adjunct Prof, University of Calgary; Langs: Persian; Farsi; (403)571-8684; Fax. (403)571-8657.

BANIK, Tapan K; William Osler HC-Brampton, NI 423-2100 Bovaird Dr E, Brampton ON L6R 3J7; Calcutta (India)'76; DPM(Lond); MRCPsy(UK); FRCPC; Psy (Affective Disorders). Staff, William Osler Health System - Brampton Civic Hospital; Langs: Bengali; (905)494-2120

BANJO, Olufemi; Yarmouth Reg Hosp, 60 Vancouver St, Yarmouth NS B5A 2P5; (Nigeria)'00; MB ChB; FRCPC; Psy. Staff, Yarmouth Regional Hospital; (902)742-3542

BANK, Ilana M; MUHC-Montreal Children's Hosp, 2300 rue Tupper, Montreal QC H3H 1P3; McG'02; FRCPC; Peds; PedEmergMed. Staff, McGill University Health Centre - Montreal Children's Hospital; (514)412-4400

BANKAY, Clarence; 576 Main St E, Hamilton ON L8M 1J2; West Indies (Jamaica)'68; (905)528-3288; Fax. (905)528-7753.

BANKS, Diana; 105-901 King St W, Toronto ON M5V 3H5; McM'09; CCFP; Staff, Halton Healthcare Services Corporation - Oakville Site; (416)599-6000

BANKS, John V; Dartmouth Med Centre, 310-46 Portland St, Dartmouth NS B2Y 1H4; Dublin (Ireland)'72; MB ChB; BAO; (902)465-4532; Fax. (902)464-4906.

BANKS, Kent D; MD Esthetics, 201-1910 Sooke Rd, Victoria BC V9B 1V7; Cal'92; CCFP; (250)478-2336; Fax. (250)478-2004.

BANKS, Malcolm R; 215 Chaplin St W, Swift Current SK S9H 0E8; Leeds (England)'67; MB ChB; Pres/Medical Staff, Cypress Regional Hospital; (306)773-6337; Fax. (306)773-1467.

BANKS, Mark D G; The Credit Valley Hosp, 2200 Eglinton Ave W, Mississauga ON L5M 2N1; McM'98; FRCPC; Anes. Staff, The Credit Valley Hospital; (905)813-2200

BANMANN, Daniel H; Chinook Reg Hosp, 960 19 St S, Lethbridge AB T1J 1W5; Alb'83; CCFP; CCFP(E.M.); FCFP; Staff, Chinook Regional Hospital; Clin Assoc Prof, University of Alberta; (403)388-6301; banmann@la.shockware.com.

BANMANN, Darin S; Pan Am Sports Med Centre, 75 Poseidon Bay, Winnipeg MB R3M 3E4; Man'98; CCFP; (204)925-1550; Fax. (204)452-5362.

BANNACH, Bernard G; Medical Examiner Bldg, 7007 116 St NW, Edmonton AB T6H 5R8; Tor'86; FRCPC; GenPath (Forensic Pathology). Asst Chief Ministry of Justice/Med Examiner, Province of Alberta; Clin Lecturer Lab Med & Path/Aj Prof, University of Alberta; (780)427-4987; bernard.bannach@gov.ab.ca.

BANNER, Laara; 117 Niven Dr, Yellowknife NT X1A 3W8; UBC'00; CCFP.

BANNER, Robert; I-620 Richmond St, London ON N6A 5J9; Sask'90; FRCPC; Anes;CCFP; FCFP; Staff, St Joseph's Hospital - St Joseph's Health Care; Staff, Tillsonburg District Memorial Hospital; (519)850-6575; Fax. (519)850-6583; banneroffice@bellnet.ca.

BANNERMAN, Alistair R E; Rosedale Med Associates, PO Box 460 13009 Rosedale Ave, Summerland BC V0H 1Z0; Manchester (England)'99; MRCGPract(UK); BSc; (250)404-4242; Fax. (250)494-3305.

BANNERMAN, S Judith; Yorston Med Clinic, 201-143 Fourth Ave S, Williams Lake BC V2G 1J8; UBC'75; (250)398-8102; Fax. (250)398-8101.

BANNISTER, Elizabeth A G; Summerhill Med Clinic, 207-130 Conception Bay Hwy, Conception Bay S NL A1W 3A6; Mem'89; Dir Assessment & Retaining Faculty of Med Professional Development & Conferencing Services, Memorial University Of Newfoundland; (709)834-2039; Fax. (709)834-9649.

BANNISTER, Leslie R; Avenue Med Clinic, 1-221 Brant Ave, Brantford ON N3T 3J2; Wes'67; CCFP; FCFP; Staff, The Brant Community Healthcare System - Brantford General Hospital Site; (519)753-8666; Fax. (519)753-6880.

BANNISTER, Susan L; Alberta Childrens Hosp, 2888 Shaganappi Trail NW, Calgary AB T3B 6A8; Cal'96; MEd; FRCPC; Peds. Staff, Alberta Children's Hospital; (403)955-7049

BANNO, Dean; Royal Columbia Hosp, 330 Columbia St E, New Westminster BC V3L 3W7; UBC'90; FRCPC; Anes (Cardiac Anesthesia). Staff, Eagle Ridge Hospital & Health Care Centre; Staff, Royal Columbian Hospital; (604)520-4602; dsbanno@telus.net.

BANNON, David; Prince County Hosp, PO Box 3000 Stn Main 65 Roy Boates Ave, Summerside PE C1N 2A9; Staff, Prince County Hospital; (902)432-2500

BANNOUR, Leila; Clinique Med du Richelieu, 200-500 Rte Marie-Victorin, Sorel-Tracy QC J3R 1K7; Tunis (Tunisia)'00; (450)742-5638

BANO, Ather; Misericordia Community Hosp, 16940 87 Ave NW, Edmonton AB T5R 4H5; Punjab (Pakistan)'88; FRCPC; AnatPath. Staff, Covenant Health - Misericordia Community Hospital; Staff, University of Alberta Hospital; (780)271-5529

BANON, Elisabeth; SMBD Jewish Gen Hosp, A532-3755 ch Cote-St-Catherine, Montreal QC H3T 1E2; McG'91; FRCPC; Psy (Depression). Staff Institute of Commun & Family Psy, Sir Mortimer B Davis Jewish General; adj Prof Psy, McGill University; Langs: English; French; (514)340-8222 x5895; Fax. (514)340-8126.

BANOS, Manuel; Clinique Med des Sommets, 1070 rue Principale, Ste-Agathe-des-Mts QC J8C 1L6; Laval'99; Staff, Centre Hospitalier Laurentien; (819)321-1212; Fax. (819)321-3232.

BANOUB, Tahany D; The Credit Valley Hosp, 2200 Eglinton Ave W, Mississauga ON L5M 2N1; Ain Shams (Egypt)'84; FRCPC; Psy (Adolescent & Adult Medicine). Staff, The Credit Valley Hospital; (905)813-2398; Fax. (905)813-1594.

BANSAL, Atul; Markham Stouffville Hosp, PO Box 1800 Stn Main 381 Church St, Markham ON L3P 7P3; St Maarten (Jamaica)'00; FRCPC; IntMed (Critical Care Medicine). Staff, Markham Stouffville Hospital; (905)472-7000

BANSAL, Deepak; Alberta Children's Hosp, 2888 Shaganappi Trail NW, Calgary AB T3B 6A8; (India)'94; Staff, Alberta Children's Hospital; (403)955-7203

BANSAL, Nina-Karen; 4067 Oak St, Vancouver BC V6H 2M7; Man'06; FRCPC; Peds. (604)875-1118

BANSAL, Praveen; Heart Lake Med Centre, 101-10425 Kennedy Rd, Brampton ON L6Z 0A4; Tor'89; CCFP; FCFP; (905)846-7611; Fax. (905)846-7753.

BANSAL, Sundeep K; 6970 Lisgar Dr, Mississauga ON L5N 8C8; Tor'90; (905)824-4441; Fax. (905)824-4431.

BANSAL, Vikas K; Holland Centre, 43 Wellesley St E, Toronto ON M4Y 1G7; Tor'03; CCFP; (416)967-8500

BANTA, Gregory A; RCMP Pacific Region Hlth Ctre, 1101-45337 Calais Cres, Chilliwack BC V2R 0N6; UBC'88; CCFP; Staff, Royal Canadian Mounted Police Region Health Centre; Staff, Cedar Medical Centre; (604)703-2588; Fax. (604)703-2595.

BANTOCK, Ivan M G; Nicola Med Dental Bldg, 200-321 Nicola St, Kamloops BC V2C 6G6; Southampton (England)'85; (250)372-5522; Fax. (250)372-8412.

BANTON, Keith J; PO Box 6047 Stn Main, Saskatoon SK S7K 4E4; Birmingham (England)'68; MB ChB; FFARCS(Eng); FRCPC; Anes. Court Staff, Royal University Hospital; Ac Staff Anes, Saskatoon City Hospital; Clin Assoc Prof, University of Saskatchewan.

BANVILLE, Christine; Clinique Med Ste-Catherine, 4570 rte de Fossambault, Ste-Cath-D-L-J-Car QC G3N 2T6; Laval'76; (418)875-4356; Fax. (418)875-1446.

BANVILLE, Francois; Clinique Med de Matane, 101-548 av Du Phare E, Matane QC G4W 1A7; Laval'88; Staff, Centre Hospitalier de Matane; (418)562-4532; Fax. (418)562-4532.

BANVILLE, Marie-Claire; Centre De L'Osteoporose, 101-1200 av de Germain-des-Pre, Quebec QC G1V 3M7; Laval'82; (418)650-2671; Fax. (418)650-3916; marie-claire.banville@grmo.net.

BANVILLE, Nathalie; 2898 North Tetagouche Rd, North Tetagouche NB E2A 4Y7; Laval'93; FRCPC; Anes.

BANWATT, Sundeep S; Southdown Med Centre, 1375 Southdown Rd, Mississauga ON L5J 2Z1; Tor'97; CCFP; (905)822-2900

BANWELL, Brenda L; The Hosp for Sick Children, 555 University Ave, Toronto ON M5G 1X8; Wes'91; FRCPC; Peds; Neur. Staff Neurol, The Hospital For Sick Children; (416)813-6660; Fax. (416)813-6334; brenda.banwell@sickkids.ca.

BANWELL, Brian R; Hotel-Dieu Grace Hosp, 1030 Ouellette Ave, Windsor ON N9A 1E1; Tor'94; FRCPC; Anes. Staff, Hôtel-Dieu Grace Hospital; (519)973-4444 x2208

BANWELL, Michael A; 831 Anders Rd, West Kelowna BC V1Z 1K1; Qns'76; CCFP; Staff, Kelowna General Hospital; (250)769-4911; Fax. (250)769-5757.

BAPAT, Archana; 201-1110 Sheppard Ave E, North York ON M2K 2W2; Jabalpur (India)'67; (416)225-7956

BAPTISTA, Luis C; Fort Med Clinic, 101-6603 132 Ave NW, Edmonton AB T5C 2A4; Alb'72; Langs: Portuguese; Spanish; (780)476-1388; Fax. (780)473-3530.

BAPTISTE-DESRUISSEAU, Dinah; CSSSG-Hop de Hull, 116 boul Lionel-Emond, Gatineau QC J8Y 1W7; Montpellier (France)'78; FRCPC; MedMicrobiol; InfectDis. Ac Staff, Hull Hospital; (819)966-6200; Fax. (819)966-6067.

BAQI, S Mahin; 207-100 Humber College Blvd, Etobicoke ON M9V 5G4; Wes'92; FRCPC; IntMed (AIDS/HIV); InfectDis. Staff, William Osler Health System - Etobicoke General Hospital; Langs: Bengali; (416)742-6377; mahin_baqi@oslerhc.org.

BAR-OR, Amit; MUHC-Montreal Neurology Inst, 111-3801 rue University, Montreal QC H3A 2B4; McG'93; AB; FRCPC; Neur. Staff, McGill University Health Centre - Montreal Neurological Hospital; (514)398-5132; Fax. (514)398-7371.

BAR-SHLOMO, Benny; Richmond Health Science Ctre, 750-6091 Gilbert Rd, Richmond BC V7C 5L9; Hadassah (Israel)'74; ABIM; ABC; FRCPC; IntMed; Cardiol. Ac Staff, Richmond Hospital; (604)273-1555; Fax. (604)273-2969.

BARABAS, Dezso; CSSS de Chicoutimi, 305 rue Saint-Vallier, Chicoutimi QC G7H 5H6; Tirgu-Mures (Romania)'87; Staff, Complexe hospitalier de la Sagamie; (418)541-1000

BARABAS, Julianna-Melinda; Cardiology Associates, 314-874 boul de l'Universite E, Chicoutimi QC G7H 6B9; Tirgu-Mures (Romania)'87; Cardiol (P.Q.). (418)541-3502

BARABE, Frederic; Ctr Hosp Affilie-Enfant-Jesus, 1401 18e rue, Quebec QC G1J 1Z4; Laval'98; FRCPC; IntMed; Hem. Staff, Centre Hospitalier Affilié Universitaire de Québec - Hôpital De L'Enfant Jésus; (418)649-0252; Fax. (418)649-5879; frederic.barabe@crchul.ulaval.ca.

BARABE, Patrick; Hop du Sacre-Coeur de Mtl, 5400 boul Gouin O, Montreal QC H4J 1C5; Mon'98; Psy. Staff, Hôpital du Sacre-Coeur de Montréal; (514)338-2070

BARABE, Pierre-Luc; Ctr Hosp du Centre la Mauricie, 50 119e rue E, Shawinigan QC G9P 5K1; Laval'06; CCFP; CCFP(E.M.); Staff, Centre Hospitalier du Centre la Mauricie; (819)536-7500

BARABE, Serge; Ctr Hosp du Centre la Mauricie, 50 119e rue, Shawinigan-Sud QC G9P 5K1; Laval'85; Staff, Centre Hospitalier du Centre la Mauricie; Assoc Member, Association of Psychiatry in Canada; (819)536-7500

BARABTARLO, Jack; 505-15 Wertheim Crt, Richmond Hill ON L4B 3H7; (Mexico)'78; DABPN; FRCPC; Psy. Langs: Spanish; (905)882-7828; Fax. (905)882-9248.

BARAC, Ivan; St Boniface Gen Hosp, Y3020-409 Tache Ave, Winnipeg MB R2H 2A6; Belgrade (Serbia)'91; ABIM; Staff, St Boniface General Hospital; Staff, Health Sciences Centre; Asst Prof IntMed/Asst Prof Cardiol WRHA Cardiac Sciences Prog Bergen Cardiac Care Centre, University of Manitoba; Langs: Serbian; Croatian; (204)258-1282; Fax. (204)233-2157.

BARAC, Snezana; Winnipeg Clinic, 425 St Mary Ave, Winnipeg MB R3C 0N2; Belgrade (Serbia)'89; FRCPC; IntMed.

BARAKAT, Samia M; Psychealth Centre, PZ439-771 Bannatyne Ave, Winnipeg MB R3E 3N4; Cairo (Egypt)'69; MB ChB; FRCPC; Psy (Gender Issues). Head Psy, Health Sciences Centre; Head Psy, St Boniface General Hospital; Med Dir, Winnipeg Regional Health Authority; Prof Psy/Assoc Dean Professionalism & Diversity, University of Manitoba; Langs: Arabic; (204)787-3051; Fax. (204)787-4879; sbarakat@hsc.mb.ca.

BARAKAT, Sammy W; Halton Healthcare Services, 6F-700 Dorval Dr, Oakville ON L6K 3V3; Man'99; FRCPC; Psy. Staff, Sunnybrook Health Sciences Centre; (905)338-4630

BARAKETT, William; Clinique méd Brome-Missiquoi, RR 1 280 Victoria St, Knowlton QC J0E 1V0; McG'71; ASAM; CCFP; FCFP; pers Chef Dept of General Med, Hôpital Brome-Missisquoi-Perkins; Physician, Union Carbide Canada; Conférencier Family Med, McGill University; (450)243-5043; Fax. (450)243-0537.

BARAKJI, Nazir; The Dr G B Cross Mem Hosp, 67 Manitoba Dr, Clarenville NL A5A 1K3; (Egypt)'79; Staff, Central Newfoundland Regional Health Centre; Locum Tenens, The Dr G B Cross Memorial Hospital; (709)292-2500

BARALE, Anthony E; Mental Health & Addiction Serv, PO Box 949 5542 Sunshine Coast Hwy, Sechelt BC V0N 3A0; Witwatersrand (South Africa)'82; MB BCh; FRCPC; Psy (Consultation-Liaison). Consultant Psy, Victoria General Hospital; Consultant Psy, Royal Jubilee Hospital; Langs: Afrikaans; (604)885-6101

BARAM, Rola; Cite Sante Saint-Laurent, 1-1077 rue Decarie, Saint-Laurent QC H4L 3M8; Mon'01; Langs: Arabic; (514)747-5556; Fax. (514)747-5557.

BARAMA, Azemi A; CHUM-Hop Notre-Dame, 1560 rue Sherbrooke E, Montreal QC H2L 4M1; (Algeria)'79; GenSurg (P.Q.). Staff, Centre Hospitalier l'Université de Montréal (CHUM) - Hôpital Notre-Dame; (514)890-8000

BARAN, Dana; MUHC-Royal Victoria Hosp, 687 av des Pins O, Montreal QC H3A 1A1; McG'79; FRCPC; IntMed (Nephrology). Staff, McGill University Health Centre - Royal Victoria Hospital; assoc Prof Med, McGill University; Langs: English; French; (514)934-1934 x35208; Fax. (514)843-2815.

BARAN, Gregory P; Portsmouth Med Clinic, 902 Portsmouth Ave, Kingston ON K7M 1W9; Qns'91; BSc(Hon); CCFP; FCFP; Staff, Hotel-Dieu Hospital; Staff, Kingston General Hospital; (613)546-2321; drbaran@kingston.net.

BARANCHUK, Adrian M; Kingston Gen Hosp, FAPC3 310-76 Stuart St, Kingston ON K7L 2V7; Buenos Aires (Argentina)'90; FRCPC; Neur. Staff Arrhythmia Services, Kingston General Hospital; Langs: Spanish; Italian; Portuguese; (613)549-6666 x3377

BARANICK, Peter; Appletree Med Clinic, 2575A Baseline Rd, Ottawa ON K2H 7B3; Ott'73; MCFP(EM); Staff, Queensway Carleton Hospital; (613)726-3558

BARANKIN, Benjamin; 400-4256 Bathurst St, North York ON M3H 5Y8; Wes'01; FRCPC; Derm (Cosmetic Dermatology). Staff, Toronto Dermatology Centre; Langs: Russian; (416)633-0001; Fax. (416)633-0002; info@torontodermatologycentre.com.

BARANKIN, Tatyana; Bayview-Finch Med Clinic, 304-3292 Bayview Ave, North York ON M2M 4J5; Leningrad (Russia (Federation))'73; DPsy(Tor); FRCPC; Psy (Child Psychiatry). Staff Psy, Centre for Addiction & Mental Health (CAMH) - College Street Site; Staff Psy, The Hospital For Sick Children; Langs: Russian; (416)223-9635

BARANOFF, Oleg; Royal Columbian Hosp, 330 Columbia St E, New Westminster BC V3L 3W7; Jaroslavl (Russia (Federation))'85; Staff, Royal Columbian Hospital; (604)520-4001

BARANOWSKI, Susan L; Riley Park Health Centre, 144-1402 8 Ave NW, Calgary AB T2N 1B9; Cal'99; MPH; FRCSC; ObstGyn. Staff, Foothills Medical Centre; (403)289-8996; Fax. (403)289-8956; sbaranowski@shaw.ca.

BARANYI, Katherine A; Northeast Mental Health Team, 222-2750 Hastings St E, Vancouver BC V5K 1Z9; UBC'85; (604)675-3890

BARATZ, Ari Y; Create Fertility Centre, 1100-790 Bay St, Toronto ON M5G 1N8; Wes'01; FRCSC; ObstGyn. (416)323-7727; Fax. (416)323-7334.

BARBANT, Andre D; 1000 rue Chabot, St-Mathieu-Beloeil QC J3G 4S5; Mon'86; Staff, Centre Hospitalier l'Université de Montréal (CHUM) - Hôpital Notre-Dame; (450)467-1710

BARBARESE, Gabrielle; Hop Charles Lemoyne, 3120 boul Taschereau, Greenfield Park QC J4V 2H1; Mon'10; CCFP; Staff, Hopital Charles LeMoyne; (450)466-5000

BARBAROSIE, Michaela; CSSS d'Antoine Labelle-l'Annon, 1525 rue de l'Annonciation, Riviere-Rouge QC J0T 1T0; Mon'05; Psy. Staff, Centre de L'Annonciation; (819)275-2118

BARBAROSIE, Teodor P; CSSS d'Antoine-Labelle-Mt Laur, RR 1 2561 ch de la Lievre S, Mont-Laurier QC J9L 3G3; Bucharest (Romania)'66; CCFP; Fam Med, CSSS d'Antoine-Labelle; (819)623-1234; Fax. (819)623-5278.

BARBEAU, Brynlea; Algoma Univ Campus Med Clinic, 617B Queen St E, Sault Ste. Marie ON P6A 2A6; McM'02; CCFP; (705)946-7362; Fax. (705)575-4429.

BARBEAU, David; CLSC des Faubourgs, 1250 rue Sanguinet, Montreal QC H2X 3E7; Sher'92; (514)527-2361

BARBEAU, Francine; Hotel-Dieu de Levis, 143 rue Wolfe, Levis QC G6V 3Z1; Laval'69; FRCPC; Derm. Dermatology, Hôtel-Dieu de Lévis; (418)835-7121 x3673

BARBEAU, Gerald; Hôpital Laval, 2725 ch Sainte-Foy, Quebec QC G1V 4G5; Laval'74; FACC; CSPQ; FRCPC; IntMed (Interventional Cardiology); Cardiol. Staff, Hôpital Laval; (418)656-8711; Fax. (418)656-4562; gerald.barbeau@med.ulaval.ca.

BARBEAU, Jean-Jacques; Clinique méd Brome-Missiquoi, 280 rue Victoria, Knowlton QC J0E 1V0; Mon'70; Langs: English; (450)243-5043; barbeau_j@videotron.ca.

BARBEAU, Mathilde; Ctr de Read en Deficience Phys, 9500 boul du Centre-Hospitalie, Charny QC G6X 0A1; Mon'99; Staff, Centre Hospitalier Paul-Gilbert; (418)380-2064 x6306

BARBEAU, Paul-Emile; 451 ch Notre-Dame S, Duhamel-Ouest QC J9V 1X1; Mon'78; Prés Med Staff, CSSS du Témiscamingue; Staff Community & Occup Med, Centre Sante St Famille Ville-Marie; (819)622-0157; paul-emile_barbeau@ssss.gouv.qc.ca.

BARBER, Claire; 436-3330 Hospital Dr NW, Calgary AB T2N 4N1; Dal'06; FRCPC; IntMed; Rheum. Staff, Health Research Innovation Centre; (403)210-6077; Fax. (403)210-9717.

BARBER, Darren C A; Ridgeview Med Centre, 212-1240 Railway Ave, Canmore AB T1W 1P4; Trinity (Ireland)'03; MB BCh; BAO; CCFP.

BARBER, David T S; Queen's Family Med Centre, PO Box 8888 Stn Main 220 Bagot St, Kingston ON K7L 5E9; Ott'96; CCFP; (613)533-9303

BARBER, Duane F; Calgary Lab Services, 9-3535 Research Rd NW, Calgary AB T2L 2K8; Sask'84; FRCPC; AnatPath (Cytopath). Staff, Calgary Laboratory Services; Clinical Asst Prof, University of Calgary; (403)770-3673; Fax. (403)770-3295; duane.barber@cls.ab.ca.

BARBER, George P; Seymour Med Clinic, 1530 7th Ave W, Vancouver BC V6J 1S3; Cal'75; (604)738-2151; gbarber@gov.nu.ca.

BARBER, Jeffrey L; 318B Duncan Ave, Courtenay BC V9N 2M5; Sask'94; FRCPC; Psy. Staff, St Joseph's General Hospital; (250)331-9200; Fax. (250)331-9201.

BARBER, Kirk A; 510-1100 1 St SE, Calgary AB T2G 1B1; Alb'75; FRCPC; Derm. Staff, Alberta Children's Hospital; Clin Assoc Prof, University of Calgary; (403)299-5800

BARBER, Lorne E; Assiniboine Clinic, 633 Lodge Ave, Winnipeg MB R3J 0S9; Man'74; FRCSC; GenSurg. Staff, The Salvation Army Grace Hospital; (204)958-6725; Fax. (204)888-1750.

BARBER, Neil K; Family Med Centre, PO Box 8888 Stn Main 220 Bagot St, Kingston ON K7L 5E9; London (England)'72; MRCS(Eng); LRCP(Lond); MB BS; CCFP; FCFP; Assoc Staff Family Med, Hotel-Dieu Hospital; Assoc Staff, Kingston General Hospital; Clin Instructor Family Med, Queen's University; (613)533-9300

BARBER, Philip A; 3330 Hospital Dr NW, Calgary AB T2N 4N1; Sheffield (England)'91; MB ChB; FRCPC; Neur (Stroke). Staff, Foothills Medical Centre; Assoc Prof, University of Calgary; (403)210-3881; pabarber@ucalgary.ca.

BARBERA, Joseph; The Sleep & Alertness Clinic, 259-750 Dundas St W, Toronto ON M6J 3S3; Wes'97; BSc(HonsBiophysics); FRCPC; Psy (Sleep Medicine). Med Dir, Youthdale Child & Adolescent Sleep Centre; (416)603-5800 x2988; joseph.barbera@utoronto.ca.

BARBERA, Lisa C; Sunnybrook Hlth Sciences Ctre, 2075 Bayview Ave, Toronto ON M4N 3M5; Ott'95; FRCPC; RadOncol. Staff, Sunnybrook Health Sciences Centre; (416)480-4974

BARBERIE, John E; A-1804 Bowen Rd, Nanaimo BC V9S 5W4; UBC'95; FRCPC; DiagRad. (250)753-4351

BARBERO, Joseph; Trent Hills Family Health Team, RR 2 119 Isabella St, Campbellford ON K0L 1L0; Tor'08; (705)653-1801

BARBES-MORIN, Guillaume; Ctr Hosp Rouyn Noranda, 4 9e rue, Rouyn-Noranda QC J9X 2B2; Mon'01; FRCPC; Psy. Staff, Centre Hospitalier Rouyn-Noranda; (819)764-5131

BARBETTA, Timothy P; Southlake Reg Health Centre, 596 Davis Dr, Newmarket ON L3Y 2P9; Tor'78; Staff, Southlake Regional Health Centre; (905)895-4521

BARBEZIEUX, Maurice-C.; Inst Albert Prevost, 6555 boul Gouin O, Montreal QC H4K 1B3; Paris (France)'66; FRCPC; Psy. Staff, Hôpital du Sacre-Coeur de Montréal; (514)338-4356; Fax. (514)338-4357.

BARBIER, Alexandre; MUHC-Royal Victoria Hosp, 687 av des Pins O, Montreal QC H3A 1A1; Staff, McGill University Health Centre - Royal Victoria Hospital; (514)934-1934 x34876; Fax. (514)843-1741.

BARBIERI, Norma; BC Cancer Agency-Abbotsford Ct, 32900 Marshall Rd, Abbotsford BC V2S 0C2; Litoral (Argentina)'81; LMCC; FRCPC; Psy (Psychoanalysis). Staff, Abbotsford Regional Hospital & Cancer Centre; Langs: French; Spanish; (604)851-4733

BARBOSA, Rubens; Hop Reg D'Edmundston, 275 Hebert Blvd, Edmundston NB E3V 4E4; Pontificia (Chile)'92; Staff, Hôpital regional d'Edmundston; (506)739-2360

BARBOUR, Kathryn A; Vancouver Gen Hosp, 855 12th Ave W, Vancouver BC V5Z 1M9; UBC'86; Staff Hospital's Office, Vancouver General Hospital - Centennial Pavillion; (604)822-7121

BARBOUR, Sean J; 5F-2775 Laurel St, Vancouver BC V5Z 1M9; UBC'05; FRCPC; IntMed; Nephrol. Staff, Toronto General Hospital - UHN; (604)875-5950

BARBOUR-JONES, Elizabeth; Slocan Park Med Clinic, PO Box 24 3120 Slocan Park Rd, Slocan Park BC V0G 2E0; UBC'80; Ac Staff, Kootenay Lake General Hospital; Physician, Slocan Park Medical Clinic; Consultant, Regional Eating Disorder Clinic; Langs: Bilingual(English/French); (250)226-7111; Fax. (250)226-7101.

BARBOZA, Milan K; The Credit Valley Hosp, 2200 Eglinton Ave W, Mississauga ON L5M 2N1; Tor'07; FRCPC; IntMed. Staff, The Credit Valley Hospital; (905)813-2200

BARBRICK-CROZIER, Elizabeth; Summerside Med Centre, 1-475 Granville St, Summerside PE C1N 3N9; Dal'97; BSc; FRCSC; ObstGyn. Staff, Prince County Hospital; (902)432-8181; Fax. (902)432-8167.

BARBUIO, Luciana; Clinique Metro Cote-Vertu, 3-1077 rue Decarie, Saint-Laurent QC H4L 3M8; Mon'80; (514)747-0432; Fax. (514)747-6304.

BARC, Jennine M; St Boniface Gen Hosp, 409 Tache Ave, Winnipeg MB R2H 2A6; Man'85; FRCPC; Anes. Staff, St Boniface General Hospital; (204)233-8563; Fax. (204)231-0640.

BARCELO RODRIGUEZ, Enrique; Clinique Med de Lavaltrie, 200-1400 rue Notre-Dame, Lavaltrie QC J5T 1M6; Havana (Cuba)'96; CCFP; (450)586-1033; Fax. (450)586-4498.

BARCHAN, Olexander; O K Medical Centre, 1278 The Queensway, Etobicoke ON M8Z 1S3; Kiev (Ukraine)'93; FRCPC; IntMed. (416)848-9795

BARCHECHAT, Claude; CSSS du Sud de Lanaudière, 911 montee des Pionniers, Terrebonne QC J6V 2H2; Laval'03; FRCPC; Anes. Staff, Centre Hospitalier Pierre le Gardeur; (450)654-7525

BARCHET, Paul M; Selkirk Mental Health Centre, PO Box 9600 Stn Main 825 Manitoba Ave, Selkirk MB R1A 2B5; Man'87; FRCPC; Psy (Forensic Psychiatry). Staff Psy, Selkirk Mental Health Centre; Consultant, Selkirk & Interlake Crisis Stabilization Unit & Mobile Crisis Team; Asst Prof, University of Manitoba; (204)482-3810; pbarchet@mts.net.

BARCLAY, Alasdair L; Anaesthesia Associates, 2108-700 Bay St, Toronto ON M5G 1Z6; Glasgow (Scotland)'69; MB ChB; DObstRCOG; DA; FAB; FRCPC; Anes. Staff, Mount Sinai Hospital; (416)977-0186

BARCLAY, Amanda D; Victoria Gen Hosp, 1 Hospital Way, Victoria BC V8Z 6R5; McM'96; FRCPC; Peds (Intensive Care). Staff, Victoria General Hospital; (250)727-4212; Fax. (250)727-4012.

BARCLAY, John W; 307-8425 120 St, Delta BC V4C 6R2; Tor'73; CCFP; (604)597-1949; Fax. (604)597-1954; johnw._barclay@telus.net.

BARCLAY, Justin L; 6896-1796 Summer St PO Box 9000 Rpo Csc, Halifax NS B3K 6A3; Aberdeen (Scotland)'99; MB ChB; (902)473-2220

BARCLAY, Neil G; Royal Columbian Hosp, 330 Columbia St E, New Westminster BC V3L 3W7; Alb'00; CCFP; CCFP(E.M.); Staff, Royal Columbian Hospital; (604)520-4253

BARCLAY, Shane B; Kings Lane Med Clinic, 101-164 Kings Lane, Salt Spring Island BC V8K 2P7; Sask'84; Chief Staff, Vancouver Island Health Authority; (250)537-1828; Fax. (250)537-1848.

BARCLAY, Spencer L; Trenton Med Associates Ltd, PO Box 29 6 Pleasant St, Trenton NS B0K 1X0; Dal'72; Ac Staff, Aberdeen Regional Hospital; (902)752-4176; Fax. (902)755-1917.

BARCO, Cynthia C; Peace River School Div No 10, 10018 101 St, Peace River AB T8S 2A5; McM'02; CCFP; (780)532-6463

BARCZA, Lawrence Z; 80 Holland St E PO Box 1510 Stn Main, Bradford ON L3Z 2B8; Wes'73; (905)775-7411; Fax. (905)775-7666.

BARD, Celine; CHUM-Hotel-Dieu, 3840 rue Saint-Urbain, Montreal QC H2W 1T8; Ott'79; FRCPC; DiagRad. Staff, Centre Hospitalier l'Université de Montréal (CHUM) - Hôtel-Dieu; (514)890-8000; celine.bard.chum@ssss.gouv.qc.ca.

BARD, Leon; 410-125 13th St E, North Vancouver BC V7L 2L3; UBC'66; CCFP; CCFP(E.M.); (604)987-3244; Fax. (604)987-7270.

BARD, Robert J; Health Sciences Centre, AD203-820 Sherbrook St, Winnipeg MB R3A 1R9; Man'83; FRCSC; Urol (Urodynamics). Staff/Dir Urodynamic Lab, Health Sciences Centre; Asst Prof, University of Manitoba; (204)787-3170; Fax. (204)787-3040.

BARD, Timothy D; West Street Health Centre, 204-216 West St, Simcoe ON N3Y 1S8; UBC'98; FRCPC; IntMed. (519)428-9992; Fax. (519)428-0823.

BARDAGI, Victor; 1531-1 Place Ville-Marie, Montreal QC H3B 2B5; Mon'65; Assoc Staff, Centre Hospitalier Fleury; Assoc Staff, McGill University Health Centre - Montreal General Campus; (514)397-1370; Fax. (514)397-9899.

BARDAI, Sadrudin; 207-1615 Dundas St E, Whitby ON L1N 2L1; Manchester (England)'63; DCH(Glas); MRCP(Lond); (905)576-5512; Fax. (905)728-3651.

BARDAI, Zahra; Woodbridge Med Centre, A13-9600 Islington Ave, Woodbridge ON L4H 2T1; McM'97; CCFP; FCFP; (905)893-8085

BARDAKJI, Zaim; Groupe Sante Physimed, 121-6363 rte Transcanadienne, Saint-Laurent QC H4T 1Z9; Aleppo (Syria)'81; Chief GenMed, Hôpital Santa Cabrini Ospedale; Langs: Italian; French; Arabic; (514)747-8888; bardaji@videotron.ca.

BARDANA, Davide D; Kingston Gen Hosp, 76 Stuart St, Kingston ON K7L 2V7; Cal'94; Dip SportMed; FRCSC; OrthSurg (Arthroscopy). Staff, Kingston General Hospital; Asst Prof, Queen's University; Langs: Italian; (613)549-6666 x6333

BARDELL, Andrea; Royal Jubilee Hosp, 1952 Bay St, Victoria BC V8R 1J8; UBC'05; FRCPC; Psy. Staff, Royal Jubilee Hospital; (250)370-8000

BARDELL, Trevor; Belleville Queen's Univ-FMC, 101-145 Station St, Belleville ON K8N 2S9; Qns'03; FRCSC; GenSurg (Endoscopy). Staff, QHC Belleville General; Asst Prof, Queen's University; (613)210-3105; Fax. (613)210-3145.

BARDHAN, Ashit; University Hosp of Northern BC, 1475 Edmonton St, Prince George BC V2M 1S2; Rajshahi (Bangladesh)'89; Anes. Staff, University Hospital of Northern British Columbia; (250)565-2000

BARDIN, Claudette L; MUHC-Montreal Children's Hosp, 2300 rue Tupper, Montreal QC H3H 1P3; Miami (USA)'84; Peds (Neonatology). Staff, McGill University Health Centre - Montreal Children's Hospital; assoc Prof, McGill University; Langs: English; French; (514)412-4400 x22593

BAREFOOT, Judith A; Saanich Plaza Med Clinic, 3544 Blanshard St, Victoria BC V8X 1W3; Man'73; MHSc; (250)475-1101

BARER, Daniel J; Royal Alexandra Hosp, CSC 5F-10240 Kingsway NW, Edmonton AB T5H 3V9; Alb'78; Staff, Royal Alexandra Hospital; Clin Lecturer Family Med, University of Alberta; (780)735-5374; Fax. (780)735-4916.

BARETTE, Marie; CLSC Lasalle, 8550 boul Newman, LaSalle QC H8N 1Y5; Mon'79; (514)364-2572; Fax. (514)364-6365.

BARETTE, Rene; Quinte HC Corp-Belleville Gen, 265 Dundas St E, Belleville ON K8N 5A9; Sher'86; FRCPC; NuclearMed. Staff, QHC Belleville General; (613)969-7400 x2418; Fax. (613)969-1307.

BAREZPOUR, Mohammad Reza; Ctr Hosp de Lachine, 650 16e av, Lachine QC H8S 3N5; Tehran (Iran)'96; CCFP; Staff, CSSS de Dorval-Lachine-Lasalle; (514)637-2351 x77325

BARFOOT, Alison H; 2000-1415 1st Ave W, Owen Sound ON N4K 4K8; McM'08; CCFP; (519)470-3030

BARG, Stefani S N; PO Box 63210 Rpo Stadium, Calgary AB T2N 4S5; UBC'03; CCFP.

BARGH, Gordon J M; Anson Gen Hosp, 58 Anson Dr, Iroquois Falls ON P0K 1E0; Tor'09; CCFP; Staff, Anson General Hospital; (705)258-3911

BARGMAN, Howard B; 302-1137 Centre St, Thornhill ON L4J 3M6; Tor'71; FRCPC; Derm (Laser Dermatology). Court Staff, Sunnybrook Health Sciences Centre; (905)695-2020

BARGMAN, Joanne M; 8N 840-200 Elizabeth St, Toronto ON M5G 2C4; Tor'78; DABIM; DAB; FRCPC; IntMed (Nephrology). Staff, Toronto General Hospital - UHN; (416)340-4804; Fax. (416)340-4999.

BARI, Basel; Milliken Medical Centre, 17-5651 Steeles Ave E, Scarborough ON M1V 5P6; McM'91; (416)291-6323; Fax. (416)291-0890.

BARIA, Kaikhushroo; Winnipeg Clinic, 425 St Mary Ave, Winnipeg MB R3C 0N2; Karachi (Pakistan)'64; MB BS; AB; FRCSC; OrthSurg (Foot & Ankle Surgery). Staff, Seven Oaks General Hospital; (204)957-3260; Fax. (204)942-2671.

BARIA, Niloofer; 1283 Nanaimo St, Vancouver BC V5L 4T5; UBC'87; CCFP; (604)251-6313; Fax. (604)251-1311.

BARIANA, Sam S; Bramalea Med Centre, 306-18 Kensington Rd, Brampton ON L6T 4S5; (Netherlands Antilles)'03; CCFP; (905)463-2095; Fax. (905)463-2096.

BARIBAULT, Jean-P.; Ctr Hosp Affilie-Enfant-Jesus, 1401 18e rue, Quebec QC G1J 1Z4; Laval'69; CSPQ; FRCPC; Anes. Ac Staff, Centre Hospitalier Affilié Universitaire de Québec - Hôpital De L'Enfant Jésus; Université Laval; (418)649-0252

BARIBEAU, Genevieve; CLSC de Jonquiere, 3667 boul Harvey, Jonquiere QC G7X 3A9; Sher'00; Staff, Centre Hospitalier Jonquiere; (418)695-8217; Fax. (418)695-8282.

BARIBEAU, Sylvia; Clinique Medicale, 2600 rue Victoria, Lachine QC H8S 1Z3; Mon'80; (514)634-0592; Fax. (514)634-6558.

BARIBEAULT, Alain; Le Ctr de Physiatrie de Quebec, 100-700 boul Lebourgneuf, Quebec QC G2J 1E2; Sher'85; FRCPC; PhysMed&Rehab (Electromyography). Staff, Centre Hospitalier Affilié Universitaire de Québec - Hôpital De L'Enfant Jésus; Langs: English; (418)622-3371; Fax. (418)622-9004.

BARICIAK, Erika D; Children's Hosp Eastern Ont, 401 Smyth Rd, Ottawa ON K1H 8L1; Wes'99; FRCPC; Peds (Neonatology). Staff Neonatol, The Ottawa Hospital - General Campus; Staff Neonatol, Children's Hospital of Eastern Ontario (CHEO); (613)737-7600 x2415; Fax. (613)738-4847; bariciak@cheo.on.ca.

BARICIAK, Mark D; 1-677 Great Northern Rd, Sault Ste. Marie ON P6B 5A1; Ott'92; FRCSC; Ophth (Cataract Surgery). Staff, Sault Area Hospital - Sault Ste Marie; (705)949-5182; Fax. (705)251-9969.

BARIL, Bruno; Hop Charles Lemoyne, 3120 boul Taschereau, Greenfield Park QC J4V 2H1; Laval'87; FRCPC; EmergMed (P.Q.). Staff, Hopital Charles LeMoyne; (450)466-5050; Fax. (450)466-5051.

BARIL, Chantale; GMF Venta et Marees, 201-391 av Brochu, Sept-Iles QC G4R 4S7; Sher'90; CCFP; Staff, Centre Hospitalier Regional de Sept-Iles; Langs: Bilingual(French/English); (418)968-1234

BARIL, Claude; Hotel-Dieu d'Arthabaska, 5 rue des Hospitalieres, Victoriaville QC G6P 6N2; Sher'86; GenSurg. Ac Staff, Hotel-Dieu d'Arthabaska; adj Prof, Centre Hospitalier Universitaire de Sherbrooke-Hopital Fleurimont; Langs: Bilingual(French/English); (819)357-2030 x2108

BARIL, Francois; Clinique de Med Familiale, 500-106 boul Notre-Dame, Clermont QC G4A 1C7; Mon'84; Staff, Hôpital de la Malbaie; (418)439-3935; Fax. (418)439-4548.

BARIL, Helene; CHUS-Hop Hotel-Dieu, 580 rue Bowen S, Sherbrooke QC J1G 2E8; Sher'85; FRCPC; DiagRad. Staff, Centre Hospitalier Universitaire de Sherbrooke-Hôpital Hôtel-Dieu; (819)346-1110 x22450

BARIL, Jean-Francois; 203-140 rue Champlain, Dieppe NB E1A 1N8; Sher'95; LMCC; FRCPC; IntMed; Cardiol. Cardiol/Internal Med, Dr Georges-L-Dumont University Hospital Centre; (506)862-1098; jefbaril@hotmail.com.

BARIL, Jean-Guy; Clinique Med du Quartier Latin, 905 boul Rene-Levesque E, Montreal QC H2L 5B1; Mon'81; Staff, Centre Hospitalier l'Université de Montréal (CHUM) - Hôpital Notre-Dame; (514)285-5500; Fax. (514)285-2226.

BARIL, Joelle; Clin Dermatologie de Longueuil, 501 rue Adoncour, Longueuil QC J4G 2M6; Mon'93; FRCPC; Derm. Langs: Bilingual(French/English); (450)651-8707; Fax. (450)651-8708.

BARIL, Josee; CSSS de Quebec Nord, 3666 ch Royal, Quebec QC G1E 1X5; Laval'81; (418)663-3099; Fax. (418)663-2939; josee.baril@ssss.gouv.qc.ca.

BARIL, Louise M C; 209-688 rue Prospect, Sherbrooke QC J1H 1A8; Sher'85; Staff, Centre Hospitalier Universitaire de Sherbrooke-Hopital Fleurimont; Prof Family Med, Universite de Sherbrooke; (819)347-3773; louise.baril@chus.qc.ca.

BARIL, Marie-Claire; Royal Inland Hosp, 311 Columbia St, Kamloops BC V2C 2T1; Mon'87; FRCPC; Psy (Geriatric Psychiatry). Staff, Royal Inland Hospital; (250)314-2700

BARIL, Melanie; CSSS Haut-Richelieu-Rouville, 920 boul du Seminaire N, St-Jean-sur-Richel QC J3A 1B7; Mon'04; FRCPC; MedMicrobiol. Staff, Hôpital du Haut-Richelieu; (450)359-5000 x5205

BARIL, Nicole; Clinique Med Place Beaumont, 1200 boul de Rome, Brossard QC J4W 3H3; Mon'69; (450)671-6170; Fax. (450)672-6814.

BARIL, Pierre; 1401 18e rue, Quebec QC G1J 1Z4; Laval'85; EmergMed (P.Q.) (Trauma). Emergency Medicine, Centre Hospitalier Affilié Universitaire de Québec - Hôpital De L'Enfant Jésus; Teach Staff, Université Laval; Langs: English; (418)649-5632; Fax. (418)649-5975; pierre.baril3@gmail.com.

BARIL, Pierre; Polyclinique Med de Terrebonne, 201-901 Boul des Seigneurs, Terrebonne QC J6W 1T8; Mon'75; (450)471-1117; Fax. (450)471-8043.

BARIL, Rejean; Clin Med Centre-Ville, 1652 rue Royale, Trois-Rivieres QC G9A 4K3; Laval'77; (819)691-1024

BARIL, Serge; 155 Terrasse Cascade, Shawinigan-Sud QC G9P 2V4; Laval'82; Staff Emerg, CSSS de Trois-Rivières; (819)536-4217

BARIL-GRAHAM, Suzanne; Clinique Med Place Beaumont, 1200 boul de Rome, Brossard QC J4W 3H3; Mon'73; (450)671-6170; Fax. (450)672-6814.

BARIL-GUERARD, Genevieve; Kootenay Lake Gen Hosp, 3 View St, Nelson BC V1L 2V1; Sher'07; Staff, Kootenay Lake General Hospital; Langs: Spanish; French; (250)352-3111

BARISIC, Dusan; Windsor Reg Hosp-Metropolitan, 1995 Lens Ave, Windsor ON N8W 1L9; Wayne State University (USA)'06; Staff, Windsor Regional Hospital - Metropolitan Site; (519)985-2631

BARKAS, William J; MUHC-Montreal Neurology Inst, 3801 rue University, Montreal QC H3A 2B4; McG'75; FRCPC; Neur (P.Q.). Ac Staff, McGill University Health Centre - Montreal Neurological Hospital; (514)398-1931; Fax. (514)398-7454.

BARKATI, Maroie; CHUM-Hop Notre-Dame, 1560 rue Sherbrooke E, Montreal QC H2L 4M1; Mon'03; FRCPC; RadOncol. Staff, Centre Hospitalier l'Université de Montréal (CHUM) - Hôpital Notre-Dame; (514)890-8254

BARKER, Andrew P; Royal Alexandra Hosp, 541-10240 Kingsway Ave, Edmonton AB T5H 3V9; Dal'04; FRCPC; EmergMed; Anes. Staff Community Services Centre, Royal Alexandra Hospital; Att Staff Anes, University of Alberta Hospital; (780)735-5374

BARKER, Charles P G; Fort St John Hosp & Hlth Ctre, 9636 100 Ave, Fort St. John BC V1J 1Y3; London (England)'75; Staff, Fort St John Hospital & Health Centre; (250)262-5200

BARKER, Collin C; Children's & Women's HC of BC, K4 181-4480 Oak St, Vancouver BC V6H 3V4; Alb'94; FRCPC; Peds (Pediatric Gastroenterology); Gastroent. Staff, BC Children's Hospital; (604)875-2345

BARKER, David J; Glazier Med Centre, 11 Gibb St, Oshawa ON L1H 2J9; Qns'78; CCFP; Ac Staff, Lakeridge Health - Oshawa Site; (905)579-1212

BARKER, Edmund A; Associate Clinic, 4620 50 Ave, Innisfail AB T4G 1A6; London (England)'81; Staff, Innisfail Health Centre; (403)227-3301; Fax. (403)227-2856; ebarker@dthr.ab.ca.

BARKER, Elliott T; 200-288 King St, Midland ON L4R 3M6; Tor'58; DPsy; Psy (Adolescent Psychiatry). (705)526-0740

BARKER, Eric J; Grey Bruce Health Services, PO Box 591 201-369 Mary St, Wiarton ON N0H 2T0; Tor'72; CCFP; FCFP; Ac Staff, Grey Bruce Health Services - Owen Sound; Asst Prof Family & Commun Med, University of Toronto; (519)534-2412; Fax. (519)534-2413; sbpfhg@bmts.com.

BARKER, Horace R M A; Victoria Hosp, PO Box 3000 Stn Main 1200 24 St W, Prince Albert SK S6V 5T4; Staff, Victoria Hospital; (306)765-6267; Fax. (306)765-6206.

BARKER, Joanne; Welland McMaster Family Hlth Team, 555 Prince Charles Ave, Welland ON L3C 6B5; Cape Town (South Africa)'98; MB ChB; CCFP; Langs: Afrikaans; (905)734-9699

BARKER, Katherine L K; Washington Park Med Clinic, E-310 8th St, Courtenay BC V9N 1N3; Alb'87; (250)334-9241; Fax. (250)897-0225.

BARKER, Kim; 404-1 St Clair Ave W, Toronto ON M4V 1K6; McM'96; CCFP; (416)924-0777

BARKER, Kimberly L; Hamilton HS-General Site, 237 Barton St E, Hamilton ON L8L 2X2; Tor'98; CCFP; CCFP(E.M.); Staff, Hamilton Health Sciences Centre - Hamilton General Hospital; (905)527-4322 x46368

BARKER, Leslie K; Burlington Walk-In Clinic, 183-2025 Guelph Line, Burlington ON L7P 4M8; Oxford (England)'57; BMus; BCh; LRCP; MRCS; (905)681-7755; Fax. (905)333-1960.

BARKER, Mark F; Sterling Lyon Health Centre, 201-1020 Lorimer Blvd, Winnipeg MB R3P 1C7; Man'85; FRCSC; Otol (Laryngology). Medical Staff, St Boniface General Hospital; Assoc Medical Staff, Victoria General Hospital; Assoc Medical Staff Children's Hosp, Health Sciences Centre; Asst Member Otol, University of Manitoba; (204)943-0629; Fax. (204)956-1559.

BARKER, Michael I; University of Alberta Hosp, 8440 112 St NW, Edmonton AB T6G 2B7; Dal'97; FRCPC; Anes. Staff, University of Alberta Hospital; (780)407-7035; Fax. (780)407-8529.

BARKER, Nancy; Western Mem Reg Hosp, PO Box 2005 Stn Main 1 Brookfield Ave, Corner Brook NL A2H 6J7; Mem'07; CCFP; Staff, Health Sciences Centre; Staff, Western Memorial Regional Hospital; (709)637-5000

BARKER, Sarah; Medical Arts Bldg, 17 Dunedin St, Orillia ON L3V 5T3; Ott'00; FRCPC; Peds. Staff Peds, Orillia Soldiers' Memorial Hospital; Court Staff, Collingwood General & Marine Hospital; (705)327-9188; Fax. (705)327-9189.

BARKER, Sharon L; Transcona Access, 845 Regent Ave W, Winnipeg MB R2C 3A9; Man'81; CCFP; FCFP; Ac Staff, St Boniface General Hospital; (204)938-5700

BARKEY, Janice L; Children's Hosp Eastern Ont, 401 Smyth Rd, Ottawa ON K1H 8L1; Wes'95; BSc(Biology); MSc; FRCPC; Peds; Gastroent. Staff/Asst Prof Peds, Children's Hospital of Eastern Ontario (CHEO); (613)737-7600; Fax. (613)738-4854.

BARKHOUSE, Lana B; 220 Water St, Charlottetown PE C1A 9M5; Dal'90; CCFP; (902)620-2037

BARKHUIZEN, Frederick; Medical Clinic, 100-2210 Main St, Penticton BC V2A 5H8; Pretoria (South Africa)'87; MB ChB; Langs: Afrikaans; (250)493-0513; Fax. (250)493-0514.

BARKIN, Jack; 404-960 Lawrence Ave W, North York ON M6A 3B5; Tor'77; FICS; FACS; DAB; FRCS; FRCSC; Urol (Infertility). Chief of Staff, Humber River Regional Hospital - Finch Avenue Site; Dir, Can-Am HIFU; Asst Prof Surg, University of Toronto; (416)256-2737; Fax. (416)256-9098; j.barkin@rogers.com.

BARKIN, Marshall P; Hydro Place Bldg, 3025-700 University Ave, Toronto ON M5G 1Z5; Tor'75; FRCSC; ObstGyn. Staff, Mount Sinai Hospital; (416)586-4648

BARKLEY, Sarah E; 201A-175 Longwood Rd, Hamilton ON L8P 0A1; McM'09; CCFP; (905)525-9140

BARKMAN, Carla N; Atikokan Family Health Team, PO Box 1450 123 Marks St, Atikokan ON P0T 1C0; Sask'99; CCFP; (807)597-2721; Fax. (807)597-4632; carlamilo@hotmail.com.

BARKMAN, Frederick; Weeneebayko Gen Hosp, PO Box 34 19 Hospital Dr, Moose Factory ON P0L 1W0; McM'05; CCFP; Staff, Weeneebayko General Hospital; (705)658-4544

BARKMAN, Jayson M J; Bethesda Hosp Steinbach, 316 Henry St, Steinbach MB R5G 0P9; Man'05; CCFP; Staff, Bethesda Hospital Steinbach; Staff, Thompson General Hospital; (204)326-6411; jbarkman@sehealth.mb.ca.

BARKOVA, Eva; Queen Elizabeth II HSC, 1276 South Park St, Halifax NS B3H 2Y9; Dal'07; DiagRad. Staff, Queen Elizabeth II Health Sciences Centre - Victoria General Site; (902)473-5453

BARKUN, Alan N G; MUHC-Montreal Gen Hosp, D7.346-1650 av Cedar, Montreal QC H3G 1A4; McG'83; MSc; DABIM; FACP; CSPQ; DABIM; FACG; FRCP; FRCPC; IntMed (Endoscopy); Gastroent. Prof Med, McGill University; Langs: German; (514)934-8233; Fax. (514)934-8375; alan.barkun@muhc.mcgill.ca.

BARKUN, Jeffrey S T; MUHC-Royal Victoria Hosp, S930-687 av des Pins O, Montreal QC H3A 1A1; McG'83; MSc(Epidemiol.); FRCSC; GenSurg (Hepatobiliary Surgery). Head Hepatobiliary Oncol, McGill University Health Centre - Royal Victoria Hospital; assoc Prof, McGill University; Langs: German; English; (514)934-1934 x35964; Fax. (514)843-1434; jeffrey.barkun@muhc.mcgill.ca.

BARKWELL, Robert G; Annapolis Collaborative Practi, PO Box 573 821 St George St, Annapolis Royal NS B0S 1A0; Tor'71; CCFP; FCFP; Clinical Asst Prof FamMed, Dalhousie University; (902)532-2324; Fax. (902)532-5424; robert.barkwell@doctorsns.com.

BARLAS, Joanna; Women's College Hosp, 76 Grenville St, Toronto ON M5S 1B2; Mem'98; FRCPC; Psy. Staff, Women's College Hospital; (416)323-6400

BARLOW, Amanda J; 304-250 Keary St, New Westminster BC V3L 5E7; Adelaide (Australia)'84; MB BS; FRACP; FRCPC; Peds (Adult Congenital Heart Disease); Cardiol. Staff Ped Cardiol, Royal Columbian Hospital; Staff Cardiol, Providence Health Care - St Paul's Hospital; (604)521-5020

BARLOW, Jane M; Ottawa Eating Disorders Clinic, 03-1309 Carling Ave, Ottawa ON K1Z 7L3; Dal'78; FRCPC; Psy (Eating Disorders). (613)729-0801; cbtottawa@me.com.

BARLOW, Joseph R; The Hosp For Sick Children, 555 University Ave, Toronto ON M5G 1X8; Tor'93; FRCPC; Anes. Staff, The Hospital For Sick Children; (416)813-7500; Fax. (416)813-7445.

BARLOW, Karen M; Alberta Children's Hosp, C1 332-2888 Shaganappi Trail, Calgary AB T3B 6A8; North Dakota (USA)'89; MB ChB; MRC(UK); Staff Ped Neurol, Alberta Children's Hospital; Clinical Asst Prof, University of Calgary; (403)955-7816; Fax. (403)955-7609; karenbarlow@calgaryhealthregion.ca.

BARMAN, Mira; Taddle Creek Family Health Team, 302-790 Bay St, Toronto ON M5G 1N8; Tor'94; BSc; CCFP; FCFP; Staff, Women's College Hospital; (416)585-9555; Fax. (416)585-5815.

BARMANIA, Yacoob E; 202-567 College St, Toronto ON M6G 1B2; RCS (Ireland)'71; LRCP; LRCS; (416)967-4967

BARNABE, Cheryl C M; Heritage Med Res Bldg, 3330 Hospital Dr NW, Calgary AB T2N 4N1; Man'03; FRCPC; IntMed; Rheum. Staff, Foothills Medical Centre; (403)220-7725; Fax. (403)283-5666.

BARNABE, Gerard; 600 rue Benoit, Saint-Hyacinthe QC J2S 1L6; Mon'58; AB; Peds. Staff, Centre Hospitalier Honore-Mercier; Consultant, Hôpital Ste-Justine; (450)773-7386; Fax. (450)773-0086.

BARNABE, Patrick; 4001-381 Kent St, Ottawa ON K2P 2A8; Ott'72; (613)238-2698; Fax. (613)238-7731.

BARNABI, Francesco; 100-145 Station St, Belleville ON K8N 2S9; Tor'00; FRCSC; GenSurg., QHC Belleville General; Langs: Italian.

BARNARD, Alan D; East Kootenay Reg Hosp, 13 24th Ave N, Cranbrook BC V1C 3H9; Pretoria (South Africa)'83; CCFP; FCFP; Staff, East Kootenay Regional Hospital; (250)426-5281

BARNARD, Chantelle B; Alberta Children's Hosp, 2888 Shaganappi Trail NW, Calgary AB T3B 6A8; Sask'01; FRCPC; Peds (Hospitalist). Staff, Alberta Children's Hospital; Asst Prof Clinical, University of Calgary; (403)955-2953; chantelle.barnard@calgaryhealthregion.ca.

BARNARD, Corlia E; South Calgary Med Clinic, 118-40 Sunpark Plaza SE, Calgary AB T2X 3X7; (South Africa)'99; MB ChB; (403)254-4000

BARNARD, Cornel; Chase Medical Clinic, PO Box 410, Chase BC V0E 1M0; Orange Free State (South Africa)'04; LMCC; MB ChB; CCFP; Langs: Afrikaans; (250)679-1422; Fax. (250)679-8815.

BARNARD, D Kelly; BC Coroners Service-Med Unit, 5F-910 Government St, Victoria BC V8W 1X3; UBC'83; (250)387-1636

BARNARD, Eduard; Red Deer Reg Hosp Centre, 3942 50A Ave, Red Deer AB T4N 4E7; Orange Free State (South Africa)'91; MB ChB; FRCPC; Anes. Staff, Red Deer Regional Hospital Centre; (403)356-0121; Fax. (403)356-0124.

BARNARD, Esther; Grande Cache Med Centre, PO Box 540, Grande Cache AB T0E 0Y0; (South Africa)'88; (780)827-2540; Fax. (780)827-5698; jageb@telus.net.

BARNARD, Isabel H; Burris Clinic, 300-275 Lansdowne St, Kamloops BC V2C 6J3; Stellenbosch (South Africa)'83; MB ChB; LMCC; CCFP; Langs: Afrikaans; German; (250)551-3363; Fax. (250)551-3360; drihbarnard@hotmail.com.

BARNARD, Johan J H; 35707 St Andrews Crt, Abbotsford BC V3G 2Z3; Pretoria (South Africa)'96; MB ChB; Staff, Abbotsford Regional Hospital & Cancer Centre; (604)556-2467

BARNARD, Johannes M; The Lighthouse Med Clinic, 205-2903 32 Ave, Vernon BC V1T 2L6; Stellenbosch (South Africa)'96; MB ChB; CCFP; CCFP(E.M.); (250)545-2552; Fax. (250)545-2545.

BARNARD, Louis; Polyclinique Boreale, 668 rue de Parfondeval, Baie-Comeau QC G5C 3R3; Laval'83; Staff, Centre Hospitalier Régional Baie-Comeau; (418)589-3701

BARNARD, Maja; North York Gen Hosp, 4SE 111-4001 Leslie St, North York ON M2K 1E1; Tor'94; FRCPC; AnatPath. Staff Path, North York General Hospital; Langs: Croatian; (416)756-6455

BARNARD, Thomas; 2430 Dougall Ave, Windsor ON N8X 1T2; Rochester (USA)'77; FAAFP(Geriatrics); MPH; MSc(Metab&Nutrition); CCFP; CCFP(E.M.); FCFP; Teacher Faculty, Fellowship in Anti-Aging & Functional Medicine; Aj Prof Human Biology & Nutritional Sciences, University Of Guelph; Clin Prof Family Med, University of Western Ontario; (519)967-8400; Fax. (519)967-1276; barnardue@illnesscentre.medirect.net.

BARNARD, Werner J; 2342 9th Ave N, Regina SK S4R 8C5; Pretoria (South Africa)'89; MB BS; LMCC; Langs: Afrikaans; (306)584-2305; Fax. (306)584-2334; allergy.doctor@sasktel.net.

BARNARD-THOMPSON, Kathleen; 5-1060 Burnham St, Cobourg ON K9A 5V9; Tor'02; BSc(Hon); MHA; CCFP; Staff, Northumberland Hills Hospital; (905)373-8333

BARNARDO, Georgina C; Lakeside Med Clinic, 3919 8th St E, Saskatoon SK S7H 5M7; Sask'03; CCFP; (306)374-6884; Fax. (306)374-2552; gcbarnardo@lakeside.ca.

BARNES, Belinda; The Ottawa Hosp-Gen Campus, 501 Smyth Rd, Ottawa ON K1H 8L6; Ott'88; CCFP; FCFP; Staff, The Ottawa Hospital - General Campus; (613)737-8560; Fax. (613)737-8828.

BARNES, Charlene A; Westgate Family Med Clinic, 192-17010 90 Ave NW, Edmonton AB T5T 1L6; Man'96; BSc; FRCSC; ObstGyn. (780)483-2901; Fax. (780)483-2910.

BARNES, Christopher; The Ottawa Hosp-Gen Campus, 5235-501 Smyth Rd, Ottawa ON K1H 8L6; Qns'08; CCFP; Staff, The Ottawa Hospital - General Campus; (613)737-8940

BARNES, Chris H; Family Health Clinic, PO Box 1540 527 Causley St, Blind River ON P0R 1B0; Tor'83; (705)356-1666; Fax. (705)356-2403.

BARNES, Daphne; Bow River Prof Centre, 226-4411 16 Ave NW, Calgary AB T3B 0M3; Manchester (England)'73; MRCPsy; MSc; FRCPC; Psy. (403)270-0590

BARNES, David C; Queen Elizabeth II HSC, 308-1276 South Park St, Halifax NS B3H 2Y9; Mem'81; FRCPC; DiagRad; NuclearMed. Ac Staff, Queen Elizabeth II Health Sciences Centre - Victoria General Site; Dean Radiology/Asst Prof, Dalhousie University; (902)473-5452

BARNES, Ekow N B; Sioux Lookout Meno-Ya-Win H C, PO Box 1500 Stn Main, Sioux Lookout ON P8T 1C2; (Ghana)'96; CCFP; Staff, Sioux Lookout Meno-Ya-Win Health Centre; (807)737-5191; Fax. (807)737-7176.

BARNES, Elizabeth A; Sunnybrook Odette Cancer Centr, 2075 Bayview Ave, Toronto ON M4N 3M5; Cal'96; FRCPC; RadOncol. Staff, Sunnybrook Health Sciences Centre; (416)480-4951; Fax. (416)480-6002.

BARNES, Jeffrey G; St Boniface Clinic, 343 Tache Ave, Winnipeg MB R2H 2A5; Man'03; FRCPC; Neur.

BARNES, Lisa M; Pender Community Health Centre, 59 Pender St W, Vancouver BC V6B 1R3; Mem'90; CCFP; Staff, Vancouver General Hospital - Centennial Pavillion; Staff, BC Children's Hospital; Physician/Prof, Sexual Assault; Staff, Pender Community Health Centre; (604)669-9181

BARNES, Patrick T; PES Provis Endoscopy, 7-3095 Glen Erin Dr, Mississauga ON L5L 1J3; Ott'68; BA; GenSurg (Gastroenterology). Consultant GenSurg, Mackenzie Richmond Hill Hospital; (905)607-0022

BARNES, Penny J; Queen Elizabeth II HSC, 718-5788 University Avenue, Halifax NS B3H 1V8; Mem'88; FRCPC; AnatPath. Staff Path, Queen Elizabeth II Health Sciences Centre - Victoria General Site; Assoc Prof Med, Dalhousie University; (902)473-2832

BARNES, Peter B J; Dr Hugh Twomey Hlth Care Ctre, PO Box 250 25 Twomey Dr, Botwood NL A0H 1E0; Mem'07; BA; BSc; CCFP; Staff, Dr Hugh Twomey Health Care Centre; (709)257-2999; Fax. (709)257-4687; peter.barnes@centralhealth.nl.ca.

BARNES, Robert D; MUHC-Montreal Children's Hosp, E315-2300 rue Tupper, Montreal QC H3H 1P3; McG'91; ABPeds; MD; FRCP; MSc; FRCPC; Peds (Pediatric Endocrinology & Metabolism); Endocrin (P.Q.); Endocrin&Metab. Att Physician Endocrin&Metab & Biochemical Genetics, McGill University Health Centre - Montreal Children's Hospital; Asst Prof Peds, McGill University; (514)412-4315; robert.barnes@muhc.mcgill.ca.

BARNES, William R; St James Street Med Clinic, 1600 Portage Ave, Winnipeg MB R3J 0C6; Man'81; CCFP; Med Advisor Occupational Disease Unit, Workers' Comp Board of MB; Examiner Clinical Assessment & Enhancement Prog, University of Manitoba; (204)774-1868; Fax. (204)774-7303; william.barnes@reveraliving.com.

BARNETT, Aaron D; 200-100 Colborne St W, Orillia ON L3V 2Y9; McM'02; CCFP; CCFP(E.M.); (705)327-3330; Fax. (705)327-7675.

BARNETT, Carly A; PO Box 62023 Rpo Westmount, Edmonton AB T5M 4B5; Alb'10; CCFP; (780)761-9796

BARNETT, Carmen E; 1433 Ontario St, Burlington ON L7S 1G5; Ott'07; FRCSC; GenSurg. (905)333-0622

BARNETT, Diane L; 4313 Gallant Ave, North Vancouver BC V7G 2C1; UBC'84; (604)929-5222; Fax. (604)929-3256.

BARNETT, Harold B; 202-200 James St S, Hamilton ON L8P 3A9; Dal'83; CCFP; (905)522-3357; Fax. (905)522-0032.

BARNETT, Kim E; Minoru Residence, 6111 Minoru Blvd, Richmond BC V6Y 1Y4; Cal'92; BSc; FRCPC; IntMed; GeriatricMed. Ac Medical Staff Geriatrician, Richmond Hospital; (604)244-5300; Fax. (604)244-5305.

BARNETT, Kimberly A; 6-940 Murphy Rd, Sarnia ON N7S 5C4; Mem'79; Ac Staff, Bluewater Health - Mitton Site; (519)542-7721; Fax. (519)542-7723.

BARNETT, Michael G; St Joseph's Health Centre, PO Box 630, Ile-a-la-Crosse SK S0M 1C0; Sask'10; CCFP; Staff, St Joseph's Hospital; (306)833-2016; Fax. (306)833-3020; mbarnett@sasktel.net.

BARNETT, Michael J; Leukemia BMT Program, 10F-2775 Laurel St, Vancouver BC V5Z 1M9; Nottingham (England)'77; BMus; BSc; FRCPC; Hem; IntMed. Staff, Vancouver General Hospital - Centennial Pavillion; (604)875-4863; Fax. (604)875-4763.

BARNETT, Thomas W; Lions Gate Hosp, 231 15th St E, North Vancouver BC V7L 2L7; McM'75; FRCPC; Psy. Staff, Lions Gate Hospital; Ac Staff Adolescent Psy, Vancouver General Hospital - Centennial Pavillion; Asst Prof, University of British Columbia; (604)988-3131

BARNETT, William H; London HSC-University Hosp, PO Box 5339 Stn B ALL 132A-399 Windermere Rd, London ON N6A 5A5; National (Ireland)'79; LRCPSI; FRCPC; IntMed; Gastroent. Consultant Gastroent, London Health Sciences Centre - University Hospital; Assoc Prof Med, University of Western Ontario; (519)663-3757; Fax. (519)663-3232; william.barnett@lhsc.on.ca.

BARNHILL, Byron B; Vanier Med Centre, 6-325 Vanier Blvd, Bathurst NB E2A 3N1; Dal'70; Ac Staff, Hopital Regional Chaleur; (506)546-9166; Fax. (506)546-3339; barnhill@nbnet.nb.ca.

BARNHILL, John A; Dr G B Cross Mem Hosp, 67 Manitoba Dr, Clarenville NL A5A 1K3; Wes'96; FRCSC; CCFP; GenSurg. Staff, The Dr G B Cross Memorial Hospital; (709)466-3411

BARNHILL, Thomas A; 301-1113 Regent St, Fredericton NB E3B 3Z2; Dal'87; FRCSC; OrthSurg (Upper Extremity Surgery). Ac Staff, Dr Everett Chalmers Regional Hospital; Lecturer Surg, Dalhousie University; (506)458-0494; Fax. (506)458-0496.

BARNOR, Nah-Amakuma; 2545 Eglinton Ave W, Toronto ON M6M 1T2; Tor'74; BSc; FACP; FRCPC; Peds (Developmental Pediatrics). Staff, Humber River Regional Hospital - Church Street Site; Ac Staff, Women's College Hospital; (416)652-0482

BARNOUTI-CALOTTI, Maya; Postmaster Med Clinic, 2540 Postmaster Dr, Oakville ON L6M 0N2; Saddam (Iraq)'93; MB ChB; CCFP; Langs: Arabic; (905)844-1700; mahanaief@yahoo.ca.

BARNSDALE, Christopher A; Greenwood Fam Physicians, PO Box 5 709 1 St NE, Sundre AB T0M 1X0; (United Kingdom)'98; MB BS; CCFP; (403)638-2424; Fax. (403)638-3580.

BARNSDALE, Emily R; Mission Oaks Med Clinic, 32136 Lougheed Hwy, Mission BC V2V 1A4; Leicester (United Kingdom)'96; (604)826-7111; Fax. (604)826-8507.

BARNSDALE, Peter H; Mission Oaks Med Clinic, 32136 Lougheed Hwy, Mission BC V2V 1A4; Leicester (England)'98; MB ChB; CCFP; (604)826-7111; Fax. (604)826-4467.

BARNSLEY, G Philip; Harbour City Health Centre, 204-1125 Dufferin Cres, Nanaimo BC V9S 2B5; Dal'01; FRCSC; PlasSurg. (250)591-0701

BARNWELL, Donna M; Medical Centre C08-3000 Lawrence Ave E, Scarborough ON M1P 2V1; (Jamaica)'87; FRCSC; ObstGyn (Prenatal Care). Staff, The Scarborough Hospital - General Campus; (416)431-2797; Fax. (416)431-2891.

BARODIA, Rajiv P; 3050G Portage Ave, Winnipeg MB R3K 0Y1; Gujarat (India)'88.

BAROLET, Alan W; Mount Sinai Hosp, 1609-600 University Ave, Toronto ON M5G 1X5; Tor'92; FRCPC; FRCPC; Cardiol; IntMed. Staff, Mount Sinai Hospital; (416)586-4800 x8495; Fax. (416)586-5360; abarolet@mtsinai.on.ca.

BAROLET, Daniel; Clinique Dr Daniel Barolet Inc, 200-3333 100e av, Laval QC H7T 0G3; Laval'87; FRCPC; Derm (P.Q.) (Cutaneous Laser Surgery). Ac Member, Centre Hospitalier l'Université De Montréal (CHUM) - Hôpital Saint-luc; Dir, Roselab Skin Optics Research Lab; Aj Prof Derm, McGill University; Universite de Montreal; Langs: Bilingual(English/French); (450)686-4744; barolet@videotron.ca.

BARON, Cynthia M; Health Sciences Centre, 820 Sherbrook St, Winnipeg MB R3A 1R9; Man'88; FRCPC; Anes. Staff Anes, Health Sciences Centre; Lecturer, University of Manitoba; (204)774-6511

BARON, Deneen D; PO BOX 75504 Rpo Edgemont Vill, North Vancouver BC V7R 4X1; UBC'92; CASM.

BARON, Emmanuelle; UMF Charles Lemoyne, 201-299 boul Sir-Wilfrid-Lauri, Saint-Lambert QC J4R 2L1; Mon'98; Dip SportMed; CCFP; Langs: Bilingual(French/English); (450)466-5630; Fax. (450)466-5631; emmanuelle.baron@usherbrooke.ca.

BARON, Genevieve; ASSS de l'Estrie, 300-300 rue King E, Sherbrooke QC J1G 1B1; Sher'95; FRCPC; CommunMed. (819)829-3400; g.baron@rrsss16.gouv.qc.ca.

BARON, Jeffrey J; Hys Med Centre, 202-11010 101 St NW, Edmonton AB T5H 4B9; Alb'99; FRCPC; DiagRad. (780)426-1121

BARON, Kenneth I; Health Sciences Ctr Gen Hosp, 700 William Ave, Winnipeg MB R3E 0Z3; Man'79; FRCPC; Anes. Staff Anes, Health Sciences Centre; Staff Anes, St Boniface General Hospital; (204)774-6511

BARON, Leonard B; Misericordia Community Hosp, 16940 87 Ave NW, Edmonton AB T5R 4H5; Alb'77; FRCPC; Anes. Staff, Covenant Health - Grey Nuns Community Hospital; Consultant, Leduc Community Hospital; Staff, Covenant Health - Misericordia Community Hospital; (780)735-2863; Fax. (780)735-2967.

BARON, Marie-Helene; CSSS de Chicoutimi, 305 rue Saint-Vallier, Chicoutimi QC G7H 5H6; Mon'02; Staff, Complexe hospitalier de la Sagamie; (418)541-1000 x3140

BARON, Michel; ASSS de l'Estrie, 300-300 rue King E, Sherbrooke QC J1G 1B1; Sher'71; GeriatricMed (P.Q.); IntMed. (819)829-3400 x42508

BARON, Mireille; Clin de Perinatalite de Trois-, 100-4900 boul des Forges, Trois-Rivieres QC G8Y 1X1; Mon'07; CCFP; (819)373-2303

BARON, Murray; SMBD Jewish Gen Hosp, A725-3755 ch Cote-Sainte-Cathe, Montreal QC H3T 1E2; McG'72; FRCPC; IntMed; Rheum. Staff, Sir Mortimer B Davis Jewish General; Staff, McGill University Health Centre - Montreal General Campus; adj Prof, McGill University; (514)340-8231; Fax. (514)340-7906; mbaron@rhu.jgh.mcgill.ca.

BARON, Tara; 1485 Bancroft Dr, Sudbury ON P3B 1R6; McM'95; FAAP; FRCPC; Peds. Prog Dir Pediatrics/Asst Prof, Northern Ontario School of Medicine; (705)523-7120; Fax. (705)523-8232; tara.baron@normed.ca.

BARONIA, Benedicto; Hamilton HS-McMaster Site, PO Box 2000 Stn Lcd 1 4E5-1200 Main St W, Hamilton ON L8N 3Z5; Manila (Philippines)'84; Staff, Hamilton Health Sciences Centre - McMaster Children's Hospital; (905)521-2100

BAROZZINO, Tony; St Michael's Health Centre, 2F-61 Queen St E, Toronto ON M5C 2T2; Qns'89; FRCPC; Peds (Neonatology). Staff, Mount Sinai Hospital; Chief Peds, St Michael's Hospital; Assoc Staff Peds, The Hospital For Sick Children; Langs: Italian; (416)867-3655; Fax. (416)867-3736; barozzinot@smh.toronto.on.ca.

BARR, Cameron; Boyle McCauley Health Centre, 103-10628 96 St NW, Edmonton AB T5H 2J2; Alb'06; CCFP; (780)422-7333; Fax. (780)422-7343.

BARR, Charlie; 125 Lakeview Ave, Kingston ON K7M 3T6; Ott'89; (613)384-4664

BARR, David B; Springbank Med Centre, 309-460 Springbank Dr, London ON N6J 0A8; Wes'88; BSc(Hon); (519)858-0013; Fax. (519)858-3713; dbmd@rogers.com.

BARR, George W; Midnapore Mall, 33-240 Midpark Way SE, Calgary AB T2X 1N4; Alb'76; CCFP; (403)256-2355; Fax. (403)256-4852.

BARR, Jennifer; London HSC-University Hosp, PO Box 5339 Stn B A10 218-399 Windermere Rd, London ON N6A 5A5; UBC'03; FRCPC; Psy. Staff, London Health Sciences Centre - South Street; (519)685-8500

BARR, Richard E; Rockyview Gen Hosp, 6618-7007 14 St SW, Calgary AB T2V 1P9; Qns'82; FRCSC; Urol. Staff, Rockyview General Hospital; (403)943-8960; Fax. (403)943-8962.

BARR, Ronald D; Hamilton HS-McMaster Site, PO Box 2000 Stn Lcd 1 1200 Main St W, Hamilton ON L8N 3Z5; Glasgow (Scotland)'66; MB ChB; MD(Hons); FRCPath; FACP; FRCPCH; FRCPC; IntMed (Hematology). Ped Hem Oncol, Hamilton Health Sciences Centre - McMaster University Medical Centre; Prof, McMaster University; (905)521-2100 x73464; Fax. (905)521-1703.

BARR, Ronald G; F507-4480 Oak St, Vancouver BC V6H 3V4; McG'73; MA; MDCM; FRCPC; Peds (Developmental Pediatrics). Staff, BC Children's Hospital; Head Developmental Neurosciences & Child Health, Child & Family Research Institute; Langs: French; (604)875-3568; Fax. (604)875-3569.

BARR, Scott K M; Barr Plastic Surgery Centre, 205 Douglas St, Sudbury ON P3E 1E9; Tor'88; FRCSC; PlasSurg (Cosmetic Surgery). Staff, Health Sciences North-St Joseph's Health Centre; Staff, Health Sciences North - Memorial Site; Staff, Health Sciences North-Laurentian Site; (705)523-4900; Fax. (705)523-4720; info@barrplasticsurgery.com.

BARR, Susan G; HSC-Faculty Of Med, 3280 Hospital Dr NW, Calgary AB T2N 4Z6; Qns'90; BSc(Hon); MSc; FRCPC; IntMed; Rheum. Assoc Prof Med, University of Calgary; (403)220-7038; Fax. (403)210-7367.

BARR, Susan L; Festubert Family Practice, 350 Festubert St, Duncan BC V9L 3S9; UBC'92; CCFP; Staff, Cowichan District Hospital; (250)746-7720; Fax. (250)748-4839.

BARRA, Lillian; St Joseph's Health Care, PO Box 5777 Stn B 268 Grosvenor St, London ON N6A 4V2; Wes'05; FRCPC; IntMed; Rheum. Staff, St Joseph's Hospital - St Joseph's Health Care; (519)646-5986; Fax. (519)646-6072.

BARRAL, Myrlinda V; Chatham-Kent Health Alliance, PO Box 2030 Stn Main 80 Grand Ave W, Chatham ON N7M 5L9; Santo Tomas (Philippines)'69; FRCPC; Psy (Adolescent Psychiatry). Ac Staff, Chatham-Kent Health Alliance; Aj Prof Psy, University of Western Ontario; (519)351-6144 x5744; Fax. (519)351-0450; mbarral@ckha.on.ca.

BARRE, Nicole M; 250 16th St, West Vancouver BC V7V 3R5; UBC'03; CCFP; (604)926-1510

BARRE, Paul E; MUHC-Royal Victoria Hosp, R236-687 av des Pins O, Montreal QC H3A 1A1; UBC'66; DABIM(IntMed); FRCP(Nephrol); FRCPC; Nephrol (P.Q.) (Clinical Nephrology); IntMed. Dir Hemodialysis, McGill University Health Centre - Royal Victoria Hospital; assoc Prof, McGill University; Langs: English; (514)934-1934 x35208; Fax. (514)843-2815; paul.barre@muhc.mcgill.ca.

BARRECA, Peter A; The Two Hundred, 314-200 St Clair Ave W, Toronto ON M4V 1R1; Tor'73; BSc(Hons.); CCFP; FCFP; Staff, St Michael's Hospital; Chair Med Advisory Committee/Chief Med Staff, St Joseph's Infirmary; (416)923-2509; Fax. (416)923-1265.

BARRENECHEA, Ana-Maria; 404-360 Bloor St W, Toronto ON M5S 1X1; (Chile)'69; FRCPC; Psy. Court Staff, Women's College Hospital; Langs: Spanish; (416)964-3418; Fax. (416)964-3418; am.barrenechea@utoronto.ca.

BARRERO GARCIA, Miguel A; CSSS de Trois-Rivieres, 1991 boul du Carmel, Trois-Rivieres QC G8Z 3R9; Santiago (Chile)'93; Staff, CSSS de Trois-Rivières; (819)697-3333

BARRESE, Carol A; Joseph Brant Mem Hosp, 1230 North Shore Blvd E, Burlington ON L7S 1W7; Tor'86; Anes. Staff, Joseph Brant Memorial Hospital; (905)336-4135

BARRESE, Nancy; Oshawa Clinic, 117 King St E, Oshawa ON L1H 1B9; Tor'99; FRCPC; IntMed; Nephrol. Staff, Lakeridge Health - Oshawa Site; (905)721-3546

BARRETH, C Angela; 15-9701 84 Ave, Grande Prairie AB T8V 4Z8; Dal'99; CCFP; (780)532-2205; Fax. (780)532-0037.

BARRETH, Drew; 208-9815 97 St, Grande Prairie AB T8V 8B9; Alb'00; FRCSC; ObstGyn. (780)538-2190; Fax. (780)538-2191.

BARRETT, Alison P; Stevenson Mem Hosp, PO Box 4000 Stn Main 200 Fletcher Cres, Alliston ON L9R 1W7; Tor'91; ObstGyn. Staff, Stevenson Memorial Hospital; (705)435-6281

BARRETT, Brendan J; Health Sciences Centre, 300 Prince Philip Dr, St. John's NL A1B 3V6; National (Ireland)'83; MB ChB; MRC; MSc(ClinEpidem); FRCPC; IntMed; Nephrol. Staff Nephrol, Health Sciences Centre; Prof Nephrol, Memorial University Of Newfoundland; (709)777-8073; Fax. (709)777-6995; bbarrett@mun.ca.

BARRETT, David J; Regent Med Clinic, 102-2737 Keele St, North York ON M3M 2E9; (Jamaica)'92; DAB; (416)398-4500; Fax. (416)398-4700.

BARRETT, Elizabeth A; Algoma District Med Group, 240 McNabb St, Sault Ste. Marie ON P6B 1Y5; McM'86; FRCPC; Psy;CCFP; FCFP; (705)759-1234; Fax. (705)541-2224.

BARRETT, J Alison; Health Sciences Centre, 300 Prince Philip Dr, St. John's NL A1B 3V6; Mem'00; FRCPC; Anes. Staff, Health Sciences Centre; (709)777-6540

BARRETT, Jeffrey R; Grey Bruce Health Services, 203-369 Mary St, Wiarton ON N0H 2T0; McM'98; CASM; CCFP; Staff, Grey Bruce Health Services - Wiarton Site; (519)534-5220; Fax. (519)534-1024.

BARRETT, Jon F R; Sunnybrook Hlth Sciences Ctre, M4 172-2075 Bayview Ave, Toronto ON M4N 3M5; Witwatersrand (South Africa)'83; MB ChB; MRC; FRCSC; ObstGyn (Maternal Fetal Medicine). Staff Aubrey & Marla Dan Program, Sunnybrook Health Sciences Centre; (416)480-4920; Fax. (416)480-4933; jon.barrett@sw.ca.

BARRETT, Lisa; 750 Great Northern Rd, Sault Ste. Marie ON P6B 0A8; Mem'05; FRCPC; IntMed; InfectDis. (705)759-3434

BARRETT, Scott R; 106-107 Edward St, St Thomas ON N5P 1Y8; Mem'98; BSc; (519)637-3877

BARRETT, Thomas A; 211-2223 Broadway W, Vancouver BC V6K 2E4; Cork (Ireland)'71; Ac Staff, Vancouver General Hospital - Centennial Pavillion; Vis Staff, BC Women's Hospital & Health Centre; Vis Staff, UBC Hospital - Koerner Pavillion; Clin Instructor, University of British Columbia; (604)736-6301

BARRETTARA, Giuliano; Medical Clinic, 460 King St W, Oshawa ON L1J 2K9; Tor'81; Langs: Italian; (905)725-4002; Fax. (905)725-0702.

BARRETTE, Andree; 2222 rue Saint-Jean-Baptiste, Jonquiere QC G8A 1V8; Laval'84; Staff Family Planning, Centre Hospitalier Jonquiere; (418)542-8808

BARRETTE, Gaetan; Hop Maisonneuve-Rosemont, 5415 boul de l'Assomption, Montreal QC H1T 2M4; Mon'84; DiagRad. Staff, Hopital Maisonneuve-Rosemont; Pres, Federation Medecins Specialistes Quebec; (514)252-3535

BARRETTE, Ian; CSSSG-Hop de Hull, 116 boul Lionel-Emond, Gatineau QC J8Y 1W7; Ott'93; CCFP; FCFP; Staff Privil, Hull Hospital; Staff Privil, Stevenson Memorial Hospital; Langs: English; French; (819)595-6000

BARRETTE, Louis-Rene; Clinique Urologie, 316 rue Saint-Vallier, Chicoutimi QC G7H 4J1; Laval'65; FRCSC; Urol (Adult Urology). Chef urologie, Complexe hospitalier de la Sagamie; Assoc Member, Administration de la Regie Regionale(Saguenay-Lac Saint-Jean); Prof, Universite de Sherbrooke; Langs: Bilingual(French/English); (418)549-7811; Fax. (418)549-7821; urolrbarrette@bellnet.ca.

BARRETTE, Marie; CLSC du Richelieu, 300 ch de Marieville, Richelieu QC J3L 3V8; Mon'85; (450)658-7561; Fax. (450)658-4390.

BARRETTE, Michelle; CLSC des Seigneuries, 160 boul De Montarville, Boucherville QC J4B 6S2; Mon'94; (450)655-3630; Fax. (450)655-8530.

BARRETTE, Pierre; CSSS du Suroît, 150 rue Saint-Thomas, Salaber-de-Valleyf QC J6T 6C1; Mon'99; GenSurg. Staff, Centre Hospitalier Régional du Suroît; (450)371-9920

BARRETTE, Real; CHUM-Hop Notre-Dame, 1560 rue Sherbrooke E, Montreal QC H2L 4M1; Mon'93; Staff, Centre Hospitalier l'Université de Montréal (CHUM) - Hôpital Notre-Dame; (514)890-8000

BARRETTE, Serge; 170 ch de Plaisance, Cap-aux-Meules QC G4T 1M5; Mon'79; Langs: English; (418)986-3443

BARRETTE, Stephane; Ctr Hosp de Verdun, 4000 boul Lasalle, Verdun QC H4G 2A3; Laval'90; Hem; Peds (Medical Oncology). Staff, Centre Hospitalier de Verdun; adj Prof, Universite de Montreal; Langs: Bilingual(French/English); French; (514)362-1000

BARRETTE-DELORME, Michelle; CSSS de la Vallée de l'Or, 725 6e rue, Val-d'Or QC J9P 3Y1; Laval'72; Ophth. Ophthalmology, Centre de Sante Vallee-de-l'Or; Staff, Centre Hospitalier de Val d'Or; (819)825-6711

BARRETTO, Ignacio J M; PO Box 640, Ponteix SK S0N 1Z0; Glasgow (Scotland)'60; DTMH(Liverpool); CAFCI; Vis Staff, Cypress Regional Hospital; Vis Staff, Prairie View Health Centre; (306)625-3382; Fax. (306)625-3764.

BARRIAULT, Jocelyn; Ctr Hosp de Verdun, 4000 boul Lasalle, Verdun QC H4G 2A3; Mon'84; Staff, Centre Hospitalier de Verdun; (514)765-7337; Fax. (514)765-7333.

BARRIAULT, Ronald J; 326 Chaleur St, Charlo NB E8E 2G2; Dal'68; CCFP; FCFP; Staff, Hôpital Régional Campbellton; (506)789-5035

BARRIE, Gordon; 405-60 St Clair Ave E, Toronto ON M4T 1N5; Aberdeen (Scotland)'68; MB ChB; DABPN; MRCPsy; FRCPC; Psy. Assoc Psychiatrist CAPS, University of Toronto; (416)929-9824; Fax. (416)929-2062.

BARRIE, James R; University of Alberta Hosp, 8440 112 St NW, Edmonton AB T6G 2B7; Alb'88; FRCPC; DiagRad. Staff, University of Alberta Hospital; (780)407-1210; Fax. (780)407-1202.

BARRIE, Michael A; Northumberland Hills Hosp, 1000 Depalma Dr, Cobourg ON K9A 5W6; Cal'01; CCFP; Staff, Northumberland Hills Hospital; (905)373-6811

BARRIE, William J; Maple Leaf Clinic, 301-14 College St, Toronto ON M5G 1K2; Sask'79; BSc(Hon.Biochem.); Court Staff, St Michael's Hospital; (416)465-3252

BARRIEAU, Andre; 105-185 av Acadie, Dieppe NB E1A 1G6; Sher'07; CCFP; (506)862-4182; Fax. (506)862-4179.

BARRIEAU, Louise; Villa Medica Inc, 225 rue Sherbrooke E, Montreal QC H2X 1C9; Mon'85; Gen Practice, Hôpital de réadaptation Villa Medica; (514)288-8201; Fax. (514)288-6370.

BARRIENTOS, Lorena; Doctor's Office Atrium on Bay, 52-595 Bay St, Toronto ON M5G 2C2; Concepcion (Chile)'00; CCFP; (416)598-1703; Fax. (416)598-1778.

BARRIER, Alain; CHUM-Hotel-Dieu, 3840 rue Saint-Urbain, Montreal QC H2W 1T8; Paris (France)'99; Staff, Centre Hospitalier l'Université de Montréal (CHUM) - Hôtel-Dieu; (514)890-8000

BARRIER, France; CHUM-Hop Notre-Dame, 1560 rue Sherbrooke E, Montreal QC H2L 4M1; Nice-Sophia-Antipolis (France)'95; Staff, Centre Hospitalier l'Université de Montréal (CHUM) - Hôpital Notre-Dame; (514)890-8000

BARRIERAS, Diego; Hôpital Ste-Justine, 3175 ch Cote-Sainte-Catherine, Montreal QC H3T 1C5; Mon'91; FRCSC; Urol (Pediatric Urology). Staff, Hôpital Ste-Justine; (514)345-4716; Fax. (514)345-4824.

BARRIERE, Ginette; Carrefour Sante Le St-Laurent, 140-5300 boul Saint-Laurent, Sainte-Catherine QC J5C 1A8; Mon'80; (450)638-6383; Fax. (450)638-5023.

BARRIGA, Peter C; Hop Santa Cabrini Ospedale, 5655 rue Saint-Zotique E, Montreal QC H1T 1P7; McG'90; FRCPC; IntMed; InfectDis; MedMicrobiol. Staff, Hôpital Santa Cabrini Ospedale; Langs: Bilingual(English/French); (514)252-6000 x7203

BARRIGAR, Diana; South Vancouver Med Clinic, 350 Marine Dr SE, Vancouver BC V5X 2S5; Qns'01; BSc; MA; CCFP; (604)323-0077; dianabarrigar@gmail.com.

BARRINGTON, Keith J; Hôpital Ste-Justine, 3175 ch Cote Sainte-Catherine, Montreal QC H3T 1C5; Liverpool (England)'79; Peds (Neonatology). Staff, Hôpital Ste-Justine; Langs: English; French; (514)345-4931 x5929

BARRINGTON, Michelle R; PO Box 11648, Iqaluit NU X0A 1H0; Mem'05.

BARRINGTON, Thomas W; One Med Place, 109-20 Wynford Dr, North York ON M3C 1J4; Tor'56; FACS; FRCSC; OrthSurg. (416)441-1060; Fax. (416)441-1061.

BARRIO, Sally E; 107-15240 56 Ave, Surrey BC V3S 5K7; UBC'89; CCFP; Staff, Surrey Memorial Hospital; (778)574-1414

BARRIOS, Albaro; University of Alberta Hosp, 8440 112 St NW, Edmonton AB T6G 2B7; Guatemala (Guatemala)'84; Staff, University of Alberta Hospital; (780)407-8407

BARRIOS, Rolando A; St Paul's Hosp, 533-1081 Burrard St, Vancouver BC V6Z 1Y6; San Carlos (Guatemala)'81; FRCPC; CommunMed. Staff BC Centre for Excellence in HIV, Providence Health Care - St Paul's Hospital; Aj Prof School of Population & Public Health, University of Alberta; Langs: Spanish; (604)806-8060; Fax. (604)806-9311.

BARRON, Alexander C; North York Gen Hosp, 4001 Leslie St, North York ON M2K 1E1; Wes'94; FRCPC; Peds. Staff, North York General Hospital; (416)756-6000

BARRON, Jane R; Health Sciences Centre, 300 Prince Philip Dr, St. John's NL A1B 3V6; Mem'93; FRCPC; NeurPath. Staff, Health Sciences Centre; (709)777-7711

BARRON, Laurie W; Pan Am Clinic, 75 Poseidon Bay, Winnipeg MB R3M 3E4; Sask'96; FRCSC; OrthSurg. (204)927-2772

BARRON, Lesley K; Georgetown Prof Arts Bldg, 204-99 Sinclair Ave, Georgetown ON L7G 5G1; Wes'96; FRACS; GenSurg. Surgeon, Halton Healthcare Services Corporation - Georgetown Hospital; (905)873-3344

BARRON, Philip T; 207-267 O'Connor St, Ottawa ON K2P 1V3; Aberdeen (Scotland)'62; MB ChB; FRCS; GenSurg. Assoc Prof, University of Ottawa; (613)567-8000; Fax. (613)567-8022; ptbarron@sympatico.ca.

BARRON, Stanley P; Rouge Valley-Centenary HC, 2867 Ellesmere Rd, Scarborough ON M1E 4B9; Tor'64; DABPN; FRCPC; Psy. Staff, Rouge Valley Health System - Centenary Health Centre Site; (416)281-7318

BARRON, Stephen R; Wilson Centre Family Practice, 1-2185 Wilson Ave, Port Coquitlam BC V3C 6C1; Mem'78; CCFP; FCFP; Assoc Staff, Royal Columbian Hospital; Assoc Staff, Eagle Ridge Hospital & Health Care Centre; (604)942-7227; Fax. (604)942-7058.

BARRON, Teresa; Clinique Med des Sommets, 1070 rue Principale, Ste-Agathe-des-Mts QC J8C 1L6; Baylor(Texas) (USA)'85; FRCPC; Peds. (819)321-1212; Fax. (819)321-3232.

BARRON-KLAUNINGER, Kathryn; Appletree Med Centre, 1582 Bank St, Ottawa ON K1H 7Z5; Ott'86; CCFP; FCFP; Staff, The Ottawa Hospital - General Campus; (613)731-0497

BARROW, John L; 10-6213 Centre St NW, Calgary AB T2K 0V2; Durham (England)'63; MB BS; ACLS; ATLS; LMCC; BAAnth; DObstRCOG; CCFP; Staff, Peter Lougheed Centre; (403)274-2231

BARROWS, Tammy L; The Ottawa Hosp-Gen Campus, CCW 1401-501 Smyth Rd, Ottawa ON K1H 8L6; Mem'99; FRCPC; Anes. Staff, The Ottawa Hospital - General Campus; (613)737-8899 x8187; Fax. (613)737-8189.

BARRS, Gary B; Clinique Med Verdun-Lasalle, 5989 rue De Verdun, Verdun QC H4H 1M6; Tor'72; Staff, St Mary's Hospital Centre; (514)766-3574; Fax. (514)766-6462; garybarrs@videotron.ca.

BARRY, Anne E; Valley Reg Hosp, 150 Exhibition St, Kentville NS B4N 5E3; Dal'83; BSc(Hons); Med Staff, Valley Regional Hospital; (902)678-7381

BARRY, Colin A; Saint John Reg Hosp, PO Box 2100 Stn Main 400 University Ave, Saint John NB E2L 4L2; Mem'97; BSc; FRCPC; IntMed (Interventional Cardiology); Cardiol. Staff, Saint John Regional Hospital; Langs: French; (506)648-6101; Fax. (506)648-6110; colinabarry@hotmail.com.

BARRY, David M; Burnside Fam Med Clinic, 2-101 Burnside Rd W, Victoria BC V9A 1B7; Oxford (England)'73; BMus; BCh; MRC(UK); CCFP; Ac Staff Privil, Victoria General Hospital; Ac Staff Privil, Royal Jubilee Hospital; (250)381-8901; Fax. (250)381-6773.

BARRY, Frances J; MUHC-Royal Victoria Hosp, 687 av des Pins O, Montreal QC H3A 1A1; Sask'75; CSPQ; FRCPC; Anes. Staff, McGill University Health Centre - Royal Victoria Hospital; adj Prof, McGill University; (514)934-1934 x34880

BARRY, Keith R; PO Box 95001 Rpo Whyte, Edmonton AB T6E 0E5; Alb'10; CCFP.

BARRY, Michael H; Saint John Reg Hosp, PO Box 2100 Stn Main 400 University Ave, Saint John NB E2L 4L2; Dal'82; FRCPC; DiagRad. Staff, Saint John Regional Hospital; (506)648-6918; Fax. (506)648-6925.

BARRY, Patricia E; 526 Guelph Line, Burlington ON L7R 3M4; McM'78; BSc; CGPP; CCFP; FCFP; (905)639-0772; Fax. (905)639-7897.

BARRY, Sean P; Univ Hlth Network-Toronto Western Hosp, WW 432-399 Bathurst St, Toronto ON M5T 2S8; Dal'06; Neursurg. Staff, Toronto Western Hospital - University Health Network; (416)603-5675

BARRY, Thomas J; 203-640 Prospect St, Fredericton NB E3B 9M7; Dal'74; CCFP; FCFP; Staff, Dr Everett Chalmers Regional Hospital; Teach Staff Family Pract, Dalhousie University; (506)459-8580

BARSAUSKAS, Algis J; Inst U Geriatrie de Montreal, 4565 ch Queen-Mary, Montreal QC H3W 1W5; Ott'71; Staff, Institut Universitaire de Gériatrie de Montréal; (514)340-1424; Fax. (514)340-2832.

BARSKE, Heather L; Pan Am Clinic, 75 Poseidon Bay, Winnipeg MB R3M 3E4; Man'04; FRCSC; OrthSurg.

BARSKY, Jacob B; South Calgary Urgent Care Ctre, 31 Sunpark Plaza SE, Calgary AB T2X 3W5; Sask'79; CCFP; CCFP(E.M.); FCFP; Ac Staff, Chinook Regional Hospital; Court Staff, Covenant Health - St Michael's Health Centre; Staff, South Calgary Urgent Care Centre; (403)943-9476

BARSKY, Michael F; The Credit Valley Hosp, 2200 Eglinton Ave W, Mississauga ON L5M 2N1; Sask'83; FRCPC; DiagRad. Staff Diagnostic Imaging, The Credit Valley Hospital; (905)813-3978; Fax. (905)813-3042.

BARSKY, Stephen; Scarborough Hosp-Birchmount, OPMH-3030 Birchmount Rd, Scarborough ON M1W 3W3; Sask'83; FRCPC; Psy (General Psychiatry). Chief Psy/Med Dir Mental Health Services, The Scarborough Hospital - General Campus; Chief Psy/Med Dir Mental Health Services, The Scarborough Hospital - Birchmount Campus; Lecturer, University of Toronto; (416)495-2563; Fax. (416)495-2426; sbarsky@tsh.to.

BARSOOM, Laith M; Nymark Medical Centre, 4839 Leslie St, North York ON M2J 2K8; Baghdad (Iraq)'96; MB ChB; CCFP; Court Member Family Physician, Rouge Valley Health System - Centenary Health Centre Site; Langs: Arabic; (416)498-3600

BARSOUM, Milad K; Markham College Med Clinic, 408-474 College St, Toronto ON M6G 1A4; Cairo (Egypt)'62; MB ChB; FRCSC; Urol. Ac Staff, Mackenzie Richmond Hill Hospital; Langs: French; Arabic; (416)961-5160

BARSOUM, Nabila J; Mackenzie Richmond Hill Hosp, 10 Trench St, Richmond Hill ON L4C 4Z3; Ein Shams (Egypt)'64; FRCPC; GenPath. Staff, Mackenzie Richmond Hill Hospital; (905)883-1212; Fax. (905)883-2161.

BARSOUM, Randa M K; 10 Royal Orchard Blvd, Thornhill ON L3T 3C3; Cairo (Egypt)'93; CCFP; (905)771-7600

BARSS, Alex; 2135 Norris Ave PO Box 247, Lumby BC V0E 2G0; Alb'87; Staff, Vernon Jubilee Hospital; (250)547-2127

BARSS, David H; David Barss Inc, 58 York St, Bridgewater NS B4V 1P9; Dal'74; CCFP; FCFP; Ac Staff/Head Med, South Shore Regional Hospital; (902)543-7824; Fax. (902)543-5624.

BARSS, Kenneth A; Little Current Med Association, PO Box 549 15 Meredith St E, Little Current ON P0P 1K0; Dal'87; CCFP; FCFP; (705)368-2450; Fax. (705)368-2480.

BARSS, Peter G; Salmon Arm Health Unit, PO Box 627 851 16 St NE, Salmon Arm BC V1E 4N7; Chicago (USA)'71; FAB; DSc; MPH; DTMH; FRCPC; CommunMed (Injury Epidemiology). Langs: Spanish; Portuguese; French; (250)833-4149

BART, Bevin B; Rockyview Gen Hosp, 7007 14 St SW, Calgary AB T2V 1P9; Wes'91; FRCPC; Anes (Pediatric Anesthesia). Staff, Rockyview General Hospital; Clinical Asst Prof, University of Calgary; (403)943-3410; Fax. (403)943-8590.

BART, John L; 5987 Bathurst St, North York ON M2R 1Z3; London (England)'69; MB BS; LRCP; MRCS; Ac Staff, North York General Hospital - Branson Division; Court Staff, Sunnybrook Health Sciences Centre; (416)642-1282; Fax. (416)642-1284.

BARTEL, Douglas W; Ridge Meadows Hosp & Hlth CC, PO Box 5000 Stn Del Ctr 11666 Laity St, Maple Ridge BC V2X 7G5; Alb'89; BSc; CCFP; CCFP(E.M.); Physician Emerg Room, Ridge Meadows Hospital & Health Care Centre; (604)463-1823; Fax. (604)463-1888.

BARTEL, S Alexander; Hodgins Prof Bldg, 101-45625 Hodgins Ave, Chilliwack BC V2P 1P2; UBC'75; Ac Staff, Chilliwack General Hospital; Langs: German; (604)792-2721; Fax. (604)792-3404.

BARTELLAS, Elias I; 320 Freshwater Rd, St. John's NL A1B 1C2; Hebrew (Israel)'76; MD; DAB; FRCSC; ObstGyn. Staff, Health Care Corporation Of St John's; Clin Asst, Memorial University Of Newfoundland; (709)579-1813; Fax. (709)722-9012.

BARTELS, Ute K; The Hosp For Sick Children, 555 University Ave, Toronto ON M5G 1X8; Frankfurt (Germany)'89; Staff, The Hospital For Sick Children; (416)813-5249

BARTER, Ola J; Dr Charles A Janeway Child HC, 300 Prince Philip Dr, St. John's NL A1B 3V6; Mem'89; BMedSci; FRCPC; Peds (Pediatric Critical Care); Critical Care Medicine. Staff, Janeway Children's Health & Rehabilitation Centre; Asst Prof, Memorial University Of Newfoundland; Langs: French; (709)777-4769; Fax. (709)778-4333.

BARTER, Richard B; Health Sciences Centre, 300 Prince Philip Dr, St. John's NL A1B 3V6; RCS (Ireland)'79; LRCPS; ACLS; ATLS; Staff Emerg, Health Sciences Centre; Med Examiner, Aerolife Medevac Services; Med Examiner, Province of Newfoundland & Labrador; Pres Medical Staff, Health Care Corporation Of St John's; Clin Associate Family Med, Memorial University Of Newfoundland; (709)777-6335

BARTER LEYVA, Maria T; Ctr Hosp Affilie-St-Sacrement, 1050 ch Sainte-Foy, Quebec QC G1S 4L8; Santiago (Cuba)'95; CCFP; Staff, Centre Hospitalier Affilié Universitaire de Québec - Hôpital du St-Sacrement; (418)682-7511

BARTFELD, Naama; Summerridge Health Centre, 26-8707 Dufferin St, Thornhill ON L4J 0A2; Tor'07; CCFP; (905)764-0005; Fax. (905)764-0044.

BARTH, Bernard A; Oakdale Med Bldg, 205-2065 Finch Ave W, North York ON M3N 2V7; Tor'67; Staff, Humber River Regional Hospital - Finch Avenue Site; (416)746-0022; Fax. (416)746-0027.

BARTH, David; Univ Hlth Network-Toronto Gen, 11E 410-200 Elizabeth St, Toronto ON M5G 2C4; Tor'96; FRCPC; FRCPC; FRCPC; HemPath; Hem; IntMed (Apheresis Medicine). Staff, Princess Margaret Hospital - University Health Network; Staff, Toronto General Hospital - UHN; (416)340-4914; Fax. (416)340-5543; david.barth@uhn.on.ca.

BARTHA, David J; Claridge House, 304-11027 87 Ave NW, Edmonton AB T6G 2P9; Alb'03; FRCPC; IntMed. (780)735-2000

BARTHA, Lillian J; UCMC Sunridge, 2685 36 St NE, Calgary AB T1Y 5S3; (403)943-5000; Fax. (403)476-8784.

BARTHEL, Jennifer E; Sioux Lookout First Nations H, PO Box 1300 Stn Main 61 Queen St, Sioux Lookout ON P8T 1B8; Cal'09; CCFP.

BARTHELEMY, Bernard F; CSSS du Haut Saint-Maurice, 885 boul Ducharme, La Tuque QC G9X 3C1; Staff, Centre Hospitalier Saint-Joseph de la Turque; (819)523-4581

BARTHÉLÉMY, Lucie A; CSSS Alphonse Desjardins-UMF, 100-1205 boul de la Rive-Sud, Saint-Romuald QC G6W 0J4; (Other Foreign)'02; (418)380-8597; Fax. (418)380-8596.

BARTHOLOMEW, Julie-Anne; SMBD Jewish Gen Hosp, 3755 ch Cote-Sainte-Catherine, Montreal QC H3T 1E2; Saba (Netherlands Antilles)'06; Peds. Staff, Sir Mortimer B Davis Jewish General; (514)340-8222

BARTIE, Darryl C; 102-9814 97 St, Grande Prairie AB T8V 8H5; (South Africa)'99; MB ChB; (780)538-0129; Fax. (780)532-6997.

BARTLEMAN, Anne-Pascale; Perth Family Medicine, 39 Drummond St, Perth ON K7H 2J9; Ott'07; CCFP.

BARTLEMAN, Betty P; Oceanview Paediatrics, 101-1650 Terminal Ave N, Nanaimo BC V9S 0A3; Qns'88; FRCPC; Peds. Staff, BC Children's Hospital; (250)591-1906; Fax. (250)591-1913.

BARTLETT, Clark G; 1-1501 Boundary Cres, Nanaimo BC V9S 4P1; UBC'06; FRCSC; Otol. (250)753-2142

BARTLETT, Eric S; Univ Hlth Network-Princess M, 3 956-610 University Ave, Toronto ON M5G 2M9; Oklahoma(OK) (USA)'98; Staff, Princess Margaret Hospital - University Health Network; (416)946-4501 x6320

BARTLETT, J Andrew; 201-7031 Westminster Hwy, Richmond BC V6X 1A3; Qns'82; AB; AB; FRCSC; Otol (Facial Plastic Surgery). Staff, Richmond Hospital; Staff, Delta Hospital; Clin Prof, University of British Columbia; (604)273-4353; Fax. (604)273-4323.

BARTFELT, John M; London Road Diagnostic Clinic, 8-481 London Rd, Sarnia ON N7T 4X3; London (England)'70; (519)344-1121; Fax. (519)344-0115.

BARTLETT, Krista; Halton Hills FHT-Guelph Street, 171 Guelph St, Georgetown ON L7G 4A1; Mem'97; CCFP; (905)877-4123; Fax. (905)873-8882.

BARTLETT, Leah D; 208-1 Quarry Ridge Rd, Barrie ON L4M 7G1; McM'05; FRCPC; Peds. (705)728-3766

BARTLETT, Lewis J; Valley Med Imaging, 404A-2151 McCallum Rd, Abbotsford BC V2S 3N8; UBC'79; FRCPC; DiagRad. (604)855-0112

BARTLETT, Lloyd C; Medical Arts Bldg, 1620-233 Kennedy St, Winnipeg MB R3C 3J5; Wes'41; FACN; FRCSC; GenSurg. (204)942-8388; Fax. (204)947-8086.

BARTLETT, Lynsey E; Carling-Broadview Med Bldg, 205-770 Broadview Ave, Ottawa ON K2A 3Z3; Dal'06; CCFP; (613)729-1324

BARTLETT, Norman R; Campbellford Mem Hosp, PO Box 1027 146 Oliver Rd, Campbellford ON K0L 1L0; Tor'94; BSc; MSc; CCFP; CCFP(E.M.); FCFP; Head EmergMed, Campbellford Memorial Hospital; (705)653-1140 x2194

BARTLETT, Penelope; 173 Fern Rd W, Qualicum Beach BC V9K 1S4; Birmingham (England)'86; MB ChB; (250)752-6907; Fax. (250)752-6918.

BARTLETT, Peter J; Health Sciences Centre, 300 Prince Philip Dr, St. John's NL A1B 3V6; Mem'84; FRCPC; DiagRad. Staff General Hosp, Health Sciences Centre; Clinical Asst Prof Radiol, Memorial University Of Newfoundland; (709)777-7944; Fax. (709)777-7383.

BARTLETT, R Paul; Star FHT-Tavistock Comm Hlth I, PO Box 310 80 Maria St, Tavistock ON N0B 2R0; Alb'71; CCFP; Staff, Stratford General Hospital - Huron Perth Healthcare Alliance; Teach Staff Family Practice, University of Western Ontario; (519)655-2322; Fax. (519)655-3073.

BARTLETT, Robert L; 170 Paradox Point, Bocabec NB E5B 3X1; Dal'74; Staff, Saint John Regional Hospital; (506)529-8666; bartlett.robert@jdirving.com.

BARTLETT, Sarah K B; PO Box 19508 Rpo Ctre Point Ma, Vancouver BC V5T 4E7; Dal'05; CCFP; (604)872-8441

BARTLETT, Steven; Clin Familiale de Coaticook, 206-18 rue du Manege, Coaticook QC J1A 3B3; Sher'91; CCFP; Staff, Centre Hospitalier de Coaticook; (819)849-4808; Fax. (819)849-7400.

BARTLETT, Wayne C; Keystone Place, 303-270 Douglas Ave, Bathurst NB E2A 1M9; Mem'85; GenSurg. Med Staff, Hopital Regional Chaleur; (506)548-9960; Fax. (506)548-1898.

BARTLEY, Debra; London HSC-Victoria Hosp, B1 182-800 Commissioners Rd E, London ON N6A 5W9; Tor'99; FRCSC; OrthSurg. Staff, London Health Sciences Centre - Victoria Campus; (519)685-8021

BARTLEY, Simon D K; 224 Glen Cres PO Box 5111 Stn Main, Banff AB T1L 1G3; UBC'99; CCFP; CCFP(E.M.); Staff, Covenant Health - Banff Mineral Springs Hospital.

BARTOL, Stephen W; Windsor Reg Hosp-Western Camp, 1453 Prince Rd, Windsor ON N9C 3Z4; Dal'83; FRCSC; OrthSurg. Staff, Windsor Regional Hospital - Tayfour Site; Staff, Henry Ford Hospital-Detroit, Michigan(USA); (519)257-5294; Fax. (519)253-9967; sbartol@medaccesssolutions.com.

BARTOLUCCI, Giampiero; 2F-152 Hester St, Hamilton ON L9A 2N8; Rome (Italy)'58; FRCPC; Psy (Brain Injury Psychiatry). Staff, St Joseph's Healthcare - Charlton Campus; Locum Tenens, Thunder Bay Regional Health Sciences Centre; Locum Tenens, St Joseph's Care Group - St Joseph's Hospital; Emeritus Prof Psy, McMaster University; Langs: Italian; (905)540-1308; Fax. (905)540-8061.

BARTON, Anise C; Nicola Med Dental Bldg, 400-321 Nicola St, Kamloops BC V2C 6G6; Alb'01; BSc; FRCSC; GenSurg. Staff, Royal Inland Hospital; Langs: Bilingual(English/French); (250)828-2848

BARTON, Douglas G; Brockville Gen Hosp, 75 Charles St, Brockville ON K6V 1S8; Qns'04; CCFP; CCFP(E.M.); Staff, Brockville General Hospital - Charles Street; (613)345-5649

BARTON, Guy J; Oshawa Clinic, 117 King St E, Oshawa ON L1H 1B9; Sheffield (England)'67; MB ChB; DMRD; FFR(E); FRCPC; DiagRad. (905)721-4300

BARTON, James W; Saskatoon Nephrology Group, 434-230 Avenue R S, Saskatoon SK S7M 2Z1; Mem'94; FRCPC; IntMed; Nephrol. Clin Prof Med, University of Saskatchewan; (306)934-3300; Fax. (306)934-3355.

BARTON, Jason J S; UBC Eye Care Centre, 2550 Willow St, Vancouver BC V5Z 3N9; UBC'84; FRCPC; Neur (Neuro Ophthalmology). Staff, Vancouver General Hospital - Centennial Pavillion; Prof/Chair Canada Research, University of British Columbia; (604)875-4339

BARTON, Jeffrey D; 206-640 Prospect St, Fredericton NB E3B 9M7; Dal'96; CCFP; FCFP; Staff, Dr Everett Chalmers Regional Hospital; (506)457-4784; Fax. (506)457-4786.

BARTON, Michele C; Hamilton Comm Health Centre, M1-414 Victoria Ave N, Hamilton ON L8L 5G8; McM'87; DOHS; BSc(Hon); Physician, Karmax Heavy Stamping; (905)529-5221; Fax. (905)546-0361.

BARTON, Nicola A; Park Avenue Med Centre, 4634 Park Ave, Terrace BC V8G 1V7; Ott'80; BSc; LMCC; (250)615-5030; nikibarton@telus.net.

BARTON, Pamela M; Chronic Pain Centre, 160-2210 2 St SW, Calgary AB T2S 3C3; Cal'76; ABPMR; ABNEM; BSc; LMCC; BSc(Hons); FRCPC; PhysMed&Rehab (Pain Medicine). Staff Consultant, Foothills Medical Centre; Consultant Calgary Pain Program, Alberta Health Services; Clin Assoc Prof Div of PhysMed&Rehab, University of Calgary; Fax. (403)508-7441.

BARTON, Rachel K; 3106 Gibbins Rd, Duncan BC V9L 1E8; Cal'91; FRCSC; GenSurg. Staff, Cowichan District Hospital; (250)737-1020

BARTON, Ronald T; Northgate Centre, 1038-9499 137 Ave NW, Edmonton AB T5E 5R8; Manchester (England)'73; MB ChB; (780)377-4050

BARTON, William F; Dartmouth Gen Hosp, 325 Pleasant St, Dartmouth NS B2Y 4G8; Dal'73; FRCPC; DiagRad. Staff, Dartmouth General Hospital; Lecturer Radiol Div, Dalhousie University; (902)465-8323; Fax. (902)465-8360.

BARTOSIK, Lidia M; Trillium Hlth Ctr-Mississauga, 100 Queensway W, Mississauga ON L5B 1B8; Cracow (Poland)'71; FRCPC; Anes. Staff, Trillium Health Centre - Mississauga; Asst Prof Anes, University of Toronto; Langs: Polish; (905)848-7628; Fax. (905)848-0328; lidia.bartosik@sympatico.ca.

BARTOSIK, Lukasz P; Montfort Hosp, 713 Montreal Rd, Ottawa ON K1K 0T2; Tor'05; FRCPC; Anes. Staff, Montfort Hospital; (613)746-4621

BARTS, Agnieszka D; Columbia Med Bldg, 311-301 Columbia St E, New Westminster BC V3L 3W5; UBC'01; BSc; MHSc; FRCPC; IntMed; Endocrin&Metab. Clin Instructor, University of British Columbia; (604)787-8808; Fax. (604)787-8806.

BARTSCH, Margaret; Associate Family Phys Clinic, 262 2nd Ave NE, Swift Current SK S9H 2C8; Man'74; CCFP; Staff, Cypress Regional Hospital; Physician, Palliser Regional Care Centre; (306)773-1555; Fax. (306)773-6817.

BARTUCCI, Michael; Health For All Family Health T, 202-379 Church St, Markham ON L6B 0T1; Tor'09; BSc; CCFP; Lecturer, University of Toronto; Langs: Italian; (905)472-2200; Fax. (905)472-5662; michael.bartucci@utoronto.ca.

BARTUCZ, John P; Trillium Hlth Ctr-Mississauga, 100 Queensway W, Mississauga ON L5B 1B8; Tor'68; DMRD; DiagRad. Ac Staff, Trillium Health Centre - Mississauga; (905)848-7523

BARUCH, Philippe; Inst U en Sante Mentale de QC, H1121-2601 ch de la Canardiere, Quebec QC G1J 2G3; Paris (France)'86; Psy (P.Q.). Dir-Enseigement, Institut Universitaire Sante; (418)663-5321; Fax. (418)663-5758.

BARUCH, Ruth; Toronto East Gen Hosp Inc, 825 Coxwell Ave, Toronto ON M4C 3E7; Man'76; FRCPC; Psy. Staff, Toronto East General Hospital Inc; (416)469-6198; Fax. (416)469-6805.

BARUCHEL, Sylvain; The Hosp For Sick Children, 555 University Ave, Toronto ON M5G 1X8; Renes (France)'83; MedOncol (P.Q.). Staff, The Hospital For Sick Children; (416)813-7795; Fax. (416)813-5327; sylvain.baruchel@sickkids.ca.

BARWELL, Jean; Dixie Road Med Associates, 2200 Dixie Rd, Mississauga ON L4Y 1Z4; McM'98; CCFP; (905)279-1700; Fax. (905)897-9167.

BARWICH, Doris B A; Fraser Health Authority, 400-13450 102 Ave, Surrey BC V3T 0H1; Man'79; CCFP; Physician Palliative Care, BC Cancer Agency Fraser Valley Centre; Langs: German; (604)587-4669; colleen.poore@fraserhealth.ca.

BARWIN, B Norman; Carling-Broadview Med Bldg, 108-770 Broadview Ave, Ottawa ON K2A 3Z3; Belfast (Ireland)'65; MD; FACOG; FRCOG; FSOGC; Consultant Gyn, Royal Ottawa Mental Health Centre - Royal Ottawa Health Care Group; Teach Staff, University of Ottawa; Langs: Afrikaans; (613)728-5104; Fax. (613)728-3497.

BARWITZKI, Gary W; Bluewater Methadone Clinic, 118 Victoria St N, Sarnia ON N7T 5W9; Wes'89; CCFP; CCFP(E.M.); Emerg Med, Bluewater Health - Mitton Site; Instructor Emerg & Family Med, University of Western Ontario; (519)337-5000

BARYLA, Yuliya; Leaside Health Centre, 795 Eglinton Ave E, Toronto ON M4G 4E4; Belarussian (Russia (Federation))'01; CCFP; (416)424-3145; Fax. (416)424-2611.

BARYSHNIK, Devra B; Dixon Med Centre, 407-531 Davis Dr, Newmarket ON L3Y 6P5; Tor'00; FRCPC; Neur (Neuromuscular Diseases). Court Staff EMG Lab, Sunnybrook Health Sciences Centre; (905)895-6673; Fax. (905)895-8676.

BARYSHNIK, Sheldon M; Dixon Med Centre, 407-531 Davis Dr, Newmarket ON L3Y 6P5; Wes'71; FRCPC; Neur. Staff, Southlake Regional Health Centre; (905)895-6673; Fax. (905)895-8765.

BARZELAI, Laurence P; 203-1448 Commercial Dr, Vancouver BC V5L 3X9; Dal'78; CCFP; (604)255-6565; Fax. (604)255-6559.

BASAPPA, Naveen S; Cross Cancer Institute, 11560 University Ave NW, Edmonton AB T6G 1Z2; Alb'03; FRCPC; IntMed; MedOncol. Staff, Cross Cancer Institute; (780)432-8762; Fax. (780)432-8888.

BASATI, Raghmeet; West Winds Med Clinic, 2120-4818 Westwinds Dr NE, Calgary AB T3J 3Z5; Alb'02; CCFP; Langs: Punjabi; (403)568-2295; Fax. (403)568-2247.

BASCARON, Marie-Eve; Ctr Hosp de Verdun, 4000 boul Lasalle, LaSalle QC H4G 2A3; Mon'05; CCFP; Staff, Centre Hospitalier de Verdun; (514)362-1000

BASCO, Debbie E; Burnaby Hosp, 3935 Kincaid St, Burnaby BC V5G 2X6; UBC'98; Staff, Burnaby Hospital; (604)434-4211

BASECQZ, Guy M; Aberdeen Hosp, 835 East River Rd, New Glasgow NS B2H 3S6; Louvain (Belgium)'61; MD; FRCPC; Psy (Infant Psychiatry). Staff, Aberdeen Regional Hospital; (902)752-7600

BASFORD, Tavis J; James Street Med Walk-In Clini, 1-179 James St S, Hamilton ON L8P 3A3; Qns'04; CCFP; (905)575-0808

BASHAGHA, Ahmed; Excellent Care Medical Centre, 3885 Duke of York Blvd, Mississauga ON L5B 0E4; Al-Fateh (Libya)'03; CCFP; (905)270-3885; abashaga@yahoo.com.

BASHALA, Roger; Clinique Medicale, 157 Water St, Campbellton NB E3N 3L4; Kinshasa (Congo (Democratic Republic))'95; LMCC; CCFP; Dir Palliative Care, Hôpital Régional Campbellton; Prof adj clin, Universite de Sherbrooke; Langs: Lingala; Swahili; French; (506)753-7727; Fax. (506)753-7711.

BASHIR, Abdelnasir; London HSC-Victoria Hosp, PO Box 5010 Stn B D2 521-800 Commissioners Rd E, London ON N6A 5W9; Gezira (Sudan)'95; FRCPC; IntMed. Staff, London Health Sciences Centre - Victoria Campus; (519)685-8500

BASHIR, Bashir M; CancerCare Manitoba, 300 McTavish Ave E, Brandon MB R7A 2B2; Al Fateh (Libya)'00; FRCPC; RadOncol.

BASHIR, Jamil G; St Paul's Hosp, CVT 458-1081 Burrard St, Vancouver BC V6Z 1Y6; Alb'91; FRCSC; CardSurg (Cardiac & Vascular Surgery). Staff, Providence Health Care - St Paul's Hospital; (604)806-9668

BASHIR, Khalid; Victoria Med Bldg, 316-1669 Victoria St, Prince George BC V2L 2L5; Karachi (Pakistan)'92; MB BS; ABIM; FRCPC; IntMed; Nephrol. Langs: Urdu; Punjabi; (250)564-3451; Fax. (250)564-3458.

BASHOUR, Mounir; Lasik MD, 1250 rue Rene-Levesque O, Montreal QC H3B 4W8; McG'93; BSc(Eng); FACS; ABOph; CSPQ; DABOph; PhDEng; FAAO; FICS; MCh; FRCSC; Ophth (Cosmetic Surgery). Langs: Arabic; French; (514)933-0133; Fax. (514)845-0600; mbashour@lasikmd.com.

BASI, Raviqubal S; 21st Medical Clinic, 502-402 21st St E, Saskatoon SK S7K 0C3; Sask'92; FRCPC; IntMed. Staff, Battlefords Union Hospital; (306)956-3444; Fax. (306)956-3577.

BASIAN, Herbert; 206-360 College St, Toronto ON M5T 1S6; Tor'54; DABS; FRCSC; GenSurg (Vascular Surgery). Teach Staff/Hon Consultant, Toronto General Hospital - UHN; Pt-Time Consultant Vascular Surg, University of Toronto; (416)923-9318; Fax. (416)923-8067.

BASIC, Doris; Cardiology Consultants, 103-803A 1 Ave NE, Calgary AB T2E 7C5; Tor'97; BSc; MSc; FRCPC; IntMed (Echocardiography); Cardiol. Clinical Asst Prof, University of Calgary; (403)571-8600; Fax. (403)215-2213.

BASIK, Mark; SMBD Jewish Gen Hosp, 3755 ch Cote-Sainte-Catherine, Montreal QC H3T 1E2; McG'85; FRCSC; GenSurg. Staff, Sir Mortimer B Davis Jewish General; (514)340-8222; Fax. (514)340-8302.

BASILE, Fadi; CHUM-Hotel-Dieu, 3840 rue Saint-Urbain, Montreal QC H2W 1T8; Beirut (Lebanon)'71; AB(Cardiovasc&ThorSurg; FRCSC; GenSurg; Cardiovasc&ThorSurg. Chef cardio-vas/chir thor/Chef chir thorac, Centre Hospitalier l'Université de Montréal (CHUM) - Hôtel-Dieu; Clin Assoc Prof, Universite de Montreal; Langs: Arabic; (514)890-8131

BASILE, Vincenzo S; Sunnybrook Hlth Sciences Ctre, A233-2075 Bayview Ave, Toronto ON M4N 3M5; McM'04; FRCPC; Neur. Staff, Sunnybrook Health Sciences Centre; (416)480-4475; Fax. (416)480-4674.

BASILIJ, Robert; Hanover Med Associates, 118 7th Ave, Hanover ON N4N 2G9; Wes'82; CCFP; Staff, South Bruce Grey Health Centre - Durham Site; Preceptor, University of Western Ontario; (519)364-2820; Fax. (519)364-3965; hmabobb@wightman.ca.

BASINGER, Marilyn R; Heritage Hill Medicentre, 110-8180 Macleod Trail SE, Calgary AB T2H 2B8; Alb'78; CCFP; FCFP; Ac Staff, Rockyview General Hospital; (403)259-3256

BASINSKI, Antoni; Univ Hlth Network-Toronto Western Hosp, 2W404-399 Bathurst St, Toronto ON M5T 2S8; Qns'85; PhD; Staff, Toronto Western Hospital - University Health Network; Ac Staff, Toronto General Hospital - UHN; Teach Staff Public Health Services, University of Toronto; (416)603-5888 x1; Fax. (416)603-5821.

BASKER, Ivor G W; City Centre Fam Physicians, 100-514 Queen St, Saskatoon SK S7K 0M5; Cape Town (South Africa)'63; MB ChB; DA; (306)244-3016; Fax. (306)244-4737.

BASKER, Rajasekar; Hotel-Dieu Grace Hosp, 1030 Ouellette Ave, Windsor ON N9A 1E1; Tamil Nadu (India)'99; Staff, Hôtel-Dieu Grace Hospital; (519)973-4411

BASKERVILLE, Leon; Grand River Hosp-KW Hlth Ctre, PO Box 9056 Stn C 835 King St W, Kitchener ON N2G 1G3; Qns'70; Staff, Grand River Hospital - Kitchener/Waterloo Health Centre; (519)742-3611

BASKETT, Roger J F; Queen Elizabeth II HSC-Halifax, 2269-1796 Summer St, Halifax NS B3H 3A7; Dal'97; FRCSC; CardSurg. Staff, Queen Elizabeth II Health Sciences Centre - Halifax Infirmary Site; (902)473-3808; Fax. (902)473-4448.

BASKIN, Leland B; Calgary Lab Services, 9-3535 Research Rd NW, Calgary AB T2L 2K8; San Antonio(TX) (USA)'86; ABPath(AP&CP); Staff, Foothills Medical Centre; Staff, Peter Lougheed Centre; Staff, Rockyview General Hospital; Staff, Calgary Laboratory Services; Clin Assoc Prof Path & LabMed, University of Calgary; (403)770-3758; leland.baskin@cls.ab.ca.

BASKIND, Roy D; 273-5 Fairview Mall Dr, North York ON M2J 2Z1; (USA)'01; FRCPC; Neur. (416)502-8100; Fax. (416)502-8110.

BASMADJIAN, Arsene J; Institut de Cardiologie de Mtl, 5000 rue Belanger, Montreal QC H1T 1C8; Mon'92; MSc; CSPQ; FACC; FRCPC; IntMed (Echocardiography); Cardiol. Chief Echocardiography, Institut de Cardiologie de Montréal; assoc Prof, Universite de Montreal; Langs: Armenian; English; French; (514)376-3330 x3800; Fax. (514)593-2567.

BASMADJIAN, Girair; Clinique Domus Medica, 5601 rue Belanger, Montreal QC H1T 1G3; Alexandria (Egypt)'65; FRCSC; Ophth (Retinal Disease). Staff, Hôpital Santa Cabrini Ospedale; Staff, St Mary's Hospital Centre; Langs: Armenian; Arabic; French; (514)256-5011; Fax. (514)256-6000; gbasmadjian@videotron.ca.

BASMAJIAN, Haig; Port Hope Med Centre, 209-249 Ontario St, Port Hope ON L1A 3Y9; Qns'75; FACS; FRCSC; GenSurg. Ac Staff, Northumberland Hills Hospital; (905)885-8949; Fax. (905)885-0716.

BASQUE, Andre-Denis; Ctr Hosp Pierre-Janet, 20 rue Pharand, Gatineau QC J9A 1K7; Mon'04; FRCPC; Psy. Psychiatre, Centre Hospitalier Pierre-Janet; (819)771-7761; Fax. (819)771-2908.

BASQUE, Eric J Y; Clinique Med de la Pointe, 7496 Route 11, Pte-Robichaud NB E1X 1K9; Mon'96; CCFP; FCFP; (506)393-5000; Fax. (506)393-5050.

BASQUE, Marie-Helene; CLSC de Paspebiac, CP 7000 273 boul Gerard-D-Levesque, Paspebiac QC G0C 2K0; Mon'99; Staff, CLSC de Paspebiac; (418)752-2572

BASQUE-ARSENAULT, Lorraine; Dr Georges-L Dumont Reg Hosp, 330 Av Universite, Moncton NB E1C 2Z3; Laval'91; Staff, Dr Georges-L-Dumont University Hospital Centre; (506)862-4000; Fax. (506)862-4135.

BASRAN, Jenny F S; Saskatoon City Hosp, 7601-701 Queen St, Saskatoon SK S7K 0M7; Sask'98; BSc; FRCPC; IntMed; GeriatricMed. Staff, Saskatoon City Hospital; Head Div of Geriatric Med., Dept of Med, University of Saskatchewan; (306)655-8925; Fax. (306)655-8929; jenny.basran@saskatoonhealthregion.ca.

BASRAN, Rashpal S; Royal University Hosp, 3666-103 Hospital Dr, Saskatoon SK S7N 0W8; Sask'95; FRCPC; IntMed; Cardiol. Staff, Royal University Hospital; (306)655-1504; Fax. (306)655-1506.

BASRAN, S K Cindy; The Ottawa Hosp-Civic Campus, B310-1053 Carling Ave, Ottawa ON K1Y 4E9; Sask'96; FRCPC; Anes. Staff, The Ottawa Hospital - Civic Campus; (613)986-4961

BASRUR, Vasanth R; Grand River Hosp-Kw Hlth Ctre, PO Box 9056 Stn C 835 King St W, Kitchener ON N2G 1G3; Tor'61; PhD; DMRT; FRCPC; RadOncol. Staff, Grand River Hospital - Kitchener/Waterloo Health Centre; (519)749-4370 x5489

BASS, Adam; Foothills Med Centre, 1403 29 St NW, Calgary AB T2N 2T9; Cal'06; FRCPC; IntMed; Nephrol. Staff, Foothills Medical Centre; (403)944-3962; Fax. (403)944-3199.

BASS, Bryan C; Ingram Family Physicians, 103-149 Ingram St, Duncan BC V9L 1N8; UBC'85; Staff, Cowichan District Hospital; (250)746-4401; Fax. (250)746-4473.

BASS, Catherine J; Canadian Forces Hlth Services, PO Box 1000 Stn Main Training Centre Bldg 0166, Borden ON L0M 1C0; (Other Foreign)'02; CCFP.

BASS, Juan A; Children's Hosp Eastern Ont, 401 Smyth Rd, Ottawa ON K1H 8L1; del Rosario Bogota (Colombia)'79; FRCSC; GenSurg; PedGenSurg. Asst Prof PedSurg, Children's Hospital of Eastern Ontario (CHEO); Asst Prof PedSurg, University of Ottawa; (613)737-7600 x2670; Fax. (613)738-4849; bass@cheo.on.ca.

BASS, Shana; 17 rue Baronscourt, Hampstead QC H3X 1H1; McG'90; CCFP; Staff, Sir Mortimer B Davis Jewish General; (514)488-0028

BASS, Stephanie J; Musquodoboit Harbour Med Clin, 7907 Highway 7, Musquodoboit Harbr NS B0J 2L0; Dal'03; CCFP; (902)889-2650

BASS, Sydney; 415 14 St NW, Calgary AB T2N 2A1; UBC'73; FRCPC; IntMed; Gastroent. (403)270-9555; Fax. (403)270-7479.

BASSAL, Christine; Centre Med Saint-Charles, 102-1740 ch Saint-Charles, Terrebonne QC J6W 3R3; Mon'87; Physician, Centre Medical St-Charles; (450)492-2277; Fax. (450)492-1030.

BASSARATH, Lindley E; Addiction & Mental Hlth-Clarke, 307-250 College St, Toronto ON M5T 1R8; Tor'87; FRCPC; Psy (Child Psychiatry). Staff, St Michael's Hospital; Staff Family Court Clinic, Centre for Addiction & Mental Health (CAMH) - College Street Site; (416)535-8501 x4856

BASSER, Wilma V; 375 Kingston Rd, Pickering ON L1V 1A3; Tor'63; FRCPC; IntMed (Gastroenterology). Ac Staff, The Scarborough Hospital - General Campus; (905)509-6888

BASSETT, Anne; Addiction & Mental Hlth-ARF Di, 1F-33 Russell St, Toronto ON M5S 2S1; UBC'82; FRCPC; Psy (Schizophrenia Genetics). Dir Clinical Genetics Research Prog, Centre for Addiction & Mental Health (CAMH) - Russell Street Site; Prof Psy, University of Toronto; (416)535-8501 x2734; Fax. (416)535-7199.

BASSETT, Kenneth L; Therapeutics Initiative, 2176 Health Sciences Mall, Vancouver BC V6T 1Z3; UBC'77; Staff Office of Health, UBC Hospital - Koerner Pavillion; (604)822-3130

BASSETT, Michael C; 104-15111 Russell Ave, White Rock BC V4B 2P4; UBC'71; BSc; MSc; Ac Staff, Peace Arch Hospital; (604)542-9831

BASSI, Amrik S; Martindale Med Clinic, 200-126 Martindale Dr NE, Calgary AB T3J 3G5; Punjab (India)'70; Langs: Punjabi; Hindi; Urdu; English; (403)293-7443; Fax. (403)293-7306.

BASSIL, Brian; Portage Prof Bldg, 601-5400 Portage Rd, Niagara Falls ON L2G 5X7; London (England)'65; MB BS; MRCP; DCH; Ac Staff, Niagara Health System - Greater Niagara General Site; (905)356-6333; Fax. (905)356-4166.

BASSILIOUS, Ereny; McMaster University, HSC 3A-1280 Main St W, Hamilton ON L8S 4K1; McM'05; FRCPC; Peds; Endocrin&Metab. (905)521-2100

BASSINGTHWAIGHTE, Mary; Nelson Mental Health Centre, 333 Victoria St, Nelson BC V1L 4K3; Seattle (USA)'85; Staff, Nelson Mental Health Centre; (250)505-7248

BASSON, Anel; Dr C W Wiebe Med Centre, 385 Main St, Winkler MB R6W 1J2; (Other Foreign)'06; (204)325-4312

BASSON, Denise I; North Shore Stress & Anxiety C, 330-145 Chadwick Crt, North Vancouver BC V7M 3K1; Cape Town (South Africa)'84; MB ChB; FRCPC; Psy. Staff Psy, Royal Ottawa Mental Health Centre - Royal Ottawa Health Care Group; (604)985-3535; Fax. (604)985-2670.

BASSON, Hendrik J; Dr C W Wiebe Med Centre, 385 Main St, Winkler MB R6W 1J2; (South Africa)'77; MB ChB; MD; (204)325-4312; Fax. (204)325-4594; basson@winklerclinic.com.

BASSON, Nico; South Hill Med Place, 5-2685 2 Ave W, Prince Albert SK S6V 5E3; Stellenbosch (South Africa)'95; MB ChB; (306)922-9570; Fax. (306)922-2513; bassonnico@hotmail.com.

BASSON, Nicol; East Hill Walk-In Clinic, 610-3020 22 St, Red Deer AB T4R 3J5; (South Africa)'87; MB ChB; LMCC; CCFP; Staff, Red Deer Regional Hospital Centre; (403)343-0115; Fax. (403)343-8551.

BASSON, Paul J; 100F-6640 Vedder Rd, Chilliwack BC V2R 0J2; Stellenbosch (South Africa)'87; MB ChB; Langs: Afrikaans; (604)858-2246; Fax. (604)858-4498; drpaulbasson@shawcable.com.

BASSON, Ronel C; Life Medical Clinic, PO Box 1406 Stn Main 4740 50 Ave, Whitecourt AB T7S 1P3; (South Africa)'95; MB ChB; LMCC; Staff, Whitecourt Healthcare Centre; (780)706-7080; Fax. (780)706-7064; jaimie@lifemedclinic.ca.

BASSON, Rosemary J; Purdy Pavilion, 2221 Wesbrook Mall, Vancouver BC V6T 1Z9; London (England)'71; MRCP; FRCP(UK); MD; Staff, Vancouver General Hospital - Centennial Pavillion; Court Staff, Lions Gate Hospital; Clin Prof/Dir Sexual Medicine, University of British Columbia; (604)827-1323; rosemarybasson@vch.ca.

BASSOON, Felix; Humber River Reg Hosp-Finch, 2111 Finch Ave W, North York ON M3N 1N1; McG'85; FRCPC; Anes. Staff, Humber River Regional Hospital - Finch Avenue Site; (416)747-3835; Fax. (416)747-3773.

BASSOON-ZALTZMAN, Caroline; Bathurst-Steeles Health Centre, 6257 Bathurst St, North York ON M2R 2A5; McG'85; ABIM; FRCPC; IntMed (Endocrinology). (416)223-9791; Fax. (416)223-9558.

BASSYOUNI, Hanan A; Peter Lougheed Centre, 3500 26 Ave NE, Calgary AB T1Y 6J4; Cal'98; MD; FRCPC; Endocrin&Metab; IntMed (Endocrinology). Consultant, Peter Lougheed Centre; Langs: Arabic; (403)943-5425

BASTA, Ayman F; Carberry Plain Health Centre, PO Box 2000 210 First Ave, Carberry MB R0K 0H0; Cairo (Egypt)'98; CCFP; Fam Med, Carberry Plains Health Centre; (204)834-2144

BASTA, Magdy N; Queen Elizabeth II HSC-Halifax, 2501E-1796 Summer St, Halifax NS B3H 3A7; Assiut (Egypt)'82; MB ChB; Staff, Queen Elizabeth II Health Sciences Centre - Halifax Infirmary Site; Staff, Queen Elizabeth II Health Sciences Centre - Victoria General Site; (902)473-4417; Fax. (902)473-3158.

BASTA, Mourad M; Bayshore Med Bldg, 202-3029 Carling Ave, Ottawa ON K2B 8E8; Cairo (Egypt)'72; MB ChB; CCFP; FCFP; Langs: Arabic; (613)726-1839; Fax. (613)726-9733.

BASTA, Sally; North York Total Rehab, 5292 Yonge St, North York ON M2N 5P9; Ott'07; CCFP; (416)223-6666; Fax. (416)223-5591.

BASTARACHE, Annie; Groupe Med de Trois-Rivieres, 225-1900 boul des Recollets, Trois-Rivieres QC G8Z 4K4; Laval'88; Staff, Centre de santé Cloutier-du-Rivage; (819)375-6666; Fax. (819)373-3423; abasta@hotmail.com.

BASTARACHE, Patrice; CHUS-Hop Fleurimont, 3001 12e Av N, Sherbrooke QC J1H 5N4; Sher'96; CCFP; CCFP(E.M.); Staff, Centre Hospitalier Universitaire de Sherbrooke-Hopital Fleurimont; (819)346-1110

BASTARRIKA ALEMAN, Gorka; Sunnybrook Hlth Sciences Ctre, 2075 Bayview Ave, Toronto ON M4N 3M5; Pamplona (Spain)'98; Staff, Sunnybrook Health Sciences Centre; (416)480-6100

BASTEDO, Clare; Ctr Hosp de LaSalle, 8585 Tsse Champlain, LaSalle QC H8P 1C1; Wes'05; FRCPC; Gastroent; IntMed. Staff, Centre Hospitalier de LaSalle; (514)362-8000

BASTEDO, Paul A; 201-29 Main St E, Huntsville ON P1H 2C6; Tor'74; CCFP; FCFP; Staff, Huntsville District Memorial Hospital - Muskoka Algonquin Healthcare; (705)789-2345; Fax. (705)789-5977; pbastedo@gmail.com.

BASTEDO, Timothy P; 1882 Niagara Stone Rd, Niagara-on-the-Lke ON L0S 1T0; Tor'10; CCFP; (905)468-3275

BASTI, Peyvand A; 199-5 Fairview Mall Dr, North York ON M2J 2Z1; (Iran)'96; CCFP; Langs: Farsi; (416)619-5995

BASTIAN, Elizabeth J; Bulkley Valley Dist Hosp, PO Box 370 3950 8th Ave, Smithers BC V0J 2N0; McG'75; Staff, Bulkley Valley District Hospital; (250)847-6219; Fax. (250)847-6230.

BASTIAN, James S; Nu Image Medispa, 101-2631 28th Ave, Regina SK S4S 6X3; Sask'84; BSc(Physiol); BA(Hons.)(P; DAB; FACOG; FRCSC; ObstGyn (Cosmetic Surgery). (306)790-8500; Fax. (306)790-8501.

BASTIANELLI, Francesco E; Nepean Med Centre, 211-1 Centrepointe Dr, Nepean ON K2G 6E2; Ott'81; FRCSC; Ophth. Ac Staff, The Ottawa Hospital - Riverside Campus; (613)226-1919; Fax. (613)226-2803.

BASTIANON, Todd M; Casselman Med Centre, PO Box 380 629 Principal St, Casselman ON K0A 1M0; Tor'90; CCFP; (613)764-5440; Fax. (613)764-9974.

BASTIANON, William A; Tecumseh Med Centre, 104-11811 Tecumseh Rd E, Windsor ON N8N 4M7; Wes'92; Court Staff, Hôtel-Dieu Grace Hospital; (519)979-3355; Fax. (519)979-1429.

BASTIDE, Adrien; CHUQ-Ctr Hosp Univ Laval, 2705 boul Laurier, Quebec QC G1V 4G2; Bordeaux (France)'60; ObstGyn (P.Q.) (Perinatal Medicine). Staff, Centre Hospitalier Universitaire de Quebec-CHUL; adj Prof, Université Laval; (418)656-4141; adrien.bastide@ogy.ulaval.ca.

BASTIEN, Francine; CLSC Pte-aux-Trembles Mtl Est, 13926 rue Notre-Dame E, Pte-aux-Trembles QC H1A 1T5; Mon'88; (514)642-4050; Fax. (514)642-5438.

BASTIEN, Francois; Clinique Med Havre Sante, 521 boul Du Havre, Salaber-de-Valleyf QC J6S 4Z5; Mon'67; Staff, Centre Hospitalier Régional du Suroît; Physician, Asten Hill Assurance; (450)371-6444 x260; Fax. (450)371-5315.

BASTIEN, Gilles Simon; 1385 rue Jean-Talon E, Montreal QC H2E 1S6; McG'79; MHSA(Ed); CCFP; Staff, CSSS du Coeur de l'Isle Hôpital Jean-Talon; Langs: French; English; (514)495-6767 x6234; Fax. (514)495-6783; gilles.bastien@videotron.ca.

BASTIEN, Marie-Claude; Polyclinique Saint-Eustache, 75 rue Grignon, Saint-Eustache QC J7P 4J2; Mon'89; Staff Ped & Obst, Hôpital de Saint-Eustache; Langs: English; (450)623-6170

BASTIEN, Marie-Helene; CHUQ-Ctr Hosp Univ Laval, 1207-2705 boul Laurier, Quebec QC G1V 4G2; Laval'02; IntMed. Staff, Centre Hospitalier Universitaire de Quebec-CHUL; (418)525-4444

BASTIEN, Nancy; GMF Lafontaine, 242 rue Lafontaine, Riviere-du-Loup QC G5R 3A7; Sher'89; Staff, Centre Hospitalier Regional du Grand-Portage; Langs: Bilingual(French/English); (418)862-3110; Fax. (418)862-9656.

BASTIEN, Pascal; North York Gen Hosp, 4001 Leslie St, North York ON M2K 1E1; Ott'08; FRCPC; IntMed. Staff, North York General Hospital; (416)756-6000

BASTIEN, Pierre; CSSS d'Antoine-Labelle-Mt Laur, RR 1 2561 ch de la Lievre S, Mont-Laurier QC J9L 3G3; Mon'73; ObstGyn. Ac Staff, Hopital de la Cite de la santé; Langs: English; (819)623-1234

BASTIEN, Sylvie; Clin Familiale du Boulevard, 19-300 boul Saint-Luc, St-Jean-Sur-Richel QC J2W 2A3; Mon'85; (450)349-3333; Fax. (450)349-1155.

BASTIEN, Yves; CSSS de Saint-Jerome, 290 rue de Montigny, Saint-Jerome QC J7Z 5T3; Sher'74; ABIM; IntMed. Ac Staff, Hôtel-Dieu de Saint-Jérôme; Langs: English; (450)431-8200

BASTIEN-CHRETIEN, Christine; CSSS de Rimouski-Neigette, CP 3150 succ A 150 av Rouleau, Rimouski QC G5L 5T1; Laval'07; Psy. Staff, Hôpital Regional Rimouski; (418)724-8441

BASTIN, Gauthier; Centre Med St-Leonard, 360 rue Béliveau, St-Leonard-d'Aston QC J0C 1M0; Sher'88; ac Staff, Hôpital Sainte-croix; adj Prof, Centre Hospitalier Universitaire de Sherbrooke-Hopital Fleurimont; (819)399-2030; Fax. (819)399-2343; gauthier_bastin@gmf.gouv.qc.ca.

BASUR, Roshan L; 102-2425 Tecumseh Rd E, Windsor ON N8W 1E6; Srinagar (India)'68; LRCP; MRCS; FRCS; Ac Staff, Windsor Regional Hospital - Metropolitan Site; (519)944-1344; Fax. (519)944-7220.

BASWICK, Brenda; The Credit Valley Hosp, 2200 Eglinton Ave W, Mississauga ON L5M 2N1; McM'09; CCFP; Staff, The Credit Valley Hospital; (905)813-2200

BATA, Iqbal R; Queen Elizabeth II HSC-Halifax, 2149-1796 Summer St, Halifax NS B3H 3A7; Newcastle-Upon-Tyne (England)'82; FRCPC; IntMed; Cardiol. Staff, Queen Elizabeth II Health Sciences Centre - Halifax Infirmary Site; Staff Cardiol & Med, Queen Elizabeth II Health Sciences Centre - Victoria General Site; Assoc Prof Med, Dalhousie University; (902)473-8623; Fax. (902)473-2434.

BATALION, Hyman; Hop Ste-Anne, 305 boul Anciens-Combattants, Ste-Anne-de-Bellev QC H9X 1Y9; McG'61; Staff Dept of Veterans Affairs, Hopital Ste-Anne; (514)457-3440; Fax. (514)457-8466.

BATARSEH, Samir J; Albany Medical Clinic, 807 Broadview Ave, Toronto ON M4K 2P9; Cairo (Egypt)'62; MB ChB; FRCSC; ObstGyn (Infertility). Chief Dept of ObstGyn & Dir, Toronto East General Hospital Inc; Co-Dir, I V F Canada; Langs: Bilingual(English/French); (416)461-9471

BATAY-CSORBA, Peter A; Health & Wellness, 303-250 Harding Blvd W, Richmond Hill ON L4C 9M7; Tor'87; BSc; PhD; Ac Staff, Mackenzie Richmond Hill Hospital; Langs: Spanish; Hungarian; (905)737-3071

BATCHELOR, Bret E; 864 Old Loop Rd, Vanderhoof BC V0J 3A2; Cal'08; CCFP; (250)567-2201

BATCHRA, Nandita; 5-1435 Plains Rd E, Burlington ON L7R 3P9; Tor'93; FRCSC; Otol. Ac Staff, Joseph Brant Memorial Hospital; Langs: Punjabi; Hindi; (905)681-3663; Fax. (905)681-4510.

BATEJKO, Oksana; St Joseph's Health Ctre, 30 The Queensway, Toronto ON M6R 1B5; Saba (Netherlands Antilles)'02; Staff, St Joseph's Health Centre; (416)530-6000

BATEMAN, Gail E; Red Deer Reg Hosp Centre, PO Box 5030 Stn Postal Box Ctr 3942 50A Ave, Red Deer AB T4N 6R2; Dal'98; FRCPC; DiagRad. Staff, Red Deer Regional Hospital Centre; (403)343-4792; Fax. (403)343-4433.

BATEMAN, Kendall H; Grey Nun's Community Hosp & HC, 1100 Youville Drive West NW, Edmonton AB T6L 5X8; Dal'01; FRCPC; Anes. Staff, Covenant Health - Grey Nuns Community Hospital; (780)450-7020

BATEMAN, William A; Medcan Health Mgmt Inc, 1500-150 York St, Toronto ON M5H 3S5; Qns'83; DAvMed; Staff Emerg, Niagara Health System - Douglas Memorial Hospital Site; Staff Emerg, Humber River Regional Hospital - Finch Avenue Site; Consultant Aerospace & Diving Med, DRDC Toronto; Staff, Medcan Health Management Inc; (416)340-5900; Fax. (416)350-5981; william.bateman@drdc-rddc.gc.ca.

BATER, Marilyn G; Royal Jubilee Hosp, KW162-1952 Bay St, Victoria BC V8R 1J8; Alb'86; FRCPC; IntMed; GeriatricMed. Staff, Royal Jubilee Hospital; Med Dir, Seniors Health, Vancouver Island Health Authority; Clin Instructor, University of British Columbia; (250)370-8752; Fax. (250)370-8285.

BATES, Carol E; York Medical, 123-14800 Yonge St, Aurora ON L4G 1N3; Tor'86; CCFP; Staff, Southlake Regional Health Centre; (905)713-0404; Fax. (905)713-6341.

BATES, Douglas R; University Downs Fam Practice, 425 University Ave E, Waterloo ON N2K 4C9; Cal'78; CCFP; FCFP; Staff, Grand River Hospital - Kitchener/Waterloo Health Centre; Staff, St Mary's General Hospital; (519)569-8821; Fax. (519)569-8823.

BATES, J Terence; Anne Johnston Health Station, 2398 Yonge St, Toronto ON M4P 2H4; Tor'69; MPH; DABPM(OccupMed); CCFP; Ac Staff, North York General Hospital; Court Staff, Sunnybrook Health Sciences Centre; Physician, Anne Johnston Health Station; Asst Prof, University of Toronto; (416)486-8666; Fax. (416)486-8660; tbates@toronto.ca.

BATES, J Wayne; Orillia Soldiers Mem Hosp, 170 Colborne St W, Orillia ON L3V 2Z3; Qns'69; Staff, Orillia Soldiers' Memorial Hospital; (705)325-2201

BATES, Janet M; Scotch Creek Medical Clinic, 2-3874 Squilax-Anglemont Rd, Scotch Creek BC V0E 1M5; Alb'90; (250)955-0660

BATES, Joanna M; Ctre for Hlth Educ Scholarship, 3326-910 10th Ave W, Vancouver BC V5Z 1M9; McG'76; CCFP; FCFP; Dir Med Educ, Providence Health Care - St Paul's Hospital; Dep Registrar, College of Physicians & Surgeons of British Columbia; Asst Prof/Dir Centre for Hlth Educ Scholarship, University of British Columbia; (604)875-5185

BATES, K Stephen; Avenue Med Centre, 1-221 Brant Ave, Brantford ON N3T 3J2; McM'79; FRCSC; ObstGyn. Staff, The Brant Community Healthcare System - Brantford General Hospital Site; Clin Assoc Prof ObstGyn, McMaster University; (519)753-8666; Fax. (519)753-3109; stephen.bates@sympatico.ca.

BATES, Kenneth R J; North Shuswap Medical, 2-3974 Squilax-Anglemont Rd, Scotch Creek BC V0E 1M5; Cal'80; CCFP; (250)955-0660; Fax. (250)679-5518.

BATES, Robert; 2B-150 Sidney St, Belleville ON K8P 5E2; Tor'81; Staff Med & Family Practice, QHC Belleville General.

BATES, Sarah L; Sheldon Chumir Centre, 1213 4 St SW, Calgary AB T2R 0X7; Cal'00; CCFP; (780)436-0020; Fax. (780)436-0603.

BATES, Shannon M; McMaster University Med Ctre, HSC 3W11-1200 Main St W, Hamilton ON L8N 3Z5; McG'91; BSc; MSc; FRCPC; IntMed (Thromboembolism); Hem. Staff Thromboembolism Unit, Hamilton Health Sciences Centre-Juravinski Site; Staff Thromboembolism Unit, Hamilton Health Sciences Centre - McMaster Children's Hospital; Assoc Prof Med, McMaster University; (905)521-2100 x73928

BATES, Susan J; Complexe Sante Reine-Elizabeth, 335-2100 av de Marlowe, Montreal QC H4A 3L5; McG'78; (514)868-9710; Fax. (514)868-9710.

BATES, W Paul; 16 Longbow Rd, London ON N6G 1Y4; Tor'70; CCFP; FCFP; Court Staff, London Health Sciences Centre - Victoria Campus; Court Staff, St Joseph's Hospital - St Joseph's Health Care; Med Examiner, Civil Aviation Canada; Med Examiner Marine Medicine, Transport Canada; batesp@tc.gc.ca.

BATES, William F; 267 County Rd 3 RR 1 Stn Main, Belleville ON K8N 4Z1; Qns'64; Hon Staff, QHC Belleville General; (613)966-5000; Fax. (613)962-0688.

BATH, Navdeep; Trelawny Medical Centre, 10-3899 Trelawny Circle, Mississauga ON L5N 6S3; Punjab (India)'90; MB BS; CCFP; FCFP; Langs: Punjabi; Hindi; Urdu; (905)785-9449

BATH, Parvinder S; 14 Ostrander Blvd, Brampton ON L6X 0G8; Punjab (India)'88; MB BS; CCFP; FCFP; (905)566-9449

BATHALON, Sebastien; CSSS Drummond-Hop Sainte-Croix, 570 rue Heriot, Drummondville QC J2B 1C1; Sher'00; FRCSC; Otol. Staff, Hôpital Sainte-croix; (819)478-6464

BATHE, Oliver F; Tom Baker Cancer Centre, 1331 29 St NW, Calgary AB T2N 4N2; Cal'90; MSc; FACS; FRCSC; GenSurg (Gastrointestinal Surgery). Staff, Foothills Medical Centre; Staff Div of SurgOncol, Tom Baker Cancer Centre; University of Calgary; Langs: German; (403)521-3275; Fax. (403)944-3926; bathe@ucalgary.ca.

BATHINA, Sudheer; Upper River Valley Hosp, 11300 130 Rte, Watervil-Carleton NB E7P 0A4; Andhra (India)'97; Staff, Upper River Valley Hospital - Waterville; (506)375-8488

BATIST, Gerald; SMBD Jewish Gen Hosp, 3755 ch Cote-Sainte-Catherine, Montreal QC H3T 1E2; McG'77; FRCPC; MedOncol; IntMed (P.Q.). Staff Oncol, Sir Mortimer B Davis Jewish General; Head Centre for Translational Research, McGill University; (514)340-8222 x5527; gbatist@jgh.mcgill.ca.

BATOHI, Pravin; St Joseph's Health Care, PO Box 5777 Stn B 268 Grosvenor St, London ON N6A 4V2; Natal (South Africa)'83; MB ChB; LMCC(SA); BSc; DA; FRCP; Anes. Staff, St Joseph's Hospital - St Joseph's Health Care; Staff, London Health Sciences Centre - University Hospital; Asst Prof Anes & Perioperative Med, University of Western Ontario; Langs: Afrikaans; Zulu; (519)646-6000 x64219; Fax. (519)646-6116.

BATOOL, Muqadas; Stonebridge Med & Cosmetics Ct, 2-303 Stonebridge Blvd, Saskatoon SK S7T 0G3; CCFP; (306)382-6666; Fax. (306)382-6686.

BATOOL, Tahira; McMaster University, MDCL 3101A-1280 Main St W, Hamilton ON L8S 4K1; Punjab (India)'05; IntMed.

BATRA, Gurumukh D; 303-168 Charlotte St, Ottawa ON K1N 8K6; Vikram (India)'62; MB BS; MD; FAAP; FRCPC; Peds (Clinical Pediatrics). Ac Staff, Children's Hospital of Eastern Ontario (CHEO); Asst Prof, University of Ottawa; (613)789-0238

BATT, Jane A E; St Michael's Hosp, 30 Bond St, Toronto ON M5B 1W8; McM'91; FRCPC; IntMed; Respir. Staff, St Michael's Hospital; (416)864-6060 x77645

BATT, Nathan; 236 Hastings St E, Vancouver BC V6A 1P1; UBC'66; Vis Staff, Vancouver General Hospital - Centennial Pavillion; Clin Instructor, University of British Columbia; (604)669-8377

BATTAD, Anthony B; St Boniface Gen Hosp, C5012-409 Tache Ave, Winnipeg MB R3T 2E8; Man'99; FRCPC; IntMed. Staff, St Boniface General Hospital; (204)269-3570

BATTAGLIA, Donna; St Thomas-Elgin Gen Hosp, PO Box 2007 Stn Main 189 Elm St, St Thomas ON N5P 3W2; Tor'83; FRCPC; AnatPath. Staff, St Thomas Elgin General Hospital; (519)631-2030; Fax. (519)637-3222.

BATTCOCK, Natalie R; Western Mem Reg Hosp, PO Box 2005 Stn Main 1 Brookfield Ave, Corner Brook NL A2H 6J7; Mem'85; ACLS; ATLS; CCFP; Staff, Health Sciences Centre; Staff, Western Memorial Regional Hospital; Staff, Eastern Health Corporate Office; (709)777-6300

BATTCOCK, Stephen G; St Clare's Mercy Hosp, 154 Lemarchant Rd, St. John's NL A1C 5B8; Mem'83; DiagRad. Staff Radiol, St Clare's Mercy Hospital; (709)777-5602; Fax. (709)777-5210.

BATTEL, Luigi A; Kingston Family Health Team, 200-2437 Princess St, Kingston ON K7M 3G1; Tor'92; CCFP; FCFP; Staff Family & EmergMed, Sault Area Hospital - Sault Ste Marie; Langs: Italian; (613)546-6652; Fax. (613)546-5292.

BATTEN, Adrian P; Grand River Hosp-Kw Hlth Ctre, PO Box 9056 Stn C 835 King St W, Kitchener ON N2G 1G3; McG'83; FRCPC; AnatPath; GenPath. Staff, Grand River Hospital - Kitchener/Waterloo Health Centre; (519)749-4300 x3900

BATTEN, Brian K; Ross Mem Hosp, 10 Angeline St N, Lindsay ON K9V 4M8; McM'85; Staff, Ross Memorial Hospital; (705)328-6143

BATTEN, Jane S; Family Practice 535, 535 Montreal Rd, Ottawa ON K1K 0V1; McG'86; BSc(Hons); MSc(Anatomy); CCFP; Langs: English; French; (613)746-5350; Fax. (613)746-5340.

BATTEN, Tony F; ENT Consultants, 219-1 Paton St, St. John's NL A1B 4S8; Mem'90; FRCSC; Otol. Staff Head & Neck Surg, Health Care Corporation Of St John's; (709)579-1003; Fax. (709)579-1708.

BATTERSHILL, Peter M; BC Cancer Agency-Vanc Isl Ctr, 2410 Lee Ave, Victoria BC V8R 6V5; UBC'81; Staff, BC Cancer Agency Vancouver Island Centre; Fam Med, Dawson Creek & District Hospital; (250)519-5572

BATTH, Sue K; 1-3 Catalina Dr, Nepean ON K2H 7X2; Ott'75; BSc(Hons); FRCPC; Psy (Tourette's Disorder). Consultant, Royal Ottawa Mental Health Centre - Royal Ottawa Health Care Group; Clinical Asst Prof Med, University of Ottawa; Langs: Punjabi; (613)596-2858; Fax. (613)596-3293; sbatth.tait@gmail.com.

BATTHISH, Michelle; The Hosp for Sick Children, 555 University Ave, Toronto ON M5G 1X8; Tor'05; FRCPC; Peds; Rheum. Staff, The Hospital For Sick Children; (416)813-7500

BATTIGELLI, Marino; The Credit Valley Hosp, 2200 Eglinton Ave W, Mississauga ON L5M 2N1; McM'76; FRCPC; Psy (Administrative Psychiatry). Affil Staff, Joseph Brant Memorial Hospital; Chief Psy, The Credit Valley Hospital; (905)813-4421

BATTISTA, Renaldo N; Fonds de Recherche du Quebec-S, 800-500 rue Sherbrooke O, Montreal QC H3A 3C6; Mon'72; MPH(Harvard); DSc(Harvard); FRCPC; CommunMed. Staff, McGill University Health Centre - Montreal General Campus; Pres, Agency for Health Services & Technology Assessment; Dir Health Administration, Universite de Montreal; Prof, McGill University; Langs: Italian; Spanish; (514)873-2114

BATTISTUZZI, Susan C; St Boniface Gen Hosp, 409 Tache Ave, Winnipeg MB R2H 2A6; Man'94; BSc; MSc; FRCPC; AnatPath. Staff, St Boniface General Hospital; (204)632-7133; sbattistuzzi@sogh.mb.ca.

BATTY, Helen P; Women's College Hosp, 76 Grenville St, Toronto ON M5S 1B2; Tor'73; MEd; CCFP; FCFP; Staff Family Practice Health Centre, Women's College Hospital; Teach Staff, University of Toronto; (416)323-6244

BATUYONG, Eldridge D; Red Deer Reg Hosp Centre, PO Box Stn Postal Box Centre 3942 50A Ave, Red Deer AB T4N 6R2; Wes'06; FRCSC; OrthSurg. Staff, Red Deer Regional Hospital Centre; (403)343-4422; Fax. (403)343-4866.

BAU, Alan L; The Credit Valley Hosp, 2200 Eglinton Ave W, Mississauga ON L5M 2N1; Tor'94; FRCPC; DiagRad. Staff, The Credit Valley Hospital; (905)813-3978; Fax. (905)813-3042.

BAUER, Christopher A; Valley Reg Hosp, 150 Exhibition St, Kentville NS B4N 5E3; Alb'88; Staff, Valley Regional Hospital; Langs: American Sign Language; German; (902)678-7381; Fax. (902)679-1206.

BAUER, Robert; Humber River Reg Hosp-Church, 200 Church St, Toronto ON M9N 1N8; McG'86; FACC; FRCPC; IntMed; Cardiol. Staff, Humber River Regional Hospital - Church Street Site; Langs: English; French; Italian; (416)245-1150; Fax. (416)245-1166.

BAUERMEISTER, Senta; 2205 Millar Rd W RR 4, Spencerville ON K0E 1X0; Ott'90; (613)658-1200

BAUGHAN, James G; 209-300 Columbia St, Kamloops BC V2C 6L1; Alb'98; BMedSci; FRCSC; GenSurg. Staff GenSurg, Royal Inland Hospital; (250)374-0574; Fax. (250)374-5584; baughan2@telus.net.

BAUGNIET, Jessica L; Dixie Road Med Associates, 2200 Dixie Rd, Mississauga ON L4Y 1Z4; Wes'00; CCFP; (905)279-1700

BAULD GIFFIN, Dawn; London HSC-Victoria Hosp, 800 Commissioners Rd E, London ON N6A 5W9; Wes'95; FRCPC; EmergMed. Staff, London Health Sciences Centre - Victoria Campus; (519)667-6538; Fax. (519)667-6769.

BAUM, Joseph B; Medical Clinic Bldg, 201-89 Humber College Blvd, Etobicoke ON M9V 4B8; Tor'76; FRCSC; PlasSurg. Staff, William Osler Health System - Etobicoke General Hospital; (416)746-0138

BAUM, Sol; Bathurst-Steeles Health Centre, 6257 Bathurst St, North York ON M2R 2A5; Ott'76; CCFP; FCFP; Staff, Mount Sinai Hospital; Staff, North York General Hospital - Branson Division; Staff, North York General Hospital; (416)223-9791; Fax. (416)223-9558.

BAUMAN, Gary T; Vancouver Native Health Clinic, 449 Hastings St E, Vancouver BC V6A 1P5; UBC'85; Assoc Staff, Providence Health Care - St Paul's Hospital; Staff, Street Health Outreach Program; (604)255-9766; Fax. (604)254-5750.

BAUMAN, Glenn S; London Reg Cancer Centre, 790 Commissioners Rd E, London ON N6A 4L6; Wes'90; FRCPC; RadOncol. Chief/Dept Chair Oncol, University of Western Ontario; (519)685-8500; Fax. (519)685-8739.

BAUMAN, John; 500-1060 7 St SW, Calgary AB T2R 0C4; Sydney (Australia)'67; FRCS(E); FRCSC; OrthSurg (Disability Assessment). Staff, Rockyview General Hospital; Staff, Peter Lougheed Centre; Clinical Asst Prof, University of Alberta; (403)777-2244; Fax. (403)777-2241.

BAUMAN, Kent; Beechwood Forest Med Centre, 2-890 Glasgow St, Kitchener ON N2N 3G6; Wes'87; CCFP; FCFP; Court Staff, Grand River Hospital - Kitchener/Waterloo Health Centre; Court Staff, St Mary's General Hospital; (519)744-4293; Fax. (519)744-6424.

BAUMAN, Nicholaus L L; 41 Frederick St, Orillia ON L3V 5W6; McM'03; FRCSC; GenSurg. (705)481-1419; Fax. (705)327-3284.

BAUMAN, Shannon; Sports Med and Rehab Ctre, 104-480 Huronia Rd Box 15, Barrie ON L4N 6M2; McM'03; Dip SportMed; CCFP; Family Medicine, Royal Victoria Regional Health Centre; (705)734-3340; Fax. (705)734-9210.

BAUMANN, Paul O; 64A River Street, Parry Sound ON P2A 2T6; Qns'10; FRCPC; Peds; (416)442-5600.

BAUMANDER, Donald; Bramalea City Centre, 387-25 Peel Centre Dr, Brampton ON L6T 3R5; Tor'82; Staff, William Osler Health System - Brampton Civic Hospital; (905)793-7077; Fax. (905)793-7506.

BAUMGARD, Godfrey M; Burrard Health Bldg, 604-1160 Burrard St, Vancouver BC V6Z 2E8; Manchester (England)'69; MB ChB; FRCPC; Peds. Assoc Staff, Providence Health Care - St Paul's Hospital; Ac Staff, BC Children's Hospital; Ac Staff, BC Women's Hospital & Health Centre; Clin Prof Peds, University of British Columbia; (604)685-6161

BAUNEMANN, Heiko; Port Arthur Health Centre Inc, 194 Court St N, Thunder Bay ON P7A 4V7; Muenster (Germany)'60; FACOG; MD; FRCSC; ObstGyn. Court Staff Gyn (All Sites), Thunder Bay Regional Health Sciences Centre; Langs: German; (807)346-1000; Fax. (807)346-6251.

BAUR, Martin; 205-9148 23 Ave NW, Edmonton AB T6N 1H9; UBC'02; FRCPC; IntMed. Staff, University of Alberta Hospital; (780)462-3010

BAUR, Nicole; 206-1650 Terminal Ave, Nanaimo BC V9S 0A3; UBC'07; FRCPC; IntMed; Rheum. (250)591-4293

BAUSET, Richard; Southlake Reg Health Centre, 596 Davis Dr, Newmarket ON L3Y 2P9; Sher'83; Cardiovasc&ThorSurg; GenSurg (P.Q.). Staff, Southlake Regional Health Centre; (905)895-4521

BAUSMER, Tracy A; New Vision Family Health Team, 421 Greenbrook Dr, Kitchener ON N2M 4K1; Tor'02; CCFP; (519)578-3510; Fax. (519)578-6040.

BAUTISTA, Alberto; Nineteen-O-Nine Med Centre, 1909 Tecumseh Rd E, Windsor ON N8W 1C9; Manila (Philippines)'62; FRCPC; IntMed. (519)255-9217; Fax. (519)255-1039.

BAUTISTA, Dorothy V; Dr Charles A Janeway Child HC, 300 Prince Philip Dr, St. John's NL A1B 3V6; Mem'85; FRCSC; Ophth (Pediatric Ophthalmology & Strabismus). Staff, Janeway Children's Health & Rehabilitation Centre; (709)777-4696

BAUTISTA, Elizabeth M; Killick Health Services Inc, 129 Lincoln Rd, Grnd-Falls-Windsor NL A2A 1P3; Mem'99; CCFP; (709)292-8400

BAUTISTA, Filomena M; 315-3024 Hurontario St, Mississauga ON L5B 4M4; Santo Tomas (Philippines)'81; CCFP; Ac Staff, Trillium Health Centre - Mississauga; (905)566-8250; Fax. (905)566-0676.

BAUTISTA, Michael J; Dr L A Miller Centre, 100 Forest Rd, St. John's NL A1A 1E5; Mem'81; AB; FRCPC; Anes. Staff, St Clare's Mercy Hospital; Clinical Asst Prof, Memorial University Of Newfoundland; (709)777-6555

BAVAKUTTY MOHAMMED, Sheeja; 8-700 Markham Rd, Scarborough ON M1H 2A7; (India)'91; CCFP; (416)264-3443

BAVERSTOCK, Marcus B; 2012 2nd St N, Cranbrook BC V1C 4M5; London (England)'62; MB BS; MRCP(Lond); FRCPC; IntMed. Staff, East Kootenay Regional Hospital; (250)426-2610; Fax. (250)489-2612.

BAVERSTOCK, Richard J; Rockyview Gen Hosp, 6608-7007 14 St SW, Calgary AB T2V 1P9; UBC'98; BSc; FRCSC; Urol (Incontinence). Staff, Rockyview General Hospital; (403)943-8980; Fax. (403)943-8979.

BAW, Bandar A I; Hamilton HS-General Campus, 237 Barton St E, Hamilton ON L8L 2X2; Jeddah (Saudi Arabia)'00; FRCPC; EmergMed. Staff, Hamilton Health Sciences Centre - Hamilton General Hospital; (905)527-4322

BAWA, Faizal I; Bracebridge Med Centre, 2-55 Muskoka Rd 118 W, Bracebridge ON P1L 1T2; Wes'96; CCFP; Asst Prof, Northern Ontario School of Medicine-Laurentian University; (705)645-1027; Fax. (705)646-2543.

BAWA, Hussam-Ul H; 200-2580 32 St NE, Calgary AB T1Y 7M8; Karachi (Pakistan)'80; MB BS; MRCPsy(U.K.); MCPS(Pakistan); DPM(Ireland); FRCPC; Psy. Staff, Peter Lougheed Centre; Clinical Asst Prof Psy, University of Calgary; Langs: Urdu; Punjabi; Bengali; (403)944-9700

BAWA, Jameet; Etobicoke Walk-In & Family Phy, 106-100 Humber College Blvd, Etobicoke ON M9V 5G4; Tor'02; CCFP; (416)742-9449; Fax. (416)742-6963.

BAWA, Yusuf E; PO Box 48114, New Westminster BC V3M 0A7; Natal (South Africa)'84; MB ChB; Med Dir, Langley Memorial Hospital; (604)526-9633

BAWANGOANWALA, Asifa; 3350 Smoke Tree Rd, Mississauga ON L5N 7M5; Amravati (India)'96; MB BS; CCFP; Langs: Urdu; Gujarati; Marathi; (905)566-1414

BAWAZEER, Mohammed A; St Michael's Hosp, 30 Bond St, Toronto ON M5B 1W8; Jeddah (Saudi Arabia)'02; FRCSC; GenSurg. Staff, St Michael's Hospital; (416)685-4996

BAWDEN, Carole A; 202-1865 Marine Dr, West Vancouver BC V7V 1J7; UBC'93; FRCPC; Psy. (604)926-6670

BAX, Kevin; London HSC-Victoria Hosp, B1 164-800 Commissioners Rd E, London ON N6A 5W9; Indiana (USA)'01; FAAP; Staff, London Health Sciences Centre - Victoria Campus; (519)685-8354; Fax. (519)685-8156.

BAXENDALE, Gary R; 203-3825 Sunset St, Burnaby BC V5G 1T4; UBC'92; CCFP; CCFP(E.M.); Staff, Burnaby Hospital; (604)434-9515

BAXTER, Alan D; The Ottawa Hosp-Gen Campus, 501 Smyth Rd, Ottawa ON K1H 8L6; Oxford (England)'71; BMus; BSc; FFARCS; FRCPC; Anes. Staff, The Ottawa Hospital - General Campus; Clin Assoc Prof, University of Ottawa; (613)737-8187

BAXTER, Brian; 425 Cecelia St, Pembroke ON K8A 1S7; UBC'76; (613)735-3188; Fax. (613)735-2296.

BAXTER, Cecilia I; Royal Alexandra Hosp, 2F-10240 Kingsway NW, Edmonton AB T5H 3V9; Cal'80; BSc; FRCPC; Peds. Staff Children's Pavillon, Royal Alexandra Hospital; Emeritus Prof, University of Alberta; (780)735-4605; Fax. (780)735-4071; cecilia.baxter@albertahealthservices.ca.

BAXTER, Colin H; Yorkview Med Centre, 104-3695 Keele St, North York ON M3J 1N2; Aberdeen (Scotland)'66; MB ChB; Ac Staff, Humber River Regional Hospital - Finch Avenue Site; (416)633-3711; Fax. (416)633-0521.

BAXTER, Cynthia L; Sunridge Prof Centre, 201-2675 36 St NE, Calgary AB T1Y 6H6; Alb'99; FRCPC; Psy. Staff, Peter Lougheed Centre; (403)943-5656

BAXTER, Daniel J G; Montfort Hosp, 713 Montreal Rd, Ottawa ON K1K 0T2; McG'05; FRCPC; DiagRad. Staff, Montfort Hospital; (613)746-4621

BAXTER, Edith M; Family Practice Associates, 200-6155 North St, Halifax NS B3K 5R3; Dal'04; CCFP; (902)453-3511; Fax. (902)454-9010.

BAXTER, Frederick J; St Joseph's Healthcare, 50 Charlton Ave E, Hamilton ON L8N 4A6; McM'74; FRCPC; Anes;CCFP; CCFP(E.M.); Chief Anes, St Joseph's Healthcare - Charlton Campus; Court Staff, Hamilton Health Sciences Centre - McMaster University Medical Centre; Clin Assoc Prof Anes, McMaster University; (905)522-4941 x3853; Fax. (905)521-6019.

BAXTER, Heather A; Maternity Care Clinic, 109-178 96 Ave NE, Calgary AB T3K 6G4; Tor'83; CCFP; FCFP; Physician, Maternity Care Clinic; (403)735-4922; Fax. (403)735-4901.

BAXTER, Kathy L; Harbour Centre, 706-133 Prince William St, Saint John NB E2L 2B5; Mem'92; FRCPC; Derm. Assoc Prof, Saint John Regional Hospital; (506)634-2622; Fax. (506)634-2627.

BAXTER, Keith A; 4211-2775 Laurel St, Vancouver BC V5Z 1M9; UBC'99; FRCSC; GenSurg; VascSurg. (604)875-5538

BAXTER, Kenneth L; Royal Court Med Centre, 301-1 Quarry Ridge Rd, Barrie ON L4M 7G1; Tor'60; Staff Family Practice Affiliate, Royal Victoria Regional Health Centre; (705)726-2991

BAXTER, Mary L S; Dartmouth Med Centre, 301-46 Portland St, Dartmouth NS B2Y 1H4; McM'84; BSc; FRCPC; Derm (Gynecologic Dermatology). Consultant, Dartmouth General Hospital; Consultant, Queen Elizabeth II Health Sciences Centre - Victoria General Site; Lecturer, Dalhousie University; (902)465-8720; Fax. (902)465-8712.

BAXTER, Maureen; Emerg Preparedness & Occup Hlth, PL3712-171 Slater St, Ottawa ON K1P 5H7; McG'79; FRCSC; OrthSurg (Diving Medicine). Medical Officer Occupational Health Workplace Health & Safety Prog/Med Dir Hlth Safety & Emerg Preparedness, Health Canada; Langs: French; Bilingual(English/French); (613)946-6583; Fax. (613)990-9397; peggy.baxter@hc-sc.gc.ca.

BAXTER, Nancy N; St Michael's Hosp, 16CC 040-30 Bond St, Toronto ON M5B 1W8; Tor'90; PhD; FRCSC; GenSurg (Colon & Rectal Surgery). Staff, St Michael's Hospital; (416)864-5168; Fax. (416)360-0637.

BAXTER, P Janine; Driftwood Family Medicine, 11-450 Westheights Dr, Kitchener ON N2N 2B9; Qns'86; (519)725-4070; Fax. (519)725-4071.

BAXTER, Stephanie A; Hotel-Dieu Hosp, 166 Brock St, Kingston ON K7L 5G2; Dal'98; FRCSC; Ophth (Cornea/External Disease). Staff, Hotel-Dieu Hospital; Att Staff, Kingston General Hospital; Langs: French; (613)544-3400 x3203; Fax. (613)544-1454; sbaxter@baxtereyemd.com.

BAXTER, W L Miranda; Hermitage Medicentre, 12747 50 St NW, Edmonton AB T5A 4L8; Alb'85; CCFP; (780)473-2102

BAY, Ariel M; Rouge Valley-Centenary HC, 2867 Ellesmere Rd, Scarborough ON M1E 4B9; McM'04; Critical Care Medicine; IntMed. Staff, Rouge Valley Health System - Centenary Health Centre Site; (416)284-8131

BAY, Dennis; Chatham-Kent Health Alliance, PO Box 2030 Stn Main 80 Grand Ave W, Chatham ON N7M 5L9; Dal'02; CCFP; CCFP(E.M.); Staff, Chatham-Kent Health Alliance; (519)352-6400

BAY, Trevor A; Manitoba X-Ray Clinic, 3263 Portage Ave, Winnipeg MB R3K 0W6; Man'72; FRCPC; DiagRad. Ac Staff, St Boniface General Hospital; (204)832-0273

BAYARDELLE, Paul; CHUM-Hop Notre-Dame, 1560 rue Sherbrooke E, Montreal QC H2L 4M1; Strasbourg (France)'72; FRCPC; MedMicrobiol. ac Staff, Centre Hospitalier l'Université de Montréal (CHUM) - Hôpital Notre-Dame; Langs: English; (514)890-8000 x25103; paul.bayardelle.chum@ssss.gouv.qc.ca.

BAYAT, Muhammad R H; Valley Medical Imaging, 102-32475 Simon Ave, Abbotsford BC V2T 5E3; Cape Town (South Africa)'99; FRCPC; DiagRad. (604)859-8988

BAYCROFT, Sur J; Ambulatory Surgical Centre, 700-1200 Burrard St, Vancouver BC V6Z 2C7; UBC'96; FRCPC; Anes. Staff Anes, Richmond Hospital; (604)669-6181

BAYDA, Michael C; La Ronge Health Centre, PO Box 6000 Bag 6900, La Ronge SK S0J 1L0; Sask'09; CCFP; (306)425-2422; Fax. (306)425-8516.

BAYDALA, Lola T; Misericordia Community Hosp, 2-16940 87 Ave NW, Edmonton AB T5R 4H5; Alb'81; FRCPC; Peds. Staff, Covenant Health - Misericordia Community Hospital; (780)735-2731; Fax. (780)735-2794.

BAYDOCK, Bradley M S; Legacy Sport Med Clinic, 14-160 Meadowood Dr, Winnipeg MB R2M 5L6; Man'95; BSc; CCFP; FCFP; (204)667-1550; bbaydock@ahwc.ca.

BAYDOCK, Sandra A; Southside Women's Health Centr, 120-3017 66 St NW, Edmonton AB T6K 4B2; Man'98; FRCSC; ObstGyn (Urogynecology). Staff, Covenant Health - Grey Nuns Community Hospital; (780)461-6220; Fax. (780)461-4197.

BAYER, Judith L; Cobourg Clinic, PO Box 86 Stn Main 44 University Ave E, Cobourg ON K9A 4K4; McG'86; BSc; CCFP; (905)372-3323; Fax. (905)372-3692.

BAYER, Michael W; Cobourg Clinic, PO Box 86 Stn Main 44 University Ave E, Cobourg ON K9A 4K4; McG'86; CCFP; CCFP(E.M.); FCFP; Ac Staff, Northumberland Hills Hospital; Queen's University; (905)372-3323; Fax. (905)372-3692.

BAYER, Nessa A; Medical & Dental Bldg, 404-586 Eglinton Ave E, Toronto ON M4P 1P2; Tor'99; FRCPC; Peds. (416)489-3273; Fax. (416)489-1510; nessa.bayer@rogers.com.

BAYFIELD, David J; Georgian Bay Gen Hosp, PO Box 760 Stn Main 1112 St Andrews Dr, Midland ON L4R 4P4; McM'92; CCFP; CCFP(E.M.); FCFP; Staff, Georgian Bay General Hospital - Midland; (705)526-3751

BAYFIELD, Sofia T; Foremed Clinic, 115 16th St W, North Vancouver BC V7M 1T3; UBC'96; CCFP; (604)904-8804; Fax. (604)904-0972.

BAYLE, Marie-Noelle; CSSS d'Antoine-Labelle-Mt Laur, 2561 ch de la Lievre S, Mont-Laurier QC J9L 3G3; Bordeaux (France)'91; Staff, CSSS d'Antoine-Labelle; (819)275-2118

BAYLEY, Andrew J S; Univ Hlth Network-Princess M, 610 University Ave, Toronto ON M5G 2M9; Qns'92; FRCPC; RadOncol. Staff RadOncol, Princess Margaret Hospital - University Health Network; (416)946-2919

BAYLEY, Mark T; Toronto Rehab Inst-Univ Ctr, 3 131-550 University Ave, Toronto ON M5G 2A2; Qns'88; FRCPC; PhysMed&Rehab (Acquired Brain Injury Rehabilitation). Consultant, West Park Healthcare Centre; Med Dir Neurorehabilitation Prog, Toronto Rehabilitation Institute - University Centre; Clin Assoc Prof, McMaster University; Langs: English; French; (416)597-3422; Fax. (416)597-0678.

BAYLEY, T Arnold; Bickle Ctre Toronto Rehab Inst, 130 Dunn Ave, Toronto ON M6K 2R7; Tor'55; FACP; FRCPC; IntMed; Endocrin&Metab; NuclearMed. Hon Consultant, St Joseph's Health Centre; Hon Consultant, St Michael's Hospital; (416)597-3422; Fax. (416)595-1222.

BAYLEY, Valerie A; 6A-145 Carlton St, St Catharines ON L2R 1R5; Tor'83; CCFP; FCFP; Ad Staff Privil, Niagara Health System - St Catharines General Site; (905)685-4866; Fax. (905)685-8162.

BAYLIS, Barry W; HSC Faculty of Med, 3330 Hospital Dr NW, Calgary AB T2N 4N1; Cal'83; FRCPC; IntMed (Endocrinology). Staff, Foothills Medical Centre; (403)220-2859

BAYLIS, Penny Jane; McGill Sports Med Clinic, 475 av des Pins O, Montreal QC H2W 1S4; (Other Foreign)'02; CCFP; (514)398-7007; Fax. (514)398-4035.

BAYLISS, Michael; Credit Valley Med Arts Centre, 202-2000 Credit Valley Rd, Mississauga ON L5M 4N4; McM'04; FRCPC; IntMed; Cardiol. Staff, The Credit Valley Hospital; (905)569-8631; Fax. (905)569-3836.

BAYLISS, Ann; The Southcom Bldg, 301-2227 South Millway, Mississauga ON L5L 3R6; Tor'86; FRCPC; Peds (Consultant Pediatrics). Staff, The Credit Valley Hospital; (905)569-9798; Fax. (905)569-8630.

BAYLY, Kenneth E; 701 Avenue P N, Saskatoon SK S7L 2W1; Sask'80; (306)382-5854; Fax. (306)382-7477.

BAYLY, Peter L; Lively Med Centre, 2-204 Sixth Ave, Lively ON P3Y 1M4; Tor'63; Hon Staff, Health Sciences North-Laurentian Site; (705)692-4774; Fax. (705)692-0528.

BAYNE, J Laura; Sexual Health Center, 179 Clarence St, Ottawa ON K1N 5P7; Cal'99; CCFP; Staff, The Ottawa Hospital - General Campus; Staff, Kingston General Hospital; Lecturer, University of Ottawa; (613)580-2424

BAYNE, Jason P; 205-3017 66 St NW, Edmonton AB T6K 4B2; Man'03; FRCSC; GenSurg; VascSurg. (780)461-6012; Fax. (780)461-5442.

BAYNE, John M; 206-1077 56 St, Delta BC V4L 2A2; Qns'75; FRCSC; Ophth. Staff, Delta Hospital; (604)943-1411

BAYOUMI, Ahmed M M; 30 Bond St, Toronto ON M5B 1W8; Tor'89; FRCPC; IntMed (HIV). Staff, St Michael's Hospital; (416)864-5728; Fax. (416)864-5558; ahmed.bayoumi@utoronto.ca.

BAYOUMI, Imaan M; Napanee Area Community H C, 6 Dundas St E, Napanee ON K7R 1H6; Qns'87; CCFP; FCFP; Staff, Kingston General Hospital; Staff, Hotel-Dieu Hospital; Aj Staff Family Med, Queen's University; (613)354-8937; Fax. (613)354-8940.

BAZ, Bechara; Ctr Hosp Rouyn-Noranda, 4 9e rue, Rouyn-Noranda QC J9X 2B2; (Lebanon)'97; Staff, Centre Hospitalier Rouyn-Noranda; (819)764-5131

BAZ, Rami; Hop Reg D'Edmundston, 275 boul Hebert, Edmundston NB E3V 4E4; (Lebanon)'01; Staff, Hôpital regional d'Edmundston; (506)739-2200

BAZARJANI, Sadrollah S; The Ottawa Hosp-Civic Campus, 1053 Carling Ave, Ottawa ON K1Y 4E9; Tehran (Iran)'82; FRCPC; NuclearMed. Staff, The Ottawa Hospital - Civic Campus; (613)761-4221; Fax. (613)761-4041.

BAZELEY, Peter A; Western Mem Reg Hosp, PO Box 2005 1 Brookfield Ave, Corner Brook NL A2H 6J7; Mem'10; CCFP; Locum Tenens, Western Memorial Regional Hospital.

BAZIANY, Azaad A; 505 4th Ave N, Saskatoon SK S7K 2M5; Baghdad (Iraq)'86; FRCPC; Psy. (306)668-0505

BAZILE, Marie Y; CLSC Fort-Coulonge, CP 430 160 ch de la Chute, Fort-Coulonge QC J0X 1V0; (Haiti)'89; CCFP; (819)683-3000; Fax. (819)683-2008.

BAZILLI, Catherine J; Northmount Med Centre, 401-145 13th St E, North Vancouver BC V7L 2L4; Cal'90; MHSc; Ac Staff Family Pactice, Lions Gate Hospital; Clin Staff Family Practice, University of British Columbia; (604)980-4808; Fax. (604)985-5959.

BAZIN, Anne-Marie; Ctr Hosp de Verdun, 4000 boul Lasalle, Verdun QC H4G 2A3; Mon'85; FRCPC; IntMed. Staff, Centre Hospitalier de Verdun; (514)322-1000

BAZIN, Genevieve; Polyclinique de Trois-Rivieres, 250-1900 boul des Recollets, Trois-Rivieres QC G8Z 4K4; Sher'88; Ophth (P.Q.). (819)375-4040

BAZIN, Marc; Service Sante ALCOA, 100 Rte Maritime, Baie-Comeau QC G4Z 2L6; Laval'84; PhD; CST; Med Consultant, Alcoa De Baie-Comeau; (418)296-7055; Fax. (418)294-7729.

BAZIN, Richard; Ctr Hosp Affilie-St-Sacrement, 1050 ch Sainte-Foy, Quebec QC G1S 4L8; Laval'79; Ophth. Consultant, Centre Hospitalier Universitaire De Québec - Pavillon De St-françois-d'assise; Prof, Centre Hospitalier Affilié Universitaire de Québec - Hôpital du St-Sacrement; Teach Staff, Université Laval; (418)682-7573

BAZIN, Sylvie; Centre de Obst/Gyn, 4250 1re av, Quebec QC G1H 2S5; Laval'87; FRCSC; ObstGyn (Echography). Ac Member, Centre Hospitalier Universitaire De Québec - Pavillon De St-françois-d'assise; Langs: English; (418)654-0555 x283; Fax. (418)654-1898.

BAZINET, Andree; Institut Philippe Pinel de Mon, 10905 boul Henri-Bourassa E, Montreal QC H1C 1H1; Mon'90; Psy. Staff, Institut Philippe-Pinel de Montreal; (514)648-8461

BAZINET, Brigitte; Ctr Physiatrie Val-des-Arbres, 500-1600 boul Saint-Martin E, Laval QC H7G 4R8; Mon'83; FACP; FRCPC; PhysMed&Rehab (Sports Medicine). Staff Med, Hopital de la Cite de la santé; Physician Med, Centre de Physiatrie Val-des-Arbres Inc.; Langs: English; (450)669-5396; Fax. (450)669-5138.

BAZINET, Emilie; 202-185 rue Acadie, Dieppe NB E1A 1G6; Sher'10; CCFP.

BAZINET, Jocelyn; Hotel-Dieu de Levis, 143 rue Wolfe, Levis QC G6V 3Z1; Laval'99; FRCSC; Urol. Staff, Hôtel-Dieu de Lévis; (418)835-7121

BAZINET, Lucie; Clinique Med Monteuil, 200-4650 boul des Laurentides, Laval QC H7K 2J4; Mon'84; Staff, Hopital de la Cite de la santé; Médecin, Clinique Med Monteuil; (450)628-8717; Fax. (450)628-5305.

BAZINET, Sara; 202-387 Main St, Shediac NB E4P 2B5; Sher'07; CCFP; Langs: Bilingual(English/French); (506)532-6946; Fax. (506)532-1569.

BAZINET, Stephan; CLSC Caplan, CP 208 96 rte 132 O, Caplan QC G0C 1H0; Mon'91; (418)388-2572; Fax. (418)388-5646.

BAZIOS, Sofia; Davisville Med & Dental Centre, 216-1849 Yonge St, Toronto ON M4S 1Y2; Tor'98; CCFP; Langs: Greek; (416)487-9309

BAZIUK, Natalie; 1-491 Simcoe St S, Oshawa ON L1H 4J9; Tor'83; BSc; FRCSC; Ophth (Retina Vitreous Surgery). Staff, Lakeridge Health - Oshawa Site; Langs: Ukrainian; (905)434-2669; Fax. (905)434-3807.

BAZLEY, Kynan P; Kynan Bazley, PO Box 2053, Rossland BC V0G 1Y0; Otago (New Zealand)'06; MB ChB; (250)231-6327

BAZOS, Michael J; 202-658 Danforth Ave, Toronto ON M4J 5B9; Tor'85; BSc; Assoc Staff, The Scarborough Hospital - Birchmount Campus; Court Staff, Toronto East General Hospital Inc; Langs: Greek; (416)466-3921; Fax. (416)466-1169; drbazos@healthcoachmd.com.

BAZZO, Jean-Pierre; Clinique Medimax, CP 62 Succ Pl-Desjardins 303-4 Complexe Desjardins, Montreal QC H5B 1B2; Sher'84; Staff, Hôtel-Dieu de Saint-Jérôme; (514)287-2683

BEACH, Anne E; Healthworks, 3F-24 Bellair St, Toronto ON M5R 2C7; Wes'74; (416)962-2263; Fax. (416)962-2548.

BEACH, Craig; Regional Mental HC-St Thomas, 467 Sunset Dr, St Thomas ON N5P 3V9; McM'03; Staff, Regional Mental Health Care-St Joseph's Health Care; (519)631-8510; Fax. (519)531-2361.

BEACH, David A; Picton Clinic, 5C-389 Main St, Picton ON K0K 2T0; Qns'81; CCFP; FCFP; Staff, QHC Prince Edward County Memorial; Assoc Prof FamMed, Queen's University; (613)476-7870; Fax. (613)476-6482.

BEACH, Jeremy R; 5-30 University Terrace, 8303 112 St NW, Edmonton AB T6G 1K4; Newcastle-Upon-Tyne (England)'83; MB BS; FRCP; FRCPC; OccupMed. Assoc Prof/Dir Residency Prog, University of Alberta; (780)492-6291; Fax. (780)492-9677.

BEACH, Renee A; Women's College Hosp, 76 Grenville St, Toronto ON M5S 1B2; McM'07; Staff, Women's College Hospital; (416)323-6400

BEACH, Scott F; Westbrook Prof Bldg, 203-1610 37 St SW, Calgary AB T3C 3P1; UBC'01; CCFP; (403)246-4431

BEACOM, Rosalind M; The Malone Med Clinic, 4955 41 Ave, Drayton Valley AB T7A 1V4; Queen's (Ireland)'77; (780)542-3366; Fax. (780)542-6207.

BEAIRSTO, Susan E; Foothills Med Centre, 58-1403 29 St NW, Calgary AB T2N 2T9; Cal'85; CCFP; Staff, Foothills Medical Centre; (403)944-4258

BEAIRSTO, W Art D; 77 Parklea Dr, Toronto ON M4G 2J7; Tor'77; DBact; CCFP; (416)422-3501; Fax. (416)422-3170.

BEAL, John R; Nashwaaksis Med Clinic, 475 Brookside Dr, Fredericton NB E3A 8V4; Qns'79; Staff, Dr Everett Chalmers Regional Hospital; (506)458-9447; Fax. (506)458-1326.

BEAL, Timothy; Child & Parent Resource Inst, 201-600 Sanatorium Rd, London ON N6H 3W7; The Univ of Rochester (USA)'04; Gen Practice, Child & Parent Resource Institute; (519)858-2774

BEALER, Rodney E; Malone Med Clinic, 4955 41 Ave, Drayton Valley AB T7A 1V4; London (England)'70; MB BS; DA; LMCC; (780)542-3366; Fax. (780)542-6207.

BEALL, Franklin R; 290-546 St Paul St, Kamloops BC V2C 5T1; Tor'70; DABIM; FRCPC; IntMed. Ac Staff, Royal Inland Hospital; (250)372-7535; bismarck23@shaw.ca.

BEALLOR, Carrie R; The Beallor Travel Hlth Clinic, 206-2900 Steeles Ave E, Thornhill ON L3T 4X1; Tor'95; DTMH; CCFP; Langs: Bilingual(English/French); (905)882-7575; Fax. (905)731-1298.

BEAMISH, Gregory H; 6-3600 Ellesmere Rd, Scarborough ON M1C 4Y8; Wes'80; CCFP; (416)282-2282; Fax. (416)282-4762.

BEAMISH, John J; 201-170 Simcoe St, Peterborough ON K9H 2H7; McM'79; CCFP; FCFP; (705)748-5632; Fax. (705)742-2036; john.beamish@peterboroughfht.com.

BEAMISH, Judith M; Sun Life Financial, 150 King St W, Toronto ON M5H 1J9; Tor'76; FRCPC; IntMed; Cardiol. VP/Chief Med Dir, Sun Life Assurance Co; (416)979-6077; Fax. (416)979-4070; judy.beamish@sunlife.com.

BEAMISH, Stephen R; Upper Grand Family Health Team, PO Box 460 70 Victoria St, Elora ON N0B 1S0; Wes'91; CCFP; CCFP(E.M.); FCFP; Staff, Groves Memorial Community Hospital; (519)846-5841; Fax. (519)846-8453; stephen.beamish@fpae.ca.

BEAN, Sharon H; Scarborough Radiology, G03-3000 Lawrence Ave E, Scarborough ON M1P 2V2; Witwatersrand (South Africa)'92; FRCPC; DiagRad. (416)438-6636

BEAN, Warren A; Mackenzie Richmond Hill Hosp, 10 Trench St, Richmond Hill ON L4C 4Z3; Witwatersrand (South Africa)'86; MB ChB; Anes. Staff, Mackenzie Richmond Hill Hospital; (905)883-1212

BEANLANDS, Donald S; 33 Waterford Dr, Nepean ON K2E 7V4; Dal'58; FACC; FACP; IntMed (Cardiology). Dep Dir Ottawa Heart Inst, The Ottawa Hospital - Civic Campus; Emeritus Prof, University of Ottawa; (613)727-8277

BEANLANDS, Rob S B; Univ of Ottawa Heart Institute, 3409-40 Ruskin St, Ottawa ON K1Y 4W7; Ott'83; ABIM; ABIM(Cardiol); AB; FRCPC; IntMed (Nuclear Cardiology); Cardiol. Staff, University of Ottawa Heart Institute; Staff, The Ottawa Hospital - Civic Campus; Asst Prof Med & Radiol, University of Ottawa; (613)761-5296

BEARD, D Glenn; Credit Valley Prof Bldg, 412-2300 Eglinton Ave W, Mississauga ON L5M 2V8; Wes'76; ABOtol; FRCSC; Otol. Ac Staff, The Credit Valley Hospital; (905)820-8344; Fax. (905)820-9699; d.glenn.beard@sympatico.ca.

BEARD, Jonathan D; South Mississauga SW Etobicoke, 300-2085 Hurontario St, Mississauga ON L5A 4G1; West Indies (Jamaica)'00; (905)848-7484; Fax. (905)804-7912.

BEARD, Lisa L; Bramalea Med Group, 500-18 Kensington Rd, Brampton ON L6T 4S5; Qns'92; CCFP; FCFP; Ac Staff, William Osler Health System - Brampton Civic Hospital; (905)791-7575; Fax. (905)791-7532.

BEARDSLEY, Jennifer K; Catherine Booth Hosp, 4375 av Montclair, Montreal QC H4B 2J5; Mon'02; CCFP; Chief méd interne, Catherine Booth Hospital; (514)481-0431; Fax. (514)481-0029.

BEARDSLEY, Robin M; The Westend Family Care Clinic, 80 Michael Cowpland Dr, Kanata ON K2M 1P6; Tor'87; CCFP; FCFP; Staff, Westend Family Care Clinic Family Health Team; (613)599-3321; Fax. (613)599-3366; robin.beardsley@sympatico.ca.

BEARSS, Erin; The Joseph & Wolf Lebovic Bldg, 4F-60 Murray St, Toronto ON M5T 3L9; McM'02; CCFP; CCFP(E.M.); Staff, Mount Sinai Hospital; (416)586-5158

BEARSS, Luke; Mount Sinai Hosp, 206-600 University Ave, Toronto ON M5G 1X5; Wes'05; CCFP; CCFP(E.M.); Staff, Mount Sinai Hospital; (416)586-5058

BEASLEY, Debra E; 200A-672 Brant St, Burlington ON L7R 2H3; McM'81; CCFP; Staff, Joseph Brant Memorial Hospital; (905)333-1343; Fax. (905)333-6467.

BEASLEY, Kenneth A; 100-34 McMurray St, Brantford ON N3R 4J1; Qns'97; BSc(Hons); FRCSC; Urol (Laparoscopy). (519)754-2111

BEATON, Blaine G; Lunenburg Med Clinic, PO Box 1450 42 High St, Lunenburg NS B0J 2C0; Dal'85; CCFP; Staff, Fishermen's Memorial Hospital; (902)634-7226; Fax. (902)634-4944; bbeaton@bwr.eastlink.ca.

BEATON, Jessica J; Fort William Clinic, 117 McKellar St S, Thunder Bay ON P7E 1H5; Ott'09; CCFP.

BEATON, Melanie; London HSC-University Hosp, PO Box 5339 Stn B ALL132B-339 Windermere Rd, London ON N6A 5A5; Ott'00; FRCPC; IntMed; Gastroent. Staff, London Health Sciences Centre - University Hospital; (519)663-3344; Fax. (519)663-3232.

BEATON, William N; 200-300 Columbia St, Kamloops BC V2C 6L1; Cal'76; FRCSC; OrthSurg (Adult Reconstructive Surgery). Staff, Royal Inland Hospital; (250)374-1448; Fax. (250)374-2663.

BEATTIE, Anne M; Victoria Med Centre, 503-304 Victoria Ave N, Hamilton ON L8L 5G4; Wes'85; FRCSC; Ophth (General Ophthalmic Surgery). Court Staff, Hamilton Health Sciences Centre - McMaster University Medical Centre; Ac Staff, St Joseph's Healthcare - Charlton Campus; (905)525-7907; Fax. (905)525-9186.

BEATTIE, B Lynn; UBC Hosp, 2211 Wesbrook Mall, Vancouver BC V6T 2B5; UBC'65; FRCPC; IntMed; GeriatricMed. Assoc Staff Alzheimer Clinic, UBC Hospital - Koerner Pavillion; Emeritus Prof Div of Geriatric Med, University of British Columbia; (604)822-7176; Fax. (604)822-7191; lbeattie@mail.ubc.ca.

BEATTIE, Beverly A; Tecumseh Urgent Care, 11811 Tecumseh Rd E, Windsor ON N8N 4M7; Wes'73; (519)979-2831; Fax. (519)979-1429.

BEATTIE, David; Upper Canada Fam Hlth Team, 4-5 Home St, Brockville ON K6V 0A5; Flinders (Australia)'05; CCFP; (613)423-1111

BEATTIE, Erin D; C01 B-310 Bridge St W, Napanee ON K7R 0A4; McM'09; CCFP; (613)354-7640

BEATTIE, Joan K; The Doctor's Office, 3599 Sheppard Ave E, Scarborough ON M1T 3K8; Qns'65; DPH; FACPrevMed; FRCP; FRCPC; CommunMed (Family Medicine). (416)321-2643

BEATTIE, Robert A; Arkona Med Centre, PO Box 99 14 Union St, Arkona ON N0M 1B0; Wes'75; Court Staff, Strathroy Middlesex General Hospital - Middlesex Hospital Alliance; (519)828-3821; Fax. (519)828-3429.

BEATTIE, William; Univ Hlth Network-Toronto Gen, EN3 464-200 Elizabeth St, Toronto ON M5G 2C4; McM'82; FRCPC; Anes. Staff, Toronto General Hospital - UHN; (416)340-3111

BEATTY, Dorothy L; Queen Elizabeth II HSC-Halifax, 355-1796 Summer St, Halifax NS B3H 3A7; Dal'07; FRCPC; EmergMed. Staff, Queen Elizabeth II Health Sciences Centre - Halifax Infirmary Site; (902)473-4220; Fax. (902)473-3617.

BEATTY, Gary L; Woodstock Med Clinic, 6-110 Chapel St, Woodstock NB E7M 1H1; Dal'75; BSc; CCFP; FCFP; (506)328-2042; Fax. (506)328-6848.

BEATTY, Myles F; Glazier Med Centre, 11 Gibb St, Oshawa ON L1H 2J9; Wes'75; FRCSC; ObstGyn. Court Staff, Lakeridge Health - Port Perry Site; Leader Phys Maternal Newborn, Lakeridge Health - Oshawa Site; Teach. Assoc., Queen's University; (905)579-1212; Fax. (905)579-2021.

BEATTY, Steven E; York Prof Bldg, 307-679 Davis Dr, Newmarket ON L3Y 5G8; Tor'80; FRCSC; PlasSurg (Hand Surgery). Staff PlasSurg, Southlake Regional Health Centre; Court Staff, Markham Stouffville Hospital; Court Staff, Mackenzie Richmond Hill Hospital; (905)853-6644; Fax. (905)853-1898.

BEAU, Jean-Michel; 1141 rue Royale CP 800, Malartic QC J0Y 1Z0; Lyon (France)'83; DPsy(Lyon,Fr.); Psychiatre, Hôpital psychiatrique de Malartic; Staff Psy, Centre Hospitalier de Val d'Or; Staff Psy, CH Hôtel-Dieu d'Amos; Langs: English; (819)825-5858 x8296; Fax. (819)825-7726; jeanmichel_beau@ssss.gouv.qc.ca.

BEAUBIEN, Eliot R; Peterborough Reg Nephrology, 239 Charlotte St, Peterborough ON K9J 2V2; Cal'97; FRCPC; IntMed; Nephrol. Staff, Northumberland Hills Hospital; Staff, Peterborough Regional Health Centre - Hospital Drive; Staff, Ross Memorial Hospital; (705)750-1786; Fax. (705)750-0591.

BEAUBIEN, Guy; Hop du Sacre-Coeur de Mtl, 5400 boul Gouin O, Montreal QC H4J 1C5; Mon'95; CSPQ; FRCPC; Anes. Staff, Hôpital du Sacre-Coeur de Montréal; (514)338-2222 x2680; Fax. (514)338-2009.

BEAUBIEN, Jean; CHUQ-Hotel-Dieu de Quebec, 11 Cote Du Palais, Quebec QC G1R 2J6; Laval'96; CSPQ; Critical Care Medicine (P.Q.); Anes. Staff, Centre Hospitalier Universitaire de Québec (CHUQ) - Siege Social; Chef Anesthesiology, Université Laval.

BEAUBIEN, Lise B; 535 Montreal Rd, Ottawa ON K1K 0V1; Ott'82; BSc; CCFP; FCFP; Court Staff Privileges, The Ottawa Hospital - General Campus; Clinical Asst Prof Family Med, University of Ottawa; Langs: Bilingual(English/French); (613)746-5350; Fax. (613)746-5340.

BEAUCAGE, Clement; Centre de Sante Publique, 2400 av D'Estimauville, Quebec QC G1E 7G9; Laval'74; CommunMed. Ac Staff, Centre Hospitalier Universitaire de Quebec-CHUL; (418)666-7000 x356; Fax. (418)666-2776.

BEAUCAGE, France; CSSS de Trois-Rivieres, 155 rue Toupin, Trois-Rivieres QC G8T 3Z8; Mon'82; Staff, Centre de santé Cloutier-du-Rivage; Geriatric Medicine, CHSLD Le Trifluvien; Physician, Centre de Sante des Femmes de la Mauricie; (819)370-2200 x3437; Fax. (819)370-1508.

BEAUCAGE, Francois; Hop du Sacre-Coeur de Mtl, 5400 boul Gouin O, Montreal QC H4J 1C5; Mon'01; FRCPC; IntMed; Respir. Staff, Hôpital du Sacre-Coeur de Montréal; (514)338-2162

BEAUCAGE, Gilles; CSSS Pierre Boucher, 1333 boul Jacques-Cartier E, Longueuil QC J4M 2A5; Mon'87; ACLS; ATLS; FRCPC; EmergMed (P.Q.). Staff, Centre Hospitalier Pierre Boucher; (450)468-8111; Fax. (450)468-8114.

BEAUCAGE, Jennifer K; 130 Ted Commanda Dr, Sturgeon Falls ON P2B 3J9; Qns'05; CCFP; (705)753-1661; Fax. (705)753-9669.

BEAUCE, Catherine; Ctre Hosp Reg Chisasibi, CP 250, Chisasibi QC J0M 1E0; McG'05; CCFP; Staff, Cree Board of Health & Social Services James Bay; (819)855-9001

BEAUCHAMP, Andre; Centre Med St-Louis, 100-900 boul Moody, Terrebonne QC J6W 3K8; Mon'82; (450)471-1212; Fax. (450)471-5795.

BEAUCHAMP, Aude; 302-301 Columbia St E, New Westminster BC V3L 3W5; McG'99; FRCSC; ObstGyn. Staff, Royal Columbian Hospital; Staff, Eagle Ridge Hospital & Health Care Centre; Langs: French; (604)759-0241; Fax. (604)759-0310.

BEAUCHAMP, Chantal; CSSS du Lac-des-Deux-Montagnes, 520 boul Arthur-Sauve, Saint-Eustache QC J7R 5B1; Laval'08; CCFP; CCFP(E.M.); Staff, Hôpital de Saint-Eustache.

BEAUCHAMP, Coralie; Clinique Fertilite Ovo, 8000 boul Decarie, Montreal QC H4P 2S4; Laval'98; FRCSC; ObstGyn. (514)798-2000; Fax. (514)798-2001.

BEAUCHAMP, Daniel; Hop Maisonneuve-Rosemont, 5415 boul de l'Assomption, Montreal QC H1T 2M4; Mon'71; DiagRad. Ac Staff, Hopital Maisonneuve-Rosemont; (514)252-3535; Fax. (514)252-3537.

BEAUCHAMP, Elizabeth; MUHC-Royal Victoria Hosp, H4.24-687 av des Pins O, Montreal QC H3A 1A1; McG'06; MDCM; MedMicrobiol; InfectDis; IntMed. Staff, McGill University Health Centre - Royal Victoria Hospital; (514)934-1934

BEAUCHAMP, Gilles; Hop Maisonneuve-Rosemont, 5415 boul de l'Assomption, Montreal QC H1T 2M4; Mon'72; FACS; FRCSC; GenSurg; ThorSurg. Staff, Hopital Maisonneuve-Rosemont; Prof, Universite de Montreal; Langs: English; (514)252-3400 x4426; Fax. (514)252-3488; gilles.beauchamp@umontreal.ca.

BEAUCHAMP, Jacques; GMF Concorde, 300 boul de la Concorde E, Laval QC H7G 2E6; Mon'72; Langs: English.

BEAUCHAMP, Marc; 112-6100 av du Boise, Montreal QC H3S 2W1; Mon'88 Université de Montreal; FRCS; FRCSC; OrthSurg (Shoulder). Staff, Centre Hospitalier l'Université de Montréal (CHUM) - Hôtel-Dieu; assoc Chercheur Research Centre, Hop Du Sacre-Coeur De Montreal; Staff, Hôpital Santa Cabrini Ospedale; adj Prof, Universite de Montreal; Langs: English; French; Portuguese; Italian; (514)737-6100; info@beauchamportho.com.

BEAUCHAMP, Martine; CSSS de la Baie-des-Chaleurs, RR 2 419 boul Perron, Maria QC G0C 1Y0; Mon'04; CCFP; Staff, CSSS de la Baie-des-Chaleurs; (418)752-2572

BEAUCHAMP, Richard D; Children's & Women's HC of BC, A205-4480 Oak St, Vancouver BC V6H 3V4; UBC'71; FRCSC; OrthSurg (Pediatric Orthopedics). Ac Staff, BC Children's Hospital; Med Dir, Shriners Gait Lab; Clin Prof Orth, University of British Columbia; (604)875-2627; Fax. (604)875-2275.

BEAUCHAMP, Robert J; Bluewater Health-Norman Site, 89 Norman St, Sarnia ON N7T 6S3; Wes'84; FRCPC; Anes. Staff, Bluewater Health - Mitton Site; Staff, Bluewater Health - Norman Site; (519)464-4408

BEAUCHAMP, Yvon; Hop du Sacre-Coeur de Mtl, 5400 boul Gouin O, Montreal QC H4J 1C5; Mon'71; CCFP; Staff, Hôpital du Sacre-Coeur de Montréal; (514)338-2050

BEAUCHEF, Jean-P; Clinique Camu, 101-2984 boul Taschereau, Greenfield Park QC J4V 2G9; Rennes (France)'73; IntMed; Endocrin (P.Q.). (450)466-4333

BEAUCHEMIN, Annie; Clinique medicale Notre-Dame, 120-504 rue Notre-Dame, Repentigny QC J6A 2T8; Mon'04; CCFP; (450)585-3232

BEAUCHEMIN, Christiane; Regie de l'Assurance Maladie Q, Q26-1125 Grande Allee O, Quebec QC G1S 1E7; Laval'86; VP, Regie de l'Assurance Maladie du Quebec; (418)682-5129; Fax. (418)644-8193.

BEAUCHEMIN, Dany; 10A rue Georges, Pierreville QC J0G 1J0; Sher'09; CCFP; Médecin, Cooperative de solidarité et de santé Shoomer-Jauvin; (450)568-3296; Fax. (450)568-0333.

BEAUCHEMIN, David; 10A rue Georges, Pierreville QC J0G 1J0; Sher'09; CCFP; Médecin, Cooperative de solidarité et de santé Shoomer-Jauvin; (450)568-3296; Fax. (450)568-0333.

BEAUCHEMIN, Denise; Clinique Med Centre-Ville, 1652 rue Royale, Trois-Rivieres QC G9A 4K3; Mon'77; (819)379-4521; Fax. (819)379-4615.

BEAUCHEMIN, Eric; Hop Ste-Anne-De-Beaupre, 11000 rue des Montagnards RR 1, Beaupre QC G0A 1E0; Sher'97; CCFP; Staff, Hôpital Sainte Anne de Beaupré; Langs: English; (418)827-3726; Fax. (418)827-6861.

BEAUCHEMIN, Francine; CSSS de Laval, 280 boul du Roi-du-Nord, Laval QC H7L 4L2; Mon'92; (450)622-5110; Fax. (450)622-4150.

BEAUCHEMIN, Jean-Pierre; UMF Laval, 2690 ch des Quatre-Bourgeois, Quebec QC G1V 0B7; Laval'82; CCFP; FCFP; GeriatricMed (P.Q.). Staff, Hôpital Laval; Staff, CLSC CHSLD Hauteville des Rivieres; Prof FamMed, Université Laval; (418)656-8711; Fax. (418)656-4503; jean-pierre.beauchemin@fmed.ulaval.ca.

BEAUCHEMIN, Julie; Hop Charles Lemoyne, 3120 boul Taschereau, Greenfield Park QC J4V 2H1; Mon'99; FRCPC; IntMed; Rheum. Staff, Hopital Charles LeMoyne; (450)466-5000

BEAUCHEMIN, Kim; Ctr Hosp Laurentien, 234 rue Saint-Vincent, Ste-Agathe-des-Mts QC J8C 2B8; Sher'97; Staff, Centre Hospitalier Laurentien; (819)324-4000

BEAUCHEMIN, Lyne; CSSS de l'Energie-Ste-Therese, 1705 av Georges, Shawinigan QC G9N 2N1; Laval'97; FRCPC; Psy. Staff, CH du Centre-de-la-Mauricie (Ste-Thérèse de Shawinigan); (819)536-7575; lyne_beauchemin@ssss.gouv.qc.ca.

BEAUCHEMIN, Marie-Andree; Clinique Externe des Moulins, 101-1355 Grande Allée, Terrebonne QC J6W 4K6; Mon'97; FRCPC; Psy. Langs: English; (450)964-6418; Fax. (450)964-9260.

BEAUCHEMIN, Marie-Claude; CHUM-Hop Notre-Dame, 1560 rue Sherbrooke E, Montreal QC H2L 4M1; Sher'96; RadOncol. Staff, Centre Hospitalier l'Université de Montréal (CHUM) - Hôpital Notre-Dame; (514)890-8254

BEAUCHEMIN, Marie-Josee; Inst U en Sante Mentale de QC, 2601 de la Canardiere, Quebec QC G1J 2G3; Mon'02; FRCPC; Psy. Staff, Institut Universitaire Sante.

BEAUCHEMIN, Michel; Ctr Hosp Affilie-St-Sacrement, 1050 ch Sainte-Foy, Quebec QC G1S 4L8; Mon'97; CSPQ; FRCPC; AnatPath. Staff, Centre Hospitalier Affilié Universitaire de Québec - Hôpital du St-Sacrement; (418)682-7805

BEAUCHEMIN, Nathalie; Hop Charles Lemoyne, 3120 boul Taschereau, Greenfield Park QC J4V 2H1; Mon'86; Psy. Staff, Hopital Charles LeMoyne; (450)466-5200

BEAUCHEMIN, Pierre; Clinique Medi-Plus, 4100 av 3E O, Quebec QC G1H 6E1; Laval'72; Dip SportMed; Langs: English; (418)622-6969; Fax. (418)622-2037; medica@videotron.ca.

BEAUCHEMIN, Suzanne M; AIM Orleans Hlth & Wellness Cl, 3-1605 Orleans Blvd, Orleans ON K1C 7E2; Ott'85; BSc; CCFP; Court Staff, The Ottawa Hospital - Riverside Campus; Att Staff, The Ottawa Hospital - Civic Campus; Medical Staff, Dr Bernstein Health & Diet Clinic; Langs: English; French; (613)830-6890; Fax. (613)837-6312.

BEAUCHESNE, Andre; Centre Med Saint-Jacques, 1364 rue Saint-Jacques, L'Ancienne-Lorette QC G2E 2X1; Laval'78; (418)877-7727

BEAUCHESNE, Christian; Centre Med Robinson Inc, 4 rue Robinson N, Granby QC J2G 8Z9; Sher'78; Ac Staff, Centre Hospitalier de Granby; Langs: English; (450)378-8435; Fax. (450)375-8832.

BEAUCHESNE, Luc M; Univ of Ottawa Heart Institute, 40 Ruskin St, Ottawa ON K1Y 4W7; McG'88; FRCPC; IntMed (Adult Congenital Heart Disease); Cardiol. Staff, University of Ottawa Heart Institute; Asst Prof Med, University of Ottawa; Langs: English; French; (613)761-4422

BEAUCHESNE, Pierre; CSSS de Rimouski-Neigette, CP 3150 Succ A 150 av Rouleau, Rimouski QC G5L 5T1; Laval'72; DiagRad (P.Q.). Staff, Hôpital Regional Rimouski; (418)724-8581; Fax. (418)724-8654.

BEAUCLAIR, Linda; 1025 av des Pins O, Montreal QC H3A 1A1; Laval'79; FRCPC; Psy (Psycho Pharmacology). adj Prof, McGill University; Langs: Bilingual(French/English); (514)843-1672; Fax. (514)843-2898.

BEAUDET, Anne-Marie; Windsor Reg Hosp-Metropolitan, 1995 Lens Ave, Windsor ON N8W 1L9; Tor'05; FRCPC; DiagRad. Staff, Windsor Regional Hospital - Metropolitan Site; (519)254-5577

BEAUDET, Christine; CSSS de Rimouski-Neigette, CP 3150 Succ A 150 av Rouleau, Rimouski QC G5L 5T1; Laval'03; FRCSC; ObstGyn. Staff, Hôpital Regional Rimouski; (418)724-3000

BEAUDET, Francois; Hop du Sacre-Coeur de Mtl, 92-5400 boul Gouin O, Montreal QC H4J 1C5; Mon'73; FRCPC; IntMed; Rheum. Clin Asst Staff Rheum, Hôpital du Sacre-Coeur de Montréal; adj Prof, Universite de Montreal; (514)338-2050

BEAUDET, Isabelle-Pascale; CHUQ-Hotel-Dieu de Quebec, 11 Cote du Palais, Quebec QC G1R 2J6; Sher'03; FRCPC; IntMed; Gastroent. Staff, Centre Hospitalier Universitaire de Québec (CHUQ) - Siege Social; (418)525-4444

BEAUDET, Julie; Hop Maisonneuve-Rosemont, 5415 boul de l'Assomption, Montreal QC H1T 2M4; Mon'93; FRCPC; IntMed; MedOncol; Hem. Staff, Hopital Maisonneuve-Rosemont; (514)252-3404; jbeaudet.hmr@ssss.gouv.qc.ca.

BEAUDET, Louis-D.; Polyclinique de Trois-Rivieres, 330-1900 boul des Recollets, Trois-Rivieres QC G8Z 4K4; Sher'73; AB; Derm. Staff, Centre Hospitalier Regional de Trois-Rivieres; (819)379-3141

BEAUDET, Louis-Edmond; Centre Med Mailloux, 130-1900 av Mailloux, Quebec QC G1J 5B9; Laval'75; Ac Staff, Centre Hospitalier Affilié Universitaire de Québec - Hôpital De L'Enfant Jésus; Teach Staff Psy, Université Laval; (418)667-7014; Fax. (418)667-5808.

BEAUDET, Luc; 190 Ingram St, Duncan BC V9L 1P1; UBC'01; FRCSC; ObstGyn. Staff, BC Women's Hospital & Health Centre; (250)748-2422

BEAUDET, Lynn; CHUS-Hop Hotel-Dieu, 580 rue Bowen S, Sherbrooke QC J1G 2E8; Sher'80; Ac Staff, Centre Hospitalier Universitaire de Sherbrooke-Hôpital Hôtel-Dieu; (819)346-1110 x21000; Fax. (819)565-2116.

BEAUDET, Marie-France; 880 av Painchaud, Quebec QC G1S 0A3; Mon'99; CCFP; Staff, CSSS de la Vielle Capitale; Staff, Centre Hospitalier Universitaire de Quebec-CHUL; Langs: English; (418)688-1221; Fax. (418)688-0105; beaudem@yahoo.com.

BEAUDET, Nathalie; 305-111 Echo Dr, Ottawa ON K1S 5K8; Mon'77; MSc; (613)422-9478

BEAUDET, Pierre; Clinique Med Familiale, 2185 boul de Tadoussac, Chicoutimi QC G7G 4X2; Laval'70; (418)698-2414; Fax. (418)698-2413.

BEAUDET, Veronique; CHUM-Hop St-Luc, 1058 rue Saint-Denis, Montreal QC H2X 3J4; Mon'02; FRCPC; Anes. Staff, Centre Hospitalier l'Université De Montréal (CHUM) - Hôpital Saint-luc.

BEAUDET-PLESZCZYNSKA, C Chantal; Direction de la Sante Publique, 300 rue King E, Sherbrooke QC J1G 1B1; Sher'71; Langs: English; (819)829-3400 x42435; Fax. (819)569-8894; cbeaudet.agence05@ssss.gouv.qc.ca.

BEAUDETTE, Katherine N; Family Med Associates, 500-267 O'Connor St, Ottawa ON K2P 1V3; Alb'97; MSc; CCFP; FCFP; (613)760-3725

BEAUDETTE, Roxanne M; South Sherbrook Health Centre, B-88 Sherbrook St, Winnipeg MB R3C 2B3; Man'91; CCFP; Staff, Victoria General Hospital.

BEAUDIN, Gabriel; Groupe Sante Medisys Inc, 1110-500 rue Sherbrooke O, Montreal QC H3A 3C6; Mon'72; Staff, Hopital Charles LeMoyne; (514)845-1211

BEAUDIN, Genevieve; Ctr Hosp Anna-Laberge, 200 boul Brisebois, Chateauguay QC J6K 4W8; Mon'07; CCFP; Staff, Hôpital Anna-Laberge; (450)699-2425

BEAUDIN, Jean-Hugues; Clinique Psychiatrie, 190 rue Labonte, Longueuil QC J4H 2P7; Sher'01; FRCPC; Psy. Staff, Hopital Charles LeMoyne; (450)466-5000

BEAUDIN, Julie; Clinique Med Pierre-Boucher, 1615 boul Jacques-Cartier E, Longueuil QC J4M 2X1; Sher'96; (450)468-6223

BEAUDOIN, Andre; Hop du Sacre-Coeur de Mtl, 5400 boul Gouin O, Montreal QC H4J 1C5; Mon'68; IntMed. Staff, Hôpital du Sacre-Coeur de Montréal; adj Prof, Universite de Montreal; (514)338-2050

BEAUDOIN, Angele C; 10565 124 St NW, Edmonton AB T5N 1R8; Alb'90; (780)432-1261; Fax. (780)438-6549.

BEAUDOIN, Anne; Centre Francois-Charon, 525 boul Wilfrid-Hamel, Quebec QC G1M 2S8; Laval'82; Ac Staff, Hôtel-Dieu de Lévis; (418)529-9141; Fax. (418)649-3703.

BEAUDOIN, Annie; CHUS-Hop Hotel-Dieu, 580 rue Bowen S, Sherbrooke QC J1G 2E8; Sher'98; FRCPC; IntMed; Gastroent. Staff, Centre Hospitalier Universitaire de Sherbrooke-Hôpital Hôtel-Dieu; Langs: English; French; (819)346-1110; Fax. (819)822-6797.

BEAUDOIN, C Gabriel; 224 rue Monseigneur-Charbonnea, Boucherville QC J4B 2G6; Laval'57; CSPQ; Anes. (450)449-0258

BEAUDOIN, Catherine; CSSS de Trois-Rivieres, 1991 boul du Carmel, Trois-Rivieres QC G8Z 3R9; Mon'02; Staff, CSSS de Trois-Rivières; Langs: English; (819)697-3333

BEAUDOIN, Daniel; Polyclinique Med de Terrebonne, 201-901 boul des Seigneurs, Terrebonne QC J6W 1T8; Mon'75; LMCC; (450)471-1117; Fax. (450)471-8043; beaudoin.daniel@sympatico.ca.

BEAUDOIN, Danielle; 110-2880 ch des Quatre-Bourgeo, Quebec QC G1V 4X7; Laval'86; FRCSC; Otol. Staff, Centre Hospitalier Affilié Universitaire de Québec - Hôpital De L'Enfant Jésus; Staff, Centre Hospitalier Affilié Universitaire de Québec - Hôpital du St-Sacrement; (418)653-8717; Fax. (418)653-7199.

BEAUDOIN, Denise; Clinique Med Robinson Inc, 4 rue Robinson N, Granby QC J2G 8Z9; Sher'79; (450)378-8435; Fax. (450)375-8832.

BEAUDOIN, Eddy; 5155 rue Sainte-Catherine E, Montreal QC H1V 2A5; Mon'53; (514)255-2833; Fax. (514)255-1277.

BEAUDOIN, Francois; Ctre d'Obstetrique-Gynecologie, 203-1361 av Beaumont, Mont-Royal QC H3P 2W3; Mon'81; FRCSC; ObstGyn. Ac Staff, Hôpital Ste-Justine; (514)344-4411; Fax. (514)344-1991.

BEAUDOIN, Gaetan; CRSSS Baie-James-Chibougamau, 51 3e rue, Chibougamau QC G8P 1N1; Mon'85; FRCSC; GenSurg. Staff, CRSSS de la Baie-James; (418)748-2676

BEAUDOIN, Guylaine; C S S T, 1199 rue de Bleury, Montreal QC H3B 3J1; Sher'85; (514)906-3003 x2318; Fax. (514)906-3001.

BEAUDOIN, Jacques; Centre Med Laennec, 200-1750 av De Vitre, Quebec QC G1J 1Z6; Laval'68; CSPQ; Cardiol (P.Q.). ac Staff Cardiol, Centre Hospitalier Affilié Universitaire de Québec - Hôpital De L'Enfant Jésus; (418)663-2858; Fax. (418)663-2352; clinic.desilets@qc.aira.com.

BEAUDOIN, Jacques; Clinique Med Hickson, 3805 rue De Verdun, Verdun QC H4G 1K8; Mon'73; Staff, Centre Hospitalier de Verdun; (514)769-9671; Fax. (514)769-9676.

BEAUDOIN, Jean-Louis; 110-1 Place du Commerce, Verdun QC H3E 1A2; Mon'70; FRCSC; PlasSurg. (514)769-8809

BEAUDOIN, Jean-Pierre; Clinique Med Antoine-Labelle, 200-555 boul Saint-Antoine, Saint-Jerome QC J7Z 3B8; Mon'85; Staff, Hôpital de Saint-Eustache; (450)438-1252; Fax. (450)438-6441.

BEAUDOIN, Jonathan; Hôpital Laval, 2725 ch Sainte-Foy, Quebec QC G1V 4G5; Laval'03; FRCPC; IntMed; Cardiol. Staff, Hôpital Laval; (418)656-8711

BEAUDOIN, Julie; Clinique Med de Levis, 100-4975 boul de la Rive-Sud, Levis QC G6V 4Z5; Laval'04; (418)833-5810; Fax. (418)833-2720.

BEAUDOIN, Karine; Medi-Centre Chomedey, 610 boul Cure-Labelle, Laval QC H7V 2T7; Mon'07.

BEAUDOIN, Marc; CHUM-Hop Notre-Dame, 1560 rue Sherbrooke E, Montreal QC H2L 4M1; Mon'65; FRCPC; IntMed; Gastroent (P.Q.). Chef gastro, Centre Hospitalier l'Université de Montréal (CHUM) - Hôpital Notre-Dame; (514)890-8000 x27057

BEAUDOIN, Melanie; Hotel-Dieu de Levis, 143 rue Wolfe, Levis QC G6V 3Z1; Mon'05; Psy. Staff, Hôtel-Dieu de Lévis; (418)835-7141

BEAUDOIN, Michel; Carrefour Med Vallee Richelieu, 665 boul Sir-Wilfrid-Laurier, Beloeil QC J3G 4J1; Sher'92; Staff, Hôpital de l'Archipel; (450)467-0088; Fax. (450)467-4936.

BEAUDOIN, Nathalie; CHUM-Hotel-Dieu, 3840 rue Saint-Urbain, Montreal QC H2W 1T8; Mon'93; FRCSC; GenSurg; VascSurg. Staff, Centre Hospitalier l'Université de Montréal (CHUM) - Hôtel-Dieu; (514)890-8000

BEAUDOIN, Nicole; Inst de Readaptation de Mtl, 6300 av De Darlington, Montreal QC H3S 2J4; Mon'82; FRCPC; PhysMed&Rehab. Staff, Institut de Réadaptation Gingras-Lindsay de Montréal; assoc Prof, Universite de Montreal; Langs: Bilingual(French/English); (514)340-2084; Fax. (514)340-2775.

BEAUDOIN, Rene; CHUS-Hop Fleurimont, 3001 12e Av N, Sherbrooke QC J1H 5N4; Sher'77; EmergMed (P.Q.). Ac Staff Emerg Dept, Centre Hospitalier Universitaire de Sherbrooke-Hopital Fleurimont; Assoc Prof Family Med, Universite de Sherbrooke; Langs: English; (819)346-1110 x14274; Fax. (819)564-5386; rene.beaudoin@usherbrooke.ca.

BEAUDOIN, Richard; Clinique Medi-Plus, 4100 av 3E O, Quebec QC G1H 6E1; Laval'72; ac Staff, Centre Hospitalier Universitaire De Québec - Pavillon De St-françois-d'assise; (418)622-6969; Fax. (418)622-2037.

BEAUDOIN, Richard; Clinique Med St-Henri, 223 rue Commerciale RR 1, St-Henri-De-Levis QC G0R 3E0; Laval'75; Ac Staff, Hôtel-Dieu de Lévis; (418)882-2268; Fax. (418)882-3561.

BEAUDOIN, Robert; 3495A rue Hochelaga, Montreal QC H1W 1H6; Mon'76; Langs: Spanish; English; (514)529-3663; Fax. (514)529-7175.

BEAUDOIN, Simon; Clin de Chirurgie Orthopedique, 10445 1re av, Saint-Georges QC G5Y 6X8; Laval'02; FRCSC; OrthSurg. (418)228-2899

BEAUDRY, Caroline; Hotel-Dieu de Levis, 143 rue Wolfe, Levis QC G6V 3Z1; Laval'04; FRCPC; Peds. Staff, Hôtel-Dieu de Lévis; (418)835-7121

BEAUDRY, Claude; Hop Maisonneuve-Rosemont, 5415 boul de l'Assomption, Montreal QC H1T 2M4; Mon'69; Peds. Staff, Hopital Maisonneuve-Rosemont; (514)252-3400

BEAUDRY, Constant; RSRY Pavillon Hotel-Dieu, 1800 des Saules, Saint-Hyacinthe QC J2S 2T2; Mon'70; Staff, Centre Hospitalier Honore-Mercier; (450)771-3333

BEAUDRY, Daniel; Dr Georges-L Dumont Reg Hosp, 330 av Universite, Moncton NB E1C 2Z3; Mon'69; Respir (Pneumology). Staff, Dr Georges-L-Dumont University Hospital Centre; Langs: Bilingual(French/English); (506)858-8985; Fax. (506)383-4492; daniel.beaudry@bellaliant.net.

BEAUDRY, Daniel; Ctr Hosp de Lachine, 650 16e av, Lachine QC H8S 3N5; Mon'93; Staff, CSSS de Dorval-Lachine-Lasalle; (514)637-2351

BEAUDRY, Florent; 229 av Proulx, Quebec QC G1M 1W6; Laval'70; Obstetrics, CSSS de Quebec-Sud; (418)681-3348

BEAUDRY, Gaetan; Polyclinique Med Fabreville, 380 boul Cure-Labelle, Laval QC H7P 5L3; Mon'76; (450)628-5800; Fax. (450)628-0217.

BEAUDRY, Genevieve; CSSS du Sud de Lanaudière, 911 montée des Pionniers, Terrebonne QC J6V 2H2; Sher'01; ObstGyn. Staff, Centre Hospitalier Pierre le Gardeur; (450)654-7525

BEAUDRY, J Pierre; MUHC-Royal Victoria Hosp, S4.41-687 av des Pins O, Montreal QC H3A 1A1; McG'74; BA; MDCM; Cardiol; IntMed (Interventional Cardiology). Staff, McGill University Health Centre - Royal Victoria Hospital; Langs: Bilingual(English/French); (514)934-1934 x34632; Fax. (514)843-1694.

BEAUDRY, Jacques; 1652 rue Royale, Trois-Rivieres QC G9A 4K3; Laval'67; (819)379-4521; Fax. (819)379-4615.

BEAUDRY, Jean-Marc; Commission des Lesions Prof, 700-900 Pl D'Youville, Quebec QC G1R 3P7; Laval'75; FRCPC; IntMed. Langs: English; (418)644-7777; Fax. (418)644-6078.

BEAUDRY, Josianne E; CFB Borden, PO Box 1000 Stn Forces, Borden ON L0M 1C0; Laval'05; CCFP; Langs: Spanish; English; (705)424-1200

BEAUDRY, Line; CSSS de Laval, 1755 boul Rene-Laennec, Laval QC H7M 3L9; Mon'88; CCFP; Staff, Hopital de la Cite de la santé; (450)668-1010

BEAUDRY, Louise F; Ctr Hosp Pierre-Janet, 20 rue Pharand, Gatineau QC J9A 1K7; Mon'74; FRCPC; Psy. Psychiatre, Centre Hospitalier Pierre-Janet; (819)776-8086; Fax. (819)771-4727.

BEAUDRY, Louise; CLSC Laurier-Station, 135 rue de la Station Ss 1, Laurier-Station QC G0S 1N0; Laval'82; CCFP; FCFP; (418)728-3435; Fax. (418)728-3477.

BEAUDRY, Luce; CSSS du Nord de Lanaudière, 1000 boul Sainte-Anne, Joliette QC J6E 6J2; Mon'70; Staff, Centre Hospitalier Régional de Lanaudière; (450)759-8222

BEAUDRY, Marie-Eve; CSSS du Lac-des-Deux-Montagnes, 520 boul Arthur-Sauve, Saint-Eustache QC J7R 5B1; Sher'02; FRCPC; Anes. Staff, Hôpital de Saint-Eustache; (450)473-6811; Fax. (450)473-6966.

BEAUDRY, Mathieu; CHUS-Hop Fleurimont, 3001 12e Av N, Sherbrooke QC J1H 5N4; Sher'99; CSPQ; FRCPC; Anes. Staff, Centre Hospitalier Universitaire de Sherbrooke-Hopital Fleurimont; (819)346-1110

BEAUDRY, Melanie; Inst Albert Prevost, 6555 boul Gouin O, Montreal QC H4K 1B3; Mon'05; Psy. (514)338-2222; Fax. (514)338-4215.

BEAUDRY, Michel G; Polyclinique, 215-874 boul de l'Universite E, Chicoutimi QC G7H 6B9; Sher'82; MSc(Epidemiol); DABSM; FRCPC; Neur; Electroenceph (P.Q.). Staff, Complexe hospitalier de la Sagamie; Langs: Spanish; English; (418)549-9571; Fax. (418)549-8631.

BEAUDRY, Nicole; Ctr Hosp De Verdun, 4000 boul Lasalle, Verdun QC H4G 2A3; Mon'86; Clin Instructor, Universite de Montreal; (514)362-1000

BEAUDRY, P Paul; Alberta Children's Hosp, 2888 Shaganappi Trail NW, Calgary AB T3B 6A8; Cal'98; FRCSC; GenSurg; PedGenSurg. Staff Surg, Alberta Children's Hospital; (403)955-2850; Fax. (403)955-7634.

BEAUDRY, Paul; 22-41 rue de l'Eglise, Verdun QC H4G 2L8; Sher'77; FRCPC; Psy (Psychoanalysis). Clin Staff Psy, McGill University Health Centre - Royal Victoria Hospital; adj Prof, McGill University; (514)769-2943; Fax. (514)769-0602.

BEAUDRY, Philippe R; 303-720 Guelph Line, Burlington ON L7R 4E2; Sher'76; ABCD; ABIM; NBME; FACC; FRCPC; IntMed (Adult Cardiology); Cardiol. Staff, Joseph Brant Memorial Hospital; Langs: Bilingual(English/French); (905)333-3300

BEAUDRY, Pierre; Clinique Med Fam des Recollets, 101-940 boul des Recollets, Trois-Rivieres QC G8Z 3W9; Laval'71; CSPQ; Cardiol. (819)373-0303

BEAUDRY, Veronique; Hop du Sacre-Coeur de Mtl, 5400 boul Gouin O, Montreal QC H4J 1C5; Mon'03; CCFP; CCFP(E.M.); Staff, Hôpital du Sacre-Coeur de Montréal; (514)338-2222

BEAUDRY, Veronique; CSSS de Sept-Iles, 45 rue du Pere-Divet, Sept-Iles QC G4R 3N7; Mon'99; FRCPC; Psy. Staff, Centre Hospitalier Regional de Sept-Iles; (418)962-9761

BEAUDRY, Yves; MUHC-Royal Victoria Hosp, 687 av des Pins O, Montreal QC H3A 1A1; McG'83; CSPQ; FRCPC; IntMed; Cardiol. Staff, McGill University Health Centre - Royal Victoria Hospital; (514)934-1934

BEAUDRY-NEHME, Angele; Clinique Med Centrale, 2050 rue Regent, Saint-Hubert QC J4T 3R5; Sher'75; (450)678-9194; Fax. (450)678-0915.

BEAUDRY-REMILLARD, Janine; 1756 Route 241, Waterloo QC J0E 2N0; Ott'63; Psy (P.Q.). (514)539-2060; Fax. (514)539-3838.

BEAUFIELD, Gary S; Wentworth Limeridge Med Ctre, 201-849 Upper Wentworth St, Hamilton ON L9A 5H4; Mem'85; (905)389-9099; Fax. (905)389-5755; gbeaufield@yahoo.ca.

BEAULAC, Emilie; CHUS-Hop Hotel-Dieu, 580 rue Bowen S, Sherbrooke QC J1G 2E8; Laval'07; CCFP; Staff, Centre Hospitalier Universitaire de Sherbrooke-Hôpital Hôtel-Dieu; (819)346-1110

BEAULE, Caroline; Ctr Hosp du Centre la Mauricie, 50 119e rue, Shawinigan-Sud QC G9P 5K1; Laval'95; FRCPC; IntMed. Staff, Centre Hospitalier du Centre la Mauricie; (819)536-7500; Fax. (819)536-7649.

BEAULE, Paul E; The Ottawa Hosp-Gen Campus, 1646-501 Smyth Rd, Ottawa ON K1H 8L6; Ott'92; FRCSC; OrthSurg. Staff, The Ottawa Hospital - General Campus; (613)737-8899 x73265

BEAULIEU, Andre; Ctr de Rhumatologie St-Louis, 360-3165 ch Saint-Louis, Quebec QC G1W 4R4; Mon'72; FRCPC; Rheum. Langs: Bilingual(French/English); (418)659-5757; Fax. (418)659-5758.

BEAULIEU, Andree; Clinique Med Montfort, 2185 rue de Montfort, Jonquiere QC G7X 4P6; Laval'81; (418)547-4783

BEAULIEU, Andree-Anne; Centre Hosp Honore-Mercier, 2750 boul Laframboise, Saint-Hyacinthe QC J2S 4Y8; Sher'06; FRCPC; MedMicrobiol (P.Q.). Staff, Centre Hospitalier Honore-Mercier; (450)771-3333 x3205

BEAULIEU, Catherine; Hotel-Dieu de Levis, 143 rue Wolfe, Levis QC G6V 3Z1; Laval'05; CCFP; CCFP(E.M.); Staff, Hôtel-Dieu de Lévis; (418)835-7121

BEAULIEU, Celina; CSSS du Nord de Lanaudière, 1000 boul Sainte-Anne, St-Charles-Brromee QC J6E 6J2; Sher'00; Gastroent; IntMed. Staff, Centre Hospitalier Régional de Lanaudière; (450)759-8222

BEAULIEU, Chantal; Centre Med Ste Anne, 500 Old St. Patrick St, Ottawa ON K1N 9G4; Sher'92; FRCSC; GenSurg (Breast Cancer). (613)241-3013; Fax. (613)241-4482.

BEAULIEU, Claude A; Villa Marconi Nursing Home, 1026 Baseline Rd, Ottawa ON K2C 0A6; Ott'68; Att Physician, Glebe Center; Att Physician, Medex Nursing Home; Att Physician, Villa Marconi Nursing Home; (613)727-6201; beaulieulabelle@sympatico.ca.

BEAULIEU, Claude; CSSS Les Eskers de l'Abitibi, 622 4e rue O, Amos QC J9T 2S2; Laval'99; CCFP; Staff, CH Hôtel-Dieu d'Amos; (819)732-3341

BEAULIEU, David S; Stikine Health Centre, PO Box 386, Dease Lake BC V0C 1L0; UBC'96; CCFP; (250)771-4444

BEAULIEU, Denis; CSSS des Basques, 550 rue Notre-Dame E RR 1, Trois-Pistoles QC G0L 4K0; Laval'76; Staff, Centre Hospitalier Trois-Pistoles; (418)851-3700 x319; Fax. (418)851-2944.

BEAULIEU, Denis; Clinique Med Val-Belair, 202-1147 boul Pie-XI N, Quebec QC G3K 2P8; Laval'84; Langs: Bilingual(French/English); (418)843-2473; Fax. (418)843-0224.

BEAULIEU, Gaston; CSSS du Nord de Lanaudière, 1000 boul Sainte-Anne, St-Charles-Brromee QC J6E 6J2; Laval'72; GenSurg (Psychiatry). Staff, Centre Hospitalier Régional de Lanaudière; (450)759-8222; Fax. (450)759-0011.

BEAULIEU, Genevieve; Centre médicale Centrale, 4-135 rue Saint-Antoine N, Granby QC J2G 5G7; Sher'04; CCFP; (450)372-6006; Fax. (450)372-4174.

BEAULIEU, Genevieve; CHUS-Hop Fleurimont, 3001 12e av N, Sherbrooke QC J1H 5N4; Sher'00; FRCPC; Peds. Staff, Centre Hospitalier Universitaire de Sherbrooke-Hopital Fleurimont; (819)346-1110

BEAULIEU, Guylaine; CLSC Malauze, 14 boul Perron E CP 190, Matapedia QC G0J 1V0; Laval'81; (819)865-2221

BEAULIEU, Helene; GMF du Chatel, 200-9465 boul de l'Ormiere, Quebec QC G2B 3K7; Laval'86; (418)843-5141; Fax. (418)843-5343.

BEAULIEU, J Marc-Andre; Direction de la Sante au Trava, CP 40 M5 03-73 Prom Leikin, Ottawa ON K1A 0R2; Ott'82; BSc; FRCPC; Neur (Epilepsy). (613)843-6463

BEAULIEU, Michel F; Clinique Med Asclepios, 2-750 Taylor Creek Dr, Orleans ON K1C 1T1; Laval'77; LMCC; Ac Member, Montfort Hospital; Clin Prof, University of Ottawa; Langs: Bilingual(French/English).

BEAULIEU, Jean-Yves; Clinique Med Desy, 5636 boul Henri-Bourassa E, Montreal-Nord QC H1G 2T2; Mon'87; Physician, Clinique Medical Desy; Langs: English; (514)326-9060; Fax. (514)326-0919; cliniquedesy@qc.aira.com.

BEAULIEU, Joelle; Clinique Med Fleur de Lys, 8 rue Du Terminus E, Rouyn-Noranda QC J9X 3B4; Sher'98; Ac Member ObstGyn, Centre Hospitalier Rouyn-Noranda; (819)764-6185

BEAULIEU, Josee; Clinique Med de Coaticook, 206-18 rue du Manege, Coaticook QC J1A 3B3; Laval'91; Staff, Centre Hospitalier de Coaticook; (819)849-4808; Fax. (819)849-7400.

BEAULIEU, Julie; GMF La Cigogne, 420-3141 boul Taschereau, Greenfield Park QC J4V 2H2; Mon'00; CCFP; Staff, Hopital Charles LeMoyne; (450)466-7892; Fax. (450)466-9602.

BEAULIEU, Linda; Centre Med Saint-Francois, 200-2125 boul Lemire, Drummondville QC J2B 8N8; Sher'86; Ac Staff, Hôpital Sainte-croix; (819)477-6793; Fax. (819)477-6962.

BEAULIEU, Louise; CSSS de Rimouski-Neigette, CP 3150 Succ A 150 av Rouleau, Rimouski QC G5L 5T1; Laval'80; CSPQ; FRCPC; Anes. Staff, Hôpital Regional Rimouski; (418)724-8282; Fax. (418)724-8748.

BEAULIEU, Lucie; 230-365 rue Normand, St-Jean-sur-Richel QC J3A 1T6; Sher'80; FRCPC; Psy. Staff, Hôpital du Haut-Richelieu; (450)359-9537

BEAULIEU, Lucie; 405-5811 boul Taschereau, Brossard QC J4Z 1A5; Laval'92; FRCPC; Peds. Chief Dept of Ped, Centre Hospitalier Pierre Boucher; (450)443-6585; Fax. (450)443-9002.

BEAULIEU, Lucie; Centre Med Saint-Jacques, 1364 rue Saint-Jacques, Quebec QC G2E 2X1; Laval'89; Staff, Centre Hospitalier Affilié Universitaire de Québec - Hôpital De L'Enfant Jésus; (418)877-7727; Fax. (418)877-2781.

BEAULIEU, Lysanne; CLSC de la Region-Sherbrooke, 50 rue Camirand, Sherbrooke QC J1H 4J5; Sher'88; (819)565-1330; Fax. (819)565-8196.

BEAULIEU, Marcella J; Seabird Island Health, PO Box 765 2895 Chowat Rd, Agassiz BC V0M 1A0; Man'04; CCFP; (604)796-2165; Fax. (604)796-1124.

BEAULIEU, Marie-Claude; CLSC de la Region-Sherbrooke, 50 rue Camirand, Sherbrooke QC J1H 4J5; Sher'81; CCFP; Consultant, Centre Hospitalier Universitaire de Sherbrooke-Hôpital Hôtel-Dieu; (819)565-1330; Fax. (819)565-8196.

BEAULIEU, Marie-D.; 10.083-2021 av Union, Montreal QC H3A 2S9; Laval'76; MSc; CCFP; FCFP; Chef Family Med, Centre Hospitalier l'Université de Montréal (CHUM) - Hôpital Notre-Dame; Prof, Universite de Montreal; (514)873-2563

BEAULIEU, Marie-Pier; 3605 rue Foucher, Trois-Rivieres QC G8Y 1L1; Laval'06; FRCSC; OrthSurg (P.Q.). Staff, CSSS de Trois-Rivières; (819)693-8389

BEAULIEU, Monica C; Burrard Health Bldg, 602-1160 Burrard St, Vancouver BC V6Z 2E8; UBC'01; FRCPC; IntMed; Nephrol. (604)681-7191

BEAULIEU, Nathalie; Unite de Med Familiale Laval, 2690 ch des Quatre-Bourgeois, Quebec QC G1V 0B7; Mon'93; (418)656-4795

BEAULIEU, Pascale; CLSC-CHSLD La Pommeraie, 34 rue Saint-Joseph, Bedford QC J0J 1A0; Laval'93; Staff, CLSC-CHSLD La Pommeraie - Centre hospitalier de Bedford; (450)248-4304; pascale_beaulieu@rrsss16.gouv.qc.ca.

BEAULIEU, Pierre; Clinique Med Soleil, 64 1re Av O, Amos QC J9T 1T8; Laval'85; Staff, CH Hôtel-Dieu d'Amos; (819)732-8341; Fax. (819)732-1642.

BEAULIEU, Pierre; CSSS des Îles, 430 ch Principal, Cap-aux-Meules QC G4T 1R9; Bordeaux (France)'87; FRCPC; Anes. Staff, Hôpital de l'Archipel; (418)986-2121 x8117

BEAULIEU, Pierre-Andre; 203-404 St. George St, Moncton NB E1C 1X6; Mon'97; CCFP; Langs: English; (506)853-1820; Fax. (506)854-2136.

BEAULIEU, R Claude; 598 rue Victoria CP 36568 Csp Victoria, Saint-Lambert QC J4P 3S8; Laval'78; FRCSC; GenSurg (P.Q.) (Thoracic Surgery); Cardiovasc&ThorSurg. Staff, Hopital Charles LeMoyne; McGill University; Universite de Sherbrooke; (450)466-5000; Fax. (450)466-5081; lrt116@sympatico.ca.

BEAULIEU, Raymond; CHUM-Hotel-Dieu, 3840 rue Saint-Urbain, Montreal QC H2W 1T8; Mon'67; FRCPC; HemPath; Hem (P.Q.); MedOncol (P.Q.). Chef hématol, Centre Hospitalier l'Université de Montréal (CHUM) - Hôtel-Dieu; Prof Med, Universite de Montreal; (514)890-8197

BEAULIEU, Rene; CLSC Simonne-Monet-Chartrand, 1303 boul Jacques-Cartier E, Longueuil QC J4M 2Y8; Mon'70; ac Membre, Centre Hospitalier Pierre Boucher; Affil Member, Hôpital Santa Cabrini Ospedale; Langs: Italian; English; (450)463-2850; Fax. (450)647-0163.

BEAULIEU, Richard; CSSS de Saint-Jerome, 290 rue de Montigny, Saint-Jerome QC J7Z 5T3; Mon'87; Staff, Hôtel-Dieu de Saint-Jérôme; (450)431-8200; Fax. (450)431-8244.

BEAULIEU, Richard; Polyclinique de la Capitale, 14-4225 av 4E O, Quebec QC G1H 6P3; Laval'68; ac Staff, Centre Hospitalier Universitaire De Québec - Pavillon De St-françois-d'assise; (418)628-9921; Fax. (418)628-3203.

BEAULIEU, Roland G; Scarborough Prof Centre, 409-1371 Neilson Rd, Scarborough ON M1B 4Z8; Alb'78; FRCPC; Peds (Fetal Anomalies); Cardiol. Consultant, Rouge Valley Health System - Centenary Health Centre Site; Consultant, The Scarborough Hospital - Birchmount Campus; Consultant, North York General Hospital; (416)282-9198; Fax. (416)282-9897; rbeaul@sympatico.ca.

BEAULIEU, Samuel; Ctr Hosp Affilie-Enfant-Jesus, 1401 18e rue, Quebec QC G1J 1Z4; Laval'99; CCFP; CCFP(E.M.); Staff, Centre Hospitalier Affilié Universitaire de Québec - Hôpital De L'Enfant Jésus; (418)649-5632

BEAULIEU, Serge; Douglas Mental Hlth Univ Inst, 6875 boul Lasalle, Verdun QC H4H 1R3; Laval'88; BSc; MSc; PhD; FRCPC; Psy (Bipolar Disease). Staff, Douglas Mental Health University Institute; assoc Prof, McGill University; Langs: English; (514)761-6131 x3301; Fax. (514)888-4462.

BEAULIEU, Sophie; Clinique Med Pierre-Bertrand, 212-303 boul Pierre-Bertrand, Quebec QC G1M 3L7; Laval'98; (418)683-2724; Fax. (418)683-8861.

BEAULIEU, Sophie; Clin d'Ophtalmologie du Saguen, 150 boul Barette, Chicoutimi QC G7H 7W8; Sher'07; Ophth. (418)545-2571

BEAULIEU, Sylvain; Hop Maisonneuve-Rosemont, 5415 boul de l'Assomption, Montreal QC H1T 2M4; Laval'95; FRCPC; NuclearMed. Staff, Hopital Maisonneuve-Rosemont; (514)252-3400

BEAULIEU, Yanick; Hop du Sacre-Coeur de Mtl, 5400 boul Gouin O, Montreal QC H4J 1C5; McG'96; CSPQ; FRCPC; IntMed; Critical Care Medicine (P.Q.); Cardiol. Staff, Hôpital du Sacre-Coeur de Montréal; (514)338-2200; Fax. (514)338-2381.

BEAULIEU, Yohan; Ctr de Sante Paul-Gilbert, 9330 boul du Centre-Hospitalie, Charny QC G6X 1L6; Laval'99; CCFP; CCFP(E.M.); Staff, Centre Hospitalier Paul-Gilbert; (418)380-8993 x2064

BEAULIEU, Yves; 12021 15e av, Montreal QC H1E 0A1; Mon'77; (514)648-5070; Fax. (514)648-8634.

BEAULIEU, Yves; Clin Med Vingt Quatre Juin, 105-1055 12e Av N, Sherbrooke QC J1E 2X4; Sher'76; (819)821-2142; Fax. (819)821-0248; cmf24juin@hotmail.com.

BEAULIEU-BOIRE, Genevieve; CSSS du Suroît, 150 rue Saint-Thomas, Salaber-de-Valleyf QC J6T 6C1; Sher'06; FRCPC; IntMed (P.Q.). Staff, Centre Hospitalier Régional du Suroît; (450)371-9920

BEAULIEU-DENAULT, Camille; CSSS Drummond-Hop Sainte-Croix, 570 rue Heriot, Drummondville QC J2B 1C1; Laval'10; CCFP; Staff, Hôpital Sainte-croix; (819)478-6464

BEAULIEU JR., David; GMF de Grand-Mere, 200-1050 8e rue, Grand-Mere QC G9T 4L4; Laval'76; (819)538-5870

BEAUMIER, Alain; UMF Laval, 2690 ch des Quatre-Bourgeois, Quebec QC G1V 0B7; Laval'80; Ac Staff, Hôpital Laval; (418)656-4795; Fax. (418)656-4503.

BEAUMIER, Isabelle; Centre Med Robinson Inc, 4 rue Robinson N, Granby QC J2G 8Z9; Mon'96; Staff, Centre Hospitalier de Granby; (450)378-8435; Fax. (450)375-8832.

BEAUMIER, Louis; MUHC-Montreal Children's Hosp, C920-2300 rue Tupper, Montreal QC H3H 1P3; Laval'88; FRCPC; Peds (Neonatal & Perinatal Medicine). Staff, McGill University Health Centre - Montreal Children's Hospital; (514)412-4452; Fax. (514)412-4356.

BEAUMONT, Charl G; 157A Minnesota Dr, Stephenville NL A2N 3Y3; Witwatersrand (South Africa)'99; MB BCh; Staff, Sir Thomas Roddick Hospital.

BEAUMONT, Cyril; Centre Medical St-Jean, 202-1018 rue de la Prairie O, St-J-Chrysostome QC G6Z 0A7; Laval'72; Staff, Hôtel-Dieu de Lévis; (418)839-4433; Fax. (418)839-3574.

BEAUMONT, Denis; Clinique Med de Mont-Joli, 1385 boul Benoit-Gaboury, Mont-Joli QC G5H 4B1; Laval'72; Staff, Hôpital Regional Rimouski; (418)775-5353

BEAUMONT, Louis; Centre Bois De Boulogne, 425-1575 boul Henri-Bourassa O, Montreal QC H3M 3A9; Mon'65; ObstGyn. Ac Member, Hôpital du Sacre-Coeur de Montréal; adj Prof, Universite de Montreal; Langs: English; (514)334-1027; Fax. (514)336-8814.

BEAUMONT, Marie-Claude; Ctr Hosp Rouyn-Noranda, 4 9e rue, Rouyn-Noranda QC J9X 2B2; Laval'95; FRCSC; ObstGyn. Staff, Centre Hospitalier Rouyn-Noranda; (819)764-5131; mariecbeaumont@yahoo.ca.

BEAUMONT, Nancy; Mini-Urgence Chicoutimi, 715 boul Sainte-Genevieve, Chicoutimi QC G7G 4Z4; Laval'84; (418)696-2330

BEAUMONT, Nathalie; Centre médicale Centrale, 4-135 rue Saint-Antoine N, Granby QC J2G 5G7; Mon'90; Lakeshore General Hospital - Pointe Claire; (450)372-5401

BEAUMONT, Pierre; Centre Bois de Boulogne, 480-1575 boul Henri-Bourassa O, Montreal QC H3M 3A9; Laval'72; FRCSC; OrthSurg (Hand Surgery). Staff, Hôpital du Sacre-Coeur de Montréal; (514)332-6025; Fax. (514)332-4243.

BEAUNOYER, Mona; Hôpital Ste-Justine, 3175 ch Cote-Sainte-Catherine, Montreal QC H3T 1C5; McG'97; FRCSC; GenSurg (Transplantation); PedGenSurg. Staff, Hôpital Ste-Justine; Langs: English; (514)345-4915; Fax. (514)345-4964.

BEAUPRE, Alain; Hop Maisonneuve-Rosemont, 5415 boul de l'Assomption, Montreal QC H1T 2M4; Mon'74; FRC; FRCPC; Respir. Staff, Hopital Maisonneuve-Rosemont; (514)252-3822; Fax. (514)252-3434; beauprea@videotron.ca.

BEAUPRE, Andre; Ctr Hosp Fleury, 2180 rue Fleury E, Montreal QC H2B 1K3; Mon'98; FRCSC; GenSurg. Staff, Centre Hospitalier Fleury; Langs: English; (514)381-9311

BEAUPRE, Gaetane; Centre Med Saint-Raymond, 220 rue Saint-Joseph, Saint-Raymond QC G3L 1J1; Laval'89; CCFP; (418)337-2214; Fax. (418)337-3749.

BEAUPRE, Lucie M; Dr Beaupre Vein Clinic, 600-1335 Carling Ave, Ottawa ON K1Z 8N8; Mon'77; Langs: French; (613)722-0101; Fax. (613)722-5422.

BEAUPRE, Pierre; Hotel-Dieu de Levis, 143 rue Wolfe, Levis QC G6V 3Z1; Laval'87; FRCPC; EmergMed;CCFP; CCFP(E.M.); FCFP; Member Emerg Service, Hôtel-Dieu de Lévis; Teach Staff Emerg & Family Med Unit, Université Laval; (418)835-7121; pierre.beaupre@mfa.ulaval.ca.

BEAUPRE, Richard; Centre Francois-Charon, 525 boul Wilfrid-Hamel, Quebec QC G1M 2S8; Laval'77; Ac Member, Centre Francois-Charon; (418)529-9141 x6319; Fax. (418)649-3703.

BEAUPRIE, Ian G; Capital Health District Author, 5820 University Ave, Halifax NS B3H 1V7; Tor'87; FRCPC; Anes (Pain Management). Staff, Queen Elizabeth II Health Sciences Centre - Victoria General Site; Staff, Capital Health District Authority; Assoc Prof Anes & NeuroSurg, Dalhousie University; (902)473-4130; Fax. (902)473-4126.

BEAUREGARD, Carmen; CHUS-Hop Fleurimont, 3001 12e Av N, Sherbrooke QC J1H 5N4; Laval'91; FRCPC; Psy. Staff, Centre Hospitalier Universitaire de Sherbrooke-Hopital Fleurimont; (819)346-1110 x14000; carmen.beauregard@usherbrooke.ca.

BEAUREGARD, Catherine; CHUM-Hop Notre-Dame, 1560 rue Sherbrooke E, Montreal QC H2L 4M1; McG'97; FRCPC; IntMed; Endocrin&Metab. Staff, Centre Hospitalier l'Université de Montréal (CHUM) - Hôpital Notre-Dame; Langs: English; French; (514)890-8000 x25354

BEAUREGARD, Edith; CSSS Les Eskers de l'Abitibi, 622 4e rue O, Amos QC J9T 2S2; Mon'96; FRCSC; OrthSurg. Staff, CH Hôtel-Dieu d'Amos; (819)732-3341; Fax. (819)732-6422.

BEAUREGARD, Gilles N; Clinique Med de l'Est Inc, 210-8 Place du Commerce, Verdun QC H3E 1N3; Laval'69; FRCSC; GenSurg (P. Q.); PlasSurg. Staff, Centre Hospitalier l'Université de Montréal (CHUM) - Hôtel-Dieu; adj Prof, Universite de Montreal; (514)845-2828; Fax. (514)843-9937; drgillesbeauregard@qc.aira.com.

BEAUREGARD, Hugues; CHUM-Hop Notre-Dame, 1560 rue Sherbrooke E, Montreal QC H2L 4M1; Mon'66; Endocrin (P.Q.); IntMed. Chef endo, Centre Hospitalier l'Université de Montréal (CHUM) - Hôpital Notre-Dame; Prof, Universite de Montreal; (514)890-8000 x26625

BEAUREGARD, Jean-Mathieu; CHUQ-Hotel-Dieu de Quebec, 11 Cote du Palais, Quebec QC G1R 2J6; Laval'01; FRCPC; NuclearMed. Staff, Centre Hospitalier Universitaire de Québec (CHUQ) - Siege Social; (418)691-5151

BEAUREGARD, Liette; Canadian Med Protective Assn, 875 Carling Ave, Ottawa ON K1S 5P1; Sher'84; CSPQ; FRCPC; Anes. Staff, Canadian Medical Protective Association; Langs: English; (613)725-2000; lbeauregard@cmpa.org.

BEAUREGARD, Louis; CLSC Ste-Therese de Blainville, 55 rue Saint-Joseph, Sainte-Therese QC J7E 4Y5; Mon'76; Médecin, CLSC Ste-Therese de Blainville; (450)430-4553; Fax. (450)430-3859.

BEAUREGARD, Marie; CLSC Cote-des-Neiges, 500-5700 ch Cote-des-Neiges, Montreal QC H3T 2A8; Mon'88; CCFP; FCFP; Langs: Portuguese; English; Spanish; (514)731-8531; Fax. (514)731-0165; marie.beauregard.cdn@ssss.gouv.qc.ca.

BEAUREGARD, Melanie; CSSS Pierre Boucher, 1333 boul Jacques-Cartier E, Longueuil QC J4M 2A5; Mon'07; ObstGyn. Staff, Centre Hospitalier Pierre Boucher; (450)468-8111

BEAUREGARD, Michel; 54 rue Ranger, Ripon QC J0V 1V0; Laval'83; LMCC; Langs: English; (819)983-2048; Fax. (819)983-2048.

BEAUREGARD, Pascale; CSSS du Sud de Lanaudière, 911 montee des Pionniers, Terrebonne QC J6V 2H2; Mon'98; FRCSC; ObstGyn. Staff, Centre Hospitalier Pierre le Gardeur; (450)654-7525

BEAUREGARD, Patrice; CHUS-Hop Fleurimont, 3001 12e av N, Sherbrooke QC J1H 5N4; Mon'82; FRCPC; IntMed (Medical Oncology); Hem. Hématologue, Centre Hospitalier Universitaire de Sherbrooke-Hopital Fleurimont; Prof, Universite de Sherbrooke; Langs: Bilingual(French/English); (819)346-1110 x14816; Fax. (819)564-5434; patrice.beauregard@usherbrooke.ca.

BEAUREGARD, Solange; Clinique de Dermatologique, 133-1055 av 12E N, Sherbrooke QC J1E 2X4; Laval'79; FRCPC; Derm (Geriatric Dermatology). Staff, Centre Hospitalier Universitaire de Sherbrooke-Hopital Fleurimont; Staff, CSSS Institut universitaire de gériatrie de Sherbrooke; Langs: Spanish; English; (819)563-0006; Fax. (819)563-9474.

BEAUREGARD-LEPAGE, Francis; CSSS du Lac-Temiscamingue, 22 rue Notre-Dame N, Ville-Marie QC J9V 1W8; Sher'05; Staff, CSSS du Témiscamingue; (819)629-2420; francis_beauregard-lepage@ssss.gouv.qc.ca.

BEAURIVAGE, Charles; Hotel-Dieu d'Arthabaska, 5 rue des Hospitalieres, Victoriaville QC G6P 6N2; Sher'91; FRCPC; IntMed (Cardiology). Staff, Hotel-Dieu d'Arthabaska; Clin Prof, Universite de Sherbrooke; Langs: English; (819)357-2030; Fax. (819)357-6016.

BEAUSEJOUR, Denise; Direction de la Sante Publique, 300-300 rue King E, Sherbrooke QC J1G 1B1; Laval'76; (819)566-7861; Fax. (819)569-8894.

BEAUSEJOUR, Eric; Hop Charles LeMoyne, 3120 boul Taschereau, Greenfield Park QC J4V 2H1; Mon'00; CCFP; Staff, Hopital Charles LeMoyne; Langs: Bilingual(French/English); (450)466-5000

BEAUSEJOUR, Linda; Ctr Hosp Anna-Laberge, 200 boul Brisebois, Chateauguay QC J6K 4W8; Sher'88; Staff, Hôpital Anna-Laberge; (450)699-2425; Fax. (450)699-2525.

BEAUSEJOUR, Pierre; CHUS-Hop Hotel-Dieu, 580 rue Bowen S, Sherbrooke QC J1G 2E8; Ott'71; DPsy; FRCPC; Psy. Chef psychiatrie, Centre Hospitalier Universitaire de Sherbrooke-Hôpital Hôtel-Dieu; Chef Psy, Universite de Sherbrooke; Langs: English; French; (819)822-6733; Fax. (819)822-6790; pierre.beausejour@usherbrooke.ca.

BEAUSOLEIL, Caroline; Ctre Med de MBoucherville, 201-600 boul du Fort-Saint-Lou, Boucherville QC J4B 1S7; Sher'00; (450)655-7321

BEAUSOLEIL, Sebastien; CSSS de Rimouski-Neigette, CP 3150 Succ A 150 av Rouleau, Rimouski QC G5L 5T1; Laval'99; Staff, Hôpital Regional Rimouski; (418)724-8234

BEAUSOLEIL, Sylvain; 110-667 Champlain St, Dieppe NB E1A 1P6; Sher'95; FRCSC; GenSurg. (506)858-8199; Fax. (506)858-9012.

BEAUVAIS, Michel; Hôpital Laval, 2725 ch Sainte-Foy, Quebec QC G1V 4G5; Laval'87; CSPQ; FRCPC; Anes. Staff, Hôpital Laval; Langs: English; (418)656-8711 x4870

BEAUVAIS, Nicole L; White Pine Family Health Netwo, 208-38 Pine St, Timmins ON P4N 6K6; NOSM'09; CCFP; Staff, Timmins & District Hospital; (705)267-3272

BEAUVOLSK, Paul; Clinique Le Medical, 285-1750 boul Marie-Victorin, Longueuil QC J4G 1A5; Mon'72; (450)442-9531

BEAVER, David J; Grand River Hosp-KW Hlth Ctre, 835 King St W, Kitchener ON N2G 1G3; McM'09; CCFP; CCFP(E.M.); Staff, Grand River Hospital - Kitchener/Waterloo Health Centre; (519)749-4380

BEAVER, David J F; 258 Eagle Ridge Dr, Salt Spring Island BC V8K 2L1; London (England)'83; MB BS; MRC; CCFP; (250)537-1915; Fax. (250)537-1940; galianoclinic@hotmail.com.

BEAVER, John; Norfolk Gen Hosp, 365 West St, Simcoe ON N3Y 1T7; Wes'81; Staff, Norfolk General Hospital; (519)426-0750 x2205

BEAVER, Julia A L; Port Dover Med Centre, 807 St George St, Port Dover ON N0A 1N0; Tor'81; (519)583-0893; Fax. (519)583-2814.

BEAVER, Susan A; 476 Palmerston Blvd, Toronto ON M6G 2P1; Tor'88; FRCPC; Psy. (416)588-9525

BEAVIS, R Coleson; 508-750 Spadina Cres E, Saskatoon SK S7K 3H3; Sask'00; Dip SportMed; FRCSC; OrthSurg (Sports Medicine). (306)244-5561

BEBAWY, Amany; Queen's Med Center, 5A-1289 Marlborough Crt, Oakville ON L6H 2R9; Ain Shams (Egypt)'93; CCFP; (905)844-8878

BEBB, Dafydd G; Tom Baker Cancer Centre, 1331 29 St NW, Calgary AB T2N 4N2; Oxford (England)'92; MB ChB; FRCPC; IntMed; MedOncol. Staff MedOncol & Principal Investigator Translational Research Unit, Tom Baker Cancer Centre; Asst Prof Med, University of Calgary; Langs: Welsh; (403)521-3166; Fax. (403)283-1651.

BEBB, Richard A; 416-1033 Davie St, Vancouver BC V6E 1M7; UBC'85; FRCPC; IntMed; Endocrin&Metab. (604)689-1055; Fax. (604)689-2955.

BEBER, Brett; 410-790 Bay St, Toronto ON M5G 1N8; Tor'99; FRCSC; PlasSurg. Staff, Toronto East General Hospital Inc; (416)466-5023; Fax. (416)466-0947.

BECA, Sorin G; LMC Endocrinology Centres, 200-110 Copper Creek Dr, Markham ON L6B 0P9; Timisoara (Romania)'92; (905)294-0800

BECERRO GARIJO, Gloria; Clinique Medicale, 157 Water St, Campbellton NB E3N 3L4; Badajoz (Spain)'83; Langs: English; (506)753-0133; Fax. (506)753-0139.

BECH-HANSEN, Kay; Lasalle Walk In Clinic, 1813 Lasalle Blvd, Sudbury ON P3A 2A3; Tor'80; (705)560-9422; Fax. (705)560-9482.

BECHAI, Nabil R; North York Diagnostic Imaging, 4800 Leslie St, North York ON M2J 2K9; Tor'78; FRCPC; DiagRad. Langs: Arabic; (416)493-1011; Fax. (416)493-1019.

BECHAMP-THEBERGE, Marie-Pier; CSSS de Lac-Saint Jean-Est, CP 1300 Succ Bureau-Chef 300 boul Champlain, Alma QC G8B 5W3; Sher'08; Staff, CSSS de Lac-Saint Jean-Est; (418)669-2000; marie-pier.bechamp-theberge@ssss.gouv.qc.ca.

BECHARA, Robert; Hotel-Dieu Hosp, 166 Brock St, Kingston ON K7L 5G2; Tor'08; IntMed. Staff, Hotel-Dieu Hospital; (613)544-3100

BECHARD, David; CSSS du Rocher Percé, CP 3300 451 rue Mgr Ross E, Chandler QC G0C 1K0; Sher'05; FRCPC; IntMed. Staff, Centre Hospitalier de Chandler; (418)689-2261 x2168

BECHARD, Elisabeth; Clinique Laval-des-Rapides, 210-255 boul de la Concorde O, Laval QC H7N 5T1; Laval'88; (450)668-2660

BECHARD, Fannie; Clinique Med Nicolet, 1691 boul Louis-Frechette, Nicolet QC J3T 1Z6; Sher'05; CCFP; Staff Palliative Care, CSSS de Trois-Rivières; Langs: Bilingual(French/English); (819)293-2022; Fax. (819)293-2024.

BECHARD, Philippe; Hotel-Dieu de Levis, 143 rue Wolfe, Levis QC G6V 3Z1; Laval'96; MSc; PhmB; CSPQ; FRCPC; Anes (Pain Management). Staff, Hôtel-Dieu de Lévis; (418)835-7121; Fax. (418)835-3969.

BECHBACHE, Rafik R; Unionville Family Physicians, 301-10 Unionville Gate, Unionville ON L3R 0W7; Tor'83; BSc; MSc; CCFP; FCFP; Ac Staff, The Scarborough Hospital - Birchmount Campus; Court Staff, Markham Stouffville Hospital; Asst Prof Family & CommunMed, University of Toronto; Langs: English; French; (905)475-3121; Fax. (905)475-4270.

BECHER, Harald H H; University of Alberta Hosp, 0A8.32-8440 112 St NW, Edmonton AB T6G 2B7; Staff, University of Alberta Hospital; Staff, Mazankowski Alberta Heart Institute; (780)407-8504; Fax. (780)407-3489.

BECK, Allon; Dr Charles A Janeway Child HC, 300 Prince Philip Dr, St. John's NL A1B 3V6; Harvard (USA)'06; Critical Care Medicine; Peds.

BECK, Angus W; McGill Centre, PO Box 2000 Stn Central 55 McGill Ave, Charlottetown PE C1A 7N8; Dal'80; FRCPC; Psy (Bipolar Disease). (902)368-4938; Fax. (902)368-6189; clramsay@ihis.org.

BECK, Carolyn E; The Hosp for Sick Children, 555 University Ave, Toronto ON M5G 1X8; Qns'98; FRCPC; Peds. Staff Div of Ped Medicine, The Hospital For Sick Children; (416)813-8422; Fax. (416)813-8345.

BECK, Cynthia A; Foothills Med Centre, 1403 29 St NW, Calgary AB T2N 2T9; Cal'92; MASc; FRCPC; Psy. Medical Staff Dept of Psy, Foothills Medical Centre; Asst Prof, University of Calgary; (403)944-2723

BECK, David A V; The Group Health Centre, 240 Mcnabb St, Sault Ste. Marie ON P6B 1Y5; Wes'82; CCFP; (705)759-1234 x2229

BECK, Frantisek; 7155 Kingsway PO Box 54624 Rpo Highgate, Burnaby BC V5E 4J6; Sask'74; CCFP; Teach Staff Family Pract, University of British Columbia; Langs: Czech; Slovak.

BECK, Gail M; Royal Ottawa Hlth Care Group, 1145 Carling Ave, Ottawa ON K1Z 7K4; McG'78; FRCPC; Psy (Medico Legal Assessments). Staff, Royal Ottawa Mental Health Centre - Royal Ottawa Health Care Group; Member, Women's Issues, Ontario Med. Association; Langs: French; (613)722-6521 x6288; drgailbeck@rogers.com.

BECK, Gavin; Royal University Hosp, 103 Hospital Dr, Saskatoon SK S7N 0W8; Dal'07; FRCSC; GenSurg. Staff, Royal University Hospital; (306)966-8166

BECK, Gordon; Queen Elizabeth Hosp, PO Box 6600 Stn Central, Charlottetown PE C1A 8T5; Dal'78; Staff, Queen Elizabeth Hospital; (902)894-2111

BECK, Iain V; DGNP National Defence, 101 Colonel By Dr, Ottawa ON K1A 0K2; Wes'91; CCFP; FCFP; (613)996-0292

BECK, Jeremy N; Polyclinic, 203-199 Grafton St, Charlottetown PE C1A 1L2; Dal'07; FRCPC; IntMed; Gastroent.

BECK, John R; Northumberland Hills Hosp, 1000 Depalma Dr, Cobourg ON K9A 5W6; Queen's (Ireland)'64; IntMed (Oncology). Staff, Northumberland Hills Hospital; (905)372-6811 x3030; Fax. (905)373-6926.

BECK, Maxine E; Associated Radiologists, 300-140 Wall St, Saskatoon SK S7K 1N4; Sask'86; FRCPC; DiagRad. (306)244-1167; Fax. (306)244-2911; m.beck@shaw.ca.

BECK, Paul L; Heritage Sciences Centre, 1865-3330 Hospital Dr NW, Calgary AB T2N 4N1; Cal'90; FRCPC; IntMed; Gastroent. Staff, Foothills Medical Centre; (403)220-4500

BECK, Philip R; Inst of Commun & Family Psy, 4333 ch Cote-Sainte-Catherine, Montreal QC H3T 1E4; McG'64; DPsy; FAPA; CSPQ; FRCPC; Psy (Administration). Staff Senior Psy, Sir Mortimer B Davis Jewish General; Langs: Bilingual(French/English); (514)340-8303; Fax. (514)340-7507.

BECK, Raphael; Victoria Gen Hosp, 1 Hospital Way, Victoria BC V8Z 6R5; Hebrew (Israel)'76; FRCPC; Peds (Pediatric Intensive Care); Respir. Staff, Victoria General Hospital; Langs: German; Hebrew; (250)727-4186; Fax. (250)727-4012.

BECK, William J; Arbour Heights, 564 Tanner Dr, Kingston ON K7M 0C3; McM'78; CCFP; CCFP(E.M.); FCFP; (613)453-1687; Fax. (613)547-5509.

BECKER, Allan B; Children's Hosp, FE125-840 Sherbrook St, Winnipeg MB R3A 1S1; Man'69; FRCPC; Peds; ClinImmunol&Allergy. Staff, Health Sciences Centre; Fax. (204)787-5040; becker@cc.umanitoba.ca.

BECKER, Annalisa K; 505-750 Broadway W, Vancouver BC V5Z 1H1; UBC'06; DiagRad. (604)879-4177

BECKER, Erin B; Westshore Maternity & Fam Prac, 101-284 Helmcken Rd, Victoria BC V9B 1T2; Cal'90; Staff Med, Vancouver Island Health Authority; Clin Asst Prof Faculty of Med, University of Victoria; Clin Asst Prof Faculty of Med, University of British Columbia; (250)474-7715; Fax. (250)474-4659.

BECKER, Giuliano; Hop du Sacre-Coeur de Mtl, 5400 boul Gouin O, Montreal QC H4J 1C5; (Portugal)'98; Staff, Hôpital du Sacre-Coeur de Montréal; (514)338-2222

BECKER, Harold; Omega Med Associates, 304-2 Lansing Sq, North York ON M2J 4P8; Tor'75; PhD; CCFP; FCFP; Assoc Staff, Humber River Regional Hospital - Church Street Site; Vis Staff, Sunnybrook Health Sciences Centre; Med Dir, St. Hilda's Towers; (416)489-0711; info@omegamedical.ca.

BECKER, Jennifer C; 257-346 John St N, Arnprior ON K7S 2P6; Ott'06; CCFP; (613)623-2048

BECKER, Lev A; 1765 Vista Cres PO Box 607, Squamish BC V8B 0A5; Man'03; CCFP; CCFP(E.M.); (604)815-0043

BECKER, Lisa; Toronto Rehab Inst-Univ Ctr, 1028-550 University Ave, Toronto ON M5G 2A2; McM'01; FRCPC; PhysMed&Rehab (Stroke Rehabilitation). Staff, Toronto Rehabilitation Institute - University Centre; (416)597-3422

BECKER, Lisa M; Queensway-Carleton Hosp, 3045 Baseline Rd, Nepean ON K2H 8P4; Qns'98; FRCPC; DiagRad. Staff, Queensway Carleton Hospital; (613)721-2000

BECKER, Marissa; Centre for Global Public Healt, R070-771 McDermot Ave, Winnipeg MB R3E 0T6; Man'99; FRCPC; IntMed; InfectDis. Staff, St Boniface General Hospital.

BECKER, Regina; Carbonear Gen Hosp, 86 Highroad South, Carbonear NL A1Y 1A4; Mem'90; BSc; CCFP; FCFP; Staff, Carbonear General Hospital; (709)945-5111; ginabecker@nf.sympatico.ca.

BECKER, Rubin M; Jewish Rehab Hosp, 3205 Place Alton-Goldbloom, Laval QC H7V 1R2; McG'76; BSc; MDCM; FRCPC; IntMed (Palliative Care); GeriatricMed. Chef Med, Jewish Rehabilitation Hospital; Chief Div of IntMed, Sir Mortimer B Davis Jewish General; Assoc Prof Med & Family Med, McGill University; (450)688-9550 x211; Fax. (450)688-3673; rubin.becker@mcgill.ca.

BECKER, Taryn; Women's College Hosp, EW 4F-76 Grenville St, Toronto ON M5S 1B2; McM'02; FRCPC; IntMed; Endocrin&Metab. Staff, Women's College Hospital; (416)323-6400; taryn.becker@wchospital.ca.

BECKER, Werner J; Foothills Med Centre, 1403 29 St NW, Calgary AB T2N 2T9; Man'69; BSc; BSc(Med); FRCPC; Neur (Headache). Staff, Foothills Medical Centre; Staff, Calgary Headache Assessment & Management Program; Prof Dept of Clin Neurosciences, University of Calgary; (403)944-4240; Fax. (403)283-2270; wbecker@ucalgary.ca.

BECKETT, Andrew N; Sunnybrook Hlth Sciences Ctre, H170-2075 Bayview Ave, Toronto ON M4N 3M5; Man'05; FRCSC; GenSurg. Staff, Sunnybrook Health Sciences Centre; (416)480-4232

BECKETT, Linda A; 916 Princess St, Kingston ON K7L 1H1; McM'02; CCFP; (613)531-6127; Fax. (613)507-6127.

BECKIE, Gerald V; Associate Med Centre, 5016 48 Ave, Taber AB T1G 1R8; Sask'66; CCFP; FCFP; Staff, Taber Health Centre; (403)223-3525; Fax. (403)223-9020.

BECKLEY, Sunmolu A; Grand Bank Med Clinic, PO Box 190 45 Main St, Grand Bank NL A0E 1W0; (Ireland)'69; LRCS; LRCP; (709)832-2570; Fax. (709)832-1591; sbeckley@nf.aibn.com.

BECKMAN, Jeffrey H; 8209-2775 Laurel St, Vancouver BC V5Z 1M9; Wes'77; FRCPC; IntMed; Neur. Consultant, Vancouver General Hospital - Centennial Pavillion; (604)875-5319

BECKNER, Kevin; Shuswap Lake Gen Hosp, PO Box 520 Stn Main 601 10th St NE, Salmon Arm BC V1E 4N6; UBC'00; FRCPC; DiagRad. Staff, Shuswap Lake General Hospital; (250)833-3607

BECKS, Gregory; Grey Bruce HS-Owen Sound, PO Box 1800 Stn Main 1800 8th St E, Owen Sound ON N4K 6M9; Wes'79; FRCPC; IntMed; Endocrin&Metab. Staff, Grey Bruce Health Services - Owen Sound; Assoc Prof Med, University of Western Ontario; (519)371-0563; Fax. (519)371-9304.

BECKSTEAD, James E; Western Surgery Centre, 100-1020 Lorimer Blvd, Winnipeg MB R3P 1C7; Man'70; BSc(Med); FRCPC; Anes. Staff, Health Sciences Centre; Staff, Seven Oaks General Hospital; Physician, Western Surgery Centre; Assoc Prof, University of Manitoba.

BECOTTE, Annick; Hotel-Dieu d'Arthabaska, 5 rue des Hospitalieres, Victoriaville QC G6P 6N2; Sher'04; FRCPC; Anes. Staff, Hotel-Dieu d'Arthabaska; (819)357-2030

BECOTTE, Genevieve; CHUQ-Ctr Hosp Univ Laval, 2705 boul Laurier, Quebec QC G1V 4G2; Laval'01; BSc; CCFP; CCFP(E.M.); Staff, Centre Hospitalier Universitaire de Quebec-CHUL; (418)656-4141 x70554

BECOTTE, Therese; Medecine Familiale Montclair, 207-15 boul Montclair, Gatineau QC J8Y 2E2; Mon'78; Ac Staff, Hull Hospital; (819)772-2003; Fax. (819)772-4880.

BECTOR, Neel S; 16-2555 Erin Centre Blvd, Mississauga ON L5M 5H1; Man'96; (905)813-8444; Fax. (905)593-0698.

BECTOR, Neeraj S; 2039-8882 170 St NW, Edmonton AB T5T 3J7; Man'98; CCFP; (780)444-1935

BEDARD, Alain; Hotel-Dieu de Levis, 143 rue Wolfe, Levis QC G6V 3Z1; Laval'90; Psy. Staff, Hôtel-Dieu de Lévis; (418)835-7155; Fax. (418)835-7199.

BEDARD, Alain; Centre Med Quatre-Bourgeois, 300-979 av de Bourgogne, Quebec QC G1W 2L4; Laval'85; NBME; Langs: Bilingual(French/English); (418)653-4050; Fax. (418)653-4475; alain.bedard313@videotron.ca.

BEDARD, Alice M; Dominion Med Centre, 2383 111 St NW, Edmonton AB T6J 5E5; Ott'97; CCFP; (780)436-0020; Fax. (780)436-0603.

BEDARD, Andre; Clinique Med de Roberval, 714 boul Marcotte, Roberval QC G8H 1Z6; Laval'71; Staff, Hotel-Dieu de Roberval; (418)275-3833; Fax. (418)275-6747.

BEDARD, Andre V; Stroud Med Centre, 1-7869 Yonge St, Innisfil ON L9S 1K8; Ott'93; CCFP; (705)436-2251; Fax. (705)436-7991.

BEDARD, Anne-Marie; GMF La Cigogne, 420-3141 boul Taschereau, Greenfield Park QC J4V 2H2; Sher'99; Staff, Hopital Charles LeMoyne; (450)466-7892; Fax. (450)466-9602.

BEDARD, Anne-Marie; CHUQ-Ctr Hosp Univ Laval, D1211-2705 boul Laurier, Quebec QC G1V 4G2; Mon'03; FRCSC; OrthSurg (Upper Extremity Surgery). Staff, Centre Hospitalier Universitaire de Quebec-CHUL; Langs: Bilingual(French/English); (418)654-2102; Fax. (418)654-2288; orthopedie.chul@ens.chuq.qc.ca.

BEDARD, Brigitte; Centre Med Fontainebleau, 102-10 boul des Chateaux, Blainville QC J7B 1Z5; Laval'85; Staff, Centre Hospitalier Pierre le Gardeur; (450)419-8811; Fax. (450)419-7758.

BEDARD, Caroline; Clinique Medicale Angus, 101-4101 rue Molson, Montreal QC H1Y 3L1; Mon'10; CCFP; (514)807-2333

BEDARD, Caroline; I R D P Q-Site Francois-Charon, 525 boul Wilfrid-Hamel, Quebec QC G1M 2S8; Laval'05; CCFP.

BEDARD, Catherine; CSSS de Laval, 1755 boul Rene-Laennec, Laval QC H7M 3L9; Mon'99; CCFP; Staff, Hopital de la Cite de la santé; (450)668-1010

BEDARD, Chantal; CHUS-Hop Fleurimont, 3001 12e av N, Sherbrooke QC J1H 5N4; Laval'97; Staff, Centre Hospitalier Universitaire de Sherbrooke-Hopital Fleurimont; (819)346-1110

BEDARD, Christine; CSSS du Rocher-Perce, CP 3300 451 rue Mgr Ross E, Chandler QC G0C 1K0; Sher'94; FRCSC; GenSurg. Staff GenSurg, Centre Hospitalier de Chandler; (418)689-2261

BEDARD, Daniel; Clin Med Familiale Plessisvill, 1971 rue Bilodeau, Plessisville QC G6L 3J1; Laval'03; Staff, CLSC de l'Erable; Staff, Hotel-Dieu d'Arthabaska; (819)362-6337; danbedard@hotmail.com.

BEDARD, Danielle; Hop du Sacre-Coeur de Mtl, 5400 boul Gouin O, Montreal QC H4J 1C5; Laval'82; FRCPC; DiagRad. Staff, Hôpital du Sacre-Coeur de Montréal; Contrôleur, Virginia Mines; (514)338-2222; Fax. (514)338-2130; dbedard@minesvirginia.com.

BEDARD, Denis; Centre Med Quatre-Bourgeois, 300-979 av de Bourgogne, Quebec QC G1W 2L4; Laval'85; (418)653-4050; denis.bedard@ssss.gouv.qc.ca.

BEDARD, Denis; Mason de Soins Palliatifs de L, 655 rue Bellevue, Laval QC H7C 0A8; Mon'75; Staff, Hôpital du Sacre-Coeur de Montréal; (450)936-4300 x300

BEDARD, Diane; CLSC La Source, 791 rue de Sherwood, Quebec QC G2N 1X7; Laval'89; CCFP; Langs: English; (418)849-2572; Fax. (418)841-5110.

BEDARD, Elisabeth; Hôpital Laval, 2725 ch Sainte-Foy, Quebec QC G1V 4G5; Laval'99; FRCPC; IntMed; Cardiol. Staff, Hôpital Laval; (418)656-8711

BEDARD, Eric L; Royal Alexandra Hosp, 416C-10240 Kingsway NW, Edmonton AB T5H 3V9; Ott'97; MSc; FRCSC; GenSurg (Minimal Invasive Surgery); ThorSurg. Staff, Royal Alexandra Hospital; Asst Prof, University of Alberta; Langs: Bilingual(French/English); (780)735-5981; Fax. (780)735-4245.

BEDARD, Fernand; 225-1900 av Mailloux, Quebec QC G1J 5B9; Laval'72; DiagRad. Staff, Centre Hospitalier Affilié Universitaire de Québec - Hôpital De L'Enfant Jésus; (418)667-0060; Fax. (418)667-0061.

BEDARD, Francine; CHUQ-Hotel-Dieu de Quebec, 11 Cote-du-Palais, Quebec QC G1R 2J6; Laval'84; DiagRad. Staff, Centre Hospitalier Universitaire de Québec (CHUQ) - Siege Social; (418)691-5453

BEDARD, Gerry; Clinique Med Lavaltrie, 1400 rue Notre-Dame, Lavaltrie QC J5T 1M6; Mon'87; (450)586-1033; Fax. (450)586-4498.

BEDARD, Jacques; Clinique Med London, 200-1815 rue King O, Sherbrooke QC J1J 2E3; Mon'70; FRCPC; IntMed (Clinical Research). Staff, Centre Hospitalier Universitaire de Sherbrooke-Hôpital Hôtel-Dieu; Prof, Universite de Sherbrooke; (819)565-1921; Fax. (819)565-7780.

BEDARD, Jinny; CSSS de Sept-Iles, 45 rue Du Pere-Divet, Sept-Iles QC G4R 3N7; Sher'94; FRCPC; IntMed. Staff, Centre Hospitalier Regional de Sept-Iles; (418)962-9761

BEDARD, Julie; CHUQ-St-Francois d'Assise, 10 rue de l'Espinay, Quebec QC G1L 3L5; Laval'92; CSPQ; FRCPC; Anes. Staff, Centre Hospitalier Universitaire De Québec - Pavillon De St-françois-d'assise; Langs: English; French; (418)525-4340; Fax. (418)525-4434.

BEDARD, Justine; CHUS-Hop Hotel-Dieu, 580 rue Bowen S, Sherbrooke QC J1G 2E8; Sher'99; FRCPC; DiagRad. Staff, Centre Hospitalier Universitaire de Sherbrooke-Hôpital Hôtel-Dieu; (819)346-1110 x14962

BEDARD, Luc; Ctr Hosp Affilie-Enfant-Jesus, 1401 18e rue, Quebec QC G1J 1Z4; Laval'98; FRCSC; OrthSurg. Staff, Centre Hospitalier Affilié Universitaire de Québec - Hôpital De L'Enfant Jésus; (418)649-0252

BEDARD, Luc; CSSS de la Region de Thetford, 1717 rue Notre-Dame E, Thetford Mines QC G6G 2V4; Laval'96; Staff, Hopital du CSS de la Region de Thetford; Langs: French; English; (418)338-7777; Fax. (418)831-7967; lucbedard@videotron.ca.

BEDARD, Marc; Centre Med St-Raymond, 220 rue Saint-Joseph, Saint-Raymond QC G3L 1J1; Laval'74; ac Staff, Centre Hospitalier Portneuf; Langs: Bilingual(French/English); (418)337-2214; Fax. (418)337-3749.

BEDARD, Marie-Eve; Ctr Hosp Affilie-Enfant-Jesus, 1401 18e rue, Quebec QC G1J 1Z4; Laval'06; Respir; IntMed. Staff, Centre Hospitalier Affilié Universitaire de Québec - Hôpital De L'Enfant Jésus; (418)649-0252

BEDARD, Marie-Josee; 100-235 boul René-Lévesque E, Montreal QC H2X 1N8; Mon'82; FRCSC; ObstGyn. ac Staff, Centre Hospitalier l'Université de Montréal (CHUM) - Hôpital Notre-Dame; (514)866-2446; Fax. (514)866-4013.

BEDARD, Marie-Lene; CSSS de la Baie-des-Chaleurs, RR 2 419 boul Perron, Maria QC G0C 1Y0; Mon'07; Staff, CSSS de la Baie-des-Chaleurs; (418)759-3443

BEDARD, Marie-Sophie; Ctr Dermatologique du Quebec, 105-2880 ch des Quatre-Bourgeo, Quebec QC G1V 4X7; Laval'03; FRCPC; Derm. (418)650-3555; Fax. (418)650-1260.

BEDARD, Martin; Ctr Hosp Affilie-Enfant-Jesus, 1401 18e rue, Quebec QC G1J 1Z4; Laval'02; FRCSC; OrthSurg. Staff, Centre Hospitalier Affilié Universitaire de Québec - Hôpital De L'Enfant Jésus; (418)649-0252

BEDARD, Mathieu; Ctr Hosp Affilie-St-Sacrement, 1050 ch Sainte-Foy, Quebec QC G1S 4L8; Laval'05; FRCPC; Psy. Staff, Centre Hospitalier Affilié Universitaire de Québec - Hôpital du St-Sacrement; (418)682-7511

BEDARD, Michael; Manitowaning Medical Clinic, 23 Spragge St, Manitowaning ON P0P 1N0; Ott'90; (705)859-2170

BEDARD, Michele; Clinique Med Grand-Boulevard, 200-353 boul des Bois-Francs S, Victoriaville QC G6P 4T2; Laval'03; Staff, Hotel-Dieu d'Arthabaska; (819)751-3006

BEDARD, Mylene; Hop Charles Lemoyne, 3120 boul Taschereau, Greenfield Park QC J4V 2H1; Mon'87; Psy. Staff, Hopital Charles LeMoyne; (450)466-5020

BEDARD, Nadia; Dr Georges-L Dumont Reg Hosp, 330 av Universite, Moncton NB E1C 2Z3; Laval'07; CCFP; Staff, Dr Georges-L-Dumont University Hospital Centre; (506)833-2430

BEDARD, Nancy; Clin externe de Psychiatrie, 279 rue Providence, Granby QC J2G 4S7; Sher'92; FRCPC; Psy (Hospital Psychiatry). Staff Psy, Centre Hospitalier de Granby; (450)375-8001

BEDARD, Natacha; CSSS de Beauce-Etchemin, 1515 17e rue, Saint-Georges QC G5Y 4T8; Mon'07; ObstGyn. Staff, Centre Hospitalier Beauce-Etchemin; (418)228-2031

BEDARD, Nicholas; Clinique Med du Plateaux, 300-195 rue de l'Atmosphere, Gatineau QC J9A 0A3; Ott'94; Staff, Montfort Hospital; (819)776-0001

BEDARD, O'Donnell; Hotel-Dieu de Levis, 143 rue Wolfe, Levis QC G6V 3Z1; Laval'70; CSPQ; FRCPC; Anes. Staff, Hôtel-Dieu de Lévis; (418)835-7121 x3218

BEDARD, Philippe L; Univ Hlth Network-Princess M, 5 125-610 University Ave, Toronto ON M5G 2M9; Tor'03; FRCPC; IntMed; MedOncol. Staff, Princess Margaret Hospital - University Health Network; (416)946-4534; Fax. (416)946-4563.

BEDARD, Pierre-Michel; CHUQ-Ctr Hosp Univ Laval, H 1340-2705 boul Laurier, Quebec QC G1V 4G2; Laval'76; FRCPC; IntMed; ClinImmunol&Allergy. Ac Staff, Centre Hospitalier Universitaire de Quebec-CHUL; (418)654-2240; Fax. (418)654-2770.

BEDARD, Rejean; Ctr Hosp Laurentien, 234 rue Saint-Vincent, Ste-Agathe-Des-Mts QC J8C 2B8; Laval'84; Staff, Centre Hospitalier Laurentien; Langs: English; (819)324-4000; Fax. (819)324-4003; rejeanbedard@cgocable.ca.

BEDARD, Richard J; Cape Breton Hlthcare Complex, 1482 George St, Sydney NS B1P 1P3; Sask'71; FRCPC; IntMed. Staff, Cape Breton Healthcare Complex; (902)567-8060; Fax. (902)567-7800.

BEDARD, Robert; CSSS Maria-Chapdelaine, 2000 boul du Sacre-Coeur, Dolbeau-Mistassini QC G8L 2R5; Mon'70; Staff, Centre Maria-Chapdelaine - CH de Dolbeau-Mistassini; (450)276-1234

BEDARD, Sonia; Clinique de Pediatrie, 105 av Gatineau, Gatineau QC J8T 4J4; Sher'90; Peds. Staff, Hôpital de Gatineau; (819)561-4412

BEDARD, Valerie; CHUS-Hop Hotel-Dieu, 580 rue Bowen S, Sherbrooke QC J1G 2E8; Laval'99; FRCSC; GenSurg. Staff, Centre Hospitalier Universitaire de Sherbrooke-Hôpital Hôtel-Dieu; (819)346-1110

BEDARD, Valerie; CHSLD Normandie, 580 rue Du Couvent RR 1, Saint-Tite QC G0X 3H0; Mon'86; Staff, CLSC-CSSS de Port-Cartier; (418)365-5107; Fax. (450)365-7914.

BEDARD, Vanessa; Lakeview Med Clinic, 13-1945 McKercher Dr, Saskatoon SK S7N 4M4; McG'04; FRCPC; Peds (Child Maltreatment). Staff Community Ped/Staff Part-Time Ped Emerg Care, Royal University Hospital; Langs: Spanish; French; (306)653-0002

BEDARD, Veronique; CHUQ-Ctr Hosp Univ Laval, 2705 boul Laurier, Quebec QC G1V 4G2; Sher'99; FRCPC; Peds. Staff, Centre Hospitalier Universitaire de Quebec-CHUL; (418)656-4141

BEDARD, Yves; 110-4850 boul Henri-Bourassa, Quebec QC G1H 3A7; Laval'73; Ac Staff, Centre Hospitalier Universitaire De Québec - Pavillon De St-françois-d'assise; (418)661-6959; Fax. (418)661-1016.

BEDARD-CHARETTE, Kim; Inst Philippe Pinel de Mtl, 10905 boul Henri-Bourassa E, Montreal QC H1C 1H1; Mon'96; FRCPC; Psy. Staff, Institut Philippe-Pinel de Montreal; (514)648-8461 x500; Fax. (514)881-3706.

BEDDAGE, Victorine; North Bay Reg Health Centre, 50 College Dr, North Bay ON P1B 0A4; Colombo (Sri Lanka)'68; MB BS; MRC(Psy); DPM(Eng); FRCPC; Psy (Adult Psychiatry). Staff, North Bay Regional Health Centre - Regional Mental Health; (705)474-1200 x2307; Fax. (705)495-7824.

BEDDER, Phyllis M; 208-2025 Corydon Ave, Winnipeg MB R3P 0N5; Man'79; Ac Staff, Victoria General Hospital; (204)261-0162; Fax. (204)269-8848.

BEDELL, Richard A; St Pau's Hosp, 1081 Burrard St, Vancouver BC V6Z 1Y6; UBC'83; Staff, Providence Health Care - St Paul's Hospital; (604)682-2344

BEDER, Aaron L; 401-1017 Wilson Ave, North York ON M3K 1Z1; Tor'94; FRCSC; GenSurg; VascSurg. Staff Vascular Surgeon, Humber River Regional Hospital - Finch Avenue Site; (416)742-2961; Fax. (416)742-0076.

BEDFORD, H Melanie; North York Gen Hosp, 4001 Leslie St, North York ON M2K 1E1; Tor'95; BSc; MS; FAAP; FCCMG; FRCPC; Peds (Medical Genetics). Staff, North York General Hospital; (416)756-6345; Fax. (416)756-6727.

BEDFORD, Robert M; 224-329 March Rd, Kanata ON K2K 2E1; Ott'80; FRCPC; Psy. (613)592-3126

BEDI, Anil; Royal University Hosp, 2662-103 Hospital Dr, Saskatoon SK S7N 0W8; Mem'98; FRCPC; IntMed; Gastroent. Staff, Saskatoon City Hospital; Staff, Royal University Hospital; Staff, St Paul's Hospital (Grey Nuns) of Saskatoon; (306)966-7981; Fax. (306)966-1254.

BEDI, Bhupinder S; Jefferson Med Centre, 1553 Arlington St, Winnipeg MB R2X 1V3; Punjab (India)'75; MB BS; Langs: Punjabi; (204)633-1133; Fax. (204)633-0311.

BEDI, Jasbir S; Roslyn Med Bldg, 200-400 5 Ave SW, Calgary AB T2P 0L6; Man'07; (403)930-1005

BEDI, Vishal; Spesmed Med Specialist Ctre, PO Box 1540 2591 99 St, North Battleford SK S9A 3W1; (306)446-5543; Fax. (306)446-5548.

BEDKOWSKA, Alicja; Clin Medico-Chirurgicale de Ve, 55 rue de L'Eglise, Verdun QC H4G 3E7; Krakow (Poland)'71; Clin Prof, Centre Hospitalier de Verdun; Langs: Polish; English; (514)737-2496

BEDKOWSKA, Anna; GMF de Verdun au 55, 3F-55 rue de l'Église, Verdun QC H4G 3E7; Cracow (Poland)'01; Langs: Bilingual(French/English); (514)737-2496; Fax. (514)733-2759.

BEDKOWSKI, Wojciech A; Niagara Health Centre, 303-180 Vine St S, St Catharines ON L2R 7P3; Poznan (Poland)'73; FRCSC; ObstGyn. Staff, Niagara Health System - Ontario Street Site; Staff, Niagara Health System - St Catharines General Site; (905)988-1144; Fax. (905)988-3636.

BEDNAR, Drew A; Hamilton Commun Health Centre, M9-414 Victoria Ave N, Hamilton ON L8L 5G8; McG'82; DAB; FAAOS; FRCSC; OrthSurg (Adult Spine/Trauma). Clin Prof/Prog Dir Orth, McMaster University; (905)577-0639; Fax. (905)577-0178.

BEDNARSKA, Elzbieta I; Andrew Street Family Hlth Ctre, 16 Andrew St, Kitchener ON N2H 5R2; McM'09; CCFP; (519)804-9234; Fax. (519)804-2604.

BEDOYA-MEJIA, Juan; Groupe Aurores Boreales, 228 2e rue E, La Sarre QC J9Z 2G9; Antioquia (Colombia)'02; CCFP; Staff, Centre Hospitalier La Sarre; (819)339-5617; Fax. (819)339-2729.

BEDROSIAN, Kathleen E; 206-851 Fischer Hallman Rd, Kitchener ON N2M 5N8; Wes'88; Staff, Grand River Hospital - Kitchener/Waterloo Health Centre; Staff, St Mary's General Hospital; (519)745-3117; Fax. (519)749-1471.

BEDROSSIAN, Diane M; Downtown Toronto Doctors, 630-790 Bay St, Toronto ON M5G 1N8; McM'10; CCFP; (647)427-6001; Fax. (416)598-4659.

BEDROSSIAN, Roupen; Clinique Med Havre-Sante, 521 boul Du Havre, Salaber-de-Valleyf QC J6S 4Z5; St. Joseph (Lebanon)'68; FRCSC; ObstGyn. (450)370-1300

BEDROSSIAN, Taline; CSSS du Suroît, 150 rue Saint-Thomas, Salaber-de-Valleyf QC J6T 6C1; McG'03; FRCPC; Psy. Staff, Centre Hospitalier Régional du Suroît; (450)371-9920; Fax. (450)372-1372.

BEDUHN, Eitel E R; Doctors Bldg, 355-955 Queen St E, Sault Ste. Marie ON P6A 2C3; McM'73; (705)759-1234 x244

BEDWANI, Nagy C; Inst Albert Prevost, 6555 boul Gouin O, Montreal QC H4K 1B3; Alexandria (Egypt)'71; MB ChB; FRCPC; Psy. Associate Psy, Hôpital du Sacre-Coeur de Montréal; Clin Teacher, Universite de Montreal; (514)338-4280; Fax. (514)338-2222.

BEECH, Jack H; 217 Finlayson St PO Box 715, Sicamous BC V0E 2V0; UBC'74; BSc; Ac Staff, Shuswap Lake General Hospital; (250)836-2817; Fax. (250)836-2867; jhbeech@telus.net.

BEECKER, Jennifer R; 305-1919 Riverside Dr, Ottawa ON K1H 1A2; McM'99; FRCPC; Derm;CCFP; CCFP(E.M.); Staff, The Ottawa Hospital - General Campus; (613)523-4921; Fax. (613)523-5339.

BEECROFT, D John; Wellington Med Group, 303-121 Wellington St W, Barrie ON L4N 1L3; Wes'70; CCFP; Assoc Staff, Royal Victoria Regional Health Centre; (705)728-5536; Fax. (705)728-4885.

BEECROFT, J Robert D; Mount Sinai Hosp, 563-600 University Ave, Toronto ON M5G 1X5; Wes'98; FRCPC; DiagRad. Staff, Mount Sinai Hospital; (416)586-4800 x2566; Fax. (416)586-8695.

BEECROFT, James M; Niagara H System-Ontario St, 155 Ontario St, St Catharines ON L2R 5K3; McM'06; CCFP; CCFP(E.M.); Staff, Niagara Health System - Ontario Street Site; (905)378-4647

BEECROFT, Pearl R; H2 Medical Upper Level, 7020 4 St NW, Calgary AB T2K 1C4; Cal'82; (403)258-2133; Fax. (403)258-2162.

BEED, Stephen D; Queen Elizabeth II HSC, BB386-1276 South Park St, Halifax NS B3H 2Y9; Dal'87; FRCPC; Anes (Critical Care Medicine). Staff, Queen Elizabeth II Health Sciences Centre - Victoria General Site; Prof, Dalhousie University; (902)473-3608; Fax. (902)473-3610.

BEEGAN, Daniel; Peace Arch Hosp, 15521 Russell Ave, White Rock BC V4B 2R4; UBC'86; CCFP; FCFP; Staff, Peace Arch Hospital; (604)531-5512

BEEHARRY, Deegrasjsing S; Westbrook Medical Clinic, P57-1610 37 St SW, Calgary AB T3C 3P1; RCS (Ireland)'66; LRCP; LRCS; LM; Langs: English; French; (403)246-0887

BEEHARRY, Emmattee R; Westbrook Med Clinic, P57-1610 37 St SW, Calgary AB T3C 3P1; (Ireland)'95; BCh; BAO; BSc; (403)246-0887; Fax. (403)246-0422.

BEEKMAN, Richard A; 214 Med Place, 928-9909 102 St Box 27, Grande Prairie AB T8V 2V4; Alb'01; FRCSC; GenSurg. (780)539-4545; Fax. (780)532-6743.

BEEKMAN, Steven G; Fort Macleod Med Clinic, PO Box 820, Fort MacLeod AB T0L 0Z0; Alb'07; CCFP; (403)553-3351; Fax. (403)553-4774.

BEER, Darcy L; Children's Hosp, 840 Sherbrook St, Winnipeg MB R3A 1S1; Man'03; FRCPC; Peds; PedEmergMed.

BEERENS, Madelain; Pure North S'Energy Foundation, 800-326 11 Ave SW, Calgary AB T2R 0C5; Witwatersrand (South Africa)'81; (403)457-5077; Fax. (403)457-5019.

BEERMAN, Stephen B; 1450 Waddington Rd, Nanaimo BC V9S 4V9; UBC'85; CCFP; FCFP; (250)754-5545; Fax. (250)754-5954.

BEESTON, Chris; Brandon Reg Health Centre, 150 McTavish Ave E, Brandon MB R7A 2B3; CCFP; CCFP(E.M.); Staff, Brandon Regional Health Centre; (204)726-1122

BEESTON, Jeffery P; Georgian Bay Gen Hosp, PO Box 760 Stn Main 1112 St Andrew's Dr, Midland ON L4R 4P4; Tor'93; CCFP; FCFP; Staff, Georgian Bay General Hospital - Midland; (705)526-3751 x3442; Fax. (705)526-3448.

BEESTON, S William; Lansdowne Prof Bldg, 340-1641 Hillside Ave, Victoria BC V8T 5G1; London (England)'65; MB BS; LRCP; MRCS; Ac Staff, Royal Jubilee Hospital; Ac Staff, Victoria General Hospital; (250)592-2977

BEG-MIRZA, Athar; Brockville Gen Hosp, 2-75 Charles St, Brockville ON K6V 1S8; Punjab (India)'74; FRCSC; OrthSurg. Staff, Brockville General Hospital - Charles Street; (613)345-5645

BEGALKE, Annette D; Athabascan Place, 210-80 Chippewa Rd, Sherwood Park AB T8A 4W6; Alb'08; CCFP; (780)464-6300; Fax. (780)464-2120.

BEGAM, Maksuda; Miramichi Reg Hosp, 500 Water St, Miramichi NB E1V 3G5; Dhaka (India)'90; Staff, Miramichi Regional Hospital; (506)623-3000

BEGGS, Alan J; Regina Qu'Appelle HR-Regina, 1440 14th Ave, Regina SK S4P 0W5; Sask'99; BSc; MSc; FRCSC; OrthSurg (Spine Surgery). Staff Orth Spine Surg, Regina General Hospital; Asst Clin Prof, University of Saskatchewan; (306)766-6932; Fax. (306)766-6999.

BEGIN, Andre; CHUS-Hop Hotel-Dieu, 580 rue Bowen S, Sherbrooke QC J1G 2E8; Sher'04; FRCSC; GenSurg. Staff, Centre Hospitalier Universitaire de Sherbrooke-Hôpital Hôtel-Dieu; (819)346-1110

BEGIN, Catherine; CSSS de Rimouski-Neigette, CP 3150 Succ A 150 av Rouleau, Rimouski QC G5L 5T1; Laval'98; Staff, Hôpital Regional Rimouski; (418)723-7851

BEGIN, Claude; Hop Ste-Anne-de-Beaupre, RR 1 11000 rue des Montagnards, Beaupre QC G0A 1E0; Laval'86; Staff, Hôpital Sainte Anne de Beaupré; (418)827-3726

BEGIN, Eloise; Unite Med Familiale Maizerets, 2480 ch de la Canardiere, Quebec QC G1J 2G1; Laval'07; CCFP; (418)661-1413

BEGIN, Eric V; CSSSG-Hop de Gatineau, CP 2000 Succ Bureau-Chef, Gatineau QC J8P 7H2; Sher'87; MSc; FRCSC; GenSurg (Digestive Surgery). Staff, Hôpital de Gatineau; Langs: Bilingual(French/English); (819)966-6100; Fax. (819)568-9308.

BEGIN, Gaetan; Ctr Hosp du Centre la Mauricie, 50 119e rue, Shawinigan-Sud QC G9P 5K1; Mon'78; Staff, Centre Hospitalier du Centre la Mauricie; (819)536-7500 x7670; Fax. (819)536-7611.

BEGIN, Jean-Francois; Clinique d'Orthopedie de Levis, 6620 rue Saint-Georges, Levis QC G6V 4H1; Laval'97; FRCSC; OrthSurg. Staff, Hôtel-Dieu de Lévis; Langs: Bilingual(French/English); (418)837-8251; Fax. (418)837-2033.

BEGIN, Jennifer L; 300 Burns Ave E PO Box 3907, Melfort SK S0E 1A0; UBC'09; CCFP; (306)752-2818; Fax. (306)752-2926.

BEGIN, Lorraine; 575 rue Saint-Amable, Quebec QC G1R 5R4; Laval'75; (418)643-0355 x3110

BEGIN, Louis R; Hop du Sacre-Coeur de Mtl, 5400 Boul Gouin O, Montreal QC H4J 1C5; Sher'75; ABPath; CSPQ; AnatPath (Surgical Pathology). Chief Gen Path, Hôpital du Sacre-Coeur de Montréal; Assoc Prof Path & Surg, McGill University; Langs: English; French; (514)338-2222

BEGIN, M H Julie; CSSS de Vaudreuil-Soulanges, 490 boul Harwood, Vaudreuil-Dorion QC J7V 7H4; Ott'92; Staff, CSSS de Vaudreuil-Soulanges; Langs: English; French; (450)455-0507; Fax. (450)455-8162; julie_begin@rrsss16.gouv.qc.ca.

BEGIN, Marie; 575 rue Saint-Amable, Quebec QC G1R 2G4; Laval'91; (418)644-7451

BEGIN, Micheline; Social Development Canada, 5A-333 North River Rd, Ottawa ON K1A 0L1; Sher'79; IntMed (P.Q.) (Cardiology). Med Advisor Income Security Program Branch, Government Of Canada; Langs: English; (613)941-8356; Fax. (613)952-8466; micheline.begin@hrsdc-rhdcc.gc.ca.

BEGIN, Nicolas A; 5-1968 Portobello Blvd, Orleans ON K4A 4E7; Mon'96; FRCSC; ObstGyn. (613)837-7033; Fax. (613)837-5781.

BEGIN, Paul A; All Saints Springhill Hosp, PO Box 2560 10 Princess St, Springhill NS B0M 1X0; Dal'84; BSc; Staff, All Saints Springhill Hospital; (902)597-8055; Fax. (902)597-8019.

BEGIN, Paul; 644 rue Jacques-Cartier E, Chicoutimi QC G7H 2A4; Laval'75; FRCPC; IntMed (P.Q.); Respir. Staff, Complexe hospitalier de la Sagamie; Staff, Centre Hospitalier l'Université de Montréal (CHUM) - Hôpital Notre-Dame; (418)549-1512; Fax. (418)549-6965.

BEGIN, Philippe; CHUM-Hop Notre-Dame, 1560 rue Sherbrooke E, Montreal QC H2L 4M1; Mon'07; FRCPC; IntMed; ClinImmunol&Allergy. Staff, Centre Hospitalier l'Université de Montréal (CHUM) - Hôpital Notre-Dame; (514)890-8231

BEGIN, Pierre; Polyclinique Med Fabreville, 380 boul Cure-Labelle, Laval QC H7P 5L3; Laval'75; CCFP; ac Staff, Hôpital du Sacre-Coeur de Montréal; (450)628-5800; Fax. (450)628-0217.

BEGIN, Raymond O; CHUS-Hop Fleurimont, 3001 12e Av N, Sherbrooke QC J1H 5N4; Laval'68; Respir; IntMed. Staff, Centre Hospitalier Universitaire de Sherbrooke-Hopital Fleurimont; Consultant, Centre Hospitalier Universitaire de Sherbrooke-Hôpital Hôtel-Dieu; (819)346-1110; Fax. (819)820-6420.

BEGIN, Rejean; Ctr Hosp Fleury, 2180 rue Fleury E, Montreal QC H2B 1K3; Mon'82; FRCPC; IntMed. Staff, Centre Hospitalier Fleury; (514)381-9311

BEGIN, Serge A; Clinique Med Pointe-Levy, 215 rue Saint-Omer, Levis QC G6V 8N3; Sher'84; Staff, Centre Hospitalier Paul-Gilbert; Physician, CLSC Desjardins Levis; (418)835-1767

BEGIN, Simon; CSSS de Rimouski-Neigette, CP 3150 Succ A 150 av Rouleau, Rimouski QC G5L 5T1; Mon'86; FRCPC; Psy (General Psychiatry). Chef psychiatrie, Hôpital Regional Rimouski; (418)724-8315; Fax. (418)724-8652.

BEGIN, Thierry; CHUQ-St-Francois D'Assise, 10 rue de l'Espinay, Quebec QC G1L 3L5; Laval'97; CCFP; FCFP; Staff, Centre Hospitalier Universitaire De Québec - Pavillon De St-françois-d'assise; Langs: Italian; English; (418)525-4444

BEGIN, Veronique; Clin Med Familiale de Cowansvi, 499 rue du Sud, Cowansville QC J2K 2X9; Sher'04; Staff, Hôpital Brome-Missisquoi-Perkins; (450)263-6077

BEGIN, Violaine; Hop Charles Lemoyne, 3120 boul Taschereau, Greenfield Park QC J4V 2H1; Mon'96; FRCPC; IntMed; Nephrol. Staff, Hopital Charles LeMoyne; (450)466-5000; Fax. (450)466-5045.

BEGIN-LAROUCHE, Julie; Hotel-Dieu de Roberval, 450 rue Brassard, Roberval QC G8H 1B9; Laval'07; Anes. Staff, Hotel-Dieu de Roberval; (418)275-0110

BEGLEY, Gareth; Sylvain Med Centre, 5007 46 St, Sylvan Lake AB T4S 1C2; (South Africa)'02; (403)887-2221; Fax. (403)887-3777.

BEGNOCHE, Evelyne; CSSS Haut-Richelieu-Rouville, 920 boul du Seminaire N, St-Jean-Sur-Richel QC J3A 1B7; Laval'03; Staff, Hôpital du Haut-Richelieu; (450)359-5000

BEGO, Anne; CSSS de Saint-Jerome, 290 rue de Montigny, Saint-Jerome QC J7Z 5T3; Paris (France)'88; Psy. Staff, Hôtel-Dieu de Saint-Jérôme; (450)431-8200

BEGUM, Rehana; Victoria Family Pratice & Walk, 1184 Victoria Park Ave, East York ON M4B 2K6; Dacca (Bangladesh)'82; CCFP; Langs: Bengali; (416)721-5387

BEGUM, Rukhsana; Hop Reg D'Edmundston, 275 Hebert Blvd, Edmundston NB E3V 4E4; Chittagong (Bangladesh)'78; Staff, Hôpital regional d'Edmundston; (506)739-2645; Fax. (506)739-2745.

BEHAMDOUNI, Andre; 3 C1-172 Ethel St, Sturgeon Falls ON P2B 1V9; Mon'82; Staff, West Nipissing General Hospital; (705)753-3342

BEHAMDOUNI, Mounir E; 1011-3377 boul Rosemont, Montreal QC H1X 1K4; Tor'67; ObstGyn (P.Q.). ac Membre, Hôpital Santa Cabrini Ospedale; (514)844-2591

BEHAR, Beatriz M R; 903-1 St Clair Ave E, Toronto ON M4T 2V7; Buenos Aires (Argentina)'59; FRCPsy; FRCPC; Psy (Marital Therapy). Langs: Spanish; (416)960-1116; Fax. (416)265-1816.

BEHAR, Natan; Medical Centre, 200-171 Montreal Rd, Cornwall ON K6H 1B2; Istanbul (Turkey)'70; Staff, Hôpital du Sacre-Coeur de Montréal; Langs: Spanish; Turkish; (613)936-9428; Fax. (613)936-9361.

BEHARRY, Rajendra; Beharry Med Centre, 567 Bathurst St, Toronto ON M5S 2P8; West Indies (Jamaica)'78; (416)964-8572; Fax. (416)323-1662; drbeharry@rogers.com.

BEHBAHANI, Mojgan; North Road Med Centre, 435S North Rd, Coquitlam BC V3K 3V9; (Iran)'99; CCFP; (604)936-0411

BEHELAK, Youssef; West Island Health Centre, 103-3400 rue Du Marche, Dollard-D-Ormeaux QC H9B 2Y1; Ott'80; (514)685-3850; Fax. (514)685-8050.

BEHESHTI, Mojtaba N; 205-2120 North Park Dr, Brampton ON L6S 0C9; Shiraz (Iran)'75; AB; FRCSC; Urol (Female Urology). Staff, William Osler Health System - Brampton Civic Hospital; Langs: Farsi; (905)451-5802; Fax. (905)451-8199.

BEHESHTI, Parvaneh; 108-2419 Bellevue Ave, West Vancouver BC V7V 4T7; Tehran (Iran)'70; Langs: French; Farsi; Assyrian; (604)984-9641; Fax. (604)984-9651; drpbeheshti@hotmail.com.

BEHESNILIAN, Katyg; St Joseph's Health Centre, 30 The Queensway, Toronto ON M6R 1B5; Yerevan (Armenia (Republic))'77; FRCPC; Psy (General Adult Psychiatry). Ac Staff Outpatient Emerg Day Hosp/Physician Comm Mental Health Clinic, St Joseph's Health Centre; Langs: Armenian; Amharic; (416)530-6486 x3293; Fax. (416)530-6076.

BEHIE, Andrea; Maternity Care Clinic, 109-178 96 Ave NE, Calgary AB T3K 6G4; Cal'07; CCFP; Staff, Maternity Care Clinic; (403)735-4922

BEHIELS, Stewart J; 12720 66 St NW, Edmonton AB T5C 0A3; Alb'72; (780)475-3681; Fax. (780)478-7271.

BEHIYA, Ziad H; 619 Lakeshore Rd E, Mississauga ON L5G 1H9; Baghdad (Iraq)'92; CCFP; CCFP(E.M.); Staff, William Osler Health System - Brampton Civic Hospital; (905)891-2424

BEHJATI, Mohammad R; Orillia Soldiers' Mem Hosp, 170 Colborne St W, Orillia ON L3V 2Z3; Iran (Iran)'92; FRCPC; AnatPath. Staff, Orillia Soldiers' Memorial Hospital; (705)325-2201; Fax. (705)330-3225.

BEHKI, Rama R; 29 rue Ducharme, Gatineau QC J8Y 3P7; Qns'86; FAAO; FRCSC; Ophth (Cataract & Glaucoma). Ac Staff Riverside Eye Care Centre, The Ottawa Hospital - Riverside Campus; ac Staff, Hull Hospital; Asst Prof Ophth, University of Ottawa; Langs: English; French; (819)770-3663; Fax. (819)770-1066.

BEHKI, Subita; Medcan Health Mgmt Inc, 1500-150 York St, Toronto ON M5H 3S5; Qns'91; Staff, Medcan Health Management Inc; (416)350-5963; Fax. (416)350-5981.

BEHL, Monica A A; Allan Blair Cancer Centre, 300-4101 Dewdney Ave, Regina SK S4T 7T1; Sask'98; FRCPC; RadOncol;CCFP; (306)766-2203; Fax. (306)766-2688.

BEHL, Vernon; Royal University Hosp, 103 Hospital Dr, Saskatoon SK S7N 0W8; Sask'02; CCFP; CCFP(E.M.); Staff, Royal University Hospital; (306)655-1363; Fax. (306)655-1011.

BEHM, Allan R; Gulf Canada Square, 315-401 9 Ave SW, Calgary AB T2P 3C5; Sask'68; DAB; FRCPC; Derm. Staff, Foothills Medical Centre; Assoc Prof, University of Calgary; (403)263-0661; allanrbehm@shaw.ca.

BEHM, Ernest P; Mills Memorial Hosp, 4720 Haugland Ave, Terrace BC V8G 2W7; Cape Town (South Africa)'79; MB ChB; FRCPC; DiagRad. Staff, Mills Memorial Hospital; Langs: Afrikaans; (250)635-2211 x247; Fax. (250)638-4020.

BEHMANESH, Saeid; Clinical Sciences Bldg, 152 University Campus NW, Edmonton AB T6G 2G3; Johannes Gutenberg (Germany)'00; FRCPC; Anes. (780)938-2007

BEHMANESH, Sharareh; 211-1940 Lonsdale Ave, North Vancouver BC V7M 2K2; Tehran (Iran)'87; CCFP; Langs: Farsi; (604)973-0202

BEHME, Nancy A; Real Canadian Super Store, UL-1205 Oxford St W, London ON N6H 1V8; Tor'91; CCFP; FCFP; (519)672-8460; Fax. (519)672-4947.

BEHN, Darren; 203-1581 Hillside Ave, Victoria BC V8T 2C1; UBC'02; FRCSC; Ophth. (778)430-5393

BEHR, Marcellus A; MUHC-Montreal Gen Hosp, A5 156-1650 av Cedar, Montreal QC H3G 1A4; Qns'90; FRCPC; MedMicrobiol; InfectDis; IntMed. Staff, McGill University Health Centre - Montreal General Campus; adj Prof Med, McGill University; Langs: English; French; (514)934-1934 x42815

BEHRA, Tasniem; UBC Student Health Services, M334-2211 Wesbrook Mall, Vancouver BC V6T 1Z3; Qns'05; (604)822-7011

BEHRAM, Acar; Saint John Reg Hosp, PO Box 2100 Stn Main 400 University Ave, Saint John NB E2L 4L2; '91; Staff, Saint John Regional Hospital; (506)648-6000

BEHRENS, Ralph; Beaver Valley Clinic, PO Box 610, Fruitvale BC V0G 1L0; Cal'85; BSc; Staff, Kootenay Boundary Regional Hospital; (250)367-9211; Fax. (250)367-7543.

BEHRMANN, Bernard A; Richmond Health Science Ctre, 440-6091 Gilbert Rd, Richmond BC V7C 5L9; Witwatersrand (South Africa)'79; MB ChB; FRCPC; Peds. (604)270-4456; Fax. (604)273-6146.

BEHROOZI, Dara; Burrard Health Bldg, 304-1160 Burrard St, Vancouver BC V6Z 2E8; London (England)'86; MB BS; LMCC; CCFP; FCFP; Staff, Providence Health Care - St Paul's Hospital; Dir, British Columbia Medical Association; (604)681-1116; Fax. (604)689-1118.

BEHSE, Joseph H; 233 Van Norman St, Thunder Bay ON P7A 4B6; McM'79; Staff, Thunder Bay Regional Health Sciences Centre; Physician Students Health Services/Physician Independent Counselling, Lakehead University / Library; Physician Independent Counselling, Confederation College; (807)345-6699; Fax. (807)345-0366.

BEHZADI, Abdollah; The Credit Valley Hosp, 2200 Eglinton Ave W, Mississauga ON L5M 2N1; McG'95; MDCM; MBA; FRCSC; GenSurg (Thoracic Oncology); ThorSurg. Staff, The Credit Valley Hospital; Lecturer Surg, University of Toronto; Langs: French; Farsi; (905)813-2200; Fax. (905)813-4024; abehzadi@tsh.to.

BEIKO, Darren T; Kingston Gen Hosp, 76 Stuart St, Kingston ON K7L 2V7; Ott'96; BSc(Hons); FRCSC; Urol (Endourology). Att Staff Urol, Kingston General Hospital; Asst Prof Urol, Queen's University; Langs: French; (613)548-2498; Fax. (613)545-1970.

BEIKO, George H H; Niagara Health Centre, 103-180 Vine St S, St Catharines ON L2R 7P3; Oxford (England)'86; MB ChB(Hon); FRCSC; Ophth (Anterior Segment). Staff, Niagara Health System - Ontario Street Site; Langs: Ukrainian; (905)687-8322; Fax. (905)687-8766; georgebeiko@yahoo.ca.

BEIKO, Jason; Health Sciences Centre, GB103-820 Sherbrook St, Winnipeg MB R3A 1R9; Ott'04; FRCSC; Neursurg. Staff, Health Sciences Centre.

BEIMERS, Mary Ann; 318-460 Nanaimo St E, Vancouver BC V5L 4W3; McM'93; FRCPC; Peds (Eating Disorders). Clinical Asst Prof, Providence Health Care - St Paul's Hospital; Clinical Asst Prof, University of British Columbia; Langs: Dutch; German; French; (604)970-4144; mabeimers@shaw.ca.

BEINTEMA, Christena; 1F-176 St. George St, Toronto ON M5R 2M7; Tor'80; Court Staff, The Scarborough Hospital - General Campus; Staff/Physician, Runnymede Healthcare Centre; (416)921-3961; Fax. (416)921-9139.

BEIQUE, Caroline; Clinique de Med Familiale, 6F-2120 rue Sherbrooke E, Montreal QC H2K 1C3; McG'83; CCFP; ac Staff, Centre Hospitalier l'Université de Montréal (CHUM) - Hôpital Notre-Dame; (514)527-1958

BEIQUE, Francois A; SMBD Jewish Gen Hosp, 3755 ch Cote-Sainte-Catherine, Montreal QC H3T 1E2; McG'87; CSPQ; FRCPC; Anes. Dir Cardiac Anes, Sir Mortimer B Davis Jewish General; assoc Prof Anes, McGill University; (514)340-8222

BEIQUE, Marc A; MUHC-Royal Victoria Hosp, 687 av des Pins O, Montreal QC H3A 1A1; Ott'87; FRCPC; EmergMed. Staff, McGill University Health Centre - Royal Victoria Hospital; (514)843-1610; Fax. (514)843-1638.

BEITCHMAN, Joseph H; Child Youth & Family Program, 80 Workman Way, Toronto ON M6J 1H4; McG'68; DPH(Mich); MPH; DABPN; FRCPC; Psy (Child & Adolescent Psychiatry). Staff, Child Youth & Family Program (CAMH); (416)979-6813; Fax. (416)979-6820; joe.beitchman@camh.ca.

BEITEL, Allan; 2904-210 Victoria St, Toronto ON M5B 2R2; McG'76; AB; DCP; FRCPC; Psy (Psychoanalysis). (647)869-2006

BEITHOON, Ziad; Bonavista Peninsula Comm HC, PO Box 1 Hospital Rd, Bonavista NL A0C 1B0; (Other Foreign)'00; CCFP; Staff, Bonavista Peninsula Health Centre; Staff, Dr Walter Templeman Health Centre; ziad.beithoon@easternhealth.ca.

BEJERMAN, Mario; Clinique Med Luso Mtl Ltee, 1 av Du Mont-Royal E, Montreal QC H2T 1N4; Buenos Aires (Argentina)'62; DAB; FACS; FRCSC; GenSurg. Att Staff, Centre Hospitalier de LaSalle; Langs: French; Spanish; Portuguese; (514)849-2391; Fax. (514)849-2394.

BEKASIAK, P Antoni; 206-2425 Tecumseh Rd E, Windsor ON N8W 1E6; Poznan (Poland)'76; Staff, Windsor Regional Hospital - Metropolitan Site; (519)974-2244; docbekasiak@bellnet.ca.

BEKELE, Yilma; Dr Everett Chalmers Hosp, PO Box 9000 Stn A, Fredericton NB E3B 5N5; Addis Ababa (Ethiopia)'89; Staff, Dr Everett Chalmers Regional Hospital; (506)452-5400

BEKERIS, Edward; Medcan Health Mgmt Inc, 1500-150 York St, Toronto ON M5H 3S5; Wes'86; MD; BEng; Medical Staff, William Osler Health System - Etobicoke General Hospital; Staff, Medcan Health Management Inc; Physician Occupational Health Services, Air Canada Medical Clinic; Langs: Lithuanian; (416)350-5900; Fax. (416)350-5981.

BEKHECHI, Samir E; Clinique MetroMedic, 1538 rue Sherbrooke O, Montreal QC H3G 1L5; Mon'03; CCFP; Staff, Centre Hospitalier Régional du Suroît; (514)932-2122

BEKHIT, Emil T; Deerfoot Meadows Med Clinic, 7979 11 St SE, Calgary AB T2H 0B8; Cairo (Egypt); CCFP; (403)251-2690; Fax. (403)251-2695; emilbekhit@yahoo.ca.

BEKHIT, Magdy R; 2536 Keele St, North York ON M6L 2N8; Alexandria (Egypt)'75; MB ChB; CCFP; Physician, Maple Leaf Clinic; Langs: Arabic; (416)249-7772; Fax. (416)249-9978.

BEKHOR, Sabah; 220-5450 ch Cote-des-Neiges, Montreal QC H3T 1Y6; Baghdad (Iraq)'65; MB ChB; FRCPC; Neur; Electroenceph (P.Q.). Staff Neurol, St Mary's Hospital Centre; assoc Prof, McGill University; (514)739-2668; s.bekhor@bellnet.ca.

BEKHOR, Samia; SMBD Jewish Gen Hosp, 3755 ch Cote-Sainte-Catherine, Montreal QC H3T 1E2; Baghdad (Iraq)'65; DA; CSPQ; Anes (P.Q.) (Clinical Anaesthesia). Staff Anes, Sir Mortimer B Davis Jewish General; Prof, McGill University; (514)340-8232; Fax. (514)822-4547.

BEKIER, Estera; 187 St Clair Ave W, Toronto ON M4V 1P7; Lodz (Poland)'71; FRCPC; IntMed. (416)944-1016; Fax. (416)324-8251.

BEKKER, Antoinette; Medical Arts Centre, 127-770 6 St SW, Medicine Hat AB T1A 8M7; (South Africa)'90; (403)526-1551; Fax. (403)526-1505; drabekker@shawcable.com.

BEKKER, Ian S; Royal Jubilee Hosp, 1952 Bay St, Victoria BC V8R 1J8; UBC'09; CCFP; Staff Geriatric Outpatient Clinic, Royal Jubilee Hospital; (250)370-8565

BEKKER, Leon R; Loon Lake Medical Clinic, PO Box 190 506 1 St N, Loon Lake SK S0M 1L0; Pretoria (South Africa)'86; MB ChB; (306)837-2066; Fax. (306)837-2079.

BELAIR, Guy; Hop Maisonneuve-Rosemont, 5415 boul de l'Assomption, Montreal QC H1T 2M4; Mon'92; FRCSC; Urol. Staff, Hopital Maisonneuve-Rosemont; (514)252-3400; Fax. (514)252-3561.

BELAIR, Jacques D; CSSS de Beauce-Etchemin, 1515 17e rue, Saint-Georges QC G5Y 4T8; Laval'72; FACOG; CSPQ; FRCSC; ObstGyn. ac Staff, Centre Hospitalier Beauce-Etchemin; Langs: English; (418)228-2031; Fax. (418)227-1270.

BELAIR, Jean-Francois; Douglas Mental Hlth Univ Inst, 6875 boul Lasalle, Verdun QC H4H 1R3; Sher'85; FRCPC; Psy. Staff, Douglas Mental Health University Institute; Dir Inpatient & Day Hosp for Adolescent, Allan Memorial Institute; Teacher Faculty, McGill University; (514)761-6131 x2124

BELAIR, Louis; CSSSG-Hop de Hull, 116 boul Lionel-Emond, Gatineau QC J8Y 1W7; McG'90; DiagRad. Staff, Hull Hospital; (819)595-6028

BELAIR, Manon; CHUM-Hop Notre-Dame, 1560 rue Sherbrooke E, Montreal QC H2L 4M1; Mon'93; FRCPC; DiagRad. Staff, Centre Hospitalier l'Université de Montréal (CHUM) - Hôpital Notre-Dame; (514)890-8000

BELAIR, Marie-Lyne; Hop Maisonneuve-Rosemont, 5415 boul de l'Assomption, Montreal QC H1T 2M4; Mon'00; FRCSC; Ophth (Uveitis). Staff, Hopital Maisonneuve-Rosemont; Staff, Centre Hospitalier l'Université de Montréal (CHUM) - Hôpital Notre-Dame; Langs: Bilingual(French/English); (514)252-3400 x1733

BELAIR, Patricia; Hôpital de Saint-Eustache, 520 boul Arthur-Sauve, Saint-Eustache QC J7R 5B1; Mon'06; Psy. Staff, Hôpital de Saint-Eustache; (450)473-6811

BELAK, Zenon A; Regina Internal Med Specialist, 1821 Rose St, Regina SK S4P 1Z7; Katowice (Poland)'06; FRCPC; IntMed; Respir. Staff, Royal University Hospital; (306)525-1790; Fax. (306)359-1068.

BELAK, Zenon D; Medical Arts Bldg, 102-750 Spadina Cres E, Saskatoon SK S7K 3H3; Sask'62; Ac Staff, St Paul's Hospital (Grey Nuns) of Saskatoon; Ac Staff, Saskatoon City Hospital; Ac Staff, Royal University Hospital; (306)652-0011; Fax. (306)653-5940; zenon.belak@shaw.ca.

BELAND, Alain; Hotel-Dieu de Roberval, 450 rue Brassard, Roberval QC G8H 1B9; Sher'83; CSPQ; FRCPC; Anes. Staff, Hotel-Dieu de Roberval; (418)275-0110; Fax. (418)275-4091.

BELAND, Guy C; UMF Laval, 2690 ch des Quatre-Bourgeois, Quebec QC G1V 0B7; Laval'77; CCFP; FCFP; Staff, Hôpital Laval; Chef Family Med & Emerg Meg, Université Laval; (418)656-4795; Fax. (418)656-4503.

BELAND, Jacques; Nashwaaksis Med Clinic, 475 Brookside Dr, Fredericton NB E3A 8V4; Mon'87; (506)458-9449

BELAND, Marie; Hôpital Ste-Justine, 3175 ch Cote-Sainte-Catherine, Montreal QC H3T 1C5; Laval'73; Peds (Pediatric Emergency Medicine). ac Staff, Hôpital Ste-Justine; Langs: Bilingual(French/English); (514)345-4931

BELAND, Marie Josee; MUHC-Montreal Children's Hosp, D371-2300 rue Tupper, Montreal QC H3H 1P3; McG'80; CRCP; CSPQ; FRCPC; Peds (Pediatric Cardiology); Cardiol. Staff Ped Cardiol, McGill University Health Centre - Montreal Children's Hospital; assoc Prof, McGill University; Langs: Bilingual(French/English); (514)412-4400 x24423; Fax. (514)412-4391; marie.j.beland@muhc.mcgill.ca.

BELAND, Normand; CLSC Saint-Hubert, 6800 boul Cousineau, Saint-Hubert QC J3Y 8Z4; Mon'86; CCFP; FCFP; Clin Instructeur, Universite de Montreal; (450)443-7407; Fax. (450)676-3488.

BELAND, Pierre; Groupe Med de Trois-Rivieres, 225-1900 boul des Recollets, Trois-Rivieres QC G8Z 4K4; Sher'82; (819)375-0276; Fax. (819)375-3423.

BELAND, Renee L; Old Quebec Street Mall, 208-55 Wyndham St N, Guelph ON N1H 7T8; Tor'91; CCFP; FCFP; (519)837-2283; Fax. (519)767-2262.

BELAND, Therese; Ctre de Sante Psychologique, 2101 boul Edouard-Montpetit, Montreal QC H3T 1J3; Mon'81; (514)343-6452; Fax. (514)343-7236; sae-beland@exchange.umontreal.ca.

BELAND-VACHON, Helene; CSST de Longueuil, 500-25 boul La Fayette, Longueuil QC J4K 5B7; Mon'82; LMCC; Med Consultant, CSST Direction Regionale Longueuil; Langs: English; (450)442-6200 x6323; Fax. (450)442-6094; helene.beland-vachon@csst.qc.ca.

BELANGER, Anais L; Office of the Chief Coroner, 200-26 Grenville St, Toronto ON M7A 2G9; Ott'99; CCFP; Staff, Mackenzie Richmond Hill Hospital; (416)314-4100

BELANGER, Andre; 305-3030 boul Le carrefour, Laval QC H7T 2P5; Mon'71; MSc; Endocrin (P.Q.); IntMed. Dir, Centre de Recherche Clinique de Laval; (450)688-3132 x207; Fax. (450)688-4266.

BELANGER, Andre; Hotel-Dieu d'Arthabaska, 5 rue des Hospitalieres, Victoriaville QC G6P 6N2; Sher'05; Staff, Hotel-Dieu d'Arthabaska; (819)357-2030

BELANGER, Andre; Clinique Med Valcartier, 118-190 rue Dube, Courcelette QC G0A 1R1; Laval'83; assoc Staff, CSSS de Quebec-Sud; Staff, Centre Hospitalier Chauveau; (418)844-3721; Fax. (418)844-3318.

BELANGER, Bruno L; 610 boul Cure-Labelle, Laval QC H7V 2T7; Laval'73; (450)687-6452

BELANGER, Carl; CHUM-Hop Notre-Dame, 1560 rue Sherbrooke E, Montreal QC H2L 4M1; Mon'80; FRCPC; HemPath; Hem (P.Q.); MedOncol. Staff, Centre Hospitalier l'Université de Montréal (CHUM) - Hôpital Notre-Dame; Consultant, Hôpital Ste-Justine; adj Prof, Universite de Montreal; (514)890-8000 x25381; Fax. (514)412-7803.

BELANGER, Carole; CSSS de la région de Thetford, 1717 rue Notre-Dame E, Thetford Mines QC G6G 2V4; Sher'82; FRCPC; Psy. Staff, Centre Hospitalier Universitaire de Sherbrooke-Hopital Fleurimont; Staff, Hopital du CSS de la Region de Thetford; Staff, Centre Hospitalier Universitaire de Sherbrooke-Hôpital Hôtel-Dieu; Staff, Hôpital Sainte-croix; (418)338-7707; Fax. (418)338-7705.

BELANGER, Caroline; Hôpital Ste-Justine, 3175 ch Cote-Sainte-Catherine, Montreal QC H3T 1C5; Sher'03; FRCSC; Ophth. Staff, Hôpital Ste-Justine; (514)345-4931

BELANGER, Celine; Hotel Dieu de Levis, 143 rue Wolfe, Levis QC G6V 3Z1; Laval'83; FRCPC; Peds (Neonatology). Staff, Hôtel-Dieu de Lévis; assoc Membre, Centre Hospitalier Universitaire de Quebec-CHUL; Consultant, Centre Hospitalier Paul-Gilbert; (418)835-7322; Fax. (418)835-7323.

BELANGER, Chantal; Clinique Med Legendre, 201-1650 av Jules-Verne, Quebec QC G2G 2R1; Laval'94; Boursier Psychogeriatric, CSSS Vieille-Capitale; (418)872-5600; Fax. (418)872-8408.

BELANGER, Chantale; CSSS de la Baie-des-Chaleurs, RR 2 419 boul Perron, Maria QC G0C 1Y0; Mon'08; Staff, CSSS de la Baie-des-Chaleurs; (418)759-3443

BELANGER, Claude; Polyclinique Med Concorde, 300 boul de la Concorde E, Laval QC H7G 2E6; Mon'67; Otol (P.Q.) (Head & Neck Surgery). Staff, CSSS du Coeur de l'Isle Hôpital Jean-Talon; (450)667-5310; Fax. (450)667-5248.

BELANGER, Daniel; Hop Maisonneuve-Rosemont, 5415 boul de l'Assomption, Montreal QC H1T 2M4; Mon'83; ABIM; FRCPC; IntMed; MedOncol; Hem. Staff, Hopital Maisonneuve-Rosemont; Clin Prof, Universite de Montreal; (514)252-3404 x3404; Fax. (514)254-5094.

BELANGER, Danielle; CLSC Orleans, 3666 ch Royal, Quebec QC G1E 1X5; Laval'86; assoc Staff, Centre Hospitalier Affilié Universitaire de Québec - Hôpital du St-Sacrement; Physician Commun Health, CRSSS PECA; (418)663-3099

BELANGER, Eric C; The Ottawa Hosp-Gen Campus, 501 Smyth Rd, Ottawa ON K1H 8L6; Ott'00; BSc; FRCPC; AnatPath (Renal Pathology). Staff, The Ottawa Hospital - General Campus; Langs: Bilingual(French/English); (613)737-8899 x79837; eribelanger@ottawahospital.on.ca.

BELANGER, Estelle; Clin de ObstGyn de Trois-Rivie, 2237 7e av, Trois-Rivieres QC G8Z 3E2; Laval'91; FRCSC; ObstGyn. Staff, CSSS de Trois-Rivières; (819)379-5353; Fax. (819)379-2893; gynecotr@cgocable.ca.

BELANGER, Eve-Marie; CSSSG-Hop de Gatineau, CP 2000 Succ Bureau-Chef 909 boul de la Verendrye O, Gatineau QC J8P 7H2; Sher'88; Peds. Staff, Hôpital de Gatineau; (819)966-6165; Fax. (819)561-8103.

BELANGER, Francois P H; Alberta Children's Hosp, 2888 Shaganappi Trail NW, Calgary AB T3B 6A8; Ott'85; FRCPC; Peds (Pediatric Emergency Medicine). A-Head Dept of Peds, Alberta Children's Hospital; Teach Staff, University of Calgary; (403)955-7070

BELANGER, Gerald; Hotel-Dieu d'Arthabaska, 5 rue des Hospitalieres, Victoriaville QC G6P 6N2; Laval'71; DiagRad. Staff, Hotel-Dieu d'Arthabaska; (819)357-1151; Fax. (819)357-6003.

BELANGER, Guy-Alain; Carrefour Sante Le St-Laurent, 140-5300 boul Saint-Laurent, Sainte-Catherine QC J5C 1A8; Mon'76; Langs: English; (450)638-6383; Fax. (450)635-6359.

BELANGER, Helene; Ctr Hosp Affilie-St-Sacrement, 1050 ch Sainte-Foy, Quebec QC G1S 4L8; Laval'98; FRCPC; Psy. Staff, Centre Hospitalier Affilié Universitaire de Québec - Hôpital du St-Sacrement; (418)682-7898; Fax. (418)682-7959; helenbelanger@hotmail.com.

BELANGER, Huguette; Direction de la Sante Publique, 1255 rue Beauregard, Longueuil QC J4K 2M3; Mon'72; Med Consultant Dept of Public Health, Hopital Charles LeMoyne; Staff, Agence de santé et des services sociaux de la Montérégie; Langs: English; (450)928-6777 x4084; Fax. (450)928-3812.

BELANGER, Jacques; Centre Med Laval, 1110 boul Vanier, Laval QC H7C 2R8; Mon'78; (450)661-2521; Fax. (450)661-7193.

BELANGER, Jean-Francois; 54 av Bateman, Edmundston NB E3V 4A4; Ott'02; FRCSC; GenSurg. Staff, Hôpital regional d'Edmundston; (506)739-5949; Fax. (506)739-9066.

BELANGER, Jean-Francois; Hop Jean-Talon, 1385 rue Jean-Talon E, Montreal QC H2E 1S6; Mon'00; FRCPC; Psy. Staff, CSSS du Coeur de l'Isle Hôpital Jean-Talon; (514)495-6767

BELANGER, Jean-Francois; CSSS de la Mitis, 800 av du Sanatorium, Mont-Joli QC G5H 3L6; Laval'94; LMCC; Staff, CSSS de la Mitis; Langs: Spanish; English; (418)775-7261

BELANGER, Jean-Philippe; CSSS de Montmagny-L'Islet, 350 boul Tache O RR 1, Montmagny QC G5V 3R8; Laval'07; FRCSC; OrthSurg. Staff, CSSS de Montmagny-L'Islet; (418)248-0630

BELANGER, Jeannette E; 107-900 Greenbank Rd, Nepean ON K2J 1S8; Ott'03; CCFP; Staff, Children's Hospital of Eastern Ontario (CHEO); (613)825-8476

BELANGER, Josee; Ctr Hosp Laurentien, 234 rue Saint-Vincent, Ste-Agathe-des-Mts QC J8C 2B8; Laval'88; CCFP; CCFP(E.M.); Staff, Centre Hospitalier Laurentien; (819)324-4000

BELANGER, Julie; Hôtel-Dieu de Lévis, 143 rue Wolfe, Levis QC G6V 3Z1; Laval'06; Staff, Hôtel-Dieu de Lévis; (418)835-7121

BELANGER, Julie; Hôtel-Dieu de Sorel, 400 av de l'Hotel-Dieu, Sorel-Tracy QC J3P 1N5; Mon'05; FRCSC; GenSurg;CCFP; Staff, Hôtel-Dieu de Sorel; (450)746-6000

BELANGER, Liliane; Clinique Med Saint-Augustin, 220-334 route 138, Quebec QC G3A 2Y1; Laval'89; (418)878-3590

BELANGER, Lise; Hotel-Dieu de Levis, 143 rue Wolfe, Levis QC G6V 3Z1; Laval'98; FRCPC; Peds. Staff, Hôtel-Dieu de Lévis; (418)835-7121; Fax. (418)835-7239.

BELANGER, Louis; CSSS des Aurores Boreales, CP 6000 Succ Bureau-Chef 679 2e rue E, La Sarre QC J9Z 2X7; Mon'85; Staff, Centre Hospitalier La Sarre; (819)333-2311

BELANGER, Louis R; Place Barrette, 270 rue Malraux, Chicoutimi QC G7H 6R9; Laval'83; FRCSC; OrthSurg. Staff, Complexe hospitalier de la Sagamie; (418)690-1014

BELANGER, Louise; CLSC Richmond, 110 rue Barlow, Richmond QC J0B 2H0; Sher'86; (819)826-3781; Fax. (819)826-3867; louise.belanger@ssss.gouv.qc.ca.

BELANGER, Luc; CHUQ-Hotel-Dieu de Quebec, 11 Cote Du Palais, Quebec QC G1R 2J6; Laval'71; CSPQ; PhD; MedBiochem (P.Q.). Dir Research Centre & Assoc Clin Chemist, Centre Hospitalier Universitaire de Québec (CHUQ) - Siege Social; Dir/Prof, Universite Laval; (418)525-4444 x15543; Fax. (418)691-5489; luc.belanger@crhdq.ulaval.ca.

BELANGER, Lucie; CSSS du Nord de Lanaudière, 1000 boul Sainte-Anne, St-Charles-Brromee QC J6E 6J2; Laval'90; Staff, Centre Hospitalier Régional de Lanaudière; (450)759-8222 x2820

BELANGER, Lucie; CSSS du Sud de Lanaudière, 911 montee des Pionniers, Terrebonne QC J6V 2H2; Mon'99; FRCPC; DiagRad. Staff, Centre Hospitalier Pierre le Gardeur; (450)654-7525

BELANGER, Lucien; CSSS de Saint-Jerome, 290 rue de Montigny, Saint-Jerome QC J7Z 5T3; Laval'80; Staff, Hôtel-Dieu de Saint-Jérôme; (450)431-8200

BELANGER, Marc; Ctr Hosp Affilie-Enfant-Jesus, 1401 18e rue, Quebec QC G1J 1Z4; Mon'77; Staff, Centre Hospitalier Affilié Universitaire de Québec - Hôpital De L'Enfant Jésus; (418)649-5524; Fax. (418)649-5599.

BELANGER, Marcel A; CLSC du Plateau Mont-Royal, 4625 av de Lorimier, Montreal QC H2H 2B4; Laval'75; (514)521-7663; Fax. (514)521-6426.

BELANGER, Marie S G; Cornwall Comm Hosp-Mcconnell, PO Box 100 Stn Main 840 McConnell Ave, Cornwall ON K6H 5S5; Ott'05; CCFP; CCFP(E.M.); Staff, Cornwall Community Hospital; Staff, Hull Hospital; (613)938-4240

BELANGER, Marie-Eve; CHUS-Hop Fleurimont, 3001 12e Av N, Sherbrooke QC J1H 5N4; Mon'95; CCFP; CCFP(E.M.); Staff, Centre Hospitalier Universitaire de Sherbrooke-Hopital Fleurimont; (819)346-1110 x14274; Fax. (819)564-5386.

BELANGER, Mario; Hotel-Dieu de Levis, 143 rue Wolfe, Levis QC G6V 3Z1; Laval'80; MedOncol (P.Q.); Hem (P.Q.); IntMed. Staff, Centre Hospitalier Universitaire de Québec (CHUQ) - Siege Social; Staff, Hôtel-Dieu de Lévis; assoc Staff, CSSS de Quebec-Sud; (418)835-7121 x3371; Fax. (418)835-7160.

BELANGER, Martin; CSSS de Jonquiere, CP 1200 Stn Pdf Jonquiere 2230 rue de l'Hopital, Jonquiere QC G7X 7X2; Laval'96; Staff, Centre Hospitalier Jonquiere; (418)695-7700

BELANGER, Mathieu; Ctr Hosp Affilie-Enfant-Jesus, 1401 18e rue, Quebec QC G1J 1Z4; Laval'03; FRCSC; GenSurg (Family Medicine). Staff, Centre Hospitalier Affilié Universitaire de Québec - Hôpital De L'Enfant Jésus; (418)649-0252

BELANGER, Mathieu; CPM Health Centres, B22-550 Terminal Ave, Ottawa ON K1G 0Z3; Mon'07; CCFP; (613)731-4770; Fax. (613)731-6201.

BELANGER, Maud; Ctre Metropolitain de Chirurgi, 995 rue de Salaberry, Montreal QC H3L 1L2; Laval'05; FRCSC; PlasSurg. (514)288-2097; Fax. (514)288-3547.

BELANGER, Melanie; CSSS Pierre Boucher, 1333 boul Jacques-Cartier E, Longueuil QC J4M 2A5; Laval'96; FRCPC; IntMed; Gastroent. Staff, Hopital Charles LeMoyne; (450)468-8111

BELANGER, Michele; Health Canada, 6F-200 boul Rene-Levesque O, Montreal QC H2Z 1X4; McG'81; FRCPC; Psy. (514)283-1595

BELANGER, Michelle A; Cross Roads Ob/Gyn, 330-507 Broadway W, Vancouver BC V5Z 1E6; Ott'95; FRCSC; ObstGyn. (604)872-5484; Fax. (604)708-0748.

BELANGER, Monique; Centre de Santé Communautaire, 19 Frood Rd, Sudbury ON P3C 4Y9; Tor'91; BSc; CCFP; Physician, Centre de Sante Communautaire; Teach Staff, Northern Ontario School of Medicine; Langs: Bilingual(English/French); (705)670-2274; Fax. (705)670-2277; mbelanger@santesudbury.ca.

BELANGER, Norma; CHUQ-St-Francois d'Assise, 10 rue de l'Espinay, Quebec QC G1L 3L5; Laval'90; CCFP; Ac Staff, Centre Hospitalier Universitaire De Québec - Pavillon De St-françois-d'assise; (418)525-4425; Fax. (418)525-4322.

BELANGER, Pascale; Clinique Med Blainville, 519 boul du Cure-Labelle, Blainville QC J7C 2H6; Mon'88; (450)430-2221

BELANGER, Paul; Clinique Oculus, 10665 1re av, Saint-Georges QC G5Y 6X8; Sher'05; FRCSC; Ophth. (418)226-0300; Fax. (418)226-0301.

BELANGER, Philippe; CSSS Drummond-Hop Sainte-Croix, 570 rue Heriot, Drummondville QC J2B 1C1; Sher'06; Psy. Staff, CSSS de la Baie-des-Chaleurs; Staff, Hôpital Sainte-croix; (819)478-6464

BELANGER, Pierre; CSSS de Sept-Iles, 45 rue Du Pere-Divet, Sept-Iles QC G4R 3N7; Mon'77; FRCPC; Peds. Staff, Centre Hospitalier Regional de Sept-Iles; Langs: Bilingual(French/English); (418)962-1216; Fax. (418)968-2111.

BELANGER, Pierre; Clinique Med Desy, 5636 boul Henri-Bourassa E, Montreal-Nord QC H1G 2T2; Mon'85; Staff, Hopital de la Cite de la santé; (514)326-9060; Fax. (514)326-0919.

BELANGER, Pierre; Ctr Hosp Laurentien, 234 rue Saint-Vincent, Ste-Agathe-des-Mts QC J8C 2B8; Mon'63; Staff, Centre Hospitalier Laurentien; (819)324-4000

BELANGER, Raphael; 503-235 boul Rene-Levesque E, Montreal QC H2X 1N8; Mon'63; Endocrin (P.Q.); IntMed. Staff, Centre Hospitalier l'Université De Montréal (CHUM) - Hôpital Saint-luc; (514)866-3681

BELANGER, Rene-Maurice; Bureau du Coroner, 1701 rue Parthenais, Montreal QC H2K 3S7; Mon'65; MSc; (514)873-3284 x21233

BELANGER, Richard; CHUQ-Ctr Hosp Univ Laval, 1742-2705 boul Laurier, Quebec QC G1V 4G2; Mon'03; FRCPC; Peds (Adolescent Medicine). Staff, Centre Hospitalier Universitaire de Quebec-CHUL; (418)525-4444

BELANGER, Richard; Clinique Med de Mirabel, CP 1059 Succ St-Janvier 200-13714 boul du Curé-Labelle, Mirabel QC J7J 1A1; Mon'83; (450)435-7666

BELANGER, Robert; Ctr Hosp Anna-Laberge, 200 boul Brisebois, Chateauguay QC J6K 4W8; Mon'77; CSPQ; HemPath; Hem (P.Q.) (Bone Marrow Transplant). Staff, Hôpital Anna-Laberge; adj Prof, Universite de Montreal; Langs: English; (450)699-2707

BELANGER, Serge; Commission Lesion Professional, 500 boul Rene-Levesque O, Montreal QC H2Z 1W7; Mon'77; (514)873-6920

BELANGER, Stephane; CSSS De Sept-Iles, 45 rue du Pere-Divet, Sept-Iles QC G4R 3N7; Laval'07; CCFP; Staff, Centre Hospitalier Regional de Sept-Iles; (418)962-9761; Fax. (418)962-2701.

BELANGER, Sylvie; Clinique Med de Touraine, 2B-520 boul de l'Hopital, Gatineau QC J8V 2P5; Sher'91; Staff, Hôpital de Gatineau; (819)568-0212

BELANGER, Sylvie; CHUQ-Ctr Hosp Univ Laval, 2705 boul Laurier, Quebec QC G1V 4G2; Mon'89; FRCPC; Peds (Neonatal & Perinatal Medicine). Staff, Centre Hospitalier Universitaire de Quebec-CHUL; Staff, Centre Hospitalier Universitaire De Québec - Pavillon De St-françois-d'assise; (418)654-2282; Fax. (418)654-2771.

BELANGER, Yvan; Clinique de Ped de Rimouski, 161 av Rouleau, Rimouski QC G5L 5T3; Laval'72; FRCPC; Peds. Staff, Hôpital Regional Rimouski; Langs: English; (418)724-4221; Fax. (418)725-3025.

BELANGER-BONNEAU, Helene; Dir de la Sante Publique, 210-1000 rue Labelle, Saint-Jerome QC J7Z 5N6; Mon'79; MSc; MPH; FRCPC; CommunMed (Public Health). Staff, Complexe hospitalier de la Sagamie; ac Membre Dept of Public Health Clinic, CSSS de Saint-Jerome; Langs: English; (450)436-8622 x3213; Fax. (450)436-1761; helene.belanger.bonneau@ssss.gouv.qc.ca.

BELANGER DUCHARME, Frederique; CSSS de la Cote-de-Gaspe, 215 boul de York O, Gaspe QC G4X 2W2; Laval'09; CCFP; Staff, Centre Hospitalier de Gaspe; (418)368-3301

BELAU, Marianne R; Royal Court Med Centre, 204-5 Quarry Ridge Rd, Barrie ON L4M 7G1; Tor'81; CCFP; FCFP; Ac Staff, Royal Victoria Regional Health Centre.

BELBIN, Donald E; Chatham-Kent-Hlth-Sydenham, 325 Margaret Ave, Wallaceburg ON N8A 2A7; Mem'90; CCFP; Staff ER, Chatham-Kent Health Alliance - Sydenham Hospital Campus; (519)627-1461

BELCH, Andrew R; Cross Cancer Institute, 11560 University Ave NW, Edmonton AB T6G 1Z2; Tor'70; FRCPC; IntMed (Multiple Myeloma); Hem. Staff, University of Alberta Hospital; Staff MedOncol, Cross Cancer Institute; Prof, University of Alberta; (780)432-8757

BELCHER, David L; PO Box 7537 Stn Main, Drayton Valley AB T7A 1S7; Cambridge (England)'58; DA; DRCOG; Ac Staff, Drayton Valley Hospital & Care Centre; (780)542-4202; Fax. (780)542-4285; dbelcher@ccinet.ab.ca.

BELCHETZ, Brett; Rouge Valley-Centenary HC, 2867 Ellesmere Rd, Scarborough ON M1E 4B9; Tor'00; CCFP; Staff, Rouge Valley Health System - Centenary Health Centre Site; (416)281-7270

BELCHETZ, Gregory J; Osler ENT Associates, 617-2250 Bovaird Dr E, Brampton ON L6R 0W3; Tor'97; BSc; FRCSC; Otol (Facial Plastic Surgery). Staff, William Osler Health System - Brampton Civic Hospital; (905)792-6949; Fax. (905)792-6977.

BELCHETZ, Lance A; The Credit Valley Hosp, 2200 Eglinton Ave W, Mississauga ON L5M 2N1; Tor'95; CCFP; CCFP(E.M.); FCFP; Staff, The Credit Valley Hospital; (905)813-4530; Fax. (905)813-4548.

BELDA, Antonio A; 390 Rivertrace Close, London ON N6G 5J8; Lima (Peru)'74; FAAP; FAAAI; FRCPC; Peds (Clinical Immunology & Allergy). Assoc Staff, St Joseph's Care Group - St Joseph's Hospital; Assoc Staff, Thunder Bay Regional Health Sciences Centre; Assoc Staff, Kingston General Hospital; Lecturer/Assoc Prof, Queen's University; Langs: Spanish; allergy101@gmail.com.

BELDA, Patricia; 1110 4th Ave, Prince George BC V2L 3J3; McM'05; CCFP; (250)564-4422

BELDAVS, Robert A; Medical Arts Bldg, 1206-233 Kennedy St, Winnipeg MB R3C 3J5; Wes'87; DAB; FRCSC; Ophth (Anterior Segment). Ac Staff, Misericordia Health Centre; Ac Staff, Health Sciences Centre; Physician, Lasik MD; Physician, Western Surgery Centre; Asst Prof, University of Manitoba; Langs: English; French; (204)944-1628; Fax. (204)944-1629.

BELDER, Diana; University of Ottawa, 2044-451 Smyth Rd, Ottawa ON K1H 8M5; Ott'07; Peds.

BELEC, Daniel; Medecin-Psychiatrie Autonome, 310-50 rue Barnett, Dollard-D-Ormeaux QC H9G 3C7; Mon'71; Psy (P.Q.). (514)675-1085

BELEFQIH, Mounia; Clinique Med Chemin Saint-Jean, 675 ch Saint-Jean, La Prairie QC J5R 2L2; (450)444-2002

BELEJ-RAK, Timea; Procrea Fertility Centre, 955 Major Mackenzie Dr W, Vaughan ON L6A 4P9; Tor'99; BSc; MSc; FRCSC; ObstGyn (Infertility). Langs: Czech; Hungarian; Slovak; (289)357-0100; Fax. (289)357-0101.

BELEN, Jaime O; 28 James St PO Box 459, Inverness NS B0E 1N0; Santo Tomas (Philippines)'62; FRCSC; GenSurg. Staff, Inverness Consolidated Memorial Hospital; (902)258-2839; Fax. (902)258-3760.

BELENKIE, Israel; Faculty Of Med, 3280 Hospital Dr NW, Calgary AB T2N 4Z6; McG'67; FRCPC; IntMed; Cardiol. Staff, Foothills Medical Centre; Prof Med, University of Calgary; (403)220-4525; Fax. (403)210-9739; belenkie@ucalgary.ca.

BELENKY, Michael; Office of the Chief Med Examin, 4070 Bowness Rd NW, Calgary AB T3B 3R7; (Russia (Federation))'90; (403)297-8123; Fax. (403)297-3429.

BELFON, Ahmad E; Bowmanville Prof Bldg, 2101-222 King St E, Bowmanville ON L1C 1P6; Tor'04; (905)697-3607; Fax. (905)697-3645.

BELGARDT, Gerald R; Casey Med Clinic, 320 2nd Ave W, Prince Rupert BC V8J 1G6; Alb'89; Staff, Prince Rupert Regional Hospital; (250)624-4114

BELGASEM, Muftah A; Centric Health Cenior Centre, B-413 Linwell Rd, St. Catharines ON L2M 7Y2; Al Fateh (Libya)'98; CCFP; (905)938-3533; Fax. (905)938-8318.

BELGASEM, Nizar; Carbonear Gen Hosp, 86 Highroad S, Carbonear NL A1Y 1A4; (Libya)'03; Locum Tenens, Carbonear General Hospital; (709)945-5111

BELHACHMI, Samuel S; CHUM-Hop Notre-Dame, 1560 rue Sherbrooke E, Montreal QC H2L 4M1; Laval'99; Staff, Centre Hospitalier l'Université de Montréal (CHUM) - Hôpital Notre-Dame; (514)890-8000 x24592

BELHAJ, Abdelbaset; Rouge Valley-Centenary HC, 2867 Ellesmere Rd, Scarborough ON M1E 4B9; Al Fateh (Libya)'98; FRCPC; MedMicrobiol. Staff, Rouge Valley Health System - Centenary Health Centre Site; (416)284-3118; Fax. (416)281-7394.

BELHUMEUR, Celine; Hôpital Ste-Justine, 3175 ch Cote-Sainte-Catherine, Montreal QC H3T 1C5; Laval'87; FAAP; FRCPC; Peds (Developmental Pediatrics). Staff Developmental Ped, Hôpital Ste-Justine; (514)345-4789; Fax. (514)345-2321.

BELHUMEUR, Francois; Clinique Med Loretteville, 250-11000 boul de L'Ormiere, Quebec QC G2B 5S1; Sher'84; AB; FACOG; FRCSC; ObstGyn. Assoc Staff, Centre Hospitalier Chauveau; Assoc Staff, Centre Hospitalier Universitaire De Québec - Pavillon De St-françois-d'assise; (418)842-8419; Fax. (418)842-3246.

BELHUMEUR, Jacinthe S V; CSSS de Laval, 1755 boul Rene-Laennec, Laval QC H7M 3L9; Sher'04; FRCSC; GenSurg. Staff, Hopital de la Cite de la santé; (450)668-1010

BELHUMEUR, Marc; Ctr Hosp Affilie-Enfant-Jesus, 1401 18e rue, Quebec QC G1J 1Z4; Laval'89; FRCPC; EmergMed. Staff, Centre Hospitalier Affilié Universitaire de Québec - Hôpital De L'Enfant Jésus; (418)649-5632

BELIK, Jaques; The Hosp For Sick Children, 555 University Ave, Toronto ON M5G 1X8; Sao Paulo (Brazil)'76; ABPeds; FRCPC; Peds (Neonatology). Staff, The Hospital For Sick Children; Prof Peds, University of Toronto; (416)813-2165; Fax. (416)813-5771; jaques.belik@sickkids.ca.

BELISLE, Annie; CHUM-Hop Notre-Dame, 1560 rue Sherbrooke E, Montreal QC H2L 4M1; Mon'98; CSPQ; FRCPC; AnatPath. Pathologiste, Centre Hospitalier l'Université de Montréal (CHUM) - Hôpital Notre-Dame; (514)890-8000 x27054

BELISLE, Christian; Clinique Medicym, 205-876 boul du Cure-Labelle, Blainville QC J7C 2K9; Sher'86; Staff, Hôtel-Dieu de Saint-Jérôme; (450)430-0911

BELISLE, Damien; CSSS de Chicoutimi, 305 rue Saint-Vallier, Chicoutimi QC G7H 5H6; Mon'01; FRCPC; IntMed; Nephrol. Staff Nephrol, Complexe hospitalier de la Sagamie; Langs: Bilingual(French/English); (418)541-1000; Fax. (418)541-1197.

BELISLE, Denise; Le Mediclub, 201-6100 av Du Boise, Montreal QC H3S 2W1; Sher'78; Médecin, Le Medi-Club du Sanctuaire; Langs: Spanish; English; (514)739-5646; Fax. (514)739-6773; denise_belisle@rrsss16.gouv.qc.ca.

BELISLE, Dominique; Douglas Mental Hlth Univ Inst, 6875 boul Lasalle, Verdun QC H4H 1R3; Laval'03; FRCPC; Psy. Staff, Douglas Mental Health University Institute; (514)761-6131

BELISLE, Gilles-Michel; Lakeshore Gen Hosp, 160 av Stillview, Pointe-Claire QC H9R 2Y2; Sher'78; FRCSC; Otol. Staff, Lakeshore General Hospital - Pointe Claire; (514)630-2225

BELISLE, Julie; Clinique Med Saint-Eugene, 397 rue Jacques-Cartier S, St-Jean-sur-Richel QC J3B 7T1; Mon'05; CCFP; (450)347-3748

BELISLE, Marie-Claude; Hop Ste-Justine, 3175 ch Cote-Sainte-Catherine, Montreal QC H3T 1C5; Mon'88; FRCPC; Psy. Staff, Hôpital Ste-Justine; Staff, Centre Hospitalier l'Université de Montréal (CHUM) - Hôpital Notre-Dame; (514)345-3931 x5594; Fax. (514)345-4679.

BELISLE, Melanie; Medical Arts Centre, 30-650 Terminal Ave, Nanaimo BC V9R 5E2; McG'06; MDCM; CCFP; CCFP(E.M.); Staff, Nanaimo Regional General Hospital; (250)753-3431

BELISLE, Pierre; Clinique Medicale l'Achigan, 26 montee Remi-Henri, St-Roch-D'Ach QC J0K 3H0; Mon'77; Langs: Bilingual(French/English); (450)588-4321; Fax. (450)588-7466.

BELISLE, Roselyne; CSSS du Nord de Lanaudière, 1000 boul Sainte-Anne, St-Charles-Brromee QC J6E 6J2; Laval'08; CCFP; Staff, Centre Hospitalier Régional de Lanaudière; (450)759-8222

BELISLE, Serge; 100-235 boul René-Lévesque E, Montreal QC H2X 1N8; Sher'71; MSc; FRCSC; ObstGyn. Chef obst & gynécol, Centre Hospitalier l'Université De Montréal (CHUM) - Hôpital Saint-luc; VP, Surgery & Member of Council, Div. of Surg. -RCPSC; (514)866-2446; Fax. (514)866-4013.

BELISLE, Sylvain J; Institut de Cardiologie de Mtl, 5000 rue Belanger, Montreal QC H1T 1C8; Mon'82; CSPQ; FRCPC; Anes; Critical Care Medicine (P.Q.). Ac Staff, Institut de Cardiologie de Montréal; (514)376-3330; Fax. (514)376-8784.

BELISLE JR., Pierre; CSSS de Chicoutimi, 305 rue Saint-Vallier, Chicoutimi QC G7H 5H6; Sher'91; CSPQ; FRCPC; IntMed; Cardiol. Staff Cardiol, Complexe hospitalier de la Sagamie; (418)541-1000

BELIVEAU, Caroline A; ONE Fertility Clinic, 3210 Harvester Rd, Burlington ON L7N 3T1; Mem'94; FRCSC; ObstGyn. Langs: Bilingual(English/French); (905)634-4440

BELIVEAU, Claire; Hop Maisonneuve-Rosemont, 5415 boul de l'Assomption, Montreal QC H1T 2M4; Mon'80; FRCPC; MedMicrobiol. Staff, Hopital Maisonneuve-Rosemont; (514)252-3400 x4524; Fax. (514)252-3898.

BELIVEAU, Genevieve; Centre Med Boucherville, 201-600 boul du Fort-Saint-Lou, Boucherville QC J4B 1S7; Sher'01; Staff, Centre Hospitalier Pierre Boucher; Physician, Centre Medicale Boucheville; Langs: Bilingual(French/English); (450)655-7321; Fax. (450)655-6311.

BELIVEAU, James F; Frontenac Med Associates, 201-791 Princess St, Kingston ON K7L 1E9; McG'78; BSc(Hon.Biol); CCFP; FCFP; Ac Staff, Hotel-Dieu Hospital; Ac Staff, Kingston General Hospital; Langs: English; French; (613)544-2727; Fax. (613)544-7247.

BELIVEAU, Johanne A; 230-2944 boul Taschereau, Greenfield Park QC J4V 2G8; Laval'75; (450)672-3220; Fax. (450)465-1016.

BELIVEAU, Lionel; Centre Med Rene Laennec, 205-1100 av Beaumont, Mont-Royal QC H3P 3H5; Mon'60; Psy (P.Q.). Langs: English; (514)735-9810; Fax. (514)735-7924.

BELIVEAU, Melanie; CLSC de Sherbrooke, 1200 rue King E, Sherbrooke QC J1G 1E4; Sher'00; CCFP; (819)563-2572 x3378; Fax. (819)563-9912.

BELIVEAU, Patrick; CHUQ-Hotel-Dieu de Quebec, 11 Cote du Palais, Quebec QC G1R 2J6; Mon'98; CSPQ; FRCPC; IntMed; Cardiol. Staff, Centre Hospitalier Universitaire de Québec (CHUQ) - Siege Social; (418)525-4444

BELIVEAU, Peter I; Victoria Emerg Phys Mgmt Ltd, 325-1627 Fort St, Victoria BC V8R 1H8; McG'73; FRCPC; EmergMed. (250)479-1442; Fax. (250)479-1472.

BELIVEAU, Pierre; Centre de Physiatrie de Quebec, 100-700 boul Lebourgneuf, Quebec QC G2J 1E2; Laval'65; FRCPC; PhysMed&Rehab., Université Laval; Langs: Bilingual(French/English); (418)622-3371; Fax. (418)622-9004; pierrebeliveau@sympatico.ca.

BELIVEAU, Pierre; CSSS Les Eskers de l'Abitibi, 622 4e rue O, Amos QC J9T 2S2; Laval'92; Staff, CH Hôtel-Dieu d'Amos; (819)732-3341; Fax. (819)732-4646.

BELIVEAU, Robert; 5055 rue Saint-Zotique E, Montreal QC H1T 1N6; Mon'76; Staff, Institut de Cardiologie de Montréal; Langs: Bilingual(English/French); (514)374-1480 x292; meditpc@gmail.com.

BELIVEAU, Samuel; CSSS de Beauce-Etchemin, 1515 17e rue, Saint-Georges QC G5Y 4T8; Laval'05; IntMed (Pneumology). Staff Internist, Centre Hospitalier Beauce-Etchemin; Langs: Bilingual(French/English); (418)228-2031

BELIVEAU, Serge; CSSS du Haut St-Francois, 40 rue Dumoulin, La Patrie QC J0B 1Y0; Sher'75; (819)888-2811; Fax. (819)888-2489.

BELIVEAU, Sylvie; CHUQ-Ctr Hosp Univ Laval, 2705 boul Laurier, Quebec QC G1V 4G2; Sher'91; FRCPC; Peds. Staff Peds, Centre Hospitalier Universitaire de Quebec-CHUL; (418)654-2282; sylvie.beliveau@mail.chuq.qc.ca.

BELIVEAU, Vanessa; CLSC Lamater, 1317 boul des Seigneurs, Terrebonne QC J6W 5B1; Laval'98; (450)471-2881 x4056

BELIZAIRE-DA COSTA, Lise; CHSLD Biermans-Tri Est, 4900 boul Lapointe, Montreal QC H1K 4W9; Louvain (Belgium)'72; Staff, Hôpital Santa Cabrini Ospedale; (514)353-1227 x5176

BELKADI, Ahmed Z; CSSS du Nord de Lanaudière, 1000 boul Sainte-Anne, St-Charles-Brromee QC J6E 6J2; (Algeria)'93; Staff, Centre Hospitalier Régional de Lanaudière; (450)759-8222

BELKHEIR, Kamel; Pavillon Rosemont, 5689 rue Rosement, Montreal QC H1T 2H1; (Algeria)'82; FRCPC; Psy. Staff, Hôtel-Dieu de Sorel; (514)252-3400

BELKHOUS, Nacera; SMBD Jewish Gen Hosp, 3755 ch Cote-Sainte-Catherine, Montreal QC H3T 1E2; (Algeria)'82; CCFP; Staff, Sir Mortimer B Davis Jewish General; (514)340-8222 x4427

BELL, Alan; Keele Med Place, 2830 Keele St, North York ON M3M 3E5; Tor'80; CCFP; Staff, Humber River Regional Hospital - Finch Avenue Site; Asst Prof Family & Commun Med, University of Toronto; (416)633-6812; Fax. (416)633-6187.

BELL, Allan C; Quinte HC Corp-Belleville Gen, 265 Dundas St E, Belleville ON K8N 5A9; Tor'06; CCFP; CCFP(E.M.); Staff, QHC Belleville General; (613)969-7400

BELL, Amanda L; Medical Associates, 97 Charlotte St, Port Colborne ON L3K 3E2; McM'98; BSc(Arts); CCFP; FCFP; Ac Staff, Niagara Health System - Port Colborne General Site; Clin Assoc Prof, McMaster University; (905)834-4546; Fax. (905)834-3114.

BELL, B Curtis; 2539 7 Ave NW, Calgary AB T2N 1A5; Loma Linda(CA) (USA)'74; CCFP; FCFP; Ac Staff, Alberta Children's Hospital; Ac Staff, Foothills Medical Centre; Pt-Time Ass't. Prof., University of Calgary; (403)681-5632; bcbell@cvfp.com.

BELL, Barbara A; 115 Main St PO Box 260, Guysborough NS B0H 1N0; McM'87; BSc; CCFP; FCFP; Staff, Guysborough Memorial Hospital; (902)533-4040; Fax. (902)533-2040.

BELL, Benjamin R; North York Gen Hosp, 4001 Leslie St, North York ON M2K 1E1; Tor'08; FRCPC; IntMed. Staff, North York General Hospital; (416)756-6577

BELL, Bradley D; 202-180 Mccarter St PO Box 1540 Stn Main, Parksville BC V9P 2H4; UBC'89; Assoc Staff, Nanaimo Regional General Hospital; (250)954-1499; Fax. (250)954-1479.

BELL, Brian D; St Mary's Gen Hosp, 911 Queen's Blvd, Kitchener ON N2M 1B2; Wes'95; CCFP; CCFP(E.M.); Staff, St Mary's General Hospital; (519)744-3311

BELL, Caroline; CSSS de l'Energie-Ste-Therese, 1705 av Georges, Shawinigan QC G9N 2N1; Laval'01; FRCPC; Psy. Staff, CH du Centre-de-la-Mauricie (Ste-Thérèse de Shawinigan); Langs: Bilingual(French/English); (819)536-7500; caroline_bell@ssss.gouv.qc.ca.

BELL, Cecil D; St Michael's Hosp, 30 Bond St, Toronto ON M5B 1W8; Tor'64; AnatPath. Staff, St Michael's Hospital; (416)864-6060

BELL, Charles M; Mount Sinai Hosp, 433-600 University Ave, Toronto ON M5G 1X5; Tor'94; FRCPC; IntMed. Staff, Mount Sinai Hospital; (416)586-4800

BELL, Clifford D; Royal University Hosp, 103 Hospital Dr, Saskatoon SK S7N 0W8; Sask'85; CCFP; Staff, Royal University Hospital; (306)655-2371; Fax. (306)655-2370.

BELL, Courtney J; Guelph Family Health Team, 305-85 Norfolk St, Guelph ON N1H 4J4; McM'07; CCFP; (519)766-1490; cbell@gbhs.on.ca.

BELL, David D; Grey Bruce HS-Owen Sound, PO Box 1800 Stn Main 1800 8th St E, Owen Sound ON N4K 6M9; Tor'74; FRCPC; Anes. Staff Anes, Grey Bruce Health Services - Owen Sound; (519)376-2121

BELL, David E; 200-3994 Shelbourne St, Victoria BC V8N 3E2; Alb'75; CCFP; FCFP; Ac Staff, Victoria General Hospital; (250)477-7100; Fax. (250)477-4135.

BELL, David G; Urology Consultants, 620-5991 Spring Garden Rd, Halifax NS B3H 1Y6; Dal'84; FRCSC; Urol (Oncology). Att Staff, Queen Elizabeth II Health Sciences Centre - Victoria General Site; Consultant Staff, Cancer Treatment & Research Foundation of Nova Scotia; Prof/Head Urol, Dalhousie University; (902)425-3940; Fax. (902)422-0033.

BELL, David W; Perth Med Clinic, 1-500 East Riverside Dr, Perth-Andover NB E7H 1Z1; Tor'90; CCFP; FCFP; (506)273-9525; Fax. (506)273-9560.

BELL, Dean D; Health Sciences Centre, 820 Sherbrook St, Winnipeg MB R3A 1R9; Alb'84; FRCPC; Anes (Critical Care Medicine). Dir SICU, St Boniface General Hospital; Att Staff Anes, Health Sciences Centre; Asst Prof Anes/Att Physician ICU, University of Manitoba; (204)787-3112; Fax. (204)787-3069.

BELL, Douglas; Canadian Med Protective Assn, PO Box 8225 Stn T CSC 875 Carling Ave, Ottawa ON K1G 3H7; Qns'80; FRCSC; ObstGyn. Court Staff, The Ottawa Hospital - General Campus; University of Ottawa; (613)725-2000; Fax. (613)725-1300.

BELL, Georgina L; Portland Hotel Society, 20 Hastings St W, Vancouver BC V6B 1G6; Kingstown (Saint Lucia)'06; CCFP; Staff, Portland Hotel Society; (604)683-0073; Fax. (604)683-6286.

BELL, Helen F; 1019 Prince St, Truro NS B2N 1H7; Dal'78; BSc; MBA; Chief FamilyMed, Colchester East Hants Health Centre; (902)895-3501; Fax. (902)895-3502.

BELL, Ian R; Medical Sciences Bldg, 204-603 Davis Dr, Newmarket ON L3Y 2P7; Tor'85; Ac Staff, Southlake Regional Health Centre; (905)895-7447; Fax. (905)895-0119.

BELL, Jeffrey H; Medical Bldg, 1101-805 Broadway W, Vancouver BC V5Z 1K1; Sask'82; CCFP; Ac Staff, Vancouver General Hospital - Centennial Pavillion; Vis Staff, BC Women's Hospital & Health Centre; Asst Prof, University of British Columbia; (604)879-5271; Fax. (604)879-8712.

BELL, Kathleen E; Foothills Med Centre, 1403 29 St NW, Calgary AB T2N 2T9; (Ireland)'80; MB ChB; BAO; FRCR; Staff, Foothills Medical Centre; Clinical Asst Prof, University of Calgary; (403)944-1969

BELL, Kathryn A; Vancouver Gen Hosp, CP 5C-855 12 Ave W, Vancouver BC V5Z 1M9; UBC'87; FRCPC; IntMed; GeriatricMed. Staff STAT Centre, Vancouver General Hospital - Centennial Pavillion; (604)875-4414

BELL, Laura P; Southwood Med Clinic, 1700-2751 Cliffe Ave, Courtenay BC V9N 2L8; UBC'86; BSc; CCFP; FCFP; Med Staff, St Joseph's General Hospital; Langs: French; (250)334-2212; Fax. (250)334-2213.

BELL, Leslie W; PO Box 96, Fillmore SK S0G 1N0; Liverpool (England)'66; (306)722-3806; Fax. (306)722-3877.

BELL, Lisa; Flemington Health Centre, 10 Gateway Blvd, North York ON M3C 3A1; Tor'07; CCFP; Staff, Toronto East General Hospital Inc; (416)429-4991; Fax. (416)422-3573.

BELL, Lorraine E; MUHC-Montreal Children's Hosp, E222-2300 rue Tupper, Montreal QC H3H 1P3; McG'76; FAAP; FRFPS; FRCPC; Peds (P.Q.); Nephrol (P.Q.). Dir Div of Nephrol, McGill University Health Centre - Montreal Children's Hospital; assoc Prof, McGill University; Langs: French; (514)412-4461; Fax. (514)412-4359; lorraine.bell@muhc.mcgill.ca.

BELL, Marilynne L; The Duffus Health Centre, 208-7071 Bayers Rd, Halifax NS B3L 2C2; McM'77; BHSc; MSc; CCFP; FCFP; Court Staff, Queen Elizabeth II Health Sciences Centre - Halifax Infirmary Site; Court Staff, IWK Health Centre; Asst Prof, Dalhousie University; (902)453-4585; Fax. (902)453-5657; docmbell@eastlink.ca.

BELL, Mary J; Sunnybrook Hlth Sciences Ctre, M1 401-2075 Bayview Ave, Toronto ON M4N 3M5; McM'79; MSc(ClinEpi&Biostats); FRCPC; IntMed; Rheum. Staff, Sunnybrook Health Sciences Centre; (416)480-4580; Fax. (416)480-4233.

BELL, Neil R; Misericordia Community Hosp, C-16940 87 Ave NW, Edmonton AB T5R 4H5; Alb'78; CCFP; FCFP; Ac Staff, Covenant Health - Misericordia Community Hospital; Prof, University of Alberta; (780)735-2800; Fax. (780)735-2857.

BELL, Patricia; UMF Pavillon Rosemont, 5689 boul Rosemont, Montreal QC H1T 2H1; Mon'04; CCFP; Staff Preventive Med, Institut de Cardiologie de Montréal; Staff, Hopital Maisonneuve-Rosemont; (514)252-3814

BELL, Peter E; Family Medical Centre, 10240 Kingsway NW, Edmonton AB T5H 3V9; Alb'06; CCFP; (780)735-4201; Fax. (780)735-4978.

BELL, Peter W; Sharbot Lake Med Centre, PO Box 70 1005 Medical Centre Rd, Sharbot Lake ON K0H 2P0; Wes'68; CCFP; Asst Prof Pt-Time Family Med, Queen's University; (613)279-2100; Fax. (613)279-2872; slmc@frontenac.net.

BELL, Raymond A; Medical-Dental Bldg, 402-1120 Yates St, Victoria BC V8V 3M9; Qns'70; FRCSC; Ophth. (250)386-1451; Fax. (250)386-1459.

BELL, Robert B; Dept of Clin Neurosciences, 3330 Hospital Dr NW, Calgary AB T2N 4N1; Alb'80; FRCPC; Neur (Neuro Immunology). Staff Multiple Sclerosis Clinic, Foothills Medical Centre; Assoc Prof, University of Calgary; (403)944-4253; Fax. (403)283-4841.

BELL, Robert C; The Ottawa Hosp-Riverside, 41408-1967 Riverside Dr, Ottawa ON K1H 7W9; Alb'81; FRCPC; IntMed; Nephrol. Staff, The Ottawa Hospital - Riverside Campus; Assoc Prof, University of Ottawa; (613)738-8400 x82565; Fax. (613)738-8337.

BELL, Robert S; Univ Hlth Network-Princess M, 610 University Ave, Toronto ON M5G 2M9; McG'75; FRCSC; OrthSurg (Orthopedic Oncology). Pres/CEO, University Health Network; Staff, Princess Margaret Hospital - University Health Network; Ac Staff, Mount Sinai Hospital; Prof Surg, University of Toronto; (416)340-4686; Fax. (416)340-4837.

BELL, Roger R; Hamilton HS-General Site, 237 Barton St E, Hamilton ON L8L 2X2; Aberdeen (Scotland)'72; MB ChB; DA; FRCPC; Anes. Staff, Hamilton Health Sciences Centre - Hamilton General Hospital; (905)527-0271

BELL, Ruth E; Northfield Med Centre, 206-99 Northfield Dr E, Waterloo ON N2K 3P9; McM'75; (519)744-2592; Fax. (519)744-1197.

BELL, Scott C; St Paul's Hosp, 1081 Burrard St, Vancouver BC V6Z 1Y6; Dal'89; FRCPC; Anes. Staff, Providence Health Care - St Paul's Hospital; (604)806-8337

BELL, Stephen J; South Macleod Family Med, 100-15915 Macleod Trail SE, Calgary AB T2Y 3R9; Alb'87; CCFP; FCFP; (403)457-2457; Fax. (403)457-2458.

BELL, Stuart D; Rouge Valley-Centenary HC, 2867 Ellesmere Rd, Scarborough ON M1E 4B9; London (England)'85; MSc; FRCPC; DiagRad (Angiography). Staff, Rouge Valley Health System - Centenary Health Centre Site; (416)284-8131 x4134

BELL, Susan D; Caronport Med Clinic, PO Box 998, Caronport SK S0H 0S0; Sask'91; CCFP; Ac Staff, Moose Jaw Union Hospital; Assoc Staff, Providence Place; (306)756-2262; Fax. (306)756-2282; caronportmedicalclinic@live.ca.

BELL, Thomas A B; Toronto Inst. of Plastic Surg, 2F-199 Avenue Rd, Toronto ON M5R 2J3; Sask'79; FRCSC; PlasSurg (Cosmetic Surgery). Assoc Staff, Toronto General Hospital - UHN; Court Staff, The Scarborough Hospital - Birchmount Campus; Physician, The Toronto Inst. of Aesthetic Plastic Surg.; (416)961-9828; Fax. (416)961-5553; thomas.bell@drthomasbell.com.

BELL, Thomas W G; Chemong Med Centre FHT, PO Box 330 765 Ward St, Bridgenorth ON K0L 1H0; Wes'73; CCFP; FCFP; Court Staff, Peterborough Regional Health Centre - Hospital Drive; Teacher Family Med/Preceptor Rural Ontario Med Program, Queen's University; (705)292-0905; Fax. (705)292-8929; boots_bell@hotmail.com.

BELL, Tim G; Appletree Med Group, 2575B Baseline Rd, Ottawa ON K2H 7B3; Ott'87; (613)726-3558 x26; Fax. (613)726-3560.

BELL, Timothy H; B-1729 Comox Ave, Comox BC V9M 3M2; Tor'05; FRCSC; OrthSurg. (250)941-0080

BELL, Warren R; PO Box 3458 Stn Main, Salmon Arm BC V1E 4S2; McG'74; CCFP; FCFP; Staff, Shuswap Lake General Hospital; Langs: Bilingual(English/French); (250)832-7121; Fax. (250)832-7716; cppbell@web.net.

BELL-DINGWALL, Sarah; 2F-303 9 Ave SW, High River AB T1V 0H2; Wes'09; CCFP; Staff, High River General Hospital; (403)652-2929

BELL-IRVING, Kathleen A; 3034 Edgemont Blvd PO Box 75557 Rpo Edgemont Vill, North Vancouver BC V7R 4X1; Dal'83; CCFP; Ac Staff, Lions Gate Hospital; Clin Instructor Commun & Family Med, University of British Columbia; (604)929-7790; Fax. (604)608-9011.

BELLA, Anthony J; The Ottawa Hosp-Civic Campus, 1053 Carling Ave, Ottawa ON K1Y 4E9; McM'99; FRCSC; Urol. Assoc Scientist, The Ottawa Hospital - Civic Campus; (613)798-5555 x15073; abella@ohri.ca.

BELLA-LUFU, Mbuyamba; Wolseley Med Clinic, PO Box 488, Wolseley SK S0G 5H0; (Congo (Democratic Republic))'87; MB ChB; (306)698-2524; Fax. (306)698-2977; docdebella@hotmail.com.

BELLACK, Allan G; ISP-Social Development Canada, 5A-333 North River Rd, Ottawa ON K1A 0L1; Tor'71; CCFP; FCFP; Med Advisor, Canada Pension Plan; (613)941-0773; Fax. (613)952-8466; allan.bellack@hrsdc-rhdcc.gc.ca.

BELLAIRE, Jacqueline D; South East Toronto FHT, 1871 Danforth Ave, Toronto ON M4C 1J3; Wes'04; CCFP; (416)699-7775

BELLAIRE, Joan; Smithville Family Health Ctre, PO Box 218 230 Canboro St, Smithville ON L0R 2A0; McM'93; CCFP; FCFP; Staff, West Lincoln Memorial Hospital; Clin Associate Prof(Pt-Time), McMaster University; (905)957-3328; Fax. (905)957-2475; jbellaire@cogeco.ca.

BELLAMY, Christopher D; St Joseph's Gen Hosp, 2137 Comox Ave, Comox BC V9M 1P2; London (England)'71; MB BS; BSc(Pharm); MRC(UK); FRCPC; GenPath (Laboratory Medicine); AnatPath. Staff, St Joseph's General Hospital; (250)339-1455

BELLAMY, Danielle; CSSS Haute-Yamaska, 71 rue Court, Granby QC J2G 4Y7; Laval'82; LMCC; (450)776-5222

BELLAMY, Deanna D; 15-9701 84 Ave, Grande Prairie AB T8V 4Z8; Mem'06; CCFP; (780)539-1193; Fax. (780)532-0037.

BELLAN, Lorne D; Misericordia Health Centre, 271-99 Cornish Ave, Winnipeg MB R3C 1A2; Man'81; FRCSC; Ophth (Oculo Plastic Surgery). Staff, Misericordia Health Centre; Dept Head Ophth, University of Manitoba; (204)788-8563; Fax. (204)786-0978.

BELLAND, Liane M; Bridgeland Prof Centre, 305-1010 1 Ave NE, Calgary AB T2E 7W7; McM'96; BSc(Hons); MSc(MolecularVirology); FRCSC; ObstGyn (Minimal Invasive Surgery). Staff ObstGyn, Peter Lougheed Centre; Clinical Asst Prof ObstGyn Fac of Med, University of Calgary; Langs: Bilingual(English/French); (403)266-3030

BELLAS, Jonathon S; Health Sciences Centre, GG441-820 Sherbrook St, Winnipeg MB R3A 1R9; Man'03; FRCPC; IntMed. Staff, Health Sciences Centre.

BELLAVANCE, Charles; ASSS des Laurentides, 210-1000 rue Labelle, Saint-Jerome QC J7Z 5N6; Laval'71; (450)432-8700 x2326

BELLAVANCE, Colette; CHUS-Hop Fleurimont, 3001 12e Av N, Sherbrooke QC J1H 5N4; Sher'91; FRCPC; EmergMed. Staff, Centre Hospitalier Universitaire de Sherbrooke-Hopital Fleurimont; (819)346-1110; Fax. (819)820-6420.

BELLAVANCE, Ethel; Clinique Med Notre-Dame Inc, 147 rue Notre-Dame E, Victoriaville QC G6P 3Z8; Laval'94; Staff, Hotel-Dieu d'Arthabaska; Langs: Bilingual(French/English); (819)758-3664; Fax. (819)758-0745.

BELLAVANCE, Gilles B; Clinique Med Le Gardeurois, 155 rue Notre-Dame, Repentigny QC J5Z 3C4; Laval'86; Urol. (450)582-5551

BELLAVANCE, Louise; CLSC-CHSLD Rimouski-Neigette, 165 rue des Gouverneurs, Rimouski QC G5L 7R2; Laval'89; (418)727-5476; Fax. (418)727-5479.

BELLAVANCE, Marc; CHUS-Hop Fleurimont, 3001 12e Av N, Sherbrooke QC J1H 5N4; Laval'94; CSPQ; FRCPC; Peds; Cardiol. Staff, Centre Hospitalier Universitaire de Sherbrooke-Hopital Fleurimont; assoc Prof, Universite de Sherbrooke; (819)346-1110

BELLAZZI, Myriam; Clinique Med L'Or Et Des Bois, 1281 7e rue, Val-d'Or QC J9P 3S1; Mon'01; Staff, Centre Hospitalier de Val d'Or; (819)825-2222; Fax. (819)825-3333; mariazzi@yahoo.fr.

BELLE, Ralph M; 106-3825 Sunset St, Burnaby BC V5G 1T4; Wes'84; FRCSC; OrthSurg (Foot & Ankle Surgery). Staff, Burnaby Hospital; (604)437-9600; Fax. (604)437-9606.

BELLE-ISLE, Jasmin; Clinique Med Val-Belair, 202-1147 boul Pie Xi N, Quebec QC G3K 2P8; Sher'85; (418)843-2473

BELLE-ISLE, Pierre; Clinique de Med Familiale, 1971 rue Bilodeau, Plessisville QC G6L 3J1; Laval'75; Langs: English; (819)362-6337; Fax. (819)362-9147; montstan@videotron.ca.

BELLEAU, Luc; CHUM-Hop Notre-Dame, 1560 rue Sherbrooke E, Montreal QC H2L 4M1; Mon'89; Staff, Centre Hospitalier l'Université de Montréal (CHUM) - Hôpital Notre-Dame; (514)890-8000 x28011

BELLEAU-NANTEL, Jean F; Ctr de Sante du Val-St-Francoi, 23 rue Ambroise-Dearden, Windsor QC J1S 1G8; Laval'99; (819)542-2777

BELLEFEUILLE, Jacques-P.; 5555 rue Belanger, Montreal QC H1T 1G2; Mon'74; FRCPC; Derm. (514)256-5011

BELLEFEUILLE, Julie; 300-5307 Canotek Rd, Gloucester ON K1J 9M2; Mon'92; CCFP; FCFP; (613)746-6223; Fax. (613)746-6018.

BELLEFEUILLE, Patrice; Centre Med Fontainebleau, 102-10 boul des Chateaux, Blainville QC J7B 1Z5; Laval'95; Langs: Bilingual(French/English); (450)419-8811; Fax. (450)419-7758.

BELLEFLEUR, Stephanie; CSSS de Chicoutimi, 305 rue Saint-Vallier, Chicoutimi QC G7H 5H6; Sher'01; CCFP; CCFP(E.M.); Staff, Complexe hospitalier de la Sagamie; (418)541-1000

BELLEMARE, Benoit; CSSS de la Haute-Yamaska, 205 boul Leclerc O, Granby QC J2G 1T7; Mon'94; FRCSC; GenSurg. Staff, Centre Hospitalier de Granby; (450)372-5491; Fax. (450)372-7197.

BELLEMARE, France; CSSS du Lac-des-Deux-Montagnes, 520 boul Arthur-Sauve, St-Eustache QC J7R 5B1; Mon'92; Staff, Hôpital de Saint-Eustache; Physician, Centre Medicale St-Laurent; (450)473-6811; Fax. (450)473-6966.

BELLEMARE, Guy; CHUQ-Hotel-Dieu de Quebec, 11 Cote Du Palais, Quebec QC G1R 2J6; Laval'77; FRCSC; ObstGyn (Colposcopy). Dir, Centre Hospitalier Universitaire de Québec (CHUQ) - Siege Social; Staff, Centre Hospitalier Universitaire De Québec - Pavillon De St-françois-d'assise; Langs: Bilingual(French/English); (418)691-5446; Fax. (418)525-4170.

BELLEMARE, Jean-Francois; CHUQ-Hotel-Dieu de Quebec, 11 Cote du Palais, Quebec QC G1R 2J6; Mon'01; Critical Care Medicine (P.Q.); IntMed. Staff, Centre Hospitalier Universitaire de Québec (CHUQ) - Siege Social; (418)691-5151

BELLEMARE, Jean-Francois; Hop du Sacre-Coeur de Mtl, 5400 boul Gouin O, Montreal QC H4J 1C5; Laval'84; FACS; ACLS; DS; ATLS; DGS; FRCS; LMCC; LRCPS; MRCS; TraSurg; CSPQ; AddicMed; FRCSC; GenSurg (Critical Care Medicine). Staff, Hôpital du Sacre-Coeur de Montréal; Clin Prof, Universite de Montreal; Langs: Bilingual(English/French); (514)338-2050; Fax. (514)338-3139; jfbellemare@videotron.ca.

BELLEMARE, Johanne; CSSS du Suroît, 150 rue Saint-Thomas, Salaber-de-Valleyf QC J6T 6C1; Laval'85; FRCPC; Peds. Staff, Centre Hospitalier Régional du Suroît; (450)371-6444 x217; Fax. (450)371-5315.

BELLEMARE, Louis; CSSS Eskers de l'Abitibi, CP 547 622 4e rue O, Amos QC J9T 3A8; Sher'88; FRCSC; OrthSurg (Orthopedics). Assoc Member, Health Sciences North-Laurentian Site; Staff, CH Hôtel-Dieu d'Amos; Pres, Association d'Orthopedie du Quebec; Langs: English; (819)727-9325; orthobell@cableamos.com.

BELLEMARE, Marc; Clinique Medicentre, 5050 boul des Forges, Trois-Rivieres QC G8Y 1X2; Mon'80; FRCSC; ObstGyn (P.Q.). Staff, CSSS de Trois-Rivières; (819)378-1008; Fax. (819)378-5164.

BELLEMARE, Monique; CSSS de la Minganie, CP 190 1035 Prom des Anciens, Havre-Saint-Pierre QC G0G 1P0; Laval'91; Staff, CSSS de la Minganie; (418)538-2212; Fax. (418)538-2254; monique_bellemare@ssss.gouv.qc.ca.

BELLEMARE, Patrick; Hop du Sacre-Coeur de Mtl, 5400 boul Gouin O, Montreal QC H4J 1C5; Mon'93; FRCPC; IntMed; Critical Care Medicine (P.Q.); Respir. Staff, Hôpital du Sacre-Coeur de Montréal; (514)338-2162; Fax. (514)338-3699.

BELLEMARE, Remi; 3090 ch Chambly, Longueuil QC J4L 4N5; Laval'67; DiagRad. (450)646-3520

BELLEMARE, Sarah; CSSS de Memphremagog, 50 rue Saint-Patrice E, Magog QC J1X 3X3; Sher'07; CCFP; Staff, Centre Hospitalier et CLSC de Memphremagog; (819)843-3381; Fax. (819)843-8262.

BELLEMARE, Steven J Y R; Canadian Med Protective Assn, PO Box 8225 Stn T CSC, Ottawa ON K1G 3H7; Ott'00; FRCPC; Peds (Child Maltreatment). Langs: French; (613)725-2000; Fax. (613)725-1300; steven.bellemare@gmail.com.

BELLEMARE, Sylvain; CSSS du Nord de Lanaudière, 1000 boul Sainte-Anne, St-Charles-Brromee QC J6E 6J2; Mon'07; CCFP; Staff, Centre Hospitalier Régional de Lanaudière; (450)759-8222

BELLER, Albert M; 1560 Sylvan Pl, Sidney BC V8L 5L5; UBC'92; (778)426-1815; a.beller@rhcf.on.ca.

BELLEROSE, Sheri A; Royal Alex Place, 223-10106 111 Ave NW, Edmonton AB T5G 0B4; Alb'83; CCFP; (780)474-2223; s.bellerose@shaw.ca.

BELLEROSE-DUMONTIER, Marilyn; CSSS du Nord de Lanaudière, 1000 boul Sainte-Anne, St-Charles-Brromee QC J6E 6J2; Mon'07; CCFP; Staff, Centre Hospitalier Régional de Lanaudière; (450)759-8222

BELLETRUTTI, Mark J; Edmonton Clinic Health Academy, 3 511-11405 87 Ave, Edmonton AB T6G 1C9; Ott'01; FRCPC; Peds (Pediatric Hematology Oncology). Staff, University of Alberta Hospital; Staff, Edmonton Clinic Health Academy; (780)248-5490; Fax. (780)407-8821.

BELLETRUTTI, Paul J; HSC-Faculty of Med, 6D16-3280 Hospital Dr NW, Calgary AB T2N 4Z6; Tor'03; FRCPC; IntMed; Gastroent. (403)592-5089; Fax. (403)592-5090.

BELLEVILLE, Denis; Clinique Med Havre Sante, 521 boul Du Havre, Salaber-de-Valleyf QC J6S 4Z5; Mon'74; (450)371-6444; Fax. (450)371-5315.

BELLEVILLE, Martin; Ctr Hosp Affilie-St-Sacrement, 1050 ch Sainte-Foy, Quebec QC G1S 4L8; Laval'00; FRCPC; DiagRad. Staff, Centre Hospitalier Affilié Universitaire de Québec - Hôpital du St-Sacrement; (418)682-7511 x4970

BELLEY, Emmanuel; CSSS d'Antoine-Labelle-Mt Laur, RR 1 2561 ch de la Lièvre S, Mont-Laurier QC J9L 3G3; Mon'03; CCFP; Fam Med, CSSS d'Antoine-Labelle; Langs: English; (819)623-1234

BELLEY, Genevieve; MUHC-Montreal Gen Hosp, 1650 av Cedar, Montreal QC H3G 1A4; Mon'94; FRCPC; DiagRad. Staff, McGill University Health Centre - Montreal General Campus; (514)934-1934; Fax. (514)934-8263.

BELLEY, Guy; CSSS-Hopital De Hull, 116 boul Lionel-Emond, Gatineau QC J8Y 1W7; Laval'70; FRCPC; DiagRad. Ac Staff, Hull Hospital; (819)966-6000

BELLEY, Jacques; UMF Charles Lemoyne, 100-299 Boul Sir-Wilfrid-Lauri, Longueuil QC J4R 2L1; Mon'64; FRCPC; Peds (P.Q.) (General Pediatrics). Prof Peds, McGill University Health Centre - Montreal Children's Hospital; assoc Prof Pt-Time Ped, McGill University; (450)671-8221; Fax. (450)466-5631.

BELLEY, Marc; Ctr Hosp de Verdun, 4000 boul Lasalle, Verdun QC H4G 2A3; Mon'78; CCFP; Staff, Centre Hospitalier de Verdun; (514)362-1000

BELLEY, Richard J; Hotel-Dieu de Levis, 143 rue Wolfe, Levis QC G6V 3Z1; Laval'92; Staff, Hôtel-Dieu de Lévis; (418)835-7121

BELLEY, Sylvie; 930 rue Jacques-Cartier E, Chicoutimi QC G7H 7K9; Sher'88; Staff, Complexe hospitalier de la Sagamie; (418)545-4990 x414; Fax. (418)545-0835; sylvie.belley@ssss.gouv.qc.ca.

BELLEY-COTE, Emilie-Prudence; Hamilton HS-McMaster Site, PO Box 2000 Stn Lcd 1 1200 Main St W, Hamilton ON L8N 3Z5; Sher'06; Cardiol; IntMed. Staff, Hamilton Health Sciences Centre - McMaster University Medical Centre.

BELLIDO OVIEDO, Roxana; Wemindji Clinic, 10 Air Creebec, Wemindji QC J0M 1L0; Debrecen(Hungary) (Hungary)'00; CCFP; (819)978-0225 x2220; Fax. (819)978-0280.

BELLINASO, John L; Niagara H System-G Niagara, PO Box 1018 Stn Main 5546 Portage Rd, Niagara Falls ON L2E 6X2; Tor'93; FRCPC; Anes. Staff, Niagara Health System - Welland Hospital Site; Staff, Niagara Health System - Greater Niagara General Site; (905)378-4647

BELLINGAN, Jacob C; Osoyoos Medical Centre, PO Box 330 7802 Spartan Dr, Osoyoos BC V0H 1V0; (Other Foreign)'04; MB ChB; Langs: Afrikaans; (250)495-2661

BELLINGHAM, Geoff A; St Joseph's Health Care, PO Box 5777 Stn B A1 609-268 Grosvenor St, London ON N6A 4V2; Wes'03; FRCPC; Anes. Staff, St Joseph's Hospital - St Joseph's Health Care; (519)646-6100 x64218

BELLINI, Andrew B; Brampton Gastroenterology, 11-470 Chrysler Dr, Brampton ON L6S 0C1; Tor'92; FRCPC; IntMed (Hepatology); Gastroent. Staff Gastroent, William Osler Health System - Brampton Civic Hospital; Staff, Brampton Gastroenterology; (905)790-6362; Fax. (905)790-6612.

BELLISSIMO, Agostino M; St Joseph's Health Centre, 30 The Queensway, Toronto ON M6R 1B5; Tor'79; FRCPC; EmergMed;CCFP; CCFP(E.M.); Staff, St Joseph's Health Centre; Asst Prof, McMaster University; Langs: Italian; (416)530-6587; Fax. (416)530-6107; bellia@stjoe.on.ca.

BELLIVEAU, Adele M; 203-82 Tacoma Dr, Dartmouth NS B2W 3E5; Dal'89; BSc; CCFP; Affil Staff Privil OrthSurg, Queen Elizabeth II Health Sciences Centre - Victoria General Site; Physician Occupational Health, Worker's Compensation Board of NS; (902)461-0165; Fax. (902)461-1548.

BELLIVEAU, Anne C; Clinique Medicale de la Baie, 437 rue Albert, La Baie QC G7B 3L5; Mon'08; (418)544-7371; Fax. (418)544-6864.

BELLIVEAU, Daniel J; 353-7105 Chebucto Rd, Halifax NS B3L 4W8; Mon'91; FRCSC; Ophth (Refractive Surgery). Ac Staff Ophth, Queen Elizabeth II Health Sciences Centre - Victoria General Site; Langs: English; French; (902)453-3937; Fax. (902)453-3959; hvc@ns.aliantzinc.ca.

BELLIVEAU, Kevin; CSSS de Laval, 1755 boul Rene-Laennec, Laval QC H7M 3L9; Sher'94; FRCPC; DiagRad. Staff, Hopital de la Cite de la santé; (450)668-1010 x2551

BELLIVEAU, Manon; Family & Primary Care Physicia, 101-1789 ch Mountain, Moncton NB E1G 1A7; Sher'01; CCFP; Langs: Bilingual(French/English); (506)870-2815; Fax. (506)870-2817.

BELLIVEAU, Marc; CSSS de Saint-Jerome, 290 rue de Montigny, Saint-Jerome QC J7Z 5T3; Mon'06; FRCPC; Anes. Staff, Hôtel-Dieu de Saint-Jérôme; (450)432-2777

BELLIVEAU, Paul; Hotel-Dieu Hosp, 482C-166 Brock St, Kingston ON K7L 5G2; McG'74; ABS; FASCRS; FACS; MD; MPA; MS; FRCSC; GenSurg (Colon & Rectal Surgery)., Kingston General Hospital; Ac Member, Hotel-Dieu Hospital; Prof, Queen's University; Langs: Bilingual(French/English); (613)544-3400 x2410; Fax. (613)546-4854.

BELLO, Ahmed B; Prog of Assertive Comm Treatme, 490 Hargrave St, Winnipeg MB R3A 0X7.

BELLO, Aminu; University of Alberta Hosp, 8440 112 St NW, Edmonton AB T6G 2B7; (Nigeria)'98; MB BS; Staff, University of Alberta Hospital; (780)407-8822

BELLO-ESPINOSA, Luis E; Alberta Children's Hosp, 2888 Shaganappi Trail NW, Calgary AB T3B 6A8; (Colombia)'81; Staff, Alberta Children's Hospital; (403)955-2296

BELLON, Marie-Michelle; Ctr Hosp de Lasalle, 8585 Tsse Champlain, Lasalle QC H8P 1C1; Mon'94; FRCPC; IntMed. Staff, Centre Hospitalier de LaSalle; (514)362-8000

BELLONCIK, Yvan; CSSS d'Argenteuil, 145 boul de la Providence, Lachute QC J8H 4C7; Beirut (Lebanon)'67; CSPQ; Anes (P.Q.). Anesthesiste, Centre Hospitalier d'Argenteuil; (450)562-3761

BELLUZZO, Neal; Yorkview Med Centre, 104-3695 Keele St, North York ON M3J 1N2; Tor'99; BSc; CCFP; FCFP; Ac Staff, Humber River Regional Hospital - Finch Avenue Site; (416)633-3711; Fax. (416)633-0521.

BELMILI, Naima A; Bank Medical Centre, 1935 Bank St, Ottawa ON K1V 8A3; (France)'94; CCFP; (613)521-2391; Fax. (613)521-5443.

BELO, Susan E; Sunnybrook Hlth Sciences Ctre, 2075 Bayview Ave, Toronto ON M4N 3M5; Tor'84; FRCPC; Anes. Staff, Sunnybrook Health Sciences Centre; (416)480-4864; Fax. (416)480-6039.

BELOSTOTSKY, Vladimir; McMaster University, 1280 Main St W, Hamilton ON L8S 4K1; (Russia (Federation))'94; (905)521-2100; Fax. (905)308-7548.

BELOTTE, Danielle; Hop Jean-Talon, 1385 rue Jean-Talon E, Montreal QC H2E 1S6; Montpellier (France)'71; Psy (P.Q.) (Hospital Psychiatry). Staff, CSSS du Coeur de l'Isle Hôpital Jean-Talon; (514)495-6767 x6225

BELOVIC, Branislav; Oakville Med Centre, 202-331 Sheddon Ave, Oakville ON L6J 1X8; Komensky (Slovakia)'65; FRCPC; Derm (Dermatology Surgery). Affil Staff, Halton Healthcare Services Corporation - Oakville Site; Langs: Slovak; (905)842-0972; Fax. (905)842-8838.

BELSKY, Nadia M; 3-1278 The Queensway, Etobicoke ON M8Z 1S3; Los Andes (Venezuela)'64; Langs: Spanish; Ukrainian; Russian; Polish; (416)848-9795; Fax. (416)521-7216.

BELTON, Kenneth W; 210-221 Ioco Rd, Port Moody BC V3H 4H2; UBC'88; (604)469-7312; Fax. (604)469-7318.

BELTRAMI, Edouard; CSSS de la Haute-Gaspésie, 50 rue du Belvedere, Ste-Anne-des-Monts QC G4V 1X4; Mon'63; FRCPC; Psy. Staff, Centre Hospitalier des Monts; Prof Montreal Campus, University Of Quebec Mtl; (418)763-7771

BELUSKA, Dora-Lina; Centre Med Sainte-Anne, 113 rue Sainte-Anne, Ste-Anne-de-Bellev QC H9X 1M2; Mon'05; CCFP; Staff, Centre Hospitalier Regional de Sept-Iles; (514)457-2772

BELYAVSKAYA, Svetlana; The Doctor's Office, 800 Steeles Ave W, Thornhill ON L4J 7L2; Moscow (Russia (Federation))'72; PhD; Staff, North York General Hospital - Branson Division; Langs: Russian; (905)738-6699; Fax. (905)738-6073.

BELYEA, Melita; 100-240 Wharncliffe Rd N, London ON N6H 4P2; Tor'99; CCFP; Aj Prof, University of Western Ontario; (519)685-3210; Fax. (519)685-1432.

BELZBERG, Allan S; St Paul's Hosp, 1081 Burrard St, Vancouver BC V6Z 1Y6; Alb'70; ABIM; AB; FRCPC; NuclearMed. Dir, Surrey Memorial Hospital; Dir, Vernon Jubilee Hospital; Dir Dept of Nuclear Med, Providence Health Care - St Paul's Hospital; Assoc Prof, University of British Columbia; (604)806-8077

BELZIL, Jeanne M; Royal Alexandra Hosp, 10240 Kingsway NW, Edmonton AB T5H 3V9; Alb'78; FRCPC; Anes. Ac Staff, Royal Alexandra Hospital; (780)735-4010; Fax. (780)735-4386.

BELZIL, Simon-Pierre; CSSS des Etchemins, 331 rue du Sanatorium RR 1, Lac-Etchemin QC G0R 1S0; Laval'06; CCFP; Staff, CSSS des Etchemins; (418)625-8001

BELZIL, Yves; 596 Rang Saint-Francois, Blainville QC J7E 4H5; Sher'88; CCFP; (450)420-3334; Fax. (450)420-9546; yvesbelzil@videotron.ca.

BELZILE, Catherine; Clinique Med 3000, 3000 rue Belanger, Montreal QC H1Y 1A9; Mon'04; Staff, Hôpital du Sacre-Coeur de Montréal; (514)376-7702

BELZILE, Etienne; CHUQ-Hotel-Dieu de Quebec, 11 Cote Du Palais, Quebec QC G1R 2J6; McG'97; FRCSC; OrthSurg. Staff, Centre Hospitalier Universitaire de Québec (CHUQ) - Siege Social; (418)691-5370; Fax. (418)691-5020.

BELZILE, Francois; CHUS-Hop Fleurimont, 3001 12e Av N, Sherbrooke QC J1H 5N4; Sher'93; FRCPC; DiagRad (Angiography/Interventional). Staff, Centre Hospitalier Universitaire de Sherbrooke-Hopital Fleurimont; (819)346-1110

BELZILE, Gabriel; Clinique Cherrier, 837 rue Cherrier, Montreal QC H2L 1H6; Laval'58; Psy (P.Q.). Staff, Hôpital du Sacre-Coeur de Montréal; Médecin, Clinique Cherrier; Langs: Bilingual(French/English); (514)521-8282; Fax. (514)521-4898.

BELZILE, Gilles; Clinique Med St-Madeleine, 165 boul Sainte-Madeleine, Trois-Rivieres QC G8T 3L7; Laval'68; (819)379-8385

BELZILE, Marie-France; CLSC Rivieres Et Marees, 22 rue Saint-Laurent, Riviere-du-Loup QC G5R 4W5; Laval'81; (418)867-2642; Fax. (418)867-4713.

BELZILE, Mathieu; London HSC-Victoria Hosp, PO Box 5010 Stn B B3 433-800 Commissioners Rd E, London ON N6A 5W9; Laval'04; FRCSC; Otol (Head & Neck Surgery). Staff, London Health Sciences Centre - Victoria Campus; (819)346-1110 x14901

BELZILE, Mireille; Clinique Med St-Louis, 220-3165 ch Saint-Louis, Quebec QC G1W 4R4; Laval'84; (418)658-6970; Fax. (418)658-1654.

BELZILE, Robert; Clinique Sentinelle Sante, 232 boul St-Joseph, Gatineau QC J8Y 3X4; Ott'73; Langs: Bilingual(French/English); (819)778-1330; Fax. (819)778-3455; robert.belzile@videotron.ca.

BELZILE, Sylvain; CHUQ-Ctr Hosp Univ Laval, 2705 boul Laurier, Quebec QC G1V 4G2; Laval'92; FRCSC; OrthSurg. Staff, Centre Hospitalier Universitaire de Quebec-CHUL; (418)656-4141; robelz@sympatico.ca.

BEN ALI, Henda; Polyclinique Med Fabreville, 380 boul Curé-Labelle, Laval QC H7P 5L3; (450)628-5800

BEN AMOR, Hanene; North Renfrew Fam Health Team, RR 1 117 Banting Dr, Deep River ON K0J 1P0; (Other Foreign)'98; CCFP; (613)584-1037; Fax. (613)584-3107.

BEN AMOR, Ibtihel M; Shriners Hosp for Children, 1529 av Cedar, Montreal QC H3G 1A6; (Tunisia)'01; MedGenetics. Staff, Shriners Hospitals For Children - Canada; (514)842-5964

BEN AMOR, Leila; Hotel-Dieu de Levis, 143 rue Wolfe, Levis QC G6V 3Z1; Tunesia (Tunisia)'90; Clin Prof Psy, Hôtel-Dieu de Lévis; Langs: Arabic; English; (418)835-7155; Fax. (418)838-8873; leila_benamor@ssss.gouv.qc.ca.

BEN-ARIE, Oved; Sheppard Associates, 649 Sheppard Ave W, North York ON M3H 2S4; Cape Town (South Africa)'58; MB ChB; DPM; FRCPsy; FRCPC; Psy (General Psychiatry). (416)630-0610; Fax. (416)398-5712; drben@sympatico.ca.

BEN-ARON, Mark H; 655 Main St, Milton ON L9T 5E6; Tor'72; DABPN; BSc; FRCPC; Psy (Forensic Psychiatry).

BEN CHEIKH, Imen; Montfort Hosp, 00B198-713 Montreal Rd, Ottawa ON K1K 0T2; Tunis (Tunisia)'02; FRCPC; Psy. Staff, Montfort Hospital; (613)746-4621; Fax. (613)748-4938.

BEN FADEL, Nadya M; Children's Hosp of Eastern Ont, 401 Smyth Rd, Ottawa ON K1H 8L1; Al-Fateh (Libya)'92; FRCPC; Peds (Neonatal & Perinatal Medicine). Staff, Children's Hospital of Eastern Ontario (CHEO); (613)737-7000

BEN HAMED, Salah R S; Connaigre Peninsula Comm HC, PO Box 70 1 Alexander Ave, Harbour Breton NL A0H 1P0; Staff, Connaigre Peninsula Community Health Centre; (709)885-2359; Fax. (709)885-2012.

BEN-IBRAHIM, Mohamed A; Windsor Health Centre, 209-700 Tecumseh Rd E, Windsor ON N8X 4T2; Al-Fateh (Libya)'87; FRCSC; GenSurg. Staff, Hamilton Health Sciences Centre - Hamilton General Hospital; (519)946-0597

BEN ISSA, Entisar M; 72 Victoria Ave, Chatham ON N7L 3A1; Al-Fateh (Libya)'93; FRCPC; IntMed. (519)397-0790; Fax. (519)397-5535.

BEN JMAA, Wissal; CHUM-Hop St-Luc, 1058 rue Saint-Denis, Montreal QC H2X 3J4; Staff, Centre Hospitalier l'Université De Montréal (CHUM) - Hôpital Saint-luc; (514)890-8000

BEN KHEDHER, Najoua; CSSS du Suroit, 150 rue Saint-Thomas, Salaber-de-Valleyf QC J6T 6C1; (Tunisia)'05; Staff, Centre Hospitalier Régional du Suroît; (450)371-9920

BEN MANSOUR, El Hassan; Stratford Gen Hosp, 46 General Hospital Dr, Stratford ON N5A 2Y6; Paris (France)'97; Staff, Stratford General Hospital - Huron Perth Healthcare Alliance; (519)271-8120

BEN MILUD JALUTHA, Bashir; 5486 Falsbridge Dr NE, Calgary AB T3J 5H4; (Libya)'97; (403)280-2272

BEN MUSA, Sirajeddin A A; St Michael's Hosp, 30 Bond St, Toronto ON M5B 1W8; Al-Fateh (Libya)'02; IntMed. Staff, St Michael's Hospital; (416)360-4000

BEN OMRAN, Karima; 3-263 Queen St E, Brampton ON L6W 4K6; Al-Fateh (Libya)'89; FRCSC; ObstGyn. Staff, William Osler Health System - Brampton Civic Hospital; (905)453-8477

BEN SALEH, Adel Hassen; Associate Med Clinic, 400-20 14th St W, Prince Albert SK S6V 3K8; Al Fateh (Libya)'90; FRCPC; IntMed. Staff, Victoria Hospital; (306)953-1684

BEN SALEM, Bader; Clinique Med Le Plein Ciel, 475 boul de la Cote Vertu, Saint-Laurent QC H4L 1X7; (Tunisia)'99; CCFP; (514)337-3171

BEN-SHOSHAN, Moshe; MUHC-Montreal Children's Hosp, 2300 rue Tupper, Montreal QC H3H 1P3; Tel Aviv (Israel)'96; Staff, McGill University Health Centre - Montreal Children's Hospital; (514)412-4400 x22858; Fax. (514)412-4390.

BEN SMAINE, Nacera K; Hop Santa Cabrini Ospedale, 5655 rue Saint-Zotique E, Montreal QC H1T 1P7; (Algeria)'01; Staff, Hôpital Santa Cabrini Ospedale; (514)252-6444

BEN STA, Amor; 202-3177 rue Saint-Jacques, Montreal QC H4C 1G7; Lausanne (Switzerland)'69; (514)933-5762

BEN YEDDER, Naim; 555 rue Murray, Sherbrooke QC J1G 2K8; Sher'07; IntMed. (819)346-1110

BENABU, Yves; CSSS de Laval, 1755 boul Rene-Laennec, Laval QC H7M 3L9; Mon'07; DiagRad. Staff, Hopital de la Cite de la santé; (450)668-1010

BENADE, Johannes G; 2020 Sherwood Dr PO Box 57255 Rpo Eastgate, Sherwood Park AB T8A 5L7; Stellenbosch (South Africa)'88; MB ChB; MMed(CommunityHealth); CCFP; Langs: Afrikaans; German; (780)937-7567; gerhard.benade@ech.ab.ca.

BENADE, Maria N; PO Box 6370 Stn Main, Fort McMurray AB T9H 5N3; (South Africa)'93; MB ChB.

BENADE, Spinnler L; Northern Lights Health Region, 7 Hospital St, Fort McMurray AB T9H 1P2; (South Africa)'93; Staff, Northern Lights Regional Health Centre; (780)791-6161; Fax. (780)791-6029.

BENAIM, Daniel; Medicentre Lasalle, 303-1500 av Dollard, LaSalle QC H8N 1T5; Sher'81; Staff, CSSS Saint-Leonard et Saint-Michel; (514)363-5303

BENARD, Bernard; 402-2984 boul Taschereau, Greenfield Park QC J4V 2G9; Mon'60; BA; CSPQ; MSc; FRCP; FRCPC; IntMed (Diabetes); Endocrin (P.Q.). Langs: Italian; (450)466-0074; bbenard@videotron.ca.

BENARD, Francois; 301-235 boul René-Lévesque E, Montreal QC H2X 1N8; Mon'82; FRCSC; Urol (Andrology). Staff, Centre Hospitalier l'Université De Montréal (CHUM) - Hôpital Saint-luc; Langs: Bilingual(French/English); (514)861-0213; Fax. (514)861-3021.

BENARD, Francois; BC Cancer Agency Research Ctr, 4.113-675 10th Ave W, Vancouver BC V5Z 1L3; Sher'91; FRCPC; NuclearMed. Staff Molecular Oncology, BC Cancer Agency Research Centre; Langs: Bilingual(French/English); (604)675-8206; Fax. (604)675-8218.

BENARD, Magali A; 2383 111 St NW, Edmonton AB T6J 5E5; Alb'10; CCFP; (780)436-0020; Fax. (780)436-0603.

BENARD, Sylvette; CSSS de Rimouski-Neigette, CP 3150 Succ A 150 av Rouleau, Rimouski QC G5L 5T1; Montpellier (France)'86; Staff, Hôpital Regional Rimouski; (418)723-7851

BENAROCH, Thierry E; MUHC-Montreal Children's Hosp, C521-2300 rue Tupper, Montreal QC H3H 1P3; McG'85; MSc; FRCSC; OrthSurg (Pediatric Orthopedic Surgery). Consultant, Shriners Hospitals For Children - Canada; Staff, McGill University Health Centre - Montreal Children's Hospital; Asst Prof Surg, McGill University; (514)412-4437; Fax. (514)412-4353; thierry.benaroch@muhc.mcgill.ca.

BENAROIA, Mark; Grand River Hosp-KW Hlth Ctre, PO Box 9056 Stn C 835 King St W, Kitchener ON N2G 1G3; Tor'01; BSc(Hon); MHSc; FRCPC; IntMed (Nephrology); Nephrol. Staff Nephrol, Grand River Hospital - Kitchener/Waterloo Health Centre; Staff Nephrol, St Mary's General Hospital; Aj Clinical Asst Prof Med, McMaster University; (519)749-4300 x2189; Fax. (519)749-4210.

BENAROYA, Samuel H; MUHC-Royal Victoria Hosp, E261-687 av des Pins O, Montreal QC H3A 1A1; McG'75; FRCPC; IntMed. Staff, McGill University Health Centre - Royal Victoria Hospital; AVP Health Affairs & Assoc Dean Inter-Hospital Affairs, McGill University; (514)843-1515; Fax. (514)843-1676; samuel.benaroya@muhc.mcgill.ca.

BENAVENTE, Oscar R; S169-2211 Wesbrook Mall, Vancouver BC V6T 2B5; Cordoba (Argentina)'79; FRCPC; Neur. Langs: Spanish; (604)822-7979

BENAYA, Sebastian; 410-1015 Regent St, Fredericton NB E3B 6H5; (Zambia)'93; Staff, Miramichi Regional Hospital.

BENAYOUN, Serge; 220-5345 boul de l'Assomption, Montreal QC H1T 4B3; Mon'02; FRCSC; Urol. (514)255-9145

BENBIGA, Loubna; CLSC Mercier Est-Anjou, 9503 rue Sherbrooke E, Montreal QC H1L 6P2; Casablanca (Morocco)'02; (514)356-2572

BENCE-BRUCKLER, Isabelle A; The Ottawa Hosp-Gen Campus, Box 704 7209-501 Smyth Rd, Ottawa ON K1H 8L6; Ott'89; FRCPC; IntMed (Bone Marrow Transplant); Hem. Staff Hem, The Ottawa Hospital - General Campus; Asst Prof Med, University of Ottawa; Langs: Bilingual(English/French); (613)739-6021; Fax. (613)737-8861.

BENCHETRIT, Arie; Cosmedica, 813-1 av Holiday, Pointe-Claire QC H9R 5N3; Mon'82; FRCSC; GenSurg (Aesthetic Surgery); PlasSurg. Staff, Lakeshore General Hospital - Pointe Claire; Langs: English; French; (514)695-1384; Fax. (514)695-7782; nancy@plasticsurgerymontreal.com.

BENCHIMOL, Eric I; Children's Hosp Eastern Ont, 401 Smyth Rd, Ottawa ON K1H 8L1; Wes'02; FRCPC; Peds; Gastroent. Staff, Children's Hospital of Eastern Ontario (CHEO); (613)737-7600

BENCZE, Steven; Carling Respiratory Services, 601-1081 Carling Ave, Ottawa ON K1Y 4G2; Szeged (Hungary)'78; FRCPC; IntMed (Respirology). (613)729-8262; Fax. (613)729-7870.

BENDAGO, Mansour M; 1153 Ellesmere Rd, Scarborough ON M1P 2X6; Tripoli (Libya)'81; MB ChB; FRCSC; PlasSurg (Cosmetic Surgery). Staff PlasSurg, Rouge Valley Health System - Centenary Health Centre Site; Asst Prof, University of Saskatchewan; Langs: Arabic; (416)284-4420; Fax. (416)284-5543; reception@drbendago.com.

BENDALL, Michael G; Whitehorse Gen Hosp, 5 Hospital Rd, Whitehorse YT Y1A 3H7; Pretoria (South Africa)'71; MB ChB; DABOG; FRCSC; ObstGyn. Consultant Obst/Gyn, Whitehorse General Hospital; Langs: Afrikaans; (867)393-8915; zulubendall@klondiker.com.

BENDANA, Franklin; Hop Charles Lemoyne, 3120 boul Taschereau, Greenfield Park QC J4V 2H1; (Mexico)'71; FRCPC; Gastroent (P.Q.). Staff, Hopital Charles LeMoyne; (450)466-5000 x2144; Fax. (450)466-5036.

BENDAVID, Yves; Hop Maisonneuve-Rosemont, 5415 boul de l'Assomption, Montreal QC H1T 2M4; Mon'97; FRCSC; GenSurg. Staff, Hopital Maisonneuve-Rosemont; (514)252-3400

BENDER, Ash D; Addiction & Mental Hlth-Clarke, 250 College St, Toronto ON M5T 1R8; Wes'99; FRCPC; Psy (Occupational Psychiatry). Staff, Centre for Addiction & Mental Health (CAMH) - College Street Site; (416)535-8501 x7364; ash_bender@camh.net.

BENDER, J D Jacques; 1086 rue Labrosse, St. Eugene ON K0B 1P0; Laval'85; Langs: Bilingual(French/English); (450)795-3224; Fax. (450)795-3224.

BENDER, Jennifer S; St Joseph's Health Centre, 30 The Queensway, Toronto ON M6R 1B5; Tor'98; FRCPC; Anes. Staff, St Joseph's Health Centre; (416)530-6000

BENDER, Kimberley M; Smithville Family Health Ctre, PO Box 218 230 Canboro St, Smithville ON L0R 2A0; McM'99; CCFP; (905)957-3328; kbender@cogeco.ca.

BENDHEIM, Henry; 499 Oxford St E, London ON N5Y 3H8; Cape Town (South Africa)'70; CCFP; FCFP; Staff, St Joseph's Hospital - St Joseph's Health Care; (519)672-1495; Fax. (519)434-3048; hbendheim@rogers.com.

BENDIAK, Glenda N; Alberta Children's Hosp, 2888 Shaganappi Trail NW, Calgary AB T3B 6A8; Tor'05; FRCPC; Peds; Respir. Staff, Alberta Children's Hospital; (403)955-2952; Fax. (403)955-7059.

BENDOR-SAMUEL, Richard L; Landing Surgical Centre, 7A-1477 Lower Water St, Halifax NS B3J 3Z4; Man'86; FRCSC; PlasSurg. Staff, Queen Elizabeth II Health Sciences Centre - Victoria General Site; (902)492-2007

BENDZ, Oleg D; Humber River Reg Hosp-Church, 200 Church St, Toronto ON M9N 1N8; McG'81; Staff, Humber River Regional Hospital - Church Street Site; Langs: Russian; Ukrainian; French; (416)720-4687; Fax. (416)367-8845; oleg.bendz@gmail.com.

BENDZSAK, Anna M; Univ Hlth Network-Toronto Gen, 13EN 232A-200 Elizabeth St, Toronto ON M5G 2C4; UBC'04; FRCSC; GenSurg. Staff, Toronto General Hospital - UHN; (416)340-4798

BENECH-RIOPEL, Elise; Sante MRC d'Acton, 967 rue Boulay, Acton Vale QC J0H 1A0; Paris (France)'07; Langs: Bilingual(French/English); (450)546-4711; Fax. (450)546-4720.

BENEDEK, Caroline O; Vancouver Gen Hosp, 855 12th Ave W, Vancouver BC V5Z 1M9; Ott'98; CCFP; Staff, Royal Columbian Hospital; Staff, Vancouver General Hospital - Centennial Pavillion; Langs: Bilingual(English/French).

BENEDEK, Linda J; Sault College Health Centre, 443 Northern Ave, Sault Ste. Marie ON P6B 4J3; Dal'90; CCFP; FCFP; Staff, Sault Area Hospital - Sault Ste Marie; Med Dir, Celebration Medical Weight Management; (705)759-2554; info@celebrationmedical.ca.

BENEDET, Lynda; Univ of Waterloo Hlth Services, 200 University Ave W, Waterloo ON N2L 3G1; Wes'01; CCFP; (519)888-4096; Fax. (519)888-4306.

BENEDICT, Christina M; Univ Hlth Network-Toronto Western Hosp, 399 Bathurst St, Toronto ON M5T 2S8; Mem'75; Anes. Staff, Toronto Western Hospital - University Health Network.

BENEDICT, Richard R; Sudbury Med Centre, 407-65 Larch St, Sudbury ON P3E 1B8; Wes'76; FACS; MD; FRCSC; GenSurg (Surgical Oncology). Gen Surgeon, Health Sciences North-Laurentian Site; Asst Prof, Northern Ontario School of Medicine; Asst Prof Med, Laurentian University; (705)671-3094; Fax. (705)671-2174.

BENEDICTSON, Michele S; McCall Court, 150-4311 12 St NE, Calgary AB T2E 4P9; Cal'89; (403)517-6141; Fax. (403)205-8042.

BENEDIKTSSON, Hallgrimur; Foothills Med Centre, 1403 29 St NW, Calgary AB T2N 2T9; Reykjavik (Iceland)'73; MD; FRCPC; AnatPath (Renal Pathology). Staff Path, Foothills Medical Centre; Prof Dept of Path & LabMed, University of Calgary; Langs: Icelandic; Swedish; (403)944-8041; Fax. (403)944-8998; benedikt@ucalgary.ca.

BENES, Catherine; Humber River Reg Hosp-Keele, 2175 Keele St, Toronto ON M6M 3Z4; Lyon (France)'89; FRCPC; Psy (Schizophrenia). Staff, Humber River Regional Hospital - Keele Street Site; Langs: English; French; (416)658-2022; Fax. (416)658-2074.

BENFAYED, Hamdi H; Baywood Med Centre, 501-95 Bayly St W, Ajax ON L1S 7K8; Garyunis (Libya)'80; MB ChB; FRCSC; OrthSurg. Staff, Rouge Valley Health System - Ajax & Pickering Health Centre Site; (905)426-8100; Fax. (905)426-2036.

BENFEY, Bruno G; McGill University, 3655 Prom Sir-William-Osler, Montreal QC H3G 1Y6; Hamburg (Germany)'48; MD; MSc(Chemistry); Prof Pharm, McGill University; Langs: German; (514)398-3613; bruno.benfey@mcgill.ca.

BENFEY, Martin C; CSSS du Pontiac, 160 ch de la Chute CP 430, Fort-Coulonge QC J0X 1V0; McG'86; Staff, CSSS du Pontiac; Staff, Pontiac Hospital Centre; adj Prof, McGill University; (819)683-3000; Fax. (819)683-2008.

BENGA-MALULU, Francine; 3-3980 rue Principale CP 3201 Succ Bureau-Chef, Tracadie-Sheila NB E1X 1G5; Kinshasa (Congo (Democratic Republic))'88; Staff, Hôpital de Tracadie-Sheila.

BENGER, Ann M; Juravinski Cancer Centre, 699 Concession St, Hamilton ON L8V 5C2; Qns'75; FRCPC; IntMed (Oncology); Hem. Staff Hem, Hamilton Health Sciences Centre-Juravinski Site; Assoc Prof Med, McMaster University; (905)575-9827; Fax. (905)575-6340.

BENGEZI, Omar; 154 West Main St, Welland ON L3C 5A2; Garyunis (Libya)'81; FRCSC; PlasSurg (Cosmetic, Reconstructive & Hand Surgery). Staff PlasSurg, Niagara Health System - Welland Hospital Site; Staff Plastic Surg, Niagara Health System - Greater Niagara General Site; (905)788-0555; Fax. (905)788-3362.

BENGHIDA, Riad; Campbellton Reg Hosp, PO Box 880 Stn Main 189 Lily Lake Rd, Campbellton NB E3N 3H3; (Algeria)'95; Staff, Hôpital Régional Campbellton; (506)789-5000

BENGIZI, Adel A A; Hamilton HS-General Site, 237 Barton St E, Hamilton ON L8L 2X2; Al-Arab (Libya)'90; FRCPC; Anes; Critical Care Medicine. Staff, Hamilton Health Sciences Centre - Hamilton General Hospital; (905)527-0271

BENGOUGH, Michael N; Peterborough Reg HC-Hospital, 1 Hospital Dr, Peterborough ON K9J 7C6; University College Dublin (Ireland)'03; FRCPC; Anes (Intensive Care). Staff, Peterborough Regional Health Centre - Hospital Drive; (705)743-9654; Fax. (705)743-7669.

BENGUEREL, Robert; 149 route 132 O RR 1, Caplan QC G0C 1H0; Mon'83; Staff, CSSS de la Baie-des-Chaleurs; (418)388-2201

BENHADDAD, Abdeltif; Physimed, 6363 rte Transcanadienne, Saint-Laurent QC H4T 1Z9; Mon'04; CCFP; (514)747-8888

BENHAIM, Albert; Clinique Med Physimed, 121-6363 Rte Transcanadienne, Saint-Laurent QC H4T 1Z9; McG'85; Staff, Hopital Charles LeMoyne; (514)747-8888; Fax. (514)747-0655.

BENHAIM, Patrick; Inst U Geriatrie de Montreal, 26-4565 ch Queen-Mary, Montreal QC H3W 1W5; Mon'04; PhysMed&Rehab. Staff, Institut Universitaire de Gériatrie de Montréal; (514)340-2800

BENHAMRON, Elias S; Hop Jean-Talon, 1385 rue Jean-Talon E, Montreal QC H2E 1S6; Mon'84; Staff, CSSS du Coeur de l'Isle Hôpital Jean-Talon; (514)495-6767

BENHAMRON, Jaimes-S.; Clinique de Gastroenterologie, 5513 ch Queen-Mary, Montreal QC H3X 1V4; Mon'81; FRCPC; IntMed; Gastroent. Langs: Spanish; English; (514)769-7198; Fax. (514)769-1306.

BENIAR, Matityahu; CSSS de Rivière-de-Loup, 75 rue Saint-Henri, Riviere-du-Loup QC G5R 2A4; St-Petersbourg (Russia (Federation))'94; Staff Neurol, Centre Hospitalier Regional du Grand-Portage; Langs: Bilingual(French/English); (418)868-1010; mbiniar@excite.com.

BENIERAKIS, Constantin E; MUHC-Montreal Children's Hosp, 2300 rue Tupper, Montreal QC H3H 1P3; Dublin (Ireland)'57; DABPN; DPsy; FRCPC; Psy. Att Staff, McGill University Health Centre - Montreal Children's Hospital; Asst Prof Psy, McGill University; (514)412-4449; Fax. (514)412-4346.

BENISSA, Issa A; Fogo Island Health Centre, PO Box 9, Fogo NL A0G 2B0; Staff, Fogo Island Health Centre; Staff, Chapel Arm Medical Clinic; (709)266-2221

BENISTY, Jacques I; Hop Jean-Talon, 1385 rue Jean-Talon E, Montreal QC H2E 1S6; Sher'89; CSPQ; Cardiol; IntMed. Staff, CSSS du Coeur de l'Isle Hôpital Jean-Talon; (514)495-6767

BENITEZ, Bella; CSSS du Sud de Lanaudière, 911 montee des Pionniers, Terrebonne QC J6V 2H2; Mon'99; FRCSC; GenSurg. Staff, Centre Hospitalier Pierre le Gardeur; (450)654-7525

BENITEZ-GOMEZ, Antonio; Hilltop Med Clinic, 140-15321 16 Ave, Surrey BC V4A 1R6; Cordova (Spain)'79; CCFP; FCFP; Langs: Spanish; (604)531-5575; Fax. (604)535-0126.

BENITEZ-LAZO, Jose M; King George Medical Clinic, 102-9808 King George Blvd, Surrey BC V3T 2V6; (Nicaragua)'83; Langs: Spanish; (604)585-9972; Fax. (604)585-9973.

BENJAMEN, Sameera; 23-9750 Weston Rd, Woodbridge ON L4H 2Z7; Baghdad (Iraq)'87; MB ChB; Staff Family Med, Humber River Regional Hospital - Keele Street Site; Langs: Arabic; Assyrian; (905)303-4122

BENJAMIN, Alice; Seafort Med Bldg, 270-3550 ch Cote-des-Neiges, Montreal QC H3H 1V4; Delhi (India)'71; MB BS; FACS; FACOG; FRCSC; ObstGyn (Fetal & Maternal Medicine). Dir Obst, McGill University Health Centre - Royal Victoria Hospital; assoc Prof ObstGyn, McGill University; Langs: French; Hindi; Tamil; (514)937-4445; Fax. (514)937-0737.

BENJAMIN, Candice N; Koffler Student Services, 214 College St, Toronto ON M5T 2Z9; Tor'90; FRCPC; Peds. (416)978-8030

BENJAMIN, Derek S; Royal Court Med Centre, 203-1 Quarry Ridge Rd, Barrie ON L4M 7G1; Dal'97; FRCPC; IntMed; Nephrol. Clin Dir Nephrol, Royal Victoria Regional Health Centre; (705)728-9843; Fax. (705)728-8476.

BENJAMIN, Eric; CHUS-Hop Hotel-Dieu, 580 rue Bowen S, Sherbrooke QC J1G 2E8; Sher'06; CCFP; CCFP(E.M.); Staff, Centre Hospitalier Universitaire de Sherbrooke-Hôpital Hôtel-Dieu; (819)346-1110

BENJAMIN, Ilan; Kildare Family Med Associates, 8-7005 ch Kildare, Cote Saint-Luc QC H4W 1C1; McG'78; CCFP; Att Staff, Sir Mortimer B Davis Jewish General; adj Prof Med, McGill University; (514)489-5785; Fax. (514)489-5786.

BENJAMIN, Joshua; Rockyview Gen Hosp, 7007 14 St SW, Calgary AB T2V 1P9; Alb'94; FRCPC; Psy (Geriatric Psychiatry). Staff, Rockyview General Hospital; (403)943-3503; Fax. (403)212-1230.

BENJAMIN, Julie; Centre Med St-Bruno, 1435 rue Roberval, Saint-Bruno QC J3V 3P7; Sher'76; Staff, Centre Hospitalier Universitaire de Sherbrooke-Hopital Fleurimont; (450)653-3631; Fax. (450)653-5518.

BENJAMIN, Lynne A; 170 Rebecca St, Oakville ON L6K 1J6; Ott'87; BSc; Staff, Halton Healthcare Services Corporation - Milton District Hospital; (905)842-2179; Fax. (905)842-2179.

BENJAMIN, Marcia D; Royal Court Med Centre, 203-1 Quarry Ridge Rd, Barrie ON L4M 7G1; Dal'97; CCST; BSc(Hon); FRCP; FRCPC; Psy (Child & Adolescent Psychiatry). Langs: Spanish; Bilingual(French/English); Sign Language; (705)728-9843; Fax. (705)728-8476.

BENJAMIN, Matthew S; Rouge Valley-Centenary HC, 2867 Ellesmere Rd, Scarborough ON M1E 4B9; Boston(MA) (USA)'96; FRCPC; DiagRad. Staff Radiol, Rouge Valley Health System - Centenary Health Centre Site; (416)284-8131

BENJAMIN, Pierre; Westmount Square Centre Med, 550-1 Car Westmount, Westmount QC H3Z 2P9; Haiti (Haiti)'59; FRCPC; Cardiol (P.Q.). (514)934-2334 x297

BENJAMIN, Prabhu; Two Rivers Family Health Team, B12-350 Conestoga Blvd, Cambridge ON N1R 7L7; Tamil Nadu (India)'87; CCFP; (519)629-4615; Fax. (519)629-4630.

BENJELLOUN, Abdelhaq; Caremedics Med Centre, 18-1910 St Laurent Blvd, Ottawa ON K1G 1A4; (613)523-5550

BENJELLOUN, Ali; Dr Georges-L Dumont Reg Hosp, 330 av Universite, Moncton NB E1C 2Z3; Monastir (Tunisia)'99; Staff, Dr Georges-L-Dumont University Hospital Centre; (506)862-4000

BENKE, Stanley M; 1903 9 Ave S, Lethbridge AB T1J 1W8; Sask'00; BSc; FRCPC; IntMed (Benign & Malignant Hematology); Hem. (403)320-0633; sbenke@chr.ab.ca.

BENKELFAT, Chawki; 206-1033 av des Pins O, Montreal QC H3A 1A1; Rabat (Morocco)'79; MSc; Consultant CMDP, Douglas Mental Health University Institute; Staff, McGill University Health Centre - Royal Victoria Hospital; Assoc Prof Psy, McGill University; (514)398-6732; Fax. (514)398-4866.

BENKO, Andrew J; CHUS-Hop Fleurimont, 3001 12e Av N, Sherbrooke QC J1H 5N4; Sher'90; FRCPC; DiagRad. Staff, Centre Hospitalier Universitaire de Sherbrooke-Hopital Fleurimont; (819)346-1110 x14985

BENKO, Randy R; St Joseph's Healthcare, 50 Charlton Ave E, Hamilton ON L8N 4A6; Wes'02; FRCPC; Anes. Staff, St Joseph's Healthcare - Charlton Campus; (905)522-4941 x33853

BENKOCZI, Carmen L; Chinook Reg Hosp, 960 19 St S, Lethbridge AB T1J 1W5; Timisoara (Romania)'95; CCFP; Staff, Chinook Regional Hospital; Langs: Romanian; French; (403)388-6600; Fax. (403)388-6340.

BENLAMLIH, Mohamed; Hop Reg D'Edmundston, 275 Hebert Blvd, Edmundston NB E3V 4E4; Casablanca (Morocco)'88; Staff Specialized Med, Hôpital regional d'Edmundston; (506)739-2200; Fax. (506)739-2231.

BENMEBAREK, Djamila; Centre d'Urgence Saint-Laurent, 200-1605 boul Marcel-Laurin, Saint-Laurent QC H4R 0B7; Mon'02; Staff, Centre Hospitalier Fleury; (514)747-2555

BENMESSAOUD, Noura; CSSS Pierre Boucher, 1333 boul Jacques-Cartier E, Longueuil QC J4M 2A5; (Algeria)'85; Staff, Centre Hospitalier Pierre Boucher; (450)468-8111

BENMOFTAH, Osama S A; William Osler HC-Brampton, 2100 Bovaird Dr E, Brampton ON L6R 3J7; Al-Fateh (Libya)'00; FRCSC; OrthSurg. Staff, William Osler Health System - Brampton Civic Hospital; (905)494-2120

BENN, Ruth L; London Travel Clinic, 520 Sarnia Rd, London ON N6G 5A3; Wes'89; CCFP; FCFP; (519)672-2273; Fax. (519)672-2668.

BENNE, K M Tobias; North Queens Health Centre, RR 1, Caledonia NS B0T 1B0; Ott'96; CCFP; (902)682-2533; Fax. (902)682-3446.

BENNE, Margaret E; North Queens Med Centre, RR 1, Caledonia NS B0T 1B0; Dal'93; CCFP; (902)682-2533; Fax. (902)682-3446.

BENNETT, Alison M; Brameast Family Physicians, 38-2130 North Park Dr, Brampton ON L6S 0C9; Tor'10; CCFP.

BENNETT, Angus; Northfield Med Centre, 206-99 Northfield Dr E, Waterloo ON N2K 3P9; Glasgow (Scotland)'59; DRCOG; DTMH; (519)744-2592

BENNETT, Athena R; Sturgeon Community Hosp, 201 Boudreau Rd, St. Albert AB T8N 6C4; UBC'05; GenSurg. Staff, Sturgeon Community Hospital; (780)418-8200

BENNETT, Barbara F; Greater St Catherines CHC, 100-145 Queenston St, St Catharines ON L2R 2Z9; East Tennessee (USA)'88; CCFP; (905)688-2558; Fax. (905)688-4678.

BENNETT, Brian R; Laser Pain & Integrative Med C, 205 Bonnie Doon Shopping Ctre, Edmonton AB T6C 4E3; National (Ireland)'65; MB ChB; Langs: Spanish; (780)461-9248; Fax. (780)461-4812; brian@laserpainclinic.com.

BENNETT, Diana R; Health Action Centre, 640 Main St, Winnipeg MB R3B 0L8; Oxford (England)'74; MRCP(UK); CCFP; Staff, Health Action Centre - Health Sciences Centre; (204)940-1626; drbennett@wrha.mb.ca.

BENNETT, Erin A; The Ross Family Medicine Clini, 6F-100 Forest Rd, St. John's NL A1A 1E5; Mem'06; CCFP.

BENNETT, Ian; PO Box 1862 Stn Main, Lethbridge AB T1J 4K5; Durham (England)'62; Staff, Fort MacLeod Health Centre; (403)328-4107; Fax. (403)328-4107; benne@telusplanet.net.

BENNETT, Jean-Yves; Centre Med Laurier, 5661 boul Laurier, Terrebonne QC J7M 1T7; Laval'70; (450)477-5364

BENNETT, John D; 111-279 Wharncliffe Rd N, London ON N6H 2C2; McG'83; FRCPC; DiagRad. Asst Prof, St Joseph's Hospital - St Joseph's Health Care; (519)661-0275

BENNETT, Kathryn E; Surrey Mem Hosp, 13750 96 Ave, Surrey BC V3V 1Z2; UBC'02; FRCPC; Anes; Critical Care Medicine. Staff, Surrey Memorial Hospital; (604)581-2211

BENNETT, Kathryn M; Grandview Med Ctr Fam Hlth Team, 167 Hespeler Rd, Cambridge ON N1R 3H7; Mem'96; CCFP; FCFP; (519)623-4200; Fax. (519)623-2546.

BENNETT, Krista L; Liberton Med Centre, 212-31 Liberton Dr, St. Albert AB T8N 3X6; Alb'00; CCFP; Physician Family Pract, Sturgeon Community Hospital; (780)459-7760

BENNETT, Margaret H; North Toronto Med Bldg, 116-250 Lawrence Ave W, Toronto ON M5M 1B2; McM'92; CCFP; FCFP; (416)782-4447; Fax. (416)782-1284.

BENNETT, Mark S; Inverness Consolidated Mem Hos, PO Box 610, Inverness NS B0E 1N0; Dal'90; CCFP; Staff, Inverness Consolidated Memorial Hospital; (902)258-3210; Fax. (902)258-3061.

BENNETT, Mary M; BC Women's Hosp & Health Ctre, 1M2-4500 Oak St, Vancouver BC V6H 3N1; UBC'83; FRCPC; Peds. Staff, BC Women's Hospital & Health Centre; (604)875-2744

BENNETT, Matthew A; Sturgeon Community Hosp, 201 Boudreau Rd, St. Albert AB T8N 6C4; Alb'07; CCFP; CCFP(E.M.); Staff, Sturgeon Community Hospital; (780)418-8229; Fax. (780)418-7376.

BENNETT, Matthew T; Gordon & Leslie Diamond HCC, 9F-2775 Laurel Ave, Vancouver BC V5Z 1M9; UBC'02; FRCPC; IntMed; Cardiol. Staff, Gordon & Leslie Diamond Health Care Centre; Staff, Vancouver General Hospital - Centennial Pavillion; (604)875-5069

BENNETT, Nicholas; Woodstock Gen Hosp, 310 Juliana Dr, Woodstock ON N4V 0A4; Man'88; Physician Emerg, Woodstock General Hospital; Court Staff, Chatham-Kent Health Alliance - Sydenham Hospital Campus; (519)421-4211 x2118; Fax. (519)421-4256; nbennett@sympatico.ca.

BENNETT, Ogonda A; Alberta Health Services, 2948 Dunmore Rd SE, Medicine Hat AB T1A 8E3; Kuban State (Russia (Federation))'96; Staff, Alberta Health Services; (403)502-8200; Fax. (403)502-8403.

BENNETT, Peter W; Rosedale Med Associates, PO Box 460 13009 Rosedale Ave, Summerland BC V0H 1Z0; Manchester (England)'90; MB ChB; CCFP; (250)404-4242

BENNETT, Susan; Children's Hosp Eastern Ont, 401 Smyth Rd, Ottawa ON K1H 8L1; Liverpool (England)'75; MB ChB; DRCOG; DCH; DTMH; FRCPC; Peds. Staff, Children's Hospital of Eastern Ontario (CHEO); Assoc Prof Peds & Psy, University of Ottawa; (613)737-7600 x3626; Fax. (613)738-4834; bennett@cheo.on.ca.

BENNETT, Teresa Ann; Offord Centre for Child Studie, PO Box 2000 Stn Lcd 1 1200 Main St W, Hamilton ON L8N 3Z5; McM'01; FRCPC; Psy. Staff Offord Centre for Child Studies, Hamilton Health Sciences Centre - McMaster University Medical Centre; (905)521-2100

BENNETT, Vernon L; Royal University Hosp, 103 Hospital Dr, Saskatoon SK S7N 0W8; Sask'87; FRCPC; Psy (General Adult Psychiatry). Staff, Royal University Hospital; Assoc Prof Psy, University of Saskatchewan; (306)966-8229; Fax. (306)966-8237.

BENNETT-BOUTILIER, Nicole H; Canadian Forces Hlth Services, PO Box 17000 Stn Forces, Victoria BC V9A 7N2; NOSM'09; CCFP; (250)363-5646

BENNING, Gurpal; St Joseph Community Health Ctr, 280 Victoria St, Dalhousie NB E8C 2R6; (Dominica)'01; Staff, Centre de santé Communitaire - St-Joseph; (506)684-7000

BENNING, Harjit S; Newmount Med Walk-in Clinic, 624B 18th St, Brandon MB R7A 5B4; Southampton (England)'80; BMus; (204)726-0773; Fax. (204)726-0773.

BENNING, Tony B; Ridge Meadows Hosp & Hlth CC, 11666 Laity St, Maple Ridge BC V2X 5A3; Manchester (England)'95; MB ChB; FRCPC; Psy. Staff, Ridge Meadows Hospital & Health Care Centre; (604)463-4111

BENNINGEN, R Grant; Health Action Centre, 640 Main St, Winnipeg MB R3B 0L8; Man'72; (204)940-1626; Fax. (204)942-7828.

BENNINGER, Shawn J; CFB Borden, PO Box 1000 Stn Forces, Borden ON L0M 1C0; McM'07; CCFP.

BENNION, Laura; 350-1620 29 St NW, Calgary AB T2N 4L7; UBC'99; CCFP; (403)282-1245; Fax. (403)282-9545.

BENNY, Frederic; CSSS Haut-Richelieu-Rouville, 920 du Seminaire Blvd N, St-Jean-sur-Richel QC J3A 1B7; Mon'10; CCFP; Staff, Hôpital du Haut-Richelieu; (450)359-5000

BENNY, W Barrett; 810-943 Broadway Ave W, Vancouver BC V5Z 4E2; UBC'77; Hem (Apheresis Medicine). Staff Hematology Daycare Clinic, Vancouver General Hospital - Centennial Pavillion; Clin Assoc Prof Med Div of Hematology, University of British Columbia; Langs: Yiddish; (604)734-1213

BENO, Suzanne M; The Hosp for Sick Children, 555 University Ave, Toronto ON M5G 1X8; Sask'99; FRCPC; Peds. Staff, The Hospital For Sick Children; (416)813-5807

BENOHANIAN, Antranik N; 552 av Emile-Journault, Montreal QC H2M 1J7; Alexandria (Egypt)'68; FRCPC; Derm (Phototherapy). ac Staff, Centre Hospitalier l'Université De Montréal (CHUM) - Hôpital Saint-luc; adj Prof, Universite de Montreal; Langs: Arabic; Armenian; Italian; Bilingual(English/French); (514)381-7281; Fax. (514)381-7283; info@benohanian.com.

BENOIT, A Glenn; 202-1630 Pandosy St, Kelowna BC V1Y 1P7; Man'79; FRCSC; ObstGyn. Staff ObstGyn & Peds, Kelowna General Hospital; (250)861-6818

BENOIT, Andree; Clinique Med AJC, 110 rue Saint-Jean, Drummondville QC J2B 7T1; Sher'78; ac Staff, Hôpital Sainte-croix; (819)477-8321; Fax. (819)477-9865.

BENOIT, Archie G; Physician Anes Services, 303-400 Tache Ave, Winnipeg MB R2H 3C3; Man'79; DAB; FRCPC; Anes. Staff, St Boniface General Hospital; Assoc Prof, University of Manitoba.

BENOIT, Benoit; Hop du Sacre-Coeur de Mtl, 5400 boul Gouin O, Montreal QC H4J 1C5; Laval'01; FRCSC; OrthSurg. Staff, Hôpital du Sacre-Coeur de Montréal; (514)338-2222

BENOIT, Brien G; Canadian Medical Protective As, PO Box 8225 Stn T 875 Carling Ave, Ottawa ON K1G 3H7; Ott'62; MSc; FACS; FRCSC; Neursurg. Prof NeuroSurg, University of Ottawa; Langs: French; (613)725-9965 x692; Fax. (613)725-1300; bbenoit@cmpa.org.

BENOIT, Catherine; Campbellton Reg Hosp, PO Box 880 Stn Main 189 Lily Lake Rd, Campbellton NB E3N 3H3; Sher'03; CCFP; Staff, Hôpital Régional Campbellton; (506)789-5000

BENOIT, Celine; Clin Med Fam & Obst de Mistass, 6-170 av de l'Eglise, Dolbeau-Mistassini QC G8L 4W6; Mon'89; (418)276-4260; Fax. (418)276-6092.

BENOIT, Chantale; Clinique Externe de Psychiatri, 35 av Saint-Charles, Vaudreuil-Dorion QC J7V 7K8; Mon'94; Psy (P.Q.). (450)455-7967; Fax. (450)455-8631.

BENOIT, Daniel; Clinique Med Mascouche, 100-1025 Montee Masson, Mascouche QC J7K 2L9; Mon'75; (450)474-6000; Fax. (450)474-6666.

BENOIT, Diane; The Hosp for Sick Children, 555 University Ave, Toronto ON M5G 1X8; Sher'81; FRCPC; Psy (Infant Psychiatry). Staff, The Hospital For Sick Children; Asst Prof Psy, University of Toronto; (416)813-7528; Fax. (416)813-6565.

BENOIT, Elise; Clinique Saint-Leonard, 404-8000 boul Langelier, Saint-Leonard QC H1P 3K2; Mon'85; FRCPC; Psy. Staff Psy Outpatient Clinic Coord, Hopital Louis-H Lafontaine; (514)323-1617

BENOIT, Francois; 204-4534 boul St-Joseph, Saint-Nicephore QC J2A 1B5; Mon'74; ac Staff GenMed & Geriatric Unit, Hôpital Sainte-croix; (819)477-5203; Fax. (819)477-1485; francois_benoit@gmf.gouv.qc.ca.

BENOIT, Frederic; Hop Charles-Lemoyne, 3120 boul Taschereau, Greenfield Park QC J4V 2H1; Mon'95; FRCPC; Psy. Staff, Hopital Charles LeMoyne; adj Prof, Universite de Montreal; (450)466-5000

BENOIT, Genevieve; Hôpital Ste-Justine, 3175 ch Cote-Sainte-Catherine, Montreal QC H3T 1C5; Mon'03; FRCPC; Peds; Nephrol. Staff, Hôpital Ste-Justine; (514)345-4931 x4737

BENOIT, Janine L; Saskatoon City Hosp, 701 Queen St, Saskatoon SK S7K 0M7; Sask'86; AB; FRCPC; AnatPath (Cytopath). Staff, Saskatoon City Hospital; Asst Prof, University of Saskatchewan; (306)655-8205

BENOIT, Jean-Marc; Brant Community HC-Brantford, 200 Terrace Hill St, Brantford ON N3R 1G9; McM'99; CCFP; CCFP(E.M.); Staff, The Brant Community Healthcare System - Brantford General Hospital Site; (519)751-5507

BENOIT, Joanne; Clinique Fertilite Ovo, 8000 boul Decarie, Montreal QC H4P 2S4; Mon'80; FRCSC; ObstGyn. Staff, Centre Hospitalier l'Université De Montréal (CHUM) - Hôpital Saint-luc; (514)798-2000; Fax. (514)798-2001.

BENOIT, Joseph S; Red Deer Reg Hosp Centre, PO Box 5030 Stn Postal Box Ctr 3942 50A Ave, Red Deer AB T4N 6R2; Alb'73; Staff, Red Deer Regional Hospital Centre; (403)343-4444

BENOIT, Josiane; CMR Saint-Bruno, 265 boul Seigneurial O, Saint-Bruno QC J3V 2H4; Sher'99; (450)441-5503 x8424

BENOIT, Marie-Jose; 22B-550 Terminal Ave, Ottawa ON K1G 0Z3; Mon'83; Langs: French; (613)731-4770; Fax. (613)731-4979.

BENOIT, Melanie; 205-565 Elmwood Dr, Dieppe NB E1A 2X4; Laval'99; CCFP; Staff, Dr Georges-L-Dumont University Hospital Centre; (506)859-6803; Fax. (506)384-9099; bmelanie@nb.sympatico.ca.

BENOIT, Michel; 101-1251 boul Saint-Joseph e, Montreal QC H2J 1L9; Mon'67; (514)521-1223

BENOIT, Michele; Clinique Med Fleur de Lys, 8 rue Du Terminus E, Rouyn-Noranda QC J9X 3B4; Sher'89; Staff, Centre Hospitalier Rouyn-Noranda; (819)764-6185; Fax. (819)762-6079.

BENOIT, Paul R; Kilborn Med Centre, 505-1385 Bank St, Ottawa ON K1H 8N4; Ott'66; FRCSC; PlasSurg. Plastic Surgery, Canadian Forces Health Services Centre; Plastic Surgery, The Ottawa Hospital - General Campus; Ac Staff, Children's Hospital of Eastern Ontario (CHEO); Asst Prof Surg, University of Ottawa; (613)526-5945; Fax. (613)526-2391.

BENOIT, Philippe; Centre Hosp Honore-Mercier, 2750 boul Laframboise, Saint-Hyacinthe QC J2S 4Y8; Mon'03; BPharm; Staff, Centre Hospitalier Honore-Mercier; Langs: English; (450)771-3333

BENOIT, Robert; MUHC-Montreal Gen Hosp, C6 272-1650 av Cedar, Montreal QC H3G 1A4; Mon'71; ABIM(Endocrin); Endocrin&Metab (P.Q.) (Neuro Endocrinology). Staff, McGill University Health Centre - Montreal General Campus; Consultant Endocrin, Centre Hospitalier de LaSalle; adj Prof, McGill University; Langs: Bilingual(French/English); (514)934-8017; Fax. (514)934-8361.

BENOIT, Simon; CSSS Richelieu-Yamaska, 1333 boul Jacques Cartier E, Longueuil QC J4M 2A5; Mon'09; Staff, Centre Hospitalier Pierre Boucher; (450)468-8111

BENOIT, Suzanne; Inst Albert Prevost, 6555 boul Gouin O, Montreal QC H4K 1B3; Mon'82; FRCPC; Psy. Staff, Hopital Louis-H Lafontaine; (514)338-4621

BENOIT, Suzie; Clinique familiale des Hauts-B, 99 boul des Hauts-Bois, Sainte-Julie QC J3E 3J9; Sher'86; LMCC; Langs: Bilingual(French/English); (450)649-2490

BENOIT, Teresa C; Manitoba FASD Centre, 633 Wellington Cres, Winnipeg MB R3M 0A8; Man'79; FRCPC; Peds. Staff, Health Sciences Centre.

BENOIT, Yvon; Clinique Med Brien, 223 boul Brien, Repentigny QC J6A 6M4; Mon'64; FRCSC; GenSurg (Thoracic Surgery). (450)585-9810

BENOUALID, Henry A; 380-5950 ch de la Cote-des-Nei, Montreal QC H3S 1Z6; Nancy (France)'68; CSPQ; FRCPC; Cardiol (P.Q.). Staff, Sir Mortimer B Davis Jewish General; McGill University; (514)737-1175; Fax. (514)340-7510; henribenoualid@hotmail.com.

BENOUR, Mahmoud A; Royal Alexandra Hosp, 10240 Kingsway NW, Edmonton AB T5H 3V9; (Libya)'91; FRCSC; Neursurg. Staff, Royal Alexandra Hospital; (780)491-5116

BENRIMOH, Daniel; Polyclinique Cabrini, 200-5700 rue Saint-Zotique E, Montreal QC H1T 3Y7; Mon'85; Staff, Hôpital Santa Cabrini Ospedale; (514)256-5700; Fax. (514)256-9499.

BENSAIDANE, Soufiane; CHUQ-Hotel-Dieu de Quebec, 11 Cote du Palais, Quebec QC G1R 2J6; CCFP; Staff, Centre Hospitalier Universitaire de Québec (CHUQ) - Siege Social; (418)525-4444

BENSALEH-RATMI, Amal; 204-1789 Mountain Rd, Moncton NB E1G 5C4; Rabat (Morocco)'89; Consultant, Dr Georges-L-Dumont University Hospital Centre; Consultant, Hôpital regional d'Edmundston; Staff, The Moncton Hospital; Langs: Arabic; French; (506)860-2764; Fax. (506)860-2760.

BENSE, Michael H J; Bense Eye Centre, 102-100 Elizabeth Ave, St. John's NL A1B 1S1; Pretoria (South Africa)'70; FRCSC; Ophth. Ass't Clin Prof Surg & Ophth, Memorial University Of Newfoundland; (709)579-1447; eyecentre@bense.ca.

BENSELER, Susanne; 555 University Ave, Toronto ON M5G 1X8; Freiburg (Germany)'93; Staff, The Hospital For Sick Children; Langs: French; German; (416)813-5828; Fax. (416)813-4989; susanne.benseler@sickkids.ca.

BENSEN, William G; Charlton Med Centre, 203-25 Charlton Ave E, Hamilton ON L8N 1Y2; McM'73; ABIM; FRCPC; IntMed (Osteoporosis); Rheum. Consultant, St Joseph's Healthcare - Charlton Campus; Clin Assoc Prof, McMaster University; (905)523-7705; Fax. (905)523-6168.

BENSHABAN, Lamin Ra; Red River Med Clinic, 366 Main St, Selkirk MB R1A 2J7; (204)482-8953; Fax. (204)482-8954.

BENSIMON, Eric; 1003 boul Saint-Joseph E, Montreal QC H2J 1L2; Laval'93; FRFPS; FRCSC; PlasSurg (Cosmetic Surgery). Staff, Hôpital du Sacre-Coeur de Montréal; Langs: Bilingual(French/English); (514)288-9988; Fax. (514)288-9933; ebensimon@sympatico.ca.

BENSLER, Ernest C; Bonavista Med Clinic, 739 Lake Bonavista Dr SE, Calgary AB T2J 0N2; Cal'79; BSc; (403)278-1440; Fax. (403)271-2488.

BENSLER, Evan A; Sheldon Chumuik Centre, 1213 4 St SW, Calgary AB T2R 0X7; Cal'96; BSc; CCFP; (403)955-6011; Fax. (403)855-6023; evan.bensler@calgaryhealthregion.ca.

BENSLIMANE, Benaoumeur; CSSS Saint-Leonard, 3130 rue Larry E, Montreal QC H1Z 4N8; Mon'08; (514)722-3000

BENSON, Brian W; Sport Med Centre, 2500 University Dr NW, Calgary AB T2N 1N4; Cal'01; MSc; BPE; Dip SportMed; MCFP; LRCPS; LMCC; CCFP; (403)220-8518; bbenson@ucalgary.ca.

BENSON, Bruce D; Parkland Med Clinic, 6-5030 47 Ave, Red Deer AB T4N 3P7; Cape Town (South Africa)'87; MB ChB; CCFP; (403)346-4206; Fax. (403)346-4207.

BENSON, Gary L; West Lincoln Mem Hosp, 169 Main St E, Grimsby ON L3M 1P3; Dal'69; CCFP; FCFP; Chief/Medical Staff, West Lincoln Memorial Hospital; Family Medicine, Hamilton Health Sciences Centre - McMaster University Medical Centre; Court Staff, Joseph Brant Memorial Hospital; Asst Prof Family Practice, McMaster University; (905)945-2253; gbenson@sympatico.ca.

BENSON, Leland N; The Hosp For Sick Children, 555 University Ave, Toronto ON M5G 1X8; Chicago(IL) (USA)'74; FACC; FRCPC; Peds (Invasive & Interventional Cardiology); Cardiol. Staff, Toronto General Hospital - UHN; Staff, The Hospital For Sick Children; Prof Peds, University of Toronto; (416)813-6141; Fax. (416)813-5857; lee.benson@sickkids.ca.

BENSON, Lissa D; 101B-1771 Comox Ave, Comox BC V9M 3L9; Qns'91; CCFP; FCFP; (250)339-5780

BENSOUDA, Brahim; MUHC-Royal Victoria Hosp, 687 av des Pins O, Montreal QC H3A 1A1; Rabat (Morocco)'96; Staff, McGill University Health Centre - Royal Victoria Hospital; (514)934-1934

BENSOUSSAN, Karen; Mackenzie Richmond Hill Hosp, 10 Trench Rd, Richmond Hill ON L4C 4Z3; Tor'02; FRCPC; IntMed. Staff, Mackenzie Richmond Hill Hospital; (905)883-2064

BENSTEAD, Timothy J; Queen Elizabeth II HSC-Halifax, 3828-1796 Summer St, Halifax NS B3H 3A7; Cal'79; FRCPC; Neur. Staff, Queen Elizabeth II Health Sciences Centre - Halifax Infirmary Site; Staff Neurol, Queen Elizabeth II Health Sciences Centre - Victoria General Site; Prof, Dalhousie University; (902)473-5565; Fax. (902)473-4438; tbenstea@dal.ca.

BENT, Alfred E; Physicians Incorporated, 205-316 Willow St, Truro NS B2N 5A4; Dal'73; FRCSC; ObstGyn (Urogynecology). Prof, IWK Health Centre; (902)895-4478; Fax. (902)895-4407; abentmd@hotmail.com.

BENT, Kevin P; Dartmouth Gen Hosp, 325 Pleasant St, Dartmouth NS B2Y 4G8; Dal'94; FRCPC; Anes. Staff, Dartmouth General Hospital; (902)465-8300

BENT, Maurice A; North York Med Arts Bldg, 243-1333 Sheppard Ave E, North York ON M2J 1V1; Tor'62; FRCSC; OrthSurg (Hip & Knee Replacement). Ac Staff, North York General Hospital; (416)494-7432; Fax. (416)494-7446.

BENT, Stephen; Miramichi Reg Hosp, 500 Water St, Miramichi NB E1V 3G5; Dal'90; Staff, Miramichi Regional Hospital; (506)623-3155; stephenbent@yahoo.com.

BENTLEY, James R; Capital Health District Author, 5006-5820 University Ave, Halifax NS B3H 1V7; Leeds (England)'87; MB ChB; FRCSC; ObstGyn (Gynecologic Oncology). Staff, Capital Health District Authority; (902)473-4029; Fax. (902)473-7765; jim.bentley@dal.ca.

BENTLEY, Janna; 3293 Lakeshore Rd, Kelowna BC V1W 3S9; Alb'03; CCFP; Langs: Bilingual(English/French); (250)860-9919; janna@okanaganhealth.ca.

BENTLEY, Kenneth D M; Vernon Radiological Assoc Corp, 3100 35 Ave, Vernon BC V1T 2T1; UBC'76; FRCPC; DiagRad. Staff, Vernon Jubilee Hospital; (250)545-0747

BENTLEY, Todd C; Advanced Physiotherapy & Sport, 18-550 Fennell Ave E, Hamilton ON L8V 4S9; McM'99; MSc; BSc(Kinesiology); DABPMR; Dip SportMed; FRCPC; PhysMed&Rehab (Sports Medicine). Consultant Physiatrist Reg Rehab Center, Hamilton Health Sciences Centre - McMaster University Medical Centre; Consultant Physiatrist, St Joseph's Healthcare - Charlton Campus; Clin Assoc Prof, McMaster University; (905)304-7950; Fax. (905)304-0673.

BENTON, Claude M; Parksville Med Clinic, PO Box 250 Stn Main 154 West Memorial Ave, Parksville BC V9P 2G4; Manchester (England)'71; MB ChB; Langs: German; (250)248-5757; Fax. (250)248-2128; cjbenton@shaw.ca.

BENTOV, Yaakov H; Ctre for Advanced Reprod Techn, 210-150 Bloor St W, Toronto ON M5S 2X9; Beersheba (Israel)'96; (416)972-0110

BENTZ, Peter E; St Joseph's Care Group, 300 North Lillie St, Thunder Bay ON P7C 4Y7; Tor'61; CCFP; Ac Staff, Thunder Bay Regional Health Sciences Centre Port-Arthur; Ac Staff, St Joseph's Care Group - St Joseph's Hospital; (807)623-7677; Fax. (807)623-7697.

BENY, Majak T; Melville Med Centre, PO Box 209, Melville SK S0A 2P0; Juba (Sudan)'93; MB BS; LMCC; CCFP; Physician Emerg, Yorkton Regional Health Centre; (306)728-4466; Fax. (306)728-3183.

BENZAID, El Mostafa; Centre de Sante Valcartier, CP 1000 Bdp Succ Forces, Courcelette QC G0A 4Z0; Casablanca (Morocco)'00; CCFP; Staff, Centre de Sante Valcartier; (418)844-5000

BENZAQUEN, Bruno; Hop Maisonneuve-Rosemont, 5415 boul de l'Assomption, Montreal QC H1T 2M4; McG'98; ABIM; ABC; ACLS; BSc(Hon); CSPQ; FRCPC; Cardiol (Echography Cardiac); IntMed. Staff, Hopital Maisonneuve-Rosemont; Staff Cardiol, CSSS du Coeur de l'Isle Hôpital Jean-Talon; adj Prof Med, Universite de Montreal; Langs: Spanish; (514)252-3400 x3812; Fax. (514)252-3529; bruno.benzaquen@mail.mcgill.ca.

BENZAQUEN, Susan; 208-7330 Yonge St, Thornhill ON L4J 7Y7; Tor'86; FRCSC; ObstGyn. Ac Staff ObstGyn, Mackenzie Richmond Hill Hospital; (905)764-5040

BENZAZON, Michael; Hop Charles Lemoyne, 3120 boul Taschereau, Greenfield Park QC J4V 2H1; Laval'96; CSPQ; FRCPC; IntMed (Echocardiography & Non-Invasive Laboratory); Cardiol. Staff, Hopital Charles LeMoyne; Langs: Bilingual(French/English); (450)466-5000; Fax. (450)466-5003; michael.benzazon@gmail.com.

BENZER, Susan D; Riverside Med Clinic, 304-1101 Dewdney Ave, Trail BC V1R 4T1; UBC'86; (250)368-5656; Fax. (250)368-8811; isjrareid@telus.net.

BERALDO, Vanessa J; King West Village Med Centre, 201-626 King St W, Toronto ON M5V 1M7; (Other Foreign)'07; CCFP; (416)703-1313; Fax. (416)703-1310.

BERALL, Glenn; North York Gen Hosp, 4001 Leslie St, North York ON M2K 1E1; Ott'83; AB(ClinNutrition); FRCPC; Peds (Nutritional Disorders). Staff, Holland Bloorview Kids Rehabilitation Hospital; Staff Gastroent & Nutrition, The Hospital For Sick Children; Chief Peds, North York General Hospital; Staff, Royal Victoria Regional Health Centre; Asst Prof Peds, University of Toronto; (416)756-6222; Fax. (416)756-6853.

BERALL, Murray J; Humber River Reg Hosp-Church, 200 Church St, Toronto ON M9N 1N8; Dal'83; FRCP; FRCPC; IntMed; Nephrol. Staff, Humber River Regional Hospital - Church Street Site; (416)243-4610; Fax. (416)243-4346; mberall@hrrh.on.ca.

BERAN, Maud; University of Alberta Hosp, CSB8 120-8440 112 St NW, Edmonton AB T6G 2B7; (Belgium)'02; Staff, University of Alberta Hospital; (780)407-8822; Fax. (780)407-8529.

BERARD, Claire; CLSC de Hull, 85 rue Saint-Redempteur, Gatineau QC J8X 4E6; Mon'80; LMCC; Médecin Homecare, CLSC de Hull; Langs: Bilingual(French/English); (819)770-6908 x4268; Fax. (819)770-2489; claire_berard@ssss.gouv.qc.ca.

BERARD, Dominique; CHUS-Hop Fleurimont, 3001 12e av N, Sherbrooke QC J1H 5N4; Sher'92; CSPQ; Anes (P.Q.) (Intensive Care). Staff Anes, Centre Hospitalier Universitaire de Sherbrooke-Hopital Fleurimont; Staff Anes, Centre Hospitalier Universitaire de Sherbrooke-Hôpital Hôtel-Dieu; assoc Prof, Universite de Sherbrooke; (819)346-1110 x14403; dominique.berard@usherbrooke.ca.

BERARD, Frances C; Notre Dame Clinic, PO Box 130, Notre-Dame-Lr MB R0G 1M0; Man'89; CCFP; FCFP; Lecturer, University of Manitoba; Langs: French; (204)248-2252; Fax. (204)248-2087.

BERARD, Louis J; Inst Philippe Pinel de Mtl, 10905 boul Henri-Bourassa E, Montreal QC H1C 1H1; Mon'81; FRCPC; Psy. Dir-svcs prof, Institut Philippe-Pinel de Montreal; (514)648-8461 x304

BÉRARD, Marianik; CSSS du Nord de Lanaudière, 1000 boul Sainte-Anne, St-Charles-Brromee QC J6E 6J2; Mon'06; CCFP; CCFP(E.M.); Staff, Centre Hospitalier Régional de Lanaudière; (514)759-8222

BERARD, Roberta A; Children's Hosp of Western Ont, 800 Commissioners Rd E, London ON N6C 2V5; Tor'03; FRCPC; Peds; Rheum. Staff, Children's Hospital of Western Ontario; (519)685-8484

BERARDI, Lyndsay M; Family Med Centre, 210 Melrose Ave, Ottawa ON K1Y 4K7; NOSM'09; CCFP; (613)761-4334

BERBARI, Patricia; MedicSpa & PlasSurg Clinic, 555A boul de la Gappe, Gatineau QC J8T 8N7; Mon'95; MSc; BSc; FRCSC; PlasSurg (Cosmetic Surgery). Staff, CSSS de Gatineau; Ac Staff Pt-Time, Children's Hospital of Eastern Ontario (CHEO); University of Ottawa; Langs: Arabic; Romanian; English; (819)243-7667; Fax. (819)243-9485; drpatriciaberbari@bellnet.ca.

BERBECE, Adriana N; St Joseph's Health Centre, 332-30 The Queensway, Toronto ON M6R 1B5; Cluj (Romania)'89; FRCPC; IntMed; Nephrol. Staff, St Joseph's Health Centre; Locum Tenens IntMed, North York General Hospital; Langs: Romanian; (416)530-6227; Fax. (416)530-6233; adriananb@rogers.com.

BERBER, Mark J; Markham Stouffville Health Ctr, 408-377 Church St, Markham ON L6B 1A1; Trinity Coll. (Ireland)'79; MRCGPract; DCH; MRCPsy; FRCP; DObst; FRCPC; Psy (Anxiety & Mood Disorders). Staff, Markham Stouffville Hospital; Asst Prof, Queen's University; Lecturer, University of Toronto; (905)472-5733; Fax. (905)472-5215; mberber@cnsmedicine.com.

BERBRAYER, David; Sunnybrook Hlth Sciences Ctre, 2075 Bayview Ave, Toronto ON M4N 3M5; Man'76; BSc(Med.); DABPM; FRCPC; PhysMed&Rehab. Ac Staff, Holland Bloorview Kids Rehabilitation Hospital; Ac Staff, Sunnybrook Health Sciences Centre; Consultant, The Hospital For Sick Children; (416)480-4069; Fax. (416)480-6885.

BERCHUK, Miriam; Rockyview Gen Hosp, 7007 14 St SW, Calgary AB T2V 1P9; Ott'00; FRCPC; Anes. Staff, Rockyview General Hospital; (780)943-8720

BERCIER, Jean-Philippe; Montfort Hosp, 2D123-713 Montreal Rd, Ottawa ON K1K 0T2; Ott'10; CCFP; Staff, Montfort Hospital; (613)746-4621

BERCIK, Premysl; Hamilton HS-McMaster Site, PO Box 2000 Stn Lcd 1 1200 Main St W, Hamilton ON L8N 3Z5; Prague (Czech Republic)'91; Staff, Hamilton Health Sciences Centre - McMaster University Medical Centre; (905)521-2100; Fax. (905)521-4958.

BERCOVICI, Mark C; Sunnybrook Hlth Sciences Ctre, 2075 Bayview Ave, Toronto ON M4N 3M5; Tor'78; FRCPC; Anes. Ac Staff, Sunnybrook Health Sciences Centre; (416)480-4864; Fax. (416)480-6039.

BERCOVITCH, David D; SMBD Jewish Gen Hosp, 3755 ch Cote-Sainte-Catherine, Montreal QC H3T 1E2; McG'58; DABIM; FRCPC; IntMed; Nephrol (P.Q.). Sr Physician Nephrol, Sir Mortimer B Davis Jewish General; assoc Prof, McGill University; (514)340-7516; Fax. (514)340-8147.

BERCUSON, Judith M; Maple Med Centre, 208-955 Major Mackenzie W, Vaughan ON L6A 4P9; Man'77; CCFP; FCFP; Court Staff, St Michael's Hospital; Court Teach Staff, Toronto General Hospital - UHN; Asst Prof Family & Commun Med, University of Toronto; (289)553-7711; Fax. (289)553-7722; jmirb@rogers.com.

BERDICHEVSKY, Raul; Rosedale Med Centre, 609-600 Sherbourne St, Toronto ON M4X 1W4; (Chile)'72; FRCPC; Psy. Staff, St Michael's Hospital; (416)960-0827

BERDNIKOFF, Andre; Clinique Med Pierre-Boucher, 110-1615 boul Jacques-Cartier, Longueuil QC J4M 2X1; Mon'80; (450)468-6223; Fax. (450)468-5041.

BERDOCK, Steven E; The Hosp For Sick Children, 555 University Ave, Toronto ON M5G 1X8; Tor'83; FRCPC; Anes. Staff Anes, The Hospital For Sick Children; (416)813-7445; Fax. (416)813-7543.

BERDUSCO, Edward T M; Royal Alexandra Hosp, 541CSC-10240 Kingsway NW, Edmonton AB T5H 3V9; Tor'98; CCFP; CCFP(E.M.); Staff, Royal Alexandra Hospital; (780)735-4442; Fax. (780)735-4916.

BEREAN, Kenneth W; Surrey Mem Hosp, 13750 96 Ave, Surrey BC V3V 1Z2; Alb'82; FRCPC; AnatPath. Staff, Surrey Memorial Hospital; Staff, UBC Hospital - Koerner Pavillion; (604)585-5612

BERECZ, Steven J; Windsor Prof Centre, 200-2462 Howard Ave, Windsor ON N8X 3V6; Ott'90; (519)258-2202; Fax. (519)258-8718.

BERENBAUM, Brian; Keele Med Place, 2F-2830 Keele St, North York ON M3M 3E5; Ott'84; (416)633-6812; Fax. (416)633-6187.

BERENDT, Daniel R; Peoples Trust Plaza, 700-10216 124 St NW, Edmonton AB T5N 4A3; Alb'84; CCFP; FCFP; Staff, Royal Alexandra Hospital; Staff, Nursing Home District 24; (780)392-0715

BERENDT, Heather; Royal Alexandra Hosp, 5002 14-10240 Kingsway NW, Edmonton AB T5H 3V9; Alb'83; FRCPC; GenPath. Staff, Royal Alexandra Hospital; Staff, Caritas Health Group-Edmonton; Assoc Prof, University of Alberta; (780)735-4852; Fax. (780)735-4715.

BERENDT, Richard C; Cross Cancer Institute, 11560 University Ave NW, Edmonton AB T6G 1Z2; Alb'83; FCAP; FRCP; ABACPath; FRCPC; AnatPath; GenPath. Dir LabMed & Path, Cross Cancer Institute; Consultant, Edmonton Zone Edmonton Public Health Services; Dir-Lab Serv, Alberta Cancer Board; Clin Prof Path/Aj Prof Oncology, University of Alberta; (780)432-8454

BERES, Alana; Timmins & District Hosp, 700 Ross Ave E, Timmins ON P4N 8P2; McG'04; FRCSC; GenSurg. Staff, Timmins & District Hospital; (705)267-2131

BERESFORD, J Patricia; Lord Nelson Arcade, 250-5675 Spring Garden Rd, Halifax NS B3J 1H1; Dal'76; Court Staff, IWK Health Centre; Court Staff, Queen Elizabeth II Health Sciences Centre - Victoria General Site; Dir, Preventive Med. Centre, Halifax YMCA; (902)420-9383; Fax. (902)425-7948.

BERESFORD, Meaghen J; Women's College Hosp, W268-76 Grenville St, Toronto ON M5S 1B2; Ott'01; FRCPC; DiagRad. Staff, Women's College Hospital; (416)323-6400

BERESFORD, Peter; Columbia Med Bldg, 302-301 Columbia St E, New Westminster BC V3L 3W5; Cape Town (South Africa)'74; MB ChB; MRCOG; FRCSC; ObstGyn (High Risk Obstetrics). Staff, Eagle Ridge Hospital & Health Care Centre; Staff, Royal Columbian Hospital; Reg Head ObstGyn, Fraser Health Authority; (604)524-4441; Fax. (604)524-4425; jomobird@shaw.ca.

BERESFORD, Philip D; Michelin North America(Can)Inc, PO Box 5000, Kentville NS B4N 4M4; Mem'86.

BERETTA, Jennifer A; 95 King St W, Mississauga ON L5B 1H1; Wes'90; Staff, Trillium Health Centre - Mississauga; (905)848-2284; Fax. (905)896-7475.

BEREZA, Eugene; Biomedical Ethics Unit, 301-3647 Peel St, Montreal QC H3A 1X1; McG'88; CCFP; Staff Clin Ethicist, McGill University Health Centre - Royal Victoria Hospital; Head Biomedical Ethics Unit, McGill University; (514)398-7405; Fax. (514)398-8349.

BEREZNAY, Oliver H A; Windsor Park Med Centre, 159 St Anne's Rd, Winnipeg MB R2M 2Z5; Man'95; BSc; MSc; CCFP; Staff, St Boniface General Hospital; University of Manitoba; (204)256-4343

BEREZNY, Gary M; 107-10 South Front St, Belleville ON K8N 2Y3; Qns'79; BSc; MSc; FRCPC; IntMed (Gastroenterology). Staff, QHC Belleville General; Asst Prof, Queen's University; (613)966-0455; Fax. (613)966-8175.

BEREZOWSKI, Riva E; Grey Bruce HS-Owen Sound, PO Box 1800 Stn Main 7221-1800 8th St E, Owen Sound ON N4K 6M9; Alb'81; FACOG; FRCSC; ObstGyn (Community Gynecology). Staff Consultant, Grey Bruce Health Services - Owen Sound; Staff, South Bruce Grey Health Centre - Walkerton Site; Langs: Bilingual(English/French); (519)371-2040; Fax. (519)371-8391.

BEREZOWSKYJ, Alexandra I; Harborn Med Associates, 510-89 Queensway W, Mississauga ON L5B 2V2; Tor'82; CCFP; FCFP; Ac Staff, Trillium Health Centre - Mississauga; (905)273-4380; Fax. (905)273-4335.

BEREZOWSKYJ, Jennifer; St Paul's Hosp, 1081 Burrard St, Vancouver BC V6Z 1Y6; UBC'04; FRCPC; Anes. Staff, Providence Health Care - St Paul's Hospital; (604)682-2344

BERG, Angela W Y; Allin Clinic, 10155 120 St NW, Edmonton AB T5K 2A2; Man'98; CCFP; (780)482-7551; Fax. (780)488-2056.

BERG, Cindy L; 318-1240 Kensington Rd NW, Calgary AB T2N 3P7; Alb'96; CCFP; (403)837-7800

BERG, Dale F; Meadowlark Health Centre, 184 Meadowlark Shopping Ctr NW, Edmonton AB T5R 5W9; Alb'95; FACS; FASCRS; FRCSC; GenSurg (Colon & Rectal Surgery). Staff, Covenant Health - Misericordia Community Hospital; Clinical Asst Prof, University of Alberta; (780)484-1122; Fax. (780)489-4121.

BERG, Gary R; Burnham Med Services, 104-380 Burnham St, Peterborough ON K9H 1T6; Tor'92; BSc; MSc; CCFP; (705)741-3055; Fax. (705)741-5075.

BERG, Greg; 264 McNabb St, Sault Ste. Marie ON P6B 1Y6; Man'86; FRCPC; IntMed (Sleep Medicine); Critical Care Medicine; Respir. Dir Medicine, Sault Area Hospital - Sault Ste Marie; (705)254-5980; Fax. (705)254-6969.

BERG, Jason M; Royal Oak Centre Med Clinic, 105-4442 Saanich Rd W, Victoria BC V8Z 3E9; UBC'96; (250)479-6721

BERG, Joseph M; Surrey Place Centre, 2 Surrey Place, Toronto ON M5S 2C2; Witwatersrand (South Africa)'54; MB ChB; MSc; FRCPsy; FCCMG; Psy (Clinical Genetics). (416)925-5141; Fax. (416)923-8476; j.berg@utoronto.ca.

BERG, Karen M; 142 Park Dr, Salt Spring Island BC V8K 2R7; Man'82; Staff, Lady Minto Gulf Islands Hospital; (250)537-5750; Fax. (250)537-9946; drkmberg@telus.net.

BERG, Marina; The Polyclinic, 5-4646 Dufferin St, North York ON M3H 5S4; McM'03; CCFP; (416)222-6160

BERGEN, Daryl C; Mayfair Place, 120-6707 Elbow Dr SW, Calgary AB T2V 0E3; Cal'06; FRCPC; DiagRad. (403)777-3003; Fax. (403)777-3008.

BERGEN, Dorothea; Peace Arch Hosp, 15521 Russell Ave, White Rock BC V4B 2R4; Man'78; FRCPC; Psy. Staff, Peace Arch Hospital; (604)538-4240; Fax. (604)538-8500.

BERGEN, Harry J; Headwaters Specialist Clinic, 132-150 Rolling Hills Dr, Orangeville ON L9W 4X8; Wes'70; FRCSC; GenSurg. Ac Staff, Headwaters Health Care Centre - Orangeville Site; (519)941-8357; Fax. (519)938-5641.

BERGEN, Jerry M; Springfield Hgts Medical, 4-963 Henderson Hwy, Winnipeg MB R2K 2M3; Man'84; CCFP; Ac Staff, Concordia General Hospital; (204)663-4404; Fax. (204)663-3671.

BERGENS, Joanne E; Jasper Place Med Centre, 140 Meadowlark Shopping Ctr NW, Edmonton AB T5R 5W9; Tor'93; BSc; CCFP; Staff Physician, Covenant Health - Misericordia Community Hospital; Langs: English; French; (780)489-8470; Fax. (780)484-1620.

BERGER, Aimo; Kenderdine Med Clinic, 110-1804 McOrmond Dr, Saskatoon SK S7S 0A6; Humboldt (Germany)'00; CCFP; (306)934-6606

BERGER, Alan R; St Michael's Health Centre, 801-61 Queen St E, Toronto ON M5C 2T2; McG'83; BSc; FRCSC; Ophth (Retina Vitreous Surgery). Ac Staff, Sunnybrook Health Sciences Centre; Ac Staff, Toronto Western Hospital - University Health Network; (416)867-3663

BERGER, Brian; 1B-205 Don Head Village Blvd, Richmond Hill ON L4C 7R3; Cape Town (South Africa)'80; MB ChB; FABHPM; CCFP; FCFP; Ac Staff, Mackenzie Richmond Hill Hospital; Langs: Afrikaans; (905)770-8480; Fax. (905)770-1813; doc.brian.rica@rogers.com.

BERGER, Christopher W; Canadian Forces Hlth Serv Ctr, PO Box 99000 Stn Forces, Halifax NS B3K 5X5; Ott'86; FRCPC; Anes. Staff, Queen Elizabeth II Health Sciences Centre - Victoria General Site; Staff, Canadian Forces Health Services Centre (Atlantic); Lecturer Anes, Dalhousie University; (902)721-8751; Fax. (902)721-0395; mberger@eastlink.ca.

BERGER, Elizabeth D; Toronto East Gen Hosp, 825 Coxwell Ave, Toronto ON M5G 1V7; Tor'04; FRCPC; Peds. Staff, Toronto East General Hospital Inc; (416)530-9093

BERGER, Howard P; St Michael's Hosp, 30 Bond St, Toronto ON M5B 1W8; Ben Gurion (Israel)'94; Staff, St Michael's Hospital; Langs: Hebrew; (416)864-6060 x2395; Fax. (416)864-6073.

BERGER, Joseph; 501-4430 Bathurst St, North York ON M3H 3S3; London (England)'66; MB BS(Hons); DABPN; FRCPC; Psy (Assessment). (416)630-8775; Fax. (416)221-7728.

BERGER, Kenneth J I; 360A Bloor St W PO Box 19024 Rpo Walmer, Toronto ON M5S 3C9; Tor'92; Dip SportMed; BL; CCFP; CCFP(E.M.); Staff, Bridgepoint Health Centre; Med Staff, St Joseph's Health Centre; Consultant, Sports Injury Centre, Casual David L. MacIntosh Sports Injury Clinic & Team Phys. Rugby Canada; (416)356-9919; Fax. (416)461-6711; ken.berger@utoronto.ca.

BERGER, Leo R; Clinique Neuro Rive-Sud, 250-4896 boul Taschereau, Greenfield Park QC J4V 2J2; McG'80; FRCPC; Neur (Cerebrovascular Disease). Staff, Hopital Charles LeMoyne; assoc Prof, Universite de Sherbrooke; (514)672-1931; Fax. (514)672-3308.

BERGER, Lisa; Toronto Public Health, 8F-277 Victoria St, Toronto ON M5B 1W2; Man'77; FRCPC; CCFP; CommunMed. Physician, Anne Johnston Health Station; Aj Lecturer, University of Toronto; (416)338-7983; Fax. (416)338-7870; lberger@toronto.ca.

BERGER, Lucie; CSSS de Memphremagog, 50 rue Saint-Patrice E, Magog QC J1X 3X3; Sher'83; LMCC; Staff, Centre Hospitalier et CLSC de Memphremagog; (819)843-3381; Fax. (819)843-2786.

BERGER, Michelle; Clinique Med Sainte-Claire, GD 88 boul Begin, Sainte-Claire QC G0R 2V0; Laval'90; (418)883-3336; Fax. (418)883-2890.

BERGER, Pamela S; The Ottawa Hosp-Gen Campus, 501 Smyth Rd, Ottawa ON K1H 8L6; Wes'06; ObstGyn. Staff, The Ottawa Hospital - General Campus; (613)722-7000

BERGER, Philip B; SMH Health Centre, 4F-410 Sherbourne St, Toronto ON M4X 1K2; Man'74; CCFP; FCFP; Chief Family & CommunMed/Med Dir Inner City Hlth Core Servs, St Michael's Hospital; (416)867-3728; Fax. (416)867-3726.

BERGER, Robert K; The Moncton Hosp, 135 MacBeath Ave, Moncton NB E1C 6Z8; Dal'06; Gastroent; IntMed. Staff, The Moncton Hospital; (506)857-5111

BERGER, Sam; York-Finch Med Centre, 303-2115 Finch Ave W, North York ON M3N 2V6; Tor'67; DABIM; FRCP; FRCPC; Hem (Oncology); IntMed. Ac Staff, Humber River Regional Hospital - Finch Avenue Site; Court Staff, Toronto Western Hospital - University Health Network; Lecturer, University of Toronto; (416)745-4600

BERGER, Samuel; Lady Dunn Health Centre, 17 Government Rd, Wawa ON P0S 1K0; Cal'83; (705)856-2335

BERGER, Sheldon; The Carrington On The Park, 1204-1101 Leslie St, Toronto ON M3C 4G3; Tor'69.

BERGER-PELLETIER, Elyse; Hotel-Dieu de Levis, 143 rue Wolfe, Levis QC G6V 3Z1; Laval'06; FRCPC; EmergMed. Staff, Hôtel-Dieu de Lévis; (418)835-7122

BERGERON, Alain; Polyclinique Med Pierre-Le Gar, 300-1000 Montee des Pionniers, Terrebonne QC J6V 1S8; Mon'81; (450)657-1313; Fax. (450)657-1809.

BERGERON, Andre; Clinique méd familiale Montcal, 309 rue Montcalm, Chicoutimi QC G7J 2V1; Laval'73; ac Staff, Complexe hospitalier de la Sagamie; (418)545-4211; Fax. (418)545-2920.

BERGERON, Ann; Agence de santé et SS du SLSJ, 930 rue Jacques-Cartier E, Chicoutimi QC G7H 7K9; Laval'83; Staff, Complexe hospitalier de la Sagamie; (418)545-4980; Fax. (418)549-9710; ann.bergeron@ssss.gouv.qc.ca.

BERGERON, Anne; CLSC Saint-Hubert, 6800 boul Cousineau, Saint-Hubert QC J3Y 8Z4; Laval'74; (450)443-7400

BERGERON, Anne-Catherine; CSSS de Trois-Rivieres, 1991 boul du Carmel, Trois-Rivieres QC G8Z 3R9; Laval'08; CCFP; CCFP(E.M.); Staff, CSSS de Trois-Rivières; (819)697-3333

BERGERON, Annie-Claude; CSSS du Lac-des-Deux-Montagnes, 520 boul Arthur-Sauve, Saint-Eustache QC J7R 5B1; Mon'04; Staff, Hôpital de Saint-Eustache; Langs: Bilingual(French/English); (450)473-6811

BERGERON, Anthony; Hotel-Dieu d'Arthabaska, 5 rue des Hospitalieres, Victoriaville QC G6P 6N2; Mon'04; CCFP; Staff, Hotel-Dieu d'Arthabaska; (819)357-2030

BERGERON, Antoine; 108 ch des Faucons, Stoneham QC G3C 0T9; Laval'05; Staff, Centre Hospitalier Regional du Grand-Portage; (418)912-8104

BERGERON, Brenda A; Hop Charles Lemoyne, 3120 boul Taschereau, Greenfield Park QC J4V 2H1; McG'93; CCFP; Staff Emerg, Hopital Charles LeMoyne; Langs: Spanish; (450)466-5050

BERGERON, Celine; CHUM-Hotel-Dieu, 3840 rue Saint-Urbain, Montreal QC H2W 1T8; Laval'98; FRCPC; IntMed (Pneumology); Respir. Staff, Centre Hospitalier l'Université de Montréal (CHUM) - Hôtel-Dieu; Clinical Asst Prof, Universite de Montreal; Langs: English; (514)890-8000 x15660; Fax. (514)412-7123; celine.bergeron.1@umontreal.ca.

BERGERON, Chantal; CLSC Grande Riviere, 425 rue Leguerrier, Gatineau QC J9H 6N8; Mon'94; CCFP; Staff, Hôpital de Gatineau; Langs: English; (819)966-6540 x234; chantigone@yahoo.com.

BERGERON, Christine; CSSS Pierre Boucher, 1333 boul Jacques-Cartier E, Longueuil QC J4M 2A5; McG'97; Staff, Centre Hospitalier Pierre Boucher; (450)468-8111

BERGERON, Christine; Ctr Hosp Affilie-Enfant-Jesus, 1401 18e rue, Quebec QC G1J 1Z4; Laval'76; CSPQ; FRCPC; Anes. Staff, Centre Hospitalier Affilié Universitaire de Québec - Hôpital De L'Enfant Jésus; (418)649-5807

BERGERON, Claude; CHUS-Hop Fleurimont, 3001 12e av N, Sherbrooke QC J1H 5N4; Laval'77; FRCPC; Psy. Staff, Centre Hospitalier Universitaire de Sherbrooke-Hopital Fleurimont; (819)346-1110 x14000; Fax. (819)820-6420.

BERGERON, Claudie; Hôpital Reg Rimouski, CP 3150 succ A 150 av Rouleau, Rimouski QC G5L 5T1; Sher'07; Rheum; IntMed. Staff, Hôpital Regional Rimouski; (418)724-3000

BERGERON, Cybele; CHUS-Hop Fleurimont, 3001 12e av N, Sherbrooke QC J1H 5N4; Mon'00; FRCPC; Peds; InfectDis; MedMicrobiol. Staff, Centre Hospitalier Universitaire de Sherbrooke-Hopital Fleurimont; (819)346-1110 x12568

BERGERON, Dan; Clin d'Ophtalmologie Lebourgne, 200-777 boul Lebourgneuf, Quebec QC G2J 1C3; Laval'87; FRCSC; Ophth (Ocular Oncology). ac Membre Ophth, Centre Hospitalier Universitaire de Quebec-CHUL; Langs: English; (418)628-1417

BERGERON, Danielle; Psychanalytique for Psychotiqu, 388 rue Saint-Vallier O, Quebec QC G1K 1K6; Laval'72; FRCPC; Psy. (418)522-1555; Fax. (418)522-0562; dberger@sympatico.ca.

BERGERON, Denis; CHUS-Hop Fleurimont, 3001 12e av N, Sherbrooke QC J1H 5N4; Sher'75; FRCPC; DiagRad. Staff, Centre Hospitalier Universitaire de Sherbrooke-Hopital Fleurimont; adj Prof, Universite de Sherbrooke; (819)346-1110; Fax. (819)820-6420.

BERGERON, Dino; Centre Med Familiale de Granby, 48 rue Denison E, Granby QC J2G 4C6; Sher'93; Staff, Centre Hospitalier de Granby; (450)372-3996

BERGERON, Elise; 208-2780 av Raymond, Saint-Hyacinthe QC J2S 5W7; Mon'89; FRCSC; Ophth (Medical Ophthalmology). Staff, Centre Hospitalier Honore-Mercier; (450)773-2525; Fax. (450)773-8943.

BERGERON, Emile; Clinique Med Ste-Madeleine, 165 boul Sainte-Madeleine, Trois-Rivieres QC G8T 3L7; Laval'73; ac Staff Palliative Care, CSSS de Trois-Rivières; Physician, Abbitibi Consol(Belgo); (819)379-8385; Fax. (819)379-1607.

BERGERON, Eric; Hop Charles Lemoyne, 3120 boul Taschereau, Greenfield Park QC J4V 2H1; Mon'91; FRCSC; GenSurg. Staff, Hopital Charles LeMoyne; Langs: Bilingual(French/English); (450)466-5000 x5750; Fax. (450)466-5409.

BERGERON, Gerald; 1214 rue des Topazes, Quebec QC G2L 3A2; Laval'71; CCFP; FCFP; (418)622-1330; Fax. (418)628-4424.

BERGERON, Jacquelin; CSSS de Chicoutimi, 305 rue Saint-Vallier, Chicoutimi QC G7H 5H6; Laval'72; CSPQ; Anes (P.Q.). Staff, Complexe hospitalier de la Sagamie; (418)541-1234

BERGERON, Jacques; CHUQ-Ctr Hosp Univ Laval, 2705 boul Laurier, Quebec QC G1V 4G2; Sher'72; FRCSC; ObstGyn. Staff, Centre Hospitalier Universitaire de Quebec-CHUL; (418)525-4456

BERGERON, Jacques; Centre Med Robinson Inc, 4 rue Robinson N, Granby QC J2G 8Z9; Laval'79; (450)378-8438; Fax. (450)375-8832.

BERGERON, Jean B; Ministere de la Sante, 11e-1075 ch Sainte-Foy, Quebec QC G1S 2M1; Laval'50; (418)266-6746

BERGERON, Jean; CHUQ-Ctr Hosp Univ Laval, S224-2705 boul Laurier, Quebec QC G1V 4G2; Laval'86; CSPQ; MSc; FAHA; FRCPC; MedBiochem (Lipidology). Chef Lipid Clinic Dept of Med/adj Chef Dept of Med Biochemistry, Centre Hospitalier Universitaire de Quebec-CHUL; Langs: English; (418)654-2162; Fax. (418)654-2134; jean.bergeron@crchul.ulaval.ca.

BERGERON, Jean-Pierre; CSSS de Trois-Rivieres, 155 rue Toupin, Trois-Rivieres QC G8T 3Z8; Laval'73; Dir Professional Serv, Centre de santé Cloutier-du-Rivage; Regie Regionale Mauricie Centre du Quebec; (819)370-2221; Fax. (819)370-2471; jbergero_cloutier@ssss.gouv.qc.ca.

BERGERON, Julie; Hop Maisonneuve-Rosemont, 5415 boul de l'Assomption, Montreal QC H1T 2M4; Laval'98; FRCPC; IntMed; MedOncol (P.Q.); Hem. Staff, Hopital Maisonneuve-Rosemont; Langs: Bilingual(French/English); (514)252-3404; juliebergeron.hmr@ssss.gouv.qc.ca.

BERGERON, Julie; Ctr Hosp Affilie-Enfant-Jesus, 1401 18e rue, Quebec QC G1J 1Z4; Laval'06; FRCPC; IntMed. Staff, Centre Hospitalier Affilié Universitaire de Québec - Hôpital De L'Enfant Jésus.

BERGERON, Julie; CLSC de Villeray, 1425 rue Jarry E, Montreal QC H2E 1A7; Laval'04; CCFP; (514)376-4141

BERGERON, Karine; CHUQ-St-Francois d'Assise, B524-10 rue de l'Espinay, Quebec QC G1L 3L5; Laval'97; Staff, Centre Hospitalier Universitaire De Québec - Pavillon De St-françois-d'assise; (418)525-4444

BERGERON, Leonard; Hop du Sacre-Coeur de Mtl, 5400 boul Gouin O CP 109, Montreal QC H4J 1C5; McG'02; FRCSC; PlasSurg. Staff, Hôpital du Sacre-Coeur de Montréal; (514)338-2222

BERGERON, Lyne; CSSS Pierre Boucher, 1333 boul Jacques-Cartier E, Longueuil QC J4M 2A5; Mon'95; CSPQ; FRCPC; Anes. Staff, Centre Hospitalier Pierre Boucher; (450)468-8111

BERGERON, Marc; Ctr Hosp Affilie-Enfant-Jesus, 1401 18e rue, Quebec QC G1J 1Z4; Laval'74; FRCPC; Hem (Clinical Hematology); MedOncol (P.Q.). Head Hem/Oncol, Centre Hospitalier Affilié Universitaire de Québec - Hôpital De L'Enfant Jésus; Clin Prof, Université Laval; (418)649-5726; Fax. (418)649-5720.

BERGERON, Marc; CSSS Lac-des-Deux Montagnes, 201-1 Place de la Gare, Saint-Eustache QC J7R 0B4; Laval'89; Staff, Hôpital de Saint-Eustache; (450)473-6811 x7471; Fax. (450)491-5408; mark_bergeron@videotron.ca.

BERGERON, Marc-Andre; Comm Lesion Galeries Chagnon, 250-1200 boul Alphonse-Desjard, Levis QC G6V 6Y8; Laval'71; FRCPC; Electroenceph (P.Q.) (Migraines); Neur. Med Specialist, Bureau of Medical Evaluation Section; Med Specialist, Ministry du Travail du Quebec; (418)835-1722; Fax. (418)835-7163.

BERGERON, Marc-Yves; Clinique Med de Montmagny, 100-83 av de la Fabrique, Montmagny QC G5V 2J3; Ott'89; Langs: English; (418)248-4933; Fax. (418)248-2778; marcy.bergeron@gmf.gouv.qc.ca.

BERGERON, Marie; Clinique Epiderma, 999 boul de Maisonneuve O, Montreal QC H3A 3L4; Sher'78; (514)281-6760

BERGERON, Marie-Eve; Ctr Hosp de Matane, 333 rue Thibault, Matane QC G4W 2W5; Laval'08; CCFP; Staff, Centre Hospitalier de Matane; (418)562-3135

BERGERON, Marie-Eve; CHUQ-Ctr Hosp Univ Laval, 5762-2705 boul Laurier, Quebec QC G1V 4G2; Laval'06; FRCSC; ObstGyn. Staff, Centre Hospitalier Universitaire de Quebec-CHUL; (418)654-2738

BERGERON, Marie-France; CSSS de Laval, 1.88-1755 boul Rene-Laennec, Laval QC H7M 3L9; Mon'95; Respir; IntMed. Staff, Hopital de la Cite de la santé; (450)668-1010

BERGERON, Maryse; Clinique Le Medical, 285-1750 boul Marie-Victorin, Longueuil QC J4G 1A5; Mon'87; Staff, Centre Hospitalier Pierre Boucher; (450)442-9531

BERGERON, Maurice; 102-335 rue Ellice, Beauharnois QC J6N 1X2; Mon'63; Med Dir, Rio Tinto Alcan; Langs: Bilingual(French/English); (450)429-7281; Fax. (450)429-4188.

BERGERON, Maxime; CSSS de Saint-Jerome, 290 rue de Montigny, Saint-Jerome QC J7Z 5T3; Mon'09; Staff, Hôtel-Dieu de Saint-Jérôme; (450)431-8200

BERGERON, Michel; Ctr Hosp Univ de Quebec-CHUL, 709-2705 boul Laurier, Quebec QC G1V 4G2; Laval'68; ABIM; FRCPC; IntMed (Infectious Diseases); MedMicrobiol (P.Q.). Chair InfectDis Research Centre & Specialist, Centre Hospitalier Universitaire de Quebec-CHUL; Internal Med, Hôpital Laval; Prof, Université Laval; (418)525-4444 x48753; michel.g.bergeron@crchul.ulaval.ca.

BERGERON, Nicolas; CHUM-Hotel-Dieu, 3840 rue Saint-Urbain, Montreal QC H2W 1T8; Mon'94; FRCPC; Psy (Consultant Liaison Psychiatry). Staff, Centre Hospitalier l'Université de Montréal (CHUM) - Hôtel-Dieu; (514)890-8000 x36155; nbergeron@yahoo.com.

BERGERON, Nicole; Ctr Hosp Affilie-St-Sacrement, 1050 ch Sainte-Foy, Quebec QC G1S 4L8; Laval'76; CST; Staff, Centre Hospitalier Affilié Universitaire de Québec - Hôpital du St-Sacrement; (418)682-7878

BERGERON, Paule; CRSSS Baie-James-Sante Label, 950 boul Quevillon, Lebel-s-Quevillon QC J0Y 1X0; Laval'84; Staff, Centre de santé Lebel; Physician, CLSC Antoine Rivard; (819)755-4881; Fax. (819)755-3779.

BERGERON, Pierre; Ctr Hosp Affilie-St-Sacrement, 1050 ch Sainte-Foy, Quebec QC G1S 4L8; Laval'75; CSPQ; AnatPath. Staff, Centre Hospitalier Affilié Universitaire de Québec - Hôpital du St-Sacrement; (418)682-7511

BERGERON, Pierre; Clinique Fam d'Arthabaska, 2-39 rue Laurier E, Victoriaville QC G6P 6P6; Laval'86; assoc Staff, Hôpital Sainte-croix.

BERGERON, Pierre; Cornwall Comm Hosp-Mcconnell, PO Box 100 Stn Main 840 McConnell Ave, Cornwall ON K6H 5S5; Ott'95; CCFP; CCFP(E.M.); Staff, Cornwall Community Hospital; (613)938-4240; Fax. (613)948-4069.

BERGERON, Pierre; CSSS Pierre Boucher, 1333 boul Jacques-Cartier E, Longueuil QC J4M 2A5; Laval'84; FRCPC; DiagRad. Staff Diag Imaging, Centre Hospitalier Pierre Boucher; (450)468-8157

BERGERON, Pierre; Inst Nat'l de Sante Publique, 100-190 boul Crémazie E, Montreal QC H2P 1E2; Laval'71; MSc(Epidem.); PhD(PoliticSci); FRCPC; CommunMed (P.Q.); Public Health & Preventive Med. ac Membre, Centre Hospitalier Universitaire de Québec (CHUQ) - Siege Social; Langs: English; French; (514)864-1600 x3600; Fax. (514)864-5180; pierre.bergeron@inspq.qc.ca.

BERGERON, Richard F; Clinique Ophtalmovision, 308-5995 boul Gouin O, Montreal QC H4J 2P8; Mon'80; FRCSC; Ophth (Refractive Surgery). Staff Laser Clinic, Hôpital du Sacre-Coeur de Montréal; Prof, Universite de Montreal; Langs: Bilingual(French/English); (514)335-4492; Fax. (514)335-6710.

BERGERON, Richard; Centre Med Brunswick, 401-955 boul Saint-Jean, Pointe-Claire QC H9R 5K3; Mon'80; (514)426-6677

BERGERON, Richard; Ctr Hosp Pierre-Janet, 20 rue Pharand, Gatineau QC J9A 1K7; Sher'86; FRCPC; Psy. Staff, Centre Hospitalier Pierre-Janet; (819)776-8027; Fax. (819)771-4849; rbergeron@ohri.ca.

BERGERON, Rénald; UMF Laval, 2690 ch des Quatre-Bourgeois, Quebec QC G1V 0B7; Laval'79; CCFP; FCFP; Staff, Hôpital Laval; Doyen Faculty of Med, Université Laval; (418)656-4795; renald.bergeron@mfa.ulaval.ca.

BERGERON, Sebastien; Hôpital Laval, 2725 ch Sainte-Foy, Quebec QC G1V 4G5; Mon'96; CSPQ; FRCPC; IntMed; Cardiol. Staff, Hôpital Laval; (418)656-8711; Fax. (418)656-4581.

BERGERON, Serge B; CSSS de Chicoutimi, CP 5006 305 rue Saint-Vallier, Chicoutimi QC G7H 5H6; Sher'84; Staff, Complexe hospitalier de la Sagamie; (418)541-1000

BERGERON, Solange; Aylmer-Lucerne Med Centre, 67 rue Du Couvent, Gatineau QC J9H 6A2; Laval'85; (819)684-1234 x200; Fax. (819)684-1240.

BERGERON, Sophie; Centre Cleophas-Claveau, 1000 rue Du Docteur-desgagne, La Baie QC G7B 2Y6; Laval'97; Staff, CHSLD-CLSC Cleophas-Claveau; (418)544-3381; Fax. (418)544-0770.

BERGERON, Sophie; Hotel-Dieu de Roberval, 450 rue Brassard, Roberval QC G8H 1B9; Laval'00; CSPQ; FRCPC; AnatPath. Staff, Hotel-Dieu de Roberval; (418)275-0110 x2356

BERGERON, Sophie; CSSSG-Hop de Gatineau, CP 2000 Succ Bureau-Chef 909 boul de la Verendrye, Gatineau QC J8P 7H2; Sher'06; Peds. Staff, Hôpital de Gatineau; (819)966-6100

BERGERON, Stephane; SMBD Jewish Gen Hosp, 3755 ch Côte-Sainte-Catherine, Montreal QC H3T 1E2; McG'05; FRCSC; OrthSurg. Staff, Sir Mortimer B Davis Jewish General; (514)340-8222

BERGERON, Sylvie; Clinique Med Sanctuaire, 6100 av Du Boise, Montreal QC H3S 2W1; Sher'85; Peds. (514)739-5646

BERGERON, Vincent; CHUQ-Ctr Hosp Univ Laval, 2100-2705 boul Laurier, Quebec QC G1V 4G2; Laval'75; FRCPC; DiagRad (Echography). ac Staff, Centre Hospitalier Universitaire de Quebec-CHUL; (418)654-2258

BERGERON, Vincent; CHUQ-St-Francois d'Assise, B3 540-10 rue de l'Espinay, Quebec QC G1L 3L5; Laval'05; FRCPC; IntMed. Staff, Centre Hospitalier Universitaire De Québec - Pavillon De St-françois-d'assise; (418)525-4465; Fax. (418)525-4467.

BERGERON, Viviane; CHAQ-Hôp de l'Enfant-Jésus, 1401 18e rue, Quebec QC G1J 1Z4; Laval'02; FRCPC; IntMed; Gastroent. Staff, Centre Hospitalier Affilié Universitaire de Québec - Hôpital De L'Enfant Jésus; (418)649-0252

BERGERON, Yves M; Institut de Physiatrie Quebec, 2049 rue Sherbrooke E, Montreal QC H2K 1C1; Mon'75; FACP; FRCPC; PhysMed&Rehab. Chef méd phys & réadap, Centre Hospitalier l'Université de Montréal (CHUM) - Hôpital Notre-Dame; Dir, Institut de Physiatrie Quebec; (514)527-4155; Fax. (514)598-9963.

BERGEVIN, Alain A; CSSS Haut-Richelieu-Rouville, 920 boul Du Seminaire N, St-Jean-Sur-Richel QC J3A 1B7; Mon'92; CCFP; Staff, Hôpital du Haut-Richelieu; (450)359-5000; Fax. (450)359-5251.

BERGEVIN, Marco; CSSS de Laval, SS 215-1755 boul Rene-Laennec, Laval QC H7M 3L9; Sher'02; FRCPC; IntMed; InfectDis (AIDS/HIV); MedMicrobiol. Staff, Hopital de la Cite de la santé; Langs: Spanish; French; (450)975-5558; mbergevin.csssl@ssss.gouv.qc.ca.

BERGH, Anton E; 12 West Med Clinic, 130-227 11 Ave SW, Calgary AB T2R 1R9; Cape Town (South Africa)'85; MB ChB; (403)210-0121; Fax. (403)210-0320.

BERGH, Irene C; 104-1865 Dilworth Dr, Kelowna BC V1Y 9T1; Sask'95; CCFP; Langs: Hungarian; German; (250)717-0909; Fax. (250)717-0906.

BERGH, Nikoletta; Westgrove Med Clinic, 201-505 Queen St, Spruce Grove AB T7X 2V2; Alb'10; CCFP; (780)962-9888; Fax. (780)960-5298.

BERGH, Rodney M; 160 Percy St, Ottawa ON K1R 6E5; Dal'57; FRCPC; Peds (Administration). Teacher, Children's Hospital of Eastern Ontario (CHEO); Langs: English; French; (613)231-5000; Fax. (613)231-5002.

BERGHUIS, Harold P; West End Med Centre, 510 Prince St, Truro NS B2N 1G1; Mem'90; CCFP; FCFP; Langs: Dutch; (902)893-7422; Fax. (902)893-1026.

BERGHUIS-HUMMEL, Wendy D; Manotick Med Centre, 5492 South River Dr, Manotick ON K4M 1J3; Ott'91; CCFP; FCFP; (613)692-2571; Fax. (613)692-0271.

BERGIN, Fiona A; Mumford Clinic, 265-6960 Mumford Rd, Halifax NS B3L 4P1; Dal'91; BA; LLB; CCFP; Asst Prof, Dalhousie University; (902)473-4700; Fax. (902)473-8548.

BERGIN, M Lynn; London HSC-University Hosp, PO Box 5339 Stn B C6 133D-339 Windermere Rd, London ON N6A 5A5; Ott'84; ABIM; FACC; FRCPC; IntMed (Adult Congenital Heart Disease); Cardiol. Staff, London Health Sciences Centre - University Hospital; (519)663-3486; Fax. (519)663-3487.

BERGIN, Patrick C; Queen Elizabeth Hosp, PO Box 6600 Stn Central, Charlottetown PE C1A 8T5; Dal'88; FRCPC; IntMed. Staff, Queen Elizabeth Hospital; (902)894-0114; Fax. (902)894-0117; bergin@pei.aibn.com.

BERGIN, Siobhan M; The Nova Scotia Hosp, PO Box 1004 Stn Main, Dartmouth NS B2Y 3Z9; Dal'87; FRCPC; Psy. Staff, The Nova Scotia Hospital; Lecturer, Dalhousie University; (902)466-1830; Fax. (902)466-1851.

BERGMAN, Amanda D; Agassiz Med Centre, 130-30 Stephen St, Morden MB R6M 2G3; Man'07; CCFP.

BERGMAN, Arik; North York Gen Hosp, 4001 Leslie St, North York ON M2K 1E1; Wes'02; FRCPC; IntMed; Nephrol. Staff, North York General Hospital; (416)756-6000

BERGMAN, Arthur; 1202 Pender St W PO Box 17530, Vancouver BC V6E 0B2; Yerevan (Armenia (Republic))'88; MD; CCFP; (604)436-0800

BERGMAN, Bonnie R; Jewish Rehab Hosp, 3205 Place Alton-Goldbloom, Laval QC H7V 1R2; McG'94; CCFP; Staff, Jewish Rehabilitation Hospital; (450)688-9550

BERGMAN, Elin; Assiniboine Clinic, 633 Lodge Ave, Winnipeg MB R3J 0S9; Man'84; BSc(Chem.); CCFP; (204)958-6785; Fax. (204)888-1750.

BERGMAN, Grace E; Royal Columbian Hosp, 330 Columbia St E, New Westminster BC V3L 3W7; UBC'71; FRCPC; Anes. Ac Staff, Royal Columbian Hospital; (604)520-4602; Fax. (604)520-4899.

BERGMAN, Henry S; 202-1194 Lansdowne Dr, Coquitlam BC V3E 1J7; UBC'77; (604)464-1155; Fax. (604)464-2227.

BERGMAN, Howard; SMBD Jewish Gen Hosp, 3755 ch Cote-Sainte-Catherine, Montreal QC H3T 1E2; McG'69; FRCPC; GeriatricMed (P.Q.);CCFP; FCFP; Staff Div of Geriatric Med, Sir Mortimer B Davis Jewish General; Chef Family Med/Prof Geriatric Med The Dr Joseph Kaufmann, McGill University; Langs: English; Bilingual(French/English); (514)340-8222 x4352; Fax. (514)340-8617; howard.bergman@mcgill.ca.

BERGMAN, James N; Medical Bldg, 1803-805 Broadway Ave W, Vancouver BC V5Z 1K1; Man'91; FRCPC; Peds; Derm; ClinImmunol&Allergy. (604)876-4433; Fax. (604)876-4431.

BERGMAN, Joseph W; 123-11910 111 Ave NW, Edmonton AB T5G 0E5; Cal'01; FRCSC; OrthSurg. (780)453-8985; Fax. (780)447-4537.

BERGMAN, June S; Crowfoot Village Prof Centre, 201-60 Crowfoot Cres NW, Calgary AB T3G 3J9; Tor'70; CCFP; FCFP; Chair Board, Calgary Foothills Primary Care Network; Board Member, Canadian Counsel of Health System Accrediation; Assoc Prof Emeritus, University of Calgary; (403)862-1947; Fax. (403)206-7577; bergman@ucalgary.ca.

BERGMAN, Samuel; 205-1670 Dufferin St, Toronto ON M6H 3M2; Technion (Israel)'76; (416)652-9862; Fax. (416)652-3960.

BERGMAN, Simon; SMBD Jewish Gen Hosp, 3755 ch Cote-Sainte-Catherine, Montreal QC H3T 1E2; McG'01; MSc; FACS; FRCSC; GenSurg. Staff, Sir Mortimer B Davis Jewish General; Langs: Bilingual(French/English); (514)340-8222 x4611; Fax. (514)340-7937.

BERGMANN, Terence; Concordia Gen Hosp, 1095 Concordia Ave, Winnipeg MB R2K 3S8; Man'90; Staff, Concordia General Hospital; (204)667-1560

BERGNER, Anahy; Pan Am Clinic, 75 Poseidon Bay, Winnipeg MB R3M 3E4; (Other Foreign)'08.

BERGSON, Victor S; George Pearson Centre, 700 57th Ave W, Vancouver BC V6P 1S1; Cambridge (England)'71; MB ChB; MRCP(UK); (604)321-3231

BERGSTROM, Craig L; Parkgate Med Centre, 220-3650 Mt Seymour Pky, North Vancouver BC V7H 2Y5; McG'77; Staff, Lions Gate Hospital; (604)929-1268; Fax. (604)929-7329.

BERGSTROM, Debra J; Health Sciences Centre, 300 Prince Philip Dr, St. John's NL A1B 3V6; Alb'04; FRCPC; IntMed; Hem. Staff, Health Sciences Centre; (709)777-1334; Fax. (709)777-6532.

BERGSTROM, Richard G; University of Alberta Hosp, 8440 112 St NW, Edmonton AB T6G 2B7; Alb'81; FRCPC; Anes (Cardiovascular Anesthesia). Staff, University of Alberta Hospital; Clin Assoc Prof Anes & Pain Med, University of Alberta; Langs: English; French; (780)407-8861; Fax. (780)486-4094.

BERGSTROME, Brant E; Waypoint Centre for Mental H C, 500 Church St, Penetanguishene ON L9M 1G3; Hamburg (Germany)'90; FRCP; BScChemEng; PhD; FRCPC; Psy (Forensic Psychiatry). Staff Oak Ridge Div, Waypoint Centre for Mental Health Care; Langs: German; (705)549-3181 x2043; Fax. (705)549-3652; bbergstrome@waypointcentre.ca.

BERHE, Tzeggai; 600-10014 99 St, Grande Prairie AB T8V 3N4; (Germany)'93; MRCPsy; PhD; Staff, Queen Elizabeth II Hospital; (780)538-5160; Fax. (780)538-6279.

BÉRIAULT, Karine; Hop Brome-Missisquoi-Perkins, 950 rue Principale, Cowansville QC J2K 1K3; Sher'09; CCFP; Staff, Hôpital Brome-Missisquoi-Perkins; (450)266-4342

BERIAULT, Marie-Josee; CSSS de Trois-Rivieres, 1991 boul du Carmel, Trois-Rivieres QC G8Z 3R9; Sher'05; Critical Care Medicine; IntMed. Staff, CSSS de Trois-Rivières; (819)697-3333

BERIAULT, Michael T; Foothills Anesthesia, 1409 29 St NW, Calgary AB T2N 4J8; Qns'79; FRCPC; Anes. Staff Anes, Foothills Medical Centre; Clin Assoc Prof, University of Calgary; (403)944-1430; Fax. (403)670-2425.

BERIH, Abdullahi A; 301-222 Dixon Rd, Etobicoke ON M9P 3S5; Dal'91; BSc(Hons); CCFP; Langs: Arabic; Tigrigna; Belen; (416)247-8781; Fax. (416)247-8670.

BERING, Michael P; Medical Centre, 6-1036 7 St SW, Medicine Hat AB T1A 8V7; Alb'91; FRCSC; OrthSurg. Med Staff, Medicine Hat Regional Hospital; Clin Lecturer, University of Calgary; (403)504-5463; Fax. (403)504-5468.

BERINSTEIN, Edward F; Gibsons Med Clinic, 211-1100 Sunshine Coast Hwy, Gibsons BC V0N 1V7; Man'72; CCFP; FCFP; (604)886-2868

BERINSTEIN, Neil L; Toronto Sunnybrook Reg Cancer, 2075 Bayview Ave, Toronto ON M4N 3M5; Man'78; ABIM(IntMed&MedOncol); FRCPC; IntMed (Hematological Oncology); MedOncol. Ac Staff, Sunnybrook Health Sciences Centre; (416)480-5248

BERISTAIN, Guillermo R; 845 Evergreen Ave, Courtenay BC V9N 6Y1; (Mexico)'68; FRCSC; Urol. Staff Urol, Campbell River & District General Hospital; Staff Urol, St Joseph's General Hospital; Langs: Spanish; (250)338-7292

BERJAT, B Maria; 240-4260 av Girouard, Montreal QC H4A 3C9; Bialystok (Poland)'69; (514)489-5753

BERJAT, Michel E; CHUM-Hotel-Dieu, 3840 rue Saint-Urbain, Montreal QC H2W 1T8; Paris (France)'73; FRCPC; Rheum. Staff, Centre Hospitalier l'Université de Montréal (CHUM) - Hôtel-Dieu; (514)890-8000 x14835

BERJAT, Vanessa E I; Rocky Med Clinic, PO Box 99 Stn Main 5127 49 St, Rocky-Mtn-House AB T4T 1A1; McG'07; MDCM; CCFP; (403)845-2815; Fax. (403)845-2177.

BERKA, L Jane; Nork York Fam Phys After Hours, 2801 Bayview Ave, North York ON M2K 1E6; Karlova (Czech Republic)'63; PhD(ClinGenetics); CCFP; FCFP; Ac Staff, North York General Hospital; Langs: Czech; Slovak; Polish; Russian; (416)491-6338

BERKAL, Allen B; 308-4430 Bathurst St, North York ON M3H 3S3; Man'75; FRCPC; Psy (Anxiety Disorder). (416)638-7939; Fax. (416)638-8527.

BERKMAN, Alan C; Nanaimo Reg Gen Hosp, 1200 Dufferin Cres, Nanaimo BC V9S 2B7; Pretoria (South Africa)'85; MB ChB; FRCPC; Anes. Staff, Nanaimo Regional General Hospital; (250)754-2141; Fax. (250)755-7633.

BERKMAN, Frances A; 600-1355 Bank St, Ottawa ON K1H 8K7; Tor'90; CCFP; (613)737-4809; Fax. (613)739-3723.

BERKSHIRE, Andrew J; Kings Place, 400-440 King St, Fredericton NB E3B 5H8; Dal'89; FRCSC; OrthSurg (Arthroplasty). , Dr Everett Chalmers Regional Hospital; (506)459-2655; Fax. (506)443-0881; aberkshire@nb.aibn.com.

BERKSON, Laeora; SMBD Jewish Gen Hosp, A710-3755 ch Cote-Sainte-Cathe, Montreal QC H3T 1E2; McG'79; FRCPC; IntMed (Clinical & Education); Rheum. Staff, Sir Mortimer B Davis Jewish General; Staff, McGill University Health Centre - Royal Victoria Hospital; assoc Prof, McGill University; (514)340-8222 x4840; Fax. (514)340-8222.

BERLIE, Marie C; Clinique de Waskaganish, GD, Waskaganish QC J0M 1R0; McG'90; CCFP; FCFP; (819)895-8833; Fax. (819)895-8871.

BERLIM, Marcelo T; Douglas Mental Hlth Univ Inst, F 3131 2-6875 boul Lasalle, LaSalle QC H4H 1R3; Staff, Douglas Mental Health University Institute; (514)767-6131

BERLIN, Randall J; Alexandra Comm Health Centre, 1318 Centre St NE, Calgary AB T2E 2R7; Alb'88; DABEM; CCFP; Staff, Foothills Medical Centre; University of Calgary; (403)266-2622; Fax. (403)266-2692.

BERLIN, Seymour; 18B-3200 Dufferin St, North York ON M6A 0A1; Tor'62; CCFP; FCFP; (416)783-3544; Fax. (416)783-7413.

BERLINER, Yaniv; Univ Hlth Network-Toronto Western Hosp, 399 Bathurst St, Toronto ON M5T 2S8; Wes'04; CCFP; CCFP(E.M.); Staff, Toronto Western Hospital - University Health Network; (416)603-2581

BERLINGIERI, Joseph C; 301-2951 Walker's Line, Burlington ON L7M 4Y1; Tor'90; BA; FRCPC; IntMed (Critical Care Medicine). Ac Staff, Joseph Brant Memorial Hospital; (905)331-3101; Fax. (905)319-2499.

BERLINGUET, Helene; CLSC Portneuf, 427A boul Chabot, St-Ubald QC G0A 4L0; Laval'78; Physician, CLSC St-Ubald; (418)277-2256; Fax. (418)277-2888.

BERLINGUET, Jean-Claude; 245 rue du Cure-Majeau, Joliette QC J6E 8S8; Mon'77; VascSurg; GenSurg. Staff, Centre Hospitalier Régional de Lanaudière; (450)759-1157 x4297

BERLINGUET, Marc; CHUQ-Hotel-Dieu de Quebec, 11 Cote du Palais, Quebec QC G1R 2J6; Laval'75; FRCPC; CommunMed (P. Q.); Public Health & Preventive Med. Staff, Centre Hospitalier Universitaire de Québec (CHUQ) - Siege Social; (418)691-5151

BERLYNE, Graham S; St Joseph's Health Centre, 310-30 The Queensway, Toronto ON M6R 1B5; Manchester (England)'89; FRCPC; IntMed. Staff, St Joseph's Health Centre; (416)530-6158

BERMACK, Barry A; 3050G Portage Ave, Winnipeg MB R3K 0Y1; Man'68; FRCPC; Peds. Ac Staff Children's Hosp, Health Sciences Centre; Assoc Prof Peds, University of Manitoba; (204)885-6442; Fax. (204)831-7240; bbermack@shaw.ca.

BERMAN, Hal Kenneth; Univ Hlth Network-Toronto Gen, EN11 E230-200 Elizabeth St, Toronto ON M5G 2C4; Southwestern Texas (USA)'01; Staff, Toronto General Hospital - UHN; (416)340-4902

BERMAN, Hershl; 4F-60 Murray St Box 13, Toronto ON M5T 3L9; Qns'98; BEd; BSc; FRCPC; IntMed (Palliative Care). Staff, Toronto General Hospital - UHN; Staff, Mount Sinai Hospital; Langs: Yiddish; (416)856-4800; hal.berman@uhn.on.ca.

BERMAN, Isaac; Statcare Clinic, 104-175 ch Stillview, Pointe-Claire QC H9R 4S3; McG'05; CCFP; (514)697-9976

BERMAN, Jason N; IWK Health Centre, PO Box 9700 Rpo CSC 5850-5980 University Ave, Halifax NS B3K 6R8; Tor'97; FAAP; FRCPC; Peds (Pediatric Oncology). Staff, IWK Health Centre; Langs: Hebrew; (902)470-6552; Fax. (902)470-7216; jason.berman@iwk.nshealth.ca.

BERMAN, Kevin; Worksafe BC, 104-3020 Lincoln Ave, New Westminster BC V3B 6B4; Qns'88; Staff, Maple Ridge Mental Health; Staff, Greater Vancouver Mental Health; Clin Instructor Psy, University of British Columbia; (604)232-1906; kberman@bcmhs.bc.ca.

BERMAN, Michael; 15450 Vine Ave, White Rock BC V4B 2T4; Cape Town (South Africa)'71; MB ChB; MRC(UK); FRC; FRCSC; Ophth (Oculo Plastic Surgery). Ac Staff, Vancouver General Hospital - Centennial Pavillion; Consultant, Peace Arch Hospital; Clin Assoc Prof, University of British Columbia; Langs: Afrikaans; (604)531-3212; Fax. (604)531-4012.

BERMAN-WONG, Eva; Seven Regions Health Centre, PO Box 1000, Gladstone MB R0J 0T0; Man'93; MSc; CCFP; FCFP; Staff, Seven Regions Health Centre; University of Manitoba; Langs: Czech; (204)385-2078

BERNACKI, Barry A; 204-321A 21st St E, Saskatoon SK S7K 0C1; Man'94; BSc; FRCPC; PhysMed&Rehab. Staff, Saskatoon City Hospital; (306)244-4505; Fax. (306)244-4506.

BERNADAS, Sue Anne; PO Box 22506 Rpo Southbrook, Edmonton AB T6W 0C3; Alb'95; CCFP; Staff, Fort Saskatchewan Health Centre; (780)721-1142

BERNADSKA, Ewa; St Joseph's Health Care, PO Box 5777 Stn B 268 Grosvenor St, London ON N6A 4V2; Wroclaw (Poland)'80; FRCPC; Anes. Staff, St Joseph's Hospital - St Joseph's Health Care; (519)646-6100 x64505

BERNARD, Afiya; William Osler HC-Brampton, 2100 Bovaird Dr E, Brampton ON L6R 3J7; American University of the Caribbean (St Maarten)'04; CCFP; Staff, William Osler Health System - Etobicoke General Hospital; (905)494-2120

BERNARD, Andre; 8007 boul Mathieu, Quebec QC G1G 3M1; Laval'66; (418)628-1223; Fax. (418)628-0978.

BERNARD, Andre M; Queen Elizabeth II HSC, 10W-1276 South Park St, Halifax NS B3H 2Y9; Dal'06; FRCPC; Anes. Staff, Queen Elizabeth II Health Sciences Centre - Victoria General Site; (902)473-2331; Fax. (902)423-9454.

BERNARD, Annie; Hôpital Sainte-Croix, 570 rue Heriot, Drummondville QC J2B 1C1; Laval'07; DiagRad. Staff, Hôpital Sainte-croix; (819)478-6464

BERNARD, Brigitte; MSSS, 180-1005 ch Sainte-Foy, Quebec QC G1S 4N4; Sher'81; Peds. Med Consultant, Hôpital Laval; Med Consultant, Ministry of Health-Quebec; (418)266-5993

BERNARD, Carrie D; Queen Square Doctors FHT, 201-366 Main St N, Brampton ON L6V 1P8; McM'97; CCFP; Ac Staff, William Osler Health System - Brampton Civic Hospital; (905)455-1331; Fax. (905)455-5498.

BERNARD, Chantal; MUHC-Montreal Children's Hosp, 2300 rue Tupper, Montreal QC H3H 1P3; Sher'85; CSPQ; FRCPC; AnatPath. Staff, McGill University Health Centre - Montreal Children's Hospital; Consultant, Centre Hospitalier Universitaire de Sherbrooke-Hôpital Hôtel-Dieu; (514)412-4495; chantal.bernard@muhc.mcgill.ca.

BERNARD, Charles; Centre Med Ste-Foy Inc, 802 av Du Chanoine-Scott, Quebec QC G1V 3N4; Laval'75; ac Staff, Hôpital Laval; assoc Staff, Centre Hospitalier Affilié Universitaire de Québec - Hôpital du St-Sacrement; (418)653-4931; Fax. (418)653-4797; charlesbernard@videotron.ca.

BERNARD, Claire; CSSS de la région de Thetford, 1717 rue Notre-Dame E, Thetford Mines QC G6G 2V4; Laval'74; CSPQ; FRCPC; Anes. ac Staff Anes, Hopital du CSS de la Region de Thetford; (418)338-7777

BERNARD, Claude; Ctr Hosp Pierre-Janet, 20 rue Pharand, Gatineau QC J9A 1K7; Ott'70; Psy (P.Q.) (Clinical Psychiatry). Staff, Centre Hospitalier Pierre-Janet; (819)771-7761 x8010

BERNARD, Dalia A; Haldimand Family Health Team, 334 Broad St W, Dunnville ON N1A 1T1; Al-Mustansiriyah (Iraq)'86; CCFP; Staff, Haldimand War Memorial Hospital; (905)774-7541; Fax. (905)774-4310.

BERNARD, David; CSSS du Sud de Lanaudière, 911 Montee des Pionniers, Terrebonne QC J6V 2H2; Mon'09; CCFP; Staff, Centre Hospitalier Pierre le Gardeur; (450)654-7525

BERNARD, Denis; CHUM-Hop St-Luc, 6218-1058 rue Saint-Denis, Montreal QC H2X 3J4; Mon'63; GenSurg (Colon & Rectal Surgery). Med Coord, Centre Hospitalier l'Université De Montréal (CHUM) - Hôpital Saint-luc; Prof, Universite de Montreal; (514)890-8000 x34953; Fax. (514)412-7331.

BERNARD, Diane; Ctr Hosp Trois-Riv-St-Joseph, 731 rue Sainte-Julie, Trois-Rivieres QC G9A 1Y1; Laval'09; CCFP; CCFP(E.M.); Staff, Centre Hospitalier Regional de Trois-Rivieres; (819)697-3333

BERNARD, Edmond-Jean; CHUM-Hotel-Dieu, 3840 rue Saint-Urbain, Montreal QC H2W 1T8; Mon'87; FRCPC; IntMed; Gastroent. Staff IntMed & Gastroent, Centre Hospitalier l'Université de Montréal (CHUM) - Hôtel-Dieu; (514)890-8000 x14980

BERNARD, Francis; Hop Du Sacre-Coeur De Mtl, 5400 boul Gouin O, Montreal QC H4J 1C5; Mon'98; FRCPC; IntMed; Critical Care Medicine (P.Q.). Staff, Hôpital du Sacre-Coeur de Montréal; (514)338-2222

BERNARD, Genevieve; MUHC-Montreal Children's Hosp, A506-2300 rue Tupper, Montreal QC H3H 1P3; Mon'02; FRCPC; Neur (Movement Disorders). Staff, McGill University Health Centre - Montreal Children's Hospital; Langs: Bilingual(French/English); (514)412-4400 x24446; Fax. (514)412-4373.

BERNARD, Jean; CHUQ-Ctr Hosp Univ Laval, 2705 boul Laurier, Quebec QC G1V 4G2; Laval'76; ABD; FRCPC; Derm. ac Staff, Centre Hospitalier Universitaire de Quebec-CHUL; (418)654-2160; Fax. (418)654-2187.

BERNARD, Julie; CLSC de Paspebiac, CP 7000 273 boul Gerard-D-Levesque, Paspebiac QC G0C 2K0; Mon'99; Staff, CLSC de Paspebiac; (418)752-2572

BERNARD, Kelvin J R; Albany Med Clinic, 807 Broadview Ave, Toronto ON M4K 2P8; Tor'99; BSc(Hon)Pharm; CCFP; (416)461-9471; Fax. (416)461-2710.

BERNARD, Lea; Hop Maisonneuve-Rosemont, 5415 boul de l'Assomption, Montreal QC H1T 2M4; McG'03; Hem; IntMed. Staff, Hopital Maisonneuve-Rosemont; (514)252-3404

BERNARD, Marie; Ctr Hosp de Matane, 333 rue Thibault, Matane QC G4W 2W5; Mon'08; CCFP; Staff, Centre Hospitalier de Matane.

BERNARD, Martine; Clinique Maisonneuve-Rosemont, 340-5345 boul de l'Assomption, Montreal QC H1T 4B3; Sher'95; FRCSC; ObstGyn. Staff ObstGyn, Hopital Maisonneuve-Rosemont; Affil Staff, Universite de Montreal; (514)257-0961; Fax. (514)257-1460.

BERNARD, Maryse; Hop Maisonneuve-Rosemont, 5415 boul de l'Assomption, Montreal QC H1T 2M4; Mon'04; FRCPC; RadOncol (Lymphoma). Staff, Hopital Maisonneuve-Rosemont; Langs: Bilingual(French/English); (514)252-3400; marysebernard.hmr@ssss.gouv.qc.ca.

BERNARD, Matthew D; RCH Care Clinic, 330 Columbia St E, New Westminster BC V3L 3W7; UBC'05; FRCPC; IntMed. (604)520-4898

BERNARD, Maude; Ctr Hosp Laurentien, 234 rue Saint-Vincent, Ste-Agathe-des-Mts QC J8C 2B8; Sher'07; FRCPC; IntMed. Staff, Centre Hospitalier Laurentien; (819)324-4000

BERNARD, Nicolas; Hotel-Dieu de Levis, 143 rue Wolfe, Levis QC G6V 3Z1; Laval'96; CCFP; CCFP(E.M.); Staff, Hôtel-Dieu de Lévis; (418)835-7122

BERNARD, Pascale; CHUQ-St-Francois d'Assise, 10 rue de l'Espinay, Quebec QC G1L 3L5; Laval'01; Staff, Centre Hospitalier Universitaire De Québec - Pavillon De St-françois-d'assise; (418)525-4444

BERNARD, Richard; Polyclinique des Prairies, 980 boul Thibeau, Trois-Rivieres QC G8T 7B2; Laval'89; CCFP; (819)378-3433; Fax. (819)378-9581.

BERNARD, Sophie; CHUM-Hotel-Dieu, 3840 rue Saint-Urbain, Montreal QC H2W 1T8; Lyon (France)'94; Staff, Centre Hospitalier l'Université de Montréal (CHUM) - Hôtel-Dieu; (514)890-8000 x12732

BERNARD, Sylvie; CLSC Haute-Ville, 55 ch Sainte-Foy, Quebec QC G1R 1S9; Laval'00; (418)641-2572

BERNARD-BONNIN, Anne-Claude; Hôpital Ste-Justine, 3175 ch Cote-Sainte-Catherine, Montreal QC H3T 1C5; Mon'68; FRCPC; Peds. Ac Staff, Hôpital Ste-Justine; (514)345-4675; Fax. (514)345-4822.

BERNARDIN, Bruno; MUHC-Montreal Gen Hosp, 1650 av Cedar, Montreal QC H3G 1A4; Sher'91; FRCPC; EmergMed (Trauma). Staff, McGill University Health Centre - Montreal General Campus; adj Prof, McGill University; Langs: Spanish; English; (514)934-1934 x42501; Fax. (514)934-8421.

BERNARDIN, Jeanne; 123-100 Arden St, Moncton NB E1C 4B7; Mon'98; FRCSC; ObstGyn. Staff, The Moncton Hospital; Langs: Bilingual(French/English); (506)855-0062; Fax. (506)855-0064.

BERNARDIN, Sandra R; Hop Maisonneuve-Rosemont, 5415 boul de l'Assomption, Montreal QC H1T 2M4; Mon'95; FRCPC; IntMed. Staff, Hopital Maisonneuve-Rosemont; (514)252-3822

BERNARDINI, Marcus; Univ Hlth Network-Princess M, M700-610 University Ave, Toronto ON M5G 2M9; Wes'99; FRCSC; ObstGyn. Staff, Princess Margaret Hospital - University Health Network; (416)946-4501 x4043

BERNASCONI, Andrea G; MUHC-Montreal Neurology Inst, 3801 rue University, Montreal QC H3A 2B4; Basel (Switzerland)'88; Staff, McGill University Health Centre - Montreal Neurological Hospital; (514)398-3361; andrea@bic.mni.mcgill.ca.

BERNAT, Reinhold; Panorama Village Med Clinic, 103-15157 10 Hwy W, Surrey BC V3S 9A5; Sask'78; Staff Transitional Care Unit, UBC Hospital - Koerner Pavillion; Langs: German; (604)574-0481

BERNATCHEZ, Annie; CSSS de Sept-Iles, 45 rue du Pere-Divet, Sept-Iles QC G4R 3N7; Mon'04; CCFP; Staff, Centre Hospitalier Regional de Sept-Iles; (418)962-9761

BERNATCHEZ, Harold; CSSS de Rimouski-Neigette, CP 3150 Succ A 150 av Rouleau, Rimouski QC G5L 5T1; Laval'78; FRCPC; MedMicrobiol. Staff, Hôpital Regional Rimouski; (418)724-3000 x8335

BERNATCHEZ, Jean-Pierre; 225-2590 boul Laurier, Quebec QC G1V 4M6; Laval'66; DFAPA; FRCPC; Psy (Adult & Geriatric Psychiatry). Chief Dept of Psy, Centre Hospitalier Universitaire de Quebec-CHUL; Prof Psy, Université Laval; Langs: Bilingual(English/French); (418)655-6417; Fax. (418)780-1583; jpbernatchez@videotron.ca.

BERNATCHEZ, Joelle; UMF Richelieu-Yamaska, 1005 rue Gauthier, Saint-Hyacinthe QC J2S 8T2; Sher'08; CCFP; (450)771-3333 x4972; Fax. (450)771-3427.

BERNATCHEZ, Josee; 105A-667 rue Champlain, Dieppe NB E1A 1P6; Sher'93; Peds (P.Q.). Staff, Dr Georges-L-Dumont University Hospital Centre; Langs: Bilingual(English/French).

BERNATCHEZ, Marilou; CSSS de Trois-Rivieres, 1991 boul du Carmel, Trois-Rivieres QC G8Z 3R9; Mon'10; CCFP; Staff, CSSS de Trois-Rivières; (819)697-3333

BERNATCHEZ, Michel; CSSS Pierre de Saurel, 30 rue Ferland, Sorel-Tracy QC J3P 3C7; Mon'90; Gen Practice, Hôpital Richelieu; (450)746-4545

BERNATCHEZ, Simon; CSSS des Aurores Boreales, CP 6000 Succ Bureau-Chef 679 2e rue E, La Sarre QC J9Z 2X7; Sher'02; Staff, Centre Hospitalier La Sarre; Langs: Bilingual(English/French); (819)333-2311; s_bernatchez@hotmail.com.

BERNATSKY, Sasha R; MUHC-Royal Victoria Hosp, 687 av des Pins O, Montreal QC H3A 1A1; Tor'92; FRCPC; IntMed; Rheum. Staff, McGill University Health Centre - Royal Victoria Hospital; (514)934-1934 x44710; Fax. (514)934-8239.

BERNAZZANI, Odette; Pavillon Rosemont, 5689 boul Rosemont, Montreal QC H1T 2H1; Mon'85; FRCPC; Psy (Post Partum Disorders). Staff, Hopital Maisonneuve-Rosemont; (514)252-3922; Fax. (514)252-3810.

BERNBAUM, Stanley; Foothills Med Centre, 1403 29 St NW, Calgary AB T2N 2T9; Sask'80; CCFP; CCFP(E.M.); Staff EmergMed, Foothills Medical Centre; Staff EmergMed, Peter Lougheed Centre; Clin Lecturer Family Med, University of Calgary; (403)944-1315; Fax. (403)944-2419.

BERNDL, Anne M L; McMaster University, MDCL 3101A-1280 Main St W, Hamilton ON L8S 4K1; McM'05; FRCSC; ObstGyn.

BERNER, Mark; Clinique Med Soleil des Tanner, 3767 rue Notre-Dame O, Montreal QC H4C 1P8; Alb'75; CCFP; CCFP(E.M.); FCFP; ac Staff, St Mary's Hospital Centre; Consultant, Sir Mortimer B Davis Jewish General; adj Prof Family Med, McGill University; (514)932-8441; Fax. (514)932-8944; mark.berner@ssss.gouv.qc.ca.

BERNES, Carolyn; Maple FHT-Reddendale Family HC, 125 Lakeview Ave, Kingston ON K7M 3T6; Alb'82; CCFP; FCFP; Med Staff, Kingston General Hospital; (613)384-4664; Fax. (613)384-4182.

BERNES, Kent R; Barrhead Clinic, PO Box 4540 Stn Main, Barrhead AB T7N 1A4; Alb'90; CCFP; (780)674-2231; Fax. (780)674-2447.

BERNEY, Richard T; 17A James St PO Box 250, Forest ON N0N 1J0; Wes'75; Ac Staff, Bluewater Health - Mitton Site; Ac Staff, Bluewater Health - Norman Site; (519)786-6363; Fax. (519)786-6669.

BERNHARD, Nirit; St Joseph's Health Centre, 30 The Queensway, Toronto ON M6R 1B5; Wes'03; FRCPC; Peds. Staff, St Joseph's Health Centre; (416)530-6000

BERNHOLTZ, Jeffrey J; Health First Med Centre, 9625 Yonge St, Richmond Hill ON L4C 5T2; Tor'86; Court Staff, North York General Hospital - Branson Division; Court Staff, Mackenzie Richmond Hill Hospital; Langs: Hebrew; (905)508-4114; Fax. (905)508-4116; bernholtz@iname.com.

BERNICK, Paul E; Medical Office, 203-840 Coxwell Ave, Toronto ON M4C 5T2; Tor'92; FRCSC; GenSurg (Colon & Rectal Surgery). Staff, Toronto East General Hospital Inc; (416)461-0165; Fax. (416)461-5705.

BERNIER, Andre; CSSS de Trois-Rivieres, 1991 boul du Carmel, Trois-Rivieres QC G8Z 3R9; Laval'00; LMCC; FRCPC; DiagRad. Staff, CSSS de Trois-Rivières; Langs: English; (819)697-3333; andybernier@hotmail.com.

BERNIER, Annick; CSSS de Chicoutimi, H00-305 rue Saint-Vallier, Chicoutimi QC G7H 5H6; Sher'98; Psy. Staff, Complexe hospitalier de la Sagamie; (418)541-1000 x5151

BERNIER, Carolle; CLSC La Region-Sherbrookoise, 1200 rue King E, Sherbrooke QC J1G 1E4; Sher'75; CCFP; FCFP; Staff Family Med, Centre Hospitalier Universitaire de Sherbrooke-Hôpital Hôtel-Dieu; (819)563-2572; Fax. (819)563-9912.

BERNIER, Carolyne; CLSC Ste-Therese de Blainville, 55 rue Saint-Joseph, Sainte-Therese QC J7E 4Y5; Sher'79; (450)430-4553; Fax. (450)430-3859.

BERNIER, Chantal; Ctre de Sante St-Philippe Med, 5 rue Saint-Philippe, Windsor QC J1S 1C9; Sher'92; (819)845-5005; Fax. (819)845-5010.

BERNIER, Christian; Direction de Sante Publique, 1-205 boul de York O, Gaspe QC G4X 2W5; Mon'78; Staff, Centre Hospitalier de Gaspe; Dir Public Health, Region de la Gaspesie-Iles-de-la-Madeleine; (418)368-2443; Fax. (418)368-1317; christian_bernier@ssss.gouv.qc.ca.

BERNIER, Christina; CHUM-Hotel-Dieu, 3840 rue Saint-Urbain, Montreal QC H2W 1T8; Laval'01; FRCSC; PlasSurg. Staff, Centre Hospitalier l'Université de Montréal (CHUM) - Hôtel-Dieu; (514)890-8000

BERNIER, Claude; Hop du Sacre-Coeur de Mtl, 5400 boul Gouin O, Montreal QC H4J 1C5; Sher'74; Gastroent (P.Q.). Staff, Hôpital du Sacre-Coeur de Montréal; (514)338-2050

BERNIER, Daniel; CHUQ-Ctr Hosp Univ Laval, 2705 boul Laurier, Quebec QC G1V 4G2; Laval'95; CCFP; CCFP(E.M.); Staff, Centre Hospitalier Universitaire de Quebec-CHUL; (418)656-4141 x70553

BERNIER, Danielle A; Clinique Med d'Iberville, 235 2e av, St-Jean-Sur-Richel QC J2X 2B2; Laval'78; FRCSC; ObstGyn. Staff, Centre Hospitalier Beauce-Etchemin; Obst/Gyn, Centre de santé des Côté-Nord; Assoc Staff, Obs/Gyn, Centre Hospitalier La Sarre; Langs: French; English; (450)347-5548; Fax. (450)347-4091; daniellebernier@videotron.ca.

BERNIER, David; Unite Med Familiale Maizerets, 2480 ch de la Canardiere, Quebec QC G1J 2G1; Laval'06; CCFP; Staff, Centre Hospitalier de Gaspe; (418)661-1413

BERNIER, Denyse; GMF du Chatel, 200-9465 boul de l'Ormiere, Quebec QC G2B 3K7; Laval'85; Langs: English; French; (418)843-5141; Fax. (418)843-5343; d.bernier@hotmail.com.

BERNIER, Elise; 80 rue De Vimy, Sherbrooke QC J1J 3M4; Sher'78; Langs: Bilingual(French/English); (819)822-2555; Fax. (819)563-9209; ebernier@elisebernier.ca.

BERNIER, Francois P; Alberta Children's Hosp, 2888 Shaganappi Trail NW, Calgary AB T3B 6A8; Man'93; FRCPC; MedGenetics. Staff, Alberta Children's Hospital; Dept Head Medical Genetics, University of Calgary; Langs: Bilingual(English/French); (403)955-7373; Fax. (403)955-2701.

BERNIER, Frederic; CHUS-Hop Hotel-Dieu, 580 rue Bowen S, Sherbrooke QC J1G 2E8; Sher'02; FRCPC; IntMed; Endocrin&Metab. Staff, Centre Hospitalier Universitaire de Sherbrooke-Hôpital Hôtel-Dieu; (819)346-1110 x23599

BERNIER, Gilles P; CHUM-Hop Notre-Dame, 1560 rue Sherbrooke E, Montreal QC H2L 4M1; Mon'79; FRCPC; Neur; Electroenceph (P.Q.). Consultant, Centre Hospitalier Honore-Mercier; Staff, Centre Hospitalier l'Université de Montréal (CHUM) - Hôpital Notre-Dame; Langs: English; Spanish; (514)890-8123; Fax. (514)412-7711.

BERNIER, Helene; CSSS du Sud de Lanaudière, 911 montee des Pionniers, Terrebonne QC J6V 2H2; Mon'92; FRCPC; NuclearMed. Staff, Centre Hospitalier Pierre le Gardeur; (450)654-7525

BERNIER, Helene; Regie des Rentes du Quebec, CP 5200 Succ Terminus, Quebec QC G1K 7S9; Laval'76; (418)657-8709 x4255

BERNIER, J Jean-Robert S; Cdn Forces Health Services Ctr, 1745 Alta Vista Dr, Ottawa ON K1A 0K6; McM'90; DEH; BA; MPH; Dep Surgeon General, Canadian Forces Health Services Centre; Langs: French; (613)945-6827; Fax. (613)990-1345.

BERNIER, Jacques; Pavillon Rosemont, 5689 boul Rosemont, Montreal QC H1T 2H1; Sher'78; FRCPC; Psy (Bipolar Disease). Dir University Educ, Hopital Maisonneuve-Rosemont; Prof clin agrégé, Universite de Montreal; (514)252-3400 x4776; Fax. (514)252-3810; jbernier.hmr@ssss.qc.ca.

BERNIER, Jean-Pierre; CSSSG-Hop de Hull, 116 boul Lionel-Emond, Gatineau QC J8Y 1W7; Laval'79; FRCPC; IntMed; Gastroent. Ac Staff, Hull Hospital; (819)595-6000

BERNIER, Jean-Pierre; CHUS-Hop Fleurimont, 3001 12e Av N, Sherbrooke QC J1H 5N4; Mon'72; FRCPC; Neur; Electroenceph (P.Q.). Staff, Centre Hospitalier Universitaire de Sherbrooke-Hopital Fleurimont; Consultant, Hôpital Sainte-croix; Asst Prof Neurol, Universite de Sherbrooke; (819)346-1110; Fax. (819)820-6420.

BERNIER, Joelle; Centre de Sante Valcartier, CP 1000 Bdp Succ Forces, Courcelette QC G0A 4Z0; Laval'92; FRCPC; Psy. (418)844-5000 x5802

BERNIER, Julie; Ctr Hosp du Centre la Mauricie, 50 119e rue, Shawinigan-Sud QC G9P 5K1; Sher'96; Staff, Centre Hospitalier du Centre la Mauricie; (819)536-7500

BERNIER, Karine; CSSS de Memphremagog, 50 rue Saint-Patrice E, Magog QC J1X 3X3; Laval'02; CCFP; Staff, Centre Hospitalier et CLSC de Memphremagog; (819)843-3381

BERNIER, Linda; Hotel-Dieu d'Arthabaska, 5 rue des Hospitalieres, Victoriaville QC G6P 6N2; Sher'86; FRCSC; Otol. Staff, Hotel-Dieu d'Arthabaska; (819)357-1151; Fax. (819)357-6027.

BERNIER, Manon; Clinique Med Kingsey Falls, RR 1 19 rue Comeau, Kingsey Falls QC J0A 1B0; Sher'84; Staff, Hotel-Dieu d'Arthabaska; (819)363-3030; Fax. (819)363-3030.

BERNIER, Marie-France; CSSS de la Minganie, CP 190 1035 prom des Anciens, Havre-Saint-Pierre QC G0G 1P0; Sher'08; CCFP; Staff, CSSS de la Minganie; (418)538-2212; Fax. (418)538-2365.

BERNIER, Marie-Jose; Ctr Hosp St-Joseph de la Malba, CP 340 Succ Bereau-Chef 303 rue Saint-Etienne, La Malbaie QC G5A 1T8; Laval'72; Gen Practice, Hôpital de la Malbaie; (418)665-1711

BERNIER, Mario F; Clin Chirurgie & Esthetique Me, 500-3030 boul Le carrefour, Laval QC H7T 2P5; Sher'88; FACS; FRCSC; PlasSurg (Aesthetic Surgery). ac Staff, Hôtel-Dieu de Saint-Jérôme; Staff PlasSurg, Private Cosmetic & Plastic Surgery Clinic; Langs: English; (450)686-4755; Fax. (450)686-4733; drbernier@drbernier.com.

BERNIER, Mark J; Manitoba Clinic, 504-790 Sherbrook St, Winnipeg MB R3A 1M3; Man'81; FACOG; FRCSC; ObstGyn (Gynecological Surgery). Staff Women's Hosp, Health Sciences Centre; Site Dir ObstGyn, Seven Oaks General Hospital; Att Staff, Churchill Regional Health Authority; Assoc Prof ObstGyn/Lecturer Obstgyn/Chief Service Gynecology Women's Centre HSC, University of Manitoba; (204)788-5701; Fax. (204)784-4124.

BERNIER, Martin L D; MUHC-Montreal Gen Hosp, E5 200-1650 av Cedar, Montreal QC H3G 1A4; McG'03; FRCPC; IntMed; Cardiol. Staff, McGill University Health Centre - Montreal General Campus; (514)934-1934

BERNIER, Mathieu; CSSS de la Cote-de-Gaspe, 215 boul de York O, Gaspe QC G4X 2W2; Mon'09; CCFP; Staff, Centre Hospitalier de Gaspe.

BERNIER, Mathieu; Hôpital Laval, 2725 ch Sainte-Foy, Quebec QC G1V 4G5; Mon'99; CSPQ; FRCPC; IntMed; Cardiol. Staff, Hôpital Laval; (418)656-8711; Fax. (418)656-4581.

BERNIER, Maude; CSSS de Rimouski-Neigette, CP 3150 Succ A 150 av Rouleau, Rimouski QC G5L 5T1; Laval'07; IntMed. Staff, Hôpital Regional Rimouski; (418)724-3000

BERNIER, Michel; Clinique Fam des Prairies, 310 boul Antonio-Barrette, N-D-Des-Prairies QC J6E 1G2; Laval'93; Dip SportMed; CCFP; Staff, Centre Hospitalier Régional de Lanaudière; Clin Prof, Université Laval; Langs: Bilingual(French/English); (450)752-1238; Fax. (450)752-2965.

BERNIER, Nadia; Clinique Pediatrique Ste-Foy, 295-2600 boul Laurier, Quebec QC G1V 4T3; Laval'06; Peds. (418)658-0906

BERNIER, Pascal; Clinique Med St-Raphael, 101 rue Principale, St-Raphael-Be QC G0R 4C0; Sher'96; (418)243-2115; Fax. (418)243-2054.

BERNIER, Patrick; CSSS Vieille Capitale, 900 boul Wilfrid-Hamel, Quebec QC G1M 2R9; Laval'01; CCFP; Fam Med, CSSS de Quebec-Sud; (418)682-1762; Fax. (418)682-1763; patrick.bernier@csssvc.qc.ca.

BERNIER, Philippe; Clinique Medicale, GD 197 rue du Quai, Carleton QC G0C 1J0; Mon'70; Staff, CSSS de la Baie-des-Chaleurs; (418)364-3311; Fax. (418)364-6650; lavigie@globetrotter.net.

BERNIER, Pierre-Luc; MUHC-Montreal Children's Hosp, C829-2300 rue Tupper, Montreal QC H3H 1P3; McG'05; FRCSC; CardSurg. Staff, McGill University Health Centre - Montreal Children's Hospital; (514)934-1934 x22394

BERNIER, Richard; Ctr Hosp Affilie-Enfant-Jesus, 1401 18e rue, Quebec QC G1J 1Z4; Laval'02; Staff, Centre Hospitalier Affilié Universitaire de Québec - Hôpital De L'Enfant Jésus; (418)649-5609; Fax. (418)649-5552.

BERNIER, Robert G J; PO Box 1260, Mayerthorpe AB T0E 1N0; Alb'84; Mayerthorpe Health Care Centre; (780)786-2412; Fax. (780)786-2249; robertb@mayerthorpe.ca.

BERNIER, Roch; CIM, 440 boul Rene-Levesque O, Montreal QC H2Z 1V7; Sher'72; MSc; CCFP; FCFP; Fam Med, Institut Universitaire de Geriatrie de Sherbrooke-Pavillon Argyll; Chaire Admission Committe/Prof, Universite de Sherbrooke; (819)780-2220 x47206

BERNIER, Rose-Alexie; Centre Med Centrale, 4-135 rue Saint-Antoine N, Granby QC J2G 5G7; Sher'09; (450)372-5401

BERNIER, Sandra; CSSS du Lac-des-Deux-Montagnes, 520 boul Arthur-Sauve, Saint-Eustache QC J7R 5B1; Mon'04; Staff, Hôpital de Saint-Eustache; (450)473-6811

BERNIER, Serge; Centre de Sante Valcartier, CP 1000 Bdp Succ Forces, Courcelette QC G0A 4Z0; Laval'75; (418)622-0006

BERNIER, Sophie; Clinique Med Du Lac, 296 rue Principale, Lac-Bouchette QC G0W 1V0; Sher'05; Staff, Hotel-Dieu de Roberval; Langs: Bilingual(French/English); (418)275-0110; Fax. (418)348-6781.

BERNIER, Suzanne; 207-2600 boul Laurier CP 7777 Succ Terminus, Quebec QC G1K 7T4; Laval'81; (418)657-8718

BERNIER, Sylvie; Ministere de la Sante, 707-1075 ch Sainte-Foy, Quebec QC G1S 2M1; Laval'79; (418)266-7505; Fax. (418)266-5862.

BERNIER, Vincent; CHUQ-Hotel-Dieu de Quebec, 11 Côte du Palais, Quebec QC G1R 2J6; Laval'77; CSPQ; FRCPC; AnatPath (Hematology Pathology). Staff, Centre Hospitalier Universitaire de Québec (CHUQ) - Siege Social; Prof, Université Laval; Langs: English; (418)525-4444 x23658; vincent.bernier@mail.chuq.qc.ca.

BERNIER, Yvan; Clinique Fam des Prairies, 310 Boul Antonio-Barrette, N-D-Des-Prairies QC J6E 1G2; Laval'86; CCFP; FCFP; Staff, Centre Hospitalier Régional de Lanaudière; Prof Family Med, Universite de Montreal; Clin Prof FamilyMed, Université Laval; Langs: Bilingual(French/English); (450)752-1050; Fax. (450)752-2965.

BERNIER-BUZZANGA, Jeannine; CHUM-Hop Notre-Dame, 1560 rue Sherbrooke E, Montreal QC H2L 4M1; Laval'75; Derm. Staff, Centre Hospitalier l'Université de Montréal (CHUM) - Hôpital Notre-Dame; (514)526-3783

BERNIER-DUTRISAC, Anne-Marie; CSSS Des Iles, 430 ch Principal, Cap-aux-Meules QC G4T 1R9; Laval'07; CCFP; Staff, Hôpital de l'Archipel; (418)986-2121

BERNIER-LYCKA, Lucie M; Glenora Med Clinic, 310-10230 142 St NW, Edmonton AB T5N 3Y6; Alb'83; CCFP; FCFP; Staff, Covenant Health - Misericordia Community Hospital; Staff, Capital Care - Lynwood; Clin Instructor, University of Alberta; Langs: English; French; (780)455-3311; Fax. (780)451-4404.

BERNS, Trevor A; 6-446 Hollandview Trail, Aurora ON L4G 7Z9; Tor'99; CCFP; (905)751-1642; bernstrevor@hotmail.com.

BERNSTEIN, Abraham; 1007-655 Bay St, Toronto ON M5G 2K4; Tor'51; FACOG; FRCSC; ObstGyn (Gynecology). Assoc Staff, Mount Sinai Hospital; (416)977-2184

BERNSTEIN, Charles N; John Buhler Research Centre, 804F-715 McDermot Ave, Winnipeg MB R3E 3P4; Man'85; FRCPC; IntMed (Gastrointestinal Cancer); Gastroent. Staff Physician, Health Sciences Centre; Dir IBD Clinical Research Centre/Prof, University of Manitoba; (204)789-3369; Fax. (204)789-3972.

BERNSTEIN, E Paul; Hydro Place Bldg, 3026-700 University Ave, Toronto ON M5G 1Z5; Tor'68; FRCOG; FRCSC; ObstGyn (Gynecological Infection). Ac Staff, Mount Sinai Hospital; (416)586-5236; Fax. (416)586-8612; pbernstein@mtsinai.on.ca.

BERNSTEIN, Ira; 306-960 Lawrence Ave W, North York ON M6A 3B5; Tor'90; BSc; CCFP; FCFP; Div Head Mental Health Dept of Family and Community Med Pract, Humber River Regional Hospital - Keele Street Site; Court Staff, Toronto Western Hospital - University Health Network; Lecturer Family & CommunMed, University of Toronto; (416)256-7731; Fax. (416)781-4515.

BERNSTEIN, Keevin N; Health Sciences Centre, 820 Sherbrook St, Winnipeg MB R3A 1R9; Man'78; ABIM(Nephrol); FRCPC; IntMed (Nephrology). Med Dir Manitoba Renal Prog, Health Sciences Centre; Prof, University of Manitoba; (204)787-3585; Fax. (204)787-3326; kbernstein@hsc.mb.ca.

BERNSTEIN, Mark L; IWK Health Centre, PO Box 9700 Rpo CSC 5980 University Ave, Halifax NS B3K 6R8; Albert Einstein (USA)'75; AB(Ped); AB(PehHem); FRCPC; Hem (P.Q.); MedOncol (P.Q.); Peds. Staff, IWK Health Centre; Head Dept of Peds, Dalhousie University; Langs: French; (902)470-6839; Fax. (902)470-7216.

BERNSTEIN, Mark; Univ Hlth Network-Toronto Western Hosp, WW4 451-399 Bathurst St, Toronto ON M5T 2S8; Ott'76; BSc(Hon); MHSc(Bioethics); FRCSC; Neursurg (Biomedical Ethics). Surgeon, Toronto Western Hospital - University Health Network; Prof Surg, University of Toronto; Langs: French; (416)603-6499; Fax. (416)603-5298.

BERNSTEIN, Michael N; Sunnybrook Hlth Sciences Ctre, HG40 C-2075 Bayview Ave, Toronto ON M4N 3M5; Wes'02; FRCPC; IntMed; Gastroent. Clin Associate Div of Gastroenterology, Sunnybrook Health Sciences Centre; (416)480-5495; Fax. (416)480-5977.

BERNSTEIN, Robert L; Clinique Med Les Jardins Dorva, 204-352 av Dorval, Dorval QC H9S 3H8; McG'85; pers Médecin, Jewish Rehabilitation Hospital; pers Médecin, Lakeshore General Hospital - Pointe Claire; Langs: French; (514)631-6086; Fax. (514)631-6691.

BERNSTEIN, Robert; Bridgepoint Family Hlth Team, 430 Broadview Ave, Toronto ON M4K 2N1; McG'77; CCFP; FCFP; Staff, Bridgepoint Family Health Team; (416)470-6690; rbernstein@mtsinai.on.ca.

BERNSTEIN, Stacey E; The Hosp For Sick Children, 555 University Ave, Toronto ON M5G 1X8; Tor'92; FRCPC; Peds. Staff, The Hospital For Sick Children; (416)813-5394; Fax. (416)813-8345; stacey.bernstein@sickkids.ca.

BERNSTEIN, Stanley K; B7-5095 Yonge St, North York ON M2N 6Z4; Tor'66; Staff, Mount Sinai Hospital; (416)229-6166; Fax. (416)229-4205.

BERNSTEIN, Steven C; CHUM-Hotel-Dieu, 3840 rue Saint-Urbain, Montreal QC H2W 1T8; McG'90; FRCPC; Derm (Consultation). ac Membre, Centre Hospitalier l'Université de Montréal (CHUM) - Hôtel-Dieu; Consultant, Centre Hospitalier l'Université De Montréal (CHUM) - Hôpital Saint-luc; (514)890-8000 x14961

BERNSTEIN, Steven J; Humber River Reg Hosp-Finch, 2111 Finch St W, North York ON M3N 1N1; Tor'03; FRCPC; Anes. Staff, Humber River Regional Hospital - Finch Avenue Site; (416)744-2500

BERNSTEIN, Vanessa; BC Cancer Agency-Vanc Isl Ctr, 2410 Lee Ave, Victoria BC V8R 6V5; UBC'95; MSc; FRCPC; IntMed (Breasts); MedOncol. Staff, BC Cancer Agency Vancouver Island Centre; Ac Staff, Vancouver Island Health Authority; Consultant, Nanaimo Regional General Hospital; Asst Prof Med, University of British Columbia; (250)519-5571; Fax. (250)519-2017.

BERNSTEIN, Victoria; Gordon & Leslie Diamond HCC, 9F-2775 Laurel St, Vancouver BC V5Z 1M9; Liverpool (England)'65; FRCPC; IntMed (Cardiovascular Surgery). Assoc Dir CardiovascSurg & Cons, Vancouver General Hospital - Centennial Pavillion; Staff, Gordon & Leslie Diamond Health Care Centre; Emeritus Prof Med, University of British Columbia; (604)875-5481; Fax. (604)875-5489; dr.bernstein@telus.net.

BERNTSON, Andrea M; St Michael's Hosp, 17 045-30 Bond St, Toronto ON M5B 1W8; Wes'02; FRCPC; Psy. Staff, St Michael's Hospital; (416)864-6060; Fax. (416)864-5480.

BERNTSON, Laura C; Albany Med Clinic, 807 Broadview Ave, Toronto ON M4K 2P8; McG'74; Ac Staff Family Practice, Toronto East General Hospital Inc; (416)461-9471; Fax. (416)461-2710.

BERNUCCI, Bruno; Clinique Med Langelier, 5953 rue Belanger, Saint-Leonard QC H1T 1G8; McG'86; BSc; Staff, Hôpital Santa Cabrini Ospedale; Langs: French; Italian; (514)253-9191; Fax. (514)253-5254.

BEROLO, Helen M; Health Aware, 124 Sherwood Dr, Ottawa ON K1Y 3V2; Ott'76; CCFP; FCFP; (613)236-4187; Fax. (613)236-7482.

BERRANG, Tanya S; 2400 Lee Ave, Victoria BC V8R 4X1; UBC'01; FRCPC; RadOncol. (250)519-5577

BERRIMAN, Katherine A; Care and Cure Medical Clinic, 2024C Albert St, Regina SK S4P 2T7; Sask'83; (306)522-3824; Fax. (306)522-3829.

BERRINGER, Ross G; Canadian Med Protective Assn, PO Box 8225 Stn T CSC 875 Carling Ave, Ottawa ON K1G 3H7; UBC'80; DABEM; MCFP(EM); Medical Officer, Canadian Medical Protective Association; Clin Assoc Prof, University of British Columbia; (613)725-2000 x545; berringe@interchange.ubc.ca.

BERRINGTON, Neil R; Health Sciences Centre, GB103-820 Sherbrook St, Winnipeg MB R3A 1R9; Witwatersrand (South Africa)'85; MB ChB; MMed; FRCS(Glas); Asst Prof/Head Section NeuroSurg, Health Sciences Centre; Asst Prof, University of Manitoba; Langs: Afrikaans; (204)787-7276; Fax. (204)787-3851; nberrington@hsc.mb.ca.

BERRIS, Kenneth; 2-867 boul Saint-René O, Gatineau QC J8T 7X6; Tor'73; FRCPC; IntMed. Staff, Canadian Medical Protective Association; Langs: Bilingual(English/French); (819)243-3221

BERROW, Paul J; Souris Hosp Incorporated, PO Box 640, Souris PE C0A 2B0; Birmingham (England)'82; MB ChB; MRC; Hd FamilyMed, Souris Hospital Inc; (902)687-7150

BERRY, Brian R; Royal Jubilee Hosp, 5F-1952 Bay St, Victoria BC V8R 1J8; Ott'84; FRCPC; AnatPath; HemPath. Staff/Dir Hematopathol, Royal Jubilee Hospital; (250)370-8452

BERRY, Dale C; Sheep River Med Clinic, PO Box 1560 Stn Main 1-74 Elizabeth St, Okotoks AB T1S 1B5; Cal'82; CCFP; (403)938-4421; Fax. (403)938-5657.

BERRY, David A; 9803 34 Ave NW, Edmonton AB T6E 5X9; Alb'78; FAAP; FRCPC; Peds (General). Staff, University of Alberta Hospital; (780)462-8535; dberry@shaw.ca.

BERRY, Gregory K; MUHC-Montreal Gen Hosp, 1650 av Cedar, Montreal QC H3G 1A4; McG'91; FRCSC; OrthSurg. Staff, McGill University Health Centre - Montreal General Campus; (514)934-1934; Fax. (514)934-8453.

BERRY, Henry; 1515-44 Victoria St, Toronto ON M5C 1Y2; Tor'54; FRCP(Lond); DPsy; FRCPC; IntMed (Neurology & Psychiatry); Neur. Consultant, Centre for Addiction & Mental Health (CAMH) - College Street Site; Assoc Prof, University of Toronto; (416)366-2640; Fax. (416)366-0929.

BERRY, Margaret A; MUHC-Montreal Children's Hosp, F379-2300 rue Tupper, Montreal QC H3H 1P3; McG'74; MSc(McGill); CSPQ; CAB; MRCP; FRCPC; Peds (Neonatal & Perinatal Medicine). Staff Peds, McGill University Health Centre - Montreal Children's Hospital; Asst Prof Peds, McGill University; Langs: Bilingual(French/English); (514)412-4400 x23169; Fax. (514)412-4249.

BERRY, Marian E; Kootenay Lake Hosp, 413-3 View St, Nelson BC V1L 2V1; Wes'83; BSc; FRCPC; Neur (Neuropathology). Staff, Kootenay Lake General Hospital; Langs: Dutch; French; (250)352-3111

BERRY, Raymond E; Toronto Rehab Inst, 130 Dunn Ave, Toronto ON M6K 2R7; McM'88; CCFP; FCFP; Staff, Toronto Western Hospital - University Health Network; Ac Staff, Toronto Rehabilitation Institute - Queen Elizabeth Centre; Asst Prof Dept of Family & CommunMed, University of Toronto; (416)597-3422 x2286; r.berry@utoronto.ca.

BERRY, Robert F; Queen Elizabeth II HSC, 1276 South Park St, Halifax NS B3H 2Y9; UBC'94; FRCPC; DiagRad. Staff, Queen Elizabeth II Health Sciences Centre - Victoria General Site; (902)473-7770

BERRY, Scott R; Sunnybrook Odette Cancer Ctre, T2 036-2075 Bayview Ave, Toronto ON M4N 3M5; Tor'90; BSc; MHSc; FRCPC; IntMed; MedOncol. Staff, Sunnybrook Health Sciences Centre; Prog Dir Med Oncology Training Program, University of Toronto; (416)480-4270; Fax. (416)480-6002; scott.berry@sunnybrook.ca.

BERRY, William A D; Sault Area Hosp, 750 Great Northern Rd, Sault Ste. Marie ON P6B 0A8; Cal'97; FRCPC; IntMed; Nephrol. Staff Algoma Reg Renal Program, Sault Area Hospital - Sault Ste Marie; (705)759-3862; Fax. (705)759-4999.

BERSCHEID, Bruce B; Wall Street Med Bldg, 300-140 Wall St, Saskatoon SK S7K 1N4; Sask'79; FRCPC; DiagRad;CCFP; (306)244-1167; Fax. (306)244-2911.

BERTAGNOLLI-HANSEN, Alexa; Glenrose Rehab Hosp, 3D-10230 111 Ave NW, Edmonton AB T5G 0B7; Tor'86; Staff, Glenrose Rehabilitation Hospital; (780)735-7934; Fax. (780)735-8837.

BERTELLE, Valerie; CHUS-Hop Fleurimont, 3001 12e av N, Sherbrooke QC J1H 5N4; Brest (France)'96; Staff, Centre Hospitalier Universitaire de Sherbrooke-Hopital Fleurimont; Langs: Bilingual(French/English); (819)346-1110 x14634; valerie.bertelle@usherbrooke.ca.

BERTELLI, Christiane; Inst Albert Prevost, 6555 boul Gouin O, Montreal QC H4K 1B3; Laval'69; FRCPC; Psy. Staff, Hôpital du Sacre-Coeur de Montréal; (514)338-2222 x4246; Fax. (514)338-2222; cbertelli@hotmail.com.

BERTHELET, Eric; BC Cancer Agency-Vancouver CC, 600 10th Ave W, Vancouver BC V5Z 4E6; Mon'90; FRCPC; RadOncol. Staff, BC Cancer Agency Vancouver Centre; Langs: Bilingual(English/French); (604)877-6000 x2673

BERTHELET, France; CHUM-Hop Notre-Dame, 1560 rue Sherbrooke E, Montreal QC H2L 4M1; Mon'91; CSPQ; FRCPC; AnatPath; GenPath (P.Q.). Staff, Centre Hospitalier l'Université de Montréal (CHUM) - Hôpital Notre-Dame; (514)890-8000 x27054

BERTHELOT, Christian; Ctr Hosp Affilie-Enfant-Jesus, 1401 18e rue, Quebec QC G1J 1Z4; Laval'99; FRCPC; DiagRad. Staff, Centre Hospitalier Affilié Universitaire de Québec - Hôpital De L'Enfant Jésus; (418)649-0252

BERTHELOT, Eva; CSSS de la Cote-de-Gaspe, 215 boul de York O, Gaspe QC G4X 2W2; Mon'07; CCFP; Staff, Centre Hospitalier de Gaspe; (418)368-3301; Fax. (418)368-6850.

BERTHELOT, Gilles; 1364 rue Saint-Jacques, L'Ancienne-Lorette QC G2E 2X1; Laval'79; Ac Staff, CSSS de Quebec-Sud; (418)877-7727; Fax. (418)877-2781.

BERTHELOT, Jacques; Centre Med Racine, 201-900 boul Raymond, Quebec QC G1B 3G3; Laval'83; (418)667-8066; Fax. (418)667-8131.

BERTHELOT, Simon; Foothills Med Centre, C231-1403 29 St NW, Calgary AB T2N 2T9; Laval'98; FRCPC; EmergMed. Staff, Foothills Medical Centre; Langs: Bilingual(French/English); (403)944-1315; gronigo98@yahoo.com.

BERTHIAUME, Claude; Clinique Med Havre Sante, 521 boul Du Havre, Salaber-de-Valleyf QC J6S 4Z5; Laval'78; Staff, Centre Hospitalier Régional du Suroît; Langs: English; French; (450)371-6444 x209; Fax. (450)371-5315.

BERTHIAUME, Georges; Clinique Med Jean-Talon Pie IX, 4679 rue Jean Talon E, Saint-Leonard QC H1S 1K3; Mon'74; Langs: Bilingual(French/English); (514)374-5901; Fax. (514)374-1668.

BERTHIAUME, Luc R; 3500 26 Ave NE, Calgary AB T1Y 6J4; Ott'99; FRCPC; IntMed; Critical Care Medicine; Respir. Staff, Peter Lougheed Centre; Staff, Calgary Health Region; Langs: Bilingual(English/French); (403)943-4467; Fax. (403)291-1491.

BERTHIAUME, Marc; AL 0702L Tunney's Pasture, Ottawa ON K1A 0K9; Mon'90; MCFP; CCFP; Langs: Bilingual(English/French); English; French; (613)952-6239; Fax. (613)960-9754.

BERTHIAUME, Marie-Josee; Hop Maisonneuve-Rosemont, 5415 boul de l'Assomption, Montreal QC H1T 2M4; Mon'85; DiagRad. Staff, Hopital Maisonneuve-Rosemont; (514)252-3400 x4141; Fax. (514)252-3537.

BERTHIAUME, Pierre; CSSS de Chicoutimi, 305 rue Saint-Vallier, Chicoutimi QC G7H 5H6; Ott'70; Nephrol (P.Q.). Clin Staff, Complexe hospitalier de la Sagamie; (418)541-1084; Fax. (418)541-1197.

BERTHIAUME, Renee; Clinique Med de Francheville, 111-1220 rue Jean-Nicolet, Trois-Rivieres QC G9A 1B2; Mon'86; (819)373-0947

BERTHIAUME, Sylvie; Clinique Med du Quartier Latin, 905 boul Rene-Levesque E, Montreal QC H2L 5B1; Mon'80; CCFP; FCFP; Staff Privil Obst, Centre Hospitalier l'Université De Montréal (CHUM) - Hôpital Saint-luc; Langs: English; (514)285-5500

BERTHIAUME, Yves; CHUM-Hotel-Dieu, 3840 rue Saint-Urbain, Montreal QC H2W 1T8; Sher'80; MSc; FRCPC; Respir (Cystic Fibrosis). Staff, Centre Hospitalier l'Université de Montréal (CHUM) - Hôtel-Dieu; Prof, Universite de Montreal; Langs: English; (514)890-8000 x15667; yves.berthiaume@umontreal.ca.

BERTHOLET-ANKU, Catherine L; CHUS-Hop Fleurimont, 3001 12e av N, Sherbrooke QC J1H 5N4; Lausanna (Switzerland)'96; FRCSC; ObstGyn (Echography). Staff, Centre Hospitalier Universitaire de Sherbrooke-Hopital Fleurimont; (819)346-1110 x13721

BERTI, Karen E; Niagara On The Lake Fam Hlth T, PO Box 1360 176 Wellington St, Niagara-Lk ON L0S 1J0; McM'95; CCFP; Staff, Niagara Health System - Niagara-on-the-Lake Hospital Site; (905)468-9189; Fax. (905)468-4947.

BERTLIK, Maria; William Olser HC-Brampton, 2100 Bovaird Dr E, Brampton ON L6R 3J7; Palacky (Czech Republic)'79; FRCPC; Anes (Clinical Anaesthesia). Staff, William Osler Health System - Brampton Civic Hospital; Langs: Czech; (905)494-6576

BERTOIA, Thomas; York Prof Bldg, 300-679 Davis Dr, Newmarket ON L3Y 5G8; Tor'84; FRCSC; OrthSurg. Staff, Southlake Regional Health Centre; (905)895-1361; Fax. (905)895-0561.

BERTOIA, Mauro; Saanich Plaza Med Clinic, 3544 Blanshard St, Victoria BC V8X 1W3; UBC'85; Ac Staff, Vancouver Island Health Authority; (250)475-3331; Fax. (250)475-1157.

BERTOLDI, Margaret E; 11-426 Talbot St, St Thomas ON N5P 1B9; Sask'96; FRCPC; Peds (Child Abuse). Aj Prof, University of Western Ontario; (519)637-0009; Fax. (519)637-5799.

BERTOLO, Luigia; Centre Med Nazareth, 1771 av Dollard, LaSalle QC H8N 1T9; Padua (Italy)'81; (514)368-5500; Fax. (514)368-0056.

BERTOLO, Monica; Glenridge Walk-In Clinic, 5-209 Glenridge Ave, St Catharines ON L2T 3J6; Wes'02; BSc(Hon); CCFP; Aj Prof, Queen's University; (289)362-5333; Fax. (289)362-5335.

BERTOTHY, Christine M; 103-532 Lake St, St Catharines ON L2N 4H4; Tor'87; (905)646-1266; Fax. (905)646-9900.

BERTOTHY, Michele; The Juravinski Cancer Centre, 699 Concession St, Hamilton ON L8V 5C2; Ott'88; (905)387-9495

BERTOZZI, Hugo A R; Queen Elizabeth II Hosp, 10409 98 St, Grande Prairie AB T8V 2E8; Tor'87; BSc; FRCPC; CCFP; IntMed. Ac Staff, Queen Elizabeth II Hospital; Clinical Asst Prof/Clin Assoc Prof, University of Alberta; Langs: French; Italian; (780)538-7100

BERTRAM, Barbara O B; Bluewater Health-Norman Site, 89 Norman St, Sarnia ON N7T 6S3; McM'06; FRCPC; Anes. Staff, Bluewater Health - Norman Site; (519)464-4400; Fax. (519)464-4407.

BERTRAM, Jonathan R; Addiction & Mental Hlth-ARF, 33 Russell St, Toronto ON M5S 2S1; Dublin (Ireland)'07; Staff, Centre for Addiction & Mental Health (CAMH) - Russell Street Site; (416)535-8501

BERTRAM, Kathi; 100-8160 Cook Rd, Richmond BC V6Y 1T8; McM'02; BSc; CCFP; Assoc Staff, Richmond Hospital; (604)233-5699; Fax. (604)303-1914.

BERTRAM, Susan G; Sunnybrook Hlth Sciences Ctre, 2075 Bayview Ave, Toronto ON M4N 3M5; Tor'80; FRCPC; Anes. Staff, Sunnybrook Health Sciences Centre; (416)480-4864; Fax. (416)480-6039.

BERTRAND, Annie; Hotel-Dieu de Levis, 143 rue Wolfe, Levis QC G6V 3Z1; Sher'98; GenSurg. Staff, Hôtel-Dieu de Lévis; (418)835-1721

BERTRAND, Audrey; Ctr de Sante Vallee-Gatineau, 309 boul Desjardins, Maniwaki QC J9E 2E7; Mon'09; CCFP; Staff, CSSS de la Vallée de la Gatineau; (819)449-2300

BERTRAND, C Francois; Hop Du Sacre-Coeur De Mtl, 500-5400 boul Gouin O, Montreal QC H4J 1C5; McG'81; CSPQ; MDCM; EmergMed (P.Q.) (Cardiology). Staff, Hôpital du Sacre-Coeur de Montréal; Langs: Bilingual(French/English); (514)335-1252; Fax. (514)335-1753.

BERTRAND, Carl; Active Care Med Group, A-1108 Klondike Rd, Kanata ON K2K 0G1; Ott'92; Langs: Bilingual(English/French); (613)254-9777; Fax. (613)254-9778.

BERTRAND, Carole; Hop Maisonneuve-Rosemont, 5415 boul de l'Assomption, Montreal QC H1T 2M4; Mon'92; FRCPC; IntMed; Rheum (P.Q.). Staff, Hopital Maisonneuve-Rosemont; (514)252-3400; Fax. (514)252-3889; bertrand.carole@videotron.ca.

BERTRAND, Charles; CSSS d'Antoine-Labelle-Mt Laur, RR 1 2561 ch de la Lievre S, Mont-Laurier QC J9L 3G3; Mon'98; Staff, CSSS d'Antoine-Labelle; (819)623-1234

BERTRAND, Danyelle; Ctr Hosp Pierre-Janet, 20 rue Pharand, Gatineau QC J9A 1K7; Laval'74; FRCPC; Psy. Staff, Centre Hospitalier Pierre-Janet; (819)776-8055

BERTRAND, Denys; CSSS de Montmagny-L'Islet, 350 boul Tache O RR 1, Montmagny QC G5V 3R8; Laval'72; FRCPC; DiagRad. Ac Staff, CSSS de Montmagny-L'Islet; (418)248-0630 x4472; Fax. (418)248-8497; denys.bertrand@ssss.gouv.qc.ca.

BERTRAND, Estelle; Clin d'Expertises Med du Quebe, 440-979 av de Bourgogne, Quebec QC G1W 2L4; Sher'85; FRCPC; Psy. (418)654-3268; Fax. (418)654-3271.

BERTRAND, Genevieve; Les Gynecologues Ass de Laval, 1299 boul de la Concorde O, Laval QC H7N 5T4; Mon'04; FRCSC; ObstGyn. Staff, Hopital de la Cite de la santé; (450)668-3250

BERTRAND, Helene; Dr Helene Bertrand Inc, 220-1940 Lonsdale Ave, North Vancouver BC V7M 2K2; McG'65; CCFP; Court Staff, Lions Gate Hospital; Clin Instructor Family Practice, University of British Columbia; Langs: Spanish; French; (604)985-5381; Fax. (604)985-6493; dr.hbertrand@gmail.com.

BERTRAND, Henri A; 423 rue Guerette, Maniwaki QC J9E 1N4; Ott'69; Langs: English; French; (819)449-6637; Fax. (819)449-6638.

BERTRAND, Isabelle; CHUQ-Ctr Hosp Univ Laval, 2705 boul Laurier, Quebec QC G1V 4G2; Sher'04; FRCPC; EmergMed. Staff, Centre Hospitalier Universitaire de Quebec-CHUL; Conférencier, Université Laval; Langs: Bilingual(French/English); (418)656-4141

BERTRAND, Janie; CHUS-Hop Fleurimont, 3001 12 av N, Sherbrooke QC J1H 5N4; Sher'07; FRCPC; Derm. Staff, Centre Hospitalier Universitaire de Sherbrooke-Hopital Fleurimont; (810)346-1110

BERTRAND, Jean-Claude; Hop du Sacre-Coeur de Mtl, 5400 boul Gouin O, Montreal QC H4J 1C5; Sher'96; FRCPC; Psy. Staff, Hôpital du Sacre-Coeur de Montréal; (514)338-2070

BERTRAND, Josee; CSSS du Nord de Lanaudière, 1000 boul Sainte-Anne, St-Charles-Brromee QC J6E 6J2; Mon'98; Staff, Centre Hospitalier Régional de Lanaudière; (450)759-8222

BERTRAND, Marie; Centre Medical 25, 135B 25e av, Saint-Eustache QC J7P 2V1; Sher'86; ObstGyn (P.Q.). (450)491-3533; Fax. (450)491-4842; mbertrand@cm25.ca.

BERTRAND, Michel; 101-783 rue Notre-Dame, Repentigny QC J5Y 1B4; Mon'82; Staff, Centre Hospitalier Pierre le Gardeur; Staff, Clinique Medicale Valmont; (450)582-1260

BERTRAND, Michel; CLSC Saint-Pamphile, CP 580 103 rue du Foyer N, Saint-Pamphile QC G0R 3X0; Laval'72; (418)356-3393; Fax. (418)356-2169.

BERTRAND, Michel; CHUM-Hop Notre-Dame, 1560 rue Sherbrooke E, Montreal QC H2L 4M1; Mon'84 Université de Montréal; IntMed (Lipidology). Staff, Centre Hospitalier l'Université de Montréal (CHUM) - Hôpital Notre-Dame; adj Prof, Universite de Montreal; Langs: English; (514)890-8000 x26784; Fax. (514)412-7533.

BERTRAND, Monique; London HSC-Victoria Hosp, PO Box 5010 Stn B E5 312-800 Commissioners Rd E, London ON N6A 4G5; Mem'80; FRCSC; ObstGyn (Gynecologic Oncology). Sr Med Dir Cancer Serv/Staff, London Health Sciences Centre - Victoria Campus; Langs: Bilingual(English/French); (519)685-8088; Fax. (519)685-8176.

BERTRAND, Nadia; CHUQ-St-Francois d'Assise, 10 rue de l'Espinay, Quebec QC G1L 3L5; Mon'94; CSPQ; FRCPC; Anes. Staff, Centre Hospitalier Universitaire De Québec - Pavillon De St-françois-d'assise; (418)525-4340; Fax. (418)525-4434.

BERTRAND, Nathalie; Clinique Med Sainte-Dorothee, 102-1 boul Samson, Laval QC H7X 3S5; Laval'94; Staff, Centre Hospitalier Pierre le Gardeur; (450)689-6334; Fax. (450)689-6339.

BERTRAND, Olivier; Hôpital Laval, 2725 ch Sainte-Foy, Quebec QC G1V 4G5; (Belgium)'90; PhD; Staff, Hôpital Laval; adj Prof, Université Laval; Langs: English; (418)656-4657; Fax. (418)656-4544; olivier.bertrand@crhl.ulaval.ca.

BERTRAND, Pierre E; Centre d'Urologie Maisonneuve, 220-5345 boul de l'Assomption, Montreal QC H1T 4B3; Mon'60; FRCSC; Urol. (514)255-9006

BERTRAND, Pierre; Medigestal Inc, 101-2655 boul Daniel-Johnson, Laval QC H7P 5Y2; Mon'58; OrthSurg. (450)688-5018

BERTRAND, Raymond J; Espanola Reg Hosp & Hlth Ctre, 825 McKinnon Dr, Espanola ON P5E 1R4; Tor'90; Staff, Espanola Regional Hospital and Health Centre; (705)869-1421; Fax. (705)862-7157.

BERTRAND, Real; Inst U en Sante Mentale de QC, 2601 ch de la Canardiere, Quebec QC G1J 2G3; Laval'72; Staff, Institut Universitaire Sante; (418)663-5253

BERTRAND, Robert A; 302-5995 boul Gouin O, Montreal QC H4J 2P8; Mon'58; Otol (Neuro Otology). Emeritus Membre, Centre Hospitalier l'Université de Montréal (CHUM) - Hôpital Notre-Dame; Prof Surg, Universite de Montreal; Langs: Bilingual(French/English); Spanish; (514)332-2050; info@bjainc.com.

BERTRAND, Robert G; 40 rue des Muguets, St-Denis-de-Brompt QC J0B 2P0; Mon'75; (819)846-4077

BERTRAND, Sylvie; Clinique Med Jean-Talon Pie IX, 4679 rue Jean-Talon E, Saint-Leonard QC H1S 1K3; Mon'84; FRCPC; IntMed; Endocrin (P.Q.); Endocrin&Metab. (514)374-5901; Fax. (514)374-1668.

BERTRAND-BOVET, Audrey; Centre Med Fusion, 2035 av Sainte-Anne, Saint-Hyacinthe QC J2S 5H3; Sher'10; CCFP; (450)773-6023

BERTSCH, Angelica R; Veterans Affairs, 610-234 Donald St, Winnipeg MB R3C 4G5; Man'81; BSc(Hons).

BERTSCH, Kristine L; Crowfoot Village Fam Practice, 210-600 Crowfoot Cres NW, Calgary AB T3G 0B4; Alb'08; CCFP; (403)239-9733

BERTUCCI, Vince; Columbus Med Arts Bldg, 100-8333 Weston Rd, Woodbridge ON L4L 8E2; Tor'89; ABD; FRCPC; IntMed (Cosmetic Dermatology); Derm. Staff, Women's College Hospital; Teach Staff/Co-Dir Dermatology Laser Surg & Cosmetic Dermatology Fellowship, University of Toronto; Langs: Italian; (905)850-4415; Fax. (905)850-5517.

BERUBE, Alain; 1930 rue King O, Sherbrooke QC J1J 2E2; Sher'81; BSc(BioChem.); MSc(Pharmacol.); Physician, Correctional Services of Canada; Physician, Sherbrooke Dentention Centre & Centre Jean Patrice Chiasson; Clin Teach Staff Family Med, Universite de Sherbrooke; Langs: Bilingual(French/English); (819)821-2500; Fax. (819)563-8322; aberube.crde@ssss.gouv.qc.ca.

BERUBE, Andree-Anne; Ctr Hosp Affilie-St-Sacrement, 1515 17e rue, Saint-Georges QC G5Y 4T8; Laval'07; ObstGyn (P.Q.). Staff, Centre Hospitalier Beauce-Etchemin; (418)228-2031

BERUBE, Anne; Inst U en Sante Mentale de QC, 2601 ch de la Canardiere, Quebec QC G1J 2G3; Laval'83; FRCPC; DiagRad. Staff, Centre Hospitalier Chauveau; Staff, Institut Universitaire Sante; (418)663-5778

BERUBE, Arline; CHUM-Hop Notre-Dame, 1560 rue Sherbrooke E, Montreal QC H2L 4M1; Laval'01; FRCPC; Neur. Staff, Centre Hospitalier l'Université de Montréal (CHUM) - Hôpital Notre-Dame; (514)890-8237

BERUBE, Charles; 11515 8e av, Saint-Georges QC G5Y 1J5; Mon'77; Staff, Centre d'hébergement de Beauceville; (418)228-2021

BERUBE, Claude; Clinique Chabanel, 201-1281 rue des Champs-Elysee, Chicoutimi QC G7H 5Y4; Laval'72; Assoc Member, Complexe hospitalier de la Sagamie; (418)543-9761; Fax. (418)543-1248.

BERUBE, Denis; 3175 ch Cote-Sainte-Catherine, Montreal QC H3T 1C5; McG'85; FCCP; FRCPC; Peds (Pediatric Respirology); Respir. Staff, Hôpital Ste-Justine; Langs: French; (514)345-4931 x5409; Fax. (514)345-4804.

BERUBE, Elaine; CLSC Dorval-Lachine, 1900 rue Notre-Dame, Lachine QC H8S 2G2; Sher'89; (514)639-0650; Fax. (514)639-8593; elaine.berube@sympatico.ca.

BERUBE, Felix-Antoine; Hop Louis-H Lafontaine, 7401 rue Hochelaga, Montreal QC H1N 3M5; Laval'02; FRCPC; Psy. Staff, Hopital Louis-H Lafontaine; (514)251-2158

BERUBE, Guylaine; CLSC Saint-Hubert, 6800 boul Cousineau, Saint-Hubert QC J3Y 8Z4; Mon'90; (450)443-7400; Fax. (450)676-3488.

BERUBE, Jean-D.; CLSC du Grand Chicoutimi, 411 rue de l'Hotel-Dieu, Chicoutimi QC G7H 7Z5; Laval'76; (418)543-2221; Fax. (418)543-9512.

BERUBE, Jocelyn; CSSS de Rimouski-Neigette, CP 3150 Succ A 150 av Rouleau, Rimouski QC G5L 5T1; Laval'72; ac Staff, Hôpital Regional Rimouski; Langs: English; (418)724-8578; Fax. (418)724-8512.

BERUBE, Johan; Clinique Med de l'Ouest, 2200 boul Dionne, Saint-Georges QC G5Y 3X3; Laval'99; Emergency Med, Centre Hospitalier Beauce-Etchemin; (418)228-2024; Fax. (418)228-7715.

BERUBE, Josee; Centre Med Fusion, 200-2035 av Sainte-Anne, Saint-Hyacinthe QC J2S 5H3; Sher'93; Staff, Centre Hospitalier Honore-Mercier; (450)773-6023

BERUBE, Laurie; Hotel-Dieu de Levis, 143 rue Wolfe, Levis QC G6V 3Z1; Laval'06; ObstGyn. Staff, Hôtel-Dieu de Lévis; (418)835-7121

BERUBE, Lyne; CHUM-Hotel-Dieu, 3840 rue Saint-Urbain, Montreal QC H2W 1T8; Mon'96; CSPQ; FRCPC; IntMed; Cardiol. Staff, Centre Hospitalier l'Université de Montréal (CHUM) - Hôtel-Dieu; (514)890-8174

BERUBE, Marie-Claude; Centre de Sante de Rigaud, 1 rue de l'Hotel-de-Ville, Rigaud QC J0P 1P0; Mon'83; (450)451-5336

BERUBE, Martine; Clinique Medico-Legale, 300-234 rue Dufferin, Sherbrooke QC J1H 4M2; Sher'99; FRCPC; Psy (Legal Psychiatry). Staff, Centre Hospitalier Universitaire de Sherbrooke-Hôpital Hôtel-Dieu; Langs: Spanish; English; (819)821-2297; Fax. (819)821-9917; clinique-medico-legal-med@usherbrooke.ca.

BERUBE, Michel J A; CSSS des Iles, 430 ch Principal, Cap-aux-Meules QC G4T 1R9; Ott'89; CSPQ; FRCPC; IntMed. ac Membre, Hôpital de l'Archipel; Langs: English; French; (418)986-2121 x8197; Fax. (418)986-7001.

BERUBE, Michel; CSSS de Chicoutimi, 305 rue Saint-Vallier, Chicoutimi QC G7H 5H6; Mon'93; FRCPC; DiagRad. Chef radiodiag, Complexe hospitalier de la Sagamie; (418)541-1031; Fax. (418)541-1103.

BERUBE, Michele; CLSC des Hautes Marees, 1320 rue Saint-Paul, L'Ancienne-Lorette QC G2E 1Z4; Laval'81; Université Laval; (418)651-2572; Fax. (418)872-5336.

BERUBE, Nathalie; Regie des Rentes du Quebec, CP 5200 Succ Terminus, Quebec QC G1K 7S9; Sher'95; LMCC; (418)643-5185

BERUBE, Simon; CHUS-Hop Fleurimont, 3001 12e av N, Sherbrooke QC J1H 5N4; Sher'99; CSPQ; FRCPC; IntMed; Cardiol. Staff, Centre Hospitalier Universitaire de Sherbrooke-Hopital Fleurimont; (819)346-1110

BERUBE, Suzanne; 1672 rue Principale, Chambord QC G0W 1G0; Laval'77; Staff, Hotel-Dieu de Roberval; (418)342-6281; Fax. (418)342-6282.

BERUBE-DESROSIERS, Maxime; Centre Hosp Honore-Mercier, 2750 boul Laframboise, Saint-Hyacinthe QC J2S 4Y8; Mon'07; FRCPC; Neur. Staff, Centre Hospitalier Honore-Mercier.

BERZEN, Alan; 202-441 Clark Ave W, Thornhill ON L4J 6W8; Witwatersrand (South Africa)'80; FRCPC; Peds. Staff, The Hospital For Sick Children; (905)764-5114; Fax. (905)764-9615.

BERZEN, Leon; UBC-Dept Of Psychiatry, 0007-2255 Wesbrook Mall, Vancouver BC V6T 2A1; Witwatersrand (South Africa)'83; MB ChB; FRCPC; Psy (Neurology & Psychiatry). Staff NeuroPsy, Vancouver General Hospital - Centennial Pavillion; Clin Instructor NeuroPsy, University of British Columbia; (604)822-7298; Fax. (604)822-7105.

BERZOWSKI, Anna M; Guelph Gen Hosp, 115 Delhi St, Guelph ON N1E 4J4; Gdansk (Poland)'68; FRCPC; GenPath. Staff, Guelph General Hospital; (519)837-6440 x2316; aberzowski@gghorg.ca.

BESANT, Joan E; South Calgary Mental Health Ct, 2726-31 Sunpark Plaza SE, Calgary AB T2X 3W5; Sask'84; FRCPC; Psy;CCFP; Staff, Alberta Children's Hospital; (403)943-9363

BESELT, Jeffrey K; Campbell River & Dist Gen Hosp, 375 2nd Ave, Campbell River BC V9W 3V1; Alb'02; CCFP; CCFP(E.M.); Staff, Campbell River & District General Hospital; (250)914-1969

BESEMANN, Markus; Canadian Forces Health Servic, 405-1745 Alta Vista Dr, Ottawa ON K1A 0K6; Ott'88; FRCPC; PhysMed&Rehab (Electromyography). Langs: German; French; (613)736-9117; Fax. (613)736-9771.

BESHAI, Safa; 130-3410 Geatz Ave, Red Deer AB T4N 3Y4; Cairo (Egypt)'80; Chief Dept of Psy, Red Deer Regional Hospital Centre; (403)342-9400; Fax. (403)340-8847; red.deer.psychiatry.clinic@telus.net.

BESHARA, Eren; Wheat City Med Clinic, C1-1711 Kirkcaldy Dr, Brandon MB R7A 0B9; (Other Foreign)'96; CCFP; (204)727-1711

BESHARA, Hani M N; Halton HCS Corp-Milton, 7030 Derry Rd E, Milton ON L9T 7H6; Alexandria (Egypt)'01; FRCPC; IntMed (Critical Care Medicine). Staff, Halton Healthcare Services Corporation - Milton District Hospital; (905)878-2383

BESHARA, Nasser R; Greenbank Med Centre, 202A-139 Greenbank Rd, Nepean ON K2H 9A5; Ain Shams (Egypt)'89; FRCSC; ObstGyn. Staff, Queensway Carleton Hospital; (613)721-7111; Fax. (613)721-3667.

BESHARA, Rafik A S; Grand Falls Med Clinic, 164 Goodyear Ave, Grnd-Falls-Windsor NL A2A 1M4; Cairo (Egypt)'94; MB BCh; Staff, Central Newfoundland Regional Health Centre; (709)489-7763

BESHAY, Alfi M; 905-1 St. Paul St, St Catharines ON L2R 7L2; Cairo (Egypt)'86; FRCPC; IntMed. Staff, Niagara Health System - Ontario Street Site; (905)688-1148

BESHAY, Basem; B-25 Savoie Ave, Atholville NB E3N 4A8; Assiut (Egypt)'88; (506)759-7110; Fax. (506)753-7117.

BESHAY, Hany Y; 10-5380 Terry Fox Way, Mississauga ON L5V 0A5; Alexandria (Egypt)'85; BSc; MB ChB; LMCC; CCFP; Langs: Arabic; (905)858-3030

BESHAY, Nabil M S; 112A-210 Memorial Ave, Orillia ON L3V 7V1; Ain Shams (Egypt)'81; CCFP; (705)329-1882; Fax. (705)329-0840.

BESHAY, Samy A Y; C1-2524 Third Line, Oakville ON L6M 0G8; CCFP; (905)827-7000

BESHAY, Sanaa S; 2-134 Dundas St W, Mississauga ON L5B 1H9; Cairo (Egypt)'86; MB ChB; CCFP; CCFP(E.M.); Staff, Stevenson Memorial Hospital; Staff Emerg, Halton Healthcare Services Corporation - Oakville Site; Langs: Arabic; (905)268-0188

BESHIR, Marian; Connaigre Peninsula Comm HC, PO Box 70 1 Alexander Ave, Harbour Breton NL A0H 1P0; University of Alexandria (Egypt)'06; MB ChB; Clin Associate, James Paton Memorial Hospital; Locum Tenens, Connaigre Peninsula Community Health Centre; (709)292-2500; marian.beshir@easternhealth.ca.

BESIK, Fred R; The Credit Valley Hosp, 2200 Eglinton Ave W, Mississauga ON L5M 2N1; Tor'85; Staff, The Credit Valley Hospital; Langs: Slovak; (905)813-1100 x5121; Fax. (905)813-4024.

BESLEY, Robert H; 1556 Par Four Drive, Midland ON L4R 5K4; Tor'73; BSc(Hon); MD; (705)529-4840; Fax. (705)355-0175; rbesley@rogers.com.

BESNER, Catherine; 85 rue Saint-Redempteur, Gatineau QC J8X 4E6; Laval'04; CCFP; Staff Family Med, Hôpital de Gatineau; Langs: French; (819)966-6510; Fax. (819)966-6533.

BESNER, Guy; 999 rue de Salaberry, Montreal QC H3L 1L2; Mon'80; CSPQ; FRCPC; Anes. Staff, Centre Hospitalier l'Université De Montréal (CHUM) - Hôpital Saint-luc; Universite de Montreal; (514)332-7091

BESNER, Louis; Groupe Sante Medisys, 550-500 rue Sherbrooke O, Montreal QC H3A 3C6; Mon'77; FRCSC; OrthSurg. (514)499-2777 x3267

BESROUR, Sadok; Clinique de Med Familiale, 6e-2120 rue Sherbrooke E, Montreal QC H2K 1C3; Lyon (France)'68; DAB; Staff, Centre Hospitalier l'Université de Montréal (CHUM) - Hôpital Notre-Dame; (514)527-1958; Fax. (514)527-1649.

BESSAIH, Nawal; Hotel-Dieu de Sorel, 400 av de l'Hotel-Dieu, Sorel-Tracy QC J3P 1N5; (Other Foreign)'04; Staff, Hôtel-Dieu de Sorel.

BESSETTE, Benoit J; 202-595 Montreal Rd, Ottawa ON K1K 4L2; Ott'96; BSc; MD; FRCS; FRCSC; OrthSurg (P.Q.) (Shoulder & Knee Reconstruction). Staff, Montfort Hospital; Langs: French; (613)746-6745; Fax. (613)746-6008.

BESSETTE, Isabelle; CSSS du Nord de Lanaudière, SI 1F-1000 boul Sainte-Anne, St-Charles-Brromee QC J6E 6J2; Sher'07; CCFP; Staff, Centre Hospitalier Régional de Lanaudière; Langs: French; (450)759-8222 x2945

BESSETTE, Isabelle; Clinique Med Avenir, 220-1575 boul de l'Avenir, Laval QC H7S 2N5; Mon'91; (450)696-1025; Fax. (450)696-1019.

BESSETTE, Louis; CHUQ-Ctr Hosp Univ Laval, J760-2705 boul Laurier, Quebec QC G1V 4G2; Laval'88 Laval; AddicMed; FRCPC; IntMed (Epidemiology & Clinical Epidemiology); Rheum. Staff, Centre Hospitalier Universitaire de Quebec-CHUL; Prog Dir Rheum, Université Laval; Langs: English; (418)654-2242; Fax. (418)654-2798; louis.bessette@crchul.ulaval.ca.

BESSETTE, Luc; 2055 rue Mansfield, Montreal QC H3A 1Y7; Mon'80; Staff, Centre Hospitalier l'Université De Montréal (CHUM) - Hôpital Saint-luc; (514)345-1356; Fax. (514)345-1820.

BESSETTE, Lucie; Clinique Medi-Soleil, 120-383 boul du Seminaire N, St-Jean-sur-Richel QC J3B 8C5; Sher'88; Staff, Hôpital du Haut-Richelieu; (450)349-5555

BESSETTE, Maral A; CSSS de Trois-Rivieres, 1991 boul du Carmel, Trois-Rivieres QC G8Z 3R9; Grenoble (France)'00; Staff, CSSS de Trois-Rivières; (819)697-3333

BESSETTE, Michel; CSSS des Pays-d'En-Haut, 707 boul Sainte-Adele, Sainte-Adele QC J8B 2N1; Mon'75; Langs: Bilingual(French/English); (450)229-6601; Fax. (450)229-7220.

BESSETTE, Paul; CHUS-Hop Fleurimont, 3001 12e Av N, Sherbrooke QC J1H 5N4; Mon'88; FRCSC; ObstGyn (Gynecologic Oncology). Chef GynOncol, Centre Hospitalier Universitaire de Sherbrooke-Hopital Fleurimont; Prof, Universite de Sherbrooke; Langs: English; (819)346-1110 x13056; Fax. (819)820-6434.

BESSETTE, Paule; Centre Med Dorion Vaudreuil, 600 boul Harwood, Vaudreuil-Dorion QC J7V 6A3; Mon'75; Médecin, Centre Hospitalier l'Université de Montréal (CHUM) - Hôtel-Dieu; (450)455-9301; Fax. (450)455-9549.

BESSIERE, Guillaume; CSSS du Suroît, 150 rue Saint-Thomas, Salaber-de-Valleyf QC J6T 6C1; (France)'00; Staff, Centre Hospitalier Régional du Suroît; (450)371-9920; Fax. (450)377-1372.

BESSISSOW, Talat; MUHC-Royal Victoria Hosp, 687 av des Pins O, Montreal QC H3A 1A1; McG'05; FRCPC; IntMed; Gastroent. Staff, McGill University Health Centre - Royal Victoria Hospital; (514)934-1934 x31616

BESSOUDO, Ricardo; 719 Millidge Ave, Saint John NB E2K 2N7; (Mexico)'73; FACC; FRCP; FRCPC; IntMed (Non-Invasive Cardiology); Cardiol. Staff Cardiol, Saint John Regional Hospital; Lecturer, Dalhousie University; Langs: French; Spanish; (506)634-7844; Fax. (506)635-4883; ricardobessoudo@gmail.com.

BEST, Adrienne; William Osler HC-Brampton, 2100 Bovaird Dr E, Brampton ON L6R 3J7; Qns'07; CCFP; CCFP(E.M.); Staff, William Osler Health System - Brampton Civic Hospital; (905)494-2120

BEST, Andrew K; Royal Columbian Hosp, 330 Columbia St E, New Westminster BC V3L 3W7; Tor'99; FRCPC; DiagRad. Staff, Royal Columbian Hospital; (604)520-4640

BEST, Anthony H S; Queen Elizabeth II Hosp, 10409 98 St, Grande Prairie AB T8V 2E8; Mem'86; FRCPC; IntMed; Critical Care Medicine; EmergMed. Staff, Queen Elizabeth II Hospital; (780)830-2844; Fax. (780)830-2843.

BEST, Brian R; Peel Med Arts Bldg, 500-145 Queen St E, Brampton ON L6W 3P8; Tor'72; FRCPC; Neur. (905)456-2765

BEST, C Dale; Lougheed Plaza, 282-9600 Cameron St, Burnaby BC V3J 7N3; Sask'83; CCFP; Med Staff, Royal Columbian Hospital; Med Staff, Eagle Ridge Hospital & Health Care Centre; (604)420-4264

BEST, Carolyn; Hamilton HS-McMaster Site, PO Box 2000 Stn Lcd 1 1200 Main St W, Hamilton ON L8N 3Z5; Tor'04; FRCSC; ObstGyn. Staff, Hamilton Health Sciences Centre - McMaster University Medical Centre; (905)521-2100; Fax. (905)577-8377.

BEST, Kerri L; Medical Assoc of Port Perry, 462 Paxton St, Port Perry ON L9L 1L9; McM'00; BSc; CCFP; Court Staff Privil, Southlake Regional Health Centre; Ac Staff Privil, Lakeridge Health - Port Perry Site; (905)985-2895; drkerribest@yahoo.com.

BEST, Leoncio M; Health Sciences Centre, 300 Prince Philip Dr, St. John's NL A1B 3V6; Guadalajara (Mexico)'72; FRCS; Urol (Oncology). Staff, Health Sciences Centre; Clin Assoc Prof Surg(Urol), Memorial University Of Newfoundland; Langs: Spanish; (709)576-8115; Fax. (709)576-7713; lbest@nl.rogers.com.

BEST, Robert A; Cobequid Comm Health Centre, 40 Freer Lane, Lower Sackville NS B4C 0A2; Dal'08; CCFP; CCFP(E.M.); Staff, Cobequid Community Health Centre; (902)869-6101

BEST, Sandra J; 80 King St E, Brockville ON K6V 1B5; McG'74; Staff, Brockville General Hospital - Charles Street; Staff, Providence Continuing Care Centre (PCCC) - St Vincent de Paul Hospital; (613)342-0184; Fax. (613)342-4598.

BEST, Thomas B; 104-2100 8th St E, Saskatoon SK S7H 0V1; Sask'76; FRCPC; Peds (Pediatric Endocrinology); Endocrin&Metab. Ac Staff, Saskatoon District Health Board; Clinical Asst Prof, University of Saskatchewan; (306)975-0220; Fax. (306)975-0230.

BEST, Timothy J; 504-421 Bay St, Sault Ste. Marie ON P6A 1X3; Wes'88; FRCSC; PlasSurg (Cosmetic Surgery). Staff, Sault Area Hospital - Sault Ste Marie; Asst Prof Surg, Northern Ontario School of Medicine; (705)256-6012; Fax. (705)256-7228.

BESTARD, Jennifer A; Central Alberta Prof Centre, 173-5201 43 St, Red Deer AB T4N 1C7; McM'03; FRCPC; Neur (Headache). (403)340-1553; Fax. (403)340-1765.

BESTAWROS, Alain; CHUM-Hop Notre-Dame, 6F-1560 rue Sherbrooke E, Montreal QC H2L 4M1; McG'03; FRCPC; IntMed; MedOncol; Hem. Staff, Centre Hospitalier l'Université de Montréal (CHUM) - Hôpital Notre-Dame; (514)890-8000

BESTED, Alison C; BC Women's Hosp & Health Ctre, 4500 Oak St, Vancouver BC V6H 3N1; McM'79; BSc; FRCPC; HemPath (Chronic Illness). Staff, BC Women's Hospital & Health Centre; (604)875-3060

BESTER, Belinda A; The Cottage Medical Clinic, PO Box 2140 300 Miette Ave, Jasper AB T0E 1E0; (South Africa)'03; MB ChB; CCFP; Langs: Afrikaans; (780)852-4885; Fax. (780)852-2199.

BESTER, Charles J; Central Alberta Prof Centre, 182-5201 43 St, Red Deer AB T4N 1C7; Kansas (USA)'79; (403)343-6404; Fax. (403)343-6215.

BESTER, Charlotte; BC Cancer Agency-Vanc Isl Ctr, 2410 Lee Ave, Victoria BC V8R 6V5; Cape Town (South Africa)'87; MB ChB; Staff, BC Cancer Agency Vancouver Island Centre; (250)519-5572

BESTER, Daniel J; PO Box 100, Cardston AB T0K 0K0; Witwatersrand (South Africa)'81; BCh; MB; LMCC; Ac Staff Chinook Health Region, Cardston Hospital; (403)653-4411

BESTER, Johan C; Sunridge Family Med Teaching C, 2685 36 St NE, Calgary AB T1Y 5S3; (403)943-5000

BESTER, Michiel A N; 765 Canboro Rd, Fenwick ON L0S 1C0; (905)892-8722; Fax. (905)892-8220.

BESTER, Stephanus P; 210A-6640 Vedder Rd, Chilliwack BC V2R 0J2; Stellenbosch (South Africa)'86; MB ChB; Langs: Afrikaans; (604)858-2246; Fax. (604)858-4498.

BESTER, Stephen C; Golden Mile Centre, 215-3806 Albert St, Regina SK S4S 3R2; Cape Town (South Africa)'84; MB ChB; CCFP; FCFP; Staff, Regina General Hospital; Fam Med, Pasqua Hospital; (306)789-7900; Fax. (306)789-2642.

BESTER, Urbanus F; 1-2196 Quilchena Ave PO Box 158, Merritt BC V1K 1B8; Pretoria (South Africa)'90; MB ChB; BScPharm(Hons); CCFP; FCFP; (250)378-9020; Fax. (250)378-0873.

BESTILNY, Allan D; Calgary Trail Medicentre, 1-10407 51 Ave NW, Edmonton AB T6H 0K4; Alb'77; Staff, Calgary Trail Medicentres; (780)436-8071; Fax. (780)435-6034; sbestilny@shaw.ca.

BESTMAN-SMITH, Julie; Ctr Hosp Affilie-Enfant-Jesus, 1401 18e rue, Quebec QC G1J 1Z4; Laval'06; MedMicrobiol. Staff, Centre Hospitalier Affilié Universitaire de Québec - Hôpital De L'Enfant Jésus; (418)649-0258

BETALA BELINGA, Jean-Francois; ASSS de Chicoutimi, 930 rue Jacques-Cartier E, Chicoutimi QC G7H 7K9; (418)545-4980 x454

BETCHER, Jeffrey G; Regina Qu'Appelle HR-Regina, 1440 14th Ave, Regina SK S4P 0W5; Man'89; FRCPC; Anes; Critical Care Medicine. Staff Anes & Critical Care, Regina General Hospital; Staff, Regina Health District; Clinical Asst Prof, University of Saskatchewan; (306)766-4252

BETEL, Cara B; Sunnybrook Hlth Sciences Ctre, 2075 Bayview Ave, Toronto ON M4N 3M5; Tor'99; FRCPC; DiagRad. Staff, Sunnybrook Health Sciences Centre; (416)480-4341; Fax. (416)480-5855.

BETHUNE, Cheri E H; Shea Heights Commun Hlth Ctre, PO Box 13122 Stn A 57B Linegar Ave, St. John's NL A1B 4A4; McM'80; CCFP; FCFP; Staff, Health Sciences Centre; Prof Family Med, Memorial University Of Newfoundland; (709)737-3369

BETHUNE, Donald J; Foothills Med Centre, 1403 29 St NW, Calgary AB T2N 2T9; UBC'87; CCFP; CCFP(E.M.); Staff, Foothills Medical Centre; (403)944-2419; Fax. (403)944-2419.

BETHUNE, Drew C G; Queen Elizabeth II HSC, 714-1276 South Park St, Halifax NS B3H 2Y9; Dal'74; BSc; MSc; FRCSC; GenSurg; ThorSurg. Asst Prof Surg, Queen Elizabeth II Health Sciences Centre - Victoria General Site; Asst Prof Surg, Dalhousie University; (902)473-6692; Fax. (902)473-6144; dbethune@dal.ca.

BETHUNE, Gillian C; Mount Sinai Hosp, 6 500-600 University Ave, Toronto ON M5G 1X5; Dal'07; FRCPC; AnatPath. Staff, Mount Sinai Hospital; (416)586-4800

BETHUNE, Graeme H G; Halifax Prof Centre, 375-5991 Spring Garden Rd, Halifax NS B3H 1Y6; Dal'74; BSc; CCFP; FCFP; Staff, Queen Elizabeth II Health Sciences Centre - Victoria General Site; Med Advisor, Ocean View Manor; (902)425-6131; Fax. (902)425-1366; bethuneoffice@eastlink.ca.

BETHUNE, Margaret D; Queen Elizabeth Hosp, PO Box 6600 Stn Central, Charlottetown PE C1A 8T5; Dal'86; FRCPC; Peds. Staff, Queen Elizabeth Hospital; (902)894-2111

BETHUNE, Peter N; The Ob/Gyn Suite, 403-199 Grafton St, Charlottetown PE C1A 1L2; Dal'87; ObstGyn. Staff, Queen Elizabeth Hospital; Consultant, The Ob/Gyn Suite; (902)629-8801; Fax. (902)629-8826.

BETIT, Eve; Clinique Med Notre-Dame, 147 rue Notre-Dame E, Victoriaville QC G6P 3Z8; Laval'05; (819)758-3165; Fax. (819)758-0745.

BETIT, Jean-Luc; Clinique Med Notre-Dame, 147 rue Notre-Dame E, Victoriaville QC G6P 3Z8; Laval'73; (819)758-3165; Fax. (819)758-0745.

BETLEN, Cerasela E; Lakeridge Health-Oshawa Site, 1 Hospital Crt, Oshawa ON L1G 2B9; University of Medicine and Pharmacy (Other Foreign)'95; Psy. Staff, Lakeridge Health - Oshawa Site; (905)576-8711; Fax. (905)721-4742.

BETOURNAY, Nicole; 403-895 boul du Seminaire N, St-Jean-sur-Richel QC J3A 1J2; Mon'87; AB; Ophth (P.Q.) (Retina). Ac Member Ophth, Hôpital du Haut-Richelieu; Assoc Member Ophth, Centre Hospitalier de Verdun; (450)348-8272

BETSCHEL, Stephen D; St Michael's Hosp, 30 Bond St, Toronto ON M5B 1W8; McM'98; FRCPC; IntMed; ClinImmunol&Allergy. Staff, St Michael's Hospital; (416)864-6060

BETTACHE, Nazila; CHUM-Hop St-Luc, 1058 rue Saint-Denis, Montreal QC H2X 3J4; McG'05; FRCPC; IntMed. (514)890-8000

BETTAHAR, Redouane; CSSS de Rimouski-Neigette, CP 3150 Succ A 150 av Rouleau, Rimouski QC G5L 5T1; Paris (France)'88; RadOncol; Chef radio-oncol, Hôpital Regional Rimouski; Langs: Arabic; (418)724-8362; Fax. (418)724-8247; redouane.bettahar@ssss.gouv.qc.ca.

BETTEZ, Mathieu; CSSS de Laval, 1755 boul Rene-Laennec, Laval QC H7M 3L9; Sher'07; Urol. Staff, Hopital de la Cite de la santé; (450)668-1010

BETTEZ, Nathalie; CSSS de Chicoutimi, 305 rue Saint-Vallier, Chicoutimi QC G7H 5H6; Sher'07; CCFP; Staff, Complexe hospitalier de la Sagamie; (418)541-1079; Fax. (418)541-1129.

BETTGER, Harald; Chinook Reg Hosp, 960 19 St S, Lethbridge AB T1J 1W5; Wes'95; FRCPC; Anes. Staff, Chinook Regional Hospital; (403)388-6131

BETTIN, Leane N; Saskatoon Community Clinic, 455 2nd Ave N, Saskatoon SK S7K 2C2; Sask'00; LMCC; CCFP; Staff, Saskatoon Community Health Unit; Staff Assistant Community Faculty, University of Saskatchewan; (306)652-0300; Fax. (306)664-4120; lbettin@communityclinic.sk.ca.

BETTOLLI, Marcos; Children's Hosp Eastern Ont, 401 Smyth Rd, Ottawa ON K1H 8L1; Cordoba (Argentina)'98; Staff, Children's Hospital of Eastern Ontario (CHEO); (613)737-7600

BETZ, Martin; Royal University Hosp, 103 Hospital Dr, Saskatoon SK S7N 0W8; Wes'78; FRCPC; EmergMed. Staff, Royal University Hospital; (306)655-1363; Fax. (306)655-1011.

BETZNER, Michael J; Foothills Med Centre, C231-1403 29 St NW, Calgary AB T2N 2T9; Alb'91; FRCPC; EmergMed. Staff, Foothills Medical Centre; Clin Associate, ICU & Bedside Ass't., Calgary Reg. Health Authority; (403)944-1820; Fax. (403)944-2419.

BEUERLEIN, Murray J; 300-4309 52 Ave, Red Deer AB T4N 6S4; Tor'03; MSc; FRCSC; OrthSurg (Upper Extremity Reconstruction). (403)309-2001; Fax. (403)358-5808; doctor.beuerlein@gmail.com.

BEUZERON-MANGINA, J Helene; Queen Elizabeth Health Complex, 614-2100 av Marlowe, Montreal QC H4A 3L5; Mon'87; Staff, Douglas Mental Health University Institute; (514)845-3036

BEVER, Klaus; 2523 St Johns St, Port Moody BC V3H 2B3; Ott'76; BSc; MSc; Chief Dept of General Pract & Hospitalist Prog, Eagle Ridge Hospital & Health Care Centre; Physician, Fraser Burrard Health District Board; Clin. Staff, University of British Columbia; (604)936-7277

BEVERIDGE, J Massey B; Dr Charles S Curtis Mem Hosp, 178-200 West St, St Anthony NL A0K 4S0; Qns'90; DTMH; MPhil; FRCSC; GenSurg (Burns). Staff, Charles S Curtis Memorial Hospital; (709)454-3333; massey.beveridge@lghealth.ca.

BEVERIDGE, James E; Paterson Med Centre, RR 1 Stn Main 45 Wolsley St, Kenora ON P9N 3W7; Qns'71; Staff, Lake of the Woods District Hospital; (807)468-3021; Fax. (807)468-6964.

BEVERIDGE, John A; 2403 33 Ave SW, Calgary AB T2T 2A2; Sask'78; FRCSC; PlasSurg. Staff Surg, Rockyview General Hospital; (403)509-0220; Fax. (403)509-0222.

BEVERIDGE, Paul M; 4303 10th Ave W, Vancouver BC V6R 2H6; Cal'78; CCFP; Staff, Kelowna General Hospital; (604)224-0224; Fax. (604)221-2545.

BEVERIDGE, Robert C; Brockville Gen Hosp, 400-75 Charles St, Brockville ON K6V 1S8; Qns'80; BSc; MSc; FRCPC; IntMed (Respirology); EmergMed. Aj Prof Med, Queen's University; (613)498-0365; Fax. (613)498-1479; bevro@bgh-on.ca.

BEVERIDGE, William K; Valley Prof Centre, 70 Exhibition St, Kentville NS B4N 4K9; Dal'84; FRCSC; OrthSurg. Staff, Valley Regional Hospital; (902)678-6878; Fax. (902)678-6884.

BEWICK, David J; Saint John Med Clinic, 299 Metcalf St, Saint John NB E2K 4P8; Dal'80; FRCPC; IntMed; Cardiol. Staff Atlantic Health Sciences Corp, Saint John Regional Hospital; Assoc Prof, Dalhousie University; (506)633-2099; Fax. (506)633-1487; bewickd@nbnet.nb.ca.

BEXTON, Brian G; 3150 av de Trafalgar, Montreal QC H3Y 1H7; Mon'75; FRCPC; Psy. Staff, Hôpital du Sacre-Coeur de Montréal; Pres, Assoc Med Psychiatres du Quebec; Langs: English; (514)938-2465

BEYAK, Michael J; Hotel-Dieu Hosp, 166 Brock St, Kingston ON K7L 5G2; Tor'96; FRCPC; IntMed (Gastroenterology). Staff, Kingston General Hospital; Staff, Hotel-Dieu Hospital; Assoc Prof, Queen's University; (613)544-3400

BEYANI-MULAISHO, Nambizi; 201-477 King St, Welland ON L3B 3K4; (Zambia)'79; MB BS; MRCOG; FSOGC; FACOG; FRC; AddicMed; FRCSC; ObstGyn. (905)732-1118; Fax. (905)732-1119; unzaska@hotmail.com.

BEYDOUN, Hussein K; Queen Elizabeth II HSC-Halifax, 6896F-1796 Summer St, Halifax NS B3H 3A7; Padova (Italy)'88; FRCPC; IntMed (Interventional Cardiology); Cardiol. Staff, Queen Elizabeth II Health Sciences Centre - Victoria General Site; Staff, Queen Elizabeth II Health Sciences Centre - Halifax Infirmary Site; Assoc Prof, Dalhousie University; Langs: Arabic; Italian; (902)473-2184; Fax. (902)473-6293.

BEYERS, Cornelia; Cannon Med Clinic, 4-2151 McCallum Rd, Abbotsford BC V2S 3N9; Stellenbosch (South Africa)'98; MD; (604)853-3314

BEYERS, Leslie A; Medical & Dental Bldg, 712-586 Eglinton Ave E, Toronto ON M4P 1P2; Tor'93; CCFP; Ac Staff, Women's College Hospital; (416)440-1880; Fax. (416)440-1106.

BEYTELL, Daniel; Gateway Med Clinic, 101-2051 McCallum Rd, Abbotsford BC V2S 3N5; Pretoria (South Africa)'83; MB BS; MB ChB; Langs: Afrikaans; (604)859-9084; Fax. (604)859-7494; danielbeytell@msn.com.

BEZANSON, Kevin; Temmy Latner Ctre for Palliati, 4F-60 Murray St, Toronto ON M5T 3L9; McM'97; CCFP; (416)586-4800

BEZEAU, Marc; Clinique Sante Jacques-Cartier, 200-1815 rue King O, Sherbrooke QC J1J 2E3; Sher'81; CCFP; FCFP; (819)565-7446; Fax. (819)565-7780.

BEZJAK, Andrea; Univ Hlth Network-Princess M, 610 University Ave, Toronto ON M5G 2M9; McG'85; MSc(ClinEpidem); DrMedCh; FRCPC; IntMed (Lung Cancer); RadOncol. Staff, Princess Margaret Hospital - University Health Network; Prof RadOncol, University of Toronto; Langs: Croatian; Italian; French; (416)946-2132; Fax. (416)946-6561; andrea.bezjak@rmp.uhn.on.ca.

BEZU, Kesete T; Boniface Park Med Centre, 8-700 Markham Rd, Scarborough ON M1H 2A7; Oromia (Ethiopia)'93; FRCPC; Peds. (416)264-3443; Fax. (416)264-3446.

BEZUHLY, Michael; IWK Health Centre, PO Box 9700 Rpo CSC 5850-5980 University Ave, Halifax NS B3K 6R8; Tor'03; FRCSC; PlasSurg (Pediatric Plastic Surgery). Staff, IWK Health Centre; Langs: Russian; French; (902)470-8168; Fax. (902)470-7939.

BEZUIDENHOUT, Jakobus; East Kootenay Reg Hosp, 1324 13 Ave N, Cranbrook BC V1C 3H9; Orange Free State (South Africa)'79; MB ChB; CCFP; Staff, East Kootenay Regional Hospital; (250)426-5281

BEZUIDENHOUT, Kenneth; Battlefords Family Health Cent, 103-1192 101 St, North Battleford SK S9A 0Z6; (306)937-6840; Fax. (306)445-4887.

BEZUIDENHOUT, Leon M; South Macleod Family Med, 100-15915 Macleod Trail SE, Calgary AB T2Y 3R9; Pretoria (South Africa)'80; MB ChB; (403)457-2457; Fax. (403)457-2458; leon@bezhome.com.

BHACHU, Davinder S; 11841 223 St, Maple Ridge BC V2X 5Y2; Glasgow (Scotland)'71; MB ChB; FRCSC; OrthSurg. Staff, Ridge Meadows Hospital & Health Care Centre; (604)467-1148; Fax. (604)463-5698.

BHACHU, Santokh; Royal Alexandra Hosp, 10240 Kingsway NW, Edmonton AB T5H 3V9; Man'02; FRCPC; Anes. Staff, Royal Alexandra Hospital; (780)735-4010; Fax. (780)735-4386.

BHADURI, Mousumi; London HSC-Victoria Hosp, 800 Commissioners Rd E, London ON N6A 5W9; Pune (India)'93; Staff, London Health Sciences Centre - Victoria Campus; (519)685-8500

BHAGALOO, Lanishen; Midway Walk-In Med & HC, 2102 11th Ave, Regina SK S4P 3Y6; Physician, Quance East Medical Clinic; Teach Staff, University of Regina; (306)522-3346; Fax. (306)522-3348.

BHAGAT, Ashok; York Medical, 110-1650 Elgin Mills Rd, Richmond Hill ON L4S 0B2; Bihar (India)'61; MD; MB BS; DPM(Lond); Langs: Hindi; Bengali; Urdu; (905)770-3858; Fax. (905)770-1964; bhagat60@hotmail.com.

BHAGAT, Kaushik K B; Radiology Consultants Assoc, 120-6707 Elbow Dr SW, Calgary AB T2V 0E3; (Zimbabwe)'83; MB ChB; FRCPC; DiagRad. (403)777-3003; Fax. (403)777-3008.

BHAGAVATULA, Subramanya; 680 Kirkwood Dr, Sudbury ON P3E 1X3; Delhi (India)'86; FRCPC; Psy (Addiction Psychiatry). Staff, Health Sciences North-Laurentian Site; Psychiatrist, North Bay Regional Health Centre - Kirkwood; Langs: Bengali; English; Hindi; Punjabi; Tamil; Telugu; Urdu; (705)675-5900 x8234; drbssastry@yahoo.ca.

BHAGIRATH, Chander P; Portage Prof Bldg, 401-5400 Portage Rd, Niagara Falls ON L2G 5X7; Guru Nanak (India)'76; FAAP; FRCPC; Peds (Pediatric Cardiology). Staff, Niagara Health System - Greater Niagara General Site; Clinical Asst Prof Peds, McMaster University; Langs: Hindi; Punjabi; (905)357-2423

BHAGIRATH, Kapil M; 101-8056 King George Hwy, Surrey BC V3W 5Y2; UBC'04; FRCPC; IntMed; Cardiol. Langs: Hindi; Punjabi; (604)593-5288

BHAGIRATH, Vikas C; Nation River Health Clinic, 494 Fred St, Winchester ON K0C 2K0; Wes'06; CCFP; (613)774-0915; Fax. (613)774-0916.

BHAGIRATH, Vinai C; Hamilton HS-General Site, 6F-237 Barton St E, Hamilton ON L8L 2X2; Wes'06; FRCPC; IntMed; Hem. Staff, Hamilton Health Sciences Centre - Hamilton General Hospital; (905)527-1710; Fax. (905)521-1551.

BHALERAO, Shree U; St Michael's Hosp, 4 107M-30 Bond St, Toronto ON M5B 1W8; Sask'94; BSc; FRCPC; Psy. Staff Psy, St Michael's Hospital; (416)864-6060 x2443; Fax. (416)864-5793.

BHALERAO, Uddhav K; The Tower at Midtown, 306-201 1st Ave S, Saskatoon SK S7K 1J5; Osmania (India)'57; MB BS; FACC; FRCPC; IntMed (Cardiology). Ac Staff, Saskatoon City Hospital; Ac Staff, St Paul's Hospital (Grey Nuns) of Saskatoon; Clin Prof, University of Saskatchewan; (306)244-2977; Fax. (306)665-0717.

BHALLA, Dinesh; The Moncton Hosp, 135 Macbeath Ave, Moncton NB E1C 6Z8; Delhi (India)'80; MB BS; FRCPC; Psy (Adult Psychiatry). Staff, The Moncton Hospital; Langs: Punjabi; Hindi; (506)383-4708; Fax. (506)383-4708.

BHALLA, Indu B; Trillium Hlth Ctr-Mississauga, 100 Queensway W, Mississauga ON L5B 1B8; Delhi (India)'68; Staff, Trillium Health Centre - Mississauga; (905)848-7100

BHALLA, Jaideep; Dr Charles L LeGrow Hlth Ctr, PO Box 250 1 Grand Bay Rd, Port-aux-Basques NL A0M 1C0; Jabalpur (India)'79; MB BS; Staff, Dr Charles L Legrow Health Centre; (709)695-2175

BHALLA, Jaswinder; 681 Mountain Rd, Moncton NB E1C 2P4; (India)'86; CCFP; (506)857-1006; Fax. (506)857-9484.

BHALLA, Kiran; Dr Charles L LeGrow Hlth Ctr, PO Box 250 1 Grand Bay Rd, Port-aux-Basques NL A0M 1C0; Jabalpur (India)'79; MB BS; Staff, Dr Charles L Legrow Health Centre; (709)695-2175

BHALLA, Rashmi; Hyde Park Med & Walk-In Clinic, 4-640 Hyde Park Rd, London ON N6H 3S1; McM'05; CCFP; (519)641-3627; Fax. (519)641-3628.

BHALLA, Sanjiv K; Northgate Centre, 2018-9499 137 Ave NW, Edmonton AB T5E 5R8; Wes'97; BScChemEng; FRCPC; DiagRad. Langs: Hindi; French; (780)476-9729; Fax. (780)476-9732.

BHALLA, Sunil; Health Sciences Centre, 300 Prince Philip Dr, St. John's NL A1B 3V6; Sint Eustatius (Netherlands Antilles)'04; FRCPC; IntMed; Nephrol. Staff, Health Sciences Centre; Locum Tenens, St Clare's Mercy Hospital; (709)737-6300

BHAMBHANI, Mahesh N; 209-9252 34 Ave NW, Edmonton AB T6E 5P2; Bangalore (India)'70; MB BS; FRCPC; Peds. Staff, University of Alberta Hospital; (780)462-9442; Fax. (780)439-9664.

BHAMJEE, Hassen; 1657 Dundas St, London ON N5W 3C6; Dublin (Ireland)'68; Court Staff, London Health Sciences Centre - Victoria Campus; Court Staff, St Joseph's Hospital - St Joseph's Health Care; Physician, Continental Can Ltd.; (519)455-8210; Fax. (519)455-7103.

BHAMRA, Jamie; Seema Eye Care Centre, 110-1016 68 Ave SW, Calgary AB T2V 4J2; Cal'03; FRCSC; Ophth. (403)253-5300; Fax. (403)253-8608.

BHAN, Neelma; Harbor Mental Health Clinic, PO Box 4 5 Forest Hill Pkwy, Dartmouth NS B2W 6C6; Srinagar (India)'80; (902)434-3263

BHAN, Vineet; Univ Hlth Network-Toronto Western Hosp, EW5 559-399 Bathurst St, Toronto ON M5T 2S8; Dal'07; FRCPC; IntMed. Staff, Toronto Western Hospital - University Health Network; (416)603-2581

BHAN, Virender; Queen Elizabeth II HSC-Halifax, 3827-1796 Summer St, Halifax NS B3H 3A7; Kashmir (India)'80; MB BS; FRCPC; Neur (Multiple Sclerosis). Staff, Queen Elizabeth II Health Sciences Centre - Halifax Infirmary Site; Ac Staff/Dir Dalhousie MS Research Unit, Queen Elizabeth II Health Sciences Centre - Victoria General Site; Assoc Prof/Prog Dir Neurology Residency Prog, Dalhousie University; (902)473-3731; Fax. (902)473-4438; virender.bhan@cdha.nshealth.ca.

BHANDAL, Harleen G; C-568 Christina St N, Sarnia ON N7T 5W6; Punjab (India)'95; (519)491-7775; Fax. (519)344-2727.

BHANDAL, Samarjeet K; Alberta Children's Hosp, 2888 Shaganappi Trail NW, Calgary AB T3B 6A8; Staff, Alberta Children's Hospital; (587)894-7097

BHANDARI, Mohit; Wellington Medical Co Op, 110-293 Wellington St N, Hamilton ON L8L 8E7; Tor'94; MSc; FRCSC; OrthSurg (Trauma). Staff, Hamilton Health Sciences Centre - Hamilton General Hospital; Prof, McMaster University; (905)527-4322 x44490; Fax. (905)523-8781.

BHANDARI, Rakesh; London HSC-University Hosp, PO Box 5339 Stn B 339 Windermere Rd, London ON N6A 5A5; Indore (India)'76; DA; DAB; FRCPC; Anes (Pain Management). Ac Staff, London Health Sciences Centre - University Hospital; Asst Prof Anes, University of Western Ontario; Langs: Hindi; German; (519)685-8500 x35147

BHANDHAL, Sharn; C1-2501 Prince Michael Dr, Oakville ON L6H 0E9; Pune (India)'99; MB; BSc; FRCPC; IntMed (Kidney Diseases); Nephrol. Staff, Halton Healthcare Services Corporation - Oakville Site; (905)842-9046; Fax. (905)842-9047.

BHANGU, Dalip K; Queensway Prof Centre, 315-190 Sherway Dr, Etobicoke ON M9C 5N2; Lucknow (India)'76; FRCS; FACOG; FRCSC; ObstGyn. Staff, Trillium Health Centre - West Toronto; Langs: Hindi; Punjabi; Urdu; (416)626-7250; Fax. (416)626-7252; dalipbhangu@hotmail.com.

BHANGU, Raminder K; Windsor Reg Hosp-Western Camp, 1453 Prince Rd, Windsor ON N9C 3Z4; Punjab (India)'87; FRCPC; Psy (Geriatric Psychiatry). Staff, Windsor Regional Hospital - Tayfour Site; Langs: Punjabi; Hindi; (519)257-5211

BHANGU, Sukhinder K; Synergy Sports Medicine, 235 Wallace Ave, Toronto ON M6H 1V5; Man'04; FRCPC; PhysMed&Rehab. Staff, Toronto Rehabilitation Institute - University Centre; (416)703-3525; Fax. (647)343-8073.

BHANJI, Farhan; MUHC-Montreal Children's Hosp, C808-2300 rue Tupper, Montreal QC H3H 1P3; Wes'96; FRCPC; Peds; PedEmergMed; Critical Care Medicine (P.Q.). Staff, McGill University Health Centre - Montreal Children's Hospital; (514)412-4000

BHANJI, Nadeem H; Peter Lougheed Centre, 1926-3500 26 Ave NE, Calgary AB T1Y 6J4; Alb'98; BScPharm; FRCPC; Psy (Clinical Pharmacology). Staff, Peter Lougheed Centre; Clin Asst Prof, University of Calgary; Langs: Gujarati; French; (403)943-5694

BHANJI, Nazmudin M F; 7263 Fraser St, Vancouver BC V5X 3V8; Shiraz (Iran)'78; MD; FAAP; FRCPC; Peds. Pediatrics, BC Children's Hospital; Ac Staff, Providence Health Care - Mount Saint Joseph Hospital; Clin Assoc Prof, University of British Columbia; Langs: Persian; Hindi; Gujarati; (604)322-1440; Fax. (604)322-1401.

BHANOT, Pradeep; Seven Oaks Gen Hosp, 2300 Mcphillips St, Winnipeg MB R2V 3M3; Dal'91; CCFP; Staff, Seven Oaks General Hospital; (204)632-7133

BHANOT, Raj; Mount Uniacke Med Centre, PO Box 53, Mount Uniacke NS B0N 1Z0; Dal'87; Staff, Sacred Heart Hospital; (902)256-3300; Fax. (902)256-3301.

BHANWATH, Gokul; Roslyn Med Bldg, 200-400 5th Ave SW, Calgary AB T2P 0L6; Bangalore (India)'74; MB BS; (403)275-6606; Fax. (403)730-0941; gokulbhanwath@shaw.ca.

BHARADWAJ, Steven C; St Paul's Hosp, 1702 20th St W, Saskatoon SK S7M 0Z9; Sask'04; FRCSC; GenSurg; ThorSurg. Staff, St Paul's Hospital (Grey Nuns) of Saskatoon; (306)655-0533; Fax. (306)655-5771.

BHARADWAJ, Vinod K; Belmont Prof Centre, 401-564 Belmont Ave W, Kitchener ON N2M 5N6; Jiwaji (India)'73; MB BS; MS; FRCSC; Otol. (519)741-8688; Fax. (519)741-0884; vinod533@rogers.com.

BHARAT, Winston S P; The Credit Valley Hosp, 2200 Eglinton Ave W, Mississauga ON L5M 2N1; Tor'09; CCFP; Staff, The Credit Valley Hospital; (905)813-2200; Fax. (905)813-3894.

BHARATHA, Aditya; St Michael's Hosp, 3 077CC-30 Bond St, Toronto ON M5B 1W8; Tor'03; FRCPC; DiagRad (Neuro Radiology). Staff, St Michael's Hospital; (416)864-6060; Fax. (416)864-5380.

BHARATWAL, Nirmala; Toronto Rehab Inst-Lyndhurst, 520 Sutherland Dr, Toronto ON M4G 3V9; Bombay (India)'64; MB BS; FRCPC; PhysMed&Rehab (Spinal Cord Injury). Physical Medicine & Rehab, Toronto Rehabilitation Institute - Lyndhurst Centre; Ac Staff, Sunnybrook Health Sciences Centre; Asst Prof Dept of Med & PhysMed & Rehab Div, University of Toronto; Langs: Hindi; Marathi; (416)597-3422 x6131; Fax. (416)422-5402; bharatwal.nimmi@torontorehab.on.ca.

BHARDWAJ, Ajay K; Woodbridge Med Centre, A13-9600 Islington Ave, Woodbridge ON L4H 2T1; (Other Foreign)'08; (905)893-8085

BHARDWAJ, Arun; William Osler HC-Brampton, 2100 Bovaird Dr E, Brampton ON L6R 3J7; Rajasthan (India)'87; MB BS; FRCPC; Anes. Staff, William Osler Health System - Brampton Civic Hospital; (905)796-4066; arunbhardwaj@hotmail.com.

BHARDWAJ, Asha; St Joseph's HC-Parkwood Hosp, 801 Commissioners Rd E, London ON N6C 5J1; Punjab (India)'67; AADEP; FRCPC; PhysMed&Rehab (Disability Evaluation). Staff, Parkwood Hospital - St Joseph's Health Care; Consultant, London Health Sciences Centre - Victoria Campus; Asst Prof, University of Western Ontario; Langs: Hindi; Punjabi; (519)685-4575; Fax. (519)685-4561; asha.bhardwaj@sjhc.london.on.ca.

BHARDWAJ, Divya; Halton HCS Corp-Oakville, 327 Reynolds St, Oakville ON L6J 3L7; Rajasthan (India)'88; MB BS; FRCPC; Anes. Staff, Halton Healthcare Services Corporation - Oakville Site; (905)338-4647

BHARDWAJ, Gaurav; Enhanced Care Clinic, 14872 Yonge St, Aurora ON L4G 1N2; Tor'05; CCFP; (905)505-0950; Fax. (905)841-9878; info@adelaideclinic.com.

BHARDWAJ, Rajan; Sheldon M Chumir Urgent Care, 1213 4 St SW, Calgary AB T2R 0X7; Cal'96; BSc; CCFP; Staff, Calgary Health Region; Physician, Sheldon M Chumir Urgent Care Physician Group; (403)955-6011; Fax. (403)955-6023; rajan.bhardwaj@albertahealthservices.ca.

BHARDWAJ, Sanjeev; Meridian Med Clinic, 3-4402 37 St, Stony Plain AB T7Z 2A9; Alb'99; CCFP; (780)963-7800; Fax. (780)963-0468.

BHARGAVA, Anuj; 507-595 Montreal Rd, Ottawa ON K1K 4L2; Ott'00; FRCSC; Ophth. (613)741-2020

BHARGAVA, Keshav; Leduc Comm Hosp & Health Ctr, 3F-4210 48 St, Leduc AB T9E 5Z3; All India Inst (India)'82; FRCPC; IntMed. Staff, Leduc Community Hospital; Staff/Chief IntMed, Wetaskiwin Hospital & Care Centre; Staff, Drayton Valley Hospital & Care Centre; Consultant, Workers' Comp Board of AB; (780)986-5560; Fax. (780)986-2200.

BHARGAVA, Manoj; Medical Clinic Bldg, 315-89 Humber College Blvd, Etobicoke ON M9V 4B8; Tor'92; MS; FRCSC; OrthSurg (Arthroscopic Knee & Shoulder Surgery). Staff, William Osler Health System - Etobicoke General Hospital; Langs: Hindi; (416)741-9271

BHARGAVA, Mukesh; Heart Care Cardiac Wellness Ct, 372 King St W, Oshawa ON L1J 2J9; Gandhi (India)'90.

BHARGAVA, Rakesh K; Medical Sciences Bldg, 372 King St W, Oshawa ON L1J 2J9; Bhopal (India)'71; FRCPC; IntMed; Cardiol. Dir Heart Care Research & Cardiac Rehab & Staff Cardiol, Lakeridge Health - Oshawa Site; Langs: Hindi; (905)721-1999; Fax. (905)721-8564.

BHARGAVA, Rashmi; Golden Mile Centre, 29-3806 Albert St, Regina SK S4S 3R2; Sask'91; FRCSC; ObstGyn. Med Staff Assoc, Regina General Hospital; Clin Assoc Prof, University of Saskatchewan; Langs: Hindi; (306)522-2229; Fax. (306)522-2478.

BHARGAVA, Ravi; University of Alberta Hosp, 8440 112 St NW, Edmonton AB T6G 2B7; Ott'87; FRCPC; DiagRad. Staff Radiol, University of Alberta Hospital; Staff Radiol, Royal Alexandra Hospital; Staff Radiol, Glenrose Rehabilitation Hospital; Prof Radiol & Diagnostic Imaging, University of Alberta; (780)407-1210; Fax. (780)407-1202; rbhargav@cha.ab.ca.

BHARGAVA, Reena; 510-330 Highway 7 E, Richmond Hill ON L4B 3P8; Wes'99; FRCSC; GenSurg.

BHARGAVA, Someshwar; AIM Orleans Hlth & Wellness Cl, 3-1605 Orleans Blvd, Orleans ON K1C 7E2; Rajasthan (India)'67; FRCPC; Peds (Pediatric Asthma). Staff, Children's Hospital of Eastern Ontario (CHEO); Staff, The Ottawa Hospital - Civic Campus; Staff, Montfort Hospital; Langs: Hindi; (613)830-6890

BHARGAVA, Vandana; 100-429 Exmouth St, Sarnia ON N7T 5P1; Jabalpur University (India)'95; CCFP; (519)344-3017

BHARGAVAN, Odayoth K; 203-2825 Clearbrook Rd, Abbotsford BC V2T 6S3; Calicut (India)'76; MB BS; CCFP; (604)852-1567

BHARMAL, Azim A; Dr A Bharmal Prof Corp, 301-200 Boudreau Rd, St. Albert AB T8N 6B9; Sask'82; FRCPC; IntMed; Nephrol. Staff, Sturgeon Community Hospital; (780)458-1117; Fax. (780)458-1167; bharmal@telus.net.

BHARTIA, Sanjay M; 279-20821 Fraser Hwy, Langley BC V3A 0B6; Flinders (Australia)'02; (778)319-4459

BHARUCHA, Pheroze; 2100-222 King St E, Bowmanville ON L1C 1P6; Bombay (India)'84; CCFP; (905)623-0323; Fax. (905)697-0230.

BHARWANI, Aleem M; 3330 Hospital Dr NW, Calgary AB T2N 4N1; Alb'04; FRCPC; IntMed. Staff, Foothills Medical Centre; (403)210-6196

BHARWANI, Fayaz; South Health Campus, 4448 Front St SE, Calgary AB T3M 1M4; Cal'03; FRCPC; Anes. Staff, Rockyview General Hospital.

BHARWANI, Noorali H; 1331 25 St SE, Medicine Hat AB T1A 2E9; Patna (India)'71; LRCP(Lond); FRCS(Ed & Glas); FACS; MRCS(Eng); FRCSC; GenSurg. Staff, Medicine Hat Regional Hospital.

BHASKARA, Sreenivasa M; Cobequid Commun Health Ctre, 40 Freer Lane, Lower Sackville NS B4C 0A2; Sri Venkateswara (India)'83; MB BS; DPM; MRCPsy(Lond); FRCPC; Psy. Staff, Cobequid Community Health Centre; Staff Psy, Capital Health Centre; Asst Prof Psy, Dalhousie University; (902)865-3663; Fax. (902)869-3697; smbhaska@cdha.nshealth.ca.

BHAT, K Rama; York-Med Medical Arts Centre, 401-250 Harding Blvd W, Richmond Hill ON L4C 9M7; Karnatak (India)'63; DABS; FRCSC; GenSurg (Breast Disease). Ac Staff Surg, Mackenzie Richmond Hill Hospital; Langs: Kanarese; (905)884-0888; Fax. (905)884-0889.

BHATIA, Anuj; Univ Hlth Network-Toronto Western Hosp, MCL2 405-399 Bathurst St, Toronto ON M5T 2S8; New Delhi (India)'96; FRCPC; Anes. Staff, Toronto Western Hospital - University Health Network; (416)603-2581

BHATIA, Gargi; 204-86 Angeline St S, Lindsay ON K9V 6C5; Indore (India)'68; FACOG; FRCSC; ObstGyn. Staff, Ross Memorial Hospital; (705)324-7090; Fax. (705)324-7091.

BHATIA, Jaspreet K; Brooklin Med Centre, 1A-5959 Anderson St, Whitby ON L1M 2E9; Ott'02; CCFP; (905)655-3321

BHATIA, Niti; CN Tower, 26F-10004 104 Ave NW, Edmonton AB T5J 0K1; (Belarus)'96; FRCPC; Psy. Staff Forensic Psy, Forensic Assessment & Community Services; (780)342-6400; Fax. (780)426-7272; niti.bhatia@capitalhealth.ca.

BHATIA, Pankaj; Sudbury Reg Hosp-Laurentian, 41 Ramsey Lake Rd, Sudbury ON P3E 5J1; Wes'05; FRCSC; GenSurg. Staff, Health Sciences North-Laurentian Site; Prog Dir GenSurg, Northern Ontario School of Medicine; (705)523-7100

BHATIA, Rajan S; 2075 Hadwen Rd, Mississauga ON L5K 2L3; McG'03; FRCPC; IntMed; Cardiol. Staff, Toronto Western Hospital - University Health Network.

BHATIA, Rajdeep S; Health Sciences Centre, 300 Prince Philip Dr, St. John's NL A1B 3V6; McM'91; FRCPC; DiagRad. Staff Radiol, Health Sciences Centre; (709)777-7102; rbha@yahoo.com.

BHATIA, Ranbir S; MedReach Med Centre, 400-1642 Merivale Rd, Nepean ON K2G 4A1; Punjab (India)'64; DAvMed; Langs: Punjabi; (613)228-2020

BHATIA, Sanjay; 651 Ross Ave E, Timmins ON P4N 8T4; Christian Medical College (India)'04; FRCPC; Peds. (705)264-3599; Fax. (705)264-7130.

BHATLA, Rajiv; Royal Ottawa Hlth Care Group, 1145 Carling Ave, Ottawa ON K1Z 7K4; McG'87; FRCPC; Psy. Chief Psy, Royal Ottawa Mental Health Centre - Royal Ottawa Health Care Group; Assoc Chair Psy, University of Ottawa; (613)722-6521 x6306; Fax. (613)722-7686.

BHATLA, Sanjeev; Bowmont Med Clinic, 6535 Bowness Rd NW, Calgary AB T3B 0E8; McG'87; CCFP; FCFP; Ac Staff, Foothills Medical Centre; Court Staff, Rockyview General Hospital; (403)247-9797; Fax. (403)247-0014.

BHATNAGAR, Gopal; Trillium Cardiovascular Assoc, 608-89 Queensway W, Mississauga ON L5B 2V2; Wes'86; FRCSC; GenSurg; CardiothorSurg. Chief of Staff, Trillium Health Centre - Mississauga; Lecturer Surg, University of Toronto; (905)848-7513; Fax. (905)848-7515; gbhatnagar@thc.on.ca.

BHATT, Arun; Cedar Hills Med Clinic, 12860 96th Ave, Surrey BC V3V 6A8; Glasgow (Scotland)'95; MB ChB; CCFP; (604)584-3531

BHATT, Gunvant S; Prescott Family Health Team, 555 King St W, Prescott ON K0E 1T0; Aberdeen (Scotland)'66; MB ChB; Ac Staff, Brockville General Hospital - Charles Street; Ac Staff, Providence Continuing Care Centre (PCCC) - St Vincent de Paul Hospital; (613)925-5977; Fax. (613)925-1238.

BHATT, Gunvantrai J; 2525 Roseville Garden Dr, Windsor ON N8T 3J8; Birmingham (England)'62; MB ChB; Langs: Gujarati; Hindi; Swahili; (519)944-0018

BHATT, Jayant S; Medicine Prof Corp, 53 Pine St, Brockville ON K6V 1G5; Makerere (Uganda)'70; FRCPC; IntMed. Consultant, Providence Continuing Care Centre (PCCC) - St Vincent de Paul Hospital; (613)498-1355; Fax. (613)498-1414.

BHATT, Maala; MUHC-Montreal Children's Hosp, T 122-2300 rue Tupper, Montreal QC H3H 1P3; McM'96; PedEmergMed; Peds. Staff, McGill University Health Centre - Montreal Children's Hospital; (514)412-4400 x22740; maala.bhatt@muhc.mcgill.ca.

BHATT, Manish; Plaza 33, PO Box 23122 Rpo Plaza 33, Kelowna BC V1X 7K7; McM'99; CCFP; CCFP(E.M.); (250)765-5500; manishmd@hotmail.com.

BHATT, Manjunath K; The Medical Group, 32243 Hurd St, Mission BC V2V 3J9; Cork (Ireland)'98; MB BCh; BAO; CCFP; (604)826-6231

BHATT, Nikhil; Prescott Family Health Team, 555 King St W, Prescott ON K0E 1T0; (Grenada)'05; CCFP; (613)925-5977

BHATT, Sunil K; Care Point Medical Clinics, 1123 Davie St, Vancouver BC V6E 1N2; Man'97; BSc(Med); CCFP; Langs: Hindi; (604)915-9517

BHATTACHARJEE, Debabrata B; Northside Harbor View Hosp, PO Box 399 Stn Main, North Sydney NS B2A 3M4; Calcutta (India)'57; Staff Radiol, Northside General Hospital; (902)794-8521; Fax. (902)794-1679.

BHATTACHARJEE, Rakesh; 208-586 Eglinton Ave E, Toronto ON M4P 1P2; McM'02; Respir; Peds. (416)488-6980; Fax. (416)488-3998.

BHATTACHARYA, Ashok; 202-305 Lakeshore Rd E, Oakville ON L6J 1J3; Mem'84; FRCPC; Psy (Psychotherapy). (905)844-4825

BHATTACHARYYA, Amal; Dartmouth Comm Mental Health, 500-33 Alderney Dr, Dartmouth NS B2Y 2N4; Calcutta (India)'59; Langs: Bengali; Hindi; (902)466-1830; Fax. (902)466-1851; amal.bhattacharyya@cdha.nshealth.ca.

BHATTACHARYYA, Asok K; Provis Endoscopy Services, 100-2 Gurdwara Rd, Nepean ON K2E 1A2; Calcutta (India)'62; FRCS(Ed); FRCSC; GenSurg (Gastroenterology). Staff GenSurg, Pembroke Regional Hospital Inc; Langs: Bengali; (613)216-1823; asok@sympatico.ca.

BHATTACHARYYA, Onil; St Michael's Hosp, 30 Bond St, Toronto ON M5B 1W8; Mon'99; PhD; CCFP; Staff, St Michael's Hospital; Langs: Spanish; Chinese; Mandarin; French; (416)867-7428; Fax. (416)867-7498.

BHATTI, Balbir C; 114-12578 72 Ave, Surrey BC V3W 2M6; Guru Nanak (India)'89; MB BS; CCFP; Langs: Punjabi; Hindi; Urdu; (604)590-8070

BHATTI, Harleen K; 300-2845 Cruickshank St, Abbotsford BC V2T 6X1; (Other Foreign)'09; (604)852-6659

BHATTI, Rajinder S; 300-2845 Cruickshank St, Abbotsford BC V2T 6X1; Punjab (India)'81; MB BS; Langs: Punjabi; (604)852-6659; Fax. (604)852-6708.

BHATTI, Virinder S; Westgate Med Clinic, 402-20395 Lougheed Hwy, Maple Ridge BC V2X 2P9; Punjab (India)'70; MB BS; Med VP, Ridge Meadows Hospital & Health Care Centre; Langs: Punjabi; Hindi; (604)465-3900

BHATTY, Shahzad A; Weber Med Centre, 5A-1400 Weber St E, Kitchener ON N2A 3Z8; Grace University (Belize)'99; CCFP; Staff, Grand River Hospital - Kitchener/Waterloo Health Centre; (519)748-6933

BHAVSAR, Pravin A; Grand River Hosp-Kw Hlth Ctre, PO Box 9056 Stn C 835 King St W, Kitchener ON N2G 1G3; Gujarat (India)'72; MB BS; FCAP; FRCPC; AnatPath. Staff LabMed, Grand River Hospital - Kitchener/Waterloo Health Centre; (519)749-4300 x2251; pravin.bhavsar@grhsp.on.ca.

BHAYANA, Bhooma; 207-240 Wharncliffe Rd N, London ON N6H 4P2; Wes'85; CCFP; Staff, London Health Sciences Centre - Victoria Campus; Staff, St Joseph's Hospital - St Joseph's Health Care; (519)432-1522

BHAYANA, Deepak; 300-401 9 Ave SW, Calgary AB T2P 3C5; Wes'02; FRCPC; DiagRad. (403)284-0230

BHAYANA, Rajinder K; Boyd Med Centre, 912-388 Portage Ave, Winnipeg MB R3C 0C8; Punjab (India)'68; (204)947-6747; Fax. (204)947-6904.

BHAYANA, Renu; 425 St Mary Ave, Winnipeg MB R3C 0N2; Punjab (India)'72; Langs: Hindi; (204)957-3215; Fax. (204)957-1860.

BHAYANA, Satinder K; Family Care, C310A-7700 Hurontario St, Brampton ON L6Y 4M3; Rohtak (India)'82; MB BS; CCFP; (905)455-1234

BHAYANA, Shelly; Gulf Canada Square, 352-401 9 Ave SW, Calgary AB T2P 3C5; Man'00; MSc; BSc; FRCPC; IntMed (Thyroid Diseases); Endocrin&Metab. (403)221-4476; Fax. (403)221-4418.

BHAYANA, Veena; Manitoba Clinic, 790 Sherbrook St, Winnipeg MB R3A 1M3; Punjab (India)'69; (204)774-6541

BHAYAT, Qudsiyyah; T J Medical Clinic, 152-15277 Castle Downs Rd NW, Edmonton AB T5X 3N5; Natal (South Africa)'99; LMCC; MB ChB; CCFP; (780)472-2273; Fax. (780)473-2276.

BHELLA, Sita D; Sunnybrook Hlth Sciences Ctre, 2075 Bayview Ave, Toronto ON M4N 3M5; Wes'08; IntMed.

BHELLA, Vishal S; Clinical Skills Bldg-U of West, 2F-1393 Western Rd, London ON N6G 1G9; McM'09; CCFP; (519)661-4089

BHERER, Jean-Yves; Centre Med de Beauport, 737 av Royale, Quebec QC G1E 1Z1; Laval'72; (418)667-7114; Fax. (418)667-5843.

BHERER, Luc; Centre de Sante Publique, 2400 av d'Estimauville, Quebec QC G1E 7G9; Laval'80; CST; Méd agréé Occupational Health, Ministere de la sante et des services sociaux du Quebec; Méd agréé/Médecin Occupational Med, Dir de Sante Publique de la Capitale-Nationale; Langs: English; French; (418)266-6726; Fax. (418)666-2776; luc.bherer@ssss.gouv.qc.ca.

BHERER, Serge; Clinique Med Desy, 5636 boul Henri-Bourassa E, Montreal-Nord QC H1G 2T2; Mon'78; (514)326-9060; Fax. (514)326-0919.

BHEREUR, Anne; Hop du Sacre-Coeur de Mtl, 5400 boul Gouin O, Montreal QC H4J 1C5; Mon'00; CCFP; Staff, Hôpital du Sacre-Coeur de Montréal; (514)338-2383; Fax. (514)338-3155.

BHESANIA, Teosar; Medicine Prof Corp, 104-200 Ronson Dr, Etobicoke ON M9W 5Z9; Tor'85; BSc; Cardiol; IntMed. (416)748-9183; Fax. (416)748-9184.

BHETASI, Fatima; 390 Lincoln St, Welland ON L3B 4N4; Bombay (India)'98; MB BS; FAAP; DCH; FRCPC; Peds. Aj Prof, McMaster University; Langs: Hindi; Gujarati; Urdu; (905)788-1777; wellandpeds@hotmail.com.

BHIDE, Devayanee M; Addiction & Mental Hlth-Clarke, 250 College St, Toronto ON M5T 1R8; Nagpur (India)'71; FRCPC; Psy. Staff, Centre for Addiction & Mental Health (CAMH) - College Street Site; (416)535-8501 x2180; Fax. (416)979-8501.

BHIMANI, Laila; Jim Pattison Outpatient Care, 9750 140 St, Surrey BC V3T 0G9; Aga Khan (Pakistan)'98; MB BS; CCFP; Staff, Surrey Memorial Hospital; Langs: Hindi; Urdu; (604)582-4582

BHIMANI, Munsif; London HSC-Victoria Hosp, 800 Commissioners Rd E, London ON N6A 5W9; Wes'02; CCFP; CCFP(E.M.); Staff, London Health Sciences Centre - Victoria Campus; (519)667-6538; Fax. (519)667-6769.

BHIMJI, Arif M; R J A Medicentres Cnd Inc, 204-10458 Mayfield Rd NW, Edmonton AB T5P 4P4; Sask'89; CCFP; (780)483-7115

BHIMJI, Khadija; The Ottawa Hosp-Gen Campus, 501 Smyth Rd, Ottawa ON K1H 8L6; UBC'90; BSc; MSc; MD; CCFP; Staff Consultant, The Ottawa Hospital - Civic Campus; Staff, Queensway Carleton Hospital; Staff Consultant Palliative Care Med, The Ottawa Hospital - General Campus; Asst Prof, University of Ottawa.

BHIMJI, Shamim D; BC Cancer Agency-Vancouver CC, 600 10th Ave W, Vancouver BC V5Z 4E6; Makerere (Uganda)'71; FRCR; FRCPC; DiagRad. Consultant Radiol, BC Cancer Agency Vancouver Centre; Staff Consultant, Vancouver General Hospital - Centennial Pavillion; Clin Assoc Prof, University of British Columbia; (604)877-6098; Fax. (604)877-6196; sbhimji@bccancer.bc.ca.

BHOJANI, Faizal D; 45-125 Delhi St, Guelph ON N1E 4J5; Tor'06; FRCSC; GenSurg.

BHOLA, Nereja; St Joseph's Healthcare, 50 Charlton Ave E, Hamilton ON L8N 4A6; Bhopal (India)'78; FRCPC; Anes. Staff, St Joseph's Healthcare - Charlton Campus; (905)522-1155 x3853; Fax. (905)521-6054.

BHOLA-REEBYE, Stacy C; G F Strong Rehabilitation Ctr, 4255 Laurel St, Vancouver BC V5Z 2G9; University of the West Indies (Trinidad & Tobago)'97; MB BS; MRCS; CCFP; Staff, G F Strong Rehabilitation Centre; (604)734-1313; stacybh@hotmail.com.

BHOPAL, Jaswant S; B160-8279 Saba Rd, Richmond BC V6Y 4B6; Glasgow (Scotland)'74; MB ChB; MRC; FRCPC; Psy (Geriatric Psychiatry). Consultant Psy, Richmond Hospital; Clinical Asst Prof Psy, University of British Columbia; Langs: Punjabi; Hindi; (604)273-6641; Fax. (604)276-7468.

BHUGRA, Hardeep S; Fraser Cardiology Associates, 104-33774 Marshall Rd, Abbotsford BC V2S 1L1; (604)870-8715

BHUI, Paramjit S; Surrey Med Arts Bldg, 311-13710 94A Ave, Surrey BC V3V 1N1; Bombay (India)'79; DCH; DABPed; FRCPC; Peds. Langs: Gujarati; Hindi; Marathi; Punjabi; (604)589-3999

BHUIYAN, Nazman N; Northern Med Unit, T162-770 Bannatyne Ave, Winnipeg MB R3E 0W3; Staff, Morris General Hospital; (204)789-3711; nbhuiyan@rha-central.mb.ca.

BHUIYAN, Nihat Z; Thunder Bay Reg HSC-T-Bay, 980 Oliver Rd, Thunder Bay ON P7B 6V4; Liverpool (England)'95; Staff, Thunder Bay Regional Health Sciences Centre; (807)684-6000

BHUIYAN, Omor F; 5706 50 Ave, Vermilion AB T9X 1L4; (Bangladesh)'87; Staff, Vermilion Health Centre; (780)853-2809; Fax. (780)853-2977.

BHUIYAN, Salah U; Broad Street Clinic, 2210 Broad St, Regina SK S4P 4V6; (306)781-8080

BHULLAR, Gurdit S; West Winds Med Clinic, 2130-4818 Westwinds Dr NE, Calgary AB T3J 3Z5; Guru Nanak (India)'75; MB BS; (403)293-5454

BHULLAR, Harbir S; Windsor Med Clinic, 6720 Hawthorne Dr, Windsor ON N8T 1J9; (India)'01; CCFP; (519)944-2295

BHULLAR, Sundeep; Halton HCS Corp-Oakville, 327 Reynolds St, Oakville ON L6J 3L7; RCSI (Ireland)'08; CCFP; Staff, Halton Healthcare Services Corporation - Oakville Site; (905)845-2571

BHUPAL, Vipul K; 265 Scarlett Rd, York ON M6N 4L1; Tor'88; Staff Family Pract, Rouge Valley Health System - Centenary Health Centre Site; Langs: Hindi; Urdu; (416)604-4000

BHURJI, Pargat S; 8241 120A St, Surrey BC V3W 3P5; Bombay (India)'86; DAB; FRCPC; Peds (Neonatology). Clin Teacher, BC Children's Hospital; Dir Neonatal Intensive Care Unit & Active Privil, Surrey Memorial Hospital; Langs: Gujarati; Marathi; Hindi; Punjabi; Urdu; (604)572-0055; Fax. (604)572-0191; pbhurji@hotmail.com.

BHUTANI, Mohit; University of Alberta Hosp, 2E4.44-8440 112 St NW, Edmonton AB T6G 2B7; Sask'98; FRCPC; IntMed; Critical Care Medicine; Respir. Staff, University of Alberta Hospital; (780)407-1832; Fax. (780)407-6384.

BHUTANI, Sandra; Sturgeon Community Hosp, 201 Boudreau Rd, St. Albert AB T8N 6C4; Sask'00; FRCPC; DiagRad. Staff, Sturgeon Community Hospital; (780)412-9061

BHYAT, Rashaad; Main Street Med Centre, 9-10886 Hurontario St, Brampton ON L7A 3R9; (Ireland)'04; CCFP; (905)846-9911

BIA, F Hussain F; PO Box 220, Foam Lake SK S0A 1A0; RCS (Ireland)'69; Ac Staff, Foam Lake Health Centre; (306)272-3533; Fax. (306)272-3980.

BIABI, Mohsen; CSSS du Suroit, 150 rue Saint-Thomas, Salaber-de-Valleyf QC J6T 6C1; (Portugal)'99; Staff, Centre Hospitalier Régional du Suroît; (450)371-9920; Fax. (450)377-1372.

BIAGI, James J; Cancer Ctre Southeastern Ont, 25 King St W, Kingston ON K7L 5P9; Tor'95; FRCPC; IntMed; MedOncol. A-Dept Head Oncology, Queen's University; (613)544-2630 x4174; Fax. (613)546-8209.

BIAGINI CURY, Fabio L; MUHC-Montreal Gen Hosp, D5 400-1650 av Cedar, Montreal QC H3G 1A4; (Brazil)'99; Staff, McGill University Health Centre - Montreal General Campus; (514)934-8040

BIAGIONI, Cristina; Clinique Medicale Lorraine, 99 boul de Gaulle, Sainte-Therese QC J6Z 3Z9; Mon'06; CCFP; Staff, Hôpital de Saint-Eustache; (450)621-1444

BIAGIONI, Edward J; 403-294 Main St, Toronto ON M4C 4X5; Wes'68; Assoc Staff, Mount Sinai Hospital; Assoc Staff, The Scarborough Hospital - Birchmount Campus; (416)694-9447

BIALA, Soliman E A; Rockyview Gen Hosp, 7007 14 St SW, Calgary AB T2V 1P9; Al-Fateh (Libya)'97; MB ChB; Staff, Rockyview General Hospital; (403)943-3788

BIALCZAK, Jerzy; Palisades Med Clinic, 12808 137 Ave NW, Edmonton AB T5L 4Y8; (Poland)'83; MSc; CCFP; Staff, Royal Alexandra Hospital; Langs: Polish; (780)457-1100

BIALI, Susan; PO Box 91245 Stn West Vancouve, West Vancouver BC V7V 3N9; UBC'98; Langs: Spanish; sbiali@interchange.ubc.ca.

BIALIK, Mark J; 107-900 Greenbank Rd, Nepean ON K2J 1S8; Qns'86; FRCPC; Peds. Staff Peds, Children's Hospital of Eastern Ontario (CHEO); Staff, The Ottawa Hospital - Civic Campus; Staff, Queensway Carleton Hospital; (613)825-7151; Fax. (613)825-5705.

BIALIK, Sean J; Clinic 528, 528 Dundas St, London ON N6B 1W6; Wes'89.

BIALY, Peter C; Family Med Clinic, 1-2536 Main St, Winnipeg MB R2V 4Y1; Man'08; CCFP; (204)339-1781

BIANCHI, Fernando A; Charlton Med Centre, 304-25 Charlton Ave E, Hamilton ON L8N 1Y2; Ott'59; IntMed (Rheumatology). Ac Staff, St Joseph's Healthcare - Charlton Campus; Ac Staff, Hamilton Health Sciences Centre - McMaster University Medical Centre; Clin Assoc Prof, McMaster University; Langs: Italian; French; (905)529-1232; Fax. (905)529-3656.

BIANCHINI, Antonio U; Ctr Hosp de Lasalle, 8585 Tsse Champlain, LaSalle QC H8P 1C1; McG'92; BSc; CCFP; pers Médecin Intensive Care Unit & Emerg Rm, Centre Hospitalier de LaSalle; Langs: English; French; Italian; (514)367-8619; aubianchini@gmail.com.

BIANCO, Rodolfo; 1416 Merritt Pl, Victoria BC V8P 5H5; UBC'78; Staff Chief, Bulkley Valley District Hospital; (250)477-2526

BIANCUCCI, Christina M; Taddle Creek Family Hlth Team, 522-790 Bay St, Toronto ON M5G 1N8; Tor'07; CCFP; (416)591-1222; Fax. (416)591-1227.

BIANKI, Sylvain; CLSC du Marigot, 1351 boul des Laurentides, Vimont QC H7M 2Y2; Mon'86; Ac Staff, Hôpital du Sacre-Coeur de Montréal; (450)668-1803; Fax. (450)668-1507.

BIARD, Christian; 201-181 rue Victoria, Salaber-de-Valleyf QC J6T 1A7; Mon'85; Psy. (450)373-6252; Fax. (450)371-4910.

BIARD, Wanda; 304-1150 boul Saint-Joseph E, Montreal QC H2J 1L5; Mon'87; CSPQ; Psy (Pedology Psychiatry). Assoc Member PedoPsy, Centre Hospitalier de Gaspe; Assoc Member PedoPsy, Hôpital de l'Archipel; (514)419-5354; wandabiard@msn.com.

BIBBY, Jodi D; Kamsack Med Clinic, PO Box 69, Kamsack SK S0A 1S0; Cape Town (South Africa)'07; DCH; (306)542-2623; Fax. (306)542-3782.

BIBEAU, Marc D; The Lung Health Clinic, 8737 156 St NW, Edmonton AB T5R 1Y5; Man'01; FRCPC; IntMed; Respir. Clinical Asst Prof Med, University of Alberta; Langs: Bilingual(English/French); (780)498-1800

BIBEAU, Marie-Josee; Centre Med Fusion, 200-2035 av Sainte-Anne, Saint-Hyacinthe QC J2S 5H3; Mon'87; Physician, CLSC le Minordet; (450)773-6023

BIBEAU, Marielle; Carrefour Sante-Pav St-Louis, 23 rue Ambroise-Dearden, Windsor QC J1S 1G8; Sher'82; Staff, Carrefour de Sante et Services Sociaux-Pavillon St-Louis; (819)845-2751

BIBEAU, Virginie; CHUQ-St-Francois D'Assise, 10 rue de l'Espinay, Quebec QC G1L 3L5; Sher'05; FRCPC; IntMed (Critical Care Medicine). Staff, Centre Hospitalier Universitaire De Québec - Pavillon De St-françois-d'assise; (418)525-4444

BIBERDORF, Darren J; Richmond Med Bldg, 302-2020 Richmond Rd, Victoria BC V8R 6R5; Man'94; FRCSC; GenSurg. (250)592-4313; Fax. (250)592-5020.

BIBI, Diaa E; CSSS du Suroit, 150 rue Saint-Thomas, Salaber-de-Valleyf QC J6T 6C1; (Tunisia)'89; Staff, Centre Hospitalier Régional du Suroît; (450)371-9920; Fax. (450)371-7454.

BIBI, Mariam; St Norbert Med Clinic, 3554 Pembina Hwy, Winnipeg MB R3V 1A7; (Other Foreign)'93; CCFP; Staff, DeSalaberry District Health Centre.

BIBIC, Desa; Rosedale Med Clinic, 1955 King St E, Hamilton ON L8K 1W2; McM'85; CCFP; FCFP; Ac Staff, St Joseph's Healthcare - Charlton Campus; (905)547-2533; Fax. (905)547-4402.

BIBR, Henry J; St Joseph's Healthcare, 50 Charlton Ave E, Hamilton ON L8N 4A6; Prague (Czech Republic)'80; FRCPC; Psy. Staff, St Joseph's Healthcare - Charlton Campus; Langs: Czech; (905)522-1155; Fax. (905)521-6059.

BICAMUMPAKA, Cyrille; Health Sciences Centre, 820 Sherbrook St, Winnipeg MB R3A 1R9; (Rwanda)'84; FRCPC; AnatPath. Staff, Health Sciences Centre; (204)774-8511

BICEK, Gregory S; Canmore Gen Hosp, 1100 Hospital Pl, Canmore AB T1W 1N2; Cal'04; CCFP; CCFP(E.M.); Staff, Canmore General Hospital; (403)678-5536

BICHAI, Iman G; Toronto East Gen Hosp Inc, 825 Coxwell Ave, Toronto ON M4C 3E7; Ain Shams (Egypt)'82; Staff, Toronto East General Hospital Inc; (416)469-6580 x2947; Fax. (416)469-6864.

BICHAI, W Michel; College des Med du Quebec, 2170 boul Rene-Levesque O, Montreal QC H3H 2T8; Mon'76; Staff, Hôpital Santa Cabrini Ospedale; (514)933-4441 x5452

BICHET, Daniel; Hop du Sacre-Coeur de Mtl, 5400 boul Gouin O, Montreal QC H4J 1C5; Besancon (France)'72; MSc(Mon.); FACP; IntMed; Nephrol (P.Q.). Staff, Hôpital du Sacre-Coeur de Montréal; Chair Research in Genetics & Renal Diseases, Institute of Research in Health in Canada; Prof, Universite de Montreal; Langs: English; (514)338-2486 x2173; Fax. (514)338-2694; daniel.bichet@umontreal.ca.

BICK, Lindsay; St Mary's Hosp, 4607 53 St, Camrose AB T4V 1Y5; (South Africa)'03; MB ChB; DA; Staff, Covenant Health - St Mary's Hospital; Langs: Afrikaans; French; (780)679-6100

BICKHRAM, Mahendra; Milton Medical Centre, 1225 Maple Ave, Milton ON L9T 0A5; St George's Univ (Grenada)'10; CCFP; (905)693-6400; Fax. (905)693-6405.

BICKLE, Robert; Georgian Prof Centre, 003-125 Bell Farm Rd, Barrie ON L4M 6L2; Tor'88; CCFP; CCFP(E.M.); FCFP; Staff, Royal Victoria Regional Health Centre; (705)721-5991; Fax. (705)728-5936.

BICKNELL, Ryan T; Kingston Gen Hosp, N3-76 Stuart St, Kingston ON K7L 2V7; McM'00; BSc(Hons); MSc; FRCSC; OrthSurg (Shoulder & Elbow). Staff, Hotel-Dieu Hospital; Staff, Kingston General Hospital; Asst Prof, Queen's University; (613)549-6666 x6597; Fax. (613)548-2526; bicknelr@kgh.kari.net.

BICKNELL, Simon G; North Shore Med Imaging, 139 16th St W, North Vancouver BC V7M 1T3; UBC'97; FRCPC; DiagRad. Staff, Lions Gate Hospital; (604)987-9729

BICRELL, Eric; Clinique Med Ahuntsic, 241 rue Fleury O, Montreal QC H3L 1V2; Mon'80; Langs: Italian; Spanish; English; (514)382-0062

BIDA, Adriana; Southlake Reg Health Centre, 596 Davis Dr, Newmarket ON L3Y 2P9; (Romania)'79; FRCPC; IntMed. Staff, North York General Hospital; Staff, Southlake Regional Health Centre; (905)895-4521; Fax. (905)853-2222.

BIDARI, Imane; 208-210 Centrum Blvd, Orleans ON K1E 3V7; Casablanca (Morocco)'01; CCFP; (613)824-4848

BIDDULPH, Michael P; Queen Elizabeth II HSC-Halifax, 4413-1796 Summer St, Halifax NS B3H 3A7; Dal'02; OrthSurg. Staff, Queen Elizabeth II Health Sciences Centre - Halifax Infirmary Site; (902)473-6322; Fax. (902)473-2042.

BIDNIAK, Karen K; Links Clinic, 104-11910 111 Ave NW, Edmonton AB T5G 3G6; Alb'79; CCFP; (780)454-0351; Fax. (780)452-6767.

BIEDERMAN, Jessica L M; Quinte HC Corp-Belleville Gen, 265 Dundas St E, Belleville ON K8N 5A9; Tor'06; FRCPC; DiagRad. Staff, QHC Belleville General; (613)969-7400; Fax. (613)969-5561.

BIEDERMANN, Alyson J; Aboriginal Hlth & Wellness Ctr, 181 Higgins Ave, Winnipeg MB R3B 3G1; (Other Foreign)'07.

BIEG, Ralph P; Lonsdale Med Dental Bldg, 108-1940 Lonsdale Ave, North Vancouver BC V7M 2K2; Alb'86; BSc(Hon); CCFP; (604)987-3357; Fax. (604)987-7624.

BIELAWSKA, Hanna; The Credit Valley Hosp, 2200 Eglinton Ave W, Mississauga ON L5M 2N1; Tor'08; CCFP; CCFP(E.M.); Staff, The Credit Valley Hospital; Teach Staff, University of Toronto; (905)813-1100

BIELECKI, Barbara; Stonechurch Family Hlth Ctre, 1475 Upper Ottawa St, Hamilton ON L8W 3J6; McM'07; CCFP; Physician, Stonechurch Family Health Centre; (905)575-7757

BIELINSKI, Michael; MUHC-Royal Victoria Hosp, 687 av des Pins O, Montreal QC H3A 1A1; Cracow (Poland)'06; FRCPC; IntMed. Staff, McGill University Health Centre - Royal Victoria Hospital; (514)934-1934

BIELINSKI, Raphael; Hawkesbury & District Gen Hosp, 1111 Ghislain St, Hawkesbury ON K6A 3G5; (Poland)'05; CCFP; CCFP(E.M.); Staff, Hawkesbury & District General Hospital; (613)632-1111

BIELINSKI, Stanislaw; 100 ch Rockland, Mont-Royal QC H3P 2V9; Warsaw (Poland)'64; ObstGyn (P.Q.). ac Staff, CSSS de Dorval-Lachine-Lasalle; ac Staff, Hopital de la Cite de la santé; (514)667-3383

BIEM, H Jay; Lakeshore Gen Hosp, 160 av Stillview, Pointe-Claire QC H9R 2Y2; Sask'86; MSc(Epidemiol.); ABIM; FRCPC; IntMed. Staff, McGill University Health Centre - Montreal General Campus; Staff, Lakeshore General Hospital - Pointe Claire; Aj Prof Med, McGill University; Langs: French; German; Mandarin; (514)630-2225

BIEM, Sandra R D; Brunswick Med Centre, 200-955 boul Saint-Jean, Pointe-Claire QC H9R 5K3; Sask'86; FRCSC; ObstGyn. Langs: Bilingual(English/French); (514)276-4966

BIEN-AIME, Lubraine; Clinique Med Urgence Rive-Sud, 3200 boul Taschereau, Greenfield Park QC J4V 2H3; Liege (Belgium)'85; CCFP; Langs: Bilingual(French/English); (450)672-7658

BIENENSTOCK, Audrie M; Fontbonne Hall, 334F-301 James St S, Hamilton ON L8N 4A6; London (England)'56; MB BS; DA; LRCP; MRCS; FRCPC; Psy (Consultation-Liaison). Staff, St Joseph's Healthcare - Charlton Campus; Clin Assoc Clin Assoc Prof, McMaster University; (905)522-1155 x35230; Fax. (905)521-6059.

BIENENSTOCK, Eli A; William Osler HC-Etobicoke, 101 Humber College Blvd, Etobicoke ON M9V 1R8; Tor'94; FRCPC; NuclearMed. Staff, William Osler Health System - Etobicoke General Hospital; (416)747-3400 x32460

BIENERT, Tasha N; Copeman Healthcare Centre, 400-1128 Hornby St, Vancouver BC V6Z 2L4; Cal'02; CCFP; (604)707-2273

BIENKOWSKI, Halina; Family Practice, 100-158 Robert Angus Dr, Amherst NS B4H 4R7; (Poland)'77; MD; Langs: Polish; (902)667-1622; Fax. (902)667-5970.

BIENKOWSKI, Krzysztof W; Amherst Family Health Clinic, 100-158 Robert Angus Dr, Amherst NS B4H 4R7; (Poland)'75; (902)667-3173; Fax. (902)669-5970.

BIENKOWSKI, Peter; Carling-Broadview Med Bldg, 202-770 Broadview Ave, Ottawa ON K2A 3Z3; Dal'01; FRCSC; OrthSurg (Sports Medicine). Staff, Queensway Carleton Hospital; Langs: Polish; (613)729-3310

BIENVENU, Genevieve; Clinique Med St-Alexandre, 200-2310 rue Saint-Louis, Gatineau QC J8T 5L7; Mon'96; Staff, Hôpital de Gatineau; Langs: English; (819)243-4500; Fax. (819)243-1369; gbienvenu@medecinefamiliale.com.

BIENVENU, Jean-Pierre; 200-2924 boul Taschereau, Greenfield Park QC J4V 2G8; Sher'73; Psy (Psychoanalysis). Langs: German; (514)466-8486; jeanpierre.bienvenu@videotron.ca.

BIENVENUE, Veronique; CSSS de Saint-Jerome, 290 rue de Montigny, Saint-Jerome QC J7Z 5T3; Sher'07; Nephrol; IntMed. Staff, Hôtel-Dieu de Saint-Jérôme; (450)432-2777

BIER, Anthony B; Guelph Gen Hosp, 115 Delhi St, Guelph ON N1E 4J4; Tor'95; CCFP; CCFP(E.M.); Staff, Guelph General Hospital; (519)837-6414

BIER, Michele; 1301 rue Sherbrooke E, Montreal QC H2L 1M3; Mon'73; Med Consultant InfectDis Prog, McGill University Health Centre - Montreal General Campus; (514)528-2400; Fax. (514)528-2452.

BIER, Rino; Centre Radiologique Fleury, 2320 rue Fleury E, Montreal QC H2B 1K9; Mon'72; DiagRad. Chief Dept of Radiol, Centre Hospitalier Fleury; Langs: Italian; Portuguese; English; (514)389-0816

BIERBRIER, Gordon S; Scarborough Prof Centre, 216-1371 Neilson Rd, Scarborough ON M1B 4Z8; McG'88; FACP; FRCPC; FRCPC; Gastroent; IntMed. Staff, Rouge Valley Health System - Centenary Health Centre Site; (416)208-9860; Fax. (416)208-5936; gbierbrier@rougevalley.ca.

BIERMAN, Arlene S; St Michael's Hosp, 30 Bond St, Toronto ON M5B 1W8; North Carolina(NC) (USA)'81; FRCPC; GeriatricMed; IntMed. Chair OWHC & Women's Health/Sr Scientist Li Ka Shing Knowledge Inst, St Michael's Hospital; Assoc Prof Med, University of Toronto; (416)864-6060 x5928

BIERMAN, Petrus J L; 110 3rd St, Weyburn SK S4H 0W2; Orange Free State (South Africa)'90; MB ChB; LMCC; Physician, Sun Country Health Region; (306)842-5404; Fax. (306)842-7338; peetbierman@gmail.com.

BIERNACKA, Magdalena T; Aberdeen Hosp, 835 East River Rd, New Glasgow NS B2H 3S6; Qns'98; FRCPC; DiagRad. Staff, Aberdeen Regional Hospital; (902)752-7600; Fax. (902)752-6631.

BIERTHO, Laurent; Hôpital Laval, 2725 ch Sainte-Foy, Quebec QC G1V 4G5; Liege(Belgium) (Belgium)'98; Staff, Hôpital Laval; (418)656-8711

BIGAM, David L; University of Alberta Hosp, 2D4.34WCM-8440 112 St NW, Edmonton AB T6G 2B7; Alb'91; BSc; MSc; FRCSC; GenSurg (Hepatobiliary & Pancreatic Surgery). Dir Pancreas Transplant, University of Alberta Hospital; Teach Staff, University of Alberta; (780)407-1466; Fax. (780)407-1773.

BIGAOUETTE, Andre; Polyclinique Longueuil, 1426 ch De Chambly, Longueuil QC J4J 3X3; Mon'72; Assoc Staff, Hopital Charles LeMoyne; Assoc Staff, Hopital Maisonneuve-Rosemont; (450)651-2120; Fax. (450)651-2155.

BIGELOW, Eric; Nepean Med Centre, 311-1 Centrepointe Dr, Nepean ON K2G 6E2; Ott'93; FRCSC; GenSurg (Laparoscopic Surgery). Staff, Queensway Carleton Hospital; Langs: English; French; (613)274-7457; Fax. (613)274-7535.

BIGELOW, Gayle S; Medical Arts Bldg, 611-1 Young St, Hamilton ON L8N 1T8; McM'83; BA(Hon); MSW; FRCPC; Psy. Staff, St Joseph's Healthcare - Charlton Campus; Asst Prof, McMaster University; (905)522-5455

BIGG, Cristina M; King Edward Pediatrics Clinic, 926 King Edward Ave W, Vancouver BC V5Z 2E2; UBC'06; FRCPC; Peds. (604)600-7282

BIGGAR, Ruth A; 5488 Woodeden Dr, Manotick ON K4M 1B4; Qns'80; FRCPC; Psy. Assoc Member, Royal Ottawa Mental Health Centre - Royal Ottawa Health Care Group; (613)692-0610; Fax. (613)692-1402.

BIGGAR, W Douglas; Holland Bloorview Kids Rehab, 150 Kilgour Rd, Toronto ON M4G 1R8; Qns'66; FRCPC; Peds. Staff, Holland Bloorview Kids Rehabilitation Hospital; Consultant, The Hospital For Sick Children; (416)424-3813; Fax. (416)424-3840; dbiggar@hollandbloorview.ca.

BIGGS, Eileen M; The Westend Family Care Clinic, 80 Michael Cowpland Dr, Kanata ON K2M 1P6; Dal'75; Staff, Westend Family Care Clinic Family Health Team; (613)599-3321

BIGHAM, Aaron T; 201C-600 Princess St, Woodstock ON N4S 4H4; Tor'06; FRCSC; OrthSurg.

BIGHAM, Gerald L; Oxford Med Centre, 312 Oxford St W, London ON N6H 4N7; Wes'77; (519)432-6786; Fax. (519)432-3292.

BIGHAM, J Mark; Canadian Blood Services, 4750 Oak St, Vancouver BC V6H 2N9; Qns'82; FRCPC; CommunMed (Public Health & Preventive Medicine). Staff, Fraser Health Authority Corporate Office; Staff, Canadian Blood Services; Clin Assoc Prof, University of British Columbia; (604)707-3505

BIGLAND, Karen W W; Weyburn Health Centre, 36 4th St, Weyburn SK S4H 0X7; Witwatersrand (South Africa)'86; LMCC; MB ChB; (306)842-5444 x303; Fax. (306)842-5449; k.bigland@weyburnhealthcentre.com.

BIGLOW, Clair E; 2-152 2 Ave W PO Box 670, Qualicum Beach BC V9K 1T2; UBC'85; Staff, Nanaimo Regional General Hospital; (250)752-7100

BIGNELL, Douglas C; Doctors Bldg, 230-955 Queen St E, Sault Ste. Marie ON P6A 2C3; Birmingham (England)'79; MB ChB; PhD; FRCPC; Gastroent; IntMed. Staff Med, Sault Area Hospital - Sault Ste Marie; (705)759-3098; Fax. (705)759-8477.

BIGONNESSE, Jean-Marc; La Maison Aube-Lumiere, 220 rue Kennedy N, Sherbrooke QC J1E 2E7; Sher'83; CCFP; FCFP; Staff Palliative Care Services, Centre Hospitalier Universitaire de Sherbrooke-Hopital Fleurimont; Teach Staff Family Med, Universite de Sherbrooke; Langs: English; French; (819)821-3120; Fax. (819)821-1127; jean-marc.bigonnesse@usherbrooke.ca.

BIGRAS, Gilbert; Cross Cancer Institute, 11560 University Ave NW, Edmonton AB T6G 1Z2; Mon'85; PhD; FRCPC; AnatPath. Staff, Cross Cancer Institute; (780)432-8445

BIGRAS, Jean-Luc; Hôpital Ste-Justine, 3175 ch Cote-Sainte-Catherine, Montreal QC H3T 1C5; Mon'88; CSPQ; FRCPC; Peds; Cardiol. Staff, Hôpital Ste-Justine; adj Prof, Universite de Montreal; (514)345-4654; Fax. (514)345-4896.

BIGRAS, Magali; Centre Sante Comm-St Joseph's, 1-280 rue Victoria, Dalhousie NB E8C 2R6; Sher'09; CCFP; Staff, Centre de santé Communitaire - St-Joseph; (506)684-7727

BIGSBY, Kathryn M; Queen Elizabeth Hosp, PO Box 6600 Stn Central, Charlottetown PE C1A 8T5; Sask'82; FRCPC; Peds. Pediatrics, Queen Elizabeth Hospital; (902)894-2440; Fax. (902)894-2477; pedsclinic@ihis.org.

BIGSBY, Richard J; St Paul's Hosp, 1702 20th St W, Saskatoon SK S7M 0Z9; Sask'86; FRCSC; GenSurg; ThorSurg. Staff, St Paul's Hospital (Grey Nuns) of Saskatoon; Clinical Asst Prof, University of Saskatchewan; (306)655-0533; Fax. (306)655-5771.

BIGUE, Caroline; 500-1565 Carling Ave, Ottawa ON K1Z 8R1; McG'90; (613)226-5455

BIHUN, Julia A P; Kanata Prof Centre, 204-99 Kakulu Rd, Kanata ON K2L 3C8; Qns'90; CCFP; FCFP; (613)592-1269; Fax. (613)592-1141.

BIJLSMA, Jan Jaap; Vancouver Gen Hosp, 855 12th Ave W, Vancouver BC V5Z 1M9; UBC'94; FRCPC; EmergMed;CCFP; Staff, Vancouver General Hospital - Centennial Pavillion; Langs: Dutch; German; French; (604)875-4700

BIKANGAGA, Peter M; 207-157 Queen St E, Brampton ON L6W 3X4; Makerere (Uganda)'86; FRCPC; Peds; Respir. Staff, The Hospital For Sick Children; Staff, William Osler Health System - Brampton Civic Hospital; (905)456-5656; Fax. (905)456-9572.

BILAL, Shaukat; 3236 82 St NW, Edmonton AB T6K 3Y3; (780)761-3335; Fax. (780)756-5342.

BILAN, Margaret A; Lloydminster Med Clinic, 5120 46 St, Lloydminster AB T9V 2P7; Alb'82; (780)875-2221

BILAWICH, Ana-Maria; Vancouver Gen Hosp, 855 12th Ave W, Vancouver BC V5Z 1M9; Wes'99; FRCPC; DiagRad. Staff, Vancouver General Hospital - Centennial Pavillion; (604)875-4533

BILAWSKI, Darlene; Painswick Med Clinic, 101-505 Yonge St, Barrie ON L4N 4E1; Wes'85; CCFP; Ac Staff, Royal Victoria Regional Health Centre; (705)722-7189; Fax. (705)722-7302.

BILBAO, Juan M; Sunnybrook Hlth Sciences Ctre, E419-2075 Bayview Ave, Toronto ON M4N 3M5; La Plata (Argentina)'61; NeurPath. Staff, Sunnybrook Health Sciences Centre; (416)925-7284; Fax. (416)480-4021.

BILBEY, James H; Royal Inland Hosp, 311 Columbia St, Kamloops BC V2C 2T1; Alb'74; FRCPC; EmergMed; DiagRad. Staff, Royal Inland Hospital; (250)314-2408; Fax. (250)314-2326.

BILBILY, Ghassan F Y; Maple's Endoscopy, 105-9100 Jane St, Vaughan ON L4K 0A4; Baghdad (Iraq)'80; MB ChB; FRCPC; IntMed; Gastroent. Staff, Toronto Western Hospital - University Health Network; Staff, North York Endoscopy Centre; (905)482-3387; Fax. (905)760-5587.

BILBILY, Janan F Y; Milner Health Centre, 857 Milner Ave, Scarborough ON M1B 5N6; Baghdad (Iraq)'79; CCFP; FCFP; Langs: Arabic; (416)287-3611; Fax. (416)287-2981.

BILEFSKY, Ralph; 565-5025 Sherbrooke St W, Montreal QC H4A 1S9; McG'61; BSc; FRCPC; IntMed; Nephrol (P.Q.). Sr Physician Nephrol, Sir Mortimer B Davis Jewish General; Consultant, Donald Berman Maimonides Geriatric Centre; Lecturer, McGill University; (514)739-0250; Fax. (514)739-4145.

BILGASEM, Solieman A; Sudbury Med Centre, 200A-65 Larch St, Sudbury ON P3E 1B8; Al-Fateh (Libya)'89; FRCSC; Urol. (705)673-8455; Fax. (705)673-8676; bilgasem@hotmail.com.

BILIBAJKICH, Juliana; Oasis Med Centre, 140-486 Advance Blvd, Tecumseh ON N8N 0B8; Tor'94; CCFP; (519)727-3335; Fax. (519)727-6288.

BILIBAJKICH, Mara M; 140-486 Advance Blvd, Tecumseh ON N8N 0B8; Qns'93; CCFP; (519)727-3338; Fax. (519)727-6288; maramelinda@yahoo.com.

BILINSKI, Anna; Hop Santa Cabrini Ospedale, 5655 rue Saint-Zotique E, Montreal QC H1T 1P7; Warsaw (Poland)'58; FRCPC; DiagRad. Staff, Hôpital Santa Cabrini Ospedale; (514)252-6000

BILKEY, Timothy S; Ontario Bilkey ADHD Clinics, 245-400 Bayfield St, Barrie ON L4M 5A1; Wes'78; BSc(Hons); FRCPC; Psy (Attention Deficit Hyperactivity Disorder). Dir Psy, Ontario Bilkey ADHD Clinics-Barrie; (705)726-0036; Fax. (705)726-0836.

BILLARD, Marc; College des Med du Quebec, 2170 boul Rene-Levesque O, Montreal QC H3H 2T8; Mon'80; CCFP; FCFP; Staff, College des Medecins du Quebec; (514)933-4441; Fax. (514)933-4668.

BILLETT, Alan T; Bigelow Fowler Clinic, 1605 9 Ave S, Lethbridge AB T1J 1W2; Sask'67; CCFP; FCFP; Staff, Covenant Health - St Michael's Health Centre; Staff, Chinook Regional Hospital; Physician, Lethbridge Correctional Inst. & Aviation Examiner; (403)327-3121

BILLIA, Filio; NCSB 11-1198C, 585 University Ave, Toronto ON M5G 2N2; Tor'01; FRCPC; IntMed; Cardiol. Staff, Toronto General Hospital - UHN; (416)340-4800 x8596

BILLIARD, Jean-Sebastien; CHUM-Hop St-Luc, 1058 rue Saint-Denis, Montreal QC H2X 3J4; Lyon (France)'93; DMRD; MRCP; FRCPC; DiagRad (P.Q.) (Interventional Radiology). Staff, Centre Hospitalier l'Université De Montréal (CHUM) - Hôpital Saint-luc; Langs: French; English; (514)890-8000 x36400; joubex@gmail.com.

BILLICK, Kendall; Traveller's Health Service, 100-175 av Stillview, Pointe-Claire QC H9R 4S3; Tel Aviv (Israel)'95; CSPQ; FRCPC; IntMed; InfectDis (P.Q.). Staff, McGill University Health Centre - Montreal General Campus; Staff, Lakeshore General Hospital - Pointe Claire; Langs: Spanish; French; (514)695-8784; Fax. (514)694-3610.

BILLICK, Robin C; SMBD Jewish Gen Hosp, G026-3755 ch Cote-Sainte-Cathe, Montreal QC H3T 1E2; McG'73; ABIM; AB; FRCPC; IntMed (Cosmetic & Laser Surgery); Derm. Hd Derm, Sir Mortimer B Davis Jewish General; assoc Prof Med, McGill University; Langs: French; (514)340-8272 x2865; Fax. (514)340-8222.

BILLIE, Christine; Sioux Lookout Zone Fam Phys, PO Box 4000, Sioux Lookout ON P8T 1K2; Cal'01; CCFP; Physician, Sioux Lookout First Nations Health Authority; (807)737-5161; cbillie@slmhc.on.ca.

BILLING, Kulbir S; A10-751 Victoria St S, Kitchener ON N2M 5N4; Bhopal (India)'74; FRCPC; Anes. Staff, Guelph General Hospital; (519)745-6505; Fax. (519)745-6506.

BILLING, Suzanne; Student Health Services, 146 Stuart St, Kingston ON K7L 3N6; McM'90; CCFP; Staff, Kingston General Hospital; Staff, Hotel-Dieu Hospital; Physician Student's Health Serv, Queen's University; (613)533-6000 x75612

BILLINGHURST, Katherine A; Avenida Bonavista Shopp Ctre, 12445 Lake Fraser Dr SE, Calgary AB T2J 7A4; Dal'10; CCFP; (403)723-7453; Fax. (403)723-2463.

BILLINGHURST, Lori L; AMA Physician Locum Services, 12230 106 Ave NW, Edmonton AB T5N 3Z1; Qns'01; FRCPC; Peds; Neur. (780)722-5900; Fax. (647)344-1087.

BILLINGHURST, M Robert; Queen Elizabeth Health Complex, 2111 av Northcliffe, Montreal QC H4A 3K6; McG'09; CCFP; (514)482-3311

BILLINGS, David; Saugeen Shores Med Bldg, 36 Grey St N, Southampton ON N0H 2L0; Mem'00; BSc; CCFP; CCFP(E.M.); Staff, Grey Bruce Health Services - Southampton Site; Aj Prof Family Med, University of Western Ontario; Aj Prof Family Med, University of Toronto; Langs: English; French; (519)797-9940 x1; Fax. (519)797-1225.

BILLINGSLEY, Ian; Thunder Bay Reg HSC-T-Bay, 980 Oliver Rd, Thunder Bay ON P7B 6V4; Qns'00; FRCPC; IntMed; Cardiol. Staff, Thunder Bay Regional Health Sciences Centre; (807)684-6000

BILLINGTON, Robert G; Academic Family Medicine, 3311 Fairlight Dr, Saskatoon SK S7M 3Y5; Sask'03; BSP; BSc; CCFP; (306)655-4200; Fax. (306)655-4894.

BILLINKOFF, Errol N; Billinkoff Vasectomy Centre, 311-93 Lombard Ave, Winnipeg MB R3B 3B1; Man'82; (204)338-3700; Fax. (204)338-9199.

BILLON, Eric; CHUM-Hop Notre-Dame, 1560 rue Sherbrooke E, Montreal QC H2L 4M1; Bordeaux (France)'85; Psy (P.Q.). Staff, Centre Hospitalier l'Université de Montréal (CHUM) - Hôpital Notre-Dame; (514)890-8000 x25665

BILO, John M; Central Alberta Med Imaging, 4312 54 Ave, Red Deer AB T4N 4M1; Alb'98; FRCPC; DiagRad. Staff, Valley Regional Hospital; (403)343-6172; Fax. (403)343-6159.

BILOCQ, Alain; Clinique de Neurologie, 4380 Cote Rosemont, Trois-Rivieres QC G8Y 0A5; Sher'88; FRCSC; Neursurg. Staff, CSSS de Trois-Rivières; (819)370-4757

BILODEAU, Alain; CLSC Drummond, 350 rue Saint-Jean, Drummondville QC J2B 5L4; Sher'75; assoc Staff Family Med, Centre Hospitalier Universitaire de Sherbrooke-Hopital Fleurimont; (819)474-2572

BILODEAU, Andre; Montfort Hosp, 713 Montreal Rd, Ottawa ON K1K 0T2; Laval'84; CCFP; FCFP; VP-Acad Aff, Montfort Hospital; (613)641-4621 x6013

BILODEAU, Audrey; CSSS de la Region de Thetford, 1717 rue Notre-Dame E, Thetford Mines QC G6G 2V4; Laval'00; FRCSC; GenSurg. Staff, Hopital du CSS de la Region de Thetford; (418)338-7777

BILODEAU, Carl; Clinique Med Montfort, 2185 rue de Montfort, Jonquiere QC G7X 4P6; Laval'81; (418)547-4783

BILODEAU, Denis; CSSS du Suroît, 150 rue Saint-Thomas, Salaber-de-Valleyf QC J6T 6C1; Laval'69; Psy (P.Q.). Staff, Centre Hospitalier Régional du Suroît; (450)371-9920

BILODEAU, Elizabeth; Clinique d'Obstetrique Bilodea, 943 rue des Erables RR 1, St-Lambert-de-Lauz QC G0S 2W0; Laval'96; Staff, Centre Hospitalier Universitaire de Quebec-CHUL; (418)889-0008

BILODEAU, Eric; 401-3030 boul Le carrefour, Laval QC H7T 2P5; Mon'89; FRCSC; Otol. Staff, CSSS Saint-Leonard et Saint-Michel; (450)687-1750

BILODEAU, Francois; GMF des Seigneuries, 2220 boul Rene-Gaultier, Varennes QC J3X 1E3; Sher'90; (450)652-2917; Fax. (450)652-9902.

BILODEAU, Francoise; CSSS des Sources, 475 3e Av, Asbestos QC J1T 1X6; Laval'81; Staff, CSSS des Sources d'Asbestos; (819)879-7151

BILODEAU, Genevieve; CSSS de Portneuf, 700 rue Saint-Cyrille, Saint-Raymond QC G3L 1W1; Laval'03; CCFP; Fam Med, Centre Hospitalier Portneuf; (418)337-4611

BILODEAU, Gilles; Centre Chirugical de Joliette, 203-222 rue de la Visitation, St-Charles-Brromee QC J6E 4N5; Sher'79; AB; FRCSC; Otol. (450)759-1241; Fax. (450)759-3737.

BILODEAU, Jean-Francois; CHUS-Hop Fleurimont, 3001 12e av N, Sherbrooke QC J1H 5N4; Sher'02; FRCPC; IntMed; Nephrol. Staff, Centre Hospitalier Universitaire de Sherbrooke-Hopital Fleurimont; Langs: Bilingual(French/English); (819)346-1110; jean.francois.bilodeau@usherbrook.ca.

BILODEAU, Jean-Sebastien; CSSS de Chicoutimi, CP 5006 305 rue Saint-Vallier, Chicoutimi QC G7H 5H6; Mon'03; Critical Care Medicine (P.Q.); IntMed. Staff, Complexe hospitalier de la Sagamie; (418)541-1000

BILODEAU, Josee; CSSS de Rimouski-Neigette, CP 3150 Succ A 150 av Rouleau, Rimouski QC G5L 5T1; Laval'07; FRCSC; GenSurg. Staff, Hôpital Regional Rimouski; (418)724-3000

BILODEAU, Lara; Hôpital Laval, 2725 ch Sainte-Foy, Quebec QC G1V 4G5; Mon'02; FRCPC; Respir; IntMed. Staff, Hôpital Laval; (418)656-8711

BILODEAU, Luc; MUHC-Royal Victoria Hosp, 687 av des Pins O, Montreal QC H3A 1A1; Laval'84; CSPQ; Cardiol; IntMed (Interventional Cardiology). Staff, McGill University Health Centre - Royal Victoria Hospital; Langs: English; (514)934-1934; bilodeau@bellnet.ca.

BILODEAU, Lucie; CSSS de Laval, 1755 boul Rene-Laennec, Laval QC H7M 3L9; Mon'87; FRCSC; GenSurg. Staff, Hopital de la Cite de la santé; (450)668-1010; Fax. (450)975-5545.

BILODEAU, Marc; CHUM-Hop St-Luc, 1058 rue Saint-Denis, Montreal QC H2X 3J4; Laval'86; FRCPC; IntMed (Hepatology); Gastroent. Staff, Centre Hospitalier l'Université De Montréal (CHUM) - Hôpital Saint-luc; Langs: English; (514)890-8000 x35749; Fax. (514)412-7314; marc.bilodeau@umontreal.ca.

BILODEAU, Marc; 2231 rue de l'Hopital, Jonquiere QC G7X 9Y4; Laval'79; (418)542-8897

BILODEAU, Marc; Canadian Forces Hlth Services, 101 Colonel By Dr, Ottawa ON K1A 0K2; Laval'98; ACLS; ATLS; AvMed; LMCC; SMO; CCFP; CCFP(E.M.); Emergency Family Med, Canadian Forces Health Services Centre; Physician, Ministry of National Defense; Langs: Bilingual(French/English); (613)945-1813; marc.bilodeau2@forces.gc.ca.

BILODEAU, Marie-Claude; CHUS-Hop Hotel-Dieu, 580 rue Bowen S, Sherbrooke QC J1G 2E8; Sher'06; Psy. Staff, Centre Hospitalier Universitaire de Sherbrooke-Hôpital Hôtel-Dieu; (819)346-1110

BILODEAU, Mathieu; Centre de Sante Valcartier, CP 1000 Bdp Succ Forces, Courcelette QC G0A 4Z0; Laval'06; FRCPC; Psy. (418)844-5000

BILODEAU, Ruth; CHUQ-Ctr Hosp Univ Laval, 2705 boul Laurier, Quebec QC G1V 4G2; Laval'80; CSPQ; FRCPC; Anes. Staff, Centre Hospitalier Universitaire de Quebec-CHUL; (418)656-4141; Fax. (418)654-2774.

BILODEAU, Serge; 4094 rue Morin, Jonquiere QC G8A 1A4; Laval'68; (418)547-6622; Fax. (418)542-9283.

BILODEAU, Sylvie; Hôpital Laval, 2725 ch Sainte-Foy, Quebec QC G1V 4G5; Laval'80; DiagRad. Staff, Hôpital Laval; (418)656-4512 x5; Fax. (418)656-4578.

BILODEAU, Yvonne; Clinique Med Pasteur, 770 av 1Re, Quebec QC G1L 3K2; Laval'72; Langs: Bilingual(French/English); (418)529-0042; Fax. (418)529-4924.

BILODEAU-DUBÉ, Anne-Michèle; CSSS de la Vallée de l'Or, 725 6e rue, Val-d'Or QC J9P 3Y1; Mon'06; CCFP; Staff, Centre Hospitalier de Val d'Or; (819)825-6711

BILOS, Richard J; Linden Ridge Med Centre, E-123 Scurfield Blvd, Winnipeg MB R3Y 1L6; Glasgow (Scotland)'89; (204)488-9988; Fax. (204)488-9994.

BILOTTA, Rosetta; Columbus Med Arts Bldg, 409-8333 Weston Rd, Woodbridge ON L4L 8E2; Tor'98; MD; BSc; MHSc; DABPM; PNS; FRCPC; CommunMed;CCFP; Public Health & Preventive Med. Asst Prof, University of Toronto; Langs: Italian; (647)986-4357; Fax. (416)913-4357; rose.bilotta@utoronto.ca.

BILSKI-PIOTROWSKI, Miroslaw; Community Mental Health Serv, 109-7071 Bayers Rd, Halifax NS B3L 2C2; Warsaw (Poland)'80; FRCPC; Psy. Langs: Polish; (902)454-1433; Fax. (902)454-1440.

BILSTON, Anne E; Highland Park Walk-In Clinic, 2B-6315 Horn St, Red Deer AB T4N 6H5; London (England)'83; CCFP; (403)342-2040; Fax. (403)342-7390.

BIMAN, Birubi R; 303-984 Oliver Rd, Thunder Bay ON P7B 7C7; Ott'92; FRCPC; IntMed; Respir. Ac Staff, Thunder Bay Regional Health Sciences Centre; Assoc Prof, Northern Ontario School of Medicine-Lakehead University; Asst Prof, McMaster University; Langs: French; (807)345-4500; Fax. (807)345-4501; bbiman@hotmail.com.

BIMBI-KOVACS, Agnes E; Seaforth Med Bldg, 440-3550 ch de la Cote-des-Nei, Montreal QC H3H 1V4; Brussels (Belgium)'52; FRCPC; Peds. Clin Asst Staff, McGill University Health Centre - Montreal Children's Hospital; McGill University; (514)933-7189

BIN, James; K304-650 Summon Ave, East York ON M4C 5M5; Alb'04; FRCPC; IntMed; MedOncol. Staff, Toronto East General Hospital Inc; (416)469-3325; Fax. (416)469-8221.

BINDA, Jean; Clinique Med Cite Rive, 7095 boul Gouin E, Montreal QC H1E 6N1; Mon'64; (514)329-4000

BINDEMAN, Annalene F; Family Med Clinic, 800-4615 49 Ave, Lloydminster SK S9V 0T1; Stellenbosch (South Africa)'87; (306)825-8877; Fax. (306)825-5167.

BINDER, Sara K; Foothills Med Centre, 1403 29 St NW, Calgary AB T2N 2T9; Cal'01; FRCPC; Psy. Staff, Foothills Medical Centre; (403)944-1567; Fax. (403)944-2838.

BINDLISH, Rajiv; Hopedale Mall, 210-1515 Rebecca St, Oakville ON L6L 5G8; Tor'94; DABOph; FRCSC; Ophth (Anterior Segment Surgery). Ac Staff, Halton Healthcare Services Corporation - Oakville Site; Court Staff, Joseph Brant Memorial Hospital; Court Staff, Halton Healthcare Services Corporation - Milton District Hospital; (905)469-6666; Fax. (905)469-3171; rajbindlish@hotmail.com.

BINDLISH, Vinita; 558 Belmont Ave W, Kitchener ON N2M 5E3; McM'95; BSc; PharmD; FRCSC; CCFP; Otol. Staff, Grand River Hospital - Kitchener/Waterloo Health Centre; VP Med Staff, St Mary's General Hospital; Langs: Hindi; (519)576-2200; Fax. (519)576-5675.

BINDRA, Heera S; Tuscany Med Clinic, 102-1646 McKenzie Ave, Victoria BC V8N 0A3; Alb'02; CCFP; (250)818-0001

BINEDELL, Walter; Southside Med Centre, 2-635 Water St, Miramichi NB E1N 4B9; Pretoria (South Africa)'95; MMed; Staff, Miramichi Regional Hospital; (506)623-3000; Fax. (506)627-7582.

BINET, Daniele; Clinique Med St-Benoit, 208A Route 271, St-Benoit-Labre QC G0M 1P0; Laval'84; Gen Practice, Centre Hospitalier Beauce-Etchemin; (418)228-3613; Fax. (418)228-3613.

BINET, Jacques; CLSC Vallee des Forts, 285-365 rue Normand, St-Jean-sur-Richel QC J3A 1T6; Laval'68; Langs: English; French; (450)358-2572 x3422; Fax. (450)359-8185.

BINET, Marie-Eve; Centre Hosp Honore-Mercier, 2750 boul Laframboise, Saint-Hyacinthe QC J2S 4Y8; Laval'05; Peds. Staff, Centre Hospitalier Honore-Mercier; (450)771-3333

BINET, Stephanie; CSSS de Rivière-de-Loup, 75 rue Saint-Henri, Riviere-Du-Loup QC G5R 2A4; Sher'97; FRCPC; Psy (Pediatric Psychiatry). Staff, Centre Hospitalier Regional du Grand-Portage; (418)868-1000 x284; Fax. (418)868-0530.

BINETTE, Alain; CSSS de la Vallée de l'Or, 725 6e rue, Val-d'Or QC J9P 3Y1; Sher'74; Gastroent (P.Q.). Staff, Centre Hospitalier de Val d'Or; (819)825-5858; Fax. (819)825-7921.

BINETTE, Brett A J; PO Box 6173 Stn Main, Hinton AB T7V 1X5; Alb'01; CCFP; (780)445-5770; brettbinette@yahoo.ca.

BINETTE, J Richard F; Peterborough Clinic FHT, LL02-26 Hospital Dr, Peterborough ON K9J 7C3; Ott'81; CCFP; FCFP; Langs: English; French; (705)740-6872; Fax. (705)740-6847.

BINETTE, Marcel; Campbellton Reg Hosp, PO Box 880 Stn Main 189 Lily Lake Rd, Campbellton NB E3N 3H3; Laval'65; Psy. Staff, Hôpital Régional Campbellton; (506)789-7000; Fax. (506)789-7065.

BINETTE, Nathalie; CLSC de Montreal-Nord, 11441 boul Lacordaire, Montreal-Nord QC H1G 4J9; Mon'09; CCFP; (514)384-2000

BINETTE-GAGNON, Marylyn; 1543 av du parc-Beauvoir, Quebec QC G1T 2M5; Laval'72; Psy (P.Q.) (Psychotherapy). (418)652-8629

BING-WO, Sandra; Medical Centre Bldg A, 2F-3000 Lawrence Ave, Scarborough ON M1P 2V1; Tor'80; BSc; CCFP; Ac Staff, Rouge Valley Health System - Centenary Health Centre Site; Court Staff, The Scarborough Hospital - General Campus; (416)431-8224

BINGHAM, J Lee; Woodville Med Centre PO Box 98, Woodville ON K0M 2T0; McM'79; CCFP; FCFP; Court Staff, Ross Memorial Hospital; (705)439-2411; Fax. (705)439-2770.

BINGHAM, Katherine D; Dalla Lana School of Public Hl, 6F-155 College St, Toronto ON M5T 3M7; Tor'06; CCFP; CCFP(E.M.); (647)977-4100

BINGHAM, William T; Royal University Hosp, 103 Hospital Dr, Saskatoon SK S7N 0W8; Sask'74; FRCPC; Peds. Ac Staff VP-Peds, Royal University Hospital; (306)966-8117; Fax. (306)975-3767.

BINHAMMER, Paul A; Sunnybrook Hlth Sciences Ctre, M1-2075 Bayview Ave, Toronto ON M4N 3M5; Tor'86; FRCSC; PlasSurg (Hand Surgery). Staff Div of PlasSurg, Sunnybrook Health Sciences Centre; Staff, Toronto Western Hospital - University Health Network; (416)480-6731; paul.binhammer@reveraliving.com.

BINING, Harjinder J S; 100-5791 No. 3 Rd, Richmond BC V6X 2C9; UBC'98; FRCPC; DiagRad. Langs: Punjabi; (604)278-9152

BINKHAMIS, Shagran; The Ottawa Hosp-Gen Campus, 501 Smyth Rd, Ottawa ON K1H 8L6; Riyadh (Saudi Arabia)'03; FRCPC; DiagRad. Staff, The Ottawa Hospital - General Campus.

BINKLEY, Karen E; 204-30 St Clair Ave W, Toronto ON M4V 3A1; Tor'84; FRCPC; IntMed; ClinImmunol&Allergy. Staff, Sunnybrook Health Sciences Centre; Staff, St Michael's Hospital; (416)968-7010

BINNIE, P Alexandra; St Joseph's Health Centre, 30 The Queensway, Toronto ON M6R 1B5; Harvard (USA)'07; Critical Care Medicine; IntMed. Staff, St Joseph's Health Centre; (416)530-6000

BINNIE, Rosemary C; Children's & Women's HC of BC, B321-4480 Oak St, Vancouver BC V6H 3V4; McM'03; FRCPC; Peds. Staff, BC Children's Hospital; (604)875-2345

BINNIE, William M H; Univ Hlth Network-Toronto Gen, 1182-200 Elizabeth St, Toronto ON M5G 2C4; Tor'96; FRCPC; IntMed (Telehealth); Respir. Staff, St Michael's Hospital; Clin Associate, Toronto General Hospital - UHN; (416)340-3235

BINNINGTON, Melanie E; 100 Queensway W, Mississauga ON L5B 1B8; Tor'86; FRCPC; Peds. Staff Peds, Trillium Health Centre - Mississauga; (905)848-7100

BINNS, Marichal A; True Balance, 203-52 Sioux Rd, Sherwood Park AB T8A 4X1; Alb'92; CCFP; FCFP; (780)450-4550; Fax. (780)465-1981.

BINSTED, Anthony H; Southwood Med Clinic, 80-10233 Elbow Dr SW, Calgary AB T2W 1E8; Guy's Hosp. (England)'62; MB BS; DRCOG; DCH; ahbinsted@shaw.ca.

BINTLEY, Timothy N; Gartree Medical Clinic, 510-4400 32nd St, Vernon BC V1T 9H2; Liverpool (England)'97; MB ChB; BEd(Hons); BSc; (250)545-9112

BIR, Amnit S; St Michael's Hosp, 30 Bond St, Toronto ON M5B 1W8; Saba (Netherlands Antilles)'10; CCFP; Staff, St Michael's Hospital; (416)360-4000

BIR, Karen; 604-790 Bay St, Toronto ON M5G 1N8; (Jamaica)'00; (416)204-9200

BIRBRAGER, David B I; Blackmore Med Centre, 201-9019 Bayview Ave, Richmond Hill ON L4B 3M6; Tor'83; Dip SportMed; Staff, Mackenzie Richmond Hill Hospital; (905)886-2829; Fax. (905)886-3597; mddavidb@yahoo.com.

BIRBRAGER, Donna R; 117 King St E, Oshawa ON L1H 1B9; McM'87; FRCPC; IntMed (Hypertension); Nephrol. Staff, Lakeridge Health - Whitby Site; Ac Staff, Lakeridge Health - Oshawa Site; (905)721-4064; Fax. (905)721-4061.

BIRCH, Christopher; Lakeshore Gen Hosp, 160 av Stillview, Pointe-Claire QC H9R 2Y2; Mon'98; CCFP; ac Membre Emerg, Lakeshore General Hospital - Pointe Claire; Langs: Bilingual(French/English); (514)630-2225 x1199

BIRCH, Colin; Foothills Med Centre, 1403 29 St NW, Calgary AB T2N 2T9; Newcastle (England)'83; FSOGC; FRCSC; ObstGyn (Urological Gynecology). Staff Pelvic Floor Clinic, Foothills Medical Centre; (403)944-4808

BIRCH, Corey T; Milverton & District Med Ctre, 101-50 William St, Milverton ON N0K 1M0; Adelaide (Australia)'08; CCFP; (519)595-8548; Fax. (519)595-8856.

BIRCH, Daniel W; Royal Alexandra Hosp, 10240 Kingsway NW, Edmonton AB T5H 3V9; McM'92; MSc; FRCSC; GenSurg (Laparoscopic Surgery). Staff, Royal Alexandra Hospital; Assoc Prof, University of Alberta; (780)735-4786; Fax. (780)735-4771.

BIRCH, David R; Springbank Med Centre, 305-460 Springbank Dr, London ON N6J 0A8; Tor'82; (519)963-3782; Fax. (519)963-0453.

BIRCH, J Andrew; 6690 Fraser St, Vancouver BC V5X 3T5; Cal'80; BSc; (604)879-1242; Fax. (604)879-1595.

BIRCHALL, Iain W J; University of Alberta Hosp, 8440 112 St NW, Edmonton AB T6G 2B7; Cambridge (England)'78; FRCR; MRC; MA; MB ChB; FRCPC; DiagRad. Staff, University of Alberta Hospital; Asst Prof, University of Alberta; (780)426-1121

BIRCHARD, James D; 201-274 Dundas St E, Belleville ON K8N 1E6; Qns'84; FRCSC; OrthSurg. Staff, QHC Belleville General; (613)969-8087

BIRCHARD, John G; Harbour City Health Centre, 102-1125 Dufferin Cres, Nanaimo BC V9S 2B5; Qns'86; Dip SportMed; FRCSC; OrthSurg (Sports Medicine). (250)753-2500; Fax. (250)753-2508.

BIRCHENOUGH, Brian R; Hamilton HS-General Site, 237 Barton St E, Hamilton ON L8L 2X2; McG'93; DiagRad. Staff, Hamilton Health Sciences Centre - Hamilton General Hospital; (905)527-4322 x46521

BIRCKEL, Pierre; CLSC de Saint-Henri, 3833 rue Notre-Dame, Montreal QC H4C 1P8; Strasbourg (France)'92; (514)933-7541; Fax. (514)933-1740.

BIRD, Gordon S; Delta Hosp, 5800 Mountain View Blvd, Delta BC V4K 3V6; UBC'92; BSc; CCFP; CCFP(E.M.); Staff EmergMed, Delta Hospital; (604)946-1121

BIRD, Natasha; Clinique Med de Coaticook, 206-18 rue du Manege, Coaticook QC J1A 3B3; Sher'91; Staff, CSSS - IUGS; Langs: Bilingual(English/French); French; (819)849-4876; Fax. (819)849-2115.

BIRD, Roderick A; 20 Townsend St, Sydney NS B1P 6V2; Dal'73; FRCPC; Peds. (902)562-6664

BIRD, Sally J; IWK Health Centre, PO Box 9700 Rpo CSC 5850-5980 University Ave, Halifax NS B3K 6R8; Dal'01; FRCPC; Anes. Staff, IWK Health Centre; (902)470-8251

BIRD PYPER, Cynthia J; Commercial Street Med Centre, 102-311 Commercial St, Milton ON L9T 3Z9; Alabama (USA)'82; BSc; CCFP; FCFP; Staff, Halton Healthcare Services Corporation - Oakville Site; (905)864-4747; Fax. (905)864-7099.

BIRDI, Girish; Rouge Valley-Centenary HC, 2867 Ellesmere Rd, Scarborough ON M1E 4B9; Guru Nanak Dev (India)'78; MB BS; FRCPC; Psy (Community Mental Health). Staff, Rouge Valley Health System - Centenary Health Centre Site; (416)284-8131

BIRDI, Kirandeep; Family Med Clinic, 102-2100 av de Marlowe, Montreal QC H4A 3L5; Man'03; CCFP; (514)934-8080

BIRDI, Parvinder K; Royal Inland Hosp, 311 Columbia St, Kamloops BC V2C 2T1; Gurunanak (India)'93; Staff, Royal Inland Hospital; (250)374-5111

BIRDI, Ravdeep S; University of Alberta Hosp, 1G1.50-8440 112 St NW, Edmonton AB T6G 2B7; Alb'08; CCFP; CCFP(E.M.); Staff, University of Alberta Hospital; (780)407-8432; Fax. (780)407-3695.

BIRDSELL, Dale C; 7 Glenbrook Pl SW, Calgary AB T3E 6W4; Alb'61; FRCSC; PlasSurg (Cosmetics). Clin Prof, University of Calgary; (403)571-3140; Fax. (403)571-3138.

BIRENBAUM, Adina M; Kingston Family Health Team, 200-2437 Princess St, Kingston ON K7M 3G1; Qns'00; CCFP; (613)546-6652; Fax. (613)344-1365; abirenbaum@kfhn.net.

BIRINGER, Anne B; Mount Sinai Fam Hlth Team, 4F-60 Murray St Box 25, Toronto ON M5T 3L9; Qns'79; CCFP; FCFP; Staff FPU, Mount Sinai Hospital; Langs: Swedish; Bilingual(French/English); (416)586-4800 x5158; Fax. (416)586-3175; abiringer@mtsinai.on.ca.

BIRK, Patricia E; Children's Hosp, FE009-840 Sherbrook St, Winnipeg MB R3A 1S1; Man'90; BSc(Med); FRCPC; Peds; Nephrol. Asst Prof Peds, University of Manitoba; Langs: English; French; (204)787-4947; Fax. (204)787-1666.

BIRKEN, Catherine S; The Hosp for Sick Children, 555 University Ave, Toronto ON M5G 1X8; Tor'97; MScClinEpidemiol; FRCPC; Peds (Child Obesity). Staff, The Hospital For Sick Children; (416)813-6933; catherine.birken@sickkids.ca.

BIRKETT, Barbara M; 185 Ontario St S, Milton ON L9T 2M4; McG'58; BA; MDCM; FRCPC; Derm. Court Staff Derm, Halton Healthcare Services Corporation - Oakville Site; Langs: English; French; (905)825-6000; Fax. (905)878-8797.

BIRKETT, Leanne D; Foothills Med Centre, 1403 29 St NW, Calgary AB T2N 2T9; Wes'89; FRCPC; Psy. Staff Psychiatrist, Foothills Medical Centre; (403)944-1491; Fax. (403)270-2093.

BIRKETT, Nicholas J; Univ Of Ottawa, 451 Smyth Rd, Ottawa ON K1H 8M5; McM'74; MSc(Epidem.); Assoc Prof Epidemiol & CommunMed, University of Ottawa; (613)562-5800 x8289; Fax. (613)562-5465.

BIRKILL, Richard S; Associated Med Clinic, PO Box 510 10017 101 Ave, Lac La Biche AB T0A 2C0; (South Africa)'95; CCFP; (780)623-4421; Fax. (780)623-1920.

BIRKIN, Brenda L; Medical Clinic Bldg, 233-89 Humber College Blvd, Etobicoke ON M9V 4B8; McG'71; FRCPC; IntMed. Ac Staff, William Osler Health System - Etobicoke General Hospital; (416)741-2478; Fax. (416)741-2481.

BIRMAN, Harry; Scarborough North Med Arts, 312-4040 Finch Ave E, Scarborough ON M1S 4V5; Tor'80; FRCPC; IntMed (Respirology). Court Staff, North Bay Regional Health Centre - Regional Mental Health; Court Staff, Mount Sinai Hospital; (416)298-2922; Fax. (416)298-8877; harrybirman@rogers.com.

BIRMINGHAM, Bradley W C; Belmont House for the Aged, 55 Belmont St, Toronto ON M5R 1R1; Qns'87; Med Dir, Belmont House Home For The Aged; Med Dir, Chester Village for the Aged.

BIRMINGHAM, C Laird; Student Health Services, M334-2211 Wesbrook Mall S, Vancouver BC V6T 1Z3; UBC'75; BSc; ABIM; FACP; MHSc; FRCPC; IntMed. Med Dir Eating Disorders Program, Providence Health Care - St Paul's Hospital; Med Dir, Woodstone Residential Treatment Centre; Prov Dir Eating Disorders & Epidemiol., BC, Centre for Health Evaluation & Outcome Sciences; Staff, University of British Columbia Student Health Services; Prof/Dir Eating Disorders Prog, University of British Columbia; (604)822-7011; clbirm@interchange.ubc.ca.

BIRNBAUM, Alexander; 211-2238 Dundas St W, Toronto ON M6R 3A9; Wes'77; BASc; MSc; FRCPC; Neur. Ac Staff Med & Neur, St Joseph's Health Centre; Court Staff, Toronto Western Hospital - University Health Network; Langs: Polish; (416)532-5327; Fax. (416)532-4272.

BIRNBAUM, Debra S; Bayview-Finch Med Clinic, 300-3292 Bayview Ave, North York ON M2M 4J5; Sher'81; CCFP; Ac Staff Family Med, North York General Hospital; Langs: English; French; (416)646-4455; Fax. (416)222-5722.

BIRNBAUM, Leora; MUHC-Royal Victoria Hosp, A4.23-687 av des Pins O, Montreal QC H3A 1A1; Mon'04; FRCPC; IntMed. Staff, McGill University Health Centre - Royal Victoria Hospital; (514)934-1934

BIRNBAUM, Robert J; Carling-Broadview Med Bldg, 210-770 Broadview Ave, Ottawa ON K2A 3Z3; Wes'69; CCFP; FCFP; Asst Prof Family Med, University of Ottawa; Langs: English; French; Spanish; German; (613)722-8010; Fax. (613)729-8906.

BIRNIE, Stuart A; 212A-12295 Highway 50, Bolton ON L7E 1M2; McM'84; (905)857-5052; Fax. (905)857-6960.

BIRNIE, William A; 304-1550 Bedford Hwy, Bedford NS B4A 1E6; Man'68; BSc; FRCPC; Psy (Adult ADHD). (902)835-4598; Fax. (902)445-4290.

BIRO, Andrew J; Longevity Med Aesthetics, 3-219 Fern Rd W, Qualicum Beach BC V9K 2M2; McM'92; BSc(Hon); MSc; CCFP; Med Advisor II, Worksafe BC; (250)752-6116; Andy.Biro@worksafebc.com.

BIRO, Antal; 611 Hamilton Rd, London ON N5Z 1S8; Wes'79; Staff, London Health Sciences Centre - Victoria Campus; Staff, St Joseph's Hospital - St Joseph's Health Care; (519)451-3144

BIRO, John E; Queensway Med Centre, 300-5307 Canotek Rd, Gloucester ON K1J 9M2; Ott'66; Court Staff, The Ottawa Hospital - General Campus; (613)746-6223; Fax. (613)746-6018.

BIRO, Laurence; Trillium Hlth Ctr-Mississauga, 100 Queensway W, Mississauga ON L5B 1B8; Tor'09; CCFP; Staff, Trillium Health Centre - Mississauga; (905)848-7100

BIRON, Daniel; GMF Centre de Sante, 3745 rue Georges-Couture, Drummondville QC J2B 7P4; Laval'94; CCFP; Langs: English; (819)477-2231; Fax. (819)477-1122.

BIRON, Dominique; Clinique Pediatrique Ste-Foy, 293-2600 boul Laurier, Quebec QC G1V 4T3; Laval'83; (418)658-0906; Fax. (418)652-7094.

BIRON, Guy L; CHUM-Hop Notre-Dame, 1560 rue Sherbrooke E, Montreal QC H2L 4M1; Mon'65; FRCPC; HemPath; Hem (P.Q.). Hematological Pathology, Centre Hospitalier l'Université de Montréal (CHUM) - Hôpital Notre-Dame; adj Prof, Universite de Montreal; (514)890-8000

BIRON, Linda; CLSC et CHSLD Pommeraie, 660 rue Saint-Paul, Farnham QC J2N 3B9; Sher'85; (450)293-3622; Fax. (450)293-4429.

BIRON, Marie-Helene; Ctr Hosp Anna-Laberge, 200 boul Brisebois, Chateauguay QC J6K 4W8; Mon'08; CCFP; CCFP(E.M.); (450)699-2425

BIRON, Simon; Hôpital Laval, 2725 ch Sainte-Foy, Quebec QC G1V 4G5; Laval'72; MSc; CSPQ; FRCSC; GenSurg (Bariatric Surgery). Chef chir gén, Hôpital Laval; Staff, Institut de Pneumologie de Quebec Pharmacy; Staff, Institut de Cardiologie de Montréal; Prof, Université Laval; (418)656-4810; Fax. (418)656-4825.

BIRON, Vincent; University of Alberta Hosp, 8440 112 St NW, Edmonton AB T6G 2B7; Cal'08; Staff, University of Alberta Hospital; (780)407-8822

BIROSH, Barry A; 302-111 Main St W, North Bay ON P1B 2T6; Tor'88; BASc; Staff, North Bay Regional Health Centre - Regional Mental Health; (705)497-0424; Fax. (705)497-0968.

BIRRI, Lino; CSSS du Lac-des-Deux-Montagnes, 520 boul Arthur-Sauve, Saint-Eustache QC J7R 5B1; Mon'07; IntMed. Staff, Hôpital de Saint-Eustache; (450)473-6811

BIRSS, John C; Grandview Med Ctr Fam Hlth Team, 167 Hespeler Rd, Cambridge ON N1R 3H7; Wes'73; BSc; Ac Staff, Cambridge Memorial Hospital; (519)623-4200; Fax. (519)623-2546.

BIRT, Catherine M; Sunnybrook Hlth Sciences Ctre, M1 302A-2075 Bayview Ave, Toronto ON M4N 3M5; Tor'89; BA(Hons); MA; FRCSC; Ophth (Glaucoma). Staff, Sunnybrook Health Sciences Centre; (416)480-5882; Fax. (416)480-4481.

BIRT, Douglas F; Country Club Plaza, 320-3025 Portage Ave, Winnipeg MB R3K 2E2; Man'68; FRCSC; OrthSurg. (204)831-7144; Fax. (204)888-9055.

BIRTWHISTLE, Richard; Queens Family Health Team, 115 Clarence St, Kingston ON K7L 5N6; McM'73; MSc; CCFP; FCFP; Staff, Kingston General Hospital; Staff, Hotel-Dieu Hospital; Staff, Queen's Family Health Team - Corporate Office; Prof Family Med & Ass't Prof, Queen's University; (613)533-9303

BISAILLON, Luc; Hop Jean-Talon, 1385 rue Jean-Talon E, Montreal QC H2E 1S6; McG'92; Staff, CSSS du Coeur de l'Isle Hôpital Jean-Talon; (514)495-6767

BISAILLON, Marc; Cooperative Sante Saint-Isidor, 640 rue Saint-Regis, Saint-Isidore QC J0L 2A0; Mon'93; Staff, Hôpital Anna-Laberge; (450)992-0558

BISAILLON, Norbert; CSSS d'Antoine-Labelle, RR 4 1525 rue l'Annonciation N, Riviere-Rouge QC J0T 1T0; Mon'74; Gen Practice, Centre de L'Annonciation; (819)275-2118

BISCAY, Caroline; Asclepios Med Clinic, 2-750 Taylor Creek Dr, Orleans ON K1C 1T1; Lille(Fr.) (France)'98; CCFP; (613)830-8388

BISCHOFF, Jan C; West Hill Med Clinic, 1A-2995 2nd Ave W, Prince Albert SK S6V 5V5; Stellenbosch (South Africa)'98; MB ChB; CCFP; (306)765-8500; Fax. (306)765-8501.

BISCHOFF, Markus; 201-470 Bronte St S, Milton ON L9T 2J4; McM'96; BSc; MSc; FRCSC; OrthSurg (Knee Arthroscopy). Staff OrthSurg, Halton Healthcare Services Corporation - Milton District Hospital; Langs: German.

BISCOTTI, Marilena; Lincoln Med Centre, SS 2 4413 Ontario St, Beamsville ON L0R 1B5; Tor'89; CCFP; Langs: Italian; French; (905)563-1212; Fax. (905)563-4404.

BISESSAR, Ahailya S; North Oshawa Med Centre, 103-1400 Ritson Rd N, Oshawa ON L1G 7W7; The University of the West Indies (Trinidad & Tobago)'07; BSc(Hon); MB BS; CCFP; Physician, University of Toronto; Physician, Durham College; (905)433-5026; Fax. (905)721-1366.

BISHARA, Laila D; 205-6633 Highway 7, Markham ON L3P 7P2; Ain Shams (Egypt)'85; FRCPC; IntMed (Endocrinology); Endocrin&Metab. Staff, Markham Stouffville Hospital; Langs: French; (905)201-1429; Fax. (905)201-4956.

BISHARA, Mona; Grand River Hosp-KW Hlth Ctre, PO Box 9056 Stn C 835 King St W, Kitchener ON N2G 1G3; Cairo (Egypt)'95; FRCPC; AnatPath. Staff, Grand River Hospital - Kitchener/Waterloo Health Centre; (519)749-4300

BISHARA, Phoebe R Y; 601-73 Water St N, Cambridge ON N1R 7L6; Cairo (Egypt)'91; FRCPC; IntMed; Endocrin&Metab. (519)624-8977; Fax. (519)624-2864.

BISHAY, Azhar; 22 Kingsview Blvd, Etobicoke ON M9R 1T6; Assiut (Egypt)'71; MB BCh; FRCPC; Peds (Allergy & Immunology). Ac Staff, William Osler Health System - Etobicoke General Hospital; Court Staff, Trillium Health Centre - West Toronto; Staff, The Allergy Clinic; Langs: Arabic; (416)244-3308; Fax. (416)246-9000.

BISHAY, Fekry S; Minnedosa Med Group, PO Box 810, Minnedosa MB R0J 1E0; Alexandria (Egypt)'87; MB ChB; CCFP; (204)867-2722; Fax. (204)867-2986.

BISHAY, Wagdy W S; Assiniboine Clinic, 633 Lodge Ave, Winnipeg MB R3J 0S9; CCFP; Fam Med, Tiger Hills Health District; wagdy_bishay@hc-sc.gc.ca.

BISHEL, Gerald R; Chinook Reg Hosp, 960 19 St S, Lethbridge AB T1J 1W5; Alb'76; CCFP; Staff, Chinook Regional Hospital; (403)388-6111

BISHINSKY, Jonathan; York Cardiovascular Centre, 101-50 Minthorn Blvd, Thornhill ON L3T 7X8; McG'83; MDCM; FRCPC; IntMed (Cardiology). Staff, Mackenzie Richmond Hill Hospital; (905)731-7832; Fax. (905)731-6419.

BISHOP, Allen J; Valley Reg Hosp, 150 Exhibition St, Kentville NS B4N 5E3; Dal'78; FRCPC; Anes. Staff, Valley Regional Hospital; (902)678-7381; Fax. (902)678-0098.

BISHOP, Andrew G; St Thomas-Elgin Gen Hosp, PO Box 2007 Stn Main 189 Elm St, St Thomas ON N5P 3W2; Dal'99; CCFP; CCFP(E. M.); Staff, St Thomas Elgin General Hospital; (519)631-2020

BISHOP, Brian P; Edmonton Mental Health Clinic, 9942 108 St NW, Edmonton AB T5K 2J5; Bristol (England)'70; MB ChB; DPM; MRCPsy; Staff, Alberta Hospital Edmonton; Asst Prof, University of Alberta; (780)427-4444

BISHOP, Clare E; 202-595 Montreal Rd, Ottawa ON K1K 4L2; Dal'77; CCFP; FCFP; Langs: English; French; (613)746-6745

BISHOP, David R; Cornwall Comm Hosp-McConnell, PO Box 100 Stn Main 840 McConnell Ave, Cornwall ON K6H 5S5; McG'81; FRCPC; DiagRad. Staff, Cornwall Community Hospital; (613)938-4240 x3361

BISHOP, Douglas R; 102-1335 Carling Ave, Ottawa ON K1Z 8N8; Qns'70; FRCPC; IntMed (Bariatric Medicine). Internal Med, The Perley & Rideau Veterans' Health Centre; (613)761-8015; Fax. (613)761-9585; drbishop@bellnet.ca.

BISHOP, Edward C; 8-120 Clinical Sciences Bldg, 132 University Campus NW, Edmonton AB T6G 2R7; Cape Town (South Africa)'88; MB ChB; LMCC; FRCPC; Anes. Staff, University of Alberta Hospital; (780)407-8861

BISHOP, Elizabeth; 101-730 Brant St, Burlington ON L7R 2H9; McM'81; FRCPC; Psy. (905)632-5864; Fax. (905)632-2018.

BISHOP, Graham W; 204-107 Catherwood St, Saint John NB E2M 5J7; Wes'89; FRCPC; IntMed (Critical Care Medicine); Respir. Ac Staff, Saint John Regional Hospital; Asst Prof Med, Dalhousie University; Asst Prof, Memorial University Of Newfoundland; (506)635-0480; Fax. (506)635-0716.

BISHOP, Gregory M; Peterborough Reg HC-Hospital, 1 Hospital Dr, Peterborough ON K9J 7C6; Cal'02; FRCPC; IntMed (Critical Care Medicine). Staff, Peterborough Regional Health Centre - Hospital Drive; (705)743-2121

BISHOP, Jane M; Arbutus Clinic, PO Box 1282 5713 Dolphin St, Sechelt BC V0N 3A0; Sask'86; CCFP; FCFP; Staff, St Mary's Hospital; (604)885-2384; Fax. (604)885-8876.

BISHOP, Jeffrey M S; Victoria Gen Hosp, 1 Hospital Way, Victoria BC V8Z 6R5; UBC'04; FRCPC; Peds; PedEmergMed. Staff, Victoria General Hospital; (250)727-4025

BISHOP, Jill M; Foothills Family Med Centre, PO Box 460 114 1 St SW, Black Diamond AB T0L 0H0; Alb'08; CCFP; (403)933-4368; Fax. (403)933-2026.

BISHOP, Joan E H; Waypoint Centre for Mental H C, T3 12-500 Church St, Penetanguishene ON L9M 1G3; Tor'71; MSc(Epidemiol&Biostatistics); FRCPC; Psy (Community Psychiatry). Staff, Waypoint Centre for Mental Health Care; Reg Staff Affiliate, Orillia Soldiers' Memorial Hospital; Emeritus Prof Psy, University of Western Ontario; (705)549-3181; Fax. (705)549-9294.

BISHOP, Joanne E; East End Health Centre, 2 Mount Cashel Rd, St. John's NL A1A 1X7; Mem'07; CCFP; Staff, Central Newfoundland Regional Health Centre.

BISHOP, Leigh R; 200-89 Dawson Rd, Guelph ON N1H 1B1; Mem'97; FRCSC; GenSurg. (519)836-0404

BISHOP, Michael B; Kamsack Med Clinic, PO Box 1600, Kamsack SK S0A 1S0; London (England)'61; DA(Eng.); DRCOG; Staff Chief, Kamsack Hospital & Nursing Home; (306)542-3714; Fax. (306)542-2697; michael.bishop@shr.sk.ca.

BISHOP, Paul B; Blusson Spine Centre, 6110-818 10th Ave W, Vancouver BC V5Z 1M9; Cal'91; (604)875-4549; Fax. (604)875-5858.

BISHOP, Robert W; St Clare's Mercy Hosp, 154 LeMarchant Rd, St. John's NL A1C 5B8; Mem'05; FRCPC; Anes. Staff, St Clare's Mercy Hospital; (709)777-5500

BISHOP, Winston T; University Hosp of Northern BC, 1475 Edmonton St, Prince George BC V2M 1S2; RCS (Ireland)'67; DABIM; LRCPSI; FRCPC; IntMed (Medical Oncology). Dir Regional Cancer Care Unit/Chief MedOncol, University Hospital of Northern British Columbia; Clinical Asst Prof, University of British Columbia; (250)565-2000 x2535; Fax. (250)565-2500.

BISKIN, Robert S; Inst of Community & Family Psy, 4333 ch Cote-Sainte-Catherine, Montreal QC H3T 1E4; McG'06; MDCM; FRCPC; Psy. (514)340-8210

BISMAR, Tarek A; Rockyview Gen Hosp, 7007 14 St SW, Calgary AB T2V 1P9; Damascus (Syria)'96; AB; Staff, Rockyview General Hospital; Langs: Arabic; English; (403)943-8430

BISMIL, Ramprasad; The Ottawa Hosp-Civic Campus, 1053 Carling Ave, Ottawa ON K1Y 4E9; Pune (India)'93; FRCPC; Psy. Staff, The Ottawa Hospital - Civic Campus; (613)761-4581; Fax. (613)761-4911.

BISMILLA, Fasel A; Upper Grand Family Health Team, 350 St Andrew St W, Fergus ON N1M 1N9; RCS (Ireland)'72; LRCPS(Ire); Ac Staff, Groves Memorial Community Hospital; Ac Staff, Guelph General Hospital; (519)843-2770; Fax. (519)843-4451.

BISMILLA, Zia; The Hosp For Sick Children, 555 University Ave, Toronto ON M5G 1X8; Wes'02; FRCPC; Peds. Staff, The Hospital For Sick Children; (416)813-7654

BISMONTE, Maria Dulce B; 103-127 Westmore Dr, Etobicoke ON M9V 3Y6; Santo Tomas (Philippines)'74; MD; FRCPC; Psy. Langs: Tagalog; (416)749-3933; Fax. (416)749-3936; mdbismonte@rogers.com.

BISSADA, Eric; Hop Charles LeMoyne, 3120 boul Taschereau, Longueuil QC J4V 2H1; Mon'05; FRCSC; Otol. Staff, Hopital Charles LeMoyne; (450)466-5000

BISSADA, Hany E; The Ottawa Hosp-Gen Campus, 4428-501 Smyth Rd, Ottawa ON K1H 8L6; Cairo (Egypt)'75; FRCPC; Psy (Eating Disorders). Staff Psy, The Ottawa Hospital - General Campus; Assoc Prof, University of Ottawa; Langs: French; (613)737-8042; Fax. (613)737-8085; hbissada@ottawahospital.on.ca.

BISSESSAR, Ramnaraise; 567 Bathurst St, Toronto ON M5S 2P8; (Jamaica)'61; (416)964-8572

BISSET, Lindsay J; 47 Liberty St S, Bowmanville ON L1C 2N4; McM'03; CCFP; CCFP(E.M.); (905)623-3331

BISSETT, Randall J; Sudbury Reg Hosp-Laurentian, 41 Ramsey Lake Rd, Sudbury ON P3E 5J1; Tor'82; MHSc(HealthAdmin); FRCPC; RadOncol. Clin Staff Oncol, Health Sciences North-Laurentian Site; Staff, Northeastern Ontario Regional Cancer Centre; Asst Prof, University of Ottawa; (705)522-6237 x2451; Fax. (705)523-7329.

BISSON, Cédric; Teralys Capital Inc, 1700-999 boul de Maisonneuve O, Montreal QC H3A 3L4; McG'91; LLB; CCFP; Physician, Inovia Healthcare Ventures; Langs: German; Italian; English; (514)509-2083; cbisson@inoviacapital.com.

BISSON, Danny S; Northern Medical Unit, T162-770 Bannatyne Ave, Winnipeg MB R3E 0W3; Man'06; CCFP; (204)789-3711

BISSON, Denis; 70 rue de l'Eglise, Verdun QC H4G 2L9; Laval'72; (514)761-3788; Fax. (514)761-2059; info@drbisson.com.

BISSON, Gail M; Health Park, 208-45 Weatherbee Rd, Mira Road NS B1M 0A1; Dal'83; Staff, Cape Breton Healthcare Complex; (902)539-8566; Fax. (902)567-0635.

BISSON, Guy; Agence Chaudiere-Appalaches, 363 rte Cameron, Sainte-Marie QC G6E 3E2; Sher'80; AB; FRCPC; NuclearMed. Staff, Centre Hospitalier Universitaire de Sherbrooke-Hopital Fleurimont; Prof, Universite de Sherbrooke; (418)386-3528

BISSON, Jocelyne; Hôtel-Dieu de Lévis, 143 rue Wolfe, Levis QC G6V 3Z1; Sher'90; CSPQ; FRCPC; AnatPath. Staff, Hôtel-Dieu de Lévis; (418)835-7121; jocelyne@globetrotter.net.

BISSON, Maude; Clinique Med Lavaltrie, 1400 rue Notre-Dame, Lavaltrie QC J5T 1M6; Mon'08; CCFP; (450)586-1033; Fax. (450)586-4498.

BISSON, Patrick; Hop Charles Lemoyne, 3120 boul Taschereau, Greenfield Park QC J4V 2H1; Mon'89; IntMed. Staff, Hopital Charles LeMoyne; (450)466-5000 x2880

BISSON, Robert; Clin de Med Familiale de Hull, 202-15 boul Montclair, Gatineau QC J8Y 2E2; Ott'78; ac Staff, Hull Hospital; (819)777-2752; Fax. (819)777-2269.

BISSON, Sebastien; Hop Charles Lemoyne, 3120 boul Taschereau, Greenfield Park QC J4V 2H1; Laval'05; FRCPC; GeriatricMed; IntMed. Staff, Hopital Charles LeMoyne; (450)466-5000 x2880

BISSONNETTE, Alain; CHUQ-Ctr Hosp Univ Laval, 2705 boul Laurier, Quebec QC G1V 4G2; Laval'87; Consultant Chronic Pain, Centre Hospitalier Universitaire de Quebec-CHUL; Langs: English; (418)653-4050

BISSONNETTE, Arcel; Seine Med Centre, 115-142 Centrale Ave, Ste Anne MB R5H 1C3; Man'89; (204)422-8811; Fax. (204)422-5876.

BISSONNETTE, Bernard F; Polyclinique de Montreal, 410-12245 rue Grenet, Montreal QC H4J 2J6; Mon'75; FRCPC; IntMed (P.Q.); Rheum. Ac Staff, Hôpital du Sacre-Coeur de Montréal; Langs: Italian; English; (514)334-9112; Fax. (514)334-2945; rchart@videotron.ca.

BISSONNETTE, Bertrand; Clinique Med 201, 104 rue Sainte-Agathe, Ste-Agathe-Des-Mts QC J8C 2K3; Mon'79; (819)326-2020; Fax. (819)326-8801.

BISSONNETTE, Catherine; Polyclinique St-Eustache, 18-75 rue Grignon, Saint-Eustache QC J7P 4J2; Mon'00; DiagRad. Staff, Centre Hospitalier Pierre le Gardeur; (450)430-3350; catbissonnette@hotmail.com.

BISSONNETTE, Francois; 100-8000 boul Decarie, Montreal QC H4P 2S4; Mon'80; ObstGyn. Staff, Centre Hospitalier l'Université De Montréal (CHUM) - Hôpital Saint-luc; adj Prof, Universite de Montreal; (514)798-2000; Fax. (514)798-2001.

BISSONNETTE, Guillaume; Ctr Hosp Anna-Laberge, 200 boul Brisebois, Chateauguay QC J6K 4W8; Mon'07; FRCSC; OrthSurg. Staff, Hôpital Anna-Laberge; (450)699-2425

BISSONNETTE, Jacques; Polyclinique St-Eustache, 75 rue Grignon, St-Eustache QC J7P 4J2; Mon'71; (450)473-6514; Fax. (450)473-1916.

BISSONNETTE, Jean; CSSS du Suroît, 150 rue Saint-Thomas, Salaber-de-Valleyf QC J6T 6C1; Sher'96; CSPQ; FRCPC; Anes. Staff, Centre Hospitalier Régional du Suroît; (450)371-9920 x2141

BISSONNETTE, Julien; Hop du Sacre-Coeur de Mtl, 5400 boul Gouin O, Montreal QC H4J 1C5; Mon'08; IntMed. Staff, Hôpital du Sacre-Coeur de Montréal; (514)338-2222

BISSONNETTE, Louis; Clinique Med du Village, 200-400 rue Meigs, Farnham QC J2N 2C8; Mon'82; CCFP; Staff, Hôpital Brome-Missisquoi-Perkins; Langs: English; French; (450)293-3681; Fax. (450)293-7463.

BISSONNETTE, Lucie; 105-1205 rue Ampère, Boucherville QC J4B 7M6; Mon'83; (450)650-0170; Fax. (450)641-7331.

BISSONNETTE, Lyle V; Medical Bldg, 203-18 Pine St, Kitchener ON N2H 5Z8; Ott'97; FRCP; BSc; LMCC; FRCPC; IntMed; Gastroent. Ac Staff, Grand River Hospital - Kitchener/Waterloo Health Centre; Ac Staff, St Mary's General Hospital; (519)585-1251; Fax. (519)585-7906.

BISSONNETTE, Martine; Clinique Plateau Marquette, 200-731 rue Galt O, Sherbrooke QC J1H 1Z1; Sher'91; Staff, Centre Hospitalier Universitaire de Sherbrooke-Hopital Fleurimont; Langs: English; (819)564-8662; Fax. (819)564-1294.

BISSONNETTE, Mélanie; Clarence Rockland Family, 2741 Chamberland Rd, Rockland ON K4K 0B4; Ott'08; CCFP; Staff, Montfort Hospital; (613)446-7677

BISSONNETTE, Robert; Clinique de Dermatologie, 502-1851 rue Sherbrooke E, Montreal QC H2K 4L5; Mon'88; FRCPC; Derm. adj Prof, Universite de Montreal; (514)521-4285 x210; Fax. (514)521-4175.

BISSONNETTE, Robert T; Nanaimo Reg Gen Hosp, 1200 Dufferin Cres, Nanaimo BC V9S 2B7; Wes'81; FRCPC; DiagRad. Staff, Nanaimo Regional General Hospital.

BISSOONDATH, Rohan S; Preventous Collaborative Healt, 1635 17 Ave SW, Calgary AB T2T 0E5; (Trinidad & Tobago)'97; CCFP; (403)229-0129; Fax. (403)398-0193.

BISTRITZ, Aalo; Cross Cancer Institute, 11560 University Ave NW, Edmonton AB T6G 1Z2; Sask'93; FRCPC; DiagRad (Oncology Imaging). Staff, Cross Cancer Institute; Asst Prof, University of Alberta; (780)432-8486; Fax. (780)432-8552.

BISTRITZ, Lana M; Royal Alexandra Hosp, 217-10240 Kingsway NW, Edmonton AB T5H 3V9; Alb'00; FRCPC; IntMed; Gastroent. Staff, Royal Alexandra Hospital; (780)735-4088

BISWAS, Iqbal H; Cambridge Mem Hosp, 700 Coronation Blvd, Cambridge ON N1R 3G2; Calcutta (India)'87; MB BS; DABA; FRCPC; Anes. Pres-Med/Prof Staff Association, Cambridge Memorial Hospital; Langs: Bengali; Hindi; (519)621-2333 x2100; Fax. (519)740-4906.

BISWAS, Tuhina; Women's College Hosp, 76 Grenville St, Toronto ON M5S 1B2; Wes'03; CCFP; Staff, Women's College Hospital; (416)323-6064; Fax. (416)323-6350.

BITANGCOL, John C; Grey Nuns Community Hosp & HC, 1100 Youville Drive West NW, Edmonton AB T6L 5X8; Alb'01; CCFP; CCFP(E.M.); Staff, Covenant Health - Grey Nuns Community Hospital; (780)735-7180

BITAR, Richard; Thunder Bay Reg HSC-T-Bay, 980 Oliver Rd, Thunder Bay ON P7B 6V4; Tor'01; FRCPC; DiagRad. Staff, Thunder Bay Regional Health Sciences Centre; (807)684-6000

BITCHOKA, Joseph; Hop Santa Cabrini Ospedale, 5655 rue Saint-Zotique E, Montreal QC H1T 1P7; Yaounde (Cameroon)'78; Staff Emerg, CSSS Saint-Leonard et Saint-Michel; Staff, Hôpital Santa Cabrini Ospedale; (514)252-6444

BITNUN, Sean A; The Hosp for Sick Children, 555 University Ave, Toronto ON M5G 1X8; UBC'89; FRCPC; Peds; InfectDis. Fellow, The Hospital For Sick Children; (416)813-7654 x3362

BITONTI, David; 10B Victoria St S, Kitchener ON N2G 1C5; Qns'10; CCFP; (519)783-0024

BITONTI, Rosa M; 104-3965 Kingsway, Burnaby BC V5H 1Y8; Rome (Italy)'83; CCFP; (604)434-8781; Fax. (604)434-8699.

BITTENCOURT, Henrique; Hopital Ste-Justine, A12.55-3175 ch Cote-Sainte-Cat, Montreal QC H3T 1C5; (Brazil)'90; Staff, Hôpital Ste-Justine; (514)345-4870

BITTER-SUERMANN, Bjorn F; UBC-Dept Of Anes, 2449-910 10th Ave W, Vancouver BC V5Z 1M9; Dal'96; FRCPC; Anes. (604)875-4304; Fax. (604)875-5209.

BITTING, Seth S; Riverside Med Clinic, 305-1101 Dewdney Ave, Trail BC V1R 4T1; Tor'98; FRCSC; OrthSurg. (250)364-0044

BITTIRA, Bindu; M281-865 Regent St, Sudbury ON P3E 3Y9; Dal'98; MSc; FRCSC; CardSurg. Staff Cardiac Surg, Health Sciences North - Memorial Site; Asst Prof, Northern Ontario School of Medicine-Laurentian University; Langs: French; (705)671-5353

BITTON, Alain; MUHC-Royal Victoria Hosp, 228-687 av des Pins O, Montreal QC H3A 1A1; Mon'87; FRCPC; IntMed; Gastroent. Staff, McGill University Health Centre - Royal Victoria Hospital; (514)843-1616; Fax. (514)843-1421.

BITZAN, Martin; MUHC-Montreal Children's Hosp, E-222-2300 rue Tupper, Montreal QC H3H 1P3; Bonn (Germany)'80; MD; assoc Prof/Staff, McGill University Health Centre - Montreal Children's Hospital; Langs: German; Hebrew; French; (514)412-4461; Fax. (514)412-4359.

BIYANI, Mohan B; The Ottawa Hosp-Riverside, 1967 Riverside Dr, Ottawa ON K1H 7W9; Marathwada (India)'92; MB BS; Staff Nephrol, The Ottawa Hospital - Riverside Campus; Asst Prof Med, University of Ottawa; (613)738-8400 x82890; Fax. (613)738-8384; mbiyani@ottawahospital.on.ca.

BIYONG, Issack; Montfort Hosp, 713 Montreal Rd, Ottawa ON K1K 0T2; '91; Staff, Montfort Hospital; (613)746-4621

BIZGU, Victoria; SMBD Jewish Gen Hosp, 3755 ch Cote-Sainte-Catherine, Montreal QC H3T 1E2; (Moldova)'90; Staff, Sir Mortimer B Davis Jewish General; (514)340-7598; Fax. (514)340-7566.

BJARNASON, Georg A; 2075 Bayview Ave, Toronto ON M4N 3M5; (Iceland)'79; MD; FRCPC; IntMed; MedOncol. Staff Med & Clin Pharmacology, Sunnybrook Health Sciences Centre; Staff MedOncol, Sunnybrook Health Sciences Centre - Edmond Odette Cancer Centre; (416)480-5847

BJERKE, Thomas L; The Fraser Valley Maternity Gr, 201-32310 South Fraser Way, Abbotsford BC V2T 1X1; Minnesota (USA)'75; CCFP; FCFP; Ac Staff, Abbotsford Regional Hospital & Cancer Centre; Ac Staff, Mission Memorial Hospital; Staff, The Fraser Valley Maternity Group; Staff, The Fraser Valley Maternity Group; (604)852-3707; Fax. (604)853-8028.

BJERRE, Lise M; Family Med Centre, 210 Melrose Ave, Ottawa ON K1Y 4K7; McG'99; (613)761-4334

BJORNSON, Bruce H; Children's & Women's HC of BC, K3 143-4480 Oak St, Vancouver BC V6H 3V4; Alb'81; DABPed; FRCPC; Peds; Neur. Staff, BC Children's Hospital; Asst Prof, University of British Columbia; (604)875-2121; Fax. (604)875-2285.

BJORNSON, Candice L; Alberta Children's Hosp, 2888 Shaganappi Trail NW, Calgary AB T3B 6A8; Alb'94; FRCPC; Peds (Pediatric Pulmonology); Respir. Staff Ped Respirology, Alberta Children's Hospital; (403)955-2952; Fax. (403)955-7059; candice.bjornson@calgaryhealthregion.ca.

BJORNSON, Michele E; Alberta Children's Hosp, 2888 Shaganappi Trail NW, Calgary AB T3B 6A8; Alb'87; FRCPC; Peds. Staff, Alberta Children's Hospital; (403)955-7070

BLACH, Peter H O; McConnell Med Centre, 214-820 Mcconnell Ave, Cornwall ON K6H 4M4; Mon'88; (613)933-3222; Fax. (613)933-5757.

BLACHFORD, Patricia; Brameast Family Health Org, 38-2130 North Park Dr, Brampton ON L6S 0C9; Tor'69; (905)792-2211; Fax. (905)792-2901.

BLACHOWITZ, Roy; Thornhill Med Centre, 18 Centre St, Thornhill ON L4J 1E9; Cape Town (South Africa)'85; MB ChB; CCFP; FCFP; Ac Staff, Mackenzie Richmond Hill Hospital; (905)889-3634; Fax. (905)889-3986; dr.roy@me.com.

BLACHUT, Jan P; UBC-Dept Of Anes, 910 10th Ave W, Vancouver BC V5Z 1M9; Tor'77; FRCPC; Anes. Ac Staff, Vancouver General Hospital - Centennial Pavillion; (604)875-4304

BLACHUT, Piotr A; Gordon & Leslie Diamond HCC, 3F-2775 Laurel St, Vancouver BC V5Z 1M9; Tor'79; FRCSC; OrthSurg (Orthopedic Trauma). Ac Staff, Vancouver General Hospital - Centennial Pavillion; Staff, Gordon & Leslie Diamond Health Care Centre; University of British Columbia; Langs: German; Spanish; Polish; French; (604)875-5809; Fax. (604)875-5812; piotr@interchange.ubc.ca.

BLACK, Amanda Y; The Ottawa Hosp-Gen Campus, 501 Smyth Rd, Ottawa ON K1H 8L6; Wes'96; FRCSC; ObstGyn. Staff, The Ottawa Hospital - General Campus; (613)738-8400; Fax. (613)738-8505.

BLACK, Barbara A; Westmount Med Bldg, 225-5025 rue Sherbrooke O, Montreal QC H4A 1S9; McG'86; CCFP; (514)482-6465; Fax. (514)482-3380.

BLACK, Charlyn D; 201-2206 East Mall, Vancouver BC V6T 1Z3; Man'79; Prof Dept of Health Care & Epidemiol/Sr Staff Centre for Health Services & Policy Research, University of British Columbia; (604)822-6030; Fax. (604)822-5690.

BLACK, Colleen L; 581 Hudson Ave NE, Salmon Arm BC V1E 4N8; Cal'10; CCFP; (250)832-6092

BLACK, Daniel O; Ctr Hosp Affilie-St-Sacrement, 1050 ch Sainte-Foy, Quebec QC G1S 4L8; Massachusetts (USA)'91; FRCSC; Ophth (Neuro Ophthalmology). Staff, Centre Hospitalier Affilié Universitaire de Québec - Hôpital du St-Sacrement; Langs: English; French; (418)682-7680; danielovid@mac.com.

BLACK, David R T; Scarborough Hosp-Birchmount, 3030 Birchmount Rd, Scarborough ON M1W 3W3; McM'98; Gastroent; IntMed. Staff, The Scarborough Hospital - Birchmount Campus; (416)495-2600

BLACK, Denise R A; Dakota Medical Clinic, 17-845 Dakota St, Winnipeg MB R2M 5M3; Man'89; FRCSC; ObstGyn. Staff, Health Sciences Centre.

BLACK, Dola; St Joseph's Hlth Ctr Urban FHT, 203-27 Roncesvalles Ave, Toronto ON M6R 3B2; Dublin (Ireland)'71; Court Staff, St Joseph's Health Centre; (416)533-5575; Fax. (416)785-1031; dola.black@sickkids.ca.

BLACK, Douglas M; 560-1145 Hunt Club Rd, Ottawa ON K1V 0Y3; Dundee (Scotland)'80; FRCSC; ObstGyn (Laparoscopic Surgery). Ac Staff, The Ottawa Hospital - General Campus; Assoc Consultant, Children's Hospital of Eastern Ontario (CHEO); (613)738-2378; Fax. (613)738-9032.

BLACK, Fraser; 212-2187 Oak Bay Ave, Victoria BC V8R 1G1; Cal'93; BSc; CCFP; FCFP; Staff, Royal Jubilee Hospital; Clin Instructor, University of British Columbia; (250)595-7125; fraser.black@viha.ca.

BLACK, G Brian; Children's Hosp, 840 Sherbrook St, Winnipeg MB R3A 1S1; Dal'74; FRCSC; OrthSurg.

BLACK, Gail L; Meadowlark Health Centre, 162 Meadowlark Shopping Ctr NW, Edmonton AB T5R 5W9; UBC'80; FRCSC; ObstGyn. Site Leader ObstGyn, Covenant Health - Misericordia Community Hospital; Clin Assoc Prof, University of Alberta; (780)428-9516; Fax. (780)428-0629.

BLACK, Hans P; 3655 rue Redpath, Montreal QC H3G 2W8; McG'78; Physician, Zurmont Research Corp. Inc.; (514)393-3188; hblack@interinvest.com.

BLACK, John Douglas; 75 Warwick St PO Box 820, Digby NS B0V 1A0; Dal'74; Staff, Digby General Hospital; (902)245-5470; Fax. (902)245-2144; jblack@ns.sympatico.ca.

BLACK, J Kevin; Texada Island Health Centre, PO Box 10 2603 Sandersen Rd, Gillies Bay BC V0N 1W0; Queen's (Ireland)'78; MB ChB; (604)486-7525; Fax. (604)486-7374.

BLACK, Jason T; Goodfellow Prof Bldg, 208-170 McEwan Dr E, Bolton ON L7E 4C8; Wes'97; CCFP; (905)951-3696

BLACK, Jennifer; 135 Glenmount Park Rd, Toronto ON M4E 2N3; CCFP; Staff, Regina General Hospital; (416)841-9283

BLACK, Jennifer P; 2F-2227 South Millway, Mississauga ON L5L 3R6; Queen's (Ireland)'69; MB ChB; BAO; DRCOG; Physician Healthy Sexuality Prog, Peel Region Health Department; (905)820-3663; Fax. (905)820-4372; cairns2@sympatico.ca.

BLACK, Karen J L; IWK Health Centre, PO Box 9700 Rpo CSC, Halifax NS B3K 6R8; UBC'94; FRCPC; Peds. Staff, IWK Health Centre; Langs: German; (902)470-8823; Fax. (902)428-8859.

BLACK, Karen M; Trillium Hlth Ctr-Mississauga, 100 Queensway W, Mississauga ON L5B 1B8; Qns'71; FRCSC; GenSurg. Consultant Surg, Trillium Health Centre - Mississauga; (905)848-7200

BLACK, Katharine A; Dartmouth Comm Mental Hlth, 5F-33 Alderney Dr, Dartmouth NS B2Y 2N4; Cape Town (South Africa)'88; MB ChB; FRCPC; Psy. Staff, The Nova Scotia Hospital; (902)466-1830; Fax. (902)466-1851.

BLACK, Martin J; SMBD Jewish Gen Hosp, 3755 ch Cote-Sainte-Catherine, Montreal QC H3T 1E2; McG'67; DABOT; FRCSC; Otol (Head & Neck Oncology). Staff, Sir Mortimer B Davis Jewish General; Staff, McGill University Health Centre - Royal Victoria Hospital; Staff, McGill University Health Centre - Montreal General Campus; Chief Head & Neck Surg & Oncology Program, McGill University; (514)340-8246; Fax. (514)340-7581.

BLACK, Morry; 770 Mohawk Rd W, Hamilton ON L9C 1X9; McM'06; CCFP; Staff, Hamilton Health Sciences Centre - McMaster University Medical Centre; (905)526-9661

BLACK, Peter C V; Gordon & Leslie Diamond HC Ctr, L6-2775 Laurel St, Vancouver BC V5Z 1M9; Mainz (Germany)'97; FRCSC; Urol. Staff, Gordon & Leslie Diamond Health Care Centre; (604)875-5003

BLACK, Raymond; Peterborough Reg HC-Hospital, 1 Hospital Dr, Peterborough ON K9J 7C6; Qns'06; CCFP; Staff, Peterborough Regional Health Centre - Hospital Drive; (705)743-2121

BLACK, Richard D; 770 Mohawk Rd W, Hamilton ON L9C 1X9; Tor'77; CCFP; FCFP; (905)388-4543; Fax. (905)388-4824.

BLACK, Robert C; Meadowlark Health Centre, 162 Meadowlark Shopping Ctr NW, Edmonton AB T5R 5W9; Sask'80; BSc; FACOG; FRCSC; ObstGyn (Colposcopy). Staff, Covenant Health - Misericordia Community Hospital; Clin Prof, University of Alberta; (780)428-9516; Fax. (780)428-0629.

BLACK, Robert T; The Surgeons Office, 236 Elm St, St Thomas ON N5R 1J5; Wes'89; FRCSC; GenSurg (General Practice). Staff, St Thomas Elgin General Hospital; Acad Dir Community Surg Education, University of Western Ontario; (519)631-0567; Fax. (519)631-0921.

BLACK, Ronald W; 2-1400 Lakeshore Rd W, Mississauga ON L5J 1J1; Tor'79; Staff, Halton Healthcare Services Corporation - Oakville Site; (905)823-0300; Fax. (905)823-0144.

BLACK, Sandra E; Sunnybrook Hlth Sciences Ctre, A421-2075 Bayview Ave, Toronto ON M4N 3M5; Tor'78; BSc; FRCPC; Neur (Cognitive Neurol). Chair Neurol, Sunnybrook Health Sciences Centre; (416)480-4551; Fax. (416)480-4552; sandra.black@sunnybrook.ca.

BLACK, Sandra E; Beaumont Med Clinic, 5001A 50 Ave, Beaumont AB T4X 1E7; Cal'91; (780)929-6050; Fax. (780)929-5848.

BLACK, Steven M; Malton Med Centre, 22-7330 Goreway Dr, Mississauga ON L4T 4J2; Dublin (Ireland)'68; MB ChB; BAO; (905)677-4200; Fax. (905)677-0541.

BLACK, Timothy S; Meadowlark Health Centre, 200 Meadowlark Shopp Ctr NW, Edmonton AB T5R 5W9; UBC'94; FRCPC; DiagRad. (780)489-5315; Fax. (780)486-5160.

BLACK, Tyler R; BC Women's Hosp & Hlth Ctre, P2 138-4500 Oak St, Vancouver BC V6H 3N1; Alb'03; FRCPC; Psy (Child & Adolescent Psychiatry). Staff, BC Women's Hospital & Health Centre; (604)875-2345

BLACK, William P G; Queen West Commun Health Ctre, 168 Bathurst St, Toronto ON M5V 2R4; RCS (Ireland)'72; CCFP; FCFP; Physician, West Central Community Health Centre; (416)703-8480; Fax. (416)703-8479.

BLACK, William R; Royal Alexandra Hosp, 10240 Kingsway Ave, Edmonton AB T5H 3V9; Alb'56; FRCPC; IntMed (Cardiology). Staff, Royal Alexandra Hospital.

BLACKADAR, Andrew M; 202-255 Main St PO Box 939, Liverpool NS B0T 1K0; Dal'01; CCFP; (902)354-2003; Fax. (902)354-3626.

BLACKBEARD, Rosalind; Creston Valley Hosp, PO Box 3000 312 15th Ave N, Creston BC V0B 1G0; Cape Town (South Africa)'87; MD; Staff, Creston Valley Hospital & Health Centre; Staff, Mills Memorial Hospital; (250)631-2598; Fax. (250)638-4092.

BLACKBURN, David; Clinique Opti-Soins, 550-2655 boul du Royaume, Jonquiere QC G7S 4S9; Laval'94; Staff, Hôpital Laval; (418)548-7525; Fax. (418)548-7721.

BLACKBURN, Frederic; Clinique Urologie Saguenay, RC001-475 boul Talbot, Chicoutimi QC G7H 4A3; Laval'99; FRCSC; Urol. Staff, Complexe hospitalier de la Sagamie; (418)543-3003

BLACKBURN, Graham A; Port McNeill Med Clinic, PO Box 14, Port McNeill BC V0N 2R0; UBC'06; CCFP; (250)956-3377

BLACKBURN, Jean-Frederic; CSSS de Chicoutimi, 305 rue Saint-Vallier, Chicoutimi QC G7H 5H6; Laval'97; CSPQ; FRCPC; Anes. Staff, Complexe hospitalier de la Sagamie; (418)541-1000

BLACKBURN, Karl; Centre Hosp Honore-Mercier, 2750 boul Laframboise, Saint-Hyacinthe QC J2S 4Y8; Laval'92; CSPQ; FRCPC; IntMed; Cardiol. Staff, Centre Hospitalier Honore-Mercier; (450)771-3333

BLACKBURN, Line; CSSS de Quebec-Sud, 900 boul Wilfrid-Hamel, Quebec QC G1M 2R9; Laval'85; FSOGC; FACOG; FRCSC; ObstGyn. Staff, Centre Hospitalier Universitaire de Quebec-CHUL; Staff, CSSS de Quebec-Sud; (418)529-0291; Fax. (418)529-7405.

BLACKBURN, Manon; Hop Charles Lemoyne, 3120 boul Taschereau, Greenfield Park QC J4V 2H1; Sher'91; FRCPC; CommunMed. Staff, Hopital Charles LeMoyne; (450)928-6777

BLACKBURN, Michel; Polyclinique, 201-874 boul de l'Universite E, Chicoutimi QC G7H 6B9; Laval'70; GenSurg. Staff, Complexe hospitalier de la Sagamie; (418)545-3611

BLACKBURN, Regine; Clinique Med Fleur de Lys, 8 rue du Terminus E, Rouyn-Noranda QC J9X 3B4; Laval'83; Dir-svcs prof, Centre Hospitalier La Sarre; Staff, Centre Hospitalier Rouyn-Noranda; (819)764-6185; Fax. (819)762-6079.

BLACKBURN, Robert; Ctr Hosp Affilie-Enfant-Jesus, 1401 18e rue, Quebec QC G1J 1Z4; Laval'96; FRCPC; IntMed. Staff, Centre Hospitalier Affilié Universitaire de Québec - Hôpital De L'Enfant Jésus; (418)649-0252

BLACKBURN, Robert Y; Clinique Med du Manoir, 1441 av du Manoir, Alma QC G8B 4X3; Laval'74; Staff, CSSS de Lac-Saint Jean-Est; Dir méd, Alcan; (418)662-3944; Fax. (418)662-2607; robert.blackburn@cgocable.ca.

BLACKBURN, Steve; Hôpital Laval, 2725 ch Sainte-Foy, Quebec QC G1V 4G5; Laval'96; CSPQ; FRCPC; Anes; Critical Care Medicine (P.Q.). Staff, Hôpital Laval; (418)656-8711

BLACKBURN MAILLOUX, Geneviève; 4100 boul Lasalle, Verdun QC H4G 2A3; Mon'06; CCFP; Staff, Centre Hospitalier de Verdun; (514)362-1000

BLACKIE, Barbara J; IWK Health Centre, PO Box 9700 Rpo CSC, Halifax NS B3K 6R8; Mem'98; FRCPC; Peds. Staff, IWK Health Centre; (902)470-8798

BLACKIE, Peter B; Gander Med Bldg, 177 Elizabeth Dr, Gander NL A1V 1X1; Dal'66; CHE; CCFP; FCFP; Physician, Canadian Forces Base-Greenwood; Physician, Civil Aviation Canada; (709)256-7101 x227; Fax. (709)256-7109; pbblackie@warp.nfld.net.

BLACKIE, Stephen P; Royal City Med Bldg, 103-250 Keary St, New Westminster BC V3L 5E7; Wes'80; FRCPC; IntMed; Respir. Ac Staff RespMed, Royal Columbian Hospital; Court Staff RespMed, St Mary's Hospital; (604)525-8822; Fax. (604)525-9470.

BLACKLOCK, Donald M; 202-1350 England Ave, Courtenay BC V9N 8X6; Wes'75; (250)334-4411; Fax. (250)338-1245.

BLACKLOCK, Elaine G; 1485 Bancroft Dr, Sudbury ON P3B 1R6; Wes'83; FRCPC; Peds. Staff Peds, Health Sciences North-Laurentian Site; (705)523-7120

BLACKMAN, Adam S; Northern Alberta Sleep Clinic, 30-8702 Meadowlark Rd NW, Edmonton AB T5R 5W5; Tor'92; FRCPC; Psy (Sleep Disorders Medicine). (780)487-5333; Fax. (780)487-3045; info@torontosleep.com.

BLACKMAN, Douglas H; College of Phys & Surg of BC, 300-669 Howe St, Vancouver BC V6C 0B4; UBC'69; CCFP; Dep Registrar, College of Physicians & Surgeons of British Columbia; (604)733-7758; Fax. (604)733-3503.

BLACKMAN, Eric R; Wound Care Clinic, 5-277 Welland Ave, St Catharines ON L2R 2P7; Ott'69; FAADEP(USA); FRCSC; OrthSurg (Musculoskeletal Injury). Assessor, West Park Healthcare Centre; Staff Pt-Time, Niagara Health System - Ontario Street Site; Staff Pt-Time, Niagara Health System - St Catharines General Site; Consultant Pt-Time, Hôtel Dieu Shaver Health & Rehabilitation Centre; Physician Pt-Time, Hamilton Assessment Centre; Staff Pt-Time, Niagara Rehabilitation Centre; (905)684-1588; Fax. (905)682-3610; blackman@vaxxine.com.

BLACKMAN, Lee T; Mount St Joseph Hosp, 3080 Prince Edward St, Vancouver BC V5T 3N4; UBC'76; FRCPC; Anes. Staff, Providence Health Care - Mount Saint Joseph Hospital; (604)874-1141; Fax. (604)872-4683.

BLACKMAN, Maurice; 10024 116 St NW, Edmonton AB T5K 1V6; Trinity Coll. (Ireland)'67; MB ChB; DPM; MRCPsy; FRCPC; Psy (Child Psychiatry). Ac Staff Child Psy, Royal Alexandra Hospital; Consultant Psy, Alberta Bosco Homes; Clin Prof, University of Alberta; (780)488-3737; Fax. (780)488-3755.

BLACKMER, Jeffrey E; The Ottawa Hosp-Rehab Ctr, 505 Smyth Rd, Ottawa ON K1H 8M2; Wes'95; BSc; FRCPC; PhysMed&Rehab (Spinal Cord Injury). Med Dir Neurospinal Serv & Clin Ethicist/Staff Physical Med & Rehab, The Ottawa Hospital Rehabilitation Centre; Asst Prof, University of Ottawa; (613)737-7350 x75598; Fax. (613)737-9638; jblackmer@ottawahospital.on.ca.

BLACKMORE, Elizabeth J; Quinte HC Corp-Trenton Mem, PO Box 1600 Stn Main 242 King St, Trenton ON K8V 5S6; McM'07; Staff, QHC Trenton Memorial; (613)392-2540

BLACKMORE, Michael G; Carlton & Church Med Clinic, 60 Carlton St, Toronto ON M5B 1L1; Mem'88; FRCPC; IntMed; Rheum. Affil Staff, Sunnybrook Health Sciences Centre; (416)646-1890; Fax. (416)646-1892.

BLACKMORE, Richard G; 101-20728 Fraser Hwy, Langley BC V3A 4G6; Qns'82; Dip SportMed; Staff, Langley Memorial Hospital; Physician, National Ski Team; (604)534-6838; rgblackmore@uniserve.com.

BLACKSHAW, Patricia M P; 410-15355 24th Ave, Surrey BC V4A 2H9; Wes'70; BA; CCFP; (604)531-4131

BLACKSHAW, Stella L; Royal University Hosp, 103 Hospital Dr, Saskatoon SK S7N 0W8; Man'77; LMCC; FRCPC; Psy (Eating Disorders). Staff, Royal University Hospital; Prof, University of Saskatchewan; (306)966-8232; Fax. (306)966-8237.

BLACKSHAW, W Roy; 410-15355 24th Ave, Surrey BC V4A 2H9; Wes'70; CCFP.

BLACKSTEIN, Martin; Mount Sinai Hosp, 1222-600 University Ave, Toronto ON M5G 1X5; Tor'65; PhD; FRCPC; IntMed. Staff, Mount Sinai Hospital; (416)586-4800 x5371

BLACKWELL, Margaret M; Royal City Med Bldg, 204-250 Keary St, New Westminster BC V3L 5E7; UBC'87; BSc(Microbiol); FRCPC; IntMed; Cardiol. Staff Cardiol, Royal Columbian Hospital; (604)515-2912; Fax. (604)515-2914.

BLACKWELL, Thomas E R; Dr T Blackwell Med Prof Corp, 807-201 21st St E, Saskatoon SK S7K 0B8; Sask'71; FRCSC; Ophth. Staff, St Paul's Hospital (Grey Nuns) of Saskatoon; Staff, Saskatoon City Hospital; University of Saskatchewan; (306)244-6149; Fax. (306)244-8941; tblackwell@sasktel.net.

BLACKWOOD, C Matthew; Cedar Cove Med Clinic, 104-32423 Lougheed Hwy, Mission BC V2V 7B8; UBC'73; CCFP; FCFP; Staff, Mission Memorial Hospital; (604)826-1348; Fax. (604)820-7726; pmblackwood@shaw.ca.

BLACKWOOD, Jaime S; Alberta Children's Hosp, 2888 Shaganappi Trail NW, Calgary AB T3B 6A8; Wes'03; FRCPC; Peds; Critical Care Medicine. Staff Pediatric Intensivist, Alberta Children's Hospital; (403)955-7931; Fax. (403)955-7081.

BLACKWOOD, Peter J; Central Health Consultants, 129 Lincoln Rd, Grnd-Falls-Windsor NL A2A 1P3; Mem'85; FRCSC; GenSurg. Staff, Central Newfoundland Regional Health Centre; (709)489-2700

BLACQUIERE, Dylan P V; The Ottawa Hosp-Civic Campus, 1053 Carling Ave, Ottawa ON K1Y 4E9; Dal'07; FRCPC; Neur. Staff, The Ottawa Hospital - Civic Campus; (613)761-5353

BLADOU, Franck; SMBD Jewish Gen Hosp, 3755 ch Cote-Sainte-Catherine, Montreal QC H3T 1E2; Aix-Marseille II (France)'90; Staff, Sir Mortimer B Davis Jewish General; (514)340-8222

BLAGDON, Michelle; Centre Med Lariviere, 423 av Lariviere, Rouyn-Noranda QC J9X 4H9; Laval'89; (819)762-4004; Fax. (819)762-4204.

BLAHEY, Walter B; Bridgeland Med Bldg, 204-803A 1 Ave NE, Calgary AB T2E 7C5; Sask'73; FRCPC; IntMed; Hem. Teach Staff, University of Calgary; (403)266-1246

BLAICHMAN, Shirley; 300-4269 rue Sainte-Catherine, Westmount QC H3Z 1P7; McG'76; FRCPC; Peds. hon Staff, McGill University Health Centre - Montreal Children's Hospital; adj Prof, McGill University; Langs: Bilingual(English/French); (514)931-7430; Fax. (514)931-0363; sblaichman@qc.aibn.com.

BLAIKIE, Peter G; PO Box 245, Pugwash NS B0K 1L0; Dal'92; (902)243-2521; Fax. (902)243-2897.

BLAIN, Allison M; Hamilton HS-General Site, 237 Barton St E, Hamilton ON L8L 2X2; McM'02; FRCPC; Anes. Staff, Hamilton Health Sciences Centre - Hamilton General Hospital; (905)521-2100

BLAIN, Julie; CSSS du Sud de Lanaudière, 911 montée des Pionniers, Terrebonne QC J6V 2H2; Laval'99; FRCPC; IntMed; Gastroent. Staff, Centre Hospitalier Pierre le Gardeur; (450)654-7525

BLAIN, Marie; Centre d'Urgence St-Laurent, 200-1605 boul Marcel-Laurin, Saint-Laurent QC H4R 0B7; Mon'77; (514)747-2555; Fax. (514)747-7624.

BLAIN, Marie-Helene; CSSS du Nord de Lanaudière, 1000 boul Sainte-Anne, St-Charles-Brromee QC J6E 6J2; Sher'94; CSPQ; Cardiol; IntMed (Echocardiography). Staff, Centre Hospitalier Régional de Lanaudière; (450)759-8222 x2892

BLAIN, Marie-Yanouk; CSSS de la Cote-de-Gaspe, 215 boul de York O, Gaspe QC G4X 2W2; Mon'00; FRCSC; ObstGyn (Urogynecology). Staff, Centre Hospitalier de Gaspe; Langs: Bilingual(French/English); (418)368-3301

BLAIN, Robert; Institut de Cardiologie de Mtl, 5000 rue Belanger, Montreal QC H1T 1C8; Mon'71; FRCPC; Anes. Staff Anes, Institut de Cardiologie de Montréal; (514)376-3330 x3732; Fax. (514)376-8784; blainr@videotron.ca.

BLAIN, Samuel; Ctr Hosp du Centre la Mauricie, 50 119e rue, Shawinigan-Sud QC G9P 5K1; Mon'07; CCFP; Family Med, Centre Hospitalier du Centre la Mauricie; (819)536-7500

BLAIN, Stephanie; Clinique Med Pierre-Boucher, 1615 boul Jacques-Cartier E, Longueuil QC J4M 2X1; Mon'00; (450)468-6223

BLAIN PARE, Etienne; CSSS de la Haute-Yamaska, 205 boul Leclerc O, Granby QC J2G 1T7; McG'06; MDCM; DiagRad. Staff, Centre Hospitalier de Granby; (450)375-8000

BLAINE, Donald D P; 215 Van Buren St PO Box 928, Kemptville ON K0G 1J0; Wes'69; Ac Staff, Kemptville District Hospital; (613)258-2486; Fax. (613)258-4183.

BLAINE, Kirsten Ann; The Jenny Trout Centre, 113-342 Erie St, Stratford ON N5A 2N4; Tor'92; FRCPC; Peds. Ac Staff, Stratford General Hospital - Huron Perth Healthcare Alliance; Assoc Staff, Listowel Memorial Hospital - Listowel Wingham Hospitals Alliance; Staff, The Jenny Trout Centre; (519)272-2040; Fax. (519)272-2323.

BLAINE, Sean; STAR Family Health Team, RR 5 Stn Main 700 O'Loane Ave, Stratford ON N5A 6S6; Tor'91; CCFP; CCFP(E.M.); Ac Staff, Stratford General Hospital - Huron Perth Healthcare Alliance; Associate, Mount Sinai Hospital; Asst Prof Family & Commun Med, University of Toronto; (519)273-1060; Fax. (519)273-0371; blaines@sympatico.ca.

BLAINE, William C; Ottawa Valley Family Health, 95 Spring St, Almonte ON K0A 1A0; (Australia)'07; CCFP; (613)256-9370; Fax. (613)256-0949.

BLAIR, Cynthia; D-170 Rebecca St, Oakville ON L6K 1J6; Wes'82; CCFP; Ac Staff, Halton Healthcare Services Corporation - Oakville Site; (905)842-2174; Fax. (905)842-8071; cynthialynblair@hotmail.com.

BLAIR, David J; 3825 Cadboro Bay Rd PO Box 55047, Victoria BC V8N 6L8; Sask'71; CCFP; FCFP; Staff, Vancouver Island Health Authority; (250)595-6401

BLAIR, Donald C; The Ottawa Hosp-Riverside, 1967 Riverside Dr, Ottawa ON K1H 7W9; Ott'69; FRCPC; DiagRad. Staff Diag Imaging, The Ottawa Hospital - Riverside Campus; (613)738-8400 x82260; Fax. (613)738-8538.

BLAIR, Duane; Clinique Millenia-Santei, 295-2600 boul Laurier, Quebec QC G1V 4T3; Laval'72; GenSurg. Staff, Centre Hospitalier Affilié Universitaire de Québec - Hôpital du St-Sacrement; (418)781-0480

BLAIR, Geoffrey K; Children's & Women's HC of BC, K0 106-4480 Oak St, Vancouver BC V6H 3V4; Tor'77; FRCSC; GenSurg; PedGenSurg. Gen Surgery, BC Children's Hospital; Clin Prof Surg, University of British Columbia; (604)875-2706; Fax. (604)875-2721; gblair@cw.bc.ca.

BLAIR, Jason D; 29 rue Ducharme, Gatineau QC J8Y 3P7; Qns'04; FRCSC; Ophth. (819)770-3663

BLAIR, Jean-Francois; CHUM-Hotel-Dieu, 3840 rue Saint-Urbain, Montreal QC H2W 1T8; Mon'83; FRCSC; GenSurg; VascSurg. Staff, Centre Hospitalier l'Université de Montréal (CHUM) - Hôtel-Dieu; Staff, Centre Hospitalier l'Université de Montréal (CHUM) - Hôpital Notre-Dame; (514)890-8000 x14955

BLAIR, Kenneth; 1854 Southview Dr SE, Medicine Hat AB T1A 8L9; Cal'73; DABR; FRCPC; DiagRad. Staff, Medicine Hat Regional Hospital; (403)527-7334; Fax. (403)528-7317.

BLAIR, Louis; CHUM-Hosp Notre-Dame, 1560 rue Sherbrooke E, Montreal QC H2L 4M1; Mon'87; FRCPC; IntMed; Critical Care Medicine (P.Q.). Staff, Centre Hospitalier l'Université de Montréal (CHUM) - Hôpital Notre-Dame; (514)890-8000 x24444

BLAIR, Mary-Louise; Greenbank Med Centre, 202-139 Greenbank Rd, Nepean ON K2H 9A5; Ott'79; CCFP; Staff, Queensway Carleton Hospital; Physician, Participation House; (613)820-7202; Fax. (613)820-5985.

BLAIR, N Peter; Keary Med Centre, 210-245 Columbia St E, New Westminster BC V3L 3W4; Qns'75; FRCS(Ed); FACS; FRCSC; GenSurg (Breasts). Staff Surg, Royal Columbian Hospital; Staff, Eagle Ridge Hospital & Health Care Centre; Clin Prof Surg, University of British Columbia; (604)522-7737; Fax. (604)522-1571.

BLAIR, R D Gordon; The Credit Valley Hosp, 2200 Eglinton Ave W, Mississauga ON L5M 2N1; Dal'65; FRCPC; Neur (Clinical Neurophysiology). Staff, The Credit Valley Hospital; (905)813-4545; Fax. (905)813-4046; gblair@cvh.on.ca.

BLAIR, Tony; CSSS de Rivière-de-Loup, 75 rue Saint-Henri, Riviere-du-Loup QC G5R 2A4; Laval'74; FRCSC; ObstGyn. Staff, Centre Hospitalier Regional du Grand-Portage; (418)868-1010; Fax. (418)868-1035; antoineb@cgocable.ca.

BLAIR, W Hunter; Community Health Centre, PO Box 99 3322 Highway 3, Barrington Passage NS B0W 1G0; Glasgow (Scotland)'63; MB ChB; (902)637-2705; Fax. (902)637-3639.

BLAIS, Andre; CSSS de Rimouski-Neigette, CP 3150 Succ A 150 av Rouleau, Rimouski QC G5L 5T1; Laval'88; FRCPC; IntMed (Hematological Oncology); MedOncol (P.Q.); Hem. Hematologist, Hôpital Regional Rimouski; Langs: English; (418)723-7851

BLAIS, Annie; CSSS du Haut Saint-Maurice, 889 boul Ducharme, La Tuque QC G9X 3C1; Sher'08; Staff, Centre Hospitalier Saint-Joseph de la Turque; (819)523-4581; Fax. (819)523-7992; annie_blais@ssss.gouv.qc.ca.

BLAIS, Bernard; Clinique Med Pasteur, 770 av 1Re, Quebec QC G1L 3K2; Laval'76; Ac Staff, Centre Hospitalier Affilié Universitaire de Québec - Hôpital De L'Enfant Jésus; Assoc Staff, Centre Hospitalier Universitaire De Québec - Pavillon De St-françois-d'assise; Langs: English; (418)529-0042; Fax. (418)529-4924.

BLAIS, Bruno; CSSS du Lac-des-Deux-Montagnes, 520 boul Arthur-Sauve, St-Eustache QC J7R 5B1; Mon'88; Ac Staff, Hôpital de Saint-Eustache; (450)473-6811

BLAIS, Catherine; CSSS Bordeaux-Cartierville-St-, 555 boul Gouin O, Montreal QC H3L 1K5; Laval'99; Staff, Pavillon Notre-Dame de la Merci; (514)331-3020 x1726

BLAIS, Chantal; Clinique Medicale du Village, 200-400 rue Meigs, Farnham QC J2N 2C8; Sher'84; Langs: Bilingual(French/English); (450)293-3681; Fax. (450)293-7463.

BLAIS, Christian; CHUS-Hop Hotel-Dieu, 580 rue Bowen S, Sherbrooke QC J1G 2E8; Sher'78; FRCPC; DiagRad (Echography). Staff, Centre Hospitalier Universitaire de Sherbrooke-Hôpital Hôtel-Dieu; Assoc Prof Rad, Universite de Sherbrooke; (819)346-1110 x14962; christian.blais@usherbrooke.ca.

BLAIS, Claude-Francois; 170 av de l'Eglise, Dolbeau-Mistassini QC G8L 4W6; Laval'83; Staff, Centre Maria-Chapdelaine - CH de Dolbeau-Mistassini; (418)276-7857; Fax. (418)276-2609.

BLAIS, Claudia T; CSSS de la Haute-Gaspésie, 50 rue du Belvedere, Ste-Anne-des-Monts QC G4V 1X4; Mon'10; Staff, Centre Hospitalier des Monts; (418)763-2261

BLAIS, Conrad; Montfort Hosp, 713 Montreal Rd, Ottawa ON K1K 0T2; Laval'71; DAB; CSPQ; FRCPC; Anes (Anesthesia & Reanimation). Ac Staff, Montfort Hospital; (613)746-4621 x2620; Fax. (613)748-4914.

BLAIS, Danielle; Centre de Sante Integrale, 1-160 rue Pope RR 5, Cookshire-Eaton QC J0B 1M0; Sher'73; (819)875-5535; Fax. (819)875-3631.

BLAIS, Eric; CSSS de la Baie-des-Chaleurs, RR 2 419 boul Perron, Maria QC G0C 1Y0; Laval'93; Staff, CSSS de la Baie-des-Chaleurs; (418)759-3443

BLAIS, Francine; CSSSG-Hop De Gatineau, CP 2000 Succ Bureau-Chef 909 boul de la Verendrye O, Gatineau QC J8P 7H2; Sher'78; FRCSC; ObstGyn. Staff, Hôpital de Gatineau; Langs: English; (819)776-3732; Fax. (819)776-3732.

BLAIS, Gregoire; CSSS de la Haute-Yamaska, 205 boul Leclerc O, Granby QC J2G 1T7; Mon'88; NuclearMed (P.Q.). Staff Nuclear Med, Centre Hospitalier Regional du Grand-Portage; Nuclearr Med, CH du Centre-de-la-Mauricie (Ste-Thérèse de Shawinigan); Staff, Centre Hospitalier du Centre la Mauricie; Staff, Centre Hospitalier de Granby; (450)375-8000 x2347; gregoire_blais@ssss.gouv.qc.ca.

BLAIS, Guy R; Ottewell Med Clinic, 6138 90 Ave NW, Edmonton AB T6B 0P2; Alb'81; BMedSci; CCFP; FCFP; Court Staff Privil, University of Alberta Hospital; Ac Staff Family Med, Covenant Health - Grey Nuns Community Hospital; Clin Prof FamMed, University of Alberta; Langs: French; (780)469-5533; Fax. (780)469-1261.

BLAIS, Helene-Gabrielle; Regie des Rentes du Quebec, 348-2600 boul Laurier, Quebec QC G1V 4W1; Laval'79; Ac Staff, Hôtel-Dieu de Lévis.

BLAIS, Isabelle; Ctr Hosp Pierre-Janet, 20 rue Pharand, Gatineau QC J9A 1K7; Ott'05; FRCPC; Psy. Staff, Centre Hospitalier Pierre-Janet; (819)771-7761

BLAIS, Jacques; Clinique Med Sainte-Dorothee, 102-1 boul Samson, Laval QC H7X 3S5; Mon'82; Staff, Hôpital du Sacre-Coeur de Montréal; (450)689-6334; Fax. (450)689-6339.

BLAIS, Jacques; Clinique Med St-Gedeon, 188 2e Av S, St-Ged-De-Bce QC G0M 1T0; Laval'77; Ac Staff, Centre Hospitalier Beauce-Etchemin; (418)582-3317; Fax. (418)582-3318.

BLAIS, Jean-Philippe; CSSS de Trois-Rivieres, 1991 boul du Carmel, Trois-Rivieres QC G8Z 3R9; Sher'08; CCFP; Staff, CSSS de Trois-Rivières; (819)697-3333

BLAIS, Jocelyn; Hop Maisonneuve-Rosemont, 5415 boul de l'Assomption, Montreal QC H1T 2M4; Laval'75; FRCPC; DiagRad. Staff, Hopital Maisonneuve-Rosemont; (514)252-3535; Fax. (514)252-3537.

BLAIS, Jocelyne; Centre Med Iberville, 101-235 2e Av, St-Jean-Sur-Richel QC J2X 2B2; Mon'77; Staff, Hôpital du Haut-Richelieu; (450)347-5548; Fax. (450)347-4091.

BLAIS, Johanne; CHUQ-St-Francois d'Assise, 10 rue de l'Espinay, Quebec QC G1L 3L5; Laval'89; CCFP; FCFP; Staff Family Med, Centre Hospitalier Universitaire De Québec - Pavillon De St-françois-d'assise; Clin Prof Family Med, Université Laval; Langs: English; (418)525-4425; Fax. (418)525-4322.

BLAIS, Manon; CLSC-CHSLD Pat Montreal Est, 13926 rue Notre-Dame E, Pte-aux-Trembles QC H1A 1T5; Mon'78; (514)642-4050; Fax. (514)498-7505.

BLAIS, Marianne; Centre médicale Centrale, 4-135 rue Saint-Antoine N, Granby QC J2G 5G7; Sher'06; (450)372-5401

BLAIS, Mark R; First Edmonton Place, 585-10665 Jasper Ave NW, Edmonton AB T5J 3S9; Alb'83; (780)413-7568

BLAIS, Normand; CHUM-Hop Notre-Dame, 1560 rue Sherbrooke E, Montreal QC H2L 4M1; Sher'90; FRCPC; IntMed; MedOncol; Hem. Staff, Centre Hospitalier l'Université de Montréal (CHUM) - Hôpital Notre-Dame; Langs: Bilingual(English/French); (514)890-8000 x24634; normand.blais@geoq.com.

BLAIS, P Clifford; Medicentre Lasalle, 304-1500 av Dollard, LaSalle QC H8N 1T5; McG'81; ACLS; ATLS; Staff, Centre Hospitalier Pierre Boucher; Staff, Hopital Charles LeMoyne; (514)368-7788; Fax. (514)369-0649.

BLAIS, Philippe; Clinique Med Pelletier, 300-8330 boul Taschereau, Brossard QC J4X 1C2; Mon'89; Physician, CLSC Kateri; Langs: English; (450)465-5379; Fax. (450)465-5615.

BLAIS, Rene; Centre Antipoison du Quebec, 4F-1270 ch Sainte-Foy, Quebec QC G1S 2M4; Laval'71; DABMT; FRCPC; EmergMed (Toxicology). Dir méd, Quebec Poison Control Centre; Prof, Université Laval; Langs: Bilingual(French/English); (418)654-2731 x2233; Fax. (418)654-2747.

BLAIS, Robert J D; Omni Clinique de l'Outaouais, 202-28 boul du Mont-Bleu, Gatineau QC J8Z 1J1; Ott'86; CCFP; FCFP; Langs: French; (819)777-2111; Fax. (819)771-6890.

BLAIS, Robert; Polyclinique Ile-des-Soeurs, 2010 boul Rene-Levesque, Verdun QC H3E 2A4; Laval'82; Staff, CSSS de la Basse Côté-Nord; (514)767-2683

BLAIS, Sophie; Clinique Medicale Mascouche, 100-1025 Montee Masson, Mascouche QC J7K 2L9; Mon'93; CCFP; Staff, Hopital de la Cite de la santé; (450)474-6000; Fax. (450)474-6666.

BLAIS-BOILARD, Stephanie; Centre de Sante Cookshire, RR 5 160 rue Pope, Cookshire-Eaton QC J0B 1M0; Sher'04; CCFP; CCFP(E.M.); Staff, Centre Hospitalier Universitaire de Sherbrooke-Hôpital Hôtel-Dieu; Médecin, Centre de Sante Integrale; Langs: Spanish; English; (819)875-5535

BLAIS-MORIN, Catherine; CSSS de la Cote-de-Gaspe, 215 boul de York O, Gaspe QC G4X 2W2; Sher'00; CCFP; Staff, Centre Hospitalier de Gaspe; (418)368-6663; Fax. (418)368-5358.

BLAIS-MORIN, Pascale; CSSS de Rimouski-Neigette, CP 3150 Succ A, Rimouski QC G5L 5T1; Sher'99; LMCC; Staff, Hôpital Regional Rimouski; (418)723-7851

BLAISE, Fritz; Polyclinique Cabrini, 215-5700 rue Saint-Zotique E, Montreal QC H1T 3Y7; Port-au-Prince (Haiti)'60; Peds (P.Q.). Staff, Centre de Réadaptation Marie Enfant du CHU Sainte-Justine; Consultant, Hôpital Ste-Justine; Staff Peds, Hopital Maisonneuve-Rosemont; (514)256-1700; Fax. (514)256-1700.

BLAISE, Gilbert A; CHUM-Hop Notre-Dame, FS1136-1560 rue Sherbrooke E, Montreal QC H2L 4M1; Liege (Belgium)'72; CSPQ; FRCPC; Anes. Staff, Centre Hospitalier l'Université de Montréal (CHUM) - Hôpital Notre-Dame; (514)890-8202

BLAIZEL JR., Gilbert; 94 rue Blainville O, Sainte-Therese QC J7E 1X7; Mon'68; Staff, Hôpital de Saint-Eustache; (450)435-2843

BLAJCHMAN, Morris A; McMaster University, HSC 4N67-1280 Main St W, Hamilton ON L8S 4K1; McG'64; FRCP; BSc; MD; FRCPC; IntMed; Hem (Transfusion Medicine). Affil Staff LabMed & Med, St Joseph's Healthcare - Charlton Campus; Med Dir, Centres of Canadian Blood Services Southern Ontario; Prof Med, McMaster University; (905)525-9140 x26276; Fax. (905)527-4866; blajchma@mcmaster.ca.

BLAKE, Elizabeth K; 410 Lock St W, Dunnville ON N1A 1V6; Qns'97; CCFP; (905)701-6643; Fax. (905)701-6645.

BLAKE, Erin A; Royal Columbian Hosp, 330 Columbia St E, New Westminster BC V3L 3W7; UBC'06; FRCPC; IntMed. Staff, Royal Columbian Hospital; (604)520-4253

BLAKE, Geoffrey P; MUHC-Montreal Gen Hosp, A7 117-1650 av Cedar, Montreal QC H3G 1A4; Ott'73; ABIM; FRCPC; IntMed (Laboratory Hematology); Hem. Sr Staff Hem, McGill University Health Centre - Montreal General Campus; Asst Prof MedOncol, McGill University; (514)934-1934 x42428; blakeg@videotron.ca.

BLAKE, Kim; IWK Health Centre, PO Box 9700 Rpo CSC, Halifax NS B3K 6R8; London (England)'83; MB BS; MRC; Peds (Child Protection). Staff Gen Peds/Prof Peds, IWK Health Centre; Teach Staff, Dalhousie University; (902)470-6499; kblake@dal.ca.

BLAKE, McKenzie M; Huronia Med Centre, 200-240 Penetanguishene Rd, Midland ON L4R 4P4; Ott'09; CCFP; (705)526-9119; Fax. (705)526-0239.

BLAKE, Patrick A; 200-1500 Bank St, Ottawa ON K1H 7Z2; National (Ireland)'83; Staff, The Ottawa Hospital - General Campus; (613)738-7660; Fax. (613)738-8614.

BLAKE, Peter; London HSC-Victoria Hosp, 800 Commissioners Rd E, London ON N6A 5W9; National (Ireland)'80; FRCPI(Ire); BSc; MSc(Immunol.); FRCPC; IntMed; Nephrol. Dir Peritoneal Dialysis, London Health Sciences Centre - Victoria Campus; Prof, University of Western Ontario; (519)685-8326; Fax. (519)685-8395; peter.blake@lhsc.on.ca.

BLAKE, Theodore; Royal Columbian Hosp, 330 Columbia St E, New Westminster BC V3L 3W7; UBC'06; FRCPC; DiagRad. Staff, Royal Columbian Hospital; (604)520-4253

BLAKELEY, Ellen D; Deer Lodge Centre Inc, 2109 Portage Ave, Winnipeg MB R3J 0L3; Cal'77; FRCPC; IntMed. Staff, WRHA - Deer Lodge Centre; (204)837-1301

BLAKELY, John A; Mackenzie Richmond Hill Hosp, 10 Trench St, Richmond Hill ON L4C 4Z3; Sask'58; FRCPC; IntMed (Thrombosis). Consultant, Mackenzie Richmond Hill Hospital; Hon Staff Cardiol, Sunnybrook Health Sciences Centre; (905)883-1212; Fax. (905)883-2293; john.blakely@sunnybrook.ca.

BLAKELY, Reta M; 18-3625 Shaganappi Trail PO Box 84038 Rpo Market Mall, Calgary AB T3A 5C4; Cal'07; CCFP; (403)606-2220

BLAKENEY, Jill; Parkdale Comm Health Centre, 1229 Queen St W, Toronto ON M6K 1L2; Tor'88; PhD(Cambridge); (416)537-2455; Fax. (416)537-3526; jill.blakeney@pchc.on.ca.

BLAKER, Jessica; Klondyke Med Clinic, 1-3089 3rd Ave, Whitehorse YT Y1A 5B3; Cal'07; BSc; MSc; CCFP; Staff, Klondyke Medical Clinic; (867)668-4046; Fax. (867)668-4078.

BLAKLEY, Brian W; Health Sciences Centre, GB421-820 Sherbrook St, Winnipeg MB R3A 1R9; Sask'78; FRCSC; Otol. Staff, Health Sciences Centre; Prof, University of Manitoba; (204)787-5115; Fax. (204)787-1727.

BLAKLEY, Patricia M; Kinsmen Children's Centre, 1319 Colony St, Saskatoon SK S7N 2Z1; Sask'93; BSc; PhD; FAAP; FACMG; FCCMG; FRCPC; Peds (Developmental Pediatrics). Staff Physician Peds, Royal University Hospital; Assoc Prof Peds/Div Head Developmental Peds, University of Saskatchewan; (306)655-1096; Fax. (306)655-1449; patricia.blakley@saskatoonhealthregion.ca.

BLAKSLEE, James M; 560 Albert St PO Box 790, Winchester ON K0C 2K0; Qns'86; FRCSC; GenSurg (Endoscopy). Staff, Kemptville District Hospital; Chief GenSurg, Winchester District Memorial Hospital; (613)774-1445; Fax. (613)774-1926.

BLAMPY, Janice; Children's Hosp, CK253-840 Sherbrook St, Winnipeg MB R3A 1S1; Man'90; BSc(Med); FRCPC; Peds (Child Psychiatry). Staff Children's Hosp, Health Sciences Centre.

BLANCHARD, Basil A; 9 rue des Ormes, Rogersville NB E4Y 1S6; Mem'87; BSc; BEd; Staff, Miramichi Regional Hospital; Langs: French; (506)775-2030; Fax. (506)775-2025.

BLANCHARD, Denis; Clin Med Asbestos, 605 boul Simoneau, Asbestos QC J1T 4G7; Sher'76; Staff, CSSS des Sources d'Asbestos; (819)879-7447; Fax. (819)879-7881.

BLANCHARD, Gilbert; 8224 rue St-Paul, Bas-Caraquet NB E1W 6E2; Ott'04; CCFP; (506)727-7549; Fax. (506)727-7320.

BLANCHARD, Jocelyn; CHUS-Hop Fleurimont, 3001 12e av N, Sherbrooke QC J1H 5N4; Sher'00; FRCSC; Neursurg. Staff, Centre Hospitalier Universitaire de Sherbrooke-Hopital Fleurimont; (819)346-1110

BLANCHARD, Julie; Clin de Sante Jacques-Cartier, 200-1815 rue King O, Sherbrooke QC J1J 2E3; Sher'05; CCFP; Médecin Palliative Care, Centre Hospitalier Universitaire de Sherbrooke-Hopital Fleurimont; Langs: Bilingual(French/English); (819)565-7446; Fax. (819)565-7780.

BLANCHARD, Marie-Eve; Professional Arts Bldg, 523-100 Arden St, Moncton NB E1C 4B7; Ott'05; CCFP; Staff, The Moncton Hospital; (506)857-5452; Fax. (506)857-5454.

BLANCHARD, Marie-Eve; Clinique Med Mascouche, 1025 montee Masson, Mascouche QC J7K 2L9; Mon'96; (450)474-6000; Fax. (450)474-6666.

BLANCHARD, Mark C; Parkland Med Clinic, 203-998 Parkland Dr, Halifax NS B3M 0A6; Dal'00; CCFP; (902)404-7737; Fax. (902)404-7066.

BLANCHARD, Matthew G; The Harrow H C Inc-Family Hlth, PO Box 430 1480 Erie Rd S, Harrow ON N0R 1G0; Dal'01; BSc; CCFP; (519)738-2000; blanchard_matthew@hotmail.com.

BLANCHARD, Pierre W; 932-1075 ch Sainte-Foy, Quebec QC G1S 2M1; Sher'78; ABPeds; CSPQ; LMCC; LRCPS; Peds (Neonatal & Perinatal Medicine). Consultant Physician, Ministry of Health & Social Services-Quebec; Langs: Bilingual(French/English); (418)266-6993

BLANCHARD, Pierre-Hugues; Clinique Med Warwick, 5A rue du Centre Sportif, Warwick QC J0A 1M0; Sher'05; (819)358-4600

BLANCHARD, Stephen F; 8-389 Main St, Picton ON K0K 2T0; Wes'86; CCFP; FCFP; Staff, QHC Prince Edward County Memorial; (613)476-8323; Fax. (613)476-8211.

BLANCHET, Caroline; CMF de Jonquiere, 3835 boul Harvey, Jonquiere QC G7X 2Z5; Sher'06; CCFP; (418)542-7510

BLANCHET, Catherine; Clinique Med de Lauzon, 213 rue Saint-Joseph, Levis QC G6V 1C8; Laval'09; CCFP; (418)833-5040

BLANCHET, Chantal; CHUS-Hop Hotel-Dieu, 580 rue Bowen S, Sherbrooke QC J1G 2E8; Mon'95; LMCC; Staff, Centre Hospitalier Universitaire de Sherbrooke-Hôpital Hôtel-Dieu; (819)346-1110

BLANCHET, Chantale N; CSSS du Sud de Lanaudière, 911 montee des Pionniers, Terrebonne QC J6V 2H2; Mon'95; FRCPC; Psy. Staff, Centre Hospitalier Pierre le Gardeur; (450)654-7525

BLANCHET, Florent; Clin Ortho du Haut-Richelieu, 320-900 boul Du Seminaire N, St-Jean-Sur-Richel QC J3A 1C3; Laval'68; FRCSC; OrthSurg. Ac Staff, Hôpital du Haut-Richelieu; (450)348-6966; Fax. (450)348-0664.

BLANCHET, Genevieve; The Ottawa Hosp-Gen Campus, 501 Smyth Rd, Ottawa ON K1H 8L6; Laval'07; ObstGyn. Staff, The Ottawa Hospital - General Campus; (613)798-5555

BLANCHET, Jacques; CHUQ-Ctr Hosp Univ Laval, 2705 boul Laurier, Quebec QC G1V 4G2; Laval'76; Peds. Staff, Centre Hospitalier Universitaire de Quebec-CHUL; (418)654-2282; Fax. (418)654-2771.

BLANCHET, Jean J; CHUQ-St-Francois D'assise, D1 714-10 rue de l'Espinay, Quebec QC G1L 3L5; Laval'60; ObstGyn (Gynecology). Ac Staff, Centre Hospitalier Universitaire De Québec - Pavillon De St-françois-d'assise; (418)522-8690; Fax. (418)525-4481.

BLANCHET, Luc; Child-Family Service, 7345 rue Garnier, Montreal QC H2E 2A1; Laval'67; Psy (Child Psychiatry). Chief Child & Family Serv, CSSS du Coeur de l'Isle Hôpital Jean-Talon; Consultant, Min. of Health-Public Health & Social Services, Gov't. of Quebec & Pres. of Mental Health Committee of Quebec; Langs: English; (514)729-3425 x7244; Fax. (514)495-6774.

BLANCHET, Michel; Polyclinique de la Capitale, 7-4225 av 4E O, Quebec QC G1H 6P3; Laval'66; OrthSurg (P.Q.). Ac Staff, Centre Hospitalier Universitaire De Québec - Pavillon De St-françois-d'assise; (418)623-9871; Fax. (418)623-9873.

BLANCHET, Pierre; CHUM-Hop Notre-Dame, 1560 rue Sherbrooke E, Montreal QC H2L 4M1; Mon'84; FRCPC; Neur; Electroenceph (P.Q.). Staff, Centre Hospitalier l'Université de Montréal (CHUM) - Hôpital Notre-Dame; Asst Prof Med & Dental, Universite de Montreal; (514)890-8000 x26452; Fax. (514)412-7139; pierre.j.blanchet@umontreal.ca.

BLANCHET, Pierre; Ctr Obstetrique-Gyn de la Cite, 4250 av 1Re, Quebec QC G1H 2S5; Laval'70; FRCSC; ObstGyn (Contraception). Member ObstGyn Service, Centre Hospitalier Paul-Gilbert; Clin Prof, Université Laval; Langs: Spanish; English; (418)654-0555; Fax. (418)654-1898.

BLANCHET, Raymond; CHUM-Hop Notre-Dame, 1560 rue Sherbrooke E, Montreal QC H2L 4M1; Mon'79; FRCPC; Psy. Staff, Hopital Louis-H Lafontaine; Staff, Centre Hospitalier l'Université de Montréal (CHUM) - Hôpital Notre-Dame; (514)890-8000 x25674

BLANCHET, Richard; CSSS de Rivière-de-Loup, 75 rue Saint-Henri, Riviere-Du-Loup QC G5R 2A4; Laval'76; FRCSC; GenSurg. Staff, Centre Hospitalier Regional du Grand-Portage; Langs: English; Spanish; (418)868-1000; Fax. (418)868-1032.

BLANCHET, Richard; Clinique Med Pierre-Bertrand, 212-303 boul Pierre-Bertrand, Quebec QC G1M 3L7; Laval'86; BSc; Langs: Bilingual(French/English); (418)683-2724; Fax. (418)683-8861; richard.blanchet@orlo.ulaval.ca.

BLANCHET, Sylvain; UMF Laval, 2690 ch des Quatre-Bourgeois, Quebec QC G1V 0B7; Laval'95; CCFP; Staff, Hôpital Laval; Langs: English; (418)656-4795

BLANCHETTE, Agathe; CSSSTR-Saint Joseph, 735 rue Sainte-Julie, Trois-Rivieres QC G9A 0B5; Sher'79; Staff Palliative Care, Centre de santé Cloutier-du-Rivage; (819)370-2200 x47400

BLANCHETTE, Christine; 714 boul Marcotte, Roberval QC G8H 1Z6; Laval'79; Peds (P.Q.). Staff, Hotel-Dieu de Roberval; Langs: English; (418)275-3833; Fax. (418)275-6747; christine.blanchette@sympatico.ca.

BLANCHETTE, Claudine; Hop Jean-Talon, 1385 rue Jean-Talon E, Montreal QC H2E 1S6; Mon'98; Staff, CSSS du Coeur de l'Isle Hôpital Jean-Talon; (514)495-6767; claudineblanchette@yahoo.com.

BLANCHETTE, Danielle; 760 rue Notre-Dame E, Victoriaville QC G6P 4B7; Sher'78; Assoc Staff Public Health, Hôpital Sainte-croix; (819)758-2424; Fax. (819)752-6955.

BLANCHETTE, David; Clin de Rehabilitation de l'Es, 320-5345 boul de l'Assomption, Montreal QC H1T 4B3; Sher'94; BSc; FRCSC; OrthSurg (Sports Medicine). Langs: Spanish; English; (514)254-6161; Fax. (514)254-1596.

BLANCHETTE, Donald E; Centre Pediatrique Laval, 300-1150 boul de l'Avenir, Laval QC H7N 6L2; Sher'70; Peds. Consultant, Hôpital Ste-Justine; Staff, Hôpital du Sacre-Coeur de Montréal; (450)686-0822; Fax. (450)686-2388.

BLANCHETTE, France; Clinique CAMU Longueuil, 100-1144 rue Saint-Laurent O, Longueuil QC J4K 1E2; Mon'82; Langs: English; (450)679-4333; Fax. (450)679-1672.

BLANCHETTE, Francois; Institut Prive de Chirurgie, 180-801 Grande-Allee O, Quebec QC G1S 1C1; Mon'86; FRCSC; Ophth. Langs: Bilingual(French/English); (418)687-7328

BLANCHETTE, Marie-Eve; CSSS de la Vallée de l'Or, 725 6e rue, Val-d'Or QC J9P 3Y1; Laval'99; Staff, Centre Hospitalier de Val d'Or; (819)825-6711

BLANCHETTE, Melanie; CSSS de la Matapedia, 135 av Gaetan-Archambault, Amqui QC G5J 2K5; Mon'05; Staff, CSSS de la Matapedia; (418)629-2211

BLANCHETTE, Michel-Henri; Clinique Med Giffard, 210-3333 rue du carrefour, Quebec QC G1C 5R9; Laval'79; FRCSC; OrthSurg. Ac Member, Centre Hospitalier Universitaire de Quebec-CHUL; (418)627-2868

BLANCHETTE, Nicholas S; The Credit Valley Hosp, 2200 Eglinton Ave W, Mississauga ON L5M 2N1; Tor'05; FRCPC; Peds; Rheum. Staff, The Credit Valley Hospital; (905)813-4120; Fax. (905)813-4128.

BLANCHETTE, Pierre J; CSSS de Trois-Rivieres, 1991 boul Du Carmel, Trois-Rivieres QC G8Z 3R9; Laval'74; MedOncol (P.Q.); Hem. Staff, CSSS de Trois-Rivières; Staff, Centre Hospitalier du Centre la Mauricie; Langs: English; (819)697-3333

BLANCHETTE, Suzanne; Centre Pediatrique de Laval, 300-1150 boul de l'Avenir, Laval QC H7N 6L2; Sher'72; Peds. Langs: English; (450)686-0822; Fax. (450)686-2388.

BLANCHETTE, Tania; Centre de Sante Valcartier, CP 1000 Bdp Succ Forces, Courcelette QC G0A 4Z0; Laval'97; FRCPC; Psy (Stress). Langs: English; (418)844-5000 x5802; Fax. (418)844-7606.

BLANCHETTE, Victor S; The Hosp For Sick Children, 555 University Ave, Toronto ON M5G 1X8; Cambridge (England)'70; DCH(Lond); MRC(Eng.); FRCPC; Peds; Hem. Staff Div of Hem, The Hospital For Sick Children; (416)813-5852; victor.blanchette@sickkids.ca.

BLANCO ALEMANY, Esther; The Hosp for Sick Children, 555 University Ave, Toronto ON M5G 1X8; Orihuela (Spain)'01; Staff, The Hospital For Sick Children; (416)813-7742; Fax. (416)813-5327.

BLANCQUAERT, Ingeborg; CHUS-Hop Fleurimont, 3001 12e av N, Sherbrooke QC J1H 5N4; Brussels (Belgium)'79; Staff, Centre Hospitalier Universitaire de Sherbrooke-Hopital Fleurimont; (819)346-1110 x14633

BLAND, Elaine; Family Health Clinic, 208-3625 Shaganappi Trail NW, Calgary AB T3A 0E2; Southampton (England)'91; MRCGPract; DRCOG; CCFP; Med Examiner Dept of Justice, Southwood Hospice; (403)286-9118; elaine.bland@albertahealthservices.ca.

BLAND, Jonathan D; Caledonian Med Clinic, 340 Campbell St, Nanaimo BC V9R 3G7; UBC'85; (250)753-3202; Fax. (250)753-1039.

BLAND, Roger C; University of Alberta Hosp, 1E7.07WCM-8440 112 St NW, Edmonton AB T6G 2B7; Liverpool (England)'60; MRCS; LRCP; DRCOG; FRCPsy; FRCPC; Psy. Ac Staff, University of Alberta Hospital; Ac Staff, Alberta Health Services; Emeritus Prof, University of Alberta; (780)407-6570; Fax. (780)407-6672.

BLANDO, German; 102-185 rue Acadie, Dieppe NB E1A 1G6; Cordoba (Argentina)'99; Staff, Dr Georges-L-Dumont University Hospital Centre; Langs: Spanish; French; Portuguese; (506)204-5910; Fax. (506)204-6102.

BLANE, Shale; 106-2955 Gladwin Rd, Abbotsford BC V2T 5T4; Tor'76; MCFP(EM); Staff Emerg Dept, Abbotsford Regional Hospital & Cancer Centre; (604)851-5677

BLANEY, Gregory P; 4419 10th Ave W, Vancouver BC V6R 2H8; Ott'74; (604)224-6583

BLANEY, Nancy C; Bear Street Family Physicians, PO Box 1048 Stn Main 302-220 Bear St, Banff AB T1L 1H6; Cal'86; CCFP; (403)762-4846; Fax. (403)762-2445.

BLANEY, Raynald; Ctr Hosp Rouyn-Noranda, 4 9e rue, Rouyn-Noranda QC J9X 2B2; Sher'84; CSPQ; FRCPC; Anes. Staff, Centre Hospitalier Rouyn-Noranda; (819)764-5131; Fax. (819)764-2900.

BLANK, Arthur K; Winnipeg Reg Health Authority, 102-1001 Corydon Ave, Winnipeg MB R3M 0B6; Man'74; Staff, Victoria General Hospital; Staff, Winnipeg Regional Health Authority; (204)940-2000

BLANK, David W; MUHC-Royal Victoria Hosp, C678-687 av des Pins O, Montreal QC H3A 1A1; McG'79; CSPQ; DABCC; FRCPC; MedBiochem (Lipidology). Dir Clinical Biochem, McGill University Health Centre - Royal Victoria Hospital; assoc Prof, McGill University; Langs: Bilingual(French/English); (514)934-1934 x35029; david.blank@muhc.mcgill.ca.

BLANK, Diana S; Univ Hlth Network-Toronto Western Hosp, 7F 410-399 Bathurst St, Toronto ON M5T 2S8; McM'06; FRCPC; Psy. Staff, Toronto Western Hospital - University Health Network; (416)603-5800; Fax. (416)603-5292.

BLANK, Myles K; BC Women's Hosp & Health Ctre, E6-4500 Oak St, Vancouver BC V6H 3N1; Man'84; FRCPC; Psy (Adult Psychiatry). Staff, BC Women's Hospital & Health Centre; Clinical Asst Prof, University of British Columbia; Langs: English; French; (604)875-2207

BLANKENSTEIN, Harvey; North York Family Health Team, 701-240 Duncan Mill Rd, North York ON M3B 3S6; Tor'87; CCFP; FCFP; Ac Staff, North York General Hospital; Consultant, The Hospital For Sick Children; Court Staff, Sunnybrook Health Sciences Centre; Langs: Hebrew; (416)229-6300; Fax. (416)229-6283.

BLANKIER, Joseph; Scarborough Prof Centre, 309-1371 Neilson Rd, Scarborough ON M1B 4Z8; Tor'73; BSc(Biol&MedSciences); FRCSC; ObstGyn (Ultrasound). Staff, Toronto General Hospital - UHN; Staff, Toronto Western Hospital - University Health Network; Consultant, MCTU Diagnostic Toronto; (416)287-1818

BLANKSTEIN, Kenneth C; 301-6351 197 St, Langley BC V2Y 1X8; Dal'87; BSc; DMD(Dental); Staff, Langley Memorial Hospital; University of British Columbia; (604)532-9686; Fax. (604)532-9687; jawrecon@telus.net.

BLANQUE MARTINEZ, Maria; CLSC Ahuntsic, 1165 boul Henri-Bourassa E, Montreal QC H2C 3K2; (Grenada)'82; Langs: Spanish; English; (514)381-4221 x8322; Fax. (514)389-1361.

BLAQUIERE, Martin; CHUM-Hop Notre-Dame, 1560 rue Sherbrooke E, Montreal QC H2L 4M1; Mon'94; FRCPC; IntMed; ClinImmunol&Allergy. Staff, Centre Hospitalier l'Université de Montréal (CHUM) - Hôpital Notre-Dame; (514)890-8231

BLAQUIERE, Martine; CSSS de l'Energie, 50 rue Toupin, Trois-Rivieres QC G8T 3Y5; Sher'87; Staff, Centre de santé Cloutier-du-Rivage; (819)370-2100

BLASER, Jill A; Westwinds Primary Health Ctre, 3311 Fairlight Dr, Saskatoon SK S7M 3Y5; UBC'07; CCFP; (306)655-4200; Fax. (306)655-4894.

BLASER, Susan I; The Hosp For Sick Children, 555 University Ave, Toronto ON M5G 1X8; Toledo(Ohio) (USA)'82; FRCPC; DiagRad. Staff, The Hospital For Sick Children; (416)813-6888; Fax. (416)813-8389; susan.blaser@sickkids.ca.

BLASHKO, Carl A; Cedars Prof Park, 2923 66 St NW, Edmonton AB T6K 4C1; Alb'65; FRCPC; Psy. Staff, Covenant Health - Grey Nuns Community Hospital; Aj Prof Fac of Education & Clin Prof, University of Alberta; (780)461-4794; cablashko@telus.net.

BLASHKO, Christopher D; Royal Jubilee Hosp, 1952 Bay St, Victoria BC V8R 1J8; Alb'95; FRCPC; Psy. Staff, Royal Jubilee Hospital; (250)370-8000

BLASKOVIC, Jana M; Regional Mental HC-St Thomas, PO Box 2004 Stn Main 467 Sunset Dr, St Thomas ON N5P 3V9; Prague (Czech Republic)'65; MD; Staff, Regional Mental Health Care-St Joseph's Health Care; Langs: Czech; (519)631-8510; Fax. (519)631-2512.

BLASS, Maria M; Student Health Centre, 242-401 Sunset Ave, Windsor ON N9B 3P4; Ott'79; Staff, Windsor Regional Hospital - Metropolitan Site; Counsellor Student Affairs Windsor Prog Schulich School of Med & Dent/Aj Prof Dept of Family Med Schulich School of Med & Dent, University of Western Ontario; Dir Student Health Serv, University Of Windsor; Langs: Hungarian; (519)973-7002; Fax. (519)971-3637; mblass@uwindsor.ca.

BLASTORAH, Bernard J; Alexander Prof Bldg, 214-849 Alexander Crt, Peterborough ON K9J 7H8; Ott'89; FRCSC; OrthSurg (Adult Reconstructive Surgery). Staff, Peterborough Regional Health Centre - Hospital Drive; (705)740-9690; Fax. (705)740-9689.

BLASZKOW-PORANEK, Barbara; Family Medicine Practice, 20-6960 Mumford Rd, Halifax NS B3L 4P1; Wroclaw (Poland)'73; Staff, Queen Elizabeth II Health Sciences Centre - Victoria General Site; Staff, IWK Health Centre; (902)453-5587; Fax. (902)453-3358.

BLATTEL, Ronald A; Appletree Med Centre, 1309 Carling Ave, Ottawa ON K1Z 7L3; Qns'75; CCFP; FCFP; (613)715-9419; Fax. (613)715-9278.

BLAU, Elaine M; McMaster Family Practice Unit, 690 Main St W, Hamilton ON L8S 1A4; Sask'91; CCFP; FCFP; Clinical Asst Prof Family Med, McMaster University; (905)521-5015; Fax. (905)521-5010.

BLAUER, Evan; 121-6363 rte Transcanadienne, Saint-Laurent QC H4T 1Z9; McG'06; MDCM; CCFP; CCFP(E.M.); (514)747-8888; Fax. (514)747-4705.

BLAXLAND, Joanne B; 4303 10th Ave W, Vancouver BC V6R 2H6; Dal'78; Ad Staff Privil, Vancouver General Hospital - Centennial Pavillion; (604)224-1355; Fax. (604)224-0179.

BLAYLOCK, John F; 102-2545 McCallum Rd, Abbotsford BC V2S 3R1; Ott'83; FRCSC; Ophth. Consultant, Abbotsford Regional Hospital & Cancer Centre; Consultant, Mission Memorial Hospital; (604)850-0808; Fax. (604)850-2849.

BLAYNEY, Marc P; Sudbury Reg Hosp-Laurentian, 41 Ramsey Lake Rd, Sudbury ON P3E 5J1; University Coll. (Ireland)'80; MB BCh; BAO; FRCPI; FRCPC; Peds (Neonatology). Staff, Health Sciences North-Laurentian Site; Staff, Health Sciences North-St Joseph's Health Centre; Assoc Dean Community Engagement/Sr Associate Dean East Campus, Northern Ontario School of Medicine; Langs: English; French; (705)523-7100

BLEAKNEY, Robert R; Mount Sinai Hosp, 600 University Ave, Toronto ON M5G 1X5; Belfast (Ireland)'93; FRCPC; DiagRad. Staff, Mount Sinai Hospital; (416)586-4800 x6199; Fax. (416)586-8695.

BLEAU, Pierre; Allan Memorial Institute, 1025 av des Pins O, Montreal QC H3A 1A1; Sher'86; FRCPC; Psy. Staff, Allan Memorial Institute; Langs: English; (514)934-1934 x31794; Fax. (514)934-8391.

BLEAU-GRAVEL, Genevieve; CSSS du Lac des deux Montagnes, 520 boul Arthur-Sauve, Saint-Eustache QC J7R 5B1; Mon'07; CCFP; Staff, Hôpital de Saint-Eustache; (450)473-6811; Fax. (450)473-6966.

BLECHER, David M; Dr Charles L LeGrow Hlth Ctr, PO Box 250 1 Grand Bay Rd, Port-aux-Basques NL A0M 1C0; McM'10; CCFP; Staff, Dr Charles L Legrow Health Centre; (709)695-2175

BLECHER, Peter M; CPM Health Centre Inc, SS 1 2F-1290 Keith Ross Dr, Oshawa ON L1H 7K4; McG'92; Staff, Lakeridge Health - Oshawa Site; (905)576-3444; Fax. (905)576-7980.

BLECHSCHMIDT, Donald R; 104-100 Pertosa Dr, Brampton ON L6X 0H9; Alb'77; CCFP; FCFP; Court Staff, William Osler Health System - Brampton Civic Hospital; (905)451-1244; Fax. (905)451-6955.

BLENCH, Tanis A; 217-1111 Olympic Way SE, Calgary AB T2G 0E6; Alb'76; (403)538-8881

BLEND, Ralph; Roncesvalles Xray & Ultrasound, 201-27 Roncesvalles Ave, Toronto ON M6R 3B2; London (England)'59; MB BS; DMRD; FRCPC; DiagRad. (416)533-7078

BLESZYNSKI, Maria E; Surrey Med Arts Bldg, 211-13710 94A Ave, Surrey BC V3V 1N1; Krakow (Poland)'77; FRCSC; ObstGyn. Assoc Staff, Surrey Memorial Hospital; Langs: Polish; (604)583-8334; Fax. (604)583-4138; mbl@attglobal.net.

BLEVINS, Gregg; University of Alberta Hosp, 2E3.24WMC-8440 112 St NW, Edmonton AB T6G 2B7; Sask'96; FRCPC; Neur. Staff, University of Alberta Hospital; (780)407-2643

BLEVISS, Morley; White Oaks Med Clinic, 116-12222 137 Ave NW, Edmonton AB T5L 4X5; Dal'74; BSc; MSc; PhD; Ac Staff, Royal Alexandra Hospital; Assoc Staff, University of Alberta Hospital; Med Dir, Venta Nursing Home; (780)473-9355; Fax. (780)473-2856.

BLEW, Brian D M; The Ottawa Hosp-Gen Campus, 501 Smyth Rd, Ottawa ON K1H 8L6; Tor'98; FRCSC; Urol (Renal Transplant). Staff, The Ottawa Hospital - General Campus; (613)737-8899 x73636; Fax. (613)737-8938; bblew@ottawahospital.on.ca.

BLEW, Laura J; 306-200 James St S, Hamilton ON L8P 3A9; Ott'91; CCFP; FCFP; Court Staff Privil, St Joseph's Healthcare - Charlton Campus; Court Staff Privil, Hamilton Health Sciences Centre - McMaster University Medical Centre; (289)389-1811; Fax. (289)389-1899.

BLEW, Philip G; St Joseph's Healthcare, 50 Charlton Ave E, Hamilton ON L8N 4A6; Ott'91; FRCPC; Anes. Staff, St Joseph's Healthcare - Charlton Campus; (905)522-1155 x3853; Fax. (905)521-6019.

BLEWETT, Christopher J; 204-145 Queenston St, St Catharines ON L2R 2Z9; Wes'92; FRCSC; GenSurg (Thoracic Surgery). Staff, Niagara Health System - St Catharines General Site; Clinical Asst Prof Surg, McMaster University; (905)641-0700; Fax. (905)641-0074.

BLEYENDAAL, Argia; 1550-2109 Ottawa St, Windsor ON N8Y 1R8; Wes'84; CCFP; Ac Staff Privil, Windsor Regional Hospital - Metropolitan Site; Court Staff Privil, Hôtel-Dieu Grace Hospital; (519)944-0683; Fax. (519)944-3005.

BLICHER, Brian M; 710-4060 rue Sainte-Catherine, Westmount QC H3Z 2Z3; McG'77; CCFP; FCFP; (514)935-6555; Fax. (514)935-8686.

BLICHOWSKI, Teresa D; Regional Mental HC-London, PO Box 5532 Stn B 850 Highbury Ave, London ON N6A 4H1; Cracow (Poland)'79; FRCPC; Psy. Staff, Regional Mental Health Care-St Joseph's Health Care; (519)455-5110; Fax. (519)455-2919.

BLICKER, Jamie Z; North York Gen Hosp, 1NE 126-4001 Leslie St, North York ON M2K 1E1; McG'99; FRCPC; EmergMed. Staff, North York General Hospital; (416)756-6165

BLICKER, Jeffrey A; Oakridge Centre South Tower, 228-650 41st Ave W, Vancouver BC V5Z 2M9; McG'87; DABOph; FRCSC; Ophth. Staff, Vancouver General Hospital - Centennial Pavillion; Clin Associate Prof, University of British Columbia; Langs: Bilingual(English/French); (604)267-3883; Fax. (604)267-3892.

BLIER, Claude; Hotel-Dieu de Levis, 143 rue Wolfe, Levis QC G6V 3Z1; Laval'87; FRCPC; IntMed; Rheum. Ac Member IntMed, Hôtel-Dieu de Lévis; (418)835-7121

BLIER, E Ludger; 60 av Bateman, Edmundston NB E3V 4X6; Laval'85; Staff, Hôpital regional d'Edmundston; (506)739-9183; Fax. (506)739-9050.

BLIER, Francois; Hop Charles Lemoyne, 3120 boul Taschereau, Greenfield Park QC J4V 2H1; Mon'89; PhysMed&Rehab. Staff, Hopital Charles LeMoyne; (450)466-5000

BLIER, Jean; Montfort Hosp, 713 Montreal Rd, Ottawa ON K1K 0T2; Sher'81; BSc; CSPQ; FRCPC; Anes. Anesthetist, Montfort Hospital; Langs: English; French; (613)746-4621

BLIER, Louis; Hôpital Laval, 2725 ch Sainte-Foy, Quebec QC G1V 4G5; Laval'93; CSPQ; FRCPC; IntMed; Cardiol. Staff, Hôpital Laval; (418)656-4598; Fax. (418)656-4574.

BLIER, Pierre; 6411-1145 Carling Ave, Ottawa ON K1Z 7K4; Mon'86; PhD(NeurolSciences); MSc; Staff, Royal Ottawa Mental Health Centre - Royal Ottawa Health Care Group; Langs: Bilingual(English/French); (613)722-6521 x6944; Fax. (613)761-3610.

BLIGHT, Katherine; Grey Bruce HS-Owen Sound, PO Box 1800 Stn Main 1800 8th St E, Owen Sound ON N4K 6M9; Tor'99; FRCPC; Anes. Staff, Grey Bruce Health Services - Owen Sound; (519)316-2121

BLIGNAUT, Johann; Dr C W Wiebe Med Centre, 385 Main St, Winkler MB R6W 1J2; Pretoria (South Africa)'96; MB ChB; Physician, Boundary Trails Health Centre; Langs: Afrikaans; (204)325-4312; Fax. (204)325-4594.

BLIGNAUT, Lourens P G; Avon Med Centre, 2781 Avonhurst Dr, Regina SK S4R 3J3; Pretoria (South Africa)'87; MB ChB; LMCC; Langs: Afrikaans; (306)543-4955; Fax. (306)545-7006.

BLINICK, Cheryl; 303-2797 Bathurst St, North York ON M6B 4B9; McM'77; Staff, Mount Sinai Hospital; Court Staff, St Joseph's Health Centre; (416)787-5646; Fax. (416)787-9049.

BLINKHORN, Mark T; 406-15940 Fraser Hwy, Surrey BC V4N 0X8; UBC'88; (604)502-7228; Fax. (604)502-7229.

BLINKHORN, Nina A; 102-3040 Tutt St, Kelowna BC V1Y 2H5; London (England)'87; MB BS; (250)765-2996

BLINKINA, Anna A; Cornwall Community Hosp, PO Box 100 Stn Main 840 McConnell Ave, Cornwall ON K6H 5S5; I.M. Sechenov Moscow Medical Academy (Russia (Federation))'95; CCFP; Staff, Cornwall Community Hospital; Langs: Russian; French; (613)938-4240

BLINN, Alain J; Clare Health Centre, 8539 Hwy 1, Meteghan Centre NS B0W 2K0; Sher'09; Langs: Bilingual(English/French); (902)645-2777; Fax. (902)645-2854.

BLITZ, Maurice; St Joseph's Health Centre, SW 245-30 The Queensway, Toronto ON M6R 1B5; UBC'99; MSc(Epidemiol); FRCSC; GenSurg; ThorSurg. Div Head ThorSurg, St Joseph's Health Centre; Langs: Dutch; (416)530-6182; Fax. (416)530-6620.

BLITZER, Andrey; Family Practice Centre, 10 Royal Orchard Blvd, Thornhill ON L3T 3C3; McG'82; AB; CCFP; Court Staff, Mackenzie Richmond Hill Hospital; (905)881-1661; Fax. (905)881-1710.

BLITZER, Steve; Medical Centre, 10 Royal Orchard Blvd, Thornhill ON L3T 3C3; Tor'81; DAAPM; DCAP; Staff, Mackenzie Richmond Hill Hospital; Staff, St Joseph's Health Centre; Langs: Hebrew; French; (905)881-1661; Fax. (905)881-1710.

BLOCH, Christine L; 150 Huron St, Stratford ON N5A 5S8; Wes'87; FRCSC; ObstGyn. Court Staff, Wingham & District Hospital - Listowel Wingham Hospitals Alliance; Ac Staff, Stratford General Hospital - Huron Perth Healthcare Alliance; (519)273-4200; Fax. (519)273-1009.

BLOCH, Didier; CSSS de Vaudreuil-Soulanges, 11 ch de la Cite des Jeunes, Saint-Polycarpe QC J0P 1X0; Strasbourg I (France)'87; (450)265-3771; didier_bloch@rrsss16.gouv.qc.ca.

BLOCH, Gary; SMH-Health Centre @ 410, 80 Bond St, Toronto ON M5B 1X2; UBC'02; BA; LMCC; MCFP; CCFP; Staff, St Michael's Hospital; (416)864-3011; Fax. (416)864-3099.

BLOCH, Peter; Bronte Medical Group, 78 Jones St, Oakville ON L6L 6C5; Wes'74; BSc; Ac Staff, Halton Healthcare Services Corporation - Oakville Site; (905)827-9865; Fax. (905)827-3583.

BLOCK, David N H; Hys Medical Centre, 710-11010 101 St NW, Edmonton AB T5H 4B9; Alb'70; FRCPC; Psy. Staff, Royal Alexandra Hospital; (780)453-5255; Fax. (780)453-9099.

BLOCK, Erwin; PO Box 23099 Rpo Prairie Mall, Grande Prairie AB T8V 6X2; Alb'62; Med Examiner, Erwin W Block Prof Corp; (780)538-0100; Fax. (780)538-0104.

BLOCK, Gary; St Michael's Health Centre, 80 Bond St, Toronto ON M5B 1X2; Wes'80; FRCPC; Anes (Cardiac Anesthesia). (416)864-3011

BLOCK, Haley J; 106-311 Ludlow St, Saskatoon SK S7S 1N6; Sask'04; FRCPC; Neur. (306)975-3933; Fax. (306)975-3931.

BLOCK, Jennifer K; Bank Respiratory Services, 217-1385 Bank St, Ottawa ON K1H 8N4; Ott'03; FRCPC; IntMed; Respir. Staff, The Ottawa Hospital - General Campus; (613)523-4444; Fax. (613)523-6444.

BLOCK, Stephanie K; Lakehead University, UC 1007-955 Oliver Rd, Thunder Bay ON P7B 5E1; Man'98; BSc; CCFP; Staff, Thunder Bay Regional Health Sciences Centre; Staff Student Health & Counselling Centre, Lakehead University / Library; (807)343-8361; Fax. (807)346-7740.

BLOCK, Wendell L; East End Commun Health Centre, 1619 Queen St E, Toronto ON M4L 1G4; Tor'84; CCFP; FCFP; (416)778-5858 x112

BLOCKA, Kenneth L N; Burrard Health Bldg, 204-1160 Burrard St, Vancouver BC V6Z 2E8; Sask'72; FRCPC; IntMed; Rheum. (604)669-7124; kenblocka@telus.net.

BLOEM, Linda; Downtown Med Clinic, PO Box 1866, Unity SK S0K 4L0; Pretoria (South Africa)'87; MB ChB; Langs: Afrikaans; (306)228-4450; Fax. (306)228-4277.

BLOIS, Beau; Colchester East Hants Hlth Ctr, 600 Abenaki Rd, Truro NS B2N 5A1; Dal'08; CCFP; Staff, Colchester East Hants Health Centre; (902)956-9564

BLOIS, Heather S; Sault Area Hosp-Thessalon Divi, PO Box 60 135 Dawson St, Thessalon ON P0R 1L0; Ott'90; CCFP; Staff, Sault Area Hospital - Thessalon Division; (705)842-2014; Fax. (705)842-3214; hblois@bell.net.

BLOKKER, Catherine P; Strathroy Middlesex Gen Hosp, 337-395 Carrie St, Strathroy ON N7G 3C9; Wes'84; FRCSC; OrthSurg. Staff, Strathroy Middlesex General Hospital - Middlesex Hospital Alliance; (519)245-5310; Fax. (519)245-5346.

BLOKMANIS, Andris; Fairmont Med Bldg, 1311-750 Broadway W, Vancouver BC V5Z 1J3; Melbourne (Australia)'65; MB BS; FRACS; FRCSC; Otol (Sinusitis). Ac Staff, Vancouver General Hospital - Centennial Pavillion; Clin Prof, University of British Columbia; Langs: Latvian; (604)875-1012; Fax. (604)876-5322; ablokman@telus.net.

BLOM, Charl J P; 3907 51 Ave, Lloydminster AB T9V 2Z2; Pretoria (South Africa)'64; MB ChB; MMed(Psych); Consultant Psy, Lloydminster Hospital; Langs: Afrikaans; (780)871-5848; Fax. (780)871-5849; reception@shawbiz.ca.

BLOM, Christine R; Bayside Med Centre, 3 Beck Blvd, Penetanguishene ON L9M 1B9; Pretoria (South Africa)'94; MB ChB; DA(SA); CCFP; Staff, Georgian Bay General Hospital - Midland; Langs: Afrikaans; (705)549-3939; Fax. (705)549-0029.

BLOM, Lourens; Riverview Health Centre, 1 Morley Ave, Winnipeg MB R3L 2P4; Pretoria (South Africa)'91; MB ChB; CCFP; Staff, Riverview Health Centre; Langs: Afrikaans; (204)452-3411

BLOM, Phillip P; Westwind Med Clinic, 107-755 Goldsteam Ave, Victoria BC V9B 0H9; Pretoria (South Africa)'96; MB ChB; DA(SA); CCFP; Staff, Georgian Bay General Hospital - Midland; (250)478-1764

BLOM, Rita J M; Parksville X-Ray Clinic, 546 Island Hwy W, Parksville BC V9P 1H2; Man'76; BSc(Med); AB; FRCPC; DiagRad. Langs: English; French; (250)248-3362; Fax. (250)248-3251.

BLOMBERG, Ann L; Waypoint Centre for Mental H C, 500 Church St, Penetanguishene ON L9M 1G3; McM'86; BScN; CCFP; FCFP; Court Staff, Georgian Bay General Hospital - Midland; Ac Staff, Waypoint Centre for Mental Health Care; (705)549-3181 x2540; Fax. (705)549-0266.

BLONDAL, John A; St Joseph's Health Centre, 30 The Queensway, Toronto ON M6R 1B5; Man'86; FRCPC; IntMed; MedOncol. Head Hem/Oncol, St Joseph's Health Centre; (416)530-6586; Fax. (416)530-6356.

BLONDE, J Vince; Ormstown Med Centre, GD 24 rue Gale, Ormstown QC J0S 1K0; McG'78; CCFP; Staff, Barrie Memorial Hospital; McGill University; (450)829-2331; Fax. (450)829-3636; vblondemd@hotmail.com.

BLONDE, Yvonne M; Global Health Fellowship, 3JB-43 Bruyere St, Ottawa ON K1N 5C8; Poznan (Poland)'07; CCFP.

BLONDEAU, Claude; Inst Albert Prevost, 6555 boul Gouin O, Montreal QC H4K 1B3; Mon'03; FRCPC; Psy. (514)338-2222

BLONDEAU, Fernand; UMF Laurier, 2875 boul Laurier, Quebec QC G1V 2M2; Laval'70; CCFP; FCFP; Langs: English; (418)654-2701; Fax. (418)654-2138.

BLONDEAU, Helene; Regie des Rentes Du Quebec CP 5200 Succ Terminus, Quebec QC G1K 7S9; Laval'79; Physician, CLSC La Source; Med Evaluateur, Regie des Rentes du Quebec; (418)657-8709 x3257

BLONDEAU, Jean-Philippe; CSSS de Chicoutimi, 305 rue Saint-Vallier, Chicoutimi QC G7H 5H6; Mon'98; Staff, Complexe hospitalier de la Sagamie; (418)541-1000

BLONDEAU, Lucie; CHUQ-Hotel-Dieu de Quebec, 11 Cote Du Palais, Quebec QC G1R 2J6; Sher'85; FRCPC; RadOncol. Staff, Centre Hospitalier Universitaire de Québec (CHUQ) - Siege Social; Prog Dir RadOncol, Université Laval; (418)691-5264; Fax. (418)691-5268; lucie.blondeau@chuq.qc.ca.

BLONDEAU, Pierre; 1-1732 rue Denault, Sherbrooke QC J1K 1E8; Laval'72; FRCSC; Ophth (Glaucoma). Chef, Centre Hospitalier Universitaire de Sherbrooke-Hôpital Hôtel-Dieu; Chairman Dept of Ophth, Universite de Sherbrooke; (819)564-1135; Fax. (819)346-3953.

BLONDEL-HILL, Edith M; Kelowna Gen Hosp, 2268 Pandosy St, Kelowna BC V1Y 1T2; Alb'86; FRCPC; IntMed; InfectDis; MedMicrobiol. Staff, Kelowna General Hospital; Staff Med Microbiol, Interior Health Authority Central Okanagan Kelowna Health Unit; Langs: Bilingual(English/French); (604)862-4300 x7257

BLONDIN, Claude; Ctre Rhumatologie de Montreal, 502-235 boul René-Lévesque E, Montreal QC H2X 1N8; Mon'62; ABIM; FRCPC; IntMed; Rheum (P.Q.). Staff, Centre Hospitalier l'Université De Montréal (CHUM) - Hôpital Saint-luc; Clin Assoc Prof, Universite de Montreal; (514)871-1335; Fax. (514)495-0973.

BLONDIN, David; Victoria Gen Hosp, 2340 Pembina Hwy, Winnipeg MB R3T 2E8; Cal'07; CCFP; CCFP(E.M.); Staff, Victoria General Hospital; (204)269-3570

BLONDIN, Jean; 105-1691 boul Louis-Fréchette, Nicolet QC J3T 1Z6; Laval'77; ac Staff CMDP, Hôpital de Christ-Roi; (819)293-2022; Fax. (819)293-2024.

BLONDIN, Renee; Hop Maisonneuve-Rosemont, 5415 boul de l'Assomption, Montreal QC H1T 2M4; Mon'94; Staff, Hopital Maisonneuve-Rosemont; (514)252-3400

BLOOD, Paul A; BC Cancer Agency-Vanc Isl Ctr, 2410 Lee Ave, Victoria BC V8R 6V5; Southampton (England)'84; FRCPC; RadOncol (Palliative Care). Staff, BC Cancer Agency Vancouver Island Centre; (250)519-5500; Fax. (250)519-2000.

BLOOM, Carl M; Bramalea Med Centre, 206-18 Kensington Rd, Brampton ON L6T 4S5; McG'92; FRCPC; DiagRad. (905)793-5858

BLOOM, David; Douglas Mental Hlth Univ Inst, 6875 boul Lasalle, Verdun QC H4H 1R3; Qns'77; AB; FRCPC; Psy (Schizophrenia). Staff, Douglas Mental Health University Institute; adj Prof, McGill University; (514)761-6131 x2591; Fax. (514)762-3032; blodav@douglas.mcgill.ca.

BLOOM, Hyman; 1100-1200 Bay St, Toronto ON M5R 2A5; McM'84; LLB; FRCPC; Psy (Forensic Psychiatry). Court Staff Law & Mental Health, Centre for Addiction & Mental Health (CAMH) - College Street Site; Consultant Psy, Ontario Correctional Institute; Asst Prof, McMaster University; (416)922-7222; Fax. (416)922-3188; hy.bloom@workplace.calm.to.

BLOOM, Ira M; North York Gen Hosp, 4001 Leslie St, North York ON M2K 1E1; Wes'81; FRCPC; Anes. Staff, North York General Hospital; (416)756-6000

BLOOM, Jeff; Univ Hlth Network-Toronto Western Hosp, 2W428-399 Bathurst St, Toronto ON M5T 2S8; Cal'83; CCFP; FCFP; Staff Physician, Mount Sinai Hospital; Staff Toronto Western Family Health Team, Toronto Western Hospital - University Health Network; Staff Physician, Casey House Hospice; (416)603-5888 x1; Fax. (416)603-5821.

BLOOM, Leonard; Greenboro Med Clinic, 25 Tapiola Cres, Ottawa ON K1T 2J7; McG'83; CCFP; FCFP; Court Staff Family Med, Children's Hospital of Eastern Ontario (CHEO); Staff, The Ottawa Hospital - Riverside Campus; Staff, The Ottawa Hospital - General Campus; Asst Prof Med, University of Ottawa; (613)738-0303; Fax. (613)738-6459.

BLOOM, Michael S; William Osler HC-Brampton Civi, 2100 Bovaird Dr E, Brampton ON L6R 3J7; Tor'02; FRCPC; Anes. Staff, William Osler Health System - Brampton Civic Hospital; (905)494-2120

BLOOM, Nancy A; Woodlawn Med Clinic, 92 Main St, Dartmouth NS B2X 1R5; Dal'04; CCFP; (902)434-1500

BLOOM, Seth A; Woodlawn Medical Clinic, 92 Main St, Dartmouth NS B2X 1R5; Dal'05; CCFP; Staff, Dartmouth General Hospital; (902)434-1500; Fax. (902)462-4994.

BLOOM, Tara R; 3-7700 Bathurst St, Thornhill ON L4J 7Y3; Tor'04; CCFP; (905)660-9760

BLOOM, Walter S; MUHC-Royal Victoria Hosp, 687 av des Pins O, Montreal QC H3A 1A1; Michigan (USA)'74; FRCPC; IntMed. Sr Physician Div of IntMed, McGill University Health Centre - Royal Victoria Hospital; assoc Prof Med, McGill University; (514)843-1515; Fax. (514)843-1676; walter.bloom@muhc.mcgill.ca.

BLOOMBERG, Gary B; Eau Claire Market, PO Box 182 B27-200 Barclay Parade SW, Calgary AB T2P 4R5; Witwatersrand (South Africa)'76; FACC; FAB; FCCP; FRCPC; Cardiol; IntMed. (403)261-0080

BLOOMENTHAL, Dena F; Broadway Med Centre, 230-943 Broadway W, Vancouver BC V5Z 4E1; Alb'95; BSc; FRCSC; ObstGyn (Maternal Fetal Medicine). Staff, BC Women's Hospital & Health Centre; (604)734-2712; Fax. (604)734-8572.

BLOOMFIELD, Brian G; Highland Park Shopping Centre, 5-525 Highland Rd W, Kitchener ON N2M 5K1; Wes'70; (519)584-2183; Fax. (519)584-0079.

BLOSTEIN, Mark D; SMBD Jewish Gen Hosp, 3755 ch Cote-Sainte-Catherine, Montreal QC H3T 1E2; McG'89; FRCPC; IntMed; MedOncol; Hem. Staff, Sir Mortimer B Davis Jewish General; (514)340-8214

BLOUET, Sylvie; Clin de Chirurgie de Trois-Riv, 975 rue Saint-Prosper, Trois-Rivieres QC G9A 3V7; Sher'88; GenSurg (Surgical Oncology). Staff, CSSS de Trois-Rivières; (819)375-7979; cliniquedeChirurgie@cgocable.ca.

BLOUIN, Brigitte; Centre Med Prevost, RR 1 200-1015 rte Prevost, St-Pierre-I-D'Orl QC G0A 4E0; Laval'85; Staff, Centre Hospitalier Affilié Universitaire de Québec - Hôpital du St-Sacrement; (418)828-2213; Fax. (418)828-2214.

BLOUIN, Carole; Polyclinique Med Fabreville, 209-380 boul Curé-Labelle, Laval QC H7P 5L3; Mon'87; (450)628-5800; Fax. (450)628-0217.

BLOUIN, Daniel J; CHUS-Hop Fleurimont, 3001 12e Av N, Sherbrooke QC J1H 5N4; Sher'70; ObstGyn. Staff, Centre Hospitalier Universitaire de Sherbrooke-Hopital Fleurimont; Prof ObstGyn, Universite de Sherbrooke; (819)346-1110 x14458; Fax. (819)820-6441.

BLOUIN, Danielle; Kingston Gen Hosp, 76 Stuart St, Kingston ON K7L 2V7; Laval'87; FRCPC; EmergMed;CCFP; CCFP(E.M.); FCFP; Staff, Kingston General Hospital; (613)549-6666 x2368

BLOUIN, Denis; Clinique Med Familiale Clermon, 500-106 boul Notre-Dame, Clermont QC G4A 1G3; Laval'88; CCFP; (418)439-3935; Fax. (418)439-4548.

BLOUIN, Denys; Clinique Medicale Chatel, 200-9465 boul de l'Ormiere, Quebec QC G2B 3K7; Laval'76; (418)843-5141; Fax. (418)843-5343.

BLOUIN, Elizabeth; CSSS de Montmagny-l'Islet, 430 rue Jean-Leclerc RR 1, St-Jean-Port-Joli QC G0R 3G0; Laval'90; Staff, CSSS de Montmagny-l'Islet; (418)598-3355; Fax. (418)598-9800.

BLOUIN, Francine; Ctre de Med Privee Blouin Valo, 100B-299 boul Sir-Wilfrid-Laur, Saint-Lambert QC J4R 2L1; Laval'83; (450)465-5541; Fax. (450)465-7358; centreblouinvalois@videotron.ca.

BLOUIN, Francois; Polyclinique Med des Ponts, 120-1100 boul de la Rive-Sud, Saint-Romuald QC G6W 5M6; Mon'89; (418)839-8572; Fax. (418)839-8003.

BLOUIN, Gilles; CSSS du Rocher-Perce, CP 3300 451 rue Mgr Ross E, Chandler QC G0C 1K0; Laval'67; DMRD; FRCPC; DiagRad. Staff, CSSS de la Baie-des-Chaleurs; Staff Therapeutic Radiol, Centre Hospitalier de Chandler; (418)689-2261; Fax. (418)689-5049.

BLOUIN, Guy A; Inst Albert Prevost, 6555 boul Gouin O, Montreal QC H4K 1B3; Mon'67; Psy. Staff Albert Prevost Inst, Hôpital du Sacre-Coeur de Montréal; Clin Asst, Universite de Montreal; (514)338-2100; Fax. (514)338-4402.

BLOUIN, Julie; Centre Med Fusion, 200-2035 av Sainte-Anne, Saint-Hyacinthe QC J2S 5H3; McG'99; CCFP; Langs: Bilingual(French/English); (450)773-6023; Fax. (450)773-5915.

BLOUIN, Louis; Clinique Med Loretteville, 250-11000 boul de l'Ormiere, Quebec QC G2B 5S1; Laval'70; Staff, Centre Hospitalier Chauveau; (418)842-3731; Fax. (418)842-3246; louis.blouin@ssss.gouv.qc.ca.

BLOUIN, Lucie M; Peterborough Reg HC-Hospital, 1 Hospital Dr, Peterborough ON K9J 7C6; McM'82; Staff, Peterborough Regional Health Centre - Hospital Drive; Medical Staff, Lakeridge Health - Oshawa Site; (705)740-8326; Fax. (705)740-8125.

BLOUIN, Marie; Clinique Med Barrette, 152 boul Barrette, Chicoutimi QC G7H 7W8; Laval'90; CCFP; (418)543-3838; Fax. (418)543-3216.

BLOUIN, Marie-Claude; Clinique d'Ophtalmologie, 330 av de l'Hotel-Dieu, Sorel-Tracy QC J3P 1N4; Mon'99; FRCSC; Ophth. Staff, Hôtel-Dieu de Sorel; Langs: Bilingual(French/English); (450)855-1390; Fax. (450)855-1393.

BLOUIN, Mario; Clinique Med Saint-Louis, 3165 ch Saint-Louis, Quebec QC G1W 4R4; Laval'89; (418)653-1970

BLOUIN, Nathalie; Inst U Geriatrie de Montreal, 4565 ch Queen-Mary, Montreal QC H3W 1W5; Mon'80; Staff, Institut Universitaire de Gériatrie de Montréal; (514)340-3533

BLOUIN, Odette; CSSS de la Region de Thetford, 1717 rue Notre-Dame E, Thetford Mines QC G6G 2V4; Laval'81; DiagRad. Staff, Hopital du CSSS de la Region de Thetford; (418)338-7744

BLOUIN, Patrick; CSSS de Montmagny-L'Islet, 350 boul Tache O, Montmagny QC G5V 3R8; McG'00; Staff, CSSS de Montmagny-L'Islet; (418)248-0630

BLOUIN, Patrick; Clinique Med Loretteville, 250-11000 boul de l'Ormiere, Quebec QC G2B 5S1; Laval'80; (418)843-2580; Fax. (418)843-1734.

BLOUIN, Pierre; Polyclinique Ancienne-Lorette, 204-6385 boul Wilfrid-Hamel, L'Ancienne-Lorette QC G2E 5W2; Laval'71; (418)872-2012; Fax. (418)872-2349.

BLOUIN, Rejean; Clinique Med de Matane, 548 av Du Phare E, Matane QC G4W 1A7; Laval'75; Staff, Centre Hospitalier de Matane; (418)562-4530; Fax. (418)562-4532.

BLOUIN, Sylvie; CSSS de Laval, 1755 boul Rene-Laennec, Laval QC H7M 3L9; Mon'88; Staff, Hopital de la Cite de la santé; (450)975-5444; Fax. (450)975-5497.

BLOUIN, Valerie; CSSS Pierre Boucher, 1333 boul Jacques-Cartier E, Longueuil QC J4M 2A5; Sher'06; FRCPC; IntMed; InfectDis. Staff, Centre Hospitalier Pierre Boucher; (450)468-8111

BLOUIN, Valerie; Ctr Hosp Affilie-St-Sacrement, 1050 ch Sainte-Foy, Quebec QC G1S 4L8; Laval'07; DiagRad. Staff, Centre Hospitalier Affilié Universitaire de Québec - Hôpital du St-Sacrement; (418)682-7511

BLOUIN, Yvan; CHUS-Hop Hotel-Dieu, 580 rue Bowen S, Sherbrooke QC J1G 2E8; Laval'61; DAB; FACS; FRCSC; GenSurg. Consultant, CSSS des Sources d'Asbestos; Staff, Centre Hospitalier Universitaire de Sherbrooke-Hôpital Hôtel-Dieu; Consultant, CSSS Institut universitaire de gériatrie de Sherbrooke; adj Prof, Universite de Sherbrooke; (819)346-1110

BLOUNT, Christopher; 421 Shepherdson Rd, New Liskeard ON P0J 1P0; Tor'77; Ac Staff, Temiskaming Hospital; Coroner, Province of Ontario; (705)647-6411

BLOUW, Karin J; PO Box 519, Smithers BC V0J 2N0; UBC'91; (250)847-3097

BLOUW, Marion C; Foul Bay Prof Centre, 101-1964 Fort St, Victoria BC V8R 6R3; UBC'86; BSc; CCFP; FCFP; Clin Instructor PBL Tutor/Lecturer Island Med Prog Faculty of Med, University of British Columbia; Langs: Dutch; (250)721-9494; Fax. (250)721-9493.

BLOUW, Richard H; Southwood Med Centre, 203-2385 Pembina Hwy, Winnipeg MB R3T 2H4; Man'74; CCFP; FCFP; Ac Staff, Victoria General Hospital; Asst Prof Family Med, University of Manitoba; Langs: Dutch; (204)284-3058; Fax. (204)452-3136.

BLUE, Christopher; 1083 Ouellette Ave, Windsor ON N9A 4J8; St Matthews Univ (Cayman Islands)'04; CCFP; Staff, Hôtel-Dieu Grace Hospital; (519)915-7125

BLUEMKE, Alice M; Medical Associates of Port Cre, 2F-333 Lakeshore Rd W, Mississauga ON L5H 1G9; Tor'84; CCFP; FCFP; (905)274-7055; Fax. (905)274-0227.

BLUHM, Melanie; Guelph Community Hlth Centre, 20 Shelldale Cres, Guelph ON N1H 1C8; McM'03; CCFP; Staff GP, St Joseph's Health Centre; (519)821-6638

BLUM, Seymour J; 105-5885 ch de la Cote-des-Nei, Montreal QC H3S 2T2; McG'74; FRCPC; Gastroent. Staff, Sir Mortimer B Davis Jewish General; adj Prof, McGill University; (514)738-9409

BLUMAN, Robert A; 810-943 Broadway W, Vancouver BC V5Z 4E2; UBC'77; BSc; CCFP; FCFP; Ac Staff, BC Children's Hospital; Assoc Staff, Vancouver General Hospital - Centennial Pavillion; Asst Dean Fac of Med Div of Continuing Professional Dev & Knowledge Translation/Clin Prof Family Pract, University of British Columbia; Langs: Spanish; French; (604)734-1213; Fax. (604)734-5751.

BLUMBERGER, Daniel M; Addiction & Mental Hlth-Queen, 4 301-1001 Queen St W, Toronto ON M6J 1H4; Tor'03; FRCPC; Psy. Staff, Centre for Addiction & Mental Health (CAMH) - Queen Site; (416)535-8501 x3662; Fax. (416)583-1307.

BLUME, Warren T; 211-1135 Adelaide St N, London ON N5Y 5K7; McG'62; AB; FRCPC; Neur (Epilepsy). Staff, London Health Sciences Centre - University Hospital; Emeritus Prof, University of Western Ontario; (519)433-8353; Fax. (519)433-2834; warren.blume@lhsc.on.ca.

BLUMENAUER, Barbara T; 206-300 Columbia St, Kamloops BC V2C 6L1; UBC'92; FRCPC; IntMed; Rheum. (250)434-8215; Fax. (250)434-8217.

BLUMENFELD, Aaron J; 137 Roncesvalles Ave, Toronto ON M6R 2L2; Tor'00; FRCSC; Urol. Staff Surg, Toronto East General Hospital Inc; (416)534-6699

BLUMENFELD, Renee; Markham Place Med Centre, 206-2900 Steeles Ave E, Thornhill ON L3T 4X1; Tor'89; CCFP; Staff, The Scarborough Hospital - Birchmount Campus; (905)881-6667; Fax. (905)731-1298; rblumenfeld@rogers.com.

BLUMENKRANTZ, Miriam; MUHC-Montreal Children's Hosp, 2300 rue Tupper, Montreal QC H3H 1P3; McG'94; CSPQ; FRCPC; AnatPath. Staff, McGill University Health Centre - Montreal Children's Hospital; (514)412-4400 x24495; miriam.blumenkrantz@muhc.mcgill.ca.

BLUMENTHAL, Andrea; Lakeridge Hlth Corp-Oshawa, 1 Hospital Crt, Oshawa ON L1G 2B9; Dal'95; FRCPC; MedGenetics. Staff, Lakeridge Health - Oshawa Site; Pt-Time Teacher, University of Toronto; (905)433-2733; Fax. (905)721-6122.

BLUMER, Herbert M; 220-5950 ch de la Cote-des-Nei, Montreal QC H3S 1Z5; McG'56; MSc; DAB; FRCPC; IntMed; ClinImmunol&Allergy (P.Q.). Sr Physician, Sir Mortimer B Davis Jewish General; adj Prof, McGill University; Langs: French; (514)733-7381; Fax. (514)739-5859; hblumer@videotron.ca.

BLUMER, Ian R; Baywood Med Centre, 401-95 Bayly St W, Ajax ON L1S 7K8; Qns'81; FRCPC; IntMed (Diabetes). (905)427-2678; Fax. (905)427-2679.

BLUMER, Russell D; Humber River Reg Hosp-Church, 200 Church St, Toronto ON M9N 1N8; Dal'96; FRCPC; DiagRad. Staff, Humber River Regional Hospital - Church Street Site; (416)243-4158; Fax. (416)243-4162.

BLUNDELL, Krista J M; Gander Med Clinic, 177 Elizabeth Dr, Gander NL A1V 1H6; Mem'97; CCFP; (709)256-7101; Fax. (709)256-7109.

BLUNDELL, Ross S; St Michael's Hosp, 30 Bond St, Toronto ON M5B 1W8; Qns'76; FRCPC; IntMed. Ac Staff EmergMed, St Michael's Hospital; (416)864-5095

BLUNDERFIELD, G Mark; 208-2438 Marine Dr, West Vancouver BC V7V 1L2; Cal'76; FRCPC; Psy. (604)922-2505

BLUNSTON, Shawn D; 370A-180 Madawaska ch, Grand Falls NB E3Y 1A7; Mem'93; CCFP; (506)473-9002; Fax. (506)473-5633.

BLUNT, Gerald G; Athens & Dist Family Health Te, PO Box 1110 63 5th St, Englehart ON P0J 1H0; Ott'77; Ac Staff, Englehart & District Hospital Inc; Court Staff, Kirkland & District Hospital; Langs: English; French; (705)544-2321; Fax. (705)544-5224; gblunt@edhospital.on.ca.

BLUNT, Marie E; Bluewater Health-Norman Site, 89 Norman St, Sarnia ON N7T 6S3; Qns'86; FRCSC; ObstGyn. Staff, Bluewater Health - Norman Site; (519)464-4400

BLUSANOVICS, Peter; St Mary's Hosp Centre, 3830 av Lacombe, Montreal QC H3T 1M5; Laval'94; CCFP; Staff Family Med, St Mary's Hospital Centre; (514)345-3511

BLUSTEIN, Norman S; Richmon Hill Childrens Clinic, 404-250 Harding Blvd W, Richmond Hill ON L4C 9M7; Tor'81; FRCPC; Peds. Ac Staff MacKenzie Health, Mackenzie Richmond Hill Hospital; (905)737-9898; Fax. (905)737-8583; dr.norm@rogers.com.

BLUSTEIN, Philip K; 415 14 St NW, Calgary AB T2N 2A1; Tor'75; FRCPC; IntMed (Cardiology). (403)270-9555; Fax. (403)270-7479.

BLUTHARDT, Thomas R; Providence Healthcare, 3276 St Clair Ave E, Scarborough ON M1L 1W1; Tor'74; Staff, Providence Healthcare; (416)285-3666

BLY, Eric B; The Campbell Clinic, 160 Columbia Blvd W, Lethbridge AB T1K 4J4; Cal'09; CCFP; (403)381-7000; Fax. (403)381-8250.

BLY, Jared D; Royal Alexandra Hosp, 10240 Kingsway NW, Edmonton AB T5H 3V9; Cal'03; CCFP; CCFP(E.M.); Staff, Royal Alexandra Hospital; (780)735-5374

BLYDT-HANSEN, Tom D; Lake of the Woods Dist Hosp, 21 Sylvan St W, Kenora ON P9N 3W7; McG'92; FRCPC; Peds; Nephrol. Staff, Lake of the Woods District Hospital; Fax. (807)468-9861.

BLYTH, Christine G; Vernon Jubilee Hosp, 2101 32 St, Vernon BC V1T 5L2; UBC'98; CCFP; Staff, Vernon Jubilee Hospital; (250)545-2211

BLYTH, Scott; Western Med Clinic, 144 6th St, Brandon MB R7A 3N2; Cal'81; BSc; (204)727-6451; Fax. (204)727-4150.

BOA, Olivier; Hotel-Dieu de Levis, 143 rue Wolfe, Levis QC G6V 3Z1; PlasSurg. Staff, Hôtel-Dieu de Lévis; (418)835-7145

BOACHIE, Ahmed; Southlake Reg Health Centre, 596 Davis Dr, Newmarket ON L3Y 2P9; Accra (Ghana)'89; MB ChB; MRCPsy(UK); DCH; FRCPC; Psy (Child & Adolescent Eating Disorders). Dir Eating Disorders Prog, Southlake Regional Health Centre; Staff Eating Disorders Day Hosp, The Hospital For Sick Children; Langs: Akan; Ashanti; (905)895-4521 x2780; Fax. (905)830-5970; aboachie@southlakeregional.org.

BOAFO, Addo; Children's Hosp Eastern Ont, 401 Smyth Rd, Ottawa ON K1H 8L1; (Ghana)'78; MB ChB; MBA; FRCPC; Psy (Child Psychiatry). Staff, Children's Hospital of Eastern Ontario (CHEO); Asst Prof Psy, University of Ottawa; (613)737-7600 x2507; aboafo@cheo.on.ca.

BOAG, Alexander H; Queen's University, 115 Barrack St, Kingston ON K7L 3N6; Qns'88; FRCPC; AnatPath (Cytopath). Staff, Kingston General Hospital; Queen's University; (613)548-3232 x4190

BOAG, Graham S; Alberta Children's Hosp, 2888 Shaganappi Trail NW, Calgary AB T3B 6A8; Qns'82; FRCPC; DiagRad. Staff Diag Imaging, Alberta Children's Hospital; (403)955-7985; Fax. (403)955-7656.

BOAKE, Armour I; 405-984 Oliver Rd, Thunder Bay ON P7B 7C7; McM'00; FRCPC; IntMed; Nephrol. Langs: Spanish; French; (807)345-7879

BOAN, Derek H; Physicians Plus, 239B 5th Ave N, Saskatoon SK S7K 2P2; Sask'85; MSc(CTM); CCFP; Ac Staff, Saskatoon Health Region; (306)282-4300

BOAN, Jarol L; Aspen Medical Centre, 225-3737 Wascana Pkwy, Regina SK S4S 0A2; ABIM; MPH; Assoc Prof Med, University of Saskatchewan; (306)337-2643; jarol.boan@uregina.ca.

BOATE, Brian W; Ottawa Parkdale Med Centre, 406-1081 Carling Ave, Ottawa ON K1Y 4G2; Wes'78; FRCPC; IntMed (Adult Rheumatology); Rheum. Ac Staff, The Ottawa Hospital - Civic Campus; Consultant, Carleton Place & District Memorial Hospital; Pt-Time Teach. Staff, University of Ottawa; (613)725-2882; Fax. (613)725-1138.

BOBA, Lukasz; Royal Victoria Hosp, 201 Georgian Dr, Barrie ON L4M 6M2; Krakow (Poland)'06; CCFP; CCFP(E.M.); Staff, Royal Victoria Regional Health Centre; (705)728-9802

BOBADILLA-MARTINEZ, Julio C; Amherst Family Health Clinic, 200-158 Robert Angus Dr, Amherst NS B4H 4R7; Habana (Cuba)'89; CCFP; (902)667-3330; Fax. (902)667-4176.

BOBART, Vonda A S; Penticton Reg Hosp, 550 Carmi Ave, Penticton BC V2A 3G6; Royal College of Ireland (Ireland)'94; MB BCh; BAO; Staff, Penticton Regional Hospital; (250)492-4000

BOBBA, Raja; Charlton Med Centre, 610-25 Charlton Ave E, Hamilton ON L8N 1Y2; McM'97; FRCPC; IntMed; Rheum. Staff, Charlton Medical Centre; (905)308-8319; Fax. (905)523-8466.

BOBBY, Bradley T; Family Med Centre, 387 Cedar St, Simcoe ON N3Y 2J2; Man'98; BSc; (519)426-4821

BOBBY, Rebecca J; Health Sciences Centre, 300 Prince Philip Dr, St. John's NL A1B 3V6; Mem'08; CCFP; CCFP(E.M.); Staff, Health Sciences Centre; (709)737-6300

BOBIARSKI, Jerzy J; St Michael's Hosp, 30 Bond St, Toronto ON M5B 1W8; Lodz (Poland)'95; Staff, St Michael's Hospital; (416)864-5303

BOBIK-ORCHARD, Francis J; Grey Bruce HS-Markdale, PO Box 406 Stn Main 55 Isla St, Markdale ON N0C 1H0; Tor'70; FRCPC; Anes (Emergency Medicine). Staff, Grey Bruce Health Services - Markdale; (519)986-3040

BOBROWSKI, Jacob; 901-790 Bay St, Toronto ON M5G 1N8; Tor'77; BSc; CASM; FAAFP; Staff, Toronto General Hospital - UHN; Med Consultant, Centre for Addiction & Mental Health (CAMH) - Brentcliffe Rd Site; Member, College of Physicians & Surgeons of Ontario; Med Dir, Alpha House; (416)967-4788; Fax. (416)967-6623.

BOBYN, Larry; Family Practice Associates, 230 Robson Rd W, Kelowna BC V1X 3C8; Sask'91; BSc; BA; (250)765-9777

BOBYN, Michael P; 204-3140 Lakeshore Rd, Kelowna BC V1W 3T1; Sask'83; (250)763-1131; Fax. (250)763-3455.

BOCHINSKI, Dariuz; Alberta Urology Institute, 400-11010 101 St NW, Edmonton AB T5H 4B9; Alb'97; FRCSC; Urol. Staff, Alberta Urology Institute; Langs: Polish; (780)441-2573; Fax. (780)441-2591.

BOCK, Allan R; 301-220 Dundas St W, Whitby ON L1N 8M7; Qns'71; (905)668-7899

BOCK, Dirk E; 800 Commissioners Rd E PO Box 5010 Stn B, London ON N6A 5W9; Frankfurt (Germany)'98; Staff, London Health Sciences Centre - Victoria Campus; Langs: German; (519)685-8500 x56075

BOCK, Gerhard W; Medical Arts Bldg, 202-233 Kennedy St, Winnipeg MB R3C 3J5; Man'80; FRCPC; DiagRad. (204)942-6453; Fax. (204)944-8101.

BOCK, Philip W; Dr Everett Chalmers Reg Hosp, PO Box 9000 700 Priestman St, Fredericton NB E3B 5N5; Man'09; CCFP; Staff, Dr Everett Chalmers Regional Hospital; (506)452-5400

BOCKING, Alan D; Mount Sinai Hospital, 19 308B-600 University Ave, Toronto ON M5G 1X5; Wes'77; FRCSC; ObstGyn. Chief ObstGyn, Mount Sinai Hospital; Chair ObstGyn/Prof, University of Toronto; (416)586-8406; Fax. (416)586-8649.

BOCKING, Natalie D; Dala Lana School of Public Hlt, 10F-155 College St, Toronto ON M5T 3M7; McM'09; CCFP; (416)978-0952

BOCKMUEHL, P Christoph; Crowfoot Village Fam Practice, 210-600 Crowfoot Cres NW, Calgary AB T3G 0B4; Cal'89; CCFP; FCFP; (403)239-9733

BOCKNEK, Amber L; 245-16715 Yonge St, Newmarket ON L3X 1X4; Ott'96; CCFP; Staff, The Brant Community Healthcare System - Brantford General Hospital Site; McMaster University; (905)251-9998; Fax. (905)235-0769.

BOCQUIER, Arnaud A F; Inst Univ de Cardiologie et Pn, 2725 ch Sainte-Foy, Quebec QC G1V 4G5; Laval'04; CCFP; Staff, Institut Universitaire Cardiologie & Pneumologie de Quebec; (418)656-8711

BOCTI, Christian; CHUS-Hop Fleurimont, 3001 12e av N, Sherbrooke QC J1H 5N4; Mon'97; Neur (Cognitive Neurol). Staff, Centre Hospitalier Universitaire de Sherbrooke-Hopital Fleurimont; (819)346-1110

BOCTOR, Atef H K; St Mary's Clinic, PO Box 45 110 Roe Ave, Gander NL A1V 1W5; Cairo (Egypt)'90; MB ChB; CCFP; Staff, James Paton Memorial Hospital; Langs: Arabic; (709)651-0220; Fax. (709)651-0225.

BOCTOR, Dana L; Alberta Children's Hosp, 2888 Shaganappi Trail NW, Calgary AB T3B 6A8; Tor'99; MSc; FRCPC; Peds (Nutrition); Gastroent. Staff, Alberta Children's Hospital; (403)955-7721

BODAK, Ann-Marie; 103-747 Hyde Park Rd, London ON N6H 3S3; Tor'87; FRCPC; IntMed. (519)471-5555

BODANI, Jayalakshmi P; Regina Qu'Appelle HR-Regina, 1440 14th Ave, Regina SK S4P 0W5; Bangalore (India)'73; DCH(UK); Staff Neonatol ICU, Regina General Hospital; Clinical Asst Prof, University Of Saskatchewan; (306)766-4517; Fax. (306)766-4149.

BODASING, Deo; Sheppard Associates, 649 Sheppard Ave W, North York ON M3H 2S4; Edinburgh (Scotland)'66; MB ChB; (416)630-0610; Fax. (416)923-1365.

BODENSTAB, Robert A; Caledonian Med Clinic, 340 Campbell St, Nanaimo BC V9R 3G7; Pretoria (South Africa)'72; (250)390-5200

BODENSTEIN, Christel E; 200-2003 14 St NW, Calgary AB T2M 3N4; Stellenbosch (South Africa)'80; FRCPC; Psy (General Psychiatry). (403)284-4140

BODIG, Jessica E; Renfrew Med Group, 510 Raglan St N, Renfrew ON K7V 1P5; Qns'09; CCFP; (613)433-5712; Fax. (613)433-5727.

BODKIN, Andrew C; Bodkin Medicine Prof Corp, 210-450 Central Ave, London ON N6B 2E8; Wes'80; CCFP; FCFP; (519)686-4080

BODKIN, E Anne; London Intercommunity Hlth Ctr, 659 Dundas St E, London ON N5W 2Z1; Wes'80; CCFP; FCFP; Court Staff, St Joseph's Hospital - St Joseph's Health Care; (519)660-0874; Fax. (519)642-1532.

BODKIN, R Norman; 205-535 Belmont Ave W, Kitchener ON N2M 5E9; Wes'80; Court Staff Family Pract, Grand River Hospital - Kitchener/Waterloo Health Centre; Court Staff, St Mary's General Hospital; (519)578-0941; Fax. (519)578-7331.

BODLEY, Janet; Sunnybrook Hlth Sciences Ctre, B730-2075 Bayview Ave, Toronto ON M4N 3M5; Tor'94; FRCSC; ObstGyn. Staff, Sunnybrook Health Sciences Centre; (416)480-6100 x5951

BODLEY, Steven C; North Bay Reg Health Centre, 50 College Dr, North Bay ON P1B 0A4; Wes'81; BSc(Hon); FRCPC; Anes (Chronic Pain). Ac Staff Pain Management Clinic, North Bay Regional Health Centre - Regional Mental Health; Asst Prof, Northern Ontario School of Medicine; (705)474-8600 x4047; Fax. (705)495-7983.

BODMER, A Barbara; Westmount Med Bldg, 625-5025 rue Sherbrooke O, Montreal QC H4A 1S9; McG'80; FRCSC; ObstGyn. Staff, McGill University Health Centre - Montreal General Campus; Staff, McGill University Health Centre - Royal Victoria Hospital; McGill University; Langs: French; (514)482-4964; Fax. (514)481-7704.

BODMER, Madeleine; 8808 92 St NW, Edmonton AB T6C 3R1; McG'75; Assoc Staff, Royal Alexandra Hospital; (780)469-7147; Fax. (780)469-3871.

BODNAR, Melanie R; Clinical Sciences Bldg, 13 109-11350 83rd Ave, Edmonton AB T6G 2V2; Alb'01; FRCPC; IntMed; Hem. Staff, University of Alberta Hospital; (780)407-8450; Fax. (780)407-2680.

BODNAR, Michael; Sault Area Hosp, 750 Great Northern Rd, Sault Ste. Marie ON P6B 0A8; Ott'07; CCFP; CCFP(E.M.); Staff, Sault Area Hospital - Sault Ste Marie; (705)759-3434

BODOK, Rebecca; The Royal Courtyards, E6-18 King St E, Bolton ON L7E 1E8; Tel Aviv (Israel)'92; CCFP; Court Staff, William Osler Health System - Etobicoke General Hospital; Court Staff, Headwaters Health Care Centre - Orangeville Site; Langs: English; French; Hebrew; (905)951-1173; Fax. (905)951-9716.

BODOR, Cristina; Lakeshore Gen Hosp, 160 av Stillview, Pointe-Claire QC H9R 2Y2; Bucharest (Romania)'91; Staff, Lakeshore General Hospital - Pointe Claire; (514)630-2225

BODRUZIC, Nada; 4-55 Wheatland Trail, Strathmore AB T1P 1R7; (Bosnia-Herzegovina)'78; Langs: Serbian; Croatian; (403)934-5911; Fax. (403)934-6672.

BODURTHA, Audley J; The Ottawa Hosp-Gen Campus, 501 Smyth Rd, Ottawa ON K1H 8L6; University of West Indies Jamaica (Other Foreign)'67; MB BS; FACS; FRCSC; GenSurg (Surgical Oncology). Staff Surgeon, The Ottawa Hospital - General Campus; Prof, University of Ottawa; (613)737-8544; Fax. (613)737-8371.

BOE, Corene D; 101-3960 Quadra St, Victoria BC V8X 4A3; Cal'10; (250)592-3479

BOECHLER, Mark D; McEown Med Clinic, 102-2315 McEown Ave, Saskatoon SK S7J 2H1; Sask'83; (306)374-2438; Fax. (306)374-8262.

BOEHME, Gene R; Family Med Centre, 2931 20 Ave S, Lethbridge AB T1K 3M5; Alb'72; Ac Staff, Covenant Health - St Michael's Health Centre; Ac Staff, Chinook Regional Hospital; Langs: German; (403)328-2326; Fax. (403)327-0123.

BOEKE, Jeannette; 402 Borland St, Williams Lake BC V2G 1R7; Pretoria (South Africa)'08; Langs: Afrikaans; (250)392-7221

BOEKHOUD, John W F G; Thamesview Family Health Team, 465 Grand Ave W, Chatham ON N7L 1C5; Wes'72; Staff, Chatham-Kent Health Alliance; (519)354-3200; Fax. (519)354-6132.

BOEKHOUD, Jonathan J W; Thunder Bay Reg HSC-T-Bay, 980 Oliver Rd, Thunder Bay ON P7B 6V4; Wes'06; NuclearMed. Staff, Thunder Bay Regional Health Sciences Centre; (807)684-6000; Fax. (807)684-5854.

BOERKOEL, Cornelius F; BC Women's Hosp & Health Ctre, C234-4500 Oak St, Vancouver BC V6H 3N1; Ohio (USA)'93; FRCPC; MedGenetics. Staff, BC Women's Hospital & Health Centre; (604)875-2157

BOERNER, Scott; Univ Hlth Network-Toronto Gen, 200 Elizabeth St, Toronto ON M5G 2C4; Tor'89; ABPath; FRCP; FRCPC; AnatPath. Dir Cytopathology/Staff, Toronto General Hospital - UHN; Assoc Prof, University of Toronto; (416)340-3706; Fax. (416)340-5517.

BOERSMA, J Robert; 21-346 John St N, Arnprior ON K7S 2P6; Tor'83; BSc; BPHE; Ac Staff, Arnprior & District Memorial Hospital; (613)623-0311; Fax. (613)623-4095.

BOET, Sylvain; The Ottawa Hosp-Gen Campus, 501 Smyth Rd, Ottawa ON K1H 8L6; Rouen (France)'05; Staff, The Ottawa Hospital - General Campus; (613)737-8187

BOETTCHER, Allen; Chatham Kent Health Alliance, PO Box 2030 Stn Main 80 Grand Ave W, Chatham ON N7M 5L9; Dal'76; Staff, Chatham-Kent Health Alliance; (519)437-0609

BOEY, Gerald E; Arbutus Laser Centre, 106-2025 Broadway W, Vancouver BC V6J 1Z6; Sask'78; MD; (604)731-5512; Fax. (604)731-5511; geboey@cs.com.

BOFFA, Ernest J; Edmonton Mental Health Clinic, 3F-9942 108 St NW, Edmonton AB T5K 2J5; Alb'98; FRCPC; Psy. (780)342-7700; Fax. (780)425-9317.

BOFOYA, Boyale J; Mount Royal Family Physicians, 701 Avenue P N, Saskatoon SK S7L 2W1; (306)382-5854; Fax. (306)382-7477; bofbofoya@yahoo.ca.

BOGATY, Peter M; 403-3535 ch Queen Mary, Montreal QC H3V 1H8; Liege (Belgium)'80; ABIM; ABCD(CardiovascMed); CSPQ; FRCPC; IntMed (Heart Disease); Cardiol. Researcher Cardiol, Hôpital Laval; assoc Prof, Université Laval; Langs: Spanish; (514)731-6000; Fax. (514)731-2476; peter.bogaty@med.ulaval.ca.

BOGGILD, Andrea K; Univ Hlth Network-Toronto Gen, 13F 1350-200 Elizabeth St, Toronto ON M5G 2C4; Tor'03; BSc; MSc; FRCPC; MedMicrobiol (Tropical Medicine). Staff Tropical Disease Unit, Toronto General Hospital - UHN; (416)340-3675; Fax. (416)340-3260.

BOGHEN, R Dan; CHUM-Hop Notre-Dame, 1560 rue Sherbrooke E, Montreal QC H2L 4M1; Mon'63; FRCPC; Neur (Neuro Ophthalmology). Staff, Centre Hospitalier l'Université de Montréal (CHUM) - Hôpital Notre-Dame; assoc Prof, Universite de Montreal; Langs: French; Romanian; (514)890-8000 x26357; Fax. (514)412-7233; boghend@videotron.ca.

BOGLE, Lee B; Glenbrook Med Center, 111-4306 Richmond Rd SW, Calgary AB T3E 4P6; Cal'09; CCFP; (403)685-5480

BOGO, Norman H; 407-1100 Sheppard Ave E, North York ON M2K 2W1; McG'65; FRCPC; Psy. Ac Staff, North York General Hospital; (416)226-6988

BOGOCH, Earl R; St Michael's Orthopaedic Assoc, 800-55 Queen St E, Toronto ON M5C 1R6; Alb'74; MSc; FRCSC; OrthSurg (Musculoskeletal Injury). Med Dir Mobiility(Neuromusculoskeletal), St Michael's Hospital; Langs: Bilingual(English/French); (416)864-5350; Fax. (416)359-1601.

BOGOCH, Isaac I; Univ Hlth Network-Toronto Gen, 200 Elizabeth St, Toronto ON M5G 2C4; Tor'05; FRCPC; IntMed; InfectDis. Staff, Toronto General Hospital - UHN; (416)340-4800

BOGOCH, Ruth E; Beaumont Family Med, 4-5102 49 Ave, Beaumont AB T4X 1E4; UBC'85; (780)929-5400; Fax. (780)929-2126.

BOGOMOLNY, Howard; 207-1246 Yonge St, Toronto ON M4T 1W7; Tor'74; FRCPC; Psy. (416)962-9010; Fax. (416)962-0014; howardbogo@sympatico.ca.

BOGOSYAN, Avedis; 2030 Victoria Park Ave, North York ON M1R 1V2; Istanbul (Turkey)'70; Ac Staff, North York General Hospital; Ac Staff, Leisure World Scarborough; Ac Staff, Seven Oaks Nursing Home(Toronto); Langs: Armenian; Turkish; French; (416)443-9971; Fax. (416)443-8865.

BOGUE, Lisa A; 252-759 Hyde Park Rd, London ON N6H 3S2; Wes'94; FRCPC; Psy (Psychotherapy). (519)679-3200; Fax. (519)679-3201.

BOGUSZ, Sharlene; CSSS du Nord de Lanaudière, 1000 rue Sainte-Anne, St-Charles-Brromee QC J6E 6J2; McG'94; FRCSC; OrthSurg. Staff, Centre Hospitalier Régional de Lanaudière; (450)759-8222

BOHACEK, Linda; Health Sciences Centre, 300 Prince Philip Dr, St. John's NL A1B 3V6; Tor'04; FRCSC; GenSurg. Staff, Health Sciences Centre; (709)737-6300

BOHAMED, Annie; CSSS d'Antoine-Labelle-l'Annon, 1525 rue l'Annonciation N RR 4, Riviere-Rouge QC J0T 1T0; Mon'02; Staff, Centre de L'Annonciation; (819)275-2118; Fax. (819)275-1520.

BOHAY, Jordan A W; Credit Valley Hosp, 2200 Eglinton Ave W, Mississauga ON L5M 2N1; Man'96; FRCPC; Anes. Staff, The Credit Valley Hospital; (905)813-2200 x3946

BOHDANOWICZ, Alexandre P; 4036 Catherine St GD, Dorchester ON N0L 1G0; Wes'76; Physician, Accuride of Canada & Coroner; Langs: Russian; (519)268-7301; Fax. (519)268-2397.

BOHEMIER, Robert J P; Winnipeg Reg Hlth Authority, 650 Main St, Winnipeg MB R3B 1E2; Man'09; CCFP; CCFP(E.M.).

BOHÉMIER BERNARD, Mathieu; Inuulitsivik Health Centre, GD, Povungnituq QC J0M 1P0; Sher'09; CCFP; Staff, Inuulitsivik Health Centre; (819)988-2957; Fax. (819)988-2796.

BOHM, Clara J; Health Sciences Centre, GE445-820 Sherbrook St, Winnipeg MB R3A 1R9; McM'95; BScChemEng; FRCPC; IntMed; Nephrol. Staff, Health Sciences Centre; Staff Nephrol, Winnipeg Regional Health Authority; Asst Prof, University of Manitoba; Langs: Czech; (204)774-8511

BOHM, Eric R; Concordia Hip & Knee Institute, 301-1155 Concordia Ave, Winnipeg MB R2K 2M9; McM'95; BEng; MSc; FRCSC; OrthSurg. Staff, Concordia General Hospital; Asst Prof Joint Replacement Group, University of Manitoba.

BOHN, A David; Diamond Head Med Clinic, PO Box 9200 Stn Main, Squamish BC V8B 0C1; Man'86; CCFP; FCFP; (604)892-3544; Fax. (604)892-3542.

BOHN, Mary C; Stepleford Med Clinic, 372 McCarthy Blvd N, Regina SK S4R 7M2; Sask'91; FRCPC; IntMed (Family Medicine). (306)545-3000; Fax. (306)545-5584.

BOHNEN, John M A; St Michael's Hosp, 3 044SW-30 Bond St, Toronto ON M5B 1W8; Tor'75; FACS; FRCSC; GenSurg (Hernias). Staff, St Michael's Hospital; Vice Dean Clinical Affairs, University of Toronto; (416)864-3047; Fax. (416)864-5163; bohnenj@smh.toronto.on.ca.

BOHONIS, Dianne H; PO Box 1303 Stn A, Comox BC V9M 7Z8; Alb'90; CCFP; (250)218-2831

BOHORQUEZ, Anibal F; G F Strong Rehab Centre, 4255 Laurel St, Vancouver BC V5Z 2G9; Qns'05; FRCPC; PhysMed&Rehab. Staff, G F Strong Rehabilitation Centre; Langs: Spanish; (604)734-1313

BOHORQUEZ CARDENAS, Diogenes A; Bonaventure Med Clinic, 101-12427 Bonaventure Dr SE, Calgary AB T2J 3N8; (403)225-9499

BOIES, R Robert; Clinique Med St-Francois, 201-8495 rue Adrien, Laval QC H7A 1J9; Mon'75; (450)665-1702; Fax. (450)665-1622.

BOILARD, Christiane; Centre Hosp Paul-Gilbert, 9330 boul du Centre Hospitalier, Levis QC G6X 1L6; Laval'79; CCFP; FCFP; Staff, Centre Hospitalier Paul-Gilbert; (418)380-8993 x2088; christiane.boilard@gmf.gouv.qc.ca.

BOILARD, Jessy; CSSS de Maskinongé, 450 2e rue, Louiseville QC J5V 1V3; Laval'10; CCFP; Staff, CSSS de Maskinongé; (819)228-2731

BOILARD, Yvon; GMF des Deux Rives, 1200 rue King E, Sherbrooke QC J1G 1E4; Sher'78; CCFP; FCFP; Ac Staff, Centre Hospitalier Regional du Grand-Portage; (819)780-2222

BOILARD-LAMONTAGNE, Catherine; GMF Grand-Mere, 200-1050 8e rue, Grand-Mere QC G9T 4L4; Laval'08; CCFP; (819)729-0178

BOILEAU, Bernard; Hôpital Ste-Justine, 3175 ch Cote-Sainte-Catherine, Montreal QC H3T 1C5; Ott'80; FRCPC; Psy (Child Psychiatry). Ac Staff, Hôpital Ste-Justine; Prof, Universite de Montreal; (514)345-4695; Fax. (514)345-4635.

BOILEAU, Elisabeth; CHUM-Hop Notre-Dame, 1560 rue Sherbrooke E, Montreal QC H2L 4M1; CCFP; CCFP(E.M.); Staff, Centre Hospitalier l'Université de Montréal (CHUM) - Hôpital Notre-Dame; (514)890-8000

BOILEAU, Jacques; Hop Maisonneuve-Rosemont, 5415 boul de l'Assomption, Montreal QC H1T 2M4; Mon'67; FRCPC; HemPath; Hem (P.Q.). Staff, Hopital Maisonneuve-Rosemont; Langs: English; (514)252-3741

BOILEAU, Jean; Hop Maisonneuve-Rosemont, 5415 boul de l'Assomption, Montreal QC H1T 2M4; Mon'71; Neur. Ac Staff Neurol, Hopital Maisonneuve-Rosemont; adj Prof, Universite de Montreal; (514)252-3528; Fax. (514)252-3529.

BOILEAU, Jean-Francois; SMBD Jewish Gen Hosp, 3755 ch Cote-Sainte-Chaterine, Montreal QC H3T 1E2; Mon'00; FRCSC; GenSurg; General Surgical Oncology (P.Q.). Staff, Sir Mortimer B Davis Jewish General; (514)340-8248

BOILEAU, Laurianne; Institut de Cardiologie de Mtl, 5000 rue Belanger, Montreal QC H1T 1C8; Mon'06; Cardiol; IntMed. Staff, Institut de Cardiologie de Montréal; (514)376-3330

BOILEAU, Marc A; 400-2609 Westview Dr, North Vancouver BC V7N 4M2; Alb'80; BSc; CCFP; Langs: English; French; (604)980-0012; Fax. (604)980-0063.

BOILEAU, Martin; 1105-3030 boul Le Carrefour, Laval QC H7T 2P5; Mon'91; Ophth. Staff, Centre Hospitalier Laurentien; (450)688-6574

BOILEAU, Michel; 2157 rue Fleury E, Montreal QC H2B 1K1; Mon'73; Langs: English; (514)381-5808; Fax. (514)381-9872.

BOILEAU, Robert; CHUS-Hop Fleurimont, 2616-3001 12e Av N, Sherbrooke QC J1H 5N4; Sher'74; FRCPC; Respir; IntMed (P.Q.). Staff, Centre Hospitalier Universitaire de Sherbrooke-Hopital Fleurimont; Assoc Staff, Hôpital Sainte-croix; (819)822-6735; Fax. (819)820-6420.

BOILLAT, Miriam E; St Mary's Hosp Centre, 3830 av Lacombe, Montreal QC H3T 1M5; McG'83; CCFP; FCFP; Staff, St Mary's Hospital Centre; assoc Doyen Faculty Development, McGill University; Langs: English; French; (514)734-2629; Fax. (514)734-2602.

BOILY, Anik; CSSS Cleophas-Claveau, CP 38 Succ La Baie 1000 rue Du Docteur-Desgagne, La Baie QC G7B 3P9; Mon'91; Staff, CHSLD-CLSC Cleophas-Claveau; (418)544-3381

BOILY, Camil; Polyclinique, 215-874 boul de l'Universite E, Chicoutimi QC G7H 6B9; Laval'70; Neur (P.Q.); Electroenceph (P.Q.). Ac Staff, Complexe hospitalier de la Sagamie; (418)549-9571; Fax. (418)549-8631.

BOILY, Emilie; Hotel-Dieu de Sorel, 400 av Hotel-Dieu, Sorel-Tracy QC J3P 1N5; Mon'08; CCFP; Staff, Hôtel-Dieu de Sorel; (450)746-6000

BOILY, Helene; Centre Hosp Honore-Mercier, 2750 boul Laframboise, Saint-Hyacinthe QC J2S 4Y8; Mon'95; FRCSC; GenSurg. Staff, Centre Hospitalier Honore-Mercier; (450)771-3335

BOILY, Isabelle; Centre Medical Isamed, 682 ch de Saint-Jean, La Prairie QC J5R 2L4; Sher'87; (450)659-4777; Fax. (450)659-3391.

BOILY, Jean-Claude; Clinique de Med Familiale Gati, 201-908 boul Maloney E, Gatineau QC J8P 1H5; Laval'93; CCFP; Staff, Hôpital de Gatineau; (819)663-7711; Fax. (819)663-9326.

BOILY, Karine; Polyclinique St-Eustache, 75 rue Grignon, St-Eustache QC J7P 4J2; Mon'99; FRCSC; ObstGyn. (450)491-1150

BOILY, Marcel; Ctr Hosp Pierre-Janet, 20 rue Pharand, Gatineau QC J9A 1K7; Laval'74; FRCPC; Psy. Staff, Centre Hospitalier Pierre-Janet; (819)776-8028

BOILY, Mathieu; MUHC-Montreal Gen Hosp, 1650 av Cedar, Montreal QC H3G 1A4; Sher'05; FRCPC; DiagRad. Staff, McGill University Health Centre - Montreal General Campus; (514)934-1934

BOILY, Mireille; Clinique de Med Gen d'Alma, 22 rue Melancon E, Alma QC G8B 6W3; Sher'87; Chef gériatrie, CSSS de Lac-Saint Jean-Est; Prof, Universite de Sherbrooke; Langs: Bilingual(French/English); (418)668-2377; Fax. (418)668-0873; mireille.boily@ssss.gouv.qc.ca.

BOILY, Nathalie; Clinique Med des Sommets, 1070 rue Principale, Ste-Agathe-des-Mts QC J8C 1L6; Mon'99; (819)321-1212; Fax. (819)321-3232.

BOILY, Pierre; Clinique Med La Perade, CP 250 81 Ricard, Ste-Anne-Per QC G0X 2J0; Laval'89; LMCC; (418)325-2777; Fax. (418)325-3521.

BOILY, Raynald C; Port Health Clinic, 7-600 Ontario St, St Catharines ON L2N 7H8; Man'84; (905)934-1666; Fax. (905)934-2595.

BOILY, Yves; Hotel-Dieu de Roberval, 450 rue Brassard, Roberval QC G8H 1B9; Sher'89; IntMed (P.Q.) (Echography Cardiac). Staff, Hotel-Dieu de Roberval; (418)275-0110; Fax. (418)275-2109.

BOIRE, Gilles; CHUS-Hop Fleurimont, 3858-3001 12e av N, Sherbrooke QC J1H 5N4; Sher'81; MRCP; MMedSci; FRCPC; IntMed (Adult Rheumatology); Rheum. Staff Rheum, Centre Hospitalier Universitaire de Sherbrooke-Hopital Fleurimont; Prof Med & Rheum Div, Universite de Sherbrooke; Langs: Bilingual(English/French); (819)564-5261; Fax. (819)564-5265; gilles.boire@usherbrooke.ca.

BOIRE-LAVIGNE, Anne-Marie; CHUS-Hop Fleurimont, 3001 12e Av N, Sherbrooke QC J1H 5N4; Mon'88; CCFP; Staff, Centre Hospitalier Universitaire de Sherbrooke-Hopital Fleurimont; (819)346-1110 x14273

BOIS, Aaron J; Dept of Nomadic Engineer, 2500 University Dr NW, Calgary AB T2N 1N4; Ott'05; FRCSC; OrthSurg. (403)220-5077; Fax. (403)282-6170.

BOIS, Alain; 504-76 rue Saint-Paul, Quebec QC G1K 3V9; Laval'74; Ac Staff, Hôpital Laval; (418)654-5733

BOIS, Christine; Clin Med Horizon Sante, 8 boul des Iles, Port-Cartier QC G5B 2J4; Mon'84; Staff, CLSC-CSSS de Port-Cartier; Langs: Bilingual(French/English); (418)766-4643; Fax. (418)766-4374.

BOIS, Marc-A.; Institut de Cardiologie de Mtl, 5000 rue Belanger, Montreal QC H1T 1C8; Mon'57; FACC; CSPQ; Cardiol (P.Q.). Staff, Institut de Cardiologie de Montréal; Clin Adj, Universite de Montreal; (514)376-3330 x231; Fax. (514)593-2540.

BOIS, Marie-Lou; CSSS de l'Energie-Ste-Therese, 1705 av Georges, Shawinigan QC G9N 2N1; Laval'98; FRCPC; Psy. Staff, CH du Centre-de-la-Mauricie (Ste-Thérèse de Shawinigan); (819)537-9351; marie-lou_bois@ssss.gouv.qc.ca.

BOIS, Sylvie; Ctr Hosp de Verdun, 4000 boul Lasalle, Verdun QC H4G 2A3; Mon'90; BSc; CSPQ; FRCPC; Anes. Staff Anes, Centre Hospitalier de Verdun; (514)362-1000 x2829

BOISCLAIR, Chantal; CSSS de Rivière-de-Loup, 75 rue Saint-Henri, Riviere-Du-Loup QC G5R 2A4; Laval'92; FRCPC; DiagRad. Staff, Centre Hospitalier Regional du Grand-Portage; (418)868-1010 x381; Fax. (418)868-1035.

BOISCLAIR, Philippe; CHUQ-Ctr Hosp Univ Laval, 2705 boul Laurier, Quebec QC G1V 4G2; Laval'04; CCFP; CCFP(E.M.); Staff, Centre Hospitalier Universitaire de Quebec-CHUL; (418)525-4444

BOISJOLI, Jacques; CSSS de l'Energie-Ste-Therese, 1705 av Georges, Shawinigan QC G9N 2N1; Laval'74; Staff, CH du Centre-de-la-Mauricie (Ste-Thérèse de Shawinigan); (819)336-7575; Fax. (819)537-4098; jacques_boisjoli@ssss.gouv.qc.ca.

BOISJOLY, Andre; CSSS de Laval, 1755 boul Rene-Laennec, Laval QC H7M 3L9; Mon'77; AB; FRCPC; DiagRad. Staff, Hopital de la Cite de la santé; (450)975-5406; Fax. (450)975-5545.

BOISJOLY, Helene; Hop Maisonneuve-Rosemont, 5415 boul de l'Assomption, Montreal QC H1T 2M4; Sher'77; FACS; FRCSC; Ophth. Staff, Hopital Maisonneuve-Rosemont; Dean Faculty of Med, Universite de Montreal; (514)252-3400 x1733; helene.boisjoly@umontreal.ca.

BOISJOLY, Josie-Anne; Hop Charles LeMoyne, 3120 boul Tashereau, Greenfield Park QC J4V 2H1; Sher'05; FRCPC; IntMed; MedOncol; Hem. Staff, Hopital Charles LeMoyne; (450)466-5000

BOISMENU, Celine; Clinique Med de L'Edifice, 204-31 rue King O, Sherbrooke QC J1H 1N5; Mon'85; Council Member, Centre Hospitalier Universitaire de Sherbrooke-Hôpital Hôtel-Dieu; Staff Sub-Investigator, Diex Recherche; Clinical Teaching Prof, Universite de Sherbrooke; Langs: Bilingual(French/English); (819)346-6111; Fax. (819)346-7184; cboismenu@cmdec.com.

BOISMIER, Jenny L; 1500-2109 Ottawa St, Windsor ON N8Y 1R8; Wes'04; CCFP; (519)254-0303; Fax. (519)254-8800.

BOISSE-RHEAULT, Emmanuelle; CSSS du Nord de Lanaudière, 1000 boul Sainte-Anne, St-Charles-Brromee QC J6E 6J2; Mon'98; Staff, Centre Hospitalier Régional de Lanaudière; (450)759-8222

BOISSELLE, Andree; CSSS de Rimouski-Neigette, CP 3150 Succ A, Rimouski QC G5L 5T1; Laval'73; Endocrin (P.Q.). Staff, Hôpital Regional Rimouski; (418)723-7851

BOISSELLE, Diane; Clinique Med Sillery, 1270 av William, Quebec QC G1S 4G1; Laval'78; LMCC; Psychiatre, CSSS de Quebec Nord; Langs: English; (418)688-0664; Fax. (418)688-4601.

BOISSELLE, Jacques; Clinique Med Fam Jonquiere, 3835 boul Harvey, Jonquiere QC G7X 2Z5; Sher'77; (418)572-7519; Fax. (418)542-6541.

BOISSINOT, Pierre; CSSS de Portneuf, 700 rue Saint-Cyrille, Saint-Raymond QC G3L 1W1; Laval'70; Staff, Centre Hospitalier Portneuf; (418)337-4611

BOISSONEAU, Mary-Lee; 5-12 Castleridge Dr NE, Calgary AB T3J 1V4; NOSM'09; (403)262-4472

BOISSONNAULT, Michel; Clinique Med l'Actuel, 1130-1001 Boul De Maisonneuve, Montreal QC H2L 4P9; Mon'68; (514)524-1001; Fax. (514)524-3831.

BOISSONNAULT, Pierre; 105-185 av Acadie, Dieppe NB E1A 1G6; Sher'94; CCFP; (506)862-4182; Fax. (506)862-4179.

BOISSONNEAULT, Josee; Hotel-Dieu de Sorel, 400 av de l'Hotel-Dieu, Sorel-Tracy QC J3P 1N5; Laval'91; Staff, Hôtel-Dieu de Sorel; (450)746-6000

BOISSONNEAULT, Josee; Hop du Sacre-Coeur de Mtl, 5400 boul Gouin O, Montreal QC H4J 1C5; Mon'90; Staff, Hôpital du Sacre-Coeur de Montréal; Physician, Polyclinique de Boisbriand; (514)338-2050

BOISSONNEAULT, Mario; Clinique Med Saint-Marc, 1295 boul Saint-Sacrement, Shawinigan QC G9N 3M8; Laval'88; Staff, Centre Hospitalier du Centre la Mauricie; (819)539-2999; Fax. (819)539-0078.

BOISSY, Benoit; 23F-500 boul Rene-Levesque O, Montreal QC H2Z 1W7; Mon'90; (514)873-8030 x5083

BOISVENU, Joseph A G; Royal Columbian Hosp, 330 Columbia St E, New Westminster BC V3L 3W7; McM'85; FRCPC; Anes. Staff, Royal Columbian Hospital; (604)520-4603; Fax. (604)520-4834.

BOISVENUE, Marc André; Markham Walk-In Clinic, 3603 Highway 7, Markham ON L3R 8W3; Ott'09; CCFP; (905)474-5764

BOISVERT, Anne-Marie; Coop Sante de Contrecoeur, 4915 rte Marie-Victorin, Contrecoeur QC J0L 1C0; Mon'07.

BOISVERT, Annie; CSSTR Ctre Services Les Forges, 500 rue Saint-Georges, Trois-Rivieres QC G9A 2K8; Laval'96; CCFP; (819)379-7131; Fax. (819)379-9440.

BOISVERT, Caroline; Agence de sante Laurentides, 200-1000 rue Labelle, St-Jerome QC J7Z 5N6; Mon'92; Staff, Groupe Sante Voyage Laval; Médecin, Direction Sante Publique Laurentides; Langs: French; Spanish; English; (450)436-8622 x2253; Fax. (450)569-6305.

BOISVERT, Catherine; Hôpital régional Chaleur, 1750 Sunset Dr, Bathurst NB E2A 4L7; Sher'06; FRCPC; Anes. Staff, Hopital Regional Chaleur; (506)544-3000

BOISVERT, Denis; CSSSG-Hop de Hull, 116 boul Lionel-Emond, Gatineau QC J8Y 1W7; Sher'83; FRCPC; IntMed; Nephrol. Staff, Hull Hospital; (819)595-6000

BOISVERT, Denis E; M Gen George R Pearkes Bldg, 101 Colonel By Dr, Ottawa ON K1A 0K2; Sher'78; FRCPC; Psy. Staff, Canadian Forces Health Services Centre; (613)945-1060; Fax. (613)945-1070.

BOISVERT, Emilie; Centre Hosp Honore-Mercier, 2750 boul Laframboise, Saint-Hyacinthe QC J2S 4Y8; Sher'09; CCFP; Staff, Centre Hospitalier Honore-Mercier; (450)771-3333

BOISVERT, Genevieve; Hop Charles LeMoyne, 3120 boul Taschereau, Greenfield Park QC J4V 2H1; Sher'03; DiagRad. Staff, Hopital Charles LeMoyne; (450)466-5000

BOISVERT, Glenn; CSSS Haut-Richelieu-Rouville, 920 boul du Seminaire N, St-Jean-sur-Richel QC J3A 1B7; Sher'02; FRCPC; DiagRad. Staff, Hôpital du Haut-Richelieu; (450)359-5000

BOISVERT, Guy; Barrie Memorial Hosp, GD 28 rue Gale, Ormstown QC J0S 1K0; Laval'74; FRCPC; DiagRad (Echography). Staff, Barrie Memorial Hospital; (450)829-2321 x3268; Fax. (450)829-2632; guy_boisvert@rrsss16.gouv.qc.ca.

BOISVERT, Isabelle; 75 rue Saint-Henri, Riviere-Du-Loup QC G5R 2A4; Laval'92; FRCSC; Urol. Staff, Centre Hospitalier Regional du Grand-Portage; Langs: Bilingual(French/English); (418)868-1000; Fax. (418)868-0166.

BOISVERT, Jacques; Clin de Radiologie Montreal-No, 5636 boul Henri-Bourassa E, Montreal-Nord QC H1G 2T2; Mon'65; DiagRad. Ac Staff, Hôpital Ste-Justine; (514)325-9426; Fax. (514)325-9427.

BOISVERT, Jean-Francois; CSSS du Nord de Lanaudière, 1000 boul Sainte-Anne, St-Charles-Brromee QC J6E 6J2; Laval'83; FRCPC; MedMicrobiol. Staff, Centre Hospitalier Régional de Lanaudière; (450)759-8222 x2673; jean-francois.boisvert@ssss.gouv.qc.ca.

BOISVERT, Karine E; UMF Nord de Lanaudiere, 50 ch du Golf E, St-Charles-Brromee QC J6E 2B4; Sher'95; CCFP; Staff, Centre Hospitalier Régional de Lanaudière; (450)759-3060; Fax. (450)759-7799.

BOISVERT, Laurent; Hop Charles Lemoyne, 3120 boul Taschereau, Longueuil QC J4V 2H1; Staff, Hopital Charles LeMoyne; (450)466-5000

BOISVERT, Marianne; Ctr Hosp de Verdun, 4000 boul Lasalle, Verdun QC H4G 2A3; Mon'93; BSc; FRCPC; Psy (Consultation-Liaison). Consultant Psy, Centre Hospitalier de Verdun; Staff Clin Psy, Douglas Mental Health University Institute; (514)362-1000

BOISVERT, Mariette; CSSSG-Hop de Gatineau, 909 Boul de la Verendrye O, Gatineau QC J8P 7H2; Sher'82; FRCPC; Peds (Asthma). Staff, Hôpital de Gatineau; Langs: English; (819)561-8565; Fax. (819)561-8103; mariette_boisvert@ssss.gouv.qc.ca.

BOISVERT, Martin-Pierre; CSSS d'Antoine-Labelle-Mt Laur, 2561 ch de la Lievre S, Mont-Laurier QC J9L 3G3; Mon'09; CCFP; (819)623-1234

BOISVERT, Nathalie; Hop Charles Lemoyne, 3120 boul Taschereau, Greenfield Park QC J4V 2H1; Mon'92; Staff, Hopital Charles LeMoyne; (450)466-5050

BOISVERT, Paule; Clinique Med St-Louis, 220-3165 ch Saint-Louis, Quebec QC G1W 4R4; Laval'83; CCFP; FCFP; Assoc Staff, Centre Hospitalier Affilié Universitaire de Québec - Hôpital du St-Sacrement; (418)653-1970; Fax. (418)653-9956.

BOISVERT, Philippe; CSSS du Sud de Lanaudière, 911 Montee des Pionniers, Terrebonne QC J6V 2H2; Mon'09; CCFP; Staff, Centre Hospitalier Pierre le Gardeur; (450)654-7525

BOISVERT, Pierre; CHUQ-St-Francois d'Assise, 10 rue de l'Espinay, Quebec QC G1L 3L5; Laval'71; Otol. Ac Staff, Centre Hospitalier Universitaire De Québec - Pavillon De St-françois-d'assise; Head Dept of Otol, Université Laval; (418)525-4310; Fax. (418)525-4464.

BOISVERT, Pierre; Clinique Med Chateauguay, 120 boul Saint-Jean-Baptiste, Chateauguay QC J6K 3A9; Mon'76; (450)691-8191; Fax. (450)691-8568.

BOISVERT, Rejean; Ctr Medi Soleil St-Jean-Sur-Ri, 120-383 boul du Seminaire N, St-Jean-sur-Richel QC J3B 8C5; Laval'88; (450)347-7557

BOISVERT, Rene; CSSS de la Cote-De-Gaspe, 215 boul de York O, Gaspe QC G4X 2W2; Laval'65; Psy (P.Q.). Staff, Centre Hospitalier de Gaspe; (418)368-3301 x4220; Fax. (418)368-3481; reneboisvertmd@xplornet.com.

BOISVERT, Rene; Dr Everett Chalmers Reg Hosp, PO Box 9000 Stn A, Fredericton NB E3B 5N5; Dal'05; FRCSC; GenSurg. Staff, Dr Everett Chalmers Regional Hospital; (506)452-5400

BOISVERT, Richard; CHUS-Hop Hotel-Dieu, 580 rue Bowen S, Sherbrooke QC J1G 2E8; Mon'83; MSc; FRCPC; CommunMed; Public Health & Preventive Med; EmergMed (P.Q.). Staff, Centre Hospitalier Universitaire de Sherbrooke-Hôpital Hôtel-Dieu; Community Med, Centre Hospitalier Laurentien; Staff, Hôtel-Dieu de Saint-Jérôme; (819)346-1110

BOISVERT, Wilfrid; 6796 crois Verdon, Laval QC H7L 4P9; Mon'78; (450)622-3645

BOITEAU, Étienne; CSSS Des Iles, 430 ch Principal, Cap-aux-Meules QC G4T 1R9; Mon'06; Staff, Hôpital de l'Archipel; (418)986-2121; Fax. (418)986-7010.

BOITEAU, Paul J E; Foothills Med Centre, 1403 29 St NW, Calgary AB T2N 2T9; Laval'79; ABIM(CriticalCare); FRCPC; Respir; IntMed (Critical Care Medicine). Staff, Foothills Medical Centre; Dept Head Critical Care Med, University Of Calgary; (403)944-2471; Fax. (403)283-9994.

BOIVIN, Andrée; CSSS de la Baie-des-Chaleurs, RR 2 419 boul Perron, Maria QC G0C 1Y0; Laval'09; CCFP; Staff, CSSS de la Baie-des-Chaleurs; (418)759-3443; Fax. (418)759-5063.

BOIVIN, Antoine; Ctre de Recherche Charles Lemo, 200-150 Place Charles-Le Moyne, Longueuil QC J4K 0A8; Mon'02; CCFP; Staff, Centre Hospitalier Rouyn-Noranda; (514)775-5064

BOIVIN, Daniel; The Ottawa Cardiovascular Ctre, 502-1355 Bank St, Ottawa ON K1H 8K7; Sher'89; FRCPC; IntMed. (613)738-0088

BOIVIN, Diane; Douglas Mental Hlth Univ Inst, 6875 boul Lasalle, Verdun QC H4H 1R3; Laval'85; Staff, Douglas Mental Health University Institute; (514)761-6131 x2397

BOIVIN, Eric; CSSS de Chicoutimi, 305 rue Saint-Vallier, Chicoutimi QC G7H 5H6; Sher'89; FRCSC; OrthSurg (P.Q.). Staff, Complexe hospitalier de la Sagamie; (418)541-1000

BOIVIN, Frederic; CSSS du Grand Littoral, 1205 boul de la Rive-Sud, Levis QC G6W 0J4; Laval'08; CCFP; (418)380-8597

BOIVIN, Genevieve; Inuulitsivik Health Centre, GD, Povungnituq QC J0M 1P0; Laval'09; CCFP; Staff, Inuulitsivik Health Centre; (819)988-2957; Fax. (819)988-2796.

BOIVIN, Gilles; Ctr Hosp de Charlevoix, 74 rue Ambroise-Fafard, Baie-Saint-Paul QC G3Z 2J6; Laval'84; Staff, CSSS de Charlevoix; (418)435-5150

BOIVIN, Guy; CHUQ-Ctr Hosp Univ Laval, 2705 boul Laurier, Quebec QC G1V 4G2; Laval'85; FRCPC; MedMicrobiol. Staff, Centre Hospitalier Universitaire de Quebec-CHUL; (418)654-2705; guy.boivin@crchul.ulaval.ca.

BOIVIN, Jean-François; SMBD Jewish Gen Hosp, H411-3755 ch Cote-Ste-Catherin, Montreal QC H3T 1E2; Laval'73; DSc(Harvard) - (Epidemiol; FRCPC; CommunMed. Med Consultant, McGill University Health Centre - Montreal General Campus; Researcher, Sir Mortimer B Davis Jewish General; Prof, McGill University; Langs: German; English; (514)340-8273; Fax. (514)340-8142.

BOIVIN, Johanne; 3100 av Ellendale, Montreal QC H3S 1W3; Mon'79; FRCPC; Psy. Ac Staff, Hôpital Ste-Justine; (514)345-4931 x5729

BOIVIN, Jules; 410-3165 ch Saint-Louis, Quebec QC G1W 4R4; Laval'81; FRCSC; OrthSurg. Assoc Member, Complexe hospitalier de la Sagamie; (418)681-0167

BOIVIN, Julie; CSSS de la Baie-des-Chaleurs, RR 2 419 boul Perron, Maria QC G0C 1Y0; Sher'93; Staff, CSSS de la Baie-des-Chaleurs; (418)759-3443; Fax. (418)759-1344; hippocrate@globetrotter.net.

BOIVIN, Marie-Christine; Inst Albert Prevost, 6555 boul Gouin O, Montreal QC H4K 1B3; Laval'02; Psy. (514)338-3227

BOIVIN, Michel; CHUM-Hop St-Luc, 1058 rue Saint-Denis, Montreal QC H2X 3J4; Mon'78; FRCPC; Gastroent. Staff, Centre Hospitalier l'Université De Montréal (CHUM) - Hôpital Saint-luc; (514)890-8000 x35755; Fax. (514)890-8356; michel.boivin@umontreal.ca.

BOIVIN, Michelle F; Aberfoyle Health Centre, 102-304 The East Mall, Etobicoke ON M9B 6E2; Ott'90; BSc(Hons); MSc; (416)231-7968; Fax. (416)231-7982.

BOIVIN, Pierre R; Medical Clinic, B-354 rte du Pont, Saint-Nicolas QC G7A 2V3; Laval'96; CCFP; (418)496-3091

BOIVIN RIVEROS, Marie Claire; Civic Family Med Centre, 210 Melrose Ave, Ottawa ON K1Y 4K7; Univ of Juan N Corpas (Colombia)'99; CCFP; (613)761-4334

BOJANOWSKA-MOORE, Czeslawa; Burrard Health Bldg, 201-1160 Burrard St, Vancouver BC V6Z 2E8; Lodz (Poland)'56; (604)688-0909

BOJANOWSKI, Wieslaw M; CHUM-Hop Notre-Dame, 1560 rue Sherbrooke E, Montreal QC H2L 4M1; Mon'80; FRCSC; Neursurg. Chef NeuroSurg, Centre Hospitalier l'Université de Montréal (CHUM) - Hôpital Notre-Dame; Chef NeuroSurg, Centre Hospitalier l'Université De Montréal (CHUM) - Hôpital Saint-luc; Chef NeuroSurg, Centre Hospitalier l'Université de Montréal (CHUM) - Hôtel-Dieu; Prog Dir NeuroSurg, Universite de Montreal; (514)526-8525; Fax. (514)412-7816; michel.bojanowski.chum@ssss.gouv.qc.ca.

BOJCEVSKI, Alexandra T; Hamilton HS-General Site, 8N 01-237 Barton St E, Hamilton ON L8L 2X2; Wes'07; IntMed. Staff, Hamilton Health Sciences Centre - Hamilton General Hospital.

BOJM, Morris A; A-145 Columbia St E, New Westminster BC V3L 3W2; Tor'75; FRCSC; GenSurg (Breast Surgery). Staff Surg, Royal Columbian Hospital; Staff Surg, Eagle Ridge Hospital & Health Care Centre; (604)521-5986; Fax. (604)521-9122.

BOKENFOHR, Grace M; 1931 105 St NW, Edmonton AB T6J 5V9; Alb'80; Member Med Advisory Committee, Covenant Health - St. Joseph's Auxilliary Hospital; (780)438-3241; Fax. (780)435-2511.

BOKHOUT, Maarten; 105 Shipley St PO Box 856, Clinton ON N0M 1L0; Tor'77; MHSc; CCFP; FCFP; Site Chief Attending Staff, Clinton Public Hospital - Huron Perth Healthcare Alliance; Langs: French; Dutch; German; (519)482-3000; Fax. (519)482-7648; mcbokhout@gmail.com.

BOKORE, Wasira G; Canes Family Health Team, 200-135 Queen's Plate Dr, Etobicoke ON M9W 6V1; Dar Es Salaam (Tanzania)'99; CCFP; (416)342-5140; Fax. (416)342-5148.

BOKTOR, Basem W H; Gander Medical Clinic, 177 Elizabeth Dr, Gander NL A1V 1H6; Assiut (Egypt)'03; MB ChB; CCFP; Staff, Brookfield Bonnews Health Care Centre; (709)571-0262

BOKTOR, Fekri; Oakville Med Clinic, 306A-331 Sheddon Ave, Oakville ON L6J 1X8; Ain Shams (Egypt)'76; CCFP; (905)337-1101; Fax. (905)337-0782.

BOLAJI, Yemisi I; 270-5 Fairview Mall Dr, North York ON M2J 2Z1; Ilorin (Nigeria)'90; CCFP; Staff, Sunnybrook Health Sciences Centre; (416)493-5244

BOLAND, Margaret P; Children's Hosp of Eastern Ont, 401 Smyth Rd, Ottawa ON K1H 8L1; Qns'77; FRCPC; Peds (Pediatric Gastroenterology); Gastroent. Staff Peds, Children's Hospital of Eastern Ontario (CHEO); Staff, Ottawa Children's Treatment Centre; Assoc Prof Peds, University of Ottawa; (613)737-7600 x2516; Fax. (613)738-4854.

BOLANO DEL VECCHIO, Silvana M; College Square Med Centre, 1980 Baseline Rd, Ottawa ON K2C 0C6; Ott'06; FRCPC; IntMed; Gastroent. Staff, The Ottawa Hospital - General Campus; (613)224-6606; Fax. (613)224-6162.

BOLARIA, Roxana K; Helmcken Pediatric Associates, 212-284 Helmcken Rd, Victoria BC V9B 1T2; Sask'93; FRCPC; Peds (Pediatric Rheumatology); Rheum. Staff, Victoria General Hospital; Clin Instructor, University of British Columbia; (250)881-7347; Fax. (250)881-7349.

BOLDT, Camilla L; Providence Hematology, 440-1144 Burrard St, Vancouver BC V6Z 2A5; UBC'92; FRCPC; IntMed; Hem. Staff, Lions Gate Hospital; (604)684-5794

BOLDT, Charles I; Queen Elizabeth II Hosp, 10409 98 St, Grande Prairie AB T8V 2E8; Sask'88; FRCPC; Anes. Staff, Queen Elizabeth II Hospital; (780)538-7100

BOLDT, Michael J; 401-1200 Lonsdale Ave, North Vancouver BC V7M 3H6; UBC'92; FRCPC; IntMed. Staff, Lions Gate Hospital; (778)340-0470

BOLDUC, Alain; 35 rue Providence, Moncton NB E1C 8X3; Sher'85; FRCPC; Derm. Langs: Italian; Spanish; (506)857-1420; Fax. (506)858-0519.

BOLDUC, Bruno; Clinique Med de l'Atelier, 77 boul Seigneurial O, Saint-Bruno QC J3V 2G9; Mon'84; (450)461-1751; Fax. (450)461-1602.

BOLDUC, Chantal; Clinique Med Cartier, 502-1851 rue Sherbrooke E, Montreal QC H2K 4L5; Mon'94; FRCPC; Derm. Staff, Centre Hospitalier l'Université de Montréal (CHUM) - Hôpital Notre-Dame; (514)521-8333; Fax. (514)521-4175.

BOLDUC, Francois; Edmonton Clinic Health Academy, 4 588-11405 87 Ave NW, Edmonton AB T6G 1C9; Sher'98; FRCPC; Neur (Pediatric Neurology). Staff, University of Alberta Hospital; (780)248-5569; Fax. (780)248-5627.

BOLDUC, Francois; CSSS de la Haute-Cote-Nord, RR 1 4 rue de l'Hopital, Les Escoumins QC G0T 1K0; Laval'06; Gen Practice, Centre de santé des Côté-Nord; (418)233-2931

BOLDUC, Gerard-Raymond; 3300 boul le Carrefour, Laval QC H7T 0A1; Laval'75; (450)687-3300

BOLDUC, Guy; Centre Med Sillery, 1270 av William, Quebec QC G1S 4G1; Laval'84; LMCC; Staff, Centre Hospitalier Affilié Universitaire de Québec - Hôpital du St-Sacrement; Staff, Jeffery Hale Hospital-Saint Brigid's; (418)688-0664; Fax. (418)688-4601.

BOLDUC, Jean-Philippe; Hotel-Dieu de Levis, 143 rue Wolfe, Levis QC G6V 3Z1; Laval'99; FRCPC; DiagRad. Staff, Hôtel-Dieu de Lévis; (418)656-8711

BOLDUC, Louis; CSSS du Nord de Lanaudière, 1000 boul Sainte-Anne, St-Charles-Brromee QC J6E 6J2; Mon'96; CSPQ; Anes. Staff, Centre Hospitalier Régional de Lanaudière; (450)759-8222

BOLDUC, Michel; Inst U en Sante Mentale de QC, 2601 ch de la Canardiere, Quebec QC G1J 2G3; Laval'97; FRCPC; Psy. Staff, Institut Universitaire Sante; (418)663-5000 x6782; Fax. (418)661-6891.

BOLDUC, Monique; Clinique Med De Bernieres, 479 ch St-Joseph, Saint-Nicolas QC G7A 1N3; Laval'75; Ac Staff, Centre Hospitalier Affilié Universitaire de Québec - Hôpital du St-Sacrement; Ac Staff, Centre Hospitalier Universitaire De Québec - Pavillon De St-françois-d'assise; (418)831-9228

BOLDUC, Nadia; Clinique Sante le Frontenac, 202-5200 rue Frontenac, Lac-Megantic QC G6B 1H3; Sher'09; CCFP; Staff, CSSS du Granit; (819)583-0157

BOLDUC, Philippe; CHUM-Hotel-Dieu, 3840 rue Saint-Urbain, Montreal QC H2W 1T8; Mon'65; PhD(Lond); Respir (P.Q.). Staff, Centre Hospitalier l'Université de Montréal (CHUM) - Hôtel-Dieu; adj Prof, Universite de Montreal; (514)890-8000 x15639; Fax. (514)412-7123.

BOLDUC, Renee; St Mary's Hosp Centre, 3830 av Lacombe, Montreal QC H3T 1M5; Laval'90; CSPQ; FRCPC; Anes. Staff, St Mary's Hospital Centre; (514)345-3511 x3344; renee_bolduc@yahoo.com.

BOLDUC, Richard D; 110-1926 20 Ave NW, Calgary AB T2M 1H5; Ott'75; CCFP; Ac Staff, Alberta Children's Hospital; Ac Staff, Foothills Medical Centre; University of Calgary; (403)289-9777; Fax. (403)289-4060.

BOLDUC, Sabrina; Ctre de Perinatalite l'Autre M, 575 rue Saint-Charles E, Beloeil QC J3G 0H3; Mon'09; CCFP; (450)332-9833; Fax. (450)332-0865.

BOLDUC, Sebastien; Clinique Med Privee, 201-7110 rue Marion, Trois-Rivieres QC G9A 0A7; Laval'98; (819)374-1771; Fax. (819)374-6843.

BOLDUC, Serge; CSSS de Jonquiere, CP 1200 Stn Pdf Jonquiere 2230 rue de l'Hopital, Jonquiere QC G7X 7X2; Ott'68; FRCSC; ObstGyn. Chef obst & gynécol, Centre Hospitalier Jonquiere; (418)695-7700

BOLDUC, Stephane; CHUQ-Ctr Hosp Univ Laval, R.1742-2705 boul Laurier, Quebec QC G1V 4G2; Laval'95; FAAP; FRCSC; Urol (Pediatric Urology). Staff Urol Peds, Centre Hospitalier Universitaire de Quebec-CHUL; Langs: Bilingual(English/French); (418)654-2282; Fax. (418)654-2137; sbolduc_2002@yahoo.ca.

BOLDUC, Yves; Clinique la Cite Medicale, 295-2600 boul Laurier, Quebec QC G1V 4T3; Laval'81; Staff Minister of Health & Social Services, Province of Quebec; (418)781-0480; yves_bolduc@ssss.gouv.qc.ca.

BOLESNIKOV, Grlica; New Brunswick Cancer Network, PO Box 5100 520 King St, Fredericton NB E3B 5G8; Tuzla (Bosnia-Herzegovina)'88; Staff, New Brunswick Dept of Health; Langs: Serbo-Croatian; English; (506)453-8197; Fax. (506)453-5522.

BOLESNIKOV, Zeljko; Dept of Health & Wellness, PO Box 5100 Stn A, Fredericton NB E3B 5G8; Tuzla (Bosnia-Herzegovina)'86; Member Council, College of Physicians & Surgeons of New Brunswick; Langs: German; Italian; Serbo-Croatian; Bilingual(French/English); (506)453-4294; Fax. (506)457-7671; zeljko.bolesnikov@gnb.ca.

BOLGER, J Grant W; Glazier Med Centre, 11 Gibb St, Oshawa ON L1H 2J9; McM'99; CCFP; (905)579-1212; Fax. (905)579-5548.

BOLIS, Rafik S; St Joseph's Healthcare, 50 Charlton Ave E, Hamilton ON L8N 4A6; Cairo (Egypt)'87; FRCPC; Anes;CCFP; Staff, St Joseph's Healthcare - Charlton Campus; (905)522-1155

BOLIVAR, Patricia E; 202-60 Aberdeen St, Kentville NS B4N 2N3; Dal'96; FRCPC; Peds. (902)678-1221; Fax. (902)678-2331.

BOLL, Philip R; Credit Valley Prof Bldg, 501-2300 Eglinton Ave W, Mississauga ON L5M 2V8; Dal'02; BASc(Elec.Eng); MSc(Elec. Eng); FRCPC; IntMed; Nephrol. Staff Physician, The Credit Valley Hospital; Staff Physician, Trillium Health Centre - Mississauga; (905)820-8770

BOLLAND, Mary F; 1265 Clarkson Rd N, Mississauga ON L5J 2W4; Wes'97; CCFP; (905)822-9171; Fax. (905)823-3990.

BOLLAND, Peter G; 1273 Clarkson Rd N, Mississauga ON L5J 2W4; Tor'57; CCFP; FCFP; Staff, Halton Healthcare Services Corporation - Oakville Site; Med Dir, Sheridan Villa Home For The Aged (Mississauga); (905)822-9171; Fax. (905)823-3990.

BOLLANO, Enkelejda; York Medical Green Lane, RR 1 Lcd 1 18120 Yonge St, Newmarket ON L3Y 4V8; Tirana (Albania)'97; CCFP; (905)836-1429

BOLLEDDULA, Prasad; Dalhousie University, C205-5849 University Ave, Halifax NS B3H 4H7; (India)'84; (902)473-2331

BOLLEE, Guillaume; CHUM-Hop Notre-Dame, 1560, rue Sherbrooke E, Montreal QC H2L 4M1; Staff, Centre Hospitalier l'Université de Montréal (CHUM) - Hôpital Notre-Dame; (514)890-8000

BOLLI, Peter; Ambulatory Intmed Teach Clinic, 2-80 King St, St Catharines ON L2R 7G1; Zurich (Switzerland)'62; MACP; FRCP(Edin); Staff, Ambulatory Internal Medicine Teaching Clinic; Clin Prof Med, McMaster University; Langs: German; (905)708-0050; Fax. (905)708-0040; pbolli@xenomix.com.

BOLLOZOS, Rene P; Credit Valley Med Arts Centre, 311-2000 Credit Valley Rd, Mississauga ON L5M 4N4; Cebu (Philippines)'72; Ac Staff, The Credit Valley Hospital; Court Staff, Trillium Health Centre - Mississauga; (905)828-6525; Fax. (905)828-4208.

BOLOGNA, John T; Royal Court Med Centre, 305-1 Quarry Ridge Rd, Barrie ON L4M 7G1; Wes'82; ObstGyn. Staff, Royal Victoria Regional Health Centre; (705)728-5311; Fax. (705)728-5601.

BOLOUS, Nagy; Crestview Med Clinic, 204 O'Connell Dr, Corner Brook NL A2H 5N4; (709)639-9533; Fax. (709)639-9544.

BOLSTER, Edwin L; University of Alberta Hosp, 1D1-8440 112 St NW, Edmonton AB T6G 2B7; Sask'07; FRCPC; Peds. Staff, Stollery Children's Hospital; Staff Stollery Childrens Hosp, University of Alberta Hospital; (780)407-6370; Fax. (780)407-6414.

BOLSTER, Lauren D; Clinical Sciences Bldg, 4 112-11350 83 Ave NW, Edmonton AB T6G 2P4; Sask'07; FRCPC; IntMed; Hem. (780)407-1584; Fax. (780)407-2680.

BOLTON, Charles F; 94 Stuart St, Kingston ON K7L 2V6; Qns'56; MS(Minn.); FRCPC; Neur (Electromyography). Aj Prof, Queen's University; (613)533-6000 x77813

BOLTON, Craig J; Family Med Centre, 205-145 Station St, Belleville ON K8N 2S9; Ott'08; CCFP; CCFP(E.M.); (613)771-1910

BOLTON, David R; 805-55 Garry St, Winnipeg MB R3C 4H4; McG'69; FRCPC; Psy (Psychotherapy). Assoc Staff, Health Sciences Centre; University of Manitoba; (204)942-5064

BOLTON, Gregg M; Collingwood Gen & Marine Hosp, 459 Hume St, Collingwood ON L9Y 1W9; Ott'09; CCFP; (705)445-8645

BOLTON, James E; Central North Correctional Ctr, 1501 Fuller Dr, Penetanguishene ON L9M 2H4; Tor'83; Ac Staff, The Scarborough Hospital - General Campus; (705)549-9470 x2814

BOLTON, James M S; PsycHealth Centre, PZ430-771 Bannatyne Ave, Winnipeg MB R3E 3N4; Wes'01; FRCPC; Psy.

BOMAN, Jason M; CSSS du Suroît, 150 rue Saint-Thomas, Salaber-de-Valleyf QC J6T 6C1; Mem'01; FRCSC; Urol. Staff, Centre Hospitalier Régional du Suroît; (450)371-9920

BOMAN, Jonathan C; PsycHealth Centre, PZ162-771 Bannatyne Ave, Winnipeg MB R3E 3N4; Man'03; FRCPC; Psy.

BOMAN, Robert B; Sturgeon Community Hosp, 201 Boudreau Rd, St. Albert AB T8N 6C4; Alb'74; Dir Dept of Anes, Sturgeon Community Hospital; (780)418-7310; Fax. (780)488-4823.

BOMBARDIER, Claire; The Joseph & Wolf Lebovic, 2 008-60 Murray St, Toronto ON M5T 3L9; Mon'69; FRCPC; IntMed; Rheum. Staff Rheum, Mount Sinai Hospital; (416)586-4800 x5469; claire.bombardier@utoronto.ca.

BOMBIN, Victoria E; 5001-1795 Stone Church Rd E, Stoney Creek ON L8J 0B4; McM'08; CCFP; (905)578-5959; Fax. (905)578-5953.

BOMELA, Hlwelekazi N; Children's Hosp Eastern Ont, 401 Smyth Rd, Ottawa ON K1H 8L1; Natal (South Africa)'91; FRCPC; Peds. Staff, Children's Hospital of Eastern Ontario (CHEO); (613)737-7600

BON, Lynton S; Arthur Med Clinic, PO Box 520 270 George St, Arthur ON N0G 1A0; Man'69; Court Staff, Groves Memorial Community Hospital; (519)848-3936; Fax. (519)848-3937.

BON, Richard R; Surrey Med Arts Bldg, 102-13798 94A Ave, Surrey BC V3V 1N1; UBC'98; FRCPC; IntMed (Echocardiography); Cardiol. Staff, Surrey Memorial Hospital; Langs: Bilingual(English/French); (604)588-1414

BON, Trevor J; St Joseph's Hosp, PO Box 3251 Stn P 35 Algoma St N, Thunder Bay ON P7B 5G7; Tor'94; FRCPC; IntMed; GeriatricMed. Staff, St Joseph's Care Group - St Joseph's Hospital; Staff, Thunder Bay Regional Health Sciences Centre; Prof, Northern Ontario School of Medicine-Laurentian University; (807)346-6796; Fax. (807)346-9015.

BONA, Mark D; Hotel-Dieu Hosp, 166 Brock St, Kingston ON K7L 5G2; Ott'07; FRCSC; Ophth. Staff, Hotel-Dieu Hospital; (613)544-3310; Fax. (613)544-9948.

BONACCI, Giovanni; Family First Health Centre, 4270 Innes Rd, Orleans ON K4A 5E6; Ott'08; CCFP; Staff, The Ottawa Hospital - General Campus; (613)841-7009

BONACCI, Giuseppe; Belleville Queens U Fam Med Ct, 102-145 Station St, Belleville ON K8N 2S9; Ott'08; CCFP; (613)771-1910; Fax. (613)771-1833.

BONAFEDE, Nicoletta; 121-9401 Jane St, Vaughan ON L6A 4H7; Tor'92; FRCPC; IntMed; Cardiol. (905)303-3724; Fax. (905)303-3726.

BONAN, Raoul I L; Institut de Cardiologie de Mtl, 5000 rue Belanger, Montreal QC H1T 1C8; Paris (France)'74; CSPQ; Cardiol (P.Q.). Ac Staff, Institut de Cardiologie de Montréal; Universite de Montreal; Langs: Italian; English; (514)376-3330 x3481; Fax. (514)593-2524; raoul.bonan@mmic.net.

BONANG, Lisa M; Musquodoboit Harbour Med Clin, RR 1 7907 Highway 7, Musquodbt Hbr NS B0J 2L0; Dal'93; BSc; CCFP; FCFP; Lecturer Family Med, Dalhousie University; (902)889-2650; Fax. (902)889-2577; bonangandrewy@ns.sympatico.ca.

BONAPARTE, James; 167 Sheppard Ave W, North York ON M2N 1M9; Dal'07; FRCSC; Otol. (416)229-1050

BOND, Andrew J; Weeneebayko Gen Hosp, PO Box 34 19 Hospital Dr, Moose Factory ON P0L 1W0; Ott'05; CCFP; Staff, Weeneebayko General Hospital; (705)658-4544

BOND, Anthony C; The Moncton Hosp, 135 Macbeath Ave, Moncton NB E1C 6Z8; London (England)'68; MB BS; LRCP; MRCS; FFARCS; Staff Anes, The Moncton Hospital; (506)857-5000; Fax. (506)857-5261.

BOND, David J; Mood Disorders Centre, 2C7-2255 Wesbrook Mall, Vancouver BC V6T 2A1; Mem'96; BSc; FRCPC; Psy (Mood Disorders). Consultant Psy Mood Disorders Centre-Detwiller Pavillion, UBC Hospital - Koerner Pavillion; (604)822-7512; Fax. (604)822-7922.

BOND, David M; 80 Portland St, Dartmouth NS B2Y 1H6; Cambridge (England)'75; MB BCh; MSc; DCH; MA; Anes (Chronic Pain Management). Asst Prof, Dalhousie University; (902)407-4545; Fax. (902)407-4546.

BOND, David W; Grey Nuns Community Hosp & HC, 1100 Youville Drive West NW, Edmonton AB T6L 5X8; Alb'79; Staff Emerg Dept, Covenant Health - Grey Nuns Community Hospital; Clin Instructor, University of Alberta; (780)735-7120; Fax. (780)735-7498.

BOND, Donald G; University Hosp of Northern BC, 1475 Edmonton St, Prince George BC V2M 1S2; UBC'71; CCFP; FCFP; Staff, University Hospital of Northern British Columbia; (250)565-2000

BOND, Geoffrey H; Royal Court Med Centre, 305-5 Quarry Ridge Rd, Barrie ON L4M 7G1; Qns'83; BSc(Hons); BL; CCFP; Ac Staff, Royal Victoria Regional Health Centre; Coroner, Province of Ontario; Member, College of Physicians & Surgeons of Ontario; (705)726-1788; Fax. (705)725-1601.

BOND, Lorraine; Hôtel-Dieu de Lévis, 143 rue Wolfe, Levis QC G6V 3Z1; Laval'88; FRCPC; Psy. Staff, Hôtel-Dieu de Lévis; Staff, Centre Hospitalier Affilié Universitaire de Québec - Hôpital du St-Sacrement; (418)835-7155; Fax. (418)783-5719.

BOND, Mason C; BC Women's Hosp & Health Ctre, A123-4500 Oak St, Vancouver BC V6H 3N1; UBC'86; FRCPC; Peds. Staff, BC Women's Hospital & Health Centre; (604)875-2316

BOND, Michael; SMBD Jewish Gen Hosp, 3755 ch Cote-Sainte-Catherine, Montreal QC H3T 1E2; McG'71; FRCPC; Psy. Dir Inst of Comm & Family Psy, Sir Mortimer B Davis Jewish General; Assoc Prof Psy, McGill University; (514)340-8210

BOND, R James; Surrey Med Arts Bldg, 214-13710 94A Ave, Surrey BC V3V 1N1; Cal'96; MEd; FRCSC; GenSurg; ThorSurg. Head Thoracic Surg, Surrey Memorial Hospital; (604)588-5634

BOND, Rachel L; Gulf Canada Square, 355-401 9 Ave SW, Calgary AB T2P 3C5; (Australia)'05; FRCPC; Peds. (403)221-4434

BOND, Rebecca M; Nipigon Health Centre, PO Box 870 125 Hogan Rd, Nipigon ON P0T 2J0; Sask'99; CCFP; (807)887-1644; Fax. (807)887-1645; rbond@ndmh.ca.

BOND, Stephen D; Fraserview Med Clinic, 31-665 Front St, Quesnel BC V2J 5J5; UBC'68; (250)747-0473

BONDAR, Jay S; Peace Arch Hosp, 15521 Russell Ave, White Rock BC V4B 2R4; Qns'02; FRCPC; Psy. Staff, Peace Arch Hospital; (604)541-5854

BONDAR, Roberta L; 530 Balliol St, Toronto ON M4S 1E3; McM'77; MSc(Pathol.); PhD(Neur); FRCPC; Neur (Neuro Ophthalmology). Court Staff, North York General Hospital; Scientific Staff, Sunnybrook Health Sciences Centre; (416)481-5847; Fax. (416)481-3463.

BONDAR, Steven M; The Group Health Centre, 240 Mcnabb St, Sault Ste. Marie ON P6B 1Y5; Wes'88; Ac Staff, Sault Area Hospital - Sault Ste Marie; (705)759-1234; Fax. (705)759-7487.

BONDE, Veena; King Street Med Arts Centre, 304-71 King St W, Mississauga ON L5B 4A2; Nagpur (India)'76; FRCSC; ObstGyn. (905)949-1111; Fax. (905)949-1112.

BONDER, Lauren; Group Health Centre, 240 McNabb St, Sault Ste. Marie ON P6B 1Y5; McM'09; CCFP; (905)759-1234

BONDURANT, Helen M; Royal Alexandra Hosp, 10240 Kingsway NW, Edmonton AB T5H 3V9; Alb'05; FRCPC; Psy. Staff, Royal Alexandra Hospital; (780)735-4181; Fax. (780)735-4797.

BONDY, Gregory P; St Paul's Hosp, 1081 Burrard St, Vancouver BC V6Z 1Y6; Tor'81; BSc; MSc; FRCPC; MedBiochem (Endocrinology). Ac Staff Path & LabMed, Providence Health Care - St Paul's Hospital; Clin Assoc Prof, University of British Columbia; (604)806-8192; gbondy@providencehealth.bc.ca.

BONDY, Richard J; MUHC-Montreal Gen Hosp, D10 168.3-1650 av Cedar, Montreal QC H3G 1A4; McG'85; CSPQ; FRCPC; Anes. Staff, McGill University Health Centre - Montreal General Campus; (514)934-1934 x43030

BONENFANT, Francis; CSSS du Rocher Percé, CP 3300 451 rue Mgr Ross E, Chandler QC G0C 1K0; Sher'08; IntMed. Staff, Centre Hospitalier de Chandler; (418)689-2261

BONENFANT, Guy; CSSS de Papineau, 500 rue Belanger, Gatineau QC J8L 2M4; Montpellier (France)'87; CCFP; FCFP; Staff, CH-CHSLD de Papineau - Pavillon du centre hospitalier; (819)986-3341

BONENFANT, Paul; Centre Med Prevost, CP 200 1015 rue Prevost, St-Pierre-I-D'Orl QC G0A 4E0; Laval'80; assoc Staff, Centre Hospitalier Universitaire De Québec - Pavillon De St-françois-d'assise; (418)828-2213; Fax. (418)828-2214.

BONERT, Michael; Health Sciences Centre, 300 Prince Philip Dr, St. John's NL A1B 3V6; Tor'07; FRCPC; AnatPath. Staff, Health Sciences Centre.

BONET, Jorge F; 206-301 Columbia St E, New Westminster BC V3L 3W5; Cordoba (Argentina)'73; FRCPC; Cardiol. (604)521-2148

BONGARD, Alexandra; Scarborough Hosp-General Div, 3050 Lawrence Ave E, Scarborough ON M1P 2V5; Qns'08; CCFP; CCFP(E.M.); Staff, The Scarborough Hospital - General Campus; (416)431-8200

BONGARD, Howard B; Medical Centre, 104-3000 Lawrence Ave E, Scarborough ON M1P 2V1; Qns'71; ABIM; FRCPC; IntMed (Sleep Medicine); Respir. Co-Dir Sleep Diagnostic Centre & Active Staff, The Scarborough Hospital - General Campus; (416)439-6654; Fax. (416)439-6654; bongardhb@rogers.com.

BONHAM-CARTER, Charles Riva; Change Health Care Corp, 7 Hickson Ave, Kingston ON K7K 2N4; CapeTown (South Africa)'88; MB ChB; LMCC; CCFP; (613)549-6060

BONICARD, Pierre-Alexandre; CSSS des Aurores Boreales, CP 6000 succ Bureau-Chef 679 2e rue E, La Sarre QC J9Z 2X7; Mon'08; CCFP; Staff, Centre Hospitalier La Sarre; (819)333-2311

BONIFACIO, Antonino; Niagara H System-St Catharine, PO Box 3018 Stn Main 142 Queenston St, St Catharines ON L2R 7C6; Genova (Italy)'91; Staff, Niagara Health System - St Catharines General Site; (905)378-4647

BONIFACIO, Herbert J; The Hosp for Sick Children, 555 University Ave, Toronto ON M5G 1X8; UBC'05; FRCPC; Peds (Adolescent Medicine). Staff, The Hospital For Sick Children; (416)813-4905

BONIN, Brigitte; The Ottawa Hosp-Gen Campus, 8476-501 Smyth Rd, Ottawa ON K1H 8L6; Mon'88; FRCSC; ObstGyn (Maternal Fetal Medicine). Chief ObstGyn, The Ottawa Hospital - General Campus; Asst Prof, University of Ottawa; (613)737-8968; Fax. (613)737-8070; bbonin@ottawahospital.on.ca.

BONIN, Catherine; CSSS du Lac-Des-Deux-Montagnes, 520 boul Arthur-Sauve, Saint-Eustache QC J7R 5B1; Mon'04; Staff, Hôpital de Saint-Eustache; Staff, Centre Hospitalier d'Argenteuil; (450)473-6811

BONIN, Denis M; Sudbury Reg Hosp-Laurentian Si, 41 Ramsey Lake Rd, Sudbury ON P3E 5J1; Ott'87; FRCPC; GenPath. Staff, Health Sciences North-Laurentian Site; (705)522-7100

BONIN, Diane; Clinique Ped La Courte Echelle, 101-86 boul Brien, Repentigny QC J6A 5K7; Mon'87; FRCPC; Peds. Staff, Centre Hospitalier Pierre le Gardeur; (450)657-1705; Fax. (450)657-1800.

BONIN, Frederic; Ctr Hosp Rouyn-Noranda, 4 9e rue, Rouyn-Noranda QC J9X 2B2; Laval'97; Staff, Centre Hospitalier Rouyn-Noranda; (819)764-5131; Fax. (819)764-2900.

BONIN, Jocelyne; UMF Richelieu-Yamaska, 1005 rue Gauthier, Saint-Hyacinthe QC J2S 8T2; Sher'84; CCFP; Dir UMF, Centre Hospitalier Honore-Mercier; Langs: Bilingual(French/English); Spanish; (450)771-3333 x4972; Fax. (450)771-3427.

BONIN, Melanie; Fowler-Kennedy Sport Clinic, 3M-1151 Richmond St, London ON N6A 3K7; Mon'04; Dip SportMed; CCFP; Physician, Fowler Kennedy Sport Medicine Clinic; Langs: English; (519)661-3011; Fax. (519)661-3379.

BONIN, Michel L; Sudbury Reg Hosp-Laurentian Si, 41 Ramsey Lake Rd, Sudbury ON P3E 5J1; Ott'87; GenPath. Staff, Health Sciences North-Laurentian Site; Staff Laboratory Med & Pathology, Health Sciences North-Ramsey Lake Health Center; Asst Prof, Northern Ontario School of Medicine; Langs: English; French; Fax. (705)675-4780.

BONIN, Patricia; CSSS de Manicouagan, 635 boul Joliet, Baie-Comeau QC G5C 1P1; Sher'95; FRCPC; IntMed. Staff, Centre Hospitalier Régional Baie-Comeau; (418)589-3701

BONIN, Pierre; 102-1276 Lasalle Blvd, Sudbury ON P3A 1Y8; Ott'95; CCFP; Staff, Health Sciences North-Laurentian Site; Asst Prof/Lecturer, University of Ottawa; Langs: English; French; (705)521-0753; dr.bonin@sympatico.ca.

BONIN, Richard A; CSSSG-Hop De Gatineau, CP 2000 Succ Bureau-Chef 909 boul de la Verendrye O, Gatineau QC J8P 7H2; Ott'72; BSc; CSPQ; FRCP; FRCPC; MedMicrobiol (Infection Control). Staff, Montfort Hospital; Staff, Hôpital de Gatineau; Clin Prof, University of Ottawa; Langs: Bilingual(English/French); (819)773-2236; richard@bonin.ca.

BONIN, Richard; CSSS du Nord de Lanaudière, 1000 boul Sainte-Anne, St-Charles-Brromee QC J6E 6J2; Laval'80; FRCSC; OrthSurg. Ac Staff Orthopedics, Centre Hospitalier Régional de Lanaudière; (450)759-8222; rbonin@videotron.ca.

BONIN, Sylvie; Hop Charles Lemoyne, 3120 boul Taschereau, Greenfield Park QC J4V 2H1; Mon'86; DiagRad (Echography & Doppler). Staff Radiol, Hopital Charles LeMoyne; (450)466-5000 x2030; Fax. (450)466-5071.

BONIN-CARIGNAN, Andreanne; CSSS Domaine du Roy, 450 rue Brassard, Roberval QC G8H 1B9; Mon'08; CCFP; Staff, Hotel-Dieu de Roberval; (418)275-0110

BONIOLO, Hernan; 368 College St N PO Box 1260, Durham ON N0G 1R0; Buenos Aires (Argentina)'00; CCFP; (519)369-2510; Fax. (519)369-3831.

BONISTEEL, Stephen P; New Harbour Med Clinic, PO Box 119, New Harbour Tb NL A0B 2P0; Ott'83; CCFP; FCFP; (709)582-2244; Fax. (709)582-2333.

BONN, Gary E; 105-1335 Carling Ave, Ottawa ON K1Z 8N8; Amiens (France)'73; FACS; DAB; FRCSC; Ophth (Pediatric Ophthalmology). Staff, Children's Hospital of Eastern Ontario (CHEO); Staff, Montfort Hospital; Asst Prof Dept of Ophth, University of Ottawa; (613)729-8600; Fax. (613)729-2546.

BONN, James R; Kawartha Cardiology Clinic, 327 Charlotte St, Peterborough ON K9J 0B2; Qns'71; FRCPC; Anes. (705)743-3555

BONN, John M; Quinte HC Corp-Trenton Mem, PO Box 1600 Stn Main 242 King St, Trenton ON K8V 5S6; Qns'67; LLB; Staff, QHC Trenton Memorial; Staff, QHC Belleville General; Lecturer Family Med, Queen's University; (613)392-2541

BONNARDEAUX, Alain; Hop Maisonneuve-Rosemont, 5415 boul de l'Assomption, Montreal QC H1T 2M4; Mon'86; FRCPC; IntMed (Research); Nephrol. adj Dir Clin Research/Staff, Hopital Maisonneuve-Rosemont; adj Prof, Universite de Montreal; (514)252-3400; Fax. (514)255-3026.

BONNAUD, Jeanne; CSSR Rosemere, 400 ch de la Grande-Cote, Rosemere QC J7A 1K7; Mon'85; Langs: Bilingual(French/English); (450)621-9776

BONNEAU, Andre; Maison Soins Palliatifs de Lav, 655 rue Bellevue, Laval QC H7C 0A8; Ott'80; CCFP; FCFP; Staff, Hopital de la Cite de la santé; Physician, CLSC Norman Bethune; (450)936-4300 x291

BONNEAU, Daniel; St Michael's Hosp, 8 003BW-30 Bond St, Toronto ON M5B 1W8; Sher'75; FRCSC; Cardiovasc&ThorSurg. Ac Staff Cardiovasc&ThorSurg, St Michael's Hospital; Staff/Assoc Prof Surg, University of Toronto; (416)864-5706; Fax. (416)864-5031.

BONNEAU, Francois; Clinique Familiale Pas-a-Pas, 3650 boul Henri-Bourassa E, Montreal-Nord QC H1H 1J6; Mon'88; LMCC; CCFP; Staff Privil Obst, Hôpital du Sacre-Coeur de Montréal; Langs: Spanish; (514)328-9797; Fax. (514)328-2672.

BONNEAU, Gaston; 181 av Saint-Alphonse, Roberval QC G8H 1K5; Laval'74; (418)275-5290; Fax. (418)275-5291.

BONNEAU, Richard; CSSS de Laval, 1755 boul Rene-Laennec, Laval QC H7M 3L9; Mon'78; CSPQ; FRCPC; AnatPath. Staff, Hopital de la Cite de la santé; (450)668-1010 x23437

BONNEAU, Veronique; Hop Brome-Missisquoi-Perkins, 950 rue Principale, Cowansville QC J2K 1K3; Sher'03; CCFP; Staff, Hôpital Brome-Missisquoi-Perkins; (450)266-4342

BONNELL, Weldon; Dr Charles A Janeway Child HC, 300 Prince Philip Dr, St. John's NL A1B 3V6; Mem'01; FRCPC; Psy. Staff, Janeway Children's Health & Rehabilitation Centre; (709)777-6300

BONNELL ALLANACH, Camille; 203-860 Mountain Rd, Moncton NB E1C 2N7; Dal'09; CCFP.

BONNER, Marie; CLSC du Centre de la Mauricie, 1265 rue Trudel, Shawinigan QC G9N 8T3; Laval'86; Staff PedoPsy, CH du Centre-de-la-Mauricie (Ste-Thérèse de Shawinigan); (819)539-8371 x8345; Fax. (819)537-5780; marie_bonner@ssss.gouv.qc.ca.

BONNET, Francine M; South East Ottawa Centre, 600-1355 Bank St, Ottawa ON K1H 8K7; McG'93; CCFP; Langs: French; (613)737-4809; Fax. (613)739-3723.

BONNETT, Jennifer E; 203-600 Princess St, Woodstock ON N4S 4H4; Tor'95; BSc; CCFP; FCFP; Staff Privil, Woodstock General Hospital; (519)421-7252; Fax. (519)421-9924.

BONNEVILLE, K Scott; Thunder Bay Reg HSC-T-Bay, 980 Oliver Rd, Thunder Bay ON P7B 6V4; Wes'00; FRCPC; Anes. Staff, Thunder Bay Regional Health Sciences Centre; (807)684-6000

BONNEVILLE, Nathalie; Centre Medical des Generations, 200-465 rue Bibeau, Saint-Eustache QC J7R 0C8; Mon'92; Staff Obst, Hôpital de Saint-Eustache; Langs: English; (450)472-1955; Fax. (450)472-1905; nbonneville@cm25.ca.

BONNEVILLE, Peter; CSSSG-Hop de Gatineau, CP 2000 Succ Bureau-Chef 909 boul de la Verendrye O, Gatineau QC J8P 7H2; Mon'85; Staff, Hôpital de Gatineau; (819)561-8100 x8222; Fax. (819)986-4000.

BONNI, Azad; Kingston Gen Hosp, 76 Stuart St, Kingston ON K7L 2V7; Qns'86; FRCPC; Neur. Staff, Kingston General Hospital; (613)549-6666

BONNIER-VIGER, Yves; ASSS-Chaudiere Appalaches, 363 rue Cameron, Sainte-Marie QC G6E 3E2; Laval'97; FRCPC; CommunMed. Chef Social & Preventive Med, Université Laval; Langs: Spanish; Portuguese; English; (418)386-3363

BONNINGTON, Simon P; Annapolis Valley Health, PO Box 573 15 Chipman Dr, Annapolis Royal NS B0S 1A0; Bristol (England)'90; CCFP; (902)532-2324

BONNY, A M Yvette; Hop Maisonneuve-Rosemont, 5415 boul de l'Assomption, Montreal QC H1T 2M4; (Haiti)'59; Hem (P.Q.); HemPath; Peds (P.Q.). Staff, Hopital Maisonneuve-Rosemont; (514)252-3448

BONNY, Shawn; Ctr Hosp de Verdun, 4000 boul Lasalle, Verdun QC H4G 2A3; McG'03; Cardiol; IntMed (Acute & Chronic Pain). Staff, Centre Hospitalier de Verdun; (514)362-1000

BONNYCASTLE, Michael J; St Mary's Hosp Centre, 1314-3830 av Lacombe, Montreal QC H3T 1M5; McG'80; FRCPC; IntMed; GeriatricMed. Staff, St Mary's Hospital Centre; adj Prof, McGill University; (514)734-2660; Fax. (514)734-2641.

BONSOR, Claire N; The Medical Clinic Associates, 4794 Joyce Ave, Powell River BC V8A 3B6; UBC'92; (604)485-6261; Fax. (604)485-2820.

BONSU, Peter O; 390 Lincoln St, Welland ON L3B 4N4; (Ghana)'74; MB ChB; FAAP; FRCPC; Peds (Community Pediatrics). Staff, Niagara Health System - Welland Hospital Site; Clin Asst Prof Peds, McMaster University; (905)788-1777; Fax. (905)788-1779.

BONTA, Mark J; Univ Hlth Network-Toronto Gen, 14N 206-200 Elizabeth St, Toronto ON M5G 2C4; Tor'06; FRCPC; IntMed. Staff, Toronto General Hospital - UHN; (416)640-3111

BONTHUYS, Erasmus J; The Maple Tree Med Clinic, 1181 6 Ave NE, Salmon Arm BC V1E 2S5; Pretoria (South Africa)'01; MB ChB; Langs: Afrikaans; (250)832-9361; erasmus1@telus.net.

BOOD, Timothy W; Dalhousie Univ Hlth Services, PO Box 15000 Lcd 2 6230 Coburg Rd, Halifax NS B3H 4R2; Ott'80; Staff, Dartmouth General Hospital; Staff, Centre de sante Tulattavik de l'Ungava; Langs: Spanish; French; (902)494-2171; Fax. (902)494-2727; timothy.bood@ssss.gouv.qc.ca.

BOODHOO, Jean A; Southridge Prof Centre, 7-1224 Strachan Rd SE, Medicine Hat AB T1B 4R2; (England)'82; MB BS; MRCPsy; BSc(Hon); Staff, Medicine Hat Regional Hospital; (403)527-1918

BOODHUN, Mohamed S; Central Nfld Reg Hlth Centre, 50 Union St, Grnd-Falls-Wi NL A2A 2E1; Karachi (Pakistan)'88; MB BS; Staff, Central Newfoundland Regional Health Centre; (709)292-2191; Fax. (709)292-2449.

BOODHWANI, Munir; Univ Of Ottawa Heart Institute, H3405-40 Ruskin St, Ottawa ON K1Y 4W7; Wes'01; FRCSC; CardSurg. Staff, University of Ottawa Heart Institute; (613)761-4720

BOODOOSINGH, Lal A; 103-1907 Baseline Rd, Ottawa ON K2C 0C7; Ott'67; BSc(UBC); DPsy; Psy. Dir Child & Adolescent Psy, Royal Ottawa Mental Health Centre - Royal Ottawa Health Care Group; Asst Prof, University of Ottawa; (613)244-1550; Fax. (613)244-1921.

BOOK, Howard E; 101-2900 Yonge St, Toronto ON M4N 3N8; Man'65; DPsy; FRCPC; Psy (Psychotherapy). Sr Consultant Psychotheraphy, Toronto General Hospital - UHN; Coord Brief Psychotherapy Training, Centre for Addiction & Mental Health (CAMH) - College Street Site; Assoc Prof, University of Toronto; (416)486-6541

BOOK, Robert J; Hamilton Medical Walk In Clini, 675 Upper James St, Hamilton ON L9C 2Z5; Tor'76; Chief/Medical Staff, The Brant Community Healthcare System - Willett Hospital Site; (905)769-0330

BOOK, Ronald W; Brant Community HC-Brantford, 200 Terrace Hill St, Brantford ON N3R 1G9; McM'89; BSc(Hon); FRCPC; Psy. Med Dir Psychiatry, The Brant Community Healthcare System - Brantford General Hospital Site; (519)751-5885; Fax. (519)751-5898.

BOOKATZ, Brian J; Western Med Clinic, 144 6th St, Brandon MB R7A 3N2; Witwatersrand (South Africa)'79; FRCPC; IntMed. Staff, Brandon Regional Health Centre; (204)727-6451; Fax. (204)727-4150.

BOOKER, Jeffrey D; Cornwall Prof Bldg, 701-2125 11th Ave, Regina SK S4P 3X3; Sask'03; FRCPC; IntMed; Cardiol. (306)781-7944; Fax. (306)781-6997.

BOOKMAN, Arthur A M; Univ Hlth Network-Toronto Western Hosp, 1E 452-399 Bathurst St, Toronto ON M5T 2S8; Wes'68; MD; FRCP; FRCPC; IntMed (Rheumatoid Arthritis); Rheum. Sr Staff, Toronto Western Hospital - University Health Network; Assoc Prof, University of Toronto; (416)603-5404; Fax. (416)603-4348.

BOOKMAN, Ian; St Joseph's Health Centre, 30 The Queensway, Toronto ON M6R 1B5; Tor'00; BSc; FRCPC; IntMed; Gastroent. Staff GI Unit, St Joseph's Health Centre; Med Dir, Kensington Cancer Screening Centre; Asst Prof, University of Toronto; Langs: Spanish; (416)226-2777; Fax. (416)226-2771; office@gibookman.com.

BOON, Linda A; Lennox & Addington Gen Hosp, 8 Richmond Park Dr, Napanee ON K7R 2Z4; Qns'76; Staff, Lennox & Addington County General Hospital; (613)354-3301 x261; Fax. (613)354-4331.

BOON, Peter J; North Fraser Remand Centre, 1451 Kingsway Ave, Port Coquitlam BC V3C 1S2; Newcastle-upon-Tyne (England)'77; MB BS; Staff, BC Mental Health & Addiction Service; (604)468-3455

BOONE, Andrea; Foothills Med Centre, 1403 29 St NW, Calgary AB T2N 2T9; Mem'04; FRCPC; EmergMed; PedEmergMed. Staff, Foothills Medical Centre; (613)737-7600

BOONE, Bonita L; Univ Of New Brunswick PO Box 4400 Stn A, Fredericton NB E3B 5A3; Mem'87; CCFP; FCFP; (506)453-4837; Fax. (506)452-6087.

BOONE, Darrell C; Health Sciences Centre, 300 Prince Philip Dr, St. John's NL A1B 3V6; Mem'85; FRCSC; GenSurg. Staff, Health Sciences Centre; Chair Clinical Disciplines Surg, Memorial University Of Newfoundland; (709)777-6755; dboone@morgan.ucs.mun.ca.

BOONE, Robert H; St Paul's Hosp, 478A-1081 Burrard St, Vancouver BC V6Z 1Y6; UBC'00; FRCPC; IntMed; Cardiol. Staff, Providence Health Care - St Paul's Hospital; (604)806-9922

BOONE, Sharon A; PO Box 343 RR 1, Bowen Island BC V0N 1G0; Mem'89; DABPath; JD; FRCPC; AnatPath (Forensic Pathology). (604)626-5723

BOORA, Parveen S; Family Med Clinic, 102-9425 94 Ave, Fort Saskatchewan AB T8L 1N6; Alb'05; FRCSC; GenSurg. (780)992-0666; Fax. (780)992-0673.

BOORANY, Yusuf; Royal York Med Arts Bldg, 206-1436 Royal York Rd, Etobicoke ON M9P 3A9; Tor'79; Associate, Humber River Regional Hospital - Church Street Site; (416)245-4755; Fax. (416)245-1946.

BOORMAN, David W; 124 Illingworth Close, Red Deer AB T4R 0B1; Alb'69.

BOORMAN, Lyn D; Whites Road Med Clinic, 5A-750 Oklahoma Dr, Pickering ON L1W 3G9; Tor'73; CCFP; (905)831-8666; Fax. (905)831-8749.

BOORMAN, Michael G; Rimbey Med Clinic, PO Box 650, Rimbey AB T0C 2J0; Alb'71; (403)843-2256; Fax. (403)843-2255.

BOORMAN, Richard S; University of Calgary, 2500 University Dr NW, Calgary AB T2N 1N4; Cal'94; FRCSC; OrthSurg (Shoulder). (403)220-5077; Fax. (403)282-6170.

BOOT-NEIRYNCK, Delphine; Hotel-Dieu de Sorel, 400 av de l'Hotel-Dieu, Sorel-Tracy QC J3P 1N5; Staff, Hôtel-Dieu de Sorel; (450)746-6000

BOOTH, A William; 206-220 Main St, Antigonish NS B2G 2C2; Dal'84; CCFP; FCFP; (902)863-6669; Fax. (902)863-5956.

BOOTH, Anthony D; Medical Centre, 24-1515 Dufferin Cres, Nanaimo BC V9S 2B8; London (England)'95; FRCPC; IntMed; Nephrol. Staff, Campbell River & District General Hospital; (250)753-2446

BOOTH, Bradley D; Royal Ottawa Hlth Care Group, 2F-1145 Carling Ave, Ottawa ON K1Z 7K4; Qns'00; BSc; DABPN; DABFP; FRCPC; Psy (Forensic Psychiatry). Staff, Royal Ottawa Mental Health Centre - Royal Ottawa Health Care Group; Prog Dir, University of Ottawa; (613)722-6521 x6365

BOOTH, Christopher A; 300-1200 Lonsdale Ave, North Vancouver BC V7M 3H6; Tor'91; FRCPC; Psy (Adult Psychiatry). Staff, Maples Adolescent Treatment Centre; (604)660-5812

BOOTH, Christopher M; Cancer Care of Southeastern On, 25 King St W, Kingston ON K7L 5P9; Qns'01; FRCPC; IntMed; MedOncol. Staff, Princess Margaret Hospital - University Health Network; (613)549-6666

BOOTH, Esther G; The Richmond Hosp, 7000 Westminster Hwy, Richmond BC V6X 1A2; Cal'06; CCFP; Staff, Richmond Hospital; (604)278-9711

BOOTH, Frances A; Health Sciences Centre, 820 Sherbrook St, Winnipeg MB R3A 1R9; Man'72; FRCPC; Peds (Pediatric Neurology). Ac Staff Children's Hosp, Health Sciences Centre; Prof Peds Child Health/Sec Head Pediatric Neurology, University of Manitoba; (204)787-2414; Fax. (204)787-1922; fbooth@exchange.hsc.mb.ca.

BOOTH, Gillian L; 6F-61 Queen St E, Toronto ON M5C 2T2; Tor'93; FRCPC; Endocrin&Metab; IntMed. Staff, St Michael's Hospital; Asst Prof Med, University of Toronto; (416)867-3719; Fax. (416)867-3724; boothg@smh.toronto.on.ca.

BOOTH, Janet M; CSSS de la Vallée de l'Or, 725 6e rue, Val-d'Or QC J9P 3Y1; McG'91; GenSurg. Staff, Centre Hospitalier de Val d'Or; (819)825-6711; Fax. (819)825-7921.

BOOTH, John D; LL-107 King St W, Dundas ON L9H 1V1; Tor'75; BSc; FRCPC; IntMed (Endocrinology & Metabolism). Staff, Hamilton Health Sciences Centre - McMaster University Medical Centre; Asst Prof Med, McMaster University; (905)628-5700; Fax. (905)628-5701.

BOOTH, Karen L; St Joseph Island Med Clinic, 1186 Richards St, Richards Landing ON P0R 1J0; Tor'03; CCFP; CCFP(E.M.); Staff, Sault Area Hospital - Matthews Memorial Hospital; Staff, Sault Area Hospital - Sault Ste Marie; Staff, St Joseph Island Medical Clinic; (705)246-2477

BOOTH, Richard A; 61 Coachwood Rd W, Lethbridge AB T1K 6B3; Tor'80; FRCPC; Anes. Staff, Chinook Regional Hospital; (403)388-6131; Fax. (403)328-1126.

BOOTH, Shannon; Valley Med Clinic, 335 Jubilee St, Duncan BC V9L 1W9; Pretoria (South Africa)'07; MB ChB; (250)748-8151

BOOTH, Steven A; Health Sciences Centre, 820 Sherbrook St, Winnipeg MB R3A 1R9; UBC'06; FRCPC; Anes. Staff, Health Sciences Centre; (204)774-8511

BOOTH, Susan A; Namgis Health Centre, PO Box 49, Alert Bay BC V0N 1A0; Manchester (England)'81; MB ChB; (250)974-5520

BOOTHROYD, Wendy M; Klondyke Med Clinic, 1-3089 3rd Ave, Whitehorse YT Y1A 5B3; UBC'82; Staff, Whitehorse General Hospital; Staff, Klondyke Medical Clinic; (867)668-4065; wboothroyd@yahoo.ca.

BOOTSMAN, Laurie B; Westcoast Family Practice, 3F-2775 Laurel St, Vancouver BC V5Z 1M9; Alb'79; BSc; (604)875-5691; Fax. (604)875-5694.

BOOY, Harold; Dr C W Wiebe Med Centre, 385 Main St, Winkler MB R6W 1J2; Man'77; CCFP; FCFP; (204)325-4312; Fax. (204)325-4594; hbooy@mts.net.

BOOYENS, Barend M J; Riverside Med Clinic, 28 3 St NE, Medicine Hat AB T1A 5L8; Orange Free State (South Africa)'95; CCFP; (403)528-3008

BOOYSEN, C Francois; Queen Elizabeth II Hosp, 10409 98 St, Grande Prairie AB T8V 2E8; (South Africa)'98; MB ChB; Staff OR, Queen Elizabeth II Hospital; Langs: Afrikaans; (780)538-7100; Fax. (780)538-7364.

BOOYSEN, Johan T; James Paton Mem Hosp, 125 Trans Canada Hwy, Gander NL A1V 1P7; Pretoria (South Africa)'75; MB ChB; MMed(Rad.D); Staff, James Paton Memorial Hospital; (709)256-2500

BOOZARY, Majid; Richmond Health Centre, 9206 Yonge St, Richmond Hill ON L4C 7A2; National (Iran)'80; (905)709-7716

BOPARAI, Dennis; Lakeridge Hlth Corp-Oshawa, 1 Hospital Crt, Oshawa ON L1G 2B9; UBC'04; FRCPC; DiagRad. Staff, Lakeridge Health - Oshawa Site; (905)576-8711

BOPARAI, Gurdev S; 441-5525 West Boulevard, Vancouver BC V6M 3W6; Punjab (Pakistan)'75; MB BS; (604)438-8288

BOPARAI, Shabab; Platinum Med Clinic, 3170 Eglinton Ave E, Scarborough ON M1J 2H3; Qns'03; CCFP; Langs: Hindi; Punjabi; (416)265-2255

BORA, Bishwajit; Northern Urology Centre, 101-845 Regent St, Sudbury ON P3E 4T3; Qns'93; FRCSC; Urol. Staff, Health Sciences North-Laurentian Site; (705)673-6836; Fax. (705)673-2304.

BORAS, Valerie F; PO Box 506, Coaldale AB T1M 1M5; Cal'85; FRCPC; AnatPath. Staff LabMed, Chinook Regional Hospital; (403)388-6110; Fax. (403)388-6067.

BORASTON, Suni E; Broadway Plaza Bldg, L5-601 Broadway W, Vancouver BC V5Z 4C2; UBC'85; MHSc; Dir, The Travel Clinic; (604)707-6650; suni.boraston@vch.ca.

BORCHERT, George H; Medical Clinic Associates, 200-3207 30 Ave, Vernon BC V1T 2C6; UBC'86; BSc; CCFP; Med Staff, Vernon Jubilee Hospital; (250)549-1216; Fax. (250)549-3985.

BORDALBA, Emilia M; 4107 Fraser St, Vancouver BC V5V 4E9; Santo Tomas (Philippines)'86; Langs: Tagalog; (604)708-2180; Fax. (604)708-2182.

BORDBAR, Kamran; Unicare Clinic, 401-1100 Sheppard Ave E, North York ON M2K 2W1; Innsbruck (Austria)'97; FRCPC; Psy. (416)548-9701

BORDEAUX, Patrick; Hôpital régional Chaleur, 1750 Sunset Dr, Bathurst NB E2A 4L7; Laval'04; FRCPC; Psy. Staff, Hopital Regional Chaleur; (506)739-2200

BORDELEAU, Celine; CSSS des Basques, 550 rue Notre Dame E RR 1, Trois-Pistoles QC G0L 4K0; Laval'99; LMCC; CCFP; Staff, Centre Hospitalier Trois-Pistoles; pers Prof, Université Laval; Langs: English; (418)851-1111; Fax. (418)851-4546.

BORDELEAU, Christian; Centre Hosp Honore-Mercier, 2750 boul Laframboise, Saint-Hyacinthe QC J2S 4Y8; McG'95; LMCC; CCFP; Staff, Centre Hospitalier Honore-Mercier; (450)771-3333

BORDELEAU, Daniel; Hop Louis-H Lafontaine, 7401 rue Hochelaga, Montreal QC H1N 3M5; Laval'76; Staff Psy, Hopital Louis-H Lafontaine; Asst Prof Psy, Universite de Montreal; (514)251-4000 x2021; Fax. (514)251-7527.

BORDELEAU, Denis; 12 rue St-Paul RR 2, Ste-Brigitte-D-Lav QC G0A 3K0; Laval'74; Staff, Jeffery Hale Hospital-Saint Brigid's; (418)825-2651

BORDELEAU, Edith; CSSS de Chicoutimi, 305 rue Saint-Vallier, Chicoutimi QC G7H 5H6; Mon'95; FRCPC; DiagRad. Staff, Complexe hospitalier de la Sagamie; (418)541-1000

BORDELEAU, Gabriel; Clinique Med Rock Forest, 1-4870 boul Bourque, Sherbrooke QC J1N 3S5; Mon'70; Consultant, Centre Hospitalier Universitaire de Sherbrooke-Hôpital Hôtel-Dieu; (819)820-2673; Fax. (819)820-2112.

BORDELEAU, Gilles; 354 rue Larocque, Longueuil QC J4G 2N1; Mon'86; (514)723-5745

BORDELEAU, Jacinthe; CSSS des Basques, 550 rue Notre-Dame E, Trois-Pistoles QC G0L 4K0; Mon'07; Staff, Centre Hospitalier Trois-Pistoles; Langs: Spanish; English; (418)851-1111; Fax. (418)851-4546.

BORDELEAU, Josée; CSSS de la Baie-des-Chaleurs, RR 2 B-419 boul Perron, Maria QC G0C 1Y0; Mon'92; Staff, CSSS de la Baie-des-Chaleurs; (418)759-3443

BORDELEAU, Louise J; Juravinski Cancer Centre, 699 Concession St, Hamilton ON L8V 5C2; Ott'91; FRCPC; IntMed; MedOncol. Staff, Mount Sinai Hospital; (905)387-9711 x64609; Fax. (905)575-6326.

BORDELEAU, Marie-Josee; U Of Ottawa Health Services, 300-100 Marie Curie Pvt, Ottawa ON K1N 1A2; Mon'97; CCFP; Langs: English; (613)564-3950; Fax. (613)564-6627; mbordele@uohs.uottawa.ca.

BORDELEAU, Normand J; CSSS de l'Energie, 1265 rue Trudel, Shawinigan QC G9N 8T3; Laval'65; (819)539-8371 x8290

BORDELEAU, Serge; 900 boul Wilfrid-Hamel, Quebec QC G1M 2R9; Laval'74; Prés CMDP/Chef Serv, CSSS de la Vieille-Capitale; Langs: English; French; (418)682-1711 x2506; Fax. (418)682-1768; serge.bordeleau@csssvc.qc.ca.

BORDEN, Andrew T; Guelph Gen Hosp, 115 Delhi St, Guelph ON N1E 4J4; Tor'04; FRCPC; Anes. Staff, Guelph General Hospital; (519)830-8863

BORDMAN, Joel S; 3250 Eglinton Ave E, Scarborough ON M1J 2H6; Tor'85; DAAPM; CISAM; Staff, Humber River Regional Hospital - Church Street Site; Med Dir Complex Pain Program, First Step Medical Clinic; (416)261-2111; Fax. (416)261-7771; jsb23@rogers.com.

BORDMAN, John M; Medical Bldg, 301-18 Pine St, Kitchener ON N2H 5Z8; Tor'75; Staff, Grand River Hospital - Kitchener/Waterloo Health Centre; Staff, St Mary's General Hospital; (519)742-4321; Fax. (519)742-1305.

BORDMAN, Risa B; Golden Mile Med Centre & Walk-, 152-1880 Eglinton Ave E, Scarborough ON M1L 2L1; Tor'87; CCFP; FCFP; Staff Family & Commun Med, North York General Hospital; Assoc Staff, The Scarborough Hospital - General Campus; (416)285-7575; Fax. (416)285-7574.

BORDOFF, Benjamin; 301-267 Pelissier St, Windsor ON N9A 4K4; Tor'88; DABPN; FRCPC; Psy (General Adult Psychiatry). Consultant Psychiatrist Student Health Services, University Of Windsor; (519)253-4606; Fax. (519)253-1854.

BORDUAS, Francine; Clinique Med Neufchatel, 101-2425 boul Bastien, Quebec QC G2B 1B3; Sher'77; (418)843-3771; Fax. (418)843-3865.

BORDUAS, J Andre; Lower Outaouis Family Hlth Tea, 206-1062 Ghislain St, Hawkesbury ON K6A 3B2; Sher'81; CCFP; FCFP; Staff, Hawkesbury & District General Hospital; Langs: English; (613)632-7061; Fax. (613)632-1736.

BORDUAS PAGE, Stephanie; Hop Charles LeMoyne, 3120 boul Taschereau, Greenfield Park QC J4V 2H1; Mon'05; FRCPC; Psy. Staff, Hopital Charles LeMoyne; (450)466-5453

BOREK, Robert J; 348 Lyndock St PO Box 818, Corunna ON N0N 1G0; Wes'77; (519)862-1461; Fax. (519)862-5835.

BORENSTEIN, David A; Mackenzie Richmond Hill Hosp, 10 Trench St, Richmond Hill ON L4C 4Z3; McM'02; CCFP; CCFP(E.M.); Staff, The Scarborough Hospital - General Campus; Staff, Mackenzie Richmond Hill Hospital; (905)883-1212; Fax. (905)883-2455.

BORENSTEIN, Harold B; Norfinch Med Centre, 106-2100 Finch Ave W, North York ON M3N 2Z9; Tor'86; BSc; MSc; FRCPC; IntMed; Nephrol. Staff, Humber River Regional Hospital - Finch Avenue Site; Staff, Humber River Regional Hospital - Church Street Site; (416)739-7558; Fax. (416)739-7601.

BORETSKY, Linda; Medistat Med Familiale, 4965 rue Saint-Pierre, Pierrefonds QC H9H 5M9; Tor'99; BSc(PT); CCFP; Staff Family Med, St Mary's Hospital Centre; (514)624-4774

BORG, Mary Josephine; 303-22112 52 Ave, Langley BC V2Y 2M6; Birmingham (England)'86; MB ChB; Staff, Langley Memorial Hospital; (604)530-0056; Fax. (604)530-4718.

BORGAONKAR, Joy N; Queen Elizabeth II HSC, 3228-1276 South Park St, Halifax NS B3H 2Y9; Mem'93; FRCPC; DiagRad. Staff, Queen Elizabeth II Health Sciences Centre - Victoria General Site; (902)473-3438; Fax. (902)473-3482.

BORGAONKAR, Mark R; Health Sciences Centre, 300 Prince Philip Dr, St. John's NL A1B 3V6; Mem'94; FRCPC; IntMed; Gastroent. Staff, Health Sciences Centre; (709)777-8072

BORGAONKAR, Ram D; Medical Consultants, 193 Lemarchant Rd, St. John's NL A1C 2H5; Indore (India)'59; MB BS; LMCC; FRCPC; IntMed (Endocrinology). Clinical Asst Prof Med, Memorial University Of Newfoundland; (709)579-4191; drrdborgaonkar@medicalconsultants.nf.net.

BORGEAT, Francois; Hop Louis-H Lafontaine, 7401 rue Hochelaga, Montreal QC H1N 3M5; Laval'66; MSc; FRCPC; Psy (Anxiety Disorder). Staff, Hopital Louis-H Lafontaine; Clin Prof, Universite de Montreal; Langs: English; (514)354-1261; Fax. (514)354-5935; francois.borgeat@umontreal.ca.

BORGER, Jonathan R; London HSC-University Hosp, PO Box 5339 Stn B 339 Windermere Rd, London ON N6A 5A5; Man'06; FRCPC; Anes. Staff, London Health Sciences Centre - University Hospital; (519)685-8500

BORGER, Margaret A; Whitemud Crossing Med Centre, 127-4211 106 St NW, Edmonton AB T6J 6L7; Alb'87; BSc; (780)435-7555; Fax. (780)436-0582.

BORGERSEN, Kaj; 205-10230 142 St NW, Edmonton AB T5N 3Y6; Witwatersrand (South Africa)'75; IntMed. (780)454-3340; Fax. (780)454-3360.

BORGHESAN, Penelope J; South Health Campus, 4448 Front St SE, Calgary AB T3M 1M4; Cal'96; CCFP; (403)956-2300

BORGIA, Sergio M; William Osler HC-Brampton, N.I.194-2100 Bovaird Dr E, Brampton ON L6R 3J7; Qns'01; MSc; BSc; FRCPC; IntMed (Tuberculosis); InfectDis. Staff, William Osler Health System - Brampton Civic Hospital; Clinical Asst Prof, McMaster University; Langs: Spanish; Italian; (905)494-2120 x57658; Fax. (905)494-6506.

BORGONO, Claudio M; Clairhurst Med Centre, 306-1466 Bathurst St, Toronto ON M5R 3S3; Tor'92; Langs: Spanish; (416)536-5555; Fax. (416)536-3352.

BORGUNDVAAG, Bjug; Mount Sinai Hosp, 206-600 University Ave, Toronto ON M5G 1X5; Tor'92; CCFP; CCFP(E.M.); Staff Physician Emerg, Mount Sinai Hospital; (416)586-5058; Fax. (416)586-4719.

BORICI-MAZI, Rozita; Hotel-Dieu Hosp, S3 012-166 Brock St, Kingston ON K7L 5G2; Albania (Albania)'88; FRCPC; IntMed; ClinImmunol&Allergy. Staff, Hotel-Dieu Hospital; (613)544-3310; Fax. (613)546-1572.

BORIDY, Illya C; Radiology Consultants Assoc, 120-6707 Elbow Dr SW, Calgary AB T2V 0E3; McG'93; FRCPC; DiagRad (Magnetic Resonance Imaging). Staff, Peter Lougheed Centre; Staff, Rockyview General Hospital; Langs: English; French; (403)777-3003; Fax. (403)777-3008.

BORIGHT, Andrew; LMC Diabetes & Endo Centre, 107-1929 Bayview Ave, Toronto ON M4G 3E8; Mem'92; DPhil; BA; FRCP; BSc; MB; FRCPC; IntMed; Endocrin&Metab. Staff, Toronto General Hospital - UHN; Staff, LMC Diabetes & Endocrinology Centres-Eglinton; Staff, LMC Diabetes & Endocrinology Centres-Bayview; (416)645-2929; andrew.boright@uhn.on.ca.

BORIGHT, William R; Niagara H System-St Catharines, PO Box 3018 Stn Main 142 Queenston St, St Catharines ON L2R 7C6; McG'82; FRCPC; Anes. Staff Anes, Niagara Health System - St Catharines General Site; Staff, Niagara Health System - Ontario Street Site; (905)685-1379

BORINS, Carolyn A; Queen's Student Health, 146 Stuart St, Kingston ON K7L 3N6; Qns'94; CCFP; FCFP; (613)533-2506; Fax. (613)533-6740.

BORINS, Elaine; 6 Connable Dr, Toronto ON M5R 1Z8; Tor'62; DCAP; FRCPC; Psy (Post Traumatic Stress Disorder). Asst Prof Psy & Staff CAPS Counselling & Psycho Serv, University of Toronto; (416)921-1432; efborins@gmail.com.

BORINS, Melvin; St Joseph's Hlth Ctr Urban FHT, 404-27 Roncesvalles Ave, Toronto ON M6R 3B2; Tor'73; CCFP; FCFP; Staff, St Joseph's Health Centre; Assoc Prof Family & CommunMed, University of Toronto; (416)533-6488; Fax. (416)533-9204; melvin.borins@sickkids.ca.

BORJA, Enrique; Dr G B Cross Mem Hosp, 67 Manitoba Dr, Clarenville NL A5A 1K3; (Philippines)'79; Staff, The Dr G B Cross Memorial Hospital; (709)466-3411

BORKAR-AGGARWAL, Monica D; Brampton Urgent Care, 8-51 Mountainash Rd, Brampton ON L6R 1W4; Qns'96; CCFP; FCFP; Staff, The Credit Valley Hospital; (905)799-2722

BORKENHAGEN, Rainer H; George Pearson Centre, 700 57th Ave W, Vancouver BC V6P 1S1; McG'74; CCFP; FCFP; Ac Staff, Vancouver General Hospital - Centennial Pavillion; Asst Prof, University of British Columbia; Langs: English; French; German; (604)321-3231

BORKENT, Amy J; 10134 111 Ave NW, Edmonton AB T5G 0B3; Alb'86; Staff, Glenrose Rehabilitation Hospital; Med Staff, Royal Alexandra Hospital; Staff, The Capital Care Group; Physician, Edmonton Institute for Women; Clin Associate Pharmacology, University of Alberta; Langs: Dutch; (780)474-3712; Fax. (780)474-7032.

BORKENT, Herman A; Misericordia Community Hosp, 16940 87 Ave NW, Edmonton AB T5R 4H5; Alb'73; CCFP; Ac Staff Emerg., Covenant Health - Misericordia Community Hospital; Asst Prof, University of Alberta; (780)735-2512; Fax. (780)486-2917.

BORMANIS, Janis; Civic Parkdale Clinic, 464-737 Parkdale Ave, Ottawa ON K1Y 1J8; Ott'69; FRCP; FRCPC; Hem (Laboratory & Clinical Hematology). Chief Hem, The Ottawa Hospital - Civic Campus; (613)761-4127

BORN, Abraham; 302-4800 Leslie St, Toronto ON M2J 2K9; McG'76; FACP; FCCP; FRCPC; IntMed (Respiratory Disease) (Respirology). Ac Staff, North York General Hospital; Assoc Staff, Mount Sinai Hospital; Asst Prof, University of Toronto; Langs: Yiddish; (416)225-9299; Fax. (416)225-7304.

BORN, Trevor M; 199 Avenue Rd, Toronto ON M5R 2J3; McM'90; FRCSC; PlasSurg (Cosmetic Surgery). Staff, Toronto Western Hospital - University Health Network; University of Toronto; (416)921-7546; Fax. (416)921-8603.

BORNAIS, Pierre; Centre Med de la Vallee, 1-22 rue du Pont, Amqui QC G5J 3T5; Laval'77; Staff, CSSS de la Matapedia; Langs: French; (418)629-3244; Fax. (418)629-4484; bornaisamqui@hotmail.com.

BORNEMISZA, Susan A; Sheldon Chumuik Centre, 1213 4 St SW, Calgary AB T2R 0X7; Cal'01; CCFP.

BORNSTEIN, Jason; Kingston Gen Hosp, 76 Stuart St, Kingston ON K7L 2V7; Qns'06; EmergMed. Staff, Kingston General Hospital; (613)548-2368

BORNSTEIN, Ronald J; 216-180 Steeles Ave W, Thornhill ON L4J 2L1; Tor'76; Ac Staff, North York General Hospital; Court Staff, North York General Hospital - Branson Division; (905)886-0116; Fax. (905)886-0117.

BOROD, Manuel; MUHC-Montreal Gen Hosp, 1650 av Cedar, Montreal QC H3G 1A4; McG'76; CCFP; Staff, McGill University Health Centre - Montreal General Campus; (514)934-1934 x43920

BORODITSKY, Mark A; Pritchard Farm Health Centre, 5-3014 Henderson Hwy, East St Paul MB R2E 0H9; Man'06; CCFP; Staff, Seven Oaks General Hospital; (204)632-7133

BORODITSKY, Michael L; Manitoba Clinic, 790 Sherbrook St, Winnipeg MB R3A 1M3; Man'00; BSc(Med); BSc; FRCSC; ObstGyn. (204)788-5707; Fax. (204)788-8092.

BORON, Susan P; Hanover Med Associates, 118 7th Ave, Hanover ON N4N 2G9; Tor'74; CCFP; FCFP; Clin Assoc Prof, University of Western Ontario; (519)364-2820

BORONOWSKI, Peter W; Inuvik Reg Hosp, PO Box 2 285 MacKenzie Rd, Inuvik NT X0E 0T0; UBC'71; BSc; CCFP; FCFP; Staff, Inuvik Regional Hospital; Langs: German; (867)777-8000; Fax. (867)777-8036.

BOROOMAND-RASHTI, Kayoomars; Richmond Health Science Ctre, 750-6091 Gilbert Rd, Richmond BC V7C 5L9; Shiraz (Iran)'70; FRCPC; IntMed; Cardiol. (604)273-1555; Fax. (604)273-2969.

BOROTO, Kahimano; Yorkton Reg Health Centre, 270 Bradbrooke Dr, Yorkton SK S3N 2K6; Staff, Yorkton Regional Health Centre; (306)786-0248; Fax. (306)786-0424.

BOROUJERDI, Mehrnaz; East Toronto Health Centre, 1496 Danforth Ave, Toronto ON M4J 1N4; Islamic Azad University (Iran)'00; Staff, Sunnybrook Health Sciences Centre; (416)778-1496

BOROWIEC, Anna M; Misericordia Community Hosp, 16940 87 Ave NW, Edmonton AB T5R 4H5; Tor'04; FRCSC; GenSurg. Staff, Covenant Health - Misericordia Community Hospital; (780)735-2000

BOROWKA, Derek D; Abbotsfield Shoppers Mall, 214-3210 118 Ave NW, Edmonton AB T5W 4W1; Alb'93; BSc; Langs: Polish; (780)471-2071; Fax. (780)474-8001.

BOROWOY, Alan M; Rebecca Macdonald Centre, 2001-60 Murray St, Toronto ON M5T 3L9; Wes'08; IntMed. (416)586-4800

BOROWSKA, Anna M; St Paul's Hosp, 4F-1081 Burrard St, Vancouver BC V6Z 1Y6; UBC'89; FRCPC; Psy. Staff, Providence Health Care - St Paul's Hospital; (604)682-2344 x62896

BOROWSKI, Irwin F M; Addiction Centre of Toronto, 1288 Danforth Ave, Toronto ON M4J 1M6; Man'82; (416)462-0228; Fax. (416)461-7690.

BORREMAN, Stephane; MUHC-Royal Victoria Hosp, 687 av des Pins O, Montreal QC H3A 1A1; McG'98; CCFP; CCFP(E.M.); Staff, McGill University Health Centre - Royal Victoria Hospital; (514)934-1934

BORRETT, Donald S; Medical Office, 221-840 Coxwell Ave, Toronto ON M4C 5T2; Tor'78; FRCPC; Neur. Staff, Toronto East General Hospital Inc; (416)462-9449; Fax. (416)462-9826.

BORRETT, George F J; Salvation Army Grace Gen Hosp, 300 Booth Dr, Winnipeg MB R3J 3M7; Dublin (Ireland)'68; Staff, The Salvation Army Grace Hospital; (204)837-8311

BORRIE, Michael; St Joseph's HC-Parkwood Hosp, A280-801 Commissioners Rd E, London ON N6C 5J1; Otago (New Zealand)'76; MB ChB; FRCPC; IntMed (Dementia); GeriatricMed. Staff, Parkwood Hospital - St Joseph's Health Care; Consultant Geriatric, London Health Sciences Centre - Victoria Campus; Consultant Geriatric, St Joseph's Hospital - St Joseph's Health Care; Prog Dir, Regional Geriatric Prog., SWO; (519)685-4021; Fax. (519)685-4093.

BORSANYI, Jean-Pierre; CSSS St-Jerone, 290 rue de Montigny, Saint-Jerome QC J7Z 5T3; Laval'77; FRCSC; PlasSurg. adj Prof, Centre Hospitalier l'Université de Montréal (CHUM) - Hôpital Notre-Dame; Staff, Hôtel-Dieu de Saint-Jérôme; (450)431-8201; jpborsanyi@videotron.ca.

BORSATO, Garry W; Mayfair Place, 120-6707 Elbow Dr SW, Calgary AB T2V 0E3; Wes'89; FRCSC; GenSurg; DiagRad; CardSurg. (403)777-3007; Fax. (403)777-3008.

BORSATO, Stephanie A; Rainbow Med Clinic, 36 McIntyre St, Nairn Centre ON P0M 2L0; Tor'99; CCFP; (705)869-1112; Fax. (705)869-1132.

BORSCH, Roman N; 840-10 Saint Mary St, Toronto ON M4Y 1P9; Tor'57; ABNP; FAPA; FRCPC; Psy (Psychoanalysis). Faculty Memb., Toronto Psychoanalytic Inst.; (416)925-0056; Fax. (416)925-0056. Semi-Retired.

BORSCHEL, Debaroti M; Women's College Hosp, 614-76 Grenville St, Toronto ON M5S 1B2; Baltimore (USA)'97; Staff, Women's College Hospital; (416)323-6400

BORSCHEL, Gregory H; The Hosp for Sick Children, 555 University Ave, Toronto ON M5G 1X8; Staff, The Hospital For Sick Children; (416)813-7654 x28197; Fax. (416)813-6637; gregory.borschel@sickkids.ca.

BORSCHNECK, Daniel P; Kingston Gen Hosp, V3 354A-76 Stuart St, Kingston ON K7L 2V7; Qns'91; FRCSC; OrthSurg (Pediatric Orthopedics). Staff OrthSurg, Hotel-Dieu Hospital; Staff OrthSurg, Kingston General Hospital; Staff, QHC Belleville General; Asst Prof, Queen's University; (613)549-6666 x3351; Fax. (613)548-2390; borschnd@kgh.kari.net.

BORSOOK, Cathi; 504-1110 Sheppard Ave E, North York ON M2K 2W2; Tor'79; FRCPC; Psy (Psychotherapy). (416)226-4294

BORST, Sjoerd A; 610-5991 Spring Garden Rd, Halifax NS B3H 1Y6; McG'04; FRCPC; Psy. (902)407-4410; Fax. (902)407-4411.

BORSTLAP, Jeanne; Walk-In Med Clinic @ Southpoin, 9368 Southfort Dr, Fort Saskatchewan AB T8L 0C5; Cape Town (South Africa)'86; MB ChB; (780)997-0177

BORSUK, Daniel E; Hop Maisonneuve-Rosemont, 5415 boul de l'Assomption, Montreal QC H1T 2M4; McG'06; MDCM; FRCSC; PlasSurg. Staff, Hopital Maisonneuve-Rosemont; (514)252-3400

BORSUK, Ronnie M; Clinique Med Plateau Mont-Roya, 1374 av du Mont-Royal E, Montreal QC H2J 1Y7; McG'05; FRCSC; PlasSurg. (514)527-3997

BORTEN, Odelia; Kildare Family Med Associates, 14-7005 ch Kildare, Cote Saint-Luc QC H4W 1C1; McG'10; MDCM; CCFP; (514)397-0777

BORTH, Christopher S; Kitchener Urology Associates, 313-751 King St W, Kitchener ON N2G 1E5; Qns'99; BSc; FRCSC; Urol. Att Staff, Kingston General Hospital; Att Staff, Hotel-Dieu Hospital; Aj Prof, Queen's University; (519)954-2370

BORTHISTLE, Bruce K; Kelowna Gastroent Associates, 564 Leon Ave, Kelowna BC V1Y 6J6; Man'69; ABIM; FRCPC; IntMed. Chief Gastroenterology, Kelowna General Hospital; (250)763-6433; Fax. (250)763-3818.

BORTHWICK, Murray J; Royal Inland Hosp, 311 Columbia St, Kamloops BC V2C 2T1; McG'06; MDCM; CCFP; CCFP(E.M.); Staff, Royal Inland Hospital; (250)374-5111

BORTNICK, Jessica E; The Doctor's Office, 13-205 Marycroft Ave, Woodbridge ON L4L 5X8; McM'04; CCFP; (905)856-2100; jbortnick@mcimed.com.

BORTOLUSSI, Robert A; IWK Health Centre, PO Box 9700 Rpo Csc, Halifax NS B3K 6R8; Tor'70; MRCP; FRCPC; Peds (Pediatric Infectious Diseases). Consultant, IWK Health Centre; Prof Peds, Dalhousie University; (902)470-8498; Fax. (902)470-7232; robert.bortolussi@dal.ca.

BORTOLUZZI, Patricia; Hop Ste-Justine, 7908-3175 ch Cote-Sainte-Cathe, Montreal QC H3T 1C5; Mon'86; FRCSC; PlasSurg. Staff, Hôpital Ste-Justine; (514)345-4771; Fax. (514)345-4964.

BORTS, David; Osler Cardiology Associates, 200-3 Conestoga Dr, Brampton ON L6Z 4N5; McG'80; ABIM; FACC; FRC; FRCPC; IntMed; Cardiol. Staff, William Osler Health System - Brampton Civic Hospital; Langs: French; (905)495-4278; Fax. (905)452-1052.

BORUCH, Nadia; 305-2299 Dundas St W, Toronto ON M6R 1X7; Tor'68; CCFP; Staff, St Joseph's Health Centre; (416)766-0761

BORYS, Andrew E; Movement Disorder Clinic, 200 Woodlawn St, Winnipeg MB R3J 2H7; Man'95; FRCPC; Neur;CCFP; Fam Med, WRHA - Deer Lodge Centre; (204)940-8400; Fax. (204)940-8414.

BORYS, Thomas J; 100 Highland Rd W, Kitchener ON N2M 3B5; Tor'85; PhD; Court Staff, Grand River Hospital - Kitchener/Waterloo Health Centre; Court Staff, St Mary's General Hospital; (519)742-3600; Fax. (519)742-3386.

BORZECKI, Mark P; Arnprior & Dist Mem Hosp, 350 John St N, Arnprior ON K7S 2P6; Ott'91; MA; CCFP; CCFP(E.M.); Staff, Arnprior & District Memorial Hospital; Staff, The Ottawa Hospital - Civic Campus; Staff, The Ottawa Hospital - General Campus; (613)623-3166; Fax. (613)623-5703.

BOS, Carlo; Peterborough Reg HC-Hospital, 1 Hospital Dr, Peterborough ON K9J 7C6; Qns'74; BA; FRCSC; ObstGyn. Staff, Peterborough Regional Health Centre - Hospital Drive; Lecturer ObstGyn, Queen's University; (705)876-5036; Fax. (705)740-6891.

BOS, David C; Shelbourne Med Clinic Inc, 150-3200 Shelbourne St, Victoria BC V8P 5G8; Alb'03; CCFP.

BOS, Hayley B; Admirals Walk Health Centre, 275 Island Hwy, Victoria BC V9B 1G4; Wes'03; FRCSC; ObstGyn (Maternal Fetal Medicine). Staff, St Joseph's Hospital - St Joseph's Health Care; (250)380-9002

BOSCAN, Alejandra; South Health Campus, 4448 Front St SE, Calgary AB T3M 1M4; Zulia (Venezuela)'00; IntMed. (403)956-3800; Fax. (403)956-3836.

BOSCH, J Douglas; 262-1632 14 St NW, Calgary AB T2N 1M7; Alb'82; FACS; FRCSC; Otol (Head & Neck). Consultant, Foothills Medical Centre; Ac Staff, Peter Lougheed Centre; Consultant, Rockyview General Hospital; Prog Dir Otol Residency Prog, University of Calgary; (403)282-0054; Fax. (403)282-0059.

BOSCH, Mark J; Foothills Med Centre, C215-1403 29 St NW, Calgary AB T2N 2T9; Sask'07; FRCPC; IntMed; Hem. Staff, Foothills Medical Centre; (403)944-1993; Fax. (403)270-7891.

BOSE, Sabyasachi; Bose & Hafezi Med Specialists, 140B Idylwyld Dr N, Saskatoon SK S7L 0Y7; Calcutta (India)'75; MB BS; MRCP(UK); FRCPC; IntMed (Lipidology). Associate Clin Prof, University of Saskatchewan; (306)933-3004

BOSE, Tarun K; Complete Med Centres, 15-630 Peter Robertson Blvd, Brampton ON L6R 1T4; Dhaka (Bangladesh)'88; CCFP; (905)793-8868; Fax. (905)793-8957.

BOSE, Teertha J; Mackenzie Richmond Hill Hosp, 10 Trench St, Richmond Hill ON L4C 4Z3; McM'02; Staff, Mackenzie Richmond Hill Hospital; (905)883-2041

BOSEMBO ILONDJO, Maurice; 65 Wilson Cres CP 7333, Grand Falls NB E3Z 3E7; Kinshasa (Congo (Democratic Republic))'88; Staff, Hôpital Général de Grand-Falls; (506)473-6440; Fax. (506)473-6006; bosembo@hotmail.com.

BOSENBERG, Craig H; Royal Jubilee Hosp, 1952 Bay St, Victoria BC V8R 1J8; Cape Town (South Africa)'93; MB ChB; FRCPC; Anes. Staff, Royal Jubilee Hospital; (250)370-8000

BOSENBERG, Marc H; Central Saanich Med Clinic, 1932 Mount Newton Cross Rd, Saanichton BC V8M 2B1; Cape Town (South Africa)'77; MB ChB; DCH; (250)652-2041; Fax. (250)652-0738.

BOSEOVSKI, James; Kingston Gen Hosp, 76 Stuart St, Kingston ON K7L 2V7; Qns'07; FRCPC; IntMed. Staff, Kingston General Hospital; (613)549-6666

BOSER, Stacey R; Mosaic Womens Clinic, 1-2681 36 St NE, Calgary AB T1Y 6H6; Cal'03; CCFP; (403)250-5066; Fax. (403)250-5244; srboser@shaw.ca.

BOSEY, Gregory J; Niagara H System-St Catharine, PO Box 3018 Stn Main 142 Queenston St, St Catharines ON L2R 7C6; UBC'02; FRCPC; Anes. Staff, Niagara Health System - St Catharines General Site; (905)684-7271

BOSHOFF, Hendrik C; Glenvalley Health Centre, 207-437 Glenmore Rd, Kelowna BC V1V 1Y5; (South Africa)'97; MB ChB; (250)860-5811; hennieboshoff@hotmail.com.

BOSHOFF, Johan A; 700 3rd St SS 3, Keremeos BC V0X 1N3; Pretoria (South Africa)'94; MB ChB; CCFP; Staff, South Similkameen Health Centre; Langs: Afrikaans; (250)499-3000

BOSHOFF, Johannes C; Medical Dental Building, 109-9181 Main St, Chilliwack BC V2P 4M9; (South Africa)'72; MB ChB; (604)795-7811

BOSHOFF, Pieter; Caledonian Clinic, 340 Campbell St, Nanaimo BC V9R 3G7; Pretoria (South Africa)'90; MB ChB; (250)753-3202

BOSHOUWERS, Marie-Louise; CSSS des Iles, 430 ch Principal, Cap-aux-Meules QC G4T 1R9; Mon'85; Staff, Hôpital de l'Archipel; (418)986-2121 x8167; Fax. (418)986-6845.

BOSILJCIC-STOJANOVIC, Svetlana; Westboro Med Centre, 190 Richmond Rd, Ottawa ON K1Z 6W6; Belgrade (Serbia)'92; CCFP; Physician, Westboro Medical Centre; (613)719-7837; Fax. (613)719-7807.

BOSISIO, Bruno; Clinique Med St-Sulpice, 12-1420 rue Legendre E, Montreal QC H2M 1H5; Mon'84; Staff, Hôpital du Sacre-Coeur de Montréal; (514)382-0552

BOSKOVIC, Radinka R; Clarington FHO, 3100-222 King St E, Bowmanville ON L1C 1P6; Tuzla (Bosnia-Herzegovina)'84; CCFP; (905)623-2355

BOSKOVIC PETROVIC, Jasmina; Ctr Hosp de Lachine, 650 16e av, Lachine QC H8S 3N5; Belgrade (Serbia)'85; CCFP; Staff, Centre Hospitalier de Lachine; (514)637-2351

BOSLEY, Laurence A; Victoria Mental Health Clinic, 2328 Trent St, Victoria BC V8R 4Z3; Alb'92; FRCPC; Psy. (250)370-8175

BOSMA, Karen; London HSC-University Hosp, PO Box 5339 Stn B B2 194D-339 Windermere Rd, London ON N6A 5A5; McM'98; BA; FRCPC; IntMed; Critical Care Medicine; Respir. Asst Prof, London Health Sciences Centre - University Hospital; (519)685-8500

BOSMA, Mark A; Abbie J Lane Bldg, 6513-5909 Veterans Memorial La, Halifax NS B3H 2E2; Man'00; FRCPC; Psy (Geriatric Psychiatry). Staff, St Boniface General Hospital; Asst Prof Psy, Queen Elizabeth II Health Sciences Centre - Victoria General Site; (902)473-2935; Fax. (902)473-1422; Bosmam@cdha.nshealth.ca.

BOSMA, Peter A; Concordia Gen Hosp, 1095 Concordia Ave, Winnipeg MB R2K 3S8; Man'94; CCFP; Staff, Concordia General Hospital; (204)667-1560

BOSMA, Tymen L; St Paul's Hosp, 1081 Burrard St, Vancouver BC V6Z 1Y6; UBC'05; FRCPC; Anes. Staff, Providence Health Care - St Paul's Hospital; (604)682-2344

BOSMAN, Amanda; 101-436 Lorne St, Kamloops BC V2C 1W3; Pretoria (South Africa)'95; MB ChB; LMCC; CCFP; Langs: Afrikaans; (250)372-2112

BOSMAN, Francois M; Gabriola Commun Med Clinic, 695 Church St, Gabriola BC V0R 1X3; Cape Town (South Africa)'83; MB ChB; (250)247-9922; Fax. (250)247-9162.

BOSMAN, Jan C; Central Saanich Med Clinic, 1932 Mt Newton X Rd, Saanichton BC V8M 2B1; Orange Free State (South Africa)'86; MB ChB; Staff, Saanich Peninsula Hospital; (250)652-2041; Fax. (250)652-0738.

BOSMAN, Kylie A; Collingwood Gen & Marine Hosp, 459 Hume St, Collingwood ON L9Y 1W9; Tor'03; CCFP; CCFP(E.M.); Staff, Collingwood General & Marine Hospital; (705)445-2550

BOSS, Kenneth; Developmental Disabilities Ser, 200-1164 Devonshire Ave, North Bay ON P1B 6X7; Dal'00; FRCPC; Psy. Staff, North Bay Regional Health Centre - Regional Mental Health; (705)474-5885; Fax. (705)497-5350.

BOSSE, Charles; CSSS Les Eskers de l'Abitibi, 622 4e rue O, Amos QC J9T 2S2; Sher'94; LMCC; FRCSC; GenSurg. Staff, CH Hôtel-Dieu d'Amos; (819)732-3341; cbossemac@hotmail.com.

BOSSE, Danielle; Centre Hebergement Manicougan, 340 rue Clement-Lavoie, Baie-Comeau QC G4Z 3B8; Laval'80; Physician, Medicale Corporation Quno; (418)296-2572

BOSSE, Elizabeth; Clinique familiale des Hauts-B, CP 54 Succ Bureau-Chef 99 boul des Hauts-Bois, Boucherville QC J4B 5E6; Sher'87; Staff, Centre de santé des Côté-Nord; (450)649-2490; Fax. (450)649-2218.

BOSSE, Genevieve; CSSS de Rivière-de-Loup, 75 rue Saint-Henri, Riviere-Du-Loup QC G5R 2A4; Laval'98; FRCPC; Psy. Staff, Centre Hospitalier Regional du Grand-Portage; (418)868-1000 x4; Fax. (418)868-0530.

BOSSE, Isabelle; CSSS de Sept-Iles, 45 rue Du Pere-Divet, Sept-Iles QC G4R 3N7; Mon'96; ABOG; FRCSC; ObstGyn. Staff, Centre Hospitalier Regional de Sept-Iles; (418)962-9761; Fax. (418)962-2701.

BOSSE, Marilyn; Hôpital régional Chaleur, 1750 Sunset Dr, Bathurst NB E2A 4L7; Mon'03; FRCSC; OrthSurg. Staff, Hopital Regional Chaleur; Langs: Bilingual(French/English); (506)544-3000

BOSSE, Paul-Aime; Clinique Med de Mirabel, CP 1059 Succ St-Janvier 13714 boul Cure Labelle, Mirabel QC J7J 1A1; Mon'71; (450)435-7666; Fax. (450)435-1716.

BOSSERT, Kerri L; Mineral Springs Hosp, PO Box 1050 Stn Main 301 Lynx St, Banff AB T1L 1H7; Cal'06; CCFP; CCFP(E.M.); Staff, Covenant Health - Banff Mineral Springs Hospital; (403)762-2222

BOSTINARIU, Anca Ioana; 204-3825 Sunset St, Burnaby BC V5G 1T4; Bucharest (Romania)'70; FRCPC; Psy. Staff, BC Mental Health & Addiction Service; (604)726-3059

BOSTON, Francis M; MUHC-Royal Victoria Hosp, 687 av des Pins O, Montreal QC H3A 1A1; Cambridge (England)'59; MB ChB; DMRD; LMCC; DiagRad (P.Q.) (Gastrointestinal Radiology). Staff Radiol, McGill University Health Centre - Royal Victoria Hospital; Staff, McGill University Health Centre - Montreal General Campus; Radiologist, Westmount Square Medical Imaging; adj Prof, McGill University; Langs: Swedish; French; Norwegian; (514)843-1545; Fax. (514)843-1517.

BOSTWICK, Joanna; The Ottawa Hosp-Civic Campus, 1053 Carling Ave, Ottawa ON K1Y 4E9; McM'08; CCFP; CCFP(E.M.); Staff, The Ottawa Hospital - Civic Campus; (613)722-7000

BOSWALL, Guy J; West Royalty Med Centre, 591 North River Rd, Charlottetown PE C1E 1J7; Dal'88; FRCSC; Ophth. Staff, Queen Elizabeth Hospital; (902)892-3200; Fax. (902)892-5364; gboswall@islandtelecom.com.

BOSWALL, Margaret; Dept of Veteran's Affairs, PO Box 7700 Stn Central, Charlottetown PE C1A 8M9; Dal'88; Staff, Queen Elizabeth Hospital; Staff, Veterans Affairs Canada; (902)566-8888

BOSWELL, Valerie L; Colon Cancer Screening Ctre, 3280 Hospital Dr NW, Calgary AB T2N 4Z6; McM'85; (403)592-5100

BOSZKO, Andres; Westlaw Bldg, 210-1920 Weston Rd, York ON M9N 1W4; Madrid (Spain)'67; FRCSC; GenSurg (Thoracic Surgery). Staff, Humber River Regional Hospital - Church Street Site; (416)244-9731; Fax. (416)241-3830.

BOSZKO, Michael A; Victoria Gen Hosp, 2340 Pembina Hwy, Winnipeg MB R3T 2E8; Man'00; CCFP; CCFP(E.M.); Staff, Victoria General Hospital.

BOTA, Gary; Sudbury Reg Hosp-Laurentian, 41 Ramsey Lake Rd, Sudbury ON P3E 5J1; McM'79; FRCPC; EmergMed. Staff, Health Sciences North-Laurentian Site; (705)522-2200

BOTES, Roelof J; Claro Family Practice, 107-4930 55 Ave, Drayton Valley AB T7A 1W2; (South Africa)'00; (780)621-0202; Fax. (780)621-0213.

BOTEZ, Stephan; CHUM-Hop Notre-Dame, 1560 rue Sherbrooke E, Montreal QC H2L 4M1; Geneva (Switzerland)'99; FRCPC; Neur. Staff, Centre Hospitalier l'Université de Montréal (CHUM) - Hôpital Notre-Dame; (514)890-8000; Fax. (514)412-7554; stephan.botez@mail.mcgill.ca.

BOTHA, Adriana; Agassiz Med Centre, 130-30 Stephen St, Morden MB R6M 2G3; Pretoria (South Africa)'88; CCFP; (204)822-4474; Fax. (204)822-6886.

BOTHA, Andre J; PO Box 8460 Rpo Marine Lake, Cold Lake AB T9M 1N2; Stellenbosch (South Africa)'83; (780)639-4757; Fax. (780)639-3366.

BOTHA, Andries J; Mountainside Med Clinic, PO Box 1169 2010 129 St, Blairmore AB T0K 0E0; (South Africa)'91; MB ChB; (403)562-2292; Fax. (403)562-2293.

BOTHA, Andries N; Grimshaw Med Clinic, PO Box 1250, Grimshaw AB T0H 1W0; Stellenbosch (South Africa)'82; (780)332-4644; Fax. (780)332-1020; anbotha@telus.net.

BOTHA, Benjamin J A S; 3310 32 Ave, Vernon BC V1T 2M6; Orange Free State (South Africa)'96; MB ChB; CCFP; Staff, Prince Rupert Regional Hospital; (250)545-5321; Fax. (250)545-0450.

BOTHA, Daniel J; Victoria Gen Hosp, 2340 Pembina Highway, Winnipeg MB R3T 2E8; Orange Free State (South Africa)'81; Staff, Victoria General Hospital; (204)269-3570

BOTHA, Daniel J; 1025 103 Ave, Dawson Creek BC V1G 2G6; Limpopo (South Africa)'08; MB ChB; Langs: Afrikaans; (250)782-1186; Fax. (250)782-9447.

BOTHA, Daniel J N; Rhythm Health, 601 67 Ave SW, Calgary AB T2V 0M3; Orange Free State (South Africa)'83; MB ChB; Staff, Rockyview General Hospital; (403)255-5868; Fax. (403)252-7442; familydoc@shaw.ca.

BOTHA, Daniel J P; 1300 111 Ave, Dawson Creek BC V1G 2X5; Orange Free State (South Africa)'82; MB ChB; CCFP; Langs: Afrikaans; (250)782-8604; Fax. (250)782-3318; drbotha@hotmail.com.

BOTHA, David; 222 Wallace St PO Box 400, Hope BC V0X 1L0; Stellenbosch (South Africa)'87; MB ChB; Staff, Fraser Canyon Hospital; Langs: Afrikaans; (604)869-5621; Fax. (604)869-5620; david.botha@fraserhealth.ca.

BOTHA, Deon; 201-300 Veterans Blvd NE, Airdrie AB T4B 3P2; Orange Free State (South Africa)'97; MB ChB; (403)948-4168

BOTHA, Diederick F; Hardisty Med Clinic, PO Box 250, Hardisty AB T0B 1V0; (South Africa)'77; MB ChB; Langs: Afrikaans; (780)888-3662; Fax. (780)888-2666.

BOTHA, Francois; Westgate Med Clinic, 140-20395 Lougheed Hwy, Maple Ridge BC V2X 2P9; Pretoria (South Africa)'77; MB ChB; (604)465-1066; Fax. (604)465-7776; fbotha@crossroadmc.org.

BOTHA, Idelette; 101-595 Columbia St, Kamloops BC V2C 1K7; Orange Free State (South Africa)'04; (250)372-1080

BOTHA, Jan-Beyers; Dr Beyers Botha Med Prof Corp, 106-111 Fairford St E, Moose Jaw SK S6H 7X5; Orange Free State (South Africa)'95; FRCSC; Ophth (Cataract). (306)693-4005; Fax. (306)693-0223; beyers.botha@shaw.ca.

BOTHA, Johannes J; 6236 Gurmit Rd, Prince George BC V2K 0A2; Pretoria (South Africa)'90; MB ChB; CCFP; CCFP(E.M.); (250)962-7078

BOTHA, Johannes; Gibbons Family Med Centre, PO Box 130 4719 50 Ave, Gibbons AB T0A 1N0; Pretoria (South Africa)'84; MB ChB; (780)923-3566; drbothaj@gmail.com.

BOTHA, Lachelle G; Prince Albert Commun Clinic, 110 8th St E, Prince Albert SK S6V 0V7; (306)763-6464; Fax. (306)763-2101.

BOTHA, Maria M; Killarney Med Centre, 220-3425 26 Ave SW, Calgary AB T3E 0N3; Pretoria (South Africa)'01; MB ChB; (403)685-3350; Fax. (403)685-3370.

BOTHA, Mattheus J; Battlefords Union Hosp, 1092 107th St, North Battleford SK S9A 1Z1; (South Africa)'92; Staff, Battlefords Union Hospital; (306)446-6600; Fax. (306)446-7397.

BOTHA, Nicolaas C; Oxbow Family Med Clinic, PO Box 780, Oxbow SK S0C 2B0; Pretoria (South Africa)'84; MB ChB; LMCC; Langs: Afrikaans; Zulu; (306)483-2332; Fax. (306)483-2741.

BOTHA, Nicolaas J; Fairview Medical Clinic, 10624 110 St, Fairview AB T0H 1L0; Orange Free State (South Africa)'83; MB ChB; CCFP; Staff, CFB Health Services Centre; Langs: Afrikaans; (780)835-4255; Fax. (780)835-5009.

BOTHA, Noreen M; PO BOX 219, St Paul AB T0A 3A0; (780)645-4411; Fax. (780)645-4566.

BOTHA, Stephanus S; 1-2168 McCallum Rd, Abbotsford BC V2S 6R6; Pretoria (South Africa)'02; FRCPC; Neur. (604)504-7181

BOTHA, Vincenzo; 8888 Country Hills Blvd PO Box 91023 Rpo Royal Oak, Calgary AB T3G 5W6; (South Africa)'70; MB ChB; Northern Lights Regional Health Centre; (780)791-6161; Fax. (780)791-6042.

BOTHMA, Daniel P J; Wellington Med Clinic, 84C-3200 Island Hwy N, Nanaimo BC V9T 1W1; Stellenbosch (South Africa)'92; MB ChB; CCFP; Langs: German; Afrikaans; (250)740-2100; Fax. (250)740-2114.

BOTHWELL, Jody N; CSSSG-Hop de Gatineau, CP 2000 Succ Bureau-Chef 909 boul de l'Verendrye, Gatineau QC J8P 7H2; McG'93; FRCSC; GenSurg. Staff, Hôpital de Gatineau; (819)561-8100

BOTHWELL, Stuart M; 208-189 Kent St W, Lindsay ON K9V 5G6; Wes'08; CCFP; (705)328-9853; Fax. (705)328-9401.

BOTROS, Mary; Credit River Med Clinic, F001B-6045 Creditview Rd, Mississauga ON L5V 2A8; Ain Shams (Egypt)'93; CCFP; (905)826-6095; Fax. (905)826-9219.

BOTROS, Ussama A; Hotel-Dieu de Sorel, 400 av de l'Hotel-Dieu, Sorel-Tracy QC J3P 1N5; Staff, Hôtel-Dieu de Sorel.

BOTROS, Wagdy; Sleep Clinic, 824 King St W, Kitchener ON N2G 1G1; Ain Shams (Egypt)'75; MB ChB; DPM; MRCPsy; LMCC; FRCPC; Psy (Mood Disorders). Med Dir, Sleep Clinic; Langs: Arabic; (519)579-2002; Fax. (519)579-9371.

BOTROS, Yasser; 301-4800 Leslie St, North York ON M2J 2K9; Ain Shams (Egypt)'89; FRCSC; GenSurg (Laparoscopic Surgery). Ac Staff GenSurg, North York General Hospital; Lecturer, University of Toronto; Langs: Arabic; (416)494-0123; Fax. (416)494-9021.

BOTROUS, Mary; Medicine in Motion Med Clinic, 5-121 Ilsley Ave, Dartmouth NS B3B 1S4; Cairo (Egypt)'00; MB BCh; CCFP; Staff, Medicine in Motion Medical Centre; (902)468-2774

BOTSCHNER, Monika K; East Elgin Family Health Team, 3-418 Talbot St W, Aylmer ON N5H 1K9; Munich (Germany)'73; (519)773-9834

BOTSFORD, Deke J; 1-2380 South Island Hwy, Campbell River BC V9W 1C3; Tor'91; FRCSC; OrthSurg (Adult Reconstructive Surgery). Staff Surgeon, Campbell River & District General Hospital; (250)923-2854; botsford.orthopaedics@gmail.com

BOTTAS, Alexandra; Alberta Mental Health Board, PO Box 307 Stn Main, Edmonton AB T5J 2J7; Alb'98; FRCPC; Psy. Staff, Alberta Hospital Edmonton; Staff, Alberta Mental Health Board; (780)342-5438; bottas@telusplanet.net.

BOTTEGA, Natalie A; MUHC-Royal Victoria Hosp, H4.42-687 av des Pins O, Montreal QC H3A 1A1; McG'99; FRCPC; IntMed; Cardiol. Staff, McGill University Health Centre - Royal Victoria Hospital; (514)934-1934 x42691

BOTTEGA, Remo; 3-41 Caithness St W, Caledonia ON N3W 2J2; Tor'94; CCFP; Court Staff, Norfolk General Hospital; (905)765-9111; Fax. (905)765-9114.

BOTTEN, David L; Dalhousie Health Services, 6230 Coburg Rd, Halifax NS B3H 4J5; Dal'00; CCFP; (902)494-2171; Fax. (902)494-6872.

BOTTENHEIM, Olivia; South Riverdale Commun Hlth Ct, 955 Queen St E, Toronto ON M4M 3P3; McG'05; CCFP; (416)461-2493

BOTTING, Catherine E; South Shore Med Clinic, 620 Cassils Rd E, Brooks AB T1R 1M6; (South Africa)'95; CCFP; (403)793-8111; Fax. (403)793-8118.

BOTTING, Douglas A; 24000 Fern Cres, Maple Ridge BC V4R 2R7; UBC'72; (604)467-3768

BOTTING, Emily F; 15-555 12th Ave W PO Box 47122, Vancouver BC V5Z 3X7; UBC'10; CCFP; (604)872-0821

BOTTOMLEY, Michael G; Carbonear Gen Hosp, 86 Highroad South, Carbonear NL A1Y 1A4; Liverpool (England)'62; MB ChB; PhD; GenSurg. Staff, Carbonear General Hospital; (709)945-5111

BOTTON, Edouard; CSSS de Sept-Iles, 45 rue Du Pere-Divet, Sept-Iles QC G4R 3N7; Laval'92; FRCPC; DiagRad. Staff, Centre Hospitalier Regional de Sept-Iles; (418)962-9761 x2510; Fax. (418)962-2816.

BOTTUM, Norman E; Haliburton Family Med Centre, PO Box 870 7217 Gelert Rd, Haliburton ON K0M 1S0; Wes'85; Dip SportMed; CCFP; FCFP; Ac Staff, Haliburton Highlands Health Services - Haliburton Site; Clin Teacher, University of Toronto; (705)457-1212; Fax. (705)457-3955.

BOU FARAH, Charles; Hotel-Dieu de Sorel, 400 av de l'Hotel-Dieu, Sorel-Tracy QC J3P 1N5; Beirut (Lebanon)'98; Staff OrthSurg, Centre Hospitalier Pierre Boucher; Staff, Hôtel-Dieu de Sorel; Langs: Arabic; English; (450)746-6000

BOU KARAM, Christian E; Hop Maisonneuve-Rosemont, 5415 boul de l'Assomption, Montreal QC H1T 2M4; Mon'01; RadOncol (Oncology). Staff RadOncol, Hopital Maisonneuve-Rosemont; (514)252-3425; Fax. (514)252-3556; cboukaram.hmr@ssss.gouv.qc.ca.

BOU-MERHI, Joseph; CHUM-Hop Notre-Dame, 1560 rue Sherbrooke E, Montreal QC H2L 4M1; Mon'03; PlasSurg. Staff, Centre Hospitalier l'Université de Montréal (CHUM) - Hôpital Notre-Dame; (514)890-8000 x24444; Fax. (514)412-7575.

BOUALI, Redouane; CHUM-Hotel-Dieu, 3840 rue Saint-Urbain, Montreal QC H2W 1T8; (Nigeria)'87; Critical Care Medicine (P.Q.). Staff, Centre Hospitalier l'Université de Montréal (CHUM) - Hôtel-Dieu; Staff, CSSS de Gatineau; Prof Critical Care Med, Universite de Montreal; (514)890-8000 x12657; Fax. (514)412-7161; redouanebouali@hotmail.com.

BOUALLEGUE, Abdelkader; CSSS Bordeaux-Cartierville-St-, 555 boul Gouin O, Montreal QC H3L 1K5; Tunis (Tunisia)'76; Staff, Pavillon Notre-Dame de la Merci; (514)331-3025

BOUAYED, Rita; CSSS Pierre Boucher, 1333 boul Jacques-Cartier E, Longueuil QC J4M 2A5; Laval'02; Psy. Staff, Centre Hospitalier Pierre Boucher; (450)468-8111

BOUAZRA, Ahlem; CLSC Paspebiac, 273 rue Gerard-d-Levesque O, Paspebiac QC G0C 2K0; (Other Foreign)'01; Staff, CLSC de Paspebiac; (418)752-2572

BOUBALOS, Anastasios; Cornwall Comm Hosp-Mcconnell, PO Box 100 Stn Main 840 McConnell Ave, Cornwall ON K6H 5S5; McG'87; BSc(Chemistry); FRCPC; DiagRad (Emergency Medicine). Staff, Cornwall Community Hospital; (613)988-4240; boubalos@sympatico.ca.

BOUBEKEUR, Fadila; CSSS Bordeaux-Cartierville-St-, 555 boul Gouin O, Montreal QC H3L 1K5; (Algeria)'81; Staff, Pavillon Notre-Dame de la Merci; (514)331-3020

BOUBEZ, Ghassan; CHUM-Hop Notre-Dame, 1560 rue Sherbrooke E, Montreal QC H2L 4M1; Sher'86; OrthSurg. Staff, Centre Hospitalier l'Université de Montréal (CHUM) - Hôpital Notre-Dame; (514)890-8000 x25900; Fax. (514)412-7619.

BOUBEZ, Walid I; CSSS du Coeur-de-l'Ile, 1385 rue Jean-Talon E, Montreal QC H2E 1S6; Tartu (Estonia)'94; FRCPC; IntMed. Staff, CSSS du Coeur de l'Isle Hôpital Jean-Talon; (514)495-6767

BOUCH, Peter J; Piper Creek Med Clinic, 200-3215 49 Ave, Red Deer AB T4N 0M8; Pretoria (South Africa)'88; CCFP; (403)986-7265; Fax. (403)986-7604.

BOUCHAL, Hachemi; Hôtel-Dieu de Sorel, 400 av de l'Hotel-Dieu, Sorel-Tracy QC J3P 1N5; Staff, Hôtel-Dieu de Sorel; (450)746-6000 x7623

BOUCHARD, Alexandre; CHUQ-St-Francois D'Assise, 10 rue de l'Espinay, Quebec QC G1L 3L5; Laval'02; FRCSC; GenSurg (Colorectal Surgery). Staff, Centre Hospitalier Universitaire De Québec - Pavillon De St-françois-d'assise; (418)525-4444 x54160

BOUCHARD, Amelie; Centre Med St-Redempteur, 210-600 Rte 116, Saint-Nicolas QC G7A 4X8; Laval'08; (418)831-3677; amelie.bouchard@gmf.gouv.qc.ca.

BOUCHARD, Andre; Clinique Med Pierre-Bertrand, 212-303 boul Pierre-Bertrand, Quebec QC G1M 3L7; Laval'75; (418)683-2724; Fax. (418)683-8861; andre.bouchard@orlo.ulaval.ca.

BOUCHARD, Andre; Clinique de Med Fam de la Malb, 515 rue Saint-Etienne, La Malbaie QC G5A 1W7; Laval'88; Chef cabinet, Hôpital de la Malbaie; Langs: English; (418)665-2533; Fax. (418)665-7766; andre.bouchard.cmlm@ssss.gouv.qc.ca.

BOUCHARD, Anne-Marie; Inst Philippe Pinel de Mtl, 10905 boul Henri-Bourassa E, Montreal QC H1C 1H1; Mon'95; Psy. Staff, Institut Philippe-Pinel de Montreal; (514)648-8461; Fax. (514)881-4505.

BOUCHARD, Anne-Sylvie; Hop du Haut-Richelieu, 920 boul du Seminaire N, St-Jean-sur-Richel QC J3A 1B7; Mon'90; Staff, Hôpital du Haut-Richelieu; (450)359-5000

BOUCHARD, Annie; Centre de Sante Valcartier, CP 1000 Bdp Succ Forces, Courcelette QC G0A 4Z0; Mon'93; Staff, Centre de Sante Valcartier; (418)844-5000 x4203; bouchard.amc@forces.gc.ca.

BOUCHARD, Ariane; Clinique Med Nepisiguit, 950 av Picot, Bathurst NB E2A 4Z9; Sher'03; CCFP; Staff, Hopital Regional Chaleur; (506)546-6696

BOUCHARD, Caroline; Clinique d'ORL, 101-867 boul Saint-Joseph, Roberval QC G8H 2L8; Laval'95; FRCSC; Otol (Allergy). Staff, Hotel-Dieu de Roberval; (418)275-3266; Fax. (418)275-9152.

BOUCHARD, Catherine; CSSS de la Vallee de l'Or, 725 6e rue, Val-d'Or QC J9P 3Y1; Mon'06; CCFP; (819)825-6711; Fax. (819)825-7909.

BOUCHARD, Celine; Centre Med Sante Femme, 304-1000 ch Sainte-Foy, Quebec QC G1S 2L6; Laval'78; FRCSC; ObstGyn (Colposcopy). ac Staff, Centre Hospitalier Affilié Universitaire de Québec - Hôpital du St-Sacrement; (418)266-1616; Fax. (418)650-1374.

BOUCHARD, Chantale; Institut Philippe Pinel de Mtl, 10905 boul Henri-Bourassa E, Montreal QC H1C 1H1; Mon'92; FRCPC; Psy. Staff, Institut Philippe-Pinel de Montreal; (514)648-8461; Fax. (514)881-3784.

BOUCHARD, Christiane; Centre Med Racine, 201-900 boul Raymond, Quebec QC G1B 3G3; Laval'84; (418)667-8066; Fax. (418)667-8131.

BOUCHARD, Cindy; Hop du CSS de la Region Thetfo, 1717 rue Notre-Dame E, Thetford Mines QC G6G 2V4; Laval'09; Staff, CSSS de la Matapedia; Staff, Hopital du CSS de la Region de Thetford; (418)338-7777

BOUCHARD, Claire; CHUQ-Ctr Hosp Univ Laval, 2705 boul Laurier, Quebec QC G1V 4G2; Laval'77; ac Staff, Centre Hospitalier Universitaire de Quebec-CHUL; (418)654-2255; Fax. (418)654-2757.

BOUCHARD, Claude A; CSSS du Haut Saint-Maurice, 885 boul Ducharme, La Tuque QC G9X 3C1; Laval'70; Staff, Centre Hospitalier Saint-Joseph de la Turque; (819)523-3084

BOUCHARD, Claude; Clinique de Med Gen d'Alma, 22 rue Melancon E, Alma QC G8B 6W3; Mon'90; (418)668-2377; claude.bouchard@ssss.gouv.qc.ca.

BOUCHARD, Claude; Clinique du Vieux Gatineau, 3B-520 boul de l'Hopital, Gatineau QC J8V 2P5; Mon'83; Urol. (819)568-3224

BOUCHARD, Claude M; SAAQ, 333 boul Jean-Lesage, Quebec QC G1K 8Z2; Laval'69; Médecin, Societe Assurance Automobile du Quebec; (418)528-3881

BOUCHARD, Claude R; CLSC-CHSLD Rimouski-Neigette, 165 rue des Gouverneurs, Rimouski QC G5L 7R2; Laval'70; Physician, Programme de Sante Mentale; (418)724-7204; Fax. (418)727-5494.

BOUCHARD, Clermont; Clinique Med Chateauguay, 120 boul Saint-Jean-Baptiste, Chateauguay QC J6K 3A9; Laval'67; Langs: Bilingual(French/English); (450)691-8191; Fax. (450)691-8568.

BOUCHARD, Denis; Institut de Cardiologie de Mtl, 5000 rue Belanger, Montreal QC H1T 1C8; McG'92; FRCSC; Cardiovasc&ThorSurg (P.Q.); CardSurg. Staff, Institut de Cardiologie de Montréal; (514)376-3330; Fax. (514)376-4766.

BOUCHARD, Denyse; 200-2924 boul Taschereau, Greenfield Park QC J4V 2G8; Mon'77; Psy. Staff, Hopital Charles LeMoyne; (450)466-8486 x261; Fax. (450)466-8789.

BOUCHARD, Elise; CSSS Maria-Chapdelaine, 2000 boul du Sacre-Coeur, Dolbeau-Mistassini QC G8L 2R5; Laval'02; IntMed. Staff, Centre Maria-Chapdelaine - CH de Dolbeau-Mistassini; (418)276-1234

BOUCHARD, Francois; CSSS de Laval, CP 170 1755 boul Rene-Laennec, Laval QC H7M 3L9; Mon'90; CSPQ; FRCPC; Anes. Staff, Hopital de la Cite de la santé; (450)668-1010; Fax. (450)975-5545.

BOUCHARD, Francois; Clinique de Dermatologie, 101-937 av du Pont S, Alma QC G8B 2V5; Laval'86; FRCPC; Derm. (418)668-7616; Fax. (418)668-5011.

BOUCHARD, Francoise; Ctre de Sante Tulattavik l'Ung, CP 149, Kuujjuaq QC J0M 1C0; Laval'74; MPH(Harvard); FRCPC; CommunMed. Staff, Centre de sante Tulattavik de l'Ungava; Gen Dir Health Sevices, Correctional Services of Canada; Langs: English; (514)602-0689; bouchardfr@csc-scc.gc.ca.

BOUCHARD, Genevieve; Clinique Med Familiale Saguena, 220-874 boul de l'Universite E, Chicoutimi QC G7H 6B9; Laval'08; (418)545-1217; Fax. (418)545-4782.

BOUCHARD, Gilles; CHUQ-St-Francois d'Assise, 10 rue de l'Espinay, Quebec QC G1L 3L5; Laval'80; FRCPC; DiagRad. ac Staff, Centre Hospitalier Universitaire De Québec - Pavillon De St-françois-d'assise; (418)525-4309 x3188; Fax. (418)525-4180.

BOUCHARD, Gilles R; 370 rue Dufferin RR 4, Stanstead QC J0B 3E2; Mon'63; Langs: Bilingual(French/English); (819)876-2127; Fax. (819)876-2197; camado@sympatico.ca.

BOUCHARD, Ginette; 330 rang de la Montagne, Rougemont QC J0L 1M0; Mon'80; Med Consultant Program "Sante Parent-Enfant" & "Vivre avec Coeur", CLSC Suzor-Cote-Victoriaville; (450)469-3780; ginette_bouchard@ssss.gouv.qc.ca.

BOUCHARD, Guillaume; CSSS de Laval, 1755 boul Rene-Laennec, Laval QC H7M 3L9; Sher'00; NuclearMed. Staff, Hopital de la Cite de la santé; (450)668-1010 x2435

BOUCHARD, Guylain; Ctr Hosp Affilie-St-Sacrement, 1050 ch Sainte-Foy, Quebec QC G1S 4L8; Laval'90; Psy. Staff, Centre Hospitalier Affilié Universitaire de Québec - Hôpital du St-Sacrement; (418)682-7511

BOUCHARD, Henri-Louis; Clinique Med Saint-Louis, 220-3165 ch Saint-Louis, Quebec QC G1W 4R4; Laval'65; OrthSurg (P.Q.) (Oncology). Staff, Centre Hospitalier Universitaire de Québec (CHUQ) - Siege Social; Université Laval; (418)653-6000; hlbouch@sympatico.ca.

BOUCHARD, Hugues; Hopital de Chicoutimi, CP 5006 305 rue Saint-Vallier, Chicoutimi QC G7H 5H6; Sher'07; Nephrol; IntMed. Staff, Complexe hospitalier de la Sagamie; (418)541-1131

BOUCHARD, Isabelle; CHUQ-Ctr Hosp Univ Laval, R 1742-2705 boul Laurier, Quebec QC G1V 4G2; Laval'94; FRCPC; Peds (Diabetology). Staff, Centre Hospitalier Universitaire de Quebec-CHUL; Langs: English; (418)656-4141; Fax. (418)654-2137.

BOUCHARD, Isabelle; CSSS de Jonquiere, 2230 rue de l'Hopital, Jonquiere QC G7X 4H6; Laval'04; CCFP; Staff, Centre Hospitalier Jonquiere; (418)695-7700

BOUCHARD, J Jacques A; Foothills Med Centre, G33-1403 29 St NW, Calgary AB T2N 2T9; Ott'83; DABOS; FRCSC; OrthSurg (Spine Surgery). Staff, Foothills Medical Centre; Clin Assoc Prof, University of Calgary; Langs: Bilingual(French/English); (403)944-8236; Fax. (403)270-3587; jacques.bouchard@calgaryhealthregion.ca.

BOUCHARD, Jacques; Clin Med Fam de la Malbaie, 515 rue Saint-Etienne, La Malbaie QC G5A 1W7; Laval'79; (418)665-2533; Fax. (418)665-7766.

BOUCHARD, Jacques; 110-1 Place Du Commerce, Verdun QC H3E 1A2; Mon'68; FRCSC; PlasSurg. ac Staff, Centre Hospitalier de Verdun; (514)769-8809; Fax. (514)769-1452.

BOUCHARD, Jacques; 5-85 rue Saint-Charles O, Longueuil QC J4H 1C5; Laval'71 Laval; FRCP; Psy (Trauma). Langs: English; (450)674-9455; Fax. (450)674-9051; bouchardja@videotron.ca.

BOUCHARD, Jasmin; CHUS-Hopital Hotel-Dieu, 580 rue Bowen S, Sherbrooke QC J1G 2E8; Laval'09; CCFP; CCFP(E.M.); Staff, Centre Hospitalier Universitaire de Sherbrooke-Hôpital Hôtel-Dieu; (819)346-1110

BOUCHARD, Jean; CSSS de Trois-Rivieres, 1991 boul du Carmel, Trois-Rivieres QC G8Z 3R9; Laval'80; MedMicrobiol. Staff, CSSS de Trois-Rivières; (819)697-3333 x64022

BOUCHARD, Jean-Benoit; Clinique Pediatrie du Saguenay, 475 rue Talbot, Chicoutimi QC G7H 4A3; Laval'05; FRCPC; Peds. Staff, Complexe hospitalier de la Sagamie; (418)549-1034; Fax. (418)696-4673.

BOUCHARD, Jean-Claude; Clinique Cherbourg, 1190 boul Louis-XIV, Quebec QC G1H 6P2; Laval'71; Médecin, Centre Medicale Cherbourg Inc; (418)781-1591; Fax. (418)781-1595.

BOUCHARD, Jean-Guy; C-2 rue Jeanne D'Arc, Kedgwick NB E8B 1G3; Laval'66; (506)284-2032; Fax. (506)284-1991.

BOUCHARD, Jean-Pierre L; Ctr Hosp Affilie-Enfant-Jesus, 1401 18e rue, Quebec QC G1J 1Z4; Laval'65; CSPQ; FRCPC; Neur (Neuro Genetics). ac Staff, Centre Hospitalier Affilié Universitaire de Québec - Hôpital De L'Enfant Jésus; Prof Emeritus, Université Laval; Langs: Bilingual(French/English); (418)649-0252; Fax. (418)649-5511.

BOUCHARD, Jean-Simon; Centre Med Medford, 1 Place de l'Estrie, Bedford QC J0J 1A0; Laval'70; Staff, Hôpital du Haut-Richelieu; (450)248-3336; Fax. (450)248-7751; jean-simon_bouchard@rrsss16.gouv.qc.ca.

BOUCHARD, Josee; CLSC des Frontieres, RR 2 1922 rue Saint-Vallier, Pohenegamook QC G0L 1J0; Mon'87; Staff, Centre Hospitalier Regional du Grand-Portage; Staff, CSSS de Quebec Nord; Staff, Centre Hospitalier Notre-Dame-du-Lac; Langs: English; (418)859-2450; joseebouchard_21@hotmail.com.

BOUCHARD, Josee; Hop du Sacre-Coeur de Mtl, 5400 boul Gouin O, Montreal QC H4J 1C5; Mon'01; FRCPC; IntMed; Nephrol. Staff, Hôpital du Sacre-Coeur de Montréal; (514)338-2222

BOUCHARD, Julien; CSSS de Chicoutimi, CP 5006 305 rue Saint-Vallier, Chicoutimi QC G7H 5H6; Mon'09; CCFP; CCFP(E.M.); Staff, Complexe hospitalier de la Sagamie; (418)541-1234

BOUCHARD, Laurent; Centre Med Durocher, 140 rue Saint-Vallier O, Quebec QC G1K 1K1; Laval'77; ac Staff, CSSS de Quebec-Sud; (418)529-0291; Fax. (418)529-7405.

BOUCHARD, Laurier; 200-394 rue Saint-Vallier, Chicoutimi QC G7H 4J1; Laval'76; FRCSC; ObstGyn. Staff, Complexe hospitalier de la Sagamie; Langs: Bilingual(English/French); (418)545-2666; Fax. (418)545-3924.

BOUCHARD, Louis; CHUM-Hop St-Luc, 1058 rue Saint-Denis, Montreal QC H2X 3J4; Mon'95; FRCPC; DiagRad. Staff, Centre Hospitalier l'Université De Montréal (CHUM) - Hôpital Saint-luc; (514)890-8000 x35622

BOUCHARD, Louis M; Ctr Hosp de Lachine, 650 16e av, Lachine QC H8S 3N5; Ott'68; CSPQ; BSc(Biol.); FRCPC; AnatPath (Cytology). Chef Path, CSSS de Dorval-Lachine-Lasalle; (514)637-2351 x77382

BOUCHARD, Lucie; Clinique Med Mellon, 303-2075 boul Mellon, Jonquiere QC G7S 5Z8; Laval'95; CCFP; (418)548-1121; Fax. (418)548-5345.

BOUCHARD, Lucie; Clinique Med Fam Jonquiere, 3835 boul Harvey, Jonquiere QC G7X 2Z5; Laval'92; (418)542-7519; Fax. (418)542-6541.

BOUCHARD, Ludovic; Clinique de Chirurgie du Litto, 111-822 boul Sainte-Anne, Rimouski QC G5M 1J5; Laval'04; FRCSC; OrthSurg. (418)723-0194

BOUCHARD, M Josee; CSSS de Saint-Jerome, 290 rue de Montigny, Saint-Jerome QC J7Z 5T3; Mon'99; Cardiol; IntMed. Staff, Hôtel-Dieu de Saint-Jérôme; (450)431-8200

BOUCHARD, Manon; Hôtel-Dieu de Lévis, 143 rue Wolfe, Levis QC G6V 3Z1; Laval'04; FRCPC; Neur (Movement Disorders). Staff, Hôtel-Dieu de Lévis; Langs: English; Spanish; (418)835-7121 x7158; Fax. (418)835-7212.

BOUCHARD, Marc; CHUQ-Hotel-Dieu du Quebec, 11 Cote Du Palais, Quebec QC G1R 2J6; Laval'97; FRCSC; OrthSurg. Staff, Centre Hospitalier Universitaire de Québec (CHUQ) - Siege Social; Langs: Bilingual(French/English); (418)691-5370; Fax. (418)691-5020.

BOUCHARD, Marc; Clinique Med du Sud-Ouest, 103-4475 rue Bannantyne, Verdun QC H4G 1E2; Laval'80; Langs: Bilingual(French/English); (514)765-3600; Fax. (514)765-9625.

BOUCHARD, Marcel; CSSS de Chicoutimi, CP 264 305 rue Saint-Vallier, Chicoutimi QC G7H 5H6; Laval'72; Psy (P.Q.). Staff, Complexe hospitalier de la Sagamie; Staff, Institut Roland-Saucier; (418)549-5477; Fax. (418)549-7604.

BOUCHARD, Marie; 60 av Bateman, Edmundston NB E3V 4X6; Laval'85; Langs: English; (506)739-9183; Fax. (506)739-9050.

BOUCHARD, Marie-Claude; Salvus Family Med Clinic, 62-143 Liberton Dr, St. Albert AB T8N 6A7; Sher'99; CCFP; Langs: Bilingual(French/English); (780)460-4562; Fax. (780)460-4550; mobpinky@yahoo.ca.

BOUCHARD, Maryse L; St Michael's Hosp, 30 Bond St, Toronto ON M5B 1W8; McG'06; MDCM; FRCSC; OrthSurg. Staff, St Michael's Hospital.

BOUCHARD, Maurice; CHUQ-Ctr Hosp Univ Laval, 2705 boul Laurier, Quebec QC G1V 4G2; Laval'60; FAAP; FRCPC; Peds. Clin Prof, Centre Hospitalier Universitaire de Quebec-CHUL; Université Laval; Langs: English; Spanish; (418)656-4141; Fax. (418)654-2137.

BOUCHARD, Michel; Clinique Med Dr Michel Bouchar, CP 520 54 Notre-Dame, Cap-Chat QC G0J 1E0; Laval'72; (418)786-5565; Fax. (418)786-5585.

BOUCHARD, Michel R; CSSS Pierre Boucher, 1333 boul Jacques-Cartier E, Longueuil QC J4M 2A5; Mon'72; MSc(O.M.); Staff, Centre Hospitalier Pierre Boucher; (450)468-8111

BOUCHARD, Michele; Clinique Med de Levis, 100-4975 boul de la Rive-Sud, Levis QC G6V 4Z5; Laval'84; (418)833-5810; Fax. (418)833-2720.

BOUCHARD, Myriam; 210 rue Principale, St-Nazaire-D-L-S-J QC G0W 2V0; Mon'07; (418)668-8122

BOUCHARD, Myriam; CHUS-Hop Fleurimont, 3001 12e av N, Sherbrooke QC J1H 5N4; Laval'01; FRCPC; RadOncol. Staff, Centre Hospitalier Universitaire de Sherbrooke-Hopital Fleurimont; (819)346-1110 x14602

BOUCHARD, Nadine; CSSS Les Eskers de l'Abitibi, 622 4e rue O, Amos QC J9T 2S2; Laval'99; CSPQ; FRCPC; Anes. Staff, CH Hôtel-Dieu d'Amos; (819)732-3341; Fax. (819)732-7622.

BOUCHARD, Nadine; CSSS de Lac-Saint Jean-Est, CP 1300 Succ Bureau-Chef 300 boul Champlain, Alma QC G8B 5W3; Laval'99; CSPQ; FRCPC; Anes. Anesthesiste, CSSS de Lac-Saint Jean-Est; (418)669-2000 x2224

BOUCHARD, Nicole; CHUS-Hop Fleurimont, 2616-3001 12e av N, Sherbrooke QC J1H 5N4; Sher'00; FRCPC; IntMed; Respir. Staff, Centre Hospitalier Universitaire de Sherbrooke-Hopital Fleurimont; (819)822-6735; Fax. (819)822-6763.

BOUCHARD, Nicole; Dir de la Sante Publique, 1 9e rue, Rouyn-Noranda QC J9X 2A9; Mon'77; Staff, Centre Hospitalier Rouyn-Noranda; (819)764-3264 x49411; Fax. (819)764-4537; nbouchar@ssss.gouv.qc.ca.

BOUCHARD, Normand; Clinique Med de la Baie, 437 rue Albert, La Baie QC G7B 3L5; Laval'78; Staff, Complexe hospitalier de la Sagamie; (418)544-6863; Fax. (418)544-6864.

BOUCHARD, Patrick; CSSS de Laval, 1755 boul Rene-Laennec, Laval QC H7M 3L9; Mon'96; GenSurg. Staff, Hopital de la Cite de la santé; (450)668-1010

BOUCHARD, Patrick; Clinique Med Mellon, 203-2075 boul Mellon, Jonquiere QC G7S 5Z8; Laval'76; ac Staff, Centre Hospitalier Jonquiere; Physician, Secal & Alcan; (418)548-8281

BOUCHARD, Philippe; CHUQ-St-Francois D'Assise, 10 rue de l'Espinay, Quebec QC G1L 3L5; Laval'02; FRCSC; GenSurg. Staff, Centre Hospitalier Universitaire De Québec - Pavillon De St-françois-d'assise; (418)525-4160

BOUCHARD, Pierre; Clinique Med Fam Jonquiere, 3835 boul Harvey, Jonquiere QC G7X 2Z5; Laval'75; Langs: Bilingual(French/English); (418)542-7519; Fax. (418)542-6541.

BOUCHARD, Pierre; CLSC du Richelieu, 300 ch de Marieville, Richelieu QC J3L 3V8; Mon'88; (450)658-7561; Fax. (450)658-4390.

BOUCHARD, Raymond D; 101-150 Saint Paul St, Collingwood ON L9Y 3P2; Man'82; CCFP; FCFP; Staff, Collingwood General & Marine Hospital; (705)444-1239; Fax. (705)444-8421; rbouch2560@rogers.com.

BOUCHARD, Remi; 610 boul Du Seminaire N, St-Jean-Sur-Richel QC J3B 7B4; Mon'80; Staff, Hôpital du Haut-Richelieu; (450)348-9218; Fax. (450)348-0377.

BOUCHARD, Remi; Clinique Med Fam Jonquiere, 3835 boul Harvey, Jonquiere QC G7X 2Z5; Laval'94; (418)542-7519; Fax. (418)542-6541; remi.bouchard.cmj@ssss.gouv.qc.ca.

BOUCHARD, Remi; Clin des Medecins d'Urgence, 632 rue Bowen S, Sherbrooke QC J1G 2E9; Sher'84; CCFP; CCFP(E.M.); ac Staff, Centre Hospitalier Universitaire de Sherbrooke-Hôpital Hôtel-Dieu; (819)822-2700; Fax. (819)822-2027.

BOUCHARD, Remi W; Ctr Hosp Affilie-Enfant-Jesus, 1401 18e rue, Quebec QC G1J 1Z4; Laval'66; MSc(Physiol.); CSPQ; CRCPC; Electroenceph (P.Q.); Neur (Behavioural Neurology). ac Staff, Centre Hospitalier Affilié Universitaire de Québec - Hôpital De L'Enfant Jésus; Consultant, Hôpital Laval; Clin Assoc Prof, Université Laval; Langs: Bilingual(English/French); (418)649-0252 x3262; Fax. (418)649-5541.

BOUCHARD, Reynald; Hotel-Dieu de Roberval, 450 rue Brassard, Roberval QC G8H 1B9; Laval'65; DiagRad. Staff, Hotel-Dieu de Roberval; (418)275-0110

BOUCHARD, Roch H; Clin Notre-Dame-des-Victoires, 40-70 rue Dalhousie, Quebec QC G1K 4B2; Laval'82; Psy. Staff, Institut Universitaire Sante; (418)694-2223; Fax. (418)694-2003.

BOUCHARD, Roger; Clin de Gynecologie St-Germain, 101-180 rue des Gouverneurs, Rimouski QC G5L 8G1; Laval'77; FACOG; CSPQ; ObstGyn (Menopause). ac Membre, Hôpital Regional Rimouski; Langs: English; (418)722-4333; Fax. (418)722-8714.

BOUCHARD, Sarah; Hôpital Ste-Justine, 3175 ch Cote-Sainte-Catherine, Montreal QC H3T 1C5; McG'92; FRCS; FRCSC; GenSurg; PedGenSurg. Staff, Hôpital Ste-Justine; assoc Prof Surg, Universite de Montreal; Langs: French; (514)345-4915; Fax. (514)345-4964; sarah.bouchard.hsj@ssss.gouv.qc.ca.

BOUCHARD, Simon; CHUM-Hop St-Luc, 1058 rue Saint-Denis, Montreal QC H2X 3J4; Mon'07; Gastroent; IntMed. Staff, Centre Hospitalier l'Université De Montréal (CHUM) - Hôpital Saint-luc; (514)890-8000

BOUCHARD, Suzanne; Unite de Med Familiale, 100-500 boul de l'Hopital, Gatineau QC J8V 2P5; Laval'87; CCFP; ac Staff, Hôpital de Gatineau; (819)561-8107 x254

BOUCHARD, Sylvain; Clinique Med Centre-Ville, 95 av Rouleau, Rimouski QC G5L 5S4; Sher'90; Staff, Hôpital Regional Rimouski; Médecin, Clinique Medicale Centre-Ville; (418)722-6816; Fax. (418)721-3262.

BOUCHARD, Sylvie; Lakeshore Gen Hosp, 160 av Stillview, Pointe-Claire QC H9R 2Y2; Laval'98; CCFP; Staff, Lakeshore General Hospital - Pointe Claire; VP, Clinical Research Laboratories Pharm Inc.; (514)630-2225; sylbouc@hotmail.com.

BOUCHARD, Sylvie; Hop du Sacre-Coeur de Mtl, 5400 boul Gouin O, Montreal QC H4J 1C5; Sher'84; Staff, Hôpital du Sacre-Coeur de Montréal; Teach Staff, Universite de Montreal; (514)338-2000

BOUCHARD, Thomas P; Deer Valley Family Med Centre, 101-83 Deerpoint Rd SE, Calgary AB T2J 6W5; Cal'10; CCFP; (403)271-5123; Fax. (403)225-1276.

BOUCHARD, Yves; Clin Med Bourg-Royal, 1289 boul Louis-XIV, Quebec QC G2L 1M1; Laval'88; Staff, Jeffery Hale Hospital-Saint Brigid's; (418)627-7129; Fax. (418)627-7145.

BOUCHARD, Yves; Polyclinique St-Jerome, 102-200 rue Durand, Saint-Jerome QC J7Z 7E2; Mon'84; (450)431-7666; Fax. (450)431-1275.

BOUCHARD, Yvon; Hotel-Dieu de Roberval, 450 rue Brassard, Roberval QC G8H 1B9; Laval'78; Chef psychiatrie, Hotel-Dieu de Roberval; (418)275-3195; Fax. (418)275-4829; ybouchardmd@videotron.ca.

BOUCHARD-ARSLANIAN, Celine; 50-1405 boul Henri-Bourassa O, Montreal QC H3M 3B2; Mon'79; Instructor Advanced Cardiac Life Support, Quebec Heart Foundation; (514)336-2966; Fax. (514)336-7434.

BOUCHARD-RICHARD, Marie-Claude; Clinique Sante Femme, 31 rue Drummond, Granby QC J2G 2S3; Sher'05; ObstGyn. (450)372-4008; Fax. (450)372-0068.

BOUCHARD-ROCHETTE, Marie-Eve; CSSS de la Haute-Gaspésie, 50 rue du Belvedere, Ste-Anne-des-Monts QC G4V 1X4; Laval'10; CCFP; Staff, Centre Hospitalier des Monts; (418)763-2261

BOUCHEK, Belkacem; CSSS les Eskers de l'Abitibi, 6221 4e rue O, Amos QC J9T 2S2; (Algeria)'77; DPsy(Paris); Psychiatre, Hôpital psychiatrique de Malartic; Staff, CH Hôtel-Dieu d'Amos; Langs: German; Arabic; English; (819)732-3341 x2210; belkacem_bouchek@ssss.gouv.qc.ca.

BOUCHER, Andre J; Centre de Services de Sante, 33 rue Main, Rexton NB E4W 0E5; Laval'65; (506)523-7940; Fax. (506)523-7949.

BOUCHER, Andree; CHUM-Hop Notre-Dame, 1560 rue Sherbrooke E, Montreal QC H2L 4M1; Mon'82; FRCPC; IntMed; Endocrin (P.Q.); Endocrin&Metab. Staff, Centre Hospitalier l'Université de Montréal (CHUM) - Hôpital Notre-Dame; vice Doyen Pedagogy & Continuing Prof Development, Universite de Montreal; (514)890-8000 x25603

BOUCHER, Andree-Anne; GMF de l'Assomption, 814 boul l'Ange-Gardien N, L'Assomption QC J5W 4M9; Mon'10; (450)589-5342

BOUCHER, Anne; Hop Maisonneuve-Rosemont, 5415 boul de l'Assomption, Montreal QC H1T 2M4; Sher'79; FRCPC; IntMed (Formation Nephrology); Nephrol. Chef néphrol, Hopital Maisonneuve-Rosemont; Prof, Universite de Montreal; Langs: English; (514)252-3489; Fax. (514)255-3026; aboucher.hmr@ssss.gouv.qc.ca.

BOUCHER, Anne-Louise; Clinique Med Sainte-Madeleine, 165 boul Sainte-Madeleine, Trois-Rivieres QC G8T 3L7; Laval'89; LMCC; (819)379-8385; Fax. (819)379-1607; anne-louie_boucher@gmf.gouv.qc.ca.

BOUCHER, C Benjamin; 402 Granville St, Port Hawkesbury NS B9A 2M7; Dal'78; (902)625-3707; Fax. (902)625-1842.

BOUCHER, Carl; CSSS du Nord de Lanaudière, 1000 boul Sainte-Anne, St-Charles-Brromee QC J6E 6J2; Mon'95; CSPQ; Anes (P.Q.). Staff, Centre Hospitalier Régional de Lanaudière; (450)759-8222

BOUCHER, Carl; CSSSG-Hop de Hull, 116 boul Lionel-Emond, Gatineau QC J8Y 1W7; Sher'94; FRCSC; Otol. Staff, Hull Hospital; Hd Otol, Hopital Regional Chaleur; Langs: Bilingual(French/English); (819)966-6200; Fax. (819)966-6039; carlboucher@hotmail.com.

BOUCHER, Carl; 8224 rue St-Paul, Bas-Caraquet NB E1W 6E2; Sher'07; CCFP; (506)727-7549; Fax. (506)727-7320.

BOUCHER, Catherine; Readaptation Chaudiere-Appalac, 9500 boul Centre-Hospitalier, Charny QC G6X 0A1; Laval'07; BSc; CCFP; Médecin Family Med, Centre Hospitalier Paul-Gilbert; Langs: Bilingual(French/English); (418)380-2064

BOUCHER, Catherine; Royal Ottawa Hosp, 1145 Carling Ave, Ottawa ON K1Z 7K4; Sher'87; Psy (P.Q.) (Pediatric Psychiatry). Staff, Royal Ottawa Mental Health Centre - Royal Ottawa Health Care Group; Physician, Family Court Clinic; Langs: English; (613)722-6521 x6400; Fax. (613)724-6554.

BOUCHER, Chantale; CSSS Pierre Boucher, 1333 boul Jacques-Cartier E, Longueuil QC J4M 2A5; Laval'88; FRCPC; Peds (Public Health). Staff, Centre Hospitalier Pierre Boucher; Langs: Bilingual(French/English); (450)468-8111; Fax. (450)649-2218.

BOUCHER, Claude; GMF du Chatel, 200-9465 boul de l'Ormiere, Quebec QC G2B 3K7; Laval'73; Langs: Bilingual(French/English); (418)843-5141; Fax. (418)843-5343.

BOUCHER, Daniel A; CSST, CP 1200 Succ Terminus 280-524 rue Bourdages, Quebec QC G1K 7E2; Laval'86; CSPQ; AnatPath (Renal Pathology). (418)266-4670; Fax. (418)266-4672.

BOUCHER, Daniel A; 5-105 Progress Cres, Kapuskasing ON P5N 3J4; Ott'08; IntMed.

BOUCHER, Daniel; CP 5679 Stn Main, Caraquet NB E1W 1B7; Mon'87; Staff, Hôpital de l'Enfant-Jésus RHSJ; (506)727-7768

BOUCHER, Danny; Ctr Hosp Rouyn-Noranda, 4 9e rue, Rouyn-Noranda QC J9X 2B2; McG'93; CSPQ; FRCPC; GenPath; AnatPath. Staff, Centre Hospitalier Rouyn-Noranda; (819)764-5131 x43114; Fax. (819)764-2911; danny.boucher@ssss.gouv.qc.ca.

BOUCHER, Denis; Centre Med St-Jean, 202-1018 rue de la Prairie O, St-J-Chrysostome QC G6Z 0A7; Laval'78; (418)839-4158; Fax. (418)839-3574; denis_boucher@videotron.ca.

BOUCHER, Denis N; CSSS de la Matapedia, 135 av Gaetan-Archambault, Amqui QC G5J 2K5; Laval'04; CCFP; Staff, CSSS de la Matapedia; (418)629-2211

BOUCHER, Francois; CHUQ-Ctr Hosp Univ Laval, 1753.2-2705 boul Laurier, Quebec QC G1V 4G2; Dijon (France)'81; ABPeds; FRCPC; Peds (Infectious Diseases). ac Staff Peds, Centre Hospitalier Universitaire de Quebec-CHUL; assoc Prof Peds, Université Laval; Langs: French; English; (418)656-4141 x48169; Fax. (418)654-2786; francois.boucher@crchul.ulaval.ca.

BOUCHER, Francois-Gilles; Bruyere Academic Fam Hlth Team, 75 Bruyere St, Ottawa ON K1N 5C7; Ott'75; CCFP; FCFP; Ac Staff, The Ottawa Hospital - General Campus; Ac Staff, Bruyère Continuing Care; Asst Prof Family Med, University of Ottawa; Langs: Bilingual(French/English); (613)241-3344

BOUCHER, Gilbert; MUHC-Royal Victoria Hosp, C4.17-687 av des Pins O, Montreal QC H3A 1A1; McG'98; FRCPC; EmergMed. Staff, McGill University Health Centre - Royal Victoria Hospital; (514)934-1934 x31610; marcil2288@yahoo.ca.

BOUCHER, Gilberte; Clinique Med Colombus, 1140 rue Jean-Talon E, Montreal QC H2R 1V9; Mon'72; (514)270-2141; Fax. (514)270-6920.

BOUCHER, Guy; CSSS de Rimouski-Neigette, CP 3150 Succ A 150 av Rouleau, Rimouski QC G5L 5T1; Sher'96; Cardiol (P.Q.); IntMed. Staff, Hôpital Regional Rimouski; Langs: Bilingual(French/English); (418)723-7851; Fax. (418)724-8632.

BOUCHER, Henri; Ctr Hosp Trois-Riv-St-Joseph, 731 rue Sainte-Julie, Trois-Rivieres QC G9A 1Y1; Mon'83; Psy. Staff, Centre Hospitalier Regional de Trois-Rivieres; (819)697-3333

BOUCHER, Isabelle; Ctr Hosp Laurentien, 234 rue Saint-Vincent, Ste-Agathe-Des-Mts QC J8C 2B8; Mon'01; CCFP; Staff, Centre Hospitalier Laurentien; (819)324-4000

BOUCHER, Jacques A; Clinique de Ped de Rimouski, 161 av Rouleau, Rimouski QC G5L 5T3; Laval'73; FRCPC; Peds. Staff Peds, Hôpital Regional Rimouski; (418)724-4221; Fax. (418)725-3025; jacogin@globetrotter.net.

BOUCHER, Jean; Clinique Med de Thurso, 156 rue Galipeau, Thurso QC J0X 3B0; Mon'78; (819)985-3080; Fax. (819)985-5651; climso@bellnet.ca.

BOUCHER, Jean-Louis; Hotel-Dieu de Levis, 143 rue Wolfe, Levis QC G6V 3Z1; Laval'72; CSPQ; FRCPC; DiagRad (General Radiology Ultrasound & Mammography). assoc Membre, Hopital du CSS de la Region de Thetford; ac Membre Dept of Radiol, Hôtel-Dieu de Lévis; assoc Membre Radiol, CSSS de Montmagny-L'Islet; Langs: Bilingual(French/English); (418)835-7101; Fax. (418)833-4645; jl.boucher@videotron.ca.

BOUCHER, Jean-Pierre; Clinique Med Lanaudiere, 222 rue Bernard, St-Charles-Brromee QC J6E 2C5; Mon'82; Staff, Centre Hospitalier Régional de Lanaudière; (450)755-1033; Fax. (450)753-5558.

BOUCHER, Julie A; 1-105 Progress Cres, Kapuskasing ON P5N 3J4; Ott'99; CCFP; Staff, Sensenbrenner Hospital; Langs: French; (705)335-8148; Fax. (705)335-6013.

BOUCHER, Julie; CSSS de Trois-Rivières, 1991 boul du Carmel, Trois-Rivieres QC G8Z 3R9; Laval'01; ObstGyn. Staff, CSSS de Trois-Rivières; (819)697-3333

BOUCHER, Julie M; 1333 boul Jacques-Cartier E, Longueuil QC J4M 2A5; Mon'97; CCFP; Staff, Centre Hospitalier Pierre Boucher; Langs: English; (450)468-8111; jbouchermd@hotmail.com.

BOUCHER, Karine; Hop du Sacre-Coeur de Mtl, 5400 boul Gouin O, Montreal QC H4J 1C5; Mon'00; Staff FamMed, Hôpital du Sacre-Coeur de Montréal; (514)338-2383; Fax. (514)338-3155.

BOUCHER, Liza; Office of the Chief Coroner, 26 Grenville St, Toronto ON M7A 2G9; Mon'04; FRCPC; AnatPath (Forensic Pathology). (416)314-4040

BOUCHER, Lorraine; 4000 av Marcil, Montreal QC H4A 2Z6; Mon'80; FRCPC; Psy. (514)485-4587; Fax. (514)485-6747.

BOUCHER, Louis B; 204-2903 32 Ave, Vernon BC V1T 2L6; Stellenbosch (South Africa)'92; MB ChB; DA(UK); LMCC; CCFP; Langs: Afrikaans; (250)549-2266; Fax. (250)545-1503; louis_boucher@hotmail.com.

BOUCHER, Louis P; Clinique Med de Courville, 1049 av Larue, Quebec QC G1C 1J5; Laval'86; Staff, Centre Hospitalier Affilié Universitaire de Québec - Hôpital du St-Sacrement; Staff, Centre Hospitalier Universitaire de Québec (CHUQ) - Siege Social; (418)661-0097; Fax. (418)661-0307; lboucher@dr.com.

BOUCHER, Louis-Martin; MUHC-Montreal Gen Hosp, C5. 118-1650 av Cedar, Montreal QC H3G 1A4; Tor'01; DiagRad. Staff, McGill University Health Centre - Montreal General Campus; (514)934-8084

BOUCHER, Luc; CHUM-Hotel-Dieu, 3840 rue Saint-Urbain, Montreal QC H2W 1T8; Mon'93; FRCPC; NuclearMed. Staff, Centre Hospitalier l'Université de Montréal (CHUM) - Hôtel-Dieu; (514)890-8180

BOUCHER, Luce; Clinique Med Duberger, 2810 boul Pere-Lelievre, Quebec QC G1P 2Y1; Laval'88; ac Staff, Centre Hospitalier Universitaire de Quebec-CHUL; (418)688-8414; Fax. (418)688-4273.

BOUCHER, Lucie; CHUM-Hop St-Luc, 1058 rue Saint-Denis, Montreal QC H2X 3J4; Laval'88; FRCPC; IntMed; GeriatricMed. Staff, Centre Hospitalier l'Université De Montréal (CHUM) - Hôpital Saint-luc; (514)890-8000 x34979; Fax. (514)412-7376.

BOUCHER, Marc; Hôpital Ste-Justine, 3175 ch Cote-Sainte-Catherine, Montreal QC H3T 1C5; Mon'77; DABOG; DMat/FetMed; FRCSC; ObstGyn (Maternal Fetal Medicine). ac Staff, Hôpital Ste-Justine; Prof, Universite de Montreal; Langs: Bilingual(French/English); (514)345-4706; Fax. (514)345-4648.

BOUCHER, Marcel M; CLP Monteregie, 14001-150 Place Charles Lemoyn, Longueuil QC J4K 0A8; Mon'76; EmergMed (P.Q.). (450)928-7719

BOUCHER, Marie Carole; Hop Maisonneuve-Rosemont, 5415 boul de l'Assomption, Montreal QC H1T 2M4; Mon'75; AB; FRCSC; Ophth (Cataract). Staff, Hopital Maisonneuve-Rosemont; adj Prof, Universite de Montreal; (514)252-3400 x4954

BOUCHER, Marie-Claude; CSSS de Vaudreuil-Soulanges, RR 1 11 ch de la Cite-des-Jeunes, Saint-Polycarpe QC J0P 1X0; Mon'04; CCFP; Staff, Centre Hospitalier Régional du Suroît; Langs: English; (450)265-3771; marie-claude_boucher@rrsss16.gouv.qc.ca.

BOUCHER, Marie-Danielle R; Clinique Ped Sainte-Foy, 293-2600 boul Laurier, Quebec QC G1V 4T3; Ott'93; Peds. (418)658-0906

BOUCHER, Mario; Clinique Med Optimum, 158-1 Place Laval, Laval QC H7N 1A1; Mon'85; Staff, Hopital de la Cite de la santé; (450)668-7400

BOUCHER, Martin; Ctr Hosp Affilie-Enfant-Jesus, 1401 18e rue, Quebec QC G1J 1Z4; Laval'96; LMCC; CCFP; CCFP(E.M.); FCFP; Staff, Centre Hospitalier Affilié Universitaire de Québec - Hôpital De L'Enfant Jésus; Langs: Bilingual(French/English); (418)649-5632; Fax. (418)649-5975.

BOUCHER, Martine; 110-4850 boul Henri-Bourassa, Quebec QC G1H 3A7; Laval'81; (418)628-3517; Fax. (418)628-0000.

BOUCHER, Maryse; Centre Med Christ-Roi, 102-40 rue Kennedy, Levis QC G6V 6C4; Laval'09; CCFP; Staff, Centre Medical Christ-Roi; (418)833-4977

BOUCHER, Michael; Burlington Pain Care, 24-1960 Appleby Line, Burlington ON L7L 0B7; McM'00; CCFP; Staff Surg, Hamilton Health Sciences Centre - Hamilton General Hospital; Staff, Joseph Brant Memorial Hospital; Staff, Niagara Health System - St Catharines General Site; (905)315-8802; burlingtonpaincare@cogeco.net.

BOUCHER, Michele E; CLSC Longueuil-Ouest, 201 boul Cure-Poirier O, Longueuil QC J4J 2G4; Laval'78; Staff, CSSS Pierre-Boucher; (450)651-9831; Fax. (450)651-0924; michele.boucher@rrsss16.gouv.qc.ca.

BOUCHER, Paul E; McCaig Tower, 0447-3134 Hospital Dr SW, Calgary AB T2N 5A1; Ott'95; FRCPC; IntMed; Critical Care Medicine. Staff, Foothills Medical Centre; (403)944-2471; Fax. (403)283-9994.

BOUCHER, Paule; CSSS du Sud de Lanaudière, 911 montee des Pionniers, Terrebonne QC J6V 2H2; Mon'87; FRCPC; DiagRad. Staff, Centre Hospitalier Pierre le Gardeur; (450)654-7525 x31203; Fax. (450)581-6313.

BOUCHER, Pierre; Recherche Invascor Inc, 203-1760 boul Jacques-Cartier, Longueuil QC J4N 1C2; Mon'90; CCFP; CCFP(E.M.); Staff, Centre Hospitalier Pierre Boucher; Langs: Bilingual(English/French); (450)468-2946; pierre.boucher@invascor.com.

BOUCHER, Pierre R; CHUM-Hop Notre-Dame, 1560 rue Sherbrooke E, Montreal QC H2L 4M1; Mon'88; Staff, Centre Hospitalier l'Université de Montréal (CHUM) - Hôpital Notre-Dame; (514)890-8000 x26767; Fax. (514)896-4751.

BOUCHER, Rejean; Centre Med Racine, 102-2880 ch des Quatre-Bourgeo, Quebec QC G1V 4X7; Laval'96; Staff, Centre Lafleche Grand-Mere; Langs: English; (418)657-6363

BOUCHER, Renee-Myriam; CHUQ-Ctr Hosp Univ Laval, A1808-2705 boul Laurier, Quebec QC G1V 4G2; Laval'99; FRCPC; Neur (Pediatric Neurology). Staff, Centre Hospitalier Universitaire de Quebec-CHUL; Langs: Bilingual(French/English); (418)654-2708

BOUCHER, Roger; Medicentre Lasalle, 206-1500 av Dollard, Lasalle QC H8N 1T5; Mon'72; CSPQ; Cardiol (P.Q.).

BOUCHER, Serge S B; CHUQ-Hotel-Dieu de Quebec, 350-11 Cote Du Palais, Quebec QC G1R 2J6; Laval'70; MPH(Harvard); FRCPC; Respir (Clinical Immunology & Allergy). Chef Pneumology Serv Committee of Med & Dental Evaluation/Prof, Centre Hospitalier Universitaire de Québec (CHUQ) - Siege Social; Prof, Université Laval; Langs: English; (418)691-5386 x5386; Fax. (418)692-5755.

BOUCHER, Serge; CSSSG-Hop de Hull, 116 boul Lionel-Emond, Gatineau QC J8Y 1W7; Sher'94; Staff, Hull Hospital; (819)595-6222

BOUCHER, Serge; 403-895 boul Du Seminaire N, St-Jean-Sur-Richel QC J3A 1J2; Mon'69; FRCSC; Ophth. Staff, Hôpital du Haut-Richelieu; (450)348-6155; Fax. (450)348-6156.

BOUCHER, Stephen A; Carnat Ctr Sunridge Med Galler, 3063-2580 32 St NE, Calgary AB T1Y 7M8; Liverpool (England)'78; FRCS(Lond); MRCGPract; MB ChB; FRCPC; Psy (Post Traumatic Stress Disorder). Staff, Peter Lougheed Centre; Med Dir, Operational Stress Injury Clinic; Clinical Asst Prof, University of Calgary; (403)944-9800; Fax. (403)944-9850.

BOUCHER, Suzanne; Clinique de Med Familiale, 300 rue Paradis, Sorel-Tracy QC J3P 3G6; Mon'76; Staff, CHSLD du Bas-Richelieu; Staff, Hôtel-Dieu de Sorel; (450)742-0485; Fax. (450)742-6965; suzanne@medecinefamiliale.com.

BOUCHER, Suzanne; 2005-1050 boul Casavant O, Saint-Hyacinthe QC J2S 8B9; Mon'84; Staff, Hopital Maisonneuve-Rosemont; (450)778-5675

BOUCHER, Yvan; CSSS de Rimouski-Neigette, CP 3150 Succ A 150 av Rouleau, Rimouski QC G5L 5T1; Mon'89; NuclearMed (P. Q.). Staff, Hôpital Regional Rimouski; (418)724-8318; Fax. (418)724-8633.

BOUCHER-ARSENEAU, Yannick; Hôpital de la cite de la santé, 1755 boul Rene-Laennec, Laval QC H7M 3L9; Mon'05; Psy. Staff, Hopital de la Cite de la santé; (450)668-1010

BOUCHER-GAGNE, Emilie; CSSS du Rocher-Perce, CP 3300 451 rue Mgr Ross, Chandler QC G0C 1K0; Sher'05; Staff, Centre Hospitalier de Chandler; Langs: Spanish; English; (418)689-2261

BOUCHER-PILON, Amélie; CSSS de Trois-Rivieres, 1991 boul du Carmel, Trois-Rivieres QC G8Z 3R9; Mon'06; CCFP; Staff, CSSS de Trois-Rivières; (819)697-3333

BOUCHER-ROBICHAUD, Micheline; 105-185 av Acadie, Dieppe NB E1A 1G6; Laval'88; LMCC; CCFP; (506)862-4182; Fax. (506)862-4179.

BOUCHEREAU, Yves; Clinique Med Rock Forest, 4870 boul Bourque, Sherbrooke QC J1N 3S5; Strasbourg (France)'82; Staff, CSSS des Sources d'Asbestos; (819)820-2673

BOUCHEREAU-EYEGUE, Mila-Denise; Centre Hosp Pierre Legardeur, 911 montee des Pionniers, Terrebonne QC J6V 2H2; Mon'06; GenSurg. Staff, Centre Hospitalier Pierre le Gardeur; (450)654-7525

BOUCHEZ, Stephane M; CSSS du Nord de Lanaudière, 1000 boul Sainte-Anne, St-Charles-Brromee QC J6E 6J2; Bruxelles (Belgium)'90; Staff, Centre Hospitalier Régional de Lanaudière; (450)759-8222 x2004

BOUDAKIAN, Avidis H; Markham Stouffville Health Ctr, 309-377 Church St, Markham ON L6B 1A1; Tor'86; FRCSC; Urol (Oncology). Staff Urol, Markham Stouffville Hospital; Langs: Armenian; (905)472-7120; Fax. (905)472-2971.

BOUDANA, David A; CSSS de Chicoutimi, 305 rue Saint-Vallier, Chicoutimi QC G7H 5H6; Staff, Complexe hospitalier de la Sagamie; (418)541-1000

BOUDIFFA, Mustapha; Groupe Sante Physimed, 121-6363 Rte Transcanadienne, Saint-Laurent QC H4T 1Z9; (Algeria)'81; CCFP; Staff, Institut Universitaire de Gériatrie de Montréal; (514)747-8888

BOUDON, Emilie; CLSC Ste-Therese de Blainville, 55 rue Saint-Joseph, Sainte-Therese QC J7E 4Y5; Mon'98; Staff, Centre Drapeau et Deschambault; Staff, CLSC Ste-Therese de Blainville; (450)430-4553

BOUDREAU, Andre D; Dartmouth Gen Hosp, 325 Pleasant St, Dartmouth NS B2Y 4G8; Dal'07; Staff, Dartmouth General Hospital; (902)448-6550

BOUDREAU, Anne; Pavilion Rosemont, 5689 boul Rosemont, Montreal QC H1T 2H1; Mon'82; FRCPC; Psy (Consultation-Liaison). Staff, Hopital Maisonneuve-Rosemont; (514)252-3922

BOUDREAU, Bernard; UMF Haute-Ville, 55 ch Sainte-Foy, Quebec QC G1R 1S9; Laval'97; BSc(MedSci); CCFP; assoc Membre, Centre Hospitalier Affilié Universitaire de Québec - Hôpital du St-Sacrement; ac Membre, CSSS Haute-Ville; Prof clin agrégé, Université Laval; Langs: Bilingual(French/English); (418)641-2572 x5547; Fax. (418)522-5437; bernard.boudreau@irdpq.qc.ca.

BOUDREAU, Christine; CSSS de Rivière-de-Loup, 75 rue Saint-Henri, Riviere-du-Loup QC G5R 2A4; Laval'00; Staff, Centre Hospitalier Regional du Grand-Portage; (418)868-1000

BOUDREAU, Cindy L; 211-615 Main St, Yarmouth NS B5A 1K1; Dal'84; Staff Diagnostic, Digby General Hospital; Staff, Yarmouth Regional Hospital; (902)742-9293; Fax. (902)742-4709.

BOUDREAU, D Todd; Aberdeen Hosp, 835 East River Rd, New Glasgow NS B2H 3S6; Dal'94; FRCSC; OrthSurg. Staff, Aberdeen Regional Hospital; (902)752-7971; Fax. (902)752-0215.

BOUDREAU, Daniel; PO Box 132, Arichat NS B0E 1A0; CCFP; CCFP(E.M.).

BOUDREAU, Dany; CSSS du Sud de Lanaudière, 911 montee des Pionniers, Terrebonne QC J6V 2H2; Mon'94; FRCPC; Psy (Consultation-Liaison). Staff, Centre Hospitalier Pierre le Gardeur; (450)654-7525 x11223; Fax. (450)582-3588.

BOUDREAU, Eve M; Clinique Medicale Nepisiguit, 950 Picot Ave, Bathurst NB E2A 4Z9; Sher'08; CCFP; Langs: Bilingual(English/French); (506)546-6696; Fax. (506)545-7723.

BOUDREAU, France P; 12-585 Montreal Rd, Ottawa ON K1K 4K4; Ott'06; CCFP; Staff, Montfort Hospital; Langs: Bilingual(English/French); (613)702-0382

BOUDREAU, Ghislain; CHSLD-Hop General de Quebec, 260 boul Langelier, Quebec QC G1K 5N1; Laval'93; CCFP; Staff, Hôpital général de Québec - CHSLD; Médecin, Pharmanet Canada Inc; (418)529-0931

BOUDREAU, Ghyslain; Clinique Med Loretteville, 250-11000 boul de l'Ormiere, Quebec QC G2B 5S1; Sher'85; Staff Emerg, Centre Hospitalier Chauveau; (418)842-3731; Fax. (418)842-3246; ghyslain.boudreau@ssss.gouv.qc.ca.

BOUDREAU, Guy; CHUM-Hop Notre-Dame, 1560 rue Sherbrooke E, Montreal QC H2L 4M1; Mon'74; adj Staff Neurol Serv, Centre Hospitalier l'Université de Montréal (CHUM) - Hôtel-Dieu; Staff, Centre Hospitalier l'Université de Montréal (CHUM) - Hôpital Notre-Dame; (450)890-8000; Fax. (450)412-7097.

BOUDREAU, J Donald; MUHC-Montreal Chest Institute, 3650 rue Saint-Urbain, Montreal QC H2X 2P4; Dal'80; FRCPC; IntMed; Respir. Staff, McGill University Health Centre - Montreal Chest Institute; adj Prof, McGill University Health Centre - Royal Victoria Hospital; Dir Curriculum Development & Physicianship Prog, McGill University; (514)849-5201; Fax. (514)843-2088.

BOUDREAU, Janice; Clinique Med Pierre-Boucher, 1615 boul Jacques-Cartier E, Longueuil QC J4M 2X1; Mon'93; Staff, Centre d hebergement de l Hôtel-Dieu de Saint-Hyacinthe; (450)468-6223; Fax. (450)468-5041.

BOUDREAU, Julie; Unite de Med Familiale, 80 118e rue, Shawinigan QC G9P 3E4; Mon'10; CCFP; (819)536-7511

BOUDREAU, Luc; Dr Georges-L Dumont Reg Hosp, 330 av Universite, Moncton NB E1C 2Z3; Sher'07; FRCSC; Urol. Staff, Dr Georges-L-Dumont University Hospital Centre; (506)384-9715; Fax. (506)384-5788.

BOUDREAU, Marc; CSSS Pierre Boucher, 1333 boul Jacques-Cartier E, Longueuil QC J4M 2A5; Mon'93; Staff, Centre Hospitalier Pierre Boucher; (450)468-8111

BOUDREAU, Marie; Clinique Med Duberger, 2810 boul Pere-Lelievre, Quebec QC G1P 2Y1; Laval'79; Langs: Bilingual(French/English); (418)688-8414

BOUDREAU, Marie-Claude; Centre Med de Cowansville, 101-370 rue de la Riviere, Cowansville QC J2K 1N3; Mon'92; (450)263-0774; Fax. (450)263-6457.

BOUDREAU, Marie-Helene; Clin Sante Immigrants & Refugi, 3108 ch Sainte-Foy, Quebec QC G1X 1P8; Laval'05; CCFP; (418)651-2572 x8378

BOUDREAU, Nathalie M; ForeMed Clinics Inc, 420 Columbia St, New Westminster BC V3L 1B1; Dal'04; BSc(Hon); CCFP; Langs: Bilingual(English/French); (604)522-2206; Fax. (604)522-7206.

BOUDREAU, Pierre-Olivier; CSSS de Manicouagan, 635 boul Jolliet, Baie-Comeau QC G5C 1P1; Mon'09; Staff, Centre Hospitalier Régional Baie-Comeau; (418)589-3701

BOUDREAU, Rheal; 203-387 Main St, Shediac NB E4P 2B5; Sher'94; CCFP; Staff, Dr Georges-L-Dumont University Hospital Centre; (506)533-8347; Fax. (506)533-8039.

BOUDREAU, Richard; CSSS de Rivière-de-Loup, 75 rue Saint-Henri, Riviere-du-Loup QC G5R 2A4; Sher'70 Johns Hopkins (USA); MPH; CommunMed (P.Q.). Staff Public Health, Centre Hospitalier Regional du Grand-Portage; ac Membre, Hôpital Regional Rimouski; Med Consultant, Agence de Sante Services Sociaux-St Laurent; Langs: English; Bilingual(French/English); (418)868-1010 x2534; Fax. (418)868-1033; richard.boudreau.asss01@ssss.gouv.qc.ca.

BOUDREAU, Robert; Univ de Sherbrooke, 2500 boul de l'Universite, Sherbrooke QC J1K 2R1; Sher'78; Staff Services Sante, Universite de Sherbrooke; (819)821-7667; Fax. (819)821-7577.

BOUDREAU, Serge; Centre Med Charles-Lemoyne, 3125 boul Taschereau, Greenfield Park QC J4V 2H2; Laval'90; CCFP; Staff, Centre Hospitalier Pierre Boucher; (450)672-2250; Fax. (450)923-4252.

BOUDREAU, Suzanne; Hotel-Dieu d'Arthabaska, 5 rue des Hospitalieres, Victoriaville QC G6P 6N2; Sher'80; CSPQ; FRCPC; AnatPath. Staff Anat Path, Hotel-Dieu d'Arthabaska; (819)357-6039 x2349

BOUDREAU-POISSANT, Karele; CSSS Haut-Richelieu-Rouville, 920 boul du Seminaire N, St-Jean-sur-Richel QC J3A 1B7; Sher'07; CCFP; Staff, Hôpital du Haut-Richelieu; (450)359-5000

BOUDREAULT, Alexandre; CHUM-Hotel-Dieu de Quebec, 11 Cote du Palais, Quebec QC G1R 2J6; Laval'04; MedMicrobiol. Staff, Centre Hospitalier Universitaire de Québec (CHUQ) - Siege Social; (418)525-4444 x15131

BOUDREAULT, Annie; Centre Med Fusion, 200-2035 av Sainte-Anne, Saint-Hyacinthe QC J2S 5H3; Laval'01; CCFP; Staff, Centre Hospitalier Honore-Mercier; (450)773-6023; Fax. (450)773-5915.

BOUDREAULT, Daniel; CHUM-Hop Notre-Dame, 1560 rue Sherbrooke E, Montreal QC H2L 4M1; Mon'84; CSPQ; FRCPC; Anes. Staff, Centre Hospitalier l'Université de Montréal (CHUM) - Hôpital Notre-Dame; (514)890-8000 x26876

BOUDREAULT, Dorice; CLSC Chateauguay, 95 av de la Laverdure, Chateauguay QC J6K 5G4; Mon'81; Med Consultant Environmental Health/Reg Dir, Public Health of la Monteregie; (450)699-3333; Fax. (450)699-2325; dorice.boudreault@rrsss16.gouv.qc.ca.

BOUDREAULT, Ghislain A; Laser Visuel de Quebec, 240-801 rue Grande Alle O, Quebec QC G1S 1C1; Laval'75; FRCSC; Ophth. (418)683-7999

BOUDREAULT, Isabelle; Centre de Med Fam de Gatineau, 201-908 Boul Maloney E, Gatineau QC J8P 1H5; Laval'94; Staff, Hôpital de Gatineau; Langs: English; (819)663-7711; Fax. (819)663-9326.

BOUDREAULT, Jean-Roch; Hôpital Laval, 2725 ch Sainte-Foy, Quebec QC G1V 4G5; Mon'72; CSPQ; FACC; Cardiol (P.Q.) (Hemodynamics). Staff, Hôpital Laval; (418)656-8711 x4657; Fax. (418)656-4544.

BOUDREAULT, Johannie; CLSC des Maskoutains, 1015 rue Gauthier, Saint-Hyacinthe QC J2S 8T2; Mon'09; (450)778-2572

BOUDREAULT, Melanie; CSSS Cleophas-Claveau, CP 38 Succ La Baie 1000 av du Docteur-Desgagne, La Baie QC G7B 3P9; Laval'07; CCFP; Staff, CHSLD-CLSC Cleophas-Claveau; (418)544-0070

BOUDREAULT, Nathalie; Universite Laval, 3690-1050 av de la Medecine, Quebec QC G1V 0A6; Sher'93; Staff, Centre Hospitalier Universitaire de Quebec-CHUL; (418)656-2131

BOUDREAULT, Nicolas; CSSS des Etchemins, 331 rue du Sanatorium, Lac-Etchemin QC G0R 1S0; Laval'99; Staff, CSSS des Etchemins; (418)625-8001; Fax. (418)625-3109.

BOUDREAULT, Pascal; Polyclinique, 209-874 boul de l'Universite E, Chicoutimi QC G7H 6B9; Laval'71; (418)545-2998; Fax. (418)545-4782.

BOUDREAULT, Roberto; Centre Med de St-Felicien, 1013 boul du Sacré-Coeur, Saint-Felicien QC G8K 1R5; Laval'87; Staff, Hotel-Dieu de Roberval; (418)679-0943; Fax. (418)679-4066.

BOUDREAULT-LAROCHELLE, Samuel; CSSS du Nord de Lanaudière, 1000 boul Sainte-Anne, Joliette QC J6E 6J2; Laval'09; CCFP; Staff, Centre Hospitalier Régional de Lanaudière; (450)759-8222

BOUDRIAS, Alain; Clinique Med Ste-Julienne, 1270 Rte 125, Ste-Julienne QC J0K 2T0; Mon'76; (450)831-8383; Fax. (450)831-8957.

BOUDRIAS, Claude; CSSS du Lac-des-Deux-Montagnes, 520 boul Arthur-Sauve, St-Eustache QC J7R 5B1; Laval'84; DiagRad. Staff, Hôpital de Saint-Eustache; (450)473-6811 x2211

BOUDRIAS, Louis-David; Clinique Med de Rawdon, 201-3240 1ere av, Rawdon QC J0K 1S0; Mon'07; CCFP; Staff, Centre Hospitalier Régional Baie-Comeau; (450)834-2304; Fax. (450)834-3345.

BOUFASSA, Meriem; CSSS de Gatineau, 777 boul de la Gappe, Gatineau QC J8T 8R2; Mon'06; IntMed. Staff, CSSS de Gatineau; (819)966-6550

BOUFFARD, Anne-Pierre; Inst U en Sante Mentale de QC, 2601 de la Canardiere, Quebec QC G1J 2G3; Laval'04; FRCPC; Psy. Staff, Institut Universitaire Sante; (418)663-5321

BOUFFARD, Audrey; CSSS de la Baie-des-Chaleurs, RR 2 419 boul Perron, Maria QC G0C 1Y0; Mon'08; CCFP; Staff, CSSS de la Baie-des-Chaleurs; (418)759-3443

BOUFFARD, Danielle; CHUM-Hop Notre-Dame, 1560 rue Sherbrooke E, Montreal QC H2L 4M1; Sher'87; CSPQ; FRCPC; AnatPath. Staff Path, Centre Hospitalier l'Université de Montréal (CHUM) - Hôpital Notre-Dame; (514)890-8000 x27054

BOUFFARD, Gerald; Clin Med Place St-Redempteur, PO Box 2020 Succ Bureau-Chef 1310 1re Av, St-Redempteur QC G6K 1N7; Laval'68; CCFP; FCFP; Médecin, CRSSS de la Baie-James; pers Prof, Centre Hospitalier Universitaire de Quebec-CHUL; Médecin, CSSS Grand Littoral; Langs: English; (418)831-4705; Fax. (418)831-8656.

BOUFFARD, Michel; 100-311 McArthur Ave, Vanier ON K1L 8M3; Ott'81; (613)748-1111

BOUFFARD, Jean; Centre Med Quatre-Bourgeois, 300-979 av de Bourgogne, Quebec QC G1W 2L4; Sher'74; assoc Staff, Hôpital Laval; (418)653-4050; Fax. (418)653-4475; jean.bouffard@videotron.ca.

BOUFFARD, Karine; Dr Georges-L Dumont Reg Hosp, 330 av Universite, Moncton NB E1C 2Z3; Laval'02; CCFP; Staff, Dr Georges-L-Dumont University Hospital Centre; (506)862-4000

BOUFFARD, Odette; Clinique Med du Manoir, 1441 av du Manoir, Alma QC G8B 4X3; Mon'94; (418)662-3944; Fax. (418)662-2607.

BOUFFARD, Rachelle E; Queen Alexandra Ctre Children, 2400 Arbutus Rd, Victoria BC V8N 1V7; UBC'85; FRCPC; Psy (Consultation-Liaison). Staff, Queen Alexandra Centre for Children's Health; (250)721-6820

BOUFFARD-DUMAIS, Catherine; Unite Med Familiale Maizerets, 2480 ch de la Canardière, Quebec QC G1J 2G1; Laval'01; CCFP; Fam Med, Centre de santé des Côté-Nord; (418)661-2428; Fax. (418)661-7504.

BOUFFET, Eric; 555 University Ave, Toronto ON M5G 1X8; Lyon (France)'86; FRCPC; Peds (Brain Tumors). Dir Brain Tumor Program, The Hospital For Sick Children; Langs: Italian; French; (416)813-7654 x28973; Fax. (416)813-8024; eric.bouffet@sickkids.ca.

BOUGANIM, Nathaniel; MUHC-Royal Victoria Hosp, 687 av des Pins O, Montreal QC H3A 1A1; McG'05; FRCPC; IntMed; MedOncol. Staff, McGill University Health Centre - Royal Victoria Hospital; (514)934-1934

BOUGARD, Jean; Clinique Med Pierre-Boucher, 1615 boul Jacques-Cartier E, Longueuil QC J4M 2X1; Mon'74; Staff, Centre Hospitalier Pierre Boucher; (450)468-6223; Fax. (450)468-5041.

BOUGHEN, Gregory C; 3-4402 37 St, Stony Plain AB T7Z 2A9; Cal'84; Staff, Westview Health Centre; (780)963-7800; Fax. (780)963-0468; gboughen@shaw.ca.

BOUGHEN, Paul F; 101-2020 Richmond Rd, Victoria BC V8R 6R5; Tor'83; Staff, Vancouver Island Health Authority; (250)477-6939; Fax. (250)477-6921; paul.boughen@shaw.ca.

BOUGHNER, Derek R; London HSC-University Hosp, PO Box 5339 Stn B 339 Windermere Rd, London ON N6A 5A5; Wes'65; PhD(Biophysics); FRCPC; IntMed (Cardiology). Staff, London Health Sciences Centre - University Hospital; Prof, University of Western Ontario; (519)663-3262

BOUGHTON, Keith G; 390 Centre Ave, Kamloops BC V2C 1V5; Tor'66; CCFP; Assoc Staff, Royal Inland Hospital; (250)851-4331; Fax. (250)851-4343.

BOUGIE, Rejean; Centre Med Chaudiere, 102 18e rue, Saint-Georges QC G5Y 4T9; Laval'77; (418)228-6820

BOUHADANA, Michael J; SMBD Jewish Gen Hosp, Pav H-3755 ch Cote-Sainte-Cath, Montreal QC H3T 1E2; McG'95; CCFP; Att Staff, Sir Mortimer B Davis Jewish General; Prof Faculty, McGill University; Langs: Hebrew; English; (514)340-8213; Fax. (514)340-7579; michael.bouhadana@mcgill.ca.

BOUHAIRIE, Torik; Centre Med For Infants, 527 rue Sainte-Helene, Longueuil QC J4K 3R5; Paris (France)'70; Peds (P. Q.). (450)646-6363; Fax. (450)463-0984.

BOUHROUR, Souad; CLSC Saint-Michel, 7950 boul Saint-Michel, Montreal QC H1Z 3E1; (Algeria)'87; CCFP; (514)374-8223; Fax. (514)374-9180.

BOUILLON, Karine; CSSS de Trois-Rivieres, 1991 boul du Carmel, Trois-Rivieres QC G8Z 3R9; Mon'02; Staff, CSSS de Trois-Rivières; (819)697-3333 x63319

BOUILLY, Michel; Clinique Medicale, 6716 rue Saint-Denis, Montreal QC H2S 2S2; Mon'69; (514)274-3561

BOUIN, Mickael; Pavillon Edouard-Asselin, 264 boul Rene-Levesque E, Montreal QC H2X 1P1; (France)'97; Langs: German; English; (514)890-8000 x35708; Fax. (514)412-7377; mickael.bouin@umontreal.ca.

BOUISSET, Jeanne; CLSC des Faubourgs, 2260 rue Parthenais, Montreal QC H2K 3T5; Mon'96; CCFP; Staff, CSSS Jeanne Mance; (514)527-2361; Fax. (514)527-6016; jeanne_bouisset@ssss.gouv.qc.ca.

BOUKHALFA, Amokrane; Hôpital Sainte-Croix, 570 rue Heriot, Drummondville QC J2B 1C1; Staff, Hôpital Sainte-croix; (819)478-6464

BOUKHOUDMI, Soraya; CSSS du Nord de Lanaudière, 1000 boul Sainte-Anne, St-Charles-Brromee QC J6E 6J2; Mon'05; FRCPC; MedMicrobiol. Staff, Centre Hospitalier Régional de Lanaudière; (450)759-8222; Fax. (450)759-7861.

BOULAD, Aladin E; Cite de la Sante Laval, 1755 boul Rene-Laennec, Laval QC H7M 3L9; Cairo (Egypt)'81; MD; MB BCh; Staff, Hopital de la Cite de la santé; Langs: Arabic; English; (450)668-1010

BOULAIS, Genevieve; CSSS Haut-Richelieu-Rouville, 920 boul du Seminaire N, St-Jean-sur-Richel QC J3A 1B7; Sher'04; FRCSC; GenSurg. Staff, Hôpital du Haut-Richelieu; (450)349-5000

BOULAIS, Isabelle; CHUS-Hopital Hotel-Dieu, 580 rue Bowen S, Sherbrooke QC J1G 2E8; Sher'03; FRCPC; IntMed. Staff, Hotel-Dieu d'Arthabaska; (819)346-1110

BOULANGER, Aline; CHUM-Hotel-Dieu, 3840 rue Saint-Urbain, Montreal QC H2W 1T8; Laval'83; CSPQ; FRCPC; Anes (Clinical Research). Dir Pain Management Clinic/Staff, Centre Hospitalier l'Université de Montréal (CHUM) - Hôtel-Dieu; assoc Prof, Universite de Montreal; (514)890-8000 x15126; Fax. (514)412-7132.

BOULANGER, Caroline; Centre Med de l'Hetriere, 201-3520 rue de l'Hetriere, St-Augustin-D-Desm QC G3A 0B4; Laval'98; Langs: Bilingual(French/English); (418)651-3933

BOULANGER, Claude; Clinique d'Ophth Lebourgneuf, 200-777 boul Lebourgneuf, Quebec QC G2J 1C3; Laval'70; Ophth (P.Q.). (418)628-1417; Fax. (418)623-4517.

BOULANGER, Dany; CSSS de Quebec Nord, 3666 ch Royal, Quebec QC G1E 1X5; Laval'88; LMCC; (418)663-2572; Fax. (418)663-2624; dany.boulanger@ssss.gouv.qc.ca.

BOULANGER, Emilie; CSSS de Jonquiere, CP 1200 Succ Pdf Jonquiere 2230 rue de l'Hopital, Jonquiere QC G7X 7X2; Mon'06; Staff, Centre Hospitalier Jonquiere; (418)695-7700

BOULANGER, Isabelle; Clinique Med Saint-Lazare, 1771 ch Sainte-Angelique, Saint-Lazare QC J7T 2X7; Laval'93; LMCC; CCFP; (450)424-9557

BOULANGER, Jean; Clinique de Vinci, 101-2880 ch des Quatre-Bourgeo, Quebec QC G1V 4X7; Laval'76; FRCPC; Derm (Esthetic Dermatology). assoc Staff, Centre Hospitalier Universitaire de Québec (CHUQ) - Siege Social; Langs: English; (418)650-3109

BOULANGER, Jean-Martin; Clinique Neuro Rive-Sud, 250-4896 boul Taschereau, Greenfield Park QC J4V 2J2; Sher'99; FRCPC; Neur (Neuro Vascular). Staff Neurol, Hopital Charles LeMoyne; adj Prof, Universite de Sherbrooke; Langs: Bilingual(French/English); (450)672-1931

BOULANGER, Jocelyn; CSSS de L'Hematite, GD 1 rue de l'Aquilon, Fermont QC G0G 1J0; Laval'96; Staff, CLSC de l'Hématite; Langs: Bilingual(French/English); (418)287-5461; Fax. (418)287-5465.

BOULANGER, Julie; CSSS de la Haute-Cote-Nord, CP 1000 4 rue de l'Hopital, Les Escoumins QC G0T 1K0; McG'97; CCFP; Staff, Centre de santé des Côté-Nord; Langs: Spanish; French; (418)233-2931; Fax. (418)233-3335.

BOULANGER, Marianne; Clinique Med Les Gres, 104-190 rue St-Honore, St-Etienne-de-Gres QC G0X 2P0; Laval'06; CCFP; Staff, Centre Hospitalier du Centre la Mauricie; (819)535-6512; Fax. (819)535-1627.

BOULANGER, Maude; 14872 Yonge St, Aurora ON L4G 1N2; Ott'10; CCFP; (905)505-0950

BOULANGER, Michelle; Clinique Med Cap-St-Ignace, 40 ch des Pionniers E RR 1, Cap-Saint-Ignace QC G0R 1H0; Laval'83; (418)246-5347; Fax. (418)246-3325; michelle.boulanger@gmf.gouv.qc.ca.

BOULANGER, Nathalie; Ungava Tulattavik Health Ctr, CP 149, Kuujjuaq QC J0M 1C0; Mon'89; CCFP; Dir-svcs prof, Centre de sante Tulattavik de l'Ungava; (819)964-2905; Fax. (819)964-2270; nathalie.boulanger@ssss.gouv.qc.ca.

BOULANGER, Pascal; CSSS du Sud de Lanaudière, 911 montee des Pionniers, Terrebonne QC J6V 2H2; Sher'01; Staff, Centre Hospitalier Pierre le Gardeur; (450)654-7525; Fax. (450)470-2618.

BOULANGER, Yves; CHUS-Hopital Hotel-Dieu, 580 rue Bowen S, Sherbrooke QC J1G 2E8; Mon'92; Staff, Centre Hospitalier Universitaire de Sherbrooke-Hôpital Hôtel-Dieu; (819)346-1110

BOULANGER-DORVAL, Jean-Philippe; Hopital Regional de Rimouski, 150 av Rouleau, Rimouski QC G5L 5T1; McG'05; IntMed. Staff, Hôpital Regional Rimouski; (418)724-3000 x8122

BOULANGER JR., Michel J; Misericordia Community Hosp, 16940 87 Ave NW, Edmonton AB T5R 4H5; Alb'78; FACEP; FRCPC; EmergMed. Staff Physician Emerg Dept, Covenant Health - Misericordia Community Hospital; Staff, Alberta Health Services; Clinical Asst Prof EmergMed & Family Med, University of Alberta; Langs: English; French; (780)735-2819; Fax. (780)735-2966; mboulang@ualberta.ca.

BOULARD-GONDOLFF, Annick; CSSS de Chicoutimi, 305 rue Saint-Vallier, Chicoutimi QC G7H 5H6; Bordeaux (France)'89; Staff, Complexe hospitalier de la Sagamie; (418)541-1000; Fax. (418)541-1190.

BOULAY, Danielle; Hop Maisonneuve-Rosemont, 5415 boul de l'Assomption, Montreal QC H1T 2M4; Mon'85; Staff, Hopital Maisonneuve-Rosemont; (514)252-3400

BOULAY, Jacques A; Centre Prof Montee Masson, 880 Montee Masson, Mascouche QC J7K 2L7; Mon'75; (450)474-2493; Fax. (450)966-0156.

BOULAY, Remi; Centre Hosp Honore-Mercier, 2750 boul Laframboise, Saint-Hyacinthe QC J2S 4Y8; Laval'07; Peds. Staff, Centre Hospitalier Honore-Mercier; (450)771-3333

BOULAY, Robert M; Professional Corp Inc, 2 Johnson Ave, Miramichi NB E1N 3B7; Dal'89; CCFP; Staff, Miramichi Regional Hospital; (506)778-8994; Fax. (506)778-8719.

BOULD, Matthew; Children's Hosp of Eastern Ont, 401 Smyth Rd, Ottawa ON K1H 8L1; Leeds (United Kingdom)'97; Staff, Children's Hospital of Eastern Ontario (CHEO); (613)737-2431

BOULDING, Rachel A; 214-1717 3rd Ave, Prince George BC V2L 3G7; McM'99; FRCPC; Psy. (250)563-1156

BOULE, Christopher J; The Credit Valley Hosp, 2200 Eglinton Ave W, Mississauga ON L5M 2N1; Tor'98; CCFP; CCFP(E.M.); Staff, The Credit Valley Hospital; (905)813-4141

BOULE, Francine; CSSS de Chicoutimi, 305 rue Saint-Vallier, Chicoutimi QC G7H 5H6; Sher'82; CCFP; FCFP; Staff, Complexe hospitalier de la Sagamie; (418)541-1079; Fax. (418)541-1129; fboule@videotron.ca.

BOULE, Marie-Eve; CSSS du Nord de Lanaudière, 1000 boul Sainte-Anne, St-Charles-Brromee QC J6E 6J2; Sher'02; FRCPC; IntMed; Nephrol. Staff, Centre Hospitalier Régional de Lanaudière; (450)759-8222

BOULE, Richard; CHUS-Hop Fleurimont, 3001 12e av N, Sherbrooke QC J1H 5N4; Laval'78; MScEd; CCFP; FCFP; Clin Prof, Centre Hospitalier Universitaire de Sherbrooke-Hopital Fleurimont; Prof, Universite de Sherbrooke; Langs: Bilingual(English/French); (819)346-1110 x13201; Fax. (819)566-8059.

BOULES, Isaac; Mississauga Med Centre, 418-1420 Burnhamthorpe Rd E, Mississauga ON L4X 2Z9; Cairo (Egypt)'99; CCFP; (905)629-1006

BOULET, Daniel; Ctr Hosp Affilie-Enfant-Jesus, 1401 18e rue, Quebec QC G1J 1Z4; Laval'69; AB; FRCPC; PhysMed&Rehab (Electromyography). Dept Head, Centre Hospitalier Affilié Universitaire de Québec - Hôpital De L'Enfant Jésus; Ac Member, I R D P Q; Langs: English; (418)649-5751; Fax. (418)649-5879; daniel.boulet@irdpq.qc.ca.

BOULET, Daniel; Hotel-Dieu de Sorel, 400 av de l'Hotel-Dieu, Sorel-Tracy QC J3P 1N5; Sher'84; Psy. Staff, Hôtel-Dieu de Sorel; (450)746-6150

BOULET, Louis-Philippe; Hopital Laval, 2725 ch Sainte-Foy, Quebec QC G1V 4G5; Laval'76; FRCPC; Respir (Pneumology). Staff Respirologist, Hôpital Laval; Prof Med, Université Laval; Langs: Bilingual(English/French); (418)656-4747; Fax. (418)656-4762; lpboulet@med.ulaval.ca.

BOULET, Marc; CHUM-Hop Notre-Dame, 1560 rue Sherbrooke E, Montreal QC H2L 4M1; Mon'83; EmergMed (P.Q.). Staff, Centre Hospitalier l'Université de Montréal (CHUM) - Hôpital Notre-Dame; (514)890-8000

BOULET, Melanie; Ctr Hosp Affilie-Enfant-Jesus, 1401 18e rue, Quebec QC G1J 1Z4; Laval'00; FRCPC; PhysMed&Rehab. Staff, Centre Hospitalier Affilié Universitaire de Québec - Hôpital De L'Enfant Jésus; (418)649-5751

BOULET, Sylvie; CLSC de Cote-des-neiges, 1271 av Van Horne, Montreal QC H2V 1K5; McG'89; CCFP; FCFP; Staff Gen & Family Med, St Mary's Hospital Centre; assoc Prof Family Med, McGill University; (514)270-1536; Fax. (514)270-8731.

BOULET-ROUSSIN, Genevieve; Clinique Med Place Beaumont, J-1200 boul Rome, Longueuil QC J4W 3H3; Mon'76; (450)671-6170

BOULIANE, Martin J; 10150 121 St NW, Edmonton AB T5N 1K4; Alb'94; FRCSC; OrthSurg. (780)434-3668; Fax. (780)434-4859.

BOULIANNE, Annie; CSSS des Basques, 550 rue Notre-Dame E RR 1, Trois-Pistoles QC G0L 4K0; Mon'00; Staff, Centre Hospitalier Trois-Pistoles; (418)851-1111; Fax. (418)851-4546.

BOULIANNE, Donald; Clinique Med Dr Donald Boulian, 2245 rue Liri, Jonquiere QC G7S 1G1; Sher'89; Staff, Centre Hospitalier Jonquiere; (418)548-7671; Fax. (418)548-0712; donald.boulianne@ssss.gouv.qc.ca.

BOULIANNE, Louise; Centre Med le Mesnil, 300-1300 boul Lebourgneuf, Quebec QC G2K 2N1; Laval'00; Investigator, Province of Quebec; (418)624-1800; louise_boulianne@ssss.gouv.qc.ca.

BOULIANNE, Marc; CSSS de la Region de Thetford, 1717 rue Notre-Dame E, Thetford Mines QC G6G 2V4; Mon'91; IntMed. Staff, Hopital du CSS de la Region de Thetford; (418)338-7777; Fax. (418)338-7406.

BOULIANNE, Marie-France; Clinique Med Donnacona, 420 Route 138, Sainte-Therese QC J7E 4Y5; Mon'98; Staff, Hôtel-Dieu de Saint-Jérôme; (418)285-1122; Fax. (418)285-0006.

BOULIANNE, Pierre A; Hop Maisonneuve-Rosemont, 5415 boul de l'Assomption, Montreal QC H1T 2M4; Mon'67; DiagRad. Staff, Hopital Maisonneuve-Rosemont; Clin Adj, Universite de Montreal; (514)252-3535; Fax. (514)252-3537.

BOULIANNE, Sylvie; Hop du Sacre-Coeur de Mtl, 5400 boul Gouin O, Montreal QC H4J 1C5; Mon'93; CCFP; Staff, Hôpital du Sacre-Coeur de Montréal; (514)338-2383; Fax. (514)338-3155.

BOULIAS, Christos; West Park Healthcare Centre, 82 Buttonwood Ave, Toronto ON M6M 2J5; Tor'97; FRCPC; PhysMed&Rehab. Langs: Greek; (416)243-3680; Fax. (416)243-1177.

BOULOS, Carolyn M; Sunnybrook Hlth Sciences Ctre, 2075 Bayview Ave, Toronto ON M4N 3M5; Mem'83; FRCPC; Psy. Staff, Sunnybrook Health Sciences Centre; Staff, Mackenzie Richmond Hill Hospital; Asst Prof, University of Toronto; (416)480-4208

BOULOS, Mark I; Sunnybrook Hlth Sciences Ctre, A233-2075 Bayview Ave, Toronto ON M4N 3M5; Tor'06; FRCPC; Neur. Staff, Sunnybrook Health Sciences Centre; (416)480-4473; Fax. (416)480-4833.

BOULOS, Patrick R; CHUS-Hotel-Dieu, 580 rue Bowen S, Sherbrooke QC J1G 2E8; Mon'98; ACLS; ABOph; FRCS; LMCC; NBME; AddicMed; FRCSC; Ophth (Oculo Plastic Surgery). adj Prof, Centre Hospitalier Universitaire de Sherbrooke-Hôpital Hôtel-Dieu; Prof adj clin, Hopital Maisonneuve-Rosemont; Langs: English; Arabic; Bilingual(French/English); Spanish; French; Portuguese; (819)346-1110

BOULOS, Pauline; 201-17 King St E, Hamilton ON L9H 1B7; McG'95; FRCPC; IntMed; Rheum. Clin Teacher Rheum, St Joseph's Healthcare - Charlton Campus; Asst Prof Rheumatol, McMaster University; Langs: French; Greek; (289)238-9999; Fax. (289)238-9992.

BOULOS, Shahira; 200-372 Hollandview Trail, Aurora ON L4G 0A5; Asyut (Egypt)'86; MB ChB; CCFP; (905)726-9111; Fax. (905)726-9171.

BOULOS, Youssef R; Kendallwood Clinic, 1801 Dundas St E, Whitby ON L1N 7C5; Ain Shams (Egypt)'81; MB ChB; CCFP; (905)404-9191

BOULT, Ian F; Medical Arts Bldg, 202-233 Kennedy St, Winnipeg MB R3C 3J5; Man'71; FRCPC; DiagRad. Staff, Health Sciences Centre; (204)942-6453; Fax. (204)944-8101.

BOULTON, Anthony J; UBC-Dept of Anes, 2449-910 10th Ave W, Vancouver BC V5Z 1M9; Manchester (England)'72; MB BS; MRCP(UK); FRCPC; Anes. Ac Staff Anes, Vancouver General Hospital - Centennial Pavillion; (604)875-4304

BOULTON, Jill E; Foothills Med Centre, 780-1403 29 St NW, Calgary AB T2N 2T9; Man'82; LMCC; FRC; FRCPC; Peds (Neonatology). Staff, Foothills Medical Centre; Clin Prof/Acad Head Neonatol, University of Calgary; (403)944-4938; Fax. (403)944-4892; jill.boulton@albertahealthservices.ca.

BOULTON, Melfort R; London HSC-University Hosp, PO Box 5339 Stn B C7 124-339 Windermere Rd, London ON N6A 5A5; Tor'02; PhD; FRCSC; Neursurg. Staff, London Health Sciences Centre - University Hospital; (519)663-3602

BOULTON, Peter G; 324-1964 Fort St, Victoria BC V8R 6R3; Alb'03; FRCPC; Neur. (778)265-6533

BOULVA, Geneviève; CLSC des Faubourgs, 2260 rue Parthenais, Montreal QC H2K 3T5; Mon'09; CCFP; (514)527-2361

BOUMAN, Helen L A; PO Box 1044, Bragg Creek AB T0L 0K0; Cal'94; BSc; CCFP; Langs: French; (403)221-8797; Fax. (403)221-8785.

BOUNATIRO, Ibrahim; Lakeshore Gen Hosp, 1882-160 av Stillview, Pointe-Claire QC H9R 2Y2; (Algeria)'73; Staff Nephrol, Lakeshore General Hospital - Pointe Claire; Langs: Arabic; English; (514)630-2225 x1898; Fax. (514)630-2136.

BOURASSA, Amelie; Ctr Hosp Affilie-St-Sacrement, 1050 ch Sainte-Foy, Quebec QC G1S 4L8; Mon'03; FRCPC; EmergMed. Staff, Centre Hospitalier Affilié Universitaire de Québec - Hôpital du St-Sacrement; (418)682-7511; Fax. (418)682-7977.

BOURASSA, Anne-Marie; CSSS de Chicoutimi, 305 rue Saint-Vallier, Chicoutimi QC G7H 5H6; Mon'91; DiagRad. Staff, Complexe hospitalier de la Sagamie; (418)541-1031; Fax. (418)541-1103.

BOURASSA, Claude E; 314 rue Principale, Mansonville QC J0E 1X0; Ott'71; CCFP; Médecin Family Med, Centre Hospitalier et CLSC de Memphremagog; Langs: English; (450)292-3376; Fax. (450)292-4404.

BOURASSA, Dominique; CSSS de Rimouski-Neigette, CP 3150 Succ A 150 av Rouleau, Rimouski QC G5L 5T1; Mon'93; Staff, Hôpital Regional Rimouski; Langs: English; (418)724-8578; Fax. (418)724-8512.

BOURASSA, François; Hopital Notre-Dame de la Merci, 555 boul Gouin O, Montreal QC H3L 1K5; McG'09; CCFP; Staff, Pavillon Notre-Dame de la Merci; (514)331-3020

BOURASSA, Helene; CLSC de Gatineau-Le Guerrier, 425 rue Leguerrier, Gatineau QC J9H 6N8; Sher'94; CCFP; (819)684-2251; Fax. (819)966-6541.

BOURASSA, Marie-Claude; Clin externe de Psychiatrie, 279 rue Providence, Granby QC J2G 4S7; Mon'95; FRCPC; Psy (Pediatric Psychiatry). Langs: English; (450)375-8002; Fax. (450)372-2235.

BOURASSA, Marie-Lyne; 751 Peter Morand Cres, Ottawa ON K1G 6S9; McG'88; Ac Member, Montfort Hospital; (613)739-0909; Fax. (613)739-4667.

BOURASSA, Pierre; Human Resources Skills Devt Ca, 5e 009-355 North River Rd, Ottawa ON K1A 0L1; Laval'85; ac Staff, Hôpital de Gatineau; Med Advisor Div of Medical Expertise & Safety Prog, Human Resources Skills Development Canada; Lecturer, University of Ottawa; McGill University; Langs: Bilingual(French/English); (613)952-5340; Fax. (613)952-8466; pierre-bourassa@hrsdc-rhdcc.gc.ca.

BOURASSA, Sylvie; UMF du Nord de Lanaudiere, 50 ch du Golf E, Joliette QC J6E 2B4; Mon'09; (450)759-3060

BOURASSA, Viviane; CSSS Saint-Jérôme, 290 reu de Montigny, Saint-Jerome QC J7Z 5T3; Sher'07; CCFP; CCFP(E.M.); Staff, Centre Hospitalier Jonquiere; Staff, Hôtel-Dieu de Saint-Jérôme; (450)432-2777; viviane.bourassa@ssss.gouv.qc.ca.

BOURASSA-FULOP, Caroline; Hôpital Anna-Laberge, 200 boul Brisebois, Chateauguay QC J6K 4W8; Mon'09; CCFP; CCFP(E.M.); Staff, Hôpital Anna-Laberge; (450)699-2425

BOURBEAU, Jean; MUHC-Montreal Chest Institute, 3650 rue Saint-Urbain, Montreal QC H2X 2P4; Laval'80; MSc(Epidemiol); ABIM; MRCP; Respir; IntMed (Adult & Pediatric Respirology). Staff, McGill University Health Centre - Royal Victoria Hospital; Staff, McGill University Health Centre - Montreal Chest Institute; assoc Prof, McGill University; Langs: English; (514)934-1934 x32185; Fax. (514)843-2083; jean.bourbeau@mcgill.ca.

BOURBEAU, Jean-Luc; Clinique Med Lacordaire, 201-5650 rue Jean-Talon E, Saint-Leonard QC H1S 1M1; Sher'76; (514)255-9090; Fax. (514)255-8550.

BOURBEAU, Michel; CSSS Pierre-Boucher, 1901 rue Claude, Longueuil QC J4G 1Y5; Mon'77; Staff, Hopital Maisonneuve-Rosemont; Staff, CSSS Pierre-Boucher; Staff, CHSLD Rene-Levesque; Universite de Montreal; (450)651-2210

BOURBEAU, Sophie; Clin de Med Fam Cowansville, 499 rue du Sud, Cowansville QC J2K 2X9; McG'88; (450)263-8890; Fax. (450)263-9737.

BOURBONNAIS, Anne; Clinique Med du Village, 200-400 rue Meigs, Farnham QC J2N 2C8; Sher'87; CCFP; adj Prof, Universite de Sherbrooke; (450)293-3681; Fax. (450)293-7463; anne.bourbonnais@rrsss16.gouv.qc.ca.

BOURBONNAIS, David; Centre Hosp Pierre le Gardeur, 911 montee des Pionniers, Terrebonne QC J6V 2H2; Mon'07; GenSurg. Staff, Centre Hospitalier Pierre le Gardeur; (450)654-7525

BOURBONNIERE, Andre; GMF Concorde, 300 boul de la Concorde E, Laval QC H7G 2E6; Sher'76; ac Staff/Membre Continuing Med Educ, Hopital de la Cite de la santé; Langs: English; (450)667-5310; Fax. (450)667-5248.

BOURBONNIERE, Christine; CHSLD de Hull-Res La Pieta, 273 rue Laurier, Gatineau QC J8X 3W8; McG'80; CCFP; Staff, Centre d'hébergement - La Pietà; Langs: English; French; (819)966-6420; Fax. (819)966-6425; christine_bourbonniere@ssss.gouv.qc.ca.

BOURCHIER, Takashi D; 200-101 16th St W, North Vancouver BC V7M 1T3; UBC'04; FRCPC; IntMed. (604)904-0810

BOURCIER, Joanne D; Cornwall Comm Hosp-McConnell, PO Box 100 Stn Main 840 McConnell Ave, Cornwall ON K6H 5S5; Qns'89; CCFP; CCFP(E.M.); FCFP; Staff, Cornwall Community Hospital; (613)938-4240

BOURCIER, Marc; Clinique De Dermatologie, 35 rue Providence, Moncton NB E1C 8X3; Mon'78; FRCPC; Derm. Staff, Dr Georges-L-Dumont University Hospital Centre; Staff, The Moncton Hospital; (506)857-1421; marc.bourcier@vitalitenb.ca.

BOURDAGES, Macha; CHUQ-Ctr Hosp Univ Laval, 2705 boul Laurier, Quebec QC G1V 4G2; Laval'98; FRCPC; Peds; Critical Care Medicine (P.Q.). Staff, Centre Hospitalier Universitaire de Quebec-CHUL; (418)654-2282

BOURDAGES, Marie-Claude; 2-1 av de l'Eglise, Saint-Antoine NB E4V 1L6; Sher'06; CCFP; (506)525-2409

BOURDAGES, Raymond; Hotel-Dieu de Levis, 143 rue Wolfe, Levis QC G6V 3Z1; Laval'69; FRCPC; IntMed; Gastroent (P.Q.). Staff, Hôtel-Dieu de Lévis; Langs: English; (418)835-7182; Fax. (418)835-7218; raymondbourdages@sympatico.ca.

BOURDEAU, Danielle; 4125-100 Stokes St, Toronto ON M6J 1H4; Laval'87; FRCPC; Psy (Anxiety & Mood Disorders). Staff, Centre for Addiction & Mental Health (CAMH) - College Street Site; Langs: English; French; (416)979-6819; Fax. (416)979-6853; danielle_bourdeau@camh.net.

BOURDEAU, Gilles; 406-595 Montreal Rd, Ottawa ON K1K 4L2; Ott'70; FRCSC; Urol. Consultant, The Ottawa Hospital - General Campus; Ac Staff, Montfort Hospital; (613)745-1008; Fax. (613)744-0525.

BOURDEAU, Guillaume; CSSS de Beauce-Etchemin, 1515 17e rue, Saint-Georges QC G5Y 4T8; Laval'05; DiagRad. Staff, Centre Hospitalier Beauce-Etchemin; (418)228-2031

BOURDEAU, Isabelle; Centre de Recherche, 3850 rue Saint-Urbain, Montreal QC H2W 1T7; Mon'95; FRCPC; IntMed; Endocrin (P.Q.); Endocrin&Metab. adj Prof Med, Universite de Montreal; (514)890-8000 x14086; Fax. (514)412-7204.

BOURDEAU, Line; Coop de Solidarite Sante La Pr, 675 ch Saint-Jean, La Prairie QC J5R 2L2; Laval'03; CCFP; (450)444-2002

BOURDON, Christopher; Sudbury Reg Hosp-Laurentian Si, 41 Ramsey Lake Rd, Sudbury ON P3E 5J1; Ott'89; CCFP; CCFP(E.M.); Staff, Health Sciences North-Laurentian Site; Staff, Health Sciences North-St Joseph's Health Centre; (705)523-7095; Fax. (705)523-7041.

BOURDON, Gilles; 135-175 av Stillview, Pointe-Claire QC H9R 4S3; Mon'82; FRCSC; GenSurg. ac Staff, Lakeshore General Hospital - Pointe Claire; (514)695-6822; Fax. (514)695-7105.

BOURDUA, Isabelle; CHUS-Hop Fleurimont, 3001 12e Av N, Sherbrooke QC J1H 5N4; Sher'92; CSPQ; Anes. Staff, Centre Hospitalier Universitaire de Sherbrooke-Hopital Fleurimont; (819)346-1110; Fax. (819)820-6420.

BOURDUA, Mathilde; CSSS Pierre Boucher, 1333 boul Jacques-Cartier E, Longueuil QC J4M 2A5; Mon'98; CCFP; Staff, Centre Hospitalier Pierre Boucher; (450)468-8111

BOURDY, Christian; 5400 boul Gouin O, Montreal QC H4J 1C5; Mon'77; Staff, Hôpital du Sacre-Coeur de Montréal; vice Doyen Undergraduates Studies, Universite de Montreal; Langs: English; French; (514)338-2070; Fax. (514)338-3187; christian.bourdy@umontreal.ca.

BOURE, Benoit; Hop du Sacre-Coeur de Mtl, 5400 boul Gouin O, Montreal QC H4J 1C5; Mon'84; CSPQ; FRCPC; Anes (Adult Anesthesia). ac Membre Anes, Hôpital du Sacre-Coeur de Montréal; Clin Prof/Staff, Universite de Montreal; (514)338-2680; Fax. (514)338-2009.

BOURGAULT, Andre; Laboratoire de Med Legale, 1701 rue Parthenais, Montreal QC H2K 3S7; Mon'81; CSPQ; FRCPC; AnatPath. Staff, Laboratory Sciences Judiciairies & Medico Legal; (514)873-3300

BOURGAULT, Anne-Marie; CUSM-Hopital Royal Victoria, 687 av des Pins O, Montreal QC H3A 1A1; Sher'73; FRCPC; IntMed; InfectDis; MedMicrobiol. Staff, McGill University Health Centre - Royal Victoria Hospital; ac Staff, Centre Hospitalier l'Université De Montréal (CHUM) - Hôpital Saint-luc; (514)934-1934

BOURGAULT, Christine; Hopital Laval, 2725 ch Sainte-Foy, Quebec QC G1V 4G5; Laval'01; FRCPC; IntMed; Critical Care Medicine; Cardiol. Staff, Hôpital Laval; (418)656-8711

BOURGAULT, Francois; Clin Pediatrique Sainte-Foy, 295-2600 boul Laurier, Quebec QC G1V 4T3; Laval'72; Peds. ac Staff, Centre Hospitalier Universitaire De Québec - Pavillon De St-françois-d'assise; (418)658-0906

BOURGAULT, Josee; CLSC Montcalm, 110 rue Saint-Isidore RR 1, Saint-Esprit QC J0K 2L0; Mon'98; CCFP; (450)839-3676 x4225; Fax. (450)839-6603.

BOURGAULT, Judith; CSSS du Haut Saint-Maurice, 885 boul Ducharme, La Tuque QC G9X 3C1; Laval'83; CST; Staff, Centre Hospitalier Saint-Joseph de la Turque; CH du Centre-de-la-Mauricie (Ste-Thérèse de Shawinigan); Langs: English; (819)523-4581 x2147; Fax. (819)523-6176.

BOURGAULT, Klere; 11790 Highway 64 PO Box 28, Verner ON P0H 2M0; Ott'98; BSc(Kinanthropology); CCFP; Staff ER, West Nipissing General Hospital; Staff, North Bay Regional Health Centre - Regional Mental Health; Langs: English; French; (705)594-2338; Fax. (705)594-1361.

BOURGAULT, Louise A; B1060-801 Aviation Pkwy, Ottawa ON K1K 4R3; Ott'93; BSc(Agr); Langs: French; (613)742-2483

BOURGAULT, Robert F; RCMP Med Centre, 215-440 Coventry Rd, Ottawa ON K1A 0T1; Ott'87; Langs: French; (613)993-1922

BOURGEAU, Pierre; Centre Bois de Boulogne, 370-1575 boul Henri-Bourassa O, Montreal QC H3M 3A9; Mon'67; Neur. Ac Staff, Hôpital du Sacre-Coeur de Montréal; Langs: Bilingual(French/English); (514)337-8672; Fax. (514)337-8285.

BOURGEAULT, Jacques; CSSS du Nord de Lanaudière, 1000 boul Sainte-Anne, St-Charles-Brromee QC J6E 6J2; Mon'69; DiagRad. Staff, Centre Hospitalier Régional de Lanaudière; (450)759-8222 x2844; Fax. (450)759-2133.

BOURGEOIS, Daniel J; Peterborough Reg HC-Hospital, 1 Hospital Dr, Peterborough ON K9J 7C6; McG'84; FRCPC; DiagRad (Interventional Radiology). Staff, Ross Memorial Hospital; Ac Staff, Peterborough Regional Health Centre - Hospital Drive; Consultant, Campbellford Memorial Hospital; Langs: French; (705)876-5039; Fax. (705)743-1713.

BOURGEOIS, Gilles; Clinique Med Lavaltrie, 89C ch Lavaltrie, Lavaltrie QC J5T 2H5; Mon'78; (450)586-1033

BOURGEOIS, Jacqueline J; Humboldt Med Clinic, PO Box 220, Humboldt SK S0K 2A0; Sask'00; BSc(Hons); CCFP; (306)682-2618; Fax. (306)682-4499.

BOURGEOIS, Jacqueline M; Cambridge Mem Hosp, 700 Coronation Blvd, Cambridge ON N1R 3G2; McM'92; FRCPC; AnatPath (Pediatric Pathology). Staff Path, Cambridge Memorial Hospital; Assoc Prof, McMaster University; (519)621-2330

BOURGEOIS, Jacques; Institute of Mental Health Que, 2601 ch de la Canardiere, Quebec QC G1J 2G3; Laval'82; IntMed. Staff, Hôtel-Dieu de Lévis; Staff, Institut Universitaire Sante; Staff, Jeffery Hale Hospital-Saint Brigid's; (418)663-5000

BOURGEOIS, James; St Joseph's Mountain H Service, PO Box 585 Stn Lcd 1 100 5th St W, Hamilton ON L8N 3K7; Uniformed Services Univ (Other Foreign)'89; Staff Psy, St Joseph's Healthcare Hamilton - West 5th Campus; Staff, Hamilton Health Sciences Centre - Chedoke Hospital; (905)522-1155; Fax. (905)575-6085.

BOURGEOIS, Patrick; CSSSG-Hop de Gatineau, CP 2000 Succ Bureau-Chef 909 bou de la Verendrye O, Gatineau QC J8P 7H2; Mon'90; Staff, Hôpital de Gatineau; (819)561-8625 x3083; Fax. (819)561-8313.

BOURGEOIS, Ronald L J; 626-100 Arden St, Moncton NB E1C 4B7; Sher'95; FRCPC; IntMed (Cardiology); Cardiol. Chief Cardiology/Med Dir Heart Function Clinic, The Moncton Hospital; Langs: French; (506)855-2528; Fax. (506)855-6528.

BOURGEOIS, Stephanie; CSSS de la Haute-Yamaska, 205 boul Leclerc O, Granby QC J2G 1T7; Laval'97; FRCPC; IntMed. Staff, Centre Hospitalier de Granby; (450)375-8000

BOURGEOIS-LAW, Gisele; Royal Jubilee Hosp, 107-1952 Bay St, Victoria BC V8R 1J8; Man'79; MEd; FRCSC; ObstGyn (Menopause). Staff, Royal Jubilee Hospital; Assoc Dean Professional Development, University of British Columbia; (250)370-8111 x13713

BOURGET, Amelie; Hop Charles LeMoyne, 3120 boul Taschereau, Greenfield Park QC J4V 2H1; Mon'02; FRCSC; PlasSurg. Staff, Hopital Charles LeMoyne; (450)466-5000

BOURGET, Catherine; CHUQ-Ctr Hosp Univ Laval, 2705 boul Laurier, Quebec QC G1V 4G2; Laval'05; FRCPC; DiagRad. Staff, Centre Hospitalier Universitaire de Quebec-CHUL; (418)525-4444

BOURGET, Danny; Clinique Med St-Louis, 220-3165 ch Saint-Louis, Quebec QC G1W 4R4; Laval'89; (418)653-1970; Fax. (418)653-9956.

BOURGET, Dominique; Royal Ottawa Hlth Care Group, 1145 Carling Ave, Ottawa ON K1Z 7K4; Mon'83; FRCPC; Psy (Forensic Psychiatry). Staff, Royal Ottawa Mental Health Centre - Royal Ottawa Health Care Group; Assoc Prof Psy, University of Ottawa; (613)722-6521 x6366; Fax. (613)798-2992.

BOURGET, Gaetan; CLSC La Petite-Patrie, 6520 rue De Saint-Vallier, Montreal QC H2S 2P7; Mon'87; (514)273-4508; Fax. (514)272-6278.

BOURGET, Martine; CHUQ-Ctr Hosp Univ Laval, 2705 boul Laurier, Quebec QC G1V 4G2; Laval'86; FRCPC; Psy. Staff, Centre Hospitalier Universitaire de Quebec-CHUL; (418)654-4141; Fax. (418)691-5717.

BOURGET, Nathalie; Clinique Med St-Henri, 223 rue Commerciale RR 1, St-Henri-De-Levis QC G0R 3E0; Laval'96; CCFP; Physician, CHSLD Chanoine-Audet; (418)882-2268; Fax. (418)882-3561.

BOURGET, Philippe; Direction de Sante Publique, 205 boul de York O, Gaspe QC G4X 2W5; Sher'08; IntMed. (418)368-3301

BOURGET, Sandrine; Hotel-Dieu de Levis, 143 rue Wolfe, Levis QC G6V 3Z1; Laval'02; CCFP; CCFP(E.M.); Staff, Hôtel-Dieu de Lévis; (418)835-7121

BOURGET, Yves; CSSS de la Haute-Yamaska, 205 boul Leclerc O, Granby QC J2G 1T7; Mon'91; FRCPC; Psy. Staff, Centre Hospitalier de Granby; (450)372-5491; Fax. (450)372-2235.

BOURGIE, Jacques R; Mediclub du Sanctuaire, 203-6100 rue du Boise, Montreal QC H3S 2W1; Mon'68; FRCPC; DiagRad. ac Staff Radiol, Hopital de la Cite de la santé; adj Prof Clin Radiol, Universite de Montreal; (514)739-6301; Fax. (514)739-6792.

BOURGOIN, Michel; 105-140 rue Champlain, Dieppe NB E1A 1N8; Laval'98; FRCSC; GenSurg (Intensive Care); VascSurg. Staff, Dr Georges-L-Dumont University Hospital Centre; Langs: English; (506)854-6273; Fax. (506)854-5945.

BOURGOIN, Yves; CLSC Laurier-Station, 135 rue de la Station SS 1, Laurier-Station QC G0S 1N0; Laval'92; (418)728-3435; Fax. (418)728-2233.

BOURGOIN-COUILLARD, Sylvie; GMF de l'Assomption, 814 boul de l'Ange-Gardien N, L'Assomption QC J5W 4M9; Laval'00; LMCC; (450)589-5778

BOURGON, Luc N; 4424-501 Smyth Rd, Ottawa ON K1H 8L6; Ott'73; DABPN; FRCPC; Psy (Electroconvulsive Therapy). Ac Staff, The Ottawa Hospital - General Campus; Asst Prof, University of Ottawa; Langs: Bilingual(English/French); (613)737-8010; Fax. (613)737-8115; lbourgon@ottawahospital.on.ca.

BOURGOUIN, Daniel; CSSS de Trois-Rivieres, 1991 boul du Carmel, Trois-Rivieres QC G8Z 3R9; Laval'76; FRCSC; GenSurg; VascSurg. Staff, CSSS de Trois-Rivières; Langs: Bilingual(French/English); (819)697-3333

BOURGOUIN, Jean; CHUM-Hotel-Dieu, 3840 rue Saint-Urbain, Montreal QC H2W 1T8; Mon'70; MSc; Staff, Centre Hospitalier l'Université de Montréal (CHUM) - Hôtel-Dieu; cadre VP/Chef Medical Officer, Wex Pharmaceuticals Inc; (514)890-8000 x14240

BOURGOUIN, Paul-A.; St Mary's Hosp Centre, 5327-3830 av Lacombe, Montreal QC H3T 1M5; Laval'67; Nephrol (P.Q.); IntMed. Staff, St Mary's Hospital Centre; Staff, McGill University Health Centre - Montreal General Campus; McGill University; (514)345-3511 x3564; Fax. (514)734-2637.

BOURGOUIN, Pierre; CHUM-Hop Notre-Dame, 1560 rue Sherbrooke E, Montreal QC H2L 4M1; Mon'81; FRCPC; DiagRad. Staff, McGill University Health Centre - Montreal General Campus; Staff, Centre Hospitalier l'Université de Montréal (CHUM) - Hôpital Notre-Dame; assoc Prof, McGill University; Exec Vice-Dean & Clin Affairs, Universite de Montreal; (514)890-8250; Fax. (514)934-8263; pbourgouin@sympatico.ca.

BOURGOUIN, Pierre T; CSSS Pierre Boucher, 1333 boul Jacques-Cartier E, Longueuil QC J4M 2A5; McG'77; Staff, Centre Hospitalier Pierre Boucher; (450)468-8111 x82140

BOURKAS, Angelo E; 202-7200 rue Hutchison, Montreal QC H3N 1Z2; McG'83; MSc; CCFP; Staff, Sir Mortimer B Davis Jewish General; Staff, Donald Berman Maimonides Geriatric Centre; adj Prof Family Med, McGill University; (514)495-2555; Fax. (514)495-7932.

BOURKE, Kevin E; Lifemark Sport Med & Hlth Ctre, 182-26 Thomas Raddall Dr, Halifax NS B3S 0E2; Dal'86; BSc; Langs: English; French; (902)404-3888; Fax. (902)422-0547.

BOURKE, Michael A E; Hilltop Med Clinic, 240-15321 16 Ave, Surrey BC V4A 1R6; Dublin (Ireland)'70; MB ChB; BAO; (604)536-5656; Fax. (604)538-5670.

BOURKE, Michael E; Univ of Ottawa Heart Institute, H2410-40 Ruskin St, Ottawa ON K1Y 4W7; Ott'75; FRCPC; Anes (Cardiac Intensive Care Unit). Att Staff Anes Cardiac Div, University of Ottawa Heart Institute; Asst Prof, University of Ottawa; (613)761-4379; Fax. (613)761-4925; mbourke@ottawaheart.ca.

BOURKE, Richard A; South Walkerville Med Ctre, 340-2224 Walker Rd, Windsor ON N8W 5L7; RCS (Ireland)'67; LRCPS(Ire); FRCSC; ObstGyn. Staff, Hôtel-Dieu Grace Hospital; Staff, Windsor Regional Hospital - Metropolitan Site; (519)258-1592; Fax. (519)258-7350.

BOURNE, Mary; Aurora Newmarket Family Hlth Team, 405-531 Davis Dr, Newmarket ON L3Y 6P5; Wes'74; CCFP; FCFP; Assoc Staff, Southlake Regional Health Centre; Coroner, City of Newmarket; (905)898-2240; Fax. (905)898-2253.

BOURNS, Amy E; Sherbourne Health Centre, 333 Sherbourne St, Toronto ON M5A 2S5; Ott'08; CCFP.

BOURNS, Robert E; Halton Hills Family Health, 171 Guelph St, Georgetown ON L7G 4A1; Qns'75; CCFP; Staff, Halton Healthcare Services Corporation - Georgetown Hospital; (905)877-0233; Fax. (905)877-1229.

BOURON DAL SOGLIO, Dorothee; Hôpital Ste-Justine, 3175 ch Cote-Sainte-Catherine, Montreal QC H3T 1C5; Paris VI (France)'00; Staff, Hôpital Ste-Justine; (514)345-4931 x5352

BOURQUE, Andre; Clinique Med Familiale du Sud, 4475 rue Bannantyne, LaSalle QC H4G 1E2; Ott'72; (514)765-3600

BOURQUE, Berthier; Clinique Med Chaudiere, 102 18e rue, Saint-Georges QC G5Y 4T9; Laval'72; BSc(Biol); MSc; ac Staff, Centre Hospitalier Beauce-Etchemin; Langs: English; (418)228-6820; Fax. (418)226-0358.

BOURQUE, Christine; Dr Georges-L Dumont Reg Hosp, 330 av Universite, Moncton NB E1C 2Z3; Sher'07; FRCPC; MedMicrobiol. Staff, Dr Georges-L-Dumont University Hospital Centre; (506)862-4000

BOURQUE, Christopher N; Markham Prof Centre, 303-2265 Pembina Hwy, Winnipeg MB R3T 5J3; Man'75; FRCPC; IntMed (Neurology). Staff, Victoria General Hospital; Asst Prof IntMed, University of Manitoba; (204)269-5848; Fax. (204)269-5857.

BOURQUE, Daniel; Hop du Sacre-Coeur de Mtl, 5400 boul Gouin O, Montreal QC H4J 1C5; Mon'02; FRCPC; EmergMed. Staff, Hôpital du Sacre-Coeur de Montréal; (514)338-2222; Fax. (514)338-2384.

BOURQUE, Isabelle; CLSC de Paspebiac, CP 7000 273 boul Gerard-D-Levesque, Paspebiac QC G0C 2K0; Laval'03; Staff, CLSC de Paspebiac; (418)752-2572

BOURQUE, Jacques; Centre Med ObstGyn, 203-1361 av Beaumont, Mont-Royal QC H3P 2W3; Mon'79; FRCSC; ObstGyn. ac Staff, Centre Hospitalier l'Université de Montréal (CHUM) - Hôtel-Dieu; ac Staff, Hôpital Ste-Justine; (514)344-4411; Fax. (514)344-1991.

BOURQUE, Jean-Andre; 86 rue Du Portage, Caraquet NB E1W 1A8; Sher'94; Langs: English; French; (506)726-2169; Fax. (506)727-4418.

BOURQUE, Jean-Louis; Clinique Med Hickson, 3805 rue De Verdun, Verdun QC H4G 1K8; Mon'68; FRCSC; Urol. (514)769-9671

BOURQUE, Jean-Marc; Douglas Mental Hlth Univ Inst, 6875 boul Lasalle, Verdun QC H4H 1R3; Mon'67; FRCPC; Psy. Ac Staff, Douglas Mental Health University Institute; Consultant, Hôpital Ste-Justine; Assoc Member, Centre Hospitalier Universitaire de Sherbrooke-Hopital Fleurimont; (514)761-6131 x2085; Fax. (514)888-4077.

BOURQUE, Luc; 125-667 rue Champlain, Dieppe NB E1A 1P6; Sher'83; FRCSC; OrthSurg. Staff, Dr Georges-L-Dumont University Hospital Centre; (506)855-2922; Fax. (506)855-6603.

BOURQUE, Manon; Horizon Feminin, 206-200 rue Durand, Saint-Jerome QC J7Z 7E2; Mon'97; FRCSC; ObstGyn. (450)436-4228; Fax. (450)436-5488.

BOURQUE, Marie-Claude; CSSS Gatineau-Hop de Hull, 116 boul Lionel Emond, Gatineau QC J8Y 1W7; Mon'05; Staff, Hull Hospital; (819)966-6200; Fax. (819)966-6055.

BOURQUE, Marjolaine; CSSS des Iles, 430 ch Principal, Cap-aux-Meules QC G4T 1R9; McG'05; FRCSC; GenSurg. Staff, Hôpital de l'Archipel; (418)986-2121; Fax. (418)986-6845.

BOURQUE, Pierre R; The Ottawa Hosp-Civic Campus, C2200-1053 Carling Ave, Ottawa ON K1Y 4E9; Ott'81; FRCPC; Neur (Neuromuscular Diseases). Ac Staff, The Ottawa Hospital - Civic Campus; Assoc Prof Med, University of Ottawa; Langs: Bilingual(French/English); (613)761-5353; Fax. (613)761-5360.

BOURQUE, Rachel; Ungava Tulattavik Hosp, CP 149, Kuujjuaq QC J0M 1C0; Sher'08; CCFP; Staff, Centre de sante Tulattavik de l'Ungava; (819)964-2905 x217; Fax. (819)964-2270.

BOURQUE, Solange; CSSS de Trois-Rivieres, 1991 boul du Carmel, Trois-Rivieres QC G8Z 3R9; Sher'06; FRCPC; IntMed; Nephrol. Staff, CSSS de Trois-Rivières; (819)697-3333

BOURQUE, Sonia; CSSS de la Cote-De-Gaspe, 215 boul de York O, Gaspe QC G4X 2W2; Laval'96; CCFP; Staff, Centre Hospitalier de Gaspe; (418)368-3301; Fax. (418)368-6850.

BOURQUE, Stephane; 130-500 ch Mapleton, Moncton NB E1G 0N3; Sher'07; CCFP; Staff, Dr Georges-L-Dumont University Hospital Centre.

BOURQUE, Suzanne; CLSC Saint-Henri, 3833 rue Notre-Dame O, Montreal QC H4C 1P8; Mon'85; (514)933-7541

BOURQUE, Sylvie A; Surrey Mem Hosp, 13750 96 Ave, Surrey BC V3V 1Z2; Dal'03; FRCPC; IntMed; MedOncol. Staff, Surrey Memorial Hospital; (604)930-2098

BOURRE TESSIER, Josiane; CHUM-Hop Notre-Dame, 1560 rue Sherbrooke E, Montreal QC H2L 4M1; Mon'04; FRCPC; IntMed; Rheum. Staff, Centre Hospitalier l'Université de Montréal (CHUM) - Hôpital Notre-Dame; (514)890-8000; Fax. (514)412-7630.

BOURRELLE, Dominique; CHUM-Hop Notre-Dame, 1560 rue Sherbrooke E, Montreal QC H2L 4M1; Mon'83; FRCPC; IntMed; Rheum. Staff, Centre Hospitalier l'Université de Montréal (CHUM) - Hôpital Notre-Dame; adj Prof Med, Universite de Montreal; (514)890-8000 x28800; Fax. (514)412-7630.

BOURRELLIS, Sonia; Ctr Hosp Anna-Laberge, 200 boul Brisebois, Chateauguay QC J6K 4W8; Mon'94; FRCPC; IntMed. Staff, Hôpital Anna-Laberge; (450)699-2425 x4570; Fax. (450)699-2525.

BOURRET, Andre; CSSS Bordeaux-Cartierville-St-, 555 boul Gouin O, Montreal QC H3L 1K5; Mon'63; Staff, Pavillon Notre-Dame de la Merci; (514)331-3020

BOURRET, Danielle; College des Med du Quebec, 2170 boul Rene-Levesque O, Montreal QC H3H 2T8; Mon'79; Staff, College des Medecins du Quebec; (514)933-4441 x5373; dbourret@cmq.org.

BOURRIER, Robert G; Sandy Hill Comm Health Centre, 221 Nelson St, Ottawa ON K1N 1C7; Ott'88; CCFP; FCFP; Langs: French; (613)789-8458; Fax. (613)789-8710; rbourrier@sandyhillchc.on.ca.

BOURSIER, Manon; CSSS de laval, 2790-1755 Boul Rene-Laennec, Laval QC H7M 3L9; Laval'83; Hem (P.Q.). Staff, Hopital de la Cite de la santé; (450)668-1010; manonboursier@videotron.ca.

BOURSIQUOT, Jean-Nicolas; CHUQ-Hop Laval, 2705 rue Laurier, Quebec QC G1V 4G2; Laval'04; FRCPC; ClinImmunol&Allergy; IntMed. Staff, Centre Hospitalier Universitaire de Quebec-CHUL; (418)525-4444

BOURY-SIMOES, Delphine; CSSS d'Antoine-Labelle-Mt Laur, RR 1 2561 ch de la Lievre S, Mont-Laurier QC J9L 3G3; Staff, CSSS d'Antoine-Labelle; (819)623-1234

BOUSHEY, Edward; Montfort Hosp, 713 Montreal Rd, Ottawa ON K1K 0T2; Ott'98; CCFP; CCFP(E.M.); Staff Emer Med, Montfort Hospital; (613)746-4621

BOUSHEY, Robin P; The Ottawa Hosp-Gen Campus, W1617-501 Smyth Rd, Ottawa ON K1H 8L6; Tor'95; BSc; PhD; FRCSC; GenSurg (Colon & Rectal Surgery). Staff, The Ottawa Hospital - General Campus; (613)737-8899 x71724; Fax. (613)739-6646.

BOUSHRA, Rasha G I; Western Mem Reg Hosp, PO Box 2005 Stn Main 1 Brookfield Ave, Corner Brook NL A2H 6J7; Ain Shams (Egypt)'97; MB ChB; Staff, Western Memorial Regional Hospital; (709)637-5000

BOUSHY, David; Royal Victoria Hosp, 201 Georgian Dr, Barrie ON L4M 6M2; Tor'96; CCFP; CCFP(E.M.); Staff, Royal Victoria Regional Health Centre; (705)728-9090

BOUSQUET, Jean; Clinique Med Saint-Jerome, 102-450 boul Monseigneur-Duboi, Saint-Jerome QC J7Y 3L8; Mon'75; (450)438-1518

BOUSTANI, Elie; Hôpital de Saint-Eustache, 520 boul Arthur-Sauve, Saint-Eustache QC J7R 5B1; Laval'09; Staff, Hôpital de Saint-Eustache; (450)473-6811

BOUSTCHA, Elizabeth M; St Boniface Gen Hosp, 409 Tache Ave, Winnipeg MB R2H 2A6; McG'71; MSc(HealthAdmin.); FRCPC; IntMed (Medical Administration); GeriatricMed. Staff, St Boniface General Hospital; (204)237-2410

BOUTALEB, Asmae; Clinique Medicale, 202-5855 boul Gouin O, Montreal QC H4J 1E5; Mon'82; Langs: Arabic; English; (514)745-3030; Fax. (514)621-9161.

BOUTET, Annie; Clinique Med de la Rive, 169 rue du Prince-Albert, Otterburn Park QC J3H 1L4; Sher'05; (450)446-7333

BOUTET, Bernard; Clinique Med de Pintendre, 5-792 Rte Du President-Kennedy, Pintendre QC G6C 1C8; Laval'87; (418)837-6943; Fax. (418)837-0487.

BOUTET, Jacques; 301 rue Dufort, La Prairie QC J5R 2X6; Laval'66; Staff, Hopital Charles LeMoyne; (450)659-9193; Fax. (450)659-7090.

BOUTET, Jean-Yves; Clinique Med Soleil, 64 1re Av O, Amos QC J9T 1T8; Laval'82; Staff Trauma Team, CH Hôtel-Dieu d'Amos; Coord Medical and Administrative, GMF Les Eskers; (819)732-8341; Fax. (819)732-1642.

BOUTET, Kim; Hop du Sacre-Coeur de Mtl, 5400 boul Gouin O, Montreal QC H4J 1C5; Mon'01; FRCPC; IntMed; Respir. Staff, Hôpital du Sacre-Coeur de Montréal; (514)338-2222

BOUTET, Marianne; St Michael's Hosp, 30 Bond St, Toronto ON M5B 1W8; Laval'04; FRCSC; ObstGyn. Staff, St Michael's Hospital; (416)864-6060

BOUTET, Pierre; Hop Ste-Anne-de-Beaupre, 11000 rue des Montagnards RR 1, Beaupre QC G0A 1E0; Mon'98; Staff, Hôpital Sainte Anne de Beaupré; (418)827-3726

BOUTET, Sylvain; Centre Medical de l'Hetriere, 201-3520 rue Hetriere, St-Augustin-D-Desm QC G3A 0B4; Laval'86; (418)651-3933; Fax. (418)651-0256.

BOUTH, Jean-Claude; Clinique Med St-Andre, 102-8133 av André-Ampère, Montreal QC H1E 3J9; (Haiti)'68; (514)648-6888; Fax. (514)564-6757.

BOUTHAT, Alain; CSSS Pierre Boucher, 1333 boul Jacques-Cartier E, Longueuil QC J4M 2A5; Mon'76; Staff, Centre Hospitalier Pierre Boucher; Langs: English; (450)468-8401; Fax. (450)468-8403; bouthat@videotron.ca.

BOUTHIETTE, Pierre; 359 rue Perreault E, Rouyn-Noranda QC J9X 3C5; Mon'74; ObstGyn. (819)764-5131; Fax. (819)764-3054.

BOUTHILLIER, Alain; CHUM-Hop Notre-Dame, 1560 rue Sherbrooke E, Montreal QC H2L 4M1; Mon'87; FRCSC; Neursurg. Staff, Centre Hospitalier l'Université de Montréal (CHUM) - Hôpital Notre-Dame; (514)890-8000 x26869; Fax. (514)412-7816.

BOUTHILLIER, Annie; CLSC Riviere des Prairies, 8655 boul Perras, Montreal QC H1E 4M7; Mon'97; (514)494-4924

BOUTHILLIER, Catherine; Clinique Med Bromont, C101-89 boul de Bromont, Bromont QC J2L 2K5; Mon'02; CCFP; Staff, CSSS la Pommeraie; (450)534-5474

BOUTHILLIER, Claude; CHUM-Hop Notre-Dame, 1560 rue Sherbrooke E, Montreal QC H2L 4M1; Mon'89; FRCPC; PhysMed&Rehab. Staff, Centre Hospitalier l'Université de Montréal (CHUM) - Hôpital Notre-Dame; (514)890-8000

BOUTHILLIER, Genevieve; 397 av Laurier O, Montreal QC H2V 2K3; Mon'97; FRCPC; Psy. (514)271-9991; Fax. (514)271-8260.

BOUTHILLIER, Jean; 220-214 boul de la Cite-des-Je, Gatineau QC J8Y 6S8; Mon'76; Ac Staff, Hull Hospital; Langs: English; (819)770-2565; Fax. (819)595-0422.

BOUTHILLIER, Luc; Centre Med Maricourt, 3995 Montee Saint-Hubert, Saint-Hubert QC J3Y 4K2; Sher'78; (450)676-6911; Fax. (450)676-4097.

BOUTHILLIER, Renee; Hôpital Ste-Justine, 3175 ch Cote-Sainte-Catherine, Montreal QC H3T 1C5; Sher'80; Peds (Emergency Pediatrics). Ac Staff EmergPed, Hôpital Ste-Justine; Langs: English; (514)345-4931; Fax. (514)731-4408.

BOUTILIER, Nicole A; Aberdeen Hosp, 835 East River Rd, New Glasgow NS B2H 3S6; Dal'95; BSc; CCFP; Staff, Aberdeen Regional Hospital; (902)752-7600

BOUTILIER, Robert G; Colchester East Hants Hlth Ctr, 600 Abenaki Rd, Truro NS B2N 5A1; Dal'97; FRCPC; AnatPath., Colchester East Hants Health Centre; (902)893-5554 x2185

BOUTILIER-THOMAS, Carol M; Sterling Mall Med Clinic, 105-3 Sterling Rd, Glace Bay NS B1A 3X2; Dal'85; BSc; MSc; (902)842-1500; Fax. (902)842-1500.

BOUTIN, Carmen; Clinique Med St-Agapit, 1125 rue Principale RR 1, Saint-Agapit QC G0S 1Z0; Laval'78; (418)888-3951; Fax. (418)888-3952.

BOUTIN, Caroline; CSSS de Rimouski-Neigette, CP 3150 Succ A 150 av Rouleau, Rimouski QC G5L 5T1; Laval'99; FRCPC; Peds. Staff, Hôpital Regional Rimouski; (418)724-3000; Fax. (418)725-3025.

BOUTIN, Christine; Hôpital Ste-Justine, 3175 ch Cote-Sainte-Catherine, Montreal QC H3T 1C5; Sher'84; CSPQ; FRCPC; Peds (Echography); Cardiol. Staff, Hopital Charles LeMoyne; Staff, Hôpital Ste-Justine; Langs: English; (514)345-4931 x3977; Fax. (514)345-4896; christine_boutin@ssss.gouv.qc.ca.

BOUTIN, Guy; Cabinet Med Prive Danville, CP 570 45 rue Elm, Danville QC J0A 1A0; Sher'77; ac Staff/Prof Family Med, Institut Universitaire de Geriatrie de Sherbrooke-Pavillon Argyll; Physician Students Health Services, Bishop's College-Lennoxville; (819)839-1464

BOUTIN, Guy R; 401-3030 boul Le carrefour, Laval QC H7T 2P5; Mon'66; Otol. Ac Staff, Hopital de la Cite de la santé; Prof, Universite de Montreal; (450)687-1750; Fax. (450)687-7797; guyboutin@cgocable.ca.

BOUTIN, Helene A; 205-323 Wilson St E, Ancaster ON L9G 4A8; Alb'85; CCFP; FCFP; Ac Staff Family Med, Hamilton Health Sciences Centre - McMaster University Medical Centre; (905)648-8786; Fax. (905)648-7730.

BOUTIN, Helene; Clinique St-Barnabe, 307-176 av Rouleau, Rimouski QC G5L 8W1; Mon'82; FRCSC; Urol (Incontinence). Staff, Centre Hospitalier Régional Baie-Comeau; Staff, Hôpital Regional Rimouski; (418)724-6262; Fax. (418)722-6265.

BOUTIN, Isabelle; Hôpital Laval, 2725 ch Sainte-Foy, Quebec QC G1V 4G5; Mon'02; Respir; IntMed. Staff, Hôpital Laval; (416)656-4747

BOUTIN, Isabelle; Clinique Med de Warwick, 5A rue du Centre Sportif, Warwick QC J0A 1M0; Laval'07; CCFP; (819)358-4600

BOUTIN, Jean-Marie; CHUM-Hotel-Dieu, 3840 rue Saint-Urbain, Montreal QC H2W 1T8; Sher'80; MSc; PhD; Endocrin (P.Q.) (Laboratory Medicine). Staff, Centre Hospitalier l'Université de Montréal (CHUM) - Hôtel-Dieu; adj Prof, Universite de Montreal; (514)890-8000 x14726; jm.boutin@umontreal.ca.

BOUTIN, Manon; MUHC-Montreal Children's Hosp, 2300 rue Tupper, Montreal QC H3H 1P3; Mon'76; Peds. Staff, McGill University Health Centre - Montreal Children's Hospital; Physician, CLSC Jolimon St-Michel-des-Saints; (514)412-4499; Fax. (514)412-4399.

BOUTIN, Marie; CHUQ-Hotel-Dieu de Quebec, 11 ch Côte du Palais, Quebec QC G1R 2J6; Laval'98; CCFP; Staff, Centre Hospitalier Universitaire de Québec (CHUQ) - Siege Social; (418)360-3744

BOUTIN, Mario; Clinique Med des Promenades, A220-3333 rue du Carrefour, Quebec QC G1C 5R9; Mon'88; CCFP; FCFP; (418)663-6345; Fax. (418)663-8621.

BOUTIN, Mario; Clinique Med St Sauveur, 70 rue Principale RR 6, Saint-Sauveur QC J0R 1R6; Mon'85; BSc; (450)227-8436; Fax. (450)227-7222.

BOUTIN, Yannick; Clin Ophtalmologique de la Cit, 010-2600 boul Laurier, Quebec QC G1V 4T3; Laval'01; FRCSC; Ophth. Boursier, Centre Hospitalier Regional de Sept-Iles; (418)650-5065

BOUTIS, Kathy; The Hosp For Sick Children, 555 University Ave, Toronto ON M5G 1X8; Tor'91; FRCPC; Peds. Staff, The Hospital For Sick Children; (416)813-8982; Fax. (416)813-5043; kleanthi.boutis@sickkids.ca.

BOUTROS, Cecile; 202-500 boul Gouin E, Montreal QC H3L 3R9; Ein Shams (Egypt)'66; Physician, CLSC Saint-Laurent; Langs: Arabic; (514)382-5999

BOUTROS, Farid S A; SGH Medical Mall, 308-3030 Lawrence Ave E, Scarborough ON M1P 2T7; Ain Shams (Egypt)'90; MB ChB; ABIM; FACP; FRCPC; IntMed (Endocrinology); Endocrin&Metab. Staff GenMed & Endocrin, The Scarborough Hospital - General Campus; (416)439-8353; Fax. (416)438-6503.

BOUTROS, Gebran E; Cite de la Sante de Laval, 1755 boul Rene-Laennec, Laval QC H7M 3L9; St. Joseph (Lebanon)'84; CSPQ; FRCPC; IntMed; Cardiol. Staff, Hopital de la Cite de la santé; (450)668-1010; Fax. (450)975-5550.

BOUTROS, Hedy N; Victoria Medical Group, 205-1719 Lawrence Ave E, Scarborough ON M1R 2X7; Cairo (Egypt)'68; MB BCh; FRCPC; AnatPath (Hematology Pathology). Physician Courtesy Privil, The Scarborough Hospital - General Campus; Physician Courtesy Privil, Markham Stouffville Hospital; Physician Courtesy Privil, The Scarborough Hospital - Birchmount Campus; Langs: Arabic; (416)609-1100; Fax. (416)609-1102.

BOUTROS, Jacqueline L; 34 King St E, Stoney Creek ON L8G 1J8; Ain Shams (Egypt)'91; MB ChB; CCFP; (905)664-3838; Fax. (905)664-8633.

BOUTROS, John; Postgrad Med Educ-U of Toronto, 602-500 University Ave, Toronto ON M5G 1V7; Mon'04; FRCSC; GenSurg.

BOUTROSS-TADROSS, Odette; McMaster University HSC, PO Box 2000 Stn Lcd 1 1200 Main St W, Hamilton ON L8N 3Z5; Ain Shams (Egypt)'80; MB ChB; MSc; FRCPC; AnatPath. Staff Path, Hamilton Health Sciences Centre - McMaster University Medical Centre; Asst Prof, McMaster University; (905)521-2100 x76224; Fax. (905)820-3312.

BOUTTELL, Elaine S; Grand River Reg Cancer Centre, PO Box 9056 Stn C 835 King St W, Kitchener ON N2G 1G3; Wes'97; FRCPC; IntMed (Gastrointestinal Cancer); MedOncol. Staff, Grand River Hospital - Kitchener/Waterloo Health Centre; Staff MedOncol, Grand River Regional Cancer Centre; (519)749-4370

BOUVET, Luc; Polyclinique 55, 4825 av Bouvet, Becancour QC G9H 1X5; Laval'79; ac Staff, Hôpital de Christ-Roi; (819)233-3123; Fax. (819)233-3124.

BOUVET, Sylvie; Clin Med GMA du Camel, 200-1785 boul du Camel, Trois-Rivieres QC G8Z 3R8; Laval'84; ObstGyn (P.Q.). (819)379-8385

BOUVIER, Anne-Marie; UMF de la Laurier, 4F-2875 boul Laurier, Quebec QC G1V 2M2; Sher'99; CCFP; Staff, Centre Hospitalier Universitaire de Quebec-CHUL; (418)654-2701; Fax. (418)654-2138.

BOUVIER, Gilles; 15380 av Bourdages S, Saint-Hyacinthe QC J2T 3P7; Ott'71; Assoc Staff, Centre Hospitalier Honore-Mercier; Langs: Bilingual(French/English); (450)773-7770; Fax. (450)773-2731.

BOUVIER, Helene; Hop Riviere-des-Prairies, 7070 boul Perras, Montreal QC H1E 1A4; Sher'89; Psy (Pedology Psychiatry). Staff, Hôpital Riviere des Prairies; (514)323-7260; Fax. (514)328-3501.

BOUWER, Elizma; 4825 50th St PO Box 939, Stettler AB T0C 2L0; (South Africa)'96; CCFP; Langs: Afrikaans; (403)742-4742; Fax. (403)742-4013.

BOUWER, Hester A; Stapleford Med Clinic, 372 McCarthy Blvd N, Regina SK S4R 7M2; Stellenbosch (South Africa)'86; MB ChB; (306)545-3000; Fax. (306)545-5584.

BOUWER, Johannes C; Upper Level River City Centre, 615A-8600 Franklin Ave, Fort McMurray AB T9H 4G8; (South Africa)'92; (780)742-2352; Fax. (780)788-2034.

BOUWER, Pieter A; PO Box 939, Stettler AB T0C 2L0; (South Africa)'96; CCFP; Staff FamMed Maternity Clinic, Medicine Hat Regional Hospital; (403)742-4742; Fax. (403)742-4013.

BOUZAYEN, Renda; IWK Health Centre, PO Box 9700 Rpo Csc, Halifax NS B3K 6R8; Tunis (Tunisia)'91; FRCSC; ObstGyn (Infertility). Staff, IWK Health Centre; Langs: French; (902)470-7098; Fax. (902)425-1125.

BOVARD, James A P; Lonsdale Place, 403-1200 Lonsdale Ave, North Vancouver BC V7M 3H6; UBC'84; (604)984-9594; Fax. (604)984-6881; drbovard@shaw.ca.

BOVELL, Frank M; St Boniface Gen Hosp, 409 Tache Ave, Winnipeg MB R2H 2A6; Tor'98; BSc; MSc; FRCPC; IntMed; InfectDis. Staff, St Boniface General Hospital; (204)233-8563

BOVELL, Keith T; 201-49 Emma St, Guelph ON N1E 6X1; London (England)'75; MB BS; MRCP(UK); MD; FACG; FRCPC; IntMed; Gastroent. Ac Staff, Guelph General Hospital; (519)763-1220; Fax. (519)763-2144; ktbovell@bellnet.ca.

BOVETT, Geoffrey P; Sunnybrook Hlth Sciences Ctre, 2075 Bayview Ave, Toronto ON M4N 3M5; McM'97; Staff, Sunnybrook Health Sciences Centre; (416)480-4244

BOVO, Christiane; Clinique Med des Generations, 200-465 rue Bibeau, Saint-Eustache QC J7R 0C8; Mon'85; Staff, Hôpital de Saint-Eustache; (450)472-1955; Fax. (450)472-1905.

BOVO, Michel; 102-3090 ch de Chambly, Longueuil QC J4L 4N5; Mon'66; FRCPC; DiagRad. Staff, Centre Hospitalier Pierre Boucher; (450)646-3520

BOW, Eric J; Cancer Care Manitoba, 2081-675 McDermot Ave, Winnipeg MB R3E 0V9; Cal'76; FRCPC; IntMed; InfectDis; Hem. Staff, Health Sciences Centre; Staff, CancerCare Manitoba; Prof Med Microbiol & IntMed, University of Manitoba; (204)787-2197; ejbow@cancercare.mb.ca.

BOW, Jennifer K; Kingston Gen Hosp, V3 300-76 Stuart St, Kingston ON K7L 2V7; Wes'02; FRCSC; OrthSurg. Staff, Kingston General Hospital; (613)549-6666

BOW, Michael R; Tawa Centre, 120-3017 66 St NW, Edmonton AB T6K 4B2; Cal'80; BSc; FRCSC; ObstGyn (Family Medicine). Clin Prof ObstGyn, University of Alberta; (780)461-6220; Fax. (780)461-4197.

BOWDEN, Helen G; The Allin Clinic, 10155 120 St NW, Edmonton AB T5K 2A2; Tor'76; Staff, Lloydminster Hospital; (780)482-7551; Fax. (780)482-3533; hbowden4@shaw.ca.

BOWDEN, Lois; PO Box 380, Port Williams NS B0P 1T0; Mem'85; CCFP; FCFP; Staff, Valley Regional Hospital; (902)542-0537; Fax. (902)542-0530.

BOWDEN, Scott H; Fredericton Med Clinic, 406-1015 Regent St, Fredericton NB E3B 6H5; Mem'90; FRCS; BMedSci; BEng; LMCC; FRCSC; OrthSurg (Adult Orthopaedics). Att Staff OrthSurg, Dr Everett Chalmers Regional Hospital; Att Staff OrthSurg, Oromocto Public Hospital; Consultant OrthSurg, Carleton Memorial Hospital; (506)458-0490; Fax. (506)457-4710.

BOWDEN, William F; East Kootaney Reg Hosp, 13 24th Ave N, Cranbrook BC V1C 3H9; Alb'06; CCFP; CCFP(E.M.); Staff, East Kootenay Regional Hospital; (250)426-5281

BOWDIN, Sarah C C; The Hosp for Sick Children, 940-555 University Ave, Toronto ON M5G 1X8; Southampton (United Kingdom)'96; Staff, The Hospital For Sick Children; (416)813-6390

BOWDRIDGE, Gilda A; Medical Arts Bldg, 307-5880 Spring Garden Rd, Halifax NS B3H 1Y1; Tirgu-Mures (Romania)'82; CCFP; Staff, Cape Breton Healthcare Complex; Preceptor Family Med., Dalhousie University; Langs: Romanian; Hungarian; (902)425-4990; Fax. (902)425-5243.

BOWEN, A Scott L; Amherst Family Health Clinic, 158 Robert Angus Dr, Amherst NS B4H 4R7; Dal'97; BSc; FRCPC; IntMed (Cardiology). (902)667-4144; Fax. (902)667-4176.

BOWEN, C Vaughan A; Division of Orthopaedic Surger, 3134 Hospital Dr NW, Calgary AB T2N 5A1; Edinburgh (Scotland)'74; MD; MB ChB; FRCSC; OrthSurg (Hand & Reconstructive Microvascular Surgery). Staff, Foothills Medical Centre; Clin Prof, University of Calgary; (403)944-2112; Fax. (403)270-8004.

BOWEN, Debra S; Health & Counseling Services, 1125 Colonel By Dr, Ottawa ON K1S 5B6; Tor'82; CCFP; (613)520-2600; Fax. (613)520-3851.

BOWEN, Francis A; Regina Qu'Appelle HR-Regina, 1440 14th Ave, Regina SK S4P 0W5; Sask'85; CCFP; CCFP(E.M.); FCFP; Staff Emerg Dept, Regina General Hospital; (306)766-4213; Fax. (306)766-4357.

BOWEN, James D; PO Box 84, Norris Point NL A0K 3V0; Ott'85; Chief of Staff, Bonne Bay Health Centre; Preceptor, Memorial University Of Newfoundland; (709)458-3001; Fax. (709)458-3002; jamesbowen@westernhealth.nl.ca.

BOWEN, Julie L; Sudbury Reg Hosp-Laurentian, 41 Ramsey Lake Rd, Sudbury ON P3E 5J1; Sask'80; FRCPC; RadOncol. Staff Regional Cancer Prog, Health Sciences North-Laurentian Site; Assoc Prof, Laurentian University; Assoc Prof, University of Ottawa; (705)522-6237 x2451; Fax. (705)523-7329; jbowen@hrsrh.on.ca.

BOWEN, Nadia; Sault Area Hosp, 750 Great Northern Rd, Sault Ste. Marie ON P6B 0A8; Sask'07; CCFP; Staff, Sault Area Hospital - Sault Ste Marie; (705)759-3434; Fax. (705)759-3731.

BOWEN, Richard A; 1651 Boundary Ave, Nanaimo BC V9S 5R8; Alb'64; FRCSC; Ophth. (250)753-8415

BOWEN, Rudradeo C; Royal University Hosp, 103 Hospital Dr, Saskatoon SK S7N 0W8; McG'67; BSc; FRCPC; Psy (Anxiety Disorder). Staff Psy, Royal University Hospital; Ac Staff, Saskatchewan District Health; Prof, University of Saskatchewan; (306)966-8226; Fax. (306)966-8177.

BOWEN, Steven E; 313-6707 Elbow Dr SW, Calgary AB T2V 0E5; Sask'85; CCFP; (403)252-6022; Fax. (403)253-1923.

BOWEN, Thomas J; 217-5809 Macleod Trail SW, Calgary AB T2H 0J9; Alb'75; DAB; FRCPC; Peds (Clinical Immunology & Allergy). Clin Prof Med & Peds, University of Calgary; Clin Prof Peds, University of British Columbia; (403)283-8291; Fax. (403)287-6085.

BOWER, Neil L; 1019 Prince St, Truro NS B2N 1H7; Dal'88; (902)897-2626; Fax. (902)897-1660.

BOWERING, C Keith; Baker Clinic, 290-10405 Jasper Ave NW, Edmonton AB T5J 3N4; Mem'77; ABIM; FACP; FRCPC; IntMed (Diabetes). Clin Prof Med, University of Alberta; (780)944-9589; Fax. (780)944-1165.

BOWERING, David; Northern Health Services, 211-3228 Kalum St, Terrace BC V8G 2N1; UBC'70; Med Officer of Hlth, Northern Health Services; (250)631-4261; david.bowering@northernhealth.ca.

BOWERING, John B; St Paul's Hosp, 1081 Burrard St, Vancouver BC V6Z 1Y6; UBC'87; FRCPC; Anes (Cardiovascular Anesthesia). Staff, Providence Health Care - St Paul's Hospital; (604)682-2344 x62813; Fax. (604)806-5487.

BOWERING, M Rex; Nanaimo Mental Hlth & Addictio, 3F-528 Wentworth St, Nanaimo BC V9R 3E4; Mem'86; FRCPC; Psy (Child & Adolescent Psychiatry). Staff, Nanaimo Regional General Hospital; (250)739-5868

BOWERING, Tricia A; Sherbrooke Centre, 4F-260 Sherbrooke St, New Westminster BC V3L 3M2; UBC'98; FRCPC; Psy. (604)520-4662; Fax. (604)520-4871; tbowering@bucior.com.

BOWERMAN, Brian; Kenora Med Centre, 45 Wolsley St, Kenora ON P9N 3W7; Man'84; BSc(Med); Staff, Lake of the Woods District Hospital; Med Advisor, Birchwood Terrace Nursing Home; (807)468-3021

BOWERS, Richard J; Trillium Health Centre-Mississ, 100 Queensway W, Mississauga ON L5B 1B8; Tor'74; Staff, Trillium Health Centre - Mississauga; (905)848-7600

BOWES, B Lynette; Dr Charles A Janeway Child HC, 300 Prince Philip Dr, St. John's NL A1B 3V6; Mem'95; FRCPC; Peds (Pediatric Hematology Oncology). Staff, Janeway Children's Health & Rehabilitation Centre; (709)777-4945; Fax. (709)777-4941; lynette.bowes@easternhealth.ca.

BOWES, David M C; Nova Scotia Cancer Centre, 5820 University Ave, Halifax NS B3H 1V7; Dal'05; FRCPC; RadOncol. Staff, Nova Scotia Cancer Centre; (902)473-6096; Fax. (902)473-7205; david.bowes@cdha.nshealth.ca.

BOWES, Matthew J; Centre for Forensic Medicine, 51 Garland Ave, Dartmouth NS B3B 0J2; Qns'98; BSc; FRCPC; AnatPath (Forensic Pathology). Lecturer Path, Dalhousie University; (902)424-2955; Fax. (902)424-0607.

BOWES, R Carla; Thompson Gen Hosp, 871 Thompson Dr, Thompson MB R8N 0C8; Sask'94; FRCPC; Peds. Staff, Thompson General Hospital; (204)677-2381

BOWIE, Paul R; Children's Hosp Eastern Ont, 401 Smyth Rd, Ottawa ON K1H 8L1; McG'75; FRCPC; Peds (Emergency Medicine). Medical Officer Emerg, Children's Hospital of Eastern Ontario (CHEO); (613)737-7600 x2318; Fax. (613)738-4885; bowie@cheo.on.ca.

BOWINS, Brad E; 1700-2200 Yonge St, Toronto ON M4S 2C6; Tor'89; FRCPC; Psy. (416)322-7935

BOWKER, Blair M; Medical & Dental Bldg, 408-1221 Algonquin Ave, North Bay ON P1B 4Y3; Alb'73; FRCPC; IntMed; Endocrin (P. Q.); Endocrin&Metab. Staff Consultant, North Bay Regional Health Centre - Regional Mental Health; Teach Staff Northern Ontario Family Med Prog, University of Ottawa; (705)476-1223; Fax. (705)476-3723; blairbowker@hotmail.com.

BOWLAND, M Anne; Misericordia Community Hosp, 1NW 15-16940 87 Ave NW, Edmonton AB T5R 4H5; Alb'77; CCFP; Staff, Covenant Health - Misericordia Community Hospital; (780)735-2585; Fax. (780)735-2591.

BOWLE-EVANS, Jo Ann; 9 Elizabeth St E GD, Creemore ON L0M 1G0; Qns'67; CGPP; BA; (705)466-5013 x0; Fax. (705)466-5828; dr.jody@rogers.com.

BOWLER, Adrian P; 211 Dundas St E, Trenton ON K8V 1L8; London (England)'69; Ac Staff, QHC Trenton Memorial; (613)392-9228; Fax. (613)392-2768.

BOWLER, David F; Comox Med Clinic, 100-1695 Comox Ave, Comox BC V9M 3M1; Cape Town (South Africa)'81; MB ChB; MRCP; CCFP; Staff, St Joseph's General Hospital; Langs: Afrikaans; (250)339-2266

BOWLER, Jannice; Comox Med Clinic, 100-1695 Comox Ave, Comox BC V9M 3M1; Cape Town (South Africa)'82; MB ChB; CCFP; (250)339-2266; Fax. (250)339-0985.

BOWLER, Kathleen J; Regina Qu'Appelle HR-Pasqua, 4101 Dewdney Ave, Regina SK S4T 1A5; Ott'89; FRCPC; Anes. Staff, Regina General Hospital; Staff, Pasqua Hospital; Teach Staff Med, University of Saskatchewan; (306)766-2295

BOWLER, Kenneth A; 855 Harrington Crt, Burlington ON L7N 3P3; McM'80; FRCPC; PhysMed&Rehab (Musculoskeletal). Med Dir, Joseph Brant Memorial Hospital; (905)681-7577; Fax. (905)681-0855.

BOWLER, Lynne; Queen Elizabeth Hosp, PO Box 6600 Stn Central 60 Riverside Dr, Charlottetown PE C1A 8T5; Wes'92; BSc; MSc; FRCPC; AnatPath. Staff, Queen Elizabeth Hospital; (902)894-2300

BOWLER, W Blake; 139 Main St, Lucan ON N0M 2J0; Wes'82; (519)227-1163

BOWLES, Alan K; Queensway-Carleton Hosp, 3045 Baseline Rd, Nepean ON K2H 8P4; Ott'72; Staff, Queensway Carleton Hospital; (613)721-2000

BOWLES, M Jean; Temiskaming Hosp, PO Box 4040 421 Shepherdson Rd, New Liskeard ON P0J 1P0; Wes'82; CCFP; FCFP; Ac Staff, Temiskaming Hospital; (705)647-8121

BOWLES, Norm R; Ottawa West Med Centre, PO Box 45013 Rpo Bridlewood 701 Eagleson Rd, Kanata ON K2M 2Y1; McG'84; (613)592-9081; Fax. (613)592-6554.

BOWLING, Sheila D; Village Med Clinic, PO Box 130 Stn Fort Langley 1-9089 Glover Rd, Langley BC V1M 2R5; Alb'92; CCFP; FCFP; (604)888-8300

BOWLSBY, Glenn O; Kerrisdale Station Med Clinic, 2077 42nd Ave W, Vancouver BC V6M 2B4; UBC'83; (604)261-9494

BOWLSBY, Jeffrey K; Care Point Med Centre, 1123 Davie St, Vancouver BC V6E 1N2; UBC'80; (604)915-9517

BOWMAN, Cameron C; 480-999 Broadway W, Vancouver BC V5Z 1K5; UBC'99; FRCSC; PlasSurg (Breast Reconstruction). Clinical Asst Prof Div of PlasSurg, University of British Columbia; (604)734-1416; dr.bowman@telus.net.

BOWMAN, Caroline; West End Family Practice, 2-30 45th St S, Wasaga Beach ON L9Z 0A6; McM'03; CCFP; (705)429-9445

BOWMAN, Collin P; Queen Street Med Group, 502 Queen St, Saskatoon SK S7K 0M5; Sask'92; Assoc Staff Family Med, Saskatoon District Health Board; (306)652-9145; Fax. (306)652-1531.

BOWMAN, Denise M; Crowfoot West Business Ctre, 600 Crowfoot Cres NW, Calgary AB T3G 0B4; Cal'00; BSc; MSc; PhD; CCFP; Staff, Strathmore District Health Services; (403)452-0999

BOWMAN, John L; Collingwood Sport Medicine, 105-10 Keith Ave, Collingwood ON L9Y 0W5; Wes'72; Dip SportMed; Med Dir, Collingwood Sport Medicine & Rehabilitation Centre; (705)444-5303; Fax. (705)444-0723.

BOWMAN, Jonathan R; Northern Lights Health Region, 7 Hospital St, Fort McMurray AB T9H 1P2; Alb'89; CCFP; Staff Emerg Med, Northern Lights Regional Health Centre; (780)791-7535; Fax. (780)791-4149.

BOWMAN, M Nancy; Manitoba Clinic, 790 Sherbrook St, Winnipeg MB R3A 1M3; Man'77; FRCPC; Peds. Staff, Health Sciences Centre.

BOWMAN, Michael E; 9803 34 Ave NW, Edmonton AB T6E 5X9; Ott'06; FRCPC; Peds; InfectDis. (780)461-9299; Fax. (780)465-7267.

BOWMAN, Sylvia A; Edmonton Mental Health Clinic, 5F-9942 108 St NW, Edmonton AB T5K 2J5; Alb'91; FRCPC; Psy. Staff, Alberta Hospital Edmonton; (780)427-4444

BOWMAN, Tom; Salvation Army Grace Gen Hosp, 300 Booth Dr, Winnipeg MB R3J 3M7; Man'89; Staff, The Salvation Army Grace Hospital; (204)837-8311; Fax. (204)831-0029.

BOWMER, Michael I; St Clare's Mercy Hosp, 435-154 LeMarchant Rd, St. John's NL A1C 5B8; McG'69; FRCPC; IntMed. Staff, St Clare's Mercy Hospital; (709)777-5276

BOWRY, Ashna D K; St Michael's Health Centre, 80 Bond St, Toronto ON M5B 1X2; Bristol (United Kingdom)'06; CCFP; (416)864-3011; Fax. (416)864-3099.

BOWRY, Richard; North York Gen Hosp, 4001 Leslie St, North York ON M2K 1E1; London (England)'94; FRCPC; Anes. Staff, North York General Hospital; (416)756-6000

BOWSER, R Daniel; Victoria Med Centre, 404-304 Victoria Ave N, Hamilton ON L8L 5G4; McM'78; FRCSC; GenSurg. Staff, Hamilton Health Sciences Centre - Hamilton General Hospital; Asst Prof, McMaster University; (905)522-0262; Fax. (905)522-0268; drdan34@hotmail.com.

BOXALL, Janice M; 212-400 Bronte St S, Milton ON L9T 0H7; Qns'82; CCFP; CCFP(E.M.); FCFP; Ac Staff Family Med, Halton Healthcare Services Corporation - Milton District Hospital; (905)876-4490; Fax. (905)876-4878.

BOXEN, Izzie; Brampton Nuclear Services, 28-470 Chrysler Dr, Brampton ON L6S 0C1; Tor'74; BSc; MSc; FRCPC; NuclearMed (Cardiology). Physician, Brampton Nuclear Services; Langs: Yiddish; (905)791-3458; Fax. (905)791-3460.

BOXER, Alvin A; The Doctor's Office, 203-300 John St, Thornhill ON L3T 5W4; UBC'60; (905)764-0188; Fax. (905)764-0189; aboxer@mcimed.com.

BOXER, Jack; 301-8425 120 St, Delta BC V4C 6R2; UBC'77; Vis Staff, Vancouver General Hospital - Centennial Pavillion; (604)597-8800

BOYANG, Winston F; Northern Med Unit Grand Rapids, General Delivery, Easterville MB R0C 0V0.

BOYAR, M Avis; Rockyview Gen Hosp, 5A253-7007 14 St SW, Calgary AB T2V 1P9; Cal'79; BScN; AB(Hospice&PalliativeM; CCFP; Staff, Rockyview General Hospital; Consultant Palliative Care, Alberta Health Services; (403)943-3223; Fax. (403)253-1362.

BOYCE, David W; 303-3330 Richter St, Kelowna BC V1W 4V5; Dal'84; FRCSC; OrthSurg (Hip & Knee Arthroplasty). (250)763-0908; Fax. (250)862-5842; dboycemd@shaw.ca.

BOYCE, Debra E; Partners In Pregnancy Clinic, 302-170 Simcoe St, Peterborough ON K9H 2H7; Tor'88; BSc; CCFP; FCFP; Staff, Peterborough Regional Health Centre - Hospital Drive; (705)741-1191; Fax. (705)741-1192.

BOYCE, Frank G; Quinte HC Corp-Belleville Gen, 265 Dundas St E, Belleville ON K8N 5A9; Tor'66; Staff Emerg Med, QHC Belleville General; (613)969-5511; frankboyce100@hotmail.com.

BOYCHUK, Lesia R; Misericordia Community Hosp, 16940 87 Ave NW, Edmonton AB T5R 4H5; Sask'78; BSc(Hon); DABIM; FRCPC; IntMed; InfectDis. Ac Staff, Covenant Health - Misericordia Community Hospital; Ac Staff, Royal Alexandra Hospital; Clin Assoc Prof Med, University of Alberta; Langs: Ukrainian; (780)735-2949

BOYCOTT, Kym; Children's Hosp Eastern Ont, 401 Smyth Rd, Ottawa ON K1H 8L1; Cal'00; BSc(Hon); PhD; FRCPC; MedGenetics. Staff, Children's Hospital of Eastern Ontario (CHEO); Assoc Prof, University of Ottawa; (613)737-7600 x3223; kboycott@cheo.on.ca.

BOYCZUM, Julie; GMF Montee de la Baie, 3942 ch Oka, St-Joseph-du-Lac QC J0N 1M0; Laval'99; Staff, Hôpital de Saint-Eustache; Langs: Bilingual(English/French); (450)473-3930; Fax. (450)473-2160.

BOYD, Alyssa; West End Family Practice, 2-30 45th St S, Wasaga Beach ON L9Z 0A6; McM'03; MCFP; BSc; CCFP; Medical Staff, Collingwood General & Marine Hospital; Assoc Staff, Royal Victoria Regional Health Centre; Clin Assoc Prof, McMaster University; (705)429-9445; Fax. (705)429-9588.

BOYD, April J; Health Sciences Centre, 820 Sherbrook St, Winnipeg MB R3A 1R9; Tor'99; MSc; PhD; FRCSC; GenSurg (Vascular & Interventional Radiology); VascSurg. Assoc Prof, Health Sciences Centre; (204)787-8889; Fax. (204)787-3201; aboyd2@exchange.hsc.mb.ca.

BOYD, Barbara J; 204-99 Kakulu Rd, Kanata ON K2L 3C8; Alb'86; CCFP; FCFP; (613)592-1269; Fax. (613)592-1141.

BOYD, Brian K; Deerfoot Meadows Med Clinic, 7979 11 St SE, Calgary AB T2H 0B8; Alb'72; BScPharm; (403)251-2690; Fax. (403)251-2695.

BOYD, Bryan A; 315 St. Laurent Blvd, Ottawa ON K1K 2Z5; Tor'79; (613)248-0811

BOYD, Cameron L; The Medical Centre FHT, PO Box 4200 Stn Main 707 Charlotte St, Peterborough ON K9J 7B3; Qns'80; BSc(Hons.); Staff Flight Surgeon, Canadian Forces Health Services Centre; Med Dir, Peterborough Regional Health Centre - Hospital Drive; (705)876-4545; Fax. (705)740-8391.

BOYD, Gordon J; Queen Elizabeth II HSC, 1276 South Park St, Halifax NS B3H 2Y9; Dal'93; FRCPC; DiagRad; NuclearMed. Staff, Queen Elizabeth II Health Sciences Centre - Victoria General Site; (902)473-6150; Fax. (902)473-3482.

BOYD, Hugh F; 250 Dundas St E, Waterdown ON L0R 2H4; Tor'08; CCFP; (905)689-8242

BOYD, Jeanette E; Cedar Family Med Clinic, 203-518 Lake St, Nelson BC V1L 4C6; Cal'03; CCFP; (250)354-4414; Fax. (250)354-1912.

BOYD, Jennifer A; Inner City Family Health Team, 4F-69 Queen St E, Toronto ON M5C 1R8; Tor'09; CCFP; (416)368-5666; Fax. (416)368-2679.

BOYD, John G; Kingston Gen Hosp, C7-76 Stuart St, Kingston ON K7L 2V7; Qns'06; Neur. Staff, Kingston General Hospital; (613)549-6666

BOYD, John; St Paul's Hosp, 166-1081 Burrard St, Vancouver BC V6Z 1Y6; Wes'98; FRCPC; IntMed (Critical Care Medicine); Respir. Staff, Providence Health Care - St Paul's Hospital; (604)806-8346

BOYD, Karen L; Markham Prof Centre, 200-2265 Pembina Hwy, Winnipeg MB R3T 5J3; Man'75; Ac Staff, Victoria General Hospital; (204)989-4200; Fax. (204)989-4205.

BOYD, Kerry E; 3280 Schmon Pky, Thorold ON L2V 4Y6; Wes'88; FRCPC; Psy. Staff, Hamilton Health Sciences Centre - McMaster University Medical Centre; (905)684-6918; Fax. (905)684-5866.

BOYD, Kirsty U; The Ottawa Hosp-Civic Campus, 1053 Carling Ave, Ottawa ON K1Y 4E9; Qns'04; FRCSC; PlasSurg. Staff, The Ottawa Hospital - Civic Campus; (613)798-5555; Fax. (613)761-4635.

BOYD, Mark E; 210-1255 av Greene, Westmount QC H3Z 2A4; Sask'57; FRCOG; FACOG; FRCSC; ObstGyn (Gynecological Surgery). (514)938-5535; Fax. (514)488-1790.

BOYD, Matthew; St Martha's Reg Hosp, 25 Bay St, Antigonish NS B2G 2G5; Dal'07; Respir; IntMed. Staff, St Martha's Regional Hospital; (902)863-4500

BOYD, Michael C; Blusson Spinal Cord Centre, 6F-818 10th Ave W, Vancouver BC V5Z 1M9; Sask'80; MSc(Eng); FRCSC; Neursurg (Spine). Staff, Providence Health Care - St Paul's Hospital; Staff/Dir Combine NeuroSurgical & Orth Spine Prog, Vancouver General Hospital - Centennial Pavillion; (604)875-4746; Fax. (604)875-8223.

BOYD, Michael J; Kingsway Plaza Phase III, 503-4980 Kingsway, Burnaby BC V5H 4K7; Alb'79; FRCSC; Ophth. (604)430-9560; Fax. (604)430-5578.

BOYD, Michele; Hotel-Dieu Hosp, 166 Brock St, Kingston ON K7L 5G2; Qns'96; FRCPC; Psy. Staff Psychiatrist, Kingston Regional Treatment Centre; Staff Psychiatrist, Hotel-Dieu Hospital; (613)536-6926; Fax. (613)536-4623.

BOYD, Norman F; Univ Hlth Network-Princess M, 10 406-610 University Ave, Toronto ON M5G 2M9; London (England)'63; MD; MB BS; DSc; FRCPC; FRCPC; Hem; IntMed. Staff, Princess Margaret Hospital - University Health Network; Sr Scientist, Campbell Family Inst For Breast Cancer Research; (416)946-2942; Fax. (416)946-2024; boyd@uhnres.utoronto.ca.

BOYD, R Bruce; Great-West Life Assurance Co, 60 Osborne St N, Winnipeg MB R3C 3A5; Man'75; DLIM; BLIM; CCFP; FCFP; Med Consultant, Great West Life Assurance Company; Med Dir, Western Life Assurance Co; Med Dir, Wawanesa Life Insurance; Med Consultant, Manulife Financial; Med Dir Insurance, Gamma-Dynacare Medical Lab; (204)946-7316; Fax. (204)946-7506.

BOYD, R James; St Boniface Gen Hosp, E6003-409 Tache Ave, Winnipeg MB R2H 2A6; Man'72; BSc; CCFP; FCFP; Staff, St Boniface General Hospital; Prof/Dept Head Family Med, University of Manitoba; (204)235-3655; Fax. (204)231-0302; jaboyd@sbgh.mb.ca.

BOYD, Shelley R; 800-61 Queen St E, Toronto ON M5C 2T2; Tor'92; FRCSC; Ophth (Retina). Staff, St Michael's Hospital; (416)360-4000

BOYD, Stephanie; Grand River Hosp-KW Hlth Ctre, PO Box 9056 Stn C 835 King St W, Kitchener ON N2G 1G3; '05; CCFP; CCFP(E.M.); Staff, Grand River Hospital - Kitchener/Waterloo Health Centre.

BOYDEN, Sheri N; 16 Green St, Nepean ON K2J 3R2; McM'01; CCFP; (613)825-9799; Fax. (613)825-5963.

BOYER, David K; Windsor Reg Hosp-Metropolitan, 1995 Lens Ave, Windsor ON N8W 1L9; Wes'84; CCFP; CCFP(E.M.); FCFP; Staff, Windsor Regional Hospital - Metropolitan Site; Staff, Hôtel-Dieu Grace Hospital; (519)254-1661

BOYER, Dory; Fraser Orthopaedic Institute, 403-233 Nelson's Cres, New Westminster BC V3L 0E4; Wes'99; FRCSC; OrthSurg (Sports Injuries). Staff, Eagle Ridge Hospital & Health Care Centre; Staff, Royal Columbian Hospital; (604)523-1110; dr.boyer@telus.net.

BOYER, Francois; Ctr Frederick-Georges-Heriot, 75 rue Saint-Georges, Drummondville QC J2C 4G6; Sher'83; Staff, CHSLD Coeur-du-Québec; (819)477-0544; Fax. (819)477-1409; fboyer@9bit.qc.ca.

BOYER, Helene; CSSS Jeanne-Mance, 100-15 av du Mont-Royal O, Montreal QC H2T 2R9; Mon'87; (514)286-2600 x4354; hboyer@ssss.gouv.qc.ca.

BOYER, J Andre; 101-560 boul Henri-Bourassa O, Montreal QC H3L 1P4; Ott'64; Sec, Henri-Bourassa Medical Laboratory Inc; (514)335-1050; Fax. (514)335-5797.

BOYER, Julie; Centre Hospitalier Fleury, 2180 rue Fleury E, Montreal QC H2B 1K3; Mon'96; CCFP; CCFP(E.M.); Staff, Centre Hospitalier Fleury; Staff, Hôtel-Dieu de Saint-Jérôme; (514)384-2000

BOYER, Liette; CSSS Les Eskers de l'Abitibi, 622 4e rue O, Amos QC J9T 2S2; Sher'75; MedOncol (P.Q.); IntMed (P.Q.) (Palliative Care). Chef Dept of Med Specialist/Staff Medical Oncology, CH Hôtel-Dieu d'Amos; Langs: Bilingual(French/English); (819)732-3341 x2368; Fax. (819)732-2278.

BOYER, Marc; CSSS du Sud de Lanaudière, 911 montee des Pionniers, Terrebonne QC J6V 2H2; Mon'86; Staff, Centre Hospitalier Pierre le Gardeur; (450)654-7525; Fax. (450)585-5939.

BOYER, Michael E; The Medical Centre, 707 Charlotte St, Peterborough ON K9J 2X5; Tor'74; FRCPC; Peds. Ac Staff, Peterborough Regional Health Centre - Hospital Drive; Assoc Staff, Peterborough Regional Health Centre - Rogers St Site; (705)743-6222; Fax. (705)876-4526.

BOYER, Micheline; National Defence, 101 Colonel By Dr, Ottawa ON K1A 0K2; Ott'83; CCFP; FCFP; (613)945-1340

BOYER, Philippe L; Clinique Med St-Louis, 504 rue Saint-Louis, Joliette QC J6E 2Z2; McG'84; Staff Emerg, Centre Hospitalier Régional de Lanaudière; (450)759-0581; Fax. (450)759-0584.

BOYER, Rene; Comm Lesions Prof, 2F-505 rue des Forges, Trois-Rivieres QC G9A 6H1; Mon'61; MSc(McGill); GenSurg (Coloscopy). hon Staff Surg, Centre Hospitalier Regional de Trois-Rivieres; Med Consultant, Ministry of Labour & Solidarite(Quebec); (819)371-4928; Fax. (819)371-4430; rene.boyer@clp.gouv.qc.ca.

BOYER, Sandra; CSSS Lac-des-Deux-Montagnes, 520 boul Arthur-Sauve, Saint-Eustache QC J7R 5B1; Laval'08; CCFP; Staff, Hôpital de Saint-Eustache; Langs: Bilingual(French/English); (450)473-6811; Fax. (450)473-6966.

BOYER, Suzanne; CLSC Simone Monnet Chartrand, 1303 boul Jacques-Cartier E, Longueuil QC J4M 2Y8; Laval'96; (450)463-2850

BOYINGTON, Curtiss R; Grey Nuns Community Hosp & HC, 1100 Youville Drive West NW, Edmonton AB T6L 5X8; Sask'03; FRCPC; IntMed. Staff, Covenant Health - Grey Nuns Community Hospital; (780)735-7236

BOYKO, Boris W; 580-10665 Jasper Ave NW, Edmonton AB T5J 3S9; Alb'79; CCFP; Staff, Royal Alexandra Hospital; Staff, Glenrose Rehabilitation Hospital; Physician, Edmonton Eskimos; Glen Sather Sports Medical Clinic; Consultant Phy, Edmonton Oilers; Clin Prof Family Pract, University of Alberta; (780)761-3115; Fax. (780)761-3118.

BOYKO, Mark J; Foothills Medical Centre, 1403 29 St NW, Calgary AB T2N 2T9; Wes'07; CCFP; CCFP(E.M.); Staff, Foothills Medical Centre; (403)944-1110

BOYKO, Robert M; 142 Nahani Way, Mississauga ON L4Z 3J1; Tor'87; CCFP; CCFP(E.M.); FCFP; Staff, The Credit Valley Hospital; Coroner, Ministry of Community Safety and Correctional Services; Asst Prof Family & Commun Med, University of Toronto; (905)568-0355; Fax. (905)568-0307.

BOYLAN, Colm E; St Joseph's Healthcare, 50 Charlton Ave E, Hamilton ON L8N 4A6; Cork (Ireland)'92; Staff, St Joseph's Healthcare - Charlton Campus; (905)522-1155

BOYLAN, Declan P; Sudbury Reg Hosp-Kirkwood Site, 680 Kirkwood Dr, Sudbury ON P3E 1X3; National (Ireland)'87; FRCPC; Psy. Psychiatrist, Health Sciences North-Kirkwood Site; dboylan@hrsrh.on.ca.

BOYLAN, Khrista R A; Hamilton HS-McMaster Site, PO Box 2000 Stn Lcd 1, Hamilton ON L8N 3Z5; Dal'99; FRCPC; Psy (Child Psychiatry). Staff, Hamilton Health Sciences Centre - McMaster University Medical Centre; (905)521-2100

BOYLAN, Maureen F; Formation Health Serv Unit, PO Box 17000 Stn Forces, Victoria BC V9A 7N2; McM'87; CCFP; FCFP; Fam Med, Canadian Forces Health Services - Pacific Centre; (250)363-5641

BOYLE, Allison M; A-255 Connell St, Woodstock NB E7M 1L2; London (England)'93; MB BS; (506)324-8000; Fax. (506)324-8010; mchandra@nb.sympatico.ca.

BOYLE, Anne B; St Joseph's Healthcare, 50 Charlton Ave E, Hamilton ON L8N 4A6; McM'88; CCFP; Staff, St Joseph's Healthcare - Charlton Campus; (905)522-1155 x3529

BOYLE, Carol A J; Workers' Compensation Board, PO Box 1879 Stn Main 9912 107 St, Edmonton AB T5J 2P2; Sask'79; BSc; FRCPC; Neur. (780)498-4029; Fax. (780)498-7807.

BOYLE, David A; Alexander Prof Bldg, 202-849 Alexander Crt, Peterborough ON K9J 7H8; Queen's (Ireland)'67; MB ChB; MRCP; FRCPC; IntMed (Endocrinology & Metabolism). Ac Staff, Peterborough Regional Health Centre - Hospital Drive; (705)743-5858; Fax. (705)743-5729; drboylesoffice@gmail.com.

BOYLE, David L; Sudbury Reg Hosp-Laurentian, 910-41 Ramsey Lake Rd, Sudbury ON P3E 5J1; Ott'80; FRCPC; Anes. Staff, Health Sciences North-Laurentian Site; (705)523-7113; Fax. (705)523-7112.

BOYLE, James C; Broadway Med Centre, 350-943 Broadway W, Vancouver BC V5Z 4E1; UBC'78; FRCSC; PlasSurg (Burns). Ac Staff, Vancouver General Hospital - Centennial Pavillion; Ac Staff, BC Children's Hospital; Clin Assoc Prof, University of British Columbia; (604)737-7492; Fax. (604)737-0851; jc_boyle@telus.net.

BOYLE, James C; Southlake Reg Health Centre, 596 Davis Dr, Newmarket ON L3Y 2P9; Tor'76; CCFP; FCFP; Ac Staff, Southlake Regional Health Centre; (905)895-4521 x2321

BOYLE, Loree L; The Ottawa Hosp-Gen Campus, LM18-501 Smyth Rd, Ottawa ON K1H 8L6; Dal'05; FRCPC; IntMed. Staff, The Ottawa Hospital - General Campus; (613)737-8899

BOYLE, Marc R; 327-1641 Lonsdale Ave, North Vancouver BC V7M 2J5; Ott'73; OrthSurg. Langs: Bilingual(English/French); (604)988-4285

BOYLE, Michael; Anson Gen Family Health Team, PO Box 189 58 Anson Dr, Iroquois Falls ON P0K 1E0; Queen's (Ireland)'68; MB ChB; BAO(Belfast); (705)258-3318; Fax. (705)258-4330.

BOYLE, Neil G H; Victoria Gen Hosp, 1 Hospital Way, Victoria BC V8Z 6R5; Ott'80; BSc; CCFP; FCFP; Staff, Royal Jubilee Hospital; Staff, Victoria General Hospital; (250)727-4212

BOYLE, Patrick; Rapids Family Health Team, 4-1150 Pontiac Dr, Sarnia ON N7S 3A7; Edinburgh (Scotland)'74; BSc(Hon); MB ChB; MRCGPract; CCFP; Langs: French; (519)339-8949; pboyle@rapidsfhteam.ca.

BOYLE, Stefan R; CFB Petawawa Base Med Clinic, PO Box 9999 Stn Main, Petawawa ON K8H 2X3; Ott'94; CCFP; FCFP; Assoc Staff, Pembroke Regional Hospital Inc; Physician, Department Of National Defence; Langs: English; French; (613)687-5511 x5392; Fax. (613)687-1499.

BOYLES, Peter; The Ottawa Hosp-Civic Campus, 1053 Carling Ave, Ottawa ON K1Y 4E9; Dal'87; FRCPC; Psy. Staff, The Ottawa Hospital - Civic Campus; (613)761-4581; Fax. (613)761-5328.

BOYNE, Timothy S; Bridgeland Med Bldg, 2F-803A 1 Ave NE, Calgary AB T2E 7C5; McM'86; FRCPC; IntMed; Cardiol. (403)571-6962; Fax. (403)571-8657.

BOYNTON, Erin L; 280 Britannia Rd E, Mississauga ON L4Z 1S6; Tor'85; DAB; FRCSC; OrthSurg (Research & Clinical Orthopedics). Researcher, Mount Sinai Hospital; University of Toronto; erin.boynton@rogers.com.

BOYRAZIAN, Hagob A; 406-2130 Lawrence Ave E, Scarborough ON M1R 3A6; Erevan State (Armenia (Republic))'79; Staff, The Scarborough Hospital - Birchmount Campus; Staff, North York General Hospital - Branson Division; Staff, Rouge Valley Health System - Centenary Health Centre Site; Langs: Arabic; Russian; Turkish; (416)298-0666; Fax. (416)298-7807.

BOZDECH, Lumir; Country Hills Village, 234-5149 Country Hills Blvd NW, Calgary AB T3A 5K8; Prague (Czech Republic)'68.

BOZDECH, Miloslav B; 120-5002 55 St, Red Deer AB T4N 7A4; Sask'96; BSc; FRCSC; Ophth. Staff, Red Deer Regional Hospital Centre; Staff, Innisfail Health Centre; Langs: Czech; (403)342-2020

BOZEK, Christopher B; Burnaby Hosp, 3935 Kincaid St, Burnaby BC V5G 2X6; Tor'80; FRCPC; Neur. Staff, Burnaby Hospital; (604)412-6405

BOZEK, Nancy L; Huntsville Prof Bldg, 202-348 Muskoka Rd 3 N, Huntsville ON P1H 1H8; McM'91; CCFP; FCFP; Staff, Huntsville District Memorial Hospital - Muskoka Algonquin Healthcare; (705)788-3623; Fax. (705)788-3624.

BOZIC, Katarina; Grey Nuns Community Hosp & HC, 1100 Youville Drive West NW, Edmonton AB T6L 5X8; Belgrade (Serbia)'91; CCFP; Staff, Covenant Health - Grey Nuns Community Hospital; Langs: Serbo-Croatian; (780)735-7000

BOZINOVSKI, Jovan; 106-2020 Richmond Rd, Victoria BC V8R 6R5; Qns'98; BScChemEng; MSc; FRCSC; CardSurg.

BOZORGZADEH, Minoo; York Finch Med Centre, 101-2115 Finch Ave W, North York ON M3N 2V6; Iran (Iran)'84; FRCPC; DiagRad. Staff, QHC Belleville General; (416)744-2655

BOZYK, Kevin S; PO Box 5580 Stn Main, High River AB T1V 1M6; Sask'78; (403)652-2929; Fax. (403)652-1510.

BOZZER, Cristine; MUHC-Montreal Gen Hosp, D10.144-1650 av Cedar, Montreal QC H3G 1A4; McG'98; CSPQ; FRCPC; Anes. Staff, McGill University Health Centre - Montreal General Campus; (514)934-1934 x43261; Fax. (514)934-8549.

BRAAM, Geert B; Clinical Sciences Bldg, 11 132CSB-132 University Campu, Edmonton AB T6G 2R7; (Netherlands)'90; MD; PhD; Langs: Dutch; (780)407-3322; Fax. (780)407-7771.

BRAATEN, Jan T; 525 Golden Ave, Ottawa ON K2A 2E6; Oslo (Norway)'62; DABIM; Endocrin&Metab; IntMed (Diabetology). Staff Physician Endocrin & Metab, The Ottawa Hospital - Civic Campus; Assoc Prof Med, University of Ottawa; (613)722-4066

BRABANT, Angele Y; Riverside Cardiac Clinic, 2147 Armstrong St, Sudbury ON P3E 4W2; Ott'04; FRCPC; IntMed. Langs: Bilingual(English/French); (705)670-0654; Fax. (705)670-9348.

BRABANT, Francois; Poly Med Pierre-Le-Gardeur, 310-1000 montee des Pionniers, Terrebonne QC J6V 1S8; Mon'98; Staff, Centre Hospitalier Pierre le Gardeur; (450)657-1313

BRABANT, Gordon V; Clinique Villa Marie, 1000-1538 rue Sherbrooke O, Montreal QC H3G 1L5; McG'81; FRCSC; GenSurg. (514)933-2778

BRABANT, Jean; Ctr Hosp Affilie-St-Sacrement, 1050 ch Sainte-Foy, Quebec QC G1S 4L8; Laval'73; FRCPC; DiagRad. Staff, Centre Hospitalier Affilié Universitaire de Québec - Hôpital du St-Sacrement; Staff, Centre Hospitalier Universitaire De Québec - Pavillon De St-françois-d'assise; assoc Staff, CSSS de Quebec-Sud; (418)682-7700

BRABANT, Michel; 520 rue Notre-Dame, Repentigny QC J6A 2T8; Mon'67; (450)585-1620

BRABANT, Michel R; CHUM-Hop St-Luc, 1058 rue Saint-Denis, Montreal QC H2X 3J4; Mon'73; Staff, Centre Hospitalier l'Université De Montréal (CHUM) - Hôpital Saint-luc; (514)890-8316; Fax. (514)412-7295; michel.brabant.chum@ssss.gouv.qc.ca.

BRACALENTI, Ivan A; 206-325 Winterberry Dr, Stoney Creek ON L8J 0B6; Wes'61; DOHS(McM); CCFP; Court Staff, Hamilton Health Sciences Centre - McMaster Children's Hospital; Med Adjuster, FBA Ministry of Community & Social Services; Langs: Italian; (905)575-9004

BRACCO, David; MUHC-Montreal Gen Hosp, D10 145.3-1650 av Cedar, Montreal QC H3G 1A4; Lausanne (Switzerland)'90; Critical Care Medicine (P.Q.); Anes. Staff, McGill University Health Centre - Montreal General Campus; Assoc Prof Anes, Universite de Montreal; Assoc Prof Anes, McGill University; Langs: German; Italian; Bilingual(French/English); (514)934-1934 x43030; Fax. (514)934-8249; david.bracco@McGill.ca.

BRACE, Alec W; Memorial U-Counselling Center, PO Box 4200 Stn C, St. John's NL A1C 5S7; Mem'75; FRCPC; Psy (Forensic Psychiatry).

BRACHE, M Lou-Jacques; Lion's Gate Hosp, 231 15th St E, North Vancouver BC V7L 2L7; Cal'90; CCFP; Staff, Lions Gate Hospital; (604)988-3131 x4404; 73751.733@compuserve.com.

BRACHEMI, Soumeya; CHUM-Hop St-Luc, 1058 rue Saint-Denis, Montreal QC H2X 3J4; Laval'99; FRCPC; IntMed; Nephrol. Staff, Centre Hospitalier l'Université De Montréal (CHUM) - Hôpital Saint-luc; (514)890-8000 x32588

BRACKA, Michel C; CLSC Mercier-Est/Anjou, 9503 rue Sherbrooke E, Montreal QC H1L 6P2; Mon'86; NBME; CCFP; FCFP; Staff, Hopital Maisonneuve-Rosemont; (514)356-2572; Fax. (514)356-1839.

BRACKEN, John H; St Boniface Gen Hosp, 409 Tache Ave, Winnipeg MB R2H 2A6; Man'90; BSc; FRCSC; GenSurg. Staff GenSurg, St Boniface General Hospital; Asst Prof Surg, University of Manitoba; (204)237-2329; Fax. (204)237-3429; drbracken@hotmail.com.

BRACKEN, John; Medical Arts Bldg, 1518-233 Kennedy St, Winnipeg MB R3C 3J5; Man'66; FRCSC; Ophth. (204)943-2136

BRACKEN, Keyna J; Stonechurch Family Hlth Ctre, 1475 Upper Ottawa St, Hamilton ON L8W 3J6; McM'89; BSc; CCFP; Board Member Discipline Committee & Fitness to Pract Committee, College of Physicians & Surgeons of Ontario; Dir, Maternity Centre of Hamilton; (905)575-1300; brackenk@mcmaster.ca.

BRACKENREED, Nolan L E; Deloraine Clinic, PO Box 429, Deloraine MB R0M 0M0; Man'10; CCFP.

BRACKSTONE, Muriel; London Reg Cancer Program, A3 931-790 Commissioners Rd E, London ON N6A 4L6; Wes'99; MSc; PhD; FRCSC; GenSurg (Surgical Oncology). Asst Prof Surg & Oncol, University of Western Ontario; (519)685-8712; Fax. (519)685-8744.

BRADBURY, Bernadette; 2-4665 Central Blvd, Burnaby BC V5H 4J5; McG'96; CCFP; Langs: Bilingual(English/French); (604)558-1175

BRADBURY, Catherine M; Eleven Elizabeth Family Practi, 201-11 Elizabeth Ave, St. John's NL A1A 1W6; Mem'82; Staff, St Clare's Mercy Hospital; Staff, Health Sciences Centre.

BRADBURY, Penelope A; Cancer Research Institute, 10 Stuart St, Kingston ON K7L 3N6; (Wales)'94; (613)533-6430

BRADE, Anthony M; Univ Hlth Network-Princess M, 5 912-610 University Ave, Toronto ON M5G 2M9; McG'96; PhD; FRCPC; RadOncol. Staff, Princess Margaret Hospital - University Health Network; (416)946-6513

BRADEL, Theresa M; Allan Blair Cancer Centre, 300-4101 Dewdney Ave, Regina SK S4T 7T1; Sask'83; CCFP; FCFP; Clin Associate, Allan Blair Cancer Centre; (306)766-2032; Fax. (306)766-2688.

BRADEN, Harold P; St Joseph's Health Centre, 30 The Queensway, Toronto ON M6R 1B5; Qns'85; CCFP; FCFP; Anes. Staff, St Joseph's Health Centre; (416)530-6000

BRADETTE, Isabelle; CSSS de la Haute-Yamaska, 205 boul Leclerc O, Granby QC J2G 1T7; McG'07; MDCM; CCFP; CCFP(E.M.); Staff, Centre Hospitalier de Granby; (450)375-8000

BRADETTE, Marc; CHUQ-Hotel-Dieu de Quebec, 11 Cote Du Palais, Quebec QC G1R 2J6; Laval'85; FRCPC; IntMed (Clinical Research); Gastroent. Staff Clin Research, Centre Hospitalier Universitaire de Québec (CHUQ) - Siege Social; Prof, Université Laval; (418)691-5252; Fax. (418)691-5348.

BRADFIELD, Jane G; McMaster Campus Health Centre, MUSC B101-1280 Main St W, Hamilton ON L8S 4K1; Dal'83; Teach Staff, McMaster University; (905)525-9140 x27700

BRADFORD, John M W; Brockville Mental Health Ctre, PO Box 1050 Stn Main 1804 Highway 2 E, Brockville ON K6V 5W7; Cape Town (South Africa)'71; MB ChB; DPM; DABPN; FACPsy; FFPsy; FRCPsy; FRCPC; Psy (Forensic Psychiatry). Staff, Brockville Mental Health Centre - Royal Ottawa Health Care Group; Prof Psy, Queen's University; Prof & Head Div of Forensic Psy/Prof Dept of Criminology, University of Ottawa; Langs: Afrikaans; (613)345-1461; Fax. (613)345-4318; john.bradford@rohcg.on.ca.

BRADFORD, John P; LL104-720 Guelph Line, Burlington ON L7R 4E2; McM'80; Ac Staff, Joseph Brant Memorial Hospital; (905)632-9771; Fax. (905)632-4656.

BRADFORD, Marc S; Family Health Clinic, PO Box 1450 527 Causley St, Blind River ON P0R 1B0; McG'90; Ac Staff, Blind River District Health Centre; (705)356-1666; Fax. (705)356-2403; mbradford@brdhc.on.ca.

BRADFORD, Moira; 4349 Hastings St, Burnaby BC V5C 2J8; UBC'84; (604)299-4388; Fax. (604)299-1405.

BRADFORD, Paul; Hotel-Dieu Grace Hosp, 1030 Ouellette Ave, Windsor ON N9A 1E1; Qns'93; CCFP; CCFP(E.M.); FCFP; Staff, Hôtel-Dieu Grace Hospital; (519)973-4401

BRADFORD, Steven R; William Osler HC-Brampton, 2100 Bovaird Dr E, Brampton ON L6R 3J7; Qns'83; BSc; Staff, William Osler Health System - Brampton Civic Hospital; (905)494-2120; brast@pmh.on.ca.

BRADLEY, Barry D; Physician Anes Services, 303-400 Tache Ave, Winnipeg MB R2H 3C3; Man'86; FRCPC; Anes. (204)233-3413; Fax. (204)233-9763.

BRADLEY, Carl A; The Oakville Corporate Center, 6F-700 Dorval Dr, Oakville ON L6K 3V3; Mem'81; FRCPC; Psy (Forensic Psychiatry). Ac Staff, Halton Healthcare Services Corporation - Oakville Site; (905)815-5140; Fax. (905)815-5076.

BRADLEY, Christine A; Victoria Med Centre, 208-304 Victoria Ave N, Hamilton ON L8L 5G4; Man'83; FRCPC; IntMed; Respir. Assoc Prof, McMaster University; (905)546-9993; Fax. (905)546-1466.

BRADLEY, Douglas L; Caledonian Med Clinic, 340 Campbell St, Nanaimo BC V9R 3G7; Wes'69; (250)753-3202; Fax. (250)753-1039.

BRADLEY, Elspeth A; Surrey Place Centre, 2 Surrey Pl, Toronto ON M5S 2C2; London (England)'79; MB BS; BSc(Hons); PhD; FRCPsy(UK); FRCPC; Psy (Intellectual Disability Psy). Consultant Psy, Centre for Addiction & Mental Health (CAMH) - College Street Site; Psychiatrist-in-Chief/Chief Medical Staff/VP Medical Affairs, Surrey Place Centre; Assoc Prof Psy, University of Toronto; (416)925-5141 x261; Fax. (416)923-8476; e.bradley@utoronto.ca.

BRADLEY, Jeffrey A; Foothils Med Centre, 1403 29 St NW, Calgary AB T2N 2T9; Alb'07; FRCPC; EmergMed. Staff, Foothills Medical Centre; (403)944-1110

BRADLEY, Jeffrey; Northwest Walk-In-Clinic, 300A-595 Arthur St W, Thunder Bay ON P7E 5R5; Qns'83; ATLS; ACLS; (807)623-7101; Fax. (807)623-1625.

BRADLEY, Joelle M; 104-1015 Columbia St, New Westminster BC V3M 6V3; Cal'02; BSc; CCFP; (604)764-1029; joellebradleymd@yahoo.ca.

BRADLEY, John; 205-9148 23 Ave NW, Edmonton AB T6N 1H9; Qns'99; FRCPC; IntMed; Nephrol. Clin Prof Med, University of Alberta; (780)468-3377; Fax. (780)468-9353.

BRADLEY, John S; Carewest Glenmore Park, 2-6909 14 St SW, Calgary AB T2V 1P8; Qns'69; CCFP; FCFP; Staff, Carewest Glenmore Park; Ac Staff, Carewest Long Term Care; Clinical Asst Prof, University of Calgary; (403)258-7672; Fax. (403)252-7616; jsbsr.md2009@yahoo.ca.

BRADLEY, Krista A; North Shore Treatment Centre, 20A-700 Tranquille Rd, Kamloops BC V2B 3H9; McM'96; MSc; CCFP; FCFP; (250)554-4265

BRADLEY, Lindsay A; 3844 Albion Rd, Ottawa ON K1T 1B1; Ott'10; CCFP; (613)737-0340

BRADLEY, Shannon; Queen Elizabeth II HSC, WV10-1276 South Park St, Halifax NS B3H 2Y9; Dal'07; Anes. Staff, Queen Elizabeth II Health Sciences Centre - Victoria General Site; (902)473-7736; Fax. (902)423-9454.

BRADLEY, T Douglas; Univ Hlth Network-Toronto Gen, 9N 943-200 Elizabeth St, Toronto ON M5G 2C4; Alb'78; MD; FRCPC; IntMed (Sleep Apnea); Respir. Dir Respiratory Sleep Lab, Toronto General Hospital - UHN; Staff, Mount Sinai Hospital; Prof Med, University of Toronto; (416)340-4719; Fax. (416)340-4197; douglas.bradley@utoronto.ca.

BRADLEY, Timothy J; The Hosp For Sick Children, 555 University Ave, Toronto ON M5G 1X8; Otago (New Zealand)'90; Staff, The Hospital For Sick Children; Assoc Staff, Toronto General Hospital - UHN; (416)813-7610; timothy.bradley@sickkids.ca.

BRADLEY, William R; Cole Harbour Commun Mental Hlt, 4-51 Forest Hills Pky, Dartmouth NS B2W 6C6; McM'89; BSc; MA; CCFP; Lecturer Med & Family Med, Dalhousie University; Langs: English; French; (902)434-3263; Fax. (902)434-0181.

BRADSHAW, Candace D; Tuxedo Fam Med Centre, 981 Corydon Ave, Winnipeg MB R3M 0X1; Man'99; BSc; CCFP; FCFP; (204)988-6040

BRADSTOCK, Robert W; Bradstock Med Clinic, 101-11020 53 Ave NW, Edmonton AB T6H 0S4; Alb'74; BMedSci; CCFP; FCFP; Chief Medical Staff, Covenant Health - St. Joseph's Auxilliary Hospital; Ac Staff, Covenant Health - Grey Nuns Community Hospital; Chief of Staff, Millwoods Shephard Care Centre & Kensington Shephard's Care(Edmonton); Hon. Clin. Instr., University of Alberta; Langs: English; French; (780)434-0939; Fax. (780)434-0939.

BRADWEJN, Jacques; Royal Ottawa Hlth Care Group, 1145 Carling Ave, Ottawa ON K1Z 7K4; Sher'78; DABPN(Psy); FRCPC; Psy (Research). Staff Psy, Royal Ottawa Mental Health Centre - Royal Ottawa Health Care Group; Vice Dean Research, University of Ottawa; Langs: English; French; (613)722-6521 x6546; jbradwej@rohcg.on.ca.

BRADWELL, Peter J; 585 University Ave, Toronto ON M5G 2N2; Birmingham (England)'67; FFARCS; FRCPC; Anes. Staff, Toronto General Hospital - UHN; University of Toronto; (416)340-3242

BRADY, Annick M; Ctr Hosp du Centre la Mauricie, 50 119e rue, Shawinigan-Sud QC G9P 5K1; Sher'91; FRCPC; Psy. Staff, Centre Hospitalier du Centre la Mauricie; (819)536-7629; Fax. (819)536-7685.

BRADY, Jolene N; Cumberland Reg Hlth Care Ctre, RR 6 19428 Hwy 2, Amherst NS B4H 1N6; Tor'02; CCFP; DiagRad. (902)667-3361

BRADY, Stephen C; Richmond Health Science Ctre, 770-6091 Gilbert Rd, Richmond BC V7C 5L9; Wes'74; DAB; FRCSC; PlasSurg. Consultant, Richmond Hospital; Consultant, Delta Hospital; Consultant, Cambie Surgery Centre; (604)270-3313; Fax. (604)270-8298.

BRAGA, Luis H P; Hamilton HS-McMaster Site, PO Box 2000 Stn Lcd 1 4E19-1200 Main St W, Hamilton ON L8N 3Z5; Minas Gerais (Brazil)'94; Staff/Asst Prof Surg, Hamilton Health Sciences Centre - McMaster Children's Hospital; Langs: Portuguese; French; (905)521-2100; Fax. (905)521-9992.

BRAGA, Manoela F B; St Joseph's Healthcare, 5F-50 Charlton Ave E, Hamilton ON L8N 4A6; Federal Univ of Minas Gerais (Brazil)'99; Staff/Asst Prof, St Joseph's Healthcare - Charlton Campus; (905)522-1155

BRAGA-MELE, Rosa M; 200-245 Danforth Ave, Toronto ON M4K 1N2; Ott'93; FRCSC; Ophth. Assoc Staff, Mount Sinai Hospital; Assoc Prof, University of Toronto; Langs: Italian; Portuguese; (416)462-0393; Fax. (416)462-3612; rbragamele@rogers.com.

BRAGAGLIA, Pauline J; The Group Health Centre, 240 Mcnabb St, Sault Ste. Marie ON P6B 1Y5; Alb'78; (705)759-1234; Fax. (705)541-2302.

BRAGANZA, John A C; PO Box 20083 Mountview Postal, Red Deer AB T4N 6X5; (India)'86; MSc(Psy); MRCPsy(UK); CCST(Child&AdolescentPsy; MB BS; Consulting Staff Privil, Red Deer Regional Hospital Centre; (403)314-3387; Fax. (403)314-9307.

BRAGANZA, Joseph S R; 111-21 Queensway W, Mississauga ON L5B 1B6; National (Ireland)'60; MB ChB; BAO; FRCS(Eng); FRCSC; GenSurg (Urology). Fax. (905)897-9229; jrsbraganza@yahoo.ca.

BRAGER, Nancy P D; Foothills Med Centre, 1403 29 St NW, Calgary AB T2N 2T9; Cal'81; FRCPC; Psy (Consultation-Liaison). Staff, Foothills Medical Centre; University of Calgary; (403)270-8737; Fax. (403)270-3451.

BRAGG, Paul R G; The Ottawa Hosp-Civic Campus B308-1053 Carling Ave, Ottawa ON K1Y 4E9; Mem'81; FRCPC; Anes. Staff Anes, The Ottawa Hospital - Civic Campus; Vice Dean Postgraduate Med Education(interim), University of Ottawa; (613)761-4169; Fax. (613)761-5209.

BRAHA-WYSZOGRODSKI, Linda; 202-3400 rue Du Marche, Dollard-D-Ormeaux QC H9B 2Y1; McG'79; (514)683-1262; Fax. (514)683-5528.

BRAHIM, Asad; 16515 88 Ave NW, Edmonton AB T5R 0A4; (Jamaica)'68; MB BS; Physician Geriatric Psy/Med Dir Mental Health Clinic, Alberta Hospital Edmonton; Consultant, Royal Alexandra Hospital; Staff, Edmonton Mental Health Clinic; (782)342-6551; Fax. (780)342-6579; asad.brahim@capitalhealth.ca.

BRAHM, Evan J; Inst of Commun & Family Psy, 4333 ch Cote-Sainte-Catherine, Montreal QC H3T 1E4; McG'69; DPsy; Psy (Adolescent & Family Psychiatry). Dir Youth Services & Sr Psychiatry/Coord Psychoanalytic & Psychotherapy Service, Sir Mortimer B Davis Jewish General; Physician, Canadian Institute of Psychoanalysis; adj Prof, McGill University; Langs: French; (514)340-8210 x1219; evan.brahm@mcgill.ca.

BRAHMBHATT, Rajmayur; James Paton Mem Hosp, 125 Trans Canada Hwy, Gander NL A1V 1P7; Kasturba Medical College (India)'98; MB BS; Staff, James Paton Memorial Hospital; (709)256-5467

BRAIDA, Raymond L; 3 Paisley St, Guelph ON N1H 2N5; Tor'64; DPsy; FRCPC; Psy (Affective & Anxiety Disorders). (519)836-1622; Fax. (519)836-0065.

BRAIDEK, Catherine M; Royal Ottawa Hlth Care Group, 1145 Carling Ave, Ottawa ON K1Z 7K4; Sask'86; FRCPC; Psy (Geriatric Psychiatry). Staff, Royal Ottawa Mental Health Centre - Royal Ottawa Health Care Group; (613)722-6521 x6905; Fax. (613)798-2999.

BRAIDWOOD, Danielle; Bruyere Family Med Clinic, 75 Bruyere St, Ottawa ON K1N 5C7; McG'08; CCFP; (613)241-3344

BRAIDY, Joseph F; Clinique Pheumologie, 240-2944 boul Tashereau, Longueuil QC J4V 2G8; Beirut (Lebanon)'72; FACP; FRCPC; IntMed (Sleep Medicine); Critical Care Medicine (P.Q.); Respir. Asst Staff, Centre Hospitalier l'Université De Montréal (CHUM) - Hôpital Saint-luc; Asst Staff, Hopital Charles LeMoyne; assoc Prof, Universite de Montreal; Langs: Arabic; French; (450)465-4606

BRAIG, Florian G A; 470 Dundas St E, Belleville ON K8N 1G1; Munich (Germany)'76; FRCSC; Otol (Facial Plastic Surgery). Staff, QHC Belleville General; Langs: German; (613)966-4045

BRAIL, Jerrald N; Walk In Medical Centre, 901 Eglinton Ave W, Toronto ON M6C 2C1; UBC'64; Staff, William Osler Health System - Etobicoke General Hospital; (416)781-8100

BRAILEY, David A; Sea Cove Med Clinic, 201-1757 Beaufort Ave, Comox BC V9M 1R8; UBC'87; BSc; Assoc Staff, St Joseph's General Hospital; (250)339-5335; Fax. (250)339-1898.

BRAIN, Daryl A; Timmins & District Hosp, 700 Ross Ave E, Timmins ON P4N 8P2; Tor'95; CCFP; FCFP; Staff, Timmins & District Hospital; Assoc Prof, Northern Ontario School of Medicine-Laurentian University; (705)267-2131

BRAIN, Philippa H; Foothills Med Centre, 1403 29 St NW, Calgary AB T2N 2T9; Qns'88; FRCSC; ObstGyn. Staff, Foothills Medical Centre; Asst Prof, University of Calgary; Langs: Bilingual(English/French); (403)944-2017; Fax. (403)270-4249.

BRAIS, Bernard; MUHC-Montreal Neurology Inst, 658-3801 rue University, Montreal QC H3A 2B4; McG'85; FRCPC; Neur (P.Q.). Staff, McGill University Health Centre - Montreal Neurological Hospital; (514)398-1507

BRAIS, Marie-France; Centre Med Fusion, 200-2035 av Sainte-Anne, Saint-Hyacinthe QC J2S 5H3; Mon'91; (450)773-6023; Fax. (450)773-5915.

BRAIS, Nathalie; Clinique Med Grn St-Jean, CP 100, St-Jean-Sur-Richel QC J0J 1R0; Sher'92; (450)358-7099 x7680; Fax. (450)358-7947.

BRAIS, Pierre M; Clin Ophtalmologique de l'Oues, 1503-625 av Du President-Kenne, Montreal QC H3A 1K2; Mon'65; Ophth (Glaucoma). assoc Staff, Centre Hospitalier l'Université de Montréal (CHUM) - Hôpital Notre-Dame; adj Prof, Universite de Montreal; (514)849-9215; Fax. (514)849-5115.

BRAITHWAITE, Debra; Royal Jubilee Hosp, 1952 Bay St, Victoria BC V8R 1J8; Cal'81; CCFP; FCFP; Staff, Royal Jubilee Hospital; Staff, Victoria Hospice Society; (250)370-8715; Fax. (250)370-8843; deb.braithwaite@viha.ca.

BRAITHWAITE, Desmond L; Trinity Common Mall Optical, 150 Great Lakes Dr, Brampton ON L6R 2K7; McG'62; Ophth. (905)458-5120

BRAITHWAITE, Nicholas D J; William Osler HC-Brampton, S3. 056-2100 Bovaird Dr E, Brampton ON L6R 3J7; Tor'80; FRCSC; ObstGyn. Staff, William Osler Health System - Brampton Civic Hospital; (905)494-2120 x57985; Fax. (905)494-6508.

BRAITHWAITE, Philip; Chinook Reg Hosp, 960 19 St S, Lethbridge AB T1J 1W5; (Scotland)'80; Staff, Chinook Regional Hospital; Staff, Lethbridge Cancer Centre; (403)388-6191

BRAITHWAITE-WALTON, Heather J; Niagara HS-Welland Site, 65 Third St, Welland ON L3B 4W6; McM'05; CCFP; Staff, Niagara Health System - Welland Hospital Site; (905)378-4647 x33250

BRAKE, David J; Cape Breton Hlthcare Complex, 1482 George St, Sydney NS B1P 1P3; Mem'91; FRCPC; IntMed (Respirology); Critical Care Medicine. Staff, Cape Breton Healthcare Complex; Lecturer, Dalhousie University; (902)567-8020; Fax. (902)567-8086.

BRAKE, Heather L; PO Box 87034 Rpo Douglas Sq, Calgary AB T2Z 3V7; Mem'97; CCFP; CCFP(E.M.).

BRAKE, Heidi D; Dr Charles L Legrow Hlth Ctr, PO Box 250 1 Grand Bay Rd, Port-aux-Basques NL A0M 1C0; Mem'10; CCFP; Locum Tenens, Dr Charles L Legrow Health Centre; (709)695-2175

BRAKE, Jonathan A; IWK Health Centre, PO Box 9700 Rpo CSC 5980 University Ave, Halifax NS B3K 6R8; Dal'07; Psy. Staff, IWK Health Centre.

BRAKE, Robert J; Cox's Cove Medical Clinic, General Delivery, Coxs Cove NL A0L 1C0; Dal'66; Ac Staff, Western Memorial Regional Hospital; (709)688-2801

BRAKEL, Gillian; Ramblewood Medical Clinic, 101-14 Ramblewood Dr, Wasaga Beach ON L9Z 0C4; McM'01; MSc; BA; CCFP; (705)429-2101; Fax. (705)429-7611.

BRAMBILLA, Christa C; Cornerstone Family Med Centre, 106-100 Strowger Blvd, Brockville ON K6V 5J9; Cal'02; CCFP; Staff, Brockville General Hospital - Charles Street; (613)498-0444

BRAMSTRUP, Mary Ann; PO Box 1010, Nackawic NB E6G 2N1; Dal'81; BSc; Langs: Danish; (506)575-2460; Fax. (506)575-8687.

BRAMWELL, Lori A; Dr Charles A Janeway Child HC, 300 Prince Philip Dr, St. John's NL A1B 3V6; Mem'05; FRCSC; Ophth. Staff, Janeway Children's Health & Rehabilitation Centre; (709)777-6300

BRAMWELL-WESLEY, Vivien H C; Tom Baker Cancer Centre, 1331 29 St NW, Calgary AB T2N 4N2; London (England)'72; MB BS; PhD; MRC(UK); FRCP; FRCPC; IntMed (Breast Cancer). Dir Dept of Med/Head MedOncol, Tom Baker Cancer Centre; Ac Staff, Foothills Medical Centre; Prof Med & Oncol, University of Calgary; (403)521-3707; Fax. (403)283-1651.

BRANCH, Frederic; CHUS-Hop Fleurimont, 3001 12e av N, Sherbrooke QC J1H 5N4; Mon'07; CCFP; CCFP(E.M.); Staff, Centre Hospitalier Universitaire de Sherbrooke-Hopital Fleurimont; (819)346-1110

BRANCH, Jacques V M; Foothills Family Med Centre, PO Bag 460 114 1 St SW, Black Diamond AB T0L 0H0; Wes'00; BSc(Hon); CCFP; (403)933-4368

BRANCH, Neil; Keystone Place, 405-270 Douglas Ave, Bathurst NB E2A 1M9; Laval'91; ABIME; FRCSC; OrthSurg (Independent Medical Evaluations). VP Medical Affairs, Vitalite Health Network; Langs: Bilingual(French/English); (506)546-3325; Fax. (506)546-3996; nbranch@nbnet.nb.ca.

BRANCH, Robert G; Clinique Med East Angus, 1A-150 rue Angus S GD, East Angus QC J0B 1R0; Sher'76; Ac Staff, Centre Hospitalier Universitaire de Sherbrooke-Hôpital Hôtel-Dieu; (819)832-2438; Fax. (819)832-2104.

BRANCO, Joao; 219 Main St E, Hawkesbury ON K6A 1A1; McG'01; CCFP; (613)632-4185; Fax. (613)632-5469.

BRAND, Christopher P; 2263 Hwy 12 PO Box 184, Brechin ON L0K 1B0; Tor'78; BSc; CCFP; Ac Staff, Orillia Soldiers' Memorial Hospital; Med Dir, Leacock Care Centre; (705)484-5352; Fax. (705)484-5400.

BRAND, Engela; Fort St John Med Clinic, 10011 96 St, Fort St John BC V1J 2B2; Stellenbosch (South Africa)'05; MB ChB; (250)793-8741

BRAND, Johannes E; Associate Clinic, 5215 49 Ave, Wetaskiwin AB T9A 0R1; Pretoria (South Africa)'84; MB ChB; CCFP; (780)352-7157; Fax. (780)352-2273.

BRAND, Lukas J; ABC Med Clinic, 9842 101 Ave, Fort St. John BC V1J 2B2; Orange Free State (South Africa)'04; MB ChB; (250)785-1220

BRANDAO, Leonardo R; The Hosp For Sick Children, 555 University Ave, Toronto ON M5G 1X8; Sao Paulo (Brazil)'90; Staff, The Hospital For Sick Children; (416)813-7758

BRANDES, Jack S; 423 Spadina Rd, Toronto ON M5P 2W3; Johns Hopkins (USA)'67; PhD; FAPA; AB; FRCPC; Psy (Intensive Psychotherapy). Staff Psy, Toronto Western Hospital - University Health Network; Asst Prof Psy, University of Toronto; Langs: Hebrew; French; (416)489-6315; Fax. (416)489-6049; jack.brandes@utoronto.ca.

BRANDES, Lorne J; Cancercare Manitoba, 2086-675 McDermot Ave, Winnipeg MB R3E 0V9; Wes'68; FRCPC; IntMed (Medical Oncology). Att Staff, Health Sciences Centre; Att Staff/Researcher Manitoba Inst of Cell Biology, CancerCare Manitoba; Researcher, Manitoba Institute of Cell; Prof Med Pharmacology & Therapeutics, University of Manitoba; (204)787-2139; Fax. (204)787-1345.

BRANDON, J Bradley; Queen Elizabeth Hosp, PO Box 6600 Stn Central, Charlottetown PE C1A 8T5; UBC'83; BSc; CCFP; FCFP; Ac Staff EmergMed, Queen Elizabeth Hospital; (902)894-2200; Fax. (902)628-6470.

BRANDON, Jennifer E; Glenmore Landing, A301-1600 90 Ave SW, Calgary AB T2V 5A8; Cal'06; CCFP; Staff, Rockyview General Hospital; (403)246-0200; Fax. (403)301-0046.

BRANDON, Nicholas C; Southlake Family Health Team, 201-581 Davis Dr, Newmarket ON L3Y 2P6; Ott'10; CCFP; (905)853-3103

BRANDON, Teresa E; Alberta Prof Bldg, 303-320 23 Ave SW, Calgary AB T2S 0J2; Cal'91; CCFP; FCFP; (403)686-2150; Fax. (403)209-1299.

BRANDS, Ralph H; Dept Of Health Care & Epidem, 2206 East Mall, Vancouver BC V6T 1Z3; Wes'81; MHSc; Clin Assoc Prof Health Care & Epidemiol, University of British Columbia; (604)822-2772; rbrands@mail.ubc.ca.

BRANDSCHWEI, Frank H; Radiology Consultants Assoc, 120-6707 Elbow Dr SW, Calgary AB T2V 0E3; Alb'77; FRCPC; DiagRad. (403)777-3001; Fax. (403)777-3008.

BRANDT, E Lorne; Child & Adolescent Program, 200-6100 Bowling Green Rd, Richmond BC V6Y 4G2; Man'76; BSc; BCh(Ed.); FRCPC; CCFP; Psy (Child & Adolescent Psychiatry). Med Leader Child & Youth Team, Richmond Mental Health Centre; Lecturer Psy/Child's Adolescent Div, University of British Columbia; Langs: German; (604)207-2511 x230

BRANDT, Michael G; 412-2300 Eglinton Ave W, Mississauga ON L5M 2V8; Wes'05; FRCSC; Otol. (905)820-8484

BRANDT VEGAS, Daniel; St Joseph's Healthcare, F533-50 Charlton Ave E, Hamilton ON L8N 4A6; (Venezuela)'04; IntMed. Staff, St Joseph's Healthcare - Charlton Campus; (905)521-6068; Fax. (905)521-6146.

BRANDWEIN, Joseph; 5 109-610 University Ave, Toronto ON M5G 2M9; McG'83; BSc; FRCPC; IntMed (Leukemia); Hem. Staff, Princess Margaret Hospital - University Health Network; Assoc Prof Med, University of Toronto; (416)946-2824; Fax. (416)946-6546; joseph.brandwein@uhn.ca.

BRANDYS, Timothy M; The Ottawa Hosp-Civic Campus A2 80-1053 Carling Ave, Ottawa ON K1Y 4E9; Dal'89; MEd; FRCSC; GenSurg; VascSurg. Staff, The Ottawa Hospital - Civic Campus; (613)761-4766; Fax. (613)761-5362; tbrandys@ottawahospital.on.ca.

BRANIGAN, Monica A; Temmy Latner Ctre for Palliati, 60 Murray St, Toronto ON M5T 3L9; Ott'82; Staff, St Joseph's Health Centre.

BRANIGAN, Sheena M; Huntsville Prof Bldg, 104-348 Muskoka Rd 3 N, Huntsville ON P1H 1H8; Wes'88; CCFP; Ac Staff, Huntsville District Memorial Hospital - Muskoka Algonquin Healthcare; (705)789-2355; Fax. (705)789-1051.

BRANKOVIC, Aleksandra; 400 The East Mall, Etobicoke ON M9B 3Z9; Wes'09; CCFP; (416)621-2220

BRANKSTON, Edwin R; Courtice Health Centre, 1450 Highway 2, Courtice ON L1E 3C3; Qns'76; BSc; CCFP; CCFP(E.M.); Staff, Haliburton Highlands Health Services - Haliburton Site; Staff, Lakeridge Health - Oshawa Site; (905)721-4999

BRANNAN, Mark A; Dr G B Cross Mem Hosp, 67 Manitoba Dr, Clarenville NL A5A 1K3; Glasgow (Scotland)'78; MB ChB; FFARCSI; FFARCS; Staff Anes, The Dr G B Cross Memorial Hospital; (709)466-3411; Fax. (709)466-5553.

BRANSON, Helen M; 555 University Ave, Toronto ON M5G 1X8; Sydney (Australia)'97; Staff, The Hospital For Sick Children; (416)813-7654 x2956; Fax. (416)813-7591.

BRANSON, Richard L; Stratford Gen Hosp, 46 General Hospital Dr, Stratford ON N5A 2Y6; UBC'80; FRCPC; Anes. Chief Anes, Stratford General Hospital - Huron Perth Healthcare Alliance; (519)271-2120

BRAR, Adarshdip; Legacy Sport Medicine, 14-160 Meadowood Dr, Winnipeg MB R2M 5L6; Punjab (Pakistan)'93; FRCPC; IntMed; Rheum.

BRAR, Amandeep S; 3905 34 St NW, Edmonton AB T6T 1L5; (Other Foreign)'10; CCFP; (780)448-1166

BRAR, Anmol; Coral Spring Medical, 5070 68 St NE, Calgary AB T3J 4J1; (Other Foreign)'99; (403)397-1725

BRAR, Avneet S; Crowfoot Village Fam Practice, 210-600 Crowfoot Cres NW, Calgary AB T3G 0B4; Alb'08; CCFP.

BRAR, Balpreet S; 302-3029 Carling Ave, Ottawa ON K2B 8E8; Qns'06; FRCSC; GenSurg. (613)820-9403; Fax. (613)820-3738.

BRAR, Darshan S; 407 Marlborough Way NE, Calgary AB T2A 7E7; Santo Tomas (Philippines)'75; Langs: Tagalog; Punjabi; (403)272-2211; Fax. (403)248-4906.

BRAR, Deepinderjit S; Peterborough Reg HC-Hospital, 1 Hospital Dr, Peterborough ON K9J 7C6; Qns'87; Staff, Peterborough Regional Health Centre - Hospital Drive; (705)876-5022

BRAR, Harinderpal S; Vancouver Gen Hosp, 2447-855 12 Ave W, Vancouver BC V5Z 1M9; UBC'08; Staff, Vancouver General Hospital - Centennial Pavillion; (604)825-0970

BRAR, Harpreet S; Brar Med Clinic, 102-1090 Peter Robertson Blvd, Brampton ON L6R 3B3; Guru Nanak Dev (India)'85; CCFP; (905)790-8400; Fax. (905)799-3700.

BRAR, Jagdeep; 2704 48 St NW, Edmonton AB T6L 6B8; FRCPC; Peds. Staff, University of Alberta Hospital; (780)756-9677; Fax. (780)756-9676.

BRAR, Kanwaljit S; Pritchard Farm Health Centre, 5-3014 Henderson Hwy, East St Paul MB R2E 0H9; Man'10; CCFP.

BRAR, Mantaj S; Foothills Med Centre, 1403 29 St NW, Calgary AB T2N 2T9; Tor'06; FRCSC; GenSurg. Staff, Foothills Medical Centre; (403)670-1110

BRAR, Nirmala K; 6-1109 Summerside Dr SW, Edmonton AB T6X 0H5; (India)'85; (780)249-2727; Fax. (780)466-2726.

BRAR, Parminder S; 103-140 Niagara St, St Catharines ON L2R 4L4; Poona (India)'82; MB BS; FAAP; FRCPC; Peds. Chief Dept of Peds & Active Staff, Niagara Health System - St Catharines General Site; Langs: Hindi; Punjabi; (905)684-7787

BRAR, Pawandeep K; Temmy Latner Ctr for Palliativ, 4F-60 Murray St, Toronto ON M5T 3L9; Man'06; CCFP; (416)586-4800; Fax. (416)586-4804.

BRAR, Savtaj S; Univ Hlth Network-Princess M, 3 130-610 University Ave, Toronto ON M5G 2M9; Wes'04; GenSurg. Staff, Princess Margaret Hospital - University Health Network; (416)946-2000

BRAR, Simrit K; Foothills Med Centre, 1403 29 St NW, Calgary AB T2N 2T9; Man'04; FRCSC; ObstGyn. Staff, Foothills Medical Centre; (403)944-2645

BRAR, Simuran K; Univ Hlth Network-Toronto Western Hosp, 399 Bathurst St, Toronto ON M5T 2S8; Tor'99; FRCPC; Psy. Staff, Toronto Western Hospital - University Health Network; (416)603-5809; simuran.brar@uhn.ca.

BRAR, Sukhpal S; Clinical Sciences Bldg, 8 120-152 University Campus NW, Edmonton AB T6G 2G3; Wes'05; FRCPC; Anes. (780)407-8861; Fax. (780)407-3200.

BRASCH, Jennifer S; St Joseph's Healthcare, 50 Charlton Ave E, Hamilton ON L8N 4A6; Qns'91; BSc; FRCPC; Psy (Emergency Psychiatry). Dir Emerg Psy, St Joseph's Healthcare - Charlton Campus; Assoc Prof Psy, McMaster University; (905)522-1155 x34358; Fax. (905)521-6059.

BRASHER, Jane E M; Royal Victoria Hosp, 201 Georgian Dr, Barrie ON L4M 6M2; Wes'79; FRCPC; Anes. Staff, Royal Victoria Regional Health Centre; (705)728-9090 x4207

BRASS, Neil S; Hys Med Centre, 350-11010 101 St NW, Edmonton AB T5H 4B9; Tor'87; FRCPC; IntMed; Cardiol. Staff, Royal Alexandra Hospital; Clin Teacher, University of Alberta; (780)428-3246; Fax. (780)425-0487.

BRASSARD, Alain; Glen Sather Sport Med Clinic, 3C 101-11400 University Campus, Edmonton AB T6G 1Z1; McG'89; FRCPC; Derm (Clinical Research). Langs: French; (780)407-1257; Fax. (780)407-3003; alain.brassard@ualberta.ca.

BRASSARD, Anne; CSSS de Chicoutimi, 305 rue Saint-Vallier, Chicoutimi QC G7H 5H6; Sher'84; NuclearMed (P.Q.). Staff, Complexe hospitalier de la Sagamie; (418)541-1034; Fax. (418)541-1101.

BRASSARD, Catherine; Inst U en Sante Mentale de QC, 2601 ch de la Canardiere, Quebec QC G1J 2G3; Laval'94; FRCPC; Psy. Staff, Institut Universitaire Sante; (418)663-5321

BRASSARD, Danielle; Cornwall Health Care Centre, 208-820 McConnell Ave, Cornwall ON K6H 4M4; Laval'07; (613)936-1564

BRASSARD, Graeme M; 192-17010 90 Ave NW, Edmonton AB T5T 1L6; Alb'06; FRCSC; ObstGyn. (780)483-2901; Fax. (780)483-2910.

BRASSARD, Jean; Ctr Hosp Affilie-Enfant-Jesus, 1401 18e rue, Quebec QC G1J 1Z4; Laval'80; CSPQ; Anes. Ac Staff, Centre Hospitalier Universitaire De Québec - Pavillon De St-françois-d'assise; Ac Staff, Centre Hospitalier Affilié Universitaire de Québec - Hôpital De L'Enfant Jésus; (418)649-5807

BRASSARD, Josee; CRSSS Baie-James-Chibougamau, 51 3e rue, Chibougamau QC G8P 1N1; Laval'96; CCFP; Staff, CRSSS de la Baie-James; (418)748-2676; Fax. (418)748-6983.

BRASSARD, Liliane; CSSS Drummond-Hop Sainte-Croix, 570 rue Heriot, Drummondville QC J2B 1C1; Sher'07; ObstGyn. Staff, Hôpital Sainte-croix; (819)478-6464

BRASSARD, Liza; Clin de Med Familiale Saguenay, 220-874 boul de l'Universite E, Chicoutimi QC G7H 6B9; Laval'96; Staff, Complexe hospitalier de la Sagamie; Langs: Bilingual(English/French); (418)545-1217; Fax. (418)545-4782.

BRASSARD, Marc-Andre; CSSS de Chicoutimi, 305 rue Saint-Vallier, Chicoutimi QC G7H 5H6; Mon'95; FRCPC; RadOncol. Staff, Complexe hospitalier de la Sagamie; (418)541-1032; Fax. (418)541-1128; mabrassard@yahoo.com.

BRASSARD, Maryse; CHUQ-Ctr Hosp Univ Laval, 2705 boul Laurier, Quebec QC G1V 4G2; Laval'04; FRCPC; IntMed (Thyroid Cancer); Endocrin&Metab. Staff, Centre Hospitalier Universitaire de Quebec-CHUL; (418)656-4444; marysebrassard@hotmail.com.

BRASSARD, Michel P; Centre Med Racine, 201-900 boul Raymond, Quebec QC G1B 3G3; Laval'74; ac Staff, Centre Hospitalier Universitaire De Québec - Pavillon De St-françois-d'assise; Langs: English; (418)667-8066; Fax. (418)667-8131.

BRASSARD, Myriam; Hôpital Ste-Justine, 6E9-3175 ch Cote-Sainte-Cather, Montreal QC H3T 1C5; McG'92; CSPQ; FRCPC; Peds (Fetal Cardiology); Cardiol. Staff Cardiol, Hôpital Ste-Justine; Prof, Universite de Montreal; Langs: Bilingual(English/French); (514)345-4931 x5401; Fax. (514)345-4896; myriam_brassard@ssss.gouv.qc.ca.

BRASSARD, Nathalie; CSSS de Chicoutimi, CP 264 305 rue St-Vallier, Chicoutimi QC G7H 5H6; Laval'88; Psy (P.Q.). Staff, Complexe hospitalier de la Sagamie; (418)549-5474 x5292; Fax. (418)549-7604.

BRASSARD, Normand; CHUQ-Ctr Hosp Univ Laval, A1385-2705 boul Laurier, Quebec QC G1V 4G2; Laval'72; FRCSC; ObstGyn. Staff, Centre Hospitalier Universitaire de Quebec-CHUL; Prof, Université Laval; (418)525-4456; Fax. (418)577-2024.

BRASSARD, Paul; MUHC-Royal Victoria Hosp, R4 29-687 av des Pins O, Montreal QC H3A 1A1; Mon'87; MSc(Epidemiol); MSc(Parasitol.); FRCPC; CommunMed (Tuberculosis). adj Médecin, McGill University Health Centre - Royal Victoria Hospital; adj Médecin, McGill University Health Centre - Montreal General Campus; Prof Epidemiol & Biostatistics, McGill University; Universite de Montreal; (514)340-8222 x8373; Fax. (514)340-7563.

BRASSARD, Pierre J; 995 rue de Salaberry, Montreal QC H3L 1L2; Laval'84; FRCSC; PlasSurg. Staff PlasSurg, Centre Metropolitan de Chirurgie Plastique; (514)288-2097; Fax. (514)288-3547; info@grsmontreal.com.

BRASSARD, Richard; Clinique Med de l'Anse, 78 rue Lemaire, Sept-Iles QC G4S 1A3; Laval'75; Staff, Centre Hospitalier Regional de Sept-Iles; Langs: English; (418)962-1236; Fax. (418)962-6327.

BRASSARD, Roland; Ctr Hosp Anna-Laberge, 200 boul Brisebois, Chateauguay QC J6K 4W8; Mon'84; DiagRad. Staff, Hôpital Anna-Laberge; (450)699-2425

BRASSEUR, Marie-Helene; CLSC de Therese-de-Blainville, 55 rue Saint-Joseph, Sainte-Therese QC J7E 4Y5; Laval'03; Staff, CLSC Ste-Therese de Blainville; (450)430-4553; Fax. (450)430-0140.

BRASSEUR, Yves; Clinique Med Chemin Chambly, 101-3090 ch Chambly, Longueuil QC J4L 4N5; Mon'77; (450)670-5700; Fax. (450)670-8830.

BRATCH, Anita N; 51 Armadale Ave, Toronto ON M6S 3W9; McM'90; (416)762-2211

BRATHWAITE, Shirley N; Royal Ottawa Hlth Care Group, 1145 Carling Ave, Ottawa ON K1Z 7K4; (Jamaica)'71; FRCPC; Psy (Forensic Psychiatry). Dir Outpatient Unit, Royal Ottawa Mental Health Centre - Royal Ottawa Health Care Group; Asst Prof, University of Ottawa; (613)722-6521 x6365; Fax. (613)722-5048; sbrathwa@rohcg.on.ca.

BRATTMAN, David P; True North Imaging, 120-7330 Yonge St, Thornhill ON L4J 7Y7; Dublin (Ireland)'57; FRCPC; DiagRad. (905)707-1777

BRATTY, Joan E M; Medical Clinic, PO Box 730 Stn Main, Salmon Arm BC V1E 4N8; UBC'93; CCFP; (250)832-2321

BRATU, Ioana; University of Alberta Hosp, 2C3 56WMC-8440 112 St NW, Edmonton AB T6G 2B7; Alb'96; MSc; FACS; FRCSC; GenSurg; PedGenSurg. Staff, University of Alberta Hospital; Langs: French; Romanian; (780)407-1162; Fax. (780)407-2004.

BRATVOLD, Jeffrey S; Carry Drive Branch, 104-116 Carry Dr SE, Medicine Hat AB T1B 3Z8; Sask'94; CCFP; Staff, Medicine Hat Regional Hospital; (403)502-8925; Fax. (403)528-3866.

BRAUDE, Andrew; 204-1110 Sheppard Ave E, North York ON M2K 2W2; Cape Town (South Africa)'76; ABIM; FACCP; MMed; FRCPC; IntMed (Sleep Medicine); Respir. Staff Consultant, Holland Bloorview Kids Rehabilitation Hospital; Staff Consultant, North York General Hospital; (416)229-2315; Fax. (416)223-9828.

BRAUDE, Bernard M; The Hosp For Sick Children, 555 University Ave, Toronto ON M5G 1X8; Witwatersrand (South Africa)'74; FRCPC; Anes. Staff, The Hospital For Sick Children; (416)813-7445; bernard.braude@sickkids.ca.

BRAUDE, Laurence; Univ Hlth Network-Toronto Gen, 200 Elizabeth St, Toronto ON M5G 2C4; Witwatersrand (South Africa)'76; FRCSC; Ophth. Staff, Toronto General Hospital - UHN.

BRAUDE, Paul R; Markham Place Med Centre, 206-2900 Steeles Ave E, Thornhill ON L3T 4X1; Cape Town (South Africa)'74; MB ChB; (905)881-6667; Fax. (905)731-1298.

BRAUER, Barbara J; Mills Mem Hosp, 4720 Haugland Ave, Terrace BC V8G 2W7; Witwatersrand (South Africa)'86; Staff, Mills Memorial Hospital; (250)641-1858

BRAUER, Carmen A; Alberta Children's Hosp, 2888 Shaganappi Trail NW, Calgary AB T3B 6A8; Cal'96; FRCSC; OrthSurg. Staff, Alberta Children's Hospital; (403)955-2850; Fax. (403)955-7634.

BRAULT, David; Elora Med Group, 71 James St, Elora ON N0B 1S0; Ott'09; CCFP; (519)846-5345

BRAULT, Jacques-Christian; CLSC des Frontieres, 1922 rue Saint-Vallier, Pohenegamook QC G0L 1J0; Sher'84; Langs: English; (418)859-2450

BRAULT, Jennifer; The Ottawa Hosp-Gen Campus, 501 Smyth Rd, Ottawa ON K1H 8L6; Ott'07; Psy.

BRAULT, Jocelyne; Inst Philippe Pinel de Mtl, 10905 boul Henri-Bourassa E, Montreal QC H1C 1H1; Mon'82; FRCPC; Psy (General Psychiatry). Psychiatre, Institut Philippe-Pinel de Montreal; (514)648-8461 x475; Fax. (514)881-3782.

BRAULT, Lucie; CSSS Pierre Boucher, 1333 boul Jacques-Cartier E, Longueuil QC J4M 2A5; Mon'06; CCFP; Staff, Centre Hospitalier Pierre Boucher; Langs: Bilingual(French/English); (514)468-8111; Fax. (514)468-8274; lucie.brault@usherbrooke.ca.

BRAULT, Serge; Ctr Medi Soleil St-Jean-Sur-Ri, 120-383 boul du Seminaire N, St-Jean-sur-Richel QC J3B 8C5; Mon'71; (450)347-7557; Fax. (450)347-3099.

BRAULT, Sophie; CSSS du Nord de Lanaudière, 1000 boul Sainte-Anne, St-Charles-Brromee QC J6E 6J2; Mon'96; CSPQ; Anes. Staff, Centre Hospitalier Régional de Lanaudière; (450)759-8222 x2960

BRAULT, Suzanne; Centre Med Robinson Inc, 4 rue Robinson N, Granby QC J2G 8Z9; Sher'74; (450)378-8435; Fax. (450)375-8832; suzbra@yahoo.ca.

BRAULT, Yves; Ctr Hosp Affilie-Enfant-Jesus, 1401 18e rue, Quebec QC G1J 1Z4; Laval'69; DAAPM; FRCPC; PhysMed&Rehab. Staff, Centre Hospitalier Affilié Universitaire de Québec - Hôpital De L'Enfant Jésus; assoc Staff, Centre Hospitalier Universitaire De Québec - Pavillon De St-françois-d'assise; Staff, Centre Francois-Charon; Prof Med, Université Laval; Langs: English; (418)649-5751; Fax. (418)649-5879.

BRAUN, David F; 204-53 Stadacona St W, Moose Jaw SK S6H 1Z2; Sask'90; CCFP; (306)693-4005; Fax. (306)692-5363.

BRAUN, E Anne; Brant Community HC-Brantford, 200 Terrace Hill St, Brantford ON N3R 1G9; McM'85; FACP; BSc; MSc; FRCPC; IntMed (Geriatric Psychiatry); GeriatricMed. Staff, Niagara Health System - Ontario Street Site; Staff, St Joseph's Healthcare - Charlton Campus; Staff, Hamilton Health Sciences Centre - McMaster Children's Hospital; Chief Geriatrics & Complex Continuing Care, The Brant Community Healthcare System - Brantford General Hospital Site; Clin Assoc Prof Med & Psy, McMaster University; (519)752-7871

BRAUN, Erwin A; Rivergrove Med Clinic, 2-2605 Main St, Winnipeg MB R2V 4W3; Man'67; CCFP; FCFP; Medical Staff Geriatric Rehab, Seven Oaks General Hospital; Langs: German; (204)632-0024; Fax. (204)697-2047.

BRAUN, Jeanelle F; Agassiz Med Centre, 130-30 Stephen St, Morden MB R6M 2G3; Man'98; CCFP; Fam Med, Carman Memorial Hospital; (204)822-4474

BRAUN, Jennifer L; Guelph Community Health Centre, 176 Wyndham St N, Guelph ON N1H 8N9; McM'06; CCFP; (519)821-6638; Fax. (519)821-5834.

BRAUN, Karen Y; Charleswood Med Clinic, 3360 Roblin Blvd, Winnipeg MB R3R 0C5; Man'91; CCFP; FCFP; (204)889-7200

BRAUN, Martin E; Fairmont Med Bldg, 309-750 Broadway W, Vancouver BC V5Z 1H2; UBC'84; CCFP; CCFP(E.M.); FCFP; Langs: German; (604)708-9891; Fax. (604)708-9803; info@vancouverlaser.com.

BRAUN, Raymond I; 884 Parleeville Rd, Parleeville NB E5P 3Y8; Sask'84; MD; BAP; CCFP; FCFP; (506)512-1199

BRAUN, Theodore J; Royal Alexandra Hosp, 10240 Kingsway NW, Edmonton AB T5H 3V9; Sask'87; CCFP; CCFP(E.M.); Staff, Royal Alexandra Hospital; (780)735-4443

BRAUNBERGER, Peter; Sister Margaret Smith Centre, 301 Lillie St N, Thunder Bay ON P7C 0A6; McM'00; FRCPC; Psy. (807)684-5100

BRAUNSTEIN, Jonathan; Royal Columbian Hosp, 330 Columbian Hosp, New Westminster BC V3L 3W7; Qns'07; CCFP; CCFP(E.M.); Staff, Royal Columbian Hospital; (604)520-4000

BRAUNSTEIN, Ronald E; BC Women's Hosp & Health Ctre, P4 207-4500 Oak St, Vancouver BC V6H 3N1; Man'65; FRCPC; Psy (Child Psychiatry). Staff, BC Women's Hospital & Health Centre; (604)875-2345 x6590

BRAVERMAN, Aliza S; Wilderman Medical Clinic, 8054 Yonge St, Thornhill ON L4J 1W3; Philadelphia (USA)'00; (905)886-1212; Fax. (905)886-0248.

BRAVERMAN, Jennifer R; Univ Hlth Network-Toronto Gen, EN 233-200 Elizabeth St, Toronto ON M5G 2C4; Ott'04; FRCPC; Psy. (416)340-3043; Fax. (416)340-4198.

BRAVERMAN, Nancy; PT 406 2-4060 rue Sainte-Cathe, Montreal QC H3Z 2Z3; Tulane (USA)'87; (514)934-1934 x23404; Fax. (519)412-4478.

BRAVO, Frank; 604 Garden St, Whitby ON L1N 7B3; Barcelona (Spain)'76; FRCSC; Otol. Staff, Lakeridge Health - Oshawa Site; Langs: Spanish; Italian; (905)665-9311; Fax. (905)665-9711.

BRAY, Frederick T; Woodroffe South Med Bldg, 102-1637 Woodroffe Ave, Nepean ON K2G 1W2; McG'89; MDCM; FRCPC; IntMed; Gastroent. (613)739-7753; Fax. (613)739-7808.

BRAY, Heather J; BC Women's Hosp & Health Ctre, 1N77-4500 Oak St, Vancouver BC V6H 3N1; Sask'87; FRCPC; DiagRad. Staff, BC Women's Hospital & Health Centre; (604)875-2131

BRAY, John C; 230-175 av Stillview, Pointe-Claire QC H9R 4S3; McG'76; FACOG; CSPQ; MDCM; FRCSC; ObstGyn (Prenatal Care). Asst ObstGyn, McGill University Health Centre - Royal Victoria Hospital; adj Prof, McGill University; Langs: English; French; (514)694-5313; Fax. (514)694-5313.

BRAY, Peter W; Univ Hlth Network-Toronto Western Hosp, 2E 400-399 Bathurst St, Toronto ON M5T 2S8; Tor'94; MSc; FRCS; LMCC; FRCSC; PlasSurg (Cosmetic Surgery). Ac Staff Surg, Toronto Western Hospital - University Health Network; Staff Cosmetic Plastic Surgeon, Elements Wellness & Medispa; Asst Prof Surg, University of Toronto; (416)603-5691; Fax. (416)603-5297.

BRAY, Riina I; Unimedico Family Practice, 110-955 Major MacKenzie Dr, Maple ON L6A 4P9; Tor'94; CCFP; FCFP; Staff Environmental Health Clinic, Women's College Hospital; Langs: Spanish; (289)553-3300

BRAY, Robert C; Heritage Research Bldg, 436-3330 Hospital Dr NW, Calgary AB T2N 4N1; Cal'80; MSc; FRCSC; OrthSurg (Knee Surgery). Staff, Foothills Medical Centre; Staff, Alberta Children's Hospital; (403)220-4244

BRAY, Thomas B; Fort Med Clinic, 101-6603 132 Ave NW, Edmonton AB T5C 2A4; London (England)'69; DObstRCOG; Ac Staff, Royal Alexandra Hospital; (780)476-1388; Fax. (780)473-3530.

BRAY, Veronique; Clin Med des Trois Lacs, 160-585 av Saint-Charles, Vaudreuil-Dorion QC J7V 8P9; Sher'03; (450)455-3322

BRAZEAU, Daniel; CSSS de Rimouski-Neigette, CP 3150 Succ A 150 av Rouleau, Rimouski QC G5L 5T1; Mon'96; CCFP; Staff, Hôpital Regional Rimouski; (418)724-8574

BRAZEAU, Nathalie; CP 2450 Bdp Beebe, Stanstead QC J0B 1E0; Sher'93; CCFP; Staff, Centre Hospitalier de Matane; (819)434-1777

BRAZEAU, Serge; Inst U Geriatrie Sherbrooke, 375 rue Argyll, Sherbrooke QC J1J 3H5; Mon'93; FRCPC; IntMed; GeriatricMed. Staff, Institut Universitaire de Geriatrie de Sherbrooke-Pavillon Argyll; (819)821-1150; Fax. (819)829-7145.

BRAZEAU, Lucie; CHUS-Hop Fleurimont, 6213-3001 12e Av N, Sherbrooke QC J1H 5N4; Sher'73; FRCPC; DiagRad. Ac Staff, Centre Hospitalier Universitaire de Sherbrooke-Hopital Fleurimont; Assoc Staff, Centre Hospitalier Universitaire de Sherbrooke-Hôpital Hôtel-Dieu; (819)346-1110 x14985; Fax. (819)820-6423.

BRAZEL, Sheila M; West Toronto Eye Care, 308-2238 Dundas St W, Toronto ON M6R 3A9; Tor'87; FRCSC; Ophth (Glaucoma). (416)760-8777; Fax. (416)760-0748.

BRCIC, Branimir; Don Valley Med Associates, 144-1333 Sheppard Ave E, North York ON M2J 1V1; Tor'91; CCFP; FCFP; Ac Staff, North York General Hospital; (416)491-5900; Fax. (416)491-1149.

BRCIC, Vanessa E; PO Box 88006, Vancouver BC V6A 4A4; McM'06.

BREAKEY, Vicky; McMaster Univ, HSC 3N27A-1280 Main St W, Hamilton ON L8S 4K1; Cal'02; FRCPC; Peds (Pediatric Hematology Oncology). Teach Staff, McMaster University; (905)521-2100; Fax. (905)521-1703.

BREARLEY, Donald T; 155 Bleecker Ave, Belleville ON K8N 3T8; Qns'70; Staff, QHC Belleville General; (613)968-3136

BREARS, Sarah L; 101-1912 Enterprise Way, Kelowna BC V1Y 9S9; Alb'95; BSc; CCFP; (250)868-0700; Fax. (250)868-3003; s.brears@telus.net.

BREAU, Marie-Josee; 220-500 Mapleton Rd, Moncton NB E1G 0N3; Sher'07; CCFP; Langs: Bilingual(English/French); (506)870-2521

BREAU, Rodney H; The Ottawa Hosp-Gen Campus, L2154-501 Smyth Rd, Ottawa ON K1H 8L6; Dal'03; FRCSC; Urol. Staff, The Ottawa Hospital - General Campus; (613)737-8899

BREAULT, Annie; 200-2924 boul Taschereau, Greenfield Park QC J4V 2G8; Laval'94; FRCPC; Psy. (450)466-5496

BREAULT, Christiane; Clinique Medicale, 584 boul Manseau, Joliette QC J6E 3E4; Sher'88; CCFP; Physician, CLSC de Schette; (450)753-9234; Fax. (450)755-1157.

BREAULT, Guy; 205-185 av Acadie, Dieppe NB E1A 1G6; Mon'03; FRCSC; Urol. Staff, Dr Georges-L-Dumont University Hospital Centre; Langs: Bilingual(French/English); (506)872-4243; Fax. (506)872-2324.

BREAULT, Jacques; CSSS de Rivière-de-Loup, 75 rue Saint-Henri, Riviere-du-Loup QC G5R 2A4; Mon'65; Psy (P.Q.). Staff, Centre Hospitalier Regional du Grand-Portage; (418)868-1000

BREAULT, Marie D; CSSS du Rocher-Perce, CP 3300 451 rue Monseigneur Ross E, Chandler QC G0C 1K0; Laval'09; CCFP; CCFP(E.M.); Staff, Centre Hospitalier de Chandler; (418)689-2261

BREBION, Carol M J; Ctre Readaptation Lisette-Dupr, 8000 rue Notre-Dame, LaSalle QC H8R 1H2; McG'93; FRCPC; Psy. Staff, Lakeshore General Hospital - Pointe Claire; Langs: French; (514)364-2282 x2173

BRECKMAN, David K; Assiniboine Clinic, 633 Lodge Ave, Winnipeg MB R3J 0S9; Man'88; (204)958-6705; Fax. (204)888-1750.

BRECKMAN, Gillian L F; Assiniboine Clinic, 633 Lodge Ave, Winnipeg MB R3J 0S9; Dartmouth(NH) (USA)'88; MD; ABIM; (204)958-6714; Fax. (204)888-1750.

BRECKON, Sidney L W; University Hosp of Northern BC, 1475 Edmonton St, Prince George BC V2M 1S2; Dal'73; FRCPC; DiagRad. Ac Staff, University Hospital of Northern British Columbia; (250)565-2000; Fax. (250)565-2414.

BREDEN, Michael A; Chilliwack Gen Hosp, 45600 Menholm Rd, Chilliwack BC V2P 1P7; Wes'94; FRCPC; Anes. Staff, Chilliwack General Hospital; (604)795-4141

BREDENKAMP, Andries P; Windsor Square Shopp Centre, 240-1959 152 St, Surrey BC V4A 9E3; Pretoria (South Africa)'91; MB ChB; LMCC; CCFP; Langs: Afrikaans; (604)531-0888; windsor5@telus.net.

BREDENKAMP, Barend J; 203-1040 Shoppers Row, Campbell River BC V9W 2C6; Stellenbosch (South Africa)'74; MB ChB; MMed(Psych); FRCPC; Psy (Child & Adolescent Psychiatry). Staff, Penticton Regional Hospital; Langs: Afrikaans; (250)286-6230

BREDENKAMP, Lynne; Tumbler Ridge Med Clinic, 220 Front St, Tumbler Ridge BC V0C 2W0; Stellenbosch (South Africa)'05; MB ChB; (250)242-4251; Fax. (250)242-4076.

BREDENKAMP, Thomas L; PO Box 2983 Stn Main, Wainwright AB T9W 1S8.

BREDENOORD, Steven; Rocky Med Clinic, PO Box 99 Stn Main, Rocky-Mtn-House AB T4T 1A1; Stellenbosch (South Africa)'83; CCFP; (403)845-2815; Fax. (403)845-2177.

BREDESEN, Leif-Erik; Smith Clinic, 1-6601 48 Ave, Camrose AB T4V 3G8; Queen's (Ireland)'80; DA(Lond); Staff, Covenant Health - St Mary's Hospital; Langs: Norwegian; (780)672-2425; Fax. (780)608-5895.

BREDO, Lance K; 300-4309 52 Ave, Red Deer AB T4N 6S4; Alb'76; FRCSC; OrthSurg. (403)309-2001

BREE, Teresa L; 203-728 Spadina Cres E, Saskatoon SK S7K 3H2; Sask'86; FRCPC; IntMed; Cardiol. (306)975-0600; Fax. (306)978-5254; terry.bree@gmail.com.

BREEN, Carson F; Fort Vermilion Med Clinic, PO Box 306, Fort Vermilion AB T0H 1N0; UBC'64; (780)927-3213

BREEN, Corinne H L; Oakmed Family Health Team, 110-231 Oak Park Blvd, Oakville ON L6H 7S8; McM'01; DipCE; BA; BSc(Hon); CCFP; Staff Privil, Halton Healthcare Services Corporation - Oakville Site; (905)901-5111; Fax. (905)901-5122.

BREGER, Barry; Centre De Medecine Familiale, 1141 boul Saint-Joseph E, Montreal QC H2J 1L3; Grenoble (France)'81; BSc; MB; Langs: Bilingual(English/French); (514)277-1141; Fax. (514)277-0061.

BREGER, Laurie T; Group Med Stillview, 245-175 av Stillview, Pointe-Claire QC H9R 4S3; McG'78; CCFP; FCFP; hon Membre, Lakeshore General Hospital - Pointe Claire; Assoc Med Dir, Kells Medical Research; Langs: French; (514)697-1525; Fax. (514)697-4418.

BREGMAN, Isaiah D; Broadway Plaza Family Practice, 6-601 Broadway W, Vancouver BC V5Z 4C2; UBC'09; CCFP; (604)872-2558

BREIKSS, Karlina A; 302-4420 Chatterton Way, Victoria BC V8X 5J2; UBC'95; FRCPC; Peds. Staff Ped, Victoria General Hospital; Clin Instructor, University of British Columbia; Langs: English; French; German; (250)727-2156

BREINER, Ariel; Toronto East Gen Hosp, C304-825 Coxwell Ave, Toronto ON M4C 3E7; McG'05; FRCPC; Neur. Staff, Toronto East General Hospital Inc; (416)469-6406

BREITKREUTZ, Cindy E; Whitehorse Med Services Ltd, 406 Lambert St, Whitehorse YT Y1A 1Z7; Alb'84; CCFP; FCFP; Ac Staff, Whitehorse General Hospital; Staff, Whitehorse Medical Services Ltd; (867)393-6600; Fax. (867)393-6601.

BREITLING, Magnus K; Clinical Sciences Bldg, 8 120-152 University Campus NW, Edmonton AB T6G 2G3; Cal'06; FRCPC; Anes. (780)407-8861; Fax. (780)407-3200.

BREITMAN, Deanne R; Victoria Reg Forensic Clinic, 2840 Nanaimo St, Victoria BC V8T 4W9; Alb'01; FRCPC; Psy. (250)213-4500

BREMANG, Joseph A; St Joseph's Health Centre, 30 The Queensway, Toronto ON M6R 1B5; (Ghana)'72; MB ChB; FRCPC; Anes (Intensive Care & Anesthesia). Ac Staff, St Joseph's Health Centre; (416)530-6000 x6090; Fax. (416)530-6300.

BREMERMANN, R Danielle M; Dorval Med Assoc Fam Hlth Team, 465 Morden Rd, Oakville ON L6K 3W6; Dal'95; CCFP; FCFP; (905)842-7154; Fax. (905)842-3604; dbremermann@dorvalmedical.ca.

BREMNER, Kyla; The Medical Clinic Associates, 4794 Joyce Ave, Powell River BC V8A 3B6; Sydney (Australia)'07; MB BS; (604)223-3205

BREMNESS, Andrew B; Child & Adolescence Serv Assoc, 10645 63 Ave NW, Edmonton AB T6H 1P7; Alb'72; AB(Psy.); AB(ChildPsy); Consultant Child Psy, Covenant Health - Misericordia Community Hospital; Staff Psy, Alberta Health Services; Clin Prof Psy, University of Alberta; (780)438-0011; Fax. (780)437-6133.

BRENCHLEY, Reginald; Lindsay Prof Bldg, 14-65 Angeline St N, Lindsay ON K9V 5N7; Wes'69; Court Staff, Ross Memorial Hospital; Pres., Victoria County Med Association; (705)324-1811

BRENCKMANN, Christine; 5-1230 Alward St, Prince George BC V2M 7B1; Cal'06; MPH; MSc; BSc; CCFP; Staff, University Hospital of Northern British Columbia; Langs: Swedish; German; (250)562-2644; Fax. (250)563-3585.

BRENEMAN, Christopher D; Hamiota Dist Health Centre, 177 Birch Ave, Hamiota MB R0M 0T0; Man'95; CCFP; FCFP; Fam Med, Hamiota District Health Centre; (204)764-2412; Fax. (204)764-2325; cbreneman@arha.ca.

BRENHOUSE, Michelle; Herzl CRIU Walk-In Clinic, 500-5858 ch Cote-des-Neiges, Montreal QC H3S 1Z1; McG'08; CCFP; (514)340-8311; Fax. (514)340-8316.

BRENKEN, Ernst G; The Two Hundred, 402-200 St Clair Ave W, Toronto ON M4V 1R1; Tor'85; FRCPC; Psy (Individual Psychotherapy). Langs: German; (416)515-7538; Fax. (416)515-7538.

BRENNAGH, Michael C; 183 Simcoe Ave, Keswick ON L4P 3S7; Qns'71; DABPN; FRCP; FRCPC; Psy (Psycho Pharmacology). Consultant Psy, The Southdown Institute; Consultant Psy, Southlake Regional Health Centre; (905)476-1800; mbrennagh@southlakeregional.org.

BRENNAN, Alison T; Anaesthetic Services, 213-2186 Oak Bay Ave, Victoria BC V8R 1G3; Monash (Australia)'67; MB BS; Anes. (250)595-7211

BRENNAN, Amy M; 220-500 Mapleton Rd, Moncton NB E1G 0N3; Dal'08; CCFP; (506)870-2521; Fax. (506)870-2978.

BRENNAN, Barbara G; Hamilton HS-Chedoke Site, PO Box 2000 Stn Lcd 1, Hamilton ON L8N 3Z5; McM'83; FRCSC; ObstGyn. Staff, Hamilton Health Sciences Centre - McMaster University Medical Centre; Asst Prof, McMaster University; (905)521-2100 x76254; Fax. (905)527-2675.

BRENNAN, Brenda; Osgoode Village Health Centre, 3192 Logan Farm Dr, Osgoode ON K0A 2W0; Cal'90; CCFP; FCFP; Physician, Township of Osgoode Care Centre(Long-Term Care Facility); Physician, Osgoode Village Health Centre; (613)826-2502; Fax. (613)826-1682.

BRENNAN, Elizabeth B; 220 Main St, Antigonish NS B2G 2C2; UBC'82; (902)863-3737; Fax. (902)863-5956.

BRENNAN, F James; Kingston Gen Hosp, 76 Stuart St, Kingston ON K7L 2V7; Qns'67; FRCPC; Cardiol. Att Staff, Kingston General Hospital; Att Staff, Hotel-Dieu Hospital; Assoc Prof Med(Cardiology), Queen's University; (613)549-6666 x4547; Fax. (613)548-1387; brennanj@kgh.kari.net.

BRENNAN, Gerald D G; Children's Hosp, 840 Sherbrook St, Winnipeg MB R3A 1S1; Man'00; FRCPC; Peds; PedEmergMed.

BRENNAN, John P; The Wright Clinic, 57 James St, Parry Sound ON P2A 1T6; Wes'86; Dip SportMed; BASc(EnvEng); CCFP; Med Dir, Honda of Canada Manufacturing; (705)746-2181; Fax. (705)746-4753.

BRENNAN, Michael B; St Martha's Doctor's Offices, G26-23 Bay St, Antigonish NS B2G 2G7; Dal'82; FRCSC; PlasSurg. Ac Staff, St Martha's Regional Hospital; (902)863-5555; Fax. (902)863-1396.

BRENNAN, Michael C; Niagara H System-St Catharines, PO Box 3018 Stn Main 142 Queenston St, St Catharines ON L2R 7C6; Dal'86; DABPath; FRCPC; GenPath (Hematology Pathology). Staff, Niagara Health System - St Catharines General Site; (905)684-7271 x46226; Fax. (905)984-5578.

BRENNAN, Michael; North York Gen Hosp, 4001 Leslie St, North York ON M2K 1E1; Qns'84; FRCPC; AnatPath; GenPath. Staff, North York General Hospital; (416)756-6253; Fax. (416)756-4294.

BRENNAN, Peter G; 30 Farnham Gate Rd, Halifax NS B3M 3W8; Dal'90; (902)443-8388; Fax. (902)443-9887.

BRENNAN, Stefan D; Medical Arts Bldg, 104-750 Spadina Cres E, Saskatoon SK S7K 3H3; Sask'00; FRCPC; Psy. (306)653-4843; Fax. (306)653-3190.

BRENNAN, Terence P A; 3192 Logan Farm Dr, Osgoode ON K0A 2W0; Ott'85; CCFP; Asst Prof, University of Ottawa; Langs: Bilingual(English/French); (613)826-2502; Fax. (613)826-1682.

BRENNAN, Terrance E; Dr Everett Chalmers Reg Hosp, PO Box 9000 Stn A, Fredericton NB E3B 5N5; Dal'74; FRCPC; DiagRad. Staff, Dr Everett Chalmers Regional Hospital; (506)452-5136; Fax. (506)452-5673.

BRENNAND, Erin A; Foothills Med Centre, 1403 29 St NW, Calgary AB T2N 2T9; Alb'06; ObstGyn. Staff, Foothills Medical Centre; (403)944-1636; Fax. (403)270-4249.

BRENNEIS, Fraser R; Royal Alexandra Hosp, 10240 Kingsway NW, Edmonton AB T5H 3V9; Alb'82; CCFP; FCFP; Staff Family Med Centre, Royal Alexandra Hospital; Vice Dean Educ Fac of Med & Dentistry, University of Alberta; (780)735-4201; Fax. (780)735-4978.

BRENNEMAN, Frederick D; Sunnybrook Hlth Sciences Ctre, H170-2075 Bayview Ave, Toronto ON M4N 3M5; Tor'88; FRCSC; GenSurg. Vis Prof, Health Sciences Centre; Staff, Sunnybrook Health Sciences Centre; Teach Staff Surg, University of Toronto; (416)480-4232; Fax. (416)480-4225.

BRENNER, Jennifer L; Alberta Children's Hosp, 2888 Shaganappi Trail NW, Calgary AB T3B 6A8; McM'96; FRCPC; Peds. Staff, Alberta Children's Hospital; (403)955-2953

BRENNER, Rudy H; Complexe Sante Reine-Elizabeth, 115-2100 av de Marlowe, Montreal QC H4A 3L5; McG'74; CCFP; Staff, McGill University Health Centre - Royal Victoria Hospital; (514)731-1186

BRENT, Henry P; One Med Place, 312-20 Wynford Dr, North York ON M3C 1J4; Tor'54; MA(Physiol); FRCSC; Ophth (Glaucoma). Court Staff Sr, The Hospital For Sick Children; Asst Prof, University of Toronto; (416)441-3535; Fax. (416)441-9116.

BRENT, Michael H; Univ Hlth Network-Toronto Western Hosp, 6EW 423-399 Bathurst St, Toronto ON M5T 2S8; McM'83; BSc; FRCSC; Ophth (Cataract Surgery). Ac Staff, Toronto Western Hospital - University Health Network; Ac Staff, Mount Sinai Hospital; Asst Prof, University of Toronto; (416)603-5444; Fax. (416)603-5903.

BRENTNALL, David M; 8B Shoal Harbour Dr, Clarenville NL A5A 2C4; Mem'95; CCFP; Staff, The Dr G B Cross Memorial Hospital; (709)466-4355; Fax. (709)466-4356.

BRERETON, Sheila M; Credit Valley Prof Bldg, 205-2300 Eglinton Ave W, Mississauga ON L5M 2V8; (Ireland)'85; Staff, The Credit Valley Hospital; (905)820-8144; Fax. (905)820-1631.

BRERETON, Teresa; CFB Trenton, PO Box 1000 Stn Forces 24 CFHVC, Northbrook ON K0H 2G0; Wes'70; Staff Med Clinic, Canadian Forces Base Trenton; (613)336-8888

BRESLIN, Calvin W; 311-3101 Bloor St W, Etobicoke ON M8X 2W2; Ott'69; FRCSC; Ophth. Att Staff Ophth, Toronto Western Hospital - University Health Network; Prof, University of Toronto; (416)239-4623; Fax. (416)239-0510.

BRESSLER, Brian L; Pacific Gastroenterology Assoc, 770-1190 Hornby St, Vancouver BC V6Z 2K5; UBC'00; ABIM(Epidemiol); FRCP; MSc; FRCPC; Gastroent (Hepatology); IntMed. Clinical Asst Prof, Providence Health Care - St Paul's Hospital; (604)688-6332 x245; Fax. (604)689-2004.

BRESSLER, Hartley B; Nymark Med Centre, 4839 Leslie St, North York ON M2J 2K8; McM'93; Staff, Mount Sinai Hospital; Langs: American Sign Language; (416)498-3600; Fax. (416)498-1211.

BRET, Patrice M; N C S B, 1C550-585 University Ave, Toronto ON M5G 2N2; Lyons (France)'80; FRCPC; DiagRad. Teach Staff Medical Imaging, University of Toronto; (416)340-4800 x6558

BRETECHER, Gilbert J; Dauphin Med Clinic, 622 3rd St SW, Dauphin MB R7N 1R5; Man'77; BSc; Ac Staff, Dauphin Regional Health Centre; Physician/Med Officer of Hlth, Correctional Institute; (204)638-6445; Fax. (204)638-5670.

BRETHES, Jean-Ianic; Hotel-Dieu d'Arthabaska, 5 rue des Hospitalieres, Victoriaville QC G6P 6N2; Sher'00; FRCPC; Psy. Staff, Hotel-Dieu d'Arthabaska; (819)357-2030; Fax. (819)357-6035.

BRETHOLZ, Adam; Dr Adam Bretholz Inc, 12A-4643 rue Sherbrooke O, Montreal QC H3Z 1G2; McM'04; FRCPC; Peds (Pediatric Emergency Medicine). Staff, McGill University Health Centre - Montreal Children's Hospital; (514)691-0010

BRETON, Chantal; Clinique Statcare, 104-175 av Stillview, Pointe-Claire QC H9R 4S3; Mon'86; CCFP; FCFP; Physician, Statcare Centre; Médecin Loyola Campus, Concordia University Health Services; Langs: English; French; (514)694-9282

BRETON, Claude; Clinique Med Loretteville, 250-11000 boul de L'Ormiere, Quebec QC G2B 5S1; Laval'80; (418)842-3731; Fax. (418)842-3246; claude.breton@ssss.gouv.qc.ca.

BRETON, Denys; CSSS du Granit, 3569 rue Laval, Lac-Megantic QC G6B 1A5; Laval'71; GenSurg. Staff, Carrefour Sante Granit; (819)583-0330; Fax. (819)583-5364.

BRETON, Donald; Hop Maisonneuve-Rosemont, 5415 boul de l'Assomption, Montreal QC H1T 2M4; Mon'90; FRCPC; IntMed; Endocrin (P.Q.); Endocrin&Metab. Staff, Hopital Maisonneuve-Rosemont; (514)252-3400

BRETON, Esther; CHUQ-Hotel-Dieu de Levis, 11 ch Cote du Palais, Quebec QC G1R 2J6; Laval'00; CSPQ; Anes. Staff, Centre Hospitalier Universitaire de Québec (CHUQ) - Siege Social; Staff, Centre Hospitalier Universitaire De Québec - Pavillon De St-françois-d'assise; (418)691-5323

BRETON, Gail; SMBD Jewish Gen Hosp, 3755 ch Cote-Sainte-Catherine, Montreal QC H3T 1E2; Mon'88; FRCSC; GenSurg (P.Q.). Staff, Sir Mortimer B Davis Jewish General; (514)340-8222 x5598

BRETON, Genevieve; Clin externe de Psychiatrie, 279 rue de la Providence, Granby QC J2G 4S7; Sher'97; FRCPC; Psy. Staff, Centre Hospitalier de Granby; (450)375-8000

BRETON, Guy; Universite de Montreal, H401-2900 boul Edouard-Montpet, Montreal QC H3T 1J4; Sher'74; FRCPC; DiagRad. Chef de radiologie, Centre Hospitalier l'Université De Montréal (CHUM) - Hôpital Saint-luc; Rector, Universite de Montreal; (514)343-6991; guy.berthiaume@umontreal.ca.

BRETON, J Jacques; Hop Riviere-des-Prairies, 7070 boul Perras, Montreal QC H1E 1A4; Laval'65; DPsy; MSc; Psy (Mood Disorders). Staff Mood Disorders Clinic, Hôpital Riviere des Prairies; (514)323-7260; Fax. (514)323-4163; jj.breton.hrdp@ssss.gouv.qc.ca.

BRETON, Janie; UMF de Levis, 100-1205 boul de la Rive-Sud, Levis QC G6W 0J4; Sher'06; Staff, Hôpital de Christ-Roi; (418)380-8597 x2648

BRETON, Jeannot; Clinique de Med Familiale, 1971 rue Bilodeau, Plessisville QC G6L 3J1; Laval'75; Médecin, CLSC de l'Erable; (819)362-6337; Fax. (819)362-9147.

BRETON, Lyne; Clinique Med Haute-Ville, 785 av De Salaberry, Quebec QC G1R 2T8; Laval'78; Physician, CLSC de Limoilou; (418)525-7664; Fax. (418)525-9106.

BRETON, Martin A M; Glenmore Landing, 271A-1600 90 Ave SW, Calgary AB T2V 5A8; Tor'93; CCFP; FCFP; Langs: English; French; (403)571-5019; Fax. (403)571-5025.

BRETON, Michel; Centre Med Laval, 1110 boul Vanier, Laval QC H7C 2R8; Mon'79; Staff, Hopital de la Cite de la santé; Staff, Hopital Marie Clarac; (450)661-2521; Fax. (450)661-7193.

BRETON, Pierre; Regie des Rentes du Quebec, 348-2600 boul Laurier, Quebec QC G1V 4T3; Laval'79; LMCC; Teach Staff, Université Laval; (418)657-8739 x3806; Fax. (418)644-8237.

BRETON, Robert; Polyclinique, 314-874 boul de l'Universite E, Chicoutimi QC G7H 6B9; Sher'89; CSPQ; FRCPC; IntMed; Cardiol. (418)545-0539; Fax. (418)545-1032.

BRETON, Robert; CLSC Kateri-Sante au Travail, 210-87B boul Marie-Victorin, Candiac QC J5R 1C3; Mon'91; CCFP; (450)444-1154; Fax. (450)444-4396.

BRETON, Serge; CSSS de la Baie-des-Chaleurs, RR 2 419 boul Perron, Maria QC G0C 1Y0; Laval'76; Psy. Staff, CSSS de la Baie-des-Chaleurs; (418)759-3443; Fax. (418)759-3679.

BRETON, Sophie; CHUQ-St-Francois d'Assise, 10 rue de l'Espinay, Quebec QC G1L 3L5; Mon'96; CCFP; CCFP(E.M.); Emergency Med, Centre Hospitalier Universitaire De Québec - Pavillon De St-françois-d'assise; (418)525-4444 x21000

BRETON, Steve; CSSS de la Region de Thetford, 1717 rue Notre-Dame E, Thetford Mines QC G6G 2V4; Laval'95; CCFP; Staff, Hopital du CSS de la Region de Thetford; (418)338-7777; Fax. (418)335-9309.

BRETON-FORTIN, Julie; West Nipissing Commun Hlth Ctr, M100-145 Main St, Sturgeon Falls ON P2B 1N8; Ott'08; CCFP; Staff Fam Physician Hospitalist, West Nipissing General Hospital; Langs: Bilingual(English/French); (705)753-0151; Fax. (705)753-5253.

BRETON-THIBODEAU, Marianne; CSSS de Chicoutimi, 305 av Saint-Vallier, Chicoutimi QC G7H 5H6; Sher'00; FRCPC; IntMed; Nephrol. Staff, Complexe hospitalier de la Sagamie; (418)541-1000

BRETT, Kelly R; Univ of Calgary Sport Med Ctr, 2500 University Ave NW, Calgary AB T2N 1N4; Cal'90; (403)220-8518; Fax. (403)282-6170.

BRETT, Matthew J M; Dr C W Wiebe Med Centre, 385 Main St, Winkler MB R6W 1J2; (Other Foreign)'08; CCFP; (204)325-4312

BREUGEM, Dirk J; Maple Tree Med Clinic, 1181 6 Ave NE, Salmon Arm BC V1E 2S5; Stellenbosch (South Africa)'84; MB ChB; CCFP; CCFP(E.M.); FCFP; (250)832-9361

BREWARD, Arthur; Lakeridge HC-Bowmanville Site, 47 Liberty St S, Bowmanville ON L1C 2N4; Birmingham (England)'53; MB ChB; FFARCS(Eng); LMCC; FRCPC; Anes (Pain Management). Staff, Lakeridge Health - Bowmanville Site; Langs: German; (905)623-3331 x1700

BREWER, John T; Family Med Centre, 210 Melrose Ave, Ottawa ON K1Y 4K7; Ott'83; CCFP; FCFP; (613)761-4334; Fax. (613)761-4200.

BREWER, Monica P; Family Med Centre, 210 Melrose Ave, Ottawa ON K1Y 4K7; Ott'84; CCFP; FCFP; (613)761-4334; mbrewer@toh.on.ca.

BREWER, Timothy F; 1020 av des Pins O, Montreal QC H3A 1A2; New York(NY) (USA)'85; (514)398-6271

BREWERTON, Conway N; HBOT Clinics Inc, G100-2210 2 St SW, Calgary AB T2S 3C3; Alb'77; BSc; MPH; (403)509-4740

BREWERTON, Lee J; Chinook Reg Hosp, 960 19 St S, Lethbridge AB T1J 1W5; Alb'06; FRCPC; DiagRad. Staff, Chinook Regional Hospital; (403)388-6111

BREWSTER, C Francis; PO Box 905 Stn Main, Orillia ON L3V 6K8; Tor'74; CCFP; Staff (Term), Royal Victoria Regional Health Centre; Ac Staff, Orillia Soldiers' Memorial Hospital; Fax. (705)326-3850.

BREZDEN-MASLEY, Christine; St Michael's Hosp, 2079-30 Bond St, Toronto ON M5B 1W8; Tor'00; BSc; MSc; PhD; FRCPC; IntMed (Breast Cancer); MedOncol. Staff MedOncol/Head Oncology Clinical Research Group, St Michael's Hospital; Asst Prof, University of Toronto; Langs: Ukrainian; (416)864-5734; Fax. (416)864-3073.

BREZINA, Jeanie Shkimba; 324-398 Avenue Rd, Toronto ON M4V 2H4; Tor'62; LMCC; Langs: Slavic; Ukrainian; Polish; Russian; (416)324-5351; Fax. (416)324-5351.

BRIAND, Alain; CSSS de Chicoutimi, 305 rue Saint-Vallier, Chicoutimi QC G7H 5H6; Mon'73; CSPQ; FRCPC; Anes. Staff, Complexe hospitalier de la Sagamie; (418)541-1000 x2628

BRIAND, Claude; Clinique Med Cabano, GD 101-825 rue Commerciale N, Cabano QC G0L 1E0; Laval'74; Staff, Centre Hospitalier Notre-Dame-du-Lac; (418)854-2762; Fax. (418)854-7498.

BRIARD, Raymond; GMF de Mascouche, 100-880 Montee Masson, Mascouche QC J7K 2L7; Mon'79; (450)474-2493

BRICAULT, Yvon; Polyclinique Med Fabreville, 380 boul Cure-Labelle, Laval QC H7P 5L3; Mon'72; LMCC; Langs: English; (450)628-5800; Fax. (450)628-0217.

BRICK, R Andrew; Min of Health & Long Term Care, 370 Select Dr, Kingston ON K7M 8B6; Tor'81; CCFP; FCFP; CCFP(E.M.); Fax. (613)536-3184.

BRICKELL, Sandra E; Grand River Hosp-KW Hlth Ctre, PO Box 9056 Stn C 835 King St W, Kitchener ON N2G 1G3; McM'95; FRCPC; IntMed. Assoc Staff, Grand River Hospital - Kitchener/Waterloo Health Centre; (519)749-4300

BRICKER, David J; 2909 Grandview St, Windsor ON N8T 2L5; Wes'94; BSc; CCFP; FCFP; (519)251-1878; Fax. (519)251-1665.

BRIDEAU, Diane; CSSS de la Pointe-de-l'ile, 13926 rue Notre-Dame E, Pte-aux-Trembles QC H1A 1T5; Sher'86; (514)642-4050; Fax. (514)498-7505.

BRIDEAU, Eric; 247 University Ave, Moncton NB E1C 5K4; Mon'00; FRCPC; IntMed; Respir. Staff Pneumology, Dr Georges-L-Dumont University Hospital Centre; Prof, Universite de Sherbrooke; (506)855-6607; Fax. (506)855-7381.

BRIDEAU, Jean-Rene; 203-185 av Acadie, Dieppe NB E1A 1G6; Sher'07; CCFP; (506)853-7855; Fax. (506)853-7363.

BRIDGE, Kathleen E G; Queensway Prof Centre, 310-190 Sherway Dr, Etobicoke ON M9C 5N2; Glasgow (Scotland)'70; Staff, Trillium Health Centre - West Toronto; (416)620-7950; Fax. (416)620-0753.

BRIDGE, Margaret Ann; Charlton Med Centre, 101-25 Charlton Ave E, Hamilton ON L8N 1Y2; McM'74; CCFP; Ac Staff, St Joseph's Healthcare - Charlton Campus; Court Staff, Hamilton Health Sciences Centre - McMaster University Medical Centre; (905)521-3762; Fax. (905)521-4299.

BRIDGE, Michael A; 303-3330 Richter St, Kelowna BC V1W 4V5; UBC'03; FRCSC; OrthSurg. (250)861-1221

BRIDGE, Suzanne K; Lakeridge Hlth Corp-Oshawa, 2F-1 Hospital Crt, Oshawa ON L1G 2B9; Tor'05; FRCPC; IntMed; Critical Care Medicine. Staff, Lakeridge Health - Oshawa Site; (905)576-8711

BRIDGEO, David B; Royal Windsor Terrace, 105-380 Pelissier St, Windsor ON N9A 6W8; Mem'97; LMCC; CCFP; Member Exec Section on Gen & Family Pract, Ontario Medical Association; Treas, Essex County Medical Society; (519)974-1862; cutedrdave@gmail.com.

BRIDGER, Ian M; Burnside Family Med Clinic, 4-101 Burnside Rd W, Victoria BC V9A 1B7; London (England)'82; MB BS; (250)383-3153; Fax. (250)383-2431.

BRIDGER, Keith C; The Medical Assoc Clinic, 806 Vernon St, Nelson BC V1L 4G5; McM'83; CCFP; FCFP; (250)352-6611; Fax. (250)352-6624.

BRIDGER, Natalie A; Dr Charles A Janeway Child HC, 300 Prince Philip Dr, St. John's NL A1B 3V6; Mem'04; FRCPC; Peds; InfectDis. Staff, Janeway Children's Health & Rehabilitation Centre; (709)777-4307

BRIDGER, Tracey L; Dr Charles A Janeway Child HC, 2J745-300 Prince Philip Dr, St. John's NL A1B 3V6; Mem'94; FRCPC; Peds; Endocrin&Metab. Staff, Janeway Children's Health & Rehabilitation Centre; Full-Time Teach. Staff, Memorial University Of Newfoundland; (709)777-4387; Fax. (709)777-4726; tracey.bridger@easternhealth.ca.

BRIDGES, Eileen J; McGill Sports Med Centre, 475 av des Pins O, Montreal QC H2W 1S4; Ott'90; MSc; Dip SportMed; (514)398-7007; Fax. (514)398-4035.

BRIDGES, Ronald J; TRW Bldg, 7F-3280 Hospital Dr NW, Calgary AB T2N 4Z6; Cal'81; BSc; FRCPC; IntMed (Adult Gastroenterology); Gastroent. A-Head Div of Gatroent, Calgary Health Region; Clin Prof Med/Sr Associate Dean Clinical Affairs, University of Calgary; (403)220-4245; Fax. (403)283-5594.

BRIDGLAND, Lindsay J; University of Alberta Hosp, 8440 112 St NW, Edmonton AB T6G 2B7; Alb'07; FRCPC; IntMed. Staff, University of Alberta Hospital; (780)407-8822

BRIDLE, H Terrance; Muskoka Cosmetic Laser & Vein, 3 Willis St, Bracebridge ON P1L 2E1; Tor'76; (705)645-9888; Fax. (705)645-7580.

BRIE, Michele; CSSS de Manicouagan, 635 boul Jolliet, Baie-Comeau QC G5C 1P1; Laval'83; FRCSC; GenSurg. Staff, Centre Hospitalier Régional Baie-Comeau; (418)589-3701

BRIEDIS, Dalius J; MUHC-Royal Victoria Hosp, A4 03-687 av des Pins O, Montreal QC H3A 1A1; Johns Hopkins (USA)'72; BA; FRCP; FRCPC; IntMed (Infectious Diseases). Sr Physician InfectDis, McGill University Health Centre - Royal Victoria Hospital; Langs: Lithuanian; Bilingual(French/English); (514)398-3925; dalius.briedis@mcgill.ca.

BRIEMBERG, Hannah R; Diamond Health Care Center, 8F-2775 Laurel St, Vancouver BC V5Z 1M9; McM'94; FRCPC; Neur. Staff, Vancouver General Hospital - Centennial Pavillion; (604)875-4247

BRIEN, Chantal; CSST, CP 100 Succ Bureau-Chef 145 boul Saint-Joseph, St-Jean-sur-Richel QC J3B 6Z1; Mon'92; (450)359-2100 x2117

BRIEN, Donald M; Health Park, 302-45 Weatherbee Rd, Mira Road NS B1M 0A1; Dal'93; FRCSC; OrthSurg. (902)539-5954; Fax. (902)539-5804.

BRIEN, Erin; Saint John Reg Hosp, PO Box 2100 Stn Main 400 University Ave, Saint John NB E2L 4L2; McM'05; CCFP; Staff, Saint John Regional Hospital; (506)648-6000

BRIEN, Gilles; Centre Hosp Honore-Mercier, 2750 boul Laframboise, Saint-Hyacinthe QC J2S 4Y8; Mon'67; Méd légiste, Centre Hospitalier Honore-Mercier; (450)771-3333 x4782; Fax. (450)771-3745.

BRIEN, Heather; Argus Med Centre, 201-581 Argus Rd, Oakville ON L6J 3J4; Mem'90; BSc(PhysTher); FRCSC; OrthSurg. Staff, Halton Healthcare Services Corporation - Oakville Site; Staff, Halton Healthcare Services Corporation - Milton District Hospital; Associate Clin Prof, McMaster University; (905)339-2498; Fax. (905)339-1886.

BRIEN, Julie; Hop Charles-Lemoyne, 3120 boul Taschereau, Greenfield Park QC J4V 2H1; Sher'97; FRCPC; DiagRad. Staff, Hopital Charles LeMoyne; (450)466-5000

BRIEN, Louis; Centre Med Quatre-Bourgeois, 300-979 av de Bourgogne, Quebec QC G1W 2L4; Laval'64; Psy (P.Q.). (418)653-4050; Fax. (418)658-6465.

BRIEN, Marie-Chantal; Ctr Hosp Affilie-St-Sacrement, 1050 ch Sainte-Foy, Quebec QC G1S 4L8; Sher'92; FRCSC; ObstGyn. Staff, Centre Hospitalier Affilié Universitaire de Québec - Hôpital du St-Sacrement; (418)682-7511

BRIEN, Steven R; Peterborough Clinic, 301-26 Hospital Dr, Peterborough ON K9J 7C3; Qns'80; FRCPC; IntMed; Gastroent. Staff, Peterborough Regional Health Centre - Hospital Drive; (705)740-6851; Fax. (705)740-6899.

BRIEN, Susan E; CSSS-Hopital De Hull, 116 boul Lionel-Emond, Gatineau QC J8Y 1W7; Dal'86; FRCSC; Neursurg (Neuro Oncology). Staff, Hull Hospital; (819)966-6200

BRIEN, Thomas A; Long Pond Med Clinic, PO Box 14097 Manuels Stn Main 88 Conception Bay Hwy, Conception Bay S NL A1W 3J1; Mem'87; BSc; BMedSci; (709)834-5511; Fax. (709)834-4397.

BRIEN, William F; The Hosp for Sick Children, 3659-555 University Ave, Toronto ON M5G 1X8; Wes'77; FRCPC; HemPath. Staff HemPath, The Hospital For Sick Children; Assoc Prof Path & Med, University of Toronto; (416)813-7736; Fax. (416)813-6257; william.brien@sickkids.ca.

BRIENZ, Deborah D; Mill Bay Med Centre, 230-2720 Mill Bay Rd RR 1, Mill Bay BC V0R 2P1; Ohio (USA)'78; FAAP; FRCPC; Peds. Consultant, Victoria General Hospital; Pediatrics, Chemainus Health Care Centre; Consultant, Cowichan District Hospital; (250)743-3211; Fax. (250)743-2800.

BRIERE, Claude; Polyclinique de Trois-Rivieres, 100-1900 boul des Recollets, Trois-Rivieres QC G8Z 4K4; Laval'85; FRCPC; IntMed; Gastroent. Staff, CSSS de Trois-Rivières; (819)373-1538; Fax. (819)373-2138.

BRIERE, Claude; CLSC Joliette, 380 boul Base-de-Roc, Joliette QC J6E 9J6; Mon'76; (450)755-2211 x3305; claude.briere@ssss.gouv.qc.ca.

BRIERE, Dominique; CLSC Hochelaga-Maisonneuve, 4201 rue Ontario E, Montreal QC H1V 1K2; Mon'08; (514)253-2181 x15324; Fax. (514)253-4580.

BRIERE, Josee; CLSC Seigneurie de Beauharnois, 142 rue Saint-Laurent, Beauharnois QC J6N 1V9; Mon'96; Langs: English; Spanish; (450)429-6455

BRIERE, Luc F; Cornwall Comm Hosp-McConnell S, PO Box 100 Stn Main 840 McConnell Ave, Cornwall ON K6H 5S5; Ott'90; CCFP; Staff, Cornwall Community Hospital; (613)938-4240

BRIERE, Michel; Polyclinique St-Eustache, 75 rue Grignon, St-Eustache QC J7P 4J2; Laval'74; (450)473-6943; Fax. (450)473-1916; michelbriere@hotmail.com.

BRIERE, Nicole; Centre de Read Lucie-Bruneau, 2275 av Laurier E, Montreal QC H2H 2N8; Mon'80; (514)527-4527

BRIERE, Raymond; 105C-411 av Sirois, Rimouski QC G5L 8B2; Mon'79; Staff, Hôpital de l'Archipel; (418)722-6816

BRIERLEY, James D; Univ Hlth Network-Princess M, 610 University Ave, Toronto ON M5G 2M9; London (England)'80; BSc; MB; MRC; FRCR; FRCPC; RadOncol. Staff Radiol, Princess Margaret Hospital - University Health Network; Asst Prof, University of Toronto; (416)946-2124; Fax. (416)946-6566.

BRIERLEY, Lawrence A; 101-4450 Chatterton Way, Victoria BC V8X 5J2; Sask'74; FRCSC; Ophth (Cataract & Refractive). Consultant, Vancouver Island Health Authority; (250)384-2622; Fax. (250)384-5660; lawrence@visionrejuvenation.com.

BRIERLEY, Yann; Vernon Jubilee Hosp, 2101 32 St, Vernon BC V1T 5L2; UBC'03; FRCPC; GenPath. Staff, Vernon Jubilee Hospital; (250)558-4115

BRIGDEN, Malcolm L; Chinook Reg Hosp, 960 19 St S, Lethbridge AB T1J 1W5; McG'71; DABIM; DABHem; DABOncol; DABPHemPath(HemPath); FACP; FRCPC; IntMed (Laboratory Hematology); Hem. Staff Oncology/Hematology, Chinook Regional Hospital; Langs: Bilingual(English/French); (403)388-6800; Fax. (403)327-4160; malcolm.brigden@albertahealthservices.ca.

BRIGEL, Paul H; Medical Arts Bldg, 120-1105 Pandora Ave, Victoria BC V8V 3P9; Tor'70; CCFP; Staff, Victoria General Hospital; Staff, Royal Jubilee Hospital; Clin Asst Prof Family Pract Residents, University of British Columbia; (250)383-9533; Fax. (250)383-0312.

BRIGGS, Alice E; North Toronto Med Bldg, 114-250 Lawrence Ave W, Toronto ON M5M 1B2; Tor'55; FRCPC; IntMed (Clinical Immunology & Allergy). Court Staff, Sunnybrook Health Sciences Centre; (416)590-0956; Fax. (416)590-0957; draebriggs@bellnet.ca.

BRIGGS, Deborah E; 1-106 Drynan Way PO Box 70, Seeleys Bay ON K0H 2N0; UBC'88; CCFP; FCFP; (613)387-3120; Fax. (613)387-2842.

BRIGGS, Martha M; Queen City Obstretrics & Gynec, 3271 Quance St E, Regina SK S4V 2V2; Qns'06; FRCSC; ObstGyn. Staff, Regina General Hospital; (306)585-9565

BRIGGS, Paul S; 204-600 Princess St, Woodstock ON N4S 4H4; Tor'82; Staff, Woodstock General Hospital; (519)537-7921; Fax. (519)421-9924.

BRIGGS, Robert P; Coronation Plaza, 104-14310 111 Ave NW, Edmonton AB T5M 3Z7; Wes'92; CCFP; FCFP; (780)342-0256

BRIGHAM, Sarah I; Riverside Family Health Team, 1967 Riverside Dr, Ottawa ON K1H 7W9; Qns'05; CCFP; (613)738-8219

BRIGHOUSE, M Ruth; PO Box 2770 Stn Main, Salmon Arm BC V1E 4R6; UBC'91; BSc; DTMH; Staff, Royal Inland Hospital; Staff, Shuswap Lake General Hospital; Staff, Kelowna General Hospital; (250)804-1666; Fax. (250)832-4400; ruthbrighouse@attglobal.net.

BRIGHT, Britt; Haney Health Associates, 22338 Selkirk Ave, Maple Ridge BC V2X 2X5; Dublin (Ireland)'71; FRCPC; Psy. Consultant, Ridge Meadows Hospital & Health Care Centre; Langs: Norwegian; (604)477-7202

BRIGHT, Howard L; 47515 Mountain Park Dr, Chilliwack BC V2P 7P7; UBC'77; CCFP; CCFP(E.M.); Ac Staff, Chilliwack General Hospital; Clin Assoc Prof Family Pract, University of British Columbia; (604)793-8137

BRIGHT, Hugh G J; Kingston After Hours Med Clini, 4-775 Strand Blvd, Kingston ON K7P 2S7; Tor'68; (613)389-1251

BRIGHT, Julia M; 9146 Mary St, Chilliwack BC V2P 4J1; UBC'05; CCFP; (604)792-5966; Fax. (604)792-5961.

BRIGHT, Michael A; 22315 Mcintosh Ave, Maple Ridge BC V2X 3C2; RCS (Ireland)'72; DAB; FRCSC; Ophth. Staff, Ridge Meadows Hospital & Health Care Centre; (604)467-1541; Fax. (604)467-1454.

BRIGHT, Phillip A; Kinetic Centre, 2-25 Bruce St, Kitchener ON N2B 1Y4; Bristol (England)'76; MB ChB; MRC; DRCOG; Aj Prof Kinesiology, University of Waterloo; (519)725-2640; Fax. (519)725-4064; drphilbright@kinetecrehab.com.

BRIGHT, Priscilla M; Bank Med Centre, 1935 Bank St, Ottawa ON K1V 8A3; Durham (England)'64; (613)521-2391 x140; Fax. (613)521-5443.

BRIGHT, Rachel E; George Street Fam Practice, 1-1400 George St, White Rock BC V4B 4A3; UBC'03; CCFP; (604)536-1686

BRIGHT, Susan E; BC Women's Hosp & Health Ctre, 4500 Oak St, Vancouver BC V6H 3N1; Wes'74; FRCPC; Anes. Staff, BC Women's Hospital & Health Centre; (604)875-2424

BRIJLALL, Shashi; Victoria Hosp, PO Box 3000 Stn Main 1200 24 St W, Prince Albert SK S6V 5T4; OrthSurg. Staff, Victoria Hospital; (306)953-8972; Fax. (306)953-8976.

BRIL, Vera; Div of Neurology UHN/MSH, 5 EC 309-200 Elizabeth St, Toronto ON M5G 2C4; Tor'74; FRCPC; Neur (Electromyography). Staff Neurol & Med, Toronto General Hospital - UHN; Staff Neurol & Med, Mount Sinai Hospital; Prof Med, University of Toronto; (416)340-3315; vera.bril@utoronto.ca.

BRILL, Francine; 302-30 Prospect St, Newmarket ON L3Y 3S9; McM'86; FRCPC; Psy (Child & Adolescent Psychiatry). Staff Child & Family Clinic, Southlake Regional Health Centre; Langs: Hebrew; (289)803-2533

BRILL, Herbert; McMaster University, 1280 Main St W, Hamilton ON L8S 4K1; Wes'01; FRCPC; Peds; Gastroent. Staff, Hamilton Health Sciences Centre - McMaster Children's Hospital; (905)521-2100

BRILL, Stephanie; North Bay Reg Health Centre, 50 College Dr, North Bay ON P1B 0A4; McG'06; MDCM; CCFP; CCFP(E.M.); Staff, North Bay Regional Health Centre - Regional Mental Health; (705)474-7525

BRILL, Yoav; Medical Office, 208-840 Coxwell Ave, Toronto ON M4C 5T2; Tor'98; FRCSC; ObstGyn (Laparoscopy). Langs: Hebrew; (416)425-0112; Fax. (416)425-0229.

BRILL-EDWARDS, Michele; Children's Hosp Eastern Ont, 401 Smyth Rd, Ottawa ON K1H 8L1; Tor'73; FRCPC; Peds. Staff, Children's Hospital of Eastern Ontario (CHEO); (613)737-2328

BRILZ, Anthony P; Saskatoon City Hosp, 701 Queen St, Saskatoon SK S7K 0M7; Sask'91; CCFP; CCFP(E.M.); FCFP; Staff, Saskatoon City Hospital; (306)655-8230

BRILZ, Beverly V; 201 9 St, Wainwright AB T9W 1C5; Cal'80; BSc; CCFP; FCFP; Staff, Wainwright Health Centre; (780)842-5829

BRIMBLE, Scott; St Joseph's Healthcare, 50 Charlton Ave E, Hamilton ON L8N 4A6; Tor'96; MSc; FRCPC; FRCPC; Nephrol; IntMed. Staff, St Joseph's Healthcare - Charlton Campus; Staff, Hamilton Health Sciences Centre - McMaster Children's Hospital; Asst Prof Med, McMaster University; (905)522-1155 x33787; Fax. (905)521-6153.

BRIMO, Fadi; MUHC-Montreal Gen Hosp, D3.253-1650 av Cedar, Montreal QC H3G 1A4; Damascus (Syria)'01; FRCPC; AnatPath. Staff, McGill University Health Centre - Montreal General Campus; (514)934-1934 x43843

BRIND'AMOUR, Thomas; SMBD Jewish Gen Hosp, 3755 ch Cote-Sainte-Catherine, Montreal QC H3T 1E2; Sher'08; CCFP; Staff, Sir Mortimer B Davis Jewish General; (514)340-8213

BRINDLE, Mary E; Alberta Children's Hosp, 2888 Shaganappi Trail NW, Calgary AB T3B 6A8; Dal'98; FRCSC; GenSurg; PedGenSurg. Staff, Alberta Children's Hospital; (403)955-2848

BRINDLEY, Peter G; University of Alberta Hosp, 3C1.12-8440 112 St NW, Edmonton AB T6G 2B7; UBC'96; FRCPC; IntMed; Critical Care Medicine. Staff, University of Alberta Hospital; (780)407-7381; Fax. (780)407-6018.

BRINK, Anette; Chilliwack Gen Hosp, 45600 Menholm St, Chilliwack BC V2P 1P7; Stellenbosch (South Africa)'75; MB ChB; Staff, Chilliwack General Hospital; (604)795-4121

BRINK, Christiaan; 101-436 Lorne St, Kamloops BC V2C 1W3; Pretoria (South Africa)'95; MB ChB; CCFP; (250)372-3828; Fax. (250)372-3835; chrisbrink90@msn.com.

BRINK, Johann H; Forensic Psychiatric Hosp, 70 Colony Farm Rd, Coquitlam BC V3C 5X9; Cape Town (South Africa)'74; MB BS; FFPsy(S.A.); FRCPC; Psy (Forensic Psychiatry). Dir-Research, Forensic Psychiatric Hospital; Clin Dir, Regional Treatment Centre & Pacific Institution; Dir Clinical Services/Scientific, Forensic Psychiatric Services Commission-Kamloops; Clin Prof Psy, University of British Columbia; Asst Prof School of Criminology, Simon Fraser University; Langs: Afrikaans; Dutch; (604)524-7702; Fax. (604)524-7905; jbrink@forensic.bc.ca.

BRINK, Rosemary L; 10830 Dallain Pl, North Saanich BC V8L 5M7; Cape Town (South Africa)'88; MB ChB; (250)655-4569

BRINKERHOFF, John; Beach Avenue Med Clinic, RR 7 5848D Beach Ave, Peachland BC V0H 1X7; Alb'88; CCFP; FCFP; (250)767-3432; Fax. (250)767-2993; beachmed@telus.net.

BRINKMAN, Shauna E; Selkirk & District Gen Hosp, PO Box 5000 Stn Main 100 Easton Dr, Selkirk MB R1A 2M2; Man'07; FRCPC; DiagRad. Staff, Selkirk & District General Hospital; (204)482-5800

BRIONES-URBINA, Rosario; Women's College Hosp, 446-76 Grenville St, Toronto ON M5S 1B2; Central (Ecuador)'78; FRCPC; IntMed; Endocrin&Metab. Staff, Women's College Hospital; Asst Prof Med, University of Toronto; Langs: Spanish; (416)323-6088; Fax. (416)323-6093.

BRIOUX, Joseph E; 203-600 Princess St, Woodstock ON N4S 4H4; Tor'88; Med Staff, Woodstock General Hospital; (519)421-7252; Fax. (519)421-9924.

BRISBIN, Donald P; 202-857 Grand Ave W, Chatham ON N7L 4T1; Qns'80; BScChemEng; MSc; FRCPC; IntMed. Consultant IntMed, Chatham-Kent Health Alliance; (519)351-9277; Fax. (519)351-9278.

BRISCO, E Bertha; 211-125 13th St E, North Vancouver BC V7L 2L3; UBC'73; (604)988-0209; Fax. (604)988-0453.

BRISCO, Eric J; 211-125 13th St E, North Vancouver BC V7L 2L3; UBC'70; (604)988-5526; Fax. (604)988-0453.

BRISCOE, Natalie K; Nepean Med Centre, 401-1 Centrepointe Dr, Nepean ON K2G 6E2; Ott'05; FRCPC; Neur. (613)225-3014; Fax. (613)321-8369.

BRISEBOIS, Amanda J; Grey Nuns Community Hosp & HC, 1100 Youville Drive West NW, Edmonton AB T6L 5X8; Cal'95; MSc; FRCPC; IntMed. Med Staff, Covenant Health - Grey Nuns Community Hospital; Clinical Asst Prof, University of Alberta; (780)407-6632

BRISEBOIS, Johnny D; Kanata Prof Centre, 103-99 Kakulu Rd, Kanata ON K2L 3C8; Alb'93; CCFP; Staff Emerg, Kemptville District Hospital; Staff Emerg, Deep River & District Hospital; Langs: Spanish; French; (613)592-1448; Fax. (613)591-3778.

BRISEBOIS, Ronald J; University of Alberta Hosp, 2D4 48 WCM-8440 112 St NW, Edmonton AB T6G 2B7; Sask'88; FRCSC; GenSurg (Critical Care Medicine). Staff, University of Alberta Hospital; Asst Prof, University of Alberta; Langs: Bilingual(English/French); (780)407-6632; ronaldbrisebois@shaw.ca.

BRISKIN, Alexander; St Joseph's Health Care, PO Box 5777 Stn B 268 Grosvenor St, London ON N6A 4V2; Jerusalem (Israel)'97; Staff, St Joseph's Hospital - St Joseph's Health Care; (519)646-6000 x64218

BRISKIN, Jonathan K; Brant Community HC-Brantford, 200 Terrace Hill St, Brantford ON N3R 1G9; Tufts(MA) (USA)'89; FRCPC; Psy (Forensic Psychiatry). Staff, The Brant Community Healthcare System - Brantford General Hospital Site; (519)751-5885

BRISON, Meghan L; Vancouver Gen Hosp, 3300-855 12th Ave W, Vancouver BC V5Z 1M9; McM'08; Staff, Vancouver General Hospital - Centennial Pavillion; (604)875-5242

BRISON, Robert J; Kingston Gen Hosp, 76 Stuart St, Kingston ON K7L 2V7; Qns'77; FRCPC; EmergMed;CCFP; Staff, Kingston General Hospital; (613)548-2368; Fax. (613)548-1381.

BRISSEAU, Guy F; IWK Health Centre, PO Box 9700 Rpo CSC 5980 University Ave, Halifax NS B3K 6R8; Dal'89; FRCSC; GenSurg; PedGenSurg. Staff, IWK Health Centre; (902)470-8114

BRISSETTE, Alain; CHUM-Hop St-Luc, 1058 rue Saint-Denis, Montreal QC H2X 3J4; Mon'74; Staff, Centre Hospitalier l'Université De Montréal (CHUM) - Hôpital Saint-luc; (514)890-8000 x36360

BRISSETTE, Claude; Clinique Med St-Jerome, 102-450 boul Monseigneur-Duboi, Saint-Jerome QC J7Y 3L8; Mon'80; Staff, Hôtel-Dieu de Saint-Jérôme; Langs: English; (450)438-1776; Fax. (450)438-6119.

BRISSETTE, Suzanne; CHUM-Hop St-Luc, 1058 rue Saint-Denis, Montreal QC H2X 3J4; Mon'84; Staff, Centre Hospitalier l'Université De Montréal (CHUM) - Hôpital Saint-luc; (514)890-8000 x36553; Fax. (514)412-7295.

BRISSETTE, Sylvie; Clinique Med Adoncour, 505 rue Adoncour, Longueuil QC J4G 2M6; Laval'82; (450)646-4445; Fax. (450)646-5526.

BRISSON, Dennis A T; 401-1368 Ouellette Ave, Windsor ON N8X 1J9; Ott'57; Otol (Head & Neck). Staff, Windsor Regional Hospital - Metropolitan Site; Staff, Hôtel-Dieu Grace Hospital; Langs: Bilingual(English/French); (519)253-2710

BRISSON, Fernand; Clinique Med Lauzon, 213 rue Saint-Joseph, Levis QC G6V 1C8; Laval'73; LMCC; (418)833-5040; Fax. (418)833-6954.

BRISSON, Guy; 303-1600 boul Curé-Labelle, Laval QC H7V 2W2; Mon'78; (450)681-4213; Fax. (450)681-7673; drguybrisson@bellnet.ca.

BRISSON, Henri; CSSS Pierre Boucher, 1333 boul Jacques-Cartier E, Longueuil QC J4M 2A5; McM'98; FRCPC; Psy. Staff, Centre Hospitalier Pierre Boucher; Langs: English; French; (450)468-8401; Fax. (450)468-8403.

BRISSON, Jacques; U de Laval-Pav Ferdinand-Vandr, 1050 av de la Medecine, Quebec QC G1K 7P4; Laval'73; (418)682-7392

BRISSON, Jacynthe; CSSS de la Mitis, 800 av du Sanatorium, Mont-Joli QC G5H 3L6; Laval'78; Médecin, CSSS de la Mitis; (418)775-7261 x3145; Fax. (418)775-1989.

BRISSON, Kathleen; Clinique Med Familiale, 101 rue Lavoie, Rimouski QC G5L 5Y2; Laval'91; (418)723-5272; Fax. (418)725-2030.

BRISSON, Louis J; Windsor Reg Hosp-Metropolitan, 1995 Lens Ave, Windsor ON N8W 1L9; Ott'88; FRCPC; DiagRad. Staff, Windsor Regional Hospital - Metropolitan Site; (519)254-5577

BRISSON, Mario; Sante Saguenay-lac-Saint-Jean, 412 rue Brassard, Roberval QC G8H 3P7; Sher'77; (418)275-4980; Fax. (418)275-6670.

BRISSON, Melanie; CHUQ-St-Francois-D'Assise, 10 rue de l'Espinay, Quebec QC G1L 3L5; Laval'02; CCFP; Staff FamMed, Centre Hospitalier Universitaire De Québec - Pavillon De St-françois-d'assise; (418)525-4351

BRISSON, Melanie; Ctr Hosp Affilie-Enfant-Jesus, 1401 18e rue, Quebec QC G1J 1Z4; Laval'02; FRCPC; DiagRad. Staff, Centre Hospitalier Affilié Universitaire de Québec - Hôpital De L'Enfant Jésus; (418)649-0252

BRISSON, Michel; Unite Med Familiale Maizerets, 2480 ch de la Canardiere, Quebec QC G1J 2G1; Laval'87; Clin Prof Family Med & Clin Monitor, Centre Hospitalier Affilié Universitaire de Québec - Hôpital De L'Enfant Jésus; assoc Staff, Centre Hospitalier Universitaire De Québec - Pavillon De St-françois-d'assise; Langs: English; (418)661-1413; Fax. (418)661-7504; mibrisson42@hotmail.com.

BRISSON, Nancy; Ctr Hosp Rouyn-Noranda, 4 9e rue, Rouyn-Noranda QC J9X 2B2; Laval'06; CCFP; Staff, Centre Hospitalier Rouyn-Noranda; (819)764-5131

BRISSON, Paul; 18-6497 Jeanne D'Arc Blvd N, Orleans ON K1C 2R1; Ott'70; DAB; FRCPC; Derm (Administration). Consultant, The Ottawa Hospital - General Campus; Asst Prof Derm, University of Ottawa; Langs: English; French; (613)841-8500

BRISSON, Pierre; CLSC Hochelaga-Maisonneuve, 4201 rue Ontario E, Montreal QC H1V 1K2; Mon'73; (514)253-2181; Fax. (514)253-4550.

BRISSON, Sonia L; CSSSG-Hop de Gatineau, CP 2000 Succ Bureau-Chef 909 boul de la Verendrye, Gatineau QC J8P 7H2; Laval'90; FRCPC; MedOncol (P.Q.). Staff, Hôpital de Gatineau; (819)966-6100; Fax. (819)966-6289.

BRISSON, Suzanne; Dir de la Sante Publique de Mt, 1301 rue Sherbrooke E, Montreal QC H2L 1M3; Mon'80; ac Staff, Hopital Maisonneuve-Rosemont; (514)528-2400

BRISSON, Vincent; CSSS de Rimouski-Neigette, CP 3150 Succ A 150 av Rouleau, Rimouski QC G5L 5T1; Laval'06; FRCSC; GenSurg. Staff, Hôpital Regional Rimouski; (418)724-3000

BRISSON-JOSEPH, Andre; Clinique Med St-Andre, 102-8133 av André-Ampère, Montreal QC H1E 3J9; (Mexico)'80; ac Staff, CSSS Saint-Leonard et Saint-Michel; (514)648-6888

BRISTER, Stephanie J; Univ Hlth Network-The Toronto, 4N 472-200 Elizabeth St, Toronto ON M5G 2C4; Cal'79; FRCSC; GenSurg (Cardiac Surgery); Cardiovasc&ThorSurg. Staff, Toronto General Hospital - UHN; Assoc Prof, University of Toronto; (416)340-4945; Fax. (416)340-4946; stephanie.brister@uhn.ca.

BRISTOL, Roger; Royal University Hosp, 103 Hospital Dr, Saskatoon SK S7N 0W8; Sask'06; CCFP; CCFP(E.M.); Staff, Royal University Hospital; (306)655-1364; Fax. (306)655-1258.

BRISTOL, Sean G; Gordon & Leslie Diamond HCC, L3-2775 Laurel St, Vancouver BC V5Z 1M9; UBC'01; FRCSC; PlasSurg (Peripheral Nerve Surgery). Ac Staff, Providence Health Care - St Paul's Hospital; Ac Staff, Vancouver General Hospital - Centennial Pavillion; Staff, BC Children's Hospital; Staff, Gordon & Leslie Diamond Health Care Centre; (604)875-5866; Fax. (604)875-5861; sean.bristol@vch.ca.

BRISTOW, Kristin M; St Boniface Gen Hosp, South M1-409 Tache Ave, Winnipeg MB R2H 2A6; Cal'02; FRCPC; Psy (Anxiety Disorder). Staff Child & Adolescent Mental Health Prog, St Boniface General Hospital; Asst Prof Psy Faculty of Med, University of Manitoba; (204)237-2677; Fax. (204)235-3852.

BRISTOW, Robert G; Univ Hlth Network-Princess M, 923-610 University Ave, Toronto ON M5G 2M9; Tor'92; PhD; FRCPC; RadOncol. Scientist, Princess Margaret Hospital - University Health Network; Staff, Toronto General Hospital - UHN; Scientist, Ontario Cancer Institute; Asst Prof RadOncol & Med Biophysics, University of Toronto; (416)946-4501 x2129; Fax. (416)946-4442; rbristow@uhnres.utoronto.ca.

BRISTOW, Stanley G; PO Box 1227 Stn Main, Rocky-Mtn-House AB T4T 1A9; Alb'72; Staff, Rocky Mountain House Health Centre; (403)845-6227

BRISTOWE, J R Bruce; Radiology Consultants Assoc, 120A-6707 Elbow Dr SW, Calgary AB T2V 0E3; Tor'71; FRCPC; DiagRad. Staff Radiol, Peter Lougheed Centre; (403)777-3003; Fax. (403)777-3008.

BRITS, Annalie W; South Hill Med Practice, 5-2685 2nd Ave W, Prince Albert SK S6V 5E3; Pretoria (South Africa) MB ChB; (306)922-9570; Fax. (306)922-2513.

BRITS, Bernice; Saunte Medical Clinic, 101-15850 26th Ave, Surrey BC V3S 2N6; Pretoria (South Africa)'82; MB ChB; CCFP; Langs: Afrikaans; German.

BRITS, Nico; Saskatoon City Hosp, 5518-701 Queen St, Saskatoon SK S7K 0M7; Pretoria (South Africa)'90; MB ChB; MMed(Path); FRCPC; AnatPath. Staff, Saskatoon City Hospital; Staff, St Paul's Hospital (Grey Nuns) of Saskatoon; Clinical Asst Prof, University of Saskatchewan; Langs: Afrikaans; (306)655-8717; Fax. (306)655-8399; nbrits@paphr.sk.ca.

BRITT-COTE, Maxime S R; 31 CF Health Services Centre, PO Box 1000 Stn Main 30 rte Ortona Rd, Borden ON L0M 1C0; Ott'10; CCFP; (705)424-1200

BRITTAIN, Rodney W; Canadian Forces Supp Unit HCC, 1745 Alta Vista Dr, Ottawa ON K1A 0K6; Mem'89; MPH; CCFP; Staff Directorate Health Services Operations, Canadian Forces Health Services Centre; (613)945-6595; Fax. (613)945-6668.

BRITTEN, Heather F; Teen Health Centre, 1585 Ouellette Ave, Windsor ON N8X 1K5; McM'94; CCFP; FCFP; Langs: French; Fax. (519)253-8481; gmichie1@ford.com.

BRITTO, Ericka L; Community Health Centre, PO Box 627 851 16 St NE, Salmon Arm BC V1E 4N7; Madras (India)'87; MB BS; FRCPC; Psy (Adult General Psychiatry). Staff, Shuswap Lake General Hospital; Langs: Tamil; Telugu; (250)833-4102

BRITTO, Santosh A; Shuswap Lake Gen Hosp, PO Box 520 Stn Main 601 10 St NE, Salmon Arm BC V1E 4N6; Bangalore (India)'84; MB BS; FRCSC; GenSurg (Oncology). General Surgery, Kootenay Lake General Hospital; Staff, Boundary Hospital; Staff, Kootenay Boundary Regional Hospital; Langs: Hindi; Kanarese; Konkani; Tamil; (250)803-8177; santosh.britto@interiorhealth.ca.

BRITTON, Brian H; 504-825 Granville St, Vancouver BC V6Z 1K9; Sask'82; (604)569-0550

BRITTON, Emmanuelle; Southeast Toronto Family HT, 1871 Danforth Ave, Toronto ON M4C 1J3; McG'08; CCFP; Staff, Toronto Western Hospital - University Health Network; (416)699-7775; Fax. (416)699-7776.

BRITTON, Robert J; Nepean Med Centre, 206-1 Centrepointe Dr, Nepean ON K2G 6E2; Ott'80; FRCSC; Ophth. (613)226-3335; Fax. (613)226-3337.

BRITTON, Stephen E A; Natawihin/Nakasuwenik Clinic, GD, Ile-A-La-Crosse SK S0M 1C0; Dal'84; BSc; CCFP; Staff Family Med, St Joseph's Hospital; Clin Lecturer Family Med, University of Saskatchewan; (306)833-2044; Fax. (306)833-2041.

BRITTON-FOSTER, Michael B; Elliot Lake Family Health Team, 31 Nova Scotia Walk, Elliot Lake ON P5A 1Y9; Cal'82; Ac Staff, St Joseph's General Hospital Elliot Lake; (705)848-3673; Fax. (705)848-3449; mbf@inorth.on.ca.

BRITTON-FOSTER, Timothy S; Hillside Med Centre, PO Box 700 Stn Main 541 3 Ave, Ladysmith BC V9G 1A5; Cal'85; CCFP; (250)245-2235; Fax. (250)245-3094.

BRITTON JR, William A A; The Retina Centre of Ottawa, 500-1565 Carling Ave, Ottawa ON K1Z 8R1; Ott'79; AB; FRCSC; Ophth. Staff, The Ottawa Hospital - General Campus; Staff, Children's Hospital of Eastern Ontario (CHEO); Staff, The Ottawa Hospital - Civic Campus; University of Ottawa; (613)722-1517; Fax. (613)722-4811.

BRIZARD, Frederic; CSSS du Nord de Lanaudière, 1000 boul Sainte-Anne, St-Charles-Brromee QC J6E 6J2; Mon'02; Staff, Centre Hospitalier Régional de Lanaudière; (450)759-8222; Fax. (450)759-7776.

BRIZARD, Martin; GMF Concorde, 300 boul de la Concorde E, Laval QC H7G 2E6; Mon'84; Staff, Hopital de la Cite de la santé; Universite de Montreal; (450)667-5310; Fax. (450)667-5248.

BRIZARD, Michele; Maison Aube-Lumiere, 220 rue Kennedy N, Sherbrooke QC J1E 2E7; Sher'73; Staff Employees Health Serv, Centre Hospitalier Universitaire de Sherbrooke-Hopital Fleurimont; (819)821-3120

BRKOVICH, Andrea; 511 Erie St E, Windsor ON N9A 3X8; Wes'95; FRCSC; ObstGyn. Prof, University of Western Ontario; Langs: Bilingual(English/French); (519)253-6033; Fax. (519)253-6866.

BRNA, Paula M; IWK Health Centre, PO Box 9700 Rpo CSC 5850-5980 University Ave, Halifax NS B3K 6R8; Dal'01; FRCPC; Peds (Epilepsy); Neur. Staff, IWK Health Centre; (902)470-8888; Fax. (902)470-8486.

BROAD, Karyn D; Dr Everett Chalmers Hosp, PO Box 9000 Stn A, Fredericton NB E3B 5N5; Mem'87; Ac Staff, Dr Everett Chalmers Regional Hospital; (506)452-5400

BROAD, Robert W; University of Alberta Hosp, 2D1.02 WCM-8440 112 St NW, Edmonton AB T6G 2B7; Alb'76; FRCSC; Neursurg. Staff, University of Alberta Hospital; Clinical Asst Prof, University of Alberta; (780)407-8296; Fax. (780)407-8203.

BROADERS, Marguerite A; St Clare's Mercy Hosp, 154 Lemarchant Rd, St. John's NL A1C 5B8; Mem'98; FRCPC; Psy. Staff, St Clare's Mercy Hospital; (709)777-5390; Fax. (709)777-5093.

BROADY, Raewyn C; Gordon & Leslie Diamond HCC, 10F-2775 Laurel St, Vancouver BC V5Z 1M9; Otago (New Zealand)'90; MB ChB; Staff, Vancouver General Hospital - Centennial Pavillion; Staff, Gordon & Leslie Diamond Health Care Centre; (604)875-4952

BROCHET, Francois; CSSS de Chicoutimi, 305 rue Saint-Vallier, Chicoutimi QC G7H 5H6; Nancy (France)'77; RadOncol(Fr); Chef radio-oncol, Complexe hospitalier de la Sagamie; Langs: Italian; English; (418)541-1032; Fax. (418)541-1128.

BROCHET, Nicolas; CSSS de Chicoutimi, 305 rue Saint-Vallier, Chicoutimi QC G7H 5H6; Mon'98; FRCPC; RadOncol. Staff Service de Radio-Oncologie, Complexe hospitalier de la Sagamie; (418)541-1032

BROCHU, Annie; CHUQ-St-Francois d'Assise, 10 rue de l'Espinay, Quebec QC G1L 3L5; Laval'94; CCFP; Staff, Centre Hospitalier Universitaire De Québec - Pavillon De St-françois-d'assise; Staff Family Med, CSSS de la Vielle Capitale; Langs: Bilingual(French/English); (418)525-4351; Fax. (418)525-4322.

BROCHU, Bernard; CSSS de la Cote-de-Gaspe, 215 boul de York O, Gaspe QC G4X 2W2; Laval'98; DiagRad. Staff, Centre Hospitalier de Gaspe; (418)368-3301

BROCHU, Caroline; CLSC Point de Service Camirand, 50 rue Camirand, Sherbrooke QC J1H 4J5; Sher'04; (819)565-5370

BROCHU, Chantal; Clinique Med St-Etienne, 2-965 Rte Lagueux, St-Etienne-de Lauz QC G6J 1T5; Sher'98; Langs: Bilingual(French/English); (418)831-9538; Fax. (418)831-8552; chantalbrochu@hotmail.com.

BROCHU, Daniel; Clinique Med Lac-Megantic, 101-5256 rue Frontenac, Lac-Megantic QC G6B 1H3; Laval'71; Staff, Carrefour Sante Granit; (819)583-3347; Fax. (819)583-3347.

BROCHU, Gaetan; CHUQ-Ctr Hosp Univ Laval, 2211-2705 boul Laurier, Quebec QC G1V 4G2; Laval'91; BSc; FRCSC; GenSurg (Laparoscopic Surgery). Staff Surgeon, Centre Hospitalier Universitaire de Quebec-CHUL; Clin Prof Surg, Université Laval; Langs: Bilingual(French/English); (418)654-2259; gaetan.brochu@chg.ulaval.ca.

BROCHU, Gilles B; Clinique Med Chemin St-Jean, 102-675 ch de Saint-Jean, La Prairie QC J5R 2L2; Laval'68; (450)444-2002; Fax. (450)444-4920.

BROCHU, Ian; Gynecology Associates, 100-235 boul René-Lévesque E, Montreal QC H2X 1N8; Mon'03; FRCSC; ObstGyn. (514)866-2446

BROCHU, Isabelle; CSSS de la Matapedia, 135 av Gaetan-Archambault, Amqui QC G5J 2K5; Laval'97; CCFP; Staff, CSSS de la Matapedia; (418)629-2211

BROCHU, Jacques; Ctr Hosp Affilie-Enfant-Jesus, 1401 18e rue, Quebec QC G1J 1Z4; Laval'82; CSPQ; FRCPC; Anes. Staff, Centre Hospitalier Affilié Universitaire de Québec - Hôpital De L'Enfant Jésus; (418)649-5807; Fax. (418)649-5936.

BROCHU, Jean E; Bureau de Coroner, 11F-1701 rue Parthenais, Montreal QC H2K 3S7; Sher'78; Coroner, Government Of Quebec; (514)873-3284; Fax. (514)873-8943.

BROCHU, Jean-Guy; Clinique Medicale Nicolet, 106-1691 boul Louis-Frechette, Nicolet QC J3T 1Z6; Laval'67; Staff, Hôpital de Christ-Roi; (819)293-2022; Fax. (819)293-2024.

BROCHU, Jocelyne; Clinique d'Ophtalmologie Belle, 4135 rue de Rouen, Montreal QC H1V 1G5; Mon'71; FRCSC; Ophth. Staff, Centre Hospitalier de Verdun; Langs: English; (514)256-0007

BROCHU, Lise; Clinique Sud-Est, 7070 boul Perras, Montreal QC H1E 1A4; Laval'67; Psy (P.Q.) (Adult Psychiatry). Staff Child Psy, Hôpital Riviere des Prairies; adj Prof, Universite de Montreal; Langs: Bilingual(English/French); (514)323-7260 x4519; lise.brochu.hrdp@ssss.gouv.qc.ca.

BROCHU, Marie-Claude; CHUS-Hop Fleurimont, 3001 12e Av N, Sherbrooke QC J1H 5N4; Sher'95; FRCPC; IntMed; Cardiol. Staff, Centre Hospitalier Universitaire de Sherbrooke-Hopital Fleurimont; (819)346-1110; Fax. (819)820-6897.

BROCHU, Marie-Claude; CHUQ-St-Francois d'Assise, 10 rue de l'Espinay, Quebec QC G1L 3L5; Laval'02; FRCPC; DiagRad. Staff, Centre Hospitalier Universitaire De Québec - Pavillon De St-françois-d'assise; (418)525-4444

BROCHU, Michel; 150-930 ch Sainte-Foy, Quebec QC G1S 2L4; Laval'85; FRCPC; Psy. Ac Staff, Hôtel-Dieu de Lévis; (418)688-7272; Fax. (418)527-0053.

BROCHU, Michele; CSSS du Haut-Saint-Francois, 40 rue Dumoulin, La Patrie QC J0B 1Y0; Sher'90; Dir-svcs prof, Carrefour Sante Granit; (819)888-2811

BROCHU, Pierre; Ctr Hosp Affilie-Enfant-Jesus, 1401 18e rue, Quebec QC G1J 1Z4; Laval'70; EmergMed (P.Q.). Ac Staff, Centre Hospitalier Affilié Universitaire de Québec - Hôpital De L'Enfant Jésus; (418)649-5555

BROCHU, Pierre; Hôpital Ste-Justine, 3175 ch Cote-Sainte-Catherine, Montreal QC H3T 1C5; Mon'67; CSPQ; GenPath (P.Q.) (Pediatric Pathology). Ac Staff Path, Hôpital Ste-Justine; Clin Assoc Prof, Universite de Montreal; (514)345-4649; pierre_brochu@ssss.gouv.qc.ca.

BROCHU, Richard; Clin de Med Familiale de Hull, 202-15 boul Montclair, Gatineau QC J8Y 2E2; Laval'83; Ac Staff, Hull Hospital; (819)777-7668; Fax. (819)777-2269; richardbrochu@videotron.ca.

BROCHU, Stephanie; Centre Hosp Honore-Mercier, 2750 boul Laframboise, Saint-Hyacinthe QC J2S 4Y8; Laval'96; FRCPC; Psy. Staff, Centre Hospitalier Honore-Mercier; (450)771-3333; Fax. (450)771-3273.

BROCHU-BLAIN, Annie; Inst U en Sante Mentale de QC, 2601 ch de la Canardiere, Quebec QC G1J 2G3; Mon'00; FRCPC; Psy. Staff, Institut Universitaire Sante; (418)663-5321 x6525

BROCK, A Jeffrey; 210-750 boul Marcel-Laurin, Saint-Laurent QC H4M 2M4; McG'83; Med Dir, Med Extra; (514)522-8000; Fax. (514)526-4521; jbrock@medextra.com.

BROCK, Carol A; North York Med Arts Bldg, 225-1333 Sheppard Ave E, North York ON M2J 1V1; Wes'72; CGPP; Court Staff, North York General Hospital; (416)494-7431; Fax. (416)494-7796.

BROCK, Gerald B; St Joseph's Health Care, PO Box 5777 Stn B 268 Grosvenor St, London ON N6A 4V2; McG'86; MDCM; FRCSC; Urol (Erectile Dysfunction). Staff, St Joseph's Hospital - St Joseph's Health Care; (519)646-6042; Fax. (519)646-6037.

BROCK, Gordon I; Ctr de Sante de Temiscaming, 180 rue Anvik CP 760, Temiscaming QC J0Z 3R0; Qns'76; CCFP; FCFP; Staff, Centre de santé de Témiscaming; adj Prof Family Med/Conférencier Anes, McGill University; Langs: English; French; (819)627-3385 x1238; Fax. (819)627-9932; gordon_brock@ssss.gouv.qc.ca.

BROCK, Jo-Ann K; IWK Health Centre, PO Box 9700 Rpo Csc 5850-5980 University Ave, Halifax NS B3K 6R8; Dal'03; FRCSC; ObstGyn (Maternal Fetal Medicine). Staff, IWK Health Centre; (902)470-8888; Fax. (902)425-1125.

BROCK, Jonathan H; Surrey Mem Hosp, 13750 96 Ave, Surrey BC V3V 1Z2; Qns'97; CCFP; CCFP(E.M.); Staff, Surrey Memorial Hospital; (604)588-3369; Fax. (604)588-3377.

BROCK, Robert M; North York Med Arts Bldg, 225-1333 Sheppard Ave E, North York ON M2J 1V1; Wes'71; DAB; Dip SportMed; FACS; FRCSC; OrthSurg (Sports Medicine). Staff, North York General Hospital; (416)494-7431; Fax. (416)494-7796.

BROCKEN, Arno A L; Grandin Med Clinic, 1 St Anne St, St. Albert AB T8N 2E8; (Netherlands)'87; (780)459-5581; Fax. (780)458-7515.

BROCKER, Johann F; Prince Rupert Reg Hosp, 227-1305 Summit Ave, Prince Rupert BC V8J 2A6; Stellenbosch (South Africa)'75; MB ChB; MMedIntMed; LMCC; Staff, Prince Rupert Regional Hospital; (250)622-6207; Fax. (250)622-6209.

BROCKLEY, Graham H; Ladysmith Family Practice Clin, PO Box 699 1111 4 Ave, Ladysmith BC V9G 1A5; Cal'90; MSc; CCFP; CCFP(E.M.); FCFP; (250)245-6540; Fax. (250)245-6541.

BROCKMAN, Angie; CSSS de Laval, 1755 boul Rene-Laennec, Laval QC H7M 3L9; Mon'10; CCFP; Staff, Hopital de la Cite de la santé; (450)975-5444

BROCKWAY, Andrew G; 270 Riddell St, Woodstock ON N4S 6N6; Wes'88; Staff, Woodstock General Hospital; Staff, Stratford General Hospital - Huron Perth Healthcare Alliance; Staff, Alexandra Hospital.

BROCKWAY, Wade; Montfort Hosp, 713 Montreal Rd, Ottawa ON K1K 0T2; Ott'07; CCFP; Staff, Montfort Hospital; (613)945-1460

BRODA, Russell J; Bannatyne Med Clinic, 101-825 Sherbrook St, Winnipeg MB R3A 1M5; Man'84.

BRODAREC, Ivan; Atlantic Ear Nose & Throat Ins, 39 John St, Yarmouth NS B5A 3H4; Zagreb (Croatia)'73; Staff, Roseway Hospital; Staff Otol/Gen Surg, Yarmouth Regional Hospital; Staff, Digby General Hospital; Langs: Croatian; German; (902)742-2994; Fax. (902)742-2994.

BRODE, Sarah K; Univ of Toronto, 6263-1 King's College Cir, Toronto ON M5S 1A8; Tor'07; FRCPC; IntMed; Respir.

BRODER, Sarah L; Penticton Reg Hosp, 102-550 Carmi Ave, Penticton BC V2A 3G6; McM'90; FRCPC; IntMed (Intensive Care); Respir. Staff IntMed, Penticton Regional Hospital; Clinical Asst Prof, University of British Columbia; (250)493-0887; Fax. (250)493-7484.

BRODERICK, David J; Cobourg Med Centre, 5-1060 Burnham St, Cobourg ON K9A 5V9; Qns'84; BMechEng; Chief of Staff, Northumberland Hills Hospital; (905)373-8333; Fax. (905)373-9333.

BRODERICK, Vina L; Health Sciences Centre, 300 Prince Philip Dr, St. John's NL A1B 3V6; Mem'86; CCFP; FCFP; Staff Family Practice Unit, Health Sciences Centre; (709)777-6112

BRODERSEN, Anne F; CLSC St-Leonard, 5540 rue Jarry E, Saint-Leonard QC H1P 1T9; Mon'85; (514)328-3460; Fax. (514)328-8954.

BRODEUR, Andre; Bureau Reg CSST Laval, 200-1700 boul Laval, Laval QC H7S 2G6; Mon'66; PlasSurg. Ac Staff, Hôpital du Sacre-Coeur de Montréal; adj Prof, Universite de Montreal; (450)967-3209; Fax. (450)662-8898.

BRODEUR, Anne; Clinique Ped Ste-Foy, 295-2600 boul Laurier, Quebec QC G1V 4T3; Sher'81; Peds. Ac Staff, Centre Hospitalier Universitaire de Quebec-CHUL; Ac Staff, Centre Hospitalier Affilié Universitaire de Québec - Hôpital du St-Sacrement; Consultant, CSSS de Quebec-Sud; (418)658-0906

BRODEUR, Benoit; Ctr Hosp Fleury, 2180 rue Fleury E, Montreal QC H2B 1K3; Mon'94; MCFP(EM); CCFP; Staff, Centre Hospitalier Fleury; (514)381-9311

BRODEUR, Catherine; MUHC-Montreal Gen Hosp, D17 173-1650 av Cedar, Montreal QC H3G 1A4; Sher'98; FRCPC; IntMed; GeriatricMed. Staff, McGill University Health Centre - Montreal General Campus; (514)934-8015; Fax. (514)934-8286; cbrodeur.iugs@ssss.gouv.qc.ca.

BRODEUR, Guillaume; Centre Hosp Honore-Mercier, 2750 boul Laframboise, Saint-Hyacinthe QC J2S 4Y8; Sher'03; Gastroent; IntMed. Staff, Centre Hospitalier Honore-Mercier; (450)771-3333

BRODEUR, Isabelle; Clinique Med du Luc, 33 rue Saint-Patrice E, Magog QC J1X 5B7; Mon'95; Staff, Centre Hospitalier et CLSC de Memphremagog; (819)843-3353; Fax. (819)843-7217.

BRODEUR, Jennifer F; SCOHS-Elisabeth Bruyere Hosp, 284J-43 Bruyere St, Ottawa ON K1N 5C8; Ott'09; CCFP; Staff, SCO Health Service - Élisabeth Bruyère Hospital; (613)562-6262

BRODEUR, Jules; 5584 boul Maurice-Duplessis, Montreal-Nord QC H1G 1X9; Mon'61; MSc(Pharm.); PhD(Pharm); Consultant Commun Med, Hopital Charles LeMoyne; Consultant Commun Med, Hopital Maisonneuve-Rosemont; Emeritus Prof Med, Universite de Montreal; brodej@videotron.ca.

BRODEUR, Marie-Claude; Hop Charles LeMoyne, 3120 boul Taschereau, Greenfield Park QC J4V 2H1; Mon'02; CCFP; CCFP(E.M.); Staff, Hopital Charles LeMoyne; (450)466-5000

BRODEUR, Michel; Clinique Med La Providence, 16405 av Bourdages S, Saint-Hyacinthe QC J2T 4G9; Mon'84; Staff, Centre Hospitalier Honore-Mercier; (450)773-6734; Fax. (450)773-9909.

BRODEUR-GIRARD, Sophie; Clinique Med 3000 Inc, 3000 rue Belanger, Montreal QC H1Y 1A9; Sher'98; (514)376-7702; Fax. (514)376-2639.

BRODIE, Beverly L; 11 Stratford Rd, Stratford PE C1B 1T4; Cal'80; BSc; MD; FRCSC; ObstGyn (Reproductive Endocrinology & Infertility). Ac Staff Div of Reproductive Endocrinology, Queen Elizabeth Hospital; (902)569-9133; Fax. (902)569-9188; twodocs@eastlink.ca.

BRODIE, Brian D; 100F-6640 Vedder Rd, Chilliwack BC V2R 0J2; Cal'86; Dir-Res Serv, Burnslake Christian Support Services; Clin Preceptor Family Training Prog, University of British Columbia; (604)858-2246; Fax. (604)858-4498.

BRODIE, Deborah J; Lakeside Med Clinic, 3919 8th St E, Saskatoon SK S7H 5M7; Ott'82; CCFP; FCFP; Assoc Staff ObstGyn & Peds, Royal University Hospital; Court Staff, Saskatoon City Hospital; Ac Staff, St Paul's Hospital (Grey Nuns) of Saskatoon; Staff Med, Saskatoon District Health Board; Asst Prof, University of Saskatchewan; (306)374-6884; Fax. (306)374-2552.

BRODIE, Dennis J T; Halton-McMaster Fam Health Ctr, 208-3155 Harvester Rd, Burlington ON L7N 3V2; Ott'73; BSc; CCFP; FCFP; Ac Staff Family Med, Joseph Brant Memorial Hospital; Assoc Prof Family Med, McMaster University; Langs: Bilingual(English/French); (905)333-8222; Fax. (905)333-9343.

BRODIE, Douglas W; Stouffville Med Centre, 34 Civic Ave, Stouffville ON L4A 1H2; Tor'54; CCFP; Ac Staff, Rouge Valley Health System - Centenary Health Centre Site; (905)640-3100

BRODIE, Glen; 540 St George Blvd, Moncton NB E1E 2B5; Dal'68; FRCSC; ObstGyn. Prog Dir Maternal Child Health, The Moncton Hospital; Asst Prof, Dalhousie University; (506)857-2166; Fax. (506)854-4472; jbrodie9386@rogers.com.

BRODIE, Lauren; Cape Breton Healthcare Complex, 1482 George St, Sydney NS B1P 1P3; Dal'09; CCFP; Staff, Cape Breton Healthcare Complex; (902)565-2441

BRODIE, Richard J; 546 Brimley Rd, Scarborough ON M1J 1A8; Tor'86; DAAPM; CCFP; Ac Staff Family Pract, The Scarborough Hospital - General Campus; Clin Instructor Family & CommunMed, University of Toronto; (416)267-6961; Fax. (416)267-2475.

BRODIE-BROWN, William F; Weber Medical Centre, 5A-1400 Weber St E, Kitchener ON N2A 3Z8; Edinburgh (Scotland)'63; MB ChB; DObstRCOG; MFPHM; (519)748-6933; Fax. (519)748-9733.

BRODKIN, Elizabeth J; 400-13450 102 Ave, Surrey BC V3T 0H1; Tor'88; FRCPC; CommunMed;CCFP; FCFP; Staff, Office of the Medical Health Officer; Langs: English; French; (604)587-7894

BRODOVSKY, Sidney A; Guelph Gen Hosp, 115 Delhi St, Guelph ON N1E 4J4; Man'93; CCFP; FCFP; Staff Hospitalist, Guelph General Hospital; (519)822-5350

BRODOVSKY, Stephen C; 235-444 St Mary Ave, Winnipeg MB R3C 3T1; Man'88; FRCSC; Ophth (Cataract). Att Staff, Misericordia Health Centre; Asst Prof Ophth, University of Manitoba; Langs: English; French; (204)942-4479; Fax. (204)943-8558.

BRODSKY, Mark B; The Polyclinic, 4646 Dufferin St, North York ON M3H 5S4; Lvov (Ukraine)'60; Langs: Russian; Ukrainian; (416)222-6160; Fax. (416)222-9604.

BRODY, Daniel; MUHC-Montreal Children's Hosp, T131-2300 rue Tupper, Montreal QC H3H 1P3; McG'06; MDCM; FRCPC; Peds; PedEmergMed. Staff, McGill University Health Centre - Montreal Children's Hospital; (514)412-4400 x23039; Fax. (514)412-4397.

BRODZIAK, Helene E; 301-2500 Bathurst St, Toronto ON M6B 2Y8; Melbourne (Australia)'71; MB BS; FRCPC; Psy. (416)487-5089; h48b@aol.com.

BROEKHUYSE, Henry M; Gordon & Leslie Diamond HCC, 3F-2775 Laurel St, Vancouver BC V5Z 1M9; Tor'82; FRCSC; OrthSurg (Orthopedic Trauma Surgery). Ac Staff Orthopedic Trauma, Vancouver General Hospital - Centennial Pavillion; Staff, Gordon & Leslie Diamond Health Care Centre; Clin Prof, University of British Columbia; (604)875-5809; Fax. (604)875-5812.

BROEMLING, Natasha V; BC Children's Hosp, 4480 Oak St, Vancouver BC V6H 3V4; Alb'03; FRCPC; Anes. Staff, BC Children's Hospital; (604)875-2345 x2711

BROEMLING, Sunita R; Royal Alexandra Hosp, 10240 Kingsway NW, Edmonton AB T5H 3V9; Alb'03; FRCPC; Anes. Staff, Royal Alexandra Hospital; (780)735-4010

BROERE, James J; Chemainus Med Clinic, 9892 Esplanade St RR 1, Chemainus BC V0R 1K1; Cal'91; CCFP; FCFP; Staff, Chemainus Health Care Centre; (250)246-3261

BROEREN, Willi M J; 210-206 Rookwood Ave, Fredericton NB E3B 2M2; Dal'86; (506)458-0220

BROHOVICI, Sorel L; 203-5655 av du Parc, Montreal QC H2V 4H2; Paris (France)'69; Staff, Centre Hospitalier l'Université De Montréal (CHUM) - Hôpital Saint-luc; Staff, Hôpital du Sacre-Coeur de Montréal; Langs: Italian; English; Romanian; (514)276-5301

BROKENSHIRE, James; Queen Elizabeth II HSC-Halifax, 355-1796 Summer St, Halifax NS B3H 3A7; Wes'07; CCFP; CCFP(E.M.); Staff, Queen Elizabeth II Health Sciences Centre - Halifax Infirmary Site; (902)473-8292

BROKENSHIRE, Jennifer S; South Muskoka Mem Hosp, 75 Ann St, Bracebridge ON P1L 2E4; McM'01; CCFP; CCFP(E.M.); Staff, South Muskoka Memorial Hospital - Muskoka Algonquin Healthcare; (705)645-4400

BROKER, Hayley M; 230-150 Esplanade St W, North Vancouver BC V7M 1A3; UBC'86; CCFP; Ad Staff Privil, Lions Gate Hospital; (604)980-2128; Fax. (604)998-1335.

BROMBERG, Irwin L; Mount Sinai Hosp, 600 University Ave, Toronto ON M5G 1X5; Man'77; MedBiochem. Staff, Mount Sinai Hospital; (416)586-4499; Fax. (416)586-8628.

BROMBERG, Rudy M; Enhanced Care Clinic, 14872 Yonge St, Aurora ON L4G 1N2; Tor'07; CCFP; (905)505-0950

BROMILOW, Sarah L; 435 North Rd, Coquitlam BC V3K 3V9; Alb'08; CCFP; (604)936-0411

BROMLEY, Amy B; Foothills Med Centre, 1403 29 St NW, Calgary AB T2N 2T9; Mem'07; FRCPC; AnatPath. Staff, Foothills Medical Centre; (403)944-5055

BROMLEY, John E; Associate Med Group, 4705 48 Ave, Red Deer AB T4N 3T1; Cal'75; CCFP; Staff, Red Deer Regional Hospital Centre; Physician, Associate Medical Group; M.O., Michener Centre; Co-Dir Rural Alberta North, University of Alberta; (403)346-2057; Fax. (403)347-2989.

BROMLEY, Lisa A; Sandy Hill Comm Health Centre, 221 Nelson St, Ottawa ON K1N 1C7; Qns'92; CCFP; FCFP; Langs: English; French; (613)789-8458; Fax. (613)789-8710.

BROMLEY, Mark A; Foothills Med Centre, 231-1403 29 St NW, Calgary AB T2N 2T9; Cal'04; FRCPC; EmergMed. Staff, Foothills Medical Centre; (403)289-5663

BROMLEY, Peter J; Valley Reg Hosp, 150 Exhibition St, Kentville NS B4N 5E3; Alb'93; FRCPC; DiagRad. Staff, Valley Regional Hospital; (902)678-7381

BROMWICH, Carl R; CHUS-Hop Fleurimont, 3001 12e av N, Sherbrooke QC J1H 5N4; Dartmouth(New Hampshire) (USA)'89; FRCPC; IntMed (Palliative Medicine). Staff, Centre Hospitalier Universitaire de Sherbrooke-Hopital Fleurimont; (819)346-1110

BROMWICH, Matthew A; Children's Hosp of Eastern Ont, 401 Smyth Rd, Ottawa ON K1H 8L1; Qns'02; FRCSC; Otol. Staff, Children's Hospital of Eastern Ontario (CHEO); (613)737-7600

BRONAUGH, Thomas; Queen Elizabeth Hosp, PO Box 6600 Stn Central, Charlottetown PE C1A 8T5; Staff, Queen Elizabeth Hospital; (902)894-2111

BRONET, Sandra; 200-6100 ch de la Cote-des-Nei, Montreal QC H3S 1Z7; McG'79; (514)342-1020; Fax. (514)342-1024.

BRONIEWSKA, Marta; University of Alberta Hosp, 8440 112 St NW, Edmonton AB T6G 2B7; Cal'08; Staff, University of Alberta Hospital; (780)407-8822

BRONIEWSKI, Michal; Sunridge Med Walk In Clinic, 1288-2525 36 St NE, Calgary AB T1Y 5T4; Szczecin (Poland)'68; Peds(Poland); PedsHem(Poland); Langs: Polish; Russian; French; Spanish; (403)280-7744

BRONSON, David W; 202-11 Rea St N, Timmins ON P4N 4Z5; Tor'81; (705)264-2021

BROOK, David R; 116-2187 Oak Bay Ave, Victoria BC V8R 1G1; Sask'77; MRCGPract; CCFP; Clin Associate Commun Geriatrics & Family Med, University of British Columbia; (250)595-5562; Fax. (250)370-2858.

BROOK, Edward; 617B-330 Sparks St, Ottawa ON K1A 0N8; Ott'78; ABPM; MPH; BA(Geog.Psych.); Sr Consultant Education & Training, Civil Aviation Canada; Langs: French; (613)990-1307; Fax. (613)990-6623; edward.brook@tc.gc.ca.

BROOK, J Roger; Pelham After Hours Clinic, 202-245 Pelham Rd, St Catharines ON L2S 1X8; London (England)'53; MB BS; MRCS; LRCP; CCFP; (905)988-1933

BROOK, Shelley C; St Michael's Hosp, 17056-30 Bond St, Toronto ON M5B 1W8; Sask'82; FRCPC; Psy. Staff, St Michael's Hospital; University of Toronto; (416)864-6060

BROOK-WILLIAMS, Penelope; Brockville Mental Health Centr, PO Box 1050 Stn Main 1804 Hwy 2 E, Brockville ON K6V 5W7; London (England)'64; MB BS; BSc; FRCPC; IntMed; Psy., Brockville Mental Health Centre - Royal Ottawa Health Care Group; (613)345-1461; penelope.brook-williams@rohcg.on.ca.

BROOKE, Michael; University of Alberta Hosp, 8440 112 St NW, Edmonton AB T6G 2B7; Cambridge (England)'59; FAAN; MB ChB; ABNP; Neur (Muscle Disease). Staff, University of Alberta Hospital; (780)492-4019

BROOKER, Gary M; Portage Dist Gen Hosp, 524 5th St SE, Portage la Prairie MB R1N 3A8; Man'78; FRCPC; DiagRad (Diagnostic Imaging). Consultant Radiol, MacGregor & District Health Centre; Consultant Radiol, Portage District General Hospital; Consultant Radiol, Seven Regions Health Centre; (204)239-2268; Fax. (204)857-4580; gbrooker@shaw.ca.

BROOKES, James T; Alberta Children's Hosp, 2888 Shaganappi Trail NW, Calgary AB T3B 6A8; UBC'00; FRCSC; Otol. Staff, Alberta Children's Hospital; (403)955-2534; Fax. (403)955-7415.

BROOKES, Jonathan; London HSC-University Hosp, PO Box 5339 Stn B 339 Windermere Rd, London ON N6A 5A5; Manchester (England)'98; Staff, London Health Sciences Centre - University Hospital; (519)663-3270

BROOKS, Brenda; Cambridge Mem Hosp, 700 Coronation Blvd, Cambridge ON N1R 3G2; Ott'81; FRCPC; AnatPath. Staff, Cambridge Memorial Hospital; (519)621-2330 x2280; Fax. (519)740-4916.

BROOKS, Caleb E; St Mary's Hosp Centre, 3344-3830 av Lacombe, Montreal QC H3T 1M5; Dal'61; FRCSC; OrthSurg. Staff, St Mary's Hospital Centre; (514)345-3511

BROOKS, Christopher P; Royal Victoria Hosp, 201 Georgian Dr, Barrie ON L4M 6M2; Wes'03; FRCPC; Anes; Critical Care Medicine. Staff, Royal Victoria Regional Health Centre; (705)728-9802

BROOKS, David A; 1031 Pat Burns Ave, Gabriola BC V0R 1X2; Qns'83; Dip SportMed; (250)325-7373; Fax. (877)825-7926.

BROOKS, David H; King Street Med Arts Centre, 407-71 King St W, Mississauga ON L5B 4A2; McM'80; Ac Staff, Trillium Health Centre - Mississauga; Affil Staff, The Credit Valley Hospital; (905)279-1342; Fax. (905)279-0382.

BROOKS, Donald G; Upper Canada Med Group, 7758 Kent Blvd, Brockville ON K6V 7J9; Ott'81; Staff, Brockville General Hospital - Charles Street; Staff, Providence Continuing Care Centre (PCCC) - St Vincent de Paul Hospital; (613)498-2211; Fax. (613)345-1979.

BROOKS, Douglas; 205-974 Queen St E, Sault Ste. Marie ON P6A 2C5; Qns'73; Ac Staff, Sault Area Hospital - Sault Ste Marie; Coroner District 19, City Of Sault Ste Marie; (705)759-1234; Fax. (705)942-7332; d.brooks@cityssm.on.ca.

BROOKS, J Hamilton; Canadian National Tower, 26F-10004 104 Ave NW, Edmonton AB T5J 0K1; Manchester (England)'64; MB ChB; DPM; MRCPsy; FACS; FRCPC; Psy (Forensic Psychiatry). Staff/Consultant Psy, Alberta Hospital Edmonton; Teach Staff, University of Alberta; (780)342-6400; Fax. (780)426-7272.

BROOKS, James I; The Ottawa Hosp-Civic Campus, 1053 Carling Ave, Ottawa ON K1Y 4E9; Wes'95; BSc; FRCPC; IntMed; InfectDis. Staff, The Ottawa Hospital - Civic Campus; (613)761-4155

BROOKS, James S; Greater St Catherines CHC, 100-145 Queenston St, St Catharines ON L2R 2Z9; Tor'64; Court Staff, St Michael's Hospital; (905)688-2558; Fax. (905)688-5108; jbrooksmd@rogers.com.

BROOKS, Jane C D; Brooks & Balser Med Inc, PO Box 1599, Middleton NS B0S 1P0; Dal'97; BSc(Hons); CCFP; Staff Chief, Soldiers Memorial Hospital; Asst Prof Family Med, Dalhousie University; (902)825-2101

BROOKS, Kathleen M; 316 King St E, Cobourg ON K9A 5R8; Tor'86; FRCPC; Psy. (905)377-9925

BROOKS, Laurene J; 9937 113 St NW, Edmonton AB T5K 1N7; Alb'92; CCFP; Staff, Glenrose Rehabilitation Hospital; Langs: Spanish; French; (780)488-2232; Fax. (780)488-2479.

BROOKS, Lisa H; Scarborough Hosp-General Div, 3050 Lawrence Ave E, Scarborough ON M1P 2V5; Chicago (USA)'08; Staff, The Scarborough Hospital - General Campus; (416)495-2400

BROOKS, Marni A; First Step Med Oshawa, 32 Simcoe St S, Oshawa ON L1H 4G2; Tor'99; CCFP; Staff, North York General Hospital; (905)720-0506

BROOKS, Paul A; BC Children's Hosp, 4480 Oak St, Vancouver BC V6H 3V4; (Other Foreign)'97; Staff Children's Heart Centre, BC Children's Hospital; (604)875-2295

BROOKS, Peter J; C-59 Lorne Ave E, Stratford ON N5A 6S4; Qns'98; CCFP; (519)271-7172

BROOKS, Ruth E; Women's College Hosp, 76 Grenville St, Toronto ON M5S 1B2; Tor'85; BSc; CCFP; FCFP; Staff, Women's College Hospital; Asst Prof, University of Toronto; (416)323-6060; Fax. (416)323-6332; ruth.brooks@utoronto.ca.

BROOKS, Simon A L; South Shore Reg Hosp, 90 Glen Allan Dr, Bridgewater NS B4V 3S6; Aberdeen (Scotland)'74; MB ChB; MRCPsy; FRCPC; Psy. Staff, South Shore Regional Hospital; Asst Prof Psy, Dalhousie University; (902)543-5400

BROOKS, Steven C; Kingston Gen Hosp, E3-76 Stuart St, Kingston ON K7L 2V7; Qns'01; FRCPC; EmergMed. Staff, Kingston General Hospital; (613)549-6666

BROOKS, Tyler D P; 31 CF Health Services Centre, PO Box 1000 20 Ortona Rd, Borden ON L0M 1C0; Qns'08; CCFP; (705)424-1200

BROOKS-HILL, Robin; Revelstoke Mental Health, PO Bag 5000 1200 Newlands Rd, Revelstoke BC V0E 2S0; Tor'72; DABPN; FRCPC; Psy (Developmental Disability). Consultant Psy, Queen Victoria Hospital; Physician Developmental Disability Mental Health, Interior Health Authority Corpoate Office; (250)814-2241; Fax. (250)814-2242.

BROOKS-LIM, Elizabeth W L; Office of the Chief Med Examin, 4070 Bowness Rd NW, Calgary AB T3B 3R7; (403)297-8123; Fax. (403)297-3429.

BROOKS-HILL, Alexandra L; Sea to Sky Orthopaedics, PO Box 1275, Whistler BC V0N 1B0; Tor'00; Dip SportMed; BPHE; FRCSC; OrthSurg (Sports Medicine). Staff Orth Surg, Squamish General Hospital / Hilltop House; Staff Orth Surg, Whistler Health Care Centre; Chief Medical-Alpine Skiing, Vancouver Olympic Committee; Delbrook Surgical Centre; Cambie Surgery Centre; Langs: Bilingual(English/French); (604)905-4075

BROOKSTONE, Alan J; Alliance Clinic Ltd, 10085 Whalley Blvd, Surrey BC V3T 4G1; Witwatersrand (South Africa)'81; MB BCh; (604)813-6729

BROOME, E Alan; 486 Cadder Ave, Kelowna BC V1Y 5N3; UBC'69; (250)762-2740

BROOME, Samuel J; Eye Care Centre, 2550 Willow St, Vancouver BC V5Z 3N9; Otago (New Zealand)'74; MB ChB; DABOph; FRCSC; Ophth (General Ophthalmic Surgery). Consultant Low Vision Eye Care Centre, Vancouver General Hospital - Centennial Pavillion; Staff, UBC Eye Care Centre; Clin Assoc Prof, University of British Columbia; (604)875-5076

BROOYMANS, Corinne A M; 121-1200 Markham Rd, Scarborough ON M1H 3C3; Wes'86; CCFP; FCFP; (416)431-3800

BROPHY, James M; MUHC-Royal Victoria Hosp, R4.12-687 av des Pins O, Montreal QC H3A 1A1; McM'79; FRCPC; Cardiol. Staff, McGill University Health Centre - Royal Victoria Hospital; (514)934-1934 x36771

BROPHY, Jason C; Children's Hosp of Eastern Ont, 401 Smyth Rd, Ottawa ON K1H 8L1; Mem'99; FRCPC; Peds; InfectDis. Staff, Children's Hospital of Eastern Ontario (CHEO); (613)737-7600

BROSE, Kelsey M J; Royal University Hosp, 103 Hospital Dr, Saskatoon SK S7N 0W8; Alb'03; FRCPC; IntMed; Hem. Staff, Royal University Hospital; (306)655-1483; Fax. (306)655-1809.

BROSE, Sylva A; North York Gen Hosp, 4001 Leslie St, North York ON M2K 1E1; Mem'76; FRCPC; Anes. Staff, North York General Hospital; Asst Prof 1, University of Toronto; (416)756-6265

BROSH-KATZ, Nirit; Holland Bloorview Kids Rehab, 150 Kilgour Rd, Toronto ON M4G 1R8; Tel Aviv (Israel)'98; Staff, Holland Bloorview Kids Rehabilitation Hospital; (416)425-6220

BROSKI, Anthony P; Niagara H System-Ontario Site, 2C-155 Ontario St, St Catharines ON L2R 5K3; Ott'86; FRCPC; IntMed; Nephrol. Staff Renal Clinic, Niagara Health System - Ontario Street Site; (905)682-6411 x63186; Fax. (905)682-2751.

BROSKY, Gerald M; Cowie Family Med Centre, 16 Dentith Rd, Halifax NS B3R 2H9; Tor'77; CCFP; Staff, Queen Elizabeth II Health Sciences Centre - Victoria General Site; Assoc Prof, Dalhousie University; (902)473-1234; Fax. (902)473-4353; gerry.brosky@dal.ca.

BROSS, Pnina W; Family Physicians, 1-390 Steeles Ave W, Thornhill ON L4J 6X2; Tor'86; MSc; CCFP; FCFP; Court Staff Family Practice, North York General Hospital; Ac Staff Fam Pract, Mackenzie Richmond Hill Hospital; Langs: Hebrew; (905)881-3984; Fax. (905)881-3198.

BROSSARD, Claude F; 476 boul Marie-Victorin, Boucherville QC J4B 1W6; Mon'74; (450)655-2077

BROSSARD, Jean-Hugues; CHUM-Hop St-Luc, 2314D-1058 rue Saint-Denis, Montreal QC H2X 3J4; Mon'86; FRCPC; IntMed; Endocrin (P.Q.); Endocrin&Metab. Staff, Centre Hospitalier l'Université De Montréal (CHUM) - Hôpital Saint-luc; (514)890-8000 x36393

BROSSARD, Josee; CHUS-Hop Fleurimont, 6213-3001 12e Av N, Sherbrooke QC J1H 5N4; Sher'87; FRCPC; Peds; Hem. Staff, Centre Hospitalier Universitaire de Sherbrooke-Hopital Fleurimont; (819)346-1110 x13147

BROSSARD, Martin; Hop Jean-Talon, 1385 rue Jean-Talon E, Montreal QC H2E 1S6; Mon'96; CCFP; Staff, CSSS du Coeur de l'Isle Hôpital Jean-Talon; (514)495-6767

BROSSARD, Michel; Clinique familiale de Thetford, 1001-926 rue Labbe, Thetford Mines QC G6G 2A8; Sher'76; Staff, Hopital du CSS de la Region de Thetford; Langs: English; (418)338-3521; Fax. (418)338-4580; michel.brossard@sympatico.ca.

BROSSARD, Yves; CHUM-Hop Notre-Dame, 1560 rue Sherbrooke E, Montreal QC H2L 4M1; Mon'71; CSPQ; FRCPC; Anes. Anesthesiste, Centre Hospitalier l'Université de Montréal (CHUM) - Hôpital Notre-Dame; adj Prof, Universite de Montreal; (514)890-8000 x6876; Fax. (514)412-7653.

BROSSEAU, Isabelle; CSSS de Trois-Rivieres, 1991 boul du Carmel, Trois-Rivieres QC G8Z 3R9; Mon'03; FRCSC; GenSurg. Staff, CSSS de Trois-Rivières; (819)697-3333

BROSSEAU, Jacques; 167 rue Champlain, St-Jean-Sur-Richel QC J3B 6V5; Sher'77; Staff, Hôpital du Haut-Richelieu; (450)347-3733

BROSSEAU, Marie-Bri; CSSS de Memphremagog, 50 rue Saint-Patrice E, Magog QC J1X 3X3; Sher'01; CCFP; Staff, Centre Hospitalier et CLSC de Memphremagog; (819)843-3381

BROSSEAU, Martine; UMF Richelieu-Yamaska, 1005 rue Gauthier, Saint-Hyacinthe QC J2S 8T2; Mon'07; CCFP.

BROSSEAU-ROBERGE, Anais; Clinique Obst-Gyn Visitation, 102-222 rue de la Visitation, St-Charles-Brromee QC J6E 4N5; Sher'01; FRCSC; ObstGyn. Staff, Centre Hospitalier Régional de Lanaudière; Langs: Spanish; English; (450)759-1665; Fax. (450)759-3919.

BROSSEUK, Daniel T; Cariboo Mem Hosp, 401-517 Sixth Ave N, Williams Lake BC V2G 2G8; Qns'87; FRCSC; GenSurg (Gastrointestinal Disorders). Staff, Cariboo Memorial Hospital and Health Centre; Clin Instructor Surg, University of British Columbia; (250)398-8280; Fax. (250)398-8287; daniel_brosseuk@telus.net.

BROSSOIT, Real; Ctr Hosp de Lasalle, 8585 Tsse Champlain, LaSalle QC H8P 1C1; Mon'78; IntMed (P.Q.). Staff, Centre Hospitalier de LaSalle; (514)362-8000 x31622

BROSTER, Brett S; St Paul's Hosp, 1081 Burrard St, Vancouver BC V6Z 1Y6; UBC'96; FRCPC; Psy. Staff, Providence Health Care - St Paul's Hospital; (604)682-2344 x63636

BROTEA, Alina R; Anxiety Treatment & Research C, F609-301 James St S, Hamilton ON L8P 3B6; McM'01; FRCPC; Psy. (905)522-1155

BROTHERS, Alexander B; 100-4636 Elk Lake Dr, Victoria BC V8Z 5M1; Cal'94; CCFP; CCFP(E.M.); (250)508-8194

BROTMAN, Michael C; 170 Walmer Rd, Toronto ON M5R 2X9; Man'74; DCPsy; FRCPC; Psy (Adolescent Psychiatry). Lecturer Child & Adolescen Psy, University of Toronto; (416)968-6392; Fax. (416)929-9816.

BROUGHTON, Catherine M; City of Toronto Health Clinic, 160 Borough Dr, Scarborough ON M1P 4N8; Tor'69; (416)338-7439; Fax. (416)338-6100.

BROUGHTON, Steven A; Copeman Healthcare Centre, 400-1128 Hornby St, Vancouver BC V6Z 2L4; Wes'81; Assoc Staff, Providence Health Care - St Paul's Hospital; Asst Prof, University of British Columbia; (604)707-2273; steven.broughton@vch.ca.

BROUGHTON WILKINSON, Vanessa; 205-1875 rue Maurice-Gauvin, Laval QC H7S 2M5; Geneva (Switzerland)'04; CCFP; Staff, Hopital de la Cite de la santé; (450)902-9980; Fax. (450)902-9979.

BROUILLARD, Daniel D; Kingston Heart Clinic, 460 Princess St, Kingston ON K7L 1C2; Ott'87; FRCPC; IntMed; Rheum. (613)544-0555; Fax. (613)546-4487.

BROUILLARD, Daniel; Ctr Hosp Affilie-Enfant-Jesus, 1401 18e rue, Quebec QC G1J 1Z4; Laval'99; FRCPC; EmergMed. Staff, Centre Hospitalier Affilié Universitaire de Québec - Hôpital De L'Enfant Jésus; (418)649-5632; Fax. (418)649-5975.

BROUILLARD, Gaetan; 100-2840 boul Saint-Martin E, Laval QC H7E 5A1; Mon'75; Clin Teacher, Hopital Maisonneuve-Rosemont; (450)661-4865; Fax. (450)661-8825.

BROUILLARD, Michel; 12831 boul Rideau GD, Rollet QC J0Z 3J0; Sher'74; (819)493-5381

BROUILLET, Louise; Clinique Med Adoncour, 200-505 rue Adoncour, Longueuil QC J4G 2M6; Mon'81; (450)646-4445

BROUILLET, Mathieu; Clinique Med du Phare, 101-822 boul Sainte-Anne, Rimouski QC G5M 1J5; Mon'00; Staff, Hôpital Regional Rimouski; (418)723-5135; Fax. (418)724-2251.

BROUILLET, Michel; 50 rue Camirand, Sherbrooke QC J1H 4J5; Mon'88; adj Prof, Universite de Sherbrooke; Langs: English; French; (819)780-2222 x48332; Fax. (819)565-8196; mbrouillet.gf@gmf.gouv.qc.ca.

BROUILLET, Serge; Clinique Med Lanaudiere, 222 rue Bernard, St-Charles-Brromee QC J6E 2C5; Mon'86; Staff, Centre Hospitalier Régional de Lanaudière; (450)755-1033; Fax. (450)753-5558.

BROUILLETTE, Bernard; Centre Med Sillery, 1270 av William, Quebec QC G1S 4G1; Laval'72; Staff, Jeffery Hale Hospital-Saint Brigid's; (418)688-0664; Fax. (418)688-4601.

BROUILLETTE, Charles; CHUQ-Hotel-Dieu de Quebec, 11 Cote du Palais, Quebec QC G1R 2J6; Laval'07; CCFP; Staff, Centre Hospitalier de Matane; Staff, Centre Hospitalier Universitaire de Québec (CHUQ) - Siege Social; (418)525-4444

BROUILLETTE, Denis; CSSS de la Vallée de l'Or, 725 6e rue, Val-d'Or QC J9P 3Y1; Mon'93; FRCSC; GenSurg (Laparoscopy). Staff, Centre Hospitalier de Val d'Or; Langs: Bilingual(French/English); (819)825-5858; Fax. (819)825-7906.

BROUILLETTE, France; Clin Med Montreal-Est P A T, 201-11370 rue Notre-Dame E, Montreal-Est QC H1B 2W6; Mon'83; Langs: English; (514)645-7426; Fax. (514)645-7420.

BROUILLETTE, Genevieve; CSSS Pierre Boucher, 1333 boul Jacques-Cartier E, Longueuil QC J4M 2A5; Mon'04; FRCPC; Anes. Staff, Centre Hospitalier Pierre Boucher; (450)468-8111

BROUILLETTE, Gilles; Medicentre LaSalle, 308-1500 av Dollard, LaSalle QC H8N 1T5; Mon'71; (514)363-3545; Fax. (514)363-4021.

BROUILLETTE, Johanne; Centre Med Christ-Roi, 102-40 Rte du Président-Kenned, Levis QC G6V 6C4; Laval'74; FRCPC; Psy (Adolescent Psychiatry). Langs: English; (418)833-4977; Fax. (418)833-9557.

BROUILLETTE, Lyne; 340 rue Clement-Lavoie, Baie-Comeau QC G4Z 3B8; Sher'88; CCFP; Physician Family Med, Centre Hospitalier Régional Baie-Comeau; Langs: Bilingual(French/English); (418)296-2572; Fax. (418)294-2862.

BROUILLETTE, Marie-Helene; CSSS Baie des Chaleurs, 419 boul Perron, Maria QC G0C 1Y0; Laval'09; CCFP; Staff, CSSS de la Baie-des-Chaleurs; (418)759-3443

BROUILLETTE, Marie-Josee; Allan Memorial Institute, 1025 av des Pins O, Montreal QC H3A 1A1; Sher'86; FRCPC; Psy (Consultation). Staff, McGill University Health Centre - Royal Victoria Hospital; McGill University; (514)934-1934 x35502; Fax. (514)843-1477.

BROUILLETTE, Nancy; CSSS Drummond-Hop Sainte-Croix, 570 rue Heriot, Drummondville QC J2B 1C1; Sher'94; Staff, Hôpital Sainte-croix; (819)478-6464

BROUILLETTE, Robert T; MUHC-Montreal Children's Hosp, C508-2300 rue Tupper, Montreal QC H3H 1P3; Washington (USA)'74; Dir Ped Sleep Lab, McGill University Health Centre - Montreal Children's Hospital; Prof Peds, McGill University; (514)412-4321; Fax. (514)412-4234; robert.brouillette@muhc.mcgill.ca.

BROUSSEAU, Claude; Ctr Hosp Affilie-Enfant-Jesus, 1401 18e rue, Quebec QC G1J 1Z4; Laval'70; CSPQ; Anes. Staff, Centre Hospitalier Affilié Universitaire de Québec - Hôpital De L'Enfant Jésus; (418)649-5807; Fax. (418)649-5918.

BROUSSEAU, Ghislain; CHUQ-Ctr Hosp Univ Laval, 2705 boul Laurier, Quebec QC G1V 4G2; Laval'86; FRCPC; DiagRad. Staff, Centre Hospitalier Universitaire de Quebec-CHUL; Prof, Université Laval; (418)654-2258; Fax. (418)654-2262.

BROUSSEAU, Gilles D; Clinique Med St-Alexandre, 200-2310 rue Saint-Louis, Gatineau QC J8T 5L7; Mon'82; Staff, Hôpital de Gatineau; Asst Prof Famiy Med, McGill University; (819)243-4500; Fax. (819)243-1369.

BROUSSEAU, Marie-Claude; Clinique Pediatrique Ste-Foy, 293-2600 boul Laurier, Quebec QC G1V 4T3; Laval'01; FRCPC; Peds. Staff, CSSS de Trois-Rivières; (418)658-0906

BROUSSEAU, Nicholas; Dir Sante Publique-Mauricie QC, 50 rue Bonaventure, Trois-Rivieres QC G9A 2B5; Laval'06; FRCPC; Public Health & Preventive Med. (819)693-3636; Fax. (819)373-1627.

BROUSSEAU, Valerie J; Hotel-Dieu D'arthabaska, 5 rue des Hospitalieres, Victoriaville QC G6P 6N2; McG'04; FRCSC; Otol (Head & Neck Surgery). Staff, Hotel-Dieu d'Arthabaska; (819)357-2030

BROUSSEAU, Yves F; Ctr de Readaptation Marie Enfa, 5200 rue Bélanger, Montreal QC H1T 1C9; Laval'66; FRCPC; Peds. Staff NeuroMuscular Diseases, Centre de Réadaptation Marie Enfant du CHU Sainte-Justine; (514)374-1710x8312; Fax. (514)723-7255.

BROUSSEAU-TREMBLAY, Isabelle; Hopital de Hull, 116 boul Lionel-Emond, Gatineau QC J8Y 1W7; Laval'05; FRCPC; IntMed; GeriatricMed. Staff, Hull Hospital; (819)966-6200

BROUSSON, Michelle A; 1512 Rena Cres W, West Vancouver BC V7V 2Z3; McG'92; CCFP; FCFP; (604)224-0224; Fax. (604)221-2545.

BROUW, Maryleen; Clinique Med du Vieux-Limoilou, 755 3e Av, Quebec QC G1L 2W7; Laval'89; BACC(Psych)(Psychol); Physician, CLSC Basse-Ville-Limoilou; Physician, Clinique Medico-Esthetique Trois-Rivieres; Langs: English; French; Dutch; (418)266-0500; Fax. (418)266-0501.

BROUW, Stefan; Clinique Med du Vieux-Limoilou, 755 3e Av, Quebec QC G1L 2W7; Laval'92; CCFP; Staff, Hôpital Laval; (418)266-0500; Fax. (418)266-0501.

BROUWER, Grace J; 12720 66 St NW, Edmonton AB T5C 0A3; Alb'81; CCFP; (780)477-3681

BROVENDER, Andrea L; Trillium Hlth Ctre-Mississauga, 100 Queensway W, Mississauga ON L5B 1B8; UBC'05; FRCPC; Anes. Staff, Trillium Health Centre - Mississauga; (905)848-7100

BROW, Jim R; Listowel Mem Hosp, 255 Elizabeth St E, Listowel ON N4W 2P5; Wes'60; BSc; FRCPC; IntMed (Gastroenterology). Court Staff, Listowel Memorial Hospital - Listowel Wingham Hospitals Alliance; (519)291-3201; jbrow@rogers.com.

BROWER, Annette A; Towne Centre Medical, 19-2475 Dobbin Rd, West Kelowna BC V4T 2E9; (USA)'86; (250)768-8315; Fax. (250)768-8326.

BROWMAN, Catherine; Ctr Hosp Anna-Laberge, 200 boul Brisebois, Chateauguay QC J6K 4W8; Mon'89; FRCSC; OrthSurg. Staff, Hôpital Anna-Laberge; (450)699-2425; Fax. (450)699-2490.

BROWMAN, George P; BC Cancer Agency-Vanc Isl Ctr, 2410 Lee Ave, Victoria BC V8R 6V5; McG'71; FRCPC; IntMed (Medical Oncology); Hem. Staff, BC Cancer Agency Vancouver Island Centre; (250)519-5500

BROWMAN, Morris W; Groupe Medical Ville Marie, 1538 rue Sherbrooke O, Montreal QC H3G 1L5; McG'90; FRCPC; DiagRad. (518)933-2778

BROWN, Aaron D; 301-2151 McCallum Rd, Abbotsford BC V2S 3N8; Man'03; FRCSC; PlasSurg. (604)850-0750

BROWN, Adrian R H; North York General Hosp, 2S 191-4001 Leslie St, North York ON M2K 1E1; Tor'90; BSc; FRCSC; ObstGyn. Ac Staff, North York General Hospital; Asst Prof/Dir Distributed Med Education Fac of Med, University of Toronto; (416)756-6680; Fax. (416)756-6355; abrown@nygh.on.ca.

BROWN, Alan D; Oakville Med Centre, 301-331 Sheddon Ave, Oakville ON L6J 1X8; McM'79; BSc; MSc; AB; FRCPC; Psy (Child & Adolescent Psychiatry). Med Dir Child & Adolescent Psy Inpatient Service, Halton Healthcare Services Corporation - Oakville Site; (905)339-0956; Fax. (905)339-0452.

BROWN, Alexander B; Royal Alexandra Hosp, 10240 Kingsway NW, Edmonton AB T5H 3V9; Dal'02; FRCPC; Anes. Staff, Royal Alexandra Hospital; (780)735-4010

BROWN, Alexander M; Links Clinic Ltd, 104-11910 111 Ave NW, Edmonton AB T5G 3G6; Alb'89; FRCSC; ObstGyn. (780)454-0351; Fax. (780)453-9815.

BROWN, Allan; The Market Place, 1881 Steeles Ave W, North York ON M3H 5Y4; Tor'88; CCFP; FCFP; (416)665-2900; Fax. (416)665-2021.

BROWN, Andrew R; Huntsville District Mem Hosp, 100 Frank Miller Dr, Huntsville ON P1H 1H7; Qns'08; CCFP; Staff, Huntsville District Memorial Hospital - Muskoka Algonquin Healthcare; (705)789-2311

BROWN, Anthony L; Medical Assoc Of Port Perry, 462 Paxton St, Port Perry ON L9L 1L9; Wes'88; Staff, Lakeridge Health - Port Perry Site; (905)985-9758; Fax. (905)985-8931.

BROWN, Basil S; Digby Gen Hosp, PO Box 820 75 Warwick St, Digby NS B0V 1A0; London (England)'51; MB BS; CRCP; FRCPC; RadOncol; DiagRad. Staff, Digby General Hospital; Langs: English; French; (902)245-2501; Fax. (902)245-1301.

BROWN, Bernard H; Medi Centre Saint-Jean, 610 boul du Seminaire N, St-Jean-Sur-Richel QC J3B 7B4; Mon'80; (450)348-9218

BROWN, Bethel; 80 Valleybrook Dr, North York ON M3B 2S9; Ott'07; (416)442-5600

BROWN, Brittany J; Groves Mem Commun Hosp, 235 Union St E, Fergus ON N1M 1W3; McM'10; CCFP; Staff, Groves Memorial Community Hospital; (519)843-2010

BROWN, Bruce P; St Mary's Hosp Centre, 1304-3830 av Lacombe, Montreal QC H3T 1M5; McG'73; MPH; CCFP; CCFP(E. M.); FCFP; VP Professional Services, St Mary's Hospital Centre; (514)734-2610; Fax. (514)734-2688.

BROWN, Bryce K; Thunder Bay Reg HSC-T-Bay, 980 Oliver Rd, Thunder Bay ON P7B 6V4; Man'01; FRCPC; EmergMed; Critical Care Medicine. Staff, Thunder Bay Regional Health Sciences Centre; (807)684-6000

BROWN, C Elizabeth A; Brockville Gen Hosp, 75 Charles St, Brockville ON K6V 1S8; Tor'97; MD; MA; BA(Hons); CCFP; CCFP(E.M.); Staff Emerg Phys Services, Brockville General Hospital - Charles Street; Langs: English; French; (613)345-5645 x1160

BROWN, C Donald; Appletree Medical Clinic, C153-240 Sparks St, Ottawa ON K1P 6Z9; Qns'64; MPA; FRCPC; Psy (Botox Injection). (613)482-0118

BROWN, Carl J; St Paul's Hosp, C313-1081 Burrard St, Vancouver BC V6Z 1Y6; McM'98; FRCSC; GenSurg. Staff, Providence Health Care - St Paul's Hospital; (604)682-2344

BROWN, Carolyn E; Peterborough Clinic FHT, 202-26 Hospital Dr, Peterborough ON K9J 7C3; Tor'77; CCFP; (705)740-6859; cbrown@ptboclinic.com.

BROWN, Carolyn J; Bancroft Family Health Team, PO Box 578 16 Billa St, Bancroft ON K0L 1C0; Qns'84; CCFP; Staff Family Med, QHC North Hastings; Preceptor Family Practice, University of Ottawa; (613)332-1565; Fax. (613)332-0526; cbrown@bancroftfht.com.

BROWN, Cathryn M; 1-3801 28A St, Vernon BC V1T 9T6; UBC'00; CCFP; (250)542-9950

BROWN, Charles A; Valley Professional Center, 70 Exhibition St, Kentville NS B4N 4K9; Dal'65; FRCPC; Peds. Chief Peds/Consultant, Soldiers Memorial Hospital; Ac Staff, Valley Regional Hospital; (902)678-2525; Fax. (902)678-4550.

BROWN, Christina A; 146-148 Forest Rd PO Box 9000 Stn A, St. John's NL A1A 3B8; Mem'95.

BROWN, Christopher B; Tom Baker Cancer Centre, 1331 29 St NW, Calgary AB T2N 4N2; Ott'81; FRCPC; IntMed (Bone Marrow Transplant); Hem. Prof Med, Foothills Medical Centre; Staff, Tom Baker Cancer Centre; Prof Med, University of Calgary; (403)521-3706; Fax. (403)521-3743; cbrown@ucalgary.ca.

BROWN, Christopher W; Nepean Med Centre, 1 Centrepointe Dr, Ottawa ON K2G 6E2; Ott'02; FRCSC; OrthSurg. (613)225-1188

BROWN, Ciara E; Belleville & Quite West Commun, 161 Bridge St W, Belleville ON K8P 1K2; Newcastle-Upon-Tyne (England)'05; CCFP; (613)962-0000

BROWN, Craig; Saint John Reg Hosp, PO Box 2100 Stn Main 400 University Ave, Saint John NB E2L 4L2; Man'84; MD; FACS; FRCSC; Cardiovasc&ThorSurg (Cardiac Surgery). Ac Staff New Brunswick Heart Centre, Saint John Regional Hospital; Lecturer Surg, Dalhousie University; Asst Prof, Memorial University Of Newfoundland; (506)648-7020; Fax. (506)648-6110.

BROWN, D Ross G; Vancouver Gen Hosp, 855 12th Ave W, Vancouver BC V5Z 1M9; McM'88; FACS; MA; TraSurg; FRCSC; GenSurg (Trauma). Staff Trauma Services, Vancouver General Hospital - Centennial Pavillion; Physician, National Defence Headquarters; Staff, Dr D Ross Brown Inc; Clin Prof, University of British Columbia; (604)875-5746; Fax. (604)875-5348; ross.brown@vch.ca.

BROWN, D Stephen; Professional Arts Bldg, 105-100 Arden St, Moncton NB E1C 4B7; Ott'81; FRCSC; GenSurg; VascSurg. Staff, The Moncton Hospital; Court Staff, Dr Georges-L-Dumont University Hospital Centre; Clin Teacher Surg, Dalhousie University; Langs: English; French; (506)857-5809; Fax. (506)857-5808.

BROWN, D O Chester; Min of Hlth Monitoring & Contr, 370 Select Dr, Kingston ON K7M 8T4; Qns'77; Consultant, OHIP Head office; (613)536-3101

BROWN, Dale H; Univ Hlth Network-Princess M, 3 950-610 University Ave, Toronto ON M5G 2M9; RCS (Ireland)'82; MB ChB; BAO; LRCPSI; LMCC; FRCSC; Otol (Head & Neck Surgery & Oncology). Staff Otol/Head & Neck/Surgeon Oncology, Princess Margaret Hospital - University Health Network; Staff, Toronto General Hospital - UHN; Prof, University of Toronto; (416)946-2147; dale.brown@uhn.on.ca.

BROWN, David E; 4-1180 Place D'Orleans Dr, Orleans ON K1C 7K3; Qns'79; (613)834-0553

BROWN, David J L; Village Park Med Clinic, 110-937 Fir St, Sherwood Park AB T8A 4N6; Manchester (England)'72; MB ChB; (780)467-8886; Fax. (780)467-6763.

BROWN, David S; Surrey Med Arts Bldg, 101-13798 94A Ave, Surrey BC V3V 1N1; Dal'98; FRCSC; OrthSurg. (604)588-5634

BROWN, David S L; 1600-150 King St W, Toronto ON M5H 1J9; Belfast (Ireland)'77; MB ChB; BAO; CCBOM; Med Dir, Canadian Imperial Bank of Commerce; (416)410-1096

BROWN, Dean V; 202-520 17th St, West Vancouver BC V7V 3S8; Cal'76; CCFP; CCFP(E.M.); FCFP; Staff, Lions Gate Hospital; Langs: English; French; (604)913-8183; Fax. (604)913-8804.

BROWN, Deborah S; Business Bldg, 200-1200 Burrard St, Vancouver BC V6Z 2C7; Cal'75; BSc; Assoc Staff FamMed, BC Children's Hospital; Assoc Staff, Providence Health Care - St Paul's Hospital; (604)685-4398; Fax. (604)685-7110.

BROWN, Deirdre K; 786 Goderich St SS 3, Port Elgin ON N0H 2C3; Tor'95; CCFP; (519)832-4998

BROWN, Denis R C; Rosedale Med Clinic, PO Box 460, Summerland BC V0H 1Z0; Cape Town (South Africa)'82; MB ChB; BSc; CCFP; Staff, Penticton Regional Hospital; (250)404-4242

BROWN, Dennis B; Nicola Med Dental Bldg, 207-321 Nicola St, Kamloops BC V2C 6G6; Wes'77; FRCSC; Ophth. (250)314-1073

BROWN, Deron J; North Scarborough Prof Bldg, 306-3420 Finch Ave E, Scarborough ON M1W 2R6; Tor'97; FRCSC; Otol (Facial Plastic Surgery). Clin Instructor, Toronto General Hospital - UHN; Clin Instructor, The Scarborough Hospital - General Campus; Ac Staff, The Scarborough Hospital - Birchmount Campus; Lecturer, University of Toronto; (416)913-8738; Fax. (416)913-8739; torontoent@yahoo.ca.

BROWN, Donald C; Halifax Professional Centre, 720-5991 Spring Garden Rd, Halifax NS B3H 1Y6; Dal'59; BSc; AB; Staff Consultant, Queen Elizabeth II Health Sciences Centre - Victoria General Site; Staff Consultant, IWK Health Centre; (902)429-7890; Fax. (902)446-7856.

BROWN, E J Peter; Northland Clinic, PO Box 1600 233 8th St, Cochrane ON P0L 1C0; McG'71; FRCSC; GenSurg. Staff, Lady Minto Hospital Cochrane; (705)272-4276; Fax. (705)272-2676.

BROWN, Edward; 108-235 St Clair Ave W, Toronto ON M4V 1R4; Man'65; BSc(Med); FRCPC; Psy (Psychoanalysis). Langs: Yiddish; (416)922-2028; Fax. (416)928-2993; edbrown1@bellnet.ca.

BROWN, Edward M; 1100-105 Moatfield Dr, North York ON M3B 0A2; Tor'84; CCFP; CCFP(E.M.); Staff, Sunnybrook Health Sciences Centre; (416)446-4113

BROWN, Elizabeth A; The Westend Family Care Clinic, 80 Michael Cowpland Dr, Kanata ON K2M 1P6; Manchester (England)'86; MB ChB; CCFP; FCFP; Staff, Westend Family Care Clinic Family Health Team; (613)599-3321; Fax. (613)599-3366.

BROWN, Elwyn J; 8-2111 Centre St NW, Calgary AB T2E 2T2; Cal'80; BSc(PhysTher); CCFP; Ac Staff Family Pract, Foothills Medical Centre; (403)277-3333; Fax. (403)277-5540; elwyn@arttech.ab.ca.

BROWN, Eric E; Grey Bruce HS-Owen Sound, PO Box 1800 Stn Main 1800 8th St E, Owen Sound ON N4K 6M9; Qns'93; FRCPC; Anes. Staff, Grey Bruce Health Services - Owen Sound; (519)376-2121

BROWN, Erik D; Polyclinique l'Orelle St-Hyaci, 2113 boul Casavant O, Saint-Hyacinthe QC J2S 7E5; McG'05; Otol. (450)773-7824; Fax. (450)773-1826.

BROWN, Erin E; Gordon & Leslie Diamond HCC, 3F-2775 Laurel Street, Vancouver BC V5Z 1M9; UBC'96; PhD; FRCSC; PlasSurg (Hand Surgery). Med Dir Critical Care Emerg & Trauma Services, Vancouver General Hospital - Centennial Pavillion; Clin Assoc Prof PlasticSurg, University of British Columbia; (604)875-5866; Fax. (604)875-5861; natalia.kouznetsova@vch.ca.

BROWN, Glenn; Family Med Health Unit, PO Box 8888 Stn Main 220 Bagot St, Kingston ON K7L 5E9; McM'81; BSc; CCFP; CCFP(E.M.); FCFP; Med Staff, Lennox & Addington County General Hospital; Dept Head Family Med, Queen's University; (613)533-9300

BROWN, Gordon W; Rocky Med Clinic, PO Box 99 Stn Main, Rocky-Mtn-Hse AB T4T 1A1; Cal'73; CCFP; (403)845-3315; Fax. (403)845-2177.

BROWN, Gregory; Mood and Anxiety Division, 4F-100 Stokes St, Toronto ON M6J 1H4; Tor'59; PhD(Rochester NY); DPsy; FAPA; FRCPC; Psy. Staff, Centre for Addiction & Mental Health (CAMH) - College Street Site; (416)535-8501

BROWN, Gregory S; Health Sciences Centre, 300 Prince Philip Dr, St. John's NL A1B 3V6; Mem'99; CCFP; CCFP(E.M.); Staff Emerg, Health Sciences Centre; (709)777-6300

BROWN, Harry; Dr Poon's Metabolic Diet Clini, 201-343 Wilson Ave, North York ON M3H 1T1; Qns'60; (416)636-3237; Fax. (416)636-3236.

BROWN, Heather J; University of Manitoba, 104-65 Chancellors Cir, Winnipeg MB R3T 2N2; Man'89; Staff, Manitoba Adolescent Treatment Centre; hbrown@matc.ca.

BROWN, Helene; Clinique Med de Bernieres, 479 ch Saint-Joseph, Saint-Nicolas QC G7A 1N3; Mon'80; (418)831-9228; Fax. (418)831-0249.

BROWN, Ian R; 306-5673 North St, Niagara Falls ON L2G 1J4; Dal'90; FRCSC; Urol. Staff, Niagara Health System - Greater Niagara General Site; (905)356-1695; Fax. (905)356-5304.

BROWN, Irving H; 669 St Clair Ave W, Toronto ON M6C 1A7; Tor'76; PhD.

BROWN, J Donovan; Avon Med Centre, 2781 Avonhurst Dr, Regina SK S4R 3J3; Queen's (Ireland)'56; DPH; CCFP; FCFP; Assoc Staff, Pasqua Hospital; Assoc Staff, Regina General Hospital; (306)543-4955; Fax. (306)545-7006; donlee@sasktel.net.

BROWN, J Terence; Industrial Health Services, 101-375 Finley Ave, Ajax ON L1S 2E2; London (England)'64; MB BS; MRCS; LRCP; DObstRCOG; (905)686-6000; Fax. (905)686-1491.

BROWN, Jacqueline A; St Paul's Hosp, 1081 Burrard St, Vancouver BC V6Z 1Y6; UBC'88; FRCPC; DiagRad. Staff, Providence Health Care - St Paul's Hospital; (604)682-2344

BROWN, Jacques; CHUQ-Ctr Hosp Univ Laval, H1361-2705 boul Laurier, Quebec QC G1V 4G2; Laval'77; FRCPC; Rheum (Internal Medicine). Ac Staff, Centre Hospitalier Universitaire de Quebec-CHUL; Clin Prof, Université Laval; assoc Prof, McGill University; (418)654-2242; Fax. (418)654-2798; jacques.brown@crchul.ulaval.ca.

BROWN, James C; Rothbart Ctre for Pain Care Lt, 9-4646 Dufferin St, North York ON M3H 5S4; Saba (Netherlands Antilles)'03; (416)512-6407

BROWN, James E; London HSC-University Hosp, PO Box 5339 Stn B B6 121-339 Windermere Rd, London ON N6A 5A5; Qns'74; FRCPC; Cardiol. Staff Cardiac Invest Unit, London Health Sciences Centre - University Hospital; Prof Med & Pharmacol, University of Western Ontario; (519)663-3662; Fax. (519)434-3278; jim.brown@lhsc.on.ca.

BROWN, James K; Clarkside Med Centre, 155 Clarke Rd, London ON N5W 5C9; London (England)'61; MB BS; FRCS(Eng); FACS; FRCSC; GenSurg. (519)455-1100

BROWN, James R; Victoria Hosp, 1200 24th St W, Prince Albert SK S6V 5T4; Sask'06; CCFP; Staff, Victoria Hospital; (306)765-6200; Fax. (306)765-6224.

BROWN, Jamie C; Peterborough Reg HC-Hospital, 1 Hospital Dr, Peterborough ON K9J 7C6; Dal'04; FRCPC; IntMed; Critical Care Medicine. Staff, Peterborough Regional Health Centre - Hospital Drive; (705)743-2121

BROWN, Jeffrey K; 230 Robson Rd W, Kelowna BC V1X 3C8; Wes'96; BSc; CCFP; Preceptor Rural Family Practice Prog, University of British Columbia; (250)765-9777; Fax. (250)765-1350.

BROWN, Jeffrey M; 220-10 Disera Dr, Thornhill ON L4J 0A7; Tor'87; BSc; (905)771-7771

BROWN, Jim J; Misericordia Community Hosp, 16940 87 Ave NW, Edmonton AB T5R 4H5; Alb'79; FRCPC; EmergMed. Staff, Covenant Health - Misericordia Community Hospital; (780)735-2819; jimjbrown@shaw.ca.

BROWN, Jodie S B; Hope Centre, 240 Powers St, Winnipeg MB R2W 5L1; Man'09; CCFP.

BROWN, John K; Newmarket Med Place, 311-712 Davis Dr, Newmarket ON L3Y 8C3; Glasgow (Scotland)'73; MB ChB; Ac Staff, Southlake Regional Health Centre; (905)895-9088; Fax. (905)895-9097; john.k.brown@ontariomd.ca.

BROWN, Jordan S I; York-Med Medical Arts Centre, 202-250 Harding Blvd W, Richmond Hill ON L4C 9M7; RCS (Ireland)'91; (905)737-8346; Fax. (905)737-5245.

BROWN, Karen A; MUHC-Montreal Children's Hosp, 2300 rue Tupper, Montreal QC H3H 1P3; Tor'80; CSPQ; FRCPC; Anes (Pediatric Anesthesia). Anesthesiste, McGill University Health Centre - Montreal Children's Hospital; adj Prof, McGill University; (514)412-4463

BROWN, Kathryn; Klondyke Med Clinic, 1-3089 3rd Ave, Whitehorse YT Y1A 5B3; Perth (Australia)'90; FRACGP; CCFP; Staff, Klondyke Medical Clinic; (867)668-4046

BROWN, Kenneth E; Polyclinique Ile-des-Soeurs, 2010 boul Rene-Levesque, Verdun QC H3E 2A4; Tor'70; CCFP; FCFP; Langs: French; (514)767-2683; Fax. (514)767-7351.

BROWN, Kenneth L B; Children's & Women's HC of BC, A207-4480 Oak St, Vancouver BC V6H 3V4; Man'76; BSc; MSc; FRCSC; OrthSurg (Musculo Skeletal Oncology). Staff, BC Children's Hospital; Clin Prof, University of British Columbia; Langs: Bilingual(English/French); (604)875-2642; Fax. (604)875-2275.

BROWN, Kenneth S; F W Green Med Centre, 1629 Baker St, Cranbrook BC V1C 1B4; Alb'91; CCFP; FCFP; (250)426-6601; Fax. (250)426-6470.

BROWN, Kevin P; LAMP Comm Health Centre, 185 Fifth St, Etobicoke ON M8V 2Z5; Tor'96; CCFP; FCFP; (416)252-6475; Fax. (416)252-6395.

BROWN, Krista D; Wedgewood Med Centre, 304-12 Gleneyre St, St. John's NL A1A 2M7; Mem'03; FRCSC; ObstGyn. (709)579-2606

BROWN, Kristen; 1265 Onondaga St, Oromocto NB E2V 2P8; Dal'05; CCFP.

BROWN, Lanying; Hotel-Dieu Grace Hosp, 1030 Ouellette Ave, Windsor ON N9A 1E1; Dayton (USA)'92; Staff, Hôtel-Dieu Grace Hospital; (519)973-4411

BROWN, Lennox N; Park Avenue Med Centre, 4F-4634 Park Ave, Terrace BC V8G 1V7; Queen's (Ireland)'72; MB BCh; Ac Staff, Mills Memorial Hospital; (250)615-5040; Fax. (250)615-5049.

BROWN, Leslie N; 100-8171 Cook Rd, Richmond BC V6Y 3T8; UBC'91; (604)279-1942

BROWN, Margaret A; Wilson Centre Family Practice, 1-2185 Wilson Ave, Port Coquitlam BC V3C 6C1; Dal'90; (604)942-7227; Fax. (604)942-7058.

BROWN, Mark T; 201-53 Stadacona St W, Moose Jaw SK S6H 1Z2; Cape Town (South Africa)'95; MB ChB; (306)694-4090; Fax. (306)694-4095; drmtbrown@sasktel.net.

BROWN, Marty H; 201-211 Dundas St E, Belleville ON K8N 1E2; Dal'06; CCFP; (613)968-6300; Fax. (613)968-6303.

BROWN, Mary M; Queensway-Carleton Hosp, 3045 Baseline Rd, Nepean ON K2H 8P4; Aberdeen (Scotland)'72; MB ChB; FRCPC; Psy. Ac Staff, Queensway Carleton Hospital; (613)721-4708; Fax. (613)721-4773.

BROWN, Maura J; Vancouver Gen Hosp, 855 12th Ave W, Vancouver BC V5Z 1M9; UBC'89; FRCPC; DiagRad (Chest Radiology). Staff, Vancouver General Hospital - Centennial Pavillion; (604)875-4355; maura.brown@vch.ca.

BROWN, Meagan L; Grace Maternal Child Care, 130-1402 8 Ave NW, Calgary AB T2N 1B9; Alb'09; CCFP; (403)289-9051; Fax. (403)284-3129.

BROWN, Melanie L; 100-200 Keary St, New Westminster BC V3L 0A6; Sask'06; FRCPC; IntMed; Nephrol. (604)516-7774

BROWN, Merrilee G; Medical Assoc of Port Perry, 462 Paxton St, Port Perry ON L9L 1L9; Wes'95; CCFP; FCFP; Staff, Lakeridge Health - Port Perry Site; Preceptor Rural Family Med, Queen's University; Preceptor Rural Family Med, University of Toronto; Langs: Spanish; (905)985-2895 x5420; Fax. (905)985-3464.

BROWN, Michael S; CHUQ-Ctr Hosp Univ Laval, 2705 boul Laurier, Quebec QC G1V 4G2; London (England)'66; LRCP; MRCS; FRCPC; Peds; Nephrol (P.Q.). Staff Ped Nephrol, Centre Hospitalier Universitaire de Quebec-CHUL; (418)656-4141

BROWN, Mijin; William Osler HC-Brampton, 2100 Bovaird Dr E, Brampton ON L6R 3J7; Wes'96; FRCPC; Peds (Surgical Assistant). Staff, William Osler Health System - Brampton Civic Hospital; Langs: Korean; (905)494-2120; Fax. (905)494-6569; planetbrown@sympatico.ca.

BROWN, Mitchell H; 410-790 Bay St, Toronto ON M5G 1N8; Wes'88; FRCS; MEd; BSc; FRCSC; PlasSurg (Cosmetic Surgery). Ac Staff, North York General Hospital; Ac Staff, Women's College Hospital; Asst Prof Surg, University of Toronto; (416)323-6336; Fax. (416)323-6325; info@torontoplasticsurgery.com.

BROWN, Mitchell S; Quinte HC Corp-Belleville Gen, 265 Dundas St E, Belleville ON K8N 5A9; National U. (Ireland)'01; FRCPC; Anes. Staff, QHC Belleville General; (613)969-7400

BROWN, Murray C; Burnside Medical Clinic, 101 Burnside Rd W, Victoria BC V9A 1B7; Mem'94; CCFP; (250)381-4353

BROWN, Nadia K; Univ of Western Ontario, LL11-1151 Richmond St, London ON N6A 3K7; McM'95; BA(Hons); (519)661-3771

BROWN, Nancy-Shira E; Niagara H System-Welland Site, 65 Third St, Welland ON L3B 4W6; Man'01; CCFP; Staff, Niagara Health System - Welland Hospital Site; (905)378-4647

BROWN, Nathan J D; South Health Campus, 4448 Front St E, Calgary AB T3M 1M4; Alb'06; Anes. Staff, Foothills Medical Centre; Staff, South Health Campus; (403)956-2465

BROWN, Neil E; University of Alberta Hosp, 2E4.44WCM-8440 112 St NW, Edmonton AB T6G 2B7; Tor'71; BSc; FCCP; FRCPC; Respir (Cystic Fibrosis). Ac Staff, University of Alberta Hospital; Prof Med, University of Alberta; (780)407-6448; Fax. (780)407-6384.

BROWN, Owen H; Dr O Brown & Dr A Van Zyl Inc, 4556 Gertrude St, Port Alberni BC V9Y 6K1; Stellenbosch (South Africa)'97; MB ChB; CCFP; Staff, West Coast General Hospital; Langs: Afrikaans; (250)724-0166; brownvanzyl@shaw.ca.

BROWN, Paul K; Discovery Medical Centre, 1477 Island Hwy, Campbell River BC V9W 8E5; Man'75; (250)850-4505

BROWN, Peter Grant; 84 Chestnut Ave, Hamilton ON L8L 6K9; Man'95.

BROWN, Peter J; Oakridge Wellness Centre, 254-759 Hyde Park Rd, London ON N6H 3S2; Ott'96; BSc(Hon)(Kinesiol); (519)777-0366; peterjohnbrown@rogers.com.

BROWN, Peter M; Kingston Gen Hosp, 76 Stuart St, Kingston ON K7L 2V7; Wes'75; DAB; FRCSC; GenSurg; VascSurg. Staff, Kingston General Hospital; Att Staff, Hotel-Dieu Hospital; Assoc Prof Surg, Queen's University; (613)548-3232 x4732; Fax. (613)548-6153; brownp2@kgh.kari.net.

BROWN, Pierre; ADRLSSSS de 'Outaouais, 296-104 rue Lois, Gatineau QC J8Y 3R7; Ott'74; LMCC; Med Consultant, Outaouais Public Health; Consultant, Regional Public Health & Social Services; Langs: English; (819)776-7604; Fax. (819)770-5490; pierre_brown@ssss.gouv.qc.ca.

BROWN, Rea A; CUSM-Montreal Gen Hosp, L9 512-1650 av Cedar, Montreal QC H3G 1A4; McG'62; FRCSC; GenSurg. Sr Staff Surg, McGill University Health Centre - Montreal General Campus; Prof, McGill University; (514)934-1934 x43050; Fax. (514)934-8235.

BROWN, Richard N; MUHC-Royal Victoria Hosp, 687 av des Pins O, Montreal QC H3A 1A1; London (England)'89; Staff, McGill University Health Centre - Royal Victoria Hospital; (514)934-1934

BROWN, Robert A; AE203-671 William Ave, Winnipeg MB R3E 0Z2; Man'87; FRCPC; Anes (Acute Pain Management). Dir Acute Pain Service, Health Sciences Centre; Dir Undergraduate Prog, University of Manitoba; rabrown@hsc.mb.ca.

BROWN, Robert H; 207-2537 Beacon Ave, Sidney BC V8L 1Y3; Sask'77; CCFP; (250)656-4114

BROWN, Robert I G; Keary Med Centre, 102-245 Columbia St E, New Westminster BC V3L 3W4; Wes'79; FRCPC; IntMed; Cardiol. (604)524-9571; Fax. (604)524-5322.

BROWN, Robert L; Duffus Health Centre, 208-7071 Bayers Rd, Halifax NS B3L 2C2; Dal'63; (902)453-4585; Fax. (902)453-5657.

BROWN, Robyn; Maple Key Clinic Family Hlth Team, D2-1036 Princess St, Kingston ON K7L 1H2; Ott'88; CCFP; FCFP; (613)546-9721; Fax. (613)546-2799.

BROWN, Roger T A; Alberta Hosp Edmonton, PO Box 307 Stn Main, Edmonton AB T5J 2J7; Alb'99; FRCPC; Psy. Staff, The East Coast Forensic Psychiatry Hospital; Staff Forensyc Psy Services, Alberta Hospital Edmonton; (780)472-5555; Fax. (780)472-5350; roger.brown@cdha.nshealth.ca.

BROWN, Ronald D; SMBD Jewish Gen Hosp, 3755 ch Cote-Sainte-Catherine, Montreal QC H3T 1E2; McG'69; FRCPC; Psy (Disability Evaluation). Pres, Testmetrix Inc & Evaluation Medicale Inc.; Asst Prof Psy, McGill University; (514)340-8210; Fax. (514)938-5268.

BROWN, Ronald J; Tawa Centre, 120-3017 66 St NW, Edmonton AB T6K 4B2; Alb'81; FRCSC; ObstGyn. Ac Staff, Covenant Health - Grey Nuns Community Hospital; (780)461-6220; Fax. (780)461-4197.

BROWN, Ronald T; Washington Park Med Clinic, PO Box 3100 Stn Main, Courtenay BC V9N 5N3; Alb'76; Staff, St Joseph's General Hospital; (250)334-9241; Fax. (250)897-0225.

BROWN, Roy A; St Paul's Hosp, 1081 Burrard St, Vancouver BC V6Z 1Y6; Alb'80; Staff, Providence Health Care - St Paul's Hospital; Staff, Richmond Hospital; (604)682-2344

BROWN, Russell J; Sturgeon Community Hosp, 201 Boudreau Rd, St. Albert AB T8N 6C4; Ott'83; Anes. Staff, Sturgeon Community Hospital; Asst Prof Anes, University of Alberta; Langs: Bilingual(French/English); (780)418-7310; Fax. (780)418-7346; russelljbrown@shaw.ca.

BROWN, Sara; Selkirk Med Clinic, PO Box 590, Revelstoke BC V0E 2S0; UBC'02; BSc; CCFP; (250)837-9321; Fax. (250)837-9444.

BROWN, Sheryl E Z; 1600 Steeles Ave W, Concord ON L4K 4M2; RCS (Ireland)'91; (905)760-1415; Fax. (905)760-2735.

BROWN, Simon E; Malton Med Centre, 22-7330 Goreway Dr, Mississauga ON L4T 4J2; Glasgow (Scotland)'72; MB ChB; LMCC; Ac Staff, William Osler Health System - Etobicoke General Hospital; (905)677-4200; Fax. (905)677-0541.

BROWN, Stanley E; 105-645 Commissioners Rd E, London ON N6C 2T9; Wes'73; BSc; FRCSC; ObstGyn. Assessment Specialist Schulich School of Med & Dentistry, University of Western Ontario; (519)963-0232; Fax. (519)963-0233; stabrown@rogers.com.

BROWN, Stephen C; The Hosp for Sick Children, 555 University Ave, Toronto ON M5G 1X8; Wes'81; FRCPC; Anes (Pediatric Pain Management). Assoc Staff, The Hospital For Sick Children; Lecturer Anes, University of Toronto; (416)813-7445; stephen.brown@sickkids.ca.

BROWN, Stephen C; Briarwood Cosmetic Surgical Ct, 1-406 North Service Rd E, Oakville ON L6H 5R2; Wes'82; FRCSC; PlasSurg. Staff, Halton Healthcare Services Corporation - Oakville Site; Court Staff, Halton Healthcare Services Corporation - Milton District Hospital; Court Staff, Joseph Brant Memorial Hospital; (905)849-4282; Fax. (905)849-4630; info@briarwoodsurgical.com.

BROWN, Stephen D; William Osler HC-Brampton, 2100 Bovaird Dr E, Brampton ON L6R 3J7; McM'94; FRCPC; Anes. Staff, William Osler Health System - Brampton Civic Hospital; (905)494-2120

BROWN, Stuart M; Abbotsford Reg Hosp & Cancer C, 14-32900 Marshall Rd, Abbotsford BC V2S 0C2; London (England)'74; MRC(UK); Gen Practice, Abbotsford Regional Hospital & Cancer Centre; (604)851-4700

BROWN, Stuart Z; Dynalife Diagnostic Lab Servic, 200-10150 102 St NW, Edmonton AB T5J 5E2; Man'95; FRCPC; GenPath (Hematology Pathology). Staff, Covenant Health - Misericordia Community Hospital; Clinical Asst Prof, University of Alberta; (780)451-3702; stuart.brown2@albertahealthservices.ca.

BROWN, Tanya; Allan Blair Cancer Centre, 4101 Dewdney Ave, Regina SK S4T 7T1; (306)766-2203

BROWN, Theodorah N; Rochdale Crossing Med Clinic, 7-5875 Rochdale Blvd, Regina SK S4X 2P9; (Other Foreign)'04; (306)205-8020; Fax. (306)205-8023.

BROWN, Thomas C; Peterborough Reg HC-Hospital, 1 Hospital Dr, Peterborough ON K9J 7C6; McG'67; FRCPC; DiagRad. Staff, Peterborough Regional Health Centre - Hospital Drive; (705)876-5039

BROWN, Timothy F E; Queen Elizabeth II HSC, 1276 South Park St, Halifax NS B3H 2Y9; McM'99; FRCSC; Otol (Head & Neck Surgery). Staff, Queen Elizabeth II Health Sciences Centre - Victoria General Site; (902)473-2914; Fax. (902)473-4304.

BROWN, Vivien P; 1001-2200 Yonge St, Toronto ON M4S 2C6; McG'79; CCFP; FCFP; Assoc Staff, Mount Sinai Hospital; Clin Asst, Toronto Western Hospital - University Health Network; (416)481-1173; Fax. (416)481-7431.

BROWN, W Lorne; Richmond Health Science Ctre, 830-6091 Gilbert Rd, Richmond BC V7C 5L9; UBC'71; FICS; FRCSC; PlasSurg. Court Staff, Richmond Hospital; Court Staff, Delta Hospital; (604)273-6449; Fax. (604)273-1422; drlbrown@axion.net.

BROWN, W Mark; 3-715 Coronation Blvd, Cambridge ON N1R 7R1; Wes'87; CCFP; (519)740-1700; Fax. (519)740-8487.

BROWN, Wanda G G; Arthur Street Med Centre, 29 Arthur St, Truro NS B2N 1X7; Mem'87; (902)893-8798; Fax. (902)897-0464.

BROWN, Wayne C; Musquodoboit Harbour Med Clin, RR 1 7907 Highway 7, Musquodbt Hbr NS B0J 2L0; Dal'74; (902)889-2650; Fax. (902)889-2577.

BROWN, Wendy; Balmoral Med Arts Facility, 309-1366 Yonge St, Toronto ON M4T 3A7; Tor'75; (416)966-3061; Fax. (416)966-3095.

BROWN, William F E; McMaster Univ Medical Centre, 4V1-1200 Main St W, Hamilton ON L8N 3Z5; Wes'63; FRCPC; Neur (Neuromuscular Diseases). Staff, St Joseph's Care Group - St Joseph's Hospital; Prof Neurol, Hamilton Health Sciences Centre; (905)521-2100 x76417; Fax. (905)521-2652; browneaton@aol.com.

BROWN, William S; Royal Inland Hosp, 311 Columbia St, Kamloops BC V2C 2T1; Mem'09; Staff, Royal Inland Hospital; (250)314-2100

BROWN, Windy M; Fort Family Practicce, PO Box 99 Stn Fort Langley, Langley BC V1M 2R4; UBC'06; CCFP; (604)888-2433

BROWN-BRAKE, Sonya L; Churchill Square Med Clinic, PO Box 23205 Rpo Churchill Sq 209-10 Rowan St, St. John's NL A1B 4J9; Mem'05; CCFP.

BROWN-JOHNSON, Anita Marie; MUHC-Montreal Gen Hosp, D16 108-1650 av Cedar, Montreal QC H3G 1A4; McG'88; DrMedCh; FCFP; BSc(Hon); CCFP; FCFP; Dir Secondary Care Div Family Med & Dir Transition Care Services, McGill University Health Centre - Montreal General Campus; Asst Prof Faculty of Med Div of Geriatrics, McGill University; Langs: Spanish; French; (514)934-1934 x43945; Fax. (514)934-8281; anita.brownjohnson@muhc.mcgill.ca.

BROWN-MAHER, Tracey D; 290 LeMarchant Rd, St. John's NL A1E 1R2; Mem'01; FRCPC; Derm.

BROWN-SHREVES, Danielle N; 201-222 King St E, Bowmanville ON L1C 1P6; West Indies (Other Foreign)'06; CCFP; (905)440-3584

BROWN-THOMSON, Linda D; Kingston Gen Hosp, 76 Stuart St, Kingston ON K7L 2V7; Qns'77; CCFP; FCFP; Assoc Staff, Kingston General Hospital; Assoc Staff, Hotel-Dieu Hospital; Langs: English; French; (613)548-3232 x4088

BROWNBRIDGE, Brian R; Royal University Hosp, 103 Hospital Dr, Saskatoon SK S7N 0W8; Sask'87; FRCPC; Anes. Staff, Royal University Hospital; (306)655-1183

BROWNE, Candice; Seymour Health Centre, 1530 7th Ave W, Vancouver BC V6J 1S3; Pretoria (South Africa)'07; MB ChB; Langs: Afrikaans; (604)739-5614

BROWNE, Gregory N; The Health Plex, 114 Empire Ave, St. John's NL A1C 3G2; Mem'93; FRCSC; GenSurg; VascSurg. Att Staff Surg, St Clare's Mercy Hospital; Att Surgeon, Healthcare Corp of St. John's; Fax. (709)738-7180; gbrowne@fitforwork.com.

BROWNE, Janis L; North Toronto Med Bldg, 216-250 Lawrence Ave W, Toronto ON M5M 1B2; McM'85; CCFP; FCFP; Assoc Staff, North York General Hospital; Assoc Prof, University of Toronto; (416)785-5001; Fax. (416)785-6539.

BROWNE, Kevin P; 1714 Cranbrook St N, Cranbrook BC V1C 3S8; Sask'89; FRCPC; IntMed. Staff, East Kootenay Regional Hospital; (250)489-5423

BROWNE, Michael; Queensway-Carleton Hosp, 3045 Baseline Rd, Nepean ON K2H 8P4; Aberdeen (Scotland)'70; MB ChB; MRCPsy; FRCPC; Psy. Staff/Chief Psychiatrist, Queensway Carleton Hospital; Consultant, Royal Ottawa Mental Health Centre - Royal Ottawa Health Care Group; Psychiatrist, Carleton Place & District Memorial Hospital; Asst Prof, University of Ottawa; (613)721-2000

BROWNE, Moira M A; 201-190 Wellington St, Kingston ON K7L 3E4; Qns'88; BSc; CCFP; FCFP; Ad Staff Privil, Kingston General Hospital; Ad Staff Privil, Hotel-Dieu Hospital; (613)542-4181; Fax. (613)547-0004.

BROWNE, Noel J; Cornwall Clinic, 325 Hamilton Ave, St. John's NL A1E 1K1; Dublin (Ireland)'66; MB ChB; CCFP; (709)579-0055; Fax. (709)579-0766.

BROWNE, Philip M; 1022 20 St S, Lethbridge AB T1K 2C9; Sask'93; BSc; FRCSC; CCFP; ObstGyn. (403)381-4410; Fax. (403)381-4402; pabrowne@shaw.ca.

BROWNELL, A Keith W; Rockyview Gen Hosp, 5A211-7007 14 St SW, Calgary AB T2V 1P9; Qns'64; FRCPC; Neur (Neuromuscular Diseases). Staff Calgary Health Region, Rockyview General Hospital; Prof Clin Neurosciences, University of Calgary; (403)943-8653; Fax. (403)640-7615.

BROWNELL, Laurence G; Physician Anes Services, 303-400 Tache Ave, Winnipeg MB R2H 3C3; Man'76; FRCPC; Anes. Ac Staff, St Boniface General Hospital; (204)233-3413; Fax. (204)233-9763.

BROWNELL, Susan M; Rockyview Gen Hosp, 7007 14th St SW, Calgary AB T2V 1P9; Cal'05; FRCPC; Psy. Staff, Rockyview General Hospital; (403)943-3614; Fax. (403)943-3624.

BROWNING, Andrew D; Royal Court Med Centre, 305-1 Quarry Ridge Rd, Barrie ON L4M 7G1; McM'89; FRCSC; ObstGyn. Obstetrics & Gynecology, Royal Victoria Regional Health Centre; (705)728-5311; Fax. (705)728-5601.

BROWNING, Craig J; Georgetown Med Associates, 1A Princess Anne Dr, Georgetown ON L7G 4W4; Man'72; FRCPC; IntMed; Hem. Staff, Halton Healthcare Services Corporation - Georgetown Hospital; (905)877-8117

BROWNING, David P; 2032 Kingsway, Vancouver BC V5N 2T3; Orange Free State (South Africa)'04; (604)874-5555

BROWNLEE, Carolyn J; Montfort Hosp, 713 Montreal Rd, Ottawa ON K1K 0T2; Cal'92; CCFP; FCFP; Staff, Montfort Hospital; (613)746-4621

BROWNLEE, Richard D; 101-474 Columbia St, Kamloops BC V2C 2T5; Cal'90; BSc; MSc; FRCSC; Neursurg (Spine). Shareholder NeuroSurg, Kamloops Surgical Center; Pres, Welcome Back MRI Pain Management; (250)828-1842; Fax. (250)828-1493.

BROWNOFF, Rene; Misericordia Community Hosp, 16940 87 Ave NW, Edmonton AB T5R 4H5; Alb'74; CCFP; FCFP; Ac Staff, Covenant Health - Misericordia Community Hospital; Assoc Prof, University of Alberta; (780)735-2800; Fax. (780)735-2857.

BROWNRIGG, Peter J; 608-1525 Carling Ave, Ottawa ON K1Z 8R9; Ott'80; Otol (Facial Plastic Surgery). Consultant, The Ottawa Hospital - Riverside Campus; Staff, The Ottawa Hospital - Civic Campus; Consultant, The Ottawa Hospital - General Campus; Teach Staff Otol, University of Ottawa; (613)724-1214; Fax. (613)724-1240.

BROWNSCOMBE, Annette M; Clinic 528, 528 Dundas St E, London ON N6B 1W6; Wes'91; (519)645-1533

BROWNSCOMBE, Larry; London HSC-Victoria Hosp, 800 Commissioners Rd E, London ON N6A 5W9; Wes'79; FRCPC; IntMed. Ac Staff, London Health Sciences Centre - Victoria Campus; Asst Prof, University of Western Ontario; (519)685-8166; Fax. (519)685-8308.

BROWNSTEIN, Michael P; Nelson Mental Health Centre, 333 Victoria St, Nelson BC V1L 4K3; Qns'79; FRCPC; Psy. Staff, UBC Hospital - Koerner Pavillion; Staff, Nelson Mental Health Centre; Asst Prof, University of British Columbia; (250)354-6322

BROWNSTEIN, Seymour; The Ottawa Hosp-Gen Campus, W6213-501 Smyth Rd, Ottawa ON K1H 8L6; McG'65; FRCSC; Ophth (Ocular Pathology). Associate Ophthalmologist, The Ottawa Hospital - General Campus; Assoc Scientist, Ottawa Hosp Research Institute; Prof Ophth & Lab Med, University of Ottawa; Langs: Bilingual(English/French); (613)737-8824; Fax. (613)737-8826.

BROWNSTONE, Desi Y; 203B Regent St, London ON N6A 2G9; Wes'82; FRCPC; Psy (Psychotherapy). (519)663-0878; Fax. (519)663-0990.

BROWNSTONE, Robert M; Queen Elizabeth II HSC-Halifax, 3816-1796 Summer St, Halifax NS B3H 3A7; Man'89; PhD; FRCSC; Neursurg. Staff, Queen Elizabeth II Health Sciences Centre - Halifax Infirmary Site; Staff, Queen Elizabeth II Health Sciences Centre - Victoria General Site; (902)473-6850; Fax. (902)473-6852; rob.brownstone@dal.ca.

BROX, Alan G; Ctr Hosp de Lachine, 650 16e av, Lachine QC H8S 3N5; Mon'76; Hem (P.Q.); IntMed. Staff, CSSS de Dorval-Lachine-Lasalle; (514)637-2351 x77250; Fax. (514)637-0951.

BROX, Anya C; The Centreville Clinic, 301-3210 25th Ave, Vernon BC V1T 1P1; UBC'05; CCFP.

BROX, Dianne E; Weinlos Clinic, 15508 87 Ave NW, Edmonton AB T5R 4G5; Alb'67; CCFP; FCFP; Ac Staff, Covenant Health - Misericordia Community Hospital; (780)484-8151; Fax. (780)483-1435.

BROZEK, Jan Ludwik; McMaster University, HSC 2C19-1280 Main St W, Hamilton ON L8S 4K1; Krakow (Poland)'95; (905)525-9140; Fax. (905)524-3841.

BRUBACHER, Jeffrey R; Vancouver Gen Hosp, 855 12th Ave W, Vancouver BC V5Z 1M9; McG'87; FRCPC; EmergMed. Staff, Vancouver General Hospital - Centennial Pavillion; (604)875-4995; Fax. (604)875-4284.

BRUBACHER, Lloyd; Ilderton Med Clinic, PO Box 160 36 Heritage Dr, Ilderton ON N0M 2A0; Wes'65; CCFP; Ac Staff Family Med, St Joseph's Hospital - St Joseph's Health Care; Court Staff Family Med, London Health Sciences Centre - Victoria Campus; Assoc Prof Family Med, University of Western Ontario; (519)666-1610

BRUCE, Aisha A K; Edmonton Clinic Health Academy, 11405 87 Ave NW, Edmonton AB T6G 1C9; UBC'03; FRCPC; Peds; PedHemaOncol. Staff, University of Alberta Hospital; (780)248-5519

BRUCE, Barry W; West Carleton Med Centre, PO Box 218 119 Langstaff Dr, Carp ON K0A 1L0; Wes'72; CCFP; FCFP; Ac Staff, Queensway Carleton Hospital; Clin Instructor, University of Ottawa; (613)839-3271; Fax. (613)839-3273.

BRUCE, Calvin D; 43 Ascot Crt, Fredericton NB E3B 6C4; Dal'75; Ac Staff, Dr Everett Chalmers Regional Hospital; (506)458-0236; Fax. (506)457-4706.

BRUCE, Cameron; Kings County Med Centre Po Box 817, Montague PE C0A 1R0; Cape Town (South Africa)'97; MB ChB.

BRUCE, Carol E; West Carleton Med Centre, PO Box 218 119 Langstaff Dr, Carp ON K0A 1L0; Wes'72; Staff, Queensway Carleton Hospital; (613)839-3271; Fax. (613)839-3273.

BRUCE, Dean E; Hys Med Centre, 11010 101 St NW, Edmonton AB T5H 4B9; Alb'01; FRCPC; DiagRad. (780)426-1121

BRUCE, Garth A; Royal University Hosp, 103 Hospital Dr, Saskatoon SK S7N 0W8; Sask'70; FRCPC; Peds (Pediatric Gastroenterology). Vis Consultant Ped, Regina General Hospital; Staff, Royal University Hospital; Assoc Prof, University of Saskatchewan; (306)966-8136; Fax. (306)966-8640; g.bruce@usask.ca.

BRUCE, Helen E; Bishops Falls Med Clinic, PO Box 580, Bishops Falls NL A0H 1C0; Mem'85; (709)258-6666; Fax. (709)258-5356.

BRUCE, Jane; Orleans Family Health Clinic, 101-210 Centrum Blvd, Orleans ON K1E 3V7; Tor'86; (613)837-5454; Fax. (613)837-3781.

BRUCE, Lori E; Alexandra Hosp, 29 Noxon St, Ingersoll ON N5C 3V6; Wes'88; Ac Staff, Alexandra Hospital; (519)425-9000

BRUCE, Robert D; Finch Warden Xray & Ultrasound, 308-3443 Finch Ave E, Scarborough ON M1W 2S1; McM'76; FRCPC; DiagRad. (416)466-4152

BRUCE, Rodney R; 202-749 King St W, Kitchener ON N2G 1E4; Ott'98; BSc; MD; CCFP; FCFP; (519)576-4910; Fax. (519)576-3836.

BRUCE, Simon; St Paul's Hosp, 1081 Burrard St, Vancouver BC V6Z 1Y6; Ott'07; Anes. Staff, Providence Health Care - St Paul's Hospital; (604)806-8337 x62813

BRUCE, Tracey L; Hamilton HS-Mcmaster Site, PO Box 2000 Stn Lcd 1 1200 Main St W, Hamilton ON L8N 3Z5; McM'03; FRCPC; Anes. Staff, Hamilton Health Sciences Centre - McMaster Children's Hospital; (905)521-2100

BRUCE, W Robert; Dept of Nutritional Sciences, 150 College St, Toronto ON M5S 3E2; Chicago (USA)'58; PhD; FRSC; FRCPC; MedScient(Med) (Clinical Trials in Cancer Prevention). (416)978-5425; wr.bruce@utoronto.ca.

BRUCE-HOULE, Gwen G; Caledonian Med Clinic, 340 Campbell St, Nanaimo BC V9R 3G7; Mem'83; (250)753-3202

BRUCHET, Melvin R; Lynn Valley Med & Travel Clin, 102-1200 Lynn Valley Rd, North Vancouver BC V7J 2A2; UBC'67; Pres, North Shore Medical Associates; (604)988-0411; Fax. (604)988-5339; mbruchet@providencehealth.bc.ca.

BRUCHOVSKY, Nicholas; Vancouver Prostate Centre, 250A-2660 Oak St, Vancouver BC V6H 3Z6; Tor'61; PhD; FRCPC; MedScient(Med). (604)675-2571

BRUCKERT, Barbara A; Hop Santa Cabrini Ospedale, 5655 rue Saint-Zotique E, Montreal QC H1T 1P7; McG'05; CCFP; Staff, Hôpital Santa Cabrini Ospedale; (514)252-6000

BRUCKSCHWAIGER, Christian; 209-460 Springbank Dr, London ON N6J 0A8; Wes'74; BSc(Hon); CCFP; Ac Staff, London Health Sciences Centre - Victoria Campus; Court Staff, St Joseph's Hospital - St Joseph's Health Care; (226)781-0850

BRUCKSCHWAIGER, Dieter; Springbank Med Centre, 209-460 Springbank Dr, London ON N6J 0A8; Wes'81; CCFP; FCFP; Assoc Staff, London Health Sciences Centre - Victoria Campus; Coroner, Province of Ontario; (519)659-2002; Fax. (519)781-0852.

BRUCKSCHWAIGER, Mary L H; 637 Wellington St, London ON N6A 3R8; Wes'75; (519)679-6394; mbruck@rogers.com.

BRUDER, Eric A; Kingston Gen Hosp, 76 Stuart St, Kingston ON K7L 2V7; Wes'04; FRCPC; EmergMed. Staff, Kingston General Hospital; (613)549-6666

BRUECKS, Andrea K; Calgary Lab Services, 9-3535 Research Rd NW, Calgary AB T2L 2K8; Hamburg (Germany)'83; FRCPC; AnatPath. Staff, Calgary Laboratory Services; (403)770-3674

BRUEMMER, Aurel T; Kateri Mem Hosp Centre, PO Box 10, Kahnawake QC J0L 1B0; McM'96; Staff, Kateri Memorial Hospital Centre; (450)638-3930; Fax. (450)638-4634.

BRUFF, Karl J; Sir Thomas Roddick Hosp, PO Box 5000 Stn Main 142 Minnesota Dr, Stephenville NL A2N 2V6; Mem'00; CCFP; Staff, Sir Thomas Roddick Hospital; (709)643-5111

BRUI, Nathalie; Ctr Hosp du Centre la Mauricie, 50 119e rue, Shawinigan-Sud QC G9P 5K1; Mon'93; CCFP; Staff, Centre Hospitalier du Centre la Mauricie; Langs: Bilingual(French/English); (819)536-7500; Fax. (819)537-5596.

BRUIN, Gerard; The Credit Valley Hosp, 2200 Eglinton Ave W, Mississauga ON L5M 2N1; Tor'83; FRCPC; Anes (Chronic Pain Management). Staff, The Credit Valley Hospital; Asst Prof Anes, McMaster University; (905)813-4466

BRUINSMA, David; Hamilton HS-General Site, 237 Barton St E, Hamilton ON L8L 2X2; McM'08; CCFP; CCFP(E.M.); Staff, Hamilton Health Sciences Centre - Hamilton General Hospital; (905)527-4322

BRULE, Michele F M; Sudbury Med Centre, 401-65 Larch St, Sudbury ON P3E 1B8; Tor'86; FRCSC; GenSurg (Breasts). Staff, Health Sciences North-St Joseph's Health Centre; Staff, Little Current Health Centre; Langs: Bilingual(English/French); (705)673-8391; Fax. (705)673-7330.

BRULE, Sylvie M; Clarence-Rockland Fam Hlth Team, 2741 Chamberland St, Rockland ON K4K 0B4; Ott'95; CCFP; CCFP(E.M.); FCFP; Langs: French; (613)446-7677; Fax. (613)446-5737.

BRULL, Richard T; Univ Hlth Network-Toronto Western Hosp, 399 Bathurst St, Toronto ON M5T 2S8; Cal'99; FRCPC; Anes. Staff, Toronto Western Hospital - University Health Network; (416)603-5118; Fax. (416)603-6494.

BRULOTTE, Cory A; Foothills Med Centre, C231-1403 29 St NW, Calgary AB T2N 2T9; Ott'05; FRCPC; EmergMed. Staff, Foothills Medical Centre; (403)944-1596; Fax. (403)944-2419.

BRULOTTE, Michel; Clinique Med St-Jacques, 160 rue Principale, Saint-Jacques NB E7B 1W4; Laval'81; Staff, Hôpital regional d'Edmundston; Langs: Bilingual(French/English); (506)739-7708; Fax. (506)739-5839.

BRULOTTE, Steeve; Hotel-Dieu de Levis, 143 rue Wolfe, Levis QC G6V 3Z1; Laval'02; Cardiol; IntMed. Staff, Hôtel-Dieu de Lévis; (418)835-7121

BRULOTTE, Veronique; Hop Maisonneuve-Rosemont, 5415 boul de l'Assomption, Montreal QC H1T 2M4; Mon'06; Anes. Staff, Hopital Maisonneuve-Rosemont; (514)252-3400

BRULOTTE-LAPOINTE, Lise; Hôpital Laval, 2725 ch Sainte-Foy, Quebec QC G1V 4G5; Laval'71; FRCPC; Derm. ac Staff, Hôpital Laval; (418)656-8711

BRUM, Virginia; Clinique Metro Medic, 100-1538 rue Sherbrooke O, Montreal QC H3G 1L5; Moscow (Russia (Federation))'69; (514)932-2122

BRUMA, Cleopatra V; 280 Queenston Rd, Hamilton ON L8K 1H1; Bucharest (Romania)'96; CCFP; (905)547-0508

BRUMWELL, Anne K; Medicalwest, 212-3001 Gordon Ave, Coquitlam BC V3C 2K7; UBC'89; (604)944-4077; Fax. (604)944-0677.

BRUMWELL, Mary L; St Paul's Hosp, 1081 Burrard St, Vancouver BC V6Z 1Y6; Alb'79; ThorSurg; GenSurg. Staff, Providence Health Care - St Paul's Hospital; (604)682-2344

BRUN, Dominique; Clinique Pierre Bertrand, 303 boul Pierre-Bertrand, Quebec QC G1M 3L7; Laval'94; Staff, Centre Hospitalier Universitaire De Québec - Pavillon De St-françois-d'assise; (418)683-2724; Fax. (418)683-8861.

BRUN DEL RE, Renato; 4A-128 Queen St S, Mississauga ON L5M 1K8; Ott'79; BSc; Langs: Italian; (905)997-7711; Fax. (905)997-7714.

BRUNDAGE, Michael D; Kingston Reg Cancer Centre, 25 King St W, Kingston ON K7L 5P9; Qns'83; FRCPC; RadOncol. Staff, Kingston General Hospital; Asst Prof, Queen's University; (613)546-8201

BRUNEAU, Anne; CSSS Jeanne Mance, 1250 rue Sanguinet, Montreal QC H2X 3E7; Mon'86; CCFP; Staff Emerg, Centre Hospitalier l'Université De Montréal (CHUM) - Hôpital Saint-luc; Consultant InfectDis & Public Health, McGill University Health Centre - Montreal General Campus; Clin Prof Social & Preventive Med, Universite de Montreal; (514)527-9565

BRUNEAU, Anne; Clinique de Med Familiale, 6F-2120 rue Sherbrooke E, Montreal QC H2K 1C3; Laval'79; (514)527-1958

BRUNEAU, Claude; Clin Med Chutes de Chaudiere, 170-1310 1e Av, Saint-Redempteur QC G6K 1A5; Laval'82; Langs: Italian; English; (418)831-6226; Fax. (418)831-7698.

BRUNEAU, Danielle; Siege Social-Hydro Quebec, 75 boul Rene-Levesque O, Montreal QC H2Z 1A4; Mon'88; CCFP; FCFP; Staff, Centre Hospitalier Pierre Boucher; Médecin, CLSC Cote-des-Neiges; (514)289-3836

BRUNEAU, Genevieve; CLSC des Faubourgs, 1705 rue de la Visitation, Montreal QC H2L 3C3; Mon'04; CCFP; (514)527-2361; Fax. (514)527-3134.

BRUNEAU, Johanne; CLSC Mercier-Est-Anjou, 9503 rue Sherbrooke E, Montreal QC H1L 6P2; Mon'82; (514)356-2574 x3142

BRUNEAU, Julie; 312-264 boul Rene-Levesque E, Montreal QC H2X 1P1; Mon'79; Staff, Centre Hospitalier l'Université De Montréal (CHUM) - Hôpital Saint-luc; (514)890-8321

BRUNEAU, Luc; CHUM-Hotel-Dieu, 3840 rue Saint-Urbain, Montreal QC H2W 1T8; Mon'58; GenSurg (P.Q.). Staff, Centre Hospitalier l'Université de Montréal (CHUM) - Hôtel-Dieu; (514)890-8000

BRUNEAU, Marie-Andree; Inst U Geriatrie de Montreal, 4565 ch Queen-Mary, Montreal QC H3W 1W5; Mon'96; FRCPC; Psy. Staff, Institut Universitaire de Gériatrie de Montréal; Staff, Centre Hospitalier l'Université de Montréal (CHUM) - Hôpital Notre-Dame; (514)340-2800; Fax. (514)340-3542.

BRUNEAU, Michel R; Lac du Bonnet District Hlth Ct, PO Box 700 89 McIntosh Ave, Lac du Bonnet MB R0E 1A0; Man'94; CCFP; Staff, Lorne Memorial Hospital.

BRUNEAU, Nathalie; Hop Brome-Missisquoi-Perkins, 950 rue Principale, Cowansville QC J2K 1K3; Mon'90; OrthSurg. Staff, Hôpital Brome-Missisquoi-Perkins; Langs: Bilingual(French/English); (450)266-4342; Fax. (450)263-8669.

BRUNEAU, Rachel; CHUQ-Ctr Hosp Univ Laval, 2705 boul Laurier, Quebec QC G1V 4G2; Laval'02; CCFP; CCFP(E.M.); Staff, Centre Hospitalier Universitaire de Quebec-CHUL; (418)656-4141

BRUNEAU, Serge; Polyclinique Med Buckingham, 147 rue Joseph, Gatineau QC J8L 1G3; Mon'80; Langs: Bilingual(French/English); (819)986-1034; Fax. (819)986-3308; bruneau@videotron.ca.

BRUNEAU, Virginie; CSSS de Trois-Rivieres, 1991 boul du Carmel, Trois-Rivieres QC G8Z 3R9; Sher'02; FRCPC; NuclearMed. Staff, CSSS de Trois-Rivières; (819)697-3333

BRUNEL-GUITTON, Catherine; Hôpital Ste-Justine, 3175 ch de la Côte-Sainte-Catherine, Montreal QC H3T 1C5; Mon'03; FRCPC; MedGenetics. Staff, Hôpital Ste-Justine; (514)345-4931; Fax. (514)345-4766.

BRUNELLE, Genevieve; Centre Sante des Femmes, 3409 av de Lorimier, Montreal QC H2K 3X5; Mon'89; (514)270-6113; Fax. (514)270-6115.

BRUNELLE, Jacques; Clinique Drs Brunelle & Goyett, 10690 av Peloquin, Montreal QC H2C 2K3; Mon'65; (514)384-0861; Fax. (514)384-3300.

BRUNELLE, Marylene; CSSS Pierre Boucher, 1333 boul Jacques-Cartier E, Longueuil QC J4M 2A5; Sher'01; Staff, Centre Hospitalier Pierre Boucher; (450)468-8111

BRUNELLE, Sarah; Ctr Hosp Fleury, 2180 rue Fleury E, Montreal QC H2B 1K3; Mon'06; FRCPC; Psy. Staff, Centre Hospitalier Fleury; (514)384-2000

BRUNER, Harvey; Bramalea Med Group, 500-18 Kensington Rd, Brampton ON L6T 4S5; Tor'67; Court Staff, William Osler Health System - Brampton Civic Hospital; (905)791-7575; Fax. (905)791-7532.

BRUNET, Aileen S; Eastcoast Forensic Psy Hosp, 88 Gloria McCluskey Ave, Dartmouth NS B3B 2B8; Tor'93; FRCPC; Psy. Staff, The East Coast Forensic Psychiatry Hospital; (902)460-7331; Fax. (902)460-7343; aileen.brunet@cdha.nshealth.ca.

BRUNET, Andre; Hop Jean-Talon, 1385 rue Jean-Talon E, Montreal QC H2E 1S6; Mon'62; LMCC; Psy (P.Q.) (Psycho Geriatrics). Chief Psychogeriatrics, CSSS du Coeur de l'Isle Hôpital Jean-Talon; (514)495-6767 x6203; Fax. (514)495-6749.

BRUNET, Anne-Marie; Montfort Hosp, 713 Montreal Rd, Ottawa ON K1K 0T2; Ott'09; CCFP; Staff, Montfort Hospital; (613)746-4621

BRUNET, Bryan L; Country Hills Village, Box 418 234-5149 Country Hills Blvd NW, Calgary AB T3A 5K8; Alb'87; MBA; FRCPC; RadOncol.

BRUNET, Claire-Lucie; Ctr De Sante Commun De Grand S, 26 Main St E, Chelmsford ON P0M 1L0; Ott'83; BSc; MSc; CCFP; FCFP; Langs: Bilingual(French/English); (705)855-1513; Fax. (705)855-2510; cbrunet@santesudbury.ca.

BRUNET, Daniel; CSSS de Rivière-de-Loup, 75 rue Saint-Henri, Riviere-du-Loup QC G5R 2A4; Laval'76; FRCPC; IntMed (Cardiology). ac Staff, Centre Hospitalier Regional du Grand-Portage; (418)868-1000; Fax. (418)868-1032.

BRUNET, Denis; Ctr Hosp Affilie-Enfant-Jesus, 1401 18e rue, Quebec QC G1J 1Z4; Laval'79; FRCPC; Neur (Neuromuscular Diseases). Staff, Centre Hospitalier Affilié Universitaire de Québec - Hôpital De L'Enfant Jésus; assoc Prof, Université Laval; Langs: English; (418)649-5734; Fax. (418)649-5988; denis.brunet.cha@ssss.gouv.qc.ca.

BRUNET, Donald G; Kingston Gen Hosp, 76 Stuart St, Kingston ON K7L 2V7; Qns'73; FRCPC; IntMed; Neur., Kingston General Hospital; Prof Med, Queen's University; (613)548-2488; Fax. (613)548-1341.

BRUNET, Fabrice; Hop Ste-Justine, 3175 ch Cote-Ste-Catherine, Montreal QC H3T 1C5; Paris (France)'79; Cardiol (P.Q.). Staff, Hôpital Ste-Justine; (514)345-4665

BRUNET, Francois; CSSS de Portneuf, 700 rue Saint-Cyrille, Saint-Raymond QC G3L 1W1; Laval'79; Staff, Centre Hospitalier Portneuf; (418)337-4611 x426

BRUNET, Francois; Centre Med Haut Richelieu, 210-900 boul du Seminaire N, St-Jean-Sur-Richel QC J3A 1C3; Sher'73; Staff, Hôpital du Sacre-Coeur de Montréal; (450)348-1118

BRUNET, Gilles; Clinique Med Adoncour, 200-505 rue Adoncour, Longueuil QC J4G 2M6; Mon'74; (450)646-4445; Fax. (450)646-5526.

BRUNET, Herve J; Clinique Externe Sante Mentale, 26 rue Saint-Pierre, Saint-Constant QC J5A 1B8; Curie (France)'87; (450)635-8807; Fax. (450)635-3689.

BRUNET, Jacques A; Smyth Med Centre, 104-1929 Russell Rd, Ottawa ON K1G 4G3; Ott'73; MSc(ExpSurg,McG); FRCSC; OrthSurg (Foot & Ankle Surgery). Ac Staff, The Ottawa Hospital - General Campus; Assoc Prof, University of Ottawa; (613)521-3100

BRUNET, Jacques R; 865 rue Notre Dame PO Box 1259, Embrun ON K0A 1W0; Ott'77; Staff, Montfort Hospital; (613)443-3311; Fax. (613)443-0142.

BRUNET, Jocelyn; Centre Hosp Honore-Mercier, 2750 boul Laframboise, Saint-Hyacinthe QC J2S 4Y8; Mon'93; CCFP; Staff, Centre Hospitalier Honore-Mercier; (450)771-3333

BRUNET, Matthieu; 610 boul Du Seminaire N, St-Jean-Sur-Richel QC J3B 7B4; Mon'82; (450)348-9218

BRUNET, Nadine; CLSC du Plateau-Mont-Royal, 4625 av de Lorimier, Montreal QC H2H 2B4; Sher'03; (514)521-7663

BRUNET, Richard; Cabinet Medical, 35 rue Saint-Andre, Beauharnois QC J6N 2Y8; Mon'71; (450)395-0555; Fax. (450)395-0596.

BRUNET, Robert; 22-41 rue de l'Eglise, Verdun QC H4G 2L8; Mon'66; Psy (P.Q.). (514)769-2943; Fax. (514)769-0602.

BRUNET, Suzanne M; Hôpital Ste-Justine, 3175 ch Cote-Sainte-Catherine, Montreal QC H3T 1C5; Laval'75; FAAP; FRCPC; Peds. Ac Staff, Hôpital Ste-Justine; (514)345-4931; Fax. (514)345-4744; suzanne_brunet@ssss.gouv.qc.ca.

BRUNET, Sylvain; Centre Hosp Honore-Mercier, 2750 boul Laframboise, Saint-Hyacinthe QC J2S 4Y8; Mon'93; Nephrol; IntMed. Staff, Centre Hospitalier Honore-Mercier; Langs: English; (450)771-3333; Fax. (450)771-3306.

BRUNET, W Grant; Foothills Med Centre, 1403 29 St NW, Calgary AB T2N 2T9; Qns'83; FRCPC; DiagRad. Staff, Foothills Medical Centre; (403)944-1969; Fax. (403)670-1687.

BRUNETTA, Jason M; Maple Leaf Med Arts, 501-14 College St, Toronto ON M5G 1K2; Cal'00; BSc; BEd; CCFP; Physician, Maple Leaf Medical Clinic; (416)465-0756; Fax. (416)465-8344.

BRUNETTE, Isabelle; Hop Maisonneuve-Rosemont, 5415 boul de l'Assomption, Montreal QC H1T 2M4; Mon'83; Ophth (Cornea). Staff, Hopital Maisonneuve-Rosemont; Prof, Universite de Montreal; (514)252-3400 x4959; Fax. (514)252-3905.

BRUNETTE, Veronique; Hop du Sacre-Coeur De Montreal, 5400 boul Gouin O, Montreal QC H4J 1C5; Mon'07; IntMed. Staff, Hôpital du Sacre-Coeur de Montréal; (514)338-2222

BRUNHAM, Liam R; 1199 Lynn Valley Rd PO Box 16011, North Vancouver BC V7J 3S9; UBC'08; FRCPC; IntMed.

BRUNHAM, Robert C; BC Centre For Disease Control, 2077-655 12th Ave W, Vancouver BC V5Z 4R4; UBC'72; FRCPC; IntMed; InfectDis. Staff, Vancouver General Hospital - Centennial Pavillion; Staff, BC Centre For Disease Control; University of British Columbia; (604)707-2409; Fax. (604)707-2401.

BRUNI, Christopher A; 303-170 East St, Sault Ste. Marie ON P6A 3C6; Qns'85; FCFP; CCFP; FCFP; Ac Staff, Sault Area Hospital - Sault Ste Marie; Lecturer Family Med & Residency Prog, University of Toronto; Lecturer Family Med & Residency Prog, University of Ottawa; (705)759-1234; Fax. (705)759-6299.

BRUNI, Ida; London HSC-Victoria Hosp, PO Box 5010 Stn B 800 Commissioners Rd E, London ON N6A 5W9; Wes'05; FRCPC; Anes. Staff, London Health Sciences Centre - Victoria Campus; (519)685-8500

BRUNI, Joseph; 927-55 Queen St E, Toronto ON M5C 1R6; McG'69; BSc; FRCPC; IntMed (Neuro Epilepsy); Neur. Staff, St Michael's Hospital; COO, Moydow Mines International Inc; (416)864-5501; Fax. (416)864-5631.

BRUNI, Teresa; 588 Arthur St W, Thunder Bay ON P7E 5R7; Tor'90; FRCPC; Peds (Consultant Pediatrics). Chief Peds, Thunder Bay Regional Health Sciences Centre Port-Arthur; Teach Staff, Northern Ontario School of Medicine-Laurentian University; (807)766-3370; Fax. (807)766-3374.

BRUNIAU, Jean-Theo; Faubourg Giffard, 2321 ch de la Canardiere, Quebec QC G1J 0A3; Laval'68; ac Staff, Centre Hospitalier Universitaire De Québec - Pavillon De St-françois-d'assise; (418)661-4141

BRUNIER, Jean-Louis; Hop Louis-H Lafontaine, 7401 rue Hochelaga, Montreal QC H1N 3M5; Poitiers (France)'77; Staff, Hopital Louis-H Lafontaine; (514)251-4000

BRUNNER, Karen V; 1710B 20 St PO Box 309, Didsbury AB T0M 0W0; (South Africa)'93; LMCC; Langs: Afrikaans; (403)335-8895; Fax. (403)335-8867.

BRUNNER, Monica; PO Box 4288 Stn Terminal Main, Vancouver BC V6B 3Z7; UBC'98; FRCSC; ObstGyn.

BRUNNER, Reinhard; King West Medical, 505 King St W, Hamilton ON L8P 1B9; Zurich (Switzerland)'98; CCFP; Langs: German; (905)525-3501; office@kingwestmedical.ca.

BRUNNER, Roger; St Mary's Hosp Centre, 3830 av Lacombe, Montreal QC H3T 1M5; Wes'98; CCFP; CCFP(E.M.); FCFP; Staff, St Mary's Hospital Centre; (514)345-3511

BRUNO, Deanna M E; Women's College Hosp, 966-76 Grenville St, Toronto ON M5S 1B2; Ott'03; FRCPC; Psy. Staff, Women's College Hospital; (416)323-6400

BRUNO, Giovanni F; Stevenson Mem Hosp, PO Box 2000 Stn Main 200 Fletcher Cres, Alliston ON L9R 1W7; Padua (Italy)'80; BSc(Hon); MSc(Physics); MD; DABR; FRCPC; DiagRad (Interventional Radiology). Chief Radiologist, Stevenson Memorial Hospital; Langs: Italian; French; (705)435-6281

BRUNO, Tania R; 345 Rumsey Ave, Toronto ON M4G 1R7; Qns'01; FRCPC; PhysMed&Rehab. (416)597-3422 x5370; Fax. (416)597-7160.

BRUNS, Alessandra; CHUS-Hop Hotel-Dieu, 580 rue Bowen S, Sherbrooke QC J1G 2E8; Gama Filho (Brazil)'97; Staff, Centre Hospitalier Universitaire de Sherbrooke-Hôpital Hôtel-Dieu; Langs: Portuguese; English; Italian; (819)346-1110 x15261

BRUNSDON, Peta L; Wellness Centre, 221 Ellerdale St, Saint John NB E2J 3S4; Dal'85; (506)634-7877; Fax. (506)634-7878.

BRUNSKILL, Megen; 22 Peninsula Rd PO Box 399, Marathon ON P0T 2E0; McM'04; CCFP; (807)229-3243; m.brunskill@rogers.com.

BRUNT, Margaret E; Burnaby Hosp, 5A ACE-3935 Kincaid St, Burnaby BC V5G 2X6; UBC'79; FRCPC; IntMed. Staff, Burnaby Hospital; (604)434-4211

BRUNT, Susan; Balmoral Med Arts Facility, 405-1366 Yonge St, Toronto ON M4T 3A7; Ott'86; CCFP; Staff, Women's College Hospital; (416)923-5767; Fax. (416)923-5125.

BRUNTON, Gillian M; Newcastle Village Med Assoc, 87 Mill St N, Newcastle ON L1B 1H8; West Indies (Other Foreign)'98; CCFP; (905)987-1896; Fax. (905)987-3183.

BRUNTON, James E; 68 Symons St, Etobicoke ON M8V 1T9; Tor'52; (416)251-6901

BRUNTON, Jane A; 250 Dundas St E, Waterdown ON L0R 2H4; McM'84; CCFP; FCFP; Clinical Asst Prof Family Med, McMaster University; (905)690-6748; Fax. (905)690-6750; brunton@mcmaster.ca.

BRUNTRUP-TAYLOR, Jennifer; West Hill Medical Clinic, 1A-2995 2nd Ave W, Prince Albert SK S6V 5V5; (306)765-8500; Fax. (306)765-8501.

BRUSHETT, Frederick J; St Clare's Mercy Hosp, 154 LeMarchant Rd, St. John's NL A1C 5B8; Mem'93; CCFP; Staff, St Clare's Mercy Hospital; (709)777-5000

BRUSKY, Janna D; Royal University Hosp, 103 Hospital Dr, Saskatoon SK S7N 0W8; Sask'04; FRCPC; Peds. Staff, Royal University Hospital; (306)966-2922; Fax. (306)966-8640.

BRUSSOW, Heinrich D; High Level Med Clinic, 11202 100 Ave SS 1, High Level AB T0H 1Z0; Pretoria (South Africa)'78; MB ChB; Langs: German; Afrikaans; (780)926-2286; Fax. (780)926-3550.

BRUSSOW, Jacques E; 1300 111 Ave, Dawson Creek BC V1G 2X5; Stellenbosch (South Africa)'03; MB ChB; Langs: Afrikaans; (250)782-7525; jebrussow@gmail.com.

BRUSSOW, Waldemar H; ABC Medical Clinic, 9842 101 Ave, Fort St. John BC V1J 2B2; Pretoria (South Africa)'78; (250)785-1220

BRUTUS, Jean-Paul; L'Institut Chirurgie Special d, 112-6100 av du Boise, Montreal QC H3S 2W1; Bruxelles (Belgium)'96; PlasSurg. Staff, Centre Hospitalier l'Université de Montréal (CHUM) - Hôpital Notre-Dame; (514)737-6100; Fax. (514)737-6158.

BRUUN-MEYER, Sturla E; 800-180 Bloor St W, Toronto ON M5S 2V6; Witwatersrand (South Africa)'72; MB ChB; MRCPsy(UK); FRCPC; Psy. Staff, Centre for Addiction & Mental Health (CAMH) - College Street Site; Asst Prof Med, University of Toronto; Langs: Afrikaans; Norwegian; (416)964-0370; Fax. (416)964-6606; sbmconsulting@rogers.com.

BRUWER, Anna D B; PO Box 23021 Rpo St Mikes, Lethbridge AB T1J 4P5; Orange Free State (South Africa)'82; Staff, Chinook Regional Hospital; Langs: Afrikaans; (403)388-6111

BRUYERE, Helene A T; Cytogenetics Laboratory, 1800J-899 12th Ave W, Vancouver BC V5Z 1M9; Saint-Etienne (France)'95; Dir Cytogenetics Lab, Vancouver General Hospital - Centennial Pavillion; (604)875-4129

BRYAN, Colin F; Tilbury District Family Hlth Team, PO Box 760 22 Mills St W, Tilbury ON N0P 2L0; London (England)'66; MB BS; MD; MRCS; LRCP; Med Dir, Kent-Chatham Community Care Access; (519)682-2307

BRYAN, Susan C; Thunder Bay Reg HSC-T-Bay, 980 Oliver Rd, Thunder Bay ON P7B 6V4; McM'74; Ac Staff, St Joseph's Care Group - St Joseph's Hospital; Ac Staff Anes & Family Pract, Thunder Bay Regional Health Sciences Centre; (807)684-6000

BRYAN, Tracey L; Grey Nuns Community Hosp & HC, Box 36 1100 Youville Drive West NW, Edmonton AB T6L 5X8; Alb'05; FRCPC; Respir; IntMed. Staff, Covenant Health - Grey Nuns Community Hospital; (780)735-7000; Fax. (780)735-9921.

BRYANS, Franklin C; 252 Swiss Meadows Blvd RR 2, Ravenna ON N0H 2E0; Wes'70; MSc(NeuroPhysiol); (705)445-8755; febryans@georgian.net; Semi-Retired.

BRYANS, John; Thames Valley FHT-Windermere S, 301-460 Wellington St, St Thomas ON N5R 6H9; Wes'81; Staff, St Thomas Elgin General Hospital; (519)635-7630; Fax. (519)631-8570.

BRYANT, J Scott; 331C 6th St, Courtenay BC V9N 1M2; Wes'83; CCFP; FCFP; (250)338-1333

BRYANT, William H; The Village of Winston Park, 695 Block Line Rd, Kitchener ON N2E 3K1; Wes'64; CCFP; FCFP.

BRYCE, Cicely J; Faculty of Med-UBC, 2110-2775 Laurel St, Vancouver BC V5Z 1M9; UBC'82; FRCPC; IntMed (Breast Cancer); MedOncol. (604)875-4111 x67895

BRYCE, Elizabeth A; Vancouver Gen Hosp, JPN 1111-855 12th Ave W, Vancouver BC V5Z 1M9; Sask'83; FRCPC; IntMed (Infection Control); MedMicrobiol. Staff, Vancouver General Hospital - Centennial Pavillion; Clin Prof, University of British Columbia; (604)875-4759; Fax. (604)875-4359; elizabeth.bryce@vch.ca.

BRYDEN, Patricia A M; Alberta Prof Bldg, 300-320 23 Ave SW, Calgary AB T2S 0J2; Alb'83; (403)229-4423; Fax. (403)228-9828.

BRYDEN, Patricia L; Fredericton Med Clinic, 406-1015 Regent St, Fredericton NB E3B 6H5; Ott'86; FRCSC; GenSurg. (506)458-0475; Fax. (506)458-0479.

BRYDIE, Alan D; Queen Elizabeth II HSC-Halifax, 3511-1796 Summer St, Halifax NS B3H 3A7; Glasgow (Scotland)'94; MB ChB; FRCPC; DiagRad. Staff, Queen Elizabeth II Health Sciences Centre - Halifax Infirmary Site; Staff, Queen Elizabeth II Health Sciences Centre - Victoria General Site; (902)473-7770

BRYDIE, Sarah E; Fenwick Med Centre, 211-5595 Fenwick St, Halifax NS B3H 4M2; Glasgow (Scotland)'92; CCFP; (902)423-3323; Fax. (902)442-5593.

BRYDON, Kyle W; St Thomas Family Health Centre, 110-230 First Ave, St Thomas ON N5R 4P5; Wes'94; FRCSC; Ophth. (519)633-9846; Fax. (519)633-8321.

BRYDON, Lizabeth A; Regina Qu'Appelle HR-Regina, 1440 14th Ave, Regina SK S4P 0W5; Alb'79; FRCSC; ObstGyn (Gynecology). Staff, Regina General Hospital; Staff, Allan Blair Cancer Centre; Staff, Regina Health District; Teach Staff/Admn Staff, University of Saskatchewan; Langs: English; French; (306)766-0557

BRYDON, Marni E; Rideau Med & Dental Centre, 101-1711 4 St SW, Calgary AB T2S 1V8; McG'01; CCFP; (403)228-3667; Fax. (403)228-3660.

BRYER, Mark A; York-Finch Med Centre, 216B-2115 Finch Ave W, North York ON M3N 2V6; Witwatersrand (South Africa)'88; Neur. (416)744-0000; Fax. (416)744-0077.

BRYK, Caroline M; Colborne Family Med Centre, 612 Colborne St, London ON N6B 2V2; Tor'86; CCFP; FCFP; (519)673-1962; Fax. (519)673-3758.

BRYMER, Christopher D; London HSC-University Hosp, PO Box 5339 Stn B 339 Windermere Rd, London ON N6A 5A5; Tor'87; MSc; FRCPC; IntMed; GeriatricMed. Staff Internist, London Health Sciences Centre - University Hospital; Assoc Prof Med, University of Western Ontario; (519)663-3922; Fax. (519)663-3472; cbrymer@uwo.ca.

BRYNIAK, Christopher S; Mental Health Services, 55 Union St, Saint John NB E2L 5B7; Mem'04; FRCPC; Psy. (506)658-3737

BRYNIAK, Steven; 95 Coburg St, Saint John NB E2L 3J8; Qns'73; FRCSC; Urol (Erectile Dysfunction). Ac Staff, Saint John Regional Hospital; Ac Staff, Sussex Health Centre; Ac Staff, St Joseph's Hospital; Lecturer, Dalhousie University; (506)634-8636; Fax. (506)634-1755.

BRYNJOLFSON, John R; 4041 200B St, Langley BC V3A 1P1; UBC'69; (604)530-1181; Fax. (604)530-5609.

BRYON, Terry F; 202-29 Toronto St S, Uxbridge ON L9P 1V9; Tor'75; (905)852-6101; Fax. (905)852-0618.

BRYSKI, Lisa M; Health Sciences Centre, 820 Sherbrook St, Winnipeg MB R3A 1R9; Man'93; CCFP; CCFP(E.M.); Staff, Health Sciences Centre; (204)774-6511

BRYSON, Gregory L; The Ottawa Hosp-Civic Campus, 1053 Carling Ave, Ottawa ON K1Y 4E9; Man'89; MSc(Epidemiol.); FRCPC; Anes. Staff, The Ottawa Hospital - Civic Campus; Asst Prof Anes, University of Ottawa; (613)761-4169; Fax. (613)761-5209.

BRYSON, Julie C; Conner House Family Practice, 240 Pinnacle St, Belleville ON K8N 3A6; Wes'07; CCFP; (613)968-9840

BRYSON, Malcolm J; Medical Associates Sechelt, PO Box 638 5531 Inlet Ave, Sechelt BC V0N 3A0; UBC'90; (604)885-2257; Fax. (604)885-4718.

BRYSON, S C Peter; Kingston Gen Hosp, V4-76 Stuart St, Kingston ON K7L 2V7; McM'78; FACOG; FRCSC; ObstGyn (Gynecologic Oncology). Staff GynOncol, Kingston General Hospital; Assoc Prof, Queen's University; (613)548-6071; Fax. (613)548-1330; bryson@queensu.ca.

BRYSON, Thomas W; Bow River Med Clinic, 202-1205 Bow Valley Trail, Canmore AB T1W 1P5; Glasgow (Scotland)'67; FRCS(Glas); Ac Staff, Canmore General Hospital; (403)609-2136; Fax. (403)609-2149.

BRZESKI, Jerzy T; Lakeview Med Clinic, 10-6449 Crowchild Trail SW, Calgary AB T3E 5R7; Warsaw (Poland)'61; PhD; Langs: Polish; (403)242-4172; Fax. (403)242-4296.

BRZEZINSKA-PYTLAK, Hanna G; 278 O'Connor St, Ottawa ON K2P 1V4; Wroclaw (Poland)'80; FRCPC; Psy. Staff, The Ottawa Hospital - Civic Campus; (613)233-1565; Fax. (613)233-1851.

BRZEZINSKI, Alex E; SMBD Jewish Gen Hosp, E 938-3755 ch Cote-Ste-Catheri, Montreal QC H3T 1E2; Ott'73; FRCSC; Urol. Ac Staff, Sir Mortimer B Davis Jewish General; Ac Staff, McGill University Health Centre - Montreal Children's Hospital; adj Prof, McGill University; (514)340-7558

BRZEZINSKI, Jack J; Univ of Toronto, 602-500 University Ave, Toronto ON M5G 1V7; Tor'09.

BRZEZINSKI, Wanda T; Westmount Square Med Centre, C180-1 Car Westmount, Westmount QC H3Z 2P9; Warsaw (Poland)'63; LMCC; Physician Interim Federal Health Prog, Citizenship & Immigration Canada; Langs: English; Polish; French; Russian; (514)934-2334; Fax. (514)934-5559; wanda.brzezinski@cic.gc.ca.

BRZEZINSKI, Wojciech S; 439 6 Ave SW, Medicine Hat AB T1A 5A9; Warsaw (Poland)'80; FRCSC; GenSurg (Surgical Oncology). Consultant Surg, Brooks Health Centre; Staff Surg, Medicine Hat Regional Hospital; Consultant surg, Tom Baker Cancer Centre; Langs: Polish; Italian; French; (403)487-5151

BRZOZOWSKI, Michael S; Sunnybrook Hlth Sciences Ctre, 2075 Bayview Ave, Toronto ON M4N 3M5; Tor'88; FRCPC; EmergMed. Staff, Sunnybrook Health Sciences Centre; (416)480-4037

BSATA-PARENT, Aida; Ctre Sante Medicentre Pincourt, 88 5e av, Pincourt QC J7V 5K7; Mon'78; (514)425-1000

BSHOUTY, Zoheir; Respiratory Unit, RS105-810 Sherbrook St, Winnipeg MB R3A 1R8; Technion (Israel)'82; FRCPC; IntMed (Critical Care Medicine); Respir. Att Staff IntMed, Health Sciences Centre; Att Staff, St Boniface General Hospital; Assoc Prof Med, University of Manitoba; Langs: French; German; Hebrew; (204)787-1059; Fax. (204)787-1220; zbshouty@hsc.mb.ca.

BUBBAR, Vikrant K; 108-2626 Croydon Dr, Surrey BC V3S 0S8; McM'99; BScN; BEd; FRCSC; OrthSurg (Lower Extremity Reconstruction). (604)535-5345

BUBELA, Constantine B; Lakeridge Hlth Corp-Oshawa, 1 Hospital Crt, Oshawa ON L1G 2B9; Qns'77; DAB; FRCPC; Anes. Staff Anes, Lakeridge Health - Oshawa Site; (905)433-2800; Fax. (905)697-4696.

BUCCI, Clotilde; Pavillon Rosemont, 5689 boul Rosemont, Montreal QC H1T 2H1; Sher'82; FRCPC; Psy (General Psychiatry). (514)252-3400; Fax. (514)252-3810.

BUCCI, Raffaele; 8470 boul Lacordaire, Saint-Leonard QC H1R 2A5; Sher'80; Langs: English; French; Italian; (514)325-6160; Fax. (514)325-6160.

BUCH, Mark; SMBD Jewish Gen Hosp, 3755 ch Cote Sainte-Catherine, Montreal QC H3T 1E2; McG'07; MDCM; CCFP; CCFP(E.M.); Staff, Sir Mortimer B Davis Jewish General; (514)340-8222

BUCHAN, Shelley M; Central Reg Health Authority, 180 Centennaire Dr, Southport MB R0H 1N1; Sask'85; FRCPC; CommunMed; Public Health & Preventive Med. Med Officer of Hlth, Central Regional Health Authority; Shelley.Buchan@gov.mb.ca.

BUCHAN, Susan M; Sunwood Medical, 3000 Lougheed Hwy, New Westminster BC V3B 1C5; UBC'94; CCFP; (604)464-0345

BUCHANAN, G Stuart; 120 B rue Principale GD, St-Andre-Avellin QC J0V 1W0; McG'87; (819)983-7919

BUCHANAN, Kenneth D; Victoria Emerg Phys Mgmt Ltd, 325-1627 Fort St, Victoria BC V8R 1H8; Alb'74; FRCPC; EmergMed. Staff, Victoria General Hospital; (250)479-1442

BUCHANAN, Michael L; HSBC Tower, 1010-299 Victoria St, Prince George BC V2L 5B8; Wes'89; FRCPC; IntMed (Rheumatology). Staff, University Hospital of Northern British Columbia; Clin Instructor, University of British Columbia; (250)563-7373; Fax. (250)563-8741.

BUCHANAN, R Alan; 519-1489 Marine Dr, West Vancouver BC V7T 1B8; Cal'78; FRCPC; Psy (Mood Disorders). Clin Prof Psy, University of British Columbia; (604)922-3570

BUCHANAN, Stephanie; Whitehorse Med Services Ltd, 406 Lambert St, Whitehorse YT Y1A 1Z7; UBC'00; CCFP; Ac Staff, Whitehorse General Hospital; Staff, Whitehorse Medical Services Ltd; (867)393-6600; Fax. (867)393-6601.

BUCHANAN, Suzanne C; The Court Med Health Centre, 312-2863 Ellesmere Rd, Scarborough ON M1E 5E9; Qns'86; BSc; CCFP; Staff Family Med, Rouge Valley Health System - Centenary Health Centre Site; Langs: Spanish; French; (416)281-9055; Fax. (416)281-9006; scbuchanan@hotmail.com.

BUCHAR, Helena; F W Green Med Centre, 1629 Baker St, Cranbrook BC V1C 1B4; Prague (Czech Republic)'96; CCFP; Langs: Czech; (250)426-6601; Fax. (250)426-6470.

BUCHEL, Albert M; St Boniface Gen Hosp, 409 Tache Ave, Winnipeg MB R2H 2A6; Man'94; CCFP; CCFP(E.M.); Staff, St Boniface General Hospital; (204)632-7133

BUCHEL, Christine R; Aboriginal Hlth & Wellness Ctr, 215-181 Higgins Ave, Winnipeg MB R3B 3G1; Man'97; CCFP.

BUCHEL, Edward W; Health Sciences Centre, GC401-820 Sherbrook St, Winnipeg MB R3A 1R9; Man'92; BSc; ABS; ABPS; Med Dir/Surg/Prog Dir-Plast Su, Health Sciences Centre; Staff, Maples Surgical Centre; Staff, University of Manitoba; (204)787-7224; Fax. (204)787-5064.

BUCHEL, Tamara L; Manitoba Coll of Family Physic, 240-1695 Henderson Hwy, Winnipeg MB R2G 1P1; CCFP; Staff, Seven Oaks General Hospital; (204)668-3667

BUCHHALTER, Jeffrey R; Alberta Children's Hosp, 2888 Shaganappi Trail NW, Calgary AB T3B 6A8; Staff, Alberta Children's Hospital; (403)955-7211

BUCHHOLZ, Craig J; University of Alberta Hosp, 1E6. 13WCM-8440 112 St NW, Edmonton AB T6G 2B7; Alb'94; FRCPC; Psy. Staff, University of Alberta Hospital; (780)407-6564; Fax. (780)407-6672.

BUCHHOLZ, Holger W; University of Alberta Hosp, 3H2. 16WMC-8440 112 St NW, Edmonton AB T6G 2B7; (Germany)'03; Staff, University of Alberta Hospital; (780)407-1789; Fax. (780)407-1787.

BUCHHOLZ, Kenneth P W; Annapolis Family Practice Asso, PO Box 623 9745 St George St, Annapolis Royal NS B0S 1A0; Dal'80; CCFP; FCFP; Ac Staff, Soldiers Memorial Hospital; Ac Staff, Digby General Hospital; Sr Physician Advisor, Nova Scotia Dept of Health; Med Oversight Phys, Emergency Health Services Nova Scotia; Preceptor Family Med, Dalhousie University; Langs: German; (902)532-1670; Fax. (902)532-1674; kbuchholz@afpa.co.

BUCHIK, Glenda M; County Club Plaza, 210-3025 Portage Ave, Winnipeg MB R3K 2E2; Man'85; FRCPC; Psy. Staff, St Boniface General Hospital; University of Manitoba.

BUCHINSKI, Michael B; Villa Caritas, 16515 88 Ave NW, Edmonton AB T5R 0A4; Sask'93; FRCPC; Psy. Staff, Alberta Hospital Edmonton; (780)342-6556; Fax. (780)342-6579.

BUCHKO, Gregory M L; Banff Sport Medicine, PO Box 1300 Stn Main 207-303 Lynx St, Banff AB T1L 1B3; Sask'89; FRCSC; OrthSurg (Arthroscopic Surgery). Consultant Orth, Lifemark Springborough Physiotherapy Clinic; (403)760-2897; Fax. (403)760-8234.

BUCHLER, Brian; Stanton Terr Health Authority, PO Box 10 Stn Main 550 Byrne Rd, Yellowknife NT X1A 2N1; Laval'88; FRCSC; GenSurg. Staff, Stanton Territorial Health Authority; (867)669-4122

BUCHMAN, Ellen J; 400-1 Valleybrook Dr, North York ON M3B 2S7; McM'78; CCFP; FCFP; Ac Staff, Mount Sinai Hospital; University of Toronto; (416)386-9761

BUCHMAN, Stephen; Mount Sinai Fam Hlth Team, 4F-60 Murray St Box 13, Toronto ON M5T 3L9; McM'81; FCFP; CCFP; FCFP; Physician Palliative Care, Mount Sinai Hospital; Physician Palliative Care Unit, Baycrest Centre for Geriatric Care; Asst Prof Family Med, McMaster University; Teach Staff Family & Commun Med, University of Toronto; (416)586-4800 x1537; Fax. (416)586-4804; sandy.buchman@tlcpc.org.

BUCHNER, Eduard; 142 Queenston St, St. Catharines ON L2R 2Z7; Pretoria (South Africa)'94; MB ChB; CCFP; Langs: Afrikaans; (905)684-1468

BUCHOLTZ, Ann; Medical Examiners Bldg, 7007 116 St NW, Edmonton AB T6H 5R8; (780)427-4987; Fax. (780)422-1265.

BUCHSTEIN, Miriam L; Malton Med Centre, 22-7330 Goreway Dr, Mississauga ON L4T 4J2; Tor'75; Ac Staff, William Osler Health System - Etobicoke General Hospital; (905)677-4200; Fax. (905)677-0541.

BUCK, Brian H; Grey Nuns Comm Hosp & HC, 1100 Youville Drive West NW, Edmonton AB T6L 5X8; Tor'00; FRCPC; Neur (Neuro Vascular). Staff, University of Alberta Hospital; Staff, Covenant Health - Grey Nuns Community Hospital; Asst Prof, University of Alberta; (780)735-9626; Fax. (780)735-9631.

BUCK, Erica A M; North Bay Reg Health Centre, 50 College Dr, North Bay ON P1B 0A4; Tor'91; CCFP; FCFP; Staff, North Bay Regional Health Centre - Regional Mental Health; (705)474-8600

BUCK, Michael; CSSS du Suroit, 150 rue Saint-Thomas, Salaber-de-Valleyf QC J6T 6C1; McG'07; MDCM; Hem (P.Q.); IntMed. Staff Hematol & Oncol, Centre Hospitalier Régional du Suroit; (450)371-9920

BUCK, Richard M; Chinook Reg Hosp, 960 19 St S, Lethbridge AB T1J 1W5; Man'01; CCFP; CCFP(E.M.); Staff, Chinook Regional Hospital; (403)388-6301

BUCKE, Rodney J; 201-520 17th St, West Vancouver BC V7V 3S8; Pretoria (South Africa)'76; MB ChB; FRCPC; Peds. Consultant Peds, Lions Gate Hospital; Clin Asst Neonatol, BC Children's Hospital; (604)913-8183

BUCKENHAM, Sandra W; 3036 Route 620, Cardigan NB E6B 1M1; Tor'86; FRCPC; Anes; Critical Care Medicine. Staff, Dr Everett Chalmers Regional Hospital; (506)367-1889; Fax. (506)367-1880.

BUCKERIDGE, David L; 1140 av des Pins O, Montreal QC H3A 1A3; Qns'95; FRCPC; CommunMed. (514)934-1934 x32991; Fax. (514)843-1551.

BUCKETT, William; MUHC-Royal Victoria Hosp, 687 av des Pins O, Montreal QC H3A 1A1; Birmingham (England)'88; Staff, McGill University Health Centre - Royal Victoria Hospital; McGill University; (514)934-1934; Fax. (514)843-1678.

BUCKINGHAM, Robert A; Univ Hlth Network-Toronto Gen, 200 Elizabeth St, Toronto ON M5G 2C4; Wes'68; FRCPC; Psy (General Psychiatry). Staff Psy/Clin Dir, Toronto General Hospital - UHN; Assoc Prof, University of Toronto; (416)340-3037; Fax. (416)340-4198; robert.buckingham@uhn.ca.

BUCKLE, Patricia M; Grey Nuns Community Hosp & HC, 1100 Youville Drive West NW, Edmonton AB T6L 5X8; Alb'85; IntMed. Staff, Covenant Health - Grey Nuns Community Hospital; (780)735-7000; Fax. (780)433-0512.

BUCKLER, Philip M; Southlake Reg Health Centre, 596 Davis Dr, Newmarket ON L3Y 2P9; Tor'03; FRCPC; DiagRad. Staff, Southlake Regional Health Centre; (905)895-4521

BUCKLEY, Alan B; 309-1990 Fort St, Victoria BC V8R 6V4; Dal'78; FRCPC; IntMed; Gastroent. Staff, Royal Jubilee Hospital; (250)383-5403; Fax. (250)381-7820.

BUCKLEY, Anne R; Vancouver Gen Hosp, 855 12th Ave W, Vancouver BC V5Z 1M9; National (Ireland)'79; MB BCh; FFR(RCSI); FRCR; BAO; FRCPC; DiagRad (Abdominal Imaging). Chief Section of Ultrasound/Head, Vancouver General Hospital - Centennial Pavillion; Assoc Prof Radiol, University of British Columbia; (604)875-4340

BUCKLEY, Brian J; Guardian Med Arts Bldg, 203-1950 Algonquin Ave, North Bay ON P1B 4Z2; Qns'80; BSc; Staff, North Bay Regional Health Centre - Regional Mental Health; (705)474-3010; Fax. (705)474-6591.

BUCKLEY, Niall J; 59 Payzant Dr PO Box 398, Windsor NS B0N 2T0; Cork (Ireland)'78; BSc(Hons); MB ChB; BAO; Staff, Hants Community Hospital; (902)798-1033; Fax. (902)798-1978; niallbuckley@hfx.eastlink.ca.

BUCKLEY, Charles K R; 203-101 10th Ave S, Cranbrook BC V1C 2N1; Ott'79; FRCSC; OrthSurg. Staff, East Kootenay Regional Hospital; Staff, Creston Valley Hospital & Health Centre; (250)426-9081

BUCKLEY, D Norman; McMaster University, 2U1-1280 Main St W, Hamilton ON L8S 4K1; McM'82; BAP; FRCPC; Anes (Pain Management). Staff, Hamilton Health Sciences Centre - McMaster Children's Hospital; Dept Head Anes/Prof, McMaster University; (905)521-2100 x75166; Fax. (905)523-1224; buckleyn@mcmaster.ca.

BUCKLEY, David J; Dr Charles A Janeway Child HC, 300 Prince Philip Dr, St. John's NL A1B 3V6; Sheffield (England)'78; MB ChB; FRACP(Peds); FRCPC; Neur. Staff Ped Neurol, Janeway Children's Health & Rehabilitation Centre; Asst Prof, Memorial University Of Newfoundland; (709)778-4421; Fax. (709)778-4361.

BUCKLEY, Gillian L; Centennial Med Centre, 299 Lake Ave E, Carleton Place ON K7C 1J3; Wes'94; CCFP; CCFP(E.M.); FCFP; Staff, The Ottawa Hospital - Civic Campus; (613)257-2311

BUCKLEY, Heather; Delta Health Sciences Centre, 202-4515 Harvest Dr, Delta BC V4K 4L1; UBC'98; CCFP; FCFP; Physician, Delta Health Sciences Centre; (604)946-6411

BUCKLEY, Leslie L; Univ Hlth Network-Toronto Western Hosp, 399 Bathurst St, Toronto ON M5T 2S8; McM'98; FRCPC; Psy. Staff, Toronto Western Hospital - University Health Network; (416)603-5800 x3672

BUCKLEY, M Joyce B R; 204-1305 Richmond Rd, Ottawa ON K2B 7Y4; Ott'74; ObstGyn (Age Management). (613)688-2978

BUCKLEY, Miriam R E; Vancouver Mammography, 505-750 West Broadway, Vancouver BC V5Z 1H4; Belfast (Ireland)'94; MB BCh; BAO; FRCPC; DiagRad. (604)879-4177

BUCKLEY, Richard E; 3134 Hospital Dr, Calgary AB T2N 5A1; Cal'83; FRCSC; OrthSurg (Orthopedic Trauma). Staff, Foothills Medical Centre; Prof, University of Calgary; (403)944-8371; Fax. (403)270-8004.

BUCKLEY, Roger; North York Med Arts Bldg, 222-1333 Sheppard Ave E, North York ON M2J 1V1; Tor'80; FRCSC; Urol (Prostate Cancer). Staff, The Scarborough Hospital - Birchmount Campus; Staff, North York General Hospital; Staff, Rouge Valley Health System - Centenary Health Centre Site; Staff, North York General Hospital - Branson Division; (416)499-1333; Fax. (416)499-1322.

BUCKO, Jacqueline E; Saskatoon Community Clinic, 455 2nd Ave N, Saskatoon SK S7K 2C2; Sask'09; CCFP; (306)652-0300; Fax. (306)664-4120.

BUCKRIDAN, Al-Beruni S; 104-688 Coxwell Ave, Toronto ON M4C 3B7; (Jamaica)'73; (416)465-1007

BUCKSTEG, Ute; The Brickyard Clinic, 6010 Brickwood Rd, Nanaimo BC V9V 1S5; Witwatersrand (South Africa)'88; MB ChB; (250)390-5300

BUCKSTEIN, Rena; Toronto Sunnybrook Reg Cancer, 2075 Bayview Ave, Toronto ON M4N 3M5; Boston(MA) (USA)'89; FRCPC; IntMed (Lymphoma); Hem. Staff, Sunnybrook Health Sciences Centre - Edmond Odette Cancer Centre; Asst Prof Med, University of Toronto; Langs: Hebrew; (416)480-5847; rena.buckstein@sunnybrook.ca.

BUCKTON, William A; 109-704 Mara St, Point Edward ON N7V 1X4; Tor'68; CCFP; FCFP; Ac Staff, Bluewater Health - Mitton Site; Ac Staff, Bluewater Health - Norman Site; Coroner, City of Point Edward; (519)332-2715; Fax. (519)332-5200.

BUCONJIC, Tomislav; 516-509 Commissioners Rd W, London ON N6J 1Y5; Tor'96.

BUCUR, Daniela; CHSLD Emilie Gamelin, 1440 rue Dufresne, Montreal QC H2K 3J3; Cluj (Romania)'78; Langs: Romanian; English; (514)527-8921; Fax. (514)527-3587.

BUCUR, Mirela S M; Special Services Unit, 90 John St S, Stratford ON N5A 2Y8; Cluj (Romania)'83; FRCPC; Psy. Staff Special Services, Stratford General Hospital - Huron Perth Healthcare Alliance; (519)272-8249

BUCYK, Brent J; Royal Alexandra Hosp, 10240 Kingsway NW, Edmonton AB T5H 3V9; Alb'83; FRCPC; Anes. Chair Dept of Anes, Royal Alexandra Hospital; Clin Assoc Prof, University of Alberta Hospital; (780)735-4010

BUCZEK, Malgorzata J; Carling-Broadview Med Bldg, 103-770 Broadview Ave, Ottawa ON K2A 3Z3; Cracow (Poland)'74; CCFP; FCFP; Court Staff, The Ottawa Hospital - Civic Campus; Langs: Polish; Russian; (613)729-9463; Fax. (613)729-5989.

BUCZKOWSKI, Andrzej K; Gordon & Leslie Diamond HCC, 5F-2775 Laurel St, Vancouver BC V5Z 1M9; Szczecin (Poland)'83; FRCSC; GenSurg. Staff, Gordon & Leslie Diamond Health Care Centre; Langs: Polish; (604)875-5431; Fax. (604)875-5869.

BUDAI, Balint L; South Vancouver Med Clinic, 350 Marine Dr SE, Vancouver BC V5X 2S5; McG'02; CCFP; Langs: Hungarian; Spanish; French; (604)323-0077

BUDAU, Heinz E; 109-20103 40 Ave, Langley BC V3A 2W3; UBC'87; (604)530-5221; Fax. (604)530-1335.

BUDDEN, Heidi L; 20 Townsend St, Sydney NS B1P 6V2; Dal'02; FRCPC; Peds. (902)562-6664; Fax. (902)539-0080; drheidibudden@eastlink.ca.

BUDGE, Stephen F; Westboro Med Centre, 2F-190 Richmond Rd, Ottawa ON K1Z 6W6; Dal'98; CCFP; Staff, Westboro Medical Centre; (613)719-7837; Fax. (613)719-7813.

BUDHIRAJA, Inderpreet S; Bramalea & Bovaird Walk-In Cli, 107-10095 Bramalea Rd, Brampton ON L6R 0K1; (India)'01; CCFP; (905)793-3311

BUDHOO, Salesh K S; 9-1150 Lorne Park Rd, Mississauga ON L5H 3A5; Medunsa (South Africa)'00; MB ChB; CCFP; (905)271-5717

BUDISIN, Branko; G03-3000 Lawrence Ave E, Scarborough ON M1P 2V1; Qns'02; FRCPC; DiagRad. Staff, The Scarborough Hospital - General Campus; (416)438-6636

BUDNING, Andrew S; Credit Valley Prof Bldg, 305-2300 Eglinton Ave W, Mississauga ON L5M 2V8; McG'87; FRCSC; Ophth (General Ophthalmic Surgery). Staff, The Credit Valley Hospital; Staff, The Hospital For Sick Children; (905)820-5464; Fax. (905)569-2377.

BUDUHAN, Gordon P; Queen Elizabeth II HSC, 7-1276 South Park St, Halifax NS B3H 2Y9; Tor'00; FRCSC; GenSurg; ThorSurg. Staff, Queen Elizabeth II Health Sciences Centre - Victoria General Site; (902)473-8337; Fax. (902)423-4547.

BUDZIANOWSKA-KWIATKOWSKI, Margret; 350-2755 Lougheed Hwy, Port Coquitlam BC V3B 5Y9; Wroclaw (Poland)'82; CCFP; Staff, Eagle Ridge Hospital & Health Care Centre; Staff, Fraser Canyon Hospital; Staff, Royal Columbian Hospital; University of British Columbia; Langs: Polish; German; Russian; (604)941-6659; Fax. (604)941-9289; margret.budzianowska-kwiatkowski@fraserhealth.ca.

BUECKERT, Hartmut; Guelph Gen Hosp, 115 Delhi St, Guelph ON N1E 4J4; Wes'95; CCFP; CCFP(E.M.); FCFP; Staff, Guelph General Hospital; (519)837-1401; hnbueckert@sympatico.ca.

BUEDDEFELD, H Dieter; Altona Clinic, PO Box 999 217 5th Ave NE, Altona MB R0G 0B0; Man'81; CCFP; FCFP; (204)324-6447; Fax. (204)324-5694.

BUEHNER, Sharon E; The Group Health Centre, 240 Mcnabb St, Sault Ste. Marie ON P6B 1Y5; McG'92; CCFP; CCFP(E.M.); FCFP; Langs: English; French; (705)759-1234

BUENAFE, Jay R; Buenafe Clinic, 203-930 Jefferson Ave, Winnipeg MB R2P 1W1; CCFP; (204)697-9013; Fax. (204)697-9017.

BUENGER, Usha R; The Ottawa Hosp-Rehab Ctr, 505 Smyth Rd, Ottawa ON K1H 8M2; Cal'88; FRCPC; PhysMed&Rehab. Staff Physical Med & Rehab, The Ottawa Hospital Rehabilitation Centre; (613)737-7350 x75627; Fax. (613)737-9638.

BUENO, Antonio D; 3438 Main St, Vancouver BC V5V 3N2; Santo Tomas (Philippines)'64; Langs: Tagalog; (604)873-6541

BUENO PATINO, Mario; South Huron Hosp, SS 2 Stn Main 24 Huron St W, Exeter ON N0M 1S2; Santander (Colombia)'92; CCFP; Staff, South Huron Hospital Association; (519)235-2700

BUETI, Giuseppe A; Health Sciences Centre, GG621B-820 Sherbrook St, Winnipeg MB R3A 1R9; Man'98; BSc; FRCPC; IntMed; Nephrol. Staff, Health Sciences Centre; (204)787-2300; Fax. (204)787-3326.

BUETOW, Candice L; Garden City Family Health Team, 7-145 Carlton St, St Catharines ON L2R 1R5; Wes'95; Staff, Niagara Health System - Ontario Street Site; (905)988-1548; Fax. (905)988-3769.

BUFFAM, Frank V; UBC Eye Care Centre, H-2550 Willow St, Vancouver BC V5Z 3N9; McG'68; FRCSC; Ophth (Oculo Plastic Surgery). Ac Staff, Vancouver General Hospital - Centennial Pavillion; Clin Prof, University of British Columbia; Langs: Bilingual(English/French); (604)874-4333; Fax. (604)875-5070; fbuffam@eyecarecentre.org.

BUFFETT, Bernard R; Highlands Med Clinic, GD Stn Main, Neils Harbour NS B0C 1N0; Dal'84; Staff, Buchanan Memorial Hospital; (902)336-2300; Fax. (902)336-2228; buffettb@cbdha.nshealth.ca.

BUFFO SEQUEIRA, Ilan; Variety Childrens Heart Centre, FE241-685 William Ave, Winnipeg MB R3E 0Z2; Anahuac (Mexico)'97.

BUGADA, Nadia; Glen Erin Med-Dental Centre, 11-2318 Dunwin Dr, Mississauga ON L5L 1C7; Tor'86; CCFP; Staff, The Credit Valley Hospital; (905)828-1145

BUGDAHN, Margaret B; 202-10 Unionville Gate, Unionville ON L3R 0W7; Tor'80; BSc; CCFP; FCFP; Staff, Markham Stouffville Hospital; Langs: Polish; (905)305-7655; Fax. (905)305-8571.

BUGDEN, Gena N; Health Sciences Centre, 300 Prince Philip Dr, St. John's NL A1B 3V6; Mem'05; CCFP; CCFP(E.M.); Staff, Health Sciences Centre; (709)777-6300

BUGEAUD, Eric; Clinique de Psychiatrie, 250-2012 boul René-Laennec, Laval QC H7M 4J8; Mon'98; FRCPC; Psy. Staff, Hopital de la Cite de la santé; (450)662-3665 x2

BUGEAUD, Ronald; Clinique Med Notre-Dame, 120-504 rue Notre-Dame, Repentigny QC J6A 2T8; Laval'07; (450)585-3232; Fax. (450)582-9763.

BUGEJA, Ann L; The Ottawa Hosp-Riverside, 1967 Riverside Dr, Ottawa ON K1H 7W9; Tor'01; ABIM; FRCPC; IntMed; Nephrol. Staff Nephrol, The Ottawa Hospital - Riverside Campus; Asst Prof Med, University of Ottawa; (613)738-8400 x82730

BUGEJA, Francis X; 1-3260 Edgemont Blvd, North Vancouver BC V7R 2P2; Alb'88; (604)988-2444; Fax. (604)987-0483.

BUGIS, Samuel P; Dr Samuel P Bugis Prof Corp, 1665 West Broadway, Vancouver BC V6J 5A4; Alb'78; FACS; FRCSC; GenSurg (Head & Neck Surgery). Consultant Surg Oncol, BC Cancer Agency Vancouver Centre; Assoc Staff, Providence Health Care - St Paul's Hospital; Assoc Staff, Vancouver Coastal Health; Ac Staff, Fraser Health Authority; Clin Assoc Prof Surg, University of British Columbia; (604)638-2843; Fax. (604)638-6054; sbugis@mail.ubc.ca.

BUGLASS, Tiffany D; Associated Radiologists, 15-2685 2nd Ave W, Prince Albert SK S6V 5E3; Sask'92; FRCPC; DiagRad. (306)763-8595; Fax. (306)763-7054.

BUGLASS, Todd D; South Hill Med Centre, 7-2685 2nd Ave W, Prince Albert SK S6V 5E3; Sask'92; FRCSC; Ophth. Clinical Asst Prof Ophth & Rural Family Med, University of Saskatchewan; (306)922-7400; Fax. (306)922-7450; toddoffice@sasktel.net.

BUGWANDIN, Suria K; Forest Glade Med Centre, 3145 Forest Glade Dr, Windsor ON N8R 1W6; Utkal (India)'88; (519)739-2888; Fax. (519)739-2848.

BUHARIWALLA, Farokh R; Pier Med Clinic, 788 Victoria Rd, Sydney NS B1N 1J7; Dal'83; CCFP; CCFP(E.M.); FCFP; Ac Staff, Cape Breton Healthcare Complex; Teach Staff, Dalhousie University; (902)564-8361; Fax. (902)567-6161.

BUHAS, Daniela C; MUHC-Montreal Children's Hosp, 2300 rue Tupper, Montreal QC H3H 1P3; Craiova (Romania)'96; FRCPC; MedGenetics. Staff, McGill University Health Centre - Montreal Children's Hospital; (514)412-4427

BUHLER, Karen I; Laurel Med Centre Ltd, 304-888 8th Ave W, Vancouver BC V5Z 3Y1; UBC'80; CCFP; Head Dept of Family Practice, BC Women's Hospital & Health Centre; Clinical Asst Prof Family Practice, University of British Columbia; (604)874-0261; Fax. (604)874-3099.

BUHR, Lori A; PO Box 383 Stn Main, St. Albert AB T8N 7A2; Sask'03; CCFP.

BUHRMANN, Ralf R; The Ottawa Hosp-Gen Campus, W6283-501 Smyth Rd, Ottawa ON K1H 8L6; McG'89; MPH; PhD; FRCSC; Ophth (Glaucoma). Staff Ottawa Eye Institute, The Ottawa Hospital - General Campus; Asst Prof Ophth, University of Ottawa; Langs: German; French; (613)737-8706; Fax. (613)737-8836; rbuhrmann@ottawahospital.on.ca.

BUI, Duong X; 664 Gerrard St E, Toronto ON M4M 1Y3; (Vietnam)'77; (416)461-7198; Fax. (416)461-5071.

BUI, Esther; Sunnybrook Hlth Sciences Ctre, A442-2075 Bayview Ave, Toronto ON M4N 3M5; Tor'02; FRCPC; Neur (Epilepsy). Staff Neurol, Sunnybrook Health Sciences Centre; Staff, Toronto Western Hospital - University Health Network; (416)480-5200; Fax. (416)480-4992.

BUI, Helen; MUHC-Montreal Children's Hosp, E315-2300 rue Tupper, Montreal QC H3H 1P3; Sher'97; Endocrin&Metab; Peds. Staff, McGill University Health Centre - Montreal Children's Hospital; (514)412-4400 x22482

BUI, John T; 3-3033 Palstan Rd, Mississauga ON L4Y 4E7; Medical and Pharmaceutical University (Other Foreign)'92; CCFP; (905)270-4567; Fax. (905)270-4521.

BUI, Linh-Khue; CSSS Pierre Boucher, 1333 boul Jacques-Cartier E, Longueuil QC J4M 2A5; Laval'90; Electroenceph (P.Q.); Neur (P.Q.). Staff, Centre Hospitalier Pierre Boucher; Langs: Vietnamese; English; (450)468-8111

BUI, Luke L Q; 10023 Yonge St, Richmond Hill ON L4C 1T7; Tor'01; BSc; FRCSC; GenSurg (Minimal Invasive Surgery). Ac Staff, Mackenzie Richmond Hill Hospital; (905)918-0243

BUI, Ngoc Yen G; 1255 rue Beauregard, Longueuil QC J4K 2M3; Sher'86; CCFP; (450)928-6777; Fax. (450)928-3021.

BUI, Paul; St Paul's Hosp, 1081 Burrard St, Vancouver BC V6Z 1Y6; UBC'97; FRCSC; CardSurg. Staff, Providence Health Care - St Paul's Hospital; (604)682-2344

BUI, T D N Dominique; Hop de Readaptation Lindsay, 6363 ch Hudson, Montreal QC H3S 1M9; Saigon (Vietnam)'75; LMCC; Staff, Institut de Réadaptation Gingras-Lindsay de Montréal; (514)737-3661 x4124; Fax. (514)345-5220; dbui@ssss.gouv.qc.ca.

BUI, Tam Cong; 10904B 107 Ave NW, Edmonton AB T5H 0X5; Saigon (Vietnam)'78; (780)429-1813; Fax. (780)424-0195.

BUI, The-Bao; CHUS-Hop Fleurimont, 3001 12e Av N, Sherbrooke QC J1H 5N4; Laval'85; FRCPC; DiagRad. Staff, Centre Hospitalier Universitaire de Sherbrooke-Hopital Fleurimont; Chef Radiol, Universite de Sherbrooke; (819)346-1110 x14985; Fax. (819)829-3240.

BUIE, Anne E; Lougheed Plaza, 240-9600 Cameron St, Burnaby BC V3J 7N3; Cal'92; (604)421-1027

BUIE, Daniel A; 203-1711 Cook St, Victoria BC V8T 3P2; UBC'69; Staff, Victoria General Hospital; (250)382-9731; Fax. (250)386-7672; docbuie@shaw.ca.

BUIE, Robert; 400 Rock Chapel Rd, Dundas ON L9H 5E2; Laval'53; Psy (Psychotherapy). Court Staff, Hamilton Health Sciences Centre - McMaster University Medical Centre; Langs: English; French.

BUIE, W Donald; Foothills Med Centre, 1403 29 St NW, Calgary AB T2N 2T9; Alb'84; MSc; FRCSC; GenSurg (Colon & Rectal Surgery). Staff, Foothills Medical Centre; Staff, Tom Baker Cancer Centre; (403)944-2020; Fax. (403)944-1277.

BUITENDAG, Ernest; Charles S Curtis Mem Hosp, 200 West St, St Anthony NL A0K 4S0; Pretoria (South Africa)'91; Staff, Charles S Curtis Memorial Hospital; (709)454-3333

BUITHIEU, Jean; MUHC-Royal Victoria Hosp, M4 76-687 av des Pins O, Montreal QC H3A 1A1; Mon'86; ABIM(IntMed); FRCP; Cardiol; IntMed (Echography Cardiac). Staff, McGill University Health Centre - Royal Victoria Hospital; (514)843-1505; Fax. (514)843-2813.

BUITHIEU, Maria; Hôpital Ste-Justine, 3175 ch Cote-Sainte-Catherine, Montreal QC H3T 1C5; Mon'81; FRCPC; Peds (Diabetology). Ac Staff, Hôpital Ste-Justine; Universite de Montreal; Langs: Bilingual(English/French); (514)345-4675; Fax. (514)345-4822.

BUJAK, Matthew C; Rosedale Med Centre, 812-600 Sherbourne St, Toronto ON M4X 1W4; Tor'04; FRCSC; Ophth. (416)551-6325

BUJOLD, Alexis; Hop Maisonneuve-Rosemont, 5415 boul de l'Assomption, Montreal QC H1T 2M4; Mon'03; FRCPC; RadOncol. Staff, Hopital Maisonneuve-Rosemont; (514)252-3425

BUJOLD, Emmanuel; CHUQ-Ctr Hosp Univ Laval, 2705 boul Laurier, Quebec QC G1V 4G2; Mon'96; FSOGC; DMat/FetMed; FABOG; FRCSC; ObstGyn (Cerebral Palsy). Staff, Centre Hospitalier Universitaire de Quebec-CHUL; (418)525-4456

BUJOLD, Louis; 3-396 William St, Dalhousie NB E8C 2X2; Laval'90; CCFP; FCFP; Staff, Hôpital Régional Campbellton; Langs: Bilingual(English/French); (506)684-3770; Fax. (506)684-3772.

BUJOLD, Marie-Claire; Cumberland Med Clinic, 11-900 Watters Rd, Orleans ON K4A 0B4; Ott'98; CCFP; FCFP; Staff Privil, Montfort Hospital; Med Dir, Maison Accueil Sagesse-Notre-Dame; Langs: English; French; (613)830-3837

BUJOLD, Rachel; CHUS-Hop Fleurimont, 3001 12e Av N, Sherbrooke QC J1H 5N4; Sher'81; BSc; MSc; FRCPC; RadOncol. Staff RadOncol, Centre Hospitalier Universitaire de Sherbrooke-Hopital Fleurimont; assoc Prof, Universite de Sherbrooke; (819)346-1110; Fax. (819)820-6445; rachel.bujold@usherbrooke.ca.

BUKA, Irena S; Misericordia Community Hosp, 231-16940 87 Ave NW, Edmonton AB T5R 4H5; Dundee (Scotland)'75; MB ChB; FRCPC; Peds. Ac Staff, Covenant Health - Misericordia Community Hospital; (780)735-2731; Fax. (780)735-2794.

BUKALA, Bernard P; Medical Arts Bldg, 2-93 St Vincent St N, Stratford ON N5A 6H5; Tor'96; FRCSC; Urol. Staff, Stratford General Hospital - Huron Perth Healthcare Alliance; Staff, Clinton Public Hospital - Huron Perth Healthcare Alliance; Staff, Wingham & District Hospital - Listowel Wingham Hospitals Alliance; Langs: Polish; (519)272-0064; Fax. (519)272-0447.

BUKCZYNSKI, Jacob M; 405-1366 Yonge St, Toronto ON M4T 3A7; Tor'09; CCFP; (416)923-5767; Fax. (416)923-5125.

BUKHANOV, Karina; Mount Sinai Hosp, 1275-600 University Ave, Toronto ON M5G 1X5; Tor'88; FRCPC; DiagRad. Head Div of Breast Imaging, Mount Sinai Hospital; Dept Head Div of Breast Imaging, Toronto General Hospital - UHN; Langs: Russian; (416)586-4800 x4805; Fax. (416)586-4714.

BUKHARI, Rukhsana N; 175 Glen Rd, Toronto ON M4W 2W8; Punjab (Pakistan)'73; MB BS; FRCPC; Psy (Psychoanalysis). (416)929-1510; Fax. (416)920-2230.

BUKMUZ, Nadine M; MCI The Doctor's Office, PO Box 134 LR8-200 Bay St, Toronto ON M5J 2J3; Cape Town (South Africa)'82; MB ChB; Court Staff, Markham Stouffville Hospital; Langs: Hebrew; Afrikaans; (416)368-6787; Fax. (416)368-7632; nadine.bukmuz@sympatico.ca.

BUKMUZ, Rica; 1B-205 Don Head Village Blvd, Richmond Hill ON L4C 7R3; Cape Town (South Africa)'80; MB ChB; Ac Staff Privil, Mackenzie Richmond Hill Hospital; (905)770-8480; Fax. (905)770-1813; doc.brian.rica@rogers.com.

BUKOVY, Brent E; The Spence Clinic, 500-1265 Arthur St E, Thunder Bay ON P7E 5H7; Tor'90; (807)626-1138; Fax. (807)626-1142.

BUKOWSKYJ, Maria; Canadian Med Protective Assn, PO Box 8225 Stn T CSC 875 Carling Ave, Ottawa ON K1G 3H7; Wes'76; FCCP; FRCPC; IntMed; Respir. Staff, Kingston General Hospital; Lecturer, Queen's University; (613)725-2000

BUKSAK, Raena D; St Boniface Gen Hosp, L1202-409 Tache Ave, Winnipeg MB R2H 2A6; Man'02; FRCPC; AnatPath. Staff, St Boniface General Hospital; (204)233-8563

BULAEV, Yury; Misericordia Community Hosp, 16940 87 Ave NW, Edmonton AB T5R 4H5; (Russia (Federation))'77; MD; Staff, Covenant Health - Misericordia Community Hospital; Langs: Russian; French; (780)930-5611; Fax. (780)930-5774.

BULAI, Bianca A; GMF des Aurores Boreales, 228 2e rue E, La Sarre QC J9Z 2G9; (Other Foreign)'95; CCFP; (819)339-5617

BULAJIC, Ranka; Health Park, LL01-45 Weatherbee Rd, Mira Road NS B1M 0A1; Kragujevac (Serbia)'01; (902)567-3626; Fax. (902)567-3624.

BULAKHTINA, Elena A; Hamilton HS-General Site, 237 Barton St E, Hamilton ON L8L 2X2; Moscow (Russia (Federation))'97; FRCPC; AnatPath. Staff, Hamilton Health Sciences Centre - Hamilton General Hospital; (905)527-4322

BULAMBO YOGOLELO, Willy; Labrador South Health Centre, PO Box 70 1 Main St, Forteau NL A0K 2P0; Universite de Kisangani (Congo (Brazzaville))'96; MB BS; Staff, Labrador South Health Centre; (709)931-2450

BULANSKI, Emily M; Can Amera Family Hlth Network, B7A-350 Conestoga Blvd, Cambridge ON N1R 7L7; Alb'90; CCFP; Staff, Waypoint Centre for Mental Health Care; Staff, St Joseph's Healthcare - Charlton Campus; Langs: Polish; French; (519)620-7122; Fax. (519)620-3234.

BULAT, Duane C; Victoria Square Med Clinic, PO Box 5700 Stn Main 217-2345 10th Ave W, Prince Albert SK S6V 7V6; Alb'98; FRCPC; Peds. (306)953-5664; Fax. (306)922-9394.

BULATOVIC-STAJKOVIC, Sladjana; Mount Sinai Hosp, 775-600 University Ave, Toronto ON M5G 1X5; University of Nis (Other Foreign)'86; Staff, Mount Sinai Hospital; (416)586-8379

BULAWKA, Craig; Boyle McCauley Health Centre, 10628 96 St NW, Edmonton AB T5H 2J2; Alb'06; Staff, University of Alberta Hospital; (780)422-7343; Fax. (780)422-7333.

BULDO, George P; Lakeridge Health-Oshawa, 1 Hospital Crt, Oshawa ON L1G 2B9; Tor'91; FRCPC; IntMed; Nephrol. Chief Med, Lakeridge Health - Oshawa Site; Langs: Italian; (905)576-8711 x6201; Fax. (905)743-5315.

BULGER, Maureen A; PO Box 2071 Stn Terminal, Richmond BC V6X 8V6; Tor'79; weissell@telus.net.

BULGER, James; 12 Mckay St, Cayuga ON N0A 1E0; Tor'80; Staff, West Haldimand General Hospital; (905)772-3581; Fax. (905)772-3582.

BULK, Mahamed A; Placentia Health Centre, PO Box 480, Placentia NL A0B 2Y0; Al Fateh (Libya)'99; MB BCh; CCFP; Staff, Placentia Health Centre; Staff, Dr William H Newhook Health Centre; (709)227-2061; bulk@mun.ca.

BULL, Duncan; East Wellington Family Hlth Team, 6 Thompson Cres, Erin ON N0B 1T0; Qns'77; CCFP; FCFP; (519)833-9396; Fax. (519)833-9838.

BULL, Ronald K; 9090 Newman Rd, Chilliwack BC V2P 3Z8; Cal'74; (604)702-4739

BULLARD, Jared M P; Cadham Provincial Lab, 750 William Ave, Winnipeg MB R3E 3J7; Man'04; FRCPC; Peds; MedMicrobiol; InfectDis.

BULLARD, Michael; University of Alberta Hosp, 1G1.58WCM-8440 112 St NW, Edmonton AB T6G 2B7; Alb'72; FRCPC; EmergMed. Staff, University of Alberta Hospital; Dept Chair Emerg Med (Acting), University of Alberta; (780)407-8856; Fax. (780)407-3314.

BULLEID, Barbara A; Dr Everett Chalmers Reg Hosp, PO Box 9000 Stn A, Fredericton NB E3B 5N5; Tor'74; FRCPC; Peds. Staff/Dir Nurseries, Dr Everett Chalmers Regional Hospital; (506)452-5286; Fax. (506)447-4421.

BULLEN, Sandra; Oakfield Med Clinic, 201-1021 Court Ave, Winnipeg MB R2P 1V7; Man'92; CCFP; FCFP.

BULLEN KESTY, Cynthia L; Near North Med Clinic, 1-66 Josphine St, North Bay ON P1B 0A7; McM'78; BSc; FRCSC; Ophth (Cornea/External Disease). Staff, North Bay Regional Health Centre - Regional Mental Health; Instructor, Mayo Clinic; (705)472-4782; Fax. (705)472-1848.

BULLER, Christopher E H; St Michael's Hosp, CC7 152-30 Bond St, Toronto ON M5B 1W8; Wes'84; FRCPC; IntMed (Interventional Cardiology); Cardiol. Dir Cardiac Catheterization & Intervention, St Michael's Hospital; Prof Med, University of Toronto; (416)864-3050

BULLER, Kurt W; Kamloops Mental Health Centre, 100-235 Lansdowne St, Kamloops BC V2C 1X8; Man'83; FRCPC; Psy. Ac Staff, Royal Inland Hospital; (250)377-6500; Fax. (250)377-6503.

BULLEY, Sean R; Etobicoke Med Ctr Fam Hlth Team, 400 The East Mall, Etobicoke ON M9B 3Z9; Tor'97; MSc; FRCPC; IntMed; ClinImmunol&Allergy. Staff Physician, Hamilton Health Sciences Centre - McMaster Children's Hospital; Consultant, Adult & Pediatric Allergy; (416)621-2220; Fax. (416)621-2357.

BULLOCK, Colin A J; PO Box 1205, Comox BC V9M 7Z8; UBC'05; CCFP; Staff, University Hospital of Northern British Columbia; Staff, St Joseph's General Hospital; (250)339-2242

BULLOCK, David; 1673 Ridgewood Dr, Castlegar BC V1N 2L5; Alb'79; CCFP; (250)365-2889; Fax. (250)365-0347; bullock@telus.net.

BULLOCK, Graham L; Queen Elizabeth II HSC-Halifax, 3021-1796 Summer St, Halifax NS B3H 3A7; Mem'86; FRCPC; EmergMed. Staff, Queen Elizabeth II Health Sciences Centre - Halifax Infirmary Site; (902)473-2020

BULLOCK, Lana; McMaster Family Practice, 690 Main St W, Hamilton ON L8S 1A4; UBC'04; CCFP; (905)521-5015; Fax. (905)521-5010.

BULLOCK, Martin J; DJ Mackenzie Bldg, 716-5788 University Ave, Halifax NS B3H 1V8; Mem'88; FRCPC; AnatPath. Staff, Queen Elizabeth II Health Sciences Centre - Victoria General Site; Asst Prof Med, Dalhousie University; (902)473-3148; Fax. (902)473-1049; martin.bullock@cdha.nshealth.ca.

BULLOCK, R Wayne; Hamilton HS-General Site, 237 Barton St E, Hamilton ON L8L 2X2; McM'84; BPHE; CCFP; CCFP(E.M.); Staff, Hamilton Health Sciences Centre - Hamilton General Hospital; Staff, West Haldimand General Hospital; (905)527-4322 x46368; rwbullock@hotmail.com.

BULLOCK, William R; Central Park Medical, 302-1711 Cook St, Victoria BC V8T 3P2; McM'81; (250)383-3443; Fax. (250)383-5721.

BULLOCK PRIES, Karen R; Bethesda Hosp Steinbach, 316 Henry St, Steinbach MB R5G 0P9; McM'87; CCFP; CCFP(E.M.); FCFP; Staff, Bethesda Hospital Steinbach; (204)326-6411

BULOTA, Veronique; Clin Med La Cite Place du Parc, 900-300 rue Léo-Pariseau, Montreal QC H2X 4B3; Mon'78; Staff, Centre Hospitalier l'Université de Montréal (CHUM) - Hôtel-Dieu; (514)281-1722; Fax. (514)281-6697.

BULTERYS, Octaaf S P J; 1225 113 Ave, Dawson Creek BC V1G 2Y9; Brussels (Belgium)'80; Langs: Afrikaans; (250)782-8209

BUMA, Nicolaas H; Thames Valley FHT-Strathroy Me, 74 Front St E, Strathroy ON N7G 1Y7; Wes'71; Ac Staff, Strathroy Middlesex General Hospital - Middlesex Hospital Alliance.

BUNCE, Paul E; Univ Hlth Network-Toronto Gen, 13EN 216-200 Elizabeth St, Toronto ON M5G 2C4; Tor'05; FRCPC; IntMed; InfectDis. Staff, Toronto General Hospital - UHN; (416)340-3111

BUNCIC, J Raymond; The Hosp for Sick Children, 555 University Ave, Toronto ON M5G 1X8; McG'65; BA; FRCSC; Ophth (Neuro Ophthalmology). Staff, Holland Bloorview Kids Rehabilitation Hospital; Staff Ophth, The Hospital For Sick Children; Staff, Toronto General Hospital - UHN; Prof Ophth, University of Toronto; (416)813-8919; Fax. (416)813-5159.

BUNEA, Mioara; CSSS de Gatineau, 777 boul de la Gappe, Gatineau QC J8T 8R2; Mon'07; FRCPC; Psy. Staff, CSSS de Gatineau; (819)966-6550

BUNEA, Ruxandra; SMBD Jewish Gen Hosp, 3755 ch Cote-Sainte-Catherine, Montreal QC H3T 1E2; McG'94; FRCPC; IntMed. Staff IntMed, Sir Mortimer B Davis Jewish General; Staff IntMed, McGill University Health Centre - Montreal General Campus; (514)340-8232

BUNGASH, Arif; Saint John Reg Hosp, PO Box 2100 Stn Main 400 University Ave, Saint John NB E2L 4L2; (Other Foreign)'91; Staff, Saint John Regional Hospital; (506)648-6000

BUNGE, Martin K; Health Sciences Centre, 820 Sherbrook St, Winnipeg MB R3A 1R9; Pretoria (South Africa)'87; MB ChB; MSc; FRCPC; DiagRad (Neuro Radiology). Staff, Health Sciences Centre; Diagnostic-Radiology, Ste Rose General Hospital; University of Manitoba; Langs: Afrikaans; German; Zulu; (204)787-2288

BUNI, Reeda; 604-8600 Franklin Ave, Fort McMurray AB T9H 4G8; (Libya)'84; Staff, Northern Lights Regional Health Centre; (780)743-3262; Fax. (780)743-3278.

BUNN, Roger C; Bramalea Med Group, 500-18 Kensington Rd, Brampton ON L6T 4S5; Qns'75; CCFP; FCFP; Ac Staff, William Osler Health System - Brampton Civic Hospital; (905)791-7575; Fax. (905)791-7532.

BUNN, Steven E; 15121 121 St NW, Edmonton AB T5X 3C8; UBC'86; (780)472-7171; Fax. (780)478-9179.

BUNSTON, Sarah; North York Gen Hosp, 4001 Leslie St, North York ON M2K 1E1; Dal'05; CCFP; Staff, North York General Hospital; (416)756-6000

BUNTEN, Earle R; Plaza 33, PO Box 23122 Rpo Plaza 33, Kelowna BC V1X 7K7; Alb'82; Staff, Vernon Jubilee Hospital; (250)765-5500

BUNTING, Brendan J; Family Health Clinic, PO Box 4127 Stn Main 10-5011 48 Ave, Ponoka AB T4J 1R5; Queen's (Ireland)'74; MB ChB; BAO; Med Staff, Ponoka Hospital & Care Centre; (403)783-5305; Fax. (403)783-8722; buntingb@telusplanet.net.

BUNTING, Hal G; Peace Arch Hosp, 15521 Russell Ave, White Rock BC V4B 2R4; UBC'95; Staff, Peace Arch Hospital; (604)531-5512

BUNTING, Howard; The Hosp for Sick Children, 555 University Ave, Toronto ON M5G 1X8; London (England)'00; Clin Fellow Ophth, The Hospital For Sick Children; (416)813-7654

BUONASSISI, Thomas J; Lonsdale Place, 307-1200 Lonsdale Ave, North Vancouver BC V7M 3H6; UBC'95; FRCSC; Otol (Facial & Cosmetic Surgery). Staff, Buonassisi Facial Cosmetic Surgery; (604)904-4245; Fax. (604)904-4235; info@drbuonassisi.com.

BURAK, A John; College of Phys & Surg of BC, 300-69 Howe St, Vancouver BC V6C 0B4; UBC'76; CCFP; FCFP; Staff, College of Physicians & Surgeons of British Columbia; Clin Assoc Prof, University of British Columbia; (604)733-7758; Fax. (604)733-3503.

BURAK, Kelly W; Univ of Calgary Med Clinic, A2-3330 Hospital Dr NW, Calgary AB T2N 4N1; Sask'94; FRCPC; IntMed (Hepatology); Gastroent. Assoc Prof Med, University of Calgary; (403)944-6555

BURBACK, Darren C; Rockyview Gen Hosp, 5A 142-7007 14 St SW, Calgary AB T2V 1P9; Sask'93; FRCPC; IntMed; GeriatricMed. Staff, Rockyview General Hospital; Clinical Asst Prof Med, University of Calgary; (403)943-3453; Fax. (403)212-1230.

BURBACK, Lisa M; PO Box 307 Stn Main, Edmonton AB T5J 2J7; Alb'07; FRCPC; Psy. Staff, University of Alberta Hospital; (780)342-5473; Fax. (780)342-5411.

BURBRIDGE, Brent E; Royal University Hosp, 103 Hospital Dr, Saskatoon SK S7N 0W8; Sask'85; AB; FRCPC; DiagRad (Angiography & Interventional Radiology). Asst Prof, Royal University Hospital; (306)655-2402; Fax. (306)655-2370.

BURCH, Karen A; 100 Station Lane, Kentville NS B4N 0A3; Virginia (USA)'05; FRCPC; IntMed. Staff, Valley Regional Hospital; (902)681-9410; Fax. (902)681-1058.

BURCHETT, Glenn M; Links Clinic, 104-11910 111 Ave NW, Edmonton AB T5G 3G6; UBC'91; (780)454-0351; Fax. (780)452-6767.

BURCHETT, Lisa K; Links Clinic, 104-11910 111 Ave NW, Edmonton AB T5G 3G6; Alb'92; BSc; (780)454-0351; Fax. (780)452-6767.

BURCHILL, Luke; Toronto Congenital Cardiac Ctr, 5N 519-585 University Ave, Toronto ON M5G 2N2; Melbourne (Australia)'99; Clin Fellow, Toronto General Hospital - UHN; (416)340-4871

BURDAN, Lyudmila N; Med Point Health Care Centre, 233-355 Wellington St, London ON N6A 3N7; Kiev (Ukraine)'68; FRCPC; Psy. Staff, London Health Sciences Centre - Victoria Campus; (519)432-1919

BURDEN, George M; Elmsdale Med Centre, 106 Elmsdale Rd, Elmsdale NS B2S 1K6; Dal'78; Court Staff, Queen Elizabeth II Health Sciences Centre - Victoria General Site; Langs: French; (902)883-2216 x105; Fax. (902)883-1734.

BURDEN, Julia K; 5-52 Abbott St, Smiths Falls ON K7A 1W3; Wes'07; CCFP; Teach Staff, University of Western Ontario; (613)205-1025; Fax. (613)205-1026.

BURDETT, Rachel L; Leamington District Mem Hosp, 194 Talbot St W, Leamington ON N8H 1N9; Alb'02; BSc; LLB; FRCPC; Psy. Staff, Leamington District Memorial Hospital; Staff, Chatham-Kent Health Alliance; (519)326-2373 x4179

BUREAU, Anne-Marie; CLSC de Hull, 85 rue Saint-Redempteur, Gatineau QC J8X 4E6; Mon'86; (819)770-6900; Fax. (819)770-8707.

BUREAU, Benoit; Ctr Hosp Rouyn-Noranda, 4 9e rue, Rouyn-Noranda QC J9X 2B2; Sher'90; Staff, Centre Hospitalier Rouyn-Noranda; (819)764-5131; Fax. (819)797-3869.

BUREAU, Etienne; Clinique du Dr Etienne Bureau, 3605 rue Foucher, Trois-Rivieres QC G8Y 1L1; Laval'98; FRCSC; OrthSurg. (819)693-8389

BUREAU, Helene; Clinique Med St-Alexandre, 200-2310 rue Saint-Louis, Gatineau QC J8T 5L7; Sher'87; Staff, Hôpital de Gatineau; (819)243-4500; Fax. (819)243-1369; hbureau@medecinefamiliale.com.

BUREAU, Marc; CSSS de la Cote-de-Gaspe, 215 boul de York O, Gaspe QC G4X 2W2; Laval'76; FRCSC; ObstGyn. Staff, Centre Hospitalier de Gaspe; (418)368-3301

BUREAU, Marie-Pierre; Centre Hosp Honore-Mercier, 2750 boul Laframboise, Saint-Hyacinthe QC J2S 4Y8; Laval'02; CCFP; CCFP(E.M.); Staff, Centre Hospitalier Honore-Mercier; (450)771-3333

BUREAU, Nathalie J; CHUM-Hop St-Luc, 1058 rue Saint-Denis, Montreal QC H2X 3J4; Mon'87; FRCPC; DiagRad (Musculoskeletal). Staff, Centre Hospitalier l'Université De Montréal (CHUM) - Hôpital Saint-luc; adj Prof, Universite de Montreal; (514)890-8350 x35304; Fax. (514)412-7359.

BUREAU, Nathalie; Inst Philippe Pinel de Mtl, 10905 boul Henri-Bourassa E, Montreal QC H1C 1H1; Mon'92; FRCPC; Psy. Staff, Centre Hospitalier Regional de Sept-Iles; Staff, Institut Philippe-Pinel de Montreal; (514)648-8461 x449

BUREAU, Yanick; Coop Temiscavie, 19 rue Dollard, Ville-Marie QC J9V 1L1; Laval'91; Langs: Spanish; English; (819)622-2433

BUREAU, Yves-Andre; 220-620 rue King E CP 21509 CSP Ste-Famille, Sherbrooke QC J1G 5K2; McG'89; FRCSC; ObstGyn. (819)563-3343

BUREAU MORIN, Marie-Andree; Clinique Familiale, 13555 boul Lacroix, Saint-Georges QC G5Y 1P1; Mon'10; CCFP; (418)228-8001

BUREAU-MORIN, Marie-Helene; CSSS des Etchemins, RR 1 331 rue du Sanatorium, Lac-Etchemin QC G0R 1S0; Laval'05; Staff, CSSS des Etchemins; (418)625-3101; Fax. (418)625-3020.

BUREAU-MORIN, Veronique; CSSS de Beauce-Etchemin, 1515 17e rue, Saint-Georges QC G5Y 4T8; Laval'05; Staff, Centre Hospitalier Beauce-Etchemin; (418)228-2031

BURECHAILO, Leta R; 7019 Alberni St, Powell River BC V8A 2C2; UBC'00; CCFP; (604)485-9213

BURELLE, Denis; Institut de Cardiologie de Mtl, 5000 rue Belanger, Montreal QC H1T 1C8; Sher'74; DABIM; Cardiol (P.Q.); IntMed. Ac Staff, Institut de Cardiologie de Montréal; Chief Cardiol, Hopital Maisonneuve-Rosemont; (514)376-3330; Fax. (514)593-2540.

BURELLE, Sebastien; 1295 boul Saint-Sacrement, Shawinigan QC G9N 3M8; Mon'07; Staff, Centre Hospitalier du Centre la Mauricie; (819)539-2999

BURES, Nicole F; Foothills Med Centre, 1403 29 St NW, Calgary AB T2N 2T9; Cal'07; FRCPC; AnatPath. Staff, Foothills Medical Centre; (403)944-4752; Fax. (403)944-4748.

BURESI, Michelle; South Health Campus, 7E GI-4448 Front St SE, Calgary AB T3M 1M4; Cal'06; FRCPC; IntMed; Gastroent. Staff, Foothills Medical Centre; (403)956-3804

BUREY, Sharon T A; 13390 Lanoue St, Windsor ON N8N 5E1; Dal'83; BSc; FRCPC; Peds (Behavioural Pediatrics). (519)979-5260; dr.burey@bellnet.ca.

BURG, Jan B; 104-1569 6th Ave, Prince George BC V2L 3N4; Pretoria (South Africa)'73; Staff, University Hospital of Northern British Columbia; (250)562-1674

BURGA ALVARADO, Alfonso; Cornwall Comm Hosp-McConnell, PO Box 100 Stn Main 840 McConnell Ave, Cornwall ON K6H 5S5; Lima (Peru)'01; FRCPC; EmergMed. Staff, Cornwall Community Hospital; (613)938-4240

BURGE, Frederick I; Abbie J Lane Mem Bldg, 5909 Veterans Memorial Lane, Halifax NS B3H 2E2; Qns'81; MSc(Epidemiol); CCFP; FCFP; Staff, Queen Elizabeth II Health Sciences Centre - Victoria General Site; Prof, Dalhousie University; (902)473-4742; Fax. (902)473-4760.

BURGE, Jonathan A; The Hosp for Sick Children, 1524-555 University Ave, Toronto ON M5G 1X8; Auckland (New Zealand)'99; Clin Fellow Plastic Surg, The Hospital For Sick Children; (416)813-6448

BURGEL, Sonja H; North Lambton Comm Hlth Ctre, 3-59 King St W, Forest ON N0N 1J0; Wes'83; CCFP; FCFP; (519)786-4545; sburgel@nlchc.com.

BURGER, Jasper G W; 202-8425 120 St, Delta BC V4C 6R2; Stellenbosch (South Africa)'89; MB ChB; MBA; LMCC; CCFP; (604)596-5391; Fax. (604)596-5091.

BURGER, Jeinien; Community Medi Centre, 2707 50 Ave, Lloydminster SK S9V 2A8; Stellenbosch (South Africa)'98; MB ChB; (306)825-4427; Fax. (306)825-2028.

BURGER, Leon E; Family Health Centre, 4918 52 St, Athabasca AB T9S 1G9; Stellenbosch (South Africa)'75; MB ChB; LMCC; Staff, Athabasca Healthcare Centre; Langs: Afrikaans; (780)675-5018; Fax. (780)675-5028.

BURGER, Lydia A; Riverside Med Clinic, 28 3 St NE, Medicine Hat AB T1A 5L8; Orange Free State (South Africa)'95; CCFP; FCFP; Physician, Hummingbird Medical Spa; Langs: Afrikaans; (403)528-3008; Fax. (403)528-9648.

BURGER, Michael B; Family Health Centre, 4918 52 St, Athabasca AB T9S 1G9; Orange Free State (South Africa)'00; MB ChB; (780)675-5018; Fax. (780)675-5028.

BURGER, Michael; 301-180 Vine St S, St Catharines ON L2R 7P3; McG'77; FRCPC; Peds. Ac Staff, Niagara Health System - St Catharines General Site; Asst Prof Peds, McMaster University; Langs: English; French; (905)682-9234; Fax. (905)682-9235.

BURGER, Tobias J L; 1025 103rd Ave, Dawson Creek BC V1G 2G6; Pretoria (South Africa)'09; MB BCh; Langs: Afrikaans; (250)782-1186

BURGESS, Ellen D; Foothills Med Centre, 1403 29 St NW, Calgary AB T2N 2T9; Man'76; MD; FRCPC; IntMed (Hypertension); Nephrol. Ac Staff, Foothills Medical Centre; Dir-Research, Hypertension Research Clinic; Staff, Calgary Health Region; (403)944-1598; Fax. (403)283-2494; ellen.burgess@albertahealthservices.ca.

BURGESS, Gavin; Alberta Children's Hosp, 2888 Shaganappi Trail NW, Calgary AB T3B 6A8; Cape Town (South Africa)'96; MB ChB; FRCPC; Peds; PedEmergMed. Staff, Alberta Children's Hospital; (403)955-7070

BURGESS, John D; Palliser Health Authority, 666 5 St SW, Medicine Hat AB T1A 4H6; (403)529-8024; Fax. (403)529-8998.

BURGESS, John J; Foothills Med Centre, 880-1403 29 St NW, Calgary AB T2N 2T9; Dublin (Ireland)'71; MB ChB; BAO; FRCSC; GenSurg; Cardiovasc&ThorSurg. Staff, Foothills Medical Centre; (403)944-2405; Fax. (403)270-3715.

BURGESS, Kenneth G; Crown Point Family Health Ctre, 67 Kenilworth Ave N, Hamilton ON L8H 4R6; McM'77; CCFP; CCFP(E.M.); Ac Staff, Hamilton Health Sciences Centre - McMaster Children's Hospital; Court Staff, St Joseph's Healthcare - Charlton Campus; Asst Prof FamilyMed, McMaster University; (905)547-2302; Fax. (905)548-9722.

BURGESS, Lorraine T; Soldiers Mem Hosp, PO Box 730 462 Main St, Middleton NS B0S 1P0; Dal'86; Court Staff Privil, Western Kings Memorial Health Centre; Staff, Soldiers Memorial Hospital; (902)825-6160; Fax. (902)825-3812.

BURGESS, Robert D; Whistler Health Care Centre, 201-4380 Lorimer Rd RR 4, Whistler BC V0N 1B4; Tor'74; (604)932-3977; Fax. (604)932-0660.

BURGESS, Stephen M; St Joseph's Gen Hosp, 2137 Comox Ave, Comox BC V9M 1P2; UBC'08; CCFP; Staff, St Joseph's General Hospital; (250)339-2242

BURGESS, Susan C; Downtown Comm Health Centre, 569 Powell St, Vancouver BC V6A 1G8; Qns'80; MA; CCFP; Ac Staff, Providence Health Care - St Paul's Hospital; Vis Staff, Vancouver General Hospital - Centennial Pavillion; Staff, Downtown Community Health Clinic; Clin Assoc Prof, University of British Columbia; Langs: English; French; (604)255-3151; Fax. (604)255-0314; burgnesb@interchange.ubc.ca.

BURGESS, Terrance D; Plaza 33, PO Box 23122 Rpo Plaza 33, Kelowna BC V1X 7K7; Alb'91; CCFP; CCFP(E.M.); (250)765-5500

BURGESS, Tracy A; Orleans Family Health Clinic, 101-210 Centrum Blvd, Orleans ON K1E 3V7; Tor'82; BSc; CCFP; FCFP; Langs: English; French; (613)837-5454; Fax. (613)837-3781.

BURGET, Nancy E; Kingston Family, 202-275 Bagot St, Kingston ON K7L 3G4; McM'86; BScN; CCFP; CCFP(E.M.); FCFP; Assoc Staff, Kingston General Hospital; (613)549-7477; Fax. (613)549-4920.

BURGGRAF, Gary W; FAPC3-76 Stuart St, Kingston ON K7L 2V7; McG'66; BSc; FACC; MD; Cardiol. Att Staff, Hotel-Dieu Hospital; Att Staff, Kingston General Hospital; Prof Med, Queen's University; (613)549-6666 x3722; Fax. (613)548-1387.

BURGHARDT, Margaret; Active Health Sports Med Ctre, 102-115 Bell Farm Rd, Barrie ON L4M 5G1; Tor'88; BSc; CCFP; Staff, Orillia Soldiers' Memorial Hospital; Staff, Royal Victoria Regional Health Centre; Asst Prof Clinical Family Med, McMaster University; (705)725-1050

BURGMANN, Allan J F; Lion's Gate Hosp, 231 15th St E, North Vancouver BC V7L 2L7; UBC'92; FRCPC; Psy. Staff, Lions Gate Hospital; (604)988-3131

BURGMANN, Twila; 405-275 Lansdowne St, Kamloops BC V2C 1X8; UBC'00; FRCPC; IntMed; Gastroent. (250)372-9700; Fax. (250)372-9983.

BURGOYNE, Glen D; 432 Ellis St, Penticton BC V2A 4M2; Cal'74; CCFP; FCFP; (250)492-4066; Fax. (250)492-2299.

BURHAN, Amer M A; Addiction & Mental Hlth-Queen, 4 303-1001 Queen St W, Toronto ON M6J 1H4; Baghdad (Iraq)'93; FRCPC; Psy. Staff, Centre for Addiction & Mental Health (CAMH) - Queen Site; Langs: Arabic; (416)535-8501

BURILOSKI-CHKIPOVA, Anita; Care Point Medical Centres, 140-777 Royal Oak Dr, Victoria BC V8X 4V1; Zagreb (Croatia)'91; Langs: Croatian; (250)479-7147

BURJORJEE, Jessica E; Kingston Gen Hosp, 76 Stuart St, Kingston ON K7L 2V7; Qns'99; FRCPC; Anes. Staff, Hotel-Dieu Hospital; Staff, Providence Care - St Mary's of the Lake Hospital Site; Staff, Providence Care - Mental Health Services; Staff, Kingston General Hospital; (613)548-7827

BURK, Keith W; 7-420 Erb St W, Waterloo ON N2L 6H6; Dal'83; (519)884-6707; Fax. (519)884-0631.

BURK-VASSALLO, Jane L; 30-100 Fourth Ave, St Catharines ON L2S 3P1; Dal'88; BSc(Pharm); CCFP; FCFP; (905)704-1216; Fax. (905)704-0739; drburkvassallo@contursmd.com.

BURKART, Brian C; Life Mark Health Centre, 2225 Macleod Trail SE, Calgary AB T2G 5B6; Alb'84; FRCSC; OrthSurg (Arthritis & Joint Replacement). Clinical Asst Prof Surg, University of Calgary; (403)291-0045; Fax. (403)291-0552.

BURKART, Layton D; University of Alberta Hosp, 1G1. 62WCM-8440 112 St NW, Edmonton AB T6G 2B7; Alb'96; FRCPC; EmergMed. Staff, University of Alberta Hospital; (780)407-8860

BURKE, Bonnie A; Office of the Chief Coroner, 200-26 Grenville St, Toronto ON M7A 2G9; McM'94; FRCSC; GenSurg. Staff, Sunnybrook Health Sciences Centre; Staff, Office of the Chief Coroner; (416)314-4100; Fax. (416)314-0888.

BURKE, Bradley D; PO Box 52009, Windsor ON N8X 0A1; Qns'95; BSc; FRCPC; PhysMed&Rehab. Staff, Windsor Regional Hospital - Tayfour Site; Staff, Hôtel-Dieu Grace Hospital.

BURKE, Brian J; Hants Community Hosp, 89 Payzant Dr, Windsor NS B0N 2T0; Dal'91; FRCPC; Psy. Staff Mental Health Services, Hants Community Hospital; (902)792-2042; Fax. (902)798-0709.

BURKE, Brian R; Windsor Health Unit, 269-1720 Howard Ave, Windsor ON N8X 5A6; Tor'84; FRCPC; Psy. Staff Psy, Windsor Regional Hospital - Tayfour Site; Staff, Hôtel-Dieu Grace Hospital; Staff, Windsor Regional Hospital - Metropolitan Site; Staff, St Joseph's Hospital - St Joseph's Health Care; (519)252-5250; Fax. (519)252-3439.

BURKE, Bruce R; Atrium Prof Bldg, 201-190 Cundles Rd E SS 103, Barrie ON L4M 4S5; Ott'81; ABIM; FACC; FRCPC; IntMed; Cardiol. Court Staff Cardiol, Southlake Regional Health Centre; Cardiology, Royal Victoria Regional Health Centre; Court Staff, Stevenson Memorial Hospital; (705)722-8090; Fax. (705)722-7142.

BURKE, Clarissa; Ilderton Med Clinic, 36 Heritage Dr, Ilderton ON N0M 2A0; Wes'08; CCFP; Teach Staff, University of Western Ontario.

BURKE, Donald G; Abbotsford Reg Hosp & Cancer C, 14-32900 Marshall Rd, Abbotsford BC V2S 0C2; Tor'89; FRCPC; IntMed (Critical Care Medicine). Internal Medicine, Abbotsford Regional Hospital & Cancer Centre; (604)851-4811

BURKE, Emory; North York Med Arts Bldg, 241-1333 Sheppard Ave E, North York ON M2J 1V1; Tor'66; FRCPC; Cardiol. Consultant Div of Cardiol, North York General Hospital; Court Staff Cardiol, Sunnybrook Health Sciences Centre; Asst Prof Med, University of Toronto; (416)494-7500; Fax. (416)494-7575.

BURKE, Graham H; 1-1 Spencer St PO Box 6942, Picton ON K0K 2T0; Mem'77; MSc; BMedSci; BA; DBIM; Med Dir Palliative Care Service, QHC Prince Edward County Memorial; Med Advisor, Community Living Belleville; Med Advisor, Picton Manor Nursing Home; Med Advisor, Children's Aid Society; Med Advisor, Kentwood Park; Med Advisor, Prince Edward Children's Aid Society; (613)476-5766; Fax. (613)476-1559.

BURKE, Howard M; Bowmanville Prof Bldg, 2100-222 King St E, Bowmanville ON L1C 1P6; Tor'88; CCFP; FCFP; Ac Staff, Lakeridge Health - Bowmanville Site; Court Staff, The Scarborough Hospital - General Campus; Coroner, City of Bowmanville Area; Asst Prof, University of Toronto; (905)623-0323; Fax. (905)697-0230.

BURKE, John H; 11380 Pachena Pl, North Saanich BC V8L 5J5; Sydney (Australia)'67; MB BS; FFARCS; DA; Staff, Victoria General Hospital; Staff, Royal Jubilee Hospital; Staff, Saanich Peninsula Hospital; (250)656-1402

BURKE, John; 560 Albert St PO Box 520, Winchester ON K0C 2K0; McG'83; Staff, Winchester District Memorial Hospital; Langs: Gaelic; (613)774-2730; Fax. (613)774-3698.

BURKE, John W; Cobequid Commun Health Centre, 40 Freer Lane, Lower Sackville NS B4C 0A2; Mem'93; FRCPC; DiagRad. Staff, Cobequid Community Health Centre; Staff, Queen Elizabeth II Health Sciences Centre - Victoria General Site; (902)869-6527; Fax. (902)869-6121.

BURKE, Judith L; 4640 17 Ave NW, Calgary AB T3B 0P3; Cal'78; CCFP; FCFP; (403)202-2727; Fax. (403)202-2733.

BURKE, Morris E; 1501-200 Tuxedo Blvd, Winnipeg MB R3P 0R3; Man'51; CCFP; Ac Staff, Concordia General Hospital; Ac Staff, Misericordia Health Centre; Med Dir, Beacon Hill Lodges; (204)489-8585

BURKE, Peggy; Lefebre & Burke Weight Loss &, 100-10655 Southport Rd SW, Calgary AB T2W 4Y1; Alb'83; (403)278-3411; Fax. (403)278-3414; lefebreclinic@telus.net.

BURKE, Robert C; 300-1011 Glenmore Trail SW, Calgary AB T2V 4R6; Man'75; DAB; FACS; FRCSC; Otol. Staff, Rockyview General Hospital; Staff, Alberta Children's Hospital; Staff, Tom Baker Cancer Centre; (403)571-5201; Fax. (403)571-5202; roburke@arczone.com.

BURKE-PERRY, Rosemary; PEI College of Family Physicia, 14 Royalty Rd, Charlottetown PE C1E 1T8; (902)894-2605; Fax. (902)894-3975.

BURKES, Ronald; Mount Sinai Hosp, 1221-600 University Ave, Toronto ON M5G 1X5; Tor'78; FRCPC; IntMed (Colon Cancer). Staff, Toronto General Hospital - UHN; Staff, Toronto Western Hospital - University Health Network; Consultant Oncology, Baycrest Centre for Geriatric Care; Staff, Princess Margaret Hospital - University Health Network; Prof Med, University of Toronto; (416)586-5117; Fax. (416)586-3228.

BURKHART, Chadwick T; 60 Albert St, Southampton ON N0H 2L0; Mem'00; CCFP; (519)483-6000

BURKHOLDER, Charles L; New Denver Med Clinic, PO Box 9, New Denver BC V0G 1S0; Wes'88; CCFP; Staff GP, Slocan Community Health Centre; (250)358-7211; Fax. (250)358-7213; cburkholder@cw.bc.ca.

BURKHOLDER, Lee M; Alberta Children's Hosp, C4 317-2888 Shaganappi Trail N, Calgary AB T3B 6A8; Alb'04; FRCPC; PhysMed&Rehab (Pediatric Rehabilitation). Staff, Alberta Children's Hospital; (403)955-7251; Fax. (403)955-3045.

BURKHOLDER, Shauna C; Alberta Children's Hosp, 2888 Shaganappi Trail NW, Calgary AB T3B 6A8; Alb'04; BSc(MedSci); Critical Care Medicine; Peds. Staff Pediatric Intensivist, Alberta Children's Hospital; Clinical Asst Prof, University of Calgary; (403)955-7931; Fax. (403)955-7081; shauna.burkholder@albertahealthservices.ca.

BURKO, Benjamin; Club Tiny Tots, 3550-6900 boul Decarie, Cote Saint-Luc QC H3X 2T8; McG'88; BSc; Peds (Emergency & General Pediatrics). Staff, Lakeshore General Hospital - Pointe Claire; Staff Emerg Dept, McGill University Health Centre - Montreal Children's Hospital; Att Staff, Sir Mortimer B Davis Jewish General; CEO, Timing Corp. & Med. Dir., Tiny Tots Med Centre; adj Prof Med, McGill University; (514)342-9911 x287; benjamin.burko@videotron.ca.

BURKO, Thomas; MedVisit, 206-3910 Bathurst St, North York ON M3H 5Z3; Tor'80; BSc; MSc; Med Dir, MedVisit - Housecall Service; (416)631-0298; Fax. (416)631-0613; drburko@medvisit.ca.

BURLEY, H Joseph; Sharbot Lake Med Clinic, PO Box 70 1005 Medical Centre Rd, Sharbot Lake ON K0H 2P0; McM'78; BSc; FRCPC; Psy. Staff, Hotel-Dieu Hospital; Staff, Kingston General Hospital; Staff, Providence Care - Mental Health Services; Asst Prof Psy, Queen's University; Asst Prof Psy, Dalhousie University; (613)279-2100; jburley20@cogeco.ca.

BURLIN, Robert M; Stein Med Clinic, 188-550 Burrard St, Vancouver BC V6C 2B5; UBC'77; Staff, St Mary's Hospital; (604)688-5924

BURLING, William W; Westgate Medicentre, 9540 163 St NW, Edmonton AB T5P 3M7; Man'78; CCFP; (780)489-4976

BURMAN, Dmitriy K; Jane Medical Clinic, 101-2780 Jane St, Downsview ON M3N 2J2; (Latvia)'93; (416)745-8500; Fax. (416)748-8730.

BURMAN, Mark L; MUHC-Montreal Gen Hosp, B5 159-1650 av Cedar, Montreal QC H3G 1A4; McG'92; FRCSC; OrthSurg. Staff, McGill University Health Centre - Montreal General Campus; Langs: Bilingual(English/French); (514)934-1934 x42568; Fax. (514)934-8283.

BURN, Robert A F; The Doctors Office at Nose Hil, 137-1829 Ranchlands Blvd NW, Calgary AB T3G 2A7; Cambridge (England)'71; MB BCh; FRCS(Eng); CCFP; Langs: Bilingual(English/French); (403)239-8888; Fax. (403)241-1506.

BURNELL, Colin D; Concordia Hip & Knee Institute, 301-1155 Concordia Ave, Winnipeg MB R2K 2M9; Man'97; FRCSC; OrthSurg. Staff Joint Replacement Group, Concordia General Hospital; (204)661-7459; Fax. (204)661-7420.

BURNELL, Margot J; Saint John Reg Hosp, PO Box 2100 Stn Main 400 University Ave, Saint John NB E2L 4L2; Wes'80; FRCPC; IntMed; MedOncol. Ac Staff, Saint John Regional Hospital; Asst Prof RadOncol & IntMed, Dalhousie University; (506)648-6884; Fax. (506)648-6880.

BURNEO DE LAS CASAS, Jorge G; London HSC-University Hosp, PO Box 5339 Stn B 339 Windermere Rd, London ON N6A 5A5; Lima (Peru)'96; Staff, London Health Sciences Centre - South Street; Staff, London Health Sciences Centre - Victoria Campus; Staff, St Joseph's Hospital - St Joseph's Health Care; Staff, London Health Sciences Centre - University Hospital; (519)663-3464 x13431

BURNET, Neil M; 38 Main St PO Box 70, Lundar MB R0C 1Y0; Sydney (Australia)'69; Staff, Elizabeth M Crowe Memorial Hospital; (204)762-5609; Fax. (204)762-5939; nburnet@irha.mb.ca.

BURNETT, Andrew J; Foul Bay Prof Centre, 322-1964 Fort St, Victoria BC V8R 6R3; Dal'79; FRCSC; Ophth (Vitreo Retinal Surgery). (250)595-0122; Fax. (250)595-6562.

BURNETT, Charles E; 12409 109A Ave NW, Edmonton AB T5M 4A7; Edinburgh (Scotland)'61; DObstRCOG; ObstGyn. Staff, Royal Alexandra Hospital; Clin Assoc Prof, University of Alberta; (780)489-0333

BURNETT, Christopher J; Niverville Med Clinic, PO Box 538 111 Second Ave S, Niverville MB R0A 1E0; Dundee (Scotland)'81; Langs: Lingala; French; (204)388-6626; Fax. (204)388-5091.

BURNETT, Judith; Guelph Gen Hosp, 115 Delhi St, Guelph ON N1E 4J4; Mem'84; FRCPC; Anes (Critical Care Medicine). Staff, Homewood Health Centre; Staff Anes, Guelph General Hospital; (519)822-5350

BURNETT, Mairi; Niverville Med Clinic, PO Box 538 111 Second Ave S, Niverville MB R0A 1E0; Dundee (Scotland)'81; Langs: French; (204)388-6626; Fax. (204)388-5091.

BURNETT, Margaret A; RS4-810 Sherbrook St, Winnipeg MB R3A 1R8; Man'81; FRCSC; ObstGyn. Med Staff, Health Sciences Centre; University of Manitoba.

BURNETT, Patricia J; PO Box 670, Fernie BC V0B 1M0; Cincinnati(Ohio) (USA)'83; FRCPC; IntMed; Gastroent. (250)423-4442

BURNETT, R Stephen J; Rebalance MD, 104-3551 Blanshard St, Victoria BC V8Z 0B9; Wes'94; FRCSC; OrthSurg. (250)940-4444

BURNETT, Ralph H; The Moncton Hosp, 135 MacBeath Ave, Moncton NB E1C 6Z8; Dal'72; FRCSC; GenSurg; VascSurg; ThorSurg. Staff, The Moncton Hospital; (506)860-2170; Fax. (506)857-5088; rhburnett@hotmail.com.

BURNETTE, David M; Brandon Reg Health Centre, 150 McTavish Ave E, Brandon MB R7A 2B3; Alb'74; DiagRad. Staff, Brandon Regional Health Centre; (204)578-4000

BURNHAM, Robert S; 1-6220 Highway 2A, Lacombe AB T4L 2G5; Alb'80; MSc; AB; AB(ElectrodiagnosticMe; FRCPC; PhysMed&Rehab (Musculoskeletal Rehabilitation). Clin Assoc Prof, University of Alberta; (403)782-6555; Fax. (403)782-6511; rburnham@telusplanet.net.

BURNIER, Miguel N; MUHC-Royal Victoria Hosp, H7 53-687 av des Pins O, Montreal QC H3A 1A1; Parana (Brazil)'74; MSc; Staff Dept of Ophth, McGill University Health Centre - Royal Victoria Hospital; Staff, McGill University Health Centre - Montreal General Campus; Staff, Sir Mortimer B Davis Jewish General; McGill University; Langs: Spanish; Portuguese; French; (514)843-1544; Fax. (514)843-1624.

BURNS, A George; 7561 Main St, Louisbourg NS B1C 1J7; Cal'97; BSc(Hon); BAP; LMCC; CCFP; Staff, Cape Breton Healthcare Complex; Langs: French; (902)733-3232; Fax. (902)733-3371.

BURNS, Andrew R; Credit Valley Clinic, 2207 Dunwin Dr, Mississauga ON L5L 1X1; Tor'99; FRCSC; GenSurg (Surgical Oncology). Staff, The Credit Valley Hospital; Staff, Trillium Health Centre - Mississauga; Staff, William Osler Health System - Brampton Civic Hospital; (905)820-4481

BURNS, Anthony S; Toronto Rehab Inst-Lyndhurst, 520 Sutherland Dr, Toronto ON M4G 3V9; Yale University (USA)'94; MD; MSc; Staff, Toronto Rehabilitation Institute - Lyndhurst Centre; Lyndhurst Centre; (416)597-3422; Fax. (416)597-7156.

BURNS, Brenda R; Peterborough Reg HC-Hospital, 1 Hospital Dr, Peterborough ON K9J 7C6; Tor'06; CCFP; Staff, Lakeridge Health - Port Perry Site; Staff, Peterborough Regional Health Centre - Hospital Drive; (705)876-5022

BURNS, Bruce F; The Ottawa Hosp-Gen Campus, 4258-501 Smyth Rd, Ottawa ON K1H 8L6; Alb'76; FRCPC; AnatPath. Staff, The Ottawa Hospital - Civic Campus; Staff, The Ottawa Hospital - General Campus; Prof, University of Ottawa; (613)737-8899 x79041; bfburns@ottawahospital.on.ca.

BURNS, Emma; IWK Health Centre, PO Box 9700 Rpo CSC 5850-5980 University Ave, Halifax NS B3K 6R8; Dal'06; FRCPC; Peds; PedEmergMed. Staff, IWK Health Centre; (902)470-8823; Fax. (902)470-7248.

BURNS, Gerard M; Active Care Med Group, 1108 Klondike Rd, Kanata ON K2K 0G1; Laval'64; BA; Langs: English; French; (613)254-9777; Fax. (613)254-9778.

BURNS, Graham B; Vancouver Comm Coll Hlth Serv, 1155 Broadway E, Vancouver BC V5T 4V5; McM'81; Dir Health Services, Vancouver Community College; (604)871-7186; Fax. (604)871-7190.

BURNS, Jonathan A; Cannon Med Clinic, 4-2151 McCallum Rd, Abbotsford BC V2S 3N9; UBC'91; CCFP; CCFP(E.M.); FCFP; Staff, Abbotsford Regional Hospital & Cancer Centre; (604)853-3314

BURNS, Karen E A; St Michael's Hosp, QW4045-30 Bond St, Toronto ON M5B 1W8; Wes'94; FRCPC; IntMed (Critical Care Medicine); Respir. Staff, St Michael's Hospital; (416)864-6060 x3567

BURNS, Karen L M; Queensway-Carleton Hosp, 3045 Baseline Rd, Nepean ON K2H 8P4; Ott'88; FRCPC; AnatPath. Staff, Queensway Carleton Hospital; (613)721-1000

BURNS, Kenneth J; 402-20395 Lougheed Hwy, Maple Ridge BC V2X 2P9; UBC'78; Dir Med Undergrad & Post Grad Prog, Ridge Meadows Hospital & Health Care Centre; Instructor, University of British Columbia; (604)465-3900

BURNS, Kevin D; The Ottawa Hosp-Riverside, 535A-1967 Riverside Dr, Ottawa ON K1H 7W9; McG'84; BSc; MDCM; FRCPC; IntMed; Nephrol. Staff Nephrol/Prof, The Ottawa Hospital - Riverside Campus; Prof Med, University of Ottawa; Langs: English; French; (613)738-8400 x82580; Fax. (613)562-5487; kburns@ottawahospital.on.ca.

BURNS, Kyle D; Deaf Well Being Program, 300-4211 Kingsway, Burnaby BC V5H 1Z6; UBC'04; FRCPC; Psy. Staff, Providence Health Care - St Paul's Hospital; Staff, BC Mental Health & Addiction Services; (604)456-0900; kburns@forensic.bc.ca.

BURNS, Margaret J; Trillium Hlth Ctr-West Toronto, 150 Sherway Dr, Etobicoke ON M9C 1A5; Tor'69; FRCPC; DiagRad (Nuclear Medicine). Ac Staff, Trillium Health Centre - West Toronto; (416)521-4047 x5517; Fax. (416)521-4014.

BURNS, Michael A; Evergreen Commun Health Ctre, 3425 Crowley Dr, Vancouver BC V5R 6G3; UBC'91; Staff Immunodefiency Clinic, Providence Health Care - St Paul's Hospital; (604)707-3639

BURNS, Michele A; Rockyview Gen Hosp, 7007 14 St SW, Calgary AB T2V 1P9; Cal'92; FRCPC; IntMed. Staff, Rockyview General Hospital; (403)943-3000; michele.burns@shaw.ca.

BURNS, Paulette E; 5 Armstrong Point Rd PO Box 416, Port Carling ON P0B 1J0; McM'82; Staff, South Muskoka Memorial Hospital - Muskoka Algonquin Healthcare; (705)765-5349; Fax. (705)765-5377.

BURNS, Stephen R; The Medical Clinic Associates, 4794A Joyce Ave, Powell River BC V8A 3B6; UBC'92; CCFP; Staff Emerg & Family Pract, Powell River General Hospital; (604)485-6261; Fax. (604)485-2820.

BURNS, Timothy; 103-460 Wellington St, St Thomas ON N5R 6H9; Tor'75; FRCPC; IntMed. Ac Staff, St Thomas Elgin General Hospital; (519)637-9879; Fax. (519)631-6143.

BURNS LACHANCE, Jennifer L; Hammonds Plains Fam Practice, 2120 Hammonds Plains Rd, Hammonds Plains NS B4B 1P3; McM'02; BSc; CCFP; (902)832-9233; Fax. (902)832-7409.

BURNSTEIN, Marcus J; St Michael's Hosp, 16 046-30 Bond St, Toronto ON M5B 1W8; Dal'79; AB; MSc; DABCRS; FRCSC; GenSurg (Colon & Rectal Surgery). Staff, St Michael's Hospital; Assoc Prof, University of Toronto; (416)864-6050; Fax. (416)864-5668; burnstein@smh.ca.

BURNSTEIN, Matthew D; Public Gardens Med Clinic, 200-5675 Spring Garden Rd, Halifax NS B3J 1H1; Dal'83; Court Staff, Queen Elizabeth II Health Sciences Centre - Victoria General Site; (902)425-5440; Fax. (902)482-6019.

BURRA, Tara A R; St Joseph Health Centre, 30 The Queensway, Toronto ON M6R 1B5; Tor'06; Psy. Staff, St Joseph's Health Centre; (416)530-6486; Fax. (416)530-6076.

BURRAGE, Kenneth J; ENT Consultants, 219-1 Paton St, St. John's NL A1B 4S8; Mem'81; FRCSC; Otol (Head & Neck Surgery & Oncology). Assoc Prof Otol, Memorial University Of Newfoundland; (709)579-1003; Fax. (709)579-1708.

BURRELL, Althea A; Univ of Toronto, 1 KIng's College Cir, Toronto ON M5S 1A8; Tor'07; IntMed.

BURRELL, Erin C; Petersen Health Centre, 3800 Finnerty Rd, Victoria BC V8N 1M5; Cal'07; Psy. (250)721-8492

BURRELL, John; Sault Area Hosp, 750 Great Northern Rd, Sault Ste. Marie ON P6B 0A8; Qns'75; FRCSC; OrthSurg. Staff, Sault Area Hospital - Sault Ste Marie; (705)759-3434; burrellj@sah.on.ca.

BURRELL, Steven C; Queen Elizabeth II HSC, 1276 South Park St, Halifax NS B3H 2Y9; Dal'95; FRCPC; DiagRad; NuclearMed. Staff, Queen Elizabeth II Health Sciences Centre - Victoria General Site.

BURRILL, Dean E; Royal Columbian Hosp, 330 Columbia St E, New Westminster BC V3L 3W7; UBC'83; FRCPC; Anes. Staff, Royal Columbian Hospital; (604)520-4602

BURRILL, Joshua H P; BC Children's Hosp, 4480 Oak St, Vancouver BC V6H 3V4; London (England)'99; MB BS; Staff, BC Children's Hospital; (604)875-0507

BURRILL, Randy S; Pictou Med Clinic, PO Box 520 222 Haliburton Rd, Pictou NS B0K 1H0; Dal'83; (902)485-5151; Fax. (902)485-4049.

BURRIS, David M; St Paul's Hosp, 1702 20th St W, Saskatoon SK S7M 0Z9; UBC'79; BSc; FRCPC; Anes. Staff, St Paul's Hospital (Grey Nuns) of Saskatoon; (306)655-5241

BURRIS, H Alan; Burris Clinic, 300-275 Lansdowne St, Kamloops BC V2C 6J3; Adelaide (Australia)'80; MB BS; (250)377-3347

BURRIS, Robert J; Family Med Associates, 15-9701 84 Ave, Grande Prairie AB T8V 4Z8; Dal'78; FRCPC; IntMed (Diabetology). Staff, Queen Elizabeth II Hospital; Asst Prof, University of Alberta; (780)538-9420; Fax. (780)532-0037.

BURRON, Ian S; Lake of the Woods Dist Hosp, 21 Sylvan St, Kenora ON P9N 3W7; Man'10; CCFP; Staff, Lake of the Woods District Hospital; (807)468-9861; Fax. (807)468-3939.

BURROW, Sarah R; McMaster University HSC, PO Box 2000 Stn Lcd 1 1200 Main St W, Hamilton ON L8N 3Z5; Ohio (USA)'91; MSc; FRCSC; OrthSurg (Pediatric Orthopedic Surgery). Staff, Hamilton Health Sciences Centre - McMaster University Medical Centre; Assoc Prof, McMaster University; (905)521-2100 x73177; Fax. (905)521-9992.

BURROWES, Paul W; 265-1632 14 Ave NW, Calgary AB T2N 1M7; UBC'75; FRCPC; DiagRad. Staff, Foothills Medical Centre; Assoc. Clin. Prof., Med., University of Calgary; (403)944-1969; Fax. (403)670-1687; paul.burrowes@calgaryhealthreg.ca.

BURROWS, David R; The Group Health Centre, 240 Mcnabb St, Sault Ste. Marie ON P6B 1Y5; Liverpool (England)'76; FRCPC; Peds. Staff, Thunder Bay Regional Health Sciences Centre; Staff, Sault Area Hospital - Sault Ste Marie; (705)759-1234; Fax. (705)541-2304.

BURROWS, Gary T; 411-401 Richmond St W, Toronto ON M5V 3A8; UBC'82; FRCPC; Psy (Psychotherapy). Consultant, Centre for Addiction & Mental Health (CAMH) - College Street Site; (416)598-4188; Fax. (416)598-4055.

BURROWS, George M; Georgina Med Clinic, PO Box 140, Sutton West ON L0E 1R0; Tor'54; CCFP; Staff, Southlake Regional Health Centre; (905)722-3251; Fax. (905)722-3422.

BURROWS, Jason B; J P Outpatient Care & Surgical, 9450 140th St, Surrey BC V3T 0G9; UBC'05; FRCSC; ObstGyn (Maternal Fetal Medicine). (604)582-4558

BURROWS, Kim J; 208-3330 Richter St, Kelowna BC V1W 4V5; McM'86; FRCPC; Peds. (250)762-0466; Fax. (250)762-0477.

BURROWS, Simon L M; Abbotsford Reg Hosp & Cancer C, 32900 Marshall Rd, Abbotsford BC V2S 0C2; Staff, Abbotsford Regional Hospital & Cancer Centre; (604)851-4700

BURRY, Andrea F; Moncton Med Clinic, 301-860 Mountain Rd, Moncton NB E1C 2N7; Tor'02; CCFP; (506)853-5150

BURRY, Dana L; Valley Care Med Centre, E-310 8th St, Courtenay BC V9N 1N3; Mem'96; CCFP; (250)331-0500

BURS, Simona C; Rockyview Health Centre, 210-1016 68 Ave SW, Calgary AB T2V 4J2; (Romania)'91; FRCPC; IntMed. Staff, Cardiometabolic Evaluation & Risk Assessment Centre; Langs: Romanian; German; (403)541-0033

BURSEY, Brandy R; Queensway-Carleton Hosp, 3045 Baseline Rd, Ottawa ON K2H 8P4; UBC'08; CCFP; CCFP(E.M.); Staff, Queensway Carleton Hospital; (613)721-2000

BURSEY, R Ford; Health Sciences Centre, 300 Prince Philip Dr, St. John's NL A1B 3V6; Mem'82; FACP; MD; FRCPC; IntMed (Gastroenterology); Gastroent. Staff, Health Sciences Centre; Asst Dean Continuing Med Educ/Prof Med, Memorial University Of Newfoundland; (709)777-6960; Fax. (709)777-6931; ford.bursey@med.mun.ca.

BURSTEIN, Irving J; Decarie Square Office Tower, 3025-6900 boul Decarie, Cote Saint-Luc QC H3X 2T8; McG'74; Sr Physician Family Med, Sir Mortimer B Davis Jewish General; Asst Prof Family Med, McGill University; Langs: Bilingual(English/French); (514)733-1000; Fax. (514)733-4555.

BURSTEIN, Jason M; Scarborough Prof Centre, 406-1371 Neilson Rd, Scarborough ON M1B 4Z8; Tor'98; FRCPC; IntMed; Cardiol. Staff, Rouge Valley Health System - Ajax & Pickering Health Centre Site; (416)281-9499; Fax. (416)283-5705.

BURSTEIN, Lili M; Aurora Med Centre, 200-15017 Yonge St, Aurora ON L4G 1M5; Tor'86; CCFP; Staff, Southlake Regional Health Centre; (905)727-9481; Fax. (905)727-6280.

BURT, Christiana C; Univ Hlth Network-Toronto Gen, EN3 462-200 Elizabeth St, Toronto ON M5G 2C4; Cambridge (England)'01; Clin Fellow Anes, Toronto General Hospital - UHN; (416)340-4800

BURT, David W; Rideau Family Health Team, 5-3635 Rivergate Way, Ottawa ON K1V 2A4; UBC'80; (613)739-3700; Fax. (613)739-7043.

BURTON, Beverly A; The Associate Clinic, PO Box 549 1222 Bev McLachlin Dr, Pincher Creek AB T0K 1W0; Cal'06; CCFP; (403)627-3321

BURTON, Corey; 407-860 Mountain Rd, Moncton NB E1C 2N7; Mem'01; CCFP; (506)853-5168; Fax. (506)854-8909.

BURTON, Elizabeth A; Lacewood Medical Center, 200-366 Lacewood Dr, Halifax NS B3S 1M7; Dal'06; CCFP; Staff, Dartmouth General Hospital; (902)445-9400; Fax. (902)445-7108.

BURTON, Jeffrey R; University of Alberta Hosp, 2C2WCM-8440 112 St NW, Edmonton AB T6G 2B7; Tor'66; FRCPC; Cardiol. Consultant, University of Alberta Hospital; Prof Med, University of Alberta; Langs: French; (780)407-1421; Fax. (780)407-6452.

BURTON, Jennifer; 100 Mile House Dist Gen Hosp, PO Box 399, 100 Mile House BC V0K 2E0; Man'94; Staff, 100 Mile House District General Hospital; (250)395-7600

BURTON, Jodie M; Health Sciences Centre, 1007-3330 Hospital Dr NW, Calgary AB T2N 4N1; Tor'00; FRCPC; Neur. Staff, Rockyview General Hospital; (403)210-7419

BURTON, Philip J; 301-1113 Regent St, Fredericton NB E3B 3Z2; Dal'89; BSc; FRCSC; OrthSurg (Arthroscopic Knee & Shoulder Surgery). Staff, Everett Chalmers Regional Hospital-Atlantic Health Sciences Corp-Region 3; (506)457-2755; Fax. (506)443-9183; pjburton@rogers.com.

BURTON, Tracy L; Associate Med Clinic, PO Box 549, Pincher Creek AB T0K 1W0; Cal'06; CCFP; (403)627-3321; Fax. (403)627-2280; tburton@pinchermedical.ca.

BURTON, Wayne P; Family Med Clinic, 2931 20 Ave S, Lethbridge AB T1K 3M5; Utah (USA)'04; MD; BSc; CCFP; (403)328-2326

BURTON-MACLEOD, Rebecca L; Foothills Med Centre, 1403 29 St NW, Calgary AB T2N 2T9; Dal'03; FRCPC; EmergMed. Staff, Foothills Medical Centre; (403)944-1315

BURTON-MACLEOD, Sarah M; Grey Nuns Community Hosp, 4011-1100 Youville Drive West, Edmonton AB T6L 5X8; Dal'02; CCFP; Staff Reg Palliative Care Prog, Covenant Health - Grey Nuns Community Hospital; (780)735-7834

BURUIANA, Manole; Cabbagetown Women's Clinic, 302 Gerrard St E, Toronto ON M5A 2G7; Timisoara (Romania)'62; Med Dir, Cabbagetown Women's Clinic; (416)323-0642; Fax. (416)323-3099; lica1938@yahoo.ca.

BURUL, Claude J; Shouldice Hosp, 7750 Bayview Ave, Thornhill ON L3T 4A3; Tor'72; FRCSC; GenSurg. Gen Surgery, Shouldice Hospital; (905)889-1125

BURWASH, Ian G; Univ of Ottawa Heart Institute, 40 Ruskin St, Ottawa ON K1Y 4W7; Qns'85; FRCPC; IntMed (Echocardiography); Cardiol. Staff, University of Ottawa Heart Institute; Staff, The Ottawa Hospital - Civic Campus; Assoc Prof Med, University of Ottawa; (613)761-5490; Fax. (613)761-5081.

BURWELL, G Scott; Whitby Clinic, 200 Brock St N, Whitby ON L1N 4H5; Qns'81; BSc; CCFP; (905)668-3378; Fax. (905)668-3807; sburwell@hotmail.com.

BURWELL, M Shayne; Medical Arts Bldg, 427-750 Spadina Cres E, Saskatoon SK S7K 3H3; Sask'93; FRCSC; PlasSurg (Hand Surgery). Langs: English; French; (306)653-7117; Fax. (306)653-7127.

BURY, Jeffrey H; Strathcona Med Dental Bldg, 200-8225 105 St NW, Edmonton AB T6E 4H2; Cal'87; FRCSC; OrthSurg. (780)439-5858; Fax. (780)433-1344.

BURY, Katherine D; Rathburn Healthplex Medical, 2-452 Rathburn Rd, Etobicoke ON M9C 3S8; Tor'62; FACS; MSc; FRCSC; GenSurg (Family Medicine). Langs: Polish; (416)621-2323; Fax. (416)621-2321.

BURYM, Craig J; St Boniface Gen Hosp, 409 Tache Ave, Winnipeg MB R2H 2A6; Man'00; FRCSC; ObstGyn. Staff, St Boniface General Hospital; (204)237-2713

BURZYNSKI, Jeffrey H; Children's Hosp, 840 Sherbrook St, Winnipeg MB R3A 1S1; Man'99; FRCPC; Peds; Critical Care Medicine.

BUS, Judith I; Business Bldg, 510-1200 Burrard St, Vancouver BC V6Z 2C7; UBC'83; Ac Staff, Providence Health Care - St Paul's Hospital; Clin Teacher, University of British Columbia; Langs: Hungarian; (604)681-9022

BUSAHMEN, Waleed E; Tacoma Family Practice, 101-58 Tacoma Dr, Dartmouth NS B2W 3E5; Al-Fateh (Libya)'01; MB BCh.

BUSCHE, Karen L; Brant Community HC-Brantford, 200 Terrace Hill St, Brantford ON N3R 1G9; McM'08; CCFP; CCFP(E.M.); Staff, The Brant Community Healthcare System - Brantford General Hospital Site; (519)751-5544

BUSCHE, Kevin D; Rockyview Gen Hosp, 7007 14 St SW, Calgary AB T2V 1P9; Wes'97; FRCPC; Neur. Ac Staff Neurol, Rockyview General Hospital; Clin Assoc Prof, University of Calgary; (403)943-3214; Fax. (403)640-7615; kdbusche@ucalgary.ca.

BUSCHMANN, Donald K; Canadian Forces Hlth Services, PO Box 99000 Stn Forces, Halifax NS B3K 5X5; Sask'83; CCFP; (902)427-8700

BUSH, Haydn; 108-450 Central Ave, London ON N6B 2E8; London (England)'67; PhD; MRCP(UK); DMRT; FRCP; MB BS; FRCPC; RadOncol (Psycho Oncology); Psy. Staff/Chief Psy/Physician Leader, Regional Mental Health Care-St Joseph's Health Care; Assoc Prof Psy, Schulich School of Medicine-University of Western Ontario; (519)672-3020; Fax. (519)672-6090.

BUSH, Keith J; Bayvalley Med Arts Bldg, 206-145 Queenston St, St Catharines ON L2R 2Z9; Wes'90; FRCSC; PlasSurg. (905)685-8400; Fax. (905)685-8401.

BUSH, Kevin L; 808-1200 Burrard St, Vancouver BC V6Z 2C7; UBC'84; BSc; FRCSC; PlasSurg (Reconstructive Surgery). Ac Staff, UBC Hospital - Koerner Pavillion; Ac Staff, Providence Health Care - St Paul's Hospital; Ac Staff, Vancouver General Hospital - Centennial Pavillion; Ac Staff, Squamish General Hospital / Hilltop House; Clin Prof, University of British Columbia; (604)806-3676; Fax. (604)806-0926; info.kbush@telus.net.

BUSH, Robert P; Rob Bush MD Incorporated, PO Box 40 110 Blair Ave, Tatamagouche NS B0K 1V0; Qns'91; CCFP; Med Staff, Lillian Fraser Memorial Hospital / Primary Health Care Centre; (902)657-3517; Fax. (902)657-3513.

BUSH, Shirley H; SCOHS-Elizabeth Bruyere Hosp, 43 Bruyere St, Ottawa ON K1N 5C8; London (England)'87; Staff, SCO Health Service - Élisabeth Bruyère Hospital; (613)562-6262

BUSHBY, Barbara J; Maple Lodge Bldg, PO Box 2018 115-54 Ridge Rd, Deep River ON K0J 1P0; Wes'88; CCFP; FCFP; (613)584-3238; Fax. (613)584-3239.

BUSHRA, Ambreen; 21-429 Tranquille Rd, Kamloops BC V2B 3G9; Rawalpindi (Pakistan)'94; MB BS; (250)376-7242

BUSHUK, Michael B; Medical Bldg C, C12-3000 Lawrence Ave E, Scarborough ON M1P 2V1; Tor'80; MSc; FAAOS; FRCSC; OrthSurg (Musculoskeletal Injury). Ac Staff, The Scarborough Hospital - General Campus; (416)438-6400; Fax. (416)438-6420.

BUSING, Nicholas M W; Primrose Family Med Centre, 35 Primrose Ave, Ottawa ON K1R 0A1; Qns'72; CCFP; FCFP; Court Staff, The Ottawa Hospital - Civic Campus; Ac Staff, SCO Health Service - Élisabeth Bruyère Hospital; Pres/CEO, Association of Faculty of Medicine of Canada; Prof, University of Ottawa; Langs: Bilingual(English/French); (613)230-7788

BUSKI, Z John; Landmark Prof Centre, 103-2731 Hewes Way NW, Edmonton AB T6L 6W6; Alb'69; FRCSC; Ophth. Ac Staff, Royal Alexandra Hospital; Ac Staff, Covenant Health - Grey Nuns Community Hospital; Asst Prof, University of Alberta; (780)450-3335; Fax. (780)461-9430.

BUSLETTA, Angela V; 21561 Old Yale Rd, Langley BC V3A 4M9; Alb'93; FRCSC; ObstGyn. Staff, Langley Memorial Hospital; (604)534-4441; Fax. (604)534-4491.

BUSQUE, Denis; 790 4e rue, Grand-Mere QC G9T 4T8; Laval'65; Langs: English; (819)538-1742; Fax. (819)538-9002; dbusque1@hotmail.com.

BUSQUE, Lambert; Hop Maisonneuve-Rosemont, 5415 boul de l'Assomption, Montreal QC H1T 2M4; Mon'86; FRCPC; IntMed; Hem. Staff, Hopital Maisonneuve-Rosemont; adj Prof Med, Universite de Montreal; (514)252-3404

BUSQUE, Nadia; Hopital Laval, 2725 ch Sainte-Foy, Quebec QC G1V 4G5; Laval'03; Staff, Hôpital Laval; Staff, Centre Hospitalier Universitaire de Québec (CHUQ) - Siege Social; (418)656-8711

BUSS, Mandy R; Northern Connections Centre, LL-425 Elgin Ave, Winnipeg MB R3A 1P2; Man'09.

BUSS, Michael I; Clinical Sciences Bldg, 8 120-152 University Campus, Edmonton AB T6G 2G3; Man'86; BSc; FRCPC; Anes (Cardiovascular Anesthesia). Staff, University of Alberta Hospital; (780)407-8861; Fax. (780)407-3200.

BUSSE, Erhard W; 217 Main St E, Milton ON L9T 1N9; Tor'66; FRCPC; Psy (Disability Psychiatry). Staff, Halton Healthcare Services Corporation - Oakville Site; The Great-West Life Assurance; Consultant Psy, Manulife Financial; Consultant Psy, Sun Life Assurance Co; Staff, North Halton Mental Health Clinic; Hon. Clin. Lect., University of Toronto; Langs: German; (905)693-4240; Fax. (905)693-0596; erhardbusse@yahoo.ca.

BUSSE, Justin E; Halton HCS Corp-Georgetown, 1 Princess Anne Dr, Georgetown ON L7G 2B8; McM'98; CCFP; CCFP(E.M.); Staff, Halton Healthcare Services Corporation - Georgetown Hospital; (905)873-3000

BUSSER, James R; Gordon & Leslie Diamond HCC, 7192-2775 Laurel St, Vancouver BC V5Z 1M9; Wes'84; MHSc; FRCPC; IntMed. Ac Staff, Vancouver General Hospital - Centennial Pavillion; Staff, Gordon & Leslie Diamond Health Care Centre; Clinical Asst Prof, University of British Columbia; (604)875-5907; Fax. (604)875-5906.

BUSSEY, Lynn-Ann; Cowie Family Med Centre, 16 Dentith Rd, Halifax NS B3R 2H9; Dal'02; CCFP; (902)473-1234; Fax. (902)473-4353.

BUSSIERE, Marc-Alain; CSSS de Lac-Saint Jean-Est, CP 1300 succ Bureau-chef 300 boul Champlain S, Alma QC G8B 5W3; Mon'04; Staff, CSSS de Lac-Saint Jean-Est; (418)669-2000

BUSSIERE, Miguel E; 222-3017 66 St NW, Edmonton AB T6K 4B2; Qns'01; FRCPC; Neur. Staff, The Ottawa Hospital - Civic Campus; (780)735-9626; Fax. (780)735-9631.

BUSSIERE, Veronique; Clinique de Gyn et d'Obst, 2237 7e av, Trois-Rivieres QC G8Z 3E2; Mon'01; FRCSC; ObstGyn. Staff, CSSS de Trois-Rivières; (819)379-5353

BUSSIERES, Claude; 216-2780 av Raymond, Saint-Hyacinthe QC J2S 5W7; Mon'81; FRCSC; PlasSurg. Staff Plastic Surg, Centre Hospitalier Honore-Mercier; (450)773-5115; Fax. (450)250-5115.

BUSSIERES, Helene; Inst U en Sante Mentale de QC, 2601 ch de la Canardiere, Quebec QC G1J 2G3; Laval'93; FRCPC; Psy (Anxiety Disorder). Ac Member, Institut Universitaire Sante; Assoc Member, Centre Hospitalier Affilié Universitaire de Québec - Hôpital De L'Enfant Jésus; (418)663-5020; Fax. (418)663-0494.

BUSSIERES, Jean S; Hôpital Laval, 2725 ch Sainte-Foy, Quebec QC G1V 4G5; Laval'78; CSPQ; DAB; FRCPC; Anes. Staff Anes, Hôpital Laval; Prof Anes, Université Laval; (418)656-4565; jean.bussieres@anr.ulaval.ca.

BUSSIERES, Josee; CSSSG-Hop de Hull, 116 boul Lionel-Emond, Gatineau QC J8Y 1W7; Mon'95; Staff, Hull Hospital; (819)595-6000

BUSSIERES, Nicolas; Hop Charles Lemoyne, 3120 boul Taschereau, Greenfield Park QC J4V 2H1; Sher'97; CCFP; CCFP(E.M.); FCFP; Staff, Hopital Charles LeMoyne; (450)466-5000 x5050

BUSSIERES, Richard; CHUQ-Hotel-Dieu de Quebec, 11 Cote Du Palais, Quebec QC G1R 2J6; Laval'97; FRCSC; Otol (Ears). Staff, Centre Hospitalier Universitaire de Québec (CHUQ) - Siege Social; Langs: Bilingual(English/French); (418)691-5151; ricbussieres@hotmail.com.

BUSSIERES-LABRECQUE, Audrey; CSSS de Trois-Rivieres, 1991 boul du Carmel, Trois-Rivieres QC G8Z 3R9; Laval'08; Staff, CSSS de Trois-Rivières; (819)697-3333

BUSTAMANTE, Helene; Hop du Sacre-Coeur de Mtl, 5400 boul Gouin O, Montreal QC H4J 1C5; Mon'07; Staff, Hôpital du Sacre-Coeur de Montréal; (514)338-2222 x2383

BUSTANI, Laith A; Queensway-Carleton Hosp, 3045 Baseline Rd, Nepean ON K2H 8P4; Wes'03; CCFP; Staff, Queensway Carleton Hospital; Langs: Bilingual(English/French); (613)721-2000

BUSTIN, Robin G; 131-121 Orchard St PO Box 700, Berwick NS B0P 1E0; Dal'80; CCFP; Staff, Western Kings Memorial Health Centre; Staff, Valley Regional Hospital; (902)538-7381

BUSTROS-LUSSIER, Genevieve; ASSS de la Monteregie, 1255 rue Beauregard, Longueuil QC J4K 2M3; Sher'08; CCFP; Staff, Unite de Medicine Familiale; (450)928-6777

BUSUIOC, Ruxandra; CLSC Notre Dame-de-Grace, 2525 boul Cavendish, Montreal QC H4B 2Y4; Sher'07; CCFP; (514)484-7878; Fax. (514)485-6406.

BUTALIA, Sonia; Richmond Road Diag & Trmt Ctre, 1820 Richmond Rd SW, Calgary AB T2T 5C7; Tor'04; FRCPC; IntMed (Endocrinology); Endocrin&Metab. (403)955-8327; Fax. (403)955-8249.

BUTAN, Radu; Peterborough Reg Nephrology, 239 Charlotte St, Peterborough ON K9J 2V2; Wes'03; FRCPC; IntMed; Nephrol. (705)750-1786

BUTANY, Jagdish; Univ Hlth Network-Toronto Gen, E11 443-200 Elizabeth St, Toronto ON M5G 2C4; Mysore (India)'70; FRCPC; AnatPath (Cardiovascular Pathology). Staff, Toronto General Hospital - UHN; Staff, Sunnybrook Health Sciences Centre; (416)340-3003; jagdish.butany@uhn.on.ca.

BUTANY, Vidya J; Medical & Dental Bldg, 704-586 Eglinton Ave E, Toronto ON M4P 1P2; Punjab (India)'68; FRCPC; Psy. Asst Prof, University of Toronto; (416)544-0147; Fax. (416)544-0261.

BUTCHART, Michael K; Ridge Meadows Hosp & Hlth CC, 11666 Laity St, Maple Ridge BC V2X 5A3; UBC'97; FRCPC; DiagRad., Ridge Meadows Hospital & Health Care Centre; Staff, Langley Memorial Hospital; (604)463-1824

BUTCHER, Douglas S; 100-300 Main St N, Brampton ON L6V 4H6; Tor'69; Court Staff, William Osler Health System - Brampton Civic Hospital; (905)450-0151; Fax. (905)450-7152.

BUTCHER, Kenneth S; University of Alberta Hosp, 2E3. 27WMC-8440 112 St NW, Edmonton AB T6G 2B7; Wes'97; BSc; PhD; FRCPC; Neur (Stroke). Asst Prof, University of Alberta Hospital; (780)407-2171; Fax. (780)407-1325.

BUTCHER, Matthew S; Regina Qu'Appelle HR-Regina, 1440 14th Ave, Regina SK S4P 0W5; Alb'04; FRCPC; DiagRad. Staff, Regina General Hospital; (306)766-4444

BUTCHER, Shaun S; PO Box 360, McLennan AB T0H 2L0; (South Africa)'04; (780)767-3941

BUTCHEY, Janki; Aims Health Group, 1051 Wonderland Rd S, London ON N6K 3X4; Lodz (Poland)'70; FRCPC; Psy (Career Counselling). Langs: Polish; Dutch; Ukrainian; (519)474-6568; Fax. (519)471-7299; mbutch2832@rogers.com.

BUTCHEY, Joseph K; Scarborough Hosp-Birchmount, 3030 Birchmount Rd, Scarborough ON M1W 3W3; Wes'92; CCFP; CCFP(E.M.); Ac Staff EmergMed, The Scarborough Hospital - Birchmount Campus; Ac Staff, Rouge Valley Health System - Centenary Health Centre Site; Staff Emerg Dept, The Scarborough Hospital - General Campus; (416)495-2550

BUTCHEY, Joseph R K; 205-450 Central Ave, London ON N6B 2E8; London (England)'67; MB BS; MRCS; LRCP; FAAAI; FRCPC; IntMed (Asthma). Staff Consultant, London Health Sciences Centre - Victoria Campus; Ac Staff, St Joseph's Hospital - St Joseph's Health Care; Staff Consultant, London Health Sciences Centre - University Hospital; Assoc Prof Med, University of Western Ontario; (519)673-1491; Fax. (519)673-0275; jbutchey@uwo.ca.

BUTCHEY, Maurice R S; 1051 Wonderland Rd S, London ON N6K 3X4; Glasgow (Scotland)'70; Staff, St Joseph's Hospital - St Joseph's Health Care; Elgin-Middlesex Detention Centre; (519)472-2060; Fax. (519)471-7299; mbutchey@aimhealthgroup.com.

BUTCHEY, Robert; Tillsonburg Med Clinic, 154 Rolph St, Tillsonburg ON N4G 3Z1; West Indies (Jamaica)'01; CCFP; (519)842-3682

BUTEAU, Chantal; Hôpital Ste-Justine, 3175 ch Cote-Sainte-Catherine, Montreal QC H3T 1C5; Laval'94; FRCPC; Peds; InfectDis (P.Q.). Staff, Hôpital Ste-Justine; (514)345-4931 x5566; Fax. (514)345-4908.

BUTEAU, Dominique; Hotel-Dieu de Levis, 143 rue Wolfe, Levis QC G6V 3Z1; Sher'93; Staff, Hôtel-Dieu de Lévis; (418)834-7121

BUTEAU, Francois-Alexandre; Cross Cancer Institute, 11560 University Ave NW, Edmonton AB T6G 1Z2; Laval'06; FRCPC; NuclearMed. Staff, Cross Cancer Institute; (780)432-8771

BUTEAU, Gaston; CSSS de Rimouski-Neigette, CP 3150 Succ A 150 av Rouleau, Rimouski QC G5L 5T1; Laval'77; CSPQ; FRCPC; Anes. Staff, Hôpital Regional Rimouski; (418)724-8282

BUTEAU, Genevieve; CSSS de Rivière-de-Loup, 75 rue Saint-Henri, Riviere-du-Loup QC G5R 2A4; Laval'03; FRCPC; DiagRad. Staff, Centre Hospitalier Regional du Grand-Portage; (418)686-1010

BUTEAU, Jacques; 200-4 Beechwood Ave, Vanier ON K1L 8L9; Mon'91; FRCPC; Psy. (613)741-7174; Fax. (613)741-0176.

BUTLER, Anna L; Peel Children's Centre, 85A Aventura Crt, Mississauga ON L5T 2Y6; Wes'87; FRCPC; Psy (Child Psychiatry). (905)795-3500

BUTLER, Blair W E; BC Women's Hosp & Health Ctre, IU25-4500 Oak St, Vancouver BC V6H 3N1; Mem'99; FRCSC; ObstGyn (Perinatology). Clinical Asst Prof ObstGyn, BC Women's Hospital & Health Centre; (604)875-3075

BUTLER, Brian T; Halton Healthcare Services, 6F-700 Dorval Dr, Oakville ON L6K 3V3; Tor'73; DABFP; DABPN; LLB; FRCPC; Psy. (905)338-4630; Fax. (905)845-6419; bthomasbutler@sympatico.ca.

BUTLER, Clay K; 143 Commercial St PO Box 145 Stn Main, Glace Bay NS B1A 5V2; Dal'85; BSc; FRCSC; GenSurg (Gastroenterology). Staff GenSurg, Cape Breton Healthcare Complex; (902)842-0030; Fax. (902)842-0499.

BUTLER, Craig R; University of Alberta Hosp, 2C2-8440 112 St NW, Edmonton AB T6G 2B7; Dal'01; FRCPC; IntMed; Cardiol. Staff, University of Alberta Hospital; (780)407-8822; Fax. (780)407-6452.

BUTLER, David M; Medical Bldg, 1401-805 Broadway W, Vancouver BC V5Z 1K1; Dal'72; FRCSC; Ophth. Consultant, Vancouver General Hospital - Centennial Pavillion; (604)876-6016; Fax. (604)879-1122.

BUTLER, Deborah J; 401-73 Water St N, Cambridge ON N1R 7L6; Ott'87; FRCSC; ObstGyn (Laparoscopic Surgery). Staff, Cambridge Memorial Hospital; University of Toronto; (519)620-2223; Fax. (519)620-7183.

BUTLER, Gary C; Westview Health Centre, 4405 South Park Dr, Stony Plain AB T7Z 2M7; Cal'03; CCFP; CCFP(E.M.); Staff, Westview Health Centre; (780)968-3600

BUTLER, Geoffrey W; St Clair Beach Health Centre, 6-500 Manning Rd, Windsor ON N8N 5H3; Wes'98; (519)979-7314; Fax. (519)739-2816.

BUTLER, Gregory J; 150 Exhibition St, Kentville NS B4N 5E3; Dal'76; FRCP; FACR; FRCPC; DiagRad. Staff, Valley Regional Hospital; (902)678-7381 x2742; Fax. (902)678-0098; butlergj@avdha.nshealth.ca.

BUTLER, James B; 675 Mcdermot Ave, Winnipeg MB R3E 0V9; McG'94; BA; DrMedCh; LMCC; FRC; FRCPC; RadOncol (Cancer Head & Neck). Staff, Health Sciences Centre; Assoc Prof, University of Manitoba; (204)787-2175; Fax. (204)786-0194.

BUTLER, Jared J; Central Nfld Reg Health Centre, 50 Union St, Grnd-Falls-Windsor NL A2A 2E1; (Ireland)'08; CCFP; Staff, Central Newfoundland Regional Health Centre; (709)292-2500

BUTLER, Jeremy R; Halton HSC-Oakville Site, 327 Reynolds Dr, Oakville ON L6J 3L8; Columbia University (USA)'02; Staff, Halton Healthcare Services Corporation - Oakville Site; (905)845-2571

BUTLER, Jessica M; Carleton Sports Med Clinic, 1125 Colonel By Dr, Ottawa ON K1S 5B6; Dal'08; CCFP; Staff, The Ottawa Hospital - Civic Campus; (613)520-3510

BUTLER, John S; 431 King St PO Box 640, Petrolia ON N0N 1R0; Mem'99; CCFP; Staff, Bluewater Health - Charlotte Eleanor Englehart Hospital; (519)882-2500; Fax. (519)882-4321.

BUTLER, Kimberly A; Fredericton Med Clinic, 304-1015 Regent St, Fredericton NB E3B 6H5; Dal'03; FRCSC; ObstGyn. (506)457-2113

BUTLER, Marcus O; Univ Hlth Network-Princess M, 610 University Ave, Toronto ON M5G 2M9; Yale University (USA)'92; Staff, Princess Margaret Hospital - University Health Network; (416)946-2000

BUTLER, Matthew R; Dr Charles L Legrow Hlth Ctr, PO Box 250 1 Grand Bay Rd, Port-aux-Basques NL A0M 1C0; Mem'08; CCFP; Staff, Dr Charles L Legrow Health Centre; (709)695-2175

BUTLER, Matthew S; Plains Surgical Associates, MOW 2F-1440 14th Ave, Regina SK S4P 0W5; Tor'04; FRCSC; GenSurg., Plains Surgical Associates; (306)766-6911; Fax. (306)766-6917.

BUTLER, Michael T W; 303-6411 Nelson Ave, Burnaby BC V5H 4H3; Cal'05; Ophth. (604)433-1258

BUTLER, Nicolaas M J; The Brandon Clinic, 620 Dennis St, Brandon MB R7A 5E7; (Other Foreign)'93; CCFP; (204)728-4440

BUTLER, Olivia M; Shouldice Hosp, 7750 Bayview Ave, Thornhill ON L3T 4A3; RCS (Ireland)'77; Anes. Staff, Shouldice Hospital; (905)889-1125; Fax. (905)889-4216.

BUTLER, Robert F; Family Practice Clinic, 84 Memorial Ave, Grnd-Falls-Wi NL A2A 1R9; Mem'76; Ac Staff, Central Newfoundland Regional Health Centre; (709)489-6688; Fax. (709)489-7523.

BUTLER, Robert J; London HSC-University Hosp, PO Box 5339 Stn B 339 Windermere Rd, London ON N6A 5A5; Qns'07; DiagRad. Staff, London Health Sciences Centre - University Hospital; (519)685-8500

BUTLER, Roger G; Ross Family Med Clinic, 622-100 Forest Rd, St. John's NL A1A 3Z9; Mem'77; CCFP; FCFP; Staff, Health Sciences Centre; Assoc Prof Med, Memorial University Of Newfoundland; (709)777-6301; Fax. (709)777-8323; rbutler@mun.ca.

BUTLER, Ronald J; London HSC-University Hosp, PO Box 5339 Stn B 339 Windereme Rd, London ON N6A 5A5; Wes'90; MSc; FRCPC; Anes; Critical Care Medicine. Staff ICU & Anes, London Health Sciences Centre - University Hospital; Asst Prof Med, University of Western Ontario; (519)663-3030; Fax. (519)663-3150.

BUTLER, Trevor J; Valley Prof Centre, 145-70 Exhibition St, Kentville NS B4N 4K9; Dal'01; FRCSC; Urol. (902)678-1130; Fax. (902)678-4020.

BUTLER, William J; Mackenzie Richmond Hill Hosp, 10 Trench St, Richmond Hill ON L4C 4Z3; UBC'71; FRCPC; Anes. Staff, Mackenzie Richmond Hill Hospital; (905)883-2110

BUTLER-JONES, David A; Public Hlth Agency of Canada, 1015 Arlington St, Winnipeg MB R3E 3P6; Tor'78; MHSc; FACPrevMed; FRCPC; CommunMed;CCFP; Chief Public Health Officer, Public Health Agency of Canada; Prof Faculty of Med, University of Manitoba; Clin Assoc Prof, University of Saskatchewan; (204)789-7058; Fax. (204)784-5939.

BUTRIS, Jaclin; Highland Med Group, 40-875 Highland Rd W, Kitchener ON N2N 2Y2; Baghdad (Iraq)'93; CCFP; (519)579-8181; Fax. (519)579-8180.

BUTT, Debra A; Ellesmere Health Care Center, 1-2060 Ellesmere Rd, Scarborough ON M1H 2V6; Tor'97; BSc; MSc; CCFP; FCFP; Staff, The Scarborough Hospital - General Campus; (416)439-2273; Fax. (416)439-2244; dbutt@tsh.to.

BUTT, Donald F; Sun Life Assurance, 740-1100 Melville St, Vancouver BC V6E 4A6; Tor'60; BScPharm; CCFP; FCFP; Med Consultant, Sunlife Assurance.

BUTT, John C; Pathfinder Forum, 400-1681 Chestnut St, Vancouver BC V6J 4M6; Alb'60; FRCPath; (604)738-0878

BUTT, Kimberly D; Dr Everett Chalmers Reg Hosp, PO Box 9000 Stn A, Fredericton NB E3B 5N5; Mem'93; FRCSC; ObstGyn (Maternal Fetal Medicine). Staff, Dr Everett Chalmers Regional Hospital; Dalhousie University; Langs: Bilingual(French/English); (506)452-5286; Fax. (506)447-4421.

BUTT, Mohammad I; Peace Arch Hosp, 15521 Russell Ave, White Rock BC V4B 2R4; Lahore (Pakistan)'60; FRCPC; IntMed. Staff Consultant Internal Med, Peace Arch Hospital; (604)531-5512

BUTT, Peter R; Mental Health & Addictions Ser, 314 Duchess St, Saskatoon SK S7K 0R1; McM'81; BA; CCFP; CCFP(E.M.); FCFP; Med Dir/Staff Saskatoon Health Region, Northern Medical Services; Assoc Prof Family Med, University of Saskatchewan; (306)655-0452; Fax. (306)655-0457; butt.nms@sasktel.net.

BUTT, Robinette D; Queen Elizabeth II HSC, 1276 South Park St, Halifax NS B3H 2Y9; Mem'99; FRCPC; DiagRad. Staff, Queen Elizabeth II Health Sciences Centre - Victoria General Site; (902)473-2700

BUTT, Shehbaz; Markham Stouffville Hosp, PO Box 1800 Stn Main 381 Church St, Markham ON L3P 7P3; Ott'97; FRCPC; Anes. Staff, Markham Stouffville Hospital; (905)472-7074

BUTT, Sheldon L; 23CF Health Services Centre, PO Box 17000 Stn Forces, Winnipeg MB R3J 3Y5; Mem'08; CCFP; (204)833-2500

BUTT, Shyla Imdad; William Osler HC-Etobicoke, 101 Humber College Blvd, Etobicoke ON M9V 1R8; Lahore (Pakistan)'95; Staff, William Osler Health System - Etobicoke General Hospital; (416)747-3400; Fax. (416)747-8608.

BUTTAR, Sonia D; 210-7110 120 St, Surrey BC V3W 3M8; McG'91; Langs: French; Punjabi; (604)502-5155; Fax. (604)502-5199.

BUTTENSCHOEN, Klaus; University of Alberta Hosp, 2D3. 78-8440 112 St NW, Edmonton AB T6G 2B7; (Germany)'88; Staff, University of Alberta Hospital; (780)407-2927; Fax. (780)407-2926.

BUTTER, Andreana M; Children's Hosp of Western Ont, B1 188-800 Commissioners Rd E, London ON N6C 2V5; Ott'98; BSc(Hon); MSc; FRCSC; GenSurg (Minimal Invasive Surgery); PedGenSurg. Staff Ped Gen Surg, St Joseph's Hospital - St Joseph's Health Care; Staff Ped GenSurg, London Health Sciences Centre - Victoria Campus; Asst Prof, University of Western Ontario; Langs: French; (519)685-8401; Fax. (519)685-8421.

BUTTERS, Stacey L; Medical Clinic Associates, 3591 31 St, Vernon BC V1T 5J4; UBC'89; (250)542-1215; Fax. (250)542-0160.

BUTTERWORTH, Peter J; 3970 Lakeshore Rd, Kelowna BC V1W 1V5; Cal'94; BSc; (250)764-8878

BUTTERWORTH, Sonia A; Children's & Women's HC of BC, KO 113-4480 Oak St, Vancouver BC V6H 3V4; UBC'97; FRCSC; GenSurg; PedGenSurg. Staff, BC Children's Hospital; (604)875-2667

BUTTINGER, Chris S; Lakeside Med Clinic, 3919 8th St E, Saskatoon SK S7H 5M7; Sask'96; CCFP; FCFP; (306)374-6884; Fax. (306)374-2552; cbuttinger@hotmail.com.

BUTTLE, Jeffrey W; Lower Mainland Drug Freedom In, 25 Blackwood St, New Westminster BC V3L 2R3; Dal'88; ABAM; FRCPC; Psy. (604)738-5414; mail@drbuttle.com.

BUTTON, Cheryl L; Sudbury Reg Hosp-Laurentian, 41 Ramsey Lake Rd, Sudbury ON P3E 5J1; Mem'88; BMedSci; MSc; BSc; FRCPC; Anes (Intensive Care). Staff, Health Sciences North-Laurentian Site; (705)671-5492; cbutton@hrsrh.on.ca.

BUTTON, Eric G; Gander Med Clinic, 177 Elizabeth Dr, Gander NL A1V 1H6; Dal'74; CCFP; FCFP; (709)256-7101; Fax. (709)256-7109.

BUTTON, Erica A; Hinton Med Clinic, 102 Allen Cove, Hinton AB T7V 2A6; Sask'98; CCFP; (780)865-3338; Fax. (780)865-2024; clinic@hintonmedical.com.

BUTTON, John R; Chatham-Kent Family Hlth Team, 68 Main St E, Ridgetown ON N0P 2C0; Tor'77; (519)674-2882; Fax. (519)674-0597.

BUTTON, Lonzel; Harbour Grace Med Centre, PO Box 280, Harbour Grace NL A0A 2M0; Dal'73; CCFP; FCFP; (709)596-6604; Fax. (709)596-6153.

BUTTON, Walter W; Cowan Topsail Med Clinic, 201-496 Topsail Rd, St. John's NL A1E 2C2; Mem'79; (709)368-2120; Fax. (709)368-2444.

BUTTOO, Ajit S; 1813 Lasalle Blvd, Sudbury ON P3A 2A3; Manchester (England)'58; (705)560-9422

BUTTOO, Kenneth; Ajax Med Arts Bldg, 201-601 Harwood Ave S, Ajax ON L1S 2J5; Manchester (England)'76; MB ChB; FCCP; FACP; ABIM; FRCPC; IntMed (Critical Care Medicine); ClinImmunol&Allergy. Consultant Med, Rouge Valley Health System - Ajax & Pickering Health Centre Site; (905)427-8817; Fax. (905)427-2028.

BUTTS, Charles A; Cross Cancer Institute, 11560 University Ave NW, Edmonton AB T6G 1Z2; Dal'85; FRCPC; IntMed; MedOncol., Cross Cancer Institute; (780)432-8513; Fax. (780)432-8888.

BUTZELAAR, Joris Y; Allin Clinic, 10155 120 St NW, Edmonton AB T5K 2A2; (780)482-7551; Fax. (780)488-2056.

BUTZNER, J Decker; Alberta Children's Hosp, 2888 Shaganappi Trail NW, Calgary AB T3B 6A8; Virginia (USA)'76; FRCPC; Peds (Pediatric Gastroenterology). Staff Ped Gastroenterology & Nutrition, Alberta Children's Hospital; Prof Peds, University of Calgary; (403)955-7747; Fax. (403)955-7639; butzner@ucalgary.ca.

BUU, C Dung Anh; 212-8260 boul Maurice-Duplessi, Montreal QC H1E 3A3; Sher'95; Peds. Staff, Hopital Charles LeMoyne; (514)643-1113; Fax. (514)643-1767.

BUU, Michael M; Vaughan Comm Health Centre, 206-9401 Jane St, Vaughan ON L6A 4H7; Hue (Vietnam)'80; CCFP; (905)303-8490

BUU, Natalie T; MUHC-Montreal Children's Hosp, C1114-2300 rue Tupper, Montreal QC H3H 1P3; McG'99; CSPQ; FRCPC; Anes. Staff, McGill University Health Centre - Montreal Children's Hospital; (514)412-4400 x22463

BUWEMBO, Joseph E; Regina Qu'Appelle HR-Regina, 2F MOW-1440 14th Ave, Regina SK S4P 0W5; Makerere (Uganda)'79; MB ChB; MMed; FRCSC; Neursurg. Staff, Regina General Hospital; Consultant Neurosurg, Regina Health District; Assoc Prof Section of Neurosurg & Surg, University of Saskatchewan; Langs: Luganda; (306)565-3940; Fax. (306)565-2325.

BUXTON, H Max; Calabogie Med Centre, PO Box 40, Calabogie ON K0J 1H0; Qns'84; BSc; CCFP; CCFP(E.M.); Staff, Renfrew Victoria Hospital; Assoc Prof, University of Ottawa; Langs: Bilingual(English/French); (613)752-2323; Fax. (613)752-2323.

BUXTON, Jane A; School of Population & Public, 2206 East Mall, Vancouver BC V6T 1Z3; London (England)'79; MB BS; FRCPC; CommunMed. Staff, School of Population & Public Health; (604)827-4001; jane.buxton@bccdc.ca.

BUYS, Lecia; Family Health Centre, 4918 52 St, Athabasca AB T9S 1G9; Pretoria (South Africa)'07; (780)675-5018; Fax. (780)675-5028.

BUYS, Stephanus; 205 St Laurent Ave, Quesnel BC V2J 2C8; Pretoria (South Africa)'03; MB ChB; Langs: Afrikaans; (250)992-8948

BUYS, Yvonne M; Univ Hlth Network-Toronto Western Hosp, EW6 405-399 Bathurst St, Toronto ON M5T 2S8; Tor'88; FRCSC; Ophth (Glaucoma)., Toronto Western Hospital - University Health Network; Physician Non-Ecomomic Loss, Worker's Safety & Insurance Board; Assoc Prof Ophth, University of Toronto; (416)603-5682; Fax. (416)603-5682; y.buys@utoronto.ca.

BUZAGLO, Karen; Clinique OVO, 8000 boul Decarie, Montreal QC H4P 2S4; McG'04; FRCSC; ObstGyn. (514)798-2000

BUZAID, Amin M; Cape Breton Healthcare Complex, 1482 George St, Sydney NS B1P 1P3; Dammam (Saudi Arabia)'01; FRCPC; IntMed; Cardiol. Staff, Cape Breton Healthcare Complex; (902)567-8000

BUZATU, Liliana; Kelown Gen Hosp, 2268 Pandosy St, Kelowna BC V1Y 1T2; (Romania)'95; (250)862-4000

BUZON, Antonio A; Finch-Midland Med Centre, 314-4190 Finch Ave E, Scarborough ON M1S 4T7; Santo Tomas (Philippines)'74; DABUrol; FACS(C); FRCSC; Urol. Ac Staff, The Scarborough Hospital - Birchmount Campus; Court Staff, Rouge Valley Health System - Centenary Health Centre Site; Locum Tenens, North York General Hospital; Langs: Tagalog; (416)293-6622; Fax. (416)293-7363.

BWENGE, Alexandra S; Physiotherapie du Sport du QC, 1000 av Emile-Journault, Montreal QC H2M 2E7; Mon'07; CCFP; (514)385-5682

BYAM, R Flayne; 300B Village Ave PO Box 40023 Rpo Southridge, Okotoks AB T1S 2G2; Cal'78; (403)938-7707; Fax. (403)938-1406.

BYCZKO, Beata J; Willow Women's Clinic, 1013-750 Broadway W, Vancouver BC V5Z 1H9; Dal'92; Clin Instructor Family Practice, University of British Columbia; (604)709-5603

BYERS, David S; 544 Palmerston Blvd, Toronto ON M6G 2P5; Tor'67; DABPN; FRCPC; Psy (Forensic Psychiatry). (416)532-1582

BYERS, Jean E F; Ontario Shores Ctr Mental HS, 700 Gordon St, Whitby ON L1N 5S9; Tor'67; DABPN(GeriatricPsy.); FRCPC; Psy (Geriatric Psychiatry). Staff, Ontario Shores Centre for Mental Health Sciences; Staff, Sault Area Hospital - Sault Ste Marie; Asst Prof Psy, University of Toronto; (905)668-5881 x6297; Fax. (905)430-4032.

BYERS, Susan D; Biqelow Fowler Clinic, 1605 9 Ave S, Lethbridge AB T1J 1W2; Cal'04; CCFP; (403)327-3121

BYERS, Trevor J; Smyth Associate Clinic, 4904 48 St, Leduc AB T9E 6V1; Alb'97; CCFP; (780)986-2712; Fax. (780)986-0356.

BYFORD, Larry J; The Ottawa Hosp-Civic Campus, 1053 Carling Ave, Ottawa ON K1Y 4E9; Qns'80; FRCPC; Anes. Staff Anes, The Ottawa Hospital - Civic Campus; Assoc Prof, University of Ottawa; (613)761-4169; Fax. (613)761-5209; lbyford@ottawahospital.on.ca.

BYKER, Leonard; Medical Arts Clinic, 780 Central Ave N, Swift Current SK S9H 0M3; (306)773-2811; Fax. (306)778-4081.

BYKERK, Vivian; The Joseph & Wolf Lebovic Bldg, 2005-60 Murray St, Toronto ON M5T 3L9; McM'81; BSc(Hons); FRCPC; IntMed (Clinical Research); Rheum. Staff, Mount Sinai Family Health Team; (416)586-8648; Fax. (416)586-8766.

BYLES, Nancy I A; Orillia Soldiers' Mem Hosp, 170 Colborne St W, Orillia ON L3V 2Z3; Cal'96; FRCPC; IntMed; GeriatricMed. Staff, Orillia Soldiers' Memorial Hospital; (705)325-2201

BYLSMA-HOWELL, Margaret I; Royal Columbian Hosp, 330 Columbia St E, New Westminster BC V3L 3W7; UBC'78; FRCPC; Anes. Staff, Royal Columbian Hospital; (604)520-4602

BYMAN, Andrea L; Lions Gate Hosp, 231 15th St E, North Vancouver BC V7L 2L7; UBC'90; Staff, Lions Gate Hospital; (604)988-3131

BYMAN, Vickie A; Burnaby Hosp, 3935 Kincaid St, Burnaby BC V5G 2X6; UBC'93; CCFP; CCFP(E.M.); Staff, Burnaby Hospital; (604)434-4211

BYNKOSKI, Stacey A; Family Matters Med Centre, X-730 St Anne's Rd, Winnipeg MB R2N 0A2; Man'07.

BYRICK, Robert J; St Michael's Hosp, 30 Bond St, Toronto ON M5B 1W8; Wes'71; FRCPC; Anes. Staff, St Michael's Hospital; (416)864-5071; Fax. (416)864-6014.

BYRNE, Aidan P; 108-2360 Beacon Ave, Sidney BC V8L 1X3; Cal'90; CCFP; FCFP; Staff, Royal Jubilee Hospital; (250)655-3838

BYRNE, Alan J; Oakville Med Arts Bldg, 5-358 Reynolds St, Oakville ON L6J 3L9; Dublin (Ireland)'76; LRCS; LRCP; FRCSI; FRCSC; GenSurg (Consultation). Langs: English; French; (905)842-1168; Fax. (905)842-4118.

BYRNE, Brendan J O; Panorama Village Med Clinic, 103-15157 56th Ave, Surrey BC V3S 9A5; McG'90; BSc; MDCM; Fax. (604)574-0481.

BYRNE, Damien F; 402-2151 Mccallum Rd, Abbotsford BC V2S 3N8; Alb'94; FRCSC; GenSurg. (604)859-3117; Fax. (604)850-3791.

BYRNE, Doris M; 5-358 Reynolds St, Oakville ON L6J 3L9; Dublin (Ireland)'85; MB ChB; BAO; Staff, Halton Healthcare Services Corporation - Oakville Site; (905)845-2571

BYRNE, John; The Abberfoyce Health Centre, 102-304 The East Mall, Etobicoke ON M9B 6E2; National (Ireland)'75; MB ChB; BAO; CCFP; CCFP(E.M.); Staff, Toronto General Hospital - UHN; Med Examiner, Civil Aviation Canada; (416)231-7968

BYRNE, Kelly P A; Univ of Alberta Hosp, 8440 112 St NW, Edmonton AB T6G 2B7; (New Zealand)'02; Staff, University of Alberta Hospital; (780)407-7361; Fax. (780)407-3200.

BYRNE, Michael F; Gordon & Leslie Diamond HCC, 5153-2775 Laurel St, Vancouver BC V5Z 1M9; Liverpool (England)'92; MB ChB; MRCP; MD; BA; MA; FRCPC; IntMed (Pancreatic Biliary Disease); Gastroent. Clin Prof, Vancouver General Hospital - Centennial Pavillion; Staff, Gordon & Leslie Diamond Health Care Centre; Clin Prof, University of British Columbia; (604)875-5640; Fax. (604)875-5447.

BYRNE, Miriam R; 3F-250 College St, Toronto ON M5T 1R8; National (Ireland)'77; MB ChB; BAO; FRCPC; Psy. (416)535-8501

BYRNE, Paul G; 35-1600 Steeles Ave W, Concord ON L4K 4M2; National (Ireland)'74; MB ChB; BAO; FRCS; FRCSC; GenSurg (Colon & Rectal Surgery). (905)669-7578; Fax. (905)669-8737.

BYRNE, Paul J; University of Alberta Hosp, 3A3 WMC-8440 112 St NW, Edmonton AB T6G 2B7; National (Ireland)'76; BAO; DCH; FAAP; FRCPC; Peds (Neonatology). Staff Neonatol, University of Alberta Hospital; Clin Assoc Prof Peds & Co-Dir, University of Alberta; (780)407-1305; Fax. (780)407-3030.

BYRNE, Paul J; Brampton East Health Centre, 200-300 Main St N, Brampton ON L6V 4H6; Tor'75; Ac Staff, William Osler Health System - Brampton Civic Hospital; (905)451-1806; Fax. (905)451-8272.

BYRNE, Tara; Markham Stouffville Hosp, PO Box 1800 Stn Main 381 Church St, Markham ON L3P 7P3; Wes'96; CCFP; CCFP(E.M.); Staff, Markham Stouffville Hospital; (905)472-7111

BYRNES, Jennifer R; 1-3801 28A St, Vernon BC V1T 9T6; McM'01; CCFP; (250)542-9950

BYRNS, Katherine; Hotel-Dieu de Levis, 143 rue Wolfe, Levis QC G6V 3Z1; Laval'01; FRCSC; Ophth. Staff, Hôtel-Dieu de Lévis; (418)835-7121; Fax. (418)835-7213.

BYRON, Kevin; Seawatch Med Clinic, 203-2276 South Island Hwy, Campbell River BC V9W 1C4; McM'07; CCFP; (250)923-1189

BYSTRIN, Irina; Queen-Spadina Med Centre, 455 Queen St W, Toronto ON M5V 2A9; Moscow (Russia (Federation))'53; (416)869-3627 Semi-Retired.

BYSTROM, Ryan S; Town Centre Medical, 19-2475 Dobbin Rd, Westbank BC V4T 2E9; UBC'97; BSc; CCFP; (250)768-8315; Fax. (250)768-8326.

BYSZEWSKI, Anna M; The Ottawa Hosp-Civic Campus, 1053 Carling Ave, Ottawa ON K1Y 4E9; Ott'83; BSc(Hon); FRFPS; MEd; FRCPC; IntMed; GeriatricMed. Staff, The Ottawa Hospital - Civic Campus; Assoc Prof Med, University of Ottawa; Langs: French; Polish; (613)761-4195; Fax. (613)761-5334; abyszewski@ottawahospital.on.ca.

BZONEK, Peter; Carlisle Med Centre, PO Box 311 1493 Centre Rd, Carlisle ON L0R 1H0; Tor'87; BSc; CCFP; FCFP; Court Staff Privil Family Med, Hamilton Health Sciences Centre - McMaster Children's Hospital; Ac Staff Privil Family Med, Joseph Brant Memorial Hospital; (905)689-3301; Fax. (905)689-5772.

CABALO, Eve C; St Paul's Hosp, 1081 Burrard St, Vancouver BC V6Z 1Y6; Alb'04; FRCPC; Psy. Staff, Providence Health Care - St Paul's Hospital; (604)682-2344

CABANA, Caroline; Clinique Med Mascouche, 1025 Montee Masson, Mascouche QC J7K 2L9; Mon'93; CCFP; Staff Palliative Care, Centre Hospitalier Pierre le Gardeur; (450)474-6000; Fax. (450)474-6666.

CABANA, Diane T; Clinique Med Mercier, 101-464 boul Saint-Jean-Baptis, Mercier QC J6R 2B1; Sher'77; ObstGyn (P.Q.). Langs: Bilingual(English/French); (450)699-0539; Fax. (450)699-8438.

CABANA, Francois; 3001 12e Av N, Sherbrooke QC J1H 5N4; Laval'91; OrthSurg (Spine Surgery). Staff, Centre Hospitalier Universitaire de Sherbrooke-Hopital Fleurimont; Langs: English; (819)346-1110; Fax. (819)820-6410; orthopedie-med@usherbrooke.ca.

CABANA, Louise; Clinique Med St-Vincent, 250 rue King E, Sherbrooke QC J1G 1A9; Sher'88; CCFP; Physician, Sherbrooke Geriatric University Institute; Langs: English; (819)563-0510; Fax. (819)564-6889.

CABATU, Moises D; 218 Stanley St, Fredericton NB E3B 3A3; Santo Tomas (Philippines)'52; Court Staff, Dr Everett Chalmers Regional Hospital; Med Examiner, Ministry of Transportation; Langs: Tagalog; (506)455-4092

CABIGON, Enrico F; Regina Qu'Appelle HR-Pasqua, 100-4101 Dewdney Ave, Regina SK S4T 1A5; Santo Tomas (Philippines)'68; DABAP; MD; BA; FRCPC; AnatPath. Ac Staff AnatPath, Pasqua Hospital; Asst Prof, University of Saskatchewan; Langs: Tagalog; Waray; Ilonggo; (306)766-2422; Fax. (306)766-2752.

CABILIO, Nora; Queen Elizabeth Hosp, PO Box 6600 Stn Central, Charlottetown PE C1A 8T5; Cal'09; CCFP; Staff, Queen Elizabeth Hospital; (902)894-2111

CABOT, Julie; Clinique Sante Thetford, 2000-926 rue Labbe, Thetford Mines QC G6G 2A8; Laval'96; pers Chef méd fam, Hopital du CSS de la Region de Thetford; (418)338-4581; Fax. (418)338-4584; julie.cabot@gmf.gouv.qc.ca.

CABRAL, David A; Children's & Women's HC of BC, K4 119-4480 Oak St, Vancouver BC V6H 3V4; Perth (Australia)'78; MB BS; FRCPC; Peds (Pediatric Rheumatology). A-Prog Dir Clinical Fellowship, BC Children's Hospital; Assoc Prof, University of British Columbia; (604)875-2437; Fax. (604)875-3141.

CABRERA, Anthony E; 112 Queenston St, St Catharines ON L2R 2Z4; Mem'89; BMedSci; DABOph; CSPQ; FRCSC; Ophth (Cornea & Refractive Surgery). Langs: Italian; French; Spanish; (905)684-0181; Fax. (905)684-7579.

CABRERA, Maria Linda T; 120-6180 Blundell Rd, Richmond BC V7C 4W7; (Philippines)'99; (604)271-1314; Fax. (604)241-8615.

CABRERA-ABREU, Casimiro J; Providence Care-Mental Health, PO Box 603 Stn Main 752 King St W, Kingston ON K7L 4X3; (Spain)'82; MRCPsy; Staff, Providence Care - Mental Health Services; (613)548-5567; Fax. (613)548-5563.

CABRERA-ALEKSANDROVA, Tatiana; hMUHC-Royal Victoria Hosp, 687 av des Pins O, Montreal QC H3A 1A1; (Mexico)'95; Staff, McGill University Health Centre - Royal Victoria Hospital; (514)934-1934

CABURAO, Isaac C; Broad Street Med Clinic, 2210 Broad St, Regina SK S4P 4V6; (Philippines)'73; Staff, Regina General Hospital; Staff, Pasqua Hospital; (306)359-3966; Fax. (306)359-3906.

CACCIA, Nicolette C; 204 Church St, Weston ON M9N 1N7; Tor'92; BSc; MEd; FRCSC; ObstGyn (Adolescent Gynecology). Staff Part Time Gynecology, The Hospital For Sick Children; Staff, Humber River Regional Hospital - Church Street Site; (416)438-2727; Fax. (416)438-2713.

CACES, Rebecca F; Women's Hosp, WR004C-735 Notre Dame Ave, Winnipeg MB R3E 0L8; Santo Tomas (Philippines)'74; FAAP; FRCPC; Peds (Neonatology). Staff Neonatol, Health Sciences Centre; Med Dir, Manitoba Neonatal Transport Program; Assoc Prof, University of Manitoba; (204)787-4218; Fax. (204)787-1587.

CACIC, Ivan; The Credit Valley Hosp, 2200 Eglinton Ave W, Mississauga ON L5M 2N1; McM'06; FRCPC; Anes. Staff, The Credit Valley Hospital; (905)813-3946; Fax. (905)813-3340.

CACO, Christopher C; Guelph Imaging Centre, 206-55 Wyndham St N, Guelph ON N1H 7T8; Tor'78; FRCPC; DiagRad. (519)767-0220

CADA, Michaela; The Hosp for Sick Children, 555 University Ave, Toronto ON M5G 1X8; Ott'03; FRCPC; Peds (Pediatric Hematology Oncology). Staff, The Hospital For Sick Children; (416)813-1500 x8335

CADDICK, Robert; 540 St. George Blvd, Moncton NB E1E 2B5; Durham (England)'66; BMus; BSc; DRCOG; FRCSC; ObstGyn. (506)853-1187; Fax. (506)854-2556.

CADDIGAN, Deborah; Inuit Med Centre, 300-24 Selkirk St, Vanier ON K1L 0A4; Mem'80; (613)740-0999; dr.deborahcaddigan@gmail.com.

CADDY, Sheila C; Hys Med Centre, 207-11010 101 St, Edmonton AB T5H 4B9; Alb'06; FRCSC; ObstGyn. Staff, University of Alberta Hospital; Staff Lois Hole Hospital for Women Robbins Pavilion, Royal Alexandra Hospital; (780)420-1771; Fax. (780)425-9299.

CADEDDU, Margherita O; St Joseph Healthcare, G810-50 Charlton Ave E, Hamilton ON L8N 4A6; Wes'94; FRCSC; GenSurg (Colon & Rectal Surgery). Ac Staff, St Joseph's Healthcare - Charlton Campus; Ac Staff, Hamilton Health Sciences Centre - McMaster Children's Hospital; Langs: Italian; French; (905)522-0677; Fax. (905)522-0864.

CADEGAN, Perry K; Sterling Prof Centre, PO Box 569 Stn Main 65 Minto St, Glace Bay NS B1A 6G4; Dal'75; BSc; CCFP; FCFP; Staff, Cape Breton Healthcare Complex; Exec Officer, Canadian Federation of Clinical Hypnosis; Lecturer Family Med, Dalhousie University; (902)849-3138; Fax. (902)849-2218.

CADENHEAD, Kathleen; Oakridge Centre South Tower, 312-650 41st Ave W, Vancouver BC V5Z 2M9; UBC'81; CCFP; FCFP; Staff, BC Women's Hospital & Health Centre; Ac Staff, BC Children's Hospital; Chair Nutrition Committee, British Columbia Medical Association; Clin Assoc Prof Family Practice, University of British Columbia; (604)261-8177; Fax. (604)261-9607.

CADER, Shifaya; East York Town Centre, 27E-45 Overlea Blvd, East York ON M4H 1C3; Peradeniya (Sri Lanka)'80; CCFP; (416)696-9836; Fax. (416)696-8080.

CADER, Sonia; University of Alberta Hosp, 2D2 08-8440 112 St NW, Edmonton AB T6G 2B7; UBC'05; FRCSC; GenSurg. Staff, University of Alberta Hospital; (780)407-2906; Fax. (780)407-3492.

CADESKY, Eric; The Doctors' Office, 101-777 Broadway W, Vancouver BC V5Z 4J7; McG'04; MDCM; CCFP; Clin Instructor, University of British Columbia; Langs: Spanish; French; (604)734-8252

CADESKY, Kenneth I; 18F-655 Bay St, Toronto ON M5G 2K4; Tor'78; FRCSC; ObstGyn (Gynecology). Staff, Mount Sinai Hospital; (416)348-9030; Fax. (416)348-0828.

CADET, Sylvie; Clinique Med Rene-Gaultier, 15-2020 boul Rene-Gaultier, Varennes QC J3X 1N9; Alb'83; Langs: Bilingual(French/English); (450)652-2222; Fax. (450)652-3970; sylviecadet@ymail.com.

CADGER, Ewan M; 2425 Bevan Ave, Sidney BC V8L 4R5; Cal'81; Ac Staff, Saanich Peninsula Hospital; (250)656-1164; Fax. (250)656-7870.

CADIEU, Travis M; Vancouver Gen Hosp, 505-855 12th Ave W, Vancouver BC V5Z 1M9; UBC'02; FRCPC; EmergMed. Staff, Vancouver General Hospital - Centennial Pavillion; (604)875-5242

CADIEUX, Pierre; Clin de Varices Dr Pierre Cadi, 159 ch Watchorn, Morin-Heights QC J0R 1H0; Mon'80; (450)226-8346

CADIEUX, Roger; Clin Med Physerqo Sud Ouest, 5260 rue De Verdun, Verdun QC H4H 1K1; Mon'59; CommunMed (P.Q.). Staff, Centre Hospitalier de Verdun; (514)766-1696; Fax. (514)766-3472.

CADILI, Abdul Mujib A K M; Liberton Med Centre, 106-31 Liberton Dr, St. Albert AB T8N 3X6; Baghdad (Iraq)'74; MB ChB; FRCS(Ed); FRCSC; GenSurg. Chief Surg, Sturgeon Community Hospital; Langs: Arabic; German; (780)460-8655; drcadili@hotmail.com.

CADILI, Ali; 503-111 Fairford St E, Moose Jaw SK S6H 7X5; Sask'04; FRCSC; GenSurg. Staff, University of Alberta Hospital; (306)693-3638; Fax. (306)693-3774.

CADIVY, Alexandre; Centre Hosp Pierre-Janet, 20 rue Pharand, Gatineau QC J9A 1K7; Lyon (France)'94; Staff, Centre Hospitalier Pierre-Janet; (819)771-7761; Fax. (819)771-2908.

CADMAN, David T; Bayridge Family Centre, 1295 North Service Rd, Burlington ON L7R 4M2; Qns'74; MSc(MedSci.); FRCPC; Peds (Developmental/Behavioural Pediatrics). Ac Staff, Hamilton Health Sciences Centre - McMaster University Medical Centre; Med Dir, Bayridge Family Centre; (905)319-1488; Fax. (905)319-3670.

CADOGAN, George I; Donway X-Ray, 402-75 The Donway W, North York ON M3C 2E9; Alb'58; BSc; DMRD; FRCPC; DiagRad. (416)449-2635; Fax. (416)449-0108.

CADORET, Louise; CLSC Chateauguay, 95 av de la Verdure, Chateauguay QC J6K 0E8; Laval'89; Staff, CLSC Chateauguay; Langs: English; French; (450)699-3333

CADORET, Pierre; Clinique Med de l'Assomption, CP 3406 814 boul de l'Ange-Gardien N, L'Assomption QC J5W 4M9; Mon'75; Fax. (450)589-5779.

CADORETTE, Martin; CSSS de Trois-Rivieres, 1991 boul du Carmel, Trois-Rivieres QC G8Z 3R9; Laval'96; Staff, CSSS de Trois-Rivières; Langs: French; (819)697-3333; martin.cadorette@gmail.com.

CADORETTE, Sebastien; CSSS de l'Energie-Lafleche, 1650 6e av, Grand-Mere QC G9T 2K4; Laval'93; CCFP; Staff, Centre Lafleche Grand-Mere; (819)533-2525

CADOTTE, Helene; Children's Hosp Eastern Ont, 401 Smyth Rd, Ottawa ON K1H 8L1; Sher'87; FRCPC; Psy. Staff, Children's Hospital of Eastern Ontario (CHEO); (613)738-6990 x241; Fax. (613)738-4891.

CADOTTE, Lucie; Clinique Med Fam des Recollets, 101-940 boul des Recollets, Trois-Rivieres QC G8Z 3W9; Mon'85; assoc Membre Gen Med, Centre Hospitalier Regional de Trois-Rivieres; (819)373-0303; Fax. (819)373-8431.

CADOTTE, Marcel; CSSS Bordeaux-Cartierville-St-, 555 boul Gouin O, Montreal QC H3L 1K5; Mon'62; MSc; GenPath (P.Q.) (Cytogenetics). Staff, Pavillon Notre-Dame de la Merci; (514)331-3020

CADOTTE, Richard N; Clin Radiologique de Verdun, 50 rue de l'Eglise, Verdun QC H4G 2L9; Mon'75; DiagRad. Staff, Centre Hospitalier de LaSalle; (514)769-8828; Fax. (514)769-3791.

CADRIN, Camille; Ctr Hosp Chauveau, 11999 rue de l'Hôpital, Quebec QC G2A 2T7; Laval'72; LMCC; CSPQ; FRCPC; IntMed (Cardiology). assoc Membre, Centre Hospitalier Affilié Universitaire de Québec - Hôpital du St-Sacrement; Staff, Centre Hospitalier Chauveau; assoc Membre, Institut Universitaire Sante; (418)842-3651; Fax. (418)842-8660; cadrinc@videotron.ca.

CADRIN, Christine; Hop Brome-Missisquoi-Perkins, 950 rue Principale, Cowansville QC J2K 1K3; Laval'86; FRCSC; ObstGyn. Staff, Hôpital Brome-Missisquoi-Perkins; (450)266-4342

CADRIN, Danielle; CSSS des Basques, 550 rue Notre-Dame E RR 1, Trois-Pistoles QC G0L 4K0; Laval'76; Staff, Centre Hospitalier Trois-Pistoles; (418)851-1111; Fax. (418)851-2944.

CADRIN, Robert; Clin Med Mont Ste-Anne, RR 1 100-10974 boul Ste-Anne, Beaupre QC G0A 1E0; Laval'80; Staff, Hôpital Sainte Anne de Beaupré; (418)827-4022; Fax. (418)827-4964.

CADRIN-CHENEVERT, Alexandre; Ctr Hosp Reg de Lanaudiere, 1000 boul Sainte-Anne, St-Charles-Brromee QC J6E 6J2; Mon'04; FRCPC; DiagRad. Staff, Centre Hospitalier Régional de Lanaudière; (450)759-8222

CADSKY, Otakar; Alberta Hosp Edmonton, PO Box 307 Stn Main, Edmonton AB T5J 2J7; London (England)'74; MB BS; LRCP; MRCS; MRCPsy; Staff Forensic Psy., Alberta Hospital Edmonton; Asst Prof, University of Alberta; (780)342-5577; Fax. (780)342-5182.

CAETANO, Helen M; 604-5400 Portage Rd, Niagara Falls ON L2G 5X7; Tor'95; FRCSC; Otol. (905)358-8008; Fax. (905)358-0665.

CAETANO, Melanie G; Islington Med Clinic, 601-1243 Islington Ave, Etobicoke ON M8X 1Y9; Tor'98; FRCSC; ObstGyn (Infertility). Staff, St Joseph's Health Centre; Langs: Portuguese; (416)231-7878; Fax. (416)231-7801.

CAFFARO, Leslie E; Garneau Prof Centre, 407-11044 51 Ave NW, Edmonton AB T6H 5B4; Alb'94; FRCPC; Psy. (780)438-6181; Fax. (780)437-3499.

CAFFARO, Michael J; Hillcrest Med Associates, 117 Jasper St, Hinton AB T7V 2A8; Alb'90; CCFP; FCFP; Med Pres, Hinton Healthcare Centre; Asst Prof Family Med., University of Alberta; (780)865-2203; Fax. (780)865-7383.

CAFFARO, Paul A; Associate Med Clinic, PO Box 510, Slave Lake AB T0G 2A0; Alb'74; (780)849-5240; Fax. (780)849-4574.

CAFFIN, Pierre-Yves; CSSSG-Hop De Gatineau, CP 2000 Succ Bureau-Chef 909 boul de la Verendrye O, Gatineau QC J8P 7H2; Montpellier (France)'04; Staff, Hôpital de Gatineau; (819)561-8100

CAGIANNOS, Catherine; The Ottawa Hosp-Civic Campus, 1053 Carling Ave, Ottawa ON K1Y 4E9; Wes'92; FRCSC; GenSurg; VascSurg. Staff, The Ottawa Hospital - Civic Campus; (613)798-5555

CAGIANNOS, Ilias; The Ottawa Hosp-Civic Campus, B3-1053 Carling Ave, Ottawa ON K1Y 4E9; Tor'95; FRCSC; Urol (Urological Oncology). Staff, The Ottawa Hospital - Civic Campus; Assoc Prof, University of Ottawa; Langs: Greek; (613)761-4500; Fax. (613)761-5305.

CAGLAR, Derin; MUHC-Montreal Gen Hosp, D3.229-1650 av Cedar, Montreal QC H3G 1A4; Ankara (Turkey)'93; Staff, McGill University Health Centre - Montreal General Campus; (514)934-1934 x43837; Fax. (514)934-8296.

CAHALAN, Alan D; 100-240 Wharncliffe Rd N, London ON N6H 4P2; Tor'91; BSc; CCFP; (519)685-3210; Fax. (519)685-1432.

CAHILL, Eugene John(Sean); Synergy Wellness Centre, 221-501 Bethel Dr, Sherwood Park AB T8H 0N2; Galway (Ireland)'75; MB ChB; BAO; MRCGPract; (780)464-0123; Fax. (780)449-6993.

CAHILL, Gabriel T; Tera Losa Med Centre, 9760 170 St NW, Edmonton AB T5T 5L4; National (Ireland)'69; (780)486-3660; Fax. (780)486-3673.

CAHILL, Mark K; Family Med Centre, 2931 20 Ave S, Lethbridge AB T1K 3M5; Alb'05; BSc; CCFP; (403)328-2326

CAILHIER, Jean-Francois; CHUM-Hop St-Luc, 1058 rue Saint-Denis, Montreal QC H2X 3J4; Mon'96; FRCPC; IntMed; Nephrol. Staff, Centre Hospitalier l'Université De Montréal (CHUM) - Hôpital Saint-luc; (514)890-8000 x32588; jfcailhier@hotmail.com.

CAILLE, Francois-Xavier; CHUS-Hop Fleurimont, 3001 12e av N, Sherbrooke QC J1H 5N4; Sher'06; Staff, Centre Hospitalier Universitaire de Sherbrooke-Hopital Fleurimont; (819)346-1110

CAILLIER, Lisa A; Sirona Med Clinic, 1464 56 St, Delta BC V4L 2A7; UBC'03; FRCPC; PhysMed&Rehab. Staff, G F Strong Rehabilitation Centre; (604)943-9843

CAIN, John P; Kingston Gen Hosp, 76 Stuart St, Kingston ON K7L 2V7; Wes'67; FRCPC; IntMed (Critical Care Medicine); Anes. Staff, Kingston General Hospital; (613)548-7827; Fax. (613)548-1375; cainj@kgh.kari.net.

CAIN, Michael H; Health & Wellness Centre, B22-550 Terminal Ave, Ottawa ON K1G 0Z3; Ott'76; CCFP; (613)731-4770; Fax. (613)731-4979.

CAIN, Michelle R; 302C-50 Vancouver St, Yarmouth NS B5A 2P4; Dal'92; (902)742-1687; Fax. (902)742-7085.

CAIN, Patricia; Cumberland Med Clinic, 11-900 Watters Rd, Orleans ON K4A 0B4; Sher'92; CCFP; (613)830-3837

CAIN, Richard S; Valley Reg Hosp, 150 Exhibition St, Kentville NS B4N 5E3; Dal'67; Anes (Intensive Care). Staff, Valley Regional Hospital; (902)678-7381 x3201; brcain@accesswave.ca.

CAIN, Ryan A; 800 Baker St, Cranbrook BC V1C 1A2; UBC'02; FRCSC; Otol. (250)489-3323; Fax. (250)489-5233.

CAINE, J Douglas; Oak Bay Med Centre, 159-2515 90 Ave SW, Calgary AB T2V 0L8; McG'92; CCFP; (403)281-2020; Fax. (403)281-7785.

CAINE, Sean P; North York Gen Hosp, 1NE 126-4001 Leslie St, North York ON M2K 1E1; Tor'06; CCFP; CCFP(E.M.); Staff, North York General Hospital; (416)756-6000

CAINES, Angela E; Jenny Trout Centre, 110-342 Erie St, Stratford ON N5A 2N4; Wes'05; FRCPC; IntMed. (519)273-0100; Fax. (519)273-0675.

CAINES, Judy S W; Queen Elizabeth II HSC, 3212-1276 South Park St, Halifax NS B3H 2Y9; Dal'73; FRCPC; DiagRad. Staff, Queen Elizabeth II Health Sciences Centre - Victoria General Site; (902)473-3678; Fax. (902)473-2018.

CAINES, Nadean M; 203-61 Riverside Dr PO Box 808, Corner Brook NL A2H 6G7; Mem'06; FRCSC; ObstGyn. Staff, Western Memorial Regional Hospital.

CAINES, Sarah R; 500-20 Marr Rd, Rothesay NB E2E 2R5; Mem'06; CCFP; Staff, Saint John Regional Hospital; (506)849-9339; Fax. (506)849-8834.

CAIRE FON, Nathalie M T; Inst U Geriatrie de Montreal, 4565 ch Queen-Mary, Montreal QC H3W 1W5; Mon'90; CCFP; Staff, Institut Universitaire de Gériatrie de Montréal; (514)340-1424

CAIRNCROSS, Sarah W; UHS-MacEwan Student Centre, 2500 University Dr NW, Calgary AB T2N 1N4; Wes'86; BSc(Hons.); CCFP; FCFP; (403)210-9355

CAIRNEY, A Elizabeth; 800 Commissioners Rd E, London ON N6A 5W9; Tor'76; FRCPC; Peds (Pediatric Oncology). Ac Staff London Hlth Sciences Ctr, London Health Sciences Centre - Victoria Campus; University of Western Ontario; (519)685-8494; Fax. (519)685-8384; beth.cairney@lhsc.on.ca.

CAIRNS, Alan J; PO Box 1760, Sechelt BC V0N 3A0; Glasgow (Scotland)'69; MB ChB; DObstRCOG; Staff, St Mary's Hospital; (604)885-5196; Fax. (604)885-5193; alancairns@dccnet.com.

CAIRNS, Anne; Grand Manan Hosp, 196 Route 776, Grand Manan Island NB E5G 1A3; McM'92; CCFP; FCFP; Staff, Grand Manan Hospital; (506)662-4060

CAIRNS, Bonnie J; Bronte Med Group, 78 Jones St, Oakville ON L6L 6C5; McM'89; CCFP; FCFP; Court Staff, Halton Healthcare Services Corporation - Oakville Site; (905)827-9865; Fax. (905)827-3583.

CAIRNS, Brenda D; Brooklin Med Centre, 1A-5959 Anderson St, Brooklin ON L1M 2E9; Wes'79; Ac Staff, Lakeridge Health - Oshawa Site; (905)655-3321; Fax. (905)655-4848.

CAIRNS, Heather M; 120-1641 Hillside Ave, Victoria BC V8T 5G1; UBC'79; Ac Staff, Royal Jubilee Hospital; Assoc Staff, Victoria General Hospital; (250)592-4212

CAIRNS, John A; 9113-2775 Laurel St, Vancouver BC V5Z 1M9; UBC'68; FRCP; FACC; FRCPC; Cardiol (Cardiovascular Medicine); IntMed. Prof Med, University of British Columbia; (604)875-4111 x66708; jacairns@medd.med.ubc.ca.

CAIRNS, Patricia D; Medisys, LL 6-1849 Yonge St, Toronto ON M4S 1Y2; Tor'86; BSc; FRCPC; DiagRad. (416)485-9155; Fax. (416)485-9532.

CAIRNS, Robyn A; BC Women's Hosp & Health Ctre, 4500 Oak St, Vancouver BC V6H 3N1; UBC'85; FRCPC; DiagRad. Staff, BC Women's Hospital & Health Centre; (604)875-2132

CAISSIE, Mathieu; CHUQ-Hop Saint-Sacrement, 1050 ch Sainte-Foy, Quebec QC G1S 4L8; Sher'04; FRCSC; Ophth. Staff, Centre Hospitalier Affilié Universitaire de Québec - Hôpital du St-Sacrement; (418)682-7511

CAISSIE, Romeo; CSSS de Rivière-de-Loup, 75 rue Saint-Henri, Riviere-Du-Loup QC G5R 2A4; Laval'78; FRCPC; Peds (Hospitalist). Staff, Centre Hospitalier Regional du Grand-Portage; (418)868-1010 x2835; Fax. (418)868-3338.

CAIT, Ted A; Baywood Med Centre, 503-95 Bayly St W, Ajax ON L1S 7K8; Tor'88; CCFP; FCFP; Court Staff, Rouge Valley Health System - Ajax & Pickering Health Centre Site; Physician Retirment Home, Amica at Whitby; (905)427-0597; Fax. (905)427-3710.

CAJAL, Stefan I; Clinique de Medecine, 3/F-1665 rue Sainte-Catherine, Montreal QC H3H 1L9; Bucharest (Romania)'73; Staff, Providence Notre-Dame-de-Lourdes Inc; (514)931-0801

CAJEE, Ismail; Queen Elizabeth II HSC-Halifax, 3021-1796 Summer St, Halifax NS B3H 3A7; Natal (South Africa)'75; MB ChB; CCFP; CCFP(E.M.); Staff, Queen Elizabeth II Health Sciences Centre - Victoria General Site; Staff, Queen Elizabeth II Health Sciences Centre - Halifax Infirmary Site; (902)473-3383; Fax. (902)473-3617.

CAKAREVIC, Svetlana; Appletree Med Centre, 2575B Baseline Rd, Ottawa ON K2H 7B3; Belgrade (Serbia)'91; CCFP; Langs: Serbian; (613)482-0118

CALABRESE, Julie; Hop Charles Lemoyne, 3120 boul Taschereau, Greenfield Park QC J4V 2H1; Sher'99; FRCPC; Peds. Staff, Hopital Charles LeMoyne; (450)466-5000

CALABRESE, Stephane; CSSS d'Antoine-Labelle-Mt Laur, 2561 ch de Lievre S, Mont-Laurier QC J9L 3G3; Aix-Marseille II (France)'02; Staff, CSSS d'Antoine-Labelle; (819)623-1234; Fax. (819)440-4299.

CALAM, Betty; St Paul's Hosp, 1081 Burrard St, Vancouver BC V6Z 1Y6; UBC'79; MClSc; CCFP; FCFP; Staff, Providence Health Care - St Paul's Hospital; Assoc Prof Family Med, University of British Columbia; (604)806-8569; Fax. (604)806-8556; bcalam@providencehealth.bc.ca.

CALARCO, Mary Jo; 24 Elora St S PO Box 398, Harriston ON N0G 1Z0; McM'86; Staff, North Wellington Health Care - Palmerston & District Hospital; (519)338-2505; Fax. (519)510-2507.

CALDARERI, Carmelo; Centre Prof Belanger, 404-3871 rue Belanger, Montreal QC H1X 3M7; Sher'79; CCFP; (514)374-3140; Fax. (514)374-3142; carmelo@pharmaciegabriel.com.

CALDARONE, Christopher A; The Hosp for Sick Children, 1525-555 University Ave, Toronto ON M5G 1X8; Columbia (Colombia)'88; FRCSC; CardSurg. Fellow, The Hospital For Sick Children; (416)813-6420; Fax. (416)813-7984; christopher.caldarone@sickkids.ca.

CALDER, C Jill; Royal Inland Hosp, 311 Columbia St, Kamloops BC V2C 2T1; Qns'86; FRCPC; PhysMed&Rehab (Emergency Medicine). Staff/Head PhysMed&Rehab, Royal Inland Hospital; Clin Dir Rehab Services, Interior Health West Service Area; (250)374-0750; Fax. (250)374-0454; drcalder@chaw.ca.

CALDER, Douglas; 237 Hastings St N PO Box 1390, Bancroft ON K0L 1C0; McM'79; Staff Family Med, QHC North Hastings; (613)332-1157; Fax. (613)332-3357; calderd@hastingscourt.com.

CALDER, Lisa A; The Ottawa Hosp-Civic Campus, F654-1053 Carling Ave, Ottawa ON K1Y 4E9; Wes'00; FRCPC; EmergMed. Staff, The Ottawa Hospital - Civic Campus; (613)798-5555 x14784; lcalder@ohri.ca.

CALDER, Suzanne; Mississauga Med Centre, 205-1420 Burnhamthorpe Rd E, Mississauga ON L4X 2Z9; Belfast (Ireland)'79; Staff, Trillium Health Centre - Mississauga; (905)625-4016; Fax. (905)625-7721.

CALDER, Tammy R; Rockyview Gen Hosp, 7007 14 St SW, Calgary AB T2V 1P9; UBC'96; CCFP; Staff, Rockyview General Hospital; (403)943-3000

CALDERON, Gerardo G; Scarborough Med Centre, 2680 Lawrence Ave E, Scarborough ON M1P 4Y4; Manila (Philippines)'63; Court Staff, The Scarborough Hospital - General Campus; Langs: Tagalog; (416)755-2242; Fax. (416)755-8412.

CALDERON-GRANDE, Henry E; Kenaston Mall Walk In Clinic, 1859A Grant Ave, Winnipeg MB R3N 1Z2; (El Salvador)'80; (204)487-8009; Fax. (204)487-8011.

CALDIS, Efstratios V; 221-11118 Homer St, Vancouver BC V6B 6L5; Cape Town (South Africa)'79; MB ChB; FRCPC; Psy. (604)669-0568

CALDWELL, Chalmers W; Langley Mem Hosp, 22051 Fraser Hwy, Langley BC V3A 4H4; London (England)'71; MB BS; FRCPC; Anes. Staff, Langley Memorial Hospital; (604)534-4121; Fax. (604)533-6411; cwincald@telus.net.

CALDWELL, Forrest H; U of Guelph Student Hlth Serv, 110-50 Stone Rd E, Guelph ON N1G 2W1; Tor'81; Dip SportMed; CCFP; FCFP; Staff Family & Emerg Med, Guelph General Hospital; Langs: English; French; (519)824-4120 x52131; Fax. (519)836-7431; fcaldwel@uoguelph.ca.

CALDWELL, J Paul; Cobourg Clinic, PO Box 86 Stn Main 44 University Ave E, Cobourg ON K9A 4K4; Tor'71; CCFP; FCFP; Staff, Northumberland Hills Hospital; (905)372-3323; Fax. (905)372-3692.

CALDWELL, Lyle H; Foothills Med Centre, 1403 29 St NW, Calgary AB T2N 2T9; Cal'74; FRCPC; Psy. Ac Staff Psy., Foothills Medical Centre; (403)944-1273; Fax. (403)270-2093.

CALDWELL, Steven Stewart; Clinical Sciences Bldg, 11 107-152 University Campus N, Edmonton AB T6G 2G3; Edinburgh (Scotland)'89; BSc(Hon); MB BS(Hons); LMCC; FRCP; FRCPC; IntMed (Clinical Nephrology); Nephrol. Staff Nephrol, University of Alberta Hospital; Clin Assoc Prof, University of Alberta; (780)407-7779; Fax. (780)407-7771.

CALHOUN, Erin; PO Box 160, Trochu AB T0M 2C0; Sask'07; CCFP; (403)442-3814; Fax. (403)442-3816.

CALHOUN, Kevin W; Bowmanville Prof Bldg, 3100-222 King St E, Bowmanville ON L1C 1P6; Wes'81; Staff, Lakeridge Health - Bowmanville Site; Staff, Lakeridge Health - Oshawa Site; (905)623-2355; Fax. (905)623-9607; kcal@rogers.com.

CALHOUN, Laura L; Psychealth Centre, PZ443-771 Bannatyne Ave, Winnipeg MB R3E 3N4; Alb'86; FRCPC; Psy.

CALHOUN, Todd C R; North York Gen Hosp, 4001 Leslie St, North York ON M2K 1E1; Ott'96; FRCPC; Anes. Staff, North York General Hospital; Langs: English; French; (416)756-6002; todd@toronto-home.com.

CALIFARETTI, Nadia B; Grand River Hosp-KW Hlth Ctre, PO Box 9056 Stn C 835 King St W, Kitchener ON N2G 1G3; Tor'93; FRCPC; IntMed; MedOncol. Staff MedOncol, Grand River Hospital - Kitchener/Waterloo Health Centre; (519)749-4370 x5715; Fax. (519)749-4378.

CALITZ, Jaco; Life Medical Clinic, PO Box 1406 Stn Main 4740 50 Ave, Whitecourt AB T7S 1P3; (South Africa)'91; MB ChB; Langs: Afrikaans; (780)706-7080; Fax. (780)706-7064.

CALITZ, Johannes J; 110-2504 Skaha Lake Rd, Penticton BC V2A 6G1; Stellenbosch (South Africa)'99; (250)492-3511

CALKIN, Cynthia V; Abbie J Lane Mem Bldg, 5909 Veterans Memorial Lane, Halifax NS B3H 2E2; Dal'93; FRCPC; Psy;CCFP; (902)473-2585

CALLAGHAN, Denis J; 700 Main St E, Hamilton ON L8M 1K7; McM'83; Staff, Hamilton Health Sciences Centre - Hamilton General Hospital; Staff, Hamilton Health Sciences Centre-Juravinski Site; (905)544-9889; Fax. (905)544-9189.

CALLAGHAN, Maximilian; 33 CF Health Services Centre, PO Box 17000 Stn Forces, Kingston ON K7K 7B4; Cal'02; CCFP; (613)541-5010

CALLAGHAN, Sarah; Beaches Family Practie & Walk, 116 Glen Manor Dr, Toronto ON M4E 2X2; National University (Ireland)'02.

CALLAGHAN, Siobhan; Langs Comm Hlth Centre, 1145 Cocession Rd, Cambridge ON N3H 4L5; McM'94; BSc; CCFP; Staff, Langs Farm Village Association; (519)653-1470; Fax. (519)653-6277; smcallaghan@yahoo.com.

CALLAGHAN, W Bryan; Greenbank Med Centre, 200-139 Greenbank Rd, Nepean ON K2H 9A5; Qns'72; CSPQ; FRCSC; PlasSurg (Cosmetic Surgery). Ac Staff, Queensway Carleton Hospital; Court Staff, Carleton Place & District Memorial Hospital; Lecturer Surg, University of Ottawa; (613)721-6463; Fax. (613)721-9899; drwbcallaghan@gmail.com.

CALLAGHAN, Wayne D; 1096 Goyeau St, Windsor ON N9A 1J1; Wes'88; FRCPC; IntMed; Nephrol. Ac Staff IntMed, Hôtel-Dieu Grace Hospital; Med Staff, Windsor Regional Hospital - Tayfour Site; (519)977-5364; Fax. (519)977-5651.

CALLAHAN, David J; Meadowlark Health Centre, 166 Meadowlark Shopping Ctr NW, Edmonton AB T5R 5W9; Qns'82; FRCSC; GenSurg (Breasts). Asst Prof Clinical, University of Alberta; (780)486-5030; Fax. (780)486-1035.

CALLAHAN, Elizabeth A; Midtown Med Clinic, 35 Campbell Ave, St. John's NL A1E 2Z3; Mem'77; CCFP; FCFP; (709)579-0703; Fax. (709)579-1477.

CALLAHAN, Justine E; Family Practice 535, 535 Montreal Rd, Ottawa ON K1K 0V1; Ott'05; CCFP; (613)746-5350; Fax. (613)746-5340.

CALLAHAN, Peter J; Broadway Family Health Centre, PO Box 900 Stn Main 3 Herald Ave, Corner Brook NL A2H 6J2; Mem'94; BSc(Hon); BMedSci; CCFP; Staff, Western Memorial Regional Hospital; (709)639-5920

CALLAHAN-DYER, Deborah M; Major's Path Family Practice, 301-35 Major's Path, St. John's NL A1A 4Z9; Mem'82; CCFP; FCFP; Staff, St Clare's Mercy Hospital; (709)579-2324; Fax. (709)579-3419.

CALLAN, Nicole; 203-331 Sheddon Ave, Oakville ON L6J 1X8; Ott'05; FRCSC; GenSurg. Staff, Halton Healthcare Services Corporation - Oakville Site; (905)618-0098

CALLANAN, Terrence S; St Clare's Mercy Hosp, 154 Lemarchant Rd, St. John's NL A1C 5B8; Mem'76; BMedSci; DPsy; FRCPC; Psy (Psychological Social Rehabilitation). Staff START Clinic, St Clare's Mercy Hospital; Staff Mental Health Program, Health Care Corporation Of St John's; Chair Clinical Disciplines Psy, Memorial University Of Newfoundland; Langs: English; French; (709)777-5111; ts.callanan@mun.ca.

CALLARY, Eva; Health Canada, PL3712-171 Slater St, Ottawa ON K1P 5H7; Bonn (Germany)'76; MD; FRCPC; CommunMed (Occupational Health). Langs: German; Bilingual(French/English); (613)946-6583; Fax. (613)990-9397; eva.callary@hc-sc.gc.ca.

CALLEGARI, Peter R; Vancouver Island Hlth Authorit, 1952 Bay St, Victoria BC V8R 1J8; Edinburgh (Scotland)'66; MB ChB; MRCP(UK); Staff, Vancouver Island Health Authority; Clinical Asst Prof, University of British Columbia; (250)370-8509; Fax. (250)370-8285.

CALLEIA, Sarah G E; Brockville Mental Health Ctre, PO Box 1050 Stn Main, Brockville ON K6V 5W7; McG'62; FRCPC; Psy (Child & Adolescent Psychiatry). Staff, Brockville Mental Health Centre - Royal Ottawa Health Care Group; (613)345-1461

CALLEJO, Sonia A; MUHC-Montreal Gen Hosp, L4 221-1650 rue Cedar, Montreal QC H3G 1A4; Buenos Aires (Argentina)'94; FRCSC; Ophth. Staff, McGill University Health Centre - Montreal General Campus; (514)934-1934 x44079

CALLEN, David J A; McMaster University, 3A52-1280 Main St W, Hamilton ON L8S 4K1; McM'02; FRCPC; Neur. Staff, Hamilton Health Sciences Centre - McMaster Children's Hospital; (905)521-2100

CALLERY, Christopher J; 28 Sovereign St PO Box 910, Waterford ON N0E 1Y0; Galway (Ireland)'70; MB ChB; BAO; Staff, Norfolk General Hospital; (519)443-8695; Fax. (519)443-8695.

CALLES, Jose; 4573 rue Sherbrooke O, Westmount QC H3Z 1E9; (Mexico)'74; ClinImmunol&Allergy (P.Q.) (Internal Medicine). Staff, Centre Hospitalier de Verdun; Staff, St Mary's Hospital Centre; Staff, CSSS de Dorval-Lachine-Lasalle; (514)933-4336; Fax. (514)933-0392.

CALLOW, John A; Lakeridge Hlth Corp-Oshawa, 1 Hospital Crt, Oshawa ON L1G 2B9; Tor'78; CCFP; Ac Staff Emerg, Lakeridge Health - Oshawa Site; (905)576-8711

CALLUM, Jeannie L; Sunnybrook Hlth Sciences Ctre, B204-2075 Bayview Ave, Toronto ON M4N 3M5; Tor'93; FRCPC; IntMed (Transfusion Medicine); Hem. Dir Blood Bank, Sunnybrook Health Sciences Centre; Teach Staff, University of Toronto; (416)480-4757; Fax. (416)480-6035; jeannie.callum@sunnybrook.ca.

CALMAN, Arla S; 2002D Comox Ave, Comox BC V9M 3M6; Alb'81; (250)339-7115

CALNEN, Charlotte A; Duffus Health Centre, 208-7071 Bayers Rd, Halifax NS B3L 2C2; Dal'01; CCFP; (902)453-4585; Fax. (902)453-5657.

CALOIA, David V; William Osler HC-Brampton Civi, 2100 Bovaird Dr E, Brampton ON L6R 3J7; Tor'97; FRCSC; ObstGyn. Staff, William Osler Health System - Brampton Civic Hospital; (905)494-2120

CALOUCHE, Sonia; Clinique Psy de St-Eustache, 111 rue Saint-Laurent, Saint-Eustache QC J7P 3Z5; Ain Shams (Egypt)'82; FRCPC; Psy (General Psychiatry). Staff, Hopital de la Cite de la santé; (450)473-1720

CALPIN, Carolyn; The Westway Children's Clinic, 4-1723 Kipling Ave, Etobicoke ON M9R 2Y8; Wes'90; FRCPC; Peds. Staff, The Hospital For Sick Children; (416)244-8404; carolyn.calpin@sickkids.ca.

CALUGAROIU, Dariu; St Joseph's Health Centre, 1-280 Victoria St, Dalhousie NB E8C 2R6; Cluj-Napoca (Romania)'99; Staff, Centre de santé Communitaire - St-Joseph; (506)684-7000

CALUSERIU, Oana; Medical Sciences Bldg, 8 42B-131 University Campus NW, Edmonton AB T6G 2H7; Tirgu-Muras (Romania)'96; FRCPC; MedGenetics. (780)407-2993; Fax. (780)407-6845.

CALVA, Anne-Marie; CLSC des Patriotes, 10-50 ch de la Rabastaliere E, Saint-Bruno QC J3V 2A5; Mon'97; Physician, CHSLD Montarville; Langs: Bilingual(French/English); (450)461-1012; Fax. (450)461-3088.

CALVERLEY, Virginia C; IWK Health Centre, PO Box 9700 Rpo CSC 5850-5980 University Ave, Halifax NS B3K 6R8; Qns'81; FRCSC; GenSurg (Breast Cancer). Staff, IWK Health Centre; Staff Surgeon, Capital Health District Authority; Asst Prof, Dalhousie University; (902)470-3826; Fax. (902)470-6696.

CALVERT, Chrystella K; 109 King St W, Dundas ON L9H 1V1; McM'85; FRCPC; Peds (Attention Deficit Hyperactivity Disorder). Langs: Bilingual(English/French); (905)628-9200; Fax. (905)628-9600.

CALVERT, Erik; Richmond Health Science Ctre, 310-6091 Gilbert Rd, Richmond BC V7C 5L9; UBC'01; FRCSC; OrthSurg. Staff, UBC Hospital - Koerner Pavillion; (604)273-6148; Fax. (604)273-3421.

CALVERT, Lynn C; Halton Family Health Centre, 2951 Walker's Line, Burlington ON L7M 4Y1; Tor'97; BSc; MSc; Langs: English; French; (905)336-3437

CALVERT, Robert A; Grey Nuns Community Hosp, 1100 Youville Drive West NW, Edmonton AB T6L 5X8; Cal'01; FRCPC; Anes. Staff, Covenant Health - Grey Nuns Community Hospital; (780)735-7000

CALVIN, Brian C; The Medical Arts Centre, 103-650 South Terminal Ave, Nanaimo BC V9R 5E2; UBC'90; BSc; CCFP; Staff Palliative Med, Nanaimo Regional General Hospital; (250)753-3431; Fax. (250)754-6897.

CALVO BALLESTEROS, M Eugenia; Hamilton Hs Corp-Mcmaster Site, PO Box 2000 Stn Lcd 1 HSC 2U1-1200 Main St W, Hamilton ON L8N 3Z5; (Costa Rica)'97; Staff, Hamilton Health Sciences Centre - McMaster University Medical Centre; (905)521-2100

CALVY, Christian; Dr Georges-L Dumont Reg Hosp, 330 av Universite, Moncton NB E1C 2Z3; Marseille (France)'77; Staff, Dr Georges-L-Dumont University Hospital Centre; Langs: Bilingual(French/English); (506)862-4177; Fax. (506)862-4325.

CALZONETTI, Elizabeth A; Joseph Brant Mem Hosp, 1230 North Shore Blvd E, Burlington ON L7S 1W7; McM'90; FRCPC; DiagRad. Staff, Joseph Brant Memorial Hospital; (905)632-3730

CAMACHO MALDONADO, Pedro; Dr Camacho & Dr Humphreys Clin, 1822B Comox Ave, Comox BC V9M 3M7; (Colombia)'95; ABIM; FRCPC; IntMed. Staff, St Joseph's General Hospital; Langs: Spanish; (250)339-2242

CAMAZZOLA, Daniele; 208-22 Richmond St, Richmond Hill ON L4C 3Y1; Ott'96; BSc; FRCSC; OrthSurg (Hip & Knee Reconstruction). Ac Staff OrthSurg, Mackenzie Richmond Hill Hospital; Langs: Italian; (905)883-4443; Fax. (905)883-4477.

CAMBRIDGE, Mary J; Couchiching Family Health Team, 201-119 Memorial Ave, Orillia ON L3V 5X1; Ott'91; CCFP; FCFP; Staff, Orillia Soldiers' Memorial Hospital; (705)326-2208; Fax. (705)325-9498.

CAMBRIDGE, Robert M; Soldiers Mem Hosp, 170 Colborne St W, Orillia ON L3V 2Z3; Ott'92; BSc; CCFP; FCFP; Staff, Orillia Soldiers' Memorial Hospital; Assoc Teach Staff, University of Toronto; (705)325-2201

CAMBRIDGE, Rosemarie T P; 106-9193 Main St, Chilliwack BC V2P 7S5; Limpopo (South Africa)'09; MB ChB; (604)858-8343

CAMBRIDGE, Sean L O; 106-9193 Main St, Chilliwack BC V2P 7S5; Limpopo (South Africa)'05; MB ChB; (604)858-8343

CAMBRON, Helene; CSSS de Temiscouata, 58 rue de l'Eglise CP 310, Notre-Dame-du-Lac QC G0L 1X0; Mon'94; Staff, Centre Hospitalier Notre-Dame-du-Lac; (418)899-6751

CAMBRON-GOULET, Evelyne; Sante Serv Sociaux Monteregie, 1255 rue Beauregard, Longueuil QC J4K 2M3; Mon'05; FRCPC; CommunMed. Staff, Agence de santé et des services sociaux de la Montérégie; (450)928-6777

CAMDEN, Marie-Christine; Ctr Hosp Affilie-Enfant-Jesus, 1401 18e rue, Quebec QC G1J 1Z4; Laval'05; FRCPC; Neur. Staff, Centre Hospitalier Affilié Universitaire de Québec - Hôpital De L'Enfant Jésus; (418)649-0252

CAMERLAIN, Monique; Clinique Med Belvedere, 202-2235 rue Galt O, Sherbrooke QC J1K 1K6; Mon'68; FRCPC; Rheum (Pharmacology). Staff Member Rheum, Centre Hospitalier Universitaire de Sherbrooke-Hopital Fleurimont; (819)563-4244; Fax. (819)563-8924.

CAMERON, Billie-Rose H; 102-751 Victoria St S, Kitchener ON N2G 1E5; Qns'97; FRCSC; Otol. (519)954-6938; Fax. (519)954-6940.

CAMERON, Bonnie J; 305-2238 Dundas St W, Toronto ON M6R 3A9; McM'80; FRCPC; Peds (Pediatric Rheumatology); Rheum. Ac Staff, The Hospital For Sick Children; Asst Prof Peds, University of Toronto; (416)538-8512; Fax. (416)538-8513.

CAMERON, Brian H; Hamilton HS-McMaster Site, 4E7-1200 Main St W, Hamilton ON L8N 3Z5; Qns'80; MD; FACS; FRC; FRCSC; GenSurg; PedGenSurg. Staff, Hamilton Health Sciences Centre - McMaster Children's Hospital; (905)521-2100 x75231; Fax. (905)521-9992; cameronb@mcmaster.ca.

CAMERON, Brian W; North Burlington Med Centre, 18-1960 Appleby Line, Burlington ON L7L 0B7; Cal'82; CCFP; Ac Staff, Joseph Brant Memorial Hospital; Ac Staff, South Muskoka Memorial Hospital - Muskoka Algonquin Healthcare; (905)319-2000; Fax. (905)319-6292.

CAMERON, Bruce C; Peterborough Clinic FHT, LL02-26 Hospital Dr, Peterborough ON K9J 7C3; Tor'80; CCFP; Staff, Peterborough Regional Health Centre - Hospital Drive; (705)740-6840; Fax. (705)740-6847; bcameron@ptboclinic.com.

CAMERON, Bruce D; Dr Georges-L.-Dumont Reg Hosp, 330 av Universite, Moncton NB E1C 2Z3; Wes'98; FRCPC; HemPath. Staff, Dr Georges-L-Dumont University Hospital Centre; (506)862-4000

CAMERON, Catherine; The Start Clinic, 32 Park Rd, Toronto ON M4W 2N4; Tor'91; CCFP; (416)598-9344; Fax. (416)598-8198; cathycameron@sympatico.ca.

CAMERON, Christopher D; 1135 Dufferin Cres, Nanaimo BC V9S 2B5; UBC'83; DAB; FRCSC; OrthSurg (General Orthopedics). Staff, Nanaimo Regional General Hospital; (250)754-3727; Fax. (250)754-1447.

CAMERON, Clare R A; Grandview Med Ctr Fam Hlth Team, 167 Hespeler Rd, Cambridge ON N1R 3H7; McM'80; CCFP; FCFP; (519)623-4200; Fax. (519)623-2546.

CAMERON, Colin J; Royal Ottawa Health Care, PO Box 1050 Stn Main 1804 Highway 2 E, Brockville ON K6V 5W7; McG'87; FRCPC; Psy (General Psychiatry). Clin Dir Integrated Forensic Prog Secure Treatment Unit, Brockville Mental Health Centre - Royal Ottawa Health Care Group; Asst Prof Psy, University of Ottawa; Langs: French; Spanish; (613)341-2870 x1218; colin.cameron@rohcg.on.ca.

CAMERON, Cynthia; CLSC Grand Littoral, 200-1205 boul de la Rive-Sud, Saint-Romuald QC G6W 0J6; Laval'07; CCFP; (418)380-8597; Fax. (418)380-8596.

CAMERON, D William; The Ottawa Hosp-Gen Campus, 501 Smyth Rd Box 228, Ottawa ON K1H 8L6; Qns'79; FACP; FRCPC; IntMed (Infectious Diseases). Staff, The Ottawa Hospital - General Campus; Prof Med, University of Ottawa; Aj Prof, Queen's University; (613)737-8923; Fax. (613)737-8925.

CAMERON, Daniel J; Parkdale Med Tower, 607-1081 Carling Ave, Ottawa ON K1Y 4G2; Tor'90; CCFP; Staff Family Pract/Asst Surg, The Ottawa Hospital - Riverside Campus; Langs: Bilingual(English/French); (613)725-3117; Fax. (613)725-3237.

CAMERON, David A; Brant Community HC-Brantford, 200 Terrace Hill St, Brantford ON N3R 1G9; Tor'87; CCFP; Staff, The Brant Community Healthcare System - Willett Hospital Site; Staff, The Brant Community Healthcare System - Brantford General Hospital Site; (519)751-5544

CAMERON, David J; Nith Valley Family Practice, 1-10 Waterloo St, New Hamburg ON N3A 1V5; Wes'83; (519)662-1551; Fax. (519)662-1402.

CAMERON, Donald A; 210-125 13th St E, North Vancouver BC V7L 2L3; Qns'82; FRCPC; Neur (Traumatic Brain Injuries). Consultant, UBC Hospital - Koerner Pavillion; Ac Staff, Lions Gate Hospital; Consultant, Vancouver General Hospital - Centennial Pavillion; Clin Instructor Med, University of British Columbia; (604)986-7002; Fax. (604)986-7013; info@lghfoundation.com.

CAMERON, Donna M; Lakeside Med Clinic, 3919 8th St E, Saskatoon SK S7H 5M7; Sask'02; CCFP; (306)374-6884

CAMERON, Douglas A; Univ Hlth Network-Toronto Gen, 3PMCC 560-200 Elizabeth St, Toronto ON M5G 2C4; Dal'74; FACC; FRCPC; IntMed (Electrophysiology); Cardiol. Staff Electrophysiologist, Toronto General Hospital - UHN; (416)340-4339

CAMERON, Elizabeth A; 6-1230 Alward St, Prince George BC V2M 7B1; Cal'07; CCFP; (250)563-3024

CAMERON, Elizabeth A; Northgate Med Centre, 2711 Avonhurst Dr, Regina SK S4R 3J3; (England) BSc(Hon); MB ChB; (306)543-4566; Fax. (306)543-4441.

CAMERON, Estelle E A; Sydney Family Practice, 196 Kings Rd, Sydney NS B1S 1A1; Dal'77; (902)567-0040; Fax. (902)539-9250.

CAMERON, G Stuart; Foul Bay Prof Centre, 324-1964 Fort St, Victoria BC V8R 6R3; Sask'61; AB; MSc; FRCSC; Neursurg. Assoc Staff, Victoria General Hospital; (250)592-2822; Fax. (250)592-2181.

CAMERON, Glenn G; Waypoint Centre for Mental H C, 500 Church St, Penetanguishene ON L9M 1G3; Tor'70; FRCPC; Psy;CCFP; FCFP; Staff, Waypoint Centre for Mental Health Care; Langs: French; (705)549-3181 x2679; Fax. (705)549-0266.

CAMERON, Glenna G; 7575 16 Sideroad RR 1, Bolton ON L7E 5R7; Ott'76; DiagRad (Ultrasound). (905)707-1777

CAMERON, Hugh U; Sunnybrook Holland Ortho Arthr, 318-43 Wellesley St E, Toronto ON M4Y 1H1; St. Andrews (Scotland)'69; MB ChB; DAB; FAAOS; FRCSC; OrthSurg (Orthopedics) (Joint Replacement). Staff, Sunnybrook Health Sciences Centre - Holland Orthopaedic & Arthritic Centre; Assoc Prof, University of Toronto; (416)967-8734; Fax. (416)975-2679.

CAMERON, Ian A; St Mary's Med Clinic, PO Box 297, Sherbrooke NS B0J 3C0; Dal'69; CCFP; FCFP; Staff, Queen Elizabeth II Health Sciences Centre - Victoria General Site; (902)522-2275

CAMERON, Ian B; 205-6440 Royal Oak Ave, Burnaby BC V5H 3P2; Tor'88; (604)432-1654; Fax. (604)430-1936.

CAMERON, James A; 410-2255 Carling Ave, Ottawa ON K2B 7Z5; Ott'78; Ophth (Anterior Segment). Staff, The Ottawa Hospital - General Campus; (613)596-0300

CAMERON, James P; University of Alberta Hosp, 8440 112 St NW, Edmonton AB T6G 2B7; Staff, University of Alberta Hospital; (780)407-8896; Fax. (780)407-3200.

CAMERON, Jane L; Kensington Mews 1, 403-2 14 St NW, Calgary AB T2N 1Z4; Alb'91; MSc; BPE; BMedSci; (403)270-9505; Fax. (403)270-9790; jaca@telusplanet.net.

CAMERON, Jean M; A-26 Market St, Antigonish NS B2G 3B4; Dal'85; (902)863-3003

CAMERON, John C; Sunnybrook Holland Ortho Arthr, 343-43 Wellesley St E, Toronto ON M4Y 1H1; Tor'70; FRCSC; OrthSurg. Staff, Sunnybrook Health Sciences Centre - Holland Orthopaedic & Arthritic Centre; University of Toronto; (416)928-3279; Fax. (416)967-8705.

CAMERON, Judith M; Seaforth Med Bldg, 680-3550 ch de la Cote-des-Nei, Montreal QC H3H 1V4; McG'74; FAAD; BSc; MDCM; FRCPC; Derm. Sr Staff Derm, McGill University Health Centre - Montreal General Campus; assoc Prof Med, McGill University; Langs: Bilingual(English/French); (514)939-2954

CAMERON, Karen A; New Vision Family Health Team, 421 Greenbrook Dr, Kitchener ON N2M 4K1; Dal'94; CCFP; Ac Staff, Grand River Hospital - Kitchener/Waterloo Health Centre; Court Staff, St Mary's General Hospital; (519)578-3510; Fax. (519)578-6040.

CAMERON, Kelsey; Dr Everett Chalmers Reg Hosp, PO Box 9000 Stn A, Fredericton NB E3B 5N5; Dal'08; Staff, Dr Everett Chalmers Regional Hospital; (506)452-5400

CAMERON, Kenneth M; 105-375 Pleasant St, Dartmouth NS B2Y 4N4; Edinburgh (Scotland)'76; CCFP; FCFP; Ac Staff, Dartmouth General Hospital; (902)469-9564; Fax. (902)469-2449; kcameron@ns.aliantzinc.ca.

CAMERON, Kristjana G; UBC Mood Disorders Centre, 2C7-2255 Wesbrook Mall, Vancouver BC V6T 2A1; Alb'07; FRCPC; Psy. (604)822-7512

CAMERON, Lauren M; Southwest Family Health Ctre, 204-200 James St S, Hamilton ON L8P 3A9; McM'84; CCFP; FCFP; Assoc Staff, St Joseph's Healthcare - Charlton Campus; (905)526-1606; Fax. (905)526-7692.

CAMERON, Marianne C; Dartmouth Gen Hosp, 325 Pleasant St, Dartmouth NS B2Y 4G8; Dal'05; CCFP; Staff, Dartmouth General Hospital; (902)465-8300

CAMERON, Marilyn J; 103-6935 120 St, Delta BC V4E 2A8; Sask'79; CCFP; FCFP; (604)590-4443; Fax. (604)590-5192.

CAMERON, Mark H; Broad Street Med Clinic, 2210 Broad St, Regina SK S4P 4V6; Sask'88; CCFP; FCFP; Ac Staff, Pasqua Hospital; Ac Staff, Regina General Hospital; Asst Prof, University of Saskatchewan; (306)781-8080; Fax. (306)781-5644.

CAMERON, Mary M; Guelph Gen Hosp, 115 Delhi St, Guelph ON N1E 4J4; Qns'98; CCFP; CCFP(E.M.); Staff, Guelph General Hospital; (519)837-6440

CAMERON, Murray R; St Boniface Gen Hosp, 409 Tache Ave, Winnipeg MB R2H 2A6; Man'71; FRCPC; Anes;CCFP; FCFP; Staff, St Boniface General Hospital; (204)233-8563

CAMERON, Nancy E; 77722B London Rd RR 5, Clinton ON N0M 1L0; Wes'77; MHSc; DOHS(McM); Med Officer of Hlth, Huron Country Health Unit; (519)482-3416; Fax. (519)482-7820.

CAMERON, Nancy; CSSS de Portneuf, 700 rue Saint-Cyrille, Saint-Raymond QC G3L 1W1; Sher'93; Staff, Centre Hospitalier Portneuf; (418)337-4611

CAMERON, Paul E; PO Box 284, Bragg Creek AB T0L 0K0; Qns'78; (403)949-3488; Fax. (403)949-3486.

CAMERON, Peter P G; Huronia Med Centre, PO Box 790 Stn Main, Midland ON L4R 4P4; London (England)'71; MB BS; MRCS; LRCP; (705)526-3921; Fax. (705)526-5757.

CAMERON, Reid S; Hornepayne Comm Hosp, PO Box 190 278 Front St, Hornepayne ON P0M 1Z0; McM'96; CCFP; Chief of Staff, Hornepayne Community Hospital; (807)868-2442; Fax. (807)868-3145; reid9906@hotmail.com.

CAMERON, Robert A; Associate Med Clinic, PO Box 549, Pincher Creek AB T0K 1W0; Alb'89; (403)627-3321; Fax. (403)627-2280.

CAMERON, Robert D A; Regina Qu'Appelle HR-Regina, 1440 14th Ave, Regina SK S4P 0W5; Sask'70; FACS; FRCSC; GenSurg. Ac Staff, Regina General Hospital; Ac Staff, Pasqua Hospital; Ac Staff, Regina Health District; Clin Prof Surg, University of Saskatchewan; (306)766-6911; Fax. (306)766-6917.

CAMERON, Robert; Sandwich Med Clinic, 3211 Sandwich St, Windsor ON N9C 1A9; Wes'77; DLIM; Court Staff, London Health Sciences Centre - University Hospital; (519)682-3699; Fax. (519)682-9570.

CAMERON, Roderick H; X-Ray Associates, B02-250 Harding Blvd W, Richmond Hill ON L4C 9M7; Wes'80; FRCPC; DiagRad. Staff, Mackenzie Richmond Hill Hospital; (905)737-0595

CAMERON, Roderick J; Royal Inland Hosp, 311 Columbia St, Kamloops BC V2C 2T1; UBC'88; FRCPC; Anes. Staff, Royal Inland Hospital; (250)374-5111

CAMERON, Ronald J; 303-1101 Dewdney Ave, Trail BC V1R 4T1; Nat'l. (Ireland)'89; MB ChB; BAO; FRCSC; GenSurg. (250)364-1188; Fax. (250)364-1399.

CAMERON, Sandra J; Sudbury Reg Hosp-Mem Site, 865 Regent St, Sudbury ON P3E 3Y9; Qns'79; FRCPC; IntMed; Respir. Ac Staff/Chief Medical Staff, Health Sciences North - Memorial Site; (705)671-5277

CAMERON, Scott B; 4092 Shelbourne St, Victoria BC V8N 4P6; Man'07; ClinImmunol&Allergy; Peds. (250)595-8111

CAMERON, Scott L; Prince County Hosp, PO Box 3000 Stn Main 65 Roy Boates Ave, Summerside PE C1N 2A9; Dal'87; Staff Chief EmergMed, Prince County Hospital; Preceptor Northumberland Teaching Unit, Dalhousie University; (902)436-9131 x175

CAMERON, Stephanie A; Riverside Med Clinic, 304-1101 Dewdney Ave, Trail BC V1R 4T1; UBC'91; CCFP; FCFP; (250)368-5656; Fax. (250)368-8811.

CAMERON, Stewart M; Dalhousie Family Med Mumford, 265-6960 Mumford Rd, Halifax NS B3L 4P1; Dal'79; MEd; CCFP; FCFP; Staff, Queen Elizabeth II Health Sciences Centre - Victoria General Site; Staff For Women Children and Families, IWK Health Centre; Assoc Prof Family Med, Dalhousie University; (902)473-4700; Fax. (902)473-8548; stewart.cameron@dal.ca.

CAMERON-ROSS, Lorien; British Army Training Unit Suf, PO BOX 5000 LCD 1, Medicine Hat AB T1A 8K7.

CAMFIELD, Carol S; IWK Health Centre, PO Box 9700 Rpo CSC, Halifax NS B3K 6R8; Michigan (USA)'70; Peds. Staff, IWK Health Centre; (902)470-8479; Fax. (902)470-8486; camfield@dal.ca.

CAMFIELD, Peter R; IWK Health Centre, PO Box 9700 Rpo CSC 5850 University Ave, Halifax NS B3K 6R8; Harvard(MA) (USA)'70; Neur; Peds. Staff, IWK Health Centre; Langs: English; French; (902)470-8479; Fax. (902)470-8486.

CAMICIOLI, Joseph R M; Glenrose Rehab Hosp, E223-10230 111 Ave NW, Edmonton AB T5G 0B7; McG'87; FRCPC; Neur. Staff, Glenrose Rehabilitation Hospital; (780)474-8840; Fax. (780)474-8804.

CAMIRAND, Louis; Clinique Med du Cuivre, 12 rue Gamble E, Rouyn-Noranda QC J9X 3B7; Sher'92; Staff, Centre Hospitalier Rouyn-Noranda; Langs: German; (819)764-9434

CAMIRAND, Michel; Centre de Sante Sutton, CP 630 33 rue Principale S, Sutton QC J0E 2K0; Sher'79; Staff, Hôpital Brome-Missisquoi-Perkins; (450)538-3983; Fax. (450)538-8396; mcamirand@aol.com.

CAMIRAND, Yannick; Ctr Hosp Charlevoix, 74 rue Ambroise-Fafard, Baie-Saint-Paul QC G3Z 2J6; Laval'00; FRCPC; Psy. Staff, CSSS de Charlevoix; (418)435-5150

CAMIRE, Bruno; Centre Obst/Gyn de la Cite, 4250 av 1Re, Quebec QC G1H 2S5; Laval'99; FRCSC; ObstGyn. Staff, Centre Hospitalier Universitaire De Québec - Pavillon De St-françois-d'assise; (418)654-0555

CAMIRE, Eric; CHUQ-Hotel-Dieu de Quebec, 11 Cote du Palais, Quebec QC G1R 2J6; Laval'02; Critical Care Medicine (P.Q.); Anes. Staff, Centre Hospitalier Universitaire de Québec (CHUQ) - Siege Social; (418)525-4444

CAMIRE, Jean-Sebastien; Ctr Hosp Laurentien, 234 rue Saint-Vincent, Ste-Agathe-des-Mts QC J8C 2B8; Sher'07; GenSurg. Staff, Centre Hospitalier Laurentien; (819)324-4000

CAMIRE, Laurent; Centre de Med Familiale, 189 av Damase-Potvin, Baie-Comeau QC G4Z 2Y9; Sher'71; Staff, Centre Hospitalier Régional Baie-Comeau; (418)296-9119; Fax. (418)296-9446.

CAMIRE, Marcel; 110-2880 ch des Quatre-Bourgeo, Quebec QC G1V 4X7; Laval'85; FRCSC; Otol (Oncology). Staff, Centre Hospitalier Affilié Universitaire de Québec - Hôpital du St-Sacrement; (418)653-8717; Fax. (418)653-7199.

CAMIRE, Michel; CSSS Drummond-Hop Sainte-Croix, 570 rue Heriot, Drummondville QC J2B 1C1; Laval'95; OrthSurg (P.Q.) (Arthroplasty). Staff, Hôpital Sainte-croix; (819)478-6464; camiremi@hotmail.com.

CAMIRE, Myriam; CHUQ-Hotel-Dieu de Quebec, 11 Cote Du Palais, Quebec QC G1R 2J6; Mon'99; FRCPC; DiagRad. Staff, Centre Hospitalier Universitaire de Québec (CHUQ) - Siege Social; (418)525-4444

CAMIRE, Pierre; Clinique Med 3000 Inc, 3000 rue Belanger, Montreal QC H1Y 1A9; Mon'79; Langs: English; (514)376-7702; Fax. (514)376-2639; pcamire@videotron.ca.

CAMIRE, Raymond D; CLSC Saint-Romuald, 200-1205 boul de la Rive-Sud, Saint-Romuald QC G6W 0J6; Laval'76; (418)380-8991; Fax. (418)839-4190; raymond_camire@ssss.gouv.qc.ca.

CAMIRE, Sophie; Clinique Med Nepisiguit, 950 av Picot, Bathurst NB E2A 4Z9; Mon'98; CCFP; Langs: English; (506)546-6696; Fax. (506)545-7723; cmni@nbnet.nb.ca.

CAMIRE, Valerie; Clinique Med de la Marconi, 201-3525 boul Saint-Joseph, Drummondville QC J2B 0H3; Laval'04; CCFP; (819)850-0476

CAMLIOGLU, Errol B; SMBD Jewish Gen Hosp, 3755 ch Cote-Sainte-Catherine, Montreal QC H3T 1E2; Ott'01; FRCPC; DiagRad. Staff, Sir Mortimer B Davis Jewish General; (514)340-8233

CAMMISULI, Salvatore; 4F-117 King St E, Oshawa ON L1H 1B9; Tor'98; FRCPC; Peds; Derm. (905)721-4356; Fax. (905)721-4342.

CAMORIANO NOLASCO, Gerardo; Kingston Eye Institute, 725 Arlington Park Pl, Kingston ON K7M 7E4; McG'06; MDCM; Ophth. (613)546-1858

CAMPANA, Bruce; Victoria Gen Hosp, 1 Hospital Way, Victoria BC V8Z 6R5; McG'82; FACEP; FRCPC; EmergMed (Hyperbaric Medicine). Staff, Victoria General Hospital; Clinical Asst Prof, University of British Columbia; (250)727-4105

CAMPANARO, Judith M; Medical Bldg, 400-18 Pine St, Kitchener ON N2H 5Z8; Qns'88; FRCSC; ObstGyn (Infertility). Court Staff Privil, Grand River Hospital - Kitchener/Waterloo Health Centre; (519)570-0090; Fax. (519)570-3202; jcss@karmaobgyn.com.

CAMPANARO, Roberto M; Atikokan Family Health Team, PO Box 1450 123 Marks St, Atikokan ON P0T 1C0; Alb'90; BSc; Staff, Atikokan General Hospital; Langs: Spanish; French; (807)597-2721; Fax. (807)597-4632; campanaror@aghospital.on.ca.

CAMPBELL, Aaron; Kingston Gen Hosp, 308-76 Stuart St, Kingston ON K7L 2V7; Sask'99; FRCSC; OrthSurg (Knee Surgery). Staff, Kingston General Hospital; Staff, Hotel-Dieu Hospital; Asst Prof Surg, Queen's University; (613)549-6666 x6802

CAMPBELL, Alan D; 100 Queensway W, Mississauga ON L5B 1B8; Tor'71; FACEP; Chief EmergMed, Trillium Health Centre - Mississauga; Asst Prof Med & Part Time Continuing Med Ed, University of Toronto; (905)848-7600

CAMPBELL, Alisha H; Meadowlands Family Hlth Clinic, 888 Meadowlands Dr, Ottawa ON K2C 3R2; Ott'07; CCFP; (613)228-2882; Fax. (613)228-2856.

CAMPBELL, Andrew I M; Children's & Women's HC of BC, AB307-4480 Oak St, Vancouver BC V6H 3V4; Ott'93; FRCSC; CardSurg. Staff, BC Children's Hospital; (604)875-3165

CAMPBELL, Andrew S; Vancouver Gen Hosp, 855 12th Ave W, Vancouver BC V5Z 1M9; Ott'04; FRCPC; EmergMed. Staff, Vancouver General Hospital - Centennial Pavillion; (604)875-4995

CAMPBELL, Audrey C; BC Centre For Disease Control, 655 12th Ave W, Vancouver BC V5Z 4R4; McM'05; FRCPC; Public Health & Preventive Med. (778)865-1240

CAMPBELL, Barbara E; Cross Cancer Institute, 11560 University Ave NW, Edmonton AB T6G 1Z2; Alb'74; FRCPC; DiagRad. Staff, Cross Cancer Institute; (780)432-8744; Fax. (780)432-8552.

CAMPBELL, Barbara E; Greenwood Med Centre, 10-496 Discovery Ave, Kingston ON K7K 7E9; Ott'84; CCFP; (613)507-7003; Fax. (613)507-7006.

CAMPBELL, Barry I; St Boniface Gen Hosp, M5-409 Tache Ave, Winnipeg MB R2H 2A6; Man'84; FRCPC; Psy (Geriatric Psychiatry). Dir Geriatric Psy, St Boniface General Hospital; Consultant, WRHA - Deer Lodge Centre; Consultant, Riverview Health Centre; Physician, Tache Nursing Centre; Assoc Prof Psy, University of Manitoba; (204)233-8563; Fax. (204)231-0640.

CAMPBELL, Bruce A; St Mary's Hosp Centre, 3830 av Lacombe, Montreal QC H3T 1M5; Dal'98; FRCPC; IntMed. Staff, St Mary's Hospital Centre; (514)345-3500 x3460; Fax. (514)734-2641.

CAMPBELL, Bryan G; Niagara H System-Welland Site, 65 Third St, Welland ON L3B 4W6; Dal'00; FRCPC; DiagRad (Abdominal Radiology). Staff, Niagara Health System - Welland Hospital Site; (905)378-4647

CAMPBELL, Carolyn N J; Grand River Hosp-KW Hlth Ctre, PO Box 9056 Stn C 835 King St, Kitchener ON N2G 1G3; McM'88; BSc(Hons); FRCPC; IntMed; MedOncol. Staff Grand River Reg Cancer Ctre, Grand River Hospital - Kitchener/Waterloo Health Centre; Aj Prof Oncol, McMaster University; (519)749-4380; Fax. (519)749-4378.

CAMPBELL, Carolyne A; 249 McLeod St, Ottawa ON K2P 1A1; McG'90; FRCPC; Psy. (613)567-7267; Fax. (613)233-9710.

CAMPBELL, Catherine J M; Women's College Hosp, 10W-76 Grenville St, Toronto ON M5S 1B2; McM'83; Dip SportMed; CCFP; FCFP; Staff, Women's College Hospital; (416)323-6479; Fax. (416)323-6487.

CAMPBELL, Catherine W; Marketed Health Product, AL 0701C-200 Tunney's Pasture, Ottawa ON K1A 0K9; McG'81; Staff, Marketed Hlth Products Directoral; (613)946-6347

CAMPBELL, Christina S F; Bayswater Family Practice, 200-2475 Bayswater St, Vancouver BC V6K 4N3; UBC'06; CCFP; (604)731-0091

CAMPBELL, Craig E; 201-1919 Riverside Dr, Ottawa ON K1H 1A2; McG'75; FSOGC; FACOG; FRCSC; ObstGyn (Urological Gynecology). Ac Staff, The Ottawa Hospital - Civic Campus; Asst Prof, University of Ottawa; (613)729-1096; Fax. (613)728-4480.

CAMPBELL, Craig G N; London HSC-Victoria Hosp, PO Box 5010 Stn B 800 Commissioners Rd E, London ON N6A 5W9; Ott'96; FRCPC; Peds (Pediatric Neurology); Neur. Staff Ped Neurol, London Health Sciences Centre - Victoria Campus; Asst Prof, University of Western Ontario; (519)685-8332

CAMPBELL, Crystal R; Family Practice Associates, PO Box 2010 223 16 Ave N, Creston BC V0B 1G0; Cal'07; CCFP; (250)428-9371; Fax. (250)428-9350.

CAMPBELL, Curtis; Grey Nuns Community Hosp & HC, 1100 Youville Drive West NW, Edmonton AB T6L 5X8; Man'03; CCFP; CCFP(E.M.); Staff, Covenant Health - Grey Nuns Community Hospital; Physician, CFB Health Services Centre; (780)973-4011; curtis.campbell@canadianforces.gc.ca.

CAMPBELL, D Paula; VGH-Diamond Centre, 8F-2775 Laurel St N, Vancouver BC V5Z 1M9; UBC'95; BSc; FRCPC; Psy. Staff, Providence Health Care - St Paul's Hospital; (604)875-4139

CAMPBELL, D Robert; Regional Mental HC-London, PO Box 5532 Stn B 850 Highbury Ave, London ON N6A 4H1; Wes'67; FRCPC; Psy (Eating Disorders). Staff, Regional Mental Health Care-St Joseph's Health Care; Physician Lead Moods & Anxiety & Assessment Program, Regional Mental Health Care-St Joseph's Health Care; Pres, Eating Disorder Foundation of Canada; Assoc Prof Schulich School of Med & Dentistry, University of Western Ontario; (519)455-5110 x47401; Fax. (519)455-2919.

CAMPBELL, David C; Royal University Hosp, 103 Hospital Dr, Saskatoon SK S7N 0W8; Dal'88; MSc; FRCPC; Anes (Cardiac Anesthesia). Dir Obstetric Anes, Royal University Hospital; Dept Head Anes/Prof, University of Saskatchewan; (306)655-1183; Fax. (306)655-1279; david.campbell@saskatoonhealthregion.ca.

CAMPBELL, David D; Meadowlark Health Centre, 176 Meadowlark Shopping Ctr NW, Edmonton AB T5R 5W9; Alb'73; FRCSC; PlasSurg. Staff Chief Div of PlasSurg, Royal Alexandra Hospital; Ac Staff, Glenrose Rehabilitation Hospital; Court Staff, University of Alberta Hospital; Assoc Prof Med, University of Alberta; (780)428-7737; Fax. (780)425-7679.

CAMPBELL, David Scott; Kings County Med Centre, PO Box 877, Montague PE C0A 1R0; BSc; MSc; CCFP; (902)838-0830; Fax. (902)838-0834.

CAMPBELL, Deanna L; 201-6628 Crowchild Trail SW, Calgary AB T3E 5R8; Alb'92; BSc(Med); CCFP; FCFP; Staff Privil Obstetrics, Rockyview General Hospital; (403)240-9350; Fax. (403)240-9783.

CAMPBELL, Derek S; 5998 Salish Rd, Duncan BC V9L 0B3; Ott'73; FRCPC; Anes (Pain Management). (250)748-4191

CAMPBELL, Derek W; 401-2031 McCallum Rd, Abbotsford BC V2S 3N5; UBC'96; FRCPC; Anes. Staff, Abbotsford Regional Hospital & Cancer Centre; (604)854-1558

CAMPBELL, Donald C; 166 Currie Rd PO Box 263, Dutton ON N0L 1J0; Wes'57; Consultant, St Thomas Elgin General Hospital; (519)762-2740

CAMPBELL, Donald M; Albro Lake Med Clinic, 6 Primrose St, Dartmouth NS B3A 4C5; Glasgow (Scotland)'60; MB ChB; (902)463-2717; ay171@chebucto.ns.ca.

CAMPBELL, Donald M; Humber River Reg Hosp-Church, 200 Church St, Toronto ON M9N 1N8; Wes'79; FRCPC; AnatPath. Staff, Humber River Regional Hospital - Church Street Site; (416)243-4698; Fax. (416)243-4296.

CAMPBELL, Doreen J; 807-123 Edward St, Toronto ON M5G 1E2; Sheffield (England)'69; MB ChB; FRCPC; Rheum; PhysMed&Rehab; IntMed. Att Staff, St Michael's Hospital; University of Toronto; (416)408-1010; Fax. (416)408-2828.

CAMPBELL, Douglas M; St Michael's Hosp, 15 014CC-30 Bond St, Toronto ON M5B 1W8; Cal'97; MSc; FRCPC; Peds (Neonatal & Perinatal). Staff, St Michael's Hospital; Staff Pt-Time, The Hospital For Sick Children; Staff Pt-Time, Rouge Valley Health System - Ajax & Pickering Health Centre Site; University of Toronto; Langs: Bilingual(English/French); (416)867-3655; Fax. (416)867-3736.

CAMPBELL, Duncan A; Lemarchand Mansion, 401-11523 100 Ave NW, Edmonton AB T5K 0J8; Qns'70; ABIM; IntMed. Ac Staff, Royal Alexandra Hospital; Staff Teacher Med, University of Alberta; Langs: French; (780)488-6868

CAMPBELL, Earl A D; Gulf Canada Square, 330-401 9 Ave SW, Calgary AB T2P 3C5; Cal'93; FRCSC; PlasSurg (Cosmetic Surgery). Staff, Foothills Medical Centre; Staff, Alberta Children's Hospital; (403)221-4459; Fax. (403)221-4419.

CAMPBELL, Elroy S; Queen Elizabeth II Hosp, 10409 98 St, Grande Prairie AB T8V 2E8; Staff, Queen Elizabeth II Hospital; (780)538-7656; Fax. (780)538-7277.

CAMPBELL, Fiona A; The Hosp for Sick Children, 555 University Ave, Toronto ON M5G 1X8; McM'84; Staff, The Hospital For Sick Children; (416)813-7445

CAMPBELL, Garth; Beausejour Prof Centre, PO Box 1208, Beausejour MB R0E 0C0; Man'84; Staff/Chief Medical Staff, Beausejour District Hospital; (204)268-2288; Fax. (204)268-4194.

CAMPBELL, Garth L; Queen Elizabeth II Hosp, 10409 98 St, Grande Prairie AB T8V 2E8; Alb'89; Staff, Queen Elizabeth II Hospital; (780)538-7588; Fax. (780)532-9120.

CAMPBELL, Genevieve M; Woodlawn Medical Clinic, 92 Main St, Dartmouth NS B2X 1R5; Cal'82; CCFP; (902)434-1500; Fax. (902)462-8464.

CAMPBELL, Glenn R; North End Community Health Ctr, 2165 Gottingen St, Halifax NS B3K 3B5; UBC'98; CCFP; (902)420-0303; Fax. (902)422-0859.

CAMPBELL, Gordon S; Polyclinic, 308-199 Grafton St, Charlottetown PE C1A 1L2; UBC'83; FACS; FAAOS; MPH; BSc; FRCSC; OrthSurg (Hand & Upper Extremity Surgery). (902)298-8894; Fax. (902)629-8824.

CAMPBELL, Graham M C; Canada Diagnostics Centre, 1-6020 1A St SW, Calgary AB T2H 0G3; Cal'98; FRCPC; DiagRad. (403)253-4666; Fax. (403)253-4669.

CAMPBELL, Grant K; Links Clinic, 104-11910 111 Ave NW, Edmonton AB T5G 3G6; Alb'82; (780)454-0351; Fax. (780)452-6767; drgcampbell@shaw.ca.

CAMPBELL, Gregory J; 75 Bruyere St, Ottawa ON K1N 5C7; Dal'09; CCFP; (613)683-4365; Fax. (613)241-2755.

CAMPBELL, Gwen A M; Selkirk Family Medicine, 307-1101 Dewdney Ave, Trail BC V1R 4T1; Glasgow (Scotland)'83; MB ChB; (250)368-5656

CAMPBELL, Helen; 1119 Pembroke St, Victoria BC V8T 1J5; UBC'88; FRCPC; Psy. Consultant, Saanich Peninsula Hospital; (250)213-4400

CAMPBELL, Holly A; Saint John Reg Hosp, PO Box 2100 Stn Main 400 University Ave, Saint John NB E2L 4L2; Dal'95; BSc; FRCPC; RadOncol (Brachy Therapy). Staff, Saint John Regional Hospital; (506)648-6885; Fax. (506)648-6880; holly.campbell@horizon.nb.ca.

CAMPBELL, Ian G; London Road Diagnostic Clinic, 481 London Rd, Sarnia ON N7T 4X3; McM'81; CCFP; FCFP; Ac Staff, Bluewater Health - Norman Site; Ac Staff, Bluewater Health - Mitton Site; (519)339-0990; Fax. (519)339-0915.

CAMPBELL, Ian H; 245-175 av Stillview, Pointe-Claire QC H9R 4S3; Dal'85; CCFP; (514)697-4017; Fax. (514)697-4418.

CAMPBELL, J Daniel; Bayview Business Centre, 217-16700 Bayview Ave, Newmarket ON L3X 1W1; Tor'82; FRCSC; GenSurg; VascSurg. Staff, Southlake Regional Health Centre; (905)853-2401; Fax. (905)853-3278.

CAMPBELL, James A; 202-16 O'Brien St, Orillia ON L3V 5S2; Qns'80; FRCSC; GenSurg. Staff, Orillia Soldiers' Memorial Hospital; (705)325-4936; Fax. (705)325-7574.

CAMPBELL, James; Commissioners Walk-In Clinic, 111-1 Commissioners Rd E, London ON N6C 5Z3; Wes'81; (519)668-2400

CAMPBELL, Janis P; Southland Court Med Clinic, 150-10601 Southport Rd SW, Calgary AB T2W 3M6; Jefferson(PA) (USA)'79; FRCPC; Derm. Teach Staff, University of Calgary; (403)286-6888

CAMPBELL, Joan P; CML Healthcare, 5400 Portage Rd, Niagara Falls ON L2G 5X7; Tor'81; FRCPC; DiagRad. (905)356-6101; Fax. (905)356-9937.

CAMPBELL, John A; St Mary's Gen Hosp, 911 Queens Blvd, Kitchener ON N2M 1B2; Tor'91; Staff, St Mary's General Hospital; Staff, Grand River Hospital - Kitchener/Waterloo Health Centre; Staff, Grand River Hospital - Freeport Site; (519)744-3311

CAMPBELL, John A; Killick Health Services Inc, 129 Lincoln Rd, Grnd-Falls-Windsor NL A2A 1P3; Mem'02; CCFP; CCFP(E.M.); Staff, Central Newfoundland Regional Health Centre; (709)292-8400

CAMPBELL, John D; 87 Mill St N, Newcastle ON L1B 1H8; Tor'57; (905)987-1778

CAMPBELL, John; The Polyclinic, 307-199 Grafton St, Charlottetown PE C1A 1L2; Dal'00; FRCSC; OrthSurg (Sports Medicine). Staff, Queen Elizabeth Hospital; Preceptor Family Resident, Dalhousie University; (902)629-8856; Fax. (902)368-1694.

CAMPBELL, Joseph A L J; Dundas Med Centre, 303-274 Dundas St E, Belleville ON K8N 1E6; Ott'97; FRCPC; IntMed; Cardiol. Staff, QHC Belleville General; (613)966-4377; Fax. (613)966-4730; joecampbellmd@hotmail.com.

CAMPBELL, Judith M; Seven Oaks Gen Hosp, 2300 McPhillips St, Winnipeg MB R2V 3M3; Man'79; CCFP; Staff, Seven Oaks General Hospital; (204)632-7133

CAMPBELL, Karin M A; 3461 Cook St, Victoria BC V8X 1B3; Tor'89; CCFP; FCFP; (250)386-6161; Fax. (250)382-0613.

CAMPBELL, Latoya L; Ungava Tulattavik Hosp, CP 149, Kuujjuaq QC J0M 1C0; McG'08; CCFP; Staff, Centre de sante Tulattavik de l'Ungava; (819)964-2905; Fax. (819)964-6353.

CAMPBELL, Laurence; Inst Albert Prevost, 6555 boul Gouin O, Montreal QC H4K 1B3; Mon'05; FRCPC; Psy. Staff, Hôpital du Sacre-Coeur de Montréal; (514)338-2222

CAMPBELL, Louise; Deer Lake Medical Clinic, 1-4 Clinic Dr, Deer Lake NL A8A 1E2; (Ireland)'04; MB BCh; (709)635-5150

CAMPBELL, Malcolm S; 444-7620 Elbow Dr SW, Calgary AB T2V 1K2; Glasgow (Scotland)'74; MB ChB; (403)988-5401

CAMPBELL, Martin; Montfort Hosp, 713 Motnreal Rd, Ottawa ON K1K 0T2; Laval'06; FRCPC; Psy. Staff, Montfort Hospital; (613)746-4621

CAMPBELL, Mary-Anne; Sydney Family Practice, 196 Kings Rd, Sydney NS B1S 1A1; Dal'86; (902)567-0040; Fax. (902)539-9250.

CAMPBELL, Michael D; Gateway Med Clinic, 207-2051 McCallum Rd, Abbotsford BC V2S 3N5; Tor'88; (604)859-0777; Fax. (604)859-0767.

CAMPBELL, Milena K; Gateway Hlth & Wellness Ctre, 203-2051 McCallum Rd, Abbotsford BC V2S 3N5; UBC'96; BSc; CCFP; Langs: Italian; (604)854-3441

CAMPBELL, Morgan R; 31956 Lougheed Hwy, Mission BC V2V 0C6; Sask'84; BSc; (604)820-7751

CAMPBELL, Nicole; St Thomas-Elgin Gen Hosp, PO Box 2007 Stn Main 189 Elm St, St Thomas ON N5P 3W2; Wes'02; FRCPC; Anes. Staff, St Thomas Elgin General Hospital; (519)631-2020

CAMPBELL, Norman R; Faculty Of Med, GE 86-3280 Hospital Dr NW, Calgary AB T2N 4Z6; Mem'80; BMedSci; FRCPC; IntMed. Teach Staff, University of Calgary; (403)210-7961; Fax. (403)210-9837.

CAMPBELL, Pamela C; Gulf Canada Square, 330-401 9 Ave SW, Calgary AB T2P 3C5; Tor'64; CCFP; Langs: English; French; (403)221-4459; Fax. (403)221-4406.

CAMPBELL, Patricia M; Foothills Med Centre, 1403 29 St NW, Calgary AB T2N 2T9; Staff, Foothills Medical Centre; (403)944-1381

CAMPBELL, Patricia M; Clinical Sciences Bldg, 11 107-152 University Campus N, Edmonton AB T6G 2G3; Edinburgh (Scotland)'86; MB ChB; MRC; FRCPC; IntMed (Transplantation); Nephrol. Staff, University of Alberta Hospital; (780)407-7579; Fax. (780)407-7771; trish.campbell@ualberta.ca.

CAMPBELL, Peter J; Baywood Med Centre, 505-95 Bayly St W, Ajax ON L1S 7K8; London (England)'79; MRC(UK); FRCPC; IntMed (Gastroenterology). Staff, Rouge Valley Health System - Ajax & Pickering Health Centre Site; (905)683-1236; Fax. (905)683-1271.

CAMPBELL, Rebecca M; Royal Victoria Hosp, 201 Georgian Dr, Barrie ON L4M 6M2; Dal'76; FRCPC; IntMed; Anes. Staff, Royal Victoria Regional Health Centre; (705)728-9802

CAMPBELL, Robert; Hotel-Dieu Hosp, J2 019-166 Brock St, Kingston ON K7L 5G2; Ott'99; FRCSC; Ophth (Glaucoma). Staff, Hotel-Dieu Hospital; (613)544-3310x3189; Fax. (613)533-6667.

CAMPBELL, Ronald M; 200-5503 206 St, Langley BC V3A 2C6; Wes'71; FRCPC; DiagRad. (604)534-4114

CAMPBELL, Samuel G; Queen Elizabeth II HSC-Halifax, 355-1796 Summer St, Halifax NS B3H 3A7; Witwatersrand (South Africa)'87; CHE; CCFP; CCFP(E.M.); Chief Dept of Emergency Med, Queen Elizabeth II Health Sciences Centre - Halifax Infirmary Site; Assoc Prof, Dalhousie University; (902)473-3871; Fax. (902)473-3617; emsgc@cdha.nshealth.ca.

CAMPBELL, Susan L; Baker Clinic, 100-10405 Jasper Ave NW, Edmonton AB T5J 3N4; Alb'84; (780)944-9585; Fax. (780)944-9534.

CAMPBELL, Susan M; Killick Health Services Inc, 129 Lincoln Rd, Grnd-Falls-Windsor NL A2A 1P3; Mem'02; CCFP; Staff, Central Newfoundland Regional Health Centre; (709)292-8400

CAMPBELL, Susan M C; 1058-200 Taunton Rd W, Whitby ON L1R 3H8; Tor'94; BSc; MSc; FAAP; FRCPC; Peds. Court Staff, Rouge Valley Health System - Ajax & Pickering Health Centre Site; (905)444-9636; Fax. (905)444-9853.

CAMPBELL, Suzanne M; Omineca Med Clinic, 3348 Hospital Rd, Vanderhoof BC V0J 3A2; UBC'98; CCFP; (250)567-2201

CAMPBELL, T Malcolm; Centennial CMH & Brain Injury, PO Box 1000 Stn Main, Ponoka AB T4J 1R8; Queen's (Ireland)'74; MB ChB; DRCOG; Pres Med Advisory Committee, Centennial Centre for Mental Health & Brain Injury; (403)783-7600; tmcmb@telusplanet.net.

CAMPBELL, Thomas A; Quinte HC Corp-Belleville Gen, 265 Dundas St E, Belleville ON K8N 5A9; Tor'66; FRCSC; Urol. Staff, QHC Belleville General; Staff, QHC Trenton Memorial; (613)966-9383; Fax. (613)968-5808.

CAMPBELL, Thomas; Trillium Hlth Ctr-Mississauga, 100 Queensway W, Mississauga ON L5B 1B8; Wes'92; Staff, Trillium Health Centre - Mississauga; (905)848-7191

CAMPBELL, Vern; St Michael's Hosp, 7 073 BW-30 Bond St, Toronto ON M5B 1W8; Man'76; FACS; FRCSC; VascSurg. Staff Div of Surg & Vascular Surgeon, St Michael's Hospital; Lecturer, University of Toronto; (416)864-5236; Fax. (416)864-6052.

CAMPBELL, Wayne H; Toronto East Gen Hosp Inc, 825 Coxwell Ave, Toronto ON M4C 3E7; McG'74; FRCPC; Psy. Staff, Toronto East General Hospital Inc; (416)469-6580 x2684; Fax. (416)469-6805.

CAMPBELL, William G; 11807 Jasper Ave NW, Edmonton AB T5K 0N8; Alb'81; Fam Med, Covenant Health - Edmonton General Continuing Care Centre; (780)488-1222

CAMPBELL, William G; Sheldon Chumir Centre, 2131-1213 4 St SW, Calgary AB T2R 0X7; Alb'73; CCFP; Staff, Foothills Medical Centre; (403)240-2221

CAMPBELL-MOSCROP, Alan J; 201-200 James St S, Hamilton ON L8P 3A9; Durham (England)'64; MB BS; FRCSC; PlasSurg (Cutaneous Malignancy). Ac Staff, St Joseph's Healthcare - Charlton Campus; Asst Prof, McMaster University; Langs: French; (905)525-8460; Fax. (905)525-9944.

CAMPBELL-SCHERER, Denise L; Grey Nuns Fam Med Cedars Prof, 2927 66 St NW, Edmonton AB T6K 4C1; Tor'00; CCFP; Att Physician, Covenant Health - Grey Nuns Community Hospital; Assoc Prof, University of Alberta; Langs: German; French; (780)342-1470

CAMPEAU, Denise L; Leamington Dist Mem Hosp, 3F-194 Talbot St W, Leamington ON N8H 1N9; Wes'94; FRCSC; ObstGyn;CCFP; FCFP; Staff, Leamington District Memorial Hospital; (519)326-2373

CAMPEAU, Gilles; GMF Centre de santé, 3745 rue Georges-Couture, Drummondville QC J2B 7P4; Laval'69; ac Staff, Hôpital Sainte-croix; (819)477-2231; Fax. (819)477-1122.

CAMPEAU, Jean; CSSS de la Region de Thetford, 1717 rue Notre-Dame E, Thetford Mines QC G6G 2V4; Sher'84; FRCPC; IntMed. Staff, Hopital du CSS de la Region de Thetford; (418)338-7777

CAMPEAU, Marie-Pierre; CHUM-Hop Notre-Dame, 1560 rue Sherbrooke E, Montreal QC H2L 4M1; Mon'02; FRCPC; RadOncol. Staff, Centre Hospitalier l'Université de Montréal (CHUM) - Hôpital Notre-Dame; (514)890-8254

CAMPEAU, Rejean; Clinique Med Desy, 5636 boul Henri-Bourassa E, Montreal-Nord QC H1G 2T2; Mon'78; (514)326-9060; Fax. (514)326-0919.

CAMPFENS, Lisa C; Foothills Med Centre, 231-1403 29 St NW, Calgary AB T2N 2T9; Qns'88; FRCP; FRCPC; EmergMed (Trauma). Staff, Foothills Medical Centre; (403)944-1635; Fax. (403)944-2419.

CAMPILLO, Sarah; MUHC-Montreal Children's Hosp, C504-2300 rue Tupper, Montreal QC H3H 1P3; McG'98; FRCPC; Peds; Rheum. Staff, McGill University Health Centre - Montreal Children's Hospital; (514)412-4268; Fax. (514)412-4365; sarah.campillo@muhc.mcgill.ca.

CAMPISI, Paolo; The Hosp for Sick Children, 6EW-555 University Ave, Toronto ON M5G 1X8; Wes'97; FRCSC; Otol. Staff, The Hospital For Sick Children; (416)813-2192; Fax. (416)813-5036; paolo.campisi@sickkids.ca.

CAMPLING, M Ruth; 306-125 13th St E, North Vancouver BC V7L 2L3; UBC'81; Staff, Lions Gate Hospital; (604)985-2712; Fax. (604)988-8193.

CAMPOS, Alfredo; Summerside Med Centre, 101-475 Granville St, Summerside PE C1N 3N9; Pontificia (Colombia)'99; FRCSC; Otol. Otolaryngology, Prince County Hospital; Langs: Spanish; (902)432-8181; Fax. (902)436-9660; alfredocampos@eastlink.ca.

CAN, T Bich Dao; Hotel-Dieu de Sorel, 400 av de l'Hotel-Dieu, Sorel-Tracy QC J3P 1N5; Laval'91; Respir (P.Q.); IntMed. Staff, Hôtel-Dieu de Sorel; Langs: Vietnamese; (450)746-6000; Fax. (450)746-6082.

CAN THI, Bich Ngoc; Hop Jean-Talon, 1385 rue Jean-Talon E, Montreal QC H2E 1S6; Mon'90; Staff, CSSS du Coeur de l'Isle Hôpital Jean-Talon; (514)495-6767

CANAAN, Julie; Ctr Hosp de Verdun, 4000 boul Lasalle, Verdun QC H4G 2A3; Mon'07; CCFP; Staff, Centre Hospitalier de Verdun; (514)362-1000

CANADAS, Luis A; Four Rivers Med Clinic, 878 Main St, Winnipeg MB R2W 3P1; (El Salvador)'81; Langs: Spanish; (204)586-5592

CANAKIS, Anne-Marie; MUHC-Montreal Children's Hosp, D380-2300 rue Tupper, Montreal QC H3H 1P3; McG'95; FRCPC; Peds; Respir. Staff, McGill University Health Centre - Montreal Children's Hospital; (514)412-4444

CANAVAN, Joycelin; BC Cancer Centre, 2410 Lee Ave, Victoria BC V8R 6V5; Dublin (Ireland)'06; MB BCh; FRCPC; RadOncol. Staff, BC Cancer Agency Vancouver Island Centre; (250)519-5599

CANCADE, Edward M; Caledonian Med Clinic, 340 Campbell St, Nanaimo BC V9R 3G7; Man'76; CCFP; Staff, Nanaimo Regional General Hospital; (250)753-3202; Fax. (250)753-1039.

CANDERLE, Frank; Com El Med Bldg, 301-2620 Commercial Dr, Vancouver BC V5N 4C4; Ott'95; BSc; CCFP; (604)438-8288

CANDIA, Pascual R; Medica One, 2019 Caroline St, Burlington ON L7R 1L1; (Venezuela)'85; CCFP; (905)333-0911; Fax. (905)333-0311.

CANDLER, David C; Cross Cancer Institute, 11560 University Ave NW, Edmonton AB T6G 1Z2; Alb'89; Staff, Cross Cancer Institute; (780)432-8771

CANDUSSO, Cathryn A; Orangeville Family Med Centre, M1-32 First St, Orangeville ON L9W 2E1; Ott'90; (519)938-8000; Fax. (519)938-8080.

CANELLA, Louis F; 209-1246 Yonge St, Toronto ON M4T 1W7; Tor'83; FRCPC; Psy. Teacher, University of Toronto; Langs: Italian; (416)929-0896

CANERS, Dennis T; Plessis Med Centre, 12-801 Regent Ave W, Winnipeg MB R2C 3A7; Man'79; CCFP; FCFP; (204)222-4200; Fax. (204)222-8181.

CANETE, Yuri C; Hantsport Medical Clinic, 27 Main St, Hantsport NS B0P 1P0; Cebu (Philippines)'89; CCFP; Staff, Western Memorial Regional Hospital; (902)684-3325; Fax. (902)684-0182.

CANFIELD, Joyce; MUHC-Montreal Children's Hosp, D567-2300 rue Tupper, Montreal QC H3H 1P3; Dal'66; FRCPC; Psy (P.Q.) (Child Psychiatry). Staff, McGill University Health Centre - Montreal Children's Hospital; (514)412-4449; Fax. (514)412-4346.

CANGE, Sylvie; 324 boul Notre-Dame-des-Champs, Repentigny QC J6A 3B6; Mon'79; PlasSurg. (450)654-9124

CANHAM, Hal B; Grey Nuns Community Hosp & HC, 1100 Youville Drive West NW, Edmonton AB T6L 5X8; Alb'83; CCFP; CCFP(E.M.); Staff Emerg Phys, Covenant Health - Grey Nuns Community Hospital; (780)735-2180; Fax. (780)735-7498; hal.canham@gov.ab.ca.

CANIL, Christina M B; The Ottawa Hosp-Gen Campus, 501 Smyth Rd, Ottawa ON K1H 8L6; Tor'96; BSc; FRCPC; IntMed; MedOncol. Staff, The Ottawa Hospital - General Campus; (613)737-7700

CANIL, Katherine A; Qikiqtani Gen Hosp, PO Box 1000, Iqaluit NU X0A 0H0; McM'90; BSc; FRCSC; GenSurg. Staff, Baffin Regional Hospital; (867)979-7347; Fax. (867)979-7346; kcanil@gov.nu.ca.

CANISIUS, Elisabeth M; Hamilton HS-McMaster Site, PO Box 2000 Stn Lcd 1 3N10-1200 Main St W, Hamilton ON L8N 3Z5; McM'04; FRCPC; Peds. Staff, Hamilton Health Sciences Centre - McMaster Children's Hospital; (905)521-2100

CANNIFF, Wayne W; 233 Chamberlain St PO Box 713 Stn Main, Pembroke ON K8A 6X9; Ott'71; FRCSC; Ophth (Neuro Ophthalmology). Staff, Pembroke Regional Hospital Inc; (613)735-0503; Fax. (613)735-4227.

CANNING, Aidan W N; 145 Wellington St, Sarnia ON N7T 1G4; National (Ireland)'66; MB ChB; BAO; (519)337-5600; Fax. (519)337-0439.

CANNING, G Anne; Professional Arts Bldg, 525-100 Arden St, Moncton NB E1C 4B7; National (Ireland)'77; MB ChB; BAO; FRCPC; Peds. Staff, Dr Georges-L-Dumont University Hospital Centre; (506)855-7711; Fax. (506)853-8465.

CANNING, K Alexander; Dr K A Canning Inc, 102-3040 Tutt St, Kelowna BC V1Y 2H5; Ott'86; (250)763-7701; Fax. (250)763-7849.

CANNING, Roderick O; Professional Arts Bldg, 521-100 Arden St, Moncton NB E1C 4B7; National (Ireland)'77; MB ChB; BAO; FRCPC; Peds (Neonatology). (506)857-5451; Fax. (506)857-5891.

CANNITELLI, Albert; 10-9591 Weston Rd, Woodbridge ON L4H 3A5; Tor'89; FRCPC; Peds. Assoc Staff, William Osler Health System - Etobicoke General Hospital; Court Staff, Humber River Regional Hospital - Finch Avenue Site; (905)832-8400

CANNON, Crystal E; St Joseph's Hosp, PO Box 3251 Stn P 35 Algoma St N, Thunder Bay ON P7B 5G7; Tor'76; CCFP; Ac Staff, St Joseph's Care Group - St Joseph's Hospital; (807)346-2358

CANNON, John E; St Boniface Gen Hosp, 409 Tache Ave, Winnipeg MB R2H 2A6; Man'79; FRCPC; Anes. Staff, St Boniface General Hospital; Asst Prof, University of Manitoba; (204)237-2580; Fax. (204)231-0425.

CANO, Pablo O; Northeastern On Reg Cancer Ctr, 41 Ramsey Lake Rd, Sudbury ON P3E 5J1; San Marcos (Peru)'72; FRCPC; Rheum (Medical Oncology); IntMed. Staff N E Oncol Program, Health Sciences North-Laurentian Site; Asst Prof, University of Ottawa; Langs: Spanish; French; (705)522-6237 x2305; Fax. (705)523-7329; pcano@hrsrh.on.ca.

CANO, Paul B; Smithville Family Health Ctre, PO Box 218 230 Canboro St, Smithville ON L0R 2A0; McM'88; CCFP; FCFP; Ac Staff, West Lincoln Memorial Hospital; (905)957-3328; Fax. (905)957-2475; pcano@cogeco.ca.

CANT, Jennifer A; Peace Arch Hosp, 15521 Russell Ave, White Rock BC V4B 2R4; Mem'78; FRCPC; Anes. Staff Anes, Peace Arch Hospital; (604)535-4500

CANTAROVICH, Marcelo; MUHC-Royal Victoria Hosp, PR2. 58-687 av des Pins O, Montreal QC H3A 1A1; Buenos Aires (Argentina)'80; CSPQ; FRCPC; Nephrol (Transplantation). Asst Physician, McGill University Health Centre - Royal Victoria Hospital; adj Prof, Universite de Montreal; Langs: English; French; Spanish; (514)843-1708; Fax. (514)843-1689.

CANTARUTTI, Paul G; Medical Arts Bldg, 201-581 Davis Dr, Newmarket ON L3Y 2P6; Tor'87; CCFP; FCFP; Staff Family & CommunMed, Humber River Regional Hospital - Finch Avenue Site; Staff Family & CommunMed, Mackenzie Richmond Hill Hospital; Langs: Italian; (905)853-3103; Fax. (905)853-9136.

CANTIN, Aline; Polyclinique St-Jerome, 304-200 rue Durand, Saint-Jerome QC J7Z 7E2; Laval'77; Urol. (450)436-7173

CANTIN, Andre M; CHUS-Hop Fleurimont, 3001 12e Av N, Sherbrooke QC J1H 5N4; Sher'78; FRCPC; Respir (Pneumology). Staff Pulmonary, Centre Hospitalier Universitaire de Sherbrooke-Hopital Fleurimont; Prof, Universite de Sherbrooke; Langs: Bilingual(French/English); (819)346-1110; Fax. (819)564-5377.

CANTIN, Bernard; Hôpital Laval, 2725 ch Sainte-Foy, Quebec QC G1V 4G5; Laval'95; FRCPC; IntMed; Cardiol. Staff, Hôpital Laval; (418)656-4657; Fax. (418)646-4544.

CANTIN, Caroline; CSSS d'Argenteuil, 145 av de la Providence, Lachute QC J8H 4C7; Sher'10; CCFP; Staff, Centre Hospitalier d'Argenteuil; (450)562-3761

CANTIN, Celine; Centre Med Saint-Raymond, 220 rue Saint-Joseph, Saint-Raymond QC G3L 1J1; Laval'81; (418)337-2214; Fax. (418)337-3749.

CANTIN, Craig P; Prince Albert Med Clinic, 681 15th St W, Prince Albert SK S6V 7H9; Pretoria (South Africa)'98; MB ChB; CCFP; (306)764-1505; Fax. (306)764-7775.

CANTIN, Guy; Ctr Hosp Affilie-Enfant-Jesus, 1401 18e rue, Quebec QC G1J 1Z4; Laval'77; FRCPC; Hem (Hematological Oncology); MedOncol. Staff, Centre Hospitalier Affilié Universitaire de Québec - Hôpital De L'Enfant Jésus; Chef Hematology Serv, Hôpital Laval; Consultant Hem, CSSS de Montmagny-L'Islet; Clin Prof, Université Laval; (418)649-5727

CANTIN, Isabelle; Ctr Hosp Affilie-Enfant-Jesus, 1401 18e rue, Quebec QC G1J 1Z4; Laval'83; CSPQ; Anes. Staff, Centre Hospitalier Affilié Universitaire de Québec - Hôpital De L'Enfant Jésus; (418)649-0252

CANTIN, Jean-Claude; Clinique Ped Laurier, 3-39 rue Laurier E, Victoriaville QC G6P 6P6; Laval'72; FRCPC; Peds. assoc Staff, Hotel-Dieu d'Arthabaska; (819)357-2259; Fax. (819)357-2303.

CANTIN, Jerome; Ctr Hosp du Centre la Mauricie, 50 119e rue, Shawinigan-Sud QC G9P 5K1; Laval'01; FRCSC; ObstGyn. Staff, Centre Hospitalier du Centre la Mauricie; Langs: Spanish; English; (819)536-7500 x2168

CANTIN, Julie; CSSS de Chicoutimi, 123-305 rue Saint-Vallier, Chicoutimi QC G7H 5H6; Mon'97; CCFP; CCFP(E.M.); Staff, Complexe hospitalier de la Sagamie; (418)541-1000

CANTIN, Leo; Ctr Hosp Affilie-Enfant-Jesus, 1401 18e rue, Quebec QC G1J 1Z4; Laval'81; FRCSC; Neursurg (Neuro Oncology). Staff, Centre Hospitalier Affilié Universitaire de Québec - Hôpital De L'Enfant Jésus; (418)649-5734; Fax. (418)649-5915; leo.cantin.cha@ssss.gouv.qc.ca.

CANTIN, Luce; Hôpital Laval, 2725 ch Sainte-Foy, Quebec QC G1V 4G5; Mon'02; FRCPC; DiagRad. Staff, Hôpital Laval; (418)656-8711

CANTIN, Marie-Andree; Hôpital Ste-Justine, 3175 ch Cote-Sainte-Catherine, Montreal QC H3T 1C5; Laval'84; FRCSC; OrthSurg (Pediatric Orthopedics). Ac Staff, Hôpital Ste-Justine; Ac Staff, Shriners Hospitals For Children - Canada; adj Prof, Universite de Montreal; Langs: English; (514)345-4876; Fax. (514)345-4755.

CANTIN, Mireille; CSSS Becancour-Nicolet-Yamaska, 216 rue Principale GD, Fortierville QC G0S 1J0; Mon'95; (819)287-4442; Fax. (819)287-4017.

CANTIN, Real; Clinique Med Ste-Croix, 6350 rue Principale, Sainte-Croix QC G0S 2H0; Laval'72; LMCC; Langs: Bilingual(French/English); (418)926-3260; Fax. (418)926-2014; real.cantin@gmf.gouv.qc.ca.

CANTIN, Rejean; CSSS de Rivière-de-Loup, 75 rue Saint-Henri, Riviere-du-Loup QC G5R 2A4; Laval'74; CSPQ; AnatPath (Cytology). Staff, Centre Hospitalier Regional du Grand-Portage; Clin Teach Staff Med School, Université Laval; Langs: Bilingual(French/English); (418)868-1010 x2435

CANTIN, Simon; 1055 av Du Pont S, Alma QC G8B 2V7; Laval'88; FRCSC; OrthSurg (Hip & Knee Reconstruction). Staff, CSSS de Lac-Saint Jean-Est; (418)662-9472; Fax. (418)662-2660.

CANTIN, Sylvie M D; Lorraine Wing Tower C, 2F-201 Deacon St, Pembroke ON K8A 2J6; Mon'01; BSc; MCFP; CCFP; Langs: Bilingual(English/French); (613)732-3422; Fax. (866)837-8902.

CANTON, Toni J; GF C1-473 Dupont St, Toronto ON M5G 1Y6; San Diego (USA)'09; (416)588-1888

CANTOR, Elliott J F; Royal Health Care Centre, 130 Adelaide St W Box 92, Toronto ON M5H 3P5; Ott'09; CCFP; (416)361-6142; Fax. (416)361-1200.

CANTOR, Kenneth Z; 4677 av Roslyn, Montreal QC H3W 2L3; McG'63; DABIM; FRCPC; IntMed; Cardiol (P.Q.). Langs: Bilingual(English/French); (514)935-1197; Fax. (514)935-1310.

CANTOR, Michael J; John Buhler Research Centre, 804E-715 McDermot Ave, Winnipeg MB R3E 3P4; Man'97; FRCPC; IntMed; Gastroent.

CANTOR, Warren; PACE-Partners Advance Evaluati, 602-581 Davis Dr, Newmarket ON L3Y 2R2; Wes'91; ABC; FRFPS; ABIM; FRCPC; IntMed (Interventional Cardiology); Cardiol. Staff, Southlake Regional Health Centre; (905)898-5800; Fax. (905)898-5808.

CANTWELL, Lorraine M; Shoppers Drug Mart Bldg, 250 LeMarchant Rd, St. John's NL A1E 1P7; Ott'85; BSc(Hons).

CANTY, Andrea A; 707 Millidge Ave, Saint John NB E2K 2N7; Dal'90; BSc(Hon); MSc; CCFP; FCFP; Med Staff, Saint John Regional Hospital; Court Staff, St Joseph's Hospital; Lecturer, Dalhousie University; Assoc Prof, Memorial University Of Newfoundland; (506)696-0567; Fax. (506)696-0787; dr.a.canty@hb.aibn.com.

CANUEL, Jean-Pierre; Le Centre Med St-Jean, 202-1018 rue de la Prairie O, St-J-Chrysostome QC G6Z 0A7; Sher'82; Staff, Centre Hospitalier Affilié Universitaire de Québec - Hôpital du St-Sacrement; (418)839-4433; Fax. (418)839-3574.

CANZANI, Genevieve; Ctr Hosp de Verdun, 4000 boul Lasalle, Verdun QC H4G 2A3; Mon'92; FRCPC; IntMed. Staff, Centre Hospitalier de Verdun; (514)765-8121

CAO, Jeffrey Q; BC Cancer Agency-Vancouver CC, 600 10th Ave W, Vancouver BC V5Z 4E6; Alb'05; FRCPC; RadOncol. Staff, BC Cancer Agency Vancouver Centre; (604)877-6000

CAO, Y Kathy; 407-2115 Finch Ave W, North York ON M3N 2V6; Tor'06; FRCSC; Ophth. (416)748-2020

CAOUETTE, Benoit; Clin Med Plateau Marquette, 731 rue Galt O, Sherbrooke QC J1H 1Z1; Mon'96; Staff, Centre Hospitalier Universitaire de Sherbrooke-Hopital Fleurimont; (819)346-1110

CAOUETTE, Christine; CHUQ-Hotel-Dieu de Quebec, 11 Cote Du Palais, Quebec QC G1R 2J6; Laval'95; Staff, Centre Hospitalier Universitaire de Québec (CHUQ) - Siege Social; (418)525-4444 x15808; Fax. (418)691-5019; christine.caouette@chuq.qc.ca.

CAOUETTE, Georges; CHUQ-Hop Laval, 2705 boul Laurier, Quebec QC G1V 4G2; Laval'90; FRCPC; Peds (General Pediatrics). Staff, Centre Hospitalier Universitaire de Quebec-CHUL; (418)525-4444

CAOUETTE, Helene; CSSS de Montmagny-L'Islet, 350 boul Tache O RR 1, Montmagny QC G5V 3R8; Laval'81; Otol. Staff, CSSS de Montmagny-L'Islet; (418)248-0630

CAOUETTE, Marie-Josee; Ctr Hosp Laurentien, 234 rue Saint-Vincent, Ste-Agathe-Des-Mts QC J8C 2B8; Mon'95; CCFP; Staff, Centre Hospitalier Laurentien; (819)324-4000; Fax. (819)324-4017.

CAOUETTE, Pascale; Ctr Hosp Affilie-Enfant-Jesus, 1401 18e rue, Quebec QC G1J 1Z4; Laval'96; FRCPC; IntMed; Gastroent. Gastroent/Int'l Med, Centre Hospitalier Affilié Universitaire de Québec - Hôpital De L'Enfant Jésus; (418)649-0252; Fax. (418)649-5570.

CAOUETTE, Richard; CSSSG-Hop de Gatineau, CP 2000 Succ Bureau-Chef 909 boul de la Verendrye O, Gatineau QC J8P 7H2; Laval'00; FRCSC; Otol. Staff, Hôpital de Gatineau; (819)561-8100

CAOUETTE-LABERGE, Louise; Hôpital Ste-Justine, 7907-3175 ch Cote-Sainte-Cathe, Montreal QC H3T 1C5; Laval'77; FRCSC; PlasSurg (Pediatric General Surgery). Staff, Hôpital Ste-Justine; Prof, Universite de Montreal; Langs: English; (514)345-4771; Fax. (514)345-4964; louise_laberge@ssss.gouv.qc.ca.

CAPE, Steven D; St Mary's Hosp Centre, 3830 av Lacombe, Montreal QC H3T 1M5; McG'91; assoc Membre Family Med & Gen Med, St Mary's Hospital Centre; Staff Fam Med, McGill University Health Centre - Montreal Chest Institute; Aj Prof Family Med, McGill University; (514)345-3511

CAPELLE, Lisa R; Cross Cancer Institute, 11560 University Ave NW, Edmonton AB T6G 1Z2; Auckland (New Zealand)'99; FRCPC; RadOncol. Staff, Cross Cancer Institute; (780)432-8771

CAPELLO, Timothy A; Carling-Broadview Med Bldg, B4-770 Broadview Ave, Ottawa ON K2A 3Z3; Tor'88; (613)725-6260; Fax. (613)725-6243.

CAPELLO-DESJARDINS, Nancy; Queensway-Carleton Hosp, 3045 Baseline Rd, Nepean ON K2H 8P4; Ott'94; CCFP; CCFP(E.M.); Staff EmergMed, Queensway Carleton Hospital; Staff EmergMed, Carleton Place & District Memorial Hospital; (613)721-4710

CAPES, Sarah E; 308-1990 Fort St, Victoria BC V8R 6V4; Ott'91; MSc; ABIM; FRCPC; IntMed (Adult Endocrinology); Endocrin&Metab. Staff, Victoria General Hospital; Staff, Royal Jubilee Hospital; (250)595-6210; Fax. (250)595-6240.

CAPISONDA, S Rhona B; Chinook Paediatric Clinic, 951 19 St S, Lethbridge AB T1J 3H5; Manila Central (Philippines)'89; Staff Peds, Chinook Regional Hospital; Langs: Tagalog; (403)320-7825; Fax. (403)320-8613; rhona_capisonda@yahoo.com.

CAPLAN, Aubrey H; Kelvin Prof Centre, 139 Carmen Ave, Winnipeg MB R2L 0E5; Man'62; FRCPC; Peds (Behavioural Medicine). Staff, St Boniface General Hospital; Staff Children's Hosp, Health Sciences Centre; Asst Prof Peds, University of Manitoba; (204)661-3885; Fax. (204)663-2869; caplan@cc.umanitoba.ca.

CAPLAN, David J; Rexdale Med Centre, 2-123 Rexdale Blvd, Etobicoke ON M9W 1P1; Tor'92; CCFP; FCFP; Ac Staff, William Osler Health System - Etobicoke General Hospital; (416)743-5853; Fax. (416)743-1358.

CAPLAN, Deborah; The Brandon Clinic, 620 Dennis St, Brandon MB R7A 5E7; Sask'90; CCFP; FCFP; Fam Med, Brandon Regional Health Centre; (204)728-4440; Fax. (204)726-1765.

CAPLAN, Jason A; 110-164 Queen St E, Brampton ON L6V 1B4; Cal'99; CCFP; Ad Staff Privil, Sunnybrook Health Sciences Centre; (905)456-6816; Fax. (905)456-0490.

CAPLAN, Joseph; 506-1110 Finch Ave W, North York ON M3J 2T2; Glasgow (Scotland)'57; DPsy; FRCPC; Psy. Consultant Psy, North York General Hospital - Branson Division; Clin Lecturer, University of Toronto; (416)663-3829

CAPLAN, Shari G; 1940 Avenue Rd, North York ON M5M 4A1; Tor'90; CCFP; FCFP; Ac Staff, Women's College Hospital; Clin Teacher, University of Toronto; (416)385-9277; Fax. (416)385-9266.

CAPLAN, Stephen N; SMBD Jewish Gen Hosp, 3755 ch Cote-Sainte-Catherine, Montreal QC H3T 1E2; McG'71; FRCP; FRCPC; Hem (Blood Transfusion). Dir Div of Hematol, Sir Mortimer B Davis Jewish General; Assoc Prof Med & Oncology, McGill University; (514)340-8207; Fax. (514)340-8733; scaplan@lab.jgh.mcgill.ca.

CAPOLICCHIO, Gianpaolo; MUHC-Montreal Children's Hosp, C527-2300 rue Tupper, Montreal QC H3H 1P3; McG'92; FRCSC; Urol (Laparoscopy). Staff, McGill University Health Centre - Montreal Children's Hospital; Staff, Shriners Hospitals For Children - Canada; Aj Prof Surg, McGill University; (514)412-4400 x22875; Fax. (514)412-4384.

CAPPELLANI, Ronald B; Associated Anaes of Winnipeg, 849 Notre Dame Ave, Winnipeg MB R3E 0M4; Ott'83; FRCPC; Anes;CCFP; Staff Anes, Health Sciences Centre; Prof Anes, University of Manitoba; (204)775-6967; Fax. (204)775-6967.

CAPPELLO, Emma M; Hamilton HS-General Site, 237 Barton St E, Hamilton ON L8L 2X2; McM'06; FRCPC; Anes. Staff, Hamilton Health Sciences Centre - Hamilton General Hospital; (905)521-2100 x46698

CAPPELLO, Marie L; Fort William Clinic, 117 McKellar St S, Thunder Bay ON P7E 1H5; Tor'04; CCFP; (807)626-1234; Fax. (807)623-8832.

CAPPON, Ian D; Gateway Med Clinic, 101-2051 McCallum Rd, Abbotsford BC V2S 3N5; Dal'83; MSc; PhD; Staff, Abbotsford Regional Hospital & Cancer Centre; (604)859-9084; Fax. (604)859-7494; idcappon@telus.net.

CAPPON, Paul S; 278 O'Connor St, Ottawa ON K2P 1V4; McM'80; CSPQ; BA; CCFP; CommunMed (P.Q.) (Psychotherapy). Langs: English; French; Italian; German; (613)233-1565; Fax. (613)233-1851.

CAPRICCI, Arlene P; The Spence Clinic, 500-1265 Arthur St E, Thunder Bay ON P7E 5H7; McG'79; Court Staff, Thunder Bay Regional Health Sciences Centre; (807)626-1114; Fax. (807)626-1121.

CAPSTICK, James; Nanaimo Reg Gen Hosp, 1200 Dufferin Cres, Nanaimo BC V9S 2B7; Cal'02; FRCPC; Anes. Staff, Nanaimo Regional General Hospital; (250)755-7605

CAPSTICK, Valerie A; Cross Cancer Institute, 11560 University Ave NW, Edmonton AB T6G 1Z2; Alb'83; BMedSci; FSOGC; FRCSC; ObstGyn (Gynecologic Oncology). Ac Staff, Royal Alexandra Hospital; Ac Staff Gyn, Cross Cancer Institute; Assoc Prof, University of Alberta; (780)432-8560; Fax. (780)432-8333.

CAPUSAN, Gheorghe V; CSSS du Haut Saint-Maurice, 885 boul Ducharme, La Tuque QC G9X 3C1; Craiova (Romania)'84; Staff, Centre Hospitalier Saint-Joseph de la Turque; Langs: Romanian; (819)523-4581; Fax. (819)523-5019.

CAPUSTEN, Bernice M; Central Alberta Med Imaging, 4312 54 Ave, Red Deer AB T4N 4M1; Sask'76; FRCPC; DiagRad. Chief, Central Zone David Thompson Health Region; Asst Prof Rad, University of Calgary; Langs: English; French; (403)755-1056; Fax. (403)342-1088; capusten@telusplanet.net.

CARABOTT, Paul; Bramalea Med Group, 500-18 Kensington Rd, Brampton ON L6T 4S5; (Malta)'69; (905)791-7575

CARAISCOS, Valerie B; Univ Hlth Network-Toronto Gen, 9N 927-200 Elizabeth St, Toronto ON M5G 2C4; Tor'08; CCFP; (416)340-4800; Fax. (416)340-4823.

CARAVAGGIO, Robert J; 305-474 College St, Toronto ON M6G 1A4; Tor'91; Staff, Toronto General Hospital - UHN; Lecturer, University of Toronto; (416)323-1996; Fax. (416)323-1665.

CARAVAN, Christine L; Waterford Hosp, PO Box 4810 306 Waterford Bridge Rd, St. John's NL A1E 4J8; Mem'91; FRCPC; Psy. Staff, Waterford Hospital; (709)777-3311; Fax. (709)777-3011.

CARBERY, Michael; Ctr Hosp du Centre la Mauricie, 50 119e rue, Shawinigan QC G9P 5K7; Mon'08; Staff, Centre Hospitalier du Centre la Mauricie; (819)536-7500

CARBIN, Robert J; 202-2200 Fairview St, Burlington ON L7R 4H9; Tor'62; OrthSurg. Staff, Joseph Brant Memorial Hospital; (905)333-3668; Fax. (905)333-3255.

CARBONNEAU, Annie; SMBD Jewish Gen Hosp, 3755 ch Cote-Sainte-Catherine, Montreal QC H3T 1E2; Laval'03; FRCPC; RadOncol (Lung Cancer). Staff, Sir Mortimer B Davis Jewish General; Langs: Bilingual(French/English); (514)340-8222; Fax. (514)340-7510.

CARBONNEAU, Diane; Clinique Med Saint-Louis, 220-3165 ch Saint-Louis, Quebec QC G1W 4R4; Laval'89; Staff, Institut Universitaire Sante; (418)653-1970

CARBONNEAU, Louise; Centre Hosp Honore-Mercier, 2750 boul Laframboise, Saint-Hyacinthe QC J2S 4Y8; Laval'09; CCFP; Staff, Centre Hospitalier Honore-Mercier; (450)771-3333

CARBONNEAU, Marjorie; CHUS-Hop Hotel-Dieu, 580 rue Bowen S, Sherbrooke QC J1G 2E8; Laval'06; FRCSC; Ophth. Staff, Centre Hospitalier Universitaire de Sherbrooke-Hôpital Hôtel-Dieu; (819)346-1110 x28008

CARBONNEAU GIROUARD, Maxime; CSSS du Sud de Lanaudière, 911 montee des Pionniers, Terrebonne QC J6V 2H2; Mon'08; CCFP; Staff, Centre Hospitalier Pierre le Gardeur; (450)654-7525

CARBYN, Kevin M; 1040-5991 Spring Garden Rd, Halifax NS B3H 1Y6; Dal'92; (902)444-8253; Fax. (902)444-8251.

CARCAO, Manuel; The Hosp for Sick Children, 555 University Ave, Toronto ON M5G 1X8; Tor'90; FRCPC; Peds (Pediatric Hematology Oncology); Hem. Staff Physician, The Hospital For Sick Children; Asst Prof, University of Toronto; Langs: Portuguese; (416)813-5367; Fax. (416)813-5327.

CARCELLER, Ana M; Hôpital Ste-Justine, 3175 ch Cote-Sainte-Catherine, Montreal QC H3T 1C5; Barcelona (Spain)'78; PhD; MS; AB; FRCPC; Peds. Staff, Hôpital Ste-Justine; (514)345-4931; Fax. (514)345-4822; ana_carceller@ssss.gouv.qc.ca.

CARD, Annika M; Plastic Surgery Associates, 602-750 Spadina Cres E, Saskatoon SK S7K 3H3; Sask'05; FRCSC; PlasSurg. (306)653-7766; Fax. (306)653-7768.

CARD, Bradley D; Star FHT-Tavistock Comm Hlth I, PO Box 310 80 Maria St, Tavistock ON N0B 2R0; Wes'80; BSc; CCFP; FCFP; Ac Physician, Stratford General Hospital - Huron Perth Healthcare Alliance; Clin Teacher Family Med, University of Western Ontario; (519)655-2322; Fax. (519)655-3073.

CARD, Cynthia M; Tom Baker Cancer Centre, 1331 29 St NW, Calgary AB T2N 4N2; Mem'97; MSc(MedEduc); FRCPC; IntMed (Thoracic Cancer); MedOncol. Staff, Tom Baker Cancer Centre; Clinical Asst Prof, University of Calgary; (403)521-3688; Fax. (403)283-1651.

CARD, James; Mackenzie Health Centre, PO Box 2410, Mackenzie BC V0J 2C0; UBC'08; CCFP; Staff, University Hospital of Northern British Columbia; (250)997-4342; Fax. (250)997-3940.

CARD, Robert T; 103 Hospital Dr, Saskatoon SK S7N 0W8; Qns'64; MSc; FRCPC; IntMed; Hem. Staff, Royal University Hospital; (306)655-0655; Fax. (306)655-6426.

CARD, Sharon E; Royal University Hosp, 103 Hospital Dr, Saskatoon SK S7N 0W8; Qns'90; FRCPC; IntMed. Staff, Royal University Hospital; (306)966-7961; Fax. (306)966-1943.

CARDAMORE, Robin; Montfort Hosp, 713 Montreal Rd, Ottawa ON K1K 0T2; Ott'07; FRCPC; EmergMed. Staff, Montfort Hospital; (613)746-4621

CARDELLA, Carl J; 11C 1258-585 University Ave, Toronto ON M5G 2N2; Tor'67; BSc; FRCPC; IntMed (Nephrology). Prof Med, University of Toronto; (416)340-4480; Fax. (416)340-5244.

CARDELLA, Jonathan A; 408-1017 Wilson Ave, North York ON M3K 1Z1; Tor'04; FRCSC; GenSurg; VascSurg.

CARDEW, Savannah S C R; Women's College Hosp, 690-76 Grenville St, Toronto ON M5S 1B2; UBC'04; FRCPC; IntMed. Staff, Women's College Hospital; (416)323-6400

CARDIN, Gabrielle; CLSC Jean-Olivier-Chenier, 29 ch d'Oka, Saint-Eustache QC J7R 1K6; Sher'10; CCFP; (450)934-3145

CARDIN, Louise; Clinique Med Ste-Therese, 101-233 rue Turgeon, Sainte-Therese QC J7E 3J8; Mon'74; ac Staff, Hôpital du Sacre-Coeur de Montréal; (450)430-1030

CARDIN, Michel; Polyclinique St-Eustache, 75 rue Grignon, Saint-Eustache QC J7P 4J2; Mon'74.

CARDIN, Michel; Base Militaire de Longue Point, 6560 rue Hochelaga, Montreal QC H1N 1X9; Mon'77; Staff, National Defence Montreal Detachment Services Group; (514)252-2777 x4926

CARDIN-LANGLOIS, Etienne; CHUS-Hop Hotel-Dieu, 580 rue Bowen S, Sherbrooke QC J1G 2E8; Sher'07; FRCSC; PlasSurg. Staff, Centre Hospitalier Universitaire de Sherbrooke-Hôpital Hôtel-Dieu; (819)346-1110

CARDIN ST-ANTOINE, Annie; Centre Med Vaudreuil-Dorion, 600 boul Harwood, Vaudreuil-Dorion QC J7V 6A3; Mon'04; CCFP; (450)455-9301 x258

CARDINAL, Alain; Clinique Med Le Mesnil, 300-1300 boul LeBourgneuf, Quebec QC G2K 2N1; Laval'89; (418)624-1800

CARDINAL, Andree; Ctr Hosp Affilie-Enfant-Jesus, 1401 18e rue, Quebec QC G1J 1Z4; Laval'89; FRCPC; Psy. Staff, Centre Hospitalier Affilié Universitaire de Québec - Hôpital De L'Enfant Jésus; (418)649-5769; Fax. (418)649-5934.

CARDINAL, Bernard; GMF Concorde, 300 boul de la Concorde E, Laval QC H7G 2E6; Mon'72; (450)667-5310; Fax. (450)667-5248.

CARDINAL, Bernard; CSSS de Quebec Nord, 3666 ch Royal, Quebec QC G1E 1X5; Laval'84; (418)663-3099; Fax. (418)663-2939; bernard.cardinal@ssss.gouv.qc.ca.

CARDINAL, Celine; Clinique Med Ahuntsic, 241 rue Fleury O, Montreal QC H3L 1V2; Sher'87; LMCC; (514)382-0062

CARDINAL, Francine; 1427 rue Fleury E, Montreal QC H2C 1R9; Mon'91; FRCPC; Derm. (514)728-3376; Fax. (514)728-9046.

CARDINAL, Godefroy A; CSSS des Aurores Boreales, CP 6000 Succ Bureau-Chef 679 2e rue E, La Sarre QC J9Z 2X7; McG'86; FRCPC; Peds. Staff, Centre Hospitalier La Sarre; (819)333-2311

CARDINAL, Heloise; CHUM-Hop Notre-Dame, 1560 rue Sherbrooke E, Montreal QC H2L 4M1; Sher'95; FRCPC; IntMed; Nephrol. Staff, Centre Hospitalier l'Université de Montréal (CHUM) - Hôpital Notre-Dame; Staff, Centre Hospitalier l'Université De Montréal (CHUM) - Hôpital Saint-luc; Langs: Italian; English; (514)890-8000

CARDINAL, Katharina B; 6426 28 Ave NW, Edmonton AB T6L 6N3; Cal'98; BSc; CCFP; Staff, Covenant Health - Grey Nuns Community Hospital; (780)462-3491; Fax. (780)461-2650.

CARDINAL, Lise; Centre de Sante Publique, 2400 av d'Estimauville, Quebec QC G1E 7G9; Laval'82; FRCPC; CommunMed. Ac Staff, Centre Hospitalier Affilié Universitaire de Québec - Hôpital De L'Enfant Jésus; (418)666-7000 x476; Fax. (418)666-2776.

CARDINAL, Michel; Clinique Med St-Alexandre, 200-2310 rue Saint-Louis, Gatineau QC J8T 5L7; Ott'84; Staff, Hôpital de Gatineau; (819)243-4500; Fax. (819)243-1369; mcardinal@medecinefamiliale.com.

CARDINAL, Nadine; CSSS Jeanne-Mance, 100-15 av du Mont-Royal O, Montreal QC H2T 2R9; Mon'05; CCFP; (514)286-9657

CARDINAL, Patrice-Etienne; Radiologie Laennec, 104-1100 av Beaumont, Mont-Royal QC H3P 3H5; Mon'87; FRCPC; DiagRad. (514)738-6866

CARDINAL, Pierre; The Ottawa Hosp-Gen Campus, W0528-501 Smyth Rd, Ottawa ON K1H 8L6; Ott'82; FRCPC; IntMed; Respir. Staff, The Ottawa Hospital - General Campus; Asst Prof, University of Ottawa; (613)737-7777

CARDINAL, Stephanie; GMF Concorde, 300 boul de la Concorde E, Laval QC H7G 2E6; Mon'02; (450)667-5310

CARDINAL, Valerie; Ctr Hosp du Centre la Mauricie, 50 119e rue, Shawinigan-Sud QC G9P 5K1; Sher'00; CSPQ; FRCPC; Anes. Staff, Centre Hospitalier du Centre la Mauricie; (819)536-7500

CARDISH, Robert J; 33 Russell St, Toronto ON M5S 2S1; Tor'73; FRCPC; Psy. Staff, Centre for Addiction & Mental Health (CAMH) - Russell Street Site; Asst Prof, University of Toronto; (416)595-6878

CARDONA, Caroline A; MUHC-Royal Victoria Hosp, 687 av des Pins O, Montreal QC H3A 1A1; McG'04; CCFP; Staff, McGill University Health Centre - Royal Victoria Hospital; (514)934-1934 x34277

CARDOSO, Manuel R; Clinique Med Luso Mtl Ltee, 1 av Du Mont-Royal E, Montreal QC H2T 1N4; Mon'84; MSc; ABIM; FRCPC; IntMed (Hypertension). Langs: Portuguese; French; Spanish; (514)849-2391; Fax. (514)849-2394.

CARDOSO, Marguerite; Clinique Domus Medica, 303-5601 rue Belanger E, Montreal QC H1T 1G3; Mon'81; assoc Staff, Hôpital Santa Cabrini Ospedale; (514)256-5011; Fax. (514)253-1691.

CARDOSO, Reynaldo; Regina Qu'Appelle HR-Regina, MOW-1440 14th Ave, Regina SK S4P 0W5; (Mexico)'71; DAB; FRCSC; ObstGyn (Maternal Fetal Medicine). Ac Staff Maternal-Fetal Med & Gyn, Regina General Hospital; Clin Prof, University of Saskatchewan; Langs: Spanish; (306)586-5800; Fax. (306)586-2990; dr_cardoso@sasktel.net.

CARDOSO, Tatiana; 1530 7th Ave W, Vancouver BC V6J 1S3; (Other Foreign)'00; CCFP; (604)739-5613; Fax. (604)738-2143.

CARDWELL, Starr E M; 10-8180 MacLeod Trail SW, Calgary AB T2H 2B8; Sask'89; FRCPC; Peds. Clinical Asst Prof Peds, University of Calgary; (403)252-6651

CARDY, Vanessa L; Wakefield Family Med Centre, 777 ch Riverside RR 2, Wakefield QC J0X 3G0; Dal'04; CCFP; Staff, Centre Hospitalier Gatineau Mémorial; (819)459-2363

CAREAU, Dominique; Clinique Med du Vieux Fort, 7777 boul de la Rive-Sud, Levis QC G6V 6Z1; Laval'83; (418)835-5612; Fax. (418)835-3927.

CARERE, Ronald; Burrard Bldg, 479-1081 Burrard St, Vancouver BC V6Z 1Y6; Ott'84; FACC; FRCPC; IntMed (Coronary Care); Cardiol. Assoc Staff, Vancouver General Hospital - Centennial Pavillion; Physician Program Dir, Providence Health Care - St Paul's Hospital; Reg Dir Cardiac Sciences Prog, Vancouver Coastal Health; Clin Assoc Prof Med, University of British Columbia; (604)806-9922

CARETTE, Marie-Eve; Les Gynecologues Ass de Laval, 1299 boul de la Concorde O, Laval QC H7N 5T4; Mon'02; FRCSC; ObstGyn. Staff ObstGyn, Hopital de la Cite de la santé; Langs: Bilingual(French/English); (450)668-3250; mecarette@yahoo.ca.

CARETTE, Simon; Univ Hlth Network-Toronto Western Hosp, EW1 422-399 Bathurst St, Toronto ON M5T 2S8; Laval'75; FRCPC; IntMed; Rheum. Ac Staff, Toronto Western Hospital - University Health Network; Ac Staff, Mount Sinai Hospital; Prof Med, University of Toronto; Langs: Bilingual(French/English); (416)603-6751; Fax. (416)603-4348; simon.carette@uhn.on.ca.

CAREW, Daniel A; Klondyke Med Clinic, 1-3089 3rd Ave, Whitehorse YT Y1A 5B3; Sask'91; CCFP; FCFP; Staff, Klondyke Medical Clinic; (867)668-4060; Fax. (867)668-4067.

CAREW, Heidi E; Anderson Avenue Family Pract, 25 Anderson Ave, St. John's NL A1B 3E4; Mem'07; CCFP; (709)726-5065; Fax. (709)579-0347.

CAREW, Marjorie C; 152-759 Hyde Park Rd, London ON N6H 3S2; Mem'79; FRCPC; Psy. (519)663-0985

CAREW, Maureen T; Canadian Forces Supp Unit HCC, 1745 Alta Vista Dr, Ottawa ON K1A 0K6; Mem'88; FRCPC; CommunMed. Community Medicine, Canadian Forces Health Services Centre; (613)945-6600; Fax. (613)945-6823.

CAREY, Aidan G; Lockview Med Clinic, 203-159 Cobequid Rd, Lower Sackville NS B4C 2N1; Dublin (Ireland)'81; MB ChB; CCFP; (902)865-7545; Fax. (902)865-7546.

CAREY, Colleen M; Foothills Med Centre, C231-1403 29 St NW, Calgary AB T2N 2T9; UBC'04; CCFP; CCFP(E.M.); Staff, Foothills Medical Centre; (403)944-8430

CAREY, Mark S; 6F-2775 Laurel St, Vancouver BC V5Z 1M9; Wes'81; FRCSC; ObstGyn (Gynecologic Oncology). (604)875-4268

CAREY, Paul D; 1440 14 Ave, Vernon BC V1B 2T1; Stellenbosch (South Africa)'95; MB ChB; (250)549-5737

CAREY, Timothy; London HSC-Victoria Hosp, B1 184-800 Commissiners Rd E, London ON N6A 5W9; Ott'83; FRCSC; OrthSurg (Pediatric Orthopedic Surgery). Ac Staff, London Health Sciences Centre - Victoria Campus; Assoc Prof Surg, University of Western Ontario; (519)685-8021; Fax. (519)685-8038.

CAREY, Wayne D; 100-4 car Westmount, Westmount QC H3Z 2S6; Alb'76; AB; FRCPC; Derm (Cosmetic Surgery). Chief Derm, McGill University Health Centre - Royal Victoria Hospital; adj Prof, McGill University; (514)394-1394 x34648; Fax. (514)788-3202.

CARFAGNINI, Gregory P; Thunder Bay Reg HSC-T-Bay, 980 Oliver Rd, Thunder Bay ON P7B 6V4; Man'06; CCFP; CCFP(E.M.); Staff, Thunder Bay Regional Health Sciences Centre; (807)684-6100

CARGILL, Darren C; Hospice of Windsor & Essex Cty, 6038 Empress St, Windsor ON N8T 1B5; Wes'03; BSc; CCFP; Consultant Palliative Care, Windsor Regional Hospital - Metropolitan Site; (519)974-7100; dcargill@hospicewindsoressex.com.

CARGILL, Yvonne M; Harmony Med Centre, 101-152 Cleopatra Dr, Nepean ON K2G 5X2; Sask'85; FRCSC; ObstGyn (Ultrasound). Ac Staff, The Ottawa Hospital - Civic Campus; Asst Prof, University of Ottawa; (613)728-6212

CARICEVIC, Bogdan; Polyclinique Masson, 200-3425 rue Masson, Montreal QC H1X 1R6; McG'78; BSc; MDCM; (514)376-9961

CARIGNAN, Alex; CHUS-Hop Fleurimont, 3001 12e av N, Sherbrooke QC J1H 5N4; Mon'03; FRCPC; MedMicrobiol. Staff, Centre Hospitalier Universitaire de Sherbrooke-Hopital Fleurimont; (819)346-1110 x16455

CARIGNAN, Benoit; Ctre d'Hebergement St-Joseph, 611 boul Queen-Victoria, Sherbrooke QC J1H 3R6; Sher'86; Staff, Centre Hospitalier et CLSC de Memphremagog; Médecin, Centre d'Hebergement St-Joseph; Langs: Bilingual(French/English); (819)780-2222; Fax. (819)564-2006.

CARIGNAN, Jacqueline; Clinique d'Ophth Lebourneuf, 200-777 boul Lebourgneuf, Quebec QC G2J 1C3; Laval'72; Ophth. Staff, Centre Hospitalier Chauveau; Langs: English; (418)628-1417; Fax. (418)623-4517.

CARIGNAN, Lucie; UMF Maizerets, 2480 ch de la Canardiere, Quebec QC G1J 2G1; Laval'87; Staff, Hôpital Laval; (418)661-1413

CARIGNAN, Marisol; CSSS de la Region de Thetford, 1717 rue Notre-Dame E, Thetford Mines QC G6G 2V4; Sher'01; FRCSC; Otol. Staff, Hopital du CSS de la Region de Thetford; (418)338-7777 x4093

CARIGNAN, Pierre; CSSS de la Baie-des-Chaleurs, RR 2 419 boul Perron, Maria QC G0C 1Y0; Laval'91; IntMed (P.Q.). Staff, CSSS de la Baie-des-Chaleurs; (418)759-3443 x2421

CARIGNAN, Renee; 209-12245 rue Grenet, Montreal QC H4J 2J6; Mon'88; AB; FRCSC; Ophth (Cataract). Staff, Hôpital du Sacre-Coeur de Montréal; Staff Ophth, Hopital Maisonneuve-Rosemont; Universite de Montreal; (514)332-4009

CARIGNAN, Sebastien; Clinique ALHP, 114-475 boul Talbot, Chicoutimi QC G7H 4A3; Mon'01; FRCSC; GenSurg (Endoscopic Surgery). Staff, Complexe hospitalier de la Sagamie; Langs: Bilingual(French/English); (418)549-4598; Fax. (418)549-9948.

CARIGNAN, Stephane; Hop Maisonneuve-Rosemont, 5415 boul de l'Assomption, Montreal QC H1T 2M4; Mon'89; FRCPC; DiagRad. Staff, Hopital Maisonneuve-Rosemont; (514)252-3400 x4234

CARIGNAN, Suzanne; CSSS de Rivière-de-Loup, 75 rue Saint-Henri, Riviere-Du-Loup QC G5R 2A4; Laval'86; FRCPC; IntMed. Staff, Centre Hospitalier Regional du Grand-Portage; (418)862-8261; Fax. (418)868-1035.

CARKNER, Robert M; 101-1032 Austin Ave, Coquitlam BC V3K 3P3; UBC'89; Staff, Royal Columbian Hospital; Staff, Eagle Ridge Hospital & Health Care Centre; (604)939-2441; Fax. (604)939-2420.

CARLE, Henri L; Coronation Plaza, 102E-14310 111 Ave NW, Edmonton AB T5M 3Z7; Alb'78; FRCPC; Anes. (780)455-2372; Fax. (780)452-7157.

CARLE, Jean; CSSS de Montmagny-L'Islet, 350 boul Tache O RR 1, Montmagny QC G5V 3R8; Laval'84; Staff, CSSS de Montmagny-L'Islet; (418)248-0630

CARLE, Michelle V; Coronation Plaza, 102-14310 111 Ave NW, Edmonton AB T5M 3Z7; Alb'06; FRCSC; Ophth.

CARLE, Roger; 555 rue Murray, Sherbrooke QC J1G 2K8; Laval'64; Psy. Psychiatre, Centre Hospitalier Universitaire de Sherbrooke-Hôpital Hôtel-Dieu; assoc Prof Psy, Universite de Sherbrooke; (819)822-6760; Fax. (819)822-6768.

CARLEN, Peter L; Univ Hlth Network-Toronto Western Hosp, 5W 442-399 Bathurst St, Toronto ON M5T 2S8; Tor'67; FRCP; FRCPC; Neur (Epilepsy). Neurologist, Toronto Western Hospital - University Health Network; Sr Scientist, Toronto Western Research Institute; Prof Med Neurol & Physiol, University of Toronto; Langs: French; Hebrew; (416)603-5017; Fax. (416)603-5768; carlen@uhnres.utoronto.ca.

CARLETON, Susan A; 127 Park St, Waterloo ON N2L 1Y4; Ott'71; FRCPC; Neur (Electromyography). (519)743-1451; Fax. (519)743-8220.

CARLI, Francesco; MUHC-Montreal Gen Hosp, 1650 av Cedar, Montreal QC H3G 1A4; Turin (Italy)'73; FRCPC; Anes. Staff, McGill University Health Centre - Montreal General Campus; (514)934-1934 x43261

CARLI BUTTENSCHOEN, Brigitte D; Extended Med Treatment Bldg, 1090 Youville Drive West NW, Edmonton AB T6L 0A3; (780)735-7834

CARLIER, Maureen T; Montfort Hosp, 713 Montreal Rd, Ottawa ON K1K 0T2; Andhra (India)'61; FRCPC; AnatPath. Chief Gen Path & Labs, Montfort Hospital; Langs: English; French; (613)746-4621 x4401; Fax. (613)748-4921.

CARLIER, Michelle A; Impact, 304-489 College St, Toronto ON M6G 1A5; Wes'97; FRCPC; Psy. Staff, Centre for Addiction & Mental Health (CAMH) - Queen Site; (416)925-3350

CARLILE, John B; Limestone City Sleep Laborator, 1-235 Brock St, Kingston ON K7L 1S3; Witwatersrand (South Africa)'72; MB BCh; PhD; FRCPC; Psy (Sleep Medicine). (613)547-9172; Fax. (613)547-9910; jbcarlile@gmail.com.

CARLIN, Robert C; CLSC Metro, 300-1801 boul De Maisonneuve O, Montreal QC H3H 1J9; McG'95; CCFP; FCFP; Physician, Queen Elizabeth Urgent Care Clinic; Staff Public Health, Cree Board of Health and Social Services Montreal; Prof Faculty Family Med, McGill University; Langs: English; French; (514)934-0354; Fax. (514)934-6155.

CARLING-CHAMBERS, Lucille B; 2104 Old Lakeshore Rd, Burlington ON L7R 1A3; Qns'79; BSc; FRCPC; IntMed; Cardiol. Staff Physician CCU/ICU & Active Med-Cardiol, Joseph Brant Memorial Hospital; Langs: Bilingual(English/French); (905)632-3531; Fax. (905)632-1126.

CARLINI, Ryan J; 113-2462 Howard Ave, Windsor ON N8X 3V6; Saba (Netherlands Antilles)'10; CCFP; (519)946-0160

CARLISLE, Corine E; Addiction & Mental Hlth-ARF, 3109-33 Russell St, Toronto ON M5S 2S1; UBC'97; FRCPC; Psy. Fellow, The Hospital For Sick Children; (416)535-8501

CARLISLE, Euan; St Joseph's Healthcare, 50 Charlton Ave E, Hamilton ON L8N 4A6; Queen's (Ireland)'80; FRCP(UK); MD; FRCPC; IntMed; Nephrol. Staff Nephrol, St Joseph's Healthcare - Charlton Campus; Assoc Prof, McMaster University; (905)522-1155 x3741; Fax. (905)521-6088; euan@mcmaster.ca.

CARLISLE, Maxine A; Lake of the Woods Dist Hosp, RR 1 Stn Main 21 Sylvan St, Kenora ON P9N 3W7; Man'04; CCFP; Staff, Lake of the Woods District Hospital; (807)468-9861

CARLOS, Joseph M; 1F-3850 Finch Ave E, Scarborough ON M1T 1T6; Santo Tomas (Philippines)'71; (416)299-6063

CARLOS, Mary Anne; Petitcodiac Health Centre PO Box 2501 Stn Main, Petitcodiac NB E4Z 6H4; Dal'82; (506)756-3400; Fax. (506)756-3406.

CARLSEN, Lloyd N; SGH Medical Mall, 501-3030 Lawrence Ave E, Scarborough ON M1P 2T7; Qns'57; FACS; FRCSC; PlasSurg (Cosmetic Surgery). Chief PlasSurg, Cosmetic Surgery Hospital; Staff, The Scarborough Hospital - General Campus; Asst Prof Surg, McMaster University; (416)289-7100; Fax. (416)289-4256.

CARLSON, Barbara A; Midtown Med Clinic, 35 Campbell Ave, St. John's NL A1E 2Z3; Mem'76; (709)579-0703

CARLSON, Brian D; North Road Med Centre, S-435 North Rd, Coquitlam BC V3K 3V9; Mem'74; Staff, Royal Columbian Hospital; (604)936-0411

CARLSON, Britt I; Halton HCS Corp-Oakville, 327 Reynolds St, Oakville ON L6J 3L7; Wes'95; CCFP; FCFP; CCFP(E.M.); Court Staff, Halton Healthcare Services Corporation - Oakville Site; (905)845-2571

CARLSON, Catherine A; 101-3960 Quadra St, Victoria BC V8X 4A3; McM'87; BSc(Hons); CCFP; FCFP; Staff, Island Sexual Health Society; (250)592-3479; ccarlson@islandsexualhealth.org.

CARLSON, Christopher G; Glen Sather Sports Med Clinic, 1A. 102-11400 University Ave NW, Edmonton AB T6G 1Z1; Alb'06; CCFP; Staff, University of Alberta Hospital; (780)407-7755; Fax. (780)407-1828.

CARLSON, Erin P V; University Hosp of Northern BC, 1475 Edmonton St, Prince George BC V2M 1S2; UBC'10; CCFP; Staff, University Hospital of Northern British Columbia; (250)565-2000

CARLSON, Kevin V; Rockyview Gen Hosp, 6608-7007 14 St SW, Calgary AB T2V 1P9; UBC'94; FRCSC; Urol (Incontinence). Staff, Rockyview General Hospital; Southern Alberta Institute of Urology; Clin Prof, University of Calgary; (403)943-8978; Fax. (403)943-8979.

CARLSON, Malcolm L; Stratford Gen Hosp, 46 General Hospital Dr, Stratford ON N5A 2Y6; McM'78; GenPath. Lab Mgr, Stratford General Hospital - Huron Perth Healthcare Alliance; (519)271-2120 x2521; malcolm.carlson@hpha.ca.

CARLSON, Robert F; J2-925 Main St, West Vancouver BC V7T 2Z3; UBC'82; Med Staff, Abbotsford Regional Hospital & Cancer Centre; (604)922-7372

CARLSON, Ryan G; Univ Hlth Network-Princess M, 610 University Ave, Toronto ON M5T 2M9; Alb'07; FRCPC; RadOncol. Fellow, Princess Margaret Hospital Pharmacy-University Health Network; (416)946-6560; ryan.carlson@uhn.on.ca.

CARLSON, William H; 21-1523 Dufferin Cres, Nanaimo BC V9S 5H6; UBC'06; FRCSC; Urol. (250)591-2214

CARLSON-REID, Heidi M; West Main Plaza, 106C-1600 Main St W, Moncton NB E1E 1G5; McG'96; FRCPC; Peds. Staff, The Moncton Hospital; Langs: Bilingual(English/French); (506)857-5830; Fax. (506)857-5832; hccarlso@wrha.ca.

CARLSSON, Anthony M; 175 6 St SE, Medicine Hat AB T1A 1G7; Dal'99; FCASS; FRCSC; Ophth (Cornea & Anterior Segment). (403)458-3937; Fax. (403)488-7987.

CARLSTEN, Christopher R; Diamond Health Care Centre, 7F-2775 Laurel St, Vancouver BC V5Z 1M9; Stanford (USA)'00; Respir; OccupMed; IntMed. (604)875-4122

CARLTON, Joseph A; SMBD Jewish Gen Hosp, E005-3755 ch Cote-Sainte-Cathe, Montreal QC H3T 1E2; Johns Hopkins (USA)'72; FRCPC; Neur. Ac Staff Neurol, Sir Mortimer B Davis Jewish General; (514)340-8222 x5849; Fax. (514)340-7567.

CARLTON, Timothy J; Avenue Med Clinic, 221 Brant Ave, Brantford ON N3T 3J3; McM'87; FRCPC; IntMed (Sleep Disorders); Respir. Ac Staff, The Brant Community Healthcare System - Brantford General Hospital Site; (519)753-8666; Fax. (519)753-5672.

CARLYLE, Robert W; Northumberland Hills Hosp, 1000 DePalma Dr, Cobourg ON K9A 5W6; Tor'63; FRCPC; Psy. Staff, Northumberland Hills Hospital; (905)377-9891

CARMAN, Wayne W; Cosmetic Surgery Institute, 101-325 Eglinton Ave E, Toronto ON M4P 1L7; Tor'75; BSc; MSc; FRCSC; PlasSurg (Cosmetic Surgery). Ac Staff, The Scarborough Hospital - General Campus; Dir, Cosmetic Surgery Institute; (416)322-7108; Fax. (416)322-7110.

CARMANT, Lionel; Hôpital Ste-Justine, 3175 ch Cote-Sainte-Catherine, Montreal QC H3T 1C5; Sher'86; FRCPC; Electroenceph (P.Q.); Neur. Staff EEG Lab, Hôpital Ste-Justine; (514)345-4894

CARMEL, Luc; CSSS de Laval, 1755 boul Rene-Laennec, Laval QC H7M 3L9; Mon'85; Staff, Hopital de la Cite de la santé; (450)668-1010; Fax. (450)975-5545.

CARMEL, Michel; CHUS-Hop Fleurimont, 3001 12e Av N, Sherbrooke QC J1H 5N4; Sher'77; FRCS; FRCSC; Urol (Erectile Dysfunction). Chef Urology Servicew, Centre Hospitalier Universitaire de Sherbrooke-Hopital Fleurimont; Prof Dept of Surg & Urol, Universite de Sherbrooke; Langs: Bilingual(English/French); (819)346-1110 x14595; Fax. (819)820-6411; michel.carmel@usherbrooke.ca.

CARMICHAEL, Catherine A; The Concourse Bldg, 702-100 Adelaide St W, Toronto ON M5H 1S3; McM'87; CCFP; FCFP; Staff, Halton Healthcare Services Corporation - Oakville Site; (416)935-1962; Fax. (416)966-0837.

CARMICHAEL, Frederick J; William Osler HC-Etobicoke, 101 Humber College Blvd, Etobicoke ON M9V 1R8; Tor'78; Anes. Staff, William Osler Health System - Etobicoke General Hospital; (416)747-3500

CARMICHAEL, Paula A; 1794 Route 640, Hanwell NB E3C 2A8; Dal'99; BSc; CCFP; Staff, Digby General Hospital; (506)455-4233; carmichaelpaula@hotmail.com.

CARMICHAEL, Rejean; Clinique Opti-Soins, 550-2655 boul Du Royaume, Jonquiere QC G7S 4S9; Laval'85; (418)548-1211; Fax. (418)548-7721.

CARMICHAEL, Richard W; 20-1450 O'Connor Dr, Toronto ON M4B 2T8; Tor'70; MD; Assoc Staff, Toronto East General Hospital Inc; (647)722-2370; Fax. (416)367-4301; rich.car@sympatico.ca.

CARMODY, Douglas E; Summerside Med Centre, 1-475 Granville St, Summerside PE C1N 3N9; Dal'87; IntMed. (902)432-8109

CARMONA, Rajendra; Charlton Med Centre, 708-25 Charlton Ave E, Hamilton ON L8N 1Y2; West Indies (Jamaica)'00; MB BS; FRCPC; IntMed; Rheum. Staff, Charlton Medical Centre; Teach Staff, McMaster University; (905)521-9034; Fax. (905)521-8099.

CARNAT, Toby A; King Street Med Arts Centre, 400-71 King St W, Mississauga ON L5B 4A2; Dal'02; FRCSC; Urol. (905)276-4484; Fax. (905)272-0647.

CARNE, Nicole A P; CSSS du Haut-Saint-François, 460 2e Avenue, Weedon QC J0B 3J0; Staff, CSSS du Haut-Saint-François; (819)877-3434

CARNEY, Dominic P; The Lung Health Clinic, 8737 156 St NW, Edmonton AB T5R 1Y5; Alb'04; FRCPC; IntMed (Family Medicine); Critical Care Medicine; Respir. Staff, University of Alberta Hospital; (780)498-1800; Fax. (780)498-7774.

CARNOIS, Isabelle; CLSC Longueuil Ouest, 201 boul Cure-Poirier O, Longueuil QC J4J 2G4; Mon'92; (450)651-9831; Fax. (450)651-0924.

CARO, Jonathan; 3026-3080 Yonge St, Toronto ON M4N 3N1; Wes'83; FRCPC; Psy. (416)932-9096

CARO GALVIS, Luisa F; Westbrook Shopping Centre, 28-1200 37 St SW, Calgary AB T3C 1S2; (Other Foreign)'01; (403)944-1110

CARO GUZMAN, Alexis H; Charles S Curtis Mem Hosp, 178-200 West St, St Anthony NL A0K 4S0; Pontificia Universidad (Chile)'99; CCFP; Staff, Charles S Curtis Memorial Hospital; (709)454-3333

CAROL, Angela M; Urban Core Commun Health Ctre, 71 Rebecca St, Hamilton ON L8R 1B6; McM'96; CCFP; FCFP; Staff, St Joseph's Healthcare - Charlton Campus; Staff, Hamilton Health Sciences Centre - McMaster University Medical Centre; (905)522-3233; Fax. (905)522-3706.

CAROLAN, Hannah; BC Cancer Agency-Vancouver CC, 600 10th Ave W, Vancouver BC V5Z 4E6; UBC'00; FRCPC; RadOncol. Staff, BC Cancer Agency Vancouver Centre; (604)877-6000 x2668

CAROM, Donald P; Windsor Health Centre, 205-700 Tecumseh Rd E, Windsor ON N8X 4T2; Tor'63; Court Staff, Hôtel-Dieu Grace Hospital; (519)258-4771; Fax. (519)258-4793.

CARON, Andre B; Polyclinique Med Concorde, 300 boul de la Concorde E, Laval QC H7G 2E6; Mon'75; FRCPC; IntMed; ClinImmunol&Allergy. ac Staff, Centre Hospitalier l'Université de Montréal (CHUM) - Hôpital Notre-Dame; (450)667-5310

CARON, Andrew; 165 boul Sainte-Madeleine, Trois-Rivieres QC G8T 3L7; Sher'10; (819)379-8385

CARON, Carole; CSSS de Lac-Saint Jean-Est, CP 1300 Succ Bureau-Chef 300 boul Champlain, Alma QC G8B 5W3; Mon'89; CSPQ; FRCPC; AnatPath. Chief Med Biology, CSSS de Lac-Saint Jean-Est; Anatomical Pathology, Hotel-Dieu de Roberval; Langs: English; (418)669-2000 x3338; carole.caron.clj@ssss.gouv.qc.ca.

CARON, Catherine; Ctre Hosp de Matane, 333 rue Thibault, Matane QC G4W 2W5; Laval'08; Staff, Centre Hospitalier de Matane; (418)562-3135

CARON, Catherine; CSSS de Temiscouata, CP 310 58 rue de l'Eglise, Notre-Dame-du-Lac QC G0L 1X0; Sher'05; CCFP; Staff, Centre Hospitalier Notre-Dame-du-Lac; (418)899-6751

CARON, Catherine M; Bruyere Academic Fam Hlth Team, 75 Bruyere St, Ottawa ON K1N 5C7; Wes'89; BSc; MSc; CCFP; FCFP; Asst Prof, University of Ottawa; Langs: French; (613)241-1154; Fax. (613)241-1971.

CARON, Chantal; Hop Riviere-Des-Prairies, 7070 boul Perras, Montreal QC H1E 1A4; Laval'83; MSc(Epidemiol); FRCPC; Psy (Pediatric Psychiatry). Staff Child Psy Inpatient & Day Care Unit, Hôpital Riviere des Prairies; Clin Researcher, Université Laval; (514)323-7260; Fax. (514)328-3530.

CARON, Chantal; Ctr Hosp Affilie-St-Sacrement, 1050 ch Sainte-Foy, Quebec QC G1S 4L8; Laval'78; CSPQ; AnatPath. Staff Path, Centre Hospitalier Affilié Universitaire de Québec - Hôpital du St-Sacrement; (418)682-7805; Fax. (418)682-7383.

CARON, Charles; CHUM-Hop St-Luc, 1058 rue Saint-Denis, Montreal QC H2X 3J4; Mon'81; CSPQ; FRCPC; Anes. Staff, Centre Hospitalier l'Université De Montréal (CHUM) - Hôpital Saint-luc; (514)890-8358; Fax. (514)281-9271.

CARON, Christine; 597 av Notre-Dame, Saint-Lambert QC J4P 2K8; Mon'95; Langs: English; (450)766-0766; Fax. (450)766-0767.

CARON, Daniel C; Hop Maisonneuve-Rosemont, 5415 boul de l'Assomption, Montreal QC H1T 2M4; Mon'75; CSPQ; Endocrin (P.Q.) (Diabetology). Chief Endocin & Metab, Hopital Maisonneuve-Rosemont; Dir, Diabetes Education Center; Clinical Asst Prof, Universite de Montreal; Langs: English; (514)252-3400; Fax. (514)252-3561; ensendo.hmr@ssss.gouv.qc.ca.

CARON, Denis F; CHUQ-Hotel-Dieu de Quebec, 11 Cote Du Palais, Quebec QC G1R 2J6; Laval'67; DiagRad. Staff, Centre Hospitalier Universitaire de Québec (CHUQ) - Siege Social; Head Dept of Radiol, Université Laval; (418)691-5453; Fax. (418)691-5394.

CARON, Dominique; Clinique Med de l'Atelier, 77 boul Seigneurial O, Saint-Bruno QC J3V 2G9; Laval'89; CCFP; FCFP; Langs: Spanish; English; (450)461-1751

CARON, Edith; CSSS de Saint-Jerome, 290 rue de Montigny, Saint-Jerome QC J7Z 5T3; Laval'88; Psy (Emergency Psychiatry). Staff, Hôtel-Dieu de Saint-Jérôme; (450)431-8392; Fax. (450)431-8244.

CARON, Elaine; Clinique Med Chateauguay, 120 boul Saint-Jean-Baptiste, Chateauguay QC J6K 3A9; Mon'84; Staff, Centre Hospitalier de Verdun; (450)691-8191; Fax. (450)691-8568.

CARON, Francine; CHUQ-Ctr Hosp Univ Laval, 2705 boul Laurier, Quebec QC G1V 4G2; Laval'74; FRCPC; Derm (Pediatric Dermatology). Ac Staff, Centre Hospitalier Universitaire de Quebec-CHUL; (418)654-2160; Fax. (418)654-2187.

CARON, Francois; Ctr Hosp Affilie-Enfant-Jesus, 1401 18e rue, Quebec QC G1J 1Z4; Laval'86; CSPQ; Anes (Intensive Care). Staff, Centre Hospitalier Affilié Universitaire de Québec - Hôpital De L'Enfant Jésus; Université Laval; (418)649-5803

CARON, Gilles J; CSSS de la Region de Thetford, 1717 rue Notre-Dame E, Thetford Mines QC G6G 2V4; Mon'90; Staff, Hopital du CSS de la Region de Thetford; (418)842-0790

CARON, Jacques; Clinique Med Frontenac, 24 rue Frontenac, Riviere-du-Loup QC G5R 1S5; Laval'77; LMCC; (418)862-0333; Fax. (418)868-0505.

CARON, Jean-Francois; Clinique Med Humani, 120-30 boul Bouthillier, Rosemere QC J7A 4B4; Laval'05; (450)951-3010

CARON, Jerome; Centre Med Dorion Vaudreuil, 600 boul Harwood, Vaudreuil-Dorion QC J7V 6A3; Mon'80; (450)455-9301; Fax. (450)455-8964.

CARON, Joanna M; UMF St-Mary, 3777 rue Jean-Brillant, Montreal QC H3T 1M5; McG'05; CCFP; (514)734-2631

CARON, Johanne; CSSS de Trois-Rivieres, 1991 boul du Carmel, Trois-Rivieres QC G9A 1Y1; Laval'91; FRCPC; IntMed; MedOncol; Hem. Staff HemOncol, CSSS de Trois-Rivières; (819)697-3333 x63337

CARON, Josee; Tribunal Admin du Quebec, 22F-500 boul Rene-Levesque O, Montreal QC H2Z 1W7; Mon'83; GenSurg. Langs: English; (514)873-7154 x5080

CARON, Louis; Ctr Hosp Affilie-St-Sacrement, 1050 ch Sainte-Foy, Quebec QC G1S 4L8; Laval'03; Ophth. Staff, Centre Hospitalier Affilié Universitaire de Québec - Hôpital du St-Sacrement; (418)682-7511 x4650; Fax. (418)862-7554.

CARON, Louise; Clinique Med St Louis, 220-3165 ch Saint-Louis, Quebec QC G1W 4R4; Laval'97; Physician, Groupe Sante Medisys; (418)653-1970

CARON, Lucie; Hotel-Dieu Du Sacre-Coeur, 413N-1 av Du Sacre-Coeur, Quebec QC G1N 2W1; Laval'74; FRCPC; Psy. Staff, Hotel-Dieu du Sacre-Coeur de Jesus de Quebec; (418)529-6851; Fax. (418)691-0750.

CARON, Marcel; Clinique Med de l'Est, 106-437 rue King E, Sherbrooke QC J1G 1B7; Sher'71; FRCSC; ObstGyn. Staff, Centre Hospitalier Universitaire de Sherbrooke-Hopital Fleurimont; Chef obst & gyn, Centre Hospitalier Universitaire de Sherbrooke-Hôpital Hôtel-Dieu; (819)563-9087

CARON, Marie C; CSSS de Saint-Jerome, 290 rue de Montigny, Saint-Jerome QC J7Z 5T3; Laval'64; Psy (P.Q.). Staff, Hôtel-Dieu de Saint-Jérôme; (450)431-8392

CARON, Marie-Josee; CSSS de Saint-Jerome, 290 rue de Montigny, Saint-Jerome QC J7Z 5T3; Mon'00; CSPQ; FRCPC; Anes. Staff, Hôtel-Dieu de Saint-Jérôme; (450)431-8200

CARON, Marie-Josee; Hop du Sacre-Coeur de Mtl, 5400 boul Gouin O, Montreal QC H4J 1C5; Mon'88; CCFP; Chef Palliative Care Services, Hôpital du Sacre-Coeur de Montréal; Langs: Bilingual(French/English); (514)338-2222 x2591; Fax. (514)338-2359.

CARON, Marilyn; Centre Hosp Beauce-Etchemin, 1515 17e rue, Saint-Georges QC G5Y 4T8; Laval'07; FRCPC; Derm. Staff, Centre Hospitalier Beauce-Etchemin; (418)228-2031

CARON, Marjolaine; GMF Val-Belair, 202-1147 boul Pie-XI N, Quebec QC G3K 2P8; Mon'96; Staff, Centre Hospitalier Chauveau; (418)843-0001; Fax. (418)843-0224.

CARON, Matthieu; Medicentre Benjamin-Papineau, 106-1600 boul Curé-Labelle, Laval QC H7V 2W2; Laval'78; (450)973-3781; Fax. (450)967-7453.

CARON, Maurice; Multi Clin Personnes Accidentr, 1465 rue Belanger, Montreal QC H2G 1A5; Mon'73; MScA; Langs: Bilingual(French/English); (514)728-2264; Fax. (514)728-7076; dr.maurice.caron@gmail.com.

CARON, Michel; Clinique Medicale du Faubourg, 145-1160 boul Saint-Joseph, Gatineau QC J8Z 1T3; Laval'83; Staff, Hôpital de Gatineau; Staff, Centre Hospitalier Pierre-Janet; Langs: English; (819)595-1991

CARON, Michel; Clinique Med Nepisiguit, 950 av Picot, Bathurst NB E2A 4Z9; Sher'00; FRCSC; OrthSurg. (506)546-6699; Fax. (506)548-4124.

CARON, Michelle; CSSS Pierre Boucher, 1333 boul Jacques-Cartier E, Longueuil QC J4M 2A5; Laval'89; FRCPC; NuclearMed. Staff, Centre Hospitalier Pierre Boucher; (450)468-8174

CARON, Michelle; Centre Hosp Beauce-Etchemin, 1515 17e rue, Saint-Georges QC G5Y 4T8; Laval'07; FRCSC; ObstGyn. Staff, Centre Hospitalier Beauce-Etchemin; (418)228-2031

CARON, Nadia; CHUS-Hop Fleurimont, 3001 12e av N, Sherbrooke QC J1H 5N4; Laval'98; FRCPC; IntMed. Staff, Centre Hospitalier Universitaire de Sherbrooke-Hopital Fleurimont; (819)346-1110

CARON, Nadine; 308-1669 Victoria St, Prince George BC V2L 2L5; UBC'97; FRCSC; GenSurg (Endocrinology Surgery). Staff, University Hospital of Northern British Columbia; (250)564-5324; Fax. (250)564-5393.

CARON, Olivier; CP 5533, Caraquet NB E1W 1B7; Sher'07; CCFP; (506)726-2100

CARON, Patricia; Clinique Med St-Gedeon, 188 2e Av S, St-Gedeon-d-Beauce QC G0M 1T0; Laval'10; CCFP; (418)582-3317

CARON, Patricia-Anne; Centre Hosp Honore-Mercier, 2750 boul Laframboise, Saint-Hyacinthe QC J2S 4Y8; Mon'91; FRCSC; GenSurg. Staff, Centre Hospitalier Honore-Mercier; (450)771-3333

CARON, Paul L J; Residence pour Aines Lev-Tov, 6900 rue Sherbrooke O, Montreal QC H4B 1P9; McG'71; (514)489-4448

CARON, Paul; Hop Brome-Missisquoi-Perkins, 950 rue Principale, Cowansville QC J2K 1K3; Mon'75; CSPQ; FRCPC; Anes. Staff, Hôpital Brome-Missisquoi-Perkins; (450)266-4342 x55546

CARON, Renee; 7320 Rue Germain, Charlesbourg QC G1H 5P8; Laval'89; (819)821-7667

CARON, Renee; Service de Sante, 2500 boul de l'Universite, Sherbrooke QC J1K 2R1; Sher'87; Médecin Service de Sante, Universite de Sherbrooke; Langs: Bilingual(French/English); (819)821-7667

CARON, Sandrine; 1-3980 rue Principale CP 3603 Succ Bureau-Chef, Tracadie-Sheila NB E1X 1G5; Laval'03; CCFP; (506)395-2554; Fax. (506)395-2443.

CARON, Serge; Clinique Med La Pocatiere, 202-1200 6e Av, La Pocatiere QC G0R 1Z0; Mon'72; Staff, Centre Hospitalier des Monts; ac Membre, CSSS de Kamouraska; (418)856-4647; Fax. (418)856-3211.

CARON, Sophie; GMF du Carrefour, 210-3333 rue du carrefour, Quebec QC G1C 5R9; Laval'01; (418)663-6345 x1015

CARON, Stephane; Dir de la Sante Pub Cote-Nord, 691 rue Jalbert, Baie-Comeau QC G5C 2A1; Mon'89; (418)589-9845 x2384; stephane_caron@ssss.gouv.qc.ca.

CARON, Stephanie; Ctr Hosp Affilie-Enfant-Jesus, 1401 18e rue, Quebec QC G1J 1Z4; Mon'02; FRCPC; IntMed; GeriatricMed. Staff, Centre Hospitalier Affilié Universitaire de Québec - Hôpital De L'Enfant Jésus; (418)649-0252

CARON, Suzanne; Hotel-Dieu de Levis, 143 rue Wolfe, Levis QC G6V 3Z1; Laval'94; Psy. Staff, Hôtel-Dieu de Lévis; (418)835-7155

CARON, Valerie; CSSSG-Hop de Hull, 116 boul Lionel-Emond, Gatineau QC J8Y 1W7; Laval'99; CCFP; Staff, Hull Hospital; (819)966-6222

CARON, Vincent; 198 av de la Greve O, Riviere-Ouelle QC G0L 2C0; Laval'71; Staff, Centre Hospitalier Regional du Grand-Portage; (418)371-0877

CARON-BOULET, Nicole M; Veteran's Affairs, 610-234 Donald St, Winnipeg MB R3C 4G5; Man'84; CCFP; FCFP; Staff, St Boniface General Hospital.

CARON-FAUCONNIER, Genevieve; Clinique Familiale, 13555 boul Lacroix, Saint-Georges QC G5Y 1P1; Sher'98; CCFP; Médecin, Centre Hospitalier Beauce-Etchemin; Clin Prof Med, Université Laval; Langs: English; (418)228-8001; Fax. (418)228-5583.

CAROTHERS, Melanie; Grand River Hosp-Freeport HC, 3570 King St E, Kitchener ON N2A 2W1; Ott'72; Med Staff, St Mary's General Hospital; Staff, Grand River Hospital - Freeport Site; Med Dir, Nithview Home for the Aged; (519)749-4300 x7357

CARPENITO, Gerardo; Kingsway Plaza Phase III, 600-4980 Kingsway, Burnaby BC V5H 4K7; UBC'94; FRCPC; IntMed; Nephrol. Staff, Burnaby Hospital; (604)432-9114

CARPENTER, David C; Canadian Forces Supp Unit HCC, 213-1745 Alta Vista Dr, Ottawa ON K1A 0K6; Ott'79; BSc(Hon); MScPharm; MHSc(OccupationalMed.); DTMH(Lond); Staff, Canadian Forces Health Services Centre; Langs: German; French; (613)945-6705; Fax. (613)945-5887.

CARPENTER, Frederick J; Hilden Med Clinic, RR 1 1174 Hwy 2, Brookfield NS B0N 1C0; Dal'73; FRCSC; Ophth. (902)893-8066; Fax. (902)895-2389; redbird@ns.sympatico.ca.

CARPENTER, Jennifer L; Kingston Reg Cancer Centre, 25 King St W, Kingston ON K7L 5P9; Qns'97; FRCPC; CCFP; EmergMed. (613)548-2368

CARPENTER, Jillian A; R A Pollett Bldg, PO Box 808 203-61 Riverside Dr, Corner Brook NL A2H 6G7; Mem'04; FRCSC; ObstGyn. Staff, Western Memorial Regional Hospital.

CARPENTER, Noah H; The Brandon Clinic, 620 Dennis St, Brandon MB R7A 5E7; Man'71; BSc(Med); FCCP; FRCS(Ed); GenSurg (Thoracic Surgery). Gen Surgery, Brandon Regional Health Centre; Court Staff, Winnipeg Regional Health Authority; Langs: French; (204)728-4440; ncarpenter@wrha.mb.ca.

CARPENTER, Susan P C; Arnika Centre, 3304 33 St NW, Calgary AB T2L 2A6; Cal'74; FRCPC; Psy (Intellectual Disability Psy). Med Dir, Arnika Centre; Associate Clin Prof, University Of Calgary; (403)284-1121 x373; Fax. (403)267-1241.

CARPENTIER, Andre; CHUS-Hop Fleurimont, 3001 12e Av N, Sherbrooke QC J1H 5N4; Sher'91; FRCPC; IntMed; Endocrin (P.Q.); Endocrin&Metab. Staff, Centre Hospitalier Universitaire de Sherbrooke-Hopital Fleurimont; (819)564-5244; Fax. (819)564-5292.

CARPENTIER, Daniel; CLSC La Source, 791 rue de Sherwood, Quebec QC G2N 1X7; Laval'89; Staff, CSSS de Quebec Nord; (418)628-5630 x3319; Fax. (418)841-5110.

CARPENTIER, Frederic; Clinique Med De Montmagny, 100-83 av de la Fabrique, Montmagny QC G5V 2J3; Laval'97; LMCC; Staff, CSSS de Montmagny-L'Islet; (418)248-4933; Fax. (418)248-2778; frederic.carpentier@gmf.gouv.qc.ca.

CARPENTIER, Louis; Clinique Med Deux-Montagnes, 201 9e Av, Deux-Montagnes QC J7R 3M1; Mon'72; (450)472-7520; Fax. (450)472-0886.

CARPENTIER, Louis; Ctr Hosp Affilie-St-Sacrement, 1050 ch Sainte-Foy, Quebec QC G1S 4L8; Mon'90; CCFP; Staff Emerg, Centre Hospitalier Affilié Universitaire de Québec - Hôpital du St-Sacrement; (418)682-7515

CARPENTIER, Marie-Pierre; Montfort Hosp, 713 Montreal Rd, Ottawa ON K1K 0T2; Sher'97; CCFP; CCFP(E.M.); Staff, Montfort Hospital; Langs: English; Spanish; (613)746-4621; mpcarpentier@sympatico.ca.

CARPENTIER, Veronique; CLSC Jardin-du-Quebec, 2 rue Sainte-Famille, Saint-Remi QC J0L 2L0; Mon'05; CCFP; (450)454-4671

CARPINETA, Lucia; MUHC-Montreal Children's Hosp, C343-2300 rue Tupper, Montreal QC H3H 1P3; McG'95; FRCPC; DiagRad (Pediatric Radiology). Staff, McGill University Health Centre - Montreal Children's Hospital; (514)412-4450; Fax. (514)412-4347.

CARR, Anthony C; Mission Services, 293 Wellington St N, Hamilton ON L8L 8E7; London (England)'69; MB BS; MRCPsy; MRC; Psy. Staff, St Joseph's Healthcare Hamilton - West 5th Campus; Assoc Prof Psy, McMaster University; (905)528-4211

CARR, Brendan S J; Royal Jubilee Hosp, 3F-1952 Bay St, Victoria BC V8R 1J8; Dal'89; MBA; CCFP; CCFP(E.M.); Staff, Royal Jubilee Hospital; (250)519-1867

CARR, David; Univ Hlth Network-Toronto Gen, 200 Elizabeth St, Toronto ON M5G 2C4; Ott'01; CCFP; CCFP(E.M.); Staff, Toronto General Hospital - UHN; (416)340-3947

CARR, G David A; The Medical Centre FHT, 707 Charlotte St, Peterborough ON K9J 7B3; Qns'03; CCFP; CCFP(E.M.); Physician Emerg, Peterborough Regional Health Centre - Hospital Drive; (705)876-4592; Fax. (705)742-7076.

CARR, Jane C; 584 Riverbend Square PO Box 21044 Rpo Terwillegar, Edmonton AB T6R 2V4; Alb'90; FRCPC; Psy. Staff, Covenant Health - Misericordia Community Hospital.

CARR, Janice D; Town Plaza Med Clinic, 40-4314 Main St RR 4, Whistler BC V0N 1B4; Man'78; (604)905-7089; Fax. (604)905-7039.

CARR, John A; Harbour City Health Centre, 202-1125 Dufferin Cres, Nanaimo BC V9S 2B5; UBC'84; FRCSC; GenSurg (Endoscopy). Ac Staff, Nanaimo Regional General Hospital; (250)754-1523; Fax. (250)754-6423.

CARR, Jonathan D; 410-4800 Leslie St, North York ON M2J 2K9; Tor'83; CCFP; FCFP; Staff, Mount Sinai Hospital; Staff, North York General Hospital - Branson Division; Staff, North York General Hospital; Teach Staff Family Practice, University of Toronto; (416)497-9900; Fax. (416)497-6992.

CARR, Jordan P; North York Gen Hosp, 4001 Leslie St, North York ON M2K 1E1; Cal'98; FRCPC; Peds. Staff, North York General Hospital; (416)756-6000

CARR, Lesley K; Sunnybrook Hlth Sciences Ctre, MG501-2075 Bayview Ave, Toronto ON M4N 3M5; Tor'89; FRCSC; Urol. Ac Staff, Sunnybrook Health Sciences Centre; Asst Prof, University of Toronto; (416)480-5113; Fax. (416)480-5116.

CARR, Lindsay A; The Ottawa Hosp-Civic Campus, M206-1053 Carling Ave, Ottawa ON K1Y 4E9; Ott'08; CCFP; CCFP(E.M.); Staff, The Ottawa Hospital - Civic Campus; (613)789-5555

CARR, Melanie L; 1010-170 Bloor St W, Toronto ON M5S 1T9; Tor'85; FRCPC; Psy. (416)545-1541; Fax. (416)545-1686.

CARR, Nicholas J; Skinworks Clinic, 3578 41st Ave W, Vancouver BC V6N 3E6; UBC'83; BSc; FRCSC; PlasSurg (Cosmetic Surgery). Head PlasticSurg/Ac Staff, Vancouver General Hospital - Centennial Pavillion; Head PlasticSurg, University of British Columbia; (604)733-9711; Fax. (604)733-7957.

CARR, Padraic E; Cedars Prof Park, 2915 66 St NW, Edmonton AB T6K 4C1; Alb'90; BMedSci; FRCPC; Psy (General Adult Psychiatry). Staff Outpatient Psy, Alberta Hospital Edmonton; Leader, Covenant Health - Grey Nuns Community Hospital; Clin Prof Med, University of Alberta; (780)450-9453; Fax. (780)461-6190.

CARR, Sean A; 106-2100 Finch Ave W, North York ON M3N 2Z9; Wes'06; Respir; IntMed. Staff, Humber River Regional Hospital - Finch Avenue Site; (416)739-7558; Fax. (416)739-7601.

CARR, Stuart N; College Plaza, 903-8215 112 St NW, Edmonton AB T6G 2C8; Alb'93; FRCPC; Peds; ClinImmunol&Allergy. Staff Admitting, University of Alberta Hospital; Asst Prof Clin Peds, University of Alberta; (780)413-6689; allergydoc@telusplanet.net.

CARR, Thomas J; Northeastern On Reg Cancer Ctr, 41 Ramsey Lake Rd, Sudbury ON P3E 5J1; Wes'77; FRCPC; NuclearMed. Staff Nuclear Med, Health Sciences North-St Joseph's Health Centre; (705)523-7100; tcarr@hrsrh.on.ca.

CARRANZA, Ruben G; MUHC-Montreal Children's Hosp, 2300 rue Tupper, Montreal QC H3H 1P3; (Philippines)'71; ac Staff, McGill University Health Centre - Montreal Children's Hospital; (514)412-4400

CARRANZA MAMANE, Belina; CHUS-Hop Fleurimont, 3001 12e av N, Sherbrooke QC J1H 5N4; Sher'02; FRCSC; ObstGyn (Gynecological Reproductive Endocrinology). Staff, Centre Hospitalier Universitaire de Sherbrooke-Hopital Fleurimont; (819)346-1110 x13120

CARRE, Valerie; Clinique Gyneco Saguenay, 200-394 rue Saint-Vallier, Chicoutimi QC G7H 4J1; Mon'99; FRCSC; ObstGyn. (418)545-2666

CARRE DESROSIERS, M Genevieve N; CSSS de Trois-Rivieres, 1991 boul du Carmel, Trois-Rivieres QC G8Z 3R9; (Haiti)'91; Staff, CSSS de Trois-Rivières; (819)697-3333

CARREIRO, Stephen R; Ctre Hosp de Lachine, 650 16e av, Lachine QC H8S 3N5; McG'03; CCFP; Staff, CSSS de Dorval-Lachine-Lasalle; (514)637-2351

CARRERAS, Francisco J; CSSS de Rivière-du-Loup, 75 rue Saint-Henri, Riviere-du-Loup QC G5R 2A4; Buenos Aires (Argentina)'02; Staff, Centre Hospitalier Regional du Grand-Portage; (418)868-1000; Fax. (418)868-1032.

CARRET, Anne-Sophie; Hôpital Ste-Justine, 3175 ch Cote-Sainte-Catherine, Montreal QC H3T 1C5; Nancy (France)'92; Staff, Hôpital Ste-Justine; (514)345-4931 x4870

CARRETERO, Antonio P; Moose Jaw Union Hosp, 455 Fairford St E, Moose Jaw SK S6H 1H3; Lyceum Northwestern University (Philippines) BS; MSc; MD; FRCPC; AnatPath (Cytopath). Associate Path, Moose Jaw Union Hospital; Langs: Bicol; Tagalog; (306)694-0345; Fax. (306)694-0283; antonio.carretero@fhhr.ca.

CARREY, Normand J; IWK Health Centre, PO Box 9700 Rpo CSC, Halifax NS B3K 6R8; Tor'82; AB; FRCPC; Psy. Staff, IWK Health Centre; (902)470-8375

CARRIE, Douglas W; Royal Columbian Hosp, 330 Columbia St E, New Westminster BC V3L 3W7; Wes'86; FRCPC; Anes. Staff, Royal Columbian Hospital; Clin Instructor, University of British Columbia; (604)520-4253; dcarrie@msn.com.

CARRIER, Alexis; CSSS de Montmagny-L'Islet, 350 boul Tache O, Montmagny QC G5V 3R8; Laval'02; IntMed. Staff, CSSS de Montmagny-L'Islet; (418)248-0630

CARRIER, Annie; Ctr Hosp Reg de Lanaudiere, 1000 boul Sainte-Anne, St-Charles-Brromee QC J6E 6J2; Sher'90; Staff, Centre Hospitalier Régional de Lanaudière; (450)759-8222; Fax. (450)759-7969.

CARRIER, Christian; CSSS de Trois-Rivieres, 1991 boul du Carmel, Trois-Rivieres QC G8Z 3R9; Laval'90; FRCPC; IntMed (Hematological Oncology); MedOncol (P.Q.); Hem. Staff, CSSS de Trois-Rivières; Langs: English; (819)697-3333

CARRIER, Daniel A; Polyclinique des Ponts, 120-1100 boul de la Rive-Sud, Levis QC G6W 5M6; Laval'89; CCFP; Staff, Centre Hospitalier Paul-Gilbert; Langs: English; (418)834-1177

CARRIER, Daniel; Clinique Med Saint-Prime, 581 rue Coulombe, Saint-Prime QC G8J 1P2; Sher'88; CCFP; ac Staff, Hotel-Dieu de Roberval; (418)251-9080; Fax. (418)251-9073; janic.beaumont.lml@ssss.gouv.qc.ca.

CARRIER, Daniel J; CSSS Drummond-Hop Sainte-Croix, 570 rue Heriot, Drummondville QC J2B 1C1; Sher'89; FRCPC; IntMed. Staff, Hôpital Sainte-croix; (819)478-6464; Fax. (819)472-6453.

CARRIER, Francois-Martin; CHUM-Hop St-Luc, 1058 rue Saint-Denis, Montreal QC H2X 3J4; Laval'03; FRCPC; Anes; Critical Care Medicine (P.Q.). Staff, Centre Hospitalier l'Université De Montréal (CHUM) - Hôpital Saint-luc; (514)890-8000 x36581; Fax. (514)412-7310.

CARRIER, Gaetan; Public Health Program, 100-190 boul Crémazie E, Montreal QC H2P 1E2; Mon'82; (514)864-1600 x3248

CARRIER, Gaëtan; Hop Charles Lemoyne, 3120 boul Taschereau, Greenfield Park QC J4V 2H1; Mon'79; BSc; MBA; CSPQ; FRCPC; MedBiochem. Staff, Hopital Charles LeMoyne; (450)466-5000 x2691; gaetan.carrier@rrsss16.gouv.qc.ca.

CARRIER, Guy; Hôpital de la Malbaie, 303 rue Saint-Etienne, La Malbaie QC G5A 1T8; Sher'80; DiagRad. Staff, Hopital du CSS de la Region de Thetford; Chef Med Imaging, Hôpital Laval; Staff, Hôpital de la Malbaie; Physician Clinique Radiol, Secar Quebec; Prof, Université Laval; (418)665-1700

CARRIER, Guyta; 401 Grand Blvd, L'Ile-Perrot QC J7V 4X3; Laval'83; CCFP; FCFP; (514)453-1100; Fax. (514)453-2339.

CARRIER, Heather N; Stratford Gen Hosp, 46 General Hospital Dr, Stratford ON N5A 2Y6; Wes'01; CCFP; CCFP(E.M.); Staff, Stratford General Hospital - Huron Perth Healthcare Alliance; (519)272-8200

CARRIER, Isabelle; CSSS de Beauce-Etchemin, 1515 17e rue, Saint-Georges QC G5Y 4T8; Laval'00; FRCSC; Otol. Staff, Centre Hospitalier Beauce-Etchemin; (418)228-2031; Fax. (418)227-1270.

CARRIER, Jean-Sebastien; CSSS de Saint-Jerome, 290 rue de Montigny, Saint-Jerome QC J7Z 5T3; Laval'07; FRCPC; IntMed; Respir (P.Q.). Staff, Hôtel-Dieu de Saint-Jérôme; (450)432-2777

CARRIER, Jerome; CSSS de Montmagny-L'Islet, 350 boul Tache O RR 1, Montmagny QC G5V 3R8; Laval'89; IntMed (Cardiology). Staff, CSSS de Montmagny-L'Islet; (418)248-0630 x2442; Fax. (418)234-5512.

CARRIER, Johanne; CHUS-Hop Fleurimont, 3001 12e Av N, Sherbrooke QC J1H 5N4; Sher'93; CSPQ; FRCPC; Anes. Staff, Centre Hospitalier Universitaire de Sherbrooke-Hopital Fleurimont; (819)346-1110; Fax. (819)564-3552.

CARRIER, Jude; Hop de Baie-Saint-Paul, 74 rue Ambroise-Fafard, Baie-Saint-Paul QC G3Z 2J6; Laval'70; LMCC; GenSurg (Administrative Medicine). Staff, CSSS de Charlevoix; Staff, Centre Hospitalier Affilié Universitaire de Québec - Hôpital De L'Enfant Jésus; Université Laval; (418)435-5150

CARRIER, Julie; Moncton Med Clinic, 207-860 Mountain Rd, Moncton NB E1C 2N7; Sher'03; CCFP; Staff, The Moncton Hospital; Langs: English; (506)853-5133; Fax. (506)853-5126.

CARRIER, Julie; Ctr de Sante Paul-Gilbert, 9330 boul du Centre-Hospitalie, Charny QC G6X 1L6; Laval'01; Staff, Centre Hospitalier Paul-Gilbert; (418)380-8993; Fax. (418)832-1848.

CARRIER, Julie; CHUS-Hop Fleurimont, 3001 12e Av N, Sherbrooke QC J1H 5N4; Sher'93; FRCPC; IntMed; Gastroent. Staff Gastroent, Centre Hospitalier Universitaire de Sherbrooke-Hopital Fleurimont; (819)346-1110 x12336

CARRIER, Louise; Geriatric Psy Commun Services, 131Y-75 Bruyere St, Ottawa ON K1N 5C7; Sher'85; FRCPC; Psy (Geriatric Psychiatry). (613)562-0283; Fax. (613)562-0497.

CARRIER, Lucie; CSSS Pierre Boucher, 1333 boul Jacques-Cartier E, Longueuil QC J4M 2A5; Mon'77; NuclearMed. Staff Nuclear Med, Centre Hospitalier Pierre Boucher; (450)468-8111

CARRIER, Marc; The Ottawa Hosp-Gen Campus, 501 Smyth Rd Box 201A, Ottawa ON K1H 8L6; Ott'02; MSc(Epidemiol); FRCPC; IntMed (Thrombosis); Hem. Staff, Montfort Hospital; Asst Prof, The Ottawa Hospital - General Campus; Assoc Scientist, The Ottawa Hospital-Research Institute; Langs: Bilingual(English/French); (613)737-8899 x73034

CARRIER, Marc; CSSS de Laval, 1755 boul Rene-Laennec, Laval QC H7M 3L9; Laval'07; MedMicrobiol. Staff, Hopital de la Cite de la santé; (450)668-1010 x24613

CARRIER, Marie-Andree; Hôtel-Dieu de Sorel, 400 av de l'Hotel-Dieu, Sorel-Tracy QC J3P 1N5; Mon'98; FRCPC; MedMicrobiol. Staff, Centre Hospitalier Pierre Boucher; Staff, Hôtel-Dieu de Sorel; (450)746-6000

CARRIER, Marie-Eve; CSSS du Suroît, 150 rue Saint-Thomas, Salaber-de-Valleyf QC J6T 6C1; Mon'04; DiagRad. Staff, Centre Hospitalier Régional du Suroît; (450)371-9920

CARRIER, Marie-France; Hotel-Dieu du Sacre-Coeur, 1 av Du Sacre-Coeur, Quebec QC G1N 2W1; Laval'76; Psy. ac Staff, Hotel-Dieu du Sacre-Coeur de Jesus de Quebec; (418)529-6851 x20451; Fax. (418)691-0750.

CARRIER, Mathieu; CSSS de Saint-Jerome, 290 rue de Montigny, Saint-Jerome QC J7Z 5T3; Mon'03; FRCSC; OrthSurg. Staff, Hôtel-Dieu de Saint-Jérôme; (450)431-8200

CARRIER, Michel; 100-347 rue Saint-Georges, Saint-Jerome QC J7Z 5A8; Laval'76; Médecin, Centre Hospitalier Laurentien; (450)432-3303; Fax. (450)432-3099; michelcarrierdr@bellnet.ca.

CARRIER, Michel; Institut de Cardiologie de Mtl, 5000 rue Belanger, Montreal QC H1T 1C8; Sher'78; FRCSC; GenSurg; Cardiovasc&ThorSurg. Consultant, Hôpital Ste-Justine; ac Staff, Institut de Cardiologie de Montréal; (514)376-3330

CARRIER, Pierre; C S S S Charlevoix, B408-303 rue Saint-Etienne, La Malbaie QC G5A 1T1; Laval'74; Dir Prof Services, Hôpital de la Malbaie; Médecin, C S S S Charlvoix; (418)665-1713; Fax. (418)665-1706; pierre.carrier@ssss.gouv.qc.ca.

CARRIER, Pierre; Clinique Med du Coteau, 100-440 boul Saint-Luc, St-Jean-sur-Richel QC J2W 1C1; Mon'88; Staff, Hôpital du Haut-Richelieu; Langs: Bilingual(French/English); (450)359-6819; Fax. (450)359-3247; pcarrier@videotron.ca.

CARRIER, Serge; SMBD Jewish Gen Hosp, E208-3755 ch Cote-Sainte-Cathe, Montreal QC H3T 1E2; Laval'87; FRCSC; Urol (Andrology). Staff, Sir Mortimer B Davis Jewish General; assoc Prof Div of Urol, McGill University; (514)340-8222 x7558; Fax. (514)340-7559.

CARRIER, Simon; Centre Obst/Gyn Loretteville, 250-11000 boul de l'Ormiere, Quebec QC G2B 5S1; Laval'70; FACOG; FSOGC; FRCSC; ObstGyn. ac Staff, Centre Hospitalier Universitaire De Québec - Pavillon De St-françois-d'assise; Chef obst & gyn, Centre Hospitalier Chauveau; (418)842-8419; Fax. (418)842-3246.

CARRIER, Stephane; Clinique Med Hôp de Jonquière, CP 1200 Succ Pdf Jonquiere 2230 rue de l'Hopital, Jonquiere QC G7X 7X2; Sher'83; FRCPC; IntMed (Cardiology). Staff, Centre Hospitalier Jonquiere; (418)695-7700; stephane.carrier@ssss.gouv.qc.ca.

CARRIER, Yves C; Clin Med Du Haut-Madawaska A-809 rue Principale, Clair NB E7A 2H7; Sher'73; Staff, Hôpital regional d'Edmundston; (506)992-0041; Fax. (506)992-0042.

CARRIERE, Benoit; Hôpital Ste-Justine, 3175 ch Cote-Sainte-Catherine, Montreal QC H3T 1C5; Mon'96; FRCPC; Peds. Staff, Hôpital Ste-Justine; (514)345-4931 x2294

CARRIERE, Brigitte; CSSS de Lac-Saint Jean-Est, CP 1300 Succ Bureau-Chef 300 boul Champlain S, Alma QC G8B 5W3; Mon'87; Peds (General Pediatrics). ac Staff, CSSS de Lac-Saint Jean-Est; (418)669-2000 x6662; Fax. (418)662-8003; brigitte.carriere@ssss.gouv.qc.ca.

CARRIERE, Christopher G; CFB Petawawa, PO Box 9999 Stn Main 2 Field Ambulance, Petawawa ON K8H 2X3; Ott'09.

CARRIERE, Isabelle; Clinique Med Vieux Aylmer, 101-204 ch d'Aylmer, Gatineau QC J9H 1A1; Ott'10; CCFP; (819)682-5464

CARRIERE, Jacques; Inst U en Sante Mentale de QC, 2601 de la Canardière, Quebec QC G1J 2G3; Ott'79; FRCPC; Psy. Staff, Institut Universitaire Sante; Langs: English; French; (418)663-5000

CARRIERE, Marc; Clinique Ophtalmologie Alma, 209 av Du Pont S, Alma QC G8B 2T7; Sher'89; FRCSC; Ophth. (418)668-2234; Fax. (418)668-0988.

CARRIERE, Nicole; CSST-Dir des Services Medicaux, 1199 rue De Bleury, Montreal QC H3B 3J1; Mon'76; Psy. (514)906-3003 x2323; Fax. (514)906-3001.

CARRIM, Ebrahim; Torbay Mall Med Clinic, 141 Torbay Rd, St. John's NL A1A 2H1; RCSI (Ireland)'75; MB BS; (709)579-4400; Fax. (709)579-2929.

CARROLL, Alan M; Glenrose Rehab Hosp, 327-10230 111 Ave NW, Edmonton AB T5G 0B7; Dublin (Ireland)'68; DPM; MRCPsy; FRCPC; Psy (Child Psychiatry). Dir Child & Family Psy, Glenrose Rehabilitation Hospital; Dir ChildPsy, Royal Alexandra Hospital; Clin Prof, University of Alberta; (780)735-7939; Fax. (780)735-8246.

CARROLL, Allison B; Children's & Women's HC of BC, 215-4480 Oak St, Vancouver BC V6H 3N1; Mem'06; Critical Care Medicine; Peds. Staff, BC Children's Hospital; (604)875-2345

CARROLL, Bronwyn N; Nipawin Medical Group, PO Box 2135 200 1st Ave E, Nipawin SK S0E 1E0; (306)862-4626; Fax. (306)862-3522.

CARROLL, Bryan W; Family Medical Village, 209-197 Talbot St W, Leamington ON N8H 1N8; Wes'69; BA; ABOG; ObstGyn (Gynecology). Staff, Leamington District Memorial Hospital; Physician, Women's Health Care Centre; (519)326-2910; Fax. (519)326-7824.

CARROLL, Cathie W; Mill Cove Plaza, 207-967 Bedford Hwy, Bedford NS B4A 1A9; Exec Dir, Nova Scotia College of Family Physicians; (902)499-0303; Fax. (902)457-2584.

CARROLL, Cory J; Tottenham Med Centre, PO Box 2000 119 Queen St N, Tottenham ON L0G 1W0; Mem'01; CCFP; (905)936-4211

CARROLL, John R; Rufus Guinchard Health Centre, PO Box 40, Port Saunders NL A0K 4H0; Minnesota (USA)'87; MD.

CARROLL, Julia M; Compass Dermatology, 8-650 Mount Pleasant Rd, Toronto ON M4S 2N5; Dal'01; FRCPC; Derm. (647)351-9277; Fax. (647)351-9077.

CARROLL, June C; Granovsky Gluskin Fam Med Ctre, 4F-60 Murray St Box 25, Toronto ON M5T 3L9; Tor'75; CCFP; FCFP; Staff, Mount Sinai Hospital; Assoc Prof, University of Toronto; (416)586-4800 x5158; Fax. (416)586-3175; jcarroll@mtsinai.on.ca.

CARROLL, Paul J; CLSC Metro, 1801 boul de Maisonneuve O, Montreal QC H3H 1J9; Mon'92; CCFP; Physician, Clinique Urgence Pincourt; Langs: Spanish; (514)934-0354; pjcarroll1998@yahoo.com.

CARRUTHERS, Angela M; Ross Mem Hosp, 10 Angeline St N, Lindsay ON K9V 4M8; Ott'91; BMedSci; CCFP; CCFP(E.M.); Staff, Ross Memorial Hospital; (705)324-6111; Fax. (705)328-6164.

CARRUTHERS, Benjamin C; 6-460 Brant St, Burlington ON L7R 4B6; McM'76; Coroner, Province of Ontario; Med Dir, Reliable Life Insurance Co; (905)639-4214; Fax. (905)639-3935.

CARRUTHERS, D Barry; Worker's Comp Board, 6951 Westminster Hwy, Richmond BC V7C 1C6; Dal'73; FCBOM; CCFP; Physician, Workers' Comp Board of BC; (604)232-8369; Barry.Carruthers@worksafebc.com.

CARRUTHERS, Danny E; 102-535 Belmont Ave W, Kitchener ON N2M 5E9; Wes'71; FSOGC; FACOG; FRCSC; ObstGyn. Chief ObstGyn, Grand River Hospital - Kitchener/Waterloo Health Centre; (519)578-2210; Fax. (519)578-0392.

CARRUTHERS, George H; Parkdale Med Centre, 20 St Peter's Rd, Charlottetown PE C1A 5N1; Dal'91; CCFP; FCFP; (902)894-7087; Fax. (902)894-5012.

CARRUTHERS, J Alastair; Carruthers Dermatology Centre, 820-943 Broadway W, Vancouver BC V5Z 4E1; Oxford (England)'69; BMus; BCh; MA; FRCPC; Derm. Ac Staff, Vancouver General Hospital - Centennial Pavillion; Clin Prof Div of Derm, University of British Columbia; (604)714-0222; Fax. (604)714-0223.

CARRUTHERS, Jean D A; 820-943 Broadway W, Vancouver BC V5Z 4E1; UBC'71; FRCS(Eng); DAB(CosmeticSurg); FRCSC; Ophth (Aesthetic Facial Ophth). Ac Staff, Vancouver General Hospital - Centennial Pavillion; Clin Prof Ophth & Research/Assoc Member, University of British Columbia; (604)714-0222; Fax. (604)714-0223.

CARRUTHERS, Joan M; Oak Bay Family Phys Ltd, 101-1640 Oak Bay Ave, Victoria BC V8R 1B2; UBC'85; (250)598-6744; Fax. (250)598-6778.

CARRUTHERS, Robert G; Surrey Mem Hosp, 13750 96 Ave, Surrey BC V3V 1Z2; Qns'84; FRCPC; Anes. Staff Anes & Pain Med, Surrey Memorial Hospital; (604)588-3367

CARRUTHERS, Robert J; Bayview Med Clinic, 102-1650 Terminal Ave N, Nanaimo BC V9S 0A3; UBC'80; Medical Staff, Nanaimo Regional General Hospital; (250)591-3040; Fax. (250)591-3033.

CARSCADDEN, John A; Hys Med Centre, 202-11010 101 St NW, Edmonton AB T5H 4B9; Alb'02; FRCPC; DiagRad. (780)426-1121

CARSCADDEN, Terence R; Lively Med Centre, 204 Sixth Ave, Lively ON P3Y 1M4; Qns'64; (705)692-4774

CARSLEY, Holly H; Lillian Fraser Mem Hosp, PO Box 40 110 Blair Ave, Tatamagouche NS B0K 1V0; Qns'93; Staff, Lillian Fraser Memorial Hospital / Primary Health Care Centre; (902)657-2382; Fax. (902)657-3745.

CARSLEY, John K; Vancouver Coastal Hlth Authori, 800-601 Broadway W, Vancouver BC V5Z 4C2; McG'77; MSc(Epidem&Biostat.); FRCPC; CommunMed;CCFP; FCFP; Public Health & Preventive Med. Med Officer of Hlth, Vancouver Coastal Health; Langs: French; (604)675-3863

CARSON, B G Craig; Halton Hills Family Health Team, 204-99 Sinclair Ave, Georgetown ON L7G 5G1; McM'95; CCFP; FCFP; (905)873-3344

CARSON, Brent J W; Madrona Imaging Westhill Ctre, A-1804 Bowen Rd, Nanaimo BC V9S 5W4; Alb'87; FRCPC; DiagRad. (250)753-4351; Fax. (250)753-0856.

CARSON, Derek L; 33 Fifth St E, Cornwall ON K6H 2L5; Dal'87; Staff, Cornwall Community Hospital - Second Street Site; Staff, Cornwall Community Hospital; (613)936-2106

CARSON, George D; Regina Qu'Appelle HR-Regina, 3C 55-1440 14th Ave, Regina SK S4P 0W5; Qns'68; FACOG; FSOGC; FRCSC; ObstGyn (Maternal Fetal Medicine). Staff, Regina General Hospital; Clin Prof, University of Saskatchewan; (306)766-0540; Fax. (306)766-4453; george.carson@rqhealth.ca.

CARSON, James B; J A Hildes Northern Med Unit, T162-770 Bannatyne Ave, Winnipeg MB R3E 0W3; Man'75; FRCPC; Peds. carsonjb@cc.umanitoba.ca.

CARSON, James D; 255 Main St, Unionville ON L3R 2H3; Tor'80; Dip SportMed; CCFP; FCFP; Staff, The Scarborough Hospital - Birchmount Campus; Staff, Markham Stouffville Hospital; Staff, Sunnybrook Health Sciences Centre; (905)477-0027; Fax. (905)477-0065.

CARSON, John H; Saint John Reg Hosp, PO Box 2100 Stn Main 400 University Ave, Saint John NB E2L 4L2; Dal'73; AB; FRCPC; RadOncol (Lung). Staff, Saint John Regional Hospital; Assoc Prof, Dalhousie University; (506)648-6884 x7407; Fax. (506)648-6880; john.carson@horizonnb.ca.

CARSON, Joseph M; 201-300 Veterans Blvd NE, Airdrie AB T4B 3P2; (Ireland)'83; (403)948-4168

CARSON, Julie-Ann; Calgary Lab Services, 9-3535 Research Rd NW, Calgary AB T2L 2K8; Man'03; FRCPC; MedMicrobiol. Staff, Calgary Laboratory Services; (403)770-3338

CARSON, Katharine D; Conroy Med Centre, 100-2 Lorry Greenberg Dr, Ottawa ON K1G 5H6; Ott'82; CCFP; FCFP; Langs: English; French; (613)737-0654; Fax. (613)737-3265.

CARSON, Margaret E; 105-599 Main St, Hampton NB E5N 6C2; Dal'06; (506)832-2900

CARSON, Rachel C C; 11-1599 Dufferin Cres, Nanaimo BC V9S 5L5; Qns'99; BEng; FRCPC; IntMed (End of Life Care); Nephrol. Site Chief Nephrology/Staff, Nanaimo Regional General Hospital; (250)591-1895; Fax. (250)591-1897.

CARSON, Sharon K; 4-700 Guelph Line, Burlington ON L7R 3M8; Tor'96; FRCPC; Peds. (289)288-0061

CARSTENS, Derek J; Kitimat Gen Hosp & Health Ctr, 920 Lahakas Blvd S, Kitimat BC V8C 2S3; Stellenbosch (South Africa)'84; MB ChB; LMCC; Staff, Kitimat Hospital & Health Centre; (250)632-2121

CARSTENSEN, H Michael; Stratford Gen Hosp, 46 General Hospital Dr, Stratford ON N5A 2Y6; Mem'08; Staff, Stratford General Hospital - Huron Perth Healthcare Alliance; (519)272-8210

CARSTONIU, Jan K; Headache & Pain Management, 101-124 Merton St, Toronto ON M4S 2Z2; Cal'83; FRCPC; Anes (Chronic Pain Management). Langs: French; (416)322-7539; Fax. (416)322-6935; nopain06@rogers.com.

CARSWELL, Brian A; Alder Med Centre, 277 Evergreen Rd, Campbell River BC V9W 5Y4; Alb'74; Ac Staff, Campbell River & District General Hospital; (250)287-7441; Fax. (250)287-4384.

CARSWELL, David J; The Harrow Clinic, PO Box 100 32 Munger St W, Harrow ON N0R 1G0; Wes'70; Ac Staff, Hôtel-Dieu Grace Hospital; Langs: Bilingual(French/English); (519)738-3555; Fax. (519)738-3990.

CARTAGENA, Ricardo A; The Brandon Clinic, 620 Dennis St, Brandon MB R7A 5E7; (El Salvador)'79; FRCPC; IntMed. (204)728-4440; Fax. (204)726-1765.

CARTAN, Stephen J; Medical Clinic Bldg, 215-89 Humber College Blvd, Etobicoke ON M9V 4B8; Tor'69; OrthSurg. Staff, William Osler Health System - Etobicoke General Hospital; (416)745-8793; Fax. (416)745-9987.

CARTER, Alexandra J E; Queen Elizabeth II HSC-Halifax, 3021-1796 Summer St, Halifax NS B3H 3A7; Wes'01; FRCPC; EmergMed. Staff, Queen Elizabeth II Health Sciences Centre - Halifax Infirmary Site; (902)473-2164; Fax. (902)473-3617.

CARTER, Allister W; Pleasant Street Med Clinic, 1-250 Pleasant St, Miramichi NB E1V 1Y5; Dal'71; BSc; (506)622-3231; Fax. (506)622-5866.

CARTER, Beverley A; Health & Community Services, PO Box 8700 Stn A 57 Margaret's Pl, St. John's NL A1B 4J6; Mem'89; FRCPC; AnatPath. Dir Path & Lab Med, Province of Newfoundland & Labrador; (709)729-2300

CARTER, Cedric J; UBC Hospital, 2211 Wesbrook Mall, Vancouver BC V6T 2B5; London (England)'69; MB BS; FRCP(Lond); FRCPC; IntMed; Hem. Ac Staff Path, UBC Hospital - Koerner Pavillion; (604)822-7275; cjcarter@mail.ubc.ca.

CARTER, Christine M; 3-11220 76 Ave NW, Edmonton AB T6G 0K1; Alb'92; FRCPC; Psy (Psychotherapy). Staff, University of Alberta Hospital; (780)988-4206; Fax. (780)758-6378.

CARTER, Christopher J; CSSSG-Hop de Hull, 116 boul Lionel-Emond, Gatineau QC J8Y 1W7; Qns'74; BSc; FRCSC; OrthSurg. Staff, Hull Hospital; Langs: English; French; (819)966-6200; Fax. (819)595-6326.

CARTER, Clifford S; Garneau Prof Centre, 401-11044 82 Ave NW, Edmonton AB T6G 0T2; Alb'71; BSc; FRCSC; Otol. Ac Staff, University of Alberta Hospital; Ac Staff, Royal Alexandra Hospital; Prog Dir Div of Otol/Clin Prof, University of Alberta; (780)433-1996; Fax. (780)439-2789; cscarter@telusplanet.net.

CARTER, Diana M G; BC Women's Hosp & Health Ctre, RMH-4500 Oak St, Vancouver BC V6H 3N1; London (England)'73; MB BS; FRCPC; Psy (Reproductive Psy). Court Staff Psy, Providence Health Care - St Paul's Hospital; Staff, BC Women's Hospital & Health Centre; Clin Assoc Prof Psy, University of British Columbia; (604)875-2025; Fax. (604)875-3115; dcarter@cw.bc.ca.

CARTER, Erin; Women's College Hosp, 946-76 Grenville St, Toronto ON M5S 1B2; McM'05; BEd; BA(Hons); Psy. Staff Women's Mental Health Prog, Women's College Hospital; Lecturer, University of Toronto; (416)323-6400; Fax. (416)323-6356.

CARTER, J Ann; Atwood Med Clinic, 101-143 Fourth Ave S, Williams Lake BC V2G 1J8; UBC'81; BSc; Anesthetist, Cariboo Memorial Hospital and Health Centre; Langs: German; (250)398-5162; Fax. (250)398-5673; ann_carter@telus.net.

CARTER, James W; Regina Qu'Appelle HR-Regina, 1440 14th Ave, Regina SK S4P 0W5; Dal'77; FRCSC; GenSurg (Oncology). Staff, Regina General Hospital; Clin Assoc Prof, University of Saskatchewan; (306)766-6911; Fax. (306)766-6917.

CARTER, John E; Dartmouth Gen Hosp, 325 Pleasant St, Dartmouth NS B2Y 4G8; Dal'99; CCFP; CCFP(E.M.); Staff, Dartmouth General Hospital; (902)465-8300

CARTER, John R H; Chaparral Corner Plaza, 216-10 Chaparral Dr SE, Calgary AB T2X 3R7; Sask'98; LMCC; CCFP; (403)201-3003; Fax. (403)201-3009.

CARTER, Julia H G; Gulf Canada Square, 370-401 9 Ave SW, Calgary AB T2P 3C5; Cal'94; BSc(Hon); CCFP; FCFP; (403)221-4467; Fax. (403)221-4442.

CARTER, Kerryn J; Alberta Children's Hosp, 2888 Shaganappi Trail NW, Calgary AB T3B 6A8; (New Zealand)'95; Staff, Alberta Children's Hospital; (403)955-7810

CARTER, Kevin C A; Queensway-Carleton Hosp, 3045 Baseline Rd, Ottawa ON K2H 8P4; Tor'01; CCFP; Staff, Queensway Carleton Hospital; (613)721-2000

CARTER, Linda J; Walk-In Med Clinic, 9368 Southfort Dr, Fort Saskatchewan AB T8L 0C5; Alb'96; CCFP; (780)997-0177; Fax. (780)992-2065.

CARTER, Lorna J; Dartmouth Med Centre, 44-46 Portland St, Dartmouth NS B2Y 1H4; Dal'79; CCFP; FCFP; Staff, Dartmouth General Hospital; (902)465-4534; Fax. (902)464-4908.

CARTER, Melissa T; The Hosp for Sick Children, 555 University Ave, Toronto ON M5G 1X8; McM'04; MSc; BSc; FRCPC; MedGenetics (Clinical Genetics). Consultant Child Development, Holland Bloorview Kids Rehabilitation Hospital; Staff, The Hospital For Sick Children; (416)813-6390; Fax. (416)813-5345; mcarter@hollandbloorview.ca.

CARTER, Michael D; 200-550 West Ave, Kelowna BC V1Y 4Z4; UBC'84; FRCSC; Urol (Male Infertility). (250)469-7763; Fax. (250)763-8220.

CARTER, Michael G R; UBC Hospital, 2211 Wesbrook Mall, Vancouver BC V6T 2B5; Liverpool (England)'71; DCH(Eng); MRC; DObstRCOG; MCFP(EM); Staff, UBC Hospital - Koerner Pavillion; Ac Staff, Vancouver General Hospital - Centennial Pavillion; Clinical Asst Prof EmergMed, University of British Columbia; (604)822-7662; Fax. (604)822-7573.

CARTER, Norma C; Dixon Medical, 101-531 Davis Dr, Newmarket ON L3Y 6P5; Qns'02; CCFP; (905)830-9933; Fax. (905)830-0154.

CARTER, Robert B; 3132 50A Ave, Sylvan Lake AB T4S 1A7; Alb'73; PlasSurg. Staff, Red Deer Regional Hospital Centre; (403)887-7366

CARTER, Robert M; 611 Wonderland Rd N, London ON N6H 4V6; Mem'00; (519)471-6686

CARTER, Robert T M; Gateway Med Clinic, 950-3803 Gateway Blvd NW, Edmonton AB T6J 7A9; Alb'80; CCFP; Ac Staff, Covenant Health - Grey Nuns Community Hospital; Clinical Asst Prof, University of Alberta; (780)436-7240; Fax. (780)436-8142.

CARTER, Robin G; Carman Community Health Centre, PO Box 1570, Carman MB R0G 0J0; Man'75; CCFP; FCFP.

CARTER, Teresa A; McMaster University, 1280 Main St W, Hamilton ON L8S 4K1; London (England)'83; FRCPC; Peds. Staff, Hamilton Health Sciences Centre - McMaster Children's Hospital; Teach Staff, McMaster University; (905)521-2100 x73508

CARTER, W Joel; Near North Med Clinic, 201-66 Josephine St, North Bay ON P1B 0A7; Ott'95; BSc; CCFP; Staff, North Bay Regional Health Centre - Regional Mental Health; Site Coord FamMed Residency, Northern Ontario School of Medicine; Asst Prof, Northern Ontario School of Medicine-Laurentian University; (705)495-2685; Fax. (705)495-4128.

CARTHY, J Michael; Glover Med Clinic, 101-5796 Glover Rd, Langley BC V3A 4H9; Qns'71; AB; FRCPC; EmergMed. (604)530-3233; Fax. (604)534-4580.

CARTIER, Andre; Hop du Sacre-Coeur de Mtl, 5400 boul Gouin O, Montreal QC H4J 1C5; Mon'74; FAAAAI; FRCPC; Respir (Asthma). Staff Chest Phys, Hôpital du Sacre-Coeur de Montréal; Clin Prof Med, Universite de Montreal; Langs: English; (514)338-2162; Fax. (514)338-3699; andre.cartier@umontreal.ca.

CARTIER, Benoit; CSSS du Suroît, 150 rue Saint-Thomas, Salaber-de-Valleyf QC J6T 6C1; Mon'81; GenSurg (P.Q.). ac Staff Vasc & GenSurg, Centre Hospitalier Régional du Suroît; (450)371-9920; bcartier@sympatico.ca.

CARTIER, Georges-Etienne; Hop Louis-H Lafontaine, 1237-7401 rue Hochelaga, Montreal QC H1N 3M5; Mon'65; Psy (P.Q.) (Emergency Consultant). Staff, Hopital Louis-H Lafontaine; adj Prof, Universite de Montreal; (514)251-4000 x3385

CARTIER, Kim; Centre Prof Belanger, 402-3871 rue Belanger, Montreal QC H1X 3M7; Mon'01; (514)722-1166; Fax. (514)722-6022.

CARTIER, Louis-Jacques; The Moncton Hosp, 135 MacBeath Ave, Moncton NB E1C 6Z8; Laval'94; CSPQ; FRCPC; MedBiochem. Staff, The Moncton Hospital; (450)759-8222 x2617

CARTIER, Marie; GMF Centre Med du Parc, 101-84 rue Court, Granby QC J2G 4Y5; Mon'97; Staff, Centre Hospitalier de Granby; Langs: Spanish; English; (450)375-1161; Fax. (450)375-7740.

CARTIER, Pierre; CSSS de Saint-Jerome, 290 rue de Montigny, Saint-Jerome QC J7Z 5T3; Mon'71; MSc; FRCPC; IntMed; Nephrol (P.Q.). ac Membre, Hôtel-Dieu de Saint-Jérôme; assoc Membre, Centre Hospitalier La Sarre; assoc Membre, CSSS d'Antoine-Labelle; assoc Membre, Hôpital du Sacre-Coeur de Montréal; assoc Membre, CSSS de Rouyn-Noranda; Prof, Universite de Montreal; Langs: Bilingual(English/French); (450)431-8420; Fax. (450)431-8743; pcartier47@sympatico.ca.

CARTIER, Raymond; Institut de Cardiologie de Mtl, 5000 rue Belanger, Montreal QC H1T 1C8; Mon'79; FRCSC; GenSurg (Cardiovascular Surgery); Cardiovasc&ThorSurg; VascSurg. Ac Staff Cardiac Surg, Institut de Cardiologie de Montréal; Clin Prof Surg, Universite de Montreal; Langs: Bilingual(French/English); (514)376-3330 x3715; Fax. (514)593-2157; rc2910@aol.com.

CARTIER, Richard; CLSC Arthur Buies, 1000 rue Labelle, Saint-Jerome QC J7Z 5N6; Mon'87; (450)431-8001

CARTIER, Yannick; Hop du Sacre-Coeur de Mtl, 5400 boul Gouin O, Montreal QC H4J 1C5; Mon'92; FRCPC; DiagRad. Staff, Hôpital du Sacre-Coeur de Montréal; (514)338-2222 x2853; Fax. (514)338-3541.

CARTOTTO, Robert C; Sunnybrook Hlth Sciences Ctre, D712-2075 Bayview Ave, Toronto ON M4N 3M5; Qns'86; FRCSC; PlasSurg (Burns). Ac Staff Ross Tilley Burn Unit, Sunnybrook Health Sciences Centre; Assoc Prof, University of Toronto; (416)480-6706; Fax. (416)480-6708.

CARTWRIGHT, Pierre; Clinique Med de L'Archipel, 3-539 ch Principal, Cap-aux-Meules QC G4T 1E7; Laval'88; Staff, Hôpital de l'Archipel; Langs: Bilingual(French/English); (418)986-6768; Fax. (418)986-6848.

CARULEI, Victor A; PO Box 220, Assiniboia SK S0H 0B0; Cape Town (South Africa)'75; MB ChB; Staff, Assiniboia Union Hospital; (306)642-3364; vcarulei@fhr.ca.

CARUSO, Andrew; Keele Med Place, 301-2830 Keele St, North York ON M3M 3E5; Tor'74; Sr Staff, Humber River Regional Hospital - Church Street Site; (416)630-1615; Fax. (416)630-5720.

CARUSO, Andrew; Sudbury Reg Hosp-Laurentian, 41 Ramsey Lake Rd, Sudbury ON P3E 5J1; Wes'95; CCFP; CCFP(E.M.); Staff, Health Sciences North-Laurentian Site; (705)675-4700

CARVALHAL, Adriana S; St Michael's Hosp, 17 042-30 Bond St, Toronto ON M5B 1W8; De Pelotas (Brazil)'90; Staff, St Michael's Hospital; (416)864-6337; Fax. (416)864-5480.

CARVALHO, Anna-Maria; MUHC-Montreal Gen Hosp, B2 117 3-1650 av Cedar, Montreal QC H3G 1A4; UBC'00; FRCPC; EmergMed. Staff, McGill University Health Centre - Montreal General Campus; (514)934-1934 x42501

CARVALHO, George F; MUHC-Royal Victoria Hosp, S5 05-687 av des Pins O, Montreal QC H3A 1A1; Wes'00; CSPQ; FRCPC; Anes. Staff, McGill University Health Centre - Royal Victoria Hospital; (514)934-1934 x34880

CARVALHO, Gustavo J; Ackroyd Medical Centre, 135-8291 Ackroyd Rd, Richmond BC V6X 3K5; Alb'88; BSc; (604)276-9550; gjcarvalhomd@aol.com.

CARVALHO, Jean-Christopher; CSSS de Rimouski-Neigette, CP 3150 Succ A 150 av Rouleau, Rimouski QC G5L 5T1; Sher'03; FRCPC; IntMed; Cardiol. Staff, Hôpital Regional Rimouski; (418)724-3000

CARVALHO, Jose C A; Mount Sinai Hosp, 781-600 University Ave, Toronto ON M5G 1X5; Sao Paulo (Brazil)'78; FRCPC; Anes. Staff, Mount Sinai Hospital; (416)586-4800

CARVALHO, Preston M M A; William Osler HC-Brampton, 2100 Bovaird Dr E, Brampton ON L6R 3J7; London (England)'81; MB BS; MRC; FRCR; FRCPC; DiagRad. Staff, William Osler Health System - Brampton Civic Hospital; (905)494-2120 x58627

CARVALHO, Raul A J; Steveston Med Group, 204-3811 Chatham St, Richmond BC V7E 2Z4; RCS (Ireland)'71; Ac Staff, Richmond Hospital; Ac Staff, Providence Health Care - Mount Saint Joseph Hospital; Ac Staff, Providence Health Care - St Vincent's Hospital-Langara Site; Ac Staff, Providence Health Care - Holy Family Hospital; Clin Teacher Family Practice, University of British Columbia; Langs: Portuguese; Swahili; (604)277-7166; Fax. (604)277-3811; rcarvalho@providencehealth.bc.ca.

CARVER, Daniel J; 2605-5955 Veterans Memorial La, Halifax NS B3H 2E1; Dal'86; FRCPC; IntMed; GeriatricMed. Asst Prof, Dalhousie University; (902)473-2561; Fax. (902)473-7133.

CARVER, Glenn E; 375 Daniel St S, Arnprior ON K7S 3K6; Ott'69; (613)623-7773

CARVER, Rachel D; Group One Med Associates, 1111 Springfield Rd, Kelowna BC V1Y 8R7; Dal'79; Med Staff, Kelowna General Hospital; (250)762-4006; Fax. (250)762-4290; drrcarver@groupmedical.ca.

CARY, Paul S; 86 St Andrews St, Cambridge ON N1S 1M4; London (England)'70; MB BS; MRCS; LRCP; DObstRCOG; (519)623-3200; Fax. (519)623-3200.

CASACALENDA, Nicola; Inst of Commun & Family Psy, 4333 ch Cote-Sainte-Catherine, Montreal QC H3T 1E4; Sher'92; FRCPC; Psy. Staff, Sir Mortimer B Davis Jewish General; McGill University; Langs: French; Italian; (514)340-8210; ncasacal@icfp.jgh.mcgill.ca.

CASALE, Joseph A; Queenston Med & Dental Centre, 205-631 Queenston Rd, Hamilton ON L8K 6R5; Qns'76; CCFP; Ac Staff, St Joseph's Healthcare - Charlton Campus; (905)573-7878; Fax. (905)573-6594; drjcasale@gmail.com.

CASALE, Maria; Univ of Guelph Student Hlth Se, 50 Stone Rd E, Guelph ON N1G 2W1; Ott'98; BSc; CCFP; Physician Student's Health Services, University Of Guelph; Langs: Italian; Spanish; (519)824-4120; Fax. (519)836-7431.

CASAUBON, Leanne K; Univ Hlth Network-Toronto Western Hosp, WW5 448-399 Bathurst St, Toronto ON M5T 2S8; Dal'99; MSc; FRCPC; Neur (Stroke). Staff Neurologist, Toronto Western Hospital - University Health Network; Asst Prof Med, University of Toronto; Langs: Bilingual(French/English); (416)603-5685; Fax. (416)603-5768.

CASAULT, David J R; CFHSTC Banting Coy-CFB Borden, PO Box 1000 Stn Forces, Borden ON L0M 1C0; Ott'04; CCFP.

CASE, Allison M; Royal University Hosp, 4544-103 Hospital Dr, Saskatoon SK S7N 0W8; Tor'93; BSc; FRCSC; ObstGyn. Dir Assisted Reproduction Unit & Active Staff, Royal University Hospital; Assoc Prof, University of Saskatchewan; (306)966-1953; Fax. (306)966-8040; allison.case@usask.ca.

CASE, Bruce W; MUHC-Montreal Gen Hosp, C3 165-1650 av Cedar, Montreal QC H3G 1A4; McG'72; CSPQ; MSc(Epidem); DOHS; FRCPC; AnatPath (Epidemiology). Asst Pathologist, McGill University Health Centre - Montreal General Campus; assoc Prof Path/assoc Membre Epidemiol/Biostatistics/Occupational Health, McGill University; Teach Staff Environmental Epidemiol, Universite de Montreal; Prof Environmental Epidemiol, Institut Armand Frappier; Langs: French; (514)934-1934 x44398

CASELLA, Luigi; St Michael's Hosp, 3 052-30 Bond St, Toronto ON M5B 1W8; Naples (Italy)'53; FACC; FRCPC; IntMed (Cardiology). Staff, St Michael's Hospital; Langs: Italian; Spanish; (416)864-5394; Fax. (416)864-5472.

CASELLA, Tesha E; Lakeridge Health Port Perry, 451 Paxton St, Port Perry ON L9L 1L9; McM'10; CCFP; (905)985-7321

CASEY, Alan R; The Rehabilitation Centre, RR141-800 Sherbrook St, Winnipeg MB R3A 1M4; Sask'96; FRCPC; PhysMed&Rehab. Staff, The Rehabilitation Centre; (204)787-2270; acasey@cc.umanitoba.ca.

CASEY, Ann P; St Clare's Mercy Hosp, 154 Lemarchant Rd, St. John's NL A1C 5B8; Mem'78; FRCPC; Anes. Staff Anes, St Clare's Mercy Hospital; (709)777-5520

CASEY, Brett M; BC Women's Hosp & Health Ctre, 2J40-4500 Oak St, Vancouver BC V6H 3N1; Texas (USA)'87; (604)875-2852; Fax. (604)875-2707; bcasey@cw.bc.ca.

CASEY, Carmel; Gander Med Clinic, 177 Elizabeth Dr, Gander NL A1V 1H6; Mem'88; CCFP; FCFP; (709)256-7101; Fax. (709)256-7109.

CASEY, Carolyn; 291 Donlands Ave, East York ON M4J 3R5; Dal'93; Fax. (416)510-6870.

CASEY, Deborah K; Univ Hlth Network-Toronto Western Hosp, E7 457-399 Bathurst St, Toronto ON M5T 2S8; McG'07; MDCM; FRCPC; IntMed; Respir. Staff, Toronto Western Hospital - University Health Network; (416)603-2581

CASEY, J Stephanie; Dawson Center Level 2, 197 Dufferin St, Bridgewater NS B4V 2G9; Dal'82; FRCPC; Psy (Eating Disorders). Staff Psy, IWK Health Centre; (902)543-5400; Fax. (902)527-5292; stephanie.casey@iwk.ns.health.ca.

CASEY, Janel B; 4F-260 Sherbrooke St, New Westminster BC V3L 3M2; UBC'06; FRCPC; Psy. (604)520-4662

CASEY, Linda M; Children's & Women's HC of BC, K4 218-4480 Oak St, Vancouver BC V6H 3V4; Alb'84; FRCPC; Peds. Staff, BC Children's Hospital; (604)875-2345 x5113

CASEY, Maitias D; Avon Med Centre, 2781 Avonhurst Dr, Regina SK S4R 3J3; National (Ireland)'67; Ac Staff, Pasqua Hospital; Ac Staff, Regina General Hospital; (306)543-4955; Fax. (306)545-7006.

CASEY, Michael J; 106-501 Krug St, Kitchener ON N2B 1L3; Qns'79; CCFP; FCFP; Ac Staff, Grand River Hospital - Kitchener/Waterloo Health Centre; Ac Staff, St Mary's General Hospital; (519)742-8866; Fax. (519)742-4757.

CASEY, Michelle; St Lawrence Med Clinic, 1012 Prince St, Lansdowne ON K0E 1L0; Laval'09; CCFP; Langs: Bilingual(English/French); (613)659-2525; Fax. (613)659-2278.

CASEY, Patrick J; Queen Elizabeth II HSC-Halifax, 2288-1796 Summer St, Halifax NS B3H 3A7; Dal'97; FRCSC; GenSurg; VascSurg. Staff, Queen Elizabeth II Health Sciences Centre - Halifax Infirmary Site; (902)473-2829; Fax. (902)473-2841.

CASEY, Richard W; Trafalgar Prof Centre, 407-1235 Trafalgar Rd, Oakville ON L6H 3P1; Wes'77; FRCSC; Urol. Ac Staff, Halton Healthcare Services Corporation - Oakville Site; Ac Staff, The Credit Valley Hospital; (905)842-1393; Fax. (905)338-3150; drcasey@malehealth.com.

CASEY, Robin E; Alberta Children's Hosp, 2888 Shaganappi Trail NW, Calgary AB T3B 6A8; Sask'84; MSc; Staff Med Genetics & Peds, Alberta Children's Hospital; (403)955-7587; Fax. (403)955-3091; tworobins@xplornet.com.

CASEY, William E; Western Mem Reg Hosp, PO Box 2005 Stn Main 1 Brookfield Ave, Corner Brook NL A2H 6J7; Ott'80; FRCPC; DiagRad. Staff, Western Memorial Regional Hospital; (709)637-5000 x5583; Fax. (709)637-5327; billcasey@westernhealth.nl.ca.

CASEY-CAMPBELL, Mildred; CFB 8 Wing Trenton, PO Box 1000 Stn Forces 50 Yukon St, Astra ON K0K 3W0; Mon'09; CCFP; Staff, Canadian Forces Base; (613)392-2811

CASH, Rebecca L; Thistlewood Prof Centre, 207-8077 Islington Ave, Woodbridge ON L4L 7X7; Wes'04; FRCSC; ObstGyn. (905)850-0004; Fax. (905)850-0006.

CASHA, Steven; Foothills Med Centre, 1403 29 St NW, Calgary AB T2N 2T9; Tor'93; FRCSC; Neursurg (Spine). Staff, Foothills Medical Centre; (403)944-3405; Fax. (403)283-2270.

CASHIN, Megan S; London HSC-Victoria Campus, PO Box 5010 Stn B 800 Commissioners Rd E, London ON N6A 5W9; Mem'04; FRCSC; OrthSurg. Staff, London Health Sciences Centre - Victoria Campus; (519)658-8500

CASHMAN, Frank E; 120 Eglinton Ave E, Toronto ON M4P 1E2; McG'69; FRCPC; Psy. (416)640-4614; Fax. (647)341-2836; fcashman@smh.toronto.on.ca.

CASHMAN, Neil R; UBC Hosp, F137-2211 Wesbrook Mall, Vancouver BC V6T 2B5; Worchester(MA) (USA)'78; FRCPC; Neur. Staff, UBC Hospital - Koerner Pavillion; (604)822-2135; Fax. (604)822-7299.

CASIANO, Hygiea; Manitoba Adolescent Trmt Ctre, 120 Tecumseh St, Winnipeg MB R3E 2A9; Man'03; FRCPC; Psy. Staff, Manitoba Adolescent Treatment Centre; (204)477-6391; hcasiano@matc.ca.

CASILLA, Vanbric R; Penticton Reg Hosp, 550 Carmi Ave, Penticton BC V2A 3G6; Alb'06; FRCPC; IntMed; Nephrol. Staff, Penticton Regional Hospital; (250)492-4000

CASIMIR-TORDJMAN, Euphrosyne; Douglas Mental Hlth Univ Inst, 6875 boul Lasalle, Verdun QC H4H 1R3; Paris (France)'73; Psy (P.Q.). Staff, Douglas Mental Health University Institute; (514)761-6131

CASIRO, Oscar G; Univ of Victoria Med Sciences, PO Box 1700 Stn CSC, Victoria BC V8W 2Y2; Buenos Aires (Argentina)'74; FRCPC; Peds (Neonatology). Staff, Victoria General Hospital; Prof, University of Victoria; Reg Associate Dean Vancouver Island Faculty of Med/Prof, University of British Columbia; Langs: Spanish; (250)472-5500; Fax. (250)472-5505; impadmin@uvic.ca.

CASKEY, Elizabeth R B; Kanata North Med Centre, 832 March Rd, Kanata ON K2W 0C9; Tor'97; CCFP; (613)599-5599; Fax. (613)599-1005.

CASKEY, William A; White Clinic Associates, 100-383 Ellis St, Penticton BC V2A 4L9; Tor'74; Staff, Penticton Regional Hospital; (250)492-3024; Fax. (250)492-2761.

CASOLA, Paul G; 510-586 Eglinton Ave E, Toronto ON M4P 1P2; Tor'84; BSc(Hons Biochem); PhD(Biochem); ASAM; FRCPC; Psy (Addiction Medicine). Court Staff, Centre for Addiction & Mental Health (CAMH) - Russell Street Site; Court Staff, St Michael's Hospital; Med Dir, Salvation Army Harbour Light Centre; Psychiatrist/Consultant, Salvation Army Addictions & Rehabilitation Centre; Lecturer Psy, University of Toronto; (416)277-8361

CASPAR-BELL, Gudrun M; Royal University Hosp, 3654-103 Hospital Dr, Saskatoon SK S7N 0W8; Staff, Royal University Hospital; (306)966-2044; Fax. (306)966-7926.

CASPARI, David A; Medcan Health Mgmt Inc, 1500-150 York St, Toronto ON M5H 3S5; Tor'76; FACP; AB; FRCPC; EmergMed (Internal Medicine). Staff, Medcan Health Management Inc; (416)350-5684

CASPER, Robert F J; Toronto Ctre Adv Reprod Tech, 210-150 Bloor St W, Toronto ON M5S 2X9; Wes'73; FRCSC; ObstGyn (Reproductive Endocrinology). Prof ObstGyn, University of Toronto; (416)972-0777; Fax. (416)972-0036.

CASPERS, Jennifer M; Guelph Med Place, 202-83 Dawson Rd, Guelph ON N1H 1B1; McM'81; CCFP; Court Staff, Homewood Health Centre; Chief FamilyMed, Guelph General Hospital; (519)767-1512; Fax. (519)767-1513; jcaspers@rogers.com.

CASPIN, Shirley L; 303-294 Main St, Toronto ON M4C 4X5; McG'77; CCFP; FCFP; Staff Family Pract, Toronto East General Hospital Inc; Langs: Bilingual(English/French); (416)699-2667; Fax. (416)699-8791.

CASS, Aaron I; Surrey Med Arts Bldg, 113-13798 94A Ave, Surrey BC V3V 1N1; Ott'98; FRCPC; IntMed; Nephrol. (604)582-6606

CASS, Daniel E; Office of the Chief Coroner, 2F-26 Grenville St, Toronto ON M7A 2G9; Tor'88; FRCPC; EmergMed. Assoc Prof Med, University of Toronto; (416)314-6808; Fax. (416)212-1797; das.cass@ontario.ca.

CASS, J Charles; 312-200 St Clair Ave W, Toronto ON M4V 1R1; Tor'81; (416)968-2277; Fax. (416)968-2270; dr.c.cass@rogers.com.

CASS, William; 1028-790 Bay St Box 50, Toronto ON M5G 1N8; Tor'68; DABIM; BASc; FRCPC; IntMed. Ac Staff Internal Med, Sunnybrook Health Sciences Centre - Holland Orthopaedic & Arthritic Centre; University of Toronto; (416)929-9955; Fax. (416)929-7312.

CASSAM, Humaira; College Square Med Centre, 1980 Baseline Rd, Ottawa ON K2C 0C6; Wes'89; (613)224-6606; Fax. (613)224-6162.

CASSAN, Philippe; Ctr Hosp Reg de Lanaudiere, 1000 boul Sainte-Anne, St-Charles-Brromee QC J6E 6J2; Paris V (France)'78; Staff, Centre Hospitalier Régional de Lanaudière; (450)759-8222; Fax. (450)759-0011.

CASSANO-BAILEY, Alessandra; Health Sciences Centre, 820 Sherbrook St, Winnipeg MB R3A 1R9; Man'05; FRCPC; DiagRad. Staff, Health Sciences Centre; (204)774-8511

CASSAR, Louis J; 200-72 boul Saint-Jean-Baptist, Chateauguay QC J6K 4Y7; McG'53; (450)692-7282

CASSAR, Nagib L; Westmount Med Bldg, 625-5025 rue Sherbrooke O, Montreal QC H4A 1S9; Cairo (Egypt)'61; MB ChB; FACOG; FRCSC; ObstGyn. Staff, McGill University Health Centre - Royal Victoria Hospital; adj Prof, McGill University; (514)481-4728; Fax. (514)481-7744.

CASSAR, Stephen L; Gaslight Plaza, 220-579 3 St SE, Medicine Hat AB T1A 0H2; Cal'87; FRCSC; PlasSurg. Chief Dept of Surg, Medicine Hat Regional Hospital; (403)529-1770; Fax. (403)529-1178.

CASSAR-DEMAJO, Wilfred A; Univ Hlth Network-Toronto Western Hosp, MCL2 411J-399 Bathurst St, Toronto ON M5T 2S8; (Malta)'67; FRCPC; IntMed; Anes. Staff, Toronto Western Hospital - University Health Network; Asst Prof, University of Toronto; (416)603-5800 x2388; Fax. (416)603-1068.

CASSELL, Krista; The Ob/Gyn Suite, 403-199 Grafton St, Charlottetown PE C1A 1L2; Dal'98; BSc(Hon); FRCSC; ObstGyn. Consultant, The Ob/Gyn Suite; (902)629-8801; Fax. (902)629-8826.

CASSELMAN, Charles W; East Kootenay Reg Hosp, 13 24th Ave N, Cranbrook BC V1C 3H9; Tor'92; CCFP; FCFP; Staff, East Kootenay Regional Hospital; (250)426-5281

CASSELMAN, Ronald C; Bayvalley Med Arts Bldg, 502-145 Queenston St, St Catharines ON L2R 2Z9; Wes'67; FRCSC; Urol. Staff Urol, Hotel-Dieu Hospital; Staff Urol, Niagara Health System - St Catharines General Site; (905)687-4004; Fax. (905)687-6664; medi4004@bellnet.ca.

CASSES, Alberto; Georgian Prof Centre, 303-125 Bell Farm Rd, Barrie ON L4M 6L2; Del Rosario (Colombia)'83; FRCSC; OrthSurg (Arthroplasty). Staff, Royal Victoria Regional Health Centre; Staff, Stevenson Memorial Hospital; Langs: Spanish; (705)735-4550; Fax. (705)735-4535.

CASSES, Fernando; 2795 Chelsea Close, West Vancouver BC V7S 3E9; Del Rosario (Colombia)'81; FRCSC; GenSurg. Langs: Spanish; (604)913-1697

CASSIANI, Nadine; Hop Maisonneuve-Rosemont, 5415 boul de l'Assomption, Montreal QC H1T 2M4; Mon'98; Staff, Hopital Maisonneuve-Rosemont; (514)252-3400

CASSIDY, Beverley; Wolfville Prof Centre, 7-4 Little Rd, Wolfville NS B4P 1P4; Dal'90; FRCPC; Psy. (902)542-4392

CASSIDY, Brighid; Lions Gate Hosp, 231 15th St E, North Vancouver BC V7L 2L7; Tor'06; CCFP; CCFP(E.M.); Staff, Lions Gate Hospital; (604)988-3131

CASSIDY, Darby J; 1624 7th Ave, Prince George BC V2L 3P6; Man'03; FRCSC; Urol. (250)596-9180

CASSIDY, Keri-Leigh; Senior's Mental Health, 6516-5909 Veterans Memorial La, Halifax NS B3H 2E2; Dal'96; FRCPC; Psy. (902)473-2927; Fax. (902)473-5713.

CASSIDY, Michael R; Peter Lougheed Centre, 2260-3500 26 Ave NE, Calgary AB T1Y 6J4; Alb'81; FRCPC; Anes. Ac Staff, Peter Lougheed Centre; Clin Associate, University of Calgary; (403)943-5554; Fax. (403)943-4474.

CASSIDY, Myles J A; Children's & Women's HC of BC, 1L7-4480 Oak St, Vancouver BC V6H 3V4; Glasgow (Scotland)'02; Staff, BC Children's Hospital; (604)875-2711

CASSIDY, Walter J; 42 Hanna St E, Windsor ON N8X 2M8; Qns'64; FRCPC; Psy. Chief/Dir Psy, Hôtel-Dieu Grace Hospital; Chief Psy, Windsor Regional Hospital - Metropolitan Site; (519)977-9157; Fax. (519)977-9274.

CASSIE, Scott G; Univ Hlth Network-Toronto Gen, EG001-200 Elizabeth St, Toronto ON M5G 2C4; Cal'07; GenSurg. Staff, Toronto General Hospital - UHN; (416)340-4800

CASSIM, Essop M; Kingston Med Arts Centre, 202-800 Princess St, Kingston ON K7L 5E4; RCS (Ireland)'68; LRCPS(Ire); Physician, Coach Canada; Langs: Afrikaans; Gujarati; (613)544-6455; Fax. (613)544-2621.

CASSIM, Mohamed R H; Lloydminster Hosp, 3820 43rd Ave, Lloydminster SK S9V 1Y5; Natal (South Africa)'81; MB ChB; Staff, Lloydminster Hospital; (306)820-6090; Fax. (306)825-6516.

CASSIM, Nasreen; 547 Michigan St, Victoria BC V8V 1S5; Natal (South Africa)'83; (250)388-6811

CASSIS, Chantal; Hop Jean-Talon, 1385 rue Jean-Talon E, Montreal QC H2E 1S6; McG'03; FRCPC; IntMed; Hem. Staff, CSSS du Coeur de l'Isle Hôpital Jean-Talon; (514)495-6767 x6115

CASSIS, Irene M; 5010 43 St, Red Deer AB T4N 6H2; Alb'85; FRCSC; ObstGyn. Staff/Chief ObstGyn, Red Deer Regional Hospital Centre; (403)342-6377; Fax. (403)342-6479.

CASSIS, Mona; 1269 5 Ave N, Lethbridge AB T1H 0M9; Alb'89; CCFP; (403)328-8507; Fax. (403)381-6920.

CASSITY, Sheri-Lynn E; Foothills Med Centre, 704-1403 29 St NW, Calgary AB T2N 2T9; Alb'01; FRCPC; Psy. Staff, Foothills Medical Centre; (403)944-5872

CASSOFF, Joseph; SMBD Jewish Gen Hosp, 3755 ch Cote-Sainte-Catherine, Montreal QC H3T 1E2; McG'69; FRCPC; DiagRad. Staff, Sir Mortimer B Davis Jewish General; Asst Prof DiagRad, McGill University; (514)340-8222 x3758; Fax. (514)340-7907; jcassoff@rad.jgh.mcgill.ca.

CASSON, Alan G; Saskatoon City Hosp, 2F-701 Queen St, Saskatoon SK S7K 0M7; Manchester (England)'81; MB ChB; MSc(Med.); FACS; FRCSC; GenSurg (Surgical Oncology); ThorSurg. Head Dept of Surg/Staff, Royal University Hospital; Staff, Saskatoon City Hospital; Prof/Dept Head Surg, University of Saskatchewan; (306)655-8997; Fax. (306)655-8269; surgery.dept@usask.ca.

CASSON, R Ian; Family Med Centre, PO Box 8888 Stn Main 220 Bagot St, Kingston ON K7L 5E9; Tor'76; CCFP; CCFP(E.M.); FCFP; Ac Staff, Kingston General Hospital; Ac Staff, Hotel-Dieu Hospital; Asst Prof Family Med, Queen's University; (613)533-9303 x73905; Fax. (613)544-9899.

CASTAGNA, Avril E; Medical Centre, 415-3030 Lawrence Ave E, Scarborough ON M1P 2T7; Dublin (Ireland)'84; MB BCh; BAO; MRCP(Paeds); MD; FRCPC; Neur (Pediatrics). Staff Peds, The Scarborough Hospital - General Campus; (416)431-4848; Fax. (416)431-5940.

CASTAGNA, Luigi A; SGH Medical Mall, 415-3030 Lawrence Ave E, Scarborough ON M1P 2T7; Tor'82; FRCPC; Peds (Behavioural Pediatrics). Staff Peds, The Scarborough Hospital - Birchmount Campus; Langs: Italian; German; Spanish; (416)431-4848; Fax. (416)431-5940.

CASTAN, Rafael E; Centre Med Jean-Talon, 102-1392 rue Jean-Talon E, Montreal QC H2E 1S4; (Dominican Republic)'64; Cardiol (P.Q.). Staff Cardiol Services, CSSS du Coeur de l'Isle Hôpital Jean-Talon; (514)273-2805; Fax. (514)273-8352.

CASTANEDA-BUCCI, Cristina; Medicentre Chomedy, 610 boul Cure-Labelle, Laval QC H7V 2T7; Mon'08; CCFP; (450)687-6452 x231

CASTANO, Roberto; Hop du Sacre-Coeur de Mtl, J.3185-5400 boul Gouin O, Montreal QC H4J 1C5; Bogota (Colombia)'83; Staff, Hôpital du Sacre-Coeur de Montréal; (514)338-2222 x7271; Fax. (514)338-3123; roberto.castano@umontreal.ca.

CASTANO HERRERA, Elkin D; Grand River Hosp-KW Hlth Centr, PO Box 9056 Stn C 835 King St W, Kitchener ON N2G 1G3; Pontificia (Colombia)'93; FRCPC; Anes. Staff, Grand River Hospital - Kitchener/Waterloo Health Centre; (519)744-7361

CASTEL, Helene; CHUM-Hop St-Luc, 1058 rue Saint-Denis, Montreal QC H2X 3J4; Caen (France)'04; Staff, Centre Hospitalier l'Université De Montréal (CHUM) - Hôpital Saint-luc; (514)890-8000

CASTEL, Josette; CLSC-UMF Haue-Ville, 55 ch Sainte-Foy, Quebec QC G1R 1S9; Brest (France)'82; MSc(Epidemiol); CCFP; FCFP; Staff, CSSS Haute-Ville; Prof, Université Laval; (418)641-2572; Fax. (418)641-0282; josette.castel@irdpq.qc.ca.

CASTEL, Saulo; Sunnybrook Hlth Sciences Ctre, FG03-2075 Bayview Ave, Toronto ON M4N 3M5; Sao Paulo (Brazil)'84; FRCPC; Psy (Concurrent Disorders). Dir Inpatient Services, Sunnybrook Health Sciences Centre; Langs: Portuguese; (416)480-6832 x4202; saulo.castel@sunnybrook.ca.

CASTELLI, Mario F; Castelli Endoscopy Clinic, PO Box 11 320-790 Bay St, Toronto ON M5G 1N8; Wes'68; FRCPC; IntMed (Gastroenterology). Langs: Italian; (416)613-5050; Fax. (416)613-5051; info@castelliclinic.com.

CASTELLUCCI, Lana A; The Ottawa Hosp-Civic Campus, 1053 Carling Ave, Ottawa ON K1Y 4E9; Ott'06; FRCPC; IntMed; Critical Care Medicine. Staff, The Ottawa Hospital - Civic Campus; (613)798-5555

CASTIGLIONE, Alberto; All In One Med Clinic, 100-10083 Keele St, Maple ON L6A 3Y8; Tor'93; CCFP; Ac Staff, Mackenzie Richmond Hill Hospital; (905)832-4644; Fax. (905)832-7717.

CASTIGLIONE, John S; 203-1615 Dufferin St, Toronto ON M6H 4H4; McM'73; Court Staff, Humber River Regional Hospital - Keele Street Site; Langs: Italian; (416)656-0080; Fax. (416)656-2010.

CASTILLO, Eliana; HSC-Faculty of Med, 1440-3330 Hospital Dr NW, Calgary AB T2N 4N1; Javeriana (Colombia)'97; FRCPC; IntMed. Langs: Spanish; (403)220-6376; ecastillo@mac.com.

CASTILLO, Guillermo I; 201-540 College St, Toronto ON M6G 1A6; (Mexico)'72; FACS; FRCSC; Otol. Staff, The Scarborough Hospital - General Campus; (416)923-3663

CASTILLO, Heather M; 201 Deacon St, Pembroke ON K8A 2J6; Ott'05; CCFP; (613)732-3422

CASTILLO ABADIA, Maria D; Cedars Professional Park, 2931 66 St NW, Edmonton AB T6K 4C1; (Colombia)'01; Staff, Covenant Health - Grey Nuns Community Hospital; (780)463-4555

CASTILLOUX, Jean-Francois; CHUS-Hop Fleurimont, 300 12 av N, Sherbrooke QC J1H 5N4; Sher'02; FRCPC; IntMed (Hemophilia); MedOncol; Hem. Staff, Centre Hospitalier Universitaire de Sherbrooke-Hopital Fleurimont; Langs: Bilingual(French/English); (819)346-1110 x16236

CASTILLOUX, Julie; Ctr Hosp Univ de Quebec-CHUL, 2705 boul Laurier, Quebec QC G1V 4G2; Laval'02; Gastroent; Peds. Staff, Centre Hospitalier Universitaire de Quebec-CHUL; Langs: Bilingual(French/English); (418)656-4141 x48424; Fax. (418)654-2137.

CASTNER, R Paul; Nanaimo Reg Gen Hosp, 1200 Dufferin Cres, Nanaimo BC V9S 2B7; Tor'84; BSc; MSc; FRCPC; Anes. Staff, Nanaimo Regional General Hospital; Instructor, University of British Columbia; (250)754-2141

CASTONGUAY, Andre; Centre Med de Dolbeau, 1530 rue des Erables, Dolbeau-Mistassini QC G8L 2W7; Laval'71; (418)276-0111; Fax. (418)276-6298.

CASTONGUAY, Benoit; Clinique Med Centre-Ville, 95 av Rouleau, Rimouski QC G5L 5S4; Sher'90; (418)722-6816; Fax. (418)721-3262.

CASTONGUAY, Claude; CLSC-GMF des Deux-Rives, 1200 rue King E, Sherbrooke QC J1G 1E4; Sher'90; Staff Palliative Care, Centre Hospitalier Universitaire de Sherbrooke-Hôpital Hôtel-Dieu; Prof adj clin, Universite de Sherbrooke; (819)563-2572

CASTONGUAY, Danny; Clin Med Familiale Notre-Dame, 2120 rue Sherbrooke E, Montreal QC H2K 1C3; Sher'09; CCFP; (514)527-1958

CASTONGUAY, J D Gilles; A-8371 boul Newman, LaSalle QC H8N 1Y4; Mon'76; (514)366-4280; Fax. (514)363-3231.

CASTONGUAY, Julie; 41 Av Mgr Plourde, Edmundston NB E3V 4M1; Sher'97; LMCC; CCFP; Langs: English; (506)739-4417; Fax. (506)735-5223.

CASTONGUAY, Leslie A; The Doctor's Office, 1011 Upper Middle Rd E, Oakville ON L6H 4L5; UBC'89; (905)849-7007; Fax. (905)849-7883.

CASTONGUAY, Mathieu C; MacKenzie Bldg, 5788 University Ave, Halifax NS B3H 1V8; Dal'06; FRCPC; AnatPath. (902)473-2266; Fax. (902)473-1049.

CASTONGUAY, Stephanie; CSSS de Laval, 1755 boul Rene-Laennec, Laval QC H7M 3L9; Mon'04; FRCPC; MedMicrobiol. Staff, Hopital de la Cite de la santé; (450)668-1010

CASTONGUAY, Vincent; Univ Hlth Network-Princess M, 610 University Ave, Toronto ON M5G 2M9; Laval'04; MedOncol; Hem; IntMed. Fellow, Princess Margaret Hospital - University Health Network; (416)946-2000

CASTOR, Schiller; CSSS du Sud de Lanaudière, 911 montee des Pionniers, Terrebonne QC J6V 2H2; (Haiti)'90; MSc; CCFP; Staff, Centre Hospitalier Pierre le Gardeur; (450)654-7525

CASTRO, Denise A; The Hosp for Sick Children, 555 University Ave, Toronto ON M5G 1X8; Severino Sombra (Brazil)'97; Staff, The Hospital For Sick Children; (416)813-6025

CASTRO-CONTRERAS, Nestor E; Hotel-Dieu de Sorel, 400 av de l'Hotel-Dieu, Sorel-Tracy QC J3P 1N5; University Nacional de Colombia (Colombia)'93; Staff, Hôtel-Dieu de Sorel; (450)746-6000

CASTRODALE, Joseph; Grace Med Centre, 302-2830 Keele St, North York ON M3M 3E5; Tor'76; Ac Staff, Humber River Regional Hospital - Church Street Site; Ac Staff, Humber River Regional Hospital - Finch Avenue Site; Langs: Italian; (416)638-7269; Fax. (416)638-7455.

CASTURA, Christina; Oakmed Family Health Team, 110-231 Oak Park Blvd, Oakville ON L6H 7S8; Qns'05; CCFP; Staff, Halton Healthcare Services Corporation - Oakville Site; (905)901-5111; Fax. (905)901-5122; dr.castura@oakmed.ca.

CASULLO, Joseph; MUHC-Montreal Gen Hosp, 1650 av Cedar, Montreal QC H3G 1A4; McG'85; FRCPC; DiagRad. Staff DiagRad, McGill University Health Centre - Montreal General Campus; (514)934-1934 x42889

CASWELL, Sherri L; Richmond Health Science Ctre, 560-6091 Gilbert Rd, Richmond BC V7C 5L9; UBC'94; FRCPC; IntMed. (604)270-3484

CASWILL, Melissa E; Dr C W Wiebe Medical Centre, 385 Main St, Winkler MB R6W 1J2; Man'06; CCFP; (204)325-4312

CATAFORD, Jean; Centre Med de la Piniere, 100-3395 boul de la Piniere, Terrebonne QC J6X 4N1; Mon'80; (450)477-2683; Fax. (450)477-1234; j_cataford@hotmail.com.

CATANIA, Philip J J; East Street Med Arts Centre, 301-170 East St, Sault Ste. Marie ON P6A 3C6; Wes'79; Assoc Staff, Sault Area Hospital - Sault Ste Marie; (705)541-2313; Fax. (705)759-5936; catania_p@ghc.on.ca.

CATAPHARD, Isabelle; Clinique de l'Oreille Seminair, 300-900 boul du Seminaire N, St-Jean-sur-Richel QC J3A 1C3; Mon'99; FRCSC; Otol. Staff, Hôpital du Haut-Richelieu; (450)376-1300

CATAUDELLA, Julia A; Coxwell Med Bldg, 100-688 Coxwell Ave, Toronto ON M4C 3B7; Qns'01; BSc; CCFP; Court Staff, The Scarborough Hospital - General Campus; (416)465-2868; Fax. (416)465-3538.

CATCHING, John D; The Ottawa Hosp-Gen Campus, 501 Smyth Rd, Ottawa ON K1H 8L6; Wisconsin (USA)'68; FRCPC; Cardiol; IntMed. Staff, The Ottawa Hospital - General Campus; Consultant, Almonte General Hospital; (613)737-8165; Fax. (613)739-6727; jcatching@ottawahospital.on.ca.

CATCHLOVE, Richard F H; Clinique Plaza Cote-des-Neiges, 6700 ch Cote-des-Neiges, Montreal QC H3S 2B2; Sydney (Australia)'63; MB BS; MSc; FFARCS; Sr Staff Anes, McGill University Health Centre - Royal Victoria Hospital; Assoc Prof Anes, McGill University; Langs: English; French; (514)342-2941; rcatch@videotron.ca.

CATELIN, Celine; CHUS-Hop Fleurimont, 3001 12e av N, Sherbrooke QC J1H 5N4; Brest (France)'04; Staff, Centre Hospitalier Universitaire de Sherbrooke-Hopital Fleurimont; (819)346-1110 x13354

CATELLIER, Priscilla; CHUQ-Ctr Hosp Univ Laval, 2705 boul Laurier, Quebec QC G1V 4G2; Laval'90; Respir; Peds. Staff, Centre Hospitalier Universitaire de Quebec-CHUL; (418)656-4141

CATFORD, Erika A; 400-100 Colborne St W, Orillia ON L3V 2Y9; Tor'05; CCFP; (705)330-3520; Fax. (705)330-3521.

CATHERALL, Malcolm S; Red Deer Reg Hosp Centre, PO Box 5030 Stn Postal Box Ctr 3942 50A Ave, Red Deer AB T4N 6R2; Liverpool (England)'72; Staff, Red Deer Regional Hospital Centre; (403)343-4422

CATHERS, Christopher R; Near North Med Clinic, 201-66 Josephine St, North Bay ON P1B 0A7; (Other Foreign)'09; CCFP; Staff, North Bay Regional Health Centre - Regional Mental Health; (705)495-2685

CATO, Shani A; Grey Bruce HS-Owen Sound, PO Box 1800 Stn Main 8228-1800 8th St E, Owen Sound ON N4K 6M9; Mona Campus (Jamaica)'98; MB BS; FAAP; FRCPC; Peds. Staff, Grey Bruce Health Services - Owen Sound; (519)376-2121

CATON, Brent W; Royal Jubilee Hosp, 1952 Bay St, Victoria BC V8R 1J8; Alb'97; FRCPC; Anes. Staff, Royal Jubilee Hospital; (250)370-8441

CATONA, Tamara; 301-1676 Martin Dr, Surrey BC V4A 6E7; Bucharest (Romania)'73; MD; FRCPC; Psy (General Adult Psychiatry). Staff, Peace Arch Hospital; Langs: Romanian; Italian; (604)535-1338

CATRE, Melanio G; 304-840 Coxwell Ave, East York ON M4C 5T2; Tor'93; BSc; MSc; FRCSC; OrthSurg (Sports Medicine). Staff, Toronto East General Hospital Inc; Lecturer Orth, University of Toronto; Langs: Tagalog; (416)461-4761; Fax. (416)461-5574.

CATTAN, Candice; Lakeshore Gen Hosp, 160 av Stillview, Pointe-Claire QC H9R 2Y2; Laval'99; FRCPC; Psy. Staff, Lakeshore General Hospital - Pointe Claire; (514)630-2225

CATTAN, Edward F E; 6-2530 St. Joseph Blvd, Orleans ON K1C 1G1; Alexandria (Egypt)'77; CSPQ; FRCPC; Psy (Psycho Pharmacology). Staff, Montfort Hospital; Langs: French; Arabic; Italian; (613)830-1004; Fax. (613)830-9689.

CATTANEO, Matteo; Burris Clinic, 300-275 Lansdowne St, Kamloops BC V2C 6J3; Stellenbosch (South Africa)'92; MB ChB; CCFP; (250)372-3303; Fax. (250)377-7300.

CATTANI, Lynnsey A; Concordia Health Associates, 102-1155 Concordia Ave, Winnipeg MB R2K 2M9; Man'09; CCFP; (204)654-6030

CATTON, Charles N; Univ Hlth Network-Princess M, 5 991-610 University Ave, Toronto ON M5G 2M9; Ott'76; ABIM; AB(T); FRCPC; IntMed (Genito Urinary Oncology); RadOncol. Staff, Princess Margaret Hospital - University Health Network; Prof, University of Toronto; (416)946-2121; Fax. (416)946-4586; charles.catton@rmp.uhn.on.ca.

CATTON, Lienne L; Timmins & District Hosp, 700 Ross Ave E, Timmins ON P4N 8P2; McM'04; CCFP; CCFP(E.M.); Staff, Timmins & District Hospital; (705)267-2131

CATTON, Pamela A; Univ Hlth Network-Princess M, 5 948-610 University Ave, Toronto ON M5G 2M9; Ott'77; FRCPC; RadOncol. Staff, Princess Margaret Hospital - University Health Network; Prof RanOncol, University of Toronto; (416)946-4457; Fax. (416)946-4442.

CATTRAL, Mark S; 11C-1232 585 University Ave, Toronto ON M5G 2N2; Alb'83; MSc; FACS; FRCSC; GenSurg (Hepatobiliary Surgery). Sr Scientist, Toronto General Hospital - UHN; Prof Surg, University of Toronto; (416)340-3760; Fax. (416)340-4039.

CATTRAN, Charles B; Univ of Ottawa Heart Institute, H2410-40 Ruskin St, Ottawa ON K1Y 4W7; Qns'76; FRCPC; Anes (Critical Care Medicine). Ac Staff, The Ottawa Hospital - Civic Campus; Asst Prof Div of Cardiac Anes, University of Ottawa Heart Institute; (613)761-4379; Fax. (613)761-4925; ccattran@ottawaheart.ca.

CATTRAN, Daniel C; N C S B11-1256, 585 University Ave, Toronto ON M5G 2N2; Tor'66; FACP; FRCPC; IntMed; Nephrol. Sr Scientist, Toronto General Hospital - UHN; (416)340-4187; Fax. (416)340-3714; daniel.cattran@uhn.on.ca.

CATTRAN, Meeka L; Sandy Hill Community Health Ct, 221 Nelson St, Ottawa ON K1N 1C7; Ott'07; CCFP; (613)789-8450; Fax. (613)789-8710.

CATURAY, Michael J; Markham Med Clinic, 200 Bullock Dr, Markham ON L3P 1W2; Wes'95; CCFP; (905)294-7111; Fax. (905)294-0750.

CATY, Veronique; Hop Maisonneuve-Rosemont, 5415 boul l'Assomption, Montreal QC H1T 2M4; Mon'05; FRCPC; DiagRad. Staff, Hôtel-Dieu de Saint-Jérôme; Staff, Hopital Maisonneuve-Rosemont; (450)252-3533

CATZ-BIRO, Laura; 211-250 Lawrence Ave W, Toronto ON M5M 1B2; McG'92; MSc; CCFP; Staff, Centre for Addiction & Mental Health (CAMH) - Russell Street Site; Langs: Spanish; (416)787-3771

CATZAVELOS, G Charles; Cornwall Com Hosp-McConnell, PO Box 100 Stn Main 840 McConnell Ave, Cornwall ON K6H 5S5; Cape Town (South Africa)'77; MD; DABPath; FRCPC; AnatPath (Research). Staff, Cornwall Community Hospital; Langs: Afrikaans; (613)938-4240 x4539; charles.catzavelos@mac.com.

CAUCHI, Mario M; CPM Ctre for Pain Management, 9-6400 Millcreek Dr, Mississauga ON L5N 3E7; Wes'69; PhC; (905)288-1045; Fax. (905)858-2144; mariocauchi@hay.net.

CAUCHOIS, Emmanuel; Douglas Mental Hlth Univ Inst, 6875 boul Lasalle, Verdun QC H4H 1R3; Paris (France)'80; Psy (P.Q.) (Child & Adolescent Psychiatry). Staff, Douglas Mental Health University Institute; Langs: Spanish; (514)761-6131

CAUCHON, Guy; Polyclinique Sante-Plus, 459 rue Principale, Granby QC J2G 2W9; Laval'95; Staff, Centre Hospitalier de Granby; (450)777-3221

CAUCHON, Michel; Unite Med Familiale Maizerets, 2480 ch de la Canardiere, Quebec QC G1J 2G1; Laval'86; CCFP; FCFP; Staff, Centre Hospitalier Affilié Universitaire de Québec - Hôpital De L'Enfant Jésus; Prof Family Med, Université Laval; Langs: Bilingual(French/English); (418)661-1413; Fax. (418)661-7504.

CAUCHON, Natalie; Dr Nathalie Caucon Corp Prof, 950 av Picot, Bathurst NB E2A 4Z9; Sher'92; CCFP; Staff, Fam Med, Hopital Regional Chaleur; Langs: Bilingual(French/English); (506)546-6696; Fax. (506)545-7723; cmni@nbnet.nb.ca.

CAUDLE, Jaelyn M; Kingston Gen Hosp, 76 Stuart St, Kingston ON K7L 2V7; Qns'03; FRCPC; EmergMed. Staff, Kingston General Hospital; (613)549-6666

CAUDRELIER, Jean-Michel; The Ottawa Hosp-Gen Campus, 501 Smyth Rd, Ottawa ON K1H 8L6; Lille (France)'93; FRCPC; RadOncol. Staff, The Ottawa Hospital - General Campus; (613)737-7700 x70217

CAUGHEY, Sharon C; Riverside Prof Centre, 212-1919 Riverside Dr, Ottawa ON K1H 1A2; Qns'86; FRCSC; ObstGyn. Court Staff, Children's Hospital of Eastern Ontario (CHEO); Ac Staff, The Ottawa Hospital - General Campus; Asst Prof ObstGyn, University of Ottawa; (613)739-4711

CAUGHEY, William G; 7-95 Manitoba St PO Box 1360 Stn Main, Bracebridge ON P1L 1V5; Qns'67; FRCPC; IntMed. Ac Staff Cardiol, South Muskoka Memorial Hospital - Muskoka Algonquin Healthcare; Hon Consultant, Huntsville District Memorial Hospital - Muskoka Algonquin Healthcare; (705)645-3255; Fax. (705)645-8658; caughey@muskoka.com.

CAUGHLIN, Cori E; Gulf Canada Square, 300-401 9 Ave SW, Calgary AB T2P 3C5; Sask'04; FRCPC; DiagRad. (403)284-0230; Fax. (403)284-0240.

CAULFEILD, Jonathan D; Grey Bruce HS-Owen Sound, PO Box 1800 Stn Main 7205-1800 8th St E, Owen Sound ON N4K 6M9; Tor'01; FRCSC; GenSurg. Staff, Grey Bruce Health Services - Owen Sound; (519)372-1807; Fax. (519)372-2401; jon.caulfeild@utoronto.ca.

CAULFEILD, Roddy T; 148 Rainbow Beach Rd RR 2, Annan ON N0H 1B0; Tor'70; CCFP; Court Staff, Stratford General Hospital - Huron Perth Healthcare Alliance; Court Staff, Grey Bruce Health Services - Owen Sound; (519)372-2082; Fax. (519)372-2401.

CAULFIELD, Joanne H; Royal Alexandra Hosp, 10240 Kingsway NW, Edmonton AB T5H 3V9; Alb'90; CCFP; FCFP; Staff, Royal Alexandra Hospital; (780)735-4201; Fax. (780)735-4978.

CAULFORD, Paul G; The Scarborough Academic Famil, 1125 Markham Rd, Scarborough ON M1H 2Y5; Tor'78; MSc; CCFP; FCFP; Med Dir, The Community Volunteer Clinic for Medically Uninsured Immigrants & Refugees; Asst Prof Med, University of Toronto; (416)264-4446; Fax. (416)264-4456.

CAULLEY, Emmanuel N N; Grey Bruce HS-Owen Sound, PO Box 1800 Stn Main 8238-1800 8th St E, Owen Sound ON N4K 6M9; U of Ghana (Ghana)'81; MB ChB; FRCSC; ObstGyn (Colposcopy). Staff, Grey Bruce Health Services - Owen Sound; (519)370-2112; Fax. (519)370-2125.

CAUMARTIN, Marie-Celine; Clin Pediatrie de Trois-Rivier, 110-5725 boul des Forges, Trois-Rivieres QC G8Y 5L5; Sher'77; FRCPC; Peds. Assoc Staff, CSSS de Trois-Rivières; (819)375-0504; Fax. (819)375-0686.

CAUMARTIN, Yves; Centre Med Berger Inc, 416-1000 ch Sainte-Foy, Quebec QC G1S 2L6; Laval'01; FRCSC; Urol (Transplantation). Staff, Centre Hospitalier Universitaire de Québec (CHUQ) - Siege Social; (418)266-2876

CAUSER, Petrina A; North York Gen Hosp, 4001 Leslie St, North York ON M2K 1E1; Tor'95; FRCPC; DiagRad. Staff, North York General Hospital; (416)756-6000

CAUSEY, Shannon E; Atrium Prof Bldg, 201-190 Cundles Rd E, Barrie ON L4M 4S5; McM'99; FRCSC; ObstGyn. (705)737-2347

CAUSSIGNAC, Yves; CHUM-Hop Notre-Dame, 1560 rue Sherbrooke E, Montreal QC H2L 4M1; Mon'72; Gastroent (P.Q.); IntMed. Staff Med, Centre Hospitalier l'Université de Montréal (CHUM) - Hôpital Notre-Dame; Clinical Asst Prof Med, Universite de Montreal; (514)890-8000 x27450; Fax. (514)412-7671.

CAUSTON, Norman D; Medical Dental Building, 207-9181 Main St, Chilliwack BC V2P 4M9; UBC'82; DAB; FRCSC; GenSurg (Endoscopy). Ac Staff, Chilliwack General Hospital; Clin Instructor, University of British Columbia; (604)792-1556; Fax. (604)792-4413.

CAUVIER, Andree-Anne; 410 Route 273 CP 206, St-Apollinaire QC G0S 2E0; Laval'85; assoc Staff, Centre Hospitalier Universitaire De Québec - Pavillon De St-françois-d'assise; (418)881-2736; Fax. (418)881-2735.

CAVACUITI, Christopher A; St Jamestown Health Centre, 1F-410 Sherbourne St, Toronto ON M4X 1K2; Tor'95; MHSc; ASAM; CCFP; FCFP; Staff Physician Family & CommunMed, St Michael's Hospital; Asst Prof Family & CommunMed, University of Toronto; (416)864-3096; Fax. (416)864-6035.

CAVALCANTI, Rodrigo B; Univ Hlth Network-Toronto Western Hosp, EW8 420-399 Bathurst St, Toronto ON M5T 2S8; Tor'97; MSc; FRCPC; IntMed. Staff, Toronto Western Hospital - University Health Network; (416)603-6412; Fax. (416)603-6495.

CAVALIER, Lisa L; York Med Hlth Clinic, 17215 Leslie St, Newmarket ON L3Y 8E4; Wes'87; BSc(Hon.); (905)853-0404

CAVALLE-GARRIDO, Maria T; MUHC-Montreal Children's Hosp, D369-2300 rue Tupper, Montreal QC H3H 1P3; Valencia (Spain)'88; FRCPC; Peds; Cardiol. Staff, McGill University Health Centre - Montreal Children's Hospital; (514)412-4423; Fax. (514)412-4273.

CAVANAGH, Annik; Centre Med Robinson, 4 rue Robinson N, Granby QC J2G 8Z9; Mon'05; (450)378-8435

CAVANAGH, Marie-Pier; CSSS Sainte-Croix, 570 rue Heriot, Drummondville QC J2B 1C1; Sher'09; CCFP; Staff, Hôpital Sainte-croix; (819)478-6464

CAVANAGH, Matthew N; Sudbury Reg Hosp-Laurentian, 41 Ramsey Lake Rd, Sudbury ON P3E 5J1; Wes'06; FRCPC; IntMed; Critical Care Medicine. Staff, Health Sciences North-Laurentian Site; (705)532-9872

CAVANAGH, Patricia D; Richmond Street Clinic, 201-862 Richmond St W, Toronto ON M6J 1C9; McM'89; MA(Ire); BA; MD; FRCPC; Psy (Assertive Commun Treatment). Clin Head Outpatients, Centre for Addiction & Mental Health (CAMH) - Queen Site; Asst Prof, University of Toronto; (416)535-8501; Fax. (416)583-1279; patricia.cavanagh@camh.ca.

CAVANAGH, Thomas L; 5120 46 St, Lloydminster AB T9V 2P7; Alb'77; CCFP; (780)875-2221; Fax. (780)875-0605.

CAVANAUGH, David V; Springbank Med Centre, 302-460 Springbank Dr, London ON N6J 0A8; Qns'85; Staff, Parkwood Hospital - St Joseph's Health Care; Physician, Wortley Village Medical Centre; (519)672-6443; Fax. (519)672-9411.

CAVE, Andrew J; Edmonton Clinic, 1A.102-11400 University Ave, Edmonton AB T5G 1Z1; Manchester (England)'71; MB ChB; MRCGPract; CCFP; FCFP; Staff Phys & Co-Site Chief Family Med Clinic, University of Alberta Hospital; Prof Family Med & Research Dir, University of Alberta; (780)407-7755; Fax. (780)407-1828.

CAVE, Anita L; London HSC-University Hosp, PO Box 5339 Stn B 339 Windermere Rd, London ON N6A 5A5; Ott'05; Anes. Staff, London Health Sciences Centre - University Hospital; (519)685-8300

CAVE, Cathy L; Royal Alexandra Hosp, 10240 Kingsway NW, Edmonton AB T5H 3V9; Sask'86; Anes. Staff, Royal Alexandra Hospital; (780)735-4111

CAVE, Dean B; Students Union Bldg, 2-66 University Campus NW, Edmonton AB T6G 2J7; Alb'81; Ac Staff, Hinton Healthcare Centre; (780)492-2612; Fax. (780)492-0172.

CAVE, Dominic A; University of Alberta Hosp, WMC 1C1.04-8440 112 St NW, Edmonton AB T6G 2B7; London (England)'94; FRCPC; Anes; Critical Care Medicine. Staff, University of Alberta Hospital; (780)407-7035

CAVE, Donna M; 2-220 Student's Union Bldg, 66 University Campus NW, Edmonton AB T6G 2J7; Alb'83; (780)492-2612

CAVENO, Jordan W J; Foothills Med Centre, C222-1403 29 St NW, Calgary AB T2N 2T9; UBC'02; FRCPC; Anes. Staff, Foothills Medical Centre; (403)944-1430; Fax. (403)270-2268.

CAVERS, Kenneth J; Victoria Gen Hosp, 2340 Pembina Hwy, Winnipeg MB R3T 2E8; Alb'96; CCFP; FCFP; Staff, Victoria General Hospital; (204)269-3570

CAVERS, William J R; Westside Integrated Hlth Ctre, 130-180 Wilson St, Victoria BC V9A 7N6; UBC'77; CCFP; FCFP; Ac Staff, Royal Jubilee Hospital; Assoc Staff, Victoria General Hospital; (250)592-3122

CAVETT, Teresa D; Dept of Family Med-U of Manito, T158-770 Bannatyne Ave, Winnipeg MB R3E 0W3; Man'84; CCFP.

CAVILLA, Benjamin; 1625 Fort St PO Box 5414, Victoria BC V8R 6S4; Alb'06; CCFP; (250)661-9353

CAWADIAS, Alexander C; Montfort Hosp, 713 Montreal Rd, Ottawa ON K1K 0T2; Ott'83; FRCPC; Anes. Staff, Montfort Hospital; (613)746-4621; Fax. (613)748-4914.

CAWKWELL, Margaret E; Sheddon Avenue Med Assoc, 308-331 Sheddon Ave, Oakville ON L6J 1X8; Tor'87; CCFP; FCFP; Assoc Staff, Halton Healthcare Services Corporation - Oakville Site; (905)845-8771; Fax. (905)845-8379.

CAYA, Joanne; CSSS de Lac-Saint Jean-Est, CP 1300 Succ Bureau-Chef 300 boul Champlain S, Alma QC G8B 5W3; Sher'89; DiagRad. Diag Radiol, CSSS de Lac-Saint Jean-Est; (418)662-3421

CAYA, Nathalie; Clinique Medical, 3-39 rue Laurier E, Victoriaville QC G6P 6P6; Sher'87; Peds. (819)357-2259; Fax. (819)357-2303.

CAYA, Valerie; Groupe Med de Trois-Rivieres, 1900 boul des Recollets, Trois-Rivieres QC G8Z 4K4; Sher'10; (819)375-6666

CAYCEDO, Antonio J; Sudbury Reg Hosp-Laurentian, 41 Ramsey Lake Rd, Sudbury ON P3E 5J1; El Bosque (Spain)'97; FRCSC; GenSurg. Staff, Health Sciences North-Laurentian Site; (705)523-7100

CAYEN, Barry; Downsview Orth & Arthritis Ctr, 810 Wilson Ave, North York ON M3K 1E5; Tor'03; MSc; MPH; FRCSC; OrthSurg (Hip & Knee Arthroplasty). Staff OrthSurg, Humber River Regional Hospital - Church Street Site; (416)479-8969; Fax. (416)981-7675.

CAYER, Alexandra; Ctr Hosp Rouyn-Noranda, 4 9e rue, Rouyn-Noranda QC J9X 2B2; Sher'09; CCFP; Staff, Centre Hospitalier Rouyn-Noranda; (819)764-5131

CAYER, Julie; Hop Charles Lemoyne, 3120 boul Taschereau, Greenfield Park QC J4V 2H1; Laval'00; Staff, Hopital Charles LeMoyne; (450)466-5000

CAYER, Marie-Michelle; Centre Hosp Pierre-Boucher, 1333 boul Jacques-Cartier E, Longueuil QC J4M 2A5; Sher'05; FRCSC; Ophth. Staff, Centre Hospitalier Pierre Boucher; (450)468-8111

CAYER, Nathalie; Centre Med de la Malbaie, 515 rue Saint-Etienne, La Malbaie QC G5A 1W7; McG'92; CCFP; FCFP; Staff, Hôpital de la Malbaie; Langs: Bilingual(French/English); (418)665-2366; Fax. (418)665-7766.

CAYER, Suzanne; UMF Laval, 2690 ch des Quatre-Bourgeois, Quebec QC G1V 0B7; Laval'81; ac Staff, Hôpital Laval; ac Staff, CSSS Haute-Ville; (418)656-4795; Fax. (418)656-4503; suzanne.cayer@irdpq.qc.ca.

CAYER, Sylvie; CHUQ-Ctr Hosp Univ Laval, 2705 boul Laurier, Quebec QC G1V 4G2; Laval'91; FRCPC; Peds (Neonatology); Gastroent. Staff Gastroenterol Peds, Centre Hospitalier Universitaire de Quebec-CHUL; Langs: Bilingual(French/English); (418)654-2282; Fax. (418)654-2137.

CAYOUETTE, Marie-Claude; Clinique Med De La Marconi, 201-3525 boul Saint-Joseph, Drummondville QC J2B 0H3; Laval'04; CCFP; (819)850-0476; Fax. (819)850-0197.

CAYOUETTE, Maryse; Ctr Hosp Reg de Lanaudiere, 1000 boul Sainte-Anne, St-Charles-Brromee QC J6E 6J2; Sher'91; FRCPC; IntMed; MedMicrobiol. Staff, Centre Hospitalier Régional de Lanaudière; (450)759-8222; maryse_cayouette@ssss.gouv.qc.ca.

CAYTAK, Joseph; The Ottawa Hosp-Gen Campus, 501 Smyth Rd, Ottawa ON K1H 8L6; McG'79; CCFP; CCFP(E.M.); FCFP; Staff, The Ottawa Hospital - General Campus; (613)737-8000

CAZA, France; CSSS de Laval, 280 boul Du Roi-Du-Nord, Laval QC H7L 4L2; Mon'86; (450)622-5110; Fax. (450)622-4150.

CAZA, Genevieve; Polyclinique St-Eustache, 2F-75 rue Grignon, St-Eustache QC J7P 4J2; Mon'95; CCFP; Staff Family Med, Hôpital de Saint-Eustache; (450)623-6677

CAZA, Gregoire F; Renfrew Victoria Hosp, 499 Raglan St N, Renfrew ON K7V 1P6; Ott'98; CCFP; Staff, Renfrew Victoria Hospital; (613)432-4851; Fax. (613)432-4851.

CAZEAUX, Myriam; Clinique Med Riel, 455 boul Riel, Gatineau QC J8Z 2J8; Mon'87; (819)777-7416; Fax. (819)777-5061.

CEALICU TOMA, Florina; Ctr Hosp Pierre-Janet, 20 rue Pharand, Gatineau QC J9A 1K7; Craiova (Romania)'86; Psy (P.Q.) (Legal Psychiatry). Médecin Psy, Centre Hospitalier Pierre-Janet; Assoc Prof, University of Ottawa; Langs: Romanian; English; (819)776-8066; Fax. (819)776-8004.

CEAPCHI, Nora C; 2-832 March Rd, Kanata ON K2W 0C9; Bucharest (Romania)'95; CCFP; (613)599-5599; Fax. (613)599-1005.

CEASER, Jack; City of Lakes Family Hlth Team, C-960 Notre Dame Ave, Sudbury ON P3A 2T4; McM'02; BSc; Dip SportMed; CCFP; Family Physician Focusing in Sport & Exercise Med, Strive Sport Medicine Centre; Family Phys Focusing on Sport & Exercise Med, Northern Ontario School of Medicine; (705)560-1018

CEBALLOS, Katherine M; BC Cancer Agency-Vancouver CC, 600 10th Ave W, Vancouver BC V5Z 4E6; Dal'96; FRCPC; AnatPath. Staff, BC Cancer Agency Vancouver Centre; Fax. (604)873-5384.

CEBRIAN, Clara; St Joseph's Healthcare, 50 Charlton Ave E, Hamilton ON L8N 4A6; Sask'89; FRCPC; Psy (Inpatient Psychiatry). Ac Staff, St Joseph's Healthcare - Charlton Campus; Clinical Asst Prof, McMaster University; (905)522-1155 x34370; Fax. (905)540-6595; cebriac@mcmaster.ca.

CEBULIAK, David N; Rockyview Gen Hosp, 7007 14 St SW, Calgary AB T2V 1P9; Alb'82; CCFP; CCFP(E.M.); Staff, Rockyview General Hospital; (403)943-3449

CECCHERINI-NELLI, Alfonso; Alberta Hosp Edmonton, PO Box 307 Stn Main, Edmonton AB T5J 2J7; Pisa (Italy)'82; Staff, Alberta Hospital Edmonton; Langs: Italian; (780)342-5473; Fax. (780)342-5411; alfonso.ceccherini@albertahealthservices.ca.

CECERE, Assunta; St Mary's Hosp Centre, 3830 av Lacombe, Montreal QC H3T 1M5; Mon'02; Staff, St Mary's Hospital Centre; (514)345-3511

CECERE, Renzo; MUHC-Royal Victoria Hosp, S8.76-687 av des Pins O, Montreal QC H3A 1A1; McG'90; FRCSC; GenSurg; CardiothorSurg; Cardiovasc&ThorSurg (P.Q.). Staff, McGill University Health Centre - Royal Victoria Hospital; (514)843-1463

CECUTTI, William A; Family Care Med Centre, 104-3050 Garden St, Whitby ON L1R 2G7; Tor'88; (905)430-5305; Fax. (905)430-6416.

CEDENO ROJAS, Mary Y; South Health Campus, 4F-4448 Front St SE, Calgary AB T3M 1M4; (Other Foreign)'95; CCFP; (403)956-2300

CEJIC, Sonny S; Thames Valley FHT-Byron Fam Me, 1228 Commissioners Rd W, London ON N6K 1C7; Tor'96; MSc; BEd; CCFP; FCFP; Staff Family Med, London Health Sciences Centre - University Hospital; Asst Prof, University of Western Ontario; (519)472-9670; Fax. (519)657-1766; scejic@uwo.ca.

CEKAN, Daniel F; 5-246 Dundas St S, Cambridge ON N1R 5S2; (Czech Republic)'00; MD; CCFP; (519)740-6111; Fax. (519)623-5300.

CELESTIN, Kathlyn; Medisys, 11F-500 rue Sherbrooke O, Montreal QC H3A 3C6; Mon'97; CCFP; Langs: English; (514)845-1211; Fax. (514)845-4842.

CELESTIN-NOEL, S Marie; CSSS d'Antoine-Labelle-Mt Laur, RR 1 2561 ch de la Lievre S, Mont-Laurier QC J9L 3G3; (Haiti)'01; FRCSC; GenSurg. gén Chirurgien, CSSS d'Antoine-Labelle; (819)623-1234; Fax. (819)440-4299.

CELIKER, Mahmut Y; IWK Health Centre, PO Box 9700 Rpo CSC 5850-5980 University Ave, Halifax NS B3K 6R8; Istanbul (Turkey)'87; Staff, IWK Health Centre; (902)470-8888

CELIS, M Lourdes M; 230-151 Walden Gate SE, Calgary AB T2X 0R2; Manila (Philippines)'90; CCFP; Physician Palliative Care, Southwood Hospice; Physician, Sheldon M Chumir Urgent Care Physician Group; Langs: Tagalog; (403)264-6372; Fax. (403)264-6399; lourdes.celis@albertahealthservices.ca.

CELLARIUS, Victor; Temmy Latner Centre, 60 Murray St, Toronto ON M5T 3L9; Cal'99; BSc; CCFP; Staff Temmy Latner Centre for Palliative Care, Mount Sinai Hospital; (416)586-4800 x2411; Fax. (416)586-4804.

CELLIERS, Andre; Harbourside Family Health Ctre, 243 Harbour Dr, Summerside PE C1N 5R1; Orange Free State (South Africa)'90; Staff, Prince County Hospital; Langs: Afrikaans; (902)432-2600; Fax. (902)432-2610.

CELLOT, Sonia; 3175 ch de la Côte-Sainte-Cath, Montreal QC H3T 1C5; Mon'97; Hem; Peds. Staff, Hôpital Ste-Justine; (514)345-4931 x6026; Fax. (514)345-4884; sonia.cellot@umontreal.ca.

CELLUCCI, Tanya; McMaster Children's Hosp, 3A 74-1280 Main St W, Hamilton ON L8S 4K1; Tor'05; FRCPC; Peds; Rheum. (905)521-2100

CELLUPICA, Umberto; Maple Kidz Clinic, 215-955 Major Mackenzie Dr, Maple ON L6A 4P9; Qns'96; FRCPC; Peds. Staff Peds, Children's Treatment Network of Simcoe-York; (905)303-0304; Fax. (905)303-3035.

CEMBROWSKI, George S; University of Alberta Hosp, 4B1. 24WCM-8440 112 St NW, Edmonton AB T6G 2B7; Cal'78; BSc(Hon); AB; Dir Med Biochemistry, University of Alberta Hospital; Assoc Prof LabMed & Path, University of Alberta; (780)407-3185; Fax. (780)407-8599; cembr001@cha.ab.ca.

CENAIKO, David F; Sunridge Prof Centre, 302-2675 36 St NE, Calgary AB T1Y 6H6; Sask'85; FRCSC; ObstGyn. Staff, Foothills Medical Centre; Staff, Peter Lougheed Centre; Asst Prof, University of Calgary; (403)250-6922; Fax. (403)250-6951.

CENCIG, Agnes; Clinique Med du Quartier, 1191 av Cartier, Quebec QC G1R 2S9; Laval'79; Ac Staff, CLSC-CHSLD Haute-Ville-Des-Rivieres; (418)522-1911; agnes.cencig@ssss.gouv.qc.ca.

CENGARLE-SAMAK, Alexandre; CSSS de Laval, 1755 boul Rene-Laennec, Laval QC H7M 3L9; McG'07; MDCM; FRCPC; DiagRad. Staff, Hopital de la Cite de la santé; (450)668-1010

CENIC, Aleksa; Hamilton HS-General Site, 715-237 Barton St E, Hamilton ON L8L 2X2; McM'02; BSc; MSc; FRCSC; Neursurg (Spine Surgery). Staff, Hamilton Health Sciences Centre - Hamilton General Hospital; (905)527-4322

CENKOWSKI, Barbara A; Mount Carmel Clinic, 886 Main St, Winnipeg MB R2W 5L4; Cracow (Poland)'78; CCFP; Langs: Polish; Russian; (204)582-2311; Fax. (204)582-1341.

CENTAZZO, Sophie I; Queensway-Carleton Hosp, 3045 Baseline Rd, Nepean ON K2H 8P4; Mon'95; FRCPC; DiagRad. Staff, Queensway Carleton Hospital; (613)721-4700 x2701

CENTER, Richard P; Sault Area Hosp, 750 Great Northern Rd, Sault Ste. Marie ON P6B 0A8; Tor'79; Staff, Sault Area Hospital - Sault Ste Marie; (705)759-3434

CENTIS, Tajana M; Health Sciences North-Laurenti, 41 Ramsey Lake Rd, Sudbury ON P3E 5J1; Qns'09; Staff, Health Sciences North-Laurentian Site; (705)523-7100

CEOLIN-WIETFELDT, Sandra; Thistlewood Prof Centre, 306-8077 Islington Ave, Woodbridge ON L4L 7X7; McM'94; CCFP; FCFP; Court Staff, Humber River Regional Hospital - Finch Avenue Site; (905)856-8714; Fax. (905)856-4036.

CEPEDA, Rolando; Hart Fertility Centre, 102-1057 Main St W, Hamilton ON L8S 1B7; Mexico (Mexico)'81; FRCSC; ObstGyn. Clinical Asst Prof ObstGyn, McMaster University; (905)972-8382; Fax. (905)972-8600.

CEPICA ANGEL, Denisa; Fall River Family Practice, PO Box 2160 3425 Highway 2, Fall River NS B2T 1K6; Dal'02; CCFP; (902)861-2237; Fax. (902)861-1914; dcepica@dal.ca.

CEPONIS, Peter J M; CFB Shilo, PO Box 5000, Shilo MB R0K 2A0; Tor'08; CCFP; (204)765-3000

CERAT, Jean; Polyclinique Med Pierre Le Gar, 370-950 montee des Pionniers, Terrebonne QC J6V 1S8; Sher'85; FRCSC; Otol. Staff, Centre Hospitalier Pierre le Gardeur; (450)582-0333

CERAT, Jean-Michel; CSSS Haut-Richelieu-Rouville, 920 boul du Seminaire N, St-Jean-Sur-Richel QC J3A 1B7; Mon'02; Staff, Hôpital du Haut-Richelieu; (450)359-5000

CERAT, Nathalie; Serv Externe de Psychiatrie, 230-383 boul du Seminaire N, St-Jean-sur-Richel QC J3B 8C5; Mon'90; FRCPC; Psy. Staff, Hôpital du Haut-Richelieu; (450)346-2222; Fax. (450)346-2311.

CERAT, Suzanne; CLSC du Richelieu, 300 ch de Marieville, Richelieu QC J3L 3V8; Sher'86; (450)658-7561; Fax. (450)658-4390.

CERAT, Yves; Clin Gyn-Obst Pierre-Boucher, 200-1760 boul Jacques-Cartier, Longueuil QC J4N 1C2; Mon'83; FRCSC; ObstGyn. Staff, Centre Hospitalier Pierre Boucher; (450)468-2151; Fax. (450)468-3309.

CERESIA, Patrick J; Canadian Med Protective Assn, PO Box 8225 Stn T CSC 875 Carling Ave, Ottawa ON K1G 3H7; Ott'75; (613)725-2000 x666; Fax. (613)725-1300; pceresia@cmpa.org.

CERESNE, Lance A; 200-236 Avenue Rd, Toronto ON M5R 2J4; Tor'99; CCFP; Ac Staff, Sunnybrook Health Sciences Centre; Lecturer, University of Toronto; (416)922-2000; Fax. (416)922-2005.

CERESNEY, Maureen N; Meadowlark Prof Bldg, 302-8702 Meadowlark Rd NW, Edmonton AB T5R 5W5; UBC'97; FRCPC; Psy. (780)487-5333

CERINO, Michel; Ctr Hosp Reg de Lanaudiere, 1000 boul Sainte-Anne, St-Charles-Brromee QC J6E 6J2; Mon'77; FRCPC; NuclearMed. Staff, Centre Hospitalier Régional de Lanaudière; (450)759-8222 x2689; Fax. (450)759-9075.

CERKVENIK, Majda; Golfdale Walk Inc Clinic, 3750 Lawrence Ave E, Scarborough ON M1G 1R1; Tor'89; (416)438-1664; Fax. (416)438-3646.

CERMIGNANI, Monica S; MUHC-Montreal Gen Hosp, B2117-1650 av Cedar, Montreal QC H3G 1A4; Qns'97; FRCPC; EmergMed;CCFP; Staff Emerg Phys, McGill University Health Centre - Montreal General Campus; (514)934-1934 x42501; Fax. (514)934-8421.

CERNAT, Geta; 8-9301 Bathurst St, Richmond Hill ON L4C 9S2; (Other Foreign)'92; CCFP; (905)237-7472; Fax. (905)237-2854.

CERNEA, Carmen D; CLSC Saint-Henri, 3833 rue Notre-Dame O, Montreal QC H4C 1P8; (Other Foreign)'97; CCFP; (514)933-7541

CERNICA, Maria; Polyclinique de L'Ile-des-Soeu, 2010 boul Rene-Levesque, Verdun QC H3E 2A4; Bucharest (Romania)'65; Langs: Romanian; English; (514)767-2683

CERNOHORSKY, Karel; Univ of Alberta Hosp, 8440 112 St NW, Edmonton AB T6G 2B7; Alb'91; FRCPC; IntMed. Staff, University of Alberta Hospital; (780)407-8822

CERNY, Kristina G; 1512 Hastings Cres SE, Calgary AB T2G 4C9; Cal'06; CCFP; (403)243-7468; Fax. (403)243-7498.

CERNY, Vladimir; Queen Elizabeth II HSC, 10W-1276 South Park St, Halifax NS B3H 2Y9; Charles (Other Foreign)'85; Staff, Queen Elizabeth II Health Sciences Centre - Victoria General Site; (902)473-2700

CERSKUS, Timothy R; Humber River Reg Hosp-Church, 200 Church St, Toronto ON M9N 1N8; Tor'80; Staff, Humber River Regional Hospital - Church Street Site; (416)249-8111

CERVANTES, Jaime; Greenwood Med Clinic, 9804A 104 St, Fort Saskatchewan AB T8L 2E6; (Mexico)'72; (780)998-9400; Fax. (780)998-9410.

CERVANTES, Pablo; 650-3550 ch Cote-des-Neiges, Montreal QC H3H 1V4; (Mexico)'72; FRCPC; Psy (Mood Disorders). Dir Mood Disorder Unit, McGill University Health Centre - Montreal General Campus; adj Prof, McGill University; Langs: Spanish; French; (514)939-3215

CERVENKO, Paul R; CFB Kingston, PO Box 17000 Stn Forces, Kingston ON K7K 7B4; Qns'87; MHSc; CCFP; FCFP; (613)541-5010

CERVIN, Catherine K; Laurentian University-E Campus, 935 Ramsey Lake Rd, Sudbury ON P3E 2C6; Tor'77; CCFP; FCFP; Assoc Dean Postgraduate Med Educ, Northern Ontario School of Medicine; Teach Staff, Laurentian University; (705)662-7259; Fax. (705)662-7274.

CERVINI, Patrick; Hotel-Dieu Grace Hosp, 1030 Ouellette Ave, Windsor ON N9A 1E1; Tor'03; FRCPC; DiagRad. Staff, Hôtel-Dieu Grace Hospital; (519)973-4411

CERVINKA, Anthony G; St Thomas-Elgin Gen Hosp, PO Box 2007 Stn Main 189 Elm St, St Thomas ON N5P 3W2; Wes'01; FRCSC; OrthSurg. Staff, St Thomas Elgin General Hospital; (519)631-2030

CESAIRE, J Jacques; CSSS Pierre Boucher, 1333 boul Jacques-Cartier E, Longueuil QC J4M 2A5; Liege (Belgium)'70; Staff, Centre Hospitalier Pierre Boucher; (450)468-8111; cesairej@videotron.ca.

CESARI, Matthew; Sunnybrook Hlth Sciences Ctre, E425A-2075 Bayview Ave, Toronto ON M4N 3M5; McG'04; FRCPC; AnatPath. Staff, Sunnybrook Health Sciences Centre; (416)480-4600

CESARZ, John A; Queen Street Med Clinic, 102A-505 Queen St, Spruce Grove AB T7X 2V2; Sask'02; FRCPC; IntMed. (780)960-4102; Fax. (780)962-8176.

CESCON, Amelio O; New Vision Family Health Team, 421 Greenbrook Dr, Kitchener ON N2M 4K1; Tor'74; BSc(Hon); CCFP; Staff, Grand River Hospital - Kitchener/Waterloo Health Centre; Staff, St Mary's General Hospital; (519)578-3510; Fax. (519)578-6040.

CESCON, David W; Univ Hlth Network-Toronto Gen, 200 Elizabeth St, Toronto ON M5G 2C4; Tor'05; FRCPC; IntMed; MedOncol. Staff, Toronto General Hospital - UHN; (416)790-0929

CESCON, Maria A; Woodville Med Centre, PO Box 98, Woodville ON K0M 2T0; McM'79; CCFP; FCFP; Staff, Ross Memorial Hospital; (705)439-2411; Fax. (705)439-2770.

CHA, Charlie Y K; Sunnyside Med Arts Centre, 411-27 Roncesvalles Ave, Toronto ON M6R 3B2; Tor'87; BSc(Med); Staff, St Joseph's Health Centre; Lecturer Family & CommunMed, University of Toronto; (416)533-6807

CHA, James Y M; Oshawa Med Arts Bldg, 203-300 King St W, Oshawa ON L1J 2K1; Man'84; DABIM; FRCPC; IntMed (Cardiology). Staff, Lakeridge Health - Oshawa Site; (905)725-8632; Fax. (905)725-2348.

CHA, Lily S L; 1020 Wilson Ave, North York ON M3K 1G6; Man'82; BSc(Med); FRCSC; ObstGyn. Ac Staff, Humber River Regional Hospital - Church Street Site; Langs: Mandarin; (416)633-7201; Fax. (416)633-8576; lilycha@rogers.com.

CHAABANE, Sonia; Polyclinique Med Pierre Le Gar, 300-1000 montée des Pionniers, Terrebonne QC J6V 1S8; Lyon (France)'94; Staff, Centre Hospitalier Pierre le Gardeur; (450)657-1313

CHAALALA, Chiraz; CHUM-Hopital Notre-Dame, 1560 rue Sherbrooke E, Montreal QC H2L 4M1; Sher'96; FRCSC; Neursurg. Staff, Centre Hospitalier Universitaire de Sherbrooke-Hopital Fleurimont; Staff, Centre Hospitalier l'Université de Montréal (CHUM) - Hôpital Notre-Dame; Langs: Bilingual(French/English); (514)890-8000

CHABA, Todd P; University of Alberta Hosp, 5B4.46WCM-8440 112 St NW, Edmonton AB T6G 2B7; Alb'93; FRCPC; IntMed; AnatPath. Asst Prof, University of Alberta Hospital; Asst Prof, University of Alberta; (780)407-2758; Fax. (780)407-3009.

CHABABI ATALLAH, Myrna; CHUS-Hop Hotel-Dieu, 580 rue Bowen S, Sherbrooke QC J1G 2E8; Staff, Centre Hospitalier Universitaire de Sherbrooke-Hôpital Hôtel-Dieu; (819)346-1110

CHABAN, Roman J; 200-1017 Wilson Ave, North York ON M3K 1Z1; Tor'83; FRCSC; Otol. Staff, Humber River Regional Hospital - Keele Street Site; Staff, Humber River Regional Hospital - Church Street Site; (416)781-4000; Fax. (416)781-2414.

CHABANE-CHAOUCH, Nacera; CSSS de Laval, 1755 boul Rene-Laennec, Laval QC H7M 3L9; (Algeria)'85; CCFP; Staff, Hopital de la Cite de la santé; (450)668-1010

CHABIKULI, Sibomana S; 103-240 Penetanguishene Rd PO Box 790 Stn Main, Midland ON L4R 4P4; Medunsa (South Africa)'99; CCFP; CCFP(E.M.); (705)527-7575; Fax. (705)527-7571.

CHABOT, Bertrand; CRSSS Baie-James-Chibougamau, 51 3e rue, Chibougamau QC G8P 1N1; Laval'98; CCFP; Staff, CRSSS de la Baie-James; (418)748-3469; Fax. (418)748-2549.

CHABOT, Carol; Polyclinique Masson, A200-3425 rue Masson, Montreal QC H1X 1R6; Mon'82; ac Staff, Centre Hospitalier l'Université de Montréal (CHUM) - Hôpital Notre-Dame; (514)376-9961; Fax. (514)376-8100.

CHABOT, Celine; Regie des Rentes du Quebec, CP 5200 Succ Terminus 348-2600 boul Laurier, Quebec QC G1K 7S9; Laval'76; Staff, Regie des Rentes du Quebec; (514)657-8709 x4951

CHABOT, Christian; CRSSS Baie-James-Sante Lebel, 950 boul Quevillon, Lebel-s-Quevillon QC J0Y 1X0; Laval'91; Staff, Centre de santé Lebel; (819)755-4881 x234; Fax. (819)755-3779.

CHABOT, Danielle; Polyclinique Pierre Le Gardeur, 300-1000 Montee des Pionniers, Terrebonne QC J6V 1S8; Mon'86; (450)657-1313; Fax. (450)657-1809.

CHABOT, Denys; Centre Hosp Chauveau, 11999 rue de l'Hopital, Quebec QC G2A 2T7; Laval'80; FRCSC; PlasSurg (Aesthetic Surgery). Staff, Centre Hospitalier Chauveau; Langs: Bilingual(French/English); (418)843-9674; denyschabotmd@chirurgieplastique.ca.

CHABOT, Francois; Hotel-Dieu d'Arthabaska, 5 rue des Hospitalieres, Victoriaville QC G6P 6N2; Laval'97; CSPQ; FRCPC; Anes (Alternative Medicine). Staff, Hotel-Dieu d'Arthabaska; (819)357-2030; chabotfrancois@videotron.ca.

CHABOT, Gilles; Hôpital Ste-Justine, 3175 ch Cote-Sainte-Catherine, Montreal QC H3T 1C5; Mon'74; Peds. Ac Staff, Hôpital Ste-Justine; (514)345-4788; Fax. (514)345-4822.

CHABOT, Jacques; CHUQ-Ctr Hosp Univ Laval, 2705 boul Laurier, Quebec QC G1V 4G2; Laval'83; CSPQ; Anes. Staff, Centre Hospitalier Universitaire de Quebec-CHUL; (418)656-4141

CHABOT, Julie V; Centre Med Quatre-Bourgeois, 300-979 av de Bourgogne, Quebec QC G1W 2L4; Laval'93; CCFP; Médecin, Hôpital général de Québec - CHSLD; Langs: Bilingual(French/English); (418)653-4050; Fax. (418)653-4475.

CHABOT, Magda; CSSS de la Region de Thetford, 1717 rue Notre-Dame E, Thetford Mines QC G6G 2V4; Laval'91; ABOtol; FRCPC; Otol (Plastic Surgery). Staff, Hopital du CSS de la Region de Thetford; Staff, Centre Hospitalier Beauce-Etchemin; Langs: Bilingual(French/English); (418)338-7777; Fax. (418)338-7764.

CHABOT, Marianne; Service Medical Prive, 105-100 boul de Montarville, Boucherville QC J4B 5M4; Sher'04; (450)641-6774

CHABOT, Marie-Christine; Ctr Hosp de la Rég de L'Amiant, 1717 rue Notre-Dame E, Thetford Mines QC G6G 2V4; Laval'07; CCFP; Staff, Hopital du CSS de la Region de Thetford; (418)338-7777

CHABOT, Pierre; Hop Maisonneuve-Rosemont, 5415 boul de l'Assomption, Montreal QC H1T 2M4; Laval'81; FRCPC; RadOncol. Staff, Hopital Maisonneuve-Rosemont; Clin Instructeur Radiol, Universite de Montreal; (514)252-3425; Fax. (514)252-3556.

CHABOT, Serge; Clinique Med de Mistassini, 148 boul Saint-Michel, Dolbeau-Mistassini QC G8L 5J8; Laval'85; ac Staff, Centre Maria-Chapdelaine - CH de Dolbeau-Mistassini; Physician, Oasis Medical Clinics; (418)276-3161; Fax. (418)276-4581.

CHABOYER, Raymond; Mount Seymour Med Clinic, 2F-333 Seymour Blvd, North Vancouver BC V7J 2J4; Man'87; CCFP; FCFP; (604)904-7712; Fax. (604)904-7714.

CHABROL-JOSEPH, Elsy; CSSS de Laval, 280 boul Du Roi-Du-Nord, Laval QC H7L 4L2; Mon'88; (450)622-5110

CHACHAMOVICH, Eduardo; Douglas Mental Hlth Univ Inst, 6875 boul Lasalle, Verdun QC H4H 1R3; Rio Grande do Sul (Brazil)'98; Staff, Douglas Mental Health University Institute; (514)761-6131 x3301; Fax. (514)762-3023.

CHACKO, Mary; Medical Centre, 102-2100 Ellesmere Rd, Scarborough ON M1H 3B7; Indore (India)'81; CCFP; FCFP; Langs: Tamil; Hindi; Malay; (416)438-8517; Fax. (416)438-8518.

CHACKO, Saji A; North Ajax Medical Clinic, 475 Westney Rd, Ajax ON L1T 3H4; New Delhi (India)'01.

CHACKO, Sunita; Foothills Med Centre, 1403 29 St NW, Calgary AB T2N 2T9; Cal'07; CCFP; Staff, Foothills Medical Centre; (403)944-1110

CHACON, Danelia D; Appletree Med Centre, 3001 Carling Ave, Ottawa ON K2B 7Y6; Carabobo (Venezuela)'75; FRCPC; MedMicrobiol; Peds. (613)596-2872

CHACON-ANDRADE, Hernando E; 102-536 Laura Ave, Red Deer County AB T4E 0A5; (Colombia)'87; (403)340-3280

CHACON MERCADO, Marco; CSSS de Trois-Rivieres, 1991 boul du Carmel, Trois-Rivieres QC G8Z 3R9; Madrid (Spain)'99; Critical Care Medicine (P.Q.). Staff, CSSS de Trois-Rivières; (819)697-3333

CHAD, Anthony F; Rockyview Gen Hosp, 7007 14 St SW, Calgary AB T2V 1P9; Sask'00; CCFP; CCFP(E.M.); Staff, Rockyview General Hospital; (403)943-3449; Fax. (403)943-3220.

CHAD, Jennifer M; Lakeside Med Clinic, 3919 8th St E, Saskatoon SK S7H 5M7; Sask'09; BSc; CCFP; (306)374-6884; Fax. (306)374-2552; jmchad@lakeside.ca.

CHAD, Lawrence L; Toronto East Gen Hosp Inc, 825 Coxwell Ave, Toronto ON M4C 3E7; McG'76; FRCPC; Psy. Dep Chief Dept of Psy/Dir Out-Patient Dept of Psychiatric Emerg Services, Toronto East General Hospital Inc; University of Toronto; (416)469-6502; Fax. (416)469-6805; lchad@tegh.on.ca.

CHAD, Zave H; Clinique de Pediatrie, 105 av Gatineau, Gatineau QC J8T 4J4; McG'74; AB; AB; FRCPC; Peds (P.Q.); ClinImmunol&Allergy. Langs: Bilingual(French/English); (819)561-4412; zchad@sympatico.ca.

CHADA, Reena R; St Clair Med Clinic, 2F-50 St Clair Ave E, Toronto ON M4T 1M9; McM'07; CCFP; (416)921-1066; Fax. (416)921-8459.

CHADA, Usha; 114-2810 Victoria Park Ave, North York ON M2J 4A9; Dublin (Ireland)'71; MB ChB; BAO; Court Staff, North York General Hospital; Court Staff, Rouge Valley Health System - Centenary Health Centre Site; Court Staff, The Scarborough Hospital - Birchmount Campus; Langs: Hindi; Punjabi; Urdu; (416)497-0100; Fax. (416)497-0100.

CHADDAH, Sasha S D; 301-219 Oxford St W, London ON N6H 1S5; Tor'88; (519)432-7546; Fax. (519)679-5302.

CHADDAH, Vijay K; 206-345 8th St E, Owen Sound ON N4K 1L3; Bristol (England)'62; Staff, South Bruce Grey Health Centre - Durham Site; (519)371-1741; Fax. (519)371-8926.

CHADHA, Ashok K; Richmond Med Centre, 307 Bridge St W, Napanee ON K7R 2G3; Delhi (India)'79; (613)354-7386

CHADHA, Neil K; Children's & Women's HC of BC, 4480 Oak St, Vancouver BC V6H 3V4; Manchester (England)'99; MB ChB; Staff, BC Children's Hospital; (604)875-2345

CHADHA, Randeep K R; 2166 Mount Newton Cross Rd, Saanichton BC V8M 2B2; Leicester (England)'05; MB ChB; CCFP; CCFP(E.M.); (250)544-7676

CHADHA, Rashmi; Pacific Spirit Commun Hlth Ctr, 2110 43rd Ave W, Vancouver BC V6M 2E1; Manchester (England)'00; MB BS; CCFP; (604)261-6366

CHADHA, Rati; Women's Health Clinic, 1001 10th Ave, Calgary AB T2R 0B7; Delhi (India)'96; FACOG; FRCSC; ObstGyn (Maternal Fetal Medicine). Staff, Foothills Medical Centre; Clinical Asst Prof, University of Calgary; Langs: Hindi; Urdu; Punjabi; (403)944-4419; Fax. (403)283-0415; rati.chadha@albertahealthservices.ca.

CHADHA, Uday; South Bank Med Centre, 5-2430 Bank St, Ottawa ON K1V 0T7; Rajasthan (India)'81; FRCPC; Peds (Neonatology). Chief Div of Neonatol, The Ottawa Hospital - Civic Campus; (613)526-3377; Fax. (613)736-6948.

CHADWICK, Chris D J; The Ottawa Hosp-Civic Campus, 1053 Carling Ave, Ottawa ON K1Y 4E9; Ott'75; FRCSC; GenSurg. Ac Staff Surg, The Ottawa Hospital - Civic Campus; (613)761-4068

CHAE, Anita S; St Joseph's Health Centre, 30 The Queensway, Toronto ON M6R 1B5; Wes'99; FRCPC; DiagRad. Staff, St Joseph's Health Centre; (416)530-6010

CHAER, Sanae; Centre Med Lacordaire, 201-5650 rue Jean-Talon E, Saint-Leonard QC H1S 1M1; Sher'97; FRCPC; Peds. Langs: Bilingual(French/English); (514)255-5595; Fax. (514)255-8550.

CHAFAI, Parviz; Clinique Med Pierre-Boucher, 310-1615 boul Jacques-Cartier, Longueuil QC J4M 2X1; Bordeaux (France)'72; CSPQ; FRCSC; OrthSurg. Med Dir-Orthop Surgery, Centre Hospitalier Pierre Boucher; (450)468-5454; Fax. (514)369-9248.

CHAFE, Alfred; Dr Alfred Chafe Med Services I, 2559 Birch St, Abbotsford BC V2S 4H9; Mem'78; CCFP; Staff, Abbotsford Regional Hospital & Cancer Centre; (778)240-4091

CHAFE, Susan M J; Cross Cancer Institute, 11560 University Ave NW, Edmonton AB T6G 1Z2; Mem'86; BSc; FRCPC; RadOncol (Breasts). Staff, Cross Cancer Institute; Staff, University of Alberta Hospital; Assoc Prof, University of Alberta; Langs: Spanish; (780)432-8518; Fax. (780)432-8332.

CHAGNON, Annie; Clinique Med de la Marine, 101-303 boul de la Marine, Varennes QC J3X 2G6; Mon'88; (450)652-9616; Fax. (450)652-4345.

CHAGNON, David-Olivier; CHUM-Hopital St-Luc, 1058 rue Saint-Denis, Montreal QC H2X 3J4; Laval'04; FRCPC; DiagRad. Staff, Centre Hospitalier l'Université De Montréal (CHUM) - Hôpital Saint-luc; (514)890-8000

CHAGNON, Francois; CSSS Pierre Boucher, 1333 rue Jacques-Cartier E, Longueuil QC J4M 2A5; Laval'05; GenSurg. Staff, Centre Hospitalier Pierre Boucher; Staff, Centre Hospitalier Régional du Suroît; (450)468-8111

CHAGNON, Francoise; MUHC-Montreal Gen Hosp, C2 125-1650 av Cedar, Montreal QC H3G 1A4; McG'81; MHA; FACS; CHE; FRCSC; Otol (Laryngology & Care of the Professional Voice). Staff Otol Head and Neck Surg, St Mary's Hospital Centre; Staff Otol Head and Neck Surg, McGill University Health Centre - Montreal General Campus; Dir, Canassurance Inc; Dir, Lallemand Inc.; adj Prof Otol, McGill University; Langs: English; French; (514)934-1934 x42285; Fax. (514)934-8587.

CHAGNON, Gilles; CHUS-Hop Hotel-Dieu, 580 rue Bowen S, Sherbrooke QC J1G 2E8; Mon'83; FRCPC; Psy. Staff, Hopital Maisonneuve-Rosemont; Staff, Centre Hospitalier Universitaire de Sherbrooke-Hôpital Hôtel-Dieu; (819)346-1110 x25541; Fax. (819)829-6263.

CHAGNON, Isabelle; Hop du Sacre-Coeur de Mtl, 5400 boul Gouin O, Montreal QC H4J 1C5; Mon'96; FRCPC; IntMed. Staff, Hôpital du Sacre-Coeur de Montréal; (514)338-2050

CHAGNON, Karine; Hop Maisonneuve-Rosemont, 5415 boul de l'Assomption, Montreal QC H1T 2M4; Mon'02; FRCPC; IntMed; Respir. Staff, Hopital Maisonneuve-Rosemont; (514)252-3400

CHAGNON, Luc; Clinique de Med Familiale, 123-151 Main St E, Hawkesbury ON K6A 1A1; Sher'89; CCFP; FCFP; Chief of Staff, Hawkesbury & District General Hospital; Langs: Bilingual(English/French); (613)632-0151; Fax. (613)632-1073.

CHAGNON, Marie-Noel; Hop Brome-Missisquoi-Perkins, 950 rue Principale, Cowansville QC J2K 1K3; Sher'08; Staff, Hôpital Brome-Missisquoi-Perkins; (450)266-4342

CHAGNON, Michel; Clin Greffe de Cheveux Bedard, 301-630 rue Sherbrooke O, Montreal QC H3A 1E4; Sher'85; FRCSC; GenSurg. Langs: English; (514)842-8449; Fax. (514)842-8440.

CHAGNON, Nicolas L R; Monfort Hosp, 713 Montreal Rd, Ottawa ON K1K 0T2; McG'00; CCFP; CCFP(E.M.); Staff, Montfort Hospital; (613)748-4996

CHAGNON, Normand; Clinique Medicale Waterloo, CP 760 100-4900 rue Foster, Waterloo QC J0E 2N0; Sher'78; (514)539-1102

CHAGNON, Patrick; Hotel-Dieu d'Arthabaska, 5 rue des Hospitalieres, Victoriaville QC G6P 6N2; Laval'91; LMCC; IntMed. Staff, Hotel-Dieu d'Arthabaska; Clin Teacher, Universite de Sherbrooke; (819)357-2030; Fax. (819)357-6016.

CHAGNON, Pierre-Marc; CHUM-Hop Notre-Dame, 1560 rue Sherbrooke E, Montreal QC H2L 4M1; Mon'02; FRCPC; IntMed; Critical Care Medicine (P.Q.). Staff, Centre Hospitalier l'Université de Montréal (CHUM) - Hôpital Notre-Dame; (514)890-8000

CHAGNON-LESSARD, Marie; CSSS de la Haute-Cote-Nord, CP 1000 4 rue de l'Hopital, Les Escoumins QC G0T 1K0; Sher'07; CCFP; Staff, Centre de santé des Côté-Nord; (418)233-2931; Fax. (418)233-2631.

CHAGOYA, Leopoldo; 5 Carey Rd, Toronto ON M4S 1N9; (Mexico)'59; DPsy(McG); FRCPC; Psy (Couple Therapy). Head Family & Couple Therapy Clinic, Mount Sinai Hospital; Assoc Prof, University of Toronto; Langs: Spanish; French; (416)489-3997; Fax. (416)489-3997.

CHAHAL, Anthony M; 910 10th Ave W, Vancouver BC V5Z 1M9; Alb'03; FRCPC; EmergMed. (604)875-4700

CHAHAL, Chaman P S; 207-245 Columbia St E, New Westminster BC V3L 3W4; (Grenada)'06; FRCPC; Neur. (604)526-1848

CHAHAL, Jaskarndip S; 800-55 Queen St E, Toronto ON M5C 1R6; Man'05; OrthSurg. (416)893-1230

CHAHAL, Mangeet K; Heart Care Cardiac Wellness Ct, 372 King St W, Oshawa ON L1R 0A6; Ohio (USA)'05.

CHAHAL, Ramandeep S; Special Services Unit, 90 John St S, Stratford ON N5A 2Y8; Bangalore (India)'03; (519)272-8186; Fax. (519)272-8226.

CHAHAL, Jeevyn K; 645 Victoria St, Kamloops BC V2C 2B3; Sask'97; BSc; CCFP; Assoc Staff, Chilliwack General Hospital; Langs: Punjabi; (250)374-9917

CHAHAL, Vickramjit S; Belmont Prof Centre, 302-564 Belmont Ave W, Kitchener ON N2M 5N6; Wes'02; FRCSC; PlasSurg.

CHAHINE, Danielle A; Quinte West Med Centre, 80 Catherine St, Trenton ON K8V 6N8; McG'05; CCFP; (613)394-0770; Fax. (613)394-7079.

CHAHINE-MALUS, Natalie; Hotel-Dieu Grace Hosp, 1030 Ouellette Ave, Windsor ON N9A 1E1; McG'98; FRCPC; IntMed; Respir. Staff, Hôtel-Dieu Grace Hospital; (519)973-4411 x3100

CHAI, Brian C; Cobblestone Clinic, 1-3414A 28 Ave, Vernon BC V1T 1W9; Alb'89; FRCPC; IntMed. Med Staff, Vernon Jubilee Hospital; (250)503-0870; Fax. (250)503-0915.

CHAIBOU, Mahamadou; The Moncton Hosp, 135 MacBeath Ave, Moncton NB E1C 6Z8; Rhode Island (USA)'91; Staff, The Moncton Hospital; Langs: Dioula; (506)857-5111; mahamadou@usa.net.

CHAIMOWITZ, Gary A; St Joseph's Mountain H Service, PO Box 585 Stn Lcd 1 100 West 5th St, Hamilton ON L8N 3K7; Cape Town (South Africa)'79; MB ChB; ABNP; ABPN; MBA; FRCPC; Psy (Forensic Psychiatry). Staff, St Joseph's Healthcare Hamilton - West 5th Campus; Staff, Hamilton Health Sciences Centre - McMaster University Medical Centre; Staff, St Joseph's Healthcare - Charlton Campus; Assoc Prof, McMaster University; (905)522-1155 x35424; Fax. (905)381-5606; chaimow@mcmaster.ca.

CHAIN-CHANG, Marybelle M T; Castlemore Physician Clinique, 1-3744 Castlemore Rd, Brampton ON L6P 0W7; DBact(Tor); MSc(Tor.); CCBOM; DIH(Tor); LMCC; FCBOM; Staff, William Osler Health System - Etobicoke General Hospital; Staff, Toronto Western Hospital - University Health Network; Staff, William Osler Health System - Brampton Civic Hospital; Langs: English; French; Burmese; Chinese; (416)344-4512; Fax. (416)344-3200.

CHAINE, Claude; 20200 boul des Acadiens, Becancour QC G9H 1M8; Laval'77; (819)233-3333

CHAIT, Peter G; Ellesmere XRay Associates, 310-1333 Neilson Rd, Scarborough ON M1B 4Y9; Witwatersrand (South Africa)'80; FFR(D.S.A.); FRCR(UK); FRCPC; DiagRad (Pediatric Interventional Radiology). (416)287-1222; Fax. (416)281-2555; peter.chait@rogers.com.

CHAITON, Abraham; Dr A Chaiton Med Prof Corp, 405-2115 Finch Ave W, North York ON M3N 2V6; Tor'69; MSc; FRCPC; IntMed (Rheumatology). Court Staff Rheumatology, Lions Gate Hospital; Staff, Sunnybrook Health Sciences Centre; Staff, Humber River Regional Hospital - Finch Avenue Site; (416)741-2456; Fax. (416)741-2454; achaiton@aol.com.

CHAIZE, Eric; Clinique Med du Cuivre, 12 rue Gamble E, Rouyn-Noranda QC J9X 3B7; Sher'87; MSc; (819)764-9441; Fax. (819)764-5792.

CHAKER, Ahmad M A; Windsor Med Centre, 3-130 Ouellette Place, Windsor ON N8X 1L9; Baghdad (Iraq)'84; Dip SportMed; CCFP; Physician Emerg Rm, Leamington District Memorial Hospital; Langs: Arabic; (519)971-2901; achaker@gmail.com.

CHAKKALACKAL, Mary J; Clinic for Centred Psychotherapy, 403-265 Yorkland Blvd, North York ON M2J 5C7; Calicut Kerala (India)'76; MB BS; MD; Langs: Malayalam; (416)229-2399; Fax. (416)229-9771.

CHAKLADER, Mohsina; Main Health Care, 301-294 Main St, Toronto ON M4C 4X5; Ott'06; IntMed. (416)693-3030; Fax. (416)693-3033.

CHAKRABARTI, Anita; St Joseph's Health Centre, 710 Victoria Ave E, Thunder Bay ON P7C 5P7; McM'90; FRCPC; Psy. Staff, Lakehead Psychiatric Hospital - St. Joseph's Care Group; (807)624-3475

CHAKRABARTI, Gobinda L; 29 Castor Cres, Scarborough ON M1G 3R1; Calcutta (India)'53; FRCP(Ed); MRCPsy; FRSM(London,UK); FRCPC; Neur; Psy. (416)438-8001

CHAKRABARTI, Santabhanu; Heart Rhythm Services, 211-1033 Davie St, Vancouver BC V6E 1M7; Calcutta (India)'94; MB BS; Cardiol; Peds. (604)806-9842

CHAKRABARTI, Subrata; London HSC-University Hosp, PO Box 5339 Stn B 339 Windermere Rd, London ON N6A 5A5; Calcutta (India)'81; MB BS; PhD(Man); FRCPC; AnatPath (Gastroenterology Pathology). Staff, London Health Sciences Centre - University Hospital; Dept Chair Path/Prof, University of Western Ontario; Langs: Bengali; (519)685-8500 x36350; Fax. (519)685-8500; subrata.chakrabarti@lhsc.on.ca.

CHAKRABARTI, Sumontra; Trillium Hlth Ctr-Mississauga, 100 Queensway W, Mississauga ON L5B 1B8; Wes'05; FRCPC; IntMed; InfectDis. Staff, Trillium Health Centre - Mississauga; (905)848-7100 x4196

CHAKRABARTY, Lina S; Scarborough Hosp-General Div, 3050 Lawrence Ave E, Scarborough ON M1P 2V5; Sask'02; CCFP; CCFP(E.M.); Staff, The Scarborough Hospital - General Campus; (416)438-2911

CHAKRABO, Santanu; The Ottawa Hosp-Civic Campus, 1053 Carling Ave, Ottawa ON K1Y 4E9; Calcutta (India)'93; Staff, The Ottawa Hospital - Civic Campus; (613)761-4982

CHAKRABORTY, Amiya R; St. Boniface Gen Hosp, C5106-409 Tache Ave, Winnipeg MB R2H 2A6; Staff, St Boniface General Hospital; (204)233-8563

CHAKRABORTY, Anita R; Sunnybrook Hlth Sciences Ctre, H336-2075 Bayview Ave, Toronto ON M4N 3M5; Tor'04; CCFP; Staff, Sunnybrook Health Sciences Centre; (416)480-6100 x7255; Fax. (416)480-5146.

CHAKRABORTY, Krishna; Rexdale Medical Centre, 39A-1530 Albion Rd, Etobicoke ON M9V 1B4; Calcutta (India)'87; CCFP; (416)744-3019

CHAKRABORTY, Pranesh K; Children's Hosp Eastern Ont, 401 Smyth Rd, Ottawa ON K1H 8L1; McM'93; FRCPC; Peds; MedBiochem. Staff Metabolics, Children's Hospital of Eastern Ontario (CHEO); Dir/CEO, Newborn Screening Ontario; Asst Prof, University of Ottawa; (613)737-7600 x2821

CHAKRABORTY, Santanu; The Ottawa Hosp-Civic Campus, 1053 Carling Ave, Ottawa ON K1Y 4E9; Calcutta (India)'93; Staff, The Ottawa Hospital - Civic Campus; (613)737-8571

CHAKRABORTY, Tapash; Lions Gate Hosp, 231 15th St E, North Vancouver BC V7L 2L7; University College (United Kingdom)'95; MB BS; Staff, Lions Gate Hospital; (604)984-5783

CHAKRAVARTI, Anita; Royal University Hosp, 103 Hospital Dr, Saskatoon SK S7N 0W8; Sask'82; FRCPC; Anes (Pain Management). Staff Anes Perioperative Med & Pain Mgnt, Royal University Hospital; Asst Prof College of Med, University of Saskatchewan; (306)655-1183; Fax. (306)655-1279.

CHAKRAVARTI, Neetu; Doctors R Us, 12-205 Van Kirk Dr, Brampton ON L7A 3V4; American Univ of the Caribbean (Netherlands Antilles)'03; CCFP; (905)495-2254; Fax. (905)495-5350.

CHAKRAVARTY, Subrata; Westlock Healthcare Centre, 10220 93 St, Westlock AB T7P 2G4; Guwahati (India)'95; MD; MB BS; Staff Anes, Westlock Healthcare Centre; (780)349-3301; Fax. (780)350-3088; drsubrata@yahoo.com.

CHAKRAVERTTY, Rajesh; Mount Sinai Hosp, 600 University Ave, Toronto ON M5G 1X5; Wes'05; FRCSC; OrthSurg. Staff, Mount Sinai Hospital; (416)596-4200

CHAKROBORTY, Amitabha; Hamilton HS-Henderson Site, 711 Concession St, Hamilton ON L8V 1C3; Calcutta (India)'83; FRCPC; IntMed. Staff, Hamilton Health Sciences Centre-Juravinski Site; (905)389-4411

CHALAOUI, Jean; CHUM-Hop Notre-Dame, 1560 rue Sherbrooke E, Montreal QC H2L 4M1; Beyrouth (Lebanon)'71; AB; FACR; FRCPC; DiagRad (Thoracic Radiology). Staff, Centre Hospitalier l'Université de Montréal (CHUM) - Hôpital Notre-Dame; (514)890-8250

CHALATI, Bachar; Stewiacke Med Associates, PO Box 190, Stewiacke NS B0N 2J0; Damascus (Syria)'84; Langs: English; French; (902)639-2484; Fax. (902)639-2380; bachar@ns.sympatico.ca.

CHALCHAL, Haji I; Allan Blair Cancer Centre, 300-4101 Dewdney Ave, Regina SK S4T 7T1; Karachi (Pakistan)'90; MB BS; ABIM; Asst Prof Med, University of Saskatchewan; Langs: Urdu; (306)766-2774; Fax. (306)766-2688.

CHALFIN, Laura; Hornby Island Med Clinic, 2115 Sollans, Hornby Island BC V0R 1Z0; Columbia(NY) (USA)'83; (250)335-3036

CHALHOUB, Sarkis; Princess Centre, 105-33 Princess St, Leamington ON N8H 5C5; Damascus (Syria)'75; (519)322-5664; Fax. (519)322-5668.

CHALIFOUR, Jean-Francois; CSSS de Saint-Jerome, 290 rue de Montigny, Saint-Jerome QC J7Z 5T3; Sher'97; Respir; IntMed. Staff, Hôtel-Dieu de Saint-Jérôme; (450)431-8200; Fax. (450)431-8209.

CHALIFOUR, Robert; B22-550 Terminal Ave, Ottawa ON K1G 0Z3; Laval'79; Staff, Montfort Hospital; Langs: English; (613)731-2244; Fax. (613)731-4979.

CHALIFOUX, Marie-Pierre; Clinique Med des Sommets, 1070 rue Principale, Ste-Agathe-des-Mts QC J8C 1L6; Mon'06; CCFP; (819)321-1212; Fax. (819)321-3232.

CHALK, Colin H; MUHC-Montreal Gen Hosp, L7 313-1650 av Cedar, Montreal QC H3G 1A4; McG'84; BSc; FRCPC; Neur (Peripheral Neuropathology). Staff, McGill University Health Centre - Montreal General Campus; Assoc Prof Neurol & NeuroSurg, McGill University; Langs: English; French; (514)934-8059; Fax. (514)934-8265; colin.chalk@mcgill.ca.

CHALKLIN, Lori W; Caroline Family Hlth Team-CMG, 15-3305 Harvester Rd, Burlington ON L7N 3N2; McM'85; CCFP; FCFP; Staff, Joseph Brant Memorial Hospital; University of Toronto; Clin Assoc Prof Family Med, McMaster University; (905)632-8007; Fax. (905)632-0375.

CHALMERS, Andrew; Mary Pack Arthritis Centre, 2F-895 10th Ave W, Vancouver BC V5Z 1L7; UBC'72; BSc(Med); FRCPC; IntMed (Medical Education); Rheum. Ac Staff, Vancouver General Hospital - Centennial Pavillion; Prof Med, University of British Columbia; (604)875-5353; Fax. (604)871-4501.

CHALMERS, George R; Lonsdale Men Dental Bldg, 102-1940 Lonsdale Ave, North Vancouver BC V7M 2K2; Alb'70; BSc; Ac Staff, Lions Gate Hospital; (604)988-5291; Fax. (604)988-5298.

CHALMERS, Paula D; 3261 5th Ave W, Vancouver BC V6K 1V3; Tor'73; CCFP; FCFP; (604)736-4660; Fax. (604)736-4643.

CHALMERS-NIXON, Tara S; Sloane Square, 419-5920 1A St SW, Calgary AB T2H 0G3; Alb'98; BSc; FRCPC; IntMed; Gastroent. Clinical Asst Prof, Rockyview General Hospital; Clinical Asst Prof Div of Gastroent, University of Calgary; Langs: French; (403)984-4575; Fax. (403)228-9108.

CHALONER, Wouna M; 266 Hammond Rd PO Box 868, Shelburne NS B0T 1W0; Stellenbosch (South Africa)'88; CCFP; FCFP; (902)875-4454; Fax. (902)875-3631.

CHALOULT, Louis; Polyclinique Med Concorde, 300 boul de la Concorde E, Laval QC H7G 2E6; Laval'60; FRCPC; Psy (Anxiety Disorder). Staff, Hôpital du Sacre-Coeur de Montréal; assoc Prof, Universite de Montreal; (450)667-5310 x2617; Fax. (450)667-5248.

CHALUT, Dominic; MUHC-Montreal Children's Hosp, 2300 rue Tupper, Montreal QC H3H 1P3; Mon'91; FRCPC; Peds. Staff, McGill University Health Centre - Montreal Children's Hospital; (514)412-4400; Fax. (514)412-4397.

CHALUT, Lise; Centre Med Maricourt, 3995 Montee Saint-Hubert, Saint-Hubert QC J3Y 4K2; Sher'80; (450)676-6911; Fax. (450)676-4097.

CHALVARDJIAN, Peter G; South Common Med Centre, 3-2110 Burnhamthorpe Rd W, Mississauga ON L5L 5Z5; Tor'90; (905)820-3209

CHAM, Bonnie P; Cangene Plasma Resources, 137 Innovation Dr, Winnipeg MB R3T 6B6; Man'82; ABPeds; FRCPC; Peds (Pediatric Hematology Oncology); Hem. Assoc Prof, University of Manitoba; bcham@cangene.com.

CHAMAKHI, Ines; Hop du Sacre-Coeur de Montreal, 5400 boul Gouin O, Montreal QC H4J 1C5; Mon'99; FRCPC; IntMed; MedOncol; Hem. Staff, Hôpital du Sacre-Coeur de Montréal; (514)338-2150

CHAMARD-BERGERON, Thomas; Hop Maisonneuve-Rosemont, 5415 boul de l'Assomption, Montreal QC H1T 2M4; Mon'04; FRCPC; Psy. Staff, Hopital Maisonneuve-Rosemont; (514)252-3400 x4769

CHAMARTI, Venkata R; Saskatoon City Hosp, 701 Queen St, Saskatoon SK S7K 0M7; Staff, Saskatoon City Hospital; (306)655-8000

CHAMBERLAIN, Debbie M; Cambridge Mem Hosp, 700 Coronation Blvd, Cambridge ON N1R 3G2; McM'91; Staff, Cambridge Memorial Hospital; (519)621-2330

CHAMBERLAIN, Grant W; Group One Med Associates, 1111 Springfield Rd, Kelowna BC V1Y 8R7; Wes'88; Dip SportMed; CCFP; FCFP; (250)762-4286; Fax. (250)762-4213.

CHAMBERLAIN, Jean E; Fontbonne Bldg, 301 James St S, Hamilton ON L8P 3B6; Tor'91; BSc; FRCSC; ObstGyn (International Health). Staff, St Joseph's Healthcare - Charlton Campus; Asst Prof, McMaster University; (905)521-6041; Fax. (905)521-6089; jchamber@mcmaster.ca.

CHAMBERLAIN, Susan M; Kingston Gen Hosp, V4-76 Stuart St, Kingston ON K7L 2V7; Qns'91; FRCSC; ObstGyn. Staff ObstGyn, Kingston General Hospital; Langs: English; French; (613)548-1327; Fax. (613)548-1330.

CHAMBERLAIN, Wayne W W; Queensway-Carleton Hosp, 3045 Baseline Rd, Nepean ON K2H 8P4; Tor'91; FRCPC; Anes. Staff, Queensway Carleton Hospital; (613)721-2000 x2903; Fax. (613)721-4774.

CHAMBERLAINE, Charles H; London HSC-Victoria Campus, PO Box 5375 Stn B 800 Commissioners Rd E, London ON N6A 5W9; Dublin (Ireland)'73; FRCPC; Psy. Staff, London Health Sciences Centre - Victoria Campus; Assoc Prof, University of Western Ontario; (519)667-6869; Fax. (519)667-6836; cchamber@uwo.ca.

CHAMBERLAND, Gilles; Inst Albert Prevost, 6555 boul Gouin O, Montreal QC H4K 1B3; Mon'90; FRCPC; Psy (Administration). (514)338-4212; gbouchard@ssss.gouv.qc.ca.

CHAMBERLAND, Guy; Clinique Med de Shawinigan-Sud, 200-2355 5e av, Shawinigan-Sud QC G9P 1P4; Laval'86; Staff, Centre Hospitalier du Centre la Mauricie; (819)537-6205; Fax. (819)537-5596; guy.chamberland@gmf.gouv.qc.ca.

CHAMBERLAND, Guy; Clin de Laser et Chir Esthetiq, 1000 rue Chabanel, Chicoutimi QC G7H 2R3; Laval'89; CCFP; (418)549-0294

CHAMBERLAND, Henri; Clin de Gynecologique de Levis, 400-4975 boul de la Rive-Sud, Levis QC G6V 4Z5; Laval'69; ObstGyn. Ac Staff, Hôtel-Dieu de Lévis; (418)833-1522; Fax. (418)833-1526.

CHAMBERLAND, Manon; Clinique Med Warwick, 5A rue du Centre Sportif, Warwick QC J0A 1M0; Sher'82; (819)358-4600; Fax. (819)358-4620.

CHAMBERLAND, Martine S; CHUS-Hop Fleurimont, 3001 12e Av N, Sherbrooke QC J1H 5N4; Sher'84; FRCPC; IntMed. Ac Staff, Centre Hospitalier Universitaire de Sherbrooke-Hopital Fleurimont; Teach Staff, Universite de Sherbrooke; (819)346-1110; Fax. (819)820-6406.

CHAMBERLAND, Pierre; CSSS du Suroît, 150 rue Saint-Thomas, Salaber-de-Valleyf QC J6T 6C1; Mon'69; GenSurg. Staff, Centre Hospitalier Régional du Suroît; (450)371-9925

CHAMBERS, Danaze G; Bear Street Family Physicians, PO Box 1048 Stn Main 302-220 Bear St, Banff AB T1L 1H6; Cal'77; BA; Staff, Covenant Health - Banff Mineral Springs Hospital; (403)762-4846; Fax. (403)762-2445.

CHAMBERS, Gordon K; 4550 Bellevue Dr, Vancouver BC V6R 1E5; UBC'73; (604)307-8143

CHAMBERS, Jeffrey D; Kelowna Eye Care Centre, 1-2918 Tutt St, Kelowna BC V1Y 8Z5; McG'93; FACS; FRCSC; Ophth. Ac Staff, Kelowna General Hospital; (250)762-2003; Fax. (250)762-2563.

CHAMBERS, Karen; Clinique du Lac, 187 Johnson Rd, Ladysmith QC J0X 2A0; Mon'95; CCFP; Staff, CSSS du Pontiac; Langs: Bilingual(English/French); (819)647-3182; Fax. (819)647-3524; kchamb@allstream.net.

CHAMBERS, Michael T; Winston Park Family Physicians, 104-2315 Bristol Cir, Oakville ON L6H 6P8; Tor'71; Ac Staff, The Credit Valley Hospital; Med Dir, Trillium Health Centre - Mississauga; (905)829-2826; Fax. (905)829-2846.

CHAMBERS, Steven W; Allin Clinic, 10155 120 St NW, Edmonton AB T5K 2A2; Alb'79; Ac Staff, Royal Alexandra Hospital; Ac Staff, Glenrose Rehabilitation Hospital; Clinical Asst Prof Family Med, University of Alberta; (780)482-7551; Fax. (780)488-2056.

CHAMELIAN, Laury; CHUM-Hop Notre-Dame, 1560 rue Sherbrooke E, Montreal QC H2L 4M1; Mon'96; FRCPC; Psy. Staff, Centre Hospitalier l'Université de Montréal (CHUM) - Hôpital Notre-Dame; (514)890-8000 x25665

CHAMI, George; Regina Internal Med Specialist, 1821 Rose St, Regina SK S4P 1Z7; Wes'04; Gastroent; IntMed (Therapeutic Endoscopy). (306)352-0772; Fax. (306)359-1068.

CHAMI, Nidal; 105A-667 rue Champlain, Dieppe NB E1A 1P6; (Lebanon)'97; Staff, Dr Georges-L-Dumont University Hospital Centre.

CHAMI, Rose; Hôpital Ste-Justine, 3175 ch Cote-Sainte-Catherine, Montreal QC H3T 1C5; Beirut (Lebanon)'05; Staff, Hôpital Ste-Justine; (514)345-4931 x5344

CHAMIA, Nabil J; 201-381 Kent St, Ottawa ON K2P 2A8; Cairo (Egypt)'62; MB ChB; AB; LMCC; (613)563-0344

CHAMITOFF, Shayna E; 200B-3060 Cedar Hill Rd, Victoria BC V8T 3J5; McM'79; FRCPC; Psy. (250)592-5627; Fax. (250)592-5628; shaynachamitoff@hotmail.com.

CHAMOUN, Alain; Clinique Med MD-Plus, 301-1100 av Beaumont, Mont-Royal QC H3P 3H5; Mon'90; (514)738-4445; Fax. (514)738-8284.

CHAMOUN, Chamoun; Ottawa Cardiovascular Centre, 502-1355 Bank St, Ottawa ON K1H 8K7; Ott'96; FACC; FRCPC; IntMed (Intensive Care); Cardiol. Staff Cardiol & Intensivist/Asst Prof Med, Montfort Hospital; Staff Cardiol, University of Ottawa Heart Institute; Langs: Spanish; Arabic; Bilingual(French/English); (613)738-1584; Fax. (613)738-9097.

CHAMPAGNE, Allyson H; 299 Lake Ave E, Carleton Place ON K7C 1J3; McM'96; CCFP; (613)257-2311

CHAMPAGNE, Amelie; Clinique Med Lanaudiere, 222 rue Bernard, St-Charles-Brromee QC J6E 2C5; Laval'07; (450)755-1033; Fax. (450)753-5558.

CHAMPAGNE, Anne-Marie; Clinique med de Shawnigan-Sud, 200-2355 5e Av, Shawinigan-Sud QC G9P 1P4; Sher'97; CCFP; (819)537-6205; Fax. (819)537-5596; anne-marie.champagne@gmf.gouv.qc.ca.

CHAMPAGNE, Caro Line; St Mary's Gen Hosp, 911 Queens Blvd, Kitchener ON N2M 1B2; Sher'82; FRCPC; IntMed; NuclearMed. Staff, St Mary's General Hospital; (519)749-6495; Fax. (519)749-6997.

CHAMPAGNE, Claude; Hotel-Dieu d'Arthabaska, 5 rue des Hospitalieres, Victoriaville QC G6P 6N2; Sher'00; Staff, Hotel-Dieu d'Arthabaska; (819)357-2030; Fax. (819)357-7406.

CHAMPAGNE, Elaine M C; Club Tiny Tots, 3550-6900 boul Decarie, Cote Saint-Luc QC H3X 2T8; Sher'80; Peds. Assoc Staff, Hôpital Ste-Justine; Langs: English; French; (514)342-9911

CHAMPAGNE, Eric; Centre Hosp Paul-Gilbert, 9330 boul du Centre-Hospitalie, Levis QC G6X 1L6; Laval'99; CCFP; Staff, Centre Hospitalier Paul-Gilbert; Staff, Centre Hospitalier Chauveau; (418)380-8993

CHAMPAGNE, Francois; CSSS Drummond-Hop Sainte-Croix, 570 rue Heriot, Drummondville QC J2B 1C1; Sher'03; Staff, Hôpital Sainte-croix; Langs: English; (819)478-6464

CHAMPAGNE, Ginette; CSSS Bordeaux-Cartierville-St-, 555 boul Gouin O, Montreal QC H3L 1K5; Sher'79; Staff, Pavillon Notre-Dame de la Merci; hon Membre, Hôpital du Sacre-Coeur de Montréal; Langs: English; French; (514)331-3020; Fax. (514)331-2053; ginette585@hotmail.com.

CHAMPAGNE, Jean; Centre Med du Saint-Jovite, CP 19069 Csp Place Ouimet 992 rue de Saint-Jovite, Mont-Tremblant QC J8E 3C1; Laval'74; (819)425-2728; Fax. (819)425-8012.

CHAMPAGNE, Jean; Hôpital Laval, 2725 ch Sainte-Foy, Quebec QC G1V 4G5; Sher'89; FRCPC; IntMed (Electrophysiology); Cardiol. Staff Institute de Cardiologie de Quebec, Hôpital Laval; (418)656-4598; Fax. (418)656-4574.

CHAMPAGNE, Jean-Pierre; North York Gen Hosp, 4001 Leslie St, North York ON M2K 1E1; Tor'02; CCFP; CCFP(E.M.); Staff, Health Sciences North-Laurentian Site; (416)756-6000

CHAMPAGNE, Josette; Hôpital Ste-Justine, 3175 ch Cote-Sainte-Catherine, Montreal QC H3T 1C5; Sher'79; FRCPC; Peds (Hematological Oncology); MedOncol (P.Q.); Hem (P.Q.). Ac Staff, Hôpital Ste-Justine; adj Prof, Universite de Montreal; (514)345-4931; josette.champagne@umontreal.ca.

CHAMPAGNE, Kateri; Clinique Med le Plein-Ciel, 475 boul de la Cote-Vertu, Saint-Laurent QC H4L 1X7; Mon'89; DABSM; MSc(Epidemiol); FRCPC; IntMed (Sleep Medicine); Respir. Staff, McGill University Health Centre - Montreal Chest Institute; Langs: Bilingual(French/English); (514)699-3171; Fax. (514)332-8550.

CHAMPAGNE, Louise; UMF Hôp Charles Le Moyne, 201-299 boul Sir-Wilfrid-Lauri, Saint-Lambert QC J4R 2L1; Laval'90; CCFP; FCFP; (450)466-5630; Fax. (450)466-5631.

CHAMPAGNE, Lucie; Clinique Sante de Thetford, 2000-926 rue Labbe, Thetford Mines QC G6G 2A8; Mon'06; (418)338-4581

CHAMPAGNE, Marie-Rose; 116 boul Lionel-Emond, Gatineau QC J8Y 1W7; (Haiti)'71; CSPQ; MedBiochem (P.Q.). Ac Staff, Hull Hospital; (819)966-6200 x5236; maro.champ@sympatico.ca.

CHAMPAGNE, Martin A; Ctr Hosp de Verdun, 4000 boul Lasalle, Verdun QC H4G 2A3; Sher'85; FRCPC; IntMed (Apheresis Medicine); MedOncol; Hem. Staff, Centre Hospitalier de Verdun; assoc Prof Med, Universite de Montreal; (514)362-1000 x2615; martin.a.champagne@umontreal.ca.

CHAMPAGNE, Martin; Ctr Hosp de Verdun, 4000 boul Lasalle, Verdun QC H4G 2A3; Mon'85; Staff, Centre Hospitalier de Verdun; (514)765-7325

CHAMPAGNE, Myriam; CSSS du Sud de Lanaudière, 911 montée des Pionniers, Terrebonne QC J6V 2H2; Mon'02; CCFP; CCFP(E.M.); Staff, Centre Hospitalier Pierre le Gardeur; Langs: Spanish; English; (450)654-7525 x31184

CHAMPAGNE, Myriam; 1200 rue King E, Sherbrooke QC J1G 1E4; Sher'08; CCFP; (819)780-2222

CHAMPAGNE, Nathalie; Clinique Med de L'Or, 228 2e rue E, La Sarre QC J9Z 2G9; Laval'93; (819)333-5617; Fax. (819)339-3940.

CHAMPAGNE, Patrick; Bridgeland Medical Bldg, 3F-803 1 Ave NE, Calgary AB T2E 7C5; Ott'06; FRCPC; IntMed; Cardiol. Staff, Foothills Medical Centre; (403)944-8119

CHAMPAGNE, Paul R; Dr Georges-L Dumont Reg Hosp, 330 Av Universite, Moncton NB E1C 2Z3; Man'88; FRCPC; DiagRad. Staff, Dr Georges-L-Dumont University Hospital Centre; (506)862-4166; Fax. (506)862-4135.

CHAMPAGNE, Pierre; Clinique Med St-Joseph, 841 av Sainte-Therese RR 1, St-Joseph-D-Beauce QC G0S 2V0; Laval'74; Staff, Centre d'hébergement de Beauceville; (418)397-6891

CHAMPAGNE, Pierre; Private Institute of Surgery, 180-801 Grande Allee O, Quebec QC G1S 1C1; Laval'79; Langs: Bilingual(French/English); (418)687-7328; Fax. (418)687-6110; pchampagne@institutprivedechirurgie.com.

CHAMPAGNE, Richard S; Clinique Med Cadillac, 3435 rue Bossuet, Montreal QC H1M 2M1; Mon'75; (514)253-1211; Fax. (514)253-5091.

CHAMPAGNE, Sylvie; St Paul's Hosp, 1081 Burrard St, Vancouver BC V6Z 1Y6; Sher'78; FRCPC; Peds; MedMicrobiol. Staff, Providence Health Care - St Paul's Hospital; (604)682-2344 x62517

CHAMPION, J A Gerard; Timmins Family Health Team, 1-681 Algonquin Blvd E, Timmins ON P4N 8S6; Ott'00; CCFP; (705)267-5600; Fax. (705)268-3900.

CHAMPION, Jeffrey A; Dartmouth Med Centre, 210-46 Portland St, Dartmouth NS B2Y 1H4; Dal'85; (902)465-4555; Fax. (902)464-4903.

CHAMPION, Lois K; London HSC-University Hosp, PO Box 5339 Stn B 339 Windermere Rd, London ON N6A 5A5; Qns'81; FRCPC; Anes. Staff, London Health Sciences Centre - University Hospital; (519)663-3030; Fax. (519)663-3079.

CHAMPION, Malcolm C; The Ottawa Hosp-Civic Campus, 1053 Carling Ave, Ottawa ON K1Y 4E9; Dundee (Scotland)'74; MB ChB; MRCS; LRCP; FRCP(UK); FRCPC; Gastroent; IntMed. Staff G I Unit A-1, The Ottawa Hospital - Civic Campus; Chairman Finance Committee, Canadian Association of Gastroenterology; Assoc Prof, University of Ottawa; (613)761-4674; Fax. (613)761-5269; mchampion@ottawahospital.on.ca.

CHAMPION, Pauline; 60 Riverside Dr PO Box 6600 Stn Central, Charlottetown PE C1A 8T5; Dal'90; BSc(Hon); Ac Staff ER, Queen Elizabeth Hospital; Langs: Cantonese; Chinese; (902)620-0451

CHAMPION, Philip E; Queen Elizabeth Hosp, PO Box 6600 Stn Central 60 Riverside Dr, Charlottetown PE C1A 8T5; Dal'82; FRCPC; IntMed; MedOncol. Staff, Prince County Hospital; Staff, Queen Elizabeth Hospital; (902)894-2111

CHAMPION, Stacy; The Boardwalk Prof Centre, 220 Water St, Charlottetown PE C1A 9M5; Dal'98; (902)620-2037; stacy.champion@gmal.com.

CHAMPOUX, Genevieve; CSSS du Suroît, 150 rue Saint-Thomas, Salaber-de-Valleyf QC J6T 6C1; Sher'02; Staff, Centre Hospitalier Régional du Suroît; (450)371-9920; Fax. (450)371-5828.

CHAMPOUX, Jean-J.; Clinique Med Dagenais, 2065 boul des Laurentides, Laval QC H7M 4M2; Mon'84; Staff, Centre Hospitalier l'Université De Montréal (CHUM) - Hôpital Saint-luc; (450)975-1557

CHAMPOUX, Nathalie; Inst U Geriatrie de Montreal, 4565 ch Queen-Mary, Montreal QC H3W 1W5; Mon'88; CCFP; Staff, Institut Universitaire de Gériatrie de Montréal; Clin Staff, Universite de Montreal; (514)340-3514; Fax. (514)340-2832.

CHAMPOUX, Richard J; Clinique Med des Cantons, 1474 rue King O, Sherbrooke QC J1J 2C2; Mon'75; (819)565-1955; Fax. (819)565-5516.

CHAN, Aaron Y; Pelham Group Health Centre, 118-245 Pelham Rd, St Catharines ON L2S 1X8; Tor'94; CCFP; FCFP; Staff, Niagara Health System - St Catharines General Site; Langs: Cantonese; (905)688-9670; Fax. (905)688-6979.

CHAN, Adrien M T; Thunder Bay Reg HSC-T-Bay, 980 Oliver Rd, Thunder Bay ON P7B 6V4; Mem'96; MedOncol; IntMed. Staff Northwestern Ontario Reg Cancer Care, Thunder Bay Regional Health Sciences Centre; Langs: English; French; (807)684-7200; Fax. (807)684-5806.

CHAN, Adrienne K; St Michael's Hosp, 4-30 Bond St, Toronto ON M5B 1W8; Tor'00; FRCPC; IntMed; InfectDis. Staff, St Michael's Hospital; (416)864-5746

CHAN, Albert W; 206-301 Columbia St E, New Westminster BC V3L 3W5; Tor'94; FRCPC; IntMed (Interventional Cardiology); Cardiol. Clinical Asst Prof Med, University of British Columbia; Langs: Cantonese; (604)520-3858; Fax. (604)520-3957; albertwchan@shaw.ca.

CHAN, Alex C H; St Paul's Hosp, 5909B-1081 Burrard St, Vancouver BC V6Z 1Y6; Man'91; BSc; MPH; FRCPC; IntMed. Clin Instructor IntMed, Providence Health Care - St Paul's Hospital; Teach Staff, University of British Columbia; (604)682-2344 x63195; Fax. (604)806-8005.

CHAN, Alex D M; 160 1 St S, Cranbrook BC V1C 1B7; McM'90; BSc; MSc; FRCSC; OrthSurg (Spine Surgery). Staff, East Kootenay Regional Hospital; (250)417-0562

CHAN, Alex S L; Oak Ridge Med Centre, 100-13291 Yonge St, Richmond Hill ON L4E 4L6; Man'90; CCFP; CCFP(E.M.); FCFP; (905)773-7759

CHAN, Alex T C; G/F 3-260 Spadina Ave, Toronto ON M5T 2E4; Tor'79; Staff, Toronto Western Hospital - University Health Network; Langs: Cantonese; (416)979-9988; Fax. (416)979-8774.

CHAN, Alexander K P; Tom Baker Cancer Centre, 1331 29 St NW, Calgary AB T2N 4N2; Wes'78; DABR; FRCPC; RadOncol (Brain Malignancy). Med Staff, Foothills Medical Centre; Sr Staff RadOncol, Tom Baker Cancer Centre; Clin Assoc Prof, University of Calgary; (403)521-3077; Fax. (403)283-1651; alexc@cancerboard.ab.ca.

CHAN, Alfred T; Dr Alfred T Chan Medical Inc, 3215 31 Ave, Vernon BC V1T 2H2; UBC'75; CCFP; FCFP; Clin Prof Family Pract, University of British Columbia; Langs: Chinese; (250)545-2034; Fax. (250)545-4784.

CHAN, Alicia K J; Med Sciences Bldg-U of A, 8 53-131 University Campus NW, Edmonton AB T6G 2H7; Tor'92; FRCPC; Peds (Metabolism). Staff, University of Alberta Hospital; University of Alberta; (780)407-8314; Fax. (780)407-6845.

CHAN, Alvin; Solutions Health Care Assoc, 578 St Clair Ave W, Toronto ON M6C 1A6; Tor'88; Court Staff, St Joseph's Health Centre; (416)654-4552; Fax. (416)656-2897.

CHAN, An Wen; Women's College Hosp, 8F 842-76 Grenville St, Toronto ON M5S 1B2; Cal'00; DPhil; ABD; FRCPC; Derm (Moles Surgery). Assoc Staff, Toronto General Hospital - UHN; Staff, Women's College Hospital; (416)323-7732; Fax. (416)323-6306.

CHAN, Andrew C S; The Endoscopy Centre, 301-272 Charlotte St, Peterborough ON K9J 2V4; Liverpool (England)'88; MB ChB; MRC(UK); FRCPC; IntMed; Gastroent. Att Staff, Peterborough Regional Health Centre - Hospital Drive; Att Staff, Peterborough Regional Health Centre - Rogers St Site; Langs: Cantonese; (705)876-4516; Fax. (705)874-7300.

CHAN, Andrew Y; North York Gen Hosp, 4001 Leslie St, North York ON M2K 1E1; Tor'96; FRCPC; Anes. Staff, North York General Hospital; (416)756-6520

CHAN, Andy; UBC Faculty of Med, 317-2194 Health Sciences Mall, Vancouver BC V6T 1Z3; UBC'08; Teach Staff, University of British Columbia; (604)822-2421

CHAN, Angela S A; BC Cancer Agency-Vancouver CC, 600 10th Ave W, Vancouver BC V5Z 4E6; Qns'07; MedOncol; IntMed. Staff, BC Cancer Agency Vancouver Centre; (604)877-6000

CHAN, Angelina G J; Leamington Dist Mem Hosp, 194 Talbot St W, Leamington ON N8H 1N9; Tor'02; FRCSC; ObstGyn. Staff, Leamington District Memorial Hospital; (519)324-0705

CHAN, Angeline W L; 202-3000 Highway 7 E, Markham ON L3R 6E1; Hong Kong (Hong Kong)'67; MB; BSc; FRCPC; Psy (Child & Adolescent Psychiatry). (905)480-1050; Fax. (905)480-0898.

CHAN, Anthony K C; McMaster University, 1280 Main St W, Hamilton ON L8S 4K1; (Hong Kong)'87; MB BS; FRCPC; Peds (Hematological Oncology); Hem. Staff, Royal University Hospital; Langs: Cantonese; Chinese; (905)521-2100 x75625; akchan@mcmaster.ca.

CHAN, Anthony K H; Bayvalley Med Arts Bldg, 305-145 Queenston St, St Catharines ON L2R 2Z9; Tor'87; FRCSC; ObstGyn. Staff, Niagara Health System - St Catharines General Site; Staff, Niagara Health System - Ontario Street Site; (905)685-5506; Fax. (905)685-8558.

CHAN, Ariane C; York Prof Bldg, 210-679 Davis Dr, Newmarket ON L3Y 5G8; Tor'90; Ac Staff, Southlake Regional Health Centre; Langs: French; (905)895-6636; Fax. (905)895-6618; arianechan10@hotmail.com.

CHAN, Arlene S L; Crossways Sexual Health Clinic, 2340 Dundas St W, Toronto ON M6P 4A9; Tor'02; BSc; CCFP; (416)338-7088

CHAN, Audrey S; King West Med Associates, 505 King St W, Hamilton ON L8P 1B9; McM'04; CCFP; (905)525-3501; Fax. (905)528-5468.

CHAN, Benedict S; Guelph Gen Hosp, 115 Delhi St, Guelph ON N1E 4J4; Cal'97; CCFP; FCFP; Staff, Guelph General Hospital; (519)822-5350

CHAN, Benjamin T; Espanola Reg Hosp & Hlth Ctre, 825 McKinnon Dr, Espanola ON P5E 1R4; Tor'88; MPH; MPA; Staff, Espanola Regional Hospital and Health Centre; CEO, Ontario Health Quality Council; Langs: Cantonese; Spanish; French; (705)869-1420; ben.chan@ohqc.ca.

CHAN, Betty L; 303-1033 Bay St, Toronto ON M5S 3A5; Tor'85; FRCPC; IntMed; Endocrin&Metab. Consultant Pt-Time Div of Endocrin&Metab, St Michael's Hospital; (416)515-0007; john@baywoodclinic.com.

CHAN, Bob C C; William Osler HC-Brampton, 2100 Bovaird Dr E, Brampton ON L6R 3J7; Tor'80; FRCPC; DiagRad. Staff Diag Imaging, William Osler Health System - Brampton Civic Hospital; (905)494-2120; Fax. (905)451-6168.

CHAN, Bok Man; St Michael's Hosp, 30 Bond St, Toronto ON M5B 1W8; London (England)'87; FRCPC; Anes (Pain Management). Staff, St Michael's Hospital; Asst Prof, University of Toronto; (416)864-5071; bokman.chan@utoronto.ca.

CHAN, Bonnie F; Mackenzie Richmond Hill Hosp, 10 Trench St, Richmond Hill ON L4C 4Z3; CCFP; Staff, Mackenzie Richmond Hill Hospital; (905)883-1212

CHAN, Bowen; Health Source Med Clinic, C1-473 Dupont St, Toronto ON M6G 1Y6; Tor'05; CCFP; (416)588-1888

CHAN, Brian A; 207-4190 Finch Ave E, Scarborough ON M1S 4T7; Saba (Netherlands Antilles)'09; (416)298-3883

CHAN, Charles K N; 9N945-585 University Ave, Toronto ON M5G 2N2; Tor'81; FCCP; FACP; FRCPC; IntMed (Interstitial Lung Disease); Respir. Consultant Respirol, Mount Sinai Hospital; Staff, Toronto General Hospital - UHN; Prof Med, University of Toronto; Langs: Cantonese; (416)340-3235; charles.chan@uhn.on.ca.

CHAN, Charlton C W; Maitland Valley Family Hlth Team, 180 Cambria Rd N, Goderich ON N7A 4N8; Wes'69; (519)524-6060; Fax. (519)524-5225.

CHAN, Chin K; Shouldice Hosp, 7750 Bayview Ave, Thornhill ON L3T 4A3; McG'69; BSc; DAB; FRCSC; GenSurg (Hernias). Associate Surg, Shouldice Hospital; Langs: Chinese; (905)889-1125; Fax. (905)889-4216.

CHAN, Chris C W; Sunnybrook Hlth Sciences Ctre, 2075 Bayview Ave, Toronto ON M4N 3M5; (Other Foreign)'06; FRCPC; IntMed. Clin Fellow, Sunnybrook Health Sciences Centre; (416)480-4522

CHAN, Christopher T M; Univ Hlth Network-Toronto Gen, 8N 842-200 Elizabeth St, Toronto ON M5G 2C4; Tor'95; FRCPC; IntMed; Nephrol. Staff, Toronto General Hospital - UHN; Langs: Cantonese; French; (416)340-3073; Fax. (416)340-4999; christopher.chan@uhn.on.ca.

CHAN, Christopher W J; MedWest Med Clinic, 10 & 10A-110 Wedge Rd, Saskatoon SK S7L 6Y4; Sask'92; (306)979-6185; Fax. (306)979-6186.

CHAN, Clara C; Rosedale Med Centre, 601-600 Sherbourne St, Toronto ON M4X 1W4; Qns'05; FRCSC; Ophth (Cataract). Clin Asst, Toronto Western Hospital - University Health Network; Lecturer, University of Toronto; Langs: Cantonese; (416)960-5007

CHAN, Clifford C; Medical Arts Bldg, 1-715 Coronation Blvd, Cambridge ON N1R 7R1; Man'78; FRCSC; ObstGyn. Chief Obst, Cambridge Memorial Hospital; (519)740-1660; Fax. (519)623-6355.

CHAN, Cynthia S Y; South Community Health Centre, 6405 Knight St, Vancouver BC V5P 2V9; Man'78; CCFP; FCFP; (604)321-6151; Fax. (604)301-2272.

CHAN, Cyril F Y; 2784 Kingsway, Vancouver BC V5R 5H6; UBC'78; Vis Staff, Providence Health Care - Mount Saint Joseph Hospital; Langs: Cantonese; Mandarin; (604)433-2461; Fax. (604)439-2461.

CHAN, Danial L A; Foothills Med Centre, 1403 29 St NW, Calgary AB T2N 2T9; Cal'01; Staff, Foothills Medical Centre; (403)944-1252

CHAN, David H; Stonechurch Family Health Ctre, 1475 Upper Ottawa St, Hamilton ON L8W 3J6; Tor'83; MSc; CCFP; FCFP; Asst Prof Family Med, McMaster University; Langs: Cantonese; (905)575-1300; Fax. (905)575-0779; dchan@mcmaster.ca.

CHAN, David K W; 923-55 Queen St E, Toronto ON M5C 1R6; Tor'98; FRCPC; Neur. Staff, St Michael's Hospital; (416)864-5474; Fax. (416)864-5473.

CHAN, David Y K; 203-800 Bathurst St, Toronto ON M5R 3M8; Sydney (Australia)'71; Ac Staff, St Joseph's Health Centre; Langs: Cantonese; Mandarin; (416)535-4602; Fax. (416)532-6649; dychanmd@yahoo.com.

CHAN, Denise; Foothills Med Centre, 1403 29 St NW, Calgary AB T2N 2T9; UBC'01; FRCPC; NuclearMed; DiagRad. Staff, Foothills Medical Centre; (403)944-1252

CHAN, Denise W; 118-5811 No 3 Rd, Richmond BC V6X 4L7; Tor'06; CCFP; (604)279-8881

CHAN, Donald R; Palisades Med Clinic, 12808 137 Ave NW, Edmonton AB T5L 4Y8; Cal'87; BSc; MSc; CCFP; FCFP; (780)457-1100; Fax. (780)457-0033.

CHAN, Dora; 505-18 Wynford Dr, North York ON M3C 3S2; Wes'06; FRCSC; ObstGyn.

CHAN, Douglas S; Misericordia Community Hosp, 16940 87 Ave NW, Edmonton AB T5R 4H5; Alb'04; FRCPC; Anes. Staff, Covenant Health - Misericordia Community Hospital; (780)735-2863; Fax. (780)735-2967.

CHAN, Edmond S; Children's & Women's HC of BC, 1C31B-4480 Oak St, Vancouver BC V6H 3V4; Alb'99; FRCP; FRCPC; Peds (Pediatric Allergy); ClinImmunol&Allergy. Staff Physician, BC Children's Hospital; Clinical Asst Prof, University of British Columbia; Langs: Cantonese; (604)875-2118; Fax. (604)875-3653.

CHAN, Edward; Cambridge Med Place, 2B-695 Coronation Blvd, Cambridge ON N1R 7J9; Wes'92; FRCSC; GenSurg. Ac Staff, Cambridge Memorial Hospital; Aj Clinical Asst Prof Surg, McMaster University; (519)740-1625; Fax. (519)740-0115; echan@cmh.org.

CHAN, Edward S M; Southlake Reg Hosp, 596 Davis Dr, Newmarket ON L3Y 2P9; Ott'01; CCFP; CCFP(E.M.); Staff, Southlake Regional Health Centre; (905)895-4521

CHAN, Edward Y; Westminster Med Bldg, 505-625 Fifth Ave, New Westminster BC V3M 1X4; (Hong Kong)'67; MRC(UK); AB; ABIM; FRCPC; IntMed. Ac Staff, Royal Columbian Hospital; (604)522-6711; Fax. (604)522-6535.

CHAN, Edwin S L; 111-21 Queensway W, Mississauga ON L5B 1B6; Dundee (Scotland)'90; FRCPC; IntMed; Rheum. (905)897-9228

CHAN, Elisa K Y; BC Cancer Agency-Vancouver CC, 600 10th Ave, Vancouver BC V5Z 4E6; Tor'06; FRCPC; RadOncol. Staff, BC Cancer Agency Vancouver Centre; (604)877-6000 x2668

CHAN, Eliza K; Concordia Hosp, 1095 Concordia Ave, Winnipeg MB R2K 3S8; Man'88; CCFP; FCFP; CCFP(E.M.); Staff, Concordia General Hospital; (204)667-1560

CHAN, Emily H; Royal Victoria Hosp, 201 Georgian Dr, Barrie ON L4M 6M2; McM'06; FRCPC; Anes. Staff, Royal Victoria Regional Health Centre; (705)728-9802

CHAN, Eng Lyan; Woo Med Centre, 489 St Mary's Rd, Winnipeg MB R2M 3L1; Rangoon (Burma)'77; (204)254-2360; Fax. (204)256-3892.

CHAN, Eng-Soon; Sanofi Pasteur, 1755 Steeles Ave W, North York ON M2R 3T4; Rangoon (Burma)'88; FRCPC; CommunMed (Family Medicine). Langs: Chinese; (416)667-2722

CHAN, Erin T W; Tsh Family Med Teaching Unit, A 2F-3000 Lawrence Ave E, Scarborough ON M1P 2V1; Ott'10; CCFP; (416)431-8224

CHAN, Eugene J; Westminster Med Bldg, 206-625 Fifth Ave, New Westminster BC V3M 1X4; UBC'58; Derm. (604)524-3171; Fax. (604)524-2285.

CHAN, Eugene Y C; 553 St Clair Ave W, Toronto ON M6C 1A3; Tor'89; (416)652-3307

CHAN, Florence; Anne Johnston Health Station, 2398 Yonge St, Toronto ON M4P 2H4; Tor'04; CCFP; (416)486-8666

CHAN, Francis M Y C; Caledonian Med Clinic, 340 Campbell St, Nanaimo BC V9R 3G7; UBC'91; CCFP; (250)753-3202; Fax. (250)753-1039.

CHAN, Frank S M; Keele-Ingram Prof Centre, 303-2221 Keele St, North York ON M6M 3Z5; Wes'81; FRCPC; IntMed. Staff, Humber River Regional Hospital - Keele Street Site; (416)241-4010; Fax. (416)241-1579.

CHAN, Gabriel F P; Yee Hong Med Centre/Geriatric, 60 Scottfield Dr, Scarborough ON M1S 5T7; (Hong Kong)'82; MB BS(HK); MRCP(UK); FRCP(Edin); FRCPC; IntMed; GeriatricMed. Leader Med Elder Program, North York General Hospital; Staff Med, The Scarborough Hospital - Birchmount Campus; Consultant Geriatric, Yee Hong Centre For Geriatric Care; Langs: Chiuchow; Cantonese; Mandarin; (416)940-4818; Fax. (416)292-1709.

CHAN, Gabriel; Clin Med Maisonneuve-Rosemont, 205-5345 boul de l'Maisonneuve, Montreal QC H1T 4B3; Wes'00; FRCSC; GenSurg. Staff, Hopital Maisonneuve-Rosemont; (514)252-0606; Fax. (514)252-0896.

CHAN, Gabriel W L; Kent Place Mall, 206 2-189 Kent St W, Lindsay ON K9V 5G6; Wes'05; FRCPC; IntMed; Gastroent. Staff, London Health Sciences Centre - University Hospital; (705)878-5200; Fax. (705)878-5229.

CHAN, Gerald C B; Finch-Midland Med Centre, 306-4190 Finch Ave E, Scarborough ON M1S 4T7; (Hong Kong)'80; MB BS; MRC(UK); FRCPC; IntMed (Hepatology); Gastroent. Staff Gastroent, The Scarborough Hospital - Birchmount Campus; Langs: Cantonese; Mandarin; (416)299-3502; Fax. (416)299-3797.

CHAN, Gladys K Y; North York Med Arts Bldg, 243-1333 Sheppard Ave E, North York ON M2J 1V1; Wes'04; FRCSC; OrthSurg. (416)494-7351; Fax. (416)494-7446.

CHAN, Grace S; Sandy Hill Commun Health Ctre, 221 Nelson St, Ottawa ON K1N 1C7; Mem'03; CCFP; Staff, Canadian Forces Health Services Centre; (613)789-8458

CHAN, Gregory K; Family Health Clinic, PO Box 4127 Stn Main 10-5011 48 Ave, Ponoka AB T4J 1R5; Alb'06; CCFP; (403)783-5305; Fax. (403)783-8722.

CHAN, H B Tony; 90 Main St E, Milton ON L9T 1N3; Ott'78; CCFP; Medical Staff Family Pract, Halton Healthcare Services Corporation - Milton District Hospital; (905)878-2542; Fax. (905)878-7667.

CHAN, Helen S L; The Hosp for Sick Children, 9412-555 University Ave, Toronto ON M5G 1X8; (Hong Kong)'71; ABPeds; FAAP; FRCPC; Peds (Pediatric Oncology). Staff Peds & Ped HemOncol & Sr Scientist Research Inst, The Hospital For Sick Children; Prof Peds, University of Toronto; Langs: Cantonese; (416)813-6910; Fax. (416)813-5327.

CHAN, Henry; Atria 1, W300-2255 Sheppard Ave E, North York ON M2J 4Y1; (Hong Kong)'97; FRCSC; OrthSurg. (416)495-9902

CHAN, Herman; Sunnybrook Hlth Sciences Ctre, M3 200-2075 Bayview Ave, Toronto ON M4N 3M5; Tor'95; FRCPC; Anes. Staff, Sunnybrook Health Sciences Centre; (416)480-4864; Fax. (416)480-6039.

CHAN, Howard H W; St Joseph's Healthcare, L208-50 Charlton St E, Hamilton ON L8N 4A6; Hongkong (Hong Kong)'87; FRCPC; IntMed (Clinician Investigator Program); Hem. Staff, St Joseph's Healthcare - Charlton Campus; (905)522-1155; chanh@mcmaster.ca.

CHAN, Ian L; Lions Gate Hospital, 231 15th St E, North Vancouver BC V7L 2L7; Wes'06; FRCPC; DiagRad. Staff, Lions Gate Hospital; (604)984-5775

CHAN, Ida H T; Mayfair Place, 120-6707 Elbow Dr SW, Calgary AB T2V 0E3; UBC'05; FRCPC; DiagRad; NuclearMed. (403)777-3007; Fax. (403)777-3008.

CHAN, Irene M Y; 4123 Fraser St, Vancouver BC V5V 4E9; UBC'92; Langs: Cantonese; (604)876-8063; Fax. (604)876-8063.

CHAN, Irene O L; Queensway Carleton Hosp, 3045 Baseline Rd, Nepean ON K2H 8P4; Qns'05; CCFP; Staff, Queensway Carleton Hospital; (613)721-2000

CHAN, James W T; The Ottawa Hosp-Gen Campus, 501 Smyth Rd, Ottawa ON K1H 8L6; Tor'95; FRCPC; IntMed. Staff, The Ottawa Hospital - General Campus; (613)737-8979; Fax. (613)737-8688; jchan@ottawahospital.on.ca.

CHAN, Jean-Wen; Trillium Hlth Ctr-Mississauga, 100 Queensway W, Mississauga ON L5B 1B8; Tor'95; FRCPC; DiagRad (Neuro Radiology). Staff, Trillium Health Centre - Mississauga; (905)848-7529

CHAN, Jeanie C; Oakridge Centre South Tower, 222-650 41st Ave W, Vancouver BC V5Z 2M9; Alb'77; BMedSci; Court Staff, Providence Health Care - Mount Saint Joseph Hospital; Assoc Staff, BC Children's Hospital; Langs: Cantonese; (604)261-2633; Fax. (604)261-2687.

CHAN, Jennifer A; Foothills Med Centre, C1150B-1403 29 St NW, Calgary AB T2N 2T9; McG'98; FRCPC; NeurPath. Staff, Foothills Medical Centre; (403)944-4755

CHAN, Jennifer M; Aikens Street Comm Health Ctre, 601 Aikins St, Winnipeg MB R2W 4J5; Wes'01; CCFP; (204)940-2025; jchan@wrha.mb.ca.

CHAN, Jessica W; 234 Hastings St E, Vancouver BC V6A 1P1; UBC'03; CCFP; (604)688-0351

CHAN, John F Y; Times Medical Clinic, 96-550 Hwy 7 E, Richmond Hill ON L4B 3Z4; Tor'90; Langs: Cantonese; (905)707-8181

CHAN, John; Mackenzie Richmond Hill Hosp, 10 Trench St, Richmond Hill ON L4C 4Z3; McM'99; FRCPC; Psy. Staff, Mackenzie Richmond Hill Hospital; (905)883-1212; Fax. (905)883-2144.

CHAN, John K F; 2-2629 Cedar Park Pl, Abbotsford BC V2T 3S4; Cal'80; CCFP; FCFP; Staff, Abbotsford Regional Hospital & Cancer Centre; Langs: Chinese; Mandarin; Cantonese; (604)854-3117; Fax. (604)854-4377.

CHAN, John S; Rockyview Gen Hosp, 7007 14 St SW, Calgary AB T2V 1P9; UBC'95; BSc; FRCPC; IntMed; Respir. Staff, Rockyview General Hospital; (403)943-3283; Fax. (403)252-6471; john.chan@calgaryhealthregion.ca.

CHAN, John W L; High Point Med Centre, 405-3461 Dixie Rd, Mississauga ON L4Y 3X4; Tor'79; Langs: Chinese; (905)624-7225; Fax. (905)624-7225.

CHAN, John Y W; Chalmers Gate Med Bldg, 209-328 Highway 7 E, Richmond Hill ON L4B 3P7; (Hong Kong)'74; MB BS; MRCP(UK); FRCP(Edin); Staff, Mackenzie Richmond Hill Hospital; Langs: Chinese; (905)882-4828; Fax. (905)882-1602; johnywchan@rogers.com.

CHAN, Jonathan E K; 308-385 Silver Star Blvd, Scarborough ON M1V 0E3; McM'03; FRCSC; Urol. (416)776-3383; Fax. (416)776-3382.

CHAN, Jonathan S; Aspire Med Clinics, 4120-15 Sunpark Plaza SE, Calgary AB T2X 0M5; Alb'01; CCFP; CCFP(E.M.); (403)910-3990; Fax. (403)910-0449.

CHAN, Joseph; Chalmers Med Office, 8-360 Highway 7 E, Richmond Hill ON L4B 3Y7; Tor'81; CCFP; (905)881-0906; Fax. (905)881-0900.

CHAN, Joseph E; 202-3251 Sheppard Ave E, Scarborough ON M1T 3W5; Wes'03; FRCSC; GenSurg. (416)773-1900; Fax. (416)773-1902.

CHAN, Joseph J; Misericordia Health Centre, 99 Cornish Ave, Winnipeg MB R3C 1A2; London (England)'65; MB BS; Ac Staff Anes, Misericordia Health Centre; (204)774-6581; Fax. (204)788-8529.

CHAN, Juanita Y; Mississauga Med Centre, 205-1420 Burnhamthorpe Rd E, Mississauga ON L4X 2Z9; McG'98; BSc; CCFP; FCFP; (905)625-4016; Fax. (905)625-7721.

CHAN, K H Albert; 301-5171 221A St, Langley BC V2Y 0A2; Man'87; DABOS; FRCSC; OrthSurg (Sports Medicine). Surgeon, Abbotsford Regional Hospital & Cancer Centre; Head Dept of Surg, Langley Memorial Hospital; Surgeon, Langley Surgical Centre; (604)539-9868

CHAN, Ka Lam; Delhi Family Health Team, 105 Main St, Delhi ON N4B 2L8; Tor'08; BSc; MSc; CCFP; (519)582-2323

CHAN, Kai-Sun; 104-515 Main St, Vancouver BC V6A 2V1; UBC'67; Ac Staff, Providence Health Care - Mount Saint Joseph Hospital; Vis Staff, Providence Health Care - St Paul's Hospital; (604)685-4017; Fax. (604)685-4017.

CHAN, Kam Ming; Glenrose Rehab Hosp, 1436-10230 111 Ave NW, Edmonton AB T5G 0B7; Glasgow (Scotland)'84; ABPMR; FRCPC; PhysMed&Rehab (Neuromuscular Diseases). Staff, Glenrose Rehabilitation Hospital; Staff, Royal Alexandra Hospital; Staff, University of Alberta Hospital; Assoc Prof Div of PhyMed & Rehab/Neuroscience, University of Alberta; Langs: Chinese; (780)735-8210

CHAN, Karen B Y; Digestive Health Clinic, 510-330 Highway 7 E, Richmond Hill ON L4B 3P8; Wes'98; FRCPC; IntMed; Gastroent. (905)707-5007; Fax. (905)707-5008.

CHAN, Karl K S; 5573 Victoria Dr, Vancouver BC V5P 3W2; (Hong Kong)'63; MB BS; Staff, Providence Health Care - Mount Saint Joseph Hospital; Langs: Cantonese; Mandarin; Vietnamese; (604)877-1233; Fax. (604)877-1030.

CHAN, Katherine Y; 401-2299 Dundas St W, Toronto ON M6R 1X7; UBC'80; Staff, Humber River Regional Hospital - Finch Avenue Site; (416)769-2351; Fax. (416)769-4329; drkchan23@gmail.com.

CHAN, Kelvin H; 2450 Lancaster Rd, Ottawa ON K1B 5N3; Ott'10; CCFP; (613)738-9119

CHAN, Kelvin K; Sunnybrook Hlth Sciences Ctre, Wing T 2F-2075 Bayview Ave, Toronto ON M4N 3M5; Tor'99; FRCPC; IntMed; MedOncol. Staff, Sunnybrook Health Sciences Centre; (416)480-5000

CHAN, Kelvin; Surrey Mem Hosp, 13750 96 Ave, Surrey BC V3V 1Z2; UBC'07; CCFP; Staff, Surrey Memorial Hospital; (604)512-6329

CHAN, Kenneth H; Regent Med Bldg, 480-2184 Broadway W, Vancouver BC V6K 2E1; UBC'73; CCFP; FCFP; Ac Staff, Providence Health Care - Mount Saint Joseph Hospital; (604)736-6391; Fax. (604)736-6392.

CHAN, Kenneth; Scarborough Hosp-General Div, 3050 Lawrence Ave E, Scarborough ON M1P 2V5; Qns'92; FRCPC; Anes. Staff Anes, The Scarborough Hospital - General Campus; Locum Anes, William Osler Health System - Brampton Civic Hospital; (416)431-8133; Fax. (416)431-8192.

CHAN, Kenneth L; Hop Charles Lemoyne, 3120 boul Taschereau, Greenfield Park QC J4V 2H1; McG'89; FRCSC; ObstGyn; GynOnco (P.Q.). Staff, Hopital Charles LeMoyne; Langs: Cantonese; French; (450)466-5000

CHAN, Kerry K; Campbell Clinic, 430 Mayor Magrath Dr S, Lethbridge AB T1J 3M1; Alb'85; FRCPC; Peds (Developmental/Behavioural Pediatrics). Ac Staff, Chinook Regional Hospital; Associate, Crowsnest Pass Health Centre; Consultant, Taber Health Centre; University of Calgary; (403)328-8101; Fax. (403)328-8150; kerry@crowsnestpass.com.

CHAN, Kevin C Y; Kanata Prof Centre, 207-99 Kakulu Rd, Kanata ON K2L 3C8; Dal'99; FRCPC; Peds. (613)591-1234; Fax. (613)591-1237.

CHAN, Kevin J; The Hosp for Sick Children, 555 University Ave, Toronto ON M5G 1X8; Ott'97; FAAP; MPH; FRCPC; Peds; PedEmergMed. Asst Prof, The Hospital For Sick Children; Asst Prof, University of Toronto; Langs: Cantonese; French; (416)813-7654 x1417

CHAN, King-Sun; Chinatown Med Centre, 201-480 Dundas St W, Toronto ON M5T 1G9; Wuhan Med. Coll. (China)'60; Langs: Chinese; (416)591-3988; Fax. (416)591-6988.

CHAN, Kitty Y; Links Clinic, 104-11910 111 Ave NW, Edmonton AB T5G 3G6; Alb'89; CCFP; (780)454-0351; Fax. (780)453-9471.

CHAN, Kong; Alder Med Centre, 277 Evergreen Rd, Campbell River BC V9W 5Y4; Dublin (Ireland)'74; MB ChB; BAO; MRC; FRCOG; Ac Staff, Campbell River & District General Hospital; (250)287-7454; Fax. (250)286-3628.

CHAN, Konrad K; Joseph Brant Mem Hosp, 1230 North Shore Blvd E, Burlington ON L7S 1W7; Glasgow (Scotland)'90; FRCPC; GenPath. Staff, Joseph Brant Memorial Hospital; (905)632-3730

CHAN, Kris H K; University of Alberta Hosp, 2C2-8440 112 St NW, Edmonton AB T6G 2B7; Alb'07; FRCPC; IntMed. Staff, University of Alberta Hospital; (780)407-1857; Fax. (780)407-6452.

CHAN, Kwan-Leung; Univ of Ottawa Heart Institute, 40 Ruskin St, Ottawa ON K1Y 4W7; Man'78; FRCPC; IntMed; Cardiol. Staff Teacher, University of Ottawa Heart Institute; Staff Teacher, The Ottawa Hospital - Civic Campus; Langs: Cantonese; (613)761-4189; Fax. (613)761-4170; kchan@ottawaheart.ca.

CHAN, Kwok-Hung; 3F 307-2130 Lawrence Ave E, Scarborough ON M1R 3A6; (Hong Kong)'62; MB BS; Langs: Cantonese; (416)751-6141; Fax. (416)751-5270.

CHAN, Laura H; Sterling Lyon Health Centre, 201-1020 Lorimer Blvd, Winnipeg MB R3P 1C7; Man'01; BSc; FRCSC; Otol. Asst Prof Otol, University of Manitoba; (204)943-0629; Fax. (204)956-1559.

CHAN, Laura H Y; Royal Court Med Centre, 106-1 Quarry Ridge Rd, Barrie ON L4M 7G1; National (Ireland)'04; CCFP; Langs: Cantonese; (705)725-9922

CHAN, Lawrence K C; The Doctor's Office, 325 Bamburgh Cir, Scarborough ON M1W 3Y1; Tor'94; CCFP; FCFP; Langs: Cantonese; Mandarin; (416)492-8068; Fax. (416)497-7796.

CHAN, Leslie F; 224-555 Strathcona Blvd SW, Calgary AB T3H 2Z9; UBC'97; CCFP; (403)686-2911

CHAN, Loh Yen L; East Mississauga Comm Hlth Ctr, 7-2555 Dixie Rd, Mississauga ON L4Y 4C4; Tor'07; CCFP; Langs: Cantonese; (905)602-7723; Fax. (905)602-5432.

CHAN, Lucille S Y; Guelph Family Health Team, 101-83 Dawson Rd, Guelph ON N1H 1B1; Wes'06; CCFP; (519)766-1360

CHAN, Macky M K; Markham Stoufville Urgent Care, 100-110 Copper Creek Dr, Markham ON L6B 0P9; Tor'07; CCFP; (905)472-8911; Fax. (905)472-6081.

CHAN, Mercedes O; BC Children's Hosp, K4 119-4480 Oak St, Vancouver BC V6H 3V4; (Hong Kong)'04; FRCPC; Peds; Rheum. Staff, BC Children's Hospital; (604)875-2345

CHAN, Michael C K; 407-2863 Ellesmere Rd, Scarborough ON M1E 5E9; Qns'86; FRCSC; GenSurg; ThorSurg. Ac Staff, Rouge Valley Health System - Centenary Health Centre Site; Langs: Cantonese; (416)287-1943; Fax. (416)283-4083.

CHAN, Michael C Y; Hys Med Centre, 350-11010 101 St NW, Edmonton AB T5H 4B9; (Hong Kong)'87; DABIM(CardioVasDis); FRCS; FACC; FRCPC; IntMed (Heart Failure); Cardiol. Staff Cardiol Dept, Royal Alexandra Hospital; Staff Cardiol Dept, University of Alberta Hospital; Assoc Clin Prof, University of Alberta; (780)428-3246; Fax. (780)425-0487.

CHAN, Michael P; Providence Care-Mental Health, PO Box 603 Stn Main 752 King St W, Kingston ON K7L 4X3; (Jamaica)'81; MRCPsy; FRCPC; Psy. Staff Psy, Providence Care - Mental Health Services; Adjunct Ass't. Prof., Queen's University; (613)546-1101; Fax. (613)540-6113.

CHAN, Ming-Ka; Health Sciences Centre, AE405-820 Sherbrook St, Winnipeg MB R3A 1R9; Wes'95; BSc; FRCPC; Peds. Prog Dir Peds & Child Health, Health Sciences Centre; Site Coord Canadian Forces Phys Ass't Prog, University of Manitoba; Langs: Cantonese; (204)787-1676; Fax. (204)787-1938; mkc88@hotmail.com.

CHAN, Monica K H; 119-8787 Woodbine Ave, Markham ON L3R 9S2; Tor'98; CCFP; Langs: Chinese; (905)415-9009; Fax. (905)415-9119.

CHAN, Nancy G; London HSC-University Hosp, PO Box 5339 Stn B 339 Windermere Rd, London ON N6A 4G5; UBC'01; FRCPC; AnatPath. Staff, London Health Sciences Centre - University Hospital; (519)685-8500; Fax. (519)663-2930.

CHAN, Nathaniel I; 4825 Dalhousie Dr NW, Calgary AB T3A 6K7; UBC'04; FRCPC; Peds. Staff, Peter Lougheed Centre; (403)239-9333

CHAN, Nelson N S; St Joseph's Fam Med Centre, 346 Platt's Lane, London ON N6G 1J1; Tor'08; CCFP; (519)672-9660

CHAN, Norman G; Norman Chan Med Prof Corp, 201-83 Dawson Rd, Guelph ON N1H 1B1; McM'87; FRCPC; IntMed; Cardiol. Staff, Guelph General Hospital; (519)837-9111; Fax. (519)837-8582.

CHAN, Norman H; 1513 Main St E, Hamilton ON L8K 1E2; Tor'75; Court Staff, St Joseph's Healthcare - Charlton Campus; Court Staff, Hamilton Health Sciences Centre - McMaster Children's Hospital; (905)547-7854; Fax. (905)545-8767.

CHAN, Patricia C K; Finch-Midland Med Centre, 303-4190 Finch Ave E, Scarborough ON M1S 4T7; (Hong Kong)'81; FRCP(Edin); FACP; MB BS(HK); FRCPC; IntMed (Nephrology). Ac Staff, Toronto East General Hospital Inc; Court Staff, The Scarborough Hospital - General Campus; Staff Nephrologist, Scarborough Regional Dialysis Program; (416)335-9889; Fax. (416)335-9339.

CHAN, Patrick B; 62 Queen's Park Cres, Winnipeg MB R3P 1H9; Man'75; FRCPC; EmergMed. Staff, Misericordia Health Centre; Staff, St Boniface General Hospital; Asst Prof, University of Manitoba; (204)488-3762; Fax. (204)488-3762; patrickbwchan@shaw.ca.

CHAN, Patrick D S; 154 Meadowlark Shopping Ctr NW, Edmonton AB T5R 5W9; Alb'90; MSc; FRCSC; Neursurg. (780)429-4761; Fax. (780)425-4274.

CHAN, Patrick F; 230-150 Esplanade W, North Vancouver BC V7M 1A3; UBC'96; (604)980-2128

CHAN, Patrick S P; 58 Beverley St, Toronto ON M5T 1X9; London (England)'63; MB BS; FRCPC; Derm. Consultant Derm, Trillium Health Centre - Mississauga; Consultant Derm, Toronto Western Hospital - University Health Network; Lecturer, University of Toronto; Langs: Chinese; (416)979-1845

CHAN, Paul C; 8-1170 Burnhamthorpe Rd W, Mississauga ON L5C 4E6; (Hong Kong)'77; MRC(UK); Langs: Cantonese; Mandarin; (905)566-0092; Fax. (905)566-0946; pclchan@hotmail.com.

CHAN, Paul P; SMBD Jewish Gen Hosp, 3755 ch Cote-Sainte-Catherine, Montreal QC H3T 1E2; Tor'75; FRCPC; Psy. Staff, Douglas Mental Health University Institute; Dir Emerg Psy, Sir Mortimer B Davis Jewish General; McGill University; (514)340-8222

CHAN, Paul S H; 106-4235 Sheppard Ave E, Scarborough ON M1S 1T7; Tor'88; Langs: Cantonese; (416)292-5000; Fax. (416)292-5861.

CHAN, Paul Y H; 201-3030 Lincoln Ave, Coquitlam BC V3B 6B4; Alb'92; CCFP; Langs: Cantonese; Mandarin; (604)552-7757

CHAN, Peter A; Anaesthetic Services, 213-2186 Oak Bay Ave, Victoria BC V8R 1G3; Tor'02; FRCPC; Anes. Staff, Providence Health Care - St Paul's Hospital; (250)508-5818

CHAN, Peter K; Evergold Centre, 28-3833 Midland Ave, Scarborough ON M1V 5L6; Tor'88; (416)291-0980; Fax. (416)291-8674.

CHAN, Peter K Y; Vancouver Gen Hosp, 5F-855 12th Ave W, Vancouver BC V5Z 1M9; UBC'88; FRCPC; Psy. Staff, Vancouver General Hospital - Centennial Pavillion; (604)875-4809; Fax. (604)875-5652.

CHAN, Peter S K; 102-4631 Steeles Ave E, Scarborough ON M1V 4S5; Tor'79; Staff, The Scarborough Hospital - Birchmount Campus; (416)293-6600

CHAN, Peter T K; MUHC-Royal Victoria Hosp, S6.95-687 av des Pins O, Montreal QC H3A 1A1; McG'94; BSc; MSc; FRCSC; Urol (Erectile Dysfunction). Staff, McGill University Health Centre - Royal Victoria Hospital; (514)843-1571

CHAN, Philip; Lion's Gate Hosp, 231 15th St E, North Vancouver BC V7L 2L7; Wes'98; BSc; CCFP; Staff, Lions Gate Hospital; Langs: Cantonese; (604)988-3131

CHAN, Philip S L; St Joseph's Healthcare, D149-50 Charlton Ave E, Hamilton ON L8N 4A6; Qns'01; FRCPC; Anes. Staff, St Joseph's Healthcare - Charlton Campus; (905)522-1155; Fax. (905)521-6019.

CHAN, Raphael L; The Ottawa Hosp-Gen Campus, 5235-501 Smyth Rd, Ottawa ON K1H 8L6; UBC'98; CCFP; Staff, The Ottawa Hospital - General Campus; (613)737-8940; Fax. (613)739-6182.

CHAN, Raymond H K; 134-9450 137 Ave NW, Edmonton AB T5E 6C2; Alb'81; FRCPC; DiagRad; NuclearMed. Staff/Consultant Radiol, Westlock Healthcare Centre; (780)478-7221

CHAN, Raymond H M; 5-4646 Dufferin St, North York ON M3H 5S4; Qns'04; FRCPC; IntMed; Cardiol. Teach Staff, McMaster University; (416)222-6160

CHAN, Raymond K H; 101-420 Highway 7 E, Richmond Hill ON L4B 3K2; Tor'95; CCFP; Langs: Cantonese; Mandarin; (905)709-0777; Fax. (905)709-0776.

CHAN, Raymond P; Maple Med Centre, 102-995 Major Mackenzie Dr, Vaughan ON L6A 4P9; Tor'95; FRCPC; DiagRad. Staff, St Michael's Hospital.

CHAN, Richard C; Royal City Med Bldg, 101-250 Keary St, New Westminster BC V3L 5E7; Dallas(TX) (USA)'78; BSc; DAB; DABNS; FRCSC; Neursurg (Peripheral Nerve Surgery). Staff, Royal Columbian Hospital; Staff, Eagle Ridge Hospital & Health Care Centre; (604)526-6612; Fax. (604)520-1705.

CHAN, Richard C W; Broadview Med Centre, G/F-741 Broadview Ave, Toronto ON M4K 3Y3; Tor'78; Langs: Cantonese; Mandarin; (416)463-2438; Fax. (416)463-2526; dr.chan@rogers.com.

CHAN, Richard K; Richmond Hosp, 7000 Westminster Hwy, Richmond BC V6X 1A2; UBC'98; CCFP; CCFP(E.M.); Staff, Richmond Hospital; (604)244-5585

CHAN, Robert K W; 1502-400 Campbell Rd, St. Albert AB T8N 0R8; Cal'03; FRCSC; OrthSurg (Elbow & Wrist Surgery). Staff, Sturgeon Community Hospital; (780)569-5495; Fax. (780)569-5493; drchan2011@yahoo.ca.

CHAN, Ronnie S; 142 Queenston St, St. Catharines ON L2R 2Z7; Tor'03; FRCPC; IntMed; Gastroent. (905)378-4647

CHAN, Roy K; Huntingwood Med Clinic, 2361 Warden Ave, Scarborough ON M1T 1V7; Tor'78; CCFP; Staff, The Scarborough Hospital - General Campus; (416)299-4999; Fax. (416)299-1322; dr_roychan@hotmail.com.

CHAN, Ruby W Y; 211-1676 Martin Dr, Surrey BC V4A 6E7; Tor'88; FRCPC; Peds. Staff, Peace Arch Hospital; Staff, Langley Memorial Hospital; (604)531-7707

CHAN, Ryan; Children's & Women's HC of BC, 4480 Oak St, Vancouver BC V6H 3V4; Ott'06; FRCPC; Psy. Staff, BC Children's Hospital; (604)875-2345

CHAN, S H Sandy; Oakridge Plaza, 320-5780 Cambie St, Vancouver BC V5Z 3A7; UBC'91; (604)324-8141; Fax. (604)324-8141.

CHAN, Sammy Y; St Paul's Hosp, B180-1081 Burrard St, Vancouver BC V6Z 1Y6; UBC'84; FRCPC; IntMed; Cardiol. Staff, Providence Health Care - St Paul's Hospital; Staff, Vancouver General Hospital - Centennial Pavillion; (604)806-8605; Fax. (604)806-8590.

CHAN, Shermeen S M; 38 King St W, Dundas ON L9H 1T7; McM'06; CCFP; (905)628-5118; Fax. (905)628-1739.

CHAN, Sherry; G F Strong Rehabilitation Ctr, 4255 Laurel St, Vancouver BC V5Z 2G9; UBC'07; CCFP; Staff, G F Strong Rehabilitation Centre; (604)734-1313

CHAN, Stanley M; Royal Alexandra Hosp, 2306-10240 Kingsway NW, Edmonton AB T5H 3V9; Ott'98; FRCSC; Ophth (Cataract Surgery). Staff, Royal Alexandra Hospital; Assoc Prof, University of Alberta; (780)735-4985; Fax. (780)735-5242.

CHAN, Steven Y T; New Vision Family Health Team, 421 Greenbrook Dr, Kitchener ON N2M 4K1; Tor'05; CCFP; (519)578-3510; Fax. (519)578-6040.

CHAN, Paul; Eastwood Med Clinic, 101-1346 Kingston Rd, Scarborough ON M1N 1P9; Tor'78; Staff, Toronto East General Hospital Inc; (416)698-0883; Fax. (416)698-0917.

CHAN, Susanne M; Southlake Reg Health Centre, 596 Davis Dr, Newmarket ON L3Y 2P9; Wes'06; FRCPC; AnatPath. Staff, Southlake Regional Health Centre; (905)895-4521

CHAN, Suzanne; Medical Sciences Bldg, 8 25-131 University Campus NW, Edmonton AB T6G 2H7; Alb'96; FRCPC; AnatPath. Staff, University of Alberta Hospital; (780)407-3983

CHAN, Tak Keung; 5935 Leslie St, North York ON M2H 1J8; Tor'90; (416)491-9738

CHAN, Tak-Leung; Lakeridge Hlth Corp-Oshawa, 1 Hospital Crt, Oshawa ON L1G 2B9; Man'86; CCFP; FCFP; Staff, Lakeridge Health - Oshawa Site; (905)576-8711; Fax. (905)721-7763.

CHAN, Terence C K; Cambie Surgery Centre, 2836 Ash St, Vancouver BC V5Z 3C6; (Hong Kong)'68; FRCPC; Anes. (604)874-1349

CHAN, Terence; 203-4383 Portage Rd, Niagara Falls ON L2E 6A6; MCW(WI) (USA)'01; DABIM; FRCPC; IntMed. Chief Med, Niagara Health System - Greater Niagara General Site; (905)357-3988

CHAN, Teresa M; McMaster University, MDCL 3101A-1280 Main St W, Hamilton ON L8S 4K1; Wes'08.

CHAN, Theresa W; Surrey Mem Hosp, 13750 96 Ave, Surrey BC V3V 1Z2; UBC'03; FRCPC; IntMed; MedOncol. Staff, Surrey Memorial Hospital; (604)930-4017

CHAN, Thomas T; Scarborough Hosp-General Div, 3050 Lawrence Ave E, Scarborough ON M1P 2V5; Tor'93; CCFP; CCFP(E.M.); Staff, The Scarborough Hospital - General Campus; Lecturer, University of Toronto; (416)438-2911 x6838; Fax. (416)431-8169.

CHAN, Tiffany S; East Edmonton Health Centre, 7910 112 Ave NW, Edmonton AB T5B 0C2; UBC'09; CCFP; (780)342-4700

CHAN, Timothy; 5-555 Balmoral St, Winnipeg MB R3B 2R2; Man'84; (204)943-8705; Fax. (204)943-8705.

CHAN, Toby Y B; 411-564 Belmont Ave, Kitchener ON N2M 5N6; Ott'06; FRCSC; Ophth (Glaucoma). (519)742-1313; Fax. (519)742-3662.

CHAN, Tommy K C; 402-1017 Wilson Ave, North York ON M3K 1Z1; Wes'79; FRCSC; OrthSurg (Arthroplasty). Ac Staff, Humber River Regional Hospital - Church Street Site; Langs: Cantonese; (416)636-9963

CHAN, Tommy W; Rockyview Gen Hosp, 7007 14 St SW, Calgary AB T2V 1P9; Ott'99; FRCPC; Anes. Staff, Rockyview General Hospital; (403)943-8720

CHAN, Trevor H; Low Risk Maternity Clinic, 130-1402 8 Ave NW, Calgary AB T2N 1B9; Alb'06; CCFP; Staff, Foothills Medical Centre; (403)284-3711; Fax. (403)284-3719.

CHAN, Vanessa P S; Jackson Park Health Centre, 150-2475 McDougall St, Windsor ON N8X 3N9; Glasgow (Scotland)'99; FRCPC; IntMed. (519)252-9861

CHAN, Vicky W K; Royal Columbian Hosp, 330 Columbia St E, New Westminster BC V3L 3W7; Tor'06; FRCPC; IntMed; Hem. Staff, Royal Columbian Hospital; (604)777-8358

CHAN, Victor R; Keary Med Centre, 203-245 Columbia St E, New Westminster BC V3L 3W4; (Hong Kong)'65; FACP; FRCPC; IntMed; Nephrol. Staff, Royal Columbian Hospital; Staff, Surrey Memorial Hospital; Clin Assoc Prof Emeritus, University of British Columbia; (604)525-9666; Fax. (604)525-2173.

CHAN, Victoria M Y; 57 Major Mackenzie Dr E, Richmond Hill ON L4C 1G8; Tor'90; FRCPC; IntMed; Respir. Ac Staff, Mackenzie Richmond Hill Hospital; Langs: Chinese; (905)780-6873; Fax. (905)780-6894.

CHAN, Vincent; Univ of Ottawa Heart Institute, 3405A-40 Ruskin St, Ottawa ON K1Y 4W7; Qns'05; FRCSC; CardSurg.

CHAN, Vincent; McArthur Family Med Centre, 206-311 McArthur Ave, Vanier ON K1L 8M3; Man'90; BSc; Langs: Chinese; (613)740-0200; Fax. (613)740-0808; vchan@magma.ca.

CHAN, Vincent W S; Univ Hlth Network-Toronto Western Hosp, 399 Bathurst St, Toronto ON M5T 2S8; McG'80; FRCPC; Anes (Pain Management). Staff Anes, Toronto Western Hospital - University Health Network; Prof, University of Toronto; (416)603-5118; Fax. (416)603-6494; vincent.chan@uhn.on.ca.

CHAN, W Mun-Kam; 7-50 Lockridge Ave, Markham ON L3R 8X4; Tor'92; Langs: Chinese; (905)940-3899; Fax. (905)940-2513.

CHAN, Wai Lam W; Finch-Midland Med Centre, 205-4190 Finch Ave E, Scarborough ON M1S 4T7; (Hong Kong)'76; FRCS(Ed & Glas); Court Staff Family Pract, The Scarborough Hospital - General Campus; Langs: Chinese; (416)299-9088; Fax. (416)299-1543.

CHAN, Wai Sun; Bridlewood Medical Centre, 64 Stonehaven Dr, Kanata ON K2M 2Y2; Belfast (Ireland)'97; (613)592-0805

CHAN, Wayne W K; Tecumseh Manning Med Centre, 108-13278 Tecumseh Rd E, Windsor ON N8N 3T6; Wes'81; BSc; (519)979-2242; Fax. (519)979-9628.

CHAN, Wee Shian; BC Women's Hosp & Health Ctre, 4500 Oak St, Vancouver BC V6H 3N1; Alb'92; FRCPC; IntMed. Staff, BC Women's Hospital & Health Centre; Langs: Mandarin; (604)875-2424

CHAN, Wesley C; Health Sciences Centre, 300 Prince Philip Dr, St. John's NL A1B 3V6; Qns'06; FRCPC; DiagRad. Staff, Health Sciences Centre; (709)737-6300

CHAN, William W L; Total Care Health Centre, 3155 Eglinton Ave E, Scarborough ON M1J 2G2; Tor'76; (416)267-3191

CHAN, William Y F.; 2-2629 Cedar Park Pl, Abbotsford BC V2T 3S4; Cal'82; CCFP; FCFP; (604)854-3117; Fax. (604)854-4377.

CHAN, Wilson W; Calgary Lab Services, 9-3535 Research Rd NW, Calgary AB T2L 2K8; Alb'06; FRCPC; MedMicrobiol. Staff, Calgary Laboratory Services; (403)770-3338

CHAN, Wing Chow; Rosedale Med Centre, 601-600 Sherbourne St, Toronto ON M4X 1W4; Tor'70; DAB; FRCSC; Ophth. Court Staff, St Joseph's Health Centre; Langs: Cantonese; Mandarin; (416)960-5007; Fax. (416)960-0333.

CHAN, Wing-Shing; 103-117 Centrepointe Dr, Nepean ON K2G 5X3; New South Wales (Australia)'70; DTMH; Staff, Queensway Carleton Hospital; (613)221-9765; Fax. (613)221-9805.

CHAN, Winnie W Y; Grand River Hosp-KW Hlth Ctre, PO Box 9056 Stn C 835 King St W, Kitchener ON N2G 1G3; (Hong Kong)'85; MB BS; FRCPC; GenPath. Staff, Grand River Hospital - Kitchener/Waterloo Health Centre; Langs: Chinese; (519)749-4300 x5142; Fax. (519)749-4221; winnie.chan@grhosp.on.ca.

CHAN, Yun Kai; Niagara Falls Med Centre, 309-6453 Morrison St, Niagara Falls ON L2E 7H1; Ott'81; DABIM; FRCPC; IntMed (Cardiology). Med Consultant, Niagara Health System - Greater Niagara General Site; Langs: Chinese; (905)357-5040; Fax. (905)357-2181.

CHAN, Yvonne; 102-101 Queensway W, Mississauga ON L5B 2P7; Tor'02; FRCSC; Otol (Rhinology). Ac Staff, Trillium Health Centre - Mississauga; Langs: Cantonese; (905)277-4312; Fax. (905)277-4439.

CHAN, Zoe; Crowfoot Village Fam Practice, 210-600 Crowfoot Cres NW, Calgary AB T3G 0B4; UBC'07; CCFP; Staff, Foothills Medical Centre; (403)239-9733; Fax. (403)241-8112.

CHAN-LUI, W Y Winifred; Rehabilitation Centre for Chil, 633 Wellington Cres, Winnipeg MB R3M 0A8; (Hong Kong)'63; MB BS; FRCP(Lond); FRCP(Edin); FRCP(Glas); MD(Hong Kong); FRCPC; Peds (Pediatric Neurological Muscular Disorders); Neur. Staff PedNeurol, St Boniface General Hospital; Staff PedNeurol, Rehabilitation Center For Children; Langs: Chinese; (204)452-4311; Fax. (204)474-2387.

CHAN-TAI-KONG, A Joseph; Regina Qu'Appelle HR-Regina, 1440 14th Ave, Regina SK S4P 0W5; Aberdeen (Scotland)'79; FRCPC; Anes (Intensive Care Medicine). Staff, Pasqua Hospital; Staff, Regina General Hospital; Clin Assoc Prof, University of Saskatchewan; Langs: English; French; (306)766-4252

CHAN-TAI-KONG, Chan-San H; Lloydminster Clinic, 2F-5120 46 St, Lloydminster AB T9V 2P7; Leeds (England)'80; Langs: English; French; (780)875-8750; Fax. (780)875-8771.

CHAN-WAI-LING, Nicolas; CHUM-Hop Notre-Dame, 1560 rue Sherbrooke E, Montreal QC H2L 4M1; McG'92; CCFP; CCFP(E.M.); Staff, Centre Hospitalier l'Université de Montréal (CHUM) - Hôpital Notre-Dame; (514)890-8000 x26767

CHAN-YAN, Clifford; 308-1033 Davie St, Vancouver BC V6E 1M7; Cape Town (South Africa)'67; FRCPC; IntMed. Ac Staff, Providence Health Care - St Paul's Hospital; Clin Prof, University of British Columbia; (604)566-9982

CHAN-YAN, Sharon J; PO Box 95063 Rpo Kingsgate, Vancouver BC V5T 4S8; UBC'06; CCFP; (778)847-0696

CHANA, Hari S; 9937 113 St NW, Edmonton AB T5K 1N7; Southampton (England)'78; CCFP; (780)488-2232; Fax. (780)488-2479.

CHANA, Karam; Saanich Peninsula Hosp, 2166 Mount Newton Cross Rd, Saanichton BC V8M 2B2; Southampton (England)'82; FRCPC; Anes. Staff, Saanich Peninsula Hospital; (250)652-3911 x3358

CHANA, Mundeep S; CFB Esquimalt, PO Box 17000 Stn Forces, Victoria BC V9A 7N2; Alb'07; CCFP; (250)363-7067

CHANCEY, Ann B; 610-22470 Dewdney Trunk Rd, Maple Ridge BC V2X 5Z6; UBC'91; FRCSC; OrthSurg. (604)463-5334; Fax. (604)476-1850.

CHANCHLANI, Jayshree; 100-150 West Dr, Brampton ON L6T 4P9; Hyderabad (India)'77; Langs: Hindi; Punjabi; Gujarati; Telugu; Sindhi; (905)454-7410

CHAND, Pankaj P; Waterloo Town Sq, PO Box 40054 Rpo Waterloo Sq 75 King St S, Waterloo ON N2J 4V1; Man'90; CCFP; CCFP(E.M.); (519)749-1681; Fax. (519)749-0245.

CHAND, Pavanjeet; Moy Med Centre, 1407 Ottawa St, Windsor ON N8X 2G1; Punjab (India)'90; CCFP; Physician, Canadian Mental Health Associaton; Physician, Multicultural Council of Windsor; Langs: Hindi; Punjabi; (519)946-0443; Fax. (519)946-0553.

CHANDA, Melanie N; 304 Dundas St E, Belleville ON K8N 1E6; Qns'96; FRCSC; ObstGyn (Urological Gynecology). Staff, QHC Belleville General; (613)967-9900; Fax. (613)967-4882.

CHANDARANA, Prafulchandra C; London HSC-Victoria Hosp, PO Box 5010 Stn B 800 Commissioners Rd E, London ON N6A 5W9; Makerere (Uganda)'70; MB ChB; AB(Psy); FRCPC; Psy (General Adult Psychiatry)., London Health Sciences Centre - Victoria Campus; Assoc Prof, University of Western Ontario; Langs: Gujarati; (519)667-6511; Fax. (519)667-6539.

CHANDARANA, Shamir; Foothills Med Centre, 602-1403 29 St NW, Calgary AB T2N 2T9; Wes'03; FRCSC; Otol. Staff, Foothills Medical Centre; (403)944-3954

CHANDE, Nilesh; London HSC-Victoria Hosp, PO Box 5010 Stn B E1 423A-800 Commissioners Rd E, London ON N6A 5W9; Wes'00; FRCPC; IntMed; Gastroent. Staff, London Health Sciences Centre - Victoria Campus; (519)685-8500

CHANDE, Suryakant; St Lawrence Med Clinic, PO Box 772, Morrisburg ON K0C 1X0; Birmingham (England)'64; FRCSC; GenSurg. Consultant Active, Winchester District Memorial Hospital; Lecturer Surg, University of Ottawa; (613)543-2963; Fax. (613)543-4171.

CHANDER, Sanjeev; Ottawa Cardiovascular Centre, 502-1355 Bank St, Ottawa ON K1H 8K7; Ott'93; FRCPC; IntMed. (613)738-1584

CHANDI, Rajpal S; The Credit Valley Hosp, 2200 Eglinton Ave W, Mississauga ON L5M 2N1; UBC'97; FRCPC; IntMed. Staff, The Credit Valley Hospital; (905)813-2200

CHANDLER, Cara J; Mount Carmel Clinic, 886 Main St, Winnipeg MB R2W 5L4; Man'90; BSc(Pharm); PhD; CCFP; FCFP; (204)582-2311; Fax. (204)582-1341.

CHANDLER, Christopher J; PO Box 670, Houston BC V0J 1Z0; Sask'92; CCFP; CCFP(E.M.); (250)845-2555

CHANDLER, Colin R; Kingsland Med Clinic, 7712 Elbow Dr SW, Calgary AB T2V 1K2; Leeds (England)'56; DIH; Ac Staff, Rockyview General Hospital; Med Examiner, Ministry of Transport(Aviation); (403)252-6681; Fax. (403)252-9741.

CHANDLER, David E; 205-5503 206 St, Langley BC V3A 2C6; Manchester (England)'73; MB ChB; FACP; FRCPC; IntMed (Perioperative Care). Vis Staff, Langley Memorial Hospital; Clinical Asst Prof Community & IntMed/Ac Staff, UBC Hospital - Koerner Pavillion; (604)530-5341; Fax. (604)530-2041.

CHANDLER, Gregory M; Mount Sinai Hosp, 942-600 University Ave, Toronto ON M5G 1X5; McG'03; FRCPC; Psy. Staff, Mount Sinai Hospital; Staff, Sunnybrook Health Sciences Centre; (416)586-4800; Fax. (416)586-8654.

CHANDLER, James D; 315-615 Main St, Yarmouth NS B5A 1K1; Minnesota (USA)'83; AB; FRCPC; Psy (General Psychiatry). Med Dir Mental Health Services & Chief of Psy, Yarmouth Regional Hospital; (902)742-6661; Fax. (902)742-5303.

CHANDLER, Julie E; 315-615 Main St, Yarmouth NS B5A 1K1; Minnesota (USA)'84; Consultant Privil, Yarmouth Regional Hospital; (902)742-6661; Fax. (902)742-5303.

CHANDLER, Vania J J; Circle Med at Copperfield, 123-15566 McIvor Blvd SE, Calgary AB T2Z 4Y2; Alb'08; CCFP; (403)726-0524; Fax. (403)726-0579.

CHANDNA, Divi; 580-999 Broadway W, Vancouver BC V5Z 1K5; Wes'93; (604)739-3484

CHANDOK, Natasha; William Osler HC-Brampton, 2100 Bovaird Dr E, Brampton ON L6R 3J7; Ott'03; FRCPC; IntMed; Gastroent. Staff, William Osler Health System - Brampton Civic Hospital; (905)456-0108

CHANDOLA, Rahul; Sunnybrook Health Sciences Ctr, 2075 Bayview Ave, Toronto ON M4N 3M4; (India)'98; Clin Fellow Cardiovasc Surg, Sunnybrook Health Sciences Centre; (416)480-6073

CHANDONNET, Martin; CHUM-Hotel-Dieu, 3840 rue Saint-Urbain, Montreal QC H2W 1T8; Laval'02; FRCPC; DiagRad. Staff, Centre Hospitalier l'Université de Montréal (CHUM) - Hôtel-Dieu; (514)890-8150

CHANDRA, Devendr B; St Michael's Hosp, 30 Bond St, Toronto ON M5B 1W8; Dal'00; FRCPC; Anes. Staff, St Michael's Hospital; (416)864-6060; Fax. (416)864-6014.

CHANDRA, Mark J; Ross Mem Hosp, 10 Angeline St N, Lindsay ON K9V 4M8; Qns'00; CCFP; CCFP(E.M.); Staff, Ross Memorial Hospital; (705)324-6111; Fax. (705)328-2817.

CHANDRA, Michael M; A-255 Connell St, Woodstock NB E7M 1L2; Dal'90; BSc; CCFP; (506)324-8000; mchandra@nb.sympatico.ca.

CHANDRA, Prakash; LMC Ednocrinology Centre, 238-2130 North Park Dr, Brampton ON L6S 0C9; All India Institute of Medical Sciences (India)'03; (905)595-0560; Fax. (905)595-0562.

CHANDRA, Ranjit K; Dr R K Chandra Med Prof Corp, 100-470 Hensall Cir, Mississauga ON L5A 3V4; Punjab (India)'60; OC; MB BS; MD; MACP; DSc(Hon. Punjab); FRCPCH(Hon. UK); DrMedCh(Hon.Napoli); DrSci(Hon.Chile); FRCPC; Peds (Allergy). Langs: Hindi; Punjabi; Urdu; (905)279-6880; Fax. (905)279-6896; drrkchandra@gmail.com.

CHANDRA, Sujata; Royal Alexandra Hosp, 5S 131-10240 Kingsway NW, Edmonton AB T5H 3V9; Mem'94; FRCSC; ObstGyn (Maternal Fetal Medicine). Staff Lois Hole Hospital for Women Robbins Pav, Royal Alexandra Hospital; Asst Prof ObstGyn, University of Alberta; (780)735-4812; Fax. (780)735-4981.

CHANDRA SEKHAR, Harnahalli B; 300-80 Elizabeth Ave, St. John's NL A1A 1W7; Mysore (India)'74; MRC(UK); FRCPC; IntMed (Gastroenterology). Staff, St Clare's Mercy Hospital; Asst Prof Med, Memorial University Of Newfoundland; (709)579-2522; Fax. (709)579-2523.

CHANDRAKANTH, Soornahalli; Regina Qu'Appelle HR-Pasqua, 4101 Dewdney Ave, Regina SK S4T 1A5; Staff, Pasqua Hospital; (306)766-7800; Fax. (306)766-2752.

CHANDRAKANTHAN, Selliah; Royal University Hosp, 151 EH-103 Hospital Dr, Saskatoon SK S7N 0W8; Ceylon (Sri Lanka)'81; MB BS; FRCS(Ed); FRCSC; GenSurg (Colon & Rectal Surgery). Staff, Royal University Hospital; Assoc Prof, University of Saskatchewan; (306)966-8174; Fax. (306)966-8102.

CHANDRAKUMAR, Sandrasegaram; Trillium Hlth Ctr-Mississauga, 100 Queensway W, Mississauga ON L5B 1B8; Ceylon (Sri Lanka)'78; MB BS; MRC(E); MRC(UK); FRCPC; IntMed; GeriatricMed. Staff, Trillium Health Centre - Mississauga; Langs: Tamil; (905)848-7507

CHANDRAN, A Uma; Glenrose Rehab Hosp, 2243.5-10230 111 Ave NW, Edmonton AB T5G 0B7; Alb'98; FRCPC; MedMicrobiol (Infection Control). Staff Med, Sturgeon Community Hospital; Staff Med, Glenrose Rehabilitation Hospital; Clinical Asst Prof, University of Alberta; (780)735-6079; Fax. (780)735-8861; umachandran@albertahealthservices.ca.

CHANDRAN, Geethan J; 303-2125 11th Ave, Regina SK S4P 3X3; Sask'01; FRCSC; PlasSurg. (306)545-8001; Fax. (306)545-8013.

CHANDRAN, Indira; Peel Med Arts Bldg, 505-145 Queen St E, Brampton ON L6W 3P8; Madras (India)'61; FRCOG(UK); FRCSC; ObstGyn. Ac Staff, William Osler Health System - Brampton Civic Hospital; Langs: Chinese; Hindi; Malayalam; Tamil; (905)230-5490

CHANDRAN, Lavan; Harbourfront Hlth & Wellness C, 4-8 York St, Toronto ON M5J 2Y2; Wes'06; CCFP; (416)366-2273; Fax. (416)366-5665.

CHANDRAN, Vinod; Univ Hlth Network-Toronto Western Hosp, 1EW 416-399 Bathurst St, Toronto ON M5T 2S8; Calicut (India)'96; MB BS; MD; Staff, Toronto Western Hospital - University Health Network; Langs: Hindi; Malayalam; (416)603-5192; Fax. (416)603-9387.

CHANDRANIPAPONGSE, Weerawadee; The Hosp for Sick Children, 555 University Ave, Toronto ON M5G 1X8; Mahidol University (India)'02; Clin Fellow Clinical Pharmacology, The Hospital For Sick Children; (416)813-7654

CHANDRARAJAN, B Leonard; 410-797 Princess St, Kingston ON K7L 1G1; Jaffna (Sri Lanka)'83; MB BS; MSc(Surg.); CCFP; FCFP; Asst Prof Family Med, Queen's University; Langs: Tamil; Sinhalese; (613)544-8400; Fax. (613)544-8404.

CHANDRASEKARAN, Akila P; Kennedy Grace Med Clinic, 204-1939 Kennedy Rd, Scarborough ON M1P 2L9; Madras (India)'92; MB BS; CCFP; FCFP; Staff, The Scarborough Hospital - General Campus; Staff, The Scarborough Hospital - Birchmount Campus; Langs: Tamil; (416)285-5544; Fax. (416)285-8586.

CHANDRASENA, Chandima; Family Practice 535, 535 Montreal Rd, Ottawa ON K1K 0V1; Ott'00; BSc(Hons); CCFP; Langs: Sinhalese; (613)731-4770; Fax. (613)731-4979.

CHANDRASENA, Ranjith D; Chatham-Kent Health Alliance, PO Box 2030 Stn Main 80 Grand Ave W, Chatham ON N7M 5L9; (Sri Lanka)'72; DPM; FRANZCP; MRCPsy; DABPN; FRCPC; Psy (Medico Legal Psychiatry). Chief Psy, Chatham-Kent Health Alliance; Member, Consent & Capacity Board; Dir Scientific, Chatham-Kent Clinical Trials Research Centre; Member, Ontario Review Board; Aj Prof Psy, University of Western Ontario; Langs: Sinhalese; (519)351-6144 x5744; Fax. (519)351-0450.

CHANDRASENA, Samantha H; Thamesview Family Health Team, 465 Grand Ave W, Chatham ON N7L 1C5; (Other Foreign)'09; (519)354-5540

CHANDRASENAN, Kavitha; Misericordia Community Hosp, 16940 87 Ave NW, Edmonton AB T5R 4H5; (India)'95; MB BS; CCFP; Staff, Covenant Health - Misericordia Community Hospital; Langs: Malayalam; (780)735-2000

CHANDURKAR, Vikram; Health Sciences Centre, 300 Prince Philip Dr, St. John's NL A1B 3V6; Bombay (India)'95; MB BS; FRCPC; IntMed; Endocrin&Metab. Staff, Health Sciences Centre; Asst Prof, Memorial University Of Newfoundland; Langs: Hindi; Marathi; (709)777-8027; Fax. (709)777-6273.

CHANDY, George P; The Ottawa Hosp-Civic Campus, 1053 Carling Ave, Ottawa ON K1Y 4E9; Cal'02; MSc; BSc(H); FRCPC; Respir; IntMed. Staff, The Ottawa Hospital - General Campus; Staff, The Ottawa Hospital - Civic Campus; (613)798-5555

CHANDY, Mark J K; Univ Hlth Network-Toronto Western Hosp, EW5 559-399 Bathurst Ave, Toronto ON M5T 2S8; Pennsylvania (USA)'08; FRCPC; IntMed. Staff Cardiol, Toronto Western Hospital - University Health Network; (416)603-5815

CHANEY, Jonathan W; 200-117 10th Ave S, Cranbrook BC V1C 2N1; UBC'00; FRCSC; OrthSurg. (250)489-3415

CHANG, Adam; 101-7380 Westminster Hwy, Richmond BC V6X 1A1; Alb'04; CCFP; (604)273-9404; Fax. (604)273-3342.

CHANG, Alanna M; 341-14032 23 Ave NW, Edmonton AB T6R 3L6; (USA)'06; CCFP.

CHANG, Albert; 2775 Laurel St, Vancouver BC V5Z 1M9; Tor'06; FRCPC; IntMed; Gastroent.

CHANG, Alvin; Toronto East Gen Hosp Inc, J6100-825 Coxwell Ave, Toronto ON M4C 3E7; Tor'04; FRCPC; Anes; Critical Care Medicine. Staff, Toronto East General Hospital Inc; (416)469-6580

CHANG, Annisa; 207-7130 Warden Ave, Markham ON L3R 1S2; Tor'07; CCFP; (905)470-1117; Fax. (905)470-1115.

CHANG, B Wayne; South Calgary Med Clinic, 118-40 Sunpark Plaza SE, Calgary AB T2X 3X7; Tor'96; CCFP; Clin Lecturer Family Med, University of Calgary; (403)254-4000; Fax. (403)254-1304; waynemdchang@gmail.com.

CHANG, Benny H S; 601-14 College St, Toronto ON M5G 1K2; Tor'92; CCFP; Court Staff, St Michael's Hospital; Assoc Staff, Toronto General Hospital - UHN; University of Toronto; (416)966-9441; Fax. (416)960-0489; bennychangmd@yahoo.ca.

CHANG, Boon H; Univ Hlth Network-Toronto Gen, 200 Elizabeth St, Toronto ON M5G 2C4; Qns'05; CCFP; CCFP(E.M.); Staff, Toronto General Hospital - UHN; (416)340-3946

CHANG, Bruce H; 3770 Oak St, Vancouver BC V6H 2M3; UBC'82; Ac Staff, Providence Health Care - Mount Saint Joseph Hospital; Ac Staff, BC Women's Hospital & Health Centre; Clinical Asst Prof Family Pract, University of British Columbia; (604)873-1838; Fax. (604)873-1839.

CHANG, C Michael; Taunton Health Centre, SS 1 1290 Keith Ross Dr, Oshawa ON L1H 7K4; Tor'02; BSc(Hon); MSc; FRCSC; Urol (Endourology). Staff Urol, Lakeridge Health - Oshawa Site; Langs: Spanish; Cantonese; (905)721-4971; Fax. (905)721-6696.

CHANG, C C Nancy; Maridam Fam Med Centre, A202-3000 Highway 7, Markham ON L3R 6E1; Tor'00; BSc; MSc; CCFP; Langs: Mandarin; (905)480-1050; Fax. (905)480-0898.

CHANG, Chih-Peng; Cornwall Comm Hosp-McConnell, PO Box 100 Stn Main 840 McConnell Ave, Cornwall ON K6H 5S5; Taipei (China)'89; FRCSC; OrthSurg. Staff Ortho Surg, Cornwall Community Hospital; (613)938-4240

CHANG, Christine H Y; Health Sciences Centre, 3330 Hospital Dr NW, Calgary AB T2N 4N1; Cal'05; FRCPC; Psy. Staff, Foothills Medical Centre; (403)210-7542

CHANG, Cindy C H; 3770 Oak St, Vancouver BC V6H 2M3; UBC'83; Staff, Providence Health Care - Mount Saint Joseph Hospital; Staff, BC Women's Hospital & Health Centre; Staff, BC Children's Hospital; Clinical Asst Prof, University of British Columbia; (604)873-1838

CHANG, Daniel K M; 38-480 Chrysler Dr, Brampton ON L6S 0C1; Wes'91; FRCPC; Derm. Langs: Cantonese; (905)789-6800; Fax. (905)789-5991.

CHANG, Danny T L; 9-6400 Millcreek Dr, Mississauga ON L5N 3E7; London (England)'69; MRCP(UK); DCH(Eng); MB BS; Staff, Headwaters Health Care Centre - Orangeville Site; (905)858-1368

CHANG, David H; Toronto East Gen & Orth Hosp, 825 Coxwell Ave, Toronto ON M4C 3E7; Tor'02; FRCPC; Anes. Staff, Toronto East General Hospital Inc; (416)469-6580

CHANG, Debra C S; Royal Columbian Hosp, 330 Columbia St E, New Westminster BC V3L 3W7; Tor'00; FRCPC; DiagRad. Staff, Royal Columbian Hospital; (604)520-5900; Fax. (604)520-4120.

CHANG, Derrick; Univ Hlth Network-Toronto Western Hosp, FP1 503-399 Bathurst St, Toronto ON M5T 2S8; Tor'97; CCFP; CCFP(E.M.); Staff, Toronto Western Hospital - University Health Network; Lecturer Family Med, University of Toronto; (416)603-5405; Fax. (416)603-5324.

CHANG, Diana M; St Paul's Hosp, 1081 Burrard St, Vancouver BC V6Z 1Y6; UBC'93; CCFP; CCFP(E.M.); Staff, Providence Health Care - St Paul's Hospital; Langs: Korean; (604)682-2344

CHANG, Eddie C; Royal Alexandra Hosp, 541CSC-10240 Kingsway NW, Edmonton AB T5H 3V9; Alb'97; FRCPC; EmergMed. Staff, Royal Alexandra Hospital; (780)735-4442; Fax. (780)735-4916.

CHANG, Edward N; 300-2099 152 St, Surrey BC V4A 4N7; McG'00; BSc; MDCM; DABS; FRCSC; GenSurg. Att Surgeon, Peace Arch Hospital; (604)535-7955; Fax. (604)535-7956.

CHANG, Edward Y; Hotel-Dieu Grace Hosp, 1030 Ouellette Ave, Windsor ON N9A 1E1; Qns'95; FRCPC; NuclearMed. Staff, Hôtel-Dieu Grace Hospital; (519)973-4417

CHANG, Ernest J; 107-2349 Millstream Rd, Victoria BC V9B 3R5; UBC'70; (250)391-7554

CHANG, Gao-Nan; 1490 Danforth Ave, Toronto ON M4J 1N4; Tor'76; Staff, Mount Sinai Hospital; Staff, Toronto East General Hospital Inc; Physician, Heritage Nursing Home; (416)463-4878; Fax. (416)463-4904.

CHANG, Genevieve; 53 Prospect St, Newmarket ON L3Y 3T1; Tor'95; FRCSC; ObstGyn. (905)895-8270

CHANG, George; 214-168 13th St E, North Vancouver BC V7L 4W8; Alb'89; FRCSC; GenSurg (Head & Neck Surgery). Staff, Lions Gate Hospital; Clin Instructor, University of British Columbia; (604)924-0788

CHANG, Harvey Y; SMBD Jewish Gen Hosp, G050-3755 ch Cote-Sainte-Cathe, Montreal QC H3T 1E2; McG'83; FRCPC; IntMed. Staff, Sir Mortimer B Davis Jewish General; adj Prof, McGill University; (514)340-7596; Fax. (514)340-7541.

CHANG, Heather A; Oakridge Centre South Tower, 312-650 41st Ave W, Vancouver BC V5Z 2M9; UBC'81; (604)261-8177; Fax. (604)261-9607; heatherchang@shaw.ca.

CHANG, Hong; Univ Hlth Network-Toronto Gen, 11E 413-200 Elizabeth St, Toronto ON M5G 2C4; Jiangxi (China)'85; MD; MSc; PhD; FRCPC; HemPath. Div Head Clinical Flow Cytometry, Toronto General Hospital - UHN; Assoc Prof, University of Toronto; Langs: Chinese; (416)340-4858; hong.chang@uhn.on.ca.

CHANG, Jacqueline; Crestwood Med & Dental Bldg, 207-6051 Gilbert Rd, Richmond BC V7C 3V3; McM'91; CCFP; (604)276-0952; Fax. (604)231-0583.

CHANG, Jason H S; Royal Alexandra Hosp, 541-10240 Kingsway NW, Edmonton AB T5H 3V9; Man'00; CCFP; CCFP(E.M.); Staff, Royal Alexandra Hospital; (780)735-4442; Fax. (780)735-4916.

CHANG, Jose; RS McLaughlin Durham Cancer Ct, 2F-1 Hospital Crt, Oshawa ON L1G 2B9; Tor'86; ABIM; FRCPC; IntMed (Oncology); MedOncol. Staff Oncology Clinic, Lakeridge Health - Oshawa Site; Staff MedOncol, RS McLaughlin Durham Reg Cancer Ctre; (905)576-8711; Fax. (905)721-6103; jchang@lakeridgehealth.on.ca.

CHANG, Karen D; Rouge Valley-Centenary HC, 2867 Ellesmere Rd, Scarborough ON M1E 4B9; West Indies (Jamaica)'79; FRCPC; Peds (Neonatology). Staff Neonatol, Rouge Valley Health System - Centenary Health Centre Site; (416)281-7103

CHANG, Kathleen D K; Greenwood Clinic, 675 Greenwood Ave, Toronto ON M4J 4B3; Tor'85; CCFP; Staff, Toronto East General Hospital Inc; Staff, Greenwood Medical Clinic; Langs: Cantonese; (416)406-6440; Fax. (416)406-6439.

CHANG, Kim S; 151-4800 Kingsway, Burnaby BC V5H 4J2; UBC'97; (604)451-0079

CHANG, Lawrence J A; Newmarket Med Place, 203-712 Davis Dr, Newmarket ON L3Y 8C3; Man'74; PhD(MedSci); FAAP; AB; FRCPC; Peds (Asthma & Allergy). Court Staff Peds, Markham Stouffville Hospital; Staff Peds, Southlake Regional Health Centre; Langs: Chinese; (905)853-0600; Fax. (905)853-2868.

CHANG, Li-Hsin; Guelph Gen Hosp, 115 Delhi St, Guelph ON N1E 4J4; Ott'00; CCFP; CCFP(E.M.); Staff, Guelph General Hospital; (519)837-6420

CHANG, Lily; Humber River Reg Hosp-Church, 200 Church St, Toronto ON M9N 1N8; Santo Tomas (Philippines)'69; FRCPC; Anes. Staff, Humber River Regional Hospital - Church Street Site; (416)249-8111

CHANG, Lynn; Postgrad Med Education, MDCL 21101-1280 Main St W, Hamilton ON L8S 4K1; Tor'07; RadOncol.

CHANG, Malcolm E; Professional Bldg, 208-740 4 Ave S, Lethbridge AB T1J 0N9; McG'02; FRCSC; OrthSurg (Arthroplasty). Staff OrthSurg, Chinook Regional Hospital; (403)524-1029; Fax. (403)524-1028.

CHANG, Margaret K; North York Gen Hosp, 4001 Leslie St, North York ON M2K 1E1; Tor'94; FRCPC; DiagRad. Staff, North York General Hospital; (416)756-6233

CHANG, Maria Y; Sunnybrook Hlth Sciences Ctre, KGE 31-2075 Bayview Ave, Toronto ON M4N 3M5; McM'04; CCFP; Staff, Sunnybrook Health Sciences Centre; (416)480-4939

CHANG, Martin C; Mount Sinai Hosp, 600 University Ave, Toronto ON M5G 1X5; Tor'03; FRCPC; AnatPath. Staff Path & Lab Med, Mount Sinai Hospital; (416)586-4800 x7317; Fax. (416)586-8628.

CHANG, Michael B; 300-1333 Neilson Rd, Scarborough ON M1B 4Y9; Tor'96; DABOT; FRCSC; Otol. Ac Staff, Rouge Valley Health System - Centenary Health Centre Site; Court Staff, The Scarborough Hospital - Birchmount Campus; Court Staff, The Scarborough Hospital - General Campus; Ac Staff, Rouge Valley Health System - Ajax & Pickering Health Centre Site; (416)283-0100; Fax. (416)283-9915.

CHANG, Michael E; Dr Michael E Chang Med Prof Co, 250 Court St N, Thunder Bay ON P7A 4W1; Wes'08; CCFP; CCFP(E.M.); Staff Emerg Med, Thunder Bay Regional Health Sciences Centre.

CHANG, Mildred W M; Peace Arch Hosp, 15521 Russell Ave, White Rock BC V4B 2R4; Qns'87; BSc(Hons); CCFP; CCFP(E.M.); Staff, Peace Arch Hospital; Langs: Cantonese; (604)535-5512

CHANG, Mui Khoon; University of Alberta Hosp, 1C1. 04WMC-8440 112 St NW, Edmonton AB T6G 2B7; (New Zealand); Staff, University of Alberta Hospital; (780)407-7035; Fax. (780)407-8529.

CHANG, Na Young; CSSSG-Hop de Hull, 116 boul Lionel-Emond, Gatineau QC J8Y 1W7; Sher'02; FRCPC; DiagRad. Staff, Hull Hospital; (819)966-6200

CHANG, Neil G; Markham Stouffville Health Ctr, 210-377 Church St, Markham ON L6B 1A1; Tor'83; FRCSC; ObstGyn. Staff, Markham Stouffville Hospital; (905)471-3699; Fax. (905)471-5259.

CHANG, Patricia Y; St Michael's Fam Practice Unit, 3F-61 Queen St E, Toronto ON M5C 2T2; Man'97; BSc; CCFP; FCFP; Staff Family Practice Unit, St Michael's Hospital; Langs: Mandarin; Chinese; (416)867-7426; Fax. (416)867-7498.

CHANG, Paul T; Ctr for Advance Reproductive T, 210-150 Bloor St W, Toronto ON M5S 2X9; Tor'01; BSc; FRCSC; ObstGyn (Reproductive Endocrinology & Infertility). Staff, Toronto Centre for Advanced Reproductive Technology; Lecturer Dept of Reproductive Biology, University of Toronto; Langs: Mandarin; Chinese; (416)972-0110; Fax. (416)972-0036.

CHANG, Peter C; Abbotsford Reg Hosp & Cancer C, 32900 Marshall Rd, Abbotsford BC V2S 0C2; Wes'04; FRCPC; IntMed. Staff, Abbotsford Regional Hospital & Cancer Centre; (604)851-4700

CHANG, Peter F E; 101-10151 No. 3 Rd, Richmond BC V7A 4R6; UBC'75; BSc; Ac Staff, Richmond Hospital; (604)274-7271; Fax. (604)274-7301.

CHANG, Peter P; 607-220 Duncan Mill Rd, Toronto ON M3B 3J5; (Hong Kong)'68; MB BS; DPM; DPsy; JD; FRCPC; Psy (Legal Psychiatry). Langs: Cantonese; Mandarin; Shanghai; Chinese; (416)497-1575 x108; Fax. (416)497-2261; peterpchang@rogers.com.

CHANG, Peter S; Cornwall Prof Bldg, 605-2125 11th Ave, Regina SK S4P 3X3; Sask'78; FRCSC; CCFP; PlasSurg. Staff, Regina General Hospital; Fam Med/Plastic surgery, Pasqua Hospital; Assoc Prof, University of Saskatchewan; (306)359-7753; Fax. (306)757-3316.

CHANG, Richard; East Liberty Med Centre, 105-901 King St W, Toronto ON M5V 3H5; Qns'06; CCFP; (416)599-6000; Fax. (416)530-6160.

CHANG, Ross E; Kingsway Prof Centre, 600-4980 Kingsway, Burnaby BC V5H 4K7; UBC'79; ClinImmunol&Allergy; IntMed. Ac Staff, Burnaby Hospital; (604)433-0545; Fax. (604)433-2846; rchang@telus.net.

CHANG, Ruoh-Yeng; 104-45744 Gaetz St, Chilliwack BC V2R 3P1; Alb'08; CCFP; (604)824-1588

CHANG, Samuel Y Y; Foothills Med Centre, 1001-1403 29 St NW, Calgary AB T2N 2T9; Cal'84; FRCPC; Psy (Child & Adolescent Psychiatry). Staff Dept of Psy, Foothills Medical Centre; Dir, Adolescent Substance Abuse; Dir, Psychiatric Disorders Clinic; Clin Assoc Prof, University of Calgary; (403)944-3351; Fax. (403)944-3454.

CHANG, Silvia D; 899 12th Ave W, Vancouver BC V5Z 1M9; UBC'94; BSc; FRCPC; DiagRad (Abdominal Imaging). Staff, Vancouver General Hospital - Centennial Pavillion; Assoc Prof, University of British Columbia; (604)875-4533; Fax. (604)875-4228.

CHANG, Stanley S; 1550-4380 No. 3 Rd, Richmond BC V6X 3V7; Formosa (Taiwan)'58; Ac Staff, Richmond Hospital; (604)273-9899

CHANG, Steven; Phoenix Med Centre, 106-2155 10th Ave, Prince George BC V2M 5J6; UBC'97; CCFP; CCFP(E.M.); FCFP; Staff, University Hospital of Northern British Columbia; Course Dir Clinical Skills, University of Northern British Columbia; (250)563-5111; Fax. (250)563-3649.

CHANG, Terence A; Broadway Plaza Bldg, U6-601 Broadway W, Vancouver BC V5Z 4C2; UBC'84; Board Chair, Vancouver Division of Family Practice; Clin Assoc Prof Family Med, University of British Columbia; (604)685-7516; Fax. (604)874-6222.

CHANG, Thomas M S; McGill University, 1004-3655 Prom Sir-William-Osl, Montreal QC H3G 1Y6; McG'61; PhD(Physiol); FRCPC; MedScient(Med) (Research). hon Staff, Hôpital Chinois de Montréal; Emeritus Prof University Clinic, McGill University Health Centre - Royal Victoria Hospital; Head Artificial Cells & Organs Research Centre, McGill University; Langs: Chinese; (514)398-3512; artcell.med@mcgill.ca.

CHANG, Viviana; Chrysalis Obst & Gyn Clinic, 21-10 Richard Way SW, Calgary AB T3E 7M9; UBC'98; FRCSC; ObstGyn. Staff, Rockyview General Hospital; (403)242-0770; Fax. (403)242-0711.

CHANG, W C Iris; 404-1100 Sheppard Ave E, North York ON M2K 2W1; Tor'80; (416)222-0660; Fax. (416)222-9238.

CHANG, Walter W K; Dundas Med Centre, 401-220 Dundas St W, Whitby ON L1N 8M7; Qns'71; Court Staff, Lakeridge Health - Oshawa Site; (905)668-5871; Fax. (905)668-7781.

CHANGELA, Jayantilal J; Fairlight Plaza Med Clinic, 7-3310 Fairlight Dr, Saskatoon SK S7M 4Z1; Karnatak (India)'72; MB BS; LRCP(Glas); LRCS(Glas); LMSSA(Lond); CCFP; Staff Privil, Royal University Hospital; Staff Privil, Saskatoon City Hospital; Staff Privil, St Paul's Hospital (Grey Nuns) of Saskatoon; Langs: Gujarati; Hindi; (306)384-6911; Fax. (306)384-6920.

CHANIOTIS, Lambros N; Centre Med Brunswick, 403-955 boul Saint-Jean, Pointe-Claire QC H9R 5K3; Sorbonne (France)'69; FACC; CSPQ; Cardiol (P.Q.) (Administrative Medicine). Staff, Lakeshore General Hospital - Pointe Claire; Consultant Cardiol, McGill University Health Centre - Royal Victoria Hospital; Consultant Cardiol, Hopital Ste-Anne; Gen Dir, CHSLD Chateau Sur Le Lac; Langs: French; Greek; Italian; (514)695-5838; Fax. (514)695-1037; lchaniotis@hotmail.com.

CHANKOWSKY, Jeffrey N; MUHC-Montreal Gen Hosp, 1650 av Cedar, Montreal QC H3G 1A4; McG'93; FRCPC; DiagRad (Neuro Radiology). Staff, McGill University Health Centre - Montreal General Campus; (514)934-1934 x42924; Fax. (514)934-8263; jeffrey.chankowsky@muhc.mcgill.ca.

CHANNAN, Peter K; Trillium Health Centre-Mississ, 100 Queensway W, Mississauga ON L5B 1B8; Alb'05; FRCPC; EmergMed. Staff Emerg Med, Trillium Health Centre - Mississauga; (905)848-7100

CHANOINE, Jean-Pierre; Children's & Women's HC of BC, K4 213-4500 Oak St, Vancouver BC V6H 3N1; Brussels (Belgium)'82; MD; Clin Prof/Head Endocrinology and Diabetes Unit, BC Women's Hospital & Health Centre; Langs: Bilingual(English/French); (604)875-2624; Fax. (604)875-3231; jchanoine@cw.bc.ca.

CHANT, Chris B; St Joseph's Health Care, PO Box 5777 Stn B DO 213-268 Grosvenor St, London ON N6A 4L6; Adelaide (Australia)'06; FRCSC; OrthSurg. Staff, St Joseph's Hospital - St Joseph's Health Care; (519)646-6309

CHANTAL, Louise; Ctr Hosp Rouyn-Noranda, 4 9e rue, Rouyn-Noranda QC J9X 2B2; Mon'96; Staff, Centre Hospitalier Rouyn-Noranda; (819)764-5131

CHANUT, Florence; 10F-264 boul Rene-Levesque E, Montreal QC H2X 1P1; Sher'98; FRCPC; Psy (Addiction Psychiatry). Staff Psy, Hôpital du Sacre-Coeur de Montréal; Universite de Montreal; (514)890-8321

CHAO, Eric D; Scotia Square Med Clinic, 270-5201 Duke St, Halifax NS B3J 1N9; Transkei (South Africa)'95; MB ChB; LMCC; CCFP; FCFP; (902)431-1800; Fax. (902)431-1818.

CHAO, Erwin D; Victoria Hosp, PO Box 3000 Stn Main 1200 24 St W, Prince Albert SK S6V 5T4; Transkei (South Africa)'96; MB ChB; MD; FRCPC; Anes. Staff, Victoria Hospital; (306)765-6267; Fax. (306)765-6224; echao@paphr.sk.ca.

CHAO, Hubert Y; UBC Student Health Services, M334-2211 Wesbrook Mall, Vancouver BC V6T 2B5; Wes'95; (604)822-7011

CHAO, Kelvin C; Ackroyd Med Clinic, 135-8291 Ackroyd Rd, Richmond BC V6X 3K5; UBC'89; (604)278-7211; Fax. (604)270-6232.

CHAO, Roger W; Saskatoon City Hosp, 701 Queen St, Saskatoon SK S7K 0M7; (Other Foreign)'98; Staff, Saskatoon City Hospital; (306)655-8000

CHAO, Sonia Y; Doctors on Bayview, 15900 Bayview Ave, Aurora ON L4G 7Y3; Qns'00; CCFP; CCFP(E.M.); Staff, Southlake Regional Health Centre; (905)726-9755

CHAO, Stephen; 155-1720 Howard Ave, Windsor ON N8X 5A6; Wes'96; FRCPC; IntMed (Critical Care Medicine); Respir. Ac Staff, Windsor Regional Hospital - Metropolitan Site; Aj Prof, University of Western Ontario; (519)256-8338; Fax. (519)258-7337; lungdocs3@gmail.com.

CHAO, Te Wei; The Medical Clinic Associates, 4794 Joyce Ave, Powell River BC V8A 3B6; Witwatersrand (South Africa)'06; MB ChB; (604)485-6261

CHAOUAL, Mongi; Clinique Med L'Esperance, 4261 rue Sainte-Catherine E, Montreal QC H1V 1X5; Lausanne (Switzerland)'68; (514)254-3686

CHAOULLI, Jacques; Centre Med des Boises, 4670 boul Saint-Martin O, Laval QC H7T 2Y2; Paris (France)'78; (450)687-8585

CHAPADOS, Denyse; CSSS de la Baie-des-Chaleurs, RR 2 419 boul Perron, Maria QC G0C 1Y0; Laval'91; CCFP; Staff, CSSS de la Baie-des-Chaleurs; Staff, CLSC Chaleurs Paspebiac; (418)759-3443

CHAPADOS, Isabelle; College Plaza 3, 505-8215 112 St NW, Edmonton AB T6G 2C8; Mon'98; MSc; FRCPC; Peds (Endocrinology); Endocrin&Metab. Clinical Asst Prof Peds, University of Alberta; Langs: Bilingual(French/English); (780)432-1414

CHAPARRO GOMEZ, Luis; Kingston Gen Hosp, 76 Stuart St, Kingston ON K7L 2V7; Antioquia (Colombia)'98; Clin Fellow Anes, Kingston General Hospital; (613)985-0424; Fax. (613)548-1375.

CHAPARRO MUTIS, B Cecilia; N C S B11C-1190, 585 University Ave, Toronto ON M5G 2N2; (Colombia)'83; Staff, St Michael's Hospital; Staff Toronto Lung Transplant Prog, Toronto General Hospital - UHN; Asst Prof, University of Toronto; Langs: Spanish; (416)340-4996; Fax. (416)340-3609.

CHAPDELAINE, Hugo; CHUM-Hop Notre-Dame, D3054-1560 rue Sherbrooke E, Montreal QC H2L 4M1; Mon'06; FRCPC; IntMed; ClinImmunol&Allergy. Staff, Centre Hospitalier l'Université de Montréal (CHUM) - Hôpital Notre-Dame; (514)890-8231

CHAPDELAINE, Isabelle; Hop Sacre-Coeur De Montreal, 5400 boul Gouin O, Montreal QC H4J 1C5; Mon'06; FRCPC; IntMed; Nephrol. Staff, Hôpital du Sacre-Coeur de Montréal; (514)338-2883; Fax. (514)338-2182.

CHAPDELAINE, Joyaube; CSSS Drummond-Hop Sainte-Croix, 570 rue Heriot, Drummondville QC J2B 1C1; Sher'97; FRCSC; GenSurg; PedGenSurg. Staff, Hôpital Sainte-croix; (819)478-6464

CHAPDELAINE, Pierre; 16 rue Sainte-Anne, Ste-Anne-De-Bellev QC H9X 1K8; Mon'61; hon Membre, CSSS de Dorval-Lachine-Lasalle; (514)457-9515

CHAPDELAINE, Sylvie; CSSS de Trois-Rivieres, 1991 boul du Carmel, Trois-Rivieres QC G9A 1Y1; Laval'93; MedOncol (P.Q.); Hem; IntMed. Staff, CSSS de Trois-Rivières; (819)697-3333 x53337

CHAPELSKI, Mark B E; PO Box 12357 Rpo 10, Lloydminster AB T9V 3C5; Sask'98; LMCC; CCFP; CCFP(E.M.); (780)808-2819

CHAPESKIE, Henry H; Thorndale Lims Med Centre, PO Box 130 21816 Fairview Rd, Thorndale ON N0M 2P0; Ott'84; BSc; CCFP; FCFP; Med Examiner Civil Aviation, Transport Canada; Aj Prof, University of Western Ontario; (519)461-0776; Fax. (519)461-0991.

CHAPIN, Margaret E T; Grand River Hosp-KW Hlth Ctre, PO Box 9056 Stn C 835 King St, Kitchener ON N2G 1G3; Wes'78; Staff, Grand River Hospital - Kitchener/Waterloo Health Centre; (519)749-4300

CHAPLEAU, Denis; CSSS de Saint-Jerome, 290 rue de Montigny, Saint-Jerome QC J7Z 5T3; Mon'84; MSc(Epidemiol); FRCSC; GenSurg; VascSurg. Staff, Hôtel-Dieu de Saint-Jérôme; (450)431-8200 x2418

CHAPMAN, Allison G; Maternity Care Clinic, 109-178 96 Ave NE, Calgary AB T3K 6G4; Cal'87; CCFP; FCFP; Staff, Peter Lougheed Centre; Physician, Maternity Care Clinic; Assoc. Clin. Instr., University of Calgary; (403)735-4922; Fax. (403)735-4901.

CHAPMAN, Andrea J M; BC Women's Hosp & Health Ctre, 4500 Oak St, Vancouver BC V6H 3N1; UBC'97; FRCPC; Psy. Staff, BC Women's Hospital & Health Centre; (604)875-2424

CHAPMAN, Bryanne L; New Vision Family Health Team, 421 Greenbrook Dr, Kitchener ON N2M 4K1; Tor'88; CCFP; FCFP; (519)570-1655; Fax. (519)570-3477.

CHAPMAN, David B; Four Oaks Med Associates, 5500 206 St, Langley BC V3A 8R3; Cape Town (South Africa)'88; MB ChB; Med Staff, Langley Memorial Hospital; (604)534-4214; Fax. (604)534-6616.

CHAPMAN, Dennis R; 402-20395 Lougheed Hwy, Maple Ridge BC V2X 2P9; Wes'71; Ac Staff, Ridge Meadows Hospital & Health Care Centre; (604)465-3900

CHAPMAN, John L; PO Box 90, Hornby Island BC V0R 1Z0; Maryland (USA)'79.

CHAPMAN, Kathryn A; Ross Mem Hosp, 10 Angeline St N, Lindsay ON K9V 4M8; McM'90; Staff, Ross Memorial Hospital; (705)324-6111

CHAPMAN, Kelly S; Markham Family Health Team, 101-377 Church St, Markham ON L6B 1A1; Wes'83; Staff, Markham Stouffville Hospital; (905)471-9999; Fax. (905)471-3627.

CHAPMAN, Kenneth R; Univ Hlth Network-Toronto Western Hosp, 7EW 451-399 Bathurst St, Toronto ON M5T 2S8; Tor'77; DABIM; FACP; FRCPC; IntMed (Asthma); Respir. Staff, Toronto Western Hospital - University Health Network; Pres, Inspiration Research Limited; Staff, Asthma & Airway Centre; Prof Med, University of Toronto; (416)603-5499; Fax. (416)603-3456; kchapman@ca.inter.net.

CHAPMAN, Kristine M; Diamond Healthcare Ctre-VGH, 8/F-2775 Laurel St, Vancouver BC V5Z 1M9; UBC'97; BSc; FRCPC; Neur (Neuromuscular Diseases). Staff, Providence Health Care - St Paul's Hospital; Staff Neuromuscular Disease Unit, Vancouver General Hospital - Centennial Pavillion; Clinical Asst Prof, University of British Columbia; (604)875-5168; Fax. (604)875-4471.

CHAPMAN, Larry S; 203-300 Willow Rd, Guelph ON N1H 7C6; Padova (Italy)'81; FRCPC; IntMed. Staff, Guelph General Hospital; Langs: Italian; (519)822-7345; Fax. (519)822-0030.

CHAPMAN, Laura M; USTAT/Group Clinic, 1119 Pembroke St, Victoria BC V8T 1J3; UBC'86; FRCPC; Psy (Addiction Medicine). Staff Sleep Disorder Prog, UBC Hospital - Koerner Pavillion; Consultant Psy, Vancouver General Hospital - Centennial Pavillion; Clinical Asst Prof Psy, University of British Columbia; Langs: Hindi; (250)213-4400

CHAPMAN, Leagh T; 23 Health Services, PO Box 17000 Stn Forces 62-715 Wihuri Rd, Winnipeg MB R3J 3Y5; Alb'96; FRCPC; DiagRad.

CHAPMAN, Michael G; Rapid Access Clinic, 13750 94A Ave, Surrey BC V3V 1Z2; Man'06; FRCPC; IntMed; InfectDis. (604)587-3842

CHAPMAN, Michael T; SGH Medical Mall, 402-3030 Lawrence Ave E, Scarborough ON M1P 2T7; Ott'73; FRCSC; OrthSurg (Spine). Ac Staff/Corp Chief Surg, The Scarborough Hospital - General Campus; (416)431-5452; Fax. (416)431-6910.

CHAPMAN, Paul D; Victoria Gen Hosp, 1 Hospital Way, Victoria BC V8Z 6R5; Man'07; FRCPC; PhysMed&Rehab. Staff, Victoria General Hospital; (250)727-4212

CHAPMAN, Ronald D; Northern Health Authority, 600-299 Victoria St, Prince George BC V2L 5B8; Witwatersrand (South Africa)'83; FRCPC; CommunMed. (250)649-7653; Fax. (250)565-2620.

CHAPMAN, Sharon; Collingwood Med Clinic, 350-3150 54th Ave E, Vancouver BC V5S 1Z1; Witwatersrand (South Africa)'88; MB BCh; CCFP; (604)435-3388

CHAPMAN, William B; St Joseph's Health Centre, 30 The Queensway, Toronto ON M6R 1B5; Wes'81; FRCPC; AnatPath (Gynecological Pathology). Chief Lab Services, St Joseph's Health Centre; Chief Lab Med, University of Toronto; (416)530-6267; Fax. (416)530-6284; chapmw@stjoe.on.ca.

CHAPNICK, Cary N; 120 6 Ave PO Box 250, Gimli MB R0C 1B0; Man'86; (204)642-8561; Fax. (204)642-5860.

CHAPNIK, Jerry S; Mount Sinai Hosp, 401-600 University Ave, Toronto ON M5G 1X5; Tor'62; DAB; FRCSC; Otol. Assoc Staff, Mount Sinai Hospital; Consultant, Toronto General Hospital - UHN; Assoc Prof Otol, University of Toronto; (416)586-8669; Fax. (416)586-8600; jchapnik@mtsinai.on.ca.

CHAPNIK, Victor H; Bayview North Med Centre, 6-446 Hollandview Trail, Aurora ON L4G 7Z9; Tor'96; CCFP; (905)751-1642; Fax. (905)751-0885.

CHAPPELL, Brent W; Saskatoon Med Imaging Centre, 3-3110 8th St E, Saskatoon SK S7H 0W2; Sask'84; LMCC; FRCPC; DiagRad. (306)477-1000; Fax. (306)477-1071.

CHAPPELL, Nicola R; 100-20 Heritage Meadows Rd SE, Calgary AB T2H 3C1; Cal'90; CCFP; FCFP; (403)252-8851; Fax. (403)252-1765.

CHAPPLE, Denise L; 202-474 Columbia St, Kamloops BC V2C 2T5; Cal'97; FRCPC; Peds (Child Abuse). Clin Prof, University of British Columbia; (250)374-3300; Fax. (250)374-8837; loriruth@telus.net.

CHAPPLE, Ruhiya B; Family Med Clinic, 357 Albert St, Regina SK S4R 2N6; Vikram (India)'65; MB BS; MS; Staff, Regina General Hospital; Staff, Pasqua Hospital; (306)949-8840; Fax. (306)924-9355.

CHAPUIS, Frederic; Ctr Hosp Trois-Riv-Ste-Marie, 1991 boul du Carmel, Trois-Rivieres QC G8Z 3R9; (France)'93; Staff, CSSS de Trois-Rivières; (819)697-3333; Fax. (819)371-5001.

CHAPUT, Alan J; The Ottawa Hosp-Civic Campus, 1053 Carling Ave, Ottawa ON K1Y 4E9; Tor'01; FRCPC; Anes. Staff, The Ottawa Hospital - Civic Campus; (613)798-5555

CHAPUT, Andre; Clin Med-Ctr de Sante Lanaudie, 288 boul Larochelle, Repentigny QC J6A 8K4; Mon'71; (450)581-2120

CHAPUT, Brigitte; Hotel-Dieu d'Arthabaska, 5 rue des Hospitalieres, Victoriaville QC G6P 6N2; Sher'00; CCFP; CCFP(E.M.); Staff, Hotel-Dieu d'Arthabaska; (819)357-2030

CHAPUT, Genevieve; CLSC Cote des Neiges, 5700 ch de la Cote-des-Neiges, Montreal QC H3T 2A8; Mon'06; CCFP; (514)731-8531

CHAPUT, Gerard; Clinique Med Lac Megantic, 102-5256 rue Frontenac, Lac-Megantic QC G6B 1H3; Sher'77; Langs: Bilingual(French/English); (819)583-3345; Fax. (819)583-6045.

CHAPUT, Gilles R; 2185 rue Fleury E, Montreal QC H2B 1J9; Mon'67; Ophth. Staff, Hôpital du Sacre-Coeur de Montréal; Universite de Montreal; Langs: English; (514)387-8787; Fax. (514)387-9621.

CHAPUT, Guylaine; Clinique Med Notre-Dame, 120-504 rue Notre-Dame, Repentigny QC J6A 2T8; Mon'87; (450)585-3232; Fax. (450)582-9763.

CHAPUT, Miguel; Hopital Maisonneuve-Rosemont, 5415 boul de l'Assomption, Montreal QC H1T 2M4; McG'99; FRCSC; CardSurg; VascSurg. Staff, Hopital Maisonneuve-Rosemont; (514)252-3400; Fax. (514)252-3529.

CHAPUT, Veronique; MUHC-Montreal Gen Hosp, L10 212-1650 av Cedar, Montreal QC H3G 1A4; Mon'00; FRCSC; GenSurg. Staff, McGill University Health Centre - Montreal General Campus; (514)934-1934 x43926

CHAPUT, Yves; 230-365 rue Normand, St-Jean-sur-Richel QC J3A 1T6; McG'81; FRCPC; Psy. Staff, Douglas Mental Health University Institute; (450)359-9537

CHARACH, Alice E; The Hosp for Sick Children, 555 University Ave, Toronto ON M5G 1X8; Emory(GA) (USA)'80; DCAP; MSc; FRCPC; Psy. Staff Psy, The Hospital For Sick Children; Assoc Prof Psy, University of Toronto; (416)813-6936; Fax. (416)813-5326; alice.charach@sickkids.ca.

CHARACH, Ronald H; 554 Spadina Ave, Toronto ON M5S 2J9; Man'77; FRCPC; Psy (Adolescent Psychiatry). Editor, The Medical Post; Staff Teacher, University of Toronto; (416)968-2656

CHARAL, John M; 508-2000 Credit Valley Rd, Mississauga ON L5M 4N4; Tor'83; Ac Staff, The Credit Valley Hospital; (905)828-2837

CHARANIA, Diamondali K; Glendale Med Clinic, 10-1900 Dixie Rd, Pickering ON L1V 6M4; Makerere (Uganda)'72; (905)839-3353; Fax. (905)839-3391.

CHARANIA, Hameeda; Queen Elizabeth II HSC, BB 457C-1276 South Park St, Halifax NS B3H 2Y9; Dowe Medical College (India)'99; MB BS; Staff, Queen Elizabeth II Health Sciences Centre - Victoria General Site; (902)473-4150; Fax. (902)473-6186.

CHARANIA, Hanif; 107-900 Greenbank Rd, Nepean ON K2J 1S8; Tor'90; CCFP; CCFP(E.M.); FCFP; Staff ER, Queensway Carleton Hospital; (613)825-8476; Fax. (613)825-9045.

CHARANIA, Jahangir; 109-245 Columbia St E, New Westminster BC V3L 3W4; Alb'02; Cardiol; IntMed. (604)520-3993

CHARANIA, Naveen N; Whitby Urgent Care/Walk-In Cli, 204-1615 Dundas St E, Whitby ON L1N 2L1; (Pakistan)'81; CCFP; (905)436-2273; Fax. (905)436-2263.

CHARANIA, Sahira H; 107-900 Greenbank Rd, Nepean ON K2J 1S8; Tor'88; CCFP; FCFP; (613)825-8476; Fax. (613)825-9045; zahirdhalla@rogers.com.

CHARAPOV, Ilia A; The Ottawa Hosp-Civic Campus, B307-1053 Carling Ave, Ottawa ON K1Y 4E9; Alb'03; FRCPC; Anes. Staff, The Ottawa Hospital - Civic Campus; (613)761-4169; Fax. (613)761-5209.

CHARAPOVA, Elena G; Somerset West Comm Health Ctre, 55 Eccles St, Ottawa ON K1R 6S3; Alb'02; BSc; CCFP; Langs: Russian; (613)238-1220; Fax. (613)235-2982.

CHARBONEAU, Joan M; 1-3095 Glen Erin Dr, Mississauga ON L5L 1J3; Tor'71; CCFP; Court Staff, Trillium Health Centre - Mississauga; (905)828-5033; Fax. (905)828-5034; joan@phenixgroup.ca.

CHARBONNEAU, Alain; Polyclinique de Trois-Rivieres, 250-1900 boul des Recollets, Trois-Rivieres QC G8Z 4K4; Sher'82; FRCSC; Ophth (Cataract). Staff, CSSS de Trois-Rivières; adj Prof, Universite de Montreal; Clin Instructeur, Universite de Sherbrooke; (819)379-8888; Fax. (819)374-2598.

CHARBONNEAU, Alain; CSSS du Sud de Lanaudière, 911 montee des Pionniers, Terrebonne QC J6V 2H2; Mon'04; MedMicrobiol. Staff, Centre Hospitalier Pierre le Gardeur; (450)654-7525

CHARBONNEAU, Anne-Marie; Hop Maisonneuve-Rosemont, 5415 boul de l'Assomption, Montreal QC H1T 2M4; Mon'06; CCFP; Staff, Hopital Maisonneuve-Rosemont; (514)252-3400

CHARBONNEAU, Annie; CSSS des Basques, 550 rue Notre-Dame E RR 1, Trois-Pistoles QC G0L 4K0; Mon'95; Staff, Centre Hospitalier Trois-Pistoles; (418)851-1111

CHARBONNEAU, Benoit; Ctr de Med Familiale de Granby, 48 rue Denison E, Granby QC J2G 4C6; Sher'86; (450)372-3996; Fax. (450)372-0430.

CHARBONNEAU, Chantal; CSSS des Aurores Boreales, CP 6000 Succ Bureau-Chef 679 2e rue E, La Sarre QC J9Z 2X7; Mon'08; CCFP; Staff, Centre Hospitalier La Sarre; (819)333-2311; Fax. (819)339-2729.

CHARBONNEAU, Danielle L; West Lincoln Mem Hosp, 169 Main St E, Grimsby ON L3M 1P3; McM'02; CCFP; Staff, Halton Healthcare Services Corporation - Milton District Hospital; Staff, Halton Healthcare Services Corporation - Oakville Site; Staff, West Lincoln Memorial Hospital; Staff, Joseph Brant Memorial Hospital; (905)945-2253

CHARBONNEAU, Eric Y; Hôpital Laval, 2725 ch Sainte-Foy, Quebec QC G1V 4G5; Ott'96; FRCSC; CardSurg. Staff, Hôpital Laval; (418)656-4717

CHARBONNEAU, Fabien A; 8754 First Line RR 2, Campbellville ON L0P 1B0; Ott'87; Langs: English; French.

CHARBONNEAU, Fernand; Clin Med Maisonneuve-Rosemont, 5345 boul de l'Assomption, Montreal QC H1T 4B3; Mon'65; CSPQ; Cardiol (P.Q.) (Hemodynamics). Ac Staff, Hopital Maisonneuve-Rosemont; ac Staff, Centre Hospitalier Fleury; Clin Prof, Universite de Montreal; (514)251-8610; Fax. (450)681-2861.

CHARBONNEAU, Francois; Calgary Heart Centre, 403-3280 Hospital Dr NW, Calgary AB T2N 4Z6; Mon'87; MSc; CSPQ; FRCPC; IntMed (Clinical Cardiology); Cardiol. Staff, Foothills Medical Centre; Staff, Health Research Innovation Centre; (403)521-2227; Fax. (403)283-6360; francois.charbonneau@calgaryhealthregion.ca.

CHARBONNEAU, Guillaume; Ctr de Sante Vallee-Gatineau, 309 boul Desjardins, Maniwaki QC J9E 2E7; Mon'04; CCFP; Staff, CSSS de la Vallée de la Gatineau; (819)449-4690

CHARBONNEAU, Ivan; 7975 boul Laframboise, Saint-Hyacinthe QC J2R 1E8; Mon'65; AB; PlasSurg. Staff PlasSurg, Centre de Sante et de Services Sociaux; (450)796-3800; Fax. (450)796-2434.

CHARBONNEAU, Jacques; 302-200 rue Montcalm, Gatineau QC J8Y 3B5; Laval'80; CSPQ; FRCPC; Derm (Esthetic Dermatology). Langs: English; (819)778-3188; Fax. (819)778-8815; ilco.inc@videotron.ca.

CHARBONNEAU, Jacques; 286 rue De Normandie, Sainte-Julie QC J3E 1A7; Mon'74; (450)649-1593; Fax. (450)649-0361.

CHARBONNEAU, Jean; 208-468 boul Sir-Wilfrid-Lauri, Mont-Saint-Hilaire QC J3H 6K3; Mon'84; Langs: English; (450)813-9222

CHARBONNEAU, Katerine C; CLSC Senneterre, GD 961 rue de la Clinique, Senneterre QC J0Y 2M0; Laval'09; CCFP; (819)825-5858; Fax. (819)825-7949.

CHARBONNEAU, Louise; CLSC des Faubourgs, 1250 rue Sanguinet, Montreal QC H2X 3E7; Mon'65; MedMicrobiol. (514)844-9333; Fax. (514)847-8398.

CHARBONNEAU, Louise; Clinique Bellevue, 200-4135 rue de Rouen, Montreal QC H1V 1G5; Mon'85; FRCSC; Ophth. Staff, Centre Hospitalier l'Université De Montréal (CHUM) - Hôpital Saint-luc; (514)256-0007

CHARBONNEAU, Manon; CSSS de Sept-Iles, 45 rue Du Pere-Divet, Sept-Iles QC G4R 3N7; Mon'86; FRCPC; Psy. Staff Psy, Centre Hospitalier Regional de Sept-Iles; assoc Prof, Universite de Montreal; (418)962-9761 x2500; Fax. (418)962-2701.

CHARBONNEAU, Marc; CSSS de Laval, 1755 boul Rene-Laennec, Laval QC H7M 3L9; Sher'85; Respir (P.Q.); IntMed (Pneumology). Staff, Hopital de la Cite de la santé; adj Prof, Universite de Montreal; (450)668-1010; Fax. (450)975-5064.

CHARBONNEAU, Marcel; CSSS Pierre Boucher, 1333 boul Jacques-Cartier E, Longueuil QC J4M 2A5; Mon'79; CSPQ; Cardiol. Staff, Centre Hospitalier Pierre Boucher; (450)468-8111

CHARBONNEAU, Maxime; Centre Hosp Honore-Mercier, 2750 boul Laframboise, Saint-Hyacinthe QC J2S 4Y8; Sher'03; FRCSC; GenSurg. Staff, Centre Hospitalier Honore-Mercier; (450)771-3333; Fax. (450)771-3552.

CHARBONNEAU, Myriam; RRQ-Medical Services Evaluatio, 348-2600 boul Laurier, Quebec QC G1V 4T3; Mon'92; BSc; MSc; Médecin, Hôtel-Dieu de Lévis; Physician, Centre d'Accueil St-Gervais; Langs: English; (418)657-8709 x3941

CHARBONNEAU, Nicolas; Hop Charles LeMoyne, 3120 boul Taschereau, Greenfield Park QC J4V 2H1; Mon'04; FRCSC; Otol (Head & Neck Surgery). Staff, Hopital Charles LeMoyne; (450)466-5000

CHARBONNEAU, Pierre; Clinique Med Ahuntsic, 4-241 rue Fleury O, Montreal QC H3L 1V2; Sher'86; Staff, Centre Hospitalier Fleury; (514)382-0062

CHARBONNEAU, Richard; Clinique Medicale GMF-1851, 101-1851 rue Sherbrooke E, Montreal QC H2K 4L5; Mon'89; Staff, Hôpital de Saint-Eustache; (514)524-7564; Fax. (514)527-5251.

CHARBONNEAU, Robert; CHUQ-Hotel-Dieu de Quebec, 11 Cote Du Palais, Quebec QC G1R 2J6; Mon'80; FRCPC; IntMed; Nephrol. Staff, Centre Hospitalier Universitaire de Québec (CHUQ) - Siege Social; (418)691-5464; Fax. (418)691-5757.

CHARBONNEAU, Roland; 450-1575 boul de l'Avenir, Laval QC H7S 2N5; Mon'72; FRCSC; PlasSurg. Asst Surg, McGill University Health Centre - Royal Victoria Hospital; (450)662-9515; rolandcharbonneau@vl.videotron.ca.

CHARBONNEAU, Shannon; Bowmont Med Clinic, 6535 Bowness Rd NW, Calgary AB T3B 0E8; Ott'09; CCFP; (403)247-9797

CHARBONNEAU, Sonia; CHUM-Hop Notre-Dame, 1560 rue Sherbrooke E, Montreal QC H2L 4M1; Mon'02; FRCPC; Anes. Staff, Centre Hospitalier l'Université de Montréal (CHUM) - Hôpital Notre-Dame; (514)890-8000 x26876; Fax. (514)412-7653.

CHARBONNEAU, Suzanne; 1650 rue Michel-Gamelin, Laval QC H7M 5L7; Mon'69; MSc; Langs: Bilingual(English/French); (450)669-7845

CHARBONNEAU, Sylvia M; 405-2249 Carling Ave, Ottawa ON K2B 7E9; Ott'69; BSc; FRCPC; Psy. (613)222-8606; Fax. (613)596-3250.

CHARBONNEAU, Sylvie G; Ctr Hosp de Verdun, 4000 boul Lasalle, Verdun QC H4G 2A3; Mon'82; CSPQ; AnatPath. Staff, Centre Hospitalier de Verdun; (514)362-1000 x2216

CHARBONNEAU, Sylvie; CLSC-CHSLD de la Petite-Nation, 14 rue St-Andre, St-Andre-Avellin QC J0V 1W0; Mon'82; CCFP; (819)983-7341; Fax. (819)983-1315.

CHARBONNEAU, Yoland R; The Ottawa Hosp-Civic Campus, D6-1053 Carling Ave, Ottawa ON K1Y 4E9; Ott'87; FRCPC; Psy. Ac Staff, The Ottawa Hospital - Civic Campus; Asst Prof Psy, University of Ottawa; (613)761-4588; Fax. (613)761-4177.

CHARBONNEAU, Yves; Clinique Maisonneuve-Rosemont, 60-5345 boul de l'Assomption, Montreal QC H1T 4B3; Mon'84; Staff, Centre Hospitalier l'Université De Montréal (CHUM) - Hôpital Saint-luc; (514)257-7000; Fax. (514)257-7003.

CHARBONNEAU, Yves; Carrefour Med Vallee Richelieu, 665 boul Sir-Wilfrid-Laurier, Beloeil QC J3G 4J1; Mon'72; ABAI; FRCPC; IntMed; ClinImmunol&Allergy. adj Prof, Universite de Montreal; (450)467-3331; Fax. (450)467-6941; yveschar@videotron.ca.

CHARBONNEAU-BLOUIN, Renee; Professional Health Sorel-Trac, 330 av de l'Hotel-Dieu, Sorel-Tracy QC J3P 1N4; Sher'74; (450)742-9459; Fax. (450)742-9450.

CHARBONNEY, Emmanuel; CSSS de Trois-Rivieres, 1991 boul du Carmel, Trois-Rivieres QC G8Z 3R9; Lausanne (Switzerland)'96; Critical Care Medicine (P.Q.). Staff, CSSS de Trois-Rivières; (819)697-3333

CHARENDOFF, Jeffrey S; 404-960 Lawrence Ave W, North York ON M6A 3B5; Tor'83; BSc; FRCSC; Urol (Endoscopy Urology). Staff, Humber River Regional Hospital - Keele Street Site; Staff, Humber River Regional Hospital - Church Street Site; Assoc. Dir., The Male Health Centre; (416)256-2737; Fax. (416)256-9098.

CHARENDOFF, Morris D; 310-4430 Bathurst St, North York ON M3H 3S3; Tor'47; FRCSC; OrthSurg. Assoc Staff, St John's Rehabilitation Hospital; Staff OrthSurg, North York General Hospital - Branson Division; (416)630-1818; Fax. (416)630-1248; mdorthodoc@aol.com.

CHAREST, Andre; Medical Bldg, 205-250 Harding Blvd W, Richmond Hill ON L4C 9M7; Laval'93; FRCPC; IntMed (Hypertension); Nephrol. Staff Nephrol, Mackenzie Richmond Hill Hospital; Court Staff Nephrol, Southlake Regional Health Centre; Langs: Bilingual(French/English); (905)508-5911; Fax. (905)508-2972; yorknephrology1@rogers.com.

CHAREST, Anne-Marie; CSSS de la Haute-Gaspésie, 50 rue Belvedere, Ste-Anne-des-Monts QC G4V 1X4; Mon'96; CCFP; Staff, Centre Hospitalier des Monts; Staff, CSSS de la Baie-des-Chaleurs; (418)763-2261

CHAREST, Dhany T; Professional Arts Bldg, 504-100 Arden St, Moncton NB E1C 4B7; Sher'95; FRCSC; Neursurg (Oncology). Langs: Bilingual(French/English); (506)857-5376; Fax. (506)857-5378.

CHAREST, Eve; Hotel-Dieu de Levis, 143 rue Wolfe, Levis QC G6V 3Z1; Laval'04; FRCPC; Anes. Staff, Hôtel-Dieu de Lévis; (418)835-7121 x3218

CHAREST, Francois; CSSS du Sud de Lanaudière, 911 montee des Pionniers, Terrebonne QC J6V 2H2; Mon'86; Staff, Centre Hospitalier Pierre le Gardeur; (450)654-7525

CHAREST, Isabelle; CSSS du Lac-des-Deux-Montagnes, 520 boul Arthur-Sauve, Saint-Eustache QC J7R 5B1; Mon'99; CSPQ; FRCPC; Anes. Staff, Hôpital de Saint-Eustache; (819)623-1245

CHAREST, Jean; Hôpital Ste-Justine, 3175 ch Cote-Sainte-Catherine, Montreal QC H3T 1C5; Mon'69; CSPQ; Anes. Ac Staff, Hôpital Ste-Justine; (514)345-4733; Fax. (514)345-4829.

CHAREST, Jerome; Clinique Medicina, 298-245 rue Soumande, Quebec QC G1M 3H6; Mon'00; CCFP; (418)780-0122

CHAREST, Louise; Clinique Med L'Actuel, 1130-1001 boul de Maisonneuve, Montreal QC H2L 4P9; Mon'86; MSc; (514)524-1001; Fax. (514)524-3831.

CHAREST, Louise; Clinique Med Le Norois, 201-601 4e rue O, Amos QC J9T 2S1; Sher'83; CCFP; FCFP; Staff, CH Hôtel-Dieu d'Amos; (819)732-3368

CHAREST, Mathieu; Lakeshore Gen Hosp, 160 rue Stillview, Pointe-Claire QC H9R 2Y2; Mon'02; FRCPC; NuclearMed. Staff, Lakeshore General Hospital - Pointe Claire; (514)630-2225 x1398

CHAREST, Melanie; 202-185 av Acadie, Dieppe NB E1A 1G6; Laval'99; CCFP; Prof, Universite de Moncton; Langs: Bilingual(French/English); (506)860-7203; Fax. (506)862-1265; melanie.charest@umoncton.ca.

CHAREST, Michel; Le Mediclub, 6100 av Du Boise, Montreal QC H3S 2W1; Mon'71; Langs: English; (514)739-5646; Fax. (514)739-7085.

CHAREST, Nicole; Clinique Gynecologique, 102-39 rue Laurier E, Victoriaville QC G6P 6P6; Laval'86; FRCSC; ObstGyn. (819)357-4073; Fax. (819)357-4075.

CHAREST, Raymond; Clinique Med St-Jerome, 102-450 boul Monseigneur-Duboi, Saint-Jerome QC J7Y 3L8; Mon'79; (450)438-1518; Fax. (450)438-6119.

CHAREST, Stephane; Clinique de Neurologie, 4380 Cote Rosemont, Trois-Rivieres QC G8Y 0A5; Laval'92; FRCPC; Neur; Electroenceph (P.Q.). Staff, Centre Hospitalier Regional de Trois-Rivieres; Langs: Bilingual(French/English); (819)379-7336

CHAREST, Veronie; CSSS de Rivière-de-Loup, 75 rue Saint-Hubert, Riviere-du-Loup QC G5R 2A4; Mon'08; CSPQ; Peds. Staff, Centre Hospitalier Regional du Grand-Portage; (418)868-1010

CHAREST-LEBLANC, Mireille; 336 rue Main, Shediac NB E4P 2E5; Sher'01; Dip SportMed; CCFP; Physician SportsMed, Max Health Institute; (506)532-6696; Fax. (506)532-1543; cliniquefamilialeshediac@hotmail.ca.

CHARETTE, Christiane; Centre Hosp Honore-Mercier, 2750 rue Laframboise, Saint-Hyacinthe QC J2S 4Y8; Mon'88; FAAP; Peds. Staff Dept of Peds, Centre Hospitalier Honore-Mercier; (450)771-3333; Fax. (450)771-3557.

CHARETTE, Francois; CLSC St-Leonard, 5540 rue Jarry E, Saint-Leonard QC H1P 1T9; Mon'86; CCFP; (514)328-3460; Fax. (514)328-1468.

CHARETTE, Francois G; CAMU, 2984 boul Taschereau, Longueuil QC J4V 2G9; Mon'78; BSc(Biol.); MD; Langs: English; Spanish; (450)466-4333; Fax. (450)466-0716; francois.charette@hotmail.ca.

CHARETTE, Geneviève; Ctr Hosp de Lasalle, 8585 Tsse Champlain, LaSalle QC H8P 1C1; Mon'06; Staff, Centre Hospitalier de LaSalle; (514)362-8000

CHARETTE, Guy; GMF La Cigogne, 420-3141 boul Taschereau, Longueuil QC J4V 2H2; Mon'79; (450)466-7892

CHARETTE, Luc; Clinique de Pediatrie, 105 av Gatineau, Gatineau QC J8T 4J4; Ott'73; FRCPC; Peds. Langs: Bilingual(French/English); (819)561-4412; Fax. (819)561-0717.

CHARETTE, Marie-Christine I; Asclepios Med Clinic, 2F-750 Taylor Creek Dr, Orleans ON K1C 1T1; Ott'07; CCFP; (613)830-8388

CHARETTE, Mireille; Ctr Hosp Reg de Lanaudiere, 1000 boul Sainte-Anne, St-Charles-Brromee QC J6E 6J2; Mon'91; Staff, Centre Hospitalier Régional de Lanaudière; (450)759-8222

CHARETTE, Yannick A; 2416 Long Lake Rd, Sudbury ON P3E 5H5; NOSM'10; CCFP; (705)222-0079

CHARETTE, Yves G; City of Lakes Family Hlth Team, 1679 Main St, Val Caron ON P3N 1R8; Ott'07; CCFP; Langs: Bilingual(English/French); (705)897-1018; Fax. (705)897-2234.

CHARETTE-MARTINEAU, Amelie; CLSC Haute-Ville, 55 ch Sainte-Foy, Quebec QC G1R 1S9; Sher'02; (418)641-2572

CHARGHI, Ali; Clinique Med Nova, 3755 boul Saint-Laurent, Montreal QC H2W 1X8; Geneva (Switzerland)'57; FACS; CSPQ; Urol. Staff, Centre Hospitalier l'Université de Montréal (CHUM) - Hôtel-Dieu; Clin Assoc Prof Surg, Universite de Montreal; Langs: English; French; (514)987-0080; Fax. (514)987-0075.

CHARGHI, Parissa; St Mary's Hosp Centre, 3830 av Lacombe, Montreal QC H3T 1M5; Mon'06; CCFP; Staff, St Mary's Hospital Centre; (514)345-3511

CHARGHI, Roshanak; SMBD Jewish Gen Hosp, 3755 ch Cote-Sainte-Catherine, Montreal QC H3T 1E2; Laval'99; CSPQ; FRCPC; Anes. Staff, Sir Mortimer B Davis Jewish General; (514)340-8222

CHARI, Anish S; Troohu Medical Clinic, PO Box 160 451 Dechauney Ave, Trochu AB T0M 2C0; Alb'08; BSc; CCFP; (403)442-3814; Fax. (403)442-3816.

CHARI, Rachna A; 3F-61 Queen St E, Toronto ON M5C 2T2; Cal'09; CCFP; (416)867-7428

CHARI, Radha S; Royal Alexandra Hosp, 5S139-10240 Kingsway NW, Edmonton AB T5H 3V9; Sask'88; FRCSC; ObstGyn. Dir Div of Maternal Fetal Med, Royal Alexandra Hospital; Assoc Prof ObstGyn, University of Alberta; (780)735-4815; Fax. (780)735-4981; rchari@cha.ab.ca.

CHARI, Seshadri M; 580-190 Attwell Dr, Etobicoke ON M9W 6H8; Tor'88; (416)213-8118

CHARI, Vinjamuri R; Regional Rehabilitation Centre, 300 Wellington St N, Hamilton ON L8L 0A4; Benares (India)'76; MB BS; MD; FRCPC; PhysMed&Rehab (Stroke). Staff, Hamilton Health Sciences Centre - McMaster University Medical Centre; Staff, Regional Rehabilitation Centre; Asst Prof, McMaster University; Langs: Telugu; Hindi; (905)521-2100; Fax. (905)577-8233; chari@hhsc.ca.

CHARKHSAZ, Marjan; Careview Med Centre, 214-3001 Gordon Ave, Coquitlam BC V3C 2K7; Isfahan (Iran)'97; CCFP; (604)941-7700

CHARKOW, Steven H; 385 Fairway Rd S, Kitchener ON N2C 2N9; UBC'89; (519)748-2327

CHARLAND, Frederic; Hotel-Dieu du Sacre-Coeur, 1 av du Sacre-Coeur, Quebec QC G1N 2W1; Laval'01; FRCPC; Psy. Staff, Hotel-Dieu du Sacre-Coeur de Jesus de Quebec; (418)529-6851 x20281

CHARLAND, Nancy; Clinique Med Plaza Gatineau, 381 boul Maloney E, Gatineau QC J8P 1E3; Laval'82; (819)669-7393; Fax. (819)669-0077.

CHARLAND, Patrick; CSSS de la Matapedia, 135 av Gaetan-Archambault, Amqui QC G5J 2K5; Laval'99; BScPharm; Staff, CSSS de la Matapedia; (418)629-2211; Fax. (418)629-4498.

CHARLAND, Pierre; Clinique de Radiology Sorel-Tr, 3215 rue des Erables, Sorel-Tracy QC J3R 2W6; Mon'69; CSPQ; FRCPC; DiagRad (Echography). Staff Radiol, Hôpital Anna-Laberge; Staff, Hôtel-Dieu de Sorel; Staff, Clinique Radiologie Sorel-Tracy; Langs: English; Spanish; (450)742-0433; Fax. (450)742-0435.

CHARLAND, Raymond P; Clinique Maisonneuve-Rosemont, 145-5345 boul de l'Assomption, Montreal QC H1T 4B3; Mon'65; CSPQ; BA; FRCPC; Cardiol. Langs: English; (514)251-8610; Fax. (514)251-8610; raymondcharland@yahoo.ca.

CHARLAND, Vanessa; Centre de Peri-Maternite, 575 rue Saint-Charles E, Longueuil QC J4H 1B8; Mon'06; CCFP; (450)332-9833; Fax. (450)332-0865.

CHARLEBOIS, Alison L; Sherbourne Health Centre, 333 Sherbourne St, Toronto ON M5A 2S5; McM'10; CCFP; (416)867-3728

CHARLEBOIS, Manon; Ctr Hosp Rouyn-Noranda, 4 9e rue, Rouyn-Noranda QC J9X 2B2; Mon'02; FRCSC; ObstGyn. Staff, Centre Hospitalier Rouyn-Noranda; (819)764-5131

CHARLEBOIS, Normand S; CSSS de Laval, 1755 boul Rene-Laennec, Laval QC H7M 3L9; Mon'80; DiagRad. Staff, Hopital de la Cite de la santé; (450)975-5406; Fax. (450)975-5096.

CHARLEBOIS, Patrick; MUHC-Montreal Gen Hosp, D16 173-1650 av Cedar, Montreal QC H3G 1A4; McG'96; FRCSC; GenSurg (Colon & Rectal Surgery). Staff, McGill University Health Centre - Montreal General Campus; Asst Prof Surg, McGill University; (514)934-8486; Fax. (514)934-8487.

CHARLEBOIS, Paul B; Canadian Forces Hlth Serv Ctr, PO Box 99000 Stn Forces Specialist Services Clinic, Halifax NS B3K 5X5; Dal'95; FRCPC; IntMed;CCFP; Staff, Canadian Forces Health Services Centre (Atlantic); (902)721-7894; Fax. (902)721-8866.

CHARLEBOIS, Pierre; CSSS Haut-Richelieu-Rouville, 920 boul Du Seminaire N, St-Jean-Sur-Richel QC J3A 1B7; Mon'84; Staff, Hôpital du Haut-Richelieu; (450)359-5000

CHARLEBOIS, Sarah; 66 Broad Rd, Oromocto NB E2V 1C2; Mon'09; CCFP; Staff, Oromocto Public Hospital.

CHARLEBOIS, Simon; CHUM-Hop St-Luc, 1058 rue Saint-Denis, Montreal QC H2X 3J4; Mon'68; DiagRad (P.Q.) (Thoracic Radiology). Staff, Centre Hospitalier l'Université De Montréal (CHUM) - Hôpital Saint-luc; Asst Prof Radiol, Universite de Montreal; Langs: Bilingual(French/English); (514)890-8000 x36400

CHARLES, Guy G; Hop Louis-H Lafontaine, 7401 rue Hochelaga, Montreal QC H1N 3M5; Montpellier (France)'71; LMCC; Staff, Centre Hospitalier Pierre Boucher; Staff Emerg, Hopital Louis-H Lafontaine; (514)251-4000 x2255; Fax. (514)251-8463.

CHARLES, Jocelyn E; Sunnybrook Hlth Sciences Ctre, A100-2075 Bayview Ave, Toronto ON M4N 3M5; Wes'87; CCFP; Staff, Sunnybrook Health Sciences Centre; Asst Prof, University of Toronto; (416)480-4932; Fax. (416)480-5774.

CHARLES, Julia C; Thunder Bay Reg HSC-T-Bay, 980 Oliver Rd, Thunder Bay ON P7B 6V4; Cal'88; FRCPC; Anes. Staff, Thunder Bay Regional Health Sciences Centre; Langs: Bilingual(English/French); (807)684-6290; Fax. (807)346-8015.

CHARLES, Lesley A; Glenrose Rehab Hosp, 10230 111 Ave NW, Edmonton AB T5G 0B7; North Dakota (USA)'97; BSc; MB BS; CCFP; Staff, Glenrose Rehabilitation Hospital; Clin Lecturer Family Pract, University of Alberta; (780)474-8800; Fax. (780)474-8846; lcharles@ualberta.ca.

CHARLES, Marie-Muriel; Canadian Forces Health Service, 713 Montreal Rd, Ottawa ON K1A 0K2; Ott'93; CCFP; CCFP(E.M.); Staff, Grey Bruce Health Services - Owen Sound; Staff, Canadian Forces Health Services Centre; (613)945-1367

CHARLES, Mark N; Carling-Broadview Med Bldg, 106-770 Broadview Ave, Ottawa ON K2A 3Z3; Qns'95; FRCSC; OrthSurg (Hip & Knee Reconstruction). Staff, Queensway Carleton Hospital; (613)722-3987

CHARLES, Yolande; Clinique Avenir, 220-1575 boul de l'Avenir, Laval QC H7S 2N5; Bordeaux (France)'69; ObstGyn. (450)696-1025; Fax. (450)696-1019; yolandecharles@gmail.com.

CHARLESWORTH, J David; Royal Columbian Hosp, 330 Columbia St E, New Westminster BC V3L 3W7; Man'82; AB(AnatPath); AB(ForensicPath); FRCPC; AnatPath (Forensic Pathology). Staff Forensic Pathology Unit, Royal Columbian Hospital; Pathologist, British Columbia Coroner's Service; Vis Staff, Fraser Health Authority; (604)520-4747; Fax. (604)520-4409; david.charlesworth@fraserhealth.ca.

CHARLETON, Edmond D; 950-3803 Calgary Trail NW, Edmonton AB T6J 5M8; Queen's (Ireland)'79; MB ChB; BAO; (780)436-7240

CHARLIERS-LAZURE, Ariane; CLSC Valleyfield, 71 rue Maden, Salaber-de-Valleyf QC J6S 3V4; Laval'03; (450)371-0143

CHARLIN, Bernard D; Polyclinique de l'Oreille, 252-1111 rue Saint-Charles O, Longueuil QC J4K 5G4; Montpellier (France)'81; FRCSC; Otol. Staff, Centre Hospitalier Universitaire de Sherbrooke-Hopital Fleurimont; Consultant, Centre Hospitalier Universitaire de Sherbrooke-Hôpital Hôtel-Dieu; Dir Dept of Development Research in Educ Sciences & Health, Universite de Montreal; (450)679-1651; Fax. (450)679-1651.

CHARLOT, Lunel; Ctr Hosp Reg de Lanaudiere, 1000 boul Sainte-Anne, St-Charles-Brromee QC J6E 6J2; (Haiti)'83; Staff, Centre Hospitalier Régional de Lanaudière; (450)759-8222; Fax. (450)756-4951; lunel.charlot@ssss.gouv.qc.ca.

CHARLTON, Jeff R; Royal Alexandra Hosp, 10240 Kingsway NW, Edmonton AB T5H 3V9; Alb'90; FRCPC; Anes. Staff, Royal Alexandra Hospital; (780)735-4010

CHARLTON, Katharine; St Michael's Hosp, CCW17 033-30 Bond St, Toronto ON M5B 1W8; Qns'06; FRCPC; Psy. Staff Mental Health Centre, St Michael's Hospital; (416)864-3082; Fax. (416)864-3091.

CHARLTON, Ken J; 217-217 Talbot St, St Thomas ON N5P 1B1; Ott'90; CCFP; FCFP; (519)631-9040; Fax. (519)631-9355.

CHARLTON, Marco; SAAQ, CP 19600 Succ Terminus 333 boul Jean-Lesage, Quebec QC G1K 8J6; Mon'91.

CHARLTON, Ronald W R; 148 Markham Rd, Scarborough ON M1M 2Z8; Tor'58; (416)264-3566; Fax. (416)430-7489.

CHARLTON, Scott T; Avenue Med Clinic, 1-221 Brant Ave, Brantford ON N3T 3J2; Ott'02; CCFP; (519)753-8666; Fax. (519)753-6880.

CHARMAN, Sandra M; Medica One, 2019 Caroline St, Burlington ON L7R 1L1; (Colombia)'00; CCFP; (905)333-0911; Fax. (905)333-0311.

CHARNEAU, Manon; CSSS de Rimouski-Neigette, CP 3150 Succ A 150 av Rouleau, Rimouski QC G5L 5T1; Sher'93; Psy. Staff, Hôpital Regional Rimouski; (418)724-8315; Fax. (418)724-8652.

CHARNEUX, Marco; Hop du Sacre-Coeur de Mtl, 5400 boul Gouin O, Montreal QC H4J 1C5; Mon'93; ATLS; ACLS; ABEM; CRCP; DABEM; FACEP; FCFP; RC; CSPQ; FRCPC; EmergMed (Intensive Care); Critical Care Medicine (P.Q.). Staff Emerg & Intensive Care, Hôpital du Sacre-Coeur de Montréal; adj Prof, Universite de Montreal; Langs: English; French; (514)338-2222; marco@charneux.com.

CHARNEY, Dara A; MUHC-Montreal Gen Hosp, 1650 av Cedar, Montreal QC H3G 1A4; McG'91; FRCPC; Psy (Addiction Psychiatry). Staff Psy, McGill University Health Centre - Montreal General Campus; adj Prof, McGill University; (514)934-8311; Fax. (514)934-8262; dara.charney@mcgill.ca.

CHARNISH, Michael B; Southlake Regl Health Centre, 596 Davis Dr, Newmarket ON L3Y 2P9; Wes'06; CCFP; CCFP(E.M.); Staff, Southlake Regional Health Centre; (905)895-4521

CHARPENTIER, Anne-Marie; Univ Hlth Network-Princess M, 610 University Ave, Toronto ON M5G 2M9; Mon'06; FRCPC; RadOncol. Staff RadOncol, Princess Margaret Hospital - University Health Network; Langs: Bilingual(English/French); (416)946-4501

CHARPENTIER, Danielle; 1560 rue Sherbrooke E, Montreal QC H2L 4M1; Mon'80; FRCPC; IntMed (Breast Cancer); MedOncol; Hem. Dir méd Integrated Center for Cancer Research, Centre Hospitalier l'Université de Montréal (CHUM) - Hôpital Notre-Dame; Langs: Bilingual(French/English); (514)890-8000 x25381; danielle.charpentier.chum@ssss.gouv.qc.ca.

CHARPENTIER, Pascal; CSSS de Trois-Rivieres, 1991 rue du Carmel, Trois-Rivieres QC G8Z 3R9; Mon'97; CSPQ; FRCPC; Anes. Staff, CSSS de Trois-Rivières; (819)697-3333 x69856

CHARRIERE, Norma M E; Connor House Fam Practice, 240 Pinnacle St, Belleville ON K8N 3A6; McM'08; CCFP; (613)968-9840; Fax. (613)968-5495.

CHARROIS, Gregory J R; Dynacare Kasper Med Lab, 200-10150 102 St NW, Edmonton AB T5J 5E2; Alb'05; FRCPC; AnatPath. (780)451-3702 x3287; Fax. (780)452-8488.

CHARRON, Claire; CSSS Drummond-Hop Sainte-Croix, 570 rue Heriot, Drummondville QC J2B 1C1; Sher'89; Ac Staff, Hôpital Sainte-croix; (819)478-6464

CHARRON, Louis; Centre Med Donnacona, 420 Rte 138, Donnacona QC G3M 1C2; Laval'98; Langs: Bilingual(French/English); (418)285-1122

CHARRON, Louise F; Centre de Traitement Neurologi, 407-3875 rue Saint-Urbain, Montreal QC H2W 1V1; Sher'71; FRCPC; Neur. Staff, Hôpital du Sacre-Coeur de Montréal; Staff, Centre Hospitalier l'Université de Montréal (CHUM) - Hôtel-Dieu; Staff, McGill University Health Centre - Montreal General Campus; Universite de Montreal; (514)287-7409

CHARRON, Louise; UMF Laval, 2690 ch des Quatre-Bourgeois, Quebec QC G1V 0B7; Laval'85; Staff, Hôpital Laval; (418)656-4795; Fax. (418)656-4503.

CHARRON, Marc-Andre; Clinique Med du Quartier-Latin, 905 boul Rene-Levesque E, Montreal QC H2L 5B1; Sher'96; CCFP; Staff, Centre Hospitalier l'Université De Montréal (CHUM) - Hôpital Saint-luc; (514)285-5500

CHARRON, Martin; 555 University Ave, Toronto ON M5G 1X8; Sher'83; FRCP; FRCPC; NuclearMed (Radioisotopes). Dir Nuclear Med & Research/Staff, The Hospital For Sick Children; Prof Radiol, University of Toronto; Langs: French; (416)813-7654 x2006; Fax. (416)813-7591.

CHARRON, Maryse; Hop Louis-H Lafontaine, 7401 rue Hochelaga, Montreal QC H1N 3M5; Mon'82; FRCPC; Psy. Ac Staff, Hopital Louis-H Lafontaine; (514)251-4000; Fax. (514)251-1604.

CHARRON, Maryse; CSSS de Saint-Jerome, 290 rue de Montigny, Saint-Jerome QC J7Z 5T3; Sher'05; FRCPC; IntMed; MedOncol; Hem. Staff, Hôtel-Dieu de Saint-Jérôme; (450)431-8366

CHARRON, Nicole; 102-6955 boul Taschereau, Brossard QC J4Z 1A7; Mon'87; (450)656-2310

CHARRON, Patrick M; Windsor Prof Centre, 126-2462 Howard Ave, Windsor ON N8X 3V6; Wes'91; FRCPC; PhysMed&Rehab. Coroner, Province of Ontario; (519)255-9337; Fax. (519)255-9374.

CHARRON, Pierre; CHUS-Hop Fleurimont, 3001 12e Av N, Sherbrooke QC J1H 5N4; Laval'73; IntMed. Staff, Centre Hospitalier Universitaire de Sherbrooke-Hopital Fleurimont; (819)346-1110; Fax. (819)820-6420.

CHARRON, Robert; Clin Med de Metabetchouan, 20 rue Saint-Basile, Metab-L-A-La-Croix QC G8G 1S9; Mon'82; Staff, CSSS de Lac-Saint Jean-Est; (418)349-8933; Fax. (418)349-8082.

CHARRON, Thierry; Health Sciences North, 40 Ramseu Lake Rd, Sudbury ON P3E 5J1; Sher'97; Cardiol; IntMed. (705)671-1000

CHARRON, Yan; Hop Maisonneuve-Rosemont, 5415 boul de l'Assomption, Montreal QC H1T 2M4; Sher'02; Staff, Hopital Maisonneuve-Rosemont; (514)252-3400

CHARTERS, Jane; Chamber of Commerce Bldg, 502-345 Lakeshore Rd E, Oakville ON L6J 1J5; McM'87; Langs: French; (905)845-4511; Fax. (905)845-8133.

CHARTIER, Brenda A; West Durham Family Health Team, 200B-1105 Kingston Rd, Pickering ON L1V 1B5; Qns'83; Assoc Staff, Rouge Valley Health System - Ajax & Pickering Health Centre Site; (905)420-9999; Fax. (905)420-1090.

CHARTIER, Catherine; GMF Grandes Fourches, 50 rue Camirand, Sherbrooke QC J1H 4J5; Laval'02; CCFP; Staff, Centre Hospitalier Régional Baie-Comeau; (819)780-2222

CHARTIER, Jean-Claude; GMF du Chatel, 200-9465 boul de L'Ormiere, Quebec QC G2B 3K7; Mon'74; Staff, Centre Hospitalier Universitaire de Québec (CHUQ) - Siege Social; Langs: English; (418)843-5141

CHARTIER, Lucas; Centre medical Le Mesnil, 300-1300 boul Lebourgneuf, Quebec QC G2K 2N1; McG'09; (418)624-1800; Fax. (418)624-1820.

CHARTIER, Sophie; CLSC Samuel de Champlain, 100-5811 boul Taschereau, Brossard QC J4Z 1A5; Mon'95; Langs: Bilingual(French/English); (450)445-4452

CHARTIER, Suzanne; CHUM-Hop St-Luc, 1058 rue Saint-Denis, Montreal QC H2X 3J4; Mon'80; NBME; FRCPC; Derm. Staff, Centre Hospitalier l'Université De Montréal (CHUM) - Hôpital Saint-luc; Teach Staff, Universite de Montreal; (514)890-8000 x34401

CHARTRAND, Bernard; 207-2125 rue Jean-Talon E, Montreal QC H2E 1V4; McG'79; DU; (514)729-9333

CHARTRAND, Caroline; Hôpital Ste-Justine, 3175 ch Cote-Ste-Catherine, Montreal QC H3T 1C5; Mon'04; FRCPC; Peds. Staff, Hôpital Ste-Justine; (514)345-4931

CHARTRAND, Daniel; MUHC-Montreal Neurology Inst, 3801 rue University, Montreal QC H3A 2B4; Mon'80; FRCPC; Anes. Staff, McGill University Health Centre - Montreal Neurological Hospital; vice Chaire Dept of Anes/assoc Prof, McGill University; Langs: Bilingual(French/English); (514)398-1917; Fax. (514)398-1352.

CHARTRAND, James G H; Courtenay Health Sciences Ctr, 103-1350 England Ave, Courtenay BC V9N 8X6; Cal'77; FRCSC; Urol. Ac Staff, St Joseph's General Hospital; (250)338-1301; Fax. (250)338-9414; jcmd@telus.net.

CHARTRAND, Jean-Claude; 106-1221 rue Fleury E, Montreal QC H2C 1R2; Mon'79; Ac Staff, Hôpital du Sacre-Coeur de Montréal; Staff Emerg, Centre Hospitalier Fleury; (514)381-7808; Fax. (514)384-2218.

CHARTRAND, Jean-Pierre; Lakeshore Ophtalmologie, 240-315 boul Brunswick, Pointe-Claire QC H9R 5M7; Mon'77; ABOph; MD; CSPQ; Ophth (P.Q.) (Refractive Surgery). Consultant, Lakeshore General Hospital - Pointe Claire; Dir Contact Lens Clinic, Sir Mortimer B Davis Jewish General; adj Prof, McGill University; Langs: Bilingual(French/English); Italian; (514)694-2010; Fax. (514)694-0772.

CHARTRAND, Lisa-Marie; CSSSG-Hop De Gatineau, CP 2000 Succ Bureau-Chef 909 boul La Verendrye O, Gatineau QC J8P 7H2; Laval'04; FRCSC; ObstGyn. Staff, Hôpital de Gatineau; (819)966-6100

CHARTRAND, Louis-Andre; CSSS de Sept-Iles, 45 rue Du Pere-Divet, Sept-Iles QC G4R 3N7; Mon'79; CSPQ; Cardiol (P.Q.); IntMed. Staff, Centre Hospitalier Regional de Sept-Iles; (418)962-9761 x0; Fax. (418)962-7004.

CHARTRAND, M L Roxane; Montfort Hosp, 713 Montreal Rd, Ottawa ON K1K 0T2; Ott'77; FRCPC; Anes. Staff, Montfort Hospital; (613)746-4621 x2620

CHARTRAND, Marie-Pier; CSSS de Saint-Jerome, 290 rue de Montigny, Saint-Jerome QC J7Z 5T3; Mon'05; CCFP; Staff, Hôtel-Dieu de Saint-Jérôme; (450)431-8200

CHARTRAND, Rachel; Polyclinique St-Eustache, 75 rue Grignon, St-Eustache QC J7P 4J2; Mon'81; (450)473-5782; Fax. (450)473-1916.

CHARTRAND, Raymonde; CHUM-Hop St-Luc, 1058 rue Saint-Denis, Montreal QC H2X 3J4; Mon'65; AB; NuclearMed. Member Nuclear Med Service, Centre Hospitalier l'Université De Montréal (CHUM) - Hôpital Saint-luc; Member, Health Technologie Evaluation Council; Clin Prof, Universite de Montreal; Langs: English; (514)890-8000 x36228

CHARTRAND, Serge; U of Ottawa Health Services, 300-100 Marie Curie Pvt, Ottawa ON K1N 1A2; Sher'93; (613)564-3950

CHARTRAND-LEFEBVRE, Carl; CHUM-Hotel-Dieu, 3840 rue Saint-Urbain, Montreal QC H2W 1T8; Mon'91; FRCPC; DiagRad (Abdominal Radiology). Staff Radiologie Varad, Institut de Cardiologie de Montréal; Staff, Centre Hospitalier l'Université de Montréal (CHUM) - Hôtel-Dieu; (514)890-8150; Fax. (514)412-7193; chartrandlef@videotron.ca.

CHARUSRIPAN, Paninee; Univ Hlth Network-Toronto Gen, 8N 873-200 Elizabeth St, Toronto ON M5G 2C4; Chulalongkorn University (Other Foreign)'04; Clin Fellow Otol, Toronto General Hospital - UHN; (416)340-4630

CHARYK, Rafael; Malvern Med Arts Bldg, 100-1333 Neilson Rd, Scarborough ON M1B 4Y9; Tor'73; CCFP; FCFP; Staff, Rouge Valley Health System - Centenary Health Centre Site; (416)291-7719; Fax. (416)287-3775.

CHASE, Claudette; Sioux Lookout First Nations H, PO Box 1300 Stn Main 55B Queen St, Sioux Lookout ON P8T 1B8; McM'92; CCFP; FCFP; (807)737-4794; Fax. (807)737-7216.

CHASE, Jocelyn M; Specialized Senior's Clinic, 232 Ross Dr, New Westminster BC V3L 0B2; Alb'07; FRCPC; IntMed; GeriatricMed. (604)528-5031

CHASE, Robert M; Lamp Occupational Health Prog, 185 Fifth St, Etobicoke ON M8V 2Z5; McM'85; FRCPC; CommunMed (Occupational Health). Staff, Lamp Occupational Health Program; (416)252-6471; Fax. (416)252-9141.

CHASEN, Martin R; SCOHS-Elisabeth Bruyere Hosp, 270J-43 Bruyere St, Ottawa ON K1N 5C8; Pretoria (South Africa)'83; Staff, SCO Health Service - Élisabeth Bruyère Hospital; (613)562-6262 x4008

CHASSÉ, Claudel; CSSS de la Vallée de l'Or, 725 6e rue, Val-d'Or QC J9P 3Y1; Laval'03; Psy. Staff, Centre Hospitalier de Val d'Or; (819)825-5858

CHASSE, Daniel; CSSS de Manicouagan, 635 boul Jolliet, Baie-Comeau QC G5C 1P1; Laval'07; Staff, Centre Hospitalier Régional Baie-Comeau; (418)589-3701

CHASSE, Genevieve; GMF Centre medical AJC, 110 rue Saint-Jean, Drummondville QC J2B 7T1; Sher'05; (819)477-1800

CHASSE, Hughes; 458 Maclaren St, Ottawa ON K1R 5K6; Laval'76; FRCPC; Psy (Adult Psychiatry). Langs: English; (613)230-0192; Fax. (613)230-9204.

CHASSE, Marc; 240-2944 boul Taschereau, Greenfield Park QC J4V 2G8; Ott'76; FRCPC; IntMed; Critical Care Medicine (P.Q.); Respir. (450)465-4606; Fax. (450)465-1016.

CHASSE, Michael; CHUQ-Hotel-Dieu de Quebec, 11 Cote du Palais, Quebec QC G1R 2J6; Laval'06; FRCPC; IntMed; Critical Care Medicine. Staff, Centre Hospitalier Universitaire de Québec (CHUQ) - Siege Social; (418)525-4444

CHATEAUVERT, Marie-Rose; CSSS du Sud de Lanaudière, 911 montee des Pionniers, Terrebonne QC J6V 2H2; Sher'85; Staff, Centre Hospitalier Pierre le Gardeur; (450)654-7525; Fax. (450)585-5939.

CHATEAUVERT, Sylvie; Clinique Med Duberger, 2810 boul Pere-Lelievre, Quebec QC G1P 2Y1; Laval'90; ac Staff, Centre Hospitalier Universitaire De Québec - Pavillon De St-françois-d'assise; ac Membre CMDP, CSSS de Quebec-Sud; Langs: English; (418)688-8414; Fax. (418)688-4273.

CHATEL, Nadine L; Seine Med Centre, 135-142 Centrale Ave, Ste Anne MB R5H 1C3; Man'96; CCFP; (204)422-8811; Fax. (204)422-5876.

CHATELAIN, Pierre C; CSSS de la Vallée de l'Or, 725 6e rue, Val-d'Or QC J9P 3Y1; Sher'86; CSPQ; FRCPC; AnatPath (Dermatological Pathology). Staff AnatPath, Centre Hospitalier de Val d'Or; adj Prof, Universite de Sherbrooke; (819)825-5858 x2215; Fax. (819)825-7942.

CHATELIER, Alex; CLSC des Faubourgs, 2260 rue Parthenais, Montreal QC H2K 3T5; Mon'95; CCFP; FCFP; (514)527-2361; Fax. (514)527-6016.

CHATELOIS, Yves; CLSC Samuel De Champlain, 100-5811 boul Taschereau, Brossard QC J4Z 1A5; Mon'81; (450)445-4452; Fax. (450)445-5535.

CHATENAY, Michael P; Tawa Centre, 205-3017 66 St NW, Edmonton AB T6K 4B2; Alb'90; FRCSC; GenSurg. (780)461-6012; Fax. (780)461-5442.

CHATHA, Neel-Kamal K; Queensway-Carleton Hosp, 3045 Baseline Rd, Ottawa ON K2H 8P4; Qns'07; FRCPC; IntMed; Respir. Staff Med, Queensway Carleton Hospital; (613)721-2000

CHATHA, Prabhdeep S; CML Health Care, 418-790 Bay St, Toronto ON M5G 1N8; Tor'99; FRCPC; DiagRad. (416)260-9382

CHATILLON, Annick M; CHUM-Hop St-Luc, 1058 rue Saint-Denis, Montreal QC H2X 3J4; Ott'81; Critical Care Medicine (P.Q.); Respir; IntMed. Staff, Centre Hospitalier l'Université de Montréal (CHUM) - Hôpital Saint-luc; (514)890-8000 x34872

CHATILLON, Claude E; MUHC-Montreal Neurology Inst, 3801 rue Universite, Montreal QC H3A 2B4; McG'03; FRCSC; Neursurg. Staff, McGill University Health Centre - Montreal Neurological Hospital; (514)398-6644

CHATRATH, Vikram; Queen Elizabeth II HSC-Halifax, 4875-1796 Summer St, Halifax NS B3H 3A7; New Delhi (India)'03; Staff, Queen Elizabeth II Health Sciences Centre - Halifax Infirmary Site; (902)473-2700

CHATTERGOON, Dhurbassa S; Medical Clinic Bldg, 212-89 Humber College Blvd, Etobicoke ON M9V 4B8; West Indies (Jamaica)'85; Peds (Clinical Pharmacology). Staff, William Osler Health System - Etobicoke General Hospital; Staff, William Osler Health System - Brampton Civic Hospital; (416)745-8742

CHATTERJEE, Avijit; The Ottawa Hosp-Gen Campus, 7209C-501 Smyth Rd, Ottawa ON K1H 8L6; McG'02; FRCPC; IntMed; Gastroent. Staff, The Ottawa Hospital - General Campus; (613)737-8899

CHATTERJEE, Kali S; 102-1090 Peter Robertson Blvd, Brampton ON L6R 3B3; Calcutta (India)'64; MB BS; MS; FRCS(Ed); (905)790-8400; Fax. (905)799-3700.

CHATTERJEE, Manjula; Clinique Familiale MDM Inc, 6955 boul Taschereau, Brossard QC J4Z 1A7; Bihar (India)'71; (450)656-2310

CHATTERJEE, Sukhamay; U10-15 Elizabeth St, Orangeville ON L9W 3X3; Calcutta (India)'76; MB BS; DObstRCOG; MRC; FRCSC; ObstGyn (Consultation). Staff, Headwaters Health Care Centre - Orangeville Site; (519)942-9557; Fax. (519)942-8433.

CHATTERJEE, Suman; 247-2130 North Park Dr, Brampton ON L6S 0C9; Tor'04; FRCSC; Urol (Laparoscopy). Staff, William Osler Health System - Brampton Civic Hospital; Staff, Headwaters Health Care Centre - Orangeville Site; (905)595-1586; Fax. (905)595-0446.

CHATTERJEE, Sumeeta; Addiction & Mental Hlth-Queen, 3-1001 Queen St W, Toronto ON M6J 1H4; Ott'00; FRCPC; Psy. Staff, Centre for Addiction & Mental Health (CAMH) - Queen Site; (416)535-8501 x1117

CHATTERJEE, Surjit; Hôpital Santa Cabrini Ospedale, 5565 rue St Zotique E, Montreal QC H1T 1P7; McG'06; MDCM; CCFP; CCFP(E.M.); Staff, Hôpital Santa Cabrini Ospedale; (514)252-6000

CHATUR, Nazira; 5153-2775 Laurel St, Vancouver BC V5Z 1M9; UBC'99; FRCPC; IntMed; Gastroent. (604)875-5039; Fax. (604)875-5447.

CHATUR, Rehana; 205-11044 82 Ave NW, Edmonton AB T6G 0T2; Alb'04; FRCPC; Peds. (780)432-0970; Fax. (780)432-1011.

CHATURVEDI, Patanjali; Regina Qu'Appelle HR-Regina, 1440 14th Ave, Regina SK S4P 0W5; FRCPC; DiagRad. Staff, Regina General Hospital; (306)766-4207; Fax. (306)766-4838.

CHATURVEDI, Prabhat K; 65 Minto St PO Box 294 Stn Main, Glace Bay NS B1A 5V4; Lucknow (India)'60; MB BS; FRSM; FRCS(Eng & Ed); FACS; FRCSC; GenSurg. Consultant Surg., Glace Bay Healthcare Facility; Langs: Hindi; (902)849-2218

CHATURVEDI, Rajiv R; The Hosp For Sick Children, 555 University Ave, Toronto ON M5G 1X8; Cambridge (England)'89; Staff, The Hospital For Sick Children; (416)813-6141; Fax. (416)813-7547.

CHAU, Anthony; Dept of Anes, 3200-910 10th Ave W, Vancouver BC V5Z 1M9; UBC'08; (604)875-5855

CHAU, Edmond H L; Sunnybrook Hlth Sciences Ctre, 3200-2075 Bayview Ave, Toronto ON M4N 3M5; UBC'09; Staff anes, Sunnybrook Health Sciences Centre; (416)480-4864

CHAU, Fannie T; Clinique Angus, 4101 rue Angus, Montreal QC H1Y 3L1; Mon'10; CCFP; (514)807-2333

CHAU, Jaime K; McKenzie Towne Medical, 102-620 McKenzie Towne Dr SE, Calgary AB T2Z 0Y6; Sask'05; CCFP; (403)262-6311

CHAU, James T O; North East Specialized Geriatr, 960D Nortrea Dame Ave, Sudbury ON P3A 2T4; Qns'99; CCFP; FCFP; (705)688-3970

CHAU, Jason K; Health Sciences Centre, GB421-820 Sherbrook St, Winnipeg MB R3A 1R9; Sask'02; FRCSC; Otol. Staff, Health Sciences Centre; (204)774-8511

CHAU, Justin K C; Alberta Prof Bldg, 209-320 23 Ave SW, Calgary AB T2S 0J2; Sask'98; FRCSC; Otol (Neuro Otolaryngology). Staff, Peter Lougheed Centre; Clinical Asst Prof, University of Calgary; (403)228-3300; Fax. (403)228-3349; calgaryearcentre@gmail.com.

CHAU, Laurence K L; Oakville Med Centre, 206-331 Sheddon Ave, Oakville ON L6J 1X8; Southampton (England)'88; MSc(Epid); FRCPC; IntMed (Critical Care Medicine); Respir. Med Dir ICU, Halton Healthcare Services Corporation - Oakville Site; Langs: Cantonese; (905)842-3366; Fax. (905)842-1180.

CHAU, Luc; Ctr Hosp Affilie-Enfant-Jesus, 1401 18e rue, Quebec QC G1J 1Z4; Laval'04; FRCPC; DiagRad. Staff, Centre Hospitalier Affilié Universitaire de Québec - Hôpital De L'Enfant Jésus.

CHAU, Peter H W; 4120-15 Sunpark Plaza SE, Calgary AB T2X 0M5; Sask'76; Advisor Visa Applications, United States of America Embassy; Langs: Cantonese; Mandarin; (403)910-3990; Fax. (403)910-0449.

CHAU, Vann; Children's & Women's HC of BC, K3 180-4480 Oak St, Vancouver BC V6H 3V4; Laval'00; FRCPC; Neur. Staff, BC Children's Hospital; (604)875-2345 x5948

CHAU, Vicky; Toronto Rehabilitation Institu, 550 University Ave, Toronto ON M5G 2A2; McM'08; FRCPC; IntMed (Geriatric Medicine). Staff, Toronto Rehabilitation Institute - University Centre; (416)597-3422

CHAUBEY, Vikas P; Foothills Medical Centre, 1403 29 St NW, Calgary AB T2N 2T9; McG'05; FRCPC; IntMed; InfectDis. Staff, Foothills Medical Centre; (403)944-1110

CHAUDHARI, Prashant A; Byron Street Med Centre, 320 Byron St S, Whitby ON L1N 4P8; Wes'96; (905)668-5835; Fax. (905)668-8942.

CHAUDHARY, Mihaela; Roslyn Med Bldg, 200-400 5 Ave SW, Calgary AB T2P 0L6; McM'90; CCFP; (403)930-1005; Fax. (403)930-1004.

CHAUDHARY, Mohammad I; Excellent Care Medical Centre, C106-3885 Duke of York Blvd, Mississauga ON L5B 0E4; Lahore (Pakistan)'93; MB BS; LMCC; CCFP; Langs: Urdu; Punjabi; Hindi; (905)270-3885

CHAUDHARY, Muzumel A; BC Women's Hosp & H C, P1 228-4500 Oak St, Vancouver BC V6H 3N1; Alb'03; FRCPC; Psy. Staff, BC Women's Hospital & Health Centre; (604)875-2025

CHAUDHARY, Omer A; Thames Valley Fam Hlth Team, 74 Front St E, Strathroy ON N7G 1Y7; Wes'03; CCFP; (519)245-0430; Fax. (519)245-5870.

CHAUDHARY, Reyhan A; 1016 20 St S, Lethbridge AB T1K 2C9; Alb'04; FRCSC; OrthSurg. Staff, The Ottawa Hospital - General Campus; (403)394-3720

CHAUDHARY, Ripan; 301-623 4 St SE, Medicine Hat AB T1A 0L1; Wes'98; BSc; FRCSC; Ophth (Retina). (403)527-8545

CHAUDHARY, Varun; St Joseph Commun Health Ctre, 2757 King St E, Hamilton ON L8G 5E4; McM'02; FRCSC; Ophth. Staff, Toronto Western Hospital - University Health Network; (905)573-7777

CHAUDHRI, Arif R; 2077A Weston Rd, York ON M9N 1X7; Wes'91; (416)241-5281; Fax. (416)241-5282.

CHAUDHRY, Ijaz-Ahmed; William Osler HC-Etobicoke, 101 Humber College Blvd, Etobicoke ON M9V 1R8; Wes'93; CCFP; Physician Emerg, Humber River Regional Hospital - Church Street Site; Physician Emerg, Humber River Regional Hospital - Finch Avenue Site; Physician Emerg, William Osler Health System - Etobicoke General Hospital; (416)747-3400

CHAUDHRY, Imran S; Dynacare Kasper Med Lab, 200-10150 102 St NW, Edmonton AB T5J 5E2; (Pakistan)'00; FRCPC; GenPath. (780)447-8499

CHAUDHRY, Love R; 2-31 Steeplebush Ave, Brampton ON L6R 3B4; New Delhi (India)'86; FRCPC; IntMed. (905)458-2287

CHAUDHRY, M Usman L; Weber Med Centre, 5A-1400 Weber St E, Kitchener ON N2A 3Z8; Punjab (Pakistan)'95; FACE; FRCPC; IntMed. (519)748-6933; Fax. (519)748-9733.

CHAUDHRY, Ahsan; Foothills Med Centre, 1403 29 St NW, Calgary AB T2N 2T9; Alb'91; Staff, Foothills Medical Centre; (403)944-1157; Fax. (403)944-2714.

CHAUDHRY, Mobina A; Thickwood Med Centre, 200-108 Wolverine Dr, Fort McMurray AB T9H 4Y7; (Pakistan)'94; CCFP; Staff, Northern Lights Regional Health Centre; Staff, Primary Care Network; Langs: Urdu; Punjabi; (780)743-8629; Fax. (780)743-8962.

CHAUDHRY, Muhammad S; William Osler HC-Brampton, 2100 Bovaird Dr E, Brampton ON L6R 3J7; Lahore (Pakistan)'91; FRCPC; IntMed (Respirology). Staff, William Osler Health System - Brampton Civic Hospital; (905)494-2120

CHAUDHRY, Nadeem A; Thompson Gen Hosp, 871 Thompson Dr, Thompson MB R8N 0C8; (Other Foreign)'95; (204)677-2381

CHAUDHRY, Naheed M; 101-477 King St, Welland ON L3B 3K4; Punjab (Pakistan)'75; FRCSC; ObstGyn. (905)714-1747; Fax. (905)714-1433.

CHAUDHRY, Sajjad A; Humber River Reg Hosp-Church, 200 Church St, Toronto ON M9N 1N8; Punjab (Pakistan)'84; FRCPC; Anes (Family Practice). Staff, Humber River Regional Hospital - Church Street Site; Langs: Urdu; Punjabi; Hindi; (416)243-4154; Fax. (416)243-4194.

CHAUDHRY, Sapna; Family Practice & Women's Hlth, 2-31 Steeplebush Ave, Brampton ON L6R 3B4; Gorakhpur (India)'93; MB BS; CCFP; (905)458-2287; Fax. (905)458-2489.

CHAUDHRY, Shamsuddin; The Royal Victoria Hosp, 201 Georgian Dr, Barrie ON L4M 6M2; Multan (Pakistan)'94; CCFP; CCFP(E.M.); Staff, Royal Victoria Regional Health Centre; (705)728-9802

CHAUDHRY, Shazia; 30-5201 50 St, Leduc AB T9E 6T4; (Pakistan)'00; CCFP; (780)986-9732; Fax. (780)986-9600.

CHAUDHRY, Sukarno N; 155-1720 Howard Ave, Windsor ON N8X 5A6; Bahawalpur (Pakistan)'94; ABIM; FRCPC; IntMed (Sleep Medicine). Staff Intensivist Respirologist and Sleep Specialist, Windsor Regional Hospital - Metropolitan Site; Staff Intensivest, Brandon Regional Health Centre; Langs: Punjabi; Urdu; Hindi; (519)256-8338; Fax. (519)258-7337; anwist@gmail.com.

CHAUDHRY, Tahir S; Victoria Med Bldg, 309-1669 Victoria St, Prince George BC V2L 2L5; Punjab (India)'89; MB BS; FRCPC; Peds. (250)564-7378

CHAUDHRY, Uzma S; The Credit Valley Health Centr, 16-2555 Erin Centre Blvd, Mississauga ON L5M 5H1; Punjab (Pakistan)'01; MB BS; CCFP; (905)813-8444; Fax. (905)593-0698.

CHAUDHRY, Yash; 200-31205 MacLure Rd, Abbotsford BC V2T 5E5; Manipal University (India)'06; (604)746-4700

CHAUDHRY, Zubaida A; Mental Health Centre, PO Box 3003 Stn Main, Prince Albert SK S6V 6G1; Punjab (India)'63; Staff Psy Centre, Victoria Hospital; (306)765-6055; Fax. (306)765-6349.

CHAUDHURI, Monica M; Sioux Lookout Meno-Ya-Min HC, PO Box 909 Stn Main 69 Front St, Sioux Lookout ON P8T 1B4; Alb'98; FRCSC; GenSurg. Staff, Sioux Lookout Meno-Ya-Win Health Centre; (807)737-3030; Fax. (807)737-5142; mchaudhuri@slmhc.on.ca.

CHAUDHURY, Derek; Polyclinic, 199 Grafton St, Charlottetown PE C1A 1L2; (902)629-8810

CHAUDHURY, Prosanto K; MUHC-Royal Victoria Hosp, S10. 30-687 av des Pins O, Montreal QC H3A 1A1; McG'98; ABS; FRCSC; GenSurg (Hepatobiliary Surgery). Staff, McGill University Health Centre - Royal Victoria Hospital; Langs: French; (514)934-1934 x31951

CHAUDRY, Bushra; Perth Med Clinic, 14 Isabella St, Perth ON K7H 2W6; Punjab (Pakistan)'03; CCFP; CCFP(E.M.); Staff, SCO Health Service - Élisabeth Bruyère Hospital; (613)267-3394

CHAUFOUR, Cecile; Ctr Hosp de Verdun, 4000 boul Lasalle, LaSalle QC H4G 2A3; (France)'06; Staff, Centre Hospitalier de Verdun; (514)362-1000

CHAUHAN, Harpreet; Mount St Joseph Hosp, 3080 Prince Edward St, Vancouver BC V5T 3N4; UBC'95; FRCPC; Psy. Staff, Providence Health Care - Mount Saint Joseph Hospital; Staff, Providence Health Care - St Paul's Hospital; (604)877-8159

CHAUHAN, Jitendra; 7 Welland Ave, St Catharines ON L2R 2L8; Manchester (England)'75; MB ChB; Ac Staff, Hôtel Dieu Shaver Health & Rehabilitation Centre; (905)684-8555; Fax. (905)684-2542.

CHAUHAN, Nitin; 121-9401 Jane St, Vaughan ON L6A 4H7; Alb'06; FRCSC; Otol. (905)303-1080

CHAUHAN, Rameshchandra P; 202-595 Montreal Rd, Ottawa ON K1K 4L2; Leeds (England)'63; FRCS(Ed); FRCSC; OrthSurg. Staff Orth Surg, Montfort Hospital; Staff, Children's Hospital of Eastern Ontario (CHEO); Staff, Bruyère Continuing Care - Saint-Vincent Hospital; Langs: Gujarati; French; (613)746-6745; Fax. (613)746-6008.

CHAUHAN, Rebecca A; Kinark Child & Family Services, 475 Iroquois Shore Rd, Oakville ON L6M 1H3; McM'06; (905)944-7088

CHAUHAN, Upesh C; Medical Clinic, 5031 49 St, Innisfail AB T4G 1A4; Surat (India) MB BS; MRCGPract; CCFP; Langs: Hindi; Gujarati; (403)227-3356; Fax. (403)227-2702.

CHAUHAN, Vijay S; PMCC3 522-150 Gerrard St W, Toronto ON M5G 2C4; Ott'92; FRCPC; IntMed (Electrophysiology); Cardiol. Staff Cardiol, Toronto General Hospital - UHN; Asst Prof Med, University of Toronto; (416)340-3172

CHAULK, David C; Alberta Children's Hosp, 2888 Shaganappi Trail NW, Calgary AB T3B 6A8; Mem'00; FRCPC; Peds (Emergency Medicine); PedEmergMed. Staff, Alberta Children's Hospital; Clinical Asst Prof Peds, University of Calgary; (403)955-2461; Fax. (403)955-2777.

CHAULK, Domino R; Paradise Med Clinic, PO Box 2419 Stn Main 7 Elizabeth Dr, Paradise NL A1L 1E6; Mem'77; (709)782-3883; Fax. (709)782-0216.

CHAULK, Donald A; Western Mem Reg Hosp, PO Box 2005 Stn Main 1 Brookfield Ave, Corner Brook NL A2H 6J7; Mem'75; Staff, Western Memorial Regional Hospital; (709)637-5000

CHAUN, Hugh; 3552 41 Ave W PO Box 71067, Vancouver BC V6N 4J9; Oxford (England)'62; MA; BMus; BCh(Oxon); DTMH; FRCP(Lond); FRCPC; IntMed (Gastroenterology). (778)999-8437; hchaun@mac.com.

CHAUNY, Jean-Marc; Hop du Sacre-Coeur de Mtl, 5400 boul Gouin O, Montreal QC H4J 1C5; Mon'81; EmergMed (P.Q.). Ac Staff, Hôpital du Sacre-Coeur de Montréal; (514)338-2000

CHAURET, Denis; Montfort Hosp, 713 Montreal Rd, Ottawa ON K1K 0T2; Mon'94; FRCPC; IntMed (Diabetes). Staff Internist, Montfort Hospital; Assoc Prof Med, University of Ottawa; Langs: Bilingual(French/English); (613)746-4621; Fax. (613)748-4953; dchauret@uottawa.ca.

CHAUSSE, Luc; 814 L'Ange-Gardien N CP 3406, L'Assomption QC J5W 4M9; Ott'82; Langs: Spanish; (450)589-5778; Fax. (450)589-5779.

CHAUVETTE, Angele; Inst U Geriatrie Sherbrooke, 375 rue Argyll, Sherbrooke QC J1J 3H5; Sher'84; Staff, Institut Universitaire de Geriatrie de Sherbrooke-Pavillon Argyll; (819)780-2220

CHAUVETTE, Michel; Clinique Med du Sud-Ouest, 103-4475 rue Bannantyne, Verdun QC H4G 1E2; Mon'92; (514)765-3600; Fax. (514)765-9625.

CHAUVIN, Jean C; CLSC Saint-Hubert, 6800 boul Cousineau, Saint-Hubert QC J3Y 8Z4; Mon'80; (450)443-7407

CHAUVIN-KIMOFF, Laurel A; MUHC-Montreal Children's Hosp, 2300 rue Tupper, Montreal QC H3H 1P3; McG'79; FAAP; FRCPC; Peds. Staff, McGill University Health Centre - Montreal Children's Hospital; Assoc Prof Peds, McGill University; Langs: French; (514)412-4400; Fax. (514)939-4043.

CHAVARRIA, Cesar A; Victoria Hosp, PO Box 3000 Stn Main 1200 24 St, Prince Albert SK S6V 5T4; Sask'07; FRCPC; DiagRad. Staff, Victoria Hospital; (306)765-6200; Fax. (306)765-6224.

CHAVEZ GUERRA, Juan; Hotel-Dieu de Sorel, 400 av de l'Hotel-Dieu, Sorel-Tracy QC J3P 1N5; Monterrey (Mexico)'87; Staff, Hôtel-Dieu de Sorel; (450)746-6000

CHAVHAN, Govind B; The Hosp for Sick Children, 555 University Ave, Toronto ON M5G 1X8; Mumbai (India)'91; Staff, The Hospital For Sick Children; (416)813-6025; govind@chavhan@sickkids.ca.

CHAVOSHI, Samieh; Joseph Brant Mem Hosp, 1230 North Shore Blvd E, Burlington ON L7S 1W7; McM'90; FRCPC; Anes. Staff Anes, Joseph Brant Memorial Hospital; Langs: Persian; (905)632-3730

CHAWANE-BEKWAYO, Nomhle N; Blairmore Medical Clinic, 225 Betts Ave, Saskatoon SK S7M 1L2; (306)974-3939; Fax. (306)974-3941.

CHAWLA, Anjana; Orillia Soldiers' Mem Hosp, 170 Colborne St W, Orillia ON L3V 2Z3; Karnatak (India)'98; FRCPC; Psy. Staff, Orillia Soldiers' Memorial Hospital; (705)325-2201

CHAWLA, Ashis K; 501-2425 Bloor St W, Toronto ON M6S 4W4; Tor'01; FRCSC; Urol (Minimal Invasive Surgery). Staff Urol, St Joseph's Health Centre; Langs: French; Hindi; Punjabi; (647)435-8831

CHAWLA, Bharat B; Peterborough Reg HC-Hospital, 1 Hospital Dr, Peterborough ON K9J 7C6; New Delhi (India)'89; FRCPC; Psy. Staff, Peterborough Regional Health Centre - Hospital Drive; (705)876-5028

CHAWLA, Harmeet K; 116-100 Strowger Blvd, Brockville ON K6V 5J9; Leicester (England)'07; Peds. (613)342-2373

CHAWLA, Harvinder K; 116-100 Strowger Blvd, Brockville ON K6V 5J9; Delhi (India)'66; DABPed; FRCPC; Peds. Ac Staff, Providence Continuing Care Centre (PCCC) - St Vincent de Paul Hospital; Chief Peds, Brockville General Hospital - Charles Street; Langs: Punjabi; Hindi; Gujarati; (613)342-2373; Fax. (613)345-6559.

CHAWLA, Jasmeet S; Queensway-Carleton Hosp, 3045 Baseline Rd, Nepean ON K2H 8P4; Mangalore (India)'98; FRCPC; IntMed; Nephrol. Staff, Queensway Carleton Hospital; (613)721-2000

CHAWLA, Lalit K; Chatham-Kent Family Health Team, 207-20 Emma St, Chatham ON N7L 5K5; Alb'01; CCFP; (519)354-2172; lchawla@ckha.on.ca.

CHAWLA, Punita T; Mount Sinai Hosp, 567-600 University Ave, Toronto ON M5G 1X5; London (England)'90; MB BS; MRCP(UK); FRCR; MRCGPract; FRCPC; DiagRad (Abdominal Imaging). Staff, Toronto General Hospital - UHN; Staff, Mount Sinai Hospital; (416)586-4800 x4855; Fax. (416)586-8695.

CHAWLA, Punkuj; Alexandra Med Centre, 29 Noxon St, Ingersoll ON N5C 1B8; Cal'00; CCFP; VP, Alexandra Hospital; Staff, Southwestern Medical Centre; Aj Prof, University of Western Ontario; (519)485-9617; Fax. (519)485-9609.

CHAWLA, Rakesh K; SPAR Med Hair & Vein Clinic, 189 Fisher Dr, Hammonds Plains NS B4B 1W9; Delhi (India)'85; MB; BSc; Langs: Hindi; Punjabi; (902)446-4354; Fax. (902)446-3450.

CHAWLA, Ramandeep K; Queensway Carleton Hosp, 3045 Baseline Rd, Nepean ON K2H 8P4; Punjab(India) (India)'98; FRCPC; IntMed. Staff, Queensway Carleton Hospital; (613)721-2000

CHAWLA, Rupesh; Alberta Children's Hosp, 2888 Shaganappi Trail NW, Calgary AB T3B 6A8; Alb'93; FRCPC; Peds; InfectDis. Staff, Alberta Children's Hospital; Clinical Asst Prof, University of Calgary; (403)955-7813; Fax. (403)955-3045.

CHAWLA, Satish K; Niagara HS-Greater Niagara, PO Box 1018 Stn Main 5546 Portage Rd, Niagara Falls ON L2E 6X2; Delhi (India)'82; DAB; FRCPC; AnatPath. Staff, Niagara Health System - Greater Niagara General Site; Langs: Hindi; Punjabi; (905)378-4647

CHAWLA, Virendra S; 320 Adelaide St S, London ON N5Z 3L2; (India)'63; FRCS(E); Staff, St Joseph's Hospital - St Joseph's Health Care; Staff, Parkwood Hospital - St Joseph's Health Care; Staff, London Health Sciences Centre - Victoria Campus; (519)686-7266; Fax. (519)858-2905.

CHAYA, Jihad Y; Regional Mental HC-St Thomas, PO Box 2004 Stn Main, St Thomas ON N5P 3V9; Baghdad (Iraq)'81; FRCPC; Psy. Staff, Regional Mental Health Care-St Joseph's Health Care; Staff, Bluewater Health - Mitton Site; Langs: Arabic; French; (519)631-8510 x49309

CHAYA, Malone; Royal University Hosp, 103 Hospital Dr, Saskatoon SK S7N 0W8; (Zimbabwe)'90; MB ChB; FRCPC; Anes. Staff Anes, Royal University Hospital; Clinical Asst Prof, University of Saskatchewan; (306)655-1183; Fax. (306)655-1279.

CHAYER, Celine; Hop Maisonneuve-Rosemont, 5415 boul de l'Assomption, Montreal QC H1T 2M4; Mon'92; FRCPC; Neur (Behavioural Neurology); Electroenceph (P.Q.). Staff Movement Disorders Clinic, Centre Hospitalier l'Université de Montréal (CHUM) - Hôtel-Dieu; Staff Neurol, Institut Universitaire de Gériatrie de Montréal; Staff, Hopital Maisonneuve-Rosemont; Clinical Asst Prof, Universite de Montreal; (514)252-3528; Fax. (514)252-3529; celine.chayer@sympatico.ca.

CHAYER, Marc J; Lindsay Prof Bldg, 14-65 Angeline St N, Lindsay ON K9V 5N7; Tor'90; Staff, Ross Memorial Hospital; Langs: English; French; (705)324-9849; Fax. (705)324-8534; mchayer@nexicom.net.

CHAYER, Sebastien; CSSS du Sud de Lanaudière, 911 montee des Pionniers, Terrebonne QC J6V 2H2; Sher'97; IntMed (P.Q.). Staff, Centre Hospitalier Pierre le Gardeur; (450)654-7525; Fax. (450)582-4439.

CHAYESTEMEHR, Sacha; Hôpital Ste-Justine, 3175 ch Cote Sainte-Catherine, Montreal QC H3T 1C5; Geneva (Switzerland)'00; Staff, Hôpital Ste-Justine; (514)345-4931

CHAYKA, John; Kelowna Gen Hosp, 2268 Pandosy St, Kelowna BC V1Y 1T2; Sask'99; FRCPC; Anes. Staff, Kelowna General Hospital; (250)862-4309

CHAYTOR, E Ruth; SMBD Jewish Gen Hosp, 3755 ch Cote-Sainte-Catherine, Montreal QC H3T 1E2; Mem'86; FRCSC; OrthSurg (Foot & Ankle Surgery). Staff OrthSurg, Sir Mortimer B Davis Jewish General; Asst Prof Surg, McGill University; Langs: Bilingual(English/French); (514)340-7532; Fax. (514)340-7595; rchaytor@ort.jgh.mcgill.ca.

CHAYTOR, Janet; 8F Shoal Harbour Dr, Clarenville NL A5A 2C4; Mem'91; CCFP; (709)466-1095

CHAYTOR, Kathy L; Nova Medical, 204-496 Topsail Rd, St. John's NL A1E 2C2; Mem'99; CCFP; (709)745-6682

CHBEIR, Walif; CSSSG-Hop de Hull, 116 boul Lionel-Emond, Gatineau QC J8Y 1W7; Aix-Marseille II (France)'86; DiagRad (P.Q.). Staff, Hull Hospital; Langs: Arabic; French; (819)595-6000; Fax. (819)595-6076; walifchbeir@hotmail.com.

CHE, Claudius T K; 137 Catherine St, Fort Erie ON L2A 2H9; Tor'86; Langs: Chinese; (905)871-5077

CHE, Priscilla M; Ryerson Med Centre, W181-350 Victoria St, Toronto ON M5B 2K3; Tor'09; CCFP; Physician, Ryerson University; (416)979-5070; Fax. (416)979-5073.

CHEA, Rith; 212-10939 82 Ave NW, Edmonton AB T6G 0S7; Cal'95; FRCPC; IntMed. Staff, Royal Alexandra Hospital; Consultant, Glenrose Rehabilitation Hospital; Clin Asst Lecturer, University of Alberta; Langs: Khmer; (780)432-7272; Fax. (780)433-7232.

CHEAH, Andrew; 16-8671 No. 1 Rd, Richmond BC V7C 1V2; Sydney (Australia)'91; MB BS; FRACGP; CCFP; (604)275-5155; Fax. (604)275-5166.

CHEAH, David; Promenade Circle, 35-7700 Bathurst St, Thornhill ON L4J 7Y3; Tor'96; CCFP; FCFP; Ac Staff, Mackenzie Richmond Hill Hospital; (905)881-6510; Fax. (905)881-6513.

CHEAH, Henry K; King Street Med Arts Centre, 406-71 King St W, Mississauga ON L5B 4A2; Tor'93; LMCC; FRCSC; OrthSurg (Hip & Knee Reconstruction). Consultant, Trillium Health Centre - Mississauga; Consultant, Trillium Health Centre - West Toronto; (905)275-8688; Fax. (905)275-1094.

CHEAH, Huey; Central Health Consultants, 129 Lincoln Rd, Grnd-Falls-Windsor NL A2A 1P3; Ott'03; FRCSC; GenSurg. (709)489-2700

CHEAH, Kee Saik; 315 Herring Cove Rd, Halifax NS B3R 1V5; Dal'71; BSc; Court Staff, Queen Elizabeth II Health Sciences Centre - Victoria General Site; (902)477-5669; Fax. (902)477-4652.

CHEANG, Timothy S; Markham Stouffville Health Ctr, 402-377 Church St, Markham ON L6B 1A1; Tor'02; FRCSC; GenSurg (Minimal Invasive Surgery). (905)472-7122; Fax. (905)472-9240.

CHEBIB, Ivan A; Foothills Medical Centre, 1403 29 St NW, Calgary AB T2N 2T9; Alb'04; FRCPC; AnatPath. Staff, Foothills Medical Centre; (403)944-8041; Fax. (403)944-8998.

CHEBIL, Samir; CSSS de la Haute-Cote-Nord, CP 1000 4 rue de l'Hopital, Les Escoumins QC G0T 1K0; (Other Foreign)'03; Staff, Centre de santé des Côté-Nord; (418)233-2931

CHEDDIE, Nishaan; South Hill Med Clinic, 890A Lillooet St W, Moose Jaw SK S6H 8B4; Medunsa (South Africa)'01; MB ChB; FCP (SA); LMCC; FRCSC; GenSurg (Laparoscopy). Staff Surg, Five Hills Health Region Corporate Office; (306)691-0030; Fax. (306)694-5666; nishaancheddie@gmail.com.

CHEDEVILLE, Gaelle R S; MUHC-Montreal Children's Hosp, C-504-2300 rue Tupper, Montreal QC H3H 1P3; Tours (France)'98; Staff, McGill University Health Centre - Montreal Children's Hospital; (514)412-4268; Fax. (514)412-4365; gaelle.chedeville@muhc.mcgill.ca.

CHEDORE, Todd R; Saint John Reg Hosp, PO Box 2100 Stn Main 400 University Ave, Saint John NB E2L 4L2; Mem'94; FRCPC; Anes. Staff, Saint John Regional Hospital; Asst Clin Lecturer, Dalhousie University; (506)648-6861; Fax. (506)648-6860; tchedore@nbnet.nb.ca.

CHEE, C M Alex; South Health Campus, 480030-4448 Front St SE, Calgary AB T3M 1M4; Qns'04; FRCPC; IntMed; Respir. Staff, Foothills Medical Centre; (403)956-2435; Fax. (403)956-2991.

CHEE, Hwa Kim; 204-3825 Sunset St, Burnaby BC V5G 1T4; Tor'89; Psy. (604)436-9509

CHEE, Jung Hoon; 515-3030 Lawrence Ave E, Scarborough ON M1P 2T7; McG'00; FRCPC; IntMed (Sleep Medicine); Respir. Langs: Korean; (416)431-2300

CHEE, Peter M Y; The Richmond Hosp, 7000 Westminster Hwy, Richmond BC V6X 1A2; UBC'96; CCFP; Staff, Richmond Hospital; (604)278-9711

CHEEK, Joanna P; Univ of Victoria Health Servic, PO Box 1700 Stn CSC, Victoria BC V8W 2Y2; UBC'07; FRCPC; Psy. (250)721-8492

CHEEK, Tyler; Royal Jubilee Hosp, 1952 Bay St, Victoria BC V8R 1J8; UBC'07; CCFP; Staff, Royal Jubilee Hospital; (250)370-8000

CHEEMA, Amarjit S; 100-470 Hensall Cir, Mississauga ON L5A 3V4; Mem'82; BSc; FRCPC; IntMed (Asthma); ClinImmunol&Allergy. Langs: Punjabi; (905)566-0555; Fax. (905)566-5294.

CHEEMA, Amarpreet S; Halton HSC-Georgetown, 1 Princess Anne Dr, Georgetown ON L7G 2B8; (Other Foreign)'05; CCFP; Staff, Halton Healthcare Services Corporation - Georgetown Hospital; (905)873-0111

CHEEMA, Asim N; St Michael's Hosp, 6037Q-30 Bond St, Toronto ON M5B 1W8; Punjab (Pakistan)'90; FRCPC; IntMed (Interventional Cardiology); Cardiol. Staff Interventional Cardiologist, St Michael's Hospital; Asst Prof Med, University of Toronto; (416)864-5062

CHEEMA, Devinder P; MUHC-Montreal Gen Hosp, L4.305-1650 av Cedar, Montreal QC H3G 1A4; McG'90; FRCSC; Ophth. Staff, McGill University Health Centre - Montreal General Campus; (514)934-1934 x44078

CHEEMA, Gulzar S; 7170 120 St, Surrey BC V3W 3M8; Punjab (India)'78; MB BS; CCFP; Staff, Surrey Memorial Hospital; Langs: Hindi; Urdu; Punjabi; (604)597-1233; Fax. (604)597-7779; dr.g.cheema@telus.net.

CHEEMA, Gurnam S; Niagara Falls Med Centre, 102-6453 Morrison St, Niagara Falls ON L2E 7H1; Amritsar (India)'75; DAB; FRCSC; ObstGyn. Staff, Niagara Health System - Greater Niagara General Site; (905)374-6566; Fax. (905)374-7061.

CHEEMA, Harpaul S; Postgrad Med Education, 602-500 University Ave, Toronto ON M5G 1V7; Wes'08; FRCPC; IntMed.

CHEEMA, Kiran J; Community MD Clinic, 6-10 Earlsbridge Blvd, Brampton ON L7A 3P1; (Saint Kitts-Nevis)'06; CCFP; (905)840-4776; Fax. (905)840-2197.

CHEEMA, Navbir K; West Winds Med Clinic, 2110-4818 Westwinds Dr NE, Calgary AB T3J 3Z5; UBC'08; CCFP; (403)568-2295; Fax. (403)568-2247.

CHEEMA, Parneet K; Sunnybrook Hlth Sciences Ctre, 2075 Bayview Ave, Toronto ON M4N 3M5; Cal'06; MedOncol; IntMed. Staff, Sunnybrook Health Sciences Centre; (416)480-4757; Fax. (416)480-9002.

CHEEMA, Sohail E; St Michael's Hosp, 15F-30 Bond St, Toronto ON M5B 1W8; Punjab (Pakistan)'87; Staff Cardinal Carter Centre, St Michael's Hospital; (416)864-6073

CHEEMA, Waqar M; 3-511 Ray Lawson Blvd, Brampton ON L6Y 0N2; King Edward (Pakistan)'02; CCFP; Physician, Toronto Poly Clinic; Langs: Urdu; Punjabi; Hindi; (905)450-7427; Fax. (905)450-2535; wcheema@tpclinic.com.

CHEESEMAN, Frank D; Kingston Gen Hosp, 76 Stuart St, Kingston ON K7L 2V7; Mem'79; FRCPC; DiagRad; NuclearMed. Dir Nuclear Med, Kingston General Hospital; Asst Prof, Queen's University; (613)548-2301

CHEESEMAN, Neil R; Health Sciences Centre, 300 Prince Philip Dr, St. John's NL A1B 3V6; Mem'09; CCFP; CCFP(E.M.); Staff, Health Sciences Centre; (709)737-6300

CHEESMAN, Mark E; Medicine Hat Reg Hosp, 666 5 St SW, Medicine Hat AB T1A 4H6; UBC'97; FRCPC; Anes. Staff Palliser Health Authority, Medicine Hat Regional Hospital; (403)529-8000

CHEEVERS, Paul M; Yarmouth Reg Hosp, 311-60 Vancouver St, Yarmouth NS B5A 2P5; UBC'04; Ophth. Staff, Yarmouth Regional Hospital; (902)881-2285; Fax. (902)881-3063.

CHEFF, T Gail; 175 Twyford St, Ottawa ON K1V 0V8; Ott'87; CCFP; Physician Sclerotherapy, Dr Beaupre Vein Clinic; (613)523-3293; Fax. (613)523-3005.

CHEHADE, Nicolas; Polyclinique Med Pierre LeGard, 350-1000 Montee des Pionniers, Terrebonne QC J6V 1S8; Mon'83; FRCSC; Ophth. Staff, Polyclinique Medicale Pierre-Le-Gardeur; (450)654-6049

CHEHADE, Remi E; Clinique Remd Solution, 3943 boul St-Jean, Roxboro QC H9G 1X2; McG'94; CCFP; Staff, Hawkesbury & District General Hospital; (514)624-7363

CHEHADI, Abdel-Kareem; Shoppers Drug Mart Bldg, 250 LeMarchant Rd, St. John's NL A1E 1P7; NOSM'09.

CHEHADI, Waleed; London HSC-Victoria Hosp, PO Box 5010 Stn B D2 521-800 Commissioners Rd E, London ON N6A 5W9; Ott'08; FRCPC; IntMed. Staff, London Health Sciences Centre - Victoria Campus; (519)685-8500

CHEHAYEB, Raja; S103-2944 boul Taschereau, Greenfield Park QC J4V 2G8; Beyrouth (Lebanon)'72; CSPQ; FRCPC; Cardiol. (450)465-8679; Fax. (450)465-5095.

CHEHIL, Rakesh S; 103-7130 120 St, Surrey BC V3W 3M8; Dal'92; Langs: Punjabi; (604)572-4437; Fax. (604)572-4438.

CHEHIL, Sonia; Abbie J Lane Mem Bldg, 5909 Veterans Memorial Lane, Halifax NS B3H 2E2; Dal'98; FRCPC; Psy. (902)473-6214; Fax. (902)473-4545.

CHEHIMI, Abdul-Hamid; Salvus Family Med Clinic, 62-143 Liberton Dr, St. Albert AB T8N 6A7; (Spain)'91; CCFP; (780)460-4562; Fax. (780)460-4550.

CHEIFETZ, Arielle; 300-790 Bay St, Toronto ON M5G 1N8; Qns'10; CCFP; (416)960-1366; Fax. (416)960-1945.

CHEIFETZ, Philip N; 507-251 Bank St, Ottawa ON K2P 1X3; McG'60; FRCPC; Psy. Staff, Royal Ottawa Mental Health Centre - Royal Ottawa Health Care Group; (613)569-5222

CHEIFETZ, Rona E; Gordon & Leslie Diamond Hlth C, 5F-2775 Laurel St, Vancouver BC V5Z 1M9; Tor'84; MEd; FRCSC; GenSurg;CCFP; Consultant, BC Cancer Agency Vancouver Centre; Ac Staff, Vancouver General Hospital - Centennial Pavillion; Dir, Continuing Medical Education for Surgical Oncology Network; Asst Prof, University of British Columbia; (604)875-5880; Fax. (604)875-4315.

CHEK, Vanroeung; Carepoint Med Centre, 1060-2929 Barnet Hwy, Coquitlam BC V3B 5R5; Phnom-Penh (Cambodia)'72; (604)468-1202; Fax. (604)468-1271.

CHEKINA, Helena; Sheppard Associates, 649 Sheppard Ave W, North York ON M3H 2S4; Lvov (Ukraine)'73; MD; DPsy(McMaster); Staff, North York General Hospital - Branson Division; Staff, Waypoint Centre for Mental Health Care; Langs: Russian; Polish; Ukrainian; (416)630-0610; Fax. (416)398-5712.

CHELFI, Mustapha; CSSSG-Hop de Gatineau, 909 de la Verendrye O, Gatineau QC J8P 7H2; Paris V (France)'85; RadOncol(Paris); Chef radio-oncol, Hôpital de Gatineau; Aj Prof, McGill University; Langs: Spanish; Arabic; Berber; English; Bilingual(French/English); French; (819)966-6023; Fax. (819)966-6314; chelfmus@netscape.net.

CHELICO, Liza; William Osler HC-Brampton, 2100 Bovaird Dr E, Brampton ON L6R 3J7; Sask'03; FRCPC; Anes. Staff, William Osler Health System - Brampton Civic Hospital; (905)494-2120

CHELLEW, Matthew G; The Credit Valley Hosp, 2200 Eglinton Ave W, Mississauga ON L5M 2N1; Tor'07; CCFP; CCFP(E.M.); Staff, The Credit Valley Hospital; (905)813-4530

CHELVANA, Anushya; St Joseph's Health Care, 50 Charlton Ave E, Hamilton ON L8N 4A6; Bristol (England)'04; Staff, St Joseph's Healthcare - Charlton Campus; Staff, Firestone Institute for Respiratory Health; (905)522-1155; chelvanaa@mcmaster.ca.

CHELVANATHAN, Anjala; St Boniface Hosp, Y3015-409 Tache Ave, Winnipeg MB R2H 2A6; McM'06; Cardiol; IntMed. Staff, St Boniface General Hospital; (204)995-3068

CHELVANATHAN, Anushya; St Joseph's Healthcare, 50 Charlton Ave E, Hamilton ON L8N 4A6; Bristol (England)'00; FRCPC; IntMed; Respir. Staff, St Joseph's Healthcare - Charlton Campus; (905)522-1155

CHEMALY, Rene; Centre Bois de Boulogne, 425-1575 boul Henri-Bourassa O, Montreal QC H3M 3A9; St. Joseph (Lebanon)'71; CSPQ; FRCSC; ObstGyn. Staff Dept of Gyn & Obst, Hôpital du Sacre-Coeur de Montréal; adj Prof, Universite de Montreal; Langs: Arabic; English; (514)336-1595; Fax. (514)336-8814.

CHEMERIKA, Philip J V; 120-7404 King George Vi Hwy, Surrey BC V3W 1N6; Alb'91; (604)594-7711; Fax. (604)594-5055.

CHEMPARATHY, Joseph V; Upper Appleby Med Associates, 36-1960 Appleby Line, Burlington ON L7L 0B7; University of Calcutta (India)'80; CCFP; (905)315-9929; Fax. (905)315-9314.

CHEMPARATHY, Sheela J; Halton Family Health Centre, 2951 Walker's Line, Burlington ON L7M 4Y1; Kerala (India)'88; CCFP; (905)336-3437; Fax. (905)336-9632.

CHEMTOB, Sylvain; Hôpital Ste-Justine, 3175 ch Cote-Sainte-Catherine, Montreal QC H3T 1C5; Mon'80; FRCPC; Peds (Neonatology) (Perinatology). Ac Staff, Hôpital Ste-Justine; Prof, Universite de Montreal; (514)345-4931 x2978; Fax. (514)345-4801.

CHEN, Adam Y H; Meadowvale Prof Centre, 320-6855 Meadowvale Town Ctre, Mississauga ON L5N 2Y1; Wes'90; CCFP; Langs: Chinese; Mandarin; (905)569-2282; Fax. (905)569-6187.

CHEN, Andy Y H; Meadowvale Prof Centre, 320-6855 Meadowvale Town Ctre, Mississauga ON L5N 2Y1; Tor'92; Langs: Mandarin; (905)569-2282; Fax. (905)569-6187.

CHEN, Ann Marie C; 203-1685 Main St W, Hamilton ON L8S 1G5; Tor'96; BSc(Hon); FRCSC; ObstGyn. Staff, Hamilton Health Sciences Centre - McMaster Children's Hospital; Asst Prof ObstGyn, McMaster University; (905)308-7764; Fax. (905)308-7765.

CHEN, Anthony C; 27-420 Highway 7 E, Richmond Hill ON L4B 3K2; Tor'10; CCFP; Staff, St Joseph's Hospital - St Joseph's Health Care; (905)695-1133; Fax. (905)695-0826.

CHEN, Benjamin H; Napanee Med Specialists, 3-307A Bridge St W, Napanee ON K7R 3V3; McG'89; FACP; FRCPC; CCFP; IntMed. Staff, Lennox & Addington County General Hospital; Assoc Prof Med, Queen's University; Langs: Mandarin; French; (613)409-8888

CHEN, Betty H; Family Practice Health Centre, 76 Grenville St, Toronto ON M5S 1B2; Tor'96; CCFP; Staff, Women's College Hospital; Asst Prof Family & CommunMed, University of Toronto; (416)323-6060; Fax. (416)323-6350.

CHEN, Charlie C; Hospice Palliative Care, 218-610 6th St, New Westminster BC V3L 3C2; UBC'94; BSc; CCFP; Staff, Laurel Place Care Facility; Clin Instructor Med, University of British Columbia; Langs: Taiwanese; Mandarin; (604)777-6732

CHEN, Chee Pyn; Wellington Med Arts Bldg, 304-121 Wellington St W, Barrie ON L4N 1L2; Malaya (Malaysia)'74; MB BS; MRCP(UK); DCH(Glas); FRCP(Glas); FRCPC; Peds (Neonatology). Court Staff Peds & Neonatol, Sault Area Hospital - Sault Ste Marie; Peds & Neonatol, Royal Victoria Regional Health Centre; Lecturer, University of Toronto; Langs: Cantonese; (705)719-3066; Fax. (705)719-3086; cheechenl@yahoo.ca.

CHEN, Chi Nan; Midtown Mental Health Team, 2450 Ontario St, Vancouver BC V5T 4T7; (Singapore)'51; MB BS; FRCPC; Psy (Adult Psychiatry). Langs: Mandarin; (604)872-8441; Fax. (604)873-6071.

CHEN, C H Jerry; Kingston Gen Hosp, 8 206-76 Stuart St, Kingston ON K7L 2V7; Mon'04; FRCPC; AnatPath. Staff, Kingston General Hospital; (613)549-6666

CHEN, Chih-Chien; South Tower, 360-650 41st Ave W, Vancouver BC V5Z 2M9; (China)'82; (604)261-6000

CHEN, Christine I; Univ Hlth Network-Princess M, 5 220-610 University Ave, Toronto ON M5G 2M9; Sask'89; FRCPC; IntMed; Hem. Staff, Princess Margaret Hospital - University Health Network; (416)946-2827; Fax. (416)946-4563.

CHEN, Christine M; Health Sciences North-Laurenti, 41 Ramsey Lake Rd, Sudbury ON P3E 5J1; St Matthew's (Cayman Islands)'09; CCFP; Staff, Health Sciences North-Laurentian Site; (705)523-7100

CHEN, Connie; Rexdale Med Centre, 2-123 Rexdale Blvd, Etobicoke ON M9W 1P1; Tor'89; CCFP; FCFP; Staff, William Osler Health System - Etobicoke General Hospital; Staff Family Med, Toronto East General Hospital Inc; Lecturer Comm & Family Med, University of Toronto; Langs: Cantonese; (416)743-5853; Fax. (416)743-1358.

CHEN, Dalton T; Nanaimo Reg Gen Hosp, 1200 Dufferin Cres, Nanaimo BC V9S 2B7; Glasgow (Scotland)'88; MB ChB; CCFP; FCFP; Assoc Staff Privil, Peace Arch Hospital; Staff, Nanaimo Regional General Hospital; Clin Instructor, University of British Columbia; (250)755-7691

CHEN, Danny K; Mackenzie Richmond Hill Hosp, 10 Trench St, Richmond Hill ON L4C 4Z3; Tor'95; FRCPC; IntMed; InfectDis. Staff, Southlake Regional Health Centre; Staff, Mackenzie Richmond Hill Hospital; Langs: Mandarin; (905)883-1212 x3638; dchen@yorkcentral.on.ca.

CHEN, Danny S; Misericordia Community Hosp, 16940 87 Ave NW, Edmonton AB T5R 4H5; Sask'00; FRCPC; Anes. Staff, Covenant Health - Misericordia Community Hospital; (780)735-2863; Fax. (780)735-2967.

CHEN, Dean L H; TEGH Medical Centre, 216-840 Coxwell Ave, East York ON M4C 5T2; Tor'99; FRCPC; IntMed (Therapeutic Endoscopy); Gastroent. Staff, Toronto East General Hospital Inc; (416)778-1212; Fax. (416)778-1216.

CHEN, Edmund C F; St Joseph's Hlth Ctr Urban FHT, 205-27 Roncesvalles Ave, Toronto ON M6R 3B2; Tor'06; CCFP; (416)532-2894; edmund.chen@sickkids.ca.

CHEN, Fred S; Royal Columbian Hosp, 330 Columbia St E, New Westminster BC V3L 3W7; UBC'02; FRCPC; DiagRad. Staff, Royal Columbian Hospital; (604)520-5900

CHEN, Frederick H; Columbus Med Arts Bldg, 307-8333 Weston Rd, Woodbridge ON L4L 8E2; Tor'87; Ac Staff, Humber River Regional Hospital - Church Street Site; (905)851-2241

CHEN, Grace Y C; Meadowlark Prof Bldg, 205-8702 Meadowlark Rd NW, Edmonton AB T5R 5W5; (Taiwan)'66; (780)452-4381; Fax. (780)452-4194.

CHEN, Grant I; 214-3030 Lawrence Ave E, Scarborough ON M1P 2T7; Tor'00; BSc(Hon); FRCPC; IntMed (Gastroenterology); Gastroent. Langs: Mandarin; (416)438-5755; Fax. (416)438-3324.

CHEN, Helen Y; Regent Med Bldg, 250-2184 Broadway W, Vancouver BC V6K 2E1; UBC'98; CCFP; Consultant Staff, BC Women's Hospital & Health Centre; Langs: Mandarin; Cantonese; (604)733-5181; Fax. (604)733-5184.

CHEN, Henry J L; PO BOX 88069 Rpo Rabbit Hill, Edmonton AB T6R 0M5; Alb'87; (780)468-1884; Fax. (780)468-1868.

CHEN, Hillary J; Lakehead University, UC1007-955 Oliver Rd, Thunder Bay ON P7B 5E1; Tor'01; CCFP; Teach Staff Student Health & Counselling Centre, Lakehead University / Library; (807)343-8361

CHEN, Howard C H; Athlete's Care Sports Med Clin, 106-1971 Queen St E, Toronto ON M4L 1H9; Dal'92; Dip SportMed; CCFP; FCFP; Surg Asst, Toronto Western Hospital - University Health Network; Surgical Assistant, St Michael's Hospital; Staff Physician Sport Care, Women's College Hospital; Clin Instructor/Lecturer Family & Commun Med TEGH, University of Toronto; (416)691-6661; Fax. (416)691-6665.

CHEN, Innie; BC Women's Hosp & Health Ctre, D6-4500 Oak St, Vancouver BC V6H 3N1; UBC'05; ObstGyn. Staff, BC Women's Hospital & Health Centre; (604)875-2424

CHEN, Jacky S L; Boniface Park Med Centre, 8-700 Markham Rd, Scarborough ON M1H 2A7; Man'01; CCFP; (416)264-3443

CHEN, James C; BC Children's Hosp, 4480 Oak St, Vancouver BC V6H 3V4; Chichago (USA)'00; MD; Staff, BC Children's Hospital; (604)875-2711

CHEN, Jerry C L; 4203-2775 Laurel St, Vancouver BC V5Z 1M9; Man'88; FRCSC; GenSurg; VascSurg. Staff, Vancouver General Hospital - Centennial Pavillion; Staff, Richmond Hospital; Langs: Mandarin; Cantonese; (604)875-5535; Fax. (604)875-5542; jec@interchange.ubc.ca.

CHEN, Jia-De; 404-1100 Sheppard Ave E, North York ON M2K 2W1; Zhongshan (China)'82; MB; PhD; FRCPC; IntMed (Rheumatology). Langs: Cantonese; Mandarin; (416)222-0660; Fax. (416)222-9238.

CHEN, Jieli; L A Medical, 30-5201 50 St, Leduc AB T9E 6T4; (Other Foreign)'98; CCFP; (780)986-9600; Fax. (780)986-9732.

CHEN, John C C; 2F-4120 rue Sainte-Catherine O, Westmount QC H3Z 1P4; McG'82; FRCSC; Ophth. (514)285-8838

CHEN, John S C; William Osler HC-Brampton, 2100 Bovaird Dr E, Brampton ON L6R 3J7; Tor'88; CCFP; CCFP(E.M.); FCFP; Staff, William Osler Health System - Brampton Civic Hospital; (905)494-2120

CHEN, Joseph M; Sunnybrook Hlth Sciences Ctre, M102-2075 Bayview Ave, Toronto ON M4N 3M5; McG'85; FRCSC; Otol (Neuro Otolaryngology). Att Staff Otol, Sunnybrook Health Sciences Centre; Asst Prof Otol, University of Toronto; (416)480-4140; Fax. (416)480-5761.

CHEN, Julian C C; KMH-MRI Health Centre, 1310 Don Mills Rd, North York ON M3B 2W6; Tor'89; FRCPC; DiagRad.

CHEN, Julie L; 3-1032 17 Ave SW, Calgary AB T2T 0A5; Alb'92; CCFP; Langs: Mandarin; (403)229-1771; Fax. (403)229-1812.

CHEN, Kenneth K O; The Raxlen Clinic, B102-340 College St, Toronto ON M5T 3A9; Dal'78; (416)966-3641; Fax. (416)944-9947.

CHEN, Kim W T; Kingsway Med Clinic, 4645 Kingsway, Burnaby BC V5H 2B3; Qns'06; CCFP; (604)558-2611

CHEN, Lily F; Markham Family Health Team, 1-122 Cornell Park Ave, Markham ON L6B 1B6; Shanghai (China)'92; CCFP; (905)471-9999; Fax. (905)471-3627; lchen@msh.on.ca.

CHEN, Long; The Ottawa Hosp-Gen Campus, 501 Smyth Rd, Ottawa ON K1H 8L6; Wenzhou Medical College (China)'01; Clin Fellow Orth Surg, The Ottawa Hospital - General Campus; (613)737-6111

CHEN, Luke Y C; 10F-2775 Laurel St, Vancouver BC V5Z 1M9; Dal'03; FRCPC; IntMed; Hem. (604)875-4863

CHEN, Lydia M; 102-1111 Lonsdale Ave, North Vancouver BC V7M 2H4; UBC'81; DAB; FRCSC; Ophth (General Ophthalmic Surgery). Ac Staff, Lions Gate Hospital; Consultant, Vancouver General Hospital - Centennial Pavillion; Asst Prof, University of British Columbia; (604)988-1166; Fax. (604)988-0166.

CHEN, Marie-Luce; St Mary's Family Med Centre, 3777 rue Jean-Brillant, Montreal QC H3T 1M5; McG'09; CCFP; (514)734-2677

CHEN, Matthew M; University of Alberta Hosp, 1G1.50-8440 112 St NW, Edmonton AB T6G 2B7; Alb'04; FRCPC; EmergMed. Staff, University of Alberta Hospital; (780)407-8432

CHEN, Morie; St Joseph's Health Centre, 30 The Queensway, Toronto ON M6R 1B5; UBC'01; FRCPC; DiagRad. Staff, St Joseph's Health Centre; (416)530-6486

CHEN, Moy Fong; Lyman Duff Med Sciences Bldg, 3775 rue University, Montreal QC H3A 2B4; Monash (Australia)'68; CSPQ; MB BS; FRCPC; AnatPath (Perinatal). Staff, McGill University Health Centre - Montreal Children's Hospital; Staff, McGill University Health Centre - Montreal General Campus; Ac Staff Path, McGill University Health Centre - Royal Victoria Hospital; Assoc Prof Path, McGill University; (514)398-7192; moyfong.chen@mcgill.ca.

CHEN, Patrick Q H; The Richmond Hosp, 7000 Westminster Hwy, Richmond BC V6X 1A2; UBC'06; CCFP; CCFP(E.M.); Staff, Richmond Hospital; (604)244-5585

CHEN, Philip E; 959-999 36 St NE, Calgary AB T2A 7X6; Cal'04; FRCPC; DiagRad. Staff, Red Deer Regional Hospital Centre; (403)215-2900

CHEN, Richard Y Y; Kingsbridge Med Centre, 5-20 Kingsbridge Garden Cir, Mississauga ON L5R 3K7; Tor'86; CCFP; FCFP; Court Staff Family Med, Toronto General Hospital - UHN; Court Staff Family Med, The Credit Valley Hospital; Ac Staff Fam Med, Trillium Health Centre - Mississauga; (905)507-1111; Fax. (905)890-7102.

CHEN, Robert C C; Dr Robert C C Chen Med Prof Co, 9-2943 Major Mackenzie Dr, Maple ON L6A 3N9; Qns'98; CCFP; (905)303-4657; Fax. (905)303-3708.

CHEN, Robert E W; 7MC 411-399 Bathurst St, Toronto ON M5T 2S8; University of Cambridge (United Kingdom)'89; MB BS; MSc; FRCPC; Neur (Electromyography). Att Staff Neurol, Toronto Western Hospital - University Health Network; Assoc Prof Med, University of Toronto; Langs: Cantonese; (416)603-5207; Fax. (416)603-5004.

CHEN, Robert J B; St Michael's Hosp, 30 Bond St, Toronto ON M5B 1W8; McM'92; FRCPC; Anes. Ac Staff, St Michael's Hospital; Asst Prof, University of Toronto; Langs: French; (416)864-5071; Fax. (416)864-6014; chenr@smh.toronto.on.ca.

CHEN, Robert P; IWK Health Centre, PO Box 9700 Rpo CSC 5850-5980 University Ave, Halifax NS B3K 6R8; Dal'87; FRCPC; Peds; PedCardiol. Staff Ped Cardiol, IWK Health Centre; Assoc Prof, Dalhousie University; (902)470-8197; Fax. (902)470-6616; robert.chen@iwk.nshealth.ca.

CHEN, Roy Y; Bramalea Med Centre, 501-18 Kensington Rd, Brampton ON L6T 4S5; National (Taiwan)'66; FRCSC; Ophth. Ac Staff, William Osler Health System - Brampton Civic Hospital; (905)792-1010; Fax. (905)792-8133.

CHEN, Shin-Yee; 919-45 Holland Ave, Ottawa ON K1Y 4S3; Qns'03; FRCPC; IntMed; Cardiol. Staff, University of Ottawa Heart Institute; (613)513-8579

CHEN, Simon I; M334-2211 Wesbrook Mall, Vancouver BC V6T 1Z3; (Philippines)'99; MCFP; MCFP(EM); CCFP; CCFP(E.M.); Physician Emerg, Battlefords Union Hospital; Physician Emerg, Saskatoon Health Region Saskatoon Public Health; Langs: Mandarin; Taiwanese; (604)822-7011; Fax. (604)822-7889; simonchen_md@hotmail.com.

CHEN, Sylvia H; Eyecare Centre, D-2550 Willow St, Vancouver BC V5Z 3N9; McG'06; MDCM; FRCSC; Ophth. (604)875-4624

CHEN, Szu-Yang; Surrey Mem Hosp, 13750 96 Ave, Surrey BC V3V 1Z2; Dal'88; Staff, Surrey Memorial Hospital; (604)588-3367

CHEN, Teh-Chuen; Health Sciences North-Laurenti, 41 Ramsey Lake Rd, Sudbury ON P3E 5J1; (Taiwan)'72; DABPath; AnatPath. Ac Staff Path, Health Sciences North-St Joseph's Health Centre; Staff, Health Sciences North-Laurentian Site; (705)523-7100

CHEN, Tsai I; Trillium Hlth Ctr-Mississauga, 100 Queensway W, Mississauga ON L5B 1B8; Tor'88; CCFP; CCFP(E.M.); Staff, Humber River Regional Hospital - Church Street Site; Staff, Grand River Hospital - Kitchener/Waterloo Health Centre; Staff, Trillium Health Centre - Mississauga; (905)259-7100

CHEN, Victoria Y S; Summerville Family Health Team, 5F-101 Queensway W, Mississauga ON L5B 2P7; Tor'90; CCFP; FCFP; Ac Staff, Trillium Health Centre - Mississauga; (905)272-9700; Fax. (905)272-1416.

CHEN, Wendell E; Dr Langer & Associates, 180 Sandalwood Pky E, Brampton ON L6Z 1Y4; Tor'94; CCFP; (905)846-9255

CHEN, William C Y; Johnston Health Centre, 3-20 Bell Farm Rd, Barrie ON L4M 6E4; Wes'86; Staff, Royal Victoria Regional Health Centre; (705)728-7881

CHEN, Eric; Univ Hlth Network-Princess M, 5 719-610 University Ave, Toronto ON M5G 2M9; Tor'96; FRCPC; IntMed; MedOncol., Princess Margaret Hospital - University Health Network; Langs: Mandarin; (416)946-2263; Fax. (416)946-4467; eric.chen@uhn.on.ca.

CHEN, Yen-Fu; RH Med Rehab Centre-EMG Clinic, 15-9555 Yonge St, Richmond Hill ON L4C 9M5; McG'99; FRCPC; PhysMed&Rehab (Nerve Conduction Studies). Staff, Mackenzie Richmond Hill Hospital; Langs: Chinese; (416)760-6787

CHEN, Yu; Dr Everett Chalmers Reg Hosp, PO Box 9000 Stn A, Fredericton NB E3B 5N5; Hunan (China)'97; Staff, Dr Everett Chalmers Regional Hospital; (506)452-5435

CHEN-TOURNOUX, Annabel A; SMBD Jewish Gen Hosp, E206-3755 ch Cote-Sainte-Cathe, Montreal QC H3T 1E2; Staff, Sir Mortimer B Davis Jewish General; (514)340-8222

CHENARD, Elaine; 101-180 rue des Gouverneurs, Rimouski QC G5L 8G1; Laval'86; FRCPC; ObstGyn. (418)722-4333; Fax. (418)722-8714.

CHENARD, Helene; GMF Concorde, 300 boul de la Concorde E, Laval QC H7G 2E6; Mon'85; Clin Prof Family Med, Hopital de la Cite de la santé; Clin Prof Family Med, Universite de Montreal; Langs: Spanish; (450)667-5310; Fax. (450)667-5248.

CHENARD, Jean; CHUS-Hop Fleurimont, 3001 12e av N, Sherbrooke QC J1H 5N4; Sher'03; FRCPC; DiagRad. Staff, Centre Hospitalier Universitaire de Sherbrooke-Hopital Fleurimont; (819)346-1110

CHENARD, Marise; Ctr Hosp Affilie-Enfant-Jesus, 1401 18e rue, Quebec QC G1J 1Z4; Laval'06; FRCPC; Psy. Staff, Centre Hospitalier Affilié Universitaire de Québec - Hôpital De L'Enfant Jésus; (418)649-0252

CHENEVERT, Alain; Clinique Med Pierre-Bertrand, 212-303 boul Pierre-Bertrand, Quebec QC G1M 3L7; Laval'83; ac Staff, Centre Hospitalier Universitaire De Québec - Pavillon De St-françois-d'assise; Ac Staff, CSSS de Quebec-Sud; (418)683-2724; Fax. (418)683-8861; alain.chenevert@orlo.ulaval.ca.

CHENEVERT, Jacinthe; CHUQ-Hotel-Dieu de Quebec, 11 Cote du Palais, Quebec QC G1R 2J6; Laval'05; FRCPC; AnatPath. Staff, Centre Hospitalier Universitaire de Québec (CHUQ) - Siege Social; (418)691-5233; Fax. (418)691-5226.

CHENEVERT, Robert J; Clinique Med des Promenades, A. 222-3333 rue du Carrefour, Quebec QC G1C 5R9; Laval'89; CCFP; Ac Staff, Centre Hospitalier Universitaire De Québec - Pavillon De St-françois-d'assise; (418)663-6345

CHENG, A Lawrence; St Paul's Hosp, 1081 Burrard St, Vancouver BC V6Z 1Y6; Wes'93; CCFP; CCFP(E.M.); Staff, Providence Health Care - St Paul's Hospital; (604)806-8480

CHENG, Adam M; Alberta Children's Hosp, 2888 Shanagappi Trail NW, Calgary AB T3B 6A8; Tor'99; FRCPC; Peds; PedEmergMed. Staff, Alberta Children's Hospital; (403)955-2633

CHENG, Ah-Ling; University of Alberta Hosp, 8440 112 St NW, Edmonton AB T6G 2B7; Cal'07; DiagRad. Staff, University of Alberta Hospital; (780)407-8822

CHENG, Alan H; Royal Alexandra Hosp, 10240 Kingsway NW, Edmonton AB T5H 3V9; Qns'03; FRCPC; Anes. Staff, Royal Alexandra Hospital; (780)735-4010

CHENG, Albert S; Providence Healthcare, 3276 St Clair Ave E, Scarborough ON M1L 1W1; Wes'99; BSc; FRCPC; PhysMed&Rehab (Musculoskeletal Medicine). Staff B1 Clinics, Providence Healthcare; Staff, Toronto Rehabilitation Institute - Rumsey Centre; (416)285-3619; Fax. (416)285-3764.

CHENG, Alice Y; Credit Valley Prof Bldg, 507-2300 Eglinton Ave W, Mississauga ON L5M 2V8; Tor'98; FRCPC; IntMed; Endocrin&Metab. Staff Endocrinol, The Credit Valley Hospital; Staff Endocrinol/Asst Prof, St Michael's Hospital; Asst Prof Med, University of Toronto; Langs: Cantonese; (905)828-7622; Fax. (905)828-7769.

CHENG, Ambrose C S; 4F-260 Sherbrooke St, New Westminster BC V3L 3M2; Tor'89; FRCPC; Psy. (604)520-4662

CHENG, Amy; Royal Columbian Hosp, 330 Columbia St E, New Westminster BC V3L 3W7; Tor'06; FRCPC; EmergMed. Staff, Royal Columbian Hospital; (604)520-4257

CHENG, Andrew M; 201-145 15 St W, North Vancouver BC V7M 1R9; UBC'89; (604)988-7800; Fax. (604)988-7878.

CHENG, Anita K; Children's Hosp of Western Ont, E6 103-800 Commissioners Rd E, London ON N6C 2V5; Wes'07; FRCPC; Peds (Neonatology). Staff, Children's Hospital of Western Ontario; (519)685-8500

CHENG, Anthony; North York Cardiovascular Ctre, 307-701 Sheppard Ave E, North York ON M2K 2Z3; Tor'96; FACC; ABIM; FRCPC; IntMed (Cardiology). Dir Cardiopulmonary Lab, North York General Hospital; Langs: Cantonese.

CHENG, Bai-Sen; 2296 Eglinton Ave E, Scarborough ON M1K 2M2; Tor'94; CCFP; FCFP; Langs: Chinese; (416)615-0002

CHENG, Calvin K Y; Humber River Reg Hosp-Church, 200 Church St, Toronto ON M9N 1N8; Tor'88; BSc; FRCPC; IntMed; GeriatricMed. Staff, Humber River Regional Hospital - Church Street Site; Staff, Baycrest Centre for Geriatric Care; Staff, Mount Sinai Hospital; University of Toronto; (416)243-4629; calvin.cheng@utoronto.ca.

CHENG, Calvin W K; Delta Med Clinic, 140-4977 Trenant St, Delta BC V4K 2K5; Alb'96; CCFP; (604)946-7662; Fax. (604)940-1743; ccheng2000@hotmail.com.

CHENG, Calvino K; MacKenzie Bldg, 205-5788 University Ave, Halifax NS B3H 1V8; Cal'01; FRCPC; HemPath. Asst Prof, Dalhousie University; Langs: Chinese; French; (902)473-3140; Fax. (902)473-4113; calvino.cheng@cdha.nshealth.ca.

CHENG, Charles Y Y; Skin Matters Aesthetic Med Ctr, 5299 Arbutus St, Vancouver BC V6M 4J2; Tor'90; LMCC; Clin Examiner, Medical Council of Canada Examination Board; Clinical Asst Prof Faculty of Med, University of British Columbia; Langs: Mandarin; Taiwanese; (604)323-9588; Fax. (604)323-9558; info@skinmatters.ca.

CHENG, Chiachen; 100-28 Cumberland St N, Thunder Bay ON P7A 4K9; Qns'97; FRCPC; Psy (Child & Adolescent Psychiatry). (807)345-0060

CHENG, Davy C H; London HSC-University Hosp, PO Box 5339 Stn B C3 172-339 Windermere Rd, London ON N6A 5A5; Tor'83; MSc; FRCPC; Anes (Cardiac Anesthesia). Chief Anes, St Joseph's Hospital - St Joseph's Health Care; Chief, London Health Sciences Centre - University Hospital; University of Western Ontario; (519)663-3031; Fax. (519)663-3161; davy.cheng@lhsc.on.ca.

CHENG, Dawn M L; 2865 Woodbine Dr, North Vancouver BC V7R 2R9; UBC'92; CCFP; FCFP; (778)230-2286

CHENG, Deborah W H; 106A-100 Humber College Blvd, Etobicoke ON M9V 5G4; Tor'00; FRCPC; DiagRad.

CHENG, Edwin J; Foothills South Tower, 711-3031 Hospital Dr NW, Calgary AB T2N 2T8; Tor'07; FRCPC; IntMed; Gastroent. (403)592-5020

CHENG, Elaine V; Koffler Student Service, 111-214 College St, Toronto ON M5T 2Z9; Tor'09; CCFP; (416)978-8070; Fax. (416)978-7341.

CHENG, Erika; Bella Coola Gen Hosp, PO Box 220 1025 Elcho St, Bella Coola BC V0T 1C0; UBC'92; CCFP; Fam Med, Bella Coola General Hospital; (250)799-5342; Fax. (250)799-5991.

CHENG, Florence J; Dominion Med Centres Ltd, 9122 23 Ave NW, Edmonton AB T6N 1H9; Alb'10; (780)801-3360; Fax. (780)801-3366.

CHENG, Gemma L; Herzl CRIU Walk-In Clinic, 500-5858 ch Cote-des-Neiges, Montreal QC H3S 1Z1; Cal'79; (514)340-8311

CHENG, Gordon W; Niagara H System-St Catharines, PO Box 3018 Stn Main 142 Queenston St, St Catharines ON L2R 7C6; Qns'01; FRCPC; DiagRad. Staff, Niagara Health System - St Catharines General Site; (905)684-7271 x4570

CHENG, Henry J C K; 219-2120 North Park Dr, Brampton ON L6S 0C9; Tor'78; PhD; FRCSC; ObstGyn (Infertility). Staff Corporate ObstGyn, William Osler Health System - Brampton Civic Hospital; Staff, ISIS Regional Fertility Centre; Langs: Cantonese; (905)455-0373; Fax. (905)455-0374.

CHENG, Ivy S; Sunnybrook Hlth Sciences Ctre, 2075 Bayview Ave, Toronto ON M4N 3M5; Wes'94; FRCPC; EmergMed. Staff, Sunnybrook Health Sciences Centre; Staff, The Sports Medicine Specialists; (416)480-4207; Fax. (416)480-4704.

CHENG, James W K; Broadway Med Centre, 330-943 Broadway W, Vancouver BC V5Z 4E1; (Hong Kong)'64; MB BS; FRCPC; Peds. Vis Staff, BC Children's Hospital; Ac Staff, BC Women's Hospital & Health Centre; Consultant, Vancouver General Hospital - Centennial Pavillion; (604)731-2339

CHENG, Jenny S; 304-1125 Dufferin Cres, Nanaimo BC V9S 2B5; McG'05; FRCSC; PlasSurg. (250)591-3301

CHENG, Jerry H C; 308-1110 Sheppard Ave E, North York ON M2K 2W2; Tor'78; Court Staff, North York General Hospital; Langs: Chinese; (416)733-3500; Fax. (416)733-8083.

CHENG, Jim I; 210-2016 Sherwood Dr, Sherwood Park AB T8A 3X3; Melbourne (Australia)'70; DIH; DPH; FRCPC; CommunMed; Public Health & Preventive Med; OccupMed. Med Consultant, Workers' Comp Board of AB; Langs: Chinese; Cantonese; Shanghai; (780)416-3701; Fax. (780)416-3702.

CHENG, Joan F; Markham Stouffville Hosp, PO Box 1800 Stn Main 381 Church St, Markham ON L3P 7P3; Tor'93; BSc; CCFP; CCFP(E.M.); FCFP; Staff, Markham Stouffville Hospital; (905)472-7111

CHENG, Judy A; Meadowlark Health Centre, 140 Meadowlark Shopping Ctr NW, Edmonton AB T5R 5W9; Alb'90; (780)489-8470; Fax. (780)484-1620.

CHENG, June J; Public Health & Preventive Med, HSC 2C2-1280 Main St W, Hamilton ON L8S 4K1; McM'08; CCFP; Teach Staff, McMaster University; (905)525-9140

CHENG, Kiu-Sing; Agincourt Professional, 321-2330 Kennedy Rd, Scarborough ON M1T 0A2; Man'79; Staff, The Scarborough Hospital - Birchmount Campus; (416)299-8333

CHENG, Lucille L T; 220 Main St W, Hamilton ON L8P 1J3; Tor'79; (905)528-8088; Fax. (905)528-8096.

CHENG, M F Frederick; Oak Park Med Centre, 1-2530 Sixth Line, Oakville ON L6H 6W5; Man'99; CCFP; (905)257-1006; fcheng@mindless.com.

CHENG, Malcolm H F; Avicenna Health Centre, 100-80 Finch Ave W, North York ON M2N 2H4; Tor'92; ABPeds; BSc; MD; LMCC; FAAP; FRCP; FRCPC; Peds. Langs: Cantonese; Mandarin; (416)222-0909; Fax. (416)222-8292.

CHENG, Marshall A; 10962 Scarborough Dr, Delta BC V4C 7S5; UBC'93; FRCPC; Anes. (604)946-4045; Fax. (604)946-4035.

CHENG, Mary M L; Finch-Midland Med Centre, 316-4190 Finch Ave E, Scarborough ON M1S 4T7; (Hong Kong)'85; MB BS; FRCSC; ObstGyn. Assoc Staff ObstGyn, Rouge Valley Health System - Centenary Health Centre Site; Langs: Cantonese; Mandarin; (416)282-0644; Fax. (416)282-7835.

CHENG, Michael J C; 202 Elm St, St Thomas ON N5R 1J3; Qns'89; FRCSC; Urol. Assoc Staff, St Thomas Elgin General Hospital; Langs: Taiwanese; Mandarin; (519)633-4034; Fax. (519)633-3412.

CHENG, Michael K S; 200-311 McArthur Ave, Vanier ON K1L 8M3; Qns'96; FRCPC; Psy (Child & Family Psychiatry). Staff, Children's Hospital of Eastern Ontario (CHEO); (613)738-6990; Fax. (613)738-4891.

CHENG, Michael T W; Hillcrest Mall, 9350 Yonge St, Richmond Hill ON L4C 5G2; Mem'75; Court Staff, Mackenzie Richmond Hill Hospital; Langs: Cantonese; Mandarin; (905)883-1599; Fax. (905)883-0416.

CHENG, Michelle; Hillcrest Mall Doctor's Office, 9350 Yonge St, Richmond Hill ON L4C 5G2; Tor'08; CCFP; (905)883-1599; Fax. (905)883-0416.

CHENG, Nancy L; 2 200 Students Union Bldg, 66 University Campus NW, Edmonton AB T6G 2J7; Alb'91; CCFP; FCFP; (780)492-2612; Fax. (780)492-0172.

CHENG, Natalie Y; Dartmouth Gen Hosp, 325 Pleasant St, Dartmouth NS B2Y 4G8; Dal'05; BASc; MASc; CCFP; Staff, Dartmouth General Hospital; (902)465-8300; Fax. (902)460-4142.

CHENG, Richard S S; Pain & Sports Clinic, 303-2347 Kennedy Rd, Scarborough ON M1T 3T8; Tor'83; MSc; Dir Research & Pain Clinic, St Joseph's Health Centre; Aj Prof, Canadian Memorial Chiropractic School; Langs: Chinese; (416)321-0228

CHENG, Ronald T K; Clinical Sciences Bldg, 8 120-152 University Campus NW, Edmonton AB T6G 2G3; Alb'01; FRCPC; Anes. Staff, Queen Elizabeth II Health Sciences Centre - Victoria General Site; (780)407-8861; Fax. (780)407-3200.

CHENG, Susanna Y; Toronto Sunnybrook Reg Cancer, T2 034-2075 Bayview Ave, Toronto ON M4N 3M5; Wes'95; BSc; FRCPC; IntMed; MedOncol; Hem. Langs: Cantonese; (416)480-4928; Fax. (416)480-6002; susanna.cheng@sunnybrook.ca.

CHENG, Sylvia S; The Hosp for Sick Children, 555 University Ave, Toronto ON M5G 1X8; UBC'08; FRCPC; Peds. Staff, The Hospital For Sick Children; (416)813-7500

CHENG, Tina; Tom Baker Cancer Centre, 1331 29 St NW, Calgary AB T2N 4N2; Beijing (China)'87; FRCPC; IntMed; MedOncol. Staff, Tom Baker Cancer Centre; (403)521-3706; Fax. (403)283-1651.

CHENG, Tracy T; St Joseph's Mountain H Service, PO Box 585 Stn Lcd 1 100 5th St W, Hamilton ON L8N 3K7; Ott'03; FRCPC; Psy. Staff, St Joseph's Healthcare Hamilton - West 5th Campus; (905)522-1155

CHENG, Vivian K; Frontenac Med Associates, 201-791 Princess St, Kingston ON K7L 1E9; Alb'02; CCFP; (613)544-2727

CHENG, Willoon W M; Tillsonburg Med Centre, 13-200 Broadway St, Tillsonburg ON N4G 5A7; Alb'99; CCFP; Staff, Tillsonburg District Memorial Hospital; (519)842-4231; Fax. (519)842-7579.

CHENG, Wing K; Doctors Hosp Phase 1, 240-340 College St, Toronto ON M5T 3A9; Tor'74; ABIM; FRCPC; IntMed; Respir. (416)961-5476; Fax. (416)928-9816.

CHENG, Y Y Olivia; 459 Hume St, Collingwood ON L9Y 1W9; Tor'04; FRCSC; OrthSurg. (705)444-5533

CHENG, Yves I B; Centre d'Urgence de Salaberry, 2758 rue de Salaberry, Montreal QC H3M 1L3; Laval'86; (514)337-4772

CHENGALATH, Premkumar; Country Hills Medicentre, 220-5149 Country Hills Blvd NW, Calgary AB T3A 5K8; Bangalore (India)'72; Staff Obst, Peter Lougheed Centre; (403)241-8848; Fax. (403)241-8849; pchengal@medicentres.com.

CHENGAPA, Vinnie; Greystones Clinic Inc, 1466 Dresden Row, Halifax NS B3J 3T5; Bangalore (India)'70; MB BS; DPM(Lond); MRCPsy(UK); FRCPC; Psy (Bipolar Disease). Consultant, Queen Elizabeth II Health Sciences Centre - Victoria General Site; Asst Prof Psy, Dalhousie University; Langs: Hindi; (902)423-8333; Fax. (902)423-3133.

CHENIER, Andre; 102-1426 ch De Chambly, Longueuil QC J4J 3X3; Mon'72; (450)651-2120

CHENIER, Elisabeth; Clin Dermatologique de Lachena, 345-950 Montee des Pionniers, Terrebonne QC J6V 1S8; Mon'92; Derm. Langs: Bilingual(French/English); (450)470-1221; Fax. (450)470-1586.

CHENIER, France; Ctr Hosp Anna-Laberge, 200 boul Brisebois, Chateauguay QC J6K 4W8; Mon'98; CSPQ; FRCPC; IntMed; Anes. Staff, Hôpital Anna-Laberge; (450)699-2425 x2466

CHENIER, Martin; CSSS de Laval, 1755 boul Rene-Laennec, Laval QC H7M 3L9; Mon'83; Staff, Hopital de la Cite de la santé; (450)975-5500; Fax. (450)975-5353.

CHENIER, Sebastien; CHUS-Hop Fleurimont, 3001 12e Av N, Sherbrooke QC J1H 5N4; Mon'05; FRCPC; MedGenetics. Staff, Centre Hospitalier Universitaire de Sherbrooke-Hopital Fleurimont; (819)346-1110

CHENIER, Stephanie; CSSS des Aurores Boreales, CP 6000 Succ Bureau-Chef 679 2e rue E, La Sarre QC J9Z 2X7; Sher'97; FRCPC; DiagRad. Staff, Centre Hospitalier La Sarre; (819)333-2311 x2411

CHENIER, Veronique; Clin Dermatology de Lachenaie, 345-950 Montée des Pionniers, Terrebonne QC J6V 1S8; Mon'99; Derm. (450)470-1221

CHENKIN, Jordan S; Sunnybrook Hlth Sciences Ctre, C753-2075 Bayview Ave, Toronto ON M4N 3M5; Qns'04; FRCPC; EmergMed. Staff, Sunnybrook Health Sciences Centre; (416)480-6100

CHEOK, Andy S; 206-320 Danforth Ave, Toronto ON M4K 1N8; Tor'94; FRCPC; Psy (Anxiety Disorder). (647)269-3522

CHEONG, K M Andrew; Wilson Centre Family Practice, 1-2185 Wilson Ave, Port Coquitlam BC V3C 6C1; Singapore (Singapore)'94; MB BS; CCFP; Langs: Chinese; (604)942-7227

CHEONG, Richard A; Bluewater Health-Norman Site, 89 Norman St, Sarnia ON N7T 6S3; Ott'76; Ac Staff, Bluewater Health - Mitton Site; Ac Staff Family Med, Bluewater Health - Norman Site; (519)464-4500 x5543

CHEONG, Y Michele; Doctors Bldg, 125-955 Queen St E, Sault Ste. Marie ON P6A 2C3; Man'92; BSc; BSc(Med); FRCSC; OrthSurg (Arthroplasty). Ac Staff, Sault Area Hospital - Sault Ste Marie; (705)945-7575; Fax. (705)945-7092.

CHEONG, Yvette Y W; Mount St Joseph Hosp, 3080 Prince Edward St, Vancouver BC V5T 3N4; Tor'93; FRCPC; DiagRad (Magnetic Resonance Imaging). Staff Diag Imaging, Providence Health Care - Mount Saint Joseph Hospital; Asst Prof, University of British Columbia; (604)877-8323; Fax. (604)877-8132.

CHEPESIUK, Martin A; 92 Roncesvalles Ave, Toronto ON M6R 2K8; Tor'81; FRCPC; IntMed; Neur. Ac Staff, St Joseph's Health Centre; University of Toronto; (416)534-2115; Fax. (416)533-6791.

CHEPESIUK, William N; 92 Roncesvalles Ave, Toronto ON M6R 2K8; Qns'79; Ac Staff, St Joseph's Health Centre; (416)534-2115; Fax. (416)533-6791.

CHERAN, Sendhil K; Fitzgerald Bldg, 150 College St, Toronto ON M5S 3E2; Duke University (Other Foreign)'04; DiagRad.

CHERCOVER, David; Lions Gate Hosp, 231 15th St E, North Vancouver BC V7L 2L7; UBC'78; FRCPC; GenPath; AnatPath. Staff Path, Lions Gate Hospital; (604)984-5759

CHEREPACHA, Douglas L; Kingscross Med Group, 408-18 Kensington Rd, Brampton ON L6T 4S5; Tor'93; BPHE; CCFP; Staff, William Osler Health System - Brampton Civic Hospital; (905)792-2280; Fax. (905)792-9832; dcherepacha@hotmail.com.

CHERGUI, Assia; CSSS de Rivière-de-Loup, 75 rue Saint-Henri, Riviere-du-Loup QC G5R 2A4; Staff, Centre Hospitalier Regional du Grand-Portage; (418)868-1010

CHERIAN, Alice T; Scarborough Hosp-Birchmount, 3030 Birchmount Rd, Scarborough ON M1W 3W3; Kerala (India)'77; FRCPC; Peds. Staff, The Scarborough Hospital - Birchmount Campus; Langs: Malayalam; (416)495-2600

CHERIAN, Joe; St Joseph's Healthcare, 50 Charlton Ave E, Hamilton ON L8N 4A6; Man'93; BSc; CCFP; CCFP(E.M.); Staff, St Joseph's Healthcare - Charlton Campus; Staff, The Brant Community Healthcare System - Brantford General Hospital Site; McMaster University; (905)522-1155 x3112; jcherian3@yahoo.ca.

CHERIAN, S Rachael; Massey Med Clinic, PO Box 119 260 Cameron St, Massey ON P0P 1P0; Benin (Nigeria)'87; MB BS; CCFP; (705)865-2300; Fax. (705)865-3495.

CHERIF SLIMANE, Safia; CSSS des Aurores-Boreales, CP 6000 Succ Bureau-Chef 679 2e rue E, La Sarre QC J9Z 2X7; (Algeria)'86; CCFP; Staff, Centre Hospitalier La Sarre; (819)333-2311

CHERIGUI, Saïda; CLSC de Saint-Michel, 3355 rue Jarry E, Montreal QC H1Z 2E5; (Other Foreign)'01; (514)374-8223

CHERISOL, Remy; CSSS du Rocher-Perce, CP 3300 451 rue Mgr Ross E, Chandler QC G0C 1K0; Bruxelles (Belgium)'95; CCFP; Staff, Centre Hospitalier de Chandler; (418)689-2261

CHERIYAN, Mammen; Central Nfld Reg Hlth Centre, 50 Union St, Grnd-Falls-Wi NL A2A 2E1; Nagpur (India)'73; MB BS; MRCP(UK); FRCP(Ed); FRCPC; Peds. Staff, Central Newfoundland Regional Health Centre; (709)292-2500; Fax. (709)292-2182; mcheriyan25@hotmail.com.

CHERKEZOFF, Alexander N; Kerrisdale Commun Ctr Seniors, 5851 West Blvd, Vancouver BC V6M 3W9; UBC'57; CCFP; FCFP; Head Family Pract, Vancouver General Hospital - Centennial Pavillion; Clin Assoc Prof, University of British Columbia; (604)257-8109

CHERLA, Kiran U; Georgetown Med Associates, 199 Princess Anne Dr, Georgetown ON L7G 4W4; Tor'01; CCFP; (905)873-3000; Fax. (905)873-0800.

CHERLAND, Esther E; Royal University Hosp, 241EH-103 Hospital Dr, Saskatoon SK S7N 0W8; Sask'82; FRCPC; Psy. Staff, Royal University Hospital; (306)966-7531; Fax. (306)966-8250.

CHERNENKOFF, William; Spadina Med Clinic, 2-806 Spadina Cres E, Saskatoon SK S7K 3H4; Sask'63; FCFP; CCFP; FCFP; Staff Aviation Med, Civil Aviation Canada; Asst Prof, University of Saskatchewan; Langs: Russian; (306)955-3030; Fax. (306)955-4202; chernenkoff@sextherapists.com.

CHERNESKI, Heather M; Parkview Tertiary Mental Healt, 4950 Heather St, Vancouver BC V5Z 3L9; Cal'88; CCFP; FCFP; Staff, BC Mental Health & Addiction Service; (604)806-9565

CHERNESKY, Patricia A; Nipawin Health Centre, PO Box 1925 201 1st Ave W, Nipawin SK S0E 1E0; Sask'73; Langs: Ukrainian; (306)862-3151; Fax. (306)862-2241.

CHERNEY, David Z I; 8N 845-585 University Ave, Toronto ON M5G 2N2; McG'99; FRCPC; IntMed; Nephrol. Asst Prof Med, University of Toronto; Langs: Bilingual(English/French).

CHERNIAK, Donna A G; CLSC de Sherbrooke, 50 rue Camirand, Sherbrooke QC J1H 4J5; McM'74; FCFP; MMed; CCFP; FCFP; Staff Teacher, Universite de Sherbrooke; Langs: French; Spanish; (819)563-2572; Fax. (819)823-0238; donna.cherniak@usherbrooke.ca.

CHERNIAK, Victor; 3-715 Coronation Blvd, Cambridge ON N1R 7R1; Wes'82; Staff, Cambridge Memorial Hospital; (519)740-1700; Fax. (519)740-8487.

CHERNICK, Elisheva H; PO Box 39028 Rpo Adelaide Cent, London ON N5Y 5L1; McM'89.

CHERNICK, Grant M P; 400-1681 Chestnut St, Vancouver BC V6J 4M6; Man'77; FRCPC; Psy (Adult Psychiatry);CCFP; Psychiatrist, Vancouver Community Mental Health Services; Clinical Asst Prof, University of British Columbia; (604)737-0630; Fax. (604)737-1140.

CHERNICK, Michael; Oak Ridge Med Centre, 100-13291 Yonge St, Richmond Hill ON L4E 4L6; Witwatersrand (South Africa)'87; CCFP; FCFP; Staff Family Pract, Southlake Regional Health Centre; Langs: Afrikaans; (905)773-7759; Fax. (905)773-1325; mchernick5790@rogers.com.

CHERNIN, Jeffrey M; 403-265 Yorkland Blvd, North York ON M2J 5C7; Dal'76; MPH(Johns Hopkins); FAB; (416)921-3499

CHERNIN, Trudy R; St Michal's Hosp Academic-FHT, 300-790 Bay St, Toronto ON M5G 1N8; McM'84; BScN; CCFP; FCFP; Staff, Mount Sinai Hospital; Clin Teacher, University of Toronto; (416)960-1366; Fax. (416)960-1945.

CHERNISH, Gregory M; 627 Dudley Ave, Winnipeg MB R3M 1P5; Man'84; (204)452-4948; Fax. (204)274-2070.

CHERNISH, Robert N; 305-564 Belmont Ave W, Kitchener ON N2M 5N6; Ott'01; FRCPC; IntMed (Critical Care Medicine); Respir. Staff, St Mary's General Hospital; (519)342-0599

CHERNIWCHAN, Darin P; Fraser Valley Travel Clinic, 5-45802 Luckakuck Way, Chilliwack BC V2R 5P9; McG'91; BSc(Pharm); CM; CCFP; FCFP; Ac Staff, Abbotsford Regional Hospital & Cancer Centre; Ac Staff, Chilliwack General Hospital; Langs: English; French; (604)755-4695; Fax. (604)823-0225.

CHERNIWCHAN, Marc A; Grey Nuns Community Hosp & HC, 1100 Youville Drive West NW, Edmonton AB T6L 5X8; Alb'80; FRCPC; EmergMed. Staff, Covenant Health - Grey Nuns Community Hospital; (780)450-7180; Fax. (780)450-7498.

CHERNOFF, D Roy; Willowgrove Med Group, 2-527 Nelson Rd, Saskatoon SK S7S 1P4; Sask'80; CCFP; Staff Family Med, St Paul's Hospital (Grey Nuns) of Saskatoon; Head Family Med/Staff, Saskatoon City Hospital; Head Fam Med/Critical Care, Royal University Hospital; Physician, Cameco Inc & Cory Potash; University of Saskatchewan; (306)653-1543; Fax. (306)653-0422.

CHERNOFF, Ian W; Mount Sinai Hosp, 206-600 University Ave, Toronto ON M5G 1X5; Dal'95; BSc; CCFP; CCFP(E.M.); Staff Emerg Med, Mount Sinai Hospital; Staff, William Osler Health System - Brampton Civic Hospital; (416)586-5058; Fax. (416)586-4719; chernoff@sympatico.ca.

CHERRADI, Siham; Ungava Tulattavik Health Ctr, CP 149, Kuujjuaq QC J0M 1C0; Hassan II (Morocco)'88; CCFP; Staff, Centre de sante Tulattavik de l'Ungava; (819)964-2905; siham.cherradi@ssss.gouv.qc.ca.

CHERRY, James M; SGH Medical Mall, 202-3030 Lawrence Ave E, Scarborough ON M1P 2T7; McG'81; ABIM; FRCPC; IntMed (Adult Cardiology); Cardiol. Staff Cardiol, The Scarborough Hospital - General Campus; Staff Cardiol, Rouge Valley Health System - Centenary Health Centre Site; (416)438-8828; Fax. (416)438-2793.

CHERRY, Jason; 230-4231 Hazelbridge Way, Richmond BC V6X 3L7; UBC'00; FRCSC; Ophth. (604)270-7727

CHERRY, Mark S; Regina Qu'Appelle HR-Regina, 1440 14th Ave, Regina SK S4P 0W5; Sask'78; FRCPC; Anes. Head Dept of Anes, Regina General Hospital; Clin Assoc Teacher, University of Saskatchewan; (306)766-4252; Fax. (306)789-9270.

CHERRY, Nicola M; 5-30 University Terrace, 8303 112 St NW, Edmonton AB T6G 1K4; McG'90; FRCP(Lond); FFOM(Lond.); FRCPC; CommunMed. Physician Occup Med, University of Alberta Hospital; Teach Staff, University of Alberta; (780)492-7851; Fax. (780)492-9677.

CHERRY, Nicole A; Islington Med Clinic, 600-1243 Islington Ave, Etobicoke ON M8X 1Y9; Tor'98; FRCSC; ObstGyn. Ac Staff, St Joseph's Health Centre; Lecturer, University of Toronto; (416)231-4574; Fax. (416)231-6272.

CHERRY, Paul M H; Medical Dental Bldg, 105-1849 Yonge St, Toronto ON M4S 1Y2; London (England)'69; LRCP; FRCS(Ed); FRCS(Eng); FRCOphth(UK); MB BS; FRCSC; Ophth (Cornea and General Ophthalmology). Staff Ophth, Toronto Western Hospital - University Health Network; Asst Prof Ophth, University of Toronto; (416)481-5189; Fax. (416)241-8870.

CHERRY, Raeleen D; 14035 105 Ave NW PO Box 53013, Edmonton AB T5N 0Z1; Sask'75; FRCPC; IntMed; Gastroent. (780)489-8081; Fax. (780)489-5070.

CHERRY, Richard A; London HSC-Victoria Hosp, PO Box 5010 Stn B 800 Commissioners Rd E, London ON N6A 5W9; Wes'93; FRCPC; Anes. Staff, London Health Sciences Centre - Victoria Campus; (519)685-8500 x58525

CHERRY, Tadd Q; Peter Lougheed Centre, 3500 26 Ave NE, Calgary AB T1Y 6J4; Sask'02; FRCPC; Anes. Staff, Peter Lougheed Centre; (403)943-5554

CHERTKOW, Howard M; Smbd Jewish Gen Hosp, 3755 ch Cote-Sainte-Catherine, Montreal QC H3T 1E2; Wes'78; AB; FRCPC; Neur (Behavioural Neurology). Co- Dir Memory Clinic & Staff Neurol, Sir Mortimer B Davis Jewish General; Dir, Bloomfield Centre for Research in Aging; Prof, McGill University; (514)340-8260 x5129; Fax. (514)340-8295; howard.chertkow@mcgill.ca.

CHESEBROUGH, John N; James Street Med Walk-In Clini, 179 James St S, Hamilton ON L8P 3A3; Qns'59; (905)529-9779

CHESHENCHUK, Svitlana; Quance East Med Clinic, 49-2223 Victoria Ave E, Regina SK S4N 6E4; Vinnitza (Ukraine)'86; CCFP; Physician, Quance East Medical Clinic; Langs: Ukrainian; Polish; Russian; (306)522-2278

CHESINE, Stephen M; Carlingwood Active Care Clinic, 35B-2121 Carling Ave, Ottawa ON K2A 1H2; Wes'91; CCFP; FCFP; (613)761-6777; Fax. (613)761-7744.

CHESKES, Albert; Bochner Eye Institute, 40 Prince Arthur Ave, Toronto ON M5R 1A9; Tor'61; MSc(Ophth.); DAB; FRCSC; Ophth (Cataract Surgery). Ac Staff, Rouge Valley Health System - Centenary Health Centre Site; Ac Staff, St Michael's Hospital; Court Staff, Sunnybrook Health Sciences Centre; Asst Prof, University of Toronto; (416)921-2131; Fax. (416)966-8917.

CHESKES, Jordan W; Scarborough Eye Associates, 2941 Lawrence Ave E, Scarborough ON M1P 2V6; Tor'96; FRCSC; Ophth (Retinal Disease & Surgery). Lecturer, University of Toronto; (416)438-6000; Fax. (416)438-6206.

CHESKES, Sheldon; Queen-Lynch Med Centre, 101-157 Queen St E, Brampton ON L6W 3X4; Tor'84; CCFP; CCFP(E.M.); FCFP; Div Chief EmergMed/Ac Staff, William Osler Health System - Brampton Civic Hospital; Med Dir, Sunnybrook Osler Centre for Pre Hospital Care; (905)453-1340; Fax. (905)453-5493.

CHESKO, Jennifer C; 302-1497 Marine Dr, West Vancouver BC V7T 1B8; UBC'99; FRCPC; Psy. (604)922-0313

CHESLOCK, Carole; Capilano Med Clinic, 7905 106 Ave NW, Edmonton AB T6A 1H7; Ott'81; CCFP; FCFP; Med Staff, Queen Elizabeth II Hospital; (780)465-0951; Fax. (780)465-6928.

CHESNAY, Marylene; Clinique Med Optimum, 158-1 Place Laval, Laval QC H7N 1A1; Mon'01; Staff, Hôpital de Saint-Eustache; (450)668-7400; Fax. (450)668-5855.

CHESNEY, Alden E; Sunnybrook Hlth Sciences Ctre, B204-2075 Bayview Ave, Toronto ON M4N 3M5; Havana (Cuba)'83; Staff, Sunnybrook Health Sciences Centre; (416)480-4052; Fax. (416)480-6035.

CHESNEY, Amy L; Sunnybrook Health Sciences Ctr, M1 514-2075 Bayview Ave, Toronto ON M4N 3M5; Tor'06; PlasSurg. Staff Plastic Surg, Sunnybrook Health Sciences Centre; (416)480-6069

CHESNEY, Sarah A; F W Green Med Centre, 1629 Baker St, Cranbrook BC V1C 1B4; Alb'97; CCFP; FCFP; (250)426-6601; Fax. (250)426-6470.

CHESS, David G; St Joseph's Health Care, PO Box 5777 Stn B 268 Grosvenor St, London ON N6A 4V2; Wes'80; MSc; FRCSC; OrthSurg. Staff OrthSurg, St Joseph's Hospital - St Joseph's Health Care; Assoc Prof OrthSurg, University of Western Ontario; (519)646-6166; Fax. (519)646-6049.

CHESSER, Tracey M; The Moncton Hosp, 135 MacBeath Ave, Moncton NB E1C 6Z8; Laval'96; CCFP; CCFP(E.M.); Staff, The Moncton Hospital; Langs: English; French; (506)857-5520; traceychesser@hotmail.com.

CHESSER, W Gary; Moncton Med Clinic, 407-860 Mountain Rd, Moncton NB E1C 2N7; Dal'68; CCFP; FCFP; Ac Staff, The Moncton Hospital; Preceptor, Dalhousie University; (506)853-5168

CHESSEX, Caroline; Univ Hlth Network-Toronto Western Hosp, E5 469-399 Bathurst St, Toronto ON M5T 2S8; McG'98; FRCPC; IntMed. Staff, Toronto Western Hospital - University Health Network; (416)603-5800; Fax. (416)603-5274.

CHESSEX, Noemie; Thunder Bay Reg HSC-T-Bay, 980 Oliver Rd, Thunder Bay ON P7B 6V4; McG'05; FRCPC; IntMed; Critical Care Medicine. Staff, Thunder Bay Regional Health Sciences Centre; (807)684-6000

CHESSEX, Philippe; 311.B-4821 boul Saint-Laurent, Montreal QC H2T 1R6; Geneva (Switzerland)'75; FRCPC; Peds. Langs: English; French; (514)718-1247

CHESTNUT, Heidi A; Family Med Associates, 500-267 O'Connor St, Ottawa ON K2P 1V3; Cal'01; CCFP; (613)234-5588; Fax. (613)232-4818.

CHESTNUT, Shannon G; Lion's Gate Hosp, 231 15th St E, North Vancouver BC V7L 2L7; McM'05; CCFP; CCFP(E.M.); Staff, Lions Gate Hospital; (604)988-3131

CHETAILLE, Philippe; CHUQ-Ctr Hosp Univ Laval, 2705 boul Laurier, Quebec QC G1V 4G2; Aix-Marseille II (France)'00; Staff, Centre Hospitalier Universitaire de Quebec-CHUL; (514)654-2708; Fax. (514)654-2710.

CHETAILLE NEZONDET, Anne-Laure; CHUQ-Ctr Hosp Univ Laval, 2705 boul Laurier, Quebec QC G1V 4G2; Marseille (France)'01; MSc; MD; Ac Staff, Centre Hospitalier Universitaire de Quebec-CHUL; Clin Prof, Université Laval; (418)654-2242; Fax. (418)654-2798; anne-laure.chetaille@mail.chuq.qc.ca.

CHETE, Edwin O; St Paul's Hosp, 1081 Burrard St, Vancouver BC V6Z 1Y6; Staff, Providence Health Care - St Paul's Hospital; (604)806-8320

CHETNER, Cynthia S; 300-2580 32 St NE, Calgary AB T1Y 7M8; Cal'82; FRCPC; Psy. Staff, Peter Lougheed Centre; (403)944-9800; Fax. (403)944-9850.

CHETNER, Michael P; Hys Med Centre, 400-11010 101 St NW, Edmonton AB T5H 4B9; Alb'83; FRCSC; Urol. Staff Privil, Covenant Health - Misericordia Community Hospital; Consultant Privil, Covenant Health - Grey Nuns Community Hospital; Staff Privil, Glenrose Rehabilitation Hospital; Asst Prof, University of Alberta; (780)441-2574

CHETTAOUI, Olfa; CSSS Maria-Chapdelaine, 2000 boul du Sacre-Coeur, Dolbeau-Mistassini QC G8L 2R5; (Tunisia)'04; Staff, Centre Maria-Chapdelaine - CH de Dolbeau-Mistassini; (418)276-1234

CHETTIAR, Nataraj V; Medical Complex, 1057 St. Peter Ave, Bathurst NB E2A 2Z6; Dublin (Ireland)'79; (506)546-8313; Fax. (506)548-0917.

CHETTIAR, Ramasami V; 200-651 Boul Everard H Daigle, Gr-Sault/Gr-Falls NB E3Z 2S2; Dublin (Ireland)'74; Staff, Hôpital Général de Grand-Falls; Langs: Bilingual(English/French); (506)473-4000; Fax. (506)473-5191.

CHETTIMADA, Anil; 7-570 University Ave E, Waterloo ON N2K 4P2; Mangalore (India)'95; MB BS; CCFP; FCFP; Staff, Grand River Hospital - Kitchener/Waterloo Health Centre; (519)743-2951; Fax. (519)743-8052; achettimada@yahoo.ca.

CHETTLE, Crystal A; Brant Community HC-Brantford, 200 Terrace Hill St, Brantford ON N3R 1G9; Tor'05; FRCPC; Anes. Staff, The Brant Community Healthcare System - Brantford General Hospital Site; (519)751-5508; Fax. (519)751-5550.

CHETTY, Praven; Beach Avenue Med Clinic, 5848D Beach Ave, Peachland BC V0H 1X7; Witwatersrand (South Africa)'01; MB BCh; (250)767-3432

CHETTY, Rajendra M; 250 Patillo Rd, Windsor ON N8N 2L9; Sask'85; FRCPC; IntMed; Cardiol. Staff Cardiol, Hôtel-Dieu Grace Hospital; Staff Cardiol, Windsor Regional Hospital - Tayfour Site; (519)727-5500

CHETTY, Runjan; Univ Hlth Network-Toronto Gen, EW 11F-200 Elizabeth St, Toronto ON M5G 2C4; RCS (Ireland)'82; MB ChB; FRCPath(UK); Dir Surgical Pathologist, Toronto General Hospital - UHN; Prof Path, University of Toronto; Langs: Afrikaans; (416)340-3661; Fax. (416)340-5517.

CHETTY, Vanessa; Arya Medical Clinic, 8708 155 St NW, Edmonton AB T5R 1W2; Natal (South Africa)'97; Staff, Slave Lake Health Care Centre; (780)483-7860; Fax. (780)483-7868; slfc379@telus.net.

CHETTY, Vasudhevan; PO Box 63071 Rpo University Pl, Hamilton ON L9H 6Y3; Natal (South Africa)'85; FRCPC; MedBiochem (Diabetes). Staff, St Joseph's Healthcare - Charlton Campus.

CHEUK, Stephen T; Arid Moutain Clinic, 143-2515 90 Ave SW, Calgary AB T2V 0L8; Ott'01; FRCPC; Peds; ClinImmunol&Allergy. (403)251-6066; Fax. (403)251-6065.

CHEUNG, Alicia K F; Woodbine Med Centre, 233-8787 Woodbine Ave, Markham ON L3R 9S2; Alb'97; CCFP; FCFP; (905)415-0800; Fax. (905)415-0801.

CHEUNG, Amy H Y; Sunnybrook Hlth Sciences Ctre, 2075 Bayview Ave, Toronto ON M4N 3M5; McM'97; FRCPC; Psy. Staff, Sunnybrook Health Sciences Centre; (416)480-4073; Fax. (416)480-6878.

CHEUNG, Andrea; BC Cancer Agency, 600 10th Ave, Vancouver BC V5Z 4E6; Tor'07; CCFP; Staff, BC Cancer Agency Vancouver Centre; (604)877-6000

CHEUNG, Angela C; Univ Hlth Network-Toronto Western Hosp, 8MP 326-399 Bathurst St, Toronto ON M5T 2S8; Alb'07; FRCPC; IntMed (Family Medicine). Staff, Toronto Western Hospital - University Health Network; (416)603-5724; Fax. (416)603-5439.

CHEUNG, Angela M; Univ Hlth Network-Toronto Gen, 7EN 221-200 Elizabeth St, Toronto ON M5G 2C4; Johns Hopkins University (USA)'88; PhD; FRCPC; IntMed (Osteoporosis). Dir Osteoporosis Prog/Assoc Women's Health Prog, Toronto General Hospital - UHN; Assoc Prof Med, University of Toronto; Langs: Cantonese; (416)340-4609; Fax. (416)340-3750; angela.cheung@uhn.ca.

CHEUNG, Anita S P; 150-8220 Lansdowne Rd, Richmond BC V6X 1B9; UBC'84; CCFP; FCFP; (604)278-3322

CHEUNG, Anson W C; St Paul's Hosp, 1081 Burrard St, Vancouver BC V6Z 1Y6; Man'92; MD; FRCSC; CardSurg (Transplantation). Staff, Providence Health Care - St Paul's Hospital; Staff, Vancouver General Hospital - Centennial Pavillion; Langs: Chinese; (604)806-8282; Fax. (604)806-8375; acheung@providencehealth.bc.ca.

CHEUNG, Anthony P Y; Grace Fertility & Reproductive, 210-604 Broadway W, Vancouver BC V5Z 1G1; Sydney (Australia)'81; FRACOG; MPH; MBA; FRCSC; ObstGyn (Reproductive Endocrinology & Infertility). Staff, BC Women's Hospital & Health Centre; Asst Prof, University of British Columbia; Langs: Chinese; (604)558-4886

CHEUNG, Arthur; BC Cancer Agency-Fraser Valley, 13750 96 Ave, Surrey BC V3V 1Z2; Wes'03; FRCPC; RadOncol. Staff, BC Cancer Agency Fraser Valley Centre; (604)930-4036

CHEUNG, Bonnie; 1 Frobisher St, Richmond Hill ON L4B 4H7; Qns'90; MD; Langs: Chinese; Mandarin; (416)442-2218; Fax. (416)510-6870; jcheung@scottsinfo.com.

CHEUNG, C Y Mark; Sunnybrook Hlth Sciences Ctre, C410A-2075 Bayview Ave, Toronto ON M4N 3M5; Tor'80; FRCPC; MedBiochem; IntMed. Ac Staff Med, Sunnybrook Health Sciences Centre; Asst Prof, University of Toronto; (416)480-4991

CHEUNG, Candy M W; Crescent Heights Health Clinic, 107-233 16 Ave NW, Calgary AB T2M 0H5; UBC'08; CCFP; (403)230-3866; Fax. (403)230-5866.

CHEUNG, Carol; Univ Hlth Network-Toronto Gen, 11F-200 Elizabeth St, Toronto ON M5G 2C4; Tor'96; FRCPC; AnatPath. Staff, Toronto General Hospital - UHN; (416)340-4800

CHEUNG, Catherine Z; The Credit Valley Hosp, 2200 Eglinton Ave W, Mississauga ON L5M 2N1; Qns'00; FRCPC; IntMed; GeriatricMed. Staff Wound Healing Clinic, Women's College Hospital; The Credit Valley Hospital; (905)813-2200; Fax. (905)813-3855.

CHEUNG, Christian S G; Surrey Mem Hosp, 13750 96 Ave, Surrey BC V3V 1Z2; UBC'98; CCFP; Staff, Surrey Memorial Hospital; (604)307-8837; christian456@me.com.

CHEUNG, Christina S; Northmount Med Centre, 204-145 13 St E, North Vancouver BC V7L 2L4; Qns'06; FRCPC; Neur. (604)924-4002

CHEUNG, C L Benny; Crescent Heights Health Clinic, 107-233 16 Ave NW, Calgary AB T2M 0H5; Alb'02; CCFP; (403)230-3866

CHEUNG, Cindy H; The Peterborough Clinic, 201-26 Hospital Dr, Peterborough ON K9J 7C3; Dal'97; FRCSC; Ophth. (705)740-6854; Fax. (705)740-6865.

CHEUNG, Colleen K Y; Thornhill Med Centre, 18 Centre St, Thornhill ON L4J 1E9; Tor'97; BSc; CCFP; Staff, Mackenzie Richmond Hill Hospital; (905)889-3634; Fax. (905)889-3986.

CHEUNG, Denis K T; Rideau Valley Health Services, 1221 Greenbank Rd, Ottawa ON K2J 5V7; (Hong Kong)'70; FAAFP; DABFP; CCFP; FCFP; Staff, Children's Hospital of Eastern Ontario (CHEO); (613)258-8710

CHEUNG, Francesca T; 201-5762 Highway 7, Markham ON L3P 1A8; McM'06; CCFP; Langs: Cantonese; Mandarin; (905)471-5022; Fax. (905)471-1878.

CHEUNG, Garvin L; PO Box 4333 Stn South CRO, Edmonton AB T6E 4T3; Alb'07; CCFP.

CHEUNG, Gordon; CML Healthcare, 100-10 Kingsbridge Garden Cir, Mississauga ON L5R 3K6; Tor'83; FRCPC; DiagRad (MRI). Staff, Joseph Brant Memorial Hospital; Staff Radiol, Sunnybrook Health Sciences Centre; Asst Prof, University of Toronto; (905)568-3768; Fax. (905)568-9652.

CHEUNG, Humphrey H; Chinook Reg Hosp, 960 19 St S, Lethbridge AB T1J 1W5; Ireland (Ireland)'94; MB ChB; BAO; Staff, Chinook Regional Hospital; Langs: Cantonese; (403)388-6131; Fax. (403)388-6154.

CHEUNG, Hym D; Ashgrove Med Centre, 310-6633 Highway 7, Markham ON L3P 7P2; Qns'72; Ac Staff, The Scarborough Hospital - General Campus; (905)472-3918; Fax. (905)472-3919.

CHEUNG, Jasmine S; Scarborough Hosp-Birchmount, 3030 Birchmount Rd, Scarborough ON M1W 3W3; Tor'05; FRCPC; Anes. Staff, The Scarborough Hospital - Birchmount Campus; (416)319-8992

CHEUNG, John P; Hotel-Dieu Hosp, 166 Brock St, Kingston ON K7L 5G2; Tor'95; FRCSC; Ophth. Staff, Hotel-Dieu Hospital; (613)544-3310 x2612; Fax. (613)544-3955; jopch@hotmail.com.

CHEUNG, Joseph Y; 10917 82 Ave NW PO Box 52252, Edmonton AB T6G 0S7; Alb'09; CCFP.

CHEUNG, Justin; 410-301 Columbia St E, New Westminster BC V3L 3W5; UBC'02; FRCPC; IntMed (Gastroenterology); Gastroent. (604)525-0155

CHEUNG, Ka Wai; Vancouver Gen Hosp, 855 12th Ave W, Vancouver BC V5Z 1M9; McM'03; FRCPC; EmergMed. Staff, Vancouver General Hospital - Centennial Pavillion; (604)875-4111

CHEUNG, Kar Wing; Palisades Med Clinic, 12808 137 Ave, Edmonton AB T5L 4Y8; UBC'03; CCFP; (780)457-1100; Fax. (780)457-0033.

CHEUNG, Ken; Foothills Med Centre, 1403 29 St NW, Calgary AB T2N 2T9; UBC'94; FRCPC; Anes. Staff, Foothills Medical Centre; Asst Prof, University of Calgary; Langs: Cantonese; (403)944-1430; Fax. (403)944-2425.

CHEUNG, King; Hys Medical Centre, 11010 101 St NW, Edmonton AB T5H 4B9; (Hong Kong)'70; MB BS; FRCPC; DiagRad. Staff, Royal Alexandra Hospital; Teach Staff Radiol & Diagnostic Imaging, University of Alberta; Langs: Cantonese; (780)426-1121

CHEUNG, Lai-Keung; Lindenridge Med Centre, E-123 Scurfield Blvd, Winnipeg MB R3Y 1L6; (Taiwan)'71; GenSurg (Endoscopy). Langs: Chinese.

CHEUNG, Lawrence A; University of Alberta Hosp, 2E4. 34WCM-8440 112 St NW, Edmonton AB T6G 2B7; Alb'93; FRCPC; IntMed; Critical Care Medicine; Respir. Staff, University of Alberta Hospital; (780)407-7593; Fax. (780)407-6384.

CHEUNG, Lily S K; 3282 Douglas St, Burlington ON L7N 1G9; McG'63; DOHS; AB(OccupMed); FRCPC; IntMed; OccupMed. (905)639-5410

CHEUNG, M C Raphael; Regional Bariatric Assesstment, 1453 Prince Rd, Windsor ON N9C 3Z4; Tor'76; ABIM; FRCPC; IntMed (Diabetology); Endocrin&Metab (P.Q.). Staff, Hôtel-Dieu Grace Hospital; Staff, Windsor Regional Hospital - Metropolitan Site; Windsor Regional Hospital - Tayfour Site; Staff, Regional Bariatric Assessment & Treatment Centre; Assoc Prof, University Of Windsor; Aj Prof Med, University of Western Ontario; Langs: Chinese; (519)971-9206; Fax. (519)971-9566.

CHEUNG, Matthew C T; Sunnybrook Hlth Sciences Ctre, T2-031-2075 Bayview Ave, Toronto ON M4N 3M5; Tor'99; FRCPC; IntMed; Hem. Staff, Sunnybrook Health Sciences Centre; (416)480-4757; Fax. (416)480-6002.

CHEUNG, Ming-Tat; Westlaw Bldg, 205A-1920 Weston Rd, York ON M9N 1W4; National (Taiwan)'62; FACC; FRCPC; IntMed. Staff, Humber River Regional Hospital - Church Street Site; Staff, St Michael's Hospital; University of Toronto; (416)249-0067; Fax. (416)249-3005.

CHEUNG, Ngai Hoi; 302-2299 Dundas St W, Toronto ON M6R 1X7; Tor'76; Ac Staff, St Joseph's Health Centre; (416)535-2433; Fax. (416)535-1538.

CHEUNG, Patrick C F; Sunnybrook Odette Cancer Centr, 2075 Bayview Ave, Toronto ON M4N 3M5; Tor'95; MD; FRCPC; RadOncol (Lung Cancer). Court Staff, North York General Hospital; Ac Staff, Sunnybrook Health Sciences Centre; Staff Rad Oncologist, Toronto East General Hospital Inc; Asst Prof RadOncol, University of Toronto; Langs: Cantonese; (416)480-6165; Fax. (416)480-6002.

CHEUNG, Paul K; Credit Valley Med Arts Centre, 302-2000 Credit Valley Rd, Mississauga ON L5M 4N4; Mon'10; CCFP; (905)813-3850

CHEUNG, Po Kee; Hys Med Centre, 350-11010 101 St NW, Edmonton AB T5H 4B9; (Hong Kong)'80; FACC; FRCPC; IntMed; Cardiol. Staff, Royal Alexandra Hospital; (780)428-3246; Fax. (780)425-0487.

CHEUNG, Po-Yin; Royal Alexandra Hosp, 10240 Kingsway NW, Edmonton AB T5H 3V9; Hongkong (Hong Kong)'85; PhD; FRCPC; Peds (Neonatal & Perinatal Medicine). Staff, Royal Alexandra Hospital; Prof, University of Alberta; (780)735-6870; Fax. (780)735-4072; poyin@ualberta.ca.

CHEUNG, Raymond W; Magrath Med Clinic, 308-14127 23 Ave NW, Edmonton AB T6R 0G4; Alb'05; CCFP; (780)430-8788

CHEUNG, Roderick T F; 7-105 Progress Cres, Kapuskasing ON P5N 3J4; Tor'09; CCFP; (705)335-2051

CHEUNG, Roy L H; 401-1990 Fort St, Victoria BC V8R 6V4; McM'98; Otol. (250)590-4008; Fax. (250)590-4686.

CHEUNG, Simon S; Peel Village Med Centre, 28 Rambler Dr, Brampton ON L6W 1E2; Tor'79; CCFP; FCFP; Court Staff, William Osler Health System - Brampton Civic Hospital; (905)451-5586; Fax. (905)451-1233.

CHEUNG, Stephen S K; Surrey Med Arts Bldg, 117-13798 94A Ave, Surrey BC V3V 1N1; UBC'95; ABIM; FRCPC; IntMed; Cardiol. Staff Med, Surrey Memorial Hospital; Langs: Cantonese; (604)582-6400; Fax. (604)588-3122.

CHEUNG, Tak-Kee; Harrow H C Inc-A Family Hlth Team, PO Box 430 1480 Eric Rd S, Harrow ON N0R 1G0; Dairen (China)'55; Langs: Chinese; (519)738-2000

CHEUNG, Teresa P C; 203-316 King St E, Cobourg ON K9A 5R8; Tor'96; CCFP; (905)373-1280; Fax. (905)373-9335.

CHEUNG, Vera K F; Kingsbridge Med Center, 5-20 Kingsbridge Garden Circle, Mississauga ON L5R 3K7; Alb'04; CCFP; (905)507-1111

CHEUNG, Vincent S J; Peterborough Reg Nephrology, 239 Charlotte St, Peterborough ON K9J 2V2; Ott'94; FRCPC; IntMed (Cardiology); Nephrol. Staff, Peterborough Regional Health Centre - Hospital Drive; Court Staff, Ross Memorial Hospital; Court Staff, Northumberland Hills Hospital; Langs: English; French; (705)750-1786; Fax. (705)750-0591.

CHEUNG, W C Thomas; 3-5636 Glen Erin Dr, Mississauga ON L5M 6B1; (Hong Kong)'76; MB BS(HK); FRCS(Ed & Glas); FHKAM(Orth.); CCFP; Staff Family Med, The Credit Valley Hospital; Langs: Mandarin; Cantonese; (905)567-5991; Fax. (905)567-5435.

CHEUNG, Wendy H; Hamilton HS-McMaster Site, PO Box 2000 Stn Lcd 1 1200 Main St W, Hamilton ON L8N 3Z5; (Hong Kong)'90; FAAP; FRCPC; Peds. Staff, Hamilton Health Sciences Centre - McMaster Children's Hospital; Langs: Chinese.

CHEUNG, Winson Y T; BC Cancer Agency-Vancouver CC, 600 10th Ave W, Vancouver BC V5Z 4E6; UBC'03; FRCPC; IntMed; MedOncol. Staff, BC Cancer Agency Vancouver Centre; (604)877-6000

CHEUNG-LEE, Melody; Westgrove Prof Bldg, 325-10230 142 St NW, Edmonton AB T5N 3Y6; Alb'04; BMedSci; FRCPC; Derm. Clin Lecturer, University of Alberta; Langs: Mandarin; Cantonese; (780)757-1891; Fax. (780)757-1892.

CHEVALIER, Andree; Hop Maisonneuve-Rosemont, 5415 boul de l'Assomption, Montreal QC H1T 2M4; Mon'84; CSPQ; FRCPC; Anes. Staff, Hopital Maisonneuve-Rosemont; (514)252-3400

CHEVALIER, Christine; CSSS du Sud de Lanaudière, 911 montee des Pionniers, Terrebonne QC J6V 2H2; Sher'86; GenSurg (P.Q.). Staff, Centre Hospitalier Pierre le Gardeur; (450)654-7525

CHEVALIER, Claudia; 1600 boul Saint-Martin E, Laval QC H7G 4R8; Mon'08; Peds. (450)669-6666

CHEVALIER, Isabelle M; Hôpital Ste-Justine, 3175 ch Cote-Sainte-Catherine, Montreal QC H3T 1C5; McG'95; FAAP; ABPeds; LRCPS; MSc; FRCPC; Peds. Staff, Hôpital Ste-Justine; (514)345-4931 x5554

CHEVALIER, Jean-Francois; Dr J F Chevalier Inc, 212-300 Columbia St, Kamloops BC V2C 6L1; Laval'96; FRCSC; Neursurg (Spine Surgery). Langs: Bilingual(French/English); (250)374-1259; Fax. (250)374-1260.

CHEVALIER, Manon; Ctr Hosp Affilie-Enfant-Jesus, 1401 18e rue, Quebec QC G1J 1Z4; Sher'84; FRCPC; IntMed; GeriatricMed. Staff, Centre Hospitalier Affilié Universitaire de Québec - Hôpital De L'Enfant Jésus; (418)649-5521; Fax. (418)649-5507.

CHEVALIER, Marguerite B; Marguerite Chevalier Prof Corp, 2-1275 Walker Rd, Windsor ON N8Y 4X9; McM'95; BHSc; CCFP; FCFP; Court Staff, Hôtel-Dieu Grace Hospital; Ac Staff/Chief Family Practice, Windsor Regional Hospital - Metropolitan Site; (519)253-9116; Fax. (519)253-5404.

CHEVALIER, Natalie; Clinique Med Richelieu, 202-500 rte Marie-Victorin, Sorel-Tracy QC J3R 1K7; Mon'87; (450)742-9818; Fax. (450)742-9795.

CHEVALIER, Pierre; CSSS de Saint-Jerome, 290 rue de Montigny, Saint-Jerome QC J7Z 5T3; Mon'80; FRCPC; IntMed. Staff, Hôtel-Dieu de Saint-Jérôme; (450)431-8200; Fax. (450)431-8244.

CHEVARIE, Karine; CHUQ-Ctr Hosp Univ Laval, 2705 boul Laurier, Quebec QC G1V 4G2; Laval'99; Staff, Centre Hospitalier Universitaire de Quebec-CHUL; (418)654-2255; Fax. (418)577-4664.

CHEVERIE, Donald J; Dartmouth Gen Hosp, 325 Pleasant St, Dartmouth NS B2Y 4G8; Dal'77; FRCPC; DiagRad. Staff Radiol, Dartmouth General Hospital; Radiologist, Twin Oaks Memorial Hospital; Staff Radiol., Eastern Shore Memorial Hospital; Pt-Time Lect., DiagRad., Dalhousie University; (902)465-8321; Fax. (902)465-8360; dchev@ns.sympatico.ca.

CHEVRETTE, David; Clin d'Ophtalmologie du Saguen, 150 boul Barette, Chicoutimi QC G7H 7W8; Laval'02; FRCSC; Ophth. (418)545-2571; Fax. (418)545-0774.

CHEVRETTE, Eric; CHUQ-Ctr Hosp Univ Laval, 2705 boul Laurier, Quebec QC G1V 4G2; Laval'94; FRCPC; DiagRad. Staff, Centre Hospitalier Universitaire de Quebec-CHUL; (418)656-4141 x42258

CHEVRETTE, Evelyne; Clinique Med de Levis, 100-4975 boul de la Rive-Sud, Levis QC G6V 4Z5; Laval'06; (418)833-5810

CHEVRETTE, Karine; CSSS du Sud de Lanaudière, 911 Montee des Pionniers, Terrebonne QC J6V 2H2; Mon'96; Staff, Centre Hospitalier Pierre le Gardeur; (450)654-7525

CHEVRETTE, Line; Gladstone Medi-Centre, 4095 rue Tupper, Westmount QC H3Z 3E5; Mon'58; AB; FRCSC; Ophth (Pediatric Ophthalmology). Court Staff, Hôpital Ste-Justine; Langs: Bilingual(French/English); (514)345-4931 x5956

CHEVRETTE, Marie-Christine; Ctr Hosp Chauveau, 11999 rue de l'Hopital, Quebec QC G2A 2T7; Staff, Centre Hospitalier Chauveau; (418)842-3651; Fax. (418)842-1948.

CHEVRETTE, Maurice; CSSS de Saint-Jerome, 290 rue de Montigny, Saint-Jerome QC J7Z 5T3; Mon'67; Staff, Hôtel-Dieu de Saint-Jérôme; (450)431-8393; Fax. (450)431-8392.

CHEVRETTE, Yves; Ctr Hosp Reg de Lanaudiere, 1000 boul Sainte-Anne, St-Charles-Brromee QC J6E 6J2; Mon'85; FRCPC; DiagRad. Staff, Centre Hospitalier Régional de Lanaudière; (450)759-8222; Fax. (450)759-2133.

CHEVRIER, Pierre; CHUS-Hop Fleurimont, 3001 12e Av N, Sherbrooke QC J1H 5N4; Sher'78; CSPQ; FRCPC; MedBiochem. Staff, Centre Hospitalier Universitaire de Sherbrooke-Hopital Fleurimont; (819)346-1110 x15578

CHEVRIER, Robert L A; Medical-Surgical Eye Bldg, 879 Shefford Rd, Gloucester ON K1J 8H9; Ott'91; FRCSC; Ophth (General Ophthalmic Surgery). Ac Staff, The Ottawa Hospital - General Campus; Consultant, SCO Health Service - Élisabeth Bruyère Hospital; Ac Staff Ophth, Montfort Hospital; Lecturer Ophth, University of Ottawa; (613)741-4342; Fax. (613)741-7338.

CHEW, Ben H; Diamond Health Care Center, 6F-2775 Laurel St, Vancouver BC V5Z 1M9; UBC'98; FRCSC; Urol (Endourology). Ac Staff Vancouver Costal Health, Vancouver General Hospital - Centennial Pavillion; Ac Staff Vancouver Costal Health, UBC Hospital - Koerner Pavillion; Ac Staff Providence Health Care, Providence Health Care - St Paul's Hospital; Ac Staff Providence Health Care, Providence Health Care - Mount Saint Joseph Hospital; Asst Prof, University of British Columbia; Langs: Cantonese; (604)875-5003; Fax. (604)875-5604.

CHEW, Brian P A; Callingwood Med Centre, 454-6650 177 St NW, Edmonton AB T5T 4J5; Alb'94; BMedSci; CCFP; FCFP; Langs: Mandarin; Cantonese; (780)487-1223; Fax. (780)444-0974.

CHEW, Donald L; 5845 Ferry St, Niagara Falls ON L2G 1S5; McG'70; MBA; FRCPC; Neur. Assoc Staff, Niagara Health System - Greater Niagara General Site; Assoc Staff, Niagara Health System - St Catharines General Site; (905)357-3644; Fax. (905)357-9230; nns.niagara@sympatico.ca.

CHEW, Gilbert M M; 105-4442 West Saanich Rd, Victoria BC V8Z 3E9; UBC'74; BSc; Langs: Cantonese; (250)479-1606; Fax. (250)479-1607.

CHEW, Hall F; Sunnybrook Hlth Sciences Ctre, M1 302B-2075 Bayview Ave, Toronto ON M4N 3M5; Dal'02; FRCSC; Ophth (Cornea/External Disease). Staff, Sunnybrook Health Sciences Centre; Asst Prof Ophthalmology, University of Toronto; (416)480-5340

CHEW, Jason B; 899 12th Ave W, Vancouver BC V5Z 1M9; Auckland (New Zealand)'94; FRCPC; DiagRad. Staff, Vancouver General Hospital - Centennial Pavillion; Staff, Royal Columbian Hospital; (604)875-4000

CHEW, Jennifer P S; Fifth Avenue Court, 17-99 Fifth Ave, Ottawa ON K1S 5K4; Ott'98; CCFP; FCFP; (613)563-3670; Fax. (613)563-4124.

CHEW, Jesse; 1025-1200 Burrard St, Vancouver BC V6Z 2C7; UBC'99; FRCSC; Ophth. Langs: Cantonese; (604)682-8211

CHEW, John K H; 500-71 King St W, Mississauga ON L5B 4A2; Tor'77; (905)270-0415; Fax. (905)848-1500.

CHEW, Julian I H; West Hillhurst Health Clinic, 2128 Kensington Rd NW, Calgary AB T2N 3R7; Alb'00; CCFP; (403)270-8939; Fax. (403)270-8937.

CHEW, Roderick T; Northmount Med Centre, 100-145 13th St E, North Vancouver BC V7L 2L4; Ott'01; FRCSC; PlasSurg. Staff, Vancouver General Hospital - Centennial Pavillion; (778)340-2662

CHEW, Sander J L; 2590 Commercial Dr, Vancouver BC V5N 4C2; UBC'92; (604)871-1535

CHEW, Sen; Guildford Med Dental Centre, 28-15300 105 Ave, Surrey BC V3R 6A7; National (Taiwan)'69; MB; Assoc Medical Staff, Surrey Memorial Hospital; Langs: Mandarin; Cantonese; (604)584-6666; Fax. (604)584-9894.

CHEYNE, Robert D; 1560 George St, White Rock BC V4B 4A5; UBC'77; Chairman Emerg Dept, Peace Arch Hospital; Dir, British Columbia Medical Association; (604)531-1451

CHEYNE, William J; 1934 Ambrosi Rd, Kelowna BC V1Y 4R9; Cal'74; Dip(SportsMed); CCFP; Staff, Kelowna General Hospital; (250)860-4844

CHHABRA, Samir R; Taunton Surgical Centre, 1290 Keith Ross Dr, Oshawa ON L1H 7K7; Bombay (India)'89; FRCS(Orth&Trauma); MCh(Ortho); LMCC; FRCSC; OrthSurg. Staff, Lakeridge Health - Oshawa Site; Langs: Hindi; Punjabi; (905)721-7729; Fax. (905)721-6677; samir@writeme.com.

CHHANABHAI, Mukesh; BC Cancer Agency-Fraser Valley, 13750 96 Ave, Surrey BC V3V 1Z2; Harare (Zimbabwe)'81; FRCPC; GenPath. Staff, Surrey Memorial Hospital; Staff, BC Cancer Agency Vancouver Centre; Langs: Gujarati; (604)588-3384

CHHATWAL, Gurpreet S; Grand Bank Comm Hlth Ctre, PO Box 310, Grand Bank NL A0E 1W0; Punjabi (India)'87; MB BS; (709)832-2500; chhatwal@mun.ca.

CHHATWAL, Jasjeet K; Grand Bank Community Hlth Ctre, PO Box 310, Grand Bank NL A0E 1W0; Punjabi (India)'91; MB BS; Staff, Grand Bank Health Centre; (709)832-2500

CHHIBBER, Sameer; South Health Campus, 480042-4448 Front St SE, Calgary AB T3M 1M4; Cal'05; FRCPC; Neur. Staff, Rockyview General Hospital; (403)956-3454; Fax. (403)956-3494.

CHHINA, Tejinder S; Trillium Health Ctre-Mississau, 100 Queensway W, Mississauga ON L5B 1B8; Wes'99; FRCPC; Anes. Staff, Trillium Health Centre - Mississauga; (905)848-7628

CHHIV, Mony; 1-306 rue Jeanne-d'Arc, Quebec QC G1S 2R7; Mon'05; FRCSC; GenSurg. (418)266-3593

CHI, Frank W; 70 Spine Rd, Elliot Lake ON P5A 1X2; Ott'78; BSc; Staff, St Joseph's General Hospital Elliot Lake; Langs: Chinese; (705)848-7181; Fax. (705)848-9006; fchi@sjgh.ca.

CHI, Kim Nguyen; BC Cancer Agency-Vancouver CC, 600 10th Ave W, Vancouver BC V5Z 4E6; Ott'93; FRCPC; IntMed; MedOncol. Staff, BC Cancer Agency Vancouver Centre; Staff Surg, Vancouver General Hospital - Centennial Pavillion; Asst Prof, University of British Columbia; (604)877-6098; Fax. (604)877-0585.

CHIA, Edison W; 204 rue Principale Sud, Waterville QC J0B 3H0; Sask'74; (819)837-2668

CHIA, Shea Tzi; Dixon Med Centre, 207-531 Davis Dr, Newmarket ON L3Y 6P5; Wes'00; FRCSC; GenSurg. Ac Staff, Southlake Regional Health Centre; (905)953-8838; Fax. (905)953-8521.

CHIA, Shirline S L; PO Box 80012 Rpo Beacon Hill, Calgary AB T3R 0B2; Cal'09; CCFP.

CHIA, Stephen K L; BC Cancer Agency-Vancouver CC, 600 10th Ave W, Vancouver BC V5Z 4E6; UBC'93; FRCPC; IntMed (Breast Cancer); MedOncol. Staff, BC Cancer Agency Vancouver Centre; Asst Prof, University of British Columbia; (604)877-6000; Fax. (604)877-0585; schia@bccancer.bc.ca.

CHIAM, Benjamin T H; The Lung Health Clinic, 8737 156 St NW, Edmonton AB T5R 1Y5; Qns'99; FRCPC; IntMed; Respir. Staff, University of Alberta Hospital; (780)498-1800; Fax. (780)483-7774.

CHIAM, Tow-Foon; Millbourne Market Mall Tower 2, 330-3699 Mill Woods Rd NW, Edmonton AB T6K 3L6; (Taiwan)'72; CCFP; Staff, Royal Alexandra Hospital; (780)462-6806; Fax. (780)462-6807.

CHIAMVIMONVAT, Kanchana; Place Centrum Med Centre, 110-210 Centrum Blvd, Orleans ON K1E 3V7; Tor'84; (613)834-2828; Fax. (613)834-3227.

CHIAMVIMONVAT, Vera; 300 3-690 Dorval Dr, Oakville ON L6K 3W7; Tor'90; FRCPC; IntMed (Nuclear Cardiology); Cardiol. Staff, Women's College Hospital; Staff, Halton Healthcare Services Corporation - Oakville Site; Langs: Thai; (905)849-4567 x1; Fax. (905)845-3996.

CHIANETTA, Jean-Marc; Dr Georges-L Dumont Reg Hosp, 330 av Universite, Moncton NB E1C 2Z3; Sher'04; FRCPC; Psy. Staff, Dr Georges-L-Dumont University Hospital Centre; (506)862-4000

CHIANG, Christopher K C; Kings Cross Doctor's Office, 4-17 Kings Cross Rd, Brampton ON L6T 3V5; Tor'87; CCFP; Ac Staff, William Osler Health System - Brampton Civic Hospital; Langs: Mandarin; (905)799-0925; Fax. (905)799-4756.

CHIANG, James B; Albion-Kipling Med Centre, 207-1525 Albion Rd, Etobicoke ON M9V 5G5; Tor'62; Sr Staff, Humber River Regional Hospital - Church Street Site; (416)741-6314; Fax. (416)742-3932.

CHIANG, Lisa A; Albion-Kipling Med Centre, 207-1525 Albion Rd, Etobicoke ON M9V 5G5; Tor'89; (416)741-6314; Fax. (416)742-3932.

CHIANG, Mae S M; Lakeridge Hlth Corp-Oshawa, 1 Hospital Crt, Oshawa ON L1G 2B9; Wes'04; FRCPC; IntMed. Staff, Lakeridge Health - Oshawa Site; (905)576-8711

CHIANG, N M Sheryl; 215-9450 137 Ave NW, Edmonton AB T5E 6C2; Alb'89; BMedSci; Langs: Cantonese; Mandarin; (780)475-0502; Fax. (780)473-5493.

CHIANG, Stephen C; Iroquois Falls Family Hlth Team, 58A Anson Dr, Iroquois Falls ON P0K 1E0; American U. (Montserrat)'84; CCFP; Chief of Staff, Anson General Hospital; Lead Phys, Iroquois Falls FHT; Asst Prof Family Med, Northern Ontario School of Medicine - Laurentian University; (705)258-2818; Fax. (705)258-2828.

CHIARELLA, Angelo B; Royal Alexandra Hosp, 10240 Kingsway NW, Edmonton AB T5H 3V9; Alb'98; FRCPC; Anes. Staff, Royal Alexandra Hospital; (780)920-9744

CHIAROTTO, James A; The Court, 105-2863 Ellesmere Rd, Scarborough ON M1E 5E9; Tor'88; MSc; FRCPC; IntMed (Hematology); MedOncol. Staff, Rouge Valley Health System - Centenary Health Centre Site; Langs: Italian; French; (416)281-7483; Fax. (416)281-7228.

CHIASSON, Chantal; Figurra Med Clinic, 79 rue Sackville, Shediac NB E4P 2R1; Sher'91; ABD; AAD; FRCPC; Derm (Aesthetic Surgery). Ac Member Derm, The Moncton Hospital; Consultant Derm, Dr Georges-L-Dumont University Hospital Centre; Langs: Bilingual(English/French); (506)533-2828

CHIASSON, Darrell E; Queen Elizabeth II HSC-Halifax, 355-1796 Summer St, Halifax NS B3H 3A7; Dal'03; CCFP; CCFP(E.M.); Staff, Queen Elizabeth II Health Sciences Centre - Halifax Infirmary Site; (902)473-2700

CHIASSON, David A; The Hosp for Sick Children, 555 University Ave, Toronto ON M5G 1X8; Dal'79; BSc; MD; FRCPC; AnatPath (Forensic Medicine). Staff, Toronto General Hospital - UHN; Dir Ped Forensic Pathology Unit, The Hospital For Sick Children; Consultant Office of the Coroner Consultant Forensic & Cardiovascular Path, Province of Ontario; Asst Prof Pathobiology & LabMed, University of Toronto; (416)813-7747

CHIASSON, Eric; CHUS-Hop Hotel-Dieu, 580 rue Bowen S, Sherbrooke QC J1G 2E8; Sher'05; Psy. Staff, Centre Hospitalier Universitaire de Sherbrooke-Hôpital Hôtel-Dieu; (819)346-1110

CHIASSON, Guylaine; Dr Georges-L Dumont Reg Hosp, 330 av Universite, Moncton NB E1C 2Z3; Laval'96; FRCPC; IntMed; GeriatricMed. Staff, Dr Georges-L-Dumont University Hospital Centre; (506)862-4000; gchiasson@rogers.com.

CHIASSON, J Roland; Summerside Med Centre, 1-475 Granville St, Summerside PE C1N 3N9; Dal'73; Court Staff, Prince County Hospital; Medical Staff, Veterans Affairs Canada; Langs: English; French; (902)432-8181; Fax. (902)566-8890; jrchiass@vac-acc.gc.ca.

CHIASSON, Jean L; CHUM-Hotel-Dieu, 3840 rue Saint-Urbain, Montreal QC H2W 1T8; Laval'67; Endocrin&Metab (P.Q.) (Diabetology). Staff, Centre Hospitalier l'Université de Montréal (CHUM) - Hôtel-Dieu; Prof, Universite de Montreal; (514)890-8000 x12732

CHIASSON, Jean-P.; Clinique du Nouveau Depart Inc, 1110 av Beaumont, Mont-Royal QC H3P 3E5; Mon'68; ASAM; Langs: English; (514)521-9023; Fax. (514)521-1928; cepat@videotron.ca.

CHIASSON, John D; 203-220 Main St, Antigonish NS B2G 2C2; Dal'79; Assoc Staff, St Martha's Regional Hospital; (902)863-4070; Fax. (902)863-2575.

CHIASSON, Marie-Lise; 2A boul St-Pierre O, Caraquet NB E1W 1B6; Laval'83; Staff, Hôpital de l'Enfant-Jésus RHSJ; Langs: English; (506)727-6524; Fax. (506)727-1187.

CHIASSON, Meredith D; Queen Elizabeth II HSC-Halifax, 1796 Summer St, Halifax NS B3H 3A7; Dal'05; FRCPC; IntMed; Respir. Staff, Queen Elizabeth II Health Sciences Centre - Halifax Infirmary Site; (902)473-3698; Fax. (902)473-6202.

CHIASSON, Michel T; Cheticamp Med Clinic, PO Box 220, Cheticamp NS B0E 1H0; Dal'00; CCFP; (902)224-3110; Fax. (902)224-1905.

CHIASSON, Myriam; Hotel-Dieu de Levis, 143 rue Wolfe, Levis QC G6V 3Z1; Sher'05; FRCPC; Psy. Staff, Hôtel-Dieu de Lévis; (418)835-7121

CHIASSON, Paul J; Springdale Prof Bldg, 315-2250 Bovaird Dr E, Brampton ON L6R 0W3; Dal'94; MD; FRCSC; GenSurg (Minimal Invasive Surgery); ThorSurg. Ac Staff, William Osler Health System - Brampton Civic Hospital; Ac Staff, William Osler Health System - Etobicoke General Hospital; Court Staff, The Credit Valley Hospital; Clinical Asst Prof, McMaster University; Lecturer Surg, University of Toronto; (905)458-4520; Fax. (905)458-4080; paul.chiasson@williamoslerhs.ca.

CHIASSON, Paul; 105-185 av Acadie, Dieppe NB E1A 1G6; Laval'88; CCFP; Staff, Dr Georges-L-Dumont University Hospital Centre; Clin Prof, Universite de Sherbrooke; Langs: English; (506)862-4182; Fax. (506)862-4179; chiassp@umoncton.ca.

CHIASSON, Renelle; Dr Renelle Chiasson Corp Prof, CP 4113 Succ B 3455 Main St, Tracadie-Sheila NB E1X 1G4; Mon'96; CCFP; Langs: Spanish; English; (506)393-1050; renelle2@nb.sympatico.ca.

CHIASSON-BASQUE, Renee; 16 Allee Pointe du Jour CP 2004, Lameque NB E8T 3N3; Sher'95; Langs: English; (506)344-2258; Fax. (506)344-2383.

CHIAVARAS, Mary M; Hamilton HS-General Site, 237 Barton St E, Hamilton ON L8L 2X2; Massachusetts (USA)'02; FRCPC; DiagRad. (905)527-4322; Fax. (905)527-5761.

CHIAVARO, Hector L; 307B-77 Queensway W, Mississauga ON L5B 1B7; Cordoba (Argentina)'65; ABPeds; FRCPC; Peds (Pediatric Allergy). Court Staff, Trillium Health Centre - Mississauga; Langs: Spanish; (905)566-9809; Fax. (905)566-8665; hectorchiavaro@sympatico.ca.

CHIBA, Naoki; 105-21 Surrey St W, Guelph ON N1H 3R3; Wes'86; MSc; FRCPC; IntMed; Gastroent. Staff, Guelph General Hospital; Consultant, Groves Memorial Community Hospital; Clin Assoc Prof Med, McMaster University; Langs: Japanese; (519)836-8201; Fax. (519)836-1341; naoki.chiba@rogers.com.

CHIBBAR, Rajni; Royal University Hosp, 103 Hospital Dr, Saskatoon SK S7N 0W8; Rajasthan (India)'78; FRCPC; GenPath. Staff, Royal University Hospital; (306)655-2153; Fax. (306)655-2223.

CHIBUK, Thea K; Edmonton Clinic Health Academy, 3 596A-11405 87 Ave NW, Edmonton AB T6G 1C9; Alb'06; FRCPC; Peds. Staff, University of Alberta Hospital; (780)248-5510; Fax. (780)248-5626.

CHICHA-DZINEKU, Madeleine; Hôpital Ste-Justine, 3175 ch Cote-Sainte-Catherine, Montreal QC H3T 1C5; St. Joseph (Lebanon)'72; CSPQ; Anes (P.Q.). Staff Anes, Hôpital Ste-Justine; Langs: Italian; English; (514)345-4733; Fax. (514)345-4601.

CHICHAK, Vernon R; Weinlos Clinic, 15508 87 Ave NW, Edmonton AB T5R 4G5; Alb'76; FRCPC; IntMed. (780)484-8151; Fax. (780)487-2047; vernchichak@shaw.ca.

CHICOINE, Jean-Francois; Hôpital Ste-Justine, 3175 ch Cote-Sainte-Catherine, Montreal QC H3T 1C5; Mon'80; FRCPC; Peds. Ac Staff, Hôpital Ste-Justine; adj Prof, Universite de Montreal; (514)345-4675; Fax. (514)345-4822.

CHICOINE, Michel; Clinique Cherrier, 837 rue Cherrier, Montreal QC H2L 1H6; Sher'96; FRCPC; Psy. assoc Membre Psy, Hôpital de l'Archipel; assoc Membre Psy, Centre de L'Annonciation; (514)521-8282

CHIDAMBARAM, Malathi; North York Gen Hosp, 4001 Leslie St, North York ON M2K 1E1; Man'99; FRCPC; IntMed (Clinician Investigator Program); Nephrol. Staff, North York General Hospital; (416)756-6000

CHIDIAC, Abdallah; Cite Sante St-Laurent, 2-1077 rue Decarie, Saint-Laurent QC H4L 3M8; St-Joseph (Lebanon)'71; AB; FRCPC; Peds. Consultant, Hôpital du Sacre-Coeur de Montréal; Langs: Arabic; Spanish; French; (514)748-0111; Fax. (514)748-7224; dodychidiac@gmail.com.

CHIELLA, Antonietta A; Med Associates of Port Perry, 462 Paxton St, Port Perry ON L9L 1L9; Wes'00; CCFP; (905)985-2895

CHIEN, Karen; Bridgepoint Hosp, 14 St Matthews Rd, Toronto ON M4M 2B5; Wes'00; CCFP; Staff, Bridgepoint Health Centre; (416)461-8251

CHIEN, S M Joseph; Scarborough Prof Centre, 410-1371 Neilson Rd, Scarborough ON M1B 4Z8; Tor'87; FRCPC; IntMed; Respir. Langs: Cantonese; (416)287-1891; Fax. (416)287-8218.

CHIEN, Vincent; St Michael's Hosp, B048 1-30 Bond St, Toronto ON M5B 1W8; Tor'93; FRCPC; IntMed. Staff, St Michael's Hospital; (416)864-5431

CHIEW, S K Sean; Niagara H System-St Catharine, PO Box 3018 Stn Main 142 Queenston St, St. Catharines ON L2R 7C6; Dal'03; Cardiol; IntMed. Staff, Niagara Health System - St Catharines General Site; (905)323-3836

CHIFOR, Daniela P; 2-1836 Comox Ave, Comox BC V9M 3M7; Cluj-Napoca (Romania)'94; MD; (778)999-1316

CHIHRIN, Stephen; Westview Health Centre, 4405 South Park Dr, Stony Plain AB T7Z 2M7; Wes'08; FRCPC; IntMed. Staff, Westview Health Centre; (780)968-3600; Fax. (780)968-3791.

CHIK, Constance L; Heritage Med Research Centre, 362-107 University Campus NW, Edmonton AB T6G 2S2; Tor'78; FRCPC; IntMed; Endocrin&Metab. (780)407-3636; Fax. (780)407-6702.

CHIKUKWA, Tineyi; ENT Consulting Clinic, 607-2125 11th Ave, Regina SK S4P 3X3; (Zimbabwe)'90; MB ChB; Specialist Gen Otol, Regina Qu'Appelle Health Region; (306)565-2599; Fax. (306)565-2598.

CHILD, Dumaresq M; 169 Talbot St S, Essex ON N8M 1B7; Oxford (England)'63; BCh; MRCS; Ac Staff, Windsor Regional Hospital - Metropolitan Site; Coroner, Essex Area; Med Dir, Country Village Nursing Home; (519)776-4217

CHILD, Jeremy R; Tremont Med Clinic, 2A-2F Tremont Dr, St Catharines ON L2T 3B2; McM'98; CCFP; (905)687-8887; Fax. (905)641-3693.

CHILDS, Aaron L; Cook Street Village Health Ctr, 200-1075 Pendergast St, Victoria BC V8V 0A1; Qns'03; CCFP; (250)477-5433

CHILDS, Christopher M; Sleep Laboratory A J Lane Bldg, 4008-5909 Veterans Memorial La, Halifax NS B3H 2E2; Cambridge (England)'65; DObstRCOG; CCFP; FCFP; Staff Sleep Physician, Queen Elizabeth II Health Sciences Centre - Victoria General Site; Lecturer, Dalhousie University; (902)473-4298; Fax. (902)473-7158.

CHILDS, Timothy J; Kingston Gen Hosp, 76 Stuart St, Kingston ON K7L 2V7; Tor'97; FRCPC; AnatPath. Staff, Kingston General Hospital; (613)549-6666 x6035; childst2@kgh.kari.net.

CHILOPORA, Garvey C; Carbonear Gen Hosp, 86 Highroad S, Carbonear NL A1Y 1A4; (Malawi)'01; MB BS; Locum Tenens, Carbonear General Hospital; (709)945-5111

CHILTON, Anthony P; St Joseph's Gen Hosp, 2137 Comox Ave, Comox BC V9M 1P2; Cape Town (South Africa)'81; MB ChB; FFR(S.A.); FRCPC; DiagRad. Staff, St Joseph's General Hospital; (250)339-1423

CHILVERS, Mark A; Children's & Women's HC of BC, B321-4480 Oak St, Vancouver BC V6H 3V4; Leicester (England)'93; MB ChB; Staff, BC Children's Hospital; (604)875-2119

CHILVERS, Martyn J; London Road Diagnostic Clinic, 481 London Rd, Sarnia ON N7T 4X3; Wes'81; (519)337-7512; Fax. (519)337-3257.

CHIMICH, William T; Glenrose Rehab Hosp, 10230 111 Ave NW, Edmonton AB T5G 0B7; Alb'84; BSc(Pharm); FRCPC; Psy (Community Psychiatry);CCFP; FCFP; Ac Staff NARG Prog, Glenrose Rehabilitation Hospital; Consultant Psy, Alberta Mental Health Services; Clinical Asst Prof Psy, University of Alberta; Langs: Ukrainian; (780)735-8800; Fax. (780)735-8846.

CHIN, Ami J; Bruyere Family Med Centre, 75 Bruyere St, Ottawa ON K1N 5C8; Ott'09; CCFP; (613)562-6262

CHIN, Andy S W; Sunridge Prof Centre, 516-2675 36 St NE, Calgary AB T1Y 6H6; Alb'86; CCFP; FCFP; (403)285-2500; Fax. (403)285-2501.

CHIN, Anne S L; CHUM-Hotel-Dieu Hosp, 6 356-3840 rue Saint-Urbain, Montreal QC H2W 1T8; McG'00; FRCPC; DiagRad. Staff, Centre Hospitalier l'Université de Montréal (CHUM) - Hôtel-Dieu; Staff, Institut de Cardiologie de Montréal; (514)890-8150

CHIN, Anthony W; 407-2347 Kennedy Rd, Scarborough ON M1T 3T8; Tor'87; (416)297-8967; Fax. (416)297-9527.

CHIN, Christopher A; Children's & Women's HC of BC, 4480 Oak St, Vancouver BC V6H 3V4; London (England)'86; Staff, BC Children's Hospital; (604)875-2711

CHIN, Daniel D Y; Medical Arts Bldg, 1010-233 Kennedy St, Winnipeg MB R3C 3J5; Man'86; FRCSC; Ophth. Ac Staff, Misericordia Health Centre; Consultant, Brandon Regional Health Centre; Asst Prof Ophth, University of Manitoba; (204)942-2507; Fax. (204)957-0294.

CHIN, Dennis; 135-8120 Cook Rd, Richmond BC V6Y 1T9; UBC'74; Vis Staff, Richmond Hospital; Vis Staff, Delta Hospital; (604)278-5294

CHIN, Elaine I; Executive Health Centre, 306-4120 Yonge St, North York ON M2P 2B8; Tor'88; MBA; Court Staff, University Health Network; Staff, Trillium Health Centre - West Toronto; Langs: Cantonese; (416)222-5880; Fax. (416)222-2885; dr.chin@executivehealthcentre.com.

CHIN, Francis L; Clairhurst Med Centre, 305-1466 Bathurst St, Toronto ON M5R 3S3; (Jamaica)'71; Court Staff Visiting, North York General Hospital - Branson Division; (416)531-0123

CHIN, Gordon M; Victoria East Med Clinic, 2068 Prince of Wales Dr, Regina SK S4V 3A6; Sask'84; Staff, Regina General Hospital; (306)789-4677; Fax. (306)789-3422.

CHIN, Gregory J; 3-2650 Lawrence Ave E, Scarborough ON M1P 2S1; Tor'89; Court Staff Family Med, The Scarborough Hospital - General Campus; (416)289-0593; Fax. (416)289-7847.

CHIN, Ian D; Taunton Surgical Centre, 1300 Keith Ross Dr, Oshawa ON L1H 7K4; Tor'93; BSc; FACC; FRCSC; GenSurg (Colon & Rectal Surgery). Assoc Prof, Queen's University; (905)721-4910; Fax. (905)721-6672.

CHIN, James E; 402-1630 Pandosy St, Kelowna BC V1Y 1P7; Tor'98; BSc; FRCPC; Psy. Staff, Kelowna General Hospital; (250)712-9807

CHIN, James; Royal Alexandra Hosp, 10240 Kingsway NW, Edmonton AB T5H 3V9; Alb'07; FRCPC; Anes. Staff, Royal Alexandra Hospital; (780)735-4111

CHIN, Jeffrey M; 206-145 Sheppard Ave E, North York ON M2N 3A7; Tor'87; Staff, North York General Hospital; (416)223-4330; Fax. (416)223-4350.

CHIN, Joe Y J; City Centre Family Physicians, 100-514 Queen St, Saskatoon SK S7K 0M5; Sask'76; Ac Staff, St Paul's Hospital (Grey Nuns) of Saskatoon; Ac Staff, Saskatoon City Hospital; (306)244-3016; Fax. (306)244-4737.

CHIN, Joseph M; Agincourt X-Ray & Ultrasound, 203-4235 Sheppard Ave E, Scarborough ON M1S 1T7; RCS (Ireland)'77; LRCP; LRCPSI; FRCPC; DiagRad. (416)291-6257; Fax. (416)291-9066.

CHIN, Justin; Univ of Alberta Hosp, 8440 112 St NW, Edmonton AB T6G 2B7; Man'08; Staff, University of Alberta Hospital; (780)407-8822

CHIN, Ki Jinn; Univ Hlth Network-Toronto Western Hosp, M2 405-399 Bathurst St, Toronto ON M5T 2S8; Newcastle-Upon-Tyne (England)'96; FRCPC; Anes. Staff, Toronto Western Hospital - University Health Network; (416)603-5118

CHIN, Kwanling; LL-1107 37 St SW, Calgary AB T3C 1S5; Man'89; (403)246-7788; Fax. (403)242-8850.

CHIN, L K Joseph; London HSC-Victoria Hosp, PO Box 5010 Stn B 800 Commissioners Rd E, London ON N6A 5W9; Tor'78; FRCSC; Urol (Urological Oncology). Consultant Urol, St Joseph's Hospital - St Joseph's Health Care; Chief Surgical Oncology, London Health Sciences Centre - Victoria Campus; Consultant Urol, London Regional Cancer Centre; Prof Urol & Oncology & Chair Surg Oncol, University of Western Ontario; (519)685-8451; Fax. (519)685-8455; joseph.chin@lhsc.on.ca.

CHIN, Maxwell I; Norfinch Med Centre, 303-2100 Finch Ave W, North York ON M3N 2Z9; Ott'74; (416)661-8846; Fax. (416)661-5073.

CHIN, May K M; 5-5761 Glover Rd, Langley BC V3A 8M8; UBC'78; BSc; Med Staff, Langley Memorial Hospital; (604)530-5825

CHIN, Peter M C; Meadowvale Prof Centre, 212-6855 Meadowvale Town Ctre, Mississauga ON L5N 2Y1; Tor'78; CCFP; Court Staff, The Credit Valley Hospital; (905)821-1211; Fax. (905)821-2383.

CHIN, Stephen J; Dofasco Inc, PO Box 2460 Stn Lcd 1, Hamilton ON L8N 3J5; West Indies (Jamaica)'78; MB BS; Court Staff, Hamilton Health Sciences Centre-Juravinski Site; Court Staff, St Joseph's Healthcare - Charlton Campus; Court Staff, Hamilton Health Sciences Centre - McMaster Children's Hospital; (905)548-7130; Fax. (905)548-4345; stephen.chin@arcelormittal.com.

CHIN, Terrence B; 2-333 Mountainview Rd S, Georgetown ON L7G 6E8; Qns'01; CCFP; (905)873-4742; Fax. (905)873-1827.

CHIN, Vincent V; 407-2347 Kennedy Rd, Scarborough ON M1T 3T8; West Indies (Jamaica)'77; MB BS; FRCPC; Peds. Consultant, Rouge Valley Health System - Centenary Health Centre Site; (416)297-8967; Fax. (416)297-9527.

CHIN, Wendy W S; 101-15451 Russell Ave, White Rock BC V4B 2R5; Nottingham (United Kingdom)'01; MB BS; BMedSci; CCFP; Staff, Peace Arch Hospital; (604)531-5595

CHIN, Wu Dat N; University of Alberta Hosp, 3C1.12WMC-8440 112 St NW, Edmonton AB T6G 2B7; Witwatersrand (South Africa)'73; MB ChB; FRCPC; IntMed (Critical Care Medicine); Respir. Physician Critical Care, University of Alberta Hospital; Prof, University of Alberta; (780)407-6755; Fax. (780)407-1228.

CHIN, Y K Patrick; UBC Hospital, 2F 2C-2211 Wesbrook Mall, Vancouver BC V6T 2B5; Qns'96; FRCSC; OrthSurg. Staff, Nanaimo Regional General Hospital; Staff, UBC Hospital - Koerner Pavillion; (604)822-9985; Fax. (604)822-1999.

CHIN, Ying Wai; Victoria Heights Geriatric Cli, 232 Ross Dr, New Westminster BC V3L 0B2; HongKong (Hong Kong)'88; MB ChB; FRCPC; IntMed; GeriatricMed. Staff, Burnaby Hospital; Staff, Queen's Park Care Centre; Langs: Cantonese; (604)528-5031

CHIN CHAM, Martin; The Credit Valley Hosp, 2200 Eglinton Ave W, Mississauga ON L5M 2N1; Tor'99; CCFP; Staff, The Credit Valley Hospital; (905)813-2200

CHIN FOOK, Trevor J; Rosedale Med Centre, 812-600 Sherbourne St, Toronto ON M4X 1W4; West Indies (Jamaica)'71; MB BS; FRCSC; Ophth (Cornea/External Disease). Consultant Ophth, St Michael's Hospital; Asst Prof, University of Toronto; (416)927-0129; Fax. (416)927-0129.

CHIN-YEE, Ian; London HSC-Victoria Hosp, PO Box 5010 Stn B 800 Commissioners Rd E, London ON N6A 5W9; Cal'85; FRCPC; IntMed; Hem. Staff Hematol/Blood Bank/Chief/Chair Hematology, London Health Sciences Centre - Victoria Campus; Prof Med, University of Western Ontario; (519)685-8475; ian.chinyee@lhsc.on.ca.

CHING, Daniel H T; 102-4631 Steeles Ave E, Scarborough ON M1V 4S5; Tor'84; Court Staff, North York General Hospital; Ac Staff, The Scarborough Hospital - Birchmount Campus; (416)293-6600; Fax. (416)293-5410.

CHING, Emily K Y; GI Health Centre, 32-1960 Appleby Line, Burlington ON L7L 0B7; McM'05; FRCPC; IntMed; Gastroent. Staff, Hamilton Health Sciences Centre - McMaster Children's Hospital; Ac Consultant Gastroenterology, Baycrest Centre for Geriatric Care; Langs: Cantonese; (905)335-1888; Fax. (905)335-5656.

CHING, Joyce C Y; 105-385 Silver Star Blvd, Scarborough ON M1V 0E3; Tor'06; FRCPC; Peds; ClinImmunol&Allergy.

CHING, Karen P; Salvus Family Med Clinic, 62-143 Liberton Dr, St. Albert AB T8N 6A7; Alb'98; BSc; CCFP; Med Staff, Sturgeon Community Hospital; Langs: Cantonese; (780)460-4562; Fax. (780)460-4550; karenpching@hotmail.com.

CHINIARA, Gilles; Ctr Hosp Affilie-Enfant-Jesus, 1401 18e rue, Quebec QC G1J 1Z4; Laval'98; CSPQ; FRCPC; Anes. Staff, Centre Hospitalier Affilié Universitaire de Québec - Hôpital De L'Enfant Jésus; (418)649-5807

CHINIARA, Gisele; 150 rue Monseigneur-Ross, Gaspe QC G4X 2S7; Beirut (Lebanon)'84; FRCPC; Psy. (418)368-2291; Fax. (418)368-3481.

CHINKS, Joshua; MUHC-Montreal Gen Hosp, B2 117-1650 av Cedar, Montreal QC H3G 1A4; McG'07; MDCM; CCFP; CCFP(E.M.); Staff, McGill University Health Centre - Montreal General Campus; (514)934-1934

CHINNAPP, Vinod; Women's College Hosp, E253-76 Grenville St, Toronto ON M5S 1B2; Bangalore (India)'92; Staff, Women's College Hospital; (416)323-6008

CHINNER, Anthony J; Scarborough Prof Centre, 201-1371 Neilson Rd, Scarborough ON M1B 4Z8; Cape Town (South Africa)'63; Staff RehabMed, Rouge Valley Health System - Centenary Health Centre Site; Physician, Acute Rehabilitation Unit; Langs: Xhosa; Afrikaans; (416)284-0259; Fax. (416)284-8644; drchinner@bellnet.ca.

CHIODO, Albino; 201-840 Coxwell Ave, East York ON M4C 5T2; Tor'91; FRCSC; Otol (Endoscopic Sinus Surg). Chief of Staff, Toronto East General Hospital Inc; Staff, St Michael's Hospital; Asst Prof Otol, University of Toronto; Langs: Italian.

CHIORPEC-GEORGESCU, Margareta; CSSS d'Argenteuil, 145 av de la Providence, Lachute QC J8H 4C7; Bucharest (Romania)'85; Staff, Centre Hospitalier d'Argenteuil; Langs: Romanian; English; (450)562-8581

CHIOZZA, Stefano; 6-3603 Langstaff Rd, Woodbridge ON L4L 9G7; Modena (Italy)'93; CCFP; (905)856-0771; Fax. (905)856-1619.

CHIPETA, Daniel C; Dr Charles S Curtis Mem Hosp, 178-200 West St, St Anthony NL A0K 4S0; Staff, Charles S Curtis Memorial Hospital; (709)454-3333

CHIPMAN, Nancy L; Avenue Med Centre, 1-221 Brant Ave, Brantford ON N3T 3J2; Dal'79; Court Staff, The Brant Community Healthcare System - Brantford General Hospital Site; (519)753-8666; Fax. (519)753-6880.

CHIPPERFIELD, Katherine M; Vancouver Gen Hosp, 855 12th Ave W, Vancouver BC V5Z 1M9; Sask'96; FRCPC; IntMed; HemPath; Hem. Staff, Vancouver General Hospital - Centennial Pavillion; Med Dir, Blood Transfusion Service; (604)875-4381; Fax. (604)875-4798.

CHIPPERFIELD, Patricia M; St Paul's Hosp, 1081 Burrard St, Vancouver BC V6Z 1Y6; Sask'68; FRCPC; DiagRad. Ac Staff, Providence Health Care - St Paul's Hospital; (604)631-8006; Fax. (604)631-5283.

CHIQUETTE, Jocelyne; Ctr Hosp Affilie-St-Sacrement, 1050 ch Sainte-Foy, Quebec QC G1S 4L8; Laval'73; Staff, Centre Hospitalier Affilié Universitaire de Québec - Hôpital du St-Sacrement; (418)682-7878; Fax. (418)682-7912.

CHIQUETTE-POMAR, Annie; Clinique familiale de Thetford, 1001-926 rue Labbe, Thetford Mines QC G6G 2A8; Sher'08; CCFP; (418)338-3521; Fax. (418)338-4580.

CHIRA, Ruxandra I; CSSS Jeanne-Mance, 100-15 av du Mont-Royal O, Montreal QC H2T 2R9; CCFP; (514)286-9657

CHIRAYATH, Haiju; Dr Walter Anderson Bldg, 2251 Pandosy St, Kelowna BC V1Y 1T1; (India)'98; (250)862-4398

CHIRAYILKALAM, Shereen B; 208-114 Dundas St E, Whitby ON L1N 2H7; Kerala (India)'97; FRCSC; ObstGyn. Staff, Mount Sinai Hospital; (905)666-0500; Fax. (905)666-0400.

CHIRGWIN, Juan C L; CLSC Parc Extension, 7085 rue Hutchison, Montreal QC H3N 1Y9; McG'92; CCFP; Chef Service, CLSC Parc Extension; Langs: Spanish; (514)273-9591 x6374; Fax. (514)380-8138; juan.chirgwin@mcgill.ca.

CHIRGWIN-CAMPOS, Jerman E; St Mary's Hosp Centre, 3830 av Lacombe, Montreal QC H3T 1M5; McG'91; CCFP; CCFP(E.M.); FCFP; Staff, St Mary's Hospital Centre; (514)345-3511 x3574

CHIRICO, James C A; North Bay Parry Sound Dist H U, 681 Commercial St, North Bay ON P1B 4E7; Wes'81; MPH; FRCPC; Anes. Med Officer of Hlth/Exec Officer, North Bay Parry Sound District Health Unit Corporate Office; (705)474-1400; Fax. (705)474-8252.

CHIRICOSTA, Albert A; Polyclinique Cabrini, 204-5700 rue Saint-Zotique E, Montreal QC H1T 3Y7; Ott'64; FRCSC; Urol. ac Staff, Hôpital Santa Cabrini Ospedale; ac Staff, St Mary's Hospital Centre; (514)256-8137

CHIRITO, Edward; CLSC-CHSLD Pat Montreal Est, 13926 rue Notre-Dame E, Pte-aux-Trembles QC H1A 1T5; San Marcos (Peru)'66; Staff, Pavillon St-Joseph de la Providence; (514)642-7747

CHIRY, Samah; Ctr Hosp Anna-Laberge, 200 boul Brisebois, Chateauguay QC J6K 4W8; Mon'10; CCFP; Staff, Hôpital Anna-Laberge; (450)699-2425

CHISAMORE, Brian C; Village Park Paediatrics, 405-27 Roncesvalles Ave, Toronto ON M6R 3B2; Tor'92; Peds (Neonatal & Perinatal Medicine). Staff Follow-up Clinic, The Hospital For Sick Children; (416)516-4111; Fax. (416)516-1104; chisab@stjoe.on.ca.

CHISHOLM, Blanche T; South End Family Practice, 211-5595 Fenwick St, Halifax NS B3H 4M2; Dal'91; FRCPC; Psy. Assoc Prof, Dalhousie University; (902)423-3323; Fax. (902)442-5593.

CHISHOLM, James; Collingwood Gen & Marine Hosp, 459 Hume St, Collingwood ON L9Y 1W9; Wes'94; FRCPC; EmergMed. Staff, Collingwood General & Marine Hospital; Instructor, University of Toronto; (705)445-2550

CHISHOLM, Janice D; Queen Elizabeth II HSC, BB 379-1276 South Park St, Halifax NS B3H 2Y9; Dal'00; FRCPC; Anes. Staff, Queen Elizabeth II Health Sciences Centre - Victoria General Site; (902)473-3608; Fax. (902)473-3610.

CHISHOLM, John A; Timmins & Dist Hosp, 700 Ross Ave E, Timmins ON P4N 8P2; Wes'91; CCFP; Staff, Timmins & District Hospital; (705)267-2131

CHISHOLM, John S; Saint John Reg Hosp Facility, PO Box 2100 Stn Main 400 University Ave, Saint John NB E2L 4L2; Dal'92; FRCPC; Anes. Staff Anes, Saint John Regional Hospital; (506)648-6861; Fax. (506)648-6860.

CHISHOLM, Kenneth C; Queen Elizabeth II HSC, 1276 South Park St, Halifax NS B3H 2Y9; Dal'87; Anes. Staff, Queen Elizabeth II Health Sciences Centre - Victoria General Site; (902)473-4131; Fax. (902)473-4126.

CHISHOLM, Mary E; Capilano Med Clinic, 7905 106 Ave NW, Edmonton AB T6A 1H7; Alb'97; BSc(Hons Physiol); LMCC; CCFP; Staff Member Anes, Westview Health Centre; Staff Member Anes, Sturgeon Community Hospital; Clin Lecturer, University of Alberta; (780)465-0951; Fax. (780)465-6928.

CHISHOLM, Richard; Dr Everett Chalmers Reg Hosp, PO Box 9000 Stn A, Fredericton NB E3B 5N5; Dal'80; FRCPC; Anes. Staff, Dr Everett Chalmers Regional Hospital; (506)452-5400

CHISHOLM, Robert J; St Michael's Hosp, 7CCN 7152-30 Bond St, Toronto ON M5B 1W8; Tor'70; FACC; FRCPC; IntMed (Interventional Cardiology); Cardiol. Staff Interventional Cardiologist, St Michael's Hospital; Assoc Prof Med, University of Toronto; (416)864-5490; Fax. (416)864-5478; chisholmr@smh.toronto.on.ca.

CHISHOLM, Sherrie-Anne; Kensington Med Clinic, 6548 Hastings St, Burnaby BC V5B 1S2; Cal'81; FRCPC; IntMed. Staff, BC Mental Health & Addiction Service; (604)299-9769; Fax. (604)299-9772.

CHISVIN, Martin J; Toronto East Gen & Orth Hosp, 825 Coxwell Ave, Toronto ON M4C 3E7; Man'85; FRCPC; Psy (Geriatric Psychiatry). Staff Psy, Toronto East General Hospital Inc; (416)469-6580 x6649; Fax. (416)469-6805; mchis@tegh.on.ca.

CHITAYAT, David A; Hydro Place Bldg, 3292-700 University Ave, Toronto ON M5G 1Z5; Tel Aviv (Israel)'75; FRCPC; MedGenetics (Pediatrics). Staff, The Hospital For Sick Children; Head The Prenatal Diagnosis & Med Genetics Prog, Mount Sinai Hospital; Prof, University of Toronto; Langs: Hebrew; (416)586-4523; Fax. (416)586-4723.

CHITAYAT, Samara G; 604-25 Charlton Ave E, Hamilton ON L8N 1Y2; McG'05; FRCPC; Peds. Staff, Joseph Brant Memorial Hospital; (905)523-6766

CHITSAZ, Niloofar; Willoughby Medical, B1A-20202 66th Ave, Langley BC V2Y 1P3; Tehran (Iran)'95; MD; CCFP; Staff, Gordon & Leslie Diamond Health Care Centre; (604)514-8800

CHITSIKE, Rufaro S; Health Sciences Centre, 300 Prince Philip Dr, St. John's NL A1B 3V6; Godfrey School of Medicine (Zimbabwe)'00; MB ChB; Staff, Health Sciences Centre; (709)737-6300

CHITTAL, Dervla; University Health Services, 104-65 Chancellors Cir, Winnipeg MB R3T 2N2; Ott'05; CCFP; Staff, Portage District General Hospital; (204)474-8411; dchittal@shaw.ca.

CHITTE, Sachin A; 200-343 Preston St, Ottawa ON K1S 1N4; Qns'02; BSc; FRCSC; PlasSurg (Hand Surgery). Staff Plastic Surgeon, Queensway Carleton Hospital; (613)729-1616

CHITTLE, Andrea D; University of Guelph, 50 Stone Rd E, Guelph ON N1G 2W1; Wes'08; CCFP; (519)824-4120

CHITTOCK, Dean R; Vancouver Gen Hosp, ICU 2438-855 12th Ave W, Vancouver BC V5Z 1M9; Wes'88; BSc; FRCPC; IntMed; Critical Care Medicine; Respir. Staff, Vancouver General Hospital - Centennial Pavillion; (604)875-5949; Fax. (604)875-5957.

CHIU, Aaron; Women's Hosp, WR004-735 Notre Dame Ave, Winnipeg MB R3E 0L8; Tor'91; FAAP; FRCPC; Peds (Neonatal & Perinatal Medicine). Staff Neonatol, St Boniface General Hospital; Staff Neonatol, Health Sciences Centre; Assoc Prof Section of Neonatol, University of Manitoba; Langs: Cantonese; (204)787-1829; Fax. (204)787-1587.

CHIU, Allan Y L; Millwoods Family Med Clinic, 104-2551 Hewes Way NW, Edmonton AB T6L 6W6; Alb'85; (780)462-2767; Fax. (780)463-7025.

CHIU, Ann M; Jackson Park Health Centre, 240-2475 McDougall St, Windsor ON N8X 3N9; New South Wales (Australia)'90; FRCSC; Ophth (Cornea). Langs: Cantonese; Mandarin; (519)258-0441

CHIU, Anthony S K; 2015 Centre St NW, Calgary AB T2E 2S9; Tor'81; CCFP; FCFP; Court Staff, Foothills Medical Centre; (403)277-8777

CHIU, Anthony S Y; 308-1033 Davie St, Vancouver BC V6E 1M7; Alb'79; FRCPC; IntMed; Nephrol. Ac Staff, Providence Health Care - St Paul's Hospital; (604)566-9982

CHIU, Arthur K K; Professional Place, 305-2901 Lawrence Ave E, Scarborough ON M1P 2T3; Alb'84; FRCSC; GenSurg. Langs: Cantonese; Mandarin; (416)269-5808; Fax. (416)269-5803.

CHIU, Bobby T L; Medical Centre, 5-1939 Kennedy Rd, Scarborough ON M1P 2L9; Madras (India)'85; CCFP; (416)609-1859; Fax. (416)609-9002.

CHIU, Brendan B S; 4A-678 Guelph Line, Burlington ON L7R 3M8; Man'71; BSc(Med); Ac Staff, Joseph Brant Memorial Hospital; (905)333-3332; Fax. (905)632-0974.

CHIU, Brian K Y; University of Alberta Hosp, 5B4.14WCM-8440 112 St NW, Edmonton AB T6G 2B7; Tor'77; FRCPC; AnatPath. Staff Capital Health Authority, University of Alberta Hospital; Assoc Prof Med & Dentistry, University of Alberta; (780)407-6959; Fax. (780)407-3009.

CHIU, But-Yau; Jane-Lessard Med Clinic, 1-727 Jane St, Toronto ON M6N 4B3; Tor'75; Staff, Humber River Regional Hospital - Church Street Site; (416)767-7017; Fax. (416)762-1118.

CHIU, Chung Fok; Sheppard Med Bldg, 210-701 Sheppard Ave E, North York ON M2K 2Z3; Tor'81; BSc; Ac Staff, North York General Hospital; Court Staff, The Scarborough Hospital - Birchmount Campus; Langs: Chinese; (416)225-2177; Fax. (416)225-2678.

CHIU, Doris; Burnaby Hosp, 3935 Kincaid St, Burnaby BC V5G 2X6; UBC'07; CCFP; Staff, Burnaby Hospital; (604)434-4211

CHIU, Edward S; North York Family Health Team, 330-5 Fairview Mall Dr, North York ON M2J 2Z1; Wes'09; CCFP; (416)491-6306; Fax. (416)491-8308.

CHIU, Elizabeth M; Sheppard Med Bldg, 306-701 Sheppard Ave E, North York ON M2K 2Z3; UBC'86; Staff, North York General Hospital; Staff, The Scarborough Hospital - Birchmount Campus; (416)497-9797; Fax. (416)497-9787; echiu701@rogers.com.

CHIU, Frank K K; 125-4651 No. 3 Rd, Richmond BC V6X 2C4; Tor'91; (604)821-0006; Fax. (604)821-0006.

CHIU, Hak M; Lakeridge Hlth Corp-Oshawa, 1 Hospital Crt, Oshawa ON L1G 2B9; (Hong Kong)'65; MB BS; FRCPC; IntMed; MedOncol; Hem. Ac Staff, Lakeridge Health - Oshawa Site; Ac Staff, Lakeridge Health - Whitby Site; Ac Staff, Lakeridge Health - Bowmanville Site; Langs: Cantonese; (905)576-8711 x3279

CHIU, Isabelle; Royal Alexandra Hosp, 324CSC-10240 Kingsway NW, Edmonton AB T5H 3V9; Tor'85; ABIM(IntMed); FRCPC; IntMed; InfectDis. Med Dir OPAT, Royal Alexandra Hospital; Assoc Prof InfectDis, University of Alberta; Langs: Chinese; (780)944-2706

CHIU, Janet W C; 18220 89 Ave NW, Edmonton AB T5T 2K6; Alb'82; (780)481-8812; Fax. (780)489-7853.

CHIU, John F S; Town Centre Family Clinic, 320-6203 28 Ave NW, Edmonton AB T6L 6K3; Alb'78; CCFP; Ac Staff Family Pract, Covenant Health - Grey Nuns Community Hospital; Médecin Certified Marine, Transport Canada; Clin Prof Family Med & Psy, University of Alberta; Langs: Cantonese; (780)462-8120; Fax. (780)461-9437.

CHIU, John H C; Balmoral Med Arts Facility, 101-1366 Yonge St, Toronto ON M4T 3A7; (Hong Kong)'66; DABR; MD; FRCPC; DiagRad (Bone Densitometry). Langs: Chinese; (416)975-8951; Fax. (416)975-8610; jhcchiu@sympatico.ca.

CHIU, Leo; Lakeridge Hlth Corp-Oshawa, 1 Hospital Crt, Oshawa ON L1G 2B9; Wes'01; FRCPC; IntMed. Staff, Lakeridge Health - Oshawa Site; (905)576-8711

CHIU, Mark H N; TLC Medical Bldg, 301-5171 221A St, Langley BC V2Y 0A2; Tor'02; FRCSC; OrthSurg. (778)278-1280

CHIU, Michael S; Village Park Med Clinic, 110-937 Fir St, Sherwood Park AB T8A 4N6; Alb'76; (780)467-8889; Fax. (780)467-6763.

CHIU, Michelle; The Ottawa Hosp-Civic Campus, 1053 Carling Ave, Ottawa ON K1Y 4E9; McM'96; FRCPC; Anes. Staff, The Ottawa Hospital - Civic Campus; (613)761-4169; Fax. (613)761-5209.

CHIU, Patrick; Pacific Medical Clinic, F33-4300 Steeles Ave E, Markham ON L3R 0Y5; UBC'05; CCFP; (905)604-7889; Fax. (905)604-7890.

CHIU, Paul K; 215-9450 137 Ave NW, Edmonton AB T5E 6C2; Alb'73; AB; CAFCI; Staff, Royal Alexandra Hospital; Langs: Cantonese; Mandarin; (780)475-0502; Fax. (780)473-5493.

CHIU, Peter C H; 8-3596 27th Ave W, Vancouver BC V6S 1P8; UBC'71; Physician Emerg, Providence Health Care - Mount Saint Joseph Hospital; (604)733-7112; Fax. (604)733-0363.

CHIU, Peter L S L; Meadowlark Place Prof Centre, 404-8708 155 St NW, Edmonton AB T5R 1W2; Alb'76; FRCPC; IntMed (Musculoskeletal); Rheum. Ac Staff, Covenant Health - Misericordia Community Hospital; Ac Staff, Glenrose Rehabilitation Hospital; Clinical Asst Prof Med, University of Alberta; Langs: Cantonese; (780)489-5533; Fax. (780)489-2881.

CHIU, Priscilla P L; The Hosp for Sick Children, 1518-555 University Ave, Toronto ON M5G 1X8; Qns'91; PhD; FRCSC; GenSurg; PedGenSurg. Staff, The Hospital For Sick Children; Langs: Cantonese; (416)813-6405; Fax. (416)813-7477.

CHIU, Simon K H; 325 Bamburgh Circle, Scarborough ON M1W 3Y1; UBC'06; CCFP; (416)492-8068

CHIU, Simon S; Regional Mental HC-St Thomas, PO Box 2004 Stn Main 467 Sunset Dr, St Thomas ON N5P 3V9; Tor'85; MSc; PhD; FABPN; FRCPC; Psy (Addiction Psychiatry). Consultant Psy, Regional Mental Health Care-St Joseph's Health Care; Staff, Regional Mental Health Care-St Joseph's Health Care; Assoc Prof, University of Western Ontario; Langs: Cantonese; (519)631-8510 x49655; Fax. (519)631-9224; Simon.chiu@sjhc.london.on.ca.

CHIU, Sy-Hua; Lemarchand Med Clinic, 11503 100 Ave NW, Edmonton AB T5K 2K7; Lodz (Poland)'79; Med Constable, Workers' Comp Board; Langs: Polish; (780)488-3933; Fax. (780)488-1037; sy-hua.chiu@wcb.ab.ca.

CHIU, Sylvester S; West Haldimand Gen Hosp, 75 Parkview Rd, Hagersville ON N0A 1H0; McG'64; DABIM; FRCPC; IntMed. Dir Health Serv, Norfolk General Hospital; Consultant IntMed, West Haldimand General Hospital; (905)768-3311

CHIU, Victor W; 307-2130 Lawrence Ave E, Scarborough ON M1R 3A6; Tor'69; Staff, The Scarborough Hospital - General Campus; (416)751-6141; Fax. (416)751-5270.

CHIU, Wendy S W; MUHC-Royal Victoria Hosp, R4 01-687 av des Pins O, Montreal QC H3A 1A1; McG'94; FRCPC; IntMed; GeriatricMed. Staff, McGill University Health Centre - Royal Victoria Hospital; (514)843-1518; wendy.chiu@muhc.mcgill.ca.

CHIU, Wing-Gay; 222-633 Main St, Vancouver BC V6A 2V4; UBC'60; (604)683-4020

CHIVERS, Quinton; Univ Hlth Network-Toronto Western Hosp, 2F-399 Bathurst St, Toronto ON M5T 2S8; Cal'06; FRCSC; PlasSurg. Staff, Toronto Western Hospital - University Health Network; (416)603-5455

CHIZEN, Donna R; Royal University Hosp, 4509-103 Hospital Dr, Saskatoon SK S7N 0W8; McM'83; BSc(Hon); FRCSC; ObstGyn (Reproductive Endocrinology). Staff ObstGyn, Royal University Hospital; Assoc Prof, University of Saskatchewan; (306)966-8623; Fax. (306)966-8040.

CHIZEN, Lawrence S; Queensway Health Centre, 1214 3-1750 The Queensway, Etobicoke ON M9C 5H5; Wes'89; PhysMed&Rehab. (416)451-8538

CHKIPOV, Hristo G; CarePoint Medical Centres, 140-777 Royal Oak Dr, Victoria BC V8X 4V1; (Bulgaria)'86; (250)727-7795; Fax. (250)727-3732.

CHKREBTII, Natalia O; Glazier Med Centre, 11 Gibb St, Oshawa ON L1H 2J9; Kiev (Ukraine)'83; FRCPC; IntMed; InfectDis. (905)579-1212 x270

CHLEBAK, Anna; Katanna Laser Clinic, 306-20238 Fraser Hwy, Langley BC V3A 4E6; Tor'75; Langs: Slovak; Czech; (604)533-4544; anna@katanna.ca; Semi-Retired.

CHLEBEK, Sebastian J; Radiology Consultants Assoc, 120-6707 Elbow Dr SW, Calgary AB T2V 0E3; Man'01; FRCPC; DiagRad. (403)777-3003; Fax. (403)777-3008.

CHLEBUS, Andrew; 111-21 The Queensway W, Mississauga ON L5B 1B8; Tor'57; CRCP; FAAP; Peds (Clinical Immunology & Allergy). Hon Staff, The Hospital For Sick Children; Hon Staff, Humber River Regional Hospital - Finch Avenue Site; Hon Teach Staff Peds, University of Toronto; (905)897-0788; Fax. (905)897-9229.

CHLYSTA, Dana O; Uptown Medical Clinic, 3460 Saanich Rd, Victoria BC V8X 1W7; Man'88; CCFP; FCFP; (250)590-8375

CHLYSTA, Terry S; 14-3170 Tillicum Rd, Victoria BC V9A 7C5; Man'87; BSc(Med); (250)381-8112

CHMELICEK, John T; Alberta Med Association, 12230 106 Ave NW, Edmonton AB T5N 3Z1; Alb'85; CCFP; Member, Alberta Medical Association; (780)482-2636

CHMIEL, Agnes E; Regional Rehabilitation Centre, 300 Wellington St N, Hamilton ON L8L 0A4; McM'02; FRCPC; PhysMed&Rehab. Staff, Hamilton Health Sciences Centre - McMaster Children's Hospital; (905)521-2100

CHMIEL, Peter K; Vaughan Paediatric Clinic, 310-8333 Weston Rd, Woodbridge ON L4L 8E2; Alb'10; (905)850-3250

CHMIELEWSKA, Karolina; Hotel-Dieu de Levis, 143 rue Wolfe, Levis QC G6V 3Z1; Laval'07; FRCSC; Ophth. Staff, Hôtel-Dieu de Lévis; (418)835-7121

CHO, B C John; Univ Hlth Network-Princess M, 610 University Ave, Toronto ON M5G 2M9; Qns'95; FRCPC; RadOncol. Staff, Princess Margaret Hospital - University Health Network; (416)946-2124; jchoe@transitiontherapeutics.com.

CHO, Brian; Polaris Mental Health Clinic, 708-1243 Islington Ave, Etobicoke ON M8X 1Y9; Tor'99; FRCPC; Psy. (416)234-8241; Fax. (416)234-8422.

CHO, Brian J H; Humber River Reg Hosp-Church, 200 Church St, Toronto ON M9N 1N8; Tor'06; Critical Care Medicine; IntMed. Staff, Humber River Regional Hospital - Church Street Site; (604)875-4111

CHO, Caroline E; 715 12th Ave W, Vancouver BC V5Z 1M9; Alb'02; FRCPC; Psy. (604)875-4139

CHO, Charles Y; Southlake Reg Health Centre, 596 Davis Dr, Newmarket ON L3Y 2P9; Qns'03; FRCPC; RadOncol. Staff, Southlake Regional Health Centre; (905)895-4521

CHO, Helen Y H; 4640 17 Ave NW, Calgary AB T3B 0P3; Alb'91; BMedSci; CCFP; FCFP; Langs: Cantonese; (403)202-2727; Fax. (403)202-2733.

CHO, Jane; 17-6219 Centre St NW, Calgary AB T2K 0V2; Alb'98; CCFP; (403)274-4428; Fax. (403)274-4824.

CHO, John J W; Belmore Square, 300-1011 Glenmore Trail SW, Calgary AB T2V 4R6; UBC'07; FRCSC; Otol. Staff, Foothills Medical Centre; (403)571-5219

CHO, Kenneth M C; East Van Med Bldg, 504-1750 10th Ave E, Vancouver BC V5N 5K4; Alb'88; CCFP; (604)879-4551; Fax. (604)879-4552.

CHO, Kevin Y; 20 Drewry Ave, Toronto ON M2M 1C8; UBC'91; (416)590-7888; Fax. (416)590-7886.

CHO, Patrick A; Assiniboine Clinic, 633 Lodge Ave, Winnipeg MB R3J 0S9; Dal'93; DABU; FRCSC; Urol. Staff Urologist, The Salvation Army Grace Hospital; Staff Urologist, CancerCare Manitoba; (204)958-6739; Fax. (204)783-6769.

CHO, Roger K N; Caleo Health, 340-600 Crowfoot Cres NW, Calgary AB T3G 0B4; Sask'91; FRCSC; OrthSurg (Spine Surgery). Staff, Foothills Medical Centre; Assoc Prof, University of Calgary; Langs: Chinese; (403)452-6931; Fax. (403)452-0995.

CHO, Victoria Y W; 9912 107 St NW PO Box 2415 Stn Main, Edmonton AB T5J 2S5; Alb'85; Med Mgr, Workers' Comp Board; (780)498-4427; victoria.cho@wcb.ab.ca.

CHOBOTUK, Tara; Spryfield Pediatric Clinic, 16 Dentith Rd, Halifax NS B3R 2H9; Alb'08; FRCPC; Peds. (902)470-8043; Fax. (902)470-8137.

CHOCHINOV, Alecs H; St Boniface Gen Hosp, L1019-409 Tache Ave, Winnipeg MB R2H 2A6; Man'79; FRCPC; EmergMed. Staff, St Boniface General Hospital; Dept Head Emerg Med, University of Manitoba; (204)235-3006; Fax. (204)237-2071; achochin@sbgh.mb.ca.

CHOCHINOV, Erin M; Sunnybrook Hlth Sciences Ctre, M3 200-2075 Bayview Ave, Toronto ON M4N 3M5; Man'96; FRCPC; Anes. Staff, Sunnybrook Health Sciences Centre; (416)480-4864

CHOCHINOV, Harvey M; Cancercare Manitoba, 3017-675 McDermot Ave, Winnipeg MB R3E 0V9; Man'83; PhD(ComHealthSci); FRCPC; Psy (Psychiatric Oncology). Consultant, Manitoba Cancer Treatment & Research Foundation; Prof Dept of Psy/Chair Canada Research in Palliative Care, University of Manitoba; (204)787-4937; Fax. (204)787-4933; harvey.chochinov@cancercare.mb.ca.

CHOCHINOV, Paul; 16-1783 Plessis Rd, Winnipeg MB R3W 1N3; Man'91; (204)233-8563

CHOCRON, Charles; 230-5910 ch Cote-des-Neiges, Montreal QC H3S 1Z5; Paris (France)'69; Staff, Sir Mortimer B Davis Jewish General; Langs: Spanish; French; (514)739-1662; Fax. (514)739-5859; mayag_sonia@yahoo.ca.

CHODIRKER, Bernard N; FE231-685 William Ave, Winnipeg MB R3E 0Z2; Man'80; MSc; FRCPC; Peds; MedGenetics.

CHODIRKER, Lisa; Sunnybrook Hlth Sciences Ctre, 2075 Bayview Ave, Toronto ON M4N 3M5; Ott'03; Hem; IntMed. Staff, Sunnybrook Health Sciences Centre; (416)480-5847; Fax. (416)480-6002.

CHODKIEWICZ, Adam C; St Paul's Hosp, 1081 Burrard St, Vancouver BC V6Z 1Y6; Alb'96; FRCPC; Psy. Staff, Providence Health Care - St Paul's Hospital; (604)682-2344 x66598

CHODYRA, Anna K; Newport Family Practice, 310-205 Newport Dr, Port Moody BC V3H 5C9; Warsaw (Poland)'99; CCFP; Langs: Polish; (778)272-8550

CHOE, James; Medical Centre, 2A-1723 Kipling Ave, Etobicoke ON M9R 4E1; Tor'88; Ac Staff, William Osler Health System - Etobicoke General Hospital; Court Staff, Humber River Regional Hospital - Finch Avenue Site; Langs: Korean; (416)248-9166; Fax. (416)248-9695.

CHOE, Seong Dong; 4-2397 Finch Ave W, North York ON M9M 2X1; Kyunghee (Korea)'86; Ac Staff, Humber River Regional Hospital - Finch Avenue Site; (416)742-4646; Fax. (416)742-0138.

CHOHAN, Inderjit S; West Winds Med Clinic, 1238-4818 Westwinds Dr NE, Calgary AB T3J 3Z5; Alb'92; FRCPC; Psy. (403)293-5454; Fax. (403)407-7690.

CHOI, Abram; Queensway-Carleton Hosp, 3045 Baseline Rd, Ottawa ON K2H 8P4; McM'05; FRCPC; DiagRad. Staff, Queensway Carleton Hospital; (613)721-2000

CHOI, Antonio M F; 782 Dundas St W, Toronto ON M6J 1V1; Dublin (Ireland)'73; LRCPSI; CCFP; FCFP; Court Staff, St Joseph's Health Centre; Langs: Cantonese; (416)603-9843; Fax. (416)603-1870.

CHOI, Christine; Royal Columbian Hosp, 330 Columbia St E, New Westminster BC V3L 3W7; Tor'04; FRCPC; EmergMed. Staff, Royal Columbian Hospital; (604)520-4253

CHOI, D Young; Avicenna Health Centre, 100-80 Finch Ave W, North York ON M2N 2H4; (Korea)'65; (416)222-0909

CHOI, Edwin D; 325 Bamburgh Cir, Scarborough ON M1W 3Y1; Tor'93; MedMicrobiol. Staff, St Michael's Hospital; (416)492-8068; Fax. (416)497-7796.

CHOI, Ellen H; Dawson Road Fam Med Clinic, 83 Dawson Rd, Guelph ON N1H 1B1; Wes'94; CCFP; Staff, Guelph General Hospital; (519)766-1360; Fax. (519)763-4315.

CHOI, H David; King Street Med Arts Centre, 401-71 King St W, Mississauga ON L5B 4A2; Tor'92; CCFP; (905)273-9793; Fax. (905)273-7054.

CHOI, Heywood S; Endocrine Fellow's Office, 4F-2775 Laurel St, Vancouver BC V5Z 1M9; UBC'08; FRCPC; IntMed. (604)875-5929

CHOI, Hyon K; Arthritic Research Centre, 5591 NO. 3 Rd, Richmond BC V6X 2C7; Yonsei (Korea)'86; Rheum; IntMed. (604)207-4004

CHOI, Hyun D; Foothills Medical Centre, C231-1403 29 St NW, Calgary AB T2N 2T9; Alb'05; FRCPC; EmergMed. Staff, Foothills Medical Centre; (403)944-8430; Fax. (403)944-3684.

CHOI, James H; The Doctors Office, 245 Eglinton Ave E, Toronto ON M4P 3B7; Tor'91; CCFP; (416)488-1455; Fax. (416)485-2671.

CHOI, Julianna; Pine River Institute, 800-2 St Clair Ave E, Toronto ON M4T 2T5; Ott'94; FRCPC; Psy. Staff, Pine River Institute; (416)955-1453; jchoi@rougevalley.ca.

CHOI, Karen E; 210 Aspen Glen Landing SW PO Box 15072 Aspen Woods PO, Calgary AB T3H 0N5; Tor'07; CCFP.

CHOI, Mabel; Sunnybrook Hlth Sciences Ctre, 2075 Bayview Ave, Toronto ON M4N 3M5; Tor'99; FRCPC; Anes. Staff, Sunnybrook Health Sciences Centre; (416)480-4864

CHOI, Margaret S; Children's & Women's HC of BC, B321-4480 Oak St, Vancouver BC V6H 3V4; Ott'00; FRCPC; Peds. Staff, BC Children's Hospital; (604)875-2345 x7360

CHOI, Mark; St Paul's Hosp, 602B-1081 Burrard St, Vancouver BC V6Z 1Y6; Tor'08; IntMed. Staff, Providence Health Care - St Paul's Hospital; (604)682-2344

CHOI, Matthew C K; 125-1465 Salisbury Ave, Port Coquitlam BC V3B 6J3; Alb'92; BSc(MedSci); CCFP; Langs: Cantonese; (604)552-3001; Fax. (604)552-3701.

CHOI, Perry; Markham Stouffville Hosp, PO Box 1800 Stn Main 381 Church St, Markham ON L3P 7P3; Tor'05; FRCPC; DiagRad. Staff, Markham Stouffville Hospital; (905)472-7020

CHOI, Peter T; UBC-Dept of Anes, 3300-910 10th Ave W, Vancouver BC V5Z 1M9; UBC'93; BSc; MSc(Epid.); FRCPC; Anes (Clinical Epidemiology). Assoc Prof, University of British Columbia; Langs: Cantonese; (604)875-4575; Fax. (604)875-5344.

CHOI, Richard F Y; Bloor-Jane Med Bldg, 411-2425 Bloor St W, Toronto ON M6S 4W4; UBC'95; BSc; FRCPC; IntMed; Cardiol. Staff Cardiol, St Joseph's Health Centre; Lecturer, University of Toronto; Langs: Korean; (416)762-5521; Fax. (416)762-2154.

CHOI, Stephen B; The Ottawa Hosp-Gen Campus, 501 Smyth Rd, Ottawa ON K1H 8L6; Qns'98; FRCPC; EmergMed. Staff, The Ottawa Hospital - General Campus; (613)722-7000

CHOI, Stephen; Sunnybrook Hlth Sciences Ctre, M3200-2075 Bayview Ave, Toronto ON M4N 3M5; Wes'05; BSc; FRCPC; Anes (Regional Anesthesia). Staff, Sunnybrook Health Sciences Centre; Toronto General Hospital - UHN; (416)480-4864

CHOI, Steve C S; Oak Park Med Clinic, 1-2530 Sixth Line, Oakville ON L6H 6W5; Sydney (Australia)'00; BScPharm; MB BS; (905)257-1006; Fax. (905)257-0661.

CHOI, Tat Hung J; York Prof Bldg, 320-679 Davis Dr, Newmarket ON L3Y 5G8; Tor'81; FRCSC; GenSurg. (905)895-0624; Fax. (905)895-4690.

CHOI, W M Joyce; Collingwood Medical Clinic, 350-3150 54th Ave, Vancouver BC V5Z 0A2; UBC'07; CCFP; (604)435-3388

CHOI, Young S; 2075 Hadwen Rd, Mississauga ON L5K 2L3; Tor'91; FRCPC; IntMed. (905)855-1860 x231; Fax. (905)855-1863.

CHOI-FUNG, Betty L S; 208-1262 Don Mills Rd, North York ON M3B 2W7; Loma Linda(CA) (USA)'82; CCFP; Staff, Toronto East General Hospital Inc; Langs: Cantonese; (416)429-4110; Fax. (416)429-1564.

CHOINIERE, Andre; Ctr Hosp de Verdun, 4000 boul Lasalle, Verdun QC H4G 2A3; Mon'98; CSPQ; FRCPC; Anes. Staff, Centre Hospitalier de Verdun; (514)362-1000 x2829

CHOINIERE, Daniel; GMF de Lorraine, 99 boul De Gaulle, Lorraine QC J6Z 3Z9; Mon'86; Staff, Hopital de la Cite de la santé; Prof Family Med, Universite de Montreal; (450)621-1444; Fax. (450)621-7193.

CHOINIERE, Jean-Luc; CHUM-Hotel-Dieu, 3840 rue Saint-Urbain, Montreal QC H2W 1T8; Mon'63; CSPQ; FRCPC; Anes. Staff, Centre Hospitalier l'Université de Montréal (CHUM) - Hôtel-Dieu; (514)890-8000 x14570

CHOINIERE, Louise; Hop du Sacre-Coeur de Mtl, 5400 boul Gouin O, Montreal QC H4J 1C5; Mon'75; FRCSC; GenSurg; Cardiovasc&ThorSurg; ThorSurg. Staff, Hôpital du Sacre-Coeur de Montréal; (514)338-2050

CHOKANI, Khami; 1521 6th Ave W, Prince Albert SK S6V 5K1; Rajasthan (India)'87; MB BS; Langs: Albanian; Chichewa; Bemba; Chiyao; Hindi; Latin; Lingala; (306)765-6601; Fax. (306)765-6495; khami.chokani@cypressrha.ca.

CHOKER, Ghassan N; CHUS-Hop Fleurimont, 3001 12e av N, Sherbrooke QC J1H 5N4; (Lebanon)'98; Staff, Centre Hospitalier Universitaire de Sherbrooke-Hopital Fleurimont; (819)346-1110

CHOKKA, Pratap R; 201-2603 Hewes Way NW, Edmonton AB T6L 6W6; Alb'90; FRCPC; Psy (Anxiety Disorder). Consultant Psy, Covenant Health - Grey Nuns Community Hospital; Consultant Psy, Provincial Mental Health; Clin Assoc Prof Faculty of Med, University of Alberta; (780)465-5749; Fax. (780)465-5799.

CHOKSHI, Rashmikant G; Medical Arts Bldg, 212-336 Kings Rd, Sydney NS B1S 1A9; Mysore (India)'61; DAB; FRCSC; Otol. Staff, Cape Breton Healthcare Complex; Staff, Northside General Hospital; Staff, Glace Bay Healthcare Facility; (902)539-6040; Fax. (902)539-6041.

CHOLETTE, Pascale; CLSC Basse-Ville-Limoilou, 50 rue Saint-Joseph E, Quebec QC G1K 3A5; Laval'81; (418)529-2592; Fax. (418)529-4309.

CHOLETTE, Pierre M; Soins Palliative de l'Ouest L', 265 rue Andre-Brunet, Kirkland QC H9H 3R4; Mon'75; LMCC; (514)693-1718

CHOLIN, Brenda L; 101-11427 Railway Ave, North Battleford SK S9A 3G8; Alb'84; MPH(PublicHealth); CCFP; FCFP; (306)446-6400; Fax. (306)446-6432; brenda.cholin@pnrha.ca.

CHOLLET, Andre; 3060-5199 rue Sherbrooke E, Montreal QC H1T 3X2; Mon'82; FRCS; FRCSC; PlasSurg (Maxillo Facial Surgery). Teach Staff, Universite de Montreal; Langs: English; (514)253-5518; Fax. (514)253-3331.

CHOLUJ, Agnieszka; South Urgent Care Center, 113-31 Sunpark Plaza SE, Calgary AB T2X 3W5; Alb'05; CCFP.

CHOMEJ, Anna K; 203-1051 Upper James St, Hamilton ON L9C 3A6; McM'00; FRCSC; ObstGyn. (905)667-2600

CHOMIENNE, M Helene; Montfort Hosp, 120-713 ch Montreal, Ottawa ON K1K 0T2; Paris (France)'80; CCFP; Clin Researcher, Montfort Hospital; Assoc Prof, University of Ottawa; Langs: Bilingual(French/English); (613)746-4621 x6206; Fax. (613)748-4953; mh.chomienne@uottawa.ca.

CHOMIN, Gary L; 203-3825 Sunset St, Burnaby BC V5G 1T4; Alb'74; (604)434-9515; Fax. (604)434-5984.

CHONG, Angeline Y W; Oshawa Clinic, 117 King St E, Oshawa ON L1H 1B9; Harvard University (USA)'02; FRCPC; IntMed. (905)721-4982; Fax. (905)721-6654.

CHONG, Carolyn C; West Point Grey Med Bldg, 4570 10th Ave W, Vancouver BC V6R 2J1; UBC'90; IntMed. (604)224-0480

CHONG, Christopher A K; Lakeridge Hlth Corp-Oshawa, 1 Hospital Crt, Oshawa ON L1G 2B9; Tor'03; FRCPC; IntMed. Staff, Lakeridge Health - Oshawa Site; (905)576-8711

CHONG, Daniel N F; Orillia Soldiers Mem Hosp, 170 Colborne St W, Orillia ON L3V 2Z3; RCS (Ireland)'66; Staff, Orillia Soldiers' Memorial Hospital; (705)325-2201

CHONG, David L T; Surrey Mem Hosp, 13750 96 Ave, Surrey BC V3V 1Z2; UBC'01; BSc; CCFP; CCFP(E.M.); Staff, Surrey Memorial Hospital; Langs: Cantonese; (604)581-2211; Fax. (604)588-3382.

CHONG, Dennis K; 207-345 Lakershore Rd E, Oakville ON L6J 1J5; Leeds (England)'64; MRCS; LRCP; Elective Supervisor, McMaster University; (905)844-0864; Fax. (905)844-3212; dchong345@cogeco.ca.

CHONG, Donald T; 164 Mccaul St, Toronto ON M5T 1W4; Tor'68; (416)597-0262

CHONG, Elizabeth C; 146-6200 McKay Ave, Burnaby BC V5H 4L7; UBC'98; CCFP; (604)438-8288

CHONG, Esther; Richpoint Med Centre, 10815 Yonge St, Richmond Hill ON L4C 3E3; Tor'95; CCFP; (905)770-3004; Fax. (905)770-5663.

CHONG, Henry K H; West Point Grey Med Bldg, 4570 10th Ave W, Vancouver BC V6R 2J1; UBC'56; Ac Staff, Vancouver General Hospital - Centennial Pavillion; (604)224-0480

CHONG, John P; Sir William Osler Health Inst, 201-565 Sanatorium Rd, Hamilton ON L9C 7N4; McM'78; BASc; MSc; DOHS; FAB; FRCPC; CommunMed; Public Health & Preventive Med. Ac Staff, Hamilton Health Sciences Centre - McMaster Children's Hospital; Med Dir, Musician's Clinics of Canada; (905)574-5444; Fax. (905)574-1119; john.chong@sympatico.ca.

CHONG, Joseph M; Peace Arch Hosp, 15521 Russell Ave, White Rock BC V4B 2R4; UBC'92; Staff, Peace Arch Hospital; (604)531-5512

CHONG, Karen L; Hydro Place Bldg, 3290-700 University Ave, Toronto ON M5G 1Z5; Cal'94; FRCPC; Peds. (416)586-4523; Fax. (416)586-4723.

CHONG, Laura J; Pine Seven Med Centre, 175-4600 Highway 7, Woodbridge ON L4L 4Y7; Tor'84; Court Staff, Humber River Regional Hospital - Finch Avenue Site; (905)856-3611; Fax. (905)856-3612; chong@woodbridgemd.com.

CHONG, Michael B; Chinook Reg Hosp, 960 19 St S, Lethbridge AB T1J 1W5; London (England)'86; MB BS; FRCPC; Anes. Staff, Chinook Regional Hospital; (403)388-6131; Fax. (403)388-6154.

CHONG, Michael P; Foothills Med Centre, 1403 29 St NW, Calgary AB T2N 2T9; UBC'01; FRCPC; Anes. Staff, Foothills Medical Centre; (403)944-1430

CHONG, Nancy L; Shops On Steeles Med Centre, 206-2900 Steeles Ave E, Thornhill ON L3T 4X1; Tor'88; (905)881-6667; Fax. (905)731-1298.

CHONG, Paul W C; 203-9350 Yonge St, Richmond Hill ON L4C 5G2; (Hong Kong)'90; ABIM; FACC; FRCPC; IntMed (Invasive Cardiology); Cardiol. Court Staff Cardiol, Southlake Regional Health Centre; Staff Cardiol, Mackenzie Richmond Hill Hospital; Langs: Cantonese; (905)883-8220; Fax. (905)883-8227.

CHONG, Peter C; 101-1617 Baker St, Cranbrook BC V1C 1B4; Ott'04; FRCSC; GenSurg. (250)489-3044

CHONG, Rachel Y V; Oshawa Clinic, 117 King St E, Oshawa ON L1H 1B9; Chicago (USA)'00; FRCPC; IntMed; Endocrin&Metab. Staff, Lakeridge Health - Bowmanville Site; (905)721-4975

CHONG, Robert H; Mount Dennis Med Group, 98 Guestville Ave, Toronto ON M6N 4N6; Tor'81; Ac Staff, Humber River Regional Hospital - Church Street Site; Langs: Cantonese; (416)763-1171; Fax. (416)763-0573.

CHONG, Sophia S H; Oakridge Centre South Tower, 360-650 41st Ave W, Vancouver BC V5Z 2M9; Qns'92; Langs: Mandarin; (604)261-6000; Fax. (604)261-6667.

CHONG, Sylvia L; Headwaters Health Care Centre, 100 Rolling Hills Dr, Orangeville ON L9W 4X9; Tor'96; CCFP; FCFP; Staff, Headwaters Health Care Centre - Orangeville Site; (519)941-2410 x2214

CHONG, Tiffany L; 101-777 Broadway W, Vancouver BC V5Z 4J7; UBC'10; CCFP; (604)734-8252

CHONG, Tze-Feng; Guardian Bldg, 054-10240 124 St NW, Edmonton AB T5N 3W6; Alb'01; BSc(Hons); FRCSC; PlasSurg (Cranio Maxillofacial Surgery). Cli Care Associate, University of Alberta; (780)453-3223

CHONG, Xin; Stamford Med Centre, 201-4256 Portage Rd, Niagara Falls ON L2E 6A4; Mem'97; BSc(BioChem); MSc(Biochem); CCFP; Ac Member, Niagara Health System - Greater Niagara General Site; Asst Clin Prof Dept of Med, McMaster University; Langs: Mandarin; Chinese; (905)358-5708; Fax. (905)356-2227.

CHONG KIT, Renison; St Paul's Hosp, 1081 Burrard St, Vancouver BC V6Z 1Y6; (Jamaica)'63; MB BS; FRCPC; GenPath (Endocrinology). Physician Med Biochemist, Providence Health Care - St Paul's Hospital; (604)682-2344; rckit@dccnet.com.

CHONKO, Douglas M; 1915 Lemieux Crt NW, Edmonton AB T6R 3T5; Alb'74; (780)436-6975; Fax. (780)432-3642.

CHOO, Caroline W H; 130-8191 Westminster Hwy PO Box 707, Richmond BC V6X 1A7; UBC'87; DABPN(Psy); DABPN(GeriatricPsy); DABPN(AddictionPsy); FRCPC; Psy. Clin Prof, University of British Columbia; (604)244-5237; Fax. (604)278-4819.

CHOO, Darren W K; 6430 Main St, Vancouver BC V5W 2V4; UBC'88; Court Staff, BC Women's Hospital & Health Centre; Court Staff, BC Children's Hospital; Court Staff, Providence Health Care - Mount Saint Joseph Hospital; Langs: Cantonese; Mandarin; (604)321-4313; Fax. (604)321-4314.

CHOO, Ivan S Y; 8685 120 St, Delta BC V4C 6R4; UBC'93; BSc(Hons.); CCFP; FCFP; Langs: Cantonese; (604)591-1122; Fax. (604)591-1136; ichoo@shaw.ca.

CHOO FONE, Alan B; Health One Medical, 216-3001 Gordon Ave, Coquitlam BC V3C 2K7; Cal'91; BSc; Staff, Eagle Ridge Hospital & Health Care Centre; (604)942-3138; Fax. (604)942-6823.

CHOOI, Weng K; Valley Med Imaging, 404A-2151 McCallum Rd, Abbotsford BC V2S 3N8; Melbourne (Australia)'95; MB BS; FRCPC; DiagRad. (604)859-8998

CHOONG, Douglas K M; 101-21 Surrey St W, Guelph ON N1H 3R3; Wes'91; CCFP; FCFP; Ac Staff, Guelph General Hospital; (519)822-2188

CHOONG, Karen; McMaster University, HSC 3Y15-1280 Main St W, Hamilton ON L8S 4K1; RCS (Ireland)'91; FRCPC; Peds (Neonatology). Staff, Hamilton Health Sciences Centre - McMaster Children's Hospital; Teach Staff, McMaster University; (905)521-2100 x76610

CHOONG, Wee Kei; Delta View Rehab Centre, 9341 Burns Dr, Delta BC V4K 3N3; Cal'00; Langs: Mandarin; Cantonese; Hakka; Malay; (604)596-8842

CHOPPA, Sailaja; Windsor Prof Centre, 138-2462 Howard Ave, Windsor ON N8X 3V6; Sri Venkatesvara (India)'90; CCFP; (519)971-2726; Fax. (519)971-2711.

CHOPRA, Angeli; Hlth Sciences Ctre-Fac of Med, 3330 Hospital Dr NW, Calgary AB T2N 4N1; Baba Farid (Other Foreign)'06; Gastroent; IntMed. (403)944-1110

CHOPRA, Anil; Univ Hlth Network-The Toronto, 200 Elizabeth St, Toronto ON M5G 2C4; Tor'89; FRCPC; EmergMed. Staff Physician Emerg, Toronto General Hospital - UHN; Asst Prof, University of Toronto; (416)340-3856; Fax. (416)595-7013; anil.chopra@utoronto.ca.

CHOPRA, Ashna; Hotel-Dieu Grace Hosp, 1030 Ouellette Ave, Windsor ON N9A 1E1; Qns'91; FRCPC; Anes. Staff, Hôtel-Dieu Grace Hospital; (519)973-4421

CHOPRA, Jagdish C; Glazier Med Centre, 11 Gibb St, Oshawa ON L1H 2J9; Guru Nanak (India)'73; MB BS; Staff Family Med, Lakeridge Health - Oshawa Site; Langs: Punjabi; Hindi; Urdu; (905)579-1212; Fax. (905)571-7548.

CHOPRA, Justin A; Innovation Medical Centre, 40 Innovation Dr, Woodbridge ON L4H 0T2; McM'10; CCFP; Staff, Credit Valley Family Health Team; (905)851-2444; Fax. (905)851-4588.

CHOPRA, Kevin K; Addiction & Mental Hlth-Clarke, 1127-250 College St, Toronto ON M5T 1R8; Dal'00; FRCPC; Psy. Staff, Centre for Addiction & Mental Health (CAMH) - College Street Site; (416)535-8501 x4238

CHOPRA, Nikhil; London Medical-Dental Bldg, 411-450 Central Ave, London ON N6B 2E8; Qns'95; FRCPC; IntMed; Rheum. (519)435-0415; Fax. (519)435-1862.

CHOPRA, Priya; Springdale Prof Bldg, 611-2250 Bovaird Dr E, Brampton ON L6R 0W3; Wes'95; FRCSC; GenSurg. (905)866-6462; Fax. (905)866-5633.

CHOPRA, Raj K; Windsor Med Clinic, 1604-1608 Tecumseh Rd W, Windsor ON N9B 1T8; Rangoon (Burma)'66; (519)258-4400

CHOPRA, Sabeena B; Ryerson Med Center, 181-350 Victoria St, Toronto ON M5B 2K3; Tor'02; FRCPC; Psy. Staff, Toronto East General Hospital Inc; (416)979-5070

CHOPRA, Sachin S; Hamilton HS-General Site, 8N-237 Barton St E, Hamilton ON L8L 2X2; McM'08; Staff, Hamilton Health Sciences Centre - Hamilton General Hospital; (905)521-2100

CHOPTIANY, Philip J; Don Valley Med Associates, 330-1333 Sheppard Ave E, North York ON M2J 1V1; Tor'75; CCFP; Court Staff, Sunnybrook Health Sciences Centre; Ac Staff Emerg, North York General Hospital; (416)497-6444; Fax. (416)497-4793; pchoptiany@baycrest.org.

CHOPTIANY, Robert B W; Berrydale Family Med Centre, 417 St Anne's Rd, Winnipeg MB R2M 3C4; Man'80; Med Dir, Vista Park Lodge; (204)255-6256; Fax. (204)255-6260.

CHOQUET, Benoit; Clinique Med Olivier-Vien, 1015 boul Olivier-Vien, Roberval QC G8H 3N9; McG'87; Staff, Hotel-Dieu de Roberval; (418)275-1122; benoit@leblond.com.

CHOQUET, Julie; Clinique Med du Sub-Ouest, 4475 rue Bannantyne, Verdun QC H4G 1E2; McG'91; CCFP; ac Membre Gen Med, Centre Hospitalier de LaSalle; Staff Family Med Unit, Centre Hospitalier de Verdun; Médecin, CLSC Verdun Cote St-Paul; Langs: Spanish; (514)765-3600; Fax. (514)765-9625.

CHOQUET, Yves; Clinique Med Fabreville, 108-380 boul Curé-Labelle, Laval QC H7P 5L3; Mon'66; CSPQ; Cardiol (P.Q.). Staff, Hôpital du Sacre-Coeur de Montréal; (450)963-1961; Fax. (450)963-1205.

CHOQUETTE, Anne; Ctr Hosp Affilie-St-Sacrement, 1050 ch Sainte-Foy, Quebec QC G1S 4L8; Mon'84; CSPQ; AnatPath. Staff, Centre Hospitalier Affilié Universitaire de Québec - Hôpital du St-Sacrement; Fax. (418)682-7811.

CHOQUETTE, Claude; Clinique Med Pierre-Boucher, 1615 boul Jacques-Cartier E, Longueuil QC J4M 2X1; Sher'76; (450)468-6223; Fax. (450)468-5041; cchoq@videotron.ca.

CHOQUETTE, Denis; Institut Rhumatologie de Mtl, 1551 rue Ontario E, Montreal QC H2L 1S6; Mon'78; Rheum. (514)523-3305; Fax. (514)523-5973.

CHOQUETTE, Jean-Francois; Ctr Hosp du Centre la Mauricie, 50 119e rue, Shawinigan-Sud QC G9P 5K1; Sher'00; CSPQ; FRCPC; Anes. Staff, Centre Hospitalier du Centre la Mauricie; (819)536-7500; Fax. (819)536-7611.

CHOQUETTE, Julie; Ctr Hosp Rouyn-Noranda, 4 9e rue, Rouyn-Noranda QC J9X 2B2; Laval'03; CCFP; Staff, Centre Hospitalier Rouyn-Noranda; Langs: Bilingual(French/English); (819)764-5131

CHOQUETTE, Julie; GMF Concorde, 300 boul de la Concorde E, Laval QC H7G 2E6; Mon'02; Langs: Bilingual(French/English); (450)667-5310; Fax. (450)667-5248.

CHOQUETTE, Lise; Ctr Hosp de Verdun, 4000 boul Lasalle, Verdun QC H4G 2A3; Mon'79; Staff, Centre Hospitalier de Verdun; Langs: Bilingual(French/English); (514)765-7325

CHOQUETTE, Marie; CSSS Haut-Richelieu-Rouville, 920 boul Du Seminaire N, St-Jean-Sur-Richel QC J3A 1B7; Mon'84; FRCPC; Psy. Chef psychiatrie, Hôpital du Haut-Richelieu; (450)359-5000 x5450; Fax. (450)359-5453.

CHOQUETTE, Pierre; Clinique Med Sainte-Dorothee, 102-1 boul Samson, Laval QC H7X 3S5; Mon'74; ObstGyn. (450)689-6334

CHOR, Mark W H; Glazier Med Centre, 11 Gibb St, Oshawa ON L1H 2J9; Man'74; Staff, Lakeridge Health - Oshawa Site; Langs: Cantonese; (905)579-1212; Fax. (905)579-1583.

CHOREMIS, Johanna; SMBD Jewish Gen Hosp, 3755 ch Cote-Sainte-Catherine, Montreal QC H3T 1E2; McG'99; FRCSC; Ophth. Staff, Sir Mortimer B Davis Jewish General; (514)340-8222

CHORN, Michael; 11-4429 Kingsway, Burnaby BC V5H 2A1; Cape Town (South Africa)'80; MB ChB; (604)431-6585

CHORNELL, J Gary; St Albert Prof Bldg, 321-7 St Anne St, St. Albert AB T8N 2X4; Alb'66; FRCSC; Ophth (Aviation). Consultant, Royal Alexandra Hospital; Consultant, Occupational Health Society of Alberta; Exec Dir, Ophthalmology Society of Alberta; Consultant Teacher, University of Alberta; (780)459-9293; Fax. (780)460-0408.

CHORNEYKO, Katherine; Saskatoon City Hosp, 701 Queen St, Saskatoon SK S7K 0M7; Wes'89; FRCPC; GenPath; AnatPath. Staff Lab Med, Saskatoon City Hospital; (306)655-8398; Fax. (306)655-8399.

CHORNY, Irina; Royal Columbia Hosp, 330 Columbia St E, New Westminster BC V3L 3W7; Lvov (Ukraine)'88; MD; Staff, Royal Columbian Hospital; (604)520-4001

CHOTARD, Isabelle; Inst U en Sante Mentale de QC, 2601 ch de la Canardiere, Quebec QC G1J 2G3; Mon'97; Staff, Institut Universitaire Sante; (418)663-5253

CHOU, Alan F; 203-3825 Sunset St, Burnaby BC V5G 1T4; Tor'82; FRCPC; EmergMed. Staff, Burnaby Hospital; (604)434-9515; Fax. (604)434-5984.

CHOU, Angela; Lakeridge HC-Bowmanville Site, 47 Liberty St S, Bowmanville ON L1C 2N4; Ott'96; CCFP; FCFP; Staff, Lakeridge Health - Bowmanville Site; (905)623-3331 x1311; Fax. (905)697-5115.

CHOU, Benjamin; Valley Centre Medical Clinic, 109-20151 Fraser Hwy, Langley BC V3A 4E4; Man'79; PhD; MSc; Langs: Mandarin; Cantonese; (604)534-9284

CHOU, George C; 509-18 Kensington Rd, Brampton ON L6T 4S5; Tor'94; CCFP; (905)799-9875; Fax. (289)298-5339.

CHOU, Jean; Groupe Med de Trois-Rivieres, 225-1900 boul des Recollets, Trois-Rivieres QC G8Z 4K4; Sher'06; (819)375-6666; Fax. (819)375-3423.

CHOU, Jenny W; Surrey Med Arts Bldg, 206-13710 94A Ave, Surrey BC V3V 1N1; UBC'04; FRCPC; Peds. Langs: Mandarin; (604)585-4477

CHOU, Julie P; Peter Lougheed Centre, 3500 26 Ave NE, Calgary AB T1Y 6J4; Tor'03; FRCPC; IntMed; Respir. Staff, Peter Lougheed Centre; (403)943-4555

CHOU, Linda H; 4841 Yonge St PO Box 43036 Rpo Sheppard Ctre, North York ON M2N 6N1; Far Eastern (Philippines)'62.

CHOU, Ming Convir; Northtown Mall, 240-9450 137 Ave NW, Edmonton AB T5E 6C2; Alb'73; BMedSci; Court Staff Family Med, Royal Alexandra Hospital; (780)478-2958; Fax. (780)478-2950; mingcchou@hotmail.com.

CHOU, Queena; London HSC-Victoria Hosp, PO Box 5010 Stn B B2 443-800 Commissioners Rd E, London ON N6A 5W9; Tor'93; FSOGC; FACOG; LMCC; LRCPS; MCPS; PhC; FRCSC; ObstGyn (Urological Gynecology). Staff, St Joseph's Hospital - St Joseph's Health Care; Staff, London Health Sciences Centre - Victoria Campus; Assoc Prof Med & Dentistry, University of Western Ontario; (519)646-6343; Fax. (519)646-6253.

CHOU, Roger; Fitzgerald Bldg, 112-150 College St, Toronto ON M5S 3E2; Sydney (Australia)'00.

CHOU, Sheila; Joseph Brant Mem Hosp, 1230 North Shore Blvd, Hamilton ON L8S 1W7; Tor'96; FRCPC; DiagRad (Interventional Radiology). Staff, Hamilton Health Sciences Centre-Juravinski Site; Staff, Joseph Brant Memorial Hospital; (905)527-4322 x42261

CHOU, Shirley H Y; Children's Hosp Eastern Ont, 401 Smyth Rd, Ottawa ON K1H 8L1; Sher'78; MSc; FRCSC; GenSurg; PedGenSurg. Staff, Children's Hospital of Eastern Ontario (CHEO); Asst Prof, University of Ottawa; Langs: Mandarin; Chinese; French; (613)737-7600 x1524; Fax. (613)738-4849; chou@cheo.on.ca.

CHOU, Sophia H; Foothills Med Centre, 1403 29 St NW, Calgary AB T2N 2T9; Wes'01; FRCPC; IntMed; Nephrol. Staff, Foothills Medical Centre; (403)944-2667

CHOUDHRI, Omer H; Kanata Prof Centre, 213-99 Kakulu Rd, Kanata ON K2L 3C8; Man'91; FRCPC; IntMed. (613)592-1992

CHOUDHRY, Ashwani; Malton Med Arts Bldg, 205-3530 Derry Rd E, Mississauga ON L4T 4E3; Meerut (India)'79; MRC; LRCP(Ed); LRCS(Ed); LRCPS(Glas); ABIM; MD; FRCPC; IntMed (Echocardiography); Cardiol. Staff Cardiologist, Humber River Regional Hospital - Church Street Site; Langs: Punjabi; (905)676-0006; Fax. (905)676-9992; ashwanichoudhry@gmail.com.

CHOUDHRY, Netan; Herzig Eye Insititute, 210-131 Bloor St W, Toronto ON M5S 1R1; Georgetown University (USA)'05; FRCSC; Ophth. Staff, Herzig Eye Institute; (416)929-2020

CHOUDHRY, Sushil; 201-1090 Peter Robertson Blvd, Brampton ON L6R 3B3; Jabalpur (India)'86; MB BS; LMCC; CCFP; FCFP; Langs: Hindi; (905)494-0399; Fax. (905)494-0681.

CHOUDHURY, Anil; Mississauga Med Plex, 8-6980 Maritz Dr, Mississauga ON L5W 1Z3; Dacca (Bangladesh)'69; (905)696-0833; Fax. (905)696-7425.

CHOUDUR, Hema N; Hamilton HS-General Site, 2-237 Barton St E, Hamilton ON L8L 2X2; Andhra Pradesh (India)'89; FRCPC; DiagRad. Staff, Hamilton Health Sciences Centre - Hamilton General Hospital; (905)527-4322

CHOUERI, Georges N; Centre Med Sainte-Dorothee, 1-3 boul Samson, Laval QC H7X 3S5; St. Joseph (Lebanon)'74; FRCPC; Gastroent. Chef gastroent, Hopital de la Cite de la santé; Langs: French; Arabic; Greek; (450)969-9911; Fax. (450)969-2994.

CHOUIALI, Ahlem; CHUS-Hop Fleurimont, 3001 12e av N, Sherbrooke QC J1H 5N4; Algiers (Algeria)'96; FRCPC; MedBiochem. Staff, Centre Hospitalier Universitaire de Sherbrooke-Hopital Fleurimont; (819)346-1110

CHOUINARD, Alexandre; Clinique des Sommets, 1070 rue Principal E, Cap-aux-Meules QC G4T 1R9; Mon'98; Staff, Hôpital de l'Archipel; (819)321-1212

CHOUINARD, Catherine; CSSS de Chicoutimi, CP 5006 305 rue Saint-Vallier, Chicoutimi QC G7H 5H6; Mon'01; Psy. Staff, Complexe hospitalier de la Sagamie; (418)541-1000 x5151; Fax. (418)549-5706.

CHOUINARD, Christian; CSSS Pierre Boucher, 1333 boul Jacques-Cartier E, Longueuil QC J4M 2A5; Mon'76; GenSurg. ac Staff, Centre Hospitalier Pierre Boucher; (450)468-8111

CHOUINARD, Claude; Clinique Med du Jardin, 15094 boul Henri-Bourassa, Quebec QC G1G 3Z4; Laval'81; ac Staff, Centre Hospitalier Universitaire De Québec - Pavillon De St-françois-d'assise; (418)628-9074; Fax. (418)628-0267.

CHOUINARD, Daniel; Clinique Med le Frontenac, 202-5200 rue Frontenac, Lac-Megantic QC G6B 1H3; Sher'05; CCFP; Staff, Carrefour Sante Granit; (819)583-0157

CHOUINARD, Dany; CSSS de Saint-Jerome, 290 rue de Montigny, Saint-Jerome QC J7Z 5T3; Laval'93; CSPQ; FRCPC; Anes. Staff, Hôtel-Dieu de Saint-Jérôme; (450)431-8200

CHOUINARD, Denise; Clinique Med du Carrefour, 8585 boul Lacroix, Saint-Georges QC G5Y 5L6; Sher'99; Staff, Cree Board of Health & Social Services James Bay; (418)227-1271; denoui@hotmail.com.

CHOUINARD, Diane; Ctr Hosp Fleury, 2180 rue Fleury E, Montreal QC H2B 1K3; Mon'96; CCFP; Staff, Centre Hospitalier Fleury; (514)381-9311

CHOUINARD, Edmond E; Cambridge Mem Hosp, 700 Coronation Blvd, Cambridge ON N1R 3G2; Wes'80; FRCPC; IntMed; MedOncol. Court Staff, Hamilton Health Sciences Centre-Juravinski Site; Ac Staff, Cambridge Memorial Hospital; Court Staff, Grand River Hospital - Freeport Site; Clinical Asst Prof Dept of Oncology, McMaster University; Langs: English; French; (519)740-4940; Fax. (519)740-7722.

CHOUINARD, Gabriel; Inuulitsivik Health Centre, GD, Povungnituq QC J0M 1P0; Laval'09; CCFP; Staff, Inuulitsivik Health Centre; (819)988-2957; Fax. (819)988-2796.

CHOUINARD, Guy; Clinique Med du Jardin, 15094 boul Henri-Bourassa, Quebec QC G1G 3Z4; Laval'80; Ac Staff, Centre Hospitalier Universitaire De Québec - Pavillon De St-françois-d'assise; Langs: English; (418)628-9074; Fax. (418)628-0267.

CHOUINARD, Guy; MUHC-Royal Victoria Hosp, 687 av des Pins O, Montreal QC H3A 1A1; Mon'68; MSc(Pharm.); FAPA; FRCPC; Psy (Pharmacology). principale Staff Psy, McGill University Health Centre - Royal Victoria Hospital; Dir Clin Psychopharmacology Clinic, Allan Memorial Institute; Prof Psy, McGill University; Prof Psy & Med, Universite de Montreal; Langs: Bilingual(French/English); (514)843-1672; chouinard.g@gmail.com.

CHOUINARD, Helene; 460 rue Sainte-Helene, Longueuil QC J4K 3R2; Mon'81; (450)442-4272; Fax. (450)442-1205.

CHOUINARD, J A Jean; BCC-St Vincent Hosp, 60 Cambridge St N, Ottawa ON K1R 7A5; Ott'79; Court Staff Nephrol, The Ottawa Hospital - General Campus; Med Chief Complex Cont Care & LTC, Bruyère Continuing Care - Saint-Vincent Hospital; (613)233-4041 x3140; Fax. (613)782-2837; jchouina@scohs.on.ca.

CHOUINARD, Jean-Philippe; Clinique Med de la Rive, 169 av Prince Albert, Otterburn Park QC J3H 1L4; Mon'01; CCFP; (450)446-7333; Fax. (450)446-3420.

CHOUINARD, Jerome; CSSS de Rimouski-Neigette, CP 3150 Succ A 150 av Rouleau, Rimouski QC G5L 5T1; Mon'00; FRCSC; GenSurg. Chef chir gén, Hôpital Regional Rimouski; (418)723-7851

CHOUINARD, Josee; Clinique Pedia Courte Echelle, 101-86 boul Brien, Repentigny QC J6A 5K7; Laval'89; Peds. Staff, Centre Hospitalier Pierre le Gardeur; (450)657-1705

CHOUINARD, Lyne; Coroner's Office Bldg Delta 2, 390-2875 boul Laurier, Quebec QC G1V 5B1; Laval'88; Staff, Hôtel-Dieu de Lévis; (418)643-1845 x230

CHOUINARD, Marie-Josee; CSSS Pierre Boucher, 1333 boul Jacques-Cartier E, Longueuil QC J4M 2A5; Mon'02; FRCPC; Psy. Staff, Centre Hospitalier Pierre Boucher; (450)468-8111 x8401

CHOUINARD, Marie-Josee; Ctr Hosp Laurentien, 234 rue Saint-Vincent, Ste-Agathe-des-Mts QC J8C 2B8; Laval'99; FRCSC; ObstGyn. Staff, Centre Hospitalier Laurentien; (819)324-4000

CHOUINARD, Pascale; CHUQ-St-Francois D'Assise, 10 rue de l'Espinay, Quebec QC G1L 3L5; Laval'03; FRCPC; IntMed; Gastroent. Staff, Centre Hospitalier Universitaire De Québec - Pavillon De St-françois-d'assise; (418)525-4444

CHOUINARD, Philippe; 105A-667 rue Champlain, Dieppe NB E1A 1P6; Mon'08; CCFP; Staff, Dr Georges-L-Dumont University Hospital Centre; (506)862-4000

CHOUINARD, Raynald; CSSS de la Cote-de-Gaspe, 215 boul de York O, Gaspe QC G4X 2W2; Laval'68; CSPQ; FRCPC; Anes. Staff, Centre Hospitalier de Gaspe; (418)368-3301

CHOUINARD, Renee R; Ashgrove Med Centre, 314-6633 Highway 7, Markham ON L3P 7P2; McG'86; ObstGyn. Staff, Markham Stouffville Hospital; (905)201-9972; Fax. (905)201-9932.

CHOUINARD, Sylvain R; Hôpital Laval, 2725 ch Sainte-Foy, Quebec QC G1V 4G5; Laval'79; IntMed (P.Q.) (Nephrology). Staff, Hôpital Laval; Langs: English; (418)656-8711; Fax. (418)656-4587; tibbet@videotron.ca.

CHOUINARD, Sylvain; CHUM-Hop Notre-Dame, 1560 rue Sherbrooke E, Montreal QC H2L 4M1; Mon'90; FRCPC; Neur (Movement Disorders). Staff, Centre Hospitalier l'Université de Montréal (CHUM) - Hôpital Notre-Dame; (514)890-8123; sylvain.c@videotron.ca.

CHOUINARD, Valerie; CSSS du Suroît, 150 rue Saint-Thomas, Salaber-de-Valleyf QC J6T 6C1; Laval'93; CSPQ; FRCPC; AnatPath. Staff, Centre Hospitalier Régional du Suroît; (450)371-9920 x2091; valerie.chouinard@rrsss16.gouv.qc.ca.

CHOUINARD-CHRETIEN, Marie P; CHUQ-St-Francois-d'Assise, 10 rue de l'Espinay, Quebec QC G1L 3L5; Laval'01; CCFP; Staff, Centre Hospitalier Universitaire De Québec - Pavillon De St-françois-d'assise; (418)525-4444

CHOUINARD-ROUSSEAU, Helene; Ctr Hosp Affilie-St-Sacrement, 1050 ch Sainte-Foy, Quebec QC G1S 4L8; Sher'03; CCFP; Staff, Centre Hospitalier Affilié Universitaire de Québec - Hôpital du St-Sacrement; (418)682-7511

CHOVANEC, Milan; Guelph Gen Hosp, 115 Delhi St, Guelph ON N1E 4J4; Ott'91; FRCPC; Anes. Staff, Guelph General Hospital; (519)822-5350

CHOW, Andrew; Credit Valley Prof Bldg, 209-2300 Eglinton Ave W, Mississauga ON L5M 2V8; Tor'96; DABIM; FACRheum; FRCPC; IntMed; Rheum. Lecturer, University of Toronto; Clinical Asst Prof, McMaster University; Langs: Chinese; Cantonese; (905)607-8334; Fax. (905)607-8184.

CHOW, Barry L; Woodbridge Med Centre, A13-9600 Islington Ave, Woodbridge ON L4H 2T1; Tor'97; CCFP; FCFP; (905)893-8085; Fax. (905)893-8218.

CHOW, Benjamin J W; Univ of Ottawa Heart Institute, H1220-40 Ruskin St, Ottawa ON K1Y 4W7; Qns'96; FRCPC; IntMed (Cardiac Imaging); Cardiol. Assoc Prof, University of Ottawa Heart Institute; (613)761-4044; Fax. (613)761-4929.

CHOW, Bill P C; Demong Associate Eyecentre, 330-290 Midpark Way SE, Calgary AB T2X 1P1; Cal'90; BSc(Hon); MSc; FRCSC; Ophth. Ac Staff, Rocky Mountain Surgery Centre; Staff, Calgary Regional Health Authority; Langs: Cantonese; (403)254-2408; Fax. (403)254-5887.

CHOW, Candace S; 110 Isabel St, Winnipeg MB R3A 1G4; Man'04; CCFP; (204)786-4653

CHOW, Carlyle S H A; Baddeck Med Clinic, PO Box 130 65 High St, Baddeck NS B0E 1B0; Dal'68; Chief Med Staff, Victoria County Memorial Hospital; Preceptor, Dalhousie University; (902)295-2443; Fax. (902)295-1775.

CHOW, Chi-Ieng; 110 Isabel St, Winnipeg MB R3A 1G4; National (Taiwan)'73; Ac Staff, Misericordia Health Centre; (204)786-4653

CHOW, Chi-Ming; St Michael's Hosp, 30 Bond St, Toronto ON M5B 1W8; McG'90; ABC; ABIM; FRCP; NBEchoTestamur; FRCPC; IntMed (Echocardiography); Cardiol. Staff Echocardiographer, St Michael's Hospital; Staff, Toronto Heart Centre; Assoc Prof Med, University of Toronto; Langs: Cantonese; Mandarin; Chinese; (416)864-3024; cardio@mac.com.

CHOW, Chong J; Trillium Hlth Ctr-Mississauga, 100 Queensway W, Mississauga ON L5B 1B8; Ott'89; FRCPC; Anes (Cardiac Anesthesia). Staff, Trillium Health Centre - Mississauga; (905)848-7628; Fax. (905)848-0328; dr_chow@bigfoot.com.

CHOW, Chung Wai; 11C 1185-585 University Ave, Toronto ON M5G 2N2; Tor'89; ABIM; FRCPC; IntMed (Transplantation); Respir. Ac Physician Med, Toronto General Hospital - UHN; Asst Prof Med, University of Toronto; Langs: Cantonese; (416)340-3512; Fax. (416)340-3109; cw.chow@utoronto.ca.

CHOW, Clinton J; Chrysalis Obst & Gyn Clinic, 21-10 Richard Way SW, Calgary AB T3E 7M9; UBC'00; FRCSC; ObstGyn. (403)242-0770; Fax. (403)242-0711.

CHOW, Daliah Y L; Baywood Med Centre, 200-95 Bayly St W, Ajax ON L1S 7K8; (Hong Kong)'85; MB BS; CCFP; FCFP; Assoc Staff Family Pract, Rouge Valley Health System - Ajax & Pickering Health Centre Site; Langs: Mandarin; Cantonese; (905)686-3900; Fax. (905)686-9222.

CHOW, David R; 8 125-61 Queen St E, Toronto ON M5C 2T2; Tor'90; FRCSC; Ophth (Retina). Staff, St Michael's Hospital; Teach Staff, University of Toronto; Langs: English; French; (416)867-7447; Fax. (416)867-7445.

CHOW, Donald; The Ottawa Hosp-Civic Campus, J133-1053 Carling Ave, Ottawa ON K1Y 4E9; Qns'81; FRCSC; OrthSurg (Spine Surgery). Ac Staff, The Ottawa Hospital - Civic Campus; Consultant Rehab Ctre of Ottawa, Providence Continuing Care Centre (PCCC) - St Vincent de Paul Hospital; Asst Prof, University of Ottawa; (613)761-4258; Fax. (613)761-7751.

CHOW, Edward L W; Toronto Sunnybrook Reg Cancer, 2075 Bayview Ave, Toronto ON M4N 3M5; (Hong Kong)'88; MB BS; MSc; PhD; FRCPC; RadOncol. Staff Oncol, Sunnybrook Health Sciences Centre; Staff RadOncol, Sunnybrook Health Sciences Centre - Edmond Odette Cancer Centre; Prof, University of Toronto; Langs: Chinese; (416)480-4998; Fax. (416)480-6002.

CHOW, Esther H; 3F-799 Bloor St W, Toronto ON M6G 1L8; Tor'07; CCFP; (647)349-0053; Fax. (647)349-0063.

CHOW, Eunice Y; First Edmonton Place, 950-10665 Jasper Ave NW, Edmonton AB T5J 3S9; UBC'04; FRCPC; Derm. (780)424-4440; Fax. (780)424-8794.

CHOW, Eva W C; Addiction & Mental Hlth-ARF, 1085-33 Russell St, Toronto ON M5S 2S1; Tor'88; BSc; MPH; DABPN(Forensic/AddictonPs; JD; FRCPC; Psy (Forensic Psychiatry). Staff, Centre for Addiction & Mental Health (CAMH) - Russell Street Site; (416)535-8501

CHOW, Faye H; 3500-950 10th Ave W, Vancouver BC V5Z 1M9; UBC'96; BSc; Ac Staff, Vancouver General Hospital - Centennial Pavillion; (604)822-7121; fh_chow@yahoo.com.

CHOW, Frances L; BC Women's Hosp & Health Ctre, 4500 Oak St, Vancouver BC V6H 3N1; Sask'88; FRCPC; Anes. Staff, BC Women's Hospital & Health Centre; (604)875-2158

CHOW, Gary C H; 10-8180 MacLeod Trail SE, Calgary AB T2H 2B8; Alb'96; FRCPC; Peds. Staff, Alberta Children's Hospital; (403)252-6651

CHOW, Gilbert; North York Gen Hosp, 4001 Leslie St, North York ON M2K 1E1; Qns'96; FRCPC; DiagRad. Staff, North York General Hospital; (416)756-6000

CHOW, Harold H K; CMC Medical Centre, 5995 Steeles Ave E, Scarborough ON M1V 5P7; Tor'80; Langs: Cantonese; (416)297-5330; Fax. (416)297-9727.

CHOW, Heman; 11 Prospect St, Doaktown NB E9C 1C3; Tor'86; (506)365-6101; Fax. (506)365-6104.

CHOW, Herman; Northern Med Unit, T162-770 Bannatyne Ave, Winnipeg MB R3E 0W3; Man'09; CCFP.

CHOW, Isabel J S; Windsor Health Centre, 364-1720 Howard Ave, Windsor ON N8X 5A6; Tor'87; FRCSC; PlasSurg (Cosmetic Surgery). Staff, Hôtel-Dieu Grace Hospital; (519)971-0971; Fax. (519)971-0971.

CHOW, J Holden; 103-33774 Marshall Rd, Abbotsford BC V2S 1L1; Alb'98; CCFP; Langs: Cantonese; (604)853-5424; Fax. (604)853-6879.

CHOW, Jane; 200B-1105 Kingston Rd, Pickering ON L1V 1B5; McM'08; CCFP.

CHOW, Janet A; Carleton Univ Health Services, 1125 Colonel By Dr, Ottawa ON K1S 5B6; UBC'99; BSc; MSc; MCFP; PhC; CCFP; Physician Health & Counselling Services, Carleton University; (613)520-6674; Fax. (613)520-4059.

CHOW, Jennifer A; The Montfort Hosp, 713 Montreal Rd, Ottawa ON K1K 0T2; Qns'04; FRCPC; Anes. Staff, Montfort Hospital; (613)743-4621; Fax. (613)748-4914.

CHOW, John C; 205-9123 Mary St, Chilliwack BC V2P 4H7; UBC'84; Staff, Chilliwack General Hospital; Clinical Asst Prof Family Med, University of British Columbia; (604)795-5800; Fax. (604)795-4605.

CHOW, Jonathan S; Niagara H System-St Catharines, PO Box 3018 Stn Main 142 Queenston St, St Catharines ON L2R 7C6; Mem'91; Staff, Niagara Health System - St Catharines General Site; (905)684-7271 x5000

CHOW, Judy T; Rideau Family Health Team, 5-3635 Rivergate Way, Ottawa ON K1V 2A4; UBC'80; Langs: Chinese; (613)739-3700; Fax. (613)739-7043; dr.chow@riversidecourt.ca.

CHOW, Kan-Yan; The Medical Place, 101-178 John St, Brampton ON L6W 2A4; (Hong Kong)'64; MSc; MB BS; FACS; FRCSC; Otol. Staff, Toronto General Hospital - UHN; Staff, William Osler Health System - Brampton Civic Hospital; Asst Prof, University of Toronto; Langs: Cantonese; (905)459-3200; Fax. (905)459-3201.

CHOW, Katherine S; Mount St Joseph Hosp, 3080 Prince Edward St, Vancouver BC V5T 3N4; Cal'07; FRCPC; IntMed. Staff, Providence Health Care - Mount Saint Joseph Hospital; (604)874-1141

CHOW, Kenmau; Worksafe BC, 6951 Westminster Hwy, Richmond BC V7C 1C6; UBC'91; Staff, BC Mental Health & Addiction Service; (604)244-6260

CHOW, Kenneth C K; 5995 Steeles Ave E, Scarborough ON M1V 5P7; Wes'79; Langs: Cantonese; (416)297-5330; Fax. (416)297-9727.

CHOW, Laura C; Heart of Ottawa Med Centre, 270 Elgin St, Ottawa ON K2P 1M2; Ott'05; CCFP; (613)237-2121; Fax. (613)237-2087.

CHOW, Lawrence H; London HSC-University Hosp, PO Box 5339 Stn B B6 119-339 Windermere Rd, London ON N6A 5A5; Wes'78; FRCP; FACP; FACC; FRCPC; IntMed; Cardiol. Staff Cardiol, London Health Sciences Centre - Victoria Campus; Staff Cardiol, London Health Sciences Centre - University Hospital; Assoc Prof Med, Schulich School of Medicine-University of Western Ontario; (519)663-3992; Fax. (519)434-3278.

CHOW, Linda Y; Rockingham Ridge Medical Ctre, 30 Farnham Gate Rd, Halifax NS B3M 3W8; Cal'89; (902)457-2222; Fax. (902)443-7800.

CHOW, Lorraine; Foothills Medical Centre, C222-1403 29 St NW, Calgary AB T2N 2T9; Ott'05; FRCPC; Anes. Staff, Foothills Medical Centre; (403)944-1110; Fax. (403)944-2400.

CHOW, Mabel Y T; 2025 Caroline St, Burlington ON L7R 1L1; (Hong Kong)'71; MB BS; FRCPC; IntMed (Clinical Immunology & Allergy). Affil Staff Clinical Immunol, Hamilton Health Sciences Centre - McMaster Children's Hospital; Staff Consultant IntMed, Joseph Brant Memorial Hospital; Langs: Cantonese; (905)634-0415; Fax. (905)634-7474.

CHOW, Maria C; B6-645 Plains Rd E, Burlington ON L7T 4J5; Qns'10; CCFP; (905)681-3430

CHOW, Maria S M; Courtenay Health Science Ctre, 210-1350 England Ave, Courtenay BC V9N 8X6; Glasgow (England)'90; MB ChB; (250)334-4411

CHOW, Matthew C; BC Women's Hosp & Health Ctre, 4500 Oak St, Vancouver BC V6H 3N1; Cal'06; FRCPC; Psy. Staff, BC Women's Hospital & Health Centre; (604)875-2345

CHOW, Michael M C; University of Alberta Hosp, HSC 2D102-8440 112 St NW, Edmonton AB T6G 2B7; Qns'94; MPH; FRCSC; Neursurg (Neuro Surgery & Endovascular Therapy). Staff NeuroSurg, University of Alberta Hospital; Staff NeuroSurg, Royal Alexandra Hospital; Teach Staff, University of Alberta; (780)407-1428; Fax. (780)407-8203; michaelchow@cha.ab.ca.

CHOW, Pan Chun; 160-495 36 St NE, Calgary AB T2A 6K3; Alb'86; CCFP; FCFP; Ac Staff, Peter Lougheed Centre; Clin Lecturer, University of Calgary; (403)514-6001

CHOW, Peter H; 204-974 Queen St E, Sault Ste. Marie ON P6A 2C5; Tor'71; Ac Staff, Sault Area Hospital - Sault Ste Marie; Langs: Cantonese; (705)254-7221; Fax. (705)949-3142; phcmd3142@hotmail.com.

CHOW, Peter M; Halton HCS Corp-Georgetown, 1 Princess Anne Dr, Georgetown ON L7G 2B8; Ott'92; Staff, Halton Healthcare Services Corporation - Georgetown Hospital; (905)873-1111

CHOW, Raphael K T; 1103-123 Edward St, Toronto ON M5G 1E2; Tor'76; BSc; DABPM; FRCPC; PhysMed&Rehab. Staff, Toronto Rehabilitation Institute - University Centre; Staff, Mount Sinai Hospital; Asst Prof Med, University of Toronto; Langs: Cantonese; (416)596-7901; Fax. (416)596-0970.

CHOW, Raymond; 108-888 Kingsway, Vancouver BC V5V 3C3; UBC'77; (604)875-9555

CHOW, Roxana S; Windsor Health Centre, 103-630 Tecumseh Rd E, Windsor ON N8X 4W2; Wes'78; Ac Staff, Hôtel-Dieu Grace Hospital; Court Staff, Windsor Regional Hospital - Metropolitan Site; Court Staff, Windsor Regional Hospital - Tayfour Site; (519)258-5090; chowroxx@on.aibn.com.

CHOW, Samuel K K; Westview Health Centre, 4405 South Park Dr, Stony Plain AB T7Z 2M7; Alb'02; CCFP; CCFP(E.M.); Staff, Westview Health Centre; (780)968-3673; Fax. (780)968-3774.

CHOW, Sheung C; Finch-Midland Med Centre, 403-4190 Finch Ave E, Scarborough ON M1S 4T7; Tor'75; (416)298-4663; Fax. (416)298-3793.

CHOW, Shirley; Sunnybrook Hlth Sciences Ctre, M1400-2075 Bayview Ave, Toronto ON M4N 3M5; Wes'06; FRCPC; IntMed; Rheum. Staff, Sunnybrook Health Sciences Centre; (416)480-6100

CHOW, Sie-Chin; Norfolk Gen Hosp, 365 West St, Simcoe ON N3Y 1T7; National Defense Medical Center (Taiwan)'66; FRCPC; DiagRad. Staff, Norfolk General Hospital; (519)426-0750 x1210; Fax. (519)429-6992.

CHOW, Sing W; 290 Giles Blvd E, Windsor ON N9A 4C2; (Hong Kong)'76; MB BS; FRCPC; Peds. Ac Staff Peds, Windsor Regional Hospital - Metropolitan Site; (519)252-4888; Fax. (519)252-2823.

CHOW, Stacey A; Gateway Med Centre, 10751 King George Blvd, Surrey BC V3T 2X6; UBC'91; BSc; MD; Staff, Surrey Memorial Hospital; Langs: Cantonese; Toishan; (604)581-2611; Fax. (604)581-5069.

CHOW, Stephen S; 209-840 Coxwell Ave, Toronto ON M4C 5T2; Tor'78; MD; FRCPC; IntMed; Nephrol. Ac Staff, Toronto East General Hospital Inc; Langs: Chinese; (416)461-0939; Fax. (416)461-4717.

CHOW, Stephen; Royal Inland Hosp, 311 Columbia St, Kamloops BC V2C 2T1; (Saint Kitts-Nevis)'02; Staff, Royal Inland Hospital; (250)314-2100

CHOW, Stephen W; Dynacare Kasper Med Lab, 200-10150 102 St NW, Edmonton AB T5J 5E2; Alb'04; FRCPC; GenPath. (780)451-3702 x3225

CHOW, Susan T; Northmount Med Centre, 401-145 13th St E, North Vancouver BC V7L 2L4; UBC'92; BSc; Ac Staff, Lions Gate Hospital; (604)987-2217; Fax. (604)985-5959.

CHOW, Theresa C B; 78 Regina St N, Waterloo ON N2J 3A5; (Hong Kong)'69; DDS(UK); Staff, Grand River Hospital - Kitchener/Waterloo Health Centre; Staff, St Mary's General Hospital; (519)888-6400; Fax. (519)886-8496.

CHOW, Tiffany W; Baycrest Ctre/Geriatric Care, 3560 Bathurst St, Toronto ON M6A 2E1; Chicago(IL) (USA)'92; Scientist The Rotman Research Inst, Baycrest Centre for Geriatric Care; Staff, Baycrest Brain Health Complex; Staff, Ross Memory Clinic; Asst Prof Neurol, University of Toronto; (416)785-2444; Fax. (416)785-2484; tchow@rotman-baycrest.on.ca.

CHOW, Ting-Bong; Sudbury Med Centre, 303-65 Larch St, Sudbury ON P3E 1B8; (Taiwan)'73; Ac Staff, Health Sciences North-Laurentian Site; Ac Staff, Health Sciences North-St Joseph's Health Centre; Ac Staff, Health Sciences North - Memorial Site; (705)675-5442; Fax. (705)675-9145.

CHOW, Vance; Associated Radiologists, 300-140 Wall St, Saskatoon SK S7K 1N4; Sask'93; FRCPC; DiagRad. Staff, Royal University Hospital; Asst Prof, University of Saskatchewan; (306)244-1167; Fax. (306)244-2911.

CHOW, Victor D W; 102-123 15th St E, North Vancouver BC V7L 2P7; Qns'93; FACS; FRCSC; Urol (Male Infertility). Clinical Asst Prof, University of British Columbia; Langs: Cantonese; (604)987-8171; Fax. (604)987-8130.

CHOW, Vivian W; 108-790 Bay St, Toronto ON M5G 1N8; Tor'89; (416)921-2121; Fax. (416)929-7316; drvchowccfp@hotmail.com.

CHOW, Wai-Kwan; Medicine Hat Reg Hosp, 666 5 St SW, Medicine Hat AB T1A 4H6; (Taiwan)'71; AB; FRCPC; AnatPath; GenPath. Dir Dept of LabMed, Medicine Hat Regional Hospital; Dir, Medicine Hat Diagnostic Laboratory; (403)529-8861; Fax. (403)529-8023.

CHOW, Walter K; Central Park Medical, 304-1711 Cook St, Victoria BC V8T 3P2; UBC'86; Staff, Victoria General Hospital; Staff, Royal Jubilee Hospital; (250)382-8011; Fax. (250)360-0084.

CHOW, Y B Dominic; B8-8390 Kennedy Rd, Unionville ON L3R 0W4; (Hong Kong)'78; MRCP(UK); DCH(Glasgow); MB BS; DCH(Ire.); CCFP; FCFP; Langs: Cantonese; (905)474-5633; Fax. (905)474-5133; ybchow@hotmail.com.

CHOW, Yen; Thunder Bay Reg HSC-T-Bay, 980 Oliver Rd, Thunder Bay ON P7B 6V4; UBC'93; CCFP; Staff, Thunder Bay Regional Health Sciences Centre; Langs: Cantonese; (807)684-6100

CHOW SIET YAM, Moy Fee; Clinique Med Solumed, 1-8230 boul Taschereau, Brossard QC J4X 1C2; Mon'00; Staff, Hôpital Anna-Laberge; Langs: English; (450)466-0003

CHOWDHRY, Atif; Leamington & Area FHT-Kingsvil, 273 Main St E, Kingsville ON N9Y 1A7; Saba (Netherlands Antilles)'06; (519)733-2318

CHOWDHRY, Rajendra K; 100-651 Boul Everard H Daigle, Gr-Sault/Gr-Falls NB E3Z 2S2; Jaipur (India)'66; MB BS; FRCSC; GenSurg. Ac Staff Surg, Hôpital Général de Grand-Falls; (506)473-4840; Fax. (506)473-6377.

CHOWDHURY, Amitava D; Cancercare Manitoba, 675 McDermot Ave, Winnipeg MB R3E 0V9; Delhi (India)'81; MD; Staff, Health Sciences Centre; Staff, St Boniface General Hospital; Asst Prof Radiol, University of Manitoba; Langs: Bengali; Hindi; (204)787-2173; Fax. (204)786-0194; amit.chowdhury@cancercare.mb.ca.

CHOWDHURY, Bikash K; Tillsonburg Dist Mem Hosp, 167 Rolph St, Tillsonburg ON N4G 3Y9; Chittagong (Bangladesh)'93; CCFP; Staff, Tillsonburg District Memorial Hospital; (519)842-6311

CHOWDHURY, Dhiman; IWK Health Centre, PO Box 9700 Rpo CSC, Halifax NS B3K 6R8; (Bangladesh)'75; MB BS; MRC(UK); DCH(Dublin); FRCP(Edin); FRCPCH; Ac Staff, IWK Health Centre; Asst Prof Peds, Dalhousie University; Langs: Bengali; (902)470-7909; Fax. (902)470-6913.

CHOWDHURY, Muna; 168 Bathurst St, Toronto ON M5V 2R4; Sask'06; CCFP; (416)703-8480; Fax. (416)703-8479.

CHOWDHURY, Rezwan H; BC Cancer Ctre-Southern Interi, 399 Royal Ave, Kelowna BC V1Y 5L3; Alb'05; FRCPC; RadOncol. Staff, BC Cancer Agency Sindi Ahluwalia Hawkins Centre for the Southern Interior; (250)712-3958

CHOWDHURY, Ruma; Main Street Medical, 9-10886 Hurontario St, Brampton ON L7A 3R9; Dhaka (Bangladesh)'96; CCFP; (905)846-9911; Fax. (905)846-9299.

CHOWDHURY, Ryan H; Alberta ENT Consultants, 10130 111 St NW, Edmonton AB T5K 1K6; Alb'05; FRCSC; Otol; Critical Care Medicine. Staff, University of Alberta Hospital; (587)521-1071; Fax. (587)521-1072.

CHOWDHURY, Smriti; IWK Health Centre, PO Box 9700 Rpo CSC, Halifax NS B3K 6R8; (Bangladesh)'75; MB BS; DCH(Ire); MRCP(UK); Staff, IWK Health Centre; Langs: Bengali; (902)470-3864; Fax. (902)470-6913.

CHOWDRY, Seema; 1-170 Sandalwood Pkwy E, Brampton ON L6Z 1Y5; J J M Medical College (India)'98; CCFP; (905)846-8282; Fax. (905)846-4541.

CHOY, Alberto L; Alberta Hosp Edmonton, PO Box 307 Stn Main, Edmonton AB T5J 2J7; Alb'92; FRCPC; Psy (Forensic Psychiatry). Staff, Alberta Hospital Edmonton; (780)342-5334; Fax. (780)342-5595; alberto.choy@albertahealthservices.ca.

CHOY, Benjamin S; 203A-3636 Steeles Ave E, Markham ON L3R 1K9; Tor'94; CCFP; FCFP; Langs: Cantonese; Mandarin; (905)477-5679; Fax. (905)477-5632.

CHOY, Gregory W; Sunnybrook Hlth Sciences Ctre, M1 401-2075 Bayview Ave, Toronto ON M4N 3M5; Tor'99; FRCPC; IntMed; Rheum. Staff, Sunnybrook Health Sciences Centre; Langs: Chinese; (416)480-4580; Fax. (416)480-4233.

CHOY, Henry M T; 2-1185 Dundas St E, Mississauga ON L4Y 2C6; Tor'79; Assoc Staff, Trillium Health Centre - West Toronto; (905)896-1956; Fax. (905)896-1956.

CHOY, Jonathan B; University of Alberta Hosp, 2C2 WMC-8440 112 St NW, Edmonton AB T6G 2B7; Alb'92; FRCPC; IntMed; Cardiol. Staff, University of Alberta Hospital; (780)407-3581; Fax. (780)407-6452; jchoy@cha.ab.ca.

CHOY, Ping Fun; Sheppard Med Bldg, 218-701 Sheppard Ave E, North York ON M2K 2Z3; (Hong Kong)'73; MB BS; FACS; FRCS(Glas); CCFP; FCFP; Ac Staff, North York General Hospital; Langs: Chinese; (416)512-6126; Fax. (416)512-7331.

CHOY, Stephen C; Prichard Farm Health Centre, 5-3014 Henderson Hwy, East St Paul MB R2E 0H9; Man'10; CCFP.

CHOY, Thomas W; Scarborough Comm Mental Hlth, 301-2425 Eglinton Ave E, Scarborough ON M1K 5G8; Man'70; FRCPC; Psy. Ac Staff, The Scarborough Hospital - Birchmount Campus; (416)431-8135; Fax. (416)759-5162.

CHOY, Wesley H; Lougheed Med Clinic, 145-9855 Austin Rd, Burnaby BC V3J 1N4; Man'79; (604)421-2555

CHRAPPA, Jarmila; Western Memorial Health Clinic, 3 Herald Ave, Corner Brook NL A2H 4B8; Komensky (Slovakia)'63; FRCPC; Peds (Infectious Diseases). Langs: Czech; Slovak; French.

CHRENEK, Carson; Cabrini Centre, 3F-16811 88 Ave NW, Edmonton AB T5R 5Y6; Cal'07; BSc; MBA; FRCPC; Psy. Staff, Covenant Health - Misericordia Community Hospital; (780)735-2594; Fax. (780)735-2595.

CHRETIEN, Angelo; CSSS du Rocher-Perce, CP 3300 451 rue Mgr Ross E, Chandler QC G0C 1K0; Mon'94; CSPQ; FRCPC; Anes. Staff, Centre Hospitalier de Chandler; (418)689-2261; Fax. (418)689-5049.

CHRETIEN, Francois; Ctr Hosp du Centre la Mauricie, 50 119e rue, Shawinigan-Sud QC G9P 5K1; Sher'92; FRCPC; Peds. Staff, Centre Hospitalier du Centre la Mauricie; (819)536-7526; Fax. (819)536-7572; francois.chretien@sh.cgocable.ca.

CHRETIEN, Lizane; Clinique familiale des Pins, 1019 boul des Pins, Val-d'Or QC J9P 4T2; Sher'81; (819)825-9060; Fax. (819)825-1335.

CHRETIEN, Michel; Ottawa Research Inst, 725 Parkdale Ave, Ottawa ON K1Y 4E9; Mon'60; FRSC; FRCPC; MedScient(Med); Endocrin (P.Q.); Endocrin&Metab. Sr Scientist, The Ottawa Hospital - Civic Campus; Prof Med, University of Ottawa; Langs: French; English; (613)761-4614; Fax. (613)761-4920.

CHRETIEN, Pierre; Sante au Travail, 53 boul Comeau, Baie-Comeau QC G4Z 3A7; Mon'78; (418)294-2572 x2377; Fax. (418)296-3103.

CHRETIEN, Valerie; CLSC Chateauguay, 95 av de la Verdure, Chateauguay QC J6K 0E8; Laval'07; CCFP; (450)699-3333; Fax. (450)699-2325.

CHRIGUI, Abdelaziz; Clinique Externe Jean-Talon, 7345 rue Garnier, Montreal QC H2E 2A1; Strasbourg (France)'91; (514)729-3036; Fax. (514)495-6774.

CHRIPKO, Daniel; Windsor Reg Hosp-Metropolitan, 1995 Lens Ave, Windsor ON N8W 1L9; McG'85; CSPQ; FRCPC; Anes. Staff, Windsor Regional Hospital - Metropolitan Site; (519)254-5577

CHRIS, Allison E; Toronto Public Health, 277 Victoria St, Toronto ON M5B 1W2; Ott'03; FRCPC; CommunMed;CCFP; (416)338-7985

CHRIS, Anthony D; 153 Union St E, Waterloo ON N2J 1C4; Qns'83; FRCSC; OrthSurg. (519)570-2912; Fax. (519)570-4313.

CHRIS, Chantal E; Southgate Med Clinic, 50-45905 Yale Rd, Chilliwack BC V2P 2M6; Ott'08; CCFP; (604)792-2266

CHRIS, Stephen D; Bayview-Finch Med Clinic, 300-3292 Bayview Ave, North York ON M2M 4J5; Tor'74; (416)646-4455; Fax. (416)222-5722.

CHRISOHOU, Ramona G; Market Mall Office Centre, 208-3625 Shaganappi Trail NW, Calgary AB T3A 0E2; Cal'90; CCFP; FCFP; (403)286-9118; Fax. (403)286-3069; rchrisohou@shaw.ca.

CHRIST, Albert J L; Red Deer Reg Hosp Centre, PO Box 5030 Stn Postal Box Ctr 3942 50A Ave, Red Deer AB T4N 6R2; Sask'87; FRCPC; Anes. Staff, Red Deer Regional Hospital Centre; (403)343-4768

CHRISTAKIS, George T; Sunnybrook Hlth Sciences Ctre, H406-2075 Bayview Ave, Toronto ON M4N 3M5; Tor'81; FRCSC; GenSurg; Cardiovasc&ThorSurg. Staff Cardiovascular Surg, Sunnybrook Health Sciences Centre; Staff Surg, St Michael's Hospital; Prof Surg, University of Toronto; Langs: Greek; (416)480-6080; Fax. (416)480-6072.

CHRISTAKIS, John T; 200-245 Danforth Ave, Toronto ON M4K 1N2; Tor'82; DAB; FRCSC; Ophth. Staff Eye Clinic, Mount Sinai Hospital; Teach Staff, University of Toronto; Langs: Greek; (416)462-0393; Fax. (416)462-3612.

CHRISTAKIS, Monique S; Sunnybrook Hlth Sciences Ctre, 2075 Bayview Ave, Toronto ON M4N 3M5; Wes'90; FRCPC; DiagRad. Staff, Sunnybrook Health Sciences Centre; Asst Prof, University of Toronto; (416)480-5730

CHRISTENSEN, L Blair; Harbour City Health Centre, 201-1125 Dufferin Cres, Nanaimo BC V9S 2B5; UBC'87; BSc; FRCSC; PlasSurg. (250)753-1601; Fax. (250)753-8399.

CHRISTENSEN, Paul E L; Prince County Hosp, PO Box 3000 Stn Main 65 Roy Bates Ave, Summerside PE C1N 2A9; Dal'83; Anesthetist, Prince County Hospital; (902)888-3659

CHRISTENSON, James; University of British Columbia, 3300-910 10th Ave W, Vancouver BC V5Z 1M9; Ott'76; BSc; FRCPC; EmergMed. Staff, Vancouver General Hospital - Centennial Pavillion; Staff, Providence Health Care - St Paul's Hospital; Clin Prof/Dept Head & School Dir Emerg Med, University of British Columbia; (604)875-4284; Fax. (604)875-4872.

CHRISTENSON, Susan A; PO Box 229, Stand Off AB T0L 1Y0; (USA)'90; (403)737-8459; Fax. (403)737-2706.

CHRISTIAN, Francis T; Royal University Hosp, 103 Hospital Dr, Saskatoon SK S7N 0W8; Madras (India)'87; MB BS; FRCSC; GenSurg. Staff, Royal University Hospital; (306)966-7490; Fax. (306)966-7988.

CHRISTIAN, Keith M W; 3407 27 Ave, Vernon BC V1T 1S2; Manchester (England)'71; MB ChB; FAADEP; FRCSC; OrthSurg (Disability Evaluation). (250)545-5996; Fax. (250)545-5496; k-ch@shaw.ca.

CHRISTIAN, Michael D; Mount Sinai Hosp, 18 232-600 University Ave, Toronto ON M5G 1X5; McM'99; FRCPC; IntMed; Critical Care Medicine; InfectDis. Staff, Mount Sinai Hospital; (416)586-4800 x7943

CHRISTIANS, Neil J; Cape Breton Hlthcare Complex, 1482 George St, Sydney NS B1P 1P3; Cape Town (South Africa)'76; MB BS; FRCPC; Psy. Staff, Cape Breton Healthcare Complex; (902)849-4413

CHRISTIANSEN, Gary R; CFB Comox, PO Box 1000 Stn Main 19 Wing Comox, Lazo BC V0R 2K0; UBC'87; (250)339-8267; Fax. (250)339-8169.

CHRISTIANSEN, Henrik S; 237 Hastings St N PO Box 1270, Bancroft ON K0L 1C0; Tor'74; Ac Staff Family Med, QHC North Hastings; Court Staff, Peterborough Regional Health Centre - Hospital Drive; Court Staff, Peterborough Regional Health Centre - Rogers St Site; (613)332-1156; Fax. (613)332-3357.

CHRISTIDIS, Nickolas; North York Med Arts Bldg, 226-1333 Sheppard Ave E, North York ON M2J 1V1; Wes'92; CASM; Staff CommunMed, North York General Hospital; (416)850-4064; Fax. (416)850-6681.

CHRISTIE, Allison; Medical Centre, 2-137 King St, Estevan SK S4A 2T5; Glasgow (Scotland)'72; MB ChB; MRC(UK); DCH; (306)634-6444; Fax. (306)634-9187.

CHRISTIE, Elizabeth A; Prince Edward Family Hlth Team, 3-35 Bridge St, Picton ON K0K 2T0; McM'04; BSc; LLB; CCFP; Med Staff, QHC Prince Edward County Memorial; Asst Prof, Queen's University; (613)476-7771

CHRISTIE, Garth B; Fredericton Med Clinic, 304-1015 Regent St, Fredericton NB E3B 6H5; Dal'66; ObstGyn (Gynecology). Ac Staff, Dr Everett Chalmers Regional Hospital; (506)457-2113; Fax. (506)459-7073.

CHRISTIE, Gordon A; 313-877 Goldstream Ave, Victoria BC V9B 2X8; UBC'85; Staff, Victoria General Hospital; (250)478-4421; Fax. (250)474-6098.

CHRISTIE, Kevin M; Gibson Health Clinic, PO Box 9000 Stn A, Fredericton NB E3B 5N5; Dal'04; CCFP; Staff, Dr Everett Chalmers Regional Hospital; Assoc Prof, Dalhousie University; (506)447-4444; Fax. (506)447-4221.

CHRISTIE, Michael L; Caleo Health, 340-600 Crowfoot Cres NW, Calgary AB T3G 0B4; Alb'06; CCFP; (403)452-0999; Fax. (403)452-0995.

CHRISTIE, Sean D; Queen Elizabeth II HSC-Halifax, 3814-1796 Summer St, Halifax NS B3H 3A7; Dal'96; FRCSC; Neursurg. Staff, Queen Elizabeth II Health Sciences Centre - Halifax Infirmary Site; (902)473-2096; Fax. (902)473-8912.

CHRISTIE, Susanne C; Murakami Med Clinic, PO Box 1000 735 4 Ave, Hope BC V0X 1L0; UBC'97; BSc; CCFP; (604)869-5648; Fax. (604)869-2459.

CHRISTIE, Suzanne N; Ottawa Headache Centre, 407-1 Centrepointe Dr, Nepean ON K2G 6E2; Ott'84; FRCPC; Neur (Headache). Ac Staff, The Ottawa Hospital - General Campus; Ac Staff, Children's Hospital of Eastern Ontario (CHEO); Consultant, Montfort Hospital; Asst Prof, University of Ottawa; (613)562-6390; Fax. (613)562-6384; schristie@magma.ca.

CHRISTIE, Tyler; Sudbury Reg Hosp-Laurentian, 41 Ramsey Lake Rd, Sudbury ON P3E 5J1; Wes'08; CCFP; CCFP(E.M.); Staff, Health Sciences North-Laurentian Site; (705)522-7100

CHRISTIE-SEELY, Janet E; 3427 Greenbank Rd, Nepean ON K2J 4J1; McG'62; MSc(Exp.Med.); CCFP; FCFP; Prof Family Med, University of Ottawa; Langs: English; French; (613)823-0366

CHRISTILAW, Jan E; BC Women's Hosp & Health Ctre, B251-4500 Oak St, Vancouver BC V6H 3N1; McM'81; MHSc; FRCSC; ObstGyn. Ac Staff, Peace Arch Hospital; Head Specialized Women's Health, BC Women's Hospital & Health Centre; Clin Prof ObstGyn, University of British Columbia; (604)875-3566; Fax. (604)875-2961; jchristilaw@cw.bc.ca.

CHRISTINCK, E Rosemary; Petawawa Centennial Family HT, 154 Civic Centre Rd, Petawawa ON K8H 3H5; Tor'94; BSc; MSc; CCFP; Assoc Staff, Pembroke Regional Hospital Inc; Langs: German; (613)687-7641; Fax. (613)687-6808.

CHRISTJANSON, Lisa J; Joseph Brant Mem Hosp, 1230 North Shore Blvd E, Burlington ON L7S 1W7; McM'00; MSc; FRCPC; IntMed; Hem. Staff Cancer Clinic, Joseph Brant Memorial Hospital; (905)336-4103; Fax. (905)336-6492.

CHRISTODOULOU, Chris C; St Boniface Gen Hosp, 409 Tache Ave, Winnipeg MB R2H 2A6; Stellenbosch (South Africa)'92; FRCPC; Anes. Staff, St Boniface General Hospital; (204)233-8563

CHRISTOPOULOS, Apostolos; CHUM-Hop Notre-Dame, G 1144-1560 rue Sherbrooke E, Montreal QC H2L 4M1; Mon'01; FRCSC; Otol (Head & Neck Surgery). Staff, Centre Hospitalier l'Université de Montréal (CHUM) - Hôpital Notre-Dame; (514)890-8000

CHRISTOPOULOS, Stavroula; SMBD Jewish Gen Hosp, 3755 ch Cote-Sainte-Catherine, Montreal QC H3T 1E2; McG'99; FRCPC; IntMed; Endocrin&Metab. Staff, Sir Mortimer B Davis Jewish General; (514)340-8222 x4198

CHRISTOU, Nicolas V; Groupe Sante Phisymed, 137-6363 rte Transcanadienne, Saint-Laurent QC H4T 1Z9; McG'75; PhD; FRCSC; GenSurg (Bariatric Surgery). Prof Surg, McGill University Health Centre - Royal Victoria Hospital; Langs: Greek; French; (514)747-8888; nicolas.christou@muhc.mcgill.ca.

CHRITCHLEY, Sarah L; 200-3994 Shelbourne St, Victoria BC V8N 3E2; UBC'95; CCFP; FCFP; (250)477-7100

CHRONES, James P; Queen Charlotte Med Clinic, PO Box 9 3211 3rd Ave, Queen Charlotte BC V0T 1S0; Tor'86; CCFP; (250)559-4447; Fax. (250)559-8037.

CHRONOPOULOS, Alexandra; Cite de Sante de Laval, 1755 boul Rene-Laennec, Laval QC H7M 3L9; Mon'02; Critical Care Medicine (P.Q.); IntMed. Staff, Hôtel-Dieu de Lévis; Staff, Hopital de la Cite de la santé; (450)668-1010

CHRONOPOULOS, Julia V; Royal Alexandra Hosp, 10240 Kingsway NW, Edmonton AB T5H 3V9; Alb'06; CCFP; Staff, Royal Alexandra Hospital; Assoc Clin Lecturer, University of Alberta; (780)735-4201; julia.chronopoulos@gmail.com.

CHRUSCH, Carla A; Rockyview Gen Hosp, 7007 14 St SW, Calgary AB T2V 1P9; Man'89; MSc; FRCPC; IntMed; Critical Care Medicine; Respir. Staff, Rockyview General Hospital; (403)943-3788

CHRUSCH, Catherine M; Alberta Children's Hosp, 2888 Shaganappi Trail NW, Calgary AB T3B 6A8; Cal'85; FRCPC; DiagRad. Staff, Alberta Children's Hospital; (403)955-7985; Fax. (403)955-7656.

CHRUSCH, Maurice G; Associate Med Clinic, 400-20 14th St W, Prince Albert SK S6V 3K8; Sask'71; (306)953-1662; Fax. (306)764-3091.

CHRUSCH, Wendy M; Regina Qu'Appelle HR-Wascana, 2180 23rd Ave, Regina SK S4S 0A5; Sask'01; CSCNDiplomate(EMG); FRCPC; PhysMed&Rehab (Pediatrics). Staff Rehab Center, Wascana Rehabilitation Centre; Clin Teach Staff Med, University of Saskatchewan; Langs: French; (306)766-5585; Fax. (306)766-7442.

CHRYSLER, Bernard; MUHC-Montreal Chest Institute, 3650 rue Saint-Urbain, Montreal QC H2X 2P4; McG'72; DABIM; CSPQ; CRCP; Respir; IntMed. Staff, McGill University Health Centre - Montreal Chest Institute; Consultant, McGill University Health Centre - Royal Victoria Hospital; adj Prof, McGill University; Langs: Hungarian; French; (514)934-1934; Fax. (514)843-2088; bernard.chrysler@mcgill.ca.

CHRYSTOJA, Walter A; Cachet Family Physicians, 2-9255 Woodbine Ave, Markham ON L6C 1Y9; Tor'82; Court Staff Emerg, Rouge Valley Health System - Centenary Health Centre Site; Court Staff, Markham Stouffville Hospital; (905)877-2222; Fax. (905)887-3655.

CHRZANOWSKI, Zbigniew P; Justik Med Clinic, 8225 105 St NW, Edmonton AB T6E 4H2; Alb'62; Clin Lecturer, University of Alberta; Langs: Polish; (780)432-0211; Fax. (780)439-9349.

CHU, Agnes M C; Village Square Med Centre, 2942 Finch Ave E, Scarborough ON M1W 2T4; Tor'91; CCFP; (416)756-2725; Fax. (416)756-3898.

CHU, Alan; Foothills Med Centre, 304-1403 29 St NW, Calgary AB T2N 2T9; McM'06; FRCPC; Anes. Staff, Foothills Medical Centre; (403)944-1110

CHU, Angel K M; Foothills Med Centre, 304-1403 29 St NW, Calgary AB T2N 2T9; Alb'06; InfectDis; IntMed. Staff, Foothills Medical Centre; (403)944-2325

CHU, Ansel L; Murrayville Medical, 302-22112 52 Ave, Langley BC V2Y 2M6; Alb'90; BSc; FRCPC; PhysMed&Rehab (Electromyography). Staff, Langley Memorial Hospital; (604)533-0551; Fax. (604)533-0581.

CHU, Catherine S; Creekside Med Clinic, 4-12192 Symons Valley Rd NW, Calgary AB T3P 0A3; Alb'08; CCFP; (403)275-5488

CHU, Christopher C; Health Sciences Centre, 300 Prince Philip Dr, St. John's NL A1B 3V6; Wes'04; FRCPC; Anes. Staff, Health Sciences Centre; (709)777-6300

CHU, David K; Niagara H System-G Niagara, PO Box 1018 Stn Main 5546 Portage Rd, Niagara Falls ON L2E 6X2; Tor'87; FRCPC; DiagRad. Staff, Niagara Health System - Greater Niagara General Site; (905)358-4913

CHU, Derek D M; Royal Jubilee Hosp, 1952 Bay St, Victoria BC V8R 1J8; Alb'81; FRCPC; DiagRad; NuclearMed. Ac Staff, Royal Jubilee Hospital; Ac Staff, Vancouver Island Health Authority; (250)370-8272; Fax. (250)370-8947.

CHU, Eric K; Mackenzie Richmond Hill Hosp, 10 Trench St, Richmond Hill ON L4C 4Z3; Tor'98; FRCPC; IntMed; Critical Care Medicine; Respir. Staff, Mackenzie Richmond Hill Hospital; (905)883-1212

CHU, F Victor; Hamilton HS-General Site, 504-237 Barton St E, Hamilton ON L8L 2X2; McG'95; FRCSC; CardSurg. Staff, Hamilton Health Sciences Centre - Hamilton General Hospital; (905)523-0448; Fax. (905)523-0279.

CHU, Francis J L; Aberdeen Health Centre, 2180-4151 Hazelbridge Way, Richmond BC V6X 4J7; Sask'75; Clin Instructor, University of British Columbia; Langs: Mandarin; Cantonese; (604)233-0068

CHU, Gabriel K; 105-2190 West Railway St, Abbotsford BC V2S 2E2; Alb'03; FRCSC; Ophth. (604)853-5575

CHU, Jack Y L; Hys Med Centre, 300-11010 101 St NW, Edmonton AB T5H 4B9; Alb'88; FRCPC; Psy. Staff, Royal Alexandra Hospital; (780)424-8383; Fax. (780)424-6404.

CHU, Jacqueline; Trillium Hlth Ctr-Mississauga, 100 Queensway W, Mississauga ON L5B 1B8; McM'04; FRCPC; EmergMed. Staff, Trillium Health Centre - Mississauga; (905)848-7100

CHU, James C M; Woodside Square-Mall Level, 181-1571 Sandhurst Circle, Scarborough ON M1V 1V2; Tor'83; Langs: Cantonese; Mandarin; (416)291-9999; Fax. (416)291-7912.

CHU, Jennifer; St Michael's Hosp, 30 Bond St, Toronto ON M5B 1W8; Qns'07; FRCPC; EmergMed. Staff, St Michael's Hospital; (416)864-5095

CHU, Joseph Y C; Queensway Prof Centre, 312-190 Sherway Dr, Etobicoke ON M9C 5N2; Tor'78; FAHA; FACP; FRCPC; IntMed (Clinical Electro Physiology); Neur. Assoc Staff Neurol, Toronto Western Hospital - University Health Network; Ac Staff Neurology, William Osler Health System - Etobicoke General Hospital; Asst Prof Med, University of Toronto; Langs: Cantonese; Mandarin; Chinese; English; (416)626-0740; Fax. (416)626-0635.

CHU, Joyce C; 630 9 Ave SE, Calgary AB T2G 4V9; Alb'00; BSc; CCFP; Clinical Asst Prof Family Med, University of Calgary; (403)920-0011; Fax. (403)920-0014.

CHU, K C Dennis; Sheppard Med Bldg, 206-701 Sheppard Ave E, North York ON M2K 2Z3; Tor'85; FRCSC; ObstGyn. (416)498-1555; Fax. (416)498-9907.

CHU, Karen L; Bridgepoint Family Health Team, 430 Broadview Ave, Toronto ON M4K 2N1; Ott'97; CCFP; CCFP(E.M.); FCFP; Court Staff, Bridgepoint Health Centre; Langs: Cantonese; French; (416)470-6690; kchu@mtsinai.on.ca.

CHU, Karen P; Cross Cancer Institute, 11560 University Ave NW, Edmonton AB T6G 1Z2; Alb'04; FRCPC; RadOncol. Staff, Cross Cancer Institute; (780)432-8517

CHU, Katherine H C; Scarborough Prof Centre, 200-1371 Neilson Rd, Scarborough ON M1B 4Z8; Tor'78; FRCSC; ObstGyn (Gynecology). Langs: Chinese; Mandarin; (416)284-9215; Fax. (416)284-6995.

CHU, Kelly K-P; Lansdowne Med Treatment Ctre, 120-1641 Hillside Ave, Victoria BC V8T 5G1; Sask'75; BSc(Hon); Ac Staff, Vancouver Island Health Authority; Langs: Chinese; (250)592-4212

CHU, Kelly S; 406-89 Queensway W, Mississauga ON L5B 2V2; Cal'05; FRCSC; ObstGyn. (905)268-9928

CHU, Kim Hang; Centre de Read Lucie-Bruneau, 2275 av Laurier E, Montreal QC H2H 2N8; Saigon (Vietnam)'72; Langs: Vietnamese; (514)527-4527; Fax. (514)524-4813.

CHU, Man-Hon; Grace Med Centre, 402-2830 Keele St, North York ON M3M 3E5; Tor'85; CCFP; FCFP; Staff, North York General Hospital - Branson Division; (416)633-7337; Fax. (416)633-7337.

CHU, Marcella; Red Lake Family Health Team, PO Box 311, Red Lake ON P0V 2M0; Dal'02; CCFP; (807)727-2617; mchu@redlakehospital.ca.

CHU, Margaret; 306-1466 Bathurst St, Toronto ON M5R 3S3; Wes'00; CCFP; Staff, Sunnybrook Health Sciences Centre; Staff, Baycrest Centre for Geriatric Care; (416)536-5555; mchu@baycrest.org.

CHU, Mary P H; Aberdeen Health Centre, 2180-4151 Hazelbridge Way, Richmond BC V6X 4J7; Sask'74; Langs: Chinese; Cantonese; Mandarin; (604)233-0068; mkostashuk@hotmail.com.

CHU, Melvyn; Chalmers Gate Med Bldg, 307-328 Highway 7 E, Richmond Hill ON L4B 3P7; (Hong Kong)'75; MRCP(UK); CCFP; FCFP; Langs: Cantonese; Mandarin; (905)886-0285; Fax. (905)886-7265.

CHU, Michael W; East York Town Centre, B11-45 Overlea Blvd, Toronto ON M4H 1C3; Tor'89; CCFP; Langs: Chinese; (416)425-4122; Fax. (416)425-6583.

CHU, Michael W A; London HSC-University Hosp, PO Box 5339 Stn B B6 106-339 Windermere Rd, London ON N6A 5A5; Sask'00; MEd(UofT); FRCSC; CardSurg (Minimal Invasive Surgery). Staff Div of Cardiac Surg, London Health Sciences Centre - University Hospital; (519)663-3593; Fax. (519)663-3276.

CHU, Monica M H; 7811 Fairmount Dr SE, Calgary AB T2H 0X8; Alb'99; CCFP; (403)242-7300

CHU, Norman H Y; Scarborough Hosp-Birchmount, 3030 Birchmount Rd, Scarborough ON M1W 3W3; Tor'94; CCFP; CCFP(E.M.); Staff, The Scarborough Hospital - Birchmount Campus; Langs: Cantonese; Mandarin; (416)495-2550

CHU, P C Peter; Dundurn Med Group, 160 Dundurn St S, Hamilton ON L8P 4K3; Wes'93; CCFP; Staff, West Haldimand General Hospital; (905)528-5480; Fax. (905)289-1107.

CHU, Pamela; Tom Baker Cancer Centre, CC114B-1331 29 St NW, Calgary AB T2N 4N2; Man'97; FRCSC; ObstGyn (Gynecologic Oncology). Staff, Tom Baker Cancer Centre; (403)521-3721; Fax. (403)521-3573.

CHU, Patrick; Chalmers Gate Med Bldg, 206-328 Highway 7 E, Richmond Hill ON L4B 3P7; (Hong Kong)'81; MB BS; MRC(UK); (905)889-8322; Fax. (905)889-5017.

CHU, Robert W X; Georgetown Med Associates, 199 Princess Anne Dr, Georgetown ON L7G 4W4; Tor'94; CCFP; Assoc Staff, Halton Healthcare Services Corporation - Georgetown Hospital; (905)873-3000; Fax. (905)873-0800.

CHU, Shiron C Y; Kingsbridge Med Centre, 5-20 Kingsbridge Garden Cir, Mississauga ON L5R 3K7; Tor'89; (905)507-1111; Fax. (905)890-7102.

CHU, Sik On; Scarborough North Med Arts, 408B-4040 Finch Ave E, Scarborough ON M1S 4V5; Dal'68; Langs: Chinese; (416)754-3458; sikonchu@yahoo.com.

CHU, Siu-Chung; Cross Cancer Institute, 11560 University Ave NW, Edmonton AB T6G 1Z2; Tor'97; FRCPC; IntMed; MedOncol. Staff, Cross Cancer Institute; (780)432-8248; Fax. (780)432-8888.

CHU, Stephanie W; 1296 Pacific Blvd, Vancouver BC V6Z 2V1; (Other Foreign)'09; CCFP; (604)633-2474

CHU, Wing-Kee; 3033A Hurontario St, Mississauga ON L5A 2G9; Tor'73; (905)277-4466; Fax. (905)277-0985.

CHU, William; Sunnybrook Hlth Sciences Ctre, 2075 Bayview Ave, Toronto ON M4N 3M5; McM'03; FRCPC; RadOncol. Staff, Sunnybrook Health Sciences Centre; (416)480-6100

CHU, Yuen Mei; Rockyview Health Centre, 210-1016 68 Ave SW, Calgary AB T2V 4J2; (Venezuela)'94; FRCPC; IntMed. Staff, Foothills Medical Centre; (403)209-1115; Fax. (403)541-0073.

CHUA, Boon-Chye; North Toronto Med Bldg, 212-250 Lawrence Ave W, Toronto ON M5M 1B2; UBC'75; AB; FRCPC; Psy (Adult Psychiatry). (416)256-2880; Fax. (416)256-2870.

CHUA, Caroline L; Ellesmere Hlth Care Centre, 1-2060 Ellesmere Rd, Scarborough ON M1H 2V6; Tor'09; CCFP; (416)439-2273

CHUA, Grace L; Maple Med Centre, 214-955 Major Mackenzie Dr, Maple ON L6A 4P9; Tor'90; FACC; FRCPC; IntMed; Cardiol. Ac Staff Cardiol, Mackenzie Richmond Hill Hospital; Langs: Chinese; (905)832-8665

CHUA, Neil S; Cross Cancer Institute, 11560 University Ave NW, Edmonton AB T6G 1Z2; Wes'00; FRCPC; IntMed; MedOncol. Staff, Cross Cancer Institute; (780)432-8340; Fax. (780)432-8888.

CHUA, Robert C M; Tawa Centre, 218-3017 66 St NW, Edmonton AB T6K 4B2; Alb'82; FRCSC; ObstGyn. Ac Staff, Royal Alexandra Hospital; Ac Staff, Covenant Health - Grey Nuns Community Hospital; Clin Assoc Prof, University of Alberta; (780)468-6188; Fax. (780)468-2121.

CHUA, Therese A L; Meadowlark Health Centre, 140 Meadowlark Shopping Ctr NW, Edmonton AB T5R 5W9; Alb'90; (780)489-8470; Fax. (780)484-1620.

CHUAH, Elizabeth W T; Burnaby Hosp, 3935 Kincaid St, Burnaby BC V5G 2X6; UBC'04; FRCPC; Anes. Staff, Burnaby Hospital; (604)412-6311

CHUAH, S L Joanna; 1706 4 St SW PO Box 23055, Calgary AB T2S 3B1; Tor'08; CCFP.

CHUAH, Teong K; 6035 Martyniuk Pl, Richmond BC V7E 6K1; UBC'05; FRCSC; GenSurg. (604)450-1609

CHUANG, Ching C; 101-143 Queen St E, Brampton ON L6W 2B1; (Taiwan)'64; Ac Staff, William Osler Health System - Brampton Civic Hospital; (905)451-4810; Fax. (905)451-4810.

CHUANG, Evelyn Y; Rouge Valley HS-Ajax/Pickering, 580 Harwood Ave S, Ajax ON L1S 2J4; Wes'08; CCFP; CCFP(E.M.); Staff, Rouge Valley Health System - Ajax & Pickering Health Centre Site; (905)683-2320

CHUANG, Ian; Mackenzie Richmond Hill Hosp, 10 Trench St, Richmond Hill ON L4C 4Z3; Man'85; FRCPC; Anes. Staff, Mackenzie Richmond Hill Hospital; (905)883-1212

CHUANG, Monica M; Sunnybrook Hlth Sciences Ctre, 2075 Bayview Ave, Toronto ON M4N 3M5; Tor'06; FRCPC; Anes. Staff, Sunnybrook Health Sciences Centre; (416)480-6100

CHUANG, Ryan; Foothills Med Centre, 1403 29 St NW, Calgary AB T2N 2T9; Staff, Foothills Medical Centre; (403)944-6900; Fax. (403)944-1472.

CHUANG, Sylvester H S; The Hosp for Sick Children, 555 University Ave, Toronto ON M5G 1X8; McG'73; FRCPC; DiagRad. Head NeuroRadiol & Assoc Prof, The Hospital For Sick Children; Assoc Prof, University of Toronto; (416)813-5477; Fax. (416)813-6027.

CHUBATY, Roman A; Jefferson Med Clinic, 1553 Arlington St, Winnipeg MB R2X 1V3; Man'70.

CHUBB, P David; Hollyburn Med Centre, 108-575 16th St, West Vancouver BC V7V 4Y1; Tor'64; FRCSC; Ophth. Chief Dept of Ophth, Lions Gate Hospital; (604)926-5722; Fax. (604)926-5781.

CHUBRA-SMITH, Normandie; Chubra-Smith Anes Services Inc, 5912 Churchill St, Vancouver BC V6M 3H5; McM'79; BSc(Med.); Anes. Hd Anes, Burnaby Hospital; (604)290-3479

CHUDASAMA, Siddharaj; McMaster Univ, MDCL 3101A-1280 main St W, Hamilton ON L8S 4K1; McM'06; Teacher, McMaster University.

CHUDASAMA, Sushil; Medical House Officer, PZ262-771 Bannatyne Ave, Winnipeg MB R3E 3N4; (India)'80; (204)787-3479

CHUDLEY, Albert E; Children's Hosp, FE231-840 Sherbrook St, Winnipeg MB R3A 1S1; Man'74; FCCMG; FRCPC; Peds; MedGenetics. Consultant, St Boniface General Hospital; Consultant, Congenital Anomalies Registry; Prof Program in Genetic & Matabolism, University of Manitoba; (204)787-4370; Fax. (204)787-1419; achudley@hsc.mb.ca.

CHUDNOW, Gloria; Karmy Chronic Pain Medical Cli, 110-164 Queen St E, Brampton ON L6V 1B4; Man'83; Court Staff Privil, Mount Sinai Hospital; Physician Pain Management, Gleenspoon Pain Management Center; Staff Sclerotherapy & Cosmetic Injectables, Varicose Vein Clinic; (905)456-6816

CHUE, Pierre; Edmonton Mental Health Clinic, 3F-9942 108 St NW, Edmonton AB T5K 2J5; Cardiff (Wales)'85; MB ChB; FRCPsy; DABPN; LMCC; FRCPC; Psy (Neuro Psychiatry). Clin Prof, University of Alberta Hospital; Med Dir Community Mental Health Services, Alberta Health Services; Cons Psy Telepsychiatry, Primary Care Network; Langs: English; (780)342-7944; Fax. (780)342-7944.

CHUEN, Luan L; St Clair Med Clinic, 2F-50 St Clair Ave E, Toronto ON M4T 1M9; Qns'07; (416)921-1066; Fax. (416)921-8459.

CHUGH, Prem K; Woodlawn Med Clinic, 114 Woodlawn Rd, Dartmouth NS B2W 2S7; Rajasthan (India)'69; MB BS; Langs: Punjabi; Hindi; (902)462-7138; Fax. (902)462-3028; gurdas@eastlink.ca.

CHUGH, Taher; Enhanced Care Clinic, 14872 Yonge St, Aurora ON L4G 1N2; Tor'06; CCFP; (905)505-0950

CHUGHTAI, M Saeed; St Mary's Hosp Centre, 3830 av Lacombe, Montreal QC H3T 1M5; Punjab (Pakistan)'57; MSc; DABS; DABTS; FRCSC; GenSurg; Cardiovasc&ThorSurg (P.Q.)., St Mary's Hospital Centre; adj Prof, McGill University; (514)345-3511; Fax. (514)734-2704.

CHUGHTAI, Talat S; MUHC-Montreal Gen Hosp, L9 411-1650 av Cedar, Montreal QC H3G 1A4; McG'94; FRCSC; GenSurg; Critical Care Medicine (P.Q.). Staff, McGill University Health Centre - Montreal General Campus; (514)934-1934 x44334

CHUI, Betty K; 3054-8308 114 St NW, Edmonton AB T6G 2V2; Tor'04; FRCPC; IntMed; Nephrol. Staff, University of Alberta Hospital; (780)407-8822; Fax. (780)407-2172.

CHUI, Lica; Broadway Med Bldg, 520-943 Broadway W, Vancouver BC V5Z 4E1; UBC'99; DABOph; FRCSC; Ophth (Retina). Langs: Cantonese; Mandarin; (604)875-6985

CHUI, Mario C; One Med Place, 102-20 Wynford Dr, North York ON M3C 1J4; (Hong Kong)'71; FRCPC; DiagRad. Staff, St Michael's Hospital; (416)485-9471

CHUI, S T Thomas; Sackville Med Clinic, PO Box 8 Lcd Lower Sackville 201-667 Sackville Dr, Lower Sackville NS B4C 2S8; (Taiwan)'63; Court Staff, Queen Elizabeth II Health Sciences Centre - Victoria General Site; (902)865-9951; Fax. (902)865-6440; sackvillemedicalclinic@ns.aliantzinc.ca.

CHUI, Shyr Lin; University Hosp of Northern BC, 1475 Edmonton St, Prince George BC V2M 1S2; Oxford (England)'93; MB BS; FRCPC; DiagRad. Staff, University Hospital of Northern British Columbia; (250)565-2000

CHUI, Sze Wing; Univ Hlth Network-Toronto Gen, EN3 402-200 Elizabeth St, Toronto ON M5G 2C4; (Hong Kong)'02; Staff, Toronto General Hospital - UHN; (416)340-4800

CHUM, Elliott S; 108-2051 McCallum Rd, Abbotsford BC V2S 3N5; Alb'02; FRCPC; IntMed; Nephrol. (604)870-9886

CHUN, Kooyeon; 205-100 Humber College Blvd, Etobicoke ON M9V 5G4; Wes'92; FRCSC; ObstGyn. Staff, William Osler Health System - Etobicoke General Hospital; (416)741-5077; Fax. (416)749-3640.

CHUN, Robert; Newmarket Med Place, 105-712 Davis Dr, Newmarket ON L3Y 8C3; Witwatersrand (South Africa)'79; MB ChB; FACC; FRCPC; IntMed; Cardiol. Staff, Southlake Regional Health Centre; Asst Prof, University of Toronto; (905)953-7917; Fax. (905)953-0046.

CHUN, Rosaleen; Foothills Med Centre, 1403 29 St NW, Calgary AB T2N 2T9; Tor'96; FRCPC; Anes. Staff, Foothills Medical Centre; (403)944-1430; Fax. (403)944-2425.

CHUN, Samuel S S; 120-33 Ochterloney St, Dartmouth NS B2Y 4P5; Mem'88; FRCSC; Urol. Langs: Korean; (902)461-1258; Fax. (902)465-2740.

CHUN, Soohun; St Michael's Hosp, 30 Bond St, Toronto ON M5B 1W8; Tor'08; FRCPC; IntMed. Staff, St Michael's Hospital; (416)864-6060

CHUNDURI, Krishna V; Sheppard Med Bldg, 203-701 Sheppard Ave E, North York ON M2K 2Z3; Osmania (India)'75; CCFP; Physician, Markham Medical Clinic; Langs: Telugu; Hindi; Urdu; (416)221-0176 x7969; Fax. (647)776-7696.

CHUNG, A Maria; Gordon & Leslie Diamond Hlth C, 7F-2775 Laurel St, Vancouver BC V5Z 1M9; McG'83; FRCPC; IntMed; GeriatricMed. Staff, Vancouver General Hospital - Centennial Pavillion; Clinical Asst Prof, University of British Columbia; (604)875-5312; maria.chung@vch.ca.

CHUNG, Allison N; Nicola Med Dental Bldg, 305-321 Nicola St, Kamloops BC V2C 6G6; McM'02; CCFP; (250)374-8813

CHUNG, Andrew Y W; 103-4002 Sheppard Ave E, Scarborough ON M1S 4R5; Ott'75; CCFP; FCFP; Ac Staff, The Scarborough Hospital - Birchmount Campus; Langs: Chinese; (416)754-8080; Fax. (416)754-3646; aywchung@hotmail.com.

CHUNG, Arthur G; West Oak Medical Clinic, 2495 Old Bronte Rd, Oakville ON L6M 4J2; Wes'06; FRCPC; IntMed; ClinImmunol&Allergy. (905)582-7533

CHUNG, Brian J; Vancouver Gen Hosp, 855 12th Ave W, Vancouver BC V5Z 1M9; Tor'84; FRCPC; EmergMed. Staff, Vancouver General Hospital - Centennial Pavillion; (604)875-4700; Fax. (604)875-4872.

CHUNG, Bruce T W; Durham Med Clinic, PO Box 982 368 College St N, Durham ON N0G 1R0; (Taiwan)'66; Staff, South Bruce Grey Health Centre - Durham Site; Langs: Mandarin; (519)369-2510; Fax. (519)369-3831.

CHUNG, Carmen W H; Univ Hlth Network-Princess M, 5F-610 University Ave, Toronto ON M5G 2M9; Tor'08; IntMed. Staff, Princess Margaret Hospital - University Health Network; (416)946-4501

CHUNG, Caroline; Univ Hlth Network-Princess M, 610 University Ave, Toronto ON M5G 2M9; UBC'03; FRCPC; RadOncol. Staff, Princess Margaret Hospital - University Health Network; (416)946-2000 x2121

CHUNG, Catherine T; The Hosp for Sick Children, 555 University Ave, Toronto ON M5G 1X8; Tor'03; FRCPC; AnatPath. Staff, The Hospital For Sick Children; (416)813-1500

CHUNG, Chin K; 9 Madawaska Ave, North York ON M2M 2R1; Tor'74; BSc; CCFP; FCFP; Ac Staff, The Scarborough Hospital - General Campus; Staff, Mackenzie Richmond Hill Hospital; Staff, North York General Hospital; Staff, Humber River Regional Hospital - Finch Avenue Site; Langs: Cantonese; (416)222-4637; Fax. (416)222-3178.

CHUNG, Corinna R; Anishnawbe Mushkiki, 29 Royston Crt, Thunder Bay ON P7A 4Y7; Dal'94; MPH(Yale); CCFP; FCFP; (807)626-1221; Fax. (807)623-8832.

CHUNG, Cynthia; 113-385 Silverstar Blvd, Scarborough ON M1V 0E3; (Philippines)'03; Langs: Cantonese; (416)551-2888; Fax. (416)792-7888.

CHUNG, Dae-Gyun; Keele & Lawrence Ultrasound, 1375 Lawrence Ave W, North York ON M6L 1A4; Tor'92; PhD; FRCPC; DiagRad (Abdominal Imaging). Staff Radiol, St Michael's Hospital; University of Toronto; Langs: German; (416)243-8487

CHUNG, Edward Y C; Guelph Gen Hosp, 125 Delhi St, Guelph ON N1E 4J4; Tor'92; Staff, Guelph General Hospital; (519)837-1401; Fax. (519)837-0133.

CHUNG, Frances F T; Univ Hlth Network-Toronto Western Hosp, 2F 405-399 Bathurst St, Toronto ON M5T 2S8; (Hong Kong)'73; FRCPC; Anes. Staff, Toronto Western Hospital - University Health Network; (416)603-5118; Fax. (416)603-6494; frances.chung@uhn.on.ca.

CHUNG, Gia-Yen; Centre Med Chambly-Latour, B-5580 ch de Chambly, Saint-Hubert QC J3Y 3P5; Sher'00; (450)926-2236; Fax. (450)926-2633.

CHUNG, Han-Oh; PG Med Educ McMaster Univ, MDCL 3101A-1280 Main St W, Hamilton ON L8S 4K1; Tor'08; FRCPC; IntMed.

CHUNG, Hans T K; Sunnybrook Hlth Sciences Ctre, TW-2075 Bayview Ave, Toronto ON M4N 3M5; Tor'99; FRCPC; RadOncol. Staff, Sunnybrook Health Sciences Centre; (416)480-4834; Fax. (416)480-6002.

CHUNG, Henry V; 410-301 Columbia St E, New Westminster BC V3L 3W5; UBC'00; BScPharm; FRCPC; IntMed; Gastroent. (604)525-0155; Fax. (604)525-1699.

CHUNG, Jim J; Toronto East Gen Hosp Inc, 825 Coxwell Ave, Toronto ON M4C 3E7; Tor'95; CCFP; CCFP(E.M.); FCFP; Staff, Toronto East General Hospital Inc; (416)469-7734; Fax. (416)469-6259; jimc2270@hotmail.com.

CHUNG, Justin A; Scarborough Hosp-General Div, 3050 Lawrence Ave E, Scarborough ON M1P 2V5; Wes'08; CCFP; CCFP(E.M.); Staff, The Scarborough Hospital - General Campus; (416)438-2911

CHUNG, Kalyani; UBC Student Health Service, M334-2211 Westbrook Mall, Vancouver BC V6T 1Z3; Man'05; BSc; MSc; CCFP; (604)822-7011

CHUNG, Kin Lok; 110-470 Bronte St S, Milton ON L9T 2J4; Tor'87; CAFCI; BSc(E.E.); MSc(E.E.); (905)878-3025; Fax. (905)878-1535; kin.chung@sympatico.ca.

CHUNG, Leonard C; Hamilton HS-General Site, 237 Barton St, Hamilton ON L8L 2X2; McM'10; CCFP; Staff, Hamilton Health Sciences Centre - Hamilton General Hospital; (905)521-2100

CHUNG, Louis; Oakfield Med Clinic, 106-1021 Court Ave, Winnipeg MB R2P 1V7; London (England)'71; DCH; DA; MRC(UK); CCFP; Assoc Physician, Health Sciences Centre; Physician Family Med, Seven Oaks General Hospital; (204)338-2343; Fax. (204)339-3971.

CHUNG, Michael H; The Credit Valley Hosp, 2200 Eglinton Ave W, Mississauga ON L5M 2N1; Tor'95; CCFP; CCFP(E.M.); Staff, The Credit Valley Hospital; (905)813-4530; Fax. (905)813-4548.

CHUNG, Ngai Sang P; 111-1465 Salisbury Ave, Port Coquitlam BC V3B 6J3; Alb'76; Staff, Royal Columbian Hospital; (604)942-6011; Fax. (604)942-6099.

CHUNG, Peter W; Univ Hlth Network-Princess M, 610 University Ave, Toronto ON M5G 2M9; Sheffield (England)'90; FRCPC; RadOncol. Staff, Princess Margaret Hospital - University Health Network; (416)946-2122

CHUNG, Pin; B9-76 Arlington Dr, Keswick ON L4P 0A9; Qns'96; CCFP; Langs: Mandarin; (905)476-0308; Fax. (905)476-1079.

CHUNG, Randy D; Respiratory & Critical Care Me, 103-250 Keary St, New Westminster BC V3L 5E7; UBC'04; FRCPC; IntMed; Respir. Staff, Vancouver General Hospital - Centennial Pavillion; (604)525-8822

CHUNG, Seen Taek; Alberta Children's Hosp, 2888 Shaganappi Trail NW, Calgary AB T3B 6A8; Man'00; FRCPC; Peds; PedEmergMed. Staff, Alberta Children's Hospital; (403)955-7093

CHUNG, Shari A; Bloor Med Clinic, 844 Bathurst St, Toronto ON M5R 3G1; McG'06; MDCM; CCFP; (416)534-4214; Fax. (416)534-4582.

CHUNG, Stephen W; Gordon & Leslie Diamond Hlth C, 5F-2775 Laurel St, Vancouver BC V5Z 1M9; Tor'83; PhD; FRCSC; GenSurg (Hepatobiliary & Pancreatic Surgery). Staff, Vancouver General Hospital - Centennial Pavillion; University of British Columbia; (604)875-4459; Fax. (604)875-3973.

CHUNG, Sun Yung; Pickering Holistic Health Cent, 220-1101 Kingston Rd, Pickering ON L1V 1B5; Tor'89; CCFP; (905)831-9797 x6; Fax. (905)839-9984.

CHUNG, Tae Bong; Univ Hlth Network-Princess M, PMH3 961-610 University Ave, Toronto ON M5G 2M9; Wes'95; FRCPC; DiagRad. Staff, Princess Margaret Hospital - University Health Network; (416)946-4501 x4844; Fax. (416)946-6564.

CHUNG, Terry T H; Markham Stouffvile Hosp, PO Box 1800 Stn Main 381 Church St, Markham ON L3P 7P3; UBC'02; FRCPC; DiagRad. Staff, Markham Stouffville Hospital; (905)472-7000

CHUNG, Thomas; 3F 301-505 Highway 7 E, Thornhill ON L3T 7T1; (Hong Kong)'97; MB BS; FRCSC; Ophth. Langs: Cantonese; Mandarin; (905)709-8228; Fax. (905)709-9007.

CHUNG, Wan M; Pleasantview Prof Bldg, 304-11044 51 Ave NW, Edmonton AB T6H 5B4; Hanyang (Korea)'74; Langs: Korean; (780)434-1143; Fax. (780)989-0847.

CHUNG, Wilfred W; Kemptville District Hosp, PO Box 2007 2675 Concession Rd, Kemptville ON K0G 1J0; Tor'79; DABEM; FACEP; MCFP(EM); Staff, Kemptville District Hospital; (613)258-3435; Fax. (613)258-1896.

CHUNG, Win Yan; Superior Family Health Team, 48-44 Great Northern Rd, Sault Ste Marie ON P6B 4Y5; Edinburgh (Scotland)'04; (705)253-6599

CHUNG FOR YUEN, Kim F; 1575 Ouellette Ave, Windsor ON N8X 1K5; Edinburgh (Scotland)'72; MB ChB; DABIM; Staff, Hôtel-Dieu Grace Hospital; (519)258-4888

CHUO, Jean Y; 616-2525 Willow St, Vancouver BC V5Z 3N8; UBC'04; FRCSC; Ophth. (604)879-9311

CHUONG, Roselynn; 825 Don Mills Rd, North York ON M3C 1V4; McM'08; CCFP.

CHURCH, Brian; London HSC-Victoria Hosp, PO Box 5010 Stn B D2 315-800 Commissioners Rd E, London ON N6A 5W9; Dal'96; FRCPC; Anes. Staff, London Health Sciences Centre - University Hospital; Staff, South Huron Hospital Association; Staff, London Health Sciences Centre - Victoria Campus; Medical Officer, Canadian Forces Base; (519)685-8500 x58525

CHURCH, Christopher L; South Shore Reg Hosp, 90 Glen Allan Dr, Bridgewater NS B4V 3S6; Dal'87; FRCPC; DiagRad. Staff, South Shore Regional Hospital; (902)527-5231; Fax. (902)543-2733.

CHURCH, Deirdre L; Calgary Lab Services, 9-3535 Research Rd NW, Calgary AB T2L 2K8; Cal'78; FRCPC; IntMed (Medical Microbiology); InfectDis. Staff, Calgary Laboratory Services; Prof Path & LabMed, University of Calgary; (403)770-3281; Fax. (403)770-3347; deirdre.church@cls.ab.ca.

CHURCH, James B; McKenzie Prof Centre, 209-1595 McKenzie Ave, Victoria BC V8N 1A4; Missouri (USA)'84; CCFP; FCFP; (250)595-7772

CHURCH, Karalyn; London HSC-Victoria Hosp, PO Box 5010 St B E1 102-800 Commissioners Rd, London ON N6A 5W9; Vermont (USA)'06; FRCPC; EmergMed. Staff, London Health Sciences Centre - Victoria Campus; Teach Staff, University of Western Ontario; (519)685-8500

CHURCH, Neal G; Peter Lougheed Centre, 3500 26 Ave NE, Calgary AB T1Y 6J4; Cal'97; BSc; FRCSC; GenSurg (Upper Gastrointestinal Surgery). Staff, Peter Lougheed Centre; Clinical Asst Prof Med, University of Calgary; (403)943-5689; Fax. (403)219-3574.

CHURCH, Paige T; Sunnybrook Hlth Sciences Ctre, 2075 Bayview Ave, Toronto ON M4N 3M5; Vermont (USA)'99; Staff, Sunnybrook Health Sciences Centre; (416)480-6100; Fax. (416)480-6054.

CHURCH, Peter C; Dr Charles A Janeway Child HC, 300 Prince Philip Dr, St. John's NL A1B 3V6; Mem'06; Gastroent; Peds. Staff, Janeway Children's Health & Rehabilitation Centre; (709)777-6300

CHURCH, Rhonda L; Medavie Blue Cross, 230 Brownlow Ave, Halifax NS B3J 2S1; Dal'87; Med Consultant, Medavie Blue Cross; (902)496-7112; Fax. (902)492-2921.

CHURCH, Wayne F; Parkland Med Clinic, 6-5030 47 Ave, Red Deer AB T4N 3P7; Alb'75; CCFP; Staff, Red Deer Regional Hospital Centre; (403)346-4206; Fax. (403)346-4207.

CHURCHER, Margaret A; 110-790 Coventry Dr NE, Calgary AB T3K 4K4; Qns'79; BSc(Hons); CCFP; FCFP; Langs: English; French; (403)226-1163; Fax. (403)226-1686; mchurcher53@yahoo.ca.

CHURCHILL, Gale A; Huronia Urgent Care Clinic, 480 Huronia Rd, Barrie ON L4N 6M2; Qns'83; Staff, Royal Victoria Regional Health Centre; (705)725-7716

CHURCHILL-SMITH, Michael J; MUHC-Montreal Gen Hosp, D6 269-1650 av Cedar, Montreal QC H3G 1A4; McG'83; FRCPC; IntMed. Staff, McGill University Health Centre - Montreal General Campus; Langs: Italian; French; (514)934-1934 x4372; Fax. (514)937-6118.

CHURG, Andrew M; UBC Hospital, 2211 Wesbrook Mall, Vancouver BC V6T 2B5; Illinois (USA)'73; FRCPC; MedScient(Med). Staff, UBC Hospital - Koerner Pavillion; Staff, Vancouver General Hospital - Centennial Pavillion; (604)822-7776

CHURMAN, Mark H C; Haileybury Med Associates, PO Box 2010 494 Ferguson Ave, Haileybury ON P0J 1K0; McM'94; CCFP; Langs: English; French; (705)672-3371; Fax. (705)672-5900.

CHYCHOTA, Norman N; Associate Med Centre, 5016 48 Ave, Taber AB T1G 1R8; Man'68; BSc(Med.); FACS; Ac Staff, Taber Health Centre; Langs: Ukrainian; (403)223-3525; Fax. (403)223-9020; nchychot@telus.net.

CHYCZIJ, Harold R; 205-3017 66 St NW, Edmonton AB T6K 4B2; Ott'83; BSc; FRCSC; GenSurg (Vascular Doppler Studies); VascSurg. Sec Chief Vascular Surg Edmonton Zone, Alberta Health Services; Ac Staff Edmonton Zone, Covenant Health; Clin Prof, University of Alberta; (780)461-6012; Fax. (780)461-5442; hchyczij@surgicorp.ca.

CHYLA, Andrew; Stephenville Comm Med Clinic, 1 Washington Dr, Stephenville NL A2N 2V5; Warsaw (Poland)'63; Locum Tenens, Sir Thomas Roddick Hospital; achyla@nf.sympatico.ca.

CHYPCHAR, Tatiana; Forbes Park Med Centre, 26 Forbes St, Cambridge ON N3C 2E2; McM'93; BSc; CCFP; Staff Privil Family Med, Cambridge Memorial Hospital; Langs: Ukrainian; French; (519)658-4615; Fax. (519)658-4630.

CIABURRO, Hugo E; 5955 rue Saint-Zotique E, Saint-Leonard QC H1T 1R1; Mon'62; FRCSC; PlasSurg. ac Staff, Centre Hospitalier l'Université de Montréal (CHUM) - Hôpital Notre-Dame; adj Prof, Universite de Montreal; (514)527-3465

CIACH, Michelle; Bedford Waterfront Health Clin, 207-967 Bedford Hwy, Bedford NS B4A 1A9; Wes'06; CCFP; (902)835-6444; Fax. (902)832-1193.

CIANCIULLI, Bruno; Hop Sante Cabrini Ospedale, 5655 rue Saint-Zotique E, Montreal QC H1T 1P7; Sher'95; FRCSC; Urol. Staff, Hôpital Santa Cabrini Ospedale; (514)252-6000

CIANCIULLI, Rino; Polyclinique Cabrini, 212-5700 rue Saint-Zotique E, Montreal QC H1T 3Y7; Laval'64; FRCSC; PlasSurg (Aesthetic Surgery). ac Staff, Hôpital Santa Cabrini Ospedale; Langs: Bilingual(French/English); (514)256-3833; Fax. (514)256-7066.

CIANFRONE, Michael; Jane-Clair Med Centre, 2698 Jane St, North York ON M3L 1S5; Rome (Italy)'85; Staff, Humber River Regional Hospital - Church Street Site; Langs: Italian; (416)746-4544; Fax. (416)746-4744.

CIANFRONE, G Adrian; 200-2698 Jane St, North York ON M3L 1S5; Bologna (Italy)'75; Staff, Humber River Regional Hospital - Church Street Site; Langs: Italian; (416)746-4544; Fax. (416)746-4744; cianfronemedicine@gmail.com.

CIARALLO, Anhony; CSSS de Saint-Jerome, 290 rue de Montigny, Saint-Jerome QC J7Z 5T3; McG'08; Staff, Hôtel-Dieu de Saint-Jérôme; (450)432-2777

CIASCHINI, Patricia M; The Group Health Centre, 240 Mcnabb St, Sault Ste. Marie ON P6B 1Y5; Ott'83; FRCPC; IntMed. Ac Staff, Sault Area Hospital - Sault Ste Marie; (705)759-1234; Fax. (705)946-5241.

CIAVARELLA, Anthony L; Aldergrove Med Office, 27107 Fraser Hwy, Aldergrove BC V4W 3R2; Tor'78; (604)856-3321

CIBERE, Jolanda; Arthritis Research Centre, 5591 No. 3 Rd, Richmond BC V6X 2C7; Sask'93; PhD; FRCPC; IntMed (Clinical Research); Rheum. Asst Prof Arthritis Research Centre of Canada/Rsch Scientist, University of British Columbia; Langs: German; (604)207-4025; Fax. (604)207-4057.

CICCONE, Mario V; Timmins Family Health Team, 1-681 Algonquin Blvd E, Timmins ON P4N 8S6; Qns'85; BSc(Pharm); CCFP; CCFP(E.M.); FCFP; Staff, Timmins & District Hospital; University of Ottawa; Langs: English; French; (705)267-5600; Fax. (705)268-3900.

CICCOTELLI, William A; Grand River Hosp-KW Hlth Ctre, PO Box 9056 Stn C 835 King St W, Kitchener ON N2G 1G3; McM'02; FRCPC; IntMed; InfectDis; MedMicrobiol. Staff, Grand River Hospital - Kitchener/Waterloo Health Centre; (519)749-4348 x4348

CICORIA, Eugenio; Central Prof Bldg, 72 Brant Ave, Brantford ON N3T 5Z8; Tor'83; (519)756-0171; Fax. (519)756-0176.

CIECHANSKA, Ewa; West Carleton Family Hlth Team, 119 Langstaff Dr, Carp ON K0A 1L0; Wes'05; CCFP; (613)839-3271; Fax. (613)839-3273.

CIECIERSKI, Danuta W; Roblin Med Clinic, 200A Thompson Dr, Winnipeg MB R3J 3E1; (Other Foreign)'91; (204)895-8883; Fax. (204)895-9966.

CIESLAK, Malgorzata; 301-223 Nelson's Cres, New Westminster BC V3L 0E4; Poznan (Poland)'82; Langs: Polish; (604)524-4141; Fax. (604)525-2411; dr301223@gmail.com.

CIESLAK, Zenon; 301-223 Nelson's Cres, New Westminster BC V3L 0E4; Poznan (Poland)'82; FRCPC; Peds (Neonatal & Perinatal Medicine). Staff, Royal Columbian Hospital; Langs: Polish; (604)525-3955; Fax. (604)525-2411; zcieslak@telus.net.

CIEUTA-WALTI, Cecile; CHUS-Hop Fleurimont, 3001 12e Av N, Sherbrooke QC J1H 5N4; Paris V (France)'92; Staff, Centre Hospitalier Universitaire de Sherbrooke-Hopital Fleurimont; adj Prof, Universite de Sherbrooke; (819)346-1110 x13147

CIEZA LARA, Tomas A; Les Cardiologues Assoc, 314-874 boul de l'Universite E, Chicoutimi QC G7H 6B9; (Argentina)'98; (418)545-0539; Fax. (418)545-1032.

CIGANOVIC, Olivera; Niagara H System-G Niagara, PO Box 1018 Stn Main 5546 Portage Rd, St Catharines ON L2R 7C6; Belgrade (Serbia)'88; FRCPC; Anes. Staff, Niagara Health System - St Catharines General Site; (905)378-4647

CIL, Tulin D; Univ Hlth Network-Princess M, 3 130-610 University Ave, Toronto ON M5G 2M9; Wes'00; MEd; FRCSC; GenSurg (Surgical Oncology). Staff, Princess Margaret Hospital - University Health Network; Staff, Women's College Hospital; (416)946-4432

CILLIERS, Denise; 1025 103rd Ave, Dawson Creek BC V1G 2G6; Stellenbosch (South Africa)'76; MB ChB; MMed(Psych); FRCPC; Psy. Staff Psy, Dawson Creek & District Hospital; (250)782-8604

CILLIERS, Philip; 5500 206 St, Langley BC V3A 8R3; Cape Town (South Africa)'82; (604)534-4224; Fax. (604)534-6616.

CIMEN, Sertac; Queen Elizabeth II HSC, 1276 South Park St, Halifax NS B3H 2Y9; Unkara (Turkey)'01; MD; Staff, Queen Elizabeth II Health Sciences Centre - Victoria General Site; (902)473-2700

CIMOLAI, Nevio; BC Women's Hosp & H C, 2G6-4500 Oak St, Vancouver BC V6H 3N1; Alb'81; FRCPC; MedMicrobiol. Staff, BC Women's Hospital & Health Centre; Prof, University of British Columbia.

CIMON, Isabelle; CLSC Laurier-Station, 135 rue de la Station SS 1, Laurier-Station QC G0S 1N0; Mon'99; CCFP; (418)728-3435; Fax. (418)728-2233.

CIMON, Line; Regie des Rentes du Quebec, CP 5200 Succ Terminus, Quebec QC G1K 7S9; Laval'85; (418)657-8709 x3252

CIMON, Marie-Juie; CHUQ-Ctr Hosp Univ Laval, RC157-2705 boul Laurier, Quebec QC G1V 4G2; Laval'01; FRCPC; Psy. Staff, Centre Hospitalier Universitaire de Quebec-CHUL; Langs: Bilingual(French/English); (418)654-2121; Fax. (418)654-2132; marie-julie.cimon@mail.chuq.qc.ca.

CIMON, Michel; CSSS du Sud de Lanaudiere, 911 Montee des Pionniers, Terrebonne QC J6V 2H2; Sher'80; Staff, Centre Hospitalier Pierre le Gardeur; (450)654-7525 x23178

CIMON, Philippe; CSSSG-Hop de Gatineau, CP 2000 Succ Bureau-Chef 909 boul la Verendrye O, Gatineau QC J8P 7H2; Mon'04; Staff, Hôpital de Gatineau; (819)561-8100

CIMON-CARUFEL, Janie; CSSS de Chicoutimi, 305 rue Saint-Vallier, Chicoutimi QC G7H 5H6; Sher'08; CCFP; CCFP(E.M.); Staff, Complexe hospitalier de la Sagamie; (418)541-1000

CINA, Claudio S; York-Finch Med Centre, 411-2115 Finch Ave W, North York ON M3N 2V6; Catania (Italy)'78; MSc; VascSurg; GenSurg. Clin Assoc Prof Surg, McMaster University; Prof Surg, University of Toronto; Langs: Italian; French; (416)740-3949

CINANNI, Joseph; U of Ottawa Health Services, 300-100 Marie Curie Pvt, Ottawa ON K1N 6N5; Ott'74; (613)564-3950

CINARLI, Bahar; Khatsahlano Med Clinic, 2685 Broadway W, Vancouver BC V6K 2G2; 80Ankara (Turkey)'87; MSc(UBC); CCFP; (604)731-9187

CINATS, John G; 11202 76 Ave NW, Edmonton AB T6G 0K1; Alb'80; FRCSC; OrthSurg. (780)439-8939; Fax. (780)439-0396.

CINO, Peter J; Headwaters Health Care Centre, 100 Rolling Hills Dr, Orangeville ON L9W 4X9; Ott'90; CCFP; FCFP; Staff, Headwaters Health Care Centre - Orangeville Site; (519)941-2410

CINQ-MARS, Benoit; Ctr Hosp Affilie-St-Sacrement, 1050 ch Sainte-Foy, Quebec QC G1S 4L8; Mon'92; FRCSC; Ophth. Staff, Centre Hospitalier Affilié Universitaire de Québec - Hôpital du St-Sacrement; (418)656-4141; Fax. (418)654-1580.

CINQ-MARS, Gaetane; Clinique Med Belvedere, 202-2235 rue Galt O, Sherbrooke QC J1K 1K6; Sher'77; CCFP; FCFP; assoc Staff, Centre Hospitalier Universitaire de Sherbrooke-Hôpital Hôtel-Dieu; (819)563-4244; Fax. (819)563-8924.

CINQ-MARS, Michelle; 13950 Rte Marie-Victorin, Sorel-Tracy QC J3P 5N3; Laval'75; Med Dir, Quebec Iron & Titanium; Langs: Spanish; English; (450)561-1002; Fax. (450)746-8797.

CINQ-MARS, Suzanne; CSSS Les Eskers de l'Abitibi, 622 4e rue O, Amos QC J9T 2S2; Sher'86; CSPQ; FRCPC; Anes. Staff, CH Hôtel-Dieu d'Amos; (819)732-3341 x2456; Fax. (819)732-7622.

CIOATA, Liliana; Royal Columbian Hosp, 330 Columbia St E, New Westminster BC V3L 3W7; (Romania)'98; CCFP; Staff, Royal Columbian Hospital; (604)461-2022

CIOATA TOMSA, Elena; 201-222 King St E, Bowmanville ON L1C 1P6; (Romania)'82; CCFP; (905)440-3584

CIOFANI, Amelia; Univ of Toronto, 2F-500 University Ave, Toronto ON M5G 1V7; Tor'07; IntMed.

CIOLOFAN, Oana C; Medicale Sportive de Laval, 3095 Autoroute Laval O, Laval QC H7P 4W5; Bucharest (Romania)'99; FRCPC; Rheum; IntMed. (450)988-1026

CIOMYK, Robert; 206-3101 Bloor St W, Etobicoke ON M8X 2W2; Tor'89; (416)233-5225; Fax. (416)233-9275.

CIONA, Curtis J; Tawa Centre, 205-3017 66 St NW, Edmonton AB T6K 4B2; Alb'92; BMedSci; FRCSC; GenSurg (Colon & Rectal Surgery). Ac Staff, Covenant Health - Grey Nuns Community Hospital; Ac Staff, Cross Cancer Institute; Asst Prof Surg, University of Alberta; (780)461-6012; Fax. (780)461-5442.

CIPERA, Michelle P; CLSC Great Whale, GD, Kuujjuarapik QC J0M 1G0; Ott'93; BSc; CCFP; Langs: English; French; Czech; (819)929-3307; misa_cipera@hotmail.com.

CIPOLLETTI, Adriana A; 36 Grey St, Southampton ON N0H 2L0; Tor'02; CCFP; (519)797-9940

CIRIC, Ioana E; William Osler HC-Brampton Civi, 2100 Bovaird Dr E, Brampton ON L6R 3J7; Man'96; FRCPC; IntMed; Critical Care Medicine; Respir. Staff, William Osler Health System - Brampton Civic Hospital; (905)494-2120

CIRICILLO, Domenico; Centre Multi-Medic St-Leonard, 5953 rue Belanger, Saint-Leonard QC H1T 1G8; Sher'80; BSc; Staff, Hôpital Santa Cabrini Ospedale; (514)253-9191; Fax. (514)253-5242.

CIRKOVIC, Alain; Ctr Hosp de Verdun, 4000 boul Lasalle, Verdun QC H4G 2A3; Mon'97; FRCSC; OrthSurg (Sports Medicine). Orthopedic Surgery, Centre Hospitalier de Verdun; Langs: Bilingual(French/English); (514)362-1000

CIRONE, Robert; St Joseph's Health Centre, 30 The Queensway, Toronto ON M6R 1B5; Ott'91; FRCPC; Anes. Staff, St Joseph's Health Centre; (416)530-6090

CIRONE, Sharon L; 410-2333 Dundas St W, Toronto ON M6R 3A6; Ott'91; CCFP; CCFP(E.M.); FCFP; Consultant, St Joseph's Health Centre; Langs: English; French; (416)537-7000; Fax. (416)537-0132.

CISA, Jordi; South Hlth & Life Managment Ct, 2-2120 Regent St, Sudbury ON P3E 3Z9; Barcelona (Spain)'82; FRCSC; OrthSurg (General Orthopedics). Staff OrthSurg, Health Sciences North-Laurentian Site; Langs: Spanish; French; Catalan; (705)522-9101; Fax. (705)522-5744.

CISNEROS, Nestor F; Manitoba Clinic, 790 Sherbrook St, Winnipeg MB R3A 1M3; (El Salvador)'92; FRCPC; Peds; ClinImmunol&Allergy. Staff, Brandon Regional Health Centre; Langs: Spanish.

CISTERNAS, Felipe; Pender Community Health Centre, 59 Pender St W, Vancouver BC V6B 1R3; McG'04; CCFP; Staff, Pender Community Health Centre; Clin Instructor Family Med, University of British Columbia; Langs: Spanish; French; (604)669-9181; Fax. (604)688-9775.

CISZAK, Wojtek P; Burrard Med Bldg, 460-1144 Burrard St, Vancouver BC V6Z 2A5; Tor'81; Assoc Staff, Providence Health Care - St Paul's Hospital; University of British Columbia; Langs: Spanish; French; Russian; (604)682-5291; Fax. (604)682-5291.

CITREN, Robert M; Halton HCS Corp-Oakville, 327 Reynolds St, Oakville ON L6J 3L7; McG'71; FRCPC; DiagRad. Assoc Staff Radiol, Halton Healthcare Services Corporation - Oakville Site; (905)338-6775

CITRON, Sidney P; 40 Beverly Hills Dr, North York ON M3L 1A1; Tor'60; Assoc Staff, Humber River Regional Hospital - Church Street Site; Court Staff, Humber River Regional Hospital - Finch Avenue Site; Court Staff, St John's Rehabilitation Hospital; (416)241-4666; Fax. (416)241-4667.

CIUBOTARIU, Elena; Hop du Sacre-Coeur de Mtl, 5400 boul Gouin O, Montreal QC H4J 1C5; (Romania)'97; Rheum; IntMed. Staff, Hôpital du Sacre-Coeur de Montréal; (514)338-2222

CIUBOTARU, Sergiu; Crescent Heights Med Centre, 49 8 St NW, Medicine Hat AB T1A 6N9; (Romania)'94; CCFP; Langs: Romanian; Italian; French; (403)526-7422; Fax. (403)526-3349.

CIUNTU, Ioana; 5790 ch Cote-des-Neiges, Montreal QC H3S 1Y9; Timisoara (Romania)'99; CCFP; (514)340-8256

CIURRIA, Nicholas S; Danforth Med Centre, 1473 Danforth Ave, Toronto ON M4J 1N5; Tor'76; Langs: Italian; (416)461-0785; Fax. (416)461-0787.

CIVIDINO, Alfred A; 187 Hughson St S, Hamilton ON L8N 2B6; McM'79; FRCPC; IntMed; Rheum. Clin Prof, McMaster University; (905)528-1123; Fax. (905)528-1125; civi@cogeco.ca.

CIVIDINO, Maureen E P; St Joseph's Healthcare, 50 Charlton Ave E, Hamilton ON L8N 4A6; McM'79; DOHS; CCBOM; CCFP; FCFP; Staff, St Joseph's Healthcare - Charlton Campus; Court Staff, Hamilton Health Sciences Centre - McMaster University Medical Centre; (905)522-1155 x33344; Fax. (905)521-6111; mcividino@stjoes.ca.

CLAASEN, Cornelis J; Fairview Med Clinic, PO Box 725 10624 110 St, Fairview AB T0H 1L0; (South Africa)'92; CCFP; (780)835-4255; Fax. (780)835-5009.

CLAASEN, Izak E; Coventry Hills Family Care Ctr, 105-100 Country Village Rd NE, Calgary AB T3K 5Z2; Orange Free State (South Africa)'94; Staff, Foothills Medical Centre; (403)226-6715; Fax. (403)226-6748.

CLAASEN, J Pieter; 202-1530 Cliffe Ave, Courtenay BC V9N 2K4; Orange Free State (South Africa)'85; MB ChB; MMed(Ophth); FRCSC; Ophth (Cataract). Staff Ophth, Powell River General Hospital; Staff Ophth, St Joseph's General Hospital; Langs: Afrikaans; (250)703-2055; Fax. (250)703-2065.

CLAASSEN, Andre N; Medical Arts Clinic, 780 Central Ave N, Swift Current SK S9H 0M3; (Other Foreign)'91; Langs: Afrikaans; (306)773-2811; Fax. (306)778-4081.

CLAASSENS, Coenraad F; Associated Med Clinic, PO Box 510, Lac La Biche AB T0A 2C0; Pretoria (South Africa)'94; (780)623-4421; Fax. (780)623-1920; coendebs@yahoo.com.

CLAESSENS, E Anne; Toronto West Fertility Centre, 100-56 Aberfoyle Cres, Etobicoke ON M8X 2W4; Guy's Hosp. (England)'75; MB BS; LRCP(Lond); MRCS(Eng); FRCSC; ObstGyn (Reproductive Endocrinology). Assoc Staff ObstGyn, Mount Sinai Hospital; Asst Prof ObstGyn, University of Toronto; (416)231-3039; torontowestfertilitycenter.ryan@gmail.com.

CLAGUE, Nicholas P; Physicians Incorporated, 205-316 Willow St, Truro NS B2N 5A4; London (England)'85; MB BS; MD; BSc; FRCSC; ObstGyn. Consultant ObstGyn, Colchester East Hants Health Centre; (902)895-4477; Fax. (902)895-4407.

CLAIN, Sheryl A; 201-6628 Crowchild Trail SW, Calgary AB T3E 5R8; Dal'96; CCFP; FCFP; (403)240-9350

CLAIR, Kiran D K; MCI The Doctors Office, PO Box 134 Royal Bank Plaza 200 Bay St, Toronto ON M5J 2J3; Dal'03; CCFP; (416)368-6787

CLAIR, Veronic; School of Population & Public, 2206 East Mall, Vancouver BC V6T 1Z3; Mon'01; FRCPC; CommunMed;CCFP; Langs: Bilingual(English/French); (604)822-3282

CLAIRE, Daljit T S; Medical Centre, 117-7130 120 St, Surrey BC V3W 3M8; Alb'90; (778)578-7499

CLAIROUX, Marc I; 5775 boul Leger, Montreal-Nord QC H1G 1K7; Mon'73; FRCSC; Otol (Cervicofacial Surgery). ac Staff, Hopital Maisonneuve-Rosemont; Staff, CHSLD Paul-Gouin; assoc Staff, Centre de Réadaptation Marie Enfant du CHU Sainte-Justine; adj Prof Surg, Universite de Montreal; (514)327-4040; Fax. (514)327-5060.

CLAIROUX, Michel; CHUS-Hop Fleurimont, 3001 12e Av N, Sherbrooke QC J1H 5N4; Sher'76; CSPQ; FRCPC; Anes. Staff, Centre Hospitalier Universitaire de Sherbrooke-Hopital Fleurimont; (819)346-1110; Fax. (819)820-6420.

CLAMAN, Jeffrey M; 4420 10th Ave W, Vancouver BC V6R 2H9; UBC'82; Dip(McGill); FRCPC; Psy (Psychotherapy). Ac Staff, Vancouver General Hospital - Centennial Pavillion; Clin Assoc Prof Psy, University of British Columbia; (604)222-8277

CLAMAN, Paul; Ottawa Fertility Centre, 955 Green Valley Cres, Ottawa ON K2C 3V4; UBC'80; FRCS; BSc; ABOG; FRCSC; ObstGyn (Infertility). Prof ObstGyn & Reproductive Med Faculty of Med, University of Ottawa; Langs: Hebrew; (613)686-3378 x630; Fax. (613)225-9736.

CLAMEN, Marvin; 204-5885 ch de la Cote-des-Nei, Montreal QC H3S 2T2; McG'52; AACP; FRCPC; IntMed; Endocrin (P.Q.). Assoc Physician, Sir Mortimer B Davis Jewish General; Consultant Endocrin, Donald Berman Maimonides Geriatric Centre; McGill University; (514)739-8651; mandmclamen@gmail.com.

CLANCY, Sarah D; Green Bay Comm Health Ctre, PO Box 280 292 Main St, Springdale NL A0J 1T0; Mem'10; CCFP; Staff, Green Bay Community Health Centre; (709)673-3911

CLAPPERTON, Irma; Dir Sante Pub L'Estrie, 300-300 rue King E, Sherbrooke QC J1G 1B1; Sher'78; MSc; Public Health & Preventive Med; CommunMed (P.Q.). Med Consultant, Direction de Sante Publique de Montreal; Universite de Montreal; (819)829-3400

CLAPPERTON, Véronique; CSSS Kamouraska-Hop Notre-Dame, 1201 6e av, La Pocatiere QC G0R 1Z0; Sher'09; CCFP; Staff, CSSS de Kamouraska; (418)856-7000

CLAPSON, J Brian; Plastic Surgical Associates, 602-750 Spadina Cres E, Saskatoon SK S7K 3H3; Alb'80; FRCSC; CCFP; PlasSurg. (306)653-7766; Fax. (306)653-7768.

CLARACQ, Marine; CSSS de Manicouagan, 635 boul Joleit, Baie-Comeau QC G5C 1P1; Sher'10; CCFP; Staff, Centre Hospitalier Régional Baie-Comeau; (418)589-3701

CLARE, Michael E; Royal Inland Hosp, 311 Columbia St, Kamloops BC V2C 2T1; Alb'78; FRCPC; DiagRad. Staff, Royal Inland Hospital; (250)314-2405

CLARE, Terence P; Barriere Med Clinic, PO Box 799 537 Barriere Town Rd, Barriere BC V0E 1E0; Witwatersrand (South Africa)'83; MB ChB; Staff Chief, Barriere Medical Clinic; (250)672-9795; Fax. (250)672-9726.

CLAREMONT, Shari L; Group One Med Associates, 1111 Springfield Rd, Kelowna BC V1Y 8R7; UBC'89; CCFP; Ac Staff, Kelowna General Hospital; (250)762-4006; Fax. (250)762-4290.

CLARFIELD, Michael D; 5F-150 Eglinton Ave E, Toronto ON M4P 1E8; Tor'80; Dip SportMed; Dir The SportsMed Specialists, Toronto Western Hospital - University Health Network; Asst Prof, University of Toronto; (416)481-1601; Fax. (416)481-1267.

CLARK, Aaron T D; 202-1532 Cliffe Ave, Courtenay BC V9N 2K4; UBC'05; Urol. (250)338-7764

CLARK, Alexander J M; Queen Elizabeth II HSC, 4F-1276 South Park St, Halifax NS B3H 2Y9; Dal'74; FRCPC; Anes (Pain Management). Staff, Queen Elizabeth II Health Sciences Centre - Victoria General Site; (902)473-6428; Fax. (902)473-4126.

CLARK, Alison R; Lions Gate Hosp, 302-231 15th St E, North Vancouver BC V7L 2L7; UBC'79; BSc; MSc; CCFP; Ac Staff Maternity Clinic, Lions Gate Hospital; Clin Instructor, University of British Columbia; (604)985-6408; Fax. (604)985-6108.

CLARK, Andrew E; Professional Arts Bldg, 407-100 Arden St, Moncton NB E1C 4B7; Dal'84; FRCSC; OrthSurg (Arthroplasty). (506)858-9908; Fax. (506)858-0074.

CLARK, Andrew G; Saint John Reg Hosp, PO Box 2100 Stn Main 400 University Ave, Saint John NB E2L 4L2; Leeds (England)'79; FRCPC; Anes. Staff, Saint John Regional Hospital; (506)648-6861; Fax. (506)648-6860.

CLARK, Andrew T; Scarborough Prof Centre, 406-1371 Neilson Rd, Scarborough ON M1B 4Z8; Tor'71; CCFP; FCFP; (416)281-9319; Fax. (416)283-5705.

CLARK, Barry L; Veterans Affairs Canada, PO Box 7700 Stn Central, Charlottetown PE C1A 8M9; Wes'73; BSc; Staff, Veterans Affairs Canada; (902)566-8888

CLARK, Benjamin B; UL-2250 Fairview St, Burlington ON L7R 4C7; Ott'97; BSc; FRCPC; PhysMed&Rehab (Neuro Rehabilitation). Staff, Halton Healthcare Services Corporation - Oakville Site; Clin Dir Rehab & Assoc Memb, Joseph Brant Memorial Hospital; Evaluator, Worker's Safety & Insurance Board; (905)333-5100; Fax. (905)333-5107.

CLARK, Brenda G; Glenrose Rehab Hosp, 10230 111 Ave NW, Edmonton AB T5G 0B7; Mem'82; FRCPC; Peds. Staff, Glenrose Rehabilitation Hospital; Langs: English; French; (780)735-7921; Fax. (780)735-7907.

CLARK, C Eric; Victoria Square Med Clinic, PO Box 5700 Stn Main 216-2345 10th Ave W, Prince Albert SK S6V 7V6; Athens (Greece)'82; FRCSC; ObstGyn. (306)763-8081; Fax. (306)763-1307.

CLARK, Carl I; 200-128 Penetang St, Barrie ON L4M 1V6; Qns'84; CCFP; FCFP; Staff, Royal Victoria Regional Health Centre; (705)726-5676; Fax. (705)726-0905.

CLARK, Carolyn M; The Ottawa Hosp-Gen Campus, 501 Smyth Rd, Ottawa ON K1H 8L6; Qns'95; CCFP; Staff, The Ottawa Hospital - General Campus; (613)737-8650

CLARK, Cynthia L; 306-125 13th St E, North Vancouver BC V7L 2L3; Cal'85; BSc(Hons); CCFP; FCFP; (604)985-2712

CLARK, David A; McMaster University-HSC, 3H1E-1280 Main St W, Hamilton ON L8S 4K1; Wes'67; ABIM; PhD(Med Sci); FRCP; FRCPC; IntMed (Medical Oncology). Staff Honorary, Hamilton Health Sciences Centre - Juravinski Cancer Centre; Staff Honorary, Hamilton Health Sciences Centre - McMaster Children's Hospital; Emeritus Prof Med, McMaster University; Prof Dept of Immunology & Inst Med Sciences, University of Toronto; (905)521-2100 x64604; Fax. (905)571-4970.

CLARK, Deborah J; Rockyview Gen Hosp, 7007 14 St SW, Calgary AB T2V 1P9; Edinburgh (Scotland)'85; MRC(UK); Peds (Neonatal & Perinatal Medicine). Staff, Rockyview General Hospital; Dir Neonatology-Perinatology Fellowship Prog/Clinical Asst Prof, University of Calgary; (403)943-3563 x1615

CLARK, Donald L; Sherwood Family Med Centre, 15 Brackley Point Rd, Charlottetown PE C1A 6Y1; Dal'75; FRCPC; IntMed; Gastroent. (902)628-1801; Fax. (902)628-2021; don.clark@pei.sympatico.ca.

CLARK, Donna L; St Boniface Gen Hosp, 409 Tache Ave, Winnipeg MB R2H 2A6; Man'01; Staff, St Boniface General Hospital; (204)233-8563

CLARK, Edward G; The Ottawa Hosp-Riverside, 1967 Riverside Dr, Ottawa ON K1H 7W9; Qns'03; FRCPC; IntMed; Critical Care Medicine; Nephrol. Staff, The Ottawa Hospital - Riverside Campus; (613)738-8400; Fax. (613)738-8337.

CLARK, Eleanor J; Peace Arch Hosp, 15521 Russell Ave, White Rock BC V4B 2R4; Man'86; FRCPC; DiagRad (Mammograph). Staff, Peace Arch Hospital; (604)531-5512

CLARK, Eric A; The Ottawa Hosp-Civic Campus, 1053 Carling Ave, Ottawa ON K1Y 4E9; Qns'95; FRCPC; EmergMed; PedEmergMed. Staff, The Ottawa Hospital - Civic Campus; (613)761-4000

CLARK, Frank D; Valley Prof Centre, 140-70 Exhibition St, Kentville NS B4N 4K9; Man'86; FRCSC; GenSurg. (902)679-0488; Fax. (902)365-3585.

CLARK, Fred J S; Peace Arch Hosp, 15521 Russell Ave, White Rock BC V4B 2R4; Man'83; FRCPC; Anes. Staff, Peace Arch Hospital; (604)531-5512

CLARK, Gregory; MUHC-Royal Victoria Hosp, 687 av des Pins O, Montreal QC H3A 1A1; Ott'98; CCFP; CCFP(E.M.); Staff, McGill University Health Centre - Royal Victoria Hospital; (514)934-1934; gregclark@hotmail.com.

CLARK, Heather D; Civic Parkdale Clinic, 405-737 Parkdale Ave, Ottawa ON K1Y 1J8; McG'92; FRCPC; IntMed (Obstetric Medicine). Asst Prof, The Ottawa Hospital - Civic Campus; Ottawa Health Research Institute; Assoc Prof Med, University of Ottawa; (613)761-5164; Fax. (613)761-4036; hclark@ottawahospital.on.ca.

CLARK, Heather E; 309-1990 Fort St, Victoria BC V8R 6V4; McG'91; FRCPC; IntMed; Respir. (250)595-0700; Fax. (250)381-7820.

CLARK, Ian H; Health Sciences Centre, CE216-820 Sherbrook St, Winnipeg MB R3A 1R9; Cambridge (England)'95; FRCPC; Ophth. Staff, Health Sciences Centre; (204)774-8511

CLARK, James M; Trafalgar Pain & Headache Ctre, B9-1235 Trafalgar Rd, Oakville ON L6H 3P1; Guy's Hosp. (England)'55; FRCP(Eng); MB; BS; FRCPC; Anes (Pain Management). (905)842-7051; Fax. (905)842-8216; trafalgia@yahoo.co.uk.

CLARK, Jamieson C; Cariboo Mem Hosp, 517 Sixth Ave N, Williams Lake BC V2G 2G8; UBC'01; Gen Practice, Cariboo Memorial Hospital and Health Centre; Langs: Bilingual(English/French); (250)302-3202; jamieson_clark@telus.net.

CLARK, Jessica M; 101-115 Bell Farm Rd, Barrie ON L4M 5G1; Wes'03; FRCPC; Peds; ClinImmunol&Allergy. (705)737-3945; Fax. (705)503-1180.

CLARK, Jodie A; Crowfoot West Business Centre, 210-600 Crowfoot Cres NW, Calgary AB T3G 0B4; UBC'08; (403)239-9733

CLARK, John A; Rouge Valley-Centenary HC, 2867 Ellesmere Rd, Scarborough ON M1E 4B9; McG'88; FRCPC; DiagRad. Staff, Rouge Valley Health System - Centenary Health Centre Site; (416)281-7021; Fax. (416)281-7493.

CLARK, K Christopher; Timmins Family Health Team, 250-123 Third Ave, Timmins ON P4N 1C6; McM'99; CCFP; (705)264-1313; Fax. (705)268-7444.

CLARK, Keith M; Saskatoon East Fam Physicians, 21-2105 8th St E, Saskatoon SK S7H 0T8; Sask'88; CCFP; (306)373-5500; Fax. (306)374-9414.

CLARK, Kerr W; Hanover Care Centre, 700 19th Ave, Hanover ON N4N 3S6; Glasgow (Scotland)'65; MB ChB; Chief GenPract, Hanover & District Hospital; (519)367-3700

CLARK, Kevin; Kelowna Gen Hosp, 2268 Pandosy St, Kelowna BC V1Y 1T2; Qns'00; FRCPC; EmergMed. Staff, Kelowna General Hospital; Staff, Vancouver General Hospital - Centennial Pavillion; (250)980-1760

CLARK, Laura B; Spadina Health Centre, 404-720 Spadina Ave, Toronto ON M5S 2T9; Tor'02; CCFP; (416)928-0920; Fax. (416)928-7426.

CLARK, Linden A; Lakeland Med Clinic, 1715 Ellis St, Kelowna BC V1Y 8M9; Cal'98; MCFP; CCFP; (778)478-0277; Fax. (778)478-0279.

CLARK, Malin K; Royal University Hosp, EH 2/F-103 Hospital Dr, Saskatoon SK S7N 0W8; Sask'93; FRCP; FRCPC; Psy (Child Adolescent & Young AdultPsychiatry). Staff Child & Youth Psy, Royal University Hospital; Asst Prof Psy, University of Saskatchewan; Langs: Swedish; (306)966-7531; Fax. (306)966-8250; malin.clark@saskatoonhealthregion.ca.

CLARK, Marc; Garrison Med Clinic, PO Box 10500 Stn Forces 1 Field Ambulance, Edmonton AB T5J 4J5; (Netherlands Antilles)'06; CCFP; Staff, Edmonton Garrison Health Services Centre; (780)973-4011; marc.clark@forces.gc.ca.

CLARK, Marcia L; South Health Campus, 4448 Front St SE, Calgary AB T3M 1M4; Cal'99; MSc; FRCSC; OrthSurg (Hips Surgery). Staff, Royal Alexandra Hospital; Asst Prof, University of Alberta; (403)956-3768

CLARK, Margaret A; 1113 103 Ave, Dawson Creek BC V1G 2G8; McM'89; (250)782-2827; Fax. (250)782-2867.

CLARK, Mark A; Dauphin Med Clinic, 622 3rd St SW, Dauphin MB R7N 1R5; Man'91; CCFP; FCFP; Ac Staff, Dauphin Regional Health Centre; University of Manitoba; (204)638-6445; Fax. (204)638-5670; mark_clark25@hotmail.com.

CLARK, Mark L; 101-3040 Tutt St, Kelowna BC V1Y 2H5; Dal'78; Staff Family Med, Kelowna General Hospital; (250)868-2622; Fax. (250)868-4802.

CLARK, Peter A; Office of the Reg Coroner, 270 George St N Box D, Peterborough ON K9J 3H1; Wes'69; Staff, Office of the Regional Coroner; (705)755-5265; Fax. (705)755-5266; peter.clark@ontario.ca.

CLARK, Peter D; Royal Oak Clinic, 103-1638 Broadway E, Vancouver BC V5N 1W1; Cal'73; Physician Addiction, Evergreen Community Health Centre; (604)438-6184

CLARK, Philip A H; 369 Hilchey Rd, Campbell River BC V9W 1P8; Sask'96; CCFP; (250)923-7588

CLARK, Robert N; King Street Med Arts Centre, 202-71 King St W, Mississauga ON L5B 4A2; Tor'81; FRCPC; IntMed; Gastroent. Staff, Trillium Health Centre - Mississauga; (905)897-0305; Fax. (905)897-0306.

CLARK, Ronald R; Sparling East Med Centre, PO Box 820 1991 Brickers Rd, Fernie BC V0B 1M0; Sask'76; Staff, Elk Valley Hospital; (250)423-4442; Fax. (250)423-3424; ronald.clark@interiorhealth.ca.

CLARK, Russell P; Sports Med Clinic, 955 Oliver Rd, Thunder Bay ON P7B 5E1; Man'92; FRCSC; OrthSurg. Staff, Thunder Bay Regional Health Sciences Centre; (807)343-8936; Fax. (807)766-7226.

CLARK, Sandra G; Dauphin Med Clinic, 622 3rd St SW, Dauphin MB R7N 1R5; Man'95; BSc; CCFP; FCFP; (204)638-6445; Fax. (204)638-5670.

CLARK, Sarah A R; Lakehead University Hlth Serv, 955 Oliver Rd, Thunder Bay ON P7B 5E1; Ott'07; CCFP; Physician University Health Services, Lakehead University / Library; (807)343-8361; Fax. (807)346-7740.

CLARK, Steven M; Foothills Med Centre, C231-1403 29 St NW, Calgary AB T2N 2T9; UBC'99; BSc; CCFP; CCFP(E.M.); Staff, Foothills Medical Centre; (403)944-1596; Fax. (403)944-2419.

CLARK, Susan M; St James Street Med Clinic, 1600 Portage Ave, Winnipeg MB R3J 0C6; Qns'73; CCFP; (204)774-1868

CLARK, Tod A; Pan Am Clinic, 75 Poseidon Bay, Winnipeg MB R3M 3E4; Man'04; FRCSC; OrthSurg.

CLARK, Virginia J; Golden Med Clinic, PO Box 1170, Golden BC V0A 1H0; Cal'98; BSc; CCFP; FCFP; (250)344-2211; drvirginiaclark@shaw.ca.

CLARK, William F; London HSC-Victoria Hosp, PO Box 5010 Stn B A2 343-800 Commissioners Rd E, London ON N6A 5W9; Wes'70; FACP; FRCPC; IntMed (Nephrology). Dir Plasmapheresis Unit/Consultant, London Health Sciences Centre - Victoria Campus; Prof Med, University of Western Ontario; (519)685-8361; Fax. (519)685-8047; william.clark@lhsc.on.ca.

CLARKE, Adam C; Valley Reg Hosp, 150 Exhibition St, Kentville NS B4N 5E3; Dal'98; FRCPC; IntMed; Cardiol. Staff, Valley Regional Hospital; (902)678-1411; Fax. (902)679-1250.

CLARKE, Alison M; Valley Med Clinic, PO Bag 2931 Stn Main 231 2nd Ave, Strathmore AB T1P 1L5; Sask'90; CCFP; FCFP; (403)934-4444; Fax. (403)934-5218.

CLARKE, Allison J; Renfrew Med Group, 510 Raglan St N, Renfrew ON K7V 1P5; Dal'04; CCFP; Staff, Renfrew Victoria Hospital; (613)433-9152; Fax. (613)433-9154.

CLARKE, Andrew L; 980-1125 Howe St, Vancouver BC V6Z 2K8; UBC'86; DOHS; (604)742-0747

CLARKE, Ann E; MUHC-Montreal Gen Hosp, A6163-1650 av Cedar, Montreal QC H3G 1A4; Mem'84; FRCPC; IntMed; ClinImmunol&Allergy. Staff, McGill University Health Centre - Montreal General Campus; (514)934-8037

CLARKE, Anne I; Surrey Mem Hosp, 13750 96 Ave, Surrey BC V3V 1Z2; Tor'85; FRCPC; EmergMed. Staff, Peace Arch Hospital; Med Dir Fraser Health Emergency Program, Surrey Memorial Hospital; (604)587-3710

CLARKE, B Jean; Burrard Health Bldg, 307-1160 Burrard St, Vancouver BC V6Z 2E8; UBC'80; (604)687-7033; Fax. (604)602-0923.

CLARKE, Barry A; St Clare's Mercy Hosp, 154 Lemarchant Rd, St. John's NL A1C 5B8; Mem'88; BSc; BMedSci; FRCPC; Anes. Staff, St Clare's Mercy Hospital; Memorial University Of Newfoundland; (709)777-5520; Fax. (709)777-5210.

CLARKE, Barry S; Continuing Care Capital Health, 2056-6960 Mumford Rd, Halifax NS B3L 4P1; Dal'87; CCFP; Dir Long Term Care/Assoc Chief, Queen Elizabeth II Health Sciences Centre - Victoria General Site; Lecturer, Dalhousie University; (902)487-0814; Fax. (902)454-2684; barry.clarke@dal.ca.

CLARKE, Blaise A; Univ Hlth Network-Toronto Gen, 11EW-200 Elizabeth St, Toronto ON M5G 2C4; Witwatersrand (South Africa)'97; FRCPC; AnatPath. Staff, Toronto General Hospital - UHN; (416)340-3396

CLARKE, Brian A; Queen Elizabeth II HSC-Halifax, 2293-1796 Summer St, Halifax NS B3H 3A7; Dal'04; FRCPC; IntMed; Cardiol. Staff, Queen Elizabeth II Health Sciences Centre - Halifax Infirmary Site; (902)473-6557; Fax. (902)473-7277.

CLARKE, Collin F M; London HSC-Univesity Campus, PO Box 5339 Stn B C3 172-339 Windermere Rd, London ON N6A 5A5; Tor'05; FRCPC; Anes. Staff, London Health Sciences Centre - University Hospital; (519)685-8300

CLARKE, David B; Queen Elizabeth II HSC-Halifax, 3807-1796 Summer St, Halifax NS B3H 3A7; McG'89; BSc; PhD; DABNS; FACS; FRCSC; Neursurg. Staff, Queen Elizabeth II Health Sciences Centre - Victoria General Site; Staff, Queen Elizabeth II Health Sciences Centre - Halifax Infirmary Site; Prof Medical Neurosciences, Dalhousie University; (902)473-7214; Fax. (902)473-8917.

CLARKE, David N; Parry Sound Family Health Team, 15 James St, Parry Sound ON P2A 1T4; Wes'82; CCFP; FCFP; (705)746-9382; Fax. (705)746-7758.

CLARKE, Deirdre M; Liberton Med Centre, 205-31 Liberton Dr, St. Albert AB T8N 3X6; Galway (Ireland)'79; MB BCh; CCFP; (780)458-5505; Fax. (780)460-1479.

CLARKE, Donald H; Bayview Mall Medical Office, 50-470 Dundas St E, Belleville ON K8N 1G1; Qns'74; FAB; FRCSC; ObstGyn. (613)966-4045

CLARKE, Ellen D R; Stonechurch Family Med Ctre, 1475 Upper Ottawa St, Hamilton ON L8W 3J6; Newcastle upon Tyne (England)'01; CCFP; (905)575-1300

CLARKE, Gillian I; Summerville Condominiums, 120-7 Paton St, St. John's NL A1B 4S8; Mem'94; FRCPC; IntMed; Derm. (709)753-9800

CLARKE, Gillian L; Saint John Reg Hosp, PO Box 2100 Stn Main 400 University Ave, Saint John NB E2L 4L2; Mem'99; BCS; ABR; FRCPC; DiagRad. Staff, Saint John Regional Hospital; (506)648-6000

CLARKE, Gregory V; Valley Prof Centre, 125-70 Exhibition St, Kentville NS B4N 4K9; Dal'79; FRCSC; OrthSurg (Adult Reconstructive Surgery). Consultant, Yarmouth Regional Hospital; Consultant, Valley Regional Hospital; (902)678-7707; Fax. (902)678-1177.

CLARKE, Gwendolyn M; Royal Alexandra Hosp, 5002 3DTC-10240 Kingsway NW, Edmonton AB T5H 3V9; Alb'90; FRC; FRCPC; HemPath (Transfusion Medicine). Staff Lab Med, Royal Alexandra Hospital; Prog Dir Hematological Path Residency Training Faculty of Med, University of Alberta; (780)735-4384; Fax. (780)735-4715; gwen.clarke@albertahealthservices.ca.

CLARKE, Hance A; Univ Hlth Network-Toronto Gen, 3EB 317-200 Elizabeth St, Toronto ON M5G 2C4; Tor'03; FRCPC; Anes. Staff, Toronto General Hospital - UHN; (416)340-4800

CLARKE, Heather E; Reddendale Family Health Ctre, 125 Lakeview Ave, Kingston ON K7M 3T6; Dal'89; (613)384-4664; Fax. (613)384-4182.

CLARKE, Henry C N; 1027 Ottawa St, Windsor ON N8X 2E3; Howard(DC) (USA)'52; (519)252-1202; Fax. (519)252-1523; hclarke@netrover.com.

CLARKE, Howard; The Hosp for Sick Children, 5423-555 University Ave, Toronto ON M5G 1X8; Tor'77; PhD; FRCSC; PlasSurg. Ac Staff Surg, The Hospital For Sick Children; Assoc Staff, Toronto General Hospital - UHN; Prof Surg, University of Toronto; (416)813-6444; Fax. (416)813-6147; howard.clarke@utoronto.ca.

CLARKE, Ian M C; Bow River Prof Centre, 226-4411 16 Ave NW, Calgary AB T3B 0M3; Leeds (England)'68; MB ChB; FRCA; LMCC; Med Staff, Foothills Medical Centre; (403)270-2276

CLARKE, Ian S; Health Sciences Centre, CE216-820 Sherbrook St, Winnipeg MB R3A 1R9; Aberdeen (Scotland)'85; MB ChB; MRCPsy(UK); Staff, Health Sciences Centre; (204)774-6511

CLARKE, James R; PO Box 9000 Rpo Csc, Halifax NS B3K 6A3; Dal'01; FRCPC; DiagRad; NuclearMed. (902)473-7770; Fax. (902)473-2018.

CLARKE, Janet H; 27 Third St, Collingwood ON L9Y 1K4; McM'92; CCFP; Teach Staff, McMaster University; (705)445-4111; Fax. (705)445-8250.

CLARKE, Jo-Anne M; NE Specialized Geriatric Servi, 960D Notre Dame Ave, Sudbury ON P3A 2T4; McM'03; FRCPC; IntMed; GeriatricMed. (705)688-3970; Fax. (705)688-7720.

CLARKE, John A; Algoma District Med Group, 240 McNabb St, Sault Ste. Marie ON P6B 1Y5; London (England)'72; MB BS; DRCOG; (705)759-1234; Fax. (705)759-5683.

CLARKE, John C; Queensway-Carleton Hosp, 3045 Baseline Rd, Nepean ON K2H 8P4; Qns'98; FRCPC; DiagRad. Staff/A-Chief DiagRad, Queensway Carleton Hospital; (613)721-2000

CLARKE, John E; Liberton Med Centre, 205-31 Liberton Dr, St. Albert AB T8N 3X6; Galway (Ireland)'79; CCFP; FCFP; Fam Med, Fairview Health Complex; (780)458-5505; Fax. (780)460-1479.

CLARKE, Joseph; Family Medicine Centre, 502-168 Charlotte St, Ottawa ON K1N 8K6; West Indies (Jamaica)'79; (613)563-0320; Fax. (613)563-2211.

CLARKE, Joseph T R; The Hosp for Sick Children, 555 University Ave, Toronto ON M5G 1X8; Alb'65; FCCMG; PhD; FRCPC; Peds (Metabolic Genetics). Ac Staff, The Hospital For Sick Children; Prof Peds, University of Toronto; (416)813-5345

CLARKE, Julie L; Springbank Med Centre, 202-460 Springbank Dr, London ON N6J 0A8; Tor'86; CCFP; FCFP; CCFP(E.M.); (519)672-0060; Fax. (519)661-0597.

CLARKE, June M; Medical Clinic Bldg, 229-89 Humber College Blvd, Etobicoke ON M9V 4B8; Tor'61; FRCPC; Psy (Emergency Psychiatry). Assoc Staff, William Osler Health System - Etobicoke General Hospital; (416)746-0689; Fax. (416)746-8682.

CLARKE, Kevin D; 401-1990 Fort St, Victoria BC V8R 6V4; Dal'85; Otol (Laser Surgery). (250)595-7564; Fax. (250)595-2319.

CLARKE, Leigh L; Veteran's Affairs Canada, 1100 Pembroke St E, Pembroke ON K8A 6Y7; Tor'68; Sr Medical Officer, Veteran's Affairs Canada; Langs: English; French; (705)567-1414

CLARKE, Lloyd T; PO Box 550, Cardston AB T0K 0K0; (New Zealand)'94; MB ChB; CCFP; Chief Staff, Cardston Hospital; Physician, Kainai Continuing Care Centre; (403)653-3331; Fax. (403)653-1098.

CLARKE, Lorne A; BC Women's Hosp & Health Ctre, C234-4500 Oak St, Vancouver BC V6H 3N1; McG'84; FRCPC; Peds. Staff, BC Women's Hospital & Health Centre; (604)875-2157

CLARKE, Margaret E; Child Development Centre, 3F-3820 24 Ave NW, Calgary AB T2B 2X9; McM'84; FRCPC; Peds (Developmental Pediatrics). Staff, Alberta Children's Hospital; Prof, University of Calgary; (403)210-5000; Fax. (403)284-9298; margaret.clarke@albertahealthservices.ca.

CLARKE, Margo S; 103-20644 Eastleigh Cres, Langley BC V3A 4C4; Dal'74; DABOph; FRCSC; Ophth. Consultant, Langley Memorial Hospital; Clin Asst Prof, University of British Columbia; (604)530-3618; Fax. (604)530-1915.

CLARKE, Maxine C W; Kingston Gen Hosp, Watkins 3-76 Stuart St, Kingston ON K7L 2V7; West Indies (Jamaica)'75; MB BS; DCH; FRCPC; Peds (Neonatal Intensive Care). Staff Neonatol, Kingston General Hospital; Asst Prof, Queen's University; (613)548-7766; Fax. (613)548-1369; clarkem@kgh.kari.net.

CLARKE, Michelle B; Medical Clinic Bldg, 229-89 Humber College Blvd, Etobicoke ON M9V 4B8; Tor'90; FRCPC; Psy. (416)746-0689; Fax. (416)746-8682.

CLARKE, Michelle S; Children's & Women's HC of BC, B321-4480 Oak St, Vancouver BC V6H 3V4; Dal'99; FRCPC; Peds; PedEmergMed. Staff, BC Children's Hospital; Clin Instructor, University of British Columbia; (604)875-2045

CLARKE, Natasha C T; Finchlea Med Centre, 204-490 Bramalea Rd, Brampton ON L6T 0G1; Ott'98; BScH(Biol.); CCFP; (905)792-6500; Fax. (905)792-6853.

CLARKE, Peter V; PO Box 4, Ayton ON N0G 1C0; Tor'67; FACP; FRCPC; IntMed (Endocrinology). Ac Staff/Asst Chief IntMed, The Credit Valley Hospital; Staff Diabetes Prog, Headwaters Health Care Centre - Orangeville Site; Assoc Prof Med, University of Toronto; (519)665-2285; pclarke@cvh.on.ca.

CLARKE, Richard K; Cambridge Mem Hosp, 700 Coronation Blvd, Cambridge ON N1R 3G2; Wes'03; CCFP; CCFP(E.M.); Staff, Cambridge Memorial Hospital; (519)621-2330

CLARKE, Robert J; Delta Med Clinic, 140-4977 Trenant St, Delta BC V4K 2K5; UBC'76; Ac Staff, Delta Hospital; (604)946-7662; Fax. (604)940-1743.

CLARKE, Sharon E; Queen Elizabeth II HSC-Halifax, 3900-1796 Summer St, Halifax NS B3H 3A7; Wes'05; FRCPC; DiagRad. Staff, Queen Elizabeth II Health Sciences Centre - Halifax Infirmary Site; (902)473-1875; Fax. (902)473-1851.

CLARKE, Sophie; BC Women's Hosp & Health Ctre, 4500 Oak St, Vancouver BC V6H 3N1; Queensland (Australia)'98; Staff, BC Women's Hospital & Health Centre; (604)875-2000

CLARKE, Stephen C; Homewood Health Centre, 150 Delhi St, Guelph ON N1E 6K9; Qns'88; CCFP; Staff, Homewood Health Centre; (519)824-1010 x263; Fax. (519)767-3536.

CLARKE, Stephen D; Business Bldg, 202-1200 Burrard St, Vancouver BC V6Z 2C7; UBC'77; FRCPC; Neur. Ac Staff Neurol, Providence Health Care - St Paul's Hospital; (604)669-3586; Fax. (604)669-7387.

CLARKE, Teresa Anne; Inspire Health, 200-1330 8th Ave W, Vancouver BC V6H 4A6; UBC'81; BSc; CAFCI; Dir Outreach Services, Inspire Health; Clin Instructor Med, University of British Columbia; (604)734-7125 x224; Fax. (604)734-7105; tclarke@inspirehealth.ca.

CLARKE, Terrence; Clinique Med du Plateau, 300-195 rue de l'Atmosphere, Gatineau QC J9A 0A3; Ott'87; assoc Prof, McGill University; Langs: English; French; (819)776-0001; Fax. (819)776-2171.

CLARKE, Theresa-Ann; 241 Brant Ave, Brantford ON N3T 3J4; West Indies (Jamaica)'83; MB BS(Hons); FRCPC; Psy. Asst Prof Clinical Family Med, McMaster University; (519)753-3310; Fax. (519)753-7618.

CLARKE, W Wayne; Radiology Associates Of Regina, 6-2727 Parliament Ave, Regina SK S4S 6X5; Sask'72; FRCPC; DiagRad (Mammography). Staff, Pasqua Hospital; Staff, Regina General Hospital; Staff, Radiology Associates of Regina; Clinical Asst Prof, University of Saskatchewan; (306)352-7653; Fax. (306)522-4311.

CLARKE, William E J; Southgate Med Clinic, 1-45905 Yale Rd, Chilliwack BC V2P 2M6; Man'90; Assoc Staff, Chilliwack General Hospital; (604)795-7228

CLARKSON, Blaise D; Family Health Centre, 105-840 Coxwell Ave, East York ON M4C 5T2; Tor'03; BA; MA; BSc; CCFP; (416)469-6464; Fax. (416)469-6164.

CLARKSON, Colin A; Central Nfld Reg Hlth Centre, 50 Union St, Grnd-Falls-Windsor NL A2A 2E1; Cal'07; GenSurg. Staff, Central Newfoundland Regional Health Centre; (709)292-2500

CLARKSON, David G; Credit Valley Family Hlth Team, 105-2300 Eglinton Ave W, Mississauga ON L5M 2V8; Tor'70; MHSc; CCFP; Staff, The Credit Valley Hospital; (905)813-3850; Fax. (905)813-3851.

CLARKSON, Paul W; BC Cancer Agency-Vancouver CC, 600 10th Ave W, Vancouver BC V5Z 4E6; Otago (New Zealand)'93; MB ChB; FRCSC; OrthSurg. Staff, BC Cancer Agency Vancouver Centre; (604)877-6000 x2396

CLARREN, Sterling Keith; Children's & Women's HC of BC, F508-4480 Oak St, Vancouver BC V6H 3V4; Minnesota(MN) (USA)'73; Staff, BC Children's Hospital; (604)875-2996

CLARSON, Cheril L; Children's Hosp, 800 Commissioners Rd E, London ON N6A 5W9; Nottingham (England)'75; MB BCh; BSc; MRCP; FRCPC; Peds (Pediatric Endocrinology). Assoc Prof, London Health Sciences Centre - Victoria Campus; Staff Ped Endocrin, Children's Hospital of Western Ontario; Assoc Prof Peds, University of Western Ontario; (519)685-8138; Fax. (519)685-8105.

CLAS, David; Hop Charles Lemoyne, 3120 boul Taschereau, Greenfield Park QC J4V 2H1; McG'85; FRCSC; GenSurg. Staff, Hopital Charles LeMoyne; (450)466-5440

CLASE, Catherine M; St Joseph's Healthcare, MW 3F-50 Charlton Ave E, Hamilton ON L8N 4A6; Cambridge (England)'89; MB ChB; MSc(HRM); FRCPC; IntMed; Nephrol. Staff, St Joseph's Healthcare - Charlton Campus; Court Staff Nephrol, The Brant Community Healthcare System - Brantford General Hospital Site; Assoc Prof, McMaster University; (905)521-6094; Fax. (905)521-6153; clase@mcmaster.ca.

CLASKY, Howard J; Scarborough Hosp-General Div, 3050 Lawrence Ave E, Scarborough ON M1P 2V5; Tor'91; FRCPC; IntMed (Critical Care Medicine); EmergMed. Staff, The Scarborough Hospital - General Campus; University of Toronto; (416)438-2911 x6507; Fax. (416)787-8275.

CLASS, Sabrina F M; Mount Seymour Clinic, 2F-333 Seymour Blvd, North Vancouver BC V7J 2J4; UBC'92; BSc; (604)904-7712; Fax. (604)904-7714.

CLASSEN, Dale A; Comox Valley Surgical Centre, 2696 Windermere Ave, Cumberland BC V0R 1S0; Sask'87; FRCSC; PlasSurg (Micro Surgery). (250)336-2087

CLASSEN, Shawn C; Lakeside Med Clinic, 3919 8th St E, Saskatoon SK S7H 5M7; Sask'96; CCFP; FCFP; (306)374-6884; Fax. (306)374-2552; sclassen@hotmail.com.

CLAUDE, Sophie; CHSLD-St Augustin, 2135 Terrasse Cadieux, Quebec QC G1C 1Z2; (France)'90; Staff, Centre d'hebergement Saint-Augustin; Staff, Centre Hospitalier Chauveau; (418)667-3910 x5721; Fax. (418)667-0658.

CLAUDE-DESROCHES, Mederic; Hôpital Laval, 2725 ch Sainte-Foy, Quebec QC G1V 4G5; Laval'04; FRCPC; DiagRad. Staff, Hôpital Laval; (418)656-8711

CLAVEAU, Bernard; CSSS de Chicoutimi, 305 rue Saint-Vallier, Chicoutimi QC G7H 5H6; Laval'72; CSPQ; FRCPC; Anes. Staff, Complexe hospitalier de la Sagamie; (418)541-1234 x2217

CLAVEAU, David; CSSS de Trois-Rivieres, 1991 boul du Carmel, Trois-Rivieres QC G8Z 3R9; Laval'06; Staff, CSSS de Trois-Rivières; (819)697-3333

CLAVEAU, Denis; St Mary's Hospital Centre, 3308-3830 av Lacombe, Montreal QC H3T 1M5; Laval'73; FRCPC; Psy. Staff, St Mary's Hospital Centre; adj Prof, McGill University; Langs: Bilingual(French/English); (514)345-3511 x3998; Fax. (514)734-2609.

CLAVEAU, J Andre; Hop Santa Cabrini Ospedale, 5655 rue Saint-Zotique E, Montreal QC H1T 1P7; McG'74; Staff, Hôpital Santa Cabrini Ospedale; (514)252-6444

CLAVEAU, Jacques; 201-369 boul Fiset, Sorel-Tracy QC J3P 3R3; Laval'74; FABOG; ObstGyn (P.Q.). Langs: English; (450)742-0607

CLAVEAU, Joel; Clin Dermatology Joel Claveau, 192-2600 boul Laurier, Quebec QC G1V 4T3; Laval'88; FRCPC; Derm (Skin Cancer). Staff, Centre Hospitalier Universitaire de Québec (CHUQ) - Siege Social; Langs: Bilingual(French/English); (418)650-1222; Fax. (418)650-1224; jcl2007@videotron.ca.

CLAVEAU, Laval; Clin Med Riviere du Moulin, 1388 boul Du Saguenay E, Chicoutimi QC G7H 1G8; Laval'73; Staff, Complexe hospitalier de la Sagamie; (418)549-3564; Fax. (418)549-8463.

CLAVEAU, Michael E; Clinique Med de Roberval, 714 boul Marcotte, Roberval QC G8H 1Z6; McG'80; Staff, Hotel-Dieu de Roberval; (418)275-3833; Fax. (418)275-6747.

CLAVEAU, Richard L; NORD-ASKI Family Health Team, PO Box 1570 1403 Edward St, Hearst ON P0L 1N0; Ott'98; CCFP; Langs: English; French; (705)362-6613; Fax. (705)372-2923.

CLAVEAU, Rosaire; CSSS de Chicoutimi, CP 5006 305 rue Saint-Vallier, Chicoutimi QC G7H 5H6; Mon'89; NuclearMed (P.Q.). Staff, Complexe hospitalier de la Sagamie; (418)696-9951

CLAVEAU, Suzanne; Regie l'Assurance Maladie QC, 1125 Grande Allee O, Quebec QC G1S 1E7; Laval'75; FRCPC; IntMed; MedMicrobiol. Staff, Centre Hospitalier Universitaire de Québec (CHUQ) - Siege Social; (418)646-4636

CLAVEL, Christian; 1652 rue Royale, Trois-Rivieres QC G9A 4K3; Mon'81; (819)376-1661; Fax. (819)376-9902.

CLAVEL, Mathias; Hotel-Dieu de Sorel, 400 av de l'Hotel-Dieu, Sorel-Tracy QC J3P 1N5; Staff, Hôtel-Dieu de Sorel; (450)746-7623

CLAVEL, Natalie; The Ottawa Hosp-Gen Campus, 1401-501 Smyth Rd, Ottawa ON K1H 8L6; Ott'07; Anes. Staff Anes, The Ottawa Hospital - General Campus; (613)798-5555

CLAVEL, Sebastien; CSSS de Laval, 1755 boul Rene-Laennec, Laval QC H7M 3L9; Laval'06; FRCPC; RadOncol. (450)668-1010

CLAVET, Diane; CLSC La Region-Sherbrookoise, 1200 rue King E, Sherbrooke QC J1G 1E4; Laval'78; CCFP; FCFP; vice Doyen Pedagogue Development, Universite de Sherbrooke; (819)563-2572; Fax. (819)563-9912; diane.clavet@usherbrooke.ca.

CLAVET, Martin; Bureau du Coroner, 390-2875 boul Laurier, Quebec QC G1V 5B1; Laval'97 Laval; DAvMed; LMCC; MCFP; BASc; CCFP; FCFP; Coroner, City of Quebec; Langs: English; (418)266-4670 x5927

CLAVETTE, Carole; Clinique Med St-Jacques, 160 rue Principale, Saint-Jacques NB E7B 1W4; Laval'98; LMCC; Staff Family Med, Hôpital regional d'Edmundston; Langs: Bilingual(French/English); (506)739-7708; Fax. (506)739-5839.

CLAVETTE, Manon; Montfort Hosp, 713 Montreal Rd, Ottawa ON K1K 0T2; Sher'94; CCFP; Staff, Montfort Hospital; Langs: Bilingual(French/English); (613)746-4621

CLAVETTE, Paul F; Clinique De Med Interne, 20 rue Carrier, Edmundston NB E3V 3Y1; Laval'79; IntMed. Staff, Hôpital regional d'Edmundston; Langs: English; (506)739-9511; Fax. (506)735-8118; pclavett@mac.com.

CLAY, Jane E; Omemee Med Centre, PO Box 310 23 Wellington St, Omemee ON K0L 2W0; McM'06; BA; Physician ER, Northumberland Hills Hospital; (705)799-0000 x1; Fax. (705)799-0271.

CLAYBO, Ross A; Markham Stouffville Hosp, PO Box 1800 Stn Main 381 Church St, Markham ON L3P 7P3; Sask'80; FRCPC; EmergMed. Staff, Markham Stouffville Hospital; (905)472-7111

CLAYDEN, Gerald S; Carman Med Group, PO Box 728, Carman MB R0G 0J0; London (England)'73; MB BS; FRCS(Eng); Staff, Carman Memorial Hospital; Staff, Altona Community Memorial Health Centre/Eastview Place; Lecturer Family Med, University of Manitoba; Langs: English; French; (204)745-2024; Fax. (204)745-2151; flyindoc@mts.net.

CLAYDEN, Wesley; Fowler Kennedy Sport Med Clini, 3M-1151 Richmond St, London ON N6A 3K7; UBC'10; CCFP; Staff, Fowler Kennedy Sport Medicine Clinic; (519)661-3011

CLAYTON, Cheryl A; One Kids Place, 400 McKeown Ave, North Bay ON P1B 0B2; McM'04; FRCPC; Peds. Staff, North Bay Regional Health Centre - Regional Mental Health; (705)495-8115

CLAYTON, Dale B; 309-223 Nelson's Cres, New Westminster BC V3L 0E4; Dal'03; FRCPC; IntMed; Endocrin&Metab. Staff, Queen Elizabeth II Health Sciences Centre - Victoria General Site; Langs: Bilingual(English/French); (604)553-1557

CLAYTON, Russell P; Glover Med Clinic, 101-5796 Glover Rd, Langley BC V3A 4H9; Cape Town (South Africa)'89; MB ChB; CCFP; (604)530-3233

CLEARSKY, Lorne; Siksika Health Services, PO Box 1130, Siksika AB T0J 3W0; Man'90; FRCPC; CommunMed. (403)971-6756

CLEARY, Cynthia E; 1031 Russet Rd NE, Calgary AB T2E 5L2; Dal'95; FRCPC; IntMed (Gastroenterology). (403)277-7321; Fax. (403)277-7327.

CLEARY, Eilish; Dept Of Health & Wellness, PO Box 5100 Stn A, Fredericton NB E3B 5G8; Dublin (Ireland)'86; (506)444-2112; Fax. (506)453-8702.

CLEARY, Sean P; Univ Hlth Network-Toronto Gen, 10EN 212-200 Elizabeth St, Toronto ON M5G 2C4; Wes'99; BScChemEng; MSc; FRCSC; GenSurg. Staff, Toronto General Hospital - UHN; (416)340-5331; Fax. (416)340-3808.

CLEATOR, Iain G M; Medical Bldg, 310-943 Broadway W, Vancouver BC V5Z 4E1; Edinburgh (Scotland)'62; MB ChB; FRCS(Ed); FRCS; FACS; FRCSC; GenSurg (Haemorrhoids). Emeritus Prof Surg, University of British Columbia; (604)681-1513; Fax. (604)681-1517; cleatorclinic@shawbiz.ca.

CLEGG, Robin L; Alberta Children's Hosp, 2888 Shaganappi Trail NW, Calgary AB T3B 6A8; Man'00; FRCPC; Peds (Pediatric Cardiology); Cardiol. Staff, Alberta Children's Hospital; (403)955-7858; Fax. (403)955-7621.

CLEGHORN, Graham E; Sunnybrook Hlth Sciences Ctre, 2075 Bayview Ave, Toronto ON M4N 3M5; Cal'01; FRCPC; EmergMed. Staff, Sunnybrook Health Sciences Centre; (416)480-6100

CLEGHORN, Scott A; Oakfield Med Clinic, 104-1021 Court Ave, Winnipeg MB R2P 1V7; Man'79; FRCPC; IntMed. (204)339-1637; Fax. (204)339-0997.

CLEIMAN, Paula F; Univ Hlth Network-Toronto Gen, GS480 RFE-200 Elizabeth St, Toronto ON M5G 2C4; McG'08; CCFP; CCFP(E.M.); Staff, Toronto General Hospital - UHN; (416)340-3856; Fax. (416)340-4300.

CLELAND, David P; MUHC-Montreal Gen Hosp, D7 102-1650 av Cedar, Montreal QC H3G 1A4; McG'75; AB; Gastroent; IntMed. Staff, McGill University Health Centre - Montreal General Campus; McGill University; (514)934-8092; Fax. (514)934-8531.

CLELAND, W John D; 320-301 Victoria St, Kamloops BC V2C 2A3; Sask'82; FRCSC; Otol. (250)372-3661; Fax. (250)372-8488.

CLELLAND, Catherine A; Soc of Gen Practitioners of BC, 115-1665 Broadway W, Vancouver BC V6J 5A4; Alb'84; BMedSci; CCFP; FCFP; Exec Dir, Society of Gen. Practitioners of BC; Assoc. Clin. Instr., University of British Columbia; (604)638-2942; Fax. (604)736-6160; cclelland@bcma.bc.ca.

CLELLAND, M Jane; Port Mcneill Med Clinic, PO Box 14, Port Mcneill BC V0N 2R0; UBC'84; CCFP; (250)956-3377; Fax. (250)956-3299.

CLEMANS-GIBBON, Tracey M; Castlegar Med Associates, 1008 Columbia Ave, Castlegar BC V1N 1H2; London (England)'85; MB BS; Staff, Castlegar & District Communnity Health Centre; (250)365-2161; Fax. (250)365-2171.

CLEMENS, Kristin K; St Joseph's Health Care, PO Box 5777 Stn B 268 Grosvenor St, London ON N6A 4V2; Wes'08; FRCPC; IntMed. Staff, St Joseph's Hospital - St Joseph's Health Care.

CLEMENS, Richard S; Scarborough Hosp-General Div, 3050 Lawrence Ave E, Scarborough ON M1P 2V5; Tor'79; FRCPC; DiagRad (Interventional Radiology). Dir Dept of Diag Imaging, The Scarborough Hospital - General Campus; (416)438-8107

CLEMENT, Annie; Clinique Med Saint-Sulpice, 12-1420 rue Legendre E, Montreal QC H2M 1H5; Mon'00; CCFP; Staff, Centre Hospitalier Fleury; (514)382-0552

CLEMENT, Christine; CSSS des Aurores Boreales, CP 6000 Succ Bureau-Chef 679 2e rue E, La Sarre QC J9Z 2X7; Sher'85; Staff, Centre Hospitalier La Sarre; (819)333-2311; Fax. (819)333-4227.

CLEMENT, J C Luc; Centre Med St-Isidore, 4553 rue Ste Catherine, St Isidore ON K0C 2B0; Ott'83; CCFP; Court Staff, The Ottawa Hospital - General Campus; Ac Staff Sec, Montfort Hospital; (613)524-3225; Fax. (613)524-2513.

CLEMENT, Jacques; Hop Louis-H Lafontaine, 7401 rue Hochelaga, Montreal QC H1N 3M5; Mon'76; Staff, Hopital Louis-H Lafontaine; (514)251-4000 x3060; Fax. (514)251-1604.

CLEMENT, Jason J; St Paul's Hosp, 1081 Burrard St, Vancouver BC V6Z 1Y6; UBC'97; FRCPC; DiagRad. Staff, Providence Health Care - St Paul's Hospital; (604)261-7612

CLEMENT, Jean-Francois; 250-4896 boul Taschereau, Greenfield Park QC J4V 2J2; Mon'95; FRCPC; Neur (Epilepsy). Staff Neurol, Hopital Charles LeMoyne; Neurologue, Centre Hospitalier l'Université de Montréal (CHUM) - Hôpital Notre-Dame; (450)672-1931; Fax. (450)672-3308; jfcnrs@videotron.ca.

CLEMENT, Jean-Rene; Clinique D'Ophtalmologie, 100-2875 boul Laurier, Quebec QC G1V 2M2; Laval'69; FACS; FRCSC; Ophth (Cataract Surgery). Staff, Centre Hospitalier Chauveau; (418)654-1488; Fax. (418)658-8310.

CLEMENT, Jennifer E J; 1-523 The Queensway, Etobicoke ON M8Y 1J7; McM'04; BA; CCFP; Staff, St Joseph's Health Centre; Staff, Regional Municipality of Peel Health Department; Langs: Bilingual(English/French); (416)760-8367; Fax. (416)760-7212; clementj@peelregion.ca.

CLEMENT, John S; St Joseph's HC-Parkwood Hosp, 801 Commissioners Rd E, London ON N6C 5J1; Wes'76; CAFCI; MMedSci; MClSc; BA; MA; Assoc Staff, St Joseph's Hospital - St Joseph's Health Care; GP/Physical Medicine & Rehab, Parkwood Hospital - St Joseph's Health Care; Staff Admitting Privil Family Med, London Health Sciences Centre - University Hospital; Staff Teacher Pt-Time, University of Western Ontario; (519)685-4000; Fax. (519)685-4092; john.clement@sjhc.london.on.ca.

CLEMENT, Julien; Ctr Hosp Affilie-Enfant-Jesus, 1401 18e rue, Quebec QC G1J 1Z4; Sher'02; FRCSC; GenSurg. Staff, Centre Hospitalier Affilié Universitaire de Québec - Hôpital De L'Enfant Jésus; (418)649-0252

CLEMENT, Karine; CSSSG-Hop de Gatineau, CP 2000 succ Bureau-chef 909 boul la Verendrye, Gatineau QC J8P 7H2; Sher'06; Peds. Staff, Hôpital de Gatineau; (819)966-6100

CLEMENT, Louise; MSSS, 840-2021 av Union, Montreal QC H3A 2S9; Mon'85; Staff, Centre Hospitalier l'Université de Montréal (CHUM) - Hôtel-Dieu; (514)243-5012

CLEMENT, Marie-Helene; Clin Med Sainte-Julie, 286 rue de Normandie, Sainte-Julie QC J3E 1A7; Mon'08; CCFP; (450)649-1593

CLEMENT, Martin; Unite Med Familiale Maizerets, 2480 ch de la Canardiere, Quebec QC G1J 2G1; Laval'89; CCFP; FCFP; Staff, Centre Hospitalier Affilié Universitaire de Québec - Hôpital De L'Enfant Jésus; (418)661-1413; Fax. (418)661-7504.

CLEMENT, Maureen A; Haugen Med Group, 23C-3300 Smith Dr, Armstrong BC V0E 1B1; Tor'78; CCFP; Att Staff, Vernon Jubilee Hospital; Counsellor Clinical Scientific Section, Canadian Diabetic Associaton; Clinical Asst Prof, University of British Columbia; (250)546-8115; Fax. (250)546-2553.

CLEMENT, Nathalie; Ctr de Readaptation de l'Estri, 200-300 rue King E, Sherbrooke QC J1G 1B1; Mon'02; Staff, Centre de sante Tulattavik de l'Ungava; (819)346-8411 x43328

CLEMENT, Philip B V; Dept Of Anatomic Path, 910 10th Ave W, Vancouver BC V5Z 1M9; UBC'69; AB; FRCPC; AnatPath (Gynecological Pathology). Consultant Path, Vancouver General Hospital - Centennial Pavillion; Prof, University of British Columbia; (604)875-5555 x69775; Fax. (604)875-5685; phil.clement@vch.ca.

CLEMENT, Pierre; CSSSG-Hop de Gatineau, CP 2000 Succ Bureau-Chef, Gatineau QC J8P 7H2; Sher'84; Gastroent (P.Q.); IntMed (P.Q.). Ac Staff, Hôpital de Gatineau; (819)561-8100

CLEMENT, Pierre; South-East Ottawa Centre, 225 Donald St, Ottawa ON K1K 1N1; Ott'72; MPhil; FRCPC; Psy. Ac Staff, The Ottawa Hospital - General Campus; Asst Prof, University of Ottawa; Langs: English; (613)745-2228 Semi-Retired.

CLEMENT, Serge; CSSS de la Haute-Yamaska, 205 boul Leclerc O, Granby QC J2G 1T7; Sher'74; MedOncol (P.Q.); HemPath; IntMed (P.Q.). Staff, Centre Hospitalier de Granby; (450)375-8000 x2110; Fax. (450)375-8050.

CLEMENT, Siobhan P; Lonsdale Med Dental Bldg, 108-1940 Lonsdale Ave, North Vancouver BC V7M 2K2; UBC'97; CCFP; (604)987-3347

CLEMENT, Sylvie; CSSS Haut-Richelieu-Rouville, 920 boul Du Seminaire N, St-Jean-Sur-Richel QC J3A 1B7; Sher'87; Staff, Hôpital du Haut-Richelieu; (450)359-5000; sclement@videotron.ca.

CLEMENT MAJOR, Sebastien; CSSS de Saint-Jerome, 290 rue de Montigny, Saint-Jerome QC J7Z 5T3; Mon'99; FRCPC; IntMed. Staff, Hôtel-Dieu de Saint-Jérôme; (450)431-8200

CLEMENTS, Donna V M; Burnside Fam Med Clinic, 2-101 Burnside Rd W, Victoria BC V9A 1B7; UBC'78; (250)381-4353

CLEMENTS, Karen H; 107-490 York Rd, Guelph ON N1E 6V1; McM'87; FRCPC; Psy;CCFP; FCFP; Staff, Homewood Health Centre; (519)362-3343

CLEMENTS, L E Gotham; 402-190 Sherway Dr, Etobicoke ON M9C 5N2; Tor'67; FRCPC; IntMed (Cardiology). Ac Staff Cardiol, St Joseph's Health Centre; (416)626-1280; Fax. (416)626-6173.

CLEMENTS, Nigel D; King Street Med Arts Centre, 507-71 King St W, Mississauga ON L5B 4A2; Wes'74; FRCSC; OrthSurg (Spine). Consultant OrthSurg, Trillium Health Centre - Mississauga; (905)276-6648; Fax. (905)276-8960.

CLEMENTS, Shirley-Anne; Campbellton Reg Hosp, PO Box 880 Stn Main 189 Lily Lake Rd, Campbellton NB E3N 3H3; Laval'89; CCFP; FCFP; Staff, Hôpital Régional Campbellton; Langs: Bilingual(French/English); (506)753-2703; Fax. (506)759-7253.

CLEMENTS-BAKER, Marie I; Baywood Med Centre, 401-95 Bayly St, Ajax ON L1S 7K8; McM'06; FRCPC; IntMed; Rheum. (905)427-2678

CLEMETT, Dawn M; Foothills Med Centre, 1403 29 St NW, Calgary AB T2N 2T9; Man'98; BSc; CCFP; Staff, Foothills Medical Centre; (403)944-2800; Fax. (403)283-7365.

CLEMINSON, Douglas; Quinte HC Corp-Belleville Gen, 360-265 Dundas St E, Belleville ON K8N 5A9; Qns'86; FRCSC; GenSurg. Gen Surgeon, QHC Belleville General; Staff GenSurg, QHC Prince Edward County Memorial; (613)969-9556; Fax. (613)969-6548.

CLEMMEY, W Robert L; Somba K'E Clinic, PO Box 2637 Stn Main, Yellowknife NT X1A 2P9; London (England)'67; MB BS; MRCS; DPM; MRCPsy; FRCPC; Psy (Alternative Medicine). Consultant Psy, Stanton Territorial Health Authority; Cons Psy, Yellowknife Correctional Centre & Cons. Forensic Psy., Legal Serv. & Dept. of Justice-Gov. of Nortwest Territories; Langs: French; German; Spanish.

CLEMONS, Mark J; The Ottawa Hosp-Gen Campus, 501 Smyth Rd Box 909, Ottawa ON K1H 8L6; Newcastle (England)'91; FRCPC; MedOncol. Staff, The Ottawa Hospital - General Campus; (613)737-7700

CLENDENNING, Christine R; Northwood Hlth Care Walk-In-Cl, 1280 Lasalle Blvd, Sudbury ON P3A 1Y8; McM'91; (705)560-2227

CLENDENNING, Martha K; 65 Ellen St PO Box 1119, Blenheim ON N0P 1A0; Ott'82; CCFP; FCFP; Ac Staff/Chief FamilyMed, Chatham-Kent Health Alliance; (519)676-5592; Fax. (519)676-2228.

CLENDENNING, Robert D; Med Associates of Port Perry, 462 Paxton St, Port Perry ON L9L 1L9; Qns'88; CCFP; CCFP(E.M.); FCFP; (905)985-2895

CLERC, Doris; Inst U Geriatrie de Montreal, 4565 ch Queen-Mary, Montreal QC H3W 1W5; Sher'84; FRCPC; Psy. Staff, Institut Universitaire de Gériatrie de Montréal; (514)340-2800 x3515

CLERGET, Lionel; CSSS de Port-Cartier, 3 rue de Shelter Bay, Port-Cartier QC G5B 2W9; Staff, CLSC-CSSS de Port-Cartier; (418)766-2572

CLERK, Nilam A; Mackenzie Richmond Hill Hosp, 10 Trench St, Richmond Hill ON L4C 4Z3; Bombay (India)'69; AB; FRCPC; GenPath. Staff, Mackenzie Richmond Hill Hospital; (905)883-2580; Fax. (905)883-2160.

CLERMONT, Dawn C; Active Care Med Group, A-1108 Klondike Rd, Ottawa ON K2K 0G1; McM'92; BSc; (613)254-9777

CLERMONT, Genevieve; CSSS d'Antoine-Labelle-Mt Laur, RR 1 2561 ch de la Lievre S, Mont-Laurier QC J9L 3G3; Sher'91; CSPQ; FRCPC; IntMed. Staff, CSSS d'Antoine-Labelle; (819)623-1234 x4105

CLERMONT, Marie-Eve; IWK Health Centre, PO Box 9700 Rpo CSC 6039-5980 University Ave, Halifax NS B3K 6R8; Mon'07; FRCSC; ObstGyn. Staff, IWK Health Centre; (902)470-6788; Fax. (902)470-8640.

CLERMONT, Marie-Jose; Hôpital Ste-Justine, 3175 ch Cote-Sainte-Catherine, Montreal QC H3T 1C5; Mon'78; FRCPC; Peds (Transplantation); Nephrol (P.Q.). Chef néphrol, Hôpital Ste-Justine; Langs: English; (514)345-4737; Fax. (514)345-4838; mj.clermont@sympatico.ca.

CLERMONT, Michel; Clinique Dr Michel Clermont, 207 rue Turgeon, Sainte-Therese QC J7E 3J4; Mon'73; (450)430-0433

CLERMONT, Pierre-Andre; CSSS du Lac-des-Deux-Montagnes 520 boul Arthur-Sauve, St-Eustache QC J7R 5B1; Mon'96; FRCSC; OrthSurg. Staff, Hôpital de Saint-Eustache; (450)688-5132

CLERMONT, Richard J; CHUM-Hotel-Dieu, 3840 rue Saint-Urbain, Montreal QC H2W 1T8; Mon'61; CSPQ; FRCPC; Gastroent; IntMed. Membre Gastroent, Centre Hospitalier l'Université de Montréal (CHUM) - Hôtel-Dieu; assoc Prof, Universite de Montreal; Langs: Bilingual(French/English); (514)890-8000 x14925; Fax. (514)412-7194; richcler@ca.inter.net.

CLERSAINT, Guyrlaine; The Westend Family Care Clinic, 80 Michael Cowpland Dr, Kanata ON K2M 1P6; Ott'04; CCFP; Staff, Westend Family Care Clinic Family Health Team; (613)599-3321

CLETO, Luis F; Stratford Gen Hosp, 46 General Hospital Dr, Stratford ON N5A 2Y6; McG'85; FRCPC; Psy (General Psychiatry). Staff, Stratford General Hospital - Huron Perth Healthcare Alliance; (519)271-2120; Fax. (519)271-7137.

CLEVE, Paul D; Kelowna Gen Hosp, 2268 Pandosy St, Kelowna BC V1Y 1T2; Qns'02; EmergMed. Staff, Kelowna General Hospital; (250)862-4495

CLEVE, Richard H; Surrey Mem Hosp, 13750 96 Ave, Surrey BC V3V 1Z2; Wes'01; FRCPC; MedBiochem. Staff Lab Med, Surrey Memorial Hospital; (604)585-5666

CLEVELAND, David R; Carmi Clinic, 124-725 Carmi Ave, Penticton BC V2A 3G8; Cal'98; BSc(BioChem); FRCPC; IntMed. Staff, Penticton Regional Hospital; Langs: English; French; (250)276-9417

CLEVETTE, Nancy A; 8-5303 Canotek Rd, Ottawa ON K1J 9M1; Ott'90; BSc; CCFP; FCFP; Asst Prof, University of Ottawa; Langs: English; French; (613)746-6223

CLICHE, Bernard; Clinique Medicale St-Joseph, 841 av Sainte-Therese RR 1, St-Joseph-D-Beauce QC G0S 2V0; Laval'72; (418)397-6891; Fax. (418)397-4170.

CLICHE, Denis; Pavillon Marillac, 1075 18e rue, Saint-Georges QC G5Y 4T8; Laval'72; Psy (P.Q.). (418)228-2068; Fax. (418)227-1081.

CLICHE, Jean; 14 av Maplewood, Outremont QC H2V 2L8; Laval'67; FRCPC; DiagRad. (514)276-5536

CLICHE, Jean-Pierre; KMH Cardiology & Diagnostic Ct, 236 Avenue Rd, Toronto ON M5R 2J4; Laval'97; FRCPC; NuclearMed. Langs: French; (416)968-1278; Fax. (416)968-9709.

CLICHE, Louis; Clinique Med de Famile, 400-1200 rue des Soeurs-du-Bon, Quebec QC G1S 0B1; Laval'77; Staff, Centre Hospitalier Affilié Universitaire de Québec - Hôpital du St-Sacrement; (418)688-1385; Fax. (418)688-3249.

CLICHE, Marcel; CSSS de Manicouagan, 635 boul Jolliet, Baie-Comeau QC G5C 1P1; Laval'72; Staff, Centre Hospitalier Régional Baie-Comeau; (418)589-9631

CLICHE, Nathalie; ASSS de Mtl, 3725 rue Saint-Denis, Montreal QC H2X 3L9; Mon'85; LMCC; Staff, Hôpital de réadaptation Villa Medica; Physician, Regie Regionale Sante & Services Sociaux Montreal-Centre; Langs: Bilingual(French/English); (514)286-6500

CLICHE-FONTAINE, Marie-Michele; The Hincks Dellcrest Centre, 114 Maitland St, Toronto ON M4Y 1E1; Laval'07; Psy. Staff, Hincks-Dellcrest Centre-Gail Appel Institute; (416)972-1935

CLIFFORD, John C; 482 Regent St, London ON N5Y 4H4; McM'78; BSc; MA; FRCPC; PhysMed&Rehab (P.Q.) (Electromyography). Consultant, St Joseph's Hospital - St Joseph's Health Care; Consultant, Stratford General Hospital - Huron Perth Healthcare Alliance; Consultant, Chatham-Kent Health Alliance; (519)432-8266; Fax. (519)432-0522; drjohnclifford@bellnet.ca.

CLIFTON, Neil A; St Martha's Reg Hosp, 25 Bay St, Antigonish NS B2G 2G5; Pretoria (South Africa)'79; MB ChB; MMed; Staff Otol, St Martha's Regional Hospital; Staff Otol, Aberdeen Regional Hospital; (902)863-8393; Fax. (902)863-6750; entclinic@ns.sympatico.ca.

CLIMAN, Allan B; 407-5885 ch de la Cote-des-Nei, Montreal QC H3S 2T2; Guadalajara (Mexico)'79; ObstGyn (P.Q.). Staff, Sir Mortimer B Davis Jewish General; McGill University; (514)735-6331; Fax. (514)735-7811.

CLIMENHAGA, David B; First Edmonton Place, 390-10665 Jasper Ave NW, Edmonton AB T5J 3S9; Alb'80; FRCSC; Ophth (Anterior Segment Surgery). Consultant, Covenant Health - Grey Nuns Community Hospital; Ac Staff, Alberta Health Services; Assoc Prof, University of Alberta; (780)424-2233; Fax. (780)426-7219.

CLIMENHAGA, Harold W; 2203 TD Tower, 10088 102 Ave NW, Edmonton AB T5J 2Z1; Alb'78; FRCSC; Ophth (Cataract). Ac Staff, Royal Alexandra Hospital; Court Consultant, Wetaskiwin Hospital & Care Centre; Consultant, Westview Health Centre; Clin Assoc Prof, University of Alberta; (780)424-1020; Fax. (780)426-7632.

CLIMIE, Robert C; PO Box 159, Delta ON K0E 1G0; Qns'70; FRCPC; CommunMed. (613)928-3126

CLIMPSON-KENNEDY, L Gayle; York Prof Bldg, 101-679 Davis Dr, Newmarket ON L3Y 5G8; McM'82; Staff, Southlake Regional Health Centre; (905)898-7111; Fax. (905)898-1121.

CLINE, John C; Cline Med Centre, 233 Prideaux St, Nanaimo BC V9R 2M9; Cal'85; (250)753-3030; Fax. (250)753-3006; info@clinemedical.com.

CLINE, Leah L A; Vancouver Home Hospice, 300-999 Broadway Ave W, Vancouver BC V5Z 1K5; Glasgow (Scotland)'88; MB ChB; (604)742-4010

CLINE, Roy A; 621-10833 160 St, Surrey BC V4N 1P3; Sask'71; FAAO; FRCSC; Ophth (Adult Strabismus). Staff, BC Women's Hospital & Health Centre; Ac Staff, Vancouver General Hospital - Centennial Pavillion; Ac Staff, Delta Hospital; Clin Assoc Prof, University of British Columbia; (604)580-1008

CLINTON, Jean M; McMaster University, 1280 Main St W, Hamilton ON L8S 4K1; McM'81; FRCPC; Psy. Teach Staff, McMaster University; (905)521-2100

CLINTON, Theresa F; Atikokan Med Associates, PO Box 1450 123 Marks St, Atikokan ON P0T 1C0; McM'75; (807)597-2721; Fax. (807)597-4679.

CLINTON-BAKER, David; Burnside Medical, 4-101 Burnside Rd W, Victoria BC V9A 1B7; Auckland (New Zealand)'75; MB ChB; (250)382-3191; Fax. (250)383-2431.

CLIVE, Barbara A; The Credit Valley Hosp, 2200 Eglinton Ave W, Mississauga ON L5M 2N1; Ott'81; FRCPC; IntMed; GeriatricMed. Staff, The Credit Valley Hospital; Instructor IntMed & Geriatrics, University of Toronto; (905)813-1100 x5415; Fax. (905)813-3855; bclive@cvh.on.ca.

CLOAD, Bruce W A; Royal University Hosp, 103 Hospital Dr, Saskatoon SK S7N 0W8; Cal'03; FRCPC; EmergMed; Critical Care Medicine. Staff, Royal University Hospital; (306)655-1000

CLOETE, Nicolas G F; Caledonia Med Centre, 14 Caithness St E, Caledonia ON N3W 1L4; Pretoria (South Africa)'92; MB ChB; BSc(Hons); CCFP; Staff, Hamilton Health Sciences Centre - McMaster Children's Hospital; (905)765-4061; Fax. (905)765-0584.

CLOETE, Pieter D; 2-140 Athabascan Ave, Sherwood Park AB T8A 4E3; (South Africa)'98; (780)467-3244

CLONEY, Jacqueline F; Lockview Med Clinic, 204.1-159 Cobequid Rd, Lower Sackville NS B4C 2N1; Dal'78; (902)865-7543; Fax. (902)865-7554.

CLORY, Michael B; Cobequid Comm Health Centre, 2051-40 Freer Lane, Bedford NS B4S 0A2; McG'91; CCFP; CCFP(E.M.); (902)869-6141; Fax. (902)869-6148.

CLOSE, Alison M; 205 Turnbull Ave PO Box 1029, Biggar SK S0K 0M0; (Other Foreign)'02; CCFP.

CLOSSON, Keri L; 3-1230 Alward St, Prince George BC V2M 7B1; UBC'03; CCFP; (250)562-1231; Fax. (250)562-1207.

CLOTH, Martin I; Dufferin-Steeles Fam Med Ctre, 1881 Steeles Ave W, North York ON M3H 5Y4; Tor'76; Dip SportMed; CCFP; Physician Varsity Teams, York University; (416)665-2900

CLOTTEY, Clarence E; Bristol Family Physicians, 102-2315 Bristol Cir, Oakville ON L6H 6P8; Ghana (Ghana)'86; MB ChB; MPH(Harvard); CCFP; Langs: Akan; Ga; Portuguese; (905)287-2035; Fax. (905)287-2036.

CLOUATRE, Andre; Clin Radiologique Gatineau, 1-195 boul Greber, Gatineau QC J8T 3R1; Mon'64; FRCPC; DiagRad. Staff, Hôpital de Gatineau; (819)568-9119; Fax. (819)568-1682.

CLOUATRE, Yves J J; 24-88 Duncan Ave W, Penticton BC V2A 7J7; Mon'78; CSPQ; MHA; ABIM; FRCPC; IntMed; Nephrol. Langs: Romanian; English; (250)492-4614; Fax. (250)492-4630; yves.clouatre@shaw.ca.

CLOUTHIER, Sarah; Petawawa Centennial FHT, 154 Civic Centre Rd, Hamilton ON L8H 3H5; McM'10; CCFP; (613)687-7641

CLOUTIER, Alexis-Simon; CSSS Pierre Boucher, 1333 boul Jacques-Cartier E, Longueuil QC J4M 2A5; Mon'05; FRCSC; GenSurg. Staff, Centre Hospitalier Pierre Boucher; (450)468-8111

CLOUTIER, Anne-Marie; GMF Centre de santé, 3745 rue Georges-Couture, Drummondville QC J2B 7P4; Laval'05; CCFP; (819)477-2231

CLOUTIER, Annie; CSSS Pierre Boucher, 1333 boul Jacques-Cartier E, Longueuil QC J4M 2A5; Mon'00; Staff, Centre Hospitalier Pierre Boucher; (450)468-8111

CLOUTIER, Annie; Hotel-Dieu du Sacre-Coeur, 1 av du Sacre-Coeur, Quebec QC G1N 2W1; Laval'00; FRCPC; Psy. Staff, Hotel-Dieu du Sacre-Coeur de Jesus de Quebec; (418)529-6851

CLOUTIER, Annie-Catherine; UMF Charles LeMoyne, 201-299 boul Sir-Wilfrid-Lauri, Saint-Lambert QC J4R 2L1; Mon'97; (450)466-5630; Fax. (450)466-5631.

CLOUTIER, Christian; CHUS-Hop Fleurimont, 3001 12e Av N, Sherbrooke QC J1H 5N4; Sher'84; FRCSC; Neursurg (Pain Management). Teach Staff Surg, Centre Hospitalier Universitaire de Sherbrooke-Hopital Fleurimont; (819)346-1110; Fax. (819)820-6420; christian.cloutier@usherbrooke.ca.

CLOUTIER, Claude; CSSS du Haut-Saint-François, RR 3 460 2E Avenue, Weedon QC J0B 3J0; Sher'75; Staff, CSSS du Haut-Saint-François; Consultant, Centre Hospitalier Universitaire de Sherbrooke-Hôpital Hôtel-Dieu; (819)877-3434; Fax. (819)877-5272.

CLOUTIER, Daniel; CHUQ-Ctr Hosp Univ Laval, 2211-2705 boul Laurier, Quebec QC G1V 4G2; Sher'73; PlasSurg (Hand Surgery). Ac Staff Surg, Centre Hospitalier Universitaire de Quebec-CHUL; (418)656-2259; Fax. (418)654-2774.

CLOUTIER, Diane; Clin Laser Esthetique Quebec, 1693 rte de l'Aeroport, Quebec QC G2G 2P3; Laval'96; (418)871-3434; Fax. (418)871-7985.

CLOUTIER, Fernand; CSSS de la Vieille-Capitale, 5100-2400 av D'Estimauville, Quebec QC G1E 7G9; Laval'72; Langs: English; (418)623-1010 x226; Fax. (418)623-7513; fernand.cloutier@sssvc.qc.ca.

CLOUTIER, Frederic-Charles; 44-1480 Foster St, Victoria BC V9B 3X7; Mon'05; BSc; FRCSC; OrthSurg. (604)538-0068

CLOUTIER, Guylene; 68 av Principale, Rouyn-Noranda QC J9X 4P2; Sher'01; FRCPC; Psy (Neuro Psychiatry). Langs: English; (819)797-0397; Fax. (819)797-1836; guylene.cloutier@mac.com.

CLOUTIER, Helene; Clinique Le Medical, 285-1750 boul Marie-Victorin, Longueuil QC J4G 1A5; Mon'78; ac Staff, Centre Hospitalier l'Université de Montréal (CHUM) - Hôtel-Dieu; (450)442-9531; Fax. (450)442-1553.

CLOUTIER, Isabelle; Clinique Med St-Alexandre, 200-2310 rue Saint-Louis, Gatineau QC J8T 5L7; Mon'90; Langs: Bilingual(French/English); (819)243-4500; Fax. (819)243-1369.

CLOUTIER, Jacques; Centre Med Fafard Enr, 201-975 boul Monseigneur-De La, Baie-Saint-Paul QC G3Z 2W3; Laval'70; (418)435-6310; Fax. (418)435-3203.

CLOUTIER, Jean; 1000-1440 rue Sainte-Catherine, Montreal QC H3G 1R8; Sher'73; (514)878-1911 x251; jcloutier@fmoq.org.

CLOUTIER, Jean-Francois; Clin Medico-Chirurgicale de Ve, 43-55 rue de l'Eglise, Verdun QC H4G 3E7; Mon'02; FRCSC; Otol. Otolaryngology, Centre Hospitalier de Verdun; Staff Otol, Hopital Charles LeMoyne; Langs: Bilingual(French/English); (514)766-7171; Fax. (514)768-2507.

CLOUTIER, Jean-Marc; CHUS-Hop Fleurimont, 3001 12e Av N, Sherbrooke QC J1H 5N4; Laval'79; CSPQ; FRCPC; Anes. Staff, Centre Hospitalier Universitaire de Sherbrooke-Hopital Fleurimont; (819)346-1110; Fax. (819)820-6413.

CLOUTIER, Jennifer A; Saint John Reg Hosp, PO Box 2100 Stn Main 400 University Ave, Saint John NB E2L 4L2; Tor'03; FRCPC; Anes. Staff, Saint John Regional Hospital; (506)648-2000

CLOUTIER, Jonathan; Ctr Hosp Laurentien, 234 rue Saint-Vincent, Ste-Agathe-des-Mts QC J8C 2B8; Mon'07; IntMed. Staff, Centre Hospitalier Laurentien; (819)324-4000

CLOUTIER, Julie; Clinique Medicale Mascouche, 100-1025 Montee Masson, Mascouche QC J7K 2L9; Sher'91; CCFP; (450)474-6000

CLOUTIER, Linda; Clinique de Med Familiale, 80 118e rue, Shawinigan-Sud QC G9P 3E4; Laval'87; Staff, Centre Hospitalier du Centre la Mauricie; (819)537-8878; Fax. (819)537-3489.

CLOUTIER, M Sylvie; Conroy Med Centre, 100-2 Lorry Greenberg Dr, Ottawa ON K1G 5H6; Ott'83; (613)737-0654; Fax. (613)737-3265.

CLOUTIER, Richard; CHUQ-Hotel-Dieu de Quebec, 11 Cote Du Palais, Quebec QC G1R 2J6; Laval'68; Derm. Staff, Centre Hospitalier Universitaire de Québec (CHUQ) - Siege Social; (418)691-5200; Fax. (418)691-5048; pinault.cloutier@gmail.com.

CLOUTIER, Martin; Neuro Rive-Sud, 250-4896 boul Taschereau, Greenfield Park QC J4V 2J2; Sher'95; LMCC; FRCPC; Neur. Staff, Hopital Charles LeMoyne; Langs: Bilingual(French/English); (450)672-1931; Fax. (450)672-3308.

CLOUTIER, Michele; CLSC Vallee de la Batiscan, 90 Riviere-A-Veillette RR 4, Ste-Genev-D-Batisc QC G0X 2R0; Sher'89; (418)362-2727; Fax. (418)362-3130.

CLOUTIER, Michele; CSSS de Manicouagan, 635 boul Jolliet, Baie-Comeau QC G5C 1P1; Laval'83; Staff, Centre Hospitalier Régional Baie-Comeau; (418)589-3701

CLOUTIER, Michele; Ctr de Sante Paul-Gilbert, 9330 du Centre-Hospitalier, Charny QC G6X 1L6; Mon'89; Staff, Centre Hospitalier Paul-Gilbert; (418)380-8993

CLOUTIER, Mireille; CLSC Jardin du Quebec, 2 rue Ste-Famille, Saint-Remi QC J0L 2L0; Mon'78; Langs: Bilingual(French/English); (450)454-4671; Fax. (450)454-4538.

CLOUTIER, Nicole; Collège québécois Med Famille, 202-3210 av Jacques-Bureau, Laval QC H7P 0A9; Langs: Bilingual(French/English); (450)973-2228; Fax. (450)973-4329; cqmf@bellnet.ca.

CLOUTIER, Paul; 20 rue Carrier, Edmundston NB E3V 3Y1; Mon'84; FRCSC; GenSurg (Gastroenterology); VascSurg. Staff, Hôpital regional d'Edmundston; Langs: Bilingual(French/English); (506)735-6215; Fax. (506)735-5422.

CLOUTIER, Pierre; 328 rue A P Low CP 2340, Schefferville QC G0G 2T0; Sher'79; (418)585-2645; Fax. (418)585-3795.

CLOUTIER, Raynald; RRSSS Cote-Nord, 691 rue Jalbert, Baie-Comeau QC G5C 2A1; Laval'78; Dir admin, Regie regionale de la Cote-Nord; (418)589-9845; Fax. (418)589-8574.

CLOUTIER, Rejean; Ctr Hosp Affilie-St-Sacrement, 1050 ch Sainte-Foy, Quebec QC G1S 4L8; Laval'72; FRCSC; OrthSurg. ac Staff, Centre Hospitalier Affilié Universitaire de Québec - Hôpital du St-Sacrement; (418)682-7511

CLOUTIER, Richard; Hop Louis-H Lafontaine, 7401 rue Hochelaga, Montreal QC H1N 3M5; Mon'86; FRSC; DPsy; FRCPC; Psy (Dual Diagnosis). Chief Drug Addiction Program & Psy, Hopital Louis-H Lafontaine; Langs: English; French; (514)282-6060; Fax. (514)282-5030; clourier@videotron.ca.

CLOUTIER, Robert; Clinique Med Memphre, 200-323 rue Sherbrooke, Magog QC J1X 2R9; Sher'79; Prof Pt-Time, Universite de Sherbrooke; Langs: English; (819)847-1313; Fax. (819)847-3529; robert.cloutier@usherbooke.ca.

CLOUTIER, Réal; Hôpital Riviere des Prairies, 7070 boul Perras, Montreal QC H1E 1A4; Sher'80; MSc; Staff, Hôpital Riviere des Prairies; Langs: Bilingual(French/English); (514)323-7260 x2012; real.cloutier.pdi@ssss.gouv.qc.ca.

CLOUTIER, Sonia; Clin Radiology de la Capitale, 4225 4e av O, Quebec QC G1H 6P3; Laval'80; DiagRad. Staff Radiol, CSSS de Quebec-Sud; Langs: Bilingual(French/English); (418)628-8291; Fax. (418)628-4735.

CLOUTIER, Sophie; Polyclinique St-Eustache, 75 rue Grignon, Saint-Eustache QC J7P 4J2; Laval'94; Staff, Hôpital de Saint-Eustache; Langs: Bilingual(French/English); (450)473-6882

CLOUTIER, Stephanie; Ctr Hosp Affilie-Enfant-Jesus, B. 3000-1401 18e rue, Quebec QC G1J 1Z4; Laval'96; FRCPC; IntMed; Hem. Staff, Centre Hospitalier Affilié Universitaire de Québec - Hôpital De L'Enfant Jésus; (418)649-5726

CLOUTIER, Yvan; Clinique Musculo-Squelettique, 260-1215 ch du Tremblay, Longueuil QC J4N 1R4; Mon'73; Physician, Clinique Musculo-Squelettique; (450)442-1018

CLOUTIER-CAMIRE, France; CLSC Frontenac, 17 rue Notre-Dame O, Thetford Mines QC G6G 1J1; Laval'81; Physician, CHSLD Rene Lavoie; (418)338-3511; Fax. (418)338-1668; france_cloutier_camire@ssss.gouv.qc.ca.

CLOUTIER-MARCHAND, Francine; CHUM-Hop Notre-Dame, 1560 rue Sherbrooke E, Montreal QC H2L 4M1; Mon'71; ClinImmunol&Allergy (P.Q.). Staff, Centre Hospitalier l'Université de Montréal (CHUM) - Hôpital Notre-Dame; (514)890-8000

CLOW, David J; 586 Eglinton Ave E, Toronto ON M4P 1P2; Tor'83; BSc(Hon.); FRCPC; DiagRad (Interventional Radiology).

CLOW, Erin C; Beaverlodge Medical Clinic, PO Box 209 1030 1 Ave, Beaverlodge AB T0H 0C0; Dal'07; BSc; CCFP; (780)354-2646; Fax. (780)354-8181.

CLOW, Jennifer E; The Ottawa Hosp-Civic Campus, 1053 Carling Ave, Ottawa ON K1Y 4E9; Ott'01; CCFP; CCFP(E.M.); Staff, The Ottawa Hospital - Civic Campus; (613)798-5555

CLOWATER, Julie L; 306-40 Centre St, Chatham ON N7M 5W3; Mem'94; FRCPC; Peds. (519)352-7279

CLUETT, Helen C; 12 Prince Edward Dr, Wellington ON K0K 3L0; Qns'87; BSc; FCFP; CCFP; FCFP; (613)399-1281; Fax. (613)399-2464.

CLUETT, James A G; Tillsonburg Fam Physicians, 4-594 Broadway St, Tillsonburg ON N4G 5K9; Qns'86; FCFP; CCFP; FCFP; Staff, Tillsonburg District Memorial Hospital; (519)842-3636; Fax. (519)842-9522; vancluan@oxford.net.

CLUETT, M Joy; 121-7 Paton St, St. John's NL A1B 4S8; Mem'93; FRCSC; PlasSurg.

CLUFF, Stephen J; Southlake Reg Health Centre, 596 Davis Dr, Newmarket ON L3Y 2P9; McG'83; CCFP; CCFP(E.M.); Staff, Southlake Regional Health Centre; (905)895-4521 x2673

CLUGSTON, Timothy P; Carry Drive Med Centre, 137-116 Carry Dr SE, Medicine Hat AB T1B 3Z8; Sask'94; (403)502-8926; Fax. (403)529-2456.

CLUNIE, Michelle L; Royal University Hosp, 103 Hospital Dr, Saskatoon SK S7N 0W8; Sask'97; FRCPC; Anes. Staff, Royal University Hospital; (306)655-1183; Fax. (306)655-1279.

CLUTTERHAM, Suzanne M; 41024-2529 Shaughnessy St, Port Coquitlam BC V3C 3G1; UBC'06; CCFP; (604)760-7482

CNOOP KOOPMANS, W Michael; Lakeridge Hlth Corp-Oshawa, 1 Hospital Crt, Oshawa ON L1G 2B9; Wes'79; DABR; FRCPC; DiagRad. Staff, Lakeridge Health - Oshawa Site; (905)433-4305; Fax. (905)721-4770.

CO, Ha Thanh; CLSC Petite-Patrie, 6520 rue de Saint-Vallier, Montreal QC H2S 2P7; Mon'85; CCFP; FCFP; (514)494-4924

CO, Thanh Ngoc C; 365-1615 boul Jacques-Cartier, Longueuil QC J4M 2X1; Sher'88; FRCSC; OrthSurg. (450)463-2034; Fax. (450)463-0919.

COAD, Dwayne E; Stanton Territorial Hlth Autho, PO Box 10 Stn Main, Yellowknife NT X1A 2N1; Qns'89; CCFP; CCFP(E.M.); FCFP; Staff, Stanton Territorial Health Authority; (867)669-4100; Fax. (867)669-4171.

COADY, Catherine M; Queen Elizabeth II HSC-Halifax, 4872-1796 Summer St, Halifax NS B3H 3A7; Dal'90; FRCSC; OrthSurg (Sports Medicine). Staff, Queen Elizabeth II Health Sciences Centre - Victoria General Site; Staff, Queen Elizabeth II Health Sciences Centre - Halifax Infirmary Site; (902)473-2575; Fax. (902)473-1582.

COADY, John E; 204-274 Dundas St E, Belleville ON K8N 1E6; Qns'87; BSc; CCFP; Staff, QHC Belleville General; (613)969-7743; Fax. (613)969-7744.

COADY, Kenneth W; Parkdale Med Centre, 28 Linden Ave, Charlottetown PE C1A 5Y9; Dal'82; CCFP; (902)628-6800; Fax. (902)566-5158.

COAKLEY, Annalee; 23 McDougall Crt NE, Calgary AB T2E 8R3; Qns'01; CCFP; (403)265-3410; Fax. (403)264-3411.

COAKLEY, Arthur G; Cape Breton Hlthcare Complex, 1482 George St, Sydney NS B1P 1P3; Dal'68; BSc; BA; CCFP; CCFP(E.M.); FCFP; Staff EmergMed, Cape Breton Healthcare Complex; Teach Staff, Dalhousie University; (902)567-8000; Fax. (902)567-7904.

COATES, Allan L; The Hosp for Sick Children, 555 University Ave, Toronto ON M5G 1X8; McG'72; Peds; Respir (P.Q.) (Pediatric Pulmonology). Dir-Research Qatar Project, The Hospital For Sick Children; Prof Peds, University of Toronto; (416)813-6215; Fax. (416)813-6246.

COATES, Beverley A; Herold Road Family Physicians, 1-325 Herold Rd, Saskatoon SK S7V 1J7; Sask'75; Assoc Staff, St Paul's Hospital (Grey Nuns) of Saskatoon; (306)374-2404; Fax. (306)477-0300.

COATES, C David C; Dr D Coates Med Prof Corp, 1249 Front Rd S, Amherstburg ON N9V 2M5; Tor'86; FCFP; BSc; Coroner, Ministry of Public Safety & Security; Langs: French; (519)736-8600; Fax. (519)736-8639; drcoates@bellnet.ca.

COATES, Edward G; Laurel Med Centre Ltd, 304-888 8th Ave W, Vancouver BC V5Z 3Y1; McG'79; FRCPC; Peds (Pediatric Allergy). Langs: Spanish; French; (604)876-1020; Fax. (604)876-1070.

COATES, Geoffrey; 1200 Coronation Blvd, Cambridge ON N1R 3G2; Durham (England)'63; MB BS; MSc; FRCPC; NuclearMed. Physician Nuclear Med, Hamilton Health Sciences Centre - McMaster Children's Hospital; Staff DiagRad, Cambridge Memorial Hospital; Emeritus Prof Radiol, McMaster University; (519)621-2333; gcoates@cogeco.ca.

COATES, John R G; Windsor Family Health Team, 245-2475 McDougall St, Windsor ON N8X 3N9; Ott'94; BSc; CCFP; FCFP; (519)250-5656; Fax. (519)250-5864; jrcoatesmd@gmail.com.

COATES, Kerry J; Bayview Med Clinic, 102-1650 Terminal Ave N, Nanaimo BC V9S 0A3; UBC'80; (250)591-3040

COATES, Kevin; St Boniface Clinic, 343 Tache Ave, Winnipeg MB R2H 2A5; Man'80; CCFP; FCFP; Ac Staff, St Boniface General Hospital; Assoc Staff, Victoria General Hospital; University of Manitoba; (204)925-9597; Fax. (204)237-0779.

COATES, Pamela J K; The Credit Valley Hosp, 4F109-2200 Eglinton Ave W, Mississauga ON L5M 2N1; McG'78; FRCPC; Peds. Ac Staff, The Credit Valley Hospital; Langs: French; (905)813-1100; pcoates@cvh.on.ca.

COATTA, Erik S J; ABC Med Clinic, 9842 101 Ave, Fort St. John BC V1J 2B2; (Other Foreign)'09; CCFP; (250)785-1220

COBBIN, Paul L; 110-2504 Skaha Lake Rd, Penticton BC V2A 6G1; UBC'85; BSc; CCFP; FCFP; Staff, Penticton Regional Hospital; (250)492-3511; Fax. (250)492-3514; vicki.wood.2008@gmail.com.

COBLENTZ, Craig L; Hamilton HS-Hamiton Gen Hosp, 237 Barton St E, Hamilton ON L8L 2X2; McM'80; AB; FCCP; FRCPC; DiagRad (Pulmonary Radiology). Staff Radiol, Hamilton Health Sciences Centre - McMaster Children's Hospital; Staff, Hamilton Health Sciences Centre - Hamilton General Hospital; Prof, McMaster University; (905)527-4322; Fax. (905)527-5761.

COBOS VEGA, Haydee A; CSSS d'Antoine-Labelle-Mt Laur, RR 1 2561 ch de la Lievre S, Mont-Laurier QC J9L 3G3; Staff, CSSS d'Antoine-Labelle; (819)623-1234 x4231

COBOURN, Christopher S; First Med Place, 201-170 Queensway W, Mississauga ON L5B 3A8; Wes'83; FRCSC; GenSurg (Hepatobiliary Surgery). Chief Surg, Trillium Health Centre - Mississauga; Surgeon, Surgical Weight Loss Centre; (905)276-7211; Fax. (905)276-6486.

COBURN, Christina M; CFB Esquimalt, PO Box 17000 Stn Forces 1200 Colville Rd, Victoria BC V9A 7N2; Belfast (Ireland)'03; MB BCh; CCFP; (250)363-4120

COBURN, Harris C; Greene Clinic, 501 Mcbride St, Prince Rupert BC V8J 3G5; Belfast (Ireland)'71; MB ChB; BAO; (250)624-9121; Fax. (250)624-9359.

COBURN, John A; Colwood Med Treatment Ctr Inc, 102-1910 Sooke Rd, Victoria BC V9B 1V7; Witwatersrand (South Africa)'85; MB ChB; BPharm; CCFP; (250)474-5155

COBURN, M Ellen; 4303 10th Ave W, Vancouver BC V6R 2H6; Tor'73; Staff, BC Women's Hospital & Health Centre; Staff, UBC Hospital - Koerner Pavillion; (604)224-1355; Fax. (604)224-0179.

COBURN, Natalie S G; Sunnybrook Hlth Sciences Ctre, 2075 Bayview Ave, Toronto ON M4N 3M5; North Carolina(NC) (USA)'98; FRCSC; GenSurg. Staff, Sunnybrook Health Sciences Centre; (416)480-6916; Fax. (416)480-6002.

COBUS, Peter A; 702-1363 Lakeshore Rd, Burlington ON L7S 1B2; Ott'67; (905)634-4186; Fax. (905)633-8936.

COCHE, Edgar; GMF Concorde, 300 boul de la Concorde E, Laval QC H7G 2E6; Mon'76; assoc Staff, Hopital de la Cite de la santé; (450)667-5310; Fax. (450)667-5248.

COCHEN, Douglas A; Nepean Med Centre, 308-1 Centrepointe Dr, Nepean ON K2G 6E2; RCS (Ireland)'91; FRCSC; ObstGyn. Staff ObstGyn, Queensway Carleton Hospital; (613)274-7282; Fax. (613)274-2970.

COCHIEN, Eileen D C; Welcome Med Clinic, 105-7885 6th St, Burnaby BC V3N 3N4; UBC'98; CCFP; (604)526-8905; Fax. (604)526-1304.

COCHLIN, Joseph L; 3484 Mt Blanchard Pl, Abbotsford BC V2S 6T5; UBC'82; Ac Staff, Abbotsford Regional Hospital & Cancer Centre.

COCHRAN, Jennifer J D; Riverside Medical Clinic, 304-1101 Dewdney Ave, Trail BC V1R 4T1; Dal'04; CCFP; Staff, Squamish General Hospital / Hilltop House; (250)368-5656

COCHRANE, Christopher H; The Medical Assoc Clinic, 806 Vernon St, Nelson BC V1L 4G5; Otago (New Zealand)'82; BSc(Physiol); DIH; FRNZCGP; MB ChB; MB BS; Physician, Kootenay Lake General Hospital; (250)352-6611 x240; Fax. (250)352-6624.

COCHRANE, D Douglas; A3-216-4500 Oak St, Vancouver BC V6H 3N1; Tor'75; FRCSC; Neursurg (Pediatric Neuro Surgery). Staff, BC Women's Hospital & Health Centre; Staff Credentialing Office, Provincial Health Services Authority; Prof Div of NeuroSurg, University of British Columbia; (604)875-2094

COCHRANE, David K; 50 College Dr, North Bay ON P1B 0A4; Tor'88; FRCPC; Psy (General Psychiatry). Staff, North Bay Regional Health Centre - Regional Mental Health; Asst Prof, University of Ottawa; Reg Dir Psychiatry/Asst Prof, Northern Ontario School of Medicine; (705)474-1200 x3639; Fax. (705)495-7890; dcochrane@nbrhc.on.ca.

COCHRANE, Isabelle; Kootenay Lake Gen Hosp, 3 View St, Nelson BC V1L 2V1; Laval'05; CCFP; CCFP(E.M.); Staff, Kootenay Lake General Hospital; Langs: Bilingual(English/French); (250)352-3111

COCHRANE, Nicholas W L; University of Alberta Hosp, 8440 112 St, Edmonton AB T6G 2B7; Otago (New Zealand)'82; MB ChB; FRACR; FRCPC; DiagRad. Staff, University of Alberta Hospital; (780)407-6907

COCHRANE-BRINK, Katherine A; Youthdale Treatment Centre, 227 Victoria St, Toronto ON M5B 1T8; Tor'99; FRCPC; Psy. (416)368-3751; Fax. (416)368-5025.

COCKBURN, John E; Medisys Group, 1545 Carling Ave, Ottawa ON K1Z 8P9; Ott'87; CCFP; CCFP(E.M.); FCFP; Staff, Montfort Hospital; (613)521-8313; Fax. (613)521-8649.

COCKBURN, Lucas C; Guelph Gen Hosp, 115 Delhi St, Guelph ON N1E 4J4; Qns'06; CCFP; CCFP(E.M.); Staff, Guelph General Hospital; (519)837-6440

COCKCROFT, Donald W; Royal University Hosp, 103 Hospital Dr, Saskatoon SK S7N 0W8; UBC'70; BSc; FRCPC; IntMed (Asthma). Ac Staff RespMed/Prof RespMed, Royal University Hospital; Prof RespMed, University of Saskatchewan; (306)966-8274; Fax. (306)966-8694; don.cockcroft@usask.ca.

COCKERAM, Alan W; Hilyard Place Bldg A, 270-560 Main St, Saint John NB E2K 1J5; Cal'79; FRCP; FACG; FRCPC; IntMed (Therapeutic Endoscopy); Gastroent. Staff Gastroent, Saint John Regional Hospital; Staff Gastroent, St Joseph's Hospital; Assoc Prof, Dalhousie University; Clin Assoc Prof, Memorial University Of Newfoundland; (506)634-7742; Fax. (506)632-1107; cockera@nb.sympatico.ca.

COCKFIELD, Sandra M; University of Alberta Hosp, 11 107 CSB-8440 112 St NW, Edmonton AB T6G 2B7; Tor'82; FRCPC; IntMed (Transplantation); Nephrol. Med Dir Renal Transplant Program, University of Alberta Hospital; Prof, University of Alberta; (780)407-7239; Fax. (780)407-7771; sandra.cockfield@ualberta.ca.

COCKHILL, Leslie A; St Paul's Hosp, 1081 Burrard St, Vancouver BC V6Z 1Y6; McG'82; FRCPC; Psy (Eating Disorders). Ac Staff, Providence Health Care - St Paul's Hospital; Vis Staff, BC Women's Hospital & Health Centre; Clinical Asst Prof, University of British Columbia; Langs: English; French; (604)631-5322; Fax. (604)631-5631.

COCKWELL, Heather A; Oakville Fertility & Women's H, B-627 Lyons Lane, Oakville ON L6J 5Z7; Wes'02; FRCSC; ObstGyn (Reproductive Endocrinology & Infertility). (905)844-7238; Fax. (905)844-7256.

COCLE, Didier J; Centre Med St Basile, 101-275 boul Sir-Wilfrid-Lauri, St-Basile-Le-Grand QC J3N 1V6; Mon'77; (450)653-7323; Fax. (450)653-3021.

COCQUYT, Stuart R; Ridge Meadows Hosp & Hlth CC, PO Box 5000 Stn Del Ctr 11666 Laity St, Maple Ridge BC V2X 7G5; Alb'01; FRCPC; DiagRad. Staff, Ridge Meadows Hospital & Health Care Centre; (604)463-4111

CODDINGTON, Douglas A; PO Box 24043 Rpo Evergreen, Calgary AB T2Y 0J9; Dal'97; (403)667-4537

CODE, Catherine C; Civic Parkdale Clinic, 407B-737 Parkdale Ave, Ottawa ON K1Y 1J8; McM'98; BScN; FRCPC; IntMed. Staff, The Ottawa Hospital - General Campus; Asst Prof Med, University of Ottawa; (613)761-4473; Fax. (613)761-4036.

CODERE, Francine; CLSC du Haut St-Francois, 840 rue Papineau, Sherbrooke QC J1E 1Z2; Mon'90; Staff, Centre Hospitalier Regional de Sept-Iles; (819)829-9772 x1620; Fax. (819)829-1783.

CODERE, Francois; MUHC-Royal Victoria Hosp, 687 av des Pins O, Montreal QC H3A 1A1; Sher'76; FRCSC; Ophth. assoc Staff, Hôpital Ste-Justine; intérim Chef Ophth, McGill University Health Centre - Royal Victoria Hospital; adj Prof, Universite de Montreal; adj Prof, McGill University; (514)843-1620; Fax. (514)843-1612.

CODERRE, Amélie; CSSS du Sud de Lanaudière, 911 montee des Pionniers, Terrebonne QC J6V 2H2; Mon'09; CCFP; CCFP(E.M.); Staff, Centre Hospitalier Pierre le Gardeur; (450)654-7525

CODERRE, Sylvain P; Peter Lougheed Centre, 3500 26 Ave NE, Calgary AB T1Y 6J4; Ott'92; FRCPC; IntMed; Gastroent. Staff, Peter Lougheed Centre; (403)943-5708

CODIO, Circe; Worthington General Rehab, 33457 Cottage Lane, Abbotsford BC V2S 0B3; Mon'08; CCFP; (604)870-7999

CODSI, Marianne; Centre Med Samson, 202-4599 boul Samson, Laval QC H7W 2H2; Sher'86; CCFP; Langs: English; (450)688-7170; Fax. (450)688-3335.

CODY, Kenneth D; 110-1926 20 Ave NW, Calgary AB T2M 1H5; Cal'82; CCFP; FCFP; (403)289-1116; Fax. (403)289-4060.

COE, James Y; University of Alberta Hosp, 4C2.36WCM-8440 112 St NW, Edmonton AB T6G 2B7; Newcastle (England)'73; MB BS; MD; FACC; FAHA; FRCPC; Cardiol (Pediatric Cardiology). Consultant, Royal Alexandra Hospital; Consultant, Covenant Health - Grey Nuns Community Hospital; Staff Ped Cardiol, University of Alberta Hospital; Prof, University of Alberta; (780)407-3963; Fax. (780)407-3010.

COE, Michael J O; 102-45 St Thomas St, St. Albert AB T8N 6Z1; London (England)'74; MB BS; LRCP; MRCS; FRCSC; ObstGyn. Ac Staff, Sturgeon Community Hospital; Court Staff, Royal Alexandra Hospital; Court Staff, University of Alberta Hospital; (780)459-1105; Fax. (780)459-1107.

COELHO, Ryan M; Delhi Family Health Team, 105 Main St, Delhi ON N4B 2L8; St George (Grenada)'09; CCFP; (519)582-2323

COERTZE, Louis J; Victoria Hosp, PO Box 3000 Stn Main 1200 24th St W, Prince Albert SK S6V 5T4; Pretoria (South Africa)'98; MB ChB; CCFP; Staff Emerg Dept, Victoria Hospital; (306)765-6200; Fax. (306)765-6224.

COETZE, Hendrik A; Cook Medical Bldg, 326-1175 Cook St, Victoria BC V8V 4A1; Stellenbosch (South Africa)'84; MB ChB; Langs: Afrikaans; (250)386-2449; Fax. (250)386-2458; hcoetze@telus.net.

COETZEE, Anka; PO Box 1250, Grimshaw AB T0H 1W0; (780)332-4644; Fax. (780)332-1020.

COETZEE, Barend; Carbonear Gen Hosp, 86 Highroad S, Carbonear NL A1Y 1A4; Pretoria (South Africa)'68; MB ChB; MMed(Surg); Chief Surg/Staff, Burin Peninsula Health Care Centre; Staff, Carbonear General Hospital; (709)945-5111; barend.coetzee@easternhealth.ca.

COETZEE, Corneli M; Second Avenue Med Clinic, 330 Second Ave W, Prince Rupert BC V8J 1G6; Pretoria (South Africa)'05; MD; Langs: Afrikaans; (250)624-5500

COETZEE, Direse; La Ronge Med Clinic, PO Box 240, La Ronge SK S0J 1L0; (Other Foreign)'04; CCFP; (306)425-2174; Fax. (306)425-4199.

COETZEE, Dorothea; East Kootenay Reg Hosp, 13 24th Ave N, Cranbrook BC V1C 3H9; Pretoria (South Africa)'68; MB ChB; (250)426-5281

COETZEE, Douwette; Omineca Med Clinic, 3348 Hospital Rd, Vanderhoof BC V0J 3A2; Orange Free State (South Africa)'83; MB ChB; (250)567-2201; Fax. (250)567-2105.

COETZEE, Fanie; Associated Med Clinic, PO Box 510, Lac La Biche AB T0A 2C0; Pretoria (South Africa)'96; (780)623-4421; Fax. (780)623-1920.

COETZEE, Gillaume; Second Avenue Med Clinic, 330 Second Ave W, Prince Rupert BC V8J 1G6; Orange Free State (South Africa)'04; MB ChB; Langs: Afrikaans; (250)624-5500

COETZEE, Jacoba I; Mokala Medical, 161-31 Southridge Dr, Okotoks AB T1S 2N3; (403)995-5740; Fax. (403)995-5743.

COETZEE, Jan Adriaan; Alder Med Clinic, 277 Evergreen Rd, Campbell River BC V9W 5Y4; Pretoria (South Africa)'87; MB ChB; CCFP; FCFP; (250)287-7441

COETZEE, Louis J; Bonnyville Med Clinic, PO Box 1007 Stn Main 4610 50 St, Bonnyville AB T9N 2J7; (South Africa)'99; MB ChB; Langs: Afrikaans; Xhosa; (780)826-3346; Fax. (780)826-6362.

COETZEE, Maarten J; South Shore Med Clinic, 620 Cassils Rd E, Brooks AB T1R 1M6; Pretoria (South Africa)'89; MB ChB; Langs: Afrikaans; (403)793-8111; Fax. (403)793-8118; mcoetzee@telus.net.

COETZEE, Michelle; Associated Med Clinic, PO Box 510, Lac La Biche AB T0A 2C0; Pretoria (South Africa)'98; (780)623-4421; Fax. (780)623-1920.

COETZER, Francois W; 9711 101 Ave, Fort St. John BC V1J 6S1; Pretoria (South Africa)'79; MB ChB; FRCSC; GenSurg. General Surgery, Fort St John Hospital & Health Centre; (250)262-5282; Fax. (250)262-5331.

COETZER, Louise; The Lighthouse Medical Clinic, 205-2903 32nd Ave, Vernon BC V1T 2L6; Stellenbosch (South Africa)'96; MB ChB; CCFP; Langs: Afrikaans; (250)545-2552; Fax. (250)545-2545.

COEUGNIET, Edouard R; CHUM-Hotel-Dieu, 3840 rue Saint-Urbain, Montreal QC H2W 1T8; (France)'04; Staff, Centre Hospitalier l'Université de Montréal (CHUM) - Hôtel-Dieu; (514)890-8121

COFFEY, Alan J H; Westmount Med Bldg, 250-5025 rue Sherbrooke O, Montreal QC H4A 1S9; McG'83; FRCSC; Ophth. Assoc Staff Ophth, McGill University Health Centre - Montreal General Campus; Assoc Staff Ophth, McGill University Health Centre - Royal Victoria Hospital; Lecturer, McGill University; Langs: English; French; (514)489-4648; Fax. (514)489-6251.

COFFEY, Charles G; G R Baker Mem Hosp, 543 Front St, Quesnel BC V2J 2K7; Mem'79; DABR; FRCPC; DiagRad. Staff, Cariboo Memorial Hospital and Health Centre; Staff Medical Imaging, G R Baker Memorial Hospital; (250)985-5680

COFFEY, James; Central Nfld Reg Hlth Centre, 50 Union St, Grnd-Falls-Windsor NL A2A 2E1; Mem'03; BSc; FRCPC; Derm (Pediatrics). Staff, Central Newfoundland Regional Health Centre; (709)292-8435; Fax. (709)292-8434.

COFFEY, Joseph F; 206-496 Topsail Rd, St. John's NL A1E 2C2; Mem'02; FRCPC; Derm. Staff, Western Memorial Regional Hospital.

COFFEY, Lisa A H; Bowmont Med Clinic, 6535 Bowness Rd NW, Calgary AB T3B 0E8; Cal'00; CCFP; (403)247-9797; Fax. (403)247-0014.

COFFEY, Maitreya S; The Hosp for Sick Children, 555 University Ave, Toronto ON M5G 1X8; Chicago (USA)'01; FRCPC; Peds. Staff, The Hospital For Sick Children; (416)813-7938; Fax. (416)813-5663; trey.coffey@sickkids.ca.

COFFIN, Carla S; Health Research Innovation Ctr, 3280 Hospital Dr NW, Calgary AB T2N 4Z6; Mem'01; MSc; FRCPC; IntMed (Viral Hepatitis) (Infectious Diseases) (Liver Transplant) (Hepatology) (Liver Disease); Gastroent. Staff, Foothills Medical Centre; Staff, Health Research Innovation Centre; Staff, Calgary Health Region; Asst Prof, University of Calgary; (403)210-7563; Fax. (403)210-9345.

COGAN, Farrell S; Medcan Health Mgmt Inc, 1500-150 York St, Toronto ON M5H 3S5; Tor'76; MBA; CCFP; Ac Staff Family & Commun Med, North York General Hospital; Court Staff FamMed, The Scarborough Hospital - General Campus; Staff, Medcan Health Management Inc; Lecturer, University of Toronto; (416)350-5963; Fax. (416)350-5981.

COGAN, Samantha J; 305-1436 Royal York Rd, Etobicoke ON M9P 3A9; Tor'96; CCFP; FCFP; Staff, Women's College Hospital; Langs: English; French; (416)240-1382; Fax. (416)240-1103; sjcogan@hotmail.com.

COGAN-COLLET, M Jennifer; Institut de Cardiologie de Mtl, 5000 rue Belanger, Montreal QC H1T 1C8; McM'94; CSPQ; FRCPC; Anes. Staff, Institut de Cardiologie de Montréal; (514)376-3330

COGHLAN, John K; 2423 Apollo Rd, Westbank BC V4T 1P6; Dublin (Ireland)'68; MB ChB; BAO; FRCPC; PhysMed&Rehab (Electromyography). Staff PhysMed&Rehab, Kelowna General Hospital; (250)861-5199

COGHLAN, Matthew A; The Hosp for Sick Children, 555 University Ave, Toronto ON M5G 1X8; National University of Ireland (Ireland)'01; Clin Fellow Anes, The Hospital For Sick Children; (416)813-7445

COGLIANO, Antonio; Fowler Kennedy Sports Med Clin, 3M-1151 Richmond St, London ON N6A 3K7; Tor'93; BSc; MSc; CASM; CCFP; Court Staff Privil, Alexandra Hospital; Assoc Prof Kinesiology, University of Western Ontario; Langs: French; Italian; (519)661-3011 x88830; Fax. (519)661-3379.

COGSWELL, Arthur F; Children's & Women's HC of BC, 2L5-4480 Oak St, Vancouver BC V6H 3V4; Tasmania (Australia)'78; MB BS; FRACP(Peds); BMedSci; DCH; FRCPC; Peds (Pediatric Critical Care). Staff Physician Critical Care & Med Dir ECLS Prog, BC Children's Hospital; Clin Assoc Prof, University of British Columbia; (604)875-2729

COGSWELL, Esther M S; 66 Exhibition St, Kentville NS B4N 5J6; Dal'93; BSc; CCFP; FCFP; Ac Member, Valley Regional Hospital; (902)678-3488

COHADE, Christian; CHUM-Hotel-Dieu, 3840 rue Saint-Urbain, Montreal QC H2W 1T8; Laval'95; FRCPC; NuclearMed. Staff, Centre Hospitalier l'Université de Montréal (CHUM) - Hôtel-Dieu; (514)890-8180

COHADE, Martine; Clinique Med Ste-Dorothee, 102-1 boul Samson, Laval QC H7X 3S5; Sher'87; CCFP; Staff, Hopital de la Cite de la santé; Langs: Bilingual(French/English); (450)689-6334; Fax. (450)689-6339.

COHANE, Shannon A; Stonegate Commun Health Ctre, 150 Berry Rd, Etobicoke ON M8Y 1W3; American University of the Caribbean (St Maarten)'06; CCFP; (416)231-7070; Fax. (416)231-6903.

COHEN, Abraham; 207-1635 Lawrence Ave W, Toronto ON M6L 3C9; Tor'76; Staff, Humber River Regional Hospital - Keele Street Site; (416)249-7561

COHEN, Adrienne F; G104-3330 Hospital Dr NW, Calgary AB T2N 4N1; Alb'87; BSc(Hon); FRCPC; IntMed; GeriatricMed. Staff, Foothills Medical Centre; Clinical Asst Prof, University of Calgary; (403)944-4490; Fax. (403)944-4233.

COHEN, Albert; SMBD Jewish Gen Hosp, E110.1-3755 ch Cote-Sainte-Cat, Montreal QC H3T 1E2; Mon'85; BSc; FRCPC; IntMed; Gastroent. Staff, Sir Mortimer B Davis Jewish General; assoc Prof Med, McGill University; Langs: English; French; (514)340-8223; Fax. (514)340-8139.

COHEN, Barry A; Health Sciences Centre, GF417A-820 Sherbrook St, Winnipeg MB R3A 1R9; Dal'94; FRCPC; IntMed; Nephrol. Nephrologist, Health Sciences Centre; (204)787-1524; Fax. (204)787-3326; bcohen@hsc.mb.ca.

COHEN, C Ian; D L MacIntosh Sport Med Clinic, 55 Harbord St, Toronto ON M5S 2W6; Tor'85; Dip SportMed; CCFP; Assoc Prof Physical Educ & Health, University of Toronto; (416)978-4678; Fax. (416)971-2846; ian.cohen@utoronto.ca.

COHEN, Carole A; Sunnybrook Hlth Sciences Ctre, F307-2075 Bayview Ave, Toronto ON M4N 3M5; McG'82; FRCPC; Psy. Staff, Sunnybrook Health Sciences Centre; (416)480-4663; Fax. (416)480-5889.

COHEN, Dan A D; 563 Fairlawn Ave, North York ON M5M 1V7; Mon'92; BSc(Biol.); MSc(Neurosciences); PhD(NeuroSci); MD; CCFP; FCFP; Court Staff, North York General Hospital; Asst Prof Family & Commum Med, University of Toronto; Langs: Spanish; French; (416)789-3044; Fax. (416)789-3044; dcohen@hotmail.com.

COHEN, Dana R; Gates of Maple Med Center, 7-2200 Rutherford Rd, Vaughan ON L4K 5V2; Tor'02; FRCPC; IntMed; Rheum. Staff, Sunnybrook Health Sciences Centre; (416)849-2250

COHEN, David J; The Richmond Hosp, 2005-7000 Westminster Hwy, Richmond BC V6X 1A2; UBC'99; FRCPC; Psy. Staff, Richmond Hospital; (604)278-9711 x4361

COHEN, David R; The Moncton Hosp, 135 Macbeath Ave, Moncton NB E1C 6Z8; Dal'87; FRCPC; IntMed (Critical Care Medicine); Anes. Ac Staff Anes & Critical Care, The Moncton Hospital; (506)857-5530; Fax. (506)857-5545.

COHEN, Deborah R; Seaforth Med Bldg, 700-3550 ch de la Cote-des-Nei, Montreal QC H3H 1V4; Ott'84; FRCSC; ObstGyn. Staff, McGill University Health Centre - Royal Victoria Hospital; Asst Prof ObstGyn, McGill University; (514)933-8877; Fax. (514)933-8338.

COHEN, Dina; 2F-3205 boul Saint-Joseph E, Montreal QC H1Y 2B6; Aix-Marseille (France)'72; FRCPC; Derm. Consultant, Hopital Charles LeMoyne; (514)525-0271

COHEN, Elliott S; Central Med Bldg, 202-1105 Carling Ave, Ottawa ON K1Y 4G5; Ott'72; DABOG; FACOG; FSOGC; FRCSC; ObstGyn (Colposcopy). Staff, Almonte General Hospital; (613)729-1997; Fax. (613)729-3017.

COHEN, Eric A; Sunnybrook Hlth Sciences Ctre, D375-2075 Bayview Ave, Toronto ON M4N 3M5; Cal'83; FRCPC; IntMed (Invasive & Interventional Cardiology); Cardiol. Dir Invasive Cardiol, Sunnybrook Health Sciences Centre; Assoc Prof Med, University of Toronto; (416)480-5880; Fax. (416)480-5827; eric.cohen@sunnybrook.ca.

COHEN, Eyal; The Hosp for Sick Children, 555 University Ave, Toronto ON M5G 1X8; Tor'00; FRCPC; Peds (Hospitalist). Staff, The Hospital For Sick Children; Asst Prof Peds, University of Toronto; (416)813-5795; Fax. (416)813-5663; eyal.cohen@sickkids.ca.

COHEN, Harry; Medical Clinic for Psychotherapy, 403-265 Yorkland Blvd, North York ON M2J 5C7; Montpellier (France)'57; BSc; MSc; Langs: Yiddish; French; (416)229-2399; Fax. (416)229-9771; hhcohen@rogers.com.

COHEN, Herbert L; Claresholm Addiction & Mental, PO Box 490 139 43 Ave W, Claresholm AB T0L 0T0; McG'68; FRCPC; Psy. Psychiatrist, Claresholm Centre for Mental Health and Addictions; Consultant, Alberta Health Services Edmonton; (403)682-3583

COHEN, Howard B; The Dermatology Centre, 124 42 Ave SW, Calgary AB T2S 3B3; Lausanne (Switzerland)'61; FRCPC; Derm. Ac Staff, Foothills Medical Centre; Assoc Prof, University of Calgary; (403)299-5800; Fax. (403)299-5828.

COHEN, Howard R; Carling-Broadview Med Bldg, 207-770 Broadview Ave, Ottawa ON K2A 3Z3; Tor'74; Dip SportMed; CCFP; FCFP; Ac Staff, The Ottawa Hospital - Civic Campus; Commun Preceptor, University of Ottawa; (613)828-4198; Fax. (613)828-4895; hcohen01@rogers.com.

COHEN, Howard R; Sunnybrook Hlth Sciences Ctre, M4 146-2075 Bayview Ave, Toronto ON M4N 3M5; McG'81; FACOG; DAB; FSOGC; FRCSC; ObstGyn (Maternal Fetal Medicine). Staff Fetal Med & ObstGyn, Sunnybrook Health Sciences Centre; Asst Prof/Ac Staff ObstGyn, Women's College Hospital; Asst Prof, University of Toronto; Langs: French; (416)480-5217; Fax. (416)480-4164.

COHEN, Howard S; 12 rue Canvin, Kirkland QC H9H 4S4; McG'80; CCFP; FCFP; Assoc Staff, McGill University Health Centre - Montreal General Campus; Lecturer Family Med, McGill University; (514)697-8586; Fax. (514)697-8070.

COHEN, Ira T; St Joseph's Health Centre, 4F SSW-30 The Queensway, Toronto ON M6R 1B5; Cal'90; Staff, St Joseph's Health Centre; (416)530-6591; coheni@stjoe.on.ca.

COHEN, Irene; Thames Valley FHT-Whitehills M, 1225 Wonderland Rd N, London ON N6G 2V9; Technion (Israel)'83; CCFP; FCFP; Staff, London Health Sciences Centre - University Hospital; Staff, St Joseph's Hospital - St Joseph's Health Care; Langs: Dutch; Hebrew; (519)472-0040; Fax. (519)472-7732.

COHEN, Jack; 600-5885 ch de la Cote-des-Nei, Montreal QC H3S 2T2; McG'59; BSc; FRCSC; PlasSurg (Wound Care). Consultant IGUM Chronic Care Facility, Donald Berman Maimonides Geriatric Centre; Sr Staff, Sir Mortimer B Davis Jewish General; Consultant Jewish Eldercare Center, Mount Sinai Hospital Center; Sr Staff PlasSurg, St Mary's Hospital Centre; Lecturer, McGill University; Langs: English; French; (514)733-1472; Fax. (514)733-4857.

COHEN, Jackie; Clin Medico Chirurgicale de Ve, 55 rue de l'Eglise, Verdun QC H4G 3E7; Cracovie (Poland)'00; (514)737-2496

COHEN, James M; Cardiology Consultants, 306-803A 1 Ave NE, Calgary AB T2E 7C5; Qns'73; ABIM; FACC; FRCPC; IntMed; Cardiol. Ac Staff, Foothills Medical Centre; Asst Prof, University of Calgary; (403)571-8600; Fax. (403)571-8668.

COHEN, Janice M; SMBD Jewish Gen Hosp, 3755 ch Cote-Sainte-Catherine, Montreal QC H3T 1E2; McG'86; Staff, Sir Mortimer B Davis Jewish General; (514)340-8222 x5634; Fax. (514)340-7905.

COHEN, Jasmine S; 201-32310 South Fraser Way, Abbotsford BC V2T 1X1; Alb'96; FRCPC; Peds. Staff Peds, Abbotsford Regional Hospital & Cancer Centre; (604)853-9888; Fax. (604)853-8028.

COHEN, Jeffrey J; HIV Care Program, 2085 Tecumseh Rd E, Windsor ON N8W 1E3; McM'77; Med Dir HIV Care Prog, Windsor Regional Hospital - Metropolitan Site; Staff Hospitalist, Hôtel-Dieu Grace Hospital; Langs: Spanish; French; (519)254-6115; Fax. (519)254-3793.

COHEN, Jeremy I; Postgrad Med Education, MDCL 3101A-1280 Main St W, Hamilton ON L8S 4K1; Tor'08; IntMed.

COHEN, Joanne; St Clair Med Clinic, 2F-50 St Clair Ave E, Toronto ON M4T 1M9; Tor'83; CCFP; (416)921-8459

COHEN, Joanne P; Sexual Health Program Unit, 15 Sperling Dr, Barrie ON L4M 6K9; Tor'71; (705)721-7520; Fax. (705)721-7848.

COHEN, Jordan S; 280-1620 29 St NW, Calgary AB T2N 4L7; Cal'00; FRCPC; Psy. Staff, Foothills Medical Centre; (403)297-7345

COHEN, Lawrence B; Sunnybrook Hlth Sciences Ctre, HG63-2075 Bayview Ave, Toronto ON M4N 3M5; McM'79; FRCP; MSc; FACG; FRCPC; IntMed (Gastroenterology). Consultant Gastroent, Sunnybrook Health Sciences Centre; Consultant, Cleveland Clinic Canada; Assoc Prof Med, University of Toronto; (416)480-4725; Fax. (416)480-5977.

COHEN, Leslie S; 360-7031 Westminster Hwy, Richmond BC V6X 1A3; Cape Town (South Africa)'87; BSc(Med)Hons; MB ChB; Clin Staff Pediatric Oncol, BC Children's Hospital; Staff Privil, Richmond Hospital; (604)278-4557; Fax. (604)278-4508; llcohen@shaw.ca.

COHEN, Linda; CSSS Pierre Boucher, 1333 boul Jacques-Cartier E, Longueuil QC J4M 2A5; Mon'81; MedMicrobiol; InfectDis; IntMed. Staff Med Microbiol, Centre Hospitalier Pierre Boucher; (450)468-8111 x82256; Fax. (450)468-8201.

COHEN, M Geoffrey; Britannia Med Centre, 9-5925 Grossbeak Dr, Mississauga ON L5N 6S5; Glasgow (Scotland)'76; MB ChB; DRCOG; CCFP; Ac Staff, The Credit Valley Hospital; (905)824-2467; Fax. (905)824-2466.

COHEN, Mark D; 2085 Weston Rd, York ON M9N 1X7; Tor'79; Staff, William Osler Health System - Etobicoke General Hospital.

COHEN, Mark J; Lasik Vision, 130 King St W, Toronto ON M5X 2A2; McG'92; FRCSC; Ophth (Cornea & Refractive Surgery). Langs: English; French; (416)646-0000; Fax. (416)646-0270.

COHEN, Martin A; 209-269 boul Saint-Jean, Pointe-Claire QC H9R 3J1; McG'87; ABIM(IntMed); ABIM(Rheum.); FRCPC; IntMed; Rheum. Staff, Hôpital Anna-Laberge; Staff Med, McGill University Health Centre - Montreal General Campus; Aj Prof Med, McGill University; Langs: French; (514)697-0134; Fax. (514)697-5937.

COHEN, Matthew R; Royal Alexandra Hosp, 10240 Kingsway NW, Edmonton AB T5H 3V9; Sask'95; FRCPC; Anes. Staff, Royal Alexandra Hospital; (780)735-4010

COHEN, Michael R; The Credit Valley Hosp, 2200 Eglinton Ave W, Mississauga ON L5M 2N1; Tor'04; CCFP; CCFP(E.M.); Staff, The Credit Valley Hospital; (905)813-4530; Fax. (905)813-4548.

COHEN, Michael T; 32 Bond St, Grnd-Falls-Windsor NL A2B 1J4; Mem'79.

COHEN, Michal; The Hosp for Sick Children, 555 University Ave, Toronto ON M5G 1X8; Jerusalem (Israel)'02; Staff, The Hospital For Sick Children; (416)813-1500

COHEN, Michelle J; Brighton Quinte West FHT, 170 Main St, Brighton ON K0K 1H0; Tor'07; CCFP; (613)475-1555

COHEN, Miles A; Carlton Tower, 1703-2 Carlton St, Toronto ON M5B 1J3; Qns'84; FRCPC; Psy. (416)593-0233; Fax. (416)593-9336.

COHEN, Paul D; 306-1366 Yonge St, Toronto ON M4T 3A7; Tor'95; FRCPC; Derm. (416)487-3453; Fax. (416)487-5528; pauldcohen@rogers.com.

COHEN, Philip F; Lions Gate Hosp, 231 15th St E, North Vancouver BC V7L 2L7; Tor'76; AB; FRCPC; NuclearMed. Staff, Lions Gate Hospital; Clin Prof, University of British Columbia; Langs: Bilingual(French/English); (604)984-5954; Fax. (604)984-5781; cohen@triumf.ca.

COHEN, Rebecca A W; North York Family Health Team, 144-1333 Sheppard Ave E, North York ON M2J 1V1; Mon'08; CCFP.

COHEN, Richard S; Niagara H System-St Catharines, PO Box 3018 Stn Main 142 Queenston St, St Catharines ON L2R 7C6; Liverpool (England)'62; MB ChB; FRCSC; PlasSurg. Ac Staff, Niagara Health System - St Catharines General Site; Ac Staff, Niagara Health System - Ontario Street Site; Ac Staff, Hôtel Dieu Shaver Health & Rehabilitation Centre; (905)684-7271; Fax. (905)684-3151.

COHEN, Robert E; Medical Arts Bldg, 208-336 Kings Rd, Sydney NS B1S 1A9; Dal'72; (902)562-3133; Fax. (902)562-3217.

COHEN, Robert I; 106-51 Sunpark Dr SE, Calgary AB T2X 3V4; Dal'98; CCFP; (403)254-6663

COHEN, Sandra R A; Hop Maisonneuve-Rosemont, 5415 boul de l'Assomption, Montreal QC H1T 2M4; Sher'93; FRCPC; IntMed; Hem. Staff, Hopital Maisonneuve-Rosemont; adj Prof, Universite de Montreal; Langs: Swedish; Spanish; English; (514)252-3404; Fax. (514)254-5094.

COHEN, Sharon; Toronto Memory Program, 400-1 Valleybrook Dr, North York ON M3B 2S7; Tor'86; BA; FRCPC; Neur (Dementia). Staff Neurol, North York General Hospital; Med Dir, Toronto Memory Program; Asst Prof Med & Speech Pathol, University of Toronto; (416)386-9761; Fax. (416)386-0458; cohen@memorydisorders.ca.

COHEN, Shawn L; Drummond Med Bldg, 322-1414 rue Drummond, Montreal QC H3G 1W1; McG'94; BScPhysiol; ABOph; FRFPS; MS; FRCSC; Ophth (Glaucoma). Staff, St Mary's Hospital Centre; Staff, McGill University Health Centre; Assoc Prof Ophth, McGill University; Langs: Hebrew; Bilingual(French/English); (514)842-6510; Fax. (514)842-0777; v.cohen@sympatico.ca.

COHEN, Sherry T; North York Gen Hosp, 4001 Leslie St, North York ON M2K 1E1; Harvard (USA)'95; Psy. Staff, North York General Hospital; (416)756-6779; Fax. (416)756-6671.

COHEN, Stephen G; 206-11 Rea St N, Timmins ON P4N 4Z5; Ott'68; CCFP; FCFP; (705)267-2840

COHEN, Stephen S; Dundas Med Centre, 203-220 Dundas St W, Whitby ON L1N 8M7; McG'90; CCFP; FCFP; Staff, Rouge Valley Health System - Ajax & Pickering Health Centre Site; Staff, Rouge Valley Health System - Centenary Health Centre Site; Langs: English; French; (905)668-4571; Fax. (905)668-9781; ste1963@hotmail.com.

COHEN, Steven D; 20 Canvin St, Roxboro QC H9H 4S4; Cal'83; DOHS; CCFP; FCFP; (514)426-7156; Fax. (514)426-4578.

COHEN, Steven N; Addiction & Mental Hlth-Queen, 3-1001 Queen St W, Toronto ON M6J 1H4; Cal'02; FRCPC; Psy. Staff, Centre for Addiction & Mental Health (CAMH) - Queen Site; (416)535-8501

COHEN, Susan B; Metro Children's Aid, 250-20 De Boers St, North York ON M3J 0H1; McG'83; FRCPC; Peds. (416)924-4640 x3415; Fax. (416)324-2371.

COHEN, Sébastien; Miramichi Reg Hosp, 500 Water St, Miramichi NB E1V 3G5; Grenoble (France)'06; Staff, Miramichi Regional Hospital; (506)623-3000

COHEN, Tracey; 204-2401 Yonge St, Toronto ON M4P 3H1; Tor'00; CCFP; Att Physician, Cummer Lodge Home for the Aged; (416)485-2222; Fax. (416)485-2276.

COHEN, Trevor; 101-1964 Fort St, Victoria BC V8R 6R3; Wes'96; FRCSC; ObstGyn (Advanced Laparoscopic Surgery). (250)595-1021

COHEN, Victor; SMBD Jewish Gen Hosp, E714-3755 ch Cote-Sainte-Cathe, Montreal QC H3T 1E2; McG'95; FRCPC; IntMed; MedOncol. Staff, Sir Mortimer B Davis Jewish General; (514)340-8248; Fax. (514)340-8302.

COHEN, Zane; Mount Sinai Hosp, 451-600 University Ave, Toronto ON M5G 1X5; Tor'69; FRCSC; GenSurg (Colon & Rectal Surgery). Chairman GenSurg, University of Toronto; (416)586-4800 x8346; Fax. (416)586-8644; zcohen@mtsinai.on.ca.

COHEN BACRY, Jean-Philippe; CLSC de la Batiscan, 750 rue du Couvent, Saint-Tite QC G0X 3H0; (418)365-7555

COHEN-GELFAND, Sara N; 303-343 Wilson Ave, North York ON M3H 1T1; Tor'07; CCFP; (416)785-8412; Fax. (416)785-8324.

COHEN-NEHEMIA, Gideon; Sunnybrook Hlth Sciences Ctre, H405-2075 Bayview Ave, Toronto ON M4N 3M5; Tor'92; MSc; PhD; FRCSC; CardSurg (Cardiovascular Surgery). Staff Cardiovascular Surg, Sunnybrook Health Sciences Centre; (416)480-6077

COHN, Adam Y; Queensway Carleton Hosp, 3045 Baseline Rd, Nepean ON K2H 8P4; Ott'02; FRCPC; IntMed; Nephrol. Staff, The Ottawa Hospital - Riverside Campus; Staff, Queensway Carleton Hospital; (613)721-4842

COHN, Ronald D; The Hosp for Sick Children, 555 University Ave, Toronto ON M5G 1X8; Gesamthochschule Essen University (Other Foreign)'96; Staff Clinical & Retarolic Genetics, The Hospital For Sick Children; (416)813-7654

COHN, Tony A; Addiction & Mental Hlth-Queen, 1001 Queen St W, Toronto ON M6J 1H4; Cape Town (South Africa)'75; MB BS; MSc; FRCP; FRCPC; Psy (Chronic Psychosis). Staff, Centre for Addiction & Mental Health (CAMH) - Queen Site; (416)535-8501; Fax. (416)583-4352; tony_cohn@camh.net.

COHODAREVIC, Tea; Univ Hlth Network-Toronto Western Hosp, 4F 811-399 Bathurst St, Toronto ON M5T 2S8; Zagreb (Croatia)'81; FRCPC; PhysMed&Rehab. Staff Comprehensive Pain Prog, Toronto Western Hospital - University Health Network; (416)603-5380; Fax. (416)603-5725.

COHOLIC, Andrea A; Timmins & District Hosp, 700 Ross Ave E, Timmins ON P4N 8P2; Ott'95; CCFP; FCFP; Staff Anes, Timmins & District Hospital; (705)267-2131 x6345

COHONNER, Chantal; Clinique Med St-Francois, 201-8495 rue Adrien, Laval QC H7A 1J9; Mon'82; Langs: Bilingual(French/English); (450)665-1702; Fax. (450)665-0240.

COICOU, Yves; Clinique Sante du Nord, 100-1105 12e av N, Sherbrooke QC J1E 2X4; Sher'84; (819)565-1828; Fax. (819)565-1936.

COIMBRA, Claudia; Dr Georges-L Dumont Reg Hosp, 330 av Universite, Moncton NB E1C 2Z3; Mon'97; CSPQ; FRCPC; Anes. Staff, Dr Georges-L-Dumont University Hospital Centre; (506)862-4000

COIRE, Claire I; Trillium Hlth Ctr-Mississauga, 100 Queensway W, Mississauga ON L5B 1B8; Tor'81; FACPath; ABP; FRCPC; AnatPath (Neuropathology); GenPath. Staff, Trillium Health Centre - Mississauga; Langs: French; (905)848-7297; Fax. (905)848-8313.

COISH, Charles T; Northside Harbor View Hosp, PO Box 399 Stn Main, North Sydney NS B2A 3M4; Mem'98; CCFP; Staff, Northside General Hospital; (902)794-7250; Fax. (902)794-7259.

COISH, Donald L; Surrey Mem Hosp, 13750 96 Ave, Surrey BC V3V 1Z2; Wes'81; FRCPC; DiagRad. Staff, Surrey Memorial Hospital; (604)588-3368; don.coish@fraserhealth.ca.

COISH, Susan J; Thornhill Family Physicians, 35-7700 Bathurst St, Thornhill ON L4J 7Y3; McM'79; BSc; Staff Family Med, Mackenzie Richmond Hill Hospital; Langs: French; (905)881-6510; Fax. (905)881-6513.

COITEUX, Carl C; Clinique Domus Medica, 305-5601 rue Belanger, Montreal QC H1T 1G3; Mon'65; hon Membre, Hôpital Santa Cabrini Ospedale; Consultant Phys, Scor Life Reassurance Co; Med Consultant, Manulife and Clarica Insurance Co; (514)256-5011 x216; carlcoiteux@hotmail.com.

COITEUX, Isabelle; CHUM-Hop St-Luc, 1058 rue Saint-Denis, Montreal QC H2X 3J4; Mon'99; FRCPC; IntMed. Staff, Centre Hospitalier l'Université De Montréal (CHUM) - Hôpital Saint-luc; (514)890-8000

COJOCARU, Alice; University of Alberta Hosp, 1E7 23WCM-8440 112 St NW, Edmonton AB T6G 2B7; Bucharest (Romania)'94; MMedSci; FRCPC; Psy (Emergency Psychiatry). Staff Psy, University of Alberta Hospital; Clinical Asst Prof, University of Alberta; Langs: Romanian; French; (780)407-2194; Fax. (780)407-6672; cojocaru@ualberta.ca.

COJOCARU, Andre N; CSSS de Rivière-de-Loup, 75 rue Saint-Henri, Riviere-Du-Loup QC G5R 2A4; Mon'92; FRCSC; OrthSurg. Staff, Centre Hospitalier Regional du Grand-Portage; (418)868-1000; Fax. (418)868-1032.

COKE, William J; Univ Hlth Network-Toronto Western Hosp, EW8 415-399 Bathurst St, Toronto ON M5T 2S8; McG'74; ABIM; FRCPC; IntMed. Staff, Toronto Western Hospital - University Health Network; (416)603-5800

COKER, David A; CFB Petawawa, PO Box 9999 Stn Main 2 Field Ambulance, Petawawa ON K8H 2X3; McM'07; CCFP; Staff, Base Hospital-CFB Petawawa; (613)687-5511

COLACO, Carmen M; Rebecca Med Associates, 170 Rebecca St, Oakville ON L6K 1J6; Bangalore (India)'65; MB BS; Affil Staff, Halton Healthcare Services Corporation - Oakville Site; Langs: Portuguese; (905)845-9293; Fax. (905)845-0981.

COLACO, Carmo D D; Tillsonburg Dist Mem Hosp, 167 Rolph St, Tillsonburg ON N4G 3Y9; Bombay (India)'81; FRCSC; GenSurg. Staff, Tillsonburg District Memorial Hospital; (519)842-3611

COLAK, Errol; St Michael's Hosp, 3CC-30 Bond St, Toronto ON M5B 1W8; Tor'03; FRCPC; DiagRad. Staff, St Michael's Hospital; (416)864-5656

COLANGELO, Patricia C; Rusholme Med Clinic, 1465 Dundas St W, Toronto ON M6J 1Y7; Tor'91; FAAP; RC; FRCPC; Peds (Pediatric Neurology). Clin Asst, Toronto Western Hospital - University Health Network; Clin Asst, Mount Sinai Hospital; Langs: Italian; (416)534-1150; Fax. (416)534-9630.

COLANTONI, Guido; Polyclinique Cabrini, 211-5700 rue Saint-Zotique E, Montreal QC H1T 3Y7; Sher'82; FRCSC; ObstGyn. (514)253-1000

COLAPINTO, David A; Southlake Reg Health Centre, 596 Davis Dr, Newmarket ON L3Y 2P9; Kigezi (Uganda)'01; CCFP; Staff, Southlake Regional Health Centre; (905)895-4521

COLAPINTO, Michael N; Hamilton HS-Hamilton Gen Site, 237 Barton St E, Hamilton ON L8L 2X2; Tor'05; FRCPC; DiagRad. Staff, Hamilton Health Sciences Centre - Hamilton General Hospital; (905)521-2100

COLAPINTO, Nicholas D; North York Med Arts Bldg, 244-1333 Sheppard Ave E, North York ON M2J 1V1; Tor'67; FACS; FRCSC; GenSurg (Post-OP Complications). Staff Surg, North York General Hospital; Assoc Prof Surg, University of Toronto; (416)490-0001; Fax. (416)490-0041.

COLAS, Marie-Jose; CHUS-Hop Fleurimont, 3001 12e Av N, Sherbrooke QC J1H 5N4; Mon'84; CSPQ; FRCPC; Anes. Staff, Centre Hospitalier Universitaire de Sherbrooke-Hopital Fleurimont; Universite de Sherbrooke; (819)346-1110 x14403; Fax. (819)820-6420.

COLAS, Rolande M; 200-350 St. George St, Moncton NB E1C 1X1; (Haiti)'82; MD; LMCC; Staff, The Moncton Hospital; Langs: English; French; (506)859-0411; Fax. (506)384-1404.

COLAVINCENZO, Vincenzo A; Clin Med Familiale de LaSalle, 6-2101 av Dollard, LaSalle QC H8N 1S2; Laval'88; Staff, Centre Hospitalier de LaSalle; (514)595-8867; Fax. (514)363-9280.

COLBERT, Diane A; Health Sciences Centre, 300 Prince Philip Dr, St. John's NL A1B 3V6; Mem'97; FRCPC; DiagRad. Staff Radiol, Health Sciences Centre; (709)777-6798

COLBERT, Mariam; Ctr de Perinatalite l'Autre Ma, 575 rue Saint-Charles E, Longueuil QC J4H 1B8; Mon'03; Staff, Centre Hospitalier Pierre Boucher; (450)332-9833

COLBORNE, Brian J; Brant Community HC-Brantford, 200 Terrace Hill St, Brantford ON N3R 1G9; UBC'88; CCFP; CCFP(E.M.); Physician Emerg, The Brant Community Healthcare System - Brantford General Hospital Site; (905)751-5544; Fax. (905)752-0098.

COLBORNE, William H; North Nanaimo Med Clinic, 195-4750 Rutherford Rd, Nanaimo BC V9T 4K6; Man'69; Ac Staff, Nanaimo Regional General Hospital; (250)585-7100; Fax. (250)585-7001.

COLBOURNE, Danielle N; Churchill Square Medical, PO Box 23205 8-10 Rowan St, St. John's NL A1B 4J9; Mem'09; CCFP.

COLBOURNE, Margaret L; Children's & Women's HC of BC, B321-4480 Oak St, Vancouver BC V6H 3V4; UBC'87; FRCPC; Peds. Staff, BC Children's Hospital; (604)875-3270; Fax. (604)875-2946.

COLBOURNE, S Ann; University of Alberta Hosp, 1J2.34 WCM-8440 112 St NW, Edmonton AB T6G 2B7; Mem'87; ABIM; BMedSci; FACP; BSc(Hon); MA; BA; FRCP; IntMed; FRCPC; IntMed (Diabetes Mellitus). Staff, University of Alberta Hospital; (780)407-2774; Fax. (780)407-3132.

COLBY, Joshua; Prince Edward Family Health Te, 35 Bridge St, Picton ON K0K 2T0; Tor'04; CCFP; CCFP(E.M.); (613)476-7771; joshua.colby@sjhc.london.on.ca.

COLBY, W David; Middlesex-London Health, 101-50 King St, London ON N6A 5L7; Tor'84; FRCPC; MedMicrobiol (Tropical Diseases). Med Staff, London Health Sciences Centre - University Hospital; Coroner, Province of Ontario; Asst Prof Microbiol, University of Western Ontario; (519)663-3396; Fax. (519)663-3977; david.colby@mlhu.on.ca.

COLCLEUGH, Robert; London Med Arts Bldg, 401-746 Base Line Rd E, London ON N6C 5Z2; Wes'67; FACS; FRCSC; PlasSurg (Cosmetic Surgery). Teach Staff, London Health Sciences Centre - Victoria Campus; Prof Surg, University of Western Ontario; (519)672-6715; Fax. (519)672-9634; rcolcleugh@theplasticsurgeryclinic.com.

COLDWELL, Bobbi-Jo; Lions Gate Hosp, 231 15th St E, North Vancouver BC V7L 2L7; McM'04; FRCPC; DiagRad. Staff, Lions Gate Hospital; (604)984-5775

COLE, Basilon C; Aberdeen Hosp, 835 East River Rd, New Glasgow NS B2H 3S6; Dal'79; FRCSC; GenSurg. Ac Staff, Aberdeen Regional Hospital; (902)752-6534; Fax. (902)928-0112.

COLE, Candace C; 340 Le Page Rd, Salt Spring Island BC V8K 1N1; McM'89; Ac Staff, Cowichan District Hospital; (250)537-0022; Fax. (250)537-0034.

COLE, Christopher P; The Cole Clinic, PO Box 17 101-1344 County Rd 22, Emeryville ON N0R 1C0; Wes'85; MPH; Med Dir, The Cole Clinic for Hair Transplant; (519)727-4247; info@coleclinic.com.

COLE, Colm P; St Paul's Hosp, 1081 Burrard St, Vancouver BC V6Z 1Y6; UBC'79; FRCPC; Anes. Staff, Providence Health Care - St Paul's Hospital; (604)806-8337; Fax. (604)739-0944.

COLE, Dale L; Bowmont Med Clinic, 6535 Bowness Rd NW, Calgary AB T3B 0E8; Cal'81; CCFP; FCFP; Staff, Foothills Medical Centre; (403)247-9797; Fax. (403)247-0014.

COLE, David E C; Banting Institute, 520B-100 College St, Toronto ON M5G 1L5; Tor'75; FCCMG; PhD(McG); FRCPC; MedBiochem (Metabolic Bone Disease); MedGenetics. Staff, Women's College Hospital; Assoc Prof Peds, The Hospital For Sick Children; Prof LabMed & Med, Toronto General Hospital - UHN; Prof LabMed, University of Toronto; (416)978-6720; Fax. (416)978-5650.

COLE, Donald C; Dalla Lama Scholl of Public He, 402-155 College St, Toronto ON M5T 3M7; Tor'78; FRCPC; OccupMed (Environmental Health); CommunMed. Staff, Dalla Lana School of Public Health; Sr Scientist, Institute for Work & Health; Assoc Prof Public Health Services, University of Toronto; Langs: Spanish; French; (416)946-7870; Fax. (416)978-8299.

COLE, Edward H; R Fraser Elliott Bldg, 1S 409-200 Elizabeth St, Toronto ON M5G 2C4; FRCPC; IntMed (Renal Transplant); Nephrol. Affil Scientist, Toronto General Hospital - UHN; Prof Med, University of Toronto; (416)340-4669; Fax. (416)340-4016.

COLE, Denise; Med Professional Corp, 1004-1243 Islington Ave, Etobicoke ON M8X 1Y9; Mem'81; BSc; Ac Staff, St Joseph's Health Centre; (416)766-1349; Fax. (416)766-7310.

COLE, Howard J; 11 Elvina Gardens, Toronto ON M4P 1X7; Tor'76; DPsy; DCPsy; FRCPC; Psy (Adolescent Psychiatry). (416)487-0993; Fax. (416)487-4504.

COLE, Jeffrey S; Central Nfld Reg Hlth Centre, 50 Union St, Grnd-Falls-Wi NL A2A 2E1; Mem'93; FRCPC; Anes. Staff, Central Newfoundland Regional Health Centre; (709)292-2500

COLE, Madeleine S C; PO Box 2170, Iqaluit NU X0A 0H0; Cal'98; CCFP.

COLE, Mara; Markham Stouffville Hosp, PO Box 1800 381 Church St, Markham ON L3P 7P3; McM'06; FRCPC; Peds. Staff, Markham Stouffville Hospital; Staff, The Hospital For Sick Children; (905)472-7000

COLE, Martin G; St Mary's Hosp Centre, 3830 av Lacombe, Montreal QC H3T 1M5; McG'72; FRCPC; Psy (Geriatric Psychiatry). Staff, St Mary's Hospital Centre; Prof Psy, McGill University; Langs: French; (514)345-3511 x3349; Fax. (514)734-2609; martin.cole@ssss.gouv.qc.ca.

COLE, Martin J; 419-5920 1A St SW, Calgary AB T2H 0G3; Tor'79; FRCPC; IntMed; Gastroent., University of Calgary; (403)244-2624; Fax. (403)228-9108.

COLE, Peter N; PO Box 336 Stn A, Orangeville ON L9W 2Z7; Tor'69; MHSc; BSc(Med.); CommunMed (Public Health). Staff, Headwaters Health Care Centre - Orangeville Site; University of Toronto; (519)942-6268; Fax. (519)942-6269.

COLE, Robert D; Bridgeland Med Bldg, 206-803A 1 Ave NE, Calgary AB T2E 7C5; Cal'83; CCFP; FCFP; Ac Staff Privil, Peter Lougheed Centre; University of Calgary; (403)265-6533; Fax. (403)265-6520.

COLE, Roy V; Miramichi Reg Hosp, 500 Water St, Miramichi NB E1V 3G5; Dal'73; Staff, Miramichi Regional Hospital; (506)623-3155; Fax. (506)623-3660.

COLE, William G; University of Alberta Hosp, 2C3.65-8440 112 St NW, Edmonton AB T6G 2B7; Melbourne (Australia)'65; FRCSC; OrthSurg (Pediatric Orthopedics). Staff, University of Alberta Hospital; (780)407-7002; Fax. (780)407-7005.

COLEBROOK, John M; Red Deer Reg Hosp Centre, PO Box 5030 Stn Postal Box Ctr 3942 50A Ave, Red Deer AB T4N 6R2; Alb'98; CCFP; CCFP(E.M.); Staff, Red Deer Regional Hospital Centre; (403)343-4444; johnmcolebrook@yahoo.ca.

COLEGRAVE, Craig E; 10101 Southport Rd SW, Calgary AB T2W 3N2; UBC'90; (403)748-4448

COLELLA, Paul V; Royal Jubilee Hosp, 1952 Bay St, Victoria BC V8R 1J8; McM'98; CCFP; CCFP(E.M.); Staff, Royal Jubilee Hospital; (250)370-8000

COLEMAN, Amanda C; Elizabeth Avenue Family Practi, 116-100 Elizabeth Ave, St. John's NL A1B 1S1; Mem'07; CCFP; (709)579-5005; Fax. (709)579-5278; cmandacbennett@hotmail.com.

COLEMAN, David A; Medical Centre, 12-14 West St, Corner Brook NL A2H 2Z1; Dal'82; CCFP; FCFP; Staff, Western Memorial Regional Hospital; (709)634-7107; Fax. (709)634-0682.

COLEMAN, Douglas S; Columbia Med Bldg, 207-301 Columbia St E, New Westminster BC V3L 3W5; Cal'81; Med Dir, Western Canada Rapid Opiate Detox Centre; (604)553-2262; Fax. (604)553-2264; dcoleman61@shaw.ca.

COLEMAN, Elizabeth J; ON shores for Mental Health Se, 700 Gordon St, Whitby ON L1N 5S9; Tor'99; FRCPC; Psy. Staff, Ontario Shores Centre for Mental Health Sciences; (905)430-4055

COLEMAN, Fiona M; 2A-2379 Bevan Ave, Sidney BC V8L 4M9; Cape Town (South Africa)'86; MB ChB; (250)656-4177; Fax. (250)656-9285; dumela@shaw.ca.

COLEMAN, Gina S A; Health Canada, AL0700C-200 Tunney's Pasture D, Ottawa ON K1A 0K9; Bucharest (Romania)'80; Clin Assoc Staff, The Ottawa Hospital - Civic Campus; A-Dir Marketed Med Devices Div, Health Canada; Langs: Romanian; Bilingual(English/French); (613)948-7147; Fax. (613)946-0693; gina.coleman@hc-sc.gc.ca.

COLEMAN, Jeffrey R; Vancouver Coastal Health, 11F-601 Broadway Ave W, Vancouver BC V5Z 4C2; Wes'79; FACEP; MCFP(EM); Exec Med Dir, Vancouver Coastal Health; Clin Assoc Prof, University of British Columbia; (604)875-5269; Fax. (604)875-4750.

COLEMAN, Lomie J; Ottawa Valley Health & Wellnes, 715 Mackay St, Pembroke ON K8A 0C6; Dal'84; Staff, Pembroke Regional Hospital Inc; (613)735-1089; Fax. (613)735-2739.

COLES, Chad P; Queen Elizabeth II HSC-Halifax, 4856-1796 Summer St, Halifax NS B3H 3A7; Dal'97; FRCSC; OrthSurg (Trauma). Staff, Queen Elizabeth II Health Sciences Centre - Halifax Infirmary Site; Asst Prof, Dalhousie University; (902)473-5599; Fax. (902)473-5569.

COLES, John G; The Hosp For Sick Children, 555 University Ave, Toronto ON M5G 1X8; Wes'76; FRCSC; Cardiovasc&ThorSurg. Staff Cardiovasc Surg, The Hospital For Sick Children; Fax. (416)813-7984; john.coles@sickkids.ca.

COLES, Joyce K T; Hatchet Lake Med Centre, 2273 Prospect Rd, Hatchet Lake NS B3T 1S9; Dal'01; CCFP; (902)852-3090; Fax. (902)852-5108.

COLES, Scott R; Haliburton Family Med Centre, PO Box 870 7217 Gelert Rd, Haliburton ON K0M 1S0; Tor'94; CCFP; FCFP; (705)457-1212; Fax. (705)457-3955.

COLESHILL, Geoffrey G; Boundary Med Clinic, PO Box 400, Grand Forks BC V0H 1H0; Edinburgh (Scotland)'70; MB ChB; (250)442-8233; Fax. (250)442-3949.

COLEV, Gheorghe; 1511 Ouellette Ave, Windsor ON N8X 1K5; Jassy (Romania)'60; PhD; FRCSC; Ophth. Staff, Hôtel-Dieu Grace Hospital; (519)977-0233; Fax. (519)971-8449.

COLEY, Matthew A; St Paul's Hosp, 1081 Burrard St, Vancouver BC V6Z 1Y6; UBC'04; FRCPC; Anes. Staff, Providence Health Care - St Paul's Hospital; (604)806-8487

COLFORD, Donald F; Saint John Reg Hosp, PO Box 2100 Stn Main 400 University Ave, Saint John NB E2L 4L2; Dal'86; FRCSC; ObstGyn. Staff, Saint John Regional Hospital; (506)649-2788; Fax. (506)648-6878.

COLGAN, Simon; Highland Family Practice, C-1966 Guthrie Rd, Comox BC V9M 3X7; Belfast (Ireland)'97; MB BCh; CCFP; (250)890-0919

COLGAN, Terence J; Mount Sinai Hosp, 6 5023-600 University Ave, Toronto ON M5G 1X5; Tor'77; FCAP; FRCPC; AnatPath. Staff Path & LabMed, Mount Sinai Hospital; (416)586-4522; Fax. (416)586-8481; tcolgan@mtsinai.on.ca.

COLIMON, Leslie; Clinique Sante du Nord, 100-1105 av 12E N, Sherbrooke QC J1E 2X4; Sher'72; (819)565-1828; Fax. (819)565-1936.

COLIN, Christine; 118-5757 av Decelles, Montreal QC H3S 2C3; (France)'80; MSc; FRCPC; CommunMed (Health Promotion)., National Institute of Public Health; Vice Dean, Universite de Montreal; (514)345-2346; Fax. (514)345-7753; christine.colin@umontreal.ca.

COLIN, Francois P A; Hotel-Dieu de Sorel, 400 av de l'Hotel-Dieu, Sorel-Tracy QC J3P 1N5; Staff, Hôtel-Dieu de Sorel; (514)583-7673

COLISTRO, Robert; Royal Inland Hosp, 311 Columbia St, Kamloops BC V2C 2T1; UBC'01; FRCPC; DiagRad. Staff, Royal Inland Hospital; (250)374-2400; Fax. (250)314-2326.

COLIZZA, Franco; Ctr Cardiovasculaire Rive-Sud, 200-1615 boul Jacques-Cartier, Longueuil QC J4M 2X1; Sher'85; CSPQ; FRCPC; IntMed; Cardiol. Staff, Centre Hospitalier Pierre Boucher; (450)674-2345

COLL, Bernard; CHUS-Hop Fleurimont, 2616-3001 12e Av N, Sherbrooke QC J1H 5N4; Sher'82; Respir; IntMed. Staff, Centre Hospitalier Universitaire de Sherbrooke-Hopital Fleurimont; Assoc Staff, Hôpital Sainte-croix; (819)822-6735

COLL, Linda B; 18-6497 boul Jeanne D'Arc N, Orleans ON K1C 2R1; Qns'70; (613)841-8500; Fax. (613)841-5310.

COLL, Oisin P; 318 Gilmore Ave, Burnaby BC V5C 4R1; Alb'05; FRCSC; ObstGyn. Staff, Providence Health Care - St Paul's Hospital; (604)294-8550

COLL, Patrick G; Rockyview Gen Hosp, 7007 14 St SW, Calgary AB T2V 1P9; National (Ireland)'73; DABPN; FRCPC; Psy. Staff, Rockyview General Hospital; Assoc Prof, University of Calgary; (403)943-3614; Fax. (403)943-3624; patrick.coll@albertahealthservices.ca.

COLL, Xavier P L; CSSS du Sud de Lanaudière, 911 montee des Pionners, Terrebonne QC J6V 2H2; Staff, Centre Hospitalier Pierre le Gardeur; (450)581-3020

COLLA, Simon; Doctor's Office, 101-491 Lawrence Ave W, North York ON M5M 1C7; Tor'71; Staff, Mount Sinai Hospital; (416)787-0117; Fax. (416)787-8094.

COLLAR, Colleen A; Foothills Family Practice, 102-30 Crystalridge Dr, Okotoks AB T1S 2C3; Alb'87; CCFP; (403)938-5455; Fax. (403)938-4749.

COLLARD, S Vincent; MUHC-Montreal Children's Hosp, 2300 rue Tupper, Montreal QC H3H 1P3; McG'03; FRCPC; Anes. Staff, McGill University Health Centre - Montreal Children's Hospital; (514)412-4400

COLLARD, Stephanie; CSSS de Chicoutimi, 305 rue Saint-Vallier, Chicoutimi QC G7H 5H6; Sher'98; CCFP; Staff, Complexe hospitalier de la Sagamie; (418)541-1000; Fax. (418)541-1131.

COLLEAUX, Kevin M; 345-750 Spadina Cres E, Saskatoon SK S7K 3H3; Sask'94; FRCS; FRCSC; Ophth (Retina). Staff Eye Care Centre, Saskatoon City Hospital; Clin Assoc Prof Ophth, University of Saskatchewan; (306)933-9336; Fax. (306)933-9313; kcolleauxadmin@sasktel.net.

COLLEDGE, Eleanor M; Family Health Centre, 105-840 Coxwell Ave, Toronto ON M4C 5T2; Tor'98; CCFP; (416)469-6464; Fax. (416)469-6164.

COLLETON, Michael J; Addiction & Mental Hlth-Queen, 3-1001 Queen St W, Toronto ON M6J 1H4; Alb'97; FRCPC; Psy (Adult Psychiatry). Staff Psy, Centre for Addiction & Mental Health (CAMH) - Queen Site; Lecturer, University of Toronto; (416)535-8501 x2958; Fax. (416)583-4319; michael_colleton@camh.net.

COLLETT, F Dean; Deer Valley Centre, 33-1221 Canyon Meadows Dr, Calgary AB T2J 6G2; Alb'70; Ac Staff, Rockyview General Hospital; (403)278-2164; Fax. (403)278-3192.

COLLETT, James D; Rockyview Gen Hosp, 7007 14 St SW, Calgary AB T2V 1P9; Cal'84; CCFP; CCFP(E.M.); Staff, Rockyview General Hospital; (403)943-3449; Fax. (403)943-3220.

COLLETT, Kenneth A; Trafalgar Med Clinic, 200-1235 Trafalgar Rd, Oakville ON L6H 3P1; Wes'80; (905)844-3281; Fax. (905)849-1076.

COLLETTE, Francois; Hop du Sacre-Coeur de Mtl, 5400 boul Gouin O, Montreal QC H4J 1C5; Mon'84; EmergMed (P.Q.). Staff, Hôpital du Sacre-Coeur de Montréal; (514)338-2000

COLLETTE, Myriam; CLSC des Maskoutains, 1015 rue Gauthier, Saint-Hyacinthe QC J2S 8T2; Sher'99; (450)778-2572 x354

COLLETTE, Ronald S; 207-3825 Sunset St, Burnaby BC V5G 1T4; Alb'87; BSc(Med.); Staff, Burnaby Hospital; (604)434-1307; Fax. (604)438-6477.

COLLETTE, Sebastien; Hop Riviere-Des-Prairies, 02.429-7070 boul Perras, Montreal QC H1E 1A4; Mon'99; FRCPC; Psy (Pediatric Psychiatry). Staff Psy, Hôpital Riviere des Prairies; (514)323-7260 x2618; Fax. (514)328-3501.

COLLETTE, Stephane; A-10525 rue Principale, Saint-Louis-D-Kent NB E4X 1E7; Laval'00; CCFP; (506)876-8008; Fax. (506)876-1020.

COLLETTE, Suzon; Hop Maisonneuve-Rosemont, 5415 boul de l'Assomption, Montreal QC H1T 2M4; Mon'00; FRCPC; IntMed; Nephrol. Staff, Hopital Maisonneuve-Rosemont; (514)252-3489; csuzon.hmr@ssss.gouv.qc.ca.

COLLEY, Theresa A; M10-15 Elizabeth St, Orangeville ON L9W 3X3; Tor'69; (519)941-5670; Fax. (519)941-7321.

COLLICUTT, James A; 1-1487 George St, Sydney NS B1P 1P2; Dal'89; BSc(Hons); FRCSC; OrthSurg (Arthroplasty). Gen Consultant, Cape Breton Healthcare Complex; (902)567-0772; Fax. (902)567-2273.

COLLIER, Todd G; Nicola Med Dental Bldg, 203-321 Nicola St, Kamloops BC V2C 6G6; Tor'92; FRCPC; Neur (Electromyography). Staff, Royal Inland Hospital; (250)314-9902; Fax. (250)372-1381.

COLLIN, Emilie; CSSS Alphonse Desjardins-UMF, 100-1205 boul de la Rive-Sud, Saint-Romuald QC G6W 0J4; Sher'08; CCFP; (418)380-8597; Fax. (418)380-8596.

COLLIN, Gerard A; Montfort Hosp, 713 Montreal Rd, Ottawa ON K1K 0T2; Sher'73; FRCPC; DiagRad. Chief Dept of Radiol, Montfort Hospital; Lecturer, University of Ottawa; (613)746-4621 x4523; Fax. (613)748-4951.

COLLIN, Isabelle; UMF Laurier, ED 23-2875 boul Laurier, Quebec QC G1V 2M2; Laval'97; CCFP; Staff, Centre Hospitalier Universitaire de Quebec-CHUL; (418)654-2701; Fax. (418)654-2138.

COLLIN, Marian B; Winnipeg Clinic, 425 St Mary Ave, Winnipeg MB R3C 0N2; Oxford (USA)'98; FRCPC; Derm.

COLLIN, Marianne; Hotel-Dieu de Sorel, 400 av de l'Hotel-Dieu, Sorel-Tracy QC J3P 1N5; Ott'04; CCFP; CCFP(E.M.); Staff, Hôtel-Dieu de Sorel; (514)746-6100

COLLIN, Marie-Eve; Clinique Med Lacroix, 203-810 rte Jean-Gauvin, Quebec QC G1X 0B6; Sher'03; Staff, Centre Hospitalier Portneuf; (418)871-1911

COLLIN, Pierre; CHUQ-Ctr Hosp Univ Laval, 2705 boul Laurier, Quebec QC G1V 4G2; Laval'95; LMCC; Staff, Centre Hospitalier Universitaire de Quebec-CHUL; (418)656-4141

COLLIN, Remi; CSSSG-Hop de Gatineau, PO Box 2000 Succ Bureau-Chef 909 boul de la Verendrye O, Gatineau QC J8P 7H2; Mon'72; CSPQ; Cardiol (P.Q.). Staff, Hôpital de Gatineau; (819)966-6100

COLLINGE, Marie-Laure; CHUS-Hop Fleurimont, 3001 12e Av N, Sherbrooke QC J1H 5N4; Mon'95; Staff, Centre Hospitalier Universitaire de Sherbrooke-Hopital Fleurimont; (819)346-1110 x16535

COLLINGRIDGE, H Glenn; Cannon Clinic, 4-2151 Mccallum Rd, Abbotsford BC V2S 3N9; UBC'90; CCFP; FCFP; (604)853-3314; Fax. (604)853-2171; dcolling2@shaw.ca.

COLLINGRIDGE, Robert L; PO Box 728, Crossfield AB T0M 0S0; Alb'93; CCFP; (403)946-3988; Fax. (403)946-3990.

COLLINGS, James C; 66 Ossekeag Crt PO Box 1096 Stn Main, Hampton NB E5N 8H1; Dal'89; BSc; Ac Staff, Saint John Regional Hospital; Ac Staff, St Joseph's Hospital; Asst Prof, Dalhousie University; Asst Prof, Memorial University Of Newfoundland; (506)832-3366; Fax. (506)832-0741.

COLLINGWOOD, John M; W100-120 Torbay Rd, St. John's NL A1A 2G8; Dal'68; CCFP; Med Dir Rehab Unit, L A Miller Centre; Ac Staff, St John's Health Care Corporation; Memorial University Of Newfoundland; (709)726-8546

COLLINGWOOD, Peter W; Health Sciences Centre, 300 Prince Philip Dr, St. John's NL A1B 3V6; Mem'81; FRCPC; DiagRad. Staff, Health Sciences Centre; (709)777-6853

COLLINS, Alexandra K U; 89 Cook St, Meaford ON N4L 1N2; Bonn (Germany)'80; Staff, Grey Bruce Health Services - Meaford Site; Staff, Grey Bruce Health Services - Owen Sound; Langs: German; (519)538-5282; Fax. (519)538-2602.

COLLINS, Allison A P; Peterborough Reg HC-Hospital, 1 Hospital Dr, Peterborough ON K9J 7C6; Qns'80; FRCPC; GenPath. Staff, Peterborough Regional Health Centre - Hospital Drive; (705)743-2121; Fax. (705)876-5008; acollins@prhc.on.ca.

COLLINS, Carola J D; Avenue Med Centre, 221 Brant Ave, Brantford ON N3T 3J2; Wes'08; CCFP; (519)753-8666

COLLINS, Caroline P; Brameast Family Health Org, 38-2130 North Park Dr, Brampton ON L6S 0C9; Tor'05; CCFP; (905)792-2211; Fax. (905)792-2901.

COLLINS, Celeste; Trent Hills Family Health Team, 119 Isabella St, Campbellford ON K0L 1L0; Pretoria (South Africa)'84; MB ChB; MFGP; CCFP; Staff, Campbellford Memorial Hospital; Langs: Afrikaans; (705)653-1801; Fax. (705)653-5483.

COLLINS, Christopher A; Medical Arts Centre, 103-650 South Terminal Ave, Nanaimo BC V9R 5E2; London (England)'03; MB BS; CCFP; (250)753-3431; Fax. (250)754-6897.

COLLINS, Courtney L C; University Hosp of Northern BC, 1475 Edmonton St, Prince George BC V2M 1S2; UBC'09; CCFP; Staff, University Hospital of Northern British Columbia; (250)565-2000

COLLINS, David C; 111-210 Memorial Ave, Orillia ON L3V 7V1; Tor'69; Ac Staff, Orillia Soldiers' Memorial Hospital; Langs: English; French; (705)325-4434; Fax. (705)325-7221.

COLLINS, David J; Terrace Clinic, 204-35 Major's Path, St. John's NL A1A 4Z9; Mem'83; FRCPC; Psy. Ass't Clin Prof Psy, Memorial University Of Newfoundland; (709)777-3450

COLLINS, David R; Gordon & Leslie Diamond Hlth C, 8205B-2775 Laurel St, Vancouver BC V5Z 1M9; UBC'99; FRCPC; IntMed; Rheum. Staff, Providence Health Care - Mount Saint Joseph Hospital; Staff, Vancouver General Hospital - Centennial Pavillion; (604)875-8270

COLLINS, David S; 3B-575 West St S, Orillia ON L3V 7N6; Wes'82; FACP; FRCPC; IntMed (Adult Rheumatology); Rheum. Court Staff, Orillia Soldiers' Memorial Hospital; (705)326-1031; Fax. (705)326-9112.

COLLINS, Deborah L; Lifemark Health Centre, 230-181 Keefer Place, Vancouver BC V6B 6C1; UBC'90; Dip SportMed; MD; BScPT; CCFP; FCFP; (604)687-5911; Fax. (604)687-3944.

COLLINS, Douglas B; Sunnidale Med Centre, 2 Friesen Pl, Barrie ON L4M 4S4; Tor'94; CCFP; FCFP; (705)726-6065; Fax. (705)733-9963.

COLLINS, Edmund W; Gander Med Clinic, 177 Elizabeth Dr, Gander NL A1V 1H6; Dal'71; FRCSC; Ophth (Medical & Surgical Ophthalmology). Staff, James Paton Memorial Hospital; (709)256-7852; Fax. (709)256-1929.

COLLINS, Evan J; Immunodefiency Clinic, 13n 1300-585 University Ave, Toronto ON M5G 2N2; McM'82; FRCPC; Psy. Staff, Centre for Addiction & Mental Health (CAMH) - Queen Site; Staff, Toronto General Hospital - UHN; Staff, Immunodefiency Clinic; Head Psy/Lecturer, University of Toronto; (416)340-5077; Fax. (416)340-4890.

COLLINS, Evelyn; Hotel-Dieu du Sacre-Coeur, 1 av du Sacre-Coeur, Quebec QC G1N 2W1; Laval'80; Staff, Jeffery Hale Hospital-Saint Brigid's; Staff, Hotel-Dieu du Sacre-Coeur de Jesus de Quebec; Université Laval; (418)529-6851

COLLINS, Genevieve; CSSS de la Mitis, 800 av du Sanatorium, Mont-Joli QC G5H 3L6; Laval'83; Staff, CSSS de la Mitis; (418)775-7261; Fax. (418)775-6487.

COLLINS, James A; 1-708 Reeves St, Port Hawkesbury NS B9A 2S1; Tor'75; CCFP; Med Advisor Diab Clin & Active Staff, Strait Richmond Hospital; Med Examiner, Inverness & Richmond Counties; Physician, Stora Enso Industries; Physician, Port Hawkesbury Nursing Home; (902)625-1452; Fax. (902)625-2320.

COLLINS, Jean-Pierre; Centre Med Pierrefonds, 208-12774 boul Gouin O, Pierrefonds QC H8Z 1W5; Mon'67; DAB; FAAD; FRCPC; Derm. (514)684-8460; Fax. (514)684-1348.

COLLINS, Jessica; Hamilton HS-McMaster Site, PO Box 2000 Stn Lcd 1 4E12-1200 Main St W, Hamilton ON L8N 3Z5; McG'07; MDCM; PlasSurg. Staff, Hamilton Health Sciences Centre - McMaster University Medical Centre; (905)521-2100

COLLINS, John A; 500 Raglan St N, Renfrew ON K7V 1P5; Qns'76; (613)432-5067

COLLINS, Margaret J; PO Box 276 Stn Main, Barrie ON L4M 4T2; McM'84.

COLLINS, Marisa B; 202-4380 Lorimer Rd, Whistler BC V0N 1B4; McM'88; MHSc; CCFP; FCFP; Clinical Asst Prof Family Practice, University of British Columbia; (604)932-3202; Fax. (604)932-6953; marguerite.olding@ubc.ca.

COLLINS, Micheline; 100 boul Saint-Joseph O, Montreal QC H2T 2P6; Mon'75; FRCPC; Derm. (514)271-2594; Fax. (514)271-8594.

COLLINS, Neil D; Foothills Med Centre, 1403 29 St NW, Calgary AB T2N 2T9; Cal'90; CCFP; CCFP(E.M.); Staff, Foothills Medical Centre; (403)944-1635

COLLINS, Nelson C; 941 Pandora Ave, Victoria BC V8V 3P4; Alb'89; FRCPC; Psy. Staff, Vernon Mental Health Centre; (250)519-5181

COLLINS, Paul H; Synergy Wellness Centre, 221-501 Bethel Dr, Sherwood Park AB T8H 0N2; Cal'96; BSc; CCFP; FCFP; (780)464-0123; Fax. (780)449-1062.

COLLINS, Paul J; The Surgeons Office, 236 Elm St, St Thomas ON N5R 1J5; Wes'99; FACS; BSc(Hon); FRCSC; GenSurg., St Thomas Elgin General Hospital; Aj Prof Surg, University of Western Ontario; (519)631-0567; Fax. (519)631-0921.

COLLINS, Peter I; Addiction & Mental Hlth-Colleg, 250 College St, Toronto ON M5T 1R8; McM'83; MCA; FRCPC; Psy (Forensic Psychiatry). Staff Forensic Psy Law & Mental Health Prog, Centre for Addiction & Mental Health (CAMH) - Queen Site; Staff, Centre for Addiction & Mental Health (CAMH) - College Street Site; Coord Forensic Psy Unit & Behavioural Sciences Section, Ontario Provincial Police; Commander, Royal Canadian Navy Reserve Health Services; Assoc Prof Psy & Forensic Psy, University of Toronto; (416)979-6847; peter_collins@camh.net.

COLLINS, Rhonda L; Garden City Family Health Team, 145 Carlton St, St Catharines ON L2R 1R5; McM'07; CCFP; (905)988-5126; Fax. (905)988-6209.

COLLINS, Ronald M; Kelowna Gen Hosp, 2268 Pandosy St, Kelowna BC V1Y 1T2; UBC'84; Anes. Staff, Kelowna General Hospital; (250)862-4309; Fax. (250)862-4298.

COLLINS, Ronald W; 11-262 Oxford St E, London ON N6A 1T8; Wes'82; CCFP; FCFP; (519)438-8339; Fax. (519)438-2236.

COLLINS, Samantha M; Fredericton Med Clinic, 304-1015 Regent St, Fredericton NB E3B 6H5; Cal'04; FRCSC; ObstGyn. (506)457-2113; Fax. (506)459-7079.

COLLINS, Sharon C; Renfrew Victoria Hosp, 3F-499 Raglan St N, Renfrew ON K7V 1P6; Ott'73; BA; FRCPC; IntMed (Cardiology). Staff, Renfrew Victoria Hospital; Langs: French; (613)432-8999; Fax. (613)432-9820.

COLLINS, Sophie; Quebec Physicians Hlth Program, 200-1 boul Rene-Levesque E, Montreal QC H2X 3Z5; Laval'99; FRCPC; Anes (Physician Health). Langs: English; Spanish; (514)397-0888; Fax. (514)397-0654; scollins@pamq.org.

COLLINS, Stephen M; Hamilton HS-McMaster Site, PO Box 2000 Stn Lcd 1 2E16-1200 Main St W, Hamilton ON L8N 3Z5; London (England)'71; MB BS; MRC(UK); FRCPC; IntMed. Head Gastroent Division & Prof, Hamilton Health Sciences Centre - McMaster Children's Hospital; Prof Med, McMaster University; (905)521-2100 x75255; Fax. (905)521-4958; scollins@mcmaster.ca.

COLLINS, Stephen; Fontbonne Bldg, 4F-301 James St S, Hamilton ON L8P 3B6; Stellenbosch (South Africa)'84; FRCPC; Psy (Anxiety Disorder). Staff, Hamilton Health Sciences Centre - McMaster University Medical Centre; Ac Staff, St Joseph's Healthcare - Charlton Campus; (905)522-1155; Fax. (905)540-6533; stcollin@mcmaster.ca.

COLLINS, Timothy R; Campbell Clinic, 430 Mayor Magrath Dr S, Lethbridge AB T1J 3M1; Pretoria (South Africa)'89; MB ChB; (403)328-8101; Fax. (403)328-8150.

COLLINS, Wayne B; Family Med Clinic, PO Box 1207 484-490 Main St, Lewisporte NL A0G 3A0; Mem'85; (709)535-8617; Fax. (709)535-0172.

COLLINS, William J; 100-5791 No. 3 Rd, Richmond BC V6X 2C9; UBC'99; FRCPC; DiagRad. (604)278-9151

COLLINS-WILLIAMS, Donald J; Summerville Family Health Team, 1221 Bloor St, Mississauga ON L4Y 2N8; Tor'76; CCFP; FCFP; Ac Staff, Trillium Health Centre - Mississauga; (905)625-1241; Fax. (905)625-9514.

COLLINSON, Kathleen M; University of Alberta Hosp, 1E6. 16WCM-8440 112 St NW, Edmonton AB T6G 2B7; Alb'82; FRCPC; Psy (Liaison). Staff, University of Alberta Hospital; (780)407-6566; Fax. (780)407-6672.

COLLIS, Ernest L; Torbay Med Clinic, B-1345 Torbay Rd, Torbay NL A1K 1B2; Mem'94; CCFP; (709)437-6402; Fax. (709)437-2755.

COLLISON, Linda M; Pediatric Adolescent Clinic, 102-200 Goulet St, Winnipeg MB R2H 0R8; Man'80; FRCPC; Peds. Staff, Health Sciences Centre.

COLLISON, Susan L; Pediatric Adolescent Clinic, 410-309 Hargrave St, Winnipeg MB R3B 2J8; Man'80; Peds. Ac Staff, Health Sciences Centre; Staff, St Boniface General Hospital; Staff, Victoria General Hospital.

COLLITON, Irene E; Heritage Med Clinic, 105-2841 109 St NW, Edmonton AB T6J 6B7; Alb'77; (780)436-3790; Fax. (780)434-8378.

COLLYER, Steven J; 166-2111 Main St, Penticton BC V2A 6W6; Qns'91; Staff, Penticton Regional Hospital; (250)276-5050; Fax. (250)276-5051.

COLMAN, Jack M; Mount Sinai Hosp, 1603-600 University Ave, Toronto ON M5G 1X5; Tor'67; FACC; FRCPC; Cardiol (Adult Congenital Heart Disease); IntMed. Staff Cardiol, Mount Sinai Hospital; Staff Cardiol, Toronto General Hospital - UHN; Consultant, Baycrest Centre for Geriatric Care; Consultant Cardiol, Sunnybrook Health Sciences Centre; Prof, University of Toronto; (416)586-5288; Fax. (416)586-5968; j.colman@utoronto.ca.

COLMAN, Laurence D; A-110 Queens Plate Dr, Etobicoke ON M9V 0B4; Wes'83; MBA; MSc; FRCSC; ObstGyn. Staff, William Osler Health System - Etobicoke General Hospital; (416)741-2552; Fax. (416)741-9729.

COLMAN, Neil C; MUHC-Montreal Gen Hosp, D7.201-1650 av Cedar, Montreal QC H3G 1A4; Tor'71; FRCPC; IntMed; Respir. Sr Physician, McGill University Health Centre - Montreal General Campus; assoc Prof, McGill University; Langs: Bilingual(English/French); (514)934-1934 x43598; Fax. (514)934-8226.

COLMAN, Rebecca E; Univ of Toronto-Div of Respiro, 6263-1 King's College Cir, Toronto ON M5S 1A8; Tor'08; IntMed. Teach Staff, University of Toronto; (416)978-1562

COLMEGNA, Ines; MUHC-Royal Victoria Hosp, M11 32-687 av des Pins O, Montreal QC H3A 1A1; (El Salvador)'94; Staff, McGill University Health Centre - Royal Victoria Hospital; (514)843-1578; Fax. (514)937-0803.

COLMENARES OTERO, Maria E; Southlake Reg Health Centre, 596 Davis Dr, Newmarket ON L3Y 2P9; Pontificia (Colombia)'83; FRCPC; Anes. Staff, Southlake Regional Health Centre; (905)895-4521

COLOHAN, Desmond P; The Boardwalk Prof Centre, 220 Water St, Charlottetown PE C1A 9M5; Dal'71; MHSc(Health Admin); FRCPC; EmergMed. Staff, Queen Elizabeth Hospital; (902)367-3344; Fax. (902)367-4114.

COLOMBINI, Linda M; Hôpital Ste-Justine, 3175 de la Cote-Sainte-Catheri, Montreal QC H3T 1C5; McG'90; FRCPC; Peds (Critical Care Medicine); Respir. Staff, Hôpital Ste-Justine; (514)345-4931

COLONNE, D D Prasannajith; Joseph Brant Community H C, 1182 North Shore Blvd E, Burlington ON L7S 1C5; U.of Colombo (Sri Lanka)'85; MRCPsy(UK); FRCPC; Psy. Staff, Joseph Brant Memorial Hospital; (905)631-0694; Fax. (905)631-5804.

COLORADO, J Robert; Glenridge Walk-In Clinic, 5-209 Glenridge Dr, St. Catharines ON L2T 3J6; UBC'96; BSc(Kinesiol); LMCC; CCFP; Staff, Niagara Health System - Welland Hospital Site; Staff, Niagara Health System - Ontario Street Site; Langs: Spanish; (289)362-5333; Fax. (289)362-5335.

COLP, Jeffrey N; Community Med Centre, 2273 Prospect Rd, Hatchet Lake NS B3T 1S9; Dal'92; (902)852-3090; Fax. (902)852-5108.

COLPITTS, Anne F; 101-435 Regent St, Fredericton NB E3B 3X6; Mem'95; CCFP; FCFP; (506)458-0233; Fax. (506)457-4760.

COLPITTS, Deanna K; Bridlewood Med Centre, 64 Stonehaven Dr, Kanata ON K2M 2Y2; Tor'92; (613)592-0805; Fax. (613)592-0961.

COLPITTS, Lorraine R; Grand River Hosp-Kitchener HC, PO Box 9056 Stn C 835 King St W, Kitchener ON N2G 1G3; Ott'10; CCFP; Staff, Grand River Hospital - Kitchener/Waterloo Health Centre; (519)749-4380

COLPITTS, Melanie H; Medical Arts Bldg, 17 Dunedin St, Orillia ON L3V 5T3; Qns'06; FRCPC; Peds. (705)327-9143; Fax. (705)327-9189.

COLPRON, Louise; CHUM-Hop Notre-Dame, M3211-1560 rue Sherbrooke E, Montreal QC H2L 4M1; Mon'73; Staff, Centre Hospitalier l'Université de Montréal (CHUM) - Hôpital Notre-Dame; (514)890-8000

COLQUHOUN, James T; Port Arthur Health Centre Inc, 194 Court St N, Thunder Bay ON P7A 4V7; Tor'51; Court Staff, Thunder Bay Regional Health Sciences Centre; Ac Staff, St Joseph's Care Group - St Joseph's Hospital; (807)346-1000; Fax. (807)346-6206.

COLQUHOUN, Patrick H D; London HSC-University Hosp, PO Box 5339 Stn B C8 128-339 Windermere Rd, London ON N6A 5A5; Sask'94; MSc; FACS; FASCRS; FRCSC; GenSurg (Colon & Rectal Surgery). Staff, London Health Sciences Centre - University Hospital; (519)663-3287

COLTER, Kimberley A; Dartmouth Gen Hosp, 325 Pleasant St, Dartmouth NS B2Y 4G8; Dal'94; FRCPC; DiagRad. Staff, Dartmouth General Hospital; (902)465-8318; Fax. (902)456-8360.

COLTON, Patricia A; Univ Hlth Network-Toronto Gen, 7ES 409-200 Elizabeth St, Toronto ON M5G 2C4; Tor'96; FRCPC; Psy. Affil Scientist, Toronto General Hospital - UHN; (416)340-3477; p.colton@utoronto.ca.

COLVIN, Rolland G; Albion Med Group, 304-1525 Albion Rd, Etobicoke ON M9V 5G5; Glasgow (Scotland)'66; (416)741-1622; Fax. (416)741-2884.

COLWELL, Bruce D O; Queen Elizabeth II HSC, 455-1276 South Park St, Halifax NS B3H 2Y9; Dal'87; FRCP; BSc; FRCPC; IntMed (Colorectal Cancer); MedOncol. Staff Nova Scotia Cancer Centre, Queen Elizabeth II Health Sciences Centre - Victoria General Site; Assoc Prof Med, Dalhousie University; (902)473-6019; Fax. (902)473-6186; bruce.colwell@cdha.nshealth.ca.

COLWELL, J Randolph; South Shore Reg Hosp, 90 Glen Allan Dr, Bridgewater NS B4V 3S6; Dal'97; CCFP; CCFP(E.M.); Staff, South Shore Regional Hospital; (902)543-4603

COLWELL, Katie; 115 16th St W, North Vancouver BC V7M 1T3; Sask'09; CCFP; (604)904-8804

COLWELL, Robin L; Royal University Hosp, 103 Hospital Dr, Saskatoon SK S7N 0W8; Staff, Royal University Hospital; (306)655-1000

COLWELL, Sarah J; The Moncton Hosp, 135 MacBeath Ave, Moncton NB E1C 6Z8; Dal'93; FRCPC; AnatPath. Staff, The Moncton Hospital; (506)857-5315; dr.sarah.colwell@horizonnb.ca.

COLWILL, Richard W; Medical Centre, B2206-3000 Lawrence Ave E, Scarborough ON M1P 2V1; Tor'87; PhD; BSc; FRCPC; IntMed (Medical Oncology); Hem. Ac Staff, The Scarborough Hospital - General Campus; (416)439-5866; Fax. (416)439-8776.

COMA, Aaron L; Family Medical Center, 2931 20 Ave S, Lethbridge AB T1K 3M5; Cal'04; CCFP; (403)328-2326; Fax. (403)327-0123.

COMAMALA TORRES, Marina; Clin de Med Familiale 24 Juin, 105-1055 12e av N, Sherbrooke QC J1E 2X4; (Other Foreign)'09; CCFP; (819)821-2142

COMAN-WOOD, Lori R; 333 Lakeshore Rd W, Mississauga ON L5H 1G9; Qns'87; Staff, The Credit Valley Hospital; Langs: Sign Language; (905)274-7055; Fax. (905)274-6580.

COMANITA, Petru; Ctr Hosp de Verdun, 4000 boul Lasalle, Verdun QC H4G 2A3; Bucharest (Romania)'00; FRCPC; IntMed; Gastroent. Staff, Centre Hospitalier de Verdun; (514)362-1000

COMAY, Daniel C; Burlington Prof Centre, 314-3155 Harvester Rd, Burlington ON L7N 3V2; Tor'99; FRCPC; IntMed (Gastroenterology); Gastroent. (905)681-2036; Fax. (905)681-3740.

COMAY, Stephen A; Sheppard Med Bldg, 214-701 Sheppard Ave E, North York ON M2K 2Z3; Cape Town (South Africa)'68; MB ChB; FRCPC; Peds (Pediatric Hematology). Assoc Staff, North York General Hospital; Consultant, Rouge Valley Health System - Centenary Health Centre Site; University of Toronto; University of Western Ontario; (416)222-6011; Fax. (416)222-6706.

COMAY, Susan E; Pine Free Clinic, 1985 4th Ave W, Vancouver BC V6J 1M7; Cape Town (South Africa)'73; MB BS; (604)733-3525; Fax. (604)731-9479; susan.comay@vch.ca.

COMBDEN, Steven; Killick Health Services, 54 Union St, Grnd-Falls-Windsor NL A2A 2E2; Mem'02; CCFP; CCFP(E.M.); Staff, Health Sciences Centre; (709)292-8400

COMBRINCK, Nantes; Border City Clinic, 2707 50 Ave, Lloydminster SK S9V 2A8; Pretoria (South Africa)'00; MB ChB; (306)825-4427; Fax. (306)825-2028.

COMEAU, Alban L; PO Box 70, Saulnierville NS B0W 2Z0; Dal'78; Staff/Treating Physician South West Health Chronic Pain Prog, Yarmouth Regional Hospital; Langs: Bilingual(English/French); (902)769-3888; Fax. (902)769-3868.

COMEAU, B Keith; Fairview Med Arts Centre, 102-2200 Fairview St, Burlington ON L7R 4H9; McM'83; CCFP; Staff, Hamilton Health Sciences Centre - McMaster Children's Hospital; (905)333-0116

COMEAU, Benjamin M; Queensway Carleton Hosp, 3045 Baseline Rd, Ottawa ON K2H 8P4; Tor'06; CCFP; CCFP(E.M.); Staff, Peterborough Regional Health Centre - Hospital Drive; Staff, Queensway Carleton Hospital; (613)721-4710

COMEAU, Diane; CLSC Rimouski, 165 rue des Gouverneurs, Rimouski QC G5L 7R2; Mon'85; Staff, Hôpital Regional Rimouski; (418)723-1222

COMEAU, Emilie; CHUS-Hop Hotel-Dieu, 580 rue Bowen S, Sherbrooke QC J1G 2E8; Sher'97; FRCSC; GenSurg. Staff, Centre Hospitalier Universitaire de Sherbrooke-Hôpital Hôtel-Dieu; (819)346-1110 x23116

COMEAU, Eve-Lyne; Ctr Hosp Affilie-St-Sacrement, 1050 ch Sainte-Foy, Quebec QC G1S 4L8; Laval'07; Gastroent (P.Q.); IntMed. Staff, Centre Hospitalier Affilié Universitaire de Québec - Hôpital du St-Sacrement; (418)682-7511

COMEAU, Gisele M; 495 40th Ave W, Vancouver BC V5Y 2R5; Dal'80; (604)321-6787; Fax. (604)321-6722.

COMEAU, Laurel A; Millidge Place, 723 Millidge Ave, Saint John NB E2K 2N7; Dal'97; BSc; BEd; CCFP; FCFP; Staff, Saint John Regional Hospital; Dalhousie University; Memorial University Of Newfoundland; (506)634-6870; Fax. (506)634-6851; lpcomeau@nbnet.nb.ca.

COMEAU, Lise; Ctr Hosp Reg de Lanaudiere, 1000 boul Sainte-Anne, St-Charles-Brromee QC J6E 6J2; Mon'85; CSPQ; FRCPC; AnatPath. Staff, Centre Hospitalier Régional de Lanaudière; (450)759-8222

COMEAU, Louise M; Clin Med Obesite Pte-aux-Tembl, 201-12905 rue Sherbrooke E, Pte-aux-Trembles QC H1A 1B9; Sher'78; Langs: English; (514)642-6946; Fax. (514)642-2321; dr.louise.comeau@videotron.ca.

COMEAU, Margery; 210-1255 Greene Ave, Westmount QC H3Z 2A4; Auckland (New Zealand)'78; (514)483-2083

COMEAU, Marie-Josee; CSSSG-Hop de Hull, 116 boul Lionel-Emond, Gatineau QC J8Y 1W7; Ott'89; CCFP; FCFP; Staff, Hull Hospital; (819)595-6042

COMEAU, Nathalie; Clinique Med Mercier, 101-464 boul Saint-Jean-Baptis, Mercier QC J6R 2B1; Mon'95; Staff, Hôpital Anna-Laberge; Langs: English; (450)699-0539; Fax. (450)699-8438.

COMEAU, Paulette; Parkland Med Clinic, 6-5030 47 Ave, Red Deer AB T4N 3P7; Alb'75; Physician, Central Zone David Thompson Health Region; Langs: Spanish; (403)346-4206; Fax. (403)346-4207.

COMEAU, Raymond R; 70 Hewlett Park Landing, Red Deer County AB T4S 2J3; Alb'80; BMedSci; CCFP; Staff, Red Deer Regional Hospital Centre; (403)887-0510; Fax. (403)887-0520.

COMEAU, Reginald; CSSS de Laval, SS62-1755 boul Rene-Laennec, Laval QC H7M 3L9; Mon'02; FRCPC; IntMed; MedOncol; Hem. Staff, Hopital de la Cite de la santé; (450)431-8200

COMEAU, Scott M; West Community Health Centre, 241-2121 Marine Dr, West Vancouver BC V7V 4Y2; UBC'95; FRCPC; IntMed (Dementia); GeriatricMed. Staff, Lions Gate Hospital; (604)904-6200 x4112

COMEAU, Terrance B W; Saint John Reg Hosp, PO Box 2100 Stn Main 400 University Ave, Saint John NB E2L 4L2; Dal'89; FRCPC; IntMed; Hem. Staff, Saint John Regional Hospital; (506)648-7891; Fax. (506)638-2345.

COMEAU, Tina; 105-140 rue Champlain, Dieppe NB E1A 1N8; Laval'03; FRCSC; GenSurg. Staff, Dr Georges-L-Dumont University Hospital Centre; Langs: Bilingual(French/English).

COMERFORD, Carrie A; Workplace Health Safety, PO Box 9000 Stn A 146-148 Forest Rd, St. John's NL A1A 1E6; Mem'92; (709)778-1364

COMERFORD, Mary L; Peterborough Clinic, 1F-26 Hospital Dr, Peterborough ON K9J 7C3; McG'97; CCFP; Asst Surg, Peterborough Regional Health Centre - Hospital Drive; (705)743-2040; Fax. (705)743-4392.

COMERFORD, Thomas A; The Medical Centre, PO Box 4200 Stn Main 707 Charlotte St, Peterborough ON K9J 7B3; Ott'66; DAB; FRCPC; Peds (Clinical Immunology & Allergy). Staff, Peterborough Regional Health Centre - Hospital Drive; Staff, Peterborough Regional Health Centre - Rogers St Site; (705)876-4501; Fax. (705)743-0752.

COMERTON, Aileen; 605-267 O'Connor St, Ottawa ON K2P 1V3; Ott'81; PhD; CCFP; FCFP; Staff, The Ottawa Hospital - Civic Campus; Staff, Children's Hospital of Eastern Ontario (CHEO); (613)236-7183; Fax. (613)567-4299.

COMERTON, Mary E; 210-194 Main St, Ottawa ON K1S 1C2; Ott'81; BSc(Hon); MSc; CCFP; FCFP; (613)230-6388; Fax. (613)234-2108.

COMETTE, Melissa J; Grey Bruc HS-Owen Sound, PO Box 1800 Stn Main 8221-1800 8th St E, Owen Sound ON N4K 6M9; Dal'01; FRCSC; ObstGyn. Staff, Grey Bruce Health Services - Owen Sound; (519)372-2500; Fax. (519)372-1005.

COMEY, Robert; UBC Hosp, 6285-2211 Wesbrook Mall, Vancouver BC V6T 2B5; Cal'04; FRCPC; Psy. Staff, UBC Hospital - Koerner Pavillion; (604)822-7121

COMISAROW, Richard H; 404-960 Lawrence Ave W, North York ON M6A 3B5; Alb'68; FACS; FRCSC; Urol. Staff Urol, Humber River Regional Hospital - Church Street Site; (416)256-7473; Fax. (416)256-7535.

COMLEY, Rebecca A; Brant Community HC-Brantford, 200 Terrace Hill St, Brantford ON N3R 1G9; McM'99; CCFP; CCFP(E.M.); Staff, The Brant Community Healthcare System - Brantford General Hospital Site; (519)752-7871

COMM, D Glenn; Peter Lougheed Hosp, 3500 26 Ave NE, Calgary AB T1Y 6J4; Loma Linda (USA)'79; Anes. Staff, Peter Lougheed Centre; University of Calgary; (403)943-4555; glenncomm@shaw.ca.

COMMERFORD, Kathleen C; Ladner Centre Medical, 5132 Ladner Trunk Rd, Delta BC V4K 1W3; Cape Town (South Africa)'74; MB ChB; (604)940-0917

COMMON, Andrew A; St Michael's Hosp, 30 Bond St, Toronto ON M5B 1W8; McG'80; FAB; FRCPC; DiagRad. Chief Medical Imaging, St Michael's Hospital; (416)864-5680; Fax. (416)864-5380.

COMMONS, Amiya S; Montfort Hosp, 713 Montreal Rd, Ottawa ON K1K 0T2; Ott'85; FRCPC; AnatPath. Staff, Montfort Hospital; Staff, The Ottawa Hospital - General Campus; Asst Prof, University of Ottawa; (613)746-4621

COMPAGNA, Thomas; Lions Gate Hosp, 231 15th St E, North Vancouver BC V7L 2L7; Alb'86; CCFP; CCFP(E.M.); Staff, Lions Gate Hospital; (604)984-5813

COMPEAU, Christopher G; St Joseph's Health Centre, SSW214-30 The Queensway, Toronto ON M6R 1B5; Tor'88; MSc; FRCSC; GenSurg; ThorSurg. Staff Surgeon, Humber River Regional Hospital - Finch Avenue Site; Pres Medical Staff, St Joseph's Health Centre; Asst Prof, University of Toronto; (416)530-6530; Fax. (416)530-6529.

COMPERA-ROUAUD, Claire; CSSS de la Mitis, 800 av du Sanatorium, Mont-Joli QC G5H 3L6; Sher'08; Staff, CSSS de la Mitis; (418)775-7261

COMPTON, Amanda Y D; Family First Medical, 207-496 Topsail Rd, St. John's NL A1E 2C2; Mem'07; CCFP.

COMSTOCK, Ravneet; The Moncton Hosp, 135 MacBeath Ave, Moncton NB E1C 6Z8; Sask'99; CCFP; Staff, The Moncton Hospital; (506)857-5111

COMSTOCK, Sean A; 414-100 Arden St, Moncton NB E1C 4B7; Dal'98; FRCSC; OrthSurg. Staff, The Moncton Hospital.

COMTE, Pierre; Polyclinique d'Argenteuil, 201-551 rue Berry, Lachute QC J8H 1S4; Mon'84; CSPQ; DCH; Peds (P.Q.) (Attention Deficit). Pediatrics, Centre Hospitalier d'Argenteuil; Med Consultant, CLSC de Saint-Jerome; Langs: Bilingual(English/French); (450)562-3751; Fax. (450)562-1852; pierre_comte@cdsj.org.

COMTOIS, Amelie; 6550 av Louis-Hébert, Montreal QC H2G 2G7; Mon'10.

COMTOIS, Andre; Hotel-Dieu de Sorel, 400 av de l'Hotel-Dieu, Sorel-Tracy QC J3P 1N5; Mon'74; FRCSC; GenSurg (Thoracic). Staff, Hôtel-Dieu de Sorel; (450)746-6000; Fax. (450)746-8594; andrecomtois@acomtois.com.

COMTOIS, Hubert; CSSS de Laval, 1755 boul Rene-Laennec, Laval QC H7M 3L9; Laval'92; CSPQ; FRCPC; IntMed; Cardiol. Staff, Hopital de la Cite de la santé; (450)668-1010; Fax. (450)975-5550.

COMTOIS, J Jean-Marc; Canadian Space Agency, 6767 Rte de l'Aéroport, Saint-Hubert QC J3Y 8Y9; Wes'85; Dir Astronauts Space Life Scieces and Medicine, Canadian Space Agency; (450)926-4755; Fax. (450)926-4707.

COMTOIS, Luc; Clinique Med Rock Forest, 1-4870 boul Bourque, Sherbrooke QC J1N 3S5; Sher'86; (819)820-2673

COMTOIS, Pierre; Clinique Domus Medica, 414-5601 rue Belanger, Montreal QC H1T 1G3; Mon'73; Staff, Hôpital Santa Cabrini Ospedale; (514)256-5011

COMTOIS, Pierre; CSSS de Saint-Jerome, 290 rue de Montigny, Saint-Jerome QC J7Z 5T3; Sher'81; Psy (P.Q.). Staff, Hôtel-Dieu de Saint-Jérôme; (450)431-8200; Fax. (450)431-8207.

COMTOIS, Pierre; Coop Sante Ferme-Neuve, RR 1 70 12e rue, Ferme-Neuve QC J0W 1C0; Mon'85; (819)587-2587

COMTOIS, Robert; CSSS du Nord de Lanaudière, 1000 boul Sainte-Anne, St-Charles-Brromee QC J6E 6J2; Mon'65; FRCPC; HemPath (Hematological Oncology); Hem (P.Q.); MedOncol (P.Q.). Staff, Centre Hospitalier Régional de Lanaudière; (450)759-8222 x4065; Fax. (450)759-7861.

COMTOIS, Ronald; CHUM-Hop Notre-Dame, 1560 rue Sherbrooke E, Montreal QC H2L 4M1; Mon'76; Endocrin (P.Q.). Staff, Centre Hospitalier l'Université de Montréal (CHUM) - Hôpital Notre-Dame; (514)890-8000 x26805

CONACHER, G Neil; PCCC-Mental Health Services, 525 Montreal St, Kingston ON K7K 3H9; Dundee (Scotland)'78; MB ChB; MRCPsy(UK); FRCPC; Psy (Schizophrenia). Psychiatrist, Providence Care - Mental Health Services; Aj Associate Prof Psy, Queen's University; (613)540-6166 x4124; Fax. (613)540-6169.

CONACHER, Heather J; Knox Manse, 505 4th Ave N, Saskatoon SK S7K 2M5; Sask'93; BScAgriculture; FRCPC; CCFP; Psy. Staff Psychiatry, Royal University Hospital; (306)668-0508

CONCANNON, Michael J; Vernon Jubilee Hosp, 2101 32 St, Vernon BC V1T 5L2; McG'97; CCFP; CCFP(E.M.); FCFP; Staff, Vernon Jubilee Hospital; (250)545-2211; Fax. (250)558-1367.

CONCHIE, Robert M; Plaza 33, PO Box 23122 Rpo Plaza 33, Kelowna BC V1X 7K7; UBC'87; CCFP; CCFP(E.M.); Staff, Kelowna General Hospital; (250)765-5500

CONDE, Jean-Joseph; Clinique Familiale des Pins, 1019 boul des Pins, Val-d'Or QC J9P 4T2; Mon'86; Staff, Centre Hospitalier de Val d'Or; (819)825-8464; Fax. (819)825-1335.

CONDELLO, Adriana S; 212-284 Helmcken Rd, Victoria BC V9B 1T2; Man'01; FRCPC; Peds; PedEmergMed. (250)881-7347

CONDON, Amanda J S; River East Health Access Ctre, 975 Henderson Hwy, Winnipeg MB R2K 4L7; Man'06; CCFP; (204)938-5000

CONDON, Caroline D; Kerrisdale Station Med Clinic, 2077 42nd Ave W, Vancouver BC V6M 2B4; Liverpool (England)'72; DOphth; Clinical Asst Prof, University of British Columbia; (604)261-9494; Fax. (604)261-9405.

CONDON, Elana M; The Ottawa Hosp-Gen Campus, 501 Smyth Rd, Ottawa ON K1H 8L6; Mem'97; CCFP; FCFP; Staff, The Ottawa Hospital - General Campus; (613)737-6111; Fax. (613)737-8470.

CONDON, Richard A; 1-226 Harwood Ave S, Ajax ON L1S 2H6; National U. of Ire., U. College Cork; MB BCh; BAO; DObst; LMCC; DipA.B.H.P.M.; (905)683-8171; Fax. (905)683-8609.

CONDRUT, George M; Medteam Clinic, 103-99 Kakulu Rd, Kanata ON K2L 3C8; Wes'04; (613)592-1448

CONE, Richard L; The Medicine Cabinet, 2-3188 Barons Rd, Nanaimo BC V9T 4B5; Alb'78; CCFP; (250)751-7850

CONEYS, Marcus C D; Anesthetic Services, 213-2186 Oak Bay, Victoria BC V8R 1G3; LRCS (Ireland)'74; LRCP(Ire); LRCS(Ire); FRCPC; Anes (Pain Management). (250)595-7211

CONEYS, T David; PO Box 279, Lafleche SK S0H 2K0; Dublin (Ireland)'73; Staff, St Joseph's Hospital/Foyer d'Youville; Lafleche & District Health Centre; (306)472-5444; Fax. (306)472-5999.

CONG, Huong; MUHC-Montreal Gen Hosp, D10 144-1650 av Cedar, Montreal QC H3G 1A4; Mon'07; Anes (P.Q.). Staff, McGill University Health Centre - Montreal General Campus; (514)934-1934

CONGDON, Valerie M; Foothills Family Med Centre, PO Box 460 114 1 St SW, Black Diamond AB T0L 0H0; Cal'77; CCFP; (403)933-4368; Fax. (403)933-2026.

CONGLY, Stephen E; Health Research Innovation Ctr, 6F-3280 Hospital Dr NW, Calgary AB T2N 4Z6; Alb'06; FRCPC; IntMed; Gastroent. Physician, Health Research Innovation Centre; (403)592-5020; Fax. (403)592-5090.

CONGRAM, Sandra P; 150 Derenzy Place, Penticton BC V2A 8W7; Alb'76; Staff, Penticton Regional Hospital; (250)493-5745

CONKLIN, Robert J; 203-7031 Westminster Hwy, Richmond BC V6X 1A3; Man'69; FRCPC; Derm. Consultant, Richmond Hospital; Clin Assoc Prof, University of British Columbia; (604)273-6929

CONLEY, Douglas W; Hillsdale Terrace, 600 Oshawa Blvd N, Oshawa ON L1G 5T9; Qns'71; CCFP; FCFP; Staff, Lakeridge Health - Oshawa Site; (905)579-3313

CONLIN, Anne; The Medical Centre FHT, Ol Box 4200 Stn Main 707 Charlotte St, Peterborough ON K9J 7B3; Wes'05; FRCSC; Otol. (705)745-7607; Fax. (705)745-8679.

CONLON, M Ronan; Midwest Eye Care Institute, 341-750 Spadina Cres E, Saskatoon SK S7K 3H3; RCS (Ireland)'87; MB ChB; FRCSC; Ophth (Cataract). Clinical Asst Prof, University of Saskatchewan; (306)244-4111; Fax. (306)244-9904; mrconlon@sasktel.net.

CONLON, Patrick S J; Alexandra Marine & Gen Hosp, 120 Napier St, Goderich ON N7A 1W5; RCS (Ireland)'82; FRCPC; Psy. Chief Psy/Chief Medical Staff, Alexandra Marine & General Hospital; University of Western Ontario; (519)524-8323; Fax. (519)524-2745; dr.patrick.conlon@amgh.on.ca.

CONLY, Carly A; Bowmont Med Clinic, 6535 Bowness Rd NW, Calgary AB T3B 0E8; Sask'06; CCFP; (403)247-9797; Fax. (403)247-0014.

CONLY, John M; Foothills Med Centre, AGW5-1403 29 St NW, Calgary AB T2N 2T9; Sask'78; FRCPC; IntMed (AIDS/HIV); InfectDis. Staff, Foothills Medical Centre; Dept Head Med, University of Calgary; (403)944-8090; Fax. (403)944-2134.

CONLY, Maureen; Plaza 15 Family Practice, 100-145 15th St W, North Vancouver BC V7M 1R9; UBC'93; BSc; CCFP; Clin Instructor, University of British Columbia; (604)983-9832; Fax. (604)983-9842.

CONN, David K; Baycrest Ctre/Geriatric Care, 3560 Bathurst St, North York ON M6A 2E1; Dublin (Ireland)'76; MB ChB; BAO; FRCPC; Psy (Geriatric Psychiatry). Staff, Baycrest Centre for Geriatric Care; Staff, Mount Sinai Hospital; Assoc Prof, University of Toronto; (416)785-2456; Fax. (416)785-2450; dconn@baycrest.org.

CONN, Garson S; 315-340 College St, Toronto ON M5T 3A9; Tor'58; FAAOS; FRCSC; OrthSurg. Hon Staff, Toronto Rehabilitation Institute - University Centre; Hon Staff OrthSurg, Toronto Western Hospital - University Health Network; (416)929-5797; Fax. (416)929-9521.

CONN, Robert D; Smartrisk, 1901-400 University Avenue, Toronto ON M5G 1S5; UBC'82; FRCSC; Cardiovasc&ThorSurg. (416)597-3630; Fax. (416)595-9778; rconn@sympatico.ca.

CONNELL, Amanda E; West Carleton Family Health Te, 119 Langstaff Dr, Carp ON K0A 1L0; Ott'97; CCFP; (613)839-3271; Fax. (613)839-3273.

CONNELL, Cathy A; Dalhousie Univ Health Services, 1459 Oxford St, Halifax NS B3H 4R2; Dal'87; CCFP; FCFP; Ac Staff, IWK Health Centre; (902)494-2171; Fax. (902)494-6872; cconnell@eastlink.ca.

CONNELL, Douglas G; Victoria Gen Hosp, 1 Hospital Way, Victoria BC V8Z 6R5; Wes'73; FRCPC; DiagRad. Staff, Victoria General Hospital; (250)727-4208; Fax. (250)727-4290.

CONNELL, Ian D; 102-8584 Granville St, Vancouver BC V6P 4Z7; Tor'74; CCBOM; Consultant OccupMed, Vancouver Coastal Health; (604)266-1496; Fax. (604)266-9011; ianconnell@telus.net.

CONNELL, Norah D; Harbourview Med Clinic, 5-35 Bridge St, Picton ON K0K 2T0; Qns'74; Ac Staff, QHC Prince Edward County Memorial; (613)476-5536; Fax. (613)476-1583.

CONNELL, Stephen L; 277 Deer Rock Lake Rd RR 1, Flinton ON K0H 1P0; Auckland (New Zealand)'79; MB ChB; FRCPC; Psy (Child & Adolescent Psychiatry). (613)336-0927; Fax. (613)336-0715.

CONNELLY, Anne Marie; St Paul Family Hlth Organizati, 119-99 Wayne Gretzky Pky, Brantford ON N3S 6T6; McM'95; CCFP; FCFP; Staff, The Brant Community Healthcare System - Brantford General Hospital Site; (519)756-6400; Fax. (519)756-7343.

CONNELLY, Brendan B; 2-832 March Rd, Kanata ON K2W 0C9; Ott'02; CCFP; Lecturer Family Med, University of Ottawa; (613)599-5599; Fax. (613)599-1005.

CONNELLY, Ian H; Elora Medical Group, 71 James St, Elora ON N0B 1S0; Tor'97; CCFP; (519)846-5345

CONNELLY, Kerry L; Grey Bruce HS-Owen Sound, PO Box 1800 Stn Main 1800 8th St E, Owen Sound ON N4K 6M9; Tor'80; Staff, Grey Bruce Health Services - Owen Sound; (519)376-2121

CONNELLY, Kim A; St Michael's Hosp, QW-30 Bond St, Toronto ON M5B 1W8; Melbourne (Australia)'95; Clin Scientist, St Michael's Hospital; Asst Prof Med, University of Toronto; (416)864-5271

CONNELLY, Michael S; Peter Lougheed Centre, 3500 26 Ave NE, Calgary AB T1Y 6J4; London (England)'84; MB BS; BSc; MRC(Lond); Staff, Peter Lougheed Centre; Assoc Prof, University of Calgary; (403)943-4960; Fax. (403)250-9539.

CONNELLY, Paul J J; The Ottawa Hosp-Gen Campus, 501 Smyth Rd, Ottawa ON K1H 8L6; Tor'81; Anes. Staff, The Ottawa Hospital - General Campus; Teach Staff Anes, University of Ottawa; (613)737-8187; Fax. (613)737-8189; pconnelly@ottawahospital.on.ca.

CONNELLY, Peter; Holy Family Nursing Home, 165 Aberdeen Ave, Winnipeg MB R2W 1T9; Glasgow (Scotland)'56; CCFP; FCFP; Physician, Holy Family Nursing Home.

CONNELLY, Robert J; Kingston Gen Hosp, W3-76 Stuart St, Kingston ON K7L 2V7; Tor'90; MD; FRCPC; Peds (Neonatal & Perinatal Medicine). Med Dir NICU, Kingston General Hospital; (613)548-7766; Fax. (613)548-1369; connellr@kgh.kari.net.

CONNELLY, Ruth A; Harborn Med Associates, 510-89 Queensway W, Mississauga ON L5B 2V2; Tor'82; CCFP; (905)273-4380; Fax. (905)273-4335.

CONNELY, C Andrew; Medical Clinic, 10 Av Du Rocher, Edmundston NB E3V 4C6; Mem'83; Staff, Hôpital regional d'Edmundston; Langs: Bilingual(English/French); (506)739-6313; Fax. (506)735-7554.

CONNER, William T; 302A-200 James St S, Hamilton ON L8P 3A9; London (England)'66; MB BS; MRCP; DCH; FRCPC; Peds. Staff, Hamilton Health Sciences Centre - McMaster Children's Hospital; Staff Consultant, West Haldimand General Hospital; Clin Assoc Prof, McMaster University; Langs: Bilingual(English/French); (905)523-0531; Fax. (905)523-0871; connerw@mcmaster.ca.

CONNERS, Jennifer A; Burlington Walk In Clinic, 183-2025 Guelph Line, Burlington ON L7P 4M8; McM'80; (905)681-7755

CONNERS, John S; 185 Inkerman St E, Listowel ON N4W 2N1; Qns'64; Ac Staff, Listowel Memorial Hospital - Listowel Wingham Hospitals Alliance; (519)291-4200; Fax. (519)291-5947; conners@wightman.ca.

CONNERY, Mervin A; 372 Dundas St W, Napanee ON K7R 2B6; Qns'63; Hon Staff, Lennox & Addington County General Hospital; (613)354-5943; Fax. (613)389-6615.

CONNICK, Carol D; Misericordia Community Hosp, 16940 87 Ave NW, Edmonton AB T5R 4H5; Alb'90; Staff Professional Health Coach, Covenant Health - Misericordia Community Hospital; (780)481-7096; Fax. (780)481-2319; cconnick@telus.net.

CONNICK, Patricia L; Calgary Refugee Health Program, 23 McDougall Crt NE, Calgary AB T2E 8R3; Cal'93; CCFP; FCFP; (403)265-3410; Fax. (403)265-3411.

CONNIDIS, Stephanie A; Queen Elizabeth II HSC-Halifax, 8. 4-1796 Summer St, Halifax NS B3H 3A7; McM'88; BSc(Hons); MD; RACGP; HCOE; Staff, Queen Elizabeth II Health Sciences Centre - Halifax Infirmary Site; Medical Staff Family Med Transitional Care Unit, Queen Elizabeth II Health Sciences Centre - Victoria General Site; (902)473-6651; Fax. (902)473-4101.

CONNOLLY, Allan K; Grandview Woodlands Mht, 310-1669 Broadway E, Vancouver BC V5N 1V9; Tor'68; BPHE; (604)251-2264; Fax. (604)253-4280; allan.connolly@vcn.ca.

CONNOLLY, Bairbre L; The Hosp for Sick Children, 555 University Ave, Toronto ON M5G 1X8; Dublin (Ireland)'78; MB ChB; MCh; FRCS; FFR(RCSI); FRCPC; DiagRad (Pediatric Radiology). Staff Ped Radiol, The Hospital For Sick Children; (416)813-6034; bairbre.connolly@sickkids.ca.

CONNOLLY, Barbara S; Univ Hlth Network-Toronto Western Hosp, MCL7 43-399 Bathurst St, Toronto ON M5T 2S8; Wes'06; FRCPC; Neur. Staff, Toronto Western Hospital - University Health Network; Staff, Movement Disorder Research Centre; Staff, McGill Centre for Studies in Aging & Brain Bank; (416)603-6422

CONNOLLY, Julie A M; 1-2120 Regent St, Sudbury ON P3E 3Z9; McG'00; CCFP; (705)671-3011

CONNOLLY, Mary B C; Children's & Women's HC of BC, K3 179-4480 Oak St, Vancouver BC V6H 3V4; Dublin (Ireland)'81; MB ChB; BAO; FRCPC; Neur. Staff, BC Children's Hospital; (604)875-2121; Fax. (604)875-2285.

CONNOLLY, Mary C C; Victoria Mental Health Centre, 2328 Trent St, Victoria BC V8R 4Z3; National (Ireland)'72; MB ChB; BAO; FRCPC; Psy. (250)370-8155

CONNOLLY, Stephen H; Saint John Reg Hosp, PO Box 2100 Stn Main 400 University Ave, Saint John NB E2L 4L2; Dal'93; BSc; FRCSC; OrthSurg (Joint Arthroplasty). Staff, Saint John Regional Hospital; (506)648-6485; Fax. (506)648-6486.

CONNOLLY, Stuart J; Hamilton HS-General Site, C3 204-237 Barton St E, Hamilton ON L8L 2X2; McG'77; FRCPC; Cardiol (Clinical Electro Physiology). Ac Staff, Hamilton Health Sciences Centre - Hamilton General Hospital; Prof, McMaster University; Langs: English; French; (905)527-4322 x44563; Fax. (905)523-9165; connostu@hhsc.ca.

CONNOLLY, Thomas P; 401-2020 Richmond Ave, Victoria BC V8R 6R5; National U. (Ireland)'70; MB ChB; BAO; FRCPC; IntMed (Sleep Medicine); Respir. (250)370-9920; Fax. (250)370-9924.

CONNOLLY, Trevor W; Penticton Reg Hosp, 550 Carmi Ave, Penticton BC V2A 3G6; Sask'01; CCFP; CCFP(E.M.); Staff, Penticton Regional Hospital; (250)492-4000

CONNOLLY, W Edward S; 107-5165 rue Sherbrooke O, Montreal QC H4A 1T6; McG'75; Ophth (Cataract Surgery). Staff Consultant, Kateri Memorial Hospital Centre; Consultant staff Ophth, St Mary's Hospital Centre; assoc Prof, McGill University; Langs: Bilingual(English/French); (514)489-4911; Fax. (514)369-3088.

CONNOR, Calvin W; Amherstview Med Centre, 18 Manitou Cres W, Amherstview ON K7N 1S3; Qns'66; Court Staff, Kingston General Hospital; Physician Student Health Centre, St Lawrence College; (613)389-1604; Fax. (613)384-7359; cconnor@sl.on.ca.

CONNOR, David D; Manitoba Clinic, 790 Sherbrook St, Winnipeg MB R3A 1M3; Man'74; FRCPC; Peds. Staff Children's Hosp, Health Sciences Centre; Asst Prof, University of Manitoba; (204)788-5749; Fax. (204)772-2537.

CONNOR, Graham T; St Boniface Gen Hosp, 409 Tache Ave, Winnipeg MB R2H 2A6; Man'78; DAB; Staff, St Boniface General Hospital; Assoc Prof, University of Manitoba; (204)237-2260; Fax. (204)237-2268.

CONNOR, Marla E; Dewdney Medical, B-22195 Dewdney Trunk Rd, Maple Ridge BC V2X 3H7; UBC'91; (604)463-4102; Fax. (604)463-4686.

CONNOR, Steven A; Northumberland Travel Hlth Ctr, 202-1005 Elgin St W, Cobourg ON K9A 5J4; Dal'82; DTM; Langs: English; French; (905)373-0220; Fax. (905)373-7447.

CONNORS, Gregory; Health Research Innovation Ctr, 100-3280 Hospital Dr NW, Calgary AB T2N 4N1; Mem'83; FRCSC; ObstGyn (Obstetric Ultrasound). Staff, Health Research Innovation Centre; Assoc Prof ObstGyn, University of Calgary; (403)289-9269

CONNORS, Joseph M; BC Cancer Agency-Vancouver CC, 4431-600 10th Ave W, Vancouver BC V5Z 4E6; Yale(CT) (USA)'73; ABIM; FRCPC; IntMed (Hematology). Staff, Vancouver General Hospital - Centennial Pavillion; Clin Prof, University of British Columbia; (604)877-6000 x2746; Fax. (604)877-0585; jconnors@bccancer.bc.ca.

CONNORS, Lori A; Halifax Allergy & Asthma Assoc, 503-5657 Spring Garden Rd, Halifax NS B3J 3R4; Dal'05; FRCPC; IntMed; ClinImmunol&Allergy. (902)425-3927; Fax. (902)425-3928.

CONNORS, M Ruth; Alberta Children's Hosp, 2888 Shaganappi Trail NW, Calgary AB T3B 6A8; Mem'84; FRCPC; Anes (Critical Care Medicine). Staff Anes & Intensivist, Alberta Children's Hospital; (403)955-7605; Fax. (403)955-7506.

CONNORS, Sean P; Health Sciences Centre, 300 Prince Philip Dr, St. John's NL A1B 3V6; Mem'92; FRCPC; IntMed; Cardiol. Staff Cardiol, Health Sciences Centre; (709)777-6487

CONNORS, Shelagh; The Ob/Gyn Suite, 403-199 Grafton St, Charlottetown PE C1A 1L2; Dal'80; FRCSC; ObstGyn. Ac Staff, Queen Elizabeth Hospital; Consultant, The Ob/Gyn Suite; Clin Instructor, Dalhousie University; (902)629-8801; Fax. (902)629-8826; shelaghconnors@hotmail.com.

CONRAD, Anne R; Devon X-Ray Clinic, 102-106 Erie St S, Devon AB T9G 1A7; Alb'74; FRCPC; DiagRad. Staff Devon X-Ray Clinic, Devon General Hospital; (780)987-3900; Fax. (780)987-2000.

CONRAD, David; The Ottawa Hosp-Gen Campus, 501 Smyth Rd, Ottawa ON K1H 8L6; Ott'93; FRCPC; IntMed; Hem. Staff, The Ottawa Hospital - General Campus; (613)737-7700

CONRAD, Krzysztof; 21 Bedford Ave, Toronto ON M5R 2J9; Gdansk (Poland)'63; FRCS(Eng); FACS; AB; FRCSC; Otol (Facial Plastic Surgery). Staff, Mount Sinai Hospital; Staff, Mackenzie Richmond Hill Hospital; Physician, Nasal & Facial Plastic Surgery Institute; Assoc Prof Otol, University of Toronto; (416)961-2053; Fax. (416)962-0795; info@drkconrad.com.

CONRAD, Michael J; Cowichan District Hosp, 3045 Gibbins Rd, Duncan BC V9L 1E5; Ott'91; CCFP; CCFP(E.M.); Staff, Cowichan District Hospital; (250)746-4141

CONRAD, Sarah L; Lunenburg Family Health, PO Box 1450 42 High St, Lunenburg NS B0J 2C0; Dal'08; CCFP; (902)634-7000; Fax. (902)634-3661.

CONRADI, Alf G; University of Alberta Hosp, 3A3.04-8440 112 St NW, Edmonton AB T6G 2B7; Alb'84; FRCPC; Peds (Pediatric Intensive Care). Ac Staff Ped ICU, University of Alberta Hospital; Clin Assoc Prof, University of Alberta; (780)407-1673; Fax. (780)407-3214.

CONRADIE, Johan A; Rockyview Gen Hosp, 7007 14 St SW, Calgary AB T2V 1P9; Stellenbosch (South Africa)'90; MB ChB; MSc; BSc(Hons.); FRCPC; IntMed. Staff, Rockyview General Hospital; Langs: Afrikaans; (403)943-3000; Fax. (403)450-9931; conradie@shaw.ca.

CONRADIE, Hannes; 2268 Pandosy St, Kelowna BC V1Y 1T2; Pretoria (South Africa)'92; MB ChB; LMCC; CCFP; Staff, Kelowna General Hospital; Langs: Afrikaans; (250)862-4000

CONRADIE, Marius; Chaparral Corner Shopping Ctre, 208-803 Chaparral Dr SE, Calgary AB T2X 0E5; (South Africa)'85; MB ChB; LMCC; Langs: Afrikaans; (403)873-7734; Fax. (403)873-7735.

CONRAN, Michelle B; Avenue Med Clinic, 190 Wilson Ave, North York ON M5M 4N7; Mem'98; BASc; BEd; BSc; (416)482-2111; Fax. (416)482-2174.

CONROD, Cheryl K; PO Box 1297 Stn A, Sydney NS B1P 6K4; Dal'87; FRCSC; ObstGyn. (902)564-4460; Fax. (902)564-4468.

CONROD, Michelle A; Professional Arts Bldg, 523-100 Arden St, Moncton NB E1C 4B7; Dal'87; CCFP; FCFP; Researcher Co-Ordinator, Northumberland Family Med Teaching Unit; Lecturer, Dalhousie University; (506)857-5452; Fax. (506)857-5454; michelle.conrod@horizonnb.ca.

CONSEIL, Jean P; Urgence Med Grande-Allee, 1419 Grande Allée, Terrebonne QC J6W 5M9; Mon'75; (450)471-7066; Fax. (450)471-7254.

CONSKY, Earl S; 510-790 Bay St, Toronto ON M5G 1N8; Tor'81; FRCPC; Neur (Movement Disorders). (416)603-7904; Fax. (416)603-7929; dreconsky@bellnet.ca.

CONSTANCE, Christian M; Hop Maisonneuve-Rosemont, 5415 boul de l'Assomption, Montreal QC H1T 2M4; Mon'88; CSPQ; FRCPC; IntMed; Cardiol. Staff, Hopital Maisonneuve-Rosemont; (514)252-3400

CONSTANCE, Peter D A; 4420 10th Ave W, Vancouver BC V6R 2H9; Cape Town (South Africa)'66; MB ChB; FRCPC; Psy. (604)222-1353

CONSTANT, Yvon; Clinique Med de l'Or, 228 2e rue E, La Sarre QC J9Z 2G9; Sher'76; (819)339-5617; Fax. (819)339-2729.

CONSTANTIN, Alina D; Three Sisters Obst & Fam Med C, 106-75 Dyrgas Gate, Canmore AB T1W 0A6; Sask'00; CCFP; Staff, Canmore General Hospital; Clin Lecturer Family Med, University of Calgary; Langs: Romanian; French; (403)609-9095; Fax. (403)609-7232.

CONSTANTIN, Andre; SMBD Jewish Gen Hosp, 3755 ch Cote-Sainte-Catherine, Montreal QC H3T 1E2; Mon'85; LMCC; FRCPC; DiagRad (Interventional Radiology). Staff, Sir Mortimer B Davis Jewish General; (514)340-8233; Fax. (514)630-5954; aconstan@rad.jgh.mcgill.ca.

CONSTANTIN, Evelyn J T; MUHC-Montreal Children's Hosp, C508-2300 rue Tupper, Montreal QC H3H 1P3; McG'00; FRCPC; Peds. Staff, McGill University Health Centre - Montreal Children's Hospital; (514)412-4321

CONSTANTINE, Charles T; Surrey Med Arts Bldg, 113-13798 94A Ave, Surrey BC V3V 1N1; McG'98; BSc; MDCM; FRCPC; IntMed (Hypertension); Nephrol. Staff Fraser Health Authority, University of British Columbia; (604)870-9886; Fax. (604)864-8719.

CONSTANTINE, Maggie M; Royal Columbian Hosp, 330 Columbia St E, New Westminster BC V3L 3W7; UBC'00; FRCPC; IntMed; Hem. Staff, Royal Columbian Hospital; (604)520-4253

CONSTANTINEAU, Genevieve; CSSS de Papineau, 155 rue MacLaren E, Gatineau QC J8L 0C2; Mon'05; CCFP; Staff, Hôpital de Papineau; (819)986-4115

CONSTANTINEAU, Louise; 220-620 rue King E CP 21509 Csp Ste-Famille, Sherbrooke QC J1G 5K2; Mon'82; FRCSC; ObstGyn (Echography). Staff, Centre Hospitalier Universitaire de Sherbrooke-Hopital Fleurimont; Universite de Sherbrooke; Langs: Bilingual(French/English); (819)569-6622; Fax. (819)569-9758.

CONSTANTINESCU, Corina; Sunnybrook Hlth Sciences Ctre, 2075 Bayview Ave, Toronto ON M4N 3M5; Bucharest (Romania)'98; FRCPC; Anes. Staff, Sunnybrook Health Sciences Centre; (416)480-6100

CONSTANTINESCU, Cristina; CLSC La Petite-Patrie, 6520 rue De Saint-Vallier, Montreal QC H2S 2P7; Bucharest (Romania)'81; CCFP; Fam Med, CHSLD Paul-Gouin; Langs: Romanian; (514)273-4508; Fax. (514)272-6278.

CONSTANTINIDES, Prometheas; Hop Louis-H Lafontaine, 7401 rue Hochelaga, Montreal QC H1N 3M5; Mon'00; FRCPC; Psy. Staff, Hopital Louis-H Lafontaine; (514)251-4000; Fax. (514)251-0856.

CONSTAS-COSTOPOULOS, Nicolas; Centre Med Hochelaga, 9080 rue Hochelaga, Montreal QC H1L 2N9; Athens (Greece)'72; Langs: French; Greek; Spanish; (514)353-8742; Fax. (514)353-2351.

CONSUL, Megha; St Joseph's Health Care, PO Box 5777 Stn B 268 Grosvenor St, London ON N6A 4V2; Gandhi Medical College (India)'00; Clin Fellow Neonatal Perinatal Med, St Joseph's Hospital - St Joseph's Health Care; (519)646-6100

CONSUNJI-ARANETA, Raquel; Children's Hosp, CS516-840 Sherbrook St, Winnipeg MB R3A 1S1; Manila (Philippines)'85; Peds; Prog Dir PG Med Educ Dept of Peds & Child Health, University of Manitoba; Fax. (204)787-1944.

CONTANT, Chantal; Ctr Hosp Trois-Riv-Pav St-Jose, 731 rue Sainte-Julie, Trois-Rivieres QC G9A 1Y1; Mon'97; FRCSC; GenSurg. Staff, Centre Hospitalier Regional de Trois-Rivieres; (819)697-3333

CONTANT, Denys; Hop Jean-Talon, 1385 rue Jean-Talon E, Montreal QC H2E 1S6; Mon'95; Staff, CSSS du Coeur de l'Isle Hôpital Jean-Talon; (514)495-6767

CONTANT, Éric; Centre Hosp Reg Chisasibi, CP 250, Chisasibi QC J0M 1E0; Sher'09; CCFP; Staff, Cree Board of Health & Social Services James Bay; (819)855-9001

CONTE, Paul D; Laurentian Walk-In Clinic, 750 Ottawa St S, Kitchener ON N2E 1B6; Qns'98; CCFP; (519)748-2542; Fax. (519)748-2576.

CONTER, Howard S; Family Practice Associates, 6155 North St, Halifax NS B3K 5R3; Dal'85; (902)453-3511; Fax. (902)454-9010.

CONTI, Massimo; Hop Laval, 2725 ch Sainte-Foy, Quebec QC G1V 4G5; Pavia (Italy)'94; Staff, Hôpital Laval; (418)656-8711 x5504

CONTI, Sylvain; Polyclinique de l'Oreille, 2113 boul Casavant O, Saint-Hyacinthe QC J2S 7E5; Mon'91; FRCSC; Otol. Staff Otol, Centre Hospitalier Honore-Mercier; (450)773-7824

CONTRACTOR, Masuma M; Oak Ridge Med Centre, 100-13291 Yonge St, Richmond Hill ON L4E 4L6; (Pakistan)'83; CCFP; (905)773-7759

CONTRE, Bernard; 2530 Place des Cerisiers, Sherbrooke QC J1G 5A9; Sher'91; FRCPC; DiagRad. (819)562-6473; Fax. (819)562-0717.

CONTRERAS, Carlos E; Medical Clinic Bldg, 319-89 Humber College Blvd, Etobicoke ON M9V 4B8; (Chile)'59; Peds. Langs: Spanish; (416)743-5652

CONTRERAS DOMINGUEZ, Vladimir; Civic Parkdale Clinic, 403-737 Parkdale Ave, Ottawa ON K1Y 1J8; Madrid (Spain)'01; Staff, The Ottawa Hospital - General Campus; (613)761-5164; Fax. (613)761-4036.

CONVERY, Kevin M; Agassiz Med Centre, 130-30 Stephen St, Morden MB R6M 2G3; Ott'05; CCFP; Langs: Bilingual(English/French); (204)822-4474; Fax. (204)822-6886.

CONWAY, Aoife M; Haliburton Family Med Centre, PO Box 870 7217 Gelert Rd, Haliburton ON K0M 1S0; Cal'89; CCFP; FCFP; (705)457-1212; Fax. (705)457-3955.

CONWAY, Barry P; 302-1990 Fort St, Victoria BC V8R 6V4; Dal'76; (250)381-1444; Fax. (250)381-1585.

CONWAY, Brian; 201-1200 Burrard St, Vancouver BC V6Z 2C7; McG'82; ABIM; FRCPC; IntMed (HIV). Consultant InfectDis, Vancouver Coastal Health; Assoc Prof Pharmacol & Therapeutics, University of British Columbia; Langs: French; (604)642-6429; Fax. (604)642-6419; bconway@exchange.ubc.ca.

CONWAY, Denis M; Rosedale Med Centre, 710-600 Sherbourne St, Toronto ON M4X 1W4; Tor'77; DTMH(Lond); DA; (416)964-2295

CONWAY, Edward M; UBC Ctr for Blood Research Hem, 4306-2350 Health Sciences Mall, Vancouver BC V6T 1Z3; Tor'79; FACP; FRCPC; IntMed; Hem. Dir Centre for Blood Research, University of British Columbia; (604)822-4252

CONWAY, Emily R D; KDH Health Centre, PO Box 2113 2671 Concession Rd, Kemptville ON K0G 1J0; McM'89; CCFP; FCFP; Court Staff Privil, Kemptville District Hospital; Court Staff Privil, Children's Hospital of Eastern Ontario (CHEO); (613)258-0100; Fax. (613)258-6171.

CONWAY, James B; The Ottawa Hosp-Civic Campus, 1053 Carling Ave, Ottawa ON K1Y 4E9; McG'88; BSc; FRCPC; Anes (Critical Care Medicine). Staff, The Ottawa Hospital - Civic Campus; (613)761-4169; Fax. (613)761-5209.

CONWAY, James R; Diabetes Clinic, 218 Percy St, Smiths Falls ON K7A 4W8; Ott'72; LMCC; Consultant Staff, Sault Area Hospital - Sault Ste Marie; Ac Staff, Perth & Smiths Falls District Hospital - Perth Site (Great War Memorial Site); Dir Research, Canadian Centre Research on Diabetes; Coroner/Med Examiner, Government Of Canada; Langs: Bilingual(French/English); (613)284-0145; Fax. (613)283-9020; diabetes@diabetesclinic.ca.

CONWAY, Jennifer; The Hosp for Sick Children, 555 University Ave, Toronto ON M5G 1X8; UBC'02; FRCPC; Peds; Cardiol. Staff, The Hospital For Sick Children; (416)813-7467

CONWAY, Valentine H; Newfoundland Drive Med Clinic, 427 Newfoundland Dr, St. John's NL A1A 4A5; Dal'74; FRCSC; Ophth. (709)579-1106

CONYERS, Roop; Annapolis Comm Health Center, PO Box 573 821 St George St, Annapolis Royal NS B0S 1A0; Tor'01; BSc(Hon); PhD; CCFP; Asst Prof/Site Dir Annapolis Valley FamMed Residency Prog, Dalhousie University; (902)532-2324; Fax. (902)532-5424; rconyers@avdha.nshealth.ca.

COODIN, Michael G; Charleswood Med Clinic, 3360 Roblin Blvd, Winnipeg MB R3R 0C5; Man'05; CCFP; (204)889-4736

COOK, Alan F; Central Park Medical, 203-1711 Cook St, Victoria BC V8T 3P2; Alb'84; Staff, Royal Jubilee Hospital; (250)386-1712; Fax. (250)386-7672.

COOK, Alana; St Joseph's Hosp, 130 Bayard Dr, Saint John NB E2L 3L6; Cal'02; BSc; CCFP; Staff, St Joseph's Hospital; (506)632-5700; Fax. (506)632-5657.

COOK, Allan M; CHUS-Hop Hotel-Dieu, 580 rue Bowen S, Sherbrooke QC J1G 2E8; Dal'82; FRCPC; Psy (Neurology & Psychiatry). Staff, Centre Hospitalier Universitaire de Sherbrooke-Hôpital Hôtel-Dieu; (819)346-1110; Fax. (819)822-6790.

COOK, Andrew C; St Joseph's Gen Hosp, 2137 Comox Ave, Comox BC V9M 1P2; Witwatersrand (South Africa)'91; MB BCh; FRCPC; Anes. Staff, St Joseph's General Hospital; Langs: Afrikaans; (250)339-2242; Fax. (250)339-1432.

COOK, Anthony J; Alberta Children's Hosp, 2888 Shaganappi Trail NW, Calgary AB T3B 6A8; Wes'98; FRCSC; Urol. Staff, Rockyview General Hospital; Staff, Alberta Children's Hospital; (403)955-2266; Fax. (403)955-7634.

COOK, Ashley G; Cornwall Commun Hosp-McConnell, PO Box 100 Stn Main 840 McConnell Ave, Cornwall ON K6H 5S5; Qns'93; CCFP; Chief FamilyMed, Cornwall Community Hospital; (613)938-4240 x2217

COOK, Bruce H O; Dingwall Med Clinic, PO Box 3011 40 Goodall St, Dryden ON P8N 2Z6; NOSM'10; CCFP; (807)223-6683

COOK, Catherine; Winnipeg Reg Health Authority, 4F-650 Main St, Winnipeg MB R3B 1E2; Man'87; CCFP; FCFP; Med Officer of Hlth, Winnipeg Regional Health Authority; Assoc Dean First Nations, Metis & Inuit Health, University of Manitoba; (204)926-7000

COOK, Christopher T; Family Physicians Inc, 510 Prince St, Truro NS B2N 1G1; Dal'01; CCFP; (902)895-3433

COOK, D Roy; Rockyview Gen Hosp, 7007 14 St SW, Calgary AB T2V 1P9; Cal'77; FRCPC; IntMed. Ac Staff, Rockyview General Hospital; (403)255-7111

COOK, David B; 1570 Bay Ave, Trail BC V1R 4B3; Dal'88; FRCSC; Otol. Staff, Stanton Territorial Health Authority; (250)364-5712

COOK, Deborah J; St Joseph's Healthcare, 50 Charlton Ave E, Hamilton ON L8N 4A6; McM'85; MSc(Epid.); FCCP; FRCPC; IntMed (Critical Care Medicine). Chair Gen IntMed/Critical Care Research Prog & Internist, St Joseph's Healthcare - Charlton Campus; Acad Chair/Prof Med &Epidemiiol, McMaster University; (905)522-4941; Fax. (905)521-6022.

COOK, Dennis J A; Smith Clinic, 1-6601 48 Ave, Camrose AB T4V 3G8; Alb'77; CCFP; (780)672-2425; Fax. (780)679-2668.

COOK, Donald M; Health Sciences Centre, 300 Prince Philip Dr, St. John's NL A1B 3V6; Mem'80; DAB; FRCPC; GenPath (Laboratory Medicine). Staff Path, Health Sciences Centre; Chief, St Clare's Mercy Hospital; Clinical Asst Prof Path, Memorial University Of Newfoundland; (709)777-2106; donald.cook@easternhealth.ca.

COOK, Donald R; Rockyview Gen Hosp, 4A 194-7007 14 St SW, Calgary AB T2V 1P9; Alb'75; FRCPC; IntMed. Staff, Rockyview General Hospital; (403)943-3889

COOK, Geoffrey S; Saint John Reg Hosp, PO Box 2100 Stn Main 400 University Ave, Saint John NB E2L 4L2; Dal'99; BSc; FRCSC; PlasSurg (Hand & Wrist Surgery). Staff, Saint John Regional Hospital; Clin Lecturer, Dalhousie University; (506)648-7977; geoffcooksurgery@gmail.com.

COOK, Gregory C F; Linwell X-Ray Centre, 282 Linwell Rd, St Catharines ON L2N 6N5; Qns'77; FRCPC; DiagRad. Diag Radiol, Niagara Health System - Douglas Memorial Hospital Site; (905)935-0270; Fax. (905)935-8811.

COOK, Jolene M; Queen Elizabeth II HSC, 355-1796 Summer St, Halifax NS B3H 3A7; Dal'05; CCFP; Staff, Queen Elizabeth II Health Sciences Centre - Halifax Infirmary Site; (902)473-2220

COOK, Katherine A; 208-22 College St, Toronto ON M5G 1K2; Tor'70; FRCPC; Psy. (416)925-6170; Fax. (416)465-1426.

COOK, Laurence M; 8619 North Nechako Rd, Prince George BC V2K 4Z7; Dal'73; Ac Staff, University Hospital of Northern British Columbia; (250)561-0376

COOK, Marlyn A; Sioux Lookout Meno-Ya-Win H C, PO Box 1500 Stn Main 16-82 Seventh Ave, Sioux Lookout ON P8T 1C2; Man'87; CCFP; FCFP; Staff, Sioux Lookout Meno-Ya-Win Health Centre; (807)737-5191; Fax. (807)737-7176.

COOK, Michael I; Kitsilano Fairview Mental Hlth, 400-1212 Broadway W, Vancouver BC V6H 3V1; McM'81; FRCPC; Psy (Adult Chronic Care & Psychotherapy). Staff, University of British Columbia Student Health Services; Physician, Greater Vancouver Mental Health Service Society; Teach Staff Psy Outreach Prog/Physician Student Health Services, University of British Columbia; (604)736-2881; Fax. (604)737-4835; mcook@forensic.bc.ca.

COOK, Miles C; 300-401 9 Ave SW, Calgary AB T2P 3C5; Cal'04; FRCPC; DiagRad.

COOK, Nathalie; Children's Hosp Eastern Ont, 401 Smyth Rd, Ottawa ON K1H 8L1; Ott'92; FRCPC; Peds. Staff, Children's Hospital of Eastern Ontario (CHEO); Langs: English; French; (613)737-2393; Fax. (613)738-4878.

COOK, Peter E; Hamilton Schizophrenia Program, 102-350 King St E, Hamilton ON L8N 3Y3; UBC'74; AB; APA; BSc(Hon); FRCPC; Psy (Psychiatric Administration). Staff, St Joseph's Healthcare Hamilton - West 5th Campus; Staff, St Joseph's Healthcare - Charlton Campus; Staff, Hamilton Health Sciences Centre - McMaster Children's Hospital; Clin Assoc Prof Psy, McMaster University; (905)525-2832; Fax. (905)546-0055.

COOK, Richard C; St Paul's Hosp, 489-1081 Burrard St, Vancouver BC V6Z 1Y6; Alb'92; FRCSC; CardSurg. Staff, Providence Health Care - St Paul's Hospital; (604)806-9601

COOK, Robert D; Western Memorial Reg Hosp, PO Box 2005 Stn Main 1 Brookfield Ave, Corner Brook NL A2H 6J7; Mem'02; FRCPC; DiagRad. Staff, Western Memorial Regional Hospital; (709)637-5000

COOK, Sarah E; Emkiro Health Services, 120-70 University Ave, Toronto ON M5J 2M4; Tor'07; CCFP; (416)977-7474

COOK, Sidney D; Parry Sound Family Health Team, 57 James St, Parry Sound ON P2A 1T6; Tor'73; Ac Staff, West Parry Sound Health Centre; (705)746-2181; Fax. (705)746-4753.

COOK, Sonya M; Compass Dermatology, 8-650 Mount Pleasant Rd, Toronto ON M4S 2N5; Tor'02; FRCPC; Derm. Staff, Women's College Hospital; Staff, Sunnybrook Health Sciences Centre; (647)351-9277

COOK, Steven T; 510 Prince St, Truro NS B2N 1G1; Dal'72; Staff, Colchester East Hants Health Centre; (902)895-1556; Fax. (902)893-1026; stcook@eastlink.ca.

COOK, Timothy J; 4276 Elgin Mills Rd E, Markham ON L6C 1L4; Qns'86; DTMH; FRCPC; IntMed (Endocrinology). Assoc Staff, Mount Sinai Hospital; Dir, MDS Travel Medicine Clinic; University of Toronto; (647)228-7805

COOK, Victoria J; BC Centre For Disease Control, 655 12th Ave W, Vancouver BC V5Z 4R4; UBC'97; FRCPC; IntMed; Respir. Staff, BC Centre For Disease Control; Staff The Lung Centre, Gordon & Leslie Diamond Health Care Centre; (604)660-6108

COOK, W Douglas; Lennox & Addington Gen Hosp, 8 Richmond Park Ave, Napanee ON K7R 2Z4; Mem'76; Staff, Lennox & Addington County General Hospital; (613)354-3301

COOK, Wendy L; St Paul's Hosp, 9B-1081 Burrard St, Vancouver BC V6Z 1Y6; Tor'97; BSc(Hon); MHSc; FRCPC; IntMed; GeriatricMed. Consultant Geriatric Med, Vancouver General Hospital - Centennial Pavillion; Staff, Providence Health Care - St Paul's Hospital; Clinical Asst Prof, University of British Columbia; (604)806-8029; Fax. (604)806-8390.

COOKE, Andrew; Cancercare Manitoba, ON3245-675 McDermot Ave, Winnipeg MB R3E 0V9; Man'80; FRC; FRCPC; IntMed; RadOncol. A-Head Dept of RadOncol, St Boniface General Hospital; Physician, Manitoba Cancer Treatment & Research Foundation; Physician, Winnipeg Regional Health Authority Carlton Street Office; Physician, CancerCare Manitoba; andrew.cooke@cancercare.mb.ca.

COOKE, Breda; Foothills Med Centre, 1403 29 St NW, Calgary AB T2N 2T9; Belfast (Ireland)'90; MB BCh; Staff, Foothills Medical Centre; (403)944-1110

COOKE, C J; Rouge Valley Fertility Centre, 309-100 Consilium Pl, Scarborough ON M1H 3E3; Tor'88; MD(Hon.); FRCS; BSc(Hon); FACOG; FSOGC; FRCSC; ObstGyn (Infertility). (416)283-5539; Fax. (416)283-1636; cjcooke@rogers.com.

COOKE, Donald A; 201-7315 Edmonds St, Burnaby BC V3N 1A7; (Jamaica)'68; MB BS; FRCSC; GenSurg. Hd GenSurg, Burnaby Hospital; (604)519-3780; Fax. (604)519-3781; doncooke@telus.net.

COOKE, Donald W; 152 Dundas St E, Trenton ON K8V 1L4; Wes'75; Staff, QHC Trenton Memorial; Staff, QHC Belleville General; (613)392-3546

COOKE, Gabriel M; One Med Place, 102-20 Wynford Dr, North York ON M3C 1J4; National (Ireland)'64; DMRD; AB; FRCPC; DiagRad. Staff Radiol, St Michael's Hospital; Asst Prof, University of Toronto; (416)441-3344; Fax. (416)441-1471.

COOKE, Kathryn J; Railside Med Specialists, 4A-1306 Bow Valley Trail, Canmore AB T1W 1N6; Alb'85; BSc; FRCPC; Peds (Sports Medicine). Staff, Covenant Health - Banff Mineral Springs Hospital; Staff, Canmore General Hospital; (403)678-9600; Fax. (403)678-9467.

COOKE, Kristy A M; Reddendale Family Health Team, 7-730 Front Rd, Kingston ON K7M 6P7; Qns'06; CCFP; (613)384-4664; Fax. (613)634-8595.

COOKE, Lara J; Foothills Med Centre, F12-1403 29 St NW, Calgary AB T2N 2T9; Cal'99; FRCPC; Neur. Staff, Foothills Medical Centre; (403)944-4240

COOKE, Mary E; Mount Sinai Hosp, 1514-600 University Ave, Toronto ON M5G 1X5; Man'75; FRCPC; Anes. Staff, Mount Sinai Hospital; Asst Prof Anes, University of Toronto; (416)586-4800 x5270; Fax. (416)586-8664.

COOKE, Michael D; North Okanagan Paediatric Clin, 3-2802 34 St, Vernon BC V1T 5X1; Cal'02; FRCPC; Peds. (250)558-5506; Fax. (250)558-5108.

COOKE, Michael J; Trillium Hlth Ctr-Mississauga, 100 Queensway W, Mississauga ON L5B 1B8; Leeds (England)'65; MB ChB; FRCPC; Anes (Pain Management). Staff, Trillium Health Centre - Mississauga; (905)848-7100; Fax. (905)949-5821; mj.cooke@rogers.com.

COOKE, Raymond H; Polyclinic Prof Centre Inc, 103-199 Grafton St, Charlottetown PE C1A 1L2; Dal'89; (902)629-8844; Fax. (902)566-9251.

COOKE, Robert G; Addiction & Mental Hlth-Queen, 4215-1001 Queen St W, Toronto ON M6J 1H4; Man'76; MSc; DABPN; FRCPC; Psy (Mood Disorders). Court Staff Med, Sault Area Hospital - Sault Ste Marie; Staff, Centre for Addiction & Mental Health (CAMH) - Queen Site; (416)535-8501

COOKE, Suzette R; Alberta Children's Hosp, 2888 Shaganappi Trail NW, Calgary AB T3B 6A8; Cal'96; FRCPC; Peds. Clinical Asst Prof Hospital Ped, Alberta Children's Hospital; (403)955-3017

COOKE, T Derek V; 404-797 Princess St, Kingston ON K7L 1G1; Cambridge (England)'64; MA; MB ChB; FRCSC; OrthSurg (Arthritis Surgery). Staff, Timmins & District Hospital; Consultant Locum (All Sites), North Bay Regional Health Centre - Regional Mental Health; Prof Surg Rehab, Queen's University; (613)549-0768; Fax. (613)549-0346.

COOKEY, Benedict J; Halifax Prof Centre, 540-5991 Spring Garden Rd, Halifax NS B3H 1Y6; Dal'73; FRCPC; IntMed. Ac Staff, Queen Elizabeth II Health Sciences Centre - Victoria General Site; Dalhousie University; (902)496-3252; Fax. (902)496-0722.

COOLEN, Anna L; The Polyclinic, 199 Grafton St, Charlottetown PE C1A 1L2; Dal'06; FRCSC; ObstGyn.

COOLEN, Jillian D; IWK Health Centre, PO Box 9700 Rpo Csc 5980 University Ave, Halifax NS B3K 6R8; Dal'03; FRCSC; ObstGyn (Maternal Fetal Medicine). Staff, IWK Health Centre; (902)470-6602; Fax. (902)425-1125.

COOLICAN, Paul J; St Lawrence Med Clinic, PO Box 772 3 Thorold Lane, Ingleside ON K0C 1M0; Mem'80; CCFP; FCFP; Ac Staff, Winchester District Memorial Hospital; (613)537-2044

COOLIGAN, Terrance; Humber River Reg Hosp-Church, 200 Church St, Toronto ON M9N 1N8; Ott'75; ABIM(CriticalCare); FRCPC; IntMed (Critical Care Medicine); Respir. Staff Respirol & Intensivist, Humber River Regional Hospital - Church Street Site; Langs: English; French; (416)488-7770; Fax. (416)488-7770; tcooligan@hrrh.on.ca.

COOMARAN, Vasuki; Stapleford Med Clinic, 372 McCarthy Blvd N, Regina SK S4R 7M2; (Other Foreign)'94; (306)545-3000; Fax. (306)545-5584.

COOMBES, Robin D; Grey Bruce Hlth Serv-Owen Soun, PO Box 1800 Stn Main 1800 8th St E, Owen Sound ON N4K 6M9; Alb'00; FRCPC; Anes. Staff Anes, Grey Bruce Health Services - Owen Sound; (519)376-2121

COOMBS, Heather; St Mary's Hosp Centre, 3830 av Lacombe, Montreal QC H3T 1M5; Mem'81; CCFP; CCFP(E.M.); FCFP; EmergMed (P.Q.). Staff, St Mary's Hospital Centre; (514)734-2690

COOMBS, Jennifer M L; Manitoba Clinic, 790 Sherbrook St, Winnipeg MB R3A 1M3; Man'05; FRCPC; Peds.

COOMBS, John F; 152 Walter's Lane, Fallbrook ON K0G 1A0; Tor'71; BSc(Hon); Langs: English; French; (613)267-2523; Fax. (613)267-6216.

COOMBS, Robin R; Centre de Med de Famille, 3777 rue Jean-Brillant, Montreal QC H3T 1M5; McM'10; CCFP.

COOMBS, Susan; East Tower, 123-400 Walmer Rd, Toronto ON M5P 2X7; Tor'68; FRCPC; Peds (Consultant Pediatrics). Hon Staff, The Hospital For Sick Children; Court Staff Newborn Nursery, Sunnybrook Health Sciences Centre; (416)921-8872; Fax. (416)484-6617.

COOME, Grant E A; London HSC-Victoria Hosp, PO Box 5010 Stn B E1 102-800 Commissioners Rd E, London ON N6A 5W9; Tor'01; CCFP; CCFP(E.M.); Staff, London Health Sciences Centre - Victoria Campus; (519)685-8500

COONAN, Thomas J; Queen Elizabeth II HSC, 1276 South Park St, Halifax NS B3H 2Y9; McG'68; FRCPC; Anes. Staff Anes, Queen Elizabeth II Health Sciences Centre - Victoria General Site; (902)473-2331; Fax. (902)423-9454.

COONER, Manpreet K; Hilltop Med Clinic, 140-15321 16th Ave, Surrey BC V4A 1R6; London (England)'96; CCFP; (604)531-1626

COONEY, John A E; Villa Caritas, 16515 88 Ave NW, Edmonton AB T5R 0A4; National (Ireland)'82; MB ChB; BAO; MRCPsy; Psy (General Psychiatry). (780)342-6500

COONEY, Judy-Diane; Lansdowne Shopping Centre, 108-5124 122 St NW, Edmonton AB T6H 3S3; Alb'75; BSc; CCFP; FCFP; (780)435-3688; Fax. (780)435-3691.

COONEY, Paul R H; Huronia Urgent Care Clinic, 202-480 Huronia Rd, Barrie ON L4N 6M2; Tor'10; CCFP; (705)725-7716

COONEY, Thomas P; Royal Columbian Hosp, 330 Columbia St E, New Westminster BC V3L 3W7; National (Ireland)'73; MRC(I); MRCPath; FCCP; FRCPC; AnatPath. Staff AnatPath, Royal Columbian Hospital; Clin Assoc Prof, University of British Columbia; (604)520-4349

COOPER, Alan J; Bluewater Health-Norman Site, 89 Norman St, Sarnia ON N7T 6S3; Bristol (England)'59; Staff Psy, Bluewater Health - Mitton Site; Staff, Bluewater Health - Norman Site; (519)464-4400; Fax. (519)464-4516.

COOPER, Alfred J; 203-11 Rea St N, Timmins ON P4N 4Z5; Ott'58; (705)264-0313; Fax. (705)264-6481.

COOPER, Andrew B; William Osler Health -Brampton, 2100 Bovaird Dr E, Brampton ON L6R 3J7; UBC'88; FRCPC; Anes; Critical Care Medicine. Staff, William Osler Health System - Brampton Civic Hospital; Researcher Fellow, University of Toronto; (905)494-2120; andrew.cooper@utoronto.ca.

COOPER, Austin R; Dr Charles A Janeway Child HC, 300 Prince Philip Dr, St. John's NL A1B 3V6; Dal'69; FRCPC; Peds (Infectious Diseases). Staff, Janeway Children's Health & Rehabilitation Centre; Prof, Memorial University Of Newfoundland; (709)777-4302; Fax. (709)777-4736; acooper@mun.ca.

COOPER, Carley N; Nanaimo Reg Gen Hosp, 1200 Dufferin Cres, Nanaimo BC V9S 2B7; UBC'02; CCFP; CCFP(E.M.); Staff, Nanaimo Regional General Hospital; (250)755-7691 x52110

COOPER, Carol L; Sheddon Avenue Med Assoc, 308-331 Sheddon Ave, Oakville ON L6J 1X8; McM'85; CCFP; FCFP; Affil Staff, Halton Healthcare Services Corporation - Oakville Site; (905)845-8771; Fax. (905)845-8379.

COOPER, Christopher G; Rouge Valley-Ajax & Pickering, 580 Harwood Ave S, Ajax ON L1S 2J4; Mem'83; FRCPC; Anes. Staff, Rouge Valley Health System - Ajax & Pickering Health Centre Site; (905)683-2320 x1288

COOPER, Curtis L; The Ottawa Hosp-Gen Campus, G12-501 Smyth Rd, Ottawa ON K1H 8L6; Sask'94; FRCPC; IntMed (HIV); InfectDis. Staff Physician, The Ottawa Hospital - General Campus; Assoc Prof Med, University of Ottawa; (613)737-8899 x72296

COOPER, Donald A; BC Cancer Agency-Vancouver CC, 600 10 Ave W, Vancouver BC V5Z 4E6; UBC'78; BSc; MSc; Staff, BC Cancer Agency Vancouver Centre; (604)877-6000

COOPER, E Alexander; La Cite Medicale, 295-2600 boul Laurier, Quebec QC G1V 4T3; UBC'87; CCFP; Staff Emerg Center, Jeffery Hale Hospital-Saint Brigid's; Staff, CHSLD St Brigid's Home; Langs: French; (418)781-0480

COOPER, Gregory R; Bancroft Family Health Team, 16 Billa St, Bancroft ON K0L 1C0; Qns'84; CCFP; FCFP; Staff Family Med, QHC North Hastings; (613)332-1565; Fax. (613)332-0526; gcooper@bancroftfht.com.

COOPER, H Douglas; 19851 Willowbrook Dr, Langley BC V2Y 1A7; Cal'80; Staff, Langley Memorial Hospital; Fax. (604)534-1463.

COOPER, Jacqueline M; 301-2620 Commercial Dr, Vancouver BC V5N 4C4; UBC'10; CCFP; (604)873-6633

COOPER, James P; Univ Hlth Network-Toronto Western Hosp, 9E428-399 Bathurst St, Toronto ON M5T 2S8; Tor'84; MD; FRCPC; Psy (Geriatric Psychiatry). Staff Geriatric Psy Prog, Toronto Rehabilitation Institute - University Centre; Clin Dir Psychogeriatric Outreach Prog, Toronto Western Hospital - University Health Network; Consultant Psy, Runnymede Healthcare Centre; Asst Prof, University of Toronto; Langs: Italian; (416)603-5283; Fax. (416)603-5490.

COOPER, Jerry J I; Norfinch Med Centre, 106A-2100 Finch Ave W, North York ON M3N 2Z9; Tor'67; DPsy; FRCPC; Psy (Forensic Psychiatry). Staff Psy, Humber River Regional Hospital - Finch Avenue Site; (416)650-9082; Fax. (416)739-7601.

COOPER, Johan C; Beechy Health Centre, PO Box 40, Beechy SK S0L 0C0; Pretoria (South Africa)'96; MB ChB; (306)859-2113; Fax. (306)859-2206.

COOPER, John K; 306-2020 Richmond Rd, Victoria BC V8R 6R5; Mem'86; BSc; BMedSci; FRCSC; ObstGyn. Med Staff, Vancouver Island Health Authority; Clin Instructor, University of British Columbia; (250)592-5633; cooper@islandnet.com.

COOPER, Judith A; Queen Square Doctors FHT, 201-366 Main St N, Brampton ON L6V 1P8; Tor'87; Staff, William Osler Health System - Brampton Civic Hospital; (905)455-1455; Fax. (905)455-5498.

COOPER, Kenneth J; Canadian Forces Hlth Serv Ctr, PO Box 99000 Stn Forces, Halifax NS B3K 5X5; Dal'88; MHSc; MBA; BA; MD; FRCPC; Psy (Addiction Medicine). Staff, Canadian Forces Health Services Centre (Atlantic); Asst Prof Psy, Dalhousie University; (902)721-8376; Fax. (902)721-1295; Kenneth.Cooper@forces.gc.ca.

COOPER, Krista A; Health Canada, 0202D2-101 Tunney's Pasture Dr, Ottawa ON K1A 0K9; Qns'92; CCFP; FCFP; (613)948-8217; Fax. (613)941-1365.

COOPER, Lilanie H; Mental Health Centre, PO Box 3003 Stn Main 2345 10th Ave W, Prince Albert SK S6V 6G1; Orange Free State (South Africa)'89; MB ChB; DA; MMed(Psych); LMCC; FRCPC; Psy (Adult Psychiatry). Consultant Psy, Victoria Hospital; Consultant Psy, Kelsey Trail Health Region; (306)765-6055; Fax. (306)765-6349; lilacooper@sasktel.net.

COOPER, Linda L; Alberta Children's Hosp, 2888 Shaganappi Trail NW, Calgary AB T3B 6A8; McG'89; FRCSC; Ophth (Pediatric Ophthalmology). Staff Vision Clinic, Alberta Children's Hospital; (403)955-7940; Fax. (403)955-7672.

COOPER, Marvin; 1162 Weston Rd, Toronto ON M6M 4P4; Tor'64; FRCSC; Ophth. Assoc Staff, Humber River Regional Hospital - Keele Street Site; (416)248-1660; Fax. (416)614-0427.

COOPER, Mary Anne; Sunnybrook Hlth Sciences Ctre, HG64-2075 Bayview Ave, Toronto ON M4N 3M5; Tor'92; MEd; FRCPC; IntMed; Gastroent. Staff Gastroent, Sunnybrook Health Sciences Centre; Asst Prof, University of Toronto; (416)480-6799; Fax. (416)480-5977.

COOPER, Matthew R; Halton HCS Corp-Georgetown, 1 Princess Anne Dr, Georgetown ON L7G 2B8; McM'98; CCFP; Staff, Halton Healthcare Services Corporation - Georgetown Hospital; (905)873-0111

COOPER, Michael C; Royal Jubilee Hosp, HW140-1952 Bay St, Victoria BC V8R 1J8; UBC'82; FRCPC; Psy (Geriatric Psychiatry). Staff, Royal Jubilee Hospital; Clinical Asst Prof Psy, University of British Columbia; (250)370-8547; coopermedical@shaw.ca.

COOPER, Michael J; Hamilton HS-General Site, 237 Barton St E, Hamilton ON L8L 2X2; Mem'05; FRCSC; PlasSurg. Staff, Hamilton Health Sciences Centre - Hamilton General Hospital; (905)521-2100; Fax. (905)521-4825.

COOPER, Neil D J; 200-1632 14 Ave NW, Calgary AB T2N 1M7; Cal'90; FRCPC; Peds (Child Abuse). Med Staff, Alberta Children's Hospital; Clinical Asst Prof Med, University of Calgary; (403)284-0001; Fax. (403)284-1593.

COOPER, Pamela J; 204-6212 Main St, Stouffville ON L4A 2S5; Mem'79; FRCPC; Peds (Pediatric Neurology). Ac Staff Peds, Rouge Valley Health System - Centenary Health Centre Site; (905)640-5100; Fax. (905)640-5102; pamc@childneuro.com.

COOPER, Paul E; London HSC-University Hosp, PO Box 5339 Stn B A10 325-339 Windermere Rd, London ON N6A 5A5; Wes'73; FRCPC; Neur (Neuro Endocrinology). Consultant, St Joseph's Hospital - St Joseph's Health Care; Staff Clin Neurological Sciences, London Health Sciences Centre - University Hospital; Assoc Prof/A-Chair clin Neurological Sciences, University of Western Ontario; (519)663-2906; Fax. (519)663-2933; paul.cooper@lhsc.on.ca.

COOPER, Perry W; 490-3409 Yonge St, Toronto ON M4N 3R1; Tor'63; FRCPC; DiagRad (Neuro Radiology). Court Staff Medical Imaging, Sunnybrook Health Sciences Centre; Asst Prof Med Imaging, University of Toronto; (416)349-8199; Fax. (647)341-3507; perrycooper@rogers.com.

COOPER, Phillip W; St Martha's Doctor's Offices, 112-23 Bay St, Antigonish NS B2G 2G7; London (England)'74; MB BS; FRCS(E); DRCOG; Pres Med Staff, St Martha's Regional Hospital; (902)863-4211; Fax. (902)863-0274.

COOPER, Ruby R; Long Pond Med Clinic, PO Box 14097 Stn Main 88 Conception Bay Hwy, Conception-Bay-S NL A1W 3J1; Mem'99; CCFP; (709)834-5511; Fax. (709)834-4397.

COOPER, Richard M; 3EN 421-200 Elizabeth St, Toronto ON M5G 2C4; Tor'77; BSc; MCPS; MSc; ACLS; FRCPC; Anes (Cardiovascular Anesthesia). Staff, Mount Sinai Hospital; Staff, Toronto Western Hospital - University Health Network; Consultant Anes & Med Advisor, Toronto General Hospital - UHN; Med Dir Anes Technology, Centre for Addiction & Mental Health (CAMH) - Queen Site; Staff, Kensington Eye Institute; Assoc Prof Anes, University of Toronto; (416)340-5164; Fax. (416)340-3698; richard.cooper@uhn.ca.

COOPER, Robert A; Dufferin St Clair Comm Clinic, 1680 Dufferin St, Toronto ON M6H 3M1; Tor'92; ASAM; CCFP; FCFP; Staff, Humber River Regional Hospital - Finch Avenue Site; Staff, Humber River Regional Hospital - Church Street Site; Coun, Canadian Medical Protective Association; (416)658-6666; Fax. (416)658-8106.

COOPER, Robert C; Associate Med Group, 4705 48 Ave, Red Deer AB T4N 3T1; Sask'57; LMCC; CCFP; FCFP; Staff, Red Deer Regional Hospital Centre; Physician, Red Deer Remand Centre; Physician, Associate Medical Group; (403)346-2057; Fax. (403)347-2989.

COOPER, Robert J; PO Box 2070, Pictou NS B0K 1H0; Dal'78; CCFP; FCFP; Staff, Colchester East Hants Health Centre.

COOPER, Ryan D; Royal Alexandra Hosp, 310-10240 Kingsway NW, Edmonton AB T5H 3V9; Alb'02; FRCPC; IntMed; InfectDis (Viral Hepatitis). Staff, Royal Alexandra Hospital; (780)735-6681

COOPER, Sari D; Barrie Community Health Centre, 490 Huronia Rd, Barrie ON L4N 6M2; Qns'99; CCFP; Lecturer, University of Toronto; (705)734-9690

COOPER, Scott A; Bluewater Health-Norman Site, 89 Norman St, Sarnia ON N7T 6S3; Wes'93; BSc; AB; BSc; FRCPC; DiagRad. Staff, Bluewater Health - Norman Site; (519)464-4513; Fax. (519)336-1189.

COOPER, Stephanie L; Foothills Med Centre, F4-1403 29 St NW, Calgary AB T2N 2T9; Mem'01; ObstGyn (Maternal Fetal Medicine). Staff, Foothills Medical Centre; (403)944-4413

COOPER, Stephen C; 7020 4 St NW, Calgary AB T2K 1C4; Wes'77; (403)730-7663; Fax. (403)730-4466.

COOPER, Stephen; Little Current Med Associates, PO Box 549 15 Meredith St E, Little Current ON P0P 1K0; Cal'90; CCFP; FCFP; Chief Staff, Manitoulin Health Centre - Little Current; Fam Med, Manitoulin Health Centre - Mindemoya Site; (705)368-2450; Fax. (705)368-2480.

COOPER, Susan E; Fraser East Nephrology, 108-2051 McCallum Rd, Abbotsford BC V2S 3N5; Mem'98; FRCPC; IntMed; Nephrol. (604)870-9886

COOPER, T James; Lindsay Prof Bldg, 8-65 Angeline St N, Lindsay ON K9V 5N7; Wes'72; FRCSC; Ophth. Staff, Ross Memorial Hospital; (705)324-9404; Fax. (705)324-1944.

COOPER-ROSEN, Ethel; Woodlawn Med Clinic, 92 Main St, Dartmouth NS B2X 1R5; Dal'81; CCFP; FCFP; Assoc Staff, Dartmouth General Hospital; Assoc Staff, IWK Health Centre; Preceptor Dept. of Fam. Med., Dalhousie University; (902)434-1500; Fax. (902)434-7360.

COOPERMAN, Jonathan J; SMBD Jewish Gen Hosp, 3755 ch Cote-Sainte-Catherine, Montreal QC H3T 1E2; Haifa (Israel)'05; FRCPC; EmergMed. Staff, Sir Mortimer B Davis Jewish General; (514)340-8222 x5560

COOPERSMITH, Henry G; One Westmount Square, 550-1 Car Westmount, Westmount QC H3Z 2P9; McG'79; CHE; CCFP; Staff, Sir Mortimer B Davis Jewish General; Staff, McGill University Health Centre - Montreal General Campus; Dir Prof Services, Jewish Rehabilitation Hospital; Physician, Textiles and Manufacturing; Teacher, McGill University; (514)737-1109; Fax. (514)737-1109.

COORAY, Anurad R; William Osler HC-Etobicoke, 101 Humber College Blvd, Etobicoke ON M9V 1R8; Ukranian (Ukraine)'91; CCFP; Staff, William Osler Health System - Etobicoke General Hospital; (416)494-2120; Fax. (416)747-3611.

COP, Milorad; C242 RR 4, Shawville QC J0X 2Y0; Alexandria (Egypt)'82; Ac Staff, Pontiac Hospital Centre; (819)647-3759

COPELAND, Catherine M; Breast Centre Radiology, 7121 109 St NW, Edmonton AB T6G 1B9; Wes'76; ABR; FRCPC; DiagRad (Bone Densitometry). Clin Teacher, University of Alberta; (780)434-9147; Fax. (780)436-7650.

COPELAND, Charles L H; Anderson Med Centre, 728 Anderson St, Whitby ON L1N 3V6; Cape Town (South Africa)'84; MB ChB; CCFP; (905)666-5412; Fax. (905)665-1950.

COPELAND, David; Medical Arts Bldg, 2F-110 Sydney St, Cornwall ON K6H 3H2; McG'70; FRCPC; IntMed; ClinImmunol&Allergy. Affil Staff, McGill University Health Centre - Montreal General Campus; Affil Staff, Cornwall Community Hospital; Langs: Bilingual(English/French); (613)937-3101

COPELAND, Joseph E; BC Children's Hosp, 4480 Oak St, Vancouver BC V6H 3V4; Los Angeles (USA)'99; CCFP; FCFP; CCFP(E.M.); Staff, BC Children's Hospital; Langs: French; (604)875-2345; Fax. (604)875-2345.

COPELAND, Julie A; Thames Valley Family Hlth Team, RR 5 22262 Mill Rd, Mount Brydges ON N0L 1W0; Tor'03; CCFP; Asst Prof Family Med, University of Western Ontario; (519)264-2800; Fax. (519)264-2742; juliec@smhc.net.

COPELAND, Laura L; Humber River Reg Hosp-Church, 200 Church St, Toronto ON M9N 1N8; Ohio (USA)'01; Staff, Humber River Regional Hospital - Church Street Site; (416)249-8111

COPEN, Brenda Y K; Queen Alexandra Ctre Children, 2400 Arbutus Rd, Victoria BC V8N 1V7; Man'95; FRCPC; Psy. Staff, Queen Alexandra Centre for Children's Health; (250)519-6750

COPEN, John V W; Victoria Gen Hosp, N241-1 Hospital Way, Victoria BC V8Z 6R5; Man'95; FRCPC; Psy (Addiction Psychiatry). Staff, Victoria General Hospital; (250)727-4509

COPITHORNE, Peter G; London HSC-Victoria Hosp, PO Box 5010 Stn B E4 123-800 Commissioners Rd E, London ON N6A 5W9; Cal'06; FRCSC; OrthSurg. Staff Ortho Surg, London Health Sciences Centre - Victoria Campus; (519)685-8086

COPLAND, Michael A; Gordon & Leslie Diamond HCC, 5F-2775 Laurel St, Vancouver BC V5Z 1M9; UBC'95; FRCPC; IntMed; Nephrol. Staff, Gordon & Leslie Diamond Health Care Centre; Staff, Vancouver General Hospital - Centennial Pavillion; Clin Assoc Prof Prof, University of British Columbia; Langs: French; (604)875-5950; Fax. (604)875-5952.

COPLEY, James; Ctr Hosp Reg Chisasibi, PO Box 250, Chisasibi QC J0M 1E0; McG'10; MDCM; CCFP; Staff, Cree Board of Health & Social Services James Bay; (819)855-9001

COPPIN, Christopher M L; BC Cancer Agency-Vanc Isl Ctr, 2410 Lee Ave, Victoria BC V8R 6V5; Oxford (England)'72; BCh; MRC(UK); PhD(Oxon); ABIM(MedOncol); FRCPC; IntMed; MedOncol. Staff, BC Cancer Agency Vancouver Island Centre.

COPPIN, James A; 7860 Afton Dr, Richmond BC V7A 1A4; UBC'76; (604)274-7679

COPPOLA, John; 14-11625 Elbow Dr SW PO Box 83043, Calgary AB T2W 1G8; Alb'80; CCFP; Staff, Rockyview General Hospital.

COPPOLA, Joanne; Hinton Healthcare Centre, 1280 Switzer Dr, Hinton AB T7V 1V2; Sask'80; BSc(Hons); FRCPC; DiagRad. Staff Med Imaging, Peace Arch Hospital; Staff, Hinton Healthcare Centre; (780)865-3333

COPPOLINO, Andrew G; Grand River Hosp-KW Hlth Ctre, PO Box 9056 Stn C 835 King St W, Kitchener ON N2G 1G3; Tor'57; Psy. Staff, Grand River Hospital - Kitchener/Waterloo Health Centre; (519)743-0402

COPPS, Brenda E; 576 Main St E, Hamilton ON L8M 1J2; McM'81; CCFP; FCFP; (905)528-5292; Fax. (905)528-7753.

COPTI, Michel; Clinique Med, 102-1030 rue Berri, Montreal QC H2L 4C3; Beirut (Lebanon)'63; Electroenceph (P.Q.); Neur. Member Med Evaluation Office, Ministry of Labour & Solidarite(Quebec); Langs: Arabic; Bilingual(English/French); (514)844-1147; Fax. (514)844-7516; michelcopti@videotron.ca.

COQUET, Sean C; University of Alberta Hosp, 1C1.04-8440 112 St NW, Edmonton AB T6G 2B7; Sask'06; FRCPC; Anes. Staff, University of Alberta Hospital; (780)407-8822

COQUET-LE PAPE, Bernadette; CSSSG-Hop De Gatineau, 909 boul la Verndrye O, Gatineau QC J8P 7H2; Rennes (France)'89; Staff, Hôpital de Gatineau; (819)966-6246; Fax. (819)966-6242.

CORAZZA, Bernard; Hop Charles Lemoyne, 3120 boul Taschereau, Greenfield Park QC J4V 2H1; Mon'94; Staff, Hopital Charles LeMoyne; (450)466-5000 x2050

CORBEIL, Catherine; Clin Med Plateau Marquette, 200-731 rue Galt O, Sherbrooke QC J1H 1Z1; Sher'04; (819)822-0404

CORBEIL, Chantal P; 1485 Bancroft Dr, Sudbury ON P3B 1R6; Ott'04; FRCPC; Peds. (705)523-7120; Fax. (705)523-8232.

CORBEIL, Claude; Hop Charles LeMoyne, 3120 boul Taschereau, Greenfield Park QC J4V 2H1; Mon'79; Critical Care Medicine (P.Q.); Respir (P.Q.). Staff, Hopital Charles LeMoyne; (450)466-5000 x5053

CORBEIL, Diane; CLSC du Marigot, 1351 boul des Laurentides, Vimont QC H7M 2Y2; Mon'75; (450)668-1506; Fax. (450)668-1507.

CORBEIL, Francois; CSSS de Trois-Rivieres, 1991 boul du Carmel, Trois-Rivieres QC G8Z 3R9; Laval'83; FRCPC; IntMed; Respir. Chef Dept of Med, CSSS de Trois-Rivières; (819)697-3333

CORBEIL, Marie-Andree; CSSS Haut-Richelieu-Rouville, 920 boul du Seminaire N, St-Jean-sur-Richel QC J3A 1B7; Mon'00; FRCPC; IntMed; Endocrin&Metab. Staff, Hôpital du Haut-Richelieu; (450)359-5000

CORBEIL, Robert P; Clin des Medecins D'Urgence, 632 rue Bowen S, Sherbrooke QC J1G 2E9; Laval'78; Ac Staff, Centre Hospitalier Universitaire de Sherbrooke-Hôpital Hôtel-Dieu; (819)822-2700; Fax. (819)822-2027.

CORBEIL, Vincent; CSSS Pierre Boucher, 1333 boul Jacques-Cartier E, Longueuil QC J4M 2A5; Mon'88; FRCPC; DiagRad. Staff, Centre Hospitalier Pierre Boucher; (450)468-8157; cmvcorbeil@gmail.com.

CORBET, Kenneth J; HSC-Faculty of Med, 3330 Hospital Dr NW, Calgary AB T2N 4N1; Cal'81; FRCPC; OccupMed. Assoc Prof, University of Calgary; (403)220-3362; Fax. (403)270-7307.

CORBETT, Barbara; Dawson Road Family Med Clinic, 83 Dawson Rd, Guelph ON N1H 1B1; London (England)'80; MB BS; DRCOG; CCFP; (519)766-1360; Fax. (519)763-4315; bcorbett@cvh.on.ca.

CORBETT, Brian N; Saint John Reg Hosp, PO Box 2100 Stn Main 400 University Ave, Saint John NB E2L 4L2; Man'65; FRCPC; Cardiol. Staff, Saint John Regional Hospital; (506)648-6101; Fax. (506)648-6110.

CORBETT, Caroline A; Manitoba Clinic, 790 Sherbrook St, Winnipeg MB R3A 1M3; Man'01; FRCSC; ObstGyn.

CORBETT, Elizabeth A S; River City Centre, 609-8600 Franklin Ave, Fort McMurray AB T9H 4G8; Cork (Ireland)'83; MB ChB; BAO; MRCPsy; LMCC; (780)791-1333; Fax. (780)791-7539.

CORBETT, Peter J; Tom Baker Cancer Centre, 1331 29 St NW Box 386, Calgary AB T2N 4N2; London (England)'69; MB BS; LRCP; FRCR; FRCS; FRCPC; RadOncol (Breast Cancer). Ac Staff, Foothills Medical Centre; Sr Specialist RanOncol, Tom Baker Cancer Centre; Clin Assoc Prof, University of Calgary; (403)521-3164; peterco@cancerboard.ab.ca.

CORBETT, Shannon; Ottawa Fertility Clinic, 955 Green Valley Cres, Ottawa ON K2C 3V4; McM'06; ObstGyn. (613)686-3378

CORBETT, Thomas B; The Juravinski Cancer Centre, 699 Concession St, Hamilton ON L8V 5C2; Man'87; FRCPC; RadOncol (Genito Urinary Oncology). Med Staff Assoc, Hamilton Health Sciences Centre-Juravinski Site; Staff, The Juravinski Cancer Centre; Asst Prof Med, McMaster University; (905)387-9495 x64705; Fax. (905)575-6326; tom.corbett@jcc.hhsc.ca.

CORBETT, Thomas F X; South Side Women's Clinic, 120-3017 66 St NW, Edmonton AB T6K 4B2; National (Ireland)'79; MB ChB; MRCGPract; DABOG; FACOG; FRCSC; ObstGyn (Colposcopy). Site Leader ObstGyn, Covenant Health - Grey Nuns Community Hospital; Staff, Cross Cancer Institute; Staff ObstGyn, University of Alberta Hospital; Prof, University of Alberta; (780)468-6188

CORBEY, Leigh A; 502-2000 Credit Valley Rd, Mississauga ON L5M 4N4; Wes'00; FRCSC; ObstGyn. (905)820-8885

CORBIN, Francois; CHUS-Hop Fleurimont, 3001 12e av N, Sherbrooke QC J1H 5N4; Laval'01; CSPQ; FRCPC; MedBiochem. Staff, Centre Hospitalier Universitaire de Sherbrooke-Hopital Fleurimont; Langs: English; (819)346-1110 x15801; francois.corbin@usherbrooke.ca.

CORBIN, Jean M; 285 Whitewood Ave PO Box 1180, New Liskeard ON P0J 1P0; Mon'97; CCFP; Langs: English; (705)647-1224; Fax. (705)647-4438.

CORBIN, Jean-Francois; CHUS-Hop Hotel-Dieu, 580 rue Bowen S, Sherbrooke QC J1G 2E8; Nantes (France)'77; Staff, Centre Hospitalier Universitaire de Sherbrooke-Hôpital Hôtel-Dieu; (819)346-1110

CORBIN, Serge; 7 Carrefour De La Sante, Roxton Pond QC J0E 1Z0; Sher'82; Langs: English; (450)776-1171; Fax. (450)776-1089.

CORBY, Debora J; North Edmonton Health Centre, 14007 50 St NW, Edmonton AB T5A 5E4; Alb'04; BSc; MSc; CCFP; (780)342-4038

CORCORAN, Edan P; St Joseph's Health Centre, 710 Victoria Ave E, Thunder Bay ON P7C 5P7; Dublin (Ireland)'85; MRCPsy; FRCPC; Psy. Staff, Lakehead Psychiatric Hospital - St. Joseph's Care Group; (807)343-4300

CORCORAN, Erin L; Alberta Children's Hosp, 2888 Shaganappi Trail NW, Calgary AB T3B 6A8; Staff, Alberta Children's Hospital; (403)955-7810; Fax. (403)955-7606.

CORCORAN, Louise A; North Vancouver Med Clinic, 115 16th St W, North Vancouver BC V7M 1T3; Dublin (Ireland)'94; MB ChB; BAO; CCFP; (604)904-8804; Fax. (604)904-0972.

CORCOS, Jacques; SMBD Jewish Gen Hosp, E944-3755 ch Cote-Sainte-Cathe, Montreal QC H3T 1E2; Montpellier (France)'77; Urol (Benign Prostatic Hypertrophy). Dir Urology Services, Sir Mortimer B Davis Jewish General; Prof, McGill University; (514)340-8222 x5166; Fax. (514)340-7559.

CORD, Stephen M; Forest Hill Family Health Cent, 2F-491 Eglinton Ave W, Toronto ON M5N 1A8; Tor'92; CCFP; CCFP(E.M.); FCFP; Staff Family Practice, Mount Sinai Hospital; Staff Family Practice, Humber River Regional Hospital - Finch Avenue Site; Staff EmergMed, South Muskoka Memorial Hospital - Muskoka Algonquin Healthcare; (416)782-6111 x125; Fax. (416)782-5515; cord67@yahoo.ca.

CORDAHI, Ghassan; Hop Maisonneuve-Rosemont, 5415 boul de l'Assomption, Montreal QC H1T 2M4; St Joseph (Lebanon)'92; ABOph; assoc Prof, Hopital Maisonneuve-Rosemont; (514)252-3400

CORDEAU, Chantal; Inst Albert Prevost, 6555 boul Gouin O, Montreal QC H4K 1B3; Mon'84; Ac Staff, Hôpital du Sacre-Coeur de Montréal; (514)338-4300

CORDEAU, Eve; CSSS de Sept-Iles, 45 rue du Pere-Divet, Sept-Iles QC G4R 3N7; Sher'06; Staff, Centre Hospitalier Regional de Sept-Iles; (418)962-9761

CORDEAU, Karyne; UMF Laurier, 2875 boul Laurier, Quebec QC G1V 2M2; Laval'03; (418)654-2701

CORDEAU, Marie-Pierre; CHUM-Hotel-Dieu, 3840 rue Saint-Urbain, Montreal QC H2W 1T8; Mon'86; FRCPC; DiagRad (Thoracic Radiology). Staff, Centre Hospitalier l'Université de Montréal (CHUM) - Hôtel-Dieu; Clin Teach Staff, Universite de Montreal; (514)890-8150; mpcordeau@videotron.ca.

CORDEIRO, Erin D; Univ Hlth Network-Princess M, 610 University Ave, Toronto ON M5G 2M9; Dal'06; FRCSC; GenSurg (Surgical Oncology). Staff, Princess Margaret Hospital - University Health Network; (416)946-3583

CORDELL, Bruce A; Medical Arts Bldg, 353 St Paul Ave, Brantford ON N3R 4N3; Wes'80; FRCPC; IntMed. Ac Staff IntMed, The Brant Community Healthcare System - Brantford General Hospital Site; (519)759-4992

CORDOBA, J Carlos; CHUM-Hop Notre-Dame, 1560 rue Sherbrooke E, Montreal QC H2L 4M1; McG'93; FRCSC; PlasSurg. Staff, Centre Hospitalier l'Université de Montréal (CHUM) - Hôpital Notre-Dame; (514)890-8200

CORDON, Ian W; 103-1595 McKenzie Ave, Victoria BC V8N 1A4; Bristol (England)'77; MB ChB; FRCPC; EmergMed. (250)477-4777

CORDONI, Teresa; 350-2755 Lougheed Hwy, Port Coquitlam BC V3B 5Y9; UBC'79; CCFP; (604)941-9066; Fax. (604)941-9289; tcordoni@shaw.ca.

CORDOS, Mihaela C; York Medical Clinic, 110-1650 Elgin Mills Rd, Richmond Hill ON L4S 0B2; Cluj (Romania)'95; CCFP; (905)770-3858

CORDOVA, Juan L; 201-355 Ellice Ave, Winnipeg MB R3B 1X8; (Chile)'71; Staff, Health Sciences Centre; Langs: Spanish; French; Italian.

CORDOVA PEREZ, Francisco; St Boniface Gen Hosp, Y3005-409 Tache Ave, Winnipeg MB R2H 2A6; Staff, St Boniface General Hospital; (204)233-8563

CORDOVANI, Daniel; Sunnybrook Health Sciences Ctr, M3 200-2075 Bayview Ave, Toronto ON M4N 3M5; University of Sao Paolo (Brazil)'05; Clin Fellow Anes, Sunnybrook Health Sciences Centre; (416)480-6100; Fax. (416)480-6039.

COREN, Lee Anne H; Main West Med Group, 300-1685 Main St W, Hamilton ON L8S 1G5; McM'00; MSc; CCFP; (905)522-8915

CORENBLUM, Bernard; Richmond Road Diag & Trmt Ctr, 1888-1820 Richmond Rd SW, Calgary AB T2T 5C7; Alb'71; IntMed (Endocrinology & Metabolism). Ac Staff, Foothills Medical Centre; Staff, Richmond Road Diagnostic & Treatment Centre; (403)955-8342; Fax. (403)955-8248; corenblu@ucalgary.ca.

CORET, Alexander; St Joseph's Healthcare, 50 Charlton Ave E, Hamilton ON L8N 4A6; Haifa (Israel)'83; Staff, St Joseph's Healthcare - Charlton Campus; (905)522-1155; Fax. (905)540-6500.

CORET, Stephen D; Peace Arch Hosp, 15521 Russell Ave, White Rock BC V4B 2R4; St. Louis (USA)'77; FRCPC; GenPath; AnatPath. Staff Lab Med, Peace Arch Hospital; Staff, Mission Memorial Hospital; (604)531-5512; Fax. (604)535-4533.

CORET-SIMON, Judit; St Joseph's Healthcare, 50 Charlton Ave E, Hamilton ON L8N 4A6; Haifa (Israel)'85; Staff, St Joseph's Healthcare - Charlton Campus; (905)522-1155 x4072; Fax. (905)540-6590.

COREY, Jo Ann M; St Joseph's Mountain H Service, PO Box 585 Stn Lcd 1 100 5th St W, Hamilton ON L8N 3K7; McM'96; FRCPC; Psy. Staff, St Joseph's Healthcare Hamilton - West 5th Campus; (905)522-1155 x36602

COREY, John S; Caulfeild Village Med Clinic, 220-5317 Headland Dr, West Vancouver BC V7W 3C5; Ott'87; Staff, Lions Gate Hospital; Staff, Caulfield Village Medical Clinic; Staff, Park Royal Medical Clinic; Staff, Park Royal Village Medical Centre; (604)925-4448; Fax. (604)922-1586; drjcoreymd@aol.com.

CORIATY, Paul; Ctr Hosp de Verdun, 4000 boul Lasalle, Verdun QC H4G 2A3; Bucharest (Romania)'78; FRCSC; OrthSurg. Staff, Centre Hospitalier de Verdun; (514)362-1000

CORKAL, James F; Stanton Terr Health Authority, PO Box 10 Stn Main, Yellowknife NT X1A 2N1; Qns'78; FRCSC; OrthSurg. Staff, Stanton Territorial Health Authority; (867)669-4111

CORKERY, Douglas L J A; Conroy Med Centre, 100-2 Lorry Greenberg Dr, Ottawa ON K1G 5H6; Ott'82; (613)737-0654

CORKUM, Casey G; Trillium Summerville Fam Med U, 700-101 Queensway W, Mississauga ON L5B 2P7; Dal'09; CCFP; (905)272-9900; Fax. (905)272-9977.

CORKUM, Cheryl D; South Nepean Satellite Comm HC, 201-4100 Strandherd Dr, Ottawa ON K2J 0V2; Mem'10; CCFP; (613)288-2820; Fax. (613)288-3690.

CORKUM, Thomas P; 207-255 Lacewood Dr, Halifax NS B3M 4G2; Tor'64; FACOG; FRCSC; ObstGyn. Asst Prof, Dalhousie University; (902)457-3703; Fax. (902)457-3707.

CORLESS, Kevin J; North Oshawa Med Centre, 205-1400 Ritson Rd N, Oshawa ON L1G 7W4; RCS (Ireland)'85; Staff, Lakeridge Health - Oshawa Site; Staff, Ontario Shores Centre for Mental Health Sciences; (905)404-0372

CORLESS, William J A; 84 Dufferin Ave, Saint John NB E2K 2T8; UBC'86; BSc; (506)634-7646; Fax. (506)634-7378.

CORLEY, James B; Sundance Med Clinic, 7-402 Railway St W, Cochrane AB T4C 2B6; Alb'74; (403)932-2255; Fax. (403)932-2254.

CORMACK, Maura A; Lonsdale Med Dental Bldg, 108-1940 Lonsdale Ave, North Vancouver BC V7M 2K2; Alb'86; BSc; (604)987-3357; Fax. (604)987-7624.

CORMIER, Beatrice; CHUM-Hop Notre-Dame, 1560 rue Sherbrooke E, Montreal QC H2L 4M1; Mon'05; GynOnco; ObstGyn. Staff, Centre Hospitalier l'Université de Montréal (CHUM) - Hôpital Notre-Dame; (514)890-8000

CORMIER, Blandine; The Moncton Hosp, 135 MacBeath Ave, Moncton NB E1C 6Z8; CCFP; Staff, The Moncton Hospital; (506)857-5111

CORMIER, Chantale; Centre Hosp Honore-Mercier, 2750 boul Laframboise, Saint-Hyacinthe QC J2S 4Y8; Mon'06; FRCSC; Otol. Staff, Centre Hospitalier Honore-Mercier; (450)771-3333

CORMIER, Charles; Clinique Med Richmond, 170 rue Gouin, Richmond QC J0B 2H0; Sher'85; CCFP; (819)826-5750

CORMIER, Charline; Clinique Sante Jacques-Cartier, 200-1815 rue King O, Sherbrooke QC J1J 2E3; Sher'82; LMCC; Langs: Spanish; English; (819)565-7446 x212

CORMIER, Daniel; 201-231 Champlain St, Dieppe NB E1A 1N9; Sher'92; FRCSC; Ophth. (506)854-6333; Fax. (506)854-6474.

CORMIER, Daniel; CSSS de Trois-Rivieres, 1991 boul Du Carmel, Trois-Rivieres QC G8Z 3R9; Laval'76; CSPQ; FRCPC; Anes. Staff, CSSS de Trois-Rivières; (819)697-3333

CORMIER, David R; Fifth Avenue Med Centre, 400-14 Fifth Ave, Orangeville ON L9W 1G2; Dal'82; CCFP; Staff, Headwaters Health Care Centre - Orangeville Site; (519)941-3572; Fax. (519)941-3572.

CORMIER, Francois; CHUS-Hop Fleurimont, 3001 12e Av N, Sherbrooke QC J1H 5N4; Sher'87; CSPQ; FRCPC; Anes. Staff, Centre Hospitalier Universitaire de Sherbrooke-Hopital Fleurimont; (819)346-1110; Fax. (819)820-6420.

CORMIER, Gilles J; 201-231 Champlain St, Dieppe NB E1A 1N9; Mon'92; FRCSC; Ophth (Cataract Surgery). Staff, Beausejour & South-East Regional Health Authority - Moncton; Staff, Beausejour District Hospital; Langs: English; (506)854-6333; Fax. (506)854-6474.

CORMIER, Helene; Clinique Med de l'Ouest, 2200 boul Dionne, Saint-Georges QC G5Y 3X3; Laval'96; Staff, Centre Hospitalier Beauce-Etchemin; Langs: English; (418)228-2024; Fax. (418)228-7715.

CORMIER, Hugues; Clinique St-Leonard, 404-8000 boul Langelier, Saint-Leonard QC H1P 3K2; Sher'77; MPH; FRCPC; Psy (Public Health & Preventive Medicine). Staff, Hopital Louis-H Lafontaine; Adj Vice Dean Student Life, Universite de Montreal; (514)323-1617 x221; hugues.cormier@umontreal.ca.

CORMIER, Janice; Dr L Richard Ctre D'Oncologie, 37 rue Providence, Moncton NB E1C 8X3; Laval'91; Asst Staff Clinical Oncol, Dr Georges-L-Dumont University Hospital Centre; Langs: Bilingual(French/English); (506)862-4030; Fax. (506)862-4222.

CORMIER, Jean-Pierre; CSSS Baie des Chaleurs, RR 2 419 boul Perron, Maria QC G0C 1Y0; Laval'81; Staff, CSSS de la Baie-des-Chaleurs; (418)759-3443

CORMIER, Jules; 105-185 av Acadie, Dieppe NB E1A 1G6; Sher'05; CCFP; Clin Prof, Universite de Sherbrooke; Langs: Bilingual(French/English); (506)862-4182

CORMIER, Julie; CSSS de Rivière-de-Loup, 75 rue Saint-Henri, Riviere-du-Loup QC G5R 2A4; Laval'98; FRCPC; Psy. Staff, Centre Hospitalier Regional du Grand-Portage; (418)868-1010; Fax. (418)868-0530; julieedithcormier@hotmail.com.

CORMIER, Julie; CSSS de Portneuf, 700 rue Saint-Cyrille, Saint-Raymond QC G3L 1W1; Mon'06; CCFP; CCFP(E.M.); Staff, Centre Hospitalier Portneuf; (418)337-4611

CORMIER, Luc; CHUS-Hop Fleurimont, 3001 12 av N, Sherbrooke QC J1H 5N4; Sher'07; IntMed. Staff, Centre Hospitalier Universitaire de Sherbrooke-Hopital Fleurimont; (819)346-1110

CORMIER, M Alana; Chilliwack Gen Hosp, 45600 Menholm Rd, Chilliwack BC V2P 1P7; Dal'07; FRCP; CCFP; Staff, Chilliwack General Hospital; (604)795-4141

CORMIER, Nathalie; Clinique Med D'Amos, 641 4e rue O, Amos QC J9T 2S1; Mon'98; (819)732-1244; Fax. (819)832-4646.

CORMIER, Pascal; Hôpital régional Chaleur, 1750 Sunset Dr, Bathurst NB E2A 4L7; Paris (France)'93; Staff, Hospital Regional Chaleur; (506)544-2316; Fax. (506)544-2326.

CORMIER, Rachel M; CSSS Drummond-Hop Sainte-Croix, 570 rue Heriot, Drummondville QC J2B 1C1; Sher'04; FRCPC; Anes. Staff, Hôpital Sainte-croix; (819)478-6464

CORMIER, Renaud; 48 rue Thomas, Saint-Jacques NB E7B 1P9; Mon'99; Staff, Hôtel-Dieu St-Joseph de Saint-Quentin; Staff, Hôpital regional d'Edmundston; Fax. (506)353-0128.

CORMIER, Roberta T; Hop Maisonneuve-Rosemont, 5415 boul de l'Assomption, Montreal QC H1T 2M4; Mon'73; Clin Physician, Hopital Maisonneuve-Rosemont; Langs: Bilingual(French/English); (514)252-3945

CORMIER, Yvon F; Hôpital Laval, 2725 ch Sainte-Foy, Quebec QC G1V 4G5; Laval'71; Respir. Staff, Hôpital Laval; Consultant, CSSS de Quebec-Sud; assoc Doyen Research/Prof Med, Université Laval; Langs: French; (418)656-4747; Fax. (418)656-4762; yvon.cormier@med.ulaval.ca.

CORNE, Stephen I; Respiratory Unit, RS318-810 Sherbrook St, Winnipeg MB R3A 1R8; Man'86; FRCPC; IntMed; Respir. Staff, Health Sciences Centre.

CORNEAU, Richard; CSST, 901 boul Talbot, Chicoutimi QC G7H 6N7; Laval'72; Staff, CSSS de Lac-Saint Jean-Est; (418)696-5200 x5265

CORNEIL, Glenn G; Dr G Corneil Med Prof Corp, PO Box 1615 285 Whitewood Ave, New Liskeard ON P0J 1P0; Tor'95; CCFP; FCFP; Staff, Temiskaming Hospital; Langs: Bilingual(English/French); (705)647-4737; Fax. (705)647-4799.

CORNEIL, Trevor A; Kelowna Health Centre, 1340 Ellis St, Kelowna BC V1Y 9N1; Qns'95; FRCPC; CommunMed;CCFP; FCFP; PedEmergMed. Assoc Staff, Providence Health Care - St Paul's Hospital; Langs: Bilingual(English/French); (250)868-7729

CORNEILLE, Louise; CSSS de Laval, 1755 boul Rene-Laennec, Laval QC H7M 3L9; Mon'76; Nephrol (P.Q.) (Dialysis). Staff, Hopital de la Cite de la santé; Clin Teach Staff, Universite de Montreal; Langs: Bilingual(French/English); (450)978-8600 x8457; Fax. (450)978-2970; louisecorneille@sympatico.ca.

CORNELISSEN, Rohan; Victoria Square, 2060-2345 10th Ave W, Prince Albert SK S6V 7V6; Pretoria (South Africa)'82; MB ChB; LMCC; Langs: Afrikaans; Zulu; Portuguese; (306)764-2266; Fax. (306)764-2305.

CORNELL, I Scott; Royal Columbian Hosp, 330 Columbia St E, New Westminster BC V3L 3W7; McM'77; FRCPC; AnatPath (Dermatological Pathology). Staff, Royal Columbian Hospital; Staff, BC Biomedical Laboratories Ltd; (604)520-4348; scott.cornell@fraserhealth.ca.

CORNELL, Lilly K; 201-474 Holland Ave, Ottawa ON K1Y 0Z5; Prague (Czech Republic)'79; (613)728-1392; Fax. (613)728-4062.

CORNELL, Richard A; Collingwood Health Centre, 208-186 Erie St, Collingwood ON L9Y 4T3; Wes'90; CCFP; CCFP(E.M.); Staff, Collingwood General & Marine Hospital; Staff, Collingwood Health Centre; Langs: English; French; (705)445-0458

CORNELSON, Brian M; Health Centre at 410, 410 Sherbourne St, Toronto ON M4X 1K2; Ott'73; CCFP; FCFP; Ac Staff, St Michael's Hospital; Asst Prof, University of Toronto; (416)867-3728; Fax. (416)867-3727; cornelsonb@smh.ca.

CORNET, Anne M J; Appletree Med Centre, 2016 Ogilvie Rd, Ottawa ON K1J 7N9; Paris (France)'72; FRCP; FAAP; FRCPC; Peds (Neonatology). Langs: French; (613)482-0118; Fax. (613)749-3105.

CORNET-TOUSSAINT, Edwine; Ctr Hosp De Beauceville, 253 108 Rte, Beauceville QC G5X 2Z3; (Haiti)'78; Staff, Centre d'hébergement de Beauceville; (418)774-3304

CORNEY, Paul R; Polyclinic Prof Bldg, 199 Grafton St, Charlottetown PE C1A 1L2; Ott'08; CCFP; (902)629-8810

CORNFIELD, Mark J I; 326 Locke St S, Hamilton ON L8P 4C6; McM'76; FRCPC; Psy. (905)525-0222; Fax. (905)525-3164; marcorn88@hotmail.com.

CORNILA, Angelica M; 168 Essex St, Sarnia ON N7T 4R9; '92; FRCPC; IntMed. (519)337-7535

CORNISH, Bruce M; Royal City Centre, 228B-610 Sixth St, New Westminster BC V3L 3C2; Ott'74; Court Staff, Royal Columbian Hospital; (604)524-8228; Fax. (604)524-9318.

CORNOCK, Elizabeth; North Island Eye Centre, 201-1771 Comox Ave, Comox BC V9M 3L9; Cal'77; FRCSC; Ophth (Comprehensive Ophthalmology). (250)890-0089; Fax. (250)890-0090; drcornock.office@shawbiz.ca.

CORPUS, Rolando T; Centre for Vein Care, 501-4580 Dufferin St, North York ON M3H 5Y2; U. of the East (Philippines)'72; AB; FACS; FRCSC; GenSurg (Phlebology). Ac Staff Surg, North York General Hospital - Branson Division; Langs: Tagalog; (416)739-9123; Fax. (416)739-1238.

CORPUS, Teofilo; Bowmanville Prof Bldg, 2101-222 King St E, Bowmanville ON L1C 1P6; Tor'95; BSc; CCFP; Staff, Lakeridge Health - Bowmanville Site; (905)697-3607; Fax. (905)697-3645.

CORPUS, Todd R; Care for Vein Centre, 501-4580 Dufferin St, North York ON M3H 5Y2; Loma Linda(CA) (USA)'02; CCFP; (416)739-9123; Fax. (416)739-1238; suproc@hotmail.com.

CORR, Peter D; Campbell River & Dist Gen Hosp, 375 2nd Ave, Campbell River BC V9W 3V1; (Zimbabwe)'79; FRCPC; DiagRad. Staff, Campbell River & District General Hospital; (250)287-7111

CORRAL, Maria D R; St Paul's Hosp, 1081 Burrard St, Vancouver BC V6Z 1Y6; UBC'83; FRCPC; Psy (Reproductive Psy). Staff, Providence Health Care - St Paul's Hospital; Consultant, Vancouver General Hospital - Centennial Pavillion; Staff, BC Women's Hospital & Health Centre; Clin Prof, University of British Columbia; (604)806-8589; Fax. (604)806-8621; mcorral@providencehealth.bc.ca.

CORRALES, Jennifer; Lahey Med Centre, 2204-120 5 Ave W, Cochrane AB T4C 0A4; Cal'05; BSc; CCFP; (403)981-6000; Fax. (403)981-6001.

CORRALES MEDINA, Vincente F; The Ottawa Hosp-Civic Campus, CPC 470-1053 Carling Ave, Ottawa ON K1Y 4E9; Arequipa (Peru)'97; Staff, The Ottawa Hospital - Civic Campus; (613)761-4155; Fax. (613)761-5260.

CORREIA, Adriano J; Credit Valley Med Arts Centre, 202-2000 Credit Valley Rd, Mississauga ON L5M 4N4; Tor'06; FRCPC; IntMed; Gastroent. (905)828-6777; Fax. (905)828-6770.

CORREIA, Amelia T; 4-809 Bullivant Cres SW, Medicine Hat AB T1A 5G6; Dal'02; CCFP; Staff, Medicine Hat Regional Hospital; (403)504-8558

CORREIA, Jason D; 106-3305 Harvester Rd, Burlington ON L7N 3N2; Tor'04; FRCSC; GenSurg. (905)333-6245; Fax. (905)333-6266.

CORRIGAN, Jason R; Beaumont Family Medical, 4-5102 49 Ave, Beaumont AB T4X 1E4; Alb'04; CCFP; Staff, Ottewell Medical Clinic; (780)929-5400; Fax. (780)929-2126.

CORRIGAN, Karin Liezel; Fox Creek Med Clinic, PO Box 640, Fox Creek AB T0H 1P0; Stellenbosch (South Africa)'90; MB ChB; Langs: Afrikaans; (780)622-3010; Fax. (780)622-3474.

CORRIGAN, Mark A; Univ Hlth Network-Princess M, 3 130-610 University Ave, Toronto ON M5G 2M9; National University of Ireland (Ireland)'02; Clin Fellow Surg Oncol, Princess Margaret Hospital - University Health Network; (416)946-2000

CORRIGAN, Michael J; McConnell Med Centre, 122-820 Mcconnell Ave, Cornwall ON K6H 4M4; Glasgow (Scotland)'76; MB ChB; FRCSC; OrthSurg. (613)933-4712; Fax. (613)933-5684.

CORRIGAN, T Michael; Smith Clinic, 1-6601 48 Ave, Camrose AB T4V 3G8; Alb'70; Ac Staff, Covenant Health - St Mary's Hospital; Physician, Bethany Long Term Care; Physician, Rose Haven Care Centre; (780)672-2425; Fax. (780)679-2668.

CORRIN, Lesley S; North Toronto Med Bldg, 102-250 Lawrence Ave W, Toronto ON M5M 1B2; Man'78; (416)787-1775; Fax. (416)787-3255.

CORRIN, Murray Dean; 528 Dundas St, London ON N6B 1W6; Wes'90; (519)645-1533

CORRIN, Raymond G; The Ottawa Hosp-Gen Campus, MG-501 Smyth Rd, Ottawa ON K1H 8L6; Wes'73; DTMH; AB; EmergMed. Staff, The Ottawa Hospital - General Campus; (613)237-4899

CORRIVEAU, André E; 24F-10025 Jasper Ave NW, Edmonton AB T5J 1S6; McG'81; MBA; BSc; MDCM; FRCPC; CommunMed. Chief Med Officer of Hlth, Alberta Health & Wellness; Aj Prof, University of Calgary; Aj Prof, University of Alberta; Langs: Bilingual(English/French); (780)415-2809; Fax. (780)415-2182; andre.corriveau@gov.ab.ca.

CORRIVEAU, Christine; CHUM-Hop Notre-Dame, 1560 rue Sherbrooke E, Montreal QC H2L 4M1; Mon'79; FRCSC; Ophth. Staff Ophth, Centre Hospitalier l'Université de Montréal (CHUM) - Hôpital Notre-Dame; Prog Dir, Universite de Montreal; (514)890-8000 x27103

CORRIVEAU, Dominic; CSSS Drummond-Hop Sainte-Croix, 570 rue Heriot, Drummondville QC J2B 1C1; Mon'98; DiagRad. Staff, Hôpital Sainte-croix; (819)478-6464; Fax. (819)478-6480.

CORRIVEAU, Jean-Paul; 929 3e Av, Val-d'Or QC J9P 1T4; Mon'82; Staff, Centre Hospitalier de Val d'Or; (819)874-9111; Fax. (819)874-9191.

CORRIVEAU, Louis; CHUM-Hop Notre-Dame, 1560 rue Sherbrooke E, Montreal QC H2L 4M1; Mon'67; DAB; Ophth (Vitreo Retina). Staff, Centre Hospitalier l'Université de Montréal (CHUM) - Hôpital Notre-Dame; Consultant, Hopital de la Cite de la santé; Staff Ophth, Centre Hospitalier l'Université de Montréal (CHUM) - Hôtel-Dieu; adj Prof, Universite de Montreal; (514)890-8000

CORRIVEAU, Louis-Philippe; CHUQ-St-Francois D'Assise, 10 rue de l'Espinay, Quebec QC G1L 3L5; Laval'97; LMCC; CCFP; CCFP(E.M.); Staff, Centre Hospitalier Universitaire De Québec - Pavillon De St-françois-d'assise; (418)525-4444

CORRIVEAU, Louise; CMF Berthier, 788 av Gilles-Villeneuve, Berthierville QC J0K 1A0; Mon'78; (450)836-4212

CORRIVEAU, Louisette; RSRY Pavillon Hotel-Dieu, 1800 rue Dessaulles, Saint-Hyacinthe QC J2S 2T2; Sher'79; Staff, Centre d hebergement de l Hôtel-Dieu de Saint-Hyacinthe; (450)771-3333

CORRIVEAU, Marc M; MUHC-Royal Victoria Hosp, S10.18-687 av des Pins O, Montreal QC H3A 1A1; Mon'95; FRCS; FRCSC; GenSurg; VascSurg. Staff Vascular Surg, McGill University Health Centre - Royal Victoria Hospital; Staff Vascular Surg, McGill University Health Centre - Montreal General Campus; Langs: English; Italian; (514)843-1524; Fax. (514)843-1730.

CORRIVEAU, Marie-Noel; Centre Oculaire de Victorialle, 340 rue Notre-Dame E, Victoriaville QC G6P 4A6; Sher'78; FRCSC; Ophth. Staff, Hotel-Dieu d'Arthabaska; (819)751-5595

CORRIVEAU, Marie-Noelle; CHUQ-St-Francois D'Assise, 10 rue de l'Espinay, Quebec QC G1L 3L5; Laval'03; FRCSC; Otol. Staff, Centre Hospitalier Universitaire De Québec - Pavillon De St-françois-d'assise; (418)525-4444

CORRIVEAU, Mario; Clinique Ortho du Haut-Richeli, 320-900 boul Du Seminaire N, St-Jean-Sur-Richel QC J3A 1C3; Sher'87; FRCSC; OrthSurg (Trauma & Reconstructive Surgery). Staff OrthSurg, Hôpital du Haut-Richelieu; (450)348-6966; Fax. (450)348-0664; mariocorri@hotmail.com.

CORRIVEAU, Michael R A; Renfrew Co & Dist Health Unit, 7 International Dr RR 4, Pembroke ON K8A 6W5; Ott'77; BSc; MHSc(CommunMed&EPidemiol; Consultant, Pembroke Regional Hospital Inc; Consultant, St Francis Memorial Hospital; Med Officer of Hlth, Renfrew County & District Health Unit Corporate Office; (613)732-3629; Fax. (613)735-3067.

CORRIVEAU, Pierre; Clinique Med Ahuntsic, 117-241 rue Fleury O, Montreal QC H3L 1V2; Mon'70; (514)384-1421; Fax. (514)384-1422.

CORRIVEAU, Remi; 1033 rue Jacques-Bedard, Quebec QC G2N 1E4; Sher'82; Ac Staff, Centre Hospitalier Affilié Universitaire de Québec - Hôpital du St-Sacrement; (418)849-8253; Fax. (418)849-6618.

CORRIVEAU, Robert A; 3110 rue des Courlis, Quebec QC G1G 1V7; Laval'65; (418)622-6108

CORSER, Noel B; Hinton Medical Clinic, 102 Allen Cove, Hinton AB T7V 2A6; Cal'01; CCFP; (780)865-3338

CORSER, Sarah A; Hinton Med Clinic, 102 Allen Cove, Hinton AB T7V 2A6; Tor'04; CCFP; (780)865-3338

CORSILLI, Daniel; CHUM-Hop Notre-Dame, 1560 rue Sherbrooke E, Montreal QC H2L 4M1; Mon'03; FRCPC; IntMed; Critical Care Medicine (P.Q.). Staff, Centre Hospitalier l'Université de Montréal (CHUM) - Hôpital Notre-Dame; (514)890-8000 x24444

CORSINI, John; 201-444 Concession St, Hamilton ON L9A 1C2; Wes'69; (905)388-1483

CORSTEN, Martin J; The Ottawa Hosp-Gen Campus, S3-501 Smyth Rd, Ottawa ON K1H 8L6; Wes'92; FRCSC; Otol (Head & Neck Oncology). Staff, The Ottawa Hospital - General Campus; Staff, Children's Hospital of Eastern Ontario (CHEO); Dept Chair Otol, University of Ottawa; (613)798-5555

CORSTEN, P Gerard; IWK Health Centre, PO Box 9700 Rpo CSC, Halifax NS B3K 6R8; Dal'94; BSc(Hon); ABOtol; MEd; FRCSC; Otol (Pediatric Otolaryngology). Staff, IWK Health Centre; Staff, Queen Elizabeth II Health Sciences Centre - Victoria General Site; Dalhousie University; (902)470-8041; Fax. (902)470-8929; gerard.corsten@iwk.nshealth.ca.

CORTENS, Michael; Dryden Area Fam Hlth Team, 40 Goodall St, Dryden ON P8N 1V8; Ott'82; CCFP; FCFP; Staff, Dryden Regional Health Centre; (807)223-3737; Fax. (807)223-7282.

CORTES NINO, Maria D P; MUHC-Montreal Neurological Ins, S40A-3801 rue University, Montreal QC H3A 2B4; Javeriana (Colombia)'95; Staff, McGill University Health Centre - Montreal Neurological Hospital; adj Prof Radiology Dept, McGill University; Langs: Spanish; English; (514)398-1908; Fax. (514)398-7213; maria.cortesnino@mcgill.ca.

CORTESE, Leonardo; Windsor Reg Hosp-Western Camp, 1453 Prince Rd, Windsor ON N9C 3Z4; Rome (Italy)'86; BSc; MD; FRCPC; Psy (Schizophrenia). Clin Dir Mental Health Programs, Windsor Regional Hospital - Tayfour Site; Staff, Hôtel-Dieu Grace Hospital; Assoc Prof, University of Western Ontario; Langs: Italian; Spanish; (519)254-5577 x76970; Fax. (519)257-5109; leonardo.cortese@wrh.on.ca.

CORTEZ, Jennifer A; Highland Family Practice, 107C-1966 Guthrie Rd, Comox BC V9M 3X7; UBC'98; CCFP; (250)890-0919

CORTIN, Paul M; 41B Water St CP 125, Campbellton NB E3N 3G1; Louvain (Belgium)'67; FRCSC; Ophth. Ac Staff Ophth, Hôpital Régional Campbellton; Langs: Bilingual(French/English); (506)759-8500; Fax. (506)759-9585; cortinmd@nbnet.nb.ca.

CORUZZI, James A; Regina Qu'Appelle HR-Regina, 1440 14th Ave, Regina SK S4P 0W5; (Other Foreign)'08; CCFP; CCFP(E.M.); Staff, Regina General Hospital; (306)766-4213; Fax. (306)766-4680.

CORVALAN-GROSSLING, Veronica; PO Box 3202 Stn Terminal, Vancouver BC V6B 3X6; UBC'99; CCFP.

CORVO, Antonietta; Children's Hosp Eastern Ont, 401 Smyth Rd, Ottawa ON K1H 8L1; McG'94; FRCPC; Anes. Staff, Children's Hospital of Eastern Ontario (CHEO); (613)737-7600 x2431

CORY, Emma J; The Hosp for Sick Children, 555 University Ave, Toronto ON M5G 1X8; Wes'99; FRCPC; Peds (Medical Genetics). Staff Ped, The Hospital For Sick Children; (416)813-5794; Fax. (416)813-5846.

COSCHIZZA, Rose-Marie; BC Cancer Agency, 600 10 Ave W, Vancouver BC V5Z 4E6; UBC'93; CCFP; Staff, BC Cancer Agency Vancouver Centre; (604)877-6000

COSICO-DE JESUS, Corazon; 144 Richmond Rd, Ottawa ON K1Z 6W2; UP (Philippines)'77; FRCPC; Psy (Adolescent Psychiatry). Staff, The Ottawa Hospital - General Campus; (613)722-5680

COSIO, Ingrid; 5-1230 Alward St, Prince George BC V2M 7B1; UBC'03; CCFP; (250)562-2644

COSMA, Rodica; Kitchener Downtown CHC, 44 Francis St S, Kitchener ON N2G 2A2; McM'00; CCFP; (519)745-4404 x233; Fax. (519)745-3709; rcosma@kdchc.org.

COSMA, Yann; Clinique Med Papineau, 6930 av Papineau, Montreal QC H2G 2X7; Mon'86; (514)722-0000; Fax. (514)722-2431.

COSMAN, Catherine E; Centre Med de Cowansville, 101-370 rue de la Rivière, Cowansville QC J2K 1N3; Cal'83; Staff, Hôpital Brome-Missisquoi-Perkins; (450)263-0774; Fax. (450)263-6457.

COSMAN, Marvin S; Royal Inland Hosp, 311 Columbia St, Kamloops BC V2C 2T1; Cal'83; FRCPC; Anes. Staff, Royal Inland Hospital; (250)374-5111

COSMAN, Mitchell A; Workers' Comp Board of MB, 333 Broadway, Winnipeg MB R3C 4W3; Cal'82; Staff, Workers' Comp Board of MB.

COSMANN, Peter C; Spall Med Clinic, 150-1940 Harvey Ave, Kelowna BC V1Y 8J8; Cape Town (South Africa)'77; MB ChB; (250)860-9909

COSMIN, Nicoleta D; Georgina Family Med Centre, 201-417 The Queensway S, Keswick ON L4P 2C7; University of Medicine & Pharmacy (Other Foreign)'86; CCFP; (905)989-7800; Fax. (905)989-7803.

COSSETTE, Elise; Regie des Rentes du Quebec, CP 7777 Succ Terminus, Quebec QC G1K 7T4; Laval'86; (418)657-8709 x3633

COSSETTE, Helene; 2400-504 rue Notre-Dame, Repentigny QC J6A 2T8; Mon'88; (450)582-3992

COSSETTE, Jean; Polyclinique Med Concorde, 300 boul de la Concorde E, Laval QC H7G 2E6; Mon'92; FRCSC; Urol. (450)667-5310; Fax. (450)667-5248.

COSSETTE, Jean-Rene; CSSS de l'Energie-Ste-Therese, 1705 av Georges, Shawinigan QC G9N 2N1; Laval'69; Psy. Staff, CH du Centre-de-la-Mauricie (Ste-Thérèse de Shawinigan); (819)536-7575; Fax. (819)537-4088.

COSSETTE, Joanne; Clinique Med De Hauteville, 4435 boul De Hauteville, Terrebonne QC J6X 2Y6; Laval'76; (450)492-3153; Fax. (450)492-9380.

COSSETTE, Judith; CSSS de Trois-Rivieres, 1991 boul du Carmel, Trois-Rivieres QC G8Z 3R9; Laval'84; CSPQ; FRCPC; Anes. Staff, CSSS de Trois-Rivières; (819)697-3333

COSSETTE, Louis; CLSC de Senneterre, 961 rue de la Clinique, Senneterre QC J0Y 2M0; Ott'75; CCFP; FCFP; Fam Med, Centre de Sante Vallee-de-l'Or; Langs: Bilingual(French/English); (819)825-5858 x6121; Fax. (450)616-3745; louiscossette@hotmail.com.

COSSETTE, Luc; CSSS de Lac-Saint Jean-Est, CP 1300 Succ Bureau-Chef 300 boul Champlain S, Alma QC G8B 5W3; Laval'96; Psy (P.Q.). Staff, CSSS de Lac-Saint Jean-Est; (418)669-2000 x7221

COSSETTE, Michele; Ctre Dermatologique du QC, 105-2880 des Quatre-Bourgeois, Quebec QC G1V 4X7; Laval'83; Derm (P.Q.). (418)650-3555

COSSETTE, Patrick; CHUM-Hop Notre-Dame, 1560 rue Sherbrooke E, Montreal QC H2L 4M1; Mon'94; MSc(Neurol.); FRCPC; Neur (Epilepsy); Electroenceph (P.Q.). Staff Neurol, Centre Hospitalier l'Université de Montréal (CHUM) - Hôpital Notre-Dame; Teach Staff, Universite de Montreal; (514)890-8000 x26848; Fax. (514)890-8237.

COSSETTE, Pierre; CHUS-Hop Fleurimont, 3001 12e Av N, Sherbrooke QC J1H 5N4; Mon'91; MSc(Epidemiol.); FRCPC; IntMed. Staff, Centre Hospitalier Universitaire de Sherbrooke-Hopital Fleurimont; Doyen Fac of Med & Health Sciences, Universite de Sherbrooke; Langs: Bilingual(French/English); (819)564-5201; Fax. (819)564-5420; pierre.cossette@usherbrooke.ca.

COSSETTE, Pierre-Yves; Ctr Hosp De Verdun, 4000 boul Lasalle, Verdun QC H4G 2A3; Mon'77; Nephrol; IntMed. Nephrology, Centre Hospitalier de Verdun; (514)362-1000

COSSETTE-GAGNON, Melanie; Coop Solidarite Sante Ste-Thec, GD 115 rue Lacordaire, Sainte-Thecle QC G0X 3G0; Mon'99; CCFP; (418)289-2888

COSSETTE-POIRIER, Nicole; Hotel-Dieu de Levis, 143 rue Wolfe, Levis QC G6V 3Z1; Laval'70; LMCC; FRCPC; DiagRad. Ac Staff, Hôtel-Dieu de Lévis; Consultant, Centre Hospitalier Paul-Gilbert; Langs: English; (418)835-7101; n.cpoirier@videotron.ca.

COSSONS, Nandini H; Haliburton Family Med Centre, PO Box 870 7217 Gelert Rd, Haliburton ON K0M 1S0; Qns'01; CCFP; (705)457-1212; Fax. (705)457-3179.

COSSOY, Michael B; Health Sciences Centre, GF 543-820 Sherbrook St, Winnipeg MB R3A 1R9; Wes'99; FRCPC; Neur. Staff, Health Sciences Centre; (204)774-8511

COSTA, A Daniel; BA 110-9100 Jane St, Vaughan ON L4K 0A4; Bucharest (Romania)'70; PhD; FRCPC; Psy (Adult ADHD). (905)482-4400; Fax. (905)482-4400.

COSTA, Anthony J; University Hosp of Northern BC, 1475 Edmonton St, Prince George BC V2M 1S2; Wes'06; OrthSurg. Staff, University Hospital of Northern British Columbia; (250)564-9233

COSTA, Jean-Pascal; CHUM-Hop Notre-Dame, 1560 rue Sherbrooke E, Montreal QC H2L 4M1; Laval'05; FRCPC; IntMed. Staff, Centre Hospitalier l'Université de Montréal (CHUM) - Hôpital Notre-Dame; (514)890-8000

COSTA, Stacy L; B-2938 Finch Ave E, Scarborough ON M1W 2T4; Ott'99; BSc; PhD; FRCSC; ObstGyn (Maternal Fetal Medicine). Staff, The Scarborough Hospital - Birchmount Campus; (416)291-2205

COSTA VITALI, Atilio E; Health Sciences North-Laurenti, CT 3F-41 Ramsey Lake Rd, Sudbury ON P3E 5J1; Tucuman (Argentina)'02; Staff, Health Sciences North-Laurentian Site; (705)523-7100; Fax. (705)523-7081.

COSTACHE, Ioana; The Ottawa Hosp-Gen Campus, 501 Smyth Rd, Ottawa ON K1H 8L6; Ott'96; FRCPC; Anes. Staff, The Ottawa Hospital - General Campus; (613)737-8187

COSTACHESCU, Tudor D; CHUM-Hop Notre-Dame, 1560 rue Sherbrooke E, Montreal QC H2L 4M1; Mon'93; CSPQ; Critical Care Medicine (P.Q.); Anes. Staff, Centre Hospitalier l'Université de Montréal (CHUM) - Hôpital Notre-Dame; (514)890-8000 x26876

COSTAIN, Darren J; Doctor's Bldg, 100-955 Queen St E, Sault Ste. Marie ON P6A 2C3; Dal'02; FRCSC; OrthSurg. (705)942-5789; Fax. (705)942-5966.

COSTAIN, Gary A; Saint John Reg Hosp, PO Box 2100 Stn Main 400 University Ave, Saint John NB E2L 4L2; Dal'78; FRCPC; IntMed (Endocrinology & Metabolism). Staff, Saint John Regional Hospital; Langs: French; (506)648-6694; Fax. (506)648-6687; gary.costain@horizonnb.ca.

COSTANTINO, Anthony D; PO Box 698 Stn A, Abbotsford BC V2T 6Z8; Dal'78; FRCPC; IntMed; Neur. Staff, Abbotsford Regional Hospital & Cancer Centre; (604)853-6169; Fax. (604)853-1004.

COSTARIS, Angelos; Weston Med Centre, 1953 Weston Rd, York ON M9N 1W8; Tor'84; CCFP; Ac Staff, Humber River Regional Hospital - Church Street Site; (416)248-5539; Fax. (416)248-0520.

COSTELLO, Bernard G; PO Box 1628 Stn Main, Lethbridge AB T1J 4K3; Ott'64; FRCSC; OrthSurg (Arthroplasty). Staff OrthSurg, Chinook Regional Hospital.

COSTELLO, Fiona E; Rockview Gen Hosp, 7007 14 St SW, Calgary AB T2V 1P9; Mem'95; FRCPC; Neur. Staff, Rockyview General Hospital; (403)943-3000

COSTELLO, Kathleen A; Foothills Medical Centre, 704-1403 29 St NW, Calgary AB T2N 2T9; Alb'00; FRCPC; Psy. Staff Psy, Foothills Medical Centre; (403)944-5872; Fax. (403)944-2409.

COSTELLO, Lawrence M; Morrison Street Walk-In Clinic, 6453 Morrison St, Niagara Falls ON L2E 7H1; Dal'76; (905)374-2966; Fax. (905)374-2966.

COSTELLO, Thomas G; Wabush Med Clinic, PO Box 69, Wabush NL A0R 1B0; Mem'80; CCFP; FCFP; Med Pres/Staff Family Med, Captain William Jackman Memorial Hospital; Occup Health Phys, Scully Mines; Ass't Clin Prof Discipline of Family Med, Memorial University Of Newfoundland; (709)282-3701; Fax. (709)282-3291; costellot@crrstv.net.

COSTESCU, Dustin J W; Kingston Gen Hosp, 76 Stuart St, Kingston ON K7L 2V7; Wes'07; ObstGyn. Staff, Kingston General Hospital; (613)549-6666

COSTI, Paolo; CHUM-Hotel-Dieu, 3840 rue Saint-Urbain, Montreal QC H2W 1T8; Mon'83; CSPQ; FRCPC; Cardiol; IntMed (Electrophysiology). ac Staff, Centre Hospitalier l'Université de Montréal (CHUM) - Hôtel-Dieu; Langs: Italian; French; (514)890-8100; costi@sympatico.ca.

COSTIGAN, Norman P; 4733 49 St, Red Deer AB T4N 1T6; Alb'77; Staff, Central Alberta Cancer Centre; Staff Psy Outpatient Serv, David Thompson Health Region; Clin Prof Psy, University of Alberta; costigan@telusplanet.net.

COSTIN, Avrum; 130-10691 Shellbridge Way, Richmond BC V6X 2W8; Montpellier (France)'76; Psy. (604)644-2879

COSTIN, Ioana R; Two Rivers FHT-Hespeler Med Cl, B12-350 Conestoga Blvd, Cambridge ON N1R 7L7; Bucharest (Romania)'97; CCFP; Langs: Romanian; (519)629-4615; Fax. (519)629-4630.

COSTIN, Thomas B; Burlington Med Arts Bldg, 100-761 Brant St, Burlington ON L7R 2H7; Tor'61; Ac Staff, Joseph Brant Memorial Hospital.

COSTINIUK, Cecilia T; The Ottawa Hosp-Gen Campus, MG-501 Smyth Rd, Ottawa ON K1H 8L6; McM'06; FRCPC; IntMed; InfectDis. Staff, The Ottawa Hospital - General Campus; (613)737-8141

COSTISELLA, Marie-Agnes; 35 av Saint-Charles, Vaudreuil-Dorion QC J7V 7K8; Mon'00; Psy (Pedology Psychiatry). Staff, Centre Hospitalier Régional du Suroît; Langs: Bilingual(French/English); (450)455-3356 x222

COSTISELLA, Olivier; Pavillion Albert-Prevost, 6555 boul Gouin O, Montreal QC H4K 1B3; Lille (France)'03; (514)338-3227

COSTOM, Bruce H; 218-5858 ch de la Cote-des-Nei, Montreal QC H3S 1Z1; McG'67; FRCPC; Peds (Endocrinology). principale Médecin, Sir Mortimer B Davis Jewish General; Sr Staff, McGill University Health Centre - Montreal Children's Hospital; adj Prof, McGill University; Langs: Bilingual(French/English); (514)342-0385; Fax. (514)342-4648.

COSULICH, Elizabeth M; 245-175 av Stillview, Pointe-Claire QC H9R 4S3; UBC'84; CCFP; FCFP; (514)697-5915; Fax. (514)697-4418.

COTCHIKIAN, Rita; Clinique Med Sainte-Dorothee, 102-1 boul Samson, Laval QC H7X 3S5; McG'06; MDCM; CCFP; (450)689-6334

COTE, Agnes; Centre Med Saint-Hubert, 206-5125 boul Cousineau, Saint-Hubert QC J3Y 3K7; Mon'87; (450)678-3500; Fax. (450)678-5722.

COTE, Alain; CSSS de Laval, 280 boul Du Roi-Du-Nord, Laval QC H7L 4L2; Laval'83; (450)622-5110; Fax. (450)622-4150.

COTE, Andre; CSSS de Rivière-de-Loup, 75 rue Saint-Henri, Riviere-du-Loup QC G5R 2A4; Laval'69; DAB; FRCSC; Otol. Staff, Centre Hospitalier Regional du Grand-Portage; Langs: English; (418)868-1000

COTE, Andre; GMF Centre medical AJC, 110 rue Saint-Jean, Drummondville QC J2B 7T1; Sher'72; (819)477-1800; Fax. (819)477-9865.

COTE, Andreanne; CHUM-Hop Notre-Dame, 1560 rue Sherbrooke E, Montreal QC H2L 4M1; Mon'04; Staff, Hôpital du Sacre-Coeur de Montréal; Staff, Centre Hospitalier l'Université de Montréal (CHUM) - Hôpital Notre-Dame; Langs: Bilingual(French/English); (514)890-8000

COTE, Andree; 1900 boul des Recollets, Trois-Rivieres QC G8Z 4K4; Laval'82; Staff, CSSS de Trois-Rivières; (819)375-6666

COTE, Andree; 202-28 boul du Mont-Bleu, Gatineau QC J8Z 1J1; Ott'86; Langs: Bilingual(French/English); (819)777-2111; Fax. (819)771-6890.

COTE, Anne-Marie; CHUS-Hop Fleurimont, 3001 12e Av N, Sherbrooke QC J1H 5N4; Mon'97; FRCPC; IntMed; Nephrol. Staff, Centre Hospitalier Universitaire de Sherbrooke-Hopital Fleurimont; Langs: Bilingual(French/English); (819)564-5221; anne-marie.cote@usherbrooke.ca.

COTE, Annie; CSSS de Chicoutimi, 305 rue Saint-Vallier, Chicoutimi QC G7H 5H6; Laval'97; CCFP; Staff, Complexe hospitalier de la Sagamie; Langs: English; (418)541-1079; Fax. (418)541-1129.

COTE, Annie V; MUHC-Royal Victoria Hosp, S5 05-687 av des Pins O, Montreal QC H3A 1A1; Mon'97; CSPQ; FRCPC; Anes (Pediatric Anesthesia). adj Prof, McGill University Health Centre - Royal Victoria Hospital; adj Prof, McGill University Health Centre - Montreal Children's Hospital; Langs: Bilingual(French/English); (514)934-1934 x34880

COTE, Aurore; MUHC-Montreal Children's Hosp, D380-2300 rue Tupper, Montreal QC H3H 1P3; Laval'77; Respir (P.Q.); Peds (Pediatric Pulmonology). Dir Pediatric Network, McGill University Health Centre - Montreal Children's Hospital; assoc Prof, McGill University; Langs: Bilingual(English/French); (514)412-4444; Fax. (514)412-4364; aurore.cote@muhc.mcgill.ca.

COTE, Benoit; Clin Sante Voyage des Prairies, 310 boul Antonio-Barrette, N-D-Des-Prairies QC J6E 1G2; Mon'84; Langs: Bilingual(French/English); (450)752-3999

COTE, Benoit; Clinique Dermatologique, 1819 av Dollard, Lasalle QC H8N 1T9; Mon'85; FRCPC; Derm. Staff, Centre Hospitalier l'Université De Montréal (CHUM) - Hôpital Saint-luc; (514)366-6666; Fax. (514)366-6767.

COTE, Brigitte V; 10.083-2021 av Union, Montreal QC H3A 2S9; Mon'81; FRCPC; CommunMed; Public Health & Preventive Med. Physician-in-Charge, Montreal-Centre Region & CLSC Cote-des-Neiges; Asst Prof Family Med, McGill University; Clin Prof Social & Preventive Med, Universite de Montreal; Langs: Spanish; German; (514)864-1037

COTE, Catherine; CSSS de Laval, 1755 boul Rene-Laennec, Laval QC H7M 3L9; Mon'03; Staff, Hopital de la Cite de la santé; (450)668-1010

COTE, Chantal; CLSC Beauce-Sartigan, 763 14e Av RR 1, La Guadeloupe QC G0M 1G0; Laval'91; (418)459-3441; Fax. (418)459-3142.

COTE, Chantal; CHUQ-Ctr Hosp Univ Laval, 2705 boul Laurier, Quebec QC G1V 4G2; Laval'94; FRCPC; DiagRad. Staff, Centre Hospitalier Universitaire de Quebec-CHUL; (418)654-2258

COTE, Christian; CHUQ-St-Francois D'Assise, 10 rue de l'Espinay, Quebec QC G1L 3L5; Sher'79; AB; FRCPC; NuclearMed (Family Medicine). Staff, Centre Hospitalier Universitaire De Québec - Pavillon De St-françois-d'assise; (418)525-4444 x53618; Fax. (418)525-4350.

COTE, Christiane; CHUQ-Ctr Hosp Univ Laval, 2705 boul Laurier, Quebec QC G1V 4G2; Laval'83; Staff, Centre Hospitalier Universitaire de Quebec-CHUL; (418)656-4141

COTE, Claude; 2100 boul Labelle, Saint-Jerome QC J7Y 1S8; Mon'78; Staff, Hôtel-Dieu de Saint-Jérôme; (450)565-1227

COTE, Daniel J; CHUS-Hop Fleurimont, 3001 12e av N, Sherbrooke QC J1H 5N4; Sher'79; CSPQ; Anes. Staff, Centre Hospitalier Universitaire de Sherbrooke-Hopital Fleurimont; Prés assem Admission Committee, Universite de Sherbrooke; (819)346-1110 x75208

COTE, Danielle; 105-2880 ch des Quatre-Bourgeo, Quebec QC G1V 4X7; Laval'78; FRCPC; Derm. (418)650-3555; Fax. (418)650-1260.

COTE, Dany; Ctr Hosp Affilie-Enfant-Jesus, 1401 18e rue, Quebec QC G1J 1Z4; Sher'85; CSPQ; FRCPC; Anes. Staff, Centre Hospitalier Affilié Universitaire de Québec - Hôpital De L'Enfant Jésus; (418)649-0252

COTE, David S; Landmark Prof Center, 101-2731 Hewes Way NW, Edmonton AB T6L 6W6; Alb'79; BSc; FRCSC; Ophth (General Ophthalmic Surgery). Ac Staff, Covenant Health - Edmonton General Continuing Care Centre; Ac Staff, Covenant Health - Grey Nuns Community Hospital; Court Staff, University of Alberta Hospital; Ac Staff, Capital Health Medical Staff Association; Clin Assoc Prof, University of Alberta; (780)450-3200; Fax. (780)450-9861.

COTE, David W J; University of Alberta Hosp, 1E4 WMC-8440 112th St NW, Edmonton AB T6G 2B7; Alb'03; Otol. Staff, University of Alberta Hospital; (780)407-4491; Fax. (780)407-4490.

COTE, Denis J P; 1520 ch de la Montagne, Gatineau QC J9J 3S6; Ott'68; (819)827-1676

COTE, Elisabeth; CSSS du Lac-des-Deux-Montagnes, 520 boul Arthur-Sauve, Saint-Eustache QC J7R 5B1; Mon'02; FRCPC; DiagRad. Staff, Hôpital de Saint-Eustache; Langs: Bilingual(French/English); (450)473-6811

COTE, Elizabeth; CHSLD-Hop Gen de Quebec, 260 boul Langelier, Quebec QC G1K 5N1; Laval'99; CCFP; Staff, Hôpital général de Québec - CHSLD; (418)529-0931

COTE, Erin C; Hinton Med Clinic, 102 Allen Cove, Hinton AB T7V 2A6; Alb'09; BSc; CCFP; (780)865-3338; Fax. (780)865-2024.

COTE, Fabien; Ctr Hosp Affilie-Enfant-Jesus, 1401 18e rue, Quebec QC G1J 1Z4; Laval'87; FRCPC; IntMed; Respir. Staff RespMed, Centre Hospitalier Affilié Universitaire de Québec - Hôpital De L'Enfant Jésus; (418)649-0252; Fax. (418)649-5928.

COTE, Fanny; CSSS de Chicoutimi, CP 5006 305 av Saint-Vallier, Chicoutimi QC G7H 5H6; Laval'03; FRCPC; IntMed. Staff, Complexe hospitalier de la Sagamie; (418)541-1000

COTE, France; CRSSS Baie-James-Sante Isle-D, CP 790 130 boul Matagami, Matagami QC J0Y 2A0; Mon'93; Staff, Centre Hospitalier Regional de Trois-Rivieres; Staff, Centre de Sante Isle-Dieu Matagami; Langs: Bilingual(French/English); (819)739-2515

COTE, Francois; CHUQ-St-Francois D'Assise, 10 rue de l'Espinay, Quebec QC G1L 3L5; Laval'94; FRCPC; DiagRad. Staff, Centre Hospitalier Universitaire De Québec - Pavillon De St-françois-d'assise; (418)525-4444 x3188; Fax. (418)525-4498; francois.cote@chuq.qc.ca.

COTE, Frederic; CSSSG-Hop De Gatineau, CP 2000 Succ Bureau-Chef 909 boul La Verendrye O, Gatineau QC J8P 7H2; Laval'03; FRCSC; GenSurg. Staff, Hôpital de Gatineau; (819)561-8100

COTE, Gary; Ctr Hosp Affilie-St-Sacrement, 1050 ch Sainte-Foy, Quebec QC G1S 4L8; Laval'83; FRCPC; DiagRad. Assoc Staff, CSSS de Quebec-Sud; Consultant, Centre Hospitalier Universitaire De Québec - Pavillon De St-françois-d'assise; Ac Staff, Centre Hospitalier Affilié Universitaire de Québec - Hôpital du St-Sacrement; (418)682-7700

COTE, Gaston; Hop Ste-Anne-De-Beaupre, 11000 rue des Montagnards RR 1, Beaupre QC G0A 1E0; Laval'63; Staff, Hôpital Sainte Anne de Beaupré; (418)827-3726

COTE, Genevieve; Ctr Hosp Affilie-Enfant-Jesus, 1401 18e rue, Quebec QC G1J 1Z4; Laval'98; Staff, Centre Hospitalier Affilié Universitaire de Québec - Hôpital De L'Enfant Jésus; (418)649-5632; gen_cote@hotmail.com.

COTE, Genevieve; Hôpital Ste-Justine, 3175 ch Cote-Sainte-Catherine, Montreal QC H3T 1C5; Mon'98; CSPQ; FRCPC; Anes. Staff, Hôpital Ste-Justine; (514)345-4931 x4733

COTE, Genevieve; CSSS de Chicoutimi, 305 rue Saint-Vallier, Chicoutimi QC G7H 5H6; Sher'94; Staff, Complexe hospitalier de la Sagamie; (418)541-1079; Fax. (418)541-1129.

COTE, Genevieve L; Orleans Medical-Dental Centre, 100-2555 St. Joseph Blvd, Orleans ON K1C 1S6; Sher'97; CCFP; FCFP; Assoc Prof Family Med, University of Ottawa; Langs: English; (613)830-1298; Fax. (613)830-2170.

COTE, Genevieve M; Clinique Med Memramcook, PO Box 1560 Stn B 152 rue Centrale, Memramcook NB E4K 3V2; Sher'96; CCFP; FCFP; Staff, Dr Georges-L-Dumont University Hospital Centre; (506)758-2290; Fax. (506)758-2278.

CÔTÉ, Geneviève; Centre la Maillon de Laval, 2255 rue Bienville, Laval QC H7H 3C9; Sher'09; CCFP; (450)975-4054; Fax. (450)975-4053.

COTE, Gilles A; CSSS de la Baie-des-Chaleurs, RR 2 419 boul Perron, Maria QC G0C 1Y0; Mon'56; FRCPC; Psy (Adult Psychiatry). Staff, CSSS de la Baie-des-Chaleurs; (418)759-3443

COTE, Gilles E; CSSSG-Hop de Hull, 116 boul Lionel-Emond, Gatineau QC J8Y 1W7; Laval'80; Respir; IntMed. ac Staff, Hull Hospital; (819)595-6053

COTE, Gilles; Centre Med l'Enjeu, 1140 av Beaumont, Mont-Royal QC H3P 3E5; Laval'78; ABIM(IntMed&Cardiol.); CSPQ; FRCPC; FRCPC; Cardiol; IntMed (Interventional Cardiology). CEO, Delta Medic Inc; Med Dir/Staff Cardiologist, L'Enjeu Medical Centre; (514)288-7770 x2009; Fax. (514)288-0622; gcote@enjeucardio.com.

COTE, Gilles; 101 rue Lavoie, Rimouski QC G5L 5Y2; Laval'85; (418)723-5272

COTE, Gilles M; CSSS de Sept-Iles, 45 rue du Pere-Divet, Sept-Iles QC G4R 3N7; Laval'63; Ophth. Staff, Centre Hospitalier Regional de Sept-Iles; (418)682-7695

COTE, Guildo; Clinique Med de Cabano, 101-825 rue Commerciale N, Cabano QC G0L 1E0; Laval'93; Emergency Med, Centre Hospitalier Notre-Dame-du-Lac; (418)854-2762; Fax. (418)854-7498.

COTE, Guy; Clinique Medi-Plus, 4100 3E av O, Quebec QC G1H 6E1; Laval'72; (418)622-6969; Fax. (418)622-2037.

COTE, Guy; Clin Med l'Avenir, 200-1150 boul de l'Avenir, Laval QC H7N 6L2; Sher'84; (450)680-1150

COTE, Guylaine; 7 Carrefour de la Sante, Roxton Pond QC J0E 1Z0; Mon'85; (450)776-1171; Fax. (450)776-1089.

COTE, Isabelle; Hop Maisonneuve-Rosemont, 5415 boul de l'Assomption, Montreal QC H1T 2M4; Mon'02; Respir; IntMed. Staff, Hopital Maisonneuve-Rosemont; (514)252-3400

COTE, Isabelle; GMF Centre Med du Parc, 101-84 rue Court, Granby QC J2G 4Y5; Laval'00; Staff, Centre Hospitalier de Granby; (450)375-1161; Fax. (450)375-7740.

COTE, Isabelle; Ctr de Readaptation Interval, 3450 ch Sainte-Marguerite, Trois-Rivieres QC G8Z 1X3; Laval'06; PhysMed&Rehab. Staff, Centre Hospitalier Regional de Trois-Rivieres; (819)378-4083

COTE, Isabelle; 691 Upper James St, Hamilton ON L9C 2Z4; McG'85; FRCPC; Psy (Forensic Psychiatry). Staff, Centre for Addiction & Mental Health (CAMH) - College Street Site; University of Toronto; Langs: English; French; (905)524-2667; Fax. (905)388-6861.

COTE, Isabelle; CHUQ-Hotel-Dieu De Quebec, 11 Cote Du Palais, Quebec QC G1R 2J6; Laval'95; FRCPC; IntMed; Nephrol. Staff, Centre Hospitalier Universitaire de Québec (CHUQ) - Siege Social; (418)691-5464; Fax. (418)691-5757.

COTE, Isabelle J; Ctr Hosp Affilie-Enfant-Jesus, 1401 18e rue, Quebec QC G1J 1Z4; Laval'95; FRCPC; Psy. Staff, Centre Hospitalier Affilié Universitaire de Québec - Hôpital De L'Enfant Jésus; (418)649-5769; Fax. (418)649-5934.

COTE, Isabelle M H; I R D P Q, 525 boul Wilfrid-Hamel, Quebec QC G1M 2S8; Laval'92; FRCPC; PhysMed&Rehab (Neuropathic Pain). Physician, Centre Hospitalier Affilié Universitaire de Québec - Hôpital De L'Enfant Jésus; Physician, Institut de Readaption & Deficience Physique de Quebec; Langs: English; (418)529-9141 x3720; Fax. (418)649-3703; isabelle.cote@irdpq.qc.ca.

COTE, Jacques J; Ctr Hosp Affilie-Enfant-Jesus, 1401 18e rue, Quebec QC G1J 1Z4; Laval'74; CSPQ; FRCPC; Anes. Ac Staff, Centre Hospitalier Affilié Universitaire de Québec - Hôpital De L'Enfant Jésus; adj Prof, Université Laval; (418)649-5807; Fax. (418)649-5936.

COTE, Jacques R; Inst Nat'l de Sante Publique, 100-190 boul Cremazie E, Montreal QC H2P 1E2; Sher'73; FRCPC; CommunMed. Staff, Hopital Charles LeMoyne; Chef Community Health Sciences, Universite de Sherbrooke; (514)864-1600 x3218

COTE, Jean; Timmins Family Health Team, 1-681 Algonquin Blvd E, Timmins ON P4N 8S6; Ott'00; BSc(Biol.); CCFP; Langs: English; French; (705)267-5600; Fax. (705)268-3900.

COTE, Jean; Clinique Pediatrique Rive-Sud, 500-4975 boul de la Rive-Sud, Levis QC G6V 4Z5; Laval'72; LMCC; Peds (P.Q.). Ac Staff, Hôtel-Dieu de Lévis; (418)833-3337; Fax. (418)833-1151.

COTE, Jean; GMF Clinique Med St-Laurent, 201-200 av Saint-Laurent, Louiseville QC J5V 1J9; Laval'94; Médecin Emerg, CSSS de Maskinongé; Langs: Bilingual(French/English); (819)228-7171

COTE, Jean R; Clinique Med de Mirabel, CP 1059 Succ Stn Janvier 13714 boul Cure-Labelle, Mirabel QC J7J 1A1; Sher'77; FRCPC; IntMed; Derm. Langs: English; (450)435-7666; Fax. (450)435-1716.

COTE, Jean-F; 695 rue Poulin CP 39, Lac-Drolet QC G0Y 1C0; Sher'75; ac Staff, Carrefour Sante Granit; (819)549-2323

COTE, Jean-Francois; Ctr Hosp Affilie-Enfant-Jesus, 1401 18e rue, Quebec QC G1J 1Z4; Laval'81; Staff, Centre Hospitalier Affilié Universitaire de Québec - Hôpital De L'Enfant Jésus; (418)649-0252

COTE, Jean-Francois; Hotel-Dieu de Levis, 143 rue Wolfe, Levis QC G6V 3Z1; Laval'00; FRCPC; DiagRad. Staff, Hôtel-Dieu de Lévis; (418)835-7121

COTE, Jean-Francois; CHUQ-Ctr Hosp Univ Laval, 4221-2705 boul Laurier, Quebec QC G1V 4G2; Laval'04; FRCPC; Psy. Staff, Centre Hospitalier Universitaire de Quebec-CHUL; (418)654-2177; Fax. (418)654-2716.

COTE, Jean-Marc; CHUQ-Ctr Hosp Univ Laval, 2705 boul Laurier, Quebec QC G1V 4G2; Laval'89; CSPQ; FRCPC; Peds; Cardiol. Staff, Centre Hospitalier Universitaire de Quebec-CHUL; (418)654-2708; Fax. (418)654-2710; jean-marc.cote@chuq.qc.ca.

COTE, Jean-Paul; Clinique Orth des Bois-Francs, 5-39 rue Laurier E, Victoriaville QC G6P 6P6; Laval'62; FRCSC; OrthSurg (P.Q.). Staff, Hotel-Dieu d'Arthabaska; (819)357-8683; Fax. (819)357-2331.

COTE, Johanne; 2725 ch Sainte-Foy, Quebec QC G1V 4G5; Laval'81; LMCC; FRCPC; IntMed (Asthma); Respir. Consultant, Hopital du CSS de la Region de Thetford; Staff Pneumology, Hôpital Laval; Langs: English; (418)656-4747; Fax. (418)656-4762; johanne.cote@med.ulaval.ca.

COTE, Josee; CSSS de Rimouski-Neigette, CP 3150 Succ A 150 av Rouleau, Rimouski QC G5L 5T1; Sher'94; Staff, Hôpital Regional Rimouski; Langs: Bilingual(French/English); (418)723-7851

COTE, Joseph A M A; Univ Of Ottawa Research Inst, 5457-1145 Carling Ave, Ottawa ON K1Z 7K4; Ott'61; Langs: Bilingual(English/French); (613)715-5827; Fax. (613)715-5839.

COTE, Joseph G J; CHUQ-Hotel-Dieu De Quebec, 11 Cote Du Palais, Quebec QC G1R 2J6; Laval'80; CSPQ; Anes. Staff, Centre Hospitalier Universitaire de Québec (CHUQ) - Siege Social; Fax. (418)691-5728.

COTE, Julie; Clinique Med de Roberval, 714 boul Marcotte, Roberval QC G8H 1Z6; Mon'98; Staff, Hotel-Dieu de Roberval; Clin Prof, Universite de Sherbrooke; Langs: Bilingual(French/English); (418)275-3833; Fax. (418)275-6747.

COTE, Laurent; Ctr Hosp Fleury, 2180 rue Fleury E, Montreal QC H2B 1K3; Mon'82; Staff, Centre Hospitalier Fleury; (514)381-9311; Fax. (514)858-2435.

COTE, Leonard; CHUQ-St-Francois D'Assise, 10 rue de l'Espinay, Quebec QC G1L 3L5; Laval'76; CSPQ; Cardiol (P.Q.). Ac Staff, CSSS de Quebec-Sud; Ac Staff, Centre Hospitalier Universitaire De Québec - Pavillon De St-françois-d'assise; (418)525-4319

COTE, Lise; Clinique Med Elysee, 451 rue des Champs-Elysees, Chicoutimi QC G7H 2W3; Laval'81; Asst Staff OR, Complexe hospitalier de la Sagamie; (418)545-2323; Fax. (418)545-2756.

COTE, Louis; Queen Elizabeth Health Complex, 316-2100 av de Marlowe, Montreal QC H4A 3L5; Mon'72; FRCPC; Psy. Clin Prof, Universite de Montreal; (514)482-9804

COTE, Louise; Ctr Hosp Affilie-St-Augustin, 2135 rue de la Terrasse-Cadieu, Quebec QC G1C 1Z2; Laval'91; CCFP; Fam Med, Centre d'hebergement Saint-Augustin; Langs: English; (418)667-3910

COTE, Luc; 340 rue Martineau, Otter Lake QC J0X 2P0; Laval'78; MSc(Public Health); Public Health de l'Outaouais; (819)453-7392; cote.luc@hydro.qc.ca.

COTE, Lucie; Centre Med Disraeli, 11-25 rue Champagne, Disraeli QC G0N 1E0; Sher'89; (418)449-2655; Fax. (418)449-2415.

COTE, M E G Louise; CHUQ-Ctr Hosp Univ Laval, F 00413-2705 boul Laurier, Quebec QC G1V 4G2; Laval'74; FRCPC; MedMicrobiol; InfectDis. Clin Prof, Université Laval; (418)656-4141 x47882; Fax. (418)654-2147; cote.louise@chuq.qc.ca.

COTE, Manon; 100-1325 boul de la Cote-Vertu, Saint-Laurent QC H4L 1Z1; Laval'93; CCFP; Staff, Sir Mortimer B Davis Jewish General; Langs: German; English; (514)748-0004; Fax. (514)748-5834.

COTE, Marc-Andre; Ctr Hosp Affilie-St-Sacrement, 1050 ch Sainte-Foy, Quebec QC G1S 4L8; Laval'80; CSPQ; FRCPC; IntMed; Cardiol (P.Q.). Staff, Centre Hospitalier Affilié Universitaire de Québec - Hôpital du St-Sacrement; Staff, Centre Hospitalier Affilié Universitaire de Québec - Hôpital De L'Enfant Jésus; Clin Assoc Prof, Université Laval; (418)682-7511

COTE, Marie-Chantal; Hotel-Dieu de Levis, 143 rue Wolfe, Levis QC G6V 3Z1; Laval'95; CSPQ; FRCPC; Anes. Staff, Hôtel-Dieu de Lévis; (418)835-7121 x3218; Fax. (418)835-3969.

COTE, Marie-Claude; Institut de Cardiologie de Mon, 5000 rue Belanger, Montreal QC H1T 1C8; Mon'02; FRCPC; Psy. Staff, Institut de Cardiologie de Montréal; (514)593-2571

COTE, Marie-Eve; Clinique Med Baie St-Paul, 101-4 rue Du Moulin, Baie-Saint-Paul QC G3Z 2R8; Laval'00; CCFP; Staff Emerg Family Med, CSSS de Charlevoix; (418)435-5760; Fax. (418)435-4137.

COTE, Marie-Noelle; CHUQ-St-Francoise d'Assise, 10 rue de l'Espinay, Quebec QC G1L 3L5; Laval'05; Critical Care Medicine; IntMed. Staff, Centre Hospitalier Universitaire De Québec - Pavillon De St-françois-d'assise; (418)525-4444

COTE, Marie-Pascale; CLSC Haute-Ville, 55 ch Sainte-Foy, Quebec QC G1R 1S9; Laval'99; CCFP; Staff, Centre Hospitalier Portneuf; (418)337-4611

COTE, Mario; Hotel-Dieu de Levis, 143 rue Wolfe, Levis QC G6V 3Z1; Sher'87; CCFP; CCFP(E.M.); Staff, CSSS de Montmagny-L'Islet; Staff EmergMed, Hôtel-Dieu de Lévis; Physician, Health Canada; (418)835-7121 x6178

COTE, Mario; Clinique Familiale, 13555 boul Lacroix, Saint-Georges QC G5Y 1P1; Laval'80; (418)228-8001; Fax. (418)228-5583.

COTE, Mathieu; CHUQ-Hotel-Dieu de Quebec, 11 Cote du Palais, Quebec QC G1R 2J6; Laval'02; FRCSC; Otol. Staff, Centre Hospitalier Universitaire de Québec (CHUQ) - Siege Social; (418)525-4444

COTE, Maxime; CHUQ-Ctr Hosp Univ Laval, 2705 boul Laurier, Quebec QC G1V 4G2; Laval'84; CSPQ; FRCPC; Anes. Staff, Centre Hospitalier Universitaire de Quebec-CHUL; (418)656-4141 x47565

COTE, Mendy; CLSC Ahuntsic, 1165 boul Henri-Bourassa E, Montreal QC H2C 3K2; Mon'04; Staff, Centre Hospitalier Fleury; Langs: Bilingual(French/English); (819)697-3333

COTE, Michel C; Clinique Med St-Henri, 223 rue Commerciale RR 1, St-Henri-De-Levis QC G0R 3E0; Laval'72; Ac Staff, Hôtel-Dieu de Lévis; (418)882-2268; Fax. (418)882-3561; mcecote@globetrotter.net.

COTE, Michel J; 200A-731 rue Galt O, Sherbrooke QC J1H 1Z1; Laval'68; FRCSC; ObstGyn (Gynecology). Clin Assoc Teacher, Universite de Sherbrooke; Langs: English; (819)566-5774; Fax. (819)566-1353; mjcote69@hotmail.com.

COTE, Micheline; CLSC Basse-Ville, 50 rue Saint-Joseph E, Quebec QC G1K 3A5; Laval'77; (418)529-2572; Fax. (418)529-4309.

COTE, Mylene; Hotel-Dieu De Sorel, 400 av de l'Hotel-Dieu, Sorel-Tracy QC J3P 1N5; Sher'98; CCFP; Staff, Hôtel-Dieu de Sorel; (450)746-6000

CÔTÉ, Nancy; GMF Sud-Ouest, 119-4475 rue Bannantyne, Verdun QC H4G 1E2; Mon'09; CCFP; (514)765-3600

COTE, Nathalie; Clinique Medicale Angus, 101-4101 rue Molson, Montreal QC H1Y 3L1; Mon'90; Langs: English; (514)807-2333; Fax. (514)838-6458.

COTE, Nicole; Clinique Med Berger, 116-1000 ch Sainte-Foy, Quebec QC G1S 2L6; Laval'91; (418)688-1385; nicole_cote@ssss.gouv.qc.ca.

COTE, Patricia; Rockland MD, 110-100 ch Rockland, Mont-Royal QC H3P 2V9; Mon'06; CCFP; Langs: Bilingual(French/English); (514)667-3383; Fax. (514)667-3834.

COTE, Paul L; Medexo Inc, B301-540 boul de l'Hopital, Gatineau QC J8V 3T2; Laval'75; FRCPC; Psy. Psychiatre, Centre Hospitalier Pierre-Janet; Assoc Prof, University of Ottawa; assoc Prof, McGill University; (819)568-9578; Fax. (819)568-2967.

COTE, Peter B; 1 Clinic Crt, Manitouwadge ON P0T 2C0; McG'88; BA; AAFPhys; MCFP; MB BS; CCFP; Staff, Manitouwadge General Hospital; Langs: Spanish; French; (807)826-3333; Fax. (807)826-1215.

CÔTÉ, Philippe; Clin Externe Psychiatrique, 200-237 boul Saint-Jean-Baptis, Chateauguay QC J6K 3C3; Sher'99; FRCPC; Psy. (450)692-0002

COTE, Pierre G; CSSS de la Minganie, CP 190 1035 Prom des Anciens, Havre-Saint-Pierre QC G0G 1P0; Laval'81; Staff, CSSS de la Minganie; (418)538-2212

COTE, Pierre; Clinique Med du Quartier Latin, 905 boul Rene-Levesque E, Montreal QC H2L 5B1; Laval'87; (514)285-5500; Fax. (514)285-2226.

COTE, Pierre; Centre Med des Boulevards, 101-718 boul Frontenac E, Thetford Mines QC G6G 6H1; Laval'69; Staff, Hopital du CSS de la Region de Thetford; (418)335-7585; Fax. (418)335-7587.

COTE, Pierre R; Ctr Hosp Affilie-Enfant-Jesus, 1401 18e rue, Quebec QC G1J 1Z4; Laval'78; CSPQ; Anes. Staff, Centre Hospitalier Affilié Universitaire de Québec - Hôpital De L'Enfant Jésus; (418)649-5807

COTE, Pierre-Luc; CSSS de Rimouski-Neigette, CP 3150 Succ A 150 av Rouleau, Rimouski QC G5L 5T1; Mon'03; FRCPC; DiagRad. Staff, Hôpital Regional Rimouski; (418)723-7851

COTE, Pierre-Paul; Clinique Med St-Antoine, 609 9e rue, Saint-Jerome QC J7Z 2Z2; Mon'77; (450)432-3308; Fax. (450)432-1004.

COTE, Remi; Centre Med Chambly, 205-1101 boul Brassard, Chambly QC J3L 5R4; Sher'82; Staff, Centre Hospitalier l'Université de Montréal (CHUM) - Hôpital Notre-Dame; Langs: English; (450)658-6601; Fax. (450)658-7849.

COTE, Remi; CHUQ-Ctr Hosp Univ Laval, 2705 boul Laurier, Quebec QC G1V 4G2; Laval'75; EmergMed (P.Q.). Staff, Centre Hospitalier Universitaire de Quebec-CHUL; (418)654-2114

COTE, Remy R; Ministry du Travail-BEM, 200 ch Sainte-Foy, Quebec QC G1R 5S1; Laval'76; (418)646-0689

COTE, Rene; Clinique Med Chaudiere, 102 18e rue, Saint-Georges QC G5Y 4T9; Laval'85; (418)228-6820; Fax. (418)226-0358.

COTE, Richard; Ctr d'Hebergement Cle-des-Cham, 101 rue Collin, Saint-Cyprien QC G0L 2P0; Laval'58; Chef Community Hlth Sciences, Universite de Sherbrooke; (418)963-2018

COTE, Richard V J; Cochrane Primary Care Centre, 103-100 Grande Blvd W, Cochrane AB T4C 0S4; Alb'86; CCFP; CCFP(E.M.); (403)932-2089; Fax. (403)932-1820.

COTE, Robert; MUHC-Montreal Gen Hosp, 7854-1650 av Cedar, Montreal QC H3G 1A4; Mon'75; FRCPC; Neur. Assoc Physician Div of Neurol & Clin Epidemiology, McGill University Health Centre - Montreal General Campus; Assoc Prof Med & Neurol, McGill University; (514)934-8057; Fax. (514)934-8265.

COTE, Robin; Clin Med Fam Saint-Nazaire, 210 rue Principale, St-Nazaire-D-L-S-J QC G0W 2V0; Laval'88; Staff, CSSS de Lac-Saint Jean-Est; (418)668-8122; Fax. (418)668-5335.

COTE, Sarto R; 104-1055 av 12E N, Sherbrooke QC J1E 2X4; Sher'75; CSPQ; Cardiol (P.Q.). Assoc Staff, Centre Hospitalier Universitaire de Sherbrooke-Hôpital Hôtel-Dieu; (819)563-6588

COTE, Serge H; Centre Med AccessMed, 200-17001 aut Transcanadienne, Kirkland QC H9H 5J1; Mon'76; LMCC; (514)694-4644

COTE, Serge; CSSS de Manicouagan, 635 boul Jolliet, Baie-Comeau QC G5C 1P1; Laval'67; Psy. Staff, Centre Hospitalier Régional Baie-Comeau; (418)589-3701

COTE, Serge; CSSS de Rimouski-Neigette, CP 3150 Succ A 150 av Rouleau, Rimouski QC G5L 5T1; Laval'99; Psy. Staff, Hôpital Regional Rimouski; (418)724-8315; Fax. (418)724-8652.

COTE, Serge; 2700 ch Chambly, Longueuil QC J4L 4G9; Laval'77; PlasSurg. (450)646-4328; Fax. (450)646-4329.

COTE, Serge; 150 rue Monseigneur-Ross, Gaspe QC G4X 2S7; Sher'76; (418)368-3301

COTE, Simon J J; Hop Santa Cabrini Ospedale, 5655 rue Saint-Zotique E, Montreal QC H1T 1P7; McG'73; Gastroent; IntMed. Staff, Hôpital Santa Cabrini Ospedale; (514)252-6000; Fax. (514)252-6453.

COTE, Simon; Health Sciences North-Laurenti, 41 Ramsey Lake Rd, Sudbury ON P3E 5J1; NOSM'10; CCFP; Staff, Health Sciences North-Laurentian Site; (705)523-7100

COTE, Stephane; Clinique Medicale, 63 rue Gagne E, Sacre-Coeur QC G0T 1K0; Sher'89; (418)236-9999; Fax. (418)236-9998.

COTE, Stephane; CHUQ-Ctr Hosp Univ Laval, 2705 boul Laurier, Quebec QC G1V 4G2; Laval'02; CCFP; Staff, Centre Hospitalier Universitaire de Quebec-CHUL; (418)656-4141

COTE, Stephane; CHUQ-Ctr Hosp Univ Laval, 2705 Boul Laurier, Quebec QC G1V 4G2; Laval'98; FRCPC; IntMed. Staff, Centre Hospitalier Universitaire de Quebec-CHUL; (418)654-2160; Fax. (418)654-2187.

COTE, Stephanie J; Ctre for Personal Enhancement, 250 10th St E, Owen Sound ON N4K 1S5; Dal'03; FRCPC; Derm. (519)371-1008; Fax. (519)371-8708.

COTE, Stephanie; CHUQ-St-Francois d'Assise, 10 rue de l'Espinay, Quebec QC G1L 3L5; Laval'98; CCFP; Staff, Centre Hospitalier Universitaire De Québec - Pavillon De St-françois-d'assise; (418)525-4425; Fax. (418)525-4322.

COTE, Suzanne; Clinique Familiale MDM, 102-6955 boul Taschereau, Brossard QC J4Z 1A7; Laval'79; LMCC; Langs: Bilingual(French/English); (450)656-2310; Fax. (450)656-2619; suzanne_cote_md@videotron.ca.

COTE, Suzanne; CLSC De Pierrefonds, 13800 boul Gouin O, Pierrefonds QC H8Z 3H6; Laval'79; Staff, CLSC Pierrefonds; (514)626-2572; Fax. (514)624-7486.

COTE, Sylvain J; Sudbury Reg Hosp-Laurentian, 41 Ramsey Lake Rd, Sudbury ON P3E 5J1; Ott'89; FRCPC; Anes. Staff, Health Sciences North-Laurentian Site; (705)522-2200

COTE, Sylvain; Hotel-Dieu De Roberval, 450 rue Brassard, Roberval QC G8H 1B9; Mon'83; CSPQ; FRCPC; Anes. Staff, Hotel-Dieu de Roberval; (418)275-0110

COTE, Sylvain; Centre Med Saint-Francois, 200-2125 boul Lemire, Drummondville QC J2B 8N8; Laval'84; Ac Staff, Hôpital Sainte-croix; (819)477-6793; Fax. (819)477-6962.

COTE, Sylvie; Clinique Med Cadillac, 3435 rue Bossuet, Montreal QC H1M 2M1; Laval'85; Médecin Obst, Hopital Maisonneuve-Rosemont; Physician, CHSLD Marie-Rollet; Langs: Spanish; English; (514)253-1211

COTE, Sylvie; 3001 12e Av N, Sherbrooke QC J1H 5N4; Laval'88; FRCPC; Peds. Staff, Centre Hospitalier Universitaire de Sherbrooke-Hopital Fleurimont; Staff, Clinique Pediatrique; (819)346-1110 x74634; Fax. (819)566-5243.

COTE BECK, Martin E J; Rocky Mountain Health Centre, PO Box 2019 901 5th Ave N, Fernie BC V0B 1M0; McG'81; FRCPC; Psy. (250)423-5550

COTE-BERUBE, Janik; Hôpital Rég D'Edmundston, 275 Hebert Blvd, Edmundston NB E3V 4E4; Sher'01; CCFP; Staff, Hôpital regional d'Edmundston; (506)739-2200; nikcote@hotmail.com.

COTE-BOILEAU, Therese; CHUS-Hop Fleurimont, 3001 12e Av N, Sherbrooke QC J1H 5N4; Sher'75; CSPQ; FRCPC; Peds. Staff, Centre Hospitalier Universitaire de Sherbrooke-Hopital Fleurimont; (819)346-1110

COTE-BRISSON, Linda; CHUQ-Hotel-Dieu de Quebec, 11 Cote du Palais, Quebec QC G1R 2J6; Laval'73; FRCPC; Peds; MedOncol (P.Q.); Hem. Staff, Centre Hospitalier Universitaire de Québec (CHUQ) - Siege Social; (418)691-5151

COTE-MANTHA, Evelyne; Ctr Hosp Rouyn-Noranda, 4 9e rue, Rouyn-Noranda QC J9X 2B2; Laval'07; FRCPC; Neur. Staff, Centre Hospitalier Rouyn-Noranda; (819)764-5131 x43452

COTE-PAGE, Veronique; CSSS du Lac-des-Deux-Montagnes, 520 boul Arthur-Sauve, Saint-Eustache QC J7R 5B1; Mon'99; FRCPC; IntMed. Staff, Hôpital de Saint-Eustache; (450)473-6811

COTE-PARE, Jonathan; Ctr Hosp de LaSalle, 8585 Tsse Champlain, LaSalle QC H8P 1C1; Mon'99; Staff, Centre Hospitalier de LaSalle; (514)362-8000

COTE-RICHER, Melanie; CSSS de Chicoutimi, 305 rue Saint-Vallier, Chicoutimi QC G7H 5H6; Laval'00; FRCPC; MedBiochem. Staff, Complexe hospitalier de la Sagamie.

COTRAN, Marc E; 203-5515 rue Saint-Jacques, Montreal QC H4A 2E3; McG'03; BScH; CCFP; Staff, Cree Board of Health & Social Services James Bay; (514)483-9911; Fax. (514)483-9910.

COTTE, Celine; Clinique Med Grand-Boulevard, 200-353 boul des Bois-Francs S, Victoriaville QC G6P 4T2; Mon'92; (819)751-3006; Fax. (819)751-6625.

COTTENOIR, Nattacha; CSSS du Sud de Lanaudière, 911 montee des Pionniers, Terrebonne QC J6V 2H2; Sher'95; IntMed. Staff, Centre Hospitalier Pierre le Gardeur; (450)654-7525

COTTER, Jill E; Sandy Hill Commun Health Ctre, 221 Nelson St, Ottawa ON K1N 1C7; McM'01; CCFP; (613)789-8458; Fax. (613)789-8710.

COTTERELL, Darren S; Royal Jubilee Hosp, 1952 Bay St, Victoria BC V8R 1J8; Witwatersrand (South Africa)'98; MB ChB; Staff, Royal Jubilee Hospital; (250)519-1554

COTTERILL, Michael E; Wawa Family Health Team, PO Box 858 17 Government Rd, Wawa ON P0S 1K0; Ott'93; CCFP; FCFP; Staff, Lady Dunn Health Centre; Teach Staff, Northern Ontario School of Medicine; Langs: Bilingual(English/French); (705)856-1313; Fax. (705)856-9550.

COTTERILL, Paul C; MF-21 Bedford Rd, Toronto ON M5R 2J9; Tor'83; ABHRS; BSc; Hon Lecturer Derm, University of Toronto; (416)322-0390; Fax. (416)928-9394; paul@drcotterill.com.

COTTICK, Kimberley R; St Paul's Hosp, 1081 Burrard St, Vancouver BC V6Z 1Y6; UBC'10; CCFP; Staff, Providence Health Care - St Paul's Hospital; (604)682-2344

COTTIER, William A; All Well Primary Care Centre, 2835 Mill Woods Rd NW, Edmonton AB T6K 4A9; London (England)'69; MRCS; LRCP; (780)450-4550

COTTLE, Margaret S M; 204-625 Fifth Ave, New Westminster BC V3M 1X4; UBC'78; (604)521-3232

COTTLE, Robin W; Westminster Med Bldg, 204-625 Fifth Ave, New Westminster BC V3M 1X4; UBC'78; FRCSC; Ophth. (604)521-3232; Fax. (604)521-3824.

COTTON, David J; Royal University Hosp, 537EH-103 Hospital Dr, Saskatoon SK S7N 0W8; Man'68; FRCPC; IntMed (Sleep Medicine). Prof Med, Royal University Hospital; Prof, University of Saskatchewan; (306)966-8274; Fax. (306)966-8694; david.cotton@saskatoonhealthregion.ca.

COTTON, Marie-Eve; Hop Louis-H Lafontaine, 7401 rue Hochelaga, Montreal QC H1N 3M5; Sher'97; FRCPC; Psy. Staff, Hopital Louis-H Lafontaine; (514)251-4000

COTTON, Patrick; CLSC et CHSLD de Pommeraie, 660 rue Saint-Paul, Farnham QC J2N 3B9; Sher'08; CCFP; (450)293-3622; Fax. (450)293-4429.

COTTREAU, Alison M; 232-615 Main St, Yarmouth NS B5A 1K1; Dal'86; Staff, Yarmouth Regional Hospital; (902)742-3689; Fax. (902)742-3683.

COTTREAU, G Thomas; Queen Elizabeth Hosp, PO Box 6600 Stn Central, Charlottetown PE C1A 8T5; Laval'65; FRCSC; GenSurg (Thoracic Surgery). Staff, Queen Elizabeth Hospital; Langs: English; French; (902)894-2111

COTTRILL, Ruth A; Canadian Med Protective Assn, 875 Carling Ave, Ottawa ON K1S 5P1; Manchester (England)'69; MB ChB; DRCOG; Staff, Canadian Medical Protective Association; Fax. (613)725-1300.

COUBAN, Stephen; Queen Elizabeth II HSC, 417-1276 South Park St, Halifax NS B3H 2Y9; Dal'86; BSc(Hons); FRCPC; IntMed; Hem. Att Physician Bone Marrow Transplant Unit, Queen Elizabeth II Health Sciences Centre - Victoria General Site; Asst Prof, Dalhousie University; (902)473-7006; Fax. (902)473-4420; stephen.couban@cdha.nshealth.ca.

COUCH, Robert M; University of Alberta Hosp, 1C4-8440 112 St NW, Edmonton AB T6G 2B7; UBC'78; BSc; MSc; FRCPC; Peds (Pediatric Endocrinology). Staff, University of Alberta Hospital; Prof Peds/Dir, University of Alberta; (780)407-8249; Fax. (780)407-1509; bcouch@ualberta.ca.

COUDERT, Daniele; Clinique Med St-Nicephore, 4534 boul Saint-Joseph, Saint-Nicephore QC J2A 1B5; Mon'78; (819)472-3350; Fax. (819)472-0315.

COUET, Alain; Clin Med Du Vieux Aylmer, 101-204 ch d'Aylmer, Gatineau QC J9H 1A1; Laval'77; LMCC; Asst Prof FamilyMed, University of Ottawa; Langs: Bilingual(French/English); (819)682-5464

COUET, Hugues; Clinique Ped Sainte-Foy, 295-2600 boul Laurier, Quebec QC G1V 4T3; Laval'79; FRCPC; Peds. Ac Staff, Centre Hospitalier Universitaire de Quebec-CHUL; Ac Staff, Centre Hospitalier Affilié Universitaire de Québec - Hôpital du St-Sacrement; Consultant, CSSS de Quebec-Sud; (418)658-0906; Fax. (418)652-7094.

COUETOUX DU TERTRE, Anne; CSSS de Trois-Rivieres, 1991 boul Du Carmel, Trois-Rivieres QC G8Z 3R9; Nantes (France)'92; Staff, CSSS de Trois-Rivières; (819)697-3333 x69849

COUGHLAN, Donald W S; Credit Valley Prof Bldg, 408-2300 Eglinton Ave W, Mississauga ON L5M 2V8; Qns'85; FRCSC; GenSurg. Ac Staff GenSurg, The Credit Valley Hospital; (905)820-6233; Fax. (905)820-4947.

COUGHLIN, James R; Queen Elizabeth II Hosp, 10409 98 St, Grande Prairie AB T8V 2E8; Alb'76; FRCPC; DiagRad. Dir Dept of Med Imaging, Queen Elizabeth II Hospital; (780)538-7440; Fax. (780)538-7450.

COUGHLIN, Kevin W; London HSC-Victoria Hosp, PO Box 5010 Stn B D4 214-800 Commissioners Rd E, London ON N6A 5W9; Qns'98; BSc; MHSc; FRCPC; Peds (Neonatal & Perinatal Medicine). Staff, London Health Sciences Centre - Victoria Campus; Asst Prof, University of Western Ontario; (519)685-8500; Fax. (519)646-6123.

COUGHLIN, Larry P; Centre D'Ortho & Med Sportive, 3881 boul Saint-Jean, Dollard-D-Ormeaux QC H9G 2V1; McG'73; BSc; FACS; FRCSC; OrthSurg (Sports Medicine). Staff, McGill University Health Centre - Montreal General Campus; Staff Orthoped, St Mary's Hospital Centre; Assoc Prof Surg, McGill University; Langs: French; English; (514)624-0444; Fax. (514)624-4414.

COUGHLIN, Michael P; Medical Bldg, 344-600 Tecumseh Rd E, Windsor ON N8X 4X9; Ott'78; BSc; MSc(ExperimentSurg); FRCSC; GenSurg (Medical Oncology); ThorSurg. Ac Staff, Hôtel-Dieu Grace Hospital; Langs: English; French; German; Spanish; (519)256-3118; Fax. (519)256-3110.

COUILLARD, Fernand; Centre Med Dorion Vaudreuil, 600 boul Harwood, Vaudreuil-Dorion QC J7V 6A3; Laval'65; Psy. (450)455-9301; Fax. (450)455-8964.

COUILLARD, Martine; 18 rue Saint-Omer, Levis QC G6V 5C2; Laval'78; Staff Privil PedoPsy, Hôtel-Dieu de Lévis; Langs: Bilingual(French/English); (418)838-7155; Fax. (418)838-8873.

COUILLARD, Philippe L; Persistence Capital Partners, 500-500 rue Sherbrooke O, Montreal QC H3A 3C6; Mon'79; FRCSC; Neursurg. Chair, Health Research Foundation; (514)499-2787

COUILLARD, Philippe L; McCaig Tower, 3134 Hospital Dr NW, Calgary AB T2N 5A1; Laval'05; Critical Care Medicine; Neur. Staff, Foothills Medical Centre.

COUILLARD, Serge A J; 325 boul Greber, Gatineau QC J8T 8J3; Ott'76; (819)568-7898; Fax. (819)568-7898.

COUILLARD, Steve; CSSS de Beauce-Etchemin, 1515 17e rue, Saint-Georges QC G5Y 4T8; Laval'02; Staff, Centre Hospitalier Beauce-Etchemin; (418)228-2031; Fax. (418)227-3825.

COUILLARD JR, Bernard; Centre de Sante Valcartier, CP 1000 Bdp Succ Forces, Courcelette QC G0A 4Z0; Laval'04; CCFP; CCFP(E.M.); Langs: English; French.

COULAS, Denise P; 400-21 St Francis Memorial Dr PO Box 1030, Barrys Bay ON K0J 1B0; Tor'85; CCFP; FCFP; Ac Staff, St Francis Memorial Hospital; (613)756-0250; Fax. (613)756-9461; dr.coulas@sfmhosp.com.

COULBY, Duncan; Glazier Med Centre, 11 Gibb St, Oshawa ON L1H 2J9; Tor'82; Ac Staff, Lakeridge Health - Oshawa Site; (905)579-1212; Fax. (905)579-5548.

COULDEN, Richard A R; University of Alberta Hosp, 2C2.09 WMC-8440 112 St NW, Edmonton AB T6G 2B7; London (England)'81; Staff Diagnostic Maznkowski Hearth Institute, University of Alberta Hospital; (780)407-2787; Fax. (780)407-2929.

COULIBALY, Eva; CSSSG-Hop de Hull, 116 boul Lionel-Emond, Gatineau QC J8Y 1W7; Mon'00; FRCPC; Derm. Staff, Hull Hospital; (819)966-6100

COULL, Derek J; 104-393 Rymal Rd W, Hamilton ON L9B 1V2; Tor'10; CCFP; (905)388-4028; Fax. (905)388-3302.

COULLOUDON, Alain; CSSS de Laval, 1755 boul Rene-Laennec, Laval QC H7M 3L9; Mon'75; GenSurg (P.Q.). Ac Staff, Hopital de la Cite de la santé; (450)668-1010; Fax. (450)975-5545.

COULOMBE, Anne-Marie; CSSS de Montmagny-l'Islet, RR 1 430 rue Jean-Leclerc, St-Jean-Port-Joli QC G0R 3G0; Laval'08; Staff, CSSS de Montmagny-l'Islet; (418)598-3355

COULOMBE, Charles; 4205 4e av O, Quebec QC G1H 7A6; Sher'89; (418)624-3224; Fax. (418)844-6640; ccoulombe@plexo.ca.

COULOMBE, Denis A; Hôpital Laval, 2725 ch Sainte-Foy, Quebec QC G1V 4G5; Laval'75; CSPQ; FRCPC; Cardiol (Echocardiography). Staff Cardiol, Hôpital Laval; Teach Staff, Université Laval; Langs: Bilingual(French/English); (418)656-8711 x4598; Fax. (418)656-4581; d.coulombe@videotron.ca.

COULOMBE, François; Ctr Hosp Rouyn-Noranda, 4 9e rue, Rouyn-Noranda QC J9X 2B2; Mon'06; CCFP; Staff, Centre Hospitalier Rouyn-Noranda; (819)764-5131

COULOMBE, Genevieve; CHUM-Hop Notre-Dame, 1560 rue Sherbrooke E, Montreal QC H2L 4M1; Mon'99; FRCPC; RadOncol. Staff, Centre Hospitalier l'Université de Montréal (CHUM) - Hôpital Notre-Dame; (514)890-8254

COULOMBE, Louise A; 34 Walgate Ave, Nepean ON K2E 6M2; Ott'76; Langs: English; French; (613)656-3170; Fax. (613)224-8508; louise.coulombe@sympatico.ca.

COULOMBE, Martine; Centre Med des Laurentides, 102-1100 rue Saint-Isidore, St-Lin-Laurentides QC J5M 2V6; Laval'98; Staff, Hôtel-Dieu de Saint-Jérôme; (450)439-3870; Fax. (450)439-7849.

COULOMBE, Nicole; CLSC Ste-Therese de Blainville, 55 rue Saint-Joseph, Sainte-Therese QC J7E 4Y5; Mon'95; Physician, Clinique Med Jolibourg; (450)430-4553 x6604; Fax. (450)430-3859.

COULOMBE, Nicole; CLSC de la Haute Yamaska, 294 rue Deragon, Granby QC J2G 5J5; Laval'78; (450)375-1442; Fax. (450)375-6607.

COULOMBE, Paul; CSSS de Montmagny-l'Islet, RR 1 430 rue Jean-Leclerc, St-Jean-Port-Joli QC G0R 3G0; Laval'64; Staff, CSSS de Montmagny-l'Islet; (418)598-3355

COULOMBE, Raymond; CHUQ-Hotel-Dieu De Quebec, 11 Cote Du Palais, Quebec QC G1R 2J6; Laval'71; Endocrin (P.Q.). Ac Staff, Centre Hospitalier Universitaire de Québec (CHUQ) - Siege Social; (418)691-5016; Fax. (418)691-5757.

COULOMBE, Remy; Centre de Sante Valcartier, CP 1000 Bdp Succ Forces, Courcelette QC G0A 4Z0; Laval'86; (418)844-5000

COULOMBE, Rene C; Thunder Bay Reg HSC-T-Bay, 980 Oliver Rd, Thunder Bay ON P7B 6V4; Dal'03; CCFP; CCFP(E.M.); Staff, Thunder Bay Regional Health Sciences Centre; (807)684-6000

COULOMBE, Valerie; Clinique Med De Mont-Joli, 1385 boul Benoit-Gaboury, Mont-Joli QC G5H 4B1; Laval'96; (418)775-5353

COULOMBE-LEGAULT, Micheline; Radiologie Terrebonne Inc, 202-901 boul des Seigneurs, Terrebonne QC J6W 1T8; Mon'75; FRCPC; DiagRad. Staff, Centre Hospitalier Pierre le Gardeur; (450)471-1477

COULONG, Eric; CSSS de Beauce-Etchemin, 1515 17e rue, Saint-Georges QC G5Y 4T8; Tours (France)'88; Staff Psy, Centre Hospitalier Beauce-Etchemin; (418)228-2068; Fax. (418)227-1081.

COULSON, David B; Port Arthur Health Centre Inc, 194 Court St N, Thunder Bay ON P7A 4V7; Qns'55; MDCM; (807)346-1000 x7760; Fax. (807)346-6206.

COULSON, Pamela Chandani; Pembina Med Clinic, 104-10004 107 St, Westlock AB T7P 2K8; Alb'96; BSc; PhD; CCFP; Staff, Westlock Healthcare Centre; (780)349-4425; Fax. (780)349-4478.

COULTER, David; Lake Country Family Practice, 6-11852 97 Hwy N, Lake Country BC V4V 1E3; Cal'86; FRCPC; Psy (General Adult Psychiatry). Psychiatrist, Kitsilano Fairview Mental Health Team; (250)766-5231; dcoulter@forensic.bc.ca.

COULTER, H Joan; 73 Robin Rd, Guelph ON N1L 1H4; Tor'78; FRCPC; Psy (Psychotherapy). (519)766-4460

COULTER, Lesley A; 182-1402 8 Ave NW, Calgary AB T2N 1B9; Wes'89; CCFP; Clin Associate, Tom Baker Cancer Centre; (403)269-6111; Fax. (403)289-4377.

COULTER, Louise; Abbotsford Reg Hosp, 32900 Marshall Rd, Abbotsford BC V2S 0C2; Cal'89; BSc(Hons); FRCPC; GenPath. Staff, Abbotsford Regional Hospital & Cancer Centre; (604)585-5612

COULTER, William G; 20595 Douglas Cres, Langley BC V3A 4B6; Queen's (Ireland)'70; MB ChB; Ac Staff, Langley Memorial Hospital; (604)534-4321; Fax. (604)530-4217.

COUNIL, Francois-Pierre; CHUS-Hop Fleurimont, 3001 12e av N, Sherbrooke QC J1H 5N4; Montpellier (France)'93; Staff, Centre Hospitalier Universitaire de Sherbrooke-Hopital Fleurimont; (819)346-1110

COUPAL, Dustin J; 4010 Dewdney Ave, Regina SK S4T 1A2; Sask'00; FRCPC; Ophth. (306)566-9264

COUPAL, Gerald; 4F-5110 boul Cousineau, Saint-Hubert QC J3Y 7G5; Mon'68; Psy (Adolescent Psychiatry). Staff Child & Adolesc Psy, Hopital Charles LeMoyne; Langs: English; (450)443-2100

COUPAL, Jean F; Clinique Med Riel, 455 boul Riel, Gatineau QC J8Z 2J8; Ott'85; ac Staff, Hull Hospital; (819)777-7416; Fax. (819)777-5061.

COUPER, Janet A; Kennedy Prof Centre, 5832 St Margarets Bay Rd, Hd St Margaret Bay NS B3Z 2E4; Dal'92; (902)826-1901; Fax. (902)826-7981; janetcouper@ns.sympatico.ca.

COUPLAND, David B; Madrona Imaging Westhill Ctre, A-1804 Bowen Rd, Nanaimo BC V9S 5W4; Alb'84; FRCPC; NuclearMed; DiagRad. Staff, Nanaimo Regional General Hospital; (250)753-4351; Fax. (250)753-0856.

COUPLAND, Jason E; Strathcona Mental Health Team, 330 Heatley Ave, Vancouver BC V6A 3G3; Qns'01; FRCPC; Psy. Langs: Bilingual(English/French); (604)253-4401

COUPLAND, Nicholas J; University of Alberta Hosp, 1E7. 16WCM-8440 112 St NW, Edmonton AB T6G 2B7; (United Kingdom)'83; Staff, University of Alberta Hospital; (780)407-3369; Fax. (780)407-6672.

COUPLAND, R Steven; Sioux Lookout First Nations He, PO Box 4000, Sioux Lookout ON P8T 1K9; Tor'90; CCFP; Staff, Sioux Lookout First Nations Health Authority; (807)737-5161; Fax. (807)737-5089; scoupland@slmhc.on.ca.

COUPLAND, Robert W; Vancouver Gen Hosp, 855 12th Ave W, Vancouver BC V5Z 1M9; Alb'79; FRCPC; HemPath; AnatPath. Staff, Vancouver General Hospital - Centennial Pavillion; (604)875-5273; Fax. (604)875-4798.

COURCHENE, Robert J; Centennial Med Centre, 299 Lake Ave E, Carleton Place ON K7C 1J3; Wes'87; (613)257-2311; Fax. (613)257-4435.

COURCHESNE, Charles; Centre Med Boucherville, 201-600 boul du Fort-Saint-Lou, Boucherville QC J4B 1S7; Mon'87; (450)655-7321; Fax. (450)655-6311; courchesne1963@hotmail.com.

COURCHESNE, Cyd; Canadian Forces Supp Unit HCC, 1745 Alta Vista Dr, Ottawa ON K1A 0K6; Mon'87; BSc; DAvMed; Staff, Canadian Forces Health Services Centre; Langs: Bilingual(English/French); (613)945-6704; Fax. (613)945-6745.

COURCHESNE, Donna; Pontiac Health Centre, 200 rue Argue, Shawville QC J0X 2Y0; Laval'87; CCFP; FCFP; Staff, Pontiac Hospital Centre; (819)647-6666; Fax. (819)647-5566.

COURCHESNE, Josee; Maison Soins Palliatifs Source, 1130 rue de Montbrun, Boucherville QC J4B 8W6; Sher'79; (450)641-3165

COURCHESNE, Mathieu; 101-361 Main St E, Hawkesbury ON K6A 1A8; Sher'08; CCFP; (613)632-0605; mathieu.m.courchesne@usherbrooke.ca.

COURCHESNE, Pierre; Ctr de Med & Chirurgie Estheti, 504 boul Roland-Therrien, Longueuil QC J4H 3V9; Laval'80; ACLS; (450)677-5533; Fax. (450)677-7701.

COURCHESNE, Sophie; CSSS Drummond-Hop Sainte-Croix, 570 rue Heriot, Drummondville QC J2B 1C1; Mon'92; Staff, Hôpital Sainte-croix; (819)478-6464 x2344

COURCY, Claude; CSSS de Chicoutimi, 305 rue Saint-Vallier, Chicoutimi QC G7H 5H6; Mon'86; FRCPC; DiagRad (Angiography). Staff Radiol, Complexe hospitalier de la Sagamie; (418)541-1031

COURCY, Marie-Josee; CSSS de Trois-Rivieres, 1991 boul du Carmel, Trois-Rivieres QC G8Z 3R9; Laval'05; FRCPC; DiagRad. Staff, CSSS de Trois-Rivières; (819)697-3333

COURNOYER, Alex; Ctr Hosp Anna-Laberge, 200 boul Brisebois, Chateauguay QC J6K 4W8; Sher'90; CSPQ; Anes. Staff Anes, Hôpital Anna-Laberge; (450)699-2466

COURNOYER, Denis; MUHC-Montreal Gen Hosp, A7.127-1650 av Cedar, Montreal QC H3G 1A4; Sher'81; FRCPC; IntMed; Hem. Staff, McGill University Health Centre - Montreal General Campus; Assoc Prof Med & Oncol, McGill University; (514)934-1934 x43174

COURNOYER, Gerard; Ctr Hosp Reg de Lanaudiere, 1000 boul Sainte-Anne, St-Charles-Brromee QC J6E 6J2; Mon'78; FRCPC; Psy. Staff, Centre Hospitalier Régional de Lanaudière; adj Prof, Universite de Montreal; (450)759-8222

COURNOYER, Ghislain; CSSS de Saint-Jerome, 290 rue de Montigny, Saint-Jerome QC J7Z 5T3; Sher'99; FRCPC; IntMed; Hem; MedOncol. Staff, Hôtel-Dieu de Saint-Jérôme; Langs: Bilingual(French/English); (450)431-8200 x8500

COURNOYER, Guy; CSSS de Saint-Jerome, 290 rue Montigny, Saint-Jerome QC J7Z 5T3; Mon'79; FRCPC; Respir. Staff, Hôtel-Dieu de Saint-Jérôme; (450)431-8201

COURNOYER, Isabelle; Clin Med du Faubourg de Mt-St-, 208-468 boul Sir-Wilfrid-Lauri, Beloeil QC J3H 6K3; Laval'95; Staff, Centre d hebergement de l Hôtel-Dieu de Saint-Hyacinthe; (450)813-9222

COURNOYER, Jean C J; 116 rue Lafontaine, Riviere-du-Loup QC G5R 3A2; Mon'90; FRCSC; OrthSurg. (418)867-8989

COURNOYER, Jocelyne; Hop Louis-H Lafontaine, 7401 rue Hochelaga, Montreal QC H1N 3M5; Mon'84; FRCPC; Psy. Staff, Hopital Louis-H Lafontaine; (514)251-4084; Fax. (514)251-2498.

COURNOYER, Julie; CSSS de Papineau, 155 rue MacLaren E, Gatineau QC J8L 0C2; Mon'84; FRCSC; GenSurg (Gastroenterology). Staff, Hôpital de Papineau; Staff GenSurg, CH-CHSLD de Papineau - Pavillon du centre hospitalier; Langs: Bilingual(French/English); (819)986-4115 x4044; Fax. (819)986-4118.

COURNOYER, Serge; Hop Charles Lemoyne, 3120 boul Taschereau, Greenfield Park QC J4V 2H1; Mon'84; FRCPC; IntMed (Hemodialysis); Nephrol. Staff Nephrol, Hopital Charles LeMoyne; (450)466-5000 x2560; Fax. (450)466-5048.

COURNOYER-RODRIGUE, Genevieve; CSSS de Beauce-Etchemin, 1515 17e rue, Saint-Georges QC G5Y 4T8; Laval'09; CCFP; CCFP(E.M.); Staff, Centre Hospitalier Beauce-Etchemin; (418)228-2031

COURNOYER-ROY, Audrey; CLSC du Richelieu, 300 ch de Marieville, Richelieu QC J3L 3V8; Sher'09; CCFP; (450)658-7561

COUROUX, Peter R; Erin Mills Med Centre, E229A-5100 Erin Mills Pky, Mississauga ON L5M 4Z5; Wes'88; FRCPC; MedMicrobiol (Travel Medicine). (905)607-2600

COURSLEY, Judith F; 104-1629 Townsite Rd, Nanaimo BC V9S 1N3; Cal'86; FRCPC; Anes. (250)753-8808

COURT, Olivier; MUHC-Royal Victoria Hosp, S6 24-687 av des Pins O, Montreal QC H3A 1A1; McG'95; FRCSC; GenSurg (Bariatric Surgery); Critical Care Medicine (P.Q.). Staff, McGill University Health Centre - Royal Victoria Hospital; Langs: Bilingual(English/French); (514)934-1934 x35179; olivier.court@muhc.mcgill.ca.

COURTEAU, Claire; Medi-Centre Chomedey, 610 boul Cure-Labelle, Laval QC H7V 2T7; Mon'83; Ac Staff, Hopital de la Cite de la santé; (450)687-6452

COURTEAU, Jean-Marc; CLSC de la Region-Sherbrooke, 50 rue Camirand, Sherbrooke QC J1H 4J5; Sher'83; (819)565-1330; Fax. (819)565-8196.

COURTEAU, Jean-Pierre; 104 rue Lois, Gatineau QC J8Y 3R7; Mon'79; Public Health & Preventive Med; CommunMed (P.Q.) (Clinical Preventive Medicine). Med Consultant Public Health, Hull Hospital; Prof Epidemiol, University of Ottawa; (819)776-7660

COURTEAU, Jose; Polyclinique, 103-12905 rue Sherbrooke E, Pte-aux-Trembles QC H1A 1B9; Mon'77; (514)498-4050; Fax. (514)498-8239.

COURTEAU, Maryse; Centre Hosp Honore-Mercier, 2750 boul Laframboise, Saint-Hyacinthe QC J2S 4Y8; Mon'80; Nephrol; IntMed. Staff, Centre Hospitalier Honore-Mercier; (450)771-3333

COURTEMANCHE, Douglas J; Children's & Women's Hc Of Bc, K3 131-4480 Oak St, Vancouver BC V6H 3V4; UBC'83; MS(Melb); FRCSC; PlasSurg (Cranio Facial Surgery). Ac Staff, BC Children's Hospital; Ac Staff, Vancouver General Hospital - Centennial Pavillion; Clin Prof Surg, University of British Columbia; (604)875-2291; Fax. (604)875-2749.

COURTEMANCHE, Luc; Plexo, 6100 av du Boise, Montreal QC H3S 2W1; Mon'90; (514)739-5646

COURTEMANCHE, Marie; Clin Med Plateau Marquette, 200-731 rue Galt O, Sherbrooke QC J1H 1Z1; Sher'80; Staff, Centre Hospitalier Universitaire de Sherbrooke-Hopital Fleurimont; Langs: English; (819)564-8662; Fax. (819)564-1294.

COURTICE, Ian D; Victoria Gen Hosp, 1 Hospital Way, Victoria BC V8Z 6R5; UBC'84; FRCPC; Anes. Staff, Victoria General Hospital; (250)727-4152

COURTICE, Richard W; North Bay Reg Health Centre, 50 College Dr, North Bay ON P1B 0A4; Tor'84; FRCPC; GenPath. Staff, North Bay Regional Health Centre - Regional Mental Health; Consultant, Montfort Hospital; (705)474-8600 x2933; Fax. (705)495-7974; courtr@nbgh.on.ca.

COURTLAND, Michael R; 303-274 Dundas St E, Belleville ON K8N 1E6; Ott'81; FRCPC; IntMed (Cardiology). Staff, QHC Belleville General; (613)968-3558; Fax. (613)966-4730.

COURTNEY, Anthony O; 3001 Dewdney Ave, Regina SK S4T 0Y3; National (Ireland)'70; MB ChB; BAO; FRCSC; Ophth. Staff, Pasqua Hospital; Staff, Regina General Hospital; Asst Prof, University of Saskatchewan; (306)525-6166; Fax. (306)525-1611.

COURTNEY, Brian K; Sunnybrook Hlth Sciences Ctre, A253-2075 Bayview Ave, Toronto ON M4N 3M5; Stanford(CA) (USA)'04; FRCPC; IntMed; Cardiol. Staff, Sunnybrook Health Sciences Centre; (416)575-6531; Fax. (416)480-4745.

COURTNEY, Darren B; Royal Ottawa Mental Hlth Ctre, 1145 Carling Ave, Ottawa ON K1Z 7K4; Qns'04; FRCPC; Psy. Staff, Royal Ottawa Mental Health Centre - Royal Ottawa Health Care Group; (613)722-6521

COURTNEY, Keith; 401-919 Centre St NW, Calgary AB T2E 2P6; Staff, Foothills Medical Centre; (587)894-6558

COURTNEY, Mark J; Clinical Sciences Bldg, 11 107-152 University Campus N, Edmonton AB T6G 2G3; Ott'95; FRCPC; IntMed; Nephrol. (780)407-6153; Fax. (780)407-7771.

COURTNEY, Rosemary F; Broadway Family Physicians, 1801 Broadway Ave, Saskatoon SK S7H 2B6; Sask'04; CCFP; (306)652-2632; Fax. (306)652-2637.

COURTNEY, Susan D; Peterborough Reg HC-Hospital, 1 Hospital Dr, Peterborough ON K9J 7C6; Qns'88; Staff, Peterborough Regional Health Centre - Hospital Drive; (705)743-2121; Fax. (705)876-5012.

COURTOY, Gregory; Ctr Hosp du Centre la Mauricie, 50 119e rue, Shawinigan-Sud QC G9P 5K1; Sher'02; FRCPC; IntMed. Staff, Centre Hospitalier du Centre la Mauricie; (819)536-7575

COURVAL, Jean-Francois; Ctr Hosp de Lasalle, 8585 Tsse Champlain, LaSalle QC H8P 1C1; McG'91; CSPQ; Anes (Cardiac Anesthesia). Staff, Centre Hospitalier de LaSalle; Langs: French; (514)362-8000 x1871

COURVILLE, Ariane; 1-205 boul de York O, Gaspe QC G4X 2W5; Sher'02; FRCPC; CommunMed; Public Health & Preventive Med. Staff, Centre Hospitalier de Gaspe; (418)368-2443 x4603

COURVOISIER-GRZYWACZ, Ewa B; Foothills Med Centre, 1403 29 St NW, Calgary AB T2N 2T9; Cracow (Poland)'92; CCFP; CCFP(E.M.); Staff, Foothills Medical Centre; (403)944-1315

COUSENS, Christopher W W; Western Mem Reg Hosp, PO Box 2005 Stn Main 1 Brookfield Ave, Corner Brook NL A2H 6J7; University of Cambridge (England)'02; MB BCh; Staff, Western Memorial Regional Hospital; (709)637-5000

COUSINEAU, Antoine-Francois; 735 boul de Bromont, Bromont QC J2L 2L1; Sher'77; AB; (450)534-3140

COUSINEAU, Daniel F; CSSS du Sud de Lanaudière, 911 montee des Pionniers, Terrebonne QC J6V 2H2; Sher'73; MSc; PhD; Staff, Centre Hospitalier Pierre le Gardeur; CSST des Laurentides; (450)654-7525

COUSINEAU, Dominique; Hôpital Ste-Justine, 3175 ch Cote-Ste-Catherine, Montreal QC H3T 1C5; Mon'87; Peds (Developmental Pediatrics). Sec Chef Development, Hôpital Ste-Justine; (514)345-4931 x2852; Fax. (514)345-2321; dominique_cousineau@gouv.qc.ca.

COUSINEAU, Martin; CSSS de Rimouski-Neigette, CP 3150 Succ A 150 av Rouleau, Rimouski QC G5L 5T1; Laval'97; FRCSC; GenSurg (Digestive Surgery). Staff, Hôpital Regional Rimouski; (418)723-7851

COUSINEAU, Natalie J; Royal Victoria Hosp, 201 Georgian Dr, Barrie ON L4M 6M2; Qns'05; CCFP; CCFP(E.M.); Staff, Royal Victoria Regional Health Centre; (705)728-9802

COUSINEAU, Pierre E; Clinique Med Mont-Sainte-Anne, 100-10974 boul Sainte-Anne, Beaupre QC G0A 1E0; Mon'63; Psy (P.Q.) (Psychotherapy). Langs: Bilingual(French/English); (418)827-4022; Fax. (418)827-4964.

COUSINEAU, Sylvain; Hop du Sacre-Coeur de Mtl, 5400 boul Gouin O, Montreal QC H4J 1C5; Sher'75; CSPQ; AnatPath. Staff, Hôpital du Sacre-Coeur de Montréal; (514)338-2222 x2311

COUSINEAU, Sylvie; CSSS du Sud de Lanaudière, 911 montee des Pionniers, Terrebonne QC J6V 2H2; Mon'96; CSPQ; FRCPC; Anes. Staff, Centre Hospitalier Pierre le Gardeur; (450)654-7525; Fax. (450)470-2640.

COUSINS-CARANCI, Frances; Trillium Summerville Fam Med U, 700-101 Queensway W, Mississauga ON L5B 2P7; McM'05; CCFP; (905)272-9900 x5; Fax. (905)272-9977.

COUTELLIER, Maryse; 12523 25e av, Saint-Georges QC G5Y 5N6; Laval'78; (418)228-2244

COUTINHO, Christopher J; Southlale Reg Health Centre, 596 Davis Dr, Newmarket ON L3Y 2P0; Ott'04; FRCPC; Anes. Staff, Southlake Regional Health Centre; Staff, Lakeridge Health - Oshawa Site; (905)895-4521

COUTINHO, Jude J T; Min of Hlth & Long Term Care, 410-47 Sheppard Ave E, North York ON M2N 5N1; Tor'88; Staff, Ministry of Health & Long Term Care; (416)314-7530; Fax. (416)314-7538.

COUTLEE, Francois; CHUM-Hop Notre-Dame, 1560 rue Sherbrooke E, Montreal QC H2L 4M1; Mon'82; FRCPC; MedMicrobiol; InfectDis (P.Q.). Staff Microbiol, Centre Hospitalier l'Université de Montréal (CHUM) - Hôpital Notre-Dame; Clinical Asst Prof Med, Universite de Montreal; (514)890-8000 x25162

COUTO CHUQUER, Maria B; 2001 107 St, Blairmore AB T0K 0E0; (Brazil)'04; (403)562-5011

COUTTS, Joyce V; VISTA/Elderly Outreach Service, 2828 Nanaimo St, Victoria BC V8T 4W9; Alb'94; CCFP; Staff, Forensic Psychiatric Hospital; Staff, BC Children's Hospital; (250)953-3966; jcoutts@forensic.bc.ca.

COUTTS, Richard A; 200 Huronia Med Centre, PO Box 790 Stn Main, Midland ON L4R 4P4; Qns'78; CCFP; FCFP; Chronic Care & Rehab, Georgian Bay General Hospital - Midland; Physician, Waltec Sinkware & Bay Mills Ltd.; (705)526-9119; Fax. (705)526-0239.

COUTTS, Shelagh B; Foothills Med Centre, C1261-1403 29 St NW, Calgary AB T2N 2T9; Edinburgh (Scotland)'97; MB ChB; BSc; FRCPC; Neur (Stroke). Asst Prof Clin Neurosciences, Foothills Medical Centre; (403)944-2097

COUTTS, Stephen M; Timmins After Hours Med Clinic, 203-227 Algonquin Blvd W, Timmins ON P4N 2R8; Wes'88; (705)268-3858; Fax. (705)264-2928.

COUTU, Amelie; CSSS du Sud de Lanaudière, 911 montee des Pionniers, Terrebonne QC J6V 2H2; Mon'98; IntMed. Staff, Centre Hospitalier Pierre le Gardeur; (450)654-7525 x21300

COUTU, Benoit; CHUM-Hotel-Dieu, 3840 rue Saint-Urbain, Montreal QC H2W 1T8; Mon'81; CSPQ; FRCPC; IntMed; Cardiol. Staff, Centre Hospitalier l'Université de Montréal (CHUM) - Hôtel-Dieu; (514)890-8000 x12795

COUTU, Diane E; 200-2984 boul Taschereau, Greenfield Park QC J4V 2G9; Mon'72; GenSurg. Staff Surg, Hospital Charles LeMoyne; (450)465-9789; Fax. (450)672-4578.

COUTU, Elizabeth; CSSS du Sud de Lanaudière, 911 montee des Pionniers, Terrebonne QC J6V 2H2; Laval'09; CCFP; Staff, Centre Hospitalier Pierre le Gardeur; (450)654-7525

COUTU, Louis; Clinique Med du Sud-Ouest, 103-4475 rue Bannantyne, Verdun QC H4G 1E2; Laval'81; Staff, Centre Hospitalier de Verdun; (514)765-3600; Fax. (514)765-9625.

COUTU, Marianne; CHUS-Hop Fleurimont, 3001 12e av N, Sherbrooke QC J1H 5N4; Mon'98; FRCSC; CardSurg (Cardiology). Staff/assoc Prof, Centre Hospitalier Universitaire de Sherbrooke-Hopital Fleurimont; assoc Prof, Universite de Sherbrooke; Langs: English; (819)346-1110 x12385; Fax. (819)820-6871.

COUTU, Pierre A; 302-247 Simcoe St N, Oshawa ON L1G 4T3; Ott'74; FRCSC; GenSurg (Sclerotherapy); VascSurg. Langs: Bilingual(French/English); (905)576-5451

COUTU, Pierre; Clin Med La Cite Place du Parc, 900-300 rue Leo-Pariseau, Montreal QC H2X 4B3; Mon'79; Staff, Centre Hospitalier l'Université de Montréal (CHUM) - Hôtel-Dieu; Langs: English; (514)281-1722; Fax. (514)281-6697.

COUTU, Stephane; CHUS-Hop Fleurimont, 3001 12e Av N, Sherbrooke QC J1H 5N4; Sher'98; CSPQ; FRCPC; Anes. Staff, Centre Hospitalier Universitaire de Sherbrooke-Hopital Fleurimont; (819)346-1110 x4413

COUTURE, Caroline; CSSS de la Cote-de-Gaspe, 215 boul de York O, Gaspe QC G4X 2W2; Santo Domingo (Dominican Republic)'02; FRCPC; IntMed. Staff, Centre Hospitalier de Gaspe; (418)368-3301

COUTURE, Christian; Hôpital Laval, 2725 ch Sainte-Foy, Quebec QC G1V 4G5; Laval'96; BSc; MSc; CSPQ; FRCPC; AnatPath (Cardiovascular Pathology). Chief AnatPath & Cytology Serv, Hôpital Laval; (418)656-8711; christian.couture@ssss.gouv.qc.ca.

COUTURE, Claudine; Clinique Externe Jean-Talon, 7345 rue Garnier, Montreal QC H2E 2A1; Mon'84; Psy. Staff, Centre Hospitalier Honore-Mercier; (514)729-3425

COUTURE, Clement; Clinique Med Rochette, 2372 boul Louis-XIV, Quebec QC G1C 5K1; Laval'86.

COUTURE, Daniel C; PO Box 127, Gravelbourg SK S0H 1X0; Ott'69; (306)648-2811; Fax. (306)648-2814.

COUTURE, Daniel; 2000-3330 rue King O, Sherbrooke QC J1L 1C9; Sher'78; Langs: Bilingual(French/English); (819)820-7360

COUTURE, Denis; CSSS de Trois-Rivieres, 1991 boul du Carmel, Trois-Rivieres QC G8Z 3R9; Laval'72; FRCPC; DiagRad. Staff, CSSS de Trois-Rivières; (819)697-3333

COUTURE, Dominique; Option MD, 62 boul Labbe S, Victoriaville QC G6S 1B5; Mon'04; CCFP; Staff, Centre Hospitalier La Sarre; (819)751-1515

COUTURE, Elise; MUHC-Montreal Children's Hosp, 2300 rue Tupper, Montreal QC H3H 1P3; Mon'98; Peds. Staff, McGill University Health Centre - Montreal Children's Hospital; Langs: English; (514)412-4302; Fax. (514)412-4367; elise.couture@muhc.mcgill.ca.

COUTURE, Eva M; UMF-GMF de Chicoutimi, 305 rue Saint-Vallier, Chicoutimi QC G7H 5H6; Sher'05; CCFP; Staff, Centre Hospitalier des Monts; (418)541-1079

COUTURE, Felix; CHUQ-Hotel-Dieu de Quebec, 11 Cote Du Palais, Quebec QC G1R 2J6; Laval'85; FRCPC; IntMed (Hematological Oncology); MedOncol (P.Q.); Hem. Staff, Centre Hospitalier Universitaire de Québec (CHUQ) - Siege Social; (418)691-5225

COUTURE, Francois; 25 av Nelson, Outremont QC H2V 3Z5; Mon'72; FRCPC; IntMed; Rheum. Staff, Hopital Maisonneuve-Rosemont; Pres, Rheumatology Association of Quebec; Universite de Montreal; Langs: English; (514)271-4357; Fax. (514)271-6310; fr.couture@sympatico.ca.

COUTURE, Ghislaine; CHUQ-St-Francois D'Assise, 10 rue de l'Espinay, Quebec QC G1L 3L5; Laval'80; FRCPC; IntMed (Obstetric Medicine). Ac Staff, Centre Hospitalier Universitaire De Québec - Pavillon De St-françois-d'assise; Clin Prof, Université Laval; (418)525-4465; Fax. (418)525-4467.

COUTURE, Gilles; Centre Notre-Dame-De-Fatima, 1201 6e Av CP 460, La Pocatiere QC G0R 1Z0; Laval'70; GenSurg (P.Q.). (418)856-7000; Fax. (418)856-4737; gilcou@sympatico.ca.

COUTURE, J Dominique; Yarmouth Reg Health Centre, 304-50 Vancouver St, Yarmouth NS B5A 2P5; McG'76; Peds. Staff Ped, Yarmouth Regional Hospital; (902)742-5888; Fax. (902)742-6631; domcouture@auracom.com.

COUTURE, J G R Guy; CSSS de Laval, 1755 boul Rene-Laennec, Laval QC H7M 3L9; Mon'77; FRCSC; GenSurg; VascSurg. Staff, Hopital de la Cite de la santé; (450)668-1010; Fax. (450)629-1957.

COUTURE, Jacques A; 8734 rue Valade, Quebec QC G1G 6L5; Laval'82; ACLS; Consultant, Centre Hospitalier Affilié Universitaire de Québec - Hôpital De L'Enfant Jésus; (418)623-6908

COUTURE, Jacques; CHUQ-Hotel-Dieu de Quebec, 11 Cote Du Palais, Quebec QC G1R 2J6; Laval'77; CSPQ; FRCPC; Cardiol. Staff, Centre Hospitalier Universitaire de Québec (CHUQ) - Siege Social; (418)691-5750; Fax. (418)691-5415.

COUTURE, Jacques; CHUM-Hotel-Dieu, 3840 rue Saint-Urbain, Montreal QC H2W 1T8; Mon'63; CSPQ; FRCPC; Anes. ac Staff, Centre Hospitalier l'Université de Montréal (CHUM) - Hôtel-Dieu; assoc Prof, Universite de Montreal; (514)890-8000 x14570

COUTURE, Jean; Hotel-Dieu de Levis, 143 rue Wolfe, Levis QC G6V 3Z1; Laval'82; AB; FRCSC; GenSurg (Gastrointestinal Oncology); General Surgical Oncology (P.Q.); MedOncol (P.Q.). Staff, Gen Surg, Hôtel-Dieu de Lévis; Chief Dept of Surg, Hopital Charles LeMoyne; Clin Prof Surg, Universite de Sherbrooke; (418)835-7121

COUTURE, Josee; Pavillon Rosemont, 5689 boul Rosemont, Montreal QC H1T 2H1; Mon'93; Staff Fam Med, Hopital Maisonneuve-Rosemont; Langs: Spanish; English; (514)252-3814; Fax. (514)252-3854.

COUTURE, Julie; Le Centre Med St-Jean, 202-1018 rue de la Prairie O, St-J-Chrysostome QC G6Z 0A7; Laval'87; Ac Staff, Hôtel-Dieu de Lévis; Université Laval; (418)839-4158; Fax. (418)839-3574.

COUTURE, Julie; CHUQ-Ctr Hosp Univ Laval, 2705 boul Laurier, Quebec QC G1V 4G2; Laval'91; GeriatricMed; IntMed. Staff, Centre Hospitalier Universitaire de Quebec-CHUL; (418)525-4444 x48052; julie.couture@videotron.ca.

COUTURE, Louis; 200-72 boul Saint-Jean-Baptist, Chateauguay QC J6K 4Y7; Mon'81; Staff, Hôpital Anna-Laberge; (450)692-7282; Fax. (450)699-7788.

COUTURE, Louis P; CHUQ-Hotel-Dieu de Quebec, KO 22-11 cote du Palais, Quebec QC G1R 2J6; Laval'81; FRCPC; IntMed. Staff Dir des Services Prof, Centre Hospitalier Universitaire de Québec (CHUQ) - Siege Social; Langs: Bilingual(French/English); (450)466-5407; Fax. (418)525-4476; louis.couture@chuq.qc.ca.

COUTURE, Lyne; CSSS de Saint-Jerome, 290 rue de Montigny, Saint-Jerome QC J7Z 5T3; Mon'91; CCFP; FCFP; Staff, Hôtel-Dieu de Saint-Jérôme; (450)431-8400

COUTURE, Madeleine; CLSC Les Aboiteaux, 101-708 4e Av, La Pocatiere QC G0R 1Z0; Laval'78; Médecin, CSSS de Kamouraska; Langs: Bilingual(French/English); (418)856-7000 x6024; Fax. (418)856-5108; madeleine.couture.cssssk@ssss.gouv.qc.ca.

COUTURE, Marcel; CSSS des Îles, 430 ch Principal, Cap-aux-Meules QC G4T 1R9; Laval'88; Staff, Hôpital de l'Archipel; (418)986-2121; Fax. (418)986-6845.

COUTURE, Marie-Claude; Polyclinique Med Pierre-Le-Gar, 300-1000 Montee des Pionniers, Terrebonne QC J6V 1S8; Mon'94; Staff, Centre Hospitalier Pierre le Gardeur; (450)657-1313; Fax. (450)657-1809.

COUTURE, Marie-Maud; CHUQ-St Francois d'Assise, 10 rue de l'Espinay, Quebec QC G1L 3L5; Sher'02; FRCPC; EmergMed. Staff, Centre Hospitalier Universitaire De Québec - Pavillon De St-françois-d'assise; (418)525-4444

COUTURE, Nathalie; CSSS de Laval, 1755 boul Rene-Laennec, Laval QC H7M 3L9; Mon'07; Endocrin&Metab; IntMed. Staff, Hopital de la Cite de la santé; (450)668-1010

COUTURE, Patrick; CHUQ-Ctr Hosp Univ Laval, S102-2705 boul Laurier, Quebec QC G1V 4G2; Laval'87; PhD(Physiol); FRCPC; IntMed. Staff, Centre Hospitalier Universitaire de Quebec-CHUL; (418)654-2106; Fax. (418)654-2277; patrick.couture@crchul.ulaval.ca.

COUTURE, Pauline; Centre Med Le Carrefour, 200-3030 boul Le carrefour, Laval QC H7T 2P5; Mon'84; Chef Coronary & Intensive Care & Active Staff, Centre Hospitalier d'Argenteuil; (450)686-8899; Fax. (450)686-7466.

COUTURE, Pierre; Institut de Cardiologie de Mtl, 5000 rue Belanger, Montreal QC H1T 1C8; Mon'86; CSPQ; FRCPC; Anes., LA Maison du Peintre; Staff, Institut de Cardiologie de Montréal; (514)376-3330; Fax. (514)254-6324.

COUTURE, Simon; CHUQ-Hop Saint-Sacrement, 1050 ch Sainte-Foy, Quebec QC G1S 4L8; Mon'07; FRCSC; Ophth. Staff, Centre Hospitalier Affilié Universitaire de Québec - Hôpital du St-Sacrement; (418)682-7695

COUTURE, Sophie M; 100-65 Prestwick Close, Halifax NS B3S 0C1; Ott'01; CCFP; (902)429-2722; Fax. (902)446-3038.

COUTURE, Sophie; Radiologie Laennec Inc, 1100 av Beaumont, Mont-Royal QC H3P 3H5; Sher'07; FRCPC; DiagRad. (514)866-6146

COUTURE, Sylvain; 142 rue Saint-Laurent, Maple Grove QC J6N 1K1; Laval'92; CCFP; (514)827-2565

COUTURE, Yohann; CSSSG-Hop de Gatineau, CP 2000 Succ Bureau-Chef 909 boul la Verendrye O, Gatineau QC J8P 7H2; McG'02; Peds. Staff, Hôpital de Gatineau; (819)966-6165

COUTURE-TRUDEL, Pierre-Marc; Hop Louis-H Lafontaine, 7401 rue Hochelaga, Montreal QC H1N 3M5; Mon'01; FRCPC; Psy. Staff, Hopital Louis-H Lafontaine; (514)251-4000

COUTURE-VILLENEUVE, Francois; CSSS de Lac-Saint Jean-Est, CP 1300 Succ Bureau-Chef 300 boul Champlain S, Alma QC G8B 5W3; Laval'07; IntMed. Staff, CSSS de Lac-Saint Jean-Est; (418)669-2000

COUTURIER, Bernard L; 1760 boul Jacques-Cartier E, Longueuil QC J4N 1C2; Mon'83; FRCSC; ObstGyn. (450)468-6121; Fax. (450)468-3309.

COUTURIER, Francois; UMF Charles Lemoyne, 201-299 boul Sir-Wilfrid-Lauri, Saint-Lambert QC J4R 2L1; Mon'90; MSc(TMIH); DTMH; CCFP; FCFP; Prof, Universite de Sherbrooke; Langs: English; (450)466-5000 x3700; Fax. (450)466-5631.

COUTURIER, Jennifer L; Hamilton HS-McMaster Site, PO Box 2000 Stn Lcd 1 3A31-1200 Main St W, Hamilton ON L8N 3Z5; Wes'99; FRCPC; Psy. Staff, Hamilton Health Sciences Centre - McMaster Children's Hospital; (905)521-2100

COUTURIER, Lise Claudette; Sante Publique-Montreal, 1305 rue Sherbrooke E, Montreal QC H2L 1M3; McG'86; LRCPS; Langs: Bilingual(French/English); (514)528-2400 x3582; lcouturi@santepub.qc.ca.

COUTURIER, Mario; 409 rue Melancon, Saint-Jerome QC J7Z 4K3; Sher'81; (450)438-4848

COVALCIC, Catalina; Cambridge Mem Hosp, 700 Coronation Blvd, Cambridge ON N1R 3G2; University of Cluj (Romania)'95; Staff, Cambridge Memorial Hospital; (519)621-2333

COVARRUBIA, Kelimar C; Northern Lights Health Region, 7 Hospital St, Fort McMurray AB T9H 1P2; (Venezuela)'01; Staff, Northern Lights Regional Health Centre; (780)791-6161

COVASER, Florin; 302-8425 120 St, Delta BC V4C 6R2; Bucharest (Romania)'99; MD; CCFP; (778)593-0155

COVENDEN, Kanthan L; La Ronge Med Clinic, PO Box 240, La Ronge SK S0J 1L0; (Other Foreign)'97; (306)425-2174; Fax. (306)425-4199.

COVENDEN, Sivalingham; Oliver Med Clinic, 12018 102 Ave NW, Edmonton AB T5K 0R9; Dublin (Ireland)'67; (780)478-4631; Fax. (780)457-1711.

COVENEY, Marian L; London HSC-Victoria Campus, PO Box 5010 Stn B 800 Commissioners Rd E, London ON N6A 5W9; Dal'81; FRCPC; Anes. Staff, London Health Sciences Centre - Victoria Campus; (519)685-8500; marian.coveney@lhsc.on.ca.

COVENS, Allan L; Sunnybrook Hlth Sciences Ctre, T2051-2075 Bayview Ave, Toronto ON M4N 3M5; Tor'83; FRCSC; ObstGyn (Gynecologic Oncology). Staff, Sunnybrook Health Sciences Centre; Consultant, Princess Margaret Hospital - University Health Network; Staff, Sunnybrook Health Sciences Centre - Edmond Odette Cancer Centre; Consultant, Toronto General Hospital - UHN; Prof ObstGyn, University of Toronto; (416)480-4026; Fax. (416)480-6002.

COVERETT, Kelly O; Saskatoon Cardiol Consultants, 920-606 Spadina Cres E, Saskatoon SK S7K 3H1; Sask'99; FRCPC; IntMed (Cardiac Electrophysiology); Cardiol. Clinical Asst Prof, University of Saskatchewan; (306)975-9000; Fax. (306)975-9888.

COVERT, Caroline R; Queen Elizabeth II HSC, 1276 South Park St, Halifax NS B3H 2Y9; Dal'77; DAB; FRCPC; Anes. Staff, Queen Elizabeth II Health Sciences Centre - Victoria General Site; (902)473-2773

COVERT, Cristina; Vancouver Family Health Centre, 100-2732 Hastings St E, Vancouver BC V5K 1Z9; Ross (Dominican Republic)'02; MD.

COVERT, Earle L; Campbell Clinic, PO Box 180 Stn Main, Coaldale AB T1M 1M3; Qns'63; Staff, Chinook Regional Hospital; (403)345-3072; Fax. (403)345-2141; ecovert@telusplanet.net.

COVERT, Sabrina K; Valley Reg Hosp, 150 Exhibition St, Kentville NS B4N 5E3; Ott'02; FRCPC; DiagRad (Musculoskeletal Imaging). Staff, Valley Regional Hospital; (902)679-2657

COVINGTON, Nancy I; Halifax Sexual Health Clinic, 201-6009 Quinpool Rd, Halifax NS B3K 5J7; Qns'72; BSc; DrMedCh; (902)479-3953; nancy.covington@ns.sympatico.ca.

COWAL, Catherine A; 303-2021 Cliff Rd, Mississauga ON L5A 3N7; Tor'86; FRCSC; ObstGyn. Staff, Trillium Health Centre - Mississauga; (905)848-3711; Fax. (905)848-2463.

COWAN, Bryce J; VGH Skin Care Centre, 835 10th Ave W, Vancouver BC V5Z 4E8; Tor'99; BSc; MSc; PhD; FRCSC; PlasSurg (Mohs Micrographic Surgery). Clin Instructor Div of PlasSurg Dept of Dermatology, University of British Columbia; (604)875-4888

COWAN, Christopher J; Avenue Med Centre, 1-221 Brant Ave, Brantford ON N3T 3J2; Qns'89; FRCSC; ObstGyn (Minimal Invasive Surgery). Staff, The Brant Community Healthcare System - Brantford General Hospital Site; McMaster University; (519)753-8666; Fax. (519)753-6880; c_cowan@rogers.com.

COWAN, Cornelius C; 101-9845 Resthaven Dr, Sidney BC V8L 3E7; Alb'85; (250)656-4713; Fax. (250)655-5234.

COWAN, Daniel J; Winnipeg Clinic, 425 St Mary Ave, Winnipeg MB R3C 0N2; Man'72; AB; FRCSC; GenSurg. Ac Staff, Victoria General Hospital; Staff, Misericordia Health Centre; Staff, Seven Oaks General Hospital; (204)957-1900; Fax. (204)947-0450.

COWAN, David D; St Joseph's Ctr for Ambulatory, 2757 King St E, Hamilton ON L8G 5E4; McM'90; MIR; FRCPC; IntMed; GeriatricMed. Staff, St Joseph's Healthcare - Charlton Campus; Asst Prof Med, McMaster University; (905)573-4804; Fax. (905)573-4820.

COWAN, Gail D; Dr Charles A Janeway Child HC, 300 Prince Philip Dr, St. John's NL A1B 3V6; Mem'94; FRCPC; Anes. Staff, Janeway Children's Health & Rehabilitation Centre; (709)777-4395

COWAN, Ian G; Near North Med Clinic, 201-66 Josephine St, North Bay ON P1B 0A7; Tor'88; BSc(Hons); CCFP; Ac Staff, North Bay Regional Health Centre - Regional Mental Health; (705)495-2685; Fax. (705)495-4128.

COWAN, Ian M; Midway Walk In Med Clinic, 2102 11th Ave, Regina SK S4P 3Y6; Alb'84; (306)522-3346; Fax. (306)522-3348.

COWAN, Kyle N; Children Hosp of Eastern Ont, 401 Smyth Rd, Ottawa ON K1H 8L1; Tor'04; PedGenSurg; GenSurg. Staff, Children's Hospital of Eastern Ontario (CHEO); (613)737-7600

COWAN, Sandra L; Tamworth Med Centre, RR 1 52 Concession St S, Tamworth ON K0K 3G0; Qns'74; (613)379-2946; Fax. (613)379-5138.

COWAN, Simone S M; St Paul's Hosp, 1081 Burrard St, Vancouver BC V6Z 1Y6; Tor'03; FRCPC; IntMed; Cardiol. Staff, Providence Health Care - St Paul's Hospital; (604)682-2344

COWAN, Valerie Y; 101-9845 Resthaven Dr, Sidney BC V8L 3E7; UBC'88; (250)656-4713; Fax. (250)655-5234.

COWAN, William D; 640 Concession St, Hamilton ON L8V 1B5; McM'74; FRCSC; ObstGyn (Laparoscopic Surgery). Ac Staff, Hamilton Health Sciences Centre - McMaster Children's Hospital; Assoc Prof, McMaster University; (905)387-0621; Fax. (905)387-9954.

COWARD, Jeremy; Pemberton Med Clinic, PO Box 69, Pemberton BC V0N 2L0; London (England)'98; MB BS; (604)894-6454; Fax. (604)894-6721.

COWDEN, Elizabeth Anne M; Salvation Army Grace Gen Hosp, 300 Booth Dr, Winnipeg MB R3J 3M7; Glasgow (Scotland)'74; MB ChB; FRCP(Glas); FRCPC; MedScient(Med). VP Med Affairs, The Salvation Army Grace Hospital; (204)837-8311

COWELL, John W F; Health Quality Council of AB, 210-811 14 St NW, Calgary AB T2N 2A4; Tor'70; MSc; BSc; CCBOM; FRCPC; OccupMed;CCFP; CEO, Health Quality Council of Alberta; Clin Assoc Prof, University of Calgary; (403)297-8162; Fax. (403)297-8258; john.cowell@hqca.ca.

COWEN, Robert P; 9069 Noltowasaga Side Rd 12/13 RR 1, Glen Huron ON L0M 1L0; Pennsylvania (USA)'72; (705)466-3032

COWIE, Betty S; Piper Creek Med Clinic, 200-3215 49 Ave, Red Deer AB T4N 0M8; Cal'78; CCFP; Staff, Red Deer Regional Hospital Centre; (403)986-7255

COWIE, Neil W; 5755 Clarence Ave S, Casa Rio SK S7T 1B6; Sask'81; FRCPC; Anes. Ac Staff Anes, St Paul's Hospital (Grey Nuns) of Saskatoon; (306)655-5240; Fax. (306)655-5964.

COWIE, Robert L; HSC-Faculty Of Med, 3280 Hospital Dr NW, Calgary AB T2N 4Z6; Cape Town (South Africa)'62; MB ChB; MD; MSc; Staff TB Clinic, Foothills Medical Centre; Physician Tuberculosis Services Calgary Region, Alberta Health Services; (403)220-8981; Fax. (403)210-7944; cowie@ucalgary.ca.

COWIE, Scott E; 305-5171 221A St, Langley BC V2Y 0A2; UBC'02; FRCSC; GenSurg. (604)534-9288

COWING, Barbara L; Star FHT-Tavistock Comm Hlth I, 80 Maria St, Tavistock ON N0B 2R0; McM'07; CCFP; (519)655-2322; Fax. (519)655-3073.

COWLEY, Jennifer S; Regina Community Clinic, 1106 Winnipeg St, Regina SK S4R 1J6; Sask'89; CCFP; FCFP; (306)543-7880; Fax. (306)543-6888.

COWTAN, Edgar R; Medicine Hat Reg Hosp, 666 5 St SW, Medicine Hat AB T1A 4H6; Man'75; CCFP; CCFP(E.M.); FCFP; Ac Staff Emerg Dept, Medicine Hat Regional Hospital; (403)529-8053; Fax. (403)529-8978.

COX, Ashley R; Sunnybrook Health Sciences Ctr, A309-2075 Bayview Ave, Toronto ON M4N 3M5; Wes'06; FRCSC; Urol. Staff, Sunnybrook Health Sciences Centre; (416)480-6100

COX, Christopher J; Dr C J Cox Inc, 200-9656 King George Blvd, Surrey BC V3T 2V5; Cape Town (South Africa)'85; BSc; MB ChB; DA(Anes); Staff, Surrey Memorial Hospital; Med Dir, Hilton Villa Care Home; Staff, Laurel Place Care Facility; (604)581-4611; Fax. (604)581-2652.

COX, Christopher P; Queen Elizabeth II HSC-Halifax, 355-1796 Summer St, Halifax NS B3H 3A7; Boston (USA)'96; Staff, Valley Regional Hospital; Staff, Queen Elizabeth II Health Sciences Centre - Halifax Infirmary Site; (902)473-8921; Fax. (902)473-3617.

COX, Christopher R; St Clare's Mercy Hosp, 154 LeMarchant Rd, St. John's NL A1C 5B8; Mem'94; FRCSC; GenSurg. Staff, St Clare's Mercy Hospital; (709)777-5000

COX, Heather L; 205-3017 66 St NW, Edmonton AB T6K 4B2; Wes'03; BSc; FRCSC; GenSurg (EndovascularSurg); VascSurg. (780)461-6012; Fax. (780)461-5442; heather.cox@albertahealthservices.ca.

COX, Jafna L; Queen Elizabeth II HSC-Halifax, 2147-1796 Summer St, Halifax NS B3H 3A7; Tor'88; FRCPC; IntMed (Adult Cardiology); Cardiol. Staff, Queen Elizabeth II Health Sciences Centre - Victoria General Site; Dir Research, Div of Cardiol/Prof Med and Commun Health & Epidemiol, Dalhousie University; Langs: French; (902)473-7811; Fax. (902)473-8616.

COX, Jane E; Lively Med Centre, 2-204 Sixth Ave, Lively ON P3Y 1M4; McM'80; CCFP; FCFP; Med Staff, St Joseph's Complex Continuing Care Hospital; (705)692-4774; Fax. (705)692-0528.

COX, John O; 2055 Huron Church Rd, Windsor ON N9C 2L6; Wes'70; CCFP; (519)255-9185; Fax. (519)255-9152.

COX, Karen A; Chester Community Clinic, 17 Shoreham Village Cres, Chester NS B0J 1J0; Manchester (England)'94; MB ChB; CCFP; (902)275-5268; Fax. (902)275-5080.

COX, Katharine S; Colchester East Hants Hlth Ctr, 600 Abenaki Rd, Truro NS B2N 5A1; Dal'76; FRCPC; Peds. Staff, Colchester East Hants Health Centre; (902)893-5554; Fax. (902)893-3444.

COX, Kelly A K; 360 Wesley St, Nanaimo BC V9R 2T6; UBC'06; FRCPC; Peds. (250)591-2115

COX, Michael J; Dr Michael J Cox Inc, 340-1641 Hillside Ave, Victoria BC V8T 5G1; Cambridge (England)'69; MB ChB; FRCSC; ObstGyn. (250)383-2631; Fax. (250)383-2162.

COX, Peter N; The Hosp for Sick Children, 555 University Ave, Toronto ON M5G 1X8; Cape Town (South Africa)'77; MB ChB; FFARCS(Eng); FRCP(SA); FRCA; FRCPC; Anes (Pediatric Intensive Care). Dir PICU Dept of Critical Care Med, The Hospital For Sick Children; Prof, University of Toronto; (416)813-6484; Fax. (416)813-7299; peter.cox@sickkids.ca.

COX, Robin G; Alberta Children's Hosp, 2888 Shaganappi Trail NW, Calgary AB T3B 6A8; London (England)'76; MB BS; MRCP(UK); FRCA; FRCPC; Anes (Pediatric Anesthesia). Staff Ped Anes, Alberta Children's Hospital; Prof Anes, University of Calgary; (403)955-7260; Fax. (403)955-7606; robin.cox@albertahealthservices.ca.

COX, Ronald H; Bramalea City Centre, 387-25 Peel Centre Dr, Brampton ON L6T 3R5; Meharry(TN) (USA)'88; Staff, William Osler Health System - Brampton Civic Hospital; (905)793-7077

COX, Sinclair P; Olds Hosp & Care Centre, PO Bag 390 3901 57 Ave, Olds AB T4H 1T4; London (England)'65; MB BS; MRCS; LRCP; FRCS; Staff, Olds Hospital & Care Centre; (403)556-3381; spcox@telusplanet.net.

COX JR., J Joseph; Dir de la Sante Publique-Mtl, 1301 rue Sherbrooke E, Montreal QC H2L 1M3; Dal'95; MSc; BA; BSc; FRCPC; CommunMed;CCFP; Public Health & Preventive Med. adj Prof, McGill University; (514)528-2400 x3630; Fax. (514)528-2452.

COXON, Carol E; St Joseph's Gen Hosp, 2137 Comox Ave, Comox BC V9M 1P2; McM'97; FRCPC; Psy (Child Psychiatry). Staff, St Joseph's General Hospital; (250)339-2242

COYLE, Stephen J; Crestview Med Clinic, 3004 Portage Ave, Winnipeg MB R3K 0C8; Newcastle-upon-Tyne (England)'75; LMCC; Staff, Misericordia Health Centre; Med Examiner, Province of Manitoba; Asst Lecturer Family Med, University of Manitoba; smoncoy@shaw.ca.

CRABBE, Lindsay A; Postgrad Med Education, 4W8-1280 Main St W, Hamilton ON L8S 4K7; McM'08; FRCPC; IntMed.

CRABTREE, Marilyn J; St Lawrence Med Clinic, PO Box 772 36 Ottawa St, Morrisburg ON K0C 1X0; Tor'88; Att Staff, Winchester District Memorial Hospital; Court Staff, Cornwall Community Hospital; (613)543-2963; Fax. (613)543-4171.

CRABTREE, Paul O E; Primrose Family Med Centre, 35 Primrose Ave, Ottawa ON K1R 0A1; Ott'93; CCFP; (613)230-7788; Fax. (613)230-7778.

CRACIUNESCU, Diana; Hotel-Dieu de Sorel, 400 av de l'Hotel-Dieu, Sorel-Tracy QC J3P 1N5; Mon'09; CCFP; Staff, Hôtel-Dieu de Sorel; (450)746-6000

CRACOWER, Jill; SMBD Jewish Gen Hosp, 3755 ch Cote-Sainte-Catherine, Montreal QC H3T 1E2; McG'02; CCFP; Staff, Sir Mortimer B Davis Jewish General; (514)340-8256; Fax. (514)340-7579.

CRADDOCK, Graham N; Humber River Reg Hosp-Church, 200 Church St, Toronto ON M9N 1N8; Oxford (England)'69; BMus; BCh; MSc; FRCS; FRCSC; GenSurg (Vascular Surgery). Staff, Humber River Regional Hospital - Church Street Site; Assoc Staff, Toronto General Hospital - UHN; Head VascSurg, Humber River Regional Hospital - Keele Street Site; (416)248-9872; Fax. (416)245-6137.

CRADDOCK, Kenneth J; Univ Hlth Network-Toronto Gen, 11F-200 Elizabeth St, Toronto ON M5G 2C4; Alb'04; FRCPC; AnatPath. Staff, Toronto General Hospital - UHN; Physician, The Banting Institute; (416)340-4800

CRADDOCK, Marcy L; Southland Park 4, 120-10301 Southport Lane SW, Calgary AB T2W 1S7; UBC'99; CCFP; Staff, Kelowna General Hospital; (403)944-3413

CRAEN, Rosemary A P; London HSC-University Hosp, PO Box 5339 Stn B 339 Windermere Rd, London ON N6A 5A5; Perth (Australia)'80; MB BS; FRCPC; Anes (Neuro Anesthesia). Staff Anes, St Joseph's Hospital - St Joseph's Health Care; Staff Anes, London Health Sciences Centre - University Hospital; Assoc Prof Anes, University of Western Ontario; (519)663-3022; Fax. (519)663-2957; rosemary.craen@lhsc.on.ca.

CRAFT, Aidlee R; Baycrest Ctre/Geriatric Care, 3560 Bathurst St, North York ON M6A 2E1; McG'85; CCFP; FCFP; Staff, Baycrest Centre for Geriatric Care; Langs: Bilingual(English/French); (416)785-2500 x5399

CRAGG, Frank J; Cape Breton Hlthcare Complex, 1482 George St, Sydney NS B1P 1P3; Dal'84; FACP; FRCPC; AnatPath. Staff, Cape Breton Healthcare Complex; (902)567-7783; Fax. (902)567-7947.

CRAGGS, Rachael T; 304-888 8th Ave W, Vancouver BC V5Z 3Y1; Alb'91; (604)874-0261

CRAGO, Ronald R; Univ Hlth Network-Toronto Western Hosp, 399 Bathurst St, Toronto ON M5T 2S8; Tor'69; FRCPC; Anes. Sr Staff, Toronto Western Hospital - University Health Network; Assoc Prof, University of Toronto; (416)603-5118; Fax. (416)603-6494; ron.crago@uhn.on.ca.

CRAIB, Gordon G W; Battleford Union Hosp, 1092 107th St, North Battleford SK S9A 1Z1; Staff, Battlefords Union Hospital; (306)446-6600

CRAIG, Brian; 86 Dufferin Ave, Saint John NB E2K 2T8; Dal'84; BSc; Staff, Saint John Regional Hospital; Lecturer, Dalhousie University; (506)634-7375; Fax. (506)652-3673.

CRAIG, Catherine M; 203-17 Prince St, Dartmouth NS B2Y 4W2; Mem'89; FRCSC; ObstGyn. Ac Staff, IWK Health Centre; Consultant, Queen Elizabeth II Health Sciences Centre - Victoria General Site; Dalhousie University; (902)461-2246; Fax. (902)461-2746.

CRAIG, Cecil B; 2-16 Main St N, Markham ON L3P 1X2; Tor'65; CCFP; Ac Staff, North York General Hospital; Assoc Prof Family & Commun Med, University of Toronto; (905)471-5300; Fax. (905)471-5360; c.craig@utoronto.ca.

CRAIG, David R; Mission View Medical, 205-616 K.L.O. Rd, Kelowna BC V1Y 4X4; Man'79; FRCPC; Neur (Electrodiagnostic). Staff, Kelowna General Hospital; (250)762-7731; Fax. (250)762-7502.

CRAIG, Donald E; 47 Elizabeth Pky, Saint John NB E2H 1E8; Dal'68; Ac Staff, Saint John Regional Hospital; Lecturer Family Med Unit, Dalhousie University; (506)849-2757; Fax. (506)849-2757.

CRAIG, Dorothy M; Riverside Med Clinic, 683 Front St, Quesnel BC V2J 2K9; UBC'00; CCFP; Langs: German; (250)992-2535

CRAIG, Douglas B; MUHC-Montreal Gen Hosp, D10 144-1650 av Cedar, Montreal QC H3G 1A4; McG'65; BSc; MSc(McG.); FRCPC; Anes. Staff, McGill University Health Centre - Montreal General Campus; Langs: English; French; (514)934-1934; doug.craig@bell.net.

CRAIG, Ian D; St Thomas-Elgin Gen Hosp, PO Box 2007 Stn Main 189 Elm St, St Thomas ON N5P 3W2; Queen's (Ireland)'69; MB ChB; MD; FRCPC; AnatPath. Staff, St Thomas Elgin General Hospital; Clin Assoc Prof Path, University of Western Ontario; (519)631-2020; publicrelations@stegh.on.ca.

CRAIG, Janet E; Glenora Med Clinic, 310-10230 142 St NW, Edmonton AB T5N 3Y6; Alb'89; CCFP; FCFP; Clinical Asst Prof, University of Alberta; (780)455-3311; Fax. (780)451-4404; glenoramed@shaw.ca.

CRAIG, John C; Elmira Med Centre, 2 Park Ave W, Elmira ON N3B 1L1; Wes'80; Staff, Grand River Hospital - Kitchener/Waterloo Health Centre; Staff, St Mary's General Hospital; (519)669-5493; Fax. (519)669-5901.

CRAIG, Katherine G; Vancouver Gen Hosp, 2438-855 12th Ave W, Vancouver BC V5Z 1M9; UBC'97; FRCPC; IntMed; Critical Care Medicine. Staff, Vancouver General Hospital - Centennial Pavillion; (604)875-5949

CRAIG, Kelly L; PO BOX 76091 Rpo Southgate, Edmonton AB T6H 5Y7; Cal'05; FRCPC; IntMed; Nephrol.

CRAIG, Nancy V; 12214 82 St NW, Edmonton AB T5B 2X1; McG'86; CCFP; Langs: English; French; (780)479-1944; Fax. (780)479-1964.

CRAIG, Patricia A; 69 Abercrombie Rd, New Glasgow NS B2H 1K4; Qns'86; CCFP; FCFP; Ac Staff, Aberdeen Regional Hospital; (902)755-3000 x1; Fax. (902)752-1611.

CRAIG, William H; Westview Wellness Center, 200-2609 Westview Dr, North Vancouver BC V7N 4M2; UBC'99; FRCPC; PhysMed&Rehab (Spine). (604)904-3993; Fax. (604)904-3911.

CRAIG, William; Edmonton Clinic Health Academy, 3 515-11405 87 Ave NW, Edmonton AB T6G 1C9; McG'85; BSc; MSc; MDCM; FRCPC; Peds (Pediatric Emergency Medicine). Staff, University of Alberta Hospital; Staff, Edmonton Clinic Health Academy; Dir Div of Ped EmergMed & Assoc Prof, University of Alberta; (780)248-5575; Fax. (780)248-5625; william.craig@albertahealthservices.ca.

CRAIGEN, Gerrard P; 202-10 Alcorn Ave, Toronto ON M4V 3A9; Qns'83; BSc; LLB; FRCPC; Psy (Psycho Pharmacology & Psychotherapy). Staff, Toronto General Hospital - UHN; Lecturer Psy, University of Toronto; (416)972-1931; Fax. (416)972-7690; gerrycraigen@bellnet.ca.

CRAIGHEAD, Peter S; Tom Baker Cancer Centre, 1331 29 St NW, Calgary AB T2N 4N2; Cape Town (South Africa)'78; MB ChB; FRCPC; RadOncol (Breast Cancer). Ac Staff/Dir TBCC, Tom Baker Cancer Centre; Ac Staff, Foothills Medical Centre; Clin Prof/Dept Head Oncol, University of Calgary; (403)521-3701; Fax. (403)283-2903.

CRAIGIE, Pamela M; The Juravinski Cancer Centre, 699 Concession St, Hamilton ON L8V 5C2; Dal'88; BSc; Physician, The Juravinski Cancer Centre; (905)387-9495 x64603; Fax. (905)575-6326.

CRAIGMYLE, John W; Central Park Med Clinic, 104-3965 Kingsway, Burnaby BC V5H 1Y8; Aberdeen (Scotland)'77; MB ChB; MRC; Ac Staff, Burnaby Hospital; Clin Instructor Family Pract, University of British Columbia; (604)434-8781; Fax. (604)434-8699.

CRAM, David H; Souris Med Associates, PO Box 400, Souris MB R0K 2C0; Man'84; CCFP; Chief of Staff, Souris Health Centre; (204)483-2147; Fax. (204)483-2385; dcram@arha.ca.

CRAM, Gordon D; 102-140 Oxford St E, London ON N6A 5R9; Wes'76; BA; FRCPC; EmergMed. (519)433-4999; Fax. (519)433-4151; gord-cram@rogers.com.

CRAM, Jennifer A; 505-18 Wynford Dr, Toronto ON M3C 3S2; Tor'94; FRCSC; ObstGyn (Infertility). Staff, Toronto East General Hospital Inc; Lecturer ObstGyn, University of Toronto; (416)385-3431; Fax. (416)385-1945.

CRAM, Jennifer; Annapolis Family Practice Asso, PO Box 426 821 St George St, Annapolis Royal NS B0S 1A0; Sask'07; CCFP; (902)532-2381; Fax. (902)532-2113.

CRAMB, Robert J; Trillium Hlth Ctr-Mississauga, 100 Queensway W, Mississauga ON L5B 1B8; McM'84; FRCPC; Anes. Staff, Trillium Health Centre - Mississauga; (905)848-7100

CRAMER, Benvon; Dr Charles A Janeway Child HC, 300 Prince Philip Dr, St. John's NL A1B 3V6; National (Ireland)'74; MB ChB; MRC(UK); FRCR(UK); FRCPC; DiagRad. Staff, Janeway Children's Health & Rehabilitation Centre; Chair Clinical Disciplines Radiol, Memorial University Of Newfoundland; (709)778-4583; Fax. (709)778-4333.

CRAMER, Christine R; Wingham & District Hosp, 270 Carling Terr, Wingham ON N0G 2W0; Tor'95; CCFP; FCFP; Staff, Wingham & District Hospital - Listowel Wingham Hospitals Alliance; (519)357-3210

CRAMER, Joseph H; 312-1200 Markham Rd, Scarborough ON M1H 3C3; McG'75; BSc; FACOG; MDCM; FRCSC; ObstGyn (Infertility). Ac Staff, The Scarborough Hospital - General Campus; Langs: Hebrew; French; (416)439-9791; Fax. (416)431-1089; jcramer@pathcom.com.

CRAMER, Paul R; 201-2560 Gerrard St E, Scarborough ON M1N 1W8; Tor'84; (416)694-4944; Fax. (416)694-1285.

CRAMPTON, Susan Y; 206-480 Huronia Rd, Barrie ON L4N 6M2; Wes'05; CCFP; (705)734-1150; Fax. (705)734-6266.

CRAN, Timothy S; Westglen Med Clinic, 108-30 Springborough Blvd SW, Calgary AB T3H 0N9; UBC'94; CCFP; FCFP; Langs: French; (403)240-2221; Fax. (403)240-4670.

CRANE, Joan M G; Health Sciences Centre, 300 Prince Philip Dr, St. John's NL A1B 3V6; Mem'89; MSc; FRCSC; ObstGyn (Maternal Fetal Medicine). Staff, Health Sciences Centre; Asst Prof ObstGyn, Memorial University Of Newfoundland; (709)777-6300

CRANE, Neville; Biggar Health Centre, PO Box 70, Biggar SK S0K 0M0; (306)948-3331; Fax. (306)948-5060.

CRANFORD, Jeffrey W H; Bayvalley Med Arts Bldg, 506-145 Queenston St, St Catharines ON L2R 2Z9; Tor'77; FRCSC; GenSurg. Ac Staff, Niagara Health System - Ontario Street Site; Ac Staff, Niagara Health System - St Catharines General Site; Langs: Bilingual(English/French); (905)688-3029; Fax. (905)688-3028.

CRANMER, David J; Guelph Family Health Team, 305-85 Norfolk St, Guelph ON N1H 4J4; Wes'92; CCFP; FCFP; Ac Staff, Guelph General Hospital; Staff, Rural Ontario Medical Program; Clinical Asst Prof Family Med, McMaster University; (519)766-1490; Fax. (519)836-9530; dcranmer@gbhs.on.ca.

CRANNEY, Ann B; Canadian Med Protective Assoc, PO Box 8225 Stn T CSC, Ottawa ON K1G 3H7; RCS (Ireland)'85; FRCPC; IntMed; Rheum; GeriatricMed. Staff, The Ottawa Hospital - Riverside Campus; cranneya@kgh.kari.net.

CRANSTON, James G; Diamond Head Med Clinic, PO Box 9200, Squamish BC V8B 0C1; Cal'03; CCFP; Staff, Squamish General Hospital / Hilltop House; (604)892-3544

CRANSTON, Meghan E; Sterling Lyon Pediatrics, 401-1020 Lorimer Blvd, Winnipeg MB R3P 1C7; Man'08; Peds.

CRANSTOUN, Kelly R; North York Gen Hosp, 4001 Leslie St, North York ON M2K 1E1; Wes'90; FRCPC; FRCPC; NuclearMed; DiagRad. Dir Nuclear Med, North York General Hospital; (416)756-6183; Fax. (416)756-6370; kcransto@nygh.on.ca.

CRASWELL, Donald F; 15 Bentley Dr PO Box 818, Middleton NS B0S 1P0; Dal'69; CCFP; FCFP; (902)825-2102; Fax. (902)825-6441.

CRASWELL, Jeffrey D; Boardwalk Prof Centre, 220 Water St, Charlottetown PE C1A 9M5; Dal'97; BScChem; FRCSC; GenSurg. Staff, Queen Elizabeth Hospital; (902)628-6528; Fax. (902)367-3284.

CRATON, Neil; Legacy Sport Med Clinic, 14-160 Meadowood Dr, Winnipeg MB R2M 5L6; Man'84; BSc; Dip SportMed; MHK; Med Dir, Manitoba Public Insurance Corporation; University of Manitoba; (204)899-6158; Fax. (204)956-1593.

CRAVEN, B Catharine; Toronto Rehab Inst-Lyndhurst, 520 Sutherland Dr, Toronto ON M4G 3V9; McM'94; BA; MClSc; FRCPC; PhysMed&Rehab (Osteoporosis). Med Staff Spinal Cord Rehab Prog, Toronto Rehabilitation Institute - Lyndhurst Centre; Staff, Holland Bloorview Kids Rehabilitation Hospital; Staff, Hamilton Health Sciences Centre - McMaster University Medical Centre; Asst Prof, University of Toronto; (416)597-3422 x6122; Fax. (416)422-5402; craven.cathy@torontorehab.on.ca.

CRAVEN, Charles P; 3062 2nd Ave, Port Alberni BC V9Y 1Y9; Stellenbosch (South Africa)'78; MB ChB; (250)723-9421

CRAVEN, John L; Medical Clinic 528, 528 Dundas St, London ON N6B 1W6; Wes'82; FRCPC; Psy. (519)645-1533; Fax. (519)645-1556.

CRAVEN, Kenneth; 29 Meldrum St, Kitimat BC V8C 2L6; Man'82; DOHS; FCBOM; P/T Med Advisor, Worksafe BC; (250)639-9272; ken.craven@sympatico.ca.

CRAVEN, Marilyn A; St Joseph's Healthcare, 3F-50 Charlton Ave E, Hamilton ON L8N 4A6; McM'83; CCFP; Staff Psy, St Joseph's Healthcare - Charlton Campus; Assoc Clin Prof Psy & Behavioural NeuroSciences, McMaster University; (905)522-1155; Fax. (905)521-6059.

CRAVEN, Michelle D; Yellowbird Family Clinic, 3380 Gateway Blvd NW, Edmonton AB T6J 6V1; Man'96; CCFP; (780)434-2893

CRAVEN, Shauna C L; PO Box 4282 Stn Main, Olds AB T4H 1P8; Man'96; CCFP; FCFP.

CRAWFORD, Allison M J; Mount Sinai Hosp, 600 University Ave, Toronto ON M5G 1X5; McM'99; FRCPC; Psy. Staff, Mount Sinai Hospital; (416)586-4800 x2286

CRAWFORD, Anne-Marie; Bridgeland Prof Centre, 208-1010 1 Ave NE, Calgary AB T2E 7W7; Glasgow (Scotland)'75; MB ChB; MRCPC(UK); DABIM; FRCPC; IntMed; Rheum. Consultant Privil, Alberta Children's Hospital; Consultant Privil, Foothills Medical Centre; (403)265-5944; Fax. (403)265-5949.

CRAWFORD, Barbara; North Bay Reg Health Centre, 50 College Dr, North Bay ON P1B 0A4; Tor'99; BScN; FRCPC; Psy. Ac Staff, North Bay Regional Health Centre - Regional Mental Health; Locum Tenens Psy, Temiskaming Hospital; Lecturer, University of Toronto; Asst Prof, Northern Ontario School of Medicine; (705)474-7525; Fax. (705)495-7846.

CRAWFORD, Brent W E; Westview Hlth Ctr Stony Plain, 4405 South Park Dr, Stony Plain AB T7Z 2M7; Man'99; CCFP; CCFP(E.M.); FCFP; Staff, Westview Health Centre; (780)968-3600

CRAWFORD, Charles D; Royal Victoria Hosp, 201 Georgian Dr, Barrie ON L4M 6M2; Tor'81; FRCPC; Anes. Staff, Royal Victoria Regional Health Centre; Staff, Orillia Soldiers' Memorial Hospital; (705)728-9090 x4207; Fax. (705)739-5613.

CRAWFORD, David J; Parkview Prof Ctr, 209-2110 Main St, Winnipeg MB R2V 2C2; Man'87; CCFP; Staff, Seven Oaks General Hospital; (204)339-8132; Fax. (204)338-0812.

CRAWFORD, Frances M; Kingston Gen Hosp, 76 Stuart St, Kingston ON K7L 2V7; Wes'87; BSc; FACEP; FRCPC; EmergMed (Maritime Medicine). Ac Staff, Hotel-Dieu Hospital; Ac Staff, Kingston General Hospital; Asst Prof, Queen's University; (613)548-2368; fmc@post.queensu.ca.

CRAWFORD, Garnet C; St Boniface Gen Hosp, A8024-409 Tache Ave, Winnipeg MB R2H 2A6; Man'96; CCFP; Staff, St Boniface General Hospital; (204)233-8563

CRAWFORD, Gordon A; Georgian Prof Centre, 304-125 Bell Farm Rd, Barrie ON L4M 6L2; Cal'75; BSc; FRCSC; OrthSurg (Sports Medicine). Ac Staff, Royal Victoria Regional Health Centre; Court Staff, Orillia Soldiers' Memorial Hospital; (705)722-3172; Fax. (705)722-1065.

CRAWFORD, John G; Deep Cove Med Clinic, 4313 Gallant Ave, North Vancouver BC V7G 2C1; Glasgow (Scotland)'87; MB ChB; CCFP; (604)929-7310; Fax. (604)929-3256.

CRAWFORD, Kim R; 135 Main St PO Box 1862, Liverpool NS B0T 1K0; Dal'81; FRCPC; IntMed. Ac Staff/Chief Med, Queens General Hospital; Ac Staff, Roseway Hospital; (902)354-2282; Fax. (902)354-2089; kim.crawford@ns.sympatico.ca.

CRAWFORD, Marjorie C; Pine Med Clinic, 5110 5th Ave, Whitehorse YT Y1A 1L4; Glasgow (Scotland)'70; MB ChB; FRCA; DA(Eng.); (867)668-4353; mccyk@hotmail.com.

CRAWFORD, Mark W; The Hosp For Sick Children, 555 University Ave, Toronto ON M5G 1X8; West Indies (Jamaica)'82; FRCPC; Anes (Pediatric Anesthesia). Staff Anes, The Hospital For Sick Children; Asst Prof Anes, University of Toronto; (416)813-7445; Fax. (416)813-7543; mark.crawford@sickkids.ca.

CRAWFORD, Michelle; Clinique Med Elmwood, 206-565 Elmwood Dr, Dieppe NB E1A 2X4; Mon'91; Staff FamilyMed, Dr Georges-L-Dumont University Hospital Centre; Langs: Bilingual(English/French); (506)857-0010; Fax. (506)857-9421.

CRAWFORD, Richard I; 950 10th Ave W, Vancouver BC V5Z 1M9; UBC'87; FRCPC; GenPath; Derm; AnatPath. Staff, Providence Health Care - St Paul's Hospital; Clin Prof, University of British Columbia; (604)875-4480

CRAWFORD, Robert B; PO Box 550, Cardston AB T0K 0K0; Sask'05; CCFP; (403)653-3331; Fax. (403)653-1098.

CRAWFORD, Stephen G S; Chinook Reg Hosp, 960 19 St S, Lethbridge AB T1J 1W5; London (England)'98; MB BS; BSc; Staff, Chinook Regional Hospital; (403)388-6111

CRAWFORD, William F; Hornepayne Community Hosp, PO Box 190 278 Front St, Hornepayne ON P0M 1Z0; McM'88; Staff, Hornepayne Community Hospital; (807)868-2449; jforster@renegadeisp.com.

CRAWFORD-BOURKE, Denise; Oshawa Clinic, 117 King St E, Oshawa ON L1H 1B9; Tor'95; FRCSC; ObstGyn. Staff, Lakeridge Health - Oshawa Site; (905)721-4912; Fax. (905)721-3558.

CRAWLEY, Cinzia U; Hys Med Centre, M/F-11010 101 St NW, Edmonton AB T5H 4B9; (Ireland)'86; (780)426-1121; Fax. (780)425-5979.

CRAWLEY, Frances J M; Dr Frances Crawley Med Clinic, PO Box 2907 141 Wentworth Rd, Windsor NS B0N 2T0; Dal'83; BSc; MSc; FRCSC; GenSurg (Hernias). Staff, Hants Community Hospital; (902)798-4709; Fax. (902)798-0530.

CRAWLEY, Margaret G; Queensway Prof Centre, 112-190 Sherway Dr, Etobicoke ON M9C 5N2; Qns'80; Staff, Trillium Health Centre - West Toronto; (416)626-1066; Fax. (416)626-4775.

CRCHOVA, Melissa; Ctr Hosp Affilie-St-Sacrement, 1050 ch Sainte-Foy, Quebec QC G1S 4L8; McG'93; Staff, Centre Hospitalier Affilié Universitaire de Québec - Hôpital du St-Sacrement; (418)682-7511; Fax. (418)682-7977.

CREAGHAN, Jason D; Tungasuvvingat Inuit Family He, 24 Selkirk St, Ottawa ON K1L 6N2; Dal'95; CCFP; Langs: Bilingual(English/French); (613)740-0999

CREAN, Andrew M; N C S B I C 554, 585 University Ave, Toronto ON M5G 2N2; Southampton (England)'92; Staff, Toronto General Hospital - UHN; (416)340-4800

CREASER, Kimberley J; Queensway-Carleton Hosp, 3045 Baseline Rd, Nepean ON K2H 8P4; Dal'05; CCFP; CCFP(E.M.); Staff, Queensway Carleton Hospital; (613)721-2000

CREATCHMAN, Terrence M; 605-1 Young St, Hamilton ON L8N 1T8; McG'75; CCFP; FCFP; Asst Clin Prof Family Med, McMaster University; Langs: Bilingual(English/French); (905)547-1110; Fax. (905)547-8802.

CREBA, Aran S; St Paul's Hosp, 1081 Burrard St, Vancouver BC V6Z 1Y6; Cal'10; CCFP; Staff, Providence Health Care - St Paul's Hospital; (604)682-2344

CREE, David; 4F-10 George St, Hamilton ON L8P 1C8; Glasgow (Scotland)'71; MB ChB; CCFP; (905)529-2072; Fax. (905)529-1052.

CREEDON, Kerry; 208-125 13th St E, North Vancouver BC V7L 2L3; National (Ireland)'71; MB BCh; GenSurg. (604)987-6940; Fax. (604)987-4239.

CREEK, Kristen L B; Queen Street Medical Clinic, 1177 Queen St W, Toronto ON M6J 1J4; Man'10; CCFP; (647)350-1855; Fax. (647)350-1955.

CREERY, W David; Children's Hosp Eastern Ont, 401 Smyth Rd, Ottawa ON K1H 8L1; Wes'89; FRCPC; Peds; Critical Care Medicine. Staff, Children's Hospital of Eastern Ontario (CHEO); (613)738-3680

CREGAN, Timothy R; Ottawa West Med Clinic, 2F-760 Eagleson Rd, Kanata ON K2M 0A7; Tor'98; CCFP; (613)592-9081; Fax. (613)592-6554.

CREIGHTON, David A; Woodlawn Med Clinic, 92 Main St, Dartmouth NS B2X 1R5; Dal'83; (902)434-1500; Fax. (902)434-5011.

CREIGHTON, Paula A; Glace Bay Healthcare Complex, 300 South St, Glace Bay NS B1A 1W5; McM'93; BSc; BA; BEd; FRCPC; IntMed; GeriatricMed. Staff, Glace Bay Healthcare Facility; (902)842-2896

CREIGHTON, Robert J; 4 Colborne St PO Box 550, Walkerton ON N0G 2V0; Tor'57; Fam Med, South Bruce Grey Health Centre - Walkerton Site; (519)881-2071

CRELINSTEN, Gordon L; Seaforth Med Bldg, 660-3550 ch de la Cote-des-Nei, Montreal QC H3H 1V4; McG'70; ABIM; CSPQ; FRCPC; IntMed (Cardiovascular Medicine); Cardiol. Sr Physician, McGill University Health Centre - Royal Victoria Hospital; Assoc Physician, Sir Mortimer B Davis Jewish General; Consultant, McGill University Health Centre - Montreal Chest Institute; assoc Prof, McGill University; Langs: English; French; (514)844-0883; Fax. (514)933-5207; gcrelinsten@qc.aibn.com.

CREMIN, Denis; Burin Peninsula Hlth Care Ctr, PO Box 340, Burin NL A0E 1E0; National (Ireland)'83; MB ChB; Staff, Burin Peninsula Health Care Centre; (709)891-1040

CREPEAU, Andre; CSSS de Sept-Iles, 45 rue Du Pere-Divet, Sept-Iles QC G4R 3N7; Mon'76; FRCPC; DiagRad. Staff, Centre Hospitalier Regional de Sept-Iles; (418)962-9761 x2510

CREPEAU, Brigitte A; Penticton Reg Hosp, 550 Carmi Ave, Penticton BC V2A 3G6; McG'88; FRCPC; Anes. Staff, Penticton Regional Hospital; Langs: Bilingual(English/French); (250)492-4000

CREPEAU, Jacques; CHUS-Hop Hotel-Dieu, 580 rue Bowen S, Sherbrooke QC J1G 2E8; Laval'54; FCCP; FRCPC; IntMed; Cardiol (P.Q.). Staff, Centre Hospitalier Universitaire de Sherbrooke-Hôpital Hôtel-Dieu; (819)346-1110

CREPEAU, Jacques M; Institut de Cardiologie de Mtl, 5000 rue Belanger, Montreal QC H1T 1C8; McG'75; CSPQ; Cardiol (Hemodynamics). Ac Staff, Institut de Cardiologie de Montréal; Langs: Bilingual(French/English); (514)593-2552; Fax. (514)593-2567; jacques.crepeau@icm-mhi.org.

CREPEAU, Michel; CLSC Samuel de Champlain, 100-5811 boul Taschereau, Brossard QC J4Z 1A5; Laval'76; (450)445-4452; Fax. (450)445-5535.

CREPEAU, Rene; 1-1620 av Seaforth, Montreal QC H3H 1B7; Laval'68; FRCSC; PlasSurg. Ac Staff, McGill University Health Centre - Montreal General Campus; Ac Staff, McGill University Health Centre - Montreal Children's Hospital; Langs: English; (514)935-4472; Fax. (514)935-8803; info@renecrepeau.com.

CREPIN, Marylene; CSSS Haut-Richelieu-Rouville, 920 boul Du Seminaire N, St-Jean-Sur-Richel QC J3A 1B7; McG'97; Staff, Hôpital du Haut-Richelieu; (450)359-5000 x5176

CRERAR, Anita; St Mary's Hosp Centre, 3830 av Lacombe, Montreal QC H3T 1M5; Mon'04; CCFP; CCFP(E.M.); Staff, St Mary's Hospital Centre; (514)345-3511

CRESSEY, Christopher F; 130 Main St E PO Box 250, Palmerston ON N0G 2P0; McG'73; CCFP; Staff, North Wellington Health Care - Palmerston & District Hospital; Langs: Bilingual(English/French); (519)343-3831; Fax. (519)343-9944.

CRESSWELL, David A; Belmont Prof Centre, 408-564 Belmont Ave W, Kitchener ON N2M 5N6; Wes'88; FAAP; FRCPC; Peds (Consultant Pediatrics). Ac Staff/Chief Peds, Grand River Hospital - Kitchener/Waterloo Health Centre; Clin Asst Prof, McMaster University; (519)570-1492; Fax. (519)570-3387.

CRESSWELL, Mark E; St Paul's Hosp, 1081 Burrard St, Vancouver BC V6Z 1Y6; Witwatersrand (South Africa)'96; MB BCh; FRCR; DA; FRCPC; DiagRad. Staff, Providence Health Care - St Paul's Hospital; (604)806-8026; Fax. (604)806-8283.

CRESSWELL, Silke; Pacific Parkinson Research Ctr, M36-2221 Wesbrook Mall, Vancouver BC V6T 2B5; Ruprecht Karl University (Germany)'97; Staff, Pacific Parkinson Research Centre; (604)822-7754

CRETE, Elise; UMF Charles LeMoyne, 201-299 boul Sir Wilfrid-Lemoy, Saint-Lambert QC J4R 2L1; Mon'08; CCFP; (450)466-5630; Fax. (450)466-5631.

CRETE, Martin; Hotel-Dieu de Levis, 143 rue Wolfe, Levis QC G6V 3Z1; Laval'98; CSPQ; FRCPC; IntMed; Cardiol. Staff, Hôtel-Dieu de Lévis; (418)835-7121

CRETE, Pauline; CHUQ-Ctr Hosp Univ Laval, 2705 boul Laurier, Quebec QC G1V 4G2; Laval'92; CCFP; Staff, Centre Hospitalier Universitaire de Quebec-CHUL; (418)654-2255; Fax. (418)654-2757.

CREVIER, Jean; Ctr Hosp Reg de Lanaudiere, 1000 boul Sainte-Anne, St-Charles-Brromee QC J6E 6J2; Sher'73; Urol. Staff, Centre Hospitalier Régional de Lanaudière; (450)759-8222

CREVIER, Louis; Hôpital Ste-Justine, 3175 ch Cote-Ste-Catherine, Montreal QC H3T 1C5; Laval'00; FRCSC; Neursurg. Staff, Hôpital Ste-Justine; (514)345-4931

CREWE, Harold J; Medical Arts Clinic, 204-105 Manitoba Dr, Clarenville NL A5A 1K2; Mem'76; (709)466-2631; Fax. (709)466-3895.

CREWE, Shawn G; 9-575 West St S, Orillia ON L3V 7N6; Mem'95; FRCPC; IntMed. (705)326-9401

CREWSON, Marolyn M; Heart Lake Med Centre, 101-10425 Kennedy Rd, Brampton ON L6Z 0A4; McM'80; CCFP; Ac Staff, William Osler Health System - Brampton Civic Hospital; (905)846-7611; Fax. (905)846-7753.

CRIBB, Alina; Saskatoon City Hosp, 701 Queen St, Saskatoon SK S7K 0M7; Sask'91; CCFP; FCFP; Staff Geriatrics, Saskatoon City Hospital; (306)655-8925; Fax. (306)655-8929.

CRICH, Alexandre S; Hop Charles Lemoyne, 3120 boul Taschereau, Greenfield Park QC J4V 2H1; Sher'00; CCFP; CCFP(E.M.); Staff, Hopital Charles LeMoyne; (450)466-5050; Fax. (450)466-5051.

CRICHLOW, Allison; Regina Gen Hosp, 1440 14th Ave, Regina SK S4P 0W5; Sask'88; FRCPC; Anes. Staff, Regina General Hospital; (306)766-4444

CRICHLOW, Michael W; Regina Med Centre, 200-2550 12th Ave, Regina SK S4P 3X1; Sask'95; LMCC; FRCSC; Urol. (306)566-4146; Fax. (306)566-4158.

CRICHTON, Andrew; 102-49 Richard Way SW, Calgary AB T3E 7M8; UBC'81; FRCSC; Ophth (Cataract & Glaucoma). Staff Eye Clinic, Rockyview General Hospital; Member Ophth Fellowship Committee/Clin Prof Surg, University of Calgary; (403)245-3730; Fax. (403)245-1058; drcricht@telusplanet.net.

CRICHTON, Robert T; 111 Corbett Rd, Salt Spring Island BC V8K 2R8; (South Africa)'91; MB ChB; CCFP; (250)537-2412; Fax. (250)537-4947.

CRICHTON, Thomas P; City of Lakes Family Hlth Team, C-960 Notre Dame Ave, Sudbury ON P3A 2T4; Qns'89; CCFP; FCFP; Ac Staff, Health Sciences North-St Joseph's Health Centre; Asst Dean Family Med/Assoc Prof, Northern Ontario School of Medicine; (705)560-1018; Fax. (705)566-7617.

CRICKMER, Sean D; Peace Arch Hosp, 15521 Russell Ave, White Rock BC V4B 2R4; Qns'86; CCFP; CCFP(E.M.); Staff, Peace Arch Hospital; (604)535-4504; Fax. (604)535-4536.

CRIDLAND, Ronald G; Kelowna Sleep Clinic, 120-1856 Ambrosi Rd, Kelowna BC V1Y 4R9; Tor'82; DABSM; CCFP; Med Dir, Kelowna Sleep Clinic; (250)862-3050

CRILLY, Richard G; St Joseph's HC-Parkwood Hosp, 801 Commissioners Rd E, London ON N6C 5J1; Queen's (Ireland)'73; MB ChB; BAO; FRCP(UK); FRCPC; IntMed (Geriatric Medicine). Consultant, St Joseph's Hospital - St Joseph's Health Care; Staff Geriatric Med, Parkwood Hospital - St Joseph's Health Care; Consultant, London Health Sciences Centre - Victoria Campus; Assoc Prof Geriatric Med, University of Western Ontario; (519)685-4021; Fax. (519)685-4093; richard.crilly@sjhc.london.on.ca.

CRIPPEN, Craig A; 200-1626 Richter St, Kelowna BC V1Y 2M3; Wes'01; CCFP; (250)868-3070; Fax. (250)768-3071.

CRIPPS, John R; 241 Brock St, Gravenhurst ON P1P 1H4; Wes'82; BSc; FRCSC; Ophth (Cataract Surgery). Staff Ophth, South Muskoka Memorial Hospital - Muskoka Algonquin Healthcare; Ophthalmology, Huntsville District Memorial Hospital - Muskoka Algonquin Healthcare; Court Staff, Orillia Soldiers' Memorial Hospital; Court Staff, Royal Victoria Regional Health Centre; Clinical Asst Prof Med, Northern Ontario School of Medicine; (705)687-1256; Fax. (705)687-4353.

CRIPPS, M Christine; Ottawa Reg Cancer Centre, 501 Smyth Rd Box 913, Ottawa ON K1H 8L6; Wes'72; FRCPC; IntMed (Medical Oncology). Staff Privil, The Ottawa Hospital - Civic Campus; Educator, Ottawa Regional Cancer Centre; Assoc Prof MedOncol, University of Ottawa; (613)737-7700 x70176; Fax. (613)247-3511; ccripps@ottawahospital.on.ca.

CRIPPS, Stephanie M; 201-5171 221A St, Langley BC V2Y 0A2; Wes'95; BSc; FRCSC; Urol. Ac Staff, Langley Memorial Hospital; (604)514-8530; Fax. (604)514-8560.

CRISCI, Elisabeth M V; 7105 East Saanich Rd, Saanichton BC V8M 2B4; Ott'04; (250)652-3630

CRISP, Barbara J; Surrey Mem Hosp, 13750 96 Ave, Surrey BC V3V 1Z2; Wes'82; BSc; Staff Consultant Youth Clinic, Surrey Memorial Hospital; (604)585-5999; barbara.crisp@fraserhealth.ca.

CRISP, David T; Oshawa Clinic, 100-117 King St E, Oshawa ON L1H 1B9; Tor'78; FRCPC; IntMed; Neur. Staff, Lakeridge Health - Oshawa Site; (905)721-4300 x5414; Fax. (905)721-3585.

CRISPINO, Natascha; St Joseph's Health Centre, 30 The Queensway, Toronto ON M6R 1B5; Tor'01; CCFP; Staff, St Joseph's Health Centre; Lecturer, University of Toronto; Langs: German; Italian; (416)530-6860; Fax. (416)530-6139; n.crispino@utoronto.ca.

CRISTACHE, Aurelian; Ellendale Med Bldg, 505-5845 ch de la Cote-des-Nei, Montreal QC H3S 1Z4; Cluj (Romania)'63; (514)733-1868; Fax. (514)733-1493.

CRISTANTE, Loris; Manitoba Clinic, 790 Sherbrook St, Winnipeg MB R3A 1M3; Giessen (Germany)'79; Staff, The Salvation Army Grace Hospital; Prof Section of Surg, University of Manitoba; Langs: Italian; German; (204)788-5785; Fax. (204)783-6579; cristant@cc.umanitoba.ca.

CRISTOVEANU, Nicholas J; Frontenac Med Associates, 201-791 Princess St, Kingston ON K7L 1E9; Qns'79; BA; CCFP; FCFP; Assoc Staff, Kingston General Hospital; Assoc Staff FamilyMed, Hotel-Dieu Hospital; Med Dir, Rideaucrest Home for the Aged; Instructor Family Med, Queen's University; (613)544-2727; Fax. (613)544-7247; cristoveanu@frontenacmedical.ca.

CRITCH, Jeffrey N; Dr Charles A Janeway Child HC, 300 Prince Philip Dr, St. John's NL A1B 3V6; Mem'95; FRCPC; Peds; Gastroent. Staff Peds, Janeway Children's Health & Rehabilitation Centre; (709)777-4134; Fax. (709)777-4726.

CRITCHLEY, Carol A; Health Park, 201-45 Weatherbee Rd, Mira Road NS B1M 0A1; Dal'77; CCFP; (902)567-0555

CRITCHLEY, David D; 104-145 15th St W, North Vancouver BC V7M 1R9; Qns'87; FRCPC; Peds. (604)924-3133; Fax. (604)980-8393.

CRITCHLEY, Patrick P; Algonquin Med Centre, 3-227 Algonquin Blvd W, Timmins ON P4N 2R8; McM'88; CCFP; FCFP; Staff, Timmins & District Hospital; (705)267-5511; Fax. (705)264-6373; pcritchley@vianet.on.ca.

CRITTENDEN, Roger K; Centuria Medical, 2-1499 Gordon Dr, Kelowna BC V1Y 9R2; Cape Town (South Africa)'76; MRC(UK); Ad Staff Privil, Kelowna General Hospital; (250)762-3807

CRIVAT, C Mirela; William Osler HC-Etobicoke, 101 Humber College Blvd, Etobicoke ON M9V 1R8; Iasi (Romania)'89; CCFP; Staff, William Osler Health System - Etobicoke General Hospital; (416)747-3400; Fax. (416)747-8608.

CROCCO, Anthony G; Hamilton HS-McMaster Site, PO Box 2000 Stn Lcd 1 1200 Main St W, Hamilton ON L8N 3Z5; McM'97; FRCPC; Peds; PedEmergMed. Staff, Hamilton Health Sciences Centre - McMaster Children's Hospital; (905)521-2100

CROCHETIERE, Chantal; Hôpital Ste-Justine, 3175 ch Cote-Ste-Catherine, Montreal QC H3T 1C5; Laval'84; CSPQ; FRCPC; Anes. Ac Staff, Hôpital Ste-Justine; (514)345-4733; Fax. (514)345-4829.

CROCKER, John F S; IWK Health Centre, PO Box 9700 Rpo CSC 5850-5980 University Ave, Halifax NS B3K 6R8; Dal'66; FRCPC; Peds (Nephrology). Dir Nephrol, IWK Health Centre; Prof Peds & Dir, Dalhousie University; (902)470-8195; Fax. (902)470-8900.

CROCKER, Kenneth; Central Nfld Reg Hlth Centre, 50 Union St, Grnd-Falls-Windsor NL A2A 2E1; Mem'03; FRCPC; DiagRad. Staff, Central Newfoundland Regional Health Centre; (709)292-2500

CROCKER, Percy R; Eleven Elizabeth Family Practi, 201-11 Elizabeth Ave, St. John's NL A1A 1W6; Mem'89; CCFP; FCFP; (709)579-1106

CROCKER, Thomas C; 202-10 Alcorn Ave, Toronto ON M4V 3A9; Tor'85; FRCPC; Psy. Staff, St Michael's Hospital; (416)968-0292; Fax. (416)975-0129.

CROCKET, Jennifer A; Wetaskiwin Lung Laboratory, 5217A 50 St, Wetaskiwin AB T9A 3B8; Qns'88; FRCPC; IntMed (Pulmonary Medicine); Respir. Consultant, Leduc Community Hospital; Consultant Respirology, Wetaskiwin Lung Laboratory; (780)352-7085; Fax. (780)352-7870.

CROCKETT, Maryanne E; Basic Med Sciences Bldg, 502-745 Bannatyne Ave, Winnipeg MB R3E 0J9; Qns'92; FAAP; MPH; DCMT; FRCPC; FRCPC; InfectDis; Peds.

CROCKFORD, David N; Foothills Med Centre, C203-1403 29 St NW, Calgary AB T2N 2T9; Alb'90; BScMed; FRCPC; Psy (Addiction Psychiatry). Staff, Foothills Medical Centre; Asst Prof, University of Calgary; (403)944-4791; Fax. (403)944-2165.

CROFT, Benjamin; Southwest Family Hlth Centre, 204-200 James St S, Hamilton ON L8P 3A9; McG'06; MDCM; CCFP; Langs: Bilingual(French/English); (905)526-1606

CROFT, Dary; Ctr Hosp Affilie-Enfant-Jesus, 1401 18e rue, Quebec QC G1J 1Z4; Laval'86; CSPQ; FRCSC; GenSurg; Anes. Staff Anes & Intensive Care, Centre Hospitalier Affilié Universitaire de Québec - Hôpital De L'Enfant Jésus; (418)649-5807; Fax. (418)649-5936.

CROFT, Joan D; 3407 27 Ave, Vernon BC V1T 1S2; McG'89; BSc; CCFP; CCFP(E.M.); Staff, Vernon Jubilee Hospital; (250)545-1339; Fax. (250)545-1035.

CROFT, John A; Second Avenue Med Clinic, 330 2nd Ave W, Prince Rupert BC V8J 1G6; Orange Free State (South Africa)'88; MB ChB; CCFP; Langs: Afrikaans; (250)624-5500; Fax. (250)624-4797.

CROFT, Lorraine S; 23 McDougall Crt NE, Calgary AB T2E 8R3; Alb'84; CCFP; Staff, Foothills Medical Centre; (403)265-3410; Fax. (403)265-3411.

CROFTON, Neil; Medical Arts Bldg, 315-1105 Pandora Ave, Victoria BC V8V 3P9; UBC'85; Court Staff, Vancouver Island Health Authority; Ac Staff, Aberdeen Hospital; Staff, Mount St Mary Hospital; (250)388-5032; Fax. (250)388-5632.

CROFTS, Neil G; 152-1848 Main St, Penticton BC V2A 5H3; UBC'88; FRCSC; Urol. Staff, Penticton Regional Hospital; (250)493-4773; Fax. (250)493-4779.

CROFTS, Paul G; 102-123 15th St E, North Vancouver BC V7L 2P7; UBC'82; FRCSC; Urol. (604)987-8171; Fax. (604)987-8130.

CROFTS, Peter A; Queen Elizabeth II HSC-Halifax, 2107-1796 Summer St, Halifax NS B3H 3A7; Oxford (England)'63; MA(Oxon); BMus; BCh(Oxon); MRC(Lond); Cardiol; IntMed. Staff, Queen Elizabeth II Health Sciences Centre - Victoria General Site; Asst Prof, Dalhousie University; (902)473-3547; Fax. (902)473-2434.

CROISETIERE, Guy; Polyclinique De Trois-Rivieres, B 210-1900 boul des Recollets, Trois-Rivieres QC G8Z 4K4; Bordeaux (France)'81; (819)376-0300

CROITORU, Kendra L A; PO Box 52556 Rpo Coquitlam Ctr, New Westminster BC V3B 7J4; McM'10; CCFP; (604)941-8277

CROITORU, Kenneth; Mount Sinai Hosp, 437-600 University Ave, Toronto ON M5G 1X5; McG'81; FRCPC; IntMed; Gastroent. Staff, Mount Sinai Hospital; Prof Med, University of Toronto; Langs: English; French; (416)586-4800

CROITORU, Zenovia; Hop Jean-Talon, 1385 rue Jean-Talon E, Montreal QC H2E 1S6; Mon'01; AnatPath. Staff, CSSS du Coeur de l'Isle Hôpital Jean-Talon; (514)495-6767 x6131

CROLL, G Blair; Thunder Bay Reg HSC-T-Bay, 980 Oliver Rd, Thunder Bay ON P7B 6V4; McM'73; BASc; Staff, Thunder Bay Regional Health Sciences Centre; (807)684-6000

CROMBEZ, Jean-Charles; CHUM-Hop Notre-Dame, 1560 rue Sherbrooke E, Montreal QC H2L 4M1; Lille (France)'67; Psy (Psychosomatic Medicine). ac Staff, Centre Hospitalier l'Université de Montréal (CHUM) - Hôpital Notre-Dame; Langs: Bilingual(French/English); (514)890-8000 x27021; Fax. (514)412-7662; jean.charles.crombez@umontreal.ca.

CROMBIE, Carrie; 204-107 King St W, Dundas ON L9H 1V1; McM'95; BSc; MSc; Staff, Hamilton Health Sciences Centre - McMaster Children's Hospital; (905)627-3505; Fax. (905)627-4193.

CROMBIE, Fionnella S S; Southwest Family Health Ctre, 204-200 James St S, Hamilton ON L8P 3A9; Tor'80; CCFP; FCFP; Ac Staff, St Joseph's Healthcare - Charlton Campus; Court Staff, Hamilton Health Sciences Centre - McMaster University Medical Centre; Clin Assoc Prof Family Med, McMaster University; (905)526-1606; Fax. (905)526-7692.

CROMPTON, Daniel; University Hosp of Northern BC, 1475 Edmonton St, Prince George BC V2M 1S2; UBC'08; CCFP; CCFP(E.M.); Staff, University Hospital of Northern British Columbia; (250)565-2000

CROMPTON, John M; 740 Bateman Mill Rd, Moncton NB E1H 3T1; London (England)'76; FRCPC; Anes (Pain Management). Staff, The Moncton Hospital; Ass't. Lect., Dalhousie University; (506)857-5458; Fax. (506)857-5459.

CROMPTON, Stephanie L; 6-1230 Alward St, Prince George BC V2M 7B1; UBC'09; CCFP; (250)563-3024

CROMWELL, Korwin R; Misericordia Community Hosp, 16940 87 Ave NW, Edmonton AB T5R 4H5; Sask'89; CCFP; CCFP(E.M.); FCFP; Ac Staff, Covenant Health - Misericordia Community Hospital; (780)735-2819; Fax. (780)735-2966.

CRON, Charles C; St Margaret's Village, 5181 St Margaret's Bay Rd, Lakeside NS B3Z 4R4; Dal'70; FAAOO; FRCSC; Otol (Pediatric Otolaryngology). Ac Staff, IWK Health Centre; Ac Staff, Queen Elizabeth II Health Sciences Centre - Victoria General Site; Asst Prof Otol, Dalhousie University; (902)826-9616; Fax. (902)826-9617.

CRONIN, Catherine; 210-1815 Kirschner Ave, Kelowna BC V1Y 4N7; National (Ireland)'80; FRCP; MBA(Hons); FRCPI(Ire); FAAP; FRCPC; Peds (Neonatology). Med Dir NICU, Kelowna General Hospital; Staff Neonatol, Health Sciences Centre; Staff Neonatol, St Boniface General Hospital; Med Dir Interior Health, Perinatal & Child Health Network; Assoc Head, Winnipeg Regional Health Authority; Prof Peds, University of Manitoba; Langs: English; French; (250)870-4778; Fax. (250)870-4795.

CRONIN, Christopher P; Hamilton Comm Health Centre, M1-414 Victoria Ave N, Hamilton ON L8L 5G8; Ott'05; CCFP; (905)529-5221

CRONIN, Karen L; Yorkview Med Centre, 104-3695 Keele St, North York ON M3J 1N2; Tor'68; CCFP; Ac Staff, Humber River Regional Hospital - Finch Avenue Site; Med Dir, Kipling Acres, Metro Home for Aged; (416)633-3711; Fax. (416)633-0521; klcronin@hotmail.com.

CRONIN, Terence J; Richmond Centre, PO Box 2000 Stn Central, Charlottetown PE C1A 7N8; University Coll. (Ireland)'81; MB ChB; BAO; Psy. (902)368-4430

CRONJE, David P G; Miramichi Med Arts Centre, 679 King George Hwy, Miramichi NB E1V 1N9; Pretoria (South Africa)'71; MMed(Urol.); Langs: Afrikaans; German; (506)773-3440; Fax. (506)773-3525; davidfienie@yahoo.com.

CRONJE, J Stephen; Chinook Reg Hosp, 960 19 St S, Lethbridge AB T1J 1W5; Stellenbosch (South Africa)'82; CCFP; CCFP(E.M.); Staff, Chinook Regional Hospital; (403)328-8101; Fax. (403)328-8150.

CRONJE, Rynier; Lenore Centre Med Clinic, 4-123 Lenore Dr, Saskatoon SK S7K 7H9; 80Stellenbosch (South Africa)'83; MB ChB; (306)242-6700; Fax. (306)242-1168.

CROOK, Juanita M; BC Cancer Agency, 399 Royal Ave, Kelowna BC V1Y 5L3; Tor'78; FRCPC; RadOncol. Staff, BC Cancer Agency Sindi Ahluwalia Hawkins Centre for the Southern Interior; Langs: Bilingual(French/English); Spanish; (250)712-3900 x683979

CROOKS, Bruce N A; IWK Health Centre, PO Box 9700 Rpo CSC 5850-5980 University Ave, Halifax NS B3K 6R8; Birmingham (England)'90; BSc; MB ChB; MRCP(UK); FRCPCH; Staff, IWK Health Centre; Assoc Prof Ped Hem/Oncol, Dalhousie University; (902)470-8048; Fax. (902)470-7216; bruce.crooks@iwk.nshealth.ca.

CROOKS, Harris G; Community Med Centre, 2273 Prospect Rd, Hatchet Lake NS B3T 1S9; Dal'75; (902)852-3090; Fax. (902)852-5108.

CROOKS, Simone L; The Ottawa Hosp-Gen Campus, 501 Smyth Rd, Ottawa ON K1H 8L6; Wes'00; FRCPC; Anes. Staff, The Ottawa Hospital - General Campus; (613)737-8187

CROOKS TERON, Louisa L C; Active Care Med Group, 1108 Klonidke Rd, Kanata ON K2K 0G1; Ott'83; CCFP; FCFP; (613)254-9777; Fax. (613)254-9778.

CROOKSHANK, Emily; St Joseph's Health Centre, 30 The Queensway, Toronto ON M6R 1B5; McM'07; Neur. Staff, St Joseph's Health Centre; (416)530-6000

CROOME, Alison J G; 20-1521 Dufferin Cres, Nanaimo BC V9S 5H6; UBC'05; FRCPC; IntMed; Nephrol. (250)591-1898

CROOME, Kristopher P; London HSC-University Hosp, PO Box 5339 Stn Main C8 114-339 Windermere Rd, London ON N6A 5A5; Wes'06; FRCSC; GenSurg. Staff, London Health Sciences Centre - University Hospital; (519)685-8300

CROSBIE, Douglas R; Brigus Med Centre, GD, South River NL A0A 3W0; Mem'78; (709)528-4601

CROSBIE, Stephen H; Cape Breton Hlthcare Complex, 1482 George St, Sydney NS B1P 1P3; Dal'87; Staff, Cape Breton Healthcare Complex; (902)567-8000

CROSBIE, Victoria; Terrance on the Square, PO Box 23157 Rpo Churchill Sq, St. John's NL A1B 4J9; Mem'90; FRCPC; Peds (Developmental Disability). Staff, Janeway Children's Health & Rehabilitation Centre.

CROSBY, Amanda R; Crossroads Fam Practice, 201-5110 St Margarets Bay Rd, Upper Tantallon NS B3Z 1E2; Dal'08; BSc; CCFP; Staff Family Med Obstetrics, IWK Health Centre; Teach Staff Dept of Family Med Obstetrics, Dalhousie University; (902)826-9096; Fax. (902)820-9399.

CROSBY, Andrew J R; 1371 Greenwood St, Campbell River BC V9W 6K5; Mem'99; FRCSC; OrthSurg (Arthroplasty). Staff, Campbell River & District General Hospital; (778)346-2501; acrosby@telus.net.

CROSBY, Edward T; The Ottawa Hosp-Gen Campus, 1401-501 Smyth Rd, Ottawa ON K1H 8L6; Ott'84; FRCPC; Anes. Staff Obst Anes, The Ottawa Hospital - General Campus; Assoc Prof, University of Ottawa; (613)737-8187; Fax. (613)737-8189.

CROSBY, Jacqueline A; 17 Bear St, Tillsonburg ON N4G 1V4; Wes'89; FRCS; FACS; FRCSC; GenSurg (Surgical Oncology). Staff GenSurg, Tillsonburg District Memorial Hospital; Staff GenSurg, Alexandra Hospital; Consultant, Tillsonburg Laser Clinic; (519)842-2101; Fax. (519)842-9668; surgeons@tdmh.on.ca.

CROSBY, Janet E; 407-345 Lakeshore Rd E, Oakville ON L6J 1J5; National (Ireland)'82; MB ChB; BSc; FRCPC; Psy (Psychotherapy). (905)849-9533

CROSBY, Jason A; Manitoba Clinic, 790 Sherbrook St, Winnipeg MB R3A 1M3; Man'02; FRCSC; OrthSurg.

CROSBY, Jean D; Sydney Family Practice, 196 Kings Rd, Sydney NS B1S 1A1; Dal'79; (902)567-0040; Fax. (902)539-9250.

CROSBY, John W; 11 George St S, Cambridge ON N1S 2N3; Wes'73; FRCP; EmergMed. Med Dir, Hilltop & Riverbend Nursing Homes; Clinical Asst Prof Family Med, McMaster University; Asst Prof Med, University of Toronto; (519)621-8351; Fax. (519)621-4456; drjohncrosby@rogers.com.

CROSKERRY, Patrick; Cobequid Commun Health Centre, 40 Freer Lane, Lower Sackville NS B4C 0A2; McM'82; PhD; Staff, Cobequid Community Health Centre; (902)869-6143

CROSS, Charles H T; Canadian Forces Hlth Services, PO Box 17000 Stn Forces, Victoria BC V9A 7N2; Liverpool (England)'87; MB ChB; (250)363-2000

CROSS, David; Gulf Canada Square, 325-401 9 Ave SW, Calgary AB T2P 3C5; McG'84; ABIM; AB; FRCPC; IntMed (Asthma & Allergy); ClinImmunol&Allergy. Clinical Asst Prof Med, University of Calgary; (403)221-4470; Fax. (403)221-4406.

CROSS, James W; PO Box 130, Christopher Lake SK S0J 0N0; Sask'73; Staff EmergMed, Victoria Hospital; Med Dir, Saskatchewan Air Ambulance; (306)982-4956; jwc.cross@sk.sympatico.ca.

CROSS, Keith R; Bracebridge Med Arts Centre, 253 James St, Bracebridge ON P1L 2C2; Tor'76; DPH; CCFP; Staff, South Muskoka Memorial Hospital - Muskoka Algonquin Healthcare; Staff, Huntsville District Memorial Hospital - Muskoka Algonquin Healthcare; (705)645-2281; Fax. (705)645-0057; keith.cross@mahc.ca.

CROSS, Peter W; The Ottawa Hosp-Gen Campus, 501 Smyth Rd, Ottawa ON K1H 8L6; Qns'79; FRCPC; RadOncol. Staff, The Ottawa Hospital - General Campus; (613)737-7777

CROSS, Randolph G; 95 Hamilton St N PO Box 890, Waterdown ON L0R 2H0; McM'79; CCFP; FCFP; Assoc Staff, Joseph Brant Memorial Hospital; (905)689-6134; Fax. (905)689-5665.

CROSS, Robert; St Boniface Gen Hosp, 3036Z-409 Tache Ave, Winnipeg MB R2H 2A6; Man'87; Staff, St Boniface General Hospital; (204)233-8563

CROSS, William G; Cobourg Med Centre, 5-1060 Burnham St, Cobourg ON K9A 5V9; McG'77; CCFP; FCFP; Staff Physician, Northumberland Hills Hospital; Asst Prof, University of Toronto; Langs: English; French; (905)373-8333; Fax. (905)373-9333; bcross@eagle.ca.

CROSSEN, Nancy P; 101-147 16th St W, North Vancouver BC V7M 1T3; UBC'75; Staff, Lions Gate Hospital; (604)986-5621

CROSSLEY, John F A; Gandhi Med Clinic, 103-6935 120 St, Delta BC V4E 2A8; Sask'77; (604)590-4443; Fax. (604)590-5192.

CROSSLEY, John G; Hamilton HS-General Site, 237 Barton St E, Hamilton ON L8L 2X2; Ott'96; FRCPC; EmergMed. Staff, Hamilton Health Sciences Centre - Hamilton General Hospital; (905)527-0271

CROSSMAN, Mark W; Kerrisdale Prof Centre, 335-2025 42nd Ave W, Vancouver BC V6M 2B5; UBC'89; BSc; FRCPC; PhysMed&Rehab (Chronic Pain). Clin Instructor Div of PhysMed&Rehab, University of British Columbia; (604)261-5230; Fax. (604)261-5290.

CROSTHWAITE, Aida I; Crown Point Family Health Ctre, 67 Kenilworth Ave N, Hamilton ON L8H 4R6; Wes'91; BSc; BScN; MSc; CCFP; FCFP; Court Staff Privil, St Joseph's Healthcare - Charlton Campus; Court Staff Privil, Hamilton Health Sciences Centre - McMaster Children's Hospital; (905)540-4433; Fax. (905)540-4414.

CROTEAU, Agathe; Inst National de Sante Publiqu, 945 av Wolfe, Quebec QC G1V 5B3; Laval'84; PhD; Ac Staff, Centre Hospitalier Universitaire de Quebec-CHUL; Physician Epidemiol, Institut National de Santé Publique du Québec; Langs: Bilingual(English/French); (418)650-5115 x5244; Fax. (418)654-3136; agathe.croteau@inspq.qc.ca.

CROTEAU, Benoit; CSSS de Chicoutimi, CP 5006 305 rue Saint-Vallier, Chicoutimi QC G7H 5H6; Laval'91; Psy (P.Q.). Staff, Complexe hospitalier de la Sagamie; (418)549-5477; Fax. (418)549-7604.

CROTEAU, Bernard; Hotel-Dieu d'Arthabaska, 5 rue des Hospitalieres, Victoriaville QC G6P 6N2; Laval'10; CCFP; Staff, Hotel-Dieu d'Arthabaska; (819)357-2030

CROTEAU, Celine; Centre Med St-Bruno, 1435 rue Roberval, Saint-Bruno QC J3V 3P7; Laval'89; (450)653-7672; Fax. (450)653-8399.

CROTEAU, Christian; CSSS de Laval, 1755 boul Rene-Laennec, Laval QC H7M 3L9; Mon'95; Staff, Hopital de la Cite de la santé; Clin Teach Staff Med, Universite de Montreal; (450)668-1010

CROTEAU, Dominique; Centre Hosp Honore-Mercier, 2750 boul Laframboise, Saint-Hyacinthe QC J2S 4Y8; Mon'86; FRCPC; Psy. Staff Psy, Centre Hospitalier Honore-Mercier; (450)771-3222

CROTEAU, Francois; Clinique Med 3000 Inc, 3000 rue Belanger, Montreal QC H1Y 1A9; Laval'73; Staff, Hôpital Santa Cabrini Ospedale; (514)376-7702; Fax. (514)376-2639; mdsport@videotron.ca.

CROTEAU, Frederic; Esthetic Surg Centre Sherbrook, 100-750 13e av N, Sherbrooke QC J1E 3L7; Mon'98; DS; MRCS; DrMedCh; FRCSC; PlasSurg (Aesthetic Surgery). Staff, Centre Hospitalier Universitaire de Sherbrooke-Hôpital Hôtel-Dieu; Langs: English; (819)822-0442; Fax. (819)822-0646.

CROTEAU, Isabelle; CSSS de Laval, 1755 boul Rene-Laennec, Laval QC H7M 3L9; Mon'91; Staff EmergMed, Hopital de la Cite de la santé; (450)668-1010; Fax. (450)975-5545.

CROTEAU, Jacques; Hotel-Dieu D'Arthabaska, 5 rue des Hospitalieres, Victoriaville QC G6P 6N2; Sher'79; CSPQ; Anes. Staff, Hotel-Dieu d'Arthabaska; (819)357-2030 x2955; Fax. (819)357-6006.

CROTEAU, Louis; Clinique Med Saint-Pierre, 200-85 rue Saint-Pierre, Saint-Constant QC J5A 1G8; Mon'78; (450)845-4646; Fax. (450)845-4104.

CROTEAU, Maryse; Clinique Med Saint-Tite, 264 rue Du Moulin, Saint-Tite QC G0X 3H0; Sher'83; (418)365-5112; Fax. (418)365-3932.

CROTEAU, Myriam; CSSS de Rimouski-Neigette, CP 3150 Succ A 150 av Rouleau, Rimouski QC G5L 5T1; Laval'05; Staff, Hôpital Regional Rimouski; (418)723-7851

CROTEAU, Myriane; Centre Med Drummond, 60 rue Loring, Drummondville QC J2C 7Y9; Laval'08; CCFP; (819)477-2500

CROTEAU, Pascal; Centre de Sante du Pontiac, 200 Argue, Shawville QC J0X 2Y0; Ott'90; (819)458-2542

CROTEAU, Stephane; Inst Albert Prevost, 6555 boul Gouin O, Montreal QC H4K 1B3; Mon'95; Langs: English; (514)338-2222; crotstep@hotmail.com.

CROTEAU, Sylvain; CSSSG-Hop de Gatineau, CP 2000 Succ Bureau-Chef 909 boul de la Verendrye O, Gatineau QC J8P 7H2; Mon'88; CCFP; Staff, Hôpital de Gatineau; (819)966-6333

CROTHERS, Ivan S; Wilson Centre Family Practice, 1-2185 Wilson Ave, Port Coquitlam BC V3C 6C1; Queen's (Ireland)'78; MB ChB; BAO; DRCOG; MRC(UK); Staff, Royal Columbian Hospital; Staff, Eagle Ridge Hospital & Health Care Centre; (604)942-7227; Fax. (604)942-7058.

CROTIN, Abraham M; Scarborough Prof Centre, 317-1371 Neilson Rd, Scarborough ON M1B 4Z8; Tor'59; FRCSC; Otol (Facial & Cosmetic Surgery). Ac Staff, Rouge Valley Health System - Centenary Health Centre Site; Staff Privil, The Scarborough Hospital - General Campus; (416)284-2855; Fax. (416)284-8331.

CROUL, Sidney; Univ Hlth Network-Toronto Gen, 11E 426-200 Elizabeth St, Toronto ON M5G 2C4; Pennsylvania(PA) (USA)'77; ABNPath; ABPath; ABPN; FAAN; FCAP; BA; AddicMed; FRCPC; AnatPath (Neuro Oncology); NeurPath. Head Neuropathology, Toronto General Hospital - UHN; (416)340-3330; Fax. (416)340-5517; sidney.croul@uhn.on.ca.

CROUSE, Ettiene J; Moosomin Family Practice Ctre, PO Box 1528, Moosomin SK S0G 3N0; Orange Free State (South Africa)'89; MB ChB; CCFP; Staff Family Med, Southeast Integrated Care Centre - Moosomin; (306)435-3838; Fax. (306)435-2176; ettiene.crouse@rqhealth.ca.

CROUSE, Pierre D; 3223 17 Ave SW, Calgary AB T3E 7S1; Stellenbosch (South Africa)'82; MB ChB; DA; Langs: Afrikaans; (403)255-6196; Fax. (403)252-0444.

CROUSE, Susan; Salvus Clinic, T190-22 Church St, Moncton NB E1C 0P7; Dal'89; CCFP; FCFP; Staff, The Moncton Hospital; Preceptor, Dalhousie University; (506)384-7283; Fax. (506)384-7285.

CROUSE, Wanda J; 200B-3060 Cedar Hill Rd, Victoria BC V8T 3J5; McM'81; FRCPC; Psy (Adult Psychiatry). Staff, Royal Jubilee Hospital; (250)592-1273; Fax. (250)592-1293.

CROUZAT, Frederic B; Maple Leaf Med, GF-70 Carlton St, Toronto ON M5B 1L6; Ott'98; CCFP; (416)960-0145; Fax. (416)960-0489.

CROUZAT, Michael G; CFB Petawawa, PO Box 9999 Stn Main, Petawawa ON K8H 2X3; Wes'97; CCFP; FCFP; (613)687-5511 x7097

CROUZIER-ROUX, Emmanuelle; Ctr Hosp Laurentien, 234 rue Saint-Vincent, Ste-Agathe-des-Mts QC J8C 2B8; Sher'09; CCFP; Staff, Centre Hospitalier Laurentien; (819)324-4000

CROW, Fiona M; St Boniface Gen Hosp, 8F-409 Tache Ave, Winnipeg MB R2H 2A6; Cal'79; Att Staff, St Boniface General Hospital; Att Staff, Concordia General Hospital; Physician Palliative Care, Winnipeg Regional Health Authority; University of Manitoba; (204)233-8563

CROW, Patricia A M; CarePoint Med Clinic, 140-777 Royal Oak Dr, Victoria BC V8X 4V1; UBC'84; CCFP; FCFP; Ac Staff, Vancouver Island Health Authority; (250)479-7147

CROWCROF, Natasha S; Health Protection & Promotion, 300-480 University Ave, Toronto ON M5G 1V2; London (England)'87; (647)260-7100

CROWE, Adrian C; Niagara H System-St Catharines, PO Box 3018 Stn Main 142 Queenston St, St Catharines ON L2R 7C6; Wes'01; CCFP; CCFP(E.M.); Staff, Niagara Health System - St Catharines General Site; (905)684-7271 x4567

CROWE, Anne R; 16-385 Frederick St, Kitchener ON N2H 2P2; Tor'79; BSc; CCFP; FCFP; Grand River Hospital - Freeport Site; (519)745-7482; Fax. (519)745-1881.

CROWE, D Wayne; Courtenay Med Clinic, 788 Grant Ave, Courtenay BC V9N 2T3; UBC'82; (250)334-2445

CROWE, Marie-Josee; Hôpital Ste-Justine, 3175 ch Cote-Ste-Catherine, Montreal QC H3T 1C5; Mon'72; DAB; CSPQ; Anes (Intensive Care & Anesthesia). Anesthesiste, Hôpital Ste-Justine; Universite de Montreal; (514)345-4733; Fax. (514)345-4829; marie-josee_crowe@ssss.gouv.qc.ca.

CROWE, Robert F G; Hythe Med Clinic, PO Box 143, Hythe AB T0H 2C0; RCS (Ireland)'81; MB ChB; BAO; LRCPSI; CCFP; Staff, Beaverlodge Municipal Hospital; Clin Teacher Family Med, University of Alberta; (780)356-3869; Fax. (780)356-2969.

CROWE-BOURBONNAIS, Celine; Inst U Geriatrie de Montreal, 4565 ch Queen-Mary, Montreal QC H3W 1W5; Mon'76; Staff, Institut Universitaire de Gériatrie de Montréal; (514)340-3513; Fax. (514)340-2832.

CROWELL, Denise; Dartmouth Gen Hosp, 2862-325 Pleasant St, Dartmouth NS B2Y 4G8; Dal'02; CCFP; CCFP(E.M.); Staff, Dartmouth General Hospital; (902)465-8491; Fax. (902)460-4148.

CROWELL, Richard H; Queen Elizabeth II HSC-Halifax, 6896-1796 Summer St, Halifax NS B3H 3A7; Dal'80; FRCPC; IntMed; Cardiol. Ac Staff, Queen Elizabeth II Health Sciences Centre - Victoria General Site; Asst Prof, Dalhousie University; (902)473-3940; Fax. (902)473-6293; rcrowell@dal.ca.

CROWLEY, David; Thames Valley FHT-Strathroy Me, 74 Front St E, Strathroy ON N7G 1Y7; Tor'90; BSc(Chem); Ac Staff Privledges, Strathroy Middlesex General Hospital - Middlesex Hospital Alliance; Prin Investigator, DCTM Clinical Trials Group; (519)245-0430; Fax. (519)245-5870.

CROWLEY, John S; Medical Clinic Associates, 200-3207 30 Ave, Vernon BC V1T 2C6; RCS (Ireland)'74; LRCPSI; FRCSC; GenSurg. Staff, Vernon Jubilee Hospital; (250)260-6113; Fax. (250)260-1314.

CROWSHOE, Lynden F J; 7F-1213 4 St SW, Calgary AB T2R 0X7; Alb'95; CCFP; Teach Staff, University of Calgary; (403)955-6600; crowshoe@ucalgary.ca.

CROWSON, Jonathan B; St Joseph's Mountain H Serv, PO Box 585 Stn Lcd 1 100 5th St W, Hamilton ON L8N 3K7; Edinburgh (Scotland)'93; MRCP; Staff, St Joseph's Healthcare Hamilton - West 5th Campus; (905)522-1155; Fax. (905)575-3778.

CROWTHER, John E; 3979 Finnerty Rd, Penticton BC V2A 8W2; London (England)'87; MB BS; DA; FRCPC; Anes (Chronic Pain). Staff Anes, Penticton Regional Hospital; (250)490-4730; Fax. (250)490-4730.

CROWTHER, Mark A; St Joseph's Healthcare, L301-50 Charlton Ave E, Hamilton ON L8N 4A6; Wes'90; FRCPC; IntMed (Thrombosis); Hem. Staff, St Joseph's Healthcare - Charlton Campus; Prof Med/Chair Div of Hematol, McMaster University; (905)521-6024; Fax. (905)540-6568.

CROWTHER, Sean M; University of Alberta Hosp, 2G2. 11WMC-8440 112 St NW, Edmonton AB T6G 2B7; (Ireland)'94; Staff, University of Alberta Hospital; (780)407-6907; Fax. (780)407-3853.

CROZIER, Melanie A; 406-265 Front St N, Sarnia ON N7T 5S6; Tor'04; CCFP; (519)337-5600; Fax. (519)337-0439.

CROZIER, Robert S; 311-450 Central Ave, London ON N6B 2E8; Queen's (Ireland)'82; MB ChB; BAO; FRCPC; Psy (Individual Adult Psychotherapy). (519)679-2761; Fax. (519)679-9919.

CRUCHLEY, Jane I; Canadian Forces Hlth Services, PO Box 5000 Stn Main 23 Cdn Forces Hlth Serv Ctre, Moose Jaw SK S6H 7Z8; Dal'86; BA(Hons.); Staff, Canadian Forces Health Services - Pacific Centre; (306)694-2280

CRUCHLEY, Patricia M A; St Mary's Gen Hosp, 911 Queens Blvd, Kitchener ON N2M 1B2; UBC'75; FRCPC; Anes. Staff, St Mary's General Hospital; (519)749-6690

CRUESS, Alan F; Queen Elizabeth II HSC, 2WV 2035-1276 South Park St, Halifax NS B3H 2Y9; Qns'75; ABOph; FRCSC; Ophth (Retinal Disease). Staff, Queen Elizabeth II Health Sciences Centre - Victoria General Site; Staff Consultant, IWK Health Centre; Dist Chief Ophth, Capital Health Centre; Head Ophth & Visual Sciences/Prof, Dalhousie University; (902)473-7215; Fax. (902)473-2839.

CRUICKSHANK, Barbara; 700-250 Dundas St W, Toronto ON M5T 2Z6; Wes'77; FSOGC; FRCSC; ObstGyn (Reproductive Endocrinology & Infertility). Staff, Toronto General Hospital - UHN; Staff, Toronto Western Hospital - University Health Network; Staff, Princess Margaret Hospital - University Health Network; Staff Obst/Gyn, Mount Sinai Hospital; Asst Prof, University of Toronto; (416)586-5233; Fax. (416)586-5909.

CRUICKSHANK, Beth; Univ of Toronto, 92 College St, Toronto ON M5G 1L4; Qns'07; ObstGyn. (416)978-2668

CRUICKSHANK, Blaine; 1050 Queens Blvd, Kitchener ON N2M 1C2; Wes'76; (519)742-3588; Fax. (519)742-6379.

CRUICKSHANK, Catherine J; Lansdowne Professional Ctr II, 133-3066 Shelbourne St, Victoria BC V8R 6T9; Dal'80; CCFP; Staff, Vancouver Island Health Authority; (250)592-5900; Fax. (250)592-5398.

CRUICKSHANK, Lindsay; Prince Albert Mental Hlth Clin, PO Box 3003 Stn Main, Prince Albert SK S6V 6G1; Pretoria (South Africa)'99; MB ChB; FCP (SA); FRCPC; Psy. Consultant Psy, Victoria Hospital; (306)765-6055; Fax. (306)765-6349.

CRUICKSHANKS, Giles F; Southlake Reg Health Centre, 596 Davis Dr, Newmarket ON L3Y 2P9; Tor'95; FRCPC; Anes. Staff, Southlake Regional Health Centre; (905)895-4521

CRUICKSHANKS, Sonia M; York Prof Bldg, 308-679 Davis Dr, Newmarket ON L3Y 5G8; Tor'95; FRCPC; Psy. Staff Privil, Southlake Regional Health Centre; Langs: Slovak; (905)836-1600; Fax. (905)836-5712.

CRUISE, Charles J E; Trillium Hlth Ctr-Mississauga, 100 Queensway W, Mississauga ON L5B 1B8; Tor'78; FRCPC; Anes. Staff Anes, Trillium Health Centre - Mississauga; Langs: Bilingual(English/French); (905)848-7628

CRUISE, Lora J H; Bridgepoint Family Health Team, 430 Broadview Ave, Toronto ON M4K 2N1; McM'01; CCFP; Aj Prof DCFM, University of Toronto; (416)470-6690; lcruise@mtsinai.on.ca.

CRUM, Serena N D; Serena N Crum Prof Corp, PO Box 510, Lac La Biche AB T0A 2C0; Cal'05; CCFP; Physician, Lac La Biche Healthcare Centre - William J. Cadzow Building; (780)623-4421

CRUMLEY, Tracey L; Children's Hosp Western Ont, 800 Commissioners Rd E, London ON N6C 2V5; Wes'96; BSc; FRCSC; ObstGyn. Staff, Children's Hospital of Western Ontario; Assoc Prof, University of Western Ontario; (519)646-6401; Fax. (519)646-6010.

CRUMMEY, James M; Mount Dennis Med Group, 98 Guestville Ave, Toronto ON M6N 4N6; Tor'76; CCFP; FCFP; (416)763-1171; Fax. (416)763-0573.

CRUMMEY, Stephen; Health Sciences Centre, 300 Prince Philip Dr, St. John's NL A1B 3V6; Mem'97; BSc(Pharm); BSc(MedSci); FRCPC; Anes. Staff, Health Sciences Centre; Langs: English; French; (709)737-6300

CRUMP, Michael R; 5 209-610 University Ave, Toronto ON M5G 2M9; Tor'84; FRCPC; IntMed (Hematological Oncology); Hem. Ac Staff, Princess Margaret Hospital - University Health Network; Prof, University of Toronto; (416)946-4567; Fax. (416)946-4520; michael.crump@uhn.ca.

CRUTCHER, Rodney A; Sunridge Family Med Teaching C, 2685 36 St NE, Calgary AB T1Y 5S3; Cal'77; CCFP; CCFP(E.M.); FCFP; (403)943-5000; Fax. (403)476-8784; crutcher@ucalgary.ca.

CRUVELLIER, Paul E; St Mary's Hosp Centre, 3830 av Lacombe, Montreal QC H3T 1M5; McG'88; CCFP; FCFP; Staff, St Mary's Hospital Centre; Asst Prof Family Med, McGill University; (514)734-2677; Fax. (514)734-2663.

CRUZ, Arturo M; Woodlawn Med Centre, 114 Woodlawn Rd, Dartmouth NS B2W 2S7; Mem'83; (902)463-3937; Fax. (902)463-2011.

CRUZ, Caridad M; Rouge Valley-Centenary HC, 2867 Ellesmere Rd, Scarborough ON M1E 4B9; Santo Tomas (Philippines)'62; MD; FRCPC; Psy (Consultation). Staff, Rouge Valley Health System - Centenary Health Centre Site; Langs: Tagalog; (416)284-8131 x4226; Fax. (416)281-7320.

CRUZ, E Laura; Pivot Sport Med & Orthopaedics, 2288 Bloor St W, Toronto ON M6S 1N9; Tor'83; MSc; Dip SportMed; CCFP; Staff Physician, Women's College Hospital; Staff, St Joseph's Health Centre; Lecturer DFCM, University of Toronto; (416)767-4868; Fax. (416)763-2577; drlaura@pivotsmo.com.

CRUZ, Geraldine Z V; The Collonde Bldg, 310-3024 Hurontario St, Mississauga ON L5B 4M4; Manila Central U. (Philippines)'94; CCFP; Langs: Tagalog; (905)848-2789

CRUZ, Javier; 3859 rue Saint-Urbain, Montreal QC H2W 1T6; McG'79; PhD; (514)282-8768

CRUZ, Leo M P; Forest Hill Centre, 180 Woodbridge St, Fredericton NB E3B 4R3; (Philippines)'96; Staff, Hôpital Régional Campbellton.

CRUZ, Norman M; 203 Huron St, Stratford ON N5A 5S9; FEU (Philippines)'73; Staff, Stratford General Hospital - Huron Perth Healthcare Alliance; Langs: Tagalog; (519)271-1733; Fax. (519)271-3543.

CRUZ, Sean M; Bevan Walk-in Clinic, 207-2379 Bevan Ave, Sidney BC V8L 1Y3; Mem'95; BSc(Hons); BMedSci; (250)656-4177; Fax. (250)656-4133.

CRUZ DE PAZOS, Madelaine; Devon Med Clinic, 5-106 Erie St S, Devon AB T9G 1A7; Havana (Cuba)'89; Staff, Devon General Hospital; Langs: Spanish; (780)987-3315; Fax. (780)987-4009.

CRUZ PEREIRA, Oscar O; Balmoral Med Arts Facility, 301-1366 Yonge St, Toronto ON M4T 3A7; Alb'07; FRCPC; IntMed; Gastroent. Staff, Toronto Western Hospital - University Health Network; (416)926-0262; Fax. (416)926-0936.

CRUZ-SANTIAGO, Diane; Inst U Geriatrie de Montreal, 4565 ch Queen-Mary, Montreal QC H3W 1W5; CCFP; Staff, Institut Universitaire de Gériatrie de Montréal; (514)340-2800

CRYER, Elizabeth J; William Osler HC-Brampton, 2100 Bovaird Dr E, Brampton ON L6R 3J7; UBC'82; FRCPC; Psy. Staff, William Osler Health System - Brampton Civic Hospital; (905)494-2120

CRYSLER, John G; Niagara Health Centre, 209-180 Vine St S, St Catharines ON L2R 7P3; Qns'92; FRCPC; Peds (Endocrinology). (905)682-2709

CRYSTAL, Eugene; Sunnybrook Hlth Sciences Ctre, D382-2075 Bayview Ave, Toronto ON M4N 3M5; Vitebsk (Russia (Federation))'83; FRCPC; Cardiol. Staff, Sunnybrook Health Sciences Centre; Langs: Hebrew; Russian; (416)480-6100 x7370; Fax. (416)480-5069; tsotb_1@yahoo.ca.

CRYSTAL, Pavel; Mount Sinai Hosp, 574-600 University Ave, Toronto ON M5G 1X5; Vitebsk (Russia (Federation))'88; Staff, Mount Sinai Hospital; (416)586-4800 x4626

CRYSTAL, Sam; Dr Poon Metabolic Diet Clinic, 4-160 Main St S, Brampton ON L6W 3X4; Tor'72; Sr Staff, Humber River Regional Hospital - Church Street Site; (905)450-2700; Fax. (905)450-2707.

CSANADI, Michael A; Niagara HS-Douglas Mem Site, 7-238 Bertie St, Fort Erie ON L2A 1Z3; Tor'87; BSc(Biol.,McM); Court Staff, Niagara Health System - Douglas Memorial Hospital Site; Staff Lead Phy, Fort Erie Group Family Practice; Principal Invastigater, C & L Research; (905)871-1220; Fax. (905)871-1221.

CSANYI-FRITZ, Yvonne; University of Alberta Hosp, 1C1 04-8440 112 St NW, Edmonton AB T6G 2B7; Cal'97; FRCPC; Anes (Pediatric Anesthesia). Staff, University of Alberta Hospital; Staff, Stollery Children's Hospital; (780)407-8861; Fax. (780)407-3200.

CSERTI-GAZDEWICH, Christine M; Univ Hlth Network-Toronto Gen, 3EC 306-200 Elizabeth St, Toronto ON M5G 2C4; Tor'00; ABIM; ABP(TransfusionMed); FACP; FRCPC; IntMed (Transfusion Medicine); Hem. Staff Transfusion Medicine Specialist & Clinical Hematologist, Toronto General Hospital - UHN; Staff Clinical Hematologist, Mount Sinai Hospital; Staff Transfusion Med Spec, Sunnybrook Health Sciences Centre; Asst Prof, University of Toronto; Langs: Hungarian; (416)340-5390; Fax. (416)340-5410; christine.cserti@uhn.ca.

CSORDAS, Andrea Z; 204-325 Winterberry Dr, Hamilton ON L8J 0B6; McM'90; Staff, Hamilton Health Sciences Centre-Juravinski Site; Staff, St Joseph's Healthcare - Charlton Campus; Langs: Hungarian; (905)318-5343; Fax. (905)318-6817.

CSUPAK, Elaine M; Eveline Street Clinic, 66 Eveline St, Selkirk MB R1A 1K6; Man'06; CCFP; (204)785-5550; Fax. (204)785-5555.

CUARTERO, Julie; Cross Cancer Institute, 11560 University Ave NW, Edmonton AB T6G 1Z2; Wes'06; FRCPC; RadOncol. Staff, Cross Cancer Institute; (780)432-8749; Fax. (780)432-8380.

CUBEROVIC, Nick B; Halton HCS Corp-Milton, 7030 Derry Rd, Milton ON L9T 7H6; Tor'87; CCFP; Halton Healthcare Services Corporation - Milton District Hospital; Langs: Croatian; French; (905)878-2383

CUBITT, David; University of Alberta Hosp, 3B2.32WCM-8440 112 St NW, Edmonton AB T6G 2B7; London (England)'70; FRCPC; Anes. Staff, University of Alberta Hospital; Staff, Stollery Children's Hospital; (780)407-8861; Fax. (780)407-3200.

CUBRA, Satnam S; Viva Care Inc, 300-9855 Austin Ave, Burnaby BC V3J 1N4; Leicester (United Kingdom)'06; MB ChB; (604)422-8482

CUCAN, Elissa; Appletree Clinic, 1309 Carling Ave, Ottawa ON K1Z 7L3; Tor'08; CCFP; Staff, Collingwood General & Marine Hospital; (613)715-9816; Fax. (613)715-9278.

CUCCAROLO, Glenna; Bluewater Health-Norman Site, 89 Norman St, Sarnia ON N7T 6S3; Wes'01; FRCSC; GenSurg (Critical Care Medicine). Staff, London Health Sciences Centre - Victoria Campus; Staff, Bluewater Health - Norman Site; Staff, London Health Sciences Centre - University Hospital; (519)464-4400

CUCCINIELLO, Sandro; Niagara H System-St Catharines, 142 Queenston St, St Catharines ON L2R 7C6; Qns'73; CCFP; FCFP; Ac Staff, Niagara Health System - St Catharines General Site; Ac Staff, Niagara Health System - Ontario Street Site; (905)684-7271

CUCHUREAN, Paul; Clinique Med 6930 Papineau Inc, 6930 Av Papineau, Montreal QC H2G 2X7; Sher'87; (514)722-0000; Fax. (514)722-2431.

CUCUZZA, Marie-Jose; Clinique Med Colombus, 305-1140 rue Jean-Talon E, Montreal QC H2R 1V9; Mon'77; Langs: Italian; English; (514)270-2141; Fax. (514)270-6920.

CUDDEFORD, Cheryl M; Westwind Med Clinic, 107-755 Goldstream Ave, Victoria BC V9B 0H9; UBC'89; Staff, Vancouver Island Health Authority; (250)478-1764

CUDDIHY, Helene L; Saint Thomas Comm Health Ctre, 9040 84 Ave NW, Edmonton AB T6C 1E4; Sher'98; CCFP; FCFP; (780)434-2778; Fax. (780)466-8702.

CUDDINGTON, Gary D; The Newmark, 305-4885 Kingsway, Burnaby BC V5H 4T2; Sask'79; FRCSC; GenSurg. (604)433-9899; Fax. (604)433-0128.

CUDDINGTON, Gordon W; Regina Qu'Appelle HR-Regina, 2F-1440 14th Ave, Regina SK S4P 0W5; Sask'83; FRCSC; GenSurg. Staff, Regina General Hospital; Associate Clin Prof, University of Saskatchewan; (306)766-6911; Fax. (306)766-6917.

CUDDY, Timothy J; 100-672 Brant St, Burlington ON L7R 2H3; Tor'85; BSc; CCFP; Staff, Joseph Brant Memorial Hospital; (905)634-9012; Fax. (905)634-9904.

CUDMORE, David; Antigonish Medical Assoc, 40 Church St, Antigonish NS B2G 2C7; Dal'80; Dip SportMed; CCFP; FCFP; Physician, St. Francis Xavier University; Preceptor, Dalhousie University; (902)863-4558; Fax. (902)867-5665.

CUDMORE, Richard H; Diamond Head Med Clinic, PO Box 9200 Stn Main, Squamish BC V8B 0C1; Cambridge (England)'74; MB ChB; MRCP; CCFP; FCFP; Med Dir, Squamish General Hospital / Hilltop House; Physician, Vancouver Coastal Health; (604)892-3544; Fax. (604)892-3542.

CUDMORE, Stephen; 7-2120 Regent St, Sudbury ON P3E 3Z9; Tor'94; BSc; MSc; CCFP; Staff, Health Sciences North-St Joseph's Health Centre; (705)522-1500

CUDNOCH, P Maria; Jewish Rehabilitation Hosp, 3205 Place Alton-Goldbloom, Laval QC H7V 1R2; Lekarski (Poland)'65; CCFP; Staff, Jewish Rehabilitation Hospital; Langs: Polish; English; (450)688-9550 x3333; Fax. (450)688-6630.

CUFFE, Sinead D; UHN Princess Margaret Hosp, 610 University Ave, Toronto ON M5G 2M9; (Ireland)'00; Staff, Princess Margaret Hospital - University Health Network; (416)946-4501

CUILLERIER, Daniel J; London HSC-University Hosp, PO Box 5339 Stn B 339 Windermere Rd, London ON N6A 5A5; Sher'83; FRCPC; Anes (Neuro Anesthesia). Staff Anes, London Health Sciences Centre - University Hospital; Assoc Prof, University of Western Ontario; Langs: Bilingual(English/French); (519)685-8500 x35147; Fax. (519)663-3079; dcuiller@uwo.ca.

CUIROT, Gilles; Centre Hosp Honore-Mercier, 2750 boul Laframboise, Saint-Hyacinthe QC J2S 4Y8; Mon'68; MedOncol (P.Q.); HemPath; Hem (P.Q.). Staff Hematology/Oncology, Centre Hospitalier Honore-Mercier; (450)771-3333 x3258; Fax. (450)771-3510.

CUJEC, Bibiana; University of Alberta Hosp, 2C2 50WCM-8440 112 St NW, Edmonton AB T6G 2B7; Laval'81; FRCPC; IntMed; Cardiol. Staff, University of Alberta Hospital; Prof Med & Cardiol, University of Alberta; (780)407-3601; Fax. (780)407-6452; bibiana.cujec@ualberta.ca.

CUK, Aleksandar S; Peter Lougheed Centre, 2264-3500 26 Ave NE, Calgary AB T1Y 6J4; Cal'99; FRCPC; Anes. Staff, Peter Lougheed Centre; (403)943-5554; Fax. (403)943-4474.

CULBERT, Alison J; Sunnybrook Hlth Sciences Ctre, A103-2075 Bayview Ave, Toronto ON M4N 3M5; Ott'00; CCFP; Staff, Sunnybrook Health Sciences Centre; (416)480-4936; Fax. (416)480-6038.

CULBERT, Erin L; Medical One Oakville, 4-2501 Third Line, Oakville ON L6M 0G8; Qns'02; FRCPC; Peds. (905)618-9934; Fax. (905)901-2449.

CULBERT, Heather T; Regent Park Comm Health Centre, 465 Dundas St E, Toronto ON M5A 2B2; UBC'99; CCFP; Langs: Bilingual(English/French); (416)364-2261; Fax. (416)203-4502.

CULHAM, J A Gordon; Children's & Women's HC of BC, 1L29-4480 Oak St, Vancouver BC V6H 3V4; Man'69; FRCPC; DiagRad (Pediatric Radiology). Consultant, Vancouver General Hospital - Centennial Pavillion; Diagnostic Radiol, BC Children's Hospital; Prof Radiol, University of British Columbia; (604)875-2131; Fax. (604)875-2367.

CULHAM, Tania L; Three Bridges Comm Health Ctre, 1292 Hornby St, Vancouver BC V6Z 1W2; Cal'99; CCFP; (604)633-4220

CULIC, Cherie A; CFB Borden, PO Box 1000 Stn Forces, Borden ON L0M 1C0; McM'09; CCFP; (705)424-1200

CULL, Corine L; 10565 124 St NW, Edmonton AB T5N 1R8; Ott'02; CCFP.

CULL, Sonya M; Medical Associates of Port Per, 462 Paxton St, Port Perry ON L9L 1L9; Mem'05; CCFP; (905)985-2895

CULLEN, Angela K; Wilson Centre Family Practice, 1-2185 Wilson Ave, Port Coquitlam BC V3C 6C1; Wes'81; DA(UK); CCFP; FCFP; Staff, Royal Columbian Hospital; (604)942-7227; Fax. (604)942-7058.

CULLEN, James B; Mount Sinai Hosp, 600 University Ave, Toronto ON M5G 1X5; Tor'63; FRCPC; GenPath (Anatomical Pathology). Staff, Mount Sinai Hospital; Emeritus Prof Lab Med & Path, University of Toronto; (416)586-4800; jbcullen@sympatico.ca.

CULLEN, Nora K; West Park Healthcare Centre, 82 Buttonwood Ave, York ON M6M 2J5; Tor'94; BSc; MSc; FRCPC; PhysMed&Rehab (Brain Injury). Staff Physician, Toronto Rehabilitation Institute - University Centre; Chief of Staff, West Park Healthcare Centre; Assoc Prof, University of Toronto; (416)243-3600

CULLETON, Nancy; James Paton Mem Hosp, 125 Trans Canada Hwy, Gander NL A1V 1P7; Mem'92; CCFP; FCFP; Staff, James Paton Memorial Hospital; (709)256-2500; nculleton@nf.sympatico.ca.

CULLIGAN, Christopher J; Wellpoint Family Practice, 9F-1240 Bay St, Toronto ON M5R 2A7; Dal'98; CCFP; Staff, Toronto General Hospital - UHN; (416)969-3250

CULLIMORE, Amie J; Fontbonne Bldg, 2-301 James St S, Hamilton ON L8P 3B6; McM'94; FRCSC; ObstGyn. Staff, St Joseph's Healthcare - Charlton Campus; (905)521-6041; Fax. (905)521-6089; cullimor@mcmaster.ca.

CULLINAN, Claude A; Big Thunder Orthopaedic Assoc, 206-984 Oliver Rd, Thunder Bay ON P7B 7C7; Mem'95; FRCSC; OrthSurg. Staff, Thunder Bay Regional Health Sciences Centre; (807)344-1123; Fax. (807)344-1166.

CULLINGHAM, Andrea F L; Circle Med Clinic, 127-15566 McIvor Blvd SE, Calgary AB T2Z 4Y2; UBC'06; CCFP; (403)726-0524; Fax. (403)726-0579.

CULLITON, Margaret L; Murray Clinic, 1 Mount Bernard Ave, Corner Brook NL A2H 6Y5; Qns'86; BScEngineering; CCFP; Ac Staff Member, Western Memorial Regional Hospital; (709)785-2058; Fax. (709)785-5705.

CULLY, Gregory P; 252 Parkglen Cres SE, Calgary AB T2J 4M2; Alb'72; Staff, Peter Lougheed Centre; (403)271-5806

CULMAN, Kate N; 10-8180 Macleod Trail SE, Calgary AB T2H 2B8; Case West Reserve(Ohio) (USA)'89; FRCPC; Peds; InfectDis. Asst Prof, Alberta Children's Hospital; Asst Clin Prof Peds, University of Calgary; Langs: English; French; (403)252-6651

CULNAN, James G; Medical Bldg, 304-250 Harding Blvd W, Richmond Hill ON L4C 9M7; Tor'69; FRCPC; IntMed; Gastroent. Consultant, Mackenzie Richmond Hill Hospital; (905)884-0851

CULO, Sandi; Royal Jubilee Hosp, 1952 Bay St, Victoria BC V8R 1J8; Alb'00; BSc(Hon); FRCPC; Psy (Geriatric Psychiatry). Staff, Royal Jubilee Hospital; Staff, Peace Arch Hospital; Staff, Abbotsford Regional Hospital & Cancer Centre; Staff, Vancouver General Hospital - Centennial Pavillion; (250)519-1554

CULOS, Donald A; Rockyview Gen Hosp, 7007 14 St SW, Calgary AB T2V 1P9; Cal'85; CCFP; CCFP(E.M.); Staff Emerg, Rockyview General Hospital; (403)943-3449; Fax. (403)943-3220.

CULP, Gregory; 1200 Dufferin Cres, Nanaimo BC V9S 2B7; Ott'99; Staff, Abbotsford Regional Hospital & Cancer Centre; (250)755-7691

CULVER, Ronald L; Southern Alberta Eye Centre, 104-5340 1st St SW, Calgary AB T2H 0C8; Alb'65; FRCSC; Ophth (Cataract & Refractive). Ac Staff, Rockyview General Hospital; Ac Staff, Peter Lougheed Centre; Teach Staff, University of Calgary; (403)269-5573; Fax. (403)269-2136; drculver@culvereye.com.

CULVER, Timothy D; Foothills Med Centre, 1403 29 St NW, Calgary AB T2N 2T9; Alb'95; FRCPC; Psy. Staff, Foothills Medical Centre; (403)944-1567; Fax. (403)944-2838.

CUMBERLAND, Penny K; 301-219 Oxford St W, London ON N6H 1S5; Wes'77; (519)432-7546; Fax. (519)679-5302; pcumberland@bellnet.ca.

CUMMING, David C; Royal Alexandra Hosp, 5S131-10240 Kingsway NW, Edmonton AB T5H 3V9; Liverpool (England)'68; MB ChB; FRCOG; FRCSC; ObstGyn (Reproductive Endocrinology & Infertility). Staff ObstGyn, Royal Alexandra Hospital; Prof/A-Chair ObstGyn, University of Alberta; (780)735-5609; Fax. (780)735-4981; dcumming@ualberta.ca.

CUMMING, Gordon R; Winnipeg Clinic, 425 St Mary Ave, Winnipeg MB R3C 0N2; Man'53; BSc(Med.); FACC; FRCPC; IntMed (Cardiology). Staff Consultant, Health Sciences Centre; VP/Med Dir, The Great-West Life Assurance Co.; Prof Med & Peds, University of Manitoba; (204)957-1900; Fax. (204)957-7410.

CUMMING, Jane A K; 1051 Wonderland Rd S, London ON N6K 3X4; Wes'79; Staff, Regional Mental Health Care-St Joseph's Health Care; (519)472-2060

CUMMINGS, Bernard J; Univ Hlth Network-Princess M, 610 University Ave, Toronto ON M5G 2M9; Otago (New Zealand)'67; MB ChB; FRCR; FRANZCR; FRCPC; RadOncol. Radoncology, Princess Margaret Hospital - University Health Network; Prof RadOncol, University of Toronto; (416)946-2129; Fax. (416)946-2227.

CUMMINGS, Beth-Ann M; SMBD Jewish Gen Hosp, G 050-3755 ch Cote-Sainte-Cath, Montreal QC H3T 1E2; McG'03; FRCPC; IntMed. Staff, Sir Mortimer B Davis Jewish General; (514)340-8222 x5634

CUMMINGS, Brian E; Grand River Hosp-KW Hlth Ctre, PO Box 9056 Stn C 835 King St W, Kitchener ON N2G 1G3; Dal'95; BBA; FRCPC; AnatPath. Staff, St Mary's General Hospital; Staff, Grand River Hospital - Kitchener/Waterloo Health Centre; (519)749-4300 x2704; brian.cummings@grhosp.on.ca.

CUMMINGS, Carl; 3550-6900 boul Decarie, Cote Saint-Luc QC H3X 2T8; New York (USA)'74; FAAP; FRCPC; Peds. Asst Prof PT-Time Peds, McGill University Health Centre - Montreal General Campus; Sr Staff Peds, Sir Mortimer B Davis Jewish General; Asst Prof Peds, McGill University; Langs: Bilingual(French/English); English; French; (514)738-1770; Fax. (514)733-2234; carl. cummings@mcgill.ca.

CUMMINGS, Elizabeth A; IWK Health Centre, PO Box 9700 Rpo CSC 5850-5980 University Ave, Halifax NS B3K 6R8; Wes'90; FRCPC; Peds; Endocrin&Metab. Head Ped Endocrin, IWK Health Centre; Asst Prof Peds, Dalhousie University; (902)470-8707; Fax. (902)470-7264; eacummin@dal.ca.

CUMMINGS, Francis; GMF Concorde, 300 boul de la Concorde E, Laval QC H7G 2E6; Mon'73; ac Staff, Hopital de la Cite de la santé; Langs: Bilingual(French/English); (450)667-5310; Fax. (450)667-5248; cumfra20_siri@ssss.gouv.qc.ca.

CUMMINGS, Ina E; A809-21 ch Bord-Du-Lac Lakesho, Dorval QC H9S 5N3; McG'64; CCFP; Langs: English; French; (514)630-6922; icummings@primus.ca.

CUMMINGS, M Lee; Meadowood Med Centre, 1555 St Mary's Rd, Winnipeg MB R2M 5L9; Man'86; CCFP; (204)255-9091

CUMMINGS, Marion; 201-1466 Bathurst St, Toronto ON M5R 3S3; McG'99; MDCM; FRCPC; Peds; Nephrol. Staff, North York General Hospital; Staff, The Hospital For Sick Children; (416)531-3331

CUMMINGS, Michael B; Kingston Gen Hosp, 76 Stuart St, Kingston ON K7L 2V7; Qns'97; FRCPC; Anes. Staff, Kingston General Hospital; (613)548-7827; Fax. (613)548-1375.

CUMMINGS, Michael R; 2510 Hwy 62 PO Bag 999, Hazelton BC V0J 1Y0; South Carolina(SC) (USA)'72; (250)842-5211 x137

CUMMINGS, Suzanne; Prog Daide aux Medecins du Que, 200-1 boul Rene-Levesque E, Montreal QC H2X 3Z5; Mon'79; Langs: English.

CUMMINS, Laurence; Polyclinique St-Eustache, 75 rue Grignon, Saint-Eustache QC J7P 4J2; Mon'10; CCFP; (450)473-6777

CUMMINS, Mary G; University of Alberta Hosp, 8440 112 St NW, Edmonton AB T6G 2B7; Galway (Ireland)'81; MRCPsy; FRCPC; Psy. Staff, University of Alberta Hospital; Clinical Asst Prof, University of Alberta; (780)407-7346; Fax. (780)407-6672; mcummins@ualberta.ca.

CUMMINS, Nora R; PO Box 19137 Rpo Fourth Ave, Vancouver BC V6K 4R8; Hawaii (USA)'98; FRCPC; IntMed. (604)307-3447

CUMMINS-MCMANUS, Barbara J; Hôpital Ste-Justine, 3175 ch Cote-Ste-Catherine, Montreal QC H3T 1C5; McM'78; FRCPC; Peds. ac Staff EmergMed, Hôpital Ste-Justine; (514)345-4931 x5885

CUMYN, Annabelle L; Hôpital Ste-Justine, 3175 ch Cote-Ste-Catherine, Montreal QC H3T 1C5; McG'97; IntMed., Hôpital Ste-Justine; (514)345-4931; Fax. (514)345-4878.

CUNCIC, Cary F; Gordon & Leslie Diamond Care C, 7F-2775 Laurel St, Vancouver BC V5Z 1M9; McM'03; FRCPC; IntMed. (604)875-5181

CUNCINS, Charles; 301-111 Main St W, North Bay ON P1B 2T6; Ott'85; Langs: Latvian; French; (705)472-5670; Fax. (705)472-0137.

CUNDAL, Cory S; Crowfoot West Business Ctr, 340-600 Crowfoot Cres NW, Calgary AB T3G 0B4; Alb'93; FRCSC; OrthSurg (Spine). (403)452-6911; Fax. (403)452-8065.

CUNDIFF, Geoffrey W; Pacific Gastroenterology Assoc, 1190 Hornby St, Vancouver BC V6Z 2K5; Texas (Dallas) (USA)'89; FRCSC; PlasSurg. Staff, Providence Health Care - St Paul's Hospital; Dept Head & School Dir ObstGyn, University of British Columbia; Langs: Spanish; (604)806-9835

CUNEO, Jorge L; Ctr de Sante Vallee-Gatineau, 309 boul Desjardins, Maniwaki QC J9E 2E7; Buenos Aires (Argentina)'74; Gen Practice, CSSS de la Vallée de la Gatineau; (819)449-4690

CUNES, Jill; Alexandra Comm Health Centre, 101-1318 Centre St NE, Calgary AB T2E 2R7; McG'07; MDCM; CCFP; (403)266-2622

CUNNIFFE, Aidan M; University of Alberta Hosp, 1G1 50WMC-8440 112 St NW, Edmonton AB T6G 2B7; Tor'07; CCFP; CCFP(E.M.); Staff, University of Alberta Hospital; (780)407-8432; Fax. (780)407-3695.

CUNNIFFE, Jill J; Queen Elizabeth Hosp, PO Box 6600 Stn Central 60 Riverside Dr, Charlottetown PE C1A 8T5; Dal'98; CCFP; Staff, Queen Elizabeth Hospital; (902)894-2111

CUNNIFFE, Kathleen A; University Hosp of Northern BC, 1475 Edmonton St, Prince George BC V2M 1S2; McM'09; CCFP; CCFP(E.M.); Staff, University Hospital of Northern British Columbia; (250)565-2000

CUNNIFFE, Peter J; 39 Drummond St W, Perth ON K7H 2J9; Tor'98; CCFP; FCFP; (613)264-2868; Fax. (613)264-0454.

CUNNING, Leslie R; PO Box 425, Bragg Creek AB T0L 0K0; Cal'74; CCFP; FCFP; Staff, Oilfields General Hospital; Associate Clin Prof, University of Calgary; (403)933-4368; leslie.cunning@albertahealthservices.ca.

CUNNINGHAM, Christopher R; Centreville Clinic, 301-3210 25 Ave, Vernon BC V1T 1P1; UBC'93; BSc; CCFP; CCFP(E.M.); FCFP; Staff, Vernon Jubilee Hospital; (250)549-1245

CUNNINGHAM, Colin D B; Renfrew Victoria Hosp, 499 Raglan St N, Renfrew ON K7V 1P6; Edinburgh (Scotland)'66; MB ChB; DObstRCOG; DMRD; FRCPC; DiagRad. Consultant Radiol, Renfrew Victoria Hospital; Consultant Diagnostic Radiol, Deep River & District Hospital; (613)432-4851 x859; Fax. (613)432-3610.

CUNNINGHAM, David G; A0761-200 Tunney's Pasture Dr, Ottawa ON K1Z 0T6; Qns'76; FRCPC; Anes. Staff, London Health Sciences Centre - Victoria Campus; (613)946-5105

CUNNINGHAM, David M; 510-3535 boul Saint-Charles, Kirkland QC H9H 5B9; McG'69; BSc; MCh; FRCSC; PlasSurg (Cosmetic Surgery). Staff, Lakeshore General Hospital - Pointe Claire; Staff, McGill University Health Centre - Royal Victoria Hospital; (514)694-1425; Fax. (514)694-9889.

CUNNINGHAM, Diana M; Alexandra Comm Health Centre, 101-1318 Centre St NE, Calgary AB T2E 2R7; Cal'10; CCFP; (403)266-2622; Fax. (403)266-2692.

CUNNINGHAM, Erik; 407 185-911 Yates St, Victoria BC V8V 4Y9; UBC'87; CCFP; FCFP; Langs: German.

CUNNINGHAM, Frank N; Bonaventure Med Clinic, 101-12427 Bonaventure Dr SE, Calgary AB T2J 3N8; Cal'92; (403)225-9499; Fax. (403)225-2572.

CUNNINGHAM, Ian R; Yarmouth Reg Hosp, 60 Vancouver St, Yarmouth NS B5A 2P5; Ott'82; DiagRad. Staff, Yarmouth Regional Hospital; (902)742-3541; Fax. (902)742-0369.

CUNNINGHAM, Jane A; BC Women's Hosp & Hlth Centre, 4500 Oak St, Vancouver BC V6H 3N1; Wes'96; FRCPC; IntMed; InfectDis. Staff, BC Women's Hospital & Health Centre; (604)875-2424

CUNNINGHAM, Johann; Victoria Prof Bldg, 405-1120 Yates St, Victoria BC V8V 3M9; McG'84; BSc(Hon); MDCM; FRCSC; GenSurg (Trauma Surgery). Staff, Victoria General Hospital; Staff, Royal Jubilee Hospital; Consultant Staff, Vancouver General Hospital - Centennial Pavillion; Langs: German; (250)220-8927; Fax. (250)220-8921.

CUNNINGHAM, Karen N; London Medical-Dental Bldg, 301-450 Central Ave, London ON N6B 2E8; Wes'79; CCFP; FCFP; Ac Staff Newborns, St Joseph's Health Care, Non Teaching Family Med.; Staff Consultant, London Health Sciences Centre - University Hospital; (519)439-0346; Fax. (519)439-3400.

CUNNINGHAM, Kenneth F; 212-1940 Lonsdale Ave, North Vancouver BC V7M 2K2; Wes'84; FRCPC; IntMed (Critical Care Medicine). (604)988-0408

CUNNINGHAM, Kristopher S; 2F-26 Grenville St, Toronto ON M7A 2G9; Ott'04; FRCPC; AnatPath (General Pathology). (416)314-4040; Fax. (416)314-4060.

CUNNINGHAM, Linda D; 2816 30th Ave W, Vancouver BC V6L 1Z2; UBC'75; FRCPC; Psy. (604)228-9833

CUNNINGHAM, Randolph M; Royal Alexandra Hosp, CSC 550-10240 Kingsway NW, Edmonton AB T5H 3V9; Alb'86; CCFP; CCFP(E.M.); Staff, Royal Alexandra Hospital; (780)735-4442; Fax. (780)477-4916.

CUNNINGHAM, Sandy; 34 2nd Ave W PO Box 550, Cardston AB T0K 0K0; UBC'08; CCFP; (403)653-3331; Fax. (403)653-1098.

CUNNINGHAM, Valorie L; Cowichan Dist Hosp, 3045 Gibbins Rd, Duncan BC V9L 1E5; UBC'90; CCFP; CCFP(E.M.); Staff, Cowichan District Hospital; (250)737-2030; valorie.cunningham@viha.ca.

CUNNINGHAM, William J; Cowichan Dist Hosp, 3045 Gibbins Rd, Duncan BC V9L 1E5; McG'85; BSc; CCFP; CCFP(E.M.); Staff, Cowichan District Hospital; Langs: German; (250)709-3000 x4215

CUNNINGHAM, William L; 231 Front St, Belleville ON K8N 2Z4; Qns'76; BSc; PhD(Ed); (613)779-7304; Fax. (613)779-6960.

CUNNINGTON, John P W; McMasetr Medical Centre, HSC 3V41-1280 Main St W, Hamilton ON L8S 4K1; McM'72; FRCPC; IntMed (Respirology). Staff, Hamilton Health Sciences Centre - McMaster Children's Hospital; Assoc Prof Med, McMaster University; (905)521-2100; cunningt@mcmaster.ca.

CUPIDO, Cynthia; McMaster University, HSC 3Y-1280 Main St W, Hamilton ON L8S 4K1; McM'95; FRCPC; Peds (Pediatric Critical Care). Asst Prof/Prog Dir Ped Critical Care, McMaster University; (905)521-2100 x76610; Fax. (905)524-5707.

CUPIDO, Tracy; Kingston Gen Hosp, 76 Stuart St, Kingston ON K7L 2V7; Chicago (IL) (USA)'07; Staff, Kingston General Hospital; (613)549-6666

CUPPLES, James B; Royal Columbian Hosp, 330 Columbia St E, New Westminster BC V3L 3W7; UBC'81; FRCPC; GenPath. Staff, Peace Arch Hospital; Staff, Royal Columbian Hospital; (604)520-4352; Fax. (604)520-4409.

CUPSA, Andreea; Active Care Med Group, A-1108 Klondike Rd, Kanata ON K2K 0G1; Ott'01; CCFP; Langs: Hungarian; Romanian; (613)254-9777; Fax. (613)254-9778.

CURCIN, Nikolina; William Osler HC-Brampton, 2100 Bovaird Dr E, Brampton ON L6R 3J7; (Serbia), (Croatia)'94; FRCPC; AnatPath. Staff, William Osler Health System - Brampton Civic Hospital; (905)494-2120; Fax. (905)494-6622.

CUREA, Delia; Leslie Med Family Hlth Organiz, 311-4800 Leslie St, North York ON M2J 2K9; University of Cluj (Romania)'97; CCFP; Clin Teacher, University of Toronto; Langs: Romanian; (416)222-5439; Fax. (416)229-2513.

CURLEY, Michael A; South Health Campus, 4448 Front St SE, Calgary AB T3M 1M4; Dal'03; FRCPC; IntMed; Gastroent. Ac Staff, Queen Elizabeth II Health Sciences Centre - Victoria General Site; Physician, South Health Campus; Lecturer, Dalhousie University; (403)956-3804; Fax. (403)956-3838.

CURLEY, William F; Colchester East Hants Hlth Ctr, 600 Abenaki Rd, Truro NS B2N 5A1; Wes'92; FRCPC; Psy. Staff, Colchester East Hants Health Centre; (902)893-5526; Fax. (902)893-5551.

CURNEW, George R; Ctr Hosp De Verdun, Box 64 4000 boul Lasalle, Verdun QC H4G 2A3; McG'86; BSc; CSPQ; FRCPC; Anes (Chronic Pain Management). assoc Membre Anes, Centre de L'Annonciation; Anesthesiste, Centre Hospitalier de Verdun; Langs: French; (514)362-1000 x3200; Fax. (514)765-7306; george.curnew@mail.mcgill.ca.

CURNEW, Gregory P; M8-414 Victoria Ave N, Hamilton ON L8L 5G8; McG'84; FRCPC; IntMed; Cardiol. Staff, Hamilton Health Sciences Centre - Hamilton General Hospital; Staff IntMed & Cardiol, McMaster University; Langs: English; French; (905)667-0783; Fax. (905)667-0785.

CURPEN, Belinda N; Sunnybrook Hlth Sciences Ctre, MG160-2075 Bayview Ave, Toronto ON M4N 3M5; Sher'88; BSc; FRCPC; DiagRad (Breast Imaging). A-Head Breast Imaging, Sunnybrook Health Sciences Centre; (416)480-6100 x7051; Fax. (416)480-5266.

CURRAH, Ryan E; Medicine Hat Reg Hosp, 666 5 St SW, Medicine Hat AB T1A 4H6; Alb'05; CCFP; CCFP(E.M.); Staff, Margery E. Yuill Cancer Centre; (403)488-0610; Fax. (403)488-0226.

CURRAN, Brian M; Jackson Park Med Centre, 240-2475 McDougall St, Windsor ON N8X 3N9; National (Ireland)'80; FRCSC; Ophth (General Ophthalmic Surgery). Staff, Hôtel-Dieu Grace Hospital; Staff, Windsor Regional Hospital - Metropolitan Site; (519)258-0441; Fax. (519)258-0507.

CURRAN, Daniel E H; C01 A-310 Bridge St W, Napanee ON K7R 0A4; McM'05; CCFP; CCFP(E.M.); (613)354-2858; Fax. (613)354-6495.

CURRAN, Helen; Queen Elizabeth II HSC-Halifax, 2145-1796 Summer St, Halifax NS B3H 3A7; Ott'04; Cardiol; IntMed. Staff, Queen Elizabeth II Health Sciences Centre - Halifax Infirmary Site; (902)473-6364

CURRAN, James A; Sault Area Hosp, 750 Great Northern Rd, Sault Ste. Marie ON P6B 0A8; Ott'03; CCFP; Staff, Sault Area Hospital - Sault Ste Marie; (705)759-3434; Fax. (705)759-3651.

CURRAN, Michael J; The Ottawa Hosp-Civic Campus, 1053 Carling Ave, Ottawa ON K1Y 4E9; Tor'82; FRCPC; Anes. Staff Anes, The Ottawa Hospital - Civic Campus; Asst Prof Anes, University of Ottawa; Langs: Bilingual(English/French); (613)722-7000

CURRAN, Sean P; The Credit Valley Hosp, 2200 Eglinton Ave W, Mississauga ON L5M 2N1; Wes'98; FRCPC; Anes. Staff, The Credit Valley Hospital; (905)906-7719

CURRAN, Shelia; 6-1230 Alward St, Prince George BC V2M 7B1; Cal'07; CCFP; (250)563-3024

CURRAN-BLANEY, Nora; 540 Lakeshore Rd W, Oakville ON L6K 3P1; Ott'79; CCFP; (905)845-1544; Fax. (905)845-2024.

CURRAS, Pablo; Clinique Externe Des Moulins, 101-1355 Grande Allee, Terrebonne QC J6W 4K6; Mon'99; Psy. (450)964-6418; Fax. (450)964-9260.

CURRID, John M; York-Med Medical Arts Centre, 202-250 Harding Blvd W, Richmond Hill ON L4C 9M7; National (Ireland)'71; Staff, Mackenzie Richmond Hill Hospital; (905)737-8400; Fax. (905)737-4579.

CURRIDOR, Robert; 5-2930 Islington Ave, North York ON M9L 2K5; Tor'80; BSc; Staff, The Scarborough Hospital - Birchmount Campus; Staff, Humber River Regional Hospital - Finch Avenue Site; Langs: Italian; (416)749-8911; Fax. (416)746-2875.

CURRIE, Andrew B; Canadian Forces Hlth Services, PO Box 1000, Borden ON L0M 1C0; Sask'95; Staff, Canadian Forces Health Services Centre; Staff, Cdn Forces Base - Borden; (705)424-1200; Fax. (705)423-2088.

CURRIE, Angela S; Glenrose Rehabilitation Hosp, 10230 111 Ave NW, Edmonton AB T5G 0B7; Dal'06; FRCPC; PhysMed&Rehab. Staff, Glenrose Rehabilitation Hospital; (780)969-0748

CURRIE, Blair M; Centennial CMH & Brain Injury, PO Box 1000 Stn Main, Ponoka AB T4J 1R8; Melbourne (Australia)'64; DPM; DTMH; Serv Chief-Adult Psychiatry Provincial Prog, Centennial Centre for Mental Health & Brain Injury; (403)783-7643; Fax. (403)783-7790.

CURRIE, Heather J; Markham Family Health Team, 101-377 Church St, Markham ON L6B 1A1; McM'84; CCFP; Affil Staff, Mackenzie Richmond Hill Hospital; (905)471-9999; Fax. (905)471-3627.

CURRIE, James; Associate Clinic, 201-836 1 Ave NW, Airdrie AB T4B 0V2; Glasgow (Scotland)'73; FRCSC; ObstGyn. (403)943-6422

CURRIE, Melanie T; Westgrove Clinic, 201-505 Queen St, Spruce Grove AB T7X 2V2; Alb'96; CCFP; FCFP; (780)962-9888; Fax. (780)960-5298.

CURRIE, Richard A; Salmon Arm Med Clinic, PO Box 730 Stn Main 581 Hudson Ave NE, Salmon Arm BC V1E 4N8; Qns'04; BScChemEng; CCFP; Dept Head Emerg, Shuswap Lake General Hospital; Langs: Bilingual(English/French); (250)832-6092; Fax. (250)832-5235; rcurrie@samedicalclinic.com.

CURRIE, William R; Penticton Reg Hosp, 550 Carmi Ave, Penticton BC V2A 3G6; Man'73; BSc; FRCPC; GenPath (Forensic Pathology). Ac Staff Labs/Consultant staff, Penticton Regional Hospital; General Pathology, South Okanagan General Hospital; (250)492-4000 x2422

CURRIN, Michael R; St Joseph's Health Centre, PO Box 5777 Stn B 268 Grosvenor St, London ON N6A 4V2; Witwatersrand (South Africa)'71; Anes. Staff, St Joseph's Hospital - St Joseph's Health Care; Langs: Afrikaans; (519)646-6000

CURRY, Donald G; Foothills Med Centre, 1403 29 St NW, Calgary AB T2N 2T9; Cal'79; BAP; AB; FRC; FRCPC; EmergMed. Staff, Foothills Medical Centre; Staff, Peter Lougheed Centre; Staff, Rockyview General Hospital; Clin Asst Prof Med, University of Calgary; (403)944-8430; Fax. (403)944-3256; gilcurry@lincsat.com.

CURRY, Donald J; Burnaby Hosp, 3935 Kincaid St, Burnaby BC V5G 2X6; Cal'74; CCFP; FCFP; Staff, Burnaby Hospital; (604)434-4211; Fax. (604)412-6185.

CURRY, John J D; Beauti-Med Laser Skin Care Ctr, B210-2099 Lougheed Hwy, Port Coquitlam BC V3B 1A8; Trinity Coll. (Ireland)'67; LRCP; MRCS; DRCOG; Member, American Academy of Cosmetic Surgeons; Clin Instructor, University of British Columbia; Langs: Bilingual(English/French); (604)942-8849; Fax. (604)942-0081.

CURRY, Michael; Delta Hosp, 5800 Mountain View Blvd, Delta BC V4K 3V6; Wes'02; LLB; JD; CCFP; CCFP(E.M.); Chief Emerg Med, Delta Hospital; Staff, Alberta Health Services; Clinical Asst Prof, University of British Columbia; (604)946-1121; Fax. (604)946-6220; michael.curry@gmail.com.

CURRY, Philip L; Riverside Prof Centre, 31 Riverside Dr, Sydney NS B1S 3N1; Dal'84; FRCSC; Otol. (902)562-5135; Fax. (902)562-2605.

CURTIN, Kimberley A; The Medical Centre FHT, 707 Charlotte St, Peterborough ON K9J 2X5; McM'95; CCFP; Staff, Peterborough Regional Health Centre - Hospital Drive; Langs: Bilingual(English/French); (705)876-4597; Fax. (705)876-4599.

CURTIS, Bryan M; Health Sciences Centre, 300 Prince Philip Dr, St. John's NL A1B 3V6; Mem'97; BSc; BMedSci; FRCPC; IntMed; Nephrol. Staff Patient Research Centre, Health Sciences Centre; Asst Prof, Memorial University Of Newfoundland; (709)777-8632; Fax. (709)777-6995.

CURTIS, David; Clinique Med De Saint-Jovite, CP 19069 Csp Place Ouimet 992 rue de Saint-Jovite, Mont-Tremblant QC J8E 3C1; McG'69; (819)425-2728; Fax. (819)425-8012.

CURTIS, Glenn H; Market Mall Office Centre, 208-3625 Shaganappi Trail NW, Calgary AB T3A 0E2; Cal'94; BSc; MSc; CCFP; (403)286-9118; Fax. (403)286-3069.

CURTIS, Heather; IWK Health Centre, PO Box 9700 Rpo CSC 5850-5980 University Ave, Halifax NS B3K 6R8; Dal'03; FRCPC; DiagRad. Staff, IWK Health Centre; (902)470-8888; Fax. (902)470-7463.

CURTIS, Jacqueline R; The Hosp for Sick Children, EW 5114-555 University Ave, Toronto ON M5G 1X8; Tor'94; FRCPC; Peds; Endocrin&Metab. Staff, The Hospital For Sick Children; (416)813-7763; Fax. (416)813-6304.

CURTIS, John C; 1-1350 Bedford Hwy, Bedford NS B4A 1E1; Dal'69; AB; FRCPC; Psy (Dissociative Disorders). (902)835-8717; Fax. (902)835-1140.

CURTIS, Joseph A; Dr Charles A Janeway Child HC, 300 Prince Philip Dr, St. John's NL A1B 3V6; National (Ireland)'69; MB ChB; FRCPC; Peds. Staff, Janeway Children's Health & Rehabilitation Centre; (709)777-4626

CURTIS, M Anne; The Dematology Centre, 403-208 Bloor St W, Toronto ON M5S 3B4; Tor'82; ABIM; DABD; FRCPC; IntMed (Laser Cosmetic Surgery); Derm. Court Staff Derm, Women's College Hospital; Lecturer, University of Toronto; (416)922-9620; Fax. (416)922-4358.

CURTIS, M Shannon; Sherwood Family Med Centre, 15 Brackley Pt Rd, Charlottetown PE C1A 6Y1; Dal'08; CCFP; (902)628-3800; Fax. (902)628-3830.

CURTIS, Michael A; Lighthouse Med Centre, 3-2 Main St S, Bayfield ON N0M 1G0; Ott'05; CCFP; (519)565-4141

CURTIS, Michael J; Calgary Heart Centre, 403-3280 Hospital Dr NW, Calgary AB T2N 4Z6; Cal'85; ABIM; FRCPC; IntMed (Cardiac Catheterization); Cardiol. Ac Staff Calgary Reg Health Authority, Foothills Medical Centre; Staff, Health Research Innovation Centre; Clin Asst Prof Med, University of Calgary; (403)521-2227; Fax. (403)283-6360; michael.curtis@calgaryhealthregion.ca.

CURTIS, Michael; Health Sciences Centre, MS459-820 Sherbrook St, Winnipeg MB R3A 1R9; Man'00; FRCPC; AnatPath. Staff, Health Sciences Centre; (204)787-2829

CURTIS, Michael W; St Mary's Gen Hosp, 911 Queens Blvd, Kitchener ON N2M 1B2; Wes'88; CCFP; CCFP(E.M.); Chief, St Mary's General Hospital; Chief EmergMed, Grand River Hospital - Kitchener/Waterloo Health Centre; (519)749-6410; Fax. (519)749-6411.

CURTIS, Nickola J; 1007-655 Bay St, Toronto ON M5G 2K4; RCS (Ireland)'83; LRCP; LRCS; FACOG; FRCSC; ObstGyn (Infertility). Staff, Women's College Hospital; (416)408-1711; Fax. (416)408-1207.

CURTIS, Robin; Red Deer Reg Hosp Centre, 3942 50A Ave, Red Deer AB T4N 6R2; Sask'00; FRCPC; Anes. Staff, Red Deer Regional Hospital Centre; (403)343-4422

CURTIS, Ronald D; Wellington Med Centre, 105-126 Wellington St W, Aurora ON L4G 2N9; Wes'96; CCFP; (905)841-1633; aurorawalkinclinic@yahoo.ca.

CURTIS, Sarah J; Edmonton Clinic Health Academy, 11405 87 Ave NW, Edmonton AB T6G 1C9; Mem'00; FRCPC; Peds; PedEmergMed. Staff, Edmonton Clinic Health Academy; Asst Prof, University of Alberta; (780)248-5575; Fax. (780)248-5625.

CURTIS, Shirley L; Active Care Med Group, 1108 Klondike Rd, Ottawa ON K2K 0G1; Dal'74; (613)254-9777; Fax. (613)254-9778.

CURTIS, Tyler J; East End Community Hlth Cetre, 1619 Queen St E, Toronto ON M4L 1G4; McM'01; CCFP; (416)778-5858; Fax. (416)778-5855.

CURUVIJA, Srdjan; Montfort Hosp, 713 Montreal Rd, Ottawa ON K1K 0T2; Ott'75; FRCPC; DiagRad. Staff, Montfort Hospital; Langs: Croatian; French; (613)746-4621 x4504; Fax. (613)748-4951.

CURWIN, Julie M; CBI Health Park, 302-45 Weatherbee Rd, Sydney NS B1M 0A1; Dal'97; FRCPC; Psy. Staff, Cape Breton Healthcare Complex; (902)270-3270; Fax. (902)270-3202; jcurwin@ns.sympatico.ca.

CUSACK, Meghan M; Four Corners Med Bldg, 310-2009 Long Lake Rd, Sudbury ON P3E 6C3; Ott'08; CCFP; Physician, Regional Cancer Program HRSRH; Faculty Member, Northern Ontario School of Medicine; Langs: Bilingual(English/French); (705)222-2741; Fax. (705)222-7293; clinic-cs@hotmail.com.

CUSACK, Paul; The Boardwalk Prof Centre, 220 Water St, Charlottetown PE C1A 9M5; (902)367-4444

CUSAN, Leonello; CHUQ-Ctr Hosp Univ Laval, 2705 boul Laurier, Quebec QC G1V 4G2; Laval'85; PhD; Ac Staff Molecular Endocrin, Centre Hospitalier Universitaire de Quebec-CHUL; Prof Physiol, Université Laval; (418)654-2296; Fax. (418)654-2732; leonello.cusan@crchul.ulaval.ca.

CUSANO, Ronald E; Sunridge Prof Centre, 308-2675 36 St NE, Calgary AB T1Y 6H6; Cal'92; BSc; MSc; FRCSC; ObstGyn. (403)215-4070; Fax. (403)215-4071.

CUSHING, Sharon; The Hosp For Sick Children, BW 6103C-555 University Ave, Toronto ON M5G 1X8; Tor'03; FRCSC; Otol (Head & Neck Surgery). Staff, The Hospital For Sick Children; Langs: Bilingual(English/French); (416)813-2190

CUSHMAN JR, Robert A; HPB 7-200 Tunney's Pasture Drw, Ottawa ON K1A 0K9; McM'76; MSc(Epidem.); FRCPC; CommunMed (Infectious Diseases)., University of Ottawa; Langs: Bilingual(English/French); (613)957-8065; racushman@gmail.com.

CUSIMANO, Michael D; St Michael's Hosp, 30 Bond St, Toronto ON M5B 1W8; Tor'84; DABNS; FACS; FRCSC; Neursurg (Brain Injury). Assoc Staff, The Hospital For Sick Children; Staff NeuroSurg, St Michael's Hospital; Staff, Toronto Western Research Institute; Prof Neurosurg, University of Toronto; Langs: French; Italian; (416)864-6048; Fax. (416)864-5857.

CUSIMANO, Robert J; Univ Hlth Network-Toronto Gen, 4N 468-200 Elizabeth St, Toronto ON M5G 2C4; Cal'83; BSc; MSc; FACS; FRCSC; GenSurg (Pacemaker Surgery); Cardiovasc&ThorSurg. Staff Cardiovasc Surg, Toronto General Hospital - UHN; Assoc Prof, University of Toronto; Langs: French; Italian; (416)340-4928; Fax. (416)340-5069; robert.cusimano@uhn.ca.

CUSIMANO, Steven L; 205-132 Parkdale Ave S, Hamilton ON L8K 3P3; Wes'92; CCFP; Staff Privil, Hamilton Health Sciences Centre-Juravinski Site; Langs: Italian; French; (905)547-6331; Fax. (905)547-5755.

CUSSEN, Michael J; Hants Shore Community Hlth Ctr, RR 1 5638 Highway 215, Newport NS B0N 2A0; Dublin (Ireland)'78; MB ChB; BAO; DCH; (902)633-2110; Fax. (902)633-2332; mc2@accesswave.ca.

CUSSON, Anne-Marie; Clinique Med Richmond, 170 rue Gouin, Richmond QC J0B 2H0; Sher'87; (819)826-5750; anne-marie.cusson@ssss.gouv.qc.ca.

CUSSON, Daniel; 300 Place Juge-Desnoyers, Laval QC H7G 4R1; Mon'77; Langs: French; English; (450)951-1218; Fax. (450)951-1527.

CUSSON, Diane; Hotel-Dieu de Levis, 143 rue Wolfe, Levis QC G6V 3Z1; Laval'82; Ac Staff, Hôtel-Dieu de Lévis; Dir, Public Health Chaudiere Appalaches; (418)835-7121 x3140

CUSSON, Diane F; Clinique Med De Pintendre, 5-792 Rte Du President-Kennedy, Pintendre QC G6C 1C8; Laval'97; Langs: English; (418)837-6943; Fax. (418)837-0487.

CUSSON, Jacinthe; CLSC-d'Hebergement Valcourt, 1150 rue Champlain, Valcourt QC J0E 2L0; Sher'00; (819)542-2777; Fax. (450)532-3193.

CUSSON, Jean; Hop Charles Lemoyne, 3120 boul Taschereau, Greenfield Park QC J4V 2H1; Mon'79; ABIM; NBME; PhD; FRCPC; IntMed (Vascular Disease). Dir Centre de recherche, Hopital Charles LeMoyne; adj Prof Med, Universite de Sherbrooke; Langs: English; French; (450)466-5000 x3106; Fax. (450)466-5606.

CUSSON, Lise; Hop du Sacre-Coeur de Mtl, 5400 boul Gouin O, Montreal QC H4J 1C5; Mon'84; CCFP; FCFP; Ac Staff, Hôpital du Sacre-Coeur de Montréal; Clin Teacher, Universite de Montreal; Langs: English; (514)338-2383; Fax. (514)338-3155.

CUSSON, Sylvie; Clin Externes de Psychiatric, 230-383 boul du Seminaire N, St-Jean-sur-Richel QC J3B 8C5; Mon'91; FRCPC; Psy. Staff, Hôpital du Haut-Richelieu; (450)346-2222

CUSTEAU, Ingrid; Montfort Hosp, 713 Montreal Rd, Ottawa ON K1K 0T2; Sher'95; CSPQ; FRCPC; Anes. Staff, Montfort Hospital; Langs: Bilingual(French/English); (613)746-4621

CUTBILL, John W; 11700 Sarcee Trail NW PO Box 80010-Beacon Hill, Calgary AB T3R 0A1; Cal'92; MSc; BEng(mech); Dip SportMed; FCBOM; CCFP; FCFP; Medical Officer, Cdn Pacific Railway Company; Clinical Asst Prof, University of Calgary; (403)288-4593; Fax. (403)547-6134.

CUTBUSH, Wesley S; 205-125 Bell Farm Rd, Barrie ON L4M 6L2; Wes'75; CCFP; Ac Staff, Royal Victoria Regional Health Centre; (705)728-5261; Fax. (705)728-5265.

CUTFORTH, Dauna R; The Richmond Hosp, 7000 Westminster Hwy, Richmond BC V6X 1A2; Man'78; Staff, Richmond Hospital; (604)278-9711

CUTHBERT, Anthony L; Medical Clinic Bldg, 204-89 Humber College Blvd, Etobicoke ON M9V 4B8; Man'68; FRCPC; IntMed. (416)746-6028

CUTHBERT, Brian H; Sunnybrook Health Sciences Cen, D 108-2075 Bayview Ave, Toronto ON M4N 3M5; Aberdeen (United Kingdom)'90; Staff, Sunnybrook Health Sciences Centre; (416)480-6100 x83735

CUTHBERT, Donna A; Medical Arts Bldg, 250-1105 Pandora Ave, Victoria BC V8V 3P9; UBC'72; FRCPC; IntMed; MedOncol; HemPath; Hem. (250)383-4501; Fax. (250)360-4010.

CUTLER, Michael G; Centreville Med Clinic, PO Box 129, Wareham-Ctvle NL A0G 4P0; Mem'95; CCFP; Staff, Brookfield Bonnews Health Care Centre; (709)678-2342; Fax. (709)678-2110.

CUTLER, Paul; 4-314 Lake St, St Catharines ON L2N 4H4; Tor'65; (905)646-9301; Fax. (716)284-5159.

CUTLER, Robert L; F W Green Med Centre, 1629 Baker St, Cranbrook BC V1C 1B4; Alb'75; (250)426-6601; Fax. (250)426-6470.

CUTLER, Susan E; Eastside Health Ctr, 688A East River Rd, New Glasgow NS B2H 3S1; Dal'08; CCFP; (902)752-3632; Fax. (902)755-5532.

CUTRARA, Charles A; Trillium Cardiovascular Assoc, 608-89 Queensway W, Mississauga ON L5B 2V2; Qns'89; FRCSC; GenSurg (Cardiac Surgery); CardiothorSurg. Chief Cardiac Surg, Trillium Health Centre - Mississauga; (905)848-7513; Fax. (905)848-7515; ccutrara@thc.on.ca.

CUTT, Lorna E; 350 Festubert St, Duncan BC V9L 3S9; UBC'91; CCFP; (250)746-7720; Fax. (250)784-2405.

CUTTS, Danielle D; Victoria East Med Clinic, 2068 Prince of Wales Dr, Regina SK S4V 3A6; Sask'01; CCFP; Staff, Regina General Hospital; Associate Clin Prof, University of Saskatchewan; Langs: English; French; (306)789-4677; Fax. (306)789-3422.

CUTZ, Ernest; The Hosp For Sick Children, 555 University Ave, Toronto ON M5G 1X8; Prague (Czech Republic)'66; FRCPC; AnatPath. Sr Staff Path/Physician, The Hospital For Sick Children; Prof Path, University of Toronto; (416)813-5966; ernest.cutz@sickkids.ca.

CUTZ, Jean-Claude; St Joseph's Healthcare, LW L222-50 Charlton Ave E, Hamilton ON L8N 4A6; Tor'97; FRCPC; AnatPath. Staff, St Joseph's Healthcare - Charlton Campus; Langs: Bilingual(English/French); (905)521-6012

CUVELIER, Geoffrey; Cancer Care Manitoba, ON2062-675 Mcdermot Ave, Winnipeg MB R3E 0V9; Man'01; FRCPC; Peds (Pediatric Hematology Oncology).

CVEJIC, Elizabeth; U of Toronto-Koffler Student S, 214 College St, Toronto ON M5T 2Z9; McG'96; FRCPC; Psy. Langs: English; French; (416)978-8070; Fax. (416)978-7341.

CVEJIC, Helen; Douglas Mental Hlth Univ Inst, 6875 boul LaSalle, Verdun QC H4H 1R3; Galway (Ireland)'63; Psy (P.Q.). Staff, Douglas Mental Health University Institute; (514)761-6131 x2057; Fax. (514)762-3041.

CVETIC, Valentina; Cambridge Med Place, 1-695 Coronation Blvd, Cambridge ON N1R 7J9; Wes'98; FRCSC; ObstGyn.

CVETKOVIC, Igor; Grey Nuns Community Hosp, 1100 Youville Drive West NW, Edmonton AB T6L 5X8; Alb'07; CCFP; CCFP(E.M.); Staff, Covenant Health - Grey Nuns Community Hospital; (780)735-7000

CWAJNA, Wladyslawa; Nova Scotia Cancer Centre, 5820 University Ave, Halifax NS B3H 1V7; Silesian (Poland)'84; FRCPC; RadOncol. Staff, Cape Breton Healthcare Complex; (902)473-6018; Fax. (902)473-7205.

CWINN, A Adam; The Ottawa Hosp-Gen Campus, 501 Smyth Rd, Ottawa ON K1H 8L6; Ott'79; BSc; DABEM; MD; FRCPC; EmergMed. Head Dept of Emerg Med, The Ottawa Hospital - General Campus; Prof Dept of Emerg Med, University of Ottawa; Langs: Bilingual(French/English); (613)737-8136; acwinn@ ottawahospital.on.ca.

CYBULA, Tomasz; 103-1015 Austin Ave, New Westminster BC V3K 3N9; (South Africa)'00; (604)931-4885

CYBULSKI, Joseph B; 21 St Frances Memorial Dr PO Box 910, Barrys Bay ON K0J 1B0; Ott'71; CCFP; Ac Staff, St Francis Memorial Hospital; Langs: Polish; (613)756-2002; Fax. (613)756-0001.

CYBULSKI, Peter A; Kitchener Urology Associates, 313-751 King St W, Kitchener ON N2G 1E5; Qns'97; FRCSC; Urol. (519)954-2370

CYBULSKIE, Karen Ann; The Hosp For Sick Children, 555 University Ave, Toronto ON M5G 1X8; Tor'83; FRCPC; Anes. Staff Anes, The Hospital For Sick Children; (416)813-7445

CYBULSKY, Andrey V E; MUHC-Royal Victoria Hosp, R2 38-687 av des Pins O, Montreal QC H3A 1A1; Tor'80; FRCPC; IntMed; Nephrol. Staff, McGill University Health Centre - Royal Victoria Hospital; Prof Med, McGill University; (514)398-8148; Fax. (514)843-2815; andrey.cybulsky@mcgill.ca.

CYBULSKY, Irene J; Hamilton HS-General Site, 707-237 Barton St E, Hamilton ON L8L 2X2; Tor'84; MSc; FRCSC; GenSurg (Cardiac Surgery); Cardiovasc&ThorSurg. Ac Staff, Hamilton Health Sciences Centre - Hamilton General Hospital; Assoc Prof, McMaster University; Langs: Ukrainian; (905)777-8248; Fax. (905)527-6225.

CYBULSKY, Myron I; Univ Hlth Network-Toronto Gen, E 11-200 Elizabeth St, Toronto ON M5G 2C4; Tor'82; FRCPC; AnatPath (Cardiovascular Pathology). Staff Path, Toronto General Hospital - UHN; Prof LabMed & Path, University of Toronto; Langs: Ukrainian; (416)581-7483; myron.cybulsky@utoronto.ca.

CYMBALISTY, Christopher D; Health Sciences Centre, 820 Sherbrook St, Winnipeg MB R3A 1R9; Man'01; CCFP; CCFP(E.M.); Staff, The Salvation Army Grace Hospital; (204)837-8311

CYNGISER, Frances F; Associate Med Clinic, 25 St Michael St, St Albert AB T8N 1C7; Alb'80; (780)458-1234; Fax. (780)460-7941.

CYPEL, Marcelo; Univ Hlth Network-the Toronto, 9N 950-200 Elizabeth St, Toronto ON M5G 2C4; (Brazil)'99; Staff, Toronto General Hospital - UHN; (416)340-4800

CYPEL, Tatiana; Univ Hlth Network-Toronto Gen, 200 Elizabeth St, Toronto ON M5G 2C4; (Brazil)'00; Staff, Toronto General Hospital - UHN; (416)340-4800

CYR, Andre; Clinique Medicale du Faubourg, 145-1160 boul Saint-Joseph, Gatineau QC J8Z 1T3; Mon'97; Staff, Hull Hospital; (819)595-1991

CYR, Andreanne; Cooperative du St Robert-Clich, 291 108 Rte, Beauceville QC G5X 0C3; Laval'07; CCFP; (418)774-9891; Fax. (418)774-9878.

CYR, Anne; Clin Med Fam D'Edmundston, 50 av Bateman, Edmundston NB E3V 4A4; Laval'95; CCFP; Staff, Hôpital regional d'Edmundston; (506)735-5303

CYR, Carole; Promenades Beauport, A205-3333 rue du Carrefour, Quebec QC G1C 5R9; Laval'87; (418)660-0707; Fax. (418)667-5770.

CYR, Christian; Clinique Med St-Jerome, 102-450 Boul Monseigneur-Duboi, Saint-Jerome QC J7Y 3L8; Mon'78; (450)438-1776

CYR, Claude; Clin la Cite Medicale-Montreal, 1905-2001 av McGill College, Montreal QC H3A 1G1; Laval'93; Staff, Centre Hospitalier de Chandler; (514)788-6484

CYR, Claude; CHUS-Hop Fleurimont, 3001 12e Av N, Sherbrooke QC J1H 5N4; Sher'94; FRCPC; Peds. Staff, Centre Hospitalier Universitaire de Sherbrooke-Hopital Fleurimont; Teach Staff, Universite de Sherbrooke; (819)346-1110; Fax. (819)820-6420.

CYR, Daniel R; Polyclinique du Cap, 700 boul Thibeau, Trois-Rivieres QC G8T 7A1; Mon'95; Staff, Centre Lafleche Grand-Mere; (819)373-4771

CYR, Dominik; Ctr Hosp Affilie-St-Sacrement, 1050 ch Sainte-Foy, Quebec QC G1S 4L8; Mon'06; CCFP; Staff, Centre Hospitalier Affilié Universitaire de Québec - Hôpital du St-Sacrement; (418)682-7511

CYR, Elphege; CHUQ-St-Francois D'Assise, 10 rue de l'Espinay, Quebec QC G1L 3L5; Laval'74; FRCSC; ObstGyn (P.Q.). Ac Staff, Centre Hospitalier Universitaire De Québec - Pavillon De St-françois-d'assise; Ac Staff, CSSS de Quebec-Sud; (418)525-4444

CYR, Helene; CLSC-CHSLD-Meilleur, 410 boul de l'Ange-Gardien, L'Assomption QC J5W 1S7; Mon'85; Staff, Centre Hospitalier Pierre le Gardeur; (450)589-2101 x100

CYR, Jason; Hôpital Ste-Justine, 3175 ch Cote-Sainte-Catherine, Montreal QC H3T 1C5; Sher'07; Anes. Staff, Hôpital Ste-Justine; (514)345-4733

CYR, Jean-Francois; Hôpital Sainte-Croix, 570 rue Heriot, Drummondville QC J2B 1C1; Mon'06; Psy. Staff, Hôpital Sainte-croix; (819)478-6464

CYR, Jean-Louis; Hôpital régional Chaleur, 1750 Sunset Dr, Bathurst NB E2A 4L7; Sher'04; FRCPC; DiagRad. Staff, Hopital Regional Chaleur; (506)544-3000

CYR, Joanne; Hop Louis-H Lafontaine, 7401 rue Hochelaga, Montreal QC H1N 3M5; Mon'87; FRCPC; Psy. Staff, Hopital Louis-H Lafontaine; (514)251-4080 x3601

CYR, Jonathan; Ctr Hosp du Centre la Mauricie, 50 119e rue, Shawinigan-Sud QC G9P 5K1; Sher'01; CSPQ; GenSurg. Staff, Centre Hospitalier du Centre la Mauricie; (819)536-7505

CYR, Josiane; CLSC de Montreal-Nord, 11441 boul Lacordaire, Montreal-Nord QC H1G 4J9; Mon'07; CCFP; (514)384-2000

CYR, Luc; CSSS des Iles, 430 ch Principal, Cap-aux-Meules QC G4T 1R9; Laval'04; Staff, Hôpital de l'Archipel; Langs: Bilingual(French/English); (418)986-2121

CYR, Marc; CSSS de Rimouski-Neigette, CP 3150 succ Bureau Chef 150 av Rouleau, Rimouski QC G5L 5T1; Laval'08; Staff, Hôpital Regional Rimouski; (418)724-3000

CYR, Michael M; 301-2951 Walkers Line, Burlington ON L7M 4Y1; Ott'95; FRCPC; IntMed (Clinician Investigator Program); ClinImmunol&Allergy. Staff, Hamilton Health Sciences Centre - McMaster Children's Hospital; Clin. Scholar, McMaster University; (905)331-3101

CYR, Nathalie; Clinique Med Dr Cyr, 207-565 Promenade Elmwood, Moncton NB E1A 2X4; Sher'08; CCFP; Staff, Dr Georges-L-Dumont University Hospital Centre; (506)856-9979

CYR, Nathalie; 298-245 rue Soumande, Quebec QC G1M 3H6; Laval'93.

CYR, Nathalie; CSSS Haut-Richelieu-Rouville, 920 boul Du Seminaire N, St-Jean-Sur-Richel QC J3A 1B7; Mon'96; ObstGyn. Staff, Hôpital du Haut-Richelieu; (450)359-5000; Fax. (450)359-5251.

CYR, Pamela V; Cambridge Mem Hosp, 700 Coronation Blvd, Cambridge ON N1R 3G2; Ott'95; FRCPC; AnatPath. Staff, Cambridge Memorial Hospital; (519)621-2333 x2280; pcyr@ cmh.org.

CYR, Valerie-Anne; Dr Georges-L Dumont Reg Hosp, 330 Universite av, Moncton NB E1C 2Z3; Sher'98; Staff, Dr Georges-L-Dumont University Hospital Centre; (506)862-4000

CYR, Veronique; Hop Maisonneuve-Rosemont, 3840 rue Saint-Urbain, Montreal QC H2W 1T8; Mon'05; FRCPC; IntMed; Cardiol. Staff, Centre Hospitalier l'Université de Montréal (CHUM) - Hôtel-Dieu; (514)890-8000

CYR-HORNICK, Annie; 2-875 Dakota St, Winnipeg MB R2M 5S5; Man'98; CCFP; FCFP; (204)253-2929; Fax. (204)257-4036.

CYRENNE, Louise; Hôpital Ste-Justine, 3175 ch Cote-Ste-Catherine, Montreal QC H3T 1C5; Mon'77; CSPQ; LMCC; FRCPC; Anes (Obstetrics Anesthesia). ac Staff Anes, Hôpital Ste-Justine; Clin Instructeur, Universite de Montreal; Langs: Bilingual(French/English); (514)345-4733

CYRIAC, Jamie S; 406KW-650 Sammon Ave, East York ON M4C 5M5; Wes'00; FACS; FRCSC; GenSurg (Oncology). Staff, Toronto East General Hospital Inc; Lecturer, University of Toronto; (416)461-5155

CYRIAC, Jason P; Credit Valley Med Arts Centre, 412-2000 Credit Valley Rd, Mississauga ON L5M 4N4; Tor'96; FRCPC; IntMed; Cardiol. Staff, The Credit Valley Hospital; (905)828-4000; Fax. (905)828-7533.

CYTOWSKI, P Lorraine; Pinewood Med Centre, 1471 Hurontario St, Mississauga ON L5G 3H5; Tor'98; CCFP; FCFP; (905)274-1475; Fax. (905)274-4614.

CZAHARYN, Anthony G; Kirkland Med Center, 100-17000 Boul Hymus, Kirkland QC H9J 2W2; McG'87; BSc; AAFP; CCFP; FCFP; Langs: Bilingual(English/French); (514)693-0260

CZAJKA-FEDIRCHUK, Cynthia P; Kenora Med Associates, RR 1 Stn Main 45 Wolsley St, Kenora ON P9N 3W7; Man'07; CCFP; Staff, Lake of the Woods District Hospital; (807)468-3021; Fax. (807)468-6964.

CZAPLINSKI, Kazimierz L; St Boniface Gen Hosp, 409 Tache Ave, Winnipeg MB R2H 2A6; Wroclaw (Poland)'77; Med Officer Dept of CVT Surg, St Boniface General Hospital; (204)233-8563; Fax. (204)231-0640.

CZARLINSKA, Alina; CHUM-Hotel-Dieu, 3840 rue Saint-Urbain, Montreal QC H2W 1T8; Mon'85; FRCPC; Psy. Staff, Centre Hospitalier l'Université de Montréal (CHUM) - Hôtel-Dieu; (514)890-8000 x14218

CZARNECKA, Monika; 219 Marion St, Winnipeg MB R2H 0T5; Warsaw (Poland)'77; PhD; Staff, Victoria General Hospital.

CZARNECKI, Andrew; Sunnybrook Hlth Sciences Ctre, D 408-2075 Bayview Ave, Toronto ON M4N 3M5; Man'06; FRCPC; IntMed; Cardiol. Staff, Sunnybrook Health Sciences Centre; Langs: Polish; (416)480-6066

CZARNECKI, Cory; Alberta Hosp Edmonton, PO Box 307 Stn Main 17480 Fort Rd, Edmonton AB T5J 2J7; Man'98; FRCPC; Psy. Staff, Alberta Hospital Edmonton; Staff, Alberta Mental Health Board; (780)342-5449; Fax. (780)342-5368; czarnecki@ telusplanet.net.

CZARNECKI, Jan S C; 906 Victoria Ave E, Thunder Bay ON P7C 1B4; Tor'68; FRCSC; Ophth (Neuro Ophthalmology). Ac Staff, Thunder Bay Regional Health Sciences Centre Port-Arthur; (807)623-5747; Fax. (807)623-1645.

CZARNECKI, Wlodzimierz; Victoria Gen Hosp, G162-2340 Pembina Hwy, Winnipeg MB R3T 2E8; Warsaw (Poland)'77; PhD; FRCPC; IntMed (Clinical Cardiology); Cardiol. Staff, Victoria General Hospital; Staff, Health Sciences Centre; Staff, St Boniface General Hospital; Teach Staff Med, University of Manitoba; Langs: Polish; (204)477-3480

CZARNOTA, Gregory Jan; Sunnybrook Hlth Sciences Ctre, T2-2075 Bayview Ave, Toronto ON M4N 3M5; Tor'00; PhD; FRCP; LMCC; MB; BSc(Hon); FRCPC; RadOncol (Breast Cancer). Staff, Sunnybrook Health Sciences Centre; Langs: Polish; (416)480-6100; Fax. (416)480-6002; Gregory.Czarnota@ sunnybrook.ca.

CZARNOWSKI, Z Charles; Family Med Assoc of Ottawa, 75 Bruyere St, Ottawa ON K1N 5C7; Poznan (Poland)'78; CCFP; Staff, The Ottawa Hospital - General Campus; Asst Prof Family Med, University of Ottawa; Langs: Polish; (613)241-3344

CZAYKOWSKI, Piotr M; Cancercare Manitoba, 675 McDermot Ave, Winnipeg MB R3E 0V9; UBC'88; MSc; FRCPC; IntMed; MedOncol. Ac Staff, Health Sciences Centre; Staff Oncologist, Cancer Care Manitoba; Asst Prof IntMed & Comunity Health Sciences, University of Manitoba; (204)787-1992; piotr. czaykowski@cancercare.mb.ca.

CZECH, Eric; CSSS de Rivière-de-Loup, 75 rue Saint-Henri, Riviere-Du-Loup QC G5R 2A4; Mon'90; FRCPC; IntMed. Ac Member Internist, Centre Hospitalier Regional du Grand-Portage; Langs: Bilingual(French/English); (418)868-0466; Fax. (418)868-1059.

CZECHOWICZ, Dominika; Royal Ottawa Hlth Care Group, 1145 Carling Ave, Ottawa ON K1Z 7K4; Sask'05; FRCPC; Psy. Staff, Royal Ottawa Mental Health Centre - Royal Ottawa Health Care Group; (613)722-6521; Fax. (613)761-3602.

CZECHOWSKY, Diana; Sheldon Chumir Centre, 6F-1213 4 St SW, Calgary AB T2R 0X7; Alb'06; FRCPC; Psy. Staff, Foothills Medical Centre; (403)955-6686; Fax. (403)955-6688.

CZEMERYNSKI, Anne; Four Villages Comm Health Ctr, 1700 Bloor St W, Toronto ON M6P 4C3; Tor'84; CCFP; FCFP; Ac Staff, St Joseph's Health Centre; Lecturer, University of Toronto; Langs: Ukrainian; (416)604-3361; Fax. (416)604-3367.

CZERKAWSKI, Barbara A; BC Cancer Ctre-Southern Interl, 399 Royal Ave, Kelowna BC V1Y 5L3; McM'82; FRCPC; IntMed. Staff, Kelowna General Hospital; Staff, BC Cancer Agency Sindi Ahluwalia Hawkins Centre for the Southern Interior; Langs: Bilingual(English/French); (250)712-3930; Fax. (250)712-3911; bczerkaw@bccancer.bc.ca.

CZERNIKIEWICZ, Wojciech; St Joseph's Comm Health Centre, 2757 King St E, Hamilton ON L8G 5E4; Crackow (Poland)'02; FRCPC; Psy. Staff, St Joseph's Healthcare Hamilton - West 5th Campus; Langs: Polish; (905)573-4801; Fax. (905)573-4802.

CZIFFER, Andreas; The Group Health Centre, 240 McNabb St, Sault Ste Marie ON P6B 1Y5; Budapest (Hungary)'75; Ac Staff, Sault Area Hospital - Sault Ste Marie; Langs: Hungarian; (705)759-1234 x615; Fax. (705)759-5683.

CZIKK, Marie J; Mount Sinai Hosp, 600 University Ave, Toronto ON M5G 1X5; Tor'05; FRCSC; ObstGyn (Maternal Fetal Medicine). Staff, Mount Sinai Hospital; (416)596-4200

CZITROM, Jean-Paul; Clinique Medicale GMF-1851, 101-1851 rue Sherbrooke E, Montreal QC H2K 4L5; Mon'77; Staff, Centre Hospitalier l'Université de Montréal (CHUM) - Hôpital Notre-Dame; (514)524-7564; Fax. (514)527-5251.

CZOK, Anna A; 312-89 Humber College Blvd, Etobicoke ON M9V 4B8; Warsaw (Poland)'74; FRCPC; PhysMed&Rehab. Staff, William Osler Health System - Brampton Civic Hospital; Staff, William Osler Health System - Etobicoke General Hospital; Langs: Polish; (416)741-0921; Fax. (416)741-8498; anna_czok@ oslerhc.org.

CZOLPINSKA, Elizabeth; St Joseph's Health Centre, 710 Victoria Ave E, Thunder Bay ON P7C 5P7; Warsaw (Poland)'80; FRCPC; Psy. Staff, Thunder Bay Regional Health Sciences Centre; Psychiatrist, Lakehead Psychiatric Hospital - St. Joseph's Care Group; Langs: Polish; (807)624-3400

CZOLPINSKI, Thaddeus R; Curans Health Centre, 384 Fort William Rd, Thunder Bay ON P7B 2Z3; Warsaw (Poland)'80; FRCPC; IntMed. Langs: Polish; (807)345-3355; Fax. (807)345-0099.

CZOSNIAK, Isadore J; Dixie X-Ray Associates Ltd, 101-2115 Finch Ave W, North York ON M3N 2V6; McG'82; FRCPC; DiagRad. Ac Staff Radiol, Humber River Regional Hospital - Finch Avenue Site; (416)744-2655; Fax. (416)744-0581.

CZYZIW, Elizabeth; Health Canada, 612-200 boul Rene-Levesque O, Montreal QC H2Z 1X4; Ott'85; FCFP; Staff Teacher, Centre Hospitalier l'Université De Montréal (CHUM) - Hôpital Saint-luc; Consultant Industrial Med, SFBC Anapharm Inc.; Universite de Montreal; Langs: English; French; Ukrainian; (438)878-8035; eczyziw@gmail.com.

D'ADDARIO, Denise; Tottenham Med Centre, PO Box 2000 119 Queen St N, Tottenham ON L0G 1W0; McM'88; Ac Staff, Humber River Regional Hospital - Finch Avenue Site; (905)936-4211; Fax. (905)936-3493.

D'AGNONE, John J; 1618 9 Ave S, Lethbridge AB T1J 1W3; Alb'98; FRCPC; Psy. (403)328-3836; Fax. (403)328-3846.

D'AGOSTINO, Michael S; Sault Area Hosp, 750 Great Northern Rd, Sault Ste. Marie ON P6B 0A8; Tor'05; FRCPC; GenPath (Forensic Pathology). Staff, Health Sciences North-Laurentian Site; Staff, Sault Area Hospital - Sault Ste Marie; (705)759-3434

D'AGROSA, Raffaele; 301-1223 St Clair Ave W, Toronto ON M6E 1B5; Tor'94; MSc; CCFP; Clin Instructor Family & CommunMed, University of Toronto; Langs: Italian; (416)691-7385; Fax. (416)691-7099.

D'ALESSANDRO, Enzo; 302-1615 Dufferin St, Toronto ON M6H 4H4; Pavia (Italy)'87; FRCPC; Psy (Child & Adolescent Psychiatry). Langs: Italian; (416)651-7100

D'ALESSANDRO, Lisa C A; The Hosp for Sick Children, 555 Unviersity Ave, Toronto ON M5G 1X8; Wes'05; BSc; FRCPC; Peds; Cardiol. Staff, The Hospital For Sick Children; (416)813-1500

D'ALLAIRE, Diane; Clinique Med Physimed, 6363 Rte Transcanadienne, Saint-Laurent QC H4T 1Z9; Mon'87; (514)747-8888 x4313; Fax. (514)747-4705.

D'ALOISIO, Joseph F; 83 Larch St, Sudbury ON P3E 1B8; Ott'58; FRCSC; Urol. Staff Urol., Health Sciences North - Memorial Site; (705)522-1046; Fax. (705)522-6068.

D'AMICO, Catherine M; Nepean Med Centre, 403-1 Centrepointe Dr, Nepean ON K2G 6E2; Ott'92; BA(H); MA; CCFP; FCFP; Court Staff All Site, The Ottawa Hospital - Civic Campus; Staff, University of Ottawa; Langs: Bilingual(English/French); (613)224-6026

D'AMICO, Josiane; Hop du Sacre-Coeur de Mtl, 5400 boul Gouin O, Montreal QC H4J 1C5; Mon'99; CCFP; Chief Fam Med, Hôpital du Sacre-Coeur de Montréal; (514)338-2383; Fax. (514)338-3155.

D'AMICO, Patrick; CHUM-Hop St-luc, 1058 rue Saint-Denis, Montreal QC H2X 3J4; Mon'70; IntMed. Staff, Centre Hospitalier l'Université De Montréal (CHUM) - Hôpital Saint-luc; (514)890-8000 x32584

D'AMOUR, Monique L; CHUM-Hop Notre-Dame, 1560 rue Sherbrooke E, Montreal QC H2L 4M1; Mon'68; FRCPC; Electroenceph (P.Q.); Neur. Staff, Centre Hospitalier l'Université de Montréal (CHUM) - Hôpital Notre-Dame; (514)890-8237; Fax. (514)412-7554.

D'AMOUR, Pierre; 503-235 Boul Rene-Levesque E, Montreal QC H2X 1N8; Mon'68; Endocrin (P.Q.) (Parathyroid). Staff, Centre Hospitalier l'Université De Montréal (CHUM) - Hôpital Saint-luc; Prof, Universite de Montreal; Langs: Bilingual(French/English); (514)866-3681; Fax. (514)874-4078.

D'AMOURS, Daniel; Centre Med Laennec, 200-1750 av De Vitre, Quebec QC G1J 1Z6; Laval'72; CSPQ; FRCPC; Cardiol. Adj Cardiol, Centre Hospitalier Affilié Universitaire de Québec - Hôpital du St-Sacrement; (418)663-2858; Fax. (418)663-2352.

D'AMOURS, Denis; CHUQ-St-Francois D'Assise, 10 rue de l'Espinay, Quebec QC G1L 3L5; Laval'81; CCFP; FCFP; Staff, Centre Hospitalier Universitaire De Québec - Pavillon De St-françois-d'assise; (418)525-4425; Fax. (418)525-4322.

D'AMOURS, Georges; Clinique du Vieux Gatineau, 3B-520 boul de l'Hopital, Gatineau QC J8V 2P5; Mon'83; CSPQ; Cardiol; IntMed. (819)568-3224; Fax. (819)568-8521.

D'AMOURS, Jean-Francois; CSSS de Rivière-de-Loup, 75 rue Saint-Henri, Riviere-Du-Loup QC G5R 2A4; Sher'87; CSPQ; Anes. Staff, Centre Hospitalier Regional du Grand-Portage; (418)868-1000; Fax. (418)868-1032.

D'AMOURS, Josee; UMF Laval, 2690 ch des Quatre-Bourgeois, Quebec QC G1V 0B7; Laval'91; CCFP; (418)656-4795; Fax. (418)656-4503.

D'AMOURS, Martin; CHUQ-Ctr Hosp Univ Laval, S 27-2705 boul Laurier, Quebec QC G1V 4G2; Laval'04; PhD; FRCPC; IntMed; Endocrin&Metab., Centre Hospitalier Universitaire de Quebec-CHUL; Langs: Bilingual(French/English); (418)654-2169; Fax. (418)654-2792; martin.damours@mail.chuq.qc.ca.

D'AMOURS, Melanie; Clinique Med du Phare, 101-822 boul Sainte-Anne, Rimouski QC G5M 1J5; Laval'02; (418)723-5135

D'AMOURS, Pierre; Ctr Hosp Affilie-Enfant-Jesus, 1401 18e rue, Quebec QC G1J 1Z4; Laval'83; FRCPC; IntMed; Respir. Staff, Centre Hospitalier Affilié Universitaire de Québec - Hôpital De L'Enfant Jésus; Teach Staff Med, Université Laval; (418)649-0252; Fax. (418)649-5928.

D'AMOURS, Renee; CSSS de Matane, 349 av Saint-Jerome, Matane QC G4W 3A8; Laval'87; Staff, Centre Hospitalier de Matane; (418)562-3135; Fax. (418)562-9236.

D'AMOURS, Sonia-Sandra; Centre Med de la Vallee, 1-22 rue du Pont, Amqui QC G5J 3T5; Laval'96; Staff Family Med, CSSS de la Matapedia; (418)629-6611; Fax. (418)629-4484.

D'ANDREA, Joan W; Gates of Maple Med Center, 201-2200 Rutherford Rd, Concord ON L4K 5V2; Tor'81; CCFP; Langs: Italian; (905)303-9310; Fax. (905)303-5506.

D'ANGELO, Anthony J; Dundas Centre Med, 306-220 Dundas St W, Whitby ON L1N 8M7; Tor'88; BSc(Hon.); Court Staff Family Pract., Rouge Valley Health System - Ajax & Pickering Health Centre Site; Langs: Italian; (905)666-3373; Fax. (905)666-3575.

D'ANGELO, Antonio F; Hôpital Ste-Justine, 3175 ch Cote-Ste-Catherine, Montreal QC H3T 1C5; Qns'93; FRCPC; Peds. Staff, Hôpital Ste-Justine; (514)345-4931

D'ANGELO, Peter D; 206-145 Sheppard Ave E, North York ON M2N 3A7; Wes'78; Ac Staff, North York General Hospital; (416)223-4330; Fax. (416)223-5892.

D'ANJOU, Catherine M; Halifax Sexual Health Clinic, 201-6009 Quinpool Rd, Halifax NS B3K 5J7; McM'05; CCFP.

D'ANJOU, Guy; Hôpital Ste-Justine, 3175 ch Cote-Ste-Catherine, Montreal QC H3T 1C5; Laval'95; FRCPC; Neur. Staff, Hôpital Ste-Justine; (514)345-4894; Fax. (514)345-2572.

D'ANJOU, Jean-Maurice; Hotel-Dieu de Levis, 143 rue Wolfe, Levis QC G6V 3Z1; Laval'72; FRCPC; PhysMed&Rehab (Musculoskeletal). Ac Staff, Hôtel-Dieu de Lévis; Université Laval; (418)835-7121; Fax. (418)835-7212; jmdanjou@videotron.ca.

D'ANNUNZIO, Mario; Polyclinique St-Eustache, 75 rue Grignon, St-Eustache QC J7P 4J2; Mon'69; ac Staff Obstetrics, Hôpital de Saint-Eustache; Langs: English; (450)473-3232; Fax. (450)473-1341.

D'AOUST, Louis-Xavier; CLSC des Faubourgs, 1705 rue de la Visitation, Montreal QC H2L 3C3; Mon'10; CCFP; Staff, CLSC des Faubourgs (Visitation); (514)527-2361

D'AOUST, Louise; CHUM-Hop St-Luc, 1058 rue Saint-Denis, Montreal QC H2X 3J4; Mon'96; FRCPC; IntMed; Gastroent. Staff, Centre Hospitalier l'Université De Montréal (CHUM) - Hôpital Saint-luc; (514)890-8356

D'AOUST-BERNARD, Chantal; McArthur Med Centre, 390 McArthur Ave, Vanier ON K1L 6N6; Mon'92; CCFP; FCFP; Langs: Bilingual(French/English); (613)741-1134; Fax. (613)741-4276.

D'APICE, H Lina; CRSSS Baie-James-Sante Isle-D, CP 790 130 boul Matagami, Matagami QC J0Y 2A0; Mon'89; Staff, Centre de Sante Isle-Dieu Matagami; Langs: English; Italian; (819)739-2515; Fax. (819)739-6059; hawaling@sympatico.ca.

D'ARAGON, Frederick; CHUS-Hop Fleurimont, 3001 12e av N, Sherbrooke QC J1H 5N4; Sher'07; Anes. Staff, Centre Hospitalier Universitaire de Sherbrooke-Hopital Fleurimont; (819)346-1110

D'ARCHANGELO, Eugene S; Hawthorne Care Center, 2111 Hawthorne Ave, Port Coquitlam BC V3C 1W3; Alb'74; (604)941-4051

D'ARCY, Diane L; Public Gardens Med Clinic, 200-5675 Spring Garden Rd, Halifax NS B3J 1H1; Qns'85; CCFP; FCFP; (902)425-5440; Fax. (902)482-6019.

D'ARCY, Francis D; 120-35 Shoreham Dr, North York ON M3N 1S5; Dublin (Ireland)'63; MB ChB; BAO; Ac Staff, Humber River Regional Hospital - Finch Avenue Site; (416)551-3051

D'ARCY, Thomas M C; Burnaby Hosp, 3935 Kincaid St, Burnaby BC V5G 2X6; Dublin (Ireland)'72; FRCPC; Anes. Staff, Burnaby Hospital; (604)222-3115

D'ARGY, Marie-Claude; Clinique Med Saint-Luc, 264 boul Saint-Luc, St-Jean-Sur-Richel QC J2W 1C3; Sher'93; (450)348-6124; Fax. (450)348-4163.

D'ARSIGNY, Christine L; Richardson House, 102 Stuart St, Kingston ON K7L 2V6; McG'92; ABIM; FRCPC; IntMed (Critical Care Medicine); Critical Care Medicine (P.Q.); Respir. Staff Critical Care Med/Respirolgy, Kingston General Hospital; Assoc Prof, Queen's University; Langs: English; French; (613)548-2371; Fax. (613)549-1459.

D'ASTOUS, Helene; Hotel-Dieu de Levis, 143 rue Wolfe, Levis QC G6V 3Z1; Laval'06; CCFP; CCFP(E.M.); Staff, Hôtel-Dieu de Lévis; (418)835-7121 x6178

D'ASTOUS, Julien R; 169 Botsford St, Moncton NB E1C 4X4; Ott'70; FRCPC; IntMed (Nephrology). (506)857-3020; Fax. (506)855-2847.

D'ASTOUS, Michel; Michel D'Astous Prof Corp, 203-140 rue Champlain, Dieppe NB E1A 1N8; Laval'87; FRCPC; IntMed; Cardiol. Staff, Dr Georges-L-Dumont University Hospital Centre; Langs: Bilingual(French/English); (506)862-0110; Fax. (506)855-2324.

D'COSTA, Abelina S; William Osler HC-Brampton, 2100 Bovaird Dr E, Brampton ON L6R 3J7; Karachi (Pakistan)'99; FRCPC; Anes. Staff, William Osler Health System - Brampton Civic Hospital; (416)494-2120

D'COSTA, Darryl I; Collingwood Gen & Marine Hosp, 459 Hume St, Collingwood ON L9Y 1W9; Qns'00; BScChemEng; MSc; Staff, Collingwood General & Marine Hospital; Langs: French; (705)444-8601

D'COSTA, Joseph A; Medical & Dental Bldg, 301-3939 50A Ave, Red Deer AB T4N 4E6; Dar-Es-Salaam (Tanzania)'86; FRCPC; Psy. Staff, Red Deer Regional Hospital Centre; (403)343-2102; Fax. (403)343-2172.

D'CUNHA, Nolda M; Mariola Med Clinic, 430 Gerrard St E, Toronto ON M5A 2G9; Madras (India)'68; MB BS; MRCP(UK); FCFP; CCFP; FCFP; Assoc Staff Privil, Mount Sinai Hospital; Assoc Staff Privil, St Michael's Hospital; Langs: Hindi; Kanarese; Urdu; Tamil; (416)924-6116; Fax. (416)924-6116.

D'CUNHA REBELLO, Chrysal D E; Medical Care Clinic, 205 Markham Rd, Scarborough ON M1J 3C3; (Dominica)'98; FAAP; BSc; FRCPC; Peds. (416)265-6663; Fax. (416)265-1263.

D'EGIDIO, Gianni; The Ottawa Hosp-Gen Campus, 501 Smyth Rd, Ottawa ON K1H 8L6; Ott'06; FRCPC; IntMed (Critical Care Medicine). Staff, The Ottawa Hospital - General Campus; (613)737-8899

D'ENTREMONT, Julite; 102-26 North St, Bridgewater NS B4V 2V6; Ott'08; CCFP; (902)543-2733; Fax. (902)543-1678.

D'ENTREMONT, Lionel J; PO Box 97, Meteghan NS B0W 2J0; Ott'75; (902)645-2777; Fax. (902)645-2854.

D'EON, Jacqueline R; Pubnico Head Med Center, PO Box 40, Pubnico NS B0W 2W0; Dal'92; BSc; BA; Staff Privil, Yarmouth Regional Hospital; Langs: English; French; (902)762-2311; Fax. (902)762-0144.

D'ERRICO, Jean; Polyclinique Cabrini, 106-5700 rue Saint-Zotique E, Montreal QC H1T 3Y7; Mon'72; Staff, Hôpital Santa Cabrini Ospedale; Physician, Centre D'Accuell & Maison St Joseph; (514)253-8473

D'IGNAZIO, Giuseppe; 4309C boul Saint-Jean, Dollard-d-Ormeaux QC H9H 2A4; McG'88; Langs: Italian; (514)696-0707

D'INTINO, Yolanda M; Cape Breton Hlthcare Complex, 3F-1482 George St, Sydney NS B1P 1P3; Dal'78; FRCPC; Derm. Staff, Cape Breton Healthcare Complex; (902)567-8110; Fax. (902)567-8111.

D'IORIO, A M Michele; 324 Lakeshore Rd E, Mississauga ON L5G 1H4; Ott'74; FRCPC; Psy (Child Psychiatry). Staff, Trillium Health Centre - Mississauga; Langs: Bilingual(English/French); (905)274-8914; Fax. (905)274-1654.

D'MELLO, Jennifer; Alberta Children's Hosp, 2888 Shaganappi Trail NW, Calgary AB T3B 6A8; Cal'06; PedEmergMed (P.Q.); Peds. Staff, Alberta Children's Hospital; (403)955-7211

D'MELLO, Nisha A; Corcare Inc, 410-325 Milner Ave, Scarborough ON M1B 5N1; Ott'01; FRCPC; IntMed; Cardiol. (416)284-4744; Fax. (416)284-0141.

D'ONOFRIO, George F; 2F-2045 Dufferin St, York ON M6E 3R4; Tor'70; Court Staff, St Michael's Hospital; Langs: Italian; (416)654-0045; Fax. (416)654-5070.

D'OVIDIO, Robert G; Image One MRI, 101-3320 Richter St, Kelowna BC V1W 4V5; Tor'81; BSc; FRCPC; DiagRad (MRI). (250)860-4848; Fax. (250)860-4546; rob@imageoneonemri.ca.

D'OVIDIO, Vincent; 206-1670 Dufferin St, Toronto ON M6H 3M2; Bologna (Italy)'57; Langs: Italian; (416)652-3030

D'OYLEY, Heather M; Vancouver Gen Hosp, 855 12th Ave W, Vancouver BC V5Z 1M9; UBC'96; FRCPC; Psy. Staff, Vancouver General Hospital - Centennial Pavillion; (604)875-4111

D'SA, Alfred J; The Credit Valley Hosp, 2200 Eglinton Ave W, Mississauga ON L5M 2N1; Tor'89; Staff, The Credit Valley Hospital; (905)813-4532

D'SA, Ryan A; Niagara H System-St Catharine, 142 Queenston St, St. Catharines ON L2R 7C6; Leicester (United Kingdom)'02; FRCPC; IntMed. Staff, Niagara Health System - St Catharines General Site; (905)682-6411; Fax. (905)704-4435.

D'SILVA, Karen; St Michael's Hosp, 30 Bond St, Toronto ON M5B 1W8; Ott'07; GeriatricMed; IntMed. Staff, St Michael's Hospital; (416)864-5015

D'SOUZA, Annette M; Westminster Med Bldg, 706-625 Fifth Ave, New Westminster BC V3M 1X4; Calcutta (India)'79; FRCSC; Ophth (Anterior Segment). Staff, Ridge Meadows Hospital & Health Care Centre; Staff, Royal Columbian Hospital; Staff, Burnaby Hospital; Staff, Eagle Ridge Hospital & Health Care Centre; (604)522-8638; Fax. (604)522-3711.

D'SOUZA, David; London Reg Cancer Centre, 790 Commissioners Rd E, London ON N6A 4L6; Tor'95; DABR; FRCPC; RadOncol (Brachy Therapy). Ad Staff Privil, London Health Sciences Centre - Victoria Campus; Asst Prof, University of Western Ontario; (519)685-8650; Fax. (519)685-8627.

D'SOUZA, Irene C; 29 Gossamer Ave, North York ON M2M 2X3; Makerere (Uganda)'69; Assoc Staff, Humber River Regional Hospital - Church Street Site; Assoc Staff, St John's Rehabilitation Hospital; (416)221-3375; Fax. (416)344-2444.

D'SOUZA, Mark; Humber River Reg Hosp-Church, 200 Church St, Toronto ON M9N 1N8; Qns'09; CCFP; CCFP(E.M.); Staff, Humber River Regional Hospital - Church Street Site; (416)454-8969

D'SOUZA, Mirabelle; 107-2737 Keele St, North York ON M3M 2E9; Wes'06; FRCSC; ObstGyn. (647)346-3055; Fax. (647)346-3099.

D'SOUZA, Ryan; 106-30 Dupont St E, Waterloo ON N2J 2G9; (India)'96; CCFP; Langs: Hindi; (519)570-2321

D'SOUZA, Sameer D; William Osler HC-Brampton Civi, 2100 Bovaird Dr E, Brampton ON L6R 3J7; Tor'00; CCFP; Staff, William Osler Health System - Etobicoke General Hospital; Staff, William Osler Health System - Brampton Civic Hospital; (905)494-2120

D'SOUZA, Sudhir J A; Hamilton HS-Mcmaster Site, PO Box 2000 Stn Lcd 1 3A-1200 Main St W, Hamilton ON L8N 3Z5; McG'91; PhD; FRCPC; Peds; Nephrol. Staff, Hamilton Health Sciences Centre - McMaster Children's Hospital; (905)521-2100

D'URZO, Anthony D; 107-1670 Dufferin St, Toronto ON M6H 3M2; Tor'90; MSc; BPHE; CCFP; FCFP; Staff, Toronto Western Hospital - University Health Network; Staff, St Michael's Hospital; Asst Prof Family & CommunMed., University of Toronto; Langs: Italian; (416)652-9336; Fax. (416)652-0218; pcac@sympatico.ca.

DA COSTA, Derek; Tiny Tots Med Centre, 203-3400 rue du Marche, Dollard-D-Ormeaux QC H9B 2Y1; McG'87; BSc; Prof, St Mary's Hospital Centre; Examiner, Medical Council of Canada Examination Board; Hd Peds, Tiny Tots Med Centre; Langs: English; French; (514)685-3531; Fax. (514)685-7971.

DA COSTA, Laurington; Hotel-Dieu Hosp, 166 Brock St, Kingston ON K7L 5G2; (Jamaica)'63; FRCP(Lond); MD(Lond); FACP; FRCPC; IntMed; Gastroent. Assoc Staff, Hotel-Dieu Hospital; Assoc Staff, Kingston General Hospital; Emeritus Prof Med., Queen's University; (613)544-3310 x2291; Fax. (613)544-3114; dacostal@hdh.kari.net.

DA COSTA, Michael S; 505 Yonge St, Barrie ON L4N 4E1; Edinburgh (Scotland)'70; (705)721-1689; Fax. (705)721-0724.

DA COSTA, Rhiannon; Toronto East Gen Hosp Inc, 825 Coxwell Ave, Toronto ON M4C 3E7; Tor'95; FRCPC; IntMed; Critical Care Medicine. Staff, Toronto East General Hospital Inc; (416)465-9133; rhiannon.dacosta@tegh.on.ca.

DA COSTA JR, Leodante B; Sunnybrook Hlth Sciences Ctre, A1 37-2075 Bayview Ave, Toronto ON M4N 3M5; Minas Gerais (Brazil)'95; Staff, Sunnybrook Health Sciences Centre; Langs: Portuguese; (416)480-6820

DA CUNHA, Noel A; Associate Med Clinic, 203-10030 106 St, Westlock AB T7P 2K4; London (England)'81; MB BS; CCFP; (780)349-3341; Fax. (780)349-6686.

DA ROZA, Gerald; 101-200 Keary St, New Westminster BC V3L 0A6; UBC'99; FACP; MHSc; FRCPC; IntMed; Nephrol. Head of Medicine/Dir CTU, Royal Columbian Hospital; Clin Assoc Prof, University of British Columbia; (604)516-7774; Fax. (604)516-7764.

DA SAMY, Santhi P P; 65 Thames St, Chatham ON N7L 1S4; (Malaysia)'91; FRCSC; Otol. Staff, Chatham-Kent Health Alliance; Langs: Malay; Tamil; (519)354-1200; Fax. (519)354-1208.

DA SILVA, Anna-Maria; Protea Med Centre, 7-505 Bryne Dr, Barrie ON L4N 9P7; Witwatersrand (South Africa)'91; CCFP; Langs: Afrikaans; Portuguese; (705)735-2161; Fax. (705)735-2179.

DA SILVA, Hermano P B; Misericordia Health Centre, 99 Cornish Ave, Winnipeg MB R3C 1A2; Man'88; Staff, Misericordia Health Centre; (204)774-6581; Fax. (204)774-2075.

DA SILVA, Laurindo M; Medical Arts Bldg, 521-233 Kennedy St, Winnipeg MB R3C 3J5; Man'78; Staff, St Boniface General Hospital; Staff, Seven Oaks General Hospital.

DA SILVA, Orlando P; London HSC-Victoria Hosp, PO Box 5010 Stn B D4 210-800 Commissioners Rd E, London ON N6A 5W9; Minas Gerais (Brazil)'81; FRCPC; Peds (Neonatal Intensive Care). Staff, London Health Sciences Centre - Victoria Campus; Assoc Prof Peds/Asst Prof, University of Western Ontario; Langs: Portuguese; Spanish; (519)685-8500; Fax. (519)646-6123.

DA SILVA, Sandy C; Anchor Fam Med, 1450 Waddington Rd, Nanaimo BC V9S 4V9; UBC'91; CCFP; FCFP; (250)754-5545; Fax. (250)754-5954.

DA SILVA, Sean L; Chatham-Kent Hlth Alliance, PO Box 2030 Stn Main 80 Grand Ave W, Chatham ON N7M 5L9; (Grenada)'04; Staff, Chatham-Kent Health Alliance; (519)352-6400

DA SILVA, Sidney J; Windsor Reg Hosp-Metropolitan, 1995 Lens Ave, Windsor ON N8W 1L9; Nairobi (Kenya)'75; FRCPC; Anes. Staff, Windsor Regional Hospital - Metropolitan Site; (519)254-1661; Fax. (519)971-7924.

DA SILVA, Stefan G; Foothills Medical Centre, C231-1403 29 St NW, Calgary AB T2N 2T9; Sask'03; CCFP; CCFP(E.M.); Staff, Foothills Medical Centre; (403)944-1315

DA SILVA, Terence R; Trafalgar Med Clinic, 205-1235 Trafalgar Rd, Oakville ON L6H 3P1; Wes'75; (905)815-1330

DA SILVA, Vasco F; The Ottawa Hosp-Civic Campus, C2214-1053 Carling Ave, Ottawa ON K1Y 4E9; Lausanne (Switzerland)'74; FACS; FRCSC; Neursurg. Ac Staff, The Ottawa Hospital - Civic Campus; Court Staff Assoc, Children's Hospital of Eastern Ontario (CHEO); Asst Prof, University of Ottawa; Langs: Portuguese; Spanish; French; (613)798-5555 x19607; Fax. (613)761-4249; vdasilva@ottawahospital.on.ca.

DAABAK, Abdulghani M; South Muskoka Med Centre, 230 Manitoba St, Bracebridge ON P1L 2E1; University of Al Fateh (Libya)'01; CCFP; (705)646-7634

DAAR, Abdallah S; McLauglin Rotman Ctr for Globa, PO Box 50 406-101 College St, Toronto ON M5G 1L7; Conjoint (England)'73; DAAPhill; FRCPLon; FRCS; MRCSUK; LRCPUK; FRCSC; GenSurg. Dir Ethics & Policy, McLaughlin Centre for Molecular Medicine; Sr Scientist/Dir Program on Ethics & Commercialization, McLauglin Rotman Centre for Global Health; Chair, Global Alliance for Chronic Diseases; Prof Public Hlth Sciences & Surg/Sr Fellow Massey College, University of Toronto; Langs: Arabic; Swahili; (416)673-6573; Fax. (416)352-1606.

DABA, Ledjalem A; 19-6175 Highway 7, Woodbridge ON L4H 0P6; Addis Ababa (Ethiopia)'96; FRCPC; IntMed; Cardiol. Langs: Amharic; (905)850-3091

DABBAGH, Sufian; GMF Chapleau, 87 montee Gagnon, Bois-des-Filion QC J6Z 4C4; Cairo (Egypt)'77; CCFP; Staff, Centre Hospitalier La Sarre; (450)621-7420; Fax. (450)621-5007.

DABBOUR, Islam O; South Shore Reg Hosp, 90 Glen Allan Dr, Bridgewater NS B4V 3S6; Damascus(Syria) (Egypt)'99; Staff, South Shore Regional Hospital; (902)543-4603

DABBS, Kelly; Meadowlark Health Centre, 166 Meadowlark Shopping Ctr NW, Edmonton AB T5R 5W9; Alb'85; MD; FRCSC; GenSurg (Oncology/Breast Cancer); Critical Care Medicine. Aj Asst Prof, Cross Cancer Institute; Staff Surg, Covenant Health - Misericordia Community Hospital; Clin Assoc Prof Surg/Sr Dir Equity & Faculty Development, University of Alberta; (780)486-5030; Fax. (780)486-1035; dabbs@shaw.ca.

DABBS, Ronald H; 109-1811 Victoria St, Prince George BC V2L 2L6; McM'74; Assoc Staff, University Hospital of Northern British Columbia; (250)562-8236; Fax. (250)562-6512.

DABEE, Vassant; Children's Hosp Eastern Ont, 401 Smyth Rd, Ottawa ON K1H 8L1; Edinburgh (Scotland)'71; MB ChB; FRCPC; Peds (Pediatric Nephrology). Ac Staff Academic Peds, Children's Hospital of Eastern Ontario (CHEO); Asst Prof Peds, University of Ottawa; Langs: Bilingual(French/English); (613)737-7600 x2664; Fax. (613)738-4878.

DABHOLKAR, Shilpa; Gain Med Centre, 1199 Austin Ave, Coquitlam BC V3K 3P4; (India)'00; MB BS; CCFP; Langs: Hindi; Marathi; (604)939-7345; Fax. (604)939-7781.

DABIRZADEH, Hamidreza; The Ottawa Hosp-Civic Campus, 1053 Carling Ave, Ottawa ON K1Y 4E9; Tehran (Iran)'93; FRCPC; DiagRad. Staff, The Ottawa Hospital - Civic Campus; (613)761-4054

DABO, Sambou; Clin Med Garnison de Longue-Po, 6560 rue Hochelaga, Montreal QC H1N 1X9; (Mali)'97; (514)252-2777

DABOVAL, Thierry; Children's Hosp of Eastern On, 401 Smyth Rd, Ottawa ON K1H 8L1; Sher'92; FRCPC; Peds (Neonatal & Perinatal Medicine). Staff, Children's Hospital of Eastern Ontario (CHEO); Langs: Bilingual(French/English); (613)737-7650 x2415

DABREO, Derek E J; Medical Arts Bldg, 353 St Paul Ave, Brantford ON N3R 4N3; (Jamaica)'76; MB BS; FRCPC; IntMed (Cardiology). Consultant, The Brant Community Healthcare System - Brantford General Hospital Site; (519)759-6369

DABROWSKI, Piotr T; Misericordia Health Centre, 99 Cornish Ave, Winnipeg MB R3C 1A2; Warsaw (Poland)'68; FFARCSI; FRCPC; Anes. Staff, Misericordia Health Centre; (204)774-6581

DABRUS, Kathy; Lansdowne Prof Bldg, 310-1641 Hillside Ave, Victoria BC V8T 5G1; Man'88; Staff, Victoria Interior Health Authority; (250)592-5312; Fax. (250)592-5910.

DABRUSIN, Richard A; Mount Sinai Hospital Centre, 5690 boul Cavendish, Cote Saint-Luc QC H4W 1S7; Louvain (Belgium)'70; FACCP; Respir (P.Q.) (Pulmonary Diseases). Staff, Mount Sinai Hospital Center; Langs: English; French; (514)369-2222; Fax. (514)369-0282.

DACAMBRA, Mark; Royal Columbia Hosp, 330 Columbia St E, New Westminster BC V3L 3W7; Tor'03; FRCSC; OrthSurg. Staff, Royal Columbian Hospital; (604)520-4253

DACRE, Roger I; Balmoral Med Arts Facility, 408-1366 Yonge St, Toronto ON M4T 3A7; London (England)'82; MB BS; CCFP; FCFP; (416)924-7799; Fax. (416)924-8243; roger@doctordacre.com.

DADA, Azad; Hop Regional D'Edmundston, 275 Hebert Blvd, Edmundston NB E3V 4E4; (Tunisia)'98; Anesthetist, Hôpital regional d'Edmundston; (506)739-2200

DADA, Daniel O; Three Hills Med Clinic, PO Box 1149 779 2 St N, Three Hills AB T0M 2A0; (Nigeria)'80; MB BS; CCFP; (403)443-5522; Fax. (403)443-2873.

DADA, Nadeem; The Richmond Centre, PO Box 2000 Stn Central, Charlottetown PE C1A 7N8; Karachi (Pakistan)'89; DABPN; FRCPC; Psy (Child & Adolescent Psychiatry). Staff, Queen Elizabeth Hospital; (902)368-4430; Fax. (902)368-4427.

DADA, Olayinka; Royal Care Med Service, 505 Rymal Rd E, Hamilton ON L8W 3X1; Ilorin (Nigeria)'91; MB BS; CCFP; (905)544-2974

DADABHAI, Ambreen; Medistat Med Familiale, 4965 rue Saint-Pierre, Pierrefonds QC H9H 5M9; McG'06; MDCM; CCFP; (514)624-4774; Fax. (514)624-4704.

DADACHANJI, Shiroy; 3055 Wesbrook Mall, Vancouver BC V6T 1Z3; UBC'08; CCFP; (604)822-3614

DADJO-GUEWA, B Stephane; Ctre de Sante de L'Estrie, 1 Nation Rd, Crysler ON K0A 1R0; Shanghai (China)'00; CCFP; (613)987-2683; Fax. (613)987-9908.

DADOUN-MCHUGH, Molly; St Mary's Hosp Centre, 3830 av Lacombe, Montreal QC H3T 1M5; Montpellier (France)'80; CSPQ; Anes. Ac Staff, St Mary's Hospital Centre; (514)345-3511 x3376

DADOUR, Georges; 1385 rue Jean-Talon E, Montreal QC H2E 1S6; Lyon (France)'70; Staff, CSSS du Coeur de l'Isle Hôpital Jean-Talon; Langs: English; Arabic; French; (514)495-6767 x6235; Fax. (514)495-6772.

DAEMEN-DARVEAU, Helene; 203-352 av Dorval, Dorval QC H9S 3H8; Mon'75; MCFP(EM); Chef Med Adviser, Air Canada Centre; Langs: Bilingual(French/English); (514)422-7974; Fax. (514)422-7995; helene.darveau@aircanada.ca.

DAENINCK, Paul J; Cancer Care Manitoba, Ll 101 8-409 Tache Ave, Winnipeg MB R2H 2A6; Cal'91; DABIM; MSc; BSc; FRCPC; IntMed (Medical Oncology). Staff Coordinator Tache Site, Cancer Care Manitoba; Asst Prof Internal & Family Med, University of Manitoba; Langs: American Sign Language; (204)235-3141; Fax. (204)237-6048.

DAFNIOTIS, Olga; Clinique d'Orthopedie, 4370 Cote Rosemont, Trois-Rivieres QC G8Y 0A5; Sher'86; CSPQ; FRCSC; OrthSurg (Arthroplasty). Staff, Centre Hospitalier Regional de Trois-Rivieres; Langs: English; French; (819)374-5111; Fax. (819)374-8719.

DAFOE, Joan M; 9-65 Angeline St N, Lindsay ON K9V 5N7; Wes'03; CCFP; (705)324-8212; Fax. (705)324-8223.

DAFOE, William; Edmonton Clinic Health Academy, 2 590-11405 87 Ave NW, Edmonton AB T6G 1C9; McM'78; FACP; FACC; FRCPC; PhysMed&Rehab (Cardiac Rehabilitation). Med Dir Cardiac Rehab Division, University of Alberta Hospital; Staff, Edmonton Clinic Health Academy; (780)248-5844; Fax. (780)248-5845; williamdafoe@cha.ab.ca.

DAG-ELLAMS, Ugonwa; Kelso Lake Med Centre, 112-330 Bronte St S, Milton ON L9T 7X1; Giessen (Germany)'82; CCFP; (905)876-1011

DAGENAIS, Caroline; CSSS du Suroît, 150 rue Saint-Thomas, Salaber-de-Valleyf QC J6T 6C1; Sher'92; CSPQ; FRCPC; Anes. Staff, Centre Hospitalier Régional du Suroît; (450)371-9920

DAGENAIS, Francois; Hôpital Laval, 2725 ch Sainte-Foy, Quebec QC G1V 4G5; Mon'90; CSPQ; FRCSC; GenSurg; Cardiovasc&ThorSurg (P.Q.); CardSurg. Staff, Hôpital Laval; (418)656-4717

DAGENAIS, Gilles; Hôpital Laval, 2725 ch Sainte-Foy, Quebec QC G1V 4G5; Mon'64; CSPQ; Cardiol (P.Q.). Staff, Hôpital Laval; Head Dept of Med, Universite de Montreal; (418)656-8711; Fax. (418)656-4581.

DAGENAIS, Louis J; Clinique Med Robinson, 4 rue Robinson N, Granby QC J2G 8Z9; Sher'86; FRCS; CSPQ; Urol. Ac Member, Centre Hospitalier de Granby; Ac Member, Hôpital Brome-Missisquoi-Perkins; (450)372-1818; Fax. (450)770-8567.

DAGENAIS, Louis J; CHUM-Hop St-Luc, 1058 rue Saint-Denis, Montreal QC H2X 3J4; Mon'73; CCFP; Staff, Centre Hospitalier l'Université De Montréal (CHUM) - Hôpital Saint-luc; (514)890-8323; Fax. (514)412-7362.

DAGENAIS, Michel H; CHUM-Hop St-Luc, 1058 rue Saint-Denis, Montreal QC H2X 3J4; Mon'83; MSc; CSPQ; FRCSC; GenSurg (Liver & Pancreas Surgery). adj Chef chir gén, Centre Hospitalier l'Université De Montréal (CHUM) - Hôpital Saint-luc; assoc Prof, Universite de Montreal; Langs: Bilingual(French/English); (514)890-8000 x36146; Fax. (514)412-7380.

DAGENAIS, Michel; Phlebocentre de Vinci, 303-1991 rue Leonard-de-Vinci, Sainte-Julie QC J3E 1Y9; Mon'85; (450)649-7557

DAGENAIS, Nathalie; Clinique Fam de St-Hyacinthe, 2955 boul Laframboise, Saint-Hyacinthe QC J2S 4Z3; Mon'87; Staff, Centre Hospitalier Honore-Mercier; Langs: Bilingual(French/English); (450)774-4611; Fax. (450)773-9913.

DAGENAIS, Pierre; Clinique Med Domus Medica, 411-5601 rue Belanger, Montreal QC H1T 1G3; Mon'86; MSc(Clin.Sciences); PhD; FRCPC; IntMed; Rheum. Asst Scientific Dir, AETMIS Quebec; assoc Prof, Universite de Montreal; Langs: English; (514)256-5011; Fax. (514)259-7903.

DAGENAIS, Valerie; Ctr Hosp de Lasalle, 8585 tsse Champlain, LaSalle QC H8P 1C1; Mon'04; Staff, Centre Hospitalier de LaSalle; (514)362-8000

DAGG, Paul; Royal Inland Hosp, 417-311 Columbia St, Kamloops BC V2C 2T1; Tor'84; FRCPC; Psy. Consultant Staff, Royal Inland Hospital; Staff, Tertiary Mental Health Services; (250)314-2730

DAGHER, Alain; MUHC-Montreal Neurology Inst, 3801 rue University, Montreal QC H3A 2B4; Tor'89; FRCPC; Neur. Staff, McGill University Health Centre - Montreal Neurological Hospital; (514)398-1726; Fax. (514)398-8948.

DAGHER, Chady; CSSS de la Baie-des-Chaleurs, RR 2 419 boul Perron, Maria QC G0C 1Y0; Beirut (Lebanon)'00; Otol (P.Q.). Staff, CSSS de la Baie-des-Chaleurs; (418)759-3443; Fax. (418)759-5180.

DAGHER, Eric; CHUM-Hop St Luc, 1058 rue Saint-Denis, Montreal QC H2X 3J4; Mon'95; Staff, Centre Hospitalier l'Université De Montréal (CHUM) - Hôpital Saint-luc; (514)890-8000 x34444

DAGHISTANI, Razan; Univ Hlth Network-Toronto Western Hosp, 399 Bathurst St, Toronto ON M5T 2S8; (Saudi Arabia)'03; FRCPC; DiagRad. Staff, Toronto Western Hospital - University Health Network; (416)603-2581

DAGINAWALA, Khatija; Ctr Med L'Acadie, 101A-9825 boul de l'Acadie, Montreal QC H4N 2W2; South Gujarat (India)'76; Staff, Hôpital Sainte Anne de Beaupré; (514)336-6655; Fax. (514)336-6659.

DAGNAULT, Anne; CHUQ-Hotel-Dieu de Quebec, 11 Cote Du Palais, Quebec QC G1R 2J6; Laval'99; FRCPC; RadOncol (Breast Cancer). Staff, Centre Hospitalier Universitaire de Québec (CHUQ) - Siege Social; (418)691-5264; anne.dagnault@mail.chuq.qc.ca.

DAGNONE, A Joel; Trillium Health Centre, 406-190 Sherway Dr, Etobicoke ON M9C 5N2; Qns'98; FRCSC; Urol (Endourology). (416)622-2700; Fax. (416)622-4355.

DAGNONE, Jeffrey; Kingston Gen Hosp, 76 Stuart St, Kingston ON K7L 2V7; Wes'02; FRCPC; EmergMed. Staff, Kingston General Hospital; (613)548-2368

DAGNONE, L Eugene; Hotel-Dieu Hosp, 166 Brock St, Kingston ON K7L 5G2; Qns'68; FACEP; FRCPC; EmergMed. Staff, Hotel-Dieu Hospital; Assoc Dean Regional Education, Queen's University; (613)533-6000 x78452; Fax. (613)548-3204.

DAGNONE, R Vico; London HSC-Victoria Hosp, PO Box 5010 Stn B E1 102-800 Commissioners Rd E, London ON N6A 5W9; Qns'06; FRCPC; EmergMed. Staff, London Health Sciences Centre - Victoria Campus; (519)685-8500

DAGUIO, Glenn; Kenderdine Med Clinic, 110-1804 Mcormond Dr, Saskatoon SK S7S 0A6; (306)934-6606

DAHAN, Aime; Lakeshore Gen Hosp, 160 av Stillview, Pointe-Claire QC H9R 2Y2; Mon'92; Staff, Lakeshore General Hospital - Pointe Claire; Langs: Hebrew; English; Spanish; (514)630-2225 x1199; Fax. (514)630-2080.

DAHAN, Benjamin; Hôpital Anna-Laberge, 200 boul Brisebois, Chateauguay QC J6K 4W8; Mon'03; Neur. Staff, Hôpital Anna-Laberge; (450)699-2425; Fax. (450)699-2525.

DAHAN, Karen; Queen Elizabeth Urgent Care, 2111 av Northcliffe, Montreal QC H4A 3K6; Ott'98; CCFP; Staff, Lakeshore General Hospital - Pointe Claire; (514)481-4343

DAHAN, Karen; Ctr Hospitalier de Lasalle, 8585 Tsse Champlain, LaSalle QC H8P 1C1; Sher'06; CCFP; Centre Hospitalier de LaSalle; (514)362-8000

DAHAN, Marc-Albert; The Moncton Hosp, 135 MacBeath Ave, Moncton NB E1C 6Z8; Laval'90; CCFP; FCFP; Staff, The Moncton Hospital; (506)383-9563

DAHAN, Michael H; MUHC-Royal Victoria Hosp, F6 58-687 av des Pins O, Montreal QC H3A 1A1; Stoney Brook(N.Y.USA) (USA)'96; BA; FACOG; FRCSC; ObstGyn (Infertility Endocrinology). adj Prof, McGill University Health Centre - Royal Victoria Hospital; Langs: Spanish; French; (514)843-1650 x36813; Fax. (514)843-1496.

DAHAN, Philippe; CSSS de Laval, 1755 boul Rene-Laennec, Laval QC H7M 3L9; Mon'01; CSPQ; FRCSC; OrthSurg. Staff, Hopital de la Cite de la santé; (450)668-1010

DAHAN, Valerie; Institut de Readaptation de Mo, 6300 av de Darlington, Montreal QC H3S 2J4; Mon'01; FRCPC; PhysMed&Rehab. Staff, Institut de Réadaptation Gingras-Lindsay de Montréal; (514)340-2085

DAHCHE, Khaled M; Greenbank Med Centre, 108-139 Greenbank Rd, Ottawa ON K2H 9A5; Galway (Ireland)'03; FRCPC; IntMed. (613)695-5540

DAHCHE, Tarek; Queensway-Carleton Hosp, 3045 Baseline Rd, Ottawa ON K2H 8P4; Galway (Ireland)'03; FRCPC; IntMed. Staff, Queensway Carleton Hospital; (613)721-2000

DAHDAH, Nagib S; Hôpital Ste-Justine, 3175 ch Cote-Ste-Catherine, Montreal QC H3T 1C5; Beirut (Lebanon)'88; CSPQ; FRCPC; Cardiol. Staff, Hôpital Ste-Justine; (514)345-4931 x5403; Fax. (514)345-4896.

DAHDOUH, Elias; Hôp Ste-Justine, 3175 ch Cote-Sainte-Catherine, Montreal QC H3T 1C5; Beirut (Lebanon)'97; Staff, Hôpital Ste-Justine; (514)345-4931

DAHER, Antoine; 200 boul Brisebois, Chateauguay QC J6K 4W8; Beyrouth (Lebanon)'86; DA; Staff Anes, Hôpital Anna-Laberge; Langs: Arabic; English; (450)699-2425; Fax. (450)699-2525; antoined12@gmail.com.

DAHER, Samer; Clin la Cite Medicale-Montreal, 1905-2001 av McGill College, Montreal QC H3A 1G1; Laval'92; Staff Family Med, Centre Hospitalier de Chandler; (514)788-6484

DAHER MATTA, Giselle; Hop du Haut-Richelieu, 920 du Seminaire Blvd N, St-Jean-sur-Richel QC J3A 1B7; St Joseph (Lebanon)'87; Anes (P.Q.). Staff, Hôpital du Haut-Richelieu; Langs: Bilingual(French/English); (450)359-5000

DAHL, Eileen R; Erindale Health Centre, 2-50 Kenderdine Rd, Saskatoon SK S7N 3A1; Sask'81; CCFP; FCFP; Ac Staff, St Paul's Hospital (Grey Nuns) of Saskatoon; Ac Staff, Saskatoon City Hospital; Ac Staff, Royal University Hospital; Clin Lecturer ObstGyn, University of Saskatchewan; (306)934-6601; Fax. (306)934-6615; ehc@sasktel.net.

DAHL, Kenneth E; Dahl Clinic, PO Box 310, Magrath AB T0K 1J0; Alb'85; CCFP; (403)758-3363; Fax. (403)758-6845.

DAHL, Marshall A; 4145-2775 Laurel St, Vancouver BC V5Z 1M9; UBC'86; PhD; MD; BScPhysiol; FRCPC; IntMed; Endocrin&Metab. Staff Teacher Endocrin & Family Pract, University of British Columbia; (604)875-5577; Fax. (604)875-5188; marshall.dahl@vch.ca.

DAHLE, Colin T; Cobourg Health Centre, 203-316 King St E, Cobourg ON K9A 5R8; Sydney (Austria)'06; CCFP; Physician, Cobourg Health Centre.

DAHLGREN, Leanne S; BC Women's Hosp & Health Ctre, 2H30-4500 Oak St, Vancouver BC V6H 3N1; Sask'96; FRCSC; ObstGyn (Maternal Fetal Medicine). Staff, BC Women's Hospital & Health Centre; (604)875-2021

DAHLKE, Rita M; 1001-10 Ave SW, Calgary AB T2R 0B7; UBC'78; CCFP; FCFP; Langs: German; (403)221-8797

DAHLMANNS, Matthias; Seymour Med Clinic, 1530 7th Ave W, Vancouver BC V6G 1S3; (Germany)'91; (604)738-2151

DAHMAN, Jehad; 1058-200 Taunton Rd W, Whitby ON L1R 3H8; Damascus (Syria)'97; FAAP; Staff Pediatric Hospitalist, Humber River Regional Hospital - Finch Avenue Site; Langs: Arabic; (905)444-9636; Fax. (905)444-9853.

DAHMANE, Rafika; CSSS de Trois-Rivières, 1991 boul du Carmel, Trois-Rivieres QC G8Z 3R9; Mon'05; FRCPC; RadOncol. Staff, CSSS de Trois-Rivières; (819)371-5002

DAHMER, Mark R; Dingwall Med Group, PO Box 3011 Stn Main, Dryden ON P8N 2Z6; Wes'83; CCFP; FCFP; (807)223-2258; Fax. (807)223-4733; mdahmer@mail.drytel.net.

DAHN, Uwe; Queen Elizabeth II HSC-Halifax, 4875-1796 Summer St, Halifax NS B3H 3A7; Greifswald (Germany)'94; Staff, Queen Elizabeth II Health Sciences Centre - Halifax Infirmary Site; (902)473-4035

DAHRAB, Mishari M; IWK Health Centre, PO Box 9700 RPO CSC 5850-5980 Unviersity Ave, Halifax NS B3K 6R8; (Kuwait)'00; FRCSC; Ophth. Staff, IWK Health Centre; (902)470-8731; Fax. (902)470-7748.

DAIEN, David; Summerville Family Health Team, 211-190 Sherway Dr, Etobicoke ON M9C 5N2; McM'91; BSc; CCFP; Ac Staff, Trillium Health Centre - West Toronto; Aj Prof, University of Toronto; (416)621-9700; Fax. (416)621-4438; ddaien@thc.on.ca.

DAIGLE, Alain; 139 rue J.-Romuald Berube, Rimouski QC G0L 1B0; Laval'79.

DAIGLE, Carl; CHUM-Hotel-Dieu de Quebec, 11 Cote du Palais, Quebec QC G1R 2J6; Laval'99; CSPQ; FRCSC; GenSurg. Staff, Centre Hospitalier Universitaire de Québec (CHUQ) - Siege Social; (418)691-5370

DAIGLE, Christine; Clinique Med St-Alexandre, 200-2310 rue Saint-Louis, Gatineau QC J8T 5L7; Mon'90; BSc(Biology); Ac Staff, Hôpital de Gatineau; McGill University; (819)243-4500; Fax. (819)243-1369; cdaigle@medecinefamiliale.com.

DAIGLE, Emilien; Ctr Hosp Affilie-St-Sacrement, 1050 ch Sainte-Foy, Quebec QC G1S 4L8; Laval'65; Electroenceph (P.Q.); Neur (P.Q.). Ac Staff, Centre Hospitalier Affilié Universitaire de Québec - Hôpital du St-Sacrement; (418)682-7630; Fax. (418)682-7598.

DAIGLE, Jean-Pierre; Professional Arts Bldg, 425-100 Arden St, Moncton NB E1C 4B7; Laval'91; FRCSC; OrthSurg (Spine). (506)854-1115; Fax. (506)854-1119.

DAIGLE, Jean-Pierre; Clinique Isomed, 105-1205 rue Ampere, Boucherville QC J4B 7M6; Mon'82; FRCSC; PlasSurg (Maxillo Facial Surgery). Langs: English; (450)650-0165; Fax. (450)641-7331.

DAIGLE, Michel; Centre Hosp Honore-Mercier, 2750 boul Laframboise, Saint-Hyacinthe QC J2S 4Y8; McG'86; CSPQ; FRCSC; OrthSurg. Staff OrthSurg, Centre Hospitalier Honore-Mercier; (450)771-3366; Fax. (450)771-3553.

DAIGLE, Micheline; CSSS de Laval, 1755 boul Rene-Laennec, Laval QC H7M 3L9; Mon'73; Respir (P.Q.) (Hospitalist). Staff, Hopital de la Cite de la santé; (450)668-1010; Fax. (450)975-5545.

DAIGLE, Pierrette; 208-600 Dieppe Blvd, Dieppe NB E1A 9J8; Sher'05; CCFP; Staff, The Moncton Hospital.

DAIGLE, Robert J P; Southside Med Clinic, 640 Prospect St, Fredericton NB E3B 9M7; Laval'93; Langs: French; (506)460-1820; dr.robert.daigle@rogers.com.

DAIGLE, Samuel; 950 av Picot, Bathurst NB E2A 4Z9; Sher'98; CCFP; Staff, Hopital Regional Chaleur; Locum Tenens, Hôpital de l'Enfant-Jésus RHSJ; Locum Tenens, Hôpital de Tracadie-Sheila; Langs: English; (506)546-1018; Fax. (506)545-7723; samjulie@nb.sympatico.ca.

DAIGLE, Sebastien; Bathurst Shopping Mall, 210-1300 St. Peter Ave, Bathurst NB E2A 3A6; Sher'99; FRCSC; Urol. Langs: English; (506)546-3388; Fax. (506)548-0198.

DAIGLE, Steve; Clinique Med Belvedere, 202-2235 rue Galt O, Sherbrooke QC J1K 1K6; Sher'87; Staff, Centre Hospitalier Universitaire de Sherbrooke-Hôpital Hôtel-Dieu; Langs: English; (819)563-4244; Fax. (819)563-8924.

DAIGLE, Suzanne; Ctr Francois-Charon, 525 boul Wilfrid-Hamel, Quebec QC G1M 2S8; Laval'75; (418)529-9141; Fax. (418)649-3703.

DAIGLE, Sylvie; CSSS du Nord de Lanaudière, 1000 boul Sainte-Anne, St-Charles-Brromee QC J6E 6J2; Mon'98; CCFP; CCFP(E.M.); Staff, Centre Hospitalier Régional de Lanaudière; (450)759-8222

DAIGLE, Sylvie; 202-600 Dieppe Blvd, Dieppe NB E1A 0R9; Sher'02; CCFP; Langs: Bilingual(French/English); (506)853-3370

DAIGNAULT, Monique; Maison Mere des Soeurs de St-A, 1950 rue Provost, Lachine QC H8S 1P7; Mon'80; Staff, CSSS de Dorval-Lachine-Lasalle; (514)637-3783

DAIGNAULT, Peter G; Centre Med Brunswick, 955 boul Saint-Jean, Pointe-Claire QC H9R 5K3; McG'83; Assoc Physician Emerg & Family Med Dept, McGill University Health Centre - Montreal General Campus; Langs: French; (514)426-6677; Fax. (514)426-3323.

DAIGNAULT, Robert; CSSS de Rimouski-Neigette, CP 3150 succ Bureau Chef 150 av Rouleau, Rimouski QC G5L 5T1; Mon'68; Urol (P.Q.). Staff, Hôpital Regional Rimouski; (418)723-7851 x8491; Fax. (418)724-8615.

DAIGNEAULT, Andree; Clin des Maladies Affectives, 505-1575 boul Henri-Bourassa O, Montreal QC H3M 3A9; Sher'82; FRCPC; Psy. Chief Service des Maladies Affectives, Hôpital du Sacre-Coeur de Montréal; (514)338-4300; Fax. (514)338-4493.

DAIGNEAULT, Celine; 1211 av Bourgogne, Chambly QC J3L 1X3; Sher'83; Langs: Bilingual(French/English); (450)658-1116

DAIGNEAULT, Emilie; Clinique Med Asclepios, 750 Taylor Creek Dr, Orleans ON K1C 1T1; Ott'09; CCFP; Langs: Bilingual(English/French); (613)830-8388

DAIGNEAULT, Julie; GMF de l'Assomption, 201-814 boul L'Ange-Gardien, L'Assomption QC J5W 4M9; Mon'94; Staff, Centre Hospitalier Pierre le Gardeur; (450)589-5778

DAIGNEAULT, Linda; CLSC Olivier-Guimond, 5810 rue Sherbrooke E, Montreal QC H1N 1B2; Mon'79; (514)255-2365 x244

DAIGNEAULT, Maurice; CSSS de Saint-Jerome, 290 rue de Montigny, Saint-Jerome QC J7Z 5T3; Mon'86; CSPQ; Anes (P.Q.). Staff, Hôtel-Dieu de Saint-Jérôme; (450)431-8200

DAIGNEAULT, Patrick; CHUQ-Ctr Hosp Univ Laval, 2705 boul Laurier, Quebec QC G1V 4G2; Mon'97; FRCPC; Peds (Apnea); Respir. Staff, Centre Hospitalier Universitaire de Quebec-CHUL; (418)654-2282

DAILY, Robert F; King Street Med Arts Centre, 207-71 King St W, Mississauga ON L5B 4A2; McG'73; FRCSC; Ophth (Cataract Surgery). Ac Staff, Trillium Health Centre - West Toronto; (905)270-2621; Fax. (905)270-8669; eyeman2@rogers.com.

DAIN, Steven; London HSC-University Hosp, PO Box 5339 Stn B C3 107-339 Windermere Rd, London ON N6A 5A5; Tor'83; DABA; FRCPC; Anes (Pain Management). Staff, London Health Sciences Centre - Victoria Campus; Staff, London Health Sciences Centre - University Hospital; Staff, St Joseph's Hospital - St Joseph's Health Care; Chair Canadian Advisory Committe, ISO Technical Committee 121; Assoc Prof/Dir Anes Informatics, University of Western Ontario; (519)663-3384

DAINTON, Christopher J; Dr Christopher Dainton Med Cor, 921-650 Queens Quay W, Toronto ON M5V 3N2; Tor'07; CCFP; CCFP(E.M.); Staff, Chatham-Kent Health Alliance; Langs: Spanish.

DAITCHMAN, Julie F; 17-531 Atkinson Ave, Thornhill ON L4J 8L7; Tor'01; FRCPC; IntMed; Endocrin&Metab. Langs: Bilingual(English/French); (905)763-8660; Fax. (905)763-0708; julie.daitchman@imc.ca.

DAITER, Jeffrey; Oak Ridge Med Centre, 403-13291 Yonge St, Richmond Hill ON L4E 4L6; Wes'91; CCFP; FCFP; Staff EmergMed., Mackenzie Richmond Hill Hospital; (905)773-7759

DAITER, Ken; Whitby Medical, 4-3910 Brock St N, Whitby ON L1R 3E1; Tor'95; BSc; CCFP; (905)444-9493; Fax. (905)444-9174.

DAKE, Lauren A; Pandora Clinic, 922 Pandora Ave, Victoria BC V8V 3P3; McM'87; (250)294-6714; pandora.clinic@hotmail.cm.

DAKHIL, Christina M; Woodbridge Urgent Care Clinic, 2-4000 Hwy 7, Woodbridge ON L4L 8Z2; Tor'06; CCFP; (905)851-3777; Fax. (905)851-0682.

DAKIN, Edward B; Shouldice Hosp, 7750 Bayview Ave, Thornhill ON L3T 4A3; Otago (New Zealand)'65; MB ChB; FRCS(Ed); FRCSC; OrthSurg (Sports Medicine). Staff, Shouldice Hospital; (905)889-1174; edakin@sympatico.ca.

DAKIN HACHE, Kelly A; 720-5788 University Ave, Halifax NS B3H 1V8; Dal'00; FRCPC; AnatPath.

DAKSHINAMURTI, Shyamala L; Women's Hosp, WS012-735 Notre Dame Ave, Winnipeg MB R3E 0L8; Man'92; FRCPC; Peds (Neonatology). Staff, Health Sciences Centre.

DAKSHINAMURTI, Sowmya S; Victoria Gen Hosp, 2340 Pembina Hwy, Winnipeg MB R3T 2E8; Man'93; Staff, Victoria General Hospital; (204)269-3570

DAL CIN, Arianna; 504-304 Victoria Ave N, Hamilton ON L8L 5G4; McM'84; BSc; FRCSC; PlasSurg (Plastic & Reconstructive Surgery). Chief Plastic Surg/Associate Clinical Prof of Surgery, Hamilton Health Sciences Centre - Hamilton General Hospital; Langs: Portuguese; Italian; (905)526-0811; Fax. (905)526-0890.

DAL POZZO NIZARD, Sonia; Hôpital Ste-Justine, 3175 ch Cote-Ste-Catherine, Montreal QC H3T 1C5; paris (France)'87; Staff, Hôpital Ste-Justine; (514)345-4931 x4024

DALA, Gideon; Downtown Med Specialists, 140B Idylwyld Dr N, Saskatoon SK S7L 0Y7; Zaria (Nigeria)'78; MB BS; MSc; FCP (SA); FRCPC; IntMed (Diabetology); Endocrin&Metab. Staff, Royal University Hospital; Clinical Asst Prof Specialist Endocrinology, Saskatoon Health Region; Clinical Asst Prof Specialist Endocrinology, University of Saskatchewan; (306)933-3004; Fax. (306)244-4277.

DALAL, Bakul I; JPPN 1557-910 10th Ave W, Vancouver BC V5Z 1M9; Saurashtra (India)'77; FRCPC; GenPath. Consultant, BC Cancer Agency Vancouver Centre; Staff Path, Vancouver General Hospital - Centennial Pavillion; Associate Clin Prof, University of British Columbia; (604)875-4496

DALAL, Vikram; Thames Valley Family Hlth Team, RR 5 22262 Mill Rd, Mount Brydges ON N0L 1W0; Cal'01; CCFP; CCFP(E.M.); (519)264-2800; vikramd@symphatico.net.

DALBY, Lisa A; Tillsonburg Med Centre, 13-200 Broadway St, Tillsonburg ON N4G 5A7; Cork (Ireland)'94; CCFP; (519)842-4231; Fax. (519)842-3793.

DALCOURT, Jean-Pierre; CSSS de Trois-Rivières, 1991 boul du Carmel, Trois-Rivieres QC G8Z 3R9; Mon'68; CSPQ; Staff, CSSS de Trois-Rivières; (819)697-3333

DALE, John R; Kootenay Lake Med Clinic, 1140 Lakeside Dr, Nelson BC V1L 5Z3; (Ireland)'69; LRCPS; LM; (250)352-4666

DALENS, Bernard J; CHUQ-Ctr Hosp Univ Laval, 2206-2705 boul Laurier, Quebec QC G1V 4G2; Clemont Ferrand (France)'79; Staff, Centre Hospitalier Universitaire de Quebec-CHUL; (418)656-4141 x47565; Fax. (418)654-2774.

DALERY, Karl; CHUS-Hop Fleurimont, 3001 12e av N, Sherbrooke QC J1H 5N4; Mon'93; CSPQ; FRCPC; IntMed; Cardiol. Staff, Centre Hospitalier Universitaire de Sherbrooke-Hopital Fleurimont; Langs: Bilingual(French/English); (819)346-1110; Fax. (819)820-6897; karl.delary@usherbrooke.ca.

DALES, Robert E; The Ottawa Hosp-Gen Campus, Box 211 501 Smyth Rd, Ottawa ON K1H 8L6; Qns'78; DABSM; FRCPC; Respir (Sleep Medicine); IntMed. Prof Epidemiology & Med, University of Ottawa Heart Institute; Staff, The Ottawa Hospital - General Campus; (613)737-8198; Fax. (613)737-8537.

DALEY, Peter; Health Sciences Centre, 1J421-300 Prince Philip Dr, St. John's NL A1B 3V6; Dal'98; FRCPC; IntMed; InfectDis; MedMicrobiol. Staff, Health Sciences Centre; (709)777-2089

DALFEN, Ariel K; Mount Sinai Hosp, 600 University Ave, Toronto ON M5G 1X5; McM'98; FRCPC; Psy. Staff, Mount Sinai Hospital; (416)586-4800 x5131

DALFEN, Richard; St Mary's Hosp Centre, 3830 av Lacombe, Montreal QC H3T 1M5; McG'88; FRCPC; IntMed; Hem; MedOncol (P.Q.). Staff, St Mary's Hospital Centre; (514)345-3511 x5051

DALGARNO, S Michelle; Worksafe BC, 450-6450 Roberts St, Vancouver BC V6B 1J1; UBC'89; CCFP; (604)232-5948

DALGLEISH, P Douglas; Thornhill Square, 307-300 John St, Thornhill ON L3T 5W4; Tor'56; (905)886-3071; Fax. (905)886-3665.

DALINGHAUS, Kathleen; Klondyke Med Clinic, 1-3089 3rd Ave, Whitehorse YT Y1A 5B3; UBC'87; FRCPC; Anes. Staff, Klondyke Medical Clinic; (867)668-4065; Fax. (867)668-4067.

DALLA LANA, Eric J; Beaver Valley Clinic, PO Box 610, Fruitvale BC V0G 1L0; Alb'82; (250)367-9211; Fax. (250)367-7543.

DALLA LANA, John C; Fern Tree Clinic, PO Box 550, Qualicum Beach BC V9K 1T1; Alb'92; (250)752-6568; Fax. (250)752-6582.

DALLA LANA, Nathan G; Boundary Med Clinic, PO Box 400 7486 2nd St, Grand Forks BC V0H 1H0; Cal'07; CCFP; (250)442-8233

DALLAIRE, Annie; La Cite Medicale, 295-2600 boul Laurier, Quebec QC G1V 4M6; Sher'06; CCFP; Centre Hospitalier Beauce-Etchemin; (418)781-0480; Fax. (418)659-7072.

DALLAIRE, Chrystian; CHUQ-St-Francois d'Assise, 10 rue de l'Espinay, Quebec QC G1L 3L5; Laval'80; CSPQ; FRCPC; IntMed (Hepatology); Gastroent. Aj Chef gastro, Centre Hospitalier Universitaire De Québec - Pavillon De St-françois-d'assise; Clin Prof, Université Laval; Langs: English; (418)525-4444 x54422; Fax. (418)525-6338; c.dallaire@ens.chuq.qc.ca.

DALLAIRE, Dominic; Hop Regional D'Edmundston, 275 Hebert Blvd, Edmundston NB E3V 4E4; Laval'04; CCFP; Staff, Hôpital regional d'Edmundston; (506)739-2200

DALLAIRE, Frederic; CHUS-Hop Fleurimont, 3001 12e av N, Sherbrooke QC J1H 5N4; Laval'06; FRCPC; Peds; Cardiol. Staff, Centre Hospitalier Universitaire de Sherbrooke-Hopital Fleurimont; (819)346-1110

DALLAIRE, Gaetan; Centre Med Fafard Enr, 201-975 boul Monseigneur-de la, Baie-Saint-Paul QC G3Z 2W3; Laval'79; LMCC; Médecin traitant/Staff Cardiol Prog, CSSS de Charlevoix; (418)435-6310; Fax. (418)435-3203.

DALLAIRE, Genevieve; CSSS Haut-Richelieu-Rouville, 920 boul du Seminaire N, St-Jean-Sur-Richel QC J3A 1B7; Mon'01; MCFP(EM); ACLS; ATLS; CCFP; CCFP(E.M.); Staff Privileges, Hôpital du Haut-Richelieu; Emergency Family Med, Centre Hospitalier de Gaspe; Langs: Spanish; Arabic; Bilingual(French/English); (450)359-5000 x5175; gendallaire@hotmail.com.

DALLAIRE, Ghyslain; Hop Charles LeMoyne, 3120 boul Taschereau, Greenfield Park QC J4V 2H1; Laval'97; Staff, Hopital Charles LeMoyne; (450)466-5000

DALLAIRE, Lise; Carr Sante Le St-Laurent, 140-5300 boul Saint-Laurent, Sainte-Catherine QC J5C 1A8; Laval'81; (450)638-6383; Fax. (450)635-6359.

DALLAIRE, Louise C; CLSC de la Haute Yamaska, 294 rue Deragon, Granby QC J2G 5J5; Mon'76; (450)375-1442; Fax. (450)375-9345.

DALLAIRE, Luc; Centre Med Christ-Roi, 102-40 rte du President-Kenned, Levis QC G6V 6C4; Laval'74; ac Membre Obst, Hôtel-Dieu de Lévis; (418)833-4977; Fax. (418)833-9557.

DALLAIRE, Marie-Josee; Ctr Hosp de LaSalle, 8585 Terrasse Champlain, LaSalle QC H8P 1C1; Mon'01; FRCPC; DiagRad. Staff, Centre Hospitalier de LaSalle; (514)362-8000

DALLAIRE, Mario C; Centre Med de Baie-Comeau, 250 boul La Salle, Baie-Comeau QC G4Z 1S8; Laval'67; BSc; Assoc Member, Centre Hospitalier Régional Baie-Comeau; Consultant, Alcoa; (418)296-9681; mario.dallaire@alcoa.com.

DALLAIRE, Mario; CSSSG-Hop de Gatineau, CP 2000 Succ Bureau-Chef 909 boul de la Verendrye O, Gatineau QC J8P 7H2; Sher'88; FRCPC; IntMed. Staff, Hôpital de Gatineau; (819)561-8100; Fax. (819)561-8313; mario_dallaire@videotron.ca.

DALLAIRE, Michel H; CLSC Mer et Montagnes, 600 av William-May, Murdochville QC G0E 1W0; Laval'65; Fam Med, Installation CLSC Gaspe; (418)784-2572

DALLAIRE, Michel; CLSC Verdun, 6161 rue Laurendeau, Montreal QC H4E 3X6; Mon'80; Ac Staff, Centre Hospitalier de Verdun; Supvr, Unite de Medicine Familiale; Langs: Bilingual(French/English); (514)766-0546 x3228; Fax. (514)765-3265.

DALLAIRE, Michel; Clinique Med Saitn-Louis, 220-3165 ch Saint-Louis, Quebec QC G1W 4R4; Laval'92; Staff, CSSS de la Matapedia; (418)653-6000

DALLAIRE, Michelle; CLSC des Maskoutains, 1015 rue Gauthier, Saint-Hyacinthe QC J2S 8T2; Sher'75; Médecin Palliative Care, Centre Hospitalier l'Université de Montréal (CHUM) - Hôpital Notre-Dame; (514)287-7593

DALLAIRE, Real; Clinique Dr R Dallaire, 89 rue Industrielle, Albanel QC G8M 3H6; Laval'67; Med Staff, Centre Maria-Chapdelaine - CH de Dolbeau-Mistassini; (418)279-5563; Fax. (418)279-5563; frances@destination.ca.

DALLAIRE, Robert; 48 Saint-Cajetan, Armagh QC G0R 1A0; Sher'73; Langs: Bilingual(French/English); (418)466-2246; Fax. (418)466-3053.

DALLAIRE, Stephane; Queens Student Hlth Ontario, 146 Stuart St, Kingston ON K7L 3N6; Ott'07; CCFP; CCFP(E.M.); Staff, Brockville General Hospital - Charles Street; Langs: Bilingual(English/French); (613)533-6750; Fax. (613)533-6740.

DALLAL, Abdallah; CSSS de Saint-Jerome, 290 rue de Montigny, Saint-Jerome QC J7Z 5T3; Alexandria (Egypt)'82; MB ChB; MD; MSc; FRCPC; Psy (Clinical Research). Staff Medical Educ of Psy, Hôtel-Dieu de Saint-Jérôme; Langs: English; French; (450)431-8200; Fax. (450)431-8207.

DALLARD, Laurence-Raphaelle; CSSS de Rimouski-Neigette, CP 3150 succ Bureau Chef 150 av Rouleau, Rimouski QC G5L 5T1; Laval'05; FRCPC; Psy. Staff, Hôpital Regional Rimouski; (418)723-7851; Fax. (418)724-8616.

DALLAS, Karen; Royal Univ Hosp, 103 Hospital Dr, Saskatoon SK S7N 0W8; McG'06; MDCM; FRCPC; HemPath. Staff, Royal University Hospital; (306)655-1539

DALLING, Gordon N; Oakfield Med Clinic, 102-1021 Court Ave, Winnipeg MB R2P 1V7; Man'93; CCFP.

DALLY, Ghassan Y; South Common Med Ctr, 3-2110 Burnhamthorpe Rd W, Mississauga ON L5L 5Z5; Tor'00; MSc; CCFP; Langs: Arabic; (905)820-3209; Fax. (905)820-2576.

DALOISE, Robert A; Sturgeon Community Hosp, 201 Boudreau Rd, St. Albert AB T8N 6C4; Alb'94; Staff Emerg, Sturgeon Community Hospital; (780)460-6228; Fax. (780)460-6376.

DALOZE, Pierre M; CHUM-Hop Notre-Dame, 1560 rue Sherbrooke E, Montreal QC H2L 4M1; Louvain (Belgium)'61; CSPQ; FRCSC; GenSurg (Transplantation). Chef Dept of Surg Kidney & Pancreas, Centre Hospitalier l'Université de Montréal (CHUM) - Hôpital Notre-Dame; Fellow et AST, American Society Transplant Surgeons; Prof, Universite de Montreal; Langs: English; French; (514)890-8200; Fax. (514)412-7637.

DALOZE, Thierry; MUHC-Royal Victoria Hosp, S5.05-687 av des Pins O, Montreal QC H3A 1A1; McG'92; CSPQ; FRCPC; Anes. Staff, McGill University Health Centre - Royal Victoria Hospital; (514)934-1934 x34880; Fax. (514)843-1723.

DALPE, Linda; Hôpital de l'Enfant-Jésus RHSJ, 1 boul St-Pierre O, Caraquet NB E1W 1B6; Mon'97; CCFP; FCFP; Staff, Hôpital de l'Enfant-Jésus RHSJ; Langs: Bilingual(French/English); (506)726-2152; Fax. (506)726-2151; linda.dalpe@gmail.com.

DALPE-CHARRON, Michel H; Clinique Med de Cheneville, 34 rue Principale, Cheneville QC J0V 1E0; Ott'70; BA; Langs: English; (819)428-1222; Fax. (819)428-1223; micheldalpe-charron@hotmail.ca.

DALRYMPLE, Sharon A; Centre Med Brunswick, 203-955 Boul Saint-Jean, Pointe-Claire QC H9R 5K3; McG'83; CSPQ; MDCM; FRCSC; GenSurg (Breast Surgery). Ac Staff, Lakeshore General Hospital - Pointe Claire; Langs: English; French; (514)426-8181; Fax. (514)426-9059; cliniquedusein@bellnet.ca.

DALSHAUG, Gregory B; Royal University Hosp, 103 Hospital Dr, Saskatoon SK S7N 0W8; Sask'94; FRCSC; GenSurg; CardSurg. Staff, Royal University Hospital; (306)966-5644; Fax. (306)966-6932.

DALSIN, Judith; Victoria Mental Health Centre, 2328 Trent St, Victoria BC V8R 4Z3; Sask'84; Psy (Emergency Psychiatry). (250)370-8155; Fax. (250)370-8199.

DALTON, Douglass; CLSC Metro, 3e-1801 boul de Maisonneuve O, Montreal QC H3H 1J9; McG'81; CSPQ; CCFP; FCFP; Ac Staff G. P., St Mary's Hospital Centre; Aj Prof Family Med, McGill University; Langs: English; French; (514)934-0354; Fax. (514)934-6155.

DALTON, Shelley; James Paton Mem Hosp, 1255 Trans Canada Hwy, Gander NL A1V 1P7; Mem'94; FRCPC; DiagRad. Staff, James Paton Memorial Hospital; (709)256-2500

DALTON, Susan M; Dr L A Miller Centre, 100 Forest Rd, St. John's NL A1A 1E5; Mem'05; FRCPC; Psy. (709)777-6555

DALWADI, Bela; Central Nfld Reg Hlth Centre, 50 Union St, Grnd-Falls-Windsor NL A2A 2E1; Baroda (India)'01; MB BS; Staff, Central Newfoundland Regional Health Centre.

DALY, Andrew; Tom Baker Cancer Centre, CC 107E-1331 29th St NW, Calgary AB T2N 4N1; McG'94; BSc; FRCPC; IntMed (Bone Marrow Transplant); Hem. Staff, Peter Lougheed Centre; Staff, Foothills Medical Centre; Staff, Rockyview General Hospital; Staff, Tom Baker Cancer Centre; Langs: English; French; (403)943-2501; Fax. (403)943-5520; andrew.daly@albertahealthservices.ca.

DALY, Bruce G; 524 First Ave S, Kenora ON P9N 1W5; Man'79; (807)468-3600; Fax. (807)468-4440; bdaly@voyageur.ca.

DALY, Donald S; Medical-Dental Bldg, 303-1120 Yates St, Victoria BC V8V 3M9; Qns'66; FRCPC; IntMed; Gastroent. Staff, Royal Jubilee Hospital; (250)381-7703; Fax. (250)381-9902; dalyds@shaw.ca.

DALY, J Michael; Dr Georges-L Dumont Reg Hosp, 330 av Universite, Moncton NB E1C 2Z3; Dal'72; FRCPC; DiagRad (Interventional Radiology). Ac Staff Radiol, Dr Georges-L-Dumont University Hospital Centre; (506)862-4191; Fax. (506)862-4544.

DALY, Joyce L; Coronation Health Centre, 7-715 Coronation Blvd, Cambridge ON N1R 7R1; McM'91; BSc(PhysTher); FRCSC; OrthSurg. Staff, Cambridge Memorial Hospital; (519)622-5849; Fax. (519)622-7392.

DALY, Lanval J; St Joseph's Health Centre, 336-30 The Queensway, Toronto ON M6R 1B5; Qns'71; BSc; MD; FRCSC; ObstGyn. Staff, St Joseph's Health Centre; Teach Staff, University of Toronto; (416)530-6152; Fax. (416)530-6830.

DALY, Laura; East Wellingon Family Hlth Tea, 6 Thompson Cres, Erin ON N0B 1T0; McM'05; CCFP; (519)833-9396

DALY, Lyle F; Phoenix Med Centre, 211-2155 10th Ave, Prince George BC V2M 5J6; McM'74; FRCPC; Neur. Ac Staff, University Hospital of Northern British Columbia; (250)562-2989; Fax. (250)562-6564.

DALY, Mary M; Health Sciences Centre, 300 Prince Philip Dr, St. John's NL A1B 3V6; Mem'81; FRCPC; Anes. Staff, Health Sciences Centre; (709)777-6540

DALY, Meghan ; Women's College Hosp, 76 Grenville St, Toronto ON M5S 1B2; Ott'08; CCFP; Staff, Women's College Hospital; (416)323-6060

DALY, Patricia C; Vancouver Coastal H Authority, 800-601 Broadway W, Vancouver BC V5Z 4C2; Tor'85; FRCPC; CommunMed; Public Health & Preventive Med. (604)714-5686; Fax. (604)731-2756.

DALY, Paul A; Univ Hlth Network-Toronto Gen, 6E242-200 Elizabeth St, Toronto ON M5G 2C4; Wes'78; FRCPC; Cardiol. Ac Staff, Toronto General Hospital - UHN; Asst Prof Med, University of Toronto; (416)340-5172; Fax. (416)595-1614.

DALZIEL, Christine E; Oak Bay Family Physicians Ltd, 101-1640 Oak Bay Ave, Victoria BC V8R 1B2; Qns'77; (250)598-6744; Fax. (250)598-6778.

DALZIEL, Peter; Atrium Prof Bldg, 307-190 Cundles Rd E, Barrie ON L4M 4S5; Qns'77; Ac Staff, Royal Victoria Regional Health Centre; (705)739-1156; Fax. (705)739-9013.

DAM, Hoa Van; CP 818 Succ R, Montreal QC H2S 3M4; Saigon (Vietnam)'72; MD; Staff, Hopital Louis-H Lafontaine; Staff, Hôpital Chinois de Montréal.

DAM, Olivia; Lansdowne Professional Ctr II, 325-3066 Shelbourne St, Victoria BC V8R 6T9; Qns'00; FRCSC; Ophth. (250)598-9984; Fax. (250)598-6237; droliviadam@shaw.ca.

DAMACEN SOPLIN, Harvey I; Medicine in Motion Med Centre, 5-121 Ilsley Ave, Dartmouth NS B3B 1S4; Trujillo (Peru)'95; Staff, Medicine in Motion Medical Centre; (902)468-2774

DAMANT, Ronald W; University of Alberta Hosp, 2E437-8440 112 St NW, Edmonton AB T6G 2B7; Alb'90; BSc; FRCPC; IntMed; Respir. Staff, University of Alberta Hospital; Asst Prof Med/Dir Pre Clinical Education, University of Alberta; (780)407-3439; Fax. (780)407-6384.

DAMASO, Humbertino; Ctr Hosp de Verdun, 4000 boul Lasalle, Verdun QC H4G 2A3; Laval'93; Staff, Centre Hospitalier de Verdun; (514)362-1000

DAMBORAGAMA, Shyamali; Avenue Med Clinic, 221 Brant Ave, Brantford ON N3T 3J2; (Sri Lanka)'90; CCFP; Langs: Sinhalese; (519)753-8666 x301; Fax. (519)753-6880.

DAMBREVILLE, Etzer; Clinique Med du Boulevard, 1768 boul des Laurentides, Laval QC H7M 2P7; Guadalajara (Mexico)'79; Staff, Hôpital du Sacre-Coeur de Montréal; (450)663-8300

DAMBRY, Thierry B R; CSSS de Maskinongé, 450 2e rue, Louiseville QC J5V 1V3; Paris (France)'89; Staff, CSSS de Maskinongé; (819)228-2731

DAMESTOY, Nicole; ASSS de Laval, Tour A 2E-800 boul Chomedey, Laval QC H7V 3Y4; McG'88; FRCPC; CommunMed (Public Health). (450)978-2121 x2067; Fax. (450)978-2100.

DAMGAARD, H Neils; Associate Clinic, 4620 50 Ave, Innisfail AB T4G 1A6; Cal'76; CCFP; (403)227-3301; Fax. (403)227-2856.

DAMJI, Alkarim; 11-2687 Kipling Ave, Etobicoke ON M9V 5G6; Tor'89; CCFP; FCFP; Staff, William Osler Health System - Etobicoke General Hospital; Langs: Gujarati; Hindi; Swahili; (416)744-0461; Fax. (416)744-3356.

DAMJI, Karim F; Royal Alexandra Hosp, 2317 ATC-10240 Kingsway Ave NW, Edmonton AB T5H 3V9; UBC'87; MBA; FRCSC; Ophth (Cataract & Glaucoma). Staff, Royal Alexandra Hospital; (780)735-4200; Fax. (780)735-5242; alice.tieszen@albertahealthservices.ca.

DAMJI, Mehboob; Parkway Prof Bldg, 60 Centennial Pky S, Stoney Creek ON L8G 2C5; Ott'83; Langs: Hindi; Gujarati; Swahili; (905)662-2231; Fax. (905)662-1022.

DAMJI, Nazim F; Queensway Prof Centre, 306-190 Sherway Dr, Etobicoke ON M9C 5N2; Glasgow (Scotland)'78; DAB; FRCPC; IntMed; Hem. Staff, Trillium Health Centre - West Toronto; Langs: Gujarati; (416)695-4188

DAMJI, Rahim; Crystal Ridge Fam Med Clinic, 4-55 Wheatland Trail, Strathmore AB T1P 1R7; Alb'04; BMedSci; CCFP; Physician, Coral Springs Medical Clinic; (403)943-5911; Fax. (403)934-6672.

DAMJI, Zumil; Brockville Gen Hosp, 75 Charles St, Brockville ON K6V 1S8; McM'07; CCFP; CCFP(E.M.); CCFP; Staff, Brockville General Hospital - Charles Street; (613)345-5645

DAMLA, Garo; The Court, 301-2863 Ellesmere Rd, Scarborough ON M1E 5E9; Vienna (Austria)'82; FRCSC; ObstGyn (Hysteroscopy). Staff, Rouge Valley Health System - Centenary Health Centre Site; (416)282-0132; Fax. (416)282-2126.

DAMMERMANN, Scott; The Health Centre of Maple, 2810 Major Mackenzie Dr, Maple ON L6A 3L2; Man'90; Court Staff, Mackenzie Richmond Hill Hospital; Langs: German; (905)832-3838; Fax. (905)832-9097.

DAMODHARAN, Senthil; Child & Youth Services, 1680 Albert St, Regina SK S4P 2S6; Bharathiar (India)'95; FRCPC; Psy. (306)766-6700; Fax. (306)766-6944.

DAMPHOUSSE, Amelie; Hôpital Ste-Justine, 3175 ch cote-Sainte-Catherine, Montreal QC H3T 1C5; Mon'05; FRCPC; DiagRad. Staff, Hôpital Ste-Justine; (514)345-4931

DAMPHOUSSE, Andreanne; CSSS de Papineau, 155 rue Maclaren E, Gatineau QC J8L 0C2; Mon'09; CCFP; DiagRad. Staff, Hôpital de Papineau; Staff, CH-CHSLD de Papineau - Pavillon du centre hospitalier; (819)986-4415

DAMUDE, Leslie R; Oxford Med Centre, 312 Oxford St W, London ON N6H 4N7; Wes'80; DTMH(Liverpool); Ac Staff FamMed, St Joseph's Hospital - St Joseph's Health Care; Langs: French; (519)432-6786; Fax. (519)432-3292.

DAMUS, A Michael; Uxbridge Family Health Clinic, B-2 Elgin Park Dr, Uxbridge ON L9P 0B1; Qns'91; CCFP; FCFP; Fam Med, Markham Stouffville Hospital - Uxbridge Site; Ac Staff, Markham Stouffville Hospital; Langs: German; Spanish; (905)852-1009; Fax. (905)852-3531; damus@powergate.ca.

DAMYANOVA, Anastasiya; Hôtel-Dieu de Sorel, 400 av de l'Hôtel-Dieu, Sorel-Tracy QC J3P 1N5; (Bulgaria)'98; CCFP; CCFP(E.M.); Staff, Hôtel-Dieu de Sorel; (450)746-6000 x8

DAN, Ratna; C M L, 300 Harwood Ave S, Ajax ON L1S 2J1; (Jamaica)'79; MB BS; FRCPC; DiagRad. Langs: Spanish; French; (905)426-8947

DAN, Wai Ling; PO Box 1472 Stn A, Comox BC V9M 8A2; UBC'94; CCFP; FCFP; (250)703-3324; nature@island.net.

DANAIS BROWN, Jocelyne M; St Boniface Gen Hosp, D1048-409 Tache Ave, Winnipeg MB R2H 2A6; Man'90; CCFP; FCFP; Staff, St Boniface General Hospital; Langs: Bilingual(English/French); (204)235-3910; Fax. (204)237-9057.

DANAN, Anny; 4886 rue Jarry E, Saint-Leonard QC H1R 1X9; Grenoble (France)'72; (514)327-4440; Fax. (514)327-4364.

DANAYAN, Karoon C; Danforth Pediatrics, 100-235 Danforth Ave, Toronto ON M4K 1N2; Tor'04; FRCPC; Peds; Rheum. Langs: Armenian; (416)466-1311; Fax. (416)466-9629; 235kids@gmail.com.

DANCE, Erica A; Royal Alexandra Hosp, 541-10240 Kingsway NW, Edmonton AB T5H 3V9; Alb'98; FRCPC; EmergMed. Staff, Royal Alexandra Hospital; (780)735-4442; Fax. (780)735-4916.

DANCEA, Adrian B; MUHC-Montreal Children's Hosp, D 365-2300 rue Tupper, Montreal QC H3H 1P3; Ott'92; CSPQ; FRCPC; Peds (Pediatric Cardiology); Cardiol. div Chef, McGill University Health Centre - Montreal Children's Hospital; Langs: French; Romanian; (514)412-4423; Fax. (514)412-4391.

DANCEA, Silvia L C; Sudbury Reg Hosp-Laurentian, 41 Ramsey Lake Rd, Sudbury ON P3E 5J1; Cluj-Ivapoca (Romania)'62; PhD; FRCPC; AnatPath. Staff, Health Sciences North-Laurentian Site; Langs: Spanish; Romanian; French; (705)674-3181; Fax. (705)675-4780.

DANCEL, Mary Lou; JJ Turner Professional Bldg, 503-140 King St, Peterborough ON K9J 7Z8; Santo Tomas (Philippines)'72; DABPN; DAB; FRCPC; Psy (Child Psychiatry). Langs: Tagalog; (705)745-8705; Fax. (705)745-1055.

DANCEY, David R; Ashgrove Med Centre, 302-6633 Highway 7, Markham ON L3P 7P2; Tor'94; ABSM; FAASM; FCCP; FRCPC; IntMed (Sleep Medicine); Respir. Staff Respirology Concultant, Markham Stouffville Hospital; (905)471-4402; Fax. (905)471-1903.

DANCEY, Janet E; NCIC Clinical Trails Group, 10 Stuart St, Kingston ON K7L 2V5; Ott'88; BSc; FRCPC; IntMed; MedOncol. Staff, Hotel-Dieu Hospital; Staff, Kingston General Hospital; (613)533-6430; Fax. (613)533-6511.

DANCEY, Paul; Dr Charles A Janeway Child HC, 300 Prince Philip Dr, St. John's NL A1B 3V6; Mem'98; FRCPC; Peds; Rheum. Staff, Janeway Children's Health & Rehabilitation Centre; (709)777-4766

DANCOSE, Marc; Ctr d'Urgence Saint-Laurent, 200-1605 boul Marcel-Laurin, Saint-Laurent QC H4R 0B7; Mon'70; Staff, Hôpital du Sacre-Coeur de Montréal; (514)747-2555

DANCOSE, Robin; La Clinique Access Md, 200-17001 aut Transcanadienne, Kirkland QC H9H 5J1; McG'87; BSc; MDCM; Centre Hospitalier de LaSalle; Member, CHSLD Ste-Therese; Med Consultant en Enterprise, S A Q/Services Techniques; Clin Asst Prof Family Med, McGill University; Langs: English; French; (514)694-4644; Fax. (514)694-4646; robindancose@videotron.ca.

DANDAVINO, Andre-Hector; Ctr Medi Soleil St-Jean-Sur-Ri, 120-383 boul du Seminaire N, St-Jean-sur-Richel QC J3B 8C5; Mon'74; Ac Staff, Hôpital du Haut-Richelieu; (450)347-7557; Fax. (450)347-3099.

DANDAVINO, Mylene; MUHC-Montreal Children's Hosp, 2300 rue Tupper, Montreal QC H3H 1P3; McG'04; FRCPC; Peds. Staff, McGill University Health Centre - Montreal Children's Hospital; (514)412-4400 x53333; Fax. (514)412-4271.

DANDAVINO, Raymond; Hop Maisonneuve-Rosemont, 5415 boul de l'Assomption, Montreal QC H1T 2M4; Mon'70; Nephrol (P. Q.) (Transplantation). Ac Staff, Hopital Maisonneuve-Rosemont; Clin Prof Med, Universite de Montreal; (514)252-3489; Fax. (514)255-3026; dandavino@sympatico.ca.

DANDEKAR, Anand; Health Plus Med Centre, 1075 Autumnwood Dr, Winnipeg MB R2J 1C6; Man'04; CCFP.

DANDEKAR, Masumi; Create Fertility Centre, 108-790 Bay St, Toronto ON M5G 1N8; Sydney (Australia)'07; CCFP; (416)929-1900; Fax. (416)929-7316.

DANDENAULT, Brigitte L M; Dr Georges-L Dumont Reg Hosp, 330 av Universite, Moncton NB E1C 2Z3; Sher'96; BSc; DPsy; FRCPC; Psy (Pediatric Psychiatry). Staff Ped Psy, Dr Georges-L-Dumont University Hospital Centre; Langs: Bilingual(English/French); (506)862-4177; Fax. (506)862-4325; bdandenault@yahoo.ca.

DANDINA, Sujith K; Pain Management Clinic, 9750 140 St, Surrey BC V3T 0G9; Manipal (India)'96; Staff, Surrey Memorial Hospital; Langs: Hindi; (604)582-4587

DANDOIS, Maxime G; CSSS du Rocher-Perce, CP 3300 451 rue Mgr Ross E, Chandler QC G0C 1K0; Laval'94; Chief Emerg, Centre Hospitalier de Chandler; Staff Teacher, Université Laval; (418)689-2261; Fax. (418)689-5049.

DANDONA, Kshitij; MUHC-Royal Victoria Hosp, 687 av des Pins O, Montreal QC H3A 1A1; McG'00; Cardiol; IntMed. Staff, McGill University Health Centre - Royal Victoria Hospital; (514)934-1934

DANDUGULA, Raghu M; Riverside Med Hlth Complex, PO Box 628, Turtleford SK S0M 2Y0; (Other Foreign)'96; CCFP; (306)845-2277; Fax. (306)845-4434.

DANDURAND, Caroline; CHUS-Hop Fleurimont, 3001 12e av N, Sherbrooke QC J1H 5N4; Sher'99; CCFP; CCFP(E.M.); Staff, Centre Hospitalier Universitaire de Sherbrooke-Hopital Fleurimont; (819)346-1110

DANDURAND, Ronald; Pitt Street Med Centre, 1335 Pitt St, Cornwall ON K6J 3T7; McG'84; ABIM(Med.); ABIM(Pulmonary); FRCPC; IntMed; Respir. Staff, McGill University Health Centre - Montreal Chest Institute; Staff, McGill University Health Centre - Royal Victoria Hospital; Staff, Lakeshore General Hospital - Pointe Claire; adj Prof Med., McGill University; Langs: Bilingual(English/French); (613)932-6163

DANEAU, Suzie; CSSS de Saint-Jerome, 290 rue de Montigny, Saint-Jerome QC J7Z 5T3; Mon'83; CSPQ; Anes (P.Q.). Staff, Hôtel-Dieu de Saint-Jérôme; (450)431-8444

DANEAULT, Benoit; CHUS-Hop Fleurimont, 3001 12e av N, Sherbrooke QC J1H 5N4; Sher'03; FRCPC; IntMed; Cardiol. Staff, Centre Hospitalier Universitaire de Sherbrooke-Hopital Fleurimont; (819)823-6947

DANEAULT, Helene; Centre Med Fontainebleau, 102-10 boul des Chateaux, Blainville QC J7B 1Z5; Sher'85; (450)419-8811; Fax. (450)419-7758.

DANEAULT, Mathieu; CSSS Drummond-Hop Sainte-Croix, 570 rue Heriot, Drummondville QC J2B 1C1; Laval'04; Staff, Hôpital Sainte-croix; (819)478-6464

DANEAULT, Michel; 1270 Rte 125, Ste-Julienne QC J0K 2T0; Mon'76; Staff, Centre Hospitalier de Verdun; (450)831-3887

DANEAULT, Nicole; CHUM-Hop Notre-Dame, GR 1166-1560 rue Sherbrooke E, Montreal QC H2L 4M1; Mon'80; CSPQ; FRCPC; Neur (Neuro Vascular). Neurologue, Centre Hospitalier l'Université De Montréal (CHUM) - Hôpital Saint-luc; Staff, Centre Hospitalier l'Université de Montréal (CHUM) - Hôpital Notre-Dame; Asst Clin Prof Neurol, Universite de Montreal; Langs: Bilingual(French/English); (514)890-8000 x26260; Fax. (514)412-7556; nicole.daneault.chum@ssss.gouv.qc.ca.

DANEAULT, Serge; CHUM-Hop Notre-Dame, 1560 rue Sherbrooke E, Montreal QC H2L 4M1; Sher'80; FRCPC; CommunMed. Staff, Centre Hospitalier l'Université de Montréal (CHUM) - Hôpital Notre-Dame; Clin Teach Staff Social & Preventive Med, Universite de Montreal; (514)890-8000 x26248; Fax. (514)412-7589; serge.daneault.chum@ssss.gouv.qc.ca.

DANELICE, Michele; Surrey Mem Hosp, 13750 96 Ave, Surrey BC V3V 1Z2; Mon'93; FRCPC; Anes. Staff, Surrey Memorial Hospital; Langs: Bilingual(French/English); (604)588-3367

DANEMAN, Alan; The Hosp For Sick Children, 555 University Ave, Toronto ON M5G 1X8; Witwatersrand (South Africa)'71; MB ChB; MRACR; FRCPC; DiagRad. Staff Radiol., The Hospital For Sick Children; Prof Radiol., University Of Toronto; (416)813-6922; Fax. (416)813-7591; alan.daneman@sickkids.ca.

DANEMAN, Denis; The Hosp For Sick Children, 555 University Ave, Toronto ON M5G 1X8; Witwatersrand (South Africa)'73; MB BCh; FRCPC; Peds (Pediatric Endocrinology); Endocrin&Metab. Chief Dept of Peds, The Hospital For Sick Children; Chair Peds/Prof, University of Toronto; (416)813-6122; Fax. (416)813-7479; denis.daneman@sickkids.ca.

DANEMAN, Nick; Sunnybrook Hlth Sciences Ctre, GW 106-2075 Bayview Ave, Toronto ON M4N 3M5; Tor'01; FRCPC; IntMed; InfectDis. Staff, Sunnybrook Health Sciences Centre; (416)480-4244

DANESCU, Liviu G; 108-21 Surrey St W, Guelph ON N1H 3R3; (Romania)'02; (519)763-6201

DANESCU, Septimiu C; Tillsonburg Dist Mem Hosp, 167 Rolph St, Tillsonburg ON N4G 3Y9; (Romania)'02; Staff, Tillsonburg District Memorial Hospital; Langs: Romanian; (519)842-3611; Fax. (519)842-4113.

DANESCU, Virgil; Windermere Clinic, 204-32450 Simon Ave, Abbotsford BC V2T 4J2; Craiova (Romania)'87; CCFP; Med Staff, Abbotsford Regional Hospital & Cancer Centre; Langs: Romanian; French; (604)859-6774

DANESHMEND, Deanna J; Kingston Family Health Team, 401-800 Princess St, Kingston ON K7L 5E4; Sask'95; CCFP; CCFP(E.M.); (613)650-5471; Fax. (613)650-5473.

DANET, Ioana M; Hop du Sacre-Coeur de Mtl, 5400 boul Gouin O, Montreal QC H4J 1C4; Mon'96; FRCPC; DiagRad. Staff, Hôpital du Sacre-Coeur de Montréal; (514)388-2222; Fax. (514)338-3541.

DANFORTH, Jay A; Transport Canada, 1140-9700 Jasper Ave NW, Edmonton AB T5J 4E6; Alb'71; BSc(Med.); DAvMed(Lond); Med Officer Civil Aviation Med, Transport Canada; (780)495-3848; Fax. (780)495-4905; jay.danforth@tc.gc.ca.

DANFORTH, Leonard R; Clergy Stret Family Phys, 71 Clergy St E, Kingston ON K7L 3J3; UBC'08; CCFP; (613)542-7858

DANG, Angela N; Clinique Med de l'Est Inc, 100-30 boul Saint-Joseph E, Montreal QC H2T 1G9; Mon'91; CCFP; FCFP; Langs: Vietnamese; (514)845-4240; Fax. (514)845-5493; quydon_nguyen@yahoo.com.

DANG, Bach-Tuyet T; Markham College Med Clinic, 307-474 College St, Toronto ON M6G 1A4; Wes'79; Court Staff, Toronto General Hospital - UHN; Langs: Vietnamese; (416)537-5100; Fax. (416)537-5800.

DANG, Bao Pham N; St Joseph's Gen Hosp, 2137 Comox Ave, Comox BC V9M 1P2; Cal'03; FRCPC; IntMed; Respir. Staff, St Joseph's General Hospital; (250)339-2242

DANG, Chi Bao; Rockyview Gen Hosp, 7007 14 St SW, Calgary AB T2V 1P9; Alb'02; FRCPC; Psy. Staff Psy, Rockyview General Hospital; (403)943-8704

DANG, Dinh Quang; 2630 rue Jean-Talon E, Montreal QC H2A 1V3; Saigon (Vietnam)'78; Langs: English; French; (514)721-2333; Fax. (514)721-2333.

DANG, Dinh Thien V; Clinique Med des 2 Tours, C14-1001 rue Universite, Montreal QC H3B 4L4; Mon'00; Staff, CSSS du Coeur de l'Isle Hôpital Jean-Talon; Langs: Vietnamese; (514)954-4444

DANG, Dong My; 2520 boul de la Cote-Vertu, Saint-Laurent QC H4R 1P5; Saigon (Vietnam)'67; Médecin, Clinique Med Metro Mont Royal; Médecin, Clinique Medicale Avicenne; (514)744-1936

DANG, Francois; CSSS Haut-Richelieu-Rouville, 920 boul du Seminaire N, St-Jean-Sur-Richel QC J3A 1B7; Laval'96; Staff, Hôpital du Haut-Richelieu; (450)359-5000; Fax. (450)359-5251.

DANG, Karen; William Osler HC-Etobicoke, 101 Humber College Blvd, Etobicoke ON M9V 1R8; Tor'00; CCFP; Staff, Niagara Health System - St Catharines General Site; Staff, Niagara Health System - Greater Niagara General Site; Staff, William Osler Health System - Etobicoke General Hospital; Langs: German; (416)747-3400; Fax. (416)747-3611.

DANG, Kien Trung; St Michael's Hosp, 17F CC-30 Bond St, Toronto ON M5B 1W8; Tor'01; FRCPC; Psy. Staff, St Michael's Hospital; (416)864-5137; Fax. (416)864-5480.

DANG, Marilyne; CSSS de Memphremagog, 50 rue Saint-Patrice E, Magog QC J1X 3X3; Laval'10; Staff, Centre Hospitalier et CLSC de Memphremagog; (819)843-3381

DANG, My Hue; Centre Med Alexandre, A-8100 boul Taschereau, Brossard QC J4X 1C2; Sher'93; (450)465-5589; Fax. (450)465-0092.

DANG, Nha Khanh; CLSC-CHSLD Rosemont, 2909 rue Rachel E, Montreal QC H1W 0A9; Saigon (Vietnam)'67; pers Médecin Gen Med, CLSC-CHSLD De Rosemont; Staff Physician Gen Med, CHSLD Robert-Cliche; Staff, Centre Medical Fleury-Wilson; Langs: Bilingual(French/English); (514)524-3544; Fax. (514)524-3617.

DANG, Norman K; Kennedy Heights Med Clinic, 11944 88th Ave, Delta BC V4C 3C8; UBC'92; CCFP; Staff Privil, Surrey Memorial Hospital; (778)593-9867; Fax. (778)793-9865.

DANG, Phu An; Clin Med Rolland, 2-12315 boul Rolland, Montreal-Nord QC H1G 6A6; Saigon (Vietnam)'72; Médecin, Clinique Medical Rolland; Dir média, Centre Medical Floury Wilson; Physician-in-Charge, CLSC Saint-Laurent; Langs: Bilingual(French/English); (514)326-1919

DANG, Phuong; First Med Place, 208-170 Queensway W, Mississauga ON L5B 3A8; Alb'96; CCFP; Staff, Trillium Health Centre - West Toronto; Langs: Vietnamese; Cantonese; (905)276-2599; Fax. (905)276-7066.

DANG, Tai Huu; Turtle Mountain Med Clinic, 968 Mian St, Winnipeg MB R2W 3P5; Hue (Vietnam)'80.

DANG, Thuy Nhien; Clinique Med 8260, 212-8260 boul Maurice-Duplessi, Montreal QC H1E 3A3; Sher'93; (514)643-1113

DANG, Tommy; 205-1106 Ouellette Ave, Windsor ON N9A 1C9; Ott'98; BSc; FRCSC; Neursurg. Chief Neur, Hôtel-Dieu Grace Hospital; Langs: Vietnamese; (519)973-8771; Fax. (519)973-4690.

DANG, Yen; 3100-910 10th Ave W, Vancouver BC V5Z 4E3; Qns'06; FRCSC; GenSurg. (604)362-3895

DANG, Yen Nhi; CLSC Saint-Michel, 3355 rue Jarry E, Montreal QC H1Z 2E5; Sher'94; (514)374-8223; Fax. (514)374-3812.

DANG-TRAN, Khue-My; CSSS de la Haute-Cote-Nord, RR 1 4 rue de l'Hopital, Les Escoumins QC G0T 1K0; Bordeaux (France)'94; Staff, Centre de santé des Côté-Nord; (418)233-2931; Fax. (418)233-3335.

DANGOOR, Gail; Denison Armoury, 1 Yukon Lane, North York ON M3K 0A1; Cal'95; CCFP; FCFP; Langs: English; French; (416)633-6200; Fax. (416)635-2720.

DANGOR, Ayoub; Royal University Hosp, 103 Hospital Dr, Saskatoon SK S7N 0W8; Sask'92; FRCPC; Anes. Staff, Royal University Hospital; Staff med, Saskatoon District Health Board; Clinical Asst Prof, University of Saskatchewan; (306)655-1183; Fax. (306)655-1279.

DANI, Mukhaimer H; Miramichi Reg Hosp, 500 Water St, Miramichi NB E1V 3G5; Ain Shams (Egypt)'64; MB ChB; FRCS(Ed); FICS; Consultant ObstGyn, Miramichi Regional Hospital; Langs: Arabic; French; (506)622-5700; Fax. (506)622-5411; mukdani@yahoo.ca.

DANIAL, Amathul A; Urban Med Clinic, 105B-2603 Hewes Way NW, Edmonton AB T6L 6W6; Madras (India)'64; DRCOG; MRC; MRCS(Eng); LRCP(Lond); MRCOG(UK); Ac Staff, Covenant Health - Misericordia Community Hospital; Fam Med, Covenant Health - St. Joseph's Auxilliary Hospital; Langs: Urdu; Hindi; Tamil; Punjabi; (780)490-7427

DANIAL, Bahauddin H; Brandongate Med Clinic, 6-4025 Brandon Gate Dr, Mississauga ON L4T 3Z9; Osmania (India)'61; MB BS; FACP; FRCPC; IntMed. Langs: Hindi; Urdu; (905)678-2831; Fax. (905)678-9035.

DANIAL, Hajira F; Hys Med Centre, 604-11010 101 St NW, Edmonton AB T5H 4B9; Alb'01; BMedSci; FRCSC; ObstGyn. Associate Clin Prof, University of Alberta; (780)421-4728

DANIAL, Sarah B; Niagara Plastic Surgery Centre, 1-5668 Main St, Niagara Falls ON L2G 5Z4; Alb'91; BSc; FABPN; FRCPC; Psy (Child & Adolescent Psychiatry). Consultant Psy, Canadian Mental Health Associaton; Langs: English; French; (905)357-2360; Fax. (905)357-4714.

DANIEL, Alan B; Joseph Brant Mem Hosp, 1230 North Shore Blvd E, Burlington ON L7S 1W7; Stellenbosch (South Africa)'86; CCFP; Staff, Joseph Brant Memorial Hospital; Staff, Niagara Health System - Welland Hospital Site; (905)632-3730

DANIEL, Angus; Whitewater Bromley Comm Hlth C, 20 Robertson Dr, Beachburg ON K0J 1C0; Qns'01; CCFP; (613)582-3685

DANIEL, Antia O; Imperial Oil Resources Ltd, 18057-237 4 Ave SW, Calgary AB T2P 0H6; (Nigeria)'88; MCFP(SA); CCFP; (403)237-4557; Fax. (403)237-2137.

DANIEL, Ariadne; 3149-700 University Ave, Toronto ON M5G 1Z5; Alb'06; FRCSC; ObstGyn.

DANIEL, Arkadiusz M; 1701 Woodroffe Ave, Nepean ON K2G 1W2; Ott'96; CCFP; FCFP; Staff, Huntsville District Memorial Hospital - Muskoka Algonquin Healthcare; Langs: Polish; (613)727-5755

DANIEL, Enoch S; Petrolia Family Health Team, GD 431 King St, Petrolia ON N0N 1R0; Mem'99; CCFP; (519)882-2500

DANIEL, Geoffrey B; TRELLIS, 5-15 Brenda Blvd, Orangeville ON L9W 3Y5; Tor'87; FRCPC; Psy (Geriatric Psychiatry). Staff, Headwaters Health Care Centre - Orangeville Site; Staff, Groves Memorial Community Hospital; Consultant GeroPsy., CMHC Wellington & Dufferin Senior's Outreach Team; Staff GeroPsy, Penetanguishene Geriatric Outreach; (519)941-0465; Fax. (519)941-0580.

DANIEL, Geraldine R; 101B-2099 152 St, Surrey BC V4A 4N7; Pretoria (South Africa)'91; MB ChB; CCFP; Langs: Afrikaans; (604)538-5770; Fax. (604)531-9894.

DANIEL, Helene; CLSC Dorval-Lachine, 1900 rue Notre-Dame, Lachine QC H8S 2G2; Mon'83; Med Dir, CSSS Dorval Lachine Lasalle; Langs: English; (514)639-0650

DANIEL, J Richard; Muskoka Family Medical, PO Box 1250 Stn Main 110 Muskoka Rd S, Gravenhurst ON P1P 1V4; Cardiff(Wales) (United Kingdom)'68; MB ChB; Assoc Staff, Orillia Soldiers' Memorial Hospital; Med Dir, Huronia Regional Centre; Assoc Staff, South Muskoka Memorial Hospital - Muskoka Algonquin Healthcare; Med Advisor, Muskoka Nursing Home; Langs: Welsh; (705)684-8062; Fax. (705)684-8072; doctordcik@gmail.com.

DANIEL, James K; 400-11 Holland Ave, Ottawa ON K1Y 4S1; Qns'92; (613)829-7813; Fax. (613)829-1612.

DANIEL, Kamal M; 160-6900 Taylor Dr, Red Deer AB T4P 1K4; (Egypt)'89; MB ChB; CCFP; (403)342-2234; Fax. (403)342-2655.

DANIEL, Kimberly B; 205-3301 24 Ave, Vernon BC V1T 9S8; Cal'02; BSc; FRCSC; ObstGyn. (250)503-1717; Fax. (250)503-1715.

DANIEL, Lorretta B; Univ Hlth Network-The Toronto, 4N 494-200 Elizabeth St, Toronto ON M5G 2C4; McM'83; FACC; BSc; FRCPC; IntMed; Cardiol. Ac Staff Cardiol, Toronto General Hospital - UHN; Assoc Prof, University of Toronto; (416)340-5174; Fax. (416)340-4210; lorretta.daniel@uhn.on.ca.

DANIEL, Marie-Florence; Clin Forcemedic, 200-1021 rue Jean-Talon E, Montreal QC H2R 1V6; (Haiti)'80; (514)787-1818; Fax. (514)787-1898.

DANIEL, Peter; Orillia Med/Dental Centre, 201-16 O'Brien St, Orillia ON L3V 5S2; Wes'87; CCFP; FCFP; Med Pres Family Pract, Orillia Soldiers' Memorial Hospital; (705)326-4401; Fax. (705)326-5212.

DANIEL, Sam J; MUHC-Montreal Children's Hosp, B240-2300 rue Tupper, Montreal QC H3H 1P3; McG'96; FRCSC; Otol. Staff, McGill University Health Centre - Montreal Children's Hospital; (514)412-4304; Fax. (514)412-4342.

DANIEL, Shannon M; CSSS de la Vallée de l'Or, 725 6e rue, Val-d'Or QC J9P 3Y1; Tor'07; Ophth. Staff, Centre Hospitalier de Val d'Or; (819)825-6711

DANIEL, Shevanta G; 2-320 Harwood Ave S, Ajax ON L1S 2J1; (Russia (Federation))'99; CCFP; Langs: Russian; Sinhalese; Tamil; French; (905)231-1122

DANIELE, Pasquale; CLSC de la Petite-Nation, 14 rue St-Andre, St-Andre-Avellin QC J0V 1W0; Mon'72; (819)983-7341; Fax. (819)983-7812.

DANIELLI, Rosemary P; Guelph Family Health Team, 101-83 Dawson Rd, Guelph ON N1H 1B1; Wes'81; CCFP; FCFP; Langs: Italian; (519)766-1360; Fax. (519)766-0469.

DANIELS, Gavin R; Acadia Med Centre, 3310 8th St E, Saskatoon SK S7H 5M3; (306)373-6000; Fax. (306)477-5000.

DANIELS, James E; Medicine Hat Reg Hosp, 666 5 St SW, Medicine Hat AB T1A 4H6; Alb'93; FRCPC; DiagRad. Staff, Medicine Hat Regional Hospital; (403)529-8850; Fax. (403)529-8998.

DANIELS, Jean-Guy; CSSS des Sources, 475 3e av, Asbestos QC J1T 1X6; Laval'84; Chef Emergency Dept, CSSS des Sources d'Asbestos; Langs: Bilingual(French/English); (819)879-7151; Fax. (819)879-7433.

DANIELS, Lise; Bishop's University, 2600 rue College, Sherbrooke QC J1M 1Z7; Laval'77; Langs: English; French; (819)822-9696

DANIELS, Michel; 525 1re Av, Asbestos QC J1T 4R1; Laval'80; (819)879-5088; dianelalierca@qc.aira.com.

DANIELS, Nelson J; Burnview Clinic, 100-3225 Lawrence Ave E, Scarborough ON M1H 3C2; Tor'66; Staff, The Scarborough Hospital - General Campus; Staff, Rouge Valley Health System - Centenary Health Centre Site; (416)439-6711; Fax. (416)431-3904.

DANIELS, Peter H; 203-2276 Island Hwy S, Campbell River BC V9W 1C3; Birmingham (England)'75; MB ChB; DRCOG; Staff, Campbell River & District General Hospital; (250)923-1189; Fax. (250)923-8897.

DANIELS, Robert W; Sherwood Park Medicentre, 9-101 Bremner Dr, Sherwood Park AB T8H 0M5; Alb'86; (780)467-4717; Fax. (780)467-9316.

DANIELS, Timothy R; St Michael's Orthopaedic Assoc, 800-55 Queen St E, Toronto ON M5C 1R6; Sask'86; FRCSC; OrthSurg (Foot & Ankle Surgery). Staff, St Michael's Hospital; Assoc Prof, University of Toronto; (416)864-5392; Fax. (416)359-1601.

DANIELS, Valsa; Rehabilitation Centre, RR137-800 Sherbrook St, Winnipeg MB R3A 1M4; Mysore (India)'71; MB BS; FRCPC; PhysMed&Rehab (Neurology). Dir Stroke Program Rehab Hosp, Health Sciences Centre; Chief Stroke Serv, Winnipeg Regional Health Authority Carlton Street Office; Assoc Prof, University of Manitoba; (204)787-2206; Fax. (204)787-1476; vdaniels@hsc.mb.ca.

DANIELS, Vijay J; University of Alberta Hosp, 2F1-8440 112 St NW, Edmonton AB T6G 2B7; Man'05; FRCPC; IntMed. Staff, University of Alberta Hospital; (780)407-7675; Fax. (780)407-3132.

DANIELSON, Brita L; Cross Cancer Institute, 11560 University Ave NW, Edmonton AB T6G 1Z2; Sask'03; FRCPC; RadOncol. Staff, Cross Cancer Institute; (780)432-8518; Fax. (780)432-8380; brita.danielson@albertahealthservices.ca.

DANIELSON, Dawn A; University of Alberta Hosp, 8440 112 St NW, Edmonton AB T6G 2B7; Man'04; Peds. Staff, University of Alberta Hospital; (780)407-8822

DANIELSON, Jerry D; Regina Community Clinic, 1106 Winnipeg St, Regina SK S4R 1J6; Sask'73; (306)543-7880; Fax. (306)543-6888.

DANIELSON, Kimberly J; 90 Scollard St, Toronto ON M5R 1G2; McM'84; FRCPC; Psy. (416)975-9154; Fax. (416)969-8789.

DANILA, Alexandru-Cristian; Clin Med Saint-Nicephore, 4534 boul Saint-Joseph, Saint-Nicephore QC J2A 1B5; (Romania)'88; (819)472-3350; Fax. (819)472-0315.

DANILKEWICH, Alanna D; West Winds Primary Hlth Ctr, 3311 Fairlight Dr, Saskatoon SK S7M 3Y5; Sask'75; FCFP; CCFP; FCFP; Staff, Saskatoon City Hospital; Staff, St Paul's Hospital (Grey Nuns) of Saskatoon; Staff, Royal University Hospital; Assoc Prof Academic Family Med/Dir Faculty Development/A-Dept Head Family Med, University of Saskatchewan; (306)655-4200; Fax. (306)655-4894.

DANINO, Michel A; CHUM-Hôp Notre-Dame, 1560 rue Sherbrooke E, Montreal QC H2L 4M1; Paris (France)'99; Staff, Centre Hospitalier l'Université de Montréal (CHUM) - Hôpital Notre-Dame; (514)890-8000

DANJOUX, Cyril J E; Toronto Sunnybrook Reg Cancer, T2 158-2075 Bayview Ave, Toronto ON M4N 3M5; Hebrew (Israel)'70; DMRT; FRCP; DrMedCh; FRCPC; RadOncol (Genito Urinary Oncology). Staff, Sunnybrook Health Sciences Centre; Asst Prof RadOncol, University of Toronto; Langs: Hebrew; Bilingual(French/English); (416)480-4998; Fax. (416)480-6002; cyril.danjoux@sunnybrook.ca.

DANKOFF, Frederic J; MUHC-Royal Victoria Hosp, 687 av des Pins O, Montreal QC H3A 1A1; McG'98; CSPQ; MDCM; CCFP; Staff Emerg Research Inst, McGill University Health Centre - Royal Victoria Hospital; Clin Instructor, McGill University; Langs: French; (514)934-1934

DANKOFF, Jerrald; SMBD Jewish Gen Hosp, 3755 ch Cote-Sainte-Catherine, Montreal QC H3T 1E2; McG'78; EmergMed (P.Q.). Staff, Sir Mortimer B Davis Jewish General; (514)340-8222; Fax. (514)340-7519.

DANKWA, Essandoh K; Dr C S Curtis Mem Hospital, 178-200 West St, St Anthony NL A0K 4S0; Accra (Ghana)'80; MB ChB; MRCPath; FRCPC; AnatPath (Family Medicine). Chief Path/Assoc VP, Charles S Curtis Memorial Hospital; Clin Asst Prof, Memorial University Of Newfoundland; Langs: Fanti; (709)454-0127; Fax. (709)454-2052.

DANN, Kathleen K; Raven Song Comm Hlth Centre, 2450 Ontario St, Vancouver BC V5T 4T7; McG'78; CCFP; (604)709-6400; Fax. (604)872-5223.

DANNENBAUM, David A; 210-5450 ch de la Cote-des-Nei, Montreal QC H3T 1Y6; McG'90; CCFP; Staff, Hôpital Anna-Laberge; (514)731-3249; Fax. (514)731-0395; ddannenbaum@ssss.gouv.qc.ca.

DANS, Jody-Lynn; Formation Health Services Unit, 1200 Colville Rd, Victoria BC V9A 4P7; McM'10; CCFP; (250)363-5693

DANSEREAU, Alain; Clinique Dermato-Esthétique, 2 rue Notre-Dame, Repentigny QC J6A 2N7; Sher'81; FRCPC; Derm (Cosmetic & Laser Surgery). (450)470-1177; Fax. (450)470-1175; adansereau@videotron.ca.

DANSEREAU, Angela; The Pediclinic Hy's Centre, 505-11010 101 St NW, Edmonton AB T5H 4B9; Alb'02; BSc; FRCPC; Peds. (780)414-6812; Fax. (780)428-0852.

DANSEREAU, Benoit; Polyclinique Med des Ponts, 120-1100 boul de la Rive-Sud, Saint-Romuald QC G6W 5M6; Mon'85; CSPQ; ObstGyn (P.Q.). Chef obst & gynécol, Centre Hospitalier Beauce-Etchemin; (418)834-4943; Fax. (418)834-9275.

DANSEREAU, Danielle; Clinique Familiale, 13555 boul Lacroix, Saint-Georges QC G5Y 1P1; Laval'87; (418)228-8001; Fax. (418)228-5583.

DANSEREAU, Dominique; CSSS de Trois-Rivières, 1991 boul du Carmel, Trois-Rivieres QC G8Z 3R9; Sher'92; CSPQ; FRCPC; Anes. Staff, CSSS de Trois-Rivières; (819)697-3333

DANSEREAU, Jean-Marc; Centre Med Boucherville, 201-600 boul du Fort-St-Louis, Boucherville QC J4B 1S7; Mon'84; (450)655-7321; Fax. (450)655-6311.

DANSEREAU, Jean-Yves; Commission des Lesions, 3225 rue Cusson, Saint-Hyacinthe QC J2S 0H7; Mon'73; Rheum; IntMed (Occupational Medicine). Insp Investigator, College des Medecins du Quebec; (450)778-5672

DANSEREAU, Jerome; Victoria Gen Hosp, 1 Hospital Way, Victoria BC V8Z 6R5; Mon'80; FRCSC; ObstGyn (Maternal Fetal Medicine). Consultant, BC Women's Hospital & Health Centre; Consultant, Victoria General Hospital; Langs: Bilingual(English/French); (250)727-4127; Fax. (250)727-4254.

DANSEREAU, L Alexandra; CHUQ-Hotel-Dieu de Quebec, 11 Cote du Palais, Quebec QC G1R 2J6; Laval'89; Staff, Centre Hospitalier Universitaire de Québec (CHUQ) - Siege Social; Staff, Centre Hospitalier Affilié Universitaire de Québec - Hôpital du St-Sacrement; (418)525-4444

DANSEREAU, Luc; CSSS des Îles, 430 ch Principal, Cap-aux-Meules QC G4T 1R9; Mon'00; FRCPC; IntMed. Staff, Hôpital de l'Archipel; Langs: Bilingual(French/English); (418)986-2121

DANSEREAU, Michelle; CSSS d'Antoine-Labelle, 2561 ch Lievre St, Mont-Laurier QC J9L 3G3; Mon'80; MSc(OccMed); CCFP; Staff, CSSS d'Antoine-Labelle; Fam Med, Centre de L'Annonciation; Med Consul, DS Publique Laurentides; (819)623-1234

DANSEREAU, Pierre; Hop du Sacre-Coeur de Mtl, 5400 boul Gouin O, Montreal QC H4J 1C5; Mon'93; Staff, Hôpital du Sacre-Coeur de Montréal; (514)338-2383

DANSEREAU, Ronald; 6993 Notre Dame St, Orleans ON K1C 1H8; Ott'73; Staff, Montfort Hospital; Preceptor Clinique, University of Ottawa; Langs: Bilingual(French/English); (613)824-1613; Fax. (613)824-2663.

DANSEREAU, Yves; Clin Radiologie de Granby, 100-66 rue Court, Granby QC J2G 4Y5; Mon'81; FRCPC; DiagRad. Ac Staff, Centre Hospitalier l'Université De Montréal (CHUM) - Hôpital Saint-luc; Universite de Montreal; (450)378-0167; Fax. (450)378-0168.

DANSON, A Jeffrey; 403-5885 ch Cote-des-Neiges, Montreal QC H3S 2T2; McG'70; Att Staff Fam Pract, Sir Mortimer B Davis Jewish General; (514)342-2317; Fax. (514)342-1638; jeffreydanson@hotmail.com.

DANTER, Matthew; St Paul's Hosp, 484-1081 Burrard St, Vancouver BC V6Z 1Y6; Wes'03; FRCSC; CardSurg. Staff, Providence Health Care - St Paul's Hospital; (604)806-9307

DANTZER, Dale; 377-5 Fairview Mall Dr, North York ON M2J 2Z1; Wes'98; FRCSC; OrthSurg. Staff, Sunnybrook Health Sciences Centre; (416)492-5633; Fax. (416)495-1590.

DANYLAK, Mary; Roehampton Clinic, 89 Roehampton Ave, Toronto ON M4P 1P9; Tor'69; BSc(Hon); Staff, The Scarborough Hospital - General Campus; Staff, Rouge Valley Health System - Centenary Health Centre Site; Langs: Spanish; (416)322-3515; Fax. (416)489-7113.

DANYLEWICK, Richard; Inst for Laser & Vein Treatmen, 200-1565 boul de l'Avenir, Laval QC H7S 2N5; Sher'82; BSc; CSPQ; DAB(Phlebology); FRCSC; GenSurg (Laser Surgery); VascSurg. Staff Vascular Surg, Rockland MD; Langs: English; French; (450)668-8377; Fax. (450)668-5808.

DANYLUK, Dale E; Centennial CMH & Brain Injury, PO Box 1000 Stn Main, Ponoka AB T4J 1R8; Cal'96; FRCPC; Psy. Staff, Centennial Centre for Mental Health & Brain Injury; (403)783-7643; Fax. (403)783-7790.

DANYLUK, John M; Misericordia Community Hosp, 16940 87 Ave NW, Edmonton AB T5R 4H5; Alb'65; FRCPC; GenPath. Consultant, Cross Cancer Institute; Ac Staff Path, Covenant Health - Misericordia Community Hospital; Teach Staff, University of Alberta; (780)735-2742

DAO, Ba Anh L; Clinique Externe Psychiatrique, 11-814 boul L'Ange Gardien N, L'Assomption QC J5W 1P6; Sher'98; Psy. Staff, Centre Hospitalier Régional de Lanaudière; (450)589-2140

DAO, Ba Ngoc; CHSLD Lucille-Teasdale, 3095 rue Sherbrooke E, Montreal QC H1W 1B2; Saigon (Vietnam)'71; CCFP; FCFP; Fam Med, CHSLD Lucille-Teasdale; (514)523-1173; Fax. (514)528-2725.

DAO, Catherine T; CSSSG-Hop de Hull, 116 Boul Bionel-Emond, Gatineau QC J8Y 1W7; Sher'99; FRCPC; IntMed; Gastroent. Staff, Hull Hospital; (819)595-6200 x6030; Fax. (819)966-6218.

DAO, Chung; Main Medical, 700 Main St E, Hamilton ON L8M 1K7; (Other Foreign)'08; (905)547-3901

DAO, Hong Quyen; Centre Hospitalier des Vallées, 116 boul Lionel-Emond, Gatineau QC J8Y 1W7; Mon'96; Staff, Hull Hospital; Langs: English; Vietnamese; (819)595-6200

DAO, T Trang; Hop Santa Cabini Ospedale, 5655 rue Saint-Zotique E, Montreal QC H1T 1P7; Mon'84; Psy. Staff, Hôpital Santa Cabrini Ospedale; Vietnamese Psy. Clinic; Langs: Vietnamese; English; (514)252-6444

DAO, Thomas T H; Clinique Med 3600, 3600 rue Ontario E, Montreal QC H1W 1R7; Saigon (Vietnam)'72; (514)526-2556

DAO, Thu-Van; Clin Externe de Sante Mentale, 200-237 boul Saint-Jean-Baptis, Chateauguay QC J6K 3C3; Mon'99; Psy. Staff, Hôpital Anna-Laberge.

DAO, Tien Trong; CSSS de Laval, 1755 boul Rene-Laennec, Laval QC H7M 3L9; McG'87; CSPQ; FRCPC; DiagRad (Mammograph). Staff, Hopital de la Cite de la santé; Asst Prof DiagRad., Universite de Montreal; Langs: Vietnamese; French; (450)668-1010 x23527

DAO, Vi Vinh B; St Boniface Gen Hosp, L1 102-409 Tache Ave, Winnipeg MB R2H 2A6; Ott'03; FRCPC; IntMed; Hem. Staff, St Boniface General Hospital; (204)233-8563

DAOUD, Aida; Clinique Pediatrique Beaubien, 2301 rue Belanger, Montreal QC H2G 1C9; Damascus (Syria)'70; CSPQ; AB; MedOncol (P.Q.); Peds (P.Q.) (Pediatric Hematology Oncology). Staff Ped HemOncol, McGill University Health Centre - Montreal General Campus; (514)728-1559; Fax. (514)728-4480.

DAOUD, Eyad S A Q; Mount Sinai Hospital, 600 University Ave, Toronto ON M5G 1X5; Irkutsk State (Russia (Federation))'99; Staff, Mount Sinai Hospital; (416)596-4200; Fax. (416)586-8899.

DAOUD, Hani; Virden Med Assoc, PO Box 730 455 Frame St, Virden MB R0M 2C0; (Other Foreign)'79; MB BCh; Gen Practice, Virden Health Centre; Langs: Bilingual(English/French); (204)748-1345; Fax. (204)748-1640; daoudhani@hotmail.com.

DAOUD, Hani I K; London HSC-Victoria Hosp, PO Box 5010 Stn B 800 Commissioners Rd E, London ON N6A 5W9; (Iraq)'00; Staff, London Health Sciences Centre - Victoria Campus; (519)685-8500; Fax. (519)685-8127.

DAOUD, Maha; Hotel-Dieu de Sorel, 400 av de l'Hotel-Dieu, Sorel-Tracy QC J3P 1N5; Beirut (Lebanon)'92; Peds (P.Q.). Pediatrics, Hôtel-Dieu de Sorel; (450)746-6000; Fax. (450)746-8801.

DAOUD, Nicolas; Clin de Radiologie du Saguenay, 106-874 boul de l'Universite E, Chicoutimi QC G7H 6B9; Cairo (Egypt)'57; DA; CSPQ; FRCPC; DiagRad (Osteoporosis). Staff, Complexe hospitalier de la Sagamie; Physician, Clinique de Radiologie du Saguenay; Langs: English; Arabic; (418)545-3505; Fax. (418)545-9962.

DAOUID, Fouad; Barrie Memorial Hosp, CP 2000 28 Gale St, Ormstown QC J0S 1K0; (France)'95; Staff, Barrie Memorial Hospital; (450)829-2321

DAOUST, Danielle; CSSS du Nord de Lanaudière, 1000 boul Sainte-Anne, Joliette QC J6E 4Z1; Mon'93; Chief Intesive Care & Emerg Service, Centre Hospitalier Régional de Lanaudière; Med Consultant, Interbox Corp; (450)759-8222 x2820

DAOUST, Helene; Clinique Med des Trois Lacs, 160-585 av Saint-Charles, Vaudreuil-Dorion QC J7V 8P9; Mon'94; CCFP; Staff, Centre Hospitalier Régional du Suroît; (450)455-3322; Fax. (450)455-0756.

DAOUST, Lucie; CSSS Les Eskers de l'Abitibi, 622 4e rue O, Amos QC J9T 2S2; Mon'89; FRCPC; DiagRad. Staff, CH Hôtel-Dieu d'Amos; (819)732-3341 x2259; Fax. (819)732-6484.

DAOUST, Marguerite; Clinique Med Plaza Gatineau, 381 boul Maloney E, Gatineau QC J8P 1E3; Mon'77; (819)669-7393; Fax. (819)669-0077.

DAOUST, Raoul; Hop du Sacre-Coeur de Mtl, 5400 boul Gouin O, Montreal QC H4J 1C5; Mon'86; EmergMed (P.Q.). Ac Staff, Hôpital du Sacre-Coeur de Montréal; (514)338-2222 x3234

DAR, A Rashid; London Reg Cancer Centre, 790 Commissioners Rd E, London ON N6A 4L6; Kashmir (India)'66; DABR; DMRT; DMRD; FRCR; MB BS; FRCPC; RadOncol. Consultant, Bluewater Health - Norman Site; London Health Sciences Centre - Victoria Campus; Staff, Ontario Cancer Treatment & Research Fdn.; Asst Prof, University of Western Ontario; Langs: Hindi; Punjabi; (519)685-8650; Fax. (519)685-8627.

DAR, Shahnaz; 201-1691 McCowan Rd, Scarborough ON M1S 2Y3; Nairobi (Kenya)'76; MB ChB; Peds. Langs: Swahili; Urdu; Punjabi; Kiswahili; Gujarati; (416)293-0275; Fax. (416)293-8057.

DARAEI, Nemat A; 106-210 Memorial Ave, Orillia ON L3V 7V1; Shahid Beheshti (Iran)'95; CCFP; Langs: Farsi; (705)327-6576; Fax. (705)327-6579.

DARANI, Shaheen; Law & Mental Health Program, 3 4-1001 Queen St W, Toronto ON M6J 1H4; McM'00; FRCPC; Psy. (416)535-8501 x2984; Fax. (416)583-4327.

DARBY, Lawrence B; 201-15451 Russell Ave, White Rock BC V4B 2R5; Cork (Ireland)'89; MB ChB; BAO; Staff, Peace Arch Hospital; (604)531-5541; Fax. (604)531-2041.

DARBY, Mark C; Horizons Family Med, 5016 51 Ave, Red Deer AB T4N 4H5; Cal'02; CCFP; (403)342-7270; Fax. (403)343-2677.

DARBY, Niamh M; 201-15451 Russell Ave, White Rock BC V4B 2R5; Cork (Ireland)'87; MB ChB; BAO; Staff, Peace Arch Hospital; (604)531-5541; Fax. (604)531-2041.

DARBY, Padraig L; Addiction & Mental Hlth-Queen, 1001 Queen St W, Toronto ON M6J 1H4; Dublin (Ireland)'74; MRCPsy; MB ChB; BAO; FRCPC; Psy. Deputy Clin Dir Law & Mental Hlth Prog, Centre for Addiction & Mental Health (CAMH) - Queen Site; Asst Prof, University of Toronto; (416)979-6876; Fax. (416)583-4319.

DARBY, Peter J; Hamilton HS-McMaster Site, PO Box 2000 Stn Lcd 1 1200 Main St W, Hamilton ON L8N 3Z5; Tor'03; Anes. Staff, Hamilton Health Sciences Centre - McMaster Children's Hospital; (905)521-2100

DARBYSHIRE, James M; BC Biomedical Lab Ltd, 7455 130 St, Surrey BC V3W 1H8; Alb'75; FRCPC; AnatPath; GenPath. Ac Staff, Royal Columbian Hospital; Ac Staff, Langley Memorial Hospital; Staff, BC Biomedical Laboratories Ltd; (604)970-4005

DARBYSHIRE, Katherine R; 560 Albert St PO Box 424, Winchester ON K0C 2K0; Ott'79; CCFP; FCFP; Ac Staff/Medical Staff/Pres Med Staff, Winchester District Memorial Hospital; Teacher Voluntary Part Time, University of Ottawa; (613)774-3921; Fax. (613)774-4833.

DARCEL, Ian C; Burlington Prof Centre, 408-3155 Harvester Rd, Burlington ON L7N 3V2; Tor'82; FRCPC; IntMed; Cardiol. Ac Staff, Joseph Brant Memorial Hospital; (905)333-5077; Fax. (905)333-5078; darcel@bellnet.ca.

DARCEL, Keith R; PO Box 540, Grande Cache AB T0E 0Y0; Cal'95; CCFP; (780)827-2540; Fax. (780)827-5698.

DARCHE, Marie; RSRY Pavillon Hotel-Dieu, 1800 rue Dessaulles, Saint-Hyacinthe QC J2S 2T2; Sher'75; Gen Practice, Centre d hebergement de l Hôtel-Dieu de Saint-Hyacinthe; (450)771-3333

DARCUS, Karl L; Peter Lougheed Centre, 2264-3500 26 Ave NE, Calgary AB T1Y 6J4; Alb'01; FRCPC; Anes. Staff, Peter Lougheed Centre; (403)943-5554; Fax. (403)943-4474.

DARCY, Eve; CH Hotel-Dieu Amos, 622 4e rue O, Amos QC J9T 2S2; Mon'04; CCFP; Staff, CH Hôtel-Dieu d'Amos; (819)732-3341 x2160

DARCY, Stephen; Shea Heights Commun Hlth Ctre, PO Box 13122 Stn A 57B Linegar Ave, St. John's NL A1B 4A4; Mem'91; CCFP.

DARCZEWSKI, Irena B; Dr Barczewski Med Corp, 219 Marion St, Winnipeg MB R2H 0T5; Wroclaw (Poland)'85; CCFP; Langs: Polish; Russian; Ukrainian.

DARGAVEL, Danny A; Dargavel Medicine Prof Corp, 204-4383 Portage Rd, Niagara Falls ON L2E 6A6; McM'80; CCFP; FCFP; (905)356-3626; Fax. (905)356-5440.

DARGIE, Robin L; Chinook Prof Bldg, 409-6455 Macleod Trail SW, Calgary AB T2H 0K9; Cal'88; CCFP; Staff, Rockyview General Hospital; (403)253-5115; Fax. (403)253-3077.

DARIF, Suzan Darif Aribi; GP Med Clinic, 12225 99 St, Grande Prairie AB T8V 6X9; (South Africa)'85; MB ChB; (780)533-4444; Fax. (780)533-4443.

DARIS, Marleen; CHUQ-Ctr Hosp Univ Laval, S 762-2705 boul Laurier, Quebec QC G1V 4G2; Laval'86; CSPQ; FRCSC; ObstGyn (Colposcopy). Ac Member, Centre Hospitalier Universitaire de Quebec-CHUL; Assoc Member, Centre Hospitalier Chauveau; Asst Dir Obst/Gyn Residency, Université Laval; Langs: English; (418)654-2738; Fax. (418)525-4281; sec.gyneco@crchul.ulaval.ca.

DARLING, Colleen; 203-232A Guelph St, Georgetown ON L7G 4B1; Wes'84; (905)873-1831; Fax. (877)842-7331; sue.drdarling@yahoo.ca.

DARLING, Gail; Univ Hlth Network-The Toronto, 9N 955-200 Elizabeth St, Toronto ON M5G 2C4; Wes'81; BSc; FRCSC; GenSurg (Critical Care Medicine); ThorSurg. Consultant, Mount Sinai Hospital; Consultant, St Joseph's Health Centre; Staff, Toronto General Hospital - UHN; Prof ThorSurg/Prog Dir ThorSurg, University of Toronto; (416)340-3121; Fax. (416)340-3660; gail.darling@uhn.on.ca.

DARLING, Jennifer L; Peterborough Reg HC-Hospital, 1 Hospital Dr, Peterborough ON K9J 7C6; McM'94; CCFP; CCFP(E.M.); FCFP; Staff, Peterborough Regional Health Centre - Hospital Drive; (705)743-2121

DARLINGTON, Paul; Dalbrent Med Centre, 203-3604 52 Ave NW, Calgary AB T2L 1V9; Man'88; BSc; FRCPC; Psy (Chronic Pain). Staff, Corrections Canada; (403)232-6627

DARNELL, Timothy S; Family Med Associates, 5021 51 St, Lacombe AB T4L 2A3; Alb'92; CCFP; (403)782-3351; Fax. (403)782-5879.

DARQUES, Loïc; CSSS du Sud de Lanaudière, 911 montee des Pionniers, Terrebonne QC J6V 2H2; CCFP; Staff, Centre Hospitalier Pierre le Gardeur; (450)654-7525

DARRACOTT, John; 180 James St S PO Box 43547, Hamilton ON L8P 4V1; London (England)'63; MB BS; MB BS; MRCS; DPhysMed; FRCPC; PhysMed&Rehab (Rheumatology). Court Staff, Hamilton Health Sciences Centre; Staff, St Joseph's Healthcare - Charlton Campus; Clin Assoc Prof, McMaster University; (905)522-3700; Fax. (905)522-9614.

DARRAGH, Anne; Alexandra Comm Health Centre, 101-1318 Centre St NE, Calgary AB T2E 2R7; Cal'90; CCFP; FCFP; (403)266-2622; Fax. (403)266-2692.

DARRAH, William C; St Michael's Hosp, 30 Bond St, Toronto ON M5B 1W8; Belfast (United Kingdom)'80; MRCMRCP(UK); FFARCS; MB ChB; FRCPC; Anes (Critical Care Medicine). Staff, St Michael's Hospital; (416)864-5071; Fax. (416)864-6014.

DARRAT, Mahmoud A; Hamilton HS-General Site, 237 Barton St E, Hamilton ON L8L 2X2; Al-Arab (Libya)'90; FRCPC; Anes. Staff, Hamilton Health Sciences Centre - Hamilton General Hospital; Langs: Arabic; (905)521-2100

DARSAKLIS, Konstadina; MUHC-Royal Victoria Hosp, M4 76-687 av des Pins O, Montreal QC H3A 1A1; McG'05; FRCPC; IntMed. Staff, McGill University Health Centre - Royal Victoria Hospital; (514)934-1934 x36151

DARSAUT, Timothee E; University of Alberta Hosp, 2D1 02-8440 112 St NW, Edmonton AB T6G 2B7; Qns'02; FRCSC; Neursurg. Staff, Mazankowski Alberta Heart Institute; (780)407-1440; Fax. (780)407-8203.

DARSIGNY, Monique; CSSS Richelieu-Yamaska, 1800 rue Dessaulles, Saint-Hyacinthe QC J2S 2T2; Laval'93; Staff, Centre d hebergement de l Hôtel-Dieu de Saint-Hyacinthe; (450)771-3333

DART, Allison B; Health Sciences Centre, FE 009-840 Sherbrook St, Winnipeg MB R3A 1S1; Man'02; FRCPC; Peds (Pediatric Nephrology); Nephrol. Fellow Children's Hosp, Health Sciences Centre; Langs: French; adart@hsc.mb.ca.

DARVEAU, Michelle; Clinique Med St-Jerome, 102-450 boul Monseigneur-Dubois, Saint-Jerome QC J7Y 3L8; Laval'91; (450)438-1776; Fax. (450)438-6119.

DARVEAU, Simon; Lobe Sante Auditive Drummondvi, 110 rue Saint-Jean, Drummondville QC J2B 7T1; Sher'00; Otol. Staff, Hôpital Sainte-croix; (819)857-4777

DARVEAU, Stephane; Hôpital de Tracadie-Sheila, CP 3180 Stn Main 400 rue des Hospitalieres, Tracadie-Sheila NB E1X 1G5; Laval'97; CCFP; Staff, Hôpital de Tracadie-Sheila; (506)394-3000

DARVESH, Sultan; 1308-5955 Veterans Memorial La, Halifax NS B3H 2E1; Dal'88; BSc; MSc; PhD; FRCPC; Neur (Behavioural Neurology). Staff, Queen Elizabeth II Health Sciences Centre - Victoria General Site; Asst Prof Neurol, Dalhousie University; (902)473-2490; Fax. (902)473-7133; sultan.darvesh@dal.ca.

DARWICH, Chadi; Lakeshore Gen Hosp, 160 av Stillview, Pointe-Claire QC H9R 2Y2; Staff, Lakeshore General Hospital - Pointe Claire; (514)630-2225

DARWICH, Walid; Ctr Hosp Pierre-Janet, 20 rue Pharand, Gatineau QC J9A 1K7; Damascus (Syria)'85; Psy (P.Q.). Staff, Centre Hospitalier Pierre-Janet; (819)776-7761; Fax. (819)776-8048; darwich28@hotmail.com.

DARWISH, Nidal; Royal Oak Med Clinic, 192-8888 Country Hills Blvd NW, Calgary AB T3G 5T4; Mexico (Mexico)'90; CCFP; Langs: Spanish; (403)239-3660; Fax. (403)239-4001.

DAS, Ananya; Pacific Med Clinic, 3185 Grandview Hwy, Vancouver BC V5M 2E9; Cape Town (South Africa)'08; MB ChB; Staff, Pacific Medical Centre; (604)434-2222

DAS, Bijon; Queen Elizabeth II HSC-Halifax, 3021-1796 Summer St, Halifax NS B3H 3A7; Dal'01; CCFP; CCFP(E.M.); Staff, Queen Elizabeth II Health Sciences Centre - Halifax Infirmary Site; (902)473-8769; Fax. (902)473-3617.

DAS, Indranil; City Centre Family Physicians, 100-514 Queen St, Saskatoon SK S7K 0M5; CCFP; (306)244-3016; Fax. (306)244-4737.

DAS, Jiban; 242 Aspen Stone Pl SW, Calgary AB T3H 0H5; (Bangladesh)'76; (403)930-1005; Fax. (403)930-1004.

DAS, Jyoti N; Northgate Med Clinic, 489 Albert St N, Regina SK S4R 3C3; Calcutta (India)'59; MB; BSc; FRCS(Ed); (306)924-4727

DAS, Madhavan S; Forensic Ass & Comm Serv, 26F-1004 104 Ave NW, Edmonton AB T5J 0K1; Kerala (India)'89; MB BS; BSc; Staff, Alberta Hospital Edmonton; Langs: Hindi; Malayalam; Tamil; (780)342-6400; Fax. (780)426-7272; madhavan.das@shr.sk.ca.

DAS, Paul J; Health Centre at 80 Bond, 80 Bond St, Toronto ON M5B 1X2; Philadelphia (USA)'10; CCFP; (416)864-3011; Fax. (416)864-3099.

DAS, Pavani R; North Yoek Gen Hosp, GW33-4001 Leslie St, North York ON M2K 1E1; Chicago (USA)'00; Staff, North York General Hospital; (416)756-6130

DAS, Sharmistha; Gordon & Leslie Diamond HCC, 7F-2775 Laurel St, Vancouver BC V5Z 1M9; Qns'06; FRCPC; IntMed. (604)875-5181

DAS, Sunit; St Michael's Hosp, 30 Bond St, Toronto ON M5B 1W8; Philadelphia (USA)'01; Staff, St Michael's Hospital; (416)864-5452

DAS, Tilak; Postgrad Med Education, 602-500 University Ave, Toronto ON M5G 1V7; Oxford (United Kingdom)'04.

DASCAL, Andre; SMBD Jewish Gen Hosp, 3755 ch Cote-Sainte-Catherine, Montreal QC H3T 1E2; Mon'77; ABIM(IntMed&InfectDis); CSPQ; FRCPC; IntMed; InfectDis; Microbio & Infect Dis (P.Q.)., Sir Mortimer B Davis Jewish General; assoc Prof Med, McGill University; Langs: Romanian; French; (514)340-8294; Fax. (514)340-7548.

DASCALU, Petronela; Lakeshore Gen Hosp, 160 av Stillview, Pointe-Claire QC H9R 2Y2; Iasi University (Other Foreign)'97; FRCPC; IntMed. Staff, Lakeshore General Hospital - Pointe Claire; (514)630-2225

DASGUPTA, Bonnie; PO Box 21046 Rpo Terwillegar, Edmonton AB T6R 2V4; (India)'04; MB BS; CCFP.

DASGUPTA, Kaberi; MUHC-Royal Victoria Hosp, V1 08-687 av des Pins O, Montreal QC H3A 1A1; McG'93; MDCM; FRCPC; IntMed. Staff, McGill University Health Centre - Royal Victoria Hospital; (514)934-1934 x44715

DASGUPTA, Monidipa; St Joseph's Health Care, A3 125-268 Grosvenor St, London ON N6A 4V2; McG'92; FRCPC; IntMed; GeriatricMed. Staff All Sites, London Health Sciences Centre - University Hospital; Staff, St Joseph's Hospital - St Joseph's Health Care; Langs: Bengali; French; (519)646-6188; Fax. (519)646-6260; monidipa.dasgupta@sjhc.london.on.ca.

DASGUPTA, Mrinal; 505 Burton Close NW, Edmonton AB T6R 2B2; Calcutta (India)'61; MSc(Alb.); FACP; AddicMed; FASN; MB BS; FRCPC; IntMed (Nephrology). Consultant Nephrol, University of Alberta Hospital; Prof Med, University of Alberta; (780)430-8977; Fax. (780)430-8977; mkdg@ualberta.ca.

DASH, Satya; Univ Hlth Network-Toronto Gen, 200 Elizabeth St, Toronto ON M5G 2C4; London (England)'00.

DASHEFSKY, Sidney M; Health Sciences Centre, 820 Sherbrook St, Winnipeg MB R3A 1R9; Man'83; FRCPC; DiagRad. Ac Staff, Health Sciences Centre; (204)774-6511

DASHKOVSKY, Marina; Jewish Rehabilitation Hosp, 3205 Place Alton-Goldbloom, Laval QC H7V 1R2; (Russia (Federation))'83; CCFP; Staff, Jewish Rehabilitation Hospital; (450)688-9550

DASHTI, Abdullah; Children's Hosp Eastern Ont, 401 Smyth Rd, Ottawa ON K1H 8L1; Galway (Ireland)'00; FRCPC; Anes. Staff, Children's Hospital of Eastern Ontario (CHEO); (613)737-7600

DASHTI, Behnoosh; PG Med Educ-McMaster U, MDCL 3101A-1280 Main St W, Hamilton ON L8S 4K1; (Iran)'00.

DASKALAKIS, Zafiris; Addiction & Mental Hlth-Clarke, 7F-250 College St, Toronto ON M5T 1R8; Qns'94; PhD; FRCPC; Psy (Schizophrenia). Staff Psy., Centre for Addiction & Mental Health (CAMH) - College Street Site; Asst Prof Psy, University of Toronto; Langs: Greek; (416)535-8501 x4319; Fax. (416)979-6936.

DASKALOPOULOS, Rina; Cobourg Health Centre, 203-316 King St E, Cobourg ON K9A 5R8; Wes'06; MSc; CCFP; Physician, Northumberland Hills Hospital; Physician, Cobourg Health Centre; Langs: Greek; (905)373-1280; Fax. (905)373-9335.

DASKALOPOULOU, Styliani S; MUHC-Montreal Gen Hosp, B2 101 4-1650 av Cedar, Montreal QC H3G 1A4; (Greece)'95; Staff, McGill University Health Centre - Montreal General Campus; (514)934-1934 x42295; Fax. (514)934-8573.

DASKAREV, Albena M; Victoria Med Bldg, 515-1669 Victoria St, Prince George BC V2L 2L5; (Bulgaria)'86; (250)562-6645; Fax. (250)562-7531.

DASKAREV, Zlatin L; Victoria Med Bldg, 515-1669 Victoria St, Prince George BC V2L 2L5; Sofia (Bulgaria)'88; (250)562-6645; Fax. (250)562-7531.

DASON, Jeyapandy T; Dawson Road Family Med Clinic, 83 Dawson Rd, Guelph ON N1H 1B1; (Singapore)'87; MB BS; FRCS(Edin & Glas); DRCOG; CCFP; Staff, Guelph General Hospital; Langs: Malay; Tamil; (519)766-1360

DASSA, Justine; Club Tiny Tots, 3550-6900 boul Decarie, Montreal QC H3X 2T8; McG'03; FRCPC; Peds (Respirology). Staff, Hopital Maisonneuve-Rosemont; Langs: Bilingual(English/French); (514)342-9911

DASSYLVA, Benoit; Inst Philippe Pinel de Mtl, 10905 boul Henri-Bourassa E, Montreal QC H1C 1H1; Mon'88; FRCPC; Psy. Staff, Institut Philippe-Pinel de Montreal; (514)648-8461 x459

DASZKIEWICZ-RECIZAC, Maria; Haney Hlth Associates, 22338 Selkirk Ave, Maple Ridge BC V2X 2X5; Warsaw (Poland)'63; FRCPC; Psy (Cross-Culture Psychiatry). Staff, Ridge Meadows Hospital & Health Care Centre; Langs: Polish; (604)477-7202

DATAR, Suhasini; Labrador Grenfell Health, PO Box 7000 Stn C 227 Hamilton River Rd, Happy-Valley-Goose NL A0P 1C0; Pune (India)'75; MB BS; Staff, Labrador Health Centre; (709)897-2000

DATAR, Sunil; Grove Med Centre, Box 3850 115-187 Hwy 16A, Spruce Grove AB T7X 4P9; Delhi (India)'80; Ac Staff Privil Med, Westview Health Centre; Physician, Lendrum Medical Clinic; (780)962-4455

DATEMA, Jason; Huron Commun Family Hlth Team, PO Box 460 32B-1 Centennial Dr, Seaforth ON N0K 1W0; Qns'03; BSc; MSc; CCFP; Staff, Seaforth Community Hospital - Huron Perth Healthcare Alliance; Aj Prof, University of Western Ontario; (519)600-2273; jdatema@rogers.com.

DATH, Deepak P; Hamilton HS-Henderson Site, B3 155-711 Concession St, Hamilton ON L8V 1C3; Wes'93; FRCSC; GenSurg. Staff, Hamilton Health Sciences Centre-Juravinski Site; (905)521-2100; Fax. (905)521-6048.

DATOO, Abdulsultan A; Mackenzie Richmond Hill Hosp, 10 Trench St, Richmond Hill ON L4C 4Z3; Mysore (India)'68; MB BS; DCH(Lond); DTMH(Lond); DAB; FRCPC; Anes. Staff, Mackenzie Richmond Hill Hospital; Langs: Gujarati; Hindi; Kacchi; (905)883-2110

DATTA, Anita; Royal Univ Hosp, 103 Hospital Dr, Saskatoon SK S7N 0W8; Sask'03; FRCPC; Neur (Pediatric Neurology). Staff, Royal University Hospital; (306)966-8115; Fax. (306)975-3767.

DATTA, Biswa R; Regina Qu'Appelle HR-Regina, 2F MOW-1440 14th Ave, Regina SK S4P 0W5; Dacca (Bangladesh)'67; MB BS; DCH(Lond); DAB; FRCPC; Peds (Allergy). Staff Ped, Regina General Hospital; Clin Assoc Prof Ped, University of Saskatchewan; (306)766-6955; Fax. (306)766-6957.

DATTA, Indraneel; Suitor House, 1004 8 Ave SE, Calgary AB T2G 0M4; Cal'04; GenSurg. Staff, Foothills Medical Centre; (403)264-6720; Fax. (403)237-6646.

DATTA, Jyotirmoy; Medical Arts Bldg, 125-750 Spadina Cres E, Saskatoon SK S7K 3H3; Calcutta (India)'56; MB BS; LRCP; MRCS(Eng); Ac Staff, Saskatoon City Hospital; Ac Staff, St Paul's Hospital (Grey Nuns) of Saskatoon; Ac Staff, Royal University Hospital; Langs: Bengali; Hindi; (306)652-5414; Fax. (306)652-5554.

DATTA, Partha; Rockyview Gen Hosp, 7007 14 St SW, Calgary AB T2V 1P9; McG'95; FRCPC; IntMed. Staff, Foothills Medical Centre; Staff Int Med, Rockyview General Hospital; (403)943-8693

DATTA, Samir; Victoria East Med Clinic, 2068 Prince Wales Dr, Regina SK S4V 3A6; (Other Foreign)'09; CCFP; (306)789-4677; Fax. (306)789-3422.

DATTA, Susmita; The Court, 312-2863 Ellesmere Rd, Scarborough ON M1E 5E9; Dal'80; BSc; Staff, Rouge Valley Health System - Centenary Health Centre Site; Langs: Bengali; (416)281-9055; Fax. (416)281-9006.

DATTA, Suvomoy; Grey Nuns Comm Hosp & HC, 1100 Youville Drive West NW, Edmonton AB T6L 5X8; Sask'00; CCFP; CCFP(E.M.); Staff, Covenant Health - Grey Nuns Community Hospital; (780)735-7180

DATTANI, Indravadan D; Acadia Med Centre, 441-3310 8th St E, Saskatoon SK S7H 5M3; Mysore (India)'74; LRCP; MRCS; DRCOG; FASH; CCFP; Ac Staff, Royal University Hospital; Ac Staff, Saskatoon City Hospital; Consultant Hlth Serv Supernumerary P. O., Royal Canadian Mounted Police; Clinical Asst Prof, University of Saskatchewan; (306)373-6000; Fax. (306)477-5000; dandattani@hotmail.com.

DATTILO, Giovanni A; The Rosedale Med Centre, 607-600 Sherbourne St, Toronto ON M4X 1W4; Tor'00; CCFP; (647)261-1580

DATTILO, Joseph; South Walkerville Med Centre, 175-2224 Walker Rd, Windsor ON N8W 5L7; Wes'73; BScPharm; Court Staff, Hôtel-Dieu Grace Hospital; Court Staff, Windsor Regional Hospital - Metropolitan Site; Langs: Italian; (519)256-0379; Fax. (519)256-2734.

DATTILO, Kathleen M; Univ Hlth Network-Toronto Gen, 3EN 452-200 Elizabeth St, Toronto ON M5G 2C4; Tor'96; FRCPC; Anes (Critical Care Medicine). Staff, Toronto General Hospital - UHN; (416)340-4800

DAUD, Aamir; South Trail Crossing, 82-4307 130 Ave SE, Calgary AB T2Z 3V8; (Pakistan)'87; MB BS; (403)257-9075; Fax. (403)257-7453.

DAUDELIN, Ghislaine; CSSS de Montmagny-L'Islet, RR 1 350 boul Tache O, Montmagny QC G5V 3R8; Laval'00; FRCPC; Psy (General Psychiatry). Staff, CSSS de Montmagny-L'Islet; (418)248-0630 x5563; Fax. (418)248-8472.

DAUDELIN, Luc; Ctr Hosp de Lachine, 650 16e av, Lachine QC H8S 3N5; Mon'80; Staff, CSSS de Dorval-Lachine-Lasalle; (514)637-2351

DAUDI, Asfa; East Mississauga Comm Hlth, 7-2555 Dixie Rd, Mississauga ON L4Y 4C4; Aligarh (USA)'91; CCFP; Langs: Hindi; Urdu; (905)602-7723; Fax. (905)602-5432.

DAUDI, Faiz; Medical Clinic Bldg, 310-89 Humber College Blvd, Etobicoke ON M9V 4B8; Alb'85; FRCSC; GenSurg (Endoscopy). Langs: Urdu; French; Italian; Hindi; (416)747-7722; Fax. (416)747-1069.

DAUKSZA, Aneta; H-876 Montreal Rd, Ottawa ON K1K 4L3; Lodz (Poland)'82; CCFP; FCFP; Langs: Polish; (613)742-8182; Fax. (613)742-0430.

DAUNT, Stephen W; Danforth Med Arts, 105-235 Danforth Ave, Toronto ON M4K 1N2; Tor'03; CCFP; Staff, Humber River Regional Hospital - Finch Avenue Site; (416)462-1777; Fax. (416)462-1775.

DAUPHIN, A Marc; Clinique Med Grn St-Jean, CP 100 Succ Bureau-Chef, Richelain QC J0J 1R0; Laval'75; Langs: German; Italian; English; (450)358-7099 x6236; Fax. (450)358-7424; marcdauphin@gmail.com.

DAUPHIN, Alexandre; St Joseph's Healthcare, 50 Charlton Ave E, Hamilton ON L8N 4A6; Port-au-Prince (Haiti)'77; FRCPC; Anes. Staff, St Joseph's Healthcare - Charlton Campus; Langs: Creole; French; (905)522-4941 x3853

DAUPHIN, Linda; CSSS Pierre Boucher, 1333 boul Jacques-Cartier E, Longueuil QC J4M 2A5; Mon'87; Staff, Centre Hospitalier Pierre Boucher; (450)468-8111

DAUPHIN, Lise; Clinique Med de Verdun, 22-55 av de l'Eglise, Verdun QC H4G 3E7; Mon'82; BHSc; Staff, CSSS du Sud-Ouest Verdun; Staff, CLSC Verdun; Langs: Bilingual(French/English); (514)766-8700; Fax. (514)766-8511.

DAUPHINAIS, Christiane; 52 1/2 McGill St, Toronto ON M5B 1H2; Laval'87; CCFP; Langs: French; (416)260-2048

DAUPHINAIS, Luc; Centre Med des Laurentides, 102-1100 rue Saint-Isidore, St-Lin-Laurentides QC J5M 2V6; Sher'85; (450)439-3870; Fax. (450)439-7849.

DAUPHINAIS, Lucie; Centre Medical de Varennes, 101-2082 Rte Marie-Victorin, Varennes QC J3X 2C7; Sher'86; (450)652-2959; Fax. (450)652-3792.

DAUPHINEE, Peter A; Active Health Sports Med Ctre, 103-115 Bell Farm Rd, Barrie ON L4M 5G1; Dal'95; FRCSC; GenSurg. Staff, Royal Victoria Regional Health Centre; (705)730-6850; Fax. (705)726-1755.

DAUPHINEE-BENTLEY, Patricia K; Parrsboro & Area Professional, PO Box 638 76 Jenks Ave, Parrsboro NS B0M 1S0; Dal'82; (902)254-3760; Fax. (902)254-3617.

DAUTH, Eric; Groupe Med de Trois-Rivieres, 225-1900 boul des Recollets, Trois-Rivieres QC G8Z 4K4; Sher'88; LMCC; CCFP; (819)375-6666

DAUTH, Pierre; Clin de Med Fam Cowansville, 499 rue du Sud, Cowansville QC J2K 2X9; Laval'82; assoc Staff, Hôpital Brome-Missisquoi-Perkins; (450)263-8890; Fax. (450)263-9737.

DAUTREMONT, Kevin J; 205-53 Stadacona St W, Moose Jaw SK S6H 1Z2; Sask'83; Staff, Moose Jaw Union Hospital; Physician, Providence Place; Physician, Angus Campbell Center; (306)692-0200; Fax. (306)692-0286; kdautremont@fhhr.ca.

DAVALLOU, Mojgan; Women's College Hosp, 76 Grenville St, Toronto ON M5S 1B2; Munich (Germany)'94; FRCPC; Anes. Staff, Women's College Hospital; Langs: Farsi; (416)323-6008

DAVARI, Sara; Pavillon Rosemont, 5689 boul Rosemont, Montreal QC H1T 2H1; Mon'09; CCFP; (514)252-3400; Fax. (514)252-3854.

DAVE, Amritlal; Kings Med Clinic, 11-3340 17 Ave SE, Calgary AB T2A 0P9; Bristol (England)'62; MB ChB; DCH; MRCP; FRCPC; IntMed. Clin Asst Prof, University of Calgary; (403)273-8500; Fax. (403)569-0706.

DAVE, Hemang J; Surrey Mem Hosp, 13750 96 Ave, Surrey BC V3V 1Z2; Makerere (Uganda)'97; MB ChB; Staff, Surrey Memorial Hospital; (604)581-2211

DAVE, Kanta B; Tower Centre, 438-131 9 Ave SW, Calgary AB T2P 1K1; (India)'74; MB BS; Langs: Hindi; (403)261-8859; Fax. (403)265-0573.

DAVE, Kishorchandra M; Medical Bldg, 202-1615 Dufferin St, Toronto ON M6H 4H4; Gujarat (India)'63; CCFP; FCFP; Langs: Gujarati; Hindi; (416)652-1990; Fax. (416)652-1467.

DAVE, Mala; SFU-Health & Counselling Serv, 8888 University Dr, Burnaby BC V5A 1S6; Cal'03; CCFP; (778)782-4615; Fax. (778)782-5781.

DAVE, Malini G; Leslie Med Centre, 401-4800 Leslie St, North York ON M2J 2K9; Nagpur (India)'98; FRCPC; Peds. Langs: Hindi; Malayalam; Tamil; (416)497-1987

DAVE, Sumit; London HSC-Victoria Hosp, PO Box 5010 Stn B 800 Commissioners Rd E, London ON N6A 5W9; Jawaharlal (India)'92; Staff, London Health Sciences Centre - Victoria Campus; (519)685-8439

DAVENPORT, Anna M; Fifth Avenue Med Centre, 500-14 Fifth Ave, Orangeville ON L9W 1G2; Tor'86; Staff, Headwaters Health Care Centre - Orangeville Site; (519)942-2505; Fax. (519)941-4349.

DAVENPORT, Eric; Davenport MPC, 300B-984 Oliver Rd, Thunder Bay ON P7B 7C7; Wes'03; FRCSC; GenSurg; Critical Care Medicine. Staff, The Ottawa Hospital - Civic Campus; Langs: Bilingual(English/French); (807)285-4860; Fax. (807)285-4857.

DAVENPORT, Ethan M; CFB Petawawa CDU #2, PO Box 9999 Stn Main, Petawawa ON K8H 2X3; Dal'01; CCFP; (613)687-5511

DAVENPORT, William J; South Health Campus, 4448 Front St SE, Calgary AB T3M 1M4; Urbana(IL) (USA)'96; FRCPC; Neur. Staff, Peter Lougheed Centre; Langs: French; (403)956-2460; Fax. (403)956-2992.

DAVERNE, Heather L; ActiveCare Med Clinic, 1108 Klondike Rd, Kanata ON K2K 0G1; Sask'94; CCFP; FCFP; (613)254-9777

DAVEY, Allyson L; 202-474 Columbia St, Kamloops BC V2C 2T5; UBC'98; FRCPC; Peds. (250)374-3300

DAVEY, Cecile D; Grand River Hosp-KW Hlth Ctre, PO Box 9056 Stn C 835 King St W, Kitchener ON N2G 1G3; Jamaica (Jamaica)'92; FRCPC; Peds. Staff, Grand River Hospital - Kitchener/Waterloo Health Centre; Langs: Creole; (519)749-4300

DAVEY, Colin F; 206-159 Cobequid Rd, Lower Sackville NS B4C 2N1; Dal'88; BSc(Biol); (902)865-6817; Fax. (902)865-4942.

DAVEY, Darlene G; Rexdale Med Centre, 2-123 Rexdale Blvd, Etobicoke ON M9W 1P1; Wes'83; CCFP; FCFP; Ac Staff, William Osler Health System - Etobicoke General Hospital; (416)743-5853; darlenedavey@rogers.com.

DAVEY, E Bruce; 207-3825 Sunset St, Burnaby BC V5G 1T4; Ott'74; Ac Staff, Burnaby Hospital; Assoc Staff, Providence Health Care - Mount Saint Joseph Hospital; Assoc Staff, Providence Health Care - St Vincent's Hospital-Langara Site; (604)433-1249; Fax. (604)436-0336.

DAVEY, J Roderick; Univ Hlth Network-Toronto Western Hosp, 1E 444-399 Bathurst St, Toronto ON M5T 2S8; Tor'80; FRCSC; OrthSurg (Hip & Knee Replacement). Med Dir, Toronto Western Hospital - University Health Network; Asst Prof Surg, University of Toronto; (416)603-5732; rod.davey@uhn.on.ca.

DAVEY, Michelle A L; B-530 Main St PO Box 1148 Stn Lcd 1, Winchester ON K0C 2K0; Ott'04; FRCSC; GenSurg. Staff, Hamilton Health Sciences Centre - McMaster Children's Hospital; Langs: Bilingual(English/French).

DAVEY, P Douglas; Allin Clinic, 10155 120 St NW, Edmonton AB T5K 2A2; Alb'74; VascSurg (Bariatric Surgery); GenSurg. Chief Surg, Royal Alexandra Hospital; Associate Clin Prof, University of Alberta; (780)482-7551; Fax. (780)488-2056.

DAVEY, Phillip; Toronto Sunnybrook Reg Cancer, 2075 Bayview Ave, Toronto ON M4N 3M5; Manchester (England)'75; FRCR; DABR; MRCP; FRCPC; RadOncol. Asst Prof RadOncol, University of Toronto; (416)480-6128; Fax. (416)480-6002.

DAVEY, Robert S; PO Box 7280 Stn Main, Bonnyville AB T9N 2H6; Alb'75; FRCPC; GenPath. Staff/Pathologist, Bonnyville Healthcare Centre; (780)826-3311; Fax. (780)826-6529.

DAVEY, Ryan A; London HSC-University Hosp, PO Box 5339 Stn B 399 Windermere Rd, London ON N6A 5A5; (Ireland)'08; IntMed. Staff, London Health Sciences Centre - University Hospital; (519)685-8500

DAVEY, Stanley J; 1022 20 St S, Lethbridge AB T1K 2C9; Alb'83; FRCSC; ObstGyn. Staff ObstGyn, Tom Baker Cancer Centre; Staff ObstGyn, Chinook Regional Hospital; (403)381-4410; Fax. (403)381-4402.

DAVIAU, Marjolaine; Clinique Medicale du Village, 200-400 rue Meigs, Farnham QC J2N 2C8; Laval'01; CCFP; Staff, Hôpital Brome-Missisquoi-Perkins; Langs: English; (450)293-3681; Fax. (450)293-7463.

DAVIAULT, Elizabeth; CLSC Mercier-Est/Anjou, 9503 rue Sherbrooke E, Montreal QC H1L 6P2; Sher'89; Langs: English; Italian; (514)356-2572 x3142; Fax. (514)493-0083.

DAVID, Andrea; Sunnybrook Hlth Sciences Ctre, A103-2075 Bayview Ave, Toronto ON M4N 3M5; Tor'94; CCFP; Staff, Sunnybrook Health Sciences Centre; (416)480-4936; Fax. (416)480-6038.

DAVID, Andree; Clinique Med Monk, 6023 boul Monk, Montreal QC H4E 3H5; Mon'75; (514)761-5527

DAVID, Claude; Centre Med du Saint-Jovite, CP 19069 PL Ouimet 992 rue Saint Jovite, Mont-Tremblant QC J8E 3C1; Mon'75; Langs: English; (819)425-2728; Fax. (418)425-8012.

DAVID, Donald; 314 rue Commerciale E CP 278, Chandler QC G0C 1K0; Mon'65; (418)689-2112; Fax. (418)689-3112.

DAVID, Eleazar W; 101-8927 152 St, Surrey BC V3R 4E5; Lyceum-North (Philippines)'81; CCFP; Langs: Tagalog; (604)588-4449; eleazarwdavid@hotmail.com.

DAVID, Elizabeth N; Sunnybrook Hlth Sciences Ctre, 2075 Bayview Ave, Toronto ON M4N 3M5; Tor'97; FRCPC; DiagRad. Staff, Sunnybrook Health Sciences Centre; (416)480-4358; Fax. (416)480-5855.

DAVID, Eytan; Northmount Med Centre, 302-145 13th St E, North Vancouver BC V7L 2L4; UBC'96; FRCSC; Otol (Ear Nose & Throat Surgery). Staff, Lions Gate Hospital; (604)988-0598; Fax. (604)985-0501.

DAVID, Herve; 210-211 rue Champlain, Dieppe NB E1A 1N9; Laval'91; FRCSC; OrthSurg (Arthroplasty). Staff Orth Surg, Dr Georges-L-Dumont University Hospital Centre; (506)855-2750; Fax. (506)855-2790; dtdleppe@nb.sympatico.ca.

DAVID, Ivo; Burrard Health Bldg, 304-1160 Burrard St, Vancouver BC V6Z 2E8; Prague (Czech Republic)'82; Staff, Providence Health Care - St Paul's Hospital; (604)687-2122; Fax. (604)687-2799.

DAVID, Jacqueline; Polyclinique St-Martin, 604-1435 boul Saint-Martin O, Laval QC H7S 2C6; Mon'76; (450)668-3310; Fax. (450)668-9347.

DAVID, Julie; Clinique leger et Assoues, 201-1851 rue Sherbrooke E, Montreal QC H2K 4L5; Mon'85; FRCPC; DiagRad (Breast Imaging). Langs: English; (514)523-2121; Fax. (514)523-2318.

DAVID, Marc; MUHC-Montreal Gen Hosp, 1650 av Cedar, Montreal QC H3G 1A4; Mon'96; FRCPC; RadOncol (Palliative Care). Physician, McGill University Health Centre - Montreal General Campus; Aj Prof, McGill University; Langs: English; (514)934-1934 x48040; Fax. (514)934-8425; marc.david@muhc.mcgill.ca.

DAVID, Marc; 401-235 boul René-Lévesque E, Montreal QC H2X 1N8; Mon'78; CSPQ; Cardiol. Staff, Centre Hospitalier l'Université De Montréal (CHUM) - Hôpital Saint-luc; (514)861-1503

DAVID, Michele; 3175 ch de la Côte-Sainte-Cath, Montreal QC H3T 1C5; Mon'78; MedOncol (P.Q.); HemPath; Hem (P.Q.). Staff Hematology-Oncology, Hôpital Ste-Justine; assoc Prof, Universite de Montreal; (514)345-4639; michele.david@umontreal.ca.

DAVID, Mirla F; Winnipeg Clinic, 425 St Mary Ave, Winnipeg MB R3C 0N2; Santo Tomas (Philippines)'58; DABPed; DABACI; FRCPC; Peds (Clinical Immunology & Allergy). Ac Staff Children's Div, Health Sciences Centre; Assoc Prof Peds, University of Manitoba; (204)957-1900; Fax. (204)943-7921.

DAVID, Morton J; 1-9371 No 5 Rd, Richmond BC V7A 4E1; Dal'71; (604)272-1338

DAVID, Oliver A; 2897 17 Ave SE, Calgary AB T2A 0P7; Alb'90; DABFP; (403)272-3384; Fax. (403)272-5671.

DAVID, Pierre; Hop Louis-H Lafontaine, 7401 rue Hochelaga, Montreal QC H1N 3M5; Mon'86; FRCPC; Psy. Staff, Hopital Louis-H Lafontaine; (514)251-4084; Fax. (514)251-4027.

DAVID, Saloma; Cornerstone Med Centre, 28-1200 37 St SW, Calgary AB T3C 1S2; (India)'82; MB BS; (587)433-7015

DAVID, Sheila J; Humber River Reg Hosp, 2111 Finch Ave W, North York ON M3N 1N1; Dal'74; BSc; Staff, Humber River Regional Hospital - Finch Avenue Site; Langs: French; Spanish; (416)744-2500

DAVID, Tirone; 4N 453-200 Elizabeth St, Toronto ON M5G 2C4; Parana (Brazil)'68; FACS; FRCSC; Cardiovasc&ThorSurg. Chief Cardiovasc Surg, Toronto General Hospital - UHN; Prof Surg, University of Toronto; Langs: Portuguese; (416)340-5062; Fax. (416)340-4020; tirone.david@uhn.ca.

DAVIDMAN, Michael; SMBD Jewish Gen Hosp, 3755 ch Cote-Sainte-Catherine, Montreal QC H3T 1E2; Alb'66; FRCPC; IntMed; Nephrol (P.Q.). Ac Staff, Sir Mortimer B Davis Jewish General; assoc Prof Med, McGill University; (514)340-7516; Fax. (514)340-8147.

DAVIDOW, Jonathan; Royal Alexandra Hosp, 4228-10240 Kingsway Ave NW, Edmonton AB T5H 3V9; McG'00; FRCPC; EmergMed; Critical Care Medicine. Staff, Royal Alexandra Hospital; (780)735-5172

DAVIDS, Jonathan W; Medical Services Group, 1 President's Choice Circle, Brampton ON L6Y 5S5; McM'94; Dip SportMed; CCBOM; CCFP; FCFP; Asst Clin Prof Adjunct Family Med Faculty of Health Sciences, McMaster University; (905)861-2676; Fax. (905)861-2363.

DAVIDS, Peter; Foothills Med Centre, C231-1403 29 St NW, Calgary AB T2N 2T9; Sask'92; CCFP; CCFP(E.M.); FCFP; Staff, Foothills Medical Centre; (403)944-1596; Fax. (403)944-2419; peter.davids@calgaryhealthregion.ca.

DAVIDS, Taryn; Dixon Med Centre, 104-581 davis Dr, Newmarket ON L3Y 2P6; McM'04; FRCSC; Otol (Head & Neck Surgery). (905)898-2444

DAVIDS, Terence; Humboldt Med Clinic, PO Box 220, Humboldt SK S0K 2A0; MB ChB; Langs: Afrikaans; (306)682-2618; Fax. (306)682-4499; humboldtclinic@sasktel.net.

DAVIDSON, A George; Children's & Women's HC of BC, K3 204-4480 Oak St, Vancouver BC V6H 3V4; UBC'63; BSc; FRCPC; Peds (Cystic Fibrosis). Staff, BC Children's Hospital; Vis Staff C F Clinic, University Hospital of Northern British Columbia; Emeritus Prof, University of British Columbia; (604)875-2628

DAVIDSON, Adam; Lions Gate Hosp, 231 15th St E, North Vancouver BC V7L 2L7; UBC'06; CCFP; CCFP(E.M.); Staff, Lions Gate Hospital; (604)984-5813

DAVIDSON, Anna; Trillium Hlth Ctr-Mississauga, 100 Queensway W, Mississauga ON L5B 1B8; Wes'76; FRCPC; Anes. Staff, Trillium Health Centre - Mississauga; (905)848-7628

DAVIDSON, Cara E; Royal Court Med Centre, 208-1 Quarry Ridge Rd, Barrie ON L4M 7G1; McM'08; FRCPC; Peds. (705)728-3766

DAVIDSON, Carolyn J; Student Hlth Services, 50 George St N, Cambridge ON N1S 2M8; McM'89; CCFP; FCFP; (519)824-4120; Fax. (519)836-7431.

DAVIDSON, David; The Ottawa Hosp Academic FHT, 210 Melrose Ave, Ottawa ON K1Y 4K7; McG'76; BSc; MDCM; FCFP; CCFP; CCFP(E.M.); Att Staff, The Ottawa Hospital - Civic Campus; Asst Prof, University of Ottawa; (613)761-4334; Fax. (613)761-4200.

DAVIDSON, Derek A; Medical Clinic Person-Ctred Ps, 403-265 Yorkland Blvd, North York ON M2J 1S5; Tor'63; FACP; MDiv; BA; MA; FRCPC; IntMed (Psychotherapy); Nephrol. Hon Staff, Humber River Regional Hospital - Church Street Site; Staff, The Medical Clinic for Person-Centred Psychotherapy; (416)229-2399; Fax. (416)229-9771.

DAVIDSON, Dion; 66 Exhibition St, Kentville NS B4N 5J6; Sask'97; BSc; FACS; FRCSC; GenSurg (Critical Care Medicine); VascSurg. Consultant Vasc Surg, Yarmouth Regional Hospital; Consultant Vasc & Gen Surg/Att Staff Critical Care, Valley Regional Hospital; Consultant Vasc Surg, Fisherman's Memorial Lunenburg; (902)678-9530; Fax. (902)678-2945.

DAVIDSON, George; Pelham Group Health Centre, 205-245 Pelham Rd, St Catharines ON L2S 1X8; London (England)'79; MB BS; ASAM; NeurPath (Addiction Medicine). (905)688-3232; Fax. (905)685-4547.

DAVIDSON, Graham M; 103-7143 West Saanich Rd, Brentwood Bay BC V8M 1P7; McG'78; (250)652-9191; Fax. (250)652-5576.

DAVIDSON, J Michael; St Boniface Gen Hosp, 409 Tache Ave, Winnipeg MB R2H 2A6; Man'84; FRCPC; DiagRad. Staff, St Boniface General Hospital; (204)233-8563; Fax. (204)231-0640.

DAVIDSON, James A; Surrey Mem Hosp, 13750 96 Ave, Surrey BC V3V 1Z2; Qns'04; FRCPC; IntMed; MedOncol. Staff Fraser Valley Cancer Centre, Surrey Memorial Hospital; Langs: Bilingual(English/French); (604)930-4028

DAVIDSON, Jana-Lea; Children's & Women's Hlth Ctre, P2 307-4500 Oak St, Vancouver BC V6H 3V4; UBC'96; BSc; MSc; FRCPC; Psy (Anxiety & Mood Disorders). Staff, BC Women's Hospital & Health Centre; Clin Instructor Med, University of British Columbia; (604)875-2010

DAVIDSON, John R; North York Gen Hosp, 4001 Leslie St, North York ON M2K 1E1; Qns'77; FRCPC; Anes. Staff, North York General Hospital; Asst Prof, University of Toronto; (416)756-6265; Fax. (416)281-7453.

DAVIDSON, John S D; Hotel-Dieu Hosp, 166 Brock St, Kingston ON K7L 5G2; Qns'82; MSc; FRCSC; PlasSurg. Staff, Hotel-Dieu Hospital; (613)544-3400 x2117; Fax. (613)545-0576.

DAVIDSON, Joseph K; 2A-800 Southdown Rd, Mississauga ON L5J 2Y4; Seattle(Washington) (USA)'92; FRCSC; Ophth. Langs: English; French; (905)822-2020

DAVIDSON, Lindsay K; Kingston Gen Hosp, 76 Stuart St, Kingston ON K7L 2V7; Tor'86; MSc; MEd; FRCSC; OrthSurg (Pediatric Orthopedics). Staff, Kingston General Hospital; Staff, Hotel-Dieu Hospital; Assoc Prof, Queen's University; Langs: Bilingual(English/French); (613)544-9626; Fax. (866)545-1519.

DAVIDSON, M Jean; Sunnybrook Hlth Sciences Ctre, M1 102-2075 Bayview Ave, Toronto ON M4N 3M5; Tor'83; FRCSC; Otol (Head & Neck Surgery). Staff, Sunnybrook Health Sciences Centre; Staff, Sunnybrook Health Sciences Centre - Edmond Odette Cancer Centre; Asst Prof, University of Toronto; (416)480-6705; Fax. (416)480-5761.

DAVIDSON, Marie-Helene; CSSS Becancour-Nicolet-Yamaska, 216 rue Prinicpale, Fortierville QC G0S 1J0; Laval'01; (819)287-4442

DAVIDSON, Marilyn J; Pacific Avenue Med Centre, 300-149 Pacific Ave, Saskatoon SK S7K 1N8; Sask'85; FRCSC; ObstGyn. Associate Clin Prof ObstGyn, University of Saskatchewan; (306)653-5970; Fax. (306)653-5383.

DAVIDSON, Mark R; Meadowlark Place Prof Centre, 204-8708 155 St NW, Edmonton AB T5R 1W2; Alb'90; FRCPC; Peds. (780)489-3005; Fax. (780)489-3050.

DAVIDSON, Marla; Royal Univ Hosp, 121 EH-103 Hospital Dr, Saskatoon SK S7N 0W8; Sask'04; FRCPC; Psy. Staff, Royal University Hospital; (306)655-1000

DAVIDSON, Martha B; Smithville Family Health Ctre, PO Box 218 230 Canboro St, Smithville ON L0R 2A0; McM'86; BASc; MSc; CCFP; FCFP; Ac Staff, West Lincoln Memorial Hospital; Associate Clin Prof, McMaster University; (905)957-3870; mdavidson@cogeco.ca.

DAVIDSON, Michael H; 205-125 13th St E, North Vancouver BC V7L 2L3; Cal'73; BSc; Staff Family Pract, Lions Gate Hospital; (604)985-9551

DAVIDSON, Murray; Bloor-Jane Med Bldg, 513-2425 Bloor St W, Toronto ON M6S 4W4; Tor'61; FRCPC; IntMed (Hematology). Ac Staff, St Joseph's Health Centre; Consultant, North York General Hospital - Branson Division; Langs: Yiddish; (416)766-2365; Fax. (416)766-5076.

DAVIDSON, Niall J; Carmi Clinic, 115-725 Carmi Ave, Penticton BC V2A 3G8; Man'01; FRCPC; Neur. (250)487-2366

DAVIDSON, R Bruce; Royal Inland Hosp, 311 Columbia St, Kamloops BC V2C 2T1; UBC'92; CCFP; CCFP(E.M.); Staff, Royal Inland Hospital; (250)374-5111

DAVIDSON, Robert G; Red Deer Reg Hosp Ctr, PO Box 5030 3942 50A Ave, Red Deer AB T4N 4E7; Alb'04; CCFP; CCFP(E.M.); Staff, Red Deer Regional Hospital Centre; (403)343-4442

DAVIDSON, Ronald; Delta Health Sciences Centre, 204-4515 Harvest Dr, Delta BC V4K 4L1; Sask'70; Physician, Delta Health Sciences Centre; (604)946-0665; Fax. (604)946-0494.

DAVIDSON, Shannon; Eagle Ridge Family Health Ctre, 203-480 Huronia Rd, Barrie ON L4N 6M2; Alb'02; BScH; CCFP; (705)727-7688; Fax. (705)734-6284.

DAVIDSON, Simon I; Children's Hosp Eastern Ont, 401 Smyth Rd, Ottawa ON K1H 8L1; Witwatersrand (South Africa)'74; MB BCh; FRCPC; Psy (Child & Adolescent Psychiatry). Reg Chief Specialized Psy & Mental Hlth Services for Children & Youth, Royal Ottawa Mental Health Centre - Royal Ottawa Health Care Group; Reg Chief Specialized Psy & Mental Hlth Services for Children & Youth, Children's Hospital of Eastern Ontario (CHEO); Prof, University of Ottawa; (613)737-7600 x2723; Fax. (613)737-2257; davidson@cheo.on.ca.

DAVIDSON, Warren; Rockyview Gen Hosp, 4A 185A-7007 14 St SW, Calgary AB T2V 1P9; UBC'98; FRCPC; IntMed; Respir. Staff Resp Med, Rockyview General Hospital; Asst Prof, University of Calgary; (403)943-3345; Fax. (403)943-8666.

DAVIDSON, William; Advanced Walk-In Med Clinic, 111-21 Queensway W, Mississauga ON L5B 1B6; Glasgow (Scotland)'59; FAAP; MB ChB; Peds. Staff Physician, The Hospital For Sick Children; Lecturer, University of Toronto; Langs: French; (905)897-0788; wm.davidson@utoronto.ca.

DAVIDUCK, Wayne J; Dr Wayne J Daviduck Prof Corp, 307-200 Boudreau Rd, St. Albert AB T8N 6B9; Alb'98; BMedSci; CCFP; (780)470-3825; Fax. (780)470-3826.

DAVIES, Andrew; 123 Millennium Pkwy RR 5 Stn Main, Belleville ON K8N 4Z5; Qns'88; FRCSC; Ophth (Cataract Surgery). Court Staff, QHC Belleville General; Med Staff, QHC Trenton Memorial; Lecturer Ophth, Queen's University; (613)961-7440; Fax. (613)961-1798.

DAVIES, Andrew O; 1140 Glenwood Rd, North Bay ON P1B 4S5; Tor'70; FRCPC; Anes. Ac Staff, North Bay Regional Health Centre - Regional Mental Health; Asst Prof, University of Toronto; (705)476-3405

DAVIES, Anne-Marie; Squamish Gen Hosp, 38140 Behrner Dr, Squamish BC V8B 0J3; Tor'10; CCFP; Staff, Squamish General Hospital / Hilltop House; (604)892-5211

DAVIES, Anthony; Canora Med Clinic, PO Box 2040, Canora SK S0A 0L0; Bristol (England)'79; (306)563-5557; Fax. (306)563-4175.

DAVIES, Brian J; 185 Mitton St N, Sarnia ON N7T 6H3; Wes'85; FRCPC; IntMed (Diabetology). Staff, Bluewater Health - Norman Site; Staff, Bluewater Health - Mitton Site; Physician, Bluewater Sleep Disorder Clinic; (519)337-0011; Fax. (519)337-0522.

DAVIES, Campbell D; St Mary's Hosp Centre, 3830 av Lacombe, Montreal QC H3T 1M5; Alb'75; FRCPC; IntMed; Gastroent. Staff, St Mary's Hospital Centre; (514)345-3511 x3736; Fax. (514)734-2713.

DAVIES, Carolyn; Children's & Women's HC of BC, 1K 57-4480 Oak St, Vancouver BC V6H 3V4; UBC'88; FRCPC; Peds. Staff, BC Children's Hospital; (604)875-2045

DAVIES, Ceri J; 1A-6758 Kingston Rd, Scarborough ON M1B 1G8; Wes'91; CCFP; FCFP; (416)286-7890; Fax. (416)286-8600.

DAVIES, Christine E; Trinity Royal Clinic, 3B-28 King St, Saint John NB E2L 1G3; Dublin (Ireland)'72; CCFP; FCFP; Staff Family Med, Horizon Health Network Saint John Public Health; (506)634-7772; Fax. (506)634-7101.

DAVIES, Colleen E; 11 Murray St PO Box 1630, New Liskeard ON P0J 1P0; Ott'97; BSc(Hons); CCFP; Staff, Temiskaming Hospital; (705)647-4102; Fax. (705)647-0114.

DAVIES, Dafydd A; The Hosp for Sick Children, 1526-555 University AVe, Toronto ON M5G 1X8; Dal'04; GenSurg.

DAVIES, Dawn; Edmonton Clinic Health Academy, 3 533-11405 87 Ave NW, Edmonton AB T6G 1C9; McM'93; BScN; FRCPC; Peds (Palliative Care). Media Dir Ped Palliative Care Child Hlth Prog, University of Alberta Hospital; Staff, Edmonton Clinic Health Academy; Asst Prof Peds, University of Alberta; (780)248-5505

DAVIES, Donald; Bridgetop Med Clinic, PO Box 1630 11 Murray St, New Liskeard ON P0J 1P0; Ott'96; BSc(Hons Physiol); CCFP; Staff, Temiskaming Hospital; Asst Prof, Northern Ontario School of Medicine; (705)647-4102; Fax. (705)647-0114.

DAVIES, E Colin; Saint John Reg Hosp, PO Box 2100 Stn Main 400 University Ave, Saint John NB E2L 4L2; Dublin (Ireland)'72; MB ChB; BAO; FRCPC; Anes (Pain Management). Ac Staff, Saint John Regional Hospital; Ac Staff, St Joseph's Hospital; Assoc Prof, Dalhousie University; Langs: French; (506)648-6861; Fax. (506)648-6860.

DAVIES, Edward; London HSC-University Hosp, PO Box 5339 Stn B B8 007-339 Windermere Rd, London ON N6A 5A5; Wes'87; FRCSC; GenSurg (Hepatobiliary & Pancreatic Surgery). Staff, London Health Sciences Centre - University Hospital; Asst Prof Surg., University of Western Ontario; (519)663-3458

DAVIES, Edward G; Sgh Medical Mall, 302-3030 Lawrence Ave E, Scarborough ON M1P 2T7; Tor'90; FRCPC; IntMed (Cardiac Electrophysiology); Cardiol. Assoc Staff, The Scarborough Hospital - General Campus; (416)438-9051; Fax. (416)438-9899.

DAVIES, Grant; Calmar Med Clinic, PO Box 1079 4741 50 Ave, Calmar AB T0C 0V0; Alb'02; CCFP; (780)985-3344; Fax. (780)985-3877.

DAVIES, Gregory; Kingston Gen Hosp, 76 Stuart St, Kingston ON K7L 2V7; McM'89; FRCSC; ObstGyn (Maternal Fetal Medicine). Co-Dir Fetal Assessment Unit, Kingston General Hospital; Dir Labour & Delivery & Assoc. Prof., Queen's University; (613)548-6072; Fax. (613)548-1330; daviesg@kgh.kari.net.

DAVIES, J Bradley; South Calgary Med Clinic, 118-40 Sunpark Plaza SE, Calgary AB T2X 3X7; Alb'99; CCFP; (403)254-4000; Fax. (403)254-1282.

DAVIES, Jan M; Foothills Med Centre, 1403 29 St NW, Calgary AB T2N 2T9; Cal'75; MSc; FRCPC; Anes (Pre-Operative Assessment). Ac Staff, Foothills Medical Centre; Ac Staff, Calgary Health Region; Prof Anes, University of Calgary; Langs: English; French; (403)944-4707; Fax. (403)944-2425; jdavies@ucalgary.ca.

DAVIES, Janine; BC Cancer Ctre-Southern Interi, 399 Royal Ave, Kelowna BC V1Y 5L3; McM'03; FRCPC; IntMed; MedOncol. Staff, BC Cancer Agency Pharmacy-Centre for the Southern Interior; (250)712-3930

DAVIES, John T; Pembroke Regional Hospital Inc, 705 MacKay St, Pembroke ON K8A 1G8; Sask'97; CCFP; Staff, Pembroke Regional Hospital Inc; (613)732-2811

DAVIES, Kay M; IWK Health Centre, PO Box 9700 Rpo CSC 5850-5980 University Ave, Halifax NS B3K 6R8; London (England)'96; MB BS; Staff, IWK Health Centre; (902)470-8888

DAVIES, Laura M; Alberta Children's Hosp, 2888 Shaganappi Trail NW, Calgary AB T3B 6A8; Sask'85; FRCPC; Peds. Staff Peds, Alberta Children's Hospital; (403)955-2953

DAVIES, Martin E; Health Services Dept, 4825 Mount Royal Gate SW, Calgary AB T3E 6K6; Sask'87; CCFP; FCFP; (403)440-6326; Fax. (403)440-6759.

DAVIES, Mary P; St Joseph's Health Centre, 30 The Queensway, Toronto ON M6R 1B5; Durham (England)'62; MB BS; DObstRCOG; FFARCS; FRCPC; Anes. Ac Staff, St Joseph's Health Centre; (416)530-6000 x4090; Fax. (416)530-6300.

DAVIES, Michael J; Comox Valley Med Clinic, 3199 Cliffe Ave, Courtenay BC V9N 2L9; Sask'81; (250)334-1512; Fax. (250)334-1597.

DAVIES, Murray W; Kamsack Med Clinic, PO Box 69, Kamsack SK S0A 1S0; Sask'72; (306)542-2623

DAVIES, Nigel C M; Medical Clinic, 5031 49 St, Innisfail AB T4G 1A4; Manchester (England)'67; Ac Staff, Innisfail Health Centre; (403)227-3356; Fax. (403)227-2702; ndavies@dthr.ab.ca.

DAVIES, Nina E; Quinte Health CC-Belleville Ge, 356-265 Dundas St E, Belleville ON K8N 5A9; Ott'98; BSc; FRCSC; GenSurg. Staff GenSurg, QHC Belleville General; (613)771-1251; Fax. (613)771-1917.

DAVIES, Robert G; Pacific Place Mall, 959-999 36 St NE, Calgary AB T2A 7X6; Alb'99; BMedSci; FRCPC; DiagRad. (403)215-2900; Fax. (403)215-2920.

DAVIES, Ross; Univ of Ottawa Heart Institute, H1295A-40 Ruskin St, Ottawa ON K1Y 4W7; Tor'74; BSc; FACC; FRCPC; IntMed (Heart Transplantation); Cardiol. Pres Med & Scientific, University of Ottawa Heart Institute; Assoc Prof Med, University of Ottawa; (613)761-4593; Fax. (613)761-4877; radavies@ottawaheart.ca.

DAVIES, Sharon R; Mount Sinai Hosp, 600 University Ave, Toronto ON M5G 1X5; McM'82; FRCPC; Anes. Staff, Mount Sinai Hospital; (416)586-4800 x5270; Fax. (416)586-8664.

DAVIES, Simon J C; Geriatric Mental Hlth Prog, 5401-901 King St W, Toronto ON M5V 3H5; London (England)'93; (416)979-4749

DAVIES, Stacy J; Roslyn Med Bldg, 200-400 5 Ave SW, Calgary AB T2P 0L6; Alb'88; CCFP; (403)930-1005; Fax. (403)930-1004.

DAVIES, Ashley; 422-6880 Wallace Dr, Saanichton BC V8M 1N8; Oxford (England)'69; MA; BCh; Ac Staff, University Hospital of Northern British Columbia; (250)564-4356; Fax. (250)564-9454; ashley.davies@northernhealth.ca.

DAVIES, Thomas J; Caledonian Med Clinic, 340 Campbell St, Nanaimo BC V9R 3G7; Alb'80; Staff, Nanaimo Regional General Hospital; (250)753-3202; Fax. (250)753-1039.

DAVIES, Timothy O; Hamilton HS-Henderson Site, 711 Concession St, Hamilton ON L8V 1C3; Qns'02; FRCSC; Urol (Reconstructive Urology). Staff, Hamilton Health Sciences Centre-Juravinski Site; Asst Prof, McMaster University; (905)521-2100; Fax. (905)381-7037.

DAVIES, William M; The Doctors Bldg, 506-208 Bloor St W, Toronto ON M5S 3B4; Tor'74; FRCPC; Psy (General Adult Psychiatry). (416)603-8484

DAVIGNON, Genevieve; Orleans-Cumberland Comm FHT, 202-3095 St Joseph Blvd, Orleans ON K1E 3W6; Mon'06; CCFP; Langs: Bilingual(French/English); (613)590-0533; Fax. (613)590-7351.

DAVIGNON, Jean; Inst de Recherche Clin de Mtl, 110 av des Pins O, Montreal QC H2W 1R7; Mon'58; MSc; FACP; FRCPC; IntMed (Hyperlipidemia & Atherosclerosis). Staff, Centre Hospitalier l'Université de Montréal (CHUM) - Hôtel-Dieu; Emeritus Prof IRCM, Hyperlipidemia & Atherosclerosis Research Group, Clinical Research Inst. of Montreal(IRCM); Prof, Universite de Montreal; (514)987-5626; Fax. (514)987-5700; davignj@ircm.qc.ca.

DAVILA ACOSTA, Jorge H; Children's Hosp of Eastern Ont, 401 Smyth Rd, Ottawa ON K1H 8L1; (Peru)'02; Staff, Children's Hospital of Eastern Ontario (CHEO); (613)737-7600

DAVILMAR, Paule; Tobique Valley Comm Hlth Ctr, 120 Main St, Plaster Rock NB E7G 2E5; (506)356-6649

DAVINE, Jonathan; East Reg Mental Health Service, East Region Mental Health 2757 King St E, Hamilton ON L8G 5E4; McG'79; MDCM; FRCPC; CCFP; Psy (Adult Outpatient Psychiatry). Ac Staff, St Joseph's Healthcare - Charlton Campus; Physician, East Region Mental Health Services; Assoc Prof Psy, McMaster University; Langs: Hebrew; Bilingual(French/English); (905)573-4801; Fax. (905)573-4802.

DAVIS, Alan E; Cornwall Comm Hosp-Mcconnell, PO box 100 Stn Main 840 McConnell Ave, Cornwall ON K6H 5S5; McG'82; PhD; CCFP; CCFP(E.M.); Staff, Cornwall Community Hospital; Langs: Bilingual(English/French); (613)938-4290

DAVIS, Amie; Burlington Prof Centre, 208-3155 Harvester Rd, Burlington ON L7N 3V2; McM'05; FamilyMed. (905)333-8222; Fax. (905)634-7007.

DAVIS, Anne L; Davis Med Clinic, PO Box 99, Eastend SK S0N 0T0; Sask'88; CCFP; FCFP; (306)295-3522; Fax. (306)295-3562.

DAVIS, Beverley M; Taddle Creek Connection, B102-726 Bloor St W, Toronto ON M6G 4A1; Tor'86; CCFP; FCFP; Staff, Sunnybrook Health Sciences Centre; Langs: Bilingual(English/French); (416)964-0800; Fax. (416)964-2935.

DAVIS, Bre'el; 203-2276 Island Hwy S, Campbell River BC V9W 1C3; McM'06; CCFP; (250)923-1189

DAVIS, Breanna; Associate Med Clinic, 400-20 14th St W, Prince Albert SK S6V 3K8; Sask'07; CCFP; (306)953-1688; Fax. (306)764-3091.

DAVIS, Clive; Clive Davis Med Prof Corp, 401-304 Victoria Ave N, Hamilton ON L8L 5G4; Ott'70; BSc; FRCPC; IntMed (Critical Care Medicine). Staff IntMed.(Respirol), Hamilton Health Sciences Centre - Hamilton General Hospital; Assoc Prof Med, McMaster University; (905)522-3351; Fax. (905)522-6694.

DAVIS, Darryl R; Univ of Ottawa Heart Institute, 3409-40 Ruskin St, Ottawa ON K1Y 4W7; Ott'99; FRCPC; IntMed; Cardiol. Staff, University of Ottawa Heart Institute; Langs: Bilingual(English/French); (613)761-5000

DAVIS, Deborah J; Canadian Med Protective Assn, 875 av Carling, Ottawa ON K1S 5P1; McG'80; AB; FRCPC; Peds (Clinical Neonatology). Staff, Canadian Medical Protective Association; Langs: English; French; (613)725-2000; Fax. (613)725-1300.

DAVIS, Donna N; Whitby Clinic, 200 Brock St N, Whitby ON L1N 4H5; Mem'77; (905)668-3378

DAVIS, Geoffrey B; The Spence Clinic, 500-1265 Arthur St E, Thunder Bay ON P7E 5H7; Tor'77; Med Dir Palliative Care/Chief Medical Staff & Hospice Advisor, St Joseph's Care Group - St Joseph's Hospital; Asst Clin Prof Med, McMaster University; Asst Clin Prof Med, Northern Ontario School of Medicine-Laurentian University; (807)626-1111; Fax. (807)626-1121.

DAVIS, Heather S; 202-60 Aberdeen St, Kentville NS B4N 2N3; Dal'04; FRCPC; Peds. (902)678-1221; Fax. (902)678-2331.

DAVIS, Ian R C; Capital Health District Author, 5014-5820 University Ave, Halifax NS B3H 1V7; Tor'92; FRCPC; IntMed;CCFP; InfectDis; MedMicrobiol. (902)473-5553; Fax. (902)473-7394.

DAVIS, Janet L; The Ottawa Hosp-Riverside, 5F-1967 Riverside Dr, Ottawa ON K1H 7W9; Cal'95; FRCPC; IntMed; Nephrol. Staff, The Ottawa Hospital - Riverside Campus; (613)738-8400 x82892; Fax. (613)738-8337.

DAVIS, Jayne L; 807-123 Edward St, Toronto ON M5G 1E2; McM'93; BSc; CCFP; FCFP; (416)408-1010; Fax. (416)408-2828.

DAVIS, Jeffrey H; Children's & Women's Hlth Ctre, A123-4500 Oak St, Vancouver BC V6H 3N1; Birmingham(AL) (USA)'82; ABPeds; BEng; MD; NBME; BC Women's Hospital & Health Centre; Staff PedOncol, BC Children's Hospital; Consultant Ped Oncol, BC Cancer Agency Vancouver Centre; Clin Assoc Prof Peds, University of British Columbia; (604)875-2316; jdavis@cw.bc.ca.

DAVIS, Jennifer E; Dept of Anatomical Path, 910 10th Ave W, Vancouver BC V5Z 1M9; Adelaide (Australia)'72; MB BS; FRCPC; GenPath (Autopsy)., Vancouver General Hospital - Centennial Pavillion; Clinical Asst Prof, University of British Columbia; (604)875-4480; Fax. (604)875-5707.

DAVIS, Joann E; 255-5991 Spring Garden Rd, Halifax NS B3H 1Y6; Dal'95; FRCPC; Psy.

DAVIS, John; South Health Campus, 4448 Front St SE, Calgary AB T3M 1M4; Cal'08; FRCPC; IntMed. (403)943-2502; Fax. (403)943-4017.

DAVIS, Kathleen A; Rheumatologist Clinic, 522-267 O'Connor St, Ottawa ON K2P 1V3; Ott'78; FRCPC; IntMed; Rheum. (613)567-3767; Fax. (613)567-1481.

DAVIS, Kathleen A; Medical Bldg, 1601-805 Broadway W, Vancouver BC V5Z 1K1; Ott'89; FRCP; FRCPC; Derm. Clin Instructor Derm, University of British Columbia; (604)877-1156; Fax. (604)877-1179.

DAVIS, Kristian A M; Calabogie Med Centre, PO Box 40, Calabogie ON K0J 1H0; McM'95; Staff, Renfrew Victoria Hospital; (613)752-2323; Fax. (613)752-2323.

DAVIS, Lestrod A; 11-27 Aldershot Ave PO Box 62, Brockville ON K6V 2P7; McG'63; Ac Staff, Brockville General Hospital - Charles Street; (613)342-8036; Fax. (613)342-6537.

DAVIS, Liesl H; F W Green Clinic, 1629 Baker St, Cranbrook BC V1C 1B4; Orange Free State (South Africa)'00; MB ChB; (250)426-6601; Fax. (250)426-6470.

DAVIS, Lindsay E; St Paul's Hosp, 184-1081 Burrard St, Vancouver BC V6Z 1Y6; UBC'04; FRCPC; Psy. Staff, Providence Health Care - St Paul's Hospital; (604)806-8004

DAVIS, M Eric; Inst of Commun & Family Psy, 4333 ch Cote-Sainte-Catherine, Montreal QC H3T 1E4; McG'73; DPsy; AB; FRCPC; Psy (Geriatric Psychiatry). Staff, Sir Mortimer B Davis Jewish General; Consultant Psy, Donald Berman Maimonides Geriatric Centre; Consultant Psy, Miriam Home; Consultant Psy, Joseph Eldercare Services; Consultant Psy, Institut Canadian-Polonais; Lecturer, McGill University; (514)340-8222; Fax. (514)340-7507.

DAVIS, Martin H; Misericordia Health Centre, 99 Cornish Ave, Winnipeg MB R3C 1A2; Dublin (Ireland)'64; FFARCS; Ac Staff, Misericordia Health Centre; Ac Staff, Concordia General Hospital; (204)774-6581; Fax. (204)788-8529.

DAVIS, Mary L; Queen Elizabeth II HSC, 459 BB-1276 South Park St, Halifax NS B3H 2Y9; Burlington(VT) (USA)'77; ABIM; Staff, Queen Elizabeth II Health Sciences Centre - Victoria General Site; Teach Staff, Dalhousie University; (902)473-6054; Fax. (902)473-6186; mary.davis@cdha.nshealth.ca.

DAVIS, Meghan C; 1-67 Kenilworth Ave N, Hamilton ON L8H 4R6; McM'92; CCFP; FCFP; (905)547-2302; Fax. (905)548-9722.

DAVIS, Melinda; Foothills Med Centre, 1403 29 St NW, Calgary AB T2N 2T9; (Australia)'96; Staff, Foothills Medical Centre; (403)944-1430

DAVIS, Michael G; 103-4430 Bathurst St, North York ON M3H 3S3; Dal'75; BSc(McG); FRCPC; Derm (Cosmetic Dermatology). Staff, Mount Sinai Hospital; Med Dir, Laserderm/Spa Medica; Lecturer, University of Toronto; Langs: French; (416)638-7226; Fax. (416)638-0765.

DAVIS, Michael; Dr Everett Chalmers Hosp, PO Box 9000 Stn A 700 Priestman St, Fredericton NB E3B 5N5; Dal'05; CCFP; CCFP(E.M.); Staff, Dr Everett Chalmers Regional Hospital; (506)452-5400

DAVIS, Michael O; Western Med Clinic, 144 6th St, Brandon MB R7A 3N2; (204)727-6451

DAVIS, Neil L; Cornwall Comm Hosp-McConnell, 840 McConnell Ave, Cornwall ON K6H 5S5; (Israel)'03; Staff, Cornwall Community Hospital; (613)938-4240

DAVIS, Noelle L; Gordon & Leslie Diamond H C, 5F-2775 Laurel St, Vancouver BC V5Z 1M9; Cal'80; BSc; FRCSC; GenSurg (Surgical Oncology). Ac Staff, Vancouver General Hospital - Centennial Pavillion; Ac Staff, BC Cancer Agency Vancouver Centre; Assoc Prof Surg, University of British Columbia; (604)875-5880; Fax. (604)875-8941; noelle.davis@bccancer.bc.ca.

DAVIS, Paul; Heritage Med Research Ctr, 562-107 University Campus NW, Edmonton AB T6G 2S2; Bristol (England)'69; MB ChB; MRC; FRCPC; IntMed; Rheum. Ac Staff, University of Alberta Hospital; Assoc Dean/Dir Continuing Med Educ, University of Alberta; (780)407-6294; Fax. (780)407-6055; paul.davis@ualberta.ca.

DAVIS, Paul T; South Calgary Med Clinic, 118-40 Sunpark Plaza SE, Calgary AB T2X 3X7; Alb'72; (403)254-4000; Fax. (403)254-1282.

DAVIS, Peter V; Fort Med Clinic, 101-6603 132 Ave NW, Edmonton AB T5C 2A4; London (England)'77; DCH; DRCOG; CCFP; FCFP; Ponoka Hospital & Care Centre; (780)476-1388; Fax. (780)473-3530.

DAVIS, Philip J; Medical Arts Bldg, 305-5880 Spring Garden Rd, Halifax NS B3H 1Y1; Dal'71; (902)425-2646; Fax. (902)425-2826.

DAVIS, Randolph J; Grandview Med Ctr Fam Hlth Team, 167 Hespeler Rd, Cambridge ON N1R 3H7; Mem'87; CCFP; FCFP; (519)623-4200; Fax. (519)623-2546.

DAVIS, Richard C; Arbour Med Centre, 281 Stone Rd E, Guelph ON N1G 5J5; Tor'83; BSc; CCFP; FCFP; Assoc Staff, Homewood Health Centre; Court Staff, Guelph General Hospital; Assoc Staff, St Joseph's Health Centre; (519)823-5133; Fax. (519)827-0255.

DAVIS, Robert W; Happy Valley Family Hlth Team, PO Box 1120 Stn Main 268 Maiden Lane, St Marys ON N4X 1B7; Dublin (Ireland)'84; MB ChB; BAO; LRCPSI; CCFP; FCFP; Ac Staff, St Marys Memorial Hospital - Huron Perth Healthcare Alliance; Court Staff, Stratford General Hospital - Huron Perth Healthcare Alliance; (519)284-3450; Fax. (519)284-4471.

DAVIS, Vern; Min of Health Living & Sport, 5 2-1515 Blanshard St, Victoria BC V8W 3C8; Cal'81; BSc; MSc; DipAeroMed; BA; FCBOM; (250)952-2608

DAVIS, Victoria J; 218-4190 Finch Ave E, Scarborough ON M1S 4T7; Wes'85; BSc; MSc; FRCSC; ObstGyn (Contraception). Assoc Staff, Peterborough Regional Health Centre - Hospital Drive; Staff, The Scarborough Hospital - Birchmount Campus; Langs: Bilingual(English/French); (416)332-8128

DAVIS, William; Victoria Gen Hosp, 1 Hospital Way, Victoria BC V8Z 6R5; Witwatersrand (South Africa)'75; MB BCh; FRCPC; Anes. Staff, Royal Jubilee Hospital; Staff, Victoria General Hospital; (250)472-1617

DAVISON, Aaron; Royal Columbian Hosp, 330 Columbia St E, New Westminster BC V3L 3W7; UBC'94; FRCPC; EmergMed. Staff, Victoria General Hospital; Staff, Royal Columbian Hospital; (604)520-4253

DAVISON, Alan J; Peel Med Arts Bldg, 505-145 Queen St E, Brampton ON L6W 3P8; Tor'86; FRCSC; GenSurg. Staff, William Osler Health System - Brampton Civic Hospital; (905)451-0196; Fax. (905)451-0228.

DAVISON, Kristina; 210-92 Lakeshore Rd E, Mississauga ON L5G 4S2; Qns'99; FRCPC; Psy. (905)990-2150; Fax. (905)990-2350.

DAVISON, Michael J; Rideau Med & Dental Centre, 101-1711 4 St SW, Calgary AB T2S 1V8; UBC'01; CCFP; Dir Sarcee RCTP Program, Sarcee Carewest; (403)228-3611; Fax. (403)228-3660.

DAVISON, Patrick J; Brockville Gen Hosp, 4F-75 Charles St, Brockville ON K6V 1S8; Qns'98; FRCSC; GenSurg. Staff, Brockville General Hospital - Charles Street; (613)345-8345; Fax. (613)345-8318.

DAVISON, Peter D; Hunt Club Med Centre, 101-3328 Mccarthy Rd, Ottawa ON K1V 0H9; Queen's (Ireland)'69; MB ChB; BAO; (613)738-1564

DAVISON, Sara; Sciences Bldg 152, 11 107CSB-107 University Campu, Edmonton AB T6G 2S2; Cal'93; MHSc; FRCPC; IntMed (Biomedical Ethics); Nephrol. Staff, University of Alberta Hospital; (780)407-8716; sara.davison@ualberta.ca.

DAVITT, K Patrick; Family Care Med Centre, 112-55 Castleridge Blvd NE, Calgary AB T3J 3J8; Alb'88; (403)280-5500

DAVLOOR, Ramakrishna; Brandon Medical Arts Clinic, 339 Princess Ave, Brandon MB R7A 0N7; Madras (India)'59; MB BS; LRCP; MRCS; FRCS(Ed); FRCSC; GenSurg. Ac Staff Surg, Brandon Regional Health Centre; (204)727-2406; Fax. (204)571-0318.

DAVOINE, Emilie; Hop Brome-Missisquoi-Perkins, 950 rue Principale, Cowansville QC J2K 1K3; Laval'01; CCFP; CCFP(E.M.); Staff, Hôpital Brome-Missisquoi-Perkins; (450)266-4342

DAVOUDI, Soraya; The Ottawa Hosp-Civic Campus, 1103-1053 Carling Ave, Ottawa ON K1Y 4E9; Ott'01; FRCPC; EmergMed. Staff Emerg, The Ottawa Hospital - Civic Campus; Langs: Bilingual(English/French); (613)798-5555

DAVOUDPOUR, Parham; Southlake Reg Health Centre, 596 Davis Dr, Newmarket ON L3Y 2P9; Tehran (Iran)'00; CCFP; CCFP(E.M.); Staff, Southlake Regional Health Centre; Langs: Farsi; (905)895-4521

DAVY, Till; Medical & Dental Bldg, 202-1849 Yonge St, Toronto ON M4S 1Y2; Vienna (Austria)'77; FAAP; FRCPC; Peds. Hon Consultant, The Hospital For Sick Children; Asst Prof Peds, University of Toronto; Langs: German; (416)488-4508; Fax. (416)488-3969; till.davy@utoronto.ca.

DAVYDUKE, Daria C; Highland Family Practice, 107C-1966 Guthrie Rd, Comox BC V9M 3X7; Sask'00; CCFP; Staff, St Joseph's Care Group - St Joseph's Hospital; (250)890-0919; Fax. (250)890-0929; highlandfamily@hotmail.com.

DAW, Zohra M A; Life Labs, 3680 Gilmore Way, Burnaby BC V5G 4V8; Al Fateh (Libya)'91; MB BCh; FRCPC; HemPath (Transfusion Medicine). (604)431-5005

DAWADI, Sudhakar R; 2-1836 Comox Ave, Comox BC V9M 3M7; Hacettepe (Turkey)'91; (250)941-0041

DAWAR, Meenakshi; Vancouver Coastal Health, 800-601 Broadway W, Vancouver BC V5Z 4C2; Dal'93; BSc; MHSc; FRCPC; CommunMed;CCFP; Public Health & Preventive Med. Clinical Asst Prof Dept of Hlth Care & Epidemiology, University of British Columbia; Langs: Hindi; (604)375-3900; Fax. (604)731-2756.

DAWDY, John A; Ottawa Cardiovascular Centre, 502-1355 Bank St, Ottawa ON K1H 8K7; Wes'88; FRCPC; IntMed; Cardiol. Staff, The Ottawa Hospital - Riverside Campus; (613)738-1584

DAWE, Christiane M; Health Sciences Centre, 300 Prince Philip Dr, St. John's NL A1B 3V6; Mem'06; Staff, Health Sciences Centre; (709)777-6300

DAWE, David; Juravinski Cancer Centre, 699 Concession St, Hamilton ON L8V 5C2; Qns'07; FRCPC; IntMed; MedOncol.

DAWE, Elizabeth M; North York Family Health Team, 306-3292 Bayview Ave, North York ON M2M 4J5; McM'87; CCFP; FCFP; Staff, North York General Hospital; Assoc Prof, University of Toronto; (416)225-8499; Fax. (416)225-1089.

DAWE, Ian; Ontario Shores Ctr Mental HS, 305-700 Gordon St, Whitby ON L1N 5S9; Mem'93; BHSc; MHA; LMCC; FRCPC; Psy (Administrative Psychiatry). Staff, Ontario Shores Centre for Mental Health Sciences; (905)430-4055

DAWE, Shawna J; Tamarack Med Clinic, 191-1500 Cranbrook St, Cranbrook BC V1C 3S8; Mem'03; CCFP; (250)426-7724

DAWES, C Raymond S; 21 St Francis Memorial Dr PO Box 850, Barrys Bay ON K0J 1B0; Qns'76; CCFP; FCFP; Staff, St Francis Memorial Hospital; Dir, Ontario Medical Association; (613)756-2320; Fax. (613)756-0172.

DAWES, Jeffrey; 101-7 Glenbrook Pl SW, Calgary AB T3E 6W4; Cal'04; BSc; BComm; MBA; FRCSC; PlasSurg (Mohs Micrographic Surgery). Staff, Foothills Medical Centre; (403)571-3141; Fax. (403)571-3138; drjcdawes@me.com.

DAWES, Peter; Summerside Med Centre, 475 Granville St N, Summerside PE C1N 3N9; Witwatersrand (South Africa)'78; MB ChB; FRCSC; GenSurg (Gastroenterology). Staff, Prince County Hospital; (902)432-8181

DAWES, Simon N; Peter Lougheed Centre, 3500 26 Ave NE, Calgary AB T1Y 6J4; Ott'01; CCFP; Staff, Peter Lougheed Centre; (403)943-5461

DAWKINS, Christopher J; Crescent Beach Med Arts, 2781 Gordon Ave, Surrey BC V4A 5J5; Southampton (England)'86; (604)535-2520

DAWODU, Omotayo; Rockyview Gen Hosp, 7007 14 St SW, Calgary AB T2V 1P9; (Nigeria)'92; MB ChB; CCFP; CCFP(E.M.); Staff, Rockyview General Hospital; Langs: Yoruba; Afrikaans; (403)943-3000

DAWOOD, Ashraf M; St Joseph's Health Centre, 30 The Queensway, Toronto ON M6R 1B5; (Saudi Arabia)'03; FRCSC; ObstGyn.

DAWOOD, Dawood G; 38 Davidson Cres, Gloucester ON K1J 6M3; Shams (Egypt)'62; FRCSC; ObstGyn. Staff, Montfort Hospital; Langs: Arabic; Greek; English; (613)746-3861; Fax. (613)746-2636; drdawood@rogers.com.

DAWOOD, Isis M; Lacewood Med Centre, 200-366 Lacewood Dr, Halifax NS B3S 1M7; Cairo (Egypt)'89; MB ChB; CCFP; FCFP; (902)445-9400; Fax. (902)445-7108; isisdawood@hotmail.com.

DAWOOD, M Farouk; 902-570 University Ave E, Waterloo ON N2K 4P2; Natal (South Africa)'87; CCFP; Staff, Grand River Hospital - Kitchener/Waterloo Health Centre; Med Dir, KW Travel Clinic; (519)570-1280; Fax. (519)570-2808.

DAWOOD, Shamim; West Oak Med Clinic, 2495 Old Bronte Rd, Oakville ON L6M 4J2; Dharwar (India)'93; CCFP; Langs: Hindi; (905)582-7533; Fax. (905)582-0766.

DAWOOD-MOHAMED, Yusuf; 2251 Lawrence Ave E, Scarborough ON M1P 2P5; Bihar (India)'69; Assoc Staff, The Scarborough Hospital - General Campus; Langs: Afrikaans; (416)759-5251; Fax. (416)759-1253.

DAWRANT, Jonathan M; Alberta Children's Hosp, 2888 Shaganappi Trail NW, Calgary AB T3B 6A8; Qns'01; MSc; BSc; FRCPC; Peds (Pediatric Endocrinology); Endocrin&Metab. Staff, Alberta Children's Hospital; (403)955-7819; Fax. (403)955-5001.

DAWS, Tanja; Courtenay Med Clinic, 788 Grant Ave, Courtenay BC V9N 2T3; Pretoria (South Africa)'00; MB ChB; BSc(Hon); Langs: Afrikaans; (250)334-2445

DAWSON, Ainsley E; St Michael's Fam Practice Unit, 7F-61 Queen St E, Toronto ON M5C 2T2; McG'07; MDCM; FRCPC; IntMed; Endocrin&Metab. Langs: Italian; English; (416)867-7424; Fax. (416)867-3654.

DAWSON, Andrew S; 404-205 Newport Dr, Port Moody BC V3H 5C9; UBC'93; FRCPC; PhysMed&Rehab. Staff, G F Strong Rehabilitation Centre; (604)469-6763; Fax. (604)469-6762; ddawson@vanhosp.bc.ca.

DAWSON, Celine M; Airport Heights Med Clinic, 40 Airport Heights Dr, St. John's NL A1A 4Z7; Dal'06; CCFP; (709)237-5885

DAWSON, D Ross; Associate Med Clinic, 123 10th Ave S, Cranbrook BC V1C 2N1; UBC'81; Ac Staff, East Kootenay Regional Hospital; (250)426-4231; Fax. (250)426-4357.

DAWSON, David; Carnat Centre, 300-2580 32 St NE, Calgary AB T1Y 7M8; Cal'88; BSc; FRCPC; Psy (Schizophrenia). Staff, Peter Lougheed Centre; Med Dir Carnat Centre, Calgary Health Region; Consultant, Arnika Centre; Asst Clin. Prof. Psy., University of Calgary; (403)944-9800; Fax. (403)944-9850.

DAWSON, David F L; Cambridge Mem Hosp, 700 Coronation Blvd, Cambridge ON N1R 3G2; UBC'67; FRCPC; Psy. Staff, Cambridge Memorial Hospital; (519)621-2330

DAWSON, David J; MUHC-Royal Victoria Hosp, M10 84-687 av des Pins O, Montreal QC H3A 1A1; McG'75; BSc; ABIM; CSPQ; FRCPC; IntMed (Infectious Diseases). Chief Clinical Teaching Unit, McGill University Health Centre - Royal Victoria Hospital; Chair, Physicianship Community Centre; assoc Prof, McGill University; Langs: English; French; (514)843-1515; Fax. (514)843-1582; david.dawson@muhc.mcgill.ca.

DAWSON, David T P; Red Deer Reg Hosp Ctr, PO Box 5030 Stn Postal Box Ctr 3942 50A Ave, Red Deer AB T4N 6R2; Alb'65; FRCPC; GenPath (Administration). VP Med., Red Deer Regional Hospital Centre; Hon Teach Staff, University of Alberta; (403)343-4709; dtpdawson@shaw.ca.

DAWSON, Janet E; Rockyview Gen Hosp, 7007 14 St SW, Calgary AB T2V 1P9; Cal'78; CCFP; FCFP; Court Staff, Rockyview General Hospital; (403)943-3441; Fax. (403)943-8592; janet.dawson@calgaryhealthregion.ca.

DAWSON, Jeffrey A; Haliburton Family Hlth Center, 7217 Gelert Rd, Haliburton ON K0M 1S0; Tor'09; CCFP; (705)455-9220

DAWSON, John A; Health Wise Family Practice, 3-1499 Gordon Dr, Kelowna BC V1Y 9R2; Cal'93; CCFP; (778)484-5560

DAWSON, John E; 100-190 Main St, Ottawa ON K1S 1C2; Ott'91; (613)521-5991; Fax. (613)237-5484.

DAWSON, John; 15-9555 Yonge St, Richmond Hill ON L4C 9M5; Tor'69; BSc(Hon); CCFP; Staff Family Pract., Mackenzie Richmond Hill Hospital; Physician, Dr Bernstein Health & Diet Clinic; (905)884-6450; Fax. (905)884-3617.

DAWSON, Katharine L; Sault Area Hosp, 750 Great Northern Rd, Sault Ste. Marie ON P6B 0A8; Tor'04; CCFP; Staff, Sault Area Hospital - Sault Ste Marie; (705)759-3434

DAWSON, Keith; Ridge Meadows Hosp & Hlth CC, 11666 Laity St, Maple Ridge BC V2X 5A3; UBC'95; CCFP; Staff, Ridge Meadows Hospital & Health Care Centre; (604)463-4111

DAWSON, Keith Granger; 4197 Yuculta Cres, Vancouver BC V6N 4A9; Columbia (USA)'56; PhD; FACP; FRCPC; IntMed (Diabetes); Endocrin&Metab. Prof Med Emeritus, University of British Columbia; Langs: French; German; (604)351-5565; Fax. (604)261-8211; kdaw@mail.ubc.ca.

DAWSON, Laura A; Univ Hlth Network-Princess M, 5F-610 University Ave, Toronto ON M5G 2M9; Tor'93; FRCPC; RadOncol (Gastrointestinal Cancer). Radiation Oncologist, Princess Margaret Hospital - University Health Network; Assoc Prof, University of Toronto; (416)946-2125; Fax. (416)946-6566; laura.dawson@rmp.uhn.on.ca.

DAWSON, Lesa; Dr H Bliss Murphy Cancer Ctr, 300 Prince Philip Dr, St. John's NL A1B 3V6; Mem'94; FRCSC; ObstGyn (Gynecologic Oncology). Staff, Dr H Bliss Murphy Cancer Centre; Staff, Health Care Corporation Of St John's; Oncologist, Memorial University Of Newfoundland; Langs: English; French; (709)777-6564

DAWSON, Michael J; Maitland Valley Family Hlth Team, 180 Cambria Rd N, Goderich ON N7A 4N8; Wes'81; CCFP; Pres/Medical Staff, Alexandra Marine & General Hospital.

DAWSON, Michael P; Aurora Newmarket Family Hlth Team, 405-531 Davis Dr, Newmarket ON L3Y 6P5; Wes'79; Staff, Southlake Regional Health Centre; (905)898-2240; Fax. (905)898-2253.

DAWSON, P Colette; PO Box 1364, Bay Roberts NL A0A 1G0; Mem'08; CCFP; Staff, Health Sciences Centre.

DAWSON, Siobhan M; Gaulfield Med Clinic, 5317 Headland Dr, West Vancouver BC V7W 3C5; Stellenbosch (South Africa)'84; MB ChB; (604)925-4448

DAWSON, Susan P; Active Care Med Group, A-1108 Klondike Rd, Kanata ON K2K 0G1; Dal'92; BSc(Hon); CCFP; FCFP; (613)254-9777; Fax. (613)254-9778.

DAWSON, Wendy L M; Glenora Med Clinic, 310-10230 142 St NW, Edmonton AB T5N 3Y6; Alb'96; BSc; MA; CCFP; (780)455-3311; Fax. (780)451-4404.

DAWSON, William; London X-Ray Assoc, 105-450 Central Ave, London ON N6B 2E8; Wes'83; FRCPC; DiagRad. Staff Radiol., St Joseph's Hospital - St Joseph's Health Care; (519)672-7900

DAY, Anna; 76 Grenville St, Toronto ON M5S 1B2; Tor'76; ABIM; MD; FRFPS; FRCPC; IntMed (Respirology); Respir. Consultant, Women's College Hospital; Consultant, Mount Sinai Hospital; Staff, Sunnybrook Health Sciences Centre; Consultant, Toronto General Hospital - UHN; Staff, baycrest Centre; Assoc Prof, University of Toronto; (416)323-7346; Fax. (416)323-7550; anna.day@wchospital.ca.

DAY, Brian; Cambie Surgery Centre, 2836 Ash St, Vancouver BC V5Z 3C6; Manchester (England)'70; MRC; FRCS; MB ChB; FRCSC; OrthSurg. Consultant, UBC Hospital - Koerner Pavillion; Consultant Surg, Vancouver General Hospital - Centennial Pavillion; Assoc Prof OrthSurg, University of British Columbia; (604)874-1349; Fax. (604)874-1549.

DAY, Heather M; Ocean Walk Med Centre, 1884 Marine Dr, West Vancouver BC V7V 1J6; McM'89; BSc; FRCPC; IntMed (Rheumatology). Staff, Ocean Walk Medical Centre; (604)925-1884; Fax. (604)922-3591.

DAY, Jeremiah B; Centennial CMH & Brain Injury, PO Box 1000 Stn Main, Ponoka AB T4J 1R8; Alb'98; Staff, Centennial Centre for Mental Health & Brain Injury; (403)783-7643; Fax. (403)783-7790.

DAY, Joanna; 103-2419 Bellevue Ave, West Vancouver BC V7V 4T4; UBC'78; FRCPC; Derm (Laser Resurfacing). (604)925-9798

DAY, John C; St Clair Beach Health Centre, RR 1 6-500 Manning Rd, Windsor ON N8N 2L9; Wes'99; CCFP; (519)739-1731

DAY, Leigh A; St Mary's Gen Hosp, 911 Queens Blvd, Kitchener ON N2M 1B2; McM'04; CCFP; Staff, St Mary's General Hospital; (519)749-3311

DAY, Marilyn H; Dr CW Wiebe Med Centre, 385 Main St, Winkler MB R6W 1J2; McM'78; CCFP; FCFP; Staff, Boundary Trails Health Centre; (204)325-4312; Fax. (204)325-4594.

DAY, Michael E C; Ministry of Hlth & Long Tern C, 370 Select Dr, Kingston ON K7M 8T4; Tor'80.

DAY, Nathaniel; Centennial CMH & Brain Injury, PO Box 1000 Stn Main, Ponoka AB T4J 1R8; Alb'05; CCFP; Staff, Centennial Centre for Mental Health & Brain Injury; (403)783-7643; Fax. (403)783-7790.

DAY, Stephen C; Glover Med Clinic, 101-5796 Glover Rd, Langley BC V3A 4H9; Tor'73; DAB; MCFP(EM); (604)530-3233; Fax. (604)534-4580.

DAYA, Dean; Hamilton HS-Henderson Site, 711 Concession St, Hamilton ON L8V 1C3; Dar-Es-Salaam (Tanzania)'73; MHA; FCAP; FRCPC; AnatPath. Dir-Anatom Path, Hamilton Health Sciences Centre-Juravinski Site; Consultant Path, Hamilton Regional Cancer Centre; Prof Path., McMaster University; (905)527-4322 x42036; dayad@hhsc.ca.

DAYA, Farahnaz; 206-3530 Derry Rd e, Mississauga ON L4T 4E3; (Other Foreign)'09; CCFP; (905)672-3333

DAYA, Jayesh; LB315-60 Pearl St, Winnipeg MB R3E 1X2; (South Africa)'96; FRCPC; Anes.

DAYA, Mohamed N; Queensway Prof Centre, 306-190 Sherway Dr, Etobicoke ON M9C 5N2; Makerere (Uganda)'72; MB ChB; CCFP; FCFP; Staff, Trillium Health Centre - West Toronto; Physician, Mimico Correctional Institute; Langs: Gujarati; (416)626-1538; Fax. (416)626-1538.

DAYA, Nazim F; Westwood Mall Plaza, 5-7205 Goreway Dr, Mississauga ON L4T 2T9; Shiraz (Iran)'78; Ac Staff, William Osler Health System - Etobicoke General Hospital; (905)676-9915

DAYA, Salim H; Isis Regional Fertilty Centre, 4250 Sherwoodtowne Blvd, Mississauga ON L4Z 2G6; Manchester (England)'77; MB ChB; FRCSC; ObstGyn (Reproductive Endocrinology & Infertility). Langs: Gujarati; Kacchi; (905)896-7100; Fax. (905)896-7200; dayas@mcmaster.ca.

DAYAL, Amita; Medical Assoc of Port Perry, 462 Paxton St, Port Perry ON L9L 1L9; Wes'03; CCFP; (905)985-2895

DAYAL, Naveen R; Credit Valley Prof Bldg, 413-2300 Eglinton Ave W, Mississauga ON L5M 2V8; Bangalore (India)'75; MB BS; MRCPsy; DPM; FRCPC; Psy (Mood Disorders). Staff Psy., The Credit Valley Hospital; (905)607-4907; Fax. (905)607-4611.

DAYAL-GOSINE, Lystra; 303-5880 Spring Garden Rd, Halifax NS B3H 1Y1; RCS (Ireland)'62; LRCPSI; FRCSC; Ophth (Ophthalmology Plastic Surgery). Court Staff Ophth, Queen Elizabeth II Health Sciences Centre - Victoria General Site; Court Staff Opht, IWK Health Centre; (902)423-7595; Fax. (902)423-0853.

DAYAN, Natalie; MUHC-Royal Victoria Hosp, 687 av des Pins O, Montreal QC H3A 1A1; McG'06; MDCM; IntMed. Staff, McGill University Health Centre - Royal Victoria Hospital; (514)934-1934

DAYANANDA, Narayanappa; Dahlstrom Med Clinic, 3442 George Ferguson Way E, Abbotsford BC V2T 4Y4; Banfalore (India)'88; MB BS; (604)853-6667

DAYANANDA, Naresh; Queen Elizabeth II HSC-Halifax, 2501D-1796 Summer St, Halifax NS B3H 3A7; Queensland (Australia)'97; Staff, Queen Elizabeth II Health Sciences Centre - Halifax Infirmary Site; (902)473-4474

DAYER PASTORE, Fabienne; CSSS du Lac-des-Deux-Montagnes, 520 boul Arthur-Sauve, Saint-Eustache QC J7R 5B1; Staff, Hôpital de Saint-Eustache; (450)473-6811

DAYES, Ian S; The Juravinski Cancer Centre, 699 Concession St, Hamilton ON L8V 5C2; Tor'95; FRCPC; RadOncol. Staff, Hamilton Health Sciences Centre - Hamilton General Hospital; The Juravinski Cancer Centre; Asst Prof, McMaster University; (905)387-9495

DAYMONT, Carrie B; Children's Hosp, AE 302-671 William Ave, Winnipeg MB R3E 0Z2.

DAYO, Akinkunmi A; Drumheller Assoc Physicians, PO Box 5600, Drumheller AB T0J 0Y0; (Nigeria)'92; MB ChB; (403)823-3345; Fax. (403)823-7823.

DAYOT-VENIDA, Madeline; Brookdale Plaza, 4-871 Chemong Rd, Peterborough ON K9H 5Z5; Santo Tomas (Philippines)'70; FRCPC; Psy (General Adult Psychiatry). Court Staff, Peterborough Regional Health Centre - Hospital Drive; Langs: Tagalog; (705)743-0152; Fax. (705)743-0152.

DAYUS, Lisa E; Thames Valley Family Hlth Team, 301-460 Wellington St, St Thomas ON N5R 6H9; Wes'82; CCFP; FCFP; Staff, St Thomas Elgin General Hospital; (519)631-5670

DAZE, Pierre-Luc; CSSS de Trois-Rivières, 1991 boul du Carmel, Trois-Rivieres QC G8Z 3R9; Mon'09; Staff, CSSS de Trois-Rivières; (819)697-3333

DAZE, Yann; Lab Sciences Judiciairies, 12E-1701 rue Parthenais, Montreal QC H2K 3S7; Laval'05; FRCPC; AnatPath. (514)873-3301 x61437; Fax. (514)864-7752.

DE, Aloke; Vitallife Integrative Medicine, 205-421 Richmond Rd, Ottawa ON K2A 4H1; London (England)'95; MB BS; CCFP; (613)798-9994; Fax. (613)798-9924.

DE, Nibhas; 194 Court St N, Thunder Bay ON P7A 4V7; Calcutta (India)'61; MB BS; DCH(Lond); MRCP; FRCPC; Peds (Clinical Immunology & Allergy). Med Consultant, George Jeffrey Children's Centre; Langs: Bengali; Hindi; (807)346-1000 x7757; Fax. (807)346-6209.

DE, Sabe K; Cape Breton Hlth Care, 1482 George St, Sydney NS B1P 1P3; Dal'00; Cardiol; IntMed. Staff, Cape Breton Healthcare Complex; (902)567-6302; Fax. (902)567-3350.

DE ALBUQUERQUE, Pedro A B; MUHC-Montreal Children's Hosp, C311-2300 rue Tupper, Montreal QC H3H 1P3; Rio de Janeiro (Brazil)'95; DiagRad (P.Q.). Staff, McGill University Health Centre - Montreal Children's Hospital; (514)412-4450

DE ALWIS, Amila; The Hosp For Sick Children, 555 University Ave, Toronto ON M5G 1X8; (Pakistan)'97; Staff, The Hospital For Sick Children; (416)813-1500

DE ANDRES OTERINO, Jose A; Burin Peninsula Hlth Care Ctr, PO Box 340, Burin NL A0E 1E0; Salamanca (Spain)'87; Staff, Burin Peninsula Health Care Centre; (709)891-1040

DE ANGELIS, Dan; Ophthalmic Consultant Centers, 1880 Sismet Rd, Mississauga ON L4W 1W9; Tor'94; MD; FRCSC; Ophth (Ophthalmic Plastic & Reconstructive Surgery). Staff Ophthalmology, Mount Sinai Hospital; Staff Ophtalmology, The Hospital For Sick Children; Langs: Italian; (905)212-9482; Fax. (905)212-1012; info@retinamed.ca.

DE ANGELIS, Flavia; Hop Charles Lemoyne, 3120 boul Taschereau, Greenfield Park QC J4V 2H1; (Brazil)'02; Staff, Hopital Charles LeMoyne; (450)466-5000

DE ARANTES FROTA TAVARES, Ana C; CSSS de Rimouski-Neigette, CP 3150 succ Bureau Chef 150 av Rouleau, Rimouski QC G5L 5T1; Staff, Hôpital Regional Rimouski; (418)724-3000

DE BAKKER, Paul F; Thunder Bay Med Centre, 310-63 Algoma St N, Thunder Bay ON P7A 4Z6; McM'73; Ac Staff, Thunder Bay Regional Health Sciences Centre Port-Arthur; Ac Staff, St Joseph's Care Group - St Joseph's Hospital; (807)344-8475; Fax. (807)344-6323.

DE BANNE, Danielle M; Russell Med Centre, PO Box 70 Stn Main, Russell ON K4R 1C7; Ott'85; CCFP; FCFP; (613)445-3220; Fax. (613)445-3659.

DE BEAUMONT, Jean-Rene; Clinique Med Ste-Anne, 100-10974 boul Ste-Anne, Beaupre QC G0A 1E0; Laval'84; (418)827-4022; Fax. (418)827-4964.

DE BEER, Jan A; Vernon Jubilee Hosp, 2101 32 St, Vernon BC V1T 5L2; Orange Free State (South Africa)'97; MB ChB; CCFP; Staff, Vernon Jubilee Hospital; Langs: Afrikaans; (250)558-1201; Fax. (250)545-5602.

DE BEER, Johannes J; 36592 Auguston Parkway Rd E, Abbotsford BC V3G 3C6; Pretoria (South Africa)'97; MB ChB; (778)880-0306

DE BEER, Justin; Medical Arts Bldg, 307-1 Young St, Hamilton ON L8N 1T8; Cape Town (South Africa)'79; FRCSC; OrthSurg (Joint Replacement). Staff OrthSurg., Hamilton Health Sciences Centre-Juravinski Site; Physician, Medical Arts Bldg; (905)527-1115; Fax. (905)528-8150.

DE BEER, Nico; South Hill Med Clinic, 5-2685 2nd Ave W, Prince Albert SK S6V 5E3; MB ChB; (306)922-9570; Fax. (306)922-2513.

DE BEER, Louis N; Valleyview Med Clinic, 27-1400 Cowichan Bay Rd, Cobble Hill BC V0R 1L0; Pretoria (South Africa)'88; MB ChB; (250)743-9395

DE BELLA, Steven A; 100-3306 32 Ave, Vernon BC V1T 2M6; California (USA)'77; (250)549-1722

DE BELLE, Ross C; Centre Med for Infants, 527 rue Sainte-Helene, Longueuil QC J4K 3R5; McG'67; CSPQ; FRCPC; Peds (Gastroenterology). Att Staff Peds, McGill University Health Centre - Montreal General Campus; assoc Prof Med, McGill University; Langs: English; French; (450)646-6363; Fax. (450)463-0984.

DE BELLEFEUILLE, Claude; CSSS de Saint-Jerome, 290 rue de Montigny, Saint-Jerome QC J7Z 5T3; Mon'83; FRCPC; IntMed; Hem. Ac Member, Hôtel-Dieu de Saint-Jérôme; (450)431-8200 x2471; Fax. (450)431-8302; cdebel2@hotmail.com.

DE BELLEFEUILLE, Luc; CSSSG-Hop de Gatineau, CP 2000 Succ Bureau-Chef 909 boul de la Verendyre O, Gatineau QC J8P 7H2; Laval'86; CSPQ; FRCPC; Anes. Staff, Hôpital de Gatineau; (819)966-6100

DE BENEDETTI, Monica C; Health Sciences Bldg, 311-15 Mountain Ave S, Stoney Creek ON L8G 2V6; Mem'99; CCFP; (905)662-4911; Fax. (905)662-1688.

DE BENEDICTIS, Luigi; Hop Louis-H Lafontaine, 7401 rue Hochelaga, Montreal QC H1N 3M5; Mon'06; FRCPC; Psy. Staff, Hopital Louis-H Lafontaine; (514)251-4000

DE BIE, Isabelle; MUHC-Montreal Children's Hosp, A716A-2300 rue Tupper, Montreal QC H3H 1P3; Laval'03; FRCPC; MedGenetics. Staff, McGill University Health Centre - Montreal Children's Hospital; (514)412-4400 x22051

DE BIE, Jacques; CSSS de la Cote-De-Gaspe, 215 boul de York O, Gaspe QC G4X 2W2; Louvain (Belgium)'67; CSPQ; GenSurg. Staff, Centre Hospitalier de Gaspe; (418)368-3301

DE BILLY, Michel; Whitby Mdm Clinic, 80 Thickson Rd S, Whitby ON L1N 7T2; McG'83; CCFP; Langs: Bilingual(English/French); (905)668-6448

DE BLACAM, Killian J; Lasalle Walk In Clinic, 1813 Lasalle Blvd, Sudbury ON P3A 2A3; Dublin (Ireland)'81; CCFP; FCFP; Ac Staff, Health Sciences North-St Joseph's Health Centre; (705)560-9422; Fax. (705)560-9482.

DE BLOIS, Jonathan; Ctr Hosp Affilie-Enfant-Jesus, 1401 18e rue, Quebec QC G1J 1Z4; Laval'01; FRCPC; IntMed; Cardiol. Staff, Centre Hospitalier Affilié Universitaire de Québec - Hôpital De L'Enfant Jésus; (418)649-0252

DE BLOIS, Marc; Ctr Hosp Affilie-St-Sacrement, 1050 ch Sainte-Foy, Quebec QC G1S 4L8; Laval'92; CCFP; CCFP(E.M.); Staff, Centre Hospitalier Affilié Universitaire de Québec - Hôpital du St-Sacrement; (418)682-7511

DE BLOIS, Suzanne; Dir de la Sante Publique-Mtl, 1301 rue Sherbrooke E, Montreal QC H2L 1M3; Sher'80; FRCPC; CommunMed. Staff, Hopital Maisonneuve-Rosemont; Médecin, Agence de santé et des services sociaux de la Montérégie; Langs: Spanish; English; (514)528-2400 x3390; Fax. (514)528-2463.

DE BOECK, Thomas; Georgian Bay Gen Hosp, PO Box 760 Stn Main 1112 St Andrew's Dr, Midland ON L4R 4P4; McM'97; CCFP; Staff, Georgian Bay General Hospital - Midland; Langs: German; French; (705)526-3751

DE BOER, Aglaia K; The Ottawa Hosp-Gen Campus, Box 211 501 Smyth Rd, Ottawa ON K1H 8L6; Ott'08; IntMed. Staff, The Ottawa Hospital - General Campus; (613)737-8198

DE BOER, Cornelis; Colchester East Hants Hlth Ctr, 600 Abenaki Rd, Truro NS B2N 5A1; Amsterdam (Netherlands)'85; MRCPsy(UK); FRCPC; Psy. Child & Adolesc Psy, Colchester East Hants Health Centre; Langs: Dutch; German; (902)893-5526; Fax. (902)893-5551.

DE BOLSTER, C Leonard; Oakville Family Health Ctre, 640 Ford Dr, Oakville ON L6J 7V7; Tor'84; CCFP; Staff, The Credit Valley Hospital; (905)338-8222; Fax. (905)338-7863.

DE BONVILLE, Marianne; Ctr Hosp Affilie-Enfant-Jesus, 1401 18e rue, Quebec QC G1J 1Z4; Laval'05; Psy. Staff, Centre Hospitalier Affilié Universitaire de Québec - Hôpital De L'Enfant Jésus; (418)649-0252

DE BORTOLI, Bruno J; 220-5450 ch de la Cote-des-Nei, Montreal QC H3T 1Y6; Cracow (Poland)'00; FRCPC; IntMed; Nephrol. Staff, Hôtel-Dieu de Saint-Jérôme; (514)733-6722; Fax. (514)733-9754.

DE BORTOLI, Timothy P; Elliot Lake Family Health Team, 31 Nova Scotia Walk, Elliot Lake ON P5A 1Y9; Ott'90; Pres Med Staff/Dir EmergMed, St Joseph's General Hospital Elliot Lake; (705)461-8882; Fax. (705)848-3449.

DE BOSSET, Farideh; 1-62 Admiral Rd, Toronto ON M5R 2L5; Lausanne (Switzerland)'71; FRCPC; Psy. Asst Prof Psy, University of Toronto; Langs: French; (416)925-7906

DE BROUWER, Marie-Claude; CSSS de Temiscouata, CP 310 58 rue de l'Eglise, Notre-Dame-du-Lac QC G0L 1X0; Laval'01; Staff, Centre Hospitalier Notre-Dame-du-Lac; (418)899-6751

DE BROUWERE, Roland G; Associated Anaes of Winnipeg, 849 Notre Dame Ave, Winnipeg MB R3E 0M4; Man'90; Anes.

DE BROUX, Eric; CHUM-Hop St-Luc, 1058 rue Saint-Denis, Montreal QC H2X 3J4; Mon'96; CSPQ; MSc; BSc; FRCSC; GenSurg (Colon & Rectal Surgery). Staff, Centre Hospitalier l'Université De Montréal (CHUM) - Hôpital Saint-luc; Langs: English; (514)890-8000 x34953; Fax. (514)412-7259.

DE BROUX, Marie; Centre Med Fam de Granby, 48 rue Denison E, Granby QC J2G 4C6; Mon'86; ACLS; ATLS; CCFP; (450)372-3996; Fax. (450)372-0430.

DE BRUIN, Louis D; Alder Med Centre, 277 Evergreen Rd, Campbell River BC V9W 5Y4; (South Africa)'05; MB ChB; (250)287-7441

DE BRUIN, Maria M; Park Avenue Med Centre, 4F-4634 Park Ave, Terrace BC V8G 1V7; Orange Free State (South Africa)'89; MB ChB; Staff, Mills Memorial Hospital; Langs: Afrikaans; (250)615-5040; Fax. (250)615-5049.

DE BRUIN, Nathalia H M; Vive Medical, 6201-873 85 St SW, Calgary AB T3H 0J5; (Netherlands)'95; Langs: Dutch; (403)217-6453; Fax. (403)217-5235.

DE BRUIN, Walter; 101-8980 Mary St, Chilliwack BC V2P 4J3; Orange Free State (South Africa)'85; MB ChB; MSc; MMed; FRCSC; Ophth (Glaucoma). Langs: Dutch; Afrikaans; (604)792-2020; Fax. (604)792-2707.

DE BRUYN, Anna C; Brandon Reg Health Centre, 150 McTavish Ave E, Brandon MB R7A 2B3; Orang Free State (South Africa)'97; CCFP; CCFP(E.M.); Staff, Brandon Regional Health Centre; (204)726-1122

DE BRUYN, Jana; The Med Clinic, 10011 96 St, Fort St. John BC V1J 3P3; Stellenbosch (South Africa)'99; MB ChB; (250)785-6677; Fax. (250)787-0109.

DE BRUYN, Jeremy; Women's Health Clinic, 1001 10th Ave SW, Calgary AB T2T 0B7; Alb'03; CCFP; (403)221-8797

DE BRUYN, Jesaias P; The Medical Clinic, 10011 96 St, Fort St. John BC V1J 3P3; Stellenbosch (South Africa)'00; (250)785-6677; Fax. (250)787-0109.

DE BRUYN, Johan H; Worker's Comp Board, 150-4311 12 St NE, Calgary AB T2E 4P9; Alb'73; CCFP; (403)517-6186; Fax. (403)205-8042; johan.debruyn@wcb.ab.ca.

DE BRUYN, Jurie H; Rimbey Med Clinic, PO Box 650, Rimbey AB T0C 2J0; (South Africa)'95; CCFP; (403)843-2256; Fax. (403)843-2255; jurieivette@yahoo.ca.

DE BRUYN, Maria E; 3F-1504 15 Ave SW, Calgary AB T3C 0X9; Stellenbosch (South Africa)'89; MB ChB; CCFP; FCFP; Langs: Afrikaans; (403)245-8008; Fax. (403)245-5212; calvein@veinlaser.com.

DE BUJANDA, Marilena; CSSS Les Eskers de l'Abitibi, 622 4e rue O, Amos QC J9T 2S2; Sher'94; CSPQ; FRCPC; AnatPath. Staff Pathologiste, CH Hôtel-Dieu d'Amos; (819)732-3341

DE CABO, Cecilia; Women's Hosp, 735 Notre Dame Ave, Winnipeg MB R3E 0L8; (Argentina)'91.

DE CAEN, Allan R B; Edmonton Clinic Health Academy, 4 524-11405 87 Ave NW, Edmonton AB T6G 1C9; Cal'87; FRCPC; Peds (Pediatric Intensive Care). Staff, University of Alberta Hospital; Physician, Edmonton Clinic Health Academy; (780)248-5434

DE CAIGNY-BICEK, Catherine; Canmore Gen Hosp, 1100 Hospital Pl, Canmore AB T1W 1N2; Cal'04; BSc; CCFP; Staff Anes, Canmore General Hospital; Staff Anes, Covenant Health - Banff Mineral Springs Hospital; (403)678-5536

DE CAROLIS, Mary L; Grand River Hosp-KW Hlth Ctre, PO Box 9056 Stn C 835 King St W, Kitchener ON N2G 1G3; McM'88; Staff, Hamilton Health Sciences Centre-Juravinski Site; (905)749-4300

DE CARUFEL, France; Clinique Med La Rose des Vents, 3498 boul Sainte-Rose, Laval QC H7P 4K7; Mon'88; Staff, CLSC-Ste-Rose(Laval); (450)624-1844; Fax. (450)624-1866.

DE CARVALHO, Elda E B P; Sunnybrook Health Sciences Ctr, 2075 Bayview Ave, Toronto ON M4N 3M5; Sao Paolo (Brazil)'99; Staff, Sunnybrook Health Sciences Centre; (416)480-4336

DE CHAMPLAIN, France; Carrefour de Sante de Jonquier, CP 1200 Succ Pdf Jonquiere 2229 rue de l'Hopital, Jonquiere QC G7X 7X2; Laval'03; CCFP; Staff, Centre Hospitalier Jonquiere; (418)695-7700

DE CHAMPLAIN, Francois; MUHC-Montreal Gen Hosp, A1 113-1650 av Cedar, Montreal QC H3G 1A4; Mon'98; FRCPC; EmergMed. Staff, McGill University Health Centre - Montreal General Campus; (514)934-1934 x42501

DE CHAMPLAIN, J Paul; Richmond Med Bldg, 207-2020 Richmond Rd, Victoria BC V8R 6R5; Alb'75; ABIM; FRCPC; IntMed; Rheum. Staff, Vancouver Island Health Authority; (250)592-5434; Fax. (250)592-4097.

DE CHAMPLAIN, Marilou; CSSS St-Jerôme, 290 rue de Montigny, Saint-Jerome QC J7Z 5T3; Mon'09; CCFP; CCFP(E.M.); Staff, Hôtel-Dieu de Saint-Jérôme; (450)432-2777

DE CHAMPLAIN, Remi; Medicine Familiale Montclair, 207-15 boul Montclair, Gatineau QC J8Y 2E2; Ott'96; CCFP; Staff, Hull Hospital; Langs: English; (819)772-2003; Fax. (819)772-4880.

DE CICCIO, Maria A; Lakeshore Gen Hosp, 160 av Stillview, Pointe-Claire QC H9R 2Y2; McG'93; FRCPC; Psy. Staff, Lakeshore General Hospital - Pointe Claire; (514)630-2010; Fax. (514)630-5184.

DE COSTE, Rebecca L; 629-5991 Spring Garden Rd, Halifax NS B3H 1Y6; Dal'00; CCFP; (902)422-8488; Fax. (902)422-8494.

DE COTEAU, John F; Royal University Hosp, 103 Hospital Dr, Saskatoon SK S7N 0W8; Sask'88; FRCPC; HemPath. Staff, Royal University Hospital; (306)655-2249

DE COTEAU, W Earle; Clinical Gerontology Service, 701 Queen St, Saskatoon SK S7K 0M7; Sask'64; FRCPC; IntMed (Geriatric Medicine). Staff Clin Gerontology, Saskatoon City Hospital; Vis Staff, Providence Place; Emeritus Prof, University of Saskatchewan; (306)655-8925; Fax. (306)655-8929.

DE COUTO, John L; 140-555 Sixth St, New Westminster BC V3L 5H1; UBC'80; Assoc Staff, Royal Columbian Hospital; (604)523-1166; decoutoj@shaw.ca.

DE CROOS, J Annson B; Pringle Clinic, 728 Anderson St, Whitby ON L1N 3V6; Colombo (Sri Lanka)'70; MB BS; (905)665-5800; Fax. (905)665-5807.

DE DEMETER, Dorrit A; Humber River Reg Hosp-Church, 200 Church St, Toronto ON M9N 1N8; Tor'76; FRCSC; OrthSurg. Staff, Humber River Regional Hospital - Church Street Site; Staff, Humber River Regional Hospital - Finch Avenue Site; Med Consultant, Workplace Safety & Insurance Board; (416)243-4154; Fax. (416)747-3835.

DE DOMING, Eva N; Summit Centre, 206-200 Boudreau Rd, St. Albert AB T8N 6B9; UBC'95; FRCSC; ObstGyn. Staff, Sturgeon Community Hospital; (780)459-7390; Fax. (780)459-0128.

DE FIGUEIREDO, Antonia F; 202-622 College St, Toronto ON M6G 1B6; Tor'94; CCFP; Court Staff, St Michael's Hospital; Teacher, University of Toronto; Langs: Portuguese; (416)534-4455

DE FINA, Rachel A; Alexandra Comm Hlth Centre, 101-1318 Centre St NE, Calgary AB T2E 2R7; UBC'09; CCFP; (403)266-2622; Fax. (403)266-2692.

DE FLAMINGH, Willem J; 4904 54 Ave PO Box 90 Stn Main, Provost AB T0B 3S0; (South Africa)'07; MB ChB; (780)753-2271; Fax. (780)753-2371.

DE FOA, J Lance; Wawa Med Centre, PO Box 1218 17 Government Rd, Wawa ON P0S 1K0; Qns'92; BSc(Hon); MD; Staff, Lady Dunn Health Centre; Langs: Spanish; (705)856-1313; jldefoa@yahoo.ca.

DE FOY, Lise; CSSS Jeanne-Mance, 100-15 av du Mont-Royal O, Montreal QC H2T 2R9; Laval'79; (514)286-9657

DE FRANCE, Bryon F; Hamilton HS-McMaster Site, PO Box 2000 Stn Lcd 1 4D 14-1200 Main St W, Hamilton ON L8N 3Z5; McM'94; BSc; MSc; FRCSC; ObstGyn (Maternal Fetal Medicine). Staff, Hamilton Health Sciences Centre - McMaster Children's Hospital; Asst Prof, McMaster University; (905)521-2100 x76253; Fax. (905)577-0471.

DE FRANCESCO, Nicole J; Peterborough Reg HC-Hospital, 1 Hospital Dr, Peterborough ON K9J 7C6; Tor'96; CCFP; CCFP(E.M.); Staff, Peterborough Regional Health Centre - Hospital Drive; (705)743-2121 x5022

DE FREITAS, Brian A; 202-1130 Austin Ave, Coquitlam BC V3K 3P5; McG'76; MDCM; FRCPC; Psy. Ac Staff, Royal Columbian Hospital; (604)939-8143; Fax. (604)939-8145.

DE FREITAS, Karen D; Ontario Shores Ctr Mental HS, 700 Gordon St, Whitby ON L1N 5S9; Tor'97; FRCPC; Psy. Staff, Ontario Shores Centre for Mental Health Sciences; (905)668-5881 x6556

DE FREITAS, Leonard; Bonnyville Med Clinic, PO Box 1007 Stn Main 4610 50 St, Bonnyville AB T9N 2J7; Pretoria (South Africa)'97; MB ChB; Staff ER & Acute Care, Bonnyville Healthcare Centre; (780)826-3346; Fax. (780)826-6362.

DE FREITAS, Teresa; Rimrock Med Clinic, 14-5201 50 St, Leduc AB T9E 6T4; Alb'95; Dip(SportsMed); BSc; CCFP; Physician Emerg, Leduc Community Hospital; Consultant Sports Med, Glen Sattier Sports Med Clinic; Med Dir, Tackwando Canada; (780)986-1714

DE GANNES, Gillian C; 314-888 8th Ave W, Vancouver BC V5Z 3Y1; Wes'99; MSc; FRCPC; Derm. (604)731-5353

DE GARA, Christopher; Royal Alexandra Hosp, 208 CSC-10240 Kingsway Ave NW, Edmonton AB T5H 3V9; London (England)'77; FACS; FRCS(Eng); FRCS(Ed); MB BS; MS(Lond); FRCSC; GenSurg (Gastrointestinal Surgery). Ac Staff/Dir Bariatric Revision Clinic, Royal Alexandra Hospital; Prof Surg/Dir Phy learning Program, University of Alberta; (780)735-5544; cdgara@ualberta.ca.

DE GOIAS, Albert R; 84 Old Mill Rd, Etobicoke ON M8X 1G8; (Jamaica)'71; (416)487-3775; Fax. (416)487-9628; adegoias@prometheum.ca.

DE GOOIJER, Lisa; Broadway Med Clinic, 200-41 Broadway St W, Yorkton SK S3N 0L6; Sask'10; CCFP; (306)783-2555; Fax. (306)783-2557.

DE GRAAD, Gerben J; Associate Med Clinic, PO Box 7590 10011 101 St, Peace River AB T8S 1T2; Orange Free State (South Africa)'77; (780)624-2581

DE GRACE, Luce; CSSS Haut-Richelieu-Rouville, 920 boul du Seminaire N, St-Jean-Sur-Richel QC J3A 1B7; Mon'91; LMCC; CCFP; Staff, Hôpital du Haut-Richelieu; (450)359-5000; Fax. (450)466-0022.

DE GRACE, Marianne; CLSC la Source Nord, 791 rue de Sherwood, Quebec QC G2N 1X7; Mon'02; (418)849-2572; Fax. (418)841-5110.

DE GRACE, Michel C; Montfort Academic Family Hlth, 101B-745 Montreal Rd, Ottawa ON K1K 0T1; Ott'76; CCFP; FCFP; (613)749-4429; Fax. (613)749-7942.

DE GRACE, Raymonde F; The Moncton Hosp, 135 MacBeath Ave, Moncton NB E1C 6Z8; Laval'90; CSPQ; FRCPC; Anes (P.Q.). Staff, The Moncton Hospital; (506)857-5900

DE GRAFT-JOHNSON, Ama; Hamilton HS-General Site, 237 Barton St E, Hamilton ON L8L 2X2; Accra (Ghana)'71; FRCPC; Anes. Staff, Hamilton Health Sciences Centre - Hamilton General Hospital; Asst Prof, McMaster University; Langs: Ghanaian; (905)527-0271 x6277

DE GRANDPRE, Fernand; Clinique Med Mont-Carmel, 933 boul Rene-Levesque E, Montreal QC H2L 4S4; Mon'77; (514)282-9197; Fax. (514)282-1973.

DE GRANDPRE, Michel; Clinique Med Saint-Gabriel, 85 rue Saint-Gabriel GD, St-Gabriel-D-Brand QC J0K 2N0; Mon'77; (450)835-3431

DE GRANDPRE, Nathalie; Clin Med L'Asslomtion, RC360-5345 boul de l'Assomptio, Montreal QC H1T 4B3; Mon'86; (514)257-7000 x233; Fax. (514)788-2045.

DE GREEF, Andre; 240-8100 Rock Island Hwy, Trail BC V1R 4N7; (South Africa)'75; MB ChB; MCh; MMed; (250)368-3582; Fax. (250)368-3583; adegreef@shawcable.com.

DE GROOT, Grant G; Westbram Family Physicians, 104-100 Pertosa Dr, Brampton ON L6X 0H9; Man'98; CCFP; (905)451-1244; Fax. (905)451-6955.

DE GROOT, Janet M; 7E08-3280 Hospital Dr NW, Calgary AB T2N 4Z6; Alb'82; FRCPC; Psy (Palliative Care). Staff, Foothills Medical Centre; (403)944-1616

DE GROOT, Jean-Andre; Clinique Chirurgi Vision, 579 rue Laviolette, Trois-Rivieres QC G9A 1V6; Mon'65; FRCSC; Ophth (Strabismus). Ac Staff, Hopital Maisonneuve-Rosemont; adj Prof, Universite de Montreal; Langs: English; (819)693-5757; Fax. (819)373-9482.

DE GROOT, Wilhelmina; Martinway Plaza, 415 The Westway, Etobicoke ON M9R 1H5; Qns'90; Ac Staff Privil, William Osler Health System - Etobicoke General Hospital; Court Staff Privil, Humber River Regional Hospital - Finch Avenue Site; Langs: Dutch; (416)249-0009; Fax. (416)249-8380.

DE GUIRE, Louise; Dir de la Sante Publique-Mtl, 190 boul Crémazie E, Montreal QC H2P 1E2; Mon'75; MSc; Staff (All Sites), Centre Hospitalier l'Université de Montréal (CHUM) - Hôpital Notre-Dame; Physician, Institut National de Sante Publique du Quebec; Teach Staff Environmental & Occup Health, Universite de Montreal; Langs: Bilingual(English/French); (514)864-1600 x3210; Fax. (514)864-7646; louise.deguire@inspq.qc.ca.

DE GUIRE, Martine; CSSS Pierre Boucher, 1333 boul Jacques-Cartier E, Longueuil QC J4M 2A5; Mon'01; Staff, Centre Hospitalier Pierre Boucher; Staff, Pavillon Notre-Dame de la Merci; (450)468-8111

DE GUISE, Michele; Centre Med L'Enjeu, 1140 av Beaumont, Mont-Royal QC H3P 3E5; Mon'86; CSPQ; FRCPC; IntMed; Cardiol. ac Staff, Centre Hospitalier l'Université de Montréal (CHUM) - Hôpital Notre-Dame; (514)288-7770; Fax. (514)288-0622.

DE GUISE, Pierre; Institut de Cardiologie de Mtl, 5000 rue Belanger, Montreal QC H1T 1C8; Mon'78; CSPQ; FRCPC; IntMed; Cardiol. Staff, Institut de Cardiologie de Montréal; adj Prof, Universite de Montreal; (514)376-3330; Fax. (514)376-5241.

DE GUSSEM, Els Maria; The Salvation Army Grace Hosp, 300 Booth Dr, Winnipeg MB R3J 3M7; Erasmus (Netherlands)'99; Staff, The Salvation Army Grace Hospital; (204)837-0391

DE GUZMAN, Cecilia R; St Joseph's Healthcare, 50 Charlton Ave E, Hamilton ON L8N 4A6; (Philippines)'72; FRCPC; Anes. Court Staff, Hamilton Health Sciences Centre - McMaster University Medical Centre; Staff Pt-Time, Hamilton Health Sciences Centre - McMaster Children's Hospital; Ac Staff Anes., St Joseph's Healthcare - Charlton Campus; (905)522-4941 x3853; Fax. (905)521-6019.

DE GUZMAN, Ruby L; Strass Meditation & Healing Ho, 71 Holland Ave, Ottawa ON K1Y 0X9; Santo Tomas (Philippines)'71; FRCPC; AnatPath (Depression & Anxiety); Psy. Langs: Tagalog; (613)722-9923

DE HAAN, Melanie N; Sunnybrook Health Sciences Ctr, 2075 Bayview Ave, Toronto ON M4N 3M5; Ott'02; FRCPC; PhysMed&Rehab. Staff, Sunnybrook Health Sciences Centre; (416)480-4475; Fax. (416)480-4674.

DE HAAS, William; 102-7 Glenbrook Pl SW, Calgary AB T3E 6W4; Cal'84; BSc(Hon); FRCSC; PlasSurg (Breast Reconstruction). Chief PlasSurg, Foothills Hospital; Staff, Tom Baker Cancer Centre; Clin Asst Prof, University of Calgary; (403)571-3150; Fax. (403)217-2213.

DE JAGER, Eduard J; Abbotsford Reg Hosp & Cancer C, 14-32900 Marshall Rd, Abbotsford BC V2S 0C2; (South Africa)'97; MB ChB; CCFP; CCFP(E.M.); Staff, Abbotsford Regional Hospital & Cancer Centre; (604)851-4700

DE JAGER, Jacobus F; Regina Qu'Appelle HR-Regina, MOW 3F-1440 14th Ave, Regina SK S4P 0W5; Pretoria (South Africa)'85; MB ChB; MMed; LMCC; FRCSC; OrthSurg. Staff, Regina General Hospital; Langs: Afrikaans; (306)766-6996; Fax. (306)766-6960; reception@fdjortho.ca.

DE JAGER, Jacobus; Uptown Med Clinic, 3460 Saanich Rd, Victoria BC V8Z 0B9; Pretoria (South Africa)'77; (250)590-8375

DE JAGER, Johannes; Chetwynd Centre Med Clinic, PO Box 1485 5121 47 Ave, Chetwynd BC V0C 1J0; Pretoria (South Africa)'99; MB ChB; CCFP; Staff ER & Doctor on Call, Chetwynd General Hospital; (250)788-3234; Fax. (250)788-3237.

DE JAGER, Lodewyk P; 332 3rd St, Courtenay BC V9N 1E4; Pretoria (South Africa)'90; MB ChB; MMed; Consultant, Prince Rupert Regional Hospital; Langs: Afrikaans; (250)338-1314; Fax. (250)338-2932.

DE JAGER, Nico; Hammond Bldg, 315-310 Main St N, Moose Jaw SK S6H 3K1.

DE JESUS JR., Filemon; 144 Richmond Rd, Ottawa ON K1Z 6W2; Manila (Philippines)'77; FRCSC; Urol. Langs: Tagalog; (613)722-5680

DE JONG, Christine; 482 Burlington Ave, Burlington ON L7S 1R5; McM'92; BSc; MSc; FRCSC; ObstGyn (Urological Gynecology). Ac Staff, Joseph Brant Memorial Hospital; Associate Clin Prof, McMaster University; (905)632-8954; Fax. (905)632-9143.

DE JONG, Jennifer; J-6 Speers Blvd, Amherstview ON K7N 1Z6; Dal'07; CCFP; (613)634-4354; Fax. (613)634-0320.

DE JONGH, Heinrich L; Life Medical Clinic, PO Box 1406 Stn Main, Whitecourt AB T7S 1P3; (South Africa)'95; Langs: Afrikaans; (780)706-7080; Fax. (780)706-7064; hdj@cablerocket.com.

DE KLEER, Nancy M A; 31-1495 Cornwall Rd, Oakville ON L6J 0B2; Tor'97; FRCSC; PlasSurg. (905)901-9545; info@drdekleer.ca.

DE KLERK, Anton B; Dewdney Med Group, 22195 Dewdney Trunk Rd, Maple Ridge BC V2X 3H7; Pretoria (South Africa)'85; MB ChB; Preceptor, University of British Columbia; (604)463-4102; Fax. (604)463-4686.

DE KLERK, Barend J; Fort Vermilion Med Clinic, PO Box 306 4502 47 St, Fort Vermilion AB T0H 1N0; (South Africa)'79; MB ChB; LMCC; (780)927-3213

DE KLERK, Hein S; Southwest Med-Centre, SS 1 500-1 Springs Dr, Swift Current SK S9H 3X6; Orange Free State (South Africa)'97; MB ChB; (306)773-4681; Fax. (306)778-3449.

DE KLERK, Leon; Village Mall Med Clinic, 22-6320 50 Ave, Red Deer AB T4N 4C6; Orange Free State (South Africa)'97; Langs: Afrikaans; (403)314-5357; Fax. (403)314-5307.

DE KLERK, Ronel; Wardlaw Med Clinic, 15353-165 Osborne St, Winnipeg MB R3L 1Y7; Orange free State (South Africa)'01; (204)927-1700; Fax. (204)927-1709.

DE KLERK, Tania; Chisel Peak Med Clinic, PO Box 2769 417 10 Ave, Invermere BC V0A 1K0; Pretoria (South Africa)'97; MB ChB; (250)341-6900; Fax. (250)341-3226.

DE KLERK, Willem A; Hillcrest Clinic, 7381 Hurd St, Mission BC V2V 3H8; Stellenbosch (South Africa)'93; MB ChB; BSc; (604)826-8345; Fax. (604)826-1930.

DE KOCK, Hancke; Aberdeen Med Clinic, 1966 Harrison Way, Kamloops BC V1S 1M9; Orange Free State (South Africa)'04; MB ChB; (250)314-5311

DE KOCK, Ingrid H; Grey Nuns Community Hosp, 335 ASB-1100 Youville Drive We, Edmonton AB T6L 5X8; Pretoria (South Africa)'83; MB ChB; Staff, Covenant Health - Grey Nuns Community Hospital; Staff, Edmonton Reg Palliative Care Program; (780)450-7934; Fax. (780)450-7640.

DE KOCK, Johannes L; White Clinic, 100-383 Ellis St, Penticton BC V2A 4L9; Stellenbosch (South Africa)'93; MB ChB; (250)492-3024; Fax. (250)492-2761.

DE KOCK, Matthys J; PO Box 1250, Grimshaw AB T0H 1W0; (South Africa)'91; MB ChB; Langs: Afrikaans; (780)332-4642; Fax. (780)332-1020.

DE KOCK, Victor E; Summit Med Clinic, 4-1380 Summit Dr, Kamloops BC V2C 1T8; Stellenbosch (South Africa)'86; MB ChB; CCFP; Med Staff, Royal Inland Hospital; Langs: Afrikaans; (250)374-9800; Fax. (250)374-9876.

DE KOKER, Annemarie; Ancron Med Centre, 108-402 Baker St, Nelson BC V1L 4H8; Witwatersrand (South Africa)'05; MB ChB; (250)352-9144; Fax. (250)352-9141; jill@kristenmedical.com.

DE KOOS, Edmond B; Seaforth Med Bldg, 450-3550 ch de la Cote-des-Nei, Montreal QC H3H 1V4; McG'67; CSPQ; FRCSC; ObstGyn. Staff, McGill University Health Centre - Montreal General Campus; Staff, McGill University Health Centre - Montreal Children's Hospital; Staff, McGill University Health Centre - Royal Victoria Hospital; Teach Staff PedGyn, McGill University; (514)932-4324; Fax. (514)932-7501.

DE KOROMPAY, Victor L L; Manitoba Clinic, 75 Poseidon Bay, Winnipeg MB R3M 3E4; Sask'76; MD; FRCSC; OrthSurg (Arthroscopy). Chief Surg & Dir, The Salvation Army Grace Hospital; Teacher, University of Manitoba; (204)927-2678; Fax. (204)927-2685; vdekorompay@mts.net.

DE LA BOISSIERE, Martin; CSSS Maria-Chapdelaine, 2000 boul du Sacre-Coeur, Dolbeau-Mistassini QC G8L 2R5; Laval'86; Staff, Centre Maria-Chapdelaine - CH de Dolbeau-Mistassini; (418)276-1234; Fax. (418)276-5137.

DE LA CHEVROTIERE, Jean; 104-195 boul Greber, Gatineau QC J8T 3R1; Ott'82; Med Consultant, Produits Kruger Gatineau; Langs: Bilingual(French/English); (819)205-1600; cliniquematernite@videotron.ca.

DE LA CRUZ, Christa Lynn; 210-9719 98 Ave, Grande Prairie AB T8V 8K6; Dal'98; BSc; MSc; FRCSC; ObstGyn. Staff, Queen Elizabeth II Hospital; (780)882-8956; Fax. (780)882-8957; cldelacruz@hotmail.com.

DE LA CRUZ, Romelito; 210-9719 98 Ave, Grande Prairie AB T8V 8K6; Man'97; FRCSC; Otol. Staff, Queen Elizabeth II Hospital; (780)882-8956

DE LA HAYE DUPONSEL, Ophélie; Clinique Med du College, 1396 rye Notre-Dame, Saint-Cesaire QC J0L 1T0; Mon'06; (450)469-0505; Fax. (450)469-4554.

DE LA HUERTA, Francois; 393 boul Marcotte, Roberval QC G8H 1Z5; Mon'98; CSPQ; FRCSC; OrthSurg. (418)275-2935

DE LA MARE, Eric A; Pine Med Centre, 5110 5th Ave, Whitehorse YT Y1A 1L4; Glasgow (Scotland)'70; MSc(OccMed); DIH; DAvMed; MFOM; MB ChB; FCBOM; BVMS; Med Staff, Whitehorse General Hospital; (867)668-4353; Fax. (867)668-3899; pinemed@northwest.net.

DE LA ROCHA, Claudio; Rudd Services Limited, 825-123 Edward St, Toronto ON M5G 1E2; Mexico (Mexico)'68; FRCSC; GenSurg; Cardiovasc&ThorSurg. Staff, Shouldice Hospital.

DE LA ROCHE, Michael R P; PO Box 1491 Stn Main, Kingston ON K7L 5C7; McM'89; MSc(Epidemiol); CCFP; FCFP; Staff, QHC Belleville General; (613)547-8032; Fax. (613)547-5468.

DE LA RONDE, Sandra K; Wabano Ctre for Aboriginal Hea, 299 Montreal Rd, Ottawa ON K1L 6B8; Tor'82; BSc; FRCSC; ObstGyn (Pregnancy & Addiction). Staff, Foothills Medical Centre; Staff, Tom Baker Cancer Centre; Clin Assoc Prof, University of Calgary; Langs: French; (613)748-5999; Fax. (613)748-0550.

DE LA SABLONNIERE, Jean F; CSSS de Rivière-de-Loup, 75 rue Saint-Henri, Riviere-Du-Loup QC G5R 2A4; Sher'96; FRCPC; Psy (General Psychiatry). Staff, Institut Universitaire Sante; Staff, Centre Hospitalier Regional du Grand-Portage; (418)868-1020 x4; Fax. (418)868-0530.

DE LA SALLE, Gilles; Kemptville Dist Hosp, PO Box 2007 2675 Concession Rd, Kemptville ON K0G 1J0; Ott'72; Anes. Staff, Kemptville District Hospital; Staff, Montfort Hospital; University of Ottawa; Langs: French; (613)258-3435

DE LA TORRE, Josephine; 110-77 Westmount Rd, Guelph ON N1H 5J1; (Philippines)'85; CCFP; Langs: Tagalog; Fax. (519)829-2155.

DE LACHEVROTIERE, Hugues; UMF Le Gardeur, 135 boul Claude-David, Repentigny QC J6A 1N6; Sher'04; CCFP; Staff, Centre Hospitalier Portneuf; Langs: Bilingual(French/English); (450)654-2911 x61101

DE LACY, John L; Sunnybrook Hlth Sciences Ctre, M3-2075 Bayview Ave, Toronto ON M4N 3M5; Monash (Australia)'70; MB BS; FRCPC; Anes. Staff, Sunnybrook Health Sciences Centre; Asst Prof, University of Toronto; (416)480-4967; Fax. (416)480-6039.

DE LADURANTAYE, Alain; Hawkesbury Dist Gen Hosp, 1111 Ghislain St, Hawkesbury ON K6A 3G5; Mon'79; Staff, Hawkesbury & District General Hospital; Langs: Bilingual(French/English); (613)632-1111

DE LANGE, Hendrik; Regina Qu'Appelle HR-Pasqua, 4101 Dewdney Ave, Regina SK S4T 1A5; Staff, Pasqua Hospital; (306)766-2096; Fax. (306)766-2842.

DE LAROCHELLIERE, Robert; Hôpital Laval, 2725 ch Sainte-Foy, Quebec QC G1V 4G5; Sher'85; CSPQ; FRCPC; IntMed; Cardiol. Staff, Hôpital Laval; (418)656-8711

DE LASA, Cristina; Village Family Health Team, 102-171 East Liberty St, Toronto ON M6K 3P6; Ott'10; CCFP; (416)599-8348; Fax. (416)599-2001.

DE LEAN, Jacques; Ctr Hosp Affilie-Enfant Jesus, 1401 18e rue, Quebec QC G1J 1Z4; Laval'69; AB; Electroenceph (P.Q.); Neur. Ac Staff, Centre Hospitalier Affilié Universitaire de Québec - Hôpital De L'Enfant Jésus; Clin Prof Med, Université Laval; (418)649-0252; Fax. (418)649-7515.

DE LEEUW, Charles B; West Oaks Med Centre, 310-32700 South Fraser Way, Abbotsford BC V2T 4M5; Pretoria (South Africa)'73; MB ChB; (604)557-9938

DE LEON, Ernesto L; Hammond Bldg, 216-310 Main St N, Moose Jaw SK S6H 3K1; UST (Philippines)'67; (306)694-4377; Fax. (306)693-7728.

DE LEVIE, Melvin I; Oakridge Centre South Tower, 207-650 41st Ave W, Vancouver BC V5Z 2M9; UBC'66; Peds. Vis Staff, Providence Health Care - St Paul's Hospital; (604)266-1874; Fax. (604)266-1583.

DE LIMA, Leslie J; Workers' Comp Board, 9912 107 St NW, Edmonton AB T5K 1G5; Bombay (India)'54; (780)498-4252; Fax. (780)498-7863.

DE LOPPINOT, Anne; Clinique Med Cadillac, 3435 rue Bossuet, Montreal QC H1M 2M1; Sher'01; Staff Clinique Obstetrique, Hopital Maisonneuve-Rosemont; Langs: English; (514)253-1211; Fax. (514)253-5091.

DE LORENZI, Claudio; 150 Edna St, Kitchener ON N2H 6S1; Wes'83; FRCSC; PlasSurg (Cosmetic Surgery). Staff, St Mary's General Hospital; Staff, Grand River Hospital - Kitchener/Waterloo Health Centre; Pres, Canadian Laser Aesthetic Surgery Society; (519)570-2811; info@delorenzi.ca.

DE LOS SANTOS, Christina J; 105-901 King St W, Toronto ON M5V 3H5; Wes'07; CCFP; (416)599-6000

DE LUCA, Angelo; Polyclinique Cabrini, 110-5700 rue Saint-Zotique E, Montreal QC H1T 3Y7; Mon'92; CCFP; Staff, Hôpital Santa Cabrini Ospedale; (514)254-6282; Fax. (514)254-6282.

DE LUCA, Linda G; Burrard Health Bldg, 602-1160 Burrard St, Vancouver BC V6Z 2E8; McM'85; FRCPC; IntMed; Nephrol. Clin Asst Prof, Providence Health Care - St Paul's Hospital; Clinical Asst Prof, University of British Columbia; (604)681-7191; Fax. (604)681-4482.

DE LUCA, Marina; PO Box 2280 Stn Rpo Banks Cent, Kelowna BC V1X 4K6; McG'86; MDCM; FRCPC; Psy (Psychiatric Oncology). Staff, Kelowna General Hospital; Staff, BC Cancer Agency Sindi Ahluwalia Hawkins Centre for the Southern Interior; (250)765-3544

DE LUCA, Vincenzo; Addiction & Mental Hlth-Clarke, 250 College St, Toronto ON M5T 1R8; Naples (Italy)'98; Staff, Centre for Addiction & Mental Health (CAMH) - College Street Site; (416)979-4747

DE LUNA, Rodrigo P; Peterborough Clinic FHT, 203-26 Hospital Dr, Peterborough ON K9J 7C3; Manila (Philippines)'81; CCFP; FCFP; Langs: Tagalog; (705)740-6881; Fax. (705)743-6874.

DE MAIO, Patricia A; Qikigtani Gen Hosp, PO Box 1000 Stn 1040, Iqaluit NU X0A 0H0; McM'89; BSc(Pharm); CCFP; Staff, Qikigtani General Hospital; (867)979-7347; Fax. (867)979-7346; pdemaio@gov.nu.ca.

DE MARCHI, Ryan; Four Corners Med Bldg, 201-2009 Long Lake Rd, Sudbury ON P3E 6C3; Tor'05; BSc; FRCSC; Neursurg., Health Sciences North-Laurentian Site; Asst Prof, Northern Ontario School of Medicine; (705)522-0292; Fax. (705)522-9933.

DE MARCHI, W Gregory; 303-2021 Cliff Rd, Mississauga ON L5A 3N7; McM'76; (905)848-3712

DE MARCHIE, Michel; SMBD Jewish Gen Hosp, B300-3755 ch Cote-Sainte-Cathe, Montreal QC H3T 1E2; Laval'73; FRCPC; IntMed. Staff, Sir Mortimer B Davis Jewish General; (514)340-7500; Fax. (514)340-7554.

DE MARCO, Francis S; 1275 Walker Rd, Windsor ON N8Y 4X9; Wes'78; Staff, Hôtel-Dieu Grace Hospital; Langs: Spanish; (519)253-9116; Fax. (519)253-5404.

DE MARCO, Vincent P; 793521 3rd Line EHS RR 1, Orangeville ON L9W 2Y8; Tor'75; FRCPC; Psy (Alternative Medicine). (519)942-4978; vincedemarco@rogers.com.

DE MARGERIE, Gilles J B; CLSC Cote-des-Neiges, 500-5700 ch de la Cote-des-Nei, Montreal QC H3T 2A8; Mon'95; Staff, Hôpital de Saint-Eustache; (514)731-8531

DE MARGERIE, Michele; 107-900 Greenbank Rd, Nepean ON K2J 1S8; Sher'82; CCFP; Langs: Bilingual(French/English); (613)825-8476; Fax. (613)825-9045.

DE MARIA, Jorge; McMaster Univ Med Centre, 4E 19-1200 Main St W, Hamilton ON L8N 3Z5; National (Mexico)'71; FAAP; FRCSC; Urol (Pediatric Urology). Ac Staff Peds Surg, Hamilton Health Sciences Centre - McMaster Children's Hospital; Prof Surg & Peds, McMaster University; Langs: Spanish; (905)521-2100; Fax. (905)521-9992.

DE MARSH, John G; PO Box 9, Vernon Bridge PE C0A 2E0; McM'77; CCFP; Physician Occup Health, PEI Occupational Rehabilitation Centre; (902)651-2469

DE MAUPEOU, Michel; 679 2e rue E CP 6000 Succ Bureau-Chef, La Sarre QC J9Z 2X7; Mon'76; Anesthesiste, Centre Hospitalier La Sarre; Langs: French; English; Bilingual(French/English); (819)333-2311; Fax. (819)333-3051.

DE MEDICIS, Anne; CLSC et CHSLD de Pommeraie, 660 rue Saint-Paul, Farnham QC J2N 3B9; Sher'98; Langs: English; (450)293-3622

DE MEDICIS, Etienne; CHUS-Hop Fleurimont, 3001 12e av N, Sherbrooke QC J1H 5N4; Sher'93; CSPQ; FRCPC; Anes. Staff, Centre Hospitalier Universitaire de Sherbrooke-Hopital Fleurimont; (819)346-1110 x14956; Fax. (819)820-6413.

DE MELLO, A Joseph; The Doctor's Office at Six Poi, 1408-5230 Dundas St W, Etobicoke ON M9B 1A8; London (England)'67; MB BS; MRCS; LRCP; Hon Staff, Trillium Health Centre - Mississauga; Court Staff, St Joseph's Health Centre; (416)234-8668

DE MESTRAL, Charles; Sunnybrooke Hlth Sciences Ctr, 2075 Bayview Ave, Toronto ON M4N 3M5; McG'08; Staff, St Michael's Hospital; Staff, Sunnybrook Health Sciences Centre; (416)480-6100

DE METZ, Catherine E; Cancer Ctre of Southeastern On, 25 King St W, Kingston ON K7L 5P9; Alb'83; FRCPC; RadOncol (Lung). (613)544-2631 x4144; Fax. (613)546-8203; catherine.demetz@krcc.on.ca.

DE MEULEMEESTER, Christine; The Ottawa Hosp-Civic Campus, C2196-1053 Carling Ave, Ottawa ON K1Y 4E9; McM'92; FRCPC; Neur. Staff, The Ottawa Hospital - General Campus; Staff, The Ottawa Hospital - Civic Campus; (613)798-5555 x16234

DE MEYER, Philippe; Clinique Med L'Assomption, CP 3406 814 boul L'Ange-Gardien N, L'Assomption QC J5W 4M9; Brussels (Belgium)'83; Staff, Centre Hospitalier Pierre le Gardeur; Fax. (450)589-5779.

DE MILLE, Janet K; 999 Balmoral St, Thunder Bay ON P7B 6E7; Wes'97; CCFP; Public Health & Preventive Med. (807)625-5900

DE MINICO, Carlo; Clin Med Sainte-Dorothee, 102-1 boul Samson, Laval QC H7X 3S5; Mon'09; CCFP; (450)689-6334; Fax. (450)689-6339.

DE MOISSAC, Paul C; Seine Med Centre, 105-142 Centrale Ave, Ste Anne MB R5H 1C3; Man'83; Med Dir, Ste Anne Hospital; (204)422-8811; Fax. (204)422-5876.

DE MONTBRUN, Sandra L; St Michael's Hosp, W16 046-30 Bond St, Toronto ON M5B 1W8; Tor'04; FRCSC; GenSurg. Staff, St Michael's Hospital; (416)864-5005; Fax. (416)864-5565.

DE MONTIGNY, Catherine; CSSS de Saint-Jerome, 290 rue de Montigny, Saint-Jerome QC J7Z 5T3; Mon'99; Staff Emerg Med, Hôtel-Dieu de Saint-Jérôme; (450)431-8200; Fax. (450)431-8244.

DE MONTIGNY, Claude; 663 av Stuart, Outremont QC H2V 3H2; Mon'68; PhD; FRCPC; Psy (Mood Disorders). Staff, Royal Victoria Regional Health Centre; Staff, McGill University Health Centre - Royal Victoria Hospital; Prof, McGill University; (514)277-4687; claudedemontigny@compuserve.com.

DE MONTIGNY, Rene; 290 rue Notre-Dame, St-Germain-D-Grant QC J0C 1K0; Laval'76; Langs: English; French; (819)395-4545; Fax. (819)395-4545.

DE MOTT, Wayne T; 7774 Trentelman Pl, Saanichton BC V8M 1K9; Alb'80; Ac Staff, Royal Jubilee Hospital; Ac Staff, Victoria General Hospital; (250)652-3417

DE MUELENAERE, Philip F; Brendon Med Arts Clinic, 339 Princess Ave, Brandon MB R7A 0N7.

DE NANASSY, Joseph A; Children's Hosp Eastern Ont, 401 Smyth Rd, Ottawa ON K1H 8L1; Szeged (Hungary)'80; FRCPC; AnatPath (Pediatric Pathology). Chief Path, Children's Hospital of Eastern Ontario (CHEO); Assoc Prof, University of Ottawa; Langs: German; French; Hungarian; (613)737-7600 x2897

DE NYSSCHEN, Stefanus F; PO Box 20, Cabri SK S0N 0J0; Orange Free State (South Africa)'87; MB ChB; Langs: Afrikaans; (306)587-2286; Fax. (306)587-2311.

DE OLIVEIRA, Marcelo M; Centre D'etudes Cliniques, 225 rue Saint-Vallier, Chicoutimi QC G7H 7P2; (Brazil)'93; Staff, Complexe hospitalier de la Sagamie; (418)541-1000

DE PADUA, Felix B; Prince Albert Commun Clinic, 110 8th St E, Prince Albert SK S6V 0V7; FEU (Philippines)'72; Med Staff, Victoria Hospital; (306)763-6464; Fax. (306)763-2101.

DE PAOLI, Lorne E; Nanaimo Reg Gen Hosp, 1200 Dufferin Cres, Nanaimo BC V9S 2B7; Alb'85; FCFP; FamilyMed(EM);CCFP; Staff, Nanaimo Regional General Hospital; (250)754-2141

DE PAOLI, Maria A; Royal York Med Arts Bldg, 305-1436 Royal York Rd, Etobicoke ON M9P 3A9; Wes'91; (416)240-1382; Fax. (416)240-1103.

DE PAOLI JR., John A; Royal York Med Arts Bldg, 305-1436 Royal York Rd, Etobicoke ON M9P 3A9; Wes'94; (416)240-1382; Fax. (416)240-1103.

DE PAPE, Gregory E; 103-3949 Maple Way, Port Alberni BC V9Y 0B2; UBC'97; CCFP; (250)723-3561; Fax. (250)723-1434; gregdepape@shaw.ca.

DE PASS, Ian E; 65 Thames St, Chatham ON N7L 1S4; Mem'89; FACS; BMedSci; FRCSC; GenSurg. (519)354-1241; Fax. (519)354-1208.

DE PAUW, Anna; St Mary's Hosp Centre, 3830 av Lacombe, Montreal QC H3T 1M5; UBC'09; CCFP; Staff, St Mary's Hospital Centre; (514)734-2628

DE PERROT, Marc; Univ Hlth Network-Toronto Gen, 9N 961-200 Elizabeth St, Toronto ON M5G 2C4; Geneva (Switzerland)'94; FRCPC; DiagRad (Neuro Radiology). Scientist, Toronto General Hospital - UHN; (416)340-5549; Fax. (416)340-3478; marc.deperrot@uhn.on.ca.

DE PETRILLO, A Dennis; The Credit Valley Hosp, 2200 Eglinton Ave W, Mississauga ON L5M 2N1; Ott'66; FACOG; FRCSC; ObstGyn (Gynecologic Oncology). Staff, The Credit Valley Hospital; Pres CEO/CEO, Carepath Inc; Emeritus Prof Gyn Surg, University of Toronto; (905)813-1100; ddepetrillo@carepath.ca.

DE PIERI, Andrew P; 106-1353 Ellis St, Kelowna BC V1Y 1Z9; UBC'90; CCFP; (250)448-7408

DE PIERO, Steven A; Orillia Soldiers' Mem Hosp, 170 Colborne St W, Orillia ON L3V 2Z3; Wes'97; CCFP; CCFP(E.M.); Staff, Orillia Soldiers' Memorial Hospital; (705)325-2201

DE PLAEN, Sylvaine; Inst Albert Prevost, 6555 boul Gouin O, Montreal QC H4K 1B3; Mon'92; FRCPC; Psy. Staff, Hôpital Ste-Justine; Langs: French; Arabic; Spanish; (514)338-2222 x4638; sdeplaen@sympatico.ca.

DE POKOMANDY, Alexandra; Institut Thoracique de Montrea, J803-3650 rue Saint-Urbain, Montreal QC H2X 2P4; McG'01; MSc(Epidemiol); CCFP; Langs: English; (514)843-2090; Fax. (514)843-2092.

DE PONTE, Delta M; Humber Health Centre, H206-3199 Lakeshore Blvd W, Etobicoke ON M8V 1K8; Tor'86; MSc; Langs: Portuguese; (416)675-6622 x3234; Fax. (416)251-3416.

DE REPENTIGNY, Gaetan; Clinique De Med Familiale, 101 rue Lavoie, Rimouski QC G5L 5Y2; Mon'75; (418)723-5272; Fax. (418)725-2030.

DE RIBAUPIERRE, Sandrine; London HSC-Victoria Hosp, PO Box 5010 Stn B 800 Commissioners Rd E, London ON N6A 5W9; Geneva (Swaziland)'00; Staff, London Health Sciences Centre - Victoria Campus; Langs: Bilingual(English/French); (519)685-8500

DE RIDDER, Handre; Associated Med Clinic, PO Box 510, Lac La Biche AB T0A 2C0; Pretoria (South Africa)'94; MB ChB; CCFP; Staff GP, Lac La Biche Healthcare Centre - William J. Cadzow Building; (780)623-4421; Fax. (780)623-1920.

DE ROBLES, Paula A; Foothills South Tower, 613C-3031 Hospital Dr NW, Calgary AB T2N 2T8; (Argentina)'02; (403)944-3544; Fax. (403)944-3519.

DE ROCHE, Peter L; Mount Sinai Hosp, 600 University Ave, Toronto ON M5G 1X5; Dal'80; FRCPC; Psy (AIDS/HIV). Staff, Mount Sinai Hospital; Staff Centre for Addiction & Mental Hlth, Centre for Addiction & Mental Health (CAMH) - Brentcliffe Rd Site; Asst Prof, University of Toronto; (416)586-4800 x4595; Fax. (416)586-5970; pderoche@mtsinai.on.ca.

DE ROCQUIGNY, Andre J; Victoria Gen Hosp, 2340 Pembina Hwy, Winnipeg MB R3T 2E8; Man'67; FRCPC; Psy. Staff, Victoria General Hospital; Staff, St Boniface General Hospital; (204)477-3118; Fax. (204)269-7619.

DE ROODE, Michael; Algonquin Health Services, PO Box 520 162 Hudson St, Burks Falls ON P0A 1C0; McG'90; CCFP; Court Staff, Geraldton District Hospital; Court Staff, South Muskoka Memorial Hospital - Muskoka Algonquin Healthcare; Staff, Huntsville District Memorial Hospital - Muskoka Algonquin Healthcare; Staff, Burks Falls Hosp; Langs: French; Spanish; (705)382-1562; Fax. (705)382-2257.

DE ROSE, Gaetano; London HSC-Victoria Hosp, PO Box 5010 Stn B E2 123-800 Commissioners Rd E, London ON N6A 5W9; Wes'74; DAB; FACS; FRCSC; GenSurg (Endovasc Aortic Surg); VascSurg. Ac Staff, London Health Sciences Centre - Victoria Campus; Consultant, Ontario Cancer Clinic; University of Western Ontario; (519)667-6644; Fax. (519)667-6573; guy.derose@lhsc.on.ca.

DE RUBEIS, Andrea; Crown Point Family Hlth Ctre, 67 Kenilworth Ave N, Hamilton ON L8H 4R6; Wes'77; BSc(Hon); CCFP; FCFP; Med Staff MD, St Joseph's Care Group - St Joseph's Hospital; Langs: Italian; (905)540-4433; Fax. (905)540-4414.

DE RUBEIS, Debra A; Hamilton HS-McMaster Site, PO Box 2000 Stn Lcd 1 403-1200 Main St W, Hamilton ON L8N 3Z5; McM'93; FRCPC; Neur (Multiple Sclerosis). Staff, Hamilton Health Sciences Centre - McMaster Children's Hospital; Langs: Italian; (905)521-2100

DE RUITER, Joost M; The Hosp For Sick Children, 555 University Ave, Toronto ON M5G 1X8; Cambridge (England)'91; FRCPC; Anes. Staff, The Hospital For Sick Children; Langs: Bilingual(English/French); (416)813-5224; Fax. (416)813-7543.

DE SA, Michelle; Pickering Med Centre, 210-1885 Glenanna Rd, Pickering ON L1V 6R6; Dal'01; CCFP; (905)420-5776

DE SA, Vincent; Port Arthur Health Centre, 194 Court St N, Thunder Bay ON P7A 4V7; Makerere (Uganda)'70; FAAP; FRCPC; Peds. Langs: Swahili; (807)346-1000; Fax. (807)346-6209.

DE SAINT SARDOS, Alexandre; South Shore Med Arts Bldg, 307-42 Glen Allan Dr, Bridgewater NS B4V 3N2; Ott'04; FRCSC; Ophth. (902)543-6819

DE SAINT-VICTOR, Jean R; Hop Brome-Missisquoi-Perkins, 950 rue Principale, Cowansville QC J2K 1K3; Ott'69; FRCSC; ObstGyn. Staff, Hôpital Brome-Missisquoi-Perkins; adj Prof, McGill University; (450)266-4342

DE SALABERRY, Lara; East Ottawa Community FHT, 120-225 Donald St, Ottawa ON K1K 1N1; McM'03; CCFP; Langs: Spanish; French; (613)745-2228 x206; Fax. (613)745-9520.

DE SANCTIS, Norman; Polyclinique Med Fabreville, 380 boul Cure-Labelle, Laval QC H7P 5L3; De Pavia (Italy)'85; (450)628-5800

DE SANCTIS, Olga J; Hawkwood Village Med Clinic, 20-217 Hawksbrow Dr NW, Calgary AB T3G 3K2; Cal'89; (403)777-2757; Fax. (403)777-2755.

DE SANTIS, Teresa A; Joseph Brant Mem Hosp, 1230 North Shore Blvd E, Burlington ON L7S 1W7; McM'98; CCFP; CCFP(E.M.); Staff, Joseph Brant Memorial Hospital; (905)632-3730

DE SEQUEIRA, Carlos M G; Markham Stouffville Hosp, PO Box 1800 Stn Main 381 Church St, Markham ON L3P 7P3; Witwatersrand (South Africa)'89; MB ChB; FRCP(Rad); FRCPC; DiagRad., Markham Stouffville Hospital; (905)472-7568

DE SERRES, Gaston; Inst National de Sante Pub du, 2400 av D'Estimauville, Quebec QC G1E 7G9; Laval'80; PhD(Epidemiol); Prof d'Epidemiologie, Université Laval; (418)666-7000 x274

DE SERRES, Jean; Hema-Quebec, 4045 boul de la Cote-Vertu, Saint-Laurent QC H4R 2W7; Mon'84; MSc; LMCC; CCFP; FCFP; Langs: Bilingual(French/English); (514)832-5000 x530; Fax. (514)832-0969.

DE SERRES, Marthe; CLSC-CHSLD d'Autray, 30 rue Saint-Gabriel, St-Gabriel-D-Brand QC J0K 2N0; Sher'74; LMCC; Staff, CLSC de St-Gabriel; Langs: English; (450)835-4705; Fax. (450)835-2508.

DE SERRES, Sacha; CHUM-Hotel-Dieu de Quebec, 11 av Cote du Palais, Quebec QC G1R 2J6; Mon'02; FRCPC; IntMed; Nephrol. Staff, Centre Hospitalier Universitaire de Québec (CHUQ) - Siege Social; (418)525-5464; Fax. (418)691-5757.

DE SERRES, Sonia; Hotel Dieu d'Arthabaska, 5 rue des Hospitalieres, Victoriaville QC G6P 6N2; Sher'91; Peds. Staff, Hotel-Dieu d'Arthabaska; (819)357-2030; Fax. (819)357-2303; clinique.ped.laurier@videotron.ca.

DE SILVA, Anne; St Clair Med Centre, 1231 St Clair Ave W, Toronto ON M6E 1B5; Bombay (India)'79; MB BS; DMRD; Court Staff, St Joseph's Health Centre; Langs: Konkani; Italian; Portuguese; (416)519-7547; Fax. (416)519-7674.

DE SILVA, Lande B P; SheerHealth Med Clinic, 1560 Hydepark Rd, London ON N6H 5L5; (Sri Lanka)'99; CCFP; (519)474-7300; Fax. (519)474-7309.

DE SMET, Eric; Hôpital du Haut-Richelieu, 920 boul du Seminaire N, St-Jean-sur-Richel QC J3A 1B7; Mon'06; FRCPC; IntMed; Nephrol. Staff, Hôpital du Haut-Richelieu; (450)359-5000

DE SMET, Jan L; Clin Med La Cite Place du Parc, 900-300 rue Leo Pariseau, Montreal QC H2X 4B3; Mon'78; Staff, Centre Hospitalier l'Université de Montréal (CHUM) - Hôtel-Dieu; (514)281-1722; Fax. (514)281-6697.

DE SOUSA, Natasha; Saint John Reg Hosp, PO Box 2100 Stn Main 400 University Ave, Saint John NB E2L 4L2; UBC'07; CCFP; CCFP(E.M.); Staff, Saint John Regional Hospital; (506)648-6000

DE SOUZA, Aloysius P G C; 152-1020 McNicoll Ave, Scarborough ON M1W 2J6; RCS (Ireland)'62; LRCPSI; MRC; DCH; DObstRCOG; Ac Staff, Rouge Valley Health System - Centenary Health Centre Site; Court Staff, The Scarborough Hospital - General Campus; (416)494-9509

DE SOUZA, Claire; The Hosp For Sick Children, 555 University Ave, Toronto ON M5G 1X8; Tor'97; FRCPC; Psy (Child & Adolescent Psychiatry). Staff Psy, The Hospital For Sick Children; (416)813-6511; Fax. (416)813-5326; claire.desouza@sickkids.ca.

DE SOUZA, Darina; Halton HCS Corp-Oakville, 327 Reynolds St, Oakville ON L6J 3L7; (Ireland)'96; FRCPC; Psy. Staff, Halton Healthcare Services Corporation - Oakville Site; (905)845-2571

DE SOUZA, Dawn P; Royal University Hosp, 103 Hospital Dr, Saskatoon SK S7N 0W8; Dar es Salaam (Tanzania)'95; FRCPC; Psy. Staff, Royal University Hospital; (306)966-8232; Fax. (306)966-8237.

DE SOUZA, Duncan G; Kelowna Gen Hosp, 2268 Pandosy St, Kelowna BC V1Y 1T2; Qns'91; FRCPC; Anes. Staff, Kelowna General Hospital; (250)862-4000

DE SOUZA, Eleanor M L; 302-10 Green St, Nepean ON K2J 3Z6; Ott'87; (613)825-9192; Fax. (613)825-9192.

DE SOUZA, Francis K; Gulf Canada Square, 335-401 9 Ave SW, Calgary AB T2P 3C5; McM'91; FRCSC; OrthSurg. (403)266-4772; Fax. (403)221-4387.

DE SOUZA, Fructuoso M; 138-1140 Burnhamthorpe Rd W, Mississauga ON L5C 4E9; RCS (Ireland)'66; FACS; FICS; FRCSC; Otol (Head & Neck Surgery). Consultant Surg Staff, Trillium Health Centre - Mississauga; Asst Prof, University of Toronto; Langs: Portuguese; (905)273-9220; Fax. (905)273-6419.

DE SOUZA, Henry R; Martindale Business Centre, 21-235 Martindale Rd, St Catharines ON L2W 1A5; National (Ireland)'58; DCH(Lond); MRC(Ed.); MRC(Lond); FRCPC; IntMed (Cardiology). Staff, Niagara Health System - St Catharines General Site; (905)984-3410; Fax. (905)984-6254.

DE SOUZA, Kimberley; Univ Hlth Network-Toronto Gen, 200 Elizabeth St, Toronto ON M5G 2C4; McM'05; CCFP; CCFP(E.M.); Staff, Toronto General Hospital - UHN; (416)340-3856; Fax. (416)340-4300.

DE SOUZA, Marcelino; PO Box 3264 Stn Main, Sherwood Park AB T8H 2T2; (Zimbabwe)'83; BSc; MB ChB; Langs: Portuguese; (780)836-9316

DE SOUZA, Melissa P A; Women's College Hosp, 77 Grenville St, Toronto ON M5S 1B2; Tor'09; CCFP; (416)323-6060

DE SOUZA, Nilceia L; Dominion Med Centres Parsons R, 9122 23 Ave NW, Edmonton AB T6N 1H9; (Brazil)'91; (780)801-3360; Fax. (780)801-3366.

DE SOUZA, Selwyn X P; 101-1907 Baseline Rd, Ottawa ON K2C 0C7; Ott'90; BSc; CCFP; Langs: Bilingual(English/French); (613)723-1406; Fax. (613)723-5965.

DE SWARDT, Stefan R; 101-143 Fourth Ave S, Williams Lake BC V2G 1J8; Pretoria (South Africa)'05; MB ChB; Langs: Afrikaans; (250)398-5162

DE TINA, Donald S; PO Box 99075 Rpo Heritage Gre, Stoney Creek ON L8J 2P7; Tor'79; BSc; (905)578-9040

DE VARENNES, Benoit; MUHC-Royal Victoria Hosp, S8 86-687 av des Pins O, Montreal QC H3A 1A1; McG'84; MSc; CSPQ; FRCSC; GenSurg (Cardiac Surgery); Cardiovasc&ThorSurg. Dir Cardiac Surg, McGill University Health Centre - Royal Victoria Hospital; Assoc Prof Surg, McGill University; (514)934-1934 x34980; Fax. (514)843-1602.

DE VARENNES, Maryline; Clinique Medicale des 21, 171 6e rue, La Baie QC G7B 0A3; Sher'10; CCFP; (418)544-3331

DE VEBER, George A; York-Finch Med Centre, 316-2115 Finch Ave N, North York ON M3N 2V6; Tor'56; ABIM; FRCPC; IntMed (Nephrology). (416)920-2126; Fax. (416)920-6882; gdeveber@sympatico.ca.

DE VEBER, Hilary R H; 219-840 Coxwell Ave, East York ON M4C 5T2; McM'96; FRCPC; Peds. Staff, Toronto East General Hospital Inc; (416)696-0003; Fax. (416)696-0022.

DE VETTE, Aad; Clinique Med 3000 Inc, 3000 rue Belanger, Montreal QC H1Y 1A9; Mon'79; Staff, Hôpital Santa Cabrini Ospedale; (514)376-7702; Fax. (514)376-2639.

DE VILLA, Eileen P; Region of Peel, PO Box 630 7120 Hurontario St, Mississauga ON L5M 2C5; Tor'98; FRCPC; CommunMed;CCFP; Public Health & Preventive Med. (905)791-7800; Fax. (905)564-2683.

DE VILLA, Maria A; Bloor-Jane Med Bldg, 501-2425 Bloor St W, Toronto ON M6S 4W4; Manila (Philippines)'67; FACC; FRCPC; IntMed; Cardiol. Ac Staff/Head Cardiol, St Joseph's Health Centre; Asst Prof, University of Toronto; Langs: Tagalog; (416)766-1046

DE VILLERS, France; Clin Pediatrique Laurentienne, 106-200 rue Durand, Saint-Jerome QC J7Z 7E2; Mon'89; FRCPC; Peds (Asthma). Staff, Hôtel-Dieu de Saint-Jérôme; Staff, Hôpital Ste-Justine; Langs: English; Spanish; (450)438-1241; Fax. (450)438-3501.

DE VILLERS-SIDANI, Etienne; MUHC-Montreal Neurology Inst, 742-3801 rue University, Montreal QC H3A 2B4; McG'00; FRCPC; Neur. Staff, McGill University Health Centre - Montreal Neurological Hospital; (514)398-3390; Fax. (514)398-1338.

DE VILLIERS, Albert; Public Health Centre, 2101-10320 99 St, Grande Prairie AB T8V 6J4; Pretoria (South Africa)'93; MD; MMed(CommHealth); Med Officer Health, Alberta Health Services; Langs: Afrikaans; (780)513-7531; Fax. (780)532-4373; moh@pchr.ca.

DE VILLIERS, Annalize; Kootenay Child Hlth & Developm, 16 12th Ave S, Cranbrook BC V1C 3V7; (South Africa)'98; MB ChB; (250)426-9008

DE VILLIERS, Christie; West Hill Med Clinic, 1A-2995 2nd Ave W, Prince Albert SK S6V 5V5; (Other Foreign)'01; MB ChB; (306)765-8500; Fax. (306)765-8501.

DE VILLIERS, Frederik U; 107-437 Glenmore Rd, Kelowna BC V1V 1Y5; Orange Free (South Africa)'02; MB ChB; (250)860-5811

DE VILLIERS, Jacobus; Lakewood Common Cardiology, 411C Herold Crt, Saskatoon SK S7V 0A7; Stellenbosch (South Africa)'90; MB ChB; FRCPC; IntMed; Cardiol. Clin Assoc Prof, University of Saskatchewan; (306)374-2287; Fax. (306)374-4343.

DE VLAMING, Stanley C; Pender Community Health Centre, 59 Pender St W, Vancouver BC V6B 1R3; Man'84; Staff, Pender Community Health Centre; (604)669-9181; Fax. (604)688-9775.

DE VOS, Peter W; Omineca Clinic, 3348 Hospital Rd, Vanderhoof BC V0J 3A2; Witwatersrand (South Africa)'86; MB ChB; BSc; Staff, St John Hospital; Langs: Afrikaans; (250)567-2201; Fax. (250)567-2105.

DE VOS, Werner; 818 25 St, Wainwright AB T9W 1V8; Stellenbosch (South Africa)'93; MB ChB; LMCC; Dir Area Rep/Pharm, Therapeutics Comm Area 7; Langs: Afrikaans; (780)842-7090

DE VRIENDT, Xavier; CSSS de Rivière-de-Loup, 75 rue Saint-Henri, Riviere-du-Loup QC G5R 2A4; Laval'76; FRCPC; Psy. Staff, Centre Hospitalier Regional du Grand-Portage; (418)868-1020; Fax. (418)868-0530.

DE VRIES, Ansunette; Main Street Med Centre, PO Box 489, Oliver BC V0H 1T0; (South Africa)'99; MB ChB; (250)498-3411

DE VRIES, Gwyneth; 405-440 King St, Fredericton NB E3B 5H8; Cal'95; BSc; MSc; FRCSC; OrthSurg (Foot & Ankle Reconstruction). Staff, Dr Everett Chalmers Regional Hospital; (506)457-4733; Fax. (506)457-4778.

DE VRIES, Johannes D; Rockyview Gen Hosp, 7007 14 St SW, Calgary AB T2V 1P9; Amsterdam (Netherlands)'57; FRCPC; Psy. Staff, Rockyview General Hospital; Langs: Dutch; (403)943-3614; Fax. (403)943-3624.

DE VRIES, Matthys A; PO Box 860, Osoyoos BC V0H 1V0; Stellenbosch (South Africa)'99; MB ChB; (250)495-6565

DE VRIJER, Barbra; London HSC-Victoria Hosp, PO Box 5010 Stn B B2 412-800 Commissioners Rd E, London ON N6A 5W9; Erasmus (Netherlands)'93; Staff, London Health Sciences Centre - Victoria Campus; (519)685-8500

DE VYNCK, Willem E; Langley Mem Hosp, 22051 Fraser Hwy, Langley BC V3A 4H4; Stellenbosch (South Africa)'88; MB ChB; CCFP; CCFP(E.M.); Locum Tenens ER, Surrey Memorial Hospital; Locum Tenens ER, Langley Memorial Hospital; Langs: Afrikaans; Dutch; (604)534-4121 x74608; devynck@shaw.ca.

DE WAAL, Derick; 201-836 1 Ave NW, Airdrie AB T4B 0V2; Stellenbosch (South Africa)'90; MB ChB; CCFP; Langs: Afrikaans; (403)948-6422

DE WAAL, Egbertus B; Barrhead Clinic, PO Box 4540 Stn Main 5040 49A St, Barrhead AB T7N 1A4; (South Africa)'93; MB ChB; (780)674-2231; Fax. (780)674-2447.

DE WAAL, Philip F; 201-836 1 Ave NW, Airdrie AB T4B 0V2; (South Africa)'90; MB ChB; (403)948-6422

DE WAAL, Tonya R; Southlake Reg Health Centre, 596 Davis Dr, Newmarket ON L3Y 2P9; McM'98; FRCPC; Anes. Staff, Southlake Regional Health Centre; (905)895-4521

DE WAAL, Willem P; Haig Clinic, 601 6 Ave S, Lethbridge AB T1J 0Z2; (South Africa)'78; (403)328-6641; Fax. (403)328-6118.

DE WALS, Charlotte; Clinique Medi-Val, 100-408 rue Jeanne-Mance, Salaber-de-Valleyf QC J6T 4G1; Mon'05; (450)370-3387; Fax. (450)370-3395.

DE WALS, Phillippe; Centre De Sante Publique, 2400 av D'Estimauville, Quebec QC G1E 7G9; Louvain (Belgium)'76; PhD(PublicHealth); CSPQ; CommunMed (P.Q.). Head Social & Preventive Med, Université Laval; (418)666-7000

DE WET, Francois B; Baie Verte Peninsula Hlth Ctr, GD, Baie Verte NL A0K 1B0; Pretoria (South Africa)'91; MB ChB; CCFP; Chief Medical Staff, Baie Verte Peninsula Health Centre; (709)532-4281

DE WET, Guy A; The Maple Tree Med Clinic, 1181 6 Ave NE, Salmon Arm BC V1E 2S5; Cape Town (South Africa)'92; MB ChB; Staff, Stuart Lake Hospital; (250)832-9361; Fax. (250)833-4781.

DE WET, Johann; Southshore Med Clinic, 620 Cassils Rd E, Brooks AB T1R 1M6; (South Africa)'02; MB ChB; CCFP; Staff ER, Brooks Medical Centre; Clin Lecturer, University of Calgary; Langs: Afrikaans; (403)793-8111; Fax. (403)793-8118.

DE WET, Johannes M J; Brandon Reg Health Centre, 150 McTavish Ave E, Brandon MB R7A 2B3; Orange Free State (South Africa)'00; Staff, Brandon Regional Health Centre.

DE WET, Joseph J; Spectrum Health, 702-1080 Howe St, Vancouver BC V6Z 2T1; Pretoria (South Africa)'84; MB ChB; CCFP; (604)681-1080; Fax. (604)681-0244.

DE WET, Lourens J C; Wetaskiwin Fam Med Practice, 5107 50 St, Wetaskiwin AB T9A 1K1; (South Africa)'91; (780)352-3010; Fax. (780)352-7413.

DE WET, Pieter W; 215 Centre St PO Box 266, McLennan AB T0H 2L0; (South Africa)'87; (780)324-3054; Fax. (780)324-2009.

DE WET, Rene; Supermed Family Pract Clinic, 1D-595 Ontario Rd, Welland ON L3B 0B3; Stellenbosch (South Africa)'85; MB ChB; CCFP; Langs: Afrikaans; (905)734-8777; Fax. (905)734-4358.

DE WET, Steyn; Associate Med Clinic, PO Box 549, Pincher Creek AB T0K 1W0; (South Africa)'80; MB ChB; BSc; Staff Anes, Cardston Hospital; Langs: Afrikaans; (403)627-3321; Fax. (403)627-2280.

DE WET, Susanna A; Medical Centre, 204-595 Columbia St W, Kamloops BC V2C 1K7; Pretoria (South Africa)'93; MB ChB; Langs: Afrikaans; (250)377-8182; Fax. (250)377-8183.

DE WIT, Andre J; Port Hardy Med Associates, PO Box 2009 8785 Gray St, Port Hardy BC V0N 2P0; Pretoria (South Africa)'85; MB ChB; CCFP; (250)949-5920; Fax. (250)949-5954.

DE WIT, Christiaan C; Mills Memorial Hosp, 4720 Haughland Ave, Terrace BC V8G 2W7; Orange Free State (South Africa)'89; MB ChB; LMCC; Staff, Mills Memorial Hospital; (250)638-4060

DE WIT, Christoffel; Welland McMaster Family Hlth Team, 555 Prince Charles Dr, Welland ON L3C 6B5; Orange free (South Africa)'96; CCFP; (905)734-9699

DE WIT, Simon L; Brandon Reg Health Centre, 150 Mctavish Ave E, Brandon MB R7A 2B3; Stellenbosch (South Africa)'77; MB ChB; LMCC; FRCPC; Anes. Staff, Brandon Regional Health Centre; (204)726-1122

DE WITT, Andries J; 4-4565 Wallace St, Port Alberni BC V9Y 3Y3; Stellenbosch (South Africa)'77; MB ChB; (250)723-2222; Fax. (250)723-2270.

DE WITT, Elzaan; Desert Doctors Clinic, PO Box 860, Osoyoos BC V0H 1V0; Stellenbosch (South Africa)'06; MB ChB; (250)495-6565

DE WITT, Jacobus; Gardiner Park Med Clinic, 358 University Park Dr, Regina SK S4V 0Y8; Pretoria (South Africa)'72; MB ChB; (306)522-5671; Fax. (306)789-1588.

DE WITT, Schalk J; Tudor Glen Medicentre, 2520 Tudor Glen Market, St Albert AB T8N 3V3; Stellenbosch (South Africa)'76; MB ChB; CCFP; (780)458-5776

DE YOUNG, J Paul; McConnell Med Centre, 220-820 McConnell Ave, Cornwall ON K6H 4M4; Mem'77; BMedSci; FRCPC; IntMed (Cardiology); Endocrin&Metab. Dir ICU & CCU, Cornwall Community Hospital; Langs: French; (613)938-2332; deyoung@sympatico.ca.

DE YTURRALDE, Daniel; 4-335 rue Main, Shediac NB E4P 2B1; McG'68; CSPQ; OrthSurg (Sports Medicine). Staff, Dr Georges-L-Dumont University Hospital Centre; Langs: Spanish; English; (506)532-8880; Fax. (506)532-2715.

DEA, Nicolas; Blusson Spinal Cord Centre, 6F-818 10th Ave W, Vancouver BC V5Z 1M9; Sher'05; FRCSC; Neursurg. (604)675-2418

DEACON, Charles M A; CHUS-Hosp Fleurimont, 3001 12e av N, Sherbrooke QC J1H 5N4; Sher'96; FRCPC; Neur (Epilepsy). Staff, Centre Hospitalier Universitaire de Sherbrooke-Hopital Fleurimont; Langs: Bilingual(French/English); (819)346-1110; Fax. (819)564-5395; charles.deacon@usherbrooke.ca.

DEACON, James E; Quarry High Risk Foot Clinic, 409-797 Princess St, Kingston ON K7L 1G1; Qns'79; BSc(Hon); MD; CCFP; FCFP; Med Dir, Trillium Centre Nursing Home; (613)541-3922

DEACON, Sean D S; 303-9200 Mary St, Chilliwack BC V2P 4H6; Stellenbosch (South Africa)'89; MB ChB; FCOG(SA)FCOG; MMed(O&G); FRCSC; ObstGyn. Staff, Chilliwack General Hospital; (604)792-1986; Fax. (604)792-0149.

DEADMAN, John; Community Schizophrenia Serv, 350 King St E, Hamilton ON L8N 3Y3; Tor'57; DPsy; BA; FRCPC; Psy (Outpatient Psychiatry). Ac Medical Staff, St Joseph's Healthcare - Charlton Campus; Court Medical Staff, Hamilton Health Sciences Centre - McMaster Children's Hospital; Associate Clin Prof Dept of Psy & Behavioural Neuroscience, McMaster University; (905)527-7301; Fax. (905)648-1134; jdeadmanj@stjosham.on.ca.

DEADY, Brian L; Royal Columbian Hosp, 330 Columbia St E, New Westminster BC V3L 3W7; Cal'87; FRCPC; EmergMed. Staff, Royal Columbian Hospital; (604)520-4283; Fax. (604)520-4793.

DEAKON, R Timothy; 18-250 Wyecroft Rd, Oakville ON L6K 3T7; Ott'83; FRCSC; OrthSurg (Arthroscopy & Knee Ligament Reconstruction). Ac Staff, Halton Healthcare Services Corporation - Oakville Site; (905)849-7220; Fax. (905)849-7238.

DEAL, Cheri L; Hôpital Ste-Justine, 3175 ch Cote-Ste-Catherine, Montreal QC H3T 1C5; Mon'85; AB(PedEndo); AB; CSPQ; FRCPC; Peds (Pediatric Endocrinology); Endocrin&Metab. Staff Researcher Research Centre, Hôpital Ste-Justine; Assoc Member Experimetnal Med, McGill University; Prof Peds & Mother-Child Teaching Hosp, Universite de Montreal; Langs: English; French; (514)345-4931 x6209; cheri.l.deal@umontreal.ca.

DEALLY, Carole M R; Turtle Mountain Med Clinic, 968 Main St, Winnipeg MB R2W 3P5; Man'93; FRCPC; Peds; Critical Care Medicine.

DEAN, Erin C; RS4-810 Sherbrook St, Winnipeg MB R3A 1R9; Man'00; FRCSC; ObstGyn.

DEAN, Heather J; Children's Hosp, FE319-685 William Ave, Winnipeg MB R3E 0Z2; Qns'75; FRCPC; Peds (Diabetology). Consultant Ped Endocrin, Health Sciences Centre; Asst Dean Academic, University of Manitoba; Langs: English; French; (204)787-3337; Fax. (204)787-1655; hdean@hsc.mb.ca.

DEAN, John M; Children's & Women's HC of BC, 1C23-4480 Oak St, Vancouver BC V6H 3V4; London (England)'74; MB BS; FRCPC; Peds; ClinImmunol&Allergy. Staff Ped, BC Children's Hospital; Clinical Asst Prof Peds, University of British Columbia; Langs: Spanish; French; (604)875-2118

DEAN, Margaret S; 201-1245 Danforth Ave, Toronto ON M4J 5B5; London (England)'75; FRCPC; Psy (Adult Psychiatry). (416)463-7077; drdean@bellnet.ca.

DEAN, Naeem; Royal Alexandra Hosp, 657-10240 Kingsway NW, Edmonton AB T5H 3V9; (Pakistan)'85; Staff, Royal Alexandra Hospital; (780)944-2405; Fax. (780)491-5588.

DEANE, Brian C M; Sturgeon Community Hosp, 201 Boudreau Rd, St. Albert AB T8N 6C4; Alb'86; Staff, Sturgeon Community Hospital; (780)418-8229

DEANE, John A; Town Centre Prof Bldg, 216-6203 28 Ave NW, Edmonton AB T6L 6K3; Alb'66; BSc; (780)463-2134; Fax. (780)463-1184.

DEANE, Robert H; Dr Charles A Janeway Child Hc, 2J047-300 Prince Philip Dr, St. John's NL A1B 3V6; Cape Town (South Africa)'72; MB ChB; OrthSurg. Staff, Janeway Children's Health & Rehabilitation Centre; (709)777-4318

DEANGELIS, Matthew A; Queensway-Carleton Hosp, 3045 Baseline Rd, Nepean ON K2H 8P4; Qns'03; FRCPC; Psy. Staff, Queensway Carleton Hospital; Langs: Italian; (613)721-2000

DEANS, A Michael; Halton HSC Corp-Milton, 7030 Derry Rd, Milton ON L9T 7H6; Ott'90; CCFP; FCFP; Staff, Halton Healthcare Services Corporation - Milton District Hospital; (905)878-2383

DEANS, Gregory; St Paul's Hosp, 667-1081 Burrard st, Vancouver BC V6Z 1Y6; Man'05; FRCPC; IntMed; InfectDis. Staff, Providence Health Care - St Paul's Hospital; (604)806-8640

DEANS, James R A; 300-274 Dundas St E, Belleville ON K8N 1E6; Birmingham (England)'62; FRCSC; OrthSurg. Head Dept of Orth, QHC Belleville General; (613)966-7522; Fax. (613)966-3997; orthodeans@lks.net.

DEANS, Robin M; 4-1270 Walker Rd, Windsor ON N8Y 4T4; Ott'86; FRCSC; Ophth. Staff, Hôtel-Dieu Grace Hospital; Staff, Windsor Regional Hospital - Metropolitan Site; Langs: Bilingual(English/French); (519)256-9333; Fax. (519)256-9063.

DEAR, Richard A R; Westbrook Prof Bldg, 215-1610 37 St SW, Calgary AB T3C 3P1; (Jamaica)'72; MB BS; ABIM; FRCPC; IntMed. Consultant, Brooks Health Centre; Clin Assoc Prof, University of Calgary; (403)284-0777; Fax. (403)685-9422.

DEARMAN, Lisa M; Dr Lisa Dearman Inc, 636 Main St, Wolfville NS B4P 1E8; Dal'91; (902)697-7425; Fax. (902)697-3425.

DEASE, Murray E; Royal University Hosp, 103 Hospital Dr, Saskatoon SK S7N 0W8; Sask'98; FRCPC; Anes. Staff, Royal University Hospital; (306)655-1183; Fax. (306)655-1279.

DEATH, A Barry; 285 Commissioners Rd E, London ON N6C 2T3; Tor'67; BSc; FRCPC; PhysMed&Rehab (Amputee Rehabilitation). Staff, Parkwood Hospital - St Joseph's Health Care; Assoc Prof Dept of PhysMed & Rehab, University of Western Ontario; (519)685-4573; Fax. (519)685-4571.

DEATON, Shoshanah E C; Clarence-Rockland Fam Hlth Team, 2741 rue Chamberland, Rockland ON K4K 0B4; Ott'05; CCFP; Langs: Bilingual(English/French); (613)446-7677

DEB, Bakul; Regina Qu'Appelle HR-Regina, 1440 14th Ave, Regina SK S4P 0W5; Chittagong (Bangladesh)'85; Staff, Regina General Hospital; (306)766-6161; Fax. (306)766-4557.

DEB, Pratima; McMaster University Medical Ct, 1200 Main St W, Hamilton ON L8K 1A1; Calcutta (India)'72; FRCPC; AnatPath. Staff, St Joseph's Healthcare - Charlton Campus; Assoc Prof Pathology & Molecular Med, McMaster University; (905)521-2100

DEBAY, Badri; Hop Jean-Talon, 1385 rue Jean-Talon E, Montreal QC H2E 1S6; Damascus (Syria)'92; FRCPC; IntMed. Staff, CSSS du Coeur de l'Isle Hôpital Jean-Talon; (514)495-6767

DEBBANE, Elie G; 530-999 Broadway W, Vancouver BC V5Z 1K5; Beirut (Lebanon)'62; DPsy; FRCPC; Psy (Psychoanalysis). Staff, Lions Gate Hospital; (604)738-5386; Fax. (604)921-0794.

DEBERT, Chantel T; Foothills Med Centre, SSB AC147-1403 29 St NW, Calgary AB T2N 2T9; Cal'06; FRCPC; PhysMed&Rehab. Staff, Foothills Medical Centre; (403)944-4500

DEBERT, Francoise Amelina; CSSS d'Antoine-Labelle-l'Annon, 1525 rue l'Annonciation N, Riviere-Rouge QC J0T 1T0; Grenoble (France)'75; MSc; ac Staff, Centre de L'Annonciation; (819)275-2118; Fax. (819)275-1520.

DEBERTIN, Manfred W; St Stephen Med Clinic, 33 Wall St, St Stephen NB E3L 2L5; Dal'82; BSc; Staff, Charlotte County Hospital; (506)466-5006; Fax. (506)466-6685.

DEBLOIS, Jacques; Pavillon Ferdinand-Landry, 1050 av de la Medecine, Quebec QC G1V 0A6; Laval'84; FRCPC; EmergMed. Staff, Centre Hospitalier de Verdun; (418)656-2131

DEBLOIS, Michel; Centre medical de Cowansville, 370 rue de la Riviere, Cowansville QC J2K 1N3; Laval'73; Urol (P.Q.). (450)263-6457

DEBLONDE, Myriam; Centre Med Fusion, 200-2035 av Sainte-Anne, Saint-Hyacinthe QC J2S 5H3; Sher'79; Staff, Centre Hospitalier Honore-Mercier; (450)771-1322

DEBNATH, Pranab K; Lakewood Med Centre, 30 Lakewood Blvd, Winnipeg MB R2J 2M7; Calcutta (India)'77; MB BS; FRCSC; ObstGyn.

DEBONO, Alaine M; Collingwood Health Centre, 204-186 Erie St, Collingwood ON L9Y 4T3; Tor'87; CCFP; FCFP; Staff, Collingwood Health Centre; (705)445-5102

DEBOSZ-SZCZERBOWSKI, Grace; 208-140 Oxford St W, London ON N6H 1S1; Poznan (Poland)'67; Langs: Polish; Russian; (519)679-4737; Fax. (519)679-0497.

DEBOW, Stanley L; 602-700 Bay St, Toronto ON M5G 1Z6; Tor'64; DPsy; FRCPC; Psy. Staff, Humber River Regional Hospital - Finch Avenue Site; Staff, Mount Sinai Hospital; Teacher, University of Toronto; (416)597-0196

DEBRECENI, Andrew E; Oakville Med Arts Bldg, 6-358 Reynolds St, Oakville ON L6J 3L9; Wes'70; DABOT; FRCSC; Otol. Staff Consultant, Halton Healthcare Services Corporation - Oakville Site; Court Staff, The Credit Valley Hospital; Court Staff, Joseph Brant Memorial Hospital; Langs: Hungarian; (905)842-0752

DEBRETSION, Tadese F; Queen's Med Centre, 5A-1289 Marlborough Crt, Oakville ON L6H 2R9; (Ethiopia)'97; CCFP; Langs: Amharic; Tigrigna; (905)844-8878; Fax. (905)844-8868.

DEBRU, Estifanos O; Peter Lougheed Centre, 3500 26 Ave NE, Calgary AB T1Y 6J4; Man'96; FRCSC; GenSurg. Staff, Peter Lougheed Centre; (403)291-8555

DEBRUILLE, J Bruno; Douglas Mental Hlth Univ Inst, FBC 1105-6875 boul LaSalle, Verdun QC H4H 1R3; Paris (France)'90; PhD; FRCPC; Psy. Staff, Douglas Mental Health University Institute; Langs: Bilingual(French/English); (514)761-6131 x3405; Fax. (514)888-4099; bruno.debruille@mcgill.ca.

DEBRUYN, Jennifer C C; Alberta Children's Hosp, 2888 Shaganappi Trail NW, Calgary AB T3B 6A8; Alb'03; FRCPC; Peds (Epidemiology); Gastroent. Staff, Alberta Children's Hospital; (403)955-3071; Fax. (403)955-2922; jennifer.debruyn@albertahealthservices.ca.

DEBS, Chaouki; GMF Centre de sante, 3745 rue Georges-Couture, Drummondville QC J2B 7P4; St. Joseph (Lebanon)'71; AB; CSPQ; FRCSC; Urol. Staff Surg, Hôpital Sainte-croix; Langs: Arabic; English; (819)477-2231; Fax. (819)477-1122.

DEBS, Negib; Hop Maisonneuve-Rosemont, 5415 boul de l'Assomption, Montreal QC H1T 2M4; St. Joseph (Lebanon)'81; FRCPC; Peds. Ac Staff, Hopital Maisonneuve-Rosemont; (514)252-3400

DEC, David A; Portage Med Family Health Team, 602-5400 Portage Rd, Niagara Falls ON L2G 5X7; Tor'94; BSc; CCFP; FCFP; Staff, Niagara Health System - Greater Niagara General Site; Asst Clin Prof Family Med, McMaster University; (905)356-2228; Fax. (905)356-8161.

DECALUWE, Hélène; Hôpital Ste-Justine, 3175 ch Cote-Ste-Catherine, Montreal QC H3T 1C5; McG'99; ABPeds; FRCP; MSc; FRCPC; Peds (Immunology). Staff, Hôpital Ste-Justine; (514)345-4713; Fax. (514)345-4897.

DECARIE, Denise; Direction de la Sante Publique, 210-1000 rue Labelle, Saint-Jerome QC J7Z 5N6; Mon'72; Med Consultant InfectDis, Direction Reg. de la Sante Publique des Laurentides; Langs: English; (450)436-8622 x2292; Fax. (450)569-6305.

DECARIE, Jean Claude; Hôpital Ste-Justine, 3175 ch Cote-Ste-Catherine, Montreal QC H3T 1C5; Mon'80; DiagRad (Pediatric Neuro Radiology). Staff Ped & Radiol, Hôpital Ste-Justine; Clin Associate Prof, Universite de Montreal; Langs: English; Creole; (514)345-4931 x6977; Fax. (514)345-4762; jean-claude_decarie@ssss.gouv.qc.ca.

DECARIE, Michel; Centre Med Saint-Hubert, 206-5125 boul Cousineau, Longueuil QC J3Y 3K7; Sher'87; Staff Psy, Hopital Charles LeMoyne; Physician, CHSLD Trefle d'Or (La Prairie); (450)678-3500; Fax. (450)678-5722.

DECARIE, Paul R; Clinique Medicale Belvedere, 202-2235 rue Galt O, Sherbrooke QC J1K 1K6; Laval'69; CSPQ; OrthSurg. (819)563-4244

DECARY, Jean-Marc; Clinique Familiale la Providen, 16405 av Bourdages S, Saint-Hyacinthe QC J2T 4G9; Mon'87; (450)773-6734; Fax. (450)773-9909.

DECELL, Mary K; MUHC-Montreal Children's Hosp, 2300 rue Tupper, Montreal QC H3H 1P3; Dallas(TX) (USA)'81; Peds (P.Q.). Staff, McGill University Health Centre - Montreal Children's Hospital; (514)412-4400 x22994

DECENA, Silvino M; 203-305 Finch Ave W, North York ON M2R 1N2; (Philippines)'76; CCFP; Ac Staff, North York General Hospital - Branson Division; Langs: Tagalog; (416)222-3556; Fax. (416)222-9415.

DECHENE, Genevieve; Clinique Med du Sud-Ouest, 4475 rue Bannantyne, Verdun QC H4G 1E2; Laval'81; Staff, Centre Hospitalier de Verdun; Physician, CLSC de Verdun; Médecin, Clinique Med du Sud-Ouest; Langs: Bilingual(French/English); (514)765-3600; Fax. (514)765-9625; genevieve.dechene@sss.gouv.qc.ca.

DECHERT, K Victoria; 205 Hiram St PO Box 660, Bracebridge ON P1L 2C1; Tor'86; Ac Staff, South Muskoka Memorial Hospital - Muskoka Algonquin Healthcare; (705)645-2223; Fax. (705)645-2342.

DECK, Wilber; Direction de la Sante Publique, 1-205 boul de York O, Gaspe QC G4X 2W5; McG'90; BSc(Math); MSc; CommunMed (Public Health). Langs: Bilingual(English/French); (418)368-4622; Fax. (418)368-1317.

DECKELBAUM, Dan L E; MUHC-Montreal Gen Hosp, 1650 av Cedar, Montreal QC H3G 1A4; McG'01; FRCSC; GenSurg. Staff, McGill University Health Centre - Montreal General Campus; (514)934-1934

DECKER, Christopher; West Parry Sound Health Centre, 6 Albert St, Parry Sound ON P2A 3A4; Tor'78; MD; FRCSC; GenSurg. Staff, West Parry Sound Health Centre; Assoc Prof Surg, Northern Ontario School of Medicine; Langs: Bilingual(English/French); (705)746-9321 x3314; Fax. (705)746-2282; cdecker@nosm.ca.

DECKER, Robert F; Mill Bay Med Centre, 230-2720 Mill Bay Rd RR 1, Mill Bay BC V0R 2P1; Man'76; CCFP; Ac Staff, Cowichan District Hospital; (250)743-3211; Fax. (250)743-2800.

DECKER GOANO, Adriana; SMBD Jewish Gen Hosp, 3755 ch Cote-Sainte-Catherine, Montreal QC H3T 1E2; (Other Foreign)'10; CCFP; Staff, Sir Mortimer B Davis Jewish General; (514)340-8278

DECOBELLIS, Tania; Hop Maisonneuve-Rosemont, 5415 boul de l'Assomption, Montreal QC H1T 2M4; Mon'06; CCFP; Staff, Hopital Maisonneuve-Rosemont; (514)252-3400

DECOEUR, Isabelle; CHUM-Hop Notre-Dame, 1560 rue Sherbrooke E, Montreal QC H2L 4M1; Sher'10; CCFP; Staff, Centre Hospitalier l'Université de Montréal (CHUM) - Hôpital Notre-Dame; (514)890-8000

DECOSSE, Jillian L; Brandon Reg Hlth Centre, 150 McTavish Ave E, Brandon MB R7A 2B3; McM'10; CCFP; Staff, Brandon Regional Health Centre; (204)578-4000

DECTER, Diarmuid; Rosser Med Clinic, 841 Rosser Ave, Brandon MB R7A 0L1; Man'79; Med Staff, Brandon Regional Health Centre; (204)729-8588; Fax. (204)725-0493.

DEDUMETS, Paul; West Windsor Urgent Care, 2055 Huron Church Rd, Windsor ON N9C 2L6; Tor'69; (519)255-9185; Fax. (519)255-9152.

DEEB, Shamsa; Winchester Dist Mem Hosp, 566 Louise St, Winchester ON K0C 2K0; Al Fateh (Libya)'91; FRCSC; ObstGyn. Staff, Winchester District Memorial Hospital; (613)774-2420

DEEDO, Ryan J; Foothills Medical Centre, C231-1403 29 St NW, Calgary AB T2N 2T9; Alb'04; FRCPC; EmergMed. Staff, Foothills Medical Centre; (403)944-8430; Fax. (403)944-2419.

DEEGAN, Donald M; Orchardview Med Centre, 100-155 Main St E, Grimsby ON L3M 1P2; McM'86; CCFP; FCFP; Staff, West Lincoln Memorial Hospital; (905)945-5476; Fax. (905)945-7707.

DEEGAN, Michael F; Baldur Hlth Centre, 531 Elizabeth Ave E, Baldur MB R0K 0B0; Man'80; michael.deegan@northernhealth.ca.

DEEKS, Shelley L; Health Protection & Promotion, 300-480 University Ave, Toronto ON M5G 1V2; Tor'88; MHSc; FRCPC; CommunMed (AIDS/HIV); Public Health & Preventive Med. (647)260-7417

DEEN, Hurara; Kerr Med Centre, 344 Kerr St, Oakville ON L6K 3B8; Universidad Techologica de Santiago (Dominican Republic)'99; CCFP; (905)582-0763; Fax. (289)837-1920.

DEEN, Shajahan; 773 Dunbar Rd, Kitchener ON N2M 2X9; Qns'68; Staff, Grand River Hospital - Kitchener/Waterloo Health Centre; Staff, St Mary's General Hospital; (519)744-5943

DEERING, Susan A; Sunnybrook Hlth Sciences Ctr, KGE 31-2075 Bayview Ave, Toronto ON M4N 3M5; Cal'02; CCFP; Sec-Treas, Sunnybrook Health Sciences Centre; (416)480-4830

DEERNSTED, Eric A; Hilltop Med Clinic, 140-15321 16 Ave, Surrey BC V4A 1R6; Ott'72; (604)531-5575; Fax. (604)535-0126.

DEETH, Karen L; Halton HCS Corp-Oakville, 327 Reynolds St, Oakville ON L6J 3L7; McM'06; CCFP; CCFP(E.M.); Staff, Halton Healthcare Services Corporation - Oakville Site; (905)338-4618; Fax. (905)338-4146.

DEETLEFS, Francois; 3310 32 Ave, Vernon BC V1T 2M6; Pretoria (South Africa)'97; MB ChB; (250)392-7221; Fax. (250)392-7473.

DEFAY, J Yves; Clin Med St-Marhieu, 2571 rue Jean-Talon E, Montreal QC H2A 1T8; (Haiti)'73; (514)374-2932; Fax. (514)374-2932.

DEFOORT, Ericka N; HDH Family Med Centre, PO Box 8888 220 Bagot St, Kingston ON K7L 5E9; Wes'09; CCFP; CCFP(E.M.); (613)533-9303

DEFORGE, Daniel A; G F Strong Rehabilitation Ctre, 4255 Laurel St, Vancouver BC V5Z 2G9; Qns'84; FRCPC; PhysMed&Rehab. Staff, G F Strong Rehabilitation Centre; (604)734-1313; Fax. (604)737-6359; daniel.deforge@vch.ca.

DEFREITAS, Gina; Bathurst Med Centre, 305-4256 Bathurst St, North York ON M3H 5Y8; Tor'97; FRCSC; Urol (Female Urology). Consultant, Baycrest Centre for Geriatric Care; Staff, Humber River Regional Hospital - Finch Avenue Site; (416)630-9984; Fax. (416)630-6415.

DEGANI, Aqeel; Rideau Valley Hlth Centre, 1221 Greenbank Rd, Ottawa ON K2J 4H9; Ott'08; CCFP; Teacher, University of Ottawa; Fax. (613)258-8710.

DEGANI, Cassim T; Sheridan Centre W GTA Endoscop, 183B-2225 Erin Mills Pky, Mississauga ON L5K 1T9; Bombay (India)'64; MB BS; MS; FACS; FRCSC; GenSurg (Endoscopy). Court Staff, Humber River Regional Hospital - Finch Avenue Site; Court Staff, Rouge Valley Health System - Centenary Health Centre Site; Teach Staff, University of Toronto; Langs: Urdu; Hindi; Gujarati; (905)823-0223; Fax. (905)823-9780; postoffice@shouldice.com.

DEGANI, Naeema C; Sheridan Centre, 183-2225 Erin Mills Pky, Mississauga ON L5K 1T9; Bombay (India)'68; Co-Dir, West GTA Endoscpy Clinic; Langs: Gujarati; Hindi; (905)823-0223; Fax. (905)823-9780.

DEGEN, Eric; Univ Hlth Network-Toronto Gen, 13EN 4N456-200 Elizabeth St, Toronto ON M5G 2C4; Tor'96; CCFP; Clin Asst CardiacSurg, Toronto General Hospital - UHN; Langs: German; (416)340-4789

DEGENHART, Nathan; 21st Medical Clinic, 502-402 21st St E, Saskatoon SK S7K 0C3; Sask'06; FRCPC; IntMed. (306)956-3444; Fax. (306)956-3577.

DEGRACE, Michel F; Hotel-Dieu de Levis, 143 rue Wolfe, Levis QC G6V 3Z1; Laval'90; CSPQ; FRCPC; IntMed; Cardiol. Staff, Hôtel-Dieu de Lévis; (418)835-7121

DEGUIRE, Henri; Clinique Med Pierre-Boucher, 1615 boul Jacques-Cartier E, Longueuil QC J4M 2X1; Mon'80; CCFP; Staff, CSSS de la Minganie; (450)468-6223; henri_deguire@ssss.gouv.qc.ca.

DEGUIRE, Richard; CSSS Kamouraska-Hop-Notre Dame, 1201 6e av, La Pocatiere QC G0R 1Z0; Sher'10; CCFP; Staff, Hôpital Notre-Dame-de-Fatima; (418)856-7000

DEHAUT, Pierre; CSSS de Laval, 1755 boul Rene-Laennec, Laval QC H7M 3L9; Mon'76; FRCPC; Respir. Staff, Hopital de la Cite de la santé; Consultant, Centre Hospitalier l'Université de Montréal (CHUM) - Hôtel-Dieu; (450)668-1010; Fax. (450)975-5545.

DEHEJIA, Harsha V; 256 Elgin St, Ottawa ON K2P 1L9; Bombay (India)'60; MRC(Glas.); MRC(Lond); FCCP; FRCPC; IntMed (Clinical Immunology & Allergy). Langs: Gujarati; Hindi; Marathi; (613)233-3103; Fax. (613)233-2311.

DEHEJIA, Sudha H; 256 Elgin St, Ottawa ON K2P 1L9; Bombay (India)'60; DCH(Lond); DABPed; FRCPC; Peds. Ac Staff, Children's Hospital of Eastern Ontario (CHEO); Court Staff, The Ottawa Hospital - Civic Campus; Teacher, University of Ottawa; (613)828-9156; Fax. (613)728-5295.

DEHESHI, Benjamin; Hamilton HS-Henderson Site, B3 169B-711 Concession St, Hamilton ON L8V 1C3; Sask'00; FRCSC; OrthSurg (Sarcoma). Staff Orthopadic Surg, Hamilton Health Sciences Centre-Juravinski Site; Asst Prof, McMaster University; (905)521-2100 x43962; Fax. (905)381-7062.

DEHGHANI, Kianoush; MUHC-Montreal Gen Hosp, D144 16e-1650 av Cedar, Montreal QC H3G 1A4; Tor'02; CCFP; Public Health & Preventive Med. Staff, McGill University Health Centre - Montreal General Campus; (514)934-1934

DEHGHANI, Navid; Children's & Women's HC Of BC, 1K33-4480 Oak St, Vancouver BC V6H 3V4; UBC'96; BSc(Hon); FRCPC; Peds (Emergency Medicine); PedEmergMed. Staff EmergMed, BC Children's Hospital; Langs: Persian; (604)875-2045; Fax. (604)875-2946.

DEHGHANI, Payam; Cornwall Prof Bldg, 701-2125 11th Ave, Regina SK S4P 3X3; UBC'99; FRCPC; IntMed; Cardiol. (306)781-7944; Fax. (306)781-6997.

DEHGHANI-MOHAMMADABIDI, Payman; Scarborough Hosp-General Div, 3050 Lawrence Ave E, Scarborough ON M1P 2V5; UBC'09; CCFP; CCFP(E.M.); Staff, The Scarborough Hospital - General Campus; Langs: Farsi; (416)438-2911

DEHGHANI-YAR, Roya F; Elizabeth Village Med Clinic, 105-393 Rymal Rd W, Hamilton ON L9B 1V2; Jabalpur (India)'86; CCFP; Facilitator, McMaster University; Langs: Hindi; Persian; (905)297-2983; Fax. (905)297-2984; drroya@live.com.

DEHINBO, Olugbenga O; Cornwall Comm Hosp-Mcconnell, PO Box 100 Stn Main 840 McConnell Ave, Cornwall ON K6H 5S5; Ogun State (South Africa)'90; FRCPC; ObstGyn. Staff, Cornwall Community Hospital; Langs: Yoruba; (613)930-9419; Fax. (613)930-9423.

DEHLEN, Magdalena D; Associated Med Clinic, PO Box 510, Lac La Biche AB T0A 2C0; (South Africa)'94; (780)623-4421; Fax. (780)623-1920.

DEHNADE, Faramarze; CHUM-Hop Notre-Dame, 1560 rue Sherbrooke E, Montreal QC H2L 4M1; Montpellier (France)'68; CSPQ; OrthSurg. Staff, CSSS Saint-Leonard et Saint-Michel; Staff, Centre Hospitalier l'Université de Montréal (CHUM) - Hôpital Notre-Dame; (514)890-8000 x25900; Fax. (514)738-3879.

DEHONEY, Cameron J; 307-301 Columbia St E, New Westminster BC V3L 3W5; UBC'05; FRCPC; IntMed; Cardiol. Staff, St Michael's Hospital; (778)397-3797

DEHOUX, Eric; CSSSG-Hop de Hull, 116 boul Lionel-Emond, Gatineau QC J8Y 1W7; Mon'72; FRCPC; PhysMed&Rehab. Staff, Hull Hospital; Langs: Bilingual(French/English); (819)966-6200

DEI-BANING, Alfred; Shawmessy Med Clinic, 138-70 Shawville Blvd SE, Calgary AB T2Y 2Z3; Leningrad (Russia (Federation))'68; ABPeds; FRCPC; Peds (Pediatric Renal Diseases). Staff, Alberta Children's Hospital; Clinical Asst Prof, University of Calgary; (403)254-8703; Fax. (403)254-8609; dei-baning@shaw.ca.

DEICHERT, Kenneth; Halton Hills FHT-Guelph Street, UL-171 Guelph St, Georgetown ON L7G 4A1; Wes'89; Staff, Halton Healthcare Services Corporation - Georgetown Hospital; (905)877-4123; Fax. (905)873-8882.

DEIF, Hassan; York Radiology Consultants, 100-1333 Sheppard Ave E, North York ON M2J 1V1; Alexandria (Egypt)'74; MB ChB; FRCPC; DiagRad (Angiography). Ac Staff, North York General Hospital; Langs: Arabic; French; (416)756-6181

DEILGAT, Michel P; Agence Pablique du Canada, 065B-100 Colonnade Dr, Ottawa ON K2E 7L6; Laval'94; BA(Psy); CSPQ; PHRAM; Staff NCR & Europe Surgeon, Canadian Forces Health Services Centre; Langs: Bilingual(French/English); (613)957-6650

DEIMLING, J Peter; Couchiching Family Health Team, 206-119 Memorial Ave, Orillia ON L3V 5X1; Wes'75; CCFP; FCFP; Staff Family Med, Orillia Soldiers' Memorial Hospital; Clin Lecturer Community & FamMed, University of Toronto; (705)326-2308; Fax. (705)326-3141; pdeimling@rigers.com.

DEITCHER, Carol; Kipling Heights Med Centre, 2291 Kipling Ave, Etobicoke ON M9W 4L6; Tor'85; BA; CCFP; FCFP; Staff, William Osler Health System - Etobicoke General Hospital; Staff, Kipling Acres Home For The Aged; Staff, Kennedy Lodge Nursing Home; (416)741-4545 x214; Fax. (416)744-1484.

DEITCHER, Joseph; 308-1525 Albion Rd, Etobicoke ON M9V 5G5; UBC'62; Court Staff, William Osler Health System - Etobicoke General Hospital; (416)741-5600; Fax. (416)741-1325; joed27@hotmail.com.

DEITEL, Wayne L; St Michael's Hosp, 30 Bond St, Toronto ON M5B 1W8; Tor'93; FRCPC; DiagRad. Staff, St Michael's Hospital; (416)864-5692; Fax. (416)864-5380.

DEJOIE, Carl Louis A; Hop Jean-Talon, 1385 rue Jean-Talon E, Montreal QC H2E 1S6; (Haiti)'80; CSPQ; FRCSC; GenSurg (Gynecological Surgery). Staff, CSSS du Coeur de l'Isle Hôpital Jean-Talon; (514)495-6767

DEKANY, Eva C; 1724 Queen St W, Toronto ON M6R 1B3; Budapest (Hungary)'53; AB; FRCSC; Ophth (General Ophthalmic Surgery). Hon Staff, Women's College Hospital; Langs: Hungarian; German; (416)535-3334; Fax. (416)532-7777.

DEKETELE, Anthony G; 2-165 Manitoba St, Bracebridge ON P1L 1S3; Wes'83; FRCPC; IntMed. Staff, South Muskoka Memorial Hospital - Muskoka Algonquin Healthcare; Staff, Huntsville District Memorial Hospital - Muskoka Algonquin Healthcare; (705)645-6934; Fax. (705)645-6454.

DEKKER, Jakob J; 101-5605 55 St, Cold Lake AB T9M 1R6; (South Africa)'92; MB ChB; Staff, Cold Lake Healthcare Centre; Member Steering Comittee, Alberta Cancer Board; Med Advisor, Lakeland FASD Centre; (780)594-0025; Fax. (780)594-0011.

DEKLAJ, Tom; Windsor Reg Hosp-Metropolitan, 1995 Lens Ave, Windsor ON N8W 1L9; Tor'03; FRCPC; Urol. Staff, Windsor Regional Hospital - Metropolitan Site; (519)254-1661

DEKNA, Maisa M A; Halton HC Serv Corp-Oakville, 327 Reynolds St, Oakville ON L6J 3L7; Al Fateh (Libya)'02; Peds. Staff, Halton Healthcare Services Corporation - Oakville Site; (905)845-2571

DEKOVEN, Joel; Sunnybrook Hlth Sciences Ctre, M1 736-2075 Bayview Ave, Toronto ON M4N 3M5; Man'81; MHSc(Tor); AB; FRCPC; CommunMed (Laser Treatment); Derm. Consultant, Sunnybrook Health Sciences Centre; Consultant Occupational Disease Specialty Prog, St Michael's Hospital; Assoc Prof, University of Toronto; (416)480-4908; Fax. (416)480-6897; joel.dekoven@sunnybrook.ca.

DEKOVEN, Kathryn; Hôpital Ste-Justine, 3175 ch Cote-Ste-Catherine, Montreal QC H3T 1C5; McG'99; CSPQ; FRCPC; Anes. Staff, Hôpital Ste-Justine; (514)345-4931

DEL BEGIO, Grant R; Aberdeen Med Centre, 1966 Harrison Way, Kamloops BC V1S 1M9; Man'84; MA; Ac Staff Privil, Royal Inland Hospital; (250)314-5314; Fax. (250)372-8331.

DEL BEL, Nicole; Hamilton HS-General Site, 237 Barton St E, Hamilton ON L8L 2X2; McM'08; CCFP; CCFP(E.M.); Staff, Hamilton Health Sciences Centre - Hamilton General Hospital; (905)521-2100

DEL BIANCO, Sylvie; Centre de Med Fam de Wakefield, RR 2 CP 400, Wakefield QC J0X 3G0; Mon'90; CCFP; Staff, Centre Hospitalier Gatineau Mémorial; (819)459-2363; Fax. (819)459-2997.

DEL BIGIO, Marc R; Health Sciences Centre, MS4-820 Sherbrook St, Winnipeg MB R3A 1R9; Man'82; PhD; MD; FRCPC; NeurPath. Prof Path, University of Manitoba; (204)789-3378; Fax. (204)787-4942; delbigi@cc.umanitoba.ca.

DEL CAMPO, J C Martin; Univ Hlth Network-Toronto Western Hosp, WW5 443-399 Bathurst St, Toronto ON M5T 2S8; (Mexico)'73; FRCPC; IntMed (Epilepsy); Neur. Neurologist, Toronto Western Hospital - University Health Network; Teach Staff, University of Toronto; Langs: Spanish; (416)603-5055; Fax. (416)603-5366.

DEL CARPIO, Jaime; 700-1538 rue Sherbrooke O, Montreal QC H3G 1L5; Lima (Peru)'73; AB(IntMed&Allergy&Immu; FRCPC; IntMed; ClinImmunol&Allergy (P.Q.). Staff, McGill University Health Centre - Royal Victoria Hospital; Staff, Lakeshore General Hospital - Pointe Claire; assoc Prof, McGill University; Langs: Bilingual(English/French); Italian; Portuguese; Spanish; (514)939-1974; delcarpio@bellnet.ca.

DEL CARPIO, Raquel; MUHC-Montreal Gen Hosp, 1650 av Cedar, Montreal QC H3G 1A4; Lima (Peru)'73; MB BS; CSPQ; FRCPC; DiagRad (Neuro Radiology). Assoc Staff, McGill University Health Centre - Montreal Neurological Hospital; Assoc Dir Radiol., McGill University Health Centre - Montreal General Campus; Prof Radiology, McGill University; Langs: Spanish; Italian; French; (514)934-1934 x42873; Fax. (514)934-8263.

DEL CASTILHO, Colin; Foothills Med Centre, C 231-1403 29 St NW, Calgary AB T2N 2T9; Cal'03; CCFP; CCFP(E.M.); Staff, Foothills Medical Centre; (403)944-1635

DEL DEGAN, Sandra; La Cite Medicale, 295-2600 boul Laurier, Quebec QC G1V 4T3; Laval'90; CCFP; Staff, Centre Hospitalier Universitaire de Quebec-CHUL; (418)781-0480; Fax. (418)659-7072.

DEL GIUDICE, Lisa Maria Elisabeth; Sunnybrook Hlth Sciences Ctre, A112-2075 Bayview Ave, Toronto ON M4N 3M5; Tor'00; BSc; MSc(Epidemiol); CCFP; Staff, Sunnybrook Health Sciences Centre; Asst Prof, University of Toronto; Langs: Italian; (416)480-4939; Fax. (416)480-6038.

DEL GRANDE, Gabriella; CSSS de Laval, 1755 boul Rene-Laennec, Laval QC H7M 3L9; Mon'03; Staff, Hopital de la Cite de la santé; (450)668-1010

DEL GRANDE, Robert W; Perth-Smith Falls Dist Hosp, 33 Drummond St W, Perth ON K7H 2K1; Wes'79; FRCPC; IntMed; EmergMed. Assoc Staff, Perth & Smiths Falls District Hospital - Perth Site (Great War Memorial Site); Lecturer, Queen's University; (613)267-1500 x4286; Fax. (613)267-6614.

DEL JUNCO, Maria; 207-726 Bloor St W, Toronto ON M6G 4A1; Tor'78; (416)538-3939; Fax. (416)538-2980.

DEL MAESTRO, Rolando; MUHC-Montreal Neurology Inst, 109-3801 rue University, Montreal QC H3A 2B4; Wes'73; MD; PhD; FRCSC; Neursurg., McGill University Health Centre - Montreal Neurological Hospital; Dir, Brain Tumour Research Centre; Prof NeuroSurg & NeurOncology, McGill University; Langs: Italian; (514)398-5791; Fax. (514)398-2811; rolando.delmaestro@mcgill.ca.

DEL POZO, Rolando; Sunnyside Med Arts Centre, 501-27 Roncesvalles Ave, Toronto ON M6R 3B2; San Carlos (Guatemala)'69; Ac Staff, St Joseph's Health Centre; Trainer Med Students & Family Doctors, University of Toronto; (416)531-6403; Fax. (416)531-4244.

DEL RIZZO, Dario F; Columbus Med Arts Bldg, 405-8333 Weston Rd, Woodbridge ON L4L 8E2; McM'82; BSc; PhD; FRCSC; GenSurg (Cardiac Surgery); CardiothorSurg. Langs: French; Italian; (905)264-5977; Fax. (905)264-9686.

DEL ROSARIO, Daniel S; Pharmacita Med Clinic, 224-4810 Sheppard Ave E, Scarborough ON M1S 4N6; Santo Tomas (Philippines)'71; BSc; Langs: Tagalog; (416)282-1922; Fax. (416)609-7020.

DEL SORBO, Lorenzo; Mount Sinai Hosp, 1818-600 University Ave, Toronto ON M5G 1X5; Torino (Italy)'96; Staff, Mount Sinai Hospital; (416)340-4746

DEL VALLE-PISON, Maria; Clin Pediatrique Beaubien, 2301 rue Belanger, Montreal QC H2G 1C9; Madrid (Spain)'65; AB; Peds (P.Q.). Ac Staff, Hôpital Ste-Justine; Langs: Spanish; (514)728-1559; Fax. (514)728-4480.

DEL VALLE REBEIL, Alfonso P; Toronto Inst for Reproductive, 300-56 Aberfoyle Cres, Etobicoke ON M8X 2W4; Mexico City (Mexico)'77; FRCSC; ObstGyn (Infertility). Ac Staff, St Joseph's Health Centre; Pres/Med Dir, Repromed-The Toronto Inst for Reproductive Med; Langs: Spanish; (416)233-8111

DEL VECCHIO, Pierre; CHUM-Hop Notre-Dame, AR1001A-1560 rue Sherbrooke E, Montreal QC H2L 4M1; Mon'69; FRCPC; RadOncol. ac Staff, Centre Hospitalier l'Université de Montréal (CHUM) - Hôpital Notre-Dame; adj Prof, Universite de Montreal; (514)890-8254

DELA CRUZ, M C Armellie; 1481 Government St, Penticton BC V2A 4V9; Alb'91; BSc; FRCSC; ObstGyn. Staff, Penticton Regional Hospital; Langs: Tagalog; (250)770-1364; Fax. (250)492-3885; armellie@shaw.ca.

DELABAYS, Eugene; St Mary's Hospital Ctr, 3830 av Lacombe, Montreal QC H3T 1M5; Ott'99; FRCPC; Anes. Staff, St Mary's Hospital Centre; Staff Anes, CSSS de Trois-Rivières; Langs: Bilingual(English/French); (514)345-3511; eugenedelabays@yahoo.ca.

DELABIE, Ludovic; Churchill Reg Hlth Authority, 162 Lawrence Ave, Churchill MB R0B 0E0; Staff, Percy E Moore Hospital; Staff, Churchill Regional Health Authority; (204)675-8318; ludovic_delabie@hc-sc.gc.ca.

DELABY, Liliane; Clinique Med de la Cite, 900-300 rue Leo Parizeau, Montreal QC H2X 4B3; Mon'83; Staff, Centre Hospitalier l'Université de Montréal (CHUM) - Hôtel-Dieu; (514)281-1722

DELADOEY, Johnny Y; Hôpital Ste-Justine, 3175 ch Cote-Ste-Catherine, Montreal QC H3T 1C5; Staff, Hôpital Ste-Justine; Langs: German; French; (514)345-4735; Fax. (514)345-4988.

DELAFIELD, Mary; Centre Med Ste-Foy Inc, 802 av du Chanoine-Scott, Quebec QC G1V 3N4; McG'88; Langs: English; French; (418)653-4931; Fax. (418)653-4797.

DELAGE, Antoine; Hôpital Laval, 2725 ch Sainte-Foy, Quebec QC G1V 4G5; McG'01; CSPQ; FRCPC; IntMed; Critical Care Medicine (P.Q.); Respir. Staff, Hôpital Laval; (418)656-4747; Fax. (418)656-4762.

DELAGE, Bastien; UMF Maisonneuve-Rosemont, 5689 boul Rosemont, Montreal QC H1T 2H1; Sher'08; CCFP; (450)372-3996

DELAGE, Catherine; Centre Hosp Honore-Mercier, 2750 boul Laframboise, Saint-Hyacinthe QC J2S 4Y8; Mon'07; CCFP; CCFP(E.M.); Staff, Centre Hospitalier Honore-Mercier; (450)771-3333

DELAGE, Claude; 312-1155 Av Turnbull, Quebec QC G1R 5G3; Laval'65; FCAP; CSPQ; FRCPC; AnatPath. Staff, Centre Hospitalier Universitaire de Québec (CHUQ) - Siege Social; Asst Prof Path, Université Laval; (418)522-2235; cldelage@hotmail.com.

DELAGE, Eric; CSSS du Sud de Lanaudière, 911 montee des Pionniers, Terrebonne QC J6V 2H2; Mon'02; BSc; MSc; CSPQ; Staff, Centre Hospitalier Pierre le Gardeur; (450)654-7525

DELAGE, Francois; Clin De Cardiologie De Levis, 600-4975 boul de la Rive-Sud, Levis QC G6V 4Z5; Laval'75; CSPQ; FRCP; Cardiol (Echography Cardiac). Cardiology, Hôtel-Dieu de Lévis; (418)833-5750; Fax. (418)833-5837; fdelage@videotron.ca.

DELAGE, Gilles; Hema-Quebec, 4045 boul de la Cote-Vertu, Saint-Laurent QC H4R 2W7; Mon'69; MSc; FRCPC; MedMicrobiol (Transfusion Medicine); Microbio & Infect Dis (P.Q.). VP Affaires Medicales Microbiology, Hema-Quebec; Langs: Bilingual(French/English); (514)832-5000 x532; Fax. (514)832-1024; gilles.delage@hema-quebec.qc.ca.

DELAGE, Marie; Hôtel-Dieu de Lévis, 143 rue Wolfe, Levis QC G6V 3Z1; Mon'91; FRCPC; Psy. Staff, Hôtel-Dieu de Lévis; (418)835-7155

DELAGE, Martin E; Clinique Med St-Augustin, 220-334 Rte 138, Quebec QC G3A 1G8; Laval'79; (418)878-3590; Fax. (418)878-4876.

DELAGE, Robert; Ctr Hosp Affilie-Enfant-Jesus, 1401 18e rue, Quebec QC G1J 1Z4; Laval'83; FRCPC; IntMed; Hem. Ac Staff, Centre Hospitalier Affilié Universitaire de Québec - Hôpital De L'Enfant Jésus; assoc Prof, Université Laval; (418)649-5726

DELAGRAVE, Jacques; CSSS de l'Energie-Ste-Therese, 1705 av Georges, Shawinigan QC G9N 2N1; Laval'76; Staff, CH du Centre-de-la-Mauricie (Ste-Thérèse de Shawinigan); (819)536-7575 x4276; jacques_delagrave@ssss.gouv.qc.ca.

DELAIR, Leonard C; 307-22112 52 Ave, Langley BC V2Y 2M6; Cal'92; (604)530-2133; Fax. (604)530-2363.

DELALAY, Nathalie; Centre Hosp Honore-Mercier, 2750 boul Laframboise, Saint-Hyacinthe QC J2S 4Y8; Mon'08; Staff, Centre Hospitalier Honore-Mercier; (450)771-3333

DELAMARRE, Samuel; CHUQ-St-Francois d'Assise, 10 rue de l'Espinay, Quebec QC G1L 3L5; Laval'07; CCFP; CCFP(E.M.); Staff, Centre Hospitalier Universitaire De Québec - Pavillon De St-françois-d'assise; (418)525-4444

DELAND, Eric; CHUS-Hop Fleurimont, 3001 12e av N, Sherbrooke QC J1H 5N4; Sher'84; Critical Care Medicine (P.Q.); IntMed (Intensive Care). Staff, Centre Hospitalier Universitaire de Sherbrooke-Hopital Fleurimont; Prof, Universite de Sherbrooke; (819)346-1110 x14977; Fax. (819)820-6406.

DELAND, Pascale; CSSS de la Mitis, 800 av du Sanatorium, Mont-Joli QC G5H 3L6; Laval'98; Staff, Hôpital Regional Rimouski; Staff, CSSS de la Mitis; Langs: Bilingual(French/English); (418)775-7261; Fax. (418)775-6487.

DELANEY, Catherine; 111 Waterloo St, London ON N6B 2M4; Dublin (Ireland)'78; MB ChB; BAO; (519)670-8947

DELANEY, David A; Centre Med Via Meidca, 3943 boul Saint-Jean, Roxboro QC H9G 1X2; McG'94; CCFP; FCFP; (514)624-7363

DELANEY, Gail; Kingston Med Art Bldg, 400-800 Princess St, Kingston ON K7L 5E4; Mem'79; BMedSci; FRCPC; PhysMed&Rehab (Brain Injury). Fax. (613)353-7193.

DELANEY, J Scott; McGill Sport Med Clinic, 475 av des Pins O, Montreal QC H2W 1S4; McG'91; MDCM; CSPQ; FRCPC; EmergMed (Sports Medicine). Staff, McGill University Health Centre - Royal Victoria Hospital; Staff, McGill University Health Centre - Montreal General Campus; Assoc Prof Med & Phy, McGill University; (514)398-7007; Fax. (514)398-4035.

DELANEY, James; Georgian Prof Centre, 300-125 Bell Farm Rd, Barrie ON L4M 6L2; Tor'82; FRCSC; OrthSurg (Knee Surgery). Ac Staff OrthSurg, Royal Victoria Regional Health Centre; (705)739-8363; Fax. (705)733-8350.

DELANEY, Jesse W; Sunnybrook Health Sciences Ctr, D108-2075 Bayview Ave, Toronto ON M4N 3M5; Tor'08; IntMed. Staff, Sunnybrook Health Sciences Centre; (416)480-6100

DELANEY, Martina; Health Sciences Centre, 300 Prince Philip Dr, St. John's NL A1B 3V6; Mem'94; FRCSC; ObstGyn (Maternal Fetal Medicine). Staff, Health Sciences Centre; Assoc Prof Discipline of ObstGyn, Memorial University Of Newfoundland; (709)777-7451; Fax. (709)777-7455.

DELANEY, Perlita; Frontenac Med Associates, 201-791 Princess St, Kingston ON K7L 1E9; Ott'79; Langs: Spanish; English; (613)544-2727; Fax. (613)544-7247.

DELANEY, Peter; Grey Nuns Community Hosp & HC, 1100 Youville Drive West NW, Edmonton AB T6L 5X8; Alb'00; CCFP; CCFP(E.M.); Staff, Covenant Health - Grey Nuns Community Hospital; (780)735-7000

DELANEY, Ronald K; Shoppers Drug Mart Bldg, 250 Lemarchant Rd, St. John's NL A1E 1P8; Mem'75; (709)722-6090

DELANEY, Susan M; Dartmouth Gen Hosp, 325 Pleasant St, Dartmouth NS B2Y 4G8; Dal'00; FRCPC; DiagRad. Staff, Dartmouth General Hospital; (902)460-4526; Fax. (902)465-8360.

DELAROM, Shyah S; Westwind Med Clinic, 107-755 Goldstream Ave, Victoria BC V9B 0H9; Arhus (Denmark)'01; Langs: Danish; Farsi; (250)478-1764

DELAUNAIS, Daniel; Clin Med Fam Obs d'Mistassini, 5-170 Av de l'Eglise, Dolbeau-Mistassini QC G8L 4W6; Mon'88; (418)276-5712; Fax. (418)276-6092.

DELAVARKHAN, Morteza; Saint John Reg Hosp Facility, 400 University Ave, Saint John NB E2L 4L2; Isfahan (Iran)'86; Staff, Saint John Regional Hospital; (506)648-6000

DELBARRE, Marthe; CSSS de Saint-Jerome, 290 rue de Montigny, Saint-Jerome QC J7Z 5T3; Lille II (England)'01; Psy (P.Q.). Staff, Hôtel-Dieu de Saint-Jérôme; (450)431-8292

DELBECQ, Bernard; Royal Alexandra Hosp, 10240 Kingsway NW, Edmonton AB T5H 3V9; Alb'72; FRCPC; Anes. Staff, Royal Alexandra Hospital; (780)735-4010

DELBRIDGE, Catherine L; Queen Elizabeth II HSC, 10W-1276 South Park St, Halifax NS B3H 2Y9; Dal'06; Anes. Staff, Queen Elizabeth II Health Sciences Centre - Victoria General Site; (902)473-2331; Fax. (902)473-9454.

DELBROUCK, Nicole F L; Renfrew Victoria Hosp, 499 Raglan St N, Renfrew ON K7V 1P6; McG'84; FRCPC; IntMed; Nephrol. Med Dir Renfrew Prog, Renfrew Victoria Hospital; Consultant, Pembroke Regional Hospital Inc; Consultant, The Ottawa Hospital - General Campus; (613)432-4851 x201; Fax. (613)432-4349.

DELESPESSE, Guy J; CHUM-Hop Notre-Dame, 1560 rue Sherbrooke E, Montreal QC H2L 4M1; Brussels (Belgium)'66; FRCPC; ClinImmunol&Allergy. ac Staff, Centre Hospitalier l'Université de Montréal (CHUM) - Hôpital Notre-Dame; Prof, Universite de Montreal; (514)890-8000 x25395

DELEV, Gligor; CHUM-Hop St-Luc, 1058 rue Saint-Denis, Montreal QC H2X 3J4; Laval'83; FRCPC; EmergMed. Staff, Centre Hospitalier l'Université De Montréal (CHUM) - Hôpital Saint-luc; (514)890-8000

DELGADO, Alfonso; Hop Jean Talon, 1385 rue Jean-Talon E, Montreal QC H2E 1S6; (Colombia)'63; FRCPC; IntMed (P.Q.). Staff, CSSS du Coeur de l'Isle Hôpital Jean-Talon; (514)495-6767

DELGADO, Diego H; NCSB 11C-1201, 585 University Ave, Toronto ON M5G 2N2; Del Salvador (Argentina)'94; MSc; Staff, Toronto General Hospital - UHN; Langs: Spanish; Italian; Portuguese; (416)340-3940; Fax. (416)340-4134.

DELGADO RODRIGUEZ, Gisell; River Road Med Clinic, 671 River Rd, Gloucester ON K1V 2G2; Havana (Cuba)'93; CCFP; Langs: Spanish; (613)822-3582; fgp@eastlink.ca.

DELIAKIS, John; 411-658 Danforth Ave, Toronto ON M4J 5B9; McG'78; CCFP; Langs: Greek; French; (416)469-5550; Fax. (416)469-5536.

DELIALLISI, Ardit; Grey Bruce HS-Owen Sound, PO Box 1800 Stn Main 1800 8th St E, Owen Sound ON N4K 6M9; Tirana (Albania)'89; AnatPath. Staff, Grey Bruce Health Services - Owen Sound.

DELIALLISI, Enkelejda; Dixon Med Bldg, 203-531 Davis Dr, Newmarket ON L3Y 6P5; Tirana (Albania)'94; FRCSC; GenSurg. Staff, Southlake Regional Health Centre; Langs: Albanian; (905)715-8668; Fax. (905)715-7814.

DELIFER, Jean-Claude; 505-50 rue Crepeau, Saint-Laurent QC H4N 1M8; Beirut (Lebanon)'83; Peds. Staff, Centre Hospitalier Régional de Lanaudière; (514)892-7016

DELIGNE, Benoit; CHUM-Hop St-Luc, 1058 rue Saint-Denis, Montreal QC H2X 3J4; Louvain (Belgium)'95; IntMed (P.Q.) (AIDS/HIV). Prof Clinique, Centre Hospitalier l'Université De Montréal (CHUM) - Hôpital Saint-luc; Langs: Bilingual(French/English); (514)890-8000 x34599; Fax. (514)412-7417; benoit.deligne@umontreal.ca.

DELISLE, Bernard R; Ctr Hosp Affilie-Enfant-Jesus, 1401 18e rue, Quebec QC G1J 1Z4; Laval'82; Derm (Laser Dermatology). Staff, Centre Hospitalier Affilié Universitaire de Québec - Hôpital De L'Enfant Jésus; Dir Dept of Derm, Centre Hospitalier Universitaire de Quebec-CHUL; Chef derma, Centre de santé Cloutier-du-Rivage; (418)649-5520; Fax. (418)649-5527.

DELISLE, Caroline; GMF La Cigogne, 420-3141 boul Taschereau, Greenfield Park QC J4V 2H2; Sher'95; Staff, Hopital Charles LeMoyne; Clin Prof, Universite de Sherbrooke; Langs: English; (450)466-7892; Fax. (450)466-9602.

DELISLE, Donald; Clin Medicale Bromptonville, 201-103 rue Saint-Lambert, Sherbrooke QC J1C 0N8; Sher'79; Staff, Centre Hospitalier Universitaire de Sherbrooke-Hôpital Hôtel-Dieu; (819)846-2811; Fax. (819)846-0594.

DELISLE, Emilie; Pavillon Rosemont, 5689 boul Rosemont, Montreal QC H1T 2H1; Mon'03; CCFP; (514)252-3400

DELISLE, Francois; CSSS de Rimouski-Neigette, CP 3150 Succ A 150 av Rouleau, Rimouski QC G5L 5T1; Mon'77; Electroenceph (P.Q.); Neur. Staff, Hôpital Regional Rimouski; (418)723-7851

DELISLE, Georges; CHUQ-Ctr Hosp Univ Laval, A1842-2705 boul Laurier, Quebec QC G1V 4G2; Laval'65; CRCP; CSPQ; FRCPC; Peds; Cardiol (P.Q.). Ac Staff, Centre Hospitalier Universitaire de Quebec-CHUL; Associé, Institut Universitaire Cardiologie & Pneumologie de Quebec; Clin Assoc Prof, Université Laval; Langs: Bilingual(French/English); (418)654-2708; Fax. (418)654-2710; georges.delisle@chuq.qc.ca.

DELISLE, Gilles; CSSS de Lac-Saint Jean-Est, CP 1300 Succ Bureau-Chef 300 boul Champlain S, Alma QC G8B 5W3; Mon'95; FRCPC; Psy. Staff, CSSS de Lac-Saint Jean-Est; (418)669-2000; Fax. (418)669-0472.

DELISLE, Gilles; Centre Med Prof de Brossard, 101-2424 boul Lapiniere, Longueuil QC J4Z 2K9; Sher'82; (450)678-9033; drdelisle@duomedic.com.

DELISLE, Isabelle M G; 203-17 Prince St, Dartmouth NS B2Y 4W2; Mon'85; FRCSC; ObstGyn. Staff, Queen Elizabeth II Health Sciences Centre - Victoria General Site; Staff, IWK Health Centre; Asst Prof, Dalhousie University; Langs: French; (902)461-2246; Fax. (902)461-2746.

DELISLE, Jean-Sebastien; Hop Maisonneuve-Rosemont, 5415 boul de l'Assomption, Montreal QC H1T 2M4; McG'99; FRCPC; IntMed; Hem. Staff, Hopital Maisonneuve-Rosemont; (514)252-3404

DELISLE, Line; CHUS-Hop Fleurimont, 3001 12e av N, Sherbrooke QC J1H 5N4; Laval'79; MedOncol (P.Q.); Hem (P.Q.); IntMed. Staff, Centre Hospitalier Universitaire de Sherbrooke-Hopital Fleurimont; (819)346-1110 x6236; lise.delisle@usherbrooke.ca.

DELISLE, Lucie; Clinique Med Galt, 200-2235 rue Galt O, Sherbrooke QC J1K 1K6; Sher'88; (819)821-0088; Fax. (819)821-3901.

DELISLE, Marc; Hop Charles LeMoyne, 3120 boul Taschereau, Greenfield Park QC J4V 2H1; Laval'87; Psy (Emergency Medicine). Staff, Centre Hospitalier Affilié Universitaire de Québec - Hôpital De L'Enfant Jésus; Staff, Hopital Charles LeMoyne; (450)466-5000; delislemarc@hotmail.com.

DELISLE, Marie-Claude; Hop Louis-H Lafontaine, 7401 rue Hochelaga, Montreal QC H1N 3M5; Mon'99; FRCPC; Psy. Staff, Hopital Louis-H Lafontaine; (514)251-4000

DELISLE, Marie-France; Children's & Women's Hlth Ctre, 1U3-4500 Oak St, Vancouver BC V6H 3N1; Laval'92; FRCSC; ObstGyn (Obstetrics). Staff, BC Women's Hospital & Health Centre; University of British Columbia; Langs: English; (604)875-3075; Fax. (604)875-3864; mdelisle@cw.bc.ca.

DELISLE, Marie-Noelle; CSSS de Beauce-Etchemin, 1515 17e rue, Saint-Georges QC G5Y 4T8; Mon'05; IntMed. Staff, Centre Hospitalier Beauce-Etchemin; (418)227-3825

DELISLE, Rejean; 945 rue Saint-Jean, Roberval QC G8H 2H3; Laval'74; FRCSC; Urol. Staff, Hotel-Dieu de Roberval; (418)275-3172; Fax. (418)275-3125.

DELISLE, Rejean-Andre; CSSS de Chicoutimi, 305 rue Saint-Vallier, Chicoutimi QC G7H 5H6; Laval'78; FRCPC; Microbio & Infect Dis (P.Q.) (Infectious Diseases). ac Staff Med Biol, Complexe hospitalier de la Sagamie; Langs: Spanish; Bilingual(English/French); (418)541-1046; Fax. (418)541-1137; radeli@hotmail.com.

DELISLE, Richard J J; 31 Canadian Forces Hlth Serv C, RR 1, North Bay ON P0H 1P0; Ott'06; CCFP; (705)494-2101

DELISLE, Richard R; Clinique de Neurologie, 4380 Cote Rosemont, Trois-Rivieres QC G8Y 0A5; Laval'84; CSPQ; Neur (Adult Neurology). Neurology, Centre Hospitalier Regional de Trois-Rivieres; (819)379-7336; Fax. (819)370-6681.

DELISLE, Robert F; CHUM-Hotel-Dieu, 3840 rue Saint-Urbain, Montreal QC H2W 1T8; Mon'70; Staff, Centre Hospitalier l'Université de Montréal (CHUM) - Hôtel-Dieu; (514)890-8000 x14899; Fax. (514)412-7189; robert.delisle.chum@ssss.gouv.qc.ca.

DELISLE, Sandra; CSSS Pierre Boucher, 1333 boul Jacques-Cartier E, Longueuil QC J4M 2A5; Mon'96; Staff, Centre Hospitalier Pierre Boucher; (450)468-8111

DELISLE, Simon; CSSS des Basques, 550 rue Notre-Dame E RR 1, Trois-Pistoles QC G0L 4K0; Laval'87; ac Staff, Centre Hospitalier Trois-Pistoles; (418)851-3301; Fax. (418)851-2944; simon.delisle.asss01@ssss.gouv.qc.ca.

DELISLE, Sylvie; Regie des Rentes du Quebec, CP 7777 Succ Terminus 207-2600 boul Laurier, Quebec QC G1K 7T4; Laval'85; Physician, Regie des Rentes du Quebec; (418)657-8709 x3228; Fax. (418)644-5919.

DELIU, Enver; Springview Family Practice, 6A-5675 Spring Garden Rd, Halifax NS B3J 1H1; Sarajevo (Bosnia-Herzegovina)'78; CCFP; Langs: Albanian; Croatian; (902)423-2908; Fax. (902)429-6564; edeliu@eastlink.ca.

DELIYANNIDES, Alexandra; Capri Med Centre, 132-1835 Gordon Dr, Kelowna BC V1Y 3H4; Alb'07; CCFP; (250)717-3211

DELL, Sharon D M; The Hosp For Sick Children, 555 University Ave, Toronto ON M5G 1X8; Tor'90; FRCPC; Peds; Respir. Ac Staff, The Hospital For Sick Children; Assoc Prof/Assoc Prog Dir HPME, University of Toronto; (416)813-6248; Fax. (416)813-6246.

DELL'AQUILA, Raffaele A; Nurture North Mar Clinic, 239 Main St E, North Bay ON P1B 1B2; McG'89; CCFP; Staff, North Bay Regional Health Centre - Regional Mental Health; Langs: Bilingual(English/French); (705)478-7197; Fax. (705)478-0861; dellar@nbgh.on.ca.

DELLA SIEGA, Anthony J; Westheart Cardiology, 206-2020 Richmond Rd, Victoria BC V8R 6R5; UBC'94; FRCPC; IntMed (Interventional Cardiology); Cardiol. Staff, Royal Jubilee Hospital; (250)595-3111; Fax. (250)595-4277.

DELLA ZAZZERA, Max; Bank Med Centre, 1-1935 Bank St, Ottawa ON K1V 8A3; Mon'80; Ac Staff, Bruyère Continuing Care - Saint-Vincent Hospital; Vis Staff, The Ottawa Hospital - General Campus; Langs: Italian; French; (613)521-2391; Fax. (613)521-5443.

DELLANDREA, David A; Guardian Med Arts Bldg, 205-1950 Algonquin Ave, North Bay ON P1B 4Z2; Tor'66; DAvMed; Ac Staff, North Bay Regional Health Centre - Regional Mental Health; (705)474-4810; Fax. (705)474-3114.

DELLE DONNE, Nadia; Lakeshore Gen Hosp, 160 rue Stillview, Pointe-Claire QC H9R 2Y2; Mon'03; CCFP; CCFP(E.M.); Staff, Lakeshore General Hospital - Pointe Claire; Langs: Italian; English; (514)630-2225 x1199

DELLI COLLI, Nadia; Clin Med Belvedere, 202-2235 rue Galt O, Sherbrooke QC J1K 1K6; Mon'94; Clin Prof, Universite de Sherbrooke; (819)563-4244; Fax. (819)563-8924.

DELLI PIZZI, Andy T; Winnipeg Reg Health Authority, 496 Hargrave St, Winnipeg MB R3A 0Y7; Man'97; BSc(Gen); CCFP.

DELMONTE, Guillermo A; Ctr Med St-Sauveur, 134 rue Saint-Vallier O, Quebec QC G1K 1K1; La Habana (Cuba)'67; Assoc Staff, Centre Hospitalier Affilié Universitaire de Québec - Hôpital du St-Sacrement; (418)649-0062; Fax. (418)650-0101.

DELONG, Rachel; The Ottawa Hosp - Civic Campus, 1053 Carling Ave, Ottawa ON K1Y 4E9; UBC'09; CCFP; CCFP(E.M.); Staff, The Ottawa Hospital - Civic Campus; (613)798-5555

DELORME, Andre; CSSS de la Haute-Yamaska, 205 boul Leclerc O, Granby QC J2G 1T7; Mon'89; FRCPC; Psy (Consultation-Liaison). Staff Psy, Centre Hospitalier de Granby; (450)375-8000; Fax. (450)372-2235.

DELORME, Celine; CSST-Direction Regionale Montr, CP 3 Succ Pl-desjardins 1 Complexe Desjardins, Montreal QC H5B 1H1; Laval'82; Médecin, CSST-Direction Regionale Montreal; (514)905-3946

DELORME, Chantal; Hôpital de l'Archipel, 430 ch Principal, Cap-aux-Meules QC G4T 1R9; Mon'92; MSc(Epidemiol.); FRCSC; Ophth. Staff, Hôtel-Dieu de Lévis; Staff, Hôpital de l'Archipel; Staff, Iles-de-la-Madeleine; Langs: English; (418)986-2121

DELORME, Hugo; Ctr Hosp Rouyn-Noranda, 4 9e rue, Rouyn-Noranda QC J9X 2B2; Mon'97; FRCPC; IntMed. Staff, Centre Hospitalier Rouyn-Noranda; (819)764-5131

DELORME, Isabelle; 104-1177 despres Ave, Saint-Hyacinthe QC J2S 6L6; Mon'90; ABD; FRCPC; Derm (Botox Injection). Langs: English; (450)771-7070; Fax. (450)771-9090.

DELORME, Jacques; Clin Medicale Les Gres, 140-190 rue St-Honore, St-Etienne-Ds-Gres QC G0X 2P0; Sher'85; Staff, Centre Hospitalier du Centre la Mauricie; (819)535-6512; Fax. (819)535-1627.

DELORME, Jocelyn; Hop Maisonneuve-Rosemont, 5415 boul de l'Assomption, Montreal QC H1T 2M4; Mon'72; Microbio & Infect Dis (P.Q.). Staff, Hopital Maisonneuve-Rosemont; Langs: Italian; English; (514)252-3400 x4524

DELORME, Laurent; Hop Charles Lemoyne, 3120 boul Taschereau, Greenfield Park QC J4V 2H1; Mon'73; FRCPC; MedMicrobiol (AIDS/HIV); Microbio & Infect Dis (P.Q.). Staff, Hopital Charles LeMoyne; Member, MTS du MSSS(Quebec); (450)466-5000 x2960

DELORME, Linda; Clinique Medicym, 876 boul du Cure-Labelle, Sainte-Therese QC J7C 2K9; Mon'93; Staff, Centre Hospitalier d'Argenteuil; (450)430-0911

DELORME, Martine; Clinique Med Le Gardeurois, 155 rue Notre-Dame, Repentigny QC J5Z 3C4; Mon'04; (450)582-5551

DELORME, Michael A; 307-3330 Richter St, Kelowna BC V1W 4V5; Wes'85; FRCPC; IntMed; Hem. Ac Staff, Kelowna General Hospital; (250)869-0210; Fax. (250)869-0211.

DELORME, Mireille; CSSS Haut-Richelieu-Rouville, 920 boul du Seminaire N, St-Jean-Sur-Richel QC J3A 1B7; McG'75; CSPQ; FRCPC; Anes. Staff, Hôpital du Haut-Richelieu; (450)359-5000 x5212; Fax. (450)349-5220.

DELORME, Roger P; Clinique Med Avenir, 450-1545 boul de L'Avenir, Laval QC H7S 2N5; Mon'69; CSPQ; FRCSC; PlasSurg. Consultant, Centre Hospitalier l'Université de Montréal (CHUM) - Hôpital Notre-Dame; Consultant, Hôpital Ste-Justine; Sec, Associate of Plastic Surgeons of Quebec; (450)662-9515; Fax. (450)663-5940; rpdelorme@vl.videotron.ca.

DELORME, Sophie; Hopital Maisonneuve-Rosemont, 5415 boul de l'Assomption, Montreal QC H1T 2M4; Laval'99; FRCPC; IntMed (Diabetology); Endocrin&Metab. Med Spécialiste Endocrinologie, Hopital Maisonneuve-Rosemont; Langs: English; (514)251-3400; Fax. (514)251-5261.

DELOUYA, Guila; CHUM-Hop Notre-Dame, 1560 rue Sherbrooke E, Montreal QC H2L 4M1; Mon'05; FRCPC; RadOncol. Staff, Centre Hospitalier l'Université de Montréal (CHUM) - Hôpital Notre-Dame; (514)890-8254

DELPERO, Walter; Parkdale Med Tower, 302-1081 Carling Ave, Ottawa ON K1Y 4G2; Tor'84; DAB; FRCSC; Ophth. Ac Staff, The Ottawa Hospital - Civic Campus; Ac Staff/Head Ophth, Winchester District Memorial Hospital; Board Member Air Medical Review, Transport Canada (AARTT); Asst Prof, University of Ottawa; Langs: Italian; (613)728-0247; Fax. (613)728-7685; wdelpero@istar.ca.

DELPORT, Arend A C; The Medical Clinic Associates, 4794 Joyce Ave, Powell River BC V8A 3B6; Orange Free State (South Africa)'04; MB ChB; Langs: Afrikaans; (604)485-6261; Fax. (604)485-2820.

DELPORT, Christo; PO Box 197, La Ronge SK S0J 1L0; (South Africa)'86; MB ChB; MFGP(SA); CCFP; Physician, Northern Medical Services; (306)425-2174; Fax. (306)425-4199; tamatwes@gmail.com.

DELPORT, Johannes; University of Western Ontario, 1151 Richmond St, London ON N6A 5B7; Student, University of Western Ontario; (519)661-2030

DELRUE, Andrea N J; Niagara H System-St Catharine, PO Box 3018 Stn Main 142 Queenston St, St Catharines ON L2R 7C6; Tor'04; FRCPC; IntMed. Staff, Niagara Health System - St Catharines General Site; (905)684-7271

DELVA, M Dianne; North York Gen Hosp, 4001 Leslie St, North York ON M2K 1E1; Qns'77; CCFP; FCFP; Chief Family & Community Med, North York General Hospital; Teach Staff, University of Toronto; (902)473-1234

DELVA, Nicholas; Abbie J Lane Bldg, 8210-5909 Veterans Memorial La, Halifax NS B3H 2E2; Qns'75; FRCPC; Psy. Chief Psy, Capital Health-Halifax Infirmary; Head Psy, Dalhousie University; (902)473-2463; Fax. (902)473-4887; nicholas.delva@farmerdairy.ca.

DEMALSY, Jean-Claude; CSSS de Rimouski-Neigette, CP 3150 Succ A 150 av Rouleau, Rimouski QC G5L 5T1; Sher'79; BSc; CSPQ; FRCSC; GenSurg (Thoracic Surgery). Staff, Hôpital Regional Rimouski; (418)723-7851

DEMANCHE, Sylvie; CSSS Champlain, 50-5811 boul Taschereau, Brossard QC J4Z 1A5; Sher'86; (450)466-6084; Fax. (450)466-2283.

DEMANINS-TOWERS, Anna M; MUHC-Montreal Gen Hosp, L10 221 3-1650 Cedar Ave, Montreal QC H3G 1A4; McG'76; CCFP; FCFP; Staff, McGill University Health Centre - Montreal General Campus; Assoc Prof Oncol & Family Med, McGill University; (514)934-1934 x43964; Fax. (514)843-1471; anna.towers@muhc.mcgill.ca.

DEMARCHI, Ronald F; Prime Care Med Centre, 202-7315 Edmonds St, Burnaby BC V3N 1A7; UBC'81; (604)520-3006; Fax. (778)331-3868.

DEMARCO, James A; 4380 Lorimer Rd PO Box 1187, Whistler BC V0N 1B0; Wes'86; (604)932-4911; Fax. (604)932-4992.

DEMARCO, Thomas J; Whistler Health Care Centre, 201-4380 Lorimer Rd RR 4, Whistler BC V0N 1B4; Tor'83; Langs: English; Spanish; Italian; German; (604)932-3977; Fax. (604)932-0660; whistlermc@telus.net.

DEMARIES, Sandra; Villa Caritas, 16515 88 Ave NW, Edmonton AB T5R 0A4; Tor'03; FRCPC; Psy. Staff, Alberta Hospital Edmonton; (780)342-6552; Fax. (780)342-6579.

DEMARTY, Jennifer M; Faculty of Med, 3200-910 10th Ave W, Vancouver BC V5Z 1M9; Cal'05; Anes. (604)875-4111 x68430

DEMAS, Michael L; Grey Nuns Community Hosp & HC, 1100 Youville Drive West NW, Edmonton AB T6L 5X8; Alb'92; FRCPC; Psy. Staff, Covenant Health - Grey Nuns Community Hospital; (780)450-7496

DEMAY, Francois L; Clin D'Ophtal Sorel-Tracy, 124 rue Charlotte, Sorel-Tracy QC J3P 1H1; Lyon (France)'62; CSPQ; LMCC; FRCSC; Ophth. Assoc Staff, Hôtel-Dieu de Sorel; Langs: Bilingual(French/English); (450)742-9840; Fax. (450)742-9840.

DEMBINSKI, Brian; Horizons Family Medicine, A-5016 51 Ave, Red Deer AB T4N 4H5; Alb'08; CCFP; (403)342-7270; Fax. (403)343-2677.

DEMBO, Justine S; Sunnybrook Hlth Sciences Ctre, FG 47-2075 Bayview Ave, Toronto ON M4N 3M5; Tor'07; Psy. Staff, Sunnybrook Health Sciences Centre; (416)480-6832

DEMCHUK, Andrew M; Foothills Med Centre, 1162-1403 29 St NW, Calgary AB T2N 2T9; Sask'93; FRCPC; Neur (Stroke). Staff, Foothills Medical Centre; (403)944-8671; ademchuk@ucalgary.ca.

DEMCO, Thomas; Providence Health Care, 950-943 Broadway W, Vancouver BC V5Z 4E7; UBC'68; FRCSC; Ophth (Cataract). Ac Staff, BC Women's Hospital & Health Centre; Consultant, Vancouver General Hospital - Centennial Pavillion; Ac Staff, Providence Health Care - St Paul's Hospital; Clin Assoc Prof, University of British Columbia; (604)736-0222; Fax. (604)736-0225; tdemco@cw.bc.ca.

DEMERIA, Denny; 15912 100 Ave NW, Edmonton AB T5P 0L2; Sask'01; BSc; FRCPC; IntMed (Hepatology); Gastroent. (780)238-5599

DEMERS, Alain; Clinique médicale de Fleurimon, 210-2140 rue King E, Sherbrooke QC J1G 5G6; Laval'83; CM(FC); Staff, Centre Hospitalier Universitaire de Sherbrooke-Hopital Fleurimont; (819)563-4462; Fax. (819)563-4464.

DEMERS, Anne-Marie; Hôpital Ste-Justine, 3175 ch Cote-Ste-Catherine, Montreal QC H3T 1C5; Mon'94; FRCPC; Peds (Medical Microbiology & Infectious Diseases); MedMicrobiol; InfectDis. Staff, Hôpital Ste-Justine; (514)345-4931

DEMERS, Annie; Clinique Med Angus, 101-4101 rue Molson, Montreal QC H1Y 3L1; Mon'97; (514)807-2333

DEMERS, Annie; Service Med Prive, 105-100 boul de Montarville, Boucherville QC J4B 5M4; Laval'90; (450)641-6774

DEMERS, Annie L; UMF Grand Littorral, 1205 boul de la Rive-Sud, Saint-Romuald QC G6W 0J4; Mon'07; Staff, Hôtel-Dieu de Lévis; Physician, Coop de Sante St-Damien; (418)380-8597; Fax. (418)380-8596.

DEMERS, Bernard; CSSS du Rocher-Perce, CP 3300 451 rue Monseigneur Ross E, Chandler QC G0C 1K0; Sher'01; Staff, Centre Hospitalier de Chandler; (418)689-2261

DEMERS, Catherine; McMaster University, C4 107-1280 Main Street W, Hamilton ON L8S 4K1; Sher'91; CSPQ; FRCPC; IntMed (Heart Failure); Cardiol. Staff, Hamilton Health Sciences Centre - McMaster Children's Hospital; McMaster University; (905)521-2100 x73324; Fax. (905)577-1427.

DEMERS, Chantale; St Boniface Hosp, A8024-409 Tache Ave, Winnipeg MB R2H 2A6; Man'05; CCFP; Staff, St Boniface General Hospital; (204)233-8563

DEMERS, Charlotte; CHUS-Hop Fleurimont, 3001 12e av N, Sherbrooke QC J1H 5N4; Sher'80; FRCPC; Peds (Neonatology). Ac Staff, Centre Hospitalier Universitaire de Sherbrooke-Hopital Fleurimont; (819)346-1110 x14634; Fax. (819)564-5398.

DEMERS, Christine; Ctr Hosp Affilie-Enfant-Jesus, 1401 18e rue, Quebec QC G1J 1Z4; Laval'83; FRCPC; IntMed; Hem. Staff, Centre Hospitalier Affilié Universitaire de Québec - Hôpital De L'Enfant Jésus; (418)649-5726

DEMERS, Christine; Ctr Hosp de Verdun, 4000 boul Lasalle, Verdun QC H4G 2A3; Laval'03; CCFP; Staff, Centre Hospitalier de Verdun; (514)362-1000

DEMERS, Daniel; Clinique Med Perrier, 10-10794 rue Lajeunesse, Montreal QC H3L 2E8; Mon'80; Staff, Centre Hospitalier l'Université de Montréal (CHUM) - Hôpital Notre-Dame; (514)383-0559; Fax. (514)383-3430.

DEMERS, Donald; 287 boul de Mortagne, Longueuil QC J4B 1B4; Laval'73.

DEMERS, Francois; CSSS du Lac-des-Deux-Montagnes, 520 boul Arthur-Sauve, Saint-Eustache QC J7R 5B1; Mon'98; Staff, Hôpital de Saint-Eustache; (450)473-6811

DEMERS, Georges; CHUM-Hotel-Dieu de Quebec, 11 Cote du Palais, Quebec QC G1R 2J6; Laval'66; Otol (Oncology). Dir Dept of Otol, Centre Hospitalier Universitaire de Québec (CHUQ) - Siege Social; Prof Otol, Université Laval; (418)691-5151; geo.demers@sympatico.ca.

DEMERS, Huguette; Tribunal Administratif Du QC, 500 boul Rene-Levesque O, Montreal QC H2Z 1W7; Mon'76; DPH; CommunMed (P.Q.) (Occupational Medicine). Langs: Spanish; (514)873-8030

DEMERS, Jacques F; CSSS Kamouraska-Hop-Notre Dame, CP 460 1201 6e av, La Pocatiere QC G0R 1Z0; Laval'64; CSPQ; FRCPC; DiagRad. Staff, CSSS de Kamouraska; (418)856-7000; Fax. (418)856-4737; demersja@sympatico.ca.

DEMERS, Jacques; Hop Charles Lemoyne, 3120 boul Taschereau, Greenfield Park QC J4V 2H1; Mon'94; FRCSC; Neursurg. Staff, Hopital Charles LeMoyne; (450)466-5000; Fax. (450)466-5049.

DEMERS, Jacques; Clinique Med de l'Est Inc, 220-8 Place du Commerce, Verdun QC H3E 1N3; Laval'65; CSPQ; Anes (P.Q.). (514)281-2022; Fax. (514)281-1042.

DEMERS, Jean-P; Clin Medicale Hochelaga, 9080 rue Hochelaga, Montreal QC H1L 2N9; Mon'58; Ophth. (514)353-8742

DEMERS, Josiane; CSSS Les Eskers de l'Abitibi, 622 4e rue O, Amos QC J9T 2S2; Mon'06; Staff, CH Hôtel-Dieu d'Amos; (819)732-3241

DEMERS, Julie; Clinique Med le Mesnil, 300-1300 boul Lebourgneuf, Quebec QC G2K 2N1; Sher'96; Staff, CSSS de la Vieille-Capitale; (416)624-1800

DEMERS, Liliane; Tour Bell Canada, 3-1 Carref Alexander-Graham-Be, Montreal QC H3E 3B3; Laval'77; MSc(Occup.Health); Médecin, Bell Canada Enterprises; Langs: French; English; (514)870-3887; liliane.demers@bell.ca.

DEMERS, Louis; Clinique Med de Touraine, 2B-520 boul De l'Hopital, Gatineau QC J8V 2P5; Sher'82; Langs: English; (819)568-0212; Fax. (819)568-6310.

DEMERS, Marie-Eve; Centre Hosp Honore-Mercier, 2750 boul Laframboise, Saint-Hyacinthe QC J2S 4Y8; Sher'99; Staff, Centre Hospitalier Honore-Mercier; Staff, Family Clinic, St-Thomas d'Aquin; Langs: Bilingual(English/French); (450)771-3333 x3322; mevedem@hotmail.com.

DEMERS, Marie-Josee; CSSS de Quebec Nord, 3666 ch Royal, Quebec QC G1E 1X5; Laval'89; (418)663-3099; Fax. (418)663-2939; marie-josee.demers@ssss.gouv.qc.ca.

DEMERS, Michel C; Cabinet du Lieutenant-Governeu, RC01-1050 rue des Parlementair, Quebec QC G1A 1A1; Laval'79; Chef Service Med Assessment, Regie de l'Assurance Maladie du Quebec; Langs: Creole; English; (418)643-5385

DEMERS, Mireille; CLSC Ahuntsic, 1165 boul Henri-Bourassa E, Montreal QC H2C 3K2; Mon'06; CCFP; (514)384-2000; Fax. (514)389-1361.

DEMERS, Philippe; Institut de Cardiologie de Mtl, 5000 rue Belanger, Montreal QC H1T 1C8; Mon'95; CSPQ; FRCSC; CardSurg. Staff, Institut de Cardiologie de Montréal; (514)593-2511

DEMERS, Philippe; Hop Brome-Missisquoi-Perkins, 950 rue Prinicipale, Cowansville QC J2K 1K3; Mon'94; LMCC; CSPQ; FRACS; FRCSC; GenSurg (Digestive Surgery). Staff, Hôpital Brome-Missisquoi-Perkins; Langs: Spanish; English; (450)266-4342

DEMERS, Pierre; Lasik MD Montreal, 1250 boul Rene-Levesque O, Montreal QC H3B 4W8; McG'90; FRCSC; Ophth (Refractive Surgery). Aj Prof, Universite de Montreal; Langs: English; (514)933-0133

DEMERS, Stephanie; CSSS Haut-Richelieu-Rouville, 920 boul du Seminaire N, St-Jean-Sur-Richel QC J3A 1B7; Sher'97; Staff, Hôpital du Haut-Richelieu; (450)359-5000

DEMERS, Sylvie; Ctr Menopause-Andropause Outao, 182 rue Montcalm, Gatineau QC J8Y 3B5; Laval'96; PhD; Langs: English; (819)771-1936; Fax. (819)771-4026.

DEMERS, Vincent; CLSC du Plateau-Mont-Royal, 4625 du Plateau Mont-Royal, Montreal QC H2H 2B4; Laval'02; CCFP; Staff, CSSS de la Basse Côté-Nord; (514)521-7663

DEMERS, Yves; Groupe Med de Trois-Rivieres, 225-1900 boul Des Recollets, Trois-Rivieres QC G8Z 4K4; Laval'87; Staff, CSSS de Trois-Rivières; (819)375-6666; Fax. (819)375-3423.

DEMERS-PELLETIER, Julie; CSSS de Saint-Jerome, 290 rue de Montigny, Saint-Jerome QC J7Z 5T3; Laval'92; CSPQ; FRCPC; Anes. Staff, Hôtel-Dieu de Saint-Jérôme; (450)431-8599

DEMETER JR., Sandor; Health Sciences Centre, GG 345-820 Sherbrook St, Winnipeg MB R3A 1R9; Sask'89; BSc; AB; MHSc; FRCPC; CommunMed (Public Health); NuclearMed. Med Dir Radiology, Health Sciences Centre; Assoc Prof Commun Health Sciences Radiology/Chair Radiology/Dept Head Radiology, University of Manitoba; (204)787-3375; Fax. (204)787-3090.

DEMETRICK, Douglas; HSC-Faculty of Med, 303 HMRB-3330 Hospital Dr NW, Calgary AB T2N 4N1; Cal'86; FRCPC; AnatPath. (403)220-2890; Fax. (403)283-8727.

DEMETRICK, Jeffrey S; 3107 35 Ave, Vernon BC V1T 2T2; UBC'91; FRCSC; GenSurg. (250)545-6443

DEMEULE, Eric; CHUQ-Ctr Hosp Univ Laval, RC 219-2705 boul Laurier, Quebec QC G1V 4G2; Mon'93; CSPQ; FRCPC; IntMed; Cardiol. Staff, Centre Hospitalier Universitaire de Quebec-CHUL; (418)654-2110; Fax. (418)654-2268.

DEMIAN, Hany; Norfolk Gen Hosp, 365 West St, Simcoe ON N3Y 1T7; (Other Foreign)'00; CCFP; Staff, Norfolk General Hospital; (519)426-0750

DEMIAN, Momen; Murakami Med Clinic, PO Box 1000 735 Fouth Ave, Hope BC V0X 1L0; Egypt (Egypt)'85; CCFP; (604)869-5648

DEMIAN, Ruth A; Redwood Med Clinic, 5-8948 202 St, Langley BC V1M 4A7; Mem'86; (604)888-4472

DEMIANCZUK, Arkadiy; Business Bldg, 514-1200 Burrard St, Vancouver BC V6Z 2C7; Qns'97; FRCSC; PlasSurg (Hand Surgery). Clin Asst Prof, UBC Hospital - Koerner Pavillion; Staff, Providence Health Care - St Paul's Hospital; Staff, Vancouver General Hospital - Centennial Pavillion; Langs: Ukrainian; (604)806-6365; Fax. (604)974-0067.

DEMIANCZUK, Nestor N; Royal Alexandra Hosp, 5S117-10240 Kingsway NW, Edmonton AB T5H 3V9; Mon'74; AB; FRCSC; ObstGyn (Perinatal). Staff, Royal Alexandra Hospital; Prof, University of Alberta; Langs: French; Ukrainian; (780)735-4815; Fax. (780)735-4981; nestordemianczuk@albertahealthservices.ca.

DEMIRJIAN, Ari; 127-1320 boul Graham, Mont-Royal QC H3P 3C8; Sher'88; CSPQ; FRCPC; Derm (Laser Surgery). assoc Prof, McGill University Health Centre - Montreal General Campus; assoc Prof, McGill University; Langs: French; Spanish; Armenian; (514)344-6654; demirjian@videotron.ca.

DEMIRTAS, Ezgi; MUHC-Royal Victoria Hosp, F6 58-687 av des Pins O, Montreal QC H3A 1A1; (Turkey)'98; Staff, McGill University Health Centre - Royal Victoria Hospital; (514)934-1934 x31391; Fax. (514)843-1496.

DEMKIW-BARTEL, Coby; 205A 115th St E, Saskatoon SK S7N 2E3; Sask'00; BScPharm; BA; RT; CCFP; (306)384-7773; Fax. (306)384-7775.

DEMONG, Paige M; Sport Med Centre, 2500 University Dr NW, Calgary AB T2N 1N4; Cal'04; CCFP; (403)220-8518

DEMONG, Thaddeus; Demong Associate Eye Centre, 330-290 Midpark Way SE, Calgary AB T2X 1P1; Alb'71; AB; FRCSC; Ophth (Cornea & Refractive Surgery). Staff, Rockyview General Hospital; Med Dir, Lions Eye Bank Southern Alberta; Med Dir, Rocky Mountain Surgery Centre; Clin Instructor, University of Calgary; (403)254-2408; Fax. (403)254-5887.

DEMONTIGNY, Jillian; Associate Med Centre, 5016 48 Ave, Taber AB T1G 1R8; McM'03; CCFP; (403)223-3525

DEMOS, Michelle K; Children's & Women's Hc Of Bc, K3 176-4480 Oak St, Vancouver BC V6H 3V4; UBC'97; BSc; FRCPC; Peds; Neur. Staff, BC Children's Hospital; (604)875-2121; Fax. (604)875-2376.

DEMPSEY, G Paul; Quinte Pediatrics, 100 Station St, Belleville ON K8N 2S5; McM'91; BSc; FRCPC; Peds (Consultant Pediatrics)., QHC Belleville General; Staff, Kingston General Hospital; Staff, Hotel-Dieu Hospital; Asst Prof Peds., Queen's University; (613)966-1999; Fax. (613)966-3980.

DEMPSEY, Ian; Dartmouth ENT Associates, 100-35 Baker Dr, Dartmouth NS B2W 0H3; Dal'85; FRCSC; Otol (Rhinology). Consultant Otol., Queen Elizabeth II Health Sciences Centre - Victoria General Site; Lecturer Otol, Dalhousie University; Langs: French; (902)435-8585; Fax. (902)435-8695.

DEMPSEY, Laurel J; Verona Medical Centre, PO Box 160 6582 Hwy 38, Verona ON K0H 2W0; Tor'71; FCFP; BSc(MED); Assoc Prof Med, Queen's University; (613)374-2077; Fax. (613)374-2483.

DEMPSEY, Rose E M; Alberta Hosp Edmonton, PO Box 307 Stn Main 17480 Fort Rd, Edmonton AB T5J 2J7; (Ireland)'81; MB ChB; MRCPsy; Clin Dir Geriatric Psy, Alberta Hospital Edmonton; Clin Teacher, University of Alberta; (780)472-5355; Fax. (780)472-5342.

DEMPSEY-MCKIM, Susan R; Nashwaaksis Med Clinic, 475 Brookside Dr, Fredericton NB E3A 8V4; Dal'77; Staff, Dr Everett Chalmers Regional Hospital; (506)458-9450; Fax. (506)458-1326.

DEMPSTER, David W; PO Box 513, Burks Falls ON P0A 1C0; Tor'69; (705)382-2207; Fax. (705)382-2207.

DEMPSTER, Helen; Huntsville Prof Bldg, 202-348 Muskoka Rd 3 N, Huntsville ON P1H 1H8; Tor'02; BScEng; MSc; CCFP; Asst Prof, Northern Ontario School of Medicine; (705)788-3623; Fax. (705)788-3624.

DEMPSTER, Jeffrey J; 305-1276 South Park St, Halifax NS B3H 2Y9; McM'90; FRCSC; ObstGyn (Palliative Medicine). Court Staff, IWK Health Centre; Ac Staff, Queen Elizabeth II Health Sciences Centre - Victoria General Site; Aj Associate Prof, Dalhousie University; (902)473-4341; Fax. (902)473-6602; jeff.dempster@cdha.nshealth.ca.

DEMSAS, Habtu; Selkirk Med Centre, 353 Eveline St, Selkirk MB R1A 1N1; Bologna (Italy)'80; (204)785-2644; Fax. (204)785-8966.

DEMYTTENAERE, Sebastian V; St Mary's Hosp Ctr, 8270-3830 av Lacombe, Montreal QC H3T 1M5; McG'02; FRCSC; GenSurg (Clinical & Investigative Medicine). Staff, St Mary's Hospital Centre; (514)734-2797; Fax. (514)734-2793.

DENARDI, Franco; Niagara H System-St Catharine, 142 Queenston St, St. Catharines ON L2R 7C6; Ott'83; FRCPC; AnatPath. Staff, Niagara Health System - St Catharines General Site; Staff, Hamilton Health Sciences Centre-Juravinski Site; Langs: Italian; French; (905)378-4647

DENATH, Fareed M; Windsor Reg Hosp, 1995 Lens Ave, Windsor ON N8W 1L9; Natal (South Africa)'79; FFR(D); MB ChB; FRCPC; DiagRad. Staff, Windsor Regional Hospital - Metropolitan Site; Langs: Gujarati; (519)254-1727

DENAULT, Alexandre; Ctr Hosp Affilie-Enfant-Jesus, 1401 18e rue, Quebec QC G1J 1Z4; Laval'03; FRCSC; OrthSurg. Staff, Centre Hospitalier Affilié Universitaire de Québec - Hôpital De L'Enfant Jésus; (418)649-0252

DENAULT, Andre-Yvan; Institut de Cardiologie de Mtl, 5000 rue Belanger, Montreal QC H1T 1C8; Mon'87; CSPQ; FRCPC; IntMed; Critical Care Medicine (P.Q.); Anes. Staff, Institut de Cardiologie de Montréal; Staff, Centre Hospitalier de Verdun; (514)376-3330; Fax. (514)593-2540; denault@videotron.ca.

DENAULT, Isabelle; CSSS de Montmagny-L'Islet, RR 1 350 boul Tache O, Montmagny QC G5V 3R8; Laval'04; IntMed. Staff, CSSS de Montmagny-L'Islet; (418)248-0630

DENAULT, Jacinthe; CSSS de la Haute-Cote-Nord, RR 1 4 rue de l'Hopital, Les Escoumins QC G0T 1K0; McG'95; CCFP; Staff, Centre de santé des Côté-Nord; (418)233-2931; Fax. (418)233-3335.

DENAULT, Nathalie; Clinique Fam de St-Hyacinthe, 2955 boul Laframboise, Saint-Hyacinthe QC J2S 4Z3; Sher'85; Staff Family Med, Centre Hospitalier Honore-Mercier; (450)774-4611; Fax. (450)773-9913.

DENAULT, Pierre; Ctr Hops Affilie Enfant-jesus, 1401 18e rue, Quebec QC G1J 1Z4; Laval'70; CSPQ; Anes (Adult Anesthesia). Staff, Centre Hospitalier Affilié Universitaire de Québec - Hôpital De L'Enfant Jésus; Staff, CSSS de Montmagny-L'Islet; (418)649-5807; Fax. (418)649-5918.

DENBEIGH, Paul; 550 King St E, Kitchener ON N2G 2L8; Tor'78; CCFP; FCFP; Court Staff, Grand River Hospital - Kitchener/Waterloo Health Centre; Court Staff, St Mary's General Hospital; (519)886-6711; Fax. (519)886-6722.

DENBURG, Avram; The Hosp For Sick Children, 555 University Ave, Toronto ON M5G 1X8; McM'06; FRCPC; Peds. Staff, The Hospital For Sick Children; (416)813-7500

DENBURG, Judah; McMaster University, 3V46-1280 Main St W, Hamilton ON L8S 4K1; Hebrew (Israel)'73; FRCPC; Hem (Clinical Immunology & Allergy); IntMed. Head Div of Clinical Immunol & Allergy, Hamilton Health Sciences Centre - McMaster Children's Hospital; Prof Clinical Immunol & Allergy McMaster Univ Medical Centre, McMaster University; Langs: Yiddish; Hebrew; French; (905)521-2100 x76714; denburg@mcmaster.ca.

DENBY, John D; Trafalgar Med Clinic, 200-1235 Trafalgar Rd, Oakville ON L6H 3P1; Tor'71; BSc; Med Officer, Ministry of Correctional Services; (905)844-3281

DENEAULT, Jocelyn J; Montfort Hosp, 713 Montreal Rd, Ottawa ON K1K 0T2; Ott'67; FRCPC; IntMed; Gastroent. Assoc Staff, The Ottawa Hospital - General Campus; Ac Staff Gastroent, Montfort Hospital; Asst Clin Prof, University of Ottawa; (613)748-4904; Fax. (613)745-3115; jdeneault@uottawa.ca.

DENEAULT, Luc; CSSS Haut-Richelieu-Rouville, 920 boul du Seminaire N, St-Jean-Sur-Richel QC J3A 1B7; Sher'91; Staff, Hôpital du Haut-Richelieu; (450)459-5000; Fax. (450)245-0615.

DENEAULT, Melanie; Clinique De Med Familiale, 6F-2120 rue Sherbrooke E, Montreal QC H2K 1C3; Mon'05; CCFP; (514)527-1958; Fax. (514)527-1649.

DENEAULT, Mychele C; Clarence-Rockland Fam Hlth Team, 2741 rue Chamberland, Rockland ON K4K 0B4; Ott'96; CCFP; Langs: Bilingual(English/French); (613)446-7677; Fax. (613)446-5737.

DENEAULT-LOMBART, Emmanuelle; CSSS de Laval, 1755 boul Rene-Laennec, Laval QC H7M 3L9; Mon'08; CCFP; CCFP(E.M.); Staff, Hopital de la Cite de la santé; (450)668-1010

DENEGRI, Jorge F; Laurel Med Centre Ltd, 310-888 8th Ave W, Vancouver BC V5Z 3Y1; Buenos Aires (Argentina)'70; FRCPC; Hem (Internal Medicine). Ac Staff, Vancouver General Hospital - Centennial Pavillion; Consultant, BC Children's Hospital; Consultant, Nanaimo Regional General Hospital; Clin Assoc Prof, University of British Columbia; (604)879-6676

DENESUK, Allison; Rockyview Maternity & Family P, 258-1011 Glenmore Trail SW, Calgary AB T2V 4R6; Alb'89; BMedSci; CCFP; FCFP; Staff, Rockyview General Hospital; (403)640-0600; Fax. (403)253-0124.

DENGA, Edward T; Thickwood Family Med Ctr, 108 Wolverine Dr, Fort McMurray AB T9H 4Y7; Ibadan (Nigeria)'94; MB BS(Ibadan); MCFP(SA); CCFP; (780)713-2491; edwarddenga@yahoo.ca.

DENHEZ, Paul; Centre Oculaire de Victoriavii, 340 rue Notre-Dame E, Victoriaville QC G6P 4A6; Sher'85; FRCSC; Ophth. (819)751-5595

DENIC, Nebojsa; Health Sciences Centre, 300 Prince Philip Dr, St. John's NL A1B 3V6; Belgrade (Serbia)'82; MSc; PhD; FRCPC; AnatPath (Forensic Pathology). Staff/Clin Assoc Prof, Health Sciences Centre; Langs: Serbian; (709)737-2990; Fax. (709)777-5178; nebojsa.denic@easternhealth.ca.

DENICOURT, Marcel; Clinique Med Mont St-Hilaire, 261 boul Laurier, Mont-Saint-Hilaire QC J3H 3N8; Mon'79; Langs: English; (450)464-5151; Fax. (450)464-3703.

DENIS, Bernard; 991 Frontenac, Berthierville QC J0K 1A0; Mon'62; (450)836-0232

DENIS, Bruno; Centre Med Sillery, 1270 av William, Quebec QC G1S 4G1; Laval'89; CCFP; Staff, Jeffery Hale Hospital-Saint Brigid's; (418)688-0664; Fax. (418)688-4601.

DENIS, Francois; CSSS Cote de Gaspe, 150 rue Monseigneur-Ross, Gaspe QC G4X 2S7; Paris (France)'84; Psy (P.Q.). Psychiatre, Centre Hospitalier de Gaspe; (418)368-3301; Fax. (418)368-3481.

DENIS, Geoffroy; Dir de la Sante Publique-Mtl, 1301 Sherbrooke E, Montreal QC H2L 1M3; Mon'06; FRCPC; Public Health & Preventive Med; CommunMed (P.Q.). (514)528-2400 x3631

DENIS, Gilles; Clin Fam Basses-Laurentides, 2100 boul du Cure-Labelle, Saint-Jerome QC J7Y 1S8; Laval'75; (450)565-4320; Fax. (450)565-1099.

DENIS, Isabelle; CHUM-Hop Notre-Dame, 1560 rue Sherbrooke E, Montreal QC H2L 4M1; Mon'04; FRCPC; PhysMed&Rehab. Staff, Centre Hospitalier l'Université de Montréal (CHUM) - Hôpital Notre-Dame; (514)890-8201

DENIS, Jean-Francois; CSSS de Laval, 1755 boul Rene-Laennec, Laval QC H7M 3L9; Mon'75; CSPQ; Psy. Staff Psy, Hopital de la Cite de la santé; (450)668-1010; Fax. (450)975-5090.

DENIS, Jocelyne; Centre Med Mailloux, 130-1900 av Mailloux, Quebec QC G1J 5B9; Laval'75; Staff, Centre Hospitalier Affilié Universitaire de Québec - Hôpital De L'Enfant Jésus; (418)667-7014; Fax. (418)667-5808.

DENIS, Jocelyne M; CLSC Le Minordet, 961 rue de la Clinique, Senneterre QC J0Y 2M0; Sher'79; (819)737-2243; Fax. (819)737-3122.

DENIS, Marie-Claire; CHUQ-Ctr Hosp Univ Laval, 2705 boul Laurier, Quebec QC G1V 4G2; Laval'83; FRCPC; IntMed (P.Q.); Endocrin&Metab; Endocrin (P.Q.). Staff, Centre Hospitalier Universitaire de Quebec-CHUL; (418)654-2169; Fax. (418)654-2792.

DENIS, Ronald; 100-100 ch Rockland, Mont-Royal QC H3P 2V9; Mon'75; CSPQ; FRCSC; GenSurg (Bariatric Medicine). Staff, Hôpital du Sacre-Coeur de Montréal; Consultant, Centre Hospitalier l'Université de Montréal (CHUM) - Hôpital Notre-Dame; (514)331-4322; Fax. (514)331-8683.

DENIS, Sylvain; CSSS de Laval, 1755 boul Rene-Laennec, Laval QC H7M 3L9; Mon'83; Psy. Teacher, Hopital de la Cite de la santé; (450)668-1010; Fax. (450)975-5090.

DENIS-LEBLANC, Manon A; 4553 St Catherine St, St Isidore ON K0C 2B0; Ott'97; CCFP; Staff, Montfort Hospital; Langs: Bilingual(English/French); (613)524-3225; Fax. (613)524-2513.

DENKEMA, Raubenheimer; Grande Pririe Orthopadic Surge, 101-9815 97 St, Grande Prairie AB T8V 8B9; (South Africa)'94; MB ChB; MMed; Langs: Afrikaans; (780)402-7181; Fax. (780)402-9829.

DENKERS, Matthew R; 1280 Main St W, Hamilton ON L8S 4K1; McM'03; BHSc; FRCSC; OrthSurg (Arthroscopic Knee & Shoulder Surgery). Assoc Staff/Asst Prof Orthopaedic Surgery, Hamilton Health Sciences Centre - Hamilton General Hospital; (905)527-4322 x44158

DENNIE, Carole J; The Ottawa Hosp-Civic Campus, 1053 Carling Ave, Ottawa ON K1Y 4E9; Ott'85; FRCPC; DiagRad. Staff, The Ottawa Hospital - Civic Campus; Prof, University of Ottawa; Langs: Bilingual(French/English); (613)761-4982; Fax. (613)761-4476; cdennie@ottawahospital.on.ca.

DENNIE, Joelle; 1110 Newport Ave, Victoria BC V8S 5E4; UBC'02; FRCPC; ObstGyn. Staff, BC Women's Hospital & Health Centre; (250)590-4963

DENNIS, Jane D; Grand River Hosp-Freeport Site, PO Box 9056 3570 King St E, Kitchener ON N2A 2W1; Wes'93; BSc; FRCPC; Psy. Staff, Grand River Hospital - Freeport Site; (519)749-4300

DENNIS, John T; Main Street Med Centre, 103 Main St, Stephenville NL A2N 1H9; Birmingham (England)'58; MB ChB; (709)643-9657; Fax. (709)643-9106.

DENNIS, Kristopher; The Ottawa Hosp-Gen Camp, 501 Smyth Rd, Ottawa ON K1H 8L6; Wes'05; FRCPC; RadOncol. Staff, The Ottawa Hospital - General Campus; (613)737-7700

DENNIS, Stephen M; Queen Square Doctors FHT, 201-366 Main St N, Brampton ON L6V 1P8; Wes'63; Med Staff, William Osler Health System - Brampton Civic Hospital; (905)455-1455; Fax. (905)455-5498.

DENNISON, Heather D; Carlington Comm Hlth Services, 900 Merivale Rd, Ottawa ON K1Z 5Z8; Ott'90; CCFP; FCFP; (613)722-2161; Fax. (613)722-8471.

DENNISON, Jeffrey; Family Health Centre, 200-2462 Howard Ave, Windsor ON N8X 3V6; Ott'93; CCFP; FCFP; Assoc Staff, Windsor Regional Hospital - Metropolitan Site; Assoc Staff, Hôtel-Dieu Grace Hospital; Aj Prof, University of Western Ontario; (519)258-1156; Fax. (519)258-9774; karenandjeffrey@aol.com.

DENNY, Sarah K; Children's & Women's HC of BC, 1C31A-4480 Oak St, Vancouver BC V6H 3V4; McM'91; FRCPC; Peds. Staff Peds, BC Children's Hospital; (604)875-2729

DENOBRIGA, Lisa M; 44 Queen St, Kincardine ON N2Z 3C1; St George's (Grenada)'06; (519)396-6773

DENSMORE, Lis; Pine Med Centre, 5110 5th Ave, Whitehorse YT Y1A 1L4; Alb'74; Assoc Staff, Whitehorse General Hospital; (867)668-4353; Fax. (867)668-3899; pinemed@northwestel.net.

DENSON, Frank G; Lakehead Psychiatric Hosp, 580 North Algoma St, Thunder Bay ON P7B 5G4; Sask'88; Staff, Lakehead Psychiatric Hospital - St. Joseph's Care Group; (807)343-4368; Fax. (807)343-4327; fdenson@ptboclinic.com.

DENSON, John R; 16-260 Parsons Ave, North Bay ON P1A 1T2; Melbourne (Australia)'77; MB BS; FRCPC; Psy (Psychotherapy). (705)478-5798; Fax. (705)478-5682.

DENSON, Stephen M A; Nottingham Medical, 310-664 Wye Rd, Sherwood Park AB T8A 6G3; Alb'96; (780)416-3220; Fax. (780)416-3224.

DENSTEDT, John; St Joseph's Health Care, PO Box 5777 Stn B 268 Grosvenor St, London ON N6A 4V2; Wes'82; FRCSC; Urol. Staff, London Health Sciences Centre - South Street; Staff, St Joseph's Hospital - St Joseph's Health Care; Dept Chair Surg/Prof, University of Western Ontario; (519)646-6036; Fax. (519)646-6037.

DENT, Cynthia H; The Allin Clinic, 10155 120 St NW, Edmonton AB T5K 2A2; Ott'89; CCFP; FCFP; Staff, University of Alberta Hospital; (780)482-7551; Fax. (780)488-2056.

DENT, Peter; McMaster University, HSC 2E23-1280 Main St W, Hamilton ON L8S 4K1; Tor'60; DCH; FAAP; FRCPC; Peds (Rheumatology). Sr Staff, Hamilton Health Sciences Centre - McMaster Children's Hospital; Emeritus Prof Peds, McMaster University; (905)521-2100 x75394; Fax. (905)521-4968; dentpb@mcmaster.ca.

DENT, Robert R M; Grimes 3-1053 Carling Ave, Ottawa ON K1Y 4E9; McG'71; FRCPC; IntMed (Obesity & Weight Control). Staff Teacher, The Ottawa Hospital - Civic Campus; Asst Clin Prof, University of Ottawa; (613)798-5555 x19647; Fax. (613)761-5343; bdent@ottawahospital.on.ca.

DENT, Susan F; The Ottawa Hosp-Gen Campus, 501 Smyth Rd, Ottawa ON K1H 8L6; McM'90; FRCPC; IntMed; MedOncol. Staff, The Ottawa Hospital - General Campus; Assoc Prof, University of Ottawa; (613)737-8899 x72013; Fax. (613)247-3511; sdent@ottawahospital.on.ca.

DENTON, Andrew B; 202-943 Broadway W, Vancouver BC V5Z 4E1; Dal'95; FRCSC; Otol. (604)879-3223

DENTON, P H Omotayo; Humber River Reg Hosp-Finch, 2111 Finch Ave W, North York ON M3N 1N1; Ibadan (Nigeria)'78; MB BS; FRCPC; DiagRad. Staff, Humber River Regional Hospital - Finch Avenue Site; (416)747-3792; Fax. (416)747-3759.

DENTON, Paul D; Edmonton City Centre West, C107-10200 102 Ave NW, Edmonton AB T5J 4B7; Qns'01; FRCSC; Ophth. (780)702-0532; Fax. (780)702-0336.

DENYER, Andrew G; West Grey Med Care, PO Box 970 368 College St, Durham ON N0G 1R0; London (England)'72; MB BS; MD; Chief Staff, South Bruce Grey Health Centre - Durham Site; (519)369-2510; Fax. (519)369-3831.

DENYS, Allen P; Windsor Sleep Disorders Clinic, 1100 Ouellette Ave, Windsor ON N9A 1C9; Qns'76; FRCPC; Respir (Sleep Disorders Medicine). Consultant, Windsor Regional Hospital - Metropolitan Site; Court Staff, Hôtel-Dieu Grace Hospital; (519)258-0585; Fax. (519)258-6304.

DENYS, Jason A; Chatham-Kent Family Health Team, 209-20 Emma St, Chatham ON N7L 5K5; McM'02; CCFP; (519)354-2172; Fax. (519)354-0886; jdenys@ckha.on.ca.

DEODHARE, Sanjeev; The Credit Valley Hosp, 2200 Eglinton Ave W, Mississauga ON L5M 2N1; Bombay (India)'79; AB; AB; FRCPC; AnatPath (Hematology Pathology). Staff, The Credit Valley Hospital; Asst Prof Path, University of Toronto; Langs: Marathi; (905)813-2696; sdeodhare@cvh.on.ca.

DEOL, Janjeevan S; Royal Alexandra Hosp, 10240 Kingsway NW, Edmonton AB T5H 3V9; Alb'09; CCFP; CCFP(E.M.); Staff, Royal Alexandra Hospital; (780)735-4111

DEOL, Sandeep; Harvest Hills Med Clinic, 715-500 Country Hills Blvd NE, Calgary AB T3K 5Y7; (India)'02; MB BS; FRCPC; IntMed. Staff, Foothills Medical Centre; (403)226-8647; Fax. (403)226-8645.

DEONARAIN, Sue; Scarborough Hosp-Birchmount, 3030 Birchmount Rd, Scarborough ON M1W 3W3; McM'03; FRCSC; OrthSurg. Staff, The Scarborough Hospital - Birchmount Campus; (416)495-2400

DEONARINE, Linda A; Parkview Prof Centre, 206-2110 Main St, Winnipeg MB R2V 2C2; Man'81; FRCPC; Peds. Staff, St Boniface General Hospital; (204)334-9955

DEONG, Jean P; The Brandon Clinic, 620 Dennis St, Brandon MB R7A 5E7; Man'79; BSc; CCFP; FCFP; Staff, Brandon Regional Health Centre; Langs: Chinese; (204)728-4440; Fax. (204)726-1765.

DEPELTEAU, Helene; Hop Charles LeMoyne, 3120 boul Taschereau, Greenfield Park QC J4V 2H1; Mon'99; DiagRad. Staff, Hopital Charles LeMoyne; (450)466-5000

DEPELTEAU, Jean; Clin Med Saint-Thomas, CP 5250 830A rue Principale, Saint-Thomas QC J0K 3L0; Mon'82; Staff, Centre Hospitalier Régional de Lanaudière; (450)756-1626; Fax. (450)756-6304.

DEPETRILLO, Santino; Geraldton Medical Group, PO Box 1240 510 Hogarth Ave W, Geraldton ON P0T 1M0; Dublin (Ireland)'03; CCFP; Asst Prof, Northern Ontario School of Medicine; (807)854-0224; Fax. (807)854-0227; geraldtonmedicalclinic@yahoo.ca.

DEPEW, William T; Hotel-Dieu Hosp, 166 Brock St, Kingston ON K7L 5G2; Qns'73; FACG; BScH; FRCP; FRCPC; IntMed (Hepatology). Att Staff, Hotel-Dieu Hospital; Att Staff, Kingston General Hospital; Consultant, Providence Care - St Mary's of the Lake Hospital Site; Prof Med, Queen's University; (613)544-3310 x2483; Fax. (613)544-3114.

DEPOT, Rene; 205 rue Dunant, Laval QC H7L 2B5; Mon'61.

DEPPISCH, Linda M; Streetsville Med Centre, 8-5425 Creditview Rd, Mississauga ON L5V 2P3; McM'89; CCFP; FCFP; Ac Staff, The Credit Valley Hospital; (905)826-1164; Fax. (905)826-1214.

DEPTUCH, John M; Regina Qu'Appelle HR-Regina, 1440 14th Ave, Regina SK S4P 0W5; Sask'95; Staff, Regina General Hospital; (306)766-4444; Fax. (306)585-2102.

DEQUOY, Genevieve; Clinique De Med Familiale, 6F-2120 rue Sherbrooke E, Montreal QC H2K 1C3; Mon'05; Staff, Centre Hospitalier l'Université de Montréal (CHUM) - Hôpital Notre-Dame; (514)527-1958; Fax. (514)527-1649.

DER, Linda M; Hope Med Clinic, 12214 82 St NW, Edmonton AB T5B 2X1; Alb'87; BMedSci; CCFP; (780)479-1944; Fax. (780)479-1964.

DER, Tara-Diana; The Hosp For Sick Children, 555 University Ave, Toronto ON M5G 1X8; McM'00; FRCPC; Anes. Staff, The Hospital For Sick Children; (416)235-8724

DERAKHSHAN, Afrooz; 10171 Yonge St, Richmond Hill ON L4C 1T5; (Iran)'98; CCFP; (905)883-8183; Fax. (905)918-0037.

DERAKHSHAN, Mina; Springborough Prof Centre, 108-30 Springborough Blvd SW, Calgary AB T3H 0N9; (Iran)'91; CCFP; (403)240-2221

DERASHODIAN, Talar; Hop Charles LeMoyne, 3120 boul Taschereau, Greenfield Park QC J4V 2H1; Mon'05; RadOncol. Staff, Hopital Charles LeMoyne; (450)466-5000 x7559; Fax. (450)465-2027.

DERASPE, Amelie; Centre Jeunesse de Montreal, 12165 boul Saint-Jean-Baptiste, Montreal QC H1C 1S4; Mon'06; CCFP; (514)881-4723

DERASPE, Emmanuel; Ctr Hosp Laurentien, 234 rue Saint-Vincent, Ste-Agathe-des-Mts QC J8C 2B8; Mon'05; CCFP; Staff, Centre Hospitalier Laurentien; (819)324-4000

DERASPE, Mylene; CSSS Des Iles, 430 ch Principal, Cap-aux-Meules QC G4T 1R9; Laval'10; Staff, Hôpital de l'Archipel; (418)986-2121

DERBEKYAN, Vilma A; MUHC-Royal Victoria Hosp, 687 av des Pins O, Montreal QC H3A 1A1; McG'74; FRCPC; DiagRad; NuclearMed. Staff, McGill University Health Centre - Royal Victoria Hospital; (514)934-1934 x34102

DERBY, Ian R G; 50 Forest Ave, Hamilton ON L8N 1X1; McG'73; FRCPC; IntMed (Electromyography); Neur. Ac Staff, St Joseph's Healthcare - Charlton Campus; Clin Assoc Prof, McMaster University; (905)522-8852

DERBYSHIRE, George; West Arthur Place, 201-1265 Arthur St E, Thunder Bay ON P7E 6E7; McM'76; FRCPC; Peds (Pediatric Neurology). Chief Staff/Consultant Regional Autism Assessment Exam, Thunder Bay Regional Health Sciences Centre; (807)622-0606; Fax. (807)623-8585.

DERCKSEN, Judy A; Heiho Clinic, 697 Front St, Quesnel BC V2J 2K9; Witwatersrand (South Africa)'87; MB BCh; FamilyMed. Langs: Afrikaans; (250)992-2934; Fax. (250)992-2967.

DERDALL, Kirstin; Royal Univ Hosp, 103 Hospital Dr, Saskatoon SK S7N 0W8; Sask'07; Anes. Staff, Royal University Hospital; (306)655-1183; Fax. (306)655-1279.

DERGHAZARIAN, Chahe B; Clinique Medicale Viau, 4750 rue Jarry E, Saint-Leonard QC H1R 1X8; Beirut (Lebanon)'69; ABIM; AB; FRCPC; Hem (P.Q.); IntMed. Assoc Staff, CSSS du Coeur de l'Isle Hôpital Jean-Talon; Assoc Staff, Hopital Louis-H Lafontaine; Langs: English; French; Armenian; Spanish; (514)326-7203

DERIE-GILLESPIE, Lena; The Associate Clinic, PO Box 549 1222 Bev McLachin Dr, Pincher Creek AB T0K 1W0; Cal'08; FamilyMed. (403)627-3321; Fax. (403)627-2280.

DERIGAUD, Pascale; Clinique Familiale St-Lamber, 209 rue Woodstock, Saint-Lambert QC J4P 1W7; Mon'95; (450)466-8583

DERIS, Behado; CSSS de Temiscouata, CP 310 58 rue de l'Eglise, Notre-Dame-du-Lac QC G0L 1X0; Tehran (Iran)'89; Staff, Centre Hospitalier Notre-Dame-du-Lac; (418)899-0214

DERKACH, Peter; 82 Buttonwood Ave, Toronto ON M6M 2J5; McM'77; MSc; BSc; Staff Chief, West Park Healthcare Centre; Staff, Toronto General Hospital - UHN; Med Dir, Ukrainian Care Centre & West Park Long Term Care Centre; Langs: Ukrainian; (416)243-3600 x4100; pderkach@westpark.org.

DERKACH, Sandra E; Peninsula Village Med Clinic, PO Box 408 800-15355 24 Ave, Surrey BC V4A 2H9; UBC'09; CCFP; (604)946-6411

DERKSEN, Angela S L; Seven Oaks Gen Hosp, 2300 McPhillips St, Winnipeg MB R2V 3M3; Man'01; CCFP; CCFP(E.M.); Staff, Seven Oaks General Hospital; (204)632-7133

DERKSEN, Brent; Segue Clinic, 61 James St, St Catharines ON L2R 5B9; UBC'92; CCFP; Staff Emerg, Niagara Health System - Ontario Street Site; (905)688-1827; Fax. (905)688-7283.

DERKSEN, Kenneth J; Orangeville Family Med Centre, M1-32 First St, Orangeville ON L9W 2E1; Wes'82; CCFP; FCFP; Chief of Staff, Headwaters Health Care Centre - Orangeville Site; (519)938-8000; Fax. (519)938-8080.

DERMAN, Ryan; Bigelow-Fowler Clinic, 1605 9 Ave S, Lethbridge AB T1J 1W2; (South Africa)'06; MB BCh; (403)327-3121

DERMARKAR, Julie E; CLSC Montreal-Nord, 11441 boul Lacordaire, Montreal-Nord QC H1G 4J9; Mon'08; (514)384-2000

DERMER, Mark; Family Med Associates, 500-267 O'Connor St, Ottawa ON K2P 1V3; McG'90; CCFP; FCFP; Ac Staff, The Ottawa Hospital - General Campus; Asst Prof, University of Ottawa; (613)232-4817; Fax. (613)232-4818.

DERMER, Stanley W; S W Dermer & Associates, 302-440 Elizabeth St, Burlington ON L7R 2M1; Ott'67; FRCPC; Psy (Disability Psychiatry). (905)681-6680; Fax. (905)681-6681; drdermer@bellnet.ca.

DERMINE, Jean-Francois; Hôp Regional Rimouski, CP 3150 Succ A 150 av Rouleau, Rimouski QC G5L 5T1; Mon'06; AnatPath. Staff, Hôpital Regional Rimouski; (418)724-3000 x8535; Fax. (418)724-8637.

DEROCHE, Steven; 2372 Highway 206 PO Box 3000, Arichat NS B0E 1A0; Sher'09; CCFP; (902)226-1674; Fax. (902)226-9312.

DEROCHER, Christopher S; Duncan Mental Health Centre, 3088 Gibbins Rd, Duncan BC V9L 1E8; UBC'81; FRCPC; Psy. (250)709-3040; Fax. (250)709-3045.

DEROCHER, Mary Elizabeth; Health Centre at 410, 410 Sherbourne St, Toronto ON M5B 1W8; Qns'09; CCFP; (416)999-5217

DEROME, Gaetane; CP 1154, Cochrane ON P0L 1C0; Mon'81; Staff, Centre Hospitalier La Sarre; (705)272-3218

DEROSSIS, Anna M; SMBD Jewish Gen Hosp, E 710-3755 ch Cote-Sainte-Cath, Montreal QC H3T 1E2; McG'92; CSPQ; FRCSC; GenSurg. Staff, Sir Mortimer B Davis Jewish General; Asst Prof Surg, McGill University; (514)340-8222 x4648

DEROUIN, Kim; Associate Med Group, 4705 48 Ave, Red Deer AB T4N 3T1; Alb'89; CCFP; Staff, Associate Medical Group; (403)346-2057; Fax. (403)347-2989.

DEROY, Roma; Clin Med Bourg-Royal, 1289 boul Louis-XIV, Quebec QC G2L 1M1; Laval'87; Langs: Bilingual(French/English); (418)627-7129; Fax. (418)627-7145.

DERRICK, Susan M; Brooklin Med Centre, 1A-5959 Anderson St, Brooklin ON L1M 2E9; Qns'88; BA; CCFP; FCFP; (905)655-3321; Fax. (905)655-4848.

DERRINGTON-FRASER, Danielle; Stonechurch Family Health Ctre, 1475 Upper Ottawa St, Hamilton ON L8W 3J6; McM'06; CCFP; Physician, Stonechurch Family Health Centre; (905)575-7757

DERRY, Heather; Kelowna Gen Hosp, 2268 Pandosy St, Kelowna BC V1Y 1T2; McM'06; FRCPC; Psy. Staff, Kelowna General Hospital; (250)862-4346

DERSNAH, Douglas F; Port Hope Med Centre, 202-249 Ontario St, Port Hope ON L1A 3Y9; Qns'81; EmergMed. Staff, Northumberland Hills Hospital.

DERVAITIS, Kristina L; Newmarket Med Place, 309-712 Davis Dr, Newmarket ON L3Y 8C3; Wes'00; FRCSC; ObstGyn. (905)953-1900

DERVIN, Geoff; The Ottawa Hosp-Gen Campus, W1638-501 Smyth Rd, Ottawa ON K1H 8L6; Ott'88; FRCSC; OrthSurg. Ac Staff, The Ottawa Hospital - General Campus; Asst Prof Surg, University of Ottawa; Langs: French; (613)737-8081; Fax. (613)737-8837.

DERVISH, Greta A; 403-595 Montreal Rd, Ottawa ON K1K 4L2; Wes'91; FRCSC; GenSurg; VascSurg. Staff, Montfort Hospital; Langs: Bilingual(English/French); (613)745-8633; Fax. (613)745-8715.

DERVISH, H Zihni; Montfort Hosp, 713 Montreal Rd, Ottawa ON K1K 0T2; Liverpool (England)'64; FRCS(Eng & Ed); FRCSC; GenSurg. Ac Staff, Montfort Hospital; Court Staff, Children's Hospital of Eastern Ontario (CHEO); Langs: Turkish; French; (613)748-4621

DERY, Catherine; Clinique Med du Berger, 116-1000 ch Sainte-Foy, Quebec QC G1S 2L6; Laval'84; ac Staff, CSSS de Quebec-Sud; (418)688-1385; Fax. (418)688-3249.

DERY, Catherine; CSSS de Beauce-Etchemin, 1515 17e rue, Saint-Georges QC G5Y 4T8; Mon'91; Peds. Staff, Centre Hospitalier Beauce-Etchemin; (418)228-2031 x7670; Fax. (418)227-6246.

DERY, Claude; Clinique Med de Family, 660-2655 boul du Royaume, Jonquiere QC G7S 4S9; Laval'85; Staff, CSSS de Lac-Saint Jean-Est; (418)669-2000

DERY, Francine; CSSS de Lac-Saint Jean-Est, CP 1300 Succ Bureau-Chef 300 boul Champlain S, Alma QC G8B 5W3; Laval'94; CCFP; Staff, CSSS de Lac-Saint Jean-Est; (418)699-2000

DERY, Jean-Paul; Clinique Med 201, 104 rue Sainte-Agathe, Ste-Agathe-des-Mts QC J8C 2K3; Mon'63; FRCSC; ObstGyn. (819)326-2020; Fax. (819)326-8801.

DERY, Jean-Pierre; Hôpital Laval, 2725 ch Sainte-Foy, Quebec QC G1V 4G5; Laval'95; CSPQ; FRCPC; IntMed (Interventional Cardiology); Cardiol. Staff, Hôpital Laval; Langs: English; French; (418)656-8711; Fax. (418)656-4581; jean-pierre.dery@med.ulaval.ca.

DERY, Julie; Hôpital Ste-Justine, 3175 ch Cote-Ste-Catherine, Montreal QC H3T 1C5; Mon'01; FRCPC; DiagRad. Staff, Hôpital Ste-Justine; (514)345-4931

DERY, Lorraine; Hop Charles Lemoyne, 3120 boul Taschereau, Greenfield Park QC J4V 2H1; Sher'86; CSPQ; FRCPC; IntMed. Staff, Hopital Charles LeMoyne; (450)466-5000 x2880

DERY, Marie-Claude; CSSS de Chicoutimi, 305 rue Saint-Vallier, Chicoutimi QC G7H 5H6; Mon'91; CSPQ; FRCSC; GenSurg (Surgical Oncology). Staff, Complexe hospitalier de la Sagamie; Prof adj clin, Universite de Montreal; Prof adj clin, Universite de Sherbrooke; Langs: Bilingual(French/English); (418)615-0775; Fax. (418)615-0776; ccsinfo@utago.net.

DERY, Pierre; CHUQ-Ctr Hosp Univ Laval, R 1742-2705 boul Laurier, Quebec QC G1V 4G2; Laval'69; CSPQ; Peds (Infectious Diseases). Chef InfectDis, Centre Hospitalier Universitaire de Quebec-CHUL; Prof Dept of Peds, Université Laval; Langs: Bilingual(English/French); (418)654-2282; Fax. (418)654-2137; pierre.dery@ped.ulaval.ca.

DERY, Renee; CHUM-Hop St-Luc, 1058 rue Saint-Denis, Montreal QC H2X 3J4; Laval'78; ABR; FRCPC; DiagRad (Abdominal Imaging). adj Radiologiste, Centre Hospitalier l'Université De Montréal (CHUM) - Hôpital Saint-luc; assoc Prof, Universite de Montreal; Langs: English; French; (514)890-8000 x36400; Fax. (514)412-7359.

DERY, Richard L; CSSS de la Mitis, 800 av du Sanatorium, Mont-Joli QC G5H 3L6; Laval'82; Staff, CSSS de la Mitis; (418)775-7261; Fax. (418)775-1989.

DERY, Richard; Ctr de Sante de la Basse Cote, CP 130 1070 boul Dr Camille Marcou, Lourdes-d-Bl-Sabl QC G0G 1W0; Mon'78; Staff, CSSS de la Basse Côté-Nord; (418)461-2144

DERY, Stephane; CSSS de Chicoutimi, CO 5006 305 rue Saint-Vallier, Chicoutimi QC G7H 5H6; Sher'92; Staff, Complexe hospitalier de la Sagamie; Langs: Bilingual(French/English); (418)541-1012

DERY, Veronique; AETMIS, 10.083-2021 av Union, Montreal QC H3A 2S9; Sher'78; FRCPC; CommunMed (P.Q.) (Metabolism); Public Health & Preventive Med. Staff, Hôpital Ste-Justine; Langs: English; French; (514)873-9766; veronique.dery@aetmis.gouv.qc.ca.

DERZKO, Christine M; St Michael's Orthopaedic Assoc, 408-55 Queen St E, Toronto ON M5C 1R6; Tor'67; FRCSC; ObstGyn (Osteoporosis). Consultant Bone Marrow Transplant, Princess Margaret Hospital - University Health Network; Staff ObstGyn & Med (Endocrin), St Michael's Hospital; Assoc Prof Obstgyn & Internal Med Endocrinology, University of Toronto; Langs: Ukrainian; Polish; (416)866-7400; Fax. (416)866-7401; derzkoc@smh.ca.

DERZKO, Lydia A L; Nelson House Nursing Station, GD, Nelson House MB R0B 1A0; Man'77; Langs: Ukrainian; (204)484-2031; Fax. (204)484-2284.

DERZKO-DZULYNSKY, Larissa A; Islington Med Clinic, 903-1243 Islington Ave, Etobicoke ON M8X 1Y9; Tor'93; FRCS; FRCSC; Ophth (Uveitis). Staff, St Joseph's Health Centre; Staff, St Michael's Hospital; Asst Prof, University of Toronto; Langs: Ukrainian; Polish; French; (416)760-8763; Fax. (416)760-8627.

DES AULNIERS, Evelyne; CLSC L'Estran Grande-Vallee, 71 boul St-Francois-Xavier E, Grande-Vallee QC G0E 1K0; Mon'81; CCFP; (418)393-2001; Fax. (418)393-2767.

DES GROSEILLIERS, Sylvain; CSSS Pierre Boucher, 1333 boul Jacques-Cartier E, Longueuil QC J4M 2A5; Mon'86; FACS; CSPQ; FRCSC; GenSurg (Surgical Oncology). Staff, Centre Hospitalier Pierre Boucher; Langs: Bilingual(French/English); (450)468-8111; Fax. (450)670-8830; sdgmd@videotrun.ca.

DES LANDES, Lysanne; CSSS de Chicoutimi, 305 rue Saint-Vallier, Chicoutimi QC G7H 5H6; Sher'04; CCFP; CCFP(E.M.); Staff, Complexe hospitalier de la Sagamie; (418)541-1000

DES MARAIS, Lison; Clinique Med Du 2101, 2101 boul Edouard-Montpetit, Montreal QC H3T 1J3; Mon'81; (514)343-6452; Fax. (514)343-7236.

DES MARCHAIS, Beatrice; 1050 ch Sainte-Foy, Quebec QC G1S 4L8; Sher'91; FRCSC; Ophth (Glaucoma). Staff, Centre Hospitalier Affilié Universitaire de Québec - Hôpital du St-Sacrement; (418)682-7511 x4739; b.desmarchais@sympatico.ca.

DES MARCHAIS, Jacques E; Centre Bois De Boulogne, 350-1575 boul Henri-Bourassa O, Montreal QC H3M 3A9; Mon'64; MSc; FAAOS; MA(Ed); CSPQ; FRCSC; OrthSurg (Forensic Medical Assessment). Ac Staff, Centre Hospitalier Universitaire de Sherbrooke-Hopital Fleurimont; Chairman Central Examination Committee, Royal College Of Physicians &; Staff Teacher, Universite de Sherbrooke; Langs: Italian; (514)333-0424

DES PAROIS, Lucie; Hop Charles Lemoyne, 3120 boul Taschereau, Greenfield Park QC J4V 2H1; Sher'90; FRCPC; Psy (Electroconvulsive Therapy). Staff, Hopital Charles LeMoyne; Langs: English; (450)466-5020; Fax. (450)466-5015; ldesparois@yahoo.com.

DES ROCHES, Anne; Hôpital Ste-Justine, 3175 ch Cote-Ste-Catherine, Montreal QC H3T 1C5; Laval'90; FRCPC; Peds (Pediatric Allergy); ClinImmunol&Allergy (P.Q.). Staff, Hôpital Ste-Justine; adj Prof Med, Universite de Montreal; (514)345-4837; Fax. (514)345-2134.

DES ROCHES, Benoit P; Clinique Med Mont St-Hilaire, 261 boul Laurier, Mont-Saint-Hilaire QC J3H 3N8; Ott'85; FRCPC; Psy. Langs: Bilingual(French/English); (450)464-5151; Fax. (450)464-3703.

DES ROCHES, Renee; Hotel-Dieu de Levis, 143 rue Wolfe, Levis QC G6V 3Z1; Laval'87; FRCSC; Ophth (General). Staff Ophth, Hôtel-Dieu de Lévis; (418)835-7121

DES ROSIERS, Joel; Clin Externe Psychiatrie, 203-100 rue Grenier, Charlemagne QC J5Z 4C6; Mon'81; FRCPC; Psy (P.Q.). Staff, Centre Hospitalier Pierre le Gardeur; (450)585-9012; Fax. (450)585-9762.

DES ROSIERS, Pascale; St Mary's Hosp Centre, 3830 av Lacombe, Montreal QC H3T 1M5; Sher'85; FRCPC; Psy (AIDS/HIV). Staff, McGill University Health Centre - Montreal General Campus; Staff, St Mary's Hospital Centre; adj Prof, McGill University; (514)345-3511; desrosiep@videotron.ca.

DESAI, Dennis; Canadian Med Protective Assn, 875 Carling Ave, Ottawa ON K1S 5P1; Ott'85; FACS; FRCSC; GenSurg. Staff, Canadian Medical Protective Association; (613)725-2000; Fax. (613)725-1300.

DESAI, Devanshu; St Joseph's Health Centre, 30 The Queensway, Toronto ON M6R 1B5; Gujarat (India)'83; MB BS; FRCPC; Psy (Addiction Psychiatry). Clin Dir Day Treatment Program & Staff Psy, St Joseph's Health Centre; Consultant Psy, Centre for Addiction & Mental Health (CAMH) - Russell Street Site; Psychiatrist, Etobicoke Medical Centre Family Health Team; Teacher, University of Toronto; Langs: Gujarati; Hindi; (416)530-6486 x3019; Fax. (416)530-6076.

DESAI, Devdatta M; Mount Sinai Hosp, 1514-600 University Ave, Toronto ON M5G 1X5; Pune (India)'98; Staff, Mount Sinai Hospital; (416)586-5270

DESAI, Dushyant; 301-310 King St E, Kitchener ON N2G 2L3; Natal (South Africa)'80; FRCPC; IntMed; Cardiol. Staff, St Mary's General Hospital; Langs: Gujarati; Hindi; (519)579-8889

DESAI, Ghanshyam R; Mount Pearl Med Centre, PO Box 100 Rpo Centennial Sq 12 St David's Ave, Mount Pearl NL A1N 2C1; Dublin (Ireland)'72; MB ChB; (709)368-8381

DESAI, Heena Y; Hamilton HSC-McMaster Site, PO Box 2000 Stn Lcd 1 1200 Main St W, Hamilton ON L8N 3Z5; (USA)'03; Staff, Hamilton Health Sciences Centre - McMaster Children's Hospital; (905)521-2100

DESAI, Hiren B; 259-1720 Howard Ave, Windsor ON N8X 5A6; Bombay (India)'84; MB BS; DAB; FRCPC; Neur (Clinical Trials). Staff, Hôtel-Dieu Grace Hospital; Staff, Windsor Regional Hospital - Metropolitan Site; Langs: Gujarati; Hindi; Marathi; (519)254-4424; Fax. (866)558-2115.

DESAI, Jagdish; Brant Community HC-Brantford, 200 Terrace Hill St, Brantford ON N3R 1G9; Birmingham (England)'70; DA; Ac Staff, The Brant Community Healthcare System - Brantford General Hospital Site; Med Dir, John Noble Home for Aged; Langs: Gujarati; Hindi; (519)759-0946

DESAI, Jamsheed; Foothills Med Centre, 1162-1403 29 St NW, Calgary AB T2N 2T9; Qns'07; Neur. Staff, Foothills Medical Centre; (403)944-1110

DESAI, Milind G; B3-4640 Jane St, North York ON M3N 2K5; Gujarat (India)'83; FRCP; DABIM; Gastroent; IntMed (Hepatology). Staff, Humber River Regional Hospital - Finch Avenue Site; Langs: Marathi; Punjabi; Hindi; Gujarati; Urdu; (416)663-1250; Fax. (416)663-8561; milinddesai@rogers.com.

DESAI, Nimesh; 7A-260 Holiday Inn Dr, Cambridge ON N3C 4E8; Wes'02; FRCSC; Ophth. Associate, Cambridge Memorial Hospital; Associate, St Mary's General Hospital; Associate, Grand River Hospital - Kitchener/Waterloo Health Centre; Langs: Gujarati; (519)658-6800; Fax. (519)658-6801.

DESAI, Parag; Kingsbridge Med Centre, 5-20 Kingsbridge Garden Cir, Mississauga ON L5R 3K7; (USA)'05; (905)507-1111; Fax. (905)890-7102.

DESAI, Rashmikant J; The Credit Valley Hosp, 2200 Eglinton Ave W, Mississauga ON L5M 2N1; Birmingham (England)'65; MRCS; DAB; FRCS(Eng & Ed); FACS; FRCSC; Urol (Prostate Disorder). Staff, The Credit Valley Hospital; Ac Staff, Grey Bruce Health Services - Owen Sound; Ac Staff, Grey Bruce Health Services - Meaford Site; Langs: Gujarati; (905)813-2200; desai2341@rogers.com.

DESAI, Satish S; 101-156 Morison Ave PO Box 220 Stn Main, Parksville BC V9P 2G4; London (England)'73; DRCOG; DCH; MRCP; MB BS; Assoc Staff, Nanaimo Regional General Hospital; Langs: Hindi; Gujarati; (250)248-3133; Fax. (250)248-3178; snvdesai@shaw.ca.

DESAI, Shailesh M; Willoughby Medical Centre, B1A-20202 66 Ave, Langley BC V2Y 1P3; Natal (South Africa)'91; MB ChB; CCFP; (604)514-8800

DESAI, Shalini; Toronto East Gen Hosp Inc, 825 Coxwell Ave, Toronto ON M4C 3E7; Tor'02; FRCPC; Peds; InfectDis. Staff, Toronto East General Hospital Inc; Langs: Gujarati; (416)461-8272

DESAI, Sunil; University of Alberta, 4E2WMC-8440 112 St NW, Edmonton AB T6G 2B7; Bristol (England)'76; MB BS; DCH; MRCP; FRCPC; Peds (Pediatric Hematology Oncology). Staff, University of Alberta Hospital; Sr Specialist Peds, Cross Cancer Institute; Langs: Gujarati; (780)407-8829; Fax. (780)407-7476; sunil.desai@albertahealthservices.ca.

DESAI, Vikas R; Royal Inland Hosp, 311 Columbia St, Kamloops BC V2C 2T1; Ott'89; BSc(Hon); CCFP; CCFP(E.M.); Ac Staff, Royal Inland Hospital; Langs: French; (250)374-5111

DESAI-RANCHOD, Smeeta; 190-9040 Blundell Rd, Richmond BC V6Y 1K3; Natal (South Africa)'85; DCH; MB ChB; Staff, Providence Health Care - Mount Saint Joseph Hospital; Langs: Hindi; (604)284-5255

DESARKAR, Pushpal; Addiction & Mental Hlth-Queen, 401-1001 Queen St W, Toronto ON M6J 1H4; Calcutta (India)'00; Staff, Centre for Addiction & Mental Health (CAMH) - Queen Site; Langs: Bengali; Hindi; (416)535-8501

DESAULNIERS, Denis; 1050 avenue de la Médecine Pavillon Vandry, Quebec QC G1V 0A6; Mon'66; FACC; FACS; CSPQ; AddicMed; Cardiovasc&ThorSurg. Dir Div Anatomie Dep of GenSurg, Université Laval; Langs: Bilingual(French/English); (418)656-2131 x4516; Fax. (418)656-3821; denis.desaulniers@chg.ulaval.ca.

DESAULNIERS, Gerald; Clin Med Urgence Brossard, 7601 boul Taschereau, Brossard QC J4Y 1A2; Laval'78; Dir Prof Serv, Centre Hospitalier de Chandler; Health & Social Services, Montreal; (450)462-0863

DESAULNIERS, Gilles; Edifice Medical Fleury, 2320 rue Fleury E, Montreal QC H2B 1K9; Mon'72; DObstRCOG; FACOG; FRCS; FRCSC; ObstGyn (Laparoscopy). Staff, Centre Hospitalier Fleury; Assoc Prof ObstGyn, McGill University; adj Prof, Universite de Montreal; Langs: Bilingual(French/English); (514)336-0883; Fax. (514)336-2586; secretairegyneco@gmail.com.

DESAULNIERS, Jean; 1871 rue Royale, Trois-Rivieres QC G9A 4K7; Sher'84; CCFP; FCFP; (819)371-2522; Fax. (819)371-9744.

DESAULNIERS, Pierre; CHUM-Hotel-Dieu, 3840 rue Saint-Urbain, Montreal QC H2W 1T8; Mon'84; EmergMed (P.Q.). Staff, Centre Hospitalier l'Université de Montréal (CHUM) - Hôtel-Dieu; (514)890-8159; Fax. (514)412-7114; dsn@videotron.ca.

DESAULNIERS, Rene C; Hotel-Dieu de Levis, 143 rue Wolfe, Levis QC G6V 3Z1; Mon'68; CSPQ; GenSurg (P.Q.). Staff, Hôtel-Dieu de Lévis; Université Laval; (418)835-7121

DESAUTELS, Alex; Hop du Sacre-Coeur de Mtl, 5400 boul Gouin O, Montreal QC H4J 1C5; Mon'06; FRCPC; Neur. Staff, Hôpital du Sacre-Coeur de Montréal; (418)872-0895

DESAUTELS, Annie; CSSS Pierre Boucher, 1333 boul Jacques-Cartier E, Longueuil QC J4M 2A5; Mon'99; FRCPC; DiagRad. Staff, Centre Hospitalier Pierre Boucher; (450)468-8111

DESAUTELS, Charles; Clinique Chir Ortho C-Lemoyne, 126 rue Saint-Louis, Lemoyne QC J4R 2L5; Sher'85; CSPQ; FRCSC; OrthSurg. Staff Orth, Hopital Charles LeMoyne; (450)672-1212; Fax. (450)672-9834.

DESAUTELS, Lyne; Clinique Familiale, 140-7055 boul Taschereau, Longueuil QC J4Z 1A7; Sher'94; (450)332-2430

DESAUTELS, Michel; Clin Fam des Basses Laurentide, 2100 boul Labelle, Saint-Jerome QC J7Y 1S8; Mon'85; (450)565-1227; Fax. (450)565-1099.

DESAUTELS, Pascale; 1760 boul Jacques-Cartier E, Longueuil QC J4N 1C2; Sher'91; ObstGyn. (450)468-2151

DESAUTELS, Rene; Douglas Mental Hlth Univ Inst, 6875 boul LaSalle, Verdun QC H4H 1R3; McG'84; FRCPC; Psy (Geriatric Psychiatry). Dir Geriatric Psy, McGill University; Langs: English; (514)761-6131 x2160; Fax. (514)762-3014; rene.desautels@douglas.mcgill.ca.

DESAUTELS, Rosaire; Clinique Fam de St-Hyacinthe, 2955 boul Laframboise, Saint-Hyacinthe QC J2S 4Z3; Mon'72; Staff GP, Centre Hospitalier Honore-Mercier; (450)774-4611; Fax. (450)773-9913.

DESAUTELS, Sophie; Hop Maisonneuve-Rosemont, 5415 boul de l'Assomption, Montreal QC H1T 2M4; Laval'03; FRCPC; Psy. Staff, Hopital Maisonneuve-Rosemont; (514)252-3400 x5872

DESBIENS, Alain; Clinique Med D'Alma, 935 av du Pont S, Alma QC G8B 2V5; Laval'83; Langs: Bilingual(French/English); (418)668-6121; Fax. (418)668-5298.

DESBIENS, Christine; Ctr Hosp Affilie-St-Sacrement, 1050 ch Sainte-Foy, Quebec QC G1S 4L8; Laval'88; LMCC; CSPQ; FRCSC; GenSurg (Surgical Oncology); General Surgical Oncology (P.Q.). Staff Oncologie Surgeon, Centre Hospitalier Affilié Universitaire de Québec - Hôpital du St-Sacrement; (418)682-7511; Fax. (418)682-7956.

DESBIENS, Denis; Clinique Med Ste-Therese, 101-233 rue Turgeon, Sainte-Therese QC J7E 3J8; Sher'85; (450)430-1030

DESBIENS, France; CSSS d'Argenteuil, 145 av de la Providence, Lachute QC J8H 4C7; Laval'91; Staff, Centre Hospitalier d'Argenteuil; (450)562-3761 x8179; Fax. (450)562-2111.

DESBIENS, Francois; Centre du Sante Publique, 2400 av D'Estimauville, Quebec QC G1E 7G9; Sher'80; MPH; FRCPC; CommunMed; Public Health & Preventive Med. assoc Membre Public Health, Centre Hospitalier Affilié Universitaire de Québec - Hôpital du St-Sacrement; (418)666-7000 x400; Fax. (418)666-2766.

DESBIENS, Genevieve; CHUQ-St-Francois D'Assise, 10 rue de l'Espinay, Quebec QC G1L 3L5; Laval'08; CCFP; Staff, Centre Hospitalier Universitaire De Québec - Pavillon De St-françois-d'assise; (418)525-4351

DESBIENS, Genevieve; Ctr Hosp Fleury, 2180 rue Fleury E, Montreal QC H2B 1K3; Mon'98; FRCSC; Urol. Staff, Centre Hospitalier Fleury; (514)381-9311

DESBIENS, Isabelle; Reseau Sante Richelieu-Yamaska, 1800 rue dessaulles, Saint-Hyacinthe QC J2S 2T2; Mon'94; FRCPC; PhysMed&Rehab (Neuro Rehabilitation). Physical Med & Rehab, Centre d hebergement de l Hôtel-Dieu de Saint-Hyacinthe; Staff, Centre Montérégien De Réadaptation; Langs: Bilingual(French/English); (450)774-5003; Fax. (450)771-3667; isabelle.desbiens@rrsss16.gouv.qc.ca.

DESBIENS, Marie-Therese; Clinique Med Saint-Gabriel, 85 rue Saint-Gabriel, St-Gabriel-D-Brand QC J0K 2N0; Mon'87; (450)835-3431

DESBIENS, Paul; Clinique Med de l'Est Inc, 220-8 Place du Commerce, Verdun QC H3E 1N3; Laval'65; CSPQ; FRCPC; Anes. Staff, CSSS du Coeur de l'Isle Hôpital Jean-Talon; (514)281-2022

DESBIENS, Rene; Hop Charles LeMoyne, 3120 boul Taschereau, Greenfield Park QC J4V 2H1; Laval'65; Urol. Staff, Hopital Charles LeMoyne; (450)466-5000

DESBIENS, Richard; Ctr Hosp Affilie-Enfant-Jesus, 1401 18e rue, Quebec QC G1J 1Z4; Laval'85; FRCPC; Neur (Electroencephalography); Electroenceph (P.Q.). Ac Member, Centre Hospitalier Affilié Universitaire de Québec - Hôpital De L'Enfant Jésus; Consultant, Centre Hospitalier Universitaire de Quebec-CHUL; (418)649-5734; Fax. (418)649-5915; richard.desbiens.cha@ssss.gouv.qc.ca.

DESBIENS, Serge; CHUQ-Hotel-Dieu de Quebec, 11 Cote du Palais, Quebec QC G1R 2J6; Laval'82; Neur (Neuromuscular Diseases). Staff, Centre Hospitalier Universitaire de Québec (CHUQ) - Siege Social; (418)691-5288; Fax. (418)691-5186.

DESBOIS, Nathalie A; Carlisle Med Centre, PO Box 311 1493 Centre Rd, Carlisle ON L0R 1H0; McM'00; CCFP; Langs: French; (905)689-3301; Fax. (905)689-5772.

DESCARRIES, Laurence; CSSS de Laval, CP 144 1755 boul Rene-Laennec, Laval QC H7M 3L9; Mon'00; FRCPC; IntMed; Cardiol. Staff, Hopital de la Cite de la santé; (450)668-1010

DESCHAINTRE, Yan; CHUM-Hop Notre-Dame, GR 1166-1560 rue Sherbrooke E, Montreal QC H2L 4M1; Mon'00; FRCPC; Neur (Vasculities). Staff, Centre Hospitalier l'Université de Montréal (CHUM) - Hôpital Notre-Dame; Prof adj clin, Universite de Montreal; Langs: Bilingual(French/English); (514)890-8000 x26260; Fax. (514)412-7556.

DESCHAMBAULT, Jean; CRSSS Baie-james-Sante Isle-D, CP 790 130 boul Matagami, Matagami QC J0Y 2A0; Mon'97; Fam Med, Centre de Sante Isle-Dieu Matagami; (819)739-2515; Fax. (819)739-6059.

DESCHAMBEAULT, Julie; CSSS du Nord de Lanaudière, 1000 boul Sainte-Anne, St-Charles-Brromee QC J6E 6J2; Mon'02; Staff, Centre Hospitalier Régional de Lanaudière; (450)759-8222

DESCHAMPS, Alain; Institut de Cardiologie de Mtl, 5000 rue Belanger, Montreal QC H1T 1C8; Mon'96; CSPQ; FRCPC; Anes (Research). Staff, Institut de Cardiologie de Montréal; (514)376-3330 x3732

DESCHAMPS, Benoit; Hop Charles LeMoyne, 3120 boul Taschereau, Greenfield Park QC J4V 2H1; Mon'03; FRCPC; Psy. Staff, Hopital Charles LeMoyne; (450)466-5000

DESCHAMPS, Benoit J; St Mary's Hosp Centre, 3830 av Lacombe, Montreal QC H3T 1M5; Cal'93; Staff, St Mary's Hospital Centre; Teacher, McGill University; (514)345-3511 x3168; Fax. (514)734-2623.

DESCHAMPS, Charles; CSSS de la Haute-Yamaska, 205 boul Leclerc O, Granby QC J2G 1T7; Mon'93; Staff, Centre Hospitalier de Granby; (450)372-5491; Fax. (450)372-7197.

DESCHAMPS, Jean-Pierre; Centre Medcal l'Enjeu, 1140 av Beaumont, Mont-Royal QC H3P 3E5; Mon'81; CSPQ; FRCPC; IntMed; Cardiol (P.Q.). (514)288-7770

DESCHAMPS, Julie; CRSSS Baie-James-Chibougamau, 51 3e rue, Chibougamau QC G8P 1N1; Mon'10; CCFP; Staff, CRSSS de la Baie-James; (418)748-2676

DESCHAMPS, Lyne; 405-5811 boul Taschereau, Brossard QC J4Z 1A5; Mon'81; Peds. Ac Staff, Hopital Charles LeMoyne; Assoc Staff, Hôpital Ste-Justine; (450)443-6585

DESCHAMPS, Nicole; Clinique Medicale, 203-2200 ch de Chambly, Longueuil QC J4J 3Z3; Mon'77; FRCSC; Otol. Otolaryngology, Centre Hospitalier Pierre Boucher; (450)674-3042; Fax. (450)674-9946.

DESCHENE, Jane M; Au Chateau Home for the Aged, 100 Michaud St, Sturgeon Falls ON P2B 2Z4; Wes'81; Physician, Au Chateau Home for the Aged; (705)753-4466; Fax. (705)753-6507.

DESCHENES, Annie; Clinique Med Frontenac, 24 rue Frontenac, Riviere-du-Loup QC G5R 1S5; Sher'06; Staff, Centre Hospitalier Regional du Grand-Portage; (418)862-0333; Fax. (418)868-0505.

DESCHENES, Catherine; Ctr Hosp de Charlevoix, 74 rue Ambroise-Fafard, Baie-Saint-Paul QC G3Z 2J6; Laval'06; CCFP; (418)435-5150; Fax. (418)435-3315.

DESCHENES, Christian; CSSS de la Haute-Yamaska, 205 boul Leclerc O, Granby QC J2G 1T7; Mon'01; Staff, Centre Hospitalier de Granby; (450)375-8000

DESCHENES, Christian; 328 boul Antonio-Barrette, N-D-Des-Prairies QC J6E 1G2; Mon'86; FRCSC; Ophth (Glaucoma). ac Staff, Centre Hospitalier Régional de Lanaudière; Langs: Bilingual(French/English); (450)752-4141; Fax. (450)752-4483.

DESCHENES, Christiane S; 4-75 Spring St, Almonte ON K0A 1A0; Mon'76; Ac Staff, Almonte General Hospital; Langs: Bilingual(English/French); (613)256-1678; Fax. (613)256-4381.

DESCHENES, Dominique; 143 rue Wolfe, Levis QC G6V 3Z1; Laval'02; Respir; IntMed (Critical Care Medicine). Staff, Hôtel-Dieu de Lévis; Langs: English; French; (418)835-7121

DESCHENES, Dominique; Unite de Med Fam Laurier, 2 4F-2875 boul Laurier, Quebec QC G1V 2M2; Laval'03; CCFP; Staff, Centre Hospitalier Régional Baie-Comeau; Langs: Spanish; English; (418)654-2701; Fax. (418)654-2138.

DESCHENES, Elaine; Clinique Nos Enfants, 488 rue Centrale, Memramcook NB E4K 3S6; Sher'93; FRCPC; Peds. Staff Peds, Dr Georges-L-Dumont University Hospital Centre; Langs: Bilingual(French/English); (506)758-0440; Fax. (506)758-2615.

DESCHENES, Francois; CRSSS Baie-james-Sante Isle-D, CP 790 130 boul Matagami, Matagami QC J0Y 2A0; Mon'91; Staff, Centre de Sante Isle-Dieu Matagami; (819)739-2515

DESCHENES, Helene; CLSC Saint-Hubert, 6800 boul Cousineau, Saint-Hubert QC J3Y 8Z4; Mon'01; CCFP; (450)443-7407

DESCHENES, Isabelle; Centre Medi-Soleil, 120-383 boul du Seminaire N, St-Jean-sur-Richel QC J3B 8C5; Sher'00; FRCPC; IntMed; Rheum. Langs: English; (450)349-5555

DESCHENES, Jacques C; 12021 15e av, Montreal QC H1E 0A1; Mon'70; Langs: Bilingual(French/English); (514)648-9620; Fax. (514)648-8634.

DESCHENES, Jean; MUHC-Royal Victoria Hosp, E4 57-687 av des Pins O, Montreal QC H3A 1A1; Laval'79; FACS; FRCSC; Ophth. Staff, McGill University Health Centre - Royal Victoria Hospital; (514)843-1625; Fax. (514)843-1618.

DESCHENES, Jean L; Cross Cancer Institute, 11560 University Ave NW, Edmonton AB T6G 1Z2; Laval'86; FRCPC; AnatPath. Staff, Cross Cancer Institute; (780)432-8453; Fax. (780)432-8455.

DESCHENES, Jean-Marie; CLSC Pohenegamock, 1922 rue Saint-Vallier RR 2, Pohenegamook QC G0L 1J0; Laval'72; (418)859-2450; Fax. (418)859-3274.

DESCHENES, Jean-Pierre; CLSC-CHSLD Mrc Denis-Riverin, 50 rue du Belvedere, Ste-Anne-des-Monts QC G4V 1X4; Laval'71; IntMed (P.Q.). Staff, Centre Hospitalier des Monts; (418)763-2261; Fax. (418)763-3600.

DESCHENES, Julie; CSSS Pierre Boucher, 1333 boul Jacques-Cartier E, Longueuil QC J4M 2A5; Sher'99; FRCPC; IntMed (Pneumology); Respir. Staff, Centre Hospitalier Pierre Boucher; Langs: Bilingual(English/French); (450)468-8111

DESCHENES, Louise; CHUQ-Hotel-Dieu de Quebec, 11 Cote du Palais, Quebec QC G1R 2J6; Laval'84; MSc; FRCPC; MedMicrobiol; Microbio & Infect Dis (P.Q.). Staff Microbiol & InfectDis, Centre Hospitalier Universitaire de Québec (CHUQ) - Siege Social; (418)691-5151; louise.deschenes@chuq.qc.ca.

DESCHENES, Majorie; Ctr Hosp Affilie-Enfant-Jesus, 1401 18e rue, Quebec QC G1J 1Z4; Sher'02; FRCPC; AnatPath. Staff, Centre Hospitalier Affilié Universitaire de Québec - Hôpital De L'Enfant Jésus; (418)682-7511

DESCHENES, Marc; MUHC-Royal Victoria Hosp, R2 28-687 av des Pins O, Montreal QC H3A 1A1; McG'88; FRCPC; IntMed (Hematology Pathology); Gastroent. Staff, McGill University Health Centre - Royal Victoria Hospital; (514)843-1616; Fax. (514)843-1421.

DESCHENES, Marianne; CHUQ-Ctr Hosp Univ Laval, 2705 boul Laurier, Quebec QC G1V 4G2; Laval'98; FRCPC; Peds (Neonatal & Perinatal Medicine). Staff, Centre Hospitalier Universitaire de Quebec-CHUL; (418)656-4141

DESCHENES, Marie-Andree; CSSSM UMF Manicouagan, 340 rue Clement-Lavoie, Baie-Comeau QC G4Z 3B8; Laval'97; CCFP; (418)296-2421; Fax. (418)294-2862.

DESCHENES, Mario; College des Med du Quebec, 2170 boul Rene-Levesque O, Montreal QC H3H 2T8; Laval'85; Ac Staff, Centre Hospitalier Universitaire de Quebec-CHUL; (514)933-4441; Fax. (514)933-3112.

DESCHENES, Michel; CHUQ-Ctr Hosp Univ Laval, 2705 boul Laurier, Quebec QC G1V 4G2; Laval'75; EmergMed (P.Q.). Ac Staff, Centre Hospitalier Universitaire de Quebec-CHUL; (418)654-2114; Fax. (418)525-4564.

DESCHÊNES-LAPOINTE, Anne-Claire; Hôp Notre-Dame-du-Lac, CP 310 58 rue de l'Eglise, Notre-Dame-du-Lac QC G0L 1X0; Sher'09; CCFP; Staff, Centre Hospitalier Notre-Dame-du-Lac; (418)899-6751; Fax. (418)899-2809.

DESCHESNES, Dimitrios E; Ctr Hosp Reg Chisasibi, PO Box 250, Chisasibi QC J0M 1E0; McG'90; CCFP; CCFP(E.M.); Staff, Cree Board of Health & Social Services James Bay; (819)855-2844; Fax. (819)855-2867.

DESCHESNES, Judy; Ctr Hosp Trois-Riv-St-Joseph, 2F-731 rue St-Julie, Trois-Rivieres QC G9A 1Y1; Laval'09; Staff, Centre Hospitalier Regional de Trois-Rivieres; (819)372-3536; Fax. (819)372-3509.

DESCOINGS, Benedicte; Hop Jean-Talon, 1385 rue Jean-Talon E, Montreal QC H2E 1S6; Paris (France)'83; Staff, CSSS du Coeur de l'Isle Hôpital Jean-Talon; (514)495-6757

DESCOMBES, Andre; GMF des Seigneuries, 2220 boul Rene-Gaultier, Varennes QC J3X 1T6; Laval'86; (450)652-2917; Fax. (450)652-6418.

DESCOTEAUX, Chantal; Clinique de Sante Bagotville, CP 5000, Alouette QC G0V 1A0; Laval'91; CCFP; (418)677-4000 x7700

DESCOTEAUX, Isabelle; CSSS de la Mitis, 800 av du Sanatorium, Mont-Joli QC G5H 3L6; Laval'95; Staff, CSSS de la Mitis; (418)775-7261 x3100; Fax. (418)775-6487.

DESCOTEAUX, Jean-Gaston; Golden Med Clinic, PO Box 1170, Golden BC V0A 1H0; Ott'85; MA(MedEd); FRCSC; GenSurg. Langs: Bilingual(English/French); (250)344-2840; Fax. (250)344-2840.

DESCOTEAUX, Marc I; Hopital Jean-Talon, 1385 rue Jean-Talon E, Montreal QC H2E 1S6; Mon'91; Staff, CSSS du Coeur de l'Isle Hôpital Jean-Talon; Staff, Institut de Cardiologie de Montréal; (514)495-6733

DESFORGES, Johanne; Clin Medico Chirurgicale de Ve, 48-55 av de l'Eglise, Verdun QC H4G 3E7; Mon'87; (514)768-5833; Fax. (514)768-4447.

DESFOSSES, Annik; CSSS de Laval, 1755 boul Rene-Laennec, Laval QC H7M 3L9; Mon'00; Staff, Hopital de la Cite de la santé; (450)668-1010

DESGAGNE, Catherine; Centre Hosp Honore-Mercier, 2750 boul Laframboise, Saint-Hyacinthe QC J2S 4Y8; Sher'09; Staff, Centre Hospitalier Honore-Mercier; (450)771-3333

DESGAGNE, Luc; CHUQ-Ctr Hosp Univ Laval, 2705 boul Laurier, Quebec QC G1V 4G2; Laval'99; CSPQ; FRCPC; Anes. Staff, Centre Hospitalier Universitaire de Quebec-CHUL; (418)656-4141

DESGAGNE, Micheline; Clinique Med Caplan, 149 Rte 132 O, Caplan QC G0C 1H0; Mon'85; Langs: English; (418)388-2201; Fax. (418)388-2301.

DESGAGNES, Jean-Francois; Clinique Med Antoine-Labelle, 210-555 boul Saint-Antoine, Saint-Jerome QC J7Z 3B8; Mon'79; FRCPC; Derm (Sports Medicine). Staff, Hôtel-Dieu de Saint-Jérôme; Langs: Bilingual(French/English); (450)565-6522; Fax. (450)565-6524.

DESGAGNES, Julie; Clin Med Plateau Marquette, 200-731 rue Galt O, Sherbrooke QC J1H 1Z1; Mon'93; Staff, Centre Hospitalier Universitaire de Sherbrooke-Hôpital Hôtel-Dieu; (819)564-8542; Fax. (819)564-1294.

DESGAGNES, Marie-Christine; Centre Hosp Honore-Mercier, 2750 boul Laframboise, Saint-Hyacinthe QC J2S 4Y8; Laval'05; Anes. Staff, Centre Hospitalier Honore-Mercier; (450)771-3333

DESGRANGES, Marie-Francoise; Clinique Med Centrale, 2050 rue Regent, Saint-Hubert QC J4T 3R5; Lyon (France)'71; Peds. Chef pédiatrie, Centre Hospitalier l'Université de Montréal (CHUM) - Hôpital Notre-Dame; Asst Prof Peds, Universite de Montreal; (450)678-9194 x6884

DESGRENIERS, Guy; CLSC de Pohenegamook, 1922 rue Saint-Vallier RR 2, Pohenegamook QC G0L 1J0; Mon'87; Staff, Centre Hospitalier Regional du Grand-Portage; (418)859-2450

DESGROSEILLIERS, Anik; Inst de l'Oeil de Laurentides, 4800 rue Ambroise-Lafortune, Sainte-Therese QC J7H 1S6; Mon'07; Ophth. (450)419-6345

DESGROSEILLIERS, Denise; Clin Med L'Avenir, 200-1150 boul de l'Avenir, Laval QC H7N 6L2; Mon'87; (450)680-1150

DESGROSEILLIERS, Jean-Pierre; Bruyere Continuing Care, 75 Bruyere St, Ottawa ON K1N 5C7; Ott'65; MSc(Pharm.); FRCPC; Derm. Consultant Staff, The Ottawa Hospital - Civic Campus; Staff Photoderm Clinic, SCO Health Service - Élisabeth Bruyère Hospital; Prof Derm, University of Ottawa; Langs: French; (613)562-6354; Fax. (613)562-6022.

DESHAIES, Annie; CHUS-Hop Hotel-Dieu, 580 rue Bowen S, Sherbrooke QC J1G 2E8; Sher'01; FRCSC; OrthSurg. Staff, Centre Hospitalier Universitaire de Sherbrooke-Hôpital Hôtel-Dieu; Langs: Bilingual(French/English); (819)346-1110; Fax. (819)822-6725.

DESHAIES, Claudine; CSSS du Lac-des-Deux-Montagnes, 520 boul Arthur-Sauve, Saint-Eustache QC J7R 5B1; Mon'88; FRCPC; DiagRad (Echography). Staff Diag Imag, Hôpital de Saint-Eustache; (450)473-6811 x2211

DESHAIES, Doris; Dir de la Sante Publique-Mtl, 1301 rue Sherbrooke E, Montreal QC H2L 1M3; Laval'76; MSc; Médecin, Direction de Sante Publique de Montreal; Langs: English; (514)528-2400 x3890; Fax. (514)528-2452; ddeshaie@santepub-mtl.qc.ca.

DESHAIES, Gaetan; 1602-70 rue de la Barre, Longueuil QC J4K 5J3; Laval'61; CSPQ; FRCSC; GenSurg (Administrative). Physician, Ministry of Health & Social Services-Quebec; (450)651-7583; Fax. (450)651-2583.

DESHAIES, Isabelle; CHUQ-Hotel-Dieu de Quebec, 11 Cote du Palais, Quebec QC G1R 2J6; Laval'02; GenSurg (Oncology). Staff, Centre Hospitalier Universitaire de Québec (CHUQ) - Siege Social; Langs: Bilingual(French/English); (418)691-5370; Fax. (418)691-5020.

DESHAIES, Jean-Francois; CHUS-Hop Fleurimont, 3001 12e av N, Sherbrooke QC J1H 5N4; Sher'02; CCFP; CCFP(E.M.); Staff, Centre Hospitalier Universitaire de Sherbrooke-Hopital Fleurimont; Langs: English; (819)346-1110; jean-francois.deshaies@usherbrooke.ca.

DESHAIES, Lucie; CLSC Haute-Ville, 55 ch Sainte-Foy, Quebec QC G1R 1S9; Laval'86; (418)641-2572; Fax. (418)641-0098.

DESHAIES, Pierre; Agence SSSS-Dir Sante Publique, 12-363 Rte Cameron, Sainte-Marie QC G6E 3E2; Laval'76; MSc(Epidem.); FRCPC; CommunMed (Environmental Health). Chief-Pub Hlth, Hôtel-Dieu de Lévis; Langs: Spanish; (418)389-1563; pierre_deshaies@ssss.gouv.qc.ca.

DESHAIES, Pierre; Clin Med de Warwick, 5A ch du Centre Sportif, Warwick QC J0A 1M0; Sher'82; Staff, Hotel-Dieu d'Arthabaska; Langs: Bilingual(French/English); (819)358-4600; Fax. (819)358-4620.

DESHAIES, Pierre; Centre Med Sainte-Foy, 802 rue Du Chanoine-Scott, Quebec QC G1V 3N4; Laval'87; (418)653-4931

DESHAUER, Dorian; Brockville Mental Health Centr, PO Box 1050 1804 Hwy 2 E, Brockville ON K6V 5W7; Man'89; MSc; FRCPC; Psy (Evidence Based Medicine). Staff, Brockville Mental Health Centre - Royal Ottawa Health Care Group; Assoc Editor, Canadian Medical Association Journal; Asst Prof Psy, McMaster University; Asst Prof Psy, University of Ottawa; (613)345-1461; dorian.deshauer@cmaj.ca.

DESHPAND, Poorva P; The Hosp for Sick Children, 555 University Ave, Toronto ON M5G 1X8; Nagpur (India)'02; Staff, The Hospital For Sick Children; (416)813-6927

DESHPANDE, Amol; Univ Hlth Network-Toronto Western Hosp, 811 4 FP-399 Bathurst St, Toronto ON M5T 2S8; Tor'92; Staff, Toronto Western Hospital - University Health Network; Physician, Medipac Insurance Co.; (416)603-5380 x2603

DESHPANDE, Ashish; Windsor Health Centre, 200-700 Tecumseh Rd E, Windsor ON N8X 4T2; Bombay (India)'80; MB BS; FRCPC; Peds. Langs: Marathi; Hindi; (519)252-7008; Fax. (519)252-7002.

DESHPANDE, Maneesh; Joseph Brant Mem Hosp, 1230 North Shore Blvd, Burlington ON L7S 1W7; Qns'05; FRCPC; Anes. Staff, Joseph Brant Memorial Hospital; (905)632-3730

DESHPANDEY, Akhil; Dr Charles A Janeway Child Hlt, 300 Prince Philip Dr, St. John's NL A1B 3V6; Gandhi (India)'85; Staff, Janeway Children's Health & Rehabilitation Centre; (709)777-6300

DESHWAL, Natasha A; Bedford Basin Women Hlth Clini, 208-967 Bedford Hwy, Bedford NS B4A 1A9; Dal'95; CCFP; FCFP; (902)444-8726; Fax. (902)444-8722.

DESILETS, Alice; 205-565 Elmwood Dr, Dieppe NB E1A 2X4; Sher'86; CCFP; FCFP; (506)857-0035

DESILETS, Etienne; Hop Charles Lemoyne, 3120 boul Taschereau, Greenfield Park QC J4V 2H1; Sher'08; Gastroent (P.Q.); IntMed. Staff, Hopital Charles LeMoyne; (450)466-5000

DESILETS, Jean-Francois; Clinique Medi-Val 2000, 100-408 rue Jeanne-Mance, Salaber-de-Valleyf QC J6T 4G1; Sher'09; CCFP; (450)370-3387; Fax. (450)370-3395.

DESILETS, Joane; Dir Sante Publique Lanaudiere, 245 rue du Cure-Majeau, Joliette QC J6E 8S8; Laval'84; Staff, Centre Hospitalier Régional de Lanaudière; (450)759-1157 x4450; Fax. (450)759-0281.

DESILETS, Marie-Eve; Hop Maisonneuve-Rosemont, 5415 boul de l'Assomption, Montreal QC H1T 2M4; Mon'03; Staff, Hopital Maisonneuve-Rosemont; (514)252-3400 x4558

DESILETS, Monique; GMF de Mascouche, 100-880 Montee Masson, Mascouche QC J7K 2L7; Mon'76; Staff, Centre Hospitalier l'Université De Montréal (CHUM) - Hôpital Saint-luc; (450)474-2493; Fax. (450)966-0156.

DESILETS, Odette; La Maison Michel Sarrazin, 2101 ch Saint-Louis, Quebec QC G1T 1P5; Laval'74; Staff, Maison Michel Sarrazin; (418)688-0878; Fax. (418)681-8636.

DESILETS, Stacy A; Bridgetop Med Clinic, PO Box 1355 11 Murray St, New Liskeard ON P0J 1P0; Tor'05; CCFP; (705)647-4102; Fax. (705)647-0114.

DESILETS, Valerie; Hôpital Ste-Justine, 3175 ch Cote-Sainte-Catherine, Montreal QC H3T 1C5; Laval'90; FRCSC; ObstGyn; MedGenetics (P.Q.). Staff, Hôpital Ste-Justine; (514)345-4727; Fax. (514)345-4766.

DESILETS-COUTURE, Claudette; Centre Med Dorion Vaudreuil, 600 boul Harwood, Vaudreuil-Dorion QC J7V 6A3; Mon'76; (450)455-9301; Fax. (450)455-8964.

DESIMON, Jean-Haulis R; Family Medicine Centre, 202-3400 rue du Marche, Dollard-D-Ormeaux QC H9B 2Y1; Wisconsin (USA)'90; Langs: Bilingual(English/French); (514)683-0414; Fax. (514)683-5528.

DESINDES, Sophie; CHUS-Hop Fleurimont, 3001 12e av N, Sherbrooke QC J1H 5N4; Sher'97; FRCSC; ObstGyn (Menopause). Staff, Centre Hospitalier Universitaire de Sherbrooke-Hopital Fleurimont; Staff Teacher, Universite de Sherbrooke; (819)346-1110; Fax. (819)820-6434.

DESIR, Barbara; Hop du Sacre-Coeur de Mtl, 5400 boul Gouin O, Montreal QC H4J 1C5; Mon'96; FRCPC; IntMed; Gastroent. Staff, Hôpital du Sacre-Coeur de Montréal; (514)338-2222 x2050

DESIRE, Farah; Hop Santa Cabrini Ospedale, 5655 rue Saint-Zotique E, Montreal QC H1T 1P7; Mon'05; CCFP; Staff, Hôpital Santa Cabrini Ospedale; (514)252-6000; Fax. (514)252-6501.

DESJARDINS, Alain; Hop du Sacre-Coeur de Mtl, 5e-5400 boul Gouin O, Montreal QC H4J 1C5; Mon'83; FRCPC; IntMed; Respir. ac Staff Med, Hôpital du Sacre-Coeur de Montréal; Consultant Med, CSSS d'Antoine-Labelle; Consultant Med, Hôpital de Saint-Eustache; Langs: English; (514)338-2162; Fax. (514)338-3699; alain.desjardins@videotron.ca.

DESJARDINS, Andre L; CSSS du Sud de Lanaudière, 911 montee des Pionniers, Terrebonne QC J6V 2H2; Mon'82; CSPQ; FRCSC; OrthSurg. Staff, Centre Hospitalier Pierre le Gardeur; (450)654-7525 x21147

DESJARDINS, Anne; CHUQ-Hotel-Dieu de Quebec, 11 Cote du Palais, Quebec QC G1R 2J6; Ott'03; FRCPC; MedMicrobiol (Infectiology); Microbio & Infect Dis (P.Q.). Staff, Centre Hospitalier Universitaire de Québec (CHUQ) - Siege Social; (418)691-5131; anne.desjardins@chuq.qc.ca.

DESJARDINS, Bruce; Hotel-Dieu Grace Hosp, 1030 Ouellette Ave, Windsor ON N9A 1E1; McM'78; FRCPC; Anes. Court Staff, Leamington District Memorial Hospital; Staff Anes, Hôtel-Dieu Grace Hospital; Court Staff Anes, Windsor Regional Hospital - Metropolitan Site; (519)973-4421

DESJARDINS, Caroline; Les Gynecologues Ass Laval, 1299 boul de la Concorde O, Laval QC H7N 5T4; Mon'89; FRCSC; ObstGyn. Staff, Hopital de la Cite de la santé; Langs: Bilingual(French/English); (450)668-3250; Fax. (450)668-7595.

DESJARDINS, Celine; Clinique Ella, 601-5300 Ch de la Cote-des-Nei, Montreal QC H3T 1Y3; Mon'84; AB; MSc; FRCSC; ObstGyn (Epidemiology). Staff, St Mary's Hospital Centre; Dir Therapeutic Products, Health Canada; Clin Teacher, McGill University; Langs: English; (514)788-4504; Fax. (514)787-1458.

DESJARDINS, Daniel C J; Hop Maisonneuve-Rosemont, 5415 boul de L'Assomption, Montreal QC H1T 2M4; Sher'79; FRCSC; Ophth (Cataract). Staff, Hopital Maisonneuve-Rosemont; Staff, Universite de Montreal; Langs: English; (514)252-3878; Fax. (514)252-3905.

DESJARDINS, France; Carrefour Sante-Pav St-Louis, 23 rue Ambroise-Dearden, Windsor QC J1S 1G8; Mon'95; Staff, Centre Hospitalier Regional de Sept-Iles; (819)845-2751; Fax. (819)845-4269.

DESJARDINS, Francine C; COOP Sante Gatineau, 200 boul Greber, Gatineau QC J8T 6K2; Ott'75; (819)568-0444; Fax. (819)568-1356.

DESJARDINS, Frederic; CSSS Pierre Boucher, 1333 boul Jacques-Cartier E, Longueuil QC J4M 2A5; Mon'96; FRCPC; DiagRad. Staff, Centre Hospitalier Pierre Boucher; (450)468-8111

DESJARDINS, Gilles; CSSS de Rimouski-Neigette, CP 3150 succ Bureau Chef 150 av Rouleau, Rimouski QC G5L 5T1; Mon'73; Otol. Staff, Hôpital Regional Rimouski; (418)724-3000

DESJARDINS, Gisele; Centre D'Urgence Salaberry, 2758 rue de Salaberry, Montreal QC H3M 1L3; Mon'80; CCFP; Langs: English; (514)337-4772

DESJARDINS, J Jacques; 322 boul Antonio-Barrette, N-D-Des-Prairies QC J6E 1G2; Mon'68; Psy (P.Q.) (Child & Adolescent Psychiatry). Consultant Peds Psy, Centre Hospitalier Régional de Lanaudière; Physician, Child & Adolescent Psychotherapy Clinic; (450)759-5507

DESJARDINS, JP Jean-Pierre; 206-194 Main St, Ottawa ON K1S 1C2; Ott'64; BA; CSPQ; FRCSC; OrthSurg (Endoscopic Surgery). Staff, The Ottawa Hospital - Riverside Campus; Staff, The Ottawa Hospital - General Campus; Asst Prof, University of Ottawa; Langs: Bilingual(English/French); (613)236-7444; Fax. (613)236-5711; jpdesj@sympatico.ca.

DESJARDINS, Jacques; Res Le Renoir, 505 rue Cardinal, Laval QC H7V 3Y8; Mon'66; (450)688-8505; Fax. (450)688-1260.

DESJARDINS, Jean-Francois; CSSS de Saint-Jerome, 290 rue de Montigny, Saint-Jerome QC J7Z 5T3; Mon'91; DiagRad. Staff, Hôtel-Dieu de Saint-Jérôme; (450)431-8300; Fax. (450)431-8350.

DESJARDINS, Joanne; Plantagenet Family Health Team, PO Box 305 179 Old Highway 17, Plantagenet ON K0B 1L0; Ott'96; CCFP; Langs: French; (613)673-4318; Fax. (613)673-4480; j.desjardins@nursinghomeratings.ca.

DESJARDINS, Jocelyne; Hop Maisonneuve-Rosemont, 5415 boul de l'Assomption, Montreal QC H1T 2M4; Mon'90; ObstGyn. Staff, Hopital Maisonneuve-Rosemont; (514)252-3400

DESJARDINS, Julie; Clin Familiale des Prairies, 310 boul Antonio-Barrette, Joliette QC J6E 1G2; Sher'05; CCFP; (450)752-1050

DESJARDINS, Julie; Ungava Tulattavik Health Ctr, CP 149, Kuujjuaq QC J0M 1C0; Mon'08; CCFP; (819)964-2905; Fax. (819)964-6353.

DESJARDINS, Lyne; Clinique Fam des Prairies, 310 boul Antonio-Barrette, N-D-Des-Prairies QC J6E 1G2; Mon'89; (450)752-1050; Fax. (450)752-2965.

DESJARDINS, Marc; Clinique Med Le Gardeurois, 130-155 rue Notre-Dame, Repentigny QC J5Z 3C4; Sher'86; (450)582-5551

DESJARDINS, Marco; Direction de la Sante Publique, 550 rue Bonaventure, Trois-Rivieres QC G9A 2B5; Sher'88; LMCC; Staff, CSSS de Trois-Rivières; Consultant Med, Agence de Sante Et Des services de Sante; Langs: English; (819)693-3954; Fax. (819)373-1627.

DESJARDINS, Marie-France; Clinique Med Adoncour, 200-505 rue Adoncour, Longueuil QC J4G 2M6; Mon'74; Staff Med, Centre Hospitalier l'Université de Montréal (CHUM) - Hôtel-Dieu; (450)646-4445; Fax. (450)646-5526.

DESJARDINS, Marie-Helene; CSSS de Laval, 1755 boul Rene-Laennec, Laval QC H7M 3L9; Sher'96; Nephrol; IntMed. Staff, Hopital de la Cite de la santé; (450)668-1010

DESJARDINS, Marie-Josee; CSSS Bordeaux-Cartierville-St-, 555 boul Gouin O, Montreal QC H3L 1K5; Mon'87; Staff, Pavillon Notre-Dame de la Merci; Langs: Bilingual(English/French); (514)331-3025; mariejosee.desjardins.iles@ssss.gouv.qc.ca.

DESJARDINS, Marie-Pier; The Hosp for Sick Children, 555 University Ave, Toronto ON M5G 1X8; Laval'07; FRCPC; Peds; PedEmergMed. Staff, The Hospital For Sick Children; (416)813-1500

DESJARDINS, Maryline; MUHC-Montreal Children's Hosp, 2300 rue Tupper, Montreal QC H3H 1P3; Sher'05; ClinImmunol&Allergy; Peds. Staff, McGill University Health Centre - Montreal Children's Hospital; (514)412-4400

DESJARDINS, Michel; CP 6020 Succ Bureau-Chef, Gaspe QC G4X 2R6; Mon'76; MAT; CCFP; FCFP; Clin Prof, Université Laval; (418)368-6755

DESJARDINS, Monique; MUHC-Montreal Gen Hosp, B6 136-1650 av Cedar, Montreal QC H3G 1A4; Mon'98; FRCPC; Psy (Neuro Physiology). Staff, McGill University Health Centre - Montreal General Campus; Staff, Hôpital du Sacre-Coeur de Montréal; Langs: English; (514)338-2222

DESJARDINS, Nina; North Simoce ACT Team, 76 Nottawasaga St, Orillia ON L3V 3J4; Alb'96; FRCPC; Psy. Staff, Waypoint Centre for Mental Health Care; (705)427-3503

DESJARDINS, Pierre; Hop Charles Lemoyne, 3120 boul Taschereau, Greenfield Park QC J4V 2H1; Mon'83; ABIM; FRCPC; IntMed (Oncology); Hem. Staff, Hopital Charles LeMoyne; Langs: Bilingual(French/English); (450)466-5065

DESJARDINS, Richard; Clinique St-Barnabe, 307-176 av Rouleau, Rimouski QC G5L 8W1; Mon'75; Urol. (418)724-6262; Fax. (418)722-6265.

DESJARDINS, Sylvie; Clinique Med Blainville, 519 boul du Cure-Labelle, Sainte-Therese QC J7C 2H6; Mon'77; (450)430-2221

DESJARDINS, Valerie A; CSSS du Sud de Lanaudière, 911 montee des Pionniers, Terrebonne QC J6V 2H2; Mon'87; CSPQ; FRCPC; IntMed; Cardiol. Staff, Centre Hospitalier Pierre le Gardeur; (450)654-7525

DESJARDINS TESSIER, Amelie; Inuulitsivik Health Centre, GD, Povungnituq QC J0M 1P0; Mon'10; CCFP; Staff, Inuulitsivik Health Centre; (819)988-2957

DESLANDES, Carole; CSSS Drummond-Hop Sainte-Croix, 570 rue Heriot, Drummondville QC J2B 1C1; Mon'96; FRCPC; Psy. Staff, Hôpital Sainte-croix; (819)478-6464

DESLANDES, Isabelle; Clinique Med Pierre-Boucher, 1615 boul Jacques-Cartier E, Longueuil QC J4M 2X1; McG'93; CCFP; Staff Emerg, McGill University Health Centre - Montreal Children's Hospital; Staff Emerg, CSSS des Sources d'Asbestos; Staff, Centre Hospitalier Pierre Boucher; Staff, Hôpital de l'Archipel; (450)468-6223; Fax. (450)468-5041.

DESLANDES, Jean-Luc; Centre de Sante Valcartier, CP 1000 Bdp Succ Forces, Courcelette QC G0A 4Z0; Sher'76; (418)844-5000 x3067

DESLANDES, Melanie; CHUM-Hop Notre-Dame, 1560 rue Sherbrooke E, Montreal QC H2L 4M1; Mon'03; DiagRad. Staff, Centre Hospitalier l'Université de Montréal (CHUM) - Hôpital Notre-Dame; (514)590-8000

DESLANDES, Pierre; Clin Med Plateau Mont-Royal, 1374 av du Mont-Royal E, Montreal QC H2J 1Y7; Mon'95; Staff, Hopital Maisonneuve-Rosemont; (514)527-3997; Fax. (514)527-3994.

DESLANDRES, Colette; Hôpital Ste-Justine, 3175 ch Cote-Ste-Catherine, Montreal QC H3T 1C5; Mon'80; FRCPC; Peds (Pediatric Gastroenterology). Ac Staff, Hôpital Ste-Justine; Langs: Bilingual(French/English); (514)345-4626; Fax. (514)345-4741; colette_deslandres@ssss.gouv.qc.ca.

DESLANDRES, Erik; CHUM-Hotel-Dieu, 3840 rue Saint-Urbain, Montreal QC H2W 1T8; Mon'83; FRCPC; IntMed; Gastroent. Staff, Centre Hospitalier l'Université de Montréal (CHUM) - Hôtel-Dieu; (514)890-8000 x14980

DESLAURIERS, Daniel; Hotel-Dieu de Levis, 143 rue Wolfe, Levis QC G6V 3Z1; Laval'83; BSc(BioChem); MSc(BiolMolecul); LMCC; CSPQ; FRCPC; MedBiochem (Diabetes). Staff, Hôtel-Dieu de Lévis; Langs: Bilingual(French/English); (418)835-7121 x3263; Fax. (418)835-7139.

DESLAURIERS, Francine; 509 rue Adoncour, Longueuil QC J4G 2M6; Mon'76; FRCSC; Ophth. Ophthalmology, Centre Hospitalier Pierre Boucher; (450)646-7788; Fax. (450)646-3713.

DESLAURIERS, Gilbert E; CSSSG-Hop de Hull, 116 boul Lionel-Emond, Gatineau QC J8Y 1W7; Mon'71; FRCPC; DiagRad (Angiography). Ac Staff, Hull Hospital; (819)595-6028; Fax. (819)595-6076.

DESLAURIERS, Guy; CSSS de Saint-Jerome, 290 rue de Montigny, Saint-Jerome QC J7Z 5T3; Mon'87; Respir; IntMed. Staff, Hôtel-Dieu de Saint-Jérôme; (450)431-8201; Fax. (450)431-8209; guydeslauriers@videotron.ca.

DESLAURIERS, Guy; Clinique Fam de St-Hyacinthe, 2955 boul Laframboise, Saint-Hyacinthe QC J2S 4Z3; Sher'76; Staff, Centre d hebergement de l Hôtel-Dieu de Saint-Hyacinthe; (450)774-4611; Fax. (450)773-9913.

DESLAURIERS, J A Jean; Orleans Med Centre, 406-2555 St Joseph Blvd, Orleans ON K1C 1S8; Ott'67; (613)830-1771; Fax. (613)830-2543.

DESLAURIERS, Jean; Hôpital Laval, 2725 ch Sainte-Foy, Quebec QC G1V 4G5; Laval'68; CSPQ; Cardiovasc&ThorSurg (P.Q.); GenSurg., Hôpital Laval; Prof, Université Laval; Langs: English; (418)656-4747; Fax. (418)656-4762.

DESLAURIERS, Louis; Clinique Med de Mont-Joli, 1385 boul Gaboury, Mont-Joli QC G5H 4B1; Mon'99; Staff, CSSS de la Mitis; (418)775-5353; louis.deslauriers@cgocable.ca.

DESLAURIERS, Louis-Jean; Clinique Med des Sommets, 1070 rue Principale, Ste-Agathe-des-Mts QC J8C 1L6; McG'84; ac Staff, Centre Hospitalier Laurentien; (819)321-1212; Fax. (819)321-3232.

DESLAURIERS, Nancy; Hop Charles LeMoyne, 3120 boul Taschereau, Longueuil QC J4V 2H1; Mon'07; FRCSC; GenSurg. Staff, Hopital Charles LeMoyne; (450)466-5000

DESLAURIERS, Patrice; CSSS de Sept-Iles, 45 rue du Pere-Divet, Sept-Iles QC G4R 3N7; Sher'88; NuclearMed. Staff, Centre Hospitalier Regional de Sept-Iles; (418)962-9761 x2802; Fax. (418)968-0689.

DESLAURIERS, Robert; 110-667 Champlain St, Dieppe NB E1A 1P6; Sher'90; FRCSC; GenSurg. (506)854-6293; Fax. (506)858-9012.

DESLAURIERS, Virginie; GMF Antoine-Labelle, 200-555 boul St-Antoine, Saint-Jerome QC J7Z 3B8; Mon'09; CCFP; (450)438-1252

DESLIPPE, Helene; CSSS du Nord de Lanaudière, 1000 boul Sainte-Anne, St-Charles-Brromee QC J6E 6J2; Laval'91; CSPQ; Anes. Staff, Centre Hospitalier Régional de Lanaudière; (450)759-8222 x2960; Fax. (450)759-8289.

DESLOGES, Danielle; Clinique Chir Ortho C-Lemoyne, 126 rue Saint-Louis, Lemoyne QC J4R 2L5; Mon'84; CSPQ; FRCSC; OrthSurg. Langs: English; (450)672-1212; Fax. (450)672-9834.

DESLONGCHAMPS, Francois J; Ctr Cardiolovasculaire Rive-Su, 200-1615 boul Jacques-Cartier, Longueuil QC J4M 2X1; Sher'85; CSPQ; FRCPC; IntMed (Hemodynamics); Cardiol. Staff Cardiol Hemodynamics, Centre Hospitalier Pierre Boucher; (450)674-2345; Fax. (450)674-1622.

DESMARAIS, Dominique; Clin Pediatrique Laurentienne, 106-200 rue Durand, Saint-Jerome QC J7Z 7E2; Mon'91; FRCPC; Peds. Staff, Hôtel-Dieu de Saint-Jérôme; Langs: English; (450)438-1241; Fax. (450)438-3501.

DESMARAIS, Elaine; Clinique Med Pierre Boucher, 1615 boul Jacques-Cartier E, Longueuil QC J4M 2X1; Mon'88; Ac Staff, Centre Hospitalier Pierre Boucher; (450)468-6223

DESMARAIS, Eric; Ctr Hosp Anna-Laberge, 200 boul Brisebois, Chateauguay QC J6K 4W8; McG'98; FRCPC; DiagRad (Osteoarthritis & Osteoporosis). Staff, Hôpital Anna-Laberge; Langs: English; (450)699-2425

DESMARAIS, Jean-Anthony; Clin Med L'Avenir, 200-1150 boul de l'Avenir, Laval QC H7N 6L2; Mon'73; (450)680-1150

DESMARAIS, Jean-Luc; Hop Maisonneuve-Rosemont, 5415 boul de l'Assomption, Montreal QC H1T 2M4; Mon'73; Ac Staff, Hopital Maisonneuve-Rosemont; (514)376-9961; Fax. (514)376-8100.

DESMARAIS, Julie; Allan Memorial Institute, 1025 av des Pins O, Montreal QC H3A 1A1; McG'05; FRCPC; Psy (Clinical Pharmacology & Toxicology). Langs: Bilingual(French/English); (514)843-1672; Fax. (514)843-2898; julie.desmarais@mail.mcgill.ca.

DESMARAIS, Marc; Clinique Med Hochelaga, 9080 rue Hochelaga, Montreal QC H1L 2N9; Mon'10; (514)353-8742

DESMARAIS, Marie; Polyclinique Cabrini, 114-5700 rue Saint-Zotique E, Montreal QC H1T 3Y7; Mon'74; (514)352-6140; Fax. (514)352-5924.

DESMARAIS, Marie-Claude; Hop Louis-H Lafontaine, 7401 rue Hochelaga, Montreal QC H1N 3M5; Mon'08; CCFP; Staff Urgentologue, Hôpital Santa Cabrini Ospedale; Staff Gen Med, Hopital Louis-H Lafontaine; (514)251-4000; Fax. (514)251-4043.

DESMARAIS, Maryse; Clinique Medicale Sainte-Adele, 1150 rue du Bourg-Joli, Sainte-Adele QC J8B 1W8; Mon'91; LMCC; CCFP; Staff, Centre Hospitalier Laurentien; Staff, CSSS d'Antoine-Labelle; Staff, Hôpital Riviere des Prairies; Langs: Bilingual(French/English); (450)229-6633; Fax. (450)229-5765.

DESMARAIS, Nicole; Medicine Professional Corp, Box 23 5085 Highway 69 N, Hanmer ON P3P 1P7; Wes'95; CCFP; FCFP; Langs: English; French; (705)969-0628; Fax. (705)969-0629.

DESMARAIS, Paul-Andre; Service de Pedopsychiatrie, 6550 rue Saint-Georges, Levis QC G6V 6X2; Sher'77; FRCPC; Psy (Adolescent Psychiatry). Staff, Hôtel-Dieu de Lévis; adj Prof, Universite de Sherbrooke; (418)835-7155; Fax. (418)838-8873.

DESMARAIS, Richard; Clinique Med Richelieu, 202-500 Rte Marie-Victorin, Sorel-Tracy QC J3R 1K7; Sher'77; (450)742-9818; Fax. (450)742-9795.

DESMARAIS, Sylvie; CSSS Pierre Boucher, 1333 boul Jacques-Cartier E, Longueuil QC J4M 2A5; Mon'90; FRCPC; IntMed (Arterial Thrombosis & Vein). Staff, Centre Hospitalier Pierre Boucher; (450)468-6811; Fax. (450)468-8240.

DESMARCHAIS, Louise; Clinique Med Ville-emard, 5824 boul Monk, Montreal QC H4E 3H3; Laval'69; Peds. Ac Staff, Hôpital Ste-Justine; (514)767-5307; Fax. (514)767-0217.

DESMEULES, Jean; Centre medical de Cowansville, 101-370 rue De La Riviere, Cowansville QC J2K 1N3; Laval'65; (450)263-0774; Fax. (450)263-6457; desmeules@videotron.ca.

DESMEULES, Julie; CLSC Saint-Hubert, 6800 rue Coousineau, Longueuil QC J3Y 8Z4; McG'95; CCFP; Staff, Centre Hospitalier Honore-Mercier; (450)443-7400 x7807

DESMEULES, Julie; CLSC Basse-Ville-Limoilou, 50 rue Saint-Joseph E, Quebec QC G1K 3A5; Laval'85; (418)529-2572; Fax. (418)529-1515.

DESMEULES, Marc; Hôpital Laval, 2725 ch Sainte-Foy, Quebec QC G1V 4G5; Laval'65; FRCPC; IntMed; Respir. Staff, Hôpital Laval; Consultant, CSSS de Quebec-Sud; Consultant, Centre Hospitalier Universitaire De Québec - Pavillon De St-françois-d'assise; Teach Staff Med, Université Laval; (418)656-8711; Fax. (418)656-4762.

DESMEULES, Paul; Clin Med Nutrition D'Amaigriss, 102-475 boul Talbot, Chicoutimi QC G7H 4A3; Laval'64; FRCPC; CommunMed (P.Q.) (Public Health & Preventive Medicine). Langs: Bilingual(French/English); (418)543-1968; paul.desmeules.m.d@sympatico.ca.

DESMEULES, Simon; CHUQ-Hotel-Dieu de Quebec, 11 Cote du Palais, Quebec QC G1R 2J6; Laval'96; FRCPC; IntMed; Nephrol. Staff, Centre Hospitalier Universitaire de Québec (CHUQ) - Siege Social; (418)691-5464; Fax. (418)691-5757.

DESMOND, Gerard H; Lorne Mem Hosp, PO Box 40 2nd St N, Swan Lake MB R0G 2S0; Cape Town (South Africa)'85; MB ChB; CCFP; Staff, Lorne Memorial Hospital; (204)836-2533

DESMOND, John V; St Andrews Health Centre, 108 Sophia St, St Andrews NB E5B 2B8; Dal'06; CCFP; (506)529-9120

DESNOYERS, Elaine M; Airdrie Med Clinic, 10-620 1 Ave NW, Airdrie AB T4B 2R3; Cal'05; CCFP; (403)948-3109

DESNOYERS, Jacques; Clinique Chir Ortho C-Lemoyne, 126 rue Saint-Louis, Lemoyne QC J4R 2L5; Mon'83; CSPQ; FRCSC; OrthSurg (Knee Surgery). Staff, Hopital Charles LeMoyne; (450)672-1212 x32; Fax. (450)672-9834.

DESNOYERS, Jean-Pierre; CSSS Pierre Boucher, 1333 boul Jacques-Cartier E, Longueuil QC J4M 2A5; Mon'74; Anes. Ac Staff, Centre Hospitalier Pierre Boucher; (450)468-8111

DESNOYERS, Lyne; CHUM-Hop St-Luc, 1058 rue Saint-Denis, Montreal QC H2X 3J4; Mon'82; FRCSC; Otol. Staff, Centre Hospitalier l'Université De Montréal (CHUM) - Hôpital Saint-luc; (514)890-8000

DESNOYERS, Pierre G; Clin Med Industrielle Laurenti, 200-352 boul Labelle, Laval QC H7P 2P1; Mon'78; (450)624-9990

DESORMEAU, Isabelle; CSSS de Laval, 1755 boul Rene-Laennec, Laval QC H7M 3L9; Mon'95; CSPQ; FRCPC; Anes. Staff, Hopital de la Cite de la santé; Langs: Spanish; English; (450)668-1010

DESORMEAU, Jean; Ctr Medi Soleil St-Jean-Sur-Ri, 120-383 boul du Seminaire N, St-Jean-sur-Richel QC J3B 8C5; Mon'84; Staff, Hôpital du Haut-Richelieu; (450)349-5555

DESORMEAU, Leon M; St Martha's Reg Hosp, 25 Bay St, Antigonish NS B2G 2G5; McG'69; FRCPC; AnatPath (Forensic Pathology). Chief, St Martha's Regional Hospital, Dept. of Path/Lab.; Dalhousie University; (902)863-2830; Fax. (902)863-3708; ldesormeau@gasha.nshealth.ca.

DESORMEAUX, Julie; Hôpital de Gatineau, 909 boul de la Verendrye O, Gatineau QC J8P 7H2; Sher'09; CCFP; Staff, Hôpital de Gatineau; (819)561-8100

DESORMEAUX, Lise; CLSC Rene Cassin, 500-5800 boul Cavendish, Cote Saint-Luc QC H4W 2T5; Mon'92; CCFP; FCFP; Staff, Hôpital du Sacre-Coeur de Montréal; Langs: English; (514)484-7878; Fax. (514)485-2978.

DESORMEAUX, Yvon; Clinique Med St-Hippolyte, 780 ch des Hauteurs, Saint-Hippolyte QC J8A 1H1; Mon'80; BSc(Biol.); MSc(Path.); Langs: Bilingual(French/English); (450)224-8271; yvondesormeaux@hotmail.com.

DESPARD, Caroline; 207-648 Huron St, London ON N5Y 4J8; Tor'85; BSc; CCFP; FCFP; Staff, St Joseph's Hospital - St Joseph's Health Care; Staff, Parkwood Hospital - St Joseph's Health Care; Staff, London Health Sciences Centre - Victoria Campus; Med Examiner, Medical Council of Canada Examination Board; Adjunct Prof., University of Western Ontario; (519)667-1888; Fax. (519)667-0577.

DESPARMET, Joelle; MUHC-Montreal Children's Hosp, 2300 rue Tupper, Montreal QC H3H 1P3; Paris (France)'74; Anes (P.Q.) (Pain Management). Dir Pain Mgmt/Anaes, McGill University Health Centre - Montreal Children's Hospital; Assoc Prof Anes., McGill University; Langs: French; Italian; (514)412-4400 x22847; Fax. (514)412-4341; joelle.desparmet@muhc.mcgill.ca.

DESPATIS, Marc-Antoine; CHUS-Hop Fleurimont, 3001 12e av N, Sherbrooke QC J1H 5N4; Mon'92; BSc; MSc; CSPQ; RVT; FRCSC; GenSurg (Wound Care); VascSurg. Staff, Centre Hospitalier Universitaire de Sherbrooke-Hopital Fleurimont; (819)346-1110 x14356; Fax. (819)820-6871.

DESPOTS, Marilyne; Clinique Med des Sommets, 1070 rue Principale, Ste-Agathe-des-Mts QC J8C 1L6; Mon'07; (819)321-1212; Fax. (819)321-3232.

DESPRES, Cathy; CSSS du Sud de Lanaudière, 911 Montee des Pionniers, Terrebonne QC J6V 2H2; Sher'99; CSPQ; FRCSC; GenSurg (Endocrinology). Staff, Centre Hospitalier Pierre le Gardeur; Langs: English; (450)654-7525

DESPRES, Lise; Centre Med McMasterville, 785 rue Tetreault, McMasterville QC J3G 1A7; Mon'77; Langs: Bilingual(French/English); (450)464-1156; Fax. (450)464-1270.

DESPRES, Mylene; 101-1789 Mountain Rd, Moncton NB E1G 5C4; Ott'01; CCFP; (506)870-2905; Fax. (506)870-2817.

DESRANLEAU, Jacinthe; UMF Richelieu-Yamaska, 1005 rue Gauthier, Saint-Hyacinthe QC J2S 8T2; Mon'03; CCFP; Assoc Prof Family Med, Centre Hospitalier Universitaire de Sherbrooke-Hopital Fleurimont; (450)771-3333 x4972; Fax. (450)771-3427.

DESRANLEAU, Real; Clin Med McMasterville, 785 rue Tetreault, McMasterville QC J3G 1A7; Laval'67; BA; BTh; BRE; Langs: English; French; (450)464-1156; Fax. (450)464-1270; lyredesranleau@look.ca.

DESREUX, Michelle R; 7040 Edgemont Dr NW, Calgary AB T3A 2M1; McM'96; BSc; FRCPC; IntMed. Clin Teacher, University of Calgary; (403)685-9499; Fax. (403)685-9422.

DESROCHERS, Agnes; CHUS-Hop Fleurimont, 3001 12e av N, Sherbrooke QC J1H 5N4; Laval'79; CCFP; Staff, Centre Hospitalier Universitaire de Sherbrooke-Hopital Fleurimont; (819)346-1110; Fax. (819)820-6420.

DESROCHERS, Amelie; CHUS-Hop Fleurimont, 3001 12 av N, Sherbrooke QC J1H 5N4; Sher'08; Staff, Centre Hospitalier Universitaire de Sherbrooke-Hopital Fleurimont; (819)346-1110

DESROCHERS, Chantale; 131 rue Somerville, Montreal QC H3L 1A1; Mon'88; Staff, Hôpital du Sacre-Coeur de Montréal; Langs: Bilingual(French/English); (514)385-9687; Fax. (514)385-0800.

DESROCHERS, Charles; Clin Med Fam Chicoutimi, 2185 boul de Tadoussac, Chicoutimi QC G7G 4X2; Laval'98; Ac Member, Complexe hospitalier de la Sagamie; (418)698-2414; Fax. (418)698-2413.

DESROCHERS, Denis P; CHUQ-Hotel-Dieu de Quebec, 2440-11 Cote du Palais, Quebec QC G1R 2J6; Laval'65; CSPQ; Cardiol (Internal Medicine). Staff, Centre Hospitalier Universitaire de Québec (CHUQ) - Siege Social; Langs: Bilingual(French/English); (418)691-5750; Fax. (418)691-5415.

DESROCHERS, Diane D; Clin Medicale du Quartier, 1191 av Cartier, Quebec QC G1R 2S9; Mon'75; Staff, Institut Universitaire Sante; (418)522-1911; Fax. (418)522-1789.

DESROCHERS, Georges W; Clinique de Med Interne Laurie, 101-39 rue Laurier E, Victoriaville QC G6P 6P6; Sher'77; IntMed. Staff, Hotel-Dieu d'Arthabaska; Clin Prof Pt-Time, Universite de Sherbrooke; (819)357-3930

DESROCHERS, Jean; Hotel-Dieu de Sorel, 400 av de l'Hotel-Dieu, Sorel-Tracy QC J3P 1N5; Mon'68; Staff, Hôtel-Dieu de Sorel; (450)746-6000

DESROCHERS, Jean-Paul; Clin Medicale 201, 104 rue Sainte-Agathe, Ste-Agathe-des-Mts QC J8C 2K3; Mon'80; Langs: Spanish; English; (819)326-1555; Fax. (819)326-8801.

DESROCHERS, Josee; 131 rue Somerville, Montreal QC H3L 1A1; Mon'87; CCFP; Chief Fam Med, Hôpital du Sacre-Coeur de Montréal; Langs: English; (514)385-9687; Fax. (514)385-0800.

DESROCHERS, Natale; Haldimand Family Health Team, 334 Broad St W, Dunnville ON N1A 1T1; McM'06; FamilyMed. Langs: Bilingual(English/French); (905)774-7541

DESROCHERS, Pascal; CSSS du Nord de Lanaudière, 1000 boul Sainte-Anne, St-Charles-Brromee QC J6E 6J2; Laval'97; FRCSC; Otol. Staff, Centre Hospitalier Régional de Lanaudière; (450)759-1241

DESROCHERS, Suzon; CSSS Pierre Boucher, 1333 boul Jacques-Cartier E, Longueuil QC J4M 2A5; Mon'71; Staff Psy, Centre Hospitalier Pierre Boucher; (450)468-8401; Fax. (450)468-8403.

DESROCHES, Annie; CHUQ-Ctr Hosp Univ Laval, 2705 boul Laurier, Quebec QC G1V 4G2; Laval'01; Staff Urgentologist, Centre Hospitalier Universitaire de Quebec-CHUL; (418)656-4141; Fax. (418)577-2065.

DESROCHES, Francois; Clinique Med East Angus, 1A-150 rue Angus S GD, East Angus QC J0B 1R0; Sher'79; LMCC; Adj Clin Teach, Universite de Sherbrooke; Langs: English; (819)832-2438; Fax. (819)832-2104; francoisdesroches@hotmail.com.

DESROCHES, Gilles; 950-220 Laurier Ave W, Ottawa ON K1P 5Z9; Laval'71; FRCSC; Ophth (Retina). Ac Staff, The Ottawa Hospital - Riverside Campus; Consultant, Children's Hospital of Eastern Ontario (CHEO); Asst Prof, University of Ottawa; Langs: Bilingual(French/English); (613)236-1907; Fax. (613)236-9459; retine@magma.ca.

DESROCHES, Jacques; Clinique Med Plus St-Pie, RR 2 75 rue St-Francois, Saint-Pie QC J0H 1W0; Mon'81; Staff, Centre Hospitalier Honore-Mercier; Staff, Clinique Medical St-Francois; (450)772-2401; Fax. (450)772-6864.

DESROCHES, Jean; CSSS de Saint-Jerome, 290 rue de Montigny, Saint-Jerome QC J7Z 5T3; Mon'88; CSPQ; FRCPC; Anes. Staff, Hôtel-Dieu de Saint-Jérôme; (450)431-8200; Fax. (450)431-8208.

DESROCHES, Jean V; Medico-Centre Mont Royal, 101-4689 av Papineau, Montreal QC H2H 1V4; Mon'78; Langs: Bilingual(French/English); (514)521-5555

DESROCHES, Joel; CSSS de Trois-Rivières, 1991 boul du Carmel, Trois-Rivieres QC G8Z 3R9; McG'90; FRCPC; NuclearMed. Staff NuclearMed, CSSS de Trois-Rivières; (819)378-9854; Fax. (819)378-9814.

DESROCHES, Julie; Clin Medicale Fleur de Lys, 8 rue du Terminus E, Rouyn-Noranda QC J9X 3B4; Sher'90; CCFP; Ac Member, Centre Hospitalier Régional Baie-Comeau; Assoc Member, CSSS du Témiscamingue; (819)764-6185; julie_desroches@ssss.gouv.qc.ca.

DESROCHES, Louise A; CSSS du Nord de Lanaudière, 1000 boul Sainte-Anne, St-Charles-Brromee QC J6E 6J2; Mon'84; Staff, Centre Hospitalier Régional de Lanaudière; (450)759-8222; Fax. (450)886-1667.

DESROCHES, Olivier; Ctr Hosp Affilie-St-Sacrement, 1050 ch Sainte-Foy, Quebec QC G1S 4L8; Mon'03; CCFP; CCFP(E.M.); Staff, Centre Hospitalier Affilié Universitaire de Québec - Hôpital du St-Sacrement; (418)682-7511

DESROCHES, Valerie; Ctr Hosp de Verdun, 4000 boul Lasalle, LaSalle QC H4G 2A3; Mon'08; CCFP; Staff, Centre Hospitalier de Verdun; (514)362-1000; Fax. (514)765-7339.

DESROSIERS, Anne-Edith; Clin de Gynecologique de Levis, 100-4975 boul de la Rive-Sud, Levis QC G6V 4Z5; Mon'93; (418)833-5810

DESROSIERS, Catherine; Ctr Hospitalier le Gardeur, 911 montee des Pionniers, Terrebonne QC J6V 2H2; Mon'09; CCFP; Staff, Centre Hospitalier Pierre le Gardeur; (450)654-7525

DESROSIERS, Catherine; CLSC des Patriotes, 300 boul Serge-Pepin, Beloeil QC J3G 0B8; Sher'97; (450)536-2572

DESROSIERS, Dominique; Clinique de L'Adolescence, 305 rue Saint-Vallier, Chicoutimi QC G7H 5H6; Sher'89; Staff Clinic Adolescence, Complexe hospitalier de la Sagamie; Staff Youth Centre, Institut St-Georges Chicoutimi; Médecin, Clinique de L'Adolescence; (418)541-1059; Fax. (418)541-1157.

DESROSIERS, France; Clinique Med de la Pointe, 7496 Route 11, Pte-Robichaud NB E1X 1K9; Mon'96; CCFP; Staff Emerg & Family Med, Hôpital de Tracadie-Sheila; Langs: Bilingual(French/English); (506)393-5000; Fax. (506)393-5050.

DESROSIERS, Jacques G; Halifax Prof Centre, 420-5991 Spring Garden Rd, Halifax NS B3H 1Y6; Dal'84; (902)423-8678; Fax. (902)422-4996.

DESROSIERS, Jean-Francois; Hop Charles Lemoyne, 3120 boul Taschereau, Longueuil QC J4V 2H1; Sher'02; Staff, CHSLD-CLSC Cleophas-Claveau; Staff, Hopital Charles LeMoyne; (450)466-5000

DESROSIERS, Josee; Clin Med Saint-Thomas, CP 5250 830A rue Principale, Saint-Thomas QC J0K 3L0; Sher'90; (450)756-1626; Fax. (450)756-6304.

DESROSIERS, Karen; Professional Arts Bldg, 519-100 rue Arden, Moncton NB E1C 4B7; Sher'97; FRCSC; ObstGyn. Staff, Hopital Regional Chaleur; (506)858-0599

DESROSIERS, Line; CLSC du Marigot, 1351 boul des Laurentides, Vimont QC H7M 2Y2; Mon'89; CCFP; FCFP; Staff Fam Med/Clin Teach Staff, CLSC du Marigot; (450)668-1803; Fax. (450)668-1507.

DESROSIERS, Lucie; CSSS de Rivière-de-Loup, 75 rue Saint-Henri, Riviere-Du-Loup QC G5R 2A4; Sher'78; Peds. Consultant, CSSS de Kamouraska; (418)868-1020 x2836; Fax. (418)868-3338.

DESROSIERS, Marie-Helene; CSSSG-Hop De Gatineau, CP 2000 Succ Bureau-Chef 909 boul de la Verendyre O, Gatineau QC J8P 7H2; Sher'06; CCFP; Staff, Hôpital de Gatineau; (819)561-8100

DESROSIERS, Marie-Isabelle; Clinique Dre Marie-Isabelle, 110-210 Centrum Blvd, Orleans ON K1E 3V7; Ott'07; CCFP; Langs: Bilingual(English/French); (613)424-9077

DESROSIERS, Marie-Luce; Hop Charles Lemoyne, 3120 boul Taschereau, Greenfield Park QC J4V 2H1; Mon'85; CSPQ; Anes. Staff, Hopital Charles LeMoyne; (450)466-5000

DESROSIERS, Martin; CHUM-Hotel-Dieu, 3840 rue Saint-Urbain, Montreal QC H2W 1T8; Mon'86; FRCSC; Otol (Endoscopic Surgery). Staff, McGill University Health Centre - Montreal General Campus; Staff, Centre Hospitalier l'Université de Montréal (CHUM) - Hôtel-Dieu; Clin Instructor, Universite de Montreal; (514)890-8000 x14170; Fax. (514)412-7246.

DESROSIERS, Michel; Federation Med Omnipract du QC, 1000-1440 rue Sainte-Catherine, Montreal QC H3G 1R8; Mon'85; Dir Professional Affairs, Federation des Medecins Omnipracticiens du Quebec; Langs: French; (514)878-1911 x255; Fax. (514)878-4455; mdesrosiers@fmoq.org.

DESROSIERS, Pauline; Pavillon-Saint Joseph, 900 boul de la Cote-Vertu, Saint-Laurent QC H4L 4T9; Mon'75; CCFP; FCFP; (514)747-6132; Fax. (514)747-2726.

DESROSIERS, Sophie; CSSS du Nord de Lanaudière, 1000 boul Sainte-Anne, St-Charles-Brromee QC J6E 6J2; Mon'01; FRCSC; Otol (Facial Laser Treatment). Staff, Centre Hospitalier Régional de Lanaudière; Langs: Bilingual(French/English); (450)759-8222

DESRUISSEAUX, Annie; Centre Med Laval, 1110 boul Vanier, Laval QC H7C 2R8; Mon'02; Staff, Hopital de la Cite de la santé; (450)661-2521; Fax. (450)661-7193.

DESRUISSEAUX, Benoit; Clinique Med St-Vincent, 250 rue King E, Sherbrooke QC J1G 1A9; Sher'86; (819)563-0513; Fax. (819)564-6889.

DESSAIN, Mathieu; CSSS du Lac-des-Deux-Montagnes, 520 boul Arthur-Sauve, Saint-Eustache QC J7R 5B1; Mon'04; FRCPC; IntMed. Staff, Hôpital de Saint-Eustache; (450)473-6811; Fax. (450)473-6966.

DESSAU, Jean-Claude; Clin Med La Cite Place Du Parc, 900-300 rue Leo Pariseau, Montreal QC H2X 4B3; Mon'76; Staff, Centre Hospitalier l'Université de Montréal (CHUM) - Hôtel-Dieu; (514)281-1722; Fax. (514)281-6697.

DESSENS, Peter N; 624 Almandine Crt, Kelowna BC V1W 4Z5; Sask'82; (250)764-6337

DESSON, Sheana; Generations Family Hlth Ctr, 104-272 Lawrence Ave W, Toronto ON M5M 4M1; (Ireland)'06; MB BCh; BAO; CCFP; (416)847-9999; Fax. (416)847-8999.

DESSOUKI, Esmat A; 194 King St W, Oshawa ON L1J 2J2; Shams (Egypt)'74; MB ChB; FRCSC; OrthSurg. Ac Staff, Lakeridge Health - Oshawa Site; Ac Staff, Lakeridge Health - Whitby Site; (905)404-6611; Fax. (905)404-6612.

DESSUREAULT, Francois; 864 boul Marie-Victorin, Boucherville QC J4B 1Y5; McG'73; Langs: Italian; Greek; English; (450)655-3609

DESSUREAULT, Jacques; CMF Berthier, CP 1230 Succ Bureau-Chef 788 rue Gilles-Villeneuve, Berthierville QC J0K 1A0; Mon'78; MSc; (450)836-4212; Fax. (450)836-4814.

DESSUREAULT, Jean; CSSS Haut-Richelieu-Rouville, 920 boul du Seminaire N, St-Jean-sur-Richel QC J3A 1B7; McG'81 McGill; BSc; Urol (General Surgery). Staff, Hôpital du Haut-Richelieu; (450)359-5000; deslem@videotron.ca.

DESSUREAULT, Josee; GMF Quatre-Bourgeois, 300-979 av de Bourgogne, Quebec QC G1W 2L4; Laval'99; FRCPC; Derm. Staff, Centre Hospitalier de Val d'Or; Langs: English; (418)653-4050; Fax. (418)653-4475.

DESSUREAULT, Louise; Clinique Familiale Pas-A-Pas, 3650 boul Henri-Bourassa E, Montreal-Nord QC H1H 1J6; Mon'88; CCFP; Staff, Hôpital du Sacre-Coeur de Montréal; Langs: Bilingual(French/English); (514)328-9797

DESSUREAULT, Lucie; CSSS de l'Energie, 1265 rue Trudel, Shawinigan QC G9N 8T3; Laval'84; Staff, Centre Hospitalier du Centre la Mauricie; (819)539-0300

DESSUREAULT, M Michele; Clinique de Rhumatologie, 1119 rue Sainte-Marguerite, Trois-Rivieres QC G8Z 1Y2; Laval'83; Rheum; IntMed. Ac Member, CSSS de Trois-Rivières; Assoc Researcher, CRMS Trois-Rivieres; Clin Instructeur JMC, Universite de Montreal; Langs: English; (819)370-8106; Fax. (819)370-8120; rhumato@cgocable.ca.

DESTRADE SOSA, Lief; 340 College St, Toronto ON M5T 3A9; Mon'06; CCFP; (416)324-9697; Fax. (416)324-9490.

DESY, Delphine; 5415 boul de l'Assomption, Montreal QC H1T 2M4; Mon'04; FRCPC; AnatPath. Staff, Hopital Maisonneuve-Rosemont; (514)252-3400

DESY, Dominique; Clinique méd Brome-Missiquoi, 280 rue Victoria, Knowlton QC J0E 1V0; Laval'95; Staff, Hôpital Brome-Missisquoi-Perkins; Staff Teacher, McGill University; Langs: English; (450)243-5043; Fax. (450)243-0537.

DESY, Jean; Clinique Jean Desy, RR 2 992 av Sainte-Brigitte, Ste-Brigitte-d-Lav QC G0A 3K0; Laval'77; Staff, Cree Board of Health & Social Services James Bay; (418)825-1795

DESY, Madeleine; CSSS de Saint-Jerome, 290 rue de Montigny, Saint-Jerome QC J7Z 5T3; Mon'74; MedOncol (P.Q.); Hem (P.Q.) (Hematological Oncology). Staff, Hôtel-Dieu de Saint-Jérôme; Langs: English; (450)431-8366

DESY, Marie-Andree; CLSC du Grand Chicoutimi, 411 rue de l'Hôtel-Dieu, Chicoutimi QC G7H 7Z5; Sher'01; CCFP; (418)543-2221

DETORAKIS, Anna; 5001 50 Ave, Beaumont AB T4X 1E7; Dal'10; (780)929-6050

DETSKY, Allan S; Mount Sinai Hosp, 429-600 University Ave, Toronto ON M5G 1X5; Harvard(MA) (USA)'78; FRCPC; IntMed. Staff Int Med, Toronto General Hospital - UHN; Staff, Mount Sinai Hospital; Prof Health Policy Management & Evaluation, University of Toronto; (416)586-8507; Fax. (416)586-8350; adetsky@mtsinai.on.ca.

DETTMAN, Leah; Maternity Care Clinic, 178 96 Ave NE, Calgary AB T3K 6G4; Man'06; CCFP; Staff, Maternity Care Clinic; (403)735-4922

DETTMAN, Michael S; Vancouver Gen Hosp, 855 12th Ave W, Vancouver BC V5Z 1M9; UBC'69; DAB; FRCPC; EmergMed. Staff, Vancouver General Hospital - Centennial Pavillion; Clinical Asst Prof, University of British Columbia; (604)875-4995; Fax. (604)875-4872; mdettman@vanhosp.bc.ca.

DEUMIE, Louis; CHUM-Hop Notre-Dame, 1560 rue Sherbrooke E, Montreal QC H2L 4M1; Angers (France)'69; Psy (P.Q.). Staff, Centre Hospitalier l'Université de Montréal (CHUM) - Hôpital Notre-Dame; Asst Prof Psy, Universite de Montreal; (514)890-8000 x26746

DEUTSCH, James; Youthdale Treatment Centre, 227 Victoria St, Toronto ON M5B 1T8; Yale(CT) (USA)'83; ABPN(P); ABAP; PhD; FRCPC; Psy (Child & Adolescent Psychiatry). Staff Psy, The Hospital For Sick Children; Staff Crisis Serv, Youthdale Treatment Centres; Asst Prof Psy, University of Toronto; (416)363-3751 x2011; Fax. (416)363-7945; j.deutsch@utoronto.ca.

DEUTSCH, Margaret J; 23 Cowichan Way, Ottawa ON K2H 7E6; Dal'72; CCFP; FCFP; Staff, The Ottawa Hospital - General Campus; (613)820-1658

DEUTSCH-ANDERMANN, Eva; MUHC-Montreal Neurology Inst, 127-3801 rue University, Montreal QC H3A 2B4; McG'63; PhD; CSPQ; MedGenetics; CommunMed (P.Q.); Electroenceph (P.Q.). Head Dept of Neurogenetics & Ass't EEG, McGill University Health Centre - Montreal Neurological Hospital; Aj Prof, McGill University; (514)398-8529

DEUTSCH-LEVY, Meredith; All About Health, E-1070 Major Mackenzie Dr E, Richmond Hill ON L4S 1P3; McG'01; CCFP; Langs: Hebrew; English; (905)884-0666; Fax. (905)884-5317; mdeutsch@her.jgh.mcgill.ca.

DEUTSCHER, Clive O; Workers' Comp Board, PO Box 2415 Stn Main 9912 107 St NW, Edmonton AB T5J 2S5; Sask'67; FRCPC; Respir. (780)498-4673; Fax. (780)498-7808.

DEUTSCHER, Myles; Herold Read Family Physicians, 1-325 Herold Rd, Saskatoon SK S7V 1J7; Sask'07; CCFP; (306)374-2404; Fax. (306)477-0300.

DEUTSCHER, Raymond; Physician Anes Services, 303-400 Tache Ave, Winnipeg MB R2H 3C3; Man'79; DABA; FRCPC; Anes. Staff, St Boniface General Hospital; Asst Prof, University of Manitoba; (204)233-3413; Fax. (204)233-9763.

DEUTSCHER, Timothy R; Seafield Med Bldg, 3-1179 Seafield Cres, Nanaimo BC V9S 4S1; Alb'77; FRCPC; PhysMed&Rehab. Staff, Nanaimo Regional General Hospital; (250)741-0755; Fax. (250)741-0766.

DEV, David A; A13-9600 Islington Ave, Woodbridge ON L4H 2T1; Tor'89; (905)893-8085; Fax. (905)893-8218.

DEV, Shelly P; Sunnybrook Hlth Sciences Ctre, D112-2075 Bayview Ave, Toronto ON M4N 3M5; Tor'01; FRCPC; IntMed (Critical Care Medicine). Staff, Sunnybrook Health Sciences Centre; (416)480-6100 x7689

DEVANE, Manik; Portage Prof Bldg, 405-5400 Portage Rd, Niagara Falls ON L2G 5X7; Karnatak (India)'65; Ac Staff ObstGyn, Niagara Health System - Greater Niagara General Site; Langs: Hindi; Marathi; (905)356-6718; Fax. (905)356-6719.

DEVANESEN, Asha K; Credit Valley Med Arts Centre, 308-2000 Credit Valley Rd, Mississauga ON L5M 4N4; Madras (India)'68; Ac Staff, The Credit Valley Hospital; Langs: Hindi; (905)828-1223

DEVANESEN, Sudarshan; Credit Valley Med Arts Centre, 308-2000 Credit Valley Rd, Mississauga ON L5M 4N4; Madras (India)'68; MClSc; CCFP; FCFP; Court Staff, St Michael's Hospital; Assoc Prof Med, University of Toronto; Langs: Hindi; Tamil; Sinhalese; (905)828-1223; Fax. (905)828-5119.

DEVANI, Alim R; Market Mall Prof Bldg, 206-4935 40 Ave NW, Calgary AB T3A 2N1; Alb'07; Derm. Staff, University of Alberta Hospital; (403)271-3627; Fax. (403)284-5272.

DEVARAJ, Chikkahanumaiah; South Peel Med Arts Bldg, 302-77 Queensway W, Mississauga ON L5B 1B7; Bangalore (India)'78; FRCPC; IntMed; GeriatricMed. Ac Staff, Trillium Health Centre - Mississauga; Langs: Hindi; Kanarese; (905)281-3185; Fax. (905)281-3186.

DEVARAJAN, Sivakumaran; Chatham-Kent Health Alliance, PO Box 2030 Stn Main 80 Grand Ave W, Chatham ON N7M 5L9; (Sri Lanka)'75; MB BS; MRCPsy(UK); FRCPC; Psy. Staff, Chatham-Kent Health Alliance; Langs: Sinhalese; Tamil; (519)351-6144; Fax. (519)351-0450.

DEVASSY, Mary T; North York Family After Hours, PO Box 91130 Rpo Bayview Village 2901 Bayview Ave, North York ON M2K 2Y6; Ott'70; BScN; Staff, North York General Hospital; Langs: Malayalam; (416)491-6338

DEVAUX, Angele; CSSS Pierre Boucher, 1333 boul Jacques-Cartier E, Longueuil QC J4M 2A5; Mon'02; FRCSC; Ophth (P.Q.). Staff, Centre Hospitalier Pierre Boucher; (450)468-8111

DEVAUX, Celine; Hop Charles Lemoyne, 3120 boul Taschereau, Greenfield Park QC J4V 2H1; Mon'00; CSPQ; FRCPC; IntMed; MedOncol; Hem. Staff, Hopital Charles LeMoyne; (450)466-5065; Fax. (450)466-5066.

DEVEAU, Carole; 201-1789 Mountain Rd, Moncton NB E1G 5C4; Dal'01; MSc; BSc; CCFP; Ac Medical Staff, The Moncton Hospital; Langs: English; French; (506)870-2806; Fax. (506)870-2808.

DEVEAU, Joey; Appletree Med Group, 2948 Baseline Rd, Ottawa ON K2H 8T5; Sher'08; CCFP; (613)482-0118; Fax. (613)288-2060.

DEVEAULT, Alain; Centre Med De Gentilly, 1775 boul Becancour, Becancour QC G9H 3V4; Mon'84; CSPQ; LMCC; Emergency Med, Centre Hospitalier Regional de Trois-Rivieres; (819)298-3113; Fax. (819)298-3114.

DEVEBER, Gabrielle A; 555 University Ave, Toronto ON M5G 1X8; McM'84; ABPN; MSCHC; FRCPC; Neur (Pediatric Stroke). Staff, The Hospital For Sick Children; Staff, Child Health Evaluative Sciences Program; Assoc Prof, University of Toronto; (416)813-7721; Fax. (416)813-6334.

DEVED, Vinay; Kingsway Prof Centre, 303-10611 Kingsway NW, Edmonton AB T5G 3C8; Alb'03; FRCPC; IntMed; Nephrol. Staff Div Neph in Dept Med, Royal Alexandra Hospital; (780)496-9350; Fax. (780)425-8475.

DEVENISH, Joanne M; Dawson Med Clinic, PO Box 829, Dawson YT Y0B 1G0; Cape Town (South Africa)'88; MB ChB; (867)993-5744

DEVENYI, Paul; 50 Grangemill Cres, North York ON M3B 2J2; Budapest (Hungary)'54; FRCPC; IntMed (Addiction Medicine). Consultant, Centre for Addiction & Mental Health (CAMH) - College Street Site; Consultant, Toronto Western Hospital - University Health Network; Asst Prof, University of Toronto; Langs: Hungarian; (416)444-0246; Fax. (416)444-0246.

DEVENYI, Robert G; Univ Hlth Network-Toronto Western Hosp, 6EW 438-399 Bathurst St, Toronto ON M5T 2S8; Tor'83; DAB; FACS(Ophth); FRCSC; Ophth (Vitreo Retinal Surgery). Clinical Dept Head, Toronto Western Hospital - University Health Network; Staff, The Hospital For Sick Children; Staff, Mount Sinai Hospital; Staff Teacher, University of Toronto; (416)603-5602; Fax. (416)603-6473.

DEVERAJALU, Ramachandran; Regina Qu'Appelle HR-Regina, 1440 14th Ave, Regina SK S4P 0W5; Madras (India)'66; FRCPath; FRCPC; HemPath. Staff, Regina General Hospital; (306)766-4444; Fax. (306)766-4772.

DEVEREAUX, Emily F; Horizons Family Medicine, A-5016 51 Ave, Red Deer AB T4N 4H5; Cal'09; CCFP; (403)342-7270; Fax. (403)343-2677.

DEVEREAUX, Philip; Hamilton HS-General Site, 237 Barton St E, Hamilton ON L8L 2X2; McM'94; FRCPC; IntMed; Cardiol. Staff, Hamilton Health Sciences Centre - Hamilton General Hospital; (905)527-4322

DEVERELL, Mark A V; Family Health Clinic, PO Box 1869 525 Causley St, Blind River ON P0R 1B0; Wes'86; (705)356-2265; Fax. (705)356-2403; mdeverell@brdhc.on.ca.

DEVI, Bijayalaxmi; Baywood Med Centre, 308-95 Bayly St W, Ajax ON L1S 7K8; Sambalpur (India)'78; FRCPC; Psy. Langs: Hindi; Oriya; (905)683-0702; Fax. (905)683-8381.

DEVI, Minati; 105-266 4 St SW, Medicine Hat AB T1A 4E5; (India)'94; MB BS; Staff, Medicine Hat Regional Hospital; (403)488-0200

DEVI, Shashi P; Sheppard Med Bldg, 203-701 Sheppard Ave E, North York ON M2K 2Z3; Lucknow (India)'76; CCFP; FCFP; Court Member Family Med, Rouge Valley Health System - Centenary Health Centre Site; Staff, Toronto General Hospital - UHN; Assoc Member, North York General Hospital; Langs: Hindi; Punjabi; Urdu; Gujarati; Bengali; (416)221-0176; Fax. (647)776-7696.

DEVI, Vimla; Peter Lougheed Centre, NICU-3500 26 Ave NE, Calgary AB T1Y 6J4; (Pakistan)'95; MB BS; Staff, Peter Lougheed Centre; (403)943-4892; Fax. (403)943-2565.

DEVILLER, Genevieve; 626 boul Rene-Levesque O, Quebec QC G1S 1S8; Montpellier (France)'71; (418)687-9646; Fax. (418)683-0136.

DEVIN, Brian; Village Health Centre, 3192 Logan Farm Dr, Osgoode ON K0A 2W0; Tor'93; BSc(Hons); CCFP; FCFP; Staff, Winchester District Memorial Hospital; (613)826-2502; Fax. (613)826-1682.

DEVINE, Luke; Mount Sinai Hosp, 427-600 University Ave, Toronto ON M5G 1X5; Tor'06; FRCPC; IntMed. Staff, Mount Sinai Hospital; (416)586-4800 x8563

DEVINS, Mary; IWK Health Centre, PO Box 9700 Rpo CSC 5850-5980 Univerity Ave, Halifax NS B3K 6R8; Galway (Ireland)'95; MB BCh; BAO; Staff, IWK Health Centre; (902)470-7262; Fax. (902)470-7216.

DEVINS, Robert L; Quinte HC Corp-Belleville Gen, 265 Dundas St E, Belleville ON K8N 5A9; Qns'91; Staff, QHC Belleville General; (613)969-5511 x2434

DEVITO, Isabella; Mount Sinai Hosp, 1514-600 University Ave, Toronto ON M5G 1X5; Wes'82; FRCPC; Anes. Staff Anes, Mount Sinai Hospital; (416)586-5270

DEVITT, James H; Clinical Sciences Bldg, 8 120-152 University Campus NW, Edmonton AB T6G 2G3; Ott'77; DAB; FRCPC; Anes (Critical Care Medicine). Staff Anes, Queen Elizabeth II Health Sciences Centre - Victoria General Site; Prof, Dalhousie University; (780)407-8887; Fax. (780)407-3200.

DEVITT, Neil; Radiology Associates of Regina, 6-2727 Parliament Ave, Regina SK S4S 6X5; Wes'72; FRCPC; DiagRad. Staff, Pasqua Hospital; Staff, Radiology Associates of Regina; (306)352-7653; Fax. (306)522-4311.

DEVLIN, H Roslyn; St Michael's Hosp, 30 Bond St, Toronto ON M5B 1W8; Tor'71; FRCPC; MedMicrobiol. Staff, St Michael's Hospital; (416)864-5418; Fax. (416)854-5194.

DEVLIN, H T Michael; West Park Healthcare Centre, 3F 92-82 Buttonwood Ave, Toronto ON M6M 2J5; Tor'76; FRCPC; PhysMed&Rehab (Psychiatry). Staff, West Park Healthcare Centre; Asst Prof Div of Physiatry, University of Toronto; (416)243-3680; Fax. (416)243-1177.

DEVLIN, Paul G; 204-9656 king George Hwy, Surrey BC V3T 2V5; Dublin (Ireland)'77; MB ChB; FRCPC; Psy. Med Dir Psy, Surrey Memorial Hospital; (604)634-0500

DEVLIN, Rueben; 76 Prospect St, Newmarket ON L3Y 3T2; Tor'74; FRCSC; OrthSurg. (905)898-2384; Fax. (905)898-3021; rdevlin@rogers.com.

DEVLIN, Shane; 1031 Russet Rd NE, Calgary AB T2E 5L2; Man'99; FRCPC; IntMed (Inflammatory Bowel Disease); Gastroent. Clin Asst Prof, Peter Lougheed Centre; Physician, Health Research Innovation Centre; (403)277-7321; Fax. (403)277-7327.

DEVLIN, Timothy; 1500-150 York St, Toronto ON M5H 3S5; Tor'80; FRCPC; IntMed; Gastroent. Ac Staff, The Scarborough Hospital - Birchmount Campus; Sr Consultant, Medcan Health Management Inc; Instructor, University of Toronto; (416)350-5963; timdevlin@rogers.com.

DEVON, Jennifer L; Scarborough Hosp-General Div, 3050 Lawrence Ave E, Scarborough ON M1P 2V5; Tor'05; CCFP; CCFP(E.M.); Staff, The Scarborough Hospital - General Campus; (416)438-2911; Fax. (416)431-8204.

DEVON, Joshua G; Bramalea Med Centre, 507-18 Kensington Rd, Brampton ON L6T 4S5; Tor'73; Court Staff, William Osler Health System - Brampton Civic Hospital; (905)792-2228; Fax. (905)792-2275.

DEVON, Karen M; Women's College Hosp, 76 Grenville St, Toronto ON M5S 1B2; McG'04; FRCSC; GenSurg. Staff, Women's College Hospital; (416)323-6400

DEVONSHIRE, Virginia; 802-145 13th St E, North Vancouver BC V7L 2L4; Cal'89; FRCPC; Neur (Multiple Sclerosis). Staff, Vancouver General Hospital - Centennial Pavillion; Staff, UBC Hospital - Koerner Pavillion; (604)986-9961; Fax. (604)986-8667.

DEVOST, Nicole; Lakeridge Hlth Corp-Oshawa, 1 Hospital Crt, Oshawa ON L1G 2B9; Laval'80; CCFP; FCFP; Staff, Lakeridge Health - Oshawa Site; Langs: Bilingual(French/English); (905)576-8711 x3931

DEVRAJ-KIZUK, Rozemin P E; Palliser Med Clinic, 210-740 4 Ave S, Lethbridge AB T1J 0N9; McM'89; MSc; CCFP; Staff, Chinook Regional Hospital; Staff, Covenant Health - St Michael's Health Centre; (403)381-1013; Fax. (403)381-4011.

DEVROEDE, Ghislain J; CHUS-Hop Fleurimont, 3001 12e av N, Sherbrooke QC J1H 5N4; Louvain (Belgium)'61; DABS; MSc(Minn); DABCRS; CSPQ; FRCSC; GenSurg (Gastroenterology). Ac Staff, Centre Hospitalier Universitaire de Sherbrooke-Hopital Fleurimont; Prof Surg & Communication, Universite de Sherbrooke; Langs: Bilingual(French/English); (819)564-5231; Fax. (819)820-6871; ghislain.devroede@usherbrooke.ca.

DEW, Bernard; Humber River Reg Hosp-Church, 200 Church St, Toronto ON M9N 1N8; Tor'89; CCFP; CCFP(E.M.); FCFP; Staff, Humber River Regional Hospital - Church Street Site; (416)243-4103

DEWA, Dalisizwe M K; 203-224 Pacific Ave, Saskatoon SK S7K 1P1; (Zimbabwe)'90; FRCPC; IntMed (Echocardiography); Cardiol. Staff, Royal University Hospital; (306)975-0330; Fax. (306)975-0503.

DEWAILLY, Eric; CRCHUQ, 600-2875 boul Laurier, Quebec QC G1V 2M2; Lille (France)'82; Ac Staff, Centre Hospitalier Universitaire de Quebec-CHUL; assoc Prof Med, Université Laval; (418)656-4141 x46518; Fax. (418)654-2726.

DEWAN, Ambika; Bruyere Family Med Centre, 75 Bruyere St, Ottawa ON K1N 5C8; Tor'10; CCFP; (613)241-3344

DEWAN, Tammie J; Children's & Women's HC of BC, K1 111-4480 Oak St, Vancouver BC V6H 3V4; Dal'06; FRCPC; Peds. Staff, BC Children's Hospital; (604)875-3039

DEWAR, Catharine; 105-145 15th St W, North Vancouver BC V7M 1R9; Cal'85; PhD; FRCPC; IntMed (Adult Rheumatology); Rheum. Consultant Rheum, Lions Gate Hospital; (604)984-7617; Fax. (604)984-7672.

DEWAR, Charles M; O'Leary Hlth Centre, PO Box 550, O'Leary PE C0B 1V0; Dal'54; CCFP; FCFP; Ac Staff, Community Hospital Inc; Court Staff, Western Hospital - Health PEI; (902)859-3929; Fax. (902)859-3922.

DEWAR, Gary J; Richmond Med Bldg, 309-2020 Richmond Rd, Victoria BC V8R 6R5; Sask'71; FACS; FRCSC; GenSurg (Esophagus); ThorSurg. Staff, Royal Jubilee Hospital; Staff, Victoria General Hospital; (250)595-2820; Fax. (250)598-2850.

DEWAR, James D; Medical Assoc of Port Colborne, 97 Charlotte St, Port Colborne ON L3K 3E2; Wes'63; Staff, Niagara Health System - Port Colborne General Site; (905)834-4216; Fax. (905)834-3114.

DEWAR, Leith; Vancouver Gen Hosp, 855 12th Ave W, Vancouver BC V5Z 1M9; UBC'87; FRCSC; GenSurg; CardiothorSurg. Staff, Vancouver General Hospital - Centennial Pavillion; (604)875-4111

DEWARE, Kimberley J; Moncton Med Clinic, 203-860 Mountain Rd, Moncton NB E1C 2N7; Dal'73; CCFP; FCFP; Ac Staff, The Moncton Hospital; (506)853-5135; Fax. (506)389-2425.

DEWART, John M; Cabrini Centre, 4F-16811 88 Ave NW, Edmonton AB T5R 5Y6; Alb'83; FRCPC; Psy. Ac Staff, Covenant Health - Misericordia Community Hospital; Asst Clin Prof, University of Alberta; (780)735-2934

DEWITT, Christopher; St Paul's Hosp, 1081 Burrard St, Vancouver BC V6Z 1Y6; Colorado(CO) (USA)'98; EmergMed. Staff, Providence Health Care - St Paul's Hospital; (604)806-8480

DEWITT TALBOT, Dawn; Gordon & Leslie Health Care CC, 11F-2775 Laurel St, Vancouver BC V5Z 1M9; Harvard University (USA)'90; FRCPC; IntMed. Staff, Gordon & Leslie Diamond Health Care Centre; (604)875-4111 x66499

DEXTRAZE, Pierrette; 1629 rue St-Georges CP 100, Saint-Bernard QC G0S 2G0; Mon'75; (418)475-6615; Fax. (418)475-4369.

DEY, Chris; Sunnybrook Hlth Sciences Ctre, 2075 Bayview Ave, Toronto ON M4N 3M5; London (England)'98; Staff, Sunnybrook Health Sciences Centre; (416)480-6100

DEYELL, Marc W; Heart Rhythm Services, 211-1033 Davie St, Vancouver BC V6E 1M7; Alb'02; FRCPC; IntMed; Cardiol. (604)806-8256

DEYELL, Rebecca J; Children's & Women's HC of BC, A119C-4480 Oak St, Vancouver BC V6H 3V4; Alb'03; FRCPC; Peds (Peripheral Nerve Blocks). Staff, BC Children's Hospital; (604)875-2345 x4815; Fax. (604)875-2911.

DEYHOLOS, Michelle; Foothills Prof Bldg, 170-1620 29 St NW, Calgary AB T2N 4L7; Cal'89; Staff Privil Acute Care, Foothills Medical Centre; (403)237-6404; Fax. (403)266-4746.

DEZIEL, Annie; Hotel-Dieu de Sorel, 400 av de l'Hotel-Dieu, Sorel-Tracy QC J3P 1N5; Mon'05; CCFP; Staff, Hôtel-Dieu de Sorel; (450)746-6000

DEZIEL, Clement; Hop du Sacre-Coeur de Mtl, 5400 boul Gouin O, Montreal QC H4J 1C5; Mon'69; CSPQ; Nephrol (P.Q.). Head Nephrol, Hôpital du Sacre-Coeur de Montréal; (514)338-2050

DEZIEL, Francois; CSSS de Rivière-de-Loup, 75 rue Saint-Henri, Riviere-Du-Loup QC G5R 2A4; Mon'88; Peds. Staff, Centre Hospitalier Regional du Grand-Portage; (418)868-1010 x837; Fax. (418)868-3338.

DEZIEL, Francois; Dept of Veteran's Affairs, PO Box 7700 Stn Central, Charlottetown PE C1A 8M9; Ott'69; IntMed (Administrative Medicine). Physician, Veterans Affairs Canada; (902)566-8888; francois.deziel@vac-acc.gc.ca.

DEZIEL, Luc; Carrefour Sante Le St-Laurent, 140-5300 boul Saint-Laurent, Sainte-Catherine QC J5C 1A8; Mon'85; (450)638-6383; Fax. (450)635-6359.

DEZIEL, Marcel; Clin Med Centre-Ville, 1652 rue Royale, Trois-Rivieres QC G9A 4K3; Mon'82.

DHADLY, Pritam P S; Univ Hosp of Northern BC, 1475 Edmonton St, Prince George BC V2M 1S2; Leicester (United Kingdom)'91; MB ChB; FRCA; BMedSci; Staff, University Hospital of Northern British Columbia; (250)565-2000; Fax. (250)565-2343.

DHADWAR, Achinder K; 306-18 Kensington Rd, Brampton ON L6T 4S5; Wes'05; CCFP; (905)463-2095; Fax. (905)463-2096.

DHAITI, Magalie; Clinique Med Ste-Colette, 11520 boul Sainte-Colette, Montreal-Nord QC H1G 6J3; Sher'82; Staff, CHSLD Gouin Inc; (514)323-0430; Fax. (514)328-9643.

DHALIWAL, Amarinder S; 3-900 Ray Lawson Blvd, Brampton ON L6Y 5H7; Punjabi (India)'85; Langs: Hindi; Punjabi; (905)796-1444; Fax. (905)796-1494.

DHALIWAL, Baljinder; Vancouver Gen Hosp, 2449-855 12th Ave W, Vancouver BC V5Z 1M9; UBC'03; FRCPC; Anes. Staff, Vancouver General Hospital - Centennial Pavillion; (604)875-4304; Fax. (604)875-5344.

DHALIWAL, Gurpreet S; South Health Campus, 4448 Front St SE, Calgary AB T3M 1M4; Man'03; FRCSC; OrthSurg. (403)956-3692; Fax. (403)956-3275.

DHALIWAL, Harbhajan S; CancerCare Manitoba, 4025-675 Mcdermot Ave, Winnipeg MB R3E 0V9; Birmingham (England)'72; MB ChB; FRCP; CancerCare Manitoba; Langs: Punjabi; Hindi; Urdu; (204)787-2241; Fax. (204)787-1184.

DHALIWAL, Harinder; The Ottawa Hosp-Civic Campus, 1053 Carling Ave, Ottawa ON K1Y 4E9; UBC'04; FRCPC; IntMed; Gastroent. Staff, The Ottawa Hospital - Civic Campus; (613)798-5555

DHALIWAL, Harinder S; Foothills Medical Centre, 1403 29 St NW, Calgary AB T2N 2T9; (India)'00; Staff, Foothills Medical Centre; (403)944-1110

DHALIWAL, Harjinder S; Metrotown Med Centre, 303-6411 Nelson Ave, Burnaby BC V5H 4H3; Man'91; FRCSC; Ophth. Ophthalmology, Burnaby Hospital; Staff, Vancouver General Hospital - Centennial Pavillion; Asst Prof, University of British Columbia; Langs: Punjabi; (604)433-1258; Fax. (604)433-6154; kinder@limojetgold.com.

DHALIWAL, Harmanpreet V; 103-16033 108 Ave, Surrey BC V4N 1P2; (Senegal)'04; CCFP; Langs: Punjabi; (778)395-4446

DHALIWAL, Jagtaran S; 206-7900 Hurontario St, Brampton ON L6Y 0P6; Punjab (India)'75; FRCPC; Psy. Langs: Punjabi.

DHALIWAL, Jamit S; Harry Medovy House, 2F-671 William Ave, Winnipeg MB R3E 0Z2; Man'06; Anes.

DHALIWAL, Jaskaren K; 180 Sandalwood Parkway E, Brampton ON L6Z 1Y4; Wes'09; CCFP; University of Western Ontario; (905)846-9255; Fax. (905)846-2525.

DHALIWAL, Mandeep S; Rivers Medical Centre, PO Box 429, Rivers MB R0K 1X0; (Other Foreign)'02; (204)881-4897

DHALIWAL, Navdeep; R J A Medicentres Cnd Inc, 204-10458 Mayfield Rd NW, Edmonton AB T5P 4P4; UBC'04; CCFP; (780)483-7115; Fax. (780)484-6531.

DHALIWAL, Preet B K; 5881 Malden Rd, LaSalle ON N9H 1S5; Punjabi (India)'95; CCFP; Langs: Hindi; Urdu; Punjabi; (519)966-2473; Fax. (519)966-8961.

DHALIWAL, Rajinder; 200-3207 30 Ave, Vernon BC V1T 2C6; (Grenada)'05; CCFP; (250)549-1216

DHALIWAL, Ravinder; 117 McKellar St S, Thunder Bay ON P7E 1H5; NOSM'10; CCFP; (807)626-1234

DHALIWAL, Shannon; Ridge Meadows Hosp & Hlth CC, PO Box 5000 Stn Del Ctr 11666 Laity St, Maple Ridge BC V2X 7G5; UBC'03; Staff, Ridge Meadows Hospital & Health Care Centre; (604)875-4892

DHALIWAL, Yadvinder S; Airport Medical Centre, 127-2980 Drew Rd, Mississauga ON L4T 0A7; Manchester (England)'84; MB ChB; Langs: Punjabi; (905)678-6365

DHALLA, Aminmohamed; 309-3850 Finch Ave E, Scarborough ON M1T 3T6; Tor'89; Ac Staff Family Pract & Emerg, The Scarborough Hospital - Birchmount Campus; Langs: Gujarati; (416)292-2002; Fax. (416)292-2002.

DHALLA, Fatima; Caremedics Med Centre, 18-1910 St Laurent Blvd, Ottawa ON K1G 1A4; Makerere (Uganda)'72; MB ChB; CCFP; FCFP; Langs: Hindi; Urdu; Gujarati; (613)523-5550; Fax. (613)523-5580.

DHALLA, Irfan A N; St Michael's Hosp, 30 Bond St, Toronto ON M5B 1W8; Tor'03; FRCPC; IntMed. Staff, St Michael's Hospital; (416)864-6060

DHALLA, Mohsin N; 70 King St E, Stoney Creek ON L8G 1K2; Qns'04; CCFP; Langs: Gujarati; Hindi; Urdu; (905)667-3939; Fax. (905)662-6553.

DHALLA, Sonny; Brandon Med Arts Building, 339 Princess Ave, Brandon MB R7A 0N7; Man'83; BSc; FRCSC; GenSurg (Gastroenterology). Chief GI Unit, Brandon Regional Health Centre; (204)728-9460; Fax. (204)728-9535; varsity@westman.wave.ca.

DHALLA, Zahir A K; Nepean Med Centre, 301-1 Centrepointe Dr, Nepean ON K2G 6E2; Tor'84; FRCPC; Neur (Electromyography). (613)225-2131; Fax. (613)225-2849.

DHAMANASKAR, Kavita P; Hamilton Hs-Henderson Site, 711 Concession St, Hamilton ON L8V 1C3; Pune (India)'89; FRCPC; DiagRad. Staff Radiologist, Hamilton Health Sciences Centre-Juravinski Site; Langs: Hindi; (905)527-4322; Fax. (905)575-2660.

DHAMANASKAR, Prashant K; The Credit Valley Hosp, 200 Eglinton Ave W, Mississauga ON L5M 2N1; Pune (India)'91; FRCPC; AnatPath (General Pathology). Staff, Grand River Hospital - Kitchener/Waterloo Health Centre; Staff, The Credit Valley Hospital; (905)813-2200

DHAMI, Karan S; Queensway Med Centre, 300-5307 Canotek Rd, Ottawa ON K1J 9M2; Ott'08; CCFP; CCFP(E.M.); Langs: Hindi; Punjabi; (613)746-6223; Fax. (613)746-6018.

DHAMI, Randeep S; Height Medical, 4446 Hastings St, Burnaby BC V5C 2K2; UBC'86; CCFP; CCFP(E.M.).

DHANANI, Al-Noor; 301-101 Queensway W, Mississauga ON L5B 2P7; Tor'86; FRCP; MD; FRCPC; Neur (Neuromuscular Diseases). Staff, Trillium Health Centre - West Toronto; Med Consultant, The Credit Valley Hospital; Ac Staff, Trillium Health Centre - Mississauga; Langs: Gujarati; Kacchi; (905)270-2300; Fax. (905)270-0290.

DHANANI, Sonny; Children's Hosp Eastern Ont, 401 Smyth Rd, Ottawa ON K1H 8L1; UBC'98; Staff, Children's Hospital of Eastern Ontario (CHEO); (613)737-7600 x3654

DHANDA, Dharminder S; 200-555 Sixth St, New Westminster BC V3L 5H1; Wes'97; FRCSC; Ophth. Langs: Hindi; Punjabi; (604)521-4144

DHANI, Neesha; Univ Hlth Network-Princess M, 610 University Ave, Toronto ON M5G 2M9; Wes'01; FRCPC; IntMed; MedOncol. Staff, Princess Margaret Hospital - University Health Network; (416)946-2000

DHANIDINA, Mohammad; William Osler Hc-Etobicoke, 101 Humber College Blvd, Etobicoke ON M9V 1R8; Aberdeen (Scotland)'87; FRCPC; Anes. Staff Anes, William Osler Health System - Etobicoke General Hospital; (416)747-3554

DHANJAL, Permjeet S; St James Street Med Clinic, 1600 Portage Ave, Winnipeg MB R3J 0C6; Man'96; MD; BSc(Med); CCFP; FCFP; Langs: Punjabi; (204)774-1868; Fax. (204)774-7303; dhanjal123@aol.com.

DHANJI, Sadrudin; Madigan Shopp Centre, 48-6060 Memorial Dr NE, Calgary AB T2A 5Z5; Alb'80; BMedSci; CCFP; (403)272-8130; Fax. (403)248-1535.

DHANOA, Avtar S; Pickwick Med Clinic, 5B-1474 Pickwick Dr, Mississauga ON L5V 2G2; Mysore (India)'84; Court Staff, Trillium Health Centre - Mississauga; Langs: Hindi; Malay; Punjabi; (905)812-5552; Fax. (905)812-5553.

DHANOA, Ravijindera S; Shawnigan Village Family Pract, PO Box 240 2749 Dundas Rd, Shawnigan Lake BC V0R 2W0; London (England)'06; MB BS; (250)743-0793

DHANSAY, Aadil; 130-520 2nd Ave, Campbell River BC V9W 3V1; Cape Town (South Africa)'03; MB ChB; Staff, Campbell River & District General Hospital; (250)286-4061

DHAR, Anil; Pulmonary & Critical Care, 150-1720 Howard Ave, Windsor ON N8X 5A6; Kashmir (India)'84; FRCPC; IntMed; Critical Care Medicine; Respir. Langs: Kashmiri; Hindi; (519)255-7964; Fax. (519)255-9320; anil@dhar.org.

DHAR, Jag Mohan; 325-325 Wellington St, Sarnia ON N7T 1H4; Delhi (India)'74; MRCP(UK); DCH; FRCPC; IntMed (Nephrology). Staff Internist, Bluewater Health - Norman Site; Langs: Hindi; Kashmiri; Urdu; (519)344-4726; Fax. (519)344-4534.

DHARAMSHI, Arif; Cachet Family Phsicians, 2-9255 Woodbine Ave, Markham ON L6C 1Y9; Tor'89; Ac Staff Emerg. & Family Pract., Rouge Valley Health System - Centenary Health Centre Site; (905)887-2222; Fax. (905)887-3655.

DHARAMSHI, Shafik S N; Briarhill Med Centre, 58A-2700 Dufferin St, York ON M6B 4J3; Tor'86; Staff, The Scarborough Hospital - General Campus; (905)887-0737; Fax. (905)887-3671.

DHARAMSI, Altaf; Burnaby Hosp, 3935 Kincaid St, Burnaby BC V5G 2X6; UBC'99; CCFP; Staff, Burnaby Hospital; (604)434-4211

DHARAMSI, Nafisa; Children's Hospital, 301-840 Sherbrook St, Winnipeg MB R3A 1S1; Cal'98; FRCSC; Urol (Pediatric Urology). (204)787-4250; Fax. (204)787-2621.

DHARMALINGAM, Sudharshan; Brampton Med Bldg, 307-164 Queen St E, Brampton ON L6V 1B4; Man'96; FRCP; BSc; FRCPC; IntMed; Endocrin&Metab. Staff, William Osler Health System - Brampton Civic Hospital; Langs: Tamil; (905)451-2967; Fax. (905)450-0077.

DHARMAWARDENE, Marisa L; 710-3031 Hospital Dr NW, Calgary AB T2N 2T8; Cal'05; CCFP; (403)944-2304; Fax. (403)270-9652.

DHARSSI, Karim; 400-100 Colborne St W, Orillia ON L3V 2Y9; Man'07; CCFP; Staff, Orillia Soldiers' Memorial Hospital; (705)326-8335; Fax. (705)326-6365.

DHATT, Deepinderjit R; Northern Ontario Med Offices, B1-2009 Long Lake Rd, Sudbury ON P3E 6C3; Qns'90; CCFP; FCFP; (705)586-3601; Fax. (705)586-3602.

DHAWAN, Bal Chandra; Yarmouth Reg Hosp, 306C-60 Vancouver St, Yarmouth NS B5A 2P5; Bhopal (India)'79; Staff, Yarmouth Regional Hospital; (902)742-9234; Fax. (902)742-4365.

DHAWAN, Nishi; West Coast Women's Clinic, 3525 4th Ave W, Vancouver BC V5R 1N9; Dal'91; MB; BSc(Hons); CCFP; Co-Founder, Westcoast Women's Clinic For Midlife Health; Langs: Hindi; Punjabi; (604)738-9601; Fax. (604)738-9605.

DHAWAN, Pankaj M; 930-943 Broadway W, Vancouver BC V5Z 4E1; Gujarat (India)'80; MB BS; FRCPC; PhysMed&Rehab (Acquired Brain Injury). Staff, G F Strong Rehabilitation Centre; Staff, Vancouver General Hospital - Centennial Pavillion; Staff, UBC Hospital - Koerner Pavillion; Clinical Asst Prof Med, University of British Columbia; Langs: Hindi; Punjabi; Gujarati; (604)737-7375

DHAWAN, Shalini; Lakeshore Woods Med Clinic, 6-3420 Rebecca St, Oakville ON L6L 6W2; Tor'91; (905)847-2525

DHAWAN, Vivek; First Edmonton Place, 1370-10665 Jasper Ave NW, Edmonton AB T5J 3S9; (Russia (Federation))'00; FRCPC; IntMed; Respir. Staff IntMed, University of Alberta Hospital; (780)702-3884

DHEDA, Roshan M; Medical Clinic, 461 Holland St W, Bradford ON L3Z 0C1; Witwatersrand (South Africa)'88; MB BCh; LMCC; CCFP; FCFP; Ac Staff, Southlake Regional Health Centre; Langs: Gujarati; (905)775-3269; Fax. (905)775-0693.

DHESI, Ravinderjit K; 203-1370 Clyde Ave, Nepean ON K2G 3H8; Punjab (India)'65; FRCPC; Psy. (613)798-7954

DHESY-THIND, Sukhbinder; The Juravinski Cancer Centre, 699 Concession St, Hamilton ON L8V 5C2; Qns'96; FRCPC; IntMed (Clinician Investigator Program); MedOncol. Physician, The Juravinski Cancer Centre; (905)387-9495 x64604; Fax. (905)575-6326.

DHILLON, Anureet; 113-4515 Ebenezer Rd, Brampton ON L6P 2K7; Karnatak (India)'01; CCFP; (905)794-4088; Fax. (905)794-4259.

DHILLON, Arunbir; West Winds Med Clinic, 2130-4818 Westwinds Dr NE, Calgary AB T3J 3Z5; Ravi Shankar (India)'02; MB BS; (403)293-5454; Fax. (403)293-1511.

DHILLON, Avtar S; Gandhi Med Clinic, 203-6935 120 St, Delta BC V4E 2A8; Gurunanak (India)'90; MB BS; FRCPC; IntMed. Staff, Langley Memorial Hospital; Langs: Punjabi; (604)507-9441; Fax. (604)507-9664.

DHILLON, Baldev S; 108-7445 120 St, Delta BC V4C 0B3; Grace (Belize)'01; CCFP; Teach Staff Medical School, University of British Columbia; Langs: Hindi; Punjabi; (604)598-3936; Fax. (604)598-3935.

DHILLON, Davy; 3348 Hospital Rd, Vanderhoof BC V0J 3A2; McM'98; CCFP; (250)567-2201

DHILLON, Gagandeep S; Trillium Hlth Ctre-Mississauga, 100 Queensway W, Mississauga ON L5B 1B8; Tor'06; IntMed. Staff, Trillium Health Centre - Mississauga; (905)848-7100

DHILLON, Jasvinder; Humber River Reg Hosp-Finch, 2111 Finch Ave W, North York ON M3N 1N1; Guru Nanek Dev (India)'84; Critical Care Medicine; Peds. Staff, Humber River Regional Hospital - Finch Avenue Site; (804)747-3824; Fax. (647)435-5024.

DHILLON, Jaswinder S; Brantford Med Centre, 40 Shellington Place, Brantford ON N3S 0C5; Man'90; BSc; MHSc; CCFP; CCFP(E.M.); Staff, The Brant Community Healthcare System - Brantford General Hospital Site; Court Staff, Halton Healthcare Services Corporation - Oakville Site; Med Dir, Active Claims Management; Langs: Punjabi; Hindi; French; (519)753-9581; Fax. (519)753-9547.

DHILLON, Jatinder S; Victoria Park Clinic, 95 Darling St, Brantford ON N3T 2K7; Man'88; Staff, The Credit Valley Hospital; Langs: Punjabi; (416)720-0712; Fax. (416)720-0713.

DHILLON, Karamvir K; Oshawa Clinic, 117 King St E, Oshawa ON L1H 1B9; Pune (India)'98; MB BS; AAFP; CCFP; Langs: Hindi; Urdu; (905)721-6159; Fax. (905)721-6619.

DHILLON, Kirandeep; Niagara H System-G Niagara, 5546 Portage Rd, Niagara Falls ON L2E 6X2; (Other Foreign)'07; Staff, Niagara Health System - Greater Niagara General Site; (905)378-4647

DHILLON, Manu; Southgate Plaza, 6C-700 Balmoral Dr, Brampton ON L6T 1X2; Guru Nanak (India)'76; Langs: Hindi; Punjabi; Urdu; (905)790-2323; Fax. (905)790-6133.

DHILLON, Pawandeep K; 204-18730 Fraser Hwy, Surrey BC V3S 7Y4; Qns'04; CCFP; Langs: Punjabi; (604)575-0501; Fax. (604)575-0508.

DHILLON, Rajvir; Market Mall Office Centre, 208-3625 Shaganappi Trail NW, Calgary AB T3A 0E2; Alb'98; CCFP; (403)286-9118; Fax. (403)286-3069.

DHILLON, Rajwinder S; Niagara H System-G Niagara, 5546 Portage Rd, Niagara Falls ON L2E 6X2; Santiago (Dominican Republic)'98; FRCPC; IntMed; Rheum. Staff, Niagara Health System - Greater Niagara General Site; Langs: Punjabi; (905)358-0171

DHILLON, Ramninder; Crowfoot Primary Care, 201-60 Crowfoot Cres NW, Calgary AB T3G 3J9; Sask'07; CCFP; (403)374-0244

DHILLON, Ripple; Tauton Health Centre, SS 201 1290 Keith Ross Dr, Oshawa ON L1H 7K4; Punjab (India)'84; CCFP; FCFP; Court Staff, Lakeridge Health - Oshawa Site; Langs: Punjabi; Hindi; (905)721-4300 x5441; Fax. (905)721-6685; drdhillon@oshawaclinic.com.

DHIMAN, S Paul; Surrey Mem Hosp, 13750 96 Ave, Surrey BC V3V 1Z2; Qns'02; CCFP; CCFP(E.M.); Staff, Surrey Memorial Hospital; Langs: Punjabi; (604)581-2211

DHINDSA, Navjot; Arthritis Centre, RR 149-800 Sherbrook St, Winnipeg MB R3A 1M4; Punjab (India)'87; FRCPC; IntMed; Rheum. Staff, The Rehabilitation Centre; (204)787-2270; ndhindsa@cc.umanitoba.ca.

DHINGRA, Danny; 8171 Cook Rd, Richmond BC V6Y 3T8; (USA)'08; (604)279-1942

DHINGRA, Sanjay K; Scarborough Prof Centre, 406-1371 Neilson Rd, Scarborough ON M1B 4Z8; Sask'87; FRCPC; IntMed; Critical Care Medicine; Cardiol. (416)281-9499; Fax. (416)283-5705.

DHINGRA, Vinay K; Vancouver Gen Hosp, ICU 2438-855 12th Ave W, Vancouver BC V5Z 1M9; Sask'91; FRCPC; IntMed; Critical Care Medicine. Staff, Vancouver General Hospital - Centennial Pavillion; Staff, UBC Hospital - Koerner Pavillion; (604)875-5949; Fax. (604)875-5957.

DHIR, Achal K; London HSC-Univ Campus Site, PO Box 5339 Stn B 339 Windermere Rd, London ON N6A 5A5; Meerut (India)'78; FRCPC; Anes. Staff, London Health Sciences Centre - University Hospital; (519)663-3022

DHIR, Anita; Royal University Hosp, 103 Hospital Dr, Saskatoon SK S7N 0W8; Sask'02; FRCPC; DiagRad. Staff, Royal University Hospital; (306)655-2371

DHIRAJ, Navraj S; Hawthorne Village Med Clinic, 205-10220 Derry Rd, Milton ON L9T 7J3; Alb'99; CCFP; Asst Prof, McMaster University; Langs: Punjabi; (905)878-0676; ndhiraj@gmail.com.

DHLIWAYO, Harold K A; University of Alberta Hosp, 2A2 41-8440 112 St NW, Edmonton AB T6G 2B7; (Zimbabwe)'94; MB ChB; Staff, University of Alberta Hospital; (780)407-6907; Fax. (780)407-3853.

DHOLASANIA, Rozina N; All About Health, E-1070 Major Mackenzie Dr E, Richmond Hill ON L4S 1P3; (India)'03; CCFP; (905)884-0666; Fax. (905)884-5317.

DHUNNOO, Indra M C; College Plaza, 505-8215 112 St NW, Edmonton AB T6G 2C8; Cape Town (South Africa)'88; FRCPC; Peds (Cardiology). Clinical Asst Prof, University of Alberta; Langs: Hindi; French; Greek; (780)432-1414; Fax. (780)432-1336.

DHUNNOO, Krish; River Bend Retirement Clinic, 103 Rabbit Hill Crt NW, Edmonton AB T6R 2V3; Manchester (England)'76; MB ChB; MRC; Sec-Treas Senior Residence, Riverbend Retirement Residence; (780)438-2777

DHURJON, Leland M; Port Arthur Health Centre Inc, 194 Court St N, Thunder Bay ON P7A 4V7; (Jamaica)'81; MB BS; FRCSC; Ophth. (807)346-1000

DI CARLO, Domenico; Keele Med Place, 404-2830 Keele St, North York ON M3M 3E5; Florence (Italy)'79; BScPharm; Ac Staff, Humber River Regional Hospital - Church Street Site; Med Dir, Villa Colombo; Langs: Italian; (416)633-5558; Fax. (416)633-4264.

DI CECCO, David A; Pine-Seven Office Park, 301-4610 Hwy 7, Woodbridge ON L4L 4Y7; Tor'83; Court Staff, Humber River Regional Hospital - Finch Avenue Site; (905)265-7577; Fax. (905)265-7266.

DI CECCO, Robert; London HSC-Victoria Hosp, PO Box 5010 Stn B 800 Commissioners Rd E, London ON N6A 5W9; Tor'93; FRCSC; ObstGyn (Colposcopy). Court Staff, London Health Sciences Centre - Victoria Campus; Court Staff, Strathroy Middlesex General Hospital - Middlesex Hospital Alliance; Ac Staff, St Joseph's Hospital - St Joseph's Health Care; Assoc Prof ObstGyn, University of Western Ontario; Langs: Italian; (519)685-8500; robert.dicecco@sjhc.london.on.ca.

DI CESARE, Marie; Town Square Med Clinic, 102-8585 160 St, Surrey BC V4N 1G4; UBC'91; (604)593-5085

DI COSTANZO, Giovanni A; Markham Urology, 309-377 Church St, Markham ON L6B 1A1; McG'83; FRCSC; Urol (Infertility). Ac Staff/Hd Urol, Markham Stouffville Hospital; Langs: French; Italian; (905)472-7120; Fax. (905)472-2971.

DI DIODATO, Giulio; Royal Victoria Hosp, 201 Georgian Dr, Barrie ON L4M 6M2; McM'97; FRCPC; IntMed; Critical Care Medicine. Staff, Royal Victoria Regional Health Centre; (705)728-9802

DI FRANCESCO, Lisa M; Foothills Med Centre, CC1144 11F-1403 29 St NW, Calgary AB T2N 2T9; Cal'89; FRCPC; AnatPath. Staff, Foothills Medical Centre; (403)944-4736

DI GENOVA, Tanya; MUHC-Montreal Children's Hosp, 2300 rue Tupper, Montreal QC H3H 1P3; McG'07; MDCM; FRCPC; Peds. Staff, McGill University Health Centre - Montreal Children's Hospital; (514)412-4400

DI GRAVIO, Bruno; Belgage Med Arts Bldg, 210-525 Belmont Ave W, Kitchener ON N2M 5E2; Tor'84; FRCPC; Peds. Staff, Grand River Hospital - Kitchener/Waterloo Health Centre; (519)743-0516; Fax. (519)743-0558; bdigravio@yahoo.com.

DI IANNI, Michael; Hamilton HSC- Hamilton Gen, 237 Barton St E, Hamilton ON L8L 2X2; McM'06; FRCPC; DiagRad. Staff, Hamilton Health Sciences Centre - Hamilton General Hospital; (905)529-3732

DI IORIO, Daniela; Hop Jean-Talon, 1385 rue Jean-Talon E, Montreal QC H2E 1S6; Sher'94; FRCPC; IntMed (Medical Microbiology & Infectious Diseases); MedMicrobiol; InfectDis. Staff, CSSS du Coeur de l'Isle Hôpital Jean-Talon; Langs: Italian; English; (514)495-6767 x6135; Fax. (514)495-6782.

DI LALLA, Andrea L; 201-520 17th St, West Vancouver BC V7V 3S8; McG'94; (604)630-9601; Fax. (604)960-9501.

DI LALLO, Kate; GMF le Gardeurois, 130-155 boul Lacombe, Repentigny QC J5Z 3C4; Mon'10; CCFP; (450)582-2718

DI LENARDO, David; Hôpital de Saint-Eustache, 520 boul Arthur-Sauve, Saint-Eustache QC J7R 5B1; Laval'08; Staff, Hôpital de Saint-Eustache; (450)473-6811; Fax. (450)473-6966.

DI LIDDO, Lydia; Hôpital Ste-Justine, 3175 ch Cote-Ste-Catherine, Montreal QC H3T 1C5; Mon'00; FRCPC; Peds (Pediatric Emergency Medicine). Staff, Hôpital Ste-Justine; (514)345-4931 x4919

DI LORENZO, Maria; Hop du Sacre-Coeur de Mtl, 5400 boul Gouin O, Montreal QC H4J 1C5; McG'90; CSPQ; FRCPC; IntMed (Echocardiography); Cardiol. Staff, Hôpital du Sacre-Coeur de Montréal; Langs: English; Italian; (514)338-2200; Fax. (514)338-2381.

DI MARIA, Antoinette; Thistlewood Prof Centre, 210-8077 Islington Ave, Woodbridge ON L4L 7X7; Tor'84; CCFP; Court Staff, William Osler Health System - Etobicoke General Hospital; Langs: Italian; (905)264-2888; Fax. (905)264-2549.

DI MEGLIO, Giuseppina; Adolescent Medicine, 1040 av Atwater, Westmount QC H3Z 1X3; Mem'91; CSPQ; ABPeds; FRCPC; Peds (Adolescent Medicine). Staff, McGill University Health Centre - Montreal Children's Hospital; Langs: Italian; French; Spanish; (514)412-4481; Fax. (514)412-4319.

DI NARDO, Luciano S; Columbus Med Arts Bldg, 300-8333 Weston Rd, Woodbridge ON L4L 8E2; Tor'92; CCFP; Langs: Italian; (905)264-9859; Fax. (905)264-9311.

DI NICOLA, Vincenzo; Pavillon Rosemont, 5689 boul Rosemont, Montreal QC H1T 2H1; McM'81; DPsy; DABPN(Psy); FRCPC; Psy (Child & Adolescent Psychiatry). Staff, Hôpital Riviere des Prairies; Chief Child Psy Service, Hopital Maisonneuve-Rosemont; Prof, Universite de Montreal; Aj Prof, McGill University; Langs: Italian; Portuguese; French; Spanish; (514)252-3400 x4790; Fax. (514)252-3931.

DI NINNO, Vincent L; Crescent Heights Med Centre, 49 8 St NW, Medicine Hat AB T1A 6N9; Cal'86; CCFP; FCFP; Staff, Medicine Hat Regional Hospital; (403)526-7422; Fax. (403)526-3349.

DI PALMA, Remo A P; Bowmont Med Clinic, 6535 Bowness Rd NW, Calgary AB T3B 0E8; Cal'79; (403)247-9797

DI PAOLA, Francesca A; CAMH Addiction Med Service, 3F-100 Stokes St, Toronto ON M6J 1H4; Glasgow (Scotland)'99; CCFP; (416)535-8501

DI PAOLO, Andrea B L; 510 Raglan St N, Renfrew ON K7V 1P5; Dal'04; BA; CCFP; Staff, Renfrew Victoria Hospital; Staff Physician, Bonnechere Manor; Langs: Italian; French; (613)433-9152; Fax. (613)433-9154.

DI PAOLO, Bruno L; Di Paolo Medicine Prof Corp, 200-755 Concession St, Hamilton ON L8V 1C4; Tor'69; BSc; Staff, St Joseph's Healthcare - Charlton Campus; Court Staff, Hamilton Health Sciences Centre - Hamilton General Hospital; Langs: Italian; (905)575-2888; Fax. (905)575-9896.

DI PASQUALE, Dennis J; 410-101 Queensway W, Mississauga ON L5B 2P7; Tor'97; FRCSC; OrthSurg. (905)949-8855; Fax. (905)949-6176.

DI PERSIO, Mario B; Glenrose Rehab Hosp, 10230 111 Ave NW, Edmonton AB T5G 0B7; Dal'88; FRCPC; PhysMed&Rehab. Staff, Glenrose Rehabilitation Hospital; (780)735-8208; mdipersi@cha.ab.ca.

DI PIERDOMENICO, Anthony P; Bloor-Jane Med Bldg, 207-2425 Bloor St W, Toronto ON M6S 4W4; Sher'80; FACOG; FRCSC; ObstGyn. Ac Staff, St Joseph's Health Centre; Staff, Trillium Health Centre - West Toronto; Teacher, University of Toronto; Langs: Italian; French; (416)766-4518; Fax. (416)766-2407.

DI PIERDOMENICO, Fernando G; 290 Sandwich St S, Amherstburg ON N9V 2A8; Tor'79; Langs: Italian; (519)736-2131

DI PRIMIO, Luigia G A; The Ottawa Hosp-Gen Campus, 501 Smyth Rd, Ottawa ON K1H 8L6; Ott'93; FRCPC; DiagRad. Staff, The Ottawa Hospital - General Campus; Langs: Italian; French; (613)737-8097; Fax. (613)737-8957.

DI PRIZITO, Claudio D; Trillium Hlth Ctr-Mississauga, 100 Queensway W, Mississauga ON L5B 1B8; Buenos Aires (Argentina)'92; FRCPC; IntMed. Staff, Trillium Health Centre - Mississauga; Langs: Spanish; Italian; (905)848-7100

DI QUINZIO, Claudio; Halifax Infirmary, 1796 Summer St, Halifax NS B3H 3A7; Dal'88; FRCPC; Anes. Staff, Queen Elizabeth II Health Sciences Centre - Halifax Infirmary Site.

DI QUINZIO, Laura; Kingston Family Health Team, 200-2437 Princess St, Kingston ON K7M 3G1; Dal'04; CCFP; Assoc Prof, Queen's University; (613)546-6652

DI RENNA, Tania; The Ottawa Hosp-Gen Campus, 501 Smyth Rd, Ottawa ON K1H 8L6; Ott'03; FRCPC; Anes. Staff, The Ottawa Hospital - General Campus; Langs: Italian; French; (613)737-8899

DI SANTO, Loredana; Maple Med Centre, 201-955 Major Mackenzie Dr W, Maple ON L6A 4P9; Wes'03; CCFP; (905)417-7899; Fax. (905)419-8905.

DI SILVESTRO, Matthew; Carling-Broadview Med Bldg, 208-770 Broadview Ave, Ottawa ON K2A 3Z3; Cal'02; FRCSC; OrthSurg. Staff, Foothills Medical Centre; (613)725-9495

DI STEFANO, Joseph M; Collingwood Gen & Marine Hosp, 459 Hume St, Collingwood ON L9Y 1W9; Wes'02; CCFP; Staff, Collingwood General & Marine Hospital; (705)445-2550

DI TOMASSO, Maria; Douglas Mental Hlth Univ Inst, 6875 boul LaSalle, Verdun QC H4H 1R3; McG'90; Psy (P.Q.). Staff, Douglas Mental Health University Institute; (514)761-6131

DI TOPPA, John C; First Edmonton Place, 1215-10665 Jasper Ave NW, Edmonton AB T5J 3S9; Alb'73; FRCSC; Otol. Consultant, Covenant Health - Edmonton General Continuing Care Centre; (780)429-9911; Fax. (780)429-9926.

DI VALENTIN, Tanya; The Ottawa Hosp-General, 501 Smyth Rd, Ottawa ON K1H 8L6; Ott'04; MedOncol; IntMed. Staff, The Ottawa Hospital - General Campus; (613)737-7700

DI ZAZZO, Anne; 4577 rue Beaubien E, Montreal QC H1T 1T5; Mon'86; ObstGyn. (514)722-1162

DIACHUN, Laura L; St Joseph's HC-Parkwood Hosp, 801 Commissioners Rd E, London ON N6C 5J1; McM'93; BA; MEd; FRCPC; IntMed; GeriatricMed. Staff, Parkwood Hospital - St Joseph's Health Care; Assoc Prof, University of Western Ontario; (519)685-4021; Fax. (519)685-4093.

DIACONESCU, Razvan; Hop du Sacre-Coeur de Mtl, 5400 boul Gouin O, Montreal QC H4J 1C5; Laval'96; BSc; LMCC; CSPQ; FRCPC; IntMed (Lung Cancer); Hem. Staff Hem Oncol, Hôpital du Sacre-Coeur de Montréal; Langs: English; Italian; Spanish; Romanian; (514)338-2150

DIACONITA, Mariana; Nymark Plaza, 4839 Leslie St, North York ON M2J 2K8; (Other Foreign)'86; CCFP; Langs: Romanian; (905)668-3378

DIADORI, Paola; Hôpital Ste-Justine, 3175 ch Cote-Ste-Catherine, Montreal QC H3T 1C5; Laval'87; MSc; FRCPC; Neur (Epilepsy). Staff, Hôpital Ste-Justine; (514)345-4931 x5453; Fax. (514)345-4787.

DIAL, M Sandra; MUHC-Montreal Chest Institute, K1 14-3650 rue Saint-Urbain, Montreal QC H2X 2P4; McG'88; MRCP; CSPQ; MSc; FRCPC; IntMed; Critical Care Medicine (P.Q.); Respir. Staff, McGill University Health Centre - Montreal Chest Institute; Staff, Sir Mortimer B Davis Jewish General; (514)849-5201 x32336; Fax. (514)843-2083; sandra.dial@mcgill.ca.

DIALLO, Absa; Hop Santa Cabrini Ospedale, 5655 rue Saint-Zotique E, Montreal QC H1T 1P7; Mon'95; Staff Emerg Med, Hôpital Santa Cabrini Ospedale; VP, CMDP; Langs: Italian; Spanish; English; (514)252-6000; Fax. (514)252-6453.

DIALLO, Soraya V; Centre Hosp Honore-Mercier, 2750 boul Laframboise, Saint-Hyacinthe QC J2S 4Y8; Gamel Abdel Nasser (Guinea)'01; FRCPC; IntMed; Nephrol. Staff 1, Centre Hospitalier Honore-Mercier; (450)771-3333 x3249

DIAMANDIS, Eleftherios P; Mount Sinai Fam Hlth Team, 6 201-60 Murray St, Toronto ON M5T 3L9; Athens (Greece)'78; FRCPC; MedScient(Med); MedMicrobiol. Biochemist Chief/Chief, Mount Sinai Hospital; Staff, Toronto General Hospital - UHN; Biochemist Chief/Chief, Toronto Medical Laboratories; Prof/Head Div of Clinic Bch Dept of Laboratory Med & Pathobiology, University of Toronto; (416)586-8443

DIAMANT, Nicholas E; Kingston Gen Hosp, 76 Stuart St, Kingston ON K7L 2V7; Qns'60; DABIM; FRCPC; IntMed (Gastroenterology). Staff, Kingston General Hospital; Prof Med & Physiol, University of Toronto; Langs: Greek; French; (613)548-3232 x6553

DIAMANTOUROS, Pantelis; London HSC-University Hosp, PO Box 5339 Stn B C6 116-339 Windermere Rd, London ON N6A 5A5; Qns'99; FRCPC; IntMed; Cardiol. Staff, London Health Sciences Centre - University Hospital; Langs: Greek; (519)663-3329; Fax. (519)434-3278.

DIAMBOMBA, Yenge; 775A-600 University Ave, Toronto ON M5G 1X5; Laval'96; FRCP; FRCPC; Peds (Neonatology). Staff Neonatol., Mount Sinai Hospital; Asst Prof, University of Toronto; Langs: French; (416)586-4800 x5314; Fax. (416)586-8745; ydiambomba@mtsinai.on.ca.

DIAMOND, Aubie J; Med Care-Main Exchange, 4A-800 Steeles Ave W, Thornhill ON L4J 7L2; Man'83; Langs: Hebrew; (905)738-6699; Fax. (905)738-6073.

DIAMOND, Carolyn K; Halton Family Health Centre, 2951 Walker's Line, Burlington ON L7M 4Y1; Dal'98; CCFP; (905)336-9633; Fax. (905)336-9634.

DIAMOND, Catherine; North Bramalea Med Centre, 202-9780 Bramalea Rd, Brampton ON L6S 2P1; Qns'86; CCFP; (905)791-2390; Fax. (905)791-8476.

DIAMOND, Heather D; Manitoba Clinic, 790 Sherbrook St, Winnipeg MB R3A 1M3; Wes'97; FRCSC; ObstGyn. Fax. (204)775-6373.

DIAMOND, Ivan; Univ of Toronto, 112-150 College St, Toronto ON M5S 3E2; Qns'03; Staff, St Michael's Hospital; (416)978-8797

DIAMOND, Patrick; Clin Med Plateau Marquette, 200-731 rue Galt O, Sherbrooke QC J1H 1Z1; Sher'82; (819)564-8662; Fax. (819)564-1294.

DIAMOND, Pierre; UMF Laurier, 2875 boul Laurier, Quebec QC G1V 2M2; Laval'90; MSc; PhD; CCFP; Staff, Centre Hospitalier Universitaire de Quebec-CHUL; umf.pchul@dechuq.ulaval.ca.

DIAMOND, Rhonda; Paterson Med Centre, 45 Wolsley St, Kenora ON P9N 3W7; Man'93; CCFP; Ac Staff Privil, Lake of the Woods District Hospital; (807)468-4433; Fax. (807)468-5565; buzzrhonda68@gmail.com.

DIAMOND, Robert T; Radiology Consultants Assoc, 120-6707 Elbow Dr SW, Calgary AB T2V 0E3; Man'76; FRCPC; DiagRad. (403)777-3001; Fax. (403)777-3008.

DIAMOND, Ronald C; 804-145 13th St E, North Vancouver BC V7L 2L3; Dal'01; FRCSC; Otol. Staff, University of Alberta Hospital; (604)973-0222

DIAN, Larry; Diamond Health Care Centre, 7F-2775 Laurel St, Vancouver BC V5Z 1M9; Witwatersrand (South Africa)'78; MB BCh; FRCPC; IntMed; GeriatricMed. Staff, Vancouver General Hospital - Centennial Pavillion; Staff, Providence Health Care - St Paul's Hospital; Staff, UBC Hospital - Koerner Pavillion; (604)875-5312

DIAS, Aleksander I; 47 Santa Barbara Rd, North York ON M2N 2C1; Ott'68; Langs: Polish; (416)512-7486

DIAS, Angela C; BC Women's Hosp & HC, C234-4500 Oak St, Vancouver BC V6H 3N1; (Portugal)'01; FRCPC; MedGenetics. Staff, BC Women's Hospital & Health Centre; (604)875-2157

DIAS, Bryan F; London HSC-University Hosp, PO Box 5339 Stn B 339 Windermere Rd, London ON N6A 5A5; Sask'92; FRCPC; IntMed; Cardiol. Staff, London Health Sciences Centre - University Hospital; (519)663-3483

DIAS, E Bernice; Glace Bay Family Practice Ctr, 35 Sterling Rd, Glace Bay NS B1A 3X6; Madras (India)'77; MB BS; Staff, Glace Bay Healthcare Facility; (902)849-4601; Fax. (902)849-5119.

DIAS, Ernesto M; St James Street Med Clinic, 1600 Portage Ave, Winnipeg MB R3J 0C6; National (Ireland)'65; MB ChB; BAO; FRCS(Eng).

DIAS, Esther; Glace Bay Fam Prac, 35 Sterling Rd, Glace Bay NS B1A 3X6; Madras (India)'76; MB BS; (902)849-4601; Fax. (902)849-5119.

DIAZ, Ariel H; Ctr Hosp Trois-Riv-St-Joseph, 731 rue Sainte-Julie, Trois-Rivieres QC G9A 1Y1; (Spain)'97; Staff, Centre Hospitalier Regional de Trois-Rivieres; (819)697-3333

DIAZ, Pedro E; 153 Sackville Dr, Lower Sackville NS B4C 2R3; Havana (Cuba)'91; Langs: Spanish; (902)865-8120; Fax. (902)865-7716.

DIAZ- SANCHEZ, Liliana; CLSC du Plateau-Mont-Royal, 4625 av De Lorimier, Montreal QC H2H 2B4; CCFP; Staff, Sir Mortimer B Davis Jewish General; (514)521-7663

DIAZ-BOBADILLA, Julio F; 402-1630 Pandosy St, Kelowna BC V1Y 1P7; San Carlos (Guatemala)'80; FRCPC; Psy (Adult General Psychiatry). Staff Privil, Kelowna General Hospital; Langs: Spanish; (250)712-9807; Fax. (250)712-9805.

DIAZ DE BEDOYA, Luis Victor; CHUQ-Hotel-Dieu de Quebec, 11 Cote du Palais, Quebec QC G1R 2J6; Paris (France)'65; FRCPC; RadOncol (P.Q.). Staff RadOncol, Centre Hospitalier Universitaire de Québec (CHUQ) - Siege Social; Langs: English; Spanish; (418)691-5264; Fax. (418)691-5268.

DIAZ DE MOLNAR, Ana M; Markham College Med Clinic, 301-474 College St, Toronto ON M6G 1A4; National (Mexico)'68; Langs: Portuguese; French; (416)925-2069; Fax. (416)968-1931.

DIAZ-HERMOSILLO, Pablo; Addiction & Mental Hlth-Queen, 2 301-1001 Queen St W, Toronto ON M6J 1H4; (Mexico)'80; FRCPC; Psy (Schizophrenia). Staff, Centre for Addiction & Mental Health (CAMH) - Queen Site; Asst Prof Psy, University of Toronto; Langs: Spanish; (416)535-8501 x2555; Fax. (416)583-4601.

DIAZ-MITOMA, Francisco; AMRIC Childrens Treatment Ctr, 41 Ramsey Lake Rd, Sudbury ON P3E 5J1; Guadalajara (Mexico)'79; PhD(Alb); FRCPC; MedMicrobiol (Virology). Ac Staff, The Ottawa Hospital - General Campus; Staff Chief Lab Med, Children's Hospital of Eastern Ontario (CHEO); Prof Biochem, University of Ottawa; Langs: Spanish; (705)523-7300 x3655; Fax. (705)523-7079.

DIBARTOLO-KING, Marielena L; Alberta Children's Hosp, 2888 Shaganappi Trail NW, Calgary AB T3B 6A8; Man'02; BScMed; FRCPC; Peds; Respir. Staff, Alberta Children's Hospital; (403)955-7211; Fax. (403)955-7059.

DIBB, Maria; Dr Maria Dibb, PO Box 8000, Invermere BC V0A 1K0; UBC'87; CCFP; FCFP; (250)342-9206; Fax. (250)342-6669.

DIBBLE, Bradley J; Atrium Prof Bldg, 201-190 Cundles Rd E, Barrie ON L4M 4S5; Wes'90; FACC; FRCPC; IntMed; Cardiol. Consultant, Southlake Regional Health Centre; Consultant, Royal Victoria Regional Health Centre; (705)721-4422; Fax. (705)721-5577.

DIBDEN, Lionel; University of Alberta Hosp, 1C4 24-8440 112 St NW, Edmonton AB T6G 2B7; Witwatersrand (South Africa)'78; MB ChB; FRCPC; Peds (Child Abuse). Med Dir Child & Adolescent Protection Centre, University of Alberta Hospital; Dir Div of Gen Peds/Assoc Prof Peds/A-Chair Peds, University of Alberta; (780)407-1240; Fax. (780)407-1239.

DIBILDOX GONZALEZ, Manuel; Sunnybrook Hlth Sciences Ctr, D718-2075 Bayview Ave, Toronto ON M4N 3M5; (Spain)'02; Staff, Sunnybrook Health Sciences Centre; Langs: Spanish.

DIBSKI, Daniel; Chilliwack Gen Hosp, 45600 Menholm Rd, Chilliwack BC V2P 1P7; McG'07; MDCM; CCFP; Staff, Chilliwack General Hospital; (604)795-4141

DICAIRE, Caroline; CSSS de Trois-Rivieres, 155 rue Toupin, Trois-Rivieres QC G8T 3Z8; Mon'07; Staff, Centre de santé Cloutier-du-Rivage; (819)370-2100; Fax. (819)370-2381.

DICAIRE, Stephanie; CLSC de Paspebiac, CP 7000 273A boul Gerard-D-Levsque O, Paspebiac QC G0C 2K0; Mon'10; Staff, CLSC de Paspebiac; (418)752-2572

DICK, Alexander; Univ of Ottawa Heart Institute, H3408A-40 Ruskin St, Ottawa ON K1Y 4W7; Man'94; FRCPC; IntMed; Cardiol. Staff, University of Ottawa Heart Institute; (613)761-4231; Fax. (613)761-4338.

DICK, Barry J M; Herold Road Family Physicians, 1-325 Herold Rd, Saskatoon SK S7V 1J7; Sask'75; Staff, Maidstone Health Complex; (306)374-2404; Fax. (306)477-0300; brad@eecan.com.

DICK, Brian D; 103-139 Greenback Rd, Ottawa ON K2H 9A5; Qns'88; CCFP; (613)226-8541; Fax. (613)226-2589; melville.inc@sympatico.ca.

DICK, Donald; University of Alberta Hosp, 2C3 WCM-8440 112 St NW, Edmonton AB T6G 2B7; Sask'81; FRCSC; OrthSurg. Staff, University of Alberta Hospital; (780)407-4362; Fax. (780)407-1126.

DICK, Paul; Gray Bruce HS-Owen Sound, PO Box 1800 Stn Main 1800 8th Street E, Owen Sound ON N4K 6M9; McG'88; MSc; FRCPC; Peds. Preceptor, Rural Ontario Medical Program; Staff Teacher, University of Western Ontario; Assoc Prof Peds, University of Toronto; (519)376-2121 x2864; Fax. (519)370-2388.

DICK, Robert N B; 1872 Kingsway, Vancouver BC V5N 2S7; UBC'67; (604)876-6257

DICKE, Franciscus; Alberta Children's Hosp, 2888 Shaganappi Trail NW, Calgary AB T3B 6A8; Tor'94; FRCPC; Peds; Cardiol. Chief Div of Cardiol, Alberta Children's Hospital; Assoc Prof Peds, University of Calgary; (403)955-7858; Fax. (403)955-7621.

DICKEN, Bryan J; University of Alberta Hosp, 2C3 44WMC-8440 112 St NW, Edmonton AB T6G 2B7; Alb'00; FRCSC; GenSurg (Clinician Investigator Program); PedGenSurg. Staff, University of Alberta Hospital; (780)407-8822

DICKER, Robert A; Leslie Med Centre, 410-4800 Leslie St, North York ON M2J 2K9; Tor'52; Hon Staff, North York General Hospital - Branson Division; Langs: Hungarian; (416)497-9900; Fax. (416)497-6992.

DICKESON, Mark R C; 107-3825 Sunset St, Burnaby BC V5G 1T4; Mem'04; FRCSC; GenSurg. (604)558-3834

DICKEY, Robert L; Waypoint Centre for Mental H C, 500 Church St, Penetanguishene ON L9M 1G3; Sask'78; FRCPC; Psy (Forensic Psychiatry). Staff, Waypoint Centre for Mental Health Care; Consultant Psy, Correctional Services of Canada; Asst Prof, University of Toronto; (705)549-3181

DICKEY, Rod G; Exeter Clinic, PO Box 879, 100 Mile House BC V0K 2E0; Cal'81; BSc; (250)395-2271; Fax. (250)395-2599; rgdickey@bcinternet.net.

DICKHOFF, Peter J; Radiology Consultants Assoc, 120-6707 Elbow Dr SW, Calgary AB T2V 0E3; UBC'86; FRCPC; DiagRad. Staff, Foothills Medical Centre; (403)777-3003; Fax. (403)777-3018.

DICKHOUT, Janet S; U of Toronto-Health Services, 214 College St, Toronto ON M5T 2Z9; Tor'81; CCFP; FCFP; (416)978-8030; Fax. (416)971-2089.

DICKIE, A John; Lakeridge Hlth Corp-Oshawa, C2 160F-1 Hospital Crt, Oshawa ON L1G 2B9; Qns'91; FRCSC; GenSurg; ThorSurg. Staff, Lakeridge Health - Oshawa Site; (905)576-8711; Fax. (905)433-4577.

DICKIE, Gordon; St Joseph's HC-Parkwood Hosp, 801 Commissioners Rd E, London ON N6C 5J1; Aberdeen (Scotland)'68; MB ChB; DObstRCOG; CCFP; FCFP; Staff, Parkwood Hospital - St Joseph's Health Care; (519)685-4292; Fax. (519)685-4811.

DICKIE, Kenneth E; Royal Centre of Plastic Surger, 22 Quarry Ridge Rd, Barrie ON L4M 7G1; Alb'78; BSc; FRCSC; PlasSurg (Cosmetic Surgery). (705)726-2800; Fax. (705)726-2851.

DICKIE, Margaret J; Peterborough Clinic FHT, 303-26 Hospital Dr, Peterborough ON K9J 7C3; Qns'80; CCFP; FCFP; Staff, Peterborough Regional Health Centre - Hospital Drive; (705)740-6857; Fax. (705)740-6863; mdickie@ptboclinic.com.

DICKIE, Nadine R; Grey Bruce HS-Southampton, PO Box 310 340 High St, Southampton ON N0H 2L0; McM'92; CCFP; FCFP; Staff, Grey Bruce Health Services - Southampton Site; (519)797-3230; Fax. (519)797-1247.

DICKIE, Paul M; Spingbank Med Centre, 302-460 Springbank Dr, London ON N6J 0A8; Wes'77; BSc; (519)681-8860; Fax. (519)681-8849; pdickie@uwo.ca.

DICKIE, Sean J; Univ of Ottawa Heart Institute, H2410-40 Ruskin St, Ottawa ON K1Y 4W7; Ott'03; FRCPC; Anes. Staff, University of Ottawa Heart Institute; Langs: Bilingual(English/French); (613)761-4379; Fax. (613)761-4925.

DICKIE-CLARK, Johanna I L; Burnaby Hosp, 3935 Kincaid St, Burnaby BC V5G 2X6; Pretoria (South Africa)'73; MB ChB; FRCPC; Anes. Ac Staff, Burnaby Hospital; (604)434-4211; Fax. (604)412-6313.

DICKIESON, Andrew; Kelowna Gen Hosp, 2268 Pandosy St, Kelowna BC V1Y 1T2; Dal'99; FRCPC; Anes; Critical Care Medicine. Staff, Kelowna General Hospital; (250)862-4000

DICKIESON, Herbert P; Beechwood Comm Hlth Ctr, PO Box 9, O'Leary PE C0B 1V0; Dal'87; BSc.

DICKINSON, Andrew; Dr Everett Chalmers Reg Hosp, PO Box 9000 Stn A 700 Priestman St, Fredericton NB E3B 5N5; CCFP; Staff, Dr Everett Chalmers Regional Hospital; (506)452-5400

DICKINSON, James A; Sheldon Chumuik Centre, 8F-1213 4 St SW, Calgary AB T2R 0X7; (Australia)'73; CCFP; Vis Staff, Foothills Medical Centre; Prof Family Med, University of Calgary; (403)955-9300; Fax. (403)476-8766.

DICKINSON, John D; Queen Elizabeth II HSC, 2035-1276 South Park St, Halifax NS B3H 2Y9; Dal'89; BSc; FRCSC; Ophth (Retina Vitreous Ophthalmology). Staff, Queen Elizabeth II Health Sciences Centre - Victoria General Site; (902)473-3947; Fax. (902)473-2839.

DICKINSON, Lara; Nanaimo Reg Gen Hosp, 1200 Dufferin Cres, Nanaimo BC V9S 2B7; UBC'09; CCFP; Staff, Nanaimo Regional General Hospital; (250)754-2141

DICKINSON, Michael T; Miramichi Reg Hosp, 500 Water St, Miramichi NB E1V 3G5; Tor'91; FRCPC; Peds. Staff, Miramichi Regional Hospital; Langs: Bilingual(English/French); (506)623-3499; Fax. (506)623-3490.

DICKINSON, Peter W; 11 Canadian Forces Hlth Serv C, PO Box 5000, Shilo MB R0K 2A0; Dal'10; CCFP.

DICKMAN, John H; Prince County Hosp, PO Box 3000 Stn Main 65 Roy Boates Ave, Summerside PE C1N 2A9; Ott'73; FRCPC; EmergMed. Staff, Prince County Hospital; (902)438-4200

DICKNER, Martin; CHUM-Hop Notre-Dame, 1560 rue Sherbrooke E, Montreal QC H2L 4M1; Mon'97; CSPQ; FRCPC; Anes. Staff, Centre Hospitalier l'Université de Montréal (CHUM) - Hôpital Notre-Dame; (514)890-8000 x26876; Fax. (514)412-7653.

DICKOUT, William J; Royal Alexandra Hosp, 1108 ATC-10240 Kingsway NW, Edmonton AB T5H 3V9; Alb'75; BMedSci; FRCPC; IntMed; Respir. Staff, Royal Alexandra Hospital; Staff IntMed & RespMed, Covenant Health - Misericordia Community Hospital; Clin Assoc Prof, University of Alberta; (780)735-4111

DICKSON, Christine; 283 Westhill Ave, Ottawa ON K1Z 7H7; Qns'85; FRCPC; Psy. (613)722-7597

DICKSON, Colin; Barrie Family Medicine, 5-18 Cundles Rd E, Barrie ON L4M 2Z5; RCS (Ireland)'90; Court Staff, Royal Victoria Regional Health Centre; (705)737-1887; Fax. (705)735-6949.

DICKSON, Dann W; St Joseph's Life Care Centre, 99 Wayne Gretzky Pky, Brantford ON N3S 6T6; Cal'85; MB BCh; FRCSC; Urol. Chief Urol, The Brant Community Healthcare System - Brantford General Hospital Site; (519)751-5579; Fax. (519)751-5578.

DICKSON, David H; Brampton Med Bldg, 210-164 Queen St E, Brampton ON L6V 1B4; Wes'62; FRCSC; Ophth (Comprehensive Ophthalmology). Staff, William Osler Health System - Brampton Civic Hospital; (905)459-6710; Fax. (905)459-5085.

DICKSON, James; 550 Terminal Ave, Ottawa ON K1G 0Z3; Glasgow (Scotland)'51; MB ChB; FRCP(C); Anes (Geriatric Medicine). Langs: French; (613)731-4770; Fax. (613)731-4979.

DICKSON, Jeffrey R; St Michael's Hosp, 30 Bond St, Toronto ON M5B 1W8; Tor'98; FRCPC; Anes. Staff, St Michael's Hospital; (416)360-4000

DICKSON, John M; Fraser Valley Pediatric ENT, 303-9808 King George Blvd, Surrey BC V3T 2V6; UBC'02; BSc; FRCSC; Otol (Pediatric Otolaryngology). Staff, Surrey Memorial Hospital; Langs: Punjabi; (604)588-8883; Fax. (604)588-8877.

DICKSON, John R; 104-532 Lake St, St Catharines ON L2N 4H4; Wes'80; FRCPC; IntMed; Rheum. (905)938-3737; Fax. (905)937-4242.

DICKSON, Michael J; Victoria East Med Clinic, 2068 Prince of Wales Dr, Regina SK S4V 3A6; Belfast (Ireland)'74; MB ChB; BAO; Ac Member Family Med, Wascana Rehabilitation Centre; Med Dir, Western Canadian Headquarters-Canada Life Assurance Co.; Teach Staff Family Med, University of Saskatchewan; (306)789-4677; Fax. (306)789-3422.

DICKSON, Paul J; 220 Angeline St S, Lindsay ON K9V 4R2; Tor'70; Court Staff, Ross Memorial Hospital; Med Dir, Victoria Manor-Home For The Aged(Lindsay).

DICKSON, Robert C; PRG Med Inc, 836 Upper James St, Hamilton ON L9C 3A4; McM'73; PhD; CCFP; Ac Staff, St Joseph's Healthcare - Charlton Campus; Court Staff Hamilton Hlth Sciences, Hamilton Health Sciences Centre - McMaster University Medical Centre; Physician, Physicians Replacement Group Inc; (905)385-6777; Fax. (905)385-3939.

DICKSON, Robert I; Laurel Med Centre Ltd, 212-888 8th Ave W, Vancouver BC V5Z 3Y1; Man'64; FRCSC; Otol. Ac Staff, Vancouver General Hospital - Centennial Pavillion; Clin Assoc Prof Surg, University of British Columbia; (604)872-1231; Fax. (604)873-5951.

DICKSON, Robert; Market Mall Prof Bldg, 104-4935 40 Ave NW, Calgary AB T3A 2N1; Cal'88; CCFP; FCFP; (403)247-2253; Fax. (403)247-0669.

DICKSON, Ruth; Eli Lilly Canada, 3553 31 St NW, Calgary AB T2L 2K7; Cal'77; FRCPC; Psy. Assoc Prof, University of Calgary; (403)282-0452

DICKSON, Thomas G; Bramalea Med Centre, 400-18 Kensington Rd, Brampton ON L6T 4S5; Wes'69; FRCSC; Otol (Ear Nose & Throat Surgery). Court Staff, Trillium Health Centre - Mississauga; Ac Staff, William Osler Health System - Brampton Civic Hospital; Staff, The Credit Valley Hospital; (905)792-2311; Fax. (905)792-6931.

DICKSON, Timothy; Surrey Mem Hosp, 13750 96 Ave, Surrey BC V3V 1Z2; UBC'04; FRCPC; Anes. Staff, Surrey Memorial Hospital; (604)581-2211

DICUM, Francis D; Upper Canada Lower Bowel Clini, 301-1366 Yonge St, Toronto ON M4T 3A7; Tor'62; BA; FRCPC; IntMed (Gastroenterology). Sr Staff, Toronto East General Hospital Inc; (416)926-0262; Fax. (416)926-0936.

DICUS, Jennifer; Chaldecott Med Clinic, 4186 Dunbar St, Vancouver BC V6S 2E7; UBC'08; CCFP; (604)739-9881

DIDIER, Mijanou; Centre Med de la Vallee, 1-22 rue du Pont, Amqui QC G5J 3T5; Laval'92; Staff, CSSS de la Matapedia; Langs: English; (418)629-6611

DIDOMENICANTONIO, Gabriel; Hull Hosp, 116 boul Lionel-Emond, Gatineau QC J8Y 1W7; Laval'81; LMCC; AB(Rad.); FRCPC; DiagRad. Staff, Hull Hospital; (819)966-6029

DIDYK, Nicole E; St Mary's Gen Hosp, 911 Queens Blvd, Kitchener ON N2M 1B2; McM'96; FRCPC; IntMed; GeriatricMed. Staff, St Mary's General Hospital; Langs: Bilingual(English/French); (519)749-6578 x1043; Fax. (519)749-6566.

DIEBES, Ragaie E; Bay D'Espoir Med Clinic, PO Box 5, St Albans NL A0H 2E0; Cairo (Egypt)'65; MB ChB; (709)538-3244; Fax. (709)538-3228.

DIEC, Hung Long; CSSS Pierre Boucher, 1333 boul Jacques-Cartier E, Longueuil QC J4M 2A5; Mon'01; CSPQ; FRCSC; GenSurg. Staff, Centre Hospitalier Pierre Boucher; (450)468-8111

DIEC, Kien-Quan; Clinique Med Anjou, 8250 av de Chatillon, Anjou QC H1K 1P2; Hue (Vietnam)'77; Staff, Centre Hospitalier Fleury; (514)352-1820; Fax. (514)352-1820.

DIEC, Olivier H Q; Hop Charles LeMoyne, 3120 boul Taschereau, Greenfield Park QC J4V 2H1; Sher'02; Nephrol; IntMed. Staff, Hopital Charles LeMoyne; (450)466-5000

DIEC, Q Diana; Ctr Hosp de Verdun, 4000 boul Lasalle, Verdun QC H4G 2A3; Mon'07; Staff, Centre Hospitalier de Verdun; (514)362-1000

DIEDERICKS, Adriaan G; Bay St George Med Clinic, 129 Montana Dr, Stephenville NL A2N 2T4; Pretoria (South Africa)'81; MB BS; (709)643-6635

DIEF, Ashraf; South Simcoe Medical, 239 Holland St W, Bradford ON L3Z 1H9; Cairo (Egypt)'85; MB ChB; CCFP; Langs: Arabic; (905)775-4863; Fax. (905)775-8351; ashrafdief@hotmail.com.

DIEHL, Eberhard H; Royal Inland Hosp, 311 Columbia St, Kamloops BC V2C 2T1; Tubingen (Germany)'74; FRCPC; Anes. Staff, Royal Inland Hospital; Langs: German; (250)314-2620

DIEKMEYER, Christine; S E O C H C, 1355 Bank St, Ottawa ON K1H 8K7; Tor'90; CCFP; FCFP; Staff, The Ottawa Hospital - General Campus; Staff Teacher Pt-Time, University of Ottawa; Langs: French; (613)737-4809; Fax. (613)739-3723.

DIELEMAN, Levinus Albert; Zeidler Ledcor Centre, 2 24-130 University Campus NW, Edmonton AB T6G 2X8; (Netherlands)'83; PhD; FRCP; Assoc Prof, University of Alberta; Langs: Dutch; German; French; Swahili; (780)492-1888; Fax. (780)492-1878.

DIENA, Zeev M; Nymark Plaza, 4839 Leslie St, North York ON M2J 2K8; Tor'93; CCFP; Ac Staff, Rouge Valley Health System - Centenary Health Centre Site; Langs: Hebrew; (416)498-3600

DIENER, Tania; Population & Public Hlth Serv, 2110 Hamiton St, Regina SK S4P 2E3; Stellenbosch (South Africa)'87; MB ChB; DCH; MMed(Com.Health); MPA; DTM; Clin Lecturer Family Med, University of Saskatchewan; Langs: Afrikaans; (306)766-7770; Fax. (306)766-7607; tania.diener@rqhealth.ca.

DIEP, Bich Ngoc; 1814 boul Saint-Joseph E, Montreal QC H2H 1C7; Mon'90; (514)523-3136; Fax. (514)523-4071.

DIEP, Tung M; North Shore Eye Associates, 102-1111 Lonsdale Ave, North Vancouver BC V7M 2H4; Tor'04; FRCSC; Ophth. (604)988-1166

DIETRICH, Jaclyn N; PO Box 95024 Rpo Whyte, Edmonton AB T6E 0E5; Alb'10; CCFP.

DIETRICH, Jeanette L; Sydenham Med Clinic, 2876 Campbell Rd, Sydenham ON K0H 2T0; Qns'99; CCFP; Staff, QHC Belleville General.

DIETRICHSEN, Celeste; Bigelow-Fowler Clinic, 1605 9 Ave S, Lethbridge AB T1J 1W2; (South Africa)'98; MB ChB; Langs: Afrikaans; (403)327-3121; Fax. (403)327-3905.

DIEZ-D'AUX, Robert; 3777 Jean-Brillant, Montreal QC H3T 1M5; McG'73; MSc; AB(FamilyMed); CCFP; FCFP; Staff, St Mary's Hospital Centre; adj Prof Fac of Med, McGill University; Langs: Bilingual(English/French); (514)734-2677; Fax. (514)734-2602.

DIGBY, Aaron G; Fredericton Med Clinic, 302I-1015 Regent St, Fredericton NB E3B 6H5; Man'06; BSc; CCFP; (506)474-4622; Fax. (506)474-4624.

DIGBY, Ian J; 103-73 Delhi St, Guelph ON N1E 6L9; Cal'99; CCFP; CCFP(E.M.); Staff Emerg, Guelph General Hospital.

DIGBY, Jennifer; Dr Everett Chalmers Reg Hosp, PO Box 9000 Stn A 700 Priestman St, Fredericton NB E3B 5N5; Dal'10; CCFP; Staff, Dr Everett Chalmers Regional Hospital; (506)452-5400

DIGGES, Deborah D; The Credit Valley Hosp, 2200 Eglinton Ave W, Mississauga ON L5M 2N1; Wes'74; FRCPC; IntMed. Staff, The Credit Valley Hospital; (905)813-2200

DIGGLE, John L; Jim Pattision Outpatient Care, 9750 140 St, Surrey BC V3T 0G9; Cal'00; FRCPC; Neur. Staff, Surrey Memorial Hospital; (604)582-4550

DIGHE, Krupa H; Mackenzie Richmond Hill Hosp, 10 Trench St, Richmond Hill ON L4C 4Z3; Nanded (India)'99; GeriatricMed; IntMed. Staff, Mackenzie Richmond Hill Hospital; (905)883-1212

DIGHE, Kushal J; St Michael's Hosp, BW8 017-30 Bond St, Toronto ON M5B 1W8; Mumbai (India)'99; FRCPC; IntMed; Cardiol. Staff, St Michael's Hospital; Langs: Hindi; (416)864-6060

DIGIACOMO, Danny A; Ctr for Addiction & Mental Hlt, 60 White Squirrel Way, Toronto ON M6J 1H4; Cal'93; BSc(Hon); FRCPC; Psy. Staff, Centre for Addiction & Mental Health (CAMH) - Queen Site; Physician, Centre for Addiction & Mental Health; Lecturer, University of Toronto; (416)535-8501

DIGNAM, Jennifer; Andrew Street Family Hlth, 16 Andrew St, Kitchener ON N2H 5R2; McM'08; CCFP; (519)804-2100

DIGNAN, Thomas A; First Nations & Inuit Hlth, 981 Balmoral St, Thunder Bay ON P7B 0A6; McM'81; BScN; Board Member, Native Physicians Association in Canada; (613)299-0121

DIGNARD, Eric; CLSC Seigneurie de Beauharnois, 142 rue Saint-Laurent, Beauharnois QC J6N 1V9; Mon'93; (450)429-6455; Fax. (450)429-1119.

DIGNARD, Mario; Clin Med de l'Oir, 228 2e rue E, La Sarre QC J9Z 2G9; Laval'79; (819)339-5617

DIGNEY, Andrew; Nanaimo Reg Gen Hosp, 1200 Dufferin Cres, Nanaimo BC V9S 2B7; UBC'92; Staff, Nanaimo Regional General Hospital; (250)754-2141

DIGREGORIO, Roland C; 101-3 Wilson St E, Ancaster ON L9G 2B3; Tor'95; BSc; DDS; MSc; CCFP; (905)304-8937; Fax. (905)304-7031; rolor@bellnet.ca.

DIKE, Nwamara; Foothills Med Centre, AC142 SSB-1403 29 St NW, Calgary AB T2N 2T9; (USA)'98; BSc; Staff, Foothills Medical Centre; Staff Chronic Pain Centre, Alberta Health Services; (403)944-4224 x403; Fax. (403)283-2526; newamara.dike@albertahealthservices.ca.

DIKLICH, Roy R; Windsor Reg Hosp-Metropolitan, 1995 Lens Ave, Windsor ON N8W 1L9; Wes'84; Staff, Windsor Regional Hospital - Metropolitan Site; Langs: Croatian; Serbian; (519)985-2606

DIKSIC, Dubravka A; MUHC-Montreal Children's Hosp, 2300 rue Tupper, Montreal QC H3H 1P3; McG'94; FAAP; FRCPC; Peds (Emergency Medicine). Staff Physician Emerg, McGill University Health Centre - Montreal Children's Hospital; Assoc Prof Peds, McGill University; Langs: English; French; (514)412-4400 x23039

DIL, Pierre G; 303-1711 Cook St, Victoria BC V8T 3P2; (Zambia)'86; MB ChB; BSc; CCFP; Staff, Royal Jubilee Hospital; Staff, Victoria General Hospital; Clin Teacher, University of British Columbia; Clin Teacher, University of Victoria; (250)590-6000; Fax. (250)385-4147.

DILAY, Jocelyn E; Alberta Children's Hosp, 2888 Shaganappi Trail NW, Calgary AB T3B 6A8; Cal'95; BSc; FRCSC; PlasSurg (Pediatric Plastic Surgery). Staff, Alberta Children's Hospital; (403)955-7211

DILENGE, Marie-Emmanuelle; MUHC-Montreal Children's Hosp, A 514-2300 rue Tupper, Montreal QC H3H 1P3; Sher'93; FRCPC; Neur (Electroencephalography). Fellow NeuroRehab & Resident, McGill University Health Centre - Montreal Children's Hospital; Staff Teacher, McGill University; (514)412-4363; Fax. (514)412-4373.

DILKAS, Steven M; West Park Healthcare Centre, 3F 92-82 Buttonwood Ave, York ON M6M 2J5; Tor'04; FRCPC; PhysMed&Rehab. Staff, Toronto General Hospital - UHN; (416)243-3680; Fax. (416)243-1177.

DILL, James R; Brant Community HC-Brantford, 200 Terrace Hill St, Brantford ON N3R 1G9; Wes'97; FRCSC; OrthSurg. Staff, The Brant Community Healthcare System - Brantford General Hospital Site; (519)751-5536

DILLANE, Derek; University of Alberta Hosp, CSB8 120-8440 112 St NW, Edmonton AB T6G 2B7; (Ireland)'96; MB BCh; Staff, University of Alberta Hospital; (780)407-8861; Fax. (780)407-3200.

DILLENBURG, Rejane F; McMaster University HSC, PO Box 2000 Stn Lcd 1 3A37-1200 Main St W, Hamilton ON L8S 4J9; Porto Alegre (Brazil)'87; FRCPC; Cardiol. Staff, Hamilton Health Sciences Centre - McMaster Children's Hospital; Langs: Portuguese; (905)521-2100 x75259; Fax. (905)521-7914.

DILLI, Esma; Gordon & Leslie Diamond HCC, 8275A-2775 Laurel St, Vancouver BC V5Z 1M9; UBC'03; FRCPC; Neur. Physician, Gordon & Leslie Diamond Health Care Centre; (604)875-5574

DILLI, Melih; Fairmont Medical Bldg, 517-750 Broadway W, Vancouver BC V5Z 1H4; Belgrade (Serbia)'67; DPM(Eng); MRCPsy; FRCPC; Psy (Forensic Psychiatry). Ac Staff, Vancouver General Hospital - Centennial Pavillion; (604)876-2313; Fax. (604)733-6365.

DILLON, David A; Beaches Family Practice, 116 Glen Manor Dr, Toronto ON M4E 2X2; Milwaukee(WI) (USA)'73; (416)698-0999

DILLON, John; Pan Am Sports Med Centre, 75 Poseidon Bay, Winnipeg MB R3M 3E4; Man'98; BSc; FRCSC; OrthSurg (Arthroplasty). Staff, The Salvation Army Grace Hospital; Staff, Seven Oaks General Hospital; Physician, Pan Am Sports Med Centre; (204)927-2681; Fax. (204)789-9246; jdillon@panamclinic.com.

DILLON, Kirk F; Peterborough Reg HC-Hospital, 1 Hospital Dr, Peterborough ON K9J 7C6; Wes'89; Staff, Peterborough Regional Health Centre - Rogers St Site; Staff, Peterborough Regional Health Centre - Hospital Drive; (705)876-5022

DILLON, Lisa G; University Health Service, 104-65 Chancellors Cir, Winnipeg MB R3T 2N2; Tor'93; FCFP; CCFP; FCFP; Langs: English; French; lisaed@mts.net.

DILLON, Michael; Klinic Comm Hlth Centre, 870 Portage Ave, Winnipeg MB R3G 0P1; Qns'84; DCH; CCFP; FCFP; Ac Staff Dept of Fam Practice, Victoria General Hospital; Med Dir, Klinic Community Health Care; Asst Prof Family Med, University of Manitoba; (204)784-4090; Fax. (204)784-4013; mdillon@klinic.mb.ca.

DILWORTH, Geoffrey R; Medpoint Hlth Care Centre, 233-355 Wellington St, London ON N6A 3N7; Wes'76; BSc; DABD; FRCPC; Derm. (519)432-1919; Fax. (519)432-2566.

DILWORTH, Neil; 24 Huron St W, Exeter ON N0M 1S1; Dublin (Ireland)'07; CCFP; (519)235-5157

DIMACHKI, Saadedine; Hop Regional D'Edmundston, 275 Hebert Blvd, Edmundston NB E3V 4E4; Damascus (Syria)'88; Staff, Hôpital regional d'Edmundston; (506)739-2211

DIMAIO, Salvatore; Sir Mortimer B Davis Jewish Ge, 3755 ch Cote-Sainte-Catherine, Montreal QC H3T 1E2; McG'04; FRCSC; Neursurg. Staff, Sir Mortimer B Davis Jewish General; (514)340-8222 x5200

DIMANNO, Domenic; The Credit Valley Hosp, 2200 Eglinton Ave W, Mississauga ON L5M 2N1; Albany (NY) (USA)'05; FRCPC; Psy. Staff, The Credit Valley Hospital; (905)813-2200

DIMARZO, Laura; Univ of Ottawa Hlth Services, 300-100 Marie Curie Pvt, Ottawa ON K1N 1A2; Alb'06; CCFP.

DIMENTBERG, Ronald A; 200-5300 Ch de la Cote-des-Nei, Montreal QC H3T 1Y3; McG'84; FACS; CSPQ; FRCSC; OrthSurg (Knee Surgery). Chef Orthopadic Surg, St Mary's Hospital Centre; assoc Prof Surg, McGill University; Langs: English; French; (514)734-2728; Fax. (514)731-4634; ronald.dimentberg@ssss.gouv.qc.ca.

DIMITRAKOUDIS, Dimitrios P; Roncesvalles Med Clinic, 1-120 Roncesvalles Ave, Toronto ON M6R 2L1; Tor'96; FRCPC; Neur. Langs: Greek; (416)604-9500; Fax. (416)604-1560.

DIMITRAKOUDIS, Helena M; Roncesvalles Med Clinic, 1-120 Roncesvalles Ave, Toronto ON M6R 2L1; Tor'96; BSc; CCFP; (416)604-9500; Fax. (416)604-1560.

DIMITRY, John R; University of Alberta Hosp, 8440 112 St NW, Edmonton AB T6G 2B7; Cal'06; FRCPC; IntMed. Staff, University of Alberta Hospital; (780)407-8822

DIMITRY, Raouf; All-West Primary Care Ctr, 2-4217 23 Ave NW, Edmonton AB T6L 5Z8; Tor'73; DPsy; Dir Professional Services, Douglas Mental Health University Institute; Conférencier, McGill University; (780)462-0442

DIMOCK, John L; Nepean Med Centre, 205-1 Centrepointe Dr, Nepean ON K2G 6E2; Birmingham (England)'75; MB BS; DPsy; FAPA; LMCC; FRCPC; Psy (Disability Psychiatry). Langs: French; (613)786-3102; drdimock@rogers.com.

DIMOV, Marius; Detwiller Pavillion, 2255 Wesbrook Mall, Vancouver BC V6T 2A1; Cal'01; FRCPC; Psy. Staff, Providence Health Care - St Paul's Hospital; (604)822-7066; Fax. (604)822-7105.

DIN, Fareen; Phoenix Med Centre, 202-2155 10th Ave, Prince George BC V2M 5J6; (Ireland)'02; MB BCh; BAO; FRCPC; IntMed (Critical Care Medicine); Nephrol. Staff Renal Clinic, University Hospital of Northern British Columbia; (250)564-4225

DIN, Omar Shuja U; Grey Nuns Comm Hosp, 1100 Youville Drive West NW, Edmonton AB T6L 5X8; Alb'03; FRCPC; Psy (Sleep Medicine). Staff Outpatient Psy, Covenant Health - Grey Nuns Community Hospital; (780)450-9450; Fax. (780)461-6190.

DIN, Shamoon; King Street Med Arts Centre, 307-71 King St W, Mississauga ON L5B 4A2; Detroit (USA)'01; Langs: Urdu; Spanish; Punjabi; Hindi; (905)279-1660; Fax. (905)279-9666; family.physician@live.com.

DINDAR, Farouk; Agincourt Prof Centre, 409-2330 Kennedy Rd, Scarborough ON M1T 0A2; Witwatersrand (South Africa)'66; MB ChB; MRC(UK); AB; FRCPC; Neur (Neuromuscular Diseases). Court Staff, The Scarborough Hospital - Birchmount Campus; Langs: Gujarati; (416)282-4935; Fax. (416)282-0776.

DINDO, Luay F; 106-9648 128 St, Surrey BC V3T 2X9; Alb'84; Staff, Surrey Memorial Hospital; Langs: Arabic; (604)582-4666; Fax. (604)589-1242.

DINDO, Rashad F; Surrey Mem Hosp, 13750 96 Ave, Surrey BC V3V 1Z2; Alb'77; Ac Staff, Surrey Memorial Hospital; (604)581-2211

DINGEE, Carol K; 215-809 41st Ave W, Vancouver BC V5Z 2N6; Mem'81; FRCSC; GenSurg. Staff, Providence Health Care - Mount Saint Joseph Hospital; Consultant, BC Cancer Agency Vancouver Centre; Staff, Providence Health Care - St Paul's Hospital; (604)731-2176; Fax. (604)731-6938.

DINGEMANS, Emmanuel; CSSS de Saint-Jerome, 290 rue de Montigny, Saint-Jerome QC J7Z 5T3; McG'01; FRCPC; Anes. Staff Anes, Hôtel-Dieu de Saint-Jérôme; Langs: English; Spanish; (450)431-8599

DINGLE, Brian; 790 Commissioners Rd E, London ON N6A 4L6; Tor'74; MSc(Pharmacol.); FRCPC; IntMed (Medical Oncology); Hem. Staff, London Health Sciences Centre - University Hospital; Staff, Parkwood Hospital - St Joseph's Health Care; Asst Prof Dept. of Oncol., University of Western Ontario; (519)685-8500 x53267; brian.dingle@lhsc.on.ca.

DINGLE, Jonathan A; Hamilton HS-McMaster Site, PO Box 2000 Stn Lcd 1 1200 Main St W, Hamilton ON L8N 3Z5; McM'01; FRCPC; Anes. Staff, Hamilton Health Sciences Centre - McMaster Children's Hospital; Langs: Bilingual(English/French); (905)252-9140 x75170

DINGLE, Margaret; Halifax Infirmary, 3021-1796 Summer St, Halifax NS B3H 3A7; Dal'78; MCFP(EM); Staff, Queen Elizabeth II Health Sciences Centre - Halifax Infirmary Site; (902)473-4791; Fax. (902)473-3617.

DINH, Anh T T; 100-10924 107 Ave NW, Edmonton AB T5H 0X5; Sher'86; Langs: Vietnamese; French; (780)424-5665; Fax. (780)424-5667.

DINH, Ba-Hiep; Clinique Med Diamant, 1575 boul Henri Bourassa O, Montreal QC H3M 3A9; Saigon (Vietnam)'65; LMCC; Langs: Vietnamese; Chinese; (514)745-3827

DINH, Hoang-Diep; Clinique Med Anjou, 8250 av de Chatillon, Anjou QC H1K 1P2; Saigon (Vietnam)'68; Langs: Vietnamese; English; (514)352-1820

DINH, Laurent; The Ottawa Hosp-Gen Campus, 501 Smyth Rd, Ottawa ON K1H 8L6; Laval'87; ABNM; FRCP; LMCC; FRCPC; NuclearMed. Staff Nuclear Med, The Ottawa Hospital - General Campus; Asst Prof Med, University of Ottawa; Langs: Bilingual(English/French); (613)737-8528; Fax. (613)737-8705; ldinh@ottawahospital.on.ca.

DINH, Le Thu; Ctr Soins Prolonges Grace Dart, 5155 rue Sainte-Catherine E, Montreal QC H1V 2A5; Saigon (Vietnam)'74; (514)255-2833; Fax. (514)255-6275.

DINH, Ngoc Thuy; 2295 rue Ontario E, Montreal QC H2K 1V9; Saigon (Vietnam)'72; (514)524-1135; Fax. (514)524-1135.

DINH, Quynh-Dao; Heather Pavillion, 452D-2733 Heather St, Vancouver BC V5Z 1M9; Tor'07; InfectDis; IntMed. (604)875-4588

DINH, Rene N; CHUQ-Ctr Hosp Univ Laval, RC 106-2705 boul Laurier, Quebec QC G1V 4G2; Laval'91; FRCSC; Ophth (Cornea & Anterior Segment). Staff, Centre Hospitalier Universitaire de Quebec-CHUL; (418)654-2119; Fax. (418)654-2188.

DINH, Thi-Kien-Hoa; Clin Med Maurice-Duplessis, 8648 boul Maurice-Duplessis, Montreal QC H1E 3L1; Laval'80; (514)648-8930; Fax. (514)648-8933.

DINICOLO, Lisa; Toronto East Gen Hosp Inc, 825 Coxwell Ave, Toronto ON M4C 3E7; Ott'04; CCFP; CCFP(E.M.); Staff, Toronto East General Hospital Inc; (416)469-6580

DINNIWELL, Robert; Univ Hlth Network-Princess M, 5F-610 University Ave, Toronto ON M5G 2M9; Qns'98; FRCPC; RadOncol (Clinician Investigator Program). Staff, Princess Margaret Hospital - University Health Network; (416)946-4662

DINOVITZER, Natalie M; Greenboro Family Med Centre, 25 Tapiola Cres, Ottawa ON K1T 2J7; Ott'96; CCFP; Langs: Bilingual(English/French); (613)738-0303; Fax. (613)738-8950.

DINSA, Gurpreet S; Smyth Associate Clinic, 4904 48 St, Leduc AB T9E 6X4; Alb'01; CCFP; (780)986-2712; Fax. (780)986-0356.

DINSDALE, Henry; Kingston Gen Hosp, 725-76 Stuart St, Kingston ON K7L 2V7; Qns'55; FRSA; FACP; FRCP(Hon); FRCPC; Neur. Staff, Kingston General Hospital; Staff, Brockville General Hospital - Charles Street; Emeritus Prof Med., Queen's University; (613)548-6133; Fax. (613)548-6134; hdinsdale@cogeco.ca.

DINU, Claudia G; Continuum Med Care, 201-520 17th St, West Vancouver BC V7V 3S8; (Romania)'01; CCFP; Langs: Romanian; French; (604)913-8183

DINYARI, Kourosh; Family Medicine Associates, 7004 98 Ave NW, Edmonton AB T6A 0A5; Karachi (Pakistan)'83; MB BS; AAFP; MCFP(C); Staff, University of Alberta Hospital; Staff Hospitalist, Alberta Health Services; Teach Staff/Asst Clin Prof Family Med, University of Alberta; Langs: Persian; (780)468-6035; Fax. (780)466-9132; kourosh.dinyari@albertahealthservices.ca.

DIODATI, Jean G; Hop du Sacre-Coeur De Mtl, 136-5400 boul Gouin O, Montreal QC H4J 1C5; Mon'83; CSPQ; FRCPC; IntMed; Cardiol. Staff, Hôpital du Sacre-Coeur de Montréal; adj Prof, McGill University; (514)338-2200; Fax. (514)338-2381.

DION, Alain; Ctr Hosp Affilie-Enfant-Jesus, D3000-1401 18e rue, Quebec QC G1J 1Z4; Laval'82; FRCPC; Psy. Teacher, Centre Hospitalier Affilié Universitaire de Québec - Hôpital De L'Enfant Jésus; (418)649-5769; Fax. (418)649-5934.

DION, Andreanne; Centre Med Des Generations, 200-465 rue Bibeau, Saint-Eustache QC J7R 0C8; Laval'10; CCFP; (450)472-1955

DION, Anne-Marie; UMF Richelieu-Yamaska, 1005 rue Gauthier, Saint-Hyacinthe QC J2S 8T2; Mon'07; CCFP; (450)771-3333 x4972

DION, Bertrand R; Clin Med Fam D'Edmundston, 50 av Bateman, Edmundston NB E3V 4A4; Laval'81; Staff, Hôpital regional d'Edmundston; (506)735-4761; Fax. (506)739-1008.

DION, Chantal; CSSS de Trois-Rivières, 1991 boul du Carmel, Trois-Rivieres QC G8Z 3R9; Sher'92; FRCPC; DiagRad. Staff, CSSS de Trois-Rivières; (819)697-3333

DION, Daniel; Hop Du Sacre-Coeur De Montreal, 5400 boul Gouin O, Montreal QC H4J 1C5; Sher'02; AnatPath. Staff, Hôpital du Sacre-Coeur de Montréal; (514)338-2222 x2834

DION, Danielle; CSSS de Beauce-Etchemin, 1515 17e rue, Saint-Georges QC G5Y 4T8; Laval'86; CSPQ; FRCPC; IntMed (Clinical Cardiology); Cardiol. Staff, Centre Hospitalier Beauce-Etchemin; (418)228-2031; Fax. (418)227-8134.

DION, Dominique; 5415 boul de l'Assomption, Montreal QC H1T 2M4; Mon'84; Staff, Hopital Maisonneuve-Rosemont; Staff, St Mary's Hospital Centre; Langs: English; (514)252-3400; Fax. (514)750-2895.

DION, Francoise M; Valley Med Imaging, 102-32475 Simon Ave, Abbotsford BC V2T 5E3; Laval'80; FRCPC; DiagRad. (604)855-0112

DION, Genevieve; Hôpital Laval, 2725 ch Sainte-Foy, Quebec QC G1V 4G5; Sher'03; FRCPC; IntMed; Respir. Staff, Hôpital Laval; (418)656-8711 x5521

DION, Gerald; Clinique Mistissini, 395 boul Mistissini CP 1016, Mistissini QC G0W 1C0; Laval'78; Staff, Hôpital de l'Archipel; Physician, CLSC Inland-Mistassini; Langs: English; (418)923-3376 x322; Fax. (418)923-3240.

DION, Isabelle; Oshawa Clinic, 117 King St E, Oshawa ON L1H 1B9; Sher'97; CCFP; Langs: French; (905)723-8551; Fax. (905)721-4329.

DION, J Harold; Clinique Med l'Actuel, 1130-1001 boul de Maisonneuve, Montreal QC H2L 4P9; Ott'80; CCFP; FCFP; (514)524-1001; Fax. (514)524-3831.

DION, Janique; Ctr Hosp du Centre la Mauricie, 50 119E rue, Shawinigan-Sud QC G9P 5K1; Laval'87; CSPQ; CCFP; CCFP(E.M.); FCFP; EmergMed (P.Q.). Staff, Centre Hospitalier du Centre la Mauricie; (819)536-7579

DION, Jean D; Ctr de Sante Med Tremblant, CP 19002 201-585 rue Labelle, Mont-Tremblant QC J8E 3H2; Laval'81; Langs: English; (819)425-7070; Fax. (819)425-7008.

DION, Jean; Ctr Hosp Affilie-Enfant-Jesus, 1401 18e rue, Quebec QC G1J 1Z4; Laval'79; FRCPC; EmergMed. Staff, Centre Hospitalier Affilié Universitaire de Québec - Hôpital De L'Enfant Jésus; Asst Dir Emerg Section, Université Laval; (418)649-5632; Fax. (418)649-5975.

DION, Jean-Paul; Clin Gyn de Trois-Rivieres, 2237 7e av, Trois-Rivieres QC G8Z 3E2; Laval'75; ObstGyn (P.Q.). (819)379-5353

DION, Karine; CRSSS de la Baie-James, 51 3e rue, Chibougamau QC G8P 1N1; Laval'08; CCFP; Staff, CRSSS de la Baie-James; (418)748-2676; Fax. (418)748-2549.

DION, Louise; CHUS-Hop Hotel-Dieu, 580 rue Bowen S, Sherbrooke QC J1G 2E8; Sher'86; FRCPC; IntMed (Infectiology); Microbio & Infect Dis (P.Q.); MedMicrobiol. Staff, Centre Hospitalier de Coaticook; Clin Prof, Universite de Sherbrooke; (819)346-1110 x22508

DION, Louise; Canadian Med Protective Assn, PO Box 8225 Stn T CSC 875 Carling Ave, Ottawa ON K1G 3H7; Ott'80; AB; AB(CriticalCare); CSPQ; FRCSC; GenSurg (Critical Care Medicine). (613)725-2000

DION, Marc; Clinique Familiale, 13555 boul Lacroix, Saint-Georges QC G5Y 1P1; Laval'80; (418)228-8001; Fax. (418)228-5583.

DION, Marie-Claude; Clinique Med Caron Dion Losier, CP 3603 Succ Bureau-Chef 1-3980 rue Principale, Tracadie-Sheila NB E1X 1G5; Sher'88; CCFP; FCFP; Staff, Hôpital de Tracadie-Sheila; (506)395-2554; Fax. (506)395-2443.

DION, Marie-Helene; Hop Maisonneuve-Rosemont, 5415 boul de l'Assomption, Montreal QC H1T 2M4; Sher'02; FRCPC; Neur. Staff, Hopital Maisonneuve-Rosemont; (514)252-3400 x3528

DION, Marie-Josee; CSSS de Rimouski-Neigette, CP 3150 succ Bureau Chef 150 av Rouleau, Rimouski QC G5L 5T1; Laval'04; FRCPC; IntMed; Nephrol. Staff, Hôpital Regional Rimouski; Langs: Bilingual(French/English); (418)724-3000; Fax. (418)724-8757.

DION, Marie-Pierre; Centre de Sainte Sutton, 33 Principale S, Sutton QC J0E 2K0; Sher'03; Staff, Centre Hospitalier Régional de Lanaudière; (450)538-3983; Fax. (450)538-8396; mdion@aol.com.

DION, Marilyn; CSSS de Saint-Jerome, 290 rue de Montigny, Saint-Jerome QC J7Z 5T3; Sher'90; CSPQ; FRCPC; Anes. Staff, Hôtel-Dieu de Saint-Jérôme; (450)431-8200

DION, Maryse; 217-3591 Innes Rd, Orleans ON K1C 1T1; Sher'93; FRCPC; Psy. Langs: Bilingual(French/English); (613)830-2877; Fax. (613)830-2887.

DION, Michelle; Bathurst Shopping Mall, 202-1300 St Peter Ave, Bathurst NB E2A 3A6; Sher'98; CCFP; CCFP(E.M.); (506)546-6030; Fax. (506)546-6225.

DION, Nathalie; Polyclinique Pierre Le Gardeur, 300-1000 montée des Pionniers, Terrebonne QC J6V 1S8; Mon'93; Staff, Centre Hospitalier Pierre le Gardeur; (450)657-1313; Fax. (450)657-1809.

DION, Nicolas; Ctr Hosp Affilie-Enfant-Jesus, 1401 18e rue, Quebec QC G1J 1Z4; Laval'97; CSPQ; FRCPC; Anes. Staff, Centre Hospitalier Affilié Universitaire de Québec - Hôpital De L'Enfant Jésus; (418)649-0252

DION, Norbert; CHUQ-Hotel-Dieu De Quebec, 11 Cote du Palais, Quebec QC G1R 2J6; Mon'94; CSPQ; FRCSC; OrthSurg. Staff, Centre Hospitalier Universitaire de Québec (CHUQ) - Siege Social; (418)691-5370; Fax. (418)691-5020.

DION, Paul; Centre Prof Montee Masson, 100-880 Montee Masson, Mascouche QC J7K 2L7; Mon'78; (450)474-2493; Fax. (450)966-0156.

DION, Pierre; Clinique Med Neufchatel, 101-2425 boul Bastien, Quebec QC G2B 1B3; Laval'73; LMCC; Langs: English; (418)843-3771; Fax. (418)843-3865; pierredionmd@hotmail.com.

DION, Pierre-Luc; Hotel-Dieu de Levis, 143 rue Wolfe, Levis QC G6V 3Z1; Sher'03; FRCPC; Derm. Staff, Hôtel-Dieu de Lévis; (418)835-7121 x3672; Fax. (418)835-7238.

DION, Rejean; Lab de Sante Pub du Quebec, 20045 ch Sainte-Marie, Ste-Anne-de-Bellev QC H9X 3R5; Sher'80; Med Consul, Public Health; Langs: Bilingual(French/English); (514)457-2070 x325; Fax. (514)457-6346; rejean.dion@inspq.qc.ca.

DION, Susan; Clinique Med Champlain, GD 401 av Montcalm, Disraeli QC G0N 1E0; Laval'78; (418)449-3020; Fax. (418)449-3023.

DION, Sylvain; CLSC des Etchemis, 331 rue du Sanatorium GD, Lac-Etchemin QC G0R 1S0; Laval'86; Staff, CSSS des Etchemins; (418)625-8001; Fax. (418)625-2374; sylvaindion@ssss.gouv.qc.ca.

DION, Yves; Hotel-Dieu de Sorel, 400 av de l'Hotel-Dieu, Sorel-Tracy QC J3P 1N5; Laval'74; FRCP(Psych); CSPQ; FRCPC; Psy (General Psychiatry). Staff Psy, Hôtel-Dieu de Sorel; Staff, Centre Hospitalier l'Université de Montréal (CHUM) - Hôpital Notre-Dame; Teach Staff, Universite de Montreal; Langs: Bilingual(French/English); (450)746-6150; Fax. (450)746-6225.

DION, Yves-Marie; CHUQ-St-Francois D'Assise, 10 rue de l'Espinay, Quebec QC G1L 3L5; Laval'74; CSPQ; FRCSC; GenSurg. ac Staff, CSSS de Quebec-Sud; Chercheur, Centre Hospitalier Universitaire De Québec - Pavillon De St-françois-d'assise; Langs: English; French; (418)525-4444 x53315; dion.yves@videotron.ca.

DION-CLOUTIER, Philippe; CHUM-Hop St-Luc, 1058 rue Saint-Denis, Montreal QC H2X 3J4; Sher'08; Staff, Centre Hospitalier l'Université De Montréal (CHUM) - Hôpital Saint-luc; (514)890-8000

DIONISOPOULOS, Tassos; SMBD Jewish Gen Hosp, A505-3755 ch Cote-Sainte-Cathe, Montreal QC H3T 1E2; McG'85; FRCSC; GenSurg; PlasSurg. Staff, Sir Mortimer B Davis Jewish General; (514)340-8222 x3469; Fax. (514)340-8128.

DIONNE, Anne; 405-5811 boul Taschereau, Brossard QC J4Z 1A5; Mon'79; Peds. (450)443-6585; Fax. (450)443-9002.

DIONNE, Annie; Ctr Hosp Affilie-Enfant-Jesus, 1401 18e rue, Quebec QC G1J 1Z4; Sher'02; FRCPC; Neur (Neuromuscular Diseases). Staff, Centre Hospitalier Affilié Universitaire de Québec - Hôpital De L'Enfant Jésus; Langs: Bilingual(French/English); (418)649-0252; Fax. (418)649-5915.

DIONNE, Benoit; Ctr Hosp Laurentien, 234 rue Saint-Vincent, Ste-Agathe-Des-Mts QC J8C 2B8; Mon'89; Staff, Centre Hospitalier Laurentien; (819)234-4000

DIONNE, Christal; CSSSG-Hop de Hull, 116 boul Lionel-Emond, Gatineau QC J8Y 1W7; Sher'07; Staff, Hull Hospital; (819)966-6200

DIONNE, Christine; Ctr Hosp Affilie-Enfant-Jesus, 1401 18e rue, Quebec QC G1J 1Z4; Laval'03; FRCPC; IntMed; GeriatricMed. Staff, Centre Hospitalier Affilié Universitaire de Québec - Hôpital De L'Enfant Jésus; (418)649-5521

DIONNE, Claire L; St Boniface Gen Hosp, 409 Tache Ave, Winnipeg MB R2H 2A6; Laval'83; FRCPC; Anes. Staff, St Boniface General Hospital; (204)233-8563

DIONNE, Daniel; CSSS de Rimouski-Neigette, CP 3150 Succ A 150 av Rouleau, Rimouski QC G5L 5T1; Laval'75; AB; CSPQ; FRCPC; NuclearMed. Nuclear Med, Hôpital Regional Rimouski; (418)724-8692; Fax. (418)724-8633.

DIONNE, Gilles; CHUQ-St-Francois D'Assise, 10 rue de l'Espinay, Quebec QC G1L 3L5; Laval'72; FRCPC; DiagRad. Ac Staff, Centre Hospitalier Universitaire De Québec - Pavillon De St-françois-d'assise; (418)525-4444 x3185; Fax. (418)525-4180.

DIONNE, Guy; CHUQ-ST-Francois D'Assise, 10 rue de l'Espinay, Quebec QC G1L 3L5; Laval'80; FRCPC; DiagRad. ac Staff, Centre Hospitalier Universitaire De Québec - Pavillon De St-françois-d'assise; (418)525-4309 x3188; Fax. (418)525-4180; guyedionne@hotmail.com.

DIONNE, Jacynthe; CSSS de Jonquiere, CP 1200 Stn Pdf Jonquiere 2230 rue de l'Hopital, Jonquiere QC G7X 7X2; Laval'76; Med Dir Prof Serv, Centre Hospitalier Jonquiere; (418)695-7701; Fax. (418)695-7746; jadi707@videotron.ca.

DIONNE, Janis; Children's & Women's HC Of BC, 4480 Oak St, Vancouver BC V6H 3V4; Alb'00; FRCPC; Peds; Nephrol. Clinical Asst Prof, BC Children's Hospital; (604)875-2272; Fax. (604)875-3649; jdionne@cw.bc.ca.

DIONNE, Jean-Francois; Clinique Med Saint-Vincent, 250 rue King E, Sherbrooke QC J1G 1A9; Sher'89; Staff Emerg, Carrefour Sante Windsor; (819)563-0510; Fax. (819)564-6889; jfdionne1@videotron.ca.

DIONNE, Jean-Luc; 5415 boul de l'Assomption, Montreal QC H1T 2M4; Mon'98; FRCPC; IntMed; MedOncol; Hem. Staff, Hopital Maisonneuve-Rosemont; (514)252-3404; Fax. (514)254-5094.

DIONNE, Jeanette A C; West Carleton Family Hlth Team, PO Box 218 119 Langstaff Dr, Carp ON K0A 1L0; Dal'94; BScChemEng; BSc; CCFP; FCFP; (613)839-3271

DIONNE, Jonathan; CSSS de Jonquiere, 2230 rue de l'Hospital, Jonquiere QC G7X 7X2; Sher'03; CCFP; CCFP(E.M.); Staff, Centre Hospitalier Jonquiere; (418)695-7700; Fax. (418)695-7729.

DIONNE, Julien; Vision Pro Sante, 204-2860 boul Laframboise, Saint-Hyacinthe QC J2S 4Z1; Laval'79; CSPQ; OrthSurg (P.Q.). Assoc Member, Complexe hospitalier de la Sagamie; (450)773-8181; Fax. (450)773-8959.

DIONNE, Karla; 1590 7th Ave W, Vancouver BC V6J 1S3; UBC'91; Staff, IMC Integrative Med Centre of Canada; (604)569-0488; info@imccanada.com.

DIONNE, Langis; Medisys Quebec, 410-3165 ch Saint-Louis, Quebec QC G1W 4R4; Mon'76; Médecin, Clinique Executive Medisys; Langs: Bilingual(French/English); (418)681-0167

DIONNE, Marc; Sante Publique du Quebec, 5e-945 av Wolfe, Quebec QC G1V 5B3; Laval'71; MPH; FRCPC; CommunMed (P.Q.); Public Health & Preventive Med. Med Researcher, Centre Hospitalier Universitaire de Quebec-CHUL; Dir Scientific Risque Biologic at de la Sante at Travel, Institut National de Sante Publique du Quebec; Langs: English; (418)650-5115 x5201; Fax. (418)654-3134; marc.dionne@inspq.qc.ca.

DIONNE, Marie-Claude; Centre Med Saint-Denis, 202-620 ch des Patriotes, St-Denis-Sur-Rich QC J0H 1K0; Laval'99; CCFP; Staff, Centre Hospitalier de Val d'Or; (450)787-3233

DIONNE, Matthew L; College Square Med Centre, 1980 Baseline Rd, Ottawa ON K2C 0C6; Dal'95; CCFP; (613)224-6606

DIONNE, Melanie; CSSS du Lac-des-Deux-Montagnes, 520 boul Arthur-Sauve, Saint-Eustache QC J7R 5B1; Mon'98; Staff, Hôpital de Saint-Eustache; (450)473-6811

DIONNE, Michel; Palliative Med Residency Prog, 284J-43 rue Bruyere St, Ottawa ON K1N 5C8; Ott'00; BSc; FRCPC; AnatPath. Staff Path & Lab Med, The Ottawa Hospital - General Campus; Staff, The Ottawa Hospital - Civic Campus; Langs: French; (613)562-6262; Fax. (613)562-6371; micheldionne@hotmail.com.

DIONNE, Michele; 37 av Donegani, Pointe-Claire QC H9R 2V7; Mon'80; LMCC; Staff, CSSS de Dorval-Lachine-Lasalle; Physician, Clinique Medicale McDermott; Staff Medecin, Centre Medical St-Raphael; Langs: English; (514)697-1410; Fax. (514)697-1411.

DIONNE, Mireille; CSSS de Temiscouata, CP 310 58 rue de l'Eglise, Notre-Dame-du-Lac QC G0L 1X0; Laval'08; CCFP; Fam Med, Centre Hospitalier Notre-Dame-du-Lac; (418)899-6751; Fax. (418)899-2809.

DIONNE, Natasha P; 203-1789 Mountain Rd, Moncton NB E1G 5C4; Mon'96; CCFP; (506)388-4440; Fax. (506)387-3921.

DIONNE, Nathalie; CSSS de Rimouski-Neigette, CP 3150 Succ A 150 av Rouleau, Rimouski QC G5L 5T1; Mon'90; CSPQ; Cardiol (P.Q.); IntMed. Staff, Hôpital Regional Rimouski; (418)724-8114

DIONNE, Paul G; 607-224 boul Alexandre Tache, Gatineau QC J9A 0B8; Mon'68; CSPQ; FCAP; FRCPC; AnatPath. Langs: French; English; (514)873-1845 x236; pgdionne@hotmail.com.

DIONNE, Renee; Polyclinique de l'Oreille, 155-120 boul de l'Hopital, Gatineau QC J8T 8M2; Sher'89; FRCSC; Otol (Rhinology). Staff, Hôpital de Gatineau; Langs: English; (819)561-0002; Fax. (819)561-9644.

DIONNE, Richard; The Ottawa Hosp-Civic Campus, 1053 Carling Ave, Ottawa ON K1Y 4E9; Mon'94; CCFP; CCFP(E.M.); Staff, The Ottawa Hospital - General Campus; Langs: Bilingual(French/English); (613)761-4928

DIONNE, Suzanne; Inst U en Sante Mentale de QC, 2601 ch de la Canardiere, Quebec QC G1J 2G3; Laval'86; FRCPC; Psy. Staff, Institut Universitaire Sante; (418)663-5321

DIONNE, Suzanne; Ministere de la Sante, 12e-1075 ch Sainte-Foy, Quebec QC G1S 2M1; Laval'73; (418)266-2241

DIONNE, Sylvie; CSSS du Sud de Lanaudière, 911 Montee des Pionniers, Terrebonne QC J6V 2H2; Mon'87; CSPQ; FRCPC; Anes. Staff, Centre Hospitalier Pierre le Gardeur; (450)654-7525 x32214

DIORIO, Diane L; MUHC-Montreal Neurology Inst, 3801 rue University, Montreal QC H3A 2B4; Tor'94; Neur (P.Q.) (Neuro-Surgery). Staff, McGill University Health Centre - Montreal Neurological Hospital; (514)398-5034

DIOSY, David C; London HSC-University Hosp, PO Box 5339 Stn B 339 Windermere Rd, London ON N6A 5A5; Tor'95; BSc; FRCPC; Neur (Electroenceph/Epilepsy). Clin Associate, Health Sciences North - Memorial Site; Clin Associate EEG & Epilepsy, London Health Sciences Centre - University Hospital; Aj Prof, University of Western Ontario; Langs: French; (519)663-3248; Fax. (519)663-3152; ddiosy@uwo.ca.

DIOTALLEVI, Mark J; Mitchell Family Doctors, PO Box 790 7 Francis St, Mitchell ON N0K 1N0; McG'86; CCFP; FCFP; Staff, Stratford General Hospital - Huron Perth Healthcare Alliance; (519)348-8402; Fax. (519)348-8400.

DIOTTE, Magali; GMF de l'Assomption, CP 3406 201-814 boul l'Ange-Gardien N, L'Assomption QC J5W 4M9; Mon'09; (450)589-5778

DIPCHAND, Anne I; The Hosp For Sick Children, 555 University Ave, Toronto ON M5G 1X8; Tor'92; FRCPC; Peds (Pediatric Cardiology); Cardiol. Staff Cardiol, The Hospital For Sick Children; (416)813-6674; Fax. (416)813-7547; anne.dipchand@sickkids.ca.

DIPCHAND, Christine S; Queen Elizabeth II HSC, 5098-1276 South Park St, Halifax NS B3H 1V8; Wes'93; FRCPC; IntMed; Nephrol. Staff, Queen Elizabeth II Health Sciences Centre - Victoria General Site; (902)473-4021; Fax. (902)473-2675.

DIPPEL, Ruth G A; Student Hlth Serv, 158-50 Stone Rd E, Guelph ON N1G 2W1; Wes'95; CCFP; FCFP; (519)824-4120 x52131; Fax. (519)836-7431.

DIPPENAAR, Francois J L; The Vernon Family Pract Assoc, 3310 32 Ave, Vernon BC V1T 2M6; Pretoria (South Africa)'86; MB ChB; LMCC; (250)545-5321; Fax. (250)545-0450.

DIPPENAAR, Helgardt; Tower Prof Centre, 5520 50 Ave, Wetaskiwin AB T9A 0T3; (South Africa)'97; (780)352-9700; Fax. (780)352-9739.

DIQUINZIO, Melanie L; Valley Reg Hosp, 150 Exhibition St, Kentville NS B4N 5E3; Dal'06; InfectDis; IntMed. Staff, Valley Regional Hospital; (902)678-7381; Fax. (902)679-1904.

DIRAIMO, Louis R; 1-1678 Bank St, Ottawa ON K1V 7Y6; Ott'80; Langs: Italian; (613)230-3234; Fax. (613)230-4009; aj451@rogers.com.

DIRENFELD, Leonard; 3-3600 Ellesmere Rd, Scarborough ON M1C 4Y8; Tor'80; CCFP; Associate, The Scarborough Hospital - General Campus; Associate, Rouge Valley Health System - Centenary Health Centre Site; Ac Staff Extended Care, Sunnybrook Health Sciences Centre; Lecturer, University of Toronto; (416)282-5773; Fax. (416)282-9545.

DIRKER, Caren; Medicine Hat Reg Hosp, 666 5 St SW, Medicine Hat AB T1A 4H6; (South Africa)'04; MB BS; Staff, Medicine Hat Regional Hospital; (403)529-8000

DIRKS, Martha H; Hôpital Ste-Justine, 3175 ch Cote-Ste-Catherine, Montreal QC H3T 1C5; McG'93; LMCC; FRCPC; Peds (Pediatric Gastroenterology); Gastroent. Staff Gastroent Service, Hôpital Ste-Justine; adj Prof, Universite de Montreal; Langs: French; (514)345-4931 x7000; Fax. (514)345-4999; martha.dirks.hsj@ssss.gouv.qc.ca.

DIRKS, Peter; The Hosp For Sick Children, 1504-555 University Ave, Toronto ON M5G 1X8; Qns'89; FRCSC; Neursurg (Pediatrics). Staff NeuroSurg, The Hospital For Sick Children; Asst Prof Dept of Surg, University of Toronto; Langs: French; (416)813-6426; Fax. (416)813-4975; peter.dirks@sickkids.ca.

DIRKSCHEN VAN SCHALKWYK, Johannes; Captain William Jackman Mem Ho, 410 Booth St, Labrador City NL A2V 2K1; Pretoria (South Africa)'70; MB ChB; BSc(Med); Staff, Captain William Jackman Memorial Hospital; Langs: Afrikaans; (709)944-2632

DIRNFELD, Victor; Crestwood Med Dental, 311-6051 Gilbert Rd, Richmond BC V7C 3V3; Man'61; DABIM; FABA; FRCPC; IntMed (Cardiology). Pres Medical Staff, Richmond Hospital; (604)278-0633; Fax. (604)278-4664.

DISCEPOLA, Federico; SMBD Jewish Gen Hosp, 1202-3755 ch Cote-Sainte-Cathe, Montreal QC H3T 1E2; McG'04; FRCPC; DiagRad. Staff, Sir Mortimer B Davis Jewish General; (514)340-8222; Fax. (514)567-5580.

DISCEPOLA, Marino J; 110-1240 av Beaumont, Mont-Royal QC H3P 3E5; McG'84; DAB; FRCSC; Ophth. Staff, McGill University Health Centre - Royal Victoria Hospital; Staff, St Mary's Hospital Centre; Teacher, McGill University; Langs: Italian; French; (514)385-0530; Fax. (514)385-3039.

DISCHINGER, Heidi; Copeman Health Care Centre, 400-628 12 Ave SW, Calgary AB T2R 0H6; Cal'87; (403)686-0920; Fax. (403)217-7168.

DISCHLIEV, Spiro; Clinique Med Viau, 4750 rue Jarry E, Saint-Leonard QC H1R 1X8; Montpellier (France)'82; (514)326-7203

DISERENS, Monique M; Foothills Med Centre, 1403 29 St NW, Calgary AB T2N 2T9; McG'87; FRCPC; Anes. Staff, Foothills Medical Centre; (403)944-1430; Fax. (403)944-2425.

DISPERATI, Patricia; Toronto East Gen Hosp Inc, KW 2F-825 Coxwell Ave, Toronto ON M4C 3E7; Parana (Brazil)'00; FRCPC; IntMed; Hem. Staff, Princess Margaret Hospital - University Health Network; Staff, Toronto East General Hospital Inc; Langs: Portuguese; Spanish; (416)461-8272 x6410; Fax. (416)469-6297.

DISSANAYAKE, Chaminda; Langs Farm Village Association, 1145 Concession Rd, Cambridge ON N3H 4L5; Tor'96; CCFP; FCFP; Ac Staff, Cambridge Memorial Hospital; (519)653-1470; Fax. (519)653-6277.

DISSANAYAKE, Dilani T K; Mediplace Walk-In Clinic, 2-756 Pembina Hwy, Winnipeg MB R3M 2M7; (Sri Lanka)'79; (204)284-5408

DISTIN, Kiloran E; 800-2 St Clair Ave, Toronto ON M4T 2T5; McM'93; FRCPC; Psy (Child & Adolescent Psychiatry). (416)644-4941; Fax. (416)513-0348.

DITOMMASO, Stephen N; CLSC des Faubourgs, 1705 rue de la Visitation, Montreal QC H2L 3C3; McG'82; CCFP; FCFP; (514)527-2361; Fax. (514)527-3134.

DITOR, Allan S; Pelham Group Health Centre, 212-245 Pelham Rd, St Catharines ON L2S 1X8; Man'61; FRCPC; IntMed. Ac Staff, Niagara Health System - Ontario Street Site; Ac Staff, Niagara Health System - St Catharines General Site; (905)682-9335; Fax. (905)682-9641.

DITTBERNER, Klaus; St Amant Centre, 440 River Rd, Winnipeg MB R2M 3Z9; Man'74; Langs: German; (204)256-4301 x4247; Fax. (204)257-4349; kdittberner@stamant.mb.ca.

DIUDEA, Dana M; Royal University Hosp, 103 Hospital Dr, Saskatoon SK S7N 0W8; Cluj (Romania)'89; FRCPC; AnatPath. Staff Pathology, Royal University Hospital; (306)655-2153; Fax. (306)655-2223.

DIVAKARA MENON, Syamkumar; Hamilton HS-General Site, 237 Barton St E, Hamilton ON L8L 2X2; (India)'92; Asst Prof Arrhutmia Clinic/Staff, Hamilton Health Sciences Centre - Hamilton General Hospital; Lecturer, McMaster University; (905)521-2100 x44760; Fax. (905)577-1447; heathco@mcmaster.ca.

DIVANLI, Kemal; Hop Regional D'Edmundston, 275 Hebert Blvd, Edmundston NB E3V 4E4; Ege (Turkey)'85; Staff, Hôpital regional d'Edmundston; Consultant Phy, Centre de Sante Mentale A Kedgwick NB; Langs: Turkish; French; (506)739-2571; Fax. (506)739-2438.

DIVARIS, Dimitrios; Grand River Hosp-KW Hlth Ctre, PO Box 9056 Stn C 835 King St W, Kitchener ON N2G 1G3; Rhodesia (Zimbabwe)'81; MB ChB; LRCPS(Ed); LRCPS(Glas); FRCPC; GenPath. Med Dir Labs, Grand River Hospital - Kitchener/Waterloo Health Centre; Langs: Greek; (519)749-4300 x2323; dimitrios_divaris@grhosp.on.ca.

DIWAN, Murtaza A; Norfolk Med Centre, 310-85 Norfolk St, Guelph ON N1H 4J4; Mem'75; BSc; Otol. Staff, Groves Memorial Community Hospital; Staff, Guelph General Hospital; Langs: Gujarati; Hindi; Urdu; (519)763-1115; Fax. (519)763-1270.

DIX, David B; Children's & Women's HC of BC, A119-4480 Oak St, Vancouver BC V6H 3V4; Cape Town (South Africa)'84; MB ChB; FRCPC; Peds (Pediatric Hematology Oncology); Hem. Staff, BC Children's Hospital; (604)875-2644; Fax. (604)875-2911.

DIX, Marie D; Pratte et Whitney Canada, 1000 boul Marie-Victorin, Longueuil QC J4G 1A1; Mon'91; CCFP; (450)647-7719; Fax. (450)647-9840.

DIXIT, Radhika; 35-7700 Bathurst St, Thornhill ON L4J 7Y3; Wes'09; CCFP.

DIXIT, Sanjay; 34-1960 Appleby Line, Burlington ON L7L 0B7; Meerut (India)'96; FRCPC; IntMed; Rheum. Langs: Hindi; (905)332-9292; Fax. (905)332-9244.

DIXON, Andrew C; Edmonton Clinic Health Academy, 11405 87 Ave NW, Edmonton AB T6G 1C9; Man'03; FRCPC; Peds; PedEmergMed. Physician, Edmonton Clinic Health Academy; (780)248-5575; Fax. (780)248-5626.

DIXON, Anthony R J; Chatham-Kent Hlth Alliance, PO Box 2030 Stn Main 80 Grand Ave W, Chatham ON N7M 5L9; McM'04; CCFP; Staff, Chatham-Kent Health Alliance; (519)352-6400

DIXON, Brian L; Queen Street Diag Imaging, 200-514 Queen St, Saskatoon SK S7K 0M5; Sask'75; FRCPC; DiagRad. Assoc Staff, Royal University Hospital; (306)664-3200; Fax. (306)664-0032.

DIXON, Corinne E; 201-851 Fischer Hallman Rd, Kitchener ON N2M 5N8; Tor'86; CCFP; FCFP; Court Staff, Grand River Hospital - Kitchener/Waterloo Health Centre; Court Staff, St Mary's General Hospital; (519)743-1011; Fax. (519)743-0041.

DIXON, David; Thames Valley FHT-W London FH, 200-785 Wonderland Rd S, London ON N6K 1M6; Qns'92; MClSc; CCFP; FCFP; Aj Prof Family Med & Part Time Senior Med Consultant, University of Western Ontario; (519)641-6712; Fax. (519)641-6189.

DIXON, David J; 1103-180 Bloor St W, Toronto ON M5S 2V6; Tor'89; BSc; MA; DPhil; FRCPC; Psy. Asst Prof Psy, University of Toronto; (416)972-6161; Fax. (416)972-7539.

DIXON, Elijah; Foothills Med Centre, EG26-1403 29 St NW, Calgary AB T2N 2T9; Man'96; BSc; MSc; FACS; FRCSC; GenSurg (Hepatobiliary & Pancreatic Surgery). Staff, Foothills Medical Centre; Staff, Tom Baker Cancer Centre; Assoc Prof Surg & Oncol, University of Calgary; (403)944-3045; Fax. (403)944-1277.

DIXON, Elizabeth; Summit Family Clinic, 209-200 Boudreau Rd, St. Albert AB T8N 6B9; Alb'93; CCFP; (780)458-7000; Fax. (780)458-8484.

DIXON, Heather L; Centre for Family Medicine, 10B Victoria St S, Kitchener ON N2G 1C5; Qns'97; CCFP; FCFP; (519)783-0022; Fax. (519)783-0032.

DIXON, Kirsten; Sherbourne Health Centre, 333 Sherbourne St, Toronto ON M5A 2S5; Qns'06; (416)324-4100; Fax. (519)324-4181.

DIXON, Marjorie; First Steps Fertility, 215-4025 Yonge St, North York ON M2P 2E3; McG'97; FRCSC; ObstGyn (Fertility). Asst Prof ObstGyn, University of Toronto; Langs: Spanish; French; (416)221-7545; Fax. (416)221-9020.

DIXON, Nancy L J; Dr C W Wiebe Med Centre, 385 Main St, Winkler MB R6W 1J2; Man'04; CCFP.

DIXON, Peter F; Lakeridge Hlth Corp-Oshawa, 1 Hospital Crt, Oshawa ON L1G 2B9; Newcastle (England)'77; FRCPC; RadOncol., Lakeridge Health - Oshawa Site; (905)576-8711 x4595; Fax. (905)721-6101.

DIXON, Shannon C; Tiger Hills Med Associates, PO Box 191, Treherne MB R0G 2V0; Man'98; CCFP.

DIXON, Susan; Salveo Family Med Clinic, B8-6455 Macleod Trail SW, Calgary AB T2H 0K8; Alb'98; CCFP; (403)444-0428; Fax. (403)537-0029.

DIXON, William S; Sunnybrook Hlth Sciences Ctre, M1 302-2075 Bayview Ave, Toronto ON M4N 3M5; Tor'64; FRCSC; Ophth (Cataract Surgery). Chief Ophth, Sunnybrook Health Sciences Centre; Med Dir, Eye Bank of Canada; Prof, University of Toronto; (416)487-9100; Fax. (416)480-4481.

DIXON-WARREN, Nattana B L; Salmo Wellness Clinic, PO Box 730 423 Davies St, Salmo BC V0G 1Z0; UBC'95; BSc; CCFP; FCFP; Staff, Kootenay Boundary Regional Hospital; University of British Columbia; (250)357-2627; Fax. (250)357-2687.

DIYAEB, Mohamed A; Queentario Med Center, 4B-2325 Hurontario St, Mississauga ON L5A 4C7; Alfatah (Libya)'99; MB ChB; CCFP; Staff, South Cumberland Commun Care Center; Langs: Arabic; (905)270-8307; Fax. (905)270-6861.

DIZON, Aquilino M; Medical Clinic, GD, Melita MB R0M 1L0; UST (Philippines)'62.

DJAHANBAKHSH ASLI, Khashayar; CHUS-Hop Hotel-Dieu, 580 rue Bowen S, Sherbrooke QC J1G 2E8; Teheran (Iran)'94; Psy (P. Q.). Staff, Centre Hospitalier Universitaire de Sherbrooke-Hôpital Hôtel-Dieu; (819)346-1110

DJAIANI, George N; Univ Hlth Network-Toronto Gen, EN 3 410-200 Elizabeth St, Toronto ON M5G 2C4; USSR (Russia (Federation))'86; FRCPC; Anes. Staff, Toronto General Hospital - UHN; Langs: Latvian; Russian; (416)340-4800 x6205; george.djaiani@uhn.on.ca.

DJAKNOUN, Djaoeida; CSSS du Haut Saint-Maurice, 885 boul Ducharme, La Tuque QC G9X 3C1; (Algeria)'87; GenSurg (P.Q.). Staff, Centre Hospitalier Saint-Joseph de la Turque; (819)523-4581; Fax. (819)523-7992.

DJAN, Deborah; La Loche Health Centre, PO Box 1, La Loche SK S0M 1G0; Staff, La Loche Health Centre and Hospital; (306)822-3201; Fax. (306)822-2798; d.djan@sasktel.net.

DJEARAM, Saleena; 103-1660 Feltham Rd, Victoria BC V8N 2A1; (India)'91; MB BS; CCFP; Staff Family Practice Unit, Whitehorse General Hospital; Langs: Malayalam; Hindi; Arabic; (250)477-1858

DJERBIB, Kenza; CSSS Haut-Richelieu-Rouville, 920 du Seminaire Blvd N, St-Jean-sur-Richel QC J3A 1B7; Sher'04; DiagRad. Staff, Hôpital du Haut-Richelieu; (450)359-5000

DJEREDJIAN, Jessica; Tiny Tots Med Centre, 203-3400 rue du Marche, Dollard-D-Ormeaux QC H9B 2Y1; McG'06; MDCM; CCFP; Staff, Sir Mortimer B Davis Jewish General; (514)685-3531 x353; Fax. (514)685-7971.

DJEREDJIAN, Sarkis; Hôpital Sainte-Croix, 570 rue Heriot, Drummondville QC J2B 1C1; Mon'05; FRCPC; NuclearMed. Staff, Hôpital Sainte-croix; (819)478-6464

DJILLALI-BERKANE, Nacera; Clin Med Mont-Carmel, 933 boul Rene-Levesque E, Montreal QC H2L 4S4; Mon'05; CCFP; Staff, Hôtel-Dieu de Sorel; (514)282-9197

DJOGOVIC, Dennis; University of Alberta Hosp, 1G1 59-8440 112 St NW, Edmonton AB T6G 2B7; Alb'99; FRCPC; EmergMed (Family Medicine); Critical Care Medicine. Staff Emerg Med, University of Alberta Hospital; (780)407-8822

DJORDJEVIC, Bojana; The Ottawa Hosp-Gen Campus, 501 Smyth Rd, Ottawa ON K1H 8L6; Alb'03; FRCPC; AnatPath. Staff, The Ottawa Hospital - General Campus; Langs: Croatian; Serbian; (613)737-8899; Fax. (613)737-8853.

DJORDJEVIC, M Dragan; Wooen's College Hosp, 76 Grenville St, Toronto ON M5S 1B2; Belgrade (Serbia)'72; FRCPC; Anes. Staff, Women's College Hospital; (416)323-6008

DJURIC, Miroslav; James Paton Mem Hosp, 125 Trans Canada Hwy, Gander NL A1V 1P7; Man'03; Staff, James Paton Memorial Hospital; (709)256-2500

DJURIC, Vladimir; Rothba Centre for Pain Care, 9-4640 Dufferin St, North York ON M3H 5S4; Toledo (USA)'90; (416)612-6407

DJURICIC, Milla; Orleans Med Centre, 406-2555 St Joseph Blvd, Orleans ON K1C 1S6; (Serbia)'96; CCFP; Langs: Serbian; (613)830-1771; Fax. (613)830-2543.

DJURICKOVIC, Slobodan; Lansdowne Professional Ctr II, 305-3066 Shelbourne St, Victoria BC V8R 6T9; Wes'91; FRCSC; PlasSurg (Cosmetics). Staff, Royal Jubilee Hospital; Staff, Victoria General Hospital; Staff, Saanich Peninsula Hospital; (250)592-5510; Fax. (250)592-9601; slobodand@shaw.ca.

DLACIC, Aleksandra; North York Gen Hosp, 4001 Leslie St, North York ON M2K 1E1; Belgrade (Serbia)'96; FRCPC; Anes. Staff, North York General Hospital; Langs: Serbian; (416)756-6520; Fax. (416)756-6203.

DLIN, Arnold D; Kerrisdale Station Med Clinic, 2077 42nd Ave W, Vancouver BC V6M 2B4; Alb'73; (604)261-9494

DLIN, Ronald A; Links Med Clinic, 104-11910 111 Ave NW, Edmonton AB T5G 3G6; Alb'72; BSc; Langs: Hebrew; (780)454-0351; Fax. (780)452-6767.

DMITRIENKO, Svetlana; St Paul's Hosp, 1081 Burrard St, Vancouver BC V6Z 1Y6; (Ukraine)'86; HemPath. Staff, Providence Health Care - St Paul's Hospital; (604)682-2344

DMITRIEV, Dmitriy; 24868 130A Ave, Maple Ridge BC V4R 2C7; (Russia (Federation))'86; FRCPC; Anes. Staff, East Kootenay Regional Hospital; (778)809-7442

DMITRIEVA, Victoria; Ridge Meadows Hosp & Hlth CC, 11666 Laity St, Maple Ridge BC V2X 5A3; (Russia (Federation))'86; FRCPC; Psy. Staff, Ridge Meadows Hospital & Health Care Centre; Langs: Russian; (604)463-1814; dr.victoria.dmitrieva@interiorhealth.ca.

DMYTRYSHYN, Amie; BC Children's Hosp, 4480 Oak St, Vancouver BC V6H 3V4; St George's (Grenada)'08; Peds. Staff, BC Children's Hospital; (604)875-2345

DMYTRYSHYN, Robert; Women's College Hosp, 76 Grenville St, Toronto ON M5S 1B2; Tor'88; CCFP; Staff, Halton Healthcare Services Corporation - Milton District Hospital; Staff Family Pract, Women's College Hospital; Lecturer Fam & CommunMed, University of Toronto; Langs: Ukrainian; (416)323-6064; Fax. (416)323-6402.

DO, Anh Phuong; 407-235 Danforth Ave, Toronto ON M4K 1N2; Tor'93; FRCPC; Peds. Staff, The Hospital For Sick Children; Lecturer, University of Toronto; Langs: Vietnamese; (416)465-7421; Fax. (416)465-6588.

DO, Binh Minh; Centre Med Chambly-Latour, B-5580 ch de Chambly, Longueuil QC J3Y 3P5; Sher'96; (450)926-2236

DO, Doan Hoa; CHUS-Hop Fleurimont, 3001 12e av N, Sherbrooke QC J1H 5N4; Sher'00; FRCPC; IntMed; Cardiol. Staff, Centre Hospitalier Universitaire de Sherbrooke-Hopital Fleurimont; (819)346-1110

DO, Doan Trang; 1209 rue Belanger, Montreal QC H2S 1H7; Saigon (Vietnam)'74; (514)279-3802

DO, Duy-An; 12198 rue Notre-Dame E, Pte-aux-Trembles QC H1B 2Z1; Saigon (Vietnam)'68; Staff, CHSLD Cardinal Inc; (514)991-1807; Fax. (514)640-6267.

DO, Kiet; Family Matters Med Centre, X-730 St Annes Rd, Winnipeg MB R2N 0A2; Man'10; CCFP.

DO, Kim-Anh; Bureau Evaluation Médicale, CP 5200 Succ Terminus 348-2600 boul Laurier, Quebec QC G1K 7S9; Laval'82; Regie de l'Assurance de l'Auto du Quebec; (418)657-8709 x3229

DO, Lan Vinh; 110-667 rue Champlain, Dieppe NB E1A 1P6; Sher'00; FRCSC; GenSurg (Surgical Oncology). Staff Surg, Dr Georges-L-Dumont University Hospital Centre; Langs: Bilingual(French/English); (506)858-8199; Fax. (506)858-9012.

DO, Minh-Thu; Clin Ophtalmologique de l'Outa, 29 rue Ducharme, Gatineau QC J8Y 3P7; Mon'03; FRCSC; Ophth. (819)771-4337; Fax. (819)770-1066.

DO, Quoc-Bao; CHUM-Hotel-Dieu, 2 402-3840 rue Saint-Urbain, Montreal QC H2W 1T8; Laval'93; CSPQ; MSc; FRCSC; CardSurg (Cardiovascular & Thoracic Surgery). Staff, Centre Hospitalier l'Université de Montréal (CHUM) - Hôtel-Dieu; Langs: Vietnamese; English; (514)890-8000 x15808; Fax. (514)412-7694.

DO, Skyz; Colchester East Hants Hlth Ctr, 600 Abenaki Rd, Truro NS B2N 5A1; Ott'06; DiagRad. Staff, Colchester East Hants Health Centre; Physician, Capital Health Centre; (902)893-5554

DO, Tai Hung; CSSS de la Vallée de l'Or, 725 6e rue, Val-d'Or QC J9P 3Y1; Sher'95; FRCPC; DiagRad. Staff, Centre Hospitalier de Val d'Or; (819)825-6711; Fax. (819)825-7907.

DO, Thuan Hieu; BC Cancer Agency-Fraser Valley, 13750 96 Ave, Surrey BC V3V 1Z2; Alb'02; MSc; FRCPC; IntMed; MedOncol. Staff, BC Cancer Agency Fraser Valley Centre; (604)930-2098; Fax. (604)587-4312.

DO, Xuan Vien; Hop Charles LeMoyne, 3120 boul Taschereau, Greenfield Park QC J4V 2H1; Sher'03; FRCPC; DiagRad. Staff, Hopital Charles LeMoyne; (450)466-5000 x2030

DOAK, Gregory; Seven Oaks Gen Hosp, 2300 McPhillips St, Winnipeg MB R2V 3M3; Man'83; BSc; PhD; FRCPC; Anes. Staff, Seven Oaks General Hospital; (204)632-7133

DOAN, Julian; Lakeshore Gen Hosp, 160 av Stillview, Pointe-Claire QC H9R 2Y2; McG'04; FRCPC; Anes. Staff, Lakeshore General Hospital - Pointe Claire; (514)630-2225

DOAN, Ly Huong; Centre Bois De Boulogne, 1575 boul Henri-Bourassa O, Montreal QC H3M 3A9; Mon'00; Ac Member, Hôpital du Sacre-Coeur de Montréal; Langs: English; Vietnamese; (514)338-2383

DOAN, Quy Xuan; St Boniface Clinic, 343 Tache Ave, Winnipeg MB R2H 2A5; Man'06; CCFP; (204)925-9535

DOAN, Quynh Huong; Children's & Women's HC of BC, 4480 Oak St, Vancouver BC V6H 3V4; McG'98; MDCM; FRCPC; Peds; PedEmergMed. Staff 1, BC Children's Hospital; Langs: Vietnamese; English; (604)875-2045; q_doan@hotmail.com.

DOAN, Richard J; M D O T, 2F-125 Danforth Ave, Toronto ON M4K 1N2; Yale (USA)'82; AB(Child Psy.); AB(Psy.); FRCPC; Psy (Child Psychiatry). Staff, Centre for Addiction & Mental Health (CAMH) - College Street Site; Staff, Toronto East General Hospital Inc; Asst Prof, University of Toronto; (647)777-0130; Fax. (647)777-0134.

DOANE, Frank R; 120-2751 Gladstone St, Halifax NS B3K 4W6; Dal'77; (902)422-4555

DOANE, Paul H; Quinpool Center, 6169 Quinpool Rd, Halifax NS B3L 4P8; Dal'73; Physician, International Immunization Centre-Health Canada; (902)497-8535; Fax. (902)420-9432.

DOBBERTHIEN, Marion T; Rockyview Gen Hosp, 7007 14 St SW, Calgary AB T2V 1P9; Alb'90; FRCPC; Anes. Staff, Rockyview General Hospital; (403)943-3410; Fax. (403)943-3360.

DOBBIN, Karolyn M; Medical Assoc of Port Perry, 462 Paxton St, Port Perry ON L9L 1L9; Mem'92; FRCSC; GenSurg. (905)985-2895; Fax. (905)985-8931.

DOBBIN, Stafford; Niagara Med Group Fam Hlth Team, 4421 Queen St, Niagara Falls ON L2E 2L2; Belfast (Ireland)'67; MB ChB; BAO; CCFP; FCFP; Ac Staff, Niagara Health System - Greater Niagara General Site; Med Dir, Heart Niagara; (905)356-2236; Fax. (905)356-2568; sdobbin@niagaramedicalgroup.com.

DOBBS, Ryan C; Belleville Queen's Family Med, 103-145 Station St, Belleville ON K8N 2S9; Wes'09; CCFP; (613)771-1910; Fax. (613)771-0689.

DOBEK, Isabella; 3785 Hwy 3 PO Box 2040, Chester NS B0J 1J0; Gdansk (Poland)'75; Langs: Polish; (902)275-5625; Fax. (902)275-2032.

DOBEK, Luke; Tantallon Family Practice, 202-5110 St Margarets Bay Rd, Lakeside NS B3Z 1E2; University of Saba (Other Foreign)'06; (902)826-2744; Fax. (902)826-2887.

DOBENKO, Sheryl N; 603-320 March Rd, Kanata ON K2K 2E3; Qns'83; CCFP; FCFP; (613)591-1780; Fax. (613)591-9219.

DOBEREINER, Elisabeth F A; Alberta Children's Hosp, 2888 Shaganappi Trail NW, Calgary AB T3B 6A8; (Sweden)'96; Staff, Alberta Children's Hospital; (403)955-7810; Fax. (403)955-7606.

DOBKIN, Earl F; Bayview-Finch Med Clinic, 202-3292 Bayview Ave, North York ON M2M 4J5; Wes'69; Assoc Staff, North York General Hospital; (416)222-9955; Fax. (416)222-8088.

DOBKIN, Martin; City Centre Family Physicians, 500-71 King St W, Mississauga ON L5B 4A2; Qns'66; Ac Staff Family Med, Trillium Health Centre - Mississauga; Langs: Bilingual(English/French); (905)270-0415; Fax. (905)848-1500.

DOBKOWSKI, Wojciech B; London HSC-University Hosp, PO Box 5339 Stn B 339 Winderemer Rd, London ON N6A 5A5; Warsaw (Poland)'71; FRCPC; Anes. Staff, London Health Sciences Centre - University Hospital; Asst Prof, University of Western Ontario; Langs: Polish; (519)685-8500

DOBOSIEWICZ, Andrzej; Niagara Health Centre, 304-180 Vine St S, St Catharines ON L2R 7P3; Poznan (Poland)'77; FACOG; FSOGC; FRCS; FRCSC; ObstGyn (Laparoscopic Surgery). Staff, Niagara Health System - St Catharines General Site; Clinical Asst Prof ObstGyn Faculty of Health Sciences, McMaster University; Langs: Polish; Russian; (905)687-8648; Fax. (905)687-8877; adobosiewicz@sympatico.ca.

DOBOVICNIK, Bernard K; Riverside Med Clinic, 307-1101 Dewdney Ave, Trail BC V1R 4T1; UBC'82; BSc; MSc; Clinical Asst Prof Family Pract, University of British Columbia; Langs: English; French; German; (250)368-8802; Fax. (250)368-8813.

DOBRANOWSKI, Julian; St Joseph's Healthcare, 50 Charlton Ave E, Hamilton ON L8N 4A6; Cracow (Poland)'79; FRCPC; DiagRad. Staff, St Joseph's Healthcare - Charlton Campus; McMaster University; Langs: Polish; (905)522-4941

DOBRESCU, Otilia-Maria; Hôpital Ste-Justine, 3175 ch Cote-Ste-Catherine, Montreal QC H3T 1C5; Bucharest (Romania)'69; LMCC; Peds (General Pediatrics). ac Staff, Hôpital Ste-Justine; Universite de Montreal; Langs: English; Romanian; (514)345-4893; Fax. (514)345-4744.

DOBRINSKI, Herbert; CLSC Parc Extension, 111-7085 rue Hutchison, Montreal QC H3N 1Y9; McG'80; Langs: French; (514)273-9591 x6451; Fax. (514)273-8363.

DOBROFSKY, Shirley; Students Union Bldg, 2 200-66 University Campus NW, Edmonton AB T6G 2J7; McG'83; BSc; MSc; MDCM; FRCPC; Psy (Child Psychiatry). Staff, Glenrose Rehabilitation Hospital; Clinical Asst Prof Psy & Ped, University of Alberta; (780)492-2612; Fax. (780)492-0013.

DOBROGOWSKI, Michael J J; UBC Eye Care Centre, 2550 Willow St, Vancouver BC V5Z 3N9; UBC'84; FRCSC; Ophth. Ac Staff Eye Clinic, Providence Health Care - St Paul's Hospital; Consultant, Vancouver General Hospital - Centennial Pavillion; Prof Clinical, University of British Columbia; (604)875-5575; Fax. (604)875-5576.

DOBROUSIN, Anatoly; Canora Med Clinic, 14924 Stony Plain Rd NW, Edmonton AB T5P 3X8; (Ukraine)'92; CCFP; Langs: Russian; Ukrainian; Hebrew; (780)443-0300

DOBROWOLSKI, Marek; Ctr de Sante de la Basse Cote, CP 130 1070 boul Dr Camille Marcou, Lourdes-D-Bl-Sabl QC G0G 1W0; Lublin (Poland)'71; Staff, CSSS de la Basse Côté-Nord; Langs: Polish; French; (418)461-2144

DOBSON, Anne E; 203-1199 Bay Ave, Trail BC V1R 4A4; Ott'02; FRCSC; ObstGyn (Prolapse). (250)368-6663; Fax. (250)368-6681.

DOBSON, B Jane; King West Med Assoc, 505 King St W, Hamilton ON L8P 1B9; Tor'83; CCFP; FCFP; Staff, St Joseph's Healthcare Hamilton - West 5th Campus; (905)525-3501; Fax. (905)528-5468.

DOBSON, Clifford Larry; 33 Apache Cres, Nepean ON K2E 6H8; Alb'70; CCFP; Staff, Queensway Carleton Hospital; (613)224-0336; larrydobson@rogers.com.

DOBSON, Diana C; PO Box 433 Stn Main, North Sydney NS B2A 3M4; Dal'74; (902)794-4224

DOBSON, Gary; 4056-918 16 Ave NW, Calgary AB T2M 0K3; McG'82; FRCPC; Anes. (403)283-5324; Fax. (403)202-1240.

DOBSON, Gregory R; Queen Elizabeth II HSC-Halifax, 1796 Summer St, Halifax NS B3H 3A7; Dal'86; FRCPC; Anes. Staff, Queen Elizabeth II Health Sciences Centre - Victoria General Site; (902)473-4326

DOBSON, Ian; Thunder Bay Reg HSC-T-Bay, 980 Oliver Rd, Thunder Bay ON P7B 6V4; Tor'89; FRCPC; Anes. Chief Dept. of Anes, Thunder Bay Regional Health Sciences Centre; (807)684-6000

DOBSON, J Crawford; Trent University-Athletic Comp, 1600 West Bank Dr, Peterborough ON K9J 7B8; Wes'84; FRCSC; OrthSurg. Ac Staff Orth, Peterborough Regional Health Centre - Hospital Drive; Assoc Prof, Queen's University; (705)743-0043; Fax. (705)743-1922.

DOBSON, Joy A R; Regina Qu'Appelle HR-Regina, 1440 14th Ave, Regina SK S4P 0W5; Sask'84; FRCPC; Anes (Administrative Medicine). Staff, Regina General Hospital; (306)766-4260; Fax. (306)766-3550; joy.dobson@rqhealth.ca.

DOBSON, Malgorzata M S; 101-145 17th St W, North Vancouver BC V7M 3G4; Newcastle (England)'79; MB BS; MRCGPract; Vis Staff, Vancouver General Hospital - Centennial Pavillion; Langs: Polish; (604)980-2820; Fax. (604)980-2977.

DOBSON, Peter E; Westbram Family Practice, 104-100 Pertosa Dr, Brampton ON L6X 0H9; Tor'79; CCFP; Staff, William Osler Health System - Brampton Civic Hospital; (905)451-1244; Fax. (905)451-6955.

DOBSON, Rebecca L; Queen Elizabeth II HSC-Halifax, 1796 Summer St, Halifax NS B3H 3A7; Dal'78; AB; FRCPC; DiagRad. Ac Staff, Queen Elizabeth II Health Sciences Centre - Victoria General Site; Asst Prof, Dalhousie University; (902)473-7770; Fax. (902)473-0218.

DOBSON, Simon R M; Children's & Women's Hlth Ctre, K4 211-4500 Oak St, Vancouver BC V6H 3N1; Newcastle (England)'79; MB BS; FRCPCH; FRCPC; Peds. Staff, BC Women's Hospital & Health Centre; Clin Assoc Prof Peds, University of British Columbia; (604)875-2436; Fax. (604)875-2414.

DOBSON, Tracey; Brock University Health Centre, 500 Glenridge Ave, St Catharines ON L2S 3A1; Wes'87; Teach Staff, Brock University; (905)688-5550 x4692

DOBSON, William M; Trafalgar Med Clinic, 200-1235 Trafalgar Rd, Oakville ON L6H 3P1; Tor'80; CCFP; FCFP; Ac Staff, Halton Healthcare Services Corporation - Oakville Site; (905)844-3281; Fax. (905)849-1076.

DOBYNS, Edward; Victoria Gen Hosp, 1 Hospital Way, Victoria BC V8Z 6R5; UBC'89; CCFP; FCFP; Staff, Victoria General Hospital; (250)727-4212

DOCHERTY, Henry V; BC Cancer Ctre-Southern Interi, 399 Royal Ave, Kelowna BC V1Y 5L3; Glasgow (Scotland)'81; MB ChB; DRCOG; DCH; CCFP; FCFP; Ac Staff, Kelowna General Hospital; Staff, BC Cancer Agency Sindi Ahluwalia Hawkins Centre for the Southern Interior; (250)712-3930; Fax. (250)712-3911.

DOCHERTY, Marjorie A; Mountain-View Med Clinic, 201-1789 K. L. O. Rd, Kelowna BC V1W 3P3; Aberdeen (Scotland)'81; MB ChB; DRCOG; CCFP; FCFP; Dir Family Pract & Obst Residency Prog, Kelowna General Hospital; Assoc Prof Family Practice, University of British Columbia; Langs: English; French; (250)860-6799

DOCHERTY, Peter S; The Moncton Hosp, 135 MacBeath Ave, Moncton NB E1C 6Z8; Wes'86; FRCPC; IntMed (Pulmonary Hypertention); Rheum. Ac Staff, The Moncton Hospital; Clin Instructor, Dalhousie University; Langs: Bilingual(English/French); (506)857-5565; Fax. (506)857-5567.

DOCHEV, Atanas K; South Shore Reg Hosp, 90 Glen Allan Dr, Bridgewater NS B4V 3S6; Ukraine (Ukraine)'86; Staff Anes, South Shore Regional Hospital; Langs: Bulgarian; Russian; (902)527-5215; dotchev@hotmail.com.

DOCHEVA, Diyana S; Univ of Toronto, 602-500 University Ave, Toronto ON M5G 1V7; (Ukraine)'84; IntMed.

DOCKING, Annie E; Queensway Carleton Hosp, 3045 Baseline Rd, Ottawa ON K2H 8P4; UBC'09; CCFP; CCFP(E.M.); Staff, Queensway Carleton Hospital; (613)721-2000

DOCKING, Leanne M; Harry Medovy House, 2F-671 William Ave, Winnipeg MB R3E 0Z2; Man'01; FRCPC; Anes. Staff Anes, Health Sciences Centre.

DOCKRILL, Karen G; 207 Dundas St W, Whitby ON L1N 2M4; Dal'84; BSc; FRCPC; Peds (Neonatology). (289)634-1015; Fax. (905)666-2115; karen@momandbabydepot.ca.

DOCKRILL, Mark B; 805 Blackburn Mews, Kingston ON K7P 2N6; Qns'02; (613)634-0373

DOCKSTEADER, Brian; Sunridge Prof Centre, 301-2675 36 St NE, Calgary AB T1Y 6H6; Qns'72; FRCSC; ObstGyn. Associate/Clin Prof ObstGyn, University of Calgary; (403)291-2974; Fax. (403)250-3419.

DOCKSTEADER, Mark J; H2 Medical Centre, 7020 4 St NW, Calgary AB T2K 1C4; Alb'09; CCFP; Staff, Foothills Medical Centre; (403)730-7663; Fax. (403)730-4466.

DOCKTOR, Bobbie-Jo L; Foothills Med Centre, 1403 29 St NW, Calgary AB T2N 2T9; McM'96; FRCPC; DiagRad. Staff, Foothills Medical Centre; (403)944-1969

DOCKX, Daniel J A; Tillsonburg Med Centre, 200 Broadway St, Tillsonburg ON N4G 5A7; Wes'90; Staff, Tillsonburg District Memorial Hospital; (519)842-4231; Fax. (519)842-6955.

DOCRAT, Ahmed R; Ranchlands Fam Physicians, 12-7750 Ranchview Dr NW, Calgary AB T3G 1Y9; Dublin (Ireland)'81; MB ChB; BAO; LMCC; CCFP; Langs: French; (403)239-5822; Fax. (403)241-3530.

DOCRAT, Zohra; Brant Community Hlth Care Ctr, 1-221 Brant Ave, Brantford ON N3T 3J2; McM'85; ObstGyn. (519)753-8666 x204; Fax. (519)753-3109.

DOCTOR, Joel; Gulf Canada Square, 325-401 9 Ave SW, Calgary AB T2P 3C5; Cal'89; FRCPC; IntMed; ClinImmunol&Allergy. Asst Clin Prof Med, University of Calgary; (403)221-4479; Fax. (403)221-4403.

DOCTOR, Shaheen S; North York Gen Hosp, 4001 Leslie St, North York ON M2K 1E1; McM'95; BSc; FRCPC; Peds (Neonatology). Staff, Women's College Hospital; Staff, North York General Hospital; Asst Teacher, University of Toronto; (416)756-6444; Fax. (416)756-6817.

DODARO, Jocelyn; Centre Hosp Honore-Mercier, 2750 boul Laframboise, Saint-Hyacinthe QC J2S 4Y8; Mon'01; CCFP; Staff, Centre Hospitalier Honore-Mercier; (450)771-3333

DODD, Colin; Rockyview Gen Hosp, 7007 14 St SW, Calgary AB T2V 1P9; Cal'79; FRCPC; Anes. Staff, Rockyview General Hospital; (403)943-3410; Fax. (403)949-2201.

DODD, E Wendy; PO Box 370, Bellevue AB T0K 0C0; Cal'76; FRCPC; Anes. Ac Staff, Chinook Regional Hospital; Ac Staff, Covenant Health - St Michael's Health Centre; (403)562-8804

DODD, Faith; 35 Glenwood St, Sydney NS B1P 1V8; Dal'01; FRCSC; OrthSurg. (902)567-0509; Fax. (902)567-0529.

DODD, Graham A A; Royal Inland Hosp, 311 Columbia St, Kamloops BC V2C 2T1; UBC'92; MSc; CCFP; CCFP(E.M.); Staff Emerg, Royal Inland Hospital; (250)374-5111 x2425; Fax. (250)314-2327.

DODD, Roger F; Misericordia Community Hosp, 16940 87 Ave NW, Edmonton AB T5R 4H5; Alb'85; Staff, Covenant Health - Misericordia Community Hospital; (780)735-2000

DODD, Sharon; 180-11700 Cambie Rd, Richmond BC V6X 1L5; UBC'98; CCFP; (604)270-9833

DODD, William A H; Central Park Med Centre, 104-3965 Kingsway, Burnaby BC V5H 1Y8; UBC'60; FRCPC; Derm. Consultant, Vancouver General Hospital - Centennial Pavillion; (604)434-8781

DODDS, Christopher A; 103-12195 Harris Rd, Pitt Meadows BC V3Y 2E9; UBC'87; (604)460-2035; Fax. (604)460-2036.

DODDS, Mark; Athens District Hlth Services, PO Box 99 9 Wellington St E, Athens ON K0E 1B0; Saba Univ (Netherlands Antilles)'07; CCFP; Physician, Athens & District Family Health Team; (613)924-2623; mdodds@edhospital.on.ca.

DODDS, Martin T; Southgate Med Clinic, 1-45905 Yale Rd, Chilliwack BC V2P 2M3; UBC'90; Locum Tenens, Chilliwack General Hospital; (604)795-7228; Fax. (604)795-2535.

DODEK, Daniel Y; City Square Family Practice, 116-555 12th Ave W, Vancouver BC V5Z 3X7; UBC'99; BSc; CCFP; FCFP; Clin Instructor UBC, Providence Health Care - Mount Saint Joseph Hospital; (604)879-3900; Fax. (604)879-3969.

DODEK, Peter M; St Paul's Hosp, 1081 Burrard St, Vancouver BC V6Z 1Y6; Tor'78; FRCPC; IntMed; Respir. Ac Staff Pulmonary Research, Providence Health Care - St Paul's Hospital; (604)806-9023; Fax. (604)806-8674.

DODGE, David; The Moncton Hosp, 135 MacBeath Ave, Moncton NB E1C 6Z8; Mem'95; FRCPC; Anes. Staff, The Moncton Hospital; (506)857-5111

DODGE, Gregory T; Halton HCS Corp-Oakville, 327 Reynolds St, Oakville ON L6J 3L7; Qns'09; CCFP; CCFP(E.M.); Staff, Halton Healthcare Services Corporation - Oakville Site; (905)338-4618; Fax. (905)338-4639.

DODGSON, Bruce G; The Hosp For Sick Children, 555 University Ave, Toronto ON M5G 1X8; Wes'76; FRCPC; Anes (Pediatric Anesthesia). Staff Anes, The Hospital For Sick Children; Physician, Anesthesia Service Associates; Asst Prof, University of Toronto; (416)813-7445; Fax. (416)813-7543.

DODIG, Dubravka; Univ Hlth Network-Toronto Western Hosp, 399 Bathurst St, Toronto ON M5T 2S8; McM'00; FRCPC; Neur. Staff, Toronto Western Hospital - University Health Network; Langs: Croatian; French; (416)603-5922; Fax. (416)603-7096.

DODIN, Sylvie; CHUQ-St-Francois D'Assise, 10 rue de l'Espinay, Quebec QC G1L 3L5; Lille (France)'83; Ac Staff, Centre Hospitalier Universitaire De Québec - Pavillon De St-françois-d'assise; (418)525-4307; Fax. (418)525-4481; sylvie.dodin@ogy.ulaval.ca.

DODWELL, Emily; The Hosp For Sick Children, 555 University Ave, Toronto ON M5G 1X8; Qns'05; FRCSC; OrthSurg. Staff, The Hospital For Sick Children; (416)276-2776

DOE, Sam; 100-123 15th St E, North Vancouver BC V7L 2P7; UBC'98; FRCPC; IntMed; Cardiol. Staff, Lions Gate Hospital; (604)980-1031

DOEKSEN, Corwin N D; 1562 Lonsdale Ave PO Box 54032 Rpo Lansdale West, North Vancouver BC V7M 3L5; UBC'95; BSc(Hon)(Hons); CCFP.

DOELL, Brian; Guelph Gen Hosp, 115 Delhi St, Guelph ON N1E 4J4; Alb'97; CCFP; FCFP; Staff, Guelph General Hospital; (519)821-9260

DOELL, Donald; Kawartha Reg Memory Clinic, 168 Brock St, Peterborough ON K9H 2P4; McG'06; MDCM; FRCPC; IntMed; GeriatricMed. (705)749-3906; Fax. (705)749-2778.

DOELL, Donald V; Port Hope Comm Hlth Centre, 99 Toronto Rd, Peterborough ON K9H 2P4; McG'73; MS(Epidem.); IntMed (Respirology)., Northumberland Hills Hospital; (905)885-2626

DOELMAN, William; Kirkland & District Hosp, 145 Goverment Rd E, Kirkland Lake ON P2N 3P4; Cal'09; CCFP; Staff, Sioux Lookout Meno-Ya-Win Health Centre; Staff, Kirkland & District Hospital; (705)567-5251; wdoelman@slmhc.on.ca.

DOEPNER, Michael; CSSSSG-Hop de Gatineau, CP 2000 Succ Bureau-Chef 909 boul de la Verendrye O, Gatineau QC J8P 7H2; Ott'78; Otol (P.Q.). Ac Staff, Hôpital de Gatineau; Langs: German; (819)561-8100; Fax. (819)827-3157.

DOERING, Michele M; Regional Mental HC-London, PO Box 5532 Stn B 850 Highbury Ave, London ON N6A 4H1; Ott'93; FRCPC; Psy (Geriatric Psychiatry). Staff, Regional Mental Health Care-St Joseph's Health Care; (519)455-5110 x47374; Fax. (519)455-7151.

DOERKSEN, David C; Windsor Reg Hosp-Metropolitan, 1995 Lens Ave, Windsor ON N8W 1L9; Man'67; DAB; FRCPC; Anes. Staff, Windsor Regional Hospital - Metropolitan Site; Langs: German; (519)254-1661

DOERMER, Erroll R; Henderson Med Centre, 441 Henderson Hwy, Winnipeg MB R2K 2H5; Man'82; Asst Staff, Concordia General Hospital; Langs: German; (204)667-8650; Fax. (204)668-1928.

DOERR, Jeffrey J; Health Sciences Centre, 820 Sherbrook St, Winnipeg MB R3A 1R9; Man'84; FRCPC; Anes. Staff Anes, Health Sciences Centre; (204)774-6511

DOERSAM, Gerald B; 208-3195 Granville St, Vancouver BC V6H 3K2; Tor'78; BA; FACOG; FRCSC; ObstGyn. Ac Staff, Surrey Memorial Hospital; (604)737-7322

DOEY, Tamison; Off Site Adolescent Clinic, 3640 Wells Ave, Windsor ON N9C 1T9; McM'76; FRCPC; Psy. Ac Staff Privil, Windsor Regional Hospital - Metropolitan Site; Ac Staff Privil Psy, Hôtel-Dieu Grace Hospital; Ac Staff Privil I.O.E. Unit, Windsor Regional Hospital - Tayfour Site; (519)258-0484

DOGAR, Ghulam; The Medical Centre, 7 Pinsent Dr, Grnd-Falls-Wi NL A2A 2S8; Punjab (Pakistan)'86; MB BS; Staff, Central Newfoundland Regional Health Centre; (709)489-1200; Fax. (709)489-6724.

DOHERTY, Colleen; Southlake Reg Health Centre, 596 Davis Dr, Newmarket ON L3Y 2P9; Tor'06; FRCPC; Peds. Staff, Southlake Regional Health Centre; (905)895-4521; Fax. (905)830-5972.

DOHERTY, Delores S; 23 Cashin Ave, St. John's NL A1E 3A9; Burlington(VA) (USA)'72; FRCPC; Peds (Adolescent Health Care). Staff Child Health Prog, Janeway Children's Health & Rehabilitation Centre; Consultant, Burin Peninsula Health Care Centre; Consultant, Central Newfoundland Regional Health Centre; (709)754-2068; aspens@nfld.com.

DOHERTY, Dermot R; Children's Hosp Eastern Ont, 401 Smyth Rd, Ottawa ON K1H 8L1; National (Ireland)'94; Staff, Children's Hospital of Eastern Ontario (CHEO); (613)737-7600 x2431

DOHERTY, Edward J; 304-2 Union St, Saint John NB E2L 5A7; Dal'74; Staff, Saint John Regional Hospital; Staff, St Joseph's Hospital; Clin Researcher, Alcon; Teach Staff, Dalhousie University; (506)658-1273

DOHERTY, Geoffrey P; The Ottawa Hosp-Civic Campus, 1053 Carling Ave, Ottawa ON K1Y 4E9; Ott'01; FRCPC; DiagRad. Staff, The Ottawa Hospital - Civic Campus; Langs: French; (613)737-8899

DOHERTY, Mary A; Sunnybrook Health Sciences Ctr, 2075 Bayview Ave, Toronto ON M4N 3M5; Belfast (Ireland)'77; FRCPC; RadOncol (Lymphoma). Staff, Sunnybrook Health Sciences Centre; (416)480-4834; Fax. (416)480-6002.

DOHERTY, Mary P; 4420 10th Ave W, Vancouver BC V6R 2H9; Tor'72; FRCPC; Psy. (604)689-9474

DOHERTY, Olanrewaju J; Glenbrook Plaza Med Clinic, 136-3715 51 St SW, Calgary AB T3E 6V2; (Nigeria)'90; CCFP; (403)686-6967; Fax. (403)686-3736.

DOHERTY, Robert; South Lake Fam Health Team, 201-581 Davis Dr, Newmarket ON L3Y 2P6; Tor'79; Ac Staff, Southlake Regional Health Centre; Lecturer Family Med, University of Toronto; (905)853-3103; Fax. (905)853-9136.

DOHERTY, Timothy; St Joseph's HC-Parkwood Hosp, 404-801 Commissioners Rd E, London ON N6C 5J1; McM'96; FRCPC; PhysMed&Rehab (Electrodiagnosis). Staff, Parkwood Hospital - St Joseph's Health Care; Staff, London Health Sciences Centre - University Hospital; Staff, St Joseph's Hospital - St Joseph's Health Care; Dept Chair Physical Med & Rehab, University of Western Ontario; (519)684-4292; Fax. (519)685-4017; tim.doherty@lhsc.oc.ca.

DOHM, Brigitte H M T; 4539 Marine Ave, Powell River BC V8A 2K5; Vienna (Austria)'81; Langs: German; (604)485-7222; Fax. (604)485-7232.

DOIDGE, Mark S; 690A Queen St E, Toronto ON M4M 1G9; Tor'82; Staff, Travel Vaccine Clinic; (416)461-2419; Fax. (416)461-3129; mark_doidge@hotmail.com.

DOIDGE, Norman; 501-180 Bloor St W, Toronto ON M5S 2V6; Tor'83; FRCPC; Psy (Psychoanalysis). Member Faculty, Columbia University Centre for Psychoanalytic Training & Research; Head Long Term Psychotherapy Prog, University of Toronto; (416)925-9058; Fax. (416)516-7555.

DOIG, Anne F; City Centre Fam Physicians, 100-514 Queen St, Saskatoon SK S7K 0M5; Sask'76; CCFP; FCFP; Ac Staff, Saskatoon City Hospital; Ac Staff, Royal University Hospital; Clin Assoc Prof ObstGyn, University of Saskatchewan; (306)244-3016; Fax. (306)244-4737; adoig@ccfp.ca.

DOIG, Christopher; Faculty of Med, 3D39-3280 Hospital Dr NW, Calgary AB T2N 4Z6; Sask'88; FRCPC; IntMed; Critical Care Medicine. Staff, Foothills Medical Centre; Prof/Dept Head Community Health Sciences, University of Calgary; (403)210-7220; Fax. (403)270-7307; cdoig@ucalgary.ca.

DOIG, George; Thunder Bay Reg HSC-T-Bay, 980 Oliver Rd, Thunder Bay ON P7B 6V4; Man'70; FRCPC; Anes. Dir ICU, Thunder Bay Regional Health Sciences Centre; Section Leader Anaes, Northern Ontario School of Medicine-Laurentian University; (807)684-6000

DOIG, Pamela A; Lifemark Health Centre, 230-181 Keefer Pl, Vancouver BC V6B 6C1; Dal'85; BSc; Dip SportMed(Casem); CCFP; (604)687-5911

DOIRON, Andre; CSSS de Montmagny-L'Islet, 350 boul Tache O RR 1, Montmagny QC G5V 3R8; Laval'89; Staff, CSSS de Montmagny-L'Islet; (418)248-0630; Fax. (418)248-0820.

DOIRON, Anne; Dr Georges-L Dumont Reg Hosp, 330 av Universite, Moncton NB E1C 2Z3; Laval'92; FRCPC; DiagRad. Diagnostic Imaging, Dr Georges-L-Dumont University Hospital Centre; (506)854-6687; Fax. (506)862-4544.

DOIRON, Daniel; Riverside Med Centre, 404-2211 Riverside Dr, Ottawa ON K1H 7X5; Mem'83; LMCC; FRCPC; Psy (Child & Family Psychiatry). Consultant, Children's Hospital of Eastern Ontario (CHEO); Consultant, Royal Ottawa Mental Health Centre - Royal Ottawa Health Care Group; Asst Prof Psy, University of Ottawa; Langs: French; (613)737-2155; Fax. (613)737-4199; danieldoiron@bellnet.ca.

DOIRON, Maryjo; Superior Family Hlth Org, 470-63 Algoma St N, Thunder Bay ON P7A 4Z6; NOSM'10; CCFP; (807)344-8475; Fax. (807)344-6323.

DOIRON, Paul L; 330 av Universite, Moncton NB E1C 2Z3; Sher'90; LMCC; FRCPC; Anes. Staff, Dr Georges-L-Dumont University Hospital Centre; Langs: Bilingual(English/French); (506)862-4130

DOJA, M Asifud; Children's Hosp Eastern Ont, 401 Smyth Rd, Ottawa ON K1H 8L1; Wes'00; FRCPC; Neur. Staff, Children's Hospital of Eastern Ontario (CHEO); (613)737-2260

DOJEIJI, Suzan; The Ottawa Hosp-Rehab Ctr, 1104-505 Smyth Rd, Ottawa ON K1H 8M2; Wes'93; MD; FRCPC; PhysMed&Rehab. Staff Physical Med & Rehab, The Ottawa Hospital Rehabilitation Centre; Langs: French; (613)737-7350; Fax. (613)737-6877; sdojeiji@toh.on.ca.

DOKAINISH, Hisham; Hamilton HS-General Site, C3 111-237 Barton St E, Hamilton ON L8L 2X2; McM'95; Cardiol; IntMed. Staff, Hamilton Health Sciences Centre - Hamilton General Hospital; Langs: Italian; Spanish; French; (905)527-4322

DOLAN, James; 105-274 Dundas St E, Belleville ON K8N 1E6; Qns'64; Staff Family Med, QHC Belleville General; (613)968-3012

DOLAN, Michael C; Ottawa Valley Family Hlth, 95 Spring St SS 1, Almonte ON K0A 1A0; Ott'74; FRCPC; EmergMed. Staff, Almonte General Hospital; (613)256-9370; Fax. (613)256-0949.

DOLAN, Sean P; 201-1 Magazine St, Saint John NB E2K 5S9; Mem'83; FRCPC; IntMed (Hematology). Staff, Saint John Regional Hospital; Teacher, Dalhousie University; (506)634-1201; Fax. (506)632-6955; agsd1515@nbnet.nb.ca.

DOLATA, Wojciech; Allan Blair Cancer Centre, 4101 Dewdney Ave, Regina SK S4T 7T1; Poznaniu (Poland)'86; Staff, Allan Blair Cancer Centre; (306)766-2070; Fax. (306)766-6222.

DOLATABADI, Amir; 105-1424 Southview Dr SE, Medicine Hat AB T1B 4E7; Tehran (Iran)'90; Staff, Medicine Hat Regional Hospital; (403)487-5900; Fax. (403)487-5901.

DOLBEAR, Betty E; Headwaters Health Care Centre, 100 Rolling Hills Dr, Orangeville ON L9W 4X9; Qns'67; FRCPC; DiagRad (CT/X-Ray & Ultrasound). Staff Radiologist, Headwaters Health Care Centre - Orangeville Site; (519)941-2410 x2210; Fax. (519)941-7726.

DOLBEC, Julie; CLSC Ahuntsic, 1165 boul Henri-Bourassa E, Montreal QC H2C 3K2; Sher'06; CCFP; (514)381-2000; Fax. (514)389-1361.

DOLBEC, Luc; Complexe Hosp de la Sagamie, 305 rue Saint-Vallier, Chicoutimi QC G7H 5H6; Laval'82; CSPQ; FRCPC; Anes. Ac Staff, Complexe hospitalier de la Sagamie; (418)541-1000

DOLBEC, Pierre; CSSS de Rivière-de-Loup, 75 rue Saint-Henri, Riviere-du-Loup QC G5R 2A4; Laval'81; CSPQ; FRCPC; Anes. Staff, Centre Hospitalier Regional du Grand-Portage; (418)868-1010; Fax. (418)868-1386.

DOLCE, Patrick; CSSS de Rimouski-Neigette, CP 3150 Succ A 150 av Rouleau, Rimouski QC G5L 5T1; Laval'86; FRCPC; MedMicrobiol (Infection Control); Microbio & Infect Dis (P.Q.). Staff, Hôpital Regional Rimouski; Université Laval; (418)724-8336; Fax. (418)724-8619.

DOLDEN, Daniel A; St Mary's Hosp, PO Box 7777 5544 Sunshine Coast Hwy, Sechelt BC V0N 3A0; Wes'69; FRCPC; DiagRad. Staff, St Mary's Hospital; (604)885-2224

DOLDEN, Jennifer M; Royal Columbian Hosp, 330 Columbia St E, New Westminster BC V3L 3W7; UBC'98; FRCPC; DiagRad., Royal Columbian Hospital; Staff, Eagle Ridge Hospital & Health Care Centre; (604)520-4640; Fax. (604)520-4120; jmdolden@yahoo.com.

DOLEZALEK, Jan A; Health Sciences Centre, 300 Prince Philip Dr, St. John's NL A1B 3V6; (Slovakia)'00; FRCPC; Psy. Staff, Health Sciences Centre; (709)777-6300

DOLEZEL, Josef; 208 Huronia Med Centre PO Box 790 Stn Main, Midland ON L4R 4P4; Palacky (Czech Republic)'64; DABIM; FRCPC; IntMed (Cardiology). Internal Medicine, Georgian Bay General Hospital - Midland; (705)526-9915; Fax. (705)526-4491.

DOLHANIUK, Christina; 2925 66 St NW, Edmonton AB T6K 4C1; Alb'05; FRCSC; ObstGyn. (587)523-0235; Fax. (587)523-0237.

DOLHANTY, Dorothy A; Health Park, 310-45 Weatherbee Rd, Mira Road NS B1M 0A1; McM'91; FRCSC; ObstGyn. Staff, Cape Breton Healthcare Complex; (902)597-8115; Fax. (902)567-8119.

DOLL, Corinne M; Tom Baker Cancer Centre, 1331 29 St NW, Calgary AB T2N 4N2; UBC'94; FRCPC; RadOncol. Staff, Tom Baker Cancer Centre; (403)521-3164; Fax. (403)283-1651.

DOLLIN, Barry; Health & Counseling Services, 1125 Colonel By Dr, Ottawa ON K1S 5B6; McG'72; DPsy; FRCPC; Psy (Group Psychotherapy). Assoc Staff, Royal Ottawa Mental Health Centre - Royal Ottawa Health Care Group; Assoc Prof, University of Ottawa; (613)520-6674; Fax. (613)520-4059.

DOLLIN, Janet; Family Med Associates, 500-267 O'Connor St, Ottawa ON K2P 1V3; McG'80; CCFP; FCFP; Langs: French; (613)234-5588; jdollin@uottawa.ca.

DOLLOIS, Anne-Marie; 202-269 boul Saint-Jean, Pointe-Claire QC H9R 3J1; McG'83; CSPQ; CCFP; FCFP; Hon Staff, Lakeshore General Hospital - Pointe Claire; Chairman, CPDP Bayview Hosp.; Prospector Family Med, McGill University; Langs: English; French; (514)697-0704; Fax. (514)697-4164.

DOLMAJIAN, Jennifer; CSSS de Laval, 1755 boul Rene-Laennec, Laval QC H7M 3L9; McG'04; FRCSC; PlasSurg. Staff, Hopital de la Cite de la santé; (450)668-1010

DOLMAN, John F; Vancouver Gen Hosp, 855 12th Ave W, Vancouver BC V5Z 1M9; UBC'80; FRCPC; Anes. Ac Staff, Vancouver General Hospital - Centennial Pavillion; (604)875-4304; jdolman@vanhosp.bc.ca.

DOLMAN, Peter J; UBC Eye Care Centre, 2550 Willow St, Vancouver BC V5Z 3N9; UBC'84; FRCSC; Ophth (Orbital & Oculoplastics). Ac Staff, BC Children's Hospital; Ac Staff Ophth, Vancouver General Hospital - Centennial Pavillion; Court Staff Ophth, Providence Health Care - St Paul's Hospital; Clin Assoc Prof, University of British Columbia; Langs: English; French; (604)875-4346; Fax. (604)875-4415; peterdolman@hotmail.com.

DOLYNCHUK, Kenneth; 107-147 Provencher Blvd, Winnipeg MB R2H 0G2; Man'79; PhD; BSc; FRCP; ABPS; FRCSC; PlasSurg (Cosmetic Surgery). Att Staff Surg., St Boniface General Hospital; Associate, Western Surgery Centre; Assoc Prof Surg, University of Manitoba; (204)231-1542; Fax. (204)231-1340; contact@agelesscosmetic.com.

DOMAN, Marthinus H; PO Box 489, Boyle AB T0A 0M0; Orange Free (South Africa)'01; MB ChB; Langs: Afrikaans; (780)689-0003; Fax. (780)689-4155; thinusdoman@yahoo.ca.

DOMANKO, Wayne B; St Lawrence Med Clinic, PO Box 772, Morrisburg ON K0C 1X0; Sask'68; Med Dir, Winchester District Memorial Hospital; (613)543-2963; Fax. (613)543-4171.

DOMB, Sharon; Sunnybrook Hlth Sciences Ctre, A112-2075 Bayview Ave, Toronto ON M4N 3M5; Tor'92; CCFP; FCFP; Staff, North York General Hospital; Staff Family & CommunMed, Sunnybrook Health Sciences Centre; Asst Prof Family & CommunMed, University of Toronto; (416)480-4939; Fax. (416)480-6038; sharon.domb@sunnybrook.ca.

DOME, Valerie; Montfort Hosp, 713 Montreal Rd, Ottawa ON K1K 0T2; Sher'00; FRCSC; ObstGyn. Staff, Montfort Hospital; Langs: Bilingual(French/English); (613)746-4621

DOMENICONE, Rosaria; 201-959 Dundas St, Woodstock ON N4S 1H2; Wes'90; CCFP; Ac Staff, Woodstock General Hospital; (519)539-5621; Fax. (519)539-0628.

DOMES, Trustin; Medical Arts Bldg, 537-750 Spadina Cres E, Saskatoon SK S7K 3H3; Alb'05; FRCSC; Urol. (306)653-3255; Fax. (306)653-4386.

DOMINGUE, Claude; Clin Med L'Avenir, 200-1150 boul de l'Avenir, Laval QC H7N 6L2; Mon'78; BA(Microbiol.); Physician, Polyclinique St-Martin Laval; (450)680-1150; Fax. (450)680-1151.

DOMINGUEZ, Ada L; Regional Rehabilitation Centre, 300 Wellington St N, Hamilton ON L8L 0A4; Manila (Philippines)'96; FRCPC; IntMed. Staff, Cambridge Memorial Hospital; (905)527-0271

DOMINGUEZ, J Manuel; CHUM-Hop Notre-Dame, 1560 rue Sherbrooke E, Montreal QC H2L 4M1; Sevilla (Spain)'85; MSc(Anatomy); FRCPC; IntMed. Staff, Centre Hospitalier l'Université de Montréal (CHUM) - Hôpital Notre-Dame; (514)890-8000

DOMINGUEZ AVALOS, Jose A; CSSS du Lac-Témiscamingue, 22 rue Notre-Dame N, Ville-Marie QC J9V 1W8; (Peru)'93; Staff, CSSS du Témiscamingue; (819)629-2420; Fax. (819)629-3257; aldoava@yahoo.com.

DOMINIC, Anna; Dr Ca Janeway Child Hlth Ctr, 300 Prince Philip Dr, St. John's NL A1B 3V6; Mem'93; BSc; FRCPC; Peds (Adolescent Medicine). Staff, Janeway Children's Health & Rehabilitation Centre; Asst Prof Faculty of Med., Memorial University Of Newfoundland; (709)777-4963; Fax. (709)777-4726.

DOMINIQUE, Francis; Medical Arts Bldg, 908-233 Kennedy St, Winnipeg MB R3C 3J5; National (Ireland)'62; MB ChB; BAO; MRC(Lond); FRSM; FRCPC; Neur (Adult Neurology). Staff, St Boniface General Hospital; Neurology, Concordia General Hospital; (204)943-9443

DOMINIQUE, Lynn; Clin Med Med-Vale, 100-408 rue Jeanne-Mance, Salaber-de-Valleyf QC J6T 4G1; Sher'02; Staff GP, Centre Hospitalier Régional du Suroît; (450)370-3387; Fax. (450)370-3395.

DOMKE, Heather L; Medical Arts Bldg, 1102-233 Kennedy St, Winnipeg MB R3C 3J5; Man'83; (204)943-5495; Fax. (204)943-8282.

DOMKE, Herbert L; 101-1503 Hillside Ave, Victoria BC V8T 2C1; Loma Linda(CA) (USA)'67; BA; MPH; Assoc Staff, Royal Jubilee Hospital; (250)595-3823; Fax. (250)595-5533.

DOMKE, Sheila L; Medical Arts Bldg, 1102-233 Kennedy St, Winnipeg MB R3C 3J5; Man'77; MCFP(EM); Dir Emerg Dept, The Salvation Army Grace Hospital; Teacher Family Practice, University of Manitoba; (204)943-5495; Fax. (204)943-8282.

DOMMANN, Steven C; Northmount Med Centre, 204-145 13th St E, North Vancouver BC V7L 2L4; (South Africa)'92; (604)924-4009

DOMMISSE, Iain G; Columbia Med Bldg, 408-301 Columbia St E, New Westminster BC V3L 3W5; Cape Town (South Africa)'71; MB ChB; FICS; FRCSC; OrthSurg (Spine). Ac Staff, Royal Columbian Hospital; Ac Staff, Eagle Ridge Hospital & Health Care Centre; Clin Assoc Prof Orthopeds, University of British Columbia; (604)525-5311; Fax. (604)525-5314.

DOMOVITCH, Edward; McKenzie Prof Centre, 103-1595 McKenzie Ave, Victoria BC V8N 1A4; Tor'75; (250)477-4777; edomovit@shaw.ca.

DOMPIERRE, Gervais; SAAQ, 333 boul Jean-Lesage, Quebec QC G1K 8J6; Laval'88; Staff Emerg, Hôpital Sainte Anne de Beaupré; (418)643-7620

DOMPIERRE, Jean-Maurice; CSSS Haute Gaspésie, 50 rue du Belvedere, Ste-Anne-des-Monts QC G4V 1X4; Laval'95; Staff, Centre Hospitalier des Monts; (418)763-2261

DON, Joan; Ross Mem Hosp, 10 Angeline St N, Lindsay ON K9V 4M8; McM'89; FRCPC; Anes. Staff, Ross Memorial Hospital; Langs: Dutch; Spanish; French; (705)324-6111

DON-WAUCHOPE, Andrew; St Joseph's Healthcare, 50 Charlton Ave E, Hamilton ON L8N 4A6; Witwatersrand (South Africa)'90; FRCPC; MedBiochem. Staff, St Joseph's Healthcare - Charlton Campus; (905)522-4941

DONAGHUE, C Scott; Rouge Valley-Ajax & Pickering, 580 Harwood Ave S, Ajax ON L1S 2J4; Tor'81; CCFP; Ac Staff, Rouge Valley Health System - Ajax & Pickering Health Centre Site; (905)683-2320 x3200; Fax. (905)428-5231.

DONAGHY, John J; Alberta Hip & Knee Med Clinic, 335-401 9 Ave SW, Calgary AB T2P 3C5; Belfast (Ireland)'74; MB ChB; BAO; FRCS(Ed); FRCSC; OrthSurg. Ac Staff, Peter Lougheed Centre; Asst/Clin Prof Surg, University of Calgary; (403)266-4772; Fax. (403)221-4387.

DONAGHY, Seamus; Family Med Centre, A2-150 Main St E, Grimsby ON L3M 1P1; Galway (Ireland)'77; MB ChB; CCFP; CCFP(E.M.); FCFP; Fam Med/Anesthetist, West Lincoln Memorial Hospital; (905)945-5424; Fax. (905)945-4772.

DONAHUE, Paula C; St Thomas-Elgin Gen Hosp, PO Box 2007 Stn Main 189 Elm St, St Thomas ON N5P 3W2; Wes'76; FRCPC; IntMed. Staff, St Thomas Elgin General Hospital; (519)631-2020 x2217; Fax. (519)631-7689.

DONAIS, Guy; CarrefourSanté de Jonquiere, CP 1200 Succ Pdf Jonquiere 2230 rue de l'Hopital, Jonquiere QC G7X 7X2; Mon'76; Staff, Centre Hospitalier Jonquiere; (418)695-7700

DONAIS, Phillip; Peter Lougheed Centre, 3500 26 Ave NE, Calgary AB T1Y 6J4; Alb'99; FRCPC; Anes. Staff, Peter Lougheed Centre; (403)943-5721

DONALD, Christopher R; Mapleton Health Centre, 11 Andrews Dr W, Drayton ON N0G 1P0; Otago (New Zealand)'70; CCFP; (519)638-3088; Fax. (519)638-3982; info@mapletonhc.ca.

DONALD, Douglas N; Huronia Med Centre, PO Box 790 Stn Main, Midland ON L4R 4P4; Qns'76; Ac Staff, Georgian Bay General Hospital - Midland; (705)526-5291; Fax. (705)526-6309.

DONALD, Gregory; Moncton Med Clinic, 307-860 Mountain Rd, Moncton NB E1C 2N7; Dal'79; CCFP; FCFP; Lecturer Med School, Dalhousie University; (506)853-5140; Fax. (506)853-5141; dr. greg.donald@horizonnb.ca.

DONALD, Marion; Public Serv Occupational Hlth, 835-9700 Jasper Ave, Edmonton AB T5J 4C3; Alb'83; FCBOM; CCFP; FCFP; (780)495-5601; Fax. (780)495-2743; marion.donald@hc.sc.qc. ca.

DONALD, Shirley F; Orillia Soldiers' Mem Hosp, 170 Colborne St W, Orillia ON L3V 2Z3; Tor'78; FRCPC; Anes. Staff, Orillia Soldiers' Memorial Hospital; (705)325-2201

DONALDSON, Beth L; Copeman Healthcare Centre, 400-1128 Hornby St, Vancouver BC V6Z 2L4; Cal'02; CCFP; (604)707-2273

DONALDSON, Bruce W; 204-1676 Martin Dr, Surrey BC V4A 6E7; UBC'85; FRCPC; IntMed; Gastroent. (604)536-2188; Fax. (604)538-6317.

DONALDSON, Craig; Headwaters Hlth Care Ctr, 100 Rolling Hills Dr, Orangeville ON L9W 4X9; Wes'99; CCFP; CCFP(E.M.); (519)941-2410; Fax. (519)941-4707.

DONALDSON, Daniele; Direction Rég Sante Publique, 550 rue Bonaventure, Trois-Rivieres QC G9A 2B5; Laval'79; (819)693-3636

DONALDSON, Heather J; Vancouver Coastal Health, 220-1200 73rd Ave W, Vancouver BC V6P 6G5; UBC'99; FRCPC; Psy. Staff, Richmond Hospital; (604)266-6124

DONALDSON, Jane; Steveston Med Group, 204-3811 Chatham St, Richmond BC V7E 2Z4; UBC'89; CCFP; CCFP(E.M.); FCFP; Staff Family Pract, Richmond Hospital; (604)277-7166; Fax. (604)277-3811.

DONALDSON, Ranald R; PO Box 35038 Rpo Hillside, Victoria BC V8T 5G2; UBC'79; Ac Staff, Royal Jubilee Hospital; Ac Staff, Victoria General Hospital; (250)472-4729

DONALDSON, Suzanne C; Dr. Suzanne Donaldson Inc, 200-9656 King George Blvd, Surrey BC V3T 2V5; McM'93; CCFP; Langs: Spanish; (604)581-4611; Fax. (604)581-2652.

DONALDSON BRAMLEY, Lauren M; Project Skin MD, 1495 11th Ave W, Vancouver BC V6H 1K9; UBC'94; CCFP; (604)732-0800

DONAT, Diane J; Univ Hlth Network-Toronto Gen, 12N 214-200 Elizabeth St, Toronto ON M5G 2C4; McM'86; MSc; MEd; FRCPC; IntMed (Diabetes); Endocrin&Metab. Staff, Toronto General Hospital - UHN; Staff, Mount Sinai Hospital; Assoc Prof, University of Toronto; Langs: Hungarian; (416)340-3592; Fax. (416)340-3314; dianne.donat@uhn.on.ca.

DONAT, Jeffrey R; 202-436 Cedar Ave, Kelowna BC V1Y 4X3; Bronx(NY) (USA)'72; FRCPC; Neur. (778)436-9770

DONATELLI, Francesco; MUHC-Montreal Gen Hosp, 1650 av Cedar, Montreal QC H3G 1A4; (Italy)'96; Anes (P.Q.). Staff, McGill University Health Centre - Montreal General Campus; (514)934-1934; Fax. (514)934-8249.

DONATH, David J; CHUM-Hop Notre-Dame, 1560 rue Sherbrooke E, Montreal QC H2L 4M1; McG'82; ABR; LMCC; FRCPC; RadOncol (Brachy Therapy). Staff, Centre Hospitalier l'Université de Montréal (CHUM) - Hôpital Notre-Dame; Asst Prof Oncol, Universite de Montreal; Langs: Bilingual(French/English); (514)890-8254; Fax. (514)412-7537; david.donath.chum@ ssss.gouv.qc.ca.

DONATI, Francois; Hop Maisonneuve-Rosemont, 5415 boul de l'Assomption, Montreal QC H1T 2M4; McG'79; CSPQ; FRCPC; Anes. Staff, Hopital Maisonneuve-Rosemont; Head Dept of Anes, McGill University; (514)252-3426; Fax. (514)252-3542; francois. donati@umontreal.ca.

DONATI, Johanne; Clinique Med Pointe-du-Lac, CP 4099 Succ A 10300 ch Ste-Marguerite, Trois-Rivieres QC G9B 7Y6; Laval'75; Langs: English; (819)377-5015; Fax. (819)377-5550; cmpdl@ cgocable.ca.

DONE, Susan J; Univ Hlth Network-Toronto Gen, 11E 228-200 Elizabeth St, Toronto ON M5G 2C4; Cambridge (England)'87; PhD; FRCPC; AnatPath. Staff, Toronto General Hospital - UHN; Assoc Prof, University of Toronto; (416)946-4501; Fax. (416)340-5517.

DONEVAN, Robert H; Parry Sound Family Health Team, 15 James St, Parry Sound ON P2A 1T4; Qns'88; CCFP; Staff, West Parry Sound Health Centre; (705)746-9382; Fax. (705)746-7758.

DONG, Alice; St Michael's Hosp, 30 Bond St, Toronto ON M5B 1W8; Tor'71; FCBOM; ABPM(OccMed); Consultant Occupational Med., St Michael's Hospital; (416)864-5013; Fax. (416)864-5405.

DONG, Dennis N; 11718 Sarcee Trail NW, Calgary AB T3R 0A1; Alb'83; (403)274-1864; Fax. (403)274-9093.

DONG, Glenn L; The Richmond Hosp, 7000 Westminster Hwy, Richmond BC V6X 1A2; Wes'85; FRCPC; Anes. Staff, Richmond Hospital; Langs: Cantonese; (604)278-9711 x4200

DONG, Jay; Foothills Med Centre, C231-1403 29 St NW, Calgary AB T2N 2T9; McM'08; CCFP; CCFP(E.M.); Staff, Foothills Medical Centre; (403)944-1596

DONG, Kathyrn A; Royal Alexandra Hosp, 565CSC-10240 Kingsway NW, Edmonton AB T5H 3V9; McM'99; FRCPC; EmergMed. Staff, Royal Alexandra Hospital; (780)735-4442; Fax. (780)735-4916.

DONG, Raymond; Surrey Med Bldg, 202-9656 King George Hwy, Surrey BC V3T 2V5; UBC'81; BSc; ABIM(IntMed); ABIM(Cardiol); FRCPC; IntMed (Adult Cardiology); Cardiol. Staff, Surrey Memorial Hospital; Langs: Cantonese; Mandarin; (604)589-1882; Fax. (604)589-1896.

DONG, Sandy; 5-30 University Terrace, 8303 112 St NW, Edmonton AB T6G 1K4; Tor'97; FRCPC; EmergMed. Staff, University of Alberta Hospital; (780)492-9962; sdong@ualberta. ca.

DONG, Sunny R; Sleep Breathing Ctr, 2000-4330 Kingsway, Burnaby BC V5H 4G7; UBC'87; FRCPC; IntMed; Respir. (604)875-0333; Fax. (604)708-1934; sdong@sleep-breathing. bc.ca.

DONG, Wayne A; 1518 Westerdale Dr, Kamloops BC V1S 1Y9; Man'98; CCFP.

DONG, Wei-Feng; Cross Cancer Institute, 11560 University Ave, Edmonton AB T6G 1Z2; Nanjing (China)'82; FRCPC; AnatPath. Staff, Foothills Medical Centre; (780)432-8454

DONGIER, Maurice H J; Douglas Mental Hlth Univ Inst, 6875 boul LaSalle, Verdun QC H4H 1R3; Marseille (France)'51; FAPA; CSPQ; FRCPC; Psy. Dir Div of Clin Research, Douglas Mental Health University Institute; Consultant, McGill University Health Centre - Montreal General Campus; Staff, Allan Memorial Institute; Prof Psy, McGill University; Langs: French; (514)761-6131 x3419; Fax. (514)934-2385.

DONGIER, Suzanne; Douglas Mental Hlth Univ Inst, 6875 boul LaSalle, Verdun QC H4H 1R3; Marseille (France)'59; CSPQ; Psy (P.Q.). Clin Dir Infant Unit, Douglas Mental Health University Institute; assoc Prof, McGill University; (514)761-6131 x2032; Fax. (514)762-3041; donsuz@douglas.mcgill.ca.

DONGO JIMÉNEZ, Claudia M; CSSS du Sud de Lanaudière, 911 montee des Pionniers, Terrebonne QC J6V 2H2; Catolica de Santa Maria (Other Foreign)'99; FRCPC; AnatPath. Staff, Centre Hospitalier Pierre le Gardeur; (450)654-7525

DONKERVOORT, Laura; Parrsboro Primary Hlth Care Cl, PO Box 638 76 Jenks Ave, Parrsboro NS B0M 1S0; (Ireland)'08; MB BCh; BAO; CCFP; (902)254-3760; Fax. (902)254-3617.

DONKIN, Allan J; 6935 Harvie Ave, Powell River BC V8A 5H9; Pretoria (South Africa)'07; MB ChB; Langs: Afrikaans; (604)485-0136

DONKIN, Monia; Edson Med Centre, PO Box 6660 Stn Main, Edson AB T7E 1V1; (South Africa)'07; (780)723-3366

DONKOR, Kwame L; Niagara Falls Med Centre, 206-6453 Morrison St, Niagara Falls ON L2E 7H1; Tor'73; FRCPC; Peds (Clinical Immunology & Allergy). Ac Staff, Niagara Health System - Greater Niagara General Site; (905)357-4554; Fax. (905)357-1083; donkor@primus.ca.

DONLAN, Matthew; CHUQ-Ctr Hosp Univ Laval, 2705 boul Laurier, Quebec QC G1V 4G2; McG'06; MDCM; Peds. Staff, Centre Hospitalier Universitaire de Quebec-CHUL; (418)654-2282

DONLEVY, Mary J; PO Box 26035 Rpo Westbank, West Kelowna BC V4T 2G3; Cal'80; CCFP; FCFP; Staff, BC Women's Hospital & Health Centre; Ac Staff, Providence Health Care - Mount Saint Joseph Hospital; Vis Staff Privil, Vancouver General Hospital - Centennial Pavillion; Dir Greater Vancouver Site Residency Prog/Clin Assoc Prof, University of British Columbia.

DONN, Wayne B; St Joseph's Gen Hosp, 2137 Comox Ave, Comox BC V9M 1P2; UBC'90; BSc; FRCPC; GenPath; AnatPath. Staff, St Joseph's General Hospital; (250)339-1456; wayne. donn@sjghcomox.ca.

DONNELLAN, Fergal; 5153-2775 Laurel St, Vancouver BC V5Z 1M9; Dublin (Ireland)'00; MB BCh; BAO; (604)875-5474

DONNELLY, Bryan; Rockyview Gen Hosp, 6635-7007 14 St SW, Calgary AB T2V 1P9; Dublin (Ireland)'73; BSc(Anat.); MSc; MCh; FRCS; FRCSC; Urol. Staff, Rockyview General Hospital; Physician, Southern Alberta Institute of Urology; (403)943-8968; Fax. (403)943-8972.

DONNELLY, Carolyn P; 103-1221 Lonsdale Ave, North Vancouver BC V7M 2H5; Cal'04; FRCSC; ObstGyn. (604)980-2800

DONNELLY, J Patrick; Interlake Med Ctr, PO Box 430, Altamont MB R0G 0A0; Manchester (England)'78; BScMed(St.Andrews); DA; Staff, Misericordia Health Centre; (204)376-2781; Fax. (204)376-5956.

DONNELLY, Jocelyn; Allan Centre for Women, 707-12100 Macleod Trail SE, Calgary AB T2J 7G9; Alb'99; BMedSci; ObstGyn. (403)271-2550; Fax. (403)271-4546.

DONNELLY, M Sandra; William Osler HC-Brampton, 2100 Bovard Dr E, Brampton ON L6R 3J7; McG'82; MSc; FRCPC; IntMed; Nephrol. Chief Med, William Osler Health System - Brampton Civic Hospital; Staff, St Michael's Hospital; Asst Prof, University of Toronto; (905)494-2120 x57980; Fax. (905)494-6635.

DONNELLY, Martha L; Centennial Pavillion 5D, 855 12th Ave W, Vancouver BC V5Z 1M9; Wes'76; FRCPC; Psy (Geriatric Psychiatry). Ac Staff Geriatric Psy, Vancouver General Hospital - Centennial Pavillion; Teach Staff Family Practice & Psy, University of British Columbia; (604)875-4728; Fax. (604)875-5816.

DONNELLY, Regina; 4917 46 St, Red Deer AB T4N 1N2; Alb'66; FRCPC; IntMed. (403)343-7450; Fax. (403)342-1172.

DONNELLY, S Jane; Northmount Med Centre, 803-145 13th St E, North Vancouver BC V7L 2L4; UBC'76; (604)982-4177; Fax. (604)985-3442.

DONNELLY, Sarah; Radiology Consultants Assoc, 120-6707 Elbow Dr SW, Calgary AB T2V 0E3; Cal'03; FRCPC; DiagRad. (403)777-3003; Fax. (403)777-3008.

DONNELLY, Thomas; Trillium Hlth Ctr-Mississauga, 100 Queensway W, Mississauga ON L5B 1B8; Qns'04; FRCPC; Anes. Staff, Trillium Health Centre - Mississauga; (905)848-7100

DONNELLY WARNER, Niamh I; Rockyview Gen Hosp, 7007 14 St SW, Calgary AB T2V 1P9; UBC'01; FRCPC; Anes. Staff, Rockyview General Hospital; (403)943-3410

DONNER, Elizabeth J; The Hosp For Sick Children, 555 University Ave, Toronto ON M5G 1X8; McM'96; FRCPC; Neur (Pediatric Neurology). Staff, The Hospital For Sick Children; (416)813-7037; Fax. (416)813-6334.

DONNERY, Cara-Anne; St Joseph's Healthcare, 50 Charlton Ave E, Hamilton ON L8N 4A6; McM'03; FRCSC; ObstGyn. Staff, St Joseph's Healthcare - Charlton Campus; (905)522-1155; Fax. (905)521-6089; cara-anne@stjosesfoundation.ca.

DONOFF, Michel G; College Plaza, 205-8215 112 St NW, Edmonton AB T6G 2C8; Alb'77; CCFP; FCFP; Assoc Staff, Royal Alexandra Hospital; Prof Family Med, University of Alberta; (780)492-0780

DONOHUE, Alicia; 300-5307 Canotek Rd, Ottawa ON K1J 9M2; Ott'85; BSc; MHSc; CCFP; Langs: French; (613)746-6223; Fax. (613)746-6018.

DONOSO, Fernando; Clinique Med Luso, 1 av du Mont-Royal E, Montreal QC H2T 1N4; Santiago (Chile)'53; (514)849-2391; Fax. (514)849-2394.

DONOVAN, Andrea; Sunnybrook Hlth Sciences Ctr, AG 278-2075 Bayview Ave, Toronto ON M4N 3M5; Ott'02; FRCPC; DiagRad. Staff, Sunnybrook Health Sciences Centre; (416)480-6100; Fax. (416)480-5855.

DONOVAN, Catherine A; Health Sciences Centre, H2841-300 Prince Philip Dr, St. John's NL A1B 3V6; Mem'78; Staff, Health Sciences Centre; (709)777-8534

DONOVAN, Jeffrey; Sunnybrook Hlth Sciences Ctre, M1 700-2075 Bayview Ave, Toronto ON M4N 3M5; Ott'04; FRCPC; Derm. Staff, Sunnybrook Health Sciences Centre - Edmond Odette Cancer Centre; (416)480-4908; Fax. (416)480-6897.

DONOVAN, Keith D; London HSC-Victoria Hosp, PO Box 5010 Stn B 800 Commissioners Rd E, London ON N6A 5W9; Dal'92; FRCPC; EmergMed. Staff, London Health Sciences Centre - Victoria Campus; (519)667-6538; Fax. (519)667-6769.

DONOVAN, Kelly; Hamilton HS-McMaster Site, PO Box 2000 Stn Lcd 1 1200 Main St W, Hamilton ON L8N 3Z5; Qns'07; CCFP; Staff, Hamilton Health Sciences Centre - McMaster Children's Hospital; (905)525-9140

DONOVAN, Lois E; Richmond Road Diag & Trmt Ctre, 1820 Richmond Rd SW, Calgary AB T2T 5C7; McM'88; BSc; FRCPC; IntMed (Endocrinology Disorders in Pregnancy); Endocrin&Metab. Staff, Foothills Medical Centre; Staff, Tom Baker Cancer Centre; Clin Assoc Prof, University of Calgary; (403)955-8328; Fax. (403)955-8249.

DONOVAN, Marie-Denise; Ctr de Formation Medicine, 165 Massey Ave, Moncton NB E1A 3E9; (Ireland)'78; MFPHM; CommunMed (P.Q.)., Centre Hospitalier Universitaire de Sherbrooke-Hôpital Hôtel-Dieu; Prof, Universite de Sherbrooke; Langs: French; (506)863-2269

DONSKOY, Alex A; 8 Finch Ave W, North York ON M2N 6L1; Man'83; Langs: Russian; (416)733-3741; Fax. (416)733-3742.

DONSKY, Allan; Richmond Road Diag & Trmt Ctre, 1820 Richmond St SW, Calgary AB T2T 5C7; Cape Town (South Africa)'82; FRCPC; Peds; Psy. Clin Lecturer Psy, University of Calgary; (403)703-8628; Fax. (403)251-0284.

DONSKY, Carolyn; Kipling Heights Med Centre, 2291 Kipling Ave, Etobicoke ON M9W 4L6; Tor'92; CCFP; FCFP; Staff Family Med, William Osler Health System - Etobicoke General Hospital; (416)741-4545; Fax. (416)744-1484.

DONSKY, Geoffrey; Lakeridge Hlth Corp-Oshawa, 1 Hospital Court, Oshawa ON L1G 2B9; Ott'99; FRCPC; DiagRad. Staff, Lakeridge Health - Oshawa Site; (905)686-6411 x4305

DONSKY, Gordon; Medical & Dental Bldg, 211-1849 Yonge St, Toronto ON M4S 1Y2; Tor'61; FAAP; FRCPC; Peds (Allergy). Sr Physician Peds, The Hospital For Sick Children; Asst Prof Peds, University of Toronto; Langs: French; German; (416)488-8300; Fax. (416)488-1818.

DONSKY, Judith E; 503-1110 Sheppard Ave E, North York ON M2K 2W2; Tor'96; FRCPC; Peds; ClinImmunol&Allergy. (416)226-4294; Fax. (416)226-1928.

DONTIGNY, Andre; Ministere de la Sante, 1075 ch Sainte-Foy, Quebec QC G1S 2M1; Laval'88; FRCPC; CommunMed. (418)266-6714

DONTIGNY, Leon; Institut de Cardiologie de Mtl, 5000 rue Belanger, Montreal QC H1T 1C8; Mon'64; CSPQ; FRCSC; Cardiovasc&ThorSurg (Trauma). Staff D S P, Institut de Cardiologie de Montréal; (514)376-3330 x2502; Fax. (514)376-7782; leon_dontigny@icm-mhi.org.

DONTIGNY, Lorraine; Clin de Gyn et de Maternile, 1811 av Dollard, Lasalle QC H8N 1T9; Mon'94; FRCSC; ObstGyn. (514)364-3337; Fax. (514)364-9866.

DONWORTH, Michael; CPM-Centres for Pain Managemen, 458 Central Ave, London ON N6B 2E5; McM'79; MCFP(EM); BSc; Staff Emerg Med, Strathroy Middlesex General Hospital - Middlesex Hospital Alliance; (519)434-4727; Fax. (519)434-4700.

DOOBAY, Anand V; Markham Stouffville Hosp, PO Box 1800 Stn Main 381 Church St, Markham ON L3P 7P3; Alb'05; Critical Care Medicine; IntMed. Staff, Markham Stouffville Hospital; (905)472-7000; Fax. (905)472-7009.

DOOBAY, Budhendranauth S; 106-4256 Portage Rd, Niagara Falls ON L2E 6A4; (Jamaica)'65; FRCS; FRCS(Ed); FRCSC; GenSurg (Vascular Surgery); Cardiovasc&ThorSurg. Staff, Hamilton Health Sciences Centre - Hamilton General Hospital; Asst Prof Surg, McMaster University; (905)357-3336; Fax. (905)357-3393; b-doob@hotmail.com.

DOOBAY, Calesh D; Uxbridge Family Hlth Clinic, B-2 Elgin Park Dr, Uxbridge ON L9P 0B1; (Thailand)'01; CCFP; (905)852-1009; Fax. (905)852-3531.

DOOBAY, Dharmeandra; Uxbridge Family Hlth Clinic, B-2 Elgin Park Dr, Uxbridge ON L9P 0B1; West Indies (Jamaica)'00; CCFP; (905)852-1009; Fax. (905)852-3531.

DOOBAY, Jaya; Carleton Place & Dist Mem Hosp, 211 Lake Ave E, Carleton Place ON K7C 1J4; Qns'06; CCFP; CCFP(E.M.); Staff, Carleton Place & District Memorial Hospital; (613)253-3800

DOOKERAN, Ravi I; Winnipeg Clinic, 425 St Mary Ave, Winnipeg MB R3C 0N2; Man'99; BSc; FRCSC; Ophth (Vitreo Retinal Surgery). (204)957-3230; Fax. (204)942-0677.

DOOL, Jayson; 135-667 Champlain St, Dieppe NB E1A 1P6; Qns'98; FRCSC; PlasSurg. Staff, Rouge Valley Health System - Centenary Health Centre Site; (506)382-3665

DOOL, Nancy M; Dixon Med Centre, 403-531 Davis Dr, Newmarket ON L3Y 6P5; McM'81; Staff, Southlake Regional Health Centre; (905)853-2398

DOOLER, Deborah; Niagara H System-St Catharine, PO Box 3018 Stn Main 142 Queenston St, St Catharines ON L2R 7C6; McM'05; CCFP; Staff, Niagara Health System - St Catharines General Site; (905)684-7271

DOOLEY, Joseph; The Hugh Allen Clinic, PO Box 232 Stn Main, Sioux Lookout ON P8T 1A3; Dublin (Ireland)'79; MB ChB; BAO; CCFP; FCFP; Ac Staff Privil & Advanced Obstetrics/Chief Obstetrics, Sioux Lookout Meno-Ya-Win Health Centre; Staff, The Hugh Allen Clinic; Langs: Irish; (807)737-3803; Fax. (807)737-1771.

DOOLEY, Joseph M; IWK Health Centre, PO Box 9700 Rpo CSC 5850-5980 University Ave, Halifax NS B3K 6R8; Dublin (Ireland)'75; MB ChB; BAO; FRCPC; Peds (Pediatric Neurology). Prof, IWK Health Centre; Prof Peds, Dalhousie University; (902)470-8488; Fax. (902)470-8486.

DOOLEY, Patrick J; Petawawa Med Centre, 1121 Victoria St, Petawawa ON K8H 2E6; Tor'82; (613)687-6420; Fax. (613)687-5526.

DOONER, James; Surgical Associates, 405-1120 Yates St, Victoria BC V8V 3M9; Wes'76; FRCSC; GenSurg; VascSurg. Staff, Royal Jubilee Hospital; Staff, Victoria General Hospital; (250)384-8154; Fax. (250)384-7571.

DOORLY, Patrick; 302-125 Bell Farm Rd, Barrie ON L4M 6L2; RCS (Ireland)'78; MB ChB; BAO; DTM; LRCPSI; Court Staff, Royal Victoria Regional Health Centre; (705)737-1532; Fax. (705)737-3703.

DOPP, Philip; Sault Area Hosp, 750 Great Northern Rd, Sault Ste. Marie ON P6B 0A8; Tor'02; CCFP; Staff, Sault Area Hospital - Sault Ste Marie; (705)959-3434

DORAH, Nicholas H; 104-140 Niagara St, St Catharines ON L2R 4L4; West Indies (Jamaica)'95; FRCPC; Peds. (905)704-1281

DORAIS, Judy; CHUM-Hop Notre-Dame, 1560 rue Sherbrooke E, Montreal QC H2L 4M1; Mon'90; Gastroent (P.Q.); IntMed (Interventional Endoscopy). Staff, Centre Hospitalier l'Université de Montréal (CHUM) - Hôpital Notre-Dame; Langs: Bilingual(French/English); (514)890-8000

DORAIS, Marc; Hôpital de Saint-Eustache, 520 boul Arthur-Sauve, Saint-Eustache QC J7R 5B1; Mon'08; Staff, Hôpital de Saint-Eustache; (450)473-6811

DORAN, Brian J; Foothills Family Med Clinic, 114 1 St SW, Black Diamond AB T0L 0H0; Alb'09; CCFP; (403)933-4377

DORAN, Dale R; St Mary's Gen Hosp, 911 Queens Blvd, Kitchener ON N2M 1B2; Wes'77; FRCPC; DiagRad. Staff, St Mary's General Hospital; (519)749-6455

DORAN, James A; Southlake Reg Health Centre, 596 Davis Dr, Newmarket ON L3Y 2P9; Dublin (Ireland)'70; MB ChB; FRCR; DABR; FRCPC; DiagRad. Staff, Southlake Regional Health Centre; (905)895-4521

DORAN, Richard J; Lakeridge Hlth Corp-Oshawa, 1 Hospital Crt, Oshawa ON L1G 2B9; Ott'83; FRCPC; Anes (Pain Management). Staff, Lakeridge Health - Oshawa Site; (905)576-8711; Fax. (905)721-4773.

DORAN, Shandra A; University of Alberta Hosp, 8440 112 St NW, Edmonton AB T6G 2B7; Cal'08; Staff, University of Alberta Hospital; (780)407-8822

DORAN, Una; 509-181 First Ave W, Vancouver BC V5Y 0E3; Qns'05; CCFP; CCFP(E.M.); Staff, Abbotsford Regional Hospital & Cancer Centre; (778)788-3404

DORAN, William A L; Mud Creek Med Group, 12E Elm Ave, Wolfville NS B4P 1Z9; Man'75; CCFP; (902)542-3633; Fax. (902)542-2709.

DORAR, Jabril A; 877 Jane St, York ON M6N 4C4; Al-Fateh (Libya)'98; MB ChB; CCFP; (416)766-4444; Fax. (416)763-4442.

DORASAMY, Punginathn; Hamilton HS-General Site, 409-237 Barton St E, Hamilton ON L8L 2X2; Natal (South Africa)'82; FRCPC; IntMed. Fellow, Hamilton Health Sciences Centre - Hamilton General Hospital; (905)527-4322; Fax. (905)577-1418.

DORAY, Jean-Luc; Hop Charles Lemoyne, 3120 boul Taschereau, Greenfield Park QC J4V 2H1; Mon'80; FRCPC; Peds (Neonatology). Staff, Centre Hospitalier Pierre Boucher; Staff, Hopital Charles LeMoyne; Consultant, Hôpital Ste-Justine; (450)466-5436; Fax. (450)466-5437.

DORAY, Jean-Pierre; Hop Charles Lemoyne, 3120 boul Taschereau, Greenfield Park QC J4V 2H1; Mon'81; CSPQ; FRCPC; Peds (P.Q.). Ac Staff Ped, Hopital Charles LeMoyne; Consultant, Hôpital Ste-Justine; (450)466-5000

DORCÉLY, Amos; CSSS du Haut Saint-Maurice, 885 boul Ducharme, La Tuque QC G9X 3C1; (Other Foreign)'97; Staff, Centre Hospitalier Saint-Joseph de la Turque; (819)523-4581

DORE, Annie; Institut de Cardiologie de Mtl, 5000 rue Belanger, Montreal QC H1T 1C8; Sher'89; CSPQ; FRCPC; IntMed; Cardiol. Staff, Institut de Cardiologie de Montréal; (514)376-3330 x3666; Fax. (514)593-2541.

DORE, Francois-Guy; 1141 boul Saint-Joseph E, Montreal QC H2J 1L3; Mon'77; (514)277-1141; Fax. (514)277-0061.

DORE, Jean; Clinique Racine, 2880 ch des Quatre-Bourgeois, Quebec QC G1V 4X7; Laval'88; BSc; LMCC; CCFP; Asst Researcher, Université Laval; (418)657-6363

DORE, Marcel; Guelph Gen Hosp, 115 Delhi St, Guelph ON N1E 4J4; McG'85; Staff, Guelph General Hospital; Asst Clin Prf Family Med, McMaster University; Langs: French; Spanish; (519)837-6440 x2550; Fax. (519)837-6791.

DORE, Normand; 79 rue Leblanc O, Longueuil QC J4J 1K1; Mon'74; DAB; FAAD; CSPQ; FRCPC; Derm (Immuno Dermatology). Member, Federation Medecin Specialistes du Quebec; Adj Clin Prof Univ de Montreal Ecole d'Arch, Universite de Montreal; (450)463-3881; Fax. (450)463-0908.

DORE-BERGERON, Marie-Joelle; SMBD Jewish Gen Hosp, 3175 ch Côte-Sainte-Catherine, Montreal QC H3T 1E2; McG'03; Peds. Staff, Sir Mortimer B Davis Jewish General; (514)345-4931

DOREE, Jean-Pierre; CSSS du Sud de Lanaudière, 911 Montee des Pionniers, Terrebonne QC J6V 2H2; Grenoble (France)'88; Psy (P.Q.). Chef psychiatrie, Centre Hospitalier Pierre le Gardeur; (450)654-7525

DOREN, Denis M; 1 Hastings St N PO Box 70, Bancroft ON K0L 1C0; Ott'76; Ac Staff Privil Family Med, QHC North Hastings; Langs: Bilingual(French/English); (613)332-2626; Fax. (613)332-2125.

DORENBAUM, David; 554 Spadina Cres, Toronto ON M5S 2J9; (Mexico)'81; FRCPC; Peds; Psy. Asst Prof, University of Toronto; Langs: Hebrew; Spanish; Yiddish; (416)925-8536

DOREY, J Michael; Medical Clinic Bldg, 303-89 Humber College Blvd, Etobicoke ON M9V 4B8; Qns'66; DAB; FAAP; FRCPC; Peds. Ac Staff, William Osler Health System - Etobicoke General Hospital; Ac Staff, The Hospital For Sick Children; Asst Prof, University of Toronto; (416)743-6063; Fax. (416)743-0101; jmdorey@sympatico.ca.

DOREY, Michael W; 103-2731 Hewes Way NW, Edmonton AB T6L 6W6; Mem'01; FRCSC; Ophth. (780)450-3335; Fax. (780)461-9430.

DOREY, Sania; Saint John Reg Hosp, PO Box 2100 Stn Main 400 University Ave, Saint John NB E2L 4L2; (Russia (Federation))'86; Staff, Saint John Regional Hospital; (506)608-0487

DORFMAN, Jason K; 202-145 Sheppard Ave E, North York ON M2N 3A7; Grenada (Grenada)'82; FRCSC; Ophth. (416)635-2895; Fax. (416)635-2838.

DORIA, Andrea S; The Hosp For Sick Children, 555 University Ave, Toronto ON M5G 1X8; Para (Brazil)'92; Staff, The Hospital For Sick Children; (416)813-6079; Fax. (416)813-7591; andrea.doria@sickkids.ca.

DORIAN, Paul; St Michael's Hosp, 6-027-30 Bond St, Toronto ON M5B 1W8; McG'76; FRCPC; IntMed (Arrhythmias); Cardiol. Pres Medical Staff/Dir Div of Cardiol, St Michael's Hospital; Prof Med, University of Toronto; (416)864-5104; Fax. (416)864-5104; dorianp@smh.toronto.on.ca.

DORION, Anita; Ctr Hosp Affilie-St-Sacrement, 1050 ch Sainte-Foy, Quebec QC G1S 4L8; Laval'93; FRCPC; DiagRad. Staff, Centre Hospitalier Affilié Universitaire de Québec - Hôpital du St-Sacrement; (418)682-7511

DORION, Dominique; CHUS-Hop Hotel-Dieu, 580 rue Bowen S, Sherbrooke QC J1G 2E8; Laval'85; MSc(Tor); DABOT; FRCSC; Otol (Oncology). Staff, Centre Hospitalier Universitaire de Sherbrooke-Hôpital Hôtel-Dieu; vice Doyen Resources/adj Doyen, Universite de Sherbrooke; Langs: English; (819)346-1110 x14901; Fax. (819)564-5449; dominique.dorion@usherbrooke.ca.

DORION, Julie; Ctr Hosp Affilie-Enfant-Jesus, 1401 18e rue, Quebec QC G1J 1Z4; Laval'00; FRCPC; Psy. Staff, Centre Hospitalier Affilié Universitaire de Québec - Hôpital De L'Enfant Jésus; (418)649-5769; Fax. (418)649-5934.

DORION, Julie; Clinique Med St-Augustin, 220-334 Rte 138, Quebec QC G3A 1G8; Laval'87; LMCC; Langs: English; (418)878-3590; Fax. (418)878-4876.

DORION, Marie-Christine; CSSS du Lac-des-Deux-Montagnes, 520 boul Arthur-Sauve, Saint-Eustache QC J7R 5B1; Mon'09; CCFP; CCFP(E.M.); Staff, Hôpital de Saint-Eustache; (450)473-6811

DORION, Martin; CSSS Drummond-Hop Sainte-Croix, 570 rue Heriot, Drummondville QC J2B 1C1; Laval'93; CSPQ; OrthSurg. Staff, Hôpital Sainte-croix; (819)478-6464 x2430; Fax. (819)478-6419.

DORION, Michel; Polyclinique St-Jerome, 305-200 rue Durand, Saint-Jerome QC J7Z 7E2; Mon'77; Otol (P.Q.). (450)565-9898; Fax. (450)565-2702.

DORION, Nicole; Clinique Med St-Louis, 220-3165 ch Saint-Louis, Quebec QC G1W 4R4; Laval'97; (418)653-1970; Fax. (418)653-9956.

DORION, Pierre; 2601 ch de la Canardiere, Quebec QC G1J 2G3; Laval'66; FRCPC; Psy. Staff, Institut Universitaire Sante; Langs: Bilingual(French/English); (418)663-5321; Fax. (418)661-6891; pierre.dorion@institutsmq.qc.ca.

DORIS, C Ian; Hamilton HS-General Site, 237 Barton St E, Hamilton ON L8L 2X2; Edinburgh (Scotland)'66; MB ChB; MRC(UK); FRCPC; DiagRad. Staff, Hamilton Health Sciences Centre - Hamilton General Hospital; (905)529-3732; Fax. (905)527-5761.

DORIS, J Frederick; Alexander Prof Bldg, 207-849 Alexander Court, Peterborough ON K9J 7H8; Tor'83; FRCPC; IntMed; Rheum. Ac Staff, Peterborough Regional Health Centre - Hospital Drive; Ac Staff, Peterborough Regional Health Centre - Rogers St Site; (705)743-3851; Fax. (705)743-1330.

DORIS, Peter J; Surrey Med Bldg, 305-9656 King George Blvd, Surrey BC V3T 2V5; Qns'68; FACS; FRCSC; GenSurg. (604)583-1668; Fax. (604)583-7180; judy.drdoris@telus.net.

DORJEE, Tsering; West Winds Med Clinic, 2130-4818 Westwinds Dr NE, Calgary AB T3J 3Z5; (India)'87; (403)293-5454; Fax. (403)293-1511.

DORLAND, Katherine E; The Ottawa Hosp-Riverside, 1967 Riverside Dr, Ottawa ON K1H 7W9; Ott'10; CCFP; Staff, The Ottawa Hospital - Riverside Campus; (613)738-8400

DORNAN, John M; Saint John Reg Hosp, PO Box 2100 Stn Main 400 University Ave, Saint John NB E2L 4L2; Mem'82; FACP; FRCPC; IntMed; Endocrin&Metab. Ac Staff/Chief of Staff St John Area, HHN, Saint John Regional Hospital; Asst Teach Staff Medicial, Dalhousie University; (506)648-7304

DOROSHENKO, Alexander; Dept Of Health & Wellness, PO Box 5100 Stn A, Fredericton NB E3B 5G8; Dnepropetrovsk (Other Foreign)'94; FRCPC; Peds; InfectDis. (506)453-4294

DOROSZKIEWICZ, Nicholas W; 20 King St E PO Box 639, Hagersville ON N0A 1H0; Ott'79; CCFP; FCFP; Ac Staff, West Haldimand General Hospital; Court Staff, Norfolk General Hospital; (905)768-1277; Fax. (905)765-0817.

DOROVINI-ZIS, Catherine; Vancouver Gen Hosp, 855 12th Ave W, Vancouver BC V5Z 1M9; Athens (Greece)'69; FRCPC; AnatPath (Neuropathology). Head Neuropath/Consultant, Vancouver General Hospital - Centennial Pavillion; Prof Path & Lab Med, University of British Columbia; (604)875-4480 x63968; dorovini@interchange.ubc.ca.

DORRAN, Thomas J; Nanaimo Reg Gen Hosp, 1200 Dufferin Cres, Nanaimo BC V9S 2B7; McM'94; MBA; BSc; CCFP; CCFP(E.M.); FCFP; Staff, Nanaimo Regional General Hospital; (250)754-2141; Fax. (250)755-7633.

DORREEN, Mark S; Queen Elizabeth II HSC, 457A-1276 South Park St, Halifax NS B3H 2Y9; Cambridge (England)'74; MB BCh; FRCP; FACP; FRCPC; IntMed; MedOncol. Staff, Queen Elizabeth II Health Sciences Centre - Victoria General Site; Staff MedOncol, NS Cancer Centre; Assoc Prof Med, Dalhousie University; (902)473-3748; mark.dorreen@cdha.nshealth.ca.

DORREPAAL, Stephen; Clarity Eye Institute, 105-8800 Dufferin St, Vaughan ON L4K 0C5; Tor'06; FRCSC; Ophth (Medical Retina). (416)663-3937 x225; clarityeye@gmail.com.

DORRINGTON, Catherine L; Foothills Med Centre, C231-1403 29 St NW, Calgary AB T2N 2T9; McM'94; FRCPC; EmergMed. Staff, Foothills Medical Centre; (403)944-1405; Fax. (403)944-2419.

DORSCH, Michael F; Hys Med Centre, 350-11010 101 St NW, Edmonton AB T5H 4B9; (Germany)'94; PhD; Staff, Royal Alexandra Hospital; Langs: German; (780)428-3246; Fax. (780)425-0487.

DORSCHEID, Delbert R; St Paul's Hosp, 166-1081 Burrard St, Vancouver BC V6Z 1Y6; McG'93; MB BS; FRCPC; IntMed (Critical Care Medicine). Staff, Providence Health Care - St Paul's Hospital; Asst Prof Med, University of British Columbia; (604)682-2344 x62746; Fax. (604)806-8351.

DORT, Joseph C; Health Research Innovation Ctr, 3280 Hospital Dr NW, Calgary AB T2N 4Z6; Wes'80; FACS; FRCSC; Otol (Skull Base Surgery). Staff, Foothills Medical Centre; Staff Surg. Oncol., Tom Baker Cancer Centre; Prof Surg, University of Calgary; (403)220-4307; Fax. (403)270-3145; jdort@ucalgary.ca.

DORTAJ RABORI, Mohammad A; PO Box 2100 Rpo Banks Centre, Kelowna BC V1X 4K5; Kerman (Iran)'00; (250)862-4996

DORVAL, Gaston; Les Obst & Gyn de l'Amiante, 102-718 boul Frontenac E, Thetford Mines QC G6G 6H1; Laval'72; CSPQ; ObstGyn. Ac Staff ObstGyn, Hopital du CSS de la Region de Thetford; Langs: Bilingual(French/English); (418)338-2161; Fax. (418)338-2162.

DORVAL, Guerin; 201-2115 boul Casavant O, Saint-Hyacinthe QC J2S 7E5; Laval'69; PhD; ClinImmunol&Allergy (Allergy). Staff, Institut de Cardiologie de Montréal; Staff, Centre Hospitalier Honore-Mercier; Langs: Bilingual(French/English); (450)773-7546

DORVAL, Jacqueline; Polyclinique Med de Terrebonne, 901 boul des Seigneurs, Terrebonne QC J6W 1T8; Mon'80; (450)471-1148; Fax. (450)471-8043.

DORVAL, Jean-Francois; Institut de Cardiologie de Mtl, 5000 rue Belanger, Montreal QC H1T 1C8; Cardiol (P.Q.). Staff, Institut de Cardiologie de Montréal; (514)376-3330

DORVAL, Jean-Francois; Keary Med Centre, 103-245 Columbia St E, New Westminster BC V3L 3W4; McG'00; FRCPC; IntMed; Cardiol. (604)522-1644

DORVAL, Jean-Francois; Clinique de Med Familiale, 101 rue Lavoie, Rimouski QC G5L 5Y2; Sher'78; (418)723-5272; Fax. (418)725-2030.

DORVAL, Julie; Ctr Hosp de Charlevoix, 74 rue Ambroise-Fafard, Baie-Saint-Paul QC G3Z 2J6; Laval'00; Staff, CSSS de Charlevoix; (418)435-5150

DORVAL, Marc; Dr Georges-L Dumont Reg Hosp, 330 av Universite, Moncton NB E1C 2Z3; Mon'93; MPH; MBA; FRCPC; IntMed; Nephrol. Staff, Dr Georges-L-Dumont University Hospital Centre; (506)862-4000; Fax. (506)862-4281.

DORVAL, Nicolas; CSSS de la Region de Thetford, 1717 rue Notre-Dame E, Thetford Mines QC G6G 2V4; Laval'05; OrthSurg. Staff, Hopital du CSS de la Region de Thetford; (418)338-7777; Fax. (418)335-9191.

DORVAL, Veronique G; Hôpital Ste-Justine, 3175 ch Cote-Ste-Catherine, Montreal QC H3T 1C5; Ott'05; FRCPC; Peds (Neonatology). Staff, Hôpital Ste-Justine; (514)345-4931; Fax. (514)345-7725.

DOS SANTOS, Marlise P; The Ottawa Hosp-Civic Campus, C151-1053 Carling Ave, Ottawa ON K1Y 4E9; Fundacao (Brazil)'97; Staff, The Ottawa Hospital - Civic Campus; (613)761-4687; Fax. (613)761-4476.

DOSAJ, Arun K; 41 Lawrence Ave E PO Box 750, Madoc ON K0K 2K0; Glasgow (Scotland)'70; Court Staff, QHC Belleville General; Langs: Punjabi; Hindi; (613)473-4272; Fax. (613)473-1772.

DOSAJ, Seema; Glendale Med Clinic, 6-1101 Kingston Rd, Pickering ON L1V 1B5; Dal'90; BSc; FCFP; MCFP; CCFP; FCFP; Langs: French; Hindi; Punjabi; (905)831-1110; Fax. (905)831-1108.

DOSANI, Rehana N; The Credit Valley Hosp, 2200 Eglinton Ave W, Mississauga ON L5M 2N1; Tor'08; CCFP; Staff, The Credit Valley Hospital; Langs: Bilingual(English/French); (905)813-2200

DOSANJH, Ramneek K; 125-15299 68 Ave, Surrey BC V3S 2C1; (Other Foreign)'08; CCFP; (778)218-4100

DOSMAN, Cara F; Glenrose Rehabilitation Hosp, 10230 111 Ave NW, Edmonton AB T5G 0B7; Sask'96; FRCPC; Peds. Staff, Glenrose Rehabilitation Hospital; (780)735-7921

DOSMAN, James A H; Royal University Hosp, W3E-103 Hospital Dr, Saskatoon SK S7N 0W8; Sask'63; FRCPC; IntMed. Staff Centre for Agricultural Med, Royal University Hospital; Teach Staff, University of Saskatchewan; (306)966-8286

DOSMAN, John; Saskatoon Commun Clinic, 455 2nd Ave N, Saskatoon SK S7K 2C2; Sask'07; CCFP; (306)652-0300; Fax. (306)652-5692; jdosman@communityclinic.com.

DOSPINESCU LULIANA, Simona; GMF Medicentre Pincourt, 88 5e av, Pincourt QC J7V 5K7; CCFP; (514)425-1289

DOSS, Arulraj F; MUHC-Royal Victoria Hosp, L5 02-687 av des Pins O, Montreal QC H3A 1A1; Colombo (Sri Lanka)'62; MD; PhD(Lond); MRCP(UK); CSPQ; MB BS; CRCP; Microbio & Infect Dis (P.Q.); MedMicrobiol (Virology). Staff Microbiol, McGill University Health Centre - Royal Victoria Hospital; (514)934-1934 x35062

DOSS, Chrishanthini M; South Bank Med Centre, 3-2430 Bank St, Ottawa ON K1V 0T7; McG'90; CCFP; FCFP; (613)736-6946; Fax. (613)736-6948.

DOSS, Roshan A; Westway Med Centre, 1723 Kipling Ave, Etobicoke ON M9R 4E1; McG'96; (416)244-8404

DOSS, Sabine; CLSC de Cote-des-neiges, 1271 av Van Horne, Mont-Royal QC H2V 1K5; Mon'95; (514)731-8531

DOSSA, Fahreen A; Summitview Med Clinic, 100B-3300 Boundary Rd, Vancouver BC V5M 0A8; McM'02; CCFP; (604)437-7001

DOSSETOR, Clare B; 203-381 Kent St, Ottawa ON K2P 2A8; Alb'86; FRCPC; Derm. Langs: English; French; (613)567-8459; Fax. (613)567-4819.

DOST, Ismat Z; Central Prof Bldg, 72 Brant Ave, Brantford ON N3T 5Z8; Punjab (Pakistan)'67; DAB; MB BS; FRCPC; Peds (Clinical Immunology & Allergy). Staff, The Brant Community Healthcare System - Brantford General Hospital Site; Langs: Punjabi; Pashtu; Urdu; (519)753-2641

DOST, Rehan; 139 Grand River St N, Paris ON N3L 2M4; Tor'94; BSc; FRCPC; Neur (Hand Surgery). Langs: Punjabi; Urdu; French; (519)442-0668; Fax. (519)442-6199.

DOSTALER, Jacques P; 402-2555 St Joseph Blvd, Orleans ON K1C 1S6; Ott'72; CCFP; FCFP; Langs: Bilingual(French/English); (613)830-1693

DOSTALER, Louis-Pierre; CSSS Vieille-Capitale, 4E-2875 boul Laurier, Quebec QC G1V 2M2; Laval'82; (418)654-2701

DOSTALER, Monique R; Bluewater Health-Norman Site, 89 Norman St, Sarnia ON N7T 6S3; Ott'76; CCFP; Staff, Bluewater Health - Norman Site; Langs: Bilingual(English/French); (519)331-4264; Fax. (519)383-8532.

DOSTIE, Caroline; Ctr Hosp Trois-Riv-St-Joseph, 731 rue Sainte-Julie, Trois-Rivieres QC G9A 1Y1; Mon'93; Staff, Centre Hospitalier Regional de Trois-Rivieres; (819)372-3536

DOSTIE, Louise; Centre Med Quatre-Bourgeois, 360-979 av du Bourgogne, Quebec QC G1W 2L4; Laval'89; (418)652-1121

DOSTIE, Sarah; Polyclinique St-Eustache, 75 rue Grignon, Saint-Eustache QC J7P 4J2; Mon'01; CSPQ; FRCSC; ObstGyn. Staff, Hôpital de Saint-Eustache; Langs: Bilingual(French/English); (450)491-1150; Fax. (450)491-7470.

DOSTROVSKY, Nathaniel; 209-4430 Bathurst St, North York ON M3H 3S3; Wes'07; FRCPC; IntMed; Rheum. (416)631-6090

DOTCHIN, Stephanie A; Clinical Sciences Bldg, 2 133-152 University Campus, Edmonton AB T6G 2G3; Sask'05; FRCSC; Ophth. (780)407-6417; Fax. (780)407-7720.

DOTSIKAS, Gus; Lakeridge Hlth Corp-Oshawa, 1 Hospital Crt, Oshawa ON L1G 2B9; Tor'93; FRCPC; DiagRad. Staff, Lakeridge Health - Oshawa Site; Langs: Greek; (905)686-6411 x4305

DOTTEN, Dale A; St Michael's Hosp, 2 084-30 Bond St, Toronto ON M5B 1W8; Tor'62; FRCPC; IntMed. Staff, St Michael's Hospital; Assoc Prof Med, University of Toronto; (416)864-3054

DOTTRIDGE, Andrew H; 214-11 Hidden Creek Dr NW, Calgary AB T3A 6K6; Cape Town (South Africa)'86; CCFP; CCFP(E.M.); FCFP; (403)248-2273; Fax. (403)248-2213.

DOUCET, Albert D; 157 School St PO Box 1253, Liverpool NS B0T 1K0; Dal'76; CCFP; FCFP; Ac Staff, Queens General Hospital; Pres Med Staff, District Health Authority 1; Coord CME, Queens Co; (902)354-5556; Fax. (902)354-5599.

DOUCET, Alison M; MUHC-Montreal Chest Institute, 3650 rue Saint-Urbain, Montreal QC H2X 2P4; Ott'93; CCFP; FCFP; Staff, McGill University Health Centre - Montreal Chest Institute; Att Médecin, McGill University Health Centre - Royal Victoria Hospital; (514)934-1934; Fax. (514)529-8452.

DOUCET, Anne-Marie; Clinique Med des Bois-Francs, 101 rue Demers, Princeville QC G6L 4E8; Laval'10; (819)364-2150

DOUCET, Annie; Inst readap déficience phys, 525 boul Wilfrid-Hamel, Quebec QC G1M 2S8; Sher'87; Langs: Bilingual(French/English); (418)529-9141 x6785; Fax. (418)649-3703.

DOUCET, Audree; CSSS Maria-Chapdelaine, 2000 boul du Sacre-Coeur, Dolbeau-Mistassini QC G8L 2R5; Sher'08; CCFP; Staff, Centre Maria-Chapdelaine - CH de Dolbeau-Mistassini; (418)276-1234; Fax. (418)276-4355.

DOUCET, Caroline; CSSS de Trois-Rivières, 1991 boul du Carmel, Trois-Rivieres QC G8Z 3R9; Laval'02; FRCPC; AnatPath. Staff, CSSS de Trois-Rivières; (819)697-3333 x63568; Fax. (819)371-5007.

DOUCET, Danielle; Clinique Medicale Nepisiguit, 950 av Picot, Bathurst NB E2A 4Z9; Sher'04; CCFP; Staff, Hopital Regional Chaleur; Langs: Bilingual(French/English); (506)546-6696; Fax. (506)545-7723.

DOUCET, Gaetan; 110 rue de l'eglise, St-Casimir QC G0A 3L0; Laval'82; (418)339-3166; Fax. (418)339-2137.

DOUCET, Isabelle; CSSS de Laval, 1755 boul Rene-Laennec, Laval QC H7M 3L9; Mon'99; FRCPC; IntMed; Gastroent. Staff Gastroent, Hopital de la Cite de la santé; Staff Gastroent, Universite de Montreal; (450)668-1010; Fax. (450)975-5545.

DOUCET, Jerome; The Moncton Hosp, 135 MacBeath Ave, Moncton NB E1C 6Z8; Sher'03; FRCPC; Psy. Staff, The Moncton Hospital; (506)857-5111

DOUCET, John R; Community Mental Health, 65 Brunswick St, Fredericton NB E3B 5G5; Mem'79; FRCPC; Psy (General Adult Psychiatry). (506)453-2132; Fax. (506)453-8766.

DOUCET, Lorenne; 1100 Family Health Organizatio, 701-240 Duncan Mill Rd, North York ON M3B 3S6; Tor'07; CCFP; (416)494-7435; Fax. (416)494-4819.

DOUCET, Marc-Andre; Hôpital régional Chaleur, 1750 Sunset Dr, Bathurst NB E2A 4L7; Sher'08; CCFP; Staff, Hopital Regional Chaleur; (506)544-3000

DOUCET, Michel; Hop du Sacre-Coeur de Mtl, 5400 boul Gouin O, Montreal QC H4J 1C5; McG'93; CSPQ; FRCPC; IntMed (Interventional Cardiology); Cardiol. Staff, Hôpital du Sacre-Coeur de Montréal; (514)338-2222; Fax. (514)338-2905.

DOUCET, Paul G J; 42 Monte Carlo Cres, Moncton NB E1G 1M7; Sher'74; (506)857-4028

DOUCET, Paul M; St Boniface Gen Hosp, 409 Tache Ave, Winnipeg MB R2H 2A6; Ott'85; CCFP; CCFP(E.M.); Staff, Health Sciences Centre; Staff Emerg, St Boniface General Hospital; (204)233-8563; Fax. (204)231-0640.

DOUCET, Paul R; 805 rue Lafontaine, Drummondville QC J2B 1L8; Laval'66; ObstGyn (P.Q.). Staff, Hôpital Sainte-croix; Langs: Bilingual(English/French); (819)478-6464; paudouce@cgocable.ca.

DOUCET, Pierre L; 5 av Peronne, Outremont QC H3S 1X7; Mon'57; Psy (Psychoanalysis). Ac Staff, Hôpital du Sacre-Coeur de Montréal; Assoc Prof Psy, Universite de Montreal; (514)731-0417; Fax. (514)735-6086.

DOUCET, Rene; CHUQ-Ctr Hosp Univ Laval, 2705 boul Laurier, Quebec QC G1V 4G2; Laval'97; FRCSC; Psy. Staff, Centre Hospitalier Universitaire de Quebec-CHUL; (418)656-4141

DOUCET, Robyn T; Queen Elizabeth II HSC, 10W-1276 South Park St, Halifax NS B3H 2Y9; Dal'06; FRCPC; Anes. Staff, Queen Elizabeth II Health Sciences Centre - Victoria General Site; (902)473-2331

DOUCET, Serge; Institut de Cardiologie de Mtl, 5000 rue Belanger, Montreal QC H1T 1C8; Mon'85; CSPQ; FRCPC; IntMed (Interventional Cardiology); Cardiol. Staff, Institut de Cardiologie de Montréal; assoc Prof, Universite de Montreal; (514)376-3330 x3601; Fax. (514)593-2155.

DOUCET, Stephane; CHUM-Hop Notre-Dame, 1560 rue Sherbrooke E, Montreal QC H2L 4M1; Mon'05; MedOncol; Hem; IntMed. Staff, Centre Hospitalier l'Université de Montréal (CHUM) - Hôpital Notre-Dame; (514)890-8000

DOUCET JR., Robert J; Hotel-Dieu de Levis, 143 rue Wolfe, Levis QC G6V 3Z1; Laval'96; CCFP; CCFP(E.M.); Staff, Hôtel-Dieu de Lévis; (418)835-7121; Fax. (418)835-7263.

DOUCETTE, Jacquelyn M; 436 Waterloo St, Arva ON N0M 1C0; Wes'92; (519)438-5551

DOUCETTE, Karen E; University of Alberta Hosp, 2E4 17WMCV-8440 112 St NW, Edmonton AB T6G 2B7; Dal'96; MD; FRCPC; IntMed (Transplantation); InfectDis. Staff, University of Alberta Hospital; (780)407-1620; karen.doucette@ualberta.ca.

DOUEIK, Alexandre A; CHUS-Hop Fleurimont, 3001 12e av N, Sherbrooke QC J1H 5N4; Kharkov (Ukraine)'94; AnatPath (P.Q.). Staff, Centre Hospitalier Universitaire de Sherbrooke-Hopital Fleurimont; (819)346-1110 x15337; Fax. (819)820-6473.

DOUEK, Jennifer F; Montfort Hosp, 713 Montreal Rd, Ottawa ON K1K 0T2; McM'03; CCFP; Staff, Montfort Hospital; Langs: Bilingual(English/French); (613)746-4621

DOUEN, Andre; 303-101 Queensway W, Mississauga ON L5B 2P7; Miami(FL) (USA)'93; BSc; PhD; FRCPC; Neur (Stroke). Staff Neurol, Trillium Health Centre - Mississauga; Aj Prof Med, University of Ottawa; (905)848-2350; Fax. (905)848-8506.

DOUGALL, Alexander; HW 106-1900 Fort St, Victoria BC V8R 1J8; Glasgow (Scotland)'75; MB ChB; FRCP(Glas); Royal Jubilee Hospital; Ac Staff Geriatric Med, Vancouver Island Health Authority; Clinical Asst Prof Commun Geriatrics, University of British Columbia; (250)370-8509; Fax. (250)370-8285; alex.dougall@viha.ca.

DOUGALL, Allan M; 204-1950 Algonquin Ave, North Bay ON P1B 4Z2; McG'74; DAB; FACS; FRCSC; GenSurg. Staff, North Bay Regional Health Centre - Regional Mental Health; (705)474-5751; Fax. (705)474-6860.

DOUGALL, Hugh R; Life Mark Health Centre, 2225 Macleod Trail SE, Calgary AB T2G 5B6; Alb'79; FRCSC; OrthSurg (Foot & Ankle Reconstruction). (403)291-0045; Fax. (403)291-0552.

DOUGAN, H Sharon; PO Box 1428 Stn Main, Vernon BC V1T 6N7; UBC'69; CCFP; FCFP; (250)545-6629

DOUGHERTY, David J; 301-460 Wellington St, St Thomas ON N5R 6H9; Wes'84; Court Staff, St Thomas Elgin General Hospital; (519)631-5670; Fax. (519)631-8570.

DOUGHERTY, Elizabeth; Carrefour Med Vallee Richelieu, 665 boul Sir-Wilfrid Laurier, Beloeil QC J3G 4J1; Mon'06; CCFP; ac Membre Phy, Centre Hospitalier Honore-Mercier; Langs: Bilingual(French/English); (450)467-0088; Fax. (450)467-6941.

DOUGHERTY, Geoffrey E; MUHC-Montreal Children's Hosp, F138-2300 rue Tupper, Montreal QC H3H 1P3; McG'79; BA(Oxon); MA(Oxon); MSc(McG.); FAAP; CSPQ; FRCPC; Peds; CommunMed (P.Q.). div Chef Gen Ped, McGill University Health Centre - Montreal Children's Hospital; assoc Prof Peds & Epidemiology Biostatistics, McGill University; Langs: English; French; (514)412-4400 x23096; Fax. (514)412-4271.

DOUGHERTY, Stephen H; Douglas Square Med Clinic, 144-11520 24 St SE, Calgary AB T2Z 3E9; Wes'84; MSc; CCFP; Staff Med Deputy Reg (MCC), Council of Canada; Clin Teacher/Preceptor Residency Family Med South Campus Hosp, University of Calgary; (403)236-0211; Fax. (403)236-0261.

DOUGHTY, Paul; Strollery Childrens Hosp, 8440 112 St NW, Edmonton AB T6G 2B7; McM'06; Critical Care Medicine; Peds. Staff, Stollery Children's Hospital; (780)407-8822

DOUGLAS, Andrew; Sultherland Harris Mem Hosp, PO Box 1059 222 Haliburton Rd, Pictou NS B0K 1H0; McG'81; CCFP; Staff, Sutherland-Harris Memorial Hospital; Consultant Geriatrics, Northern Health Region; (902)485-2301; Fax. (902)485-2342.

DOUGLAS, Anne E; Brant Community HC-Brantford, 200 Terrace Hill St, Brantford ON N3R 1G9; Cal'95; BSc; CCFP; FCFP; Staff, The Brant Community Healthcare System - Brantford General Hospital Site; (519)751-5544

DOUGLAS, Datonye D O; 7090 Thunderbird Way PO Box 1619, Port Hardy BC V0N 2P0; Witwatersrand (South Africa)'01; MB BS; (250)949-7117; Fax. (250)949-7110.

DOUGLAS, Duncan R; Quinsam Med Clinic, 280-1400 Dogwood St, Campbell River BC V9W 3A6; Cape Town (South Africa)'85; MB ChB; CCFP; (250)286-0601; Fax. (250)286-0504.

DOUGLAS, Gordon R; 102-49 Richard Way SW, Calgary AB T3E 7M8; Man'66; LMCC; BSc; FRCSC; Ophth (Glaucoma). Staff, Royal Alexandra Hospital; Staff, Rockyview General Hospital; Volunteer Staff, Orbis International; (403)245-3730; Fax. (403)245-1058.

DOUGLAS, J Geoffrey; Saint John Reg Hosp Facility, PO Box 2100 Stn Main 400 University Ave, Saint John NB E2L 4L2; Dal'88; Cardiol; IntMed. Staff, Saint John Regional Hospital; (506)648-7965; Fax. (506)648-7967.

DOUGLAS, James; 3114-910 10th Ave W, Vancouver BC V5Z 1M9; UBC'07; FRCSC; OrthSurg.

DOUGLAS, M Joanne; BC Women's Hosp & Health Ctre, 1Q74-4500 Oak St, Vancouver BC V6H 3N1; Sask'67; FRCPC; Anes. Staff, BC Women's Hospital & Health Centre; (604)875-2158

DOUGLAS, Shannon; Fraser Lake Med Clinic, PO Box 98 130 Chowsunket, Fraser Lake BC V0J 1S0; UBC'00; CCFP; (250)699-6225; Fax. (250)699-6510.

DOUGLAS, Simone A; Maple Med Centre, 210-955 Major Mackenzie Dr, Vaughan ON L6A 4P9; Tor'93; BSc(Hon); CCFP; Staff, Mackenzie Richmond Hill Hospital; (905)832-2201; Fax. (905)832-2246.

DOUGLASS, Alan B; Royal Ottawa Hlth Care Group, 1145 Carling Ave, Ottawa ON K1Z 7K4; Alb'77; FRCPC; Psy (Sleep Disorders Medicine). Dir Sleep Disorders Serv, Royal Ottawa Mental Health Centre - Royal Ottawa Health Care Group; Asst Prof, University of Ottawa; Langs: French; (613)722-6521 x6226; Fax. (613)798-2980; adouglas@rohcg.on.ca.

DOUGLASS, Rebecca J; 2948 Baseline Rd, Ottawa ON K2H 8T5; Tor'06; CCFP; (613)288-2059

DOUILLARD, Helene; CSSS de Portneuf, 700 rue Saint-Cyrille, Saint-Raymond QC G3L 1W1; Laval'99; Staff, Centre Hospitalier Portneuf; (418)337-4611 x2405

DOUKAS, Kathleen; 4F-410 Sherbourne St, Toronto ON M4X 1K2; McM'08; CCFP; Staff Covenant House, St Michael's Hospital; (416)867-3728; Fax. (416)867-3726.

DOUKETIS, James D; St Joseph's Healthcare, F544-50 Charlton Ave E, Hamilton ON L8N 4A6; Tor'88; BSc; FACP; FCCP; FRCPC; IntMed (Thromboembolism). Assoc Dir Clin Teaching Unit, St Joseph's Healthcare - Charlton Campus; Prof Med & Assoc Dir Clin Teaching Unit, McMaster University; Langs: Greek; French; (905)521-6178; Fax. (905)521-6068; jdouket@mcmaster.ca.

DOULATYARIAZAR, Haleh; The Pas Clinic, PO Box 240 67 First St, The Pas MB R9A 1K1; (Azerbaijan)'97; (204)623-3334

DOULTON, Bruce C; Eleven Elizabeth Family Practi, 201-11 Elizabeth Ave, St. John's NL A1A 1W6; Cal'83; CCFP; Ac Staff, Central Newfoundland Regional Health Centre; (709)579-1106; mdoulton@nf.sympatico.ca.

DOUMIT, Maya; CSSSG-Hop de Hull, 116 boul Lionel-Emond, Gatineau QC J8Y 1W7; Ott'05; FRCPC; IntMed; Gastroent. Staff, Hull Hospital; (450)468-8111

DOUMMAR, Gilbert; CSSS Pierre Boucher, 1333 boul Jacques-Cartier E, Longueuil QC J4M 2A5; Mon'87; FRCPC; IntMed; Gastroent. Gastroenterology/Internal Med, Centre Hospitalier Pierre Boucher; (450)468-8111

DOUNAEVSKAIA, Vera; St Michael's Hosp, 4CC-30 Bond St, Toronto ON M5B 1W8; Tor'06; FRCPC; IntMed. Staff, St Michael's Hospital; (416)864-6060; Fax. (416)864-5870.

DOUPE, Lisa M; 25 Brendan Rd, East York ON M4G 2X2; Tor'71; DIH; FACOEM; DOHS; Principal, PWR Health Consultants; ldoupe@pwr.ca.

DOUROVA, Nevena; Child & Parent Resource Instit, 600 Sanatorium Rd, London ON N6H 3W7; (Bulgaria)'01; DABPN; FRCPC; Psy (Child & Adolescent Psychiatry). Asst Prof Psy, University of Western Ontario; Langs: Bulgarian; (519)858-2774; Fax. (519)858-1917.

DOUVILLE, Jocelyn; Clin Med du Faubourg de Mt-St-, 208-468 boul Sir Wilfrid-Lauri, Beloeil QC J3H 6K3; Laval'84; (450)813-9222

DOUVILLE, Linda A; 300-30 Prospect St, Newmarket ON L3Y 3S9; Tor'90; CCFP; CCFP(E.M.); FCFP; Staff, Southlake Regional Health Centre; (905)895-4156; Fax. (905)895-0740.

DOUVILLE, Lucie; CHUQ-Ctr Hosp Univ Laval, RC157-2705 boul Laurier, Quebec QC G1V 4G2; Laval'81; CSPQ; FRCPC; Psy. Staff Psy, Centre Hospitalier Universitaire de Quebec-CHUL; Teach Staff, Université Laval; (418)654-2121; Fax. (418)654-2716.

DOUVILLE, Pierre; CHUQ-Hotel-Dieu de Quebec, 11 Cote du Palais, Quebec QC G1R 2J6; Laval'78; CSPQ; FRCPC; MedBiochem (Nephrology). Consultant, Hôpital Laval; Staff, Centre Hospitalier Universitaire de Québec (CHUQ) - Siege Social; Chef, Jeffery Hale Hospital-Saint Brigid's; Consultant Med Biochemist, Centre Hospitalier Beauce-Etchemin; Langs: English; (418)691-5135; pierre.douville@chuq.qc.ca.

DOUVILLE, Veronique; CHUQ-St-Francois d'Assise, 10 rue de l'Espinay, Quebec QC G1L 3L5; Sher'03; CCFP; CCFP(E.M.); Staff Emerg Med, Centre Hospitalier Universitaire De Québec - Pavillon De St-françois-d'assise; (418)525-4444

DOUVILLE, Yvan; CHUQ-St-Francois D'Assise, 10 rue de l'Espinay, Quebec QC G1L 3L5; Laval'74; CSPQ; MMed; LMCC; DABS; FRCSC; GenSurg; VascSurg. Staff Surg, Centre Hospitalier Universitaire De Québec - Pavillon De St-françois-d'assise; Chef Surgery, Université Laval; Langs: English; (418)525-2279; Fax. (418)525-2264; yvan.douville@chg.ulaval.ca.

DOUVILLE-FRADET, Monique; Institut National de Sante Pub, U 3141-2400 av D'Estimauville, Quebec QC G1E 7G9; Laval'72; MHSc(Tor); FRCPC; CommunMed (Public Health). Ac Staff, Centre Hospitalier Universitaire de Quebec-CHUL; Langs: French; English; (418)666-7000 x313; Fax. (418)666-2776; monique.fradet@ssss.gouv.qc.ca.

DOUYON, Frantz; 424-5450 ch de la Cote-des-Nei, Montreal QC H3T 1Y3; (Haiti)'63; Nephrol (P.Q.); Peds. Staff, McGill University Health Centre - Montreal Children's Hospital; (514)735-4305; Fax. (514)735-4306.

DOUYON, Sylvie; Ctr Hosp De Verdun, 4000 boul Lasalle, LaSalle QC H4G 2A3; Mon'82; FRCSC; ObstGyn. Staff, Centre Hospitalier de Verdun; (514)362-1000

DOUYON DE AZEVEDO, Mario; Montfort Hosp, 713 Montreal Rd, Ottawa ON K1K 0T2; Laval'94; CCFP; Staff, Montfort Hospital; (613)746-4621; Fax. (613)748-4938.

DOUZIECH, Maxime; Ctr Hosp Anna-Laberge, 200 boul Brisebois, Chateauguay QC J6K 4W8; Sher'05; FRCPC; DiagRad. Staff, Hôpital Anna-Laberge; (450)699-2425

DOVE, John F C; Weeneebayko Gen Hosp, PO Box 34 19 Hospital Dr, Moose Factory ON P0L 1W0; McG'72; CCFP; FCFP; Staff, Weeneebayko General Hospital; Teacher, McMaster University; Teacher Family Med, Queen's University; Langs: English; French; (705)658-4544; dmqdocs@drytel.net.

DOVE, Marion; GMF Côté-des-Neiges, 5700 ch de la cote-des-Neiges, Montreal QC H3T 2A8; McM'94; CCFP; Staff, CSSS de la Basse Côté-Nord; Langs: English; French; German; (514)731-8531; Fax. (514)731-0563.

DOVER, Karen J; Dover Las & Cosm Med Prof Corp, 701-1081 Carling Ave, Ottawa ON K1Y 4G2; Tor'84; Langs: Bilingual(English/French); (613)715-9900; Fax. (613)715-9915; drdover@kjd-md.com.

DOW, Gordon C K; The Moncton Hosp, 135 MacBeath Ave, Moncton NB E1C 6Z8; Dal'87; BSc; MSc; FRCPC; IntMed (AIDS/HIV); InfectDis. Staff/Med Advisor New Brunswick HIV Treatment Prog, The Moncton Hospital; Clin Teacher, Dalhousie University; (506)857-5670; Fax. (506)857-5671.

DOW, Heather; 417 Connell St PO Box 9028, Woodstock NB E7M 6B5; Alb'91; CCFP; FCFP; (506)328-9986; Fax. (506)328-9980.

DOW, Jamie; Societe Ass Automobile du QC, CP 19600 Succ Terminus C4 12-333 boul Jean-Lesage, Quebec QC G1K 8J6; Laval'86; MBA; Med Consultant Road Safety, Societe Assurance Automobile du Quebec; Langs: Bilingual(French/English); (418)528-4984; Fax. (418)643-0828; jamie.dow@saaq.gouv.qc.ca.

DOW, Kimberly E; 6 303-76 Stuart St, Kingston ON K7L 2V7; Qns'77; FRCPC; Peds. Att Staff Neonatol, Kingston General Hospital; (613)548-6046; Fax. (613)548-1369; dowk@queensu.ca.

DOW, Michelle M; Clare Health Centre, PO Box 128 8559 Meteghan Ctr, Meteghan Centre NS B0W 2K0; Dal'87; CCFP; (902)645-2777; Fax. (902)645-2854; michelle.dow@ns.sympatico.ca.

DOWDALL, Timothy J; Foothills Family Med Centre, PO Box 460, Black Diamond AB T0L 0H0; (Scotland)'96; MB ChB; CCFP; (403)933-4368; Fax. (403)933-2026.

DOWDELL, Christine J; Forest Glen Plaza, 700 Strasburg Rd, Kitchener ON N2E 2M2; Nottingham (England)'75; (519)578-4450; Fax. (519)579-1142.

DOWDELL, Timothy R; St Michael's Hosp, 30 Bond St, Toronto ON M5B 1W8; Tor'85; BSc; FRCPC; DiagRad. Staff, St Michael's Hospital; (416)864-5690; Fax. (416)864-5380.

DOWDEN, Scot D; Tom Baker Cancer Centre, CC112C-1331 29 St NW, Calgary AB T2N 4N2; Mem'96; FRCPC; IntMed; MedOncol. Staff, Tom Baker Cancer Centre; (403)521-3166; Fax. (403)283-1651; drscot@shaw.ca.

DOWELL, Anthony H; 217-269 boul Saint-Jean, Pointe-Claire QC H9R 3J1; McG'80; BSc; CCFP; Ac Staff, Lakeshore General Hospital - Pointe Claire; Prin Investigator, Dynamik Research Inc; Langs: French; (514)694-6446; Fax. (514)694-1576.

DOWER, Andrea M; Hamilton HS-General Site, 237 Barton St E, Port Perry ON L9L 2X2; Mem'03; FRCPC; Anes. Staff, Hamilton Health Sciences Centre - Hamilton General Hospital; (905)201-2100

DOWER, Nancy A; Edmonton Clinic Health Academy, 11405 87 Ave NW, Edmonton AB T6G 1C9; UBC'84; BSc; PhD; FRCPC; Peds; Hem. Staff, University of Alberta Hospital; Staff, Cross Cancer Institute; Physician, Edmonton Clinic Health Academy; Asst Prof, University of Alberta; (780)407-8822; ndower@cha.ab.ca.

DOWEY, Michael T J; Surrey Mem Hosp, 13750 96 Ave, Surrey BC V3V 1Z2; Alb'90; FRCPC; NuclearMed; Psy. Staff, Surrey Memorial Hospital; (604)585-5554

DOWHANIK, Monica A; Health Sciences Centre, 820 Sherbrook St, Winnipeg MB R3A 1R9; Man'91; Staff, Health Sciences Centre; (204)774-6511

DOWHANIK, Paul B J; Seven Oaks Gen Hosp, 2300 McPhillips St, Winnipeg MB R2V 3M3; Man'91; BSc; Staff, Seven Oaks General Hospital; (204)632-7133

DOWLATSHAHI, Dariush; The Ottawa Hosp-Civic Campus, C2182B-1053 Carling Ave, Ottawa ON K1Y 4E9; McM'03; FRCPC; Neur (Clinician Investigator Program). Staff, The Ottawa Hospital - Civic Campus; (613)722-7000

DOWLING, Graeme P; Office Of Chief Med Examiner, 7007 116 St NW, Edmonton AB T6H 5R8; Man'81; FRCPC; AnatPath (Forensic Pathology). Chief Dept of Justice, Province of Alberta; Clin Assoc Prof, University of Calgary; (780)427-4987; Fax. (780)422-0546; graeme.dowling@gov.ab.ca.

DOWLING, Shawn; Foothills Med Centre, 1403 29 St NW, Calgary AB T2N 2T9; Ott'04; FRCPC; EmergMed. Staff, Foothills Medical Centre; (403)944-1596

DOWN, Hugh E; 388-1641 Hillside Ave, Victoria BC V8T 5G1; UBC'94; CCFP; (250)592-9300; Fax. (250)592-9301.

DOWN, Karin; 388-1641 Hillside Ave, Victoria BC V8T 5G1; UBC'94; CCFP; (250)592-9300; Fax. (250)592-9301.

DOWN, Nancy K; North York Med Arts Bldg, 218-1333 Sheppard Ave E, North York ON M2J 1V1; Tor'80; FACS; FRCSC; GenSurg. Staff, North York General Hospital; (416)491-0345; Fax. (416)491-7557.

DOWNAR, Eugene; Univ of Alberta Hosp, 2C2 47-8440 112 St NW, Edmonton AB T6G 2B7; Edinburgh (Scotland)'66; MB ChB; Cardiol (Electrophysiology). Staff, University of Alberta Hospital; (780)407-6946

DOWNAR, James A; Univ Hlth Network-Toronto Gen, 200 Elizabeth St, Toronto ON M5G 2C4; McG'02; FRCPC; IntMed; Palliative Care; Critical Care Medicine. Staff, Toronto General Hospital - UHN; Langs: Bilingual(English/French); (416)340-3111

DOWNAR, Jonathan; Univ Hlth Network-Toronto Western Hosp, MP7 432-399 Bathurst St, Toronto ON M5T 2S8; Cal'05; FRCPC; Psy. Staff, Toronto Western Hospital - University Health Network; Langs: Spanish; French; (416)603-5667; Fax. (416)603-5292.

DOWNAR-ZAPOLSKI, Zbigniew; Hampton Park Med Centre, 216-1419 Carling Ave, Ottawa ON K1Z 7L6; Szczecin (Poland)'71; Langs: Polish; (613)728-8880; Fax. (613)728-5295.

DOWNES, Heather F; 204-2004 14 St NW, Calgary AB T2M 3N3; Qns'91; CCFP; FCFP; (403)221-9330; Fax. (403)282-1071.

DOWNEY, Donal; Royal Inland Hosp, 311 Columbia St, Kamloops BC V2C 2T1; Dublin (Ireland)'81; FRCR; FFR(RCSI); FRCPI(Ire); MB BCh; BAO; FRCPC; DiagRad (Diagnostic Ultrasound). Staff Radiologist, Royal Inland Hospital; (250)314-2159; Fax. (250)314-2732.

DOWNEY, James F; Toronto East Gen Hosp Inc, 825 Coxwell Ave, Toronto ON M4C 3E7; McM'85; PhD; FRCPC; IntMed (AIDS); MedMicrobiol. Court Staff, Headwaters Health Care Centre - Orangeville Site; Ac Staff IntMed & Microbiol, Toronto East General Hospital Inc; Court Staff, Stevenson Memorial Hospital; (416)464-2891

DOWNEY, Mathew T; Quinte HC Corp-Belleville Gen, PO Box 428 Stn Main 265 Dundas St E, Belleville ON K8N 5A9; Qns'82; FRCPC; DiagRad., QHC Belleville General; (613)969-7400 x2523

DOWNEY, Pamela M; Rockyview Health Centre, 210-1016 68 Ave SW, Calgary AB T2V 4J2; Man'82; BSc(Med); FRCPC; EmergMed (Cardiology). Staff, Cardiometabolic Evaluation & Risk Assessment Centre; (403)541-0033

DOWNIE, David C; Avenue Med Clinic, 221 Brant Ave, Brantford ON N3T 3J2; Qns'91; FRCSC; GenSurg. Staff, The Brant Community Healthcare System - Willett Hospital Site; (519)753-8666; Fax. (519)753-5672.

DOWNIE, Elizabeth J; LL-1107 37 St SW, Calgary AB T3C 1S5; Cal'88; CCFP; (403)246-7788; Fax. (403)242-8850.

DOWNIE, Joseph A; Peter Lougheed Centre, 3500 26 Ave NE, Calgary AB T1Y 6J4; Cal'90; FRCPC; Anes. Staff, Peter Lougheed Centre; (403)943-5721

DOWNING, G Michael; Royal Jubilee Hosp, 1952 Bay St, Victoria BC V8R 1J8; Wes'73; Ac Staff Palliative Med & Research Victoria Hospice Society, Royal Jubilee Hospital; Clin Assoc Prof Family Practice, University of British Columbia; Aj Asst Prof School of Hlth Information Science, University of Victoria; (250)370-8715

DOWNING, Mark; Postgraduate Med Education, 602-500 Universiyt Ave, Toronto ON M5G 1V7; Dal'07; FRCPC; IntMed; InfectDis. Staff, Univerity of Toronto Continuing Education.

DOWNS, Allan C; Psychealth Centre, PZ155-771 Bannatyne Ave, Winnipeg MB R3E 3N4; Man'87; FRCPC; Psy (Child & Adolescent Psychiatry). Staff Psy, Health Sciences Centre; Consultant Child & Adolescent Psy., Manitoba Health; Asst Prof Psy, University of Manitoba; (204)787-7889; Fax. (204)787-4975; allan.downs@gov.mb.ca.

DOWNS, Jean-Pierre; 22 rue Saint-Michel, Vaudreuil-Dorion QC J7V 1E8; Mon'75; Staff, Centre Hospitalier l'Université de Montréal (CHUM) - Hôpital Notre-Dame; (450)455-5797; Fax. (450)455-5798.

DOWNTON, Geoffrey F; Dr Charles A Janeway Child HC, 300 Prince Philip Dr, St. John's NL A1B 3V6; Mem'77; FRCPC; Peds (Neonatal & Perinatal Medicine). Staff, Janeway Children's Health & Rehabilitation Centre; (709)777-6423

DOWSLING, Janet L; 63 Hillsdale Ave E, Toronto ON M4S 1T4; McM'75; Court Staff, North York General Hospital; Court Staff, Sunnybrook Health Sciences Centre; Consultant, The Jean Tweed Centre; (416)486-1788

DOYLE, A I Catherine; Ctr Hosp Affilie-Enfant-Jesus, 1401 18e rue, Quebec QC G1J 1Z4; Laval'88; FRCPC; IntMed (Breast Cancer); MedOncol (P.Q.); Hem. Staff, Centre Hospitalier Affilié Universitaire de Québec - Hôpital De L'Enfant Jésus; Staff, Centre Hospitalier Affilié Universitaire de Québec - Hôpital du St-Sacrement; Staff, Hôpital Laval; Université Laval; (418)649-5726

DOYLE, Aeron; St Paul's Hosp, 1081 Burrard St, Vancouver BC V6Z 1Y6; McG'92; MDCM; FRCPC; Anes. Staff, Providence Health Care - St Paul's Hospital; (604)682-2344 x62330

DOYLE, Christopher S; Innovation in Medical Helath, 1699 Lakeshore Rd W, Mississauga ON L5J 1J4; McG'93; FRCPC; Psy. Staff, The Credit Valley Hospital; Fax. (905)291-0771.

DOYLE, D Maureen; St Mary's Family Med Centre, 3777 rue Jean-Brillant, Montreal QC H3T 1M5; Qns'81; MD; CCFP; FCFP; Staff, St Mary's Hospital Centre; adj Prof, McGill University; (514)734-2677; Fax. (514)734-2602.

DOYLE, Daniel; Hôpital Laval, 3e-2725 ch Sainte-Foy, Quebec QC G1V 4G5; Mon'83; FRCS; FRCSC; GenSurg (Cardiac Surgery & Transplantation); Cardiovasc&ThorSurg. Chef chir cardio, Hôpital Laval; Clin Prof, Université Laval; Langs: Bilingual(French/English); (418)656-4717; Fax. (418)656-4707; daniel.doyle@chg.ulaval.ca.

DOYLE, David A; Children's Hosp Eastern Ont, 401 Smyth Rd, Ottawa ON K1H 8L1; Tor'69; FRCPC; Peds. Dir Child Development Serv, Children's Hospital of Eastern Ontario (CHEO); Asst Prof Peds, University of Ottawa; (613)737-0871 x2294; Fax. (613)738-4230.

DOYLE, Donna L W; Lansdowne Professional Ctr II, 235-3066 Shelbourne St, Victoria BC V8R 6T9; UBC'90; (250)592-6988; Fax. (250)592-6917.

DOYLE, Elisabete R; Health Sciences Centre, CE222-820 Sherbrook St, Winnipeg MB R3A 1R9; Man'91; FRCPC; Peds. Staff, Health Sciences Centre; (204)774-6511

DOYLE, G Tyna; Dr Charles A Janeway Child HC, 300 Prince Philip Dr, St. John's NL A1B 3V6; Mem'02; FRCPC; Peds (Developmental Pediatrics). Staff, Janeway Children's Health & Rehabilitation Centre; (709)777-6300

DOYLE, Gordon L; Burnaby Hosp, 3935 Kincaid St, Burnaby BC V5G 2X6; UBC'81; Staff, Burnaby Hospital; (604)434-4211; Fax. (604)412-6185.

DOYLE, Jason S G; Vernon Jubilee Hosp, 2101 32 St, Vernon BC V1T 5L2; Alb'94; FRCPC; GenPath. Staff Path, Vernon Jubilee Hospital; (250)558-1200 x1597; Fax. (250)558-1368.

DOYLE, Jeffrey D; St Michael's Hosp, QW 3 076-30 Bond St, Toronto ON M5B 1W8; Qns'03; Critical Care Medicine; GenSurg. Staff, St Michael's Hospital; (416)360-4000

DOYLE, John; Cancercare Manitoba, ON2021A-675 McDermot Ave, Winnipeg MB R3E 0V9; Wes'81; DABPed; FRCPC; Peds; Hem. Staff, CancerCare Manitoba; (204)787-2197

DOYLE, Judith I M; Misericordia Health Centre, 99 Cornish Ave, Winnipeg MB R3C 1A2; Dublin (Ireland)'62; Staff, Misericordia Health Centre; (204)774-6581; Fax. (204)788-8529.

DOYLE, Kenneth R; MUHC-Montreal Gen Hosp, 1650 av Cedar, Montreal QC H3G 1A4; Tor'87; FRCPC; EmergMed. Staff, McGill University Health Centre - Montreal General Campus; Langs: Bilingual(English/French); (514)934-1934 x2530

DOYLE, Leilani; The Ottawa Hosp-Civic Campus, 1053 Carling Ave, Ottawa ON K1Y 4E9; Alb'99; FRCPC; Anes;CCFP; Staff, The Ottawa Hospital - Civic Campus; (613)722-7000

DOYLE, Marijane; Ambiance Prof Centre, 2-555 Concession St, Hamilton ON L8V 1A8; Tor'75; FAAP; FRCPC; Peds (Neonatology). (905)387-0831; Fax. (905)522-0464; doyle@on.aibn.com.

DOYLE, Mary A; 204-185 Bentinck St, Sydney NS B1P 1G7; Dal'85; (902)562-2376; Fax. (902)539-5975.

DOYLE, Mary-Anne; Univ of Ottawa, 2044-451 Smyth Rd, Ottawa ON K1H 8M5; McM'05; FRCPC; IntMed; Endocrin&Metab. Teacher, University of Ottawa; Langs: Bilingual(English/French).

DOYLE, Patricia M; Credit Valley Med Arts Centre, 502-2000 Credit Valley Rd, Mississauga ON L5M 4N4; Mem'76; FRCSC; ObstGyn. Ac Staff, The Credit Valley Hospital; (905)820-8748; Fax. (905)820-0255.

DOYLE, Patrick W; 1112-899 12th Ave W, Vancouver BC V5Z 1M9; UBC'79; FRCPC; MedMicrobiol. Staff Med Microbiol & Infection Control, Vancouver General Hospital - Centennial Pavillion; (604)875-4111 x62624; pdoyle@vanhosp.bc.ca.

DOYLE, Robert; Valley Regional Hosp, 150 Exhibition St, Kentville NS B4N 5E3; Saba (Netherlands Antilles)'07; Anes. Staff, Valley Regional Hospital; (902)678-7381

DOYLE, Sharon; 2-1275 Walker Rd, Windsor ON N8Y 4X9; Wes'86; CCFP; FCFP; Consultant, Windsor Regional Hospital - Metropolitan Site; Hôtel-Dieu Grace Hospital; (519)253-9116; Fax. (519)253-5404.

DOYLE-CHAN, Wai-Kuen; 9803 34 Ave NW, Edmonton AB T6E 5X9; Manchester (England)'79; MB ChB; FRCPC; Peds. Staff Ped, Covenant Health - Grey Nuns Community Hospital; Asst Prof, University of Alberta Hospital; (780)461-1468; Fax. (780)465-7267.

DOYON, Annabelle; CSSS de Trois-Rivieres, 1991 boul du Carmel, Trois-Rivieres QC G8Z 3R9; Sher'97; CSPQ; FRCSC; GenSurg. Staff, CSSS de Trois-Rivières; (819)697-3333

DOYON, Bernard; Carrefour Med Vallee Richelieu, 665 boul Sir-Wilfrid-Laurier, Beloeil QC J3G 4J1; Laval'80; assoc Staff, Hôpital du Haut-Richelieu; (450)467-0088; Fax. (450)467-6941.

DOYON, Caroline; Hop Anna-Laberge, 200 boul Brisebois, Chateauguay QC J6K 4W8; Mon'07; GenSurg. Staff, Hôpital Anna-Laberge; (450)699-2425

DOYON, Chantal; CLSC de Sherbrooke, 1200 rue King E, Sherbrooke QC J1G 1E4; Sher'90; Ac Staff, Centre Hospitalier Universitaire de Sherbrooke-Hôpital Hôtel-Dieu; (819)563-2572; Fax. (819)563-8502.

DOYON, Elisabeth; CHUS-Hop Fleurimont, 3001 12e av N, Sherbrooke QC J1H 5N4; Sher'07; FRCPC; Anes. Staff, Centre Hospitalier Universitaire de Sherbrooke-Hopital Fleurimont; (819)346-1110 x14950

DOYON, Guy; 100-2727 rue King O, Sherbrooke QC J1L 1C2; Sher'74; MSc; FRCSC; Ophth (Cataract). Langs: English; (819)346-2727; Fax. (819)346-9367; vision@100pour100vision.qc.ca.

DOYON, Jean-Claude; Centre Med Varennes, 201-2082 Rte Marie-Victorin, Varennes QC J3X 2C7; Laval'72; (450)652-2959

DOYON, Josee; Hop Maisonneuve-Rosemont, 5415 boul de l'Assomption, Montreal QC H1T 2M4; Mon'87; CSPQ; FRCPC; AnatPath. Staff, Hopital Maisonneuve-Rosemont; (514)252-3498

DOYON, Julie; CSSS de Beauce-Etchemin, 1515 17e rue, Saint-Georges QC G5Y 4T8; Laval'05; IntMed. Staff, Centre Hospitalier Beauce-Etchemin; (418)228-2031

DOYON, Julie; Hotel-Dieu d'Arthabaska, 5 rue des Hospitalieres, Victoriaville QC G6P 6N2; Laval'00; FRCPC; Psy. Staff, Hotel-Dieu d'Arthabaska; (819)357-2030; Fax. (819)357-6035.

DOYON, Linda; GMF Centre medical AJC, 110 rue Saint-Jean, Drummondville QC J2B 7T1; Sher'89; CCFP; ac Staff, Hôpital Sainte-croix; (819)477-1800; Fax. (819)477-9865.

DOYON, Lucie P; CHSLD Emilie-Gamelin, 1440 rue Dufresne, Montreal QC H2K 3J3; Laval'83; Physician, Julius Richardson Convalescent Hosp; Médecin, Centre d'Accueil Emilie Gamelin; (514)527-8921; Fax. (514)527-3587.

DOYON, Marie-Lucie; Clinique de Radiologie, C210-1 Car Westmount, Westmount QC H3Z 2P9; Laval'83; FRCPC; DiagRad (Chest Radiology). Staff, McGill University Health Centre - Montreal General Campus; Langs: English; (514)939-9764; Fax. (514)939-9363.

DOYON, Martin; CSSS de Beauce-Etchemin, 1515 17e rue, Saint-Georges QC G5Y 4T8; Laval'95; Psy. Staff, Centre Hospitalier Beauce-Etchemin; (418)228-2068; Fax. (418)227-1081.

DOYON, Michel; Clinique Med de Terrebonne, 831 montee Masson, Terrebonne QC J6W 2C7; Mon'83; Fax. (450)492-8228.

DOYON, Yvon; CSSS de Trois-Rivieres, 155 rue Toupin, Trois-Rivieres QC G8T 3Z8; Laval'72; Staff, Centre de santé Cloutier-du-Rivage; Langs: Bilingual(French/English); (819)372-1316

DOYON-GAMACHE, Noemie; CLSC Ahuntsic, 1165 boul Henri-Bourassa E, Montreal QC H2C 3K2; Sher'10; (514)384-2000

DOYON OLIVIER, Joelle; CHUS-Hop Fleurimont, 3001 12e av N, Sherbrooke QC J1H 5N4; Sher'09; CCFP; CCFP(E.M.); Staff, Centre Hospitalier Universitaire de Sherbrooke-Hopital Fleurimont; (819)346-1110

DOYON-TROTTIER, Evelyne; Hôpital Ste-Justine, 3175 ch cote-Sainte-Catherine, Montreal QC H3T 1C5; Mon'02; FRCPC; Peds; PedEmergMed (P.Q.). Staff, Hôpital Ste-Justine; (514)345-4931 x5885

DRAB, Stephen A; 12-250 Wincott Dr, Etobicoke ON M9R 2R5; Qns'02; (416)249-0002; Fax. (416)249-0842.

DRABKIN, Rodney; Queen Alexandra Ctre Children, 2400 Arbutus Rd, Victoria BC V8N 1V7; Cape Town (South Africa)'84; MB ChB; FRCPC; Psy (Child & Adolescent Psychiatry). Staff, Queen Alexandra Centre for Children's Health; Staff Child & Adolescent Psy, Vancouver Island Health Authority; Clin Instructor, University of British Columbia; (250)519-5390; oriole1@shaw.ca.

DRACHENBERG, Darrel E; St Boniface Gen Hosp, 23036-409 Tache Ave, Winnipeg MB R2H 2A6; UBC'95; FRCSC; Urol. Staff, St Boniface General Hospital; (204)233-8563

DRACOPOULOS, Anastasios T; Family Med Clinic, 404-658 Danforth Ave, Toronto ON M4J 5B9; Athens (Greece)'89; CCFP; Langs: Greek; (416)461-0093; Fax. (416)466-3976.

DRADER, Keith S; Peter Lougheed Centre, 3500 26 Ave NE, Calgary AB T1Y 6J4; Cal'91; FRCPC; Anes. Staff, Peter Lougheed Centre; (403)943-5721

DRAGATAKIS, Leonidas N; Group Med Jean-Talon, 202-7200 rue Hutchison, Montreal QC H3N 1Z2; Athens (Greece)'72; FACC; CSPQ; FRCPC; Cardiol. Dir Cardiovasc Lab, Sir Mortimer B Davis Jewish General; Consultant, McGill University Health Centre - Royal Victoria Hospital; adj Prof Med, McGill University; (514)495-2555; Fax. (514)495-7932.

DRAGICEVICH, John T; 203-1581 Hillside Ave, Victoria BC V8T 2C1; Alb'96; FRCSC; Ophth. (778)430-5393

DRAGIN, Natacha; Centre Med Alexandre, 8100 boul Taschereau, Brossard QC J4X 1C2; Mon'97; CCFP; (450)465-5589

DRAGINDA, Anne; Fort Med Clinic, 101-6603 132 Ave NW, Edmonton AB T5C 2A4; Alb'97; CCFP; Langs: English; French; (780)476-1388; Fax. (780)473-3530; adraginda@shaw.ca.

DRAGOI-DAVID, Otilia-Elena; Ctr Hosp Rouyn-Noranda, 4 9e rue, Rouyn-Noranda QC J9X 2B2; Bucharest (Romania)'82; CCFP; Staff, Centre Hospitalier Rouyn-Noranda; (819)764-5131

DRAGOMIR, Alina R; Hamilton HS-Henderson Sie, 711 Concession St, Hamilton ON L8V 1C3; Timisoara (Romania)'92; FRCPC; IntMed (Family Medicine). Staff, Hamilton Health Sciences Centre-Juravinski Site; (905)527-4322

DRAGOMIR, Camelia C; 105-726 bloor St W, Toronto ON M6G 4A1; Bucharest (Romania)'82; CCFP; Staff MD CCFP, North Park Medical Centre; (416)534-5127; Fax. (416)534-1711.

DRAGON, Normand; CSSS Drummond-Hop Sainte-Croix, 570 rue Heriot, Drummondville QC J2B 1C1; Sher'81; BSc; MSc; FRCPC; Psy. Staff Psy, Hôpital Sainte-croix; Clin Prof, Universite de Sherbrooke; (819)478-6464 x3422; Fax. (819)478-6490.

DRAGON, Sylvie; Med Privee Notre-Dame, 597 av Notre-Dame, Longueuil QC J4P 2K8; Sher'91; CCFP; CCFP(E.M.); Staff, Hopital Charles LeMoyne; (450)766-0766; Fax. (450)766-0767.

DRAIN, Brighid; Tuxedo Park Family Med, 981 Corydon Ave, Winnipeg MB R3M 0X1; Man'05; CCFP; Staff, Seven Oaks General Hospital.

DRAISEY, Rebecca M; Tecumseh Med Centre, 11811 Tecumseh Rd E, Windsor ON N8N 4M7; Tor'86; (519)979-3355; Fax. (519)979-1429.

DRAKE, James; The Hosp For Sick Children, 1504-555 University Ave, Toronto ON M5G 1X8; Dublin (Ireland)'79; MSc; FRCSC; Neursurg. Staff, Holland Bloorview Kids Rehabilitation Hospital; Staff, The Hospital For Sick Children; Prof Surg, University of Toronto; (416)813-6125; Fax. (416)813-4975; james.drake@sickkids.ca.

DRAKE, Robert; 3-400 Cabana Rd E, Windsor ON N9G 1A3; London (England)'61; MB BS; CCFP; Coroner, Office of the Chief Coroner; (519)972-7065; Fax. (519)972-7602; dr.rmdrake@sympatico.ca.

DRAKE, Roger S; Carleton Place Mews, 44 Lansdowne Ave, Carleton Place ON K7C 2T8; Ott'81; Staff, Carleton Place & District Memorial Hospital; Staff, Almonte General Hospital; (613)257-7002; Fax. (613)257-8177.

DRAKE, Wendy T; Cobequid Commun Health Ctre, 40 Freer Lane, Lower Sackville NS B4C 0A2; Dal'96; MSc(Immunol.); CCFP; Staff, Cobequid Community Health Centre; (902)869-6101; Fax. (902)869-3699.

DRAKOS, Demetrios A; Plastic & Reconstructive Surge, 223-217 Terrace Hill St, Brantford ON N3R 1G8; Tor'96; PlasSurg. Staff, The Brant Community Healthcare System - Brantford General Hospital Site; Langs: Greek; (519)753-0085; Fax. (519)753-7399.

DRALI, Ratiba; CHSLD Jeanne le Ber, 7445 rue Hochelaga, Montreal QC H1N 3V2; (Other Foreign)'09; CCFP; (514)521-6000

DRANCE, Elisabeth; Parkview Intensice Support Uni, 4950 Heather St, Vancouver BC V5Z 3L9; UBC'84; FRCPC; Psy (Administration). Staff, Providence Health Care - Mount Saint Joseph Hospital; Staff, Vancouver General Hospital - Centennial Pavillion; Physician Prog Dir-Elder Care, Providence Health Care - St Paul's Hospital; Med Dir Older Services, Vancouver Mental Health Service; Clin Assoc Prof Psy, University of British Columbia; (604)261-9371

DRANDIC, Marijana; Rouge Valley-Ajax & Pickering, 580 Harwood Ave S, Ajax ON L1S 2J4; Wes'03; FRCPC; Psy. Staff, Rouge Valley Health System - Ajax & Pickering Health Centre Site; Langs: Serbian; Yugoslavian; (905)683-2320

DRAPEAU, Christine; CSSS de Trois-Rivières, 1991 boul du Carmel, Trois-Rivieres QC G8Z 3R9; Laval'05; FRCPC; IntMed (Respirology & Critical Care); Respir. Staff, CSSS de Trois-Rivières; (819)697-3333 x63567

DRAPEAU, Dennis; Queen Elizabeth II HSC-Halifax, 5F-1796 Summer St, Halifax NS B3H 3A7; Dal'00; FRCPC; Anes. Staff Anes, Queen Elizabeth II Health Sciences Centre - Victoria General Site.

DRAPEAU, Genevieve; 105C-411 av Sirois, Rimouski QC G5L 8B2; Mon'00; (418)722-6816; Fax. (418)721-3262; gege222@hotmail.com.

DRAPEAU, Gervais; Hotel-Dieu d'Arthabaska, 5 rue des Hospitalieres, Victoriaville QC G6P 6N2; Sher'77; CSPQ; FRCPC; NuclearMed. Chef méd nucl, Hotel-Dieu d'Arthabaska; (819)357-2030; Fax. (819)357-6003.

DRAPEAU, Jean-Claude; Clin Med Drapeau, 522 boul Saint-Germain, Rimouski QC G5L 3P9; Laval'72; (418)724-5111; Fax. (418)721-2336.

DRAPEAU, Monique; Dir Sante Pub L'Estrie, 300-300 rue King E, Sherbrooke QC J1G 1B1; Sher'78; CCFP; Staff, Centre Hospitalier Universitaire de Sherbrooke-Hopital Fleurimont; (819)829-3400 x42486; Fax. (819)564-5435; mdrapeau.agence05@ssss.gouv.qc.ca.

DRAPEAU, Nicole; CLSC Pierefonds, 13800 boul Gouin O, Pierrefonds QC H8Z 3H6; Laval'71; Staff VAD, CLSC Pierrefonds; Staff C H S P, Ctr d'Acc Denis-Benjamin Viger; Langs: Bilingual(French/English); (514)626-2572 x4441; Fax. (514)624-7486.

DRAPEAU, Sylvain; Clin Med Chandler, 60-201 boul Rene-Levesque O, Chandler QC G0C 1K0; Laval'93; (418)689-3344; Fax. (418)689-6085.

DRAPER, C Lewis W; Normanview Mall Med Clinic, 330 McCarthy Blvd N, Regina SK S4R 7M2; Glasgow (Scotland)'61; MB ChB; CCFP; FCFP; Assessor Workers Compensation Board, Saskatchewan Government Insurance; Langs: English; French; German; (306)924-6200; Fax. (306)924-6201.

DRAPER, Haley; Univ Hlth Network-Toronto Western Hosp, 8M CL433-399 Bathurst St, Toronto ON M5T 2S8; Tor'08; CCFP; Staff, Toronto Western Hospital - University Health Network; (416)603-5800

DRCA, Dragoslav; Family First Family Health Team, 4270 Innes Rd, Orleans ON K4A 5E6; Belgrade (Serbia)'99; Langs: Croatian; Serbian; (613)841-7009; Fax. (613)841-0106.

DREBIT, Robert H; Peace Hills Trust Tower, 406-10011 109 St NW, Edmonton AB T5J 3S8; Alb'82; FRCPC; Psy. Med Dir, University of Alberta Hospital; Consultant Psy., Child & Adolescent Serv. Assn.; Clin Associate Prof, University of Alberta; (780)415-6684; Fax. (780)415-6050; robert.drebit@ualberta.ca.

DRECKMANN, Robert H; Briarhill Med Centre, 58A-2700 Dufferin St, Toronto ON M6B 4J3; Tor'86; (416)256-2650; Fax. (416)256-5831.

DREIGE, Danny; CSSS de Manicouagan, 635 boul Jolliet, Baie-Comeau QC G5C 1P1; Laval'97; CSPQ; FRCSC; Ophth. Chef Ophtalmology Services, Centre Hospitalier Régional Baie-Comeau; Langs: English; Montagnais; (418)589-3701 x2698

DRESSELHUIS, Jeffrey F T; 202-7315 Edmonds St, Burnaby BC V3N 1A7; UBC'93; BSc; Med Staff, Royal Columbian Hospital; Clin Instructor Family Pract, University of British Columbia; Langs: Dutch; (604)524-1321

DRESSER, George K; London HSC-Univ Campus, PO Box 5339 Stn B ALL 144-339 Windermere Rd, London ON N6A 5A5; Wes'94; FRCPC; IntMed (Clinical Pharmacology)., London Health Sciences Centre - University Hospital; (519)663-3342; Fax. (519)663-3388; george.dresser@lhsc.on.ca.

DRESSLER, Brian B; 310 Larch St, Sudbury ON P3B 1M1; McM'88; (705)669-1111

DRESSLER, Jason D T; PO Box 143, Hythe AB T0H 2C0; Cal'10; CCFP; (780)356-3869

DREVER, Clint; South Calgary Urgent Care Ctre, 31 Sunpark Plaza SE, Calgary AB T2X 3W5; Sask'02; CCFP; CCFP(E.M.); Staff, South Calgary Urgent Care Centre; (403)943-9477

DREVER, Erin; Chinook Reg Hosp, 960 19 St S, Lethbridge AB T1J 1W5; Wes'07; Endocrin&Metab; IntMed. Staff, Chinook Regional Hospital; (403)388-6111

DREW, Brian M; Hamilton HS-General Site, 237 Barton St E, Hamilton ON L8L 2X2; McM'97; BHSc; FRCSC; OrthSurg (Spine). Asst Clinical Prof, Hamilton Health Sciences Centre - Hamilton General Hospital; (905)527-4322; Fax. (905)577-1428.

DREW-SCOTT, Ryan N; Penticton Reg Hosp, 550 Carmi Ave, Penticton BC V2A 3G6; Man'04; FRCPC; Psy. Staff, St Boniface General Hospital; (204)492-4000

DREWNIAK, Anna; Children's Hosp, FE 125-685 William Ave, Winnipeg MB R3E 0Z2; Man'07; FRCPC; Peds; ClinImmunol&Allergy.

DREWS, Tanya; Alberta Children's Hosp, 2888 Shaganappi Trail NW, Calgary AB T3B 6A8; Cal'94; Peds (Pediatric Critical Care). Staff Critical Care & PICU, Alberta Children's Hospital; (403)955-7931; Fax. (403)955-7081.

DREXLER, Jaroslav; Manitoba Clinic, 790 Sherbrook St, Winnipeg MB R3A 1M3; Komensky (Slovakia)'72; Staff, Concordia General Hospital; (204)788-5512; Fax. (204)775-6373.

DREYER, Christiaan; Dr CW Wiebe Med Centre, 385 Main St, Winkler MB R6W 1J2; Pretoria (South Africa)'84; MB ChB; DA; Physician Family Med, Boundary Trails Health Centre; Langs: Afrikaans; German; (204)325-4312; Fax. (204)325-4594; dreyer@winklerclinic.com.

DREYER, Francois; Hinton Med Clinic, 102 Allen Cove, Hinton AB T7V 2A6; Kansas (USA)'94; (780)865-3338; Fax. (780)865-2024.

DREYER, Hendrik A; Phoenix Med Centre, 205-2155 10th Ave, Prince George BC V2M 5J6; Stellenbosch (South Africa)'88; MB ChB; MMed; OrthSurg (Joint Replacement). Staff, University Hospital of Northern British Columbia; (250)563-9227; Fax. (250)563-9224.

DREYER, Jonathan; London HSC-Victoria Hosp, PO Box 5010 Stn B 800 Commissioners Rd E, London ON N6A 5W9; McG'77; BSc; LMCC; FRCPC; EmergMed. Staff Member, London Health Sciences Centre - Victoria Campus; Prof Med, University of Western Ontario; Langs: French; (519)667-6538; Fax. (519)667-6769; jonathan.dreyer@lhsc.on.ca.

DREYER, Nicolette M; 23C-3300 Smith Dr, Armstrong BC V0E 1B1; Stellenbosch (South Africa)'98; MB ChB; Member Peds & Sexual Assault Team, University Hospital of Northern British Columbia; Langs: Afrikaans; (250)546-8115; jpviljoen@webmail.co.za.

DREYFUSS, Valerie; CSSS Haut Richelieu Rouville, 230-383 boul du Seminaire N, St-Jean-sur-Richel QC J3B 8C5; Laval'97; FRCPC; Psy (Child & Adolescent Psychiatry). Langs: English; (450)346-2222; Fax. (450)346-2311.

DREYZIN, Ilona; Medcan Health Mgmt Inc, 1500-150 York St, Toronto ON M5H 3S5; Tor'91; CCFP; FCFP; Staff, North York General Hospital; Staff, Medcan Health Management Inc; (416)350-5900; Fax. (416)350-5981.

DREYZIN, Vadim; Kingsway Financial Spinal Ctr, 3F-150 Sherway Dr, Etobicoke ON M9C 1A5; Tor'94; CCFP; FCFP; Ac Staff, Mackenzie Richmond Hill Hospital; Ac Staff, North York General Hospital; Ac Staff, Humber River Regional Hospital - Church Street Site; Court Staff, Trillium Health Centre - Mississauga; Court Staff, Trillium Health Centre - West Toronto; Ac Staff, Humber River Regional Hospital - Finch Avenue Site; Langs: Russian; (416)521-4141; Fax. (416)521-4140.

DRIEDGER, Albert; London HSC-South Street Hosp, PO Box 5375 Stn B 375 South St, London ON N6A 4G5; Sask'63; PhD; ABNM; FACPE; FACP; FRCPC; IntMed (Oncology); NuclearMed. Staff, London Health Sciences Centre - Victoria Campus; Staff, London Health Sciences Centre - South Street; Prof Med, University of Western Ontario; (519)667-6570; Fax. (519)667-6734; al.driedger@lhsc.on.ca.

DRIEDGER, Bernhard E; Dr B E Driedger Inc, 107-117 10th Ave S, Cranbrook BC V1C 2N1; Alb'78; FRCSC; OrthSurg (Rehabilitation Medicine). Staff, East Kootenay Regional Hospital; (250)426-3235; Fax. (250)426-7138.

DRIEDGER, Brian D; 2-32904 Ventura Ave, Abbotsford BC V2S 6J3; Sask'90; (604)859-1211; Fax. (604)852-8466.

DRIEDGER, G Emmi; Central Alberta Prof Centre, 182-5201 43 St, Red Deer AB T4N 1C7; Qns'08; Peds. (403)343-6404

DRIJBER, Philip; Health Care Centre, PO Box 398 75 Parkview Rd, Hagersville ON N0A 1H0; Man'92; CCFP; FCFP; Staff, West Haldimand General Hospital; (905)768-1979; Fax. (905)768-3801.

DRIJBER, Shirley E; Health Care Centre, PO Box 398 1-75 Parkview Rd, Hagersville ON N0A 1H0; Wes'89; (905)768-1979; Fax. (905)768-3801.

DRIMAN, David K; London HSC-University Hosp, PO Box 5339 Stn B A3 142-339 Windermere Rd, London ON N6A 5A5; Cape Town (South Africa)'84; FRCPC; AnatPath (Gastrointestinal Pathology). Staff Path, London Health Sciences Centre - University Hospital; Prof Path, University of Western Ontario; (519)685-8500 x36378; Fax. (519)663-2930; david.driman@lhsc.on.ca.

DRIMAN, Naomi M; 303-343 Wilson Ave, North York ON M3H 1T1; Tor'08; CCFP; (416)785-8412; Fax. (416)785-8324.

DRISCOLL, Miriam A; Purdy Pavilion, M41-2221 Wesbrook Mall, Vancouver BC V6T 1Z9; UBC'96; FRCPC; Psy. Staff, Vancouver General Hospital - Centennial Pavillion; (604)822-3690

DRIVER, Katy F; 311-311 Sherbourne st, Toronto ON M5A 3Y1; Madras (India)'62; DCH; AB; FRCPC; Peds. Ac Staff, The Hospital For Sick Children; Asst Prof Peds, University of Toronto; (416)960-0072; Fax. (416)928-7546; dsvdoctors@bellnet.ca.

DRIVER, Kelly L; St Joseph's Health Centre, 4SSW-30 The Queensway, Toronto ON M6R 1B5; Qns'98; FRCPC; Psy. Staff, St Joseph's Health Centre; (416)530-6000 x4240; Fax. (416)530-6076.

DRIVOD, Marie-Laure; CHUM-Hotel-Dieu, 3840 rue Saint-Urbain, Montreal QC H2W 1T8; Mon'05; CCFP; Staff, Centre Hospitalier l'Université de Montréal (CHUM) - Hôtel-Dieu; (514)890-8000 x15010; Fax. (514)412-7114.

DRKULEC, Frank; 5115 Tecumseh Rd E, Windsor ON N8T 1C2; Wes'90; Langs: Croatian; (519)944-0005; Fax. (519)944-3731.

DROBAC, Milutin; 100-3695 Keele St, North York ON M3J 1N2; Wes'74; FRCPC; IntMed; Cardiol. Staff, Women's College Hospital; Asst Prof, University of Toronto; Langs: Serbian; (416)630-7540

DROBOT, Glen R; St Boniface Gen Hosp, C5010-409 Tache Ave, Winnipeg MB R2H 2A6; Man'96; FRCPC; IntMed. Staff, St Boniface General Hospital; (204)233-8563

DRODGE, Karen H; The Ottawa Hosp-Gen Campus, 501 Smyth Rd, Ottawa ON K1H 8L6; Mem'94; CCFP; Staff, The Ottawa Hospital - General Campus; (613)737-7700

DROHOMYRECKY, Anthony; 1-280 Manitoba St PO Box 10010 Stn Main, Bracebridge ON P1L 1W6; Tor'82; DAB; FRCSC; Urol. Urology, South Muskoka Memorial Hospital - Muskoka Algonquin Healthcare; Urology, Huntsville District Memorial Hospital - Muskoka Algonquin Healthcare; Langs: Ukrainian; (705)645-3111; droho@muskoka.com.

DROLET, Celyne; Centre d'Urgenge de Salaberry, 2758 rue de Salaberry, Montreal QC H3M 1L3; Mon'78; Langs: English; (514)337-4772; Fax. (514)337-4923.

DROLET, Christian; CHUQ-Ctr Hosp Univ Laval, 2705 boul Laurier, Quebec QC G1V 4G2; Mon'03; FRCPC; Peds; Cardiol. Staff, Centre Hospitalier Universitaire de Quebec-CHUL; (418)654-2708; christian.drolet@mail.chuq.qc.ca.

DROLET, Christine; CHUQ-Ctr Hosp Univ Laval, 2705 boul Laurier, Quebec QC G1V 4G2; Laval'04; FRCPC; Peds (Neonatal & Perinatal Medicine). Staff, Centre Hospitalier Universitaire de Quebec-CHUL; (418)525-4444

DROLET, Denise; Clinique Med de l'Atelier, 77 boul Seigneurial O, Saint-Bruno QC J3V 2G9; Laval'86; Staff Family Med, Clinique Medicale de l'Atelier; Med Consultant, VAC; Staff Med Collaborateur, Programme D'aide aux Medecine du Quebec; (450)461-1751; Fax. (450)461-1602.

DROLET, Francois; 104-201 rue Dupont, Pont-Rouge QC G3H 1N7; Laval'73; GP/Cardiol, CSSS de Portneuf; (418)873-4197; Fax. (418)873-5117; francois.drolet@ssss.gouv.qc.ca.

DROLET, Gaetan; Clinique Med des Trois Lacs, 160-585 av Saint-Charles, Vaudreuil-Dorion QC J7V 8P9; Mon'94; Staff, Centre Hospitalier de Verdun; Staff, Centre Hospitalier Régional du Suroît; Universite de Montreal; (450)455-3322

DROLET, Guillaume; CHUQ-Hotel-Dieu de Quebec, 11 Cote du Palais, Quebec QC G1R 2J6; Laval'04; FRCPC; Anes. Staff, Centre Hospitalier Universitaire de Québec (CHUQ) - Siege Social; (418)525-4444

DROLET, Isabelle; Hotel-Dieu de Levis, 143 rue Wolfe, Levis QC G6V 3Z1; Laval'98; FRCSC; Otol. Staff, Hôtel-Dieu de Lévis; (418)835-7121

DROLET, Jean-Philippe; CHUQ-Ctr Hosp Univ Laval, H1340-2705 boul Laurier, Quebec QC G1V 4G2; Laval'04; FRCPC; Peds; ClinImmunol&Allergy. Staff, Centre Hospitalier Universitaire de Quebec-CHUL; (418)654-2240; Fax. (418)654-2770.

DROLET, Manon; CSSS du Nord de Lanaudière, 1000 boul Sainte-Anne, St-Charles-Brromee QC J6E 6J2; Mon'90; Ac Staff Geriatrics, Centre Hospitalier Régional de Lanaudière; (450)759-8222

DROLET, Marianne; CSSS de Rivière-du-Loup, 75 rue St-Henri, Riviere-du-Loup QC G5R 2A4; Laval'98; Staff Med, Centre Hospitalier Regional du Grand-Portage; (418)856-4647

DROLET, Marie-Josee; ASSS-Chaudiere Appalaches, 363 Rte Cameron, Sainte-Marie QC G6E 3E2; Laval'90; MSc; FRCPC; CommunMed (Palliative Care). Staff, Hôtel-Dieu de Lévis; (418)389-1545; Fax. (418)389-1540; marie-josee.drolet@ssss.gouv.qc.ca.

DROLET, Michel J; CSSS de Portneuf, 700 rue Saint-Cyrille, Saint-Raymond QC G3L 1W1; Laval'64; Staff Chief Dept of Gen Med, Centre Hospitalier Affilié Universitaire de Québec - Hôpital du St-Sacrement; Staff, Centre Hospitalier Portneuf; Teach Staff, Université Laval; (418)337-4611

DROLET, Normand; Clinique Med Ste-Croix, 6350 rue Principale CP 370, Sainte-Croix QC G0S 2H0; Laval'72; (418)926-3260; Fax. (418)926-2014.

DROLET, Patrice; Centre de Sante Valcartier, CP 1000 Bdp Succ Forces, Courcelette QC G0A 4Z0; Laval'85; FRCPC; IntMed. (418)844-5000 x5888; Fax. (418)844-6671.

DROLET, Pierre; CHUQ-Hotel-Dieu de Quebec, 11 Cote du Palais, Quebec QC G1R 2J6; Laval'81; CSPQ; Anes. Staff, Centre Hospitalier Universitaire de Québec (CHUQ) - Siege Social; (418)691-5323; Fax. (418)691-5728.

DROLET, Pierre-A; Hop Maisonneuve-Rosemont, 5415 boul de l'Assomption, Montreal QC H1T 2M4; Laval'81; CSPQ; FRCPC; Anes. Staff, Hopital Maisonneuve-Rosemont; Dept Head Anes, Universite de Montreal; (514)252-3426; Fax. (514)252-3542.

DROLET, Renald; 479 boul Saint-Jude, Alma QC G8B 3J7; Laval'69; (418)668-3351; Fax. (418)668-5772.

DROLET, Richard; GMF Centre medical AJC, 300-110 rue Saint-Jean, Drummondville QC J2B 7T1; Laval'93; Otol. Staff, Hôpital Sainte-croix; (819)857-4777

DROLET, Sebastien; Foothills Med Ctr, 1024-1403 29 St NW, Calgary AB T2N 2T9; Laval'04; FRCSC; GenSurg (Colorectal Surgery). Staff, Foothills Medical Centre; (403)944-1110

DROLET, Sophie; CHUS-Hop Fleurimont, 3001 12e av N, Sherbrooke QC J1H 5N4; Laval'96; CSPQ; FRCPC; Anes. Staff, Centre Hospitalier Universitaire de Sherbrooke-Hopital Fleurimont; (819)346-1110 x7243

DROLET, Terrence A; Associate Clinic, 5215 49 Ave, Wetaskiwin AB T9A 0R1; Alb'60; CCFP; Ac Staff, Wetaskiwin Hospital & Care Centre; Med Examiner, Province of Alberta; (780)352-7157; Fax. (780)352-2273.

DROLET, Yvan; Hotel-Dieu de Quebec, 11 Cote du Palais, Quebec QC G1R 2J6; Laval'65; MedOncol (P.Q.); Hem (P.Q.); Peds., Centre Hospitalier Universitaire de Québec (CHUQ) - Siege Social; Clin Prof, Université Laval; (418)691-5225; yvandrolet@videotron.ca.

DROLL, Kurt P; Big Thunder Orthopaedic Assoc, 206-984 Oliver Rd, Thunder Bay ON P7B 7C7; Tor'00; FRCSC; OrthSurg. (807)344-1123

DROMEY, Edel; Sturgeon Community Hosp, 201 Boudreau Rd, St. Albert AB T8N 6C4; Alb'96; BSc; MSc; CCFP; CCFP(E.M.); Staff, Sturgeon Community Hospital; (780)418-8229

DRONE, Troy C; Grand River Hosp-KW Hlth Ctre, PO Box 9056 Stn C 835 King St W, Kitchener ON N2G 1G3; Tor'94; FRCPC; Anes. Staff, Grand River Hospital - Kitchener/Waterloo Health Centre; (519)744-7361

DROPINSKI, Jean-Pierre; Hotel-Dieu de Levis, 143 rue Wolfe, Levis QC G6V 3Z1; (Belgium)'02; Staff, Hôtel-Dieu de Lévis; (418)835-7121

DROR, Yigal; The Hosp For Sick Children, 555 University Ave, Toronto ON M5G 1X8; Hebrew (Israel)'91; FRCPC; Peds (Pediatric Oncology); Hem. Scientist Cell Biology Program/Staff Hematologist/Oncologist, The Hospital For Sick Children; Assoc Prof/Clin Scientist/Staff Hem, University of Toronto; Langs: Hebrew; (416)813-5886; yigal.dror@sickkids.ca.

DROSDOWECH, Catriona H; London Reg Cancer Centre, 790 Commissioners Rd E, London ON N6A 4L6; Man'89; CCFP; FCFP; (519)685-8600

DROSDOWECH, Darren S; St Joseph's Health Care, PO Box 5777 Stn B 268 Grosvenor St, London ON N6A 4V2; Man'89; FRCSC; OrthSurg (Shoulder). Staff, St Joseph's Hospital - St Joseph's Health Care; (519)646-6047; Fax. (519)646-6049.

DROST, Nicole Z A; St Joseph's Healthcare, T2134-50 Charlton Ave E, Hamilton ON L8N 4A6; Ott'03; FRCPC; IntMed; Respir. Staff, St Joseph's Healthcare - Charlton Campus; (905)522-1155

DROUIN, Charles; Clinique Med de Matane, 101-548 av du Phare E, Matane QC G4W 1A7; Laval'86; (418)562-4530; Fax. (418)562-4532.

DROUIN, Christian A; CSSS de Rivière-de-Loup, 75 rue Saint-Henri, Riviere-Du-Loup QC G5R 2A4; Laval'87; CSPQ; FRCPC; Derm (Geriatric Medicine). Staff Derm, Centre Hospitalier Regional du Grand-Portage; assoc Prof Derm, Université Laval; Langs: English; Spanish; German; (418)868-1000 x2627; Fax. (418)868-1032; cadrouin@videotron.ca.

DROUIN, Christine; 143 rue Wolfe, Levis QC G6V 3Z1; Laval'97; FRCPC; IntMed; Critical Care Medicine (P.Q.); Respir. Staff, Hôtel-Dieu de Lévis; Langs: Bilingual(French/English); (418)835-7121

DROUIN, Denis; Centre Med Le Mesnil, 300-1300 boul Lebourgneuf, Quebec QC G2K 2N1; Laval'75; (418)624-1800

DROUIN, Eric; Hôpital Ste-Justine, 3175 ch Cote-Ste-Catherine, Montreal QC H3T 1C5; Mon'88; CSPQ; FRCPC; Peds; Gastroent (P.Q.). Staff Ped Gastroent, Hôpital Ste-Justine; Dir Program MD, Universite de Montreal; Langs: English; (514)345-4626; Fax. (514)345-4999.

DROUIN, Francois; Clinique Fam de St-Hyacinthe, 2955 boul Laframboise, Saint-Hyacinthe QC J2S 4Z3; Sher'84; Staff, Centre Hospitalier Honore-Mercier; (450)774-4611; Fax. (450)773-9913.

DROUIN, Guy; CHUM-Hop St-Luc, 1058 rue Saint-Denis, Montreal QC H2X 3J4; Mon'62; FACS; CSPQ; FRCSC; Urol (Andrology). Staff, Centre Hospitalier l'Université De Montréal (CHUM) - Hôpital Saint-luc; Assoc Prof Surg Univ de Montreal Ecole d'Arch, Universite de Montreal; (514)890-8000

DROUIN, Guy; CSSS de la Cote-de-Gaspe, 215 boul de York O, Gaspe QC G4X 2W2; Laval'92; CCFP; FCFP; Staff, Centre Hospitalier de Gaspe; (418)368-3301; Fax. (418)368-5358.

DROUIN, Jacques; Centre Med Fafard Enr, 201-975 boul Monseigneur-de la, Baie-Saint-Paul QC G3Z 2W3; Laval'72; (418)435-6310; Fax. (418)435-3203.

DROUIN, Jacques; 7300 boul Gouin O, Montreal QC H4K 1B6; Mon'59; Psy (P.Q.) (General Psychiatry). (514)331-7995; Fax. (514)331-7995.

DROUIN, Jean; Clinique Med St-Vallier, 201-205 rue Montmagny, Quebec QC G1N 4V3; Laval'92; Staff, Hôpital général de Québec - CHSLD; Langs: English; (418)688-0872; Fax. (418)688-4951.

DROUIN, Jean; CHUQ-Ctr Hosp Univ Laval, 1185-2705 boul Laurier, Quebec QC G1V 4G2; Laval'73; LMCC; ac Staff, Centre Hospitalier Universitaire de Quebec-CHUL; Langs: Bilingual(French/English); (418)654-2167; Fax. (418)654-2172; dr.jean.drouin@chuq.qc.ca.

DROUIN, Johanne F; 110-8627 91 St NW PO Box 48025 Rpo Dynamique, Edmonton AB T6C 3N1; Ott'83; CCFP; Langs: English; French; (780)450-8635; Fax. (780)450-8602.

DROUIN, Johanne; Ctr Medi Soleil St-Jean-Sur-Ri, 120-383 boul du Seminaire N, St-Jean-sur-Richel QC J3B 8C5; Mon'95; FRCSC; Urol. Staff, Hôpital du Haut-Richelieu; Langs: Bilingual(French/English); (450)347-7557 x226; Fax. (450)347-3099.

DROUIN, Julie; Clin de Rhumatologie du Quebec, 1119 rue Sainte-Marguerite, Trois-Rivieres QC G8Z 1Y2; Laval'04; Rheum; IntMed. (819)370-8106; Fax. (819)370-8120.

DROUIN, Louis; Dir de la Sante Publique-Mtl, 1301 rue Sherbrooke E, Montreal QC H2L 1M3; Mon'72; MPH; CommunMed (P.Q.) (Environmental Health). Staff, Hopital Maisonneuve-Rosemont; Staff, Direction de Sante Publique de Montreal; (514)528-2400 x3235; Fax. (514)528-2459.

DROUIN, Michel A; 1308-12 rue des Jardins-Merici, Quebec QC G1S 4Z8; Laval'68; FRCP; DABACI; FRCPC; ClinImmunol&Allergy (P.Q.); IntMed (P.Q.) (Allergy). Langs: French; (418)527-8514; madrouin7@gmail.com.

DROUIN, Michel; CHSLD Champlain-Manoir de Verd, 1325 rue Crawford, Verdun QC H4H 2N6; Mon'79; Staff, Centre d'hébergement Champlain; (514)766-8513; Fax. (514)766-3731.

DROUIN, Michel; CLSC de Forestville, 2 7e rue CP 790, Forestville QC G0T 1E0; Laval'74; (418)587-2212; Fax. (418)587-2865.

DROUIN, Michele; FMSQ-Dir Affaires Economiques, 3000-2 Complexe Desjardins, Montreal QC H5B 1G8; Mon'82; FRCPC; DiagRad. Staff, Centre Hospitalier de Verdun; (514)350-5015; Fax. (514)350-5150.

DROUIN, Mylene; Dir de la Sante Publique-Mtl, 1301 rue Sherbrooke E, Montreal QC H2L 1M3; Sher'96; FRCPC; CommunMed; Public Health & Preventive Med. (514)528-2400 x3501; Fax. (514)528-2463.

DROUIN, Pierre; CHUM-Hop Notre-Dame, 1560 rue Sherbrooke E, Montreal QC H2L 4M1; Ott'68; CSPQ; FRCSC; ObstGyn (Gynecologic Oncology). ac Staff GynOncol, Centre Hospitalier l'Université de Montréal (CHUM) - Hôpital Notre-Dame; Prof, Universite de Montreal; Langs: Bilingual(French/English); (514)890-8000 x26793; Fax. (514)412-7604; pierre.drouin.chum@ssss.gouv.qc.ca.

DROUIN, Regen; CHUS-Hop Fleurimont, 1428-3001 12e av N, Sherbrooke QC J1H 5N4; Mon'83; AB; PhD; MedGenetics (P.Q.) (Clinical Genetics). Clin Chercheur Fac. of Med & Health Sci, Centre Hospitalier Universitaire de Sherbrooke-Hopital Fleurimont; Langs: Bilingual(French/English); (819)820-6827

DROUIN, Richard; Clin Med Mont Ste-Anne, 100-10974 boul Ste-Anne RR 1, Beaupre QC G0A 1E0; Laval'88; Staff, Hôpital Sainte Anne de Beaupré; (418)827-4022; Fax. (418)827-4964.

DROUIN, Simon; CSSS de Beauce-Etchemin, 1515 17e rue, Saint-Georges QC G5Y 4T8; Laval'93; CSPQ; FRCSC; GenSurg. GenSurg, Centre Hospitalier Beauce-Etchemin; (418)228-2031

DROUIN, Simon; Centre Hosp Honore-Mercier, 2750 boul Laframboise, Saint-Hyacinthe QC J2S 4Y8; Laval'10; CCFP; Staff, Centre Hospitalier Honore-Mercier; (450)771-3333

DROUIN, Suzanne E; Leger & Associes Radiologistes, 201-1851 rue Sherbrooke E, Montreal QC H2K 4L5; Laval'97; DABR; FRCPC; DiagRad (Diagnosis). Langs: Bilingual(French/English); (514)523-2121; Fax. (514)526-9147.

DROUIN, Sylvie; Clinique de Med Fam Montcalm, 309 rue Montcalm, Chicoutimi QC G7J 2V1; Laval'85; LMCC; ac Staff, Complexe hospitalier de la Sagamie; (418)545-4212; Fax. (418)545-2920.

DROUIN, Yves; CSSS Drummond-Hop Sainte-Croix, 570 rue Heriot, Drummondville QC J2B 1C1; Mon'91; LMCC; FRCPC; DiagRad. Staff, Hôpital Sainte-croix; Langs: English; (819)478-6464; Fax. (819)478-6480.

DROUIN-BERUBE, Nicolas; CSSS Becancour-Nicolet-Yamaska, 216 rue Principale, Fortierville QC G0S 1J0; Laval'04; CCFP; (819)287-4442; Fax. (819)287-0143.

DROVER, Aidan; Trinity Conception Health Ctre, PO Box 903 Stn Main 16 Goff Ave, Carbonear NL A1Y 1C4; Mem'74; (709)596-5136; Fax. (709)596-0212.

DROVER, Alison C; Torbay Med Clinic, B-1345 Torbay Rd, Torbay NL A1K 1B2; Bristol (England)'04; CCFP; Clinical Asst Prof Family Med, Health Sciences Centre.

DROVER, Chris; Paton Med Clinic, 219-1 Paton St, St. John's NL A1B 4S8; Mem'01; FRCSC; Otol. (709)579-0209

DROVER, Douglas N; Health Sciences Centre, 300 Prince Philip Dr, St. John's NL A1B 3V6; Mem'87; FRCSC; Urol (Incontinence). Staff Urol, Health Sciences Centre; Clin Asst Prof Surg Urology, Memorial University Of Newfoundland; (709)777-6300

DROVER, H Blair; Campbell Med Group, 39 Campbell Ave, St. John's NL A1E 2Z3; Mem'86; BMedSci; Physician Emerg, Eastern Health Corporate Office; (709)579-5001; Fax. (709)579-4499.

DROVER, John W; Kingston Gen Hosp, 76 Stuart St, Kingston ON K7L 2V7; Dal'84; BSc; FACS; FRCSC; GenSurg (Critical Care Medicine). Ac Staff, Hotel-Dieu Hospital; Asst Prof Med, Queen's University; (613)549-6666 x4159; Fax. (613)548-2456; droverj@kgh.kari.net.

DROVER, Shauna; Grey Bruce HS-Owen Sound, PO Box 1800 Stn Main 1800 8th St E, Owen Sound ON N4K 6M9; Mem'05; FRCPC; DiagRad. Supt-Fibreline, Grey Bruce Health Services - Owen Sound; (519)376-2121; Fax. (519)372-3954.

DRU, Gilbert; Medical Complex, 103-1057 St Peter Ave, Bathurst NB E2A 2Z6; Lyon (France)'83; FRCPC; Psy (Infant Psychiatry). Psychiatrist, Hopital Regional Chaleur; Dept Chief, Vitalite; Prof, University Of Sherbrooke; Langs: Bilingual(French/English); (506)546-3355; Fax. (506)546-9997.

DRUCK, Maurice N; Credit Valley Prof Bldg, 504-2300 Eglinton Ave W, Mississauga ON L5M 2V8; Tor'75; ABIM; FACC; FASN(Cardiol); FRCPC; IntMed; Cardiol. Assoc Staff, Trillium Health Centre - Mississauga; Ac Staff Cardiol, The Credit Valley Hospital; Staff Teacher, Toronto Western Hospital - University Health Network; RGA Reinsurance Co.; Assoc Prof Med, University of Toronto; Langs: Yiddish; (905)820-5525; Fax. (905)820-6342.

DRUCKER, Arnold M; Queen Elizabeth II HSC, 464-1276 South Park St, Halifax NS B3H 2Y9; Mem'02; FRCPC; IntMed; MedOncol. Staff, Queen Elizabeth II Health Sciences Centre - Victoria General Site; (902)473-6054

DRUCKER, Daniel J; Mount Sinai Hosp, TCP5 1004-600 University Ave, Toronto ON M5G 1X5; Tor'80; FRCPC; IntMed (Health Technology Assessment). Staff, Mount Sinai Hospital; Scientist, Samuel Lunenfeld Research Institute; Prof, University of Toronto; (416)361-2661; Fax. (416)361-2669; d.drucker@utoronto.ca.

DRUCKMAN, Paul B; 126-400 Walmer Rd, Toronto ON M5P 2X7; Tor'61; DPsy; Psy (Adult & Child Psychiatry). Staff, The Hospital For Sick Children; Clin Teacher, Centre for Addiction & Mental Health (CAMH) - College Street Site; Assoc Prof, University of Toronto; (416)920-9816; druckman@sympatico.ca.

DRUKER, Jennifer; Children's & Women's HC of BC, 2D18B-4480 Oak St, Vancouver BC V6H 3V4; Cape Town (South Africa)'76; MB ChB; DCH; FRCPC; Peds. Staff, BC Children's Hospital; Clin Assoc Prof, University of British Columbia; (604)875-2345; Fax. (604)875-2890.

DRUMMOND, Alan J; 20 Drummond St W, Perth ON K7H 2J5; McG'78; CCFP; CCFP(E.M.); FCFP; Ac Staff, Perth & Smiths Falls District Hospital - Perth Site (Great War Memorial Site); Clin Asst Prof Family Med/Emerg Med, University of Ottawa; Clinical Asst Prof Family Med, Queen's University; (613)267-6222; Fax. (613)267-8770.

DRUMMOND, Alasdair R; Stettler Med Clinic, PO Box 1210, Stettler AB T0C 2L0; Glasgow (Scotland)'75; MB ChB; MRC(UK); Ac Staff, Stettler Hospital and Care Centre; (403)742-3441; Fax. (403)742-3299; adrummond@dthr.ab.ca.

DRUMMOND, Derek S; Alberta Children's Hosp, 2888 Shaganappi Trail NW, Calgary AB T3B 6A8; Alb'92; BSc; MPH; FRCSC; Otol (Pediatric Otolaryngology). Staff, Alberta Children's Hospital; Asst Prof, University of Calgary; (403)955-7211

DRUMMOND, Douglas; Specialized Seniors Clinic, 232 Ross St, New Westminster BC V3L 0B2; Wes'75; BA; FCFP; CCFP; FCFP; Staff, University Hospital of Northern British Columbia; Clin Assoc Prof Family Practice, University of British Columbia; (604)528-5031

DRUMMOND, Garry T; Clinical Sciences Bldg, 2 133-152 University Campus NW, Edmonton AB T6G 2G3; Cal'82; BSc; DAB(Oph); FRCSC; Ophth (Pediatric Ophthalmology). Staff, University of Alberta Hospital; Prof, University of Alberta; (780)407-6417; Fax. (780)407-6681.

DRUMMOND, Robbie N; Royal University Hosp, 103 Hospital Dr, Saskatoon SK S7N 0W8; McG'84; CCFP; CCFP(E.M.); Staff, Royal University Hospital; (306)655-1363; Fax. (306)655-1011.

DRUMMOND, Robert; St-Mary's Hosp Centre, 3830 av Lacombe, Montreal QC H3T 1M5; McG'91; CCFP; CCFP(E.M.); FCFP; Staff, St Mary's Hospital Centre; Staff, Perth & Smiths Falls District Hospital - Perth Site (Great War Memorial Site); (514)345-3511; Fax. (514)734-2644.

DRURY, Kathryn J; Durham College Health Centre, G1030-2000 Simcoe St N, Oshawa ON L1H 7L7; Ott'95; CCFP; Staff, Rouge Valley Health System - Ajax & Pickering Health Centre Site; (905)721-3037; Fax. (905)721-3133.

DRURY, Megan B; Shuswap Lake Gen Hosp, PO Box 520 Stn Main 601 10th St NE, Salmon Arm BC V1E 4N6; Washington(WA) (USA)'96; Staff, Shuswap Lake General Hospital; (250)833-3635

DRURY, Robert; Ross Mem Hosp, 10 Angeline St N, Lindsay ON K9V 4M8; Tor'74; Staff, Ross Memorial Hospital; (705)324-6111

DRUSS, Elizabeth C; The Ottawa Hosp-Civic Campus, A6-1053 Carling Ave, Ottawa ON K1Y 4E9; Columbia(NY) (USA)'92; FRCPC; Psy. Staff, The Ottawa Hospital - Civic Campus; (613)761-4581; Fax. (613)761-5328; edruss@ottawahospital.on.ca.

DRUTZ, Harold P; The Hydro Place Bldg, 815-700 University Ave, Toronto ON M5G 1Z5; Tor'69; FACOG; FSOGC; FRCSC; ObstGyn (Reconstructive Surgery). Staff Chief UroGyn, Mount Sinai Hospital; Staff Chief UroGyn, Baycrest Centre for Geriatric Care; Prof/Head Section of UroGyn, University of Toronto; (416)586-4642; Fax. (416)586-3208.

DRUTZ, Randall A; Scarborough North Med Arts, LL3-4040 Finch Ave E, Scarborough ON M1S 4V5; Tor'77; CCFP; FCFP; Ac Staff, Rouge Valley Health System - Centenary Health Centre Site; Ac Staff, The Scarborough Hospital - General Campus; Ac Staff, The Scarborough Hospital - Birchmount Campus; (416)292-0014; Fax. (416)292-0031.

DRY, Marissa; Border City Clinic, 2707 50 Ave, Lloydminster SK S9V 2A8; Pretoria (South Africa)'01; Ac Staff, Lloydminster Hospital; Langs: Afrikaans; (306)825-4427

DRYBROUGH, Marjolein C; Signal Hill Centre, 2-5986 Signal Hill Ctr SW, Calgary AB T3H 3P8; Man'89; CCFP; FCFP; (403)240-2660; Fax. (403)242-8390.

DRYDEN, Fiona A; Beaver Valley Clinic, PO Box 610 1957 Columbia Gardens Rd, Fruitvale BC V0G 1L0; Edinburgh (United Kingdom)'89; CCFP; (250)367-9211

DRYDEN, Peter J; Rebalance MD, 104-3551 Blanchard St, Victoria BC V8Z 0B4; UBC'96; BSc; MSc; FRCSC; OrthSurg. (250)381-5424; Fax. (250)385-8150.

DRYER, Dagny E; Queen Elizabeth Hosp, PO Box 6600 Stn Central 60 Riverside Dr, Charlottetown PE C1A 8T5; Tor'72; AB; FRCPC; IntMed (Medical Oncology); Hem. Staff Dept PEI Cancer Treatment Centre & Oncology Clinic, Queen Elizabeth Hospital; Consultant, Kings County Memorial Hospital; Dir, PEI Cancer Registry; Teach Staff, Dalhousie University; (902)894-2027; Fax. (902)894-2187.

DRYER, Donna A; 205-2786 16th Ave W, Vancouver BC V5K 4M1; Brown(RI) (USA)'85; FRCPC; Psy. (604)733-4400

DRYSDALE, Anne; Linden Prof Centre, 24 Linden Ave, Charlottetown PE C1A 5Y8; Dal'78; DAB; FRCSC; Ophth. (902)628-2020; Fax. (902)566-5392.

DRYSDALE, Elaine R; BC Cancer Agency-Vancouver CC, 552-600 10th Ave W, Vancouver BC V5Z 4E6; Cal'78; FRCPC; Psy (Psychiatric Oncology). Staff, BC Cancer Agency Vancouver Centre; Ac Staff, Vancouver General Hospital - Centennial Pavillion; Clin Assoc Prof Psy, University of British Columbia; (604)877-6000 x2194; edrysdal@bccancer.bc.ca.

DRYSDALE, Ian O; The Medical Centre, PO Box 4200 Stn Main 707 Charlotte St, Peterborough ON K9J 7B3; Dal'61; FRCSC; Ophth (Comprehensive Ophthalmology). Staff Ophth, Peterborough Regional Health Centre - Hospital Drive; (705)876-4502; Fax. (705)740-8381.

DRYSDALE, John D; PO Box 1599, Middleton NS B0S 1P0; Dal'10; CCFP.

DRYSDALE, Robert A; Golden Med Clinic, PO Box 1170, Golden BC V0A 1H0; Qns'81; (250)344-6863; Fax. (250)344-7620.

DRYSDALE-BUHR, Carolyn L; Halifax Prof Centre, 425-5991 Spring Garden Rd, Halifax NS B3H 1Y6; Dal'85; (902)422-6220

DRZYMALA, Lukasz; 905-1243 Islington Ave, Etobicoke ON M8X 1Y9; Tor'03; FRCPC; IntMed; Cardiol. Staff, St Joseph's Health Centre; Langs: Polish; (416)233-4242 x3

DU CAP, Alexis; CSSS du Lac-des-Deux-Montagnes, 520 boul Arthur-Sauve, Saint-Eustache QC J7R 5B1; Mon'09; Staff, Hôpital de Saint-Eustache; (450)473-6811

DU PLESSIS, Aldine; Spesmed Med Specialist Ctr, PO Box 1540 Stn Main 2591 99 St, North Battleford SK S9A 3W1; Free State (South Africa)'92; MB ChB; LMCC; Staff, Battlefords Union Hospital; (306)446-5540; Fax. (306)446-5553.

DU PLESSIS, Catharina H; Willoughby Med Centre, B1A-20202 66 Ave, Langley BC V2Y 1P3; Pretoria (South Africa)'88; MB ChB; (604)514-8800

DU PLESSIS, Gert C; Three Sisters Obst & Fam Med C, 106-75 Dygras Gate, Canmore AB T1W 0A6; Stellenbosch (South Africa)'87; MB ChB; CCFP; CCFP(E.M.); Staff ER MD, Canmore General Hospital; Langs: Afrikaans; (403)609-9095; Fax. (403)609-7232.

DU PLESSIS, Hendrik; Spesmed Med Specialist Ctr, PO Box 1540 Stn Main 2591 99th St, North Battleford SK S9A 3W1; (South Africa)'88; FRCSC; GenSurg. (306)446-5555

DU PLESSIS, Jean G; Sleeping Beauty Med Clinic, 2715 Tetrault St, Terrace BC V8G 2W6; Stellenbosch (South Africa)'71; MB ChB; MMed(Peds); LMCC; Langs: Afrikaans; (250)638-4089; Fax. (250)615-5418; jannie@telus.net.

DU PLESSIS, Johan; Glenvalley Med Centre, 207-437 Glenmore Rd, Kelowna BC V1V 1Y5; Stellenbosch (South Africa)'86; MB ChB; CCFP; FCFP; Medical Staff, Kelowna General Hospital; Langs: Afrikaans; (250)860-5811; Fax. (250)860-2811.

DU PLESSIS, Lienki; 208-803 Chaparral Dr SE, Calgary AB T2X 0E5; (South Africa)'03; MB ChB; (403)837-7734; Fax. (403)837-7735.

DU PLESSIS, Magda; Smith Clinic, 1-6601 48 Ave, Camrose AB T4V 3G8; (South Africa)'02; MB ChB; (780)679-2425

DU PLESSIS, Marietjie; The Maple Tree Med Clinic, 1181 6 Ave NE, Salmon Arm BC V1E 2S5; Orange Free State (South Africa)'01; MB ChB; Langs: English; (250)832-9361; Fax. (250)833-4781.

DU PLESSIS, Marlie; Dakota Med Centre, 17-845 Dakota St, Winnipeg MB R2M 5M3; Orange Free State (South Africa)'99; MB ChB; CCFP; (204)254-2087

DU PLESSIS, Mia; Edson Med Centre, PO Box 6660 Stn Main 616 50th St, Edson AB T7E 1V1; (South Africa)'05; MB ChB; Langs: Afrikaans; (780)723-3366; Fax. (780)723-3437.

DU PLESSIS, Nicolaas; 102-9725 98 Ave, Grande Prairie AB T8V 8K5; Kansas (USA)'86; (780)402-6643; Fax. (780)402-6697.

DU PLESSIS, Pierre; D1-6935 Harvie Ave, Powell River BC V8A 5H9; Stekkenbosch (South Africa)'78; MB ChB; FRCSC; ObstGyn. Langs: Afrikaans; (604)485-7779

DU PLESSIS, Stephan J; Foothills Med Centre, 1403 29 St NW, Calgary AB T2N 2T9; (South Africa)'90; MB ChB; Staff, Foothills Medical Centre; (403)944-4776; Fax. (403)283-2270.

DU PLOOY, Daniel; High Level Med Clinic, 11202 100 Ave, High Level AB T0H 1Z0; (South Africa)'83; (780)926-2286; Fax. (780)923-3550.

DU PLOOY, Johan; Western Manitoba Cancer Centre, 300 McTavish Ave E, Brandon MB R7A 2B3; Pretoria (South Africa)'78; Staff, Brandon Regional Health Centre; Langs: Afrikaans.

DU PLOOY, Magarietha J; Magriet du Plooy Ped Consultin, 279-5201 43 St, Red Deer AB T4N 1C7; (South Africa)'95; MB ChB; LMCC; FCP (SA); MMed; Langs: Afrikaans; (403)986-3601; Fax. (403)986-3604; mdpadmin@shaw.ca.

DU PLOOY, Rian; Lloydminster Clinic, 5120 46 St, Lloydminster AB T9V 2P7; Stellenbosch (South Africa)'88; MB ChB; (780)875-2221; Fax. (780)875-0605.

DU PLOOY SHUEL, Sian; Alder Med Centre, 277 Evergreen Rd, Campbell River BC V9W 3R5; Man'05; CCFP; (250)287-7441; Fax. (250)287-4384.

DU PREEZ, Amelia; Bonnyville Med Clinic, PO Box 1007 Stn Main 4610 50 St, Bonnyville AB T9N 2J7; (South Africa)'90; MB ChB; Langs: Afrikaans; (780)826-3346; Fax. (780)826-6362.

DU PREEZ, Anneline; Kimberley Med Clinic, PO Box 160, Kimberley BC V1A 2Y6; Pretoria (South Africa)'98; MB ChB; CCFP; Physician Emerg Room, East Kootenay Regional Hospital; Langs: Afrikaans; (250)427-4861; Fax. (250)427-2082.

DU PREEZ, Joachim J; 100 Easton Dr PO Box 5000 Stn Main, Selkirk MB R1A 2M2; Pretoria (South Africa)'90; MB ChB; ATLS; ACLS; AddicMed; Med Officer Emerg, Selkirk & District General Hospital; Media Dir, SkyMedical Air Ambulance; Lecturer Emerg Med, University of Manitoba; Langs: Afrikaans; (204)482-5800 x20119; Fax. (204)487-7947; jdmed@mts.net.

DU PREEZ, Johannes C; Westview Hlth Ctr Stony Plain, 4405 South Park Dr, Stony Plain AB T7Z 2M7; (South Africa)'93; MB ChB; CCFP; CCFP(E.M.); Staff, Medicine Hat Regional Hospital; Staff, Westview Health Centre; (780)968-3600

DU PREEZ, Miranda; 101-595 Columbia St W, Kamloops BC V2C 1K7; Pretoria (South Africa)'98; MB ChB; FCFP; FamilyMed. Staff Family Med, Royal Inland Hospital; Langs: Afrikaans; (250)372-1080; Fax. (250)372-5236.

DU PREEZ, Quinton; The Medical Clinic, 10011 96 St, Fort St. John BC V1J 3P3; Orange Free State (South Africa)'04; MB ChB; (250)785-6677; Fax. (250)787-0109.

DU RAND, Jean; St Paul's Hosp, 1702 20th St W, Saskatoon SK S7M 0Z9; (South Africa)'05; MB ChB; Staff, St Paul's Hospital (Grey Nuns) of Saskatoon; (306)655-5280; Fax. (306)655-5914.

DU RAND, Mia; St Paul's Hosp, 1702 20th St W, Saskatoon SK S7M 0Z9; (South Africa)'05; MB ChB; Staff ICU, St Paul's Hospital (Grey Nuns) of Saskatoon; (306)655-5280; Fax. (306)655-5914.

DU RUSSEL, Michelle; Victoria Square Med Clinic, 217-2345 10th Ave W, Prince Albert SK S6V 7V6; Ott'01; BSc; FRCPC; Peds. Staff, Victoria Square Medical Clinic; Asst Prof, University of Saskatchewan; (306)953-5664; Fax. (306)922-9394.

DU SAULT, Karine; CSSS d'Argenteuil, 145 av de la Providence, Lachute QC J8H 4C7; Mon'08; CCFP; Staff, Centre Hospitalier d'Argenteuil; (450)562-3761

DU SOUICH, Bertrand; Inst de Recherche Clin de Mtl, 110 av des Pins O, Montreal QC H2W 1R7; Barcelona (Spain)'68; PhD; LMCC; ac Staff, Centre Hospitalier l'Université de Montréal (CHUM) - Hôtel-Dieu; Staff, Institut de Recherches Cliniques de Montreal; Prof, Universite de Montreal; Langs: English; Spanish; (514)987-5600

DU TOIT, Abraham; Moose Jaw Union Hosp, 455 Fairford St E, Moose Jaw SK S6H 1H3; Pretoria (South Africa)'81; MB ChB; Staff, Moose Jaw Union Hospital; (306)694-0382; Fax. (306)694-0219.

DU TOIT, Andre; Central Saanich Med Clinic, 1932 Mount Newton Cross Rd, Saanichton BC V8M 2B1; Stellenbosch (South Africa)'77; MB ChB; CCFP; (250)652-2041; Fax. (250)652-0738.

DU TOIT, Anton E; Griffiths Med Clinic, 28-5201 50 St, Leduc AB T9E 6T4; Orange Free (South Africa)'00; MB ChB; CCFP; Langs: Afrikaans; (780)986-6200; Fax. (780)986-5200.

DU TOIT, Corne; Kelowna Gen Hosp, 2268 Pandosy St, Kelowna BC V1Y 1T2; Pretoria (South Africa)'92; MB ChB; FRCPC; Anes. Staff, Kelowna General Hospital; (250)862-4000; Fax. (250)862-4020.

DU TOIT, Daniel J; Medical Arts Bldg, 206-42 Glen Allan Dr, Bridgewater NS B4V 3N2; Stellenbosch (South Africa)'98; MB ChB; (902)530-3256

DU TOIT, Daniel M; High Prairie Assoc Clinic, PO Box 1350, High Prairie AB T0G 1E0; (South Africa)'99; (780)523-2868; Fax. (780)523-2875; molsen@acp-mn.com.

DU TOIT, Dirk L; 4212 55 Ave PO Box 1340, Smoky Lake AB T0A 3C0; (780)656-2100; Fax. (780)656-2507.

DU TOIT, Elmarie; Univ of Saskatchewan, 4F-1 Campus Dr, Saskatoon SK S7N 5A3; MB ChB; Staff Student Hlth & Counselling Serv, University Of Saskatchewan; (306)966-5768; Fax. (306)966-5786.

DU TOIT, Francois J; PO Box 939, Stettler AB T0C 2L0; Bloemfontein (South Africa)'90; MB ChB; (403)742-4011; Fax. (403)742-4013.

DU TOIT, Jacobus J; Miramichi Reg Hosp, 500 Water St, Miramichi NB E1V 3G5; Pretoria (South Africa)'67; MMed; MRC(Lond); FRCOG(Lond); Staff, Miramichi Regional Hospital; Langs: Afrikaans; Sotho; (506)778-1803; Fax. (506)778-2585.

DU TOIT, Jacobus J J; 104-8980 Mary St, Chilliwack BC V2P 4J3; Pretoria (South Africa)'99; MB ChB; DA(SA); (604)392-0881

DU TOIT, Jacques H; 4539 Marine Ave, Powell River BC V8A 2K5; Stellenbosch (South Africa)'81; MB ChB; Langs: Afrikaans; (604)485-2430

DU TOIT, Linda; Dauphin Med Clinic, 622 3rd St SW, Dauphin MB R7N 1R5; Stellenbosch (South Africa)'98; MB ChB; (204)638-6445

DU TOIT, Lionel; Border City Clinic, 2707 50 Ave, Lloydminster SK S9V 2A8; Stellenbosch (South Africa)'05; BSc; MB ChB; Staff, Lloydminster Hospital; Langs: Afrikaans; (306)825-4427; Fax. (306)825-2028.

DU TOIT, Martha C; Family Health Clinic, PO Box 4127 Stn Main B10-5011 48 Ave, Ponoka AB T4J 1R5; (South Africa)'05; MB ChB; LMCC; Langs: Afrikaans; (403)783-5305; Fax. (403)783-8722.

DU TOIT, Nadia; Royal Alexandra Hosp, 10240 Kingsway NW, Edmonton AB T5H 3V9; (South Africa)'02; MB ChB; Staff, Royal Alexandra Hospital; (587)879-0278

DU TOIT, Petrus J J; 106-22838 Lougheed Hwy, Maple Ridge BC V2X 2V6; Orange Free State (South Africa)'85; MB ChB; MSc; (604)463-4165

DU TOIT, Petrus; 231 3 Ave NE SS 2, Slave Lake AB T0G 2A2; (780)849-4155; Fax. (780)849-4574.

DU TOIT, Regina M; Regional Treatment Centre, PO Box 22 560 King St W, Kingston ON K7L 4V7; Mem'00; FRCPC; Psy. (613)331-2322

DU TOIT, Stefanus E; Southwest Medi-Centre, 500-1 Springs Dr, Swift Current SK S9H 3X6; Orange Free state (South Africa)'97; MB ChB; Langs: Afrikaans; (306)773-4681; Fax. (306)778-3449.

DU TREMBLAY, Jean; Centre Med Fam de Baie-Comeau, 189 av Damase-Potvin, Baie-Comeau QC G4Z 2Y9; Laval'83; (418)296-9355

DU TREMBLAY, Pierre; Polyclinique de la Capitale, 7-4225 4e av O, Quebec QC G1H 6P3; Laval'74; CSPQ; FRCSC; OrthSurg. Ac Staff, Centre Hospitalier Universitaire De Québec - Pavillon De St-françois-d'assise; (418)623-9872; Fax. (418)623-9873.

DU TREMBLAY, Renee; Clinique Med D'Alma, 935 av du Pont S, Alma QC G8B 2V5; Laval'83; (418)668-6121; Fax. (418)668-5298.

DU VERNET, Chantal J; Perth-Smiths Falls Dist Hosp, 60 Cornelia St W, Smiths Falls ON K7A 2H9; Alb'92; CCFP; CCFP(E.M.); Staff, Perth & Smiths Falls District Hospital - Smiths Falls Site; Staff, Queensway Carleton Hospital; Langs: English; French; (613)283-2330

DUA, Hemi; Univ Hlth Network-Princess M, 610 University Ave, Toronto ON M5G 2M9; Tor'04; FRCPC; DiagRad. Staff, Princess Margaret Hospital - University Health Network; Staff, Mount Sinai Hospital; (416)946-4501

DUA, Manjula; Red Deer Med Centre, 202-3947 50A Ave, Red Deer AB T4N 6V7; Alb'86; BSc; FRCPC; Psy (Adult Psychiatry). (403)341-4303; Fax. (403)341-4322.

DUA, Mini; Yellowbird Family Clinic, 3380 Gateway Blvd NW, Edmonton AB T6J 6V1; Alb'90; (780)434-2893; Fax. (780)435-1057.

DUA, Varinder; Regional Mental HC-London, PO Box 5532 Stn B 850 Highbury Ave, London ON N6A 4H1; Punjab (India)'84; MB BS; FRCPC; Psy (Tertiary Care Psy). Staff Psy., Regional Mental Health Care-St Joseph's Health Care; Staff Psy., Regional Mental Health Care-St Joseph's Health Care; Adjunct. Prof. Psy., University of Western Ontario; Langs: Punjabi; Hindi; (519)434-9666 x47332; Fax. (519)434-9952.

DUA, Vikram; Provincal Health Services, 3644 Slocan St, Vancouver BC V5M 3E8; McM'90; FRCPC; Psy. (604)453-8300; Fax. (604)453-8390.

DUARTE DE ALMEIDA BRANDAO, Guilerme; SMBD Jewish Gen Hosp, 3755 ch Cote-Sainte-Catherine, Montreal QC H3T 1E2; (Brazil)'96; AnatPath. Staff, Sir Mortimer B Davis Jewish General; (514)340-8222 x2498

DUBARSKY, Howard B; Hunt Club Med Centre, 100-3328 McCarthy Rd, Ottawa ON K1V 0H9; Dal'89; CCFP; (613)596-5009; Fax. (613)596-5230.

DUBBERLEY, James; Pam Am Clinic, 75 Poseidon Bay, Winnipeg MB R3M 3E4; Man'96; FRCSC; OrthSurg (Trauma Surgery). Staff, Victoria General Hospital; Staff, Health Sciences Centre; (204)925-1578; Fax. (204)927-2675; jdubberley@panamclinic.com.

DUBBIN, James; Sunnybrook Hlth Sciences Ctre, A223-2075 Bayview Ave, Toronto ON M4N 3M5; Tor'75; FACC; FRCPC; Cardiol; IntMed. Staff, Sunnybrook Health Sciences Centre; Asst Prof Med, University of Toronto; (416)480-4750; Fax. (416)480-5193.

DUBE, Andre; CSSS du Nord de Lanaudière, 1000 boul Sainte-Anne, St-Charles-Brromee QC J6E 6J2; Laval'88; CSPQ; FRCPC; Anes. Staff, Centre Hospitalier Régional de Lanaudière; (450)759-8222 x2960; Fax. (450)759-8289; andre.dube@ssss.gouv.qc.ca.

DUBE, Anne; CLSC des Collines, 1884 Rte du Carrefour, Val-des-Monts QC J8N 7N5; Sher'93; Staff, Centre d'hébergement - La Pietà; Physician, CLSC Jean-Olivier-Chenier; (819)459-1112 x5119; Fax. (819)671-8257.

DUBE, Benoit; CSSS d'Antoine-Labelle, 2561 ch Lievre S, Mont-Laurier QC J9L 3G3; Laval'09; CCFP; Staff, CSSS d'Antoine-Labelle; (819)623-1234

DUBE, Chantal; Clin Imagerie des Pionniers, 130-950 montee des Pionniers, Terrebonne QC J6V 1S8; Mon'88; FRCPC; DiagRad. Staff, Centre Hospitalier Pierre le Gardeur; (450)581-1424

DUBE, Charlotte; CSSS de la Vallée de l'Or, 725 6e St, Val-d'Or QC J9P 3Y1; Mon'89; Staff, Centre Hospitalier de Val d'Or; (819)825-5858

DUBE, Christian; Ctr Hosp Rouyn-Noranda, 4 9e rue, Rouyn-Noranda QC J9X 2B2; Laval'95; FRCPC; Psy. Staff, Centre Hospitalier Rouyn-Noranda; Langs: English; (819)764-5131 x43807; Fax. (819)764-2921.

DUBE, Christine; Montfort Hosp, 713 Montreal Rd, Ottawa ON K1K 0T2; Laval'98; CCFP; CCFP(E.M.); Staff, Montfort Hospital; Langs: Bilingual(French/English); (613)746-4621 x4202

DUBE, Denis; CSSS de Maskinonge, 450 2e rue, Louiseville QC J5V 1V3; Mon'81; Staff, CSSS de Maskinongé; (819)228-2731

DUBE, Francois; Inst Univ Cardiol & Pneumologi, 2725 ch Sainte-Foy, Quebec QC G1V 4G5; Mon'83; FRCPC; IntMed (Diabetology). ac Membre, Hôpital Laval; Staff, Institut Universitaire Cardiologie & Pneumologie de Quebec; Langs: English; (418)656-4511; Fax. (418)656-4587; frandube@videotron.ca.

DUBE, Ghislain; Clinique Med St-Vallier, 201-205 rue Montmagny, Quebec QC G1N 4V3; Laval'73; LMCC; ac Staff, CHSLD Vigi Our Lady of Lourdes; (418)688-0872; Fax. (418)688-4951.

DUBE, Helene; CLSC Villeray, 1425 rue Jarry E, Montreal QC H2E 1A7; Mon'85; Langs: Bilingual(French/English); (514)376-4141 x4419; Fax. (514)376-4023; samy.mecheddal.edi@ssss.gouv.qc.ca.

DUBE, Jean; CHUS-Hop Fleurimont, 3001 12e av N, Sherbrooke QC J1H 5N4; Laval'99; CSPQ; FRCPC; MedBiochem. Staff, Centre Hospitalier Universitaire de Sherbrooke-Hopital Fleurimont; (819)346-1110 x14087

DUBE, Jean-Marie; Ctr Hosp Pierre-Janet, 20 rue Pharand, Gatineau QC J9A 1K7; Mon'82; Chef Med/Staff, Centre Hospitalier Pierre-Janet; (819)776-8047; Fax. (819)776-8048.

DUBE, Jean-Nicolas; CSSS de Trois-Rivières, 1991 boul Camel, Trois-Rivieres QC G8Z 3R9; Ott'03; FRCPC; IntMed; Critical Care Medicine (P.Q.). Staff, Centr Hosp Pavillon Sainte-Mar; (819)697-3333

DUBE, Jeanne C; Teaching Research and Wellness, 6F-3280 Hospital Dr NW, Calgary AB T2N 4N1; Mon'89; MSc(Pharmacol&Epidemiol; FRCPC; IntMed; Gastroent. Staff, Foothills Medical Centre; (403)592-5089

DUBE, Johanne; Hôpital Ste-Justine, 3175 ch Cote-Ste-Catherine, Montreal QC H3T 1C5; Mon'90; FRCSC; ObstGyn (Perinatal). Staff, Hôpital Ste-Justine; (514)345-4931 x7326

DUBE, Julie; CSSS Pierre Boucher, 1333 boul Jacques-Cartier E, Longueuil QC J4M 2A5; Sher'92; FRCPC; PhysMed&Rehab. Staff, Centre Hospitalier Pierre Boucher; (450)468-8111

DUBE, Laurier; Clinique Med Jean-Talon-Pie-IX, 4679 rue Jean-Talon E, Saint-Leonard QC H1S 1K3; Laval'82; (514)374-5901; Fax. (514)374-1668.

DUBE, Louis-Jacques; Reso-Concorde, 300 boul de la Conocrde E, Laval QC H7G 2E6; Laval'70; CSPQ; LMCC; DiagRad (Neuro Radiology). Radiologist, Radiologie Laennec Inc; (450)668-7376; Fax. (450)668-8300.

DUBE, Magalie; PO Box 74212 Rpo Beechwood, Ottawa ON K1M 2H9; Mon'91; LMCC; ABR; FRCPC; DiagRad (Ultrasound). Radiologist, Perth & Smiths Falls District Hospital - Smiths Falls Site; Physician Consultant, Canadian Medical Association; Langs: Bilingual(French/English); (613)282-7045

DUBE, Marie-Helene; GMF Les Gres, 104-190 rue Saint-Honore, St-Etienne-de-Gres QC G0X 2P0; Mon'05; (819)535-6512

DUBE, Marie-Josee; 117 Hunter St E, Hamilton ON L8N 1M5; Laval'98; FRCSC; ObstGyn. Staff, St Joseph's Healthcare - Charlton Campus; Langs: Bilingual(French/English); (905)526-0555; Fax. (905)526-0515.

DUBE, Marie-Pier; CSSS de la Haute-Yamaska, 205 boul Leclerc O, Granby QC J2G 1T7; CCFP; Staff, Centre Hospitalier de Granby; (450)375-8000

DUBE, Mark R; 1744 Oriole Dr, Sudbury ON P3E 5L7; Ott'85; CCFP; CCFP(E.M.); FCFP; Langs: Spanish; French; (705)522-2263

DUBE, Melissa; GMF Saguenay, 220-874 boul de l'Universite E, Chicoutimi QC G7H 6B9; Laval'08; (418)545-1217; Fax. (418)545-4782.

DUBE, Michel; Hop Maisonneuve-Rosemont, 5415 boul de l'Assomption, Montreal QC H1T 2M4; Mon'89; DiagRad. Staff, Hopital Maisonneuve-Rosemont; (514)252-3533; Fax. (514)252-3537.

DUBE, Michel; 220-504 rue Notre-Dame, Repentigny QC J6A 2T8; Sher'84; (450)582-8417; Fax. (450)582-6589.

DUBE, Nancy; Clinique de Med Familiale, 101 rue Lavoie, Rimouski QC G5L 5Y2; Laval'86; (418)723-5272; Fax. (418)725-2030.

DUBE, Nathalie; Regie des Rentes du Quebec, CP 5200 Succ Terminus 348-2600 boul Laurier, Quebec QC G1K 7S9; Laval'91; Physician, Regie des Rentes du Quebec; (418)657-8709 x3230; Fax. (418)528-0404.

DUBE, Normand; 200-2984 boul Taschereau, Greenfield Park QC J4V 2G9; Laval'82; FRCPC; IntMed; ClinImmunol&Allergy. ac Membre, Centre Hospitalier l'Université de Montréal (CHUM) - Hôpital Notre-Dame; Clin Staff, Universite de Montreal; (450)465-9789; Fax. (450)672-4578.

DUBE, Pascale; CSSS Les Eskers de l'Abitibi, 622 4e rue O, Amos QC J9T 2S2; McG'97; FRCSC; Ophth (Anterior Segment). Staff, CH Hôtel-Dieu d'Amos; Langs: English; (819)732-3341

DUBE, Paul; Clinique du Dr Paul Dube, CP 240 211 rue Ste-Anne, Nominingue QC J0W 1R0; Mon'74; (819)278-3322; Fax. (819)275-7381.

DUBE, Paule; Centre Oculaire de Quebec, 050-2480 ch Sainte-Foy, Quebec QC G1V 1T6; Sher'85; FRCSC; Ophth. Staff, Centre Hospitalier Affilié Universitaire de Québec - Hôpital du St-Sacrement; Staff, Centre Hospitalier Universitaire de Québec (CHUQ) - Siege Social; Langs: Bilingual(French/English); (418)780-6345

DUBE, Pierre; Hop Maisonneuve-Rosemont, 5415 boul de l'Assomption, Montreal QC H1T 2M4; Mon'89; CSPQ; FACS; FRCSC; GenSurg (Hepatobiliary Surgery); General Surgical Oncology (P.Q.). Dir GenSurg & Oncol, Hopital Maisonneuve-Rosemont; (514)252-3822; Fax. (514)252-3430.

DUBE, Rejean; CHUQ-Hotel-Dieu de Quebec, 11 Cote du Palais, Quebec QC G1R 2J6; Laval'81; FRCPC; IntMed; Gastroent. Consultant, CSSS de Quebec-Sud; Staff, Centre Hospitalier Universitaire de Québec (CHUQ) - Siege Social; Langs: English; (418)691-5252; Fax. (418)691-5484.

DUBE, Robert; Ctr Hosp Affilie-Enfant-Jesus, 1401 18e rue, Quebec QC G1J 1Z4; Laval'67; LMCC; CSPQ; FRCPC; AnatPath (P.Q.). Dir AnathPath & Otology, Centre Hospitalier Affilié Universitaire de Québec - Hôpital du St-Sacrement; Dir AnatPath, Centre Hospitalier Affilié Universitaire de Québec - Hôpital De L'Enfant Jésus; Langs: English; (418)649-5725; Fax. (418)649-5856.

DUBE, Robert; Hôpital Ste-Justine, 3175 ch Cote-Ste-Catherine, Montreal QC H3T 1C5; Sher'74; FRCPC; Peds. ac Staff, Hôpital Ste-Justine; (514)345-4789

DUBE, Roger; Polyclinique Boreale, 668 rue de Parfondeval, Baie-Comeau QC G5C 3R3; Laval'83; Staff, Centre Hospitalier Régional Baie-Comeau; (418)589-2222; Fax. (418)589-8302.

DUBE, Sampurnanand; Prairie Med Clinic, 10309 98 St, Grande Prairie AB T8V 2E7; Calcutta (India)'63; Ac Staff, Queen Elizabeth II Hospital; Langs: Hindi; (780)539-4010; Fax. (780)538-2290; samdube@telusplanet.net.

DUBE, Serge; Clinique Med Pierre-Bertrand, 212-303 boul Pierre-Bertrand, Quebec QC G1M 3L7; Laval'85; CSPQ; CCFP; FCFP; Clin Prof, Université Laval; (418)683-2724; Fax. (418)683-8861; serge.dube@orlo.ulaval.ca.

DUBE, Serge; Hop Maisonneuve-Rosemont, 5415 boul de l'Assomption, Montreal QC H1T 2M4; Mon'74; MSc; FRSM; ABS; FACS; CSPQ; FRCSC; GenSurg (Colon & Rectal Surgery). Chef Dept of Surg, Hopital Maisonneuve-Rosemont; Member, American College; Member, Canadian Society of Colon & Rectal Surgeons; Prof, Universite de Montreal; (514)252-3822

DUBE, Suzanne; MUHC-Montreal Gen Hosp, 1650 av Cedar, Montreal QC H3G 1A4; Laval'78; FRCPC; IntMed. Staff, McGill University Health Centre - Montreal General Campus; (514)934-8054

DUBE, Sylvie; CLSC des Faubourgs, 1250 rue Sanguinet, Montreal QC H2X 3E7; Mon'90; CCFP; Langs: Bilingual(French/English); (514)527-9565 x3720; Fax. (514)380-8216; sdube88@live.ca.

DUBE, Valerie; Sunnybrook Hlth Sciences Ctr, E4 32-2075 Bayview Ave, Toronto ON M4N 3M5; Laval'00; CSPQ; FRCPC; AnatPath (P.Q.). Staff, Sunnybrook Health Sciences Centre; (416)480-6100 x4014

DUBE, Valerie; CHUQ-Ctr Hosp Univ Laval, 2705 boul Laurier, Quebec QC G1V 4G2; Laval'02; FRCPC; Psy. Staff, Centre Hospitalier Universitaire de Quebec-CHUL; (418)654-2121; Fax. (418)654-2132.

DUBE, Yolande; Ctr Hosp Affilie-St-Sacrement, 1050 ch Sainte-Foy, Quebec QC G1S 4L8; Laval'74; FRCSC; Ophth. Staff, Centre Hospitalier Affilié Universitaire de Québec - Hôpital du St-Sacrement; Staff, Centre Universitaire D'Ophtamologie; Chef Ophthalmology & O R L, Université Laval; Langs: Bilingual(French/English); (418)682-7680

DUBE, Yolande; Clinique Med de Hauteviille, 4435 boul de Hauteville, Terrebonne QC J6X 2Y6; Sher'77; CCFP; (450)492-3153; Fax. (450)492-9380.

DUBEAU, Francois; MUHC-Montreal Neurology Inst, 138-3801 rue University, Montreal QC H3A 2B4; Mon'78; FRCPC; Neur (Epilepsy); Electroenceph (P.Q.). Dir EEG, McGill University Health Centre - Montreal Neurological Hospital; Assoc Prof Neurol Surg, McGill University; Langs: Bilingual(English/French); (514)398-1911; Fax. (514)398-2745; francois.dubeau@mcgill.ca.

DUBEAU, Richard A; St Mary's Gen Hosp, 911 Queens Blvd, Kitchener ON N2M 1B2; Wes'83; FRCPC; NuclearMed. Med Dir Dept of Nuclear Med, St Mary's General Hospital; (519)749-6495; Fax. (519)749-6997.

DUBEC, Jiri J; Centricare Med Clinic, 104-8140 120 St, Surrey BC V3W 3N3; UBC'00; BSc; CCFP; Langs: Tagalog; Bicol; (604)593-6616; Fax. (604)593-6617.

DUBETA, Kenneth R; Pacific Cosmetic Facial Surg I, 300-1144 Burrard St, Vancouver BC V6Z 2A5; Alb'67; FAAFPRS; FASLMS; FRCSC; Otol (Facial Plastic Surgery). Ac Staff, Providence Health Care - St Paul's Hospital; Ac Staff, Providence Health Care - Mount Saint Joseph Hospital; Vis Staff, BC Children's Hospital; Dir, Pan Asia Academy of Facial Plastic & Reconstructive Surg; Clinical Asst Prof, University of British Columbia; (604)689-1585; Fax. (604)689-1586; info@drkendubeta.com.

DUBEY, Arbind A; Allan Blair Cancer Ctr, 4101 Dewdney Ave, Regina SK S4T 7T1; FRCPC; RadOncol. Staff, Allan Blair Cancer Centre; (306)766-2288

DUBEY, Santosh; Falconridge Med Clinic, 929-5075 Falconridge Blvd NE, Calgary AB T3J 3K9; Rajasthan (India)'89; MB BS; Staff, Smart Health Medical Clinic; Langs: Hindi; Arabic; Punjabi; (403)265-5221; Fax. (403)265-5229; falconridgeclinic@gmail.com.

DUBEY, Vinita; Toronto Public Health, 10F-277 Victoria St, Toronto ON M5B 1W2; Cal'01; BSc; MPH; FRCPC; CommunMed;CCFP; Staff EmergMed, Lakeridge Health - Bowmanville Site; Staff EmergMed, Alexandra Hospital; (416)397-4696; Fax. (416)392-1482.

DUBIN, Ruth; Kingston Family Health Team, 403-800 Princess St, Kingston ON K7L 5E4; Alb'85; BSc; PhD; CCFP; FCFP; Assoc Staff, Kingston General Hospital; Staff Pain Consultant, St Mary's General Hospital; Assoc Staff Family Med., Hotel-Dieu Hospital; Court Staff, Ongwanada Resource Centre; Langs: Spanish; French; (613)549-0464; Fax. (613)549-0490; rdubin@kfhn.net.

DUBINS, Jacques H; 200-480 Lawrence Ave W, North York ON M5M 1C4; Tor'69; Ac Staff, North York General Hospital - Branson Division; Langs: French; Spanish; (416)787-1255; Fax. (416)787-1256.

DUBINSKI, William; Humber River Reg Hosp-Church, 200 Church St, Toronto ON M9N 1N8; Qns'07; AnatPath. Staff, Humber River Regional Hospital - Church Street Site; (416)249-8111

DUBINSKY, Isser L; Hay Group Ltd, 7F-121 King St W, Toronto ON M5H 3X7; Tor'75; BSc; CCFP; CCFP(E.M.); FCFP; Assoc Dir, Hay Group Hlth Care Consulting; Assoc Prof DFCM, University of Toronto; Langs: Hebrew; French; (416)815-6418; Fax. (416)868-0362; isser.dubinsky@haygroup.com.

DUBINSKY, Leslie; Veterans Affairs Canada, 4F-40 Alderney Dr, Dartmouth NS B2Y 2N5; Dal'71; Staff Regional M O, Atlantic Region Veteran Affairs Canada; (902)426-7791; Fax. (902)426-7447; leslie.dubinsky@vac-acc.gc.ca.

DUBLAND, Edward J; Collingwood Medical, 350-3150 54th Ave E, Vancouver BC V5S 1Z1; UBC'81; (604)435-3388; Fax. (604)433-2323.

DUBO, Elyse D; Sunnybrook Hlth Sciences Ctre, GF FW-2075 Bayview Ave, Toronto ON M4N 3M5; McM'88; FRCPC; Psy (Child & Adolescent Psychiatry). Staff, Sunnybrook Health Sciences Centre; Asst Prof Psy, University of Toronto; (416)480-4098; Fax. (416)480-6818.

DUBOIS, Alain; Groupe Sante Medisys, 1100-500 rue Sherbrooke O, Montreal QC H3A 3C6; Mon'70; (514)845-1211

DUBOIS, Alain; Clinique Med D'Amos, 641 4e rue O, Amos QC J9T 2S1; Mon'80; (819)732-0717; Fax. (819)732-4646.

DUBOIS, Brian J; 1569 6th Ave, Prince George BC V2L 3N4; UBC'87; FRCSC; GenSurg. (250)563-0680

DUBOIS, Chantal; Clinique Med Avenir Md, 220-1575 boul de l'Avenir, Laval QC H7S 2N5; Sher'95; FRCSC; ObstGyn. (450)696-1025

DUBOIS, Chantal; Clinique Medicale de l'Archiga, 26 mtee Remi-Henri, St-Roch-de-l'Achig QC J0K 3H0; Sher'94; CCFP; Staff, Centre Hospitalier Régional de Lanaudière; Langs: English; (450)588-4321; Fax. (450)588-7466.

DUBOIS, Claude; Hotel-Dieu du Sorel, 400 av de l'Hotel-Dieu, Sorel-Tracy QC J3P 1N5; Mon'71; FRCSC; PlasSurg (P.Q.). Staff, Hôtel-Dieu de Sorel; (450)746-6000

DUBOIS, Danielle; Regie l'Assurance Maladie QC, 1125 Grande Allee O, Quebec QC G1S 1E7; Laval'82; Peds (P.Q.). Staff, Regie de l'Assurance Maladie du Quebec; (418)682-5144 x4065

DUBOIS, David; Postgrad Med Education, M106-1151 Richmond St, London ON N6A 5B7; Laval'07; FRCPC; Anes.

DUBOIS, David; Clin Med Les Gres, 104-190 rue St Honore, St-Etienne-Ds-Gres QC G0X 2P0; Laval'95; Member Emerg, Centre Lafleche Grand-Mere; Member Emerg Med, CMCN de Shawinigan-Sud; (819)535-6512; Fax. (819)535-1627.

DUBOIS, Denise M; Brameast Family Health Org, 38-2130 North Park Dr, Brampton ON L6S 0C9; Queen's (Ireland)'79; MB ChB; MRCGPract; DObst; DRCOG; Ac Staff, William Osler Health System - Brampton Civic Hospital; (905)792-2211; Fax. (905)792-2901.

DUBOIS, Elizabeth J; Frontenac Med Associates, 201-791 Princess St, Kingston ON K7L 1E9; Pretoria (South Africa)'92; CCFP; Langs: Afrikaans; (613)544-2727; Fax. (613)544-7247.

DUBOIS, Emmanuelle; CSSS de Saint-Jerome, 290 rue de Montigny, Saint-Jerome QC J7Z 5T3; Mon'99; FRCSC; ObstGyn. Staff, Hôtel-Dieu de Saint-Jérôme; (450)431-8200

DUBOIS, Jean-Yves; Queen Elizabeth Hosp, PO Box 6600 Stn Central 60 Riverside Dr, Charlottetown PE C1A 8T5; Sher'78; CSPQ; FRCPC; Anes. Staff, Queen Elizabeth Hospital; (902)894-2111; Fax. (902)894-2146.

DUBOIS, John R; 202-717 Richmond St, London ON N6A 1S2; Ann Arbor(MI) (USA)'56; ABPN; BSc; FRCPC; Psy (Child & Adolescent Psychiatry). Emeritus Prof Psychiatry, University of Western Ontario; (519)858-5800; Fax. (519)672-7323.

DUBOIS, Josee; Hôpital Ste-Justine, 3175 ch Cote-Ste-Catherine, Montreal QC H3T 1C5; Sher'84; FRCPC; DiagRad. Chief-Radiol, Hôpital Ste-Justine; vice Doyen Postgraduate Studies, Universite de Montreal; (514)345-4637; Fax. (514)345-4816.

DUBOIS, Manon; Lakeshore Gen Hosp, 160 av Stillview, Pointe-Claire QC H9R 2Y2; Mon'98; CCFP; Staff, Lakeshore General Hospital - Pointe Claire; (514)630-2166

DUBOIS, Marc-Jacques; CHUM-Hotel-Dieu, 3840 rue Saint-Urbain, Montreal QC H2W 1T8; Mon'94; FRCPC; IntMed; Critical Care Medicine (P.Q.). Staff, Centre Hospitalier l'Université de Montréal (CHUM) - Hôtel-Dieu; (514)890-8000

DUBOIS, Marie-Eve; Hotel-Dieu de Sorel, 400 av de l'Hotel-Dieu, Sorel-Tracy QC J3P 1N5; Mon'09; CCFP; Staff, Hôtel-Dieu de Sorel; (450)746-6000

DUBOIS, Marie-Josee; Service Med Prive, 105-100 boul de Montarville, Longueuil QC J4B 5M4; Mon'95; Gen Practice, CSSS de la Minganie; (450)641-6774; marie-josee_dubois@ssss.gouv.qc.ca.

DUBOIS, Mario; Clin de Med Familiale Jonquier, 3835 boul Harvey, Jonquiere QC G7X 2Z5; Laval'76; Staff, Centre Hospitalier Jonquiere; (418)542-7510; Fax. (418)542-6541; mario.dubois.cmj@ssss.gouv.qc.ca.

DUBOIS, Marion; Carrefour de Sante de Jonquier, CP 1200 Succ PDF Jonquiere 2229 rue de l'Hopital, Jonquiere QC G7X 7X2; Laval'03; Staff, Centre Hospitalier Jonquiere; (418)695-7700; Fax. (418)695-7715.

DUBOIS, Nadine; CHUQ-St-Francois D'Assise, 10 rue de l'Espinay, Quebec QC G1L 3L5; Laval'97; CCFP; Staff, Centre Hospitalier Universitaire De Québec - Pavillon De St-françois-d'assise; (418)525-4351; Fax. (418)525-4322.

DUBOIS, Pascale; Ctr Hosp de Verdun, 4000 boul Lasalle, Verdun QC H4G 2A3; Sher'90; FRCPC; IntMed. Staff, Centre Hospitalier de Verdun; (514)362-1000; Fax. (514)765-7306.

DUBOIS, Paul M; Professional Arts Bldg, 421-100 Arden St, Moncton NB E1C 4B7; Ott'76; DAB; FACS; FRCSC; GenSurg; ThorSurg. Consultant, Dr Georges-L-Dumont University Hospital Centre; Clin Instructor, Dalhousie University; (506)857-0569; Fax. (506)855-9513; pmdubois@nbnet.nb.ca.

DUBOIS, Pierre; 945 rue Saint-Jean, Roberval QC G8H 2H3; Laval'81; CSPQ; GenSurg (P.Q.) (Gastroenterology). Staff, Hotel-Dieu de Roberval; (418)275-3125; christine291@sympatico.ca.

DUBOIS, Richard; 1543 boul des Forges, Trois-Rivieres QC G8Z 1T7; Laval'89; (819)697-2777; Fax. (819)697-1731.

DUBOIS, Robert; 650 boul de la Gappe, Gatineau QC J8T 7S8; Sher'77; FRCSC; PlasSurg (Cosmetics). (819)561-1070; Fax. (819)561-4990; dr.dubois@videotron.ca.

DUBOIS, Suzy; 200-394 rue Saint-Vallier, Chicoutimi QC G7H 4J1; Mon'91; FRCSC; ObstGyn (Vulvar Disease). Staff, CRSSS de la Baie-James; Staff, Centre Hospitalier Jonquiere; Staff, Complexe hospitalier de la Sagamie; Langs: English; (418)545-2666; Fax. (418)545-3924.

DUBORD, Greg M; 850-36 Toronto St, Toronto ON M5C 2C5; Mem'86; MPH; BMedSci; Dir, Toronto Centre For Cognitive Therapy; (416)777-6699

DUBORD, Janet Y; PO Box 18006 Rpo Kerrisdale, Vancouver BC V6M 4L3; Alb'92.

DUBORD, Paul; Medical Bldg, 1603-805 Broadway W, Vancouver BC V5Z 1K1; Alb'75; FRCSC; Ophth (Cornea). Consultant, Providence Health Care - St Paul's Hospital; Member Expert Advisory Panel on Human Cell Tissue & Organ Transpant, World Health Organization; Clin Prof, University of British Columbia; (604)875-8889; Fax. (604)879-9154.

DUBREUCQ, Jean-Luc; Inst Philippe Pinel de Mtl, 10905 boul Henri-Bourassa E, Montreal QC H1C 1H1; Lille (France)'85; FRCPC; Psy (P.Q.). Staff, Institut Philippe-Pinel de Montreal; Asst Prof Psy, Universite de Montreal; (514)648-8461; Fax. (514)881-3706.

DUBREUIL, Daniel; Hotel-Dieu de Levis, 143 rue Wolfe, Levis QC G6V 3Z1; Laval'01; FRCSC; GenSurg; ThorSurg. Staff, Hôtel-Dieu de Lévis; (418)835-7121

DUBREUIL, Martin; CSSS du Nord de Lanaudière, 1000 boul Sainte-Anne, St-Charles-Brromee QC J6E 6J2; Mon'81; Electroenceph (P.Q.); Neur (Electrodiagnostic Medicine). Staff, Centre Hospitalier Régional de Lanaudière; (450)759-8222; Fax. (450)759-7966.

DUBREUIL-MOISAN, Nathalie; CSSS Haut-Richelieu-Rouville, 920 boul du Seminaire N, St-Jean-sur-Richel QC J3A 1B7; Mon'99; Hem; Peds. Staff, Hôpital du Haut-Richelieu; (450)359-5000 x5205; Fax. (450)359-5237.

DUBROVSKY, Alexander; MUHC-Montreal Children's Hosp, 2300 rue Tupper, Montreal QC H3H 1P3; McG'04; FRCPC; Peds (P.Q.) (Pediatric Emergency Medicine). Staff, McGill University Health Centre - Montreal Children's Hospital; (514)412-4499

DUBROVSKY, Bernardo O; 1004-3445 rue Drummond, Montreal QC H3G 1X9; Buenos Aires (Argentina)'62; LMCC; Staff Teacher Psychiatry & Physiology, McGill University; (514)844-5702; Fax. (514)844-5702.

DUBRULE, Charles-Etienne; CHUQ-Ctr Hosp Univ Laval, 1207-2705 boul Laurier, Quebec QC G1V 4G2; Laval'03; FRCPC; IntMed. Staff, Centre Hospitalier Universitaire de Quebec-CHUL; (418)654-2160; Fax. (418)654-2187.

DUBUC, Benoit; CHUQ-Ctr Hosp Univ Laval, 2705 boul Laurier, Quebec QC G1V 4G2; Sher'86; Staff, Centre Hospitalier Universitaire de Quebec-CHUL; (418)525-4444

DUBUC, Elise; Le Centre D'Obstetrique-Guneco, 203-1361 av Beaumont, Mont-Royal QC H3P 2W3; Sher'06; FRCSC; ObstGyn. (514)344-4411

DUBUC, Eric; CSSS des Etchemins, 331 rue du Sanatorium, Lac-Etchemin QC G0R 1S0; Sher'08; Staff, CSSS des Etchemins; (418)625-8001; Fax. (418)625-3020.

DUBUC, Jean; CLSC Basse-Ville-Limoilou, 50 rue Saint-Joseph E, Quebec QC G1K 3A5; Mon'77; Langs: Bilingual(French/English); (418)529-2572 x4514; Fax. (418)529-8802.

DUBUC, Marc; Institut de Cardiologie de Mtl, 5000 rue Bélanger, Montreal QC H1T 1C8; Mon'80; CSPQ; FRCPC; IntMed (Electrophysiology); Cardiol. Staff, Institut de Cardiologie de Montréal; assoc Prof Med, Universite de Montreal; Langs: English; French; (514)376-3330; Fax. (514)593-2581; marc.dubuc@bellnet.ca.

DUBUC, Marie-Eve; GMF Centre Med du Parc, 84 rue Court, Granby QC J2G 4Y5; Laval'08; CCFP.

DUBUC, Mario; Clin Med Belvedere, 202-2235 rue Galt O, Sherbrooke QC J1K 1K6; Sher'79; CSPQ; CCFP; FCFP; Staff, Centre Hospitalier Universitaire de Sherbrooke-Hôpital Hôtel-Dieu; Clin Prof, Universite de Sherbrooke; (819)563-4244; Fax. (819)563-8924.

DUBUC, Michel; Centre de Medecine Industriell, 260-1215 ch du Tremblay, Longueuil QC J4N 1R4; Sher'80; BA; MSc; BSc; Consultant, Medical du Travail; (450)442-1018; Fax. (450)442-1967.

DUBUC, Myriam; CSSS de Laval, 1755 boul Rene-Laennec, Laval QC H7M 3L9; Mon'97; CSPQ; FRCPC; Anes. Staff, Hopital de la Cite de la santé; (450)668-1010 x23456

DUBUC, Richard; Clinique Metro Medic, 100-1538 rue Sherbrooke O, Montreal QC H3G 1L5; Mon'69; Derm (Immuno Dermatology). Staff, Centre Hospitalier l'Université de Montréal (CHUM) - Hôtel-Dieu; (514)932-2122

DUBUC, Sebastien; CSSS de L'Hematite, GD 1 rue de l'Aquilon, Fermont QC G0G 1J0; Sher'92; Staff, CLSC de l'Hématite; (418)287-5461; Fax. (418)287-5465.

DUBYNA, Dale S; Winnipeg Clinic, 425 St Mary Ave, Winnipeg MB R3C 0N2; Man'80; FRCSC; ObstGyn (Colposcopy). Staff, Health Sciences Centre; Staff, Misericordia Health Centre; Staff, St Boniface General Hospital; University of Manitoba; (204)957-3233; Fax. (204)943-1900.

DUCAS, Dean F; 8-30 Thirteenth St E, Cornwall ON K6H 6V9; McG'85; (613)933-9082

DUCAS, Diane A; St Boniface Gen Hosp, M5-409 Tache Ave, Winnipeg MB R2H 2A6; McG'84; FRCPC; Psy. Staff, St Boniface General Hospital; (204)237-2919; Fax. (204)237-6264.

DUCAS, John; St Boniface Gen Hosp, Y3021-409 Tache Ave, Winnipeg MB R2H 2A6; McG'76; DABIM; FRCPC; IntMed (Invasive Cardiology); Cardiol. Staff Cardiology, St Boniface General Hospital; Assoc Staff Section of Cardiol, Health Sciences Centre; Assoc Prof Med WRHA Cardiac Sciences Prog, University of Manitoba; (204)258-1274; Fax. (204)233-2157.

DUCASSE, Chantal; Centre Multi-Medic, 265-38 Place du Commerce, Verdun QC H3E 1T8; Mon'93; CCFP; Médecin, Centre Multi-Medic; (514)768-4717; Fax. (514)769-4846.

DUCCESCHI, Sylvia P; Vancouver Family Health Ctre, 100-2732 Hastings St E, Vancouver BC V5K 1Z9; Ott'87; CCFP; FCFP; Clinical Asst Prof, University of British Columbia; Langs: French; Italian; (604)253-3166; Fax. (604)253-2048.

DUCEPPE, Emmanuelle; CHUM-Hotel-Dieu, 3840 rue Saint-Urbain, Montreal QC H2W 1T8; Mon'08; IntMed. Staff, Centre Hospitalier l'Université de Montréal (CHUM) - Hôtel-Dieu; (514)890-8000

DUCHAINE, Claude; Clin Med de Metabetchouan, 20 rue Saint-Basile, Metab-L-A-La-Croix QC G8G 1S9; Mon'83; Staff, CSSS de Lac-Saint Jean-Est; Médecin, Resolute Forest Products; (418)349-8933; Fax. (418)349-8082; claude.duchaine@abitibibowater.com.

DUCHAINE, Denise; Clinique Med de la Baie, 437 rue Albert, La Baie QC G7B 3L5; Laval'78; Assoc Member, Complexe hospitalier de la Sagamie; (418)544-6863; Fax. (418)544-6864.

DUCHAINE, Sylvain; Trenton Mem Hosp, 242 King St, Trenton ON K8V 5S6; Tor'89; Staff, QHC Trenton Memorial; Langs: English; French; (613)392-2541

DUCHARME, Andre; Centre Med des Laurentides, 102-1100 rue Saint-Isidore, St-Lin-Laurentides QC J5M 2V6; Sher'74; (450)439-3870; Fax. (450)439-7849.

DUCHARME, Andree; Tribunal Administratif du QC, 4F-575 rue St-Amable, Quebec QC G1R 5R4; Laval'78; (418)643-3418

DUCHARME, Anique; Institut de Cardiologie de Mtl, 5000 rue Belanger, Montreal QC H1T 1C8; Mon'91; MSc; CSPQ; FRCPC; IntMed (Echocardiography); Cardiol. Staff, Institut de Cardiologie de Montréal; Dir, Heart Failure Clinic; Prof, Universite de Montreal; (514)376-3330 x3947; Fax. (514)593-2575.

DUCHARME, Brigitte; CSSS Pierre Boucher, 1333 boul Jacques-Cartier E, Longueuil QC J4M 2A5; Mon'90; CCFP; Staff, Centre Hospitalier Pierre Boucher; (450)468-8111

DUCHARME, Diane; CSSS du Grand Littoral, 200-1205 boul de la Rive-Sud, Levis QC G6W 0J6; Laval'85; Médecin, CSSS du Grand Littoral; (418)380-8991; Fax. (418)839-5750.

DUCHARME, Francine M; Hôpital Ste-Justine, 7939-3175 ch Cote-Ste-Catherin, Montreal QC H3T 1C5; Mon'82; MSc; FRCPC; Peds (Asthma). Staff, Hôpital Ste-Justine; Prof Peds, Universite de Montreal; (514)345-4931 x4398; Fax. (514)345-4822.

DUCHARME, J M Pierre; Phoenix Med Centre, 405-2155 10th Ave, Prince George BC V2M 5J6; Ott'81; Staff, University Hospital of Northern British Columbia; Staff Physician, Central Interior Native Health; (250)564-8018; Fax. (250)562-5253.

DUCHARME, James; Aim Health Group, 9-6400 Millcreek Dr, Mississauga ON L5N 3E7; McG'78; CSPQ; FRCPC; EmergMed. Chief Medical Officer, Aim Health Group; Clin Prof Med, McMaster University; Langs: Bilingual(English/French); (905)858-1368

DUCHARME, Jean-Luc; CSSS du Nord de Lanaudière, 1000 boul Sainte-Anne, St-Charles-Brromee QC J6E 6J2; Mon'75; Staff, Centre Hospitalier Régional de Lanaudière; (450)759-8222; Fax. (450)759-7969.

DUCHARME, Louis-Albert; Medical Complex, 1057 St Peter Ave, Bathurst NB E2A 2Z6; Mon'80; BSc; Staff, Hopital Regional Chaleur; (506)546-1500; Fax. (506)548-3427; ducharme@nb.sympatico.ca.

DUCHARME, Marie; Clinique Med Centre-Ville, 5-167 rue de la Reine, Gaspe QC G4X 2W6; Mon'86; Gen Practice, Centre Hospitalier de Gaspe; Dir, Regional Public Health Lab; (418)368-1811; Fax. (418)368-2616.

DUCHARME, Mario; CSSS Pierre Boucher, 1333 boul Jacques-Cartier E, Longueuil QC J4M 2A5; Mon'86; Electroenceph (P.Q.); Neur (P.Q.). Staff, Centre Hospitalier Pierre Boucher; (450)468-8111; Fax. (450)468-8247.

DUCHARME, Martine; CLSC Jean-Olivier Chenier, 29 ch D'Oka, St-Eustache QC J7R 1K6; Mon'87; Langs: Bilingual(French/English); (450)491-1233; Fax. (450)491-6898.

DUCHARME, Pascal; CSSS Rimouski-Neigette, CP 3150 Succ A 150 av Rouleau, Rimouski QC G5L 5T1; Sher'03; Staff, Hôpital Regional Rimouski; (418)724-3000

DUCHARME, Rene; Montfort Hosp, 713 ch Montreal, Ottawa ON K1K 0T2; Mon'77; CSPQ; FRCPC; Psy (Adult Psychiatry). Ac Member Mental Health Prog, Montfort Hospital; Asst Prof, University of Ottawa; Langs: Bilingual(French/English); (613)746-4621 x3919; Fax. (613)748-4938.

DUCHARME, Simon; MUHC-Royal Victoria Hosp, 687 av des Pins O, Montreal QC H3A 1A1; Mon'07; Psy (P.Q.). Staff, McGill University Health Centre - Royal Victoria Hospital; (514)934-1934

DUCHARME-DERY, Suzanne; Ctr de Sante Basse Cote Nord, CP 130 1070 boul Dr Camille Marcou, Lourdes-d-Bl-Sabl QC G0G 1W0; Mon'78; Staff, CSSS de la Basse Côté-Nord; (416)461-2144

DUCHASTEL, Morency; Clinique Med l'Actuel, 1130-1001 boul de Maisonneuve, Montreal QC H2L 4P9; Mon'96; Staff, Centre Hospitalier Gatineau Mémorial; Staff, Centre Hospitalier de LaSalle; Staff, Clinique Medicale l'Actuel; Langs: Spanish; English; (514)524-1001

DUCHASTEL, Paul A; 2045 Dufferin St, York ON M6E 3R4; Laval'67; CCFP; Langs: Bilingual(French/English); (416)656-7733; Fax. (416)656-6502; pduchastel@hotmail.com.

DUCHASTEL, Yves J; Centre Bois de Boulogne, 340-1575 boul Henri-Bourassa O, Montreal QC H3M 3A9; Mon'59; Electroenceph (P.Q.); Neur (P.Q.) (Alzheimer's Disease). Langs: Bilingual(French/English); (514)337-2054; Fax. (514)337-1906.

DUCHEN, Suzanne; 333 Eglinton Ave E, Toronto ON M4P 1L7; Witwatersrand (South Africa)'81; MB ChB; FRCPC; Psy (Mood Disorders). Consultant, Baycrest Centre for Geriatric Care; Lecturer, University of Toronto; (416)398-7880; Fax. (416)398-0888.

DUCHESNAY, Gaetan; CSSS de Trois-Rivières, 1991 boul du Carmel, Trois-Rivieres QC G8Z 3R9; Sher'88; Urol. Staff, CSSS de Trois-Rivières; (819)697-3333

DUCHESNE, Andre; 415-1915 rue Adoncour, Longueuil QC J4N 1R9; Sher'88; Langs: English; (450)674-4657; duchesnea@videotron.ca.

DUCHESNE, Annie; CSSSG-Hop de Hull, 116 boul Lionel-Emond, Gatineau QC J8Y 1W7; Sher'89; CSPQ; FRCSC; GenSurg. Staff, Hull Hospital; (819)595-6200; Fax. (819)595-6039.

DUCHESNE, Catherine J; 309-1580 Merivale Rd, Ottawa ON K2G 4B5; Qns'82; CCFP; CCFP(E.M.); FCFP; Ac Staff, The Ottawa Hospital - Civic Campus; (613)226-4030; Fax. (613)225-3891.

DUCHESNE, Dominique; Centre Med Brunswick, 401-955 boul Brunswick, Pointe-Claire QC H9R 5K3; Sher'97; (514)459-3428

DUCHESNE, J Luc L; Orleans Med-Dental Centre, 100-2555 St Joseph Blvd, Orleans ON K1C 1S6; Ott'81; Ac Staff, Montfort Hospital; Ac Staff, The Ottawa Hospital - General Campus; (613)830-1298; Fax. (613)830-2170; lduchesne@rogers.com.

DUCHESNE, Line; CSSS du Nord de Lanaudière, 1000 boul Sainte-Anne, Joliette QC J6E 6J2; Mon'81; Rheum; IntMed. Staff, Centre Hospitalier Régional du Suroît; Langs: English; (450)759-8222

DUCHESNE, Lloyd; Univ of Ottawa Heart Institute, 40 Ruskin St, Ottawa ON K1Y 4W7; Ott'92; BSc; FRCPC; IntMed; Cardiol. Staff Cardiol, The Ottawa Hospital - General Campus; Staff Cardiol, University of Ottawa Heart Institute; Assoc Prof, University of Ottawa; (613)761-4512; Fax. (613)761-5215.

DUCHESNE, Manon; CSSS des Aurores Boreales, CP 6000 Succ Bureau-Chef 679 2e rue E, La Sarre QC J9Z 2X7; Sher'06; Staff, Centre Hospitalier La Sarre; (819)333-2311; Fax. (819)333-3185.

DUCHESNE, Marie-Claude; CLSC Rimouski-Neigette, 165 rue des Gouverneurs, Rimouski QC G5L 7R2; Mon'97; CCFP; (418)727-5493; Fax. (418)723-7668.

DUCHESNE, Marjorie; Clin Med du Boise, 130-288 rue Pierre-Saindon, Rimouski QC G5L 9A8; Laval'00; CCFP; Staff, Hôpital Regional Rimouski; (418)724-4672; Fax. (418)724-4753.

DUCHESNE, Nathalie; Imagix-Radiologie Brossard, 2340 boul Lapiniere, Brossard QC J4Z 2K7; Laval'90; FRCPC; DiagRad. (450)656-1220; nduchesne@ottawahospital.on.ca.

DUCHESNE, Rachel; CLSC de Gatineau, 85 rue Saint-Redempteur, Gatineau QC J8X 4E6; Laval'91; CCFP; FCFP; Médecin, CLSC de Gatineau; Langs: Bilingual(French/English); (819)966-6510 x4245; Fax. (819)966-6533.

DUCHESNE, Raymond; Poluclinique Med Concorde, 300 boul de la Concorde E, Laval QC H7G 2E6; Mon'74; DAB; CSPQ; Ophth. (450)667-5310; Fax. (450)667-8329.

DUCHESNE, Robert; CSSS du Sud de Lanaudière, 911 montee des Pionniers, Terrebonne QC J6V 2H2; Mon'70; CSPQ; FRCSC; OrthSurg. Staff, Centre Hospitalier Pierre le Gardeur; Langs: Bilingual(French/English); (450)654-7525 x21147; Fax. (450)582-2051.

DUCHESNE, Sylvane; Centre Hosp Honore-Mercier, 2750 boul Laframboise, Saint-Hyacinthe QC J2S 4Y8; Laval'90; Peds. Staff, Centre d hebergement de l Hôtel-Dieu de Saint-Hyacinthe; (450)771-3425; Fax. (450)771-3626.

DUCHESNE-PANISSET, Manon; Ctr Hosp de Verdun, 4000 boul Lasalle, LaSalle QC H4G 2A3; Mon'86; Staff, Centre Hospitalier de Verdun; (514)362-1000

DUCHESNEAU, Helene; Centre d'Urgence de Salaberry, 2758 rue de Salaberry, Montreal QC H3M 1L3; Mon'80; (514)337-4772; Fax. (514)337-4923.

DUCHESNEAU, Kathleen; Centre Hosp Honore-Mercier, 2750 boul Laframboise, Saint-Hyacinthe QC J2S 4Y8; Laval'88; LMCC; CSPQ; FRCPC; Anes. Staff, Centre Hospitalier Honore-Mercier; (450)771-3333 x3353

DUCHESNEAU, Marie-Claude; CSSS Haut-Richelieu-Rouville, 920 boul du Seminaire N, St-Jean-sur-Richel QC J3A 1B7; Sher'01; CCFP; CCFP(E.M.); Staff, Hôpital du Haut-Richelieu; (450)359-5000; Fax. (450)359-5251.

DUCHOLKE, Linda M; 350-2755 Lougheed Hwy, Port Coquitlam BC V3B 5Y9; UBC'85; CCFP; (604)942-1550; Fax. (604)941-9289.

DUCHOWSKA, Helena L; 315-6051 Gilbert Rd, Richmond BC V7C 3V3; Warsaw (Poland)'57; PhD(PedRheum); Sr Staff, Richmond Hospital; Langs: Polish; French; Russian; (604)273-3218; Fax. (604)273-3224; hduchowska@gmail.com.

DUCKETT, Genevieve; Ctr Hosp de Verdun, 4000 boul Lasalle, Verdun QC H4G 2A3; Mon'84; FRCPC; DiagRad. Staff, Centre Hospitalier de Verdun; (514)765-8121 x2171

DUCKETT, Jean; Clinique Domus Medica, 401-5601 rue Belanger, Montreal QC H1T 1G3; Mon'69; Insp Examinateur, College des Medecins du Quebec; Langs: Bilingual(French/English); (514)256-5011; Fax. (514)384-1850.

DUCKITT, Kirsten; Campbell River & District Gen, 375 2nd Ave, Campbell River BC V9W 3V1; Cambridge (England)'89; FRCSC; ObstGyn. Staff, Campbell River & District General Hospital; (250)850-2141

DUCKWORTH, Geoffrey S; 1101-170 Bloor St W, Toronto ON M5S 1T9; Tor'65; DPsy; PhD; FRCPC; Psy (Adult Psychiatry). Consultant West Park Longterm Care, West Park Healthcare Centre; Consultant, Runnymede Healthcare Centre; (416)712-0584; Fax. (416)503-8305; hmcbride@oise.utoronto.ca.

DUCLOS, Alain J; CHUM-Hop St-Luc, 1058 rue Saint-Denis, Montreal QC H2X 3J4; Mon'00; FRCSC; Urol. Staff, Centre Hospitalier l'Université De Montréal (CHUM) - Hôpital Saint-luc; (514)890-8000

DUCLOS, Benoit; CSSSG-Hop de Gatineau, CP 2000 Succ Bureau-Chef 909 boul de la Verendrye O, Gatineau QC J8P 7H2; Mon'99; Urol. Staff, Hôpital de Gatineau; (819)561-8100

DUCLOS, David; CSSS Gatineau (Pav Gatineau), CP 2000 Succ Bureau-Chef 909 boul de la Verendrye O, Gatineau QC J8P 7H2; Sher'04; Staff GP, Hôpital de Gatineau; Langs: Bilingual(English/French); (819)561-6100

DUCLOS, Elizabeth; Clinique Med Deux-Montagnes, 201 9e av, Deux-Montagnes QC J7R 3M1; Sher'98; (450)472-7545; Fax. (450)472-0886.

DUCLOS, Lucie; Clin de Chirurgie Esthetique, 3350 boul Rosemont, Montreal QC H1X 1K3; Laval'89; FRCSC; PlasSurg (Esthetic Plastic Surgery). Staff, Hopital Maisonneuve-Rosemont; Staff, Centre Hospitalier Pierre le Gardeur; Staff Teacher, Universite de Montreal; Langs: English; (514)252-0912; dreduclos@dreduclos.com.

DUCLOS, Madeleine; Ctr Med Berri-Gouin, 306-500 boul Gouin E, Montreal QC H3L 3R9; Laval'92; ABPh; CCFP; Langs: English; (514)333-3396; Fax. (514)333-3496.

DUCLOS, Marie; MUHC-Montreal Gen Hosp, D5 400-1650 av Cedar, Montreal QC H3G 1A4; Laval'87; CSPQ; FRCPC; RadOncol (Gynecology). Staff, McGill University Health Centre - Montreal General Campus; Asst Prof Oncol, McGill University; Langs: Bilingual(French/English); (514)934-8040; Fax. (514)934-8392; marie.duclos@mcgill.ca.

DUCLOS, Pierre; CHUQ Hôp Saint-Francois d'Auss, 10 rue de l'Espinay, Quebec QC G1L 3L5; Laval'69; Endocrin (P.Q.); IntMed. Ac Staff, Centre Hospitalier Universitaire De Québec - Pavillon De St-françois-d'assise; (418)525-4444

DUCROS, Genevieve M; 24 Canadian Forces HSC, PO Box 1000 PO Stn Forces 50 Yukon ST, Astra ON K0K 3W0; Qns'91; BSc; CCFP; Fam Med, Hornepayne Community Hospital; Langs: English; French.

DUDA, Barbara; Hop du Sacre-Coeur de Mtl, 5400 boul Gouin O, Montreal QC H4J 1C5; Mon'88; FRCPC; IntMed; Endocrin&Metab; Endocrin (P.Q.). Staff, Hôpital du Sacre-Coeur de Montréal; Universite de Montreal; Langs: Bilingual(French/English); (514)338-2050; Fax. (514)338-3549.

DUDAR, Amber; The Port Arthur Hlth Centre, 194 Court St N, Thunder Bay ON P7A 4V7; Tor'03; BSc; FRCSC; ObstGyn. Asst Prof, Northern Ontario School of Medicine; (807)346-1000 x7756; Fax. (807)346-6206.

DUDEBOUT, Jill J; Queen's Univ Etherington Hall, 2015-94 Stuart St, Kingston ON K7L 3N6; Sask'05; FRCPC; IntMed; Hem. (613)533-2946; Fax. (613)533-6855.

DUDEK, Malgorzata; Humber River Reg Hosp-Keele, 2175 Keele St, York ON M6M 3Z4; Bialystok (Poland)'88; FRCPC; Psy. Staff, Centre for Addiction & Mental Health (CAMH) - Queen Site; Staff, Humber River Regional Hospital - Keele Street Site; Lecturer, University of Toronto; Langs: Polish.

DUDEK, Nancy L; 505 Smyth Rd, Ottawa ON K1H 8M2; Wes'99; FRCPC; PhysMed&Rehab. Assoc Staff, The Ottawa Hospital - Civic Campus; Assoc Staff, The Ottawa Hospital - General Campus; Assoc Staff Physical Med & Rehab, The Ottawa Hospital Rehabilitation Centre; Ac Staff, SCO Health Service; Assoc Prof Med, University of Ottawa; (613)737-7350 x75596; Fax. (613)739-6974; ndudek@toh.on.ca.

DUDGEON, Deborah J; 34 Barrie St, Kingston ON K7L 3J7; McM'85; FRCPC; IntMed (Pain Management); MedOncol. Staff, Kingston General Hospital; Prof Med, Queen's University.

DUDLEY, Alistair; Kamsack Med Clinic, PO Box 69, Kamsack SK S0A 1S0; (306)542-2623; Fax. (306)542-3782.

DUDLEY, Denis K L; Medical Towers, 650-1600 Carling Ave, Ottawa ON K1Z 1G3; (Jamaica)'72; MB BS; MRCOG; DABOG; FRCSC; ObstGyn (AIDS/HIV). Exec Dir, Laser Dermatology-Minister of Health; (613)722-3483; Fax. (613)722-2877; laserderm@on.aibn.com.

DUDLEY, Emer M; Chatham-Kent Family Health Team, 9-30 McNaughton Ave, Wallaceburg ON N8A 1R9; Cork (Ireland)'75; MB BCh; DCH; MRCGPract; DObst; Court Staff, Chatham-Kent Health Alliance; (519)627-1497

DUDLEY, John; Workplace Safety & Ins Board, PO Box 2099 Stn Lcd 1 120 King St W, Hamilton ON L8N 4C5; Sask'77; FRCPC; Psy. Staff Psy, St Joseph's Healthcare - Charlton Campus; Assoc Med Dir, Workplace Safety & Insurance Board; Associate Clin Prof, McMaster University; (905)521-4439; john_dudley@wsib.on.ca.

DUDON, Emmanuelle M J; CSSS de Rivière-de-Loup, 75 rue Saint-Henri, Riviere-Du-Loup QC G5R 2A4; Mon'92; CSPQ; FRCSC; OrthSurg (Hand Surgery). Staff, Centre Hospitalier Regional du Grand-Portage; Langs: Russian; English; (418)868-1010 x2456; Fax. (418)868-1032.

DUDZIC, Edyta M; Royal University Hosp, 103 Hospital Dr, Saskatoon SK S7N 0W8; Alb'88; CRCP; FRCPC; NuclearMed. Staff Nuclear Med, Royal University Hospital; Assoc Prof Nuclear Med, University of Saskatchewan; (306)655-1820; Fax. (306)655-1742; edyta.dudzic@saskatoonhealthregion.ca.

DUECK, Andrew D; Sunnybrook Hlth Sciences Ctr, H185-2075 Bayview Ave, Toronto ON M4N 3M5; Qns'99; FRCSC; GenSurg (Clinical & Investigative Medicine); VascSurg. Staff, Sunnybrook Health Sciences Centre; (416)480-6947

DUECK, Bradley J; Hodgins Prof Bldg, 101-45625 Hodgins Ave, Chilliwack BC V2P 1P2; UBC'96; CCFP; (604)792-2721; Fax. (604)792-3404.

DUECK, Darrin; Oakbank Med Clinic, PO Box 521 A-622 Main St, Oakbank MB R0E 1J0; Man'96; CCFP; Staff, Beausejour District Hospital; (204)444-2934; Fax. (204)444-3135.

DUECK, Dorie-Anna C; Thunder Bay Reg HSC-T-Bay, 980 Oliver Rd, Thunder Bay ON P7B 6V4; Man'97; FRCPC; IntMed; MedOncol. Staff, Thunder Bay Regional Health Sciences Centre; (807)684-7200; Fax. (807)684-5808.

DUECK, Gregory; BC Cancer Ctre-Southern Interi, 399 Royal Ave, Kelowna BC V1Y 5L3; Sask'03; FRCPC; IntMed; MedOncol. Staff, BC Cancer Agency Sindi Ahluwalia Hawkins Centre for the Southern Interior; (250)712-3996

DUECK, Kenneth; Gateway Hlth & Wellness Ctr, 203-2051 McCallum Rd, Abbotsford BC V2S 3N5; Man'89; CCFP; Staff Family Practice, Abbotsford Regional Hospital & Cancer Centre; Med Dir, Menno Extended Care Hospital; Clin Instructor Family Practice, University of British Columbia; (604)855-0677; Fax. (604)855-0722.

DUEMLER, Marianne R; 303-2021 Cliff Rd, Mississauga ON L5A 3N7; Alb'78; FRCSC; ObstGyn. Consultant, Trillium Health Centre - Mississauga; (905)848-3711; Fax. (905)848-2463.

DUERKSEN, Anthony J; The Credit Valley Hosp, 2200 Eglinton Ave W, Mississauga ON L5M 2N1; Man'08; CCFP; CCFP(E.M.); Staff, The Credit Valley Hospital; (905)813-4530; Fax. (905)813-4548.

DUERKSEN, Carl D; Henderson Med Centre, 441 Henderson Hwy, Winnipeg MB R2K 2H5; Man'83; CCFP; FCFP; Staff, Concordia General Hospital; (204)667-8650; Fax. (204)668-1928.

DUERKSEN, Donald R; St Boniface Gen Hosp, C5120-409 Tache Ave, Winnipeg MB R2H 2A6; Man'84; FRCPC; IntMed; Gastroent. Coord Section of Gastroenterology, St Boniface General Hospital; (204)237-2796; Fax. (204)233-7154.

DUERKSEN, Mark T; Steinbach Family Med Centre, 10-333 Loewen Blvd, Steinbach MB R5G 0C3; Man'88; CCFP; FCFP; (204)326-3401; Fax. (204)326-3899.

DUFF, Brian D; Agassiz Med Centre, 130-30 Stephen St, Morden MB R6M 2G3; Man'83; CCFP; FCFP; (204)822-4474; Fax. (204)822-6886.

DUFF, Henry; Univ of Calgary, GC73-3280 Hospital Dr NW, Calgary AB T2N 4Z6; McG'75; FRCPC; Cardiol (Cardiac Electrophysiology). Prof Med, University of Calgary; (403)220-5500; Fax. (403)283-8878; hduff@ucalgary.ca.

DUFF, John H; 1092 St Anthony Rd, London ON N6H 2P6; Tor'57; FRCSC; GenSurg. (519)657-2366; Fax. (519)657-2068; jhduff@sympatico.ca.

DUFF, Jonathan P; Edmonton Clinic Health Academy, 4 539-11405 87 Ave NW, Edmonton AB T6G 1C9; Alb'00; FRCPC; Peds; Critical Care Medicine. Staff, University of Alberta Hospital; (780)248-5445

DUFF, Melissa S; PO Box 52037 Rpo Garneau, Edmonton AB T6G 2T5; McM'05; CCFP.

DUFF, Sharon; Hamilton HS-General Site, PO Box 585 Stn Lcd 1 4N 425-237 Barton St, Hamilton ON L8L 2X2; McM'04; FRCPC; Psy. Staff, Hamilton Health Sciences Centre - Hamilton General Hospital; (905)521-2100; Fax. (905)527-3360.

DUFF, Susie; C-665 Earl Armstrong Rd, Ottawa ON K1V 2G2; Mon'79; BSc(BioChem); FRCPC; IntMed; Rheum. Staff, Clinique Medicale du Faubourg; Langs: Bilingual(English/French); (613)822-0411; Fax. (613)822-1399.

DUFF, Virginia A; St Joseph's Health Centre, 4F-30 The Queensway, Toronto ON M6R 1B5; Qns'82; FRCPC; Psy (Chronic Care). Consultant Psy, Centre for Addiction & Mental Health (CAMH) - Queen Site; Staff, St Joseph's Health Centre; Clin Asst, Toronto General Hospital - UHN; Lecturer, University of Toronto; (416)530-6000 x3101; Fax. (416)530-6363; duffg@stjoe.on.ca.

DUFFETT, Lisa D M; Ottawa Blood Disease Centre, L2248-501 Smyth Rd, Ottawa ON K1H 8L6; Mem'07; Hem; IntMed. (613)737-8899

DUFFIE, Anne F; 1501 rue Saint-Patrick, Montreal QC H3K 2B7; Mem'87; (514)731-9090 x112

DUFFIN, Jacalyn M; Queen's Univ History of Med, 78 Barrie St, Kingston ON K7L 3J7; Tor'74; PhD(Sorbonne); FRCPC; IntMed; Hem. Staff IntMed & Hem, Kingston General Hospital; Prof Hannah Professor of the History of Med, Queen's University; Langs: French; (613)533-6580; duffinj@queensu.ca.

DUFFY, Anne C; Faculty Of Med, 4F-3280 Hospital Dr, Calgary AB T2N 4Z6; Cal'91; FRCPC; Psy. Staff, IWK Health Centre; (403)210-6410

DUFFY, Charles H; Prince County Hosp, PO Box 3000 Stn Main 65 Roy Boataes Ave, Summerside PE C1N 2A9; Mem'90; CCFP; CCFP(E.M.); FCFP; Staff, Prince County Hospital; (902)432-2500

DUFFY, Ciaran; Children's Hosp of Eastern Ont, W1420-401 Smyth Rd, Ottawa ON K1H 8L1; National (Ireland)'79; MB ChB; MSc; FRCPI; FRCPC; Peds (Administration); Rheum. Staff, Children's Hospital of Eastern Ontario (CHEO); Dept Chair Peds, University of Ottawa; (613)737-7600; Fax. (613)738-4864; ciaran.duffy@muhc.mcgill.ca.

DUFFY, Deirdre A; Red Deer Reg Hosp Centre, 3942 50A Ave, Red Deer AB T4N 4E7; Cork (Ireland)'80; DCH; CCFP; CCFP(E.M.); FCFP; Staff Emerg, Red Deer Regional Hospital Centre; (403)343-4448; deirdreduffy@hotmail.com.

DUFFY, Gavin R; Health Sciences Centre, 300 Prince Philip Dr, St. John's NL A1B 3V6; Mem'87; FRCSC; Urol. Staff, Health Sciences Centre; (709)777-6300

DUFFY, Gerard; Manitoba Clinic, 790 Sherbrook St, Winnipeg MB R3A 1M3; Liverpool (England)'63; MB ChB; FRCPC; IntMed. (204)774-6541; Fax. (204)786-8092.

DUFFY, Martin; Rockyview Gen Hosp, 6628-7007 14 St SW, Calgary AB T2V 1P9; McG'97; BSc; MDCM; FRCSC; Urol (Stone Disorders). Consultant Urol., Rockyview General Hospital; (403)943-8998; Fax. (403)943-8999.

DUFFY, Patrick J; Regina Qu'Appelle HR-Regina, MOW 3F-1440 14th Ave, Regina SK S4P 0W5; Dublin (Ireland)'81; MB ChB; BAO; AB(AP&Hem); FRCPC; GenPath (Hematology); IntMed; AnatPath. Staff, Regina General Hospital; Associate Clin Prof, University of Saskatchewan; (306)766-4444

DUFFY, Paul J; Bone And Joint Clinic, 3134 Hospital Dr NW, Calgary AB T2N 5A1; Mem'97; FRCSC; OrthSurg. Staff, Foothills Medical Centre; (403)944-8215; Fax. (403)270-8004.

DUFFY, Peter J; The Ottawa Hosp-Gen Campus, 501 Smyth Rd, Ottawa ON K1H 8L6; Mem'88; Anes. Staff Anes, The Ottawa Hospital - General Campus; Asst Prof Anes, University of Ottawa; (613)737-8187; Fax. (613)247-7528.

DUFORT, Jean-Pierre; Clin Med L'Assomption, 360-5345 boul de l'Assomption, Montreal QC H1T 4B3; Mon'79; Staff, CSSS Saint-Leonard et Saint-Michel; (514)257-7000; Fax. (514)257-7003.

DUFORT, Julie; Direction de la Sante Publique, 1255 rue Beauregard, Longueuil QC J4K 2M3; Mon'00; FRCPC; CommunMed; Public Health & Preventive Med. (450)928-6777 x3177

DUFORT, Louis; CSSS de Memphremagog, 50 rue Saint-Patrice E, Magog QC J1X 3X3; Laval'99; Staff, Centre Hospitalier et CLSC de Memphremagog; (819)843-2292

DUFOUR, Alexandre; CSSS Domaine du Roy, 450 rue Brassard, Roberval QC G8H 1B9; Sher'08; Staff, Hotel-Dieu de Roberval; (418)275-0110

DUFOUR, Amelie; CSSS de Saint-Jérôme, 290 rue de Montigny, Saint-Jerome QC J7Z 5T3; Mon'08; CCFP; CCFP(E.M.); Staff, Hôtel-Dieu de Saint-Jérôme; (450)432-2777

DUFOUR, Andre; Clin Familiale Saint-Lambert, 209 rue de Woodsock, Saint-Lambert QC J4P 1W7; Laval'80; CCFP; Staff, Centre Hospitalier l'Université De Montréal (CHUM) - Hôpital Saint-luc; (450)466-8583

DUFOUR, Anne; Clin Pediatrique Sainte-Foy, 293-2600 boul Laurier, Quebec QC G1V 4T3; Laval'85; Langs: English; (418)658-0906; Fax. (418)652-7094.

DUFOUR, Claude; Ctr Hosp de Matane, 333 rue Thibault, Matane QC G4W 2W5; Laval'72; CSPQ; FRCSC; GenSurg. Chef chirg gén, Centre Hospitalier de Matane; (418)562-5356; Fax. (418)562-8530.

DUFOUR, Daniel; 33 rue Fleet, Gore QC J0V 1K0; Sher'87; Staff, Hôpital du Haut-Richelieu; (450)562-0033

DUFOUR, Daniel M; Brockville Gen Hosp, 75 Charles St, Brockville ON K6V 1S8; Cal'97; CCFP; Ac Staff, Brockville General Hospital - Charles Street; Langs: English; French; (613)345-5645; dmdufour@yahoo.com.

DUFOUR, Emilie; CSSS Pierre Boucher, 1333 boul Jacques-Cartier E, Longueuil QC J4M 2A5; Laval'04; CCFP; CCFP(E.M.); Staff, Centre Hospitalier Pierre Boucher; (450)468-8111 x82188

DUFOUR, Georges E; Ctr Hosp Fleury, 2180 rue Fleury E, Montreal QC H2B 1K3; Mon'63; Psy (P.Q.). Staff, Centre Hospitalier Fleury; (514)381-9311; Fax. (514)433-6982.

DUFOUR, Georges; Ctr Hosp du Centre la Mauricie, 50 119e rue, Shawinigan-Sud QC G9P 5K1; Laval'65; LMCC; Otol. Staff, Centre Hospitalier du Centre la Mauricie; Staff, Centre Lafleche Grand-Mere; Staff, Centre Hospitalier Saint-Joseph de la Turque; Langs: Bilingual(French/English); (819)536-7500

DUFOUR, Jean-Jacques; Bertrand-Johnson Acoustique In, 302-5995 boul Gouin O, Montreal QC H4J 2P8; Laval'68; FRCSC; Otol (Neuro Otology). ac Staff, Centre Hospitalier l'Université de Montréal (CHUM) - Hôpital Notre-Dame; Staff, Sir Mortimer B Davis Jewish General; Staff, McGill University Health Centre - Montreal Neurological Hospital; assoc Prof, Universite de Montreal; adj Prof, McGill University; (514)322-2050

DUFOUR, Jerome; CSSS de Laval, 1755 boul Rene-Laennec, Laval QC H7M 3L9; Sher'02; Staff, Hopital de la Cite de la santé; (450)975-5309

DUFOUR, Julie; Clin Med Saint-Henri, 223 rue du Commerciale, St-Henri-de-Levis QC G0R 3E0; Laval'90; LMCC; (418)882-2268

DUFOUR, Karlyne L; Moncton Med Clinic, 403-860 Mountain Rd, Moncton NB E1C 2N7; Dal'94; CCFP; FCFP; (506)853-5158; Fax. (506)853-5172.

DUFOUR, Marc E; Four Corners Med Bldg, 203-2009 Long Lake Rd, Sudbury ON P3E 6C3; Utrecht (Netherlands)'83; MRC; FRCSC; ObstGyn. Langs: Dutch; (705)674-1210; Fax. (705)674-9424.

DUFOUR, Marc; CSSS de Memphremagog, 50 rue Saint-Patrice E, Magog QC J1X 3X3; Reims (France)'78; Staff, Centre Hospitalier et CLSC de Memphremagog; (819)843-2292

DUFOUR, Marcel; Ctr hosp Affilie-Enfant-Jesus, 1401 18e rue, Quebec QC G1J 1Z4; Laval'73; CSPQ; FRCSC; OrthSurg (Transplantation). Staff, Centre Hospitalier Affilié Universitaire de Québec - Hôpital De L'Enfant Jésus; Langs: English; (418)649-0252; Fax. (418)649-5567; mdeo@videotron.ca.

DUFOUR, Marie; Hotel-Dieu De Levis, 143 rue Wolfe, Levis QC G6V 3Z1; Laval'85; LMCC; CSPQ; FRCPC; DiagRad (Magnetic Resonance). Staff, Hôtel-Dieu de Lévis; (418)835-7121

DUFOUR, Marie-Helene; UMF de la Laurier, 4F-2875 boul Laurier, Quebec QC G1V 2M2; Laval'09; CCFP; (418)654-2701

DUFOUR, Marie-Josee; CHUQ-Ctr Hosp Univ Laval, 622-2705 boul Laurier, Quebec QC G1V 4G2; Laval'96; Staff, Centre Hospitalier Universitaire de Quebec-CHUL; (418)654-2255; Fax. (418)654-2173.

DUFOUR, Natasha; CHUM-Hop Notre-Dame, 1560 rue Sherbrooke E, Montreal QC H2L 4M1; Mon'97; FRCPC; Psy. Staff, Centre Hospitalier l'Université de Montréal (CHUM) - Hôpital Notre-Dame; (514)890-8000

DUFOUR, Serge; 124 av du Parc, Granby QC J2G 2M2; Sher'81; (450)777-2343; Fax. (450)372-1119.

DUFOUR, Stefanie; Ctr de Med Familiale de Granby, 48 rue Denison E, Granby QC J2G 4C6; Mon'97; Staff, Centre Hospitalier de Granby; (450)372-3996

DUFOUR, Suzanne; CSSS de Lac-Saint Jean-Est, CP 1300 Succ Bureau-Chef 300 boul Champlain, Alma QC G8B 5W3; Mon'84; Staff, CSSS de Lac-Saint Jean-Est; Physician, CLSC En Sante Au Traval; Prof Med, Universite de Sherbrooke; Langs: Bilingual(French/English); (418)669-2000; Fax. (418)668-3487; suzanne.dufour@ssss.gouv.qc.ca.

DUFOUR, Yves; CSSS de Rimouski-Neigette, CP 3150 Succ A 150 av Rouleau, Rimouski QC G5L 5T1; Laval'98; Staff Emerg, Hôpital Regional Rimouski; (418)723-7851

DUFRESNE, Brian E; 108 Robin Cres, Fort McMurray AB T9H 2W3; UBC'87; CCFP; CCFP(E.M.); Northern Lights Regional Health Centre; (780)791-6161; Fax. (780)791-6042.

DUFRESNE, Chantal; Clinique Med Perrier, 10-10794 rue Lajeunesse, Montreal QC H3L 2E8; Sher'93; (514)383-0559; maiger@sympatico.ca.

DUFRESNE, Chantelle; CLSC Seigneurie de Beauharnois, 142 rue Saint-Laurent, Beauharnois QC J6N 1V9; Sher'98; Médecin, CLSC Seigneurie de Beauharnois; (450)429-6455; Fax. (450)429-1119.

DUFRESNE, Charles; Clinique Med de la Baie, 437 rue Albert, La Baie QC G7B 3L5; Laval'84; (418)544-6863; Fax. (418)544-6864.

DUFRESNE, Diane; Clin Orl, 101-867 boul Saint-Joseph, Roberval QC G8H 2L8; Mon'87; FRCSC; Otol (Allergy). Staff, Hotel-Dieu de Roberval; Langs: English; (418)275-3293; Fax. (418)275-9152.

DUFRESNE, Francois; Hop Charles LeMoyne, 3120 boul Taschereau, Greenfield Park QC J4V 2H1; Laval'98; FRCPC; EmergMed;CCFP; Staff, Hopital Charles LeMoyne; Staff, McGill University Health Centre - Montreal General Campus; (450)466-5050

DUFRESNE, Geneil; PO Box 67149 Rpo Northland, Calgary AB T2L 2L2; Alb'06; CCFP.

DUFRESNE, Genevieve D; 2-750 Taylor Creek Dr, Orleans ON K1C 1T1; Ott'06; CCFP; (613)830-8388; Fax. (613)830-8588.

DUFRESNE, Georges; Ctr Hosp Affilie-Enfant-Jesus, 1401 18e rue, Quebec QC G1J 1Z4; Laval'76; EmergMed (P.Q.). Staff, Centre Hospitalier Affilié Universitaire de Québec - Hôpital De L'Enfant Jésus; (418)649-5632; Fax. (418)649-5975; gdufresn@videotron.ca.

DUFRESNE, Jacques J; 624 boul du Seminaire N, St-Jean-Sur-Richel QC J3B 7B4; Mon'65; Ac Staff, Hôpital du Haut-Richelieu; (450)348-3141; Fax. (450)348-5749.

DUFRESNE, Jean; CHUS-Hop Fleurimont, 3001 12e av N, Sherbrooke QC J1H 5N4; Mon'85; FRCPC; IntMed (Oncology); Hem. Staff, Centre Hospitalier Universitaire de Sherbrooke-Hopital Fleurimont; assoc Prof, Universite de Sherbrooke; Langs: English; (819)346-1110 x14816; jean.dufresne@usherbrooke.ca.

DUFRESNE, Jean-Claude; Clin Med Dr Jean-Claude Dufres, 3540A boul Dagenais O, Laval QC H7P 1V7; Mon'78; Langs: English; (450)628-8681; Fax. (450)628-2336.

DUFRESNE, Jose; CSSS de Trois-Rivières, 1991 boul du Carmel, Trois-Rivieres QC G8Z 3R9; Mon'88; CSPQ; FRCSC; GenSurg (Thoracic Surgery); VascSurg. Staff, CSSS de Trois-Rivières; Staff, Centre Hospitalier Regional de Trois-Rivieres; (819)697-3555

DUFRESNE, Julie; Hop Charles Lemoyne, 3120 boul Taschereau, Greenfield Park QC J4V 2H1; Sher'99; Gastroent; IntMed. Staff, Hopital Charles LeMoyne; (450)466-5000; Fax. (450)466-5036.

DUFRESNE, Louis R; Ministere de la Sante, 6F-1075 ch Sainte-Foy, Quebec QC G1S 2M1; Mon'63; FRCPC; IntMed; Nephrol (P.Q.). Staff, Centre Hospitalier l'Université de Montréal (CHUM) - Hôpital Notre-Dame; Prof Med, Universite de Montreal; Langs: English; French; (418)266-7500

DUFRESNE, Louise; Clin Med St-Sauveur, 70 rue Principale, Saint-Sauveur QC J0R 1R6; Mon'97; (450)227-8436

DUFRESNE, Lucille J; CSSS du Nord de Lanaudière, 1000 boul Sainte-Anne, St-Charles-Brromee QC J6E 6J2; Mon'78; LMCC; Staff, Centre Hospitalier Régional de Lanaudière; (450)759-8222

DUFRESNE, Marc L G; Polyclinique, 300-874 boul de l'Universite E, Chicoutimi QC G7H 6B9; Laval'62; PlasSurg. Langs: Bilingual(French/English); (418)549-7270; Fax. (418)549-7438.

DUFRESNE, Marie-Claude; CHUQ-St-Francois D'Assise, 10 rue de l'Espinay, Quebec QC G1L 3L5; Laval'90; FRCPC; DiagRad (Echography & Doppler). Staff, Centre Hospitalier Universitaire De Québec - Pavillon De St-françois-d'assise; (418)525-4303

DUFRESNE, Maurice J A; AIM Health Group, B22-550 Terminal Ave, Ottawa ON K1G 0Z3; Ott'71; MBA; Langs: English; French; (613)731-4774; Fax. (613)731-4979; mdufresne0607@rogers.com.

DUFRESNE, Michel P; Hop Maisonneuve-Rosemont, 5415 boul de l'Assomption, Montreal QC H1T 2M4; Sher'82; FRCPC; DiagRad (Radiology Vascular & Intervention). Staff, Hopital Maisonneuve-Rosemont; Universite de Montreal; (514)252-3400; Fax. (514)252-3537.

DUFRESNE, Normand; Clinique Acces MD, 302-28 ch du Golf E, Joliette QC J6E 2B4; Mon'80; Staff Emerg Dept, Centre Hospitalier Régional de Lanaudière; (450)756-2626

DUFRESNE, Roger A; 306-900 av Rockand, Montreal QC H2V 3A2; Mon'55; CSPQ; FRCPC; Psy (Psychoanalysis & Psychotherapy). Med Consultant, Centre Hospitalier l'Université de Montréal (CHUM) - Hôpital Notre-Dame; Staff Training Psychoanalyst, Canadian Psychoanalyst Society & Institute; assoc Prof, Universite de Montreal; Langs: English; (514)739-6537; Fax. (514)278-8419.

DUFRESNE, Serge; Clinique Med du Quartier Latin, 905 boul Rene-Levesque E, Montreal QC H2L 5B1; Mon'85; MSc; BSc; CCFP; Staff, Centre Hospitalier l'Université De Montréal (CHUM) - Hôpital Saint-luc; Med Consultant, DSP Monteregie Ministere Santi Services Sociaux; Langs: English; (514)285-5500; Fax. (514)285-2226.

DUFRESNE, Simon; 5415 boul de l'Assomption, Montreal QC H1T 2M4; Mon'05; FRCPC; MedMicrobiol. Staff, Hopital Maisonneuve-Rosemont; (514)252-3817; Fax. (514)252-3898.

DUFRESNE, Sylvain; Clin des Trois Lacs, 160-585 av Saint-Charles, Vaudreuil-Dorion QC J7V 8P9; Mon'92; Staff, Centre Hospitalier Régional du Suroît; (450)455-3322

DUFRESNE, Sylvie; Clin les Jardins, 200-72 boul Saint-Jean-Baptist, Chateauguay QC J6K 4Y7; Mon'82; (450)692-7282; Fax. (450)699-7788.

DUFRESNE, Sylvie; CSSS de Vaudreuil-Soulanges, RR 1 11 ch de La Cite-des Jeunes, Saint-Polycarpe QC J0P 1X0; Sher'94; (450)265-3771; Fax. (450)265-3556; sylvie_dufresne@rrsss16.gouv.qc.ca.

DUFRESNE-BEAUCHAMP, Marie-Helene; Ctr Hosp Rouyn-Noranda, 4 9e rue, Rouyn-Noranda QC J9X 2B2; Mon'05; CCFP; Staff, Centre Hospitalier Rouyn-Noranda; (819)764-5131

DUFTON, John A; University Hosp of Northern BC, 1475 Edmonton St, Prince George BC V2M 1S2; UBC'07; DiagRad. Staff, University Hospital of Northern British Columbia; (250)565-2000

DUGAL, Michele; CHUQ-Hotel-Dieu de Quebec, 11 Cote du Palais, Quebec QC G1R 2J6; Laval'79; FRCPC; IntMed; ClinImmunol&Allergy (P.Q.). Staff, Centre Hospitalier Universitaire de Québec (CHUQ) - Siege Social; (418)691-5087

DUGAN, Alison K; The Ottawa Hosp-Gen Campus, 2139-501 Smyth Rd, Ottawa ON K1H 8L6; Qns'85; FRCP(Biostat); BA; MSc; FRCPC; IntMed. Staff IntMed, The Ottawa Hospital - General Campus; Asst Prof Med, University of Ottawa; Langs: French; (613)739-6739; Fax. (613)737-8688.

DUGAS, Alexandre; Hop Maisonneuve-Rosemont, 5415 boul de l'Assomption, Montreal QC H1T 2M4; McG'05; FRCPC; DiagRad. Staff, Hopital Maisonneuve-Rosemont; (514)252-3400 x4333

DUGAS, Andre; Clinique Med Memphre, 200-323 rue Sherbrooke, Magog QC J1X 2R9; Sher'79; (819)847-1313; Fax. (819)847-3529.

DUGAS, Anna-Viola M; Vanier Med Centre, 10-325 Vanier Blvd, Bathurst NB E2A 3N1; Ott'70; Ac Staff, Hopital Regional Chaleur; (506)546-3000

DUGAS, Christine; Clinique Med Val-Bélair, 202-1147 boul Pie-XI N, Quebec QC G3K 2P8; Laval'90; Staff, Hôpital Sainte Anne de Beaupré; (418)843-2473; Fax. (418)843-0224.

DUGAS, Geoffrey R; William Osler HC-Brampton, 2100 Bovaird Dr E, Brampton ON L6R 3J7; Wes'01; FRCPC; Anes. Staff, William Osler Health System - Brampton Civic Hospital; (905)494-2120

DUGAS, Gisele; CHSLD St-Antoine-de-Padoue, 521 rue Saint-Antoine, Laurentides QC J5M 3A3; Mon'90; (450)439-2609

DUGAS, Giselle; 8559 Hwy 1 PO Box 128, Meteghan Centre NS B0W 2K0; Sher'05; CCFP; Langs: Bilingual(French/English); (902)645-2777; Fax. (902)645-2854.

DUGAS, Isabelle L; Cape Breton Hlthcare Complex, 1482 George St, Sydney NS B1P 1P3; Mon'97; CCFP; Staff, Cape Breton Healthcare Complex; Langs: Bilingual(French/English); (902)567-7804; Fax. (902)567-8062.

DUGAS, Lise S; PO Box 5714 Stn Main, Caraquet NB E1W 1B7; Sher'83; CCFP; FCFP; (506)727-2278; Fax. (506)727-3893.

DUGAS, Luc-Antoine; CSST Bas-Saint-Laurent, 180 rue des Gouverneurs, Rimouski QC G5L 8G1; Laval'95; CSPQ; FRCSC; OrthSurg (Reconstructive Surgery). Langs: English; (418)725-6100

DUGAS, Ludivine; Polyclinique Med de la Lievre, 536 rue de la Madone, Mont-Laurier QC J9L 1S7; McG'02; Staff Family Phys, CSSS d'Antoine-Labelle; Langs: English; (819)440-2345; Fax. (819)440-2330.

DUGAS, Marc-Andre N; CHUQ-Ctr Hosp Univ Laval, 2705 boul Laurier, Quebec QC G1V 4G2; Laval'93; FRCPC; Peds (Pediatric Critical Care); Critical Care Medicine (P.Q.). Staff, Centre Hospitalier Universitaire de Quebec-CHUL; Chef Pediatrics, Université Laval; (418)654-2282; Fax. (418)654-2137; marc-andre.dugas@mail.chuq.qc.ca.

DUGAS, Mario; Hop du Sacre-Coeur de Mtl, 5e-5400 boul Gouin O, Montreal QC H4J 1C5; Mon'81; Respir; IntMed (Hyperbaric Medicine). Staff, Hôpital du Sacre-Coeur de Montréal; adj Prof, Universite de Montreal; (514)338-2162; Fax. (514)338-3699; mariomd@videotron.ca.

DUGAS, Michel; ChUQ-Ctr Hosp Univ Laval, 2705 boul Laurier, Quebec QC G1V 4G2; Laval'86; FRCPC; IntMed; GeriatricMed. Ac Staff, Centre Hospitalier Universitaire de Quebec-CHUL; (418)654-2255; Fax. (418)654-2757.

DUGAS, Renee; Ctr Hosp Laurentien, 234 rue Saint-Vincent, Ste-Agathe-des-Mts QC J8C 2B8; Mon'74; CSPQ; FRCSC; GenSurg. Staff, Hôtel-Dieu de Saint-Jérôme; Staff, Centre Hospitalier Laurentien; (819)324-4000; Fax. (819)324-4064.

DUGAS, Ruth; Clinique Medicale 3000, 3000 rue Belanger, Montreal QC H1Y 1A9; Mon'94; (514)376-7702

DUGDALE, Ian P; B-22195 Dewdney Trunk Rd, Maple Ridge BC V2X 3H7; UBC'92; (604)463-4102; Fax. (604)463-4686.

DUGGAL, Anil; Bluewater Surgical, 106-704 Mara St, Point Edward ON N7V 1X4; McM'01; (519)336-1555

DUGGAL, Kishan; Thompson Gen Hosp, 871 Thompson Dr, Thompson MB R8N 0C8; Punjab (India)'61; MB BS; LRCP; MRCS; FRCS; Staff, Thompson General Hospital; (204)677-2381

DUGGAL, Neil; London HSC-University Hosp, PO Box 5339 Stn B A10 307-339 Windermere Rd, London ON N6A 5A5; Ott'92; BSc; MSc; FRCSC; Neursurg (Spine). Consultant NeuroSurg, London Health Sciences Centre - University Hospital; Assoc Prof, University of Western Ontario; Langs: Bilingual(English/French); (519)663-2926; Fax. (519)663-2947.

DUGGAL, Rishi; Bluewater Health-Norman Site, 89 Norman St, Sarnia ON N7T 6S3; Ott'02; FRCPC; DiagRad. Staff, Bluewater Health - Mitton Site; Staff, Bluewater Health - Norman Site; (519)464-4400

DUGGAL, Vikas; Regional Mental HC-London, PO Box 5532 Stn B 850 Highbury Ave, London ON N6A 4H1; Ott'01; FRCPC; Psy. Staff, Regional Mental Health Care-St Joseph's Health Care; (519)455-5110 x47552

DUGGAN, Ann; Inuit Family Hlth Team, 24 Shlkirk St, Ottawa ON K1L 0A4; Qns'90; DTMH(Liverpool); MPH; DSc; CCFP; FCFP; Physician, Citizenship & Immigration Canada; (613)740-0999; ann.duggan@cic.gc.ca.

DUGGAN, Keltie; Peter Lougheed Centre, 5021-3500 26 Ave NE, Calgary AB T1Y 6J4; Cal'00; CCFP; Staff, Peter Lougheed Centre; (403)943-5461

DUGGAN, Laura; Royal Columbia Hosp, 330 Columbia St E, New Westminster BC V3L 3W7; Ott'94; FRCPC; Peds; Anes. Staff, Royal Columbian Hospital; (604)520-4253

DUGGAN, Maire; Foothills Med Centre, C1135-1403 29 St NW, Calgary AB T2N 2T9; Cork (Ireland)'78; MB ChB; BAO; FRCPC; AnatPath (Cytopath). Staff Path, Foothills Medical Centre; Prof Path & Lab Med, University of Calgary; (403)944-4763; Fax. (403)944-1460; maire.duggan@cls.ab.ca.

DUGGAN, Norah A T; Shea Heights Comm Hlth Centre, PO Box 13122 Stn A 57B Linegar Ave, St. John's NL A1B 4A4; Mem'95; BSc; CCFP; Med Officer Sr, Notre Dame Bay Memorial Health Centre; Asst Prof Family Med, Memorial University Of Newfoundland; (709)737-3369; natduggan@netscape.net.

DUGGAN, Peter R; Foothills Medical Centre, C210-1403 29 St NW, Calgary AB T2N 2T9; Mem'94; FRCPC; IntMed; Hem. Staff, Foothills Medical Centre; (403)944-4451; Fax. (403)944-1647.

DUGGAN, Robert M; 500 Raglan St N, Renfrew ON K7V 1P5; Tor'74; Ac Staff, Renfrew Victoria Hospital; (613)432-7097

DUGGAN, Scott S; Kingston Gen Hosp, 76 Stuart St, Kingston ON K7L 2V7; Cal'98; FRCPC; Anes. Staff, Kingston General Hospital; (613)549-6666 x2604; Fax. (613)548-1375.

DUGGAN, Shelley; 205-9148 23 Ave NW, Edmonton AB T6N 1H9; Alb'96; FRCPC; IntMed; Critical Care Medicine; Nephrol. Staff Nephrol, University of Alberta Hospital; Asst Clin Prof Nephrol, University of Alberta; (780)468-3377; Fax. (780)468-9353.

DUGGLEBY, Gerald E; Ridgeview Med Centre, 212-1240 Railway Ave, Canmore AB T1W 1P4; Sask'81; CCFP; (403)609-8333; Fax. (403)609-3666.

DUGRE, Bernard; Clinique Med St Vincent, 250 rue King E, Sherbrooke QC J1G 1A9; Laval'76; (819)563-0510; Fax. (819)564-6889.

DUGRE, Colette; CLSC de la Haute Yamaska, 294 rue Deragon, Granby QC J2G 5J5; Laval'81; (450)375-1442; Fax. (450)375-6607.

DUGRE, Helene; Pavillon Edouard-Asselin, 264 boul Rene-Levesque E, Montreal QC H2X 1P1; Laval'90; Staff, Centre Hospitalier l'Université De Montréal (CHUM) - Hôpital Saint-luc; Physician, Centre Medicale Brunswick; (514)890-8000 x34101; Fax. (514)499-1697.

DUGUAY, Annick; CLSC Riviere-aux-Renards, 154 Boul Benard E, Gaspe QC G4X 5R5; Laval'10; CCFP; Staff, Centre Hospitalier de Gaspe; (418)269-2572; Fax. (418)269-5162.

DUGUAY, Annie; Clinique Med Bonaventure, 103 rue Nicolas Denys GD, Bonaventure QC G0C 1E0; Laval'98; CCFP; Langs: English; (418)534-2145; Fax. (418)534-2501.

DUGUAY, Bernard E; CSSS de la Baie-des-Chaleurs, RR 2 419 boul Perron, Maria QC G0C 1Y0; Laval'81; FRCPC; DiagRad. Staff, CSSS de la Baie-des-Chaleurs; (418)753-3443 x2112

DUGUAY, Christine; CSSS du Sud de Lanaudière, 911 Montee des Pionniers, Terrebonne QC J6V 2H2; Mon'01; CCFP; Staff, Centre Hospitalier Pierre le Gardeur; (450)654-7525

DUGUAY, Claude; Clinique Ophth de Rimouski, 106-161 av Rouleau, Rimouski QC G5L 5T3; Laval'64; Ophth (P.Q.). (418)723-4514; Fax. (418)723-4519.

DUGUAY, Francois; Hop du Sacre-Coeur de Mtl, 5400 boul Gouin O, Montreal QC H4J 1C5; Mon'90; Staff Geriatrics, Hôpital du Sacre-Coeur de Montréal; Clin Teach Staff Family Med, Universite de Montreal; (514)338-2050

DUGUAY, Gary; The Moncton Hosp, 135 MacBeath Ave, Moncton NB E1C 6Z8; Mon'01; CCFP; CCFP(E.M.); Staff, The Moncton Hospital; (506)857-5353

DUGUAY, Johanne; Hop Marie-Clarac, 3530 boul Gouin E, Montreal-Nord QC H1H 1B7; Mon'89; Staff, Hopital Marie Clarac; (514)321-8800

DUGUAY, Kirk J; The Moncton Hosp, 135 MacBeath Ave, Moncton NB E1C 6Z8; Mem'98; FRCPC; Anes. Staff, The Moncton Hospital; (506)857-5258; kirkduguay@hotmail.com.

DUGUAY, Lyne; Polyclinique Med Pierre Le Gar, 300-1000 montee des Pionniers, Terrebonne QC J6V 1S8; Mon'93; Staff, Centre Hospitalier Pierre le Gardeur; (450)657-5799; Fax. (450)657-1809.

DUGUAY, Pierre; Clinique Med Pierre-Bertrand, 303 boul Pierre-Bertrand, Quebec QC G1M 3L7; Laval'87; CSPQ; FRCSC; Ophth (P.Q.) (Uveitis). Médecin, Hôtel-Dieu de Lévis; Médecin, CH St-Sacrement Ltee; Conférencier, Université Laval; Langs: Bilingual(French/English); (418)683-3348; Fax. (418)683-4448.

DUGUAY, Pierre; Centre Hosp Honore-Mercier, 2750 boul Laframboise, Saint-Hyacinthe QC J2S 4Y8; Mon'98; FRCSC; PlasSurg. Staff, Centre Hospitalier Honore-Mercier; (450)771-3333

DUGUAY, R Lester; CSSS des Iles, 430 ch Principal, Cap-aux-Meules QC G4T 1R9; Laval'69; CSPQ; FRCSC; GenSurg. Staff, Hôpital de l'Archipel; (418)986-2121

DUGUAY, Veronique; CSSS des Etchemins, RR 1 331 rue Du Sanatorium, Lac-Etchemin QC G0R 1S0; Sher'06; CCFP; Staff, CSSS des Etchemins; (418)625-8001; Fax. (418)625-3009.

DUGUAY-PICARD, Lauza; 38 rue Otho, Neguac NB E9G 4H3; Sher'01; CCFP.

DUGUAY VIBERT, Denise; Hôpital de CSC de Lamèque, 29 rue de l'Hopital, Lameque NB E8T 1C5; Laval'99; CCFP; Staff, Hôpital de CSC de Lamèque; Langs: Bilingual(French/English); (506)344-3430; Fax. (506)344-3436.

DUGUET, Nathalie; Clinique Med L'Envolee, 5025 rue de Salaberry, Montreal QC H4J 1J1; Mon'89; Staff, Hôpital du Sacre-Coeur de Montréal; (514)331-2323; Fax. (514)333-8534.

DUGUID, Murray P; Trafalgar Med Clinic, 200-1235 Trafalgar Rd, Oakville ON L6H 3P1; Tor'71; Staff, Halton Healthcare Services Corporation - Oakville Site; (905)844-3281; Fax. (905)849-1076.

DUGUID, Nigel J D; 135 Lemarchant Rd, St. John's NL A1C 2H3; Edinburgh (Scotland)'69; MB ChB; MRC; FRCPC; IntMed; Respir. Ac Staff, St Clare's Mercy Hospital; Clin Prof Med, Memorial University Of Newfoundland; (709)777-5673; Fax. (709)576-6629.

DUHAIME, Francine; Clin Med Fleur de Lys, 8 rue Du Terminus E, Rouyn-Noranda QC J9X 3B4; Sher'76; Staff, Centre Hospitalier Rouyn-Noranda; (819)764-6185; Fax. (819)762-6079.

DUHAIME, Jean-Daniel; Hop du Sacre-Coeur de Mtl, 5400 boul Gouin O, Montreal QC H4J 1C5; Mon'00; CCFP; CCFP(E.M.); Staff, Hôpital du Sacre-Coeur de Montréal; (514)338-2222

DUHAIME, Morris; Groupe d'experts en Ortho de M, 525-5450 ch de la Cote-des-Nei, Montreal QC H3T 1Y6; Mon'61; CSPQ; FRCSC; OrthSurg. Staff, Hôpital Ste-Justine; (514)739-3613; josee_boucher@ssss.gouv.qc.ca.

DUHAIME, Nancy; CLSC Antoine-Rivard, 10 rue St-Alphonse CP 39, Panet QC G0R 2J0; Sher'91; (418)249-2572; Fax. (418)831-0249.

DUIA, Sheela; Meadowbrook Med Clinic, 3907 34 St NW, Edmonton AB T6T 1L5; (India)'91; MB BS; CCFP; (780)448-1166; Fax. (780)448-2830.

DUIC, Andrew D; Dufferin Med Clinic, 2045 Dufferin St, Toronto ON M6E 3R4; Zagreb (Croatia)'56; FRCPC; Peds. Hon Staff, The Hospital For Sick Children; Asst Prof, University of Toronto; Langs: Croatian; German; Italian; (416)656-6500; Fax. (416)656-6502.

DUIGENAN, Shauna; The Ottawa Hosp-Gen Campus, 501 Smyth Rd, Ottawa ON K1H 8L6; Wes'04; FRCPC; DiagRad. Staff, The Ottawa Hospital - General Campus; Langs: Bilingual(English/French); (613)722-7000

DUJARDIN, Thiery; CHUQ-Hotel-Dieu de Quebec, 11 Cote du Palais, Quebec QC G1R 2J6; Nice (France)'90; Urol (P.Q.). Staff, Centre Hospitalier Universitaire de Québec (CHUQ) - Siege Social; (418)691-5068; Fax. (418)691-3154.

DUJON, Leighton D; Meadowlark Health Centre, 160 Meadowlark Shopping Ctr NW, Edmonton AB T5R 5W9; West Indies (Jamaica)'73; MB BS; CAFCI; LMCC; CCFP; Ac Member, Covenant Health - Misericordia Community Hospital; University of Alberta; (780)484-8806; Fax. (780)484-8873.

DUKE, Anthony S R; Toronto East Gen Hosp Inc, 825 Coxwell Ave, Toronto ON M4C 3E7; Tor'72; FRCPC; Peds. Ac Staff Peds, Toronto East General Hospital Inc; Staff Peds, The Hospital For Sick Children; Teacher, University of Toronto; (416)469-6580

DUKE, Douglas C; North Edmonton Health Centre, 14007 50 St NW, Edmonton AB T5A 5E4; Alb'76; (780)472-5036; Fax. (780)472-5187.

DUKE, Gavin G; Central Alberta Med Imaging, 4312 54 Ave, Red Deer AB T4N 4M1; Alb'73; FRCPC; DiagRad. Staff, Red Deer Regional Hospital Centre; (403)343-6172; Fax. (403)343-6159.

DUKE, Margaret H; 225-5780 Cambie St, Vancouver BC V5Z 3A7; UBC'91; FRCPC; Psy. Staff, Providence Health Care - St Paul's Hospital; (604)685-1125; Fax. (604)662-3211.

DUKE, Marin J; Waterloo Sports Med Centre, 12-65 University Ave E, Waterloo ON N2J 2V9; Man'95; BSc; Dip SportMed; CCFP; Langs: Bilingual(English/French); (519)746-2220; Fax. (519)746-2295.

DUKE, Pauline S; Health Sciences Centre, 300 Prince Philip Dr, St. John's NL A1B 3V6; Mem'79; CCFP; FCFP; Ac Staff, Health Sciences Centre; (709)777-6743

DUKE, Peter C; Children's Hosp, 2F-671 William Ave, Winnipeg MB R3E 0Z2; Man'64; FAB; FRCPC; Anes (Cardiac Anesthesia). Staff, St Boniface General Hospital; Dir Cardiac Anes, Health Sciences Centre; Prof Anes & Surg, University of Manitoba; pduke@cc.umanitoba.ca.

DUKE, Sandra M; Medicine Hat Shopping Mall, 142-3292 Dunmore Rd SE, Medicine Hat AB T1B 2R4; Mem'98; CCFP; (403)502-1466; Fax. (403)526-6448.

DUKE, Stephen M; Dartmouth Med Centre, 310-46 Portland St, Dartmouth NS B2Y 1H4; Ott'94; FRCPC; IntMed. Site Chief Int Med, Dartmouth General Hospital; Lecturer Dep of Med, Dalhousie University; (902)465-8704; Fax. (902)464-4906; drsduke-1@hotmail.com.

DUKELOW, Adam M; London HSC-Victoria Hosp, PO Box 5010 Stn B 800 Commissioners Rd E, London ON N6A 5W9; Wes'02; FRCPC; EmergMed. Staff, London Health Sciences Centre - Victoria Campus; (519)685-8500 x76538

DUKELOW, Robert H; 1754 Highway 59 RR 1, Port Rowan ON N0E 1M0; Wes'69; Ac Staff, Norfolk General Hospital; (519)596-7691; Fax. (519)586-7555.

DUKELOW, Sean P; Foothills Medical Centre, 905D-1403 29 St NW, Calgary AB T2N 2T9; Wes'03; CSCN(EMG); BSc; PhD; FRCPC; PhysMed&Rehab (Stroke). Staff, Foothills Medical Centre; (403)944-5930; Fax. (403)944-0977.

DUKESHIRE, Lauralee; Horizons Family Med, A-5016 51 Ave, Red Deer AB T4N 4H5; Alb'03; CCFP; Physician, Associate Medical Group; (403)342-7270; Fax. (403)343-2677.

DUKESZ, Yitzchok; 6-200 Davis Dr, Newmarket ON L3Y 2N4; Man'82; DAB; (905)830-4497; Fax. (905)830-4498.

DUKIC, Helena; Glazier Med Centre, 11 Gibb St, Oshawa ON L1H 2J9; Belgrade (Serbia)'98; CCFP; (905)579-1212; Fax. (905)579-5548; hdukic@yahoo.ca.

DUKSZTA, Janusz R; Create Fertility Centre, 620-790 Bay St, Toronto ON M5G 1N8; Royal Coll. (Ireland)'56; Psy. Langs: Polish.

DULAC, Kathleen; Clinique Medicale le Frontenac, 202-5200 rue Frontenac, Lac-Megantic QC G6B 1H3; Laval'09; (819)583-0157

DULAI, Gurjeet; Smyth Associate Clinic, 4904 48 St, Leduc AB T9E 6X4; Alb'03; BSc; CCFP; (780)986-2712; Fax. (780)986-0356.

DULAI, Sukhdeep K; University of Alberta Hosp, 2C3 46-8440 112 St NW, Edmonton AB T6G 2B7; Alb'98; FRCSC; OrthSurg. Staff, University of Alberta Hospital; (780)407-6198; Fax. (780)407-2004.

DULAY, Daisy; Westheart Management, 202-2020 Richmond Rd, Victoria BC V8R 6R5; Mem'02; FRCPC; IntMed; Cardiol. (250)595-3111; Fax. (250)595-4277.

DULAY, Jaspal; London HSC-South Street Hosp, PO Box 5375 Stn B N584-375 South St, London ON N6A 4G5; Tor'05; CCFP; Staff, London Health Sciences Centre - South Street; (519)685-8500

DULAY, Navdesh K; Platinum Med Clinic FHG, 3170 Eglinton Ave E, Scarborough ON M1J 2H3; McG'06; MDCM; CCFP; (416)265-2255

DULLEGE, Suzanne; Tri Area Med Centre, 52 St Lawrence St E, Madoc ON K0K 2K0; McM'08; CCFP; Staff, Caressant Care Nursing Home; (613)473-4134; Fax. (613)473-4740; sdullege@stegh.on.ca.

DULONG, Anick; CSSS du Sud de Lanaudière, 911 Montee des Pionniers, Terrebonne QC J6V 2H2; Mon'98; CCFP; Staff, Centre Hospitalier Pierre le Gardeur; (450)654-7525

DULUDE, Francois; Clinique Med Chateauguay, 120 boul Saint-Jean-Baptiste, Chateauguay QC J6K 3A9; Mon'76; (450)691-8191; Fax. (450)691-8568.

DULUDE, Michel; Clin Med St-Felix de Valois, 610 ch Joliette RR 1, St-Felix-de-Valois QC J0K 2M0; Mon'86; (450)889-5577; Fax. (450)889-4239.

DULUDE, Serge; FMOQ, 2000-3500 boul de Maisonneuve, Montreal QC H3Z 3C1; Mon'79; Staff, Hopital Ste-Anne; Chef, Universite de Montreal; (514)878-1911; sdulude@fmoq.org.

DUMAINE, Marcel; Clin Med Havre Sante, 521 boul du Havre, Salaber-de-Valleyf QC J6S 4Z5; Mon'65; (450)371-6444; Fax. (450)371-5315.

DUMAIS, Alexandre; Inst Philippe Pinel de Mtl, 10905 boul Henri-Bourassa E, Montreal QC H1C 1H1; Mon'06; FRCPC; Psy. Staff, Institut Philippe-Pinel de Montreal; (514)648-8461

DUMAIS, Alexis; CSSS Pierre Boucher, 1333 boul Jacques-Cartier E, Longueuil QC J4M 2A5; Sher'07; Staff, Centre Hospitalier Pierre Boucher; Langs: Bilingual(French/English); (450)468-8111; Fax. (450)468-8274.

DUMAIS, Carol; Place Saint-Laurent, 110-70 rue Saint-Germain E, Rimouski QC G5L 7J9; Laval'77; (418)725-5233; Fax. (418)725-5977; drcdumais@globetrotter.net.

DUMAIS, Daniel; CLSC Simonne-Monet-Chartrand, 1303 boul Jacques-Cartier E, Longueuil QC J4M 2Y8; Mon'81; (450)463-2850 x72449

DUMAIS, Dany; CSSS de Rivière-du-Loup, 75 rue Saint-Henri, Riviere-du-Loup QC G5R 2A4; Laval'05; FRCPC; DiagRad. Staff, Centre Hospitalier Regional du Grand-Portage; (418)868-1010 x2291

DUMAIS, Huguette; Comm Lesions Prof, 530 rue Notre-Dame, Joliette QC J6E 3H7; Laval'80; CSPQ; Anes (P.Q.). Staff, Centre Hospitalier Régional Baie-Comeau; (450)757-7973

DUMAIS, Gaston R J; Polyclinique de Montreal, 112-12245 rue Grenet, Montreal QC H4J 2J6; Mon'58; DABLaser Surgery; FRCPC; Derm (Laser Dermatology). Langs: Bilingual(French/English); (514)332-4545; Fax. (514)332-8664; gdumais@dr-g-dumais.com.

DUMAIS, Lynne; CSSS du Suroît, 150 rue Saint-Thomas, Salaber-de-Valleyf QC J6T 6C1; Laval'97; CSPQ; FRCPC; Anes. Staff, Centre Hospitalier Régional du Suroît; (450)371-9920

DUMAIS, Marie-Eve; CSSS de la Matapedia, 135 av Gaetan-Archambault, Amqui QC G5J 2K5; Sher'07; CCFP; Staff, CSSS de la Matapedia; (418)629-2211; Fax. (418)629-4498.

DUMAIS, Marion; MD Signature, 1313 boul Frechette, Chambly QC J3L 2Y9; Sher'99; CCFP; (450)403-4773; Fax. (450)403-4770.

DUMAIS, Michelle; 180 Route 170 RR 1, L'Anse-Saint-Jean QC G0V 1J0; Laval'93; (418)272-2112; Fax. (418)272-1464.

DUMAIS, Rejean; CHUS-Hop Hotel-Dieu, 580 rue Bowen S, Sherbrooke QC J1G 2E8; Sher'84; CSPQ; FRCSC; OrthSurg (Reconstructive Surgery). Staff, Centre Hospitalier Universitaire de Sherbrooke-Hôpital Hôtel-Dieu; Langs: Bilingual(English/French); (819)346-1110 x28304; Fax. (819)822-6725.

DUMAIS, Richard G; Dr Georges-L Dumont Reg Hosp, 330 av Universite, Moncton NB E1C 2Z3; Mon'86; FRCPC; Anes. Dir Pain Clinic/Staff Anes, Dr Georges-L-Dumont University Hospital Centre; (506)862-4721; Fax. (506)869-2130.

DUMAIS, Robert; Sudbury Reg Hosp-Laurentian, 41 Ramsey Lake Rd, Sudbury ON P3E 5J1; Ott'96; FRCPC; Anes. Staff, Health Sciences North-Laurentian Site; Staff, Health Sciences North-St Joseph's Health Centre; Langs: English; French; (705)675-4733; Fax. (705)671-5458.

DUMARAIX, Nathalie; CSSS du Lac-des-Deux-Montagnes, 520 boul Arthur-Sauve, Saint-Eustache QC J7R 5B1; Sher'87; FRCPC; Psy. Staff Psy, Hôpital de Saint-Eustache; (450)473-6811; Fax. (450)473-6966.

DUMARESQ, Cynthia; Clinique Med de Mont-Joli, 1385 boul Gaboury, Mont-Joli QC G5H 4B1; Sher'07; Staff, CSSS de la Mitis; (418)775-5353

DUMARESQ, Jeannot; Hotel-Dieu de Levis, 143 rue Wolfe, Levis QC G6V 3Z1; Laval'06; Microbio & Infect Dis (P.Q.). Staff, Hôtel-Dieu de Lévis; (418)835-7121

DUMAS, Alain; Centre Med Boucherville, 201-600 boul du Fort-St-Louis, Boucherville QC J4B 1S7; Laval'81; (450)655-7321; Fax. (450)655-6311.

DUMAS, Amelie; Ctr Hosp Affilie-Enfant-Jesus, 1401 18e rue, Quebec QC G1J 1Z4; Laval'04; FRCSC; PlasSurg. Staff, Centre Hospitalier Affilié Universitaire de Québec - Hôpital De L'Enfant Jésus; (418)649-0252

DUMAS, Bruno; Clinique Med du Phare, 101-822 boul Sainte-Anne, Rimouski QC G5M 1J5; Laval'71; Ophth. Consultant Ophth, Centre Hospitalier Saint-Joseph de la Turque; Consultant Ophth, Centre Hospitalier de Chandler; Staff, Hôpital Regional Rimouski; (418)723-4515; Fax. (418)724-0743.

DUMAS, Catherine; CHUM-Hotel-Dieu, 3840 rue Saint-Urbain, Montreal QC H2W 1T8; Mon'07; EmergMed. Staff, Centre Hospitalier l'Université de Montréal (CHUM) - Hôtel-Dieu; (514)890-8000

DUMAS, Christiane; CSSS Vieille Capitale, 900 boul Wilfrid-Hamel, Quebec QC G1M 3J6; Sher'79; DiagRad. Staff, CSSS de Quebec-Sud; (418)682-1711

DUMAS, Diane; Hop du Sacre-Coeur de Mtl, 5400 boul Gouin O, Montreal QC H4J 1C5; Mon'79; CSPQ; Anes (P.Q.). Staff, Hôpital du Sacre-Coeur de Montréal; (514)338-2222 x2140

DUMAS, Francois; CSSS de la Baie-des-Chaleurs, RR 2 419 boul Perron, Maria QC G0C 1Y0; Mon'90; FRCPC; Peds. Staff Ped, CSSS de la Baie-des-Chaleurs; Staff Ped, Centre Hospitalier Universitaire de Quebec-CHUL; Langs: English; (418)759-3443; Fax. (418)759-5890.

DUMAS, Guy; Centre Med St-Leonard, 360 rue Beliveau, St-Leonard-d'Aston QC J0C 1M0; Laval'76; ac Staff, Hôpital Sainte-croix; Admin, College des Medecins du Quebec; Clin Adj Prof Family Med/Prof, Universite de Sherbrooke; Langs: English; (819)399-2030; Fax. (819)399-2343; guy_dumas@gmf.gouv.qc.ca.

DUMAS, Jacinthe; 105-1055 12e av N, Sherbrooke QC J1E 2X4; Laval'77; (819)821-2142; Fax. (819)821-0248.

DUMAS, Jean F; Clinique Med Le Gardeurois, 130-155 rue Notre-Dame, Repentigny QC J5Z 3C4; Mon'81; Langs: English; (450)582-5546; Fax. (450)582-2718.

DUMAS, Jean-Marc; Groupe Belle Chasse Sante Inc, 8600 boul Marie-Victorin, Brossard QC J4X 1A1; Laval'65; FRCPC; DiagRad (Radiology). Prés, Groupe Belle Chasse Sante Inc; Treas, Radiologie Monteregie; Langs: Bilingual(French/English); (450)923-1810; Fax. (450)923-4488.

DUMAS, Louise; CSSS de Trois-Rivieres, 1991 boul du Carmel, Trois-Rivieres QC G8Z 3R9; Laval'90; Staff, CSSS de Trois-Rivières; (819)697-3333

DUMAS, Marie-Pierre; CSSS Vieille Capital, 55 ch Sainte-Foy, Quebec QC G1R 1S9; Laval'05; CCFP; Staff, CSSS Haute-Ville; (418)641-2572; marie-pierre.dumas@irdpq.qc.ca.

DUMAS, Mario E; CHUS-Hop Fleurimont, 3001 12e av N, Sherbrooke QC J1H 5N4; (Haiti)'83; FRCPC; Respir (P.Q.). Staff, Centre Hospitalier Universitaire de Sherbrooke-Hopital Fleurimont; (819)346-1110 x14851

DUMAS, Olivier; CHUQ-Hotel-Dieu de Quebec, 11 Cote du Palais, Quebec QC G1R 2J6; Laval'04; FRCPC; IntMed; MedOncol; HemPath. Staff, Centre Hospitalier Universitaire de Québec (CHUQ) - Siege Social; (418)652-5444

DUMAS, Richard; 305-3030 boul Le carrefour, Laval QC H7T 2P5; Sher'88; Endocrin&Metab; Endocrin (P.Q.); IntMed. (450)688-3132; Fax. (450)688-4266.

DUMAS, Serge; Centre Med Berger, 116-1000 ch Sainte-Foy, Quebec QC G1S 2L6; Laval'68; Staff, Centre Hospitalier Affilié Universitaire de Québec - Hôpital du St-Sacrement; Langs: Bilingual(French/English); (418)688-1385; Fax. (418)688-3249; serge_dumas@ssss.gouv.qc.ca.

DUMAS, Sylvie; Ctr Hosp Chauveau, 11999 rue de l'Hopital, Quebec QC G2A 2T7; Laval'84; Staff, Centre Hospitalier Chauveau; Staff, CSSS de Quebec-Sud; (418)843-2572 x7602; Fax. (418)843-3880.

DUMAS-LAVERDIERE, Martin; Hotel-Dieu de Levis, 143 rue Wolfe, Levis QC G6V 3Z1; Sher'99; CSPQ; FRCPC; Anes. Staff Anes, Hôtel-Dieu de Lévis; (418)835-7121

DUMAS-PILON, Maxine; Centre Hosp Saint-Mary, 3777 rue Jean-Brillant, Montreal QC H3T 1M5; Laval'02; CCFP; Staff, St Mary's Hospital Centre; (514)734-2631

DUMATOL-SANCHEZ, Jocelyn; Healthway Four Seasons Med Cli, 865 Portage Ave, Winnipeg MB R3G 0N8; Santo Tomas (Philippines)'86; MCFP; CCFP; Staff ER Phys, Victoria General Hospital; Physician, Northern Medical Unit; I-Prog Dir MLP IMG, University of Manitoba; Langs: Tagalog; Spanish; (204)783-6464; jsanchez@mts.net.

DUMBRAVA, Daniela; Hop Louis-H Lafontaine, 7401 rue Hochelaga, Montreal QC H1N 3M5; (Romania)'95; CCFP; Staff, Hopital Louis-H Lafontaine; (514)251-4000

DUMESNIL, Jean G; Hôpital Laval, 2725 ch Sainte-Foy, Quebec QC G1V 4G5; Mon'68; CSPQ; FRCPC; Cardiol. Staff, Hôpital Laval; Prof Med, Université Laval; (418)656-8711 x5108; Fax. (418)656-4562; medjgd@hermes.ulaval.ca.

DUMITRESCU, Corina; 101-13025 Yonge St PO Box 2639, Richmond Hill ON L4E 1A6; (Grenada)'07; CCFP; (905)773-3342; Fax. (905)881-5051.

DUMITRESCU, Luiza A A; Ctr Hosp Laurentien, 234 rue Saint-Vincent, Ste-Agathe-Des-Mts QC J8C 2B8; Jassy (Romania)'80; Psy (General Psychiatry). Staff, Centre Hospitalier Laurentien; Langs: English; Romanian; (819)324-4045; Fax. (819)324-4020.

DUMITRU, Ioana; St Paul's Hosp, Fl 3-1081 Burrard St, Vancouver BC V6Z 1Y6; McM'98; FRCPC; Anes. Staff, Providence Health Care - St Paul's Hospital; (604)682-2344 x62813

DUMKA, Evelyn; Medical Clinic, PO Box 249, Catalina NL A0C 1J0; Mem'74; (709)469-3030

DUMONT, Alain; CHUS-Hop Fleurimont, 3001 12e av N, Sherbrooke QC J1H 5N4; Sher'85; DAB; CSPQ; FRCSC; OrthSurg. Staff, Centre Hospitalier Universitaire de Sherbrooke-Hopital Fleurimont; adj Prof, Universite de Sherbrooke; (819)346-1110 x14233

DUMONT, Andre; CSSS de la Haute-Gaspésie, 50 rue du Belvedere, Ste-Anne-des-Monts QC G4V 1X4; Laval'66; LMCC; ac Staff, Centre Hospitalier des Monts; Langs: Bilingual(French/English); (418)763-2261 x2732; Fax. (418)763-7176.

DUMONT, Catherine; CSSS du Grand Littoral, 1205 boul de la Rive-Sud, Levis QC G6W 0J4; Laval'08; (418)380-8597

DUMONT, Charles H; Lakeshore Gen Hosp, 160 av Stillview, Pointe-Claire QC H9R 2Y2; Ott'68; FRCPC; IntMed. Staff, Lakeshore General Hospital - Pointe Claire; (514)630-2225

DUMONT, Daniel; 6555 boul Gouin O, Montreal QC H4K 1B3; Mon'83; MSc(Clin.Science); FRCPC; Psy. Staff, Centre Hospitalier de Chandler; Staff, Hôpital du Sacre-Coeur de Montréal; Universite de Montreal; (514)338-4621

DUMONT, Eric; Hôpital Laval, 2725 ch Sainte-Foy, Quebec QC G1V 4G5; Mon'98; CSPQ; CardSurg. Staff, Hôpital Laval; (418)656-4717

DUMONT, Guillaume; CSSS de Sept-Iles, 45 rue du Pere-Divet, Sept-Iles QC G4R 3N7; Laval'00; FRCPC; Psy. Psychiatrist, Centre Hospitalier Regional de Sept-Iles; Langs: Bilingual(French/English); (418)962-9761; Fax. (418)960-0409.

DUMONT, Guy; 2 rue des Cedres Box 2151, Pont-Rouge QC G3H 1S7; Laval'83; (418)873-3224

DUMONT, Isabelle; Rimouski Fam Med, 165 rue des Gouverneurs, Rimouski QC G5L 7R2; Laval'99; CCFP; Staff, Hôpital Regional Rimouski; Université Laval; (418)727-5493; Fax. (418)723-7668.

DUMONT, Jacques; Ctr de Readaptation Ubald-Vill, 2525 ch de la Canardiere, Quebec QC G1J 2G2; Laval'82; Ac Staff, Centre Hospitalier Universitaire De Québec - Pavillon De St-françois-d'assise; (418)663-5008; Fax. (418)687-3585.

DUMONT, Jocelyn; 60 av Bateman, Edmundston NB E3V 4X6; Laval'80; (506)735-8891; Fax. (506)739-9050.

DUMONT, Julie; 200-394 rue Saint-Vallier, Chicoutimi QC G7H 4J1; Laval'92; FRCSC; ObstGyn. Staff, Complexe hospitalier de la Sagamie; Langs: English; (418)545-2666; Fax. (418)545-3924.

DUMONT, Karine; CSSS de Laval, 1755 boul Rene-Laennec, Laval QC H7M 3L9; Laval'08; Staff, Hopital de la Cite de la santé; (450)668-1010

DUMONT, Louis; CSSS de Montmagny-L'Islet, RR 1 350 boul Tache O, Montmagny QC G5V 3R8; McG'04; FRCPC; Anes. Staff, CSSS de Montmagny-L'Islet; (418)248-0630; Fax. (418)248-6838.

DUMONT, Luc; CSSS de la Region de Thetford, 1717 rue Notre-Dame E, Thetford Mines QC G6G 2V4; Sher'93; CSPQ; FRCSC; OrthSurg. Staff, Hopital du CSS de la Region de Thetford; Langs: English; (418)338-7777

DUMONT, Marc; Clinique Med D'Alma, 935 av du Pont S, Alma QC G8B 2V5; Laval'84; (418)668-6121; Fax. (418)668-5298; marc.dumont@ssss.gouv.qc.ca.

DUMONT, Marcel; 1588 av Saint-Laurent, Plessisville QC G6L 2P6; Laval'69; PhD; MSc; (819)362-8112; Fax. (819)362-8157.

DUMONT, Marcel; CHUQ-St-Franois D'Assise, 10 rue de l'Espinay, Quebec QC G1L 3L5; Laval'79; NuclearMed (P.Q.). pers Chef Nuclear Med, Centre Hospitalier Universitaire De Québec - Pavillon De St-françois-d'assise; Consultant, Centre Hospitalier Affilié Universitaire de Québec - Hôpital du St-Sacrement; Consultant, Centre Hospitalier Affilié Universitaire de Québec - Hôpital De L'Enfant Jésus; Head Radiol, Université Laval; (418)525-4484; Fax. (418)525-4350.

DUMONT, Michelle; Pavillon Rosemont, 5689 boul Rosemont, Montreal QC H1T 2H1; Laval'77; Psy. Staff, Centre Hospitalier Universitaire De Québec - Pavillon De St-françois-d'assise; (514)252-3400 x4725

DUMONT, Randall; University Hosp of Northern BC, 1475 Edmonton St, Prince George BC V2M 1S2; UBC'04; FRCPC; GenPath. Staff, University Hospital of Northern British Columbia; (250)565-2421

DUMONT, Serge; CLSC Desjardins, 15 rue de l'Arsenal, Levis QC G6V 4P6; Laval'74; Staff Physician Mental Health & Palliative Care, CLSC de Levis; (418)835-3400 x3208; Fax. (418)835-6413.

DUMONT, Serge; CLSC Bordeaux-Cartierville, 11822 av de Bois-De-Boulogne, Montreal QC H3M 2X6; Mon'97; Staff, CLSC Bordeaux-Cartierville; (514)331-2572; Fax. (514)331-2064.

DUMONT, Tania; Carson Med Clinic, E-876 Montreal Rd, Ottawa ON K1K 4L3; Sher'05; FRCSC; ObstGyn. Staff, The Hospital For Sick Children; (613)742-8182

DUMONT, Yannick; CSSS de Trois-Rivières, 1991 boul du Carmel, Trois-Rivieres QC G8Z 3R9; Laval'04; FRCSC; GenSurg. Staff, CSSS de Trois-Rivières; (819)697-3333

DUMONT, Yves G; Groupe Sante Medisys Inc, 1100-500 rue Sherbrooke O, Montreal QC H3A 3C6; Laval'66; MSc(Lond.); FRSM; CommunMed (P.Q.). Dir, Mediys Inc., Consultants in Occup. Health & Safety; (514)845-1211; Fax. (514)845-4842.

DUMONT-MACKAY, Vincent; Institut de Cardiologie de Mtl, 5000 rue Belanger, Montreal QC H1T 1C8; Mon'00; CCFP; FCFP; Staff, Institut de Cardiologie de Montréal; (514)376-3330

DUMONTIER, Real; Centre Med Plexus, CP 189 107 ch cu Lac Millette, Saint-Sauveur QC J0R 1R0; Sher'74; (450)227-9933; Fax. (450)227-4900.

DUMOUCHEL, Richard; Clinique Med du Coteau, 100-440 boul Saint-Luc, St-Jean-sur-Richel QC J2W 0E2; Mon'88; Staff, Hôpital du Haut-Richelieu; (450)359-6819; Fax. (450)359-3247.

DUMOULIN, Joanne; CHUS-Hop Hotel-Dieu, 580 rue Bowen S, Sherbrooke QC J1G 2E8; Sher'96; Psy. Staff, Centre Hospitalier Universitaire de Sherbrooke-Hôpital Hôtel-Dieu; (819)822-6756

DUMOULIN, Lyne; Hop Louis-H Lafontaine, 7401 rue Hochelaga, Montreal QC H1N 3M5; Mon'96; FRCPC; Psy. Staff, Hopital Louis-H Lafontaine; (514)251-4000 x3039

DUMPER, Jamie W; 206-1650 Terminal Ave, Nanaimo BC V9S 0A3; Cal'04; FRCSC; Otol (Head & Neck Surgery). Staff, University of Alberta Hospital; (250)591-4405

DUNBAR, Michael; Queen Elizabeth II HSC, 4822-1796 Summer St, Halifax NS B3H 3A7; Dal'92; PhD(Sweden); FRCSC; OrthSurg (Hip & Knee Arthroplasty). Dir Orthopedic Research, Queen Elizabeth II Health Sciences Centre - Halifax Infirmary Site; Dir Ortho Research, Dalhousie University; (902)473-7337; Fax. (902)473-7370.

DUNBAR, Ross H; Westland Fam Pracitce Clinic, 144-70 McLeod Ave, Spruce Grove AB T7X 3C7; Alb'91; CCFP; FCFP; Staff, Westview Health Centre; Med Examiner, Province of Alberta; Clin Lecturer, University of Alberta; (780)962-9393; Fax. (780)962-4295; drdunbar@telus.net.

DUNBERRY, Michel; Societte Centre Chirug Joliett, 202-222 rue de la Visitation, St-Charles-Boromee QC J6E 4N5; McG'82; CSPQ; FRCSC; GenSurg. Staff, Centre Hospitalier Régional de Lanaudière; Langs: Bilingual(English/French); (450)753-7588; Fax. (450)756-6144; mdunberry@videotron.ca.

DUNCAN, Barbara R; 120-6180 Blundell Rd, Richmond BC V7C 4W7; UBC'79; (604)276-1660; Fax. (604)241-8615.

DUNCAN, Charles G; Birchley Pl, PO Box 759 209 Hwy 20 E, Fonthill ON L0S 1E0; Aberdeen (Scotland)'67; Court Staff, Niagara Health System - Welland Hospital Site; (905)892-5777; Fax. (905)892-7539.

DUNCAN, Clive; Gordon & Leslie Diamond HCC, 3F-2775 Laurel St, Vancouver BC V5Z 1M9; Dublin (Ireland)'68; MB BCh; FRCSC; OrthSurg (Hip Reconstruction). Staff, Gordon & Leslie Diamond Health Care Centre; Staff, Vancouver General Hospital - Centennial Pavillion.

DUNCAN, David A; Saskatchewan Hosp-Battleford, PO Box 39 Stn Main, North Battleford SK S9A 2X8; Witwatersrand (South Africa)'81; MB BCh; MMed(Psych); Staff, Saskatchewan Hospital - North Battleford; Consultant, Battlefords Regional Care Centre; (306)446-6800; Fax. (306)446-6867.

DUNCAN, Eric G; Credit Valley Prof Bldg, 402-2300 Eglinton Ave W, Mississauga ON L5M 2V8; Bristol (England)'79; MB ChB; BSc(Hon)Pharm; FRCS(Ed); FRCSC; Neursurg. Consultant, Trillium Health Centre - Mississauga; Court Consultant, The Credit Valley Hospital; Langs: Bilingual(English/French); (905)607-0005; Fax. (905)607-0341.

DUNCAN, Fiona C; 4186 Dunbar St, Vancouver BC V6S 2E7; UBC'99; CCFP; (604)739-9881

DUNCAN, G Stephen; Caroline Family Hlth Team-CMG, 15-3305 Harvester Rd, Burlington ON L7N 3N2; Wes'93; CCFP; FCFP; Staff, Joseph Brant Memorial Hospital; (905)632-8007; Fax. (905)681-6341.

DUNCAN, Graeme G; BC Cancer Agency-Vancouver CC, 600 10th Ave W, Vancouver BC V5Z 4E6; Edinburgh (Scotland)'81; MRC(UK); FRCPC; RadOncol. Consultant, BC Cancer Agency Vancouver Centre; Ac Staff, Vancouver General Hospital - Centennial Pavillion; Clin Prof, University of British Columbia; (604)877-6000 x2672; Fax. (604)877-0505.

DUNCAN, Jacqueline; Regional Mental HC-London, PO Box 5532 Stn B 850 Highbury Ave, London ON N6A 4H1; Galway (Ireland)'81; MB ChB; BAO; MRCPsy; DCPsy; DCH; DObst; FRCPC; Psy (Psychiatric Rehabilitation). Staff, Regional Mental Health Care-St Joseph's Health Care; (519)455-5110; jduncan@cmha-mhassc.ca.

DUNCAN, John; 5F-2775 Laurel St, Vancouver BC V5Z 1M9; Ott'95; BSc(Hons); MSc; ABIM; FRCPC; IntMed; Nephrol. Clinical Asst Prof, University of British Columbia; (604)875-5950; Fax. (604)875-5952.

DUNCAN, Mark A; 208-3330 Richter St, Kelowna BC V1W 4V5; Ott'90; FRCPC; Peds. (250)762-0466; Fax. (250)762-0477.

DUNCAN, Mary Jean; Children's Hosp of Eastern Ont, 401 Smyth Rd, Ottawa ON K1H 8L1; Qns'78; FRCSC; PlasSurg (Pediatrics). Ac Staff, The Ottawa Hospital - General Campus; Ac Staff, Children's Hospital of Eastern Ontario (CHEO); Clin Lecturer Surg, University of Ottawa; (613)737-7600; Fax. (613)738-4840; mduncan@cheo.on.ca.

DUNCAN, Peter G; Victoria Gen Hosp, 1 Hospital Way, Victoria BC V8Z 6R5; Man'70; FRCPC; Anes (Pediatric Anesthesia). Staff Locum Anes, BC Children's Hospital; Staff, Victoria General Hospital; Ac Staff, Vancouver Island Health Authority; Clin Prof, University of British Columbia; (250)727-4152; Fax. (250)727-9424.

DUNCAN, Stephen; The Brandon Clinic, 620 Dennis St, Brandon MB R7A 5E7; Man'89; (204)728-4440; Fax. (204)726-1765.

DUNCAN, Sarah L H; City of Lakes Family Hlth Team, 25 Black Lake Rd, Lively ON P3Y 1J3; McM'08; CCFP; (705)692-1018; Fax. (705)692-7156.

DUNCAN, Sharon A; Peace Arch Hosp, 15521 Russell St, White Rock BC V4B 2R4; UBC'96; CCFP; Staff, Peace Arch Hospital; (604)535-4500

DUNCAN, Stephen C; Health Sciences Centre, 1410-3330 Hospital Dr NW, Calgary AB T2N 4N1; Dal'99; FRCPC; IntMed. Staff, Foothills Medical Centre; Teacher Health Sciences Centre, University of Calgary; (403)220-8892; Fax. (403)283-6151; steve.duncan@albertahealthservices.ca.

DUNCAN, Walter; BC Children's Hosp, 1F14-4480 Oak St, Vancouver BC V6H 3V4; Sask'74; FRCPC; Peds; PedCardiol. Staff, BC Children's Hospital; Staff, BC Women's Hospital & Health Centre; (604)875-3878; wduncan@cw.bc.ca.

DUNDAS, Caroline-Ann C; The Sundance Clinic, 113-31 Sunpark Plaza SE, Calgary AB T2X 3W5; Alb'95; CCFP; (403)254-2030

DUNDAS, Kathryn J E; 240-815 17 Ave SW, Calgary AB T2T 0A1; Cal'97; Chief EmergMed & Assoc, Sundre Hospital & Care Centre; Langs: Spanish; (403)266-5585; kjekill@telusplanet.net.

DUNDAS, Susan D; The Hincks-Dellcrest Centre, 207-440 Jarvis St, Toronto ON M4Y 2H4; McM'85; FRCPC; Psy (Child Psychiatry). Staff, The Hincks-Dellcrest Centre - Toronto; Teacher, University of Toronto; (416)924-1164 x3302; Fax. (416)924-8208.

DUNDAS, Timothy; Worksafe BC, 321 Battle St, Kamloops BC V2C 6P1; London (England)'67; MRCS; LRCP; DObstRCOG; MB BS; CCFP; Med Advisor II, Workers' Compensation Board; (250)371-6017; Fax. (250)371-6036.

DUNDON, John; 11-421 Greenbrook Dr, Kitchener ON N2M 4K1; Univ College Dublin (Ireland)'90; MB ChB; BSc(Hons.); LLB; BAO; CCFP; FCFP; Assoc Staff, Grand River Hospital - Kitchener/Waterloo Health Centre; Assoc Staff, St Mary's General Hospital; (519)570-2222; Fax. (519)570-2053.

DUNFIELD, James I; Park Avenue Med Centre, 500-4634 Park Ave, Terrace BC V8G 1V7; Dal'80; FACS; FRCSC; GenSurg. (250)615-5073; Fax. (250)615-5078.

DUNGEY, Paul E; Kingston Gen Hosp, 76 Stuart St, Kingston ON K7L 2V7; Qns'88; FRCPC; EmergMed., Kingston General Hospital; (613)549-6666 x3967

DUNHAM, Christopher P; Children's & Women's HC of BC, B321-4480 Oak St, Vancouver BC V6H 3V4; Ott'01; FRCPC; NeurPath. Staff, BC Children's Hospital; (604)875-3639; Fax. (604)875-3529; cdunham@cw.bc.ca.

DUNHAM, Michael B; 202-8330 Fairmount Dr SE, Calgary AB T2H 0Y8; Alb'99; BSc(Zoology); FRCSC; GenSurg (Trauma Surgery); Critical Care Medicine. Dir, Advanced Trauma Life Support; (403)252-5674; Fax. (403)252-3938; michael.dunham@calgaryhealthregion.ca.

DUNHAM, Peter B; Foothills Prof Bldg, 170-1620 29 St NW, Calgary AB T2N 4L7; Alb'69; (403)221-9345; Fax. (403)221-9336.

DUNHIN, Anna; North Battleford Med Clinic, 102-11427 Railway Ave, North Battleford SK S9A 3G8; MB ChB; DA; Staff, Battlefords Union Hospital; Langs: Afrikaans; (306)445-4415; Fax. (306)445-5145.

DUNIEWICZ, Magdalena; Hop du Sacre-Coeur de Mtl, 5400 boul Gouin O, Montreal QC H4J 1C5; Mon'00; CCFP; CCFP(E.M.); Staff, Hôpital du Sacre-Coeur de Montréal; (514)338-2000

DUNIN-BELL, Ola H; The Credit Valley Hosp, 2200 Eglinton Ave W, Mississauga ON L5M 2N1; Qns'79; AB; FRCSC; GenSurg (Pediatric Surgery). Staff, The Credit Valley Hospital; (905)813-2200

DUNKERLEY, Heather; Wortley Village Med Centre, 205-190 Wortley Rd, London ON N6C 4Y7; Qns'07; CCFP.

DUNKERLEY, Robert; Wortley Village Med Centre, 205-190 Wortley Rd, London ON N6C 4Y7; Wes'72; Court Staff, London Health Sciences Centre - Victoria Campus; Court Staff, Parkwood Hospital - St Joseph's Health Care; (519)681-3320; Fax. (519)649-5055.

DUNKLEY, Geoffrey C; The Ottawa Hosp-Gen Campus, 501 Smyth Rd, Ottawa ON K1H 8L6; Qns'78; FRCPC; CommunMed. Staff, The Ottawa Hospital - General Campus; (613)562-5800; Fax. (613)562-5465.

DUNLAP, Hal J; Children's Hosp Eastern Ont, 401 Smyth Rd, Ottawa ON K1H 8L1; Ott'78; FRCPC; DiagRad. Court Staff, The Ottawa Hospital - General Campus; Media Dir Diagnostic Imaging, Children's Hospital of Eastern Ontario (CHEO); Asst Prof Radiol, University of Ottawa; (613)737-7600 x3224; Fax. (613)737-2306; dunlap@cheo.on.ca.

DUNLOP, R H Brett; Charlton Med Centre, 606-25 Charlton Ave E, Hamilton ON L8N 1Y2; McM'76; FRCSC; OrthSurg. Staff, St Joseph's Healthcare - Charlton Campus; Staff, Hamilton Health Sciences Centre - Hamilton General Hospital; Physician, Charlton Medical Centre; Head Div of Orthopeds, McMaster University; (905)521-5770; Fax. (905)521-8830.

DUNN, Anita Y; 209-840 Coxwell Ave, East York ON M4C 5T2; Tor'04; FRCPC; IntMed; Nephrol. Staff, St Joseph's Health Centre; (647)776-2762; Fax. (647)436-3161.

DUNN, Barbara L; Seymour Med Clinic, Stn 1 200-1530 7th Ave W, Vancouver BC V6J 1S3; Cal'80; Assoc Staff, Providence Health Care - St Vincent's Hospital-Heather Site; Vis Staff, Vancouver General Hospital - Centennial Pavillion; (604)739-5611; Fax. (604)738-2102.

DUNN, Carolyn M; Clinique Pediatrique de Longue, 105-2160 ch du Tremblay, Longueuil QC J4N 1A8; Mon'87; FRCPC; Peds. Ac Staff Peds & Prenatal, Centre Hospitalier Pierre Boucher; Langs: Bilingual(French/English); (450)448-4440; Fax. (450)448-5403.

DUNN, Celina T; Worksafe BC, PO Box 5350 Stn Terminal, Vancouver BC V6B 5L5; Cal'85; CCFP; (604)273-2266

DUNN, Charlene R; 222-495 36 St NE, Calgary AB T2A 6K3; Cal'89; CCFP; (403)235-1770; Fax. (403)272-9923.

DUNN, David; Ctr Hosp de Verdun, 4000 boul Lasalle, Verdun QC H4G 2A3; McG'75; Staff, Centre Hospitalier de Verdun; (514)362-1000 x2275; Fax. (514)362-2823.

DUNN, Desiree; Western Mem Reg Hosp, PO Box 2005 Stn Main 1 Brookfield Ave, Corner Brook NL A2H 6J7; McM'01; CCFP; Staff, Western Memorial Regional Hospital; Langs: Bilingual(English/French); (709)637-5000

DUNN, Michael; Sunnybrook Hlth Sciences Ctre, 2075 Bayview Ave, Toronto ON M4N 3M5; Tor'78; FRCPC; Peds (Neonatology). Ac Staff Peds, The Hospital For Sick Children; Staff, Sunnybrook Health Sciences Centre; Assoc Prof Peds, University of Toronto; (416)480-6100 x87777; michael.dunn@sw.ca.

DUNN, Michael P; 400-224 Esplanade W, North Vancouver BC V7M 1A4; Wes'88; (604)232-1541

DUNN, Michael V T; Valley Reg Hosp, 150 Exhibition St, Kentville NS B4N 5E3; Tor'83; FRCPC; DiagRad., Valley Regional Hospital; (902)679-2657; Fax. (902)678-0098.

DUNN, Patrice M; 300-5511 West Boulevard, Vancouver BC V6M 4H3; UBC'84; FRCPC; Psy. (604)264-9400

DUNN, Rex S; Cape Breton Healthcare Complex, 1482 George St, Sydney NS B1P 1P3; Dal'75; FRCSC; GenSurg; VascSurg. Staff, Cape Breton Healthcare Complex; (902)567-7798; Fax. (902)567-7255.

DUNN, Sheila; Women's College Hosp, 76 Grenville St, Toronto ON M5S 1B2; Tor'77; MSc; CCFP; CCFP(E.M.); FCFP; Staff, Women's College Hospital; Assoc Prof Family & Commun Med, University of Toronto; (416)323-6065 x15

DUNNE, Caitlin; St Paul's Hosp, 435-1081 Burrard St, Vancouver BC V6Z 1Y6; Wes'08; Staff, Providence Health Care - St Paul's Hospital; (604)682-2344 x66140

DUNNE, Fiona M; HSC-Faculty Of Med, 1410-3330 Hospital Dr NW, Calgary AB T2N 4N1; Cal'95; FRCPC; IntMed. (403)220-6882; Fax. (403)283-6151.

DUNNE, James V; 320-2184 Broadway W, Vancouver BC V6K 2E1; National (Ireland)'67; MB BCh; FRCPC; IntMed (Pain Management). (604)732-4993; Fax. (604)732-4984.

DUNNE, M Maureen; Shoppers Drug Mart Bldg, 250 LeMarchant Rd, St. John's NL A1E 1P7; Mem'78; (709)739-7444

DUNNE, Michel I P; Nanaimo Cancer Clinic, PO Box 190 1200 Dufferin Cres, Nanaimo BC V9S 2B7; Dublin (Ireland)'79; MB ChB; BAO; CCFP; CCFP(E.M.); (250)716-7706

DUNNE, Nancy M; Humber River Reg Hosp-Finch, 2111 Finch Ave W, North York ON M3N 1N1; Wes'80; FRCPC; Anes. Staff, Humber River Regional Hospital - Finch Avenue Site; (416)747-3835

DUNNE, Shelly M; One Med Place, 301-20 Wynford Dr, North York ON M3C 1J4; Mem'93; FRCPC; IntMed; Rheum. Staff, Toronto East General Hospital Inc; (416)441-3522; Fax. (416)441-0175.

DUNNING, Shelley; Belgage Med Arts Bldg, 103-525 Belmont Ave W, Kitchener ON N2M 5E2; Tor'84; (519)744-9806; Fax. (519)744-4012.

DUNPHY, Derek J; 193 Elizabeth Ave, St. John's NL A1B 1S9; Mem'95; FRCSC; Ophth. (709)739-8383; Fax. (709)739-8384.

DUNRAJ, Vishay; Trethewey Med Clinic, 508 Trethewey Dr, Toronto ON M6M 4C2; RCS (Ireland)'84; MB ChB; DCH; DA; CCFP; FCFP; Staff, Guelph General Hospital; Staff, Humber River Regional Hospital - Finch Avenue Site; (416)244-9293; Fax. (416)244-6606.

DUNSMORE, Sara E; Brandon Clinic, 620 Denis St, Brandon MB R7A 5E7; Man'07; FRCPC; IntMed; Nephrol.

DUNSMUIR, James T M; Brant Community HC-Brantford, 200 Terrace Hill St, Brantford ON N3R 1G9; McM'86; Anes. Staff, The Brant Community Healthcare System - Brantford General Hospital Site; (519)752-7871

DUNSTALL, Joanne M; The U of Toronto-Mississauga, 3359 Mississauga Rd N, Mississauga ON L5L 1C6; Tor'75; CCFP; FCFP; (905)828-5255

DUNSTAN-ADAMS, Elizabeth E; Caledonian Med Clinic, 340 Campbell St, Nanaimo BC V9R 3G7; UBC'89; BSc; (250)753-3202; Fax. (250)753-1039.

DUNWOODY, James M; 106-3825 Sunset St, Burnaby BC V5G 1T4; Qns'91; FRCSC; OrthSurg. (604)294-8209; jmdunwoody@telus.net.

DUONG, Alex K; M Gen George R Pearkes Bldg, 101 Colonel By Dr, Ottawa ON K1A 0K2; Wes'09; CCFP; (613)945-1444

DUONG, Catherine M H N; Ctr Hosp de LaSalle, 8585 Tsse Champlain, LaSalle QC H8P 1C1; Mon'94; LMCC; CCFP; Chief Gen Med, Centre Hospitalier de LaSalle; (514)362-8000 x1429; Fax. (514)367-8624.

DUONG, Dinh Huy; Hop Charles-LeMoyne, 3120 boul Taschereau, Greenfield Park QC J4V 2H1; Sher'84; CSPQ; Cardiol; IntMed. Staff, Hopital Charles LeMoyne; (450)466-5000

DUONG, Du Ton; 4607 50 Ave PO Box 3955 Stn Main, Olds AB T4H 1P6; Alb'05; CCFP; Staff, University of Alberta Hospital; (403)556-7130; Fax. (403)556-1944.

DUONG, Dung Ngoc; Gates of Maple Med Center, 101-2200 Rutherford Rd, Concord ON L4K 5V2; Saigon (Vietnam)'90; CCFP; Langs: Vietnamese; (905)417-5018; Fax. (905)417-5410.

DUONG, Giang Nghiep; CSSS Du Sud De Lanaudière, 911 montee des Pionniers, Terrebonne QC J6V 2H2; Mon'03; CCFP; Staff, Centre Hospitalier Saint-Joseph de la Turque; Staff, Centre Hospitalier Pierre le Gardeur; (450)654-7525

DUONG, Hoang; CSSS du Sud de Lanaudière, 911 montee des Pionniers, Terrebonne QC J6V 2H2; Mon'94; IntMed. Staff, Centre Hospitalier Pierre le Gardeur; (450)654-7525; Fax. (450)585-5939.

DUONG, Hong-Huy; GMF Centre Medical Saint-Andre, 100-8133 av Andre-Ampere, Montreal QC H1E 3J9; Saigon (Vietnam)'68; Dir serv Profesional, CSSS Lucille Teasdale; (514)648-6888

DUONG, Huu Hoang; Hotel-Dieu de Sorel, 400 av de l'Hotel-Dieu, Sorel-Tracy QC J3P 1N5; Sher'93; FRCPC; DiagRad. Staff, Hôtel-Dieu de Sorel; (450)746-6057; Fax. (450)746-6104.

DUONG, Huu Thanh; 829 Somerset St W, Ottawa ON K1R 6R4; Saigon (Vietnam)'66; Langs: Chinese; Vietnamese; French; (613)594-3392; Fax. (613)567-2789.

DUONG, Mylinh; Hamilton HS-Juravinski Site, A3 76-711 Concession Rd, Hamilton ON L8V 1C3; Adelaide (Australia)'93; Staff, Hamilton Health Sciences Centre-Juravinski Site; Teach Staff, McMaster University; (905)389-4411; Fax. (905)389-0108.

DUONG, Nguyen H; 203-302 Spadina Ave, Toronto ON M5T 2E7; Saigon (Vietnam)'78; Langs: Vietnamese; (416)596-8900; Fax. (416)596-8928.

DUONG, Nhan Hoang; Dr N Duong Med Prof Corp, 200-829 Somerset St W, Ottawa ON K1R 6R4; Tor'98; CCFP; Langs: Vietnamese; (613)594-3392; Fax. (613)567-2789.

DUONG, Thuy Long; CLSC Parc-Extension, 7085 rue Hutchison, Montreal QC H3N 1Y9; Saigon (Vietnam)'78; (514)273-9591

DUONG, Tuyet Minh; Centre Med Mira, 100-1560 boul de Rome, Brossard QC J4W 3A1; Mon'86; (450)466-1880

DUONG, Van Tinh; Dispensaire Kuujjuarapik, CP 420, Kuujjuarapik QC J0M 1G0; Saigon (Vietnam)'75; (819)929-9090

DUPERE, Audrey; 644 rue Jacques-Cartier E, Chicoutimi QC G7H 2A4; Sher'98; LMCC; FRCPC; Derm. Ac Member, Complexe hospitalier de la Sagamie; Affil Staff, Universite de Sherbrooke; Langs: French; (418)545-1542; Fax. (418)549-6965.

DUPERE, David; Queen Elizabeth II HSC, 306-1276 South Park St, Halifax NS B3H 2Y9; Dal'94; BSc; FRCPC; IntMed (Medical Oncology); Palliative Care. Staff Med & Palliative Care, Queen Elizabeth II Health Sciences Centre - Victoria General Site; Asst Prof, Dalhousie University; Langs: English; French; (902)473-6187; Fax. (902)473-6602; david.dupere@cdha.nshealth.ca.

DUPERE, Marc; Visage Clinic, 209-179 John St, Toronto ON M5T 1X4; McG'96; FRCSC; PlasSurg (General Surgery). Ac Staff, Toronto East General Hospital Inc; Langs: Spanish; English; (416)929-9800; Fax. (416)368-3113; dupere@visageclinic.ca.

DUPERE, Melissa; Hotel-Dieu St-Joseph, 21 rue Canada, Saint-Quentin NB E8A 2P6; Sher'07; CCFP; Staff, Hôtel-Dieu St-Joseph de Saint-Quentin; (506)235-2300

DUPERE, Sophie; Centre Hosp Honore-Mercier, 2750 boul Laframboise, Saint-Hyacinthe QC J2S 4Y8; Mon'04; FRCSC; PlasSurg. Staff, Centre Hospitalier Honore-Mercier; (450)771-3333; Fax. (450)771-3246.

DUPERRE, Jean A; Clin Ophtalmologique de l'Oues, 1503-625 av du President-Kenne, Montreal QC H3A 1K2; Laval'69; Ophth (Glaucoma). ac Staff, Centre Hospitalier l'Université de Montréal (CHUM) - Hôpital Notre-Dame; Langs: Bilingual(French/English); (514)849-9215; Fax. (514)849-5115.

DUPERREY, Daniel; CHUQ-St-Francois D'assise, 10 rue de l'Espinay, Quebec QC G1L 3L5; Laval'80; CSPQ; Anes. Staff, Hôpital Laval; Staff, Centre Hospitalier Universitaire De Québec - Pavillon De St-françois-d'assise; (418)525-4340

DUPERRON, Louise; Centre d'Obstetrique-Gynecolog, 203-1361 av Beaumont, Mont-Royal QC H3P 2W3; Mon'80; FRCSC; ObstGyn (Prenatal Care). ac Staff, Hôpital Ste-Justine; Langs: Bilingual(French/English); (514)344-4411; Fax. (514)344-1991.

DUPERRON, Marie-Josee; 101-254 boul Cure-Labelle, Sainte-Rose QC H7L 3A2; Sher'88; Staff, Hopital de la Cite de la santé; (450)622-3603; Fax. (450)622-3605.

DUPERVAL, Raymond; CHUS-Hop Fleurimont, 3001 12e av N, Sherbrooke QC J1H 5N4; Strasbourg (France)'70; FRCPC; IntMed (Infectious Diseases). chef Microbiologiste, Centre Hospitalier Universitaire de Sherbrooke-Hôpital Hôtel-Dieu; Langs: English; Creole; (819)346-1110 x14321; Fax. (819)822-6789.

DUPLAIN, Rejean; UMF CHRTR-Pavillon St-Joseph, 2E-731 rue Sainte-Julie, Trois-Rivieres QC G9A 1Y1; Mon'85; CCFP; Staff, Centre Hospitalier Regional de Trois-Rivieres; Staff, CSSS de Trois-Rivières; Adj Vice Dean Campus Mauricie, Universite de Montreal; (819)372-3536; Fax. (819)372-3509.

DUPLAN, Danny; CSSS de Laval, 1755 boul Rene-Laennec, Kingston ON K7M 3L9; Mon'04; FRCPC; RadOncol. Staff, Hopital de la Cite de la santé; (450)668-1010

DUPLAN, Edgard; Hop Riviere-des-Prairies, 7070 boul Perras, Montreal QC H1E 1A4; Port-au-Prince (Haiti)'71; Staff, Hôpital Riviere des Prairies; (514)323-7260; Fax. (514)323-9801.

DUPLESSIS, Marc; CSSS de Trois-Rivières, 1991 boul du Carmel, Trois-Rivieres QC G8Z 3R9; McG'88; CSPQ; FRCPC; AnatPath. Staff, CSSS de Trois-Rivières; (819)697-3333; Fax. (819)371-5007.

DUPLESSIS, Michel; Neuro Rive-Sud, 250-4896 boul Taschereau, Greenfield Park QC J4V 2J2; Sher'75; CSPQ; FRCPC; Neur; Electroenceph (P.Q.). Ac Staff Neur, Hopital Charles LeMoyne; (514)672-1931; Fax. (514)672-3308.

DUPLESSIS, Pierre; Inst de Readaptation de Mtl, 6300 av de Darlington, Montreal QC H3S 2J4; Mon'70; MPH; Public Health & Preventive Med; CommunMed (P.Q.). Staff, Institut de Réadaptation Gingras-Lindsay de Montréal; (514)340-2076; pierre.duplessis@ifrc.org.

DUPLESSIS, Veronique; CSSS Vallee de la Gatineau, 309 boul Desjardins, Maniwaki QC J9E 2E7; Mon'04; CCFP; Staff, CSSS de la Vallée de la Gatineau; (819)449-4690

DUPONT, Alain; Polyclinique du Cap, 110-700 boul Thibeau, Trois-Rivieres QC G8T 7A1; Laval'81; (819)373-4551; Fax. (819)373-6516.

DUPONT, Anik; CHUQ-St-Francois D'Assise, 10 rue de l'Espinay, Quebec QC G1L 3L5; Laval'04; Staff, Centre Hospitalier Universitaire De Québec - Pavillon De St-françois-d'assise; (418)525-4444

DUPONT, Daniele; Dir Sante Securite Hydro-Quebe, 7F-75 boul Rene-Levesque O, Montreal QC H2Z 1A4; Sher'75; Médecin, Hydro-Quebec; (514)289-2211 x4886; Fax. (514)289-2362; dupont.daniele@hydro.qc.ca.

DUPONT, Elise; SMBD Jewish Gen Hosp, 3755 ch Cote-Sainte-Catherine, Montreal QC H3T 1E2; Mon'77; CSPQ; FRCPC; Anes. Ac Staff, Sir Mortimer B Davis Jewish General; (514)340-8222 x5701

DUPONT, France; Clinique Med Duberger, 2810 boul Pere-Lelievre, Quebec QC G1P 2Y1; Laval'85; (418)688-8414; Fax. (418)688-4273.

DUPONT, Helene; Direction de la Sante Publique, 104 rue Lois, Gatineau QC J8Y 3R7; Laval'82; Dir, Direction de la Sante Publique; (819)777-3871; Fax. (819)777-0271; helene_dupont@ssss.gouv.qc.ca.

DUPONT, Jacinthe; Centre Med Rochette, 2372 boul Louis-XIV, Quebec QC G1C 5K1; Laval'87; Langs: English; (418)660-3692; Fax. (418)660-7392.

DUPONT, Jacqueline O; St Boniface Gen Hosp, C3-409 Tache Ave, Winnipeg MB R2H 2A6; Man'86; FRCPC; NuclearMed. Consultant, Health Sciences Centre; Consultant, Brandon Regional Health Centre; Med Staff Assoc, St Boniface General Hospital; Asst Prof, University of Manitoba; (204)237-2748; Fax. (204)258-1048.

DUPONT, Julie; Ctr Hosp de Verdun, 4000 boul Lasalle, Verdun QC H4G 2A3; Laval'95; Staff, Centre Hospitalier de Verdun; (514)362-1000 x2141

DUPONT, Michel; PCN Sainte-Foy, 3081 ch Sainte-Foy, Quebec QC G1X 1P9; Laval'71; LMCC; Langs: Bilingual(French/English); (418)653-1930

DUPONT, Michel; CHUQ-St-Francois d'Assise, 10 rue de l'Espinay, Quebec QC G1L 3L5; Laval'07; CCFP; CCFP(E.M.); Staff, Centre Hospitalier Universitaire De Québec - Pavillon De St-françois-d'assise; (418)525-4444

DUPONT, Micheline; Clinique Med Pelletier, 300-8330 boul Taschereau, Brossard QC J4X 1C2; Mon'81; (450)465-5379; Fax. (450)465-5615.

DUPONT, Nathalie; CSSS du Sud de Lanaudière, 911 montee des Pionniers, Terrebonne QC J6V 2H2; Laval'94; Staff, Centre Hospitalier Pierre le Gardeur; (418)654-7525

DUPONT, Robert; CSSS de la Haute-Yamaska, 205 boul Leclerc O, Granby QC J2G 1T7; Mon'95; FRCPC; DiagRad. Staff, Centre Hospitalier de Granby; (450)372-5491

DUPONT, Serge; College des Med du Quebec, 2170 boul Rene-Levesque O, Montreal QC H3H 2T8; Mon'78; Prof, College des Medecins du Quebec; (514)933-4441 x5203; Fax. (514)933-4668.

DUPONT, Stephane; CSSS de la Haute-Yamaska, 205 boul Leclerc O, Granby QC J2G 1T7; Sher'90; FRCSC; Ophth. Staff, Centre Hospitalier de Granby; Langs: Bilingual(French/English); (450)372-5491; Fax. (450)991-1664; clinique@ophtalmogranby.ca.

DUPONT-CHALAOUI, Katrie; Les Gynecologues Ass Laval, 1299 boul de la Concorde O, Laval QC H7N 5T4; Mon'02; FRCSC; ObstGyn. (450)668-3250; Fax. (450)668-7595.

DUPONT-GIRARD, Michele; Dir de la Sante Publique-Mtl, 1301 rue Sherbrooke E, Montreal QC H2L 1M3; Mon'74; Ac Staff, Hôpital du Sacre-Coeur de Montréal; (514)528-2400; Fax. (514)528-2459; mdupont@santepub-mtl.qc.ca.

DUPRAS, Annik; CHUM-Hop Notre-Dame, 1560 rue Sherbrooke E, Montreal QC H2L 4M1; Sher'94; FRCPC; IntMed; GeriatricMed. Staff, Centre Hospitalier l'Université de Montréal (CHUM) - Hôpital Notre-Dame; Universite de Montreal; Langs: Bilingual(French/English); (514)890-8000 x26769

DUPRAS, Eric; CSSS Les Eskers de l'Abitibi, 622 4e rue O, Amos QC J9T 2S2; Sher'91; CSPQ; FRCSC; GenSurg. Staff, CH Hôtel-Dieu d'Amos; (819)732-3341; Fax. (819)732-6484.

DUPRAS, Genevieve; 24 rue Gale GD, Ormstown QC J0S 1K0; Mon'99; CSPQ; FRCSC; GenSurg. Staff, Barrie Memorial Hospital; (450)829-2321; genevieve_dupras@rrsss16.gouv.qc.ca.

DUPRAS, Georges; CSSS De Saint-Jerome, 290 rue de Montigny, Saint-Jerome QC J7Z 5T3; McG'68; AB; FRCPC; NuclearMed (Radiation Protection). Staff, Hôtel-Dieu de Saint-Jérôme; (450)431-8284; Fax. (450)431-8331.

DUPRAS, Louise; Hop Charles Lemoyne, 3120 boul Taschereau, Greenfield Park QC J4V 2H1; Mon'73; Staff, Hopital Charles LeMoyne; (450)466-5000; Fax. (450)466-5012; dupraslouise@hotmail.com.

DUPRAS, Marie-Claude; CLSC des Faubourgs, 2260 rue Parthenais, Montreal QC H2K 3T5; Laval'96; CCFP; (514)527-2361; marie-claude_dupras@ssss.gouv.qc.ca.

DUPRAS, Raymonde; Clinique Argyle, 28 rue Argyle, Longueuil QC J4P 2H4; Mon'78; Staff Med, CHSLD St-Georges; Staff Med, Centre d'hébergement Champlain; Staff Med, CHSLD d'Acceuil Marcelle Ferron; Staff, Centre Dollard Cormier; Langs: Bilingual(French/English); (514)370-5555; Fax. (514)370-2074.

DUPRAT, Christine C; River East Health Access Ctre, 975 Henderson Hwy, Winnipeg MB R2K 4L7; Man'94; CCFP; FCFP; (204)938-5000

DUPRE, John; 339 Windermere Rd, London ON N6A 5A5; Oxford (England)'58; FRCP; FACP; IntMed; Endocrin (P.Q.); MedScient(Med) (Endocrinology & Metabolism). Staff, London Health Sciences Centre - University Hospital; Prof, University of Western Ontario; (519)931-5201; Fax. (519)931-5237; john.dupre@lhsc.on.ca.

DUPRE, Marc P J; St Boniface Gen Hosp, 409 Tache Ave, Winnipeg MB R2H 2A6; Ott'03; FRCPC; AnatPath. Staff, St Boniface General Hospital; Fax. (204)233-8563.

DUPRE, Marguerite; College des Med du Quebec, 2170 boul Rene-Levesque O, Montreal QC H3H 2T8; Mon'77; FRCPC; EmergMed. Med Insp, College des Medecins du Quebec; Langs: English; (514)933-4441 x5299; Fax. (514)933-4668; mdupre@cmq.org.

DUPRE, Nicolas; Ctr Hosp Affilie-Enfant-Jesus, 1401 18e rue, Quebec QC G1J 1Z4; McG'96; MSc; FRCPC; Neur (Neuro Genetics). Staff, Centre Hospitalier Affilié Universitaire de Québec - Hôpital De L'Enfant Jésus; assoc Prof, Université Laval; Langs: Bilingual(English/French); Spanish; Italian; (418)649-0252 x3177; Fax. (418)649-5915; nicdupre@aol.com.

DUPRIEZ, Anne-Frederique; Institut de Cardiologie de Mtl, 5000 eue Belanger, Montreal QC H1T 1C8; Mon'98; CCFP; Staff, Institut de Cardiologie de Montréal; (514)376-3330

DUPUIS, Celine; West Island Palliative Care, 265 rue Andre-Brunet, Roxboro QC H9H 3R4; Laval'81; CSPQ; AnatPath (P.Q.). (514)693-1718

DUPUIS, Hubert; 4813 Route 134, Cocagne NB E4R 2Y2; Sher'80; Staff, Dr Georges-L-Dumont University Hospital Centre; (506)862-4182; Fax. (506)862-4179.

DUPUIS, Isabelle; Centre de Sante, 1 rue de la Clinique, Ste-Anne-Madawaska NB E7E 1B9; Mon'89; LMCC; CCFP; FCFP; Staff Emerg, Hôpital regional d'Edmundston; Langs: English; (506)445-6200; Fax. (506)445-6201.

DUPUIS, Jean-Eric J; Moose Creek Med Centre, PO Box 40 66 Sabourin St, Moose Creek ON K0C 1W0; Ott'94; BSc(Hons.); BEd; Ac Physician, Montfort Hospital; Preceptor, University of Ottawa; Langs: Bilingual(English/French); (613)538-2710 x1; Fax. (613)538-4458.

DUPUIS, Jean-Luc; Clin Med Familiale de Malbaie, 515 rue Saint-Etienne, La Malbaie QC G5A 1W7; Mon'68; (418)665-2366; Fax. (418)665-7766.

DUPUIS, Jean-Yves; Univ of Ottawa Heart Institute, H2410-40 Ruskin St, Ottawa ON K1Y 4W7; Sher'78; CSPQ; FRCPC; Anes (Cardiovascular Anesthesia). Staff, University of Ottawa Heart Institute; Staff Ottawa Heart Inst, The Ottawa Hospital - Civic Campus; Langs: Bislama; English; (613)761-4379; Fax. (613)761-4925; jydupuis@ottawaheart.ca.

DUPUIS, Jocelyn; Institut de Cardiologie de Mtl, 5000 rue Belanger, Montreal QC H1T 1C8; Mon'86; PhD(Experi Med); CSPQ; FRCPC; IntMed (Adult Cardiology); Cardiol. Staff Cardiol, Institut de Cardiologie de Montréal; Associé Clin Prof Med, Universite de Montreal; (514)376-3330; Fax. (514)593-2567; jocelyn.dupuis@bellnet.ca.

DUPUIS, Kaitlin C; 1864 Oak Bay Ave, Victoria BC V8R 1C5; McM'09; CCFP; (250)380-1551

DUPUIS, Marie-Josee; Hotel-Dieu de Levis, 143 rue Wolfe, Levis QC G6V 3Z1; Mon'03; FRCPC; IntMed. Staff, Hôtel-Dieu de Lévis; (418)835-7121

DUPUIS, Marie-Josee; 100-235 boul Rene-Levesque E, Montreal QC H2X 1N8; Mon'86; FRCSC; ObstGyn. Prof adj clin, Centre Hospitalier l'Université de Montréal (CHUM) - Hôpital Notre-Dame; Clin Prof, Centre Hospitalier l'Université De Montréal (CHUM) - Hôpital Saint-luc; (514)866-2446; Fax. (514)866-4013.

DUPUIS, Martine; CSSS de Laval, 1755 boul Rene-Laennec, Laval QC H7M 3L9; McG'87; Staff, Hopital de la Cite de la santé; Langs: English; (450)668-1010; Fax. (450)975-5353.

DUPUIS, Martine; Clinique Med des Promenades, A222-3333 rue du carrefour, Quebec QC G1C 5R9; Laval'86; (418)663-6345; Fax. (418)663-8621.

DUPUIS, Natalie; Sudbury Reg Hosp-Laurentian, 41 Ramsey Lake Rd, Sudbury ON P3E 5J1; Ott'03; FRCPC; Anes. Staff, Health Sciences North-St Joseph's Health Centre; Staff, Health Sciences North-Laurentian Site; (705)523-4733; Fax. (705)671-5458.

DUPUIS, Paul; 2381 Amethyst Beach Site 14 Comp 13 RR 13, Thunder Bay ON P7B 5E4; McG'87; CCFP; CCFP(E.M.); FCFP; Staff, Thunder Bay Regional Health Sciences Centre; (807)768-3646; Fax. (807)768-1706.

DUPUIS, Paule; CSSS Pierre Boucher, 1333 boul Jacques-Cartier E, Longueuil QC J4M 2A5; Mon'01; FRCSC; Otol (Oncology). Staff, Centre Hospitalier Pierre Boucher; Staff, Centre ORL Rive-Sud; Langs: Bilingual(French/English); (450)468-8111

DUPUIS, Philippe; CHUQ-Ctr Hosp Univ Laval, 2705 boul Laurier, Quebec QC G1V 4G2; Laval'05; Endocrin&Metab; IntMed. Staff, Centre Hospitalier Universitaire de Quebec-CHUL; (418)654-2169

DUPUIS, Pierre R; SMBD Jewish Gen Hosp, E 003-3755 ch cote-Sainte-Cath, Montreal QC H3T 1E2; Mon'67; DAB; CSPQ; FRCSC; OrthSurg. Staff, Sir Mortimer B Davis Jewish General; (514)340-8222 x3153; Fax. (514)340-7595.

DUPUIS, Robert; CSSS de la Region de Thetford, 1717 rue Notre-Dame E, Thetford Mines QC G6G 2V4; Laval'81; FRCPC; IntMed (Clinical Cardiology). Staff, Hopital du CSSS de la Region de Thetford; Langs: English; (418)338-7777; robertdupuis@hotmail.com.

DUPUIS, Veronique; Hôpital de CSC de Lamèque, 29 rue de l'Hopital, Lameque NB E8T 1C5; Laval'05; CCFP; Staff, Hôpital de CSC de Lamèque; Langs: Bilingual(French/English); (506)344-3430; Fax. (506)344-3436; vdupuis@reg6.health.nb.ca.

DUPUIS-RIENDEAU, Emilie; CSSS de la Cote-de-Gaspe, 215 boul de York O, Gaspe QC G4X 2W2; Laval'06; CCFP; Staff, Centre Hospitalier de Gaspe; Langs: Spanish; English; (418)368-6663

DUPUY, Andre; 300 rue de longueuil, Longueuil QC J4H 1H4; Laval'66; Dir, Clinique Medico Esthetique Viens Longueuil; Langs: Bilingual(French/English); (450)646-7268; Fax. (450)670-9767.

DUQUE-RENDON, Hector A; Hanover & Dist Hosp, 325-90 7th Ave, Hanover ON N4N 1N1; Antioquia (Colombia)'89; FRCSC; GenSurg. Staff T T L, Hamilton Health Sciences Centre - Hamilton General Hospital; Staff, Hanover & District Hospital; Consultant, South Gray Howell Health Centre; Langs: Spanish; (519)364-0910; Fax. (519)364-0920; hduque@sympatico.ca.

DUQUETTE, Antoine; CHUM-Hop Notre-Dame, 1560 rue Sherbrooke E, Montreal QC H2L 4M1; Mon'02; FRCPC; Neur. Staff, Centre Hospitalier l'Université de Montréal (CHUM) - Hôpital Notre-Dame; (514)890-8000

DUQUETTE, Claude; Clinique D'Ophtalmologie, 100-2875 boul Laurier, Quebec QC G1V 2M2; Laval'65; FRCSC; Ophth. (418)658-2010; Fax. (418)658-8310.

DUQUETTE, France; Clinique Mirabel, CP 1059 Succ St-Janvier 13714 boul du Cure-Labelle, Mirabel QC J7J 1A1; Mon'91; Staff, Hôpital de Saint-Eustache; (450)435-7666

DUQUETTE, Louis; Clinique Med Saint-Patrice, 417A rue Principale, St-Patr-Beaur QC G0S 1B0; Mon'78; (418)596-2213; Fax. (418)596-2024; louiduque@hotmail.com.

DUQUETTE, Marie-Camille; CHUQ-Ctr Hosp Univ Laval, 2705 boul Laurier, Quebec QC G1V 4G2; Laval'04; FRCPC; Peds. Staff, Centre Hospitalier Universitaire de Quebec-CHUL; (418)525-4444

DUQUETTE, Maurice; Ctr Hosp Fleury, 2180 rue Fleury E, Montreal QC H2B 1K3; Mon'71; CSPQ; OrthSurg (P.Q.). Staff, Centre Hospitalier Fleury; (514)381-2000

DUQUETTE, Sebastien; CSSS Haute Gaspésie, 50 rue du Belvedere, Ste-Anne-des-Monts QC G4V 1X4; Sher'97; CSPQ; FRCPC; Anes. Staff, Centre Hospitalier des Monts; (418)763-2261

DUQUETTE, Stephane; Hop Maisonneuve-Rosemont, 5415 boul de l'Assomption, Montreal QC H1T 2M4; Mon'02; Staff, Hopital Maisonneuve-Rosemont; (514)252-3400

DURANCEAU, Alfred M; 509 rue Adoncour, Longueuil QC J4G 2M6; Mon'76; FRCSC; Ophth. Langs: Bilingual(French/English); (450)646-7788; alfred.duranceau@bellnet.ca.

DURANCEAU, Andre C H; CHUM-Hop Notre-Dame, D8051-1560 rue Sherbrooke E, Montreal QC H2L 4M1; Mon'67; CSPQ; GenSurg. ac Staff, Centre Hospitalier l'Université de Montréal (CHUM) - Hôpital Notre-Dame; Consultant, Hôpital Ste-Justine; Teach Staff, Universite de Montreal; (514)890-8000 x26252; Fax. (514)412-7855; andre.duranceau@umontreal.ca.

DURANCEAU, Caroline; 114-475 rue Talbot, Chicoutimi QC G7H 4A3; Laval'06; Endocrin&Metab; IntMed. (418)549-5987

DURANCEAU, Jacques A; Clinique Med de Bromont, D104-89 boul de Bromont, Bromont QC J2L 2K5; Mon'69; CSPQ; FRCPC; PhysMed&Rehab (Sports Medicine). Med Consultant, Institut de Cardiologie de Montréal; Med Consultant, Hôpital Ste-Justine; Asst Prof Sports Med, Universite de Montreal; Langs: English; (450)534-5474

DURANCEAU, Louise A; CHUM-Hotel-Dieu, 3840 rue Saint-Urbain, Montreal QC H2W 1T8; Ott'68; PlasSurg. Staff, Centre Hospitalier l'Université De Montréal (CHUM) - Hôpital Saint-luc; Staff, Centre Hospitalier l'Université de Montréal (CHUM) - Hôtel-Dieu; adj Prof, Universite de Montreal; (514)890-8000 x14444

DURANCEAU, Paul; 101-2810 boul Saint-Martin E, Laval QC H7E 4Y6; Mon'73; FRCSC; PlasSurg. Staff, Hôpital du Sacre-Coeur de Montréal; (450)661-5930; Fax. (450)661-5930.

DURANCEAU, Robert; Clinique Med Sainte-Rosalie, 4700 boul Laurier E, Saint-Hyacinthe QC J2R 2C2; Mon'79; Staff, Centre Hospitalier Honore-Mercier; (450)799-5511; Fax. (450)799-5517.

DURAND, Barend J; Med Arts Center, 770 6 St SW, Medicine Hat AB T1A 4J6; Orange Free State (South Africa)'81; CCFP; (403)487-5450

DURAND, Brigitte; Clinique Med de Hauteville, 4435 boul de Hauteville, Terrebonne QC J6X 2Y6; Mon'77; (450)492-3153; Fax. (450)492-9380.

DURAND, D'Arcy C; 123-11910 111 Ave NW, Edmonton AB T5G 0E5; Cal'04; FRCSC; OrthSurg. (780)453-8985; Fax. (780)447-4537.

DURAND, Daniel L; Centre Hosp Anna-Laberge, 200 boul Brisebois, Chateauguay QC J6K 4W8; McG'86; PlasSurg. Staff, Hôpital Anna-Laberge; (450)699-2425; Fax. (450)699-2525.

DURAND, Etienne; UMF Haute-Ville, 55 ch Ste-Foy, Quebec QC G1R 1S9; Mon'05; CCFP; (418)641-2572

DURAND, Isabelle; Centre Hosp Honore-Mercier, 2750 boul Laframboise, Saint-Hyacinthe QC J2S 4Y8; Bordeaux (France)'99; Staff, Centre Hospitalier Honore-Mercier; (450)778-2572

DURAND, Lorraine; 2-200 Student Union Bldg, 66 University Campus NW, Edmonton AB T6G 2J7; Alb'96; CCFP; Staff, University of Alberta Hospital; (780)492-2612; Fax. (780)492-0172.

DURAND, Madeleine; CHUM-Hotel-Dieu, 3840 rue Saint-Urbain, Montreal QC H2W 1T8; Laval'04; IntMed. Staff, Centre Hospitalier l'Université de Montréal (CHUM) - Hôtel-Dieu; (514)890-8000 x14624

DURAND, Marie-Josee; Ctr Hosp de LaSalle, 8585 Tsse Champlain, LaSalle QC H8P 1C1; Laval'98; Staff, Centre Hospitalier de LaSalle; Langs: Spanish; English; (450)759-8222

DURAND, Myriam; CHUS-Hop Hotel-Dieu, 580 rue Bowen S, Sherbrooke QC J1G 2E8; Sher'05; Psy. Staff, Centre Hospitalier Universitaire de Sherbrooke-Hôpital Hôtel-Dieu; (819)346-1110

DURAND, Nancy E; Sunnybrook Hlth Sciences Ctr, C714-2075 Bayview Ave, Toronto ON M4N 3M5; McG'86; FRCSC; ObstGyn (Colposcopy). Staff, Women's College Hospital; Staff, Sunnybrook Health Sciences Centre; Asst Prof, University of Toronto; (416)480-5183; Fax. (416)480-5204.

DURAND, Nancy; GMF Centre de santé, 3745 rue Georges-Couture, Drummondville QC J2B 7P4; Sher'05; CCFP; (819)477-2231; Fax. (819)477-1122.

DURAND, Pierre J; Ctr Hosp Affilie St-Sacremant, L2 032-1050 ch Sainte-Foy, Quebec QC G1S 4L8; Laval'77; FRCPC; CommunMed;CCFP; FCFP; GeriatricMed (P.Q.). Staff, Centre Hospitalier Affilié Universitaire de Québec - Hôpital du St-Sacrement; Community Med, Centre d'hebergement Saint-Augustin; Staff, Centre Hospitalier Universitaire de Quebec-CHUL; Med Consultant Chronic Care, Ministry of Health-Quebec; Dean Med, Université Laval; (418)682-7997; Fax. (418)682-7998.

DURAND, Sebastien; Clin de Chirurgie Orthopedique, 10445 1re av, Saint-Georges QC G5Y 6X8; Laval'03; FRCSC; OrthSurg. Staff, Centre Hospitalier Beauce-Etchemin; (418)228-2899

DURAND-MARTEL, Pascali; CSSS de Trois-Rivieres, 1991 boul du Carmel, Trois-Rivieres QC G8Z 3R9; Sher'06; FRCPC; Neur. Staff, CSSS de Trois-Rivières; (819)697-3333

DURANLEAU, Denis; Clinique Med Saint-Jacques, 5155 rue Saint-Jacques O, Montreal QC H4A 2E3; Sher'85; FACP(USA); PhysMed&Rehab. Staff, Institut de Réadaptation Gingras-Lindsay de Montréal; (514)489-8216; Fax. (514)658-4331.

DURANT, Dean; Peterborough Reg HC-Hospital, 1 Hospital Dr, Peterborough ON K9J 7C6; West Indies (Jamaica)'01; FRCPC; DiagRad. Staff, Peterborough Regional Health Centre - Hospital Drive; (705)743-2121

DURANTE, Kathleen M; Golden River Health Clinic, PO Box 400 601 Trumpeter Dr, Gold River BC V0P 1G0; Cal'00; CCFP; Fam Med, R W Large Memorial Hospital; (250)283-2626; kathleen_durante@rwlmh.ca.

DURANTE, Lino M; Port Hope Med Centre, 201-249 Ontario St, Port Hope ON L1A 3Y9; Ott'79; Ac Staff, Lakeridge Health - Bowmanville Site; Assoc Staff, Northumberland Hills Hospital; (905)885-6391; Fax. (905)885-6849.

DURAR, Mahmud; 8214 144 Ave NW, Edmonton AB T5E 2H4; (Libya)'08; MB BCh; (780)478-0975; Fax. (780)478-0946.

DURCAN, Anne M; Mount Carmel Clinic, 886 Main St, Winnipeg MB R2W 5L4; Man'92; CCFP; FCFP; (204)582-2311

DURCAN, Liam V; MUHC-Montreal Neurology Inst, 244-3801 rue University, Montreal QC H3A 2B4; Man'89; FRCPC; Neur. Staff, McGill University Health Centre - Montreal Neurological Hospital; Langs: French; (514)398-5034; Fax. (514)398-3972; liam.durcan@mcgill.ca.

DURCAN, Thomas J G; Burlington Prof Centre, 203-3155 Harvester Rd, Burlington ON L7N 3V2; Dublin (Ireland)'73; MB ChB; BAO; CCFP; (905)637-8833; Fax. (905)637-6745.

DURÉ, Marjorie; Clinique Med de Thurso, 156 rue Galipeau, Thurso QC J0X 3B0; (Mexico)'92; CCFP; (819)985-3080

DUREPOS, Christian P; Timmins Family Health Team, 1-681 Algonquin Blvd E, Timmins ON P4N 8S6; Ott'92; CCFP; FCFP; Staff, Timmins & District Hospital; Langs: Bilingual(French/English); (705)267-5600; Fax. (705)668-7244.

DURET, Jean-Sebastien; Ctr Hosp Affilie-Enfant-Jesus, 1401 18e rue, Quebec QC G1J 1Z4; Laval'98; FRCPC; DiagRad. Staff, Centre Hospitalier Affilié Universitaire de Québec - Hôpital De L'Enfant Jésus; (418)649-5782

DURHAM, James S; Gordon & Leslie Diamond Ctr EN, 4F-2775 Laurel St, Vancouver BC V5Z 1M9; Sask'80; FRCSC; Otol. Ac Staff, Vancouver General Hospital - Centennial Pavillion; Clin Instructor, University of British Columbia; (604)875-5629; Fax. (604)875-5018; sdurham@interchange.ubc.ca.

DURIE, Peter R; 555 University Ave, Toronto ON M5G 1X8; McM'74; BSc; FRCPC; Peds (Pediatric Gastroenterology). Staff, The Hospital For Sick Children; Staff, St Michael's Hospital; Prof, University of Toronto; Langs: Swahili; (416)813-6185; Fax. (416)813-6531.

DURIER, Jean-Louis M; Humber River Reg Hosp-Finch, 2111 Finch Ave W, North York ON M3N 1N1; Paris (France)'77; Urol. Staff, Humber River Regional Hospital - Finch Avenue Site; (416)664-3091

DURIVAGE, Antoine; Inst Phillippe Pinel de Mtl, 10905 boul Henri-Bourassa E, Montreal QC H1C 1H1; Mon'82; FRCPC; Psy. Staff, Institut Philippe-Pinel de Montreal; Universite de Montreal; (514)648-8461 x510; Fax. (514)881-3706.

DURIVAGE, Gidej; Hop Maisonneuve-Rosemont, 5415 boul de l'Assomption, Montreal QC H1T 2M4; Mon'98; FRCPC; IntMed; Gastroent. Staff, Hopital Maisonneuve-Rosemont; (514)252-3400

DURKIN, Chris; 3300-910 10th Ave W, Vancouver BC V5Z 1M9; UBC'08; (604)875-4111 x68430

DURNIN, Isabelle; Clinique Med Mascouche, 1025 Montee Masson, Mascouche QC J7K 2L9; Sher'94; Staff, Centre Hospitalier Pierre le Gardeur; (450)474-6000

DURNIN-GOODMAN, Eithne M; Alliance Clinic, 10085 Whalley Blvd, Surrey BC V3T 4G1; Cal'91; CCFP; Staff, Orchard Recovery Centre; Staff, Complement Health Care; (604)582-5826

DURNO, Carol A; Rouge Valley-Centenary HC, 2867 Ellesmere Rd, Scarborough ON M1E 4B9; Tor'91; MSc; FRCPC; Peds (Clinician Investigator Program). Staff, Rouge Valley Health System - Centenary Health Centre Site; Staff, The Hospital For Sick Children; Asst Prof, University of Toronto; (416)281-7476; carol.durno@rougevalley.ca.

DUROCHER, Andre; CHUM-Hop Notre-Dame, G4131-1560 rue Sherbrooke E, Montreal QC H2L 4M1; Mon'89; FRCPC; Neur. Staff, Centre Hospitalier l'Université de Montréal (CHUM) - Hôpital Notre-Dame; (514)890-8000; Fax. (514)412-7556.

DUROCHER, France; Les Gynecologues Ass Laval, 1299 boul de la Concorde O, Laval QC H7N 5T4; McG'87; ObstGyn. Staff, Hopital de la Cite de la santé; Langs: English; (450)668-3250; Fax. (450)668-7595.

DUROCHER, Gilles; Polyclinique D'Argenteuil, 201-551 rue Berry, Lachute QC J8H 1S4; Sher'76; Staff, Centre Hospitalier d'Argenteuil; (450)562-3751; Fax. (450)562-1852; gcdurocher@sympatico.ca.

DUROCHER, Jean-Guy; CSSS Drummond-Hop Sainte-Croix, 570 rue Heriot, Drummondville QC J2B 1C1; Sher'92; CSPQ; Anes. Staff, Hôpital Sainte-croix; (450)478-6464

DUROCHER, Lorraine; 3258 rue Martine RR 2, Sorel-Tracy QC J3P 5N3; Mon'71; DiagRad. Staff, Hopital Charles LeMoyne; (450)746-4743

DUROCHER, Louis-Philippe; 114-5700 rue Saint-Zotique E, Montreal QC H1T 3Y7; Mon'69; Derm (Travel Medicine). (514)352-6140; Fax. (514)352-5924.

DUROCHER, William; Kirkland & Dist Hosp, PO Box 3000 Stn Main 145 Government Rd E, Kirkland Lake ON P2N 3P4; Mem'80; Staff, Kirkland & District Hospital; Staff, Temiskaming Hospital; (705)567-5251; durocher@nt.net.

DURR, Dory G; Clinique Med Monchamp, 102-227 rue Sainte-Catherine, Saint-Constant QC J5A 2J5; St. Joseph (Lebanon)'82; FRCSC; Otol. Staff, Hôpital Anna-Laberge; (450)632-2795

DURRANI, Ahmad I; Durrani Med Prof Corp, 18 Springsyde St, Whitby ON L1N 9H5; Punjab (Pakistan)'94; CCFP; (905)579-1212 x205; Fax. (905)579-5548.

DURRANT, Timothy J; Halton HSC Corp-Oakville, 327 Reynolds St, Oakville ON L6J 3L7; Tor'88; FRCPC; DiagRad. Staff, Halton Healthcare Services Corporation - Oakville Site; (905)338-4601

DURRER, Jane K; 209 Ross Terrace, Fredericton NB E3A 8E5; Tor'81; CCFP; (506)488-2312; Fax. (506)357-6599.

DURSUN, Serdar M; Grey Nuns Comm Hosp & HC, 1810-1100 Youville Drive West, Edmonton AB T6L 5X8; Ankara (Turkey)'85; FRCPC; MedScient(Med). Staff Psy, Covenant Health - Grey Nuns Community Hospital; (780)735-7119; Fax. (780)735-7496.

DUSABLON, Manon; 1 rue des Florins, Blainville QC J7C 5P6; Mon'95; Langs: French; (450)420-1116; Fax. (450)939-4316.

DUSANG, Trent S; Synergy Wellness Centre, 221-501 Bethel Dr, Sherwood Park AB T8H 0N2; Alb'88; (780)467-4140; Fax. (780)449-5138.

DUSEVIC, Myrna M E; Rockyview Gen Hosp, 7007 14 St SW, Calgary AB T2V 1P9; Sask'81; FRCPC; Anes. Staff, Rockyview General Hospital; (403)943-3410; Fax. (403)943-8590.

DUSHENSKI, David G; Mount Sinai Hosp, 206-600 University Ave, Toronto ON M5G 1X5; Alb'92; CCFP; CCFP(E.M.); Staff, Mount Sinai Hospital; Teacher, University of Toronto; (416)586-5058; Fax. (416)586-4719; ddushenski@mtsinai.on.ca.

DUSHINSKI, John W; Rockyview Gen Hosp, 6645-7007 14 St SW, Calgary AB T2V 1P9; Alb'91; BSc; FRCSC; Urol (Endourology)., Rockyview General Hospital; Staff, Calgary Health Region; Clinical Asst Prof, University of Calgary; (403)943-8988; Fax. (403)943-8990.

DUSIK, Laureen A; Travel Medicine & Vaccination, 115C-1835 Gordon Dr, Kelowna BC V1Y 3H4; UBC'89; MSc; (250)448-7148

DUSKA, George P; Peter Lougheed Centre, 3500 26 Ave NE, Calgary AB T1Y 6J4; Cal'95; FRCPC; Psy. Staff, Peter Lougheed Centre; (403)943-5656; Fax. (403)219-3524.

DUSSAULT, Andreanne; CSSS de Portneuf, 700 rue Saint-Cyrille, Saint-Raymond QC G3L 1W1; Laval'08; CCFP; Staff, Centre Hospitalier Portneuf; (418)337-4611; Fax. (418)337-4808.

DUSSAULT, Catherine; CHUQ-Ctr Hosp Univ Laval, 2705 boul Laurier, Quebec QC G1V 4G2; Mon'04; Gastroent; IntMed. Staff, Centre Hospitalier Universitaire de Quebec-CHUL; (418)654-2104

DUSSAULT, Charles; CSSS du Nord de Lanaudière, RC D27-1000 Sainte-Anne Blvd, Joliette QC J6E 6J2; Sher'08; IntMed. Staff, Centre Hospitalier Régional de Lanaudière; (450)759-8222

DUSSAULT, Isabelle; CSSS de la Haute-Yamaska, 205 boul Leclerc O, Granby QC J2G 1T7; Sher'98; CCFP; Staff, Centre Hospitalier de Granby; (450)375-8000 x2124

DUSSAULT, Jean; CHUQ-Hotel-Dieu de Quebec, 11 Cote du Palais, Quebec QC G1R 2J6; Laval'68; CSPQ; FRCSC; GenSurg. Staff, Centre Hospitalier Universitaire de Québec (CHUQ) - Siege Social; (418)691-5151; Fax. (418)691-5020.

DUSSAULT, Louis-Martin; Hop Charles LeMoyne, 3120 boul Taschereau, Greenfield Park QC J4V 2H1; Laval'00; FRCPC; Psy. Staff Psy, Hopital Charles LeMoyne; (450)466-5453

DUSSAULT, Louise; Clinique Med de Coaticook, 206-18 rue du Manege, Coaticook QC J1A 3B3; Laval'77; Ac Staff CMDP, Centre Hospitalier de Coaticook; Consultant, Centre Hospitalier Universitaire de Sherbrooke-Hôpital Hôtel-Dieu; (819)849-4808; Fax. (819)849-7400.

DUSSAULT, Lucie; CSSSG-Hop de Gatineau, CP 2000 Succ Bureau-Chef 909 boul de la Verendrye O, Gatineau QC J8P 7H2; Mon'90; CCFP; Staff, Hôpital de Gatineau; (819)561-8100

DUSSAULT, Marie-Claude; Centre Med Donnacona, 420 Rte 138, Donnacona QC G3M 1C2; Sher'87; (418)285-1122; Fax. (418)285-0006.

DUSSAULT, Martin; Ctr Hosp de Charlevoix, 74 rue Ambroise-Fafard, Baie-Saint-Paul QC G3Z 2J6; Sher'94; FRCPC; Psy. Staff, CSSS de Charlevoix; Langs: English; (418)435-0487; Fax. (418)435-2287; martin.dussault@ssss.gouv.qc.ca.

DUSSAULT, Marylene; Clin Med Plateau Marquette, 200-731 rue Galt O, Sherbrooke QC J1H 1Z1; Laval'01; Staff Hospitalisation, Centre Hospitalier Universitaire de Sherbrooke-Hôpital Hôtel-Dieu; (819)564-8542; Fax. (819)564-1294.

DUSSAULT, Michele; CSSS Pierre Boucher, 1333 boul Jacques-Cartier E, Longueuil QC J4M 2A5; Mon'95; Staff, Centre Hospitalier Pierre Boucher; (450)468-8111

DUSSAULT, Pierre; Ctr Hosp Anna-Laberge, 200 boul Brisebois, Chateauguay QC J6K 4W8; Laval'82; FRCPC; IntMed; Gastroent. Staff Gastroent, Hôpital Anna-Laberge; (450)699-2425; Fax. (450)699-2525.

DUSSEAULT, Laurie; Andrew Street Family Hlth Ctre, 16 Andrew St, Kitchener ON N2H 5R2; Wes'03; CCFP; Staff, Sunnybrook Health Sciences Centre; Locum Tenens, North York General Hospital; (519)804-9234; Fax. (519)804-2604.

DUSSUREAULT, Martine; CSSS du Nord de Lanaudière, 1000 boul Sainte-Anne, St-Charles-Brromee QC J6E 6J2; Mon'93; CSPQ; Cardiol (P.Q.); IntMed. Staff, Centre Hospitalier Régional de Lanaudière; (450)759-8222

DUST, Nicholas; Montfort Hosp, 713 Montreal Rd, Ottawa ON K1K 0T2; Ott'06; FRCPC; Peds. Staff, Montfort Hospital; Langs: Bilingual(English/French); (613)746-4621

DUST, William N; Royal University Hosp, 103 Hospital Dr, Saskatoon SK S7N 0W8; Alb'80; FACS; FRCSC; OrthSurg (Adult Reconstructive Surgery). Head OrthSurg, Royal University Hospital; Plant Foreman Surg, University of Saskatchewan; (306)966-8199; Fax. (306)966-8196; wdust@shaw.ca.

DUTA, Daniel; 3106B Gibbins Rd, Duncan BC V9L 1E8; Man'93; FRCSC; GenSurg. (250)737-1020; Fax. (250)737-1022.

DUTA, Valentin; PO BOX 672 Stn Main, Grande Prairie AB T8V 3A8; (Romania)'98; CCFP.

DUTCHAK, Peter A; Kingston Heart Clinic, 460 Princess St, Kingston ON K7L 1C2; Sask'00; FRCPC; NuclearMed. Langs: Bilingual(English/French); (613)544-3242

DUTCHMAN, David A J; Carmi Clinic, 111-725 Carmi Ave, Penticton BC V2A 3G8; London (England)'78; MB BS; (250)492-4242; Fax. (250)492-4232.

DUTCHYN, Shannon L; 105-22314 Fraser Hwy, Langley BC V3A 8M6; UBC'99; CCFP; Staff, Langley Memorial Hospital; (604)532-9944; ladydoc@shaw.ca.

DUTCZAK, Miroslaw; Queen East Med Clinic, Queen East Med Clinic 1586 Queen St E, Toronto ON M4L 1G1; McM'82; BSc(Tor); Langs: Polish; (416)469-9900; Fax. (416)469-9960.

DUTIL, Christian; Clinique Med Blainville, 519 boul du Cure-Labelle, Blainville QC J7C 2H6; Mon'78; (450)430-2222; Fax. (450)430-1274.

DUTIL, Julie; CRSSS Baie-James-Chibougamau, 51 3e rue, Chibougamau QC G8P 1N1; CCFP; Staff, CRSSS de la Baie-James; Langs: Bilingual(French/English); (418)748-2676; Fax. (418)748-6318.

DUTIL, Maha Theresa; Albany Clinic, 807 Broadview Ave, Toronto ON M4K 2P8; Tor'82; FRCPC; Derm. Staff, Women's College Hospital; Asst Prof, University of Toronto; (416)461-9471

DUTIL, Renald; Hôp de réadaptation Villa Medi, 225 rue Sherbrooke E, Montreal QC H2X 1C9; Laval'67; Staff, Hôpital de réadaptation Villa Medica; Langs: Bilingual(French/English); (514)288-8201; Fax. (514)288-8202.

DUTKIEWICZ-STVRTECKY, Janina H; Winston Park Family Physicians, 104-2315 Bristol Cir, Oakville ON L6H 6P8; Warsaw (Poland)'75; Ac Staff, The Credit Valley Hospital; Langs: Czech; Slovak; Polish; (905)829-2826; Fax. (905)829-2846.

DUTOY, Jean-Luc; CLSC Le Minordet, 961 de la Clinique CP 4000, Senneterre QC J0Y 2M0; Louvain (Belgium)'82; (819)737-2243; Fax. (819)737-3122.

DUTRISAC, Renaud; Toronto East Gen & Orth Hosp, 825 Coxwell Ave, Toronto ON M4C 3E7; McG'08; CCFP; CCFP(E.M.); Staff, Toronto East General Hospital Inc; (416)469-6435

DUTT, Monika; Public Health Services, 235 Townsend St, Sydney NS B1P 5E7; Qns'03; FRCPC; CCFP; CommunMed. Physician, Cape Breton District Health Authority Public Health Sydney; Langs: Spanish; French; Bengali; (306)425-2174; Fax. (306)425-4199.

DUTT, Purnima; Fort Saskatchewan Med Clinic, 9421 94 Ave, Fort Saskatchewan AB T8L 1N6; Indore (India)'76; MB BS; (780)998-2231

DUTTA, Prasannajit; James Paton Mem Hosp, 125 Trans Canada Hwy, Gander NL A1V 1P7; Gauhati (India)'93; MB BS; Staff, James Paton Memorial Hospital; (709)256-2500

DUTTA, Sidharth; Bramalea & Bovaird Walk-In Cli, 210-10095 Bramalea Rd, Brampton ON L6R 0K1; Tver State Medical Academy (Other Foreign)'98; CCFP; Langs: Hindi; (905)793-5700

DUTTA, Sourabh; Hamilton HSC-McMaster Site, 4F-1200 Main St W, Hamilton ON L8N 3Z5; All-India Institute of Medical Sciences (India)'90; FRCPC; Peds. Staff, Hamilton Health Sciences Centre - McMaster Children's Hospital; (905)521-2100; Fax. (905)521-5007.

DUTTCHEN, Kaylene M; Foothills Medical Centre, 1403 29 St NW, Calgary AB T2N 2T9; Cal'04; FRCPC; Anes. Staff, Foothills Medical Centre; (403)944-1430; Fax. (403)944-2425.

DUTTON, Patricia M; 214-11 Hidden Creek Dr NW, Calgary AB T3A 6K6; Cal'06; CCFP; (403)248-2273

DUTZ, Jan P; Skin Care Centre, 835 10th Ave W, Vancouver BC V5Z 4E8; Qns'83; FRCPC; IntMed; Derm; Rheum. Langs: English; French; German; (604)875-5151; Fax. (604)873-9919.

DUVAL, Bruce J; Medical Arts Bldg, 222-750 Spadina Cres E, Saskatoon SK S7K 3H3; Man'85; FRCSC; GenSurg; VascSurg. Staff Surg, Saskatoon District Health Board; Asst Clin Prof Surg, University of Saskatchewan; (306)653-3366; Fax. (306)653-8832.

DUVAL, Carolyn R; Medical Arts Bldg, 602-750 Spadina Cres E, Saskatoon SK S7K 3H3; Man'89; FRCSC; PlasSurg (Reconstructive Surgery). (306)653-7766; Fax. (306)653-7768.

DUVAL, Cristian; Ctr Hosp du Centre la Mauricie, 50 119e rue, Shawinigan-Sud QC G9P 5K1; Mon'98; Staff, Centre Hospitalier du Centre la Mauricie; (819)536-7500

DUVAL, Douglas B; Royal Alexandra Hosp, 10240 Kingsway NW, Edmonton AB T5H 3V9; Man'77; AB; FRCPC; Anes. Ac Staff, Royal Alexandra Hospital; Ac Staff, University of Alberta Hospital; Ac Staff, Covenant Health - Grey Nuns Community Hospital; Clin Assoc Prof, University of Alberta; (780)735-4010; Fax. (780)735-5040; dduval@telusplanet.net.

DUVAL, Eve; Tour A-800 boul Chomedey, Laval QC H7V 3Y4; Mon'80; Consultant Phys, Direction de la Sante Publique de Laval; (450)978-2000; Fax. (450)978-2100; eve_duval@ssss.gouv.qc.ca.

DUVAL, Jean-Felix; CISC de Pierrefonds, 13800 boul Gouin O, Pierrefonds QC H8Z 3H6; (Haiti)'79; (514)626-2572 x4441; Fax. (514)624-7486.

DUVAL, Johanne; Centre de Med Fam de Gatineau, 201-908 boul Maloney E, Gatineau QC J8P 1H5; Laval'92; Staff, Hôpital de Gatineau; (819)663-7711; Fax. (819)663-9326.

DUVAL, Lindsay A; PO Box 355 Rpo Corydon, Winnipeg MB R3M 3V3; Man'80; FRCSC; Otol.

DUVAL, Louis; Polyclinique Med Concorde, 222-300 boul de la Concorde E, Laval QC H7G 2E6; Mon'68; Urol (P.Q.). Staff, Centre Hospitalier Fleury; (450)667-5310; Fax. (450)669-5409.

DUVAL, Louis-Rene; CSSS De Sept-Iles, 45 rue du Pere-Divet, Sept-Iles QC G4R 3N7; Mon'86; Staff, CLSC-CSSS de Port-Cartier; Staff, Centre Hospitalier Regional de Sept-Iles; Langs: English; (418)962-9761

DUVAL, Marie-Andree; CSSS de Trois-Rivières, 1991 boul du Carmel, Trois-Rivieres QC G8Z 3R9; Sher'93; CSPQ; AnatPath (P. Q.). Staff, CSSS de Trois-Rivières; (819)697-3333 x63495; Fax. (819)371-5007.

DUVAL, Michel E; 3140 rue Somerset, Montreal QC H4K 1R6; Mon'71; MSc; CommunMed (P.Q.). Staff, Hopital de la Cite de la santé; Staff, Hôpital du Sacre-Coeur de Montréal; Staff, Pavillon Notre-Dame de la Merci.

DUVAL, Michel; Hôpital Ste-Justine, 3175 ch Cote-Ste-Catherine, Montreal QC H3T 1C5; Paris (France)'93; Hem (P.Q.). Staff, Hôpital Ste-Justine; (514)345-4969; Fax. (514)345-4792; michel.duval@umontreal.ca.

DUVAL, Nicolas; Clinique Orthopedique Duval, 1487 boul des Laurentides, Vimont QC H7M 2Y3; Laval'84; CSPQ; FRCSC; OrthSurg (Hip & Knee Reconstruction). Langs: English; (450)663-3901; Fax. (450)663-0776; secretariatclinique@duval.com.

DUVAL, Pierre; Clinique Nesbitt, 215 rue du Sud, Cowansville QC J2K 2X5; Mon'93; MSc; BSc; CSPQ; FRCSC; OrthSurg. Staff, Hôpital Brome-Missisquoi-Perkins; (450)263-8551

DUVAL, Renee-Claude; CHUQ-Ctr Hosp Univ Laval, 2705 boul Laurier, Quebec QC G1V 4G2; Sher'85; FRCPC; Peds. Staff, Centre Hospitalier Universitaire de Quebec-CHUL; (418)654-2282; Fax. (418)691-5717.

DUVAL, Richard; Centre Med Seine, 130-142 Centrale Ave, Ste Anne MB R5H 1C3; Sher'74; Langs: Bilingual(French/English); (204)422-8811; Fax. (204)422-5876.

DUVALL, Anne; South Barrie Family Med, 202-480 Huronia St, Barrie ON L4N 6M2; McM'84; CCFP; FCFP; Ac Staff, Royal Victoria Regional Health Centre; Langs: Finnish; (705)722-0516; Fax. (705)722-0814.

DUVALL, Donald E; Royal Victoria Hosp, 201 Georgian Dr, Barrie ON L4M 6M2; McM'82; FRCPC; Anes (Pain Management). Staff, Royal Victoria Regional Health Centre; (705)728-9090

DUVENAGE, Jan Charles; Midtown Med Centre, 5706 50 Ave, Vermilion AB T9X 1L4; (South Africa)'85; (780)853-2809; Fax. (780)853-2970.

DUWYN, Rejean; Kincardine Family Health Team, 44 Queen St, Kincardine ON N2Z 3C1; Wes'07; CCFP; CCFP(E.M.); Staff, South Bruce Grey Health Centre - Kincardine Site; (519)396-6748; Fax. (519)396-6177; duwyn@bmts.com.

DVALI, Linda; 403-658 Danforth Ave, East York ON M4J 5B9; Wes'96; FRCSC; PlasSurg (Peripheral Nerve Injury). Chief Plastic Surg, Toronto East General Hospital Inc; Staff, Toronto Western Hospital - University Health Network; (647)346-0154; Fax. (647)346-7342; linda.dvali@uhn.on.ca.

DVORAK, Marcel F S; Blusson Spinal Cord Centre, 818 10th Ave W, Vancouver BC V5Z 1M9; Ott'84; FRCSC; OrthSurg (Spine Surgery). Staff, Vancouver General Hospital - Centennial Pavillion.

DVORAKOVA, Marie; Calgary Lab Services, 3535 Research Rd NW, Calgary AB T2L 2K8; Staff, Calgary Laboratory Services; (403)770-3569; Fax. (403)770-3788.

DVORKIN, Gary S; Ctr Hosp de Verdun, 4000 boul Lasalle, Verdun QC H4G 2A3; Alb'79; FRCPC; Neur. Staff, Centre Hospitalier de Verdun; Langs: English; French; (514)362-1000 x2489

DWIGHT, Prabo J; William Osler HS-Brampton, 2100 Bovaird Dr E, Brampton ON L6R 3J7; Qns'04; FRCPC; Peds (Neonatal & Perinatal Medicine). Staff, St Joseph's Hospital - St Joseph's Health Care; Staff, William Osler Health System - Brampton Civic Hospital; (905)494-2120

DWINNELL, Shannon; Foothills Med Centre, 4F-1403 29 St NW, Calgary AB T2N 2T9; UBC'03; FRCSC; ObstGyn (Neonatology). Staff, Foothills Medical Centre; (604)875-2424; Fax. (403)283-0415.

DWIVEDI, Shivendra; Hop Santa Cabrini Ospedale, 5655 rue Saint-Zotique E, Montreal QC H1T 1P7; McG'82; CSPQ; FRCPC; Anes. Staff, Hôpital Santa Cabrini Ospedale; (514)252-6581; Fax. (514)252-6501.

DWORAK, Andrew S C; York Medical, 3-17215 Leslie St, Newmarket ON L3Y 8E4; Tor'67; CCFP; FCFP; Staff, The Scarborough Hospital - Birchmount Campus; Staff Teacher, University of Toronto; Langs: Polish; (905)853-0404; Fax. (905)853-3702.

DWORETZ, Arthur; 102-9 av Lanning, Saint-Sauveur QC J0R 1R6; North Carolina(NC) (USA)'83; Psy (P.Q.). Langs: Bilingual(English/French); (450)822-1334; Fax. (450)227-9898.

DWORKIN, Barry; Meadowlands Fam Hlth Centre, 16-888 Meadowlands Dr, Ottawa ON K2C 3R2; McG'88; BSc; CCFP; FCFP; Teach Staff Family Med, The Ottawa Hospital - General Campus; Physician, Meadowlands Family Health Centre; Asst Prof Family Med, University of Ottawa; Langs: Bilingual(English/French); (613)228-2882; Fax. (613)228-2856.

DWORKIN, Rochelle L; Hanover Med Assoc, 118 7th Ave, Hanover ON N4N 2G9; Alb'84; CCFP; Chief Obstetrics, Hanover & District Hospital; Staff, South Bruce Grey Health Centre - Durham Site; Staff, South Bruce Grey Health Centre - Walkerton Site; (519)364-2820; Fax. (519)364-3965.

DWORKIND, Michael; SMBD Jewish Gen Hosp, 3755 Cote St Catherine Rd, Montreal QC H3T 1E2; McG'74; BSc; CCFP; FCFP; Dir/Consultant Palliative Care Services, Sir Mortimer B Davis Jewish General; Consultant Palliative Care, Mount Sinai Hospital Center; assoc Prof Family Med, McGill University; Langs: English; French; Yiddish; (514)340-8278; Fax. (514)340-8298.

DWOSH, Adam A; Bathurst-Steeles Health Centre, 2F-6257 Bathurst St, North York ON M2R 2A5; Qns'95; CCFP; FCFP; (416)223-9791; Fax. (416)223-9558.

DWOSH, Hy Avi; Mackenzie Richmond Hill Hosp, 10 Trench St, Richmond Hill ON L4C 4Z3; McM'97; FRCPC; IntMed; Critical Care Medicine. Staff, Mackenzie Richmond Hill Hospital; (905)883-1212

DWOSH, Isaac; Albany Med Clinic, 2F-807 Broadview Avenue, Toronto ON M4K 2P8; Qns'71; FRCP; FRCPC; IntMed (Adult Rheumatology). Att Staff, Kingston General Hospital; Consultant, Hotel-Dieu Hospital; Consultant, Providence Care - St Mary's of the Lake Hospital Site; Staff, Sunnybrook Health Sciences Centre - Edmond Odette Cancer Centre; Consultant, Sunnybrook Health Sciences Centre; Consultant, Albany Medical Clinic; Prof Med, Queen's University; Langs: Yiddish; (416)461-9471; Fax. (416)461-2710; dwoshi@queensu.ca.

DWYER, Desmond P; Fairmont Med Centre, 705-750 Broadway W, Vancouver BC V5Z 1H6; Cork (Ireland)'69; MB BCh; CCFP; Vis Staff, Vancouver General Hospital - Centennial Pavillion; Med Dir, Braddan Hospital; Clinical Asst Prof, University of British Columbia; (604)733-3434; Fax. (604)733-6622.

DWYER, Joseph G; 1030 Ouellette Ave, Windsor ON N9A 1E1; Wes'79; FRCSC; Otol. Staff, Hôtel-Dieu Grace Hospital; (519)973-4444; Fax. (519)973-0803.

DWYER, Kevin C J J; Brantford Med Centre, 100-40 Shellington Place, Brantford ON N3S 0C5; Tor'70; (519)753-9581

DWYER, Lynn E; Memorial U-Student Hlth Serv, PO Box 4200 Stn C, St. John's NL A1C 5S7; Mem'86; Assoc Staff, St Clare's Mercy Hospital; (709)737-7597

DWYER, Neil; Professional Arts Bldg, 620-100 Arden St, Moncton NB E1C 4B7; Mem'99; BPharm; FRCSC; Urol (Incontinence). Staff, The Moncton Hospital; Consultant Staff, Dr Georges-L-Dumont University Hospital Centre; Lecturer, Dalhousie University; (506)854-7254; Fax. (506)854-1014.

DY, Colleen; Lonsdale Women's Clinic, 1777 Lonsdale Ave, North Vancouver BC V7M 2J6; UBC'00; FRCSC; ObstGyn. (604)628-6162

DY, Hans A; 102-476 Holland Ave, Ottawa ON K1Y 0Z5; Dal'85; CCFP; FCFP; Asst Prof Dept of Family Med, University of Ottawa; (613)722-6216; Fax. (613)722-2177; hdy@sympatico.ca.

DY, Jessica G; The Ottawa Hosp-Civic Campus, D4 SD-1053 Carling Ave, Ottawa ON K1Y 4E9; Wes'99; FRCSC; ObstGyn. Staff, The Ottawa Hospital - Civic Campus; Asst Prof, University of Ottawa; (613)761-4522; Fax. (613)761-4915.

DY PAC, Emily T; 606-388 Bloor St E, Toronto ON M4W 3W9; Santo Tomas (Philippines)'72; FRCPC; Psy. Langs: Fukinese; (416)920-4604

DYACHUK, Elena; CFB Trenton, PO Box 1000 Stn Forces 190-95 RCAF Rd, Astra ON K0K 3W0; Amur State Academy of Medicine (Russia (Federation))'97; CCFP; Langs: Russian; (613)955-8714; Fax. (613)955-8656.

DYACK, Sarah; IWK Health Centre, PO Box 9700 Rpo CSC 5850-5980 University Ave, Halifax NS B3K 6R8; Dal'94; FRCPC; Peds (Clinical Genetics). Staff Med Genetics, IWK Health Centre; Asst Prof, Dalhousie University; (902)470-8592; Fax. (902)470-8709; sarah.dyack@iwk.nshealth.ca.

DYASON, Claire G; Foothills South Tower, 710-3031 Hospital Dr NW, Calgary AB T2N 2T8; Qns'09; CCFP; (403)944-2304

DYBLE, Barbara J; Univ of Victoria Hlth Services, PO Box 1700 Stn CSC, Victoria BC V8W 2Y2; Cal'85; BSc; CCFP; FCFP; (250)721-8492

DYCK, Chadwyn L; Penticton Reg Hosp, 102-550 Carmi Ave, Penticton BC V2A 3G6; Man'00; FRCPC; IntMed. Staff, Penticton Regional Hospital; (250)493-0887

DYCK, Christopher J; Niagara H System-St Catharines, PO Box 3018 Stn Main 142 Queenston St, St Catharines ON L2R 7C6; Tor'02; FRCPC; DiagRad. Staff, Niagara Health System - St Catharines General Site; (416)864-5656

DYCK, Clayton H; Kildonan Med Centre, 2300 Mcphillips St, Winnipeg MB R2V 3M3; Man'88; CCFP; FCFP; (204)632-3203

DYCK, Coreen; 401-2151 McCallum Rd, Abbotsford BC V2S 3N8; UBC'96; FRCSC; GenSurg (Gastroenterology). Staff GenSurg, Abbotsford Regional Hospital & Cancer Centre; (604)853-1918; Fax. (604)853-5027.

DYCK, David F; Foothills Med Centre, 1403 29 St NW, Calgary AB T2N 2T9; UBC'00; CCFP; CCFP(E.M.); Staff, Foothills Medical Centre; (403)944-1315; Fax. (403)944-2419.

DYCK, Frederick G; 3406 28 Ave, Vernon BC V1T 1W9; UBC'91; (250)542-5520; Fax. (250)542-8596.

DYCK, Gordon H; Clearspring Med Clinic, 1-390 Main St, Steinbach MB R5G 1Z3; Man'85; BSc(Med); BA; Langs: German; (204)326-6111; Fax. (204)326-6952.

DYCK, John D; Stollery Children's Hosp, 4C2 WMC-8440 112 St NW, Edmonton AB T6G 2B7; Alb'79; FRCPC; Peds; Cardiol. Dir Ped. Cardiol., University of Alberta Hospital; Staff, Stollery Children's Hospital; Assoc Prof, University of Alberta; (780)407-3964; Fax. (780)407-3954; jdyck@cha.ab.ca.

DYCK, Kelly; Broadway Family Physicians, 1801 Broadway Ave, Saskatoon SK S7H 2B6; Sask'03; CCFP; (306)652-2632; Fax. (306)652-2637; kf.dyck1@sasktel.net.

DYCK, Michael; 1500 Pembina Ave, Winkler MB R6W 1T4; Man'93; FRCPC; Psy (Community Psychiatry). Psychiatrist, Eden Mental Health Centre; (204)822-6764; Fax. (204)822-1909; mpdyck@mts.net.

DYCK, Roland F; Royal University Hosp, 103 Hospital Dr, Saskatoon SK S7N 0W8; Sask'72; FRCPC; IntMed; Nephrol. Staff, Royal University Hospital; Ac Staff, Saskatoon Health Region; Academic Staff, University of Saskatchewan; (306)966-7985; Fax. (306)966-7996; roland.dyck@usask.ca.

DYE, Audrey A; Professional Bldg, 222 King St E, Bowmanville ON L1C 1P6; University of Guyana (Guyana)'00; CCFP; (905)440-3600; Fax. (905)697-7745.

DYER, Alan M; PO Box 58052 Rpo Mac's Conv, Calgary AB T2X 3V2; Glasgow (Scotland)'60; MB ChB; Dip Ortho(Eng.); Ophth. (403)262-4884

DYER, Cinda R; 304-1407 Yonge St, Toronto ON M4T 1Y7; Tor'84; FRCPC; Psy;CCFP; CCFP(E.M.); (416)922-6699; Fax. (416)922-7250.

DYER, David W; 1901 Ocean Park Rd, Surrey BC V4A 3M2; McM'80; CCFP.

DYER, Erin; Univ Of Western Ontario, D1000-1151 Richmond St, London ON N6A 5C1; McM'04; FRCSC; Neursurg. Teacher, University of Western Ontario.

DYKE, A Keith; Saugeen Shores Med Bldg, 36 Grey St N, Southampton ON N0H 2L0; Mem'00; CCFP; Staff, Hanover & District Hospital; Staff, Grey Bruce Health Services - Markdale; Staff, Grey Bruce Health Services - Wiarton Site; Staff, Grey Bruce Health Services - Southampton Site; (519)797-9940; Fax. (519)797-1225; y2kmd@hotmail.com.

DYKE, Corinne H; Radiology Consultants Assoc, 120-6707 Elbow Dr SW, Calgary AB T2V 0E3; Man'87; FRCPC; DiagRad. (403)777-3003; Fax. (403)777-3008.

DYKE, Debra R; 2000-1415 1st Ave W, Owen Sound ON N4K 4K8; Mem'92; CCFP; FCFP; Ac Staff, Grey Bruce Health Services - Owen Sound; Lecturer Part Time, University of Toronto; Aj Prof, University of Western Ontario; (519)470-3030; Fax. (519)470-3035.

DYKE, George W; 3634 Walnut Grove Rd, Mississauga ON L5L 2W8; Mem'75; FRCPC; Anes. Ac Staff, The Credit Valley Hospital; (905)820-6475

DYKE, Marion E M B; The Evans Clinic, 233 Evans Ave, Etobicoke ON M8Z 1J6; Mem'77; Ac Staff Family Pract, William Osler Health System - Etobicoke General Hospital; Physician, The Evans Clinic; (416)252-1357; Fax. (416)252-3169.

DYKEMAN, F Bruce; 102-1A Marr Rd, Rothesay NB E2E 3L4; Dal'78; CCFP; FCFP; (506)847-7517; Fax. (506)847-8968.

DYKEMAN, Ronald; General Motors of Canada, 1908 Colonel Sam Dr, Oshawa ON L1H 8P7; Dal'95; FRCPC; OccupMed. Physician, General Motors Of Canada Ltd; (416)399-0406

DYKEMAN, Winston R; 2840 Main St, Hillsborough NB E4H 2Y7; Dal'71; BSc; CCFP; Ac Staff, The Moncton Hospital; (506)734-2063; Fax. (506)734-2502.

DYKHUIS, Sandra; Medistat Med Familiale, 4965 rue Saint-Pierre, Pierrefonds QC H9H 5M9; Sher'93; CCFP; CCFP(E.M.); (514)624-4774; Fax. (514)624-4704.

DYKIN, Kimberly; PO Box 3955 Stn Main, Olds AB T4H 1P6; Alb'08; CCFP; (403)556-7130; Fax. (403)556-1944.

DYLEWSKI, Irving M; St Mary's Hosp Centre, 3830 av Lacombe, Montreal QC H3T 1M5; McG'79; BSc; MBA; FRCPC; IntMed. Staff IntMed, St Mary's Hospital Centre; Teacher Faculty, McGill University; Langs: French; (514)345-3511 x3084; Fax. (514)489-9316; idlt1717@sympatico.ca.

DYLEWSKI, Joe S; St Mary's Hosp Centre, 3830 av Lacombe, Montreal QC H3T 1M5; McG'76; ABIM; MD; Microbio & Infect Dis (P.Q.); MedMicrobiol; IntMed (Infectious Diseases). Chef Lab, St Mary's Hospital Centre; assoc Prof, McGill University; Langs: French; (514)345-3511 x3075; joe.dylewski@ssss.gouv.qc.ca.

DYMENT, David A; Children's Hosp Eastern Ont, 401 Smyth Rd, Ottawa ON K1H 8L1; Cal'06; FRCPC; MedGenetics. Staff, Children's Hospital of Eastern Ontario (CHEO); (613)737-7600

DYMENT, David B; Central Park Med Clinic, 301-3965 Kingsway, Burnaby BC V5H 1Y8; McM'75; BSc(Eng); CCFP; Fam Med, Burnaby Hospital; (604)439-9300; Fax. (604)437-1770.

DYMENT, Lana W; Central Park Med Clinic, 301-3965 Kingsway, Burnaby BC V5H 1Y8; UBC'97; CCFP; FCFP; (604)437-4441; Fax. (604)439-9572.

DYMENT, Stuart Z; 125 The Queensway PO Box 15302, Toronto ON M8Y 0B4; Tor'83; (416)537-7000

DYMON, Diane A; Middlesex London Health, 101-50 King St, London ON N6A 5L7; Wes'95; CCFP; (519)663-5446; Fax. (519)663-8273.

DYMON, William A; 202-3101 Bloor St W, Etobicoke ON M8X 2W2; Tor'68; CCFP; CCFP(E.M.); FCFP; Att Staff, Toronto Western Hospital - University Health Network; Lecturer, University of Toronto; Langs: Ukrainian; (416)231-9991; Fax. (416)231-8085.

DYRDA, Katia; Institut de Cardiologie de Mtl, 5000 rue Belanger, Montreal QC H1T 1C8; Ott'03; FRCPC; IntMed; Cardiol. Staff, Institut de Cardiologie de Montréal; (514)376-3330

DYSART, Allison; Tantramar Health Centre, C-2 Main St, Sackville NB E4L 4A3; Dal'92; (506)536-4441; Fax. (506)536-0299.

DYSON, William H; Univ Of Victoria Health Serv, PO Box 1700 Stn CSC, Victoria BC V8P 5C2; McM'75; (250)721-8492; Fax. (250)472-5472.

DYTOC, Marlene T; College Plaza, 907-8215 112 St NW, Edmonton AB T6G 2C8; Tor'97; FRCPC; Derm. Clinical Asst Prof, University of Alberta; Langs: Chinese; Tagalog; (780)466-8806; Fax. (780)433-8872.

DYUB, Adel M A; Hamilton HS-General Site, 504-237 Barton St E, Hamilton ON L8L 2X2; Al-Fateh (Libya)'99; FRCSC; CardSurg. Staff, Hamilton Health Sciences Centre - Hamilton General Hospital; (905)527-0271; Fax. (905)577-8228.

DZAJA, Nancy; St Joseph's Healthcare, 50 Charlton Ave E, Hamilton ON L8N 4A6; Wes'07; ObstGyn. Staff, St Joseph's Healthcare - Charlton Campus; (905)522-4941

DZAVIK, Vladimir; Univ Hlth Network-Toronto Gen, 6EN 246-200 Elizabeth St, Toronto ON M5G 2C4; Alb'83; MD; BSc; FRFPS; FRCPC; IntMed (Interventional Cardiology); Cardiol., Toronto General Hospital - UHN; Langs: Czech; Polish; Slovak; (416)340-4800 x6265; Fax. (416)340-3390; vlad.dzavik@uhn.on.ca.

DZEVER, Olga; Etobicoke Med Centre, 400 The East Mall, Etobicoke ON M9B 3Z9; Belgrade (Serbia)'76; CCFP; Langs: Croatian; Serbian; (416)621-2220; Fax. (416)621-2203.

DZIECIOL, Gordon; 2-1701 Martin Grove Rd, Etobicoke ON M9V 4N4; Wes'84; Langs: German; (416)742-9988; Fax. (416)742-7802.

DZIEDZIC, Margaret; Trillium Hlth Ctr-West Toronto, 150 Sherway Dr, Etobicoke ON M9C 1A5; Lodz (Poland)'87; FRCPC; PhysMed&Rehab. Staff, Trillium Health Centre - West Toronto; Staff, Trillium Health Centre - Mississauga; Langs: Polish; (416)521-4037; Fax. (416)521-4093.

DZIERZANOWSKI, Martin; 655 Willow St, Truro NS B2N 5H2; Dal'00; BSc; FRCSC; GenSurg. Chief Surgery/Staff Surgeon Colchester East Hlth Authority, Colchester East Hants Health Centre; (902)895-5390; Fax. (902)895-5128; surgeon@eastlink.ca.

DZIEWALTOWSKA-GINTOWT, B; 213 Spinnaker Dr, Halifax NS B3N 3C3; Warsaw (Poland)'70; CCFP; Staff, All Saints Springhill Hospital; Med Consultant, Nova Scotia Addiction Services; Langs: Polish; (902)597-3727; Fax. (902)597-3729.

DZIKOWSKI, Dana; Family Med Centre, 305-400 Tache Ave, Winnipeg MB R2H 3E1; Man'06; FRCSC; ObstGyn. Staff, St Boniface General Hospital; (204)233-8563

DZINEKU, Frederick; Hop Maisonneuve-Rosemont, 5415 boul de l'Assomption, Montreal QC H1T 2M4; McG'06; MDCM; ObstGyn. Staff, Hopital Maisonneuve-Rosemont; (514)252-3400

DZINEKU, Jean L; Centre Med Pierrefonds, 119-12774 boul Gouin O, Pierrefonds QC H8Z 1W5; Beirut (Lebanon)'70; Ac Staff, Lakeshore General Hospital - Pointe Claire; (514)684-3884; Fax. (514)684-3891.

DZINEKU, Marie-Dominique; Clinique Med Saint-Vincent, 250 rue King E, Sherbrooke QC J1G 1A9; Sher'95; CCFP; Staff Long Term, Institut Universitaire de Geriatrie de Sherbrooke-Pavillon Argyll; Staff, Centre Jeunesse Estrie Val-du-Lac; Langs: Bilingual(French/English); (819)563-0510; Fax. (819)564-6889.

DZIURDZY, Stanley A; A-1463 Ontario St, Burlington ON L7S 1G6; Tor'63; DPsy; FRCPC; Psy. Langs: Polish; (905)632-2543

DZONGOWSKI, Peter; London East Med Centre, 295 Saskatoon St, London ON N5W 6A2; Wes'92; CCFP; FCFP; Med Staff, London Health Sciences Centre - Victoria Campus; Med Staff, St Joseph's Hospital - St Joseph's Health Care; Langs: Polish; Greek; (519)659-3747; Fax. (519)659-8575.

DZUS, Anne K; Royal University Hosp, 5513-103 Hospital Dr, Saskatoon SK S7N 0W8; Sask'81; FRCSC; OrthSurg. Staff, Royal University Hospital; (306)966-8210; Fax. (306)966-8196.

E, C Choan; The Ottawa Hosp-Gen Campus, Box 903 501 Smyth Rd, Ottawa ON K1H 8L6; Tor'93; FRCPC; RadOncol (Genito Urinary Oncology). Staff, The Ottawa Hospital - General Campus; Asst Prof Med, University of Ottawa; (613)737-7700 x70202; Fax. (613)247-3511; ce@ottawahospital.on.ca.

EADES, Barnett R; PO Box 77090 Stn Main, St Albert AB T8N 6C1; Otago (New Zealand)'62; DPsy(Tor.); Psy. Consultant Geriatric Psy Day Program, Covenant Health - Edmonton General Continuing Care Centre; (780)459-0658

EADIE, Carmen N; Formed Clinics Inc, 204-18730 Fraser Hwy, Surrey BC V3S 8E7; Man'80; CCFP; (604)575-0501

EAGLE, Christopher; Seventh Street Plaza, 14F-10030 107 St NW, Edmonton AB T5J 3E4; Cal'77; FRCPC; Anes (Cardiovascular Anesthesia). Pres/CEO, Alberta Health Services Calgary; Prof Comm Hlth Sciences/Chief Clinical Officer, University of Calgary; (780)342-2000; Fax. (780)342-2063; chris.eagle@calgaryhealthregion.ca.

EAGLESHAM, Hugh H; Misericordia Health Centre, 99 Cornish Ave, Winnipeg MB R3C 1A2; Sask'64; FRCPC; DiagRad. Consultant, St Boniface General Hospital.

EAMAN, Stanley G; Vernon Professional Group, 2505 32 Ave, Vernon BC V1T 2K8; McG'65; Psy. Staff, Vernon Jubilee Hospital; (250)549-1633; Fax. (250)549-3963.

EAPEN, Libni J; The Ottawa Hosp-Gen Campus, Box 902 501 Smyth Rd, Ottawa ON K1H 8L6; Dal'77; FRCP; FACR; FRCPC; RadOncol (Oncology). Ac Staff Ottawa Reg Cancer Centre, The Ottawa Hospital - General Campus; Asst Prof, University of Ottawa.

EAPEN, Lisbi P J V; Pringle Creek Med Office, 728 Anderson St, Whitby ON L1N 3V6; Dal'85; (905)665-5800; Fax. (905)665-5807.

EAPEN, Tamina; Montfort Hosp, 713 Montreal Rd, Ottawa ON K1K 0T2; Ott'06; FRCPC; Psy. Staff, Montfort Hospital; Langs: Bilingual(English/French); (613)746-4621

EAPEN-JOHN, Reena E; 604-165 Dundas St W, Mississauga ON L5B 2N6; Benin (Nigeria)'85; CCFP; FCFP; Staff, Trillium Health Centre - Mississauga; Langs: Hindi; Malayalam; (905)803-0078

EAPPEN, Roy; 555-5757 av Decelles, Montreal QC H3S 2C3; McG'85; FRCPC; IntMed (Diabetes); Endocrin&Metab. (514)739-7771; Fax. (514)739-5548; eapr9@rogers.com.

EARL, Kevin D; Agassiz Med Clinic, 130-30 Stephen St, Morden MB R6M 2G3; Man'08; CCFP.

EARL, Simon F; HSBC Building, 1003-299 Victoria St, Prince George BC V2L 5N8; Cape Town (South Africa)'83; MB ChB; FRCPC; Peds., University Hospital of Northern British Columbia; (250)563-2257; Fax. (250)563-3395.

EARLE, Craig C; Sunnybrook Hlth Sciences Ctre, G106-2075 Bayview Ave, Toronto ON M4N 3M5; Ott'90; FRCPC; IntMed; MedOncol. Staff, Sunnybrook Health Sciences Centre; (416)480-6047; Fax. (416)480-6046.

EARLE, Elizabeth M; Burnaby Hosp, 3935 Kincaid St, Burnaby BC V5G 2X6; Alb'78; FRCPC; GenPath. Staff Labs, Burnaby Hospital; (604)434-6357

EARLE, Harry T; Westbram Family Physicians, 208-100 Pertosa Dr, Brampton ON L6X 0H9; Mem'77; Staff, William Osler Health System - Brampton Civic Hospital; Med Dir, Peel Manor Home for Senior Citizens; (905)454-2080

EARLE, John M; 38 Water St E, Brockville ON K6V 1A2; Qns'69; FRCSC; Urol (Adult & Pediatric Urology). Ac Staff, Brockville General Hospital - Charles Street; Ac Staff, Providence Continuing Care Centre (PCCC) - St Vincent de Paul Hospital; Staff Consultant, Perth & Smiths Falls District Hospital - Smiths Falls Site; (613)342-5668; Fax. (613)345-1568.

EARLE, John M; Queensway-Carleton Hosp, 3045 Baseline Rd, Nepean ON K2H 8P4; Qns'75; MCFP(EM); Staff/Chief EmergMed, Queensway Carleton Hospital; (613)721-2000

EARLE, Lisa; Bethesda Hosp Steinbach, PO Box 939 Stn Main 316 Henry St, Steinbach MB R5G 1A3; Ott'04; CCFP; Fam Med, Bethesda Hospital Steinbach; (204)326-6411; learle@sehealth.mb.ca.

EARLE, Lynda M M; 200-215 Dominion St, Bridgewater NS B4V 2K7; Dal'01; FRCPC; Public Health & Preventive Med;CCFP; (902)543-0850

EARLY, Anita M; Lions Gate Hosp, 231 15th St E, North Vancouver BC V7L 2L7; Wes'90; Staff, Lions Gate Hospital; (604)790-6957

EARMME, Christine S Y; 104-3965 Kingsway, Burnaby BC V5H 1Y8; Tor'96; CCFP; (604)434-8781; Fax. (604)434-8699.

EASAW, Jacob C; Tom Baker Cancer Centre, 1331 29 St NW, Calgary AB T2N 4N2; Alb'00; FRCPC; IntMed; MedOncol. (403)521-3446

EASO, Hyacinth S E; Grand River Hosp-Freeport Site, PO Box 9056 3570 King St E, Kitchener ON N2A 2W1; Dal'04; FRCPC; Psy. Staff, Grand River Hospital - Freeport Site; (519)749-4300; Fax. (519)894-8308.

EASO, James; Halton HCS Corp-Milton, 7030 Derry Rd, Milton ON L9T 7H6; McM'01; CCFP; Staff, Halton Healthcare Services Corporation - Milton District Hospital; (905)876-7026

EASON, Brad D; CFB Petawawa, Z127-46 Centurian Rd, Petawawa ON K8H 2X3; Ott'06; CCFP; Langs: Bilingual(English/French); (613)687-5511

EASSON, Alexandra M; Univ Hlth Network-Princess M, 3 124-610 University Ave, Toronto ON M5G 2M9; Qns'91; MSc; FRCSC; GenSurg (Surgical Oncology). Staff, Mount Sinai Hospital; Staff, Princess Margaret Hospital - University Health Network; (416)946-2328; Fax. (416)946-4429.

EAST, Andrea J; Gane Yohs Med Centre, 1769 Chiefswood Rd, Ohsweken ON N0A 1M0; McM'80; (519)445-2251; Fax. (519)445-4679.

EAST, Nathalie; Centre Hosp-Rouyn-Noranda, 4 9e rue, Rouyn-Noranda QC J9X 2B2; Mon'01; FRCSC; ObstGyn. Staff ObstGyn, Centre Hospitalier Rouyn-Noranda; Langs: Bilingual(French/English); (819)764-5131; Fax. (819)764-2924; natheast@hotmail.com.

EAST, William; 401-3320 Richter St, Kelowna BC V1W 4V5; Sask'77; BSc(Anatomy); FRCPC; Anes. Physician, Palliser Health Authority; (250)868-9799; william.east@cls.ab.ca.

EASTABROOK, Genevieve D M; London HSC-Victoria Hosp, B2 412-800 Commissioners Rd E, London ON N6A 4G5; Cal'03; FRCSC; ObstGyn (Maternal Fetal Medicine). Staff, London Health Sciences Centre - Children's Hospital; (519)685-8500

EASTERBROOK, Mark D; Upper Grand Family Health Team, 753 Tower St S, Fergus ON N1M 2R2; Qns'99; CCFP; (519)843-4380; Fax. (519)843-3211.

EASTERBROOK, W Michael; Create Fertility Centre, 310-790 Bay St, Toronto ON M5G 1N8; Tor'65; FACS; FRCSC; Ophth (Laser Surgery). Ac Staff, Toronto Western Hospital - University Health Network; Ac Staff, St Michael's Hospital; Assoc Staff, Mount Sinai Hospital; Prof Ophth, University of Toronto; (416)926-1486; Fax. (416)926-0091; michaeleasterbrook@sympatico.ca.

EASTMURE, John J; North Muskoka Med Clinic, 202-29 Main St E, Huntsville ON P1H 2C6; McM'83; CCFP; Staff, Huntsville District Memorial Hospital - Muskoka Algonquin Healthcare; (705)789-5581; Fax. (705)788-7888.

EASTON, Alexander; DJ Mackenzie Bldg, 734B-5788 University Ave, Halifax NS B3H 1V8; London (England)'88; MB BS; BSc(Hon)(Hons.); PhD; FRCPC; NeurPath. Staff Neuropathologist, Queen Elizabeth II Health Sciences Centre - Victoria General Site; Asst Prof Paath, Dalhousie University; (902)473-8255

EASTON, David W; Health Sciences Centre, 820 Sherbrook St, Winnipeg MB R3A 1R9; Man'95; FRCPC; EmergMed; Critical Care Medicine. Staff Critical Care Med, Health Sciences Centre; (204)774-6511

EASTON, Paul A; HSC-Faculty Of Med, 223-3330 Hospital Dr NW, Calgary AB T2N 4N1; Qns'76; FRCPC; IntMed; Respir. (403)220-7045; Fax. (403)283-3615.

EASTON, William A; Scarborough Prof Centre, 203-1371 Neilson Rd, Scarborough ON M1B 4Z8; Man'76; FACOG; FRCSC; ObstGyn (Urogynecology). Assoc Staff, Mount Sinai Hospital; Ac Staff, Rouge Valley Health System - Centenary Health Centre Site; Asst Prof ObstGyn, University of Toronto; (416)287-2800; Fax. (416)287-3395.

EASTWOOD, Diane E; Regional Mental HC-London, PO Box 5532 Stn B 850 Highbury Ave, London ON N6A 4H1; Qns'79; BSc; FRCPC; Psy (Psychosis). Staff, Regional Mental Health Care-St Joseph's Health Care; (519)455-5110; diane.eastwood@sjhc.london.on.ca.

EASTWOOD, Katrina; 130 Ontario St, Kingston ON K7L 2Y4; Edinburgh (Scotland)'63; MB ChB; Langs: English; French; (613)539-9721

EASWARA MURTHI, Manjula; 102-10127 121 Ave, Grande Prairie AB T8V 7V3; Czech.Rep. (Czech Republic)'87; (780)538-0111; Fax. (780)532-0407.

EATON, Christopher J; Royal Ottawa Hlth Care Group, 1145 Carling Ave, Ottawa ON K1Z 7K4; Man'01; Psy. Staff, Royal Ottawa Mental Health Centre - Royal Ottawa Health Care Group; Langs: Bilingual(English/French); (613)722-6521 x7020; Fax. (613)798-2971.

EATON, David F; Thamesview Family Health Team, PO Box 429 26 Erie St S, Wheatley ON N0P 2P0; Ott'72; Ac Staff, Leamington District Memorial Hospital; Ac Staff, Chatham-Kent Health Alliance; (519)825-4302; Fax. (519)825-9570.

EATON, Jo-Ann; Wortley Village Med Centre, 215-190 Wortley Rd, London ON N6C 4Y7; Ott'84; Staff Occupational Med, London Health Sciences Centre - South Street; Physician, Wortley Village Medical Centre; (519)438-7666; Fax. (519)438-7418.

EATON, Robert J; Family Med Associates, 500-267 O'Connor St, Ottawa ON K2P 1V3; McM'80; Court Staff Privil, The Ottawa Hospital - General Campus; Langs: Bilingual(English/French); (613)565-7575

EATON, William H; Dr Leonard A Miller Centre, 712-100 Forest Rd, St. John's NL A1A 3Z9; Mem'74; CCFP; FCFP; Staff, Health Sciences Centre; (709)777-6301

EAVES, Allen; Stem Cell Technologies Inc, 400-570 7th Ave W, Vancouver BC V5Z 4S6; Dal'69; BSc; PhD; FACP; FRCPC; IntMed (Medical Oncology). CEO, Terry Fox Laboratory of the BC Cancer Agency; Pres/CEO, Stemcell Technologies Inc; Emeritus Prof Hematology, University of British Columbia; (604)877-0713; infoweb@stemcell.com.

EAYRS, Gertrude E; Addiction & Mental Hlth-Queen, 1001 Queen St W, Toronto ON M6J 1H4; Dal'95; FRCPC; Psy (Legal Psychiatry). Staff Psy, Centre for Addiction & Mental Health (CAMH) - Queen Site; Teach Staff Psy, University of Toronto; (416)535-8501 x2893

EBACHER, Annie; CHUS-Hop Fleurimont, 3001 12e av N, Sherbrooke QC J1H 5N4; Sher'99; FRCPC; RadOncol. Staff, Centre Hospitalier Universitaire de Sherbrooke-Hopital Fleurimont; (819)346-1110

EBAIJ, Ali M A; Abbotsford Shoppers Mall, 258-3210 118 Ave NW, Edmonton AB T5W 4W1; University of Al Fateh (Libya)'00; MB ChB; CCFP; (780)479-3318; Fax. (780)479-3302.

EBBELING-TREON, Lori R; Clinique St Boniface Clinic, 343 Tache Ave, Winnipeg MB R2H 2A5; Man'86; CCFP; FCFP.

EBBERT, Kirsten V J; King Edward Pediatrics Clinic, 926 King Edward Ave W, Vancouver BC V5Z 2E2; Cal'06; FRCPC; Peds. Staff, BC Children's Hospital; Staff, Northmount Medical Centre; (604)600-7282

EBBESON, Regan L; Northmount Med Centre, 303-145 13th St E, North Vancouver BC V7L 2L4; UBC'03; FRCPC; Peds. Staff Ped, Burnaby Hospital; Clinical Asst Prof, University of British Columbia; (604)984-8880; Fax. (604)984-8887.

EBEID, Manal; 197-5 Fairview Mall Dr, North York ON M2J 2Z1; Ain Shams (Egypt)'89; CCFP; Langs: Arabic; (416)493-0346; Fax. (416)493-0336.

EBERDT, Caroline T; St Paul's Hosp, 1081 Burrard St, Vancouver BC V6Z 1Y6; McM'07; CCFP; CCFP(E.M.); Staff, Providence Health Care - St Paul's Hospital; (604)682-2344

EBERHARD, Juliette A; Coleman Clinic, 186 Kenneth St, Duncan BC V9L 1N4; Cape Town (South Africa)'83; MB ChB; (250)746-4102; Fax. (250)746-5960.

EBERHARD, R Stuart; London HSC-Victoria Hosp, PO Box 5010 Stn B E1 308-800 Commissioners Rd E, London ON N6A 5W9; Wes'67; ABIM; FACP; FRCPC; IntMed (Gastroenterology). Ac Staff Credentials Committee, London Health Sciences Centre - Victoria Campus; Staff Consultant, Four Counties Health Services - Middlesex Hospital Alliance; Consultant, South Bruce Grey Health Centre - Kincardine Site; Aj Prof Med., University of Western Ontario; (519)685-8400; Fax. (519)685-8308.

EBERHARD, Thomas S C; 1292 Highbury Ave N, London ON N5Y 1B4; Wes'71; (519)451-1421

EBERT, Daniel; Brockville Gen Hosp, 75 rue Charles, Brockville ON K6V 1S8; McG'88; CCFP; CCFP(E.M.); FCFP; Staff, Brockville General Hospital - Charles Street; Staff, Montfort Hospital; Langs: Bilingual(English/French); (613)345-5645

EBERT, Nicole; Omineca Med Clinic, RR 2 3348 Hospital Rd, Vanderhoof BC V0J 3A2; UBC'93; CCFP; Med Staff, St John Hospital; Clin Associate, University of British Columbia; (250)567-2201; Fax. (250)567-2105.

EBERT, Sean P; Omineca Med Clinic, RR 2 3348 Hospital Rd, Vanderhoof BC V0J 3A2; UBC'93; CCFP; Clin Instructor Family Pract, University of British Columbia; (250)567-2201; Fax. (250)567-2105.

EBESH, Osama; Chilliwack Gen Hosp, L1 WB-45600 Menholm St, Chilliwack BC V2P 1P7; Aleppo (Syria)'87; Staff Specialist Pediatrician, Chilliwack General Hospital; Clin Instructor, University of British Columbia; Langs: Arabic; (604)793-4508

EBISUZAKI, Lawrence K; The Peterborough Clinic, 301-26 Hospital Dr, Peterborough ON K9J 7C3; Tor'96; BSc; MSc; DABS; FACS; FRCSC; GenSurg. Ac Staff, Peterborough Regional Health Centre - Hospital Drive; (705)740-6852; Fax. (705)740-6899.

EBRAHIM, Farouk A; 54-4550 Ebenezer Rd, Brampton ON L6P 2R2; Witwatersrand (South Africa)'86; CCFP; Langs: Afrikaans; Hindi; (905)794-4277; Fax. (905)794-7211.

EBRAHIM, Karim; 100B-3300 Boundary Rd, Burnaby BC V5M 4A4; Alb'91; (604)437-7001

EBRAHIM, Salim K; 4446 Hastings St, Burnaby BC V5C 2K2; Alb'89; (604)298-4491

EBRAHIM, Shehla; Afterglow Skin & Laser Centre, 104-2609 Westview Dr, North Vancouver BC V7N 4M2; Karachi (Pakistan)'86; CCFP; FCFP; Staff, Ambleside Dermedics & Health Centre; Langs: Urdu; (604)232-1570

EBTIA, Mahasti; Gordon & Leslie Diamond HCC, 9F-2775 Laurel St, Vancouver BC V5Z 1M9; Tehran (Iran)'00; FRCPC; IntMed. Staff, Gordon & Leslie Diamond Health Care Centre; (604)875-5302

EBY, Donald H; Grey Bruce HS-Owen Sound, PO Box 1800 Stn Main 1800 8th St E, Owen Sound ON N4K 6M9; Tor'77; MSc; CCFP; CCFP(E.M.); FCFP; Med Dir Grey Bruce Huron Paramedic, Grey Bruce Health Services - Owen Sound; (519)376-2121; Fax. (519)376-3948; d.eby@sympatico.ca.

EBY, John R; Westwind Med Ave, 107-755 Goldstream Ave, Victoria BC V9B 0H9; Sask'75; CCFP; FCFP; (250)478-1764; Fax. (250)478-1300.

EBY, Roberta J; St Joseph's Healthcare, 50 Charlton Ave E, Hamilton ON L8N 4A6; Wes'85; FRCPC; EmergMed. Staff Emerg, St Joseph's Hospital - St Joseph's Health Care; Asst Clin Prof Med, McMaster University; Lecturer Med & Surg, University of Toronto; (905)522-4941 x3112; Fax. (905)573-4842.

ECCLES, Robin C; Alberta Children's Hosp, 2888 Shaganappi Trail NW, Calgary AB T3B 6A8; Tor'79; FRACS; FRCSC; GenSurg; PedGenSurg. Med Staff, Alberta Children's Hospital; Consultant, Foothills Medical Centre; Clin Asst Prof Surg, University of Calgary; (403)955-7807; Fax. (403)955-7634; robin.eccles@albertahealthservices.ca.

ECHAVARRIA CANO, Maria; O & G Med Associates, 208-9815 97 Street, Grande Prairie AB T8V 8B9; (Argentina)'97; LMCC; Staff, Queen Elizabeth II Hospital; (780)538-2190; Fax. (780)538-2191.

ECHAVE, Pablo; CHUS-Hop Fleurimont, 3001 12e av N, Sherbrooke QC J1H 5N4; Louisiana (LA) (USA)'01; FRCPC; Anes. Staff, Centre Hospitalier Universitaire de Sherbrooke-Hopital Fleurimont; (819)346-1110

ECHENBERG, Donald; CHUS-Hop Hotel-Dieu, 580 rue Bowen S, Sherbrooke QC J1G 2E8; McG'76; BSc; MDCM; FACP; FRCPC; IntMed (Cardiology). ac Membre, Centre Hospitalier Universitaire de Sherbrooke-Hôpital Hôtel-Dieu; assoc Prof Med, Universite de Sherbrooke; Langs: Spanish; English; (819)346-1110 x28303; Fax. (819)820-6406; dechen@videotron.ca.

ECHENDU, Wegbo; St Clare's Mercy Hosp, 154 Lemarchant Rd, St. John's NL A1C 5B8; (Nigeria)'87; Staff, St Clare's Mercy Hospital; (709)777-5000

ECHEZONA, Anthony O; Parkland Med Centre, 202-10127 121 Ave, Grande Prairie AB T8V 7V3; '90; MCFP; FRACGP; (780)532-1004; Fax. (780)532-1066.

ECHLIN, Paul S; Elliot Sports Med Clinic, 102-1100 Walkers Line, Burlington ON L7N 2G3; Carribean (Montserrat)'98; CCFP; (905)336-3340; Fax. (905)336-6095.

ECHLIN, Thomas H; Medical Associates, 1909 Tecumseh Rd E, Windsor ON N8W 1C9; Qns'56; CM; CCFP; FCFP; (519)258-6602; Fax. (519)258-3282.

ECKER, George A; Fredericton Med Clinic, 411-1015 Regent St, Fredericton NB E3B 6H5; Qns'88; FRCPC; IntMed; Rheum. Staff, Dr Everett Chalmers Regional Hospital; (506)458-0314; Fax. (506)458-8623.

ECKFELDT, Charles T; Wrinch Mem Hosp, PO Box 999 2510 Hwy 62, Hazelton BC V0J 1Y0; UBC'93; CCFP; FCFP; Staff Family Med, Wrinch Memorial Hospital; (250)842-5234; Fax. (250)842-5865.

ECKHART, Martin S; Associate Med Clinic, PO Box 7590 Stn Main, Peace River AB T8S 1T2; McG'92; CCFP; FCFP; Assoc Prof Rural Teaching Site, University of Alberta; Langs: German; French; (780)624-2581; Fax. (780)624-4015; prdocs@telusplanet.net.

ECKHAUS, Allan A; Baywood Med Centre, 307-95 Bayly St W, Ajax ON L1S 7K8; Tor'00; FRCSC; PlasSurg. Staff, Rouge Valley Health System - Ajax & Pickering Health Centre Site; (905)619-9600; Fax. (905)619-9617.

ECKLAND JETZER, Shelly; Steveston Med Group, 203-3811 Chatham St, Richmond BC V7E 2Z4; UBC'08; CCFP; (604)284-5389

ECKLER, Howard; Near North Med Clinic, 202-66 Josephine St, North Bay ON P1B 0A7; Tor'66; Staff, North Bay Regional Health Centre - Regional Mental Health; (705)476-1512; Fax. (705)495-4500.

ECKLER, Nettie M; 201-1 Hesperus Rd, Thornhill ON L4J 0G9; McM'91; Staff, Mackenzie Richmond Hill Hospital; (905)882-4949; Fax. (905)882-0560.

ECKLER, Sarah J; Queen West Commun Health Ctre, 168 Bathurst St, Toronto ON M5V 2R4; Tor'98; CCFP; Langs: Bilingual(English/French); (416)703-8480

ECOB, Naomi A; Kent Place Mall, 200-189 Kent St W, Lindsay ON K9V 5G6; Wes'85; Staff, Ross Memorial Hospital; (705)878-4656; Fax. (705)878-8835.

ECONOMOPOULOS, Peter A; Toronto East Gen Hosp Inc, 825 Coxwell Ave, Toronto ON M4C 3E7; Wes'99; FRCPC; IntMed. Staff, Toronto East General Hospital Inc; (416)461-8272

EDAMURA, Arthur; 2201 Broadway W, Vancouver BC V6K 2E4; UBC'76; (604)222-2256; Fax. (604)222-2257.

EDANI, Shakibeh A; North East Comm Health Ctre, 14007 50 St NW, Edmonton AB T5A 5E4; (Iraq)'89; MB ChB; CCFP; (780)342-4038; Fax. (780)342-4192.

EDDE, Donald J; 200-5950 ch de la Cote-des-Nei, Montreal QC H3S 1Z6; Beirut (Lebanon)'80; FRCPC; DiagRad (P.Q.). ac Staff, CSSS du Coeur de l'Isle Hôpital Jean-Talon; Langs: Bilingual(French/English); (514)739-5050; Fax. (514)739-5610; mtledc@qc.aihn.com.

EDDEB, Abdurrahman A; Humber River Reg Hosp-Church, 200 Church St, Toronto ON M9N 1N8; Al-Fateh (Libya)'90; FRCPC; DiagRad. Staff, Humber River Regional Hospital - Church Street Site; Langs: Arabic; (416)243-4159; Fax. (416)243-4162.

EDDENDEN, Peter W; Oakville Health Centre, 208-1060 Speers Rd, Oakville ON L6L 2X4; Tor'81; Med Advisor Oakville Branch, Halton Diabetes Program; Member, Canadian Society of Addiction Medicine; (905)845-0825; Fax. (905)845-3636.

EDDIE, Patrick; Hôpital régional Chaleur, 1750 Sunset Dr, Bathurst NB E2A 4L7; Mon'97; CCFP; Staff Family Med & Emerg, Hopital Regional Chaleur; Staff Emerg Med Service, Reseau Sante Acadie-Bathurst; Langs: English; (506)544-3000; Fax. (506)544-2532.

EDDY, Allison A; Children's & Women's HC of BC, 2015-4480 Oak St, Vancouver BC V6H 3V4; McM'75; FRCPC; Peds (Pediatric Nephrology). Staff, BC Children's Hospital; (604)875-2315

EDDY, Andrew; 170-1620 29 St NW, Calgary AB T2N 4L7; Alb'09; CCFP; Staff, University of Alberta Hospital; (403)221-9340; Fax. (403)221-9336.

EDDY, Donald; Gain Med Centre, 1199 Austin Ave, Coquitlam BC V3K 3P4; Mem'73; CCFP; Clin Instructor Family Med, University of British Columbia; (604)939-7345; Fax. (604)939-7781.

EDDY, M Joan; Eagle Ridge Hosp & Health CC, 475 Guildford Way, Port Moody BC V3H 3W9; Mem'80; CCFP; Staff, Eagle Ridge Hospital & Health Care Centre; (604)461-2022 x54325

EDDY, Richard J; Royal Jubilee Hosp, 1952 Bay St, Victoria BC V8R 1J8; Mem'82; FRCPC; IntMed (Musculoskeletal Imaging); DiagRad. Staff Diag Imaging, Royal Jubilee Hospital; (250)370-8272

EDE, Anizor; 11855 102 Ave NW, Edmonton AB T5K 0R6; Louvain (Belgium)'70; DTMH; FRCPC; Psy. Langs: French; (780)482-3891; Fax. (780)488-7241.

EDE, Megeri; PO Box 56030 Rpo Minto Place, Ottawa ON K1R 7Z1; Edinburgh (Scotland)'64; MB ChB; DTMH(Liverpool); FACP; FRCPC; IntMed (Allergy). Pres, Solar Energy for Africa Ltd; Langs: Ibo; Hausa; Yoruba; (613)236-9441

EDELIST, Darren; High Performance Sports Med, 1604-2300 Yonge St, Toronto ON M4P 1E4; Wes'99; Dip SportMed; CCFP; Team Physician, Ryerson University; (416)486-4776; Fax. (416)486-4773.

EDELS, Margrieta; London Medical-Dental Bldg, 301-450 Central Ave, London ON N6B 2E8; Ott'80; Langs: Latvian; (519)439-0346; Fax. (519)439-3400.

EDELSTEIN, Chaim Z I; 507-5885 ch Cote-des-Neiges, Montreal QC H3S 2T2; McG'91; FRCSC; Ophth (Cataract Surgery). Asst Prof Ophth, McGill University; Langs: English; French; (514)342-5434; cedelstein@yahoo.com.

EDELSTEIN, Earl; 5151 Isabella Ave, Montreal QC H3W 1S9; McG'69; principale Médecin, Sir Mortimer B Davis Jewish General; Att Médecin, Jewish Eldercare Centre - CHSLD JUIF de Montréal; Att Médecin, CLSC Cote-des-Neiges; Conférencier, McGill University; Langs: French; Yiddish; (514)737-7582

EDELSTEIN, Eugene; 5885 ch de la Cote-des-Neiges, Montreal QC H3S 2T2 Suite 507; Alb'60; Ophth (P.Q.). Staff, Sir Mortimer B Davis Jewish General; (514)342-5434

EDELSTEIN, Jerome; 301-960 Lawrence Ave W, Toronto ON M6A 3B5; Tor'91; MD; MRCS; FRCSC; PlasSurg (Cosmetic Surgery). Ac Staff PlasSurg, Humber River Regional Hospital - Church Street Site; Ac Staff, Toronto Midtown Private Cosmetic Surgery Unit; (416)256-5614; Fax. (416)256-4194; plastic-surgery@bellnet.ca.

EDEN, David S; Reg Supervising Coroners Off, 13F-119 King St W, Hamilton ON L8P 4Y7; Wes'87; (905)546-8202; Fax. (905)546-8210.

EDEN, Silke C; South Shore Reg Hosp, 90 Glen Allan Dr, Bridgewater NS B4V 3S6; (Australia)'83; Staff, South Shore Regional Hospital; (902)543-4603

EDEN-WALKER, Michael; Kanata Prof Centre, 103-99 Kakulu Rd, Kanata ON K2L 3C8; UBC'78; (613)592-1448

EDER, Lihi; Univ Hlth Network-Toronto Western Hosp, 1E 410-399 Bathurst St, Toronto ON M5T 2S8; (Israel)'02; Staff, Toronto Western Hospital - University Health Network; (416)603-2581

EDGAR, Adrian; Primary Outreach Serv Clinic, 211-524 Powell St, Vancouver BC V6A 1G9; McM'10; (604)216-8741

EDGAR, Allison C; Collingwood Gen & Marine Hosp, 459 Hume St, Collingwood ON L9Y 1W9; Tor'08; CCFP; Staff, Collingwood General & Marine Hospital; (705)445-7667

EDGAR, John P; 105 Baldwin Ave, Cornwall ON K6H 4J1; Manchester (England)'66; MRCS; LRCP; Court Staff, Glengarry Memorial Hospital; Ac Staff, Cornwall Community Hospital - Second Street Site; Ac Staff, Cornwall Community Hospital; (613)933-8155; Fax. (613)933-0997.

EDGAR, Melvin L; 6438 Fraser St, Vancouver BC V5W 3A4; Adelaide (Australia)'61; MB BS; CCFP; Vis Staff Providence Health Group, Providence Health Care - Mount Saint Joseph Hospital; Hon Staff, Vancouver General Hospital - Centennial Pavillion; Vis Staff, BC Women's Hospital & Health Centre; Langs: English; French; (604)327-3330

EDGAR, Patricia A; Three Sisters Obst & Fam Med C, 105-75 Dyrgas Gate, Canmore AB T1W 0A6; Tor'72; BSc; Ac Staff, Covenant Health - Banff Mineral Springs Hospital; (403)609-6095; Fax. (403)609-7232.

EDGAR, Philip A; Yarmouth Reg Hosp, 60 Vancouver St, Yarmouth NS B5A 2P5; Dal'90; Staff, Yarmouth Regional Hospital; (902)742-3541

EDGCUMBE, Daniel P; PO Box219 Stn Main, Vegreville AB T9C 1R2; (780)632-6414; Fax. (780)632-6404.

EDGE, Kristen; Beaver Valley Clinic, PO Box 610, Fruitvale BC V0G 1L0; Ott'06; CCFP; (250)367-7543

EDGECUMBE, Boyd M S; Royal Alexandra Hosp, 10240 Kingsway NW, Edmonton AB T5H 3V9; Alb'01; CCFP; CCFP(E.M.); Staff, Royal Alexandra Hospital; (780)735-4442

EDGERLEY, Michael W; Danforth Birchmount Med Ctre, 34-462 Birchmount Rd, Scarborough ON M1K 1N8; Tor'86; CCFP; FCFP; Staff, The Scarborough Hospital - General Campus; Langs: Bilingual(English/French); (416)698-9988; Fax. (416)698-1055.

EDGUER, Beste; Hys Med Centre, 204-11010 101 St NW, Edmonton AB T5H 4B9; McM'94; FRCPC; Neur (Movement Disorders). Consultant, Royal Alexandra Hospital; (780)441-9880

EDINGTON, R Bruce; Hanover Med Associates, 118 7th Ave, Hanover ON N4N 2G9; Wes'81; CCFP; FCFP; Ac Staff, Hanover & District Hospital; Associate, South Bruce Grey Health Centre - Walkerton Site; Aj Prof Family Med, University of Western Ontario; (519)364-2820; Fax. (519)364-3965.

EDINGTON, Robert; Peterborough Reg Health Ctr, 1 Hospital Dr, Peterborough ON K9J 7C6; Wes'92; FRCPC; Anes. Staff, Peterborough Regional Health Centre - Hospital Drive; (705)743-2121

EDIRISINGHE, Manorie; The Westend Family Care Clinic, 80 Michael Cowpland Dr, Kanata ON K2M 1P6; Ott'90; CCFP; FCFP; Staff, Westend Family Care Clinic Family Health Team; (613)599-3321; Fax. (613)599-3366.

EDIRISINGHE, Mayuri M; Courtice Health Centre, 1450 Highway 2, Courtice ON L1E 3C3; Ott'00; BSc; CCFP; (905)721-3549; Fax. (905)721-6174.

EDMESTON, John T; Burnaby Hosp, 3935 Kincaid St, Burnaby BC V5G 2X6; Cal'00; BSc; MSc; CCFP; Staff, Burnaby Hospital; (604)434-4211; jedmeston@telus.net.

EDMISON, David R; Focus Eye Centre, 110-1565 Carling Ave, Ottawa ON K1Z 8R1; Qns'67; FRCSC; Ophth. Staff Privil, The Ottawa Hospital - Civic Campus; Staff Privil, The Ottawa Hospital - General Campus; Langs: Bilingual(English/French); (613)724-3937; Fax. (613)724-6264; edmison@focuseye.com.

EDMONDS, Colleen L; PO Box 471 Stn Ganges, Salt Spring Island BC V8K 2W1; McM'85.

EDMONDS, Diane E; Ferguson Med Incorporated, 102-26 North St, Bridgewater NS B4V 2V6; Dal'95; BSc(Hon); CCFP; FCFP; Ac Staff Family Med, South Shore Regional Hospital; (902)543-2733; deetch@bwr.eastlink.ca.

EDMONDS, Gillian; North Perth Family Health Team, 185 Inkerman St E, Listowel ON N4W 2N1; Tor'01; CCFP; Langs: Bilingual(English/French); (519)291-4200

EDMONDS, John F; The Hosp For Sick Children, 1234-555 University Ave, Toronto ON M5G 1X8; London (England)'65; MB BS; FFARCS; FRCPC; Anes (Pediatric Critical Care). Clin Dir Med Informatics, The Hospital For Sick Children; Asst Prof Anes, University of Toronto; (416)813-6480; Fax. (416)813-5372.

EDMONDS, Kenneth R; UBC Hospital, 2211 Wesbrook Mall, Vancouver BC V6T 2B5; Cal'84; CCFP; CCFP(E.M.); Clin Instructor Surg, UBC Hospital - Koerner Pavillion; Clin Instructor Surg, University of British Columbia; (604)822-7121; Fax. (604)822-7573.

EDMONDS, Marcia; London HSC-Victoria Hosp, PO Box 5010 Stn B E1 102-800 Commissioners Rd E, London ON N6A 5W9; Wes'95; FRCPC; EmergMed. Staff, London Health Sciences Centre - Victoria Campus; Staff, St Joseph's Hospital - St Joseph's Health Care; (519)685-8500

EDMONDS, Merrill W; St Joseph's Health Care, PO Box 5777 Stn B B5 115-268 Grosvenor St, London ON N6A 4V2; Wes'66; FACP; FRCPC; IntMed; Endocrin&Metab. Staff, St Joseph's Hospital - St Joseph's Health Care; Prof Med, University of Western Ontario; (519)646-6370; Fax. (519)646-6109.

EDMONDS, William; Lonsdale Med Dental Bldg, 108-1940 Lonsdale Ave, North Vancouver BC V7M 2K2; London (England)'72; MRCS; LRCP; LMCC; (604)987-3357

EDMONDSON, Nadeen; Halton HC Serv Corp-Oakville, 327 Reynolds St, Oakville ON L6J 3L7; (Japan)'95; FRCPC; AnatPath. Staff, Mount Sinai Hospital; Staff, Halton Healthcare Services Corporation - Oakville Site; (905)338-4690 x6277

EDMONDSON, Victoria J; Medical Clinic, PO Box 730 Stn Main, Salmon Arm BC V1E 4N8; Cape Town (South Africa)'99; MB ChB; (250)832-6092

EDMUNDS, Darryn J; Second Avenue Med Clinic, 320 2nd Ave W, Prince Rupert BC V8J 1G6; Orange Free (South Africa)'05; MB ChB; CCFP; Langs: Afrikaans; (250)624-4114

EDMUNDS, Nevenka; Health Point Care Centre, 1454 Hillside Ave, Victoria BC V8T 2B7; Belgrade (Serbia)'90; CCFP; (250)370-5637; Fax. (250)370-5623.

EDMUNDS, Peter M; Lonsdale Place, 403-1200 Lonsdale Ave, North Vancouver BC V7M 3H6; Stellenbosch (South Africa)'85; MB ChB; (604)984-4460; Fax. (604)984-6881.

EDNEY, James A; 351 Christie St, Toronto ON M6G 3C3; London (England)'66; MB BS; DObstRCOG; CCFP; FCFP; Media Dir Complex Continuing Care Prog/Ac Staff, Toronto Rehabilitation Institute - University Centre; Court Staff, Toronto General Hospital - UHN; Med Dir, Castleview-Wychwood Towers; Asst Prof Family & CommunMed, University of Toronto; (416)392-5750; jedney@the-wire.com.

EDNEY, Rachel E; Kipling Acres L T C, 2233 Kipling Ave, Etobicoke ON M9W 4L3; London (England)'67; MB BS; CCFP; FCFP; Staff, William Osler Health System - Etobicoke General Hospital; (416)392-2341

EDORA, Felipe T; 4-101 Burnside Rd W, Victoria BC V9A 1B7; UBC'95; CCFP; FCFP; (250)727-9932

EDSTROM, John P; Rosehaven Care Centre, 4612 53 St, Camrose AB T4V 1Y6; Mem'93; FRCPC; Psy. (780)679-3000

EDSTROM, Karen D; Dundas Dermatology Otolaryngol, 102-17 King St E, Dundas ON L9H 1B7; Mem'90; BScBiol; BScMed; FRCPC; Derm (Cosmetic Dermatology). Staff, Hamilton Health Sciences Centre - McMaster Children's Hospital; Asst Prof Med, McMaster University; (905)628-3376; Fax. (905)628-8833.

EDWARD, Girgis; Brandon Clinic Med Corporation, 620 Dennis St, Brandon MB R7A 5E7; Ain Shams (Egypt)'95; CCFP.

EDWARD, Raouf K A; 102-2160 Weston Rd, North York ON M9N 1X6; Ain Shams (Egypt)'76; MB ChB; FRCPC; Psy. Staff, Humber River Regional Hospital - Church Street Site; Langs: Arabic; (416)243-5091; Fax. (416)243-8374.

EDWARD, Rex H; Pleasant Street Med Clinic, 8-250 Pleasant St, Miramichi NB E1V 1Y5; Colombo (Sri Lanka)'73; MB BS; FRCS(Edin); FACS; FRCSC; GenSurg. Staff, Miramichi Regional Hospital; (506)627-1296; Fax. (506)627-1319.

EDWARD-CHANDRAN, Therese S; Lansdowne Professional Ctr II, 265-3066 Shelbourne St, Victoria BC V8R 6T9; Peradeniya (Sri Lanka)'72; MB BS; FRCPC; Psy (Adult General Psychiatry). Langs: Tamil; (250)590-6557

EDWARDS, Alun; Richmond Road Diagnostic Ctre, 1820 Richmond Rd SW, Calgary AB T2T 5C7; Cambridge (England)'79; MB BCh; FRCPC; IntMed; Endocrin&Metab. Chief Endocrin & Metab, Alberta Health Services-Calgary Zone; Assoc Prof/Chief Endocrin & Metab, University of Calgary; (403)955-8343; Fax. (403)955-8248.

EDWARDS, Bonnie L; West Street Health Centre, 203-216 West St, Simcoe ON N3Y 1S8; Tor'77; (519)426-2014

EDWARDS, Carla; McMaster University, 1280 Main St W, Hamilton ON L8S 4K1; Mem'00; BSc; MSc; FRCPC; Psy (Child & Adolescent Psychiatry). Consultant Psy, Guelph General Hospital; Staff, Homewood Health Centre; Staff, McMaster University; (905)525-9140; edwacarl@homewood.org.

EDWARDS, Cedric A W; The Ottawa Hosp-Riverside, 5 22-1967 Riverside Dr, Ottawa ON K1H 7W9; Ott'97; MD; FRCPC; IntMed; Nephrol. Staff, The Ottawa Hospital - Riverside Campus; Asst Prof, University of Ottawa; (613)738-8400; Fax. (613)738-8337; ceedwards@ottawahospital.on.ca.

EDWARDS, Christopher G; Nanaimo Reg Gen Hosp, 1200 Dufferin Cres, Nanaimo BC V9S 2B7; Wes'89; CCFP; FCFP; Staff, Nanaimo Regional General Hospital; (250)755-7691 x3005; Fax. (250)716-7747.

EDWARDS, D Virginia; 567 Rushton Rd, York ON M6C 2Y6; Wes'66; FRCPC; Psy. Court Staff, Toronto East General Hospital Inc; Lecturer, University of Toronto; (416)651-6009

EDWARDS, David C; Meadowlark Health Centre, 174 Meadowlark Shopping Ctr NW, Edmonton AB T5R 5W9; Alb'83; BMedSci; FRCSC; PlasSurg. Staff PlasSurg, Covenant Health - Misericordia Community Hospital; Clin Asst Prof, University of Alberta; (780)483-6400; Fax. (780)481-3002.

EDWARDS, Donna F; International Med Services, 4000 Leslie St, North York ON M2K 2R9; Tor'79; CCFP; FCFP; Langs: English; French; (416)494-7512; Fax. (416)492-3740.

EDWARDS, Elizabeth F; 100-11 Rosemount Ave, Ottawa ON K1Y 4R8; Sask'88; (613)724-5852

EDWARDS, Enid A; St Paul's Hosp, 1081 Burrard St, Vancouver BC V6Z 1Y6; Sask'81; FRCPC; GenPath. Staff, Providence Health Care - St Paul's Hospital; Staff, Providence Health Care - Mount Saint Joseph Hospital; Member Faculty, University of British Columbia; (604)806-8897; eedwards@providencehealth.bc.ca.

EDWARDS, Geoffrey B L; 202-5511 West Boulevard, Vancouver BC V6M 3W6; UBC'81; (604)263-4750

EDWARDS, Gordon L; Grey Bruce HS-Owen Sound, PO Box 1800 Stn Main 1800 8th St E, Owen Sound ON N4K 6M9; Qns'71; Staff, Grey Bruce Health Services - Owen Sound; (519)376-2121 x105; gedwards@gbhs.on.ca.

EDWARDS, Heather E; Allan Centre for Women, 707-12100 MacLeod Trail SE, Calgary AB T2J 7G9; Tor'02; PhD; BEd; MSc; BSc(Hon); FRCSC; ObstGyn. Staff, Foothills Medical Centre; (403)271-2550; Fax. (403)271-4546.

EDWARDS, James N; Office Of The Chief Coroner, 26 Grenville St, Toronto ON M7A 2G9; Wes'79; (416)314-1013; Fax. (416)314-4030; jim.n.edwards@ontario.ca.

EDWARDS, Jeremy; St Michael's Hosp, 7F-30 Bond St, Toronto ON M5B 1W8; Tor'03; FRCPC; IntMed; Cardiol. Lecturer, St Michael's Hospital; (416)360-4000

EDWARDS, John G; Elbow River Healing Lodge, 1213 4 St SW, Calgary AB T2R 0X7; Cal'76; CCFP; FCFP; (403)955-6600; Fax. (403)955-6601.

EDWARDS, Lawrence A J; Keele-Ingram Prof Centre, 105-2221 Keele St, North York ON M6M 3Z5; Tor'61; FRCPC; IntMed (Gastroenterology). Sr Consultant Gastroent, Humber River Regional Hospital - Church Street Site; (416)244-0053; Fax. (416)244-6102.

EDWARDS, Lesley C; AL0700C Tunney's Pasture, 0353-200 Tunney's Pasture Drwy, Ottawa ON K1A 0K9; Dal'73; FRCSC; ObstGyn. (613)957-4667; Fax. (613)946-0639.

EDWARDS, Lori M; Hamilton HSC-McMaster Site, PO Box 2000 Stn Lcd 1 1200 Main St W, Hamilton ON L8N 3Z5; Tor'07; FRCPC; AnatPath.

EDWARDS, Lynn; Bow Island Med Clinic, PO Box 870, Bow Island AB T0K 0G0; Alb'83; CCFP; FCFP; Staff Family Med/Obsterics, Medicine Hat Regional Hospital; Staff, Bow Island Health Centre; Clin Asst Family Med, University of Alberta; (403)545-2244; Fax. (403)545-2099.

EDWARDS, Marianne C; 310-10924 107 Ave NW, Edmonton AB T5H 0X5; Alb'95; BSc(MedSci); DAB; FRCSC; Ophth (Glaucoma). Clin Assoc Prof Ophth, University of Alberta; (780)990-0670; mceglaucoma@interbaun.com.

EDWARDS, Mark; Saultcare Med Clinic, 48-44 Great Northern Rd, Sault Ste. Marie ON P6B 4Y5; Wes'83; (705)253-1313

EDWARDS, Michelle; Ctr Hosp de Lachine, 650 16e av, Lachine QC H8S 3N5; Man'07; IntMed. Staff, Centre Hospitalier de Lachine; (514)637-2351; michelle.edwards@mail.mcgill.ca.

EDWARDS, Neil W; 33 Church St S, Ajax ON L1S 6A6; Tor'85; Staff, Rouge Valley Health System - Ajax & Pickering Health Centre Site; Staff, Ontario Shores Centre for Mental Health Sciences; (905)683-0200; Fax. (905)683-0636.

EDWARDS, Pamela V; High Prairie Med Clinic, PO Box 449, High Prairie AB T0G 1E0; Alb'79; (780)523-4501; Fax. (780)523-4800.

EDWARDS, Ralph K; North Road Med Centre, 435S North Rd, Coquitlam BC V3K 3V9; Alb'70; (604)936-0411; Fax. (604)931-7022.

EDWARDS, Raymond K F; Kingston Gen Hosp, 76 Stuart St, Kingston ON K7L 2V7; Qns'80; FRCPC; EmergMed. Staff, Kingston General Hospital; Staff, Hotel-Dieu Hospital; (613)548-2368

EDWARDS, Shawn; STAR Family Health Team, 700 O'Loane Ave, Stratford ON N5A 6S6; Wes'94; CCFP; FCFP; (519)273-1060; Fax. (519)273-0371.

EDWARDS, Susan A; St Joseph's Health Centre, 30 The Queensway, Toronto ON M6R 1B5; McM'94; CCFP; FCFP; Staff, St Joseph's Health Centre; Teacher, University of Toronto; (416)530-6860; Fax. (416)530-6139; susan.edwards@utoronto.ca.

EDWARDS, Susan L; Lansdowne Professional Ctr II, 347-3066 Shelbourne St, Victoria BC V8R 6T9; Alb'88; (250)598-0678

EDWARDS, Wayne J; Wayne J Edwards Prof Corp, 1624 9 Ave S, Lethbridge AB T1J 1W3; West Indies (Jamaica)'80; MB BS; MRCPsy(UK); FRCPC; Psy (Child & Adolescent Psychiatry). Staff, Chinook Regional Hospital; Consultant Psy., Lethbridge Mental Health Clinic; Consultant Psy, University Of Lethbridge; (403)328-1021; Fax. (403)317-2007.

EDWARDS, Wendy E; 100-202 King St W, Chatham ON N7M 1E5; McM'93; BScN; FRCPC; Peds. Staff, Chatham-Kent Health Alliance; (519)358-1880; Fax. (519)358-1586.

EDWARDS, Wesley J; Ridge Meadows Hosp & Hlth CC, 11666 Laity St, Maple Ridge BC V2X 7G5; Tasmania (Australia)'02; Staff, Ridge Meadows Hospital & Health Care Centre.

EDWORTHY, John D; Austin Family Practice, 102-1015 Austin Avenue, Coquitlam BC V3K 3N9; UBC'77; BSc; CCFP; FCFP; Staff, Royal Columbian Hospital; Clin Assoc Prof, University of British Columbia; (604)939-9251; Fax. (604)939-2592.

EDWORTHY, Steven; HSC-Faculty of Med, 3330 Hospital Dr NW, Calgary AB T2N 4N1; Cal'82; BSc; FRCPC; IntMed; Rheum. Staff Rheum., Foothills Medical Centre; Assoc Prof Med & Community Health, University of Calgary; (403)220-7740; Fax. (403)270-7349; sedworth@ucalgary.ca.

EDYE, Frances; 700-177 Lombard Ave, Winnipeg MB R3B 0W5; Man'80; FRCPC; Psy. Psychiatrist, WRHA - Deer Lodge Centre.

EDYE-ROWNTREE, James; Norway House Hosp, PO Box 730, Norway House MB R0B 1B0; Man'09; CCFP; Staff, Norway House Hospital; (204)359-8204; james.edye-rowntree@hc-sc.gc.ca.

EEK, Judy D; Rockyview Gen Hosp, 7007 14 St SW, Calgary AB T2V 1P9; Alb'72; CCFP; Staff, Rockyview General Hospital; (403)305-7611

EELES, Ruth; Canmore Associate Med Clinic, 124-1151 Sidney St, Canmore AB T1W 3G1; (United Kingdom)'99; MB ChB; (403)678-5585; Fax. (403)678-6262.

EESA, Muneer; Foothills Med Centre, 1403 29 ST NW, Calgary AB T2N 2T9; (India)'03; MB BS; Staff, Foothills Medical Centre; (403)944-1110

EFALA, Khal Mabru; 205-3500 Dufferin St, North York ON M3K 1N2; Al Fateh (Libya)'00; FRCSC; OrthSurg. (416)630-6311

EFFA, Evan; Royal Jubilee Hosp, 1952 Bay St, Victoria BC V8R 1J8; UBC'84; FRCPC; Anes. Staff, Royal Jubilee Hospital; (250)389-6577

EFFORD, Erin; Dr Everett Chalmers Reg Hosp, PO Box 9000 Stn A 700 Priestman St, Fredericton NB E3B 5N5; Mem'04; FRCPC; DiagRad. Staff, Dr Everett Chalmers Regional Hospital; (506)452-5400

EFFORD, Jason R; Spaniards Bay Med Clinic, PO Box 280, Spaniards Bay NL A0A 3X0; Mem'04; CCFP; (709)786-3171; Fax. (709)786-5257.

EFOE, Anani; Hôp Régional d'Edmundston, 275 boul Hébert, Edmundston NB E3V 4E4; Benin (Other Foreign)'95; Staff, Hôpital regional d'Edmundston; (506)739-2200

EFTEKHARI, Maryam; Quality Care Clinic, 414-250 Harding Blvd W, Richmond Hill ON L4C 9M7; Tehran (Iran)'84; CCFP; Langs: Farsi; (905)237-7723; Fax. (905)291-0768.

EGAN, Francis G; Richmond Med Bldg, 205-2020 Richmond Rd, Victoria BC V8R 6R5; (Ireland)'85; MRC; MB ChB; (250)592-8121; Fax. (250)592-8182.

EGAN, Raymond R; 103-186 Albert St, London ON N6A 1M1; Wes'86; FRCPC; Psy. (519)645-6462

EGAR, Susanne E; Inverness Consolidated Mem Hos, PO Box 610 39 James St, Inverness NS B0E 1N0; Ott'09; CCFP; Staff, Inverness Consolidated Memorial Hospital; (902)258-1956

EGBAGBE, Augustine; Canora Med Clinic, PO Box 2040, Canora SK S0A 0L0; (306)563-5557; Fax. (306)563-4175.

EGBERT, Alwyn M; Rathburn Med Centre, 600 The East Mall, Etobicoke ON M9B 4B1; (W.Indies) (Jamaica)'63; MB BS; DPH(Tor); Court Staff, Trillium Health Centre - West Toronto; (416)626-9222

EGBEWUNMI, Adeyemi T; Waypoint Centre for Mental Hlt, 500 Church St, Penetanguishene ON L9M 1G3; Ibadan (Nigeria)'98; (705)549-3181

EGBEYEMI, Olanrewaju Y; Prince Albert Commun Clinic, 110 8th St E, Prince Albert SK S6V 0V7; Ogun State (Nigeria)'91; MB ChB; CCFP; Langs: Yoruba.

EGEDY, Maud M P; CHUQ-Ctr Hosp Univ Laval, R1742-2705 boul Laurier, Quebec QC G1V 4G2; Liege (Belgium)'99; Staff, Centre Hospitalier Universitaire de Quebec-CHUL; (418)654-2282; Fax. (418)654-2137.

EGELER, R Maarten; The Hosp For Sick Children, 9402 BW-555 University Ave, Toronto ON M5G 1X8; Netherlands (Netherlands)'85; Staff, The Hospital For Sick Children; Langs: Dutch; (416)813-7654; Fax. (416)813-5327.

EGER, Robert P; Kelowna Gen Hosp, 2268 Pandosy St, Kelowna BC V1Y 1T2; UBC'88; FRCPC; Anes. Staff, Kelowna General Hospital; (250)862-4309

EGERDIE, Russell B; Urology Assoc/Urologic Med Res, 18-450 Westheights Dr, Kitchener ON N2N 2B9; Qns'83; FRCSC; Urol. Staff Urol, Grand River Hospital - Kitchener/Waterloo Health Centre; VP Medical/Staff Urol, St Mary's General Hospital; (519)578-1282; Fax. (519)578-1362.

EGERSZEGI, E Patricia; Hôpital Ste-Justine, 7908-3175 ch Cote-Ste-Catherin, Montreal QC H3T 1C5; McG'81; MSc; FACS(PlasSurg); CSPQ; FRCSC; PlasSurg (Pediatric Plastic Surgery). ac Staff Surg, Hôpital Ste-Justine; assoc Prof Surg, Universite de Montreal; Langs: Hungarian; French; (514)345-4964; Fax. (514)345-4964.

EGGER, Gian; The Credit Valley Hosp, 2200 Eglinton Ave W, Mississauga ON L5M 2N1; Geneva (Switzerland)'81; BSc; Peds (Pediatric Cardiology). Staff Peds, The Credit Valley Hospital; Langs: Bilingual(English/French); (905)813-4120; Fax. (905)813-4128.

EGGERTSON, Douglas E; Clinique St Boniface Clinic, 343 Tache Ave, Winnipeg MB R2H 2A5; Man'78; FRCPC; IntMed; Neur. Staff, St Boniface General Hospital; Consultant, Seven Oaks General Hospital; Asst Prof, University of Manitoba; Fax. (204)237-0779.

EGHTEDARI-NAMIN, Fariba; PsycHealth Centre, PZ202-771 Bannatyne Av, Winnipeg MB R3E 3N4; Isfahan University (Other Foreign)'91; FRCPC; Psy.

EGIER, Stuart; Etobicoke Med Centre, 400 The East Mall, Etobicoke ON M9B 3Z9; Tor'75; Acad Staff, Trillium Health Centre - Mississauga; Ac Staff, Trillium Health Centre - West Toronto; Med Dir, Complex Care; (416)621-2220; Fax. (416)621-2357.

EGLES, Diane E; Chesley Med Clinic, PO Box 117 32 2nd St E, Chesley ON N0G 1L0; McG'80; CCFP; Fam Med, South Bruce Grey Health Services - Chesley Site; (519)363-3220; Fax. (519)363-0385; degles@sbghc.on.ca.

EGOLF, Richard J; 103-33774 Marshall Rd, Abbotsford BC V2S 1L1; UBC'89; (604)853-5424; Fax. (604)853-6879.

EGRI, Zoltan J; Doctor's Office, 500-491 Lawrence Ave W, North York ON M5M 1C7; Tor'94; FRCPC; IntMed; Cardiol. Langs: Hungarian; (416)781-9500; Fax. (416)781-7985.

EGWARE, Oluwatomi; Pasqua South Med Centre, 3515 Pasqua St, Regina SK S4S 7G9; (Cayman Islands)'08; CCFP; Clin Assoc Prof, University of Saskatchewan; (306)205-8020; Fax. (306)205-8023; pasquasouthmedicalcentre@sasktel.net.

EHASOO, Valerie A; Seniors Outreach Team, 2828 Nanaimo St, Victoria BC V8T 4W9; Ott'97; CCFP; FCFP; (250)519-3566

EHLEN, Thomas G; Gordon & Leslie Diamond HCC, 6F-2775 Laurel St, Vancouver BC V5Z 1M9; Mainz (Germany)'83; FRCSC; ObstGyn (Gynecologic Oncology). Head/Med Mgr, Vancouver General Hospital - Centennial Pavillion; Co-Investigator, BC Cancer Agency Vancouver Centre; Ac Staff, BC Children's Hospital; Staff, Gordon & Leslie Diamond Health Care Centre; Asst Prof, University of British Columbia; Langs: German; (604)875-5608; Fax. (604)875-4869.

EHLERS, Leo G; 3-4402 37 St, Stony Plain AB T7Z 2A9; Stellenboch (South Africa)'89; MB ChB; (780)963-7800; Fax. (780)963-0468.

EHLERS, Marianne; The Pas Health Complex Inc, PO Box 240 67 1st St W, The Pas MB R9A 1K4; CCFP; Staff, St. Anthony General Hospital; (204)623-6431

EHMAN, William J; The Family Practice Clinic, 2778 104th St, Nanaimo BC V9T 2E4; Sask'77; (250)758-1711; Fax. (250)758-2802.

EHRAMDJIAN, Vagharchag; Hop Maisonneuve-Rosemont, 5415 boul de l'Assomption, Montreal QC H1T 2M4; Alexandria (Egypt)'65; DiagRad. Staff, Hopital Maisonneuve-Rosemont; (514)252-3535; Fax. (514)252-3537.

EHRAT, Caroline B; Perth Family Med, 39 Drummond St W, Perth ON K7H 2J9; Wes'94; CCFP; CCFP(E.M.); FCFP; Staff, Perth & Smiths Falls District Hospital - Perth Site (Great War Memorial Site); (613)264-2686; Fax. (613)264-0454.

EHRENSPERGER, Eric; MUHC-Montreal Gen Hosp, L7 408-1650 av Cedar, Montreal QC H3G 1A4; Wes'97; FRCPC; Neur. Staff, McGill University Health Centre - Montreal General Campus; (519)934-8057; Fax. (519)934-8265; eehren@po-box.mcgill.ca.

EHRLICH, Helga; Bruyere Academic Fam Hlth Team, 75 Bruyere St, Ottawa ON K1N 5C7; McM'85; CCFP; FCFP; Staff, SCO Health Service - Élisabeth Bruyère Hospital; Langs: German; (613)241-3344; hehrlich@bruyere.org.

EHRLICH, Lisa E; Sunnybrook Hlth Sciences Ctre, 2075 Bayview Ave, Toronto ON M4N 3M5; Dal'75; FRCPC; DiagRad; NuclearMed. Staff, Sunnybrook Health Sciences Centre; (416)480-4336; Fax. (416)480-5855.

EHRLICH, Robert M; Markham Stouffville Hosp, PO Box 1800 Stn Main 381 Church St, Markham ON L3P 7P3; Tor'55; FRCPC; Peds (Pediatric Endocrinology). Staff, Markham Stouffville Hospital; Emeritus Prof Peds, University of Toronto; (905)472-7000 x3974; rehrlich@sympatico.ca.

EIBOCK, Danielle; Centre Prof Belanger, 3871 rue Belanger, Montreal QC H1X 3M7; Sher'96; (514)722-1166; Fax. (514)722-6022; danielle@pharmaciegabriel.com.

EICHHORST, Nicolas O; Old Orchard Med Clinic, 11-4429 Kingsway, Burnaby BC V5H 2A1; Qns'98; CCFP; (604)431-6585

EICKMEIER, Daniel J; Huron Commun Family Hlth Team, PO Box 460 32B-1 Centennial Dr, Seaforth ON N0K 1W0; Wes'02; CCFP; (519)600-2273; deickmeier@rogers.com.

EID, Clovis; 155 Highfield St, Moncton NB E1C 5P1; Beirut (Lebanon)'65; FRCSC; Ophth (Glaucoma). Ac Staff Senior, Dr Georges-L-Dumont University Hospital Centre; Langs: Arabic; English; (506)383-5123; Fax. (506)383-5125; picou@rogers.com.

EID, Iyad; University of Alberta Hosp, 8440 112 St NW, Edmonton AB T6G 2B7; (Pakistan)'96; MB BS; Staff GenSurg, University of Alberta Hospital; (780)407-8822

EID, Joseph; CSSS Les Eskers de l'Abitibi, 622 4e rue O, Amos QC J9T 2S2; (Lebanon)'94; Staff, CH Hôtel-Dieu d'Amos; (819)732-3341 x2279; Fax. (819)732-6422.

EID, Jouhaina; St Mary's Hosp Centre, 5329-3830 av Lacombe, Montreal QC H3T 1M5; McG'91; ABIM; MS; Nephrol (P.Q.). Chef nephrology, St Mary's Hospital Centre; adj Prof Med, McGill University; Langs: English; French; German; Arabic; (514)345-3511 x3554; Fax. (514)734-2637.

EID, Karim E C; 2050A Lawrence Ave E, Scarborough ON M1R 2Z5; Alexandria (Egypt)'74; MSc(Mtl.); Staff, Rouge Valley Health System - Centenary Health Centre Site; Staff, The Scarborough Hospital - General Campus; Assoc Staff, Toronto Rehabilitation Institute - Lyndhurst Centre; Langs: Arabic; French; (416)752-2207

EID, Roula; Blackburn Hamlet Med Care Clin, 2575 Innes Rd, Ottawa ON K1B 3K1; Laval'01; CCFP; Langs: Bilingual(French/English); (613)590-0785; Fax. (613)824-3447.

EID, Soheil E; Clin Med de la Cite, 170-175 rue de la Visitation, St-Charles-Brromee QC J6E 4N4; Alexandria (Egypt)'71; Respir (P.Q.). Staff, Centre Hospitalier Régional de Lanaudière; (450)759-7244; Fax. (450)759-7244.

EIDELMAN, David H; MUHC-Montreal Gen Hosp, D7 177-1650 av Cedar, Montreal QC H3G 1A4; McG'79; FRCPC; IntMed; Respir. Chef Dept of Med, McGill University Health Centre - Royal Victoria Hospital; Médecin, McGill University Health Centre - Montreal General Campus; Dir adj Health & Affairs/Doyen, McGill University; Langs: Bilingual(French/English); (514)934-8014; Fax. (514)934-8226.

EIDLITZ, Carey J; Joseph Brant Mem Hosp, 1230 North Shore Blvd E, Burlington ON L7S 1W7; Tor'86; FRCPC; Anes (Intensive Care). Staff, Joseph Brant Memorial Hospital; (905)632-3730 x4135

EIDSNESS, Ryan; 4010 Dewdney Ave, Regina SK S4T 1A2; Sask'02; FRCSC; Ophth. (306)566-9264; Fax. (306)399-3739.

EIDUS, Leslie B; Rockyview Gen Hosp, 7007 14 St SW, Calgary AB T2V 1P9; Ott'77; FRCPC; AnatPath. Staff, Rockyview General Hospital; Fax. (403)943-3333.

EIGL, Bernhard; BC Cancer Agency-Vancouver CC, 600 10th Ave W, Vancouver BC V5Z 4E6; McM'98; FRCPC; IntMed; MedOncol. Staff, BC Cancer Agency Vancouver Centre; Langs: German; (604)877-6000

EIKELBOOM, John; Hamilton HS-General Site, 622-237 Barton St E, Hamilton ON L8L 2X2; Perth (Australia)'89; FRCPC; IntMed. Staff, Hamilton Health Sciences Centre - Hamilton General Hospital; (905)527-1710; Fax. (905)521-1551.

EILEY, David; 200-175 av Stillview, Pointe-Claire QC H9R 4S3; McG'90; FACS; FRCSC; Urol. adj Prof, McGill University; Langs: English; French; (514)697-5317; Fax. (514)695-0431.

EIN, Arnold L A; Yorkview Med Centre, 104-3695 Keele St, North York ON M3J 1N2; Dal'71; (416)633-3711; Fax. (416)633-0521.

EINAGEL JR., Victor; Clinique Med Mercier, 101-464 boul Saint-Jean-Baptis, Mercier QC J6R 2B1; McG'80; AB; FRCPC; EmergMed. Staff Emerg, St Mary's Hospital Centre; Asst Prof Family Med, McGill University; (450)699-0539; Fax. (450)699-8438.

EINO, Dalia M; Oakville Med Arts Bldg, 2-358 Reynolds St, Oakville ON L6J 3L9; Tor'97; FRCSC; Ophth. Asst Prof, Hamilton Health Sciences Centre - Hamilton General Hospital; Asst Prof, McMaster University; (905)845-5861; Fax. (905)845-7151.

EINSTOSS, Howard S; 203-1525 Albion Rd, Etobicoke ON M9V 5G5; Tor'70; Ac Staff, William Osler Health System - Etobicoke General Hospital; (416)741-1100; Fax. (416)741-1176.

EINTRACHT, Shaun L; SMBD Jewish Gen Hosp, 3755 ch Cote-Sainte-Catherine, Montreal QC H3T 1E2; Johannesburgh (South Africa)'90; FRCPC; MedBiochem (General Pathology). Staff, Sir Mortimer B Davis Jewish General; (514)340-8222 x2729

EIPE, Naveen; The Ottawa Hosp Civic Campus, B310-1053 Carling Ave, Ottawa ON K1Y 4E9; (India)'96; Staff, The Ottawa Hospital - Civic Campus; (613)798-5555

EIRIKSSON, Lua; Univ Hlth Network-Princess M, M700-610 University Ave, Toronto ON M5G 2M9; Dal'05; FRCSC; ObstGyn. Staff, Princess Margaret Hospital - University Health Network; (416)946-4043

EISA, Mohamed; Regina Mental Health Clinic, 2110 Hamilton St, Regina SK S4P 2E3; MRCP(UK); DPM(Ireland); DCP(Ireland); (306)766-7800; Fax. (306)766-7811.

EISEN, Andrea; Sunnybrook Odette Cancer Ctr, T2 038-2075 Bayview Ave, Toronto ON M4N 3M5; Tor'92; ABIM; FRCPC; IntMed; MedOncol. Staff, Sunnybrook Health Sciences Centre - Edmond Odette Cancer Centre; Staff, Sunnybrook Odette Cancer Centre; (416)480-4617; Fax. (416)480-6002.

EISEN, Ari B; St Hoseph's Health Centre, 30 The Queensway, Toronto ON M6R 1B5; Tor'86; FRCPC; DiagRad; NuclearMed. Head Nuclear Med, St Joseph's Health Centre; (416)530-6010; abeisen@sympatico.ca.

EISEN, David; The Acne Treatment Clinic, 406-1366 Yonge St, Toronto ON M4T 3A7; Tor'77; Court Staff, Humber River Regional Hospital - Church Street Site; (416)923-4211; Fax. (905)770-4782; nenedoc@rogers.com.

EISEN, David W; 1701 Martin Grove Rd, Etobicoke ON M9V 4N4; McM'90; LLB; MBA; BA; CCFP; FCFP; Chair Div of Med Obst/Ac Staff, North York General Hospital; Asst Prof, University of Toronto; Langs: Hebrew; (416)744-0461; Fax. (416)744-3356.

EISEN, Doron A; West Durham Family Health Team, 200B-1105 Kingston Rd, Pickering ON L1V 1B5; Tor'88; CCFP; FCFP; Staff, Rouge Valley Health System - Centenary Health Centre Site; Langs: Hebrew; (905)420-9999; Fax. (905)420-1090.

EISEN, Jeffrey S; Royal Victoria Hosp, 201 Georgian Dr, Barrie ON L4M 6M2; Qns'99; FRCPC; EmergMed. Staff, Royal Victoria Regional Health Centre; (705)728-9802; Fax. (705)728-5922.

EISEN, Joel M; Credit Valley Prof Bldg, 205-2300 Eglinton Ave W, Mississauga ON L5M 2V8; Tor'84; Court Staff, The Credit Valley Hospital; (905)820-8144; Fax. (905)820-1631.

EISEN, Joel N; York-Med Medical Arts Centre, 301-250 Harding Blvd W, Richmond Hill ON L4C 9M7; Tor'81; FRCP; FRCPC; Psy. Staff Teacher, Toronto General Hospital - UHN; Staff, Mackenzie Richmond Hill Hospital; Asst Prof, University of Toronto; (905)884-5387; joel.eisen@utoronto.ca.

EISEN, Leonard B; Mount Sinai Hosp, 1514-600 University Ave, Toronto ON M5G 1X5; Tor'85; FRCPC; Anes. Staff Anes, Mount Sinai Hospital; Asst Prof Anes, University of Toronto; (416)586-4800 x5270; Fax. (416)586-8664; len.eisen@sympatico.ca.

EISENBERG, Eric L; Dermatology Enhancement Centre, 206-3420 Hurontario St, Mississauga ON L5B 4A9; Mon'81; FRCPC; Derm (Cosmetic Surgery). Staff Derm, Toronto Western Hospital - University Health Network; Lecturer, University of Toronto; Langs: Spanish; French; (905)896-1515; Fax. (905)896-0116; ericeisenberg@rogers.com.

EISENBERG, Howard E; 411 Queen St, Newmarket ON L3Y 2G9; McG'72; MSc(Psychol.); MD; Pres, Syntrek Inc; (905)895-4488; centerformindenhancement@gmail.com.

EISENBERG, Mark J; SMBD Jewish Gen Hosp, 3755 ch Cote-Sainte-Catherine, Montreal QC H3T 1E2; Rochester(New York) (USA)'85; AB; MPH; CSPQ; Cardiol (P.Q.); IntMed (Clinical Trials). Staff Cardiol, Sir Mortimer B Davis Jewish General; adj Prof, McGill University; Langs: English; French; Hebrew; (514)340-8222 x3564; Fax. (514)340-7564.

EISENBERG, Morty; Family Physicians, 1-390 Steeles Ave W, Thornhill ON L4J 6X2; Tor'75; MSc(CH); CCFP; FCFP; Ac Staff, Mackenzie Richmond Hill Hospital; Ac Staff, St John's Rehabilitation Hospital; Asst Prof Family & CommunMed, University of Toronto; (905)881-3984; Fax. (905)881-3198.

EISENER, Barbara A; 109 King St W, Dundas ON L9H 1V1; Dal'81; CCFP; FCFP; (905)628-9200; Fax. (905)628-9600.

EISENER, Beverley M; Pleasant St Med Group, 105-375 Pleasant St, Dartmouth NS B2Y 4N4; Dal'80; Ac Staff, Dartmouth General Hospital; Court Staff, IWK Health Centre; (902)469-9564; Fax. (902)469-2449.

EISENER-PARSCHE, Pamela D; Bruyere Continuing Centre, 43 Bruyere St, Ottawa ON K1N 5C8; Qns'90; CCFP; FCFP; Physician, Bruyere Continuing Centre; Langs: Bilingual(English/French); (613)562-6262

EISENHAUER, Elizabeth A; Kingston Gen Hosp, 25 King St W, Kingston ON K7L 5P9; Qns'76; FRCPC; IntMed (Medical Oncology); Hem. Att Staff Med Oncology, Cancer Centre of Southeastern Ontario; Dir New Drug Program, NCIC Clinical Trials Group; (613)544-2630

EISENHAUER, Mary A; London Reg Cancer Centre, 790 Commissioners Rd E, London ON N6A 4L6; Qns'83; FRCPC; EmergMed. Ac Staff, London Health Sciences Centre - Victoria Campus; Staff, London Regional Cancer Center; Assoc Prof, University of Western Ontario; (519)685-8640; Fax. (519)685-8624.

EISENSTAT, L Jonathan; Lakeridge Hlth Corp-Oshawa, 1 Hospital Crt, Oshawa ON L1G 2B9; Cal'91; BSc; FRCPC; IntMed (Cardiology); Critical Care Medicine. Staff, Lakeridge Health - Oshawa Site; Clin Instructor Med, University of Toronto; (905)721-7359; Fax. (905)721-4745.

EISMAN, Harley N; MUHC-Montreal Children Hosp, 2300 Tupper St, Montreal QC H3H 1P3; McG'92; MDCM; FRCPC; Peds. Chief EmergMed, McGill University Health Centre - Montreal Children's Hospital; (514)412-4400

EISNER, Dana; 2921 Lake Shore Blvd W, Etobicoke ON M8V 1J3; Karlova (Czech Republic)'71; Court Staff, St Joseph's Health Centre; Langs: Czech; (416)252-3665; Fax. (416)252-3815.

EISNER, James R; Foothills Med Centre, G28-1403 29 St NW, Calgary AB T2N 2T9; Cal'98; CCFP; FCFP; Staff, Foothills Medical Centre; (403)944-2800

EISNER, Rhonda B; Malvern Med Arts Bldg, 100-1333 Neilson Rd, Scarborough ON M1B 4Y9; Tor'76; Staff, Rouge Valley Health System - Centenary Health Centre Site; (416)291-7719; Fax. (416)287-3775.

EJAZ, Naila; West Winds Med Clinic, 2130-4818 Westwinds Dr NE, Calgary AB T3J 3Z5; (Pakistan)'98; MB BS; (403)830-1097

EK, Daniel M; Harbour View Med Clinic, 43 Court St N, Thunder Bay ON P7A 4T5; Tor'90; CCFP; FCFP; Staff, Thunder Bay Regional Health Sciences Centre Port-Arthur; Staff General Pract, St Joseph's Care Group - St Joseph's Hospital; (807)343-4252; Fax. (807)346-8687.

EK, Nathan; Kirkland Disrict Fam Hlth Team, PO Box 10 Stn Main 2 Water Lane, Kirkland Lake ON P2N 3M6; Cal'86; Med Staff Anes, Kirkland & District Hospital; (705)567-2224; Fax. (705)567-3838.

EKANEM, Aquaeno E; Kingsway Garden Mall, 303-1 Kingsway Garden Mall NW, Edmonton AB T5G 3A6; (780)479-3699; Fax. (780)479-3399.

EKEH, Norbert I; One Step Med Centre, 1A-3585 Lawrence Ave E, Scarborough ON M1G 1P4; Nsukka (Nigeria)'84; MRC; ObstGyn. Langs: Ibo; (416)431-0736; Fax. (416)431-0648.

EKERT, Lee; Grey Nuns Community Hosp, 1100 Youville Drive West NW, Edmonton AB T6L 5X8; Sask'05; FRCSC; OrthSurg. Staff, Covenant Health - Grey Nuns Community Hospital; (780)735-7000

EKINS, Marilyn B C; Winnipeg Clinic, 425 St Mary Ave, Winnipeg MB R3C 0N2; Wes'70; FRCSC; Ophth (Cornea). Staff, Misericordia Health Centre; Staff, Children's Hospital of Eastern Ontario (CHEO); Assoc Prof Ophth, University of Manitoba; (204)957-3251; Fax. (204)947-0450.

EKOE, Jean-Marie; CHUM-Hotel-Dieu, 3840 rue Saint-Urbain, Montreal QC H2W 1T8; Lausanne (Switzerland)'76; Endocrin (P. Q.) (Diabetology). Staff, Centre Hospitalier l'Université de Montréal (CHUM) - Hôtel-Dieu; Prof Med, Universite de Montreal; (514)890-8100

EKONG, Chris E U; Regina Qu'Appelle HR-Regina, NOW 122-1440 14th Ave, Regina SK S4P 0W5; Ibadan (Nigeria)'72; MB BS; FACS; FICS; FRCSC; Neursurg. Head Neursurg, Regina General Hospital; Court Staff, Pasqua Hospital; Chair, Medi-Fax Canada Inc; Clin Prof, University of Saskatchewan; (306)781-7229; Fax. (306)352-0499.

EKONG, Enobong; Grey Bruce HS-Owen Sound, PO Box 1800 Stn M 8238-1800 8th St E, Owen Sound ON N4K 6M9; Qns'07; ObstGyn. Staff, Grey Bruce Health Services - Owen Sound; (519)371-8381; Fax. (519)371-8399.

EKSTEEN, Ben; Diamond Head Med Clinic, PO Box 9200 Stn Main, Squamish BC V8B 0C1; Stellenbosch (South Africa)'94; MB ChB; CCFP; FCFP; Langs: Afrikaans; (604)892-3544

EKSTEEN, Eduard C; University of Alberta Hosp, 2C3 59 WMC-8440 112 St NW, Edmonton AB T6G 2B7; Stellenbosch (South Africa)'85; FRCSC; Otol (Pediatric Otolaryngology). Staff, University of Alberta Hospital; (780)407-2109; Fax. (780)407-2111.

EKSTEEN, Hendrik; Holley Clinic, 348 Front St, Quesnel BC V2J 2K3; Stellenbosch (South Africa)'00; (250)992-2158

EKSTEEN, Johannes A; Health Research Innovation Ctr, 4AC66-3280 Hospital Dr NW, Calgary AB T2N 4Z6; Staff, Health Research Innovation Centre; (403)592-5080

EKSTRAND, Gayle P; Queensway Med Centre, 300-5307 Canotek Rd, Gloucester ON K1J 9M2; Ott'87; MSc; BPE(Hons); CCFP; FCFP; Langs: Bilingual(English/French); (613)746-6223; Fax. (613)746-6018.

EKWALANGA, Pauline R; Sunridge Professional Center, 501-2675 36 St NE, Calgary AB T1Y 6H6; Cal'01; MSc; BN; RN; FRCSC; ObstGyn. Staff, Peter Lougheed Centre; Chair, Perinatal Safety Committe; Langs: Bilingual(English/French); (403)263-5760; Fax. (403)263-9493.

EKWUEME, Henry; Lloydminster Hosp, 3820 43 Ave, Lloydminster SK S9V 1Y5; Staff, Lloydminster Hospital; (306)820-6194; Fax. (306)825-9880.

EL-ACHKAR, Ghassan G; 5180 ch Queen-Mary, Montreal QC H3W 3E7; Bucarest (Romania)'85; FRCSC; Ophth. (514)489-8841

EL-ADL, Mamdouh; Providence Care-Mental Health, PO Box 603 Stn Main 752 King St W, Kingston ON K7L 4X3; (Egypt)'84; Staff, Providence Care - Mental Health Services; (613)546-1101; Fax. (613)540-6114.

EL ALFY, Ahmed; Cambridge Mem Hosp, 700 Coronation Blvd, Cambridge ON N1R 3G2; Ain Shams (Egypt)'94; FRCPC; Anes. Staff, Cambridge Memorial Hospital; Langs: Arabic; (519)621-2330

EL-ASHRY, Dalia; 220-89 Queensway W, Mississauga ON L5B 2V2; Tor'96; FRCPC; IntMed (Hepatology); Gastroent. Langs: Arabic; (905)275-1133; Fax. (905)275-4535.

EL-BAILEY, Mohamed; Saint John Reg Hosp, PO Box 2100 Stn Main 400 University Ave, Saint John NB E2L 4L2; Alexandria (Egypt)'81; Staff, Saint John Regional Hospital; (506)648-6000

EL-BATNIGI, Nemer; Lakeridge Health-Oshawa Site, 1 Hospital Crt, Oshawa ON L1G 2B9; Cluj-Napoca (Romania)'99; CCFP; CCFP(E.M.); Staff, Lakeridge Health - Oshawa Site; Langs: Arabic; Romanian; (905)576-8711

EL-BAWAB, Najwa; Burntwood Comm Hlth, 50 Selkirk Ave, Thompson MB R8N 0M7.

EL-BEHEIRY, Hossam; Trillium Hlth Ctr-Mississauga, 100 Queensway W, Mississauga ON L5B 1B8; Cairo University (Egypt)'78; MB ChB; MSc; PhD; FRCPC; Anes (Critical Care Medicine). Staff Anesthesiologist, Toronto General Hospital - UHN; Staff, Trillium Health Centre - Mississauga; Langs: Arabic; (905)848-7100; Fax. (905)848-5990.

EL-BRAKEY, Mary R R; Grand River Hosp-KW Hlth Ctre, PO Box 9056 Stn C 835 King St W, Kitchener ON N2G 1G3; Cairo (Egypt)'93; FRCPC; Anes. Staff, Grand River Hospital - Kitchener/Waterloo Health Centre; Langs: Arabic; (519)749-4300

EL-CHAAR, Darine; Postgraduate Med Education, 602-500 University Ave, Toronto ON M5G 1V7; Ott'06; ObstGyn. (613)737-8566

EL DAGNI, Mohamed W M M; 12620A 132 Ave NW, Edmonton AB T5L 3P9; (Egypt)'84; (780)990-1820; Fax. (780)488-0988.

EL-DEFRAWY, Sherif; Kensington Eye Institute, 600-340 College St, Toronto ON M5T 3A9; Cal'89; FRCSC; Ophth. Staff, Hotel-Dieu Hospital; Asst Prof, Queen's University; Dept Chair Ophth & Vision Sciences, University of Toronto; (416)928-2132; Fax. (416)928-6607.

EL DEMELLAWY, Dina M S; Children's Hosp of Eastern Ont, 401 Smyth Rd, Ottawa ON K1H 8L1; Ain Shams (Egypt)'94; FRCPC; AnatPath. Staff, Children's Hospital of Eastern Ontario (CHEO); (613)737-7600

EL-FAKHARANY, Fawzia; Belle Rive MediCentre, 102-16703 82 St NW, Edmonton AB T5Z 0H5; (Egypt)'81; LMCC; MRCOG(UK); MB ChB; (780)457-7142; Fax. (780)457-7152.

EL-FAKHARANY, Mohamed M; Windsor Reg Hosp-Metropolitan, 1995 Lens Ave, Windsor ON N8W 1L9; (Egypt)'95; Staff, Windsor Regional Hospital - Metropolitan Site; (519)254-5577

EL FAKIR, Abdelghani; Clinique Metro Medic, 220-5910 ch de la Cote-des-Nei, Montreal QC H3S 1Z5; Hassan II (Morocco)'85; ObstGyn (P.Q.). Staff, Hôpital de Saint-Eustache; (514)731-1186

EL FISHAWY, Rami; CSSS de Saint-Jerome, 290 rue de Montigny, Saint-Jerome QC J7Z 5T3; Staff, Hôtel-Dieu de Saint-Jérôme; (450)431-8420

EL FITORI, Adel; Lorraine Wing Tower C, 201 Deacon St, Pembroke ON K8A 2J6; Al-Arab (Libya)'93; FRCSC; GenSurg (Endoscopy). Staff, Pembroke Regional Hospital Inc; (613)732-3675; Fax. (613)732-6347.

EL FOULADI, Nadia; CLSC La Petite Patrie, 6520 rue de Saint-Valleir, Montreal QC H2S 2P7; Sher'04; Gen Practice, Hôpital de réadaptation Villa Medica; (514)834-4614

EL-GAALY, Sherief; Victoria Gen Hosp, 2340 Pembina Hwy, Winnipeg MB R3T 2E8; FRCPC; Psy. Staff, Victoria General Hospital; (204)269-3570

EL-GABALAWY, Hani S; Arthritis Centre, RR 149-800 Sherbrook St, Winnipeg MB R3A 1M4; Cal'77; FRCPC; IntMed; Rheum. Prof Med Immunology/Chair Rheumatology Research, University of Manitoba; (204)787-2208; Fax. (204)787-4594.

EL-GADDAFI, Walid F A; The Ottawa Hosp-Civic Campus, 2F-1053 Carling Ave, Ottawa ON K1Y 4E9; (Libya)'01; Staff, The Ottawa Hospital - Civic Campus; (613)798-5555

EL GANDLI, Daw Saad; CSSS de Manicouagan, 635 boul Jolliet, Baie-Comeau QC G5C 1P1; Al Fateh (Libya)'96; Otol (P.Q.). Staff, Centre Hospitalier Régional Baie-Comeau; (418)589-3701 x2645; Fax. (418)589-8907.

EL-GAYED, Ali Abdel Halim Hussein; Saskatoon Cancer Centre, 20 Campus Dr, Saskatoon SK S7N 4H4; Cairo (Egypt)'79; MB ChB; FFR(Ire.); PhD; MSc; Staff, Saskatoon Cancer Centre; Staff, Royal University Hospital; Clin Assoc Prof, University of Saskatchewan; Langs: Arabic; (306)655-2740; Fax. (306)655-2639; ali.el-gayed@saskcancer.ca.

EL-GEHANI, Faraj E; Jack Ady Cancer Centre, 960 19 St S, Lethbridge AB T1J 1W5; (Libya)'92; MB BCh; Staff, Chinook Regional Hospital; Staff, Jack Ady Cancer Centre; (403)388-6866; Fax. (403)327-7896.

EL GENDI, Amina; Victoria Med Bldg, 212-1669 Victoria St, Prince George BC V2L 2L5; (Germany)'01; (250)614-2330

EL GHAMUDI, Abdulhakim A A; Cambridge Mem Hosp, 700 Coronation Blvd, Cambridge ON N1R 3G2; Tripoli (Libya)'90; FRCPC; Anes (Pain Management). Staff, Cambridge Memorial Hospital; Langs: Arabic; (519)621-2330 x2100; taha97@hotmail.com.

EL GOUHARY, Enas El Gouhary; The Hosp For Sick Children, 555 University Ave, Toronto ON M5G 1X8; Cairo (Egypt)'98; Peds. Staff, The Hospital For Sick Children; Langs: Arabic; (416)813-1500

EL-GOUHARY, Inas; 9312 137 Ave NW, Edmonton AB T5E 6C2; (Egypt)'00; MB BCh; CCFP; Staff, The Good Samaritan Society; (780)456-0658; Fax. (780)475-0732; inas.el-gouhary@capitalhealth.ca.

EL-GUEBALY, Nady A; Foothills Med Centre, 1403 29 St NW, Calgary AB T2N 2T9; Cairo (Egypt)'64; DPH; DPsy; FAPA; FACP; AddicMed; FRCPC; Psy (Addiction Medicine). Staff, Foothills Medical Centre; Dir, Addiction Centre od Calgary; Prof, University of Calgary; Langs: Arabic; French; (403)944-2086; Fax. (403)944-2056; nady.el-guebaly@albertahealthservices.ca.

EL GWAIDY, Nivine A F; STE112-210 Memorial Ave, Orillia ON L3V 7V1; Ain Shams (Egypt)'81; CCFP; (705)329-1882; Fax. (705)329-0840.

EL-HADDAD, Issam; CSSS des Aurores Boreales, CP 6000 Succ Bureau-Chef 679 2e rue E, La Sarre QC J9Z 2X7; Sher'99; FRCSC; GenSurg. Staff, Centre Hospitalier La Sarre; (819)333-2311

EL-HADDAD, Jacques; CHUS-Hop Hotel-Dieu, 580 rue Bowen S, Sherbrooke QC J1G 2E8; Sher'98; FRCSC; PlasSurg. Staff, Centre Hospitalier Universitaire de Sherbrooke-Hôpital Hôtel-Dieu; (819)346-1110

EL HAFFAF, Ahmed Z A; CHUM-Hotel-Dieu, 3840 rue Saint-Urbain, Montreal QC H2W 1T8; (Algeria)'85; FRCPC; MedGenetics. Staff, Centre Hospitalier l'Université de Montréal (CHUM) - Hôtel-Dieu; (514)890-8000

EL-HAJJ, Eyad O; Astotin Med Clinic, PO Box 10 5216 53 St, Lamont AB T0B 2R0; (Russia (Federation))'96; (780)895-7436; Fax. (780)985-7493.

EL-HAJJ, May I; Grey Bruce HS-Owen Sound, PO Box 1800 Stn Main 8223-1800 8th St E, Owen Sound ON N4K 6M9; Beirut (Lebanon)'95; FRCSC; ObstGyn. Staff, Grey Bruce Health Services - Owen Sound; Langs: Arabic; French; (519)371-2651; Fax. (519)371-6178.

EL-HAKIM, Assaad; 200-175 ch Stillview, Pointe-Claire QC H9R 4S3; Laval'97; FRCSC; Urol. (514)697-9658; Fax. (514)695-0431.

EL-HAKIM, Hamdy G E H; Walter Mackenzie Hlth Sciences, 2C3 57-132 University Campus N, Edmonton AB T6G 2R7; Shams (Egypt)'86; Asst Prof Dept Surg & Ped, University of Alberta Hospital; Langs: Arabic; French; (780)407-8629; Fax. (780)407-2004; haelhakim@cha.ab.ca.

EL-HALEES, Walid; St Martha's Reg Hosp, 25 Bay St, Antigonish NS B2G 2G5; (Jordan)'93; MB BS; Staff, St Martha's Regional Hospital; (902)863-1565

EL-HAMAMSY, Ismail; Institut de Cardiologie de Mtl, 5000 rue Belanger, Montreal QC H1T 1C8; Mon'00; FRCSC; CardSurg. Staff, Institut de Cardiologie de Montréal; (514)376-3330

EL HARRAM, Mohamed A; The Medical Centre, 707 Charlotte St, Peterborough ON K9J 2X5; Garyunis (Libya)'81; FRCSC; Urol. (705)876-4506; Fax. (705)743-6278.

EL-HAWARY, Rany; IWK Health Centre, PO Box 9700 Rpo CSC 5850-5980 University Ave, Halifax NS B3K 6R8; Dal'98; BSc(Med); MSc; BEng; FRCSC; OrthSurg (Pediatric Orthopedics). Staff, IWK Health Centre; Asst Prof, Dalhousie University; (902)470-7245; Fax. (902)470-7341; ron.el-hawary@iwk.nshealth.ca.

EL-HAWRANI, Amged; University of Alberta Hosp, 8440 112 St NW, Edmonton AB T6G 2B7; (Ireland)'93; MB BCh; Staff, University of Alberta Hospital; (780)407-3357

EL-HELOU, Philippe P; Charlton Med Centre, 300-25 Charlton Ave E, Hamilton ON L8N 1Y2; Ott'92; IntMed (Infectious Diseases). Staff, St Joseph's Healthcare - Charlton Campus; Langs: Arabic; French; (905)522-1155 x3998; Fax. (905)523-7352.

EL HELOU, Salhab; McMaster Univ, 1280 Main St W, Hamilton ON L8S 4K1; (Germany)'90; Teach Staff, McMaster University; Langs: Bilingual(English/French); (905)521-2100

EL HELOU, Therese; MUHC-Montreal Gen Hosp, L8 210-1650 Cedar Ave, Montreal QC H3G 1A4; (Lebanon)'00; CSPQ; FRCPC; Derm. Staff, McGill University Health Centre - Montreal General Campus; (514)934-1934 x4808; Fax. (514)934-8520.

EL JALBOUT, Ramy; Hôpital Ste-Justine, 3175 ch cote-Sainte-Caterine, Montreal QC H3T 1C5; Beirut (Lebanon)'04; DiagRad (P.Q.). Staff, Hôpital Ste-Justine; (514)345-4931

EL KARSH, Ashraf; 302-8425 120 St, Delta BC V4C 6R2; (Other Foreign)'90; CCFP; (778)593-0155

EL-KATEB, Hayam H R; Eastvale Med Clinic, 4-7 Eastvale Dr, Markham ON L3S 4N8; Cairo (Egypt)'82; CCFP; Langs: Arabic; (905)471-2007; Fax. (905)471-2056.

EL-KEEB, Rabea A H; 117 King St E, Oshawa ON L1H 1B9; Al Fateh (Libya)'00; FRCPC; IntMed; Respir. Staff, The Ottawa Hospital - General Campus; (905)721-4996; Fax. (905)721-3557.

EL KEILANI, Akram M I; Hotel-Dieu Grace Hosp, 1030 Ouellette Ave, Windsor ON N9A 1E1; Garyounis (Libya)'95; FRCPC; AnatPath. Staff, Hôtel-Dieu Grace Hospital; Langs: Arabic; (519)973-4411

EL KHATIB, Adel A M; Duggan Village Mall, 1-6601 48 AVE, Camrose AB T4V 3G8; (Egypt)'05; MB ChB; (780)608-5877; Fax. (780)608-5878.

EL-KHODARY, Mohamed A I; The Ottawa Hosp-Gen Campus, L2121 CPCR-501 Smyth Rd, Ottawa ON K1H 8L6; Cairo (Egypt)'02; Staff, The Ottawa Hospital - General Campus; (413)737-8571

EL-KHOLI, Vivian M; William Osler Hlth Ctr-Brampto, 2100 Bovaird Dr E, Brampton ON L6R 3J7; Cairo (Egypt)'82; MB ChB; FRCPC; Psy (Sleep Medicine). Staff, William Osler Health System - Brampton Civic Hospital; (905)494-2120; Fax. (905)494-6710.

EL KHOULY, Nihal; Goodfellow Prof Bldg, 206-170 McEwan Dr E, Bolton ON L7E 4C8; Alexandria (Egypt)'94; CCFP; Langs: Arabic; German; (905)857-3474; Fax. (905)951-7855.

EL KHOURY, Mona; CHUM-Hotel-Dieu, 3840 rue Saint-Urbain, Montreal QC H2W 1T8; (Lebanon)'95; DiagRad (P.Q.). Staff, Centre Hospitalier l'Université de Montréal (CHUM) - Hôtel-Dieu; (514)934-1934 x45073

EL KOUSSA, Lamis; CSSS de la Vallée de l'Or, 725 6e rue, Val-d'Or QC J9P 3Y1; (Lebanon)'90; Staff, Centre Hospitalier de Val d'Or; (819)825-6711

EL MAADAWY, Sherif S; Parkland Med Associates, 102A-505 Queen St, Spruce Grove AB T7X 2V2; Cairo (Egypt)'93; MB ChB; FRCPC; PhysMed&Rehab. Staff, Glenrose Rehabilitation Hospital; (780)960-4102; Fax. (780)666-2621.

EL-MADAH, Hesham; North Gate Med Clinic, 980 Central Park Dr, Brampton ON L6S 3L7; (Libya)'99; CCFP; Langs: Arabic; (905)458-4771; Fax. (905)458-5376.

EL-MALLAH, Medhat W; Lakeridge Hlth Corp-Oshawa, 1 Hospital Crt, Oshawa ON L1G 2B9; Minya (Turkey)'91; FRCPC; RadOncol. Staff, Lakeridge Health - Oshawa Site; Langs: Arabic; (905)576-8711

EL-MARAGHI, Robert H; Royal Victoria Hosp, 201 Georgian Dr, Barrie ON L4M 6M2; Ott'99; FRCPC; IntMed (Clinician Investigator Program); MedOncol. Staff, Royal Victoria Regional Health Centre; (705)739-5661; Fax. (705)739-5619.

EL MASRI, William S; The Endoscopy Clinic, 340-340 College St, Toronto ON M5T 3A9; Alexandria (Egypt)'75; MB ChB; FACS; FRCSC; Otol (Endoscopic Sinus Surg). Staff, Mount Sinai Hospital; Ac Staff, Toronto East General Hospital Inc; Asst Prof, University of Toronto; Langs: French; Italian; Arabic; Armenian; (416)966-1160; Fax. (416)966-9288.

EL MASRY, Amir; Flin Flon Gen Hosp, PO Box 340 Stn Main 50 Church St, Flin Flon MB R8A 1N2; (Other Foreign)'81; Fam Med, Flin Flon General Hospital Inc; Staff, Northern Health Flin-Flon Regional Office; (204)687-6130; Fax. (204)681-3462.

EL-MATARY, Wael M M; Children's Hosp, AE408-840 Sherbrook St, Winnipeg MB R3A 1S1; Alexandria (Egypt)'90; MB BCh.

EL-MESSIDI, Amira; MUHC-Royal Victoria Hosp, 687 av des Pins O, Montreal QC H3A 1A1; McG'02; FRCSC; ObstGyn (Maternal Fetal Medicine). Staff, McGill University Health Centre - Royal Victoria Hospital; Langs: Arabic; French; (514)934-1934; Fax. (514)843-1675.

EL MEZOUAR, Zineb; CLSC Riviere des Prairies, 8655 boul Perras, Montreal QC H1E 4M7; (Other Foreign)'87; CCFP; (514)494-4924

EL NAGAR, Islam; Queen Elizabeth II HSC, 4857-1796 Summer St, Halifax NS B3H 3A7; Alexandria (Egypt)'02; Staff, Queen Elizabeth II Health Sciences Centre - Halifax Infirmary Site.

EL-NAGGAR, Walid I M H; IWK Health Centre, PO Box 9700 Rpo CSC 5850-5980 University Ave, Halifax NS B3K 6R8; Cairo (Egypt)'87; MB BCh; Staff, IWK Health Centre; (902)470-7961; Fax. (902)470-5469.

EL RABAA, Hoda; 135B-1685 Main St W, Hamilton ON L8S 1G5; Cairo (Egypt)'84; CCFP; (905)521-2222; Fax. (905)521-2222.

EL RAMI, Hares; Ctr Hosp Rouyn-Noranda, 4 9e rue, Rouyn-Noranda QC J9X 2B2; (Lebanon)'89; Staff, Centre Hospitalier Rouyn-Noranda; (819)764-5131; Fax. (819)764-2900.

EL-RASSI, Roula; CSSS de Rivière-de-Loup, 75 rue Saint-Henri, Riviere-du-Loup QC G5R 2A4; Saint-Joseph (Lebanon)'91; Staff, Centre Hospitalier Regional du Grand-Portage; (418)868-1010; Fax. (418)868-1075.

EL RAYESS, Malak; Hop du Sacre-Coeur de Mtl, 5400 boul Gouin O, Montreal QC H4J 1C5; McG'06; MDCM; FRCPC; IntMed; Cardiol (P.Q.). Staff, Hôpital du Sacre-Coeur de Montréal; (514)338-2222

EL SABAWY, Mary; Gillam Hosp, PO Box 2000 115 Gillam Dr, Gillam MB R0B 0L0; MB ChB; CCFP; Staff, Gillam Hospital; (204)652-2600

EL-SADI, Salman A K; London HSC-Victoria Hosp, PO Box 5010 Stn B 800 Commissioners Rd E, London ON N6A 5W9; Jordan (Jordan)'92; CCFP; CCFP(E.M.); Staff, London Health Sciences Centre - Victoria Campus; Langs: Arabic; (519)685-8500

EL-SAHEB, Hady; MUHC-Royal Victoria Hosp, 687 av des Pins O, Montreal QC H3A 1A1; McG'05; Ophth. Staff, McGill University Health Centre - Royal Victoria Hospital; (514)934-1934

EL-SAHRIGY, Dina; Rouge Valley-Ajax & Pickering, 580 Harwood Ave S, Ajax ON L1S 2J4; Alexandria (Egypt)'92; FRCPC; AnatPath (Clinical Pathology). Staff, Rouge Valley Health System - Ajax & Pickering Health Centre Site; Langs: Arabic; (905)683-2320 x1474

EL SAIDI, Mohammed; Quinte HC Corp-Belleville Gen, 265 Dundas St E, Belleville ON K8N 5A9; (Egypt)'84; MB ChB; FRCSC; Psy. Staff, QHC Belleville General; Langs: Arabic; (613)969-7400; Fax. (613)969-8448.

EL-SALIBI, Elias; Glengarry Mem Hosp, 43-20260 Country Rd, Alexandria ON K0C 1A0; Mon'99; CCFP; Staff, Glengarry Memorial Hospital; Langs: English; Arabic; (613)525-1513; Fax. (613)525-1680.

EL-SALVITI, Gamal I; Mckinney Med Centre, 102-510 Ingersoll Ave, Woodstock ON N4S 4X9; Ain Shams (Egypt)'78; MB ChB; FRCSC; GenSurg. Staff, Woodstock General Hospital; Langs: Arabic; (519)421-1996; Fax. (519)421-3334.

EL-SAWAF, Amro; Terrace Plaza, 650-4445 Calgary Trail NW, Edmonton AB T6H 5R7; Saba (MA) (USA)'03; FRCPC; IntMed; Derm. (780)429-0222; Fax. (780)429-1222.

EL-SAWY, Reda M; 505-381 Kent St, Ottawa ON K2P 2A8; Cairo (Egypt)'63; MB ChB; DPM; ABPMR; FRCPC; PhysMed&Rehab (Spine). Consultant, Montfort Hospital; Consultant, The Ottawa Hospital - General Campus; Consultant, The Ottawa Hospital - Civic Campus; Consultant, Queensway Carleton Hospital; Langs: French; Arabic; (613)234-7780; Fax. (613)234-6636.

EL-SAYED, Assem S M; Saskatoon Cancer Centre, 20 Campus Dr, Saskatoon SK S7N 4H4; (306)655-2980; Fax. (306)655-6422.

EL SAYED, Jihan M; Medicentres, 16703 82 St NW, Edmonton AB T5Z 0H5; Cairo (Egypt)'89; (780)457-7142; Fax. (780)457-7152.

EL-SAYED, Samy M; The Ottawa Hosp-Gen Campus, 501 Smyth Rd, Ottawa ON K1H 1C4; Mansoura (Egypt)'77; FFR(Dublin); FRCR(Lond); AB; FRCPC; RadOncol (Clinical Oncology). Staff, The Ottawa Hospital - General Campus; Prof, University of Ottawa; Langs: Arabic; French; (613)737-7700 x6769; Fax. (613)247-3511.

EL-SAYED, Yasser N E M; Women's Hosp, WS012-735 Notre Dame Ave, Winnipeg MB R3E 0L8.

EL-SAYEGH, Rawieh; Huron Square Med Centre, 2500 Hurontario St, Mississauga ON L5B 1N4; Ain Shams (Egypt)'79; CCFP; Staff, Trillium Health Centre - Mississauga; Langs: Arabic; (905)897-6160; Fax. (905)897-6729.

EL SEISI, Somaya; A8-1390 Major Mackenzie Dr E, Richmond Hill ON L4S 0A1; Ain Shams (Egypt)'80; MB BCh; CCFP; Langs: Arabic; (905)884-7711

EL SHATSHAT, Mohamed; Arborg Health Centre, PO Box 430 234 Gislason Dr, Arborg MB R0C 0A0; (Libya)'96; CCFP; Fam Med, Arborg & District Health Centre; Langs: Arabic; (204)376-2781; Fax. (204)376-5356; mohamede@nursinghomeratings.ca.

EL-SHEIKH, Yasser S; 211-1333 Sheppard Ave E, North York ON M2J 1V1; McM'04; FRCSC; PlasSurg. Staff, Hamilton Health Sciences Centre - McMaster Children's Hospital.

EL-SHERBINY, Mohamed T; MUHC-Montreal Children's Hosp, C527-2300 rue Tupper, Montreal QC H3H 1P3; Mansoura (Egypt)'89; Urol (P.Q.) (Pediatric Urology). Staff, McGill University Health Centre - Montreal Children's Hospital; Langs: Arabic; Bilingual(French/English); (514)412-4366; Fax. (514)412-4384; elsherbi@yahoo.com.

EL-SHINNAWY, Ihab H; St Joseph's Healthcare, L222 5-50 Charlton Ave E, Hamilton ON L8N 4A6; Ain Shams (Egypt)'93; FRCPC; AnatPath. Staff, St Joseph's Healthcare - Charlton Campus; (905)522-4941

EL-TAKLI, Issam K; Brampton Gastroenterology, 11-470 Chrysler Dr, Brampton ON L6S 0C1; Baghdad (Iraq)'92; FRCPC; IntMed; Gastroent. Langs: Arabic; (905)790-6362; Fax. (905)790-6612.

EL-TATARI, Bassam; Family Hlth Centre, 105-2462 Howard Ave, Windsor ON N8X 3V6; (Czech Republic)'99; CCFP; Langs: Arabic; Czech; Slovak; (519)946-0705; Fax. (519)946-3265.

EL TAWIL, Basel A; Leamington District Mem Hosp, 3F-194 Talbot St W, Leamington ON N8H 1N9; Al Fateh (Libya)'86; FRCPC; IntMed (Gastroenterology). Staff, Leamington District Memorial Hospital; Langs: Arabic; (519)322-4755; Fax. (519)322-5965.

EL ZAHARNA, Ramy; ZMC Medical Centre, 2-1801 Harwood Ave, Ajax ON L1T 0K8; (Slovakia)'00; CCFP; Staff, Cape Breton Healthcare Complex; Langs: Arabic; (905)427-5444; Fax. (905)427-6444.

EL-ZEIN, Mohamad A K; University of Western Ontario, M106-1151 Richmond St, London ON N6A 5B7; (Lebanon)'91; Staff, Alberta Children's Hospital; (403)955-7985; Fax. (403)955-7656.

EL-ZIMAITY, Hala M T; Univ Hlth Network-Toronto Gen, 11E210-200 Elizabeth St, Toronto ON M5G 2C4; Ain Shams (Egypt)'82; FRCPC; AnatPath. Staff, Toronto General Hospital - UHN; Langs: Arabic; (416)340-4551

EL-ZUBEIDI, Wassim; Aberdeen Hosp, 835 East River Rd, New Glasgow NS B2H 3S6; (Montserrat)'98; ABIM; FRCPC; IntMed (Gastroenterology). Staff, Aberdeen Regional Hospital; (902)755-6639; Fax. (902)755-9349.

EL ZUWAY, Rabeh M A; Niagara H System-G Niagara, 5546 Portage Rd, Niagara Falls ON L2E 6X2; (Libya)'00; FRCPC; IntMed. Staff, Niagara Health System - Greater Niagara General Site; Langs: Arabic; (905)378-4647

ELAHI, Mohammed; 306-500 Sheppard Ave E, North York ON M2N 6H7; Wes'93; MSc; FRCSC; Otol (Trauma); PlasSurg. Staff Plastic Surg, St Michael's Hospital; Staff, The Scarborough Hospital - General Campus; Langs: Urdu; French; Punjabi; (416)221-2441; Fax. (416)221-3550.

ELAHI, Mohammed; 302-2304 Islington Ave, Etobicoke ON M9W 3W9; Tor'91; CCFP; Langs: French; Urdu; Punjabi; (416)749-4959

ELAHI, Sofia B; 302-2304 Islington Ave, Etobicoke ON M9W 3W9; Peshawar (Pakistan)'95; CCFP; (647)348-0588; Fax. (647)348-5807.

ELALEM, Abdusalam; Windsor Health Centre, 258-1720 Howard Ave, Windsor ON N8X 5A6; Al Fateh (Libya)'87; MB ChB; FRCSC; ThorSurg (Digestive Endoscopy); GenSurg. Staff, Windsor Regional Hospital - Metropolitan Site; Staff, Hôtel-Dieu Grace Hospital; Langs: Arabic; (519)256-6590; Fax. (519)256-8064; aelalem@yahoo.ca.

ELANTHOLI PARAMESWARAN, Saibishkumar; Univ Hlth Network-Princess M, 5 620-610 University Ave, Toronto ON M5G 2M9; (India)'99; FRCPC; RadOncol. Staff, Princess Margaret Hospital - University Health Network; Langs: Hindi; (416)946-2919; Fax. (416)946-4586.

ELASHAAL, Abdelrahman A B; 216-2425 Tecumseh Rd E, Windsor ON N8W 1E6; Al-Arab (Libya)'89; FRCSC; OrthSurg. Staff, Hôtel-Dieu Grace Hospital; Langs: Arabic; (519)254-5763

ELASHAAL, Abdurrahim A; St Michael's Hosp, 30 Bond St, Toronto ON M5B 1W8; Al Fateh (Libya)'93; FRCSC; Neursurg. Staff, St Michael's Hospital; Langs: Arabic; (416)864-6060

ELAVATHIL, Leelamma J; Hamilton HS-Henderson Site, 711 Concession St, Hamilton ON L8V 1C3; Kerala (India)'75; MB BS; FRCPC; GenPath; AnatPath. Staff, Hamilton Health Sciences Centre-Juravinski Site; Assoc Prof, McMaster University; Langs: Malayalam; (905)527-4322 x42038; elavathil@hhsc.ca.

ELAZHARY, Nicolas; CHUS-Hop Fleurimont, 3F-3001 12e av N, Sherbrooke QC J1H 5N4; Mon'02; CCFP; CCFP(E.M.); Staff, Centre Hospitalier Universitaire de Sherbrooke-Hopital Fleurimont; (819)346-1110 x14274

ELBARDISY, Nozahy N; Selkirk & District Gen Hosp, PO Box 5000 Stn Main 100 Easton Dr, Selkirk MB R1A 2M2; Ain Shams (Egypt)'85; MB ChB; CCFP; Staff, Selkirk & District General Hospital; (204)482-5800

ELBAROUN, Basem A O N; 101-2299 Dundas St W, Toronto ON M6R 1X7; Al Fateh (Libya)'02; (416)538-0707; Fax. (416)538-0700.

ELBAZ, Armand; 145-6000 ch de la Cote-des-Nei, Montreal QC H3S 1Z8; Toulouse (France)'75; Staff, Sir Mortimer B Davis Jewish General; (514)731-2755; Fax. (514)731-7096.

ELBAZ, Audrey; Clinique Med 910, 910 boul Saint-Joseph E, Montreal QC H2J 1K6; McG'06; MDCM; CCFP; (514)590-0910

ELBESHTI, Essam A M; GP Med Clinic, 12225 99 St, Grande Prairie AB T8V 6X9; Al-Fateh (Libya)'02; MB BCh; CCFP; (780)533-4444; Fax. (780)533-4443.

ELBREKI, Mustafa M; Jackson Park Health Centre, 210-2475 McDougall St, Windsor ON N8X 3N9; Al-Arab (Libya)'92; FRCSC; Otol. Langs: Arabic; (519)966-3888; Fax. (519)967-8882.

ELDEIRY, Azza; 7004 98 Ave NW, Edmonton AB T6A 0A5; (Egypt)'92; MB BCh; Langs: Arabic; (780)468-6035; Fax. (780)466-9132.

ELDER, Beverly A; Charlton Med Centre, 406-25 Charlton Ave E, Hamilton ON L8N 1Y2; Wes'83; (905)525-0255; Fax. (905)525-9764.

ELDER, Brian R; The Ottawa Hosp-Civic Campus, 1053 Carling Ave, Ottawa ON K1Y 4E9; Qns'88; FRCPC; EmergMed. Staff, The Ottawa Hospital - Civic Campus; (613)798-5555

ELDER, Graham M; Doctors Bldg, 120-955 Queen St E, Sault Ste. Marie ON P6A 2C3; McG'95; FRCSC; OrthSurg. Langs: French; (705)253-8536; Fax. (705)253-0048; grahamelder@shaw.ca.

ELDER, Janice L; Hamilton HS-Henderson Site, 711 Concession St, Hamilton ON L8V 1C3; Wes'88; FRCPC; DiagRad. Staff Radiol, Hamilton Health Sciences Centre-Juravinski Site; (905)577-4322 x42261; Fax. (905)575-2660.

ELDER, John R; 408-1100 Sheppard Ave E, North York ON M2K 2W1; Tor'61; Ophth (Glaucoma). Ac Staff/Consultant, North York General Hospital; (416)226-2253; Fax. (416)226-5829.

ELDRIDGE, Karen-Lee; 202-170 Simcoe St, Peterborough ON K9H 2H7; McM'89; CCFP; FCFP; Assoc Prof, Queen's University; (705)743-3804; Fax. (705)872-4357; keldridge@prhc.on.ca.

ELEASON, Sheila M; Central Alberta Prof Centre, 265-5201 43 St, Red Deer AB T4N 1C7; Alb'85; CCFP; FCFP; Staff, Red Deer Regional Hospital Centre; (403)342-1919; Fax. (403)347-4877.

ELEDRISI, Fadel; Walmart Clinic, 16940 127 St, Edmonton AB T6V 1S8; Al Fateh (Libya)'02; MB BCh; (780)665-1760

ELEFF, Michael K; Psychealth Centre, PZ263-771 Bannatyne Ave, Winnipeg MB R3E 3N4; Man'76; FRCPC; Psy (Psychotic Disorders). Staff, Health Sciences Centre; Assoc Prof, University of Manitoba; (204)787-5005; Fax. (204)787-7480.

ELEKIABY, Amr Saad; 24-1515 Dufferin Cres, Nanaimo BC V9S 2B8; Cairo (Egypt)'91; MB BCh; Staff, Nanaimo Regional General Hospital; (250)753-2446

ELEMARY, Mohamed; Saskatoon Cancer Centre, 20 Campus Dr, Saskatoon SK S7N 4H4; Staff, Saskatoon Cancer Centre; (306)655-2980

ELEMUO, Raphael E; 12-1000 Northwest Blvd RR 6, Creston BC V0B 1G6; Ibadan (Nigeria)'97; MB BS; (250)428-7887; Fax. (250)428-7171.

ELEPANO, Patricia; 104-440 Boler Rd, London ON N6K 4L2; Tor'93; CCFP; FCFP; (519)471-2929

ELEPANO, Suzanne M; City Centre Med Clinic, 130-5 Park Home Ave, North York ON M2N 6L4; Tor'97; CCFP; (416)730-9588

ELESIN, Fayisayo; Plaza 2 Shopping Ctr, 616-8600 Franklin Ave, Fort McMurray AB T9H 4G8; (Nigeria)'98; MB BS; CCFP; (780)714-6665; Fax. (780)714-5021.

ELEY, Judy M; Market Mall Office Centre, 208-3625 Shaganappi Trail NW, Calgary AB T3A 0E2; Ott'90; MSc; (403)286-9118; Fax. (403)286-3069.

ELFASSI, Emile; Le Sanctuaire, 201-6100 ave du Boise, Montreal QC H3S 2W1; Mon'96; Prof, Universite de Montreal; Langs: Bilingual(French/English); (514)739-5646

ELFASSY, Bernard; Cite Sante St-Laurent, 1-1077 rue Decarie, Saint-Laurent QC H4L 3M8; Mon'85; Staff, Centre Hospitalier l'Université de Montréal (CHUM) - Hôtel-Dieu; (514)747-5556; Fax. (514)747-5557.

ELFIKY, Ashraf M; PO Box 3560 Stn Main, Sherwood Park AB T8H 2T4; Cairo (Egypt)'67; LRCP(Lond); MRCS(Eng); Langs: Arabic; (780)464-2004

ELFIRJANI, Ali Salem B; Rouge Valley-Ajax & Pickering, 580 Harwood Ave S, Ajax ON L1S 2J4; Garyunis (Libya)'96; FRCPC; IntMed; Nephrol. Staff, Rouge Valley Health System - Ajax & Pickering Health Centre Site; Langs: Arabic; (905)683-2320

ELFORD, Rod; Copeman Health Care Centre, 400-628 12 Ave SW, Calgary AB T2R 0H6; Alb'93; BPE; MSc; CCFP; FCFP; Med Dir, Health Link Alberta; (403)270-2273; Fax. (403)521-2250.

ELFORD, Kimberly; Oakville Fertility & Women's H, B-627 Lyons Lane, Oakville ON L6J 5Z7; Cal'95; BSc; FRCSC; ObstGyn (Infertility). Staff ObstGyn, Halton Healthcare Services Corporation - Oakville Site; (905)844-7238; Fax. (905)844-7256; kelford@oakvillefertility.com.

ELFORTI, Nabil; Lessard Med Clinic, 6633 177 St NW, Edmonton AB T5T 4K3; Al Fateh (Egypt)'97; MB ChB; CCFP; (780)757-7999; Fax. (780)757-7991.

ELFOURTIA, Abdelmunem; Beverly Med Clinic, 4243 118 Ave NW, Edmonton AB T5W 1A5; (Libya)'02; MB BCh; CCFP; (780)756-7700; Fax. (780)756-7788.

ELGAMAL, Akram S; Strathroy Middlesex Gen Hosp, 318B-395 Carrie St, Strathroy ON N7G 3C9; Cairo (Egypt)'75; MB ChB; FRCSC; GenSurg. Staff, Strathroy Middlesex General Hospital - Middlesex Hospital Alliance; (519)245-8392; Fax. (519)245-8305; aelgamal@smgh.mhalliance.on.ca.

ELGERSMA, Vincent V; South Shore Med Clinic, 620 Cassils Rd E, Brooks AB T1R 1M6; Alb'93; AB; CCFP; (403)793-8111; Fax. (403)793-8118.

ELGHAMARI, Abdulmonem; Rathburn Healthplex Med, 2-452 Rathburn Rd, Etobicoke ON M9C 3S8; Tripoli (Libya)'92; MB ChB; CCFP; Langs: Arabic; (416)621-2323; Fax. (416)621-2321.

ELGHDEWI, Turia A; Lloyd Women's Clinic, 3308 50 Ave, Lloydminster AB T9V 0V6; Al-Fateh (Libya)'88; FRCSC; ObstGyn. Langs: Arabic; (780)875-8755; Fax. (780)875-5868; elghdewi@yahoo.ca.

ELGHOBARY, Tamer; Trillium Hlth Ctr-Mississauga, 100 Queensway W, Mississauga ON L5B 1B8; Ain Shams (Egypt)'95; MB BCh; FRCSC; CardSurg. Staff, Trillium Health Centre - Mississauga; Langs: Arabic; French; (905)848-7580

ELGHOL, Eimad M E; North East Med Centre, 7210 144 Ave NW, Edmonton AB T5C 2R7; Al Fateh (Libya)'03; MB BCh; CCFP; Langs: Arabic; (780)478-2995

ELGRIGNI, Hassan R; 11035 Groat Rd NW, Edmonton AB T5M 3J9; (Libya)'03; MB BCh; (780)705-4090; Fax. (780)705-4394.

ELHAJEMHMED, Abdalla; 17719 98A Ave NW, Edmonton AB T5T 5W8; (Libya)'05; MB BCh; (780)481-5555; Fax. (780)487-5666.

ELHARATHI, Hythum; PO Box 179, Swan Hills AB T0G 2C0; (Libya)'08; MB ChB; (780)333-7077; Fax. (780)333-7009.

ELHILALI, Mostafa M; MUHC-Royal Victoria Hosp, S695-687 av des Pins O, Montreal QC H3A 1A1; Cairo (Egypt)'59; MB ChB; MCh; PhD; FRCSC; Urol (Oncology). Consultant, Sir Mortimer B Davis Jewish General; Chief Urology, McGill University Health Centre - Royal Victoria Hospital; Chief Urology, McGill University Health Centre - Montreal General Campus; Head Surg, McGill University; (514)843-1516; Fax. (514)843-1552; mostafa.elhilali@muhc.mcgill.ca.

ELIA, Bashar J; Deerfoot Meadows Med Clinic, 7979 11 St SE, Calgary AB T2H 0B8; (Iraq)'89; MB ChB; (403)251-2690

ELIA, Mario F; 1A-163 Commissioners Rd W, London ON N6J 1X9; Wes'10; CCFP; (519)657-2032; Fax. (519)657-3357.

ELIA, Steven T; North York Gen Hosp, 4001 Leslie St, North York ON M2K 1E1; Tor'78; FRCPC; IntMed (Cardiology); Anes. Ac Staff Med, North York General Hospital; Langs: Macedonian; (416)635-2578

ELIAS, Cynthia G; Meadowlark Health Centre, 200 Meadowlark Shopping Ctr NW, Edmonton AB T5R 5W9; Alb'79; BMedSci; FRCPC; DiagRad. Staff, Covenant Health - Misericordia Community Hospital; (780)489-5313; Fax. (780)486-5160.

ELIAS, David A; PO Box 3033 Stn Main, Grand-Bay-Wesfld NB E5K 4V3; Dal'89; BSc(Pharm); CCFP; CCFP(E.M.); Staff, Horizon Health Network Saint John Public Health; Staff, Restigouche Hospital Centre; Med Advisor, WHSCC of New Brunswick; Teach Staff, University of New Brunswick; Langs: English; French; (506)738-4400

ELIAS, Kamelia Y R; River Park Med Centre, 4-1500 Dakota St, Winnipeg MB R2N 3Y7; Ain Shams (Egypt)'84; CCFP.

ELIAS, Suzan M; 300 Taunton Rd E, Oshawa ON L1G 7T4; University of Khartoum (Sudan)'84; CCFP; Langs: Arabic; (905)448-0457

ELIAS-LOPEZ, Esmeralda; Clinique Med des Bois-Francs, 101 rue Demers E, Princeville QC G6L 4E8; Sher'04; Staff Family Med, Hotel-Dieu d'Arthabaska; (819)364-2150

ELIASON, Barry K; 18-1710 Ellis St, Kelowna BC V1Y 2B5; Alb'77; Staff, Kelowna General Hospital; (250)763-5427; Fax. (250)763-2922.

ELIASON, Darrel G; 5927 Bowness Rd NW, Calgary AB T3B 0C7; Alb'71; BMedSci; (403)286-3035

ELIASON, Heather L; Sunridge Family Med Teaching C, 2685 36 St NE, Calgary AB T1Y 5S3; Cal'01; CCFP; (403)943-5000; Fax. (403)476-8784.

ELIASSON, Theresa; University of Alberta Hosp, 8440 112 St NW, Edmonton AB T6G 2B7; Alb'93; FRCPC; Anes. Staff, University of Alberta Hospital; (780)407-7035

ELIE, Andreanne; Clinique Psychee, 400-400 rue Laurier O, Montreal QC H2V 2K7; Laval'93; FRCPC; Psy. Staff, Centre Hospitalier l'Université de Montréal (CHUM) - Hôtel-Dieu; (514)279-4141

ELIE, John D; 130-3545 ch de la Cote-des-Nei, Montreal QC H3H 1V1; Ott'67; BSc; CSPQ; Derm. Langs: Arabic; French; (514)935-3024; Fax. (514)935-7291.

ELIE, Kathryn D; Ctr Hosp de Lachine, 650 16e av, Lachine QC H8S 3N5; Lausanne (Switzerland)'63; MedMicrobiol (P.Q.) (Infectious Diseases). Consultant, Douglas Mental Health University Institute; Ac Staff, CSSS de Dorval-Lachine-Lasalle; Langs: English; French; (514)637-2351 x5380

ELIE, Louis-Michel; St Mary's Hosp Centre, 3830 av Lacombe, Montreal QC H3T 1M5; McG'91; FRCPC; Psy. Staff, St Mary's Hospital Centre; (514)345-3511 x3349; Fax. (514)734-2609.

ELIEV, Sonia; COOP de Sante de Gracefield, 30 rue Principale, Gracefield QC J0X 1W0; Mon'90; LMCC; CCFP; Assoc Staff, CSSS de la Vallée de la Gatineau; Langs: Spanish; English; (819)463-0100; seliev@ireseau.com.

ELIMOVA, Elena; Sunnybrook Hlth Sciences Ctre, T2 036-2075 Bayview Ave, Toronto ON M4N 3M5; Mem'08; IntMed. Staff, Sunnybrook Health Sciences Centre - Edmond Odette Cancer Centre; (416)480-4270; Fax. (416)480-6002.

ELINSON, Roman; Healthcare 365, 905-1867 Yonge St, Toronto ON M4S 1Y5; Tor'01; CCFP; Langs: Russian; (416)642-9160; Fax. (416)487-3931.

ELIOSOFF, Ronald V; Appletree Med Group, 368 Slater St, Ottawa ON K1R 5C1; UBC'72; BSc; FRCPC; IntMed. (613)236-9441; Fax. (613)236-9425.

ELIT, Lorraine; The Juravinski Cancer Centre, 699 Concession St, Hamilton ON L8V 5C2; Wes'84; MSc; FRCSC; ObstGyn (Gynecologic Oncology). Court Staff, The Brant Community Healthcare System - Brantford General Hospital Site; Court Staff, Cambridge Memorial Hospital; Staff, Hamilton Health Sciences Centre-Juravinski Site; Staff, Joseph Brant Memorial Hospital; Staff, St Joseph's Healthcare - Charlton Campus; Physician Gyn Oncol, The Juravinski Cancer Centre; Assoc Prof, McMaster University; (905)389-5688; Fax. (905)575-6343.

ELIZOV, Michelle; SMBD Jewish Gen Hosp, G 050-3755 ch Cote-Sainte-Cath, Montreal QC H3T 1E2; McG'95; FRCPC; IntMed. Staff, Sir Mortimer B Davis Jewish General; (514)340-8222 x4974; Fax. (514)340-7905.

ELJAOUDI, Abdurraouf; Consort Med Centre, PO Box 58 5402 52 Ave, Consort AB T0C 1B0; Al Fateh (Libya)'03; MB BCh; CCFP; (403)577-3737; Fax. (403)577-3739.

ELKABAS, Oren S; Clin Med Hampstead, 2-5141 av Coolbrook, Montreal QC H3X 2L2; Sher'93; (514)481-6399

ELKABIR, Nabil; 12 West Med Clinic, 130-227 11 Ave SW, Calgary AB T2R 1R9; (Libya)'98; MB ChB; (403)210-0121; Fax. (403)210-0320.

ELKAMS, Sameh; Lakewood Med Centre, 30 Lakewood Blvd, Winnipeg MB R2J 2M6; (Egypt)'86; CCFP; (204)257-4900

ELKASHAB, Magdy A M H; Dufferin Subspecialty Clinic, 2F-1664 Dufferin St, Toronto ON M6H 3M1; Cairo (Egypt)'80; MB ChB; MSc; FRCPC; IntMed (Hepatology); Gastroent. Staff, Mount Sinai Hospital; (416)652-0606; Fax. (416)652-0633.

ELKASSEM, Samer; Southview Clinic, 105-1424 Southview Dr SE, Medicine Hat AB T1B 4E7; Cal'03; FRCSC; GenSurg. Langs: Arabic; (403)487-5900; Fax. (403)487-5901.

ELKELANI, Saad M A; West Lambton Community H C, 1F-481 London Rd, Sarnia ON N7T 4X3; Al-Fateh (Libya)'84; MB ChB; FRCSC; ObstGyn. Langs: Arabic; (519)344-9031; Fax. (519)344-9044.

ELKHEMRI, Abdulgader; Pine Falls Hlth Complex, PO Box 2000 37 Maple St, Pine Falls MB R0E 1M0; Fam Med, Pine Falls Health Complex; (204)367-5400

ELKHUIZEN, Carola E; 186 Marsh St PO Box 179, Clarksburg ON N0H 1J0; McM'03; BA; CCFP; (519)599-5775; Fax. (519)599-7140.

ELKIN, Eric N; Carling-Broadview Med Bldg, 209-770 Broadview Ave, Ottawa ON K2A 3Z3; Ott'70; Att Staff, Queensway Carleton Hospital; (613)729-1296

ELKIN, Jonathan A; Assiniboine Clinic, 633 Lodge Ave, Winnipeg MB R3J 0S9; Man'96; BSc; CCFP; FCFP; (204)958-6711; Fax. (204)888-1750.

ELKIN, Mark S; Charleswood Med Clinic, 3360 Roblin Blvd, Winnipeg MB R3R 0C5; Man'98; CCFP; FCFP; (204)889-7200

ELKINK, Meghan S; 3-3295 Dunmore Rd SE, Medicine Hat AB T1B 3R2; Alb'07; CCFP; (403)528-7243; Fax. (403)528-9995.

ELKOURI, Stephane; CHUM-Hotel-Dieu, 3840 rue Saint-Urbain, Montreal QC H2W 1T8; Mon'95 Mayo Clinic (USA); FACS; CSPQ; FRCSC; GenSurg (Clinical Research); VascSurg. Staff, Centre Hospitalier l'Université de Montréal (CHUM) - Hôtel-Dieu; Langs: Bilingual(French/English); (514)890-8000 x15148; stephane.elkouri@umontreal.ca.

ELKOUSSY, Moustafa A; 301-22112 52 Ave, Langley BC V2Y 2M6; Cairo (Egypt)'72; FRCSC; OrthSurg. Staff, Prince Rupert Regional Hospital; (604)514-7514; Fax. (604)514-7516.

ELKOUT, Lotfia; 206-6453 Morrison St, Niagara Falls ON L2E 7H1; Al Fateh (Liberia)'01; MB BCh; InfectDis; Peds. Staff, IWK Health Centre; (905)357-4554

ELKURBO, Mohamed; Concordia Hip & Knee Inst, 301-1155 Concordia Ave, Winnipeg MB R2K 2M9; Al Fateh (Libya)'97; FRCSC; OrthSurg. (204)926-1200

ELLABIB, Mohamed; 49 Olivia Place, Ancaster ON L9K 1R4; Al Fateh (Libya)'92; Staff, Hamilton Health Sciences Centre - Hamilton General Hospital; (905)512-6980

ELLARD, Susan L; BC Cancer Ctre-Southern Interi, 399 Royal Ave, Kelowna BC V1Y 5L3; Tor'90; FRCPC; IntMed; MedOncol. Staff, BC Cancer Agency Sindi Ahluwalia Hawkins Centre for the Southern Interior; (250)712-3996; Fax. (250)712-3911.

ELLAURIE, Isphara; 5002 51 St PO Box 1448, St Paul AB T0A 3A0; Natal (South Africa)'75; MB ChB; (780)645-7878; Fax. (780)645-7898.

ELLCHUK, Tasha; Royal University Hosp, 103 Hospital Dr, Saskatoon SK S7N 0W8; UBC'03; FRCPC; DiagRad. Staff, Royal University Hospital; (306)655-2371; Fax. (306)655-2370.

ELLEKER, M George; University of Alberta Hosp, 2E3WMC-8440 112 St NW, Edmonton AB T6G 2B7; Alb'75; FRCPC; Neur. Staff, University of Alberta Hospital; Assoc Dean Postgrad Med Educ, University of Alberta; (780)407-6528; Fax. (780)407-1325; george.elleker@ualberta.ca.

ELLEN, Ruth L B; Ellen Medicine Prof Corp, 1211 Agincourt Rd, Ottawa ON K2C 2H8; Ott'01; FRCPC; IntMed; GeriatricMed. Staff, The Ottawa Hospital - Civic Campus.

ELLERKER, Mark R; Glace Bay Family Practice Ctr, 35 Sterling Rd, Glace Bay NS B1A 3X6; Dal'94; CCFP; FCFP; (902)842-5400; Fax. (902)842-5323.

ELLERKER, Stephanie; Glace Bay Family Practice Ctr, 35 Sterling Rd, Glace Bay NS B1A 3X6; Mem'97; CCFP; Staff FamMed Faculty, Dalhousie University; (902)842-5400; Fax. (902)842-5323.

ELLESTAD, Leslie I; 204-2004 14 St NW, Calgary AB T2M 3N3; Alb'80; CCFP; Staff Community Med, Alberta Health Services; (403)221-9330

ELLETT, Robert W; Mission View Medical, 205-616 K.L.O. Rd, Kelowna BC V1Y 4X4; Man'73; FRCSC; GenSurg; VascSurg. (250)762-7731; Fax. (250)762-7502.

ELLEZAM, Benjamin; Hopital Ste-Justine, 3175 ch Cote-Sainte-Catherine, Montreal QC H3T 1C5; Mon'06; AnatPath. Staff, Hôpital Ste-Justine; (514)345-4931

ELLI, Eric R; Waterford Hosp, 306 Waterford Bridge Rd, St. John's NL A1E 4J8; Manila (Philippines)'84; Staff, Waterford Hospital; (709)777-3300

ELLINGHAM, Diana; Brock University Hlth Serv, 500 Glenridge Ave, St Catharines ON L2S 3A1; Mem'75; BMedSci; CCFP; FCFP; Physician, Brock University; Asst Clin Prof, McMaster University; (905)688-4692; Fax. (905)688-6448.

ELLINS, Mary L; Hamilton HS-General Site, 237 Barton St E, Hamilton ON L8L 2X2; McM'80; FRCPC; DiagRad (Interventional Radiology). Staff, Hamilton Health Sciences Centre - Hamilton General Hospital; (905)527-0271 x6521; Fax. (905)527-5761.

ELLIOT, David C; Piper Creek Med Clinic, 200-3215 49 Ave, Red Deer AB T4N 0M8; Wes'71; CCFP; FCFP; Staff, Red Deer Regional Hospital Centre.

ELLIOT, E Kathie; Kerrisdale Station Med Clinic, 2077 42nd Ave W, Vancouver BC V6M 2B4; UBC'63; (604)261-9494; Fax. (604)261-9405.

ELLIOT, Tracy L A; Foothills Med Centre, 1403 29 St NW, Calgary AB T2N 2T9; Wes'95; FRCPC; DiagRad (Breast Imaging). Staff, Foothills Medical Centre; Asst Prof, University of Alberta; (403)944-1110; tracyelliot@hotmail.com.

ELLIOTT, Alan; Northbrook Med Centre, 12357 Hwy 41 RR 1, Northbrook ON K0H 2G0; Qns'56; (613)336-8888; Fax. (613)336-2819.

ELLIOTT, Alari K; Queensway-Carleton Hosp, 3045 Baseline Rd, Nepean ON K2H 8P4; Ott'99; FRCPC; DiagRad. Sfty/Compl Mgr, Queensway Carleton Hospital; (613)721-2000

ELLIOTT, April S; Alberta Children's Hosp, 2888 Shaganappi Trail NW, Calgary AB T3B 6A8; McM'96; FRCPC; Peds. Staff, Alberta Children's Hospital; (403)955-7795

ELLIOTT, Brian D; Family Med Associates, 5021 51 St, Lacombe AB T4L 2A3; Alb'96; (403)782-3351; Fax. (403)782-5879.

ELLIOTT, Carl M; 1292 Weston Rd, Toronto ON M6M 4R3; Tor'51; CCFP; Staff, Humber River Regional Hospital - Church Street Site; (416)243-0700; Fax. (416)243-0624.

ELLIOTT, Catherine T; Environmental Hlth Services, 400-555 12th Ave W, Vancouver BC V5Z 3X7; UBC'04; FRCPC; CommunMed. (604)707-2462

ELLIOTT, Christopher R; 202-808 East River Rd, New Glasgow NS B2H 3S3; Dal'74; CCFP; Ac Staff, Aberdeen Regional Hospital; Preceptor, Dalhousie University; (902)752-6162

ELLIOTT, David; Nova Scotia Dept of Health, PO Box 488 Stn Central 4F-1894 Barrington St, Halifax NS B3J 2R8; Dal'81; BSc(Hons); MSc; Dir, Canadian Agency for Drugs & Technologies in Health; Aj Asst Prof, Dalhousie University; (902)424-4842; Fax. (902)424-0506.

ELLIOTT, Deborah; Providence Care DDCOT, 301-234 Concession St, Kingston ON K7K 6W6; Qns'79; FRCPC; Psy. (613)530-2400; Fax. (613)530-2212.

ELLIOTT, Denise M; Tower A, 5F-333 North River Rd, Ottawa ON K1A 0L1; Cal'96; MHA; CCFP; FCFP; Staff, Canadian Forces Health Services Centre; Langs: English; French; (613)952-3621

ELLIOTT, Elizabeth A; Guelph Gen Hosp, 115 Delhi St, Guelph ON N1E 4J4; McM'94; FRCSC; ObstGyn. Staff, Guelph General Hospital; (519)837-6440; Fax. (519)837-6452.

ELLIOTT, Jacobi; Grandview District Hosp, PO Box 399 644 Mill St, Grandview MB R0L 0Y0; Stellenbosch (South Africa)'94; CCFP; Staff, Grandview District Hospital; (204)546-2425; grandmed@mts.net.

ELLIOTT, Jacqueline M; Churchill Square Med Clinic, PO BOX 23205 Rpo Churchill Sq 209-10 Rowan St, St. John's NL A1B 4J9; Mem'03; CCFP; (709)722-8561; Fax. (709)722-7350.

ELLIOTT, James A; London HSC-Victoria Hosp, PO Box 5010 Stn B 800 Commissioners Rd E, London ON N6A 5W9; Wes'77; FRCPC; DiagRad (Interventional Radiology). Staff, London Health Sciences Centre - Victoria Campus; Asst Prof, University of Western Ontario; (519)685-8500; Fax. (519)667-6872.

ELLIOTT, Jason E; Heartland Fertility & Gyn Clin, 701-1661 Portage Ave, Winnipeg MB R3J 3T7; Man'07; FRCSC; ObstGyn.

ELLIOTT, John F; 625-2424 4 St SW, Calgary AB T2S 2T4; Alb'69; FRCPC; Psy. (403)229-1520

ELLIOTT, John F; Clinical Sciences Bldg, 2 125-11350 83 Ave NW, Edmonton AB T6G 2P4; Alb'82; BMedSci; PhD; FRCPC; Derm (Contact Dermatitis). Prof, University of Alberta; Dir Patch Test Clinic, University Dermatology Centre; (780)492-0895; Fax. (780)407-4548.

ELLIOTT, Lawrence J; Faculty of Med, S113-770 Bannatyne Ave, Winnipeg MB R3E 0W3; Man'85; FRCPC; CommunMed;CCFP; Dir Commun Med Residecy Prog/Asst Prof, University of Manitoba; Fax. (204)789-3905.

ELLIOTT, Lori T; Brantford Gen Hosp, 200 Terrace Hill St, Brantford ON N3R 1G9; McM'98; CCFP; CCFP(E.M.); FCFP; Staff, The Brant Community Healthcare System - Brantford General Hospital Site; (519)751-5507

ELLIOTT, Mary E; Univ Hlth Network-Princess M, 18 712-610 University Ave, Toronto ON M5G 2M9; Tor'84; FRCPC; Psy (Psychiatric Oncology). Prin Investigator, Princess Margaret Hospital - University Health Network; Lecturer, University of Toronto; (416)946-2897; Fax. (416)946-2284; mary.elliott@uhn.on.ca.

ELLIOTT, P Davis; Foothills Med Cetnre, 1403 29 St NW, Calgary AB T2N 2T9; Alb'67; DiagRad. Staff Diag. Imaging, Foothills Medical Centre; Asst Prof, University of Calgary; (403)944-1110

ELLIOTT, Robert D; The Ottawa Hosp-Gen Campus, 501 Smyth Rd, Ottawa ON K1H 8L6; Qns'74; FRCPC; Anes. Staff, The Ottawa Hospital - General Campus; Asst Prof, University of Ottawa; Langs: Bilingual(English/French); (613)737-8187; Fax. (613)737-8189.

ELLIOTT, Robert M; Turnbull Clinic, 201-170 Simcoe St, Peterborough ON K9H 2H7; McM'76; CCFP; FCFP; Staff, Peterborough Regional Health Centre - Hospital Drive; (705)748-2673; Fax. (705)742-8996; relliott@prhc.on.ca.

ELLIOTT, Scott H; Fairview Med Clinic, 222 Fairview Dr, Brantford ON N3R 2W9; Tor'86; CCFP; FCFP; Ac Staff, The Brant Community Healthcare System - Brantford General Hospital Site; (519)756-8340; Fax. (519)752-2256.

ELLIOTT, Stacy L; Purdy Pavilion, M41-2221 Westbrook Mall, Vancouver BC V6T 1Z9; UBC'85; Staff, Vancouver General Hospital - Centennial Pavillion; Ac Staff, G F Strong Rehabilitation Centre; Faculty, International Collaboration on Repair Discoveries; Clin Prof Psy & Urologic Sciences, University of British Columbia; (604)822-3690; Fax. (604)822-3148.

ELLIOTT, Teresa C; Alderlea Med Clinic, 101-330 Festubert St, Duncan BC V9L 3S9; Cape Town (South Africa)'91; MB ChB; CCFP; (250)748-9000; Fax. (250)748-1299.

ELLIOTT, Thomas G; Gordon & Leslie Diamond HCC, 4102-2775 Laurel St, Vancouver BC V5Z 1M9; Queensland (Australia)'82; MB BS; FRCPC; IntMed (Insurance Medicine); Endocrin&Metab. Staff, Vancouver General Hospital - Centennial Pavillion; Staff, Gordon & Leslie Diamond Health Care Centre; Assoc Prof, University of British Columbia; Langs: French; German; (604)875-5900; tom.elliott@ubc.ca.

ELLIOTT, Vance W; Synergy Wellness Centre, 113-501 Bethel Dr, Sherwood Park AB T8H 0N2; Sask'94; BSc; CCFP; (780)416-8999; Fax. (780)416-8977; info@drvanceelliott.com.

ELLIOTT, Wade C; Levy Elliott Sports Med Clinic, 102-1100 Walker's Line, Burlington ON L7N 2G3; McM'97; CCFP; (905)336-3340; Fax. (905)336-6095.

ELLIS, Anne K; Kingston Gen Hosp, Doran 1-76 Stuart St, Kingston ON K7L 2V7; Qns'99; BSc; MSc; FRCPC; IntMed (Anaphylaxis); ClinImmunol&Allergy. Att Physician, Kingston General Hospital; Clin Physician, Hôtel-Dieu Grace Hospital; Consultant Phys, St Mary's of the Lake; Assoc Prof, Queen's University; (613)548-2336; Fax. (613)546-3079.

ELLIS, Barry J; 11564 140 St NW, Edmonton AB T5M 1S7; Tor'89; CCFP; CCFP(E.M.); Staff, Royal Alexandra Hospital.

ELLIS, Catherine L; Hatchet Lake Med Centre, 2273 Prospect Rd, Brookside NS B3T 1S9; Dal'92; (902)852-3081; Fax. (902)852-5108.

ELLIS, Christine J; Rimbey Med Clinic, PO Box 650, Rimbey AB T0C 2J0; Alb'05; CCFP; (403)843-2256; Fax. (403)843-2255.

ELLIS, Connie L; Bowmont Med Clinic, 6535 Bowness Rd NW, Calgary AB T3B 0E8; Sask'91; CCFP; FCFP; Staff, Foothills Medical Centre; Clin Assoc Prof, University of Calgary; (403)247-9797; Fax. (403)247-0014; ellis@bowmont.net.

ELLIS, David A F; Art of Facial Surgery, 167 Sheppard Ave W, North York ON M2N 1M9; Tor'66; FACS; FRCSC; Otol (Facial Cosmetic). Ac Staff Facial Plastic Surg, Toronto General Hospital - UHN; Prof, University of Toronto; (416)229-1050; Fax. (416)229-1260; drface@artoffacialsurgery.com.

ELLIS, David R; Seafield Med Bldg, 1-1179 Seafield Cres, Nanaimo BC V9S 4S1; Otago (New Zealand)'67; MB ChB; FAAOS; FRCSC; OrthSurg (Arthroscopy). Ac Staff, Nanaimo Regional General Hospital; (250)754-3377; Fax. (250)754-1373.

ELLIS, Edward; 1934 Oakdean Cres, Gloucester ON K1J 6H3; San Francisco(CA) (USA)'71; MPH; FRCPC; CommunMed (Public Health & Preventive Medicine)., University of Ottawa; (613)406-8722

ELLIS, G Graham; 201-9656 King George Hwy, Surrey BC V3T 2V5; Oxford (England)'61; DPM(Lond); MRCPsy; MB BCh; MA(Oxon); FRCPC; Psy. (604)588-4644; Fax. (604)588-4644.

ELLIS, Jack M; Regional Mental HC-St Thomas, PO Box 2004 Stn Main 467 Sunset Dr, St Thomas ON N5P 3V9; Qns'81; BA(Hon); FRCPC; Psy (Forensic Psychiatry). Staff, Regional Mental Health Care-St Joseph's Health Care; (519)631-8510 x49408; Fax. (519)631-2361; jack.ellis@sjhc.london.on.ca.

ELLIS, Janet W M; Sunnybrook Health Sciences Ctr, FW 52-2075 Bayview Ave, Toronto ON M4N 3M5; Cambridge (England)'91; FRCPC; Psy. Staff, Toronto General Hospital - UHN; Staff, Sunnybrook Health Sciences Centre; (416)480-4073; Fax. (416)480-4613; janet.ellis@sunnybrook.ca.

ELLIS, Jennifer D; St Paul's Hosp, 1081 Burrard St, Vancouver BC V6Z 1Y6; UBC'99; FRCPC; DiagRad. Staff, Providence Health Care - St Paul's Hospital; (604)806-8006

ELLIS, John G; Impala Med Clinic, 111-3722 57 Ave, Red Deer AB T4N 4R7; Pretoria (South Africa)'90; MB ChB; LMCC; (403)352-7425; johngellis@hotmail.com.

ELLIS, Olga F; 201-9656 King George Hwy, Surrey BC V3T 2V5; Belfast (Ireland)'62; MB BCh; (604)588-4644; Fax. (604)588-4644.

ELLIS, Paul D; Univ Hlth Network-Toronto Gen, RFE GS 434-200 Elizabeth St, Toronto ON M5G 2C4; Tor'92; BSc; MSc; FRCPC; Neur (Emergency Medicine). Clin Associate, Toronto General Hospital - UHN; (416)340-5066; Fax. (416)340-4300.

ELLIS, Peter M; Kingston Gen Hosp, V3-76 Stuart St, Kingston ON K7L 2V7; McG'85; MSc(Exp.Surg.); FRCSC; Neursurg (Pain Management). Assoc Staff, Hotel-Dieu Hospital; Medicine Prof Corp, Kingston General Hospital; Asst Prof, Queen's University; (613)549-6666 x6029; Fax. (613)548-1346.

ELLIS, Peter; The Juravinski Cancer Centre, 699 Concession St, Hamilton ON L8V 5C2; Sydney (Australia)'88; MB BS; MMed; PhD; FRACP; FRCP; FRCPC; IntMed (Medical Oncology). Physician, The Juravinski Cancer Centre; McMaster University; (905)387-9495 x64609; Fax. (905)575-6326; peter.ellis@jcc.hhcc.ca.

ELLIS, Stephen D; Village Family Physicians, 275 Pictou Rd, Truro NS B2N 2S7; Dal'93; CCFP; (902)895-1232; Fax. (902)897-9749.

ELLIS, Susan M O; 77 Hunter St E, Hamilton ON L8N 1M4; McM'92; FRCSC; ObstGyn. Court Staff, Hamilton Health Sciences Centre - McMaster Children's Hospital; Ac Staff, St Joseph's Healthcare - Charlton Campus; Associate Clin Prof ObstGyn, McMaster University; (905)521-2788; Fax. (905)521-1127.

ELLIS GHIZ, Katherine; Queen Elizabeth Hosp, PO Box 6600 Stn Central 60 Riverside Dr, Charlottetown PE C1A 8T5; Dal'05; CCFP; Staff, Queen Elizabeth Hospital; (902)894-2111

ELLISON, Anthony K; 1-458 Reid St, Quesnel BC V2J 2M6; Witwatersrand (South Africa)'80; MB ChB; DA(Eng.); FFARCSI; (250)992-6006

ELLISON, C Andrew; 904-750 Broadway W, Vancouver BC V5Z 1H8; Cambridge (England)'67; MB BCh; MRCS; LRCP; CCFP; Ac Staff, Vancouver General Hospital - Centennial Pavillion; Court Staff, Providence Health Care - Mount Saint Joseph Hospital; Court Staff, BC Women's Hospital & Health Centre; (604)875-0282; Fax. (604)876-0323.

ELLISON, Erin; Royal Victoria Hosp, 201 Georgian Dr, Barrie ON L4M 6M2; UBC'86; FRCPC; AnatPath. Staff, Royal Victoria Regional Health Centre; (705)728-9090 x43204

ELLISON, Jason J; 22CF Health Services Centre, PO Box 6550 Stn Forces, Cold Lake AB T9M 2C6; Wes'07; CCFP; (780)840-8000

ELLISON, Philip; Univ Hlth Network-Toronto Western Hosp, 2W404-399 Bathurst St, Toronto ON M5T 2S8; Tor'78; MBA; CCFP; FCFP; Staff, Toronto Western Hospital - University Health Network; Asst Prof Family & Commun Med, University of Toronto; (416)603-5888; Fax. (416)603-5448; philip.ellison@uhn.on.ca.

ELLMAN, Jon P; McGill Mental Health Service, 5502-3600 rue McTavish, Montreal QC H3A 0G3; Ott'70; FRCPC; Psy. Staff Psy, McGill University Health Centre - Montreal General Campus; (514)398-6019

ELLS, Anna L; Ells Retina Centre, 344-933 17 Ave SW, Calgary AB T2T 5R6; Ott'87; FRCSC; Ophth (Retina). Staff, Alberta Children's Hospital; (403)245-3171; Fax. (403)245-4205.

ELLSMERE, James C D; Queen Elizabeth II HSC, 1276 South Park St, Halifax NS B3H 2Y9; Dal'99; FRCSC; GenSurg (Clinical & Investigative Medicine). Staff, Queen Elizabeth II Health Sciences Centre - Victoria General Site; (902)473-1886; Fax. (902)425-3817.

ELLSWORTH, Janet; Edmonton Clinic Hlth Academy, 4 515-11405 87 Ave NW, Edmonton AB T6G 1C9; Man'77; MD; FRCPC; Peds (Pediatric Rheumatology). Ac Staff, Glenrose Rehabilitation Hospital; Ac Staff, Stollery Children's Hospital; Staff, Edmonton Clinic Health Academy; Assoc Prof Peds, University of Alberta; (780)248-5620; Fax. (780)248-5628; janet.ellsworth@albertahealthservices.ca.

ELLTOFT, John D; 209 Church St, St Catharines ON L2R 3E8; Liverpool (England)'64; Langs: Bilingual(English/French); (905)682-5657

ELLWOOD, Amanda D; Regina Qu'Appelle HR-Regina, 1440 14th Ave, Regina SK S4P 0W5; Ott'06; FRCPC; IntMed; Nephrol. Staff, Regina General Hospital; (306)525-2404; Fax. (306)525-2553.

ELLYATT, William G; 105-750 Base Line Rd E, London ON N6C 2R5; Wes'58; CCFP; FCFP; Med Dir, Elmwood Nursing Home; (519)645-0706

ELLYSON, Josee; CSSS-IUGS-GMF-GF, 50 rue Camirand, Sherbrooke QC J1H 4J5; Sher'83; Staff, CSSS Institut universitaire de gériatrie de Sherbrooke; Staff Teacher, Universite de Sherbrooke; Langs: English; (819)780-2222; Fax. (819)562-3261; jellyson.gf@gmf.gouv.qc.ca.

ELMAN, Debra R; Sunnybrook Hlth Sciences Ctre, A101-2075 Bayview Ave, Toronto ON M4N 3M5; Tor'93; CCFP; FCFP; Assoc Staff Family & Community Med, North York General Hospital; Staff, Sunnybrook Health Sciences Centre; Teach Staff Family & Commun Med, University of Toronto; (416)480-4934; Fax. (416)480-6038; debra.elman@utoronto.ca.

ELMAN, Elyssa R; 800-1310 av Greene, Montreal QC H3Z 2B2; McG'08; CCFP; (514)780-2222; Fax. (514)780-2777.

ELMAN, Sheldon; Medisys Health Group, 1100-500 rue Sherbrooke O, Montreal QC H3A 3C6; McG'74; CCFP; (514)499-2782; Fax. (514)845-9178.

ELMANFUD, Omran R; Sunnybrook Hlth Sciences Ctr, E208-2075 Bayview Ave, Toronto ON M4N 3M5; Al Fateh (Libya)'98; FRCPC; IntMed; Cardiol. Staff, Sunnybrook Health Sciences Centre; Langs: Arabic; (416)480-4524; Fax. (416)480-4072.

ELMARAGHY, Amr W; Sunnyside Med Arts Centre, 504-27 Roncesvalles Ave, Toronto ON M6R 3B2; Tor'94; FRCSC; OrthSurg (Upper Extremity Surgery). Staff OrthSurg, St Joseph's Health Centre; Asst Prof, University of Toronto; (416)530-0400; Fax. (416)530-0692.

ELMARAGHY, Mohamed; Dr Elmaraghy Spa Surgica, 100-135 Erb St E, Waterloo ON N2J 1M3; Tor'93; FRCSC; PlasSurg (Breast Surgery). Chief PlasSurg, Grand River Hospital - Kitchener/Waterloo Health Centre; Chief Plastic Surg, St Mary's General Hospital; Physician, Spa Surgica; (519)585-0859; Fax. (519)585-7847; info@spasurgica.com.

ELMAYERGI, Nader; Mount Sinai Hosp, 600 University Ave, Toronto ON M5G 1X5; Cairo (Egypt)'98; MB ChB; FRCPC; IntMed; Cardiol. Staff, Mount Sinai Hospital; Langs: Arabic; (416)586-8472

ELMEKKAWI MOHAMED, Amir E A; The Hosp for Sick Children, 555 University Ave, Toronto ON M5G 1X8; Mansoura (Egypt)'00.

ELMER, Craig D; Prince Albert Med Clinic, 681 15th St W, Prince Albert SK S6V 7H9; Sask'81; Staff, Victoria Hospital; (306)764-1505; Fax. (306)764-7775.

ELMISTEKAWY, El Sayed M; 40 Ruskin St, Ottawa ON K1Y 4W7; (Egypt)'91; (613)761-4720; Fax. (613)761-4713.

ELMONTASER, Ghazi I A; Dr Everett Chalmers Reg Hosp, PO Box 9000 Stn A 700 Priestman St, Fredericton NB E3B 5N5; Al-Fateh (Libya)'96; FRCPC; AnatPath. Staff, Dr Everett Chalmers Regional Hospital; (506)452-5461

ELMS, Ford J; Health Sciences Centre, 300 Prince Philip Dr, St. John's NL A1B 3V6; Mem'84; FRCPC; GenPath. Staff, Health Sciences Centre; (709)737-6300

ELMSALLATI, Taher; River City Center, 605A-8600 Franklin Ave, Fort McMurray AB T9H 4G8; (Netherlands Antilles)'07; BScGeology; (780)750-5700; Fax. (780)750-5777.

ELMUSHARAF, Mohamed S; Rhema Med Clinic, 602-8600 Franklin Ave, Fort McMurray AB T9H 4G8; (Sudan)'88; CCFP; Clin Lecturer Faculty of Med & Dentistry, University of Alberta; Langs: Arabic; (780)714-9090; Fax. (780)714-9040.

ELOFF, Arnolda G; South Health Campus, 4F-4448 Front St SE, Calgary AB T3M 1M4; (South Africa)'79; MB ChB; MMed; Staff, Foothills Medical Centre; (403)956-2460; Fax. (403)956-2992.

ELOMAMI, Abdulghani; Red Deer Reg Hosp Ctr, PO Box 5030 Stn Postal Box Ctr 3942 50A Ave, Red Deer AB T4N 6R2; (Libya)'94; FRCPC; AnatPath. Staff, Red Deer Regional Hospital Centre; (403)356-4220; Fax. (403)352-7627.

ELOSKOUF, Carol M M Y; 132 The Queensway S, Keswick ON L4P 1Z7; Ain Shams (Egypt)'99; CCFP; Langs: Arabic; French; (905)989-2388; Fax. (905)989-0898.

ELOY, Laurence; CSSS du Nord de Lanaudière, 1000 boul Sainte-Anne, St-Charles-Brromee QC J6E 6J2; Sher'94; CSPQ; FRCSC; GenSurg. Staff, Centre Hospitalier Régional de Lanaudière; Langs: Bilingual(French/English); (450)759-8222; Fax. (450)756-6144.

ELREFAI, Thaer; 309-150 Montreal Rd, Ottawa ON K1L 8H2; Rostov (Russia (Federation))'96; CCFP; Staff, Dr A A Wilkinson Memorial Health Centre; Langs: Arabic; Russian; (613)695-9001; Fax. (613)695-8002.

ELRIFY, Elsaid R; Rouge Valley-Ajax & Pickering, 580 Harwood Ave S, Ajax ON L1S 2J4; Alexandria (Egypt)'89; Staff, Rouge Valley Health System - Ajax & Pickering Health Centre Site; Langs: Arabic; (905)683-2320

ELS, Charl; 154 Meadowlark Shopping Ctr NW, Edmonton AB T5R 5W9; Orange Free State (South Africa)'90; Staff, University of Alberta Hospital; (780)932-7217

ELS, Meandi; Atwood Med Clinic, 101-143 4th Ave S, Williams Lake BC V2G 1J7; Orange Free State (South Africa)'04; MB ChB; Langs: Afrikaans; (250)398-5162

ELSAWINIYA, Abdelbaset A; Misericordia Comm Hosp, 2F-16940 87 Ave NW, Edmonton AB T5R 4H5; Al-Fateh (Libya)'95; Staff, Covenant Health - Misericordia Community Hospital; Staff, Covenant Health - Grey Nuns Community Hospital; (780)735-2731; Fax. (780)735-2794.

ELSAYED, Sameer; London HSC-Victoria Hosp, 800 Commissioners Rd E, London ON N6A 5W9; Qns'95; MD; FRCPC; MedMicrobiol; IntMed; InfectDis. Staff, London Health Sciences Centre - Victoria Campus; Assoc Prof Medicine, Microbiol & Immunol & Path, University of Western Ontario; Langs: Arabic; (519)685-8726; Fax. (519)685-8109.

ELSDON, Thomas C; Windsor Health Centre, 462-1720 Howard Ave, Windsor ON N8X 5A6; Wes'83; FRCSC; Urol. Staff, Hôtel-Dieu Grace Hospital; Staff, Windsor Regional Hospital - Metropolitan Site; (519)977-5991; Fax. (519)977-9739.

ELSER, Christine; Mount Sinai Hosp, 1286-600 University Ave, Toronto ON M5G 1X5; (Germany)'95; Staff, Mount Sinai Hospital; Langs: German; (416)586-2899

ELSEY, Brent; Royal Victoria Hosp, 201 Georgian Dr, Barrie ON L4M 6M2; Tor'78; Staff, Royal Victoria Regional Health Centre; (705)792-3333; Fax. (705)728-4120.

ELSHAZLY, Shehab; University Hosp of Northern BC, 1475 Edmonton St, Prince George BC V2M 1S2; Ain Shams (Egypt)'98; DiagRad. Staff, University Hospital of Northern British Columbia; (250)565-2000

ELSHERIF, Hanan E L A; St Joseph's Hosp, 35 Algoma St N, Thunder Bay ON P7B 5G7; Cairo (Egypt)'87; Staff, St Joseph's Care Group - St Joseph's Hospital; (807)343-2463; Fax. (807)345-8177.

ELSHOBARY, Hanan M; Ctr Hosp de Lachine, 650 16e av, Lachine QC H8S 3N5; Mansoura (Egypt)'92; Staff, CSSS de Dorval-Lachine-Lasalle; (514)637-2351

ELSIDDEIG, Awatif H E; 12620A 132 Ave NW, Edmonton AB T5L 3P9; (Sudan)'94; MB BS; (780)990-1820; Fax. (780)488-0988.

ELSOBKY, Reem; St Joseph's Health Centre, 30 The Queensway, Toronto ON M6R 1B5; Ain Shams (Egypt)'94; FRCPC; IntMed. Staff, St Joseph's Health Centre; Langs: Arabic; (416)530-6084

ELSOLH, Bashar; Clinique Med Avicenne, 815 boul de la Cote-Vertu, Saint-Laurent QC H4L 1Y6; Damascus (Syria)'80; (514)748-8999; Fax. (514)748-6527.

ELSTEIN, Eleanor; MUHC-Royal Victoria Hosp, M4 76-687 av des Pins O, Montreal QC H3A 1A1; Mon'85; FACC; CSPQ; FRCPC; IntMed; Cardiol. Staff, McGill University Health Centre - Royal Victoria Hospital; (514)934-1934

ELSTEIN, Jack; 1746 ch Chambly, Longueuil QC J4J 3X5; Ott'76; ABIM; FACP; FRCPC; IntMed. Staff, McGill University Health Centre - Montreal General Campus; adj Prof, McGill University; (450)646-2900

ELSUGY, Ramadan E; 606-2250 Bovaird Dr E, Brampton ON L6R 0W3; Al Fateh (Libya)'96; ObstGyn. Langs: Arabic; (905)497-7666; Fax. (905)497-7999.

ELTAYEB, Suha; Ajax Med Arts Bldg, 202-601 Harwood Ave S, Ajax ON L1S 2J5; Tor'94; FRCSC; ObstGyn. Ac Staff ObstGyn, Rouge Valley Health System - Ajax & Pickering Health Centre Site; Langs: Arabic; French; (905)427-0558; Fax. (905)427-1268.

ELUMIR, Lizette L M; Lake Bonavista Shopping Ctr, 141-755 Lake Bonavista Dr SE, Calgary AB T2J 0N3; Tor'99; CCFP; (403)852-4946; Fax. (403)204-9078.

ELVES, Emmett J; The Brandon Clinic, 620 Dennis St, Brandon MB R7A 5E7; Man'75; BSc; FRCPC; Peds (Child Abuse). Chief Peds, Brandon Regional Health Centre; Lecturer Family Pract & Peds, University of Manitoba; (204)728-4440; Fax. (204)726-1765.

ELWELL, Leo B; 3-9 Chippewa Rd, Sherwood Park AB T8A 6J7; Alb'94; FRCPC; Psy. (780)410-8011

ELWOOD, J Mark; Cancer Research Centre, 2 109-675 10th Ave W, Vancouver BC V5Z 1L3; Queen's (Ireland)'70; DSc; MBA; MB BCh; FAFPHM; FRCPC; CommunMed (Electromagnetic Fields); Public Health & Preventive Med.

ELWOOD, Richard K; BC Centre for Disease Control, 655 12th Ave W, Vancouver BC V5Z 4R4; National (Ireland)'70; MB ChB; MRCP(UK); FRCP; FRCPC; IntMed (Tuberculosis); Respir. Clin Physician, BC Centre For Disease Control; Clin Prof, University of British Columbia; (604)707-2702; Fax. (604)707-2690; kevin.elwood@bccdc.ca.

ELYABROUDI, William; Ctr Hosp de Matane, 333 rue Thibault, Matane QC G4W 2W5; (Syria)'95; Staff, Centre Hospitalier de Matane; (418)562-3135; Fax. (418)562-1823.

ELYAS, Ausama H; Flin Flon Gen Hosp, PO Box 340 50 Church St, Flin Flon MB R8A 1N2; Baghdad (Iraq)'87; Staff Dialysis Unit, Flin Flon General Hospital Inc; Langs: Arabic; (204)687-7591

ELYSEE, Jacques S; CHUQ-Hotel-Dieu de Quebec, 11 Cote du Palais, Quebec QC G1R 2J6; (Haiti)'95; Staff, Centre Hospitalier Universitaire de Québec (CHUQ) - Siege Social; (418)691-5288; Fax. (418)691-5186.

ELZAWI, Abdul F M; 401-1590 Yonge St, Toronto ON M4T 1Z8; Al Fateh (Libya)'81; ABIM; FRCPC; IntMed (Cardiology). Staff Cardiologist, Women's College Hospital; Langs: Italian; Arabic; (416)962-5545; Fax. (416)962-6676.

ELZINGA, Christine L; Tom Baker Cancer Centre, 1331 29 St NW, Calgary AB T2N 4N2; Cal'84; CCFP; FCFP; Staff, Rockyview General Hospital; (403)521-3093

EMAMI, S Sean; 28 Langstaff Rd E, Thornhill ON L3T 3P8; Tor'00; CCFP; (905)709-9985; Fax. (905)709-4138.

EMARA, Barry; South Walkerville Med Centre, 200-2224 Walker Rd, Windsor ON N8W 5L7; Wes'95; FRCSC; Ophth (Cataract). Staff Ophth, Hôtel-Dieu Grace Hospital; Staff Ophth, Windsor Regional Hospital - Metropolitan Site; Surgeon Refractive, Lasik Centers of America; Aj Prof, University of Western Ontario; Langs: Arabic; (519)258-0162; Fax. (519)252-7223.

EMARD, Helene; CLSC Montcalm, RR 1 110 rue St-Isidore, Saint-Esprit QC J0K 2L0; Mon'88; Physician, CHSLD Montcalm-Foyer St-Jacques; (450)839-3676; Fax. (450)839-6603.

EMBER, Andrew P; Canadian Pansion Plan, 5A-333 North River Rd, Ottawa ON K1A 0L1; McG'72; MDCM; CCBOM; CCFP; FCFP; Langs: English; French; (613)952-9462; Fax. (613)954-4927.

EMBERLEY, Julie; Dr Charles A Janeway Child HC, 300 Prince Philip Dr, St. John's NL A1B 3V6; Mem'06; FRCPC; Peds (Neonatal & Perinatal Medicine). Staff, Janeway Children's Health & Rehabilitation Centre; (709)777-6300

EMBIL, John; Health Sciences Centre, MS673-820 Sherbrook St, Winnipeg MB R3A 1R9; Dal'89; FRCPC; IntMed; InfectDis (Wound Care). Consultant InfectDis, Health Sciences Centre; Prof, University of Manitoba; Langs: Spanish; Bilingual(French/English); (204)787-4654; Fax. (204)787-2989; jembil@hsc.mb.ca.

EMBREE, Joanne; 545-730 William Ave, Winnipeg MB R3E 3J7; Dal'81; FRCPC; Peds; InfectDis. Staff Children's Hosp, Health Sciences Centre; Dept Head Med Microbiol/Assoc Prof, University of Manitoba; (204)789-3619; embree@ms.umanitoba.ca.

EMELIANOVA, Svetlana; North York Gen Hosp-Branson, 2F-555 Finch Ave W, North York ON M2R 1N5; Moscow 2 (Russia (Federation))'92; FRCPC; Psy. Staff, North York General Hospital - Branson Division; Staff, Women's College Hospital; (416)632-8701; Fax. (416)632-8718.

EMERIAUD, Guillaume; Hôpital Ste-Justine, 3175 ch Cote-Ste-Catherine, Montreal QC H3T 1C5; (France)'00; Critical Care Medicine (P.Q.). Staff, Hôpital Ste-Justine; (514)345-4931 x3316; Fax. (514)345-7731.

EMERSON, Brian P; Ministry of Health, 4 2-1515 Blanshard St, Victoria BC V8W 3C8; UBC'85; MHSc; Med Officer of Hlth, Vancouver Island Health Authority; (250)952-1701

EMERSON, Kelly J; The Simcoe Clinic, 2-279 Yonge St, Barrie ON L4N 7T9; Cal'92; CCFP; FCFP; Staff, Royal Victoria Regional Health Centre; (705)728-8860; Fax. (705)737-4733.

EMERSON, Yvette; Selkirk & District Gen Hosp, PO Box 5000 Stn Main 100 Easton Dr, Selkirk MB R1A 2M2; Man'92; CCFP; Selkirk & District General Hospital; (204)482-5800

EMERY, Andrew N; Cobourg Med Centre, 5-1060 Burnham St, Cobourg ON K9A 5V9; London (England)'72; MB BS; DObstRCOG; MRCGPract; Ac Staff, Northumberland Hills Hospital; (905)373-8333

EMERY, Christopher; Envoy Med Dispatch, 481-1/2 William Ave, Winnipeg MB R3A 0J5; Man'74; Ac Staff, St Boniface General Hospital; (204)786-4444; Fax. (204)774-1157.

EMERY, Derek J; University of Alberta Hosp, 8440 112 St NW, Edmonton AB T6G 2B7; Cal'86; FRCPC; DiagRad (Neuro Radiology). Staff, University of Alberta Hospital; (780)407-6907; Fax. (780)407-6176.

EMERY, France; Clin Med du Vieux-Terrebonne, 883 rue Saint-Pierre, Terrebonne QC J6W 1E6; Mon'83; Langs: English; (450)964-9111

EMERY, Marie-Lou; CSSS de la Cote-de-Gaspe, 215 boul de York O, Gaspe QC G4X 2W2; Mon'07; CCFP; CCFP(E.M.); Staff, Centre Hospitalier de Gaspe; (418)368-3301

EMERY, William A; 16-495 36 St NE, Calgary AB T2A 6K3; Liverpool (England)'76; MB ChB; DRCOG; MRC; (403)514-6001; Fax. (403)514-6002.

EMERY, William T; Valley Med Clinic, PO Box 2932 Stn Main 231 First Ave, Strathmore AB T1P 1L5; Alb'10; CCFP; (403)934-4444

EMES, Craig E; 201-26 Bastion Sq, Victoria BC V8W 1H9; Alb'90; FRCPC; Psy. (250)381-6030

EMIL, Sherif G S; MUHC-Montreal Children Hosp, C818-2300 rue Tupper, Montreal QC H3H 1P3; McG'91; FACS; FAAP; FRCSC; GenSurg; PedGenSurg. Staff, McGill University Health Centre - Montreal Children's Hospital; Langs: Arabic; French; (514)412-4497; Fax. (514)412-4289; sherif.emil@mcgill.ca.

EMILI, Anna-Marie; Main West Med Group, 300-1685 Main St W, Hamilton ON L8S 1G5; McM'00; CCFP; Assoc Staff Family Med, Hamilton Health Sciences Centre - McMaster Children's Hospital; Physician, Main West Medical Group; (905)522-8915

EMILI, Julie-Anne; Main West Med Group, 300-1685 Main St W, Hamilton ON L8S 1G5; McM'00; FRCPC; CommunMed;CCFP; Staff, Hamilton Health Sciences Centre - McMaster Children's Hospital; Physician, Main West Medical Group; (905)522-8915; emilij@mcmaster.ca.

EMINI, Neim N; Orangeville Family Med Centre, M1-32 First St, Orangeville ON L9W 2E1; Flinders (Australia)'08; CCFP; (519)938-8000; Fax. (519)938-8080.

EMMANUEL, Majella; Univ Hlth Network-Toronto Gen, 200 Elizabeth St, Toronto ON M5G 2C4; UBC'05; CCFP; CCFP(E.M.); Staff, Toronto General Hospital - UHN; Langs: Tamil; (416)340-3111

EMMENEGGER, Urban; Sunnybrook Hlth Sciences Ctre, 2075 Bayview Ave, Toronto ON M4N 3M5; Bern (Switzerland)'92; Staff, Sunnybrook Health Sciences Centre; (416)480-4928

EMMOTT, Kirsten B; Southwood Med Clinic, 1700-2751 Cliffe Ave, Courtenay BC V9N 2L8; UBC'73; Ac Staff, St Joseph's General Hospital; (250)334-2212; kbemmott@shaw.ca.

EMOKPARE, Bernard D; Quance East Med Clinic, 1-2223 Victoria Ave E, Regina SK S4N 6E4; Benin (Nigeria)'95; MB BS; (306)522-2278; Fax. (306)522-2281.

EMON, Steven J; Active Health Sports Med Ctre, 112-115 Bell Farm Rd, Barrie ON L4M 5G1; Tor'91; FRCSC; Ophth. Ac Staff, Royal Victoria Regional Health Centre; Ac Staff, Orillia Soldiers' Memorial Hospital; (705)727-1500; Fax. (705)727-1562.

EMOND, Anne; Hop du Sacre Coeur de Mtl, 5400 boul Gouin O, Montreal QC H4J 1C5; Laval'79; FRCP; CSPQ; FRCPC; Psy. Staff Geriatric Psy, Hôpital du Sacre-Coeur de Montréal; Langs: English; (514)338-3563; Fax. (514)338-4359.

EMOND, Benoit; Ctr Hosp Laurentien, 234 rue Saint-Vincent, Ste-Agathe-des-Mts QC J8C 2B8; Laval'96; CSPQ; FRCSC; GenSurg. Staff, Centre Hospitalier Laurentien; (819)324-4000

EMOND, Carl P; St Mary's Hosp Centre, 3830 av Lacombe, Montreal QC H3T 1M5; McG'77; CSPQ; FRCSC; GenSurg (Surgical Oncology); VascSurg. Staff, St Mary's Hospital Centre; Asst Prof Surg, McGill University; Langs: Bilingual(English/French); (514)734-2698

EMOND, Daniel; Ctr Hosp de Verdun, 4000 boul Lasalle, Verdun QC H4G 2A3; Mon'95; Staff Emerg & Cardiol, Centre Hospitalier de Verdun; (514)362-1000 x2141

EMOND, Danielle; Regie l'Assurance Maladie QC, Q044-1125 Grande Allee O, Quebec QC G1S 1E7; Laval'98; Nephrol; IntMed. Staff, Hôpital Regional Rimouski; (418)682-5144 x4886

EMOND, Francois; Ctr Hosp Affilie-Enfant-Jesus, 1401 18e rue, Quebec QC G1J 1Z4; Laval'97; FRCPC; Neur (Multiple Sclerosis). Staff, Centre Francois-Charon; Staff, Centre Hospitalier Affilié Universitaire de Québec - Hôpital De L'Enfant Jésus; Langs: Bilingual(English/French); (418)649-0252; Fax. (418)649-5915.

EMOND, Gilles; Clinique Med St-Jerome, 102-450 boul Monseigneur-Duboi, Saint-Jerome QC J7Y 3L8; Mon'97; Staff, Centre Hospitalier Laurentien; Langs: Bilingual(French/English); (450)438-1776; Fax. (450)438-6119.

EMOND, Jean-Paul; Hotel-Dieu de Levis, 143 rue Wolfe, Levis QC G6V 3Z1; Laval'65; Urol. Ac Staff, Hôtel-Dieu de Lévis; (418)835-7121

EMOND, Joanne; Direction de la Sante Publique, 1255 rue Beauregard, Longueuil QC J4K 2M3; Mon'78; (450)928-6777 x5412; Fax. (450)928-6783.

EMOND, Julie; CSSS Haute Gaspésie, 50 rue du Belvedere, Ste-Anne-des-Monts QC G4V 1X4; Sher'95; FRCPC; IntMed. Staff, Centre Hospitalier des Monts; (418)763-2261

EMOND, Karine; Clinique Med du Lac, 33 rue Saint-Patrice E, Magog QC J1X 5B7; Sher'08; CCFP; (819)843-3353

EMOND, Marcel; Ctr Hosp Affilie-Enfant-Jesus, 1401 18e rue, Quebec QC G1J 1Z4; Mon'98; FRCPC; EmergMed;CCFP; CCFP(E.M.); Staff, Centre Hospitalier Affilié Universitaire de Québec - Hôpital De L'Enfant Jésus; (418)649-5632

EMOND, Michael; Kincardine Comm Med Clinic, 44 Queen St, Kincardine ON N2Z 3C1; Tor'78; DOHS; CCFP; FCFP; Physician, South Grey Bruce Health Centre; (519)396-6749; Fax. (519)396-6177; memondear@gmail.com.

EMOND, Michel; Ctr Devaluation de Sante Fonda, 1001 rue Saint-Denis, Montreal QC H2X 3H9; Mon'60; FRCPC; IntMed; Gastroent (P.Q.). ac Staff, Centre Hospitalier l'Université de Montréal (CHUM) - Hôpital Notre-Dame; (514)890-8332; Fax. (514)412-7362.

EMOND, Mutsuko; Hôpital Ste-Justine, 3175 ch Cote-Ste-Catherine, Montreal QC H3T 1C5; Toho (Japan)'90; PhD; Psy (P.Q.). Clin Prof, Hôpital Ste-Justine; Langs: Japanese; (514)345-4931 x4586

EMOND, Natalie; Polyclinique, Rc60-5345 boul de l'Assomption, Montreal QC H1T 4B3; Mon'92; CCFP; Langs: English; (514)257-7000; Fax. (514)257-7003; nemond@md-plus.ca.

EMOND, Nathalie; UMF Laval CSSSVC, 2690 ch des Quatre-Bourgeois, Quebec QC G1V 0B7; Laval'00; Staff, Hôpital Laval; (418)656-4795; Fax. (418)656-4503.

EMOND, Sylvie; Clin Med Bourg-Royal-80, 1289 boul Louis-XIV, Quebec QC G2L 1M1; Laval'88; (418)627-7129; Fax. (418)627-7145.

EMPEY, Karen E; Unionville Family Physicians, 201-10 Unionville Gate, Markham ON L3R 0W7; Tor'78; CCFP; FCFP; Court Staff, The Scarborough Hospital - Birchmount Campus; (905)305-7642; Fax. (905)305-7495.

EMRICH, A George; St Thomas Walk in Med Clinic, 230 First Ave, St Thomas ON N5R 4P5; Wes'71; (519)633-9627; Fax. (519)633-9677.

EMRICH, H Walter; Maple Family Health Team, 71 Clergy St E, Kingston ON K7L 3J3; Qns'76; CCFP; FCFP; Associate, Kingston General Hospital; Associate, Hotel-Dieu Hospital; Asst Prof Family Med, Queen's University; (613)542-7858; Fax. (613)544-9795.

EMSALEM, Abdurahman M; Grey Bruce HS-Owen Sound, PO Box 1800 Stn M 1800 8th St E, Owen Sound ON N4K 6M9; Al Fateh (Libya)'05; MB BCh; Staff, Grey Bruce Health Services - Owen Sound; (519)376-2121

EMSALEM, Ahmed M K M; Brentwood Medical, 78 Athabascan Ave, Sherwood Park AB T8A 4E3; Al Fateh (Libya)'99; MB ChB; CCFP; (780)467-0083

EMSLIE, Linda M; Regina Mental Health Clinic, 3F-2110 Hamilton St, Regina SK S4P 2E3; Glasgow (Scotland)'79; MRCPsy(UK); MB ChB; (306)766-7800; Fax. (306)766-7811.

EMSLIE, R Jim; Dr R Jim Emslie Inc, 16-1710 Ellis St, Kelowna BC V1Y 2B5; UBC'77; BSc; Staff, Kelowna General Hospital; (250)763-4111; Fax. (250)763-4112.

ENACHE, Lucian; GMF Concorde, 300 boul de la Concorde E, Laval QC H7G 2E6; Mon'09; CCFP; (450)667-5310

ENARSON, Mark; Edmonton Clinic Hlth Academy, 3 512-11405 87 Ave, Edmonton AB T6G 1C9; Alb'00; FRCPC; Peds; PedEmergMed. Staff Peds Emerg, University of Alberta Hospital; Staff Ped, Edmonton Clinic Health Academy; (780)248-5575; Fax. (780)248-5626.

ENARSON, Paul J; Children's & Women's HC of BC, 4480 Oak St, Vancouver BC V6H 3V4; Cal'06; FRCPC; Peds; PedEmergMed. Staff, BC Children's Hospital; (604)875-2345 x7333

ENCHIN, Adam M; Youthdale Treatment Centres, 227 Victoria St, Toronto ON M5T 1T8; Wes'97; FRCPC; Psy;CCFP; (461)363-3751; Fax. (416)363-7945.

ENDER, Peter; Hop Jean-Talon, 1385 rue Jean-Talon E, Montreal QC H2E 1S6; Ott'77; FRCPC; Neur (P.Q.) (Clinical Neurology). Staff Neurol, CSSS du Coeur de l'Isle Hôpital Jean-Talon; Staff Neurol, Hopital Marie Clarac; (514)495-6767; Fax. (514)495-6738; peter.ender.cdi@ssss.gouv.qc.ca.

ENDERSBY, Ryan; Chinook Reg Hosp, 960 19 St S, Lethbridge AB T1J 1W5; Alb'04; FRCPC; Anes. Staff, Chinook Regional Hospital; (403)388-6111

ENDSIN, Arnold; Workers' Compensation Board, 200-1881 Scarth St, Regina SK S4P 4L1; Sask'80; CCFP; FCFP; Med Consultant, Consumer's Co-Op Refineries Lt; Med Consultant, Saskatoon Government Insurance; Med Consultant, Worker's Comp Board of SK; (306)787-4458; Fax. (306)780-5559.

ENE, Mokelu; Regina Med Centre, 100-2550 12th Ave, Regina SK S4P 3X1; (306)566-4120; Fax. (306)566-4150.

ENENAJOR, Aweriarue G; Hys Centre, 503-11010 101 St NW, Edmonton AB T5H 4B9; (Slovakia)'80; FRCPC; IntMed. Staff, University of Alberta Hospital; (780)496-1390; Fax. (780)496-1387.

ENEPEKIDES, Danny J; Sunnybrook Hlth Sciences Ctre, M1 102-2075 Bayview Ave, Toronto ON M4N 3M5; McG'94; FRCSC; Otol. Staff, Sunnybrook Health Sciences Centre; (416)480-5125

ENG, Aik-Ping; 523 Main St, Vancouver BC V6A 2V1; Taiwan (Taiwan)'68; Assoc Staff, Vancouver General Hospital - Centennial Pavillion; Vis Staff, Providence Health Care - St Paul's Hospital; Langs: Cantonese; Fookien; Hakka; Malay; Taiwanese; Teochew; (604)683-5230

ENG, Frank; Medical Arts Bldg, 603-581 Davis Dr, Newmarket ON L3Y 2P6; McG'03; MDCM; PhD; FRCSC; GenSurg (Laparoscopic Surgery). Ac Staff, Southlake Regional Health Centre; Lecturer, University of Toronto; Langs: French; Cantonese; (905)830-3588; Fax. (905)830-3530.

ENG, Helen W K; 101-15451 Russell Ave, White Rock BC V4B 2R5; Alb'95; CCFP; Langs: Cantonese; (604)531-5595; drhelen5@yahoo.ca.

ENG, Henry S; 425-100 Richmond St W, Toronto ON M5H 3K6; Tor'80; Staff, Toronto East General Hospital Inc; (416)360-8208; Fax. (416)360-0692.

ENG, Kenneth; Sunnybrook Health Sciences Cen, M1 202B-2075 Bayview Ave, Toronto ON M4N 3M5; Tor'96; FRCSC; Ophth (Retina Vitreous Ophthalmology). Staff, Sunnybrook Health Sciences Centre; Asst Prof, University of Toronto; (416)480-4688; Fax. (416)480-4481.

ENG, Michael K; St Paul's Hosp, C319-1081 Burrard St, Vancouver BC V6Z 1Y6; Cal'02; FRCSC; Urol. Staff, Providence Health Care - St Paul's Hospital; (604)806-9610

ENG, Stanley L; Elemental Prof Health Centre, 1600 Pembina Hwy, Winnipeg MB R3T 5Z2; Man'99; CCFP; (204)475-1600; Fax. (204)475-1601; dreng@mts.net.

ENGBERS, Peter B; Woodstock Gen Hosp, 310 Juliana Dr, Woodstock ON N4V 0A4; Wes'84; AnatPath; GenPath. Staff Path, Woodstock General Hospital; (519)421-4205; pengbers@wgh.on.ca.

ENGEL, Andre; Aim Health Group, 22B-550 Terminal Ave, Ottawa ON K1G 0Z3; McG'71; AB; Peds. Ac Staff, Children's Hospital of Eastern Ontario (CHEO); Langs: Hebrew; Hungarian; French; (613)731-2244; Fax. (613)731-4979.

ENGEL, Bruce E; Greenbank Med Centre, 102-139 Greenbank Rd, Nepean ON K2H 9A5; Qns'67; FRCSC; Ophth. (613)829-2031; Fax. (613)829-2274.

ENGEL, C Jay; Kingston Reg Cancer Ctr, 25 King St W, Kingston ON K7L 5P9; Dublin (Ireland)'84; MB ChB; FACS; FRCSC; GenSurg (Surgical Oncology). Assoc Prof, Queen's University; (613)544-2361 x6651; Fax. (613)546-8221.

ENGEL, Christopher V W; Rehabilitation Centre, RR135-800 Sherbrook St, Winnipeg MB R3A 1M4; Man'72; FRCPC; PhysMed&Rehab. Staff, Health Sciences Centre; (204)787-2290; Fax. (204)787-1476; cengel@hsc.mb.ca.

ENGEL, Francis; Maternity & Gynecology Centre, 1811 av Dollard, LaSalle QC H8N 1T9; Laval'79; LMCC; ObstGyn. Ac Staff, Centre Hospitalier de LaSalle; Ac Staff, CSSS de Dorval-Lachine-Lasalle; Consultant, Hôpital Anna-Laberge; (514)364-3700

ENGEL, Jeff S; Dr C W Wiebe Med Centre, 385 Main St, Winkler MB R6W 1J2; Man'88; FRCSC; OrthSurg. (204)325-4312

ENGELBERG, David; Royal Bank Plaza Med Centre, LR8-200 Bay St, Toronto ON M5J 2J3; UBC'99; DMD; CCFP; Lecturer Family & Community Med/Aj Prof Family & Dentistry, University of Toronto; Langs: Hebrew; (416)368-6787; Fax. (416)368-7632.

ENGELBRECHT, Adele; Bigelow-Fowler Clinic, 1605 9 Ave S, Lethbridge AB T1J 1W2; (South Africa)'07; MB BCh; (403)327-3121

ENGELBRECHT, Frederik H S; PO Box 2316, Battleford SK S0M 0E0; Pretoria (South Africa)'90; MB ChB; BSc(Hon); CCFP; Staff Staff Phy, Melfort Hospital; Langs: Afrikaans; (306)937-2485; erik05@sasktel.net.

ENGELBRECHT, Jan; The Rhema Clinic, 1439 1st St, Brandon MB R7A 2Y7; Pretoria (South Africa)'87; Staff, Brandon Regional Health Centre; Med Examiner, Province of Manitoba; Langs: Afrikaans; (204)728-3600; Fax. (204)725-0414; jan.engelbrecht@gmail.com.

ENGELBRECHT, Roland; Atwood Med Clinic, 101-143 Fourth Ave S, Williams Lake BC V2G 1J8; (South Africa)'08; MB ChB; (250)398-5162

ENGELBRECHT, Stephanus J; Western Med Clinic, 144 6th St, Brandon MB R7A 3N2; Orange Free State (South Africa)'91; MB ChB; LMCC; Staff, Brandon Regional Health Centre; Langs: Afrikaans; (204)727-6451; Fax. (204)727-4150.

ENGELBRECHT, Werner; 302 Cameron St, Williams Lake BC V2G 1S9; Orange Free State (South Africa)'04; MB ChB; (250)305-1102; Fax. (250)305-1138.

ENGELBRECHT, William M; Wentworth Medical & Cosmetic, 6201-873 85 St SW, Calgary AB T3H 0J5; (South Africa)'00; (403)217-6453; Fax. (403)217-5235.

ENGELL, Anne; Creemore Med Centre, 1-15 Elizabeth St E, Creemore ON L0M 1G0; Tor'79; CCFP; FCFP; Chief of Staff, Collingwood General & Marine Hospital; (705)466-3077; Fax. (705)466-2587.

ENGELS, Holger; Tilbury District Family Hlth Team, PO Box 760 22 Mill St W, Tilbury ON N0P 2L0; Tor'85; (519)682-2307; Fax. (519)682-9979; dochoagie@tdhft.ca.

ENGELS, Paul; Royal Alexandra Hosp, 205CSC-10240 Kingsway NW, Edmonton AB T5H 3V9; Wes'03; FACS; FRCSC; GenSurg; Critical Care Medicine. Staff, Royal Alexandra Hospital; (780)735-6924; Fax. (780)735-6925.

ENGEN, Dale A; Kingston Gen Hosp, 76 Stuart St, Kingston ON K7L 2V7; Sask'99; FRCPC; Anes. Staff, Kingston General Hospital; (613)549-6666 x4914; Fax. (613)548-1375.

ENGFIELD, Marc; CSSS-Hopital De Hull, 116 boul Lionel-Emond, Gatineau QC J8Y 1W7; Ott'98; FRCPC; IntMed (Critical Care Medicine). Staff, Hull Hospital; Langs: German; French; (819)595-6000

ENGINEER, Ariz A; Fairlawn Med Centre, 209-2401 Yonge St, Toronto ON M4P 3H1; Tor'87; Langs: Gujarati; Hindi; (416)322-9933; Fax. (416)322-7097.

ENGLAND, Michael B A; 105 Dunedin Rd, Rothesay NB E2H 1P6; Tor'67; FRCPC; DiagRad. Staff Radiol, Saint John Regional Hospital; Staff Radiol, St Joseph's Hospital; Teach Staff, Dalhousie University; (506)632-5555; drengland@health.nb.ca.

ENGLAND, Ronald M; Worker's Comp Board, 150-4311 12 St NE, Calgary AB T2E 4P9; Ott'77; FRCSC; OrthSurg.

ENGLE, Fredric M; 3 335-700 University Ave, Toronto ON M5G 1Z5; Alb'69; BSc; FACOG; FRCSC; ObstGyn (Colposcopy). Assoc Staff, Mount Sinai Hospital; Asst Prof ObstGyn, University of Toronto; (416)586-5252; Fax. (416)586-8612; fred.engle@utoronto.ca.

ENGLE, John; Kincardine Commun Med Clinic, 44 Queen St, Kincardine ON N2Z 3C1; (519)396-6747; Fax. (519)396-6177.

ENGLERT, Peter S; 69 Main St PO Box 1269, Grand Bend ON N0M 1T0; McM'77; BSc(Hon); CCFP; FCFP; Ac Staff, South Huron Hospital Association; Aj Prof Family Med, University of Western Ontario; (519)238-2362; Fax. (519)238-6478; penglert@gbchc.com.

ENGLISH, Edward; 2519 Yonge St, Toronto ON M4P 2H9; Tor'66; BA; FRCSC; OrthSurg (General Orthopedics). Staff, Providence Healthcare; Ac Staff, The Scarborough Hospital - General Campus; Consultant, St John's Rehabilitation Hospital; (416)482-2399; Fax. (416)482-9904.

ENGLISH, John C; Vancouver Gen Hosp, 855 12th Ave W, Vancouver BC V5Z 1M9; Cal'84; FRCPC; AnatPath. Consultant Path, Vancouver General Hospital - Centennial Pavillion; Clinical Asst Prof, University of British Columbia; (604)875-4480; john.english@vch.ca.

ENGLISH, Jordan H; Hys Med Centre, 202-11010 101 St NW, Edmonton AB T5H 4B9; Alb'99; FRCPC; DiagRad. (780)426-1121; Fax. (780)425-5979.

ENGLISH, Keltie; Cobequid Commun Health Ctr, 40 Freer Lane, Lower Sackville NS B4C 0A2; Dal'80; BSc; Staff, Cobequid Community Health Centre; (902)865-1160

ENGLISH, Kerri E; Hamilton HS-General Site, 237 Barton St E, Hamilton ON L8L 2X2; Wes'02; CCFP; CCFP(E.M.); Staff, Hamilton Health Sciences Centre - Hamilton General Hospital; (905)521-2100

ENGLISH, Michael J; MUHC-Montreal Gen Hosp, 1650 av Cedar, Montreal QC H3G 1A4; Newcastle-upon-Tyne (England)'69; FRCA; CSPQ; FRCPC; Anes (P.Q.). Staff, McGill University Health Centre - Montreal General Campus; assoc Prof, McGill University; (514)934-1934 x4324

ENGLISH, Nicole M; Rexdale Med Centre, 2-123 Rexdale Blvd, Etobicoke ON M9W 1P1; Tor'93; CCFP; (416)743-5853; Fax. (416)743-1358.

ENGLISH, Shane; The Ottawa Hosp-Civic Campus, 1053 Carling Ave, Ottawa ON K1Y 4E9; Ott'05; FRCPC; IntMed; Critical Care Medicine., The Ottawa Hospital - General Campus; Staff, The Ottawa Hospital - Civic Campus; Langs: Bilingual(English/French); (613)737-8222

ENGMAN, Richard T; 1822 Comox Ave, Comox BC V9M 3M7; Cal'84; FRCPC; IntMed. (250)339-6222

ENGMANN, Eric C; Halton HSC Corp-Oakville, 327 Reynolds St, Oakville ON L6J 3L7; Tor'95; FRCPC; DiagRad. Staff, Halton Healthcare Services Corporation - Oakville Site; (905)338-4601

ENGO, Michael L; SMBD Jewish Gen Hosp, 3755 ch Cote-Sainte-Catherine, Montreal QC H3T 1E2; McG'93; CCFP; CCFP(E.M.); Staff Emerg, Sir Mortimer B Davis Jewish General; Staff Emerg, McGill University Health Centre - Montreal General Campus; Langs: English; French; (514)340-8222 x5568

ENIOJUKAN, Rachael; Kateri Mem Hosp Centre, PO Box 10, Kahnawake QC J0L 1B0; CCFP; Fam Med, Kateri Memorial Hospital Centre; (450)638-3930; Fax. (450)638-4634.

ENNAIFER, Atika; Clinique Med Du Sub-Ouest, 103-4475 rue Bannantyne, LaSalle QC H4G 1E2; (Tunisia)'03; CCFP; Obstetrics, Centre Hospitalier de LaSalle; Langs: Bilingual(English/French); (514)765-3600; Fax. (514)765-9625.

ENNIS, Jeffrey; Medical Arts Bldg, 710-1 Young St, Hamilton ON L8N 1T8; McM'88; MSW; BSc; FRCPC; Psy (Chronic Pain Management). PhysMed&Rehab, Hamilton Health Sciences Centre - McMaster University Medical Centre; Staff Psy/Prog Mgr, St Joseph's Healthcare - Charlton Campus; Physician, Medical Arts Bldg; Dir, Ennis Centre for Pain Management; Clinical Asst Prof Psy & PhysMed&Rehab, McMaster University; (905)627-7300; Fax. (905)627-4757.

ENNIS, Jonathan D; Ennis Medical Professional, 502-790 Bay St, Toronto ON M5G 1N8; Tor'74; FRCPC; Psy. Staff Psy, Toronto General Hospital - UHN; Asst Prof, University of Toronto; (416)922-8370; Fax. (416)922-1148.

ENNIS, Robert; Western Mem Reg Hosp, PO Box 2005 Stn Main 1 Brookfield Ave, Corner Brook NL A2H 6J7; Mem'98; Staff, Western Memorial Regional Hospital; (709)637-5000

ENNIS, Sandra E; Elizabeth Avenue Med Practice, 116-100 Elizabeth Ave, St. John's NL A1B 1S1; Mem'07; CCFP; (709)579-5005

ENNS, Charmaine L; 355 11th St, Courtenay BC V9N 1S4; Sask'91; FRCPC; CommunMed; Public Health & Preventive Med. (250)334-5461; Fax. (250)334-5467.

ENNS, Echo-Marie E; Peter Lougheed Centre, 3500 26 Ave NE, Calgary AB T1Y 6J4; UBC'90; CCFP; Staff, Peter Lougheed Centre; (403)943-4555

ENNS, Gordon B; 101-45625 Hodgins Ave, Chilliwack BC V2P 1P2; UBC'90; (604)792-2721; Fax. (604)792-3404.

ENNS, Heather-Anne S; Delta Hosp, 5800 Mountain View Blvd, Delta BC V4K 3V6; UBC'96; CCFP; CCFP(E.M.); Staff, Delta Hospital; (604)940-9695

ENNS, James P I; Health Sciences Centre, 820 Sherbrook St, Winnipeg MB R3A 1R9; Man'83; FRCPC; Anes (Cardiac Anesthesia). Staff Anes, Health Sciences Centre; (204)774-6511

ENNS, Murray W; Psychealth Centre, PZ 433-771 Bannatyne Ave, Winnipeg MB R3E 3N4; Man'87; FRCPC; Psy (Mood Disorders). Dept Head Psy/Prof, University of Manitoba; (204)787-7078; Fax. (204)787-4879; menns@cc.umanitoba.ca.

ENNS, Robert A; Pacific Gastroenterology Assoc, 770-1190 Hornby St, Vancouver BC V6Z 2K5; UBC'88; FRCPC; IntMed; Gastroent. (604)688-6332 x222; renns@interchange.ubc.ca.

ENRIGHT, Angela C; Royal Jubilee Hosp, 1952 Bay St, Victoria BC V8R 1J8; Dublin (Ireland)'70; DCH; DAB; FFARCS; MB BCh; BAO; FRCPC; Anes. Staff Anes, Royal Jubilee Hospital; Langs: Spanish; French; (250)370-8441; ape@telus.net.

ENRIGHT, Jody; 220-500 Mapleton Rd, Moncton NB E1G 0N3; Dal'07; CCFP; (506)870-2938; Fax. (506)870-2978.

ENRIGHT, Katherine A; The Credit Valley Hosp, 2200 Eglinton Ave W, Mississauga ON L5M 2N1; Wes'04; FRCPC; IntMed; MedOncol. Staff, The Credit Valley Hospital; (905)813-1100 x4471

ENRIGHT, Mark L; 8 Third St, Collingwood ON L9Y 1K3; Wes'87; CCFP; CCFP(E.M.); Staff, Collingwood General & Marine Hospital; (705)445-4334

ENRIGHT, Paula D; 43 Bruyere St, Ottawa ON K1N 5C8; Ott'05; CCFP; (613)562-6262

ENRIGHT, William M; 317 Clifton Ave PO Box 940, Windsor NS B0N 2T0; Dal'80; Ac Staff, Hants Community Hospital; (902)798-2017; Fax. (902)798-5418.

ENRIQUEZ, Carlos E; Dr Charles A Janeway Child HC, 300 Prince Philip Dr, St. John's NL A1B 3V6; Autonomous (Mexico)'78; MB BS; Staff, Janeway Children's Health & Rehabilitation Centre; (709)738-2394

ENS, Andrea R D; The Hosp for Sick Children, 555 Univesity Ave, Toronto ON M5G 1X8; Wes'07; FRCPC; Peds.

ENSENAT, Santiago; University of Alberta Hosp, 3A3 13WMC-8440 112 St NW, Edmonton AB T6G 2B7; Universidad de Buenos Aires (Argentina)'99; DrMedCh; Staff, University of Alberta Hospital; Staff, Royal Alexandra Hospital; Associate Clin Prof, University of Alberta; Langs: Spanish; (780)407-1305; Fax. (780)407-3030; santiago.ensenat@capitalhealth.ca.

ENSING, Dianne; 11-450 Westheights Dr, Kitchener ON N2N 2B9; Wes'81; CCFP; CCFP(E.M.); FCFP; (519)725-4070; Fax. (519)725-4071.

ENSWORTH, Stephanie; Mary Pack Arthritis Center, 895 10th Ave W, Vancouver BC V5Z 1L7; UBC'83; BScPharm; FRCPC; IntMed (Lupus); Rheum. Ac Staff, Vancouver General Hospital - Centennial Pavillion; Consultant, BC Women's Hospital & Health Centre; Physician Rheumatology & Autoimmune Advisory Committee Diseases Drug Benefit Adjudication, BC Ministry of Health Services; Clinical Asst Prof Rheum, University of British Columbia; (604)875-4010; Fax. (604)875-4321; ensworth@shaw.ca.

ENTAIFA, Hussein; Medicine In Motion Med Centre, 5-121 Ilsley Ave, Dartmouth NS B3B 1S4; Garyunis (Libya)'03; MB ChB; Staff, Bonavista Peninsula Health Centre; (902)468-2774; Fax. (902)468-1359; enteifa77@yahoo.com.

ENTWISTLE, Catherine M A; Kilborn Med Centre, 402-1385 Bank St, Ottawa ON K1H 8N4; Ott'84; FRCSC; Ophth. Court Staff, The Ottawa Hospital - Riverside Campus; Langs: English; French; (613)739-0074; Fax. (613)739-0946.

ENTWISTLE, Lucy M; University of Alberta Hosp, 1C1 04-8440 112 St NW, Edmonton AB T6G 2B7; Birmingham (England)'74; AB; FRCPC; Anes. Staff, University of Alberta Hospital; (780)407-7035

ENTWISTLE, Peter B; 9715 348 Ave PO Box 820, Oliver BC V0H 1T0; Dundee (Scotland)'86; MB ChB; Med Staff Phy, South Okanagan General Hospital; (250)498-2232; Fax. (250)498-0105; entwistlep@shaw.ca.

ENVER, Khalid; Groves Mem Hosp, 235 Union St E, Fergus ON N1M 1W3; Punjab (Pakistan)'80; FRCS(Ed); MB BS; FRCSC; GenSurg. Staff, Groves Memorial Community Hospital; Staff, Collingwood General & Marine Hospital; (519)843-2322; Fax. (519)843-2705.

ENWEANI, Cyprian C; Lenore Centre Med Clinic, 4-123 Lenore Dr, Saskatoon SK S7K 7H9; Sask'89; CCFP; FCFP; (306)242-6700; Fax. (306)242-1168.

ENYINGI, Juliette A; Manitoba Adolescent Trmt Ctre, 228 Maryland St, Winnipeg MB R3G 1L6; Man'95; BSc(Med); FRCPC; Psy (Child & Adolescent Psychiatry). Staff, Manitoba Adolescent Treatment Centre; Asst Prof Psy, University of Manitoba; (204)958-9600; Fax. (204)958-9618.

EOM, Minjeong; Meadowlands Family Hlth Centre, 888 Meadowlands Dr, Ottawa ON K2C 3R2; Qns'04; CCFP; Staff, The Ottawa Hospital - Civic Campus; Langs: Korean; (613)228-2882; Fax. (613)228-2856.

EPELBAUM, Mikhail; L'vov Med Institute, 10046-27 Legend Crt, Ancaster ON L9K 1P2; Lvov (Ukraine)'78; AB; FRCPC; Psy (Forensic Psychiatry). Staff, St Joseph's Healthcare Hamilton - West 5th Campus; Staff, Joseph Brant Memorial Hospital; Staff Forensic Unit, St Joseph's Healthcare - Charlton Campus; (905)921-2255; epelbaum@mcmaster.ca.

EPLETT, Catherine J; One Med Place, 310-20 Wynford Dr, North York ON M3C 1J4; McM'84; BSc; FRCSC; Ophth (Oculo Plastic Surgery). Ac Staff, Rouge Valley Health System - Centenary Health Centre Site; Ac Staff, The Scarborough Hospital - General Campus; Ac Staff, The Scarborough Hospital - Birchmount Campus; Clin Instructor, University of Toronto; (416)441-3580; Fax. (416)441-3280.

EPP, Annette M; Pacific Avenue Med Centre, 300-149 Pacific Ave, Saskatoon SK S7K 1N8; Sask'88; FRCSC; ObstGyn. (306)653-5970; Fax. (306)653-5383.

EPPEL, Alan B; St Joseph's Healthcare, 3Fl-50 Charlton Ave E, Hamilton ON L8N 4A6; Dublin (Ireland)'73; MB ChB; MRCPsy; FRCPC; Psy. Dir Communtiy Psy Services, St Joseph's Healthcare - Charlton Campus; Clin Assoc Prof, McMaster University; (905)522-1155 x3538

EPPLER, Jeffrey D; Kelowna Gen Hosp, 2268 Pandosy St, Kelowna BC V1Y 1T2; UBC'87; FRCPC; EmergMed. Staff, Kelowna General Hospital; (250)862-4485; Fax. (250)862-4361.

EPSTEIN, Ian L; Queen Elizabeth II HSC, 1276 South Park St, Halifax NS B3H 2Y9; Dal'04; FRCPC; IntMed; Gastroent. Staff, Queen Elizabeth II Health Sciences Centre - Victoria General Site; (902)473-7781; Fax. (902)473-4406.

EPSTEIN, Irvin; Start Clinic, 301-32 Park Rd, Toronto ON M4W 2N4; Genoa (Italy)'83; FRCPC; Psy (Adolescent Clinic). Staff Psy, Centre for Addiction & Mental Health (CAMH) - College Street Site; Staff Psy, Start Clinic; Asst Prof, University of Toronto; Langs: Italian; (416)535-8501 x4801; Fax. (416)979-6936; irvin_epstein@camh.net.

EPSTEIN, Michael N; Keary Med Centre, 201-245 Columbia St E, New Westminster BC V3L 3W4; Dal'84; FRCPC; IntMed; Cardiol. Staff, Royal Columbian Hospital; (604)522-8667; Fax. (604)522-8623; mepstein@shaw.ca.

EPSTEIN, Nancy E; 340-790 Bay St, Toronto ON M5G 1N8; McG'81; FRCSC; Ophth (Medical Ophthalmology). Court Staff, Sunnybrook Health Sciences Centre; Lecturer Ophth, University of Toronto; Langs: Bilingual(English/French); (416)979-9993; Fax. (416)979-9099.

EPSTEIN, Norman L; The Credit Valley Hosp, 2200 Eglinton Ave W, Mississauga ON L5M 2N1; Ott'85; CCFP; CCFP(E.M.); Staff, The Credit Valley Hospital; Teach Staff, University of Toronto; (905)813-4141

EPSTEIN, Norman; 202 St Clair Ave W, Toronto ON M4V 1R2; Dal'53; MCAA; FAB; AB; FRCPC; Peds. Consultant, St Joseph's Health Centre; (416)921-8073; Fax. (416)921-0362.

EPSTEIN, Ralph; Southwest Family Health Ctre, 305-200 James St S, Hamilton ON L8P 3A9; Witwatersrand (South Africa)'78; CCFP; FCFP; Staff, St Joseph's Healthcare - Charlton Campus; Staff, Hamilton Health Sciences Centre - McMaster University Medical Centre; (905)522-7944; Fax. (905)522-7766.

EPSTEIN, Shirley; 243 Eglinton Ave W, Toronto ON M4R 1B1; Tor'75; Court Staff, North York General Hospital; (416)489-2106

EPSTEIN, Stanley W; 240-340 College St, Toronto ON M5T 3A9; Dal'62; FCCP; FRCPC; IntMed (Respirology). Staff Outpatient, West Park Healthcare Centre; Hon Staff, Toronto Western Hospital - University Health Network; (416)961-5476; Fax. (416)928-9816.

ERAGHUBI, Milad; Medical Clinic, 10620 104 Ave, Grande Prairie AB T8V 8J8; (Libya)'93; MB BCh; (780)814-5800

ERAK, Drago; Queensway Carleton Hosp, 3045 Baseline Rd, Ottawa ON K2H 8P4; Belgrade (Serbia)'82; FRCPC; Psy. Staff, Queensway Carleton Hospital; (613)721-2000

ERAMIAN, Douglas; Ctr Hosp Affilie-Enfant-Jesus, 1401 18e rue, Quebec QC G1J 1Z4; Mon'01; FRCPC; EmergMed. Staff, Centre Hospitalier Affilié Universitaire de Québec - Hôpital De L'Enfant Jésus; (418)649-5555; Fax. (418)649-5632; douglas.eramian.1@ulaval.ca.

ERASMUS, Daniel J E; Fort Vermilion Med Clinic, PO Box 306, Fort Vermilion AB T0H 1N0; (South Africa)'82; MB ChB; (780)927-3213; Fax. (780)927-4664.

ERASMUS, Deon E; Provost Med Centre, PO Box 90 Stn Main, Provost AB T0B 3S0; Pretoria (South Africa)'80; MB ChB; (780)753-2271; Fax. (780)753-2371.

ERASMUS, Dorethea S; Group One Med Associates, 1111 Springfield Rd, Kelowna BC V1Y 8R7; Pretoria (South Africa)'86; MB ChB; LMCC; CCFP; (250)762-4246; Fax. (250)762-4041.

ERASMUS, Elizabeth A; Elbow River Healing Lodge, 7F-1213 4 St SW, Calgary AB T2R 0X7; Alb'97; BScN; CCFP; Staff Physician Casual Position, Sheldon M Chumir Urgent Care Physician Group; (403)955-6600; Fax. (403)955-6601.

ERASMUS, Jacobus F; 4904 50 Ave PO Box 1030, Redwater AB T0A 2W0; South Afirica (South Africa)'93; MB ChB; Staff, Redwater Health Centre; Langs: Afrikaans; (780)942-3199; Fax. (780)942-3144.

ERASMUS, Magda; 4904 50 Ave PO Box 1030, Redwater AB T0A 2W0; (South Africa)'93; MB ChB; Langs: Afrikaans; (780)942-3199; Fax. (780)942-3144.

ERASMUS, Marilise; Queen Elizabeth II Hosp, 10409 98 St, Grande Prairie AB T8V 2E8; (South Africa)'96; Staff, Queen Elizabeth II Hospital; (780)538-7100; Fax. (780)832-4917.

ERASMUS, Murray J; Retina Consultants of Victoria, 212-911 Yates St, Victoria BC V8V 4X3; Cape Town (South Africa)'83; MB ChB; FRCSC; Ophth (Retina Vitreous Surgery). Asst Clin Prof Ophth, University of British Columbia; (250)598-1252; Fax. (250)598-9475; retinaconsultants@shaw.ca.

ERB, Heidrun Y; Belgage Med Arts Bldg, 110-525 Belmont Ave W, Kitchener ON N2M 5E2; Qns'70; Langs: German; (519)745-3530; Fax. (519)571-0728.

ERB, Jason W; Kingston Gen Hosp, 76 Stuart St, Kingston ON K7L 2V7; Dal'03; FRCPC; Anes; Critical Care Medicine. Staff, Kingston General Hospital; (613)548-3232

ERB, John B; St Lawrence Dist Med Centre, PO Box 39 1012A Prince St, Lansdowne ON K0E 1L0; Tor'78; CCFP; FCFP; (613)659-2525; Fax. (613)659-2278.

ERB, Siegfried R; Gordon & Leslie Diamond HCC, 5153-2775 Laurel St, Vancouver BC V5Z 1M9; Wes'77; FRCPC; IntMed (Hepatology). Ac Staff, Vancouver General Hospital - Centennial Pavillion; Clinical Asst Prof/Teach Staff, University of British Columbia; Langs: German; French; (604)875-5618; Fax. (604)875-5373.

ERDELJAN, Petar; 506-3030 Lawrence Ave E, Scarborough ON M1P 2T7; Qns'04; MSc; FRCSC; Urol (Endocrinology). Langs: Serbian; (416)439-3323; Fax. (416)439-4261.

ERDELYI, Barbara; Leslie Med Centre, 410-4800 Leslie St, North York ON M2J 2K9; Tor'99; CCFP; Staff, North York General Hospital; (416)497-9900; Fax. (416)497-6992.

ERDMAN, Florence A; 258 Johnston Ave, North York ON M2N 1H6; McG'81; FRCPC; Psy (Psychotherapy). Langs: English; French; (416)225-7762

ERDSTEIN, Julius; 100-14770 boul de Pierrefonds, Pierrefonds QC H9H 4Y6; McG'86; MSc; MDCM; FRCPC; Peds. Staff, McGill University Health Centre - Montreal Children's Hospital; assoc Prof, McGill University; Langs: English; French; Spanish; Hebrew; (514)696-2442; Fax. (514)624-3099.

ERENBERG, Yale A; Ultrasound & Mammography Assoc, 111-342 Erie St, Stratford ON N5A 2N4; Man'78; FRCPC; DiagRad. Staff Rad, Stratford General Hospital - Huron Perth Healthcare Alliance; Staff, Seaforth Community Hospital - Huron Perth Healthcare Alliance; Staff, St Marys Memorial Hospital - Huron Perth Healthcare Alliance; Staff, Listowel Memorial Hospital - Listowel Wingham Hospitals Alliance; (519)273-1721; Fax. (519)273-1928; yerenberg@rogers.com.

ERENDZHINOVA, Ekaterina P; Children's & Women's HC of BC, K3 205-4480 Oak St, Vancouver BC V6H 3V4; Omsk (Russia (Federation))'92; FRCPC; Peds. Staff, BC Children's Hospital; Langs: Russian; (613)737-7707; Fax. (613)737-4867.

ERENRICH, Hedi M; Medical & Dental Bldg, 706-1849 Yonge St, Toronto ON M4S 1Y2; Tor'83; CCFP; FCFP; (416)483-4113; Fax. (416)483-4010.

EREZ, Hanna J; Credit Valley Prof Bldg, 206-2300 Eglinton Ave W, Mississauga ON L5M 2V8; Wes'74; FRCPC; Peds. Ac Staff, The Credit Valley Hospital; Ac Staff, Trillium Health Centre - Mississauga; Consultant, Mount Sinai Hospital; Langs: Hebrew; (905)820-1036; herez@cvh.on.co.

ERFAEI, Afaf A E; The Moncton Hosp, 135 MacBeath Ave, Moncton NB E1C 6Z8; Al Fateh (Egypt)'99; FRCPC; HemPath. Staff, The Moncton Hospital; (506)857-5306

ERFAN EZZAT, Omar; A M Guy Mem Hlth Ctr, PO Box 10 15 Water St, Buchans NL A0H 1G0; Staff, A M Guy Memorial Health Centre; (709)672-3304

ERFANFAR, Alireza; Russell Clinic, PO Box 549 117 Westbourne St W, Russell MB R0J 1W0; (204)773-2146; Fax. (204)773-2718.

ERGAIEY, Houda A; Belmont Prof Centre, 303-564 Belmont Ave W, Kitchener ON N2M 5N6; Tripoli (Libya)'92; ABIM; FRCPC; IntMed; Gastroent. Med Staff, Grand River Hospital - Kitchener/Waterloo Health Centre; Med Staff, St Mary's General Hospital; Langs: Arabic; (519)745-9889; Fax. (519)745-6446.

ERGINA, Patrick L; MUHC-Royal Victoria Hosp, S876B-687 av des Pins O, Montreal QC H3A 1A1; UCSD (CA) (USA)'83; MPH; ABIM; DGS; MSc; ABS; BSc; CEd; BPhil; MD; CSPQ; FRCSC; GenSurg (Adult Cardiac Surgery); CardiothorSurg; Cardiovasc&ThorSurg (P.Q.). Prog Dir Cardiac Surg & Residency, McGill University Health Centre - Royal Victoria Hospital; Dir Surg, McGill University; Langs: English; French; (514)843-1463; Fax. (514)843-1602.

ERHARD, Philippe M; Pan Am Clinic, 75 Poseidon Bay, Winnipeg MB R3M 3E4; Besancon (France)'79; Dip SportMed; CCFP; FCFP; Ac Staff, Tache Nursing Home; Lecturer, University of Manitoba; Langs: English; French; (204)927-2772; phil.erhard@gmail.com.

ERHARDT, Gunnar D; Royal Columbian Hosp, 330 Columbia St E, New Westminster BC V3L 3W7; Man'78; DABEM; DABMT; Staff, Royal Columbian Hospital; Physician, Vancouver Drug & Poison Information Centre; Langs: German; (604)520-4253; Fax. (604)520-4722.

ERHAZE, Irhuo; Weyburn Mental Health Centre, PO Box 2003, Weyburn SK S4H 2Z9; Staff, Weyburn Community Health Services (Mental Health); (306)842-8665; Fax. (306)842-8690.

ERIAN, Ragaee S; Parkland Med Associates, 205-505 Queen St, Spruce Grove AB T7X 2V2; (Egypt)'93; MB BCh; CCFP; (780)962-2001; Fax. (780)962-8176.

ERICKSEN, Marty L; PO Box 113 Stn Main, Lethbridge AB T1J 3Y3; Alb'96; CCFP.

ERICKSON, Allan M; 325-1627 Fort St, Victoria BC V8R 1H8; UBC'76; BSc; DABEM; FACEP; MCFP(EM)(EM); FAAEM; Ac Staff, Royal Jubilee Hospital; Assoc Staff, Victoria General Hospital; Physician, Victoria International Airport; Clinical Asst Prof Med, University of British Columbia; (250)479-1442; Fax. (250)479-1472.

ERICKSON, Grant B; Medicine Hat Reg Hosp, 666 5 St SW, Medicine Hat AB T1A 4H6; (USA)'03; FRCPC; GenSurg. Staff, Medicine Hat Regional Hospital; (403)529-8024; Fax. (403)529-8998.

ERICKSON, Leroy M; Dawson Creek & Dist Hosp, 11100 13 St, Dawson Creek BC V1G 3W8; Alb'64; DABR(NucMed.); FRCPC; DiagRad (General Radiology & Ultrasound). Ac Staff, Dawson Creek & District Hospital; Staff/Vis Specialist, Chetwynd General Hospital; (250)784-7321; Fax. (250)784-7302.

ERICKSON, Robin; Royal University Hosp, 103 Hospital Dr, Saskatoon SK S7N 0W8; Alb'05; FRCPC; Peds; Nephrol. Staff Pediatric Nephrology, Royal University Hospital; (306)966-7900; Fax. (306)966-8640.

ERICKSON, Timothy N; Parkland Med Associates, 205-505 Queen St, Spruce Grove AB T7X 2V2; Alb'87; Ac Staff, Westview Health Centre; Ac Staff, University of Alberta Hospital; (780)962-2001; Fax. (780)962-8176.

ERIKI, Simon P; PO Box 26, McLennan AB T0H 2L0; (South Africa)'08; MB BCh.

ERIKSEN, Guy R; Surrey Mem Hosp, 13750 96 Ave, Surrey BC V3V 1Z2; Stellenbosch (South Africa)'85; MB ChB; FRCPC; DiagRad. Staff Radiol, Surrey Memorial Hospital; Langs: Afrikaans; (604)585-5666 x2253

ERLANK, Andries G; Holley Clinic, 348 Front St, Quesnel BC V2J 2K3; Pretoria (South Africa)'05; MB ChB; CCFP; Langs: Afrikaans; (250)992-2158

ERLANK, Minette B; Holley Clinic, 348 Front St, Quesnel BC V2J 2K3; Pretoria (South Africa)'07; Langs: Afrikaans; (250)992-2158; Fax. (250)992-9391.

ERLICH, Christine M; One Med Place, 315-20 Wynford Dr, North York ON M3C 1J4; Tor'85; DAB; FRCSC; Ophth. Staff, Toronto East General Hospital Inc; Physician, Don Mills Surgical Unit; Langs: Polish; (416)445-1206; Fax. (416)445-1235.

ERLICH, Murray; 1105-20 Eglinton Ave W, Toronto ON M4R 1K8; Tor'85; FRCPC; Psy. Teach Staff, University of Toronto; (416)322-6089

ERLICK, Lawrence S; 2682 Eglinton Ave E, Scarborough ON M1K 2S3; Tor'71; CCFP; Assoc Staff, The Scarborough Hospital - General Campus; (416)269-6100; Fax. (416)269-7720.

ERLING, J Thomas; Nith Valley Family Practice, 1-10 Waterloo St, New Hamburg ON N3A 1V5; Tor'81; CCFP; (519)662-1551; Fax. (519)662-1402.

ERNEST, Gary P; 80 Gorham St PO Box 1480, Liverpool NS B0T 1K0; Dal'80; CCFP; FCFP; Staff/Site Coord Med, Queens General Hospital; Teach Staff, Dalhousie University; Langs: English; French; (902)354-2669; Fax. (902)354-2943; gpernest@ns.sympatico.ca.

ERNEST-BIZET, Florence; CSSS de la Baie-des-Chaleurs, RR 2 419 boul Perron, Maria QC G0C 1Y0; Paris (France)'87; Psy (P.Q.). Staff, CSSS de la Baie-des-Chaleurs; (418)759-3443; Fax. (418)759-5063.

ERNST, Alfred H; Rosetown Med Group, PO Box 340, Rosetown SK S0L 2V0; Sask'66; CCFP; FCFP; Med Staff, Rosetown & District Health Centre; (306)882-2631; Fax. (306)882-4488.

ERNST, Blair D; The Credit Valley Hosp, 2200 Eglinton Ave W, Mississauga ON L5M 2N1; Qns'99; FRCPC; IntMed; Hem. Head Hematology, The Credit Valley Hospital; (905)813-1100 x1841; bernst@cvh.on.ca.

ERNST, Caroline; Dundas Family Med Group, 133 King St W, Hamilton ON L9H 1V3; McM'95; BScN; FAAP; FRCPC; Peds. Ac Staff, Hamilton Health Sciences Centre - McMaster Children's Hospital; Ac Staff, St Joseph's Healthcare - Charlton Campus; Physician, Main West Medical Group; Asst Prof Peds, McMaster University; (905)521-5030; ernstc@mcmaster.ca.

ERNST, D Scott; London Reg Cancer Program, 790 Commissioners Rd E, London ON N6A 4L6; Ott'83; FRCPC; IntMed (Genito Urinary Tumors); MedOncol. Staff, London Health Sciences Centre - Victoria Campus; (519)685-8600; Fax. (519)685-8624.

ERNST, Mark A; Selk Physical Med & EMG, 104-311 Ludlow St, Saskatoon SK S7S 1N6; Sask'92; Dip SportMed; FRCSC; OrthSurg (Knee Surgery). Staff Surg, St Paul's Hospital (Grey Nuns) of Saskatoon; Staff Surg, Saskatoon City Hospital; Clin Assoc Prof, University of Saskatchewan; (306)651-0800; Fax. (306)651-0801; drmernst@sasktel.net.

ERNST, Pierre-Paul; SMBD Jewish Gen Hosp, G203-3755 ch Cote-Ste-Catherin, Montreal QC H3T 1E2; Mon'77; FRCPC; IntMed; Respir. Staff, Sir Mortimer B Davis Jewish General; (514)340-8222 x3636

EROS, Eva M; 523-100 Arden St, Moncton NB E1C 4B7; London (England)'72; MB BS; DCH; FamilyMed. Ac Staff, The Moncton Hospital; (506)857-5452; Fax. (506)857-5454.

ERRAGUNTLA, Vasudha; Saskatoon Eye Surgeons, 704-201 First Ave S, Saskatoon SK S7K 1J5; Calcutta (India)'91; Staff, Saskatoon City Hospital; (306)974-4497; Fax. (306)974-4498.

ERRETT, Lee E; St Michael's Hosp, 8003B-30 Bond St, Toronto ON M5B 1W8; Mem'77; FRCSC; GenSurg (Cardiac Surgery); Cardiovasc&ThorSurg. Staff GenSurg & Cardiovasc/ThorSurg/Prof Surg, St Michael's Hospital; Prof Surg, University of Toronto; (416)864-5303; Fax. (416)864-5185; errett@smh.toronto.on.ca.

ERROUISSI, Nizar; CSSS de Haut Saint-Maurice, 885 boul Ducharme, La Tuque QC G9X 3C1; Sousse (Tunisia)'99; Anes (P. Q.). Staff, Centre Hospitalier Saint-Joseph de la Turque; (819)523-4581; Fax. (819)523-7992.

ERRUNZA, Jennifer; McGill Student Health Centre, 3600 rue McTavish, Montreal QC H3A 0G3; McG'06; MDCM; FRCPC; Psy. (514)398-6019

ERRY, Rajeev; 6D-1450 Kingston Rd, Pickering ON L1V 1C1; Tor'92; BSc; Staff, Rouge Valley Health System - Ajax & Pickering Health Centre Site; Langs: Hindi; Punjabi; (905)420-6025; Fax. (905)837-1099.

ERSH, Gita; South Urgent Care Center, 31 Sunpark Plaza SE, Calgary AB T2X 3W5; Cal'05; CCFP.

ERSKINE, Matthew; Foothills Med Centre, C231-1403 29 St NW, Calgary AB T2N 2T9; McG'02; FRCPC; EmergMed. Staff, Rockyview General Hospital; (403)944-8430

ERTEL, Michael J; Kelowna Gen Hosp, 2268 Pandosy St, Kelowna BC V1Y 1T2; Wes'90; CCFP; CCFP(E.M.); Staff, Kelowna General Hospital; (250)862-4485

ERUM, Uzma; Peter Lougheed Centre, 3500 26 Ave NE, Calgary AB T1Y 6J4; (Pakistan)'99; Staff, Peter Lougheed Centre; (403)943-1111

ERVIN, Francis L C; 308-22230 North Ave, Maple Ridge BC V2X 2L5; Dal'79; ABIM; AB; FCCP; FRCPC; IntMed; Respir. Consultant, Ridge Meadows Hospital & Health Care Centre; Langs: English; French; (604)466-8199; Fax. (604)466-8194.

ERWEE, Franle; Tower Prof Centre, 5520 50 Ave, Wetaskiwin AB T9A 0T3; (South Africa)'06; MB ChB; (780)352-9700

ERWIN, Desmond H; 102-1910 Sooke Rd, Victoria BC V9B 1V7; Belfast (Ireland)'77; MB ChB; BAO; (250)478-8833

ERYAVEC, Erik; Hamilton HS-General Site, 237 Barton St E, Hamilton ON L8L 2X2; Tor'89; Asst Cardiac Surgical Dept of Surgery, Hamilton Health Sciences Centre - Hamilton General Hospital; Langs: Croatian; (905)527-0271 x46277; Fax. (905)577-8023.

ERYAVEC, Goran M; Seniors Health Centre, 2 Buchan Crt, North York ON M2J 5A3; Wes'87; DAB(Psy&Neurol); DAB(GeriatricPsy); FRCPC; Psy (Consultation). Staff, North York General Hospital; Lecturer Psy, University of Toronto; (416)756-6050 x8057; Fax. (416)756-1844; eryavec@sympatico.ca.

ESADEG, Souad; Kitchener Downtown CHC, 44 Francis St S, Kitchener ON N2G 2A2; Al Fateh (Libya)'89; FamilyMed. Staff, Toronto Western Hospital - University Health Network; Langs: Arabic; (519)745-4404; Fax. (519)745-3709.

ESAKIA, Elvira; Nanaimo Reg Gen Hosp, 1200 Dufferin Cres, Nanaimo BC V9S 2B7; (Other Foreign)'80; FRCPC; AnatPath. Staff, Nanaimo Regional General Hospital; (250)755-7691 x52238

ESAU, David J; Gain Med Centre, 1199 Austin Ave, New Westminster BC V3K 3P4; UBC'09; CCFP; (604)939-7345

ESBIN, Bobby E; First Step, 2681 Eglinton Ave E, Scarborough ON M1K 2S2; Tor'84; BSc; Court Staff Privil, Sunnybrook Health Sciences Centre; (416)264-1715

ESCALLON, Jaime M; Mount Sinai Hosp, 1266-600 University Ave, Toronto ON M5G 1X5; Bogota (Colombia)'73; FACS; FRCS; FRCSC; GenSurg (Surgical Oncology). Staff All Site, Princess Margaret Hospital - University Health Network; Staff, Mount Sinai Hospital; Langs: Spanish; (416)586-5163; Fax. (416)586-8847; jescallon@mtsinai.on.ca.

ESCANLAR, Vincent; CFB Gagetown BMC, PO Box 17000 Stn Forces, Oromocto NB E2V 4J5; Qns'06; (506)422-4257; Fax. (506)422-1431.

ESCHE, Bernd A; Ottawa Reg Cancer Centre, 501 Smyth Rd, Ottawa ON K1H 8L6; Tor'79; BSc; MSc; FRCPC; RadOncol. Ac Staff Ottawa Reg Cancer Centre, The Ottawa Hospital - General Campus; Asst Prof, University of Ottawa; Langs: German; French; (613)737-7700 x70201; Fax. (613)247-3511.

ESCHE, Irena; Northhill Prof Bldg, 221-1632 14 Ave NW, Calgary AB T2N 1M7; Cal'83; FRCPC; Psy (Occupational Psychiatry). (403)288-2404; Fax. (403)210-4768; irena.esche@shaw.ca.

ESCHUN, Gerald M; Foothills Med Centre, 1403 29 St NW, Calgary AB T2N 2T9; Man'92; FRCPC; Anes; Critical Care Medicine. Staff, Foothills Medical Centre; (403)944-1430; Fax. (403)270-2268.

ESCHUN, Gregg M; St Boniface Gen Hosp, BG034-409 Tache Ave, Winnipeg MB R2H 2A6; Man'93; FRCPC; IntMed (Critical Care Medicine); Respir. Staff, St Boniface General Hospital; (204)233-8563

ESCOREDO, Sandra I; Royal Alexandra Hosp, 5027-10240 Kingsway Ave NW, Edmonton AB T5H 3V9; Argentina (Argentina)'87; Staff, Royal Alexandra Hospital; Langs: French; Spanish; (780)735-4670; Fax. (780)735-4072.

ESCOTT, Heather; Dr Charles A Janeway Child HC, 300 Prince Philip Dr, St. John's NL A1B 3V6; Mem'04; FRCPC; Peds; Cardiol. Staff, Janeway Children's Health & Rehabilitation Centre; (709)777-6300

ESCOTT, Nicholas G; Thunder Bay Reg HSC-T-Bay, 980 Oliver Rd, Thunder Bay ON P7B 6V4; McM'74; FCAP; FRCPC; GenPath (Colposcopy). Staff, Thunder Bay Regional Health Sciences Centre; Consultant LabMed & ClinPath/Assoc Prof, Northern Ontario School of Medicine-Laurentian University; (807)684-6584; Fax. (807)684-5878; escottn@tbh.net.

ESCUDERO, Carolina A; BC Women's Hosp & Health Ctre, 4500 Oak St, Vancouver BC V6H 3N1; McM'07; Peds. Staff, BC Women's Hospital & Health Centre; (604)875-2120

ESCUDERO, Juan L; 202-381 Kent St, Ottawa ON K2P 2A8; Santiago (Spain)'62; Ac Staff, The Ottawa Hospital - Riverside Campus; Langs: Italian; Spanish; French; (613)234-2258

ESDAILE, David S; Family Med Associates, 306-267 O'Connor St, Ottawa ON K2P 1V3; McG'73; CCFP; FCFP; Langs: English; French; (613)233-6652; Fax. (613)233-0981.

ESELLE, Emmanuel N; University Hosp of Northern BC, 3F-1475 Edmonton St, Prince George BC V2M 1S2; (Other Foreign)'97; Staff, University Hospital of Northern British Columbia; (250)713-9144

ESGUERRA, Robert G; 103-99 Kakulu Rd, Kanata ON K2L 3C8; McG'88; BSc; LMCC; Langs: Bilingual(English/French); (613)592-1448; Fax. (613)591-3778.

ESHAFI, Kourosh; 102-1024 Ewen Ave, New Westminster BC V3M 5E1; (Other Foreign)'04; CCFP; (778)397-1655

ESHAGHIAN, Farhang; Seaforth Community Hosp, PO Box 99 24 Centennial Dr, Seaforth ON N0K 1W0; Virgen Milagrosa (Philippines)'82; Staff, Seaforth Community Hospital - Huron Perth Healthcare Alliance; (519)527-1650; feshaghian@rogers.com.

ESHAGHIAN, Reza L; Victoria Hosp, PO Box 3000 Stn Main 1200 24th St W, Prince Albert SK S6V 5T4; Wes'10; CCFP; Staff, Victoria Hospital; (306)765-6200

ESHAWESH, Abdulhamid F; Melville Med Centre, PO Box 209, Melville SK S0A 2P0; Tripoli (Libya)'97; MB ChB; CCFP; (306)728-4466

ESHGHABADI, Mashalah; Norfolk Gen Hosp, 365 West St, Simcoe ON N3Y 1T7; Tehran (Iran)'77; AB; AB; FRCPC; AnatPath (Cytopath). Med Dir, Norfolk General Hospital; (519)426-0750 x2200

ESHGHI ESFAHANI, Farid; Winnipeg Clinic, 425 St Mary Ave, Winnipeg MB R3C 0N2; Pecs (Hungary)'90; Staff, St Boniface General Hospital; fesfahani@yahoo.com.

ESHLEMAN, Paul; 1180 Walkley Rd PO Box 83065, Ottawa ON K1V 1A3; Wes'94; BSc; FRCPC; Psy. Staff, North Bay Regional Health Centre - Regional Mental Health; Staff, Timmins & District Hospital.

ESKANDAR, Monira; Addiction & Mental Hlth-Queen, 1113-1001 Queen St W, Toronto ON M6J 1H4; Cairo (Egypt)'72; MB ChB; CCFP; Staff, Centre for Addiction & Mental Health (CAMH) - Queen Site; Langs: Arabic; (416)535-8501 x2972; Fax. (416)583-1266.

ESKANDAR, Sherif N F; 1007-600 Queen Quay W, Toronto ON M5V 3M3; Cairo (Egypt)'97; FRCPC; Anes;CCFP; Staff, Centre for Addiction & Mental Health (CAMH) - Queen Site; (416)535-8501; Fax. (416)583-1291.

ESKANDAR-GERGIES, Shokry; W E Nash Clinic, 15 Hospital St, Roblin MB R0L 1P0; Alexandria (Egypt)'88; (204)937-2151

ESKANDER, Ihab; 14-450 Westheights Dr, Kitchener ON N2N 2B9; Cairo (Egypt)'86; MB ChB; CCFP; Langs: Arabic; (519)584-7411; Fax. (519)584-7967.

ESKAROUS, Soad B H; Lakewood Med Centre, 30 Lakewood Blvd, Winnipeg MB R2J 2M6; Cairo (Egypt)'81; CCFP; Staff, Pembina-Manitou Health Centre; (204)257-4900

ESKHAROUN, Magdoline; PO Box 36569 Rpo McTaggart, Edmonton AB T6R 0T4; (Sudan)'92; MB BS.

ESKICIOGLU, Cagla; 203-840 Coxwell Ave, East York ON M4C 5T2; Tor'05; FRCSC; GenSurg (Clinical & Investigative Medicine). (416)461-0165

ESLAMI, Ali; Surrey Mem Hosp, 13750 96 Ave, Surrey BC V3V 1Z2; Shahid Beheshti University (Iran)'95; Staff, Surrey Memorial Hospital; Langs: Farsi; (604)581-2211

ESLER, David J; Mount St Joseph Hosp, 3080 Prince Edward St, Vancouver BC V5T 3N4; UBC'85; CCFP; CCFP(E.M.); Staff, Providence Health Care - Mount Saint Joseph Hospital; (604)874-1141

ESMAIL, Aashif; Kingsway Garden Mall, 303-1 Kingsway Garden Mall NW, Edmonton AB T5G 3A6; Man'86; BSc(Med); CCFP; FCFP; (780)479-3699; Fax. (780)479-3399; dr.esmail@thedoxx.com.

ESMAIL, Amirali M; Concordia Gen Hosp, 1095 Concordia Ave, Winnipeg MB R2K 3S8; Man'76; FRCPC; Anes. Ac Staff, Concordia General Hospital; Ac Staff, Victoria General Hospital; (204)667-1560; Fax. (204)661-7201.

ESMAIL, Mansurali H M; Willoughby Med Centre, B1A-20202 66 Ave, Langley BC V2Y 1P3; Makerere (Uganda)'72; MB BS; (604)514-8800

ESMAIL, Salim M A; Pleasantview Prof Centre, 314-11044 51 Ave NW, Edmonton AB T6H 5B4; Alb'80; FRCSC; OrthSurg (Orthopedics). Staff, Leduc Community Hospital; (780)944-0026; Fax. (780)428-7109.

ESMAIL, Sherali G; North York Med Arts Bldg, 304-1333 Sheppard Ave E, North York ON M2J 1V1; Tor'82; FRCPC; IntMed (Neurology/Electromyography); Neur. Consultant Staff, Women's College Hospital; Consultant Neurol, North York General Hospital; (416)224-0910; Fax. (416)224-2304.

ESMAILI, Haydeh F; St Joseph's Gen Hosp, 2137 Comox Ave, Comox BC V9M 1P2; Mashhad (Iran)'77; Staff, St Joseph's General Hospital; Langs: Farsi; (250)890-3712

ESMOND, Elizabeth M; 31-301 Metcalfe St, Ottawa ON K2P 1R9; Queensland (Australia)'73; MB BS; FRCPC; Psy (Child Psychiatry). Consultant, Children's Hospital of Eastern Ontario (CHEO); Consultant, Royal Ottawa Mental Health Centre - Royal Ottawa Health Care Group; Asst Prof Med, University of Ottawa; (613)739-8388; Fax. (613)731-2248.

ESMOND, John E; Esmond Stapper Med, 404-71 King St W, Mississauga ON L5B 4A2; Tor'94; CCFP; Langs: Spanish; (905)273-3636; Fax. (905)273-9881; esmond27@me.com.

ESPER, Philip; 909 boul St-Joseph, Drummondville QC J2C 2C4; Sher'04; FRCSC; Ophth. Langs: Bilingual(French/English); (819)474-8469

ESPERANZATE, Patrick; Belleville Queen's Univ-FMC, 200-145 Station St, Belleville ON K8N 2S9; Dublin (Ireland)'03; CCFP; (613)771-1910

ESPINA, Melanie R; Base Hosp-CFB Peawawa, PO Box 9999 Stn Main, Petawawa ON K8H 2X3; Ott'08; CCFP; Staff, Base Hospital-CFB Petawawa; (613)687-5511; Fax. (613)588-4880.

ESPINAL MONTOYA, Victor; Cape Breton Healthcare Complex, 1482 George St, Sydney NS B1P 1P3; Antioquia (Colombia)'91; Staff, Cape Breton Healthcare Complex; (902)304-1899

ESPIRITU, Froilan N; Medical Centre, A3-1700 Eglinton Ave E, North York ON M4A 2X4; Manila (Philippines)'73; Langs: Tagalog; (416)285-5393

ESQUIVEL, Manuel N; Markham College Med Clinic, 205-474 College St, Toronto ON M6G 1A4; (Mexico)'69; FRCPC; IntMed. Staff, Ontario Shores Centre for Mental Health Sciences; Langs: Bilingual(English/French); (416)961-8186; Fax. (416)961-8186.

ESSA, Reda A A; Pine Faills Primary Hlth Care, PO Box 1500, Pine Falls MB R0E 1M0; Al Fateh (Libya)'96; CCFP; (204)367-2278; Fax. (204)367-2525.

ESSAADI, Aziza; Clinique Med des Trois Lacs, 585 av Saint-Charles, Vaudreuil-Dorion QC J7V 8P9; (Morocco)'04; (450)455-3322

ESSABRI, Mohyeddin; Medical Doctors Clinic, 39A-1530 Albion Rd, Etobicoke ON M9V 1B4; (Croatia)'92; CCFP; Langs: Arabic; Croatian; (416)744-3019

ESSAJI, Fakhruddin K; Mount Pearl Med Centre, PO Box 100 Rpo Centennial Sq 12 St David's Ave, Mount Pearl NL A1N 2C1; Dublin (Ireland)'79; MB ChB; (709)368-8381

ESSAK, Alexander F; 617 Belmont St PO Box 16035 Rpo Sixth Street, New Westminster BC V3M 6W6; Tor'80; (604)726-3647

ESSAK, Mark; Cobourg Health Centre, 203-316 King St E, Cobourg ON K9A 5R8; McG'87; CCFP; Physician, Cobourg Health Centre; Asst Prof, McMaster University; Langs: Bilingual(English/French); (905)373-1282; Fax. (905)373-9335.

ESSAK, Zafar M; 16050-617 Belmont St, New Westminster BC V3M 5Z8; Wes'77; Dir, Medical & Counseling Services, BCIT; (604)432-8608

ESSALAH, Abdulhafid A; Landmark Med Centre, 11-4150 Albert St, Regina SK S4S 3R8; Tripoli (Libya)'86; MB ChB; DCH; FRCPCH; FAAP; FRCPC; FRCPC; Nephrol; Peds (Pediatric Intensive Care). Att Staff Peds, Regina General Hospital; Clin Assoc Prof, University of Saskatchewan; (306)924-9110; Fax. (306)924-0888; dressalah@hotmail.com.

ESSEBAG, Vidal; MUHC-Montreal Gen Hosp, E5 200-1650 av Cedar, Montreal QC H3G 1A4; McG'97; MDCM; MSc; DPhil; ABIM; ABCD; ABCCE; FACC; FRCP; FRCPC; IntMed (Clinical & Investigative Medicine); Cardiol. Dir Cardiac Electrophysiology, McGill University; Langs: Spanish; French; Portuguese; (514)934-1934

ESSER, David; The Scarborough Hosp-Gen Div, 3050 Lawrence Ave E, Scarborough ON M1P 2V5; Wes'87; Staff, Humber River Regional Hospital - Finch Avenue Site; Staff, The Scarborough Hospital - General Campus; (416)431-8133

ESSER, Michael; Alberta Children's Hosp, 2888 Shaganappi Trail NW, Calgary AB T3B 6A8; Dal'03; FRCPC; Neur. Staff, Alberta Children's Hospital; (403)955-5735; Fax. (403)955-7609.

ESSERY, Cameron R; Penticton Reg Hosp, 101-550 Carmi Ave, Penticton BC V2A 3G6; Man'78; FRCSC; GenSurg; ThorSurg. Staff, Penticton Regional Hospital; (250)493-0134

ESSIAMBRE, Richard E; CSSS de Laval, 1755 boul Rene-Laennec, Laval QC H7M 3L9; Ott'78; CSPQ; Cardiol (P.Q.); IntMed. Staff, Hopital de la Cite de la santé; (450)668-1010; Fax. (450)975-5550.

ESSIEMBRE, Christiane; CSSS de Chicoutimi, 305 rue Saint-Vallier, Chicoutimi QC G7H 5H6; Laval'87; CSPQ; FRCPC; Anes. Staff, Complexe hospitalier de la Sagamie; (418)690-0260; Fax. (418)545-3455.

ESSOP, Ridwana; High Level Med Clinic, 11202 100 Ave, High Level AB T0H 1Z0; Pretoria (South Africa)'04; MB ChB; (780)841-3200; Fax. (780)841-3350.

ESTANBUL, Fatuma A; The Westway Med Clinic, 4-1723 Kipling Ave, Etobicoke ON M9R 2Y8; Addis Ababa (Ethiopia)'84; (416)244-8404

ESTE, Francis A; Lincoln Centre, 201-3030 Lincoln Ave, Coquitlam BC V3B 6B4; Alb'91; FRCSC; Urol. (604)552-7778; Fax. (604)552-7973.

ESTERBAUER, Ronald G; Main Street Square, 381 Main St N, Markham ON L3P 1Z3; Tor'82; CCFP; FCFP; Staff, Rouge Valley Health System - Centenary Health Centre Site; Staff, The Scarborough Hospital - Birchmount Campus; Staff, Markham Stouffville Hospital; (905)471-4795; Fax. (905)471-4796.

ESTEREZ, Philippe; 505 av Stuart, Outremont QC H2V 3H1; Mon'77; Langs: Bilingual(French/English); (514)278-8981; Fax. (514)278-9240; p.esterez@videotron.ca.

ESTERHUIZEN, Andries J; 4918 52 ST, Athabasca AB T9S 1G9; (South Africa)'06; MB ChB; (780)675-5018; Fax. (780)675-5028.

ESTERHUIZEN, Stefanus C; Fort St Johns Med Clinic, 10011 96 St, Fort St. John BC V1J 3P3; Limpopo (South Africa)'08; (250)787-0109

ESTEVEZ, Wendy; St Mary's Hosp Centre, 3830 av Lacombe, Montreal QC H3T 1M5; McG'97; CCFP; Staff, St Mary's Hospital Centre; (514)345-3511 x3460; Fax. (514)734-2605.

ESTEY, Andrea; Edmonton Clinic Health Academy, 3 512-11405 87 Ave NW, Edmonton AB T6G 1C9; Cal'06; FRCPC; Peds; PedEmergMed. (780)248-5575; Fax. (780)775-8876.

ESTEY, Eric P; 400 Hys Centre, 11010 101 St NW, Edmonton AB T5H 4B9; Dal'87; FRCSC; Urol (Minimally Invasive Laparoscopy). Staff Urol, Royal Alexandra Hospital; Staff, Alberta Urology Institute; Asst Prof, University of Alberta; (780)423-5832; Fax. (780)441-2593.

ESTEY, Frank P; Summerside Med Centre, 101-475 Granville St, Summerside PE C1N 3N5; McG'76; CCFP; (902)432-8181; Fax. (902)436-9660; frank.estey@pei.sympatico.ca.

ESTEY, Ronald H; Nisga'a Valley Health Authorit, 4920 Tait Ave, Aiyansh BC V0J 1A0; McG'70; CCFP; FCFP; (250)633-5026; Fax. (250)633-2457; ronestey@hotmail.com.

ESUFALI, Zakir H; Scarborough Hosp-Birchmount, 3030 Birchmount Rd, Scarborough ON M1W 3W3; Wes'99; Anes. Staff, The Scarborough Hospital - Birchmount Campus; (416)495-2561; Fax. (416)495-2879.

ESWAR, Shruthi; Surrey Mem Hosp, 13750 96 Ave, Surrey BC V3V 1Z2; Bangalore (India)'98; MB BS; FRCPC; Psy. Staff, Surrey Memorial Hospital; Langs: Hindi; (604)585-5666

ETALEB, Osmaa; MCI The Doctors Office, 255 Morningside Ave, Scarborough ON M1E 3E6; (Libya)'99; CCFP; (416)284-1020; Fax. (416)284-1271.

ETCHELLS, Edward; Sunnybrook Hlth Sciences Ctre, H469-2075 Bayview Ave, Toronto ON M4N 3M5; Tor'87; MSc; FRCPC; IntMed. Staff, Sunnybrook Health Sciences Centre; Assoc Prof Med, University of Toronto; (416)480-5996; Fax. (416)480-6777.

ETCHES, Duncan J; BC Women's Hosp & Health Ctre, F326-4500 Oak St, Vancouver BC V6H 3N1; UBC'74; MClSc; CCFP; FCFP; Staff, BC Women's Hospital & Health Centre; Staff, Vancouver General Hospital - Centennial Pavillion; Staff, BC Children's Hospital; Physician, Amherst Private Hospital; Clin Prof, University of British Columbia; (604)875-2029; Fax. (604)875-3197.

ETCHES, Nora J M; BC Women's Hosp & Health Ctre, F326-4500 Oak St, Vancouver BC V6H 3N1; UBC'74; CCFP; FCFP; Staff, Vancouver General Hospital - Centennial Pavillion; Staff, BC Women's Hospital & Health Centre; Staff, Providence Health Care - Mount Saint Joseph Hospital; Clin Asst Prof Family Med, University of British Columbia; (604)875-2029

ETCHES, R Ian; Five Hills Health Region, 455 Fairford St E, Moose Jaw SK S6H 1H3; Sask'80; FCAP; FRCPC; AnatPath. Dir Labs, Five Hills Health Region; (306)694-0346; ietc@fhhr.ca.

ETCHES, Vera G; Ottawa Public Health, 7W-100 Constellation Cres, Nepean ON K2G 6J8; UBC'00; MHSc; FRCPC; CommunMed;CCFP; Asst Prof, Northern Ontario School of Medicine-Laurentian University; (613)580-6744; Fax. (613)580-9641; vera.etches@ottawa.ca.

ETEMAD-REZAI, Roya; London HSC-University Hosp, PO Box 5339 Stn B 339 Windermere Rd, London ON N6A 5A5; Qns'96; ABR; LRCPS; LMCC; BSc; FRCPC; DiagRad (Body & Thoracic Cross Sectional). Staff, London Health Sciences Centre - University Hospital; Langs: German; Farsi; Bilingual(French/English); (519)685-8500 x33648; Fax. (519)663-8803; roya.etemadrezai@lhsc.on.ca.

ETHANS, Karen D; Rehabilitaion Centre, 143A-800 Sherbrook St, Winnipeg MB R3A 1M4; Dal'93; FRCPC; PhysMed&Rehab (Spinal Cord Injury). Asst Prof, University of Manitoba; (204)787-1819; Fax. (204)787-1476.

ETHERIDGE, John-Paul B; 203-437 Glenmore St, Kelowna BC V1V 1Y5; Stellenbosch (South Africa)'95; MB ChB; CCFP; Staff, Prince Rupert Regional Hospital; (250)860-9754; Fax. (250)491-8615.

ETHERINGTON, Jeremy; Interior Health Authority, 220-1815 Kirschner Rd, Kelowna BC V1Y 4N7; Cal'82; CCFP; CCFP(E.M.); FCFP; VP Med & Quality, Interior Health Authority Corpoate Office; Clin Prof Div of EmergMed, University of British Columbia; (250)862-4010; Fax. (250)862-4201; jeremy.etherington@interiorhealth.ca.

ETHIER, Dennis R; Family Med Associates, 5021 51 St, Lacombe AB T4L 2A3; Alb'79; (403)782-3351; Fax. (403)782-5879.

ETHIER, Jean; CHUM-Hop St-Luc, 3103-1058 rue Saint-Denis, Montreal QC H2X 3J4; Mon'81; FRCPC; IntMed; Nephrol. Staff Med, Centre Hospitalier l'Université De Montréal (CHUM) - Hôpital Saint-luc; Staff Med, Centre Hospitalier l'Université de Montréal (CHUM) - Hôtel-Dieu; assoc Prof, Universite de Montreal; Langs: English; (514)890-8000 x14742; Fax. (514)412-7342; jean.ethier.chum@ssss.gouv.qc.ca.

ETHIER, Jean-Francois; CHUS-Hop Hotel-Dieu, 580 rue Bowen S, Sherbrooke QC J1G 2E8; McG'06; MDCM; IntMed. Staff, Centre Hospitalier Universitaire de Sherbrooke-Hôpital Hôtel-Dieu; (819)346-1110 x14949

ETHIER, Jean-Leon; Commission Lesions Profess, 500 boul Rene-Levesque O, Montreal QC H2Z 1W7; Mon'61; LMCC; Médecin, Commission des Lesions Professionelles; (514)873-4809; Fax. (514)873-0232; jean-leon.ethier@clp.gouv.qc.ca.

ETHIER, Jean-Luc; Timmins & Dist Hosp, 1550-700 Ross Ave E, Timmins ON P4N 8P2; Ott'01; BSc; FRCSC; Otol. Staff, Timmins & District Hospital; Langs: French; (705)360-6675

ETHIER, Julie; Ctr Hosp Fleury, 2180 rue Fleury E, Montreal QC H2B 1K3; Mon'05; Staff, Centre Hospitalier Fleury; (514)381-9311

ETHIER, Lucien; Clinique Med 201, 104 rue Sainte-Agathe, Ste-Agathe-Des-Mts QC J8C 2K3; Mon'79; Staff, Centre Hospitalier Laurentien; (819)326-2020; Fax. (819)326-8801.

ETHIER, Marcel; Clinique Dr Marcel Ethier, GD 10 ch du Bout-Den-Bas, La Baleine QC G0A 2A0; Mon'70; Staff, CSSS de Charlevoix; Staff, GMF Pierre Boucher; (418)438-2381; Fax. (418)438-2580.

ETHIER, Marie-Pascale; CLSC Hochelaga-Maisonneuve, 4201 rue Ontario E, Montreal QC H1V 1K2; Mon'10; CCFP; (514)253-2181

ETHIER, Romeo; 625 ch Rockland, Mont-Royal QC H3P 2X4; Mon'55; FRCPC; DiagRad (Neuro Radiology); RadOncol (P.Q.). Consultant, Hôpital Ste-Justine; Diagnostic-Radiology, McGill University Health Centre - Montreal Neurological Hospital; Prof DiagRad, McGill University; (514)733-4344; Fax. (514)733-4344; romeoethier@minitel.net.

ETHIER, Serge; Clin Med Richmond, 170 rue Gouin, Richmond QC J0B 2H0; Sher'86; (819)826-5750

ETHIER, Serge; Institut de Cardiologie de Mtl, 5000 rue Belanger, Montreal QC H1T 1C8; Mon'65; DiagRad. Staff, Institut de Cardiologie de Montréal; Staff, Centre Hospitalier l'Université de Montréal (CHUM) - Hôtel-Dieu; (514)376-3330 x3217; Fax. (514)593-2580.

ETIENNE, Pierre E G; Douglas Mental Hlth Univ Inst, A0132 1-6875 boul Lasalle, LaSalle QC H4H 1R3; Liege (Belgium)'72; Psy. Staff, Douglas Mental Health University Institute; (514)761-6131

ETKIN, Mark S; 146 Arlington St, Winnipeg MB R3G 1Y5; Man'80; FRCPC; Psy. Staff, Misericordia Health Centre; Staff, Concordia General Hospital; Assoc Prof Med, University of Manitoba; (204)955-1929; Fax. (204)787-7701; etkin@cc.umanitoba.ca.

ETLIN, David D; 110-36 York Milld Rd PO Box 400, North York ON M2P 2E9; Tor'70; FRCPC; IntMed (Chronic Pain Management). (416)226-4722

ETOOM, Yousef A T; The Hosp for Sick Children, 555 University Ave, Toronto ON M5G 1X8; (Jordan)'00; Staff, The Hospital For Sick Children; (416)813-7467

ETTEHAD DABAGH, Mojgan; Parrsboro & Anes Professional, PO Box 638 76 Jenks Ave, Parrsboro NS B0M 1S0; (United Kingdom)'94; (902)254-3760; Fax. (902)254-3617.

ETTIN, Philip G; Belmont Prof Centre, 407-564 Belmont Ave W, Kitchener ON N2M 5N6; Pretoria (South Africa)'72; MB ChB; Langs: Afrikaans; (519)743-7545

ETTLER, Helen C; London HSC-University Hosp, PO Box 5339 Stn B 339 Windermere Rd, London ON N6A 5A5; Cape Town (South Africa)'84; MB ChB; FRCPC; GenPath; AnatPath. Staff, London Health Sciences Centre - University Hospital; University of Western Ontario; (519)685-8300 x36376

ETZKORN, William G; Chin Bldg, 303-622 College St, Toronto ON M6G 1B4; Alb'82; CCFP; FCFP; Staff, Toronto Western Hospital - University Health Network; Staff, Toronto General Hospital - UHN; Teacher, University of Toronto; Langs: Portuguese; (416)534-1143; Fax. (416)534-6131.

EUGÈNE, Alain; CSSS de la Cote-de-Gaspe, 215 boul de York O, Gaspe QC G4X 2W2; (Other Foreign)'01; Staff, Centre Hospitalier de Gaspe; (418)368-3301

EUGENE, Dardye; CHUQ-Ctr Hosp Univ Laval, 2705 boul Laurier, Quebec QC G1V 4G2; (Haiti)'95; Endocrin&Metab; Endocrin (P.Q.). Staff, Centre Hospitalier Universitaire de Quebec-CHUL; Langs: French; (418)656-4141; Fax. (418)654-2137.

EUGENIO, Arthur M; 700 Coronation Blvd, Cambridge ON N1R 3G2; Qns'04; CCFP; Staff, Mount Sinai Hospital; Langs: Portuguese; (519)621-2333 x2220

EULER, Karin E; 186 Marsh St PO Box 179, Clarksburg ON N0H 1J0; Wes'91; Staff, Collingwood General & Marine Hospital; (519)599-5775; Fax. (519)599-7140.

EUSEBIO-TORRES, Engracia D; The Credit Valley Hosp, 2200 Eglinton Ave W, Mississauga ON L5M 2N1; Manila (Philippines)'71; FRCPC; Psy (Adult Psychiatry). Med Staff Psy, The Credit Valley Hospital; Langs: Tagalog; (905)813-2398; Fax. (905)813-4284.

EUSTACE, A Veronica; 12th Avenue Med Centre, 5365 12 Ave, Delta BC V4M 2B2; Galway (Ireland)'70; MB BCh; BAO; CCFP; (604)943-1148

EUSTACE, Dominic; 12th Avenue Med Centre, 5365 12 Ave, Delta BC V4M 2B2; Galway (Ireland)'69; MB BCh; BAO; CCFP; FCFP; Head Long Term Care, Saskatoon Health Region; Staff Chief, Parkridge Centre; (604)943-1148

EUSTACE, Dominique M; Alberta Children's Hosp, 2888 Shaganappi Trail NW, Calgary AB T3B 6A8; Sask'00; FRCPC; Peds. Staff, Alberta Children's Hospital; (403)943-7211

EUSTACE, Marsha L; Health Sciences Centre, 300 Prince Philip Dr, St. John's NL A1B 3V6; Mem'02; FRCPC; Neur. Staff, Health Sciences Centre; (709)777-8682

EUVERMAN, Rachel M; 157 Yonge St, Toronto ON M5C 1X7; Tor'09; CCFP; (416)362-8822; Fax. (416)362-8877.

EVANI, Subbarao; Abbotsford Reg Hosp & Cancer C, 14-32900 Marshall Rd, Abbotsford BC V2S 0C2; Andhra (India)'68; DAB; MB BS; FRCSC; Urol (Adult Urology). Staff, Abbotsford Regional Hospital & Cancer Centre; Staff, Mission Memorial Hospital; (604)851-4700

EVANIUK, Debra A; 700 Unviersity Ave, Toronto ON M5G 1X5; Man'07; FRCSC; ObstGyn.

EVANS, Amanda; Kiwi Pediatrics, 16662 Mckenzie Lake Blvd SE, Calgary AB T2Z 1N4; (England)'99; MB BS; FRCPC; Peds. Preceptor, Peter Lougheed Centre; (403)281-2500; Fax. (403)256-2511.

EVANS, Andrew J; Univ Hlth Network-Toronto Gen, 11 444-200 Elizabeth St, Toronto ON M5G 2C4; Tor'95; FRCPC; AnatPath. Staff, Toronto General Hospital - UHN; (416)340-3833

EVANS, Arthur; Univ Hlth Network-The Toronto, GC 405-200 Elizabeth St, Toronto ON M5G 2C4; Alb'79; Staff, Women's College Hospital; Staff, Toronto General Hospital - UHN; (416)340-4450; Fax. (416)340-4481; wayne.evans@uhn.ca.

EVANS, C James; Workers' Compensation Board, PO Box 4700 Stn Terminal, Vancouver BC V6B 1J1; London (England)'64; MB BS; Staff, Workers' Compensation Board; (604)556-2058; Fax. (604)556-2075; jim.evans@worksafebc.com.

EVANS, Celyne; 101-2424 boul Lapiniere, Longueuil QC J4Z 2K9; Mon'82; (450)678-9033 x107; Fax. (450)678-5708.

EVANS, Dafydd; Halifax Infirmary, 1796 Summer St, Halifax NS B3H 3A7; (Wales)'97; MB BCh; Staff, Queen Elizabeth II Health Sciences Centre - Halifax Infirmary Site.

EVANS, David; Vancouver Gen Hosp, 855 12th Ave W, Vancouver BC V5Z 1M9; McG'88; FACS; AB; MSc(EPID); MDCM; FRCSC; GenSurg (Critical Care/Trauma). Staff Trauma Services, Vancouver General Hospital - Centennial Pavillion; Staff, Providence Health Care - St Paul's Hospital; Langs: Bilingual(English/French); (604)875-4570; Fax. (604)875-5348.

EVANS, David; Mount Sinai Hosp, 11F-600 University Ave, Toronto ON M5G 1X5; Birmingham (England)'56; Anes. Staff, Mount Sinai Hospital; Assoc Prof, University of Toronto; (416)586-4800 x8515; Fax. (416)586-5067.

EVANS, David; Lions Gate Hosp, 231 15th St E, North Vancouver BC V7L 2L7; Man'82; CCFP; FCFP; Staff, Victoria General Hospital; Staff, Lions Gate Hospital; Staff Elderly Outreach Service, Ministry of Health-British Columbia; Clin Instructor, University of British Columbia; (604)988-3131

EVANS, David; Chatham Kent Walk in Clinic, 857 Grand Ave W, Chatham ON N7L 4T1; Glasgow (Scotland)'61; (519)358-7158; Fax. (519)358-7194.

EVANS, Deborah J; The Allin Clinic, 10155 120 St NW, Edmonton AB T5K 2A2; Mem'98; CCFP; FCFP; (780)482-7551; Fax. (780)488-2056.

EVANS, Frank W; 300-25 Sheppard Ave W, North York ON M2N 6S6; Wes'81; BSc; AddicMed; AvMed; (416)848-9827

EVANS, George; The Ottawa Hosp - Civic Campus, B307-1053 Carling Ave, Ottawa ON K1Y 4E9; Ott'04; Anes. Staff, The Ottawa Hospital - Civic Campus; (613)761-4169; Fax. (613)761-5209.

EVANS, Gerald A; 3013-94 Stuart St, Kingston ON K7L 2N6; Ott'82; ABIM; FRCPC; IntMed; InfectDis. Consultant InfectDis, Hotel-Dieu Hospital; Att Physician Div of InfectDis, Kingston General Hospital; Assoc Prof Div of InfectDis, Queen's University; (613)533-6619

EVANS, H Brian; 339 Windermere Rd PO Box 5339 Stn B, London ON N6A 5A5; Wes'76; FRCSC; PlasSurg (Breasts). Staff, London Health Sciences Centre - University Hospital; Assoc Prof, University of Western Ontario; (519)663-2919; Fax. (519)663-3748.

EVANS, Holly C; The Ottawa Hosp-Gen Campus, 501 Smyth Rd, Ottawa ON K1H 8L6; Qns'95; FRCPC; Anes. Staff, The Ottawa Hospital - General Campus; Langs: Bilingual(English/French); (613)737-8187; Fax. (613)737-8189.

EVANS, Howard; Alberta Urology Institute, 400-11010 101 St NW, Edmonton AB T5H 4B9; Mem'98; FRCSC; Urol (Minimal Invasive Surgery). Asst Prof, University of Alberta; (780)441-2575; Fax. (780)441-2594.

EVANS, Jane B; 458 Maclaren St, Ottawa ON K1R 5K6; Mem'84; FRCPC; Psy. Staff, The Ottawa Hospital - General Campus; Asst Prof, University of Ottawa; (613)230-0586; Fax. (613)230-9204.

EVANS, Janet A; 2268 Pandosy St, Kelowna BC V1Y 1T2; Alb'95; BScPharm; CCFP; Staff, Kelowna General Hospital; (250)864-4026

EVANS, Jennifer B; Country Roads Comm Health Ctr, PO Box 58 4319 Cove Rd, Portland ON K0G 1V0; Qns'90; Assoc Staff, Brockville General Hospital - Charles Street; Assoc Staff, Providence Continuing Care Centre (PCCC) - St Vincent de Paul Hospital; (613)272-3302; Fax. (613)272-3024; drlarst@ripnet.com.

EVANS, John F; 2670 Highway 43 PO Box 179, Kemptville ON K0G 1J0; Ott'79; Med Staff, Kemptville District Hospital; (613)258-4947; Fax. (613)258-2799.

EVANS, John; Medical Assoc Of Port Perry, 462 Paxton St, Port Perry ON L9L 1L9; Qns'07; GenSurg. (905)985-2895; Fax. (905)985-5407.

EVANS, Katharine; 10435 Allbay Rd, Sidney BC V8L 2N8; McM'01; CCFP; Staff, Gordon & Leslie Diamond Health Care Centre; (250)656-1650

EVANS, Keith M; Ross Memorial Hosp, 10 Kent St, Lindsay ON K9V 4M8; Tor'86; Staff, Ross Memorial Hospital; (705)324-6111

EVANS, Kenneth G; Gordon & Leslie Diamond HCC, 7111-2775 Laurel St, Vancouver BC V5Z 1M9; UBC'76; FRCSC; GenSurg; ThorSurg. Head Thoracic Surg, Vancouver General Hospital - Centennial Pavillion; Staff, Gordon & Leslie Diamond Health Care Centre; Prog Dir Thoracic Surg, University of British Columbia; (604)875-5290; Fax. (604)875-5298.

EVANS, Kenneth W; 344-3750 46 Ave SE, Calgary AB T2B 0L1; Man'04; CCFP; Staff Critical Care Med, Foothills Medical Centre; Consultant, Injury Management Consultant; Med Consultant, International SOS; Staff Complaints Reviewer, College of Physicians & Surgeons of Alberta; (587)434-1204; ken.evans@fluor.com.

EVANS, Kirby J; Dixon Med Centre, 305-531 Davis Dr, Newmarket ON L3Y 6P5; Tor'83; FRCPC; IntMed. Staff, Southlake Regional Health Centre; (905)895-8863; Fax. (905)895-4804.

EVANS, Laura D; Crowfoot West Business Centre, 210-600 Crowfoot Cres NW, Calgary AB T3G 0B4; McM'05; CCFP; (403)239-9733; Fax. (403)241-8112.

EVANS, Mark; Peter Lougheed Centre, 3500 26 Ave NE, Calgary AB T1Y 6J4; Wes'00; CCFP; Staff, Peter Lougheed Centre; Clin Lecturer Faculty of Med, University of Calgary; (403)943-5461; Fax. (403)943-5438.

EVANS, Mark; University of Alberta Hosp, 2C3 61WCM-8440 112 St NW, Edmonton AB T6G 2B7; Alb'81; BSc; MSc; FRCSC; GenSurg; PedGenSurg. Staff, University of Alberta Hospital; Staff Consultant, Royal Alexandra Hospital; Clin Associate Prof. Surg., University of Alberta; (780)407-6320; Fax. (780)407-2004; mark.evans2@albertahealthservices.ca.

EVANS, Melissa; Cassandra Clinic, 2044-2048 Victoria Park Ave, North York ON M1R 1V2; (Ireland)'06; CCFP; (416)331-9111; Fax. (416)331-9050.

EVANS, Michele J; Southwood Med Centre, 3F-2385 Pembina Hwy, Winnipeg MB R3T 2H4; Man'76; CCFP; FCFP; (204)261-6300; Fax. (204)261-1390.

EVANS, Peter D; 737 King St W, Kitchener ON N2G 1E3; Wes'87; FRCSC; PlasSurg (Plastic & Reconstructive Surgery). Ac Staff, Grand River Hospital - Kitchener/Waterloo Health Centre; Ac Staff, St Mary's General Hospital; (519)578-1320; Fax. (519)578-1321.

EVANS, Robin J; 220-520 2nd Ave, Campbell River BC V9W 6G2; McM'06; FRCSC; PlasSurg. Staff, BC Children's Hospital; (250)287-8077

EVANS, Robyn M; 110-250 Lawrence Ave W, Toronto ON M5M 1B2; Tor'89; CCFP; Staff, North York General Hospital; Court Staff Wound Care, Women's College Hospital; (416)256-4707; Fax. (416)256-4710.

EVANS, Sarah; Rockyview Gen Hosp, 7007 14 St SW, Calgary AB T2V 1P9; UBC'08; CCFP; Staff, Rockyview General Hospital; (403)943-3000

EVANS, Stephen D; Main Street Med Centre, 1251 Stittsville Main St, Stittsville ON K2S 2E5; Ott'91; (613)831-7372; Fax. (613)831-6381.

EVANS, Steven M; 6237 Kootenay St PO Box 70, Oliver BC V0H 1T0; Alb'82; Langs: Punjabi; (250)498-3418; Fax. (250)498-4244.

EVANS, Terry; St Thomas-Elgin Gen Hosp, PO Box 2007 Stn Main 189 Elm St, St Thomas ON N5P 3W2; Ott'04; CCFP; CCFP(E.M.); Staff, St Thomas Elgin General Hospital; (519)631-2020

EVANS, Warwick L; Park Avenue Med Centre, 500-4634 Park Ave, Terrace BC V8G 1V7; Cape Town (South Africa)'75; MB ChB; FRCS(Edin); FRCSC; GenSurg. Staff GenSurg, Mills Memorial Hospital; (250)615-5060; Fax. (250)615-5054.

EVANS, William T; Upper Appleby Med Assoc, 36-1960 Appleby Line, Burlington ON L7L 0B7; McM'86; (905)315-9929; Fax. (905)315-9314; wevans@live.ca.

EVANS, William; The Juravinski Cancer Centre, 699 Concession St, Hamilton ON L8V 5C2; Tor'70; FRCPC; IntMed; MedOncol. Pres Juravinski Cancer Centre, Hamilton Health Sciences Centre; Physician, The Juravinski Cancer Centre; Chair Oncol/Prof, McMaster University; (905)387-9495 x63001; bill.evans@jcc.hhsc.ca.

EVANS-OLDERS, Rebecca; Bruyere Family Med Centre, 75 Bruyere St, Ottawa ON K1N 5C8; McG'10; MDCM; CCFP; (613)241-3344

EVASHUK, Kristin; North Hill Centre, 200-1632 14 Ave NW, Calgary AB T2N 1M7; Alb'08; Peds. (403)284-0001; Fax. (403)284-1593.

EVELEIGH, Bruce S; U of Ottawa Health Services, 300-100 Marie Curie Pvt, Ottawa ON K1N 1A2; McM'86; Langs: Bilingual(English/French); (613)564-3950; Fax. (613)564-6627.

EVENSON, Leonard G; Women's Health Clinics, 120-3017 66 St NW, Edmonton AB T6K 4B2; Sask'64; FSOGC; FACOG; ObstGyn. Ac Staff, Covenant Health - Grey Nuns Community Hospital; Court Staff, Royal Alexandra Hospital; Asst Prof, University of Alberta; (780)461-6220; Fax. (780)461-4197; evenson@shaw.ca.

EVERALL, Cheryl H; The Mortwood Park Hlth Ctr, 504 Edward St N, Thunder Bay ON P7C 4P9; McM'06; CCFP; (807)286-2003; Fax. (807)286-2684.

EVERED, Lisa; Edmonton Clinic Hlth Academy, 3 582D-11405 87 Ave NW, Edmonton AB T6G 1C9; Sask'95; FRCPC; Peds. Staff/Assoc Prof Peds & EmergMed, University of Alberta Hospital; Staff, Edmonton Clinic Health Academy; Langs: English; French; lisaevered@shaw.ca.

EVERETT, Andrew; Upper Canada Fam Hlth Team, 2-5 Home St, Brockville ON K6V 0A5; Cape Town (South Africa)'88; MB ChB; CCFP; CCFP(E.M.); FCFP; (613)423-1111; Fax. (613)423-1112.

EVERETT, Robert J; Fairmont Med Bldg, 1314-750 Broadway W, Vancouver BC V5Z 1J3; UBC'94; BSc; FRCPC; Peds. (604)879-4564; Fax. (604)879-5191.

EVERETT, Tobias C; The Hosp for Sick Children, 555 University Ave, Toronto ON M5G 1X8; Bristol (United Kingdom)'02; Staff, The Hospital For Sick Children.

EVERSON, Edward A; Trillium Hlth Ctr-Mississauga, 100 Queensway W, Mississauga ON L5B 1B8; Cal'98; FRCPC; EmergMed. Staff, Trillium Health Centre - Mississauga; (905)848-7100

EVERSON, Jennifer; Stonechurch Family Health Ctre, 1475 Upper Ottawa St, Hamilton ON L8W 3J6; McM'85; BScN; CCFP; FCFP; Ac Staff/Chair, Hamilton Health Sciences Centre - McMaster Children's Hospital; Court Staff, St Joseph's Healthcare - Charlton Campus; Physician, Stonechurch Family Health Centre; Physician Lead-Clinical Planning & Integration, Hamilton Niagara Haldimand Brant; Physician Lead-Clinical Planning & Integration, Legal Health Integration Network; Assoc Prof (Part Time), McMaster University; (905)575-9409

EVERSON, Jennifer M; Trillium Hlth Ctr-Mississauga, 100 Queensway W, Mississauga ON L5B 1B8; Tor'09; CCFP; Staff, Trillium Health Centre - Mississauga; (905)848-7100; Fax. (905)848-5990.

EVOY, Andrea M; Owen Sound Med Associates, 2000-1415 1st Ave W, Owen Sound ON N4K 4K8; McG'07; MDCM; CCFP; (519)470-3030

EVOY, Francois; CHUS-Hop Fleurimont, 3001 12e av N, Sherbrooke QC J1H 5N4; Sher'88; FRCPC; Neur; Electroenceph (P.Q.). Staff, Centre Hospitalier Universitaire de Sherbrooke-Hopital Fleurimont; (819)346-1110; Fax. (819)820-6420.

EVOY, Olga L; Hotel-Dieu Grace Hosp, 1030 Ouellette Ave, Windsor ON N9A 1E1; Tor'95; CCFP; Staff, Hôtel-Dieu Grace Hospital; (519)973-4444 x3319; Fax. (519)973-4897.

EWA, I Vivian; Peter Lougheed Centre, 3500 26 Ave NE, Calgary AB T1Y 6J4; (Nigeria)'90; MB BS; CCFP; Staff, Peter Lougheed Centre; (403)943-5461; Fax. (403)943-5438.

EWANCHUK, Mark A; Grey Nuns Comm Hosp & HC, 1100 Youville Drive West NW, Edmonton AB T6L 5X8; Alb'01; FRCPC; Anes; Critical Care Medicine. Staff, Covenant Health - Grey Nuns Community Hospital; (780)735-7026

EWANOWICH, Carol A; Royal Alexandra Hosp, 5002 6-10240 Kingsway NW, Edmonton AB T5H 3V9; Alb'95; PhD; FRCPC; AnatPath. Staff, Royal Alexandra Hospital; Clinical Asst Prof Path, University of Alberta; (780)735-6895; Fax. (780)477-4715.

EWART, Elizabeth J; Royal Inland Hosp, 311 Columbia St, Kamloops BC V2C 2T1; UBC'97; CCFP; FCFP; Staff, Royal Inland Hospital; (250)314-2782; Fax. (250)314-2280.

EWASCHUK, Ernest J; Isis Regional Fertility Centre, 2180 Meadowvale Blvd, Mississauga ON L5N 5S3; Wes'69; FSOGC; FRCSC; ObstGyn (Fertility). Hon Staff, Hamilton Health Sciences Centre - McMaster Children's Hospital; Assoc Staff ObstGyn, Halton Healthcare Services Corporation - Oakville Site; Partner Mississauga & Oakville on Sites, Isis Regional Fertility Centre; Hon. Teach. Staff, McMaster University; Langs: Ukrainian; (905)816-9822; Fax. (905)816-9833; ewaschuk@isisrfc.com.

EWASECHKO, M Gail; Rockyview Gen Hosp, 58-7007 14 St SW, Calgary AB T2V 1P9; Alb'87; BMedSci; CCFP; Staff, Rockyview General Hospital; Staff, CHR Family Planning Clinics; (403)943-3558; Fax. (403)253-5895.

EWEN, Alastair; Alberta Childrenl's Hosp, 2888 Shaganappi Trail NW, Calgary AB T3B 6A8; Aberdeen (Scotland)'78; MB ChB; FRCA; FRCPC; Anes. Staff Anes, Alberta Children's Hospital; Clinical Asst Prof, University of Calgary; (403)955-7810; aewen@acs.ucalgary.ca.

EWEN, W M John; 753 Tower St S, Fergus ON N1M 2R2; Tor'75; Ac Staff, Groves Memorial Community Hospital; Med Dir, Wellington Terrace; Coroner, Province of Ontario; (519)843-4380; Fax. (519)843-3211.

EWERT, Frank J; Univ Of Manitoba, 60 Pearl St, Winnipeg MB R3E 1X2; Man'74; FRCPC; Anes. Staff, Health Sciences Centre; Staff, Seven Oaks General Hospital; University of Manitoba.

EWERT, Robert D; Malton Med Arts Bldg, 204-3530 Derry Rd E, Mississauga ON L4T 4E3; Tor'73; Ac Staff, William Osler Health System - Etobicoke General Hospital; (905)676-1954; Fax. (905)676-9853.

EWING, David A; The Ottawa Hosp-Civic Campus, 1053 Carling Ave, Ottawa ON K1Y 4E9; Ott'85; FRCPC; Anes. Staff, The Ottawa Hospital - Civic Campus; (613)761-4169

EWING, David G; Mental Hlth Clinic Bldg 179, PO Box 1000 Stn Forces, Borden ON L0M 1C0; Tor'68; FRCPC; Psy. (705)424-1200 x7869; Fax. (705)423-7503; lynda_ewing@hotmail.com.

EWING, Erin; Family Practice Associates, PO Box 2010 223 16 Ave, Creston BC V0B 1G0; Alb'04; CCFP; Staff, Creston Valley Hospital & Health Centre; (250)428-9371; Fax. (250)428-9350.

EWING, Karen D; West Colchester Comm Hlth Ctre, GD, Bass River NS B0M 1B0; Mem'92; CCFP; (902)647-2656; Fax. (902)647-2356.

EWING, Kevin L; Hotel-Dieu Grace Hosp, 1030 Ouellette Ave, Windsor ON N9A 1E1; Tor'01; FRCPC; Anes. Staff, Hôtel-Dieu Grace Hospital; (519)973-4444 x4421; Fax. (519)973-0803.

EWING-BUI, T David; Sudbury Reg Hosp-Mem Site, 260-865 Regent St, Sudbury ON P3E 3Y9; Ott'94; MSc; FRCSC; ThorSurg (Esophageal Disorders). Staff Surg, Health Sciences North - Memorial Site; Staff, Northeastern Ontario Regional Cancer Centre; Asst Prof Surg, Laurentian University; Langs: Vietnamese; French; (705)671-5249; Fax. (705)671-5460; dewingbui@hrsrh.on.ca.

EXANTUS, Marjorie; CSSS d'Argenteuil, 145 av de la Porvidence, Lachute QC J8H 4C7; Monterrey (Mexico)'02; FRCPC; IntMed. Staff, Centre Hospitalier d'Argenteuil; (450)562-3761

EXLEY, Graham D; Fort William F H O, 117 McKellar St S, Thunder Bay ON P7E 1H5; McM'07; CCFP; (807)626-1234; Fax. (807)623-5155.

EXNER, Derek V; HSC-Faculty of Med, GE63-3280 Hospital Dr NW, Calgary AB T2N 4Z6; Sask'90; BSc(Med); MPH; FRCPC; IntMed (Cardiac Electrophysiology); Cardiol. Assoc Prof Med. & Community Health Sciences, University of Calgary; (403)220-3219; Fax. (403)210-8140.

EXNER, Jason; Royal Columbian Hosp, 330 Columbia St E, New Westminster BC V3L 3W7; UBC'00; FRCPC; EmergMed. Staff, Royal Columbian Hospital; (604)520-4000

EYBALIN, Marie-Claire; Hop Maisonneuve-Rosemont, 5415 boul de l'Assomption, Montreal QC H1T 2M4; Mon'79; FRCPC; NuclearMed. Staff, Hopital Maisonneuve-Rosemont; (514)252-3424; Fax. (514)252-3443.

EYBERS, Von; 279 Bradbrooke Dr, Yorkton SK S3N 3L3; (306)782-1868

EYDOUX, Patrice L; BC Children's Hosp, 2J3-4480 Oak St, Vancouver BC V6H 3V4; Paris (France)'75; Staff, BC Women's Hospital & Health Centre; Staff, BC Children's Hospital; Langs: Bilingual(English/French); (604)875-2304

EYDT, John M; Clinique Med Vieux Aylmer, 101-204 ch d'Aylmer, Gatineau QC J9H 1A1; McM'83; Staff, Centre d'Accueil Renaissance; Médecin, Clinique Medicale Vieux Aylmer; Langs: English; French; (819)682-5464

EYESTONE, G Russell; 5E Ambulance de Campagne, CP 1000 Bdp Succ Forces, Courcelette QC G0A 4Z0; McM'08; CCFP; (418)844-5000 x6472

EYMARD, Daniel; Centre Hosp Honore-Mercier, 2750 boul Laframboise, Saint-Hyacinthe QC J2S 4Y8; Sher'84; InfectDis; MedMicrobiol; IntMed (Medical Microbiology & Infectious Diseases). Staff Med Microbiol, Centre Hospitalier Honore-Mercier; (450)771-3333 x3535; Fax. (450)771-3510.

EYOLFSON, Douglas A; Health Sciences Centre, GF201-820 Sherbrook St, Winnipeg MB R3A 1R9; Man'93; FRCPC; EmergMed. Staff, Health Sciences Centre; (204)774-6511

EYRE, Alison; Centretown Comm Health Centre, 420 Cooper St, Ottawa ON K2P 2N6; McG'89; CCFP; Langs: Bilingual(English/French); (613)233-7279; Fax. (613)233-4541.

EYRE, Dean P; 361 Waverley St, Ottawa ON K2P 0W4; Otago (New Zealand)'62; MB ChB; DPM; FRC(Psy); Member, Canadian Psychoanalytic Society; (613)234-0803

EYSELE, Beverly-Ann; Casey Med Clinic, 320 2nd Ave W, Prince Rupert BC V8J 1G6; Stellenbosch (South Africa)'02; MB BS; Sec-Treas GP, Prince Rupert Regional Hospital; Langs: Afrikaans; (250)624-4114; Fax. (250)624-4166.

EZAYDI, Murad A; 138 Shawnessey Village Shop, 70 Shawville Blvd SE, Calgary AB T2Y 2Z3; Al Fateh (Libya)'03; LMCC; MB BCh; CCFP; (403)254-8703; Fax. (403)254-8609.

EZEANYA, Mary Angeleen; Family Health Centre, 23 Main St, Waterford ON N0E 1Y0; Jos (Nigeria)'87; CCFP; Staff, Connaigre Peninsula Community Health Centre; (519)443-6694

EZEKIEL, Daniel; City View Med Clinic, 2480 Heather St, Vancouver BC V5Z 3H9; Tor'88; Assoc Staff, Vancouver General Hospital - Centennial Pavillion; Clin Instructor Family Pract, University of British Columbia; Langs: Italian; (604)879-3900; drdan@mail.ubc.ca.

EZEKOWITZ, Justin A; University of Alberta Hosp, 2C2WMC-8440 112 St NW, Edmonton AB T6G 2B7; RCS (Ireland)'98; MB ChB; FRCPC; IntMed (Congestive Heart Failure); Cardiol. Staff, University of Alberta Hospital; (780)407-8719; Fax. (780)407-6452.

EZEMA, Enyinnaya; Mental Hlth Services, 690 East River Rd, New Glasgow NS B2H 3S1; (Nigeria)'98; (902)755-1137; Fax. (902)928-0297.

EZER, Nicole; MUHC-Montreal Chest Institute, 3650 rue Saint-Urbain, Montreal QC H2X 2P4; McG'07; MDCM; Respir; IntMed. Staff, McGill University Health Centre - Montreal Chest Institute; (514)934-1934

EZZAT, Ahmed M; Pacific Avenue Med Centre, 300-149 Pacific Ave, Saskatoon SK S7K 1N8; Alexandria (Egypt)'69; FRCSC; ObstGyn. (306)653-5970; Fax. (306)653-5383.

EZZAT, Hanna; 915-750 Broadway St W, Vancouver BC V5Z 1H8; Tor'06; FRCSC; ObstGyn. Staff, Providence Health Care - St Paul's Hospital; (604)875-8541

EZZAT, Hatoon M; Burrard Med Bldg, 490-1144 Burrard St, Vancouver BC V6Z 2A5; King Abdulaziz (Saudi Arabia)'95; MB BS; FRCPC; IntMed; Hem. Langs: Arabic; (604)684-5794 x2

EZZAT, Shereen Z; 9NU 986-585 University Ave, Toronto ON M5G 2N2; Man'84; FRCPC; IntMed (Neuro Endocrinology); Endocrin&Metab. Head Endocrine Oncology Site Group, Princess Margaret Hospital - University Health Network; Prof Med, University of Toronto; Head Endocrin Oncol, University Health Network; (416)340-3316; sezzat@mtsinai.on.ca.

EZZAT, Wendelin M; St Paul's Hosp, 1702 20th St W, Saskatoon SK S7M 0Z9; Aberdeen (Scotland)'76; MB ChB; DA; FRCPC; AnatPath. Staff Pathology, St Paul's Hospital (Grey Nuns) of Saskatoon; (306)655-5710; Fax. (306)655-5123.

FAASEN, Johannes; Natawihin/Nakasuwenik Clinic, GD, Ile-a-la-Crosse SK S0M 1C0; (306)833-2044; Fax. (306)833-2401.

FABBRO, Franck; CSSS d'Antoine-Labelle-l'Annon, 1525 rue l'Annonciation N, Riviere-Rouge QC J0T 1T0; (France)'95; Psy (P. Q.). Staff, Centre de L'Annonciation; (819)275-2118 x3608; Fax. (819)275-2464.

FABBRO, Julie F; 10-10 Headdon Gate, Richmond Hill ON L4C 8A3; Tor'85; FRCPC; Peds. (905)770-5661; Fax. (905)770-3381.

FABER, Anne; Centre Med de Loretteville, 250-11000 boul de l'Ormiere, Quebec QC G2B 5S1; Laval'78; LMCC; Langs: English; (418)842-3731; Fax. (418)842-3246; anne.faber@ssss.gouv.qc.ca.

FABER, Kenneth J; St Joseph's Health Care, PO Box 5777 Stn B D0 203-268 Grosvenor St, London ON N6A 4V2; Tor'90; FRCSC; OrthSurg. Staff, St Joseph's Hospital - St Joseph's Health Care; Assoc Prof Surg, University of Western Ontario; (519)646-6312; Fax. (519)646-6049.

FABER, Pierre; 616-2525 Willow St, Vancouver BC V5Z 3N8; Sydney (Australia)'76; FRCSC; Ophth. (604)879-9311; Fax. (604)879-9976.

FABIAN, Jacqueline; Uptown Health Centre, 8-9325 Yonge St, Richmond Hill ON L4C 0A8; (Israel)'04; FRCPC; IntMed. (905)508-8876; Fax. (905)508-1087.

FABIAN, James E; 302-1497 Marine Dr, West Vancouver BC V7T 1B8; Alb'94; FRCPC; Psy (Psychoanalytic & Psychotherapy). Clin Dir Assessment & Trmt Serv, Lions Gate Hospital; Staff, Assessment & Treatment Services; Clinical Asst Prof, University of British Columbia; (604)921-1130

FABIAN, Jose L; Hop Louis-H Lafontaine, 7401 rue Hochelaga, Montreal QC H1N 3M5; Mon'84; FRCPC; Psy. Staff, Hopital Louis-H Lafontaine; Universite de Montreal; (514)251-4000

FABIAN, Werner A; 105 Toronto St, Barrie ON L4N 1V1; Tubingen (Germany)'69; Langs: German; (705)739-4114; Fax. (705)739-4114.

FABREAU, Gabriel; Peter Lougheed Centre, 3500 26th Ave NE, Calgary AB T1Y 6J4; Cal'08; BSc; IntMed. Staff, Peter Lougheed Centre; Lecturer Clinical Scholar/Post Doctoral Fellow, University of Calgary; Langs: Spanish; (403)943-4555; gabriel.fabreau@albertahealthservices.ca.

FABRIEL-LECLERC, Christin A; Cast Clinic, 3F NIHU-1444 Edmonton St, Prince George BC V2M 6W5; Sask'85; CCFP; FCFP; (250)565-2666

FABRIZI, Anna; CHUM-Hop Notre-Dame, 1560 rue Sherbrooke E, Montreal QC H2L 4M1; Mon'94; CSPQ; FRCPC; Anes. Staff, Centre Hospitalier l'Université de Montréal (CHUM) - Hôpital Notre-Dame; (514)890-8000 x26876

FACCA, Sarah J; Norwest Community Hlth Centre, 525 Simpson St, Thunder Bay ON P7C 3J6; Wes'08; CCFP; Asst Prof, Northern Ontario School of Medicine; (807)622-8235; Fax. (807)622-7637.

FACCENDA, Kathryne A; University of Alberta Hosp, 8 120CSB-8440 112 St NW, Edmonton AB T6G 2B7; Aberdeen (Scotland)'85; MB ChB; FRCA; Staff, University of Alberta Hospital; (780)407-8861; Fax. (780)407-3200.

FACEY-CROWTHER, Lee-Anne G; Life Mark Health, 103-245 Pelham Rd, St Catharines ON L2S 1X8; Wes'79; Dip SportMed(SportsMed); BPHE; BEd; Site Coord, McMaster University; Med Dir Gender in Med Educ, Niagara College; (905)685-5959

FACHE, J Stephen; Royal Inland Hosp, 311 Columbia St, Kamloops BC V2C 2T1; Man'79; FRCPC; DiagRad. Staff, Royal Inland Hospital; (250)374-5111

FACLIER, Gil; Sunnybrook Hlth Sciences Ctre, 2075 Bayview Ave, Toronto ON M4N 3M5; Cape Town (South Africa)'69; MB ChB; FRCPC; Anes. Staff, Sunnybrook Health Sciences Centre; (416)480-5989

FACY, Anca; Facy Medicine, 504-123 Edward St, Toronto ON M5G 1E2; (Romania)'88; CCFP; FCFP; Langs: French; Romanian; (416)967-2700; Fax. (416)967-5506; facyc@rogers.com.

FADARE, Kayode; Spesmed Med Specialist Ctre, PO Box 1540 Stn Main 2591 99th St, North Battleford SK S9A 3W1; (306)446-5558

FADAVI, Ziba; Orillia Soldier's Mem Hosp, 170 Colborne St W, Orillia ON L3V 2Z3; Ahwaz (Iran)'80; FRCPC; AnatPath (Hematology Pathology). Staff Pathologist, Orillia Soldiers' Memorial Hospital; Langs: Persian; Farsi; (705)325-2201 x3597; Fax. (705)330-3225; zfadavi@osmh.on.ca.

FADAYOMI, Victor T; Glenbrook Plaza Med Clinic, 136-3715 51 St SW, Calgary AB T3E 6V2; (Nigeria)'91; MCFP; FCFP(SA); MB ChB; CCFP; (403)686-6967; Fax. (403)686-3736.

FADAZ, Annissa; Plantagenet Med Clinic, 179 Old Hwy Rd 17, Plantagenet ON K0B 1L0; (Togo)'06; CCFP.

FADDEGON, Stephen P; 306-321 Nicola St, Kamloops BC V2C 6G6; Cal'06; FRCSC; Urol. (778)471-7177

FADDOUL, Said F; CSSSG-Hop de Gatineau, CP 2000 Succ Bureau-Chef 909 boul de la Verendrye O, Gatineau QC J8P 7H2; St. Joseph (Lebanon)'81; FRCSC; Urol. Assoc Member, Hôpital de Gatineau; Ac Staff, Hull Hospital; (819)561-8100; bravo55@videotron.ca.

FADEEL, Khalid; Malvern Med Center, 100-1333 Neilson Rd, Scarborough ON M1B 4Y9; Al Fateh (Egypt)'97; MB ChB; CCFP; Langs: Arabic; (416)291-7719; Fax. (416)287-3775.

FADEL, Marc; Ontario Shores Ctr Mental HS, B5-700 Gordon St, Whitby ON L1N 5S9; Tor'06; FRCPC; Psy. Staff, Ontario Shores Centre for Mental Health Sciences; (905)430-4055; Fax. (905)430-4020.

FADEYI, Oludare S; Mental Hlth & Addiction Servic, 4780 Roger St, Port Alberni BC V9Y 3Z2; (Nigeria)'83; (250)720-6355

FADIN, Anne; Hop Brome-Missisquoi-Perkins, 950 rue Principale, Cowansville QC J2K 1K3; Mon'92; FRCSC; ObstGyn (Oncology). Staff, Hôpital Brome-Missisquoi-Perkins; Langs: Spanish; (450)266-4342; annefadin@yahoo.com.

FADLALLAH, Hussein; Hop Santa Cabrini Ospedale, 5655 rue Saint-Zotique E, Montreal QC H1T 1P7; Mon'96; CSPQ; BSc; MSc; FRCPC; Cardiol (P.Q.) (Hemodynamics). Staff Hemodynamics, Hopital Maisonneuve-Rosemont; Chef Cardiology/Staff, Hôpital Santa Cabrini Ospedale; Langs: Spanish; English; Italian; Lebanese; (514)252-6627; Fax. (514)252-6593; hussfadl@yahoo.com.

FADOIS, Emerson; 885 boul Ducharme, La Tuque QC G9X 3C1; (Haiti)'01; (819)523-4581; Fax. (819)523-7992.

FAFARD, Andre; CSSS du Haut Saint-Maurice, 885 boul Ducharme, La Tuque QC G9X 3C1; Laval'63; CSPQ; Anes. Staff, Centre Hospitalier Saint-Joseph de la Turque; (819)523-4581

FAFARD, Bruno; CLSC et CHSLD Pommeraie, 660 rue Saint-Paul, Farnham QC J2N 3B9; McG'86; Staff, CLSC-CHSLD La Pommeraie - Centre hospitalier de Bedford; (450)293-3622; bruno_fafard@rrsss16.gouv.qc.ca.

FAFARD, Josee; Hop Maisonneuve-Rosemont, 5415 boul de l'Assomption, Montreal QC H1T 2M4; McG'84; FRCPC; IntMed. Assoc Member, St Mary's Hospital Centre; Chief Active Staff, Hopital Maisonneuve-Rosemont; adj Prof Med, McGill University; adj Prof, Universite de Montreal; (514)252-3400

FAFARD, Judith; CSSS du Sud de Lanaudière, 911 montee des Pionniers, Terrebonne QC J6V 2H2; Laval'04; FRCPC; MedMicrobiol; Microbio & Infect Dis (P.Q.). Staff, Centre Hospitalier Pierre le Gardeur; (450)654-7525

FAFARD, Michel; Centre Hosp de Charlevoix, 74 rue Ambroise-Fafard, Baie-Saint-Paul QC G3Z 2J6; Laval'67; CSPQ; Anes. Staff, CSSS de Charlevoix; (418)435-5150; Fax. (418)435-3315.

FAFARD, Therese; Radiologie Jean-Talon Belanger, 1470 rue Belanger, Montreal QC H2G 1A7; Mon'73; DiagRad (P.Q.). (514)274-5449

FAGAN, Brian; Linday Prof Bldg, 15-65 Angeline St N, Lindsay ON K9V 5N7; Qns'72; (705)324-6433

FAGAN, John; The Medical Centre, 707 Charlotte St, Peterborough ON K9J 2X5; Qns'67; FRCSC; Otol. (705)876-4503; Fax. (705)876-4519.

FAGAN, Mitchell; Murrayville Family Practice, 204-22112 52 Ave, Langley BC V2Y 2M6; Qns'91; (604)533-1140; Fax. (604)533-1159.

FAGAN, Romana; 1-71 Howard Park Ave, Toronto ON M6R 1V7; Lvov (Poland)'69; Staff, St Joseph's Health Centre; Langs: Slovak; Polish; Ukrainian; Russian; (416)530-1073; Fax. (416)530-4865.

FAGAN, Stephen; Couchiching Family Health Team, 103-119 Memorial Ave, Orillia ON L3V 5X1; Dublin (Ireland)'03; CCFP; (705)326-3549

FAGAN, Susan M; Cardiology Consultants, 101-99 Airport Rd, St. John's NL A1A 4Y3; Mem'90; FRCPC; IntMed (Echocardiography); Cardiol. Dir Echocardiog Lab, Health Sciences Centre; Clin Asst Prof Med, Memorial University Of Newfoundland; (709)726-5311; Fax. (709)726-1028; cardiologyconsultants@nfld.net.

FAGBEMIGUN, Ayokunle; Russell Med Clinic, PO Box 549 117 Westbourne St W, Russell MB R0J 1W0; (Nigeria)'97; CCFP; (204)773-2146; Fax. (204)773-2718.

FAGBOLA, Adebola; Lisgar Med Centre, J-3945A Doug Leavens Blvd, Mississauga ON L5N 0A5; (Nigeria)'95; MB ChB; CCFP; Physician, Bramalea Community Health Centre; Langs: Yoruba; (905)785-7570; Fax. (905)785-6323; fmbola@hotmail.com.

FAGHFOURY, Hannaneh; Fred A Litwin Family Centre, 3F 400-60 Murray St, Toronto ON M5T 3L9; McG'04; FRCPC; MedGenetics. Staff, The Hospital For Sick Children; (416)586-4800 x4220; Fax. (416)619-5523.

FAGHIH, Mehrnoosh; ONE Fertility Clinic, 3210 Harvester Rd, Burlington ON L7N 3T1; Isfahan (Iran)'00; FACOG; FRCSC; ObstGyn (Infertility). Staff, Hamilton Health Sciences Centre - McMaster Children's Hospital; Langs: Farsi; (905)634-4440; Fax. (905)639-3810.

FAGNOU, John M; Radiology Consultants Assoc, 120-6707 Elbow Dr SW, Calgary AB T2V 0E3; Alb'04; FRCPC; DiagRad. (403)777-3003; Fax. (403)777-3008.

FAHEIM, Enass; 312-2000 Credit Valley Rd, Mississauga ON L5M 4N4; Alexandria (Egypt)'85; CCFP; Langs: Arabic; (905)828-6666; Fax. (905)819-8317.

FAHEY, Meriah S; Foothills Medical Centre, 1403 29 St NW, Calgary AB T2N 2T9; Cal'03; FRCSC; ObstGyn. Staff, Foothills Medical Centre; (403)944-4419

FAHIM, Galal Z; Northern RHA Med Clinic, PO Box 340, Flin Flon MB R8A 1N2; Ain Shams (Egypt)'82.

FAHIM, Lisa; Lakeridge Hlth Corp-Oshawa Sit, 1 Hospital Crt, Oshawa ON L1G 2B9; Tabriz (Iran)'99; FRCPC; AnatPath. Staff, Lakeridge Health - Oshawa Site; (905)576-8711

FAHIM, Maged I; 5-80 Clementine Dr, Brampton ON L6Y 0L8; Ain Shams (Egypt)'90; CCFP; Langs: Arabic; (905)451-1107; Fax. (905)451-0933.

FAHIM, Mohammad; Aberdeen Hosp, 835 East River Rd, New Glasgow NS B2H 3S6; Pontificia Universidad Catolica (Dominican Republic)'89; FCCP; Staff, Aberdeen Regional Hospital; Langs: Spanish; Urdu; Hindi; (902)752-3964; Fax. (902)752-7999.

FAHIM, Raouf M; Appletree Med Group, 2016 Ogilvie Rd, Ottawa ON K1J 7N9; Cairo (Egypt)'81; MS; (613)749-5549

FAHIM, Shireen; Humberwood Med Clinic, 28-680 Rexdale Blvd, Etobicoke ON M9W 0B5; Punjab (India)'78; MB BS; CCFP; Langs: Hindi; Punjabi; Urdu; (416)679-0100; Fax. (416)679-0130.

FAHIM, Simone S I; 308-1081 Carling Ave, Ottawa ON K1Y 4G2; Ain Shams (Egypt)'85; FRCPC; Derm. Assoc Prof Dermatology Div, University of Ottawa; Langs: Arabic; French; (613)722-8532

FAHIM, Sylvia; Family Care Med Centre, 12-1151 Dundas St W, Mississauga ON L5C 1C6; Ain Shams (Egypt)'84; MB ChB; CCFP; Langs: Arabic; French; (905)276-2700; Fax. (905)276-2706.

FAHIM, Ziaullah; Clover Care Med Clinic, 102-17770 56 Ave, Surrey BC V3S 1C7; Rajasthan (India)'87; MB BS; Staff, Langley Memorial Hospital; Langs: Dari; Farsi; Pashtu; Persian; Hindi; (604)574-7883; Fax. (604)574-9601.

FAHLMAN, Nicole M; 300-4010 Pasqua St, Regina SK S4S 7B9; Sask'96; FRCPC; IntMed; Rheum. (306)789-2281; Fax. (306)789-3563; fahlmann@associateclinic.com.

FAHMY, Hany; Dr Charles S Curtis Mem Hosp, 178-200 West St, St Anthony NL A0K 4S0; (Egypt)'83; CCFP; Staff, Charles S Curtis Memorial Hospital; (709)454-3333

FAHMY, Nader; St Joseph's Health Care, PO Box 5777 Stn B 268 Grosvenor St, London ON N6A 4V2; Alexandria (Egypt)'89; Urol. Staff, St Joseph's Hospital - St Joseph's Health Care; (519)646-6100

FAHMY, Nader; Ancaster Healthcare Centre, 385 Wilson St E, Ancaster ON L9G 2C1; McM'08; PhD; CCFP; (905)648-9868; Fax. (905)648-6524.

FAHMY, Yousef W; Churchill Meadows Medl Center, A301-3020 Thomas St, Mississauga ON L5M 0N7; Cairo (Egypt)'75; CCFP; Langs: Arabic; (905)858-7337; Fax. (905)858-7338.

FAHOUM, Abdulmajid; Liberton Med Centre, 106-31 Liberton Dr, St. Albert AB T8N 3X6; (Syria)'96; (780)418-8884; Fax. (780)458-0813.

FAHY, James F A; 306 First St, Midland ON L4R 3N9; Galway (Ireland)'73; FRCPC; IntMed. Langs: Gaelic; (705)527-0105; Fax. (705)527-6699.

FAHY, Maeve P; Mental Health Services, 3 Applewood Dr, Belleville ON K8P 4E3; Galway (Ireland)'79; MRCPsy; FRCPC; Psy (Child Abuse). Consultant, Brockville General Hospital - Charles Street; Consultant, Bruyère Continuing Care - Saint-Vincent Hospital; (613)544-9434; Fax. (613)968-4312.

FAHY, Mellisa J; Mood Disorder Unit, 2255 Wesbrook Mall, Vancouver BC V6T 2A1; UBC'92; FRCPC; Psy. Staff, Providence Health Care - St Paul's Hospital; (604)822-9745

FAID, Carol E; Hinton Med Clinic, 102 Allen Cove, Hinton AB T7V 2A6; Alb'93; CCFP; (780)865-3338

FAIDI, Samir A; Hamilton HS-General Site, 6N 608-237 Barton St E, Hamilton ON L8L 2X2; Al-Fateh (Libya)'89; FRCSC; GenSurg (Minimal Access Surgery). Staff, Hamilton Health Sciences Centre - Hamilton General Hospital; Langs: Arabic; (905)527-0271; Fax. (905)523-5889.

FAIERS, Alan A; 916 Queen St E, Toronto ON M4M 1J5; Tor'79; MSc; (416)778-8770; Fax. (416)778-9655.

FAIERS, Selena; MacDonald Med Centre, 205-2786 16th Ave W, Vancouver BC V6K 4M1; Dakar (Senegal)'05; (604)733-4400

FAILLE, Christiane; CSSS des Aurores Boreales, CP 6000 Succ Bureau-Chef 679 2e rue E, La Sarre QC J9Z 2X7; Mon'87; ac Staff, Centre Hospitalier La Sarre; (819)333-2311; Fax. (819)333-4227.

FAILY, Joan; Extended Med Treatment Bldg, 335D-1090 Youville Drive West, Edmonton AB T6L 5X8; (Kuwait)'90; CCFP; Staff, Covenant Health - Grey Nuns Community Hospital; (780)735-7834; Fax. (780)735-7640.

FAINGOLD, Ricardo; MUHC-Montreal Children's Hosp, 2300 rue Tupper, Montreal QC H3H 1P3; Rio de Janeiro (Brazil)'89; DiagRad (P.Q.). Staff, McGill University Health Centre - Montreal Children's Hospital; (514)412-4450; Fax. (514)412-4211.

FAINMAN, Shane E; Boyd Medical Complex, 392 Portage Ave, Winnipeg MB R3C 0C7; Man'81; DAAPM; (204)415-2740; Fax. (204)415-2825.

FAINSILBER, Toby; Clin d'Urgence du Reine Elizab, 2111 rue Northcliffe, Montreal QC H4A 3K6; McG'00; CCFP; (514)481-4343; Fax. (514)481-9673.

FAINSINGER, Robin L; 416-1090 Youville Drive West N, Edmonton AB T6L 0A3; Cape Town (South Africa)'81; CCFP; FCFP; Staff, Covenant Health - Grey Nuns Community Hospital; Clin Reg Dir Palliative Care Prog, Alberta Health Services; Dir Palliative Care Med, University of Alberta; (780)735-7727; Fax. (780)735-7302; robin.fainsinger@albertahealthservices.ca.

FAIR, William A; Gartree Med Clinic, 510-4400 32 St, Vernon BC V1T 9H2; Cal'81; BSc; Staff, Vernon Jubilee Hospital; (250)545-9112; Fax. (250)545-7556; docboots@shaw.ca.

FAIRBAIRN, James; Herzl CRIU Walk-In Clinic, 500-5858 ch de Cote-des-Neiges, Montreal QC H3S 1Z1; McG'10; MDCM; CCFP; Staff, Sir Mortimer B Davis Jewish General; (514)340-8222

FAIRBAIRN, Robert F; Chatham-Kent Hlth Alliance, PO Box 2030 Stn Main 80 Grand Ave W, Chatham ON N7M 5L9; Alb'58 Columbia University, New York; MSc; FRCPC; Psy. Staff, Chatham-Kent Health Alliance; Aj Prof Psy, University of Western Ontario; (519)351-6144; Fax. (519)351-0450; rfairbairn@ckha.on.ca.

FAIRBROTHER, Joseph; William Osler HC-Brampton, 2100 Bovaird Dr E, Brampton ON L6R 3J7; Southampton (England)'83; FRCPC; DiagRad. Staff/Chief DiagRad, William Osler Health System - Brampton Civic Hospital; Asst Clin Prof, McMaster University; (905)494-2120

FAIRCHILD, Alysa M; Cross Cancer Institute, 11560 University Ave NW, Edmonton AB T6G 1Z2; Qns'01; FRCPC; RadOncol. Staff, Cross Cancer Institute; (780)432-8518; Fax. (780)432-8380.

FAIRFIELD, Finlay M; Grandin Med Clinic, 1 St Anne St, St. Albert AB T8N 2E8; Alb'61; (780)459-5581; Fax. (780)458-7515.

FAIRFIELD, John A; Trillium Med Clinic, 307-1062 Ghislain St, Hawkesbury ON K6A 3B2; Ott'74; Langs: Bilingual(English/French); (613)632-0118; Fax. (613)632-3606.

FAIRFIELD, Sonia L; Bay Med Clinic, 65 Minto St, Glace Bay NS B1A 5B5; Ott'06; CCFP; (902)849-5521; Fax. (902)862-8117.

FAIRFULL-SMITH, Robert J; Civic Parkdale Clinic, 305-737 Parkdale Ave, Ottawa ON K1Y 1J8; Glasgow (Scotland)'70; FRCSC; GenSurg (Hepatobiliary & Pancreatic Surgery). (613)761-5015; Fax. (613)761-4029.

FAIRGRIEVE-PARK, S Michelle; Heritage Med Clinic, 105-2841 109 St NW, Edmonton AB T6J 6B7; Alb'90; CCFP; FCFP; (780)436-3790; Fax. (780)434-8378.

FAIRHEAD, Todd R; The Ottawa Hosp-Riverside Camp, 5 15-1967 Riverside Dr, Ottawa ON K1H 7W9; Qns'00; FRCPC; IntMed; Nephrol. Staff, The Ottawa Hospital - Riverside Campus; (613)738-8400; Fax. (613)738-8337.

FAIRHURST, Nicholas P A; Tillicum Mall Med Clinic, 14-3170 Tillicum Rd, Victoria BC V9A 7C5; London (England)'72; BSc; MB BS; MRCP(UK); CCFP; FCFP; (250)381-8112; Fax. (250)381-8252; tillicummedicalclinic@shaw.ca.

FAIRLEY, Henry S; Thunder Bay Obst & Gyn, 407-1265 Arthur St E, Thunder Bay ON P7E 6E7; Dundee (Scotland)'82; MB ChB; MRCOG; DA(UK); FRCSC; ObstGyn. Reg Dir ObstGyn, Northern Ontario School of Medicine-Laurentian University; (807)622-0055; Fax. (807)622-6333; tbogstaff@shawcable.com.

FAIRMAN, Paul M; Sudbury Med Centre, 305-65 Larch St, Sudbury ON P3E 1B8; Tor'73; Associate, Health Sciences North-Laurentian Site; Associate Dept of GP, Health Sciences North-St Joseph's Health Centre; (705)674-2211; Fax. (705)674-8930.

FAIRMAN-WRIGHT, M; 103-599 Main St PO Box 1069, Hampton NB E5N 8H1; Dal'04; CCFP; (506)832-2929; Fax. (506)832-9191.

FAIRWEATHER, Tanya; BC Women's Hosp & Health Ctre, F326-4500 Oak St, Vancouver BC V6H 3N1; UBC'99; CCFP; Staff, BC Women's Hospital & Health Centre; (604)875-2029

FAISAL, Shazia; 128-2462 Howard Ave, Windsor ON N8X 3V6; King Edward (England)'95; CCFP; Langs: Urdu; (519)258-7181; Fax. (519)258-3446.

FAISAL, Uzma; Royal Oak Med Clinic, 192-8888 Country Hills Blvd NW, Calgary AB T3G 5T4; (Pakistan)'90; MB BS; CCFP; (403)239-3660; Fax. (403)239-4001.

FAIZER, Mohamed B H; 135 Augustus St, Cornwall ON K6J 3V9; Colombo (Sri Lanka)'69; MB BS; FRCS(Eng & Ed); GenSurg. Langs: Sinhalese; Tamil; (613)932-5525

FAJARDO, Carlos; Peter Lougheed Centre, 3500 26th Ave NE, Calgary AB T1Y 6J4; Colombia (Colombia)'76; Staff, Peter Lougheed Centre; (403)943-4892; Fax. (403)943-2565.

FAKHIR, Shamsuddin; City Plaza Specialist Clinic, 3-330 Central Ave N, Swift Current SK S9H 0L4; MB BS; FRCPCH; DCH; CCST(UK); Staff, Cypress Regional Hospital; (306)778-3988; Fax. (306)778-3989.

FAKHRY, Yousef M S; Credit Valley Eye Centre, 3200 Erin Mills Pky, Mississauga ON L5L 1W8; Abdul Aziz (Saudi Arabia)'88; FRCSC; Ophth. Staff, Credit Valley Eye Care; Langs: Arabic; Afrikaans; (905)820-3937; Fax. (905)820-0111.

FAKIM, Abid; 1A-595 Ontario Rd, Welland ON L3B 0B3; RCS (Ireland)'73; Staff, Niagara Health System - Welland Hospital Site; (905)734-6431; Fax. (905)734-9744.

FALARDEAU, Catherine; Ctr Hosp Rouyn-Noranda, 4 9e rue, Rouyn-Noranda QC J9X 2B2; Sher'96; CCFP; ac Membre Emerg, Centre Hospitalier Rouyn-Noranda; Langs: English; Spanish; (819)764-5131

FALARDEAU, Genevieve; Medecins de Famille Marleau, 3 9e rue, Rouyn-Noranda QC J9X 2A9; Laval'97; CCFP; Staff, Centre Hospitalier Rouyn-Noranda; (819)797-4535 x33340; Fax. (819)797-4665.

FALARDEAU, Guy; 4850 boul Henri-Bourassa, Quebec QC G1H 3A7; Laval'72; Peds. Staff, Centre Hospitalier Universitaire de Quebec-CHUL; (418)977-8448

FALARDEAU, Jean; 2604 av Royale O, St-Charles-de-Bell QC G0R 2T0; Laval'79; (418)887-6603; Fax. (418)887-6643.

FALARDEAU, Julie-Anne; Hop Charles LeMoyne, 3210 boul Taschereau, Greenfield Park QC J4V 2H1; Sher'01; FRCPC; DiagRad. Staff, Hopital Charles LeMoyne; (450)466-5000

FALARDEAU, Pierre; CHUM-Hop St-Luc, 1058 rue Saint-Denis, Montreal QC H2X 3J4; Sher'72; MSc(Biochem); Nephrol (P.Q.). ac Staff, Centre Hospitalier l'Université de Montréal (CHUM) - Hôtel-Dieu; Staff, Centre Hospitalier l'Université De Montréal (CHUM) - Hôpital Saint-luc; assoc Prof Med, Universite de Montreal; Langs: English; French; (514)890-8000; falardeaupierre@videotron.ca.

FALARDEAU, Rejean; 75 rue des Lilas, Shefford QC J2M 1X4; Laval'89; Langs: English; (450)360-0524; Fax. (450)360-0853.

FALARDEAU, Simon; CSSS Drummond-Hop Sainte-Croix, 570 rue Heriot, Drummondville QC J2B 1C1; Sher'99; FRCPC; IntMed. Staff, Hôpital Sainte-croix; (819)478-6464

FALCIONI, Michael K; St Joseph's Health Centre, 30 The Queensway, Toronto ON M6R 1B5; Tor'94; CCFP; Staff, St Joseph's Health Centre; (416)530-6587

FALCK, Vincent G; Foothills Med Centre, C1133-1403 29 St NW, Calgary AB T2N 2T9; Cape Town (South Africa)'77; MB ChB; MMed; FRCPath(UK); FCAP; FRFPS; FRCPC; AnatPath (Dermatological Pathology). Staff, Foothills Medical Centre; Surgical Path., Calgary Lab. Services; Assoc Prof Path, University of Calgary; Langs: Afrikaans; (403)944-4746; vincent.falck@cls.ab.ca.

FALCO-KAZEMI, Barbara R; 305 Helena St, Dunnville ON N1A 2S9; McM'89; Ac Staff, Haldimand War Memorial Hospital; (905)774-8841; Fax. (905)774-8842.

FALCONER, Andrew T; Queensway-Carleton Hosp, 3045 Baseline Rd, Nepean ON K2H 8P4; Ott'85; CCFP; CCFP(E.M.); Chief of Staff, Queensway Carleton Hospital; (613)721-4710

FALCONER, Clark W; 301-2245 Broadway W, Vancouver BC V6K 2E4; Man'68; FRCPC; Psy. (604)733-9982

FALCONER, John B; 10-570 Sarsons Rd, Kelowna BC V1W 5H5; UBC'84; FRCPC; Neur. (250)764-4925

FALCONI, David R; Balmoral Med Clinic, 1122 LaSalle Blvd, Sudbury ON P3A 1Y4; Tor'78; MCFP(EM); Ac Staff, Health Sciences North-St Joseph's Health Centre; Ac Staff, Health Sciences North-Laurentian Site; (705)566-7737; Fax. (705)566-3366.

FALK, Annemarie L; Pacific Spirit Community HC, 2110 43rd Ave W, Vancouver BC V6M 2E1; UBC'93; BSc; CCFP; Clinical Asst Prof, Providence Health Care - St Paul's Hospital; Clinical Asst Prof, University of British Columbia; (604)267-2697; Fax. (604)261-7253; annemarie.falk@vch.ca.

FALK, David W; Agape Hospice, 1302 8 Ave NW, Calgary AB T2N 1B8; Cal'76; DTMH; CCFP; FCFP; (403)282-6588

FALK, Jason P; Southlake Reg Hlth Centre, 596 Davis Dr, Newmarket ON L3Y 2P9; Man'92; Staff, Southlake Regional Health Centre; Staff, St Michael's Hospital; (905)895-4521

FALK, Ryan G; Inuvik Reg Hosp, PO Box 2 285 Mackenzie Rd, Inuvik NT X0E 0T0; UBC'07; CCFP; Staff, Inuvik Regional Hospital; (604)703-8548

FALKENBERG, Kornelia; Child & Youth Services, 1680 Albert St, Regina SK S4P 2S6; Sask'86; FRCPC; Psy (Child & Adolescent Psychiatry). Physician, Regina Health District; Asst Clin Prof, University of Saskatchewan; Langs: German; (306)766-6700; Fax. (306)766-6944.

FALKENBERG-ANDERSEN, Christian; Market Mall Prof Bldg, 225-4935 40 Ave NW, Calgary AB T3A 2N1; Sask'93; BSc(Elect Eng); MSc; CCFP; Langs: Mandarin; Danish; (403)247-1090; Fax. (403)247-1009.

FALKSON, Conrad; Kingston Reg Cancer Centre, 25 King St W, Kingston ON K7L 5P9; Pretoria (South Africa)'83; FRCPC; RadOncol. Staff Kingston Regional Cancer Centre, Kingston General Hospital; Langs: Afrikaans; (613)544-2630; Fax. (613)546-8201.

FALLAHA, Michel; Clinique Maisonneuve-Rosemont, 320-5345 boul de l'Assomption, Montreal QC H1T 4B3; Mon'77; CSPQ; FRCSC; OrthSurg (Arthroplasty). Staff Arthropedie, Hopital Maisonneuve-Rosemont; Staff Teacher, Universite de Montreal; (514)254-6161; Fax. (514)254-1596.

FALLAHA, Nicole; Hôpital Ste-Justine, 3175 ch Cote-Ste-Catherine, Montreal QC H3T 1C5; Sher'95; FRCSC; Ophth. Staff, Hôpital Ste-Justine; (514)345-4715; Fax. (514)345-7706.

FALLAVOLLITA, Sabrina; SMBD Jewish Gen Hosp, 3755 ch Cote-Sainte-Catherine, Montreal QC H3T 1E2; McG'03; FRCPC; IntMed; Rheum. Staff, Sir Mortimer B Davis Jewish General; (514)340-8222; Fax. (514)340-7906.

FALLENBAUM, Fany; McGill Sports Med Clinic, 475 av des Pins O, Montreal QC H2W 1S4; Mon'00; CCFP; Médecin, McGill Sport Medical Clinic; (514)398-7007; Fax. (514)398-4035.

FALLETTA, Joseph S A; 531 Queenston Rd, Hamilton ON L8K 1J7; Tor'66; Gen Practice, Hamilton Health Sciences Centre - Hamilton General Hospital; Court Staff, St Joseph's Healthcare - Charlton Campus; (905)560-5680; Fax. (905)560-6787.

FALLIS, George W B; 105-840 Coxwell Ave, East York ON M4C 5T2; McM'75; CCFP; CCFP(E.M.); FCFP; Chief Dep of Fam Pract, Toronto East General Hospital Inc; Asst Prof Family & CommunMed, University of Toronto; (416)469-6464; Fax. (416)469-6164.

FALLIS, Robert R; Segue Clinic, 61 James St, St Catharines ON L2R 5B9; Alb'85; CCFP; FCFP; (905)688-1827; Fax. (905)688-7283.

FALLIS, Shari L; The Allan Clinic, 10155 120 St NW, Edmonton AB T5K 2A2; Alb'85; CCFP; FCFP; (780)482-7551; Fax. (780)701-5396.

FALLON, Katherine; Grand River Hosp-KW Hlth Ctre, PO Box 9056 Stn C 835 King St W, Kitchener ON N2G 1G3; McM'97; FRCPC; Anes;CCFP; Staff, Grand River Hospital - Kitchener/Waterloo Health Centre; (519)742-3611; katherine.fallon@sympatico.ca.

FALLONE, Carlo A; MUHC-Royal Victoria Hosp, R 228-687 av des Pins O, Montreal QC H3A 1A1; McG'88; FRCPC; IntMed; Gastroent (P.Q.). Staff, McGill University Health Centre - Royal Victoria Hospital; assoc Prof, McGill University; Langs: French; Italian; (514)843-1616; Fax. (514)843-1421.

FALLOWS, Glen A; 301-49 Elizabeth Ave, St. John's NL A1A 1W9; Dal'94; FRCPC; IntMed; Gastroent. Staff, Dr Everett Chalmers Regional Hospital; Lecturer, Dalhousie University; (709)777-5858

FALLS, Elizabeth; Clinique Med de l'Atelier, 77 boul Seigneurial O, Saint-Bruno QC J3V 2G9; McG'87; Physician, Clinique Medicale de l'Atelier; (450)461-1751; Fax. (450)461-1602.

FALLU, Angelo; Clinique Woodward, 717 rue Woodward, Sherbrooke QC J1G 1W4; Sher'89; Psy. Staff, Centre Hospitalier Universitaire de Sherbrooke-Hôpital Hôtel-Dieu; (819)565-1441 x21; Fax. (819)565-2246.

FALLU, Bernard; Clinique Med Val-Belair, 202-1147 boul Pie-XI N, Quebec QC G3K 2P8; Laval'87; (418)843-2473; Fax. (418)843-0224.

FALLU, Stephane; CSSS de Chicoutimi, 305 rue Saint-Vallier, Chicoutimi QC G7H 5H6; Laval'93; CSPQ; FRCPC; Anes. Staff, Complexe hospitalier de la Sagamie; (418)541-1000 x2217

FALODUN, Oladeji; Killarney Med Clinic, 220-3425 26 Ave SW, Calgary AB T3E 0N3; (Nigeria)'94; MB BS; CCFP; (403)685-3350

FALOON, Thomas; Canadian Forces Services Ctre, 101 Colonel By Dr, Ottawa ON K1A 0K2; Ott'77; CCFP; FCFP; Staff, Canadian Forces Health Services Centre; (613)945-1473; Fax. (613)945-1472.

FALTAOUS, El Sherif I M S; 214 Med Place, 12F-9909 102 St, Grande Prairie AB T8V 2V4; (Egypt)'82; MB BCh; Staff, Queen Elizabeth II Hospital; (780)539-0960; Fax. (780)539-3909.

FALTAS, Samy R N; Ashern Med Clinic, PO Box 110 1 Steenson Dr, Ashern MB R0C 0E0.

FALUTZ, Julian M; MUHC-Montreal Gen Hosp, 1650 av Cedar, Montreal QC H3G 1A4; McG'82; ABIM; FRCPC; IntMed. Asst Physician, McGill University Health Centre - Montreal General Campus; adj Prof, McGill University; (514)934-8070; Fax. (514)937-1424; julian.falutz@muhc.mcgill.ca.

FALVEY, Denis M; 509 King St, Bridgewater NS B4V 1B3; Dal'77; FRCSC; Ophth. (902)530-2020; Fax. (902)530-4040.

FALZ, Stefanie; East Kootenay Reg Hosp, 13 24th Ave N, Cranbrook BC V1C 3H9; Alb'02; CCFP; CCFP(E.M.); Staff, East Kootenay Regional Hospital; (250)489-6477

FAM, A P N; The Group Health Centre, 240 McNabb St, Sault Ste Marie ON P6B 1Y5; McM'90; FACOG; FRCSC; ObstGyn. Langs: Cantonese; Mandarin; (705)759-1234; Fax. (705)759-7466.

FAM, Ezz; 8113 Spires Rd, Richmond BC V6Y 1W1; Cairo (Egypt)'00; MB BCh; FRCPC; IntMed. Staff, Chilliwack General Hospital; (604)447-3109

FAM, Neil P; St Michael's Hosp, 30 Bond St, Toronto ON M5B 1W8; Tor'00; FRCPC; IntMed; Cardiol. Dir Coronary Care Unit/Staff Cardiol, St Michael's Hospital; Lecturer, University of Toronto; (416)864-5466; Fax. (416)864-5914.

FAMIL-DARDACHTI, Djahanguir; Clinique Medicale GMF-1851, 101-1851 rue Sherbrooke E, Montreal QC H2K 4L5; Lausanne (Switzerland)'69; Staff, Hôpital du Sacre-Coeur de Montréal; (514)522-3226; Fax. (514)527-5251.

FAMORCA, Leilani Casilda de Leon; Langs Comm Hlth Centre, 1145 Concession Rd, Cambridge ON N3H 4L5; (Philippines)'96; FRCPC; IntMed; Rheum. (519)743-4351; Fax. (519)653-8279.

FAMOURI, Sanaz; Clearsprings Med Clinic, 1-390 Main St, Steinbach MB R5G 1Z3; Man'11.

FAN, Eddy; Mount Sinai Hosp, 18 232-600 University Ave, Toronto ON M5G 1X5; Wes'01; FRCPC; IntMed; Critical Care Medicine. Staff, Mount Sinai Hospital; Staff, Toronto General Hospital - UHN; Asst Prof Critical Care Med, University of Toronto; (416)586-4800 x6571; Fax. (416)776-3148; efan@mtsinai.on.ca.

FAN, H I Anita; 408-1160 Burrard St, Vancouver BC V6Z 1Y6; Ott'02; FRCPC; PhysMed&Rehab. (604)646-4637

FAN, Jerome; William Osler HC-Brampton, 2100 Bovaird Dr E, Brampton ON L6R 3J7; McM'01; FRCPC; EmergMed. Staff, William Osler Health System - Brampton Civic Hospital; (905)494-2120

FAN, Lily Z; Niagara H System-St Catharine, 142 Queenstons St, St. Catharines ON L2R 7C6; Wes'06; FRCPC; DiagRad. Staff, Niagara Health System - St Catharines General Site; (905)684-7271

FAN, Michael K D; 205-174 Harwood Ave S, Ajax ON L1S 2H6; Tor'76; Assoc Staff, Rouge Valley Health System - Ajax & Pickering Health Centre Site; Langs: Chinese; (905)683-3220; Fax. (905)683-0083.

FAN, Nancy C; 313-2083 Alma St, Vancouver BC V6R 4N6; UBC'99; FRCPC; Psy. (604)222-2083

FAN-LUN, Melissa A; Sunnybrook Hlth Sciences Ctre, 3200-2075 Bayview Ave, Toronto ON M4N 3M5; McM'07; FRCPC; Anes. Staff, Sunnybrook Health Sciences Centre; (416)480-4864

FAN-LUN, Paul H K; Dundas Centre Med, 307-220 Dundas St W, Whitby ON L1N 8M7; London (England)'71; MB BS(London); MRCP(London); Langs: Bilingual(English/French); (905)668-6122; Fax. (905)668-6706; pfanlun@rogers.com.

FANARAS, Effie; 102 Stuart St, Kingston ON K7L 2V6; Qns'05; FRCPC; IntMed; Respir. Staff, Kingston General Hospital; Langs: Greek; (613)549-6666

FANCOURT-SMITH, Peter F; Victoria Gen Hosp, 1 Hospital Way, Victoria BC V8Z 6R5; Edinburgh (Scotland)'68; MB ChB; FRCPC; Anes. Staff Anes, Victoria General Hospital; (250)727-4152; Fax. (250)722-4106.

FANCY, Nicole D; Montague Hlth Centre, PO Box 877, Montague PE C0A 1R0; Dal'10; CCFP; (902)838-3681

FANELLA, Sergio T; Basic Med Sciences Bldg, 530-745 Bannatyne Ave, Winnipeg MB R3E 0J9; Ott'03; FRCPC; Peds; InfectDis.

FANG, Karen Y Y; Stein Med Clinic, 887 Dunsmuir St, Vancouver BC V6C 1N5; UBC'09; CCFP; (604)688-5924

FANG, Xueping; St. Joseph's Healthcare, 50 Charlton Ave E, Hamilton ON L8N 4A6; (China)'87; Staff, St Joseph's Healthcare - Charlton Campus; Langs: Mandarin; (905)522-1155 x34249; Fax. (905)521-6192.

FANIPOUR, Majid; Leader Med Clinic, PO Box 638, Leader SK S0N 1H0; (306)628-4584; Fax. (306)628-3998.

FANNING, J Ward; Valley Med Clinic, PO Box 2932 Stn Main, Strathmore AB T1P 1L5; Alb'83; CCFP; FCFP; Staff, Strathmore District Health Services; (403)934-4444; Fax. (403)934-5218.

FANOUS, Isis; 7004 98 Ave NW, Edmonton AB T6A 0A5; (Egypt)'75; BSc; MSc; Langs: Arabic; (780)468-6035; Fax. (780)466-9132.

FANOUS, Nabil E; Canadian Institute of Cosmetic, 1380-1 Car Westmount, Westmount QC H3Z 2P9; Cairo (Egypt)'71; ABOtol; ABCS; ABFPS; FRCSC; Otol (Cosmetic Surgery). Staff, McGill University Health Centre - Royal Victoria Hospital; Staff, CSSS de Dorval-Lachine-Lasalle; Staff, McGill University Health Centre - Montreal General Campus; Staff, Canadian Institute of Cosmetic Surgery; Dir Div of Facila Plastic Surg, McGill University; Langs: Arabic; French; (514)935-9906; Fax. (514)935-6482; cosmeticsurgery123@videotron.ca.

FANOUS, Sameh; Institut de L'Oeil de Montreal, 2300 boul Marcel-Laurin, Saint-Laurent QC H4R 1J9; Mon'78; Ophth (Glaucoma). Dir méd, Clinique de l'Oeil de Montreal; adj Prof, Universite de Montreal; (514)745-4445

FANTILLO, Vanessa; London HSC-Victoria Hosp, PO Box 5010 Stn B 800 Commissioners Rd E, London ON N6A 5W9; Sask'05; FRCPC; Anes. Staff, London Health Sciences Centre - Victoria Campus; (519)685-8500

FANTINI, Fiorella; CRAN, 3F-110 rue Prince-Arthur O, Montreal QC H2X 1S7; Laval'93; (514)527-6939; Fax. (514)527-0031.

FANTUS, Ivan G; Joseph & Wolfe Lebovic Bldg, 5 028-60 Murray St, Toronto ON M5T 3L9; McG'75; ABIM; FRCP; FRCPC; IntMed (Diabetology); Endocrin&Metab. Assoc Prof, Mount Sinai Hospital; Physician, Banting & Best Diabetes Centre; Prof Med/Dir Endocrinol & Metab, University of Toronto; Langs: Hungarian; (416)586-8665; fantus@mshri.on.ca.

FANZOLATO, Brigitte; Clinique Med Saint-Hippolyte, 201-780 ch des Hauteurs, Saint-Hippolyte QC J8A 1H1; Mon'92; Langs: Bilingual(French/English); (450)224-8271; Fax. (450)224-1985.

FARAAWI, Rafat Y; Belmont Prof Centre, 201-564 Belmont Ave W, Kitchener ON N2M 5N6; Alexandria (Egypt)'77; FRCPC; IntMed; Rheum. Ac Staff, Grand River Hospital - Kitchener/Waterloo Health Centre; Ac Staff, St Mary's General Hospital; Langs: Arabic; (519)742-4430; Fax. (519)742-4231.

FARADAY, Trent K; PO Box 45073 Rpo Dunbar, Vancouver BC V6S 2M8; Man'90; (604)839-5144

FARAG, Ashraf; Univ of Ottawa Heart Institute, 40 Ruskin St, Ottawa ON K1Y 4W7; Al Fateh (Libya)'02; Cardiol; IntMed. Staff, University of Ottawa Heart Institute; (613)761-5000

FARAG, George; London HSC-University Hosp, PO Box 5339 Stn B 339 Windermere Rd, London ON N6A 5A5; (Egypt)'98; FRCPC; IntMed. Staff, London Health Sciences Centre - University Hospital; (519)685-8500

FARAG, Hanan; Burke Mountain Med Clinic, 210-1465 Salisbury Ave, Port Coquitlam BC V3B 6J3; (Egypt)'91; CCFP; (604)941-5575

FARAG, Hani; Prince County Hosp, PO Box 3000 Stn Main 65 Roy Boates Ave, Summerside PE C1N 2A9; Ain Shams (Egypt)'83; FRCSC; ObstGyn. Staff, Prince County Hospital; (902)888-3659

FARAG, Hayam S M; 10240 Kingsway NW, Edmonton AB T5H 3V9; (Egypt)'90; MB BCh; (780)477-4111

FARAG, Mariam; Gander Med Clinic, 177 Elizabeth Dr, Gander NL A1V 1H6; Ain Shams (Egypt)'01; MB ChB; Staff, Western Memorial Regional Hospital; (709)256-7101

FARAG, Reda A; Medical Arts Bldg, 1001-1538 rue Sherbrooke O, Montreal QC H3G 1L5; Cairo (Egypt)'64; MB ChB; FACOG; FRCSC; ObstGyn (Fertility). Staff, St Mary's Hospital Centre; assoc Prof, McGill University; (514)933-2772; Fax. (514)933-9635; reda.farag@videotron.ca.

FARAG, Rose F; eMichael Med Center, C4-802 Southdown Rd, Mississauga ON L5J 2Y4; Alexandria (Egypt)'73; CCFP; Langs: Arabic; (289)628-1930; Fax. (905)855-3030.

FARAGO, Peter J; Windsor Health Centre, 205-700 Tecumseh Rd E, Windsor ON N8X 4T2; (Other Foreign)'08; (519)258-4771

FARAH, Antoine; CSSSG-Hop de Hull, 116 boul Lionel-Emond, Gatineau QC J8Y 1W7; St. Joseph (Lebanon)'73; AddicMed; Nephrol (P.Q.). Staff Nephrol, Hull Hospital; Staff Nephrologist, CH-CHSLD de Papineau - Pavillon du centre hospitalier; Langs: Lebanese; Arabic; French; (819)595-6000 x6035; Fax. (819)595-6061; a.farah@sympatico.ca.

FARAH, Christian; Winchester District Mem Hosp, 566 Louise St, Winchester ON K0C 2K0; Wes'00; FRCPC; Anes. Staff, Winchester District Memorial Hospital; (613)774-2420

FARAH, Majdeline; Ctr Hosp Rouyn-Noranda, 4 9e rue, Rouyn-Noranda QC J9X 2B2; (Lebanon)'95; Respir (P.Q.). Staff, Centre Hospitalier Rouyn-Noranda; (819)764-5131 x43427; Fax. (819)764-2946.

FARAH, Myriam; 602-1160 Burrard St, Vancouver BC V6Z 2E8; UBC'05; FRCPC; IntMed; Nephrol. (604)681-7191

FARAH, Rita; McGill Student Health Centre, 3301-3600 rue McTavish, Montreal QC H3A 0G3; McG'98; CCFP; (514)398-6017; Fax. (514)398-2559.

FARAH, Sameh S; Doctors Bldg, 115-955 Queen St E, Sault Ste. Marie ON P6A 2C3; Alexandria (Egypt)'77; FRCPC; IntMed; Endocrin&Metab. Consultant IntMed, Sault Area Hospital - Sault Ste Marie; Langs: Arabic; (705)945-9165; Fax. (705)945-9710.

FARAH ANDRAWES, Wafik; CSSS des Aurores Boreales, CP 6000 Succ Bureau-Chef 679 2e rue E, La Sarre QC J9Z 2X7; Ain Shams (Egypt)'91; Staff, Centre Hospitalier La Sarre; (819)333-2311

FARAH-LAJOIE, Claude; Centre Med Salaberry, 2758 rue de Salaberry, Montreal QC H3M 1L3; Mon'65; Staff, Hôpital du Sacre-Coeur de Montréal; Dir-svcs prof, Centre Hospitalier l'Université De Montréal (CHUM) - Hôpital Saint-luc; (514)337-4772; Fax. (514)337-4923.

FARAJI, Hamidreza; Hamilton HS-McMaster Site, PO Box 2000 Stn Lcd 1 1200 Main St W, Hamilton ON L8N 3Z5; (Iran)'94; FRCPC; AnatPath. Staff, Hamilton Health Sciences Centre - McMaster Children's Hospital; (905)521-2100

FARAND, Lambert; Inst Albert Prevost, 6555 boul Gouin O, Montreal QC H4K 1B3; Mon'78; Staff, Hôpital du Sacre-Coeur de Montréal; (514)338-4212; Fax. (514)338-4352.

FARAND, Paul; CHUS-Hop Fleurimont, 3001 12e av N, Sherbrooke QC J1H 5N4; Sher'00; FRCPC; IntMed; Cardiol. Staff, Centre Hospitalier Universitaire de Sherbrooke-Hopital Fleurimont; (819)346-1110

FARAZ, Muniba; University Hosp of Northern BC, 1475 Edmonton St, Prince George BC V2N 1S2; (Pakistan)'02; MB BS; Staff, University Hospital of Northern British Columbia; (250)565-2000

FARAZLI, Christiane; Parkdale Med Tower, 606-1081 Carling Ave, Ottawa ON K1Y 4G2; Mon'73; FRCPC; IntMed; Gastroent (P.Q.). Staff, The Ottawa Hospital - General Campus; Staff, Montfort Hospital; Staff, Arnprior & District Memorial Hospital; Langs: Arabic; French; (613)724-6739; Fax. (613)722-9574; dr.c.farazli@sympatico.ca.

FARB, Richard I; Univ Hlth Network-Toronto Western Hosp, 3 404-399 Bathurst St, Toronto ON M5T 2S8; Tor'85; FRCPC; DiagRad (Neuro Radiology). Staff, Toronto Western Hospital - University Health Network; (416)603-2581

FARBER, Bernard; Pickering Med Centre, 210-1885 Glenanna Rd, Pickering ON L1V 6R6; Tor'85; CCFP; Staff, Rouge Valley Health System - Ajax & Pickering Health Centre Site; (905)420-5776; Fax. (905)420-8523.

FARBER, David F; CSSS de Laval, 1755 boul Rene-Laennec, Laval QC H7M 3L9; McG'95; FRCPC; IntMed; Gastroent. Staff, Hopital de la Cite de la santé; Langs: Bilingual(French/English); (450)668-1010; davidfarber@sympatico.ca.

FARBER, Robert; Yonge-Eglinton Med Centre, 206-2401 Yonge St, Toronto ON M4P 3H1; Tor'48; FRCPC; Peds. Sr Physician, The Hospital For Sick Children; Prof, University of Toronto; (416)485-4419; Fax. (416)485-2936.

FARCNIK, Karl D; 209-22 College St, Toronto ON M5G 1K2; UBC'86; BSc; FRCPC; Psy. Staff, Toronto Western Hospital - University Health Network; Asst Prof, University of Toronto; (416)928-2226; Fax. (416)928-6778.

FARDY, John M; Health Sciences Centre, 300 Prince Philip Dr, St. John's NL A1B 3V6; Mem'82; FRCPC; IntMed; Gastroent. Staff Physician, Health Sciences Centre; Prof Med, Memorial University Of Newfoundland; (709)777-7064; Fax. (709)777-8044.

FARDY, Noreen; Eleven Elizabeth Family Practi, 201-11 Elizabeth Ave, St. John's NL A1A 1W6; Mem'97; BSc; CCFP; Langs: English; French; (709)579-1106

FAREAU-WEYL, Joelle M T; Trellis Mental Hlth & Dev Serv, 147 Delhi St, Guelph ON N1E 4J3; Strasbourg (France)'82; FRCPC; Psy (Office Psychiatry). Staff Psychiatrist/Admv Asst Prof, Waypoint Centre for Mental Health Care; Langs: Creole; Spanish; Bilingual(French/English); (519)821-2060

FARES, Leila; Hop Jean-Talon, 1385 rue Jean-Talon E, Montreal QC H2E 1S6; Casablanca (Morocco)'90; IntMed (P.Q.). Staff, CSSS du Coeur de l'Isle Hôpital Jean-Talon; (514)495-6767; Fax. (514)495-6771.

FARES, Oussama; CSSS de Papineau, 155 rue MacLaren E, Gatineau QC J8L 0C2; CCFP; Staff, Hôpital de Papineau; (819)986-3341

FAREWELL, John C; Toronto Rehab Inst-Univ Ctr, 550 University Ave, Toronto ON M5G 2A2; Tor'81; FRCPC; Psy. Consultant, Campbellford Memorial Hospital; Consultant, Peterborough Regional Health Centre - Hospital Drive; Staff, Centre for Addiction & Mental Health (CAMH) - College Street Site; Staff, Toronto Rehabilitation Institute - University Centre; Teacher, University of Toronto; (416)597-3422

FAREY, Ruth; Rideau Family Health Team, 5-3635 Rivergate Way, Ottawa ON K1V 2A4; Ott'98; CCFP; FCFP; Langs: Bilingual(English/French); (613)739-3700; Fax. (613)739-7043; rfarey@sympatico.ca.

FARGAS-BABJAK, Angelica M; Hamilton HS-Mcmaster Site, PO Box 2000 Stn Lcd 1 HSC 2U-1200 Main St W, Hamilton ON L8N 3Z5; Safarika (Slovakia)'67; CAFCI; FRCPC; Anes (Acupuncture). Ac Staff, Hamilton Health Sciences Centre - McMaster Children's Hospital; Affil Staff, St Joseph's Healthcare - Charlton Campus; Prof, McMaster University; Langs: Slovak; (905)521-2100 x75175; Fax. (905)523-1224; babjaka@mcmaster.ca.

FARGHER, Terence J; West Parry Sound Health Ctre, 6 Albert St, Parry Sound ON P2A 3A4; Stellenbosch (South Africa)'80; MB ChB; FCP (SA); FRCPC; IntMed (Respirology). Chief of Staff, West Parry Sound Health Centre; Langs: Afrikaans; (705)746-4540 x4216; Fax. (705)773-4065.

FARHADI, Elham; The Ottawa Hosp-Civic Campus, 1053 Carling Ave, Ottawa ON K1Y 4E9; Shiraz (Iran)'88; FRCPC; Peds. Staff, The Ottawa Hospital - Civic Campus; (613)737-8899

FARHANGPOUR, Erfan; Eagle Ridge Hosp & Hlth CC, 475 Guildford Way, Port Moody BC V3H 3W9; Witwatersrand (South Africa)'03; MB BCh; CCFP; Staff, Eagle Ridge Hospital & Health Care Centre; (604)461-2022

FARHAT, Fawzi E S; Green Bay Comm Health Ctre, PO Box 280 292 Main St, Springdale NL A0J 1T0; Al Fateh (Libya)'99; Staff, Green Bay Community Health Centre; (709)673-3911

FARHAT, Gloria; 17-1525 Cornwall Rd, Oakville ON L6J 0B2; St. Maarten (Netherlands Antilles)'01; CCFP; Langs: Bilingual(English/French); (289)291-0220; Fax. (289)291-0222.

FARHAT, Mohamed J K; Mission Med Clinic, 2303 4 St SW, Calgary AB T2S 2S7; Al Fateh (Libya)'96; Staff, James Paton Memorial Hospital; (403)229-1700; Fax. (403)229-1875.

FARHAT, Musbah S; Niagara H System-G Niagara, 5546 Portage Rd, Niagara Falls ON L2E 6X2; University of Al Fateh (Libya)'00; CCFP; CCFP(E.M.); Staff, Niagara Health System - Greater Niagara General Site; (905)358-0171

FARHAT, Najwa F; Family Med Clinic, PO Box 800 4615 49 Ave, Lloydminster SK S9V 0T1; Tripoli (Libya)'90; (306)825-8877

FARHAT, Walid A; The Hosp For Sick Children, M299-555 University Ave, Toronto ON M5G 1X8; Beirut (Lebanon)'92; FRCSC; Urol. Staff Urology Dept, The Hospital For Sick Children; Asst Prof, University of Toronto; Langs: Arabic; (416)813-6580; Fax. (416)813-6461; walid.farhat@sickkids.ca.

FARIA, Julio; SMBD Jewish Gen Hosp, G308-3755 ch Cote-Sainte-Cathe, Montreal QC H3T 1E2; McG'90; ABS; MD; ABC(RS); CSPQ; FRCSC; GenSurg (Colon & Rectal Surgery). Staff, Sir Mortimer B Davis Jewish General; Asst Prof Surg, McGill University; Langs: Portuguese; French; (514)340-8222 x4948; Fax. (514)340-7560.

FARIA, Sergio L; MUHC-Montreal Gen Hosp, D5400-1650 av Cedar, Montreal QC H3G 1A4; Sao Paulo (Brazil)'75; FRCPC; RadOncol (P.Q.). Staff, McGill University Health Centre - Montreal General Campus; (514)934-8040

FARIBAULT, Guy; Ctr Hosp Rouyn-Noranda, 4 9e rue, Rouyn-Noranda QC J9X 2B2; Sher'85; FRCPC; DiagRad. Staff, Centre Hospitalier Rouyn-Noranda; (819)764-5131; Fax. (819)764-2900.

FARID ARAKI, Keyghobad; The Ctr for Addiction & Mental, 60 White Squirrel Way, Toronto ON M6J 1H4; Tehran (Iran)'96; Psy. Staff, Centre for Addiction & Mental Health (CAMH) - Russell Street Site; Langs: Farsi; (416)535-8501; Fax. (416)425-5279.

FARIDI, Anjum; Mercantile Center, 3F-55 Union St, Saint John NB E2L 5B7; Punjab (India)'92; (506)648-6286

FARIDI, Kia; Allan Memorial Institute, 1025 av des Pins O, Montreal QC H3A 1A1; Cal'02; FRCPC; Psy. Staff, McGill University Health Centre - Royal Victoria Hospital; Staff, Allan Memorial Institute; (514)934-1934 x34567; kiafaridi@gmail.com.

FARIDI, Majid; 203-444 Victoria St, Kamloops BC V2C 2A7; Tabriz (Iran)'70; FRCSC; Neursurg (Spine). Staff, Royal Inland Hospital; (250)828-9511; Fax. (250)828-1823; majidfaridi@netscape.net.

FARINA, Dana M; Queen Elizabeth II HSC, 927-1276 South Park St, Halifax NS B3H 2Y9; Mem'96; Gastroent; IntMed. Staff, Queen Elizabeth II Health Sciences Centre - Victoria General Site; (902)473-7781; Fax. (902)473-4406.

FARINAS, Jean-Marc; 644A rue Jacques-Cartier E, Chicoutimi QC G7H 2A4; Mon'89; CSPQ; CardSurg; Cardiovasc&ThorSurg (P.Q.); GenSurg. (418)545-4456; Fax. (418)545-1449.

FARINE, Dan; Ontario Power Generation Bldg, 3914-700 University Ave, Toronto ON M5G 1Z5; Tel-Aviv (Israel)'76; FACOG; FRCSC; ObstGyn (Maternal Fetal Medicine). Staff Perinatologist, Mount Sinai Hospital; Prof/Head Maternal Fetal Med, University of Toronto; Langs: Hebrew; French; (416)586-8592; Fax. (416)586-8740.

FARINE, Michelle; 305-2238 Dundas St W, Toronto ON M6R 3A9; McG'80; FRCPC; Peds. Staff, The Hospital For Sick Children; Staff Teacher, University of Toronto; Langs: Bilingual(English/French); (416)538-8512; Fax. (416)538-8513.

FARION, Kenneth J; Children's Hosp Eastern Ont, 401 Smyth Rd, Ottawa ON K1H 8L1; Alb'93; FRCPC; EmergMed (Pediatrics). Ac Staff, Children's Hospital of Eastern Ontario (CHEO); Assoc Prof Peds & EmergMed, University of Ottawa; (613)737-7600 x2318; Fax. (613)738-4885.

FARIS, Andrea E; The Medical Arts Bldg, 610-581 Davis Dr, Newmarket ON L3Y 2P6; Qns'02; FRCPC; IntMed; Gastroent. (905)895-6500; Fax. (905)895-0121.

FARIS, Glenn D; 201-1205 56 St, Delta BC V4L 2A6; Qns'90; FRCPC; Psy (Geriatric Psychiatry). Staff, Delta Hospital; (604)943-9059

FARIS, Matthew W; Providence CCC-St Mary's, PO Box 3600 Stn Main 340 Union St, Kingston ON K7L 5A2; Qns'85; MD; FRCP; ABPMR; FRCPC; PhysMed&Rehab (Amputee Rehabilitation). Staff, Providence Care - St Mary's of the Lake Hospital Site; Staff, Kingston General Hospital; Asst Prof, Queen's University; (613)544-2322; Fax. (613)544-8640; mf3@queensu.ca.

FARIVAR-MOHSENI, Hesam; Peel Med Arts Bldg, 203-2120 North Park Dr, Brampton ON L6S 0C9; Tor'92; FRCSC; Urol. (905)451-1611

FARJALLA, Salaheddin G; 209-700 Tecumseh Rd E, Windsor ON N8X 4T2; Al-Fateh (Libya)'91; FRCPC; IntMed; Gastroent., Windsor Regional Hospital - Metropolitan Site; Staff, Hôtel-Dieu Grace Hospital; Langs: Arabic; (519)971-5364; Fax. (519)971-8639.

FARKAS, Noemi; Yonge & Clark Family Physician, 103-7368 Yonge St, Thornhill ON L4J 8H9; Tor'93; CCFP; (905)771-9807; Fax. (905)771-6436.

FARKOUH, Michael; Univ Hlth Network-Toronto Gen, 4NU-200 Elizabeth St, Toronto ON M5G 2C4; Wes'88; FRCPC; IntMed. Staff, Toronto General Hospital - UHN; (416)340-3141

FARLEY, Alain Y A; 1675 rue Champigny, Saint-Laurent QC H4L 4P9; Ott'61; Gastroent (P.Q.); IntMed. (514)747-6792; Fax. (514)866-0367.

FARLEY, John D; 1141 Main St, Vancouver BC V6A 4B6; Lagos (Nigeria)'79; MB BS; ABIM; FRCPC; IntMed (Hepatology). (604)687-1147

FARLEY, Julie; Hotel-Dieu De Levis, 143 rue Wolfe, Levis QC G6V 3Z1; Laval'96; FRCSC; ObstGyn. Staff, Hôtel-Dieu de Lévis; (418)835-7121

FARLEY-DESCHAMPS, Justine; 3830 av Lacombe, Montreal QC H3T 1M5; Mon'75; Staff, St Mary's Hospital Centre; Langs: English; (514)345-3511 x3395; Fax. (514)734-2663; justine.farley@ssss.gouv.qc.ca.

FARMER, Carl; 102-256 rue Montigny, Saint-Jerome QC J7Z 5P9; McG'90; CSPQ; FRCSC; OrthSurg. (450)565-6793

FARMER, James; Hotel-Dieu Hosp, 166 Brock St, Kingston ON K7L 5G2; Ott'79; FRCSC; Ophth (Ocular Pathology); AnatPath. Staff AnatPath & Ophyh Path, The Ottawa Hospital - Civic Campus; Staff Ophth, Providence Continuing Care Centre (PCCC) - St Vincent de Paul Hospital; Staff Ophth & Path, Hotel-Dieu Hospital; Staff Ophth & Path, Kingston General Hospital; Asst Prof Ophth & Path, University of Ottawa; (613)544-3400 x2169

FARMER, Jean-Pierre; MUHC-Montreal Children's Hosp, C1139-2300 rue Tupper, Montreal QC H3H 1P3; McG'83; FRCSC; Neursurg. Staff, McGill University Health Centre - Montreal Children's Hospital; Prof, McGill University; Langs: English; French; (514)412-4488; Fax. (514)412-4340.

FARMER, Marie; CHUS-Hop Fleurimont, 3001 12e av N, Sherbrooke QC J1H 5N4; Reims (France)'01; Staff, Centre Hospitalier Universitaire de Sherbrooke-Hopital Fleurimont; (819)346-1110 x6983

FARMER, Michael J; Oakridge Centre South Tower, 209-650 41st Ave W, Vancouver BC V5Z 2M9; UBC'88; MD; (604)261-5626

FARMER, Olivier R; CHUM-Hop Notre-Dame, 1560 rue Sherbrooke E, Montreal QC H2L 4M1; Mon'99; FRCPC; Psy. Staff, Centre Hospitalier l'Université de Montréal (CHUM) - Hôpital Notre-Dame; (514)890-8000 x25656; Fax. (514)412-7827.

FARMER, Patricia L; Kingston Gen Hosp, 76 Stuart St, Kingston ON K7L 2V7; Qns'85; FRCPC; AnatPath. Staff, Kingston General Hospital; (613)549-6666 x3146; Fax. (613)548-6076.

FARMER, R Charles; Westwood Med Clinic, 3320 Portage Ave, Winnipeg MB R3K 0Y8; Dundee (Scotland)'75; MB ChB; (204)832-1363

FARMER, Stephen R; Queen Elizabeth Hosp, PO Box 6600 Stn Central 60 Riverside Dr, Charlottetown PE C1A 8T5; Dal'92; Anes. Staff, Queen Elizabeth Hospital; (902)894-2111

FARNALLS, Raymond B; Foothills South Tower, 702-3031 Hospital Dr NW, Calgary AB T2N 2T8; Alb'60; DPsy; FRCPC; Psy. Asst Clin Prof, University of Calgary; (403)283-1241; Fax. (403)283-2936.

FARNAN, Paul A; 303-4180 Lougheed Hwy, Burnaby BC V5C 6A7; RCS (Ireland)'82; MB ChB; ASAM; CCFP; FCFP; Med Dir, HelthQuest Occupational; Assoc Prof Med & Fam Pract, University of British Columbia; (604)718-6929; p.farman@ubc.ca.

FARNCOMBE, Margaret L; Palliative Care Outreach Prog, 111-1716 Woodward Dr, Ottawa ON K2C 0P8; Ott'87.

FARNELL, Barbara A; 200-2437 Princess St, Kingston ON K7L 3G1; Tor'82; FRCPC; EmergMed. (613)546-6652

FARNELL, Brian J; Kingston Family Health Team, 200-2437 Princess St, Kingston ON K7M 3G1; Tor'85; (613)546-6652; Fax. (613)546-5292; bfarnell@kfhn.net.

FARNQUIST, Brenda; Kelowna Gen Hosp, 2268 Pandosy St, Kelowna BC V1Y 1T2; UBC'05; FRCPC; DiagRad. Staff, Kelowna General Hospital; (250)864-2218

FAROOKI, M Sarwar; 25-3360 rue Notre-Dame, Lachine QC H8T 3E2; Punjab (Pakistan)'57; MSc; FRCPC; IntMed; Nephrol (P.Q.). Staff, McGill University Health Centre - Montreal General Campus; (514)637-8122

FAROOKI, Nadia; Univ Hlth Network-Toronto Gen, GS 480-200 Elizabeth St, Toronto ON M5G 2C4; McG'04; FRCPC; EmergMed. Staff, Toronto General Hospital - UHN; (416)340-3856

FAROOQ, Ahmed U; Regina Qu'Appelle HR-Regina, 1440 14th Ave, Regina SK S4P 0W5; McM'03; FRCPC; DiagRad. Staff, Regina General Hospital; (306)766-4123; Fax. (306)766-3359.

FAROOQ, Bushra; Peel Medical Walk-in-Clinic, 475 Charolais Blvd, Brampton ON L6Y 0M2; Punhab (Pakistan)'89; CCFP; (905)454-3347; Fax. (905)454-3288.

FAROOQ, Mohammed; 105 Bentinck St PO Box 553 Stn A, Sydney NS B1P 6H4; Peshawar (Pakistan)'68; MB BS; Staff, Cape Breton Healthcare Complex; Langs: Urdu; Punjabi; (902)539-0283; Fax. (902)564-6779.

FAROOQ, Saqba; Regina Qu'Appelle HR-Regina, 1440 14th Ave, Regina SK S4P 0W5; McM'99; FRCPC; DiagRad. Staff, Regina General Hospital; (306)766-4444

FAROOQ, Tarik A; Eagle Ridge Family Health Ctre, 203-480 Huronia Rd, Barrie ON L4N 6M2; Wes'00; DDerm; CCFP; (705)727-7688; Fax. (705)734-6284.

FAROOQI, Abdulzahir S; 310 King St E, Kitchener ON N2G 2L3; Karachi (Pakistan)'85; MB BS; (519)749-9692; Fax. (519)749-8187; doczfarooqi@hotmail.com.

FAROOQI, Muna I; Dawson Road Family Med Clinic, 83 Dawson Rd, Guelph ON N1H 1B1; Karachi (Pakistan)'00; CCFP; Langs: Hindi; Urdu; (519)840-1960

FARQUHAR, Donald R E; 268 Grosvenor St, London ON N6A 4V2; Qns'82; FRCPC; IntMed; Respir. Att Staff, St Joseph's Hospital - St Joseph's Health Care; Att Staff, London Health Sciences Centre Pharmacy-Victoria Campus; Assoc Prof, University of Western Ontario; (519)646-6227; donald.farquhar@sjhc.london.on.ca.

FARQUHAR, James A; Douglas Mental Hlth Univ Inst, 6875 boul Lasalle, Verdun QC H4H 1R3; Tor'81; DPsy; FRCPC; Psy (Community Psychiatry). Staff, Douglas Mental Health University Institute; McGill University; Langs: Italian; French; (514)761-6131; Fax. (514)888-4091; farjam@douglas.mcgill.ca.

FARQUHARSON, Duncan F; Royal Columbian Hosp, 330 Columbia St E, New Westminster BC V3L 3W7; Tor'76; FACOG; FRCSC; ObstGyn (Maternal Fetal Medicine). Staff, Providence Health Care - St Paul's Hospital; Staff, Royal Columbian Hospital; Member Maternal/Fetal Med, BC Women's Hospital & Health Centre; Med Dir Maternal Fetal Med, Fraser Health Authority; Assoc Prof ObstGyn, University of British Columbia; (604)520-4132; Fax. (604)520-4140.

FARQUHARSON, Patricia A; U of Toronto Hlth Ctr-Koffer B, 214 College St, Toronto ON M5T 2Z9; Tor'87; PhD; (416)978-8030; Fax. (416)971-2089.

FARQUHARSON, Scott; Foothills Med Centre, C231-1403 29 St NW, Calgary AB T2N 2T9; Mem'95; CCFP; CCFP(E.M.); Staff, Foothills Medical Centre; (403)319-0327; Fax. (403)319-0327.

FARRAGOS, Anthony; Halton Hills FHT-Guelph Street, UL-171 Guelph St, Georgetown ON L7G 4A1; Qns'99; CCFP; (905)877-4123

FARRAH, Daniela T; Meadowlark Fam Physician, 180 Meadowlark Shopping Ctr NW, Edmonton AB T5R 5W9; Alb'96; BSc(Hon); CCFP; (780)484-7574; Fax. (780)486-4121.

FARRAHI, Siavash; Elmsdale Med Centre, 106 Elmsdale Rd, Elmsdale NS B2S 1K6; Mashhad (Iran)'07; (902)883-2216

FARRALES, Lynn L; 3495 Cambie St PO Box 291, Vancouver BC V5Z 4R3; Qns'99; MSc; CCFP.

FARRAN, Rex P; Alberta Children's Hosp, 2888 Shaganappi Trail NW, Calgary AB T3B 6A8; Cal'89; Anes (Pain Management). Staff, Alberta Children's Hospital; (403)955-7810

FARRAR, David; Clinique de Physiotherapie, 2500 boul de l'Universite, Sherbrooke QC J1K 2R1; Sher'73; Dir Med, Universite de Sherbrooke; Langs: Bilingual(French/English); (819)821-7593; Fax. (819)821-7576; cms@usherbrooke.ca.

FARRAUTO, Leonardo A; Hamilton HS-Henderson Site, 711 Concession St, Hamilton ON L8V 1C3; McM'95; FRCPC; PhysMed&Rehab. Ac Staff, Hamilton Health Sciences Centre-Juravinski Site; Clinical Asst Prof Med, McMaster University; Langs: Italian; (905)389-4411 x43655; Fax. (905)575-2598; farrauto@hhsc.ca.

FARRELL, Brian; Royal Jubilee Hosp, 1952 Bay St, Victoria BC V8R 1J8; Mem'03; CCFP; CCFP(E.M.); Staff, Royal Jubilee Hospital; (250)370-8000

FARRELL, Catherine A; Hôpital Ste-Justine, 3414-3175 ch Cote-Ste-Catherin, Montreal QC H3T 1C5; Qns'82; FRCPC; Peds (Intensive Care); Critical Care Medicine (P.Q.). Staff Intensive Care, Hôpital Ste-Justine; Associé Clin Prof, Universite de Montreal; Langs: Bilingual(English/French); (514)345-4931 x2977; Fax. (514)345-7731.

FARRELL, Christopher J; Parkdale Med Towers, 604-1081 Carling Ave, Ottawa ON K1Y 4G2; Qns'82; FACOG; DABOG; FRCSC; ObstGyn. (613)728-0461; Fax. (613)728-3816.

FARRELL, Donald H; Parrtown Place, 4B-28 King St, Saint John NB E2L 1G3; Dal'75; FRCSC; Ophth. (506)634-8484; Fax. (506)658-0157.

FARRELL, Edward S; 469 Smith St, New Waterford NS B1H 3R5; Dal'75; Ac Staff, New Waterford Consolidated Hospital; (902)862-6431; Fax. (902)862-2137.

FARRELL, Gerald E; Aberdeen Hosp, 835 East River Rd, New Glasgow NS B2H 3S6; Mem'74; Staff, Aberdeen Regional Hospital; (902)752-7600

FARRELL, Gerard; Dr H Bliss Murphy Cancer Ctr, 300 Prince Philip Dr, St. John's NL A1B 3V6; Mem'84; Staff, Dr H Bliss Murphy Cancer Centre; A-Asst Dean Undergraduate Med Education, Memorial University Of Newfoundland; (709)777-8087

FARRELL, Jamie; Health Sciences Centre, 2750D-300 Prince Philip Dr, St. John's NL A1B 3V6; Mem'04; FRCPC; IntMed; Respir. Staff, Health Sciences Centre; (709)737-6300

FARRELL, Janet C; St Joseph's Healthcare, 50 Charlton Ave E, Hamilton ON L8N 4A6; McM'79; FRCPC; Anes. Staff Anes, St Joseph's Hospital - St Joseph's Health Care; Assoc Prof, McMaster University; (905)522-4941 x3853; Fax. (905)521-6019.

FARRELL, Jerome K; 424 Azure Pl, Kamloops BC V2E 2R2; Dublin (Ireland)'68; MB BCh; Staff, Royal Inland Hospital; (250)374-0081; Fax. (250)374-0082.

FARRELL, Laura; Victoria Gen Hosp, 1 Hospital Way, Victoria BC V8Z 6R5; UBC'02; FRCPC; IntMed. Staff, Victoria General Hospital; (250)727-4212 x507; lheemskerk@chr.ab.ca.

FARRELL, Mark R; Queensway-Carleton Hosp, 3045 Baseline Rd, Ottawa ON K2H 8P4; Tor'86; FRCPC; Anes. Staff, Queensway Carleton Hospital; (613)721-2000

FARRELL, Maureen E; 23 Huron St W, Exeter ON N0M 1S2; Wes'01; MSc; CCFP; CCFP(E.M.); Staff, South Huron Hospital Association; (519)235-3343; Fax. (519)235-3845.

FARRELL, Patti M; 105-47 Athabascan Ave, Sherwood Park AB T8A 4H3; Alb'85; CCFP; FCFP; Family Med, Covenant Health - Edmonton General Continuing Care Centre; (780)449-4119; Fax. (780)449-4189.

FARRELL, Richard P; 275-546 St Paul St, Kamloops BC V2C 5T1; Belfast (Ireland)'80; MB BCh; BAO; DA; Staff, Royal Inland Hospital; Pres, Galenca Infomediary Services Ltd; (250)372-3104; pfarrell@telus.net.

FARRELL, Robert T C; Carbonear Gen Hosp, 86 Highroad South, Carbonear NL A1Y 1A4; Mem'89; FRCSC; GenSurg. Staff, Carbonear General Hospital; (709)945-5248

FARRELL, Sandra A; The Credit Valley Hosp, 2200 Eglinton Ave W, Mississauga ON L5M 2N1; McM'80; MSc; FRCPC; Peds; MedGenetics. Ac Staff, The Credit Valley Hospital; (905)813-4104; Fax. (905)813-4347.

FARRELL, Scott A; IWK Health Centre, PO Box 9700 Rpo CSC 6039-5980 University Ave, Halifax NS B3K 6R8; Dal'84; BEd; BAA; DObstRCOG; FRCSC; ObstGyn (Urological Gynecology). Staff, IWK Health Centre; Prof ObstGyn, Dalhousie University; (902)420-6788; Fax. (902)470-8640; scott.farrell@iwk.nshealth.ca.

FARRELL, Theresa; Stanton Terr Health Authority, PO Box 10 550 Byrne Rd, Yellowknife NT X1A 2N1; Cape Town (South Africa)'78; CCFP; Staff, Stanton Territorial Health Authority; (867)669-4111

FARRELL-COOK, Colleen L; Wedgewood Med Centre, 304-12 Gleneyre St, St. John's NL A1A 2M7; Mem'03; FRCSC; ObstGyn (Maternal Fetal Medicine). (709)579-2606

FARRELLY, Geraldine A; 3930 20 St SW, Calgary AB T2T 4Z9; Dublin (Ireland)'76; FRCPC; Peds (Developmental Pediatrics). Staff, Alberta Children's Hospital; Asst Prof, University of Calgary; (403)686-9300; Fax. (403)686-0627.

FARREN, Ruth P; 577 5th Ave, Kamloops BC V2C 3R1; UBC'86; BSc; (250)372-8568; Fax. (250)372-8563.

FARREN, S Blake; Royal Inland Hosp, 311 Columbia St, Kamloops BC V2C 2T1; UBC'86; FRCPC; Anes. Staff, Royal Inland Hospital; (250)314-2620; Fax. (250)314-2319.

FARRER, John P; PO Box 778, Sechelt BC V0N 3A0; London (England)'72; MB BS; Ac Staff, St Mary's Hospital; (604)885-5196; Fax. (604)885-5193; jpfarrer@telus.net.

FARRIER, Alain; Clinique Med Le Mesnil, 300-1300 boul LeBourgneuf, Quebec QC G2K 2N1; Laval'86; Staff, CSSS de Trois-Rivières; (418)624-1800; Fax. (418)624-1820.

FARRIES, Lawrence R; Medical & Dental Bldg, 4F-3939 50A Avenue, Red Deer AB T4N 4E6; Alb'85; FRCSC; GenSurg. Staff, Red Deer Regional Hospital Centre; (403)347-9037; Fax. (403)347-9038; lfarries@yahoo.ca.

FARRINGTON, Bruce; Scarborough Hosp-General Div, 3050 Lawrence Ave E, Scarborough ON M1P 2V5; Tor'73; Staff, The Scarborough Hospital - General Campus; (416)438-2911

FARROW, James M; Cool Aid Community Health Ctre, 713 Johnson St, Victoria BC V8W 1M8; McG'76; Physician, Cool Aid Community Health Centre; (250)385-1477

FARRUGGIA, Pasquale; Clinique Med Langelier, 5953 Belanger E, Saint-Leonard QC H1T 1G8; Palerme (Italy)'85; CCFP; FCFP; (514)253-9191; Fax. (514)253-5242.

FARRUGIA, Alexandra A E; PO Box 3090, Revelstoke BC V0E 2S0; Ott'95; CCFP; Staff Privil, Queen Victoria Hospital; (250)837-9321; Fax. (250)837-9444; a.farrugia.smg@gmail.com.

FARRUGIA, M Michele; 3F-700 University Ave, Toronto ON M5G 1Z5; Tor'98; BSc; MSc; MEd; FRCSC; ObstGyn. Physician ObstGyn, Mount Sinai Hospital; Asst Prof, University of Toronto; (416)586-8553; Fax. (416)586-8355.

FARRUGIA, Michael D P; Alliston Family Health, PO Box 280 36 Victoria St, Alliston ON L9R 1V5; (Other Foreign)'09; (705)435-8887

FARUQI, Faez; Clinique Medicale Gynesys, 425-1575 rue Henri-Bourassa O, Montreal QC H3M 3A9; Mon'86; FRCSC; ObstGyn. (514)781-5950; Fax. (514)336-8814.

FARUQI, Perves Z; Paediatric Consultants, 202 King St W, Chatham ON N7M 1E5; Karachi (Pakistan)'91; MB BS; (519)351-9322; Fax. (519)351-9323.

FARUQUI, Ferrukh I; Village Health Centre, PO Box 100 3192 Logan Farm Dr, Osgoode ON K0A 2W0; Man'87; CCFP; (613)826-2502

FASHHO, Ousama; Finch-Midland Med Centre, 410-4190 Finch Ave E, Scarborough ON M1S 4T7; Tor'83; Ac Staff, The Scarborough Hospital - Birchmount Campus; Ac Staff, Rouge Valley Health System - Centenary Health Centre Site; (416)293-2626; Fax. (416)293-2799; ofasho@interlog.com.

FASHIR, Baroudi; Cape Breton Hlth Care, 1482 George St, Sydney NS B1P 1P3; Khartoum (Sudan)'79; MB BS; FRCP; MRCP(UK); Staff, Cape Breton Healthcare Complex; (902)567-7284; Fax. (902)567-7285; bfashir@yahoo.com.

FASHORANTI, Oluwarotimi; Fashoranti Med Inc, PO Box 429 272 Church St, Pugwash NS B0K 1L0; Benin (Nigeria)'85; MB BS; CCFP; Staff, North Cumberland Memorial Hospital; Physician Marine Medical Examiner, Transport Canada; Med Dir, High Crest Nursing Home; Langs: Yoruba; (902)243-2580; Fax. (902)243-2257.

FASIE-NEAGOE, C F Cristina; Lakeshore Gen Hosp, 160 av Stillview, Pointe-Claire QC H9R 2Y2; Bucharest (Romania)'80; PhC; CCFP; FCFP; Staff, Lakeshore General Hospital - Pointe Claire; Staff, Clinique Medicale Pierrefonds; Physician, Brunswick Medical Clinic; Langs: Romanian; French; (514)817-9090; Fax. (514)630-4084; dr.cfasie@gmail.com.

FASIH, Najla; The Ottawa Hosp-Civic Campus, 1053 Carling Ave, Ottawa ON K1Y 4E9; Punjab (India)'97; Staff, The Ottawa Hospital - Civic Campus; Langs: Urdu; Hindi; Punjabi; (613)761-4054

FASIHY, Elham; Avecina Clinic, 100-20644 Fraser Hwy, Langley BC V3A 4G5; Cal'99; CCFP; (604)539-1744; efasihy@hotmail.com.

FASSIER, Francois; Shriners Hosp for Children, 1529 av Cedar, Montreal QC H3G 1A6; Grenoble (France)'80; MSc; CSPQ; FRCSC; OrthSurg (Pediatric Orthopedics). Chef cabinet, Shriners Hospitals For Children - Canada; Associé Clin Prof, Universite de Montreal; assoc Prof, McGill University; Langs: Bilingual(French/English); (514)282-6963; ffassier@shrinenet.org.

FAST, Diane; BC Women's Hosp & Health Ctre, Box 141 P4-4500 Oak St, Vancouver BC V6H 3N1; McG'82; PhD; FRCPC; Psy. Staff, BC Women's Hospital & Health Centre; Clin Prof Psy/Associate Ped, University of British Columbia; (604)875-2655

FAST, Eunice M; 304-4420 Chatterton Way, Victoria BC V8X 5J2; Man'91; BSc(Med); Clin Instructor, University Of Victoria; Clin Instructor, University of British Columbia; (250)727-9664; Fax. (250)727-9445.

FAST, Henry V; 102-900 Harrow St E, Winnipeg MB R3M 3Y7; Man'74; FRCPC; Psy (Child & Adolescent Psychiatry). Psychiatrist, Eden Mental Health Centre; Consultant, Community Mental Health Services; (204)475-2039; Fax. (204)453-7748.

FAST, Mallory D; St Boniface Clinic, 343 Tache Ave, Winnipeg MB R2H 2A5; Man'81; FRCPC; Neur. Ac Staff, St Boniface General Hospital; Asst Prof Med, University of Manitoba; (204)925-9553; Fax. (204)231-2283.

FAST, Richard B; Professional Services Corporat, PO Box 480 800 Warm Bay Rd, Atlin BC V0W 1A0; UBC'66; (250)651-0055

FATA, Paola M; MUHC-Montreal Gen Hosp, L9 411-1650 Cedar Ave, Montreal QC H3G 1A4; McG'95; CSPQ; FRCSC; GenSurg. Staff, McGill University Health Centre - Montreal General Campus; (514)934-1934 x44334

FATEIS, Aimen; Beverly Medical Clinic, 4243 118 Ave NW, Edmonton AB T5W 1A5; (Libya)'00; MB BCh; (780)756-7700; Fax. (780)756-7788.

FATHALLA, Hala H; Royal Alexandra Hosp, 10240 Kingsway NW, Edmonton AB T5H 3V9; (Iraq)'79; MB ChB; Staff, Royal Alexandra Hospital; (780)628-7485

FATHIMANI, Kamran; University of Alberta Hosp, 2D4 27-8440 112 St NW, Edmonton AB T6G 2B7; Alb'02; FRCSC; GenSurg. Staff, University of Alberta Hospital; (780)407-6306

FATHOLLAHZADEH, Afsoon; Trafalgar Prof Centre, 314-1235 Trafalgar Rd, Oakville ON L6H 3P1; McG'92; FRCPC; Peds (Pediatric & Adolescent Medicine). Langs: English; French; Farsi; (905)842-3993; Fax. (905)842-9260.

FATIMA, Anis; Shoppers World Med Centre, 106-499 Main St, Brampton ON L6Y 1N7; (Pakistan)'99; (905)796-6570

FATIMA, Qamar; 205-505 Queen St, Spruce Grove AB T7X 2V2; (Pakistan)'90; MB BS; CCFP; (780)962-2001; Fax. (780)962-8176.

FATOKUN, Olumide J; 321 White Earth St PO BOX 1150, Smoky Lake AB T0A 3C0; (Nigeria)'94; MB BS; (780)656-2100; Fax. (780)656-2406.

FATOYE, Adetunji; Seven Oaks Gen Hosp, 2300 McPhillips St, Winnipeg MB R2V 3M3; Lagos (Nigeria)'88; CCFP; Staff, Seven Oaks General Hospital; (204)632-3203; Fax. (204)694-5697.

FATOYE, Olubunmi; Medical Officer of Hlth, 490 Hargrave St, Winnipeg MB R3A 0A7; (Nigeria)'92; FRCPC; CommunMed;CCFP; Public Health & Preventive Med.

FATUM, Krista L; 469 William St S SS 2 Stn Main, Exeter ON N0M 1S2; McM'97; CCFP; (519)235-0910

FAUCHER, Anne; CHUS-Hop Hotel-Dieu, 580 rue Bowen S, Sherbrooke QC J1G 2E8; Sher'93; FRCSC; Ophth. Staff, Centre Hospitalier Universitaire de Sherbrooke-Hôpital Hôtel-Dieu; (819)346-1110

FAUCHER, Catherine; St Joseph Family Med Clinic, 403-2555 St Joseph Blvd, Orleans ON K1C 1S6; Mon'07; FRCSC; ObstGyn. (613)837-8396; Fax. (613)837-8398.

FAUCHER, Claire; CSSS de Laval, DS 074-1755 boul Rene Laennec, Laval QC H7M 3L9; Paris (France)'86; Nephrol (P.Q.). Staff, Hopital de la Cite de la santé; (450)668-1010 x24228

FAUCHER, Daniel; Clinique Medico-Sante, 62-1116 rue Vachon N, Sainte-Marie QC G6E 1N7; Laval'93; CCFP; (418)387-2565

FAUCHER, Daniel J; MUHC-Royal Victoria Hosp, 687 av des Pins O, Montreal QC H3A 1A1; Sher'78; CSPQ; FRCPC; Peds (P.Q.) (Neonatology). Staff, McGill University Health Centre - Montreal Children's Hospital; Staff, McGill University Health Centre - Royal Victoria Hospital; Staff, Sir Mortimer B Davis Jewish General; Assoc Prof Peds & ObstGyn, McGill University; (514)934-1934 x34876; daniel.faucher@muhc.mcgill.ca.

FAUCHER, Dorothee; CSSS de Beauce-Etchemin, 1515 17e rue, Saint-Georges QC G5Y 4T8; Laval'90; CSPQ; FRCSC; GenSurg. Staff, Centre Hospitalier Beauce-Etchemin; (418)228-2031

FAUCHER, Elise; CSSS de Rimouski-Neigette, CP 3150 succ Bureau Chef 150 av Rouleau, Rimouski QC G5L 5T1; Laval'04; FRCSC; ObstGyn. Staff, Hôpital Regional Rimouski; (418)723-7851

FAUCHER, Frederic; Hop Maisonneuve-Rosemont, 5415 boul de l'Assomption, Montreal QC H1T 2M4; Mon'93; FRCPC; Peds. Staff, Hopital Maisonneuve-Rosemont; (514)252-3400; Fax. (514)374-8101.

FAUCHER, Guy L; CH Jean la Lalande, 4255 av Papineau, Montreal QC H2H 2P6; Mon'59; FRCSC; ObstGyn. (514)526-4981

FAUCHER, Helene; Hotel-Dieu St-Joseph, 9 rue Canada, Saint-Quentin NB E8A 1J2; Sher'08; CCFP; Staff, Hôtel-Dieu St-Joseph de Saint-Quentin; (506)235-2300

FAUCHER, Jacques; Clin Med Dr Jacques Faucher, 454 rue Principale, Ham-Nord QC G0P 1A0; Laval'79; LMCC; ac Membre CMDP & Emerg, Hotel-Dieu d'Arthabaska; Med Dir, Ham-Nord Geriatric Centre; Langs: Bilingual(French/English); (819)344-2083; Fax. (819)344-2023; jack_md007@hotmail.com.

FAUCHER, Jacques; Clinique Med de Levis, 100-4975 boul de la Rive-Sud, Levis QC G6V 4Z5; Laval'67; Staff, Hôtel-Dieu de Lévis; Physician, Clinique Medicale De Levis; (418)833-5810; Fax. (418)833-2720.

FAUCHER, Jacques-Philippe; Hop Charles Lemoyne, 3120 boul Taschereau, Greenfield Park QC J4V 2H1; Mon'82; FRCPC; IntMed. Staff, Hopital Charles LeMoyne; adj Prof, Universite de Sherbrooke; (450)466-5750 x2880; Fax. (450)466-5768; jacques-philippe.faucher@usherbrooke.ca.

FAUCHER, Jocelyne; Vice-Rectorat Aux Relations In, 2500 boul de l'Universite, Sherbrooke QC J1K 2R1; Sher'85; MSc; CCFP; FCFP; Staff Family Med, CSSS - IUGS; Sec gén Vice-Rectorat International Relations, Universite de Sherbrooke; (819)821-8285; Fax. (819)821-8295; jocelyne.faucher@usherbrooke.ca.

FAUCHER, Line; CRSSS Baie-James-Chibougamau, 51 3e rue, Chibougamau QC G8P 1N1; Laval'98; CCFP; Staff, CRSSS de la Baie-James; Langs: Bilingual(French/English); (418)748-2676; Fax. (418)748-2549.

FAUCHER, Lise; Ctr Dermatologique Maskoutain, 2356 rue dessaulles, Saint-Hyacinthe QC J2S 2T8; Mon'90; FRCPC; Derm. Staff, Centre Hospitalier Honore-Mercier; Médecin, Centre Dermatologique Maskoutain; (450)778-2333; Fax. (450)778-1720.

FAUCHER, Lucien L; Montfort Hosp, 713 Montreal Rd, Ottawa ON K1K 0T2; Alb'70; MPs; FRCPC; Psy (Hospital Psychiatry). Staff, Montfort Hospital; Langs: English; French; (613)746-4621 x3919; Fax. (613)748-4938; lfaucher@rogers.com.

FAUCHER, Marc; Medicentre Pincourt, 88 5e av, Pincourt QC J7V 5K7; Mon'79; Médecin, Medicentre Pincourt; (514)425-1000; Fax. (514)425-1288.

FAUCHER, Roland; GMF du Chatel, 200-9465 boul de l'Ormiere, Quebec QC G2B 3K7; Laval'73; (418)843-5141; Fax. (418)843-5343.

FAUCHER, Sylvain; Inst U en Sante Mentale de QC, 2601 ch de la Canardiere, Quebec QC G1J 2G3; Laval'91; FRCPC; Psy. Staff, Institut Universitaire Sante; (418)663-5321; Fax. (418)661-0561.

FAUCHER, Yves J L; Ctr Medi Soleil St-Jean-Sur-Ri, 120-383 boul du Seminaire N, St-Jean-sur-Richel QC J3B 8C5; Laval'74; (450)349-5555

FAUGHNAN, Marie E; St Michael's Hosp, 6049-30 Bond St, Toronto ON M5B 1W8; Mon'93; FRCP; MSc; FRCPC; IntMed; Respir. Staff Physician, St Michael's Hospital; Asst Prof, University of Toronto; Langs: French; (416)864-5412; Fax. (416)864-5922; faughnanm@smh.toronto.on.ca.

FAUGHT, Andrea L; SCOHS-Elisabeth Bruyere Hosp, 43 Bruyere St, Ottawa ON K1N 5C8; Ott'91; Staff, SCO Health Service - Élisabeth Bruyère Hospital; (613)562-0050 x1524

FAUGHT, Carolyn R; The Ottawa Hosp-Gen Campus, 501 Smyth Rd, Ottawa ON K1H 8L6; McG'92; BSc; FRCPC; IntMed (Lymphoma); Hem. Staff Physician, The Ottawa Hospital - General Campus; Asst Prof, University of Ottawa; Langs: Bilingual(English/French); (613)737-8303

FAUGHT, J Wylam; The Ottawa Hosp-Gen Campus, 8420-501 Smyth Rd, Ottawa ON K1H 8L6; Alb'86; FRCSC; ObstGyn (Surgical Oncology). Staff, The Ottawa Hospital - General Campus; Dept Head ObstGyn, University of Ottawa; (613)737-8937; Fax. (613)739-6193.

FAUGHT, James W; 288 Dundas St E PO Box 420, Waterdown ON L0R 2H0; Wes'75; CCFP; FCFP; Ac Staff, Joseph Brant Memorial Hospital; Clinical Asst Prof Family Med, McMaster University; (905)689-8677; Fax. (905)689-8393.

FAUL, Hendri; Medicine Hat Reg Hosp, 666 5 St SW, Medicine Hat AB T1A 4H6; Orange Free State (South Africa)'92; MB ChB; CCFP; CCFP(E.M.); Staff Emerg, Medicine Hat Regional Hospital; Langs: Afrikaans; (403)529-8053; hjfaul@shaw.ca.

FAUL, John; Douglas Square Med Centre, 144-11520 24 St SE, Calgary AB T2Z 3E9; Orange Free State (South Africa)'90; MB ChB; CCFP; (403)236-0211; Fax. (403)236-0261.

FAULDER, Douglas G; Capital Care Norwood, 10410 111 Ave NW, Edmonton AB T5G 3A2; Alb'78; Dir Medical Services, Capital Care - Grandview; (780)448-2412; Fax. (780)413-4748; douglas.faulder@capitalcare.net.

FAULDS, Catherine; London Family Health Team, 200-440 Boler Rd, London ON N6K 4L2; Wes'86; CCFP; FCFP; Staff, London Health Sciences Centre - Victoria Campus; Staff, Parkwood Hospital - St Joseph's Health Care; Staff, St Thomas Elgin General Hospital; Aj Prof Family Med, University of Western Ontario; (519)473-4394; Fax. (519)472-5904.

FAULDS, Jason; 910 10th Ave W, Vancouver BC V5Z 4E3; Qns'06; FRCSC; GenSurg. (604)875-4545

FAULDS, Thomas R; St Thomas-Elgin Gen Hosp, PO Box 2007 Stn Main 189 Elm St, St Thomas ON N5P 3W2; Wes'86; CCFP; CCFP(E.M.); FCFP; Staff, Chatham-Kent Health Alliance; Ac Staff, St Thomas Elgin General Hospital; (519)631-2020 x2113

FAULKNER, Donald E; 250-8120 Cook Rd, Richmond BC V6Y 1T9; UBC'73; Staff, Richmond Hospital; Staff, BC Children's Hospital; (604)273-3643

FAULKNER, John R; 302-1100 Sheppard Ave E, North York ON M2K 2W1; Qns'72; FRCSC; OrthSurg. Staff, North York General Hospital; (416)222-5242; Fax. (416)222-1385.

FAULKNER, Paul E; Joseph Brant Mem Hosp, 1230 North Shore Blvd E, Burlington ON L7S 1W7; McM'91; CCFP; CCFP(E.M.); FCFP; Staff, Joseph Brant Memorial Hospital; (905)336-4116

FAULKNER, Stephen J; 160 Jubilee St, Duncan BC V9L 1W7; Otago (New Zealand)'78; MB ChB; Assoc Staff Member, Cowichan District Hospital; (250)709-9600

FAULKNOR, Janice Y; 45 Chester Cres, Georgetown ON L7G 5T4; Ott'96; CCFP; Langs: Creole.

FAULLEM, Ingrid; Clinique du Vieux Gatineau, 2B-520 boul de l'Hopital, Gatineau QC J8V 2P5; Sher'06; CCFP; (819)568-0212; Fax. (819)568-6310.

FAULQUES, Bernard; CHUM-Hop Notre-Dame, 1560 rue Sherbrooke E, Montreal QC H2L 4M1; Gastroent (P.Q.). Staff, Centre Hospitalier l'Université de Montréal (CHUM) - Hôpital Notre-Dame; (514)890-8000

FAURE, Christophe; Hôpital Ste-Justine, 3175 ch Cote-Ste-Catherine, Montreal QC H3T 1C5; Paris (France)'90; Gastroent (P.Q.). Staff, Hôpital Ste-Justine; (514)345-4931; Fax. (514)345-4999.

FAURE, Nacia; Lundbeck Canada Inc, 500-1000 de la Gauchetiere, Montreal QC H3B 4W5; Laval'72; Endocrin (P.Q.) (Palliative Care). Staff, West Island Palliative Care Residence; Langs: English; (514)940-9434

FAUST, Gilles; CHUS-Hop Hotel-Dieu, 580 rue Bowen S, Sherbrooke QC J1G 2E8; Sher'79; MBA; ABIM; CSPQ; FRCPC; IntMed; Gastroent. Staff, Centre Hospitalier Universitaire de Sherbrooke-Hôpital Hôtel-Dieu; Prof, Universite de Sherbrooke; Langs: English; (819)346-1110 x25501; Fax. (819)822-6797.

FAUTEUX, Jasmin; Rockyview Gen Hosp, 7007 14 St SW, Calgary AB T2V 1P9; Laval'08; CCFP; CCFP(E.M.); Staff, Rockyview General Hospital; (403)943-7000

FAUTH, Clarissa T; Red Deer Reg Hosp Centre, PO Box 5030 Stn Postal Box Ctr 3942 50A Ave, Red Deer AB T4N 4E7; Cal'04; FRCPC; AnatPath. Staff, Red Deer Regional Hospital Centre; (403)343-4735; Fax. (403)343-4877.

FAUVEL, C Terry; Rockyview Gen Hosp, 7007 14 St SW, Calgary AB T2V 1P9; Cal'84; FRCPC; Psy (Psychotherapy). Staff Psy., Rockyview General Hospital; (403)943-3614; Fax. (403)943-3624.

FAUX, Peter J; Queen-Lynch Med Centre, 211-157 Queen St E, Brampton ON L6W 3X4; Tor'68; FRCPC; Psy. (905)456-1144; Fax. (905)456-5472.

FAVA, Craig S; Royal Columbia Hosp, 330 Columbia St E, New Westminster BC V3L 3W7; UBC'98; FRCPC; IntMed; Critical Care Medicine; Respir. Staff, Royal Columbian Hospital; (604)520-4576

FAVA, Mark A; Gates of Maple Family Practice, 410-955 Major Mackenzie Dr W, Vaughan ON L6A 4P9; Wes'03; FRCSC; Ophth. (905)553-1404; Fax. (905)553-1406.

FAVERO, Kenneth J; 101-22112 52 Ave, Langley BC V2Y 2M6; UBC'80; FRCSC; OrthSurg. (604)534-5373; Fax. (604)534-5362.

FAVOT, Dean; Hotel Dieu Grace Hosp, 1030 Ouellette Ave, Windsor ON N9A 1E1; Guadalajara (Mexico)'81; Court Staff, Windsor Regional Hospital - Metropolitan Site; Staff, Hôtel-Dieu Grace Hospital; Langs: Spanish; (519)973-4401; Fax. (519)252-3632.

FAVREAU, Diane; CSST de longueuil, 500-25 boul La Fayette, Longueuil QC J4K 5B7; Mon'75; (450)442-6200 x6255

FAVREAU, Joel; CSSS de la Haute-Yamaska, 205 boul Leclerc O, Granby QC J2G 1T7; Mon'01; Staff, Centre Hospitalier de Granby; (450)375-8000

FAVREAU, Marc B; CHUM-Hotel-Dieu, 3840 rue Saint-Urbain, Montreal QC H2W 1T8; McG'71; FRCPC; IntMed; Rheum. ac Staff, Centre Hospitalier l'Université de Montréal (CHUM) - Hôtel-Dieu; adj Prof Med, Universite de Montreal; Langs: English; (514)890-8000

FAVREAU, Marie-Helene; Pratt & Whitney Canada, 1000 boul Marie-Victorin, Longueuil QC J4G 1A1; Mon'87; Physician, Pratt & Whitney Canada; (450)647-4119; Fax. (450)647-9251.

FAVREAULT, Luce; CSSS Les Eskers de l'Abitibi, 622 4e rue O, Amos QC J9T 2S2; Mon'98; Staff, CH Hôtel-Dieu d'Amos; (819)732-3341

FAVRON, Helene; Direction de la Sante Publique, 1255 rue Beauregard, Longueuil QC J4K 2M3; Mon'91; (450)928-6777 x3111

FAWAZ, Charbel S; 504-100 Arden St, Moncton NB E1C 4B7; Mon'04; FRCSC; Neursurg. Staff, Foothills Medical Centre; (506)857-5378; Fax. (506)857-5378.

FAWAZ, Nabil; Centre Med Lacordaire, 201-5650 rue Jean-Talon E, Saint-Leonard QC H1S 1M1; Alexandria (Egypt)'69; Langs: Arabic; Italian; English; (514)255-5595

FAWCETT, Arlie; Carnat Ctr Sunridge Med Galler, 300-2580 32 St NE, Calgary AB T1Y 7M8; Alb'82; FRCPC; Psy. (403)944-9800; Fax. (403)955-9850.

FAWCETT, Bruce M; Teck Cominco Trail Health Ctr, PO Box 1000, Trail BC V1R 4L8; Oxford (England)'67; MRC; Cominco Ltd.; (250)364-4321; bruce.fawcett@teckcominco.com.

FAWCETT, Wesley C; Kelowna Gen Hosp, 2268 Pandosy St, Kelowna BC V1Y 1T2; Sask'84; FRCPC; Anes. Staff, Kelowna General Hospital; (250)862-4309

FAWELL, John A; Large Med Clinic, 219 2nd Ave W, Prince Rupert BC V8J 1G4; Pretoria (South Africa)'07; MB ChB; Langs: Afrikaans; (250)624-9651

FAWELL, Sunelle; Large Med Clinic, 219 2nd Ave W, Prince Rupert BC V8J 1G4; Pretoria (South Africa)'04; MB ChB; Langs: Afrikaans; (250)624-9651

FAWOLE, Olukayode A; CBI Health Centre, 100 Signal Rd, Fort McMurray AB T9H 5A3; (Nigeria)'90; LMCC; MB ChB; MCFP(SA); Fax. (780)715-3800.

FAY, Didier; Centre Med Robinson Inc, 4 rue Robinson N, Granby QC J2G 8Z9; Mon'77; Affil Staff, Centre Hospitalier de Granby; (450)378-8435; Fax. (450)375-8832.

FAY, Donald F; 6137 Jubilee Rd, Halifax NS B3H 2E8; Dal'80; BEng; DPhil; Staff, District Digestmount Family Practice Capital Hlth; (902)422-2285; Fax. (902)422-6846.

FAY, Heather E; 4420 10th Ave W, Vancouver BC V6R 2H9; Aberdeen (Scotland)'73; MB ChB; (604)617-6570

FAY, Michel; Centre Med Fusion, 200-2035 av Sainte-Anne, Saint-Hyacinthe QC J2S 5H3; Mon'90; Staff, Centre Hospitalier Honore-Mercier; (450)773-6023

FAY, Nicholas; Deer Lake Med Clinic, 7-4 Clinic Dr, Deer Lake NL A8A 1E2; Dublin (Ireland)'05; BAO; MB BCh.

FAY, Sean Leo; Burrard Health Bldg, 707-1160 Burrard St, Vancouver BC V6Z 2E8; Dublin (Ireland)'70; Ac Staff, Providence Health Care - St Paul's Hospital; (604)687-8368; Fax. (604)687-8302.

FAY, William P; Sudbury Reg Hosp-Laurentian, 41 Ramsey Lake Rd, Sudbury ON P3E 5J1; National (Ireland)'66; FRCPC; IntMed (Nephrology). Dir Dialysis, Health Sciences North-Laurentian Site; (705)523-7004; Fax. (705)523-7161; wpfay@hsndudbury.ca.

FAYAD, Ashraf; The Ottawa Hosp-Civic Campus, 1053 Carling Ave, Ottawa ON K1Y 4E9; Al Fateh (Libya)'93; FRCPC; Anes. Staff, The Ottawa Hospital - Civic Campus; Langs: Arabic; (613)761-4940; Fax. (613)761-5209.

FAYAD, Hamideh; Bluewater Health-Norman Site, 89 Norman St, Sarnia ON N7T 6S3; Staff, Bluewater Health - Norman Site; (519)464-4400

FAYET, Cristina; The Four Villages CHC, 3446 Dundas St W, Toronto ON M6S 2S1; Tor'08; BSc; MSc; CCFP; Physician, Parkdale Community Health Centre; Langs: Portuguese; (416)604-3362; cristina.fayet@pchc.on.ca.

FAYEZ, Ibrahim; Sunnybrook Hlth Sciences Ctr, M1 700-2075 Bayview Ave, Toronto ON M4N 3M5; Ain Shams (Egypt)'92; CCFP; Staff, Sunnybrook Health Sciences Centre; Langs: Arabic; (416)480-4905

FAYEZ, Raad M; Colchester East Hants Hlth Ctr, 600 Abenaki Rd, Truro NS B2N 5A1; (Saudi Arabia)'01; MB BS; FRCSC; GenSurg. Staff, Aberdeen Regional Hospital.

FAZAL, Haydarally H; Ashgrove Med Centre, 204-6633 Highway 7, Markham ON L3P 7P2; Tor'77; FAAP; FRCPC; Peds (Allergy). Ac Staff, The Hospital For Sick Children; Court Staff, Markham Stouffville Hospital; Med Dir, Markham Travel Clinic; Lecturer, University of Toronto; Langs: Bilingual(English/French); (905)294-0907; Fax. (905)294-3926.

FAZAL KARIM, Karima; Clinique Med Joliette, 3841 rue Ontario E, Montreal QC H1W 1S5; Laval'99; CCFP; Langs: Spanish; French; (514)524-3731; Fax. (514)524-0675.

FAZEKAS, Arpad G; Westmount Med Bldg, 425-5025 rue Sherbrooke O, Montreal QC H4A 1S9; Szeged (Hungary)'60; PhD; (514)489-8070

FAZELI CHAGHOSHI, Leila; 405-1100 Sheppard Ave E, North York ON M2K 2W1; (Iran)'90; FRCPC; Peds. Langs: Azeri; (416)221-6588; Fax. (416)221-0637.

FAZHULLA, Shabeena; Edmonton Trail Med Clinic, 409 8 Ave NE, Calgary AB T2E 0R3; (India)'97; MB BS; CCFP; Langs: Hindi; Tamil; (403)276-8711

FAZIL, Mohammad A; Cowichian Internists, 3106 Gibbins Rd, Duncan BC V9L 1E8; Aga Khan (Pakistan)'90; MB BS; (250)748-1323

FAZIO, Luke M; Bathurst Med Centre, 305-4256 Bathurst St, North York ON M3H 5Y8; McG'99; FRCSC; Urol (Endourology). Staff, Humber River Regional Hospital - Finch Avenue Site; Langs: Bilingual(English/French); (416)630-1712; Fax. (416)630-6415.

FAZL, Mahmood; Sunnybrook Hlth Sciences Ctre, 138-2075 Bayview Ave, Toronto ON M4N 3M5; Shiraz (Iran)'75; FRCSC; Neursurg. Ac Staff, Sunnybrook Health Sciences Centre; Asst Prof, University of Toronto; Langs: Persian; (416)480-4741; Fax. (416)480-6085.

FAZZARI, Frank; Medical & Dental Bldg, 203-1221 Algonquin Ave, North Bay ON P1B 4Y3; Ott'52; Peds (Allergy). Ac Staff, North Bay Regional Health Centre - Regional Mental Health; Langs: Italian; (705)472-4050; Fax. (705)472-4090.

FEAGAN, Brian; Robarts Clinical Trials, PO Box 5015 Stn B 100 Perth Dr, London ON N6A 5K8; Wes'83; MSc(MedMicrobiol); FRCPC; IntMed (Gastroenterology). Consultant, London Health Sciences Centre - University Hospital; Consultant, Robarts Clinical Trials; Prof Med Epidemiol, University of Western Ontario; (519)931-5289; Fax. (519)931-5278.

FEAGAN, Nancy; 1462 Adelaide St N, London ON N5X 1J9; Wes'81; CCFP; FCFP; Ac Staff, St Joseph's Hospital - St Joseph's Health Care; (519)432-6318

FEAKINS, Martin J; Providence Care Mental Hlth, 725 King St W, Kingston ON K7M 2G3; Dublin (Ireland)'92.

FEANNY, Stephen J; 202-9780 Bramalea Rd, Brampton ON L6S 2P1; (Jamaica)'71; MB; BSc; FRCPC; Peds. (905)791-2390

FEARON, Margaret A; Canadian Blood Services Med Of, 67 College St, Toronto ON M5G 2M1; Dublin (Ireland)'82; LRCP; LRCS; FRCPC; MedMicrobiol (Infectious Diseases). Exec Med Dir, Med Micro, Canadian Blood Services; Teach Staff Lab Med & Path, University of Toronto; (416)313-4598; Fax. (416)974-9757.

FEARON, S Blair; Medicine Professional Incorpor, 603-2 St Clair Ave W, Toronto ON M4V 1L5; Dublin (Ireland)'83; FRCSC; Ophth (Glaucoma). Staff, North York General Hospital; (416)962-2023; Fax. (416)962-2029.

FEASBY, Thomas E; Calgary Heart Centre, 7 TRW-3280 Hospital Dr NW, Calgary AB T2N 4Z6; Man'69; FRCPC; Neur. Physician, Health Research Innovation Centre; Dean Faculty of Med, University of Calgary; (403)220-6842; Fax. (403)270-1828.

FEATHERSTON, Carlos R; 33 Somerset St W, Ottawa ON K2P 0H3; Buenos Aires (Argentina)'55; FRCPC; Psy. Staff, The Ottawa Hospital - General Campus; Langs: Spanish; (613)233-2308; Fax. (613)231-6852.

FEAVER, Bruce D; Limeworth X-Ray & Ultrasound, 102-849 Upper Wentworth St, Hamilton ON L9A 5H4; Wes'59; FRCPC; DiagRad. Ac Staff, Ross Memorial Hospital; (905)574-7755; Fax. (905)574-0384.

FEBBRARO, Mario A; Doctors Bldg, 240-955 Queen St E, Sault Ste. Marie ON P6A 2C3; Ott'71; Langs: Italian; (705)759-1234; Fax. (705)949-2333.

FEBER, Janusz; Children's Hosp Eastern Ont, 401 Smyth Rd, Ottawa ON K1H 8L1; Prague (Czech Republic)'86; FRCPC; Peds (Nephrology). Staff, Children's Hospital of Eastern Ontario (CHEO); University of Ottawa; Langs: German; Czech; Polish; Bilingual(French/English); (613)737-7600 x2441; Fax. (613)738-3254; jfeber@cheo.on.ca.

FEBEROVA, Jana; Univ of Ottawa, 451 Smyth Rd, Ottawa ON K1H 8M5; Prague (Czech Republic)'98; Teacher, University of Ottawa.

FEBERWEE, Jillian A; Halton HSC Corp-Oakville, 327 Reynolds St, Oakville ON L6J 3L7; Dal'98; FRCPC; DiagRad. Staff, Halton Healthcare Services Corporation - Oakville Site; (905)338-4601; Fax. (905)338-4375.

FECTEAU, Annie H; The Hosp For Sick Children, 1526-555 University Ave, Toronto ON M5G 1X8; McG'88; FRCSC; PedGenSurg (Liver Transplant); GenSurg. Staff, The Hospital For Sick Children; Staff, North York General Hospital; Asst Prof, University of Toronto; Langs: English; French; (416)813-6402; Fax. (416)813-7477; annie.fecteau@sickkids.ca.

FECTEAU, Claude; Clin Pediatrie de Trois-Rivier, 110-5725 boul des Forges, Trois-Rivieres QC G8Y 5L5; Sher'76; FRCPC; Peds. (819)375-0504

FECTEAU, David; Clinique Pediatrique Sainte-Fo, 293-2600 boul Laurier, Quebec QC G1V 4T3; Laval'02; FRCPC; CCFP; Peds. Staff, CSSS de Trois-Rivières; (418)658-0906

FECTEAU, Line; CSSS des Etchemins, 331 rue du Sanatorium, Lac-Etchemin QC G0R 1S0; Sher'04; Staff, CSSS des Etchemins; (418)625-8001

FECTEAU, Serge; I R D P Q-Site Francois-Charon, 525 boul Wilfrid-Hamel, Quebec QC G1M 2S8; Laval'79; FRCPC; PhysMed&Rehab. Staff, CSSS de Trois-Rivières; (418)529-9141; sergefecteau@videotron.ca.

FECYCZ, Taras D; 103-1300 Don Mills Rd, North York ON M3B 2W6; National (Ireland)'87; Langs: Ukrainian; (416)444-7765

FEDAK, Paul W M; Foothills Medical Centre, 880-1403 29 St NW, Calgary AB T2N 2T9; Tor'98; FRCSC; CardSurg (Clinical & Investigative Medicine). Staff, Foothills Medical Centre; (403)944-5931

FEDDER, Steven A; The Richmond Hosp, 7000 Westminster Hwy, Richmond BC V6X 1A2; Wes'92; CCFP; CCFP(E.M.); Richmond Hospital; (604)278-9711

FEDER, Stephen H; Children's Hosp Eastern Ont, 401 Smyth Rd, Ottawa ON K1H 8L1; McG'76; MPH; CCFP; Staff, Children's Hospital of Eastern Ontario (CHEO); Physician, Pinecrest-Queensway Community Health Centre; Langs: English; French; (613)737-7600; Fax. (613)738-4878.

FEDER, Victor M; North York Gen Hosp-Branson, 555 Finch Ave W, North York ON M2R 1N5; Buenos Aires (Argentina)'73; FRCPC; Psy., North York General Hospital - Branson Division; Langs: Spanish; (416)635-2421; Fax. (416)635-2428; vfeder@nygh.on.ca.

FEDERICI, Guiliana M; Burlington Prof Centre, 409-3155 Harvester Rd, Burlington ON L7N 3V2; McM'87; FRCPC; Peds. Langs: Italian; (905)333-5437; Fax. (905)333-5352.

FEDERICO, Paolo; Foothills Med Centre, C1241A-1403 29 St NW, Calgary AB T2N 2T9; Cal'96; BSc(Hon); MSc; FRCPC; Neur (Epilepsy) (Neuro Epilepsy). Staff, Foothills Medical Centre; Staff, Peter Lougheed Centre; Staff, Rockyview General Hospital; Asst Prof, University of Calgary; Langs: Italian; (403)944-3348; Fax. (403)283-2270.

FEDOR, Glenn A; Yorston Med Clinic, 201-143 Fourth Ave S, Williams Lake BC V2G 1J8; Alb'78; BSc(Hon); Ac Staff, Cariboo Memorial Hospital and Health Centre; (250)398-8102; Fax. (250)398-8101.

FEDORAK, Richard N; Zeidler Ledcor Centre, 130 University Campus NW, Edmonton AB T6G 2X8; Alb'78; FRCPC; IntMed (Inflammatory Bowel Disease); Gastroent. Prof Med Div of Gastroent, University of Alberta Hospital; Prof Med, University of Alberta; (780)492-8120; Fax. (780)492-8121.

FEDORKO, Ludwik M; Univ Hlth Network-Toronto Gen, 200 Elizabeth St, Toronto ON M5G 2C4; Warsaw (Poland)'78; FRCPC; Anes. Staff Anes, Toronto General Hospital - UHN; Asst Prof Anes, University of Toronto; (416)340-3227; Fax. (416)340-3698.

FEDORKOW, Donna M; Hamilton HS-Henderson Site, 711 Concession St, Hamilton ON L8V 1C3; Cal'84; FRCSC; ObstGyn (Urological Gynecology). Staff, Hamilton Health Sciences Centre-Juravinski Site; Staff ObstGyn, Hamilton Health Sciences Centre - McMaster Children's Hospital; Assoc Prof, McMaster University; (905)521-2100 x42409

FEDOROFF, J Paul; Royal Ottawa Hlth Care Group, 1145 Carling Ave, Ottawa ON K1Z 7K4; Sask'83; DABPN(Psy.); FRCPC; Psy (Forensic Psychiatry). Dir Sexual Behav Clin/Staff Psy, Royal Ottawa Mental Health Centre - Royal Ottawa Health Care Group; Assoc Prof Psy/Head Div of Forensic Psy, University of Ottawa; (613)722-6521; Fax. (613)798-2992; paul.fedoroff@theroyal.ca.

FEDOROW, Christine; Harry Medovy House, 2F-671 William Ave, Winnipeg MB R3E 0Z2; Alb'05; FRCPC; Anes.

FEDOROWICZ, Andrew; Radiology Consultants Assoc, 120-6707 Elbow Dr SW, Calgary AB T2V 0E3; Man'93; FRCPC; DiagRad; NuclearMed. (403)777-3007

FEDOROWICZ, Valerie; McGill Mental Hlth Service, 5500-3600 rue McTavish, Montreal QC H3A 0G3; McG'00; FRCPC; Psy (Child Psychiatry). Langs: Bilingual(French/English); (514)398-6019; Fax. (514)398-5529.

FEDORUK, James; The Urgent Care Ctr, 11811 Tecumseh Rd E, Windsor ON N8N 4M7; McM'78; AB; MCFP(EM); LLB; Lecturer Surg, University Of Windsor; Assoc Prof Med, University of Western Ontario; (519)979-3355; Fax. (519)979-1429; lawdoc@sympatico.ca.

FEDORUK, Lynn M; 106-2020 Richmond Rd, Victoria BC V8R 6R5; Alb'88; FRCSC; CardSurg. (250)595-1833; Fax. (250)595-1889.

FEDWICK, Jason; Foothills Med Centre, C231-1403 29 St NW, Calgary AB T2N 2T9; Cal'07; CCFP; CCFP(E.M.); Staff, Foothills Medical Centre; (403)944-1110

FEDYNA, Roman; Cedarcroft Retirement Home, 649 King St E, Oshawa ON L1H 8P9; Wes'71; BA; MD; Court Staff, Lakeridge Health - Oshawa Site; Med Dir, Wynfield Nursing Home; Med Dir, Sunnycrest Nursing Home Ltd; Langs: Polish; Ukrainian; (905)723-3574

FEENER, Tricia A; Western Memorial Hlth Clinic, 3 Herald Ave, Corner Brook NL A2H 4B8; Mem'95; BMedSci; FRCPC; Peds. Staff, Western Memorial Regional Hospital; Assoc Prof Ped, Memorial University Of Newfoundland; (709)637-3900; Fax. (709)634-9572.

FEERASTA, Sharmeen H; Leslie Med Centre, 212-4800 Leslie St, Toronto ON M2J 2K9; Aga Khan University (Pakistan)'99; FAAP; FRCPC; Peds (Pediatrics). Langs: Urdu; (416)497-1987; Fax. (416)497-0712; sharmeen_feerasta@yahoo.com.

FEERO, Peter G; 1071 Route 105, Fredericton NB E3G 7L2; Mem'84; DAB; FRCSC; Urol. (506)459-6601; Fax. (506)459-6667.

FEFERGRAD, Mark D; Sunnybrook Health Science Ctre, FG38-2075 Bayview Ave, Toronto ON M4N 3M5; Wes'01; FRCPC; Psy. Staff Psy, Sunnybrook Health Sciences Centre; (416)480-6100

FEGELMAN, Alan; Bayview Med Centre, 2722 Bayview Ave, North York ON M2L 1B9; Tor'81; (416)730-1212; Fax. (416)730-1216.

FEGHALI, Joseph; Clinique Med Domus Medica, 5601 rue Belanger, Montreal QC H1T 1G3; St. Joseph (Lebanon)'72; ABS; CSPQ; GenSurg (P.Q.). Staff, Hôpital Santa Cabrini Ospedale; Staff, Hôpital Ste-Justine; (514)256-5011; Fax. (514)259-4979.

FEGHALI, Marc; Polyclinique Med PAT, 103-12905 rue Sherbrooke E, Pte-aux-Trembles QC H1A 1B9; Sher'90; (514)498-4050; Fax. (514)498-8239.

FEGLER, John G; Heritage Family Med Ctr, 8330 Macleod Trail SE, Calgary AB T2H 2V2; Edinburgh (Scotland)'58; (403)258-3000

FEHLAU, Barbara C; Comox Med Clinic, 100-1695 Comox Ave, Comox BC V9M 3M1; Cal'93; CCFP; FCFP; Langs: German; (250)339-2266; bfehlau@shaw.ca.

FEHLINGS, Darcy; Holland Bloorview Kids Rehab, 150 Kilgour Rd, Toronto ON M4G 1R8; Tor'83; FRCPC; Peds. Staff Peds, The Hospital For Sick Children; Assoc Prof, University of Toronto; (416)425-6220 x3586; Fax. (416)424-3837.

FEHLINGS, Michael; Univ Hlth Network-Toronto Western Hosp, 4W 449-399 Bathurst St, Toronto ON M5T 2S8; Tor'83; PhD(NeuroSci); FRCSC; Neursurg (Spine & Spinal Cord Surgery). Dir, Toronto Western Hospital - University Health Network; Consultant, Toronto Rehabilitation Institute - Lyndhurst Centre; Prof Surg, University of Toronto; Langs: German; (416)603-5627; Fax. (416)603-5298.

FEIBEL, Robert J; The Ottawa Hosp-Gen Campus, 1652 CCW-501 Smyth Rd, Ottawa ON K1H 8L6; Qns'85; FRCSC; OrthSurg (Total Joint). Att Staff OrthSurg, The Ottawa Hospital - General Campus; Assoc Prof Surg, University of Ottawa; Langs: Bilingual(English/French); (613)737-8849; Fax. (613)737-8837.

FEICK, Elizabeth A; Caledonian Med Clinic, 340 Campbell St, Nanaimo BC V9R 3G7; Cal'79; (250)753-3202; Fax. (250)753-1039.

FEIERABEND, Martina M; Scarborough Hosp-General Div, 3050 Lawrence Ave E, Scarborough ON M1P 2V5; Tor'81; FRCPC; Anes. Staff, The Scarborough Hospital - General Campus; Langs: German; (416)431-8208; Fax. (416)431-8151.

FEIERSTEIN, Michele E; Manitoba Clinic, 790 Sherbrook St, Winnipeg MB R3A 1M3; Man'85; FRCPC; Peds (Pediatric Emergency Medicine). (204)957-1900

FEIFER, Andrew H; Credit Valley Prof Bldg, 411-2300 Eglinton Ave W, Mississauga ON L5M 2V8; McG'04; FRCSC; Urol. (905)997-2805; Fax. (905)997-2806.

FEIG, Denice S; L5 027-60 Murray St Box 14, Toronto ON M5T 3L9; McM'82; MSc; FRCPC; IntMed (Endocrinology); Endocrin&Metab. Staff, Mount Sinai Hospital; Staff, Toronto General Hospital - UHN; Assoc Prof, University of Toronto; (416)586-8590; Fax. (416)361-2657.

FEIGE, Erwin; Diagnostic Sleep Clinic, 104-60 Champlain St, North Bay ON P1B 7M4; Tor'83; DABSM; CCFP; FCFP; Staff, North Bay Regional Health Centre - Regional Mental Health; Langs: English; French; (705)472-1967; Fax. (705)472-0689.

FEIGE, Richard R R; Surrey Med Arts Bldg, 201-13798 94A Ave, Surrey BC V3V 1N1; Cal'81; ABIM; FCCP; FRCPC; IntMed; Respir. Assoc Dir ICU/Ac Staff, Royal Columbian Hospital; Dir Pulmonary Lab, Surrey Memorial Hospital; (604)581-6727; Fax. (604)581-7692.

FEIGEL, Roman; Parkdale Med Tower, 204-1081 Carling Ave, Ottawa ON K1Y 4G2; Warsaw (Poland)'70; FRCSC; ObstGyn. Ac Staff, The Ottawa Hospital - Civic Campus; Langs: Polish; (613)728-0474; Fax. (613)728-8381.

FEIGELSON, Lori; Toronto Headache & Pain Clinic, 209-801 York Mills Rd, North York ON M3B 1X7; Mon'07; FRCPC; PhysMed&Rehab (Musculoskeletal Injury). Langs: Bilingual(English/French); (416)699-8843; Fax. (416)699-6094.

FEIGENBAUM, Annette S J; 555 University Ave, Toronto ON M5G 1X8; Cape Town (South Africa)'78; FRCPC; Peds (Metabolic Genetics). Assoc Prof, The Hospital For Sick Children; Teach Staff, University of Toronto; Langs: Afrikaans; (416)813-7654 x1480; Fax. (416)813-5345.

FEIGHTNER, John W; St Mary's Hosp Campus, 21 Grosvenor St, London ON N6A 1Y6; Wes'71; MSc; CCFP; FCFP; Fam Med, St Mary's Hospital - St Joseph's Health Care London; (519)646-6100

FEINBERG, Faith P; North Med Centre, 201-7131 Bathurst St, Thornhill ON L4J 7Z1; Tor'81; CCFP; FCFP; Staff Family Med, North York General Hospital; Staff, North York General Hospital - Branson Division; Langs: Hebrew; (905)771-1778; Fax. (905)771-9833.

FEINBERG, Stanley M; North York Gen Hosp, 101-4001 Leslie St, North York ON M2K 1E1; Tor'80; ABS; FACS; DABCRS; FASCRS; FRCSC; GenSurg (Colon & Rectal Surgery). Chief Surg & Prog Med Dir, North York General Hospital; Asst Prof, University of Toronto; (416)756-6764; Fax. (416)756-6769; sfeinber@nygh.on.ca.

FEINDEL, Christopher M S; Univ Hlth Network-Toronto Gen, 4N 480-200 Elizabeth St, Toronto ON M5G 2C4; McG'76; MBA; FRCSC; GenSurg; Cardiovasc&ThorSurg. Staff, Toronto General Hospital - UHN; Assoc Prof Cardiac Surg, University of Toronto; Langs: English; French; (416)340-5909; Fax. (416)340-4476; chris.feindel@uhn.on.ca.

FEINER, Hannah L R; St Michael's Health Centre, 3F-61 Queen St E, Toronto ON M5C 2T2; Tor'09; CCFP; (416)867-7426

FEINMAN, Saya V; Mount Sinai Hosp, 1190-600 University Ave, Toronto ON M5G 1X5; Vienna (Austria)'48; FRCPC; IntMed (Gastroenterology). Att Staff Med, Mount Sinai Hospital; Prof, University of Toronto; (416)586-5301

FEINSTADT, Garry; The Doctors' Office, 101-777 Broadway W, Vancouver BC V5Z 4J7; Tor'72; CCFP; FCFP; (604)734-8252

FEINSTEIN, Anthony; Sunnybrook Hlth Sciences Ctre, FG 16-2075 Bayview Ave, Toronto ON M4N 3M5; Witwatersrand (South Africa)'80; MPhil; PhD; FRCPC; Psy (Neurology & Psychiatry). Staff, Sunnybrook Health Sciences Centre; Prof Psy, University of Toronto; (416)480-4216; Fax. (416)480-4613; ant.feinstein@utoronto.ca.

FEJER, Imre B; 100-4125 Lawrence Ave E, Scarborough ON M1E 2S2; Tor'69; BSc; Staff, Rouge Valley Health System - Centenary Health Centre Site; Langs: Hungarian; German; French; Urdu; (416)284-9111; Fax. (416)284-5077.

FEJES, Piroska R; Royal Court Med Centre, 204-5 Quarry Ridge Rd, Barrie ON L4M 7G1; McM'84; BSc; Fam Med, Royal Victoria Regional Health Centre; Lecturer, University of Toronto; Langs: Hungarian.

FEKETE, Ferenc; Ctr Hosp Affilie-Enfant-Jesus, 1401 18e rue, Quebec QC G1J 1Z4; Laval'77; IntMed. Staff, Centre Hospitalier Affilié Universitaire de Québec - Hôpital De L'Enfant Jésus; (418)649-0252

FEKETE, John F; Trillium Hlth Ctr-Mississauga, 100 Queensway W, Mississauga ON L5B 1B8; Budapest (Hungary)'51; FRCPC; GenPath. Staff Labs, Trillium Health Centre - Mississauga; (905)848-7100

FEKIR, Sami; Hotel-Dieu d'Arthabaska, 5 rue des Hospitalieres, Victoriaville QC G6P 6N2; Laval'06; FRCPC; DiagRad. Staff, Hotel-Dieu d'Arthabaska; (819)357-2030

FELCENBUCH-DACHIS, Harry L; Southlake Reg Health Centre, 596 Davis Dr, Newmarket ON L3Y 2P9; (Peru)'80; FRCPC; Psy (Adult & Child Psychiatry). Staff, Southlake Regional Health Centre; Langs: Spanish; (905)895-4521 x2166; Fax. (905)830-5987.

FELD, Jordan; Univ Hlth Network-Toronto Western Hosp, 6B 158-399 Bathurst St, Toronto ON M5T 2S8; Tor'97; FRCPC; IntMed (Hepatology & Gastroenterology); Gastroent. Staff, Toronto Western Hospital - University Health Network; Langs: Spanish; (416)603-5914; Fax. (416)603-6281.

FELD, Ronald; 610 University Ave, Toronto ON M5G 2M9; Tor'69; FACP; FRCPC; IntMed (Infectious Diseases). Staff Physician, Princess Margaret Hospital - University Health Network; (416)946-2260; Fax. (416)946-6546.

FELD, S Michael; Bathurst Walk-In Clinic, 101-4430 Bathurst St, North York ON M3H 3S3; Qns'70; (416)633-3629; Fax. (416)633-3624.

FELDBERG, Melissa R; St Clair Med Clinic, 2F-50 St Clair Ave E, Toronto ON M4T 1M9; Ott'01; BSc; CCFP; (416)921-1066; dr.feldberg@stclairmedical.ca.

FELDERHOF, Catharina A L; PO Box 1150, Pictou NS B0K 1H0; Dal'75.

FELDERHOF, Richard P; St Fx Med Center Bloomfield, PO Box 5000 305-5555 Union Blvd, Antigonish NS B2G 2W5; Dal'71; (902)867-4407

FELDMAN, Brian M; The Hosp For Sick Children, 555 University Ave, Toronto ON M5G 1X8; Wes'85; MSc; FRCPC; Peds (Clinical Epidemiology); Rheum. Prof Peds Health Policy Mgmt & Evaluation & DLSPH, University of Toronto; Head Div Rheum, The Hospital For Sick Children; (416)813-6117; Fax. (416)813-4989; brian.feldman@sickkids.ca.

FELDMAN, Debra C; 170 Rebecca St, Oakville ON L6K 1J6; Qns'83; CCFP; FCFP; Assoc Staff, Halton Healthcare Services Corporation - Oakville Site; (905)845-9293; Fax. (905)845-0981.

FELDMAN, Fredrick; 240-30 Disera Dr, Thornhill ON L4J 0A7; Tor'60; FRCSC; Ophth (Glaucoma). Assoc Staff, Mount Sinai Hospital; Prof Ophth, University of Toronto; (905)881-8050; Fax. (905)881-8050.

FELDMAN, Howard; UBC Hospital, S192-2211 Wesbrook Mall, Vancouver BC V6T 2B5; McG'78; FRCPC; Neur. Ac Staff, UBC Hospital - Koerner Pavillion; Head Div of Neurol/Prof/Exec Dean Research, University of British Columbia; (604)822-7979; Fax. (604)822-7703.

FELDMAN, Jacob; Westlaw Bldg, 213-1920 Weston Rd, York ON M9N 1W4; Jerusalem (Israel)'87; FRCPC; Peds. Langs: Hebrew; (416)249-6236; Fax. (416)249-5273.

FELDMAN, Kayla S; North York Gen Hosp, 4001 Leslie St, North York ON M2K 1E1; UBC'04; FRCPC; Peds (Neonatal & Perinatal Medicine). Staff, North York General Hospital; (416)756-6000

FELDMAN, Kimberley; Women's College Fam Hlth Team, 60 Grosvenor St, Toronto ON M5S 1B6; Qns'98; MHSc; CCFP; Staff, Women's College Hospital; (416)323-6065

FELDMAN, Liane S; MUHC-Montreal Gen Hosp, L9412-1650 av Cedar, Montreal QC H3G 1A4; McG'93; CSPQ; FRCSC; GenSurg (Laparoscopic Surgery). Staff, McGill University Health Centre - Montreal General Campus; Langs: English; (514)934-1934 x44337; Fax. (514)934-8438; liane.feldman@mcgill.ca.

FELDMAN, Marcel; Polyclinique de l'Oreille, 320-6020 rue Jean-Talon E, Saint-Leonard QC H1S 3B1; Rome (Italy)'72; Staff, Hôpital Santa Cabrini Ospedale; (514)253-2273; Fax. (514)483-3486.

FELDMAN, Mark E; St Joseph's Health Centre, 30 The Queensway, Toronto ON M6R 1B5; Ott'87; FRCPC; Peds. Staff Peds, St Joseph's Health Centre; Asst Prof Med, University of Toronto; (416)530-6000 x3630; Fax. (416)530-6294; feldmm@stjoe.on.ca.

FELDMAN, Michael; Sunnybrook Hlth Sciences Ctre, BG15-2075 Bayview Ave, Toronto ON M4N 3M5; Qns'00; FRCPC; EmergMed. Staff Emerg, Sunnybrook Health Sciences Centre; (416)480-6100

FELDMAN, Risa C; Doctor's Office, 101-491 Lawrence Ave W, North York ON M5M 1C7; Tor'82; CCFP; FCFP; Staff, Mount Sinai Hospital; (416)787-9796; Fax. (416)787-8094.

FELDMAN, Ross D; The Roberts Research Inst, PO Box 5015 Stn B 100 Perth Dr, London ON N6A 5K8; Qns'77; BSc(Hon); MD; LMCC; FRCPC; IntMed (Clinical Pharmacology). Staff, London Health Sciences Centre - South Street; Scientist, The Robarts Research Institute; (519)931-5717; Fax. (519)931-5222; feldmanr@lhsc.on.ca.

FELDMAN, Rubin M; Alder Medical Centre, 1211 8th Ave W, Vancouver BC V6H 1C7; Montpellier (France)'58; FRCPC; PhysMed&Rehab (Trauma). Langs: Bilingual(English/French); (604)862-6031; Fax. (604)687-3904.

FELDMAN, Sandra H; 243 Eglinton Ave W, Toronto ON M4R 1B1; Wes'85; CCFP; (416)489-2106; Fax. (416)489-2981.

FELDMAN, Sidney I D; Don Valley Med Associates, 330-1333 Sheppard Ave E, North York ON M2J 1V1; Tor'88; CCFP; FCFP; Staff Privil, Mount Sinai Hospital; Staff Privil, North York General Hospital; Asst Prof Family & Commun Med, University of Toronto; (416)494-7386; Fax. (416)497-4793.

FELDMAN-GLASER, Perle; North York Gen Hosp, 4S-4001 Leslie St, North York ON M2K 1E1; McG'80; CCFP; FCFP; Staff, North York General Hospital; (416)756-6980 x7; Fax. (416)756-6979.

FELDMANN, Joseph; 606-1 St Clair Ave E, Toronto ON M4T 2V7; Melbourne (Australia)'64; DPM; DPsy; FRCPC; Psy (Adolescent Psychiatry). Court Staff, Women's College Hospital; Asst Prof Psy, University of Toronto; Langs: English; French; (416)961-2282; Fax. (416)961-2282.

FELDSTEIN, N Aaron; Lakehead Psychiatric Hosp, PO Box 2930 Stn P 580 Algoma St N, Thunder Bay ON P7B 5G4; Dal'97; CCFP; Fam Med, Lakehead Psychiatric Hospital - St. Joseph's Care Group; (807)343-4300

FELEKI, Katherine J; 201-190 Wellington St, Kingston ON K7L 3E4; Tor'81; CCFP; Langs: Hungarian; (613)542-3105; Fax. (613)547-0004.

FELEMEGOS, Ioannis; Seaway Valley Comm Hlth Ctre, 353 Pitt St, Cornwall ON K6J 3R1; (Other Foreign)'07; CCFP; Langs: Greek; (613)936-0306

FELHABER, Taryl A; BC Cancer Agency-Vanc Isl Ctr, 2410 Lee Ave, Victoria BC V8R 6V5; Cape Town (South Africa)'93; MB ChB; CCFP; Staff, BC Cancer Agency Vancouver Island Centre; (250)519-5580; felstand@shaw.ca.

FELIX, James; Cook St Village Med Clinic, 101A-230 Cook St, Victoria BC V8V 3X3; Alb'03; CCFP; (250)220-9999

FELIX, John L; 309-360 Bloor St W, Toronto ON M5S 1X1; Budapest (Hungary)'50; IntMed(Hung); Langs: Hungarian; (416)925-0411; Fax. (416)923-0485.

FELIX, William A; 206 Lemarchant Rd, St. John's NL A1C 2H6; Dal'67; FRCSC; GenSurg. Ac Staff Surg, St Clare's Mercy Hospital; Staff Teacher, Memorial University Of Newfoundland; (709)777-5637; Fax. (709)754-2055; felwa@nl.rogers.com.

FELL, Charlene D; South Health Campus, 4448 Front St E, Calgary AB T3M 1M4; Tor'00; MSc; FRCPC; IntMed (Interstitial Lung Disease); Respir. Physician Respirology, Peter Lougheed Centre; (403)943-5634; Fax. (403)943-4017.

FELL, David A; Newmarket Med Place, 208-712 Davis Dr, Newmarket ON L3Y 8C3; Qns'81; FACC; FRCPC; IntMed; Cardiol. Physician Leader Regional Cardiac Care Prog, Southlake Regional Health Centre; (905)853-2888; Fax. (905)853-6607.

FELL, Heidi E; 214-11 Hidden Creek Dr NW, Calgary AB T3A 6K6; Cal'95; CCFP; FCFP; (403)248-2273

FELL, Marilyn L; White Rock Med Clinic, 101-15451 Russell Ave, White Rock BC V4B 2R5; UBC'87; (604)531-5595; Fax. (604)531-9818.

FELLEGI, Nicolette K; Greenboro Family Med Centre, 25 Tapiola Cres, Ottawa ON K1T 2J7; Ott'87; CCFP; FCFP; Langs: French; Hungarian; (613)738-0303; Fax. (613)738-8950.

FELLEGI, Vivien; East Mississauga Comm Hlth Ctr, 7-2555 Dixie Rd, Mississauga ON L4Y 4C4; Ott'89; Langs: English; French; (905)602-7723

FELLENZ, Lora G; 6507 Cosens Bay Rd, Vernon BC V1B 1N7; UBC'86; CCFP; (250)503-1558; Fax. (250)503-1582.

FELLENZ, Mathias O; 3105 27 St, Vernon BC V1T 4W4; UBC'86; FRCSC; Ophth. Langs: German; (250)549-4362; Fax. (250)549-4397.

FELLER, Andrea E; Niagara Reg Public Hlth, PO Box 1052 Stn Main, Thorold ON L2V 0A2; Maryland (USA)'00; (905)688-3762; Fax. (905)682-3901.

FELLOWS, G Fraser; London HSC-Victoria Hosp, PO Box 5010 Stn B 800 Commissioners Rd E, London ON N6A 5W9; Qns'66; FACOG; FRCSC; ObstGyn (Abortion). Court Staff, London Health Sciences Centre - Victoria Campus; Ac Staff, St Joseph's Hospital - St Joseph's Health Care; Assoc Prof, University of Western Ontario; (519)685-8500; fraser.fellows@sjhc.london.on.ca.

FELLOWS, Joanne; PO Box 4791, Rothesay NB E2E 5X5; Dal'90; CCFP; FCFP; (506)849-8509; Fax. (506)849-8777.

FELLOWS, Lesley K; MUHC-Montreal Neurology Inst, 276-3801 rue University, Montreal QC H3A 2B4; McG'96; Neur. Staff, McGill University Health Centre - Montreal Neurological Hospital; Chef Neurology & Neurosurgery, McGill University; (514)398-8980; Fax. (514)398-1338.

FELLUS, Youcef; Ctr Hosp Gatineau Memorial, PO Box 160 101 ch Burnside, Wakefield QC J0X 3G0; Strasbourg (France)'84; Staff, Centre Hospitalier Gatineau Mémorial; (819)459-1112; Fax. (819)459-1894.

FELSEN, Shim S I; Don Valley Med Associates Inc, 144-1333 Sheppard Ave E, North York ON M2J 1V1; Tor'67; CCFP; FCFP; Langs: Bilingual(English/French); (416)491-5900; Fax. (416)491-1149.

FELSTROM, Anna; Royal University Hosp, 247-103 Hospital Dr, Saskatoon SK S7N 0W8; Sask'00; BA; FRCPC; Psy (Child & Adolescent Psychiatry). Staff, Royal University Hospital; Clin Assoc Prof, University of Saskatchewan; (306)966-7027

FELTHAM, Ian C; Loyalist Family Practice, 2A-150 Sidney St, Trenton ON K8V 5S6; Mem'91; CCFP; FCFP; Staff, QHC Trenton Memorial; (613)771-0008; Fax. (613)771-1861.

FELTHAM, Ian; Brockville Mental Health Centr, PO Box 1050 Stn Main 1804 Hwy 2 E, Brockville ON K6V 5W7; Dal'82; FRCPC; Psy;CCFP; FCFP; Staff, Brockville Mental Health Centre - Royal Ottawa Health Care Group.

FELTHAM, Matthew D; 110-342 Erie St, Stratford ON N5A 2N4; Mem'03; FRCPC; IntMed. (519)273-0100; Fax. (519)273-0675.

FELTIS, J Timothy; The Credit Valley Hosp, 2200 Eglinton Ave W, Mississauga ON L5M 2N1; Qns'77; FRCPC; GenPath. General Pathology, The Credit Valley Hospital; (905)813-4241; tfeltis@cvh.on.ca.

FELTMATE, Mary F; 61 Arthur St, Truro NS B2N 1X7; Dal'78; (902)893-7231; Fax. (902)893-2406.

FELTMATE, Patrick J G; Dr Everett Chalmers Hosp, PO Box 9000 Stn A 700 Priestman St, Fredericton NB E3B 5N5; Dal'03; FRCPC; IntMed; GeriatricMed. Staff, Dr Everett Chalmers Regional Hospital; (506)452-5400

FENECH, Darlene; Sunnybrook Health Sciences Cen, 2075 Bayview Ave, Toronto ON M4N 3M5; McM'99; FRCPC; GenSurg (Colorectal Surgery). Staff, Sunnybrook Health Sciences Centre; (416)480-4027; Fax. (416)480-6002.

FENECK, Mary M; Oakville Med Centre, 300-690 Dorval Dr, Oakville ON L6K 3W7; Tor'80; FRCPC; IntMed; Cardiol. Staff, Halton Healthcare Services Corporation - Oakville Site; (905)849-4567 x2

FENG, Ann Qian; Children's & Women's HC of BC, 2D19-4480 Oak St, Vancouver BC V6H 3V4; Shanghai (China)'84; MB; FRCPC; Peds. Staff, BC Children's Hospital; Langs: Mandarin; (604)875-3177

FENG, Luming; 277 Wilson St E, Ancaster ON L9G 2B8; Qns'95; CCFP; Staff, Hamilton Health Sciences Centre - Hamilton General Hospital; Langs: Chinese; (905)648-7973; Fax. (905)648-2582.

FENG, Xiaolan; Foothills Medical Centre, 1403 29 St NW, Calgary AB T2N 2T9; (China)'00; Staff, Foothills Medical Centre; (403)944-1110

FENG, Xiumei; Rockyview Gen Hosp, 7007 14 St SW, Calgary AB T2V 1P9; Benjing (China (Republic))'90; FRCPC; IntMed. Staff, Rockyview General Hospital; Asst Prof, University of Calgary; (403)217-7880; Fax. (403)217-7828.

FENG, Z S Chris; Wardenwood Hlth Ctr, 549 Bur Oak Ave, Markham ON L6C 3E5; Tor'07; CCFP; (905)554-0199; Fax. (905)554-4834.

FENJE, Nicholas; Royal Jubilee Hosp, 1952 Bay St, Victoria BC V8R 1J8; Tor'81; FRCPC; Anes. Staff, Royal Jubilee Hospital; (250)370-8441; Fax. (250)370-8301.

FENKELL, Louis L; Southlake Reg Health Ctr, 596 Davis Dr, Newmarket ON L3Y 2P9; Qns'04; FRCPC; RadOncol. Staff, Southlake Regional Health Centre; (905)895-4521; Fax. (905)952-2818.

FENNELL, Susan D; Active Care Med Group, A-1108 Klondike Rd, Kanata ON K2K 0G1; Wes'89.

FENNER, Danuta Z; 506-2425 Bloor St W, Toronto ON M6S 4W4; Wroclaw (Poland)'64; FRCPC; Psy (Adult Psychiatry). Staff, Centre for Addiction & Mental Health (CAMH) - Queen Site; Teacher, University of Toronto; Langs: Polish; (416)604-3212; danuta_fenner@camh.net.

FENSKE, Larry E; Royal Oak Centre Med Clinic, 105-4442 Saanich Rd W, Victoria BC V8Z 3E9; Alb'74; (250)479-6721

FENSKE, Theodore K; Hys Med Centre, 350-11010 101 St NW, Edmonton AB T5H 4B9; UBC'90; FRCPC; IntMed (Cardiac Imaging); Cardiol. Staff, Royal Alexandra Hospital; Assoc Prof, University of Alberta; (780)428-3246; Fax. (780)425-0487.

FENSTER, Howard N; Gordon & Leslie Diamond HCC, L6-2775 Laurel St, Vancouver BC V5Z 1M9; McG'72; FRCSC; Urol (Voiding Dysfunction). Ac Staff, Vancouver General Hospital - Centennial Pavillion; Staff, Gordon & Leslie Diamond Health Care Centre; Consultant, University Of British Columbia; (604)875-5003; Fax. (604)875-5604.

FENSTER, Roger F; 207-5885 ch de la Cote-des-Nei, Montreal QC H3S 2T2; McG'70; FACS; MDCM; CSPQ; FRCSC; GenSurg. Associate Surg, Sir Mortimer B Davis Jewish General; Consultant, Mount Sinai Hospital Center; Consultant, Donald Berman Maimonides Geriatric Centre; Langs: French; (514)737-8615; Fax. (514)737-6911; fenster5778@videotron.ca.

FENTON, David M; St Paul's Hosp, 1081 Burrard St, Vancouver BC V6Z 1Y6; UBC'99; FRCPC; DiagRad. Staff, Providence Health Care - St Paul's Hospital; (604)806-8006; Fax. (604)806-8437.

FENTON, David W; BC Cancer Agency-Vanc Isl Ctr, 2410 Lee Ave, Victoria BC V8R 6V5; Ott'95; FRCPC; IntMed (Breast Cancer); MedOncol. Staff, Cross Cancer Institute; (250)519-5500

FENTON, John A; Oaks Plaza, 3-2140 Regent St, Sudbury ON P3E 5S8; McM'88; FRCSC; GenSurg; VascSurg. Staff Vascular Surg/Med Dir Sudbury Vascular Lab/Chief Vascular Surg, Health Sciences North - Memorial Site; Langs: French; (705)522-4611; Fax. (705)522-4158; jfenton@hrsrh.on.ca.

FENTON, Jonathan A S; 7000 Westminster Hwy, Richmond BC V6X 1A2; London (England)'62; FRCS(Eng); FRCSC; OrthSurg. Att Staff Surg, Richmond Hospital; Langs: English; French; (604)244-5141; jask61@hotmail.com.

FENTON, Mark; Royal University Hosp, 5F-103 Hospital Dr, Saskatoon SK S7N 0W8; Sask'02; FRCPC; IntMed; Respir. Staff, Royal University Hospital; (306)966-1808; Fax. (306)966-8694.

FENTON, Paul V; Kingston Gen Hosp, 76 Stuart St, Kingston ON K7L 2V7; Qns'84; FRCPC; DiagRad. Staff, Kingston General Hospital; (613)548-2301

FENTON, Peter M; 314-1849 Yonge St, Toronto ON M4S 1Y2; Tor'91; (416)483-2000; Fax. (416)483-3422.

FENTON, Ronald S; St Michael's Hosp, 8 129 CC-30 Bond St, Toronto ON M5B 1W8; London (England)'64; MB BS; LRCP; MRCS; FRCS; FRCSC; Otol. Staff Otol, St Michael's Hospital; Assoc Prof, University of Toronto; (416)864-5279; Fax. (416)864-5367; ronald.fenton@utoronto.ca.

FENTON, Shanna L; City Centre Fam Physicians, 100-514 Queen St St, Saskatoon SK S7K 0M5; Sask'99; CCFP; Asst Clin Prof Family Med, University of Saskatchewan; (306)244-3016; Fax. (306)244-4737.

FENTON, Stanley F; Columbia Med Bldg, 203-301 Columbia St E, New Westminster BC V3L 3W5; Queen's(Belfast) (Ireland)'68; MB ChB; BAO; MRC(UK); FRCPC; IntMed; Rheum. Med Consultant, Royal Columbian Hospital; Med Consultant, Eagle Ridge Hospital & Health Care Centre; Clin Instructor Rheum, University of British Columbia; (604)526-5635; Fax. (604)526-1558.

FENTON, Stanley S A; Univ Hlth Network-Toronto Gen, 8N 855-200 Elizabeth St, Toronto ON M5G 2C4; Belfast (Ireland)'61; MB BCh; BAO; MD; FRCPI; Senior Nephrologist, Toronto General Hospital - UHN; Consultant, Mount Sinai Hospital; Emeritus Prof of Med, University of Toronto; (416)340-4073; Fax. (416)340-4999.

FENTON, W James; Royal University Hosp, 5F-103 Hospital Dr, Saskatoon SK S7N 0W8; Tor'66; FACP; FRCPC; IntMed (Tuberculosis). Ac Staff, Royal University Hospital; Consultant, St Paul's Hospital (Grey Nuns) of Saskatoon; Consultant, Saskatoon City Hospital; Clin Prof Med, University of Saskatchewan; (306)933-6347; Fax. (306)933-8312.

FENTY, Pauline L; King Street Med Arts Centre, 401-71 King St W, Mississauga ON L5B 4A2; Alb'87; Ac Staff, Trillium Health Centre - Mississauga; (905)273-9793; Fax. (905)273-7054.

FENYVES, Daphna; Pavillon Edouard-Asselin, 264 boul Rene-Levesque E, Montreal QC H2X 1P1; McM'78; FRCPC; IntMed (Hepatology); Gastroent. Staff, Heptologist, Centre Hospitalier l'Université De Montréal (CHUM) - Hôpital Saint-luc; Prof, Universite de Montreal; Langs: Bilingual(English/French); (514)890-8000 x35724; Fax. (514)412-7314.

FEOCHARI, Konstantin; Cardiogenix Centre Medical, 100-8250 boul Decarie, Montreal QC H4P 2P5; McG'81; FRCSC; ObstGyn. (514)731-7717; kfeochari@sympatico.ca.

FEQUIERE, Maguie; GMF Chapleau, 87 montee Gagnon, Bois-des-Filion QC J6Z 4C4; (Haiti)'83; CCFP; Staff General Practice, Hopital de la Cite de la santé; (450)621-7420; Fax. (450)621-5007.

FERA, David J; The Group Health Centre, 240 Mcnabb St, Sault Ste. Marie ON P6B 1Y5; Wes'81; Staff, Sault Area Hospital - Sault Ste Marie; (705)541-2246

FERA, Tharwat A E; Broadway Med Centre, 910-943 Broadway W, Vancouver BC V5Z 4E1; Cairo (Egypt)'76; MB ChB; FRCPC; IntMed (Airways Disease); Respir. Staff, Providence Health Care - Mount Saint Joseph Hospital; Consultant, Vancouver General Hospital - Centennial Pavillion; Vis Staff, Providence Health Care - St Paul's Hospital; Langs: Greek; Arabic; (604)731-1123; Fax. (604)731-1179.

FERASOL, Jairie D; Malden Clinic, 5881 Malden Rd, Windsor ON N9H 1S5; Tor'97; BSc; CCFP; Ac Staff, Hôtel-Dieu Grace Hospital; Court Staff, Windsor Regional Hospital - Metropolitan Site; (519)966-2473; Fax. (519)966-8961.

FERDAIS, Francois; Clinique Med Pauze Ferdais, 303-871 rue Shefford, Bromont QC J2L 1C4; Laval'97; Staff, Centre Hospitalier de Granby; (450)919-3911

FERDAIS, Genevieve; Clinique Med de l'Quest, 4475 rue Bannantyne, Verdun QC H4G 1E2; Mon'06; CCFP; Langs: Bilingual(French/English); (514)765-3600; Fax. (514)765-9625.

FERDINAND, Jae-Marie; MUHC-Montreal Children's Hosp, F1343-2300 rue Tupper, Montreal QC H3H 1P3; Tor'84; FAAP; FRCP; LMCC; ABPeds; MRCP; FRCPC; Peds (Child Maltreatment). Staff, McGill University Health Centre - Montreal Children's Hospital; Consultant Ped, Batshaw Youth & Family Health Centre; Aj Prof, McGill University; Langs: French; (514)412-4400 x23432; Fax. (514)412-4271.

FERDINANDIS, Talpe G H C; 2939 66 St NW, Edmonton AB T6K 4C1; (780)463-2184

FERDJOUI, Zoheir; Clinique Pediatrie Chicoutimi, 475 boul Talbot, Chicoutimi QC G7H 4A3; (Algeria)'94; (418)549-1034

FERENCE, Jean L M; RCMP Health Services, 11140 109 St NW, Edmonton AB T5G 2T4; Alb'75; (780)412-5150; Fax. (780)412-5174.

FERENCZ, Joseph C; St Joseph's Mountain H Serv, PO Box 585 Stn Lcd 1 100 West 5th St, Hamilton ON L8N 3K7; McM'89; PhD(Psychol); FRCPC; Psy (Forensic Psychiatry). Dir Forensic Psy, St Joseph's Healthcare Hamilton - West 5th Campus; Asst Prof Psy, McMaster University; (905)522-1155 x6801; Fax. (905)575-6057.

FERENCZI, Zoltan T; 11-149 rue Queen, Sherbrooke QC J1M 1J7; Alb'71; (819)565-9898; Fax. (819)565-4667.

FERENCZY, Alex S; SMBD Jewish Gen Hosp, 3755 ch Cote-Sainte-Catherine, Montreal QC H3T 1E2; Mon'68; CSPQ; GenPath (P.Q.) (Gynecological Pathology). Staff, Sir Mortimer B Davis Jewish General; Langs: Bilingual(French/English); (514)340-7526; Fax. (514)340-7542.

FERG, Allison; 1284 Fairfield Rd, Victoria BC V8V 4W3; Man'84; CCFP; Staff, Victoria General Hospital; Clin Instructor Fam Pract, University of British Columbia; (250)598-5158; Fax. (250)598-6066.

FERGUSON, Alexander H; Guelph Gen Hosp, 115 Delhi St, Guelph ON N1E 4J4; Wes'07; CCFP; CCFP(E.M.); Staff, Guelph General Hospital; (519)822-2170

FERGUSON, Anne L; 500-1200 Markham Rd, Scarborough ON M1H 3C3; McM'90; FRCPC; Psy. Staff Psy, North York General Hospital; (416)289-6285; Fax. (416)289-3903.

FERGUSON, Charles A; Child Protection Centre, FW208-685 William Ave, Winnipeg MB R3E 0Z2; McG'57; Peds (Child Maltreatment). Dir Child Protection Centre, Health Sciences Centre; Prof, University of Manitoba; (204)787-2811; Fax. (204)787-2800; gmucha@hsc.mb.ca.

FERGUSON, Craig A; Ferguson Med Incorporated, 206-26 North St, Bridgewater NS B4V 2V6; Dal'93; CCFP; FCFP; Langs: English; French; Spanish; (902)543-5533; Fax. (902)543-1033.

FERGUSON, Darren B; Saint John Reg Hosp, PO Box 2100 Stn Main 400 University Ave, Saint John NB E2L 4L2; Dal'90; FRCPC; DiagRad. Staff, Saint John Regional Hospital; (506)648-6918; Fax. (506)648-6917.

FERGUSON, David J; BC Biomedical Lab Ltd, 7455 130 St, Surrey BC V3W 1H8; Alb'75; FRCPC; HemPath. Staff Path, Royal Columbian Hospital; Staff, BC Biomedical Laboratories Ltd; Clinical Asst Prof, University of British Columbia; (604)507-5077; dferguson@bcbio.com.

FERGUSON, Deborah A; Glenmore Landing, A301-1600 90 Ave SW, Calgary AB T2V 5A8; McG'92; CCFP; FCFP; Langs: English; French; (403)246-0200; Fax. (403)301-0046; drferguson@telusplanet.net.

FERGUSON, Donald H; Carleton Place & Dist Mem Hosp, 211 Lake Ave E, Carleton Place ON K7C 1J4; Qns'64; BSc; CCFP; FCFP; Court Staff, Carleton Place & District Memorial Hospital; Court Staff, Perth & Smiths Falls District Hospital - Perth Site (Great War Memorial Site); (613)257-2200

FERGUSON, Errol; 384 Paradelle Dr, Richmond Hill ON L4E 4R8; Man'67; Consultant Med, Blue Cross Canada; (289)234-0652; Fax. (289)234-0738.

FERGUSON, G Brian; 600-158 Robert Angus Dr PO Box 116 Stn Main, Amherst NS B4H 3Y6; Dal'80; (902)667-8800; Fax. (902)667-3035.

FERGUSON, Gisele M C; The Clinic on 5th, 215 5th Ave N, Saskatoon SK S7K 2P2; Sask'96; BScN; FRCPC; Psy (Child & Youth Psychiatry). Staff Child Psy, Royal University Hospital; Clinical Asst Prof, University of Saskatchewan; Langs: English; French; (306)653-0002; Fax. (306)244-5362.

FERGUSON, Gordon; West Nipissing Comm Centre, M100-145 Main St, Sturgeon Falls ON P2B 1N8; (Other Foreign)'79; (705)753-0151

FERGUSON, Ian; Providence Healthcare, 3276 St Clair Ave E, Scarborough ON M1L 1W1; UBC'74; FRCPC; Psy (Geriatric Psychiatry). Ac Staff, Providence Healthcare; Staff, Regional Geriatric Program of Toronto; Teacher, University of Toronto; (416)285-3665; Fax. (416)285-3663; iferguso@providence.on.ca.

FERGUSON, Ian K; Strathroy Med Clinic, 74 Front St E, Strathroy ON N7G 1Y7; Wes'84; FRCSC; Urol. Ac Staff/Chief Surg, Strathroy Middlesex General Hospital - Middlesex Hospital Alliance; (519)245-0430; Fax. (519)245-5870.

FERGUSON, James; Queen Elizabeth II-HSC, 377-1276 South Park St, Halifax NS B3H 2Y9; Belfast (Ireland)'91; MB ChB; Staff, Queen Elizabeth II Health Sciences Centre - Victoria General Site; (902)473-5263

FERGUSON, James M; 9th Avenue Med Centre, 2-3855 9th Ave, Port Alberni BC V9Y 4T9; Tor'76; BSc; AB; FACS; FRCSC; GenSurg. Assoc Staff GenSurg, West Coast General Hospital; (250)724-6596; Fax. (250)724-6889; docferguson@hotmail.com.

FERGUSON, James P; Hys Med Centre, 301-11010 101 St NW, Edmonton AB T5H 4B9; Alb'75; FRCPC; IntMed; Gastroent. Ac Staff, Royal Alexandra Hospital; Med Consultant, Cross Cancer Institute; Clin Assoc Prof Med, University of Alberta; (780)421-1031; Fax. (780)426-1961.

FERGUSON, Janis A; City Square Fam Pract Clinic, 116-555 12th Ave W, Vancouver BC V5Z 3X7; Wes'77; Staff, BC Women's Hospital & Health Centre; (604)879-3900; Fax. (604)879-3969; jferguson@cw.bc.ca.

FERGUSON, Joanne L; 4A-505 23rd St E, Saskatoon SK S7K 4K7; Sask'82; CCFP; (306)242-5808; Fax. (306)242-5919.

FERGUSON, Karen E; West Carleton Family Hlth Team, PO Box 218 119 Langstaff Dr, Carp ON K0A 1L0; Qns'97; CCFP; FCFP; Physician, Wabano Centre for Aboriginal Health Inc.; Langs: English; French; (613)839-3271; Fax. (613)839-3273; kef21@hotmail.com.

FERGUSON, Kathleen J; Regina Qu'Appelle HR-Pasqua, 4101 Dewdney Ave, Regina SK S4T 1A5; Sask'92; CCFP; CCFP(E.M.); Staff, Pasqua Hospital; (306)766-8484

FERGUSON, Kathleen; St Thomas-Elgin Gen Hosp, 189 Elm St, St Thomas ON N5R 5C4; Wes'86; BSc; FRCPC; IntMed (Respiratory Sleep Disorders); Respir. Staff, St Thomas Elgin General Hospital; (519)631-2030; Fax. (519)631-5464.

FERGUSON, Kathy; 169 Botsford St, Moncton NB E1C 4X4; Sher'96; FRCPC; IntMed; Nephrol. Staff Nephrol, Dr Georges-L-Dumont University Hospital Centre; (506)857-3020; Fax. (506)855-2847.

FERGUSON, Keith; 1462 Adelaide St N, London ON N5X 1J9; Wes'83; Staff, London Health Sciences Centre - Victoria Campus; Med Consultant, Canadian Blood Services; (519)432-6318

FERGUSON, Kimberley A; Medical Assoc Of Port Perry, 462 Paxton St, Port Perry ON L9L 1L9; Tor'01; CCFP; Staff, Lakeridge Health - Port Perry Site; (905)985-2895

FERGUSON, Linda M; Colchester Research Group, 68 Robie St, Truro NS B2N 1L2; Glasgow (Scotland)'88; MB ChB; Dip SportMed; CCFP; FCFP; Ac Staff, Colchester East Hants Health Centre; Ac Staff, IWK Health Centre; (902)843-3530; Fax. (902)895-6437; kotnfreedom@tru.eastlink.ca.

FERGUSON, Michelle J; Kingston Reg Cancer Centre, 25 King St W, Kingston ON K7L 5P9; Alb'03; FRCPC; IntMed. (613)544-2630

FERGUSON, Murdo E R; Colchester Research Group, 68 Robie St, Truro NS B2N 1L2; Glasgow (Scotland)'88; MB ChB; CCFP; CCFP(E.M.); FCFP; Physician Emerg, Colchester East Hants Health Centre; (902)843-3530

FERGUSON, Natasha; CHUQ-Ctr Hosp Univ Laval, 2705 boul Laurier, Quebec QC G1V 4G2; Laval'96; FRCPC; DiagRad. Staff, Centre Hospitalier Universitaire de Quebec-CHUL; (418)656-4141 x42258

FERGUSON, Niall D; Univ Hlth Network-Toronto Western Hosp, 2MCL 411M-399 Bathurst St, Toronto ON M5T 2S8; Tor'95; FRCPC; IntMed; Critical Care Medicine; Respir. Staff, Toronto Western Hospital - University Health Network; Staff Teacher, University of Toronto; (416)603-5767; Fax. (416)603-5375.

FERGUSON, Peter C; Mount Sinai Hosp, 476G-600 University Ave, Toronto ON M5G 1X5; Tor'94; MSc; FRCSC; OrthSurg (Orthopedic Oncology). Staff, Mount Sinai Hospital; (416)586-4800 x8687; Fax. (416)586-8397.

FERGUSON, Pierre A; Centre Royal Comtois, 101-444 Mcgill St, Hawkesbury ON K6A 1R2; Sher'98; FRCPC; Psy. Langs: Bilingual(English/French); (613)632-0139; Fax. (613)632-4791.

FERGUSON, Sarah E; Univ Hlth Network-Princess M, M 700-610 University Ave, Toronto ON M5G 2M9; Qns'97; FRCSC; ObstGyn. Staff, Princess Margaret Hospital - University Health Network; (416)946-4043; Fax. (416)946-2288.

FERGUSON, Sarah; Georgetown Medical Associates, 199 Princess Anne Dr, Georgetown ON L7G 0E3; Liverpool (England)'97; CCFP; Staff, Halton Healthcare Services Corporation - Georgetown Hospital; (905)873-3000; Fax. (905)783-0800.

FERGUSON, Shaun; The Ob/Gyn Suite, 403-199 Grafton St, Charlottetown PE C1A 1L2; Dal'02; FRCSC; ObstGyn. Consultant, The Ob/Gyn Suite; (902)629-8801; Fax. (902)629-8826.

FERGUSON-LOSIER, Nanette M; King Med Clinic, 380 Portland St, Dartmouth NS B2Y 1K8; Dal'93; Langs: English; French; (902)463-2306; Fax. (902)463-2945.

FERGUSSON, Sheila M; Rutland Med Arts Bldg, 205-285 Aurora Cres, Kelowna BC V1X 7N6; Sask'80; CCFP; FCFP; (250)765-4117

FERHAT, Ferroudja; CSSS des Aurores Boreales, CP 6000 Succ Bureau-Chef 679 2e rue E, La Sarre QC J9Z 2X7; Alger (Algeria)'84; Staff, Centre Hospitalier La Sarre; (819)333-2311; Fax. (819)333-3520.

FERIGUTTI, Daniela; Clinique Med Montee Paiement, 205-492 boul de l'Hopital, Gatineau QC J8V 2P4; Laval'89; CCFP; Langs: Italian; English; (819)561-5511

FERLAND, Andre; Foothills Med Centre, EG23J-1403 29 St NW, Calgary AB T2N 2T9; Sher'84; FRCPC; IntMed (Intensive Care). Ac Staff IntMed & Critical Care, Foothills Medical Centre; Clin Associate, University of Calgary; Langs: English; (403)944-1570; Fax. (403)283-9994; andreferland@calgaryhealthregion.ca.

FERLAND, Christian; Clinique Med Monchamp, 102-227 rue Sainte-Catherine, Saint-Constant QC J5A 2J5; Mon'88; CCFP; Staff, Hôpital Anna-Laberge; Langs: English; (450)632-2245; Fax. (450)632-2795.

FERLAND, Emery; CSSS Pierre Boucher, 1333 boul Jacques-Cartier E, Longueuil QC J4M 2A5; Mon'69; ABIM; FRCPC; IntMed; MedOncol (P.Q.); Hem. Hematology, Centre Hospitalier Pierre Boucher; Staff, McGill University Health Centre - Royal Victoria Hospital; (450)468-8111; Fax. (450)468-8201.

FERLAND, Louise; 1652 rue Royale, Trois-Rivieres QC G9A 4K3; Laval'70; (819)379-4521; Fax. (819)379-4615.

FERLAND, Louise M; CHUQ-Ctr Hosp Univ Laval, 2705 boul Laurier, Quebec QC G1V 4G2; Laval'68; FRCPC; Peds. Staff, Centre Hospitalier Universitaire de Quebec-CHUL; (418)654-2282

FERLAND, Lucie; Hop Charles Lemoyne, 3120 Boul Taschereau, Greenfield Park QC J4V 2H1; Mon'87; CSPQ; FRCPC; Anes. Staff, Hopital Charles LeMoyne; (450)466-5000 x2680

FERLAND, Manon; Clinique Med du Carrefour, 8585 boul Lacroix, Saint-Georges QC G5Y 5L6; Mon'90; Staff, Centre Hospitalier Beauce-Etchemin; (418)227-1271; Fax. (418)227-2781.

FERLAND, Marc-Andre; Clinique Med de Verdun, 55 av de l'Eglise, Verdun QC H4G 3E7; Mon'75; CSPQ; FRCSC; GenSurg (Thoracic Surgery). ac Staff, Centre Hospitalier de Verdun; Langs: Bilingual(French/English); (514)768-8531; Fax. (514)768-2507.

FERLAND, Mario; CSSS du Rocher-Perce, CP 3300 451 rue Mgr Ross, Chandler QC G0C 1K0; Laval'92; FRCPC; IntMed. Staff Internal Med, Centre Hospitalier de Chandler; (418)689-2261; Fax. (418)689-6131.

FERLAND, Miren; CSSS Bordeaux-Cartierville-St-, 555 boul Gouin O, Montreal QC H3L 1K5; Mon'98; Staff, Pavillon Notre-Dame de la Merci; (514)331-3020; Fax. (514)331-6937.

FERLAND, Olivier; CSSS de Chicoutimi, CP 5006 305 rue Saint-Vallier, Chicoutimi QC G7H 5H6; Laval'04; FRCSC; GenSurg. Staff, Complexe hospitalier de la Sagamie; (418)541-1000

FERLAND, Renald; CHUQ-Ctr Hosp Univ Laval, 2705 boul Laurier, Quebec QC G1V 4G2; Laval'78; FRCSC; Otol. Ac Staff, Centre Hospitalier Universitaire de Quebec-CHUL; (418)654-2118; Fax. (418)654-2214.

FERLAND, Stephanie; CSSS du Rocher-Perce, CP 3300 451 rue Mgr Ross, Chandler QC G0C 1K0; Mon'00; Staff, Centre Hospitalier de Chandler; Staff, Cree Board of Health & Social Services James Bay; (418)689-2261

FERLAND, Stephanie; CSSSG-Hop De Gatineau, CP 2000 Succ Bureau-Chef 909 boul de la Verendrye O, Gatineau QC J8P 7H2; Mon'02; FRCPC; RadOncol. Staff, Hôpital de Gatineau; (819)966-6100

FERLAND, Sylvie; Hôpital Laval, 2725 ch Sainte-Foy, Quebec QC G1V 4G5; Laval'83; DiagRad (Thoracic). Staff Radiol, Hôpital Laval; Teach Staff, Université Laval; (418)656-4512; Fax. (418)656-4578.

FERLAND, Yves; Clinique D'Orthopedie de levis, 6620 rue Saint-Georges, Levis QC G6V 4H1; Laval'92; CSPQ; FRCSC; OrthSurg. Staff, Hôtel-Dieu de Lévis; (418)837-8251; Fax. (418)837-2033.

FERLAND-LAVIGNE, Katia; Clin Externe de Psychiatrie, 203-100 rue Grenier, Charlemagne QC J5Z 4C6; Laval'95; FRCPC; Psy. Langs: Bilingual(French/English); (450)585-9010; Fax. (450)585-2709.

FERLISI, Anthony J; All In One Med Clinic, 10083 Keele St, Maple ON L6A 3Y8; Wes'70; Staff, Humber River Regional Hospital - Finch Avenue Site; (905)832-4644; Fax. (905)832-7717.

FERLISI, James R F; All in One Med Clinic, 100-10083 Keele St, Maple ON L6A 3Y8; Wes'84; MCFP; Ac Staff, Mackenzie Richmond Hill Hospital; Ac Staff, Humber River Regional Hospital - Finch Avenue Site; Med Consultant, Boeing Canada; (905)832-4644; Fax. (905)832-7717; jferlisi@idirect.com.

FERLISI, Mary-Claire; Heart Lake Med Centre, 101-10425 Kennedy Rd, Brampton ON L6Z 0A4; McM'02; CCFP; (905)846-7611; Fax. (905)846-7753.

FERMINI, Richard; Centre de Sante de Lachute, 125 av de la Providence, Lachute QC J8H 3L4; Sher'76; (450)562-8895; Fax. (450)562-1128.

FERMOR, David; Foothills Med Centre, 1403 29 St NW, Calgary AB T2N 2T9; Cal'88; FRCPC; Anes. Staff, Foothills Medical Centre; (403)944-1430; Fax. (403)944-2425.

FERN, Brian J; College Park Med Clinic, 310-2600 8th St E, Saskatoon SK S7H 0V7; Manchester (England)'61; MB; DRCOG; (306)955-2600; Fax. (306)373-1247.

FERN, Ken T C; Oshawa Clinic, 117 King St E, Oshawa ON L1H 1B9; Qns'97; BSc; FRCSC; OrthSurg (Spine Surgery). Staff, Lakeridge Health - Oshawa Site; (905)721-4928 x4928; Fax. (905)723-4691.

FERNANDES, Artur J D B; CHUS-Hop Fleurimont, 3001 12e av N, Sherbrooke QC J1H 5N4; Sao Paulo (Brazil)'79; CSPQ; FRCPC; Rheum (P.Q.). Prof Med, Centre Hospitalier Universitaire de Sherbrooke-Hopital Fleurimont; Langs: Portuguese; (819)564-5261; Fax. (819)564-5265; artur.fernandes@usherbrooke.ca.

FERNANDES, Bernard J J; Mount Sinai Hosp, 600 University Ave, Toronto ON M5G 1X5; Makerere (Uganda)'72; FRCPath; FRCPA; FRCPC; AnatPath (Blood Transfusion); HemPath. Head HemPath & Blood Tranfusion Serv, Mount Sinai Hospital; Prof, University of Toronto; (416)586-4462; Fax. (416)586-8628; b.fernandes@utoronto.ca.

FERNANDES, Brian R F; Town Centre Prof Bldg, 103-6203 28 Ave NW, Edmonton AB T6L 6K3; Edinburgh (Scotland)'77; MB ChB; (780)462-9316; Fax. (780)462-7332.

FERNANDES, Christopher M B; London HSC-Victoria Hosp, PO Box 5010 Stn B 800 Commissioners Rd E, London ON N6A 5W9; UBC'84; FACEP; Staff, London Health Sciences Centre - Victoria Campus; (519)685-8500

FERNANDES, Clarence R; Dr Clarence R Fernandes Inc, 11948 227 St, Maple Ridge BC V2X 6J3; UBC'74; Ac Staff, Ridge Meadows Hospital & Health Care Centre; Clin Instructor Family Med, University of British Columbia; (604)467-3434; Fax. (604)463-7644.

FERNANDES, David; West Lincoln Mem Hosp, 169 Main St E, Grimsby ON L3M 1P3; McM'02; CCFP; CCFP(E.M.); Staff, Niagara Health System - Welland Hospital Site; Staff, West Lincoln Memorial Hospital; Staff, Niagara Health System - Port Colborne General Site; (905)945-2253

FERNANDES, Dellano; Royal Inland Hosp, 311 Columbia St, Kamloops BC V2C 2T1; Cal'05; FRCPC; DiagRad. Staff, Royal Inland Hospital; (250)314-2400

FERNANDES, Geraldo A J; 9197 97th Dr, North Battleford SK S9A 3K3; Dublin (Ireland)'67; LRCPSI; FRCSENT; ENT Consultant, Battlefords Union Hospital; Langs: Portuguese; (306)446-0199; gerryfernandes@yahoo.ca.

FERNANDES, John L; Market Mall Prof Bldg, 303-4935 40 Ave NW, Calgary AB T3A 2N1; Cal'97; BSc; MSc; CCFP; FCFP; Staff Admin, Foothills Medical Centre; Clin Teacher, University of Calgary; (403)247-9880; Fax. (403)247-9882.

FERNANDES, John R; Hamilton HS-General Site, 237 Barton St E, Hamilton ON L8L 2X2; McG'82; BSc; MDCM; FRCPC; FRCSC; GenPath (Forensic Pathology); ObstGyn. Staff/Med Dir Reg Forensic Pathology Unit, Hamilton Health Sciences Centre - Hamilton General Hospital; Staff, St Joseph's Healthcare - Charlton Campus; Staff Teacher, McMaster University; Langs: English; French; (905)527-4322 x46530; fernandes@hhsc.ca.

FERNANDES, Julio C; Hop du Sacre-Coeur de Mtl, 5400 boul Gouin O, Montreal QC H4J 1C5; (Brazil)'88; MSc; CSPQ; MBA; FRCSC; OrthSurg (P.Q.) (Hips Surgery). Chief of Staff, Hôpital du Sacre-Coeur de Montréal; Prof Surg, Universite de Montreal; Langs: Portuguese; French; (514)338-2222 x2060; Fax. (514)338-3661.

FERNANDEZ, Alcantro B; Parkway Prof Bldg, 60 Centennial Pky S, Stoney Creek ON L8G 2C5; Dublin (Ireland)'65; MB ChB; BAO; DCH; Ac Staff, Hamilton Health Sciences Centre - Hamilton General Hospital; Court Staff, St Joseph's Healthcare - Charlton Campus; Langs: Swahili; Hindi; (905)662-2231; Fax. (905)662-2233.

FERNANDEZ, Bridget; Health Sciences Centre, 300 Prince Philip Dr, St. John's NL A1B 3V6; Mem'94; BSc; MSc; FRCPC; MedGenetics (Clinical Genetics). Med Dir Provincial Med Genetics Prog, Health Sciences Centre; Medical Staff, Eastern Health Authoriy; Assoc Prof/Chair Discipline of Genetics & Medicine, Memorial University Of Newfoundland; (709)777-4363; Fax. (709)777-4190.

FERNANDEZ, Christina D; Centennial Med Centre, 299 Lake Ave E, Carleton Place ON K7C 1J3; Ott'86; Ac Staff, Queensway Carleton Hospital; Ac Staff, Carleton Place & District Memorial Hospital; (613)257-2311; Fax. (613)253-0044.

FERNANDEZ, Conrad V; IWK Health Centre, PO Box 9700 Rpo CSC 5850-5980 University ave, Halifax NS B3K 6R8; McM'85; BSc(Hon.); FRCPC; Peds (Pediatric Hematology Oncology). Staff, IWK Health Centre; Prof, Dalhousie University; Langs: German; (902)470-6839; Fax. (902)470-7216.

FERNANDEZ, Louis A V; 206E-5788 University Ave, Halifax NS B3H 1V8; Karachi (Pakistan)'66; FACP; FRCPC; IntMed; Hem. Staff, Queen Elizabeth II Health Sciences Centre - Victoria General Site; Prof, Dalhousie University; (902)473-2168; louis.fernandez@cdha.nshealth.ca.

FERNANDEZ, Marie-Carmel; Clinique Med Viau, 204-4750 rue Jarry E, Saint-Leonard QC H1R 1X8; Politecnico (Mexico)'90; Physician Medecin, Centre Jeunesse de Montreal; Langs: Spanish; Creole; English; (514)326-7203

FERNANDEZ, Nestor D P; Bloor-Christie Clinic, 200-799 Bloor St W, Toronto ON M6G 1L8; Tor'78; Langs: Italian; Portuguese; Spanish; (416)531-5332; Fax. (416)531-1155.

FERNANDEZ, Peter G; Ambulatory IntMed Teaching Cli, 2-80 King St, St Catharines ON L2R 7G1; Sheffield (England)'63; FACP; FRCP(Glas); FRCP(UK); FRCPC; IntMed (Cardiology). Clin Prof Med, McMaster University; (905)708-0050; Fax. (905)708-0040; intmedteach@gmail.com.

FERNANDEZ, Renee; 202-179 Davie St, Vancouver BC V6Z 2Y1; UBC'05; CCFP; (604)669-7772

FERNANDEZ, Roberto; Ctr Hosp Anna-Laberge, 200 boul Brisebois, Chateauguay QC J6K 4W8; Mon'99; FRCSC; ObstGyn. Staff, Hôpital Anna-Laberge; (450)699-2436; Fax. (450)699-2525.

FERNANDEZ-CATTELAT, Patrice; Hôpital de Tracadie-Sheila, CP 3180 Stn Main 400 rue des Hospitalieres, Tracadie-Sheila NB E1X 1G5; Sher'05; CCFP; Staff, Hôpital de Tracadie-Sheila; (506)394-3018

FERNANDEZ DE LARA NIETO, Jose; 201-51 Inglewood Dr, St. Albert AB T8N 4E7; Cuba (Cuba)'93; FRCSC; ObstGyn;CCFP; Langs: Spanish; (780)459-5673; Fax. (780)459-5611.

FERNANDEZ-LLAMAZARES, Carmen; Catherine Booth Hosp, 4375 av Montclair, Montreal QC H4B 2J5; Ott'90; Staff, Catherine Booth Hospital; (514)481-0431

FERNANDO, Anna; 117 King St E, Oshawa ON L1H 1B9; (Russia (Federation))'99; CCFP; (905)721-4966; Fax. (905)721-6611.

FERNANDO, F Priyalal; Windsor Health Centre, 207-630 Tecumseh Rd E, Windsor ON N8X 4W2; Peradeniya (Sri Lanka)'75; MSc(Leeds); MB BS; DPM(Lond); MRCPsy(UK); FRCPC; Psy (Alzheimer's Disease). Staff, Windsor Regional Hospital - Metropolitan Site; Staff, Hôtel-Dieu Grace Hospital; Aj Prof Psy, University of Western Ontario; Langs: Sinhalese; (519)258-8482

FERNANDO, Joseph; 500-10235 101 St NW, Edmonton AB T5J 3G1; London (England)'60; MRCS; LRCP; MB; Court Staff Privil, University of Alberta Hospital; Medical Officer Aviation Med, Civil Aviation Canada; Langs: Sinhalese; (780)424-3042; Fax. (780)426-5682.

FERNANDO, M Lakshman; Woodstock Gen Hosp, 310 Juliana Dr, Woodstock ON N4V 0A4; Ceylon (Sri Lanka)'70; MB BS; FRSMed(UK); FRCPC; Psy (Bipolar Disease). Consultant, London Health Sciences Centre - Victoria Campus; Chief Psy, Woodstock General Hospital; Assoc Prof Psy, University of Western Ontario; Langs: Sinhalese; (519)421-4223

FERNANDO, Mary L; 11-60 Stanley Ave, Ottawa ON K1M 1P6; McM'88; (613)247-8880

FERNHOUT, Mark J; 1014 20 St S, Lethbridge AB T1K 2C9; Alb'97; FRCSC; OrthSurg. Staff, Chinook Regional Hospital; (403)942-4361

FEROE, Raquel L; Meadowlark Health Centre, 154 Meadowlark Shopping Ctr NW, Edmonton AB T5R 5W9; Darthmouth(NH) (USA)'88; FRCPC; IntMed. (780)429-4761; Fax. (780)425-4274.

FEROZE, Nicholas; Peterborough Reg HC-Hospital, 1 Hospital Dr, Peterborough ON K9J 7C6; Cracow (Poland)'08; CCFP; Staff, Emerg, Peterborough Regional Health Centre - Hospital Drive; (705)743-2121

FEROZE, Sleem; Oakville Menopause Clinic, 4-358 Reynolds St, Oakville ON L6J 3L9; London (England)'66; MB BS; BSc; FRCOG; FACOG; LRCP; FSOGC; FRCSC; ObstGyn (Menopause). Hon Staff ObstGyn, Hamilton Health Sciences Centre - McMaster Children's Hospital; Court Staff, Halton Healthcare Services Corporation - Oakville Site; Court Staff, Halton Healthcare Services Corporation - Milton District Hospital; Langs: Swahili; Punjabi; Urdu; Gujarati; (905)844-8383; Fax. (905)844-4810; sf13@hotmail.com.

FERRACUTI, Stephen; Haliburton Family Med Centre, PO Box 870, Haliburton ON K0M 1S0; Wes'86; Staff, Western Memorial Regional Hospital; (705)457-1212 x343; Fax. (705)457-3955; drstevef@gmail.com.

FERRAO, Matthew J J; Oak Bay Med Centre, 159-2515 90 Ave SW, Calgary AB T2V 0L8; Alb'87; (403)281-2020; Fax. (403)281-7785.

FERRARI, Robert; Clinical Sciences Bldg, 13 103-11350 83 Ave, Edmonton AB T6G 2P4; Alb'90; BSc; FRCPC; IntMed (Rheumatology). Clinical Asst Prof, University of Alberta Hospital; Clin Assoc Prof Med, University of Alberta; Langs: French; Italian; Spanish; Latin; (780)990-8310; Fax. (780)472-0215; rferrari@shaw.ca.

FERRARIS, Franz B; Ottawa Valley Family Hlth, 95 Spring St, Almonte ON K0A 1A0; Cape Town (South Africa)'78; Langs: Afrikaans; (613)256-9370; Fax. (613)256-0949.

FERRARO, Pasquale; CHUM-Hop Notre-Dame, 1560 rue Sherbrooke E, Montreal QC H2L 4M1; Mon'88; CSPQ; FRCSC; GenSurg (Transplantation); ThorSurg. Staff, Centre Hospitalier l'Université de Montréal (CHUM) - Hôpital Notre-Dame; Langs: English; (514)890-8000; Fax. (514)412-7855.

FERRAROTTO, Domenic; MUHC-Montreal Gen Hosp, 1650 av Cedar, Montreal QC H3G 1A4; Tor'90; CCFP; Staff, McGill University Health Centre - Montreal General Campus; (514)934-8090

FERRAZ, Jose G P; UCMC Area 2 Clinic, 3280 Hospital Dr NW, Calgary AB T2N 4Z6; (Brazil)'89; PhD; Staff Gastroenterology/Clin Assoc Prof Div of Gastroenterology, Foothills Medical Centre; Langs: Portuguese; (403)944-6551; Fax. (403)944-6548.

FERREIRA, Bernard E; 108-704 Mara St, Point Edward ON N7V 1X4; Tor'60; FACOG; ObstGyn (Infertility). Ac Staff ObstGyn, Bluewater Health - Mitton Site; Ac Staff, Bluewater Health - Norman Site; Ac Staff, Bluewater Health - Charlotte Eleanor Englehart Hospital; Langs: Italian; Creole; (519)383-1236

FERREIRA, Ivone M; Ctre for Sleep & Chronobiology, B102-340 College St, Toronto ON M5T 3A9; Santo Amaro (Brazil)'84; FRCPC; Respir (Sleep Medicine); IntMed. Clin Associate Asthma & Airways Ctr, Toronto Western Hospital - University Health Network; Asst Clin Prof, McMaster University; Langs: Portuguese; (416)966-3641

FERREIRA, Jose; Hop Maisonneuve-Rosemont, 5415 boul de l'Assomption, Montreal QC H1T 2M4; Mon'92; CSPQ; FRCPC; AnatPath. Staff, Hopital Maisonneuve-Rosemont; (514)252-3498

FERREIRA, M Thomas D; Bloor Med Clinic, 204-844 Bathurst St, Toronto ON M5R 3G1; Lisbon (Portugal)'63; (416)531-4601; Fax. (416)531-6380.

FERREIRA, Nelson D B; Sure Hair International, 401-2115 Finch Ave W, North York ON M3N 2V6; Tor'91; BSc; Staff, Sure Hair International; Staff, First Canadian Medical Centre; Langs: Portuguese; (416)747-7873; Fax. (416)747-7441; nel.ferreira@utoronto.ca.

FERREIRA, Patrick; Alberta Children's Hosp, 2888 Shaganappi Trail NW, Calgary AB T3B 6A8; London (England)'71; MB BS; MSc; FRCPC; MedBiochem (Biochemical Genetics); MedGenetics; Peds. Staff, Alberta Children's Hospital; (403)955-7172; Fax. (403)955-3091.

FERREIRA, Stephanus C; Two Rivers Med Centre, 1306 Central St E, Prince George BC V2M 3C1; Pretoria (South Africa)'82; BSc; MB ChB; CCFP; Staff, University Hospital of Northern British Columbia; Clin Asst Prof Family Practice, University of British Columbia; Clin Asst Prof Family Practice, University of Northern British Columbia; Langs: Afrikaans; (250)563-6417; Fax. (250)563-7040; stephan.ferreira@northernhealth.ca.

FERREIRA, Susan; Victoria Gen Hosp, 1 Hospital Way, Victoria BC V8Z 6R5; London (England)'71; MB BS; BSc; FFARCS; FRCPC; Anes. Staff Anes, Victoria General Hospital; (250)727-4212

FERREMI, Christian; 1105-3030 boul le Carrefour, Laval QC H7T 2P5; Laval'92; FRCSC; Ophth (Refractive Surgery). Staff, Iris Clinique D'Ophtalmologie; Langs: French; English; (450)688-6574; Fax. (450)688-9516; ophtalmo@iris.ca.

FERRI, Lorenzo E; MUHC-Montreal Gen Hosp, L9 112-1650 av Cedar, Montreal QC H3G 1A4; McG'96; CSPQ; PhD; FACS; FRCSC; GenSurg; ThorSurg. Staff, McGill University Health Centre - Montreal General Campus; (514)934-1934 x44327; Fax. (514)934-4432.

FERRI, Melanie; Hamilton HS-Juravinski Centre, 699 Concession St, Hamilton ON L8V 5C2; McM'00; FRCPC; DiagRad. Diag Radiol, Hamilton Health Sciences Centre - Juravinski Cancer Centre; (905)527-4322 x43897; Fax. (905)575-2660.

FERRI, Patricia; CLSC Bordeaux-Cartierville, 11822 av de Bois-De-Boulogne, Montreal QC H3M 2X6; Mon'81; (514)331-2572; Fax. (514)331-0137.

FERRI, R Michael; Pembroke Reg Hosp, 705 Mackay St, Pembroke ON K8A 1G8; Qns'81; FRCPC; Psy. Chief of Staff, Pembroke Regional Hospital Inc; (613)732-3675 x6125

FERRI DE BARROS, Fabio; Alberta Children's Hosp, 2888 Shaganappi Trail NW, Calgary AB T3B 6A8; (Brazil)'95; Staff, Alberta Children's Hospital; (403)955-7189; Fax. (403)955-2813.

FERRIER, C J Scott; Buckhorn Reg Health Ctr, PO Box 209 865 William St, Buckhorn ON K0L 1J0; Man'84; Staff, Peterborough Regional Health Centre - Hospital Drive; (705)657-7933; Fax. (705)657-3176.

FERRIER, Catherine; MUHC-Montreal Gen Hosp, D17 173-1650 av Cedar, Montreal QC H3G 1A4; McG'81; CCFP; FCFP; adj Médecin, McGill University Health Centre - Montreal General Campus; adj Prof Family Med, McGill University; Langs: French; Spanish; (514)934-8015; Fax. (514)934-8286; catherine.ferrier@muhc.mcgill.ca.

FERRIER, Donald J; 100-5791 No. 3 Rd, Richmond BC V6X 2C9; Cal'86; FRCPC; DiagRad. (604)278-9152; Fax. (604)278-9291.

FERRIS, Caroline R; Creekside Withdrawal Mgmt Ctre, 13790 94A Ave, Surrey BC V3V 1N1; UBC'86; CCFP; FCFP; Clin Instructor Family Med, University of British Columbia; Langs: English; French; (604)587-3755

FERRIS, Dwight A N; Kelowna Gen Hosp, 2268 Pandosy St, Kelowna BC V1Y 1T2; Qns'96; BSc; DTMH; FRCPC; IntMed; InfectDis. Consultant InfectDis, Kelowna General Hospital; (250)862-4157

FERRON, Charles; Montfort Hosp, 713 Montreal Rd, Ottawa ON K1K 0T2; Ott'05; FRCSC; PlasSurg. Staff, Montfort Hospital; (613)746-4621; Fax. (613)748-4914.

FERRON, Jean-Paul; Polyclinique de Montreal, 410-12245 rue Grenet, Montreal QC H4J 2J6; Mon'65; FRCPC; IntMed (Hospitalist). ac Staff, Hôpital du Sacre-Coeur de Montréal; Clin Assoc Prof, Universite de Montreal; (514)334-9112; Fax. (514)334-2945.

FERRON, Marcel; Centre d'Urgence St-Laurent, 200-1605 boul Marcel-Laurin, Saint-Laurent QC H4R 0B7; Mon'74; Langs: English; (514)747-2555; centre.urgence.st-laurent@gmail.com.

FERRON, Michel; CSSS de la Baie-des-Chaleurs, RR 2 419 boul Perron, Maria QC G0C 1Y0; Mon'69; Staff, CSSS de la Baie-des-Chaleurs; (418)759-3443

FERRON, Michele; Ministere Emploi et Solidarite, 3F-575 rue Saint-Amable, Quebec QC G1R 2G4; Laval'78; (800)355-6557

FERRON, Pierre; Clinique De Med Fam Mailloux, 280-1900 av Mailloux, Quebec QC G1J 5B9; Mon'64; FRCSC; Otol. Staff, Centre Hospitalier Universitaire de Québec (CHUQ) - Siege Social; Langs: Bilingual(French/English); (418)667-3427; Fax. (418)667-3428.

FERRON, Serge; Clinique Chir Ortho C-Lemoyne, 126 rue Saint-Louis, Lemoyne QC J4R 2L5; Laval'80; CSPQ; FRCSC; OrthSurg. Staff, Hopital Charles LeMoyne; (450)672-1212; Fax. (450)672-9834.

FESSER, Jennifer; Queen Elizabeth Hosp, PO Box 6600 Stn Cenral 60 Riverside Dr, Charlottetown PE C1A 8T5; Sask'03; FRCPC; GenPath. Staff, Queen Elizabeth Hospital; (902)894-2111

FETAZ, Louise K M; Gold Ears Family Practice, 140-20395 Lougheed Hwy, Maple Ridge BC V2X 2P9; Alb'82; (604)465-1066

FETHERSTON, William H; Aurora Med Centre, 201-15017 Yonge St, Aurora ON L4G 1M5; Wes'79; Staff, Southlake Regional Health Centre; (905)727-4241; Fax. (905)727-4288.

FETOURI, Fawzi M; Parkland Med Associates, 205-505 Queen St, Spruce Grove AB T7X 2V2; Al Fateh (Libya)'01; CCFP; (780)962-2001

FETTERLY, Alexander C; 205-230 First Ave, St Thomas ON N5R 4P5; Qns'73; DAB; FRCSC; Otol (General). Consultant, St Thomas Elgin General Hospital; (519)631-6391; Fax. (519)631-6393; sfetterl@stegh.on.ca.

FETTES, Ivy M; Sunnybrook Hlth Sciences Ctre, H158-2075 Bayview Ave, Toronto ON M4N 3M5; Tor'74; PhD; FRCPC; IntMed; Endocrin&Metab. Dir Div of Endocrinol, Sunnybrook Health Sciences Centre; Prof Med, University of Toronto; (416)480-4760; ivy.fettes@sunnybrook.ca.

FETTES, Lisa F; North Bay Reg Health Centre, 50 College Dr, North Bay ON P1B 0A4; Tor'84; BSc; FRCPC; Anes (Critical Care Medicine). Staff Anes, North Bay Regional Health Centre - Regional Mental Health; Langs: Bilingual(English/French); (705)474-8600 x2139

FETURI, Elaref S; Properties Med Clinic, 5102 Rundlehorn Dr NE, Calgary AB T1Y 1C1; (Libya)'90; Staff, Properties Medical Clinic; (403)280-2700; Fax. (403)285-2641.

FEUER, Catherine F; Towne Centre Med Clinic, 201-3601 Hwy 7 E, Markham ON L3R 0M3; Tor'86; Staff Privil, Markham Stouffville Hospital; (905)604-3336; Fax. (905)604-7750.

FEUERSTEIN, Erika; Bay Centre for Birth Control, 8F-790 Bay St, Toronto ON M5G 1N8; Tor'85; CCFP; Langs: Hungarian; (416)351-3726; Fax. (416)351-3727.

FEWER, H Derek; Health Sciences Centre, GF 231-820 Sherbrook St, Winnipeg MB R3A 1R9; McG'66; BSc(Cum Laude); MDCM; FRCSC; Neursurg. Ac Staff, Health Sciences Centre; Assoc. Prof. & Prog. Dir., University of Manitoba; (204)787-7265; Fax. (204)787-3851; dfewer@exchange.hsc.mb.ca.

FEWER, Karen A; PO Box 26, Midle-Musquodoboit NS B0N 1X0; Mem'90; CCFP; (902)384-2834; Fax. (902)384-2719.

FEWSTER, Robert; 302-85 Norfolk St, Guelph ON N1H 4J4; Dublin (Ireland)'07; CCFP; (519)822-1871; Fax. (519)822-1990.

FEYI, Kennedy K K; Alberni Internal Med Clinic, 3949 Port Alberni Hwy, Port Alberni BC V9Y 4S1; (Ghana)'89; MB ChB; (250)724-8800

FEYLES, Valter; A9 303-339 Windermere Rd PO Box 5339 Stn B, London ON N6A 5A5; Torino (Italy)'82; MD; MSc; PhD; FRCSC; ObstGyn (Infertility). Med Dir The Fertility Clinic, London Health Sciences Centre - University Hospital; University of Western Ontario; Langs: Italian; (519)663-3019; Fax. (519)663-3162.

FFRENCH, Cheryl; St Boniface Gen Hosp, 409 Tache Ave, Winnipeg MB R2H 2A6; Man'06; FRCPC; EmergMed. Staff, St Boniface General Hospital; (204)233-8563

FIANNI, Majed; Alexandra Marine & Gen Hosp, 120 Napier St, Goderich ON N7A 1W5; Cairo (Egypt)'85; FRCPC; IntMed. Staff, Alexandra Marine & General Hospital; Langs: Arabic; English; (519)524-8323; Fax. (519)524-5563.

FIALA, Jindrich; 700-1240 Bay St, Toronto ON M5R 2A7; Tor'73; CCFP; FCFP; Staff, Mount Sinai Hospital; Langs: Czech; (416)977-9224; Fax. (416)352-5215; fiala@osgoodehealth.com.

FIALA, Katarina; 700-1240 Bay St, Toronto ON M5R 2A7; Tor'74; DAB; FRCPC; Derm. Staff, St Michael's Hospital; Staff, Royal Victoria Regional Health Centre; Lecturer, University of Toronto; Langs: Czech; Slovak; Hungarian; (416)928-2245; Fax. (416)646-0205; fiala@sympatico.ca.

FIALKOV, Jeffrey; Sunnybrook Hlth Sciences Ctre, M1 516-2075 Bayview Ave, Toronto ON M4N 3M5; Tor'89; FRCSC; PlasSurg (Cranio Facial Surgery). Faculty Staff, Sunnybrook Health Sciences Centre; Assoc Prof, University of Toronto; (416)480-4257; Fax. (416)480-4224; fialkov.admin@sunnybrook.ca.

FIBICH, Ernst; Ctr for the North Prince Georg, 1215 Lethbridge St, Prince George BC V2M 7E9; Hannover (Germany)'93; Staff, University Hospital of Northern British Columbia; Langs: German; French; (250)645-7335

FICARA, Giuseppe; St Mary's Hosp, 3830 av Lacombe, Montreal QC H3T 1M5; McG'97; FRCPC; Peds (Vaccination). Staff, St Mary's Hospital Centre; Staff, Lakeshore General Hospital - Pointe Claire; Langs: Bilingual(English/French); French; Italian; (514)345-3511; giuseppe.ficara@mcgill.ca.

FICEK, Henrietta; Crowfoot Corner Medicentres, 217-150 Crowfoot Cres NW, Calgary AB T3G 3T2; Lublin (Poland)'64; Teacher/Staff Continuous Med Prog, University of Calgary; (403)241-8900; Fax. (403)241-8109.

FICHMAN, Anna; Centre Med Nazareth, 1771 av Dollard, LaSalle QC H8N 1T9; (Russia (Federation))'94; CCFP; (514)368-5500; Fax. (514)368-0056.

FICHMAN, Stephen H; 205-5858 ch Cote-des-Neiges, Montreal QC H3S 1Z1; McG'63; Ophth (Refractive Surgery). Dir Contact Lens Clinic, Sir Mortimer B Davis Jewish General; adj Prof, McGill University; Langs: English; French; (514)731-6896; Fax. (514)731-0958.

FIDAL, Samuil W; North Park Med Centre, D2-2355 Keele St, North York ON M6M 4A2; Alexandria (Egypt)'80; CCFP; Physician, Toronto Poly Clinic; (416)244-4377; sfidal@tpclinic.com.

FIDDLER, David; Haliburton High Hlth Serv-Mide, PO Box 30 6 McPherson St, Minden ON K0M 2K0; Chicago (USA)'83; Staff, Ross Memorial Hospital; Staff, Haliburton Highlands Health Services - Miden Site; (705)286-2288; david@hhfht.com.

FIDDLER, Douglas; Haliburton High Hlth Serv-Mide, PO Box 30 6 McPherson St, Minden ON K0M 2K0; Iowa City(IA) (USA)'84; Staff, Royal Victoria Regional Health Centre; Staff, Haliburton Highlands Health Services - Miden Site; (705)286-2288; douglas@hhfht.com.

FIDEL, Jeffrey; Western Reg Mem Hosp, PO Box 2005 Stn Main 1 Brookfield Ave, Corner Brook NL A2H 6J7; Tulane (USA)'97; Staff, Western Memorial Regional Hospital; (709)637-5000

FIDLER, Lee M; Sunnybrook Hlth Sciences Ctre, 2075 Bayview Ave, Toronto ON M4N 3M5; Tor'10; Staff, Sunnybrook Health Sciences Centre; (416)480-6100

FIDLER, Wesley; St Joseph's Hosp, PO Box 3251 Stn P 35 Algoma St N, Thunder Bay ON P7B 5G7; Qns'89; FRCPC; IntMed; Rheum. Staff Advisor-Rheum, St Joseph's Care Group - St Joseph's Hospital; Staff, Thunder Bay Regional Health Sciences Centre; Asst Prof, Northern Ontario School of Medicine; (807)346-8467; Fax. (807)346-7010.

FIEDRICH, Elsa C; Univ of Alberta Hosp, 3A3 13-8440 112 St NW, Edmonton AB T6G 2B7; UBC'07; FRCPC; Peds. Staff, University of Alberta Hospital; (780)407-8822; Fax. (780)407-3030.

FIEGHEN, Heather E; St Joseph's Health Centre, 30 The Queensway, Toronto ON M6R 1B5; Tor'07; FRCPC; IntMed. Staff, St Joseph's Health Centre; (416)408-3102

FIEL, Naiema M; Halton HCS Corp-Georgetown, 205-1 Princess Anne Dr, Georgetown ON L7G 2B8; Al-Fateh (Libya)'91; FRCSC; ObstGyn. Staff, Halton Healthcare Services Corporation - Georgetown Hospital; Langs: Arabic; (905)873-9090; Fax. (905)873-9363.

FIELD, Deanna J; West End Med Clinic, 510 Prince St, Truro NS B2N 1G1; Dal'05; CCFP; Staff ER, Colchester East Hants Health Centre; Assoc Teach Staff, Dalhousie University; (902)895-1556; Fax. (902)893-1026; westendmedicalcentre@eastlink.ca.

FIELD, Sidney W; White Rock Med Associates, 101-15451 Russell Ave, White Rock BC V4B 2R5; Pretoria (South Africa)'90; MB ChB; BMedSci; DTh; LMCC; Staff, Peace Arch Hospital; Langs: Afrikaans; (604)531-5595; Fax. (604)531-9818.

FIELD, Simon; Queen Elizabeth II HSC-Halifax, 3021-1796 Summer St, Halifax NS B3H 3A7; Witwatersrand (South Africa)'92; MB ChB; CCFP; CCFP(E.M.); FCFP; Staff Emerg Phys, IWK Health Centre; Staff Emerg Phys, Queen Elizabeth II Health Sciences Centre - Halifax Infirmary Site; Asst Prof Emerg, Dalhousie University; Langs: Afrikaans; (902)473-5451; Fax. (902)473-3617.

FIELD, Stephen K; Health Science Ctr, 3330 Hospital Dr NW, Calgary AB T2N 4N1; McG'76; ABIM; FRCPC; IntMed; Respir. Staff Med., Foothills Medical Centre; Clin Prof Med, University of Calgary; Langs: Bilingual(English/French); (403)220-8722; Fax. (403)283-6151; sfield@ucalgary.ca.

FIELDEN, Michael P; Calgary Retina Consultant, 200-5340 1 St SW, Calgary AB T2H 0C8; Tor'03; FRCSC; Ophth (Diabetic Retinopathy). Asst Prof, University of Calgary; Langs: German; French; (403)286-6802; Fax. (403)286-6819.

FIELDEN, Robert H N; Sunnybrook Hlth Sciences Ctre, SCIL-2075 Bayview Ave, Toronto ON M4N 3M5; Tor'57; FAAOS; FRCSC; OrthSurg (Orthopedics) (Limb Defiency). Assoc Staff, Sunnybrook Health Sciences Centre; Fax. (416)816-3405.

FIELDER, Brian J; St Mary's Gen Hosp, 911 Queens Blvd, Kitchener ON N2M 1B2; Ott'05; CCFP; Staff, St Mary's General Hospital; (519)744-3311

FIELDING, Allan G; Allan Memorial Institute, 1025 av des Pins O, Montreal QC H3A 1A1; McG'80; FRCPC; Psy. Staff, McGill University Health Centre - Royal Victoria Hospital; adj Prof, McGill University; Langs: French; (514)934-1934 x35550; Fax. (514)843-1643.

FIELDING, Ariane E; Ariane Fielding Professional C, 11431 78 Ave NW, Edmonton AB T6G 0N2; Cal'06; FRCPC; Anes. Staff, University of Alberta Hospital; (780)232-8218

FIELDS, Anthony L A; Cross Cancer Institute, 11560 University Ave NW, Edmonton AB T6G 1Z2; Alb'74; ABIM; FACP; FRCPC; IntMed (Gastrointestinal Oncology); MedOncol. Staff/VP Med Affairs Commun Oncol, Cross Cancer Institute; Med Staff, University of Alberta Hospital; VP Cancer Care, Alberta Health Services; Prof Oncol, University of Alberta; (780)432-8756; Fax. (780)432-8888; anthony.fields@albertahealthservices.ca.

FIELDS, David W; 10155 120 St NW, Edmonton AB T5K 2A2; Alb'95; CCFP; (780)482-7551

FIELDS, Louis; Markham Place Med Centre, 206-2900 Steeles Ave E, Thornhill ON L3T 4X1; Tor'76; (905)881-6667; Fax. (905)731-1298.

FIELDUS, Warren; Halifax Infirmary, 355-1796 Summer St, Halifax NS B3H 3A7; Ott'04; FRCPC; EmergMed. Staff, Queen Elizabeth II Health Sciences Centre - Halifax Infirmary Site; (902)473-8769; Fax. (902)473-3617.

FIENBERG, Samantha; Grand River Hosp-Kw Hlth Ctre, PO Box 9056 Stn C 835 King St W, Kitchener ON N2G 1G3; Chicago (USA)'04; FRCPC; DiagRad. Staff, Grand River Hospital - Kitchener/Waterloo Health Centre; (519)742-3611

FIESCHI, Isabelle A; Division Hlth Services, 657 37th Ave W, Vancouver BC V5Z 1K6; McG'98; CCFP; (604)264-2889

FIFI-MAH, Aurore; South Health Campus, 480144-4448 Front St SE, Calgary AB T3M 1M4; (France)'96; FRCPC; IntMed; Rheum. Staff Rheumatology Clinic, Rockyview General Hospital; Clinical Asst Prof, University of Calgary; Langs: Bilingual(English/French); (403)956-2493; Fax. (403)956-2994.

FIFIELD, Frank; TC Medical Associates, PO Box 903 Stn Main 16 Golf Ave, Carbonear NL A1Y 1C4; Mem'74; Ac Staff, Carbonear General Hospital; (709)596-5135; Fax. (709)596-0212.

FIGARO, Alexandra O; Univ of Windsopr-Stud Hlth Ser, 401 Sunset Ave, Windsor ON N9B 3P4; Ott'96; CCFP; Langs: English; French; (519)973-7002

FIGUEIREDO, Indira C; 202-622 College St, Toronto ON M6G 1B6; Goa (India)'71; Ac Staff, St Joseph's Health Centre; Langs: Konkani; Portuguese; French; (416)534-4455; Fax. (416)534-2437.

FIGUEREDO, Alvaro; The Juravinski Cancer Centre, 699 Concession St, Hamilton ON L8V 5C2; (Uruguay)'66; ABIM; FRCPC; IntMed (Medical Oncology). Affil Staff, The Brant Community Healthcare System - Brantford General Hospital Site; Affil Staff, St Joseph's Healthcare - Charlton Campus; Internal Medicine, Hamilton Health Sciences Centre-Juravinski Site; Internal Med, Cancer Care Ontario - Provincial Office; Physician, The Juravinski Cancer Centre; Asst Clin Prof, McMaster University; Langs: Spanish; (905)387-9495 x64602; Fax. (905)575-6326.

FIGUEREDO ALVAREZ, Roasana; Ctr de Sante de Temiscaming, CP 760 180 rue Anvik, Temiscaming QC J0Z 3R0; (Uruguay)'96; Staff, Centre de santé de Témiscaming; (819)627-3385 x1247; Fax. (819)627-3629.

FIGUEREDO HURTADO, Sara M; CSSS du Nord de Lanaudière, 1000 boul Sainte-Anne, St-Charles-Brromee QC J6E 6J2; (Mexico)'92; Staff, Centre Hospitalier Régional de Lanaudière; (450)759-8222; Fax. (450)759-0011.

FIGUEROA PEREZ, Mayelin; Penhorn Med Clinic, 0120-569 Portland St, Dartmouth NS B2W 2M5; (Cuba)'95; (902)469-2579

FIGURADO, Victor J; St Lucia's Med Centre, 103-160 Dundas St E, Mississauga ON L5A 1W4; Peradeniya (Sri Lanka)'79; Langs: Tamil; Sinhalese; (905)206-1966; Fax. (905)206-1635.

FIGURSKI, Michael R; PO Box45058 Stn Rutland, Kelowna BC V1P 1P3; Man'86; BSc(Hons); Staff, Nicola Valley Health Centre; (250)765-0544; Fax. (250)765-0594.

FIKE, Stanley D; 181 Bestwick Dr SW, Kamloops BC V2C 1M6; Ott'81; (250)374-7845; fikes@telus.net.

FIKRY, Sameh A A; 121 Charles St W, Kitchener ON N2G 1H6; Cairo (Egypt)'89; CCFP; (519)569-8506; Fax. (519)569-8506.

FILAFERRO, Danny L; 390-10665 Jasper Ave NW, Edmonton AB T5J 3S9; Alb'95; FRCSC; Ophth. (780)424-2233

FILAKOVIC, Zdenko; St Joseph's Health Centre, 30 The Queensway, Toronto ON M6R 1B5; Zagreb (Croatia)'79; FRCPC; DiagRad. Staff, St Joseph's Health Centre; Langs: Croatian; (416)530-6010

FILANOVSKY, Yevgeny I; Nanaimo Reg Gen Hosp, 1200 Dufferin Cres, Nanaimo BC V9S 2B7; Alb'99; CCFP; CCFP(E.M.); Staff, Nanaimo Regional General Hospital; (250)754-2141

FILANTI, Bernardo I; Primacy Med Clinic, 1792 Trans Canada Way SE, Medicine Hat AB T1B 4C6; Alb'78; Ac Staff, Medicine Hat Regional Hospital; (403)502-8929; Fax. (403)502-8955.

FILATE, Woganne; Univ of Toronto, 6263-1 King's College Cir, Toronto ON M5S 1A8; Tor'07; IntMed. Staff, University of Toronto; (416)978-1562; Fax. (416)971-2112.

FILATOV, Sergei; Northern Health Authority, 1020-299 Victoria St, Prince George BC V2L 5B8; Leningrad (Russia (Federation))'86; FRCSC; Otol. Staff, University Hospital of Northern British Columbia; (250)562-3733

FILBEY, James A; Rebalance MD, 104-3551 Blanshard St, Victoria BC V8Z 0B9; McM'95; FRCPC; PhysMed&Rehab. Staff, Vancouver Island Health Authority; (250)940-4444

FILDERMAN, Ronald B; 203-4430 Bathurst St, North York ON M3H 3S3; Tor'64; MSc(Exp.Med.); FRCPC; Peds (Clinical Immunology & Allergy). Consultant Allergy, Rouge Valley Health System - Ajax & Pickering Health Centre Site; Consultant Allergy, Mount Sinai Hospital; (416)636-1616; Fax. (416)638-9759.

FILEK, Brian J; 305-321 Nicola St, Kamloops BC V2C 6G6; Sask'01; CCFP; (250)374-8858; Fax. (250)374-7946.

FILIATRAULT, Danielle C; Clin Pediatrique Laurentienne, 106-200 rue Durand, Saint-Jerome QC J7Z 7E2; Laval'87; LMCC; FRCPC; Peds. Staff Peds, Hôtel-Dieu de Saint-Jérôme; (450)438-1241; Fax. (450)438-3501.

FILIATRAULT, Denis; Hôpital Ste-Justine, 3175 ch Cote-Ste-Catherine, Montreal QC H3T 1C5; Mon'75; CSPQ; DiagRad (Pediatrics). Staff, Hôpital Ste-Justine; Universite de Montreal; Langs: English; (514)345-4637; Fax. (514)345-4816; denis_filiatrault@ssss.gouv.qc.ca.

FILIATRAULT, Jacques; CSSS de Chicoutimi, CP 5006 305 rue Saint-Vallier, Chicoutimi QC G7H 5H6; Mon'75; Nephrol (P.Q.). Staff Nephrologie Serv, Complexe hospitalier de la Sagamie; Langs: Bilingual(French/English); (418)541-1084; Fax. (418)541-1197.

FILIATRAULT, Liliane; Clinique St-Vincent, 765 rue Roland-Forget, Laval QC H7E 4C1; Sher'99; FRCPC; Psy (Adult General Psychiatry). Staff Psy, Hopital de la Cite de la santé; Langs: English; (450)668-2620 x2; Fax. (450)668-1077.

FILIATRAULT, Lyne; Vancouver Gen Hosp, 855 12th Ave W, Vancouver BC V5Z 1M9; McG'89; FRCPC; EmergMed. Physician Emerg, Vancouver General Hospital - Centennial Pavillion; Clinical Asst Prof, University of British Columbia; Langs: English; French; Spanish; (604)875-4700; filiatra@interchange.ubc.ca.

FILIATRAULT, Marc; CHUM-Hop Notre-Dame, 1560 rue Sherbrooke E, Montreal QC H2L 4M1; Mon'89; FRCPC; PhysMed&Rehab. Staff, Centre Hospitalier l'Université de Montréal (CHUM) - Hôpital Notre-Dame; (514)890-8201; Fax. (514)412-7610.

FILIATRAULT, Michele; Clin Pediatrique De Lengueuil, 105-2160 ch du Tremblay, Longueuil QC J4N 1A8; Laval'84; FRCPC; Peds. (450)448-4440; Fax. (450)448-5403.

FILIATRAULT, Robert; Neuro Rive-Sud, 250-4896 boul Taschereau, Greenfield Park QC J4V 2J2; Mon'73; AB; Electroenceph (P.Q.); Neur. Chief Med, Hopital Charles LeMoyne; (514)672-1931; Fax. (514)672-3308.

FILIATRAULT-BROSSEAU, Carole; CLSC Ste-Therese de Blainville, 55 rue Saint-Joseph, Sainte-Therese QC J7E 4Y5; Sher'99; Staff, Hôpital de Saint-Eustache; (450)430-4553 x6604; Fax. (450)430-3859.

FILIATREAULT, Manon; Centre Hosp Honore-Mercier, 2750 boul Laframboise, Saint-Hyacinthe QC J2S 4Y8; Sher'86; FRCPC; Psy. Staff, Centre Hospitalier Honore-Mercier; (450)771-3222; Fax. (450)771-3273.

FILICE, Raffaele; Niagara Diagnostic Imaging, 589 Lake St, St Catharines ON L2N 7L6; Wes'83; FRCPC; DiagRad. (905)937-2255

FILICE, Santo; Dr L Richard Ctre D'Oncologie, 37 Providence St, Moncton NB E1C 8X3; Sher'92; FRCPC; RadOncol (Brachy Therapy). Med Dir RadOncol, Dr Georges-L-Dumont University Hospital Centre; Langs: Bilingual(French/English); (506)862-4030; Fax. (506)862-4222; santo.filice@vitalitenb.ca.

FILION, Alain; CHUQ-Hotel-Dieu de Quebec, 11 Cote du Palais, Quebec QC G1R 2J6; Laval'95; FRCPC; IntMed; MedOncol; Hem. Staff HemOncol, Centre Hospitalier Universitaire de Québec (CHUQ) - Siege Social; Staff HemOncol, Hôtel-Dieu de Lévis; Langs: English; French; (418)691-5151 x15225; alfilion@videotron.ca.

FILION, Annie; Cooperative de Sante, 206-1937 ch du Village, St-Adolphe-d'Howrd QC J0T 2B0; Laval'02; Staff, Centre Hospitalier d'Argenteuil; (819)327-3534

FILION, Annie-Joelle; CSSS Pierre Boucher, 1333 boul Jacques-Cartier E, Longueuil QC J4M 2A5; Mon'07; CCFP; CCFP(E.M.); Staff, Centre Hospitalier Pierre Boucher; (450)468-8111

FILION, Edith; CHUM-Hop Notre-Dame, 1560 rue Sherbrooke E, Montreal QC H2L 4M1; Mon'02; FRCPC; RadOncol. Staff, Centre Hospitalier l'Université de Montréal (CHUM) - Hôpital Notre-Dame; Langs: Bilingual(French/English); (514)890-8254; Fax. (514)412-7537; edith.filion.chum@ssss.gouv.qc.ca.

FILION, Gaetan; Ctr Monteregien Readaptation, 5300 ch de Chambly, Saint-Hubert QC J3Y 3N7; Mon'86; FRCPC; PhysMed&Rehab (Psychiatry). Médecin, Jewish Rehabilitation Hospital; Physician, Centre de Physiatrie Val-des-Arbres; ac Staff, Centre de Monteregien de Readaptation; (450)676-7447 x2403; Fax. (450)676-0047; gaetan.filion@rrsss16.gouv.qc.ca.

FILION, Josee; CHUM-Hop Notre-Dame, 1560 rue Sherbrooke E, Montreal QC H2L 4M1; Mon'96; FRCPC; IntMed (Movement Disorders); GeriatricMed. Staff, Institut Universitaire de Gériatrie de Montréal; Staff, Centre Hospitalier l'Université de Montréal (CHUM) - Hôpital Notre-Dame; Staff, Centre Hospitalier l'Université de Montréal (CHUM) - Hôtel-Dieu; (514)890-8000; Fax. (514)412-7506.

FILION, Lucie; Polyclinique Med Pierre Le Gar, 300-1000 montee des Pionniers, Terrebonne QC J6V 1S8; Mon'83; Staff, Centre Hospitalier Pierre le Gardeur; Langs: Bilingual(French/English); (450)657-5799; Fax. (450)657-1809.

FILION, Marie-Josee; UMF Lavas CSSSVC, 2690 ch des Quatre-Bourgeois, Quebec QC G1V 0B7; Mon'91; Staff, Hôpital Laval; Med Examiner, Occupational Health & Safety; (418)656-4795; Fax. (418)656-4503.

FILION, Robert B; Hop Maisonneuve-Rosemont, 5415 boul de l'Assomption, Montreal QC H1T 2M4; Mon'80; DiagRad. Staff, Hopital Maisonneuve-Rosemont; (514)252-3535 x4231; Fax. (514)252-3537.

FILION, Rosalie; Ctr Hosp de Lasalle, 8585 Terrasse Champlain, LaSalle QC H8P 1C1; Laval'05; FRCSC; ObstGyn. Staff, Centre Hospitalier de LaSalle; (514)362-8000

FILION, Serge; Centre Med du Haut-Richelieu, 405-900 boul du Seminaire N, St-Jean-Sur-Richel QC J3A 1C3; Sher'76; FRCPC; IntMed; Respir. Consultant, Hôpital du Haut-Richelieu; Langs: Bilingual(French/English); (450)348-9229; Fax. (450)348-9220.

FILIPCHUK, Neil G; Bridgeland Med Bldg, 306-803 1 Ave NE, Calgary AB T2E 7C5; Alb'78; FRCPC; IntMed; Cardiol. Asst Clin Prof, University of Calgary; (403)571-8600; Fax. (403)571-8659.

FILIPCZUK, Mark J; St Joseph's Health Centre, 30 The Queensway, Toronto ON M6R 1B5; Lodz (Poland)'80; FRCPC; Psy. Clin Dir Psy Serv, St Joseph's Health Centre; (416)530-6591; Fax. (416)530-6076.

FILIPENKO, J Douglas; St Paul's Hosp, 1081 Burrard St, Vancouver BC V6Z 1Y6; UBC'82; FRCPC; AnatPath; GenPath. Assoc Staff, Providence Health Care - St Paul's Hospital; (604)806-8203; Fax. (604)806-8158.

FILIPINI, Daniel L; Hop du Sacre-Coeur de Mtl, 5400 boul Gouin O, Montreal QC H4J 1C5; (Argentina)'79; Staff Psy, Hôpital du Sacre-Coeur de Montréal; Langs: French; Spanish; (514)338-2692; Fax. (514)338-2531.

FILIPOWICZ, W Adam; 204-470 Bronte St S, Milton ON L9T 2J4; Lodz (Poland)'69; Member, College Of Family Physicians Of Canada-Ontario; Langs: Polish; (905)636-1216; Fax. (905)636-1490.

FILIPPONE, Daniela G S; Temple Court Bldg, 105-845 Regent St, Sudbury ON P3E 4T3; Wes'94; Otol. (705)674-7481; Fax. (705)674-7113.

FILL, Ian H; Burnside Fam Med Clinic, 101 Burnside Rd W, Victoria BC V9A 1B7; UBC'68; Ac Staff, Royal Jubilee Hospital; Ac Staff, Victoria General Hospital; (250)381-4353

FILLER, Guido; B1-436-800 Commissioners Rd E PO Box 5010 Stn B, London ON N6A 5W9; Hanover (Germany)'85; PhD; FRCPC; Peds (Pediatric Nephrology). Staff, London Health Sciences Centre - Victoria Campus; Consultant Stf Windsor Reg Hosp, Windsor Regional Hospital - Metropolitan Site; Dept Chair Peds/Prof, University of Western Ontario; Langs: German; (519)685-8377; Fax. (519)685-8156; guido.filler@lhsc.on.ca.

FILLION, Linda; Coop de Sante Robert Cliche, 291 Rte 108, Beauceville QC G5X 2Z4; Laval'83; Medical Staff, CHSLD de Beauceville; (418)774-9878; Fax. (418)774-9891; lindafillion@hotmail.com.

FILLION, Marc; Hop Maisonneuve-Rosemont, 5415 boul de l'Assomption, Montreal QC H1T 2M4; Sher'99; FRCPC; Peds; Endocrin&Metab. Staff, Hopital Maisonneuve-Rosemont; (514)252-3400

FILLION, Mariette; PO Box 46209 Rpo Silver Berry, Edmonton AB T6T 0K8; Alb'98; CCFP; Physician, Birth Control Centre.

FILLION, Mylene; Hotel-Dieu du Sacre-Coeur, 1 av Du Sacre-Coeur, Quebec QC G1N 2W1; Laval'05; FRCPC; Psy. Staff, CSSS de la Vieille-Capitale; (418)529-6851

FILLION, Nancy; CHUQ-Hotel-Dieu de Quebec, 11 Cote du Palais, Quebec QC G1R 2J6; Laval'99; CSPQ; Cardiol; IntMed. Staff, Centre Hospitalier Universitaire de Québec (CHUQ) - Siege Social; (418)691-5750; Fax. (418)691-5415.

FILLIS, Melissa R; Nipawin Health Centre, PO Box 1925, Nipawin SK S0E 1E0; (306)862-3151; Fax. (306)862-2241.

FILLITER, Bruce D; Dartmouth Med Centre, 44-46 Portland St, Dartmouth NS B2Y 1H4; Dal'75; Staff, All Saints Springhill Hospital; Physician, Springhills Institution; (902)465-4548; Fax. (902)469-2400.

FILOSA, Thomas M; Markham Family Health Team, 101-377 Church St, Markham ON L6B 1A1; Tor'97; CCFP; FCFP; (905)471-9999; Fax. (905)471-3627.

FILOTTO, Jean-Francois; Clinique Externe de Psychiatri, 35 av Saint-Charles, Vaudreuil-Dorion QC J7V 7K8; Mon'64; FRCPC; Psy. Staff, Centre Hospitalier Régional du Suroît; (450)455-7969 x240; Fax. (450)455-8631.

FILTEAU, Chantal; Clin Med La Malbaie, 515 rue Saint-Etienne, La Malbaie QC G5A 1W7; Laval'07; CCFP; (418)665-2366 x16; Fax. (418)665-7766.

FILTEAU, Genevieve; Ctr Med Joilbourg, 649-1271 boul Jolibourg, Laval QC H7Y 1Z8; Sher'98; LMCC; CCFP; Staff, Hopital de la Cite de la santé; Langs: Bilingual(French/English); (450)689-2424; Fax. (450)689-9548.

FILTEAU, Lucie C; The Ottawa Hosp-Civic Campus, 249C-1053 Carling Ave, Ottawa ON K1Y 4E9; McM'97; FRCPC; Anes. Staff Anes, The Ottawa Hospital - Civic Campus; Langs: Bilingual(English/French); (613)761-4169

FILTEAU, Marie-Josee; Clinique Marie Fitzbach, 1085 av Louis-St-Laurent, Quebec QC G1R 2W8; Laval'87; FRCPsy; FRCPC; Psy (Adult Psychiatry-Mood & Anxiety Disorders). Langs: Spanish; English; (418)647-4272; Fax. (418)649-5115; filteaumj@hotmail.com.

FILTEAU, Pierre; Centre médicale des Carrières, RR 2 800-1000 boul Bona-Dussault, St-Mar-Des-Carr QC G0A 4B0; Laval'83; (418)268-5596; Fax. (418)268-5729.

FILTEAU, Rene; Clinique Med Le Gardeurois, 130-155 rue Notre-Dame, Repentigny QC J5Z 3C4; Mon'76; Staff, Centre Hospitalier Pierre le Gardeur; (450)582-5551; Fax. (450)582-2718.

FILYK, Maria; East Calgary Health Centre, 3F-4715 8 Ave SE, Calgary AB T2A 3N4; Cal'95; BA; CCST; FRCPC; Psy (Child & Infant Psychiatry). Consultant Psychiatrist, Alberta Children's Hospital; Langs: English; French; (403)955-1010; Fax. (403)955-1013; maria.filyk@albertahealthservices.ca.

FILYK, Zoe; Signature Park Plaza, 304-1919 Sirocco Dr SW, Calgary AB T3H 2Y3; (Peru)'92; CCFP; (403)686-3628; Fax. (403)686-3627.

FINAN, Emer A; Mount Sinai Hosp, 775-600 University Ave, Toronto ON M5G 1X5; (Ireland)'99; Staff, Mount Sinai Hospital; (416)586-4800 x8336; Fax. (416)586-8745.

FINCATI, Maria; 200 Plaza, 162-233 16 Ave NW, Calgary AB T2M 0H5; Alb'01; (403)230-3300; Fax. (403)230-3322.

FINCH, Daygen; BC Cancer Ctre-Southern Interi, 399 Royal Ave, Kelowna BC V1Y 5L3; Alb'02; FRCPC; IntMed; MedOncol. Staff Med Oncol, BC Cancer Agency Sindi Ahluwalia Hawkins Centre for the Southern Interior; (250)712-3930

FINCH, Graham C; Lakeridge Hlth Corp-Oshawa, 1 Hospital Crt, Oshawa ON L1G 2B9; Dal'66; Staff, Lakeridge Health - Oshawa Site; (905)576-8711

FINCH, Susan J; Street Health Centre, 235 Wellington St, Kingston ON K7K 0B5; McG'91; FRCPC; Psy. Staff, Hotel-Dieu Hospital; (613)453-7859

FINDING, Diane; Columbia Med Bldg, 201-301 Columbia St E, New Westminster BC V3L 3W5; UBC'89; BSc; Staff, Royal Columbian Hospital; Staff Teacher, University of British Columbia; (604)526-4655; Fax. (604)526-7656.

FINDLATER, A Ross; Population Public Health, 204-310 Idylwyld Dr N, Saskatoon SK S7L 0Z2; McG'75; BSc; MSc(Epidemiol); FRCPC; CommunMed;CCFP; CCFP(E.M.); (306)655-4338; Fax. (306)655-4414; ross.findlater@saskatoonhealthregion.ca.

FINDLAY, Brian P; 201-112 Queenston St, St Catharines ON L2R 2Z4; Tor'79; FRCPC; IntMed (Hematology); MedOncol. Staff, Niagara Health System - St Catharines General Site; Staff, Niagara Health System - Welland Hospital Site; Asst Prof, McMaster University; (905)685-8082

FINDLAY, C Edward; 1603 20 Ave NW, Calgary AB T2M 1G9; Ohio (USA)'85; CCFP; FCFP; (403)282-7165; Fax. (403)289-8269.

FINDLAY, Douglas E; Belgage Med Arts Bldg, 206-525 Belmont Ave W, Kitchener ON N2M 5E2; Wes'84; CCFP; (519)576-4070; Fax. (519)576-4109.

FINDLAY, J Max; University of Alberta Hosp, 2D1 02 WMC-8440 112 St NW, Edmonton AB T6G 2B7; UBC'82; FRCSC; Neursurg. Staff, University of Alberta Hospital; (780)407-3548; Fax. (780)407-8203; max.findlay@albertahealthsevices.ca.

FINDLAY, Peter M; Med Assoc Of Port Credit, 2F-333 Lakeshore Rd W, Mississauga ON L5H 1G9; Tor'91; CCFP; Court Staff Family Med, The Credit Valley Hospital; (905)274-7044; Fax. (905)274-0227.

FINDLAY, Sheila J; 205-1808 Bowen Rd, Nanaimo BC V9S 5W4; Sask'88; (250)753-6646

FINDLAY, Sheri; McMaster University, HSC 3A-1280 Main St W, Hamilton ON L8S 4K1; McG'92; FRCPC; Peds (Adolescent Medicine). Staff, Hamilton Health Sciences Centre - McMaster Children's Hospital; Prof, McMaster University; (905)521-2100 x5644; Fax. (905)308-7548.

FINDLAY, Timothy; Mount St Joseph Hosp, 3080 Prince Edward St, Vancouver BC V5T 3N4; UBC'09; CCFP; CCFP(E.M.); Staff, Providence Health Care - Mount Saint Joseph Hospital; (604)874-1141

FINDLAY-SHIRRAS, Nigel J; Surrey Mem Hosp, 13750 96 Ave, Surrey BC V3V 1Z2; London (England)'74; MB BS; LMCC; MRCS; DABA; FRCPC; Anes. Chief Anes, Surrey Memorial Hospital; (604)588-3367; Fax. (604)585-5644.

FINE, Barnet; 320 35e av N, Saint-Georges QC G5Z 0M6; Montpellier (France)'77; Staff, Cree Board of Health & Social Services James Bay; ac Staff, St Mary's Hospital Centre; ac Staff, Sir Mortimer B Davis Jewish General; Conférencier Faculty of Med, McGill University; Langs: French; (418)227-7748; barry.fine@mcgill.ca.

FINE, Geoffrey M; Trillium Hlth Ctr-Mississauga, 100 Queensway W, Mississauga ON L5B 1B8; Wes'94; BSc; CCFP; CCFP(E.M.); Staff EmergMed, Trillium Health Centre - Mississauga; Coroner, Province of Ontario; Langs: English; French; (905)848-7580 x6315

FINE, Jonathan P H; Quesnel Mental Hlth Services, 395 Elliott St, Quesnel BC V2J 1Y4; London (England)'75; LRCP; DRCOG; MRC; Asst Clin Prof Family Pract, University of British Columbia; (250)992-5189; avery@quesnelbc.com.

FINE, Rebecca J; 302KW-650 Sammon Ave, East York ON M4C 5M5; McM'03; FRCPC; IntMed; Endocrin&Metab. (416)915-5461; Fax. (416)915-5463.

FINE, Sheldon; The Credit Valley Hosp, 2200 Eglinton Ave W, Mississauga ON L5M 2N1; Tor'75; ABIM; FRCPC; IntMed (Oncology). Staff IntMed & Oncol, The Credit Valley Hospital; Consultant, Princess Margaret Hospital - University Health Network; (905)813-2200 x1841; Fax. (905)813-4024; sfine@s.vh.on.ca.

FINEGAN, Barry; 8 120-152 University Campus NW, Edmonton AB T6G 2G3; National (Ireland)'76; MB ChB; FFARCSI; FRCPC; Anes (Cardiac Anesthesia). Site Chief, University of Alberta Hospital; Chair Anes & Pain Med/Prof, University of Alberta; (780)407-8861; Fax. (780)407-3200; chassist@ualberta.ca.

FINELLI, Antonio; Univ Hlth Network-Princess M, 3 130-610 University Ave, Toronto ON M5G 2M9; Tor'96; FRCSC; Urol (Oncology). Urologist/Oncologist, Princess Margaret Hospital - University Health Network; (416)946-2851; Fax. (416)946-6590; antonio.finelli@uhn.on.ca.

FINEMAN, Lauren; False Creek Urgent Care Centre, 107-555 8th Ave W, Vancouver BC V5Z 1C6; Sydney (Australia)'05; MB BS; CCFP; Med Dir, False Creek Urgent Care Centre; (604)628-2822; Fax. (604)484-8141; tmuncey@nationalsurgery.com.

FINESILVER, Allan M; 209-5885 Ch de la Cote-des-Nei, Montreal QC H3S 2T2; McG'70; BSc; FRCSC; Otol. Staff, Sir Mortimer B Davis Jewish General; Teach Staff, McGill University; Langs: English; French; (514)731-9270

FINESTONE, David L; Parkdale Med Tower, 507-1081 Carling Ave, Ottawa ON K1Y 4G2; McG'75; CCFP; FCFP; Staff, The Ottawa Hospital - Civic Campus; Asst Clin Prof, University of Ottawa; Langs: French; (613)729-1165; Fax. (613)728-3083; davidf@ottawadoctors.ca.

FINESTONE, Debra S; St Mary's Hospital Centre, 3830 av Lacombe, Montreal QC H3T 1M5; McG'82; Staff, St Mary's Hospital Centre; (514)734-2690

FINESTONE, Hillel M; Bruyere Academic Fam Hlth Team, 4f-75 Bruyere St, Ottawa ON K1N 5C8; McG'83; DABPM; DAB; FRCPC; PhysMed&Rehab (Electromyography). Staff Rehabilitation Ctr, The Ottawa Hospital - Riverside Campus; Med Chief PhysMed&Rehab, SCO Health Service - Elisabeth Bruyère Hospital; Chief Physiatry, Bruyère Continuing Care - Saint-Vincent Hospital; Assoc Prof Rehab Med, University of Ottawa; Assoc Prof, University of Western Ontario; Langs: English; French; (613)562-6094; Fax. (613)562-6312.

FINGARD, Jordan E; Hys Med Centre, 202-11010 101 St, Edmonton AB T5H 4B9; Sask'98; FRCPC; DiagRad. Staff, Red Deer Regional Hospital Centre; (780)426-1121

FINGER, Elizabeth; St Joseph's HC-Parkwood Hosp, 801 Commissioners Rd E, London ON N6C 5J1; Cornell (NY) (USA)'00; Staff, Parkwood Hospital - St Joseph's Health Care; Staff, St Joseph's Hospital - St Joseph's Health Care; (519)646-6032; Fax. (519)646-6226.

FINGEROTE, Robert J; 9651 Yonge St, Richmond Hill ON L4C 1V7; Man'80; BSc; MSc; DABIM; FRCPC; IntMed (Hepatology); Gastroent. Att Physician IntMed & Gastroenterol, Mackenzie Richmond Hill Hospital; Langs: Yiddish; (905)780-9562; Fax. (905)237-4516; rfingerote@gmail.com.

FINGLAND, Robert; Lions Gate Hosp, 231 15th St E, North Vancouver BC V7L 2L7; Ott'90; FRCPC; Anes. Staff, Abbotsford Regional Hospital & Cancer Centre; Staff, Lions Gate Hospital; (604)984-5709

FINGRUT, Philip; Bayview-Finch Med Clinic, 200-3292 Bayview Ave, North York ON M2M 4J5; Dublin (Ireland)'76; MB ChB; BAO; BASc; Ac Staff, North York General Hospital; Med Dir, Thompson Home for the Aged; Langs: Italian; French; Hebrew; (416)222-8555; Fax. (416)222-6707.

FINK, Alan D; The Doctor's Office, 203-300 John St, Thornhill ON L3T 5W4; Tor'72; BSc; (905)764-0188; Fax. (905)764-0189.

FINK, Milo P; Wascana Rehabilitation Ctr, 2180 23rd Ave, Regina SK S4S 0A5; Sask'78; FRCPC; PhysMed&Rehab (Disability Evaluation). Physical Medicine & Rehab, Wascana Rehabilitation Centre; Asst Prof, University of Saskatchewan; (306)766-5405; Fax. (306)766-7442; milo.fink@rqhealth.ca.

FINKE, Stefan; Sheldon Chumir Centre, 1213 4 St SW, Calgary AB T2R 0X7; Mon'06; CCFP; Staff, Colchester East Hants Health Centre; (403)955-6200

FINKEL, Richard M; 1F-664 Broadview Ave, Toronto ON M4K 2P1; Man'77; FRCPC; Psy. (416)461-5049

FINKELBERG, Fred; 303-66 Gerrard St, Toronto ON M5B 1G3; Tor'78; PhD(Psychol); FRCPC; Psy. (416)482-6660; Fax. (416)920-1880.

FINKELBERG, Susan; Tiny Tots Med Clinic, 203-3400 rue du Marche, Dollard-D-Ormeaux QC H9B 2Y1; McG'04; CCFP; CCFP(E.M.); (514)685-3531; Fax. (514)685-7971.

FINKELMAN, Shayna R; Don Valley Med Associates, 216-1333 Sheppard Ave E, North York ON M2J 1V1; McM'07; CCFP; (416)498-9841; Fax. (416)498-3114; sfinkelman@baycrest.org.

FINKELSTEIN, David M; Medical Arts Bldg, 104-581 Davis Dr, Newmarket ON L3Y 2P6; Tor'85; FRCSC; Otol. Staff, Southlake Regional Health Centre; (905)898-2444; Fax. (905)898-5558.

FINKELSTEIN, Harvey; Bayshore Med Bldg, 204-3029 Carling Ave, Ottawa ON K2B 8E8; McG'80; FRCPC; Derm. Ac Staff, The Ottawa Hospital - Civic Campus; Consultant, Queensway Carleton Hospital; Asst Prof Med, University of Ottawa; Langs: Bilingual(English/French); (613)820-2518

FINKELSTEIN, Ian; Toronto Headache & Pain Clinic, 209-801 York Mills Rd, North York ON M3B 1X7; Tor'94; MSc; DAAPM; CCFP; (416)699-8843; Fax. (416)699-6094.

FINKELSTEIN, Joel A; Sunnybrook Hlth Sciences Ctre, MG361-2075 Bayview Ave, Toronto ON M4N 3M5; Tor'88; FRCSC; OrthSurg (Spine). Asst Prof Orth, Sunnybrook Health Sciences Centre; Assoc Prof Orth, University of Toronto; (416)480-6774; Fax. (416)480-4705; joel.finkelstein@utoronto.ca.

FINKELSTEIN, Jonathan; Groupe Sante Physimed, 121-6363 rte Transcanadienne, Saint-Laurent QC H4T 1Z9; Mon'09; CCFP; (514)747-8888; Fax. (514)747-0655.

FINKELSTEIN, Lorne; Medical Arts Bldg, 608-1 Young St, Hamilton ON L8N 1T8; Wes'71; FACC; FRCPC; Cardiol. Ac Staff, St Joseph's Healthcare - Charlton Campus; Physician, Medical Arts Bldg; (905)529-6618; Fax. (905)529-6809; lfinkelstein@cogeco.ca.

FINKELSTEIN, Michael S; Toronto Public Health, 10F-277 Victoria St, Toronto ON M5B 1W2; Ott'95; FRCPC; CommunMed. (416)392-1784; Fax. (416)392-0047; mfinkel@toronto.ca.

FINKELSTEIN, Murray M; Family Med Centre, 4F-60 Murray St, Toronto ON M5T 3L9; McG'76; MD; PhD; CCFP; Ac Staff, Mount Sinai Hospital; Clin Assoc Prof Family Med, McMaster University; Asst Prof Family Med, University of Toronto; (416)586-3190; Fax. (416)586-3175.

FINKELSTEIN, Sandy; Scarborough Hosp-Birchmount, 3030 Birchmount Rd, Scarborough ON M1W 3W3; McM'88; FRCPC; IntMed (Respirology); Critical Care Medicine. Ac Staff, The Scarborough Hospital - Birchmount Campus; (416)495-2465; Fax. (416)495-2420; sandyfinkelstein@sympatico.ca.

FINKELSTEIN, Sheldon C; 308-1428 Ouellette Ave, Windsor ON N8X 1K4; McG'74; FRCPC; Psy. (519)256-1895; Fax. (519)256-6671.

FINKELSTEIN, Sheldon; Kipling Heights Med Centre, 2291 Kipling Ave, Etobicoke ON M9W 4L6; Tor'74; Staff, William Osler Health System - Etobicoke General Hospital; Staff, Mount Sinai Hospital; (416)741-4545; Fax. (416)744-1484.

FINKELSTEIN, Yaron; The Hosp For Sick Children, 555 University Ave, Toronto ON M5G 1X8; Tel Aviv (Israel)'94; Staff Emerg Med, The Hospital For Sick Children; Langs: Hebrew; (416)813-7654 x4160

FINKLE, Simon N; Dickson Centre, 5089-5788 University Ave, Halifax NS B3H 1V8; Man'95; FRCPC; IntMed; Nephrol. Staff, Queen Elizabeth II Health Sciences Centre - Victoria General Site; (902)473-5160; Fax. (902)473-2675.

FINLAY, Jane D C; Cross Roads Pediatric Clinic, 350-507 Broadway Ave W, Vancouver BC V5Z 1E6; Alb'85; FRCPC; Peds; InfectDis. Ac Staff, BC Children's Hospital; Ac Staff Peds, Richmond Hospital; (604)568-7115

FINLAY, Karen; Hamilon HS-Henderson Site, 711 Concession St, Hamilton ON L8V 1C3; McM'91; FRCPC; DiagRad. Staff, Hamilton Health Sciences Centre-Juravinski Site; (905)389-4411 x42261; Fax. (905)575-2660.

FINLAY, Kelvin R; Metrotown Med Centre, 303-6411 Nelson Ave, Burnaby BC V5H 4H3; Otago (New Zealand)'75; MB ChB; FRCSC; Ophth (Retina Vitreous Surgery). (604)433-1258; Fax. (604)433-6154.

FINLAY, Marisa H D; The Credit Valley Hosp, 2200 Eglinton Ave W, Mississauga ON L5M 2N1; Qns'00; FRCPC; RadOncol. Staff, The Credit Valley Hospital; (905)813-1100

FINLAY, Michel; CLSC Grande-Riviere, 425 rue Leguerrier, Gatineau QC J9H 6N8; Sher'82; Staff Med, Hull Hospital; Langs: Bilingual(French/English); (819)966-6540 x263; Fax. (819)966-6542.

FINLAY, Susan; Laurentian University Helth Se, SSR G23-935 Ramsey Lake Rd, Sudbury ON P3E 2C6; McM'86; BSc; Staff Espanola Family Hlth Team, Espanola Regional Hospital and Health Centre; Physician, Shawnee Lezhit Health Centre; Langs: Bilingual(English/French); (705)673-6546; Fax. (705)675-4821.

FINLAYSON, Alexander; Dartmouth Gen Hosp, 325 Pleasant St, Dartmouth NS B2Y 4G8; Aberdeen (Scotland)'71; MB ChB; MRCGPract; DRCOG; FRCPC; Anes (Chronic Pain). Staff, Dartmouth General Hospital; (902)465-8316

FINLAYSON, Gordon N; Anesthesiology Critical Care M, 2449-910 10th Ave W, Vancouver BC V5Z 1M9; UBC'01; FRCPC; Anes; Critical Care Medicine. Staff, Vancouver General Hospital - Centennial Pavillion; (604)875-4000

FINLAYSON, Heather C; G F Strong Rehabilitation Ctr, 4255 Laurel St, Vancouver BC V5Z 2G9; McM'01; FRCPC; PhysMed&Rehab. Staff, G F Strong Rehabilitation Centre; (604)714-4113

FINLAYSON, Judith E; 610 St Charles St, Victoria BC V8S 3N7; McM'75; MA; CCFP; FCFP; Ac Staff, Vancouver Island Health Authority; Langs: Arabic; German; (250)598-8181; Fax. (250)598-0433; drfinlayson@shawbiz.ca.

FINLAYSON, Laura; 4193-1278 Tower Rd, Halifax NS B3H 1V7; Mem'81; FRCPC; Derm (Pediatric Dermatology). Chief Pediatric Derm, IWK Health Centre; Hd Chief Div Clinical Derm & Cutaneous Science, Capital Health District Authority; Chief Pediatric Derm, Dalhousie University; (902)479-7934; Fax. (902)473-2665; laura.finlayson@cdha.nshealth.ca.

FINLAYSON, Nolan A; Seven Oaks Gen Hosp, 2300 Mcphillips St, Winnipeg MB R2V 3M3; Man'01; CCFP; Staff, Seven Oaks General Hospital; (204)632-7133

FINLAYSON, Roderick J; MUHC-Montreal Gen Hosp, D10 137-1650 av Cedar, Montreal QC H3G 1A4; Sher'86; CSPQ; FRCPC; Anes. Staff, McGill University Health Centre - Montreal General Campus; (514)934-8222; Fax. (514)934-8096.

FINLAYSON, Sarah J; Diamond Health Care Centre, 6F-2775 Laurel St, Vancouver BC V5Z 1M9; Qns'98; FRCSC; ObstGyn (Gynecology). (604)875-5604; Fax. (604)875-4869.

FINLEY, Christian; St Joseph's Healthcare, T2105H-50 Charlton Ave E, Hamilton ON L8N 4A6; UBC'02; FRCSC; GenSurg; ThorSurg. Staff, St Joseph's Healthcare - Charlton Campus; (905)522-4941

FINLEY, G Allen; IWK Health Centre, PO Box 9700 Rpo CSC 5850 University Ave, Halifax NS B3K 6R8; Dal'80; BSc; FAAP; FRCPC; Anes (Pediatric Pain Management). Med Dir Centre for Pediatric Pain Research/Staff Anes, IWK Health Centre; Consultant, Queen Elizabeth II Health Sciences Centre - Victoria General Site; Prof Anes & Psychology, Dalhousie University; Langs: Bilingual(French/English); (902)470-7708; Fax. (902)470-7709.

FINLEY, John P; IWK Health Centre, PO Box 9700 Rpo CSC 5850-5980 University Ave, Halifax NS B3K 6R8; McG'73; FRCPC; PedCardiol. Staff Ped Cardiol, IWK Health Centre; Prof Peds, Dalhousie University; (902)470-6956; Fax. (902)470-6616; john.finley@iwk.nshealth.ca.

FINLEY, Richard J; 7109-2775 Laurel St, Vancouver BC V5Z 1M9; Wes'71; FRCSC; GenSurg (Esophageal Surgery); ThorSurg. Ac Staff Surg, Vancouver General Hospital - Centennial Pavillion; Prof/Head Thoracic Surg, University of British Columbia; (604)875-4150; richard.finley@vch.ca.

FINLEY, Scott G; Surrey Memorial Hosp, 13750 96 Ave, Surrey BC V3V 1Z2; McM'04; CCFP; CCFP(E.M.); Staff, Surrey Memorial Hospital; (604)581-2211

FINN, Alexander; Royal Jubilee Hosp, 5F-1952 Bay St, Victoria BC V8R 1J8; (USA)'06; Staff, Royal Jubilee Hospital; (250)370-8432

FINN, Brian R; Centre for Family Medicine, PO Box 69 3742 Nafziger Rd, Wellesley ON N0B 2T0; Ott'82; CCFP; Staff, Grand River Hospital - Kitchener/Waterloo Health Centre; Staff, St Mary's General Hospital; (519)656-2220; Fax. (519)656-3173.

FINN, Celine; CSSS des Iles, 430 rue Prinicpal, Cap-aux-Meules QC G4T 1R9; Laval'88; FRCPC; Psy. Staff, Hôpital de l'Archipel; (418)986-2121

FINN, Nicholas G; Centre D'Oncologie Dr Leon-Ric, 37 rue Providence, Moncton NB E1C 8X3; Sher'03; BSc; FRCPC; IntMed (Medical Oncology); Hem. Staff, Dr Georges-L-Dumont University Hospital Centre; (506)862-4030

FINN, Stephanie K; Dixie Road Med Association, 2200 Dixie Rd, Mississauga ON L4Y 1Z4; Tor'99; CCFP; (905)279-1700

FINN, William P; 301-1366 Yonge St, Toronto ON M4T 3A7; Tor'59; FRCSC; GenSurg (Colon & Rectal Surgery). Staff, Hamilton Health Sciences Centre - Hamilton General Hospital; Clin Assoc Prof Surg, McMaster University; (416)926-0262; Fax. (416)926-0936.

FINNAMORE, Ryan E; Chester Family Practice, PO Box 2040, Chester NS B0J 1J0; Dal'04; CCFP; (902)275-5625

FINNEGAN, A Paul J; 554 Spadina Cres, Toronto ON M5S 2J9; Tor'73; FRCPC; Psy. (416)923-8058

FINNEGAN, Martin M; 23 Gareth Crt, Moncton NB E1A 8B4; McG'90; FRCPC; DiagRad.

FINNEGAN, Stephen J; Charles Clark Med Centre, PO Box 5550 Stn Main 303 9 Ave SW, High River AB T1V 0H2; Cape Town (South Africa)'91; MB ChB; CCFP; Staff, High River General Hospital; (403)652-2929; Fax. (403)652-1510.

FINNEY, Brett; Portage Med Clinic, 140 9th St SE, Portage La Prairie MB R1N 3V5; Man'99; CCFP; (204)857-3445

FINNEY, Trevor A; Associate Med Clinic, 203-10030 106 St, Westlock AB T7P 2K4; Pretoria (South Africa)'76; MB ChB; BSc(Wits); (780)349-3341; Fax. (780)349-6686.

FINNIE, Keith; London HSC-University Hosp, PO Box 5339 Stn B 339 Windermere Rd, London ON N6A 5A5; Aberdeen (Scotland)'73; FRCPC; IntMed; Cardiol. Staff, London Health Sciences Centre - University Hospital; Prof Med, University of Western Ontario; (519)663-3504; Fax. (519)663-3501.

FINNIS, William; North Bay Reg Health Centre, 50 College Dr, North Bay ON P1B 0A4; Birmingham (England)'71; MB ChB; MRC(UK); FRCPC; IntMed. Staff, North Bay Regional Health Centre - Regional Mental Health; (705)474-7525

FINUCANE, Brendan T; Clinical Sciences Bldg, 8 120CSB-152 University Campus, Edmonton AB T5G 2G3; National (Ireland)'67; FFARCS; FRCA; FRCPC; Anes. Staff Anes, University of Alberta Hospital; Teach Staff Anes, University of Alberta; (780)407-1877; Fax. (780)407-3200; bfinucan@ualberta.ca.

FINVERS, Kimberley A; 214-11 Hidden Creek Dr NW, Calgary AB T3A 6K6; Cal'95; BSc; CCFP; FCFP; (403)248-2273

FINZER, Alan; Misericordia Comm Hosp, 16940 87 Ave NW, Edmonton AB T5R 4H5; RCS (Ireland)'88; MB ChB; BAO; Staff, Covenant Health - Misericordia Community Hospital; (780)735-2000

FINZER, John K; 116-12222 137 Ave NW, Edmonton AB T5L 4X5; Alb'88; (780)473-9355; Fax. (780)473-2856.

FIORILLO, Loretta; Edmonton Clinic Health Academy, 3 555-11405 87 Ave NW, Edmonton AB T6G 1C9; Napoli (Italy)'81; FRCPC; Peds (Pediatric Dermatology); Derm. Staff, Edmonton Clinic Health Academy; Asst Clin Prof, University of Calgary; Assoc Prof, University of Alberta; Langs: Italian; (780)248-5480; Fax. (780)248-5625; loretta.fiorillo@albertahealthservices.ca.

FIORINI, Cynthia M; Medical Arts Bldg, 8-358 Reynolds St, Oakville ON L6J 3L9; (Ireland)'88; (905)845-6181; Fax. (905)845-5924.

FIORINI, Godfrey T; 201-1670 Dufferin St, Toronto ON M6H 3M2; Royal (Malta)'55; Staff, St Joseph's Health Centre; Langs: Italian; Maltese; (416)652-1940; Fax. (416)652-1995.

FIORINO, Michael; 12720 66 St NW, Edmonton AB T5C 0A3; Alb'79; BSc; Consultant Privil, Royal Alexandra Hospital; Consultant Privil, University of Alberta Hospital; Staff Privil, Capital Care - Grandview; (780)475-3661; Fax. (780)478-7271; michael.fiorino@capitalhealth.ca.

FIORITI, Steven; CSSS du Sud de Lanaudière, 911 montee des Pionniers, Terrebonne QC J6V 2H2; Mon'03; Staff, Centre Hospitalier Pierre le Gardeur; (450)654-7525

FIRESTONE, Gail F; 38 Mill St SS 1 PO Box 40, Mount Albert ON L0G 1M0; Ott'70; Ac Staff, Southlake Regional Health Centre; Court Staff, North York General Hospital; (905)473-2422; Fax. (905)473-5099.

FIROUZABADI-DASHTI, Roya; The Brooklin Med Centre, 1A-5959 Anderson St, Whitby ON L1M 2E9; (Iran)'96; CCFP; (905)655-3321; Fax. (905)655-4848.

FIROZ, Abu T M; 212-955 Major Mackensie Dr W, Vaughan ON L6A 4P9; Dhaka (Bangladesh)'84; MB BS; CCFP; Langs: Bengali; (905)553-2655; Fax. (905)553-8655.

FIROZ, Tabassum; Centre for Complex Disorders, 34-950 28th Ave, Vancouver BC V5Z 4H4; UBC'06; FRCPC; IntMed. Staff, BC Women's Hospital & Health Centre; (604)875-2000 x2974

FIRSTBROOK, Peggy J; 2400 Arbutus Rd, Victoria BC V8N 1V7; Ott'80; FRCPC; Psy (Child & Adolescent Psychiatry). Staff, Queen Alexandra Centre for Children's Health; (250)519-6926

FIRSZT, Jose; Clinique Med Luso Mtl Ltee, 1 av du Mont-Royal E, Montreal QC H2T 1N4; Buenos Aires (Argentina)'64; FRCSC; Urol (Erectile Dysfunction). Ac Staff, CSSS du Coeur de l'Isle Hôpital Jean-Talon; CSSS Saint-Leonard et Saint-Michel; Langs: Bilingual(French/English); (514)849-2391; Fax. (514)849-2394.

FIRTH, S Terry; 225-250B Greenbank Rd, Nepean ON K2H 8X4; Qns'65; DPsy; FRCPC; Psy. Staff, The Ottawa Hospital - Civic Campus; Clin Assoc Prof Psy, University of Ottawa; (613)237-3020; Fax. (613)828-2081.

FISCH, Christiane; CHUS-Hop Fleurimont, 3001 12e av N, Sherbrooke QC J1H 5N4; Sher'79; FRCPC; DiagRad. Staff, Centre Hospitalier Universitaire de Sherbrooke-Hopital Fleurimont; (819)346-1110; Fax. (819)820-6423.

FISCH, Danielle; Clinique Med Dr Danielle Fisch, 3352 Ch Capelton, Canton-De-Hatley QC J0B 2C0; Sher'76; CCFP; Langs: Bilingual(French/English); (819)842-4295; Fax. (819)842-1130.

FISCH, Laura N; Etobicoke Med Centre, 400 The East Mall, Etobicoke ON M9B 3Z9; Ott'98; CCFP; (416)621-2220; Fax. (416)621-2357.

FISCH, Patricia A; 200-394 rue Saint-Vallier, Chicoutimi QC G7H 4J1; Sher'83; FRCSC; ObstGyn. ac Staff, Complexe hospitalier de la Sagamie; (418)545-2666; Fax. (418)545-3924.

FISCH, Paul; Etobicoke Med Centre, 400 The East Mall, Etobicoke ON M9B 3Z9; Tor'70; BA; Att Staff, Trillium Health Centre - West Toronto; (416)621-2220 x241; Fax. (416)621-2357.

FISCHBACHER, Theodore; Alliston Family Health Team, 36 Victoria St W, Alliston ON L9R 1S8; Glasgow (Scotland)'73; BSc; MB ChB; Langs: French; (705)435-8887; Fax. (705)435-8867.

FISCHER, Annette D; Red River Family Med Centre, 2F-139 Carmen Ave, Winnipeg MB R2L 0E5; Man'02; FRCPC; Peds. (204)661-3885

FISCHER, Barbara J; 204-2825 Clearbrook Rd, Abbotsford BC V2T 6S3; UBC'73; (604)859-5449

FISCHER, Barbara L; Liberton Med Centre, 212-31 Liberton Dr, St. Albert AB T8N 3X6; Alb'96; CCFP; FCFP; (780)459-7760

FISCHER, C Richard; The West Durham Fam Hlth Team, BE 200B-1105 Kingston Rd, Pickering ON L1V 1B5; Tor'85; CCFP; FCFP; Staff, Rouge Valley Health System - Ajax & Pickering Health Centre Site; Staff, Rouge Valley Health System - Centenary Health Centre Site; (905)420-9999; Fax. (905)420-0863.

FISCHER, Corinne E; St Michael's Hosp, 17 044 CCW-30 Bond St, Toronto ON M5B 1W8; Tor'93; FRCPC; Psy (Geriatric Psychiatry). Ac Staff, St Michael's Hospital; Asst Prof, University of Toronto; (416)864-5320; Fax. (416)864-5480; fischerc@stmh.ca.

FISCHER, David A; Active Health Sports Med Ctre, 108-115 Bell Farm Rd, Barrie ON L4M 5G1; Wes'92; FRCPC; IntMed; ClinImmunol&Allergy. Aj Prof, University of Western Ontario; (705)727-7650; Fax. (705)727-7670.

FISCHER, Erica G L; U Of Toronto Health Services, 2F-214 College St, Toronto ON M5T 2Z9; McM'77; (416)978-8830; Fax. (416)971-2089.

FISCHER, Gabor; St Boniface Gen Hosp, 409 Tache Ave, Winnipeg MB R2H 2A6; (Hungary)'94; FRCPC; AnatPath. Staff, St Boniface General Hospital.

FISCHER, Gerhardt E; Lockwood Diagnostics, 320-790 Bay St, Toronto ON M5G 1N8; Alb'61; BA; FRCSC; GenSurg.

FISCHER, Howard L; Mount Sinai Hosp, 600 University Ave, Toronto ON M5G 1X5; McG'97; FRCPC; Anes. Staff, Mount Sinai Hospital; (416)586-4800 x5270

FISCHER, Jason W J; The Hosp For Sick Children, 555 University Ave, Toronto ON M5G 1X8; (Grenada)'03; Staff, The Hospital For Sick Children; (416)813-1500

FISCHER, Krista L; Active Health Sports Med Ctre, 108-115 Bell Farm Rd, Barrie ON L4M 5G1; Ott'93; CCFP; (705)727-7650; Fax. (705)727-7670.

FISCHER, Lisa K; Fowler Kennedy Sport Med, 3M-1151 Richmond St, London ON N6A 3K7; Wes'93; BScPT; Dip SportMed; CCFP; Asst Prof, University of Western Ontario; (519)661-3017; Fax. (519)661-3379.

FISCHER, Marc; Medical Arts Bldg, 419-1 Young St, Hamilton ON L8N 1T8; Wes'94; FRCSC; Urol. Physician, Medical Arts Bldg; Langs: Bilingual(English/French); (905)529-5910; mfischer@cogeco.ca.

FISCHER, Sandra; Univ Hlth Network-Toronto Gen, 200 Elizabeth St, Toronto ON M5G 2C4; (Brazil)'89; Staff, Toronto General Hospital - UHN; (416)340-4800

FISCHER, Thomas I; Southwest Med Dental Centre, 1107 37 St SW, Calgary AB T3C 1S5; Man'72; FRCPC; Psy. (403)258-2391; Fax. (403)258-2563.

FISCHLER, Ilan; Ontario Shores Ctr Mental HS, 700 Gordon St, Whitby ON L1N 5S9; Tor'02; FRCPC; Psy. Staff, Ontario Shores Centre for Mental Health Sciences; (905)668-5881

FISER, Jarmila E; Lakeridge Hlth Corp-Oshawa, 1 Hospital Crt, Oshawa ON L1G 2B9; Komensky (Slovakia)'71; FRCPC; AnatPath. Staff, Lakeridge Health - Oshawa Site; Langs: Slovak; (905)576-8711 x3408; jfiser@lakeridgehealth.on.ca.

FISET, Amelie; Centre Med Saint-Francois, 201-2125 boul Lemire, Drummondville QC J2B 8N8; Laval'04; Langs: Bilingual(French/English); (819)477-6793

FISET, Caroline; Hop Charles Lemoyne, 3120 boul Taschereau, Greenfield Park QC J4V 2H1; Mon'92; Staff, Hopital Charles LeMoyne; (450)466-5050

FISET, Caroline; CLSC Haute-Ville, 55 ch Sainte-Foy, Quebec QC G1R 1S9; Laval'08; CCFP; (416)641-2572; Fax. (416)522-5437.

FISET, Caroll; Clinique Med USS St-Jean, CP 100 Succ Bureau-Chef, Richelain QC J0J 1R0; Laval'67; Langs: English; (450)358-7099 x7680

FISET, Dany; 4928 Boul Saint-Jean, Pierrefonds QC H9H 4B2; Mon'84; (514)620-9696; Fax. (514)620-8105.

FISET, Denis; Polyclinique Med Concorde, 300 boul de la Concorde E, Laval QC H7G 2E6; Laval'72; DiagRad. Ac Member, Centre Hospitalier Fleury; (450)667-2300; Fax. (450)667-2305.

FISET, Nathalie; Clinique Familiale Chateauguay, 55 boul D'Anjou, Chateauguay QC J6J 2P9; Mon'88; (450)699-1301

FISET, Pierre; MUHC-Montreal Children's Hosp, C 1119-2300 rue Tupper, Montreal QC H3H 1P3; Laval'81; CSPQ; FRCPC; Anes (Clinical Pharmacology). Chief Anes, McGill University Health Centre - Montreal Children's Hospital; Assoc Prof Anes, McGill University; (514)934-1934 x22404; Fax. (514)412-4341; pierre.fiset@muhc.mcgill.ca.

FISET, Serge; Clinique Med Racine, 201-900 boul Raymond, Quebec QC G1B 3G3; Laval'74; (418)667-8066

FISH, Douglas; Hop Maisonneuve-Rosemont, 5415 boul de l'Assomption, Montreal QC H1T 2M4; Mon'89; FRCPC; IntMed; Hem. Staff, Hopital Maisonneuve-Rosemont; (514)252-3404; Fax. (514)254-5094.

FISH, Joel; The Hosp For Sick Children, 5410-555 University Ave, Toronto ON M5G 1X8; McM'86; BSc; MSc; FRCSC; PlasSurg (Burns). Med Dir Burn Prog, The Hospital For Sick Children; Assoc Prof Surg, University of Toronto; (416)813-7654 x28198; Fax. (416)813-8569.

FISH, Rowan; Ellendale Med Bldg, 320-5845 ch de la Cote-des-Nei, Montreal QC H3S 1Z4; McG'74; BSc; MDCM; FRCPC; Derm. Consultant Derm, Alice Hyde Medical Centre, Malone, NY; Clinical Asst Prof, Sir Mortimer B Davis Jewish General; Asst Teacher, McGill University; Langs: English; French; (514)731-1239; Fax. (514)739-0047.

FISHBEIN, David L S; 507-960 Lawrence Ave W, North York ON M6A 3B5; Tor'83; FRCPC; IntMed; Respir. Assoc Staff, Humber River Regional Hospital - Church Street Site; (416)782-5589; Fax. (416)782-0595.

FISHELL, Alicja D; Women's College Hosp, 9F-76 Grenville St, Toronto ON M5S 1B2; Tor'96; BSc; FRCP; FRCPC; Psy (Reproductive Mental Health). Staff, Women's College Hospital; Staff, Sunnybrook Health Sciences Centre; Langs: Polish; (416)323-6400 x4935; Fax. (416)323-6356.

FISHER, Barbara J; London Reg Cancer Centre, 790 Commissioners Rd E, London ON N6A 4L6; Wes'78; FRCPC; RadOncol (Brain Tumors). (519)685-8650; Fax. (519)685-8627.

FISHER, Bruce W; Medical Sciences Bldg, 2F1.23-131 University Campus N, Edmonton AB T6G 2H7; Ott'81; FRCPC; IntMed. Staff, University of Alberta Hospital; Div Dir Studies in Med Educ, University of Alberta; (780)407-7290; Fax. (780)407-3132; bruce.fisher@ualberta.ca.

FISHER, Charles G; Blusson Spinal Cord Centre, 6F-818 10th Ave W, Vancouver BC V5Z 1M9; Dal'86; FRCSC; OrthSurg. Staff, Vancouver General Hospital - Centennial Pavillion; (604)875-4746; Fax. (604)875-8223.

FISHER, Christina M; Forest Hill Family Hlth Ctr, 491 Eglinton Ave W, Toronto ON M5N 1A8; McG'94; BSc; MDCM; CCFP; Staff, Sunnybrook Health Sciences Centre; Lecturer, University of Toronto; Langs: English; French; (416)782-6111; Fax. (416)782-5515.

FISHER, D Scott; Nottingham Medical, 310-664 Wye Rd, Sherwood Park AB T8A 6G3; Alb'98; (780)416-3220; Fax. (780)416-3224.

FISHER, David; The Hosp For Sick Children, 5424-555 University Ave, Toronto ON M5G 1X8; RCS (Ireland)'90; FRCSC; PlasSurg. Staff, The Hospital For Sick Children; (416)813-6445; Fax. (416)813-6147; david.fisher@utoronto.ca.

FISHER, David T; 121-2224 Walker Rd, Windsor ON N8W 5L7; Wes'71; (519)258-5825

FISHER, Deborah T; 180 Bedford Rd, Toronto ON M5R 2K9; McM'76; CCFP; Assoc Staff, Mount Sinai Hospital; (416)929-9946; Fax. (416)963-5703; debsec@rogers.com.

FISHER, Dina A; Peter Lougheed Centre, 3500 26 Ave NE, Calgary AB T1Y 6J4; Wes'95; FRCPC; IntMed (Tuberculosis); Respir. Staff, Peter Lougheed Centre; (403)943-4045; Fax. (403)943-4848.

FISHER, Gillian; PO Box 2922, Garibaldi-Hghlands BC V0N 1T0; Cal'95; CCFP.

FISHER, Gillian; SMBD Jewish Gen Hosp, E0012-3755 ch Cote-Sainte-Cath, Montreal QC H3T 1E2; Glasgow (Scotland)'66; Staff, Sir Mortimer B Davis Jewish General; Member Faculty, McGill University; Langs: Bilingual(English/French); (514)340-7501; Fax. (514)340-7547; gfisher@ger.jgh.mcgill.ca.

FISHER, Harold N; Mount Sinai Hosp, 206-600 University Ave, Toronto ON M5G 1X5; Tor'81; FACEP; MCFP(EM); Staff Emerg, Mount Sinai Hospital; Court Staff, Mackenzie Richmond Hill Hospital; Asst Prof Family & CommunMed, University of Toronto; (416)586-5058; Fax. (416)586-4719.

FISHER, Hugh S; 7567 Oberson Rd PO Box 216, Pemberton BC V0N 2L0; UBC'88; (604)894-5684

FISHER, I Morag J; Addictions Foundation of Manit, 586 River Ave, Winnipeg MB R3L 0E8; Edinburgh (Scotland)'78; MB ChB; DRCOG; (204)944-6229; Fax. (204)284-5520.

FISHER, Janet H; PO Box 1288, Rossland BC V0G 1Y0; UBC'01; CCFP; CCFP(E.M.); (250)368-5656; Fax. (250)368-8484.

FISHER, Janis M; Glenmore Clinic, 1605 Gordon Dr, Kelowna BC V1Y 3G8; UBC'86; CCFP; Staff, Kelowna General Hospital; (250)861-8838; Fax. (250)861-6838.

FISHER, Jennifer; Alberta Children's Hosp, 2888 Shaganappi Trail NW, Calgary AB T3B 6A8; Newcastle (England)'78; MB BS; MRCPsy; FRCPC; Psy (Child Psychiatry). Staff, Alberta Children's Hospital; Clin Associate Prof Dept of Psy, University of Calgary; (403)955-5900; Fax. (403)955-5896.

FISHER, Jolene H; Univ of Toronto, 6263-1 King's College Cir, Toronto ON M5S 1A8; Man'08; IntMed. Teach Staff, University of Toronto; (416)978-1562; Fax. (416)971-2112.

FISHER, Joseph A; Univ Hlth Network-Toronto Gen, 200 Elizabeth St, Toronto ON M5G 2C4; Tor'73; FRCPC; Anes; IntMed. Staff, Toronto General Hospital - UHN; (416)340-4800 x3071; Fax. (416)340-4448; joe.fisher@utoronto.ca.

FISHER, Julie; 2888 Shaganappi Trail NW, Calgary AB T3B 6A8; McM'96; DTMH; FRCPC; Peds. Staff Peds., Alberta Children's Hospital; Asst Prof, University of Calgary; (403)955-5900; Fax. (403)955-5896.

FISHER, Mark A; Kingsway Cardiac Centre, 905-1243 Islington Ave, Etobicoke ON M8X 1Y9; Tor'92; ABIM; FRCPC; IntMed; Cardiol. Staff Cardiac Cath Lab, Toronto Western Hospital - University Health Network; Staff, St Joseph's Health Centre; (416)233-4242; Fax. (416)233-4233.

FISHER, Mark M; Care Point Med Centre, 1623 Commercial Dr, Vancouver BC V5L 3Y3; Qns'65; Vis Staff, Providence Health Care - St Paul's Hospital; (604)254-5554; Fax. (604)254-9177.

FISHER, Marnie E; Kingsway Derm & Cosmetic Ctr, 1000-1243 Islington Ave, Etobicoke ON M8X 1Y9; Ott'98; FRCPC; Derm. (416)231-0100

FISHER, Michael G; 135-535 Beaverbrook Crt, Fredericton NB E3B 1X6; Dal'72; (506)474-4555; Fax. (506)474-4554.

FISHER, Michael J; Westbrook Prof Bldg, 215-1610 37 St SW, Calgary AB T3C 3P1; Cal'04; FRCPC; IntMed. Staff, Peter Lougheed Centre; (403)284-0777; Fax. (403)284-0711.

FISHER, Murray M; Upper Canada Lower Bowel Clin, 301-1366 Yonge St, Toronto ON M4T 3A7; Tor'58; PhD(Biochem); LLD(Hon); FRCPC; IntMed (Gastroenterology). (416)926-0262; Fax. (416)926-0936.

FISHER, Myles G; Glazier Med Centre, 11 Gibb St, Oshawa ON L1H 2J9; Bristol (England)'68; MB ChB; MRCP; FRCPC; IntMed (Cardiology). Court Staff, Lakeridge Health - Oshawa Site; Consultant, Oshawa Durham Sleep Laboratory; (905)579-1212; Fax. (905)579-2021.

FISHER, Nigel R; New Westminster Hlth & Addicti, 2F-403 6th St, New Westminster BC V3L 3B1; London (England)'84; MB BS; (604)777-6832

FISHER, Rachel; MUHC-Montreal's Children's Hos, 2300 rue Tupper, Montreal QC H3H 1P3; McG'06; MDCM; FRCPC; Anes. Staff, McGill University Health Centre - Montreal Children's Hospital; (514)934-1934 x23434

FISHER, Rebecca; Children's Hosp Eastern Ont, 401 Smyth Rd, Ottawa ON K1H 8L1; Ott'96; Staff, Children's Hospital of Eastern Ontario (CHEO); Langs: Bilingual(English/French); (613)737-2328

FISHER, Robert; 102-599 Main St, Hampton NB E5N 6C2; Dal'94; BSc(Hon); CCFP; FCFP; Ac Staff Family Med & EmergMed, Saint John Regional Hospital; Asst Prof Family Med, Memorial Univ of Newfoundland; Asst Prof Family Med, Dalhousie University; (506)832-3606; Fax. (506)832-3506; drbobfisher@bellaliant.net.

FISHER, Rory H G; Sunnybrook Hlth Sciences Ctre, L101B-2075 Bayview Ave, Toronto ON M4N 3M5; Trinity Coll (Ireland)'59; MB ChB; BAO; FRCP(Ed); FRCPC; IntMed. Staff, Sunnybrook Health Sciences Centre; (416)480-6858; Fax. (416)480-6068; rory.fisher@sunnybrook.ca.

FISHER, Stephanie A; Fairmont Med Bldg, 915-750 Broadway Ave W, Vancouver BC V5Z 1H8; Qns'97; FRCSC; ObstGyn (Reprod Endocrin & Fertility). Staff, BC Women's Hospital & Health Centre; Staff, Providence Health Care - St Paul's Hospital; Clinical Asst Prof, University of British Columbia; (604)875-8039

FISHER, Stephen; 7-1637 Woodroffe Ave, Ottawa ON K2G 1W2; Ott'83; CCFP; Staff, Queensway Carleton Hospital; (613)726-0774; Fax. (613)680-0526.

FISHER, Steven W W; 926 Ash St PO Box 79159 Rpo Nottingham, Sherwood Park AB T8A 5S3; Alb'05; CCFP; CCFP(E.M.); (780)735-4442; Fax. (780)735-4916.

FISHER, Susan C; U of Ottawa Health Services, 300-100 Marie Curie Pvt, Ottawa ON K1N 1A2; McM'86; CCFP; FCFP; (613)564-3950; Fax. (613)564-6627.

FISHER, Teri V; UBS Student Hlth Service, M334-2211 Wesbrook Mall, Vancouver BC V6T 1Z3; UBC'04; CCFP; (604)822-7011

FISHER, William D; MUHC-Montreal Gen Hosp, B5 158 7-1650 av Cedar, Montreal QC H3G 1A4; Glasgow (Scotland)'66; BSc; MD; FRCS; CSPQ; FRCSC; OrthSurg (P.Q.) (Reconstructive Joint Surgery). Assoc Staff, McGill University Health Centre - Montreal General Campus; Assoc Staff, Sir Mortimer B Davis Jewish General; assoc Prof, McGill University; Langs: French; (514)934-8500; Fax. (514)934-8283; wfisher@sympatico.ca.

FISHMAN, Lawrence; Winnipeg Clinic, 790 Sherbrook St, Winnipeg MB R3A 1M3; Man'84; FRCSC; Otol. Ac Staff, Victoria General Hospital; Asst Prof Otol, University of Manitoba; Langs: Hebrew; (204)788-5507; Fax. (204)789-9243; fishman2@mts.net.

FISHMAN, Martin J; Richmond Health Science Ctre, 250-6091 Gilbert Rd, Richmond BC V7C 5L9; UBC'83; FRCPC; IntMed; Gastroent. Dir Gastroent & Endoscopy Clinic/Consultant, Richmond Hospital; Clin Instructor Div of Gastroenterology, University of British Columbia; (604)273-4447; Fax. (604)273-4254.

FISHMAN, Paula N; Leslie Med Centre, 405-4800 Leslie St, North York ON M2J 2K9; Alb'03; FRCPC; IntMed; MedOncol. Staff, North York General Hospital; (416)640-0892; Fax. (416)640-1243.

FISHMAN, S Brian; 1705-2200 Yonge St, Toronto ON M4S 2C6; Man'80; FRCPC; Psy (Adolescent Psychiatry). Staff, Sunnybrook Health Sciences Centre; (416)489-4411

FISHMAN, Steven; 616-2867 Ellesmere Rd, Scarborough ON M1E 4B9; McG'84; FRCPC; Psy (Geriatric Psychiatry). Staff, Rouge Valley Health System - Centenary Health Centre Site; (416)284-8131 x5331; Fax. (416)281-7320; sfishman@rougevalley.ca.

FISHMAN-SHAPIRO, Leona; 100-1100 Sheppard Ave E, North York ON M2K 2W1; McG'80; FRCPC; Peds (Pediatric Endocrinology). Ac Staff Pt-Time Peds, The Hospital For Sick Children; Consultant, North York General Hospital; Court Staff, Rouge Valley Health System - Centenary Health Centre Site; Asst Prof Pt-Time Peds, University of Toronto; Langs: Bilingual(English/French); (416)250-9248; Fax. (416)250-8623.

FISK, Henry J; Upper River Valley Hosp, 11300 130 Rte, Waterville NB E7P 0A4; Burlington (USA)'69; Staff, Upper River Valley Hospital - Waterville; (506)375-2949; Fax. (506)375-2962.

FISMAN, David N; Dalla Lana School of Public Hl, 678-155 College St, Toronto ON M5T 3M7; Wes'94; FRCPC; IntMed.

FISMAN, Michael Z; Regional Mental Hc-London, PO Box 5532 Stn B 850 Highbury Ave, London ON N6A 4H1; Witwatersrand (South Africa)'63; MB ChB; DPM; FRCPC; Psy. Staff, Regional Mental Health Care-St Joseph's Health Care; Staff, Parkwood Hospital - St Joseph's Health Care; Assoc Prof, University of Western Ontario; (519)455-5110 x2376; Fax. (519)455-9986.

FISMAN, Sandra N; Regional Mental HC-London, PO Box 5532 Stn B A120-850 Highbury Ave, London ON N6A 4H1; Witwatersrand (South Africa)'67; MB ChB; FRCPC; Psy (Child & Adolescent Psychiatry). Chief Psy, London Health Sciences Centre - University Hospital; Physician Leader Child & Adolescent Mental Hlth, London Health Sciences Centre - Victoria Campus; Physician Leader Child & Adolescent Mental Hlth, Regional Mental Health Care-St Joseph's Health Care; Prof, University of Western Ontario; (519)455-5110; Fax. (519)455-3712; sfisman@uwo.ca.

FITCH, Kathryn; Foothills Med Centre, PCU22-1403 29 St NW, Calgary AB T2N 2T9; McM'99; FRCPC; Psy. Staff, Foothills Medical Centre; Staff, Calgary Health Region; (403)944-1322

FITCH, Nancy K; Marathon Family Health Team, PO Box 399 22 Peninsula Rd, Marathon ON P0T 2E0; Dal'96; CCFP; (807)229-3243; Fax. (807)229-2672.

FITCH, William M; Riverview Med Clinic, 2-500 Coverdale Rd, Riverview NB E1B 3K2; Dal'77; CCFP; FCFP; Ac Staff, The Moncton Hospital; (506)387-4409; Fax. (506)387-4667.

FITCHETT, David H; St Michael's Hosp, 6 032Q-30 Bond St, Toronto ON M5B 1W8; Cambridge (England)'70; MB ChB; MRCP(UK); FESC; FRCPC; Cardiol (Acute Coronary Care). Staff Cardiol/Assoc Prof Med, St Michael's Hospital; Staff Cardiologist, Whitby Cardiovascular Institute; Langs: Bilingual(English/French); (416)864-5432; Fax. (416)864-6065; fitchettd@smh.toronto.on.ca.

FITT, Nicole S; The Ottawa Hosp-Civic Campus, 1053 Carling Ave, Ottawa ON K1Y 4E9; Ott'94; FRCPC; IntMed; GeriatricMed. Staff, The Ottawa Hospital - Civic Campus; (613)737-7777

FITURE, Ali O; York-Med Medical Arts Centre, 305-250 Harding Blvd W, Richmond Hill ON L4C 9M7; Al-Fatah (Libya)'84; MB ChB; AB; FRCSC; GenSurg; VascSurg. Staff, Hamilton Health Sciences Centre - McMaster Children's Hospital; Langs: Arabic; (905)787-0303; Fax. (905)787-0404.

FITURI, Rasem L; Windsor Health Centre, 258-1720 Howard Ave, Windsor ON N8X 5A6; Al Fateh (Libya)'92; FRCPC; IntMed (Hepatology); Gastroent. Assoc Physician All Site, Windsor Regional Hospital - Metropolitan Site; Assoc Physician, Hôtel-Dieu Grace Hospital; Langs: Arabic; (519)256-2993; Fax. (519)256-8064.

FITZBACK, Guy; Clinique Med Haute-Ville, 201-785 av de Salaberry, Quebec QC G1R 2T8; Laval'76; Staff, Jeffery Hale Hospital-Saint Brigid's; (418)525-7664; Fax. (418)525-9106.

FITZCHARLES, Mary-Ann; MUHC-Montreal Gen Hosp, 1650 av Cedar, Montreal QC H3G 1A4; Cape Town (South Africa)'73; MRCP(UK); FRCPC; Rheum. Assoc Physician, McGill University Health Centre - Montreal General Campus; assoc Prof Med, McGill University; (514)934-1934

FITZGERALD, Avril; Health Science Research Centre, 3350 Hospital Dr NW, Calgary AB T2N 4Z5; Alb'76; FRCPC; IntMed; Rheum. Staff, Foothills Medical Centre; Assoc Prof, University of Calgary; (403)944-4429; Fax. (403)944-4430.

FITZGERALD, Barbara E; Sunny Hill Hlth Ctr For Child, 3644 Slocan St, Vancouver BC V5M 3E8; UBC'85; FRCPC; Peds (Child Development). Staff, Sunny Hill Health Centre for Children; Clinical Asst Prof, University of British Columbia; (604)453-8300; Fax. (604)453-8338.

FITZGERALD, Catherine A; BC Cancer Agency-Vanc Isl Ctr, 2410 Lee Ave, Victoria BC V8R 6V5; Alb'91; BSc; LMCC; ABIM; FRCPC; IntMed; MedOncol. Staff MedOncol, BC Cancer Agency Vancouver Island Centre; (250)519-5571

FITZGERALD, Charlene D; Labrador Grenfell Health, PO Box 7000 Stn C 227 Hamilton River Rd, Happy-Valley-Goose NL A0P 1C0; McM'97; CCFP; FCFP; Staff, Labrador Health Centre; Langs: English; French; (709)897-2000

FITZGERALD, Cristin A; Peter Lougheed Centre, 1926-3500 26 Ave NE, Calgary AB T1Y 6J4; Cal'04; FRCPC; Psy. Staff, Peter Lougheed Centre; (403)943-4673; Fax. (403)219-3568.

FITZGERALD, G William N; Dr Charles S Curtis Mem Hosp, 178-200 West St, St Anthony NL A0K 4S0; Tor'69; FRCSC; GenSurg., Charles S Curtis Memorial Hospital; Associate Clin Prof Surg, Memorial University Of Newfoundland; (709)454-3333; gwn.fitz@nf.sympatico.ca.

FITZGERALD, Gregory J; Westglen Med Centre, 246-30 Springborough Blvd SW, Calgary AB T3H 0N9; Alb'91.

FITZGERALD, J Mark; The Lung Centre, 7F-2775 Laurel St, Vancouver BC V5Z 1M9; Dublin (Ireland)'78; MB ChB; BAO; MRC(PL); FRCPI(Ire); FACP; FACCP; FRCPC; IntMed (Tuberculosis); Respir. Prof Med/Dir Lung Hlth, University of British Columbia; (604)875-4122

FITZGERALD, James M; Lockview Med Clinic, 203-159 Cobequid Rd, Lower Sackville NS B4C 2N1; Dal'72; (902)865-7545; Fax. (902)865-7546.

FITZGERALD, Janice; Family Wellness Place, 48 Commonwealth Ave, Mount Pearl NL A1N 5B6; Mem'94; CCFP; (709)364-6650; Fax. (709)364-6040.

FITZGERALD, Jeremy; Regina Qu'Appelle HR-Regina, 1440 14th Ave, Regina SK S4P 0W5; Sask'04; BSc; FRCPC; IntMed (Endocrinology); Endocrin&Metab. Staff, Regina General Hospital; (306)766-4540; Fax. (306)766-4178.

FITZGERALD, Laura C; Anderson Avenue Fam Practice, 25 Anderson Ave, St. John's NL A1B 3E4; Mem'07; CCFP.

FITZGERALD, M Patricia; William Osler HC-Brampton, 2100 Bovaird Dr E, Brampton ON L6R 3J7; Dublin (Ireland)'82; FRCR; MSc; MRC; FRCPC; DiagRad (Diagnostic Imaging). Staff, William Osler Health System - Brampton Civic Hospital; (905)494-2120

FITZGERALD, Michael; Virden Med Associates, PO Box 730, Virden MB R0M 2C0; Dublin (Ireland)'82; MB ChB; Gen Practice, Virden Health Centre; (204)748-1345; Fax. (204)748-1640.

FITZGERALD, Peter G; Hamilton HS-McMaster Site, PO Box 2000 Stn Lcd 1 4E2-1200 Main St W, Hamilton ON L8N 3Z5; McM'85; FRCSC; GenSurg; PedGenSurg. Pres/Staff Sur, Hamilton Health Sciences Centre - McMaster Children's Hospital; Ac Staff Service of PedSurg, St Joseph's Healthcare - Charlton Campus; Asst Prof Surg, McMaster University; (905)521-2100 x5231; Fax. (905)521-9992.

FITZGIBBON, Edward; The Ottawa Hosp, 5235-501 Smyth Rd, Ottawa ON K1H 8L6; Cork (Ireland)'82; BAO; MB ChB; MSc; MRCGPract; CCFP; Staff, The Ottawa Hospital - General Campus; Med Dir Palliative Care Program, University of Ottawa; (613)737-8940

FITZMAURICE, Brett G; UBC-Dept Of Anes, 2449-910 10th Ave W, Vancouver BC V5Z 1M9; Sask'92; FRCPC; Anes. Staff, Vancouver General Hospital - Centennial Pavillion; (604)875-4304; Fax. (604)875-5209.

FITZMAURICE, M Aingeal; Misericordia Community Hosp, 16940 87 Ave NW, Edmonton AB T5R 4H5; National (Ireland)'76; MB ChB; BAO; FRCPC; Anes. Staff Anes., Covenant Health - Misericordia Community Hospital; (780)735-2863

FITZMAURICE, Michael J; 2450 Ontario St, Vancouver BC V5T 4T7; Ott'81; CCFP; Assoc Staff, Providence Health Care - St Paul's Hospital; (604)709-6540

FITZPATRICK, Aaron; Kelowna Gen Hosp, 2268 Pandosy St, Kelowna BC V1Y 1T2; Dal'01; CCFP; CCFP(E.M.); Staff, Kelowna General Hospital; (250)862-4495

FITZPATRICK, Catherine M R; Hotel-Dieu Hosp, 5-166 Brock St, Kingston ON K7L 5G2; Galway (Ireland)'83; MRCPsy; FRCPC; Psy (Child & Adolescent Psychiatry). Consultant Child & Adolescent Psy, Hotel-Dieu Hospital; Asst Prof Psy, Queen's University; (613)544-3400

FITZPATRICK, David J; 401-9200 Mary St, Chilliwack BC V2P 4H6; Dublin (Ireland)'77; MB ChB; CCFP; FCFP; (604)793-6861; Fax. (604)793-6865.

FITZPATRICK, David J; Courtice Health Centre, 1450 Highway 2, Courtice ON L1E 3C3; Qns'77; CCFP; FCFP; (905)721-4900 x5302; Fax. (905)721-4369.

FITZPATRICK, Donald G; Health Sciences Centre, 300 Prince Philip Dr, St. John's NL A1B 3V6; Mem'95; FRCSC; PlasSurg. Staff, Health Sciences Centre; (709)754-6165

FITZPATRICK, George F; Glenridge Med Bldg, 202-1 Belton Blvd, St Catharines ON L2T 3Y4; Dublin (Ireland)'64; (905)682-8369; Fax. (905)682-0559.

FITZPATRICK, John D; Courtenay Med Associates, 201-1350 England Ave, Courtenay BC V9N 8X6; McM'73; Staff, St Joseph's General Hospital; Langs: French; (250)334-4411; Fax. (250)338-1245.

FITZPATRICK, Kelly P; 12-1300 Garth St, Hamilton ON L9C 4L7; McM'95; FAAP; FRCPC; Peds (Consultation). Staff, Hamilton Health Sciences Centre - McMaster Children's Hospital; Staff, St Joseph's Healthcare - Charlton Campus; Asst Prof, McMaster University; Langs: English; French; (905)575-0611; Fax. (905)575-7737.

FITZPATRICK, Michael F; Richardson House, 102 Stuart St, Kingston ON K7L 2V6; Dublin (Ireland)'82; MB ChB; BAO; FRCPI(Ire); FAASM; FRCPC; IntMed (Sleep Medicine); Respir. Med Dir Sleep Disorders Centre/Staff Respirol, Kingston General Hospital; Prof Resp & Critical Care Med/Prof, Queen's University; (613)548-2379; Fax. (613)549-1459; mike.fitzpatrick@queenu.ca.

FITZPATRICK, Philip; Saskatoon City Hosp, 701 Queen St, Saskatoon SK S7K 0M7; Dublin (Ireland)'08; MB BCh; BAO; CCFP; CCFP(E.M.); Staff, Saskatoon City Hospital; (306)655-8135; Fax. (306)655-8759.

FITZPATRICK, Stephen J; St Paul's Hosp, 2B 173-1081 Burrard St, Vancouver BC V6Z 1Y6; Dal'85; FRCPC; Psy. Staff Psy, Providence Health Care - St Paul's Hospital; Staff Psy Assessment Unit, Vancouver General Hospital - Centennial Pavillion; (604)682-2344 x62319

FITZPATRICK, Tania E; Raven Song Comm Hlth Ctr, 2450 Ontario St, Vancouver BC V5T 4T7; Tor'04; CCFP; (604)872-7984

FITZPATRICK, Timothy; Queen Elizabeth Hosp, PO Box 6600 Stn Central 60 Riverside Dr, Charlottetown PE C1A 8T5; Tor'90; FRCPC; Anes. Anesthetist, Queen Elizabeth Hospital; (902)894-2111; Fax. (902)894-2491.

FITZPATRICK, Wendi; 21st Medical Clinic, 502-402 21st St E, Saskatoon SK S7K 0C3; Mem'01; BSc; FRCPC; Neur. Clinical Asst Prof Dept of Medicine, University of Saskatchewan; (306)956-3444; Fax. (306)956-3577.

FITZSIMMONS, Brian P; Fairmont Med Bldg, 1208-750 Broadway W, Vancouver BC V5Z 1J2; Cal'93; FRCSC; ObstGyn. (604)872-1260

FITZSIMONS, Carrie L; Kootenay Lake Hosp, 411-3 View St, Nelson BC V1L 2V1; McM'90; MSc; FRCPC; Peds. Staff, Kootenay Lake General Hospital; Langs: Bilingual(English/French); (250)352-9766; Fax. (250)352-9757.

FJELDSTED, Fredrik H; Dauphin Med Clinic, 622 3rd St SW, Dauphin MB R7N 1R5; Man'00; CCFP; (204)638-6445

FLADELAND, Derek A; Royal University Hosp, 103 Hospital Dr, Saskatoon SK S7N 0W8; Sask'94; FRCPC; DiagRad. Staff Med Imaging, Royal University Hospital; (306)655-2371; Fax. (306)655-2370.

FLAGEOLE, Helene; Hamilton HS-McMaster Site, PO Box 2000 Stn Lcd 1 4E8-1200 Main St W, Hamilton ON L8N 3Z5; McG'88; ABC; CSPQ; FRCSC; GenSurg; PedGenSurg. Staff, Hamilton Health Sciences Centre - McMaster Children's Hospital; Langs: Bilingual(French/English); (905)521-2100; Fax. (905)521-9992.

FLAK, Borys; UBC Hospital, 2211 Wesbrook Mall, Vancouver BC V6T 2B5; Alb'74; FRCPC; DiagRad. Ac Staff, UBC Hospital - Koerner Pavillion; Clin Prof, University of British Columbia; Langs: Ukrainian; (604)822-7744; Fax. (604)822-9701; borys-flak@vch.ca.

FLAK, Edred A; Mount Sinai Hosp, 917-600 University Ave, Toronto ON M5G 1X5; Tor'71; FRCPC; Psy. Staff Psy, Mount Sinai Hospital; Assoc Prof, University of Toronto; (416)586-4800 x4662; Fax. (416)586-8654.

FLAMAND, Francois J; 202-20 Hobson St, Cambridge ON N1S 2M6; Man'89; BSc; FRCSC; GenSurg (Colon & Rectal Surgery). Staff Consultant, Cambridge Memorial Hospital; Langs: English; French; (519)624-0077; Fax. (519)624-4800.

FLAMAND, Helene; Hop du Sacre-Coeur de Mtl, 5400 boul Gouin O, Montreal QC H4J 1C5; Mon'92; CCFP; Staff, Hôpital du Sacre-Coeur de Montréal; (418)338-2222

FLAMBERT, Florence; Clinique Med St-Vallier, 201-205 rue Montmagny, Quebec QC G1N 4V3; Bruxelles (Belgium)'75; Langs: Creole; English; (418)688-0872; Fax. (418)688-4951.

FLAMENT, Martine; Royal Ottawa Health Care Group, 6429-1145 Carling Ave, Ottawa ON K1Z 7K4; Paris (France)'78; FRCPC; Psy (Child, Adolescent Stress). Gen Practitioner, Royal Ottawa Mental Health Centre - Royal Ottawa Health Care Group; Resd Dir Univ. of Ottawa Institute of Mental Health Research, Youth Unit; Prof Psy & Psychol, University of Ottawa; Langs: English; French; (613)722-6521 x6455; Fax. (613)761-3614; martine.flament@rohcg.on.ca.

FLAMER, Cara; 208 St Clair Ave W, Toronto ON M4V 1R2; Qns'06; CCFP; (647)726-4465

FLANAGAN, Amanda; Queensway Carleton Hosp, 3045 Baseline Rd, Ottawa ON K2H 8P4; McG'08; CCFP; CCFP(E.M.); Staff, Queensway Carleton Hospital; (613)721-2000

FLANAGAN, Cathy; Columbia Med Bldg, 403-301 Columbia St E, New Westminster BC V3L 3W5; McG'80; MDCM; FRCPC; IntMed; Rheum. Consultant Rheum, Royal Columbian Hospital; Langs: English; French; (604)526-2140; Fax. (604)526-2279.

FLANAGAN, Guy; CSSS de Laval, 1755 boul Rene-Laennec, Laval QC H7M 3L9; Mon'94; FRCSC; GenSurg. Staff, Hopital de la Cite de la santé; (450)668-1010

FLANAGAN, Janine; Paediatric Consult Clinic, 5E142-30 The Queensway, Toronto ON M6R 1B5; Tor'94; FRCPC; Peds (Developmental Pediatrics). Physician, Paediatric Consult Clinic; (416)530-6000; Fax. (416)530-6294.

FLANAGAN, M Barbara; Polyclinic Prof Centre Inc, 407-199 Grafton St, Charlottetown PE C1A 1L2; Dal'75; Staff, Queen Elizabeth Hospital; (902)629-8811; Fax. (902)566-9251.

FLANAGAN, Margaret J; Medical Clinic Associates, 200-3207 30 Ave, Vernon BC V1T 2C6; Ott'87; CCFP; (250)549-1216; Fax. (250)503-3917.

FLANAGAN, Sean D; Grey Nuns Community Hosp & HC, 1100 Youville Drive West NW, Edmonton AB T6L 5X8; Alb'85; Staff, Covenant Health - Grey Nuns Community Hospital; (780)735-7000; Fax. (780)450-7498.

FLANAGAN, Thomas F; Abbottsfield Shoppers Mall, 214-3210 118 Ave NW, Edmonton AB T5W 4W1; Alb'88; Gen Practice, Covenant Health - Edmonton General Continuing Care Centre; (780)471-2071; Fax. (780)474-8001.

FLANAGAN, Wayne H; 18220 89 Ave NW, Edmonton AB T5T 2K6; Alb'74; BMedSci; (780)481-8812; Fax. (780)481-7947.

FLANDERS, Daniel I; Kindercare Pediatrics, 301-491 Eglinton Ave W, Toronto ON M5N 1A8; McG'02; FRCPC; Peds (Nutrition). Staff, North York General Hospital; Lecturer Faculty of Med Dept of Ped, University of Toronto; Langs: Bilingual(French/English); (416)848-7665; Fax. (416)848-7664; admin@kindercarepediatrics.ca.

FLANDERS, Michael E; Gladstone Med Centre, 4095 Tupper St, Westmount QC H3Z 3E5; McG'70; FRCSC; Ophth (Strabismus). assoc Staff Ophth, Centre Hospitalier l'Université de Montréal (CHUM) - Hôpital Notre-Dame; Ac Staff Ophth, McGill University Health Centre - Montreal General Campus; assoc Prof, McGill University; (514)933-5050; Fax. (514)989-7204.

FLANDERS, Tamar Y; Medical & Dental Bldg, 404-586 Eglinton Ave W, Toronto ON M4P 1P2; McG'00; FRCPC; Peds. Langs: Bilingual(English/French); (416)489-3273; Fax. (416)489-1510.

FLANNERY, John F; Toronto Rehab Inst-Hillcrest, 7 141 2-550 University Ave, Toronto ON M5G 2A2; Qns'89; FRCPC; PhysMed&Rehab. Staff, Toronto Rehabilitation Institute - University Centre; Asst Prof PhysMed&Rehab, University of Toronto; Langs: English; French; (416)597-3422 x4200; Fax. (416)516-6373.

FLANNIGAN, Kelly P; PO Box 3731, Smithers BC V0J 2N0; Cal'80; FRCPC; EmergMed. Staff, Wrinch Memorial Hospital; Ac Staff, Victoria General Hospital; Ac Staff, Royal Jubilee Hospital; Summit Injury Management; (250)842-5211

FLASCHNER, David M; 250-333 Aspen Glen Landng SW, Calgary AB T3H 0N6; Wes'01; FRCPC; PhysMed&Rehab. (403)984-9025; Fax. (403)984-9029.

FLATH, Travis R; PO Box 35034 Rpo Midtown, Edmonton AB T5J 0B7; Alb'10; CCFP.

FLATTERY, Paula M; Concordia Hlth Associates, 102-1155 Concordia Ave, Winnipeg MB R2K 2M9; Man'00.

FLAVELLE, Shauna C; 100-2631 28th Ave, Regina SK S4S 6X3; Alb'07; FRCPC; Peds. (306)586-1800; Fax. (306)586-3511.

FLAVIN, Michael P; Kingston Gen Hosp, 76 Stuart St, Kingston ON K7L 2V7; National (Ireland)'76; MB ChB; DCH; DRCOG; MRC(UK); FRCPC; Peds. Att Staff, Kingston General Hospital; Att Staff, Hotel-Dieu Hospital; Assoc Prof Peds, Queen's University; (613)548-6046; Fax. (613)548-1369.

FLAX, Stanley; 222-1333 Sheppard Ave E, North York ON M2J 1V1; Witwatersrand (South Africa)'80; MB ChB; FRCSC; Urol (Adult Urology). Court Staff, William Osler Health System - Etobicoke General Hospital; Staff, William Osler Health System - Brampton Civic Hospital; (416)499-1333; Fax. (416)499-1332.

FLECK, David L; Rockyview Gen Hosp, 7007 14 St SW, Calgary AB T2V 1P9; Alb'94; Staff, Rockyview General Hospital; (403)943-3639; Fax. (403)943-8411.

FLECKENSTEIN, Martin H; Birchwood Prof Centre, 24 Kentucky Crt, New Minas NS B4N 4N2; Dal'87; (902)681-1080; Fax. (902)681-1600.

FLEET, Jane A; Invermere Med Centre, PO Box 8000 937 7th Ave, Invermere BC V0A 1K0; McM'94; CCFP; FCFP; (250)342-9206

FLEET, Richard; Hôtel-Dieu de Lévis, 143 rue Wolfe, Levis QC G6V 3Z1; Mon'03; CCFP; CCFP(E.M.); Staff, Hôtel-Dieu de Lévis; (418)835-7121

FLEETHAM, John A; Respiratory Division, 7F-2775 laurel St, Vancouver BC V5Z 1M9; London (England)'72; MRCS; LRCP; DCH; ABIM; MB BS; FRCPC; IntMed (Sleep Disorders Medicine); Respir. Prof, University of British Columbia; (604)875-5653

FLEETWOOD, Ian; CB1 Health Centre, 2F-605 Discovery St, Victoria BC V8T 5G4; Man'94; BSc(Med); FRCSC; Neursurg (Cerebrovascular Surgery). Dir Cerebrovascular Surg, Queen Elizabeth II Health Sciences Centre - Halifax Infirmary Site; Co-Dir Radiosurgery, Queen Elizabeth II Hospital; Assoc Prof, Dalhousie University; (250)383-3638 x2

FLEGAL, Collette A; Red Deer Reg Hosp Centre, 3942 50A Ave, Red Deer AB T4N 4E7; Alb'88; CCFP; CCFP(E.M.); Staff, Red Deer Regional Hospital Centre; (403)343-4448; Fax. (403)343-4459.

FLEGEL, Kenneth M; MUHC-Royal Victoria Hosp, E2 61-687 av des Pins O, Montreal QC H3A 1A1; McG'72; MSc(Epidemiol); BSc; FACP; FRCP; FRCPC; IntMed (AIDS). Sr Physician IntMed, McGill University Health Centre - Royal Victoria Hospital; Prof Med, McGill University; Langs: French; (514)843-1515

FLEGG, Carolyn; Wall Street Ent Clinic, 300-140 Wall St, Saskatoon SK S7K 1N4; Sask'00; FRCPC; DiagRad. Staff, Hamilton Health Sciences Centre-Juravinski Site; (306)244-1167; Fax. (306)244-2911.

FLEIGE-ZAHRADKA, Bettina G; 100-190 Ingram St, Duncan BC V9L 1P1; Marburg (Germany)'84; FRCSC; ObstGyn. Clin Fellow Reproductive Endocrinol/Infertility, University of British Columbia; Langs: German; (250)748-2422; Fax. (250)748-7384.

FLEISHER, William; Psychealth Centre, PZ418-771 Bannatyne Ave, Winnipeg MB R3E 3N4; Man'74; FRCPC; Psy (Child & Adolescent Psychiatry). Staff Psy, Health Sciences Centre; Dir Faculty Development & Educational Scholarship, University of Manitoba; (204)787-7779; Fax. (204)787-4879; fleisher@cc.umanitoba.ca.

FLEISZER, David M; MUHC-Royal Victoria Hosp, S10 36-687 av des Pins O, Montreal QC H3A 1A1; McG'73; FACS; CSPQ; FRCSC; GenSurg (Breast Surgery). Dir Patient Education Office, McGill University Health Centre - Royal Victoria Hospital; Associé Surgeon, McGill University; Langs: English; French; (514)934-1934 x34045; Fax. (514)843-1503.

FLEMING, Adam J; MUHC-Montreal Children's Hosp, 2300 rue tupper, Montreal QC H2H 1P3; Tor'04; FRCPC; Peds; PedHemaOncol. Staff, McGill University Health Centre - Montreal Children's Hospital; (514)412-4400

FLEMING, Angela D; Brant Community HC-Brantford, 200 Terrace Hill St, Brantford ON N3R 1G9; McM'99; FRCPC; DiagRad. Staff, The Brant Community Healthcare System - Brantford General Hospital Site; (519)752-7871

FLEMING, Ann P; Gray Bruce HS-Owen Sound, PO Box 1800 Stn Main 1800 8th St E, Owen Sound ON N4K 6M9; Tor'80; BSc; CCFP; FCFP; Staff, Grey Bruce Health Services - Owen Sound; (519)376-2122 x2029

FLEMING, Blair; 57 Margaret's Pl PO Box 8700, St. John's NL A1B 4J6; Mem'85; Asst Med Dir, Health & Community Services; Med Advisor/Staff Phy, The Agnes Pratt Home; (709)758-1501; Fax. (709)729-5238; blairfleming@gov.nl.ca.

FLEMING, Bruce; Vancouver Gen Hosp, 855 12th Ave W, Vancouver BC V5Z 1M9; UBC'78; FRCPC; EmergMed (Family Medicine). Staff, Vancouver General Hospital - Centennial Pavillion; Teach Staff/Assoc Dean MD Undergraduate Program Admissions (Interim), University of British Columbia; (604)875-4995

FLEMING, D A Barry; Polyclinic Prof Centre Inc, 199 Grafton St, Charlottetown PE C1A 1L2; Dal'79; FRCSC; GenSurg. (902)629-8813; Fax. (902)629-8813.

FLEMING, Dana A; 410 Giles Blvd E, Windsor ON N9A 4C6; UBC'78; FRCSC; OrthSurg (Arthroplasty). Staff, Windsor Regional Hospital - Metropolitan Site; Staff, Hôtel-Dieu Grace Hospital; (519)253-4451; Fax. (519)253-0271; occtech@mnsi.net.

FLEMING, Fiona L; Manitoba Clinic, 790 Sherbrook St, Winnipeg MB R3A 1M3; Qns'87; FAAP; FRCPC; Peds (Pediatric Critical Care); Critical Care Medicine. (204)788-5748

FLEMING, Ian M; Canadian Forces Hlth Services, 4050 4th Ave, Vancouver BC V6R 1P6; Dal'88; (604)225-2520 x2504; Fax. (604)225-2525.

FLEMING, Ivor M; Mount Sinai Hosp, 1514-600 University Ave, Toronto ON M5G 1X5; UBC'85; BSc(Hons.); FRCPC; Anes;CCFP; Staff, Mount Sinai Hospital; Staff, Toronto General Hospital - UHN; Asst Prof, University of Toronto; (416)586-4800 x5270; Fax. (416)586-8664.

FLEMING, Jan E; 554 Spadina Cres, Toronto ON M5S 2J9; Tor'83; FRCPC; Psy (Adult Psychiatry). Staff Psy, Centre for Addiction & Mental Health (CAMH) - Russell Street Site; Aj Prof, Ryerson University; Assoc Prof Psy, University of Toronto; Fax. (416)413-1203; jan.fleming@sympatico.ca.

FLEMING, Jonathan A E; UBC Hospital, 2211 Wesbrook Mall, Vancouver BC V6T 2B5; Dublin (Ireland)'73; DABPN; MB BCh; FRCPC; Psy (Sleep Disorders). Ac Staff/Co-Dir Sleep Disorders Prog, UBC Hospital - Koerner Pavillion; Assoc Prof Psy, University of British Columbia; (604)822-7606; Fax. (604)822-9744; fleming@interchange.ubc.ca.

FLEMING, Karen E; Medical & Dental Bldg, 586 Eglinton Ave E, Toronto ON M4P 1P2; Tor'89; MSc; CCFP; FCFP; Staff, Sunnybrook Health Sciences Centre; Teacher, University of Toronto; Langs: English; French; (416)440-1880; Fax. (416)440-1106.

FLEMING, Marcia M; Delta Laser & Skin Care Clinic, 1-6305 120 St, Delta BC V4E 2A6; UBC'87; (604)543-8965

FLEMING, Melinda C S; Kingston Gen Hosp, 76 Stuart St, Kingston ON K7L 2V7; Tor'96; FRCPC; Anes. Staff Anes, Kingston General Hospital; (613)548-3232; Fax. (613)548-1375.

FLEMING, Michael J; Fall River Family Practice, PO Box 2160 Rpo Fall River 3060 Hwy 2, Fall River NS B2T 1K6; Dal'78; BSc; CCFP; FCFP; Dir Family Phys Programs in CME, Dalhousie University; (902)861-2237; Fax. (902)861-1914; michael.fleming@dal.ca.

FLEMING, Michaele S; 1-1261 Beaverbook Ave, London ON N6H 0G6; Wes'90; Staff, St Joseph's Hospital - St Joseph's Health Care; (519)642-2077

FLEMING, Nathalie; The Ottawa Hosp-Riverside, 1967 Riverside Dr, Ottawa ON K1H 7W9; Ott'95; FRCSC; ObstGyn (Pediatric Gynecology). Staff, Children's Hospital of Eastern Ontario (CHEO); Staff, The Ottawa Hospital - Riverside Campus; Langs: Bilingual(English/French); (613)738-8400; Fax. (613)738-8505; nfleming@toh.on.ca.

FLEMING, Rachel; Univ Hlth Network-Princess M, 610 University Ave, Toronto ON M5G 2M9; (Netherlands)'05; FRCPC; DiagRad. Staff, Princess Margaret Hospital - University Health Network; Fellow, Mount Sinai Hospital; (416)946-2000

FLEMING, Russel; Waypoint Centre for Mental H C, 500 Church St, Penetanguishene ON L9M 1G3; Wes'69; FRCPC; Psy. Staff, Waypoint Centre for Mental Health Care; (705)549-3181 x2205; Fax. (705)549-3446; rfleming@mhcp.on.ca.

FLEMING, Sarah; Univ Hlth Network-Toronto Western Hosp, 2F W W-399 Bathurst St, Toronto ON M5T 2S8; Tor'05; CCFP; Staff, Toronto Western Hospital - University Health Network; (416)603-5888 x1

FLEMMING, Anne K; BC Cancer Agency-Vancouver CC, 600 10th Ave W, Vancouver BC V5Z 4E6; Dal'92; FRCPC; DiagRad. Staff, BC Cancer Agency Vancouver Centre; (604)877-6000

FLEMMING, Bruce K; Queen Elizabeth II HSC-Halifax, 3314-1796 Summer St, Halifax NS B3H 3A7; Dal'74; FACR; FRCPC; DiagRad. Asst Radiol, Queen Elizabeth II Health Sciences Centre - Victoria General Site; (902)473-2652; Fax. (902)473-3482.

FLEMMING, Jeffery P; Foothills Med Centre, 1403 29 St NW, Calgary AB T2N 2T9; UBC'04; FRCPC; DiagRad; NuclearMed. Staff, Foothills Medical Centre; (403)944-1110

FLEMONS, W Ward; Foothills Med Centre, 1403 29 St NW, Calgary AB T2N 2T9; Alb'84; FRCPC; IntMed (Sleep Medicine); Respir. Staff, Foothills Medical Centre; Clin Assoc Prof Med, University of Calgary; (403)220-8722; Fax. (403)283-6151; flemons@ucalgary.ca.

FLESHER, Michael F; Nanaimo Reg Gen Hosp, 1200 Dufferin Cres, Nanaimo BC V9S 2B7; UBC'88; Staff, Nanaimo Regional General Hospital; (250)755-7627

FLESHNER, Neil E; Univ Hlth Network-Princess M, 3 130-610 University Ave, Toronto ON M5G 2M9; Tor'88; MPH; FRCSC; Urol (Oncology). Clinical Division Head, Princess Margaret Hospital - University Health Network; (416)946-2899; Fax. (416)946-6590; neil.fleshner@utoronto.ca.

FLETCHER, Christine G; Kingsland Med Clinic, 7712 Elbow Dr SW, Calgary AB T2V 1K2; Cal'83; BSc; (403)252-6681; Fax. (403)252-9741.

FLETCHER, Colin W; Assiniboine Clinic, 633 Lodge Ave, Winnipeg MB R3J 0S9; Man'86.

FLETCHER, Daniel; Harvey Community Hosp, 2019 Route 3, Harvey Station NB E6K 3E9; Mem'10; CCFP; Staff, Harvey Health Centre; (506)366-6400

FLETCHER, David M; Maple Leaf Med Clinic, 203-14 College St, Toronto ON M5G 1K2; Tor'89; FRCPC; IntMed (AIDS/HIV). (416)595-7075; Fax. (416)595-5508.

FLETCHER, Jennifer A; Saint John Reg Hosp, PO Box 2100 Stn Main 400 University Ave, Saint John NB E2L 4L2; Dal'93; BSc; BEd; FRCSC; OrthSurg (Sports Medicine). Staff, Saint John Regional Hospital; (506)652-5113; Fax. (506)652-5112; jafletch@nbnet.nb.ca.

FLETCHER, John N; Smith Clinic, 1-6601 48 Ave, Camrose AB T4V 3G8; Man'95; FRCSC; GenSurg. Staff, Covenant Health - St Mary's Hospital; (780)672-2425

FLETCHER, John W; Victoria Gen Hosp, 1 Hospital Way, Victoria BC V8Z 6R5; Witwatersrand (South Africa)'86; BSc(Hons); MB ChB; CCFP; Staff, Port Hardy Hospital; Staff, Victoria General Hospital; Langs: Afrikaans; (250)727-4212

FLETCHER, Judith E; View Medical Inc, 1443 View Cres, Delta BC V4L 2K2; McM'86; BScN; (604)943-6999; Fax. (604)943-8344.

FLETCHER, K A Hugh; Beach Medical, 703 Beach Rd, Qualicum Beach BC V9K 1S4; Southampton (England)'80; (250)752-2080; beachmedical@shawbiz.ca.

FLETCHER, Kenneth J; Rideau-Friel Med Ctr, 421 Rideau St, Ottawa ON K1N 5Y9; Dal'85; (613)789-7707

FLETCHER, Mark A; Medicine in Motion Med Ctr, 5-121 Ilsley Ave, Dartmouth NS B3B 1S4; Dal'91; BSc(Hon); Dip SportMed; CCFP; CCFP(E.M.); Med Dir, Medicine in Motion Medical Centre; Med Dir, Family Focus Medical Clinics; Physician, Imperial Oil Ltd; Langs: French; (902)435-0731; Fax. (902)435-0612; director@thefamilyfocus.ca.

FLETCHER, Mary; McMaster University Campus, B101-1280 Main St W, Hamilton ON L8S 4K1; McM'01; CCFP; (905)525-9140 x27700

FLETCHER, Matthew D; Dawson Creek & Dist Hosp, 11100 13 St, Dawson Creek BC V1G 3W8; St Mary's (England)'96; MB BS(Hons); LMCC; MRCS(Eng); Staff, Dawson Creek & District Hospital; Staff, St John Hospital; (250)782-8501

FLETCHER, William; Rockyview Gen Hosp, 7007 14 St SW, Calgary AB T2V 1P9; Man'75; FRCPC; Neur (Neuro Ophthalmology). Staff, Rockyview General Hospital; Att Staff Clin Neurosciences & Surg, Foothills Medical Centre; Prof, University of Calgary; (403)943-3882; Fax. (403)212-1232.

FLETT, Heather L; Addiction & Mental Hlth-Clark, 1130-250 College St, Toronto ON M5T 1R8; McM'03; FRCPC; Psy. Staff, Centre for Addiction & Mental Health (CAMH) - College Street Site; (416)535-8501

FLEURANT, Micheline; 780 boul Sainte-Foy, Longueuil QC J4J 1Z3; Mon'77; ac Staff, Centre Hospitalier l'Université de Montréal (CHUM) - Hôpital Notre-Dame; (450)651-4980; Fax. (450)651-0050.

FLEURENT, Dominique; Hotel-Dieu d'Arthabaska, 5 rue des Hospitalieres, Victoriaville QC G6P 6N2; Laval'91; FRCPC; DiagRad. Staff, Hotel-Dieu d'Arthabaska; (819)357-1151

FLEURENT, Suzanne; CLSC Des Mille-Iles, 4731 boul Levesque E, Laval QC H7C 1M9; Mon'83; (450)661-2572 x27276; Fax. (450)661-9147.

FLEURIAU-CHATEAU, Philip B; 202-595 Montreal Rd, Ottawa ON K1K 4L2; Ott'93; FRCSC; OrthSurg (Trauma). Langs: German; Spanish; French; (613)746-6745; Fax. (613)746-6008.

FLEURY, Alain; Centre Chirugical de Joliette, 202-222 rue de la Visitation, St-Charles-Brromee QC J6E 4N5; Sher'83; CSPQ; FRCSC; GenSurg (Endoscopy). Staff Gen Surg, Centre Hospitalier Régional de Lanaudière; Langs: English; (450)753-7588; Fax. (450)756-6144; alain.fleury@hotmail.com.

FLEURY, Andre; 630 boul Potvin, Alma QC G8B 2P9; Laval'70; Ac Staff, CSSS de Lac-Saint Jean-Est; (418)662-9139

FLEURY, Benoit; Clinique Med Ste-Colette, 11520 boul Sainte-Colette, Montreal-Nord QC H1G 6J3; Mon'78; (514)323-0430; Fax. (514)328-9643.

FLEURY, Catherine; Inst U en Sante Mentale de QC, 2601 ch de la Canardiere, Quebec QC G1J 2G3; Laval'94; FRCPC; Psy. Staff, Institut Universitaire Sante; (418)663-5321; Fax. (418)663-5937.

FLEURY, Dominique; Clinique Orth des Bois-Francs, 5-39 rue Laurier E, Victoriaville QC G6P 6P6; Laval'90; CSPQ; FRCSC; OrthSurg (Reconstructive Surgery). Staff Orth, Hotel-Dieu d'Arthabaska; (819)357-8683; Fax. (819)357-2331.

FLEURY, Gilles; Hop Montford, 713 Montreal Rd, Ottawa ON K1K 0T2; Mon'00; FRCPC; Psy (Toxicology). Staff, Montfort Hospital; Langs: Bilingual(French/English); (613)746-4621; Fax. (613)748-4938; gfleury@montfort.on.ca.

FLEURY, Isabelle; Hop Maisonneuve-Rosemont, 5415 boul de l'Assomption, Montreal QC H1T 2M4; Mon'04; FRCPC; IntMed; MedOncol; Hem. Staff, Hopital Maisonneuve-Rosemont; (514)252-3404

FLEURY, Jean; Inst de Readaptation de Mtl, 6300 av De Darlington, Montreal QC H3S 2J4; Mon'75; FRCPC; PhysMed&Rehab. Staff, Centre Hospitalier l'Université de Montréal (CHUM) - Hôtel-Dieu; Ac Staff, Institut de Réadaptation Gingras-Lindsay de Montréal; (514)340-2084; Fax. (514)340-2775.

FLEURY, Manon; Clinique de Medecine Familiale, 760A boul Vachon N, Sainte-Marie QC G6E 1M2; Laval'92; (418)387-4965; Fax. (418)386-1592.

FLEURY, Michel; Unite Med Familiale Maizerets, 2480 ch de la Canardiere, Quebec QC G1J 2G1; Laval'76; (418)661-1413; Fax. (418)661-7504.

FLEURY, Nadine; Ctr Hosp Affilie-St-Sacrement, 1050 ch Sainte-Foy, Quebec QC G1S 4L8; Laval'00; Staff, Centre Hospitalier Affilié Universitaire de Québec - Hôpital du St-Sacrement; (418)682-7511

FLEURY, Rejean; 595 rue Collard, Alma QC G8B 1N1; Laval'77; Staff, CSSS de Lac-Saint Jean-Est; (418)668-3351

FLEXER, William; Misericordia Community Hosp, 16940 87 Ave NW, Edmonton AB T5R 4H5; McG'96; FRCPC; Anes. Staff, Covenant Health - Misericordia Community Hospital; Langs: English; French; (780)735-2000

FLICK, James T; Saint John Reg Hosp, PO Box 2100 Stn Main 400 University Ave, Saint John NB E2L 4L2; California (USA)'81; Staff, Saint John Regional Hospital; (506)648-6286

FLIESEN, Willy E J; Clinique Psy de St-Eustache, 111 rue Saint-Eustache, Saint-Eustache QC J7P 3Z5; Louvain (Belgium)'61; Psy. Staff, Hopital Louis-H Lafontaine; adj Prof, Universite de Montreal; (450)473-1720

FLINDALL, Stephen; Southlake Reg Health Centre, 596 Davis Dr, Newmarket ON L3Y 2P9; Ott'00; CCFP; CCFP(E.M.); Staff, Southlake Regional Health Centre; (905)895-4521

FLINT, Alastair J; Univ Hlth Network-Toronto Gen, 238-200 Elizabeth St, Toronto ON M5G 2C4; Auckland (New Zealand)'79; FRANZCP; MB BS; FRCPC; Psy (Geriatric Psychiatry). Sr Scientist, Toronto General Hospital - UHN; Prof Psy, University of Toronto; (416)340-4788; Fax. (416)340-4198; alastair.flint@uhn.on.ca.

FLINT, Julia D A; Vancouver Gen Hosp, 855 12th Ave W, Vancouver BC V5Z 1M9; Cape Town (South Africa)'88; MB ChB; FRCPC; AnatPath. Staff Path, Vancouver General Hospital - Centennial Pavillion; (604)875-4111 x63541; Fax. (604)875-5707; julia.flint@vch.ca.

FLOCK, Traudl E; Dundas Med Centre, 404-220 Dundas St W, Whitby ON L1N 8M7; Tor'78; BSc; MSc; CCFP; Langs: German; (905)668-5300; Fax. (905)668-5433; thetaj@live.com.

FLOH, Alejandro A; The Hosp For Sick Children, 555 University Ave, Toronto ON M5G 1X8; Tor'01; FRCPC; Peds; Critical Care Medicine; Cardiol. Staff, The Hospital For Sick Children; Langs: Spanish; (416)813-1500

FLOMEN, Marcy S; Bloor Med Clinic, 844 Bathurst St, Toronto ON M5R 3G1; Tor'91; CCFP; FCFP; Staff, Mount Sinai Hospital; (416)534-4214; Fax. (416)534-4582.

FLOOD, Catherine G; Royal Alexandra Hosp, 10240 Kingsway NW, Edmonton AB T5H 3V9; Alb'87; BSc; FRCSC; ObstGyn (Urological Gynecology). Dir UroGyn Clinic, Royal Alexandra Hospital; Assoc Prof, University of Alberta; (780)735-5290; Fax. (780)491-5896; cflood@cha.ab.ca.

FLOOD, Diane A; Credit Valley Prof Bldg, 508-2300 Eglinton Ave W, Mississauga ON L5M 2V8; Tor'85; FCCP; FRCPC; IntMed (Pulmonary Diseases); Respir. Court Staff Adult CF Clinic, St Michael's Hospital; Court Staff Adult CF Clinic, Health Sciences North-Laurentian Site; Consultant, The Credit Valley Hospital; (905)569-3883

FLOOD, Joan; Shoniker Clinic, 2877A Ellesmere Rd, Scarborough ON M1E 4C1; Man'80; BSc(Hon); CCFP; FCFP; Staff Psy & Family Pract, Rouge Valley Health System - Centenary Health Centre Site; Staff, Sunnybrook Health Sciences Centre; Med Consultant, Pine River Institute; (416)281-7301; Fax. (416)281-7465; jflood@rougevalley.ca.

FLOOD, Justin R; Kingstom Gen Hosp, 76 Stuart St, Kingston ON K7L 2V7; Mem'04; FRCPC; DiagRad. Staff, Kingston General Hospital; (613)548-2301

FLOOK, Nigel W; Kaye Edmonton Clinic, 1A 102-11400 University Ave NW, Edmonton AB T5G 1Z1; Alb'74; BMedSci; FAAFP; CCFP; FCFP; Chief Family Med, University of Alberta Hospital; Ac Staff, Covenant Health - Misericordia Community Hospital; Dir Practice Improvement, C.P.S.A.; Dir Practice Improvement, Alberta Pension Plan; Clin Prof, University of Alberta; (780)407-7755

FLOR-HENRY, Pierre; Alberta Hosp Edmonton, PO Box 307 Stn Main 17480 Fort Rd, Edmonton AB T5J 2J7; Edinburgh (Scotland)'57; MB ChB; DPM(Lond); FRCPsy; Psy (P.Q.) (Clinical Neurology). Staff Gen Adult Psy/Dir Clin Diagnostics & Research Ctr, Alberta Hospital Edmonton; Clin Prof Psy, University of Alberta; Langs: Spanish; French; (780)342-5395; Fax. (780)342-5346.

FLORA, Peter G; 401-3101 Bloor St W, Etobicoke ON M8X 2W2; Tor'72; DABOph; FRCSC; Ophth (Contact Lenses). Staff, St Joseph's Health Centre; (416)239-7053; Fax. (416)233-4763.

FLORAKAS, Christine; Continum Med Care, 201-520 17th St, North Vancouver BC V7N 3S8; Qns'96; CCFP; Staff, Sir Mortimer B Davis Jewish General; (604)913-8183

FLORAS, John; Mount Sinai Hosp, 1614-600 University Ave, Toronto ON M5G 1X5; Tor'77; FACC; FAHA; DPhil; FESC; FRCPC; Cardiol. Staff Cardiol, Mount Sinai Hospital; Staff Cardiol, Princess Margaret Hospital - University Health Network; Prof, University of Toronto; (416)586-8704; Fax. (416)586-8702; john.floras@utoronto.ca.

FLOREA, Adrian; MUHC-Montreal Gen Hosp, 1650 av Cedar, Montreal QC H3G 1A4; McG'10; MDCM; CCFP; Staff, McGill University Health Centre - Montreal General Campus; (514)934-1934

FLOREA, Anca V; Sir Mortimer B Davis Jewish Ge, 3755 ch cote-Sainte-Catherine, Montreal QC H3T 1E2; (Romania)'97; FRCPC; AnatPath. Staff, Sir Mortimer B Davis Jewish General; (514)340-8222

FLORENCE, Peter; Royal Alexandra Hosp, 10240 Kingsway NW, Edmonton AB T5H 3V9; Alb'97; FRCPC; Psy. Staff, Royal Alexandra Hospital; (780)735-4111; Fax. (780)735-4797.

FLORENCE, Ralph; Balmoral Med Arts Facility, 409-1366 Yonge St, Toronto ON M4T 3A7; Tor'55; DAB; FRCPC; Derm. Staff, Mount Sinai Hospital; (416)923-9809; Fax. (416)923-7908.

FLORENCE, Stephen H; The Credit Valley Hosp, 2200 Eglinton Ave W, Mississauga ON L5M 2N1; Wes'83; FRCPC; DiagRad. Staff, The Credit Valley Hospital; (905)813-4405; Fax. (905)813-4430.

FLORENT, Danielle; CLSC Lamater, 1317 boul des Seigneurs, Terrebonne QC J6W 5B1; Sher'84; (450)471-2881 x4056; Fax. (450)471-6763.

FLORES, Luis A; Stamford Med Centre, 302-4256 Portage Rd, Niagara Falls ON L2E 6A4; (Venezuela)'78; FRCSC; OrthSurg. Ac Staff, Niagara Health System - Greater Niagara General Site; Langs: Spanish; (905)374-7232; Fax. (905)374-6602.

FLORES-VARGAS, Alberto L; Scarborough Prof Centre, 301-1371 Neilson Rd, Scarborough ON M1B 4Z8; (Mexico)'68; Staff, The Scarborough Hospital - General Campus; Staff, Rouge Valley Health System - Centenary Health Centre Site; Langs: Portuguese; German; Italian; Spanish; English; (416)287-0790; Fax. (416)287-0792.

FLORESCU, Marie; CHUM-Hop Notre-Dame, 6F-1560 rue Sherbrooke E, Montreal QC H2L 4M1; Sher'98; CSPQ; CMQ; FRCPC; IntMed (Lung Cancer); MedOncol. Staff, Centre Hospitalier l'Université de Montréal (CHUM) - Hôpital Notre-Dame; Langs: Bilingual(French/English); (514)890-8000 x25381

FLORICA, Brandusa; West Toronto Site, 150 Sherway Dr, Etobicoke ON M9C 1A5; (Brazil)'90; FRCPC; IntMed; Rheum. Staff, Women's College Hospital; (416)521-4196

FLORIVAL, Albert; 6363 ch Hudson, Montreal QC H3S 1M9; (Haiti)'71; (514)737-3661 x4129

FLOWER, David G; Frederiction Med Clinic, 207-1015 Regent St, Fredericton NB E3B 6H5; Dal'82; Staff, Dr Everett Chalmers Regional Hospital; (506)458-0252

FLOWERS, David J; 560 Albert St PO Box 760, Winchester ON K0C 2K0; Wes'71; Med Staff, Winchester District Memorial Hospital; Advisor Phys., Dundas Manor Nursing Home; (613)774-3348; Fax. (613)774-3642.

FLOWERS, Michele A; Wingham & District Hosp, 270 Carling Terr, Wingham ON N0G 2W0; Wes'82; FRCPC; IntMed (Gastroenterology). Internal Med, Wingham & District Hospital - Listowel Wingham Hospitals Alliance; (519)357-3210 x5238; Fax. (519)357-1715.

FLOWERS, Raymond W; PO Box 879, Clinton ON N0M 1L0; Wes'56; FRCPC; IntMed. Staff, Clinton Public Hospital - Huron Perth Healthcare Alliance; Staff, Wingham & District Hospital - Listowel Wingham Hospitals Alliance; (519)482-7743

FLOWITT, Catherine; Markland Wood Med Clinic, 4335 Bloor St W, Etobicoke ON M9C 2A5; Tor'81; CCFP; (416)695-8878

FLOYD, Robert J; 107-230 First Ave, St Thomas ON N5R 4P5; Qns'64; Staff, St Thomas Elgin General Hospital; (519)633-0038; Fax. (519)633-0135.

FLUET, Bruno; Inst U Geriatrie Sherbrooke, 375 rue Argyll, Sherbrooke QC J1J 3H5; Sher'72; Staff, Institut Universitaire de Geriatrie de Sherbrooke-Pavillon Argyll; Clin Prof, Universite de Sherbrooke; (819)780-2220; Fax. (819)829-7146; bfluet.iugs@ssss.gouv.qc.ca.

FLUET, Jocelyne; Hop Charles Lemoyne, 3120 boul Taschereau, Greenfield Park QC J4V 2H1; Sher'99; Staff, Hopital Charles LeMoyne; (450)466-5000

FLUIT, Paul; Abbotsford Reg Hosp & Cancer C, 32900 Marshall Rd, Abbotsford BC V2S 0C2; Tor'04; CCFP; Staff, Abbotsford Regional Hospital & Cancer Centre; (604)851-4775

FLUKER, Margo R; Olive Fertility Centre, 300-555 12th Ave W, Vancouver BC V5Z 4X7; Alb'80; FRCSC; ObstGyn (Reproductive Endocrinology). Staff, BC Women's Hospital & Health Centre; Clin Prof ObstGyn, University of British Columbia; (604)559-9950

FLUSK, David; Aberdeen Hosp, 835 East River Rd, New Glasgow NS B2H 3S6; Dublin (Ireland)'06; MB BCh; Staff, Aberdeen Regional Hospital; (902)752-7600

FLYNN, Anne-Josee; UMF Laurien, 2e-2875 boul Laurier, Quebec QC G1V 2M2; Laval'91; LMCC; CCFP; FCFP; Langs: English; French; (418)654-2701; Fax. (418)654-2138.

FLYNN, Christopher A; The Credit Valley Hosp, 2200 Eglinton Ave W, Mississauga ON L5M 2N1; UBC'98; FRCPC; Anes. Staff, The Credit Valley Hospital; (905)813-2200

FLYNN, Colleen S; 1241 Mississauga Rd N, Mississauga ON L5H 2J1; McM'95; FRCPC; Psy. Staff, The Credit Valley Hospital; (416)574-8862

FLYNN, D Justin; Central Square Med Clinic, PO Box 3760 3830 2 Ave, Smithers BC V0J 2N0; Dal'00; CCFP; (250)847-8761

FLYNN, Ethan; Calgary Lab Services, 9-3535 Research Rd NW, Calgary AB T2L 2K8; (USA)'95; DABPath; Staff, Calgary Laboratory Services; (403)770-3569; Fax. (403)770-3788.

FLYNN, James; Health Sciences Centre, 300 Prince Philip Dr, St. John's NL A1B 3V6; Mem'80; FRCPC; Anes (Pain Management). Dir Pain Clinic & Anes Staff, Health Sciences Centre; Consultant Centre for Pain & Disability Mgmt, Dr Leonard A Miller Centre; Clin Asst Prof Anes, Memorial University Of Newfoundland; (709)777-6540; Fax. (709)777-6506.

FLYNN, Kathleen M; Trent Univ Student Health Serv, PO Box 4800 Stn Main 1600 West Bank Dr, Peterborough ON K9J 7B8; McM'94; CCFP; FCFP; (705)748-1481; Fax. (705)748-1055.

FLYNN, Leslie V; Hotel-Dieu Hosp, 166 Brock St, Kingston ON K7L 5G2; Qns'87; MMus; FRCPC; Psy (Adult General Psychiatry). Staff, Hotel-Dieu Hospital; Vice Dean Med Education, Queen's University; (613)544-3310 x2551; Fax. (613)544-9666.

FLYNN, M Dominique; 876 Montreal Rd, Ottawa ON K1K 4L3; Ott'96; CCFP; Langs: Bilingual(English/French); (613)742-8182

FLYNN, Michael S; The Nova Scotia Hosp, PO Box 1004 Stn Main 300 Pleasant St, Dartmouth NS B2Y 3Z9; Dal'85; FRCPC; Psy (Geriatric Psychiatry). Staff, The Nova Scotia Hospital; Assoc Prof Psy, Dalhousie University; (902)464-3111; Fax. (902)464-3002.

FLYNN, Paula S; Tricities Mnetal Hlth Ctr, 1-2232 Elgin Ave, Port Coquitlam BC V3C 2B2; UBC'92; CCFP; FCFP; Staff, Providence Health Care - St Paul's Hospital; Staff, Richmond Mental Health Centre; (604)777-8400

FLYNN, Sean W; Mental Health Team, 310-1669 Broadway E, Vancouver BC V5N 1V9; Cal'88; FRCPC; Psy. Staff, BC Mental Health & Addiction Service; (604)675-3990

FLYNNE, Paul R; Lifemark Health Institute, 154-15710 87 Ave NW, Edmonton AB T5R 5W9; Liverpool (England)'68; (780)429-4761; pflynne@cpsa.ab.ca.

FOCCROULLE, Ann-Stephane; Omnicique de l'Outaouais, 202-28 boul du Mont-Bleu, Gatineau QC J8Z 1J1; Laval'95; Staff Family Med, Hôpital de Gatineau; (819)777-2111; Fax. (819)771-6890.

FOCKLER, Donald F; PO Box 1555 Stn A, Comox BC V9M 8A2; UBC'73; (250)339-2242

FODA, Abdelmonem; Red River Family Med Centre, 139 Carmen Ave, Winnipeg MB R2L 0E5; Ain Shams (Egypt)'86; CCFP.

FODA, Mohamed M R; Leduc Comm Hosp & Health Ctr, 3F-4210 48 St, Leduc AB T9E 5Z3; Cairo (Egypt)'76; MB ChB; MSc; FRCS(Glas); FRCSC; Urol (Pediatric Urology). Ac Staff, Leduc Community Hospital; Ac Staff, Covenant Health - St Mary's Hospital; Vis Consultant, Wetaskiwin Hospital & Care Centre; Langs: Arabic; French; (780)980-4627; Fax. (780)980-4629.

FODEMESI, Frank J; 190 Cherryhill Cir, London ON N6H 2M3; Wes'81; Court Staff, Strathroy Middlesex General Hospital - Middlesex Hospital Alliance; Ac Staff, Parkwood Hospital - St Joseph's Health Care; Ac Staff, St Joseph's Hospital - St Joseph's Health Care; (519)433-0063; Fax. (519)433-0064.

FODIL-CHERIF, Yamina; Midpark Family Med Centre, 330-290 Midpark Way SE, Calgary AB T2X 1P1; (Algeria)'83; (403)254-2408; Fax. (403)254-5887.

FOELL, R Blaine T; 2-23 Dairy Lane, Huntsville ON P1H 1T4; Tor'95; FRCPC; Neur. (705)789-6632; Fax. (705)789-1922; rbtfoell@yahoo.ca.

FOERSTER, David R; Red River Family Med Centre, 14-160 Meadowood Dr, Winnipeg MB R2M 5L6; Man'97; FRCSC; OrthSurg.

FOERSTER, Steven G; Red Deer Reg Hosp Centre, 3942 50A Ave, Red Deer AB T4N 4E7; Man'90; CCFP; CCFP(E.M.); Staff, Red Deer Regional Hospital Centre; (403)343-4660

FOFIE, Monica; Options for Sexual Health, 3550 Hastings St E, Vancouver BC V5K 2A7; Alb'06; (604)731-4252

FOGA, Myrosia M; Trillium Hlth Ctr-Mississauga, 100 Queensway W, Mississauga ON L5B 1B8; Man'95; MSc; BSc; FRCPC; DiagRad; NuclearMed. Staff Radiol, Trillium Health Centre - Mississauga; Langs: Ukrainian; French; (905)848-7100 x3465; Fax. (905)848-7676.

FOGARTY, Doris C; Sechelt Med Clinic, PO Box 638, Sechelt BC V0N 3A0; UBC'91; CCFP; FCFP; (604)885-2257; Fax. (604)885-4718.

FOGARTY, Finola M; Dr Finola Fogarty Prof Corp, 10024 116 St NW, Edmonton AB T5K 1V6; National (Ireland)'83; MB BCh(BAO); FRCP; FRCPC; Psy (Head Injury). Clin Lecturer Dept of Psy, University of Alberta Hospital; Staff, Covenant Health - Grey Nuns Community Hospital; Clin Dir Adult Attention Deficit Disorder Treat Prg Student Hlth Serv Clinic, University of Alberta; Langs: English; French; (780)413-0360; Fax. (780)455-5308; fin555@telus.net.

FOGEL, Bernard; Bloor Med Clinic, 844 Bathurst St, Toronto ON M5R 3G1; Tor'61; CCFP; FCFP; Staff, Humber River Regional Hospital - Church Street Site; Staff, Mount Sinai Hospital; Staff, Baycrest Centre for Geriatric Care; Asst Prof Family & Commun Med, University of Toronto; (416)534-4214; Fax. (416)534-4582.

FOGEL, Martin L; 407-400 Tache Ave, Winnipeg MB R2H 3C3; Man'85; BSc(Med); MPH; CCFP; FCFP; Ac Staff, Ste Amant Centre; (204)783-7070; m-fogel@shaw.ca.

FOGL, Tomas; Royal Ottawa Hosp, 1145 Carling Ave, Ottawa ON K1Z 7K4; McG'99; FRCPC; Psy. Staff Psy, Royal Ottawa Mental Health Centre - Royal Ottawa Health Care Group; Langs: Bilingual(English/French); (613)722-6521

FOGOLIN, Jane; Thunder Bay Reg HSC-T-Bay, 980 Oliver Rd, Thunder Bay ON P7B 6V4; McM'96; FRCPC; Psy. Staff, Thunder Bay Regional Health Sciences Centre; (807)684-6430

FOGWILL, Terence R; Workplace Hlth Safety & Comp c, PO BOX 9000 Stn A 146-148 Forest Rd, St. John's NL A1A 3B8; Mem'02; CCFP; (709)778-1565

FOIDART, Stephane; 524 First Ave S, Kenora ON P9N 1W5; Ott'06; CCFP; Langs: Bilingual(English/French).

FOK, Mark; 7F-2775 Laurel St, Vancouver BC V5Z 1M9; UBC'08; IntMed. (604)875-5706

FOK, Mei Sum; Medicla Clinic, 10659A 97 St NW, Edmonton AB T5H 2L7; Alb'05; CCFP; Langs: Cantonese; (780)428-8111

FOLDES, Eva; Hop Maisonneuve-Rosemont, 5415 boul de l'Assomption, Montreal QC H1T 2M4; Budapest (Hungary)'80; FRCPC; IntMed (P.Q.). Consultant, Institut de Cardiologie de Montréal; Staff, Hopital Maisonneuve-Rosemont; Aj Prof Dept of Med, Universite de Montreal; Langs: French; Hungarian; German; (514)252-3400 x4619; Fax. (514)252-3936.

FOLESCU, Simona; Grey Nuns Comm Hosp & HC, 1100 Youville Drive West NW, Edmonton AB T6L 5X8; (Romania)'02; Psy. Staff, Covenant Health - Grey Nuns Community Hospital; (780)735-7000; Fax. (780)435-7496.

FOLEY, Anita A; 115 Main St PO Box 260, Guysborough NS B0H 1N0; Dal'75; CCFP; FCFP; Chief Medical Staff/Staff Family Med, Guysborough Memorial Hospital; (902)533-4040; Fax. (902)533-2040.

FOLEY, Brian M; Cape Breton Hlthcare Complex, 1482 George St, Sydney NS B1P 1P3; Dublin (Ireland)'78; MB ChB; BAO; MRCPsy; LRCPSI; FRCPC; Psy (Addiction Medicine). Chief Psy/Clin Dir Mental Health Serv, Cape Breton Healthcare Complex; Consultant, Northside General Hospital; (902)567-8091 x2214; Fax. (902)567-7905.

FOLEY, Colin F; Queen Elizabeth Hosp, PO Box 6600 Stn Central 60 Riverside Dr, Charlottetown PE C1A 8T5; Dal'98; FRCPC; DiagRad. Staff Diag Imag, Queen Elizabeth Hospital; (902)894-2111; Fax. (902)894-2366.

FOLEY, Finola H; McMaster Univ Student Ctr, 1280 Main St W, Hamilton ON L8S 4K1; McM'91; (905)525-9140 x27700; Fax. (905)546-0805.

FOLEY, Frank J; 210-1366 Yonge St, Toronto ON M4T 3A7; Tor'78; CCFP; FCFP; Asst Prof, University of Toronto; (416)962-6692; Fax. (416)962-3943.

FOLEY, Garrett V M; 219 Baldwin Ave, Cornwall ON K6H 4J3; Dublin (Ireland)'77; MB BS; Assoc Staff, Cornwall Community Hospital - Second Street Site; Assoc Staff, Cornwall Community Hospital; (613)936-1505; Fax. (613)936-1388.

FOLEY, Joshua F; Medicine Hat Reg Hosp, 666 5 St SW, Medicine Hat AB T1A 4H6; Mem'83; CCFP; CCFP; Staff, Medicine Hat Regional Hospital; (403)529-8817; Fax. (403)529-8007.

FOLEY, Karen A; Univ Hlth Network-Toronto Gen, 200 Elizabeth St, Toronto ON M5G 2C4; (Ireland)'98; Staff, Toronto General Hospital - UHN; (416)340-4800

FOLEY, Marie-Claude; CSSS Haut-Richelieu-Rouville, 920 boul du Seminaire N, St-Jean-sur-Richel QC J3A 1B7; Sher'07; Hem; IntMed. Staff, Hôpital du Haut-Richelieu; (450)359-5000

FOLEY, Mark; Khatsuhlano Med Clinic, 101-230 A Cook St, Victoria BC V8V 3X3; Dal'09; CCFP; (250)220-9999

FOLEY, Stephen R; Hamilton HS-Henderson Site, 711 Concession St, Hamilton ON L8V 1C3; McM'88; BSc(Hon.); FRCPC; IntMed (Clinical Immunology & Allergy); Hem. Assoc Prof LabMed, Hamilton Health Sciences Centre-Juravinski Site; (905)389-4411 x42074

FOLINSBEE, Catherine D; Physicians Incorporated, 205-316 Willow St, Truro NS B2N 5A4; Alb'77; FRCSC; ObstGyn. Obstetrics, Colchester East Hants Health Centre; (902)895-4477; Fax. (902)895-4407.

FOLK, David M; 904-141 Wellington Cres, Winnipeg MB R3M 3X3; Cape Town (South Africa)'80; CCFP; FCFP; (204)898-5385

FOLKERSON, Curtis S; Wakefield Family Med Centre, 777 Riverside Dr PO Box 400, Wakefield QC J0X 3G0; McG'80; CCFP; FCFP; Langs: English; French; (819)459-2363; Fax. (819)459-2997.

FOLLETT, Michael S; Cross Cancer Institute, 11560 University Ave NW, Edmonton AB T6G 1Z2; Alb'90; Staff, Cross Cancer Institute; (780)432-8771; Fax. (780)432-8888.

FOLLOWS, Jonathan M; 301B-6351 197 St, Langley BC V2Y 1X8; UBC'87; (604)539-1915; Fax. (604)539-1983.

FOLMAN, Raphael Ralph; First Med Place, 170 Queensway W, Mississauga ON L5B 3A8; Tor'67; FRFPS; FRCPC; Peds (Pediatric Nephrology). Ac Staff, Trillium Health Centre - Mississauga; Hon Staff, The Hospital For Sick Children; Asst Prof, University of Toronto; Langs: Hebrew; Polish; ralph.folman@utoronto.ca.

FOLSCHER, Werner; Queen Elizabeth II Hosp, 10409 98 St, Grande Prairie AB T8V 2E8; (South Africa)'94; MB ChB; Staff, Queen Elizabeth II Hospital; (780)538-7173; Fax. (780)538-7277.

FOLTON, Kenneth L; Newell Associate Clinic, PO Box 280 Stn Main, Brooks AB T1R 1B3; Alb'77; (403)362-5501; Fax. (403)362-8426.

FOLTZ, Anne-Marie; CSSS de Lac-Saint Jean-Est, CP 1300 Succ Bureau-Chef 300 boul Champlain S, Alma QC G8B 5W3; Mon'09; Staff, CSSS de Lac-Saint Jean-Est; (418)669-2000

FOLTZ, Lynda M; Burrard Med Bldg, 490-1144 Burrard St, Vancouver BC V6Z 2A5; UBC'00; FRCPC; IntMed; Hem. (604)684-5794 x2; Fax. (604)684-5705.

FOMBONNE, Eric; Div Of Child Psychiatry, 4018 rue Sainte-Catherine O, Westmount QC H3Z 1P2; Paris (France)'80; Psy (P.Q.). Dir-Research Child Psy, McGill University Health Centre - Montreal Chest Institute; Teach Staff, McGill University; (514)412-4400 x22174; Fax. (514)412-4346.

FON, Edward A; MUHC-Montreal Neurology Inst, 3801 rue University, Montreal QC H3A 2B4; Mon'89; FRCPC; Neur. Staff, McGill University Health Centre - Montreal Neurological Hospital; (514)398-8398; Fax. (514)398-5214.

FONDOP, Jean-Jacques; Hôpital régional Chaleur, 1750 Sunset Dr, Bathurst NB E2A 4L7; (Cameroon)'98; Staff, Hopital Regional Chaleur; (506)544-3000

FONG, Allan C; Weyburn Health Centre, 36 4th St, Weyburn SK S4H 0X7; Galway (Ireland)'94; MB ChB; BAO; (306)842-5444; Fax. (306)842-5449.

FONG, Andrew; 3348 Keele St, North York ON M3J 1L5; Tor'88; Langs: Chinese; (416)398-2505; Fax. (647)342-8478.

FONG, Chi Wai; 301-385 Silver Star Blvd, Scarborough ON M1V 0E3; Tor'75; Staff, Toronto East General Hospital Inc; Langs: Cantonese; Chinese; Mandarin; (416)291-0409; Fax. (416)291-8674.

FONG, Edwin M Y C; 205-250 Harding Blvd W, Richmond Hill ON L4C 9M7; Tor'04; FRCPC; IntMed; Nephrol. (905)508-5911; Fax. (905)508-2972.

FONG, George Y; 1927 105 St NW, Edmonton AB T6J 5V9; Alb'79; CCFP; FCFP; Staff, Royal Alexandra Hospital; Langs: Cantonese; Chinese; (780)473-4417; Fax. (780)439-6590.

FONG, Handrick; St Boniface Gen Hosp, 409 Tache Ave, Winnipeg MB R2H 2A6; Dal'77; FRCSC; GenSurg; VascSurg. Staff, St Boniface General Hospital; (204)233-8563

FONG, Harmon; Halton HSC-Oakville Site, 327 Reynolds St, Oakville ON L6J 3L7; Wes'09; CCFP; CCFP(E.M.); Staff, Halton Healthcare Services Corporation - Oakville Site; (866)882-5368

FONG, Harvey O; Unison Hlth & Community Servic, 1541 Jane St, North York ON M9N 2R3; Mem'83; (416)645-7575; harvey.fong@unisonhcs.org.

FONG, Ignatius W; St Michael's Hosp, 30 Bond St, Toronto ON M5B 1W8; (Jamaica)'69; FRCPC; IntMed (Infectious Diseases). Ac Staff InfectDis, St Michael's Hospital; Prof Med, University of Toronto; (416)864-5746; Fax. (416)864-5310; fongi@smh.toronto.on.ca.

FONG, Jadine H; 285 Whitewood Ave PO Box 219, New Liskeard ON P0J 1P0; Cal'80; BSc; (705)647-8411; Fax. (705)647-8411; jfong@ntl.sympatico.ca.

FONG, Justine H S; Plaza 162, 200-233 16 Ave NW, Calgary AB T2M 0H5; Alb'97; CCFP; Langs: Cantonese; (403)230-3300; Fax. (403)230-3322.

FONG, Katherine W; OPG Bldg, 3-704-700 University Ave, Toronto ON M5G 1X6; (Hong Kong)'73; MB BS; DABR; FRCPC; DiagRad. Staff, Mount Sinai Hospital; Assoc Prof, University of Toronto; Langs: Cantonese; (416)586-4800 x5102

FONG, Kathleen C; Weyburn Health Centre, 36 4th St, Weyburn SK S4H 0X7; Sask'89; (306)842-5444; Fax. (306)842-5449.

FONG, Keng Lao; 2303 41 Ave W PO Box 18126, Vancouver BC V6M 4L3; London (England)'75; MB BS; (778)387-1633

FONG, Linda D; Hawkwood Village Med Clinic, 20-217 Hawksbrow Dr NW, Calgary AB T3G 3K2; Cal'83; CCFP; FCFP; (403)777-2757; Fax. (403)777-2755.

FONG, Michael W M; Polyclinic Prof Centre Inc, 308-199 Grafton St, Charlottetown PE C1A 1L2; Tor'93; FRCSC; Otol. (902)629-8810

FONG, Peter F K; 11 Gibb St, Oshawa ON L1H 2J9; Ott'65; FRCPC; DiagRad. Court Staff, Lakeridge Health - Bowmanville Site; (905)579-1445

FONG, Peter; Saint John Reg Hosp, PO Box 2100 Stn Main, Saint John NB E2L 4L2; Dal'95; FRCPC; IntMed (Interventional Cardiology); Cardiol. Staff New Brunswick Heart Centre, Saint John Regional Hospital; (506)648-6101; Fax. (506)648-6110; Peter.Fong@Horizon.NB.ca.

FONG, S Ken; Queensway-Carleton Hosp, 3045 Baseline Rd, Nepean ON K2H 8P4; Ott'80; Anes. Staff/Chief Anesthetist, Queensway Carleton Hospital; (613)721-2000

FONG, Sharon Y C; 2516 Commercial Dr, Vancouver BC V5N 4C2; UBC'95; CCFP; (604)872-5377

FONG, Tse Chen; Calgary Heart Centre, 402-3280 Hospital Dr NW, Calgary AB T2N 4Z6; Man'77; DiagRad. Physician, Health Research Innovation Centre; University of Calgary; Langs: Chinese; (403)944-4530; Fax. (403)944-4577; chen.fong@albertahealthservices.ca.

FONG WAI CHIN, Philip A; Sun Country Health Region, PO Box 2003 Stn Main, Weyburn SK S4H 2Z9; Galway (Ireland)'58; MB ChB; BAO; Staff Med, Weyburn General Hospital; Resd Physician Tatagwa View, Sun Country Health Region; Resd Physician, Weyburn Special Care Home; Langs: Chinese; Creole; Bilingual(French/English); (306)842-8365; philip.fong@schr.sk.ca.

FONSECA, Conchita; 2F-1365 Richmond Rd, Ottawa ON K2B 6R7; Ott'04; CCFP; CCFP(E.M.); Langs: Bilingual(English/French); (613)820-2001; Fax. (613)820-2006.

FONSECA FALCAO, Marcele; CHUS-Hop Hotel-Dieu, 580 rue Bowen S, Sherbrooke QC J1G 2E8; Rio de Janeiro (Brazil)'01; Staff, Centre Hospitalier Universitaire de Sherbrooke-Hôpital Hôtel-Dieu; (819)346-1110 x28008

FONSEKA, Sujeewa D; Kelso Lake Med Centre, 112-330 Bronte St S, Milton ON L9T 7X1; Mem'00; BA; CCFP; Staff, Halton Healthcare Services Corporation - Milton District Hospital; Clinical Asst Prof, McMaster University; Asst Clin Prof, University of Western Ontario; Langs: Sinhalese; (905)876-1011; Fax. (905)876-3401; info@klmc.ca.

FONT DEL PINO, Sonia; CSSS Haut-Richelieu-Rouville, 920 boul du Seminaire N, St-Jean-Sur-Richel QC J3A 1B7; Havana (Cuba)'85; CSPQ; FRCPC; Anes. Staff, Hôpital du Haut-Richelieu; (450)359-5000 x5212

FONTAINE, Amelie; Cross Cancer Institiute, 11560 University Ave NW, Edmonton AB T6G 1Z2; Sher'01; FRCPC; IntMed; Hem. Staff Med Oncology, Cross Cancer Institute; Asst Prof Med, University of Alberta; Langs: Bilingual(English/French); (780)432-8340

FONTAINE, Daniel G; Calgary Lab Services, C422-3535 Research Rd NW, Calgary AB T2L 2K8; Mem'98; FRCPC; AnatPath. Staff, Calgary Laboratory Services; (403)770-3759; Fax. (403)770-3788.

FONTAINE, Daphne H; Medical Arts Bldg, 260-1105 Pandora Ave, Victoria BC V8V 3P9; McM'91; (250)380-1901; Fax. (250)380-1982.

FONTAINE, Francis; Centre Chiromedic, 300-1545 boul de L'Avenir, Laval QC H7S 2N5; Mon'03; CCFP; Staff, Hopital de la Cite de la santé; (450)967-0500

FONTAINE, Geneviève; Centre Hosp Honore-Mercier, 2750 boul Laframboise, Saint-Hyacinthe QC J2S 4Y8; Mon'07; CCFP; Staff, Centre Hospitalier Honore-Mercier; (450)771-3333

FONTAINE, Isabelle; Clinique Medicale St-Cyrille, B-4105 rue Principale, St-Cyrille-de-Wend QC J1Z 1C7; Mon'82; (819)781-0105; Fax. (819)397-2668.

FONTAINE, Isabelle-Anne; UMF du Grand Littoral, 1205 boul de la Rive-Sud, Saint-Romuald QC G6W 0J4; Laval'05; CCFP; Staff, CLSC Saint-Tite; (418)380-8597; Fax. (418)380-8596.

FONTAINE, Jean-Guy; CHUQ-Ctr Hosp Univ Laval, 2705 Boul Laurier, Quebec QC G1V 4G2; Laval'79; LMCC; FRCPC; IntMed; GeriatricMed. Staff, Centre Hospitalier Universitaire de Quebec-CHUL; (418)654-2255; Fax. (418)654-2757.

FONTAINE, Jean-Yves; Procrea Clinique, 401-5600 boul des Galeries, Quebec QC G2K 2H6; Laval'71; CSPQ; ABOG; RC; FRCSC; ObstGyn (Reproductive Medicine). Staff, PROCREA Cliniques; Associé Clin Prof ObstGyn, Université Laval; Langs: English; (418)260-9555; Fax. (418)260-9556; jysff@videotron.ca.

FONTAINE, Karine; CSSS Drummond-Hop Sainte-Croix, 570 rue Heriot, Drummondville QC J2B 1C1; Sher'03; Staff, Hôpital Sainte-croix; (819)478-6464

FONTAINE, Louis; Clinique Med Richelieu, 200-500 Rte Marie-Victorin, Sorel-Tracy QC J3R 1K7; Mon'86; Staff, Hôtel-Dieu de Sorel; Staff, Clinique Medicale Richelieu; (450)742-5638; Fax. (450)742-0995.

FONTAINE, Marie-Josee; CSSS du Sud de Lanaudière, 911 montee des Pionniers, Terrebonne QC J6V 2H2; Sher'96; CCFP; Staff, Centre Hospitalier Pierre le Gardeur; (450)654-7525

FONTAINE, Ronald J A; 1-6 rue de l'Eglise, Bouctouche NB E4S 2Z7; Dal'81; Staff, Hôpital Stella-Maris-de-Kent; (506)743-6545; Fax. (506)743-2889.

FONTAINE, Suzanne; Clinique Medimax, CP 91 Succ Pl-Desjardins 300-4 Complexe Desjardins, Montreal QC H5B 1B2; Mon'81; FRCPC; DiagRad. Staff, Clinique Millenia; (514)281-7955; Fax. (514)281-3906.

FONTELA, Patricia S; MUHC-Montreal Children's Hosp, C808-2300 rue Tupper, Montreal QC H3H 1P3; Staff, McGill University Health Centre - Montreal Children's Hospital; (514)412-4400 x22696

FONTEYNE, Douglas C; Town Centre Family Clinic, 320-6203 28 Ave NW, Edmonton AB T6L 6K3; Alb'92; (780)462-8120; Fax. (780)461-9437.

FONTG-WALMSLEY, Jorge A; MUHC-Montreal Gen Hosp, 1650 av Cedar, Montreal QC H3G 1A4; Alb'89; CCFP; CCFP(E.M.); Staff, McGill University Health Centre - Montreal General Campus; (514)934-1934 x42501; Fax. (514)934-8421.

FONTIGNY, Nadine J; St Boniface Clinic, 343 Tache Ave, Winnipeg MB R2H 2A5; Louvain (Belgium)'78; LLB; CCFP; FCFP; Staff, St Boniface General Hospital; Med Examiner, Province of Manitoba; (204)925-9586; Fax. (204)231-4567.

FOO, Marshall C; 408-800 Bathurst St, Toronto ON M5R 3M8; Wuhan (China)'61; Langs: Cantonese; Chinese; Mandarin; (416)530-1888

FOO, S Jo Ling; Metrohealth Clinic, 4879 Kingsway, Burnaby BC V5H 4T6; Sydney (Australia)'07; CCFP; (604)433-3341

FOO, Suan-Seh; Canterbury Clinic, 500-40 Wellesley St E, Toronto ON M4Y 1G4; Tor'90; BSc(Hons); Med Consultant, Family Adolescent Straight Talk (Fast) Gourage to Change; Med Dir, The Canterbury Clinic Toronto; (416)961-8282

FOO, Violet L Y; 302-8055 Anderson Rd, Richmond BC V6Y 1S2; UBC'87; CCFP; FCFP; (604)273-9392; Fax. (604)273-2802.

FOOLEN, Catharina H G M; Greenwood Fam Physicians, PO Box 5 709 1 St NE, Sundre AB T0M 1X0; Limburg (Netherlands)'85; CCFP; Langs: Dutch; German; (403)638-2424; Fax. (403)638-3580; careu@telus.net.

FOONG, Shu Ching; Reginal Fertility Program, 400-2000 Place Veteran's NW, Calgary AB T3B 4N2; Cal'97; FRCSC; ObstGyn (Infertility). Staff, Foothills Medical Centre; (403)284-9103

FOONG, Weng-Leong; Eglinton Square Mall, 159-1 Eglinton Sq, Scarborough ON M1L 2K1; Queen's (Ireland)'65; Staff, The Scarborough Hospital - General Campus; Staff, Rouge Valley Health System - Centenary Health Centre Site; Staff, Toronto East General Hospital Inc; Langs: Cantonese; (416)751-0465

FOOTE, John R; Mount Sinai Hosp, 206-600 University Ave, Toronto ON M5G 1X5; Tor'93; BSc; CCFP; CCFP(E.M.); Staff, The Credit Valley Hospital; Staff, Mount Sinai Hospital; Asst Prof Dept of Family & Community Med/Asst Dir Residency Prog, University of Toronto; Langs: English; French; (416)586-5058

FOOTE, Margaret J G; 11 George St S, Cambridge ON N1S 2N3; Wes'76; (519)622-7800; Fax. (519)622-7178.

FORBES, Anastasia F; Minoru Residence, 6111 Minoru Blvd, Richmond BC V6Y 1Y4; Cal'89; FRCPC; IntMed; GeriatricMed. (604)244-5300

FORBES, Andrew J; 2B-150 Sidney St, Belleville ON K8P 5E2; Wes'87; CCFP; FCFP; (613)969-1454; Fax. (613)966-5725.

FORBES, Cynthia A; Fall River Family Practice, PO Box 2160 Rpo Fall River, Fall River NS B2T 1K6; Dal'85; CCFP; FCFP; (902)861-2237; Fax. (902)861-1914.

FORBES, Frederick B T; FBT Forbes Med Pro Corp, 301A-18 Kensington Rd, Brampton ON L6T 4S5; Belfast (Ireland)'67; (905)792-2245; Fax. (905)458-0475.

FORBES, Geoffrey G A; Oakdale Med Bldg, 310-2065 Finch Ave W, North York ON M3N 2V7; McG'89; BSc; (416)745-6244

FORBES, Ian S; Willow Chest Center, 2F-2647 Willow St, Vancouver BC V5Z 1M9; Cal'86; FRCPC; CommunMed (Industrial Medicine); Psy. Staff, Vancouver General Hospital - Centennial Pavillion; (604)875-4139

FORBES, Jason K; 400-13450 102 St, Surrey BC V3T 0H1; Ott'06; FRCSC; GenSurg. (877)935-5669

FORBES, John G; Westville Med Clinic, PO Box 930, Westville NS B0K 2A0; Dal'76; Staff, Aberdeen Regional Hospital; (902)396-4142; Fax. (902)396-1707.

FORBES, Karen; Edmonton Clinic Hlth Academy, 3 579-11405 87 Ave NW, Edmonton AB T6G 1C9; Cal'99; FRCPC; Peds. (780)407-8822

FORBES, Leta M; Lakeridge Hlth Corp-Oshawa, 1 Hospital Crt, Oshawa ON L1G 2B9; McM'99; FRCPC; IntMed; MedOncol., Lakeridge Health - Oshawa Site; (905)576-8711; Fax. (905)721-6100.

FORBES, Natalie K; Kiwi Pediatrics, 16662 McKenzie Lake Blvd SE, Calgary AB T2Z 1N4; Cal'08; FRCPC; Peds. (403)281-2500; Fax. (403)256-2511.

FORBES, Patricia A; MUHC-Montreal Children's Hosp, A329-2300 rue Tupper, Montreal QC H3H 1P3; Manchester (England)'58; FAAP; Peds. Ac Staff, McGill University Health Centre - Montreal Children's Hospital; assoc Prof, McGill University; Langs: French; (514)934-4400 x22823; Fax. (514)412-4477; patricia.forbes@muhc.mcgill.ca.

FORBES, Peter J A; 300-1490 rue Sherbrooke O, Montreal QC H3G 1L3; Mon'78; (514)932-3300; Fax. (514)932-0469.

FORBES, Robert A; Riverview Med Clinic, 3-500 Coverdale Rd, Riverview NB E1B 3K2; Dal'80; CCFP; FCFP; Staff, The Moncton Hospital; (506)387-4500

FORBES, Shauna E; Scarborough Prof Centre, 308-1371 Neilson Rd, Scarborough ON M1B 4Z8; Tor'91; CCFP; FCFP; Associate, Rouge Valley Health System - Centenary Health Centre Site; Ac Staff, The Scarborough Hospital - Birchmount Campus; (416)283-7701; Fax. (416)283-7108.

FORBES, Shawn; Hamilton HS-Henderson Site, B3 162-711 Concession St, Hamilton ON L8V 1C3; McM'02; FRCSC; GenSurg (Colorectal Surgery). Staff, Hamilton Health Sciences Centre-Juravinski Site; (905)521-2100; Fax. (905)528-9388.

FORBES, Thomas; London HSC-Victoria Hosp, PO Box 5010 Stn B E2 119A-800 Commissioners Rd E, London ON N6A 5W9; Tor'90; FACS; FRCSC; GenSurg (Vasculities); VascSurg. Staff Surg, London Health Sciences Centre - Victoria Campus; Prof, University of Western Ontario; (519)667-6794; Fax. (519)667-6549.

FORBES-HOSKINS, Eleanor; Ottawa Valley Family Hlth, 95 Spring St, Almonte ON K0A 1A0; Ott'06; CCFP; Staff, Almonte General Hospital; (613)256-9370; Fax. (613)259-0949.

FORCIER, Jean-Francois; Centre Med Saint-Francois, 200-2125 boul Lemire, Drummondville QC J2B 8N8; Sher'93; CCFP; (819)477-6793; Fax. (819)477-6962.

FORCINA, Alexander E; 602 Caledonia Rd, Toronto ON M6E 4V5; Tor'92; CCFP; Langs: Italian; (416)782-2211; Fax. (416)782-2392.

FORD, Anthony J; Highland Park Walk-In Clinic, 2B-6315 Horn St, Red Deer AB T4N 6H5; Cape Town (South Africa)'81; (403)334-2204

FORD, Bryce A; 102-49 Richard Way SW, Calgary AB T3E 7M8; UBC'99; FRCSC; Ophth (Glaucoma). Clin Lecturer, University of Calgary; (403)245-3730; Fax. (403)245-1058.

FORD, David; Gastro Health Clinic, 170-4600 Hwy 7, Vaughan ON L4L 4Y7; McM'95; MSc; BSc; FRCPC; IntMed; Gastroent. Staff, William Osler Health System - Etobicoke General Hospital; (416)743-8431; Fax. (416)743-1372.

FORD, Derek; 199 Avenue Rd, Toronto ON M5R 2J3; Wes'98; BSc; FRCSC; PlasSurg (Cosmetic Surgery). Ac Staff, Lakeridge Health - Oshawa Site; Langs: Polish; (416)925-7337; info@fordplasticsurgery.com.

FORD, Gordon; 102-2675 36 St NE, Calgary AB T1Y 6H6; Cal'73; FRCPC; IntMed (Clinical Trials). Staff Respiratory Med., Rockyview General Hospital; (403)457-5864; Fax. (403)457-5860; gford@ucalgary.ca.

FORD, Jackie A; 208-99 Sinclair Ave, Georgetown ON L7G 5G1; Witwatersrand (South Africa)'70; BSc; MB ChB; FRCOG; Langs: Afrikaans; Cantonese; (905)877-8085

FORD, Jacqueline; 201-60 Hatt St, Dundas ON L9H 7T6; London (England)'64; FRCPC; DiagRad. (905)627-4625

FORD, Jason C; BC Women's Hosp & Health Ctre, 2K49-4500 Oak St, Vancouver BC V6H 3N1; UBC'96; FRCPC; GenPath. Staff, BC Women's Hospital & Health Centre; (604)875-2306; Fax. (604)875-2815.

FORD, Meredith K; Trillium Hlth Ctre-Mississauga, 100 Queensway W, Mississauga ON L5B 1B8; Wes'02; FRCPC; Anes. Staff, Trillium Health Centre - Mississauga; (905)848-7628

FORD, Michael H G; Sunnybrook Hlth Sciences Ctre, MG 375-2075 Bayview Ave, Toronto ON M4N 3M5; Tor'80; FRCSC; OrthSurg (Spine). Staff, Sunnybrook Health Sciences Centre; Asst Prof, University of Toronto; (416)480-6775; Fax. (416)480-5990.

FORD, Peter T; 204-323 Wilson St E, Ancaster ON L9G 4A8; Qns'85; CCFP; Assoc Staff, Hamilton Health Sciences Centre - McMaster University Medical Centre; (905)304-8367; Fax. (905)304-0222; ptf007@cogeco.ca.

FORD, Victor; 321 Routledge Rd NW, Edmonton AB T6R 1B9; Witwatersrand (South Africa)'79; MB ChB; FRCPC; Anes (Intensive Care & Anesthesia). Chief Anes., Covenant Health - Grey Nuns Community Hospital; (780)945-9588; Fax. (780)988-2670.

FORD-JONES, Anthony E A; The Brulington Children's Clin, B10 103-3305 Harvester Rd, Burlington ON L7N 3N2; London (England)'72; MB BS; MRCS; LRCP; FRCPC; Peds (Pediatric & Adolescent Medicine). Ac Staff Peds, Joseph Brant Memorial Hospital; Clinical Asst Prof, Hamilton Health Sciences Centre - McMaster Children's Hospital; Langs: French; (905)634-1311; Fax. (905)634-7202; afordjones@mac.com.

FORD-JONES, Elizabeth L; The Hosp For Sick Children, 1447C-555 University Ave, Toronto ON M5G 1X8; Qns'74; FRCPC; Peds (Social Pediatrics). Prof Peds, The Hospital For Sick Children; Prof Peds, University of Toronto; Langs: Bilingual(English/French); (416)813-5443; Fax. (416)813-7479; lee.ford-jones@sickkids.ca.

FORDER, Mark A; High Level Med Clinic, 11202 100 ave SS 1, High Level AB T0H 1Z0; Cape Town (South Africa)'84; MB ChB; (780)926-2286

FORDYCE, Christopher B; Gordon & Leslie Diamond Hlth C, 9F-2775 Laurel St, Vancouver BC V5Z 1M9; McG'08; FRCPC; IntMed. (604)875-5302

FORERO MANTILLA, Carlos M; St Joseph's Healthcare, 50 Charlton Ave E, Hamilton ON L8N 4A6; (Spain)'94; Staff, St Joseph's Healthcare - Charlton Campus; (905)522-4941

FOREST, Daniel; Centre Carceral St-Jerome, 2 boul de la Salette, Saint-Jerome QC J7Y 5G5; Sher'80; Langs: English; (450)436-8144; Fax. (450)436-9411; belair.forest@sympatico.ca.

FOREST, France L; Clinique du Havre, 79A rue Jacques-Cartier, Gaspe QC G4X 1M5; Mon'74; (418)368-5609; Fax. (418)368-6498.

FOREST, Genevieve; CSSS du Nord de Lanaudière, 1000 boul Sainte-Anne, St-Charles-Brromee QC J6E 6J2; Sher'99; CCFP; CCFP(E.M.); Staff, Centre Hospitalier Régional de Lanaudière; (450)759-8222

FOREST, Isabelle; 101-1355 Grande Allee, Terrebonne QC J6W 4K6; Mon'05; Psy. Staff, Centre Hospitalier Pierre le Gardeur; (450)964-6418

FOREST, Jean-Claude; CHUQ-St-Francois D'Assise, 10 rue de l'Espinay, Quebec QC G1L 3L5; Sher'75; PhD; CSPQ; FRCPC; MedBiochem (P.Q.) (Laboratory Medicine); MedScient(Med). Researcher, Centre Hospitalier Universitaire De Québec - Pavillon De St-françois-d'assise; Assoc Staff, CSSS de Quebec-Sud; Assoc Dean, Université Laval; (418)525-4438; jean-claude.forest@bcx.ulaval.ca.

FOREST, Liette; Hop Reg D'Emundston, 275 Hebert Blvd, Edmundston NB E3V 4E4; Sher'02; CCFP; Staff, Hôpital regional d'Edmundston; Langs: Bilingual(French/English); (506)739-2200; lforest@nb.sympatico.ca.

FOREST, Natacha; GMF de Lorraine, 99 boul de Gaulle, Lorraine QC J6Z 3Z9; Mon'97; (450)621-1444; Fax. (450)621-7193.

FOREST, Sophie; CLSC Grande-Riviere, 425 rue Leguerrier, Gatineau QC J9H 6N8; Mon'95; (819)684-2251

FOREST, Veronique I; 625-4141 rue Sherbrooke O, Montreal QC H3Z 1B8; Laval'01; FRCSC; Otol. (514)937-3687

FORESTELL, Clair F; Campbell Clinic, 430 Mayor Magrath Dr S, Lethbridge AB T1J 3M1; Alb'81; FRCPC; IntMed. Asst Clin Prof, University of Calgary; (403)328-8101; Fax. (403)328-8150; cforestell@campbellclinic.com.

FORESTELL, Gerald P; Huntsville Prof Bldg, 104-348 Muskoka Rd 3 N, Huntsville ON P1H 1H8; Wes'90; CCFP; CCFP(E.M.); (705)789-2355; Fax. (705)789-1051.

FORESTER, Kimberley A; Cottage Country Fam Hlth Team, 1-5 Pineridge Gate, Gravenhurst ON P1P 1Z3; NOSM'09; CCFP; (705)687-2273; Fax. (705)687-7575.

FORESTIER, Colleen A; 101 Colonel By Dr, Ottawa ON K1A 0K2; Wes'96; CCFP; FCFP; (613)945-2780

FORFAR, Katie; 705 MacKay St, Pembroke ON K8A 1G8; Qns'08; CCFP; (613)732-2811

FORGACH, Linda G; Misericordia Health Centre, 99 Cornish Ave, Winnipeg MB R3C 1A2; UBC'87; FRCPC; Anes. Staff, Misericordia Health Centre; (204)788-8364

FORGEOT D'ARC, Baudouin; Hop Riviere-des-Prairies, 7070 boul Perras, Montreal QC H1E 1A4; Staff, Hôpital Riviere des Prairies; (514)323-7260

FORGERON, M Patricia; 100-22 Marr Rd PO Box 4593, Rothesay NB E2E 5X3; Mem'97; BSc; MSc; FRCPC; PhysMed&Rehab (Disability Management & Rehabilitation). Staff, Saint John Regional Hospital; Asst Prof, Dalhousie University; Asst Prof, Memorial University Of Newfoundland; (506)849-3310; Fax. (506)849-3316.

FORGERON, Robert J; Red Deer Reg Hosp, PO Box 5030 3942 50A Ave, Red Deer AB T4N 4E7; Pennsylvania(PA) (USA)'00; CCFP; CCFP(E.M.); Staff, Red Deer Regional Hospital Centre; Staff, Ross Memorial Hospital; (403)343-4444

FORGET, Andre; CHUS-Hop Hotel-Dieu, 580 rue Bowen S, Sherbrooke QC J1G 2E8; Sher'82; CSPQ; FRCSC; GenSurg. Staff, Centre Hospitalier Universitaire de Sherbrooke-Hôpital Hôtel-Dieu; (819)346-1110

FORGET, Andre; Auteuil, 210 boul Sainte-Rose E, Laval QC H7H 1P3; Mon'73; Staff, Hopital de la Cite de la santé; (450)625-6063; Fax. (450)625-6063.

FORGET, Anne-Marie; CSSS de Sept-Iles, 45 rue du Pere-Divet, Sept-Iles QC G4R 3N7; Mon'92; FRCPC; IntMed. Staff, Centre Hospitalier Regional de Sept-Iles; (418)962-9761

FORGET, Eric J; CSSS-Hop De Hull, 116 boul Lionel-Emond, Gatineau QC J8Y 1W7; McG'01; Respir; IntMed. Staff, Hull Hospital; (819)595-6000

FORGET, Genevieve; CHUQ-Ctr Hosp Univ Laval, 2705 boul Laurier, Quebec QC G1V 4G2; Laval'06; FRCPC; IntMed; Endocrin&Metab (P.Q.). Staff, Centre Hospitalier Universitaire de Quebec-CHUL; (418)654-2169

FORGET, Guy; Hop Maisonneuve-Rosemont, 5415 boul de l'Assomption, Montreal QC H1T 2M4; Mon'62; FRCSC; Otol. Ac Member, Hopital Maisonneuve-Rosemont; adj Prof, Universite de Montreal; (514)326-1010; Fax. (514)326-6410.

FORGET, Josee; Clinique Fam des Prairies, 310 boul Antonio-Barrette, N-D-Des-Prairies QC J6E 1G2; Mon'90; Staff Obst, Centre Hospitalier Régional de Lanaudière; (450)752-1050; Fax. (450)752-2965.

FORGET, Judith; CLSC Simonne-Monet-Chartrand, 1303 boul Jacques-Cartier E, Longueuil QC J4M 2Y8; Mon'94; Staff Family Med, Residence Pour Retreates JAZZ; Staff Family Med, Residence Jardens D'Amour; Staff Family Med, Residence St-Malo; Staff Famliy Med, Residence Marie-Victorin; (450)463-2850; Fax. (450)463-8137.

FORGET, Karine; CHUS-Hop Hotel-Dieu, 580 rue Bowen S, Sherbrooke QC J1G 2E8; Sher'05; FRCPC; Psy. Staff, Centre Hospitalier Universitaire de Sherbrooke-Hôpital Hôtel-Dieu; (819)346-1110

FORGET, Marc; Inuulitsivik Health Centre, GD, Povungnituq QC J0M 1P0; Laval'93; Staff, Inuulitsivik Health Centre; (819)988-2957

FORGET, Marie-Chantal; CLSC St-Hubert, 6800 boul Cousineau, Longueuil QC J3Y 8Z4; Mon'87; LMCC; CCFP; Clin Prof Family Med, Centre Hospitalier l'Université de Montréal (CHUM) - Hôpital Notre-Dame; Langs: English; (450)443-7407; mchantal_forget@hotmail.com.

FORGET, Pierre; Clinique Med Adoncour, 200-505 rue Adoncour, Longueuil QC J4G 2M6; Mon'74; (450)646-4445; Fax. (450)646-5526.

FORGET, Robert J; Smyth Med Centre, 214-1929 Russell Rd, Ottawa ON K1G 4G3; Ott'67; CSPQ; FRCSC; OrthSurg. Langs: Bilingual(French/English); (613)521-6356; Fax. (613)521-6330.

FORGET, Sylviane; MUHC-Montreal Children's Hosp, D562-2300 rue Tupper, Montreal QC H3H 1P3; Mon'89; MSc; FRCPC; Peds (Gastroenterology); Gastroent. Staff, McGill University Health Centre - Montreal Children's Hospital; Asst Prof Peds, McGill University; Langs: English; French; (514)412-4474; Fax. (514)412-4392; sylviane.forget@muhc.mcgill.ca.

FORGET, Sylvie; Clin Externe de Psychiatrie, 203-100 rue Grenier, Charlemagne QC J5Z 4C6; Mon'94; FRCPC; Psy. Psychiatre, Centre Hospitalier Pierre le Gardeur; Langs: Bilingual(French/English); (450)585-9010 x1012; Fax. (450)585-2709.

FORGET, Yvon A; 1-5650 av Gatineau, Montreal QC H3T 1X7; Mon'62; Psy. (514)739-7340

FORGHANI, Kamran; Victoria Gen Hosp, 1 Hospital Way, Victoria BC V8Z 6R5; (Chile)'85; Staff, Victoria General Hospital; (250)727-4212

FORGHANI, Reza; SMBD Jewish Gen Hosp, C210 2-3755 ch Cote-Sainte-Cat, Montreal QC H3T 1E2; McG'01; DABR; PhD; FRCPC; DiagRad (Radiology). Staff/assoc Chef Dept of Radiology, Sir Mortimer B Davis Jewish General; Pres/CEO, Medical Imaging Centre; (514)340-8222 x5360; Fax. (514)340-7907.

FORGIE, Karen E; The Med Associates Sechelt, PO Box 638 5531 Inlet Ave, Sechelt BC V0N 3A0; Mem'90; BMedSci; MB; BN; CCFP; FCFP; Staff Intensive Care Commitee, St Mary's Hospital; Clin Instructor Family Med & Med Program, University of British Columbia; (604)885-2257; Fax. (604)885-4718.

FORGIE, Melissa A; Civic Parkdale Clinic, 465-737 Parkdale Ave, Ottawa ON K1Y 1J8; Ott'91; FRCPC; IntMed; Hem. Clin Staff, The Ottawa Hospital - Civic Campus; Vice Dean Undergraduate Med Education/Assoc Prof, University of Ottawa; Langs: English; French; (613)761-4127; Fax. (613)761-4035; mforgie@ottawahospital.on.ca.

FORGIE, Sarah; Edmonton Clinic Health Academy, 3 558D-11405 87 Ave NW, Edmonton AB T6G 1C9; Man'95; FRCPC; Peds; InfectDis. Staff, University of Alberta Hospital; Staff, Edmonton Clinic Health Academy; (780)248-5540; sarahforgie@cha.ab.ca.

FORGIE, W Rand; Saint John Reg Hosp, PO Box 2100 Stn Main 400 University Ave, Saint John NB E2L 4L2; Dal'79; FRCSC; GenSurg; Cardiovasc&ThorSurg. Staff, Saint John Regional Hospital; (506)648-6102; Fax. (506)648-6110; rforgieprofcorp@health.nb.ca.

FORGUES, Marie-Josee; Plantagenet Family Health Team, PO Box 305 179 Old Hwy 17, Plantagenet ON K0B 1L0; Mon'97; CCFP; FCFP; Langs: Bilingual(French/English); (613)673-4318; m.forgues@nursinghomeratings.ca.

FORGUES, Richard P; 360 Place des Pommiers, Laval QC H7G 1S6; Laval'59; CSPQ; FRCSC; GenSurg. Staff, Centre Hospitalier Fleury; (450)663-5774

FORKERT, Lutz; Kingston Gen Hosp, 76 Stuart St, Kingston ON K7L 2V7; Tor'70; FRCPC; Respir. Staff, Kingston General Hospital; Langs: German; (613)548-2446; Fax. (613)547-2069; forkert@post.queensu.ca.

FORKHEIM, Kevin E; Royal Jubilee Hosp, 1952 Bay St, Victoria BC V8R 1J8; Man'98; MSc; BSc; FRCPC; DiagRad; NuclearMed. Staff Radiol & Nuclear Med, Royal Jubilee Hospital; Staff Radiol & Nuclear Med, Victoria General Hospital; (250)370-8272; Fax. (250)370-8947.

FORMAN, Katherine C; Selkirk Family Med, 307-1101 Dewdney Ave, Trail BC V1R 4T1; (Mexico)'09; (250)368-8802

FORMAN, Leandra M; Summeridge Health Centre, 26-8707 Dufferin St, Thornhill ON L4J 0A2; (South Africa)'93; MB ChB; CCFP; Langs: Hebrew; Russian; (905)764-0005; Fax. (905)764-0044; summeridgehealth@gmail.com.

FORMAN, Noah A; North York Med Arts Bldg, 333-1333 Sheppard Ave E, North York ON M2J 1V1; McM'84; CCFP; FCFP; Staff, North York General Hospital; Chief Medical Officer, Toronto Fire Services; Med Dir, Toronto Maple Leafs Hockey Club; Staff Teacher, University of Toronto; Langs: Hebrew; (416)498-7007; Fax. (416)499-9669; dr.noahforman@rogers.blackberry.net.

FORMAN, Paul; Summeridge Health Centre, 26-8707 Dufferin St, Thornhill ON L4J 0A2; Witwatersrand (South Africa)'93; CCFP; (905)764-0005; Fax. (905)764-0044.

FORMAN, Rachel A; Fertility & Reproductive Med, 317-2330 Kennedy Rd, Scarborough ON M1T 0A2; Tor'96; FRCSC; ObstGyn. (416)609-8868; Fax. (416)609-8711.

FORMOSO, Alfredo F; Merivale Med Imaging Inc, 1370 Clyde Ave, Nepean ON K2G 3H8; Santo Tomas (Philippines)'72; FRCPC; DiagRad. Ac Staff, The Ottawa Hospital - Civic Campus; Consultant, Winchester District Memorial Hospital; Consultant, Arnprior & District Memorial Hospital; Teacher, University of Ottawa; Langs: Tagalog; (613)727-1072

FORNASIER, Frank; Joseph Brant Mem Hosp, 1230 North Shore Blvd, Burlington ON L7S 1W7; Ott'89; CCFP; FCFP; Staff, Joseph Brant Memorial Hospital; Langs: Italian; Spanish; French; (905)632-3737

FORNASIER, Victor; Eglinton Diagnostic Labs, 100-4040 Finch Ave E, Scarborough ON M1S 4V5; Tor'62; FACP; FRCPC; GenPath (Arthritis). Prof, St Michael's Hospital; Prof, Eglinton Medical Laboratories; Prof Lab Med & Path Physiol, University of Toronto; Langs: Italian; (416)292-0222; Fax. (416)292-5814; vmfornasier@aol.com.

FORNAZZARI, Luis R; St Michael's Hosp, 17F-30 Bond St, Toronto ON M5B 1W8; (Chile)'68; FRCPC; Neur (Memory Disorders). Consultant NeuroPsy, North Simcoe Family Health Team; Staff, St Michael's Hospital; Langs: Spanish; Italian; (416)864-6060; Fax. (416)864-5480.

FORNAZZARI, Ximena; 1206-180 Bloor St W, Toronto ON M5S 2V6; Santiago (Chile)'68; FRCPC; Psy. (416)920-4217

FOROODI, Farin; Halton HSC Corp-Oakville, 327 Reynolds St, Oakville ON L6J 3L7; McM'99; CCFP; Staff, Halton Healthcare Services Corporation - Oakville Site; Asst Clin Prof, McMaster University; Langs: Persian; (905)845-2571

FOROOGHIAN, Farzin; 300-1343 Lonsdale Ave, North Vancouver BC V7M 2H7; Alb'01; FRCSC; Ophth (Clinician Investigator Program). (604)985-0405

FOROUZANDEH, Fariba; Carberry Plain Health Centre, PO Box 2000 220 1st Ave, Carberry MB R0K 0H0; Staff, Carberry Plains Health Centre; (204)834-2144

FOROUZESH, Bahram; Cape Breton Healthcare Complex, 1482 George St, Sydney NS B1P 1P3; Tehran (Iran)'71; Staff, Cape Breton Healthcare Complex; (902)567-8000

FORREST, Christopher R; The Hosp for Sick Children, 5430-555 University Ave, Toronto ON M5G 1X8; Tor'83; FRCSC; PlasSurg (Cranio Maxillofacial & Aesthetic Surgery). Head PlasSurg/Med Dir, The Hospital For Sick Children; Staff Consultant, Sunnybrook Health Sciences Centre; Staff, Sunnybrook Health Sciences Centre - Edmond Odette Cancer Centre; Assoc Prof, University of Toronto; (416)813-8659; Fax. (416)813-6637; christopher.forrest@sickkids.ca.

FORREST, David M; Nanaimo Reg Gen Hosp, 1200 Dufferin Cres, Nanaimo BC V9S 2B7; Alb'85; BSc(Med); MHSc; FRCPC; IntMed; Critical Care Medicine; InfectDis. Dep Asst, Nanaimo Regional General Hospital; Researcher, BC Centre for Excellence in HIV/AIDS; (250)754-2141

FORREST, Donna L; 10F-2775 Laurel St, Vancouver BC V5Z 1M9; Man'89; FRCPC; IntMed; Hem. Staff, Vancouver General Hospital - Centennial Pavillion; (604)875-5270; dforrest@bccancer.bc.ca.

FORREST, Ian; 406-4430 Bathurst St, North York ON M3H 3S3; Dal'80; FRCSC; GenSurg; VascSurg. Staff Vascular Surg, Sunnybrook Health Sciences Centre; Staff Vascular & Gen Surg, North York General Hospital; (416)250-6822; Fax. (416)250-6830.

FORREST, Paul R; Abbotsford Reg Hosp & Cancer C, 32900 Marshall Rd, Abbotsford BC V2S 0C2; Tor'66; FRCPC; Anes. Assoc Staff, Abbotsford Regional Hospital & Cancer Centre; (604)851-4873; prf@uniserve.com.

FORREST, Shelley L; Rocky Mountain Health Centre, PO Box 2019, Fernie BC V0B 1M0; UBC'88; BSc; CCFP; Med Staff, Elk Valley Hospital; Clin Instructor, University of British Columbia; (250)423-4718; Fax. (250)423-6463.

FORRESTER, Dennis H G; Med Assoc Of Port Credit, 2F-333 Lakeshore Rd W, Mississauga ON L5H 1G9; Tor'78; CCFP; FCFP; Court Staff, The Credit Valley Hospital; Clin Prof Adjunct Family Med, McMaster University; Clin Prof Adjunct Dept of Family Med, University of Toronto; (905)274-7044; Fax. (905)274-0227.

FORRESTER, James C; Wellington Med Clinic, 84D-3200 North Island Hwy, Nanaimo BC V9T 1W1; Virgina (USA)'82; CCFP; (250)740-2100; Fax. (250)585-4033; strider3700@gmail.com.

FORRESTER, Robert D; Vivacare Med Clinic, 3122 Mt Lehman Rd, Abbotsford BC V2T 0C5; Edinburgh (Scotland)'75; (604)381-4102

FORSBERG, Tracy L; West Coast Family Med Clinic, 1300-6660 Sooke Rd, Sooke BC V9Z 1H4; UBC'02; BSc; CCFP; (250)642-4233; staff@sookefamilydocs.com.

FORSE, Bertram; Markham Stouffville Health Ctr, 310-377 Church St, Markham ON L6B 1A1; McG'82; Staff, Markham Stouffville Hospital; Staff, Markham Stouffville Health Centre; Langs: English; French; (905)472-5900; Fax. (905)472-2004.

FORSE, Monique I S; Markham Stouffville Health Ctr, 310-377 Church St, Markham ON L6B 1A1; McG'82; MDCM; FRCPC; IntMed (Sleep Medicine); Respir. Ac Staff, Markham Stouffville Hospital; (905)472-5900; mforse@msh.on.ca.

FORSE, Raymond A; C M P A, PO Box 8225 Stn T Csc, Ottawa ON K1G 3H7; Qns'91; FACS; FRCSC; GenSurg (Hepatobiliary & Pancreatic Surgery)., Hôtel-Dieu Grace Hospital; Langs: French.

FORSEY, Robert G P; Labrador Grenfell Health, PO Box 7000 Stn C 227 Hamilotn River Rd, Happy-Valley-Goose NL A0P 1C0; Mem'87; CCFP; FCFP; Staff, Labrador Health Centre; Clin Asst Prof, Memorial University Of Newfoundland; (709)897-2135; Fax. (709)896-4607.

FORSHNER, David; 11887 Hwy 8 PO Box 246, Pugwash NS B0K 1L0; Dal'71; Staff, All Saints Springhill Hospital; (902)243-2194; Fax. (902)257-3600.

FORSON, Agatha A; 31 Fourth St E, Cornwall ON K6H 2H7; (England)'68; (613)938-8333; Fax. (613)938-7165.

FORSON, Thomas E; 31 Fourth St E, Cornwall ON K6H 2H7; (England)'68; Langs: Ghanaian; (613)938-8333; Fax. (613)938-8336.

FORSTER, A Bruce B; UBC Dept of Radiology, 3350-950 12th Ave W, Vancouver BC V5Z 4E3; UBC'85; MSc; FRCPC; DiagRad. Staff, UBC Hospital - Koerner Pavillion; Assoc Prof/Dept Head & School Dir Radiology, University of British Columbia; (604)875-4111 x68022

FORSTER, Alan; The Ottawa Hosp-Civic Campus, 1053 Carling Ave Box 684, Ottawa ON K1Y 4E9; Ott'94; MSc; FRCPC; IntMed. Staff, The Ottawa Hospital - Civic Campus; Sr Scientist, The Ottawa Hospital-Research Institute; Assoc Prof, University of Ottawa; (613)798-5555 x12777; Fax. (613)761-5492; aforster@ohri.ca.

FORSTER, D Ian M; Meadowlark Health Centre, 154 Meadowlark Shopping Ctr NW, Edmonton AB T5R 5W9; Birmingham (England)'67; MB ChB; MRCS; LRCP; ASAM; Staff, Wainwright Health Centre; Med Dir, Lifemark Health Institute; (780)429-4761; Fax. (780)425-4274.

FORSTER, Dwight G; 1902 Richmond Rd, Victoria BC V8R 4R2; Cal'79; (250)595-7644

FORSTER, James H; E-7105 Saanich Rd W, Brentwood Bay BC V8M 1P7; Queen's (Ireland)'78; CCFP; Ac Staff, Saanich Peninsula Hospital; (250)652-4457; Fax. (250)652-4831; drjhforster@telus.net.

FORSTER, Lisa; 7A-389 Main St, Picton ON K0K 2T0; Qns'02; BSc; CCFP; Langs: Bilingual(English/French); (613)476-5744; Fax. (613)476-8773.

FORSTER-GIBSON, Cynthia; The Credit Valley Hosp, 2200 Eglinton Ave W, Mississauga ON L5M 2N1; Wes'90; PhD; Staff, The Credit Valley Hospital; (905)813-4104; Fax. (905)813-4347.

FORSYTH, Robert D; Surrey Mem Hosp, 13750 96 Ave, Surrey BC V3V 1Z2; Alb'98; CCFP; CCFP(E.M.); Staff, Surrey Memorial Hospital; (604)581-2211

FORSYTH, Sara J; 260-6180 Blundell Rd, Richmond BC V7C 4W7; UBC'02; CCFP; Clin Instructor, University of British Columbia; (604)277-3421

FORSYTH, Scott C; Oak Bay Med Centre, 159-2515 90 Ave SW, Calgary AB T2V 0L8; Cal'99; BSc; LLB; CCFP; (403)281-2020; Fax. (403)281-7785.

FORSYTHE, Caroline M; Children's & Women's HC of BC, 207-4480 Oak St, Vancouver BC V6H 3V4; Dal'05; FRCSC; OrthSurg. Staff, BC Children's Hospital; (604)875-2054

FORSYTHE, Michael E; Professional Arts Bldg, 414-100 Arden St, Moncton NB E1C 4B7; Dal'98; FRCSC; OrthSurg. (506)857-4074

FORSYTHE, Michael G; Professional Arts Bldg, 414-100 Arden St, Moncton NB E1C 4B7; Dal'71; FACS; AB; FRCSC; OrthSurg (Medico Legal Issues). Ac Staff, The Moncton Hospital; Staff, Dr Georges-L-Dumont University Hospital Centre; Staff, St Joseph's Hospital; Clin Instructor Surg, Dalhousie University; (506)857-4074; Fax. (506)857-0293.

FORSYTHE, Pamela; St John Reg Hosp, PO Box 2100 Stn Main 400 University Ave, Saint John NB E2L 4L2; Dal'78; FRCPC; Psy (Community Psychiatry). Staff, Saint John Regional Hospital; Clinical Asst Prof, Memorial University Of Newfoundland; Asst Prof/Dir Student Affairs Dalhousie Medicine New Brunswick, Dalhousie University; (506)648-7919; Fax. (506)635-1614; pamela.forsythe@horizonnb.ca.

FORT, Diana K; Penticton Reg Hosp, 550 Carmi Ave, Penticton BC V2A 3G6; Qns'98; FRCPC; EmergMed. Staff, Penticton Regional Hospital; (250)492-4000

FORT, Stephen; Cardiology Associates, 2606 Pandosy St, Kelowna BC V1Y 1V6; Leeds (England)'84; MB ChB; FRCPC; IntMed; Cardiol. Staff, Queen Elizabeth II Health Sciences Centre - Halifax Infirmary Site; (250)762-9211

FORTE, Milena F; 4F-60 Murray St Box 25, Toronto ON M5T 3L9; Wes'98; CCFP; Staff, Mount Sinai Hospital; Langs: Italian; French; (416)586-4800 x5155

FORTE, Vito; The Hosp For Sick Children, 6183-555 University Ave, Toronto ON M5G 1X8; Tor'80; FRCSC; Otol. Staff, The Hospital For Sick Children; Staff Teacher, University of Toronto; (416)813-6767; Fax. (416)813-5036; vito.forte@sickkids.ca.

FORTIER, Andre J; 200-1760 boul Jacques-Cartier, Longueuil QC J4N 1C2; Laval'77; FRCSC; ObstGyn. Staff, Centre Hospitalier Pierre Boucher; (450)468-2151; Fax. (450)468-3309; andrej.fortier@videotron.ca.

FORTIER, Anne; GMF de Saint-Donat, 377 rue du Foyer CP 760, St-Donat-De-Mtcalm QC J0T 2C0; Mon'82; (819)424-1511; Fax. (819)424-4682.

FORTIER, Anne M; 39-1111 Davis Dr, Newmarket ON L3Y 8X2; Wes'03; FRCSC; ObstGyn. Staff, Southlake Regional Health Centre; Staff, St Joseph's Healthcare - Charlton Campus; Staff, Mackenzie Richmond Hill Hospital; (905)853-1212; Fax. (905)853-1214.

FORTIER, Anne-Marie; Clin Externe Psychiatrie, 580 rue Bowen S, Sherbrooke QC J1G 2E8; Sher'95; FRCPC; Psy. Staff, Centre Hospitalier d'Argenteuil; (819)346-1110 x26535

FORTIER, Christopher; Mackenzie Richmond Hill Hosp, 10 Trench St, Richmond Hill ON L4C 4Z3; Qns'03; CCFP; CCFP(E.M.); Staff, Mackenzie Richmond Hill Hospital; (905)883-1212

FORTIER, Claude; 925 av Antonine-Maillet, Outremont QC H2V 2Y8; Mon'62; Psy (P.Q.). Staff, Hôpital du Sacre-Coeur de Montréal; (514)270-7871; Fax. (514)278-4435; cfort@videotron.ca.

FORTIER, David; CHUM-Hop Notre-Dame, 1560 rue Sherbrooke E, Montreal QC H2L 4M1; Sher'05; CCFP; Staff, Centre Hospitalier l'Université de Montréal (CHUM) - Hôpital Notre-Dame; (514)890-8000 x24444

FORTIER, Denis C J; Notre Dame Health Centre, PO Box 130 44 Rogers St, Notre-Dame-Lr MB R0G 1M0; Man'85; BSc(Med.); CCFP; FCFP; Staff/Reg Chief of Staff, Notre Dame Hospital; Teach Staff Family Med, University of Manitoba; Langs: French; (204)248-2252; Fax. (204)248-2087; dfortier@mts.net.

FORTIER, Elise; CSSS de Trois-Rivières, 1991 boul du Carmel, Trois-Rivieres QC G8Z 3R9; Mon'08; CCFP; Staff, CSSS de Trois-Rivières; (819)697-3333

FORTIER, Gerald; Clin Med R Gagnon et G Fortier, 2231 rue de l'Hopital, Jonquiere QC G7X 9Y4; Mon'70; (418)542-8153; Fax. (418)542-8151.

FORTIER, Ghyslain; CSSS du Suroît, 150 rue Saint-Thomas, Salaber-de-Valleyf QC J6T 6C1; Laval'95; CSPQ; FRCPC; Anes (General). Staff, Centre Hospitalier Régional du Suroît; Langs: Bilingual(French/English); (450)371-9920 x2141; Fax. (450)373-9239.

FORTIER, Ginette; CLSC du Marigot, 1351 boul des Laurentides, Vimont QC H7M 2Y2; Mon'74; Staff, Hôpital du Sacre-Coeur de Montréal; (450)668-1803; Fax. (450)668-1507.

FORTIER, Guylaine; CSSS Du Lac Des Deux Montagnes, 250 boul Arthur-Sauve, Saint-Eustache QC J7R 5B1; Laval'86; Staff, CSSS Du Lac Des Deux Montagnes; (450)473-6811

FORTIER, Isabelle; CSSS de Beauce-Etchemin, 1515 17e rue, Saint-Georges QC G5Y 4T8; Laval'06; Staff, Centre Hospitalier Beauce-Etchemin; (418)228-2031

FORTIER, Joanne D; Chum-Hotel-Dieu, 3840 rue Saint-Urbain, Montreal QC H2W 1T8; Mon'85; CSPQ; FRCPC; Anes. Staff, Centre Hospitalier l'Université de Montréal (CHUM) - Hôtel-Dieu; (514)890-8000 x14570; Fax. (514)412-7222.

FORTIER, Josee; Clin de Rhumatologie du Quebec, 1119 rue Sainte-Marguerite, Trois-Rivieres QC G8Z 1Y2; Laval'93; FRCPC; PhysMed&Rehab. Staff, Centre Hospitalier Regional de Trois-Rivieres; Staff, Clinique Rhumatologie du Quebec; (819)370-8106; Fax. (819)370-8120.

FORTIER, Karine; Clin Med du Grand Boulevard, 200-353 boul des Bois-Francs S, Victoriaville QC G6P 4T2; Sher'04; Staff, Hotel-Dieu d'Arthabaska; (819)751-3006; Fax. (819)751-6625.

FORTIER, Katie; 1971 rue Bilodeau, Plessisville QC G6L 3J1; Laval'08; CCFP; (819)362-6337

FORTIER, Liliane; Clinique Med McDermott, 37 av Donegani, Pointe-Claire QC H9R 2V7; Mon'81; CCFP; FCFP; (514)697-1410; Fax. (514)697-1411.

FORTIER, Louis-Philippe; Hop Maisonneuve-Rosemont, 5415 boul de l'Assomption, Montreal QC H1T 2M4; Mon'95; CSPQ; FRCPC; Anes. Staff, Hopital Maisonneuve-Rosemont; (514)252-3426; Fax. (514)252-3542.

FORTIER, Martin; Ctr Hosp du Centre la Mauricie, 50 119e rue, Shawinigan-Sud QC G9P 5K1; Sher'00; CCFP; CCFP(E.M.); Staff, Centre Hospitalier du Centre la Mauricie; (819)536-7575

FORTIER, Michel; Centre Med Berger, 304-1000 ch Sainte-Foy, Quebec QC G1S 2L6; Laval'70; FRCSC; ObstGyn (Menopause). Ac Staff, Centre Hospitalier Affilié Universitaire de Québec - Hôpital du St-Sacrement; (418)266-1616; Fax. (418)650-1374.

FORTIER, Pierre; 3C-520 boul de l'Hôpital, Gatineau QC J8V 2P5; McG'77; CCFP; Consultant Emerg, Hull Hospital; Physician, CH Chandler; Assoc Member, CH Pontiac; Assoc Member, CH Maniwaki; Langs: English; (819)777-6664; Fax. (819)777-0138.

FORTIER, Pierre-Hugues; CHUS-Hop Hotel-Dieu, 580 rue Bowen S, Sherbrooke QC J1G 2E8; Sher'99; FRCSC; Otol (Cervico Facial Oncology). Staff, Centre Hospitalier Universitaire de Sherbrooke-Hôpital Hôtel-Dieu; (819)346-1110 x14901; Fax. (819)564-5449; pierre-hugues.fortier@usherbrooke.ca.

FORTIER, Robert; CHUS-Hop Hotel-Dieu, 580 rue Bowen S, Sherbrooke QC J1G 2E8; Mon'66; Staff, Centre Hospitalier Universitaire de Sherbrooke-Hôpital Hôtel-Dieu; (819)346-1110

FORTIER, Serge; CSSS de Trois-Rivières, 1991 boul du Carmel, Trois-Rivieres QC G8Z 3R9; Laval'83; FRCSC; Urol. Staff, CSSS de Trois-Rivières; (819)697-3333 x63295; forturo@videotron.ca.

FORTIER, Simon; CSSS du Sud de Lanaudière, 911 montee des Pionniers, Terrebonne QC J6V 2H2; Mon'99; CCFP; Staff, Centre Hospitalier Pierre le Gardeur; (450)654-7525

FORTIER, Ychelle; CSSS des Îles, 430 ch Principal, Cap-aux-Meules QC G4T 1R9; Mon'08; Staff, Hôpital de l'Archipel; (418)986-2121 x8178

FORTIER, Yves; Ctr Radiology Sherbrooke Inc, 250 rue King E, Sherbrooke QC J1G 1A9; Sher'76; DiagRad (P.Q.). Staff, Centre Hospitalier Universitaire de Sherbrooke-Hôpital Hôtel-Dieu; (819)563-1443

FORTIER-RIBERDY, Annie; CSSS du Nord de Lanaudière, 1000 boul Sainte-Anne, St-Charles-Brromee QC J6E 6J2; Sher'99; Staff, Centre Hospitalier Régional de Lanaudière; (450)759-8222

FORTIER-RIBERDY, Genevieve; CHUM-Hotel-Dieu, 3840 rue Saint-Urbain, Montreal QC H2W 1T8; Mon'95; FRCPC; Derm. Staff, Centre Hospitalier l'Université de Montréal (CHUM) - Hôtel-Dieu; (514)890-8162; Fax. (514)412-7235.

FORTIN, Amanda J; 1142-41 Ramsey Lake Rd, Sudbury ON P3E 5J1; Cal'00; FRCSC; PlasSurg. Staff, London Health Sciences Centre - University Hospital; (705)523-7060; Fax. (705)523-7061.

FORTIN, Andre; CHUQ-Hotel-Dieu de Quebec, 11 Cote du Palais, Quebec QC G1R 2J6; Laval'88; FRCPC; RadOncol; DiagRad (P.Q.). Staff, Centre Hospitalier Universitaire de Québec (CHUQ) - Siege Social; (418)691-5264; Fax. (418)691-5268; afortin@videotron.ca.

FORTIN, Andre; Clinique Med Fam des Recollets, 101-940 boul des Recollets, Trois-Rivieres QC G8Z 3W9; Laval'87; Staff, CSSS de Trois-Rivières; (819)373-0303; Fax. (819)373-8431.

FORTIN, Ann; Inst Nat'l de Sante Publique, 190 boul Cremazie E, Montreal QC H2P 1E2; McG'85; Médecin, Institut National de Sante Publique du Quebec; (514)864-1600

FORTIN, Anne; Maternity & Gynecology Centre, 1811 av Dollard, Lasalle QC H8N 1T9; Sher'75; FAB; FACOG; FRCSC; ObstGyn. Staff, Centre Hospitalier de LaSalle; Staff, CSSS de Dorval-Lachine-Lasalle; Staff, McGill University Health Centre - Royal Victoria Hospital; Physician, Maternity & Gynecology Centre; Langs: English; (514)364-3700; Fax. (514)364-9866.

FORTIN, Anne-Karine; Direction de la Santé publique, 210-1000 rue Labelle, Saint-Jerome QC J7Z 5N6; McG'94; (450)436-8622 x3228; Fax. (450)436-1761.

FORTIN, Benoit; CLSC Cote-des-Neiges, 6600 ch de la Cote-des-Neiges, Montreal QC H3S 2A9; Laval'72; Médecin, CLSC Cote-des-Neiges.

FORTIN, Bernard; 5415 boul de l'Assomption, Montreal QC H1T 2M4; Mon'94; MSc; FRCPC; RadOncol (Epidemiology). Staff, Hopital Maisonneuve-Rosemont; Langs: English; French; (514)252-3400; bfortin.hmr@ssss.gouv.qc.ca.

FORTIN, Carole; CLSC Des Seigneuries de Bouche, 201-160 boul de Montarville, Boucherville QC J4B 6S2; Mon'92; CCFP; (450)655-3630; Fax. (450)449-6379.

FORTIN, Celine; CSSS de Portneuf, 3 rue du Jardin, Pont-Rouge QC G3H 0A8; Laval'92; CCFP; FCFP; Staff, Centre Hospitalier Portneuf; Langs: Bilingual(French/English); (418)873-6062; Fax. (418)873-6064; celinefortin@ssss.gouv.qc.ca.

FORTIN, Charles; Ctr Hosp Anna-Laberge, 200 boul Brisebois, Chateauguay QC J6K 4W8; Mon'05; IntMed. Staff, Hôpital Anna-Laberge; (450)699-2425

FORTIN, Christian; 2222 rue Saint-Jean-Baptiste, Jonquiere QC G8A 1V8; Laval'76; Staff, Complexe hospitalier de la Sagamie; (418)542-8808

FORTIN, Christian; La Cite Medicale, 295-2600 boul Laurier, Quebec QC G1V 4T3; Laval'73; (418)781-0635

FORTIN, Christian D; Bayrest Centre for Geriatric C, 3560 Bathurst St, Toronto ON M6A 2E1; Wes'09; (416)785-2500

FORTIN, Claude A; Maternity & Gynecology Centre, 1811 av Dollard, Lasalle QC H8N 1T9; Laval'72; FACOG; FRCSC; ObstGyn (Endoscopy). Staff, Maternity & Gynecology Centre; Teacher, McGill University; Langs: English; (514)364-3700; Fax. (514)364-9866.

FORTIN, Claude; CHUM-Hop Notre-Dame, 1560 rue Sherbrooke E, Montreal QC H2L 4M1; Mon'97; BSc(Biol.); FRCPC; MedMicrobiol (AIDS/HIV); Microbio & Infect Dis (P.Q.). Staff, Centre Hospitalier l'Université de Montréal (CHUM) - Hôpital Notre-Dame; (514)890-8000 x25103

FORTIN, Come; GMF Centre Med du Parc, 101-84 rue Court, Granby QC J2G 4Y5; Sher'79; AB; Ophth. Staff, Centre Hospitalier de Granby; (450)375-2074; Fax. (450)375-8719.

FORTIN, Dalilah; London HSC-Victoria Hosp, PO Box 5010 Stn B E-120-800 Commissioners Rd E, London ON N6A 5W9; Laval'98; FRCSC; GenSurg (Critical Care Medicine); ThorSurg. Asst Prof Surg, London Health Sciences Centre - Victoria Campus; Langs: Bilingual(English/French); (519)685-8777; Fax. (519)685-8778.

FORTIN, Daniele; CLSC Saint-Henri, 3833 rue Notre-Dame O, Montreal QC H4C 1P8; Laval'80; (514)933-7541; Fax. (514)933-1740.

FORTIN, Danielle; CSSS Maria-Chapdelaine, 2000 boul du Sacre-Coeur, Dolbeau-Mistassini QC G8L 2R5; Laval'93; FRCPC; Peds. Staff, Centre Maria-Chapdelaine - CH de Dolbeau-Mistassini; (418)276-1234; Fax. (418)276-8747.

FORTIN, David; CHUS-Hop Fleurimont, 3001 12e av N, Sherbrooke QC J1H 5N4; Sher'91; FRCSC; Neursurg (Neuro Oncology). Staff, Centre Hospitalier Universitaire de Sherbrooke-Hopital Fleurimont; assoc Prof, Universite de Sherbrooke; (819)346-1110 x13324; Fax. (819)820-6452; david.fortin@usherbrooke.ca.

FORTIN, Denis; Clinique de Gynecologie, 24 rue Melancon E, Alma QC G8B 6W3; Laval'80; ObstGyn. Staff, CSSS de Lac-Saint Jean-Est; (418)662-6553; Fax. (418)662-3731.

FORTIN, Dominique; CHUQ-Ctr Hosp Univ Laval, 2705 boul Laurier, Quebec QC G1V 4G2; Laval'85; FRCPC; DiagRad (Echography). Staff Radiol, Centre Hospitalier Universitaire de Quebec-CHUL; (418)654-2258; Fax. (418)654-2260.

FORTIN, Dominique; CHUQ-St-Francois D'Assise, 10 rue de l'Espinay, Quebec QC G1L 3L5; Laval'96; CCFP; CCFP(E.M.); FCFP; Staff Emerg, Centre Hospitalier Universitaire De Québec - Pavillon De St-françois-d'assise; Teach Staff, Université Laval; (418)525-4444; dr.fortin@videotron.ca.

FORTIN, Eric; Hop Maisonneuve-Rosemont, 5415 boul de l'Assomption, Montreal QC H1T 2M4; Laval'91; FRCSC; Ophth (Uveitis). Specialist Uveitis & Immunol Ocular, Hopital Maisonneuve-Rosemont; Staff, Hôpital Ste-Justine; Asst Prof Ophth, Universite de Montreal; (514)252-3878; Fax. (514)252-3905.

FORTIN, Frederick; CSSS Maria-Chapdelaine, 2000 boul du Sacre-Coeur, Dolbeau-Mistassini QC G8L 2R5; Mon'06; CCFP; Staff, Centre Maria-Chapdelaine - CH de Dolbeau-Mistassini; (418)276-1234; Fax. (418)276-4355.

FORTIN, Gilles; Clinique Med de Montmagny, 100-83 av de la Fabrique, Montmagny QC G5V 2J3; Laval'89; (418)248-4933; Fax. (418)248-2778; gilles.fortin@gmf.gouv.qc.ca.

FORTIN, Gilles W; CSSSG-Hop de Hull, 116 boul Lionel-Emond, Gatineau QC J8Y 1W7; Mon'70; Staff Emerg, Hull Hospital; (819)595-6000

FORTIN, Guy; CLSC-CHSLD La Source, 190 76e rue E, Quebec QC G1H 7K4; Laval'76; (418)628-2572

FORTIN, Helene; Complexe Sante Reine-Elizabeth, 337-2100 av Marlowe, Montreal QC H4A 3L5; Mon'84; FRCPC; Psy. Staff, Douglas Mental Health University Institute; (514)388-6232; hformdpsyexparb@aol.com.

FORTIN, Henriete; CSSSG-Hop de Gatineau, CP 2000 Succ Bureau-Chef 909 boul de la Verendrye O, Gatineau QC J8P 7H2; Sher'93; Peds. Staff, Hôpital de Gatineau; (819)561-8565; Fax. (819)561-8103.

FORTIN, Isabelle; Ctr de Rhum del Est du Quebec, 176 av Rouleau, Rimouski QC G5L 8W1; Mon'96; Rheum (P.Q.); IntMed. Dir serv de Rheum, Hôpital Regional Rimouski; Prés, Centre de Rhumatologie del Est des Quebec; Langs: English; (418)723-2445; Fax. (418)721-2271; creq@live.ca.

FORTIN, J B Christian; 44 av Argyle, Saint-Lambert QC J4P 2H4; Mon'73; CSPQ; Cardiol (P.Q.). Staff, Hopital Charles LeMoyne; Langs: English; (450)465-0697; Fax. (450)466-2785.

FORTIN, Jean; Clin Medicale Ciggard, 210-3333 rue du Carrefour, Quebec QC G1C 5R9; Laval'81; Clin Teach Staff, Université Laval; (418)663-6345

FORTIN, Jean-Claude; College des Med du Quebec, 2170 boul Rene-Levesque O, Montreal QC H3H 2T8; Laval'72; LMCC; Membre, College des Medecins du Quebec; (514)933-4441; Fax. (514)533-2291; jfortin@cmq.org.

FORTIN, Jean-Paul; Centre de Sante Publique, 2400 av D'Estimauville, Quebec QC G1E 7G9; Laval'70; MPH; MBA; FRCPC; CommunMed (P.Q.); Public Health & Preventive Med. Assoc Prof Social & Preventive Med, Université Laval; (418)681-8787 x3807; Fax. (418)687-9694; jpfortin@msp.ulaval.ca.

FORTIN, Jerome; Hop Maisonneuve-Rosemont, 5415 boul l'Assomption, Montreal QC H1T 2M4; Mon'07; FRCPC; EmergMed. Staff, Hopital Maisonneuve-Rosemont; (514)252-3400

FORTIN, Josee-Anne; CHUM-Hop Notre-Dame, 1560 rue Sherbrooke E, Montreal QC H2L 4M1; Mon'96; CSPQ; FRCPC; Anes. Staff, Centre Hospitalier l'Université de Montréal (CHUM) - Hôpital Notre-Dame; (514)890-8000 x26876

FORTIN, Josee-Melanie; Ctr Hosp Affilie-Enfant-Jesus, 1401 18e rue, Quebec QC G1J 1Z4; Laval'06; CCFP; Staff, Centre Hospitalier Affilié Universitaire de Québec - Hôpital De L'Enfant Jésus; (418)649-0252

FORTIN, Julie; CLSC Rimouski-Gouverneurs UMF, 165 rue des Gouverneurs, Rimouski QC G5L 7R2; Laval'90; CCFP; FCFP; Assoc Member, Hôpital Regional Rimouski; Teach Staff Family Med, Université Laval; (418)727-5493; Fax. (418)723-7668; julie.fortin@globetrotter.net.

FORTIN, Louise; CLSC Mercier-Est/Anjou, 9503 rue Sherbrooke E, Montreal QC H1L 6P2; Sher'89; (514)356-2574 x3142; Fax. (514)356-1838.

FORTIN, Louise; Ctr Hosp Fleury, 2180 rue Fleury E, Montreal QC H2B 1K3; Mon'74; FRCPC; IntMed. Assoc Member, CSSS du Coeur de l'Isle Hôpital Jean-Talon; Staff, Centre Hospitalier Fleury; adj Prof, Universite de Montreal; (514)384-2000 x5252; louisefortin2004@hotmail.com.

FORTIN, Luc; Institut de Physiatrie Quebec, 2049 rue Sherbrooke E, Montreal QC H2K 1C1; Mon'73; MSc; FRCPC; PhysMed&Rehab. ac Staff, Centre Hospitalier l'Université de Montréal (CHUM) - Hôpital Notre-Dame; Clinical Asst Prof Phys Program, Universite de Montreal; Langs: Bilingual(French/English); (514)527-4155; Fax. (514)598-9963; fortinmsc@videotron.ca.

FORTIN, Luc; CSSS de Lac-Saint Jean-Est, CP 1300 Succ Bureau-Chef 300 boul Champlain S, Alma QC G8B 5W3; Laval'90; Staff, CSSS de Lac-Saint Jean-Est; (418)669-2000

FORTIN, Lucie; Clin Ext Psych Sainte-Therese, 2F-55 rue Saint-Joseph, Sainte-Therese QC J7E 4Y5; Mon'85; FRCPC; Psy. Staff, Hôtel-Dieu de Saint-Jérôme; Langs: Bilingual(French/English); (450)430-3702; Fax. (450)430-6648; lfort44@videotron.ca.

FORTIN, Marc; 205-2075 boul Mellon, Jonquiere QC G7S 5Z8; Laval'90; (418)548-0909

FORTIN, Marc; CSSS de Chicoutimi, 305 rue Saint-Vallier, Chicoutimi QC G7H 5H6; Laval'80; CSPQ; FRCPC; Anes. Ac Staff, Complexe hospitalier de la Sagamie; (418)541-1000

FORTIN, Marcel; Clin Med de Metabetchouan, 20 rue Saint-Basile, Metab-L-A-La-Croix QC G8G 1S9; Laval'74; Staff OPD & Emerg, CSSS de Lac-Saint Jean-Est; (418)349-8757; Fax. (418)349-8082.

FORTIN, Marie-Andree; CICL-Cite de la Sante de Laval, 1895 boul Rene-Laennec, Laval QC H7M 5E2; Sher'96; FRCPC; RadOncol. Staff, Centre Hospitalier l'Université de Montréal (CHUM) - Hôpital Notre-Dame; (450)668-1010 x24683

FORTIN, Marie-Chantal; CHUM-Hop Notre-Dame, 1560 rue Sherbrooke E, Montreal QC H2L 4M1; Sher'97; FRCPC; IntMed; Nephrol. Staff, Centre Hospitalier l'Université de Montréal (CHUM) - Hôpital Notre-Dame; (514)890-8000 x26616

FORTIN, Marie-Eve; Hop Charles Lemoyne, 3120 boul Taschereau, Longueuil QC J4V 2H1; Mon'05; Psy. Staff, Hopital Charles LeMoyne; (450)466-5020

FORTIN, Marie-Pierre; Ctr Hosp Affilie-Enfant-Jesus, 1401 18e rue, Quebec QC G1J 1Z4; Laval'02; FRCPC; IntMed; GeriatricMed. Staff, Centre Hospitalier Affilié Universitaire de Québec - Hôpital De L'Enfant Jésus; (418)649-0252 x5521; Fax. (418)649-5507; mariefortin41@hotmail.com.

FORTIN, Marilyn; Hotel-Dieu de Levis, 143 rue Wolfe, Levis QC G6V 3Z1; Laval'00; FRCPC; Anes; Critical Care Medicine (P.Q.). Staff, Hôtel-Dieu de Lévis; (418)835-7121 x3218

FORTIN, Marquis; Clinique Med de Familiale, 6e-2120 rue Sherbrooke E, Montreal QC H2K 1C3; Sher'73; Staff, Centre Hospitalier l'Université de Montréal (CHUM) - Hôpital Notre-Dame; Prof, Universite de Montreal; (514)527-1958; Fax. (514)527-1649.

FORTIN, Martin; CSSS de Chicoutimi, CP 5006 DE-305 rue Saint-Vallier, Chicoutimi QC G7H 5H6; Sher'83; CCFP; FCFP; Ac Staff, Complexe hospitalier de la Sagamie; (418)511-1088; Fax. (418)511-1129.

FORTIN, Maude; CSSS du Lac-des-Deux-Montagnes, 520 boul Arthur-Sauve, Saint-Eustache QC J7R 5B1; Mon'10; CCFP; Staff, Hôpital de Saint-Eustache; (450)473-6811

FORTIN, Michel R; Ctr Hosp du Centre la Mauricie, 50 119e rue, Shawinigan-Sud QC G9P 5K1; Laval'82; ABOtol; CSPQ; FRCSC; Otol (Neuro Otology). Staff, Centre Hospitalier du Centre la Mauricie; Langs: English; (819)536-7500; Fax. (819)536-7619; m_r_fortin@yahoo.ca.

FORTIN, Michel-Andre; CSSS de la Haute Yamaska, 294 rue Deragon, Granby QC J2G 5J5; Mon'75; Assoc Staff, Centre Hospitalier de Granby; (450)375-1442; Fax. (450)375-6607.

FORTIN, Paul; CHUQ-Ctr Hosp Univ Laval, H 1365-2705 boul Laurier, Quebec QC G1V 4G2; Laval'84; MPH; FRCPC; IntMed (Systemic Lupus Erythematosus); Rheum. Clin Chercheur, Centre Hospitalier Universitaire de Quebec-CHUL; Prof, Université Laval; Langs: Bilingual(French/English); (418)654-2242; Fax. (418)654-2798; rhumatologie.chul@ens.chuq.qc.ca.

FORTIN, Pierre; Grand River Hosp-KW Hlth Ctre, PO Box 9056 Stn C 835 King St W, Kitchener ON N2G 1G3; Mon'96; FRCPC; RadOncol (Prostate Cancer). Staff Radiation Oncology, Grand River Hospital - Kitchener/Waterloo Health Centre; Langs: Bilingual(French/English); (519)749-4370 x5489; Fax. (519)749-4378.

FORTIN, Raymond; Clinique Med de Montmagny, 100-83 av de la Fabrique, Montmagny QC G5V 2J3; Laval'69; (418)248-4933; Fax. (418)248-2778; raymond.fortin@gmf.gouv.qc.ca.

FORTIN, Raymond-Yves; Serv Externe de Psychiatrie, 230-383 boul du Seminaire N, St-Jean-sur-Richel QC J3B 8C5; Mon'65; DPsy; FRCPC; Psy. Staff, Hopital Charles LeMoyne; (450)346-2222; Fax. (450)346-2311; yvanfortin@yahoo.com.

FORTIN, Richard; Polyclinique Med PAT, 103-12905 rue Sherbrooke E, Pte-aux-Trembles QC H1A 1B9; Sher'71.

FORTIN, Richard; Hotel-Dieu de Levis, 143 rue Wolfe, Levis QC G6V 3Z1; Laval'82; CSPQ; FRCPC; Anes. Staff, Hôtel-Dieu de Lévis; (418)835-7121; Fax. (418)835-3969.

FORTIN, Robin; CSSS Domaine du Roy, 450 rue Brassard, Roberval QC G8H 1B9; Sher'94; Staff, Hotel-Dieu de Roberval; (418)275-0110; Fax. (418)275-8087.

FORTIN, Simon; CSSS de Trois-Rivières, 1991 boul du Carmel, Trois-Rivieres QC G8Z 3R9; Sher'92; CSPQ; AnatPath. Staff, CSSS de Trois-Rivières; (819)697-3333 x63110; Fax. (819)371-5007.

FORTIN, Stephane; Clinique Med Chicoutimi-Nord, 2185 boul De Tadoussac, Chicoutimi QC G7G 4X2; Sher'94; (418)698-2414

FORTIN, Stephanie; CHUM-Hop Notre-Dame, 1560 rue Sherbrooke E, Montreal QC H2L 4M1; Mon'00; CCFP; CCFP(E.M.); Staff, Centre Hospitalier l'Université de Montréal (CHUM) - Hôpital Notre-Dame; (514)890-8000 x26767

FORTIN, Suzanne; Clinique Med de Touraine, 2B-520 boul de l'Hospital, Gatineau QC J8V 2P5; McG'89; Langs: English; (819)568-0212; Fax. (819)568-6310.

FORTIN, Suzanne; Hop Maisonneuve-Rosemont, 5415 boul de l'Assomption, Montreal QC H1T 2M4; Mon'03; FRCSC; ObstGyn (Gynecologic Oncology). Staff, Hopital Maisonneuve-Rosemont; (514)252-3400

FORTIN, Suzette; Centre Med Christ-Roi, 102-40 rte du President-Kenned, Levis QC G6V 6C4; Laval'81; FRCSC; ObstGyn. Staff, Hôtel-Dieu de Lévis; (418)833-4977

FORTIN, Sylvie; CSSS d'Antoine-Labelle-Mt Laur, GD 2561 ch Lievre St, Mont-Laurier QC J9L 3G3; Mon'85; Staff, CSSS d'Antoine-Labelle; (819)623-1234

FORTIN, Veronique; Clinique Med de la Baie, 437 rue Albert, La Baie QC G7B 3L5; Laval'95; (418)544-6863; Fax. (418)544-6864.

FORTIN, Veronique; Clin Med Riviere Du Moulin, 1388 boul du Saguenay E, Chicoutimi QC G7H 1G8; Laval'95; Staff, Complexe hospitalier de la Sagamie; (418)549-3564; Fax. (418)549-8463.

FORTIN, Veronique; CSSSG-Hop De Gatineau, CP 2000 Succ Bureau-Chef 909 boul de la Verendrye O, Gatineau QC J8P 7H2; Laval'05; FRCPC; Anes. Staff, Hôpital de Gatineau; (819)966-6100

FORTIN, Vincent; Hotel-Dieu de Levis, 143 rue Wolfe, Levis QC G6V 3Z1; Laval'03; DiagRad. Staff, Hôtel-Dieu de Lévis; (418)835-7121

FORTIN, William J; 103 3rd Ave SW PO Box 5322 Stn Main, High River AB T1V 1M5; Cal'05; Fam Med, High River General Hospital; (403)603-3100

FORTIN, Yvan; Westmount Square Med Centre, 300-1 Westmount Sq, Montreal QC H3Z 2P9; Ott'87; Staff, Carrefour Sante Granit; (514)934-2334

FORTIN, Yves; Clin Med Legendre, 201-1650 av Jules-Verne, Quebec QC G2G 2R1; Laval'80; (418)872-5600; Fax. (418)872-8408.

FORTIN-PELLERIN, Etienne; CHUS-Hop Fleurimont, 3001 12e av N, Sherbrooke QC J1H 5N4; Sher'07; Peds (Neonatal & Perinatal Medicine). Staff, Centre Hospitalier Universitaire de Sherbrooke-Hopital Fleurimont; (819)346-1110

FORTIN TRUCHON, Marie-Lea; Centre Hosp Rouyn-Noranda, 4 9e rue, Rouyn-Noranda QC J9X 2B2; Laval'07; CCFP; Staff, Centre Hospitalier Rouyn-Noranda; (819)764-5131

FORTUNA, Henry; Windsor Health Unit, 360-1720 Howard Ave, Windsor ON N8X 5A6; Qns'82; CCFP; FCFP; Att Staff, Hôtel-Dieu Grace Hospital; Att Staff, Windsor Regional Hospital - Metropolitan Site; (519)977-6226; Fax. (519)977-7914.

FORTUNA, Teresa; South Shore Reg Hosp, 90 Glen Allan Dr, Bridgewater NS B4V 3S6; Dal'05; Staff, South Shore Regional Hospital; (902)543-4603; Fax. (902)527-5269.

FORWARD, Karen; London HSC-Victoria Hosp, PO Box 5010 Stn B 800 Commissioners Rd E, London ON N6A 5W9; Dal'07; FRCPC; Peds. Staff, London Health Sciences Centre - Victoria Campus; (519)685-8500

FORWARD, Kevin R; Queen Elizabeth II HSC, 315-1276 South Park St, Halifax NS B3H 2Y9; Mem'75; BMedSci; FRCPC; IntMed; InfectDis; MedMicrobiol. Chief-Microbiol Infection, Queen Elizabeth II Health Sciences Centre - Victoria General Site; Prof Microbiol & Immunol Med & Path, Dalhousie University; (902)473-4109; Fax. (902)473-4432; kevin.forward@cdha.nshealth.ca.

FORWARD, Robert G; Health Sciences Centre, 300 Prince Philip Dr, St. John's NL A1B 3V6; Mem'88; FRCPC; Anes. Staff Anes, Health Sciences Centre; Clin Assoc Prof, Memorial University Of Newfoundland; (709)777-6540

FORWARD, Roland; James Paton Memorial Hosp, 125 Trans Canada Hwy, Gander NL A1V 1P7; Dal'73; Staff, James Paton Memorial Hospital; (709)256-2500

FORZLEY, Brian R; 110-2504 Skaha Lake Rd, Penticton BC V2A 6G1; Man'02; FRCPC; IntMed; Nephrol. (250)492-3511

FOSS, Sandra E; 250-8730 Country Hills Blvd NW, Calgary AB T3G 0E2; Alb'74; CCFP; FCFP; Court Staff, Foothills Medical Centre; (403)262-7787; Fax. (403)262-7786.

FOSSO SIEWE, Jean; Ctr Hosp Rouyn-Noranda, 4 9e rue, Rouyn-Noranda QC J9X 2B2; Cocody (South Africa)'99; Staff, Centre Hospitalier Rouyn-Noranda; (819)764-5131; Fax. (819)764-2929.

FOSTER, Bethany J; MUHC-Montreal Children's Hosp, 2300 rue Tupper, Montreal QC H3H 1P3; Ott'94; Nephrol; Peds. Staff, McGill University Health Centre - Montreal Children's Hospital; (514)412-4400; Fax. (514)412-4359.

FOSTER, David A; Hys Med Centre, 202-11010 101 St NW, Edmonton AB T5H 4B9; Alb'67; FRCPC; DiagRad. Staff, Royal Alexandra Hospital; (780)428-1121; Fax. (780)425-5979.

FOSTER, Heather P M; Medical Office, 219-840 Coxwell Ave, Toronto ON M4C 5T2; Mem'76; BMedSci; FRCPC; Peds. Staff Ped, Toronto East General Hospital Inc; (416)696-0003; Fax. (416)696-0022.

FOSTER, Jennifer R; London HSC-Victoria Hosp, PO Box 5010 Stn B C2 845-800 Commissioners Rd E, London ON N6A 5W9; Dal'03; FRCPC; Peds; Critical Care Medicine. Staff, London Health Sciences Centre - Victoria Campus; (519)685-8386; Fax. (519)685-8156.

FOSTER, Kenneth D; West Parry Sound Health Ctre, 6 Albert St, Parry Sound ON P2A 3A4; Wes'83; BSc; FRCSC; GenSurg (Upper Extremity Surgery). Staff, West Parry Sound Health Centre; (705)746-4540

FOSTER, Kevin J; University of Alberta Hosp, 8440 112 St NW, Edmonton AB T6G 2B7; Alb'95; CCFP; CCFP(E.M.); FCFP; Staff, University of Alberta Hospital; (780)407-8822

FOSTER, Kimberley; University Hlth Services, PO Box 1700 Stc Csc, Victoria BC V8W 2Y2; McM'97; CCFP; (250)721-8492

FOSTER, Mark B; Crown St Medical Clinic, 110 Crown St, Saint John NB E2L 2X7; Dal'85; Staff, Saint John Regional Hospital; Pres, Harbour City Medical Group; (506)658-1431; Fax. (506)634-1136.

FOSTER, Michael J; Cochrane Primary Care Centre, 103-100 Grande Blvd W, Cochrane AB T4C 0S4; Cal'77; CCFP; FCFP; Asst Clin Prof Family Med, University of Calgary; (403)932-2089; Fax. (403)932-1820.

FOSTER, Michael J; Fairview Med Arts Centre, 103-2200 Fairview St, Burlington ON L7R 4H9; Tor'76; (905)639-0884; Fax. (905)639-0824.

FOSTER, Michelle C; Guelph Imaging Centre, 206-55 Wyndham St N, Guelph ON N1H 7T8; Wes'97; FRCPC; DiagRad. (519)767-0220

FOSTER, Nicholas K; BC Cancer Agency-Vancouver CC, 600 10th Ave W, Vancouver BC V5Z 4E6; Otago (New Zealand)'86; MB ChB; Staff, BC Cancer Agency Vancouver Centre; (604)877-6000

FOSTER, Ryan; Intesive Care Unit, 2268 Pandosy St, Kelowna BC V1Y 1T2; Tor'00; FRCPC; IntMed (Critical Care Medicine). Staff, Kelowna General Hospital; (250)862-4000

FOSTER, Sandra; 50 Tamarack Circle, Etobicoke ON M9P 3T9; McM'95; FRCPC; IntMed. (416)510-6895; Fax. (416)510-6870.

FOSTER, William; CHUQ-Hotel-Dieu de Quebec, 11 Cote du Palais, Quebec QC G1R 2J6; Laval'03; FRCSC; Ophth; RadOncol. Staff, Centre Hospitalier Universitaire de Québec (CHUQ) - Siege Social; (418)691-5264; Fax. (418)691-5268.

FOSTER JR., Harry L; Sunnybrook Hlth Sciences Ctre, 2075 Bayview Ave, Toronto ON M4N 3M5; McM'77; FRCPC; Anes. Staff, Sunnybrook Health Sciences Centre; (416)480-6100 x3230

FOSTEY, Alan; Saint John Reg Hosp, PO Box 2100 Stn Main, Saint John NB E2L 4L2; Saba (Netherlands Antilles)'98; Staff, Saint John Regional Hospital; (506)648-6000

FOTHERGILL, Judith; Elaho Med Clinic, PO Box 10003 Rpo The Chieftain 1337 Pemberton Ave, Squamish BC V8B 0R1; Bristol (England)'77; MB ChB; MRCP(UK); Ac Staff, Squamish General Hospital / Hilltop House; Med Dir, Hilltop House; (604)892-5688; Fax. (604)892-9727.

FOTHERGILL, Marnie; The Alex Youth Hlth Center, 101-1318 Center St N, Calgary AB T2E 2R7; Cal'84; BSc; CCFP; Member, Southern Alberta Mental Health Review Panel; (403)520-6270; Fax. (403)920-0014; marniefothergill@smarttech.com.

FOTHERINGHAM, John M; Atikokan Family Health Team, PO Box 1450 123 Marks St, Atikokan ON P0T 1C0; Qns'05; CCFP; (807)597-2721; Fax. (807)597-4632.

FOTI, Dean J; UBC Hospital, S128-2211 Wesbrook Mall, Vancouver BC V6T 2B5; McG'89; BSc; MDCM; FRCPC; Neur (Behavioural Neurology). Ac Staff, UBC Hospital - Koerner Pavillion; Clinical Asst Prof, University of British Columbia; Langs: Bilingual(English/French); (604)822-7678; Fax. (604)822-7897.

FOTTI, Christopher; Pritchard Farm Hlth Centre, 5-3014 Henderson Hwy, East St Paul MB R2E 0H9; Man'08; CCFP.

FOTTI, Sarah A; Health Sciences Centre Psychea, PZ162-771 Bannatyne Ave, Winnipeg MB R3E 3N4; Man'01; FRCPC; Psy.

FOUAD, Magdy A M; 4485 Roger St, Port Alberni BC V9Y 3Z5; (Egypt)'77; MB ChB; MRCOG(U.K.); FRCSC; ObstGyn (Gyn Urol). Staff, West Coast General Hospital; Langs: Arabic; (250)723-4884; Fax. (250)723-4884.

FOUCAULT, Josee; Ctr de Med Familiale de Granby, 48 rue Denison E, Granby QC J2G 4C6; Sher'94; (450)372-2001; Fax. (450)372-0430.

FOUCAULT, Lynne; CHSLD de Hull, 125 boul Lionel-Emond, Gatineau QC J8Y 5S8; Mon'87; assoc Staff, Hôpital de Gatineau; Langs: Bilingual(French/English); (819)770-1880; Fax. (819)770-8624; lynne_foucault@ssss.gouv.qc.ca.

FOUCAULT, Nathalie; GMF Centre de santé, 3745 rue George-Couture, Drummondville QC J2B 7P4; Sher'93; Peds. Langs: English; (819)477-2231; Fax. (819)477-1122; nathalie.foucault@usherbrooke.ca.

FOUCHE, Nanette; PO Box 280 Stn Main, Brooks AB T1R 1B3; (South Africa)'06; MB ChB; Physician, Oasis Medical Clinics; (403)362-5501

FOUCHER, Martin; CSSS de Rimouski-Neigette, CP 3150 Succ A 150 av Rouleau, Rimouski QC G5L 5T1; Mon'90; Staff, Hôpital Regional Rimouski; (418)723-5135

FOUDA, Omayma; Cassandra Clinic Inc, 2044-2048 Victoria Park Ave, North York ON M1R 1V2; Ain Shams (Egypt)'91; CCFP; (416)331-9111; Fax. (416)331-9050.

FOUGERE, Garnet A; Lansdowne Professional Ctr II, 225-3066 Shellbourne St, Victoria BC V8R 6T9; Man'96; MSc; CCFP; (778)432-2234

FOUGERES, Annie; CHUQ-Ctr Hosp Univ Laval, 2705 boul Laurier, Quebec QC G1V 4G2; Sher'95; FRCPC; DiagRad. Staff, Centre Hospitalier Universitaire de Quebec-CHUL; (418)656-4141 x42258; Fax. (418)654-2262.

FOULKES, Ellen F; Royal Columbian Hosp, 330 Columbia St E, New Westminster BC V3L 3W7; UBC'74; FRCPC; Anes. Staff, Royal Columbian Hospital; (604)520-4602

FOULKES, William; MUHC-Montreal Gen Hosp, L10 116-1650 av Cedar, Montreal QC H3G 1A4; London (England)'84; FRCPC; MedGenetics (P.Q.) (Cancer Genetics). Assoc Staff, McGill University Health Centre - Montreal General Campus; Assoc Staff, Sir Mortimer B Davis Jewish General; assoc Prof Med, McGill University; (514)934-1934 x44121; nancy.hamel@mail.mcgill.ca.

FOULSTON, Charlotte; Professional Corp, 540 7 Ave SW, Medicine Hat AB T1A 5B9; Alb'77; FAAP; FRCPC; Peds (Adolescent Gynecology). Dir NICU, Medicine Hat Regional Hospital; Associate/Clin Prof Peds, University of Calgary; (403)527-5500; Fax. (403)529-2246.

FOUND, Margaret H; Dorval Med Assoc Fam Hlth Team, 104-465 Morden Rd, Oakville ON L6K 3W6; McM'88; CCFP; FCFP; Ac Staff, Halton Healthcare Services Corporation - Oakville Site; Coroner, Halton Region; (905)842-7154; Fax. (905)842-3604; mfound@cogeco.ca.

FOUNTAS, Panayiotis N; Hippocrates Med Clinic, 833 Coxwell Ave, Toronto ON M4C 3E8; Athens (Greece)'71; FRCPC; IntMed (Hospitalist); Cardiol. Staff, Toronto East General Hospital Inc; Staff, Toronto Western Hospital - University Health Network; Langs: Greek; (416)467-6555; Fax. (416)467-6474.

FOUQUETTE, Bertrand G; CHUQ-St-Francois D'Assise, 10 rue de l'Espinay, Quebec QC G1L 3L5; Laval'69; CSPQ; AnatPath. Asst Staff AnatPath, Centre Hospitalier Universitaire De Québec - Pavillon De St-françois-d'assise; Teacher, Université Laval; (418)525-4324

FOUQUETTE, Yves; Ctr Hosp Pierre-Le Gardeur, 911 Montee des Pionniers, Terrebonne QC J6V 2H2; Mon'94; FRCPC; Psy. Staff, Centre Hospitalier Pierre le Gardeur; Staff, McGill University Health Centre - Montreal General Campus; (450)654-7525

FOURESTIE, Emmanuelle; Centre Hosp de Verdun, 4000 boul Lasalle, Verdun QC H4G 2A3; Laval'04; Staff, Centre Hospitalier de Verdun; (514)362-1000

FOURIE, Annelie; 3-10003 100 St, Sexsmith AB T0H 3C0; Stellenbosch (South Africa)'85; MB ChB; Fam Physician, Queen Elizabeth II Hospital; Langs: Afrikaans; (780)568-2277; Fax. (780)568-2299.

FOURIE, Annerie; Vernon Family Practice Assoc, 115-3101 Hwy 6, Vernon BC V1T 9H6; Pretoria (South Africa)'98; MB ChB; CCFP; (250)545-8332

FOURIE, Clasina E; Clearbrook Family Practice, 101-2828 Cruickshank St, Abbotsford BC V2T 5M4; Orange Free State (South Africa)'04; MB ChB; DipHIV; Physician Lead Hospital Care Physicians Program, Abbotsford Regional Hospital & Cancer Centre; (604)852-8030; Fax. (604)852-4118.

FOURIE, Hendrina H C E; 4634 Park Ave, Terrace BC V8G 1V7; Pretoria (South Africa)'01; MB ChB; Langs: Afrikaans; (250)615-5030

FOURIE, Hendrina; 123 10th Ave S, Cranbrook BC V1C 2N1; Orange Free (South Africa)'96; BPharm; MB ChB; CCFP; (250)426-4231

FOURIE, Jan G; Silver Birch Med Clinic, PO Box 489 5114 3rd St, Boyle AB T0A 0M0; (South Africa)'01; (780)689-0003; Fax. (780)689-4155.

FOURIE, Jan; Regina Gen Hosp, 1440 14th Ave, Regina SK S4P 0W5; Pretoria (South Africa)'86; MB ChB; CCFP; Staff, Regina General Hospital; (306)766-4444

FOURIE, Johan-Andre V; PO Box 1391 Stn Main, Vernon BC V1T 6N7; Pretoria (South Africa)'98; MB ChB; CCFP; CCFP(E.M.).

FOURIE, Johannes L; Associate Med Clinic, 203-10030 106 St, Westlock AB T7P 2K4; Orange Free State (South Africa)'87; MB ChB; CCFP; (780)349-3341; Fax. (780)349-6686.

FOURIE, Ockert J; Humber River Reg Hosp-Church, 200 Church St, Toronto ON M9N 1N8; McM'04; FRCPC; Anes. Staff, Humber River Regional Hospital - Church Street Site; (416)243-4154; Fax. (416)243-4194.

FOURIE, Phillip J; Dr P Fourie Med Clinic, 269 Bradbrooke Dr, Yorkton SK S3N 3L3; Stellenbosch (South Africa)'95; MB ChB; Langs: Afrikaans; German; (306)783-4999; Fax. (306)783-5099; phillipfourie@hotmail.com.

FOURIE, Theo; Western Med Clinic, 144 6th St, Brandon MB R7A 3N2; Stellenbosch (South Africa)'81; CCFP; (204)727-6451; Fax. (204)727-4150.

FOURIE, Thomas M; Foothills Med Centre, C614-1403 29 St NW, Calgary AB T2N 2T9; (South Africa)'95; MB BS; FRCPC; HemPath. Staff, Foothills Medical Centre; (403)944-1566

FOURIE, W Jacobus; Mills Memorial Hosp, 4720 Haugland Ave, Terrace BC V8G 2W7; Orange Free State (South Africa)'90; MB ChB; Staff Oncol, Mills Memorial Hospital; Medical Staff Oncology BCCA, Northern Health Authority; Medical Officer Aviation, Skeena Health District; Physician, CN Rail Skeena Area; Langs: Afrikaans; Sotho; (250)638-4036; Fax. (250)638-4030.

FOURNEY, Daryl R; Royal University Hosp, Division of Neurosurgery 103 Hospital Drive, Saskatoon SK S7N 0W8; Sask'95; FRCSC; Neursurg (Brain Tumors). Prof NeuroSurg, Royal University Hospital; Prof NeuroSurg, University of Saskatchewan; (306)966-8814; Fax. (306)966-8140; daryl.fourney@usas.ca.

FOURNIER, Andre; Service ORL Saint-Jean, 300-900 boul du Seminaire N, St-Jean-Sur-Richel QC J3A 1C3; Laval'66; Otol (P.Q.). Ac Staff, Hôpital du Haut-Richelieu; Langs: English; (450)348-1133; Fax. (450)348-1134.

FOURNIER, Anne; Hôpital Ste-Justine, 3175 ch Cote-Ste-Catherine, Montreal QC H3T 1C5; Mon'80; CSPQ; FRCPC; Peds (Pediatric Cardiology); Cardiol. Ac Staff, Hôpital Ste-Justine; Staff Consultant, Hopital Maisonneuve-Rosemont; Staff Consultant, Hopital de la Cite de la santé; Clin Assoc Prof, Universite de Montreal; Langs: Bilingual(French/English); (514)345-4654; Fax. (514)345-4896; anne_fournier@ssss.gouv.qc.ca.

FOURNIER, Anne-Marie; CSSS Haut-Richelieu-Rouville, 920 boul du Seminaire N, St-Jean-Sur-Richel QC J3A 1B7; Mon'93; Staff, Hôpital du Haut-Richelieu; (450)359-5000

FOURNIER, Annick V; Children's Hosp Eastern Ont, 401 Smyth Rd, Ottawa ON K1H 8L1; Mon'94; BSc; FRCSC; Ophth (Ophthalmology Pediatrics & Adult Strabismus). Staff, Children's Hospital of Eastern Ontario (CHEO); Langs: English; (613)737-2235; Fax. (613)738-4237; afournier@cheo.on.ca.

FOURNIER, Brigitte; 363 rte Cameron, Sainte-Marie QC G6E 3E2; Laval'87; DrMedCh; Staff, Centre d'hébergement de Beauceville; Med Consultant Service clinique de santé publique, Hôtel-Dieu de Lévis; Med Officier Infectious Illness, Agence de Sante Services Sociaux de Chaudiere Appalaches; Langs: English; (418)386-3363 x1507; Fax. (418)389-1515; brigitte_fournier@ssss.gouv.qc.ca.

FOURNIER, Carl; Clinique Méd Cadillac, 3435 rue Bossuet, Anjou QC H1M 2M1; Mon'86; Clin Prof Med, Universite de Montreal; (514)253-1211

FOURNIER, Carole; 153 ch Breuleux, Sutton QC J0E 2K0; Mon'78; (450)923-5577

FOURNIER, Charles; Clinique Med D'Alma, 935 av du Pont S, Alma QC G8B 2V5; Laval'89; (418)668-6121; Fax. (418)668-5298.

FOURNIER, Christiane; Hotel-Dieu du Sacre-Coeur, 1 av du Sacre-Coeur, Quebec QC G1N 2W1; Sher'85; FRCPC; Psy (Pediatric Psychiatry). Staff, Centre Hospitalier Universitaire de Quebec-CHUL; Staff, Hotel-Dieu du Sacre-Coeur de Jesus de Quebec; Prof, Université Laval; Langs: English; (418)529-6851 x451; Fax. (418)521-6239; christane.fournier@mail.chuq.qc.ca.

FOURNIER, Christine; Ctr Monteregien Readaptation, 5300 ch Chambly, Longueuil QC J3Y 3N7; Sher'89; FRCPC; PhysMed&Rehab. Staff, Institut de Réadaptation Gingras-Lindsay de Montréal; (450)676-7447; Fax. (450)676-0047.

FOURNIER, Claire; Pavillon Edouard-Asselin, 264 boul Rene-Levesque E, Montreal QC H2X 1P1; Geneve (Switzerland)'95; (514)890-8000

FOURNIER, Claude; Centre Med Iberville, 101-235 2e av, St-Jean-Sur-Richel QC J2X 2B2; Mon'83; Staff, Hôpital du Haut-Richelieu; (450)347-5548

FOURNIER, Claude; ASSS de Chanaudiere-Appalaches, 363 Rte Cameron, Sainte-Marie QC G6E 3E2; Sher'80; Staff, Centre Hospitalier Universitaire de Québec (CHUQ) - Siege Social; (418)386-3532; Fax. (418)389-1540.

FOURNIER, Denis; Residence Christ-Roi, 900 boul Wilfrid-Hamel, Quebec QC G1M 2R9; Laval'86; LMCC; Staff, CSSS de la Vieille-Capitale; Langs: Bilingual(French/English); (418)682-1748; Fax. (418)682-1763.

FOURNIER, Emilie; CSSS de Sept-Iles, 45 rue du Pere-Divet, Sept-Iles QC G4R 3N7; Laval'08; CCFP; Staff, Centre Hospitalier Regional de Sept-Iles; (418)962-9801

FOURNIER, Gilbert; CHUM-Hop St-Luc, 1058 rue Saint-Denis, Montreal QC H2X 3J4; Laval'71; FRCPC; Psy. Staff, Centre Hospitalier l'Université De Montréal (CHUM) - Hôpital Saint-luc; (514)890-8000 x36155

FOURNIER, Gino; Ctr Hosp Laurentien, 234 rue Saint-Vincent, Ste-Agathe-des-Mts QC J8C 2B8; Sher'96; Staff, Centre Hospitalier Laurentien; (819)324-4000

FOURNIER, Guy; 805-4700 rue Sainte-Catherine, Westmount QC H3Z 1S6; Laval'63; CSPQ; OrthSurg. Langs: Spanish; English; (514)939-9733

FOURNIER, Helene; CHUM-Hotel-Dieu, 3840 rue Saint-Urbain, Montreal QC H2W 1T8; Mon'80; MPH(Pittsburgh); FRCPC; IntMed; Endocrin&Metab. ac Staff, Centre Hospitalier l'Université de Montréal (CHUM) - Hôtel-Dieu; (514)890-8000 x14444

FOURNIER, Isabelle; CSSS Pierre Boucher, 1333 boul Jacques-Cartier E, Longueuil QC J4M 2A5; Sher'95; Staff, Centre Hospitalier Pierre Boucher; (450)468-8111

FOURNIER, Jacques; CHUQ-St-Francois D'Assise, 10 rue de l'Espinay, Quebec QC G1L 3L5; Laval'67; FRCSC; Otol. Ac Staff, Centre Hospitalier Universitaire De Québec - Pavillon De St-françois-d'assise; Consultant, Centre Hospitalier Universitaire de Quebec-CHUL; (418)525-4310

FOURNIER, Jacques; Centre Med Laval, 1110 boul Vanier, Laval QC H7C 2R8; Mon'78; CCFP; Staff, Hopital de la Cite de la santé; (450)661-2521; Fax. (450)661-7193.

FOURNIER, Jean-Marie; Centre Gertruce Lafrance, 150 boul Saint-Luc, St-Jean-sur-Richel QC J3A 1G2; Mon'65; (450)359-5555 x8741; Fax. (450)348-9136.

FOURNIER, Jean-Pierre; 200-979 av de Bourgogne, Quebec QC G1W 2L4; Laval'78; FRCPC; Psy. (418)780-2379; Fax. (418)780-2382; jpfournier@videotron.ca.

FOURNIER, Jessica; Clin Med Alma, 935 av du Pont S, Alma QC G8B 2V5; Laval'06; (418)668-6121

FOURNIER, Johanne; Groupe Sante Medisys Inc, 11F-500 rue Sherbrooke O, Montreal QC H3A 3C6; Mon'94; CCFP; Langs: English; (514)499-2777 x744; Fax. (514)499-9536; johanne.fournier@medisys.ca.

FOURNIER, Karl; Clinique Chir Ortho C-Lemoyne, 126 rue Saint-Louis, Lemoyne QC J4R 2L5; Mon'93; BSc; CSPQ; FRCSC; OrthSurg. Chief Orthopatic, Hopital Charles LeMoyne; Langs: English; (450)672-1212; Fax. (450)672-9834.

FOURNIER, Louis; 825 rue Eymard, Quebec QC G1S 4A2; Laval'59; CSPQ; Anes. Ac Staff, Centre Hospitalier Universitaire de Quebec-CHUL; (418)656-4141; Fax. (418)654-2774; ls.fournier@videotron.ca.

FOURNIER, Marc; The Ottawa Hosp-Gen Campus, 501 Smyth Rd, Ottawa ON K1H 8L6; Sask'06; Gastroent; IntMed. Staff, The Ottawa Hospital - General Campus; (613)737-8899

FOURNIER, Marc R; WRHA Critical Care Program, JJ399-700 William Ave, Winnipeg MB R3E 0Z3; Cal'94; IntMed (Family Medicine).

FOURNIER, Marcel R; Queen Elizabeth Health Complex, 424-2100 av de Marlowe, Montreal QC H4A 3L5; McG'77; ABIM; ABIM(Cardiovasc); CSPQ; FRCPC; IntMed; Cardiol. Staff, St Mary's Hospital Centre; Asst Physician, McGill University Health Centre - Royal Victoria Hospital; Asst Prof Med & Family Pract, McGill University; (514)485-5103; Fax. (514)485-5001.

FOURNIER, Pascale; Ctr Hosp de Matane, 333 rue Thibault, Matane QC G4W 2W5; Laval'85; Staff, Centre Hospitalier de Matane; (418)562-3135

FOURNIER, Paul J R; Dr Paul J R Fournier, 919-300 rue Leo Pariseau, Montreal QC H2X 4B3; McG'69; DAB; FACOG; FRCSC; ObstGyn. Assoc Staff, McGill University Health Centre - Royal Victoria Hospital; Assoc Staff, McGill University Health Centre - Montreal General Campus; Assoc Prof ObstGyn, McGill University; Langs: English; French; (514)288-9472; Fax. (514)288-3218.

FOURNIER, Pierre; Clinique Med St-Louis, 220-3165 ch Saint-Louis, Quebec QC G1W 4R4; Laval'79; (418)653-1970

FOURNIER, Pierre; CSSS Pierre Boucher, 1333 boul Jacques-Cartier E, Longueuil QC J4M 2A5; Mon'91; LMCC; Staff, Centre Hospitalier Pierre Boucher; (450)468-8111 x2223; Fax. (450)468-8274.

FOURNIER, Renee; Roper Clinic, 4500 rue Sherbrooke O, Montreal QC H3Z 1E6; Mon'83; CCFP; FCFP; Staff, Strathroy Middlesex General Hospital - Middlesex Hospital Alliance; Langs: English; French; (514)937-8000

FOURNIER, Sylvie; Clinique Med de l'Ouest, 2200 6e Av, Saint-Georges QC G5Y 3X3; Laval'86; LMCC; CCFP; Staff, Clinique médicale de l'Ouest; Langs: Bilingual(French/English); (418)228-2024; Fax. (418)228-7715.

FOURNIER, Sylvie; CSSS Haut-Richelieu-Rouville, 920 boul du Seminaire N, St-Jean-Sur-Richel QC J3A 1B7; Sher'86; Nephrol (P.Q.); IntMed (P.Q.). Staff, Hôpital du Haut-Richelieu; (450)359-5000; Fax. (450)359-5079.

FOURNIER, Yolaine; Clinique Med Fleur de Lys, 3-8 rue du Terminus E, Rouyn-Noranda QC J9X 3B4; Sher'80; Staff, Centre Hospitalier Rouyn-Noranda; (819)764-6185; Fax. (819)762-6079.

FOURNIER, Yvon; 200-555 boul Saint-Antoine, Saint-Jerome QC J7Z 3B8; Mon'82; Staff, Hôtel-Dieu de Saint-Jérôme; (450)438-1252; Fax. (450)438-6441.

FOURNIER-BLAKE, Odette; Seaforth Med Bldg, 680-3550 ch de la Cote-des-Nei, Montreal QC H3H 1V4; Ott'73; DAB; FRCPC; Derm. Sr Staff Derm, McGill University Health Centre - Montreal General Campus; Teacher, McGill University; (514)933-1698; dermskin@bellnet.ca.

FOURNIER-CLOUTIER, Vincent; CSSS de Trois-Rivières, 1991 boul du Carmel, Trois-Rivieres QC G8Z 3R9; Mon'06; FRCSC; Urol. Staff, CSSS de Trois-Rivières; (819)697-3333

FOUNIER-GOSSELIN, Marie-Pierre; CHUM-Hôp Notre-Dame, 1560 rue Sherbrooke E, Montreal QC H2L 4M1; Laval'02; FRCSC; Neursurg. Staff, Centre Hospitalier l'Université de Montréal (CHUM) - Hôpital Notre-Dame; Staff, Hôpital Ste-Justine; Langs: Bilingual(French/English); (514)890-8000; Fax. (514)412-7816; marie.pierre.fournier-gosselin@umontreal.ca.

FOURNIER-GOSSELIN, Simon; Hotel-Dieu d'Arthabaska, 5 rue des Hospitalieres, Victoriaville QC G6P 6N2; Laval'05; FRCSC; OrthSurg. (819)357-2030

FOURNIER MARSHALL, Colette S; Royal University Hosp, 103 Hospital Dr, Saskatoon SK S7N 0W8; Sask'01; CCFP; CCFP(E.M.); Staff, Royal University Hospital; (306)655-1000; Fax. (306)477-8074.

FOURON, Jean-Claude; Hôpital Ste-Justine, 3175 ch Cote-Ste-Catherine, Montreal QC H3T 1C5; Port-au-Prince (Haiti)'58; CSPQ; FRCPC; Peds (Pediatric Cardiology); Cardiol (P.Q.). Med Staff Assoc, Hôpital Ste-Justine; Prof Peds, Universite de Montreal; (514)345-4654; Fax. (514)345-4896; jean-claude_fouron@ssss.gouv.qc.ca.

FOURON, Pascale; Centre de Sante Innuulitisivik, CP 29, Salluit QC J0M 1S0; Mon'99; Staff, CSSS de la Baie-des-Chaleurs; (819)255-9090

FOURS, Suliman A A; Belle Reve Medicentre, 102-16703 82 St NW, Edmonton AB T5E 5S7; (780)457-7142; Fax. (780)457-7152.

FOUSSIAS, Agoritsa T; 200-14 Prince Arthur Ave, Toronto ON M5R 1A9; Thessaloniki (Greece)'72; FRCPC; Psy. Langs: Greek; (416)968-0616; Fax. (416)968-1976.

FOUSSIAS, Athanassios; 200-14 Prince Arthur Ave, Toronto ON M5R 1A9; Thessaloniki (Greece)'71; FRCPC; Psy. Ac Staff, Centre for Addiction & Mental Health (CAMH) - Queen Site; (416)966-0640

FOUSSIAS, George; Addiction & Mental Hlth-Clarke, 722-250 College St, Toronto ON M5T 1R8; Dal'04; FRCPC; Psy. Staff, Centre for Addiction & Mental Health (CAMH) - College Street Site; Langs: Greek; (416)535-8501

FOWKE, Jane S; Alpine Med Clinic, PO Box 4000 Stn Main 201A-211 Bear St, Banff AB T1L 1J8; London (England)'82; MB BS; Staff Privil, Covenant Health - Banff Mineral Springs Hospital; (403)762-3155; Fax. (403)762-5797.

FOWLER, Erika; Wedgewood Med Centre, 304-12 Gleneyre St, St. John's NL A1A 2M7; Mem'06; FRCSC; ObstGyn.

FOWLER, Jacqueline M; 400-224 Esplanade St W, North Vancouver BC V7M 1A4; UBC'96; CCFP; Staff, Vancouver General Hospital - Centennial Pavillion; (604)232-1504

FOWLER, Mark A; Blind River Family Med Clinic, PO Box 1450, Blind River ON P0R 1B0; Sask'80; Ac Staff, Blind River District Health Centre; Coroner, Saskatoon Justice; Coroner, Ontario Justice; Staff, Carrot River Medical Clinic; Clin Teacher, Northern Ontario School of Medicine-Laurentian University; (705)356-1666 x58; Fax. (705)356-2403.

FOWLER, Nancy C; McMaster Family Practice, A-690 Main St W, Hamilton ON L8S 1A4; McM'85; CCFP; FCFP; Assoc Prof, McMaster University; (905)521-5015; Fax. (905)521-5010.

FOWLER, Peter J; Fowler Kennedy Sport Med Clin, 3M-1151 Richmond St, London ON N6A 3K7; Wes'64; DABOS; OrthSurg (Shoulder & Knee Reconstruction). (519)661-4150; Fax. (519)661-4052; pfowler@uwo.ca.

FOWLER, Peter S; 108-911 Island Hwy, Campbell River BC V9W 2C2; Dal'73; FRCSC; PlasSurg. Consultant, Campbell River & District General Hospital; (250)287-8077; Fax. (250)287-8097.

FOWLER, Robert A; Sunnybrook Hlth Sciences Ctre, D478-2075 Bayview Ave, Toronto ON M4N 3M5; McG'95; FRCPC; IntMed. Staff, Sunnybrook Health Sciences Centre; Langs: Bilingual(French/English); (416)480-6100 x7471

FOWLER, Robert D; Carbonear Gen Hosp, 6F-86 Highroad South, Carbonear NL A1Y 1A4; Mem'95; FRCSC; Otol. Staff, Carbonear General Hospital; (709)945-5111

FOWLER, Sharyle; Royal University Hosp, 103 Hospital Dr, Saskatoon SK S7N 0W8; Cal'05; FRCPC; IntMed; Gastroent. Staff, Royal University Hospital; (306)966-7799; Fax. (306)966-7996.

FOWLER, Stephen G; B1 A-223 Queen St S, Mississauga ON L5M 1L6; Tor'76; CGPP; (416)806-0788

FOWLER, William C; South Macleod Family Med, 100-15915 Macleod Trail SE, Calgary AB T2Y 3R9; Sask'87; (403)457-2457; wcfowler@shaw.ca.

FOWLIE, Frank E; PO Box 565 Stn Main, Moncton NB E1C 8L9; Dal'76; BSc; DABR; FRCPC; DiagRad. Staff Radiol, The Moncton Hospital.

FOWLIS, Ronald A F; 206-564 Belmont Ave W, Kitchener ON N2M 5N6; Glasgow (Scotland)'68; DABIM; FRCPC; IntMed (Cardiology). Staff Grand River Hosp, Grand River Hospital - Freeport Site; Ac Staff, St Mary's General Hospital; (519)742-6062; Fax. (519)742-5512.

FOWLOW, Geoffrey N; Physician PMC Inc CMD Bldg, PO Box 220 155-157 Main Rd, Arnolds Cove NL A0B 1A0; Tor'71; CCFP; FCFP; Court Staff, The Dr G B Cross Memorial Hospital; (709)463-2603; gnfowlow@nf.aibn.com.

FOX, Allan J; Sunnybrook Hlth Sciences Ctre, AG31B-2075 Bayview Ave, Toronto ON M4N 3M5; McG'70; FACR; FRCPC; DiagRad (Neuro Radiology). Staff NeuroRadiol, Sunnybrook Health Sciences Centre; Prof Med Imaging, University of Toronto; Langs: Hebrew; French; (416)480-4371; Fax. (416)480-5218; allan.fox@sunnybrook.ca.

FOX, Anthony D; Trillium Hlth Ctr-Mississauga, 100 Queensway W, Mississauga ON L5B 1B8; London (England)'52; FRCPC; GenPath. Staff, Trillium Health Centre - Mississauga; (905)848-7299; Fax. (905)848-8313.

FOX, Eric; Greenbelt Family Health Team, 3500 Fallowfield Rd, Ottawa ON K2J 4A7; McG'07; MDCM; CCFP; Staff, The Ottawa Hospital - General Campus; (613)843-1718; Fax. (613)843-0201.

FOX, George A; Health Sciences Centre, 2749A-300 Prince Philip Dr, St. John's NL A1B 3V6; Mem'83; FRCPC; IntMed; Critical Care Medicine; Respir. Staff, Health Sciences Centre; Assoc Prof, Memorial University Of Newfoundland; (709)777-8074; Fax. (709)777-8079.

FOX, Gordon S; Mount Sinai Hosp, 1514-600 University Ave, Toronto ON M5G 1X5; Tor'60; DA; CSPQ; FRCPC; Anes. Staff, Mount Sinai Hospital; (416)586-4800 x2698; Fax. (416)586-8664.

FOX, Hyman I; North Road Med Centre, S-435 North Rd, Coquitlam BC V3K 3V9; McG'76; (604)936-0411

FOX, James; Foothills Med Centre, C 231-1403 29 St NW, Calgary AB T2N 2T9; Alb'05; FRCPC; EmergMed. Staff, Foothills Medical Centre; (403)944-1110

FOX, Joanne M; Appleby College Med, 540 Lakeshore Rd W, Oakville ON L6K 3P1; Tor'84; (905)845-1544; Fax. (905)845-2024.

FOX, Joel M; Foothills Med Centre, C229-1403 29 St NW, Calgary AB T2N 2T9; Tor'84; FRCPC; Anes. Ac Staff, Foothills Medical Centre; Coord., Quality Improvement Health Information-Dept. of Anes., Calgary Health Region; Clinical Asst Prof, University of Calgary; (403)944-1430

FOX, Joel M; Group Med Stillview, 245-175 av Stillview, Pointe-Claire QC H9R 4S3; McG'78; FRCPC; IntMed; Respir. Staff, Lakeshore General Hospital - Pointe Claire; (514)697-5417

FOX, Jonathan R; Integrated Chronic Case Serv, 3064 Highway 2, Fall River NS B2T 1J5; Dal'94; BSc; CCFP; Physician, Integrated Chronic Case Serv; Langs: English; French; (902)860-0057; Fax. (902)860-2046; jonathan.fox@cdha.nshealth.ca.

FOX, Lorne M; 2311 Pandosy St, Kelowna BC V1Y 1T4; RCS (Ireland)'82; MB ChB; FRCP; FRCPC; IntMed; Respir. (250)763-8110; Fax. (250)763-9587.

FOX, Michael J; Trafalgar Prof Centre, 314-1235 Trafalgar Rd, Oakville ON L6H 3P1; Tor'95; FRCPC; Peds. Staff, The Hospital For Sick Children; (905)842-3993; Fax. (905)842-9260.

FOX, Paul; Thames Valley FHT-W London FH, 200-785 Wonderland Rd S, London ON N6K 1M6; Wes'86; BSc; (519)641-6712; Fax. (519)641-6189; pfox@uwo.ca.

FOX, Richard J; University of Alberta Hosp, 2D1WCM-8440 112 St NW, Edmonton AB T6G 2B7; Tor'91; FRCSC; Neursurg. Staff, University of Alberta Hospital; (780)407-3558; Fax. (780)407-8203.

FOX, Rick; 301-2489 Bloor St W, Toronto ON M6S 1R6; Tor'82; FRCSC; Otol (Rhinology). Ac Staff, St Joseph's Health Centre; Asst Prof, University of Toronto; (416)767-3171; Fax. (416)766-6896.

FOX, Robert G; PO Box 1039 Rpo Vedder Crossin, Chilliwack BC V2R 3N7; Alb'01; CCFP; (604)796-2165; Fax. (604)796-2165.

FOX, Roy; Integrate Chronic Care Serv, 3064 Hwy 2, Fall River NS B2T 1J5; Durham (England)'65; MES; FRCP; FACP; FRCPC; Gastroent (Environmental Medicine). Med Dir Integrated Chronic Care Services, Capital District Health Authority; (902)860-0551; Fax. (902)860-2046; roy.fox@cdha.nshealth.ca.

FOX, Susan B; Hop Charles Lemoyne, 3120 boul Taschereau, Greenfield Park QC J4V 2H1; McG'80; RC; FRCPC; IntMed (Hematological Oncology); Hem. Ac Staff, Hopital Charles LeMoyne; Ac Staff, McGill University Health Centre - Royal Victoria Hospital; McGill University; Langs: Bilingual(French/English); (450)466-5065; suzan.fox@rrsss16.gouv.qc.ca.

FOX, Susan H; Univ Hlth Network-Toronto Western Hosp, MC7 402-399 Bathurst St, Toronto ON M5T 2S8; Manchester (England)'90; Staff, Toronto Western Hospital - University Health Network; (416)603-6422

FOX, William P; Elmwood Family Hlth Centre, 3-204 First Ave, St Thomas ON N5R 4P5; Wes'06; CCFP; (519)631-3223; Fax. (519)631-8005.

FOX, William R; Huronia Med Centre, PO Box 790 Stn Main, Midland ON L4R 4P4; Dublin (Ireland)'65; (705)526-5291

FOX-ROBICHAUD, Alison E; Hamilton HS-General Site, C5 106-237 Barton St E, Hamilton ON L8L 2X2; Ott'89; BSc; MSc; FRCPC; IntMed; Critical Care Medicine. Staff TaARI David Braley Research Inst, Hamilton Health Sciences Centre - Hamilton General Hospital; Assoc Prof Med, McMaster University; (905)521-2100 x40769; Fax. (905)575-2646.

FOXCROFT, Laura C; London HSC-Victoria Hosp, PO Box 5010 Stn B 800 Commissioners Rd E, London ON N6A 5W9; McM'01; CCFP; CCFP(E.M.); Staff, London Health Sciences Centre - Victoria Campus; (519)685-8500; laura.foxcroft@lhsc.on.ca.

FOXFORD, Robert J; MUHC-Royal Victoria Hosp, 687 av des Pins O, Montreal QC H3A 1A1; Man'78; FRCPC; EmergMed. Staff, McGill University Health Centre - Royal Victoria Hospital; (514)843-2852

FOY, James J; First Edmonton Place, 390-10665 Jasper Ave NW, Edmonton AB T5J 3S9; Alb'69; FRCSC; Ophth. Ac Staff Ophth., Royal Alexandra Hospital; Asst Prof, University of Alberta; (780)424-2233; Fax. (780)426-7219; jdfoy@shaw.ca.

FOYLE, Annette; South Shore Reg Hosp, 90 Glen Allan Dr, Bridgewater NS B4V 3S6; McG'73; FCAP; FRCPC; AnatPath. Staff, South Shore Regional Hospital; Asst Prof, Dalhousie University; (902)527-5264; annfoyle@hotmail.com.

FOYLE, Catharine; PO Box 65176 Rpo North Hill, Calgary AB T2N 4T6; Ott'88; BMedSci; CCFP; Langs: English; French.

FRABONI, Theresa; IWK Health Centre, PO Box 9700 Rpo CSC 5850-5980 University Ave, Halifax NS B3K 6R8; Ott'90; FRCPC; Peds (Developmental Pediatrics). Staff, IWK Health Centre; (902)470-8951; Fax. (902)470-7284.

FRADET, Amelie; CHUQ-St-Francois D'Assise, 10 rue de l'Espinay, Quebec QC G1L 3L5; Laval'04; CCFP; Staff Med, Centre Hospitalier Universitaire De Québec - Pavillon De St-françois-d'assise; (418)525-4351 x53710; Fax. (418)525-4322.

FRADET, Anne; Clin des Medecins D'Urgence, 632 rue Bowen S, Sherbrooke QC J1G 2E9; Sher'83; CSPQ; FRCPC; IntMed; Cardiol. Assoc Member, Centre Hospitalier et CLSC de Memphremagog; Langs: Bilingual(French/English); (819)822-2700; Fax. (819)822-2027.

FRADET, Gaetan; 110-2880 ch des Quatre-Bourgeo, Quebec QC G1V 4X7; Laval'81; FRCSC; Otol (Otoneurology). Ac Staff, Centre Hospitalier Affilié Universitaire de Québec - Hôpital De L'Enfant Jésus; Ac Staff, Centre Hospitalier Affilié Universitaire de Québec - Hôpital du St-Sacrement; Prof, Université Laval; (418)653-8717; Fax. (418)653-7199.

FRADET, Guy; Dr Walter Anderson Bldg, 2F-2251 Pandosy St, Kelowna BC V1Y 1T1; Laval'79; MSc; FICS; FCCP; FACS; FRCSC; GenSurg; Cardiovasc&ThorSurg. Chief/Med Dir Card Surg Div of Cardiovasac & ThorSurg, Vancouver General Hospital - Centennial Pavillion; Staff, Providence Health Care - St Paul's Hospital; Prof, University of British Columbia; (250)862-4300 x2421

FRADET, Jean-Francois; 150-930 Ch Sainte-Foy, Quebec QC G1S 2L4; Laval'73; CSPQ; FRCSC; OrthSurg (Medico Legal Consultant). (418)682-7007; Fax. (418)527-0053.

FRADET, Robert; Ctre de Radiologie Sherbrooke, 250 rue King E, Sherbrooke QC J1G 1A9; Sher'84; FRCPC; DiagRad. Assoc Staff, Carrefour de Sante et Services Sociaux-Pavillon St-Louis; Ac Staff, Centre Hospitalier Universitaire de Sherbrooke-Hôpital Hôtel-Dieu; adj Prof, Universite de Sherbrooke; (819)563-1443; Fax. (819)563-3542.

FRADET, Vincent; Clinique d'Urologie Berger, 416-1000 ch Sainte-Foy, Quebec QC G1S 2L6; Mon'01; FRCSC; Urol. adj Prof, Université Laval; Langs: English; Spanish; (418)266-2876; Fax. (418)266-2879; vincent.fradet@fmed.ulaval.ca.

FRADET, Yves; CHQU-Hotel-Dieu de Quebec, 11 Cote du Palais, Quebec QC G1R 2J6; Laval'76; FRCSC; Urol. Staff, Centre Hospitalier Universitaire de Québec (CHUQ) - Siege Social; Head Surg, Université Laval; (418)525-4444 x15068

FRADETTE, Clermont; Clinique Med Cadillac, 3435 rue Bossuet, Montreal QC H1M 2M1; Laval'65; FRCSC; Otol. (514)253-1211; Fax. (514)253-5091.

FRADETTE, Virginie; Carrefour Sante-Pav St-Louis, 23 rue Ambroise-Dearden, Windsor QC J1S 1G8; Sher'07; Staff, Carrefour de Sante et Services Sociaux-Pavillon St-Louis; (819)542-2777; Fax. (819)845-5834.

FRAGER, Gerri; IWK Health Centre, PO Box 9700 Rpo CSC 5850 University Ave, Halifax NS B3K 6R8; McM'85; RN; BSc(Hons.); Peds (Palliative Care). Med Dir Ped Palliatice Care, IWK Health Centre; Assoc Prof Peds, Dalhousie University; (902)470-7262; Fax. (902)470-7216; gerri.frager@iwk.nshealth.ca.

FRAGISKOS, Vasilios A; Boreal Medical Clinic, PO Box 9000 1425 Front St, Hearst ON P0L 1N0; Ott'86; Chief Med Staff/Staff, Hôpital Notre Dame Hospital - Hearst; Langs: Bilingual(English/French); (705)362-7800; Fax. (705)362-8300.

FRAGOSO ALVAREZ, Zaida; Lockview Med Clinic, 203-667 Sackville Dr, Lower Sackville NS B4C 2S4; Habana (Cuba)'95; FamilyMed. (902)252-3011

FRAIN, Margaret; CSSS des Pays-d'En-Haut, 707 boul de Sainte-Adele, Sainte-Adele QC J8B 2N1; Man'84; (450)229-6601

FRALEIGH, Warren C; North York Gen Hosp, 4001 Leslie St, North York ON M2K 1E1; Qns'72; Assoc Staff, North York General Hospital; (416)410-1014; warrenfraleigh@rogers.com.

FRALICK, Richard A; Sunnybrook Health Sciences Ctr, 2075 Bayview Ave, Toronto ON M4N 3M5; Tor'72; MHSc; FRCPC; CommunMed (Medical Oncology);CCFP; FCFP; Staff, Sunnybrook Health Sciences Centre; Asst Prof Public Health Services Famil & Commun Med, University of Toronto; (416)480-6100 x82040; Fax. (416)480-6002.

FRAME, Gidon; Old Orchard Med Clinic, 11-4429 Kingsway, Burnaby BC V5H 2A1; Witwatersrand (South Africa)'86; MB BCh; CAFCI; ABAAM; FamilyMed. Ac Staff, Burnaby Hospital; Med Dir, Laser Clinic of Vancouver BC; Owner, Anti-Aging Medical of Vancouver BC; Clinical Asst Prof, University of British Columbia; Langs: Hebrew; Afrikaans; Cantonese; Russian; (604)431-6585; Fax. (604)431-0274.

FRAME, Heather A; Assiniboine Clinic, 633 Lodge Ave, Winnipeg MB R3J 0S9; Man'82; CCFP; FCFP; (204)958-6777; Fax. (204)888-1750.

FRANC-GUIMOND, Julie; Hôpital Ste-Justine, 3175 ch Cote-Sainte-Catherine, Montreal QC H3T 1C5; Sher'96; FRCSC; Urol (Pediatrics). Staff, Hôpital Ste-Justine; (514)345-4716 x4; Fax. (514)345-4824; julie.franc-guimond.hsj@ssss.gouv.qc.ca.

FRANC-LAW, Jeffrey M; University of Alberta Hosp, 8440 112 St NW, Edmonton AB T6G 2B7; Cal'94; CCFP; CCFP(E.M.); FCFP; Med Officer Emerg Med, University of Alberta Hospital; Langs: English; French; (780)407-8432; Fax. (780)407-7215.

FRANCESCUTTI, Louis; Edmonton Clinic Health Academy, 3 372 ECHA-11405 87 Ave NW, Edmonton AB T6G 1C9; Alb'87; PhD(Immunol); MPH; FAB; FRCPC; CCFP; CommunMed (Public Health). Staff EmergMed, Royal Alexandra Hospital; Staff, University of Alberta Hospital; Pres, Royal College of Physicians & Surgeons of Canada; Assoc Prof Public Hlth Sciences/Dir, University of Alberta; Langs: Italian; (780)492-6546; Fax. (780)492-2645; louis.francescutti@ualberta.ca.

FRANCHETTO, Arlene A; Hamilton HS-General Site, 237 Barton St E, Hamilton ON L8L 2X2; McM'80; FACR; FRCPC; DiagRad (Neuro Radiology). Staff Radiol, Hamilton Health Sciences Centre - Hamilton General Hospital; Associate Clin Prof, McMaster University; (905)527-4322 x46521

FRANCHI, Donald B; The Spence Clinic, 500-1265 Arthur St E, Thunder Bay ON P7E 6E7; Wes'86; (807)626-1111; Fax. (807)626-1121.

FRANCHOMME-FOSSE, Violaine; Clinique Sante Jacques-Cartier, 200-1815 rue King O, Sherbrooke QC J1J 2E3; Mon'94; CCFP; Staff Gen Med & Perinatal, Centre Hospitalier Universitaire de Sherbrooke-Hopital Fleurimont; Langs: Bilingual(French/English); (819)565-7446; Fax. (819)565-7780.

FRANCIS, Amira; E6-18 King St E, Bolton ON L7E 1E8; Alexandria (Egypt)'87; CCFP; (905)857-7469; Fax. (905)857-7959.

FRANCIS, Christopher J; Port Arthur Health Centre Inc, 194 Court St N, Thunder Bay ON P7A 4V7; Tor'88; FRCSC; Ophth. (807)346-1000; Fax. (807)346-6206.

FRANCIS, Dennis R; Westside Integrated Hlth Ctre, 130-180 Wilson St, Victoria BC V9A 7N6; UBC'92; BSc; (250)592-1110; Fax. (250)418-8879.

FRANCIS, Denyse; CSSS Cleophas-Claveau, 800 rue Aime-Gravel, La Baie QC G7B 2M4; Mon'74; Langs: Bilingual(French/English); (418)544-7316; Fax. (418)544-0052.

FRANCIS, Eleanor; Nipawin Health Centre, PO Box 1925, Nipawin SK S0E 1E0; (South Africa)'06; MB ChB; (306)862-3151; Fax. (306)862-2241; efrancis@kthr.sk.ca.

FRANCIS, Gordon A; St Paul's Hosp, 1081 Burrard St, Vancouver BC V6Z 1Y6; McG'84; FRCPC; IntMed (Cardiovascular Disease); Endocrin&Metab. Staff Med, Providence Health Care - St Paul's Hospital; Dir Health Heart Prog Prevention Clinic/Principal Investigator Heart & Lung Dinstitate/Prof Med, University of British Columbia; (604)806-9269; teddy.chan@hli.ubc.ca.

FRANCIS, Gregory J; Thunder Bay Reg HSC-T-Bay, 980 Oliver Rd, Thunder Bay ON P7B 6V4; Tor'97; CCFP; CCFP(E.M.); Staff, Thunder Bay Regional Health Sciences Centre; (807)684-6000

FRANCIS, James E; Caledonian Clinic, 340 Campbell St, Nanaimo BC V9R 3G7; Wes'93; CCFP; (250)753-3202

FRANCIS, Johanne; Polyclinique St-Eustache, 75 rue Grignon, Saint-Eustache QC J7P 4J2; Mon'86; (450)473-6882

FRANCIS, Julie-Ann R; Kingston Gen Hosp, 76 Stuart St, Kingston ON K7L 2V7; Yale (USA)'00; AB; FRCSC; ObstGyn (Surgical Oncology). Staff, Kingston General Hospital; Asst Prof, Queen's University; (613)548-6071; Fax. (613)548-1330.

FRANCIS, Marc N; Foothills Med Centre, C231-1403 29 St NW, Calgary AB T2N 2T9; Qns'03; FRCPC; EmergMed. Staff, Foothills Medical Centre; (403)944-1635; Fax. (403)944-2419.

FRANCIS, Michael J D; Ross Memorial Hosp, 10 Angeline St N, Lindsay ON K9V 4M8; Leeds (England)'00; MB ChB; BSc; CCFP; Staff, Ross Memorial Hospital; (705)328-6115; Fax. (866)220-0221.

FRANCIS, Michael L; 260 Mississaga St W, Orillia ON L3V 3B8; Wes'83; Staff, Orillia Soldiers' Memorial Hospital; (705)325-2300

FRANCIS, Michelle C; Oceanview Paediatrics, 101-1650 Terminal Ave N, Nanaimo BC V9S 0A3; Qns'04; FRCPC; Peds. (250)591-1906; Fax. (250)591-1913.

FRANCIS, Patricia K; Bram Centre Med Clinic, 16-7910 Hurontario St, Brampton ON L6Y 0P6; RCS (Ireland)'83; MB ChB; CCFP; Langs: Afrikaans; Tamil; (289)752-1571

FRANCIS, Robert; Medcan Health Mgmt Inc, 1500-150 York St, Toronto ON M5H 3S5; McG'68; Court Staff, St Michael's Hospital; Court Staff, Mount Sinai Hospital; Assoc Staff, Toronto General Hospital - UHN; Pres, Medcan Health Management Inc; Chairman, University of Toronto; (416)350-5909; Fax. (416)350-5984.

FRANCIS, Sara-Lynn D; 87 Adelaide St N, Lindsay ON K9V 4L4; McM'98; BASc; CCFP; (705)324-2581

FRANCIS, Thomas P; Family Health Clinic, PO Box 70 6173 Kootenay St, Oliver BC V0H 1T0; Wes'79; CCFP; Langs: German; (250)498-3418

FRANCISCO, Francisco C; Humber Valley Med Centre, 7-2630 Kipling Ave, Etobicoke ON M9V 4B9; Cal'92; Langs: Tagalog; (416)746-0389

FRANCK, Robert E; McGill Mental Health, 5500-3600 rue McTavish, Montreal QC H3A 0G3; McG'74; FRCPC; Psy. Dir Psychogeriatric Serv, McGill University Health Centre - Royal Victoria Hospital; (514)398-6019; Fax. (514)398-5529.

FRANCO-BARREDO, Francisco; Clin Med L'Avenir, 200-1150 boul de l'Avenir, Laval QC H7N 6L2; Valladolid (Spain)'60; Staff, Hôpital du Sacre-Coeur de Montréal; (450)680-1150

FRANCOEUR, Diane; Le Ctr D'Obstetrique-Gynecolog, 203-1361 av Beaumont, Mont-Royal QC H3P 2W3; Laval'87; FRCSC; ObstGyn (Pediatric Gynecology). Chef obst & gyn, Hôpital Ste-Justine; Prof Dept of ObstGyn Faculty of Med, Universite de Montreal; (514)344-4411; Fax. (514)344-1991; diane.francoeur.hsj@ssss.gouv.qc.ca.

FRANCOEUR, Helene; CSSS de Beauce-Etchemin, 1515 17e rue, Saint-Georges QC G5Y 4T8; Laval'91; IntMed (Cardiology). Staff Internist, Centre Hospitalier Beauce-Etchemin; (418)228-2031 x7272; Fax. (418)227-8134.

FRANCOEUR, Jacques; Ctr Hosp Affilie-Enfant-Jesus, 1401 18e rue, Quebec QC G1J 1Z4; Laval'60; MA; Neursurg (P.Q.) (Medico Legal Issues). Staff NeuroSurg, Centre Hospitalier Affilié Universitaire de Québec - Hôpital De L'Enfant Jésus; adj Prof, Université Laval; Langs: English; (418)649-0252 x4102; Fax. (418)652-3420; jacques.francoeurmd@videotron.ca.

FRANCOEUR, Jason R; Windsor Square Shopp Centre, 201-1959 152 St, Surrey BC V4A 9E3; UBC'99; FRCSC; GenSurg. (604)535-0525

FRANCOEUR, Luc; The Moncton Hosp, 135 MacBeath Ave, Moncton NB E1C 6Z8; Mon'90; FRCPC; DiagRad. Staff, The Moncton Hospital; (506)857-5280

FRANCOEUR, Marie-Alix; 1427 rue Fleury E, Montreal QC H2C 1R9; Lille (France)'70; FRCPC; Derm. (514)324-8520; Fax. (514)324-8521; mafrancoeur@hotmail.com.

FRANCOEUR, Marie-Josee; 200-2984 boul Taschereau, Greenfield Park QC J4V 2G9; Mon'95; FRCPC; Peds (Pediatric Allergy); ClinImmunol&Allergy. Staff Ped Allergy, Hopital Charles LeMoyne; Prof Ped Allergy, Universite de Sherbrooke; Langs: English; French; (450)465-9789; Fax. (450)672-4578.

FRANCOEUR, Martin; Hop Charles LeMoyne, 3120 boul Taschereau, Greenfield Park QC J4V 2H1; Mon'89; FRCPC; DiagRad. Staff, Hopital Charles LeMoyne; (450)466-5000 x2030

FRANCOEUR, Nicolas; 461 rue Notre-Dame, Saint-Tite QC G0X 3H0; Laval'53; (418)365-6567

FRANCOEUR, T Emmett; 300-4269 rue Sainte-Catherine, Westmount QC H3Z 1P7; McG'74; FRCPC; Peds (Developmental/Behavioural Pediatrics). Dir Child Development Prog, McGill University Health Centre - Montreal Children's Hospital; assoc Prof/vice Chaire Dept of Peds, McGill University; Langs: French; (514)931-7430; Fax. (514)931-0363.

FRANCOIS, Jean; Clinique Med D'Urgence Leger, 305-5900 boul Leger, Montreal-Nord QC H1G 1K9; Nantes (France)'73; (514)321-4609; Fax. (514)321-1018.

FRANCOIS, Jose M G; St Boniface Gen Hosp, D1048-409 Tache Ave, Winnipeg MB R2H 2A6; Sher'97; BSc; MMedEd; CCFP; FCFP; Staff Family Med, St Boniface General Hospital; Assoc Prof Family Med/Assoc Dean Continuing Professional Development, University of Manitoba; Langs: English; (204)235-3910; Fax. (204)237-9057; jfrancois@centredesante.mb.ca.

FRANCZAK, Edwin J; Agincourt Med Centre, 2020 Brimley Rd, Scarborough ON M1S 4R7; Wes'66; CCFP; (416)293-2404

FRANCZYK, Juliet A E; Peterborough Reg HC-Hospital, 1 Hospital Dr, Peterborough ON K9J 7C6; Tor'84; BHSc; FRCPC; DiagRad. Staff, Peterborough Regional Health Centre - Hospital Drive; (705)876-5039

FRANGOU, Evan M; CBI Health Centre, 605 Discovery St, Victoria BC V8T 5G4; Sask'05; FRCSC; Neursurg. (250)383-3638

FRANGOU, Panayiotis E; Horizon Square Med Centre, 401-3508 32 Ave NE, Calgary AB T1Y 6J2; Manchester (England)'64; LRCP; MRCS; FRCS(Ed); MB ChB; CCFP; Langs: Greek; (403)291-5588; Fax. (403)250-6783; pefrangou@hotmail.com.

FRANIC, Slobodan E; Perth-Smith Falls Dist Hosp, 33 Drummond St W, Perth ON K7H 2K1; Madrid (Spain)'80; FRCPC; DiagRad (Breast Imaging). Ac Staff, St Joseph's Healthcare - Charlton Campus; Court Staff, Hamilton Health Sciences Centre - McMaster Children's Hospital; Staff, Perth & Smiths Falls District Hospital - Perth Site (Great War Memorial Site); Assoc Prof, McMaster University; Langs: Spanish; (613)267-1500

FRANIEK, Janet N; West Coast Women's Clinic, 3525 4th Ave W, Vancouver BC V5R 1N9; UBC'92; CCFP; (604)738-9601; Fax. (604)738-9605.

FRANK, Agnes; Clinique Enfant-Medic, 3221 boul des Sources, Dollard-D-Ormeaux QC H9B 1Z6; Budapest (Hungary)'73; CCFP; (514)685-0880; Fax. (514)685-6162.

FRANK, Andrew; Memory Disorder Clinic, 261Y-75 Bruyere St, Ottawa ON K1N 5C8; UBC'00; BSc(Hon); FRCSC; Neur (Cognitive Neurol). Med Dir Memory Disorder Clinic, SCO Health Service - Élisabeth Bruyère Hospital; (613)562-6322; Fax. (613)562-6013.

FRANK, Cathy S; Southern Ont Fertility Technol, 107-555 Southdale Rd E, London ON N6E 1A2; McM'97; ObstGyn (Infertility). (519)685-5559

FRANK, Christopher C; Providence CCC-St Mary's, PO Box 3600 Stn Main 340 Union St, Kingston ON K7L 5A2; Wes'89; CCFP; FCFP; Staff Geriatrics, Providence Care - St Mary's of the Lake Hospital Site; Assoc Prof, Queen's University; (613)544-5220 x2208; Fax. (613)544-4017; frankc@providencecare.ca.

FRANK, Cyril B; Health Research Innovation Ctr, 400-3280 Hospital Dr NW, Calgary AB T2N 4Z6; Cal'76; FRCSC; OrthSurg. Staff, Peter Lougheed Centre; Prof Surg, University of Calgary; (403)220-4554; Fax. (403)283-1778; cfrank@ucalgary.ca.

FRANK, Daniel E; Inst Of Commun & Family Psy, 4333 ch Cote-Sainte-Catherine, Montreal QC H3T 1E4; McG'70; FRCPC; Psy (Forensic Psychiatry). (514)340-8210

FRANK, Eleanor M; Royal Oak Med Centre, 206-6440 Royal Oak Ave, Burnaby BC V5H 3P2; Cal'78; (604)432-9747; Fax. (604)436-0243.

FRANK, Helen; Vegreville Family Clinic, PO Box 219, Vegreville AB T9C 1R2; (South Africa)'00; MB ChB; (780)632-6414; Fax. (780)632-6404.

FRANK, J Peter; St Joseph's Healthcare, 50 Charlton Ave E, Hamilton ON L8N 4A6; Qns'67; FRCPC; EmergMed. Staff, St Joseph's Healthcare - Charlton Campus; (905)522-4941

FRANK, Jason R; The Ottawa Hosp-Gen Campus, 501 Smyth Rd, Ottawa ON K1H 8L6; Ott'97; FRCPC; EmergMed. Staff, The Ottawa Hospital - General Campus; (613)737-8000

FRANK, Nathan P; 100-13291 Yonge St, Richmond Hill ON L4E 4L6; McG'87; CCFP; FCFP; Langs: Bilingual(English/French); (905)773-7759

FRANK, Ryan C; Alberta Children's Hosp, 2888 Shaganappi Trail NW, Calgary AB T3B 6A8; Cal'04; FRCSC; PlasSurg. Staff, Alberta Children's Hospital; (403)955-7211

FRANK, Sandi C; Hys Med Centre, 300-11010 101 St NW, Edmonton AB T5H 4B9; Alb'96; BSc; FRCPC; Psy (General Adult Psychiatry). Staff, Royal Alexandra Hospital; (780)424-8383; Fax. (780)424-6404.

FRANK, Selby A; Vegreville Family Clinic, PO Box 219, Vegreville AB T9C 1R2; (South Africa)'71; MB ChB; MCFP; Chief/Staff, Covenant Health - St Joseph's General Hospital; Commun Med Dir, Alberta Health Services; Langs: Afrikaans; (780)632-6414; Fax. (780)632-6404; selby.frank@albertahealthservice.ca.

FRANK, Sheldon M; 6-420 Erb St W, Waterloo ON N2L 6H6; Wes'69; FRCSC; ObstGyn. Ac Staff, Grand River Hospital - Kitchener/Waterloo Health Centre; (519)579-5850

FRANK, William; 291 Riverside Dr, Toronto ON M6S 4B1; Glasgow (Scotland)'56; DPH; (416)236-0248; Fax. (416)236-1486.

FRANKE, Amy B; Allin Clinic, 10155 120 St NW, Edmonton AB T5K 2A2; Alb'93; CCFP; Physician Nursing Home, Capital Care - Grandview; (780)482-7551; Fax. (780)488-2056; amy.franke@capitalhealth.ca.

FRANKE, Gordon; Wall Street Ent Clinic, 230-140 Wall St, Saskatoon SK S7K 1N4; Sask'88; FRCSC; Otol. (306)244-7865; Fax. (306)244-8864.

FRANKE, Norman A; Univ Hlth Network-Princess M, 5F-610 University Ave, Toronto ON M5G 2M9; Tor'90; Staff, Princess Margaret Hospital - University Health Network; (416)946-4501 x5663

FRANKEL, Michael; Clover Care Med Clinic, 102-17770 56 Ave, Surrey BC V3S 1C7; Witwatersrand (South Africa)'86; MB ChB; Clin Asst PedOncol, BC Children's Hospital; Staff, Kerrisdale Station; (604)574-7883; Fax. (604)574-9601.

FRANKISH, Charles W; Kanata Prof Centre, 102-99 Kakulu Rd, Kanata ON K2L 3C8; Qns'83; FRCPC; IntMed; ClinImmunol&Allergy. Staff, Carleton Place & District Memorial Hospital; Staff, The Ottawa Hospital - General Campus; Staff, Arnprior & District Memorial Hospital; Clin Teacher Pt-Time, University of Ottawa; (613)599-5700; Fax. (613)599-5929.

FRANKLAND, Allan G; 720-999 Broadway St W, Vancouver BC V5Z 1K5; UBC'98; FRCPC; Psy. (778)331-0960

FRANKLIN, Angus L R; Mississauga Med Centre, 420-1420 Burnhamthorpe Rd E, Mississauga ON L4X 2Z9; Tor'89; PhD; CCFP; FCFP; Staff, Trillium Health Centre - Mississauga; (905)625-1619; Fax. (905)625-9362.

FRANKLIN, Gabriela; 8-9019 Bayview Ave, Richmond Hill ON L4B 3M6; Albany (USA)'98; CCFP; Langs: Romanian; (905)886-9660

FRANKLIN, Jason; Murray Bldg, 144 Brock St, Kingston ON K7L 5G2; Qns'98; FRCSC; Otol (Head & Neck). Staff, Hotel-Dieu Hospital; Staff, Queen's University; (613)544-3400; Fax. (613)547-5654.

FRANKLIN, John D; Fredericton Med Clinic, 507-1015 Regent St, Fredericton NB E3B 6H5; Dal'73; FRCSC; GenSurg. (506)458-0295; Fax. (506)457-4730; franklinsoffice@nb.aibn.com.

FRANKLIN, LeRoy D; Mississauga Med Centre, 330-1420 Burnhamthorpe Rd E, Mississauga ON L4X 2Z9; London (England)'62; MB BS; MRCS(Eng); LRCP(Lond); Staff, Trillium Health Centre - Mississauga; (905)625-5185

FRANKLIN, R Bernard; Lasalle Walk In Clinic, 70-1813 Lasalle Blvd, Sudbury ON P3A 2A3; Durham (England)'63; MB BS; DA; FRCOG; ObstGyn (Family Medicine). Langs: German; (905)270-8307; Fax. (905)270-6861.

FRANKLYN, Michael T; Brady Clinic, 101-359 Riverside Dr, Sudbury ON P3E 1H5; McM'91; BSc; BScChemEng; MSc; Assoc Prof Family Med, University of Ottawa Heart Institute; Staff GP & ObstGyn, Health Sciences North-St Joseph's Health Centre; Assoc Prof Fam Med, Laurentian University; (705)688-8833; Fax. (705)688-8646.

FRANKO, Evan P; GAMA Integrated Med Centre, PO Box 2060, Warman SK S0K 4S0; Sask'01; CCFP; CCFP(E.M.); (306)382-5554; Fax. (306)382-5567.

FRANKOVICH, Renata J; PSI Sport Med Centre West, 103-1000 Palladium Dr, Kanata ON K2V 1A4; Wes'94; CCFP; FCFP; (613)599-0299; Fax. (613)599-0298; rjfrankovich@hotmail.com.

FRANSEN, Donald A; Surrey Med Arts Bldg, 104-13798 94A Ave, Surrey BC V3V 1N1; Man'69; Staff Chief, Surrey Memorial Hospital; (604)581-9333; Fax. (604)581-3837.

FRANSKY, Melissa K; 1 Manor Lane PO Box 157, Bancroft ON K0C 1C0; McM'10; CCFP; (613)332-2825

FRANTSEVA, Marina; Addiction & Mental Hlth-Queen, 2 179-1001 Queen St W, Toronto ON M6J 1H4; McM'05; Psy. Staff, Centre for Addiction & Mental Health (CAMH) - Queen Site; (416)535-8501; Fax. (416)583-1263.

FRAPE, Norwynne F; Cambridge Mem Hosp, 700 Coronation Blvd, Cambridge ON N1R 3G2; Qns'76; CCFP; Ac Staff, Cambridge Memorial Hospital; (519)740-4940; Fax. (519)740-7722.

FRAPPIER, Guy; Polyclinique Med Fabreville, 104B-380 boul Cure-Labelle, Laval QC H7P 5L3; Mon'61; (450)628-5800 x337; Fax. (450)628-0217.

FRAPPIER, Jean-Yves; Hôpital Ste-Justine, 7955-3175 ch Cote-Ste-Catherin, Montreal QC H3T 1C5; Mon'73; MSc(Epidemiol); FRCPC; Peds (Adolescent Medicine). Ac Staff, Hôpital Ste-Justine; dép Chef Peds, Universite de Montreal; Langs: Bilingual(English/French); (514)345-4673; Fax. (514)345-2361; jeanyves_frappier@ssss.gouv.qc.ca.

FRAPPIER CHALIFOUX, Hamie; Polyclinique Pierre Le Gardeur, 300-1000 montee des Pionniers, Terrebonne QC J6V 1S8; Mon'04; Family Med & Obstetrique, Centre Hospitalier Pierre le Gardeur; (450)657-5799; Fax. (450)657-1809.

FRARE, Paola; Psychiatrie Consultation-Liais, DS047-1755 boul Rene-Laennec, Laval QC H7M 3L9; Mon'92; FRCPC; Psy. Staff, Hopital de la Cite de la santé; (450)975-5589

FRAS, Mary; Alberta Children's Hosp, 2888 Shaganappi Trail NW, Calgary AB T3B 6A8; Alb'05; FRCPC; Peds; Respir. Staff, Alberta Children's Hospital; (403)955-2953; Fax. (403)955-3055.

FRASER, Alan B; 9th Avenue Med Centre, 3-3855 9th Ave, Port Alberni BC V9Y 4T9; UBC'80; (250)724-1204; Fax. (250)723-7739.

FRASER, Amy B; The Ottawa Hosp-Civic Campus, B309-1053 Carling Ave, Ottawa ON K1Y 4E9; Qns'02; FRCPC; Anes. Staff, The Ottawa Hospital - Civic Campus; (613)761-4940

FRASER, Anne L; The Westend Family Care Clinic, 80 Michael Cowpland Dr, Kanata ON K2M 1P6; Ott'84; CCFP; FCFP; Staff, Westend Family Care Clinic Family Health Team; (613)596-3321

FRASER, Brian P; Doctors Bldg, 108-955 Queen St E, Sault Ste. Marie ON P6A 2C3; McM'07; FRCSC; OrthSurg. (705)450-0117; Fax. (705)450-0119.

FRASER, Brock R; 3491 Saanich Rd, Victoria BC V8X 1W8; Cal'79; Staff, Royal Jubilee Hospital; Staff, Victoria General Hospital; (250)475-2251; Fax. (250)475-3530.

FRASER, Christopher R R; Cool Aid Community Health Ctre, 713 Johnson St, Victoria BC V8W 1M8; UBC'91; Physician, Cool Aid Community Health Centre; (250)385-1466; Fax. (250)383-1327.

FRASER, David; Coalition of Family Physicians, 900-45 Sheppard Ave E, North York ON M2N 5W9; Mem'83; Psy. Staff, Coalition of Family Physicians (COFP); (416)495-8071; Fax. (416)733-2491.

FRASER, Derek; South Side Women's Hlth Ctre, 120-3017 66 St NW, Edmonton AB T6K 4B2; Alb'04; FRCSC; ObstGyn. Staff, Brockville General Hospital - Charles Street; (780)461-6220

FRASER, Donald K; Wall Street Med Bldg, 300-140 Wall St, Saskatoon SK S7K 1N4; Dal'74; FRCPC; DiagRad. (306)244-1167; Fax. (306)244-2911.

FRASER, Douglas D; London HSC-Victoria Hosp, PO Box 5010 Stn B C2 843-800 Commissioners Rd E, London ON N6A 5W9; Cal'98; FRCP; BSc; PhD; FRCPC; Peds (Neuro Trauma); Critical Care Medicine. Staff, London Health Sciences Centre - Victoria Campus; Staff, London Health Sciences Centre - Children's Hospital; (519)685-8386; Fax. (519)685-8156; fraserd@lhsc.on.ca.

FRASER, Evelyne; Polyclinique Med des Ponts, 120-1100 boul de la Rive-Sud, Saint-Romuald QC G6W 5M6; Laval'77; (418)834-4943

FRASER, Frederick; Health Sciences Bldg, 311-15 Mountain Ave S, Stoney Creek ON L8G 2V6; Dal'69; CCFP; FCFP; Ac Staff, Hamilton Health Sciences Centre; (905)662-4911; Fax. (905)662-1688.

FRASER, Garnet D; Phoenix Med Centre, 208-2155 10th Ave, Prince George BC V2M 5J6; Qns'95; CCFP; Staff, University Hospital of Northern British Columbia; (250)562-1910; Fax. (250)564-1332.

FRASER, Gordon A D; Guelph Med Place, 210-83 Dawson Rd, Guelph ON N1H 1B1; Tor'95; FRCSC; ObstGyn. (519)821-2440; Fax. (519)821-2448.

FRASER, Graeme; 3 84-699 Concession St, Hamilton ON L8V 5C2; Wes'98; BSc; MSc; FRCPC; IntMed (Oncology); Hem. Hematology, Hamilton Health Sciences Centre - Juravinski Cancer Centre; Asst Prof, McMaster University; (905)575-7820; Fax. (905)575-6340; graeme.fraser@jcc.hhsc.ca.

FRASER, Grant R I; Medical Office Centre, 108-857 Grand Ave W, Chatham ON N7L 4T1; Tor'80; AB; FRCSC; Ophth. Staff Ophth, Chatham-Kent Health Alliance; (519)354-5292

FRASER, Holly C; Canadian Forces Base Petawawa, 101 Menin Rd, Petawawa ON K8H 2X3; Man'07; CCFP; (613)687-5511

FRASER, Hughie; 203-26 North St, Bridgewater NS B4V 2V6; Cal'05; Gastroent; IntMed. Staff Gastroenterology, South Shore Regional Hospital; (902)530-3216; Fax. (902)530-3179.

FRASER, Ian; Toronto East Gen Hosp Inc, 825 Coxwell Ave, Toronto ON M4C 3E7; Ott'76; FRCPC; Respir (Critical Care Medicine); IntMed. Chief of Staff/Med Dir Prolonged-Ventilation Weaning Prov Ctr of Excellence, Toronto East General Hospital Inc; (416)469-7777; Fax. (416)469-7717; ifraser@tegh.on.ca.

FRASER, James B G; Kelligrews Medical Clinic, PO Box 17160 Stn Main, Conception Bay S NL A1X 3H1; Dal'72; (709)834-2171; Fax. (709)834-1241.

FRASER, James D; Queen Elizabeth II HSC-Halifax, 1796 Summer St, Halifax NS B3H 3A7; Dal'86; FRCPC; DiagRad. Staff, Queen Elizabeth II Health Sciences Centre - Victoria General Site; Asst Prof, Dalhousie University; (902)473-5330; Fax. (902)473-5323.

FRASER, James M; Cornwall Prof Bldg, 511-2125 11th Ave, Regina SK S4P 3X3; Sask'81; FRCSC; OrthSurg (Pediatric Orthopedic Surgery). Staff, Regina Health District; (306)569-8641; Fax. (306)924-9180; jimfraser@sasktel.net.

FRASER, John A; London HSC-University Hosp, PO Box 5339 Stn B B7 104-339 Windermere Rd, London ON N6A 5A5; Dal'03; FRCPC; Neur. Staff, London Health Sciences Centre - University Hospital; (519)663-3702; Fax. (519)663-3999.

FRASER, John R; North End Comm Health Centre, 2165 Gottingen St, Halifax NS B3K 3B5; McG'76; CCFP; FCFP; Court Staff, Queen Elizabeth II Health Sciences Centre - Victoria General Site; Court Staff, IWK Health Centre; Teacher, Dalhousie University; (902)420-0303; Fax. (902)422-0859; jrfraser@nechc.com.

FRASER, Kristin L; Rockyview Gen Hosp, 4A186-7007 14 St SW, Calgary AB T2V 1P9; Qns'92; FRCPC; IntMed (Sleep Medicine); Respir. Staff, Rockyview General Hospital; Assoc Prof, University of Calgary; (403)943-3475; Fax. (403)943-8666.

FRASER, Lisa-Ann; St Joseph's Health Care, PO Box 5777 Stn B 268 Grosvenor St, London ON N6A 4V2; Tor'04; FRCPC; IntMed; Endocrin&Metab. Staff, St Joseph's Hospital - St Joseph's Health Care; (519)646-6245; Fax. (519)646-6067.

FRASER, Lorna E; Diagnostic Care Inc, 4949 Bathurst St, Toronto ON M2R 1Y1; Tor'82; FRCPC; DiagRad. (416)223-5460; Fax. (416)223-8335.

FRASER, Louis; Foothills Med Centre, 1403 29 St NW, Calgary AB T2N 2T9; Mem'96; FRCPC; Anes (Emergency Medicine). Staff, Foothills Medical Centre; (403)944-1110; Fax. (403)944-2400.

FRASER, Margaret A; The Ottawa Hosp-Gen Campus U17-501 Smyth Rd, Ottawa ON K1H 8L6; McG'86; FRCPC; DiagRad. Staff, The Ottawa Hospital - General Campus; Langs: Bilingual(English/French); (613)737-8500; Fax. (613)737-8957.

FRASER, Margaret; Cape Breton Healthcare Complex, 1482 George St, Sydney NS B1P 1P3; Staff, Cape Breton Healthcare Complex; (902)567-8000

FRASER, Mark A; West Carleton Family Hlth Team, PO Box 218 119 Langstaff Dr, Carp ON K0A 1L0; Ott'81; CCFP; FCFP; Assoc Staff, Queensway Carleton Hospital; (613)839-3271 x131; Fax. (613)839-3273.

FRASER, Mary; Fraser & Smith Med Prof Corp, 33 Kayla Cres, Collingwood ON L9Y 5K9; McM'05; CCFP.

FRASER, Mary-Anne; Elmsdale Med Ctr, 106 Elmsdale Rd, Elmsdale NS B2S 1K6; Dal'88; BSc; (902)883-2216; Fax. (902)883-1734.

FRASER, Michael B; PO Box 172, Morris MB R0G 1K0; Man'77; (204)746-2741

FRASER, Myriam; Clinique Med Pierre-Boucher, 365-1615 boul Jacques-Cartier, Longueuil QC J4M 2X1; Sher'79; CSPQ; FRCSC; OrthSurg. Orthopedic Surgery, Centre Hospitalier Pierre Boucher; (450)463-2034; Fax. (450)463-3890.

FRASER, Peter K; Professional Corp, 1265 Onondaga St, Oromocto NB E2V 2P8; UBC'70; Court Staff, The Moncton Hospital; Staff, Oromocto Public Hospital; Med Consultant J Divsion & Health Canada, Royal Canadian Mounted Police; Lecturer, Dalhousie University; (506)357-8060; Fax. (506)357-2238; fraseroffice@nb.aibn.com.

FRASER, R Blair; Guelph Family Health Team, 301-21 Surrey St W, Guelph ON N1H 3R3; Wes'72; Ac Staff, Guelph General Hospital; (519)836-7240; Fax. (519)836-7240.

FRASER, Richard S; MUHC-Montreal Gen Hosp, 1650 av Cedar, Montreal QC H3G 1A4; McG'76; CSPQ; AnatPath (Pulmonary Pathology). Staff, McGill University Health Centre - Montreal General Campus; (514)934-1934 x43858

FRASER, Robert B; IWK Health Centre, PO Box 9700 Rpo CSC K3606-5980 University Ave, Halifax NS B3K 6R8; Dal'88; FCAP(AnatPath); ABP(PedPath); FRCPC; AnatPath (Pediatrics). Staff Path, IWK Health Centre; Prof, Dalhousie University; (902)470-8180; Fax. (902)470-7215; robert.fraser@iwk.nshealth.ca.

FRASER, Ronald I; PO Box 896 Stn Main, Dartmouth NS B2Y 3Z6; Dal'95; FRCPC; Psy. Staff, Colchester East Hants Health Centre; (902)425-2177; Fax. (902)424-7193.

FRASER, Ronald; Sault Area Hosp, 750 Great Northern Rd, Sault Ste. Marie ON P6B 0A8; Aberdeen (Scotland)'70; Staff, Sault Area Hospital - Sault Ste Marie; (705)759-3434

FRASER, Shannon A; SMBD Jewish Gen Hosp, A 510-3755 ch Cote-Sainte-Cath, Montreal QC H3T 1E2; Tor'99; CSPQ; FRCSC; GenSurg (Minimal Invasive Surgery). Staff, Sir Mortimer B Davis Jewish General; (514)340-8222 x3115; Fax. (514)340-8231; shannonfraser@mcgill.ca.

FRASER, Suzanne M; Bonaventure Med Clinic, 201-12427 Bonaventure Dr SE, Calgary AB T2J 3N8; Cal'87; FRCPC; Psy. (403)252-1529; Fax. (403)202-5028.

FRASER, Virginia H; Med Arts Bldg, 1114-233 Kennedy St, Winnipeg MB R3C 3J5; Man'77; FACS; FRCSC; FamilyMed; GenSurg. Staff, St Boniface General Hospital; Asst Prof, University of Manitoba; (204)786-5481; Fax. (204)783-3676.

FRASER, William D; Hôpital Ste-Justine, 3175 ch Cote-Sainte-Catherine, Montreal QC H3T 1C5; Dal'79; FRCSC; ObstGyn. Staff, Hôpital Ste-Justine; Prof, Universite de Montreal; Langs: English; French; (514)345-4931; Fax. (514)345-2195; william.fraser@umontreal.ca.

FRASER, Zachary R; 92 Main St, Dartmouth NS B2X 1R5; Dal'76; MD; CCFP; FCFP; Ac Staff, Dartmouth General Hospital; Staff Addiction Prevention & Treatment Services, Capital Health Centre; Teacher, Dalhousie University; (902)434-1500; Fax. (902)462-4994.

FRASER-ROBERTS, D Leigh; The Ottawa Hosp-Gen Campus, 501 Smyth Rd, Ottawa ON K1H 8L6; McM'93; FRCPC; Peds. Staff, The Ottawa Hospital - General Campus; Langs: Bilingual(English/French); (613)722-7000

FRASINSKI, Alicja; Carmi Clinic, 114-725 Carmi Ave, Penticton BC V2A 3G8; Nottingham (England)'01; BMedSci; MB BS; Staff Primary Care Maternity Clinic, Penticton Regional Hospital; (250)492-4274; Fax. (250)493-1887.

FRATESI, Sante J; Doctors Bldg, 305-955 Queen St E, Sault Ste. Marie ON P6A 2C3; Wes'74; DAB; FICS; FACS; MEd; FRCSC; GenSurg; VascSurg. Staff Consultant Surg, Sault Area Hospital - Sault Ste Marie; Asst Prof Surg, Northern Ontario School of Medicine; Langs: Italian; (705)541-2315; Fax. (705)942-8896; samfratesi@gmail.com.

FRAUENSTEIN, Giesela H; Students Union Bldg, 2 200-66 University Campus NW, Edmonton AB T6G 2J7; (South Africa)'82; MB ChB; (780)492-2612; Fax. (780)492-0172.

FRAULIN, Frankie; Alberta Childrens Hosp, B3 031-2888 Shaganappi Trail N, Calgary AB T3B 6A8; Alb'89; FRCSC; PlasSurg (Pediatric Plastic Surgery). Staff, Alberta Children's Hospital; Asst Clin Prof, University of Calgary; (403)955-2840

FRAYNE, Alister F; Fort Langley Med Clinic, PO Box 99 Stn Fort Langley 23148 96 Ave, Langley BC V1M 2R4; Cape Town (South Africa)'82; MB ChB; CCFP; Ac Staff, Langley Memorial Hospital; Clinical Asst Prof, University of British Columbia; Langs: Afrikaans; (604)888-2433; Fax. (604)888-5293.

FRAZEE, Pamela J; Tonquin Med Clinic, PO Box 189, Tofino BC V0R 2Z0; UBC'85; BSc; Staff, Tofino General Hospital; (250)725-3282; Fax. (250)725-3215.

FRAZER, Robert; Clinique Sante Jacques-Cartier, 200-1815 rue King O, Sherbrooke QC J1J 2E3; McG'81; Staff, Centre Hospitalier Universitaire de Sherbrooke-Hôpital Hôtel-Dieu; Langs: English; French; (819)565-7446; Fax. (819)565-7780.

FRECH, Robert J; Bridges Comm Hlth Ctr, 1485 Garrison Rd, Fort Erie ON L2A 1P8; Wes'76; Staff, Niagara Health System - St Catharines General Site; Staff, Niagara Health System - Ontario Street Site; (905)871-7621; Fax. (905)871-9135.

FRECHETTE, Andre; Clinique Med St-Vallier, 201-205 rue Montmagny, Quebec QC G1N 4V3; Laval'80; ac Staff, CSSS de Quebec-Sud; (418)688-0872; Fax. (418)688-4951.

FRECHETTE, Chantal A M; Centre Med Seine, 142 Centrale Ave, Ste Anne MB R5H 1C3; Sher'92; Staff, Ste Anne Hospital; Langs: Bilingual(French/English); (204)422-8811; Fax. (204)422-5876.

FRECHETTE, Claude; CSSS de Laval, 1755 boul Rene-Laennec, Laval QC H7M 3L9; Mon'96; CCFP; FCFP; Staff, Hopital de la Cite de la santé; (450)668-1010; Fax. (450)628-5305.

FRECHETTE, Denise; CLSC des Faubourgs, 1705 rue de la Visitation, Montreal QC H2L 3C3; Mon'87; CCFP; FCFP; (514)527-2361; Fax. (514)527-3074.

FRECHETTE, Dominique; CSSSG-Hop De Gatineau, CP 2000 Succ Bureau-Chef 909 boul de la Verendrye O, Gatineau QC J8P 7H2; Ott'04; FRCPC; IntMed; MedOncol. Staff, Hôpital de Gatineau; (819)966-6100; Fax. (819)966-6296.

FRECHETTE, Eric; Hôpital Laval, 2725 ch Sainte-Foy, Quebec QC G1V 4G5; Mon'95; CSPQ; FRCSC; GenSurg; ThorSurg. Staff, Hôpital Laval; (418)656-8711

FRECHETTE, France; Ctr Hosp Anna-Laberge, 200 boul Brisebois, Chateauguay QC J6K 4W8; Mon'98; LMCC; Staff EmergMed, Hôpital Anna-Laberge; Staff Gen Med, Centre Hospitalier Pierre Boucher; Langs: Spanish; English; (450)699-2425; Fax. (450)699-2525; xylo150@hotmail.com.

FRECHETTE, France; Radiologie Jean-Talon Belanger, 1470 rue Belanger, Montreal QC H2G 1A7; Sher'89; DiagRad. Staff, Complexe hospitalier de la Sagamie; (514)274-5449

FRECHETTE, Guillaume; Hotel-Dieu d'Arthabaska, 5 rue des Hospitalieres, Victoriaville QC G6P 6N2; Laval'04; FRCPC; Psy. Staff, Hotel-Dieu d'Arthabaska; Langs: Bilingual(French/English); (819)357-2030; Fax. (819)857-6035.

FRECHETTE, Jean-Rene; 2300 boul du Millenaire, St-Basile-le-Grand QC J3N 1T8; Mon'81; (450)441-1142; Fax. (450)461-3471.

FRECHETTE, Julie; CSSSTR St-Joseph, 735 rue Sainte-Julie, Trois-Rivieres QC G9A 0B5; Mon'01; Langs: Bilingual(French/English); (819)370-2200 x42401; Fax. (819)379-9440.

FRECHETTE, Marc; Marion Med Clinic, 172 Marion St, Winnipeg MB R2H 0T4; Man'04; BSc; BEd; CCFP; Langs: Bilingual(English/French); (204)221-4489; Fax. (204)233-6185; mfrech@shaw.ca.

FRECHETTE, Marc; CSSS de la Region de Thetford, 1717 rue Notre-Dame E, Thetford Mines QC G6G 2V4; Laval'81; CSPQ; FRCPC; Anes. Chief Anes, Hopital du CSS de la Region de Thetford; (418)338-7777 x4120; Fax. (418)338-7794; marc_frechette@tm.cgocable.ca.

FRECHETTE, Marie-Christine; Clinique Med des Bois-Francs, 101 rue Demers, Princeville QC G6L 4E8; Mon'09; (819)364-2150

FRECHETTE, Pierre; 6489 rue des Giroflées, Charny QC G6X 3G5; Laval'70; BA; AvMed; MCPS; CHE; DHA; EmergMed (Physical Medicine & Rehabilitation). Asst Dir Med Staff, Centre Hospitalier Affilié Universitaire de Québec - Hôpital De L'Enfant Jésus; Physician, Ordre du Quebec; Med Coord, Traumatology Services & Emerg. Hosp., Ministry of Health & Social Services of Quebec; Clin Prof, Université Laval; Langs: Bilingual(French/English); (418)832-0007; pierfrec@videotron.ca.

FRECHETTE, Robert C; 2855 Front Rd RR 2 Stn Main, Hawkesbury ON K6A 2R2; Mon'77; Staff, Hawkesbury & District General Hospital; Langs: Bilingual(French/English); (613)632-4711; Fax. (613)632-4711.

FRECHETTE, Sharon; 172 Marion St, Winnipeg MB R2H 0T4; Man'01; CCFP.

FRECHETTE, Solange; Clinique Med Saint-Nicephore, 4534 boul Saint-Joseph, Saint-Nicephore QC J2A 1B5; Sher'82; (819)472-3350

FRECHETTE-PELLETIER, Emilie; CSSS Pierre Boucher, 1333 boul Jacques-Cartier E, Longueuil QC J4M 2A5; Mon'08; Peds. Staff, Centre Hospitalier Pierre Boucher; (450)468-8111

FRECKER, Erica; Fredericton Med Clinic, 304-1015 Regent St, Fredericton NB E3B 6H5; McM'02; FRCSC; ObstGyn.

FRECKER, Richard; 107 Braemar Ave, Toronto ON M5P 2L3; Dal'66; PhD(Tor); LMCC; BSc; Prof Emeritus, University of Toronto; rick.frecker@utoronto.ca; Semi-Retired.

FREDERICK, Catherine E; Spingbank Med Centre, 310-460 Springbank Dr, London ON N6J 0A8; Wes'87; CCFP; FCFP; Physician, Parkwood Hospital - St Joseph's Health Care; Aj Prof School of Med Dentistry, Western Univ; (519)672-3509; Fax. (519)672-8621.

FREDETTE, Marie-Josee; Ctr Hosp Affilie-St-Sacrement, D2 50A-1050 ch Sainte-Foy, Quebec QC G1S 4L8; Laval'99; FRCSC; Ophth. Staff, Centre Hospitalier Affilié Universitaire de Québec - Hôpital du St-Sacrement; (418)682-7511 x4846; Fax. (418)682-7998.

FREDETTE, Patrick J L; Seine Med Centre, 145-142 Centrale Ave, Ste Anne MB R5H 1C3; Sher'92; BSc(Med); Langs: Bilingual(French/English); (204)422-8811; Fax. (204)422-5876.

FREDETTE, Paul P; Val Est Med Clinic, 8-3140 Highway 69 N, Val Caron ON P3N 1G3; Ott'96; CCFP; Staff, Health Sciences North-St Joseph's Health Centre; Langs: Bilingual(English/French); (705)897-7464; Fax. (705)897-7464.

FREDETTE, Simon; CSSS du Rocher-Perce, CP 3300 451 rue Mgr Ross E, Chandler QC G0C 1K0; Sher'05; Staff, Centre Hospitalier de Chandler; (418)689-2261; Fax. (418)689-4957.

FREDRIKSON, Diane H; Early Psychosis Intervention P, 333-2750 Hastings St E, Vancouver BC V5K 1Z9; UBC'98; FRCPC; Psy. Staff, Providence Health Care - St Paul's Hospital; (604)675-3875; dfredrikson@providencehealth.bc.ca.

FREEBURY, David R; Onefertility, 3210 Harvester Rd, Burlington ON L7N 3T1; Cardiff (Wales)'58; MB ChB; DRCOG; FRCPC; Psy (Psychotherapy). (905)634-4440; Fax. (905)639-3810.

FREED, Adam C; Grey Nuns Comm Hosp & HC, 1100 Youville Drive West NW, Edmonton AB T6L 5X8; Alb'00; FRCPC; Anes. Staff, Covenant Health - Grey Nuns Community Hospital; (780)735-7020

FREED, Darren H; I H Asper Clinical Research, CR3030-369 Tache Ave, Winnipeg MB R2H 2A6; Alb'98; FRCSC; CardSurg.

FREED, Jennene L M; Royal Alexandra Hosp, 10240 Kingsway Ave NW, Edmonton AB T5H 3V9; Alb'01; FRCPC; Psy. Staff Adult Mentall Health Prog, Royal Alexandra Hospital; (780)735-5383; Fax. (780)735-4797.

FREEDHOFF, Jonathan E; 100-575 West Hunt Club Rd, Nepean ON K2G 5W5; Tor'99; CCFP; Langs: Hebrew; (613)730-0264

FREEDMAN, Amy K; St James Town Health Centre, 410 Sherbourne St, Toronto ON M4X 1K2; Tor'95; BSc; CCFP; Staff, Baycrest Centre for Geriatric Care; Staff Family Med, St Michael's Hospital; Teacher, University of Toronto; (416)864-3096; amy.freedman@utoronto.ca.

FREEDMAN, Arthur N; Ellendale Med Bldg, 225-5845 ch de la Cote-des-Nei, Montreal QC H3S 1Z4; McG'55; MSc; DAB; FACS; CSPQ; FRCSC; GenSurg (Clinical Surgery). Sr Staff Surg, Sir Mortimer B Davis Jewish General; Chief Surg, Jewish Eldercare Centre - CHSLD JUIF de Montréal; Asst Surg, McGill University Health Centre - Royal Victoria Hospital; adj Prof, McGill University; (514)733-9433; Fax. (514)733-2442.

FREEDMAN, David; Columbia Med Bldg, 106-301 Columbia St E, New Westminster BC V3L 3W5; UBC'88; Staff, Royal Columbian Hospital; Staff, Eagle Ridge Hospital & Health Care Centre; (604)524-3899; Fax. (604)524-3866.

FREEDMAN, David M; 11-398 Steeles Ave W, Thornhill ON L4J 6X3; McG'89; FRCPC; IntMed (Consultation); Cardiol. Assoc Staff, Toronto General Hospital - UHN; Langs: Russian; French; (905)881-0334; Fax. (905)881-1721.

FREEDMAN, Dayna M; Scarborough Prof Centre, 205-1371 Neilson Rd, Scarborough ON M1B 4Z8; Tor'96; FRCSC; ObstGyn. (416)281-1588; Fax. (416)281-0939.

FREEDMAN, Fred A; Spadina Health Centre, 404-720 Spadina Ave, Toronto ON M5S 2T9; Tor'76; CCFP; FCFP; Court Staff, Toronto General Hospital - UHN; Lecturer, University of Toronto; (416)928-0920; Fax. (416)928-7426.

FREEDMAN, Glen L; 878-1641 Lonsdale Ave, North Vancouver BC V7M 2J5; Alb'94; FRCPC; Psy. Clin Researcher Psy, BC Children's Hospital; (604)949-7743

FREEDMAN, Jeffrey I; St Boniface Gen Hosp, L2035-409 Tache Ave, Winnipeg MB R2H 2A6; Cal'97; FRCPC; Anes. Staff, St Boniface General Hospital; (204)233-8563

FREEDMAN, Joel H; 509 Park St, Kitchener ON N2G 1N9; McG'87.

FREEDMAN, John S; Thornhill Square, 310-300 John St, Thornhill ON L3T 5W4; Dal'79; BSc; FAAP; FRCPC; Peds. Ad Staff Privil, The Hospital For Sick Children; Court Staff, North York General Hospital; Asst Prof, University of Toronto; (905)881-9831; Fax. (905)886-5236.

FREEDMAN, M Lee; 4-421 Eglinton Ave W, Toronto ON M5N 1A4; McG'82; FRCPC; Psy. Staff Psy, The Hospital For Sick Children; Teacher, University of Toronto; (416)913-5546

FREEDMAN, Mark; Sunnybrook Hlth Sciences Ctre, 2075 Bayview Ave, Toronto ON M4N 3M5; Tor'00; FRCPC; EmergMed. Staff EmergMed, Sunnybrook Health Sciences Centre; (416)480-6018

FREEDMAN, Mark S; 501 Smyth Rd Box 601, Ottawa ON K1H 8L6; Tor'83; BSc; MSc; FRCPC; Neur (Multiple Sclerosis). Dir Multiple Sclerosis Research Clinic, The Ottawa Hospital - General Campus; Staff, Perth & Smiths Falls District Hospital - Perth Site (Great War Memorial Site); Consultant, Brockville Mental Health Centre - Royal Ottawa Health Care Group; Consultant, Pembroke Regional Hospital Inc; University of Ottawa; Langs: Hebrew; French; (613)737-8917; Fax. (613)737-8857; mfreedman@toh.on.ca.

FREEDMAN, Melvin H; 555 University Ave, Toronto ON M5G 1X8; Dal'66; ABPeds; FRCPC; Peds (Pediatric Hematology Oncology). Staff, The Hospital For Sick Children; (416)964-0568; Fax. (416)813-7479; mel.freedman@sympatico.ca.

FREEDMAN, Michelle R; Appletree Med Centre, 4700 Keele St, North York ON M3J 1P3; McM'93; (647)722-2370; Fax. (416)736-5523.

FREEDMAN, Morris; Baycrest Ctre/Geriatric Care, 656-3560 Bathurst St, North York ON M6A 2E1; Ott'75; FRCPC; Neur. Staff Neurol, Mount Sinai Hospital; Staff, Toronto General Hospital - UHN; Prof, University of Toronto; (416)785-2444; Fax. (416)785-2484.

FREEDMAN, Orit C; Lakeridge Hlth Corp-Oshawa, 1 Hospital Crt, Oshawa ON L1G 2B9; Tor'02; FRCPC; IntMed; MedOncol. Staff, Lakeridge Health - Oshawa Site; Langs: Hebrew; (905)576-8711

FREEDMAN, Paul E; Doctor's Office, 100-491 Lawrence Ave W, North York ON M5M 1C7; Tor'70; CCFP; FCFP; Staff, Mount Sinai Hospital; Asst Prof, University of Toronto; (416)787-0117; Fax. (416)787-8094.

FREEDMAN, Stephen M; Dufferin Subspecialty Clinic, 1664 Dufferin St, Toronto ON M6H 3M1; Cal'94; BSc; FRCPC; IntMed (Cardiac Rehabilitation). Clin Associate, Toronto General Hospital - UHN; Researcher Fellow, Mount Sinai Hospital; Langs: Bilingual(English/French); (416)652-6101; Fax. (416)652-1994.

FREEDMAN, Stephen; Alberta Children's Hosp, 2888 Shaganappi Trail NW, Calgary AB T3B 6A8; McG'96; FRCPC; Peds. Staff, Alberta Children's Hospital; (403)955-7740; Fax. (403)955-7552; stephen.freedman@sickkids.ca.

FREELAND, Alison D; Royal Ottawa Health Care Group, 1145 Carling Ave, Ottawa ON K1Z 7K4; Sask'89; BSc; FRCPC; Psy. Ac Staff Schizophrenia Prog & Psy Community Mental Health Prog, Royal Ottawa Mental Health Centre - Royal Ottawa Health Care Group; Consultant, The Ottawa Hospital - General Campus; The Ottawa Hospital - Civic Campus; Assoc Prof, University of Ottawa; (613)722-6521 x6546; Fax. (613)722-7686; alison.freeland@theroyal.ca.

FREEMAN, Adele T; Westglen Med Centre, 108-30 Springborough Blvd SW, Calgary AB T3H 0N9; Glasgow (Scotland)'61; MB ChB; DObstRCOG; BSc(Hon.); (403)240-2221; Fax. (403)240-4670; adelefreeman@sprint.ca.

FREEMAN, Carolyn R; MUHC-Montreal Gen Hosp, D5 400-1650 av Cedar, Montreal QC H3G 1A4; London (England)'72; MB BS; FRCPC; RadOncol. Chief RadOncol, McGill University Health Centre - Montreal General Campus; Chair RadOncol, McGill University; Langs: Spanish; French; (514)934-8040; Fax. (514)934-8220; carolyn.freeman@muhc.mcgill.ca.

FREEMAN, Christie L; Derm Clinic, Box 63 1154 Chemong Rd, Peterborough ON K9H 7J6; McM'98; BSc(Hon); MD; DDerm; MSc(Derm); CCFP; Langs: English; French; (705)775-0127; Fax. (705)775-0134.

FREEMAN, Hugh J; UBC Hospital, S154/277-2211 Wesbrook Mall, Vancouver BC V6T 2B5; McG'72; ABIM; AB; FACP; FACG; FRCPC; IntMed (Crohn's Disease); Gastroent. Staff, UBC Hospital - Koerner Pavillion; Prof, University of British Columbia; (604)822-7216; Fax. (604)822-7236.

FREEMAN, Jeffrey; The Ottawa Hosp-Civic Campus, 1053 Carling Ave, Ottawa ON K1Y 4E9; Tor'82; Staff, The Ottawa Hospital - Civic Campus; (613)737-8136

FREEMAN, Jeffrey M; Fowler Kennedy Sport Med Clin, 3M-1151 Richmond St, London ON N6A 3K7; Wes'84; CCFP; CCFP(E.M.); (519)661-3011; Fax. (519)661-3379.

FREEMAN, Jeremy L; Mount Sinai Hosp, 401-600 University Ave, Toronto ON M5G 1X5; Tor'73; FACS; FRCSC; Otol (Head & Neck Oncology). Staff, Toronto General Hospital - UHN; Chair Head & Neck Oncol, Temmy Latner Dynacare; Ac Staff Surg Oncol, Ontario Cancer Institute; Prof Otol, University of Toronto; (416)586-4800; Fax. (416)586-8600; jfreeman@mtsinai.on.ca.

FREEMAN, Joel B; The Reimer Clinic, 1380 Old Innes Rd, Ottawa ON K2E 1A2; McG'66; FACS; FRCS; MSc; GenSurg (Colon & Rectal Surgery). Staff Provis Endoscopy, St Joseph's General Hospital Elliot Lake; (613)366-2021; Fax. (613)366-2025.

FREEMAN, Kenneth C; Lakeridge Health-Oshawa Site, 1 Hospital Crt, Oshawa ON L1G 2B9; (Brazil)'98; EmergMed. Staff, Lakeridge Health - Oshawa Site; (905)576-8711

FREEMAN, Laura M; 210-2401 Yonge St, Toronto ON M4P 3H1; (Other Foreign)'06; (416)485-9044; Fax. (416)485-8525.

FREEMAN, Marc; Univ Hlth Network-Toronto Gen, ES1 4010-200 Elizabeth St, Toronto ON M5G 2C4; Tor'00; FRCPC; DiagRad; NuclearMed. Staff, Toronto General Hospital - UHN; (416)340-4800 x3422

FREEMAN, Michael R; St Michael's Hosp, 6Q 042-30 Bond St, Toronto ON M5B 1W8; Qns'74; FACC; FRCPC; IntMed (Nuclear Cardiology); Cardiol. Med Dir Heart & Vascular Program/Dir Nuclear Cardiol, St Michael's Hospital; Assoc Prof, University of Toronto; (416)864-5892; Fax. (416)864-5989; freemanm@smh.ca.

FREEMAN, Risa F; Don Valley Med Associates, 330-1333 Sheppard Ave E, North York ON M2J 1V1; McM'88; BSc; MEd; CCFP; FCFP; Ac Staff, North York General Hospital; Assoc Prof Family & Commun Med, University of Toronto; (416)494-7533; Fax. (416)497-4793; rfreeman@baycrest.org.

FREEMAN, Roger D; BC Women's Hosp & Health Ctre, P4 111-4500 Oak St, Vancouver BC V6H 3N1; Johns Hopkins(MD) (USA)'58; DPsy(McG); DABPN; FRCPC; Psy (Child Psychiatry). Sr Psychologist Neuropsychiatry Clinic, BC Children's Hospital; Staff, BC Women's Hospital & Health Centre; (604)875-2097; Fax. (604)875-2099; rfreeman@cw.bc.ca.

FREEMAN, Sloane J; St Michael's Hosp, 30 Bond St, Toronto ON M5B 1W8; McM'03; FRCPC; Peds. Staff, St Michael's Hospital; (416)360-4000

FREEMAN, Thomas; Thames Valley FHT-Byron Fam Me, 1228 Commissioners Rd W, London ON N6K 1C7; Wes'76; MClSc; CCFP; FCFP; Chief Family Med, St Joseph's Hospital - St Joseph's Health Care; Chief Fam Med, London Health Sciences Centre - Victoria Campus; Staff, Parkwood Hospital - St Joseph's Health Care; Prof, University of Western Ontario; (519)472-9673

FREER, Janya M; Abbie J lane Mem Bldg, 6F-5909 Veterans Memorial Lane, Halifax NS B3H 2E2; UBC'99; FRCPC; Psy (Geriatric Psychiatry). Asst Prof, Dalhousie University; (902)473-5322

FREGEAU, Johanne; Clinique Sante Jacques-Cartier, 200-1815 rue King O, Sherbrooke QC J1J 2E3; Sher'84; CCFP; Staff, Centre Hospitalier Universitaire de Sherbrooke-Hopital Fleurimont; (819)565-7446; Fax. (819)565-7780.

FREGONAS, Claudio G; The Hosp for Sick Children, 555 University Ave, Toronto ON M5G 1X8; Tor'89; FRCPC; Peds (Consultant Pediatrics). Ac Staff, William Osler Health System - Etobicoke General Hospital; Assoc Staff, The Hospital For Sick Children; Court Staff, Humber River Regional Hospital - Finch Avenue Site; Langs: Italian; (416)813-1500

FREIGANG, Dolores D; Lansdowne Prof Bldg, 310-1641 Hillside Ave, Victoria BC V8T 5G1; Cal'94; CCFP; Staff, Victoria General Hospital; Staff, Royal Jubilee Hospital; (250)592-5312; Fax. (250)592-5910.

FREIMAN, Anatoli; Toronto Dermatology Centre, 400-4256 Bathurst St, North York ON M3H 5Y8; McG'02; MDCM; FRCPC; Derm (Cosmetics). Consultant Derm, Women's College Hospital; Consultant Derm, Mackenzie Richmond Hill Hospital; Staff, Toronto Dermatology Centre; Langs: French; Russian; (416)633-0001; Fax. (416)633-0002; info@torontodermatologycentre.com.

FREIRE, Veronique; CHUM-Hop Notre-Dame, 1560 rue Sherbrooke E, Montreal QC H2L 4M1; Mon'05; FRCPC; DiagRad. Staff, Centre Hospitalier l'Université de Montréal (CHUM) - Hôpital Notre-Dame; (514)890-8000

FREIRE-LIZAMA, Tatiana; St Michael's Hosp, 30 Bond St, Toronto ON M5B 1W8; McM'97; FRCSC; ObstGyn (Obstetrics). Ac Staff, St Michael's Hospital; Asst Prof ObstGyn Faculty of Med, University of Toronto; Langs: Spanish; (416)864-6060; Fax. (416)864-6073.

FREISTATTER, Ryan L; 50 College Dr, North Bay ON P1B 0A4; Wes'08; CCFP; Langs: Bilingual(English/French); (705)474-8600

FREITAG, Andreas P; McMaster University HSC, HSC 3V41-1280 Main St W, Hamilton ON L8S 4K1; McM'85; BSc(Chem.); FRCPC; IntMed (Critical Care Medicine). Staff, Hamilton Health Sciences Centre; Asst Chief Critical Care Med, Hamilton Health Sciences Centre - McMaster Children's Hospital; Med Dir Adult Cystic Fibrosis Prog, Hamilton-Wentworth; Assoc Prof Med, McMaster University; Langs: German; (905)521-2100 x76216; Fax. (905)521-5073; freitaga@mcmaster.ca.

FREKE, Sarah J; 3-397 Brunswick Ave, Toronto ON M5R 2Z2; Tor'81; (416)921-0055; Fax. (416)972-0752.

FREMES, Stephen E; Sunnybrook Hlth Sciences Ctre, H410-2075 Bayview Ave, Toronto ON M4N 3M5; Tor'79; MSc; FRCSC; GenSurg; Cardiovasc&ThorSurg. Affil Scientist, Sunnybrook Health Sciences Centre; Prof Surg, University of Toronto; (416)480-6073; Fax. (416)480-4439; stephen.fremes@sunnybrook.ca.

FREMONT, Larry E; The Hair Loss Recovery Prog In, 7-11160 Yonge St, Richmond Hill ON L4S 1H5; Tor'66; Court Staff, The Scarborough Hospital - General Campus; Court Staff, Rouge Valley Health System - Centenary Health Centre Site; (416)439-4247

FRENCH, Amy E; The Hosp for Sick Children, 555 University Ave, Toronto ON M5G 1X8; Tor'07; FRCPC; Peds. Staff, The Hospital for Sick Children; (416)813-5310

FRENCH, Anthony J; Care Point Med Centre, 1175 Denman St, Vancouver BC V6G 2N1; Oxford (England)'71; FRCS; MRCS; LRCP; MRCGPract; Langs: French; German; Spanish; (604)681-5338; Fax. (604)681-0425.

FRENCH, Christopher G; Health Sciences Centre, 300 Prince Philip Dr, St. John's NL A1B 3V6; Mem'95; BSc; FRCSC; Urol. Staff, Health Sciences Centre; (709)722-4111

FRENCH, Derek L; 3918 Olympic View Dr, Victoria BC V9C 4B2; London (England)'54; DA; MB BS; (250)478-3731; Fax. (250)478-3710.

FRENCH, Gavin D; Western Mem Reg Hosp, PO Box 2005 Stn Main 1 Brookfield Ave, Corner Brook NL A2H 6J7; Mem'99; FRCSC; GenSurg (Minimal Invasive Surgery). Gen Surgeon, Western Memorial Regional Hospital; (709)637-5000

FRENCH, Geoffrey R; South Peel Med Arts Bldg, 205-77 Queensway W, Mississauga ON L5B 1B7; Tor'68; FRCSC; OrthSurg. Ac Staff, Trillium Health Centre - Mississauga; (905)276-3185; Fax. (905)823-6788.

FRENCH, Gordon J; The Ottawa Hosp-Gen Campus U1-501 Smyth Rd, Ottawa ON K1H 8L6; McG'79; FRCPC; DiagRad. Ac Staff Radiol, The Ottawa Hospital - General Campus; Asst Prof DiagRad, University of Ottawa; Langs: Bilingual(English/French); (613)737-8503; Fax. (613)737-8501.

FRENCH, James; Saint John Reg Hosp, PO Box 2100 Stn Main 400 University Ave, Saint John NB E2L 4L2; (Malaysia)'00; Staff, Saint John Regional Hospital; (506)648-6000

FRENCH, John A; Prince Edward Family Hlth Team, 6-35 Bridge St, Picton ON K0K 2T0; Alb'87; Staff, QHC Prince Edward County Memorial; Asst Prof, Queen's University; (613)476-6661; Fax. (613)476-9294; frenchlove@sympatico.ca.

FRENCH, Justin; Western Memorial Health Clinic, 3 Herald Ave, Corner Brook NL A2H 4B8; Mem'04; FRCSC; Ophth. Staff, Western Memorial Regional Hospital.

FRENCH, Kelly M; 240-5620 152 St, Surrey BC V3S 3K2; UBC'98; BSc; FRCPC; Psy (Geriatric Psychiatry). (778)571-4263

FRENCH, M Elaine; 1440 14 Ave, Vernon BC V1B 2T1; Cal'78; Staff, Vernon Mental Health Centre; (250)549-5737; Fax. (250)549-5788.

FRENCH, Nadine; Inner Wisdom Healing Centre, 256 Broadway Ave, Orangeville ON L9W 1K7; Mem'94; BAP; CCFP; Staff Chronic Care, Headwaters Health Care Centre - Orangeville Site; Langs: French; (519)940-8100; Fax. (519)940-8130; nfrench.appt@gmail.com.

FRENCH, Robert J; Kingston Family Health Team, 200-2437 Princess St, Kingston ON K7M 3G1; Mem'77; CCFP; FCFP; (613)546-6652; rfrench@kfhn.net.

FRENCH, Rodney J; 240-5620 152 St, Surrey BC V3S 3K2; UBC'96; BSc; FRCSC; PlasSurg (Hand & Wrist Surgery). (778)571-4263

FRENCH, Stephen J; Big Thunder Orthopedics, 206-984 Oliver Rd, Thunder Bay ON P7B 7C7; Mem'99; FRCSC; OrthSurg (Sports Medicine). Asst Prof, Northern Ontario School of Medicine; (807)344-1123

FRENCH, Susan E; Thunder Bay Reg HSC-T-Bay, 980 Oliver Rd, Thunder Bay ON P7B 6V4; Mem'00; FRCPC; Anes. Staff, Thunder Bay Regional Health Sciences Centre; (807)684-6290

FRENCH MERKLEY, Veronique; SCOHS-Elisabeth Bruyere Hosp, 43 Bruyere St, Ottawa ON K1N 5C8; Ott'03; CCFP; Consultant, Montfort Hospital; Staff Bruyère Continuing Care, SCO Health Service - Élisabeth Bruyère Hospital; Langs: Bilingual(English/French); (613)562-6262 x4010; Fax. (613)562-4265; vfrench@bbruyere.org.

FRENDO, Jennifer S; Niagara Primary Hlth Care Clin, PO Box 1360 176 Wellington St, Niagara-on-the-Lke ON L0S 1J0; Ott'03; BSc; CCFP; Surg Asst, Niagara Health System - St Catharines General Site; (905)468-9189; Fax. (905)468-4947.

FRENDO, Marion; Niagara Med Prof Centre 1882 Highway 55 PO Box 10, Virgil ON L0S 1T0; Tor'82; GenPath (Family Medicine). Staff, Niagara Health System - Niagara-on-the-Lake Hospital Site; Med Dir, Chateau Gardens Nursing Home; Med Advisor, Rescare Premier (Anagram); Langs: Maltese; (905)468-3275

FRENETTE, Bernard; Clinique Med de Coaticook, 206-18 rue du Manege, Coaticook QC J1A 3B3; Laval'76; Assoc Staff, Centre Hospitalier de Coaticook; Consultant, Centre Hospitalier Universitaire de Sherbrooke-Hôpital Hôtel-Dieu; (819)849-4808; Fax. (819)849-7400.

FRENETTE, Bertrand; Clinique Med de Coaticook, 206-18 rue du Manege, Coaticook QC J1A 3B3; Laval'76; Staff, Centre Hospitalier de Coaticook; Consultant, Centre Hospitalier Universitaire de Sherbrooke-Hôpital Hôtel-Dieu; (819)849-4808; Fax. (819)849-7400.

FRENETTE, Charles H; MUHC-Montreal Gen Hosp, T8 408-1650 av Cedar, Montreal QC H3G 1A4; McG'83; FRCPC; IntMed (Medical Microbiology & Infectious Diseases); MedMicrobiol; InfectDis. Staff, McGill University Health Centre - Montreal General Campus; (514)934-1934 x42753; Fax. (514)934-8427.

FRENETTE, E Ina F; 37 Boul St-Pierre E, Caraquet NB E1W 1B6; Dal'77; (506)726-5754; Fax. (506)727-4529.

FRENETTE, Eric; CHUS-Hop Fleurimont, 3001 12e av N, Sherbrooke QC J1H 5N4; Sher'87; CSPQ; FRCPC; Electroenceph (P.Q.); Neur. Staff, Centre Hospitalier Universitaire de Sherbrooke-Hopital Fleurimont; (819)346-1110 x14586; Fax. (819)564-5395.

FRENETTE, Gilles A; 101-1656 rue Sherbrooke E, Montreal QC H2L 1M5; Mon'67; CSPQ; FRCSC; PlasSurg (Micro Surgery). ac Staff, Centre Hospitalier l'Université de Montréal (CHUM) - Hôpital Notre-Dame; Member, Montreal Inst. of Cosmetic Surgery; adj Prof, Universite de Montreal; Langs: Bilingual(French/English); (514)527-2417; Fax. (514)521-0428; gillesfrenette@videotron.ca.

FRENETTE, Guy; Clinique Guy Frenette, 38 rue de la Ronde, Cap-Sante QC G0A 1L0; Laval'74; Staff, Centre Hospitalier Portneuf; Langs: Bilingual(French/English); (418)337-4611; Fax. (418)337-8380.

FRENETTE, Guy; Maison Victor-Gadbois, 1000 rue Chabot, St-Mathieu-Beloeil QC J3G 4S5; Laval'71; Staff, Centre Hospitalier Pierre Boucher; Med Dir, Maison Victor-Gadbois; (450)467-1710; Fax. (450)467-5799; drgfrenette@maisonvictor-gadbois.com.

FRENETTE, Jacques; Ctr Med Haut Richelieu, 210-900 boul du Seminaire N, St-Jean-sur-Richel QC J3A 1C3; Mon'75; (450)348-1118; Fax. (450)348-9998.

FRENETTE, Jacques; UMF Laval, 2690 ch des Quatre-Bourgeois, Quebec QC G1V 0B7; Laval'72; CCFP; FCFP; Ac Staff Family Med, CSSS de la Vielle Capitale; Langs: English; French; (418)656-8711; Fax. (418)656-4503; jacques.frenette@fmed.ulaval.ca.

FRENETTE, Jean; Centre médicale des Carrières, 800-1000 boul Bons-Dussault RR, St-Mar-Des-Carr QC G0A 4B0; Laval'85; CCFP; (418)268-5596; Fax. (418)268-5729.

FRENETTE, Johanne; Centre Med Donnacona, 420 Rte 138, Donnacona QC G3M 1C2; Laval'85; (418)285-1122; Fax. (418)285-0006.

FRENETTE, Louise; Clin Med Plateau Marquette, 200-731 rue Galt O, Sherbrooke QC J1H 1Z1; Sher'79; (819)564-8662

FRENETTE, Luc; Clinique Med Saint-Jacques, 160 rue Principale, Saint-Jacques NB E7B 1W4; Sher'05; CCFP; Staff, Hôpital regional d'Edmundston; (506)739-7767

FRENETTE, Lucie; Clinique Medicale De Levis, 100-4975 boul de la Rive-Sud, Levis QC G6V 4Z5; Laval'95; Médecin, Clinique Medicale De Levis; Langs: English; (418)833-5810; Fax. (418)833-2720.

FRENETTE, Marc; Clinique Med Fabreville, 380 boul Cure-Labelle, Laval QC H7P 5L3; Mon'75; CSPQ; Cardiol (P.Q.). Staff, Hôpital du Sacre-Coeur de Montréal; Langs: Italian; English; (450)963-1961; Fax. (450)963-1205.

FRENETTE, Marie G L; Clinique Pediatrique Sainte-Fo, 295-2600 boul Laurier, Quebec QC G1V 4T3; Laval'86; FRCPC; Peds (Neonatology). Ac Staff, Centre Hospitalier Universitaire De Québec - Pavillon De St-françois-d'assise; Langs: Spanish; English; (418)658-0906; Fax. (418)652-7094.

FRENETTE, Michel; 2 ch de Normandie, Ste-Agathe-Des-Mts QC J8C 3B9; Mon'77; Langs: English; (819)326-2552; Fax. (819)326-8682.

FRENETTE, Remi J; Corporation Prof Inc, 3-970 rue Principale, Beresford NB E8K 2H6; Mon'88; FRCSC; OrthSurg. Orthopedic Surgeon, Hopital Regional Chaleur; Langs: Bilingual(French/English); (506)548-4183; Fax. (506)548-0889.

FRENETTE, Stephanie; Clin Med Saint-Antoine, 1 av de l'Eglise, Saint-Antoine NB E4V 1L6; Sher'10; CCFP.

FRENETTE, Thomas P; 211-44 Mapleton Rd, Moncton NB E1C 7W8; Sher'03; CCFP; Staff Family Med, The Moncton Hospital; Langs: Bilingual(English/French); (506)388-4193; Fax. (506)388-4188.

FRENKEL, Vivien J; 3045 Baseline Rd, Nepean ON K2H 8P4; McG'82; AB; FRCPC; GenPath (Laboratory Medicine). Staff Path, Queensway Carleton Hospital; Aj Prof, University of Ottawa; (613)721-7878; vivfrenkel@hotmail.com.

FRENKIEL, Saul; SMBD Jewish Gen Hosp, 903-3755 ch Cote-Sainte-Cather, Montreal QC H3T 1E2; McG'71; FRCSC; Otol (Sinusitis). Staff McGill University Health Centre, McGill University Health Centre - Montreal General Campus; Chef Otol, Sir Mortimer B Davis Jewish General; Chef Otol & Neck Surgery/Prof, McGill University; (514)340-8246; Fax. (514)340-7581.

FRETER, Susan H; Ctr For Health Care of Elderly, 1308-5955 Veterans Memorial La, Halifax NS B3H 2E1; McG'92; BSc; MSc; ABIM; LMCC; FRCPC; IntMed; GeriatricMed. Staff, Queen Elizabeth II Health Sciences Centre - Victoria General Site; Asst Prof, Dalhousie University; Langs: German; (902)473-2490; Fax. (902)473-7133.

FRETZ, Eric B; Western Cardiology Associates, 335-1900 Richmond Rd, Victoria BC V8R 4R2; Wes'85; FRCPC; IntMed (Angioplasty); Cardiol. Dir Cardiol Education, Vancouver Island Health Authority; Asst Prof Cardiol, University of British Columbia; (250)595-1551; Fax. (250)595-6793.

FRETZ, Michele T A; St Anthony's Med Centre, 206-582 Goldstream Ave, Victoria BC V9B 2W7; Wes'85; CCFP; (250)474-3311; Fax. (250)474-2783.

FRETZ, Norman; Ranger Mental Health Clinic, 200 First Ave W, North Bay ON P1B 9M3; Wes'55; FRCPC; Psy (Hospital Psychiatry). Staff, Timmins & District Hospital; Staff, North Bay Regional Health Centre - Regional Mental Health; (705)494-3050

FREUNDLICH, George; Bingham Mem Hosp, PO Box 70 Stn Main 507 8th Ave, Matheson ON P0K 1N0; Cluj (Romania)'82; BA(Hon.); SMO; CCFP; Staff, Smooth Rock Falls Hospital; Court Staff, Lady Minto Hospital Cochrane; Court Staff, Anson General Hospital; Consultant Orthopaedic & Trauma, Workers' Comp Board of ON; Langs: Romanian; Hungarian; German; French; (705)273-4500; Fax. (705)273-4502; george.freundlich@micsgroup.com.

FREW, Euan M S; Caledonian Med Clinic, 340 Campbell St, Nanaimo BC V9R 3G7; Aberdeen (Scotland)'68; MB ChB; FRCS(Ed); FACS; FRCSC; GenSurg (Gastroenterology). Consultant Surg, Nanaimo Regional General Hospital; Clin Instructor Surg, University of British Columbia; (250)753-3202; Fax. (250)753-1039; efrew@shaw.ca.

FREW, Patricia A; The Medical Group, 32243 Hurd St, Mission BC V2V 3J9; Cape Town (South Africa)'95; MB ChB; FRCPC; Psy (Child Psychiatry). Staff Infant Psy Clinic, BC Children's Hospital; Staff Developmental Disabilities, Mental Health & Addiction Services; (604)826-6231; Fax. (604)820-1174; patricia.frew@saskatoonhealthregion.ca.

FREW, Peter-John; Mission Medical Group, 32243 Hurd St, Mission BC V2V 3J9; Cape Town (South Africa)'94; MB ChB; Langs: Afrikaans; (604)826-6231; Fax. (604)820-1174.

FREWEN, Timothy C; London HSC-Victoria Hosp, PO Box 5375 Stn B E1 406C-800 Commissioners Rd, London ON N6A 5W9; McM'77; FAAP; FRCPC; Peds (Pediatric Critical Care). Chief Peds, London Health Sciences Centre - Victoria Campus; Chief Peds, St Joseph's Hospital - St Joseph's Health Care; Chair Dept of Peds, University of Western Ontario; (519)685-8377; Fax. (519)685-8156.

FREY, Benicio N; Womens Hlth Concerns Clinic, F614-301 James St S, Hamilton ON L8P 3B6; (Brazil)'99; (905)522-1155; Fax. (905)521-6098.

FREY, Lisa; North Woodlands Med Centre, 204-40 Shellington Place, Brantford ON N3S 0C5; McM'06; CCFP; Staff Hospital Privileges-Courtesy Special, The Brant Community Healthcare System - Brantford General Hospital Site; (519)759-6116; Fax. (519)759-7727.

FREY, Michael C; 201-845 Upper James St, Hamilton ON L9C 3A3; McM'92; CCFP; FCFP; (905)777-9100

FREY, Michael G; 101-8140 Cook Rd, Richmond BC V6Y 1V1; UBC'76; Assoc Staff, Richmond Hospital; Clin Instructor Faculty of Med, University of British Columbia; Langs: German; (604)278-2191; Fax. (604)279-8883.

FRIARS, Douglas G; Dawson Road Family Med Clinic, 101-83 Dawson Rd, Guelph ON N1H 1B1; Qns'84; CCFP; FCFP; Staff, Guelph General Hospital; (519)766-1360; Fax. (519)766-0469.

FRIC-SHAMJI, Elana C; Earl Bales Walk-In Family Clin, 100-4256 Bathurst St, North York ON M3H 5Y8; Ott'03; CCFP; (647)352-7188; Fax. (647)352-7190.

FRICK, Kenneth G; Haig Clinic, 601 6 Ave S, Lethbridge AB T1J 0Z2; Sask'87; CCFP; FCFP; (403)328-6641; Fax. (403)328-6118.

FRID, Pamela; 779 Base Line Rd E, London ON N6C 5Y6; Qns'82; FRCPC; Peds (Developmental Pediatrics). Staff, London Health Sciences Centre - Children's Hospital; Med Dir, Thames Valley Children's Centre; Assoc Prof, University of Western Ontario; (519)685-8680; Fax. (519)685-8707.

FRIDERICHS, Peter A; Hillside Med Centre, 360 2nd Ave, Campbell River BC V9W 3T9; Cape Town (South Africa)'83; MB ChB; CCFP; (250)287-7708; Fax. (250)287-3086.

FRIDHANDLER, Indira; Capital Hill Family Med Centre, 1603 20 Ave NW, Calgary AB T2M 1G9; Cal'82; CCFP; FCFP; Staff, Foothills Medical Centre; (403)270-8442

FRIDMAN, Ida; St Joseph's Hlth Centre, 30 The Queensway, Toronto ON M6R 1B5; Odessa (Ukraine)'71; FRCPC; Psy. Staff, St Joseph's Health Centre; (416)530-6000; Fax. (416)530-6076.

FRIDRIKSSON, Thor; Parksville Med Clinic, PO Box 250 Stn Main, Parksville BC V9P 2G4; UBC'91; (250)248-5757; Fax. (250)248-2128.

FRIED, Ben-Ari; Sunnybrook Hlth Sciences Ctre, M3200-2075 Bayview Ave, Toronto ON M4N 3M5; Tor'06; FRCPC; Anes. Staff, Sunnybrook Health Sciences Centre; (416)480-6039

FRIED, Eve L M; Thistlewood Prof Centre, 207-8077 Islington Ave, Woodbridge ON L4L 7X7; Wes'03; FRCPC; ObstGyn. Langs: Hebrew; (905)850-0004; Fax. (905)850-0006.

FRIED, Gerald M; MUHC-Montreal Gen Hosp, D6 136-1650 av Cedar, Montreal QC H3G 1A4; McG'75; CSPQ; FRCSC; GenSurg (Gastrointestinal Surgery). Sr Staff Surg, McGill University Health Centre - Montreal General Campus; Chef Surg/Prof, McGill University; (514)934-8044; Fax. (514)934-8438; gerald.fried@mcgill.ca.

FRIED, Joseph A; Community Med Center, 1000 Upper Gage Ave, Hamilton ON L8V 4R5; McM'81; BSc; PhD; (905)575-4400

FRIED, Oded P; North York Med Arts Bldg, 318-1333 Sheppard Ave E, North York ON M2J 1V1; Ott'69; BSc; Staff, North York General Hospital; Staff, The Scarborough Hospital - Birchmount Campus; Langs: French; Hebrew; (416)494-7456; Fax. (416)494-6926.

FRIED, Steven E M; 620-790 Bay St, Toronto ON M5G 1N8; McM'79; MSc(Pharm.); Ac Staff Musculoskeletal Prog, Toronto Rehabilitation Institute - University Centre; (416)927-7321; Fax. (416)927-9984.

FRIED, Veronika A; Balmoral Med Arts Facility, 305-1366 Yonge St, Toronto ON M4T 3A7; Tor'82; CCFP; Court Staff, Women's College Hospital; Langs: French; Hungarian; (416)962-2964; Fax. (416)962-2526.

FRIEDBER, Mark K; The Hosp for Sick Children, 555 University Ave, Toronto ON M5G 1X8; Negev (Israel)'97; Staff, The Hospital For Sick Children; (416)813-7239; Fax. (416)813-7547.

FRIEDBERG, A Martin; Toronto Emerg Med Services, 4330 Dufferin St, North York ON M3H 5R9; Tor'68; (416)392-2192

FRIEDBERG, Jacob; The Hosp for Sick Children, 6133-555 University Ave, Toronto ON M5G 1X8; Tor'63; FRCSC; Otol (Pediatric Otolaryngology). Consultant, The Hospital For Sick Children; Consultant, Mount Sinai Hospital; Prof Otol, University of Toronto; (416)813-2192; Fax. (416)813-5036.

FRIEDE, Juan; CHUQ-Hotel-Dieu de Quebec, 11 Cote du Palais, Quebec QC G1R 2J6; (Colombia)'68; ABNM; NuclearMed. Staff, Centre Hospitalier Universitaire de Québec (CHUQ) - Siege Social; Université Laval; (418)691-5151 x15455; friede.j@videotron.ca.

FRIEDLAND, Jess N; MUHC-Royal Victoria Hosp, 1650 av Cedar, Montreal QC H3G 1A4; Cal'06; FRCPC; Psy. Staff, McGill University Health Centre - Montreal General Campus; (514)731-3161

FRIEDLAND, Lisa B; UHS SU Wellness Ctr, MSC 370-2500 University Dr NW, Calgary AB T2N 1N4; McM'89; BSc; CCFP; Staff, Foothills Medical Centre; (403)210-9355; Fax. (403)282-5218; lbfriedland@shaw.ca.

FRIEDLAND, Michael J; Trillium Hlth Ctr-Mississauga, 100 Queensway W, Mississauga ON L5B 1B8; Witwatersrand (South Africa)'81; FRCPC; Anes (Cardiac Anesthesia). Ac Staff Med, Trillium Health Centre - Mississauga; (905)848-7628

FRIEDLAND, Rodney; 103A-11910 111 Ave NW, Edmonton AB T5G 3G6; Capetown (South Africa)'83; MB ChB; MMed(DiagRad); FRCPC; DiagRad (Interventional Radiology). Physician, CML Healthcare Inc; (780)452-9711; Fax. (780)452-3451.

FRIEDLANDER, Mark; North York Gen Hosp, 4001 Leslie St, North York ON M2K 1E1; Cape Town (South Africa)'81; FRCPC; Anes (Chronic Pain Management). Staff Anes & Cons, North York General Hospital; (416)756-6000; Fax. (416)756-6582.

FRIEDLANDER, Robin I; Developmental Disability HS, L50-4946 Canada Way, Burnaby BC V5G 4H7; Cape Town (South Africa)'78; MB ChB; FFPsy; FRCPC; Psy (Developmental Disability). Staff Psy, BC Children's Hospital; Clin Dir, Developmental Disabilities Mental Health Services; Clin Prof, University of British Columbia; Langs: Afrikaans; (604)918-7540; Fax. (604)918-7550; rfriedlander@cw.bc.ca.

FRIEDLANDER, Sam A; Medical Office, 210-840 Coxwell Ave, Toronto ON M4C 5T2; McG'75; FRCPC; Gastroent; IntMed. Ac Staff, Toronto East General Hospital Inc; Lecturer Med, University of Toronto; Langs: Yiddish; (416)778-9467; Fax. (416)778-5741; friedlandersam@hotmail.com.

FRIEDLICH, Martin S; The Ottawa Hosp-Gen Campus, W1617-501 Smyth Rd, Ottawa ON K1H 8L6; Tor'91; FRCSC; GenSurg (Colon & Rectal Surgery). Staff, The Ottawa Hospital - General Campus; (613)739-6650; Fax. (613)739-6646; mfriedlich@ottawahospital.on.ca.

FRIEDMAN, Aaron A; Downtown Doctors, 418-720 Spadina Ave, Toronto ON M5S 2T9; Tor'88; (416)929-1530; Fax. (416)929-7398.

FRIEDMAN, Esti; 110 Queens Plate Dr, Etobicoke ON M9W 0B4; Tor'86; FRCSC; ObstGyn. Staff, William Osler Health System - Etobicoke General Hospital; (416)741-5094; Fax. (416)741-9114.

FRIEDMAN, Gad; SMBD Jewish Gen Hosp, G327-3755 ch Cote-Sainte-Cathe, Montreal QC H3T 1E2; McG'92; FRCPC; IntMed; Gastroent. Staff, Sir Mortimer B Davis Jewish General; Langs: English; French; (514)340-8286; Fax. (514)340-8282.

FRIEDMAN, Gerald; 219-7330 Yonge St, Thornhill ON L4J 7Y7; Ott'88; FRCPC; Peds (Headache). Med Dir Woman & Child Program, Mackenzie Richmond Hill Hospital; Lecturer, University of Toronto; Langs: Bilingual(English/French); (905)764-5590; Fax. (905)764-6615.

FRIEDMAN, Jack; La Cliniwue Medicale VMS, 201-6260 av Victoria, Montreal QC H3W 2S3; McG'73; FACP; FRCPC; Peds. Ac Staff, McGill University Health Centre - Montreal Children's Hospital; Ac Staff, Sir Mortimer B Davis Jewish General; Vis Staff, St Mary's Hospital Centre; Langs: Bilingual(French/English); (514)344-0098; Fax. (514)344-0061.

FRIEDMAN, Jan; BC Women's Hosp & Health Ctre, C 234-4500 Oak St, Vancouver BC V6H 3N1; Tulane(LA) (USA)'71; FAAP; FABMG; PhD(Genetics); FCCMG; CCMG; FRCPC; MedGenetics. Staff, BC Women's Hospital & Health Centre; A-Exec Dir, Child & Family Research Institute; Prof Med Genetics/Assoc Dean/Dir CFRI (Acting), University of British Columbia; (604)875-2345 x5623; Fax. (604)875-3019; jan.friedman@ubc.ca.

FRIEDMAN, Jason; Herzl CRIU Walk-In Clinic, 500-5858 ch de la Cote-des-Nei, Montreal QC H3S 1Z1; McG'00; CCFP; (514)340-8311; Fax. (514)340-8316.

FRIEDMAN, Jeremy N; The Hosp For Sick Children, 555 University Ave, Toronto ON M5G 1X8; Cape Town (South Africa)'85; MB ChB; FRCPC; Peds (General Pediatrics). Div Head Ped Med/Associate Paedatric-in-Chief, The Hospital For Sick Children; Prof Ped, University of Toronto; (416)813-7500; Fax. (416)813-5663.

FRIEDMAN, Jerry A; Park Towers, 112-400 Walmer Rd, Toronto ON M5P 2X7; Tor'69; FRCPC; Psy (Hospital Consultation). Ac Staff, Toronto East General Hospital Inc; Langs: Hebrew; (416)968-0209; Fax. (416)469-6805.

FRIEDMAN, Jonathan; Rouge Valley-Centenary HC, 2867 Ellesmere Rd, Scarborough ON M1E 4B9; Qns'01; CCFP; Staff, Rouge Valley Health System - Centenary Health Centre Site; (416)284-8131

FRIEDMAN, Lawrence; North York Gen Hosp, 4001 Leslie St, North York ON M2K 1E1; Witwatersrand (South Africa)'75; FRCPC; DiagRad. Staff, North York General Hospital; (416)756-6000 x6186

FRIEDMAN, Oded; Guelph Renal Clinic, 73 Delhi St, Guelph ON N1E 6L9; Tor'02; FRCPC; IntMed; Nephrol. Staff, Southlake Regional Health Centre; (519)822-7664; Fax. (519)822-0701.

FRIEDMAN, Robert N; U of Toronto-CAPS Clinic, 214 College St, Toronto ON M5T 2Z9; Mon'89; FRCPC; Psy. Staff, North York General Hospital; Staff Psy Services, University of Toronto; Langs: Bilingual(English/French); (416)978-8070; Fax. (416)978-7341.

FRIEDMAN, Ruby; SMBD Jewish Gen Hosp, 3755 ch Cote-Sainte-Catherine, Montreal QC H3T 1E2; McG'82; CSPQ; FRCPC; GeriatricMed (P.Q.);CCFP; Staff, Sir Mortimer B Davis Jewish General; Staff, Donald Berman Maimonides Geriatric Centre; Aj Prof Med, McGill University; (514)340-7501; Fax. (514)340-7547.

FRIEDMAN, Steven; Univ Hlth Network-Toronto Western Hosp, 1F 502-399 Bathurst St, Toronto ON M5T 2S8; Tor'90; MPH(Harvard); CCFP; CCFP(E.M.); FCFP; Asst Dir (Research) Emerg Med, Toronto Western Hospital - University Health Network; Assoc Prof Faculty of Med, University of Toronto; Langs: Bilingual(French/English); (416)603-5405; Fax. (416)923-3523.

FRIEDMAN, Susan R; Friedman Med Prof Corp, 402-235 Danforth Ave, Toronto ON M4K 1N2; Tor'81; BSc; CCFP; Court Staff Privil, Toronto General Hospital - UHN; Court Staff Privil, Women's College Hospital; (416)466-4290; Fax. (416)466-4393.

FRIEDMAN, Talia; North York Med Group, 804-204 Duncan Mill Rd, North York ON M3B 3S6; Man'06; FRCPC; DiagRad. (416)391-5778

FRIEDMAN, Yael; The Credit Valley Hosp, 2200 Eglinton Ave W, Mississauga ON L5M 2N1; Tor'03; FRCPC; Neur. Staff, The Credit Valley Hospital; Langs: Hebrew; (905)813-4466; Fax. (905)813-4046.

FRIEDMAN, Zeev Z; Mount Sinai Hosp, 1514-600 University Ave, Toronto ON M5G 1X5; Tel-Aviv (Israel)'93; Staff, Mount Sinai Hospital; (416)586-4800 x5270

FRIEDMANN, Dominique; Pavillon Edouard-Asselin, 264 boul Rene-Levesque E, Montreal QC H2X 1P1; Mon'85; FRCPC; Derm. Staff, Centre Hospitalier l'Université De Montréal (CHUM) - Hôpital Saint-luc; (514)890-8000 x34401; Fax. (514)412-7269.

FRIEDRICH, Carl E; Hunter River Clinic, PO Box 9, Hunter River PE C0A 1N0; Qns'89; CCFP; FCFP; (902)621-3052

FRIEDRICH, Jan Oliver; St Michael's Hosp, 30 Bond St, Toronto ON M5B 1W8; Harvard(MA) (USA)'96; ABIM; FRCPC; IntMed; Critical Care Medicine. Staff, St Michael's Hospital; Langs: German; French; Spanish; (416)360-4000

FRIEDRICH, Matthias G W; Institut de Cardiologie de Mtl, 5000 rue Belanger, Montreal QC H1T 1C8; (Germany)'90; Cardiol (P.Q.). Staff, Institut de Cardiologie de Montréal; Langs: German; French; Italian; (514)376-3330

FRIEFELD, Joanne; Brampton Med Bldg, 307-164 Queen St E, Brampton ON L6V 1B4; McG'80; FRCPC; IntMed; Endocrin&Metab. (905)457-8428; Fax. (905)450-0077.

FRIEL, Patrick H; Yarmouth Reg Health Centre, 404-60 Vancouver St, Yarmouth NS B5A 2P5; Mem'81; Staff, Yarmouth Regional Hospital; (902)742-5064; Fax. (902)742-5066.

FRIEND, William C; Alberta Hosp Edmonton, PO Box 307 Stn Main 17480 Fort Rd, Edmonton AB T5J 2J7; McG'83; AB; MSc; FRCPC; Psy (Forensic Psychiatry). Clin Dir Forensic Psy Prog, Alberta Hospital Edmonton; Prov Med Dir Forensic Psy, Alberta Health Services; Assoc Prof Psy, University of Alberta; (780)472-5572; Fax. (780)342-5182.

FRIESEN, Brent T; Alberta Health Services, 120-10301 Southport Lane SW, Calgary AB T2W 1S7; Man'78; FRCPC; CommunMed (Public Health). Med Officer of Hlth, Calgary Regional Health Authority; Asst Clin Prof, University of Calgary; (403)943-1280; Fax. (403)943-0200; brent.friesen@calgaryhealthregion.ca.

FRIESEN, Byron P P; Hawkesbury Dist Gen Hosp, 1111 Ghislain St, Hawkesbury ON K6A 3G5; UBC'85; FRCSC; GenSurg. Ac Staff, Hawkesbury & District General Hospital; Langs: English; French; (613)632-1111

FRIESEN, Caspar Z W; 1284 Fairfield Rd, Victoria BC V8V 4W3; Man'92; CCFP; FCFP; (250)598-5158; Fax. (250)598-6066.

FRIESEN, Colleen A; Copeman Healthcare Centre, 700-10216 124 St NW, Edmonton AB T5N 4A3; Sask'91; CCFP; (780)455-2273; Fax. (780)423-2250.

FRIESEN, D Jon; Vernon Jubilee Hosp, 2101 32 St, Vernon BC V1T 5L2; Sask'99; CCFP; CCFP(E.M.); Staff, Vernon Jubilee Hospital; (250)545-2211

FRIESEN, Dale C; Peterborough Reg Hc-Hospital, 1 Hospital Dr, Peterborough ON K9J 7C6; Qns'81; Staff, Peterborough Regional Health Centre - Hospital Drive; (705)876-5022

FRIESEN, Frank R; Okotoks Hlth & Wellness Ctre, 11 Cimarron Common, Okotoks AB T1S 2E9; Man'75; FRCPC; Peds. Staff Hospitalist, Alberta Children's Hospital; Ac Staff, Peter Lougheed Centre; Clin Assoc Prof Ped, University of Calgary; (403)995-2670

FRIESEN, Graham; St Paul's Hosp, 1081 Burrard St, Vancouver BC V6Z 1Y6; Man'10; CCFP; Staff, Providence Health Care - St Paul's Hospital; (604)806-8877

FRIESEN, Janet M; Worksafe BC, PO Box 5350 Stn Terminal, Vancouver BC V6B 3V7; Man'80; Med Adjuster Disability Awards, Worksafe BC; Fax. (604)279-7408.

FRIESEN, Johan R; 246-30 Springborough Blvd SW, Calgary AB T3H 0N9; Cal'92; CCFP; Langs: Mandarin; (403)777-9935; Fax. (403)777-9938.

FRIESEN, Kevin L; St Boniface Gen Hosp, 409 Tache Ave, Winnipeg MB R2H 2A6; Man'88; CCFP; CCFP(E.M.); Staff, St Boniface General Hospital; (204)233-8563

FRIESEN, Lisa C; La Ronge Med Clinic, PO Box 240, La Ronge SK S0J 1L0; UBC'02; CCFP; (306)425-2174; Fax. (306)425-4199.

FRIESEN, Marlyce; 33111 Downes Rd, Abbotsford BC V2S 7V6; St. Louis(MO) (USA)'70; DABIM; FRCPC; IntMed (Nephrology). Clin Asst Profession Med, University of British Columbia; (604)850-9175

FRIESEN, Marvin J; Burnaby Hosp, 3935 Kincaid St, Burnaby BC V5G 2X6; UBC'85; FRCPC; Anes. Staff, Burnaby Hospital; (604)412-6311

FRIESEN, Nelson D; Sunnidale Med Centre, 2 Friesen Pl, Barrie ON L4M 4S4; Wes'78; (705)726-6065; Fax. (705)733-9963.

FRIESEN, Randall W; Victoria Square Med Clinic, PO Box 5700 Stn Main 220-2345 10th Ave W, Prince Albert SK S6V 7V6; Sask'84; FRCSC; GenSurg. Ac Staff, Victoria Hospital; (306)922-8949; Fax. (306)922-3441; r.friesen@sasktel.net.

FRIESEN, Reinhard; 172 Brock St, Peterborough ON K9H 2P4; Tor'79; CCFP; FCFP; Staff, Peterborough Regional Health Centre - Hospital Drive; Langs: German; (705)742-0443; Fax. (705)742-5569; vfriesen1@cogeco.ca.

FRIESEN, Stephen D; North Okanagan Women's Health, 301-3210 25 St, Vernon BC V1T 1P1; Alb'93; CCFP; FCFP; (250)549-1245; Fax. (250)549-1247.

FRIESEN, Wesley H; Vancouver Gen Hosp, 855 12th Ave W, Vancouver BC V5Z 1M9; Man'74; FRCPC; Psy. Ac Staff, Vancouver General Hospital - Centennial Pavillion; (604)875-4009

FRIESNER, Abraham; 200-1635 Lawrence Ave W, Toronto ON M6L 3C9; Tor'71; Staff Emerg, Humber River Regional Hospital - Keele Street Site; Staff Emerg, Humber River Regional Hospital - Church Street Site; Med Dir, Kimberly Clark/Rolland Paper-Continental Can Co. of Canada & Overland Western Ltd.; Langs: Yiddish; French; (416)245-5888; Fax. (416)245-5889.

FRIGGSTAD, Aaron K; Herold Road Family Physisians, 1-325 Herold Rd, Saskatoon SK S7V 1J7; Sask'00; BSc; CCFP; Staff, Royal University Hospital; Clinical Asst Prof Family Med, University of Saskatchewan; (306)374-2404; Fax. (306)477-0300.

FRIGON, Chantal; MUHC-Montreal Children's Hosp, 2300 rue Tupper, Montreal QC H3H 1P3; Sher'94; MSc; CSPQ; FRCPC; Anes (Pediatric Anesthesia). Staff, McGill University Health Centre - Montreal Children's Hospital; (514)412-4400 x22463; Fax. (514)412-4341.

FRIGON, Michel; Direction de Sante Publique, 2400 av D'Estimauville, Quebec QC G1E 7G9; Laval'77 Laval; MSc; LMCC; Med Consultant Public Health, Centre Hospitalier Universitaire de Quebec-CHUL; Pres Consulting Committee Travelers Health, National Institute of Public Health of Quebec; (418)666-7000 x272; Fax. (418)666-2776; michel.frigon@ssss.gouv.qc.ca.

FRIGON, Veronick; CHUS-Hop Fleurimont, 3001 12e av N, Sherbrooke QC J1H 5N4; Sher'06; FRCPC; Anes. Staff, Centre Hospitalier Universitaire de Sherbrooke-Hopital Fleurimont; (819)346-1110

FRIMER, Michael L; Medical Bldg, 150-6180 Blundell Rd, Richmond BC V7C 4W7; Tor'66; FRCSC; GenSurg (Gastroenterology). Assoc Staff, Richmond Hospital; (604)271-7844; Fax. (604)271-7874.

FRIPP, Amber G; Peter Lougheed Centre, 3500 26 Ave NE, Calgary AB T1Y 6J4; Cal'04; BSc(EXHP); FRCPC; IntMed. Staff IntMed Phys, Peter Lougheed Centre; Clin Lecturer Int Med, University of Calgary; (403)943-4555; Fax. (403)241-9174; amber.fripp@albertahealthservices.ca.

FRISCH, Gershon D; SMBD Jewish Gen Hosp, 3755 ch Cote-Sainte-Catherine, Montreal QC H3T 1E2; McG'96; FRCPC; IntMed; Nephrol. Staff, Sir Mortimer B Davis Jewish General; (514)340-8232 x4249; Fax. (514)340-8147.

FRITSCH, Christian; Ladysmith Comm Hlth Centre, PO Box 10 Stn Main 1111 4th Ave, Ladysmith BC V9G 1A1; Alb'72; Staff Chief, Ladysmith Community Health Centre; Ac Staff, Cowichan District Hospital; Court Staff, Nanaimo Regional General Hospital; Langs: German; (250)739-5777

FRITSCH, Emanuel; Ladysmith Comm Hlth Centre, PO Box 11 Stn Main 1111 4th Ave, Ladysmith BC V9G 1A1; Alb'77; Staff, Ladysmith Community Health Centre; Staff, Nanaimo Regional General Hospital; Staff, Cowichan District Hospital; Langs: German; (250)739-5784

FRITZ, Bradley A; 4303 10th Ave W, Vancouver BC V6R 2H6; UBC'75; Staff Family Pract, UBC Hospital - Koerner Pavillion; Vis Staff, BC Women's Hospital & Health Centre; Ac Staff, Vancouver General Hospital - Centennial Pavillion; Clin Assoc Prof Family Med, University of British Columbia; (604)224-0224; Fax. (604)221-2545.

FRITZ, Daniel R; The Group Health Centre, 240 McNabb St, Sault Ste. Marie ON P6B 1Y5; Tor'89; CCFP; FCFP; Staff, Sault Area Hospital - Sault Ste Marie; (705)759-1234; Fax. (705)541-2215; fritz_d@ghc.on.ca.

FRITZ, James R; 350 Cityview Centre, 2550 15th Ave, Regina SK S4P 1A5; Sask'82; DABOph; FRCSC; Otol. Staff, Regina General Hospital; (306)359-1667; Fax. (306)569-8665.

FRITZLER, Marvin J; HSC-Faculty Of Med, 414-3330 Hospital Dr NW, Calgary AB T2N 4N1; Cal'74; PhD; FRCPC; IntMed (Rheumatology & Clinical Immunology); Rheum. Chair Bd Dir, Alberta Research & Innovation Authority; Faculty Teacher, University of Calgary; (403)220-3533; Fax. (403)210-8616; fritzler@ucalgary.ca.

FRIZ, B Hansjorg; St Clair Med Associates, 401-1366 Yonge St, Toronto ON M4T 3A7; Man'00; CCFP; CCFP(E.M.); Staff, St. Anthony General Hospital; (416)966-0178; Fax. (416)929-0843.

FRIZZELL, J Bevan; Foothills Med Centre, 1403 29 St NW, Calgary AB T2N 2T9; Cal'93; FRCPC; DiagRad. Staff, Foothills Medical Centre; (403)944-1969; Fax. (403)944-2549.

FRIZZELL, J B Haldane; Properties Med Clinic, 5102 Rundlehorn Dr NE, Calgary AB T1Y 1C1; Dal'73; Staff, Properties Medical Clinic; (403)280-2700; Fax. (403)285-2641.

FRIZZLE, Tena Ann; 205-2 Lawrence St, Amherst NS B4H 3G5; Dal'98; BSc; CCFP; FCFP; Staff, Cumberland Regional Health Care Center; Staff Faculty Ass, Dalhousie University; (902)667-1869; Fax. (902)667-0559.

FROATS, Timothy R; Brockville Gen Hosp, 1F-75 Charles St, Brockville ON K6V 1S8; Qns'73; FRCSC; ObstGyn. Staff, Brockville General Hospital - Charles Street; Staff, Brockville Mental Health Centre - Royal Ottawa Health Care Group; Staff, Providence Continuing Care Centre (PCCC) - St Vincent de Paul Hospital; Clin Asst, Queen's University; (613)498-0740; Fax. (613)345-3036.

FROBB, Mark K; Ocean Park, 1661 128 St, Surrey BC V4A 3V2; Alb'75; CCFP; Staff, Peace Arch Hospital; (604)531-0444; Fax. (604)531-0421.

FROEHLICH, Kevin F; Vancouver Gen Hosp, 855 12th Ave W, Vancouver BC V5Z 1M9; Man'03; FRCPC; Anes. Staff, Vancouver General Hospital - Centennial Pavillion; (604)875-4304

FROEHLICH, Patrick; Hôpital Ste-Justine, 3175 ch Cote-Sainte-Catherine, Montreal QC H3T 1C5; (Switzerland)'92; Staff, Hôpital Ste-Justine; (514)345-4625; Fax. (514)345-4805.

FROELICH, Christine K; University of Alberta Hosp, WMC1E714-8440 112 St NW, Edmonton AB T6G 2B7; Alb'95; FRCPC; Psy. Admn Staff Privil Psy, University of Alberta Hospital; Associate Clin Prof, University of Alberta; (780)407-6599; Fax. (780)407-6672.

FROELICH, Jennifer E; Foothills Med Centre, 1403 29 St NW, Calgary AB T2N 2T9; Alb'90; FRCPC; Anes. Staff, Foothills Medical Centre; (403)944-1430; Fax. (403)944-2425; jennifer.froelich@calgaryhealthregion.ca.

FROESCHL, Michael P V; Univ of Ottawa Heart Institute, 40 Ruskin St, Ottawa ON K1Y 4W7; McG'99; FRCP; FRCPC; IntMed (Interventional Cardiology); Cardiol. Staff, University of Ottawa Heart Institute; Langs: German; French; (613)761-4049; Fax. (613)761-5212.

FROESCHL, Sandra; The Ottawa Hosp - Gen Campus, 501 Smyth Rd, Ottawa ON K1H 8L6; Hanover (Germany)'98; FRCPC; IntMed. Staff, The Ottawa Hospital - General Campus; Langs: German; (613)737-7777

FROESE, Alison B; Kingston Gen Hosp, 76 Stuart St, Kingston ON K7L 2V7; Man'68; BSc(Med); FRCPC; Anes (Clinical Anaesthesia). Staff Anes, Kingston General Hospital; Staff, Hotel-Dieu Hospital; Prof Anes Peds & Physiol, Queen's University; (613)549-6666 x4472; Fax. (613)548-1375; froesea@kgh.kari.net.

FROESE, Colleen L; UBC Hospital, G 285-2211 Wesbrook Mall, Vancouver BC V6T 2B5; UBC'82; FRCPC; Psy. Consultant, UBC Hospital - Koerner Pavillion; (604)822-7857; Fax. (604)822-9744.

FROESE, Daniel W; George Derby Centre, 7550 Cumberland St, Burnaby BC V3N 3X5; UBC'57; Staff, Burnaby Hospital; (604)527-4493; Fax. (604)263-9974.

FROESE, Danielle K; PO Box 3797 Stn Main, Courtenay BC V9N 7P2; Qns'02; CCFP.

FROESE, David F; 204-2692 Clearbrook Rd, Abbotsford BC V2T 2Y8; Sask'78; (604)854-5777; Fax. (604)854-2330.

FROESE, Nicole L; Central Square Med Clinic, PO Box 3760 1209 Main St, Smithers BC V0J 2N0; Man'06; CCFP; Staff, Bulkley Valley District Hospital; (250)847-8761

FROESE, Norbert R; Children's & Women's HC of BC, 2L5-4480 Oak St, Vancouver BC V6H 3V4; Man'84; FRCPC; Anes. Staff, BC Children's Hospital; (604)875-2711; Fax. (604)875-3221.

FROESE, Warren G; Pan Am Sports Med Centre, 75 Poseidon Bay, Winnipeg MB R3M 3E4; Man'86; FRCSC; OrthSurg (Shoulder). (204)925-1531; Fax. (204)925-1470.

FROH, John S; Royal University Hosp, 103 Hospital Dr, Saskatoon SK S7N 0W8; Sask'98; BSc; CCFP; CCFP(E.M.); Staff, Royal University Hospital; (306)655-1000

FROH, Robert G; Parklane Surgical Clinic, 320-13710 94A Ave, Surrey BC V3V 1N1; Sask'82; MD; FRCSC; OrthSurg (Adult Reconstructive Surgery). Ac Staff, Surrey Memorial Hospital; Clin Instructor, University of British Columbia; (604)585-8469; Fax. (604)585-8479; rfroh@shawcable.com.

FROHLICH, Arnold M; Manitoba Clinic, 790 Sherbrook St, Winnipeg MB R3A 1M3; Man'84; FRCSC; Otol. Ac Staff, Victoria General Hospital; Ac Staff, Children's Hospital of Winnipeg; (204)788-5508; Fax. (204)789-9244; afrohlich@manitobaclinic.com.

FROHLICH, Dean E C; Foothills Med Centre, 1403 29 St NW, Calgary AB T2N 2T9; Alb'92; FRCPC; NuclearMed; DiagRad. Staff Diag Imag, Foothills Medical Centre; (403)944-1969; Fax. (403)944-1687.

FROHLICH, Jiri; St Paul's Hosp, B180-1081 Burrard St, Vancouver BC V6Z 1Y6; Prague (Czech Republic)'65; FRCPC; MedBiochem (Lipidology). Staff Lipid Clinic & Atherosclerosis Specialty Lab, Providence Health Care - St Paul's Hospital; Acad Dir, Healthy Heart Program; Prof Path, University of British Columbia; Langs: Czech; (604)806-8612; Fax. (604)806-8590.

FROLIC, Natasha K; St Joseph's Gen Hosp, 2137 Comox Ave, Comox BC V9M 1P2; Sask'97; BSc; FRCPC; Psy (Geriatric Medicine). Ac Member, St Joseph's General Hospital; Consultant Older Adult Team, Mental Health & Addiction Services; (250)890-3712; Fax. (250)339-1578.

FROM, Lynn; Women's College Hosp, 840-76 Grenville St, Toronto ON M5S 1B2; Tor'63; FRCPC; Derm; AnatPath. Staff Derm, Women's College Hospital; Prof Med, University of Toronto; (416)323-6629; Fax. (416)323-6306; lynn.from@sw.ca.

FROMBERG, P Mark; Mission Med Centre, 102-3320 Richter St, Kelowna BC V1W 4V5; UBC'85; (250)868-8222; Fax. (250)868-8269; fromberg@telus.net.

FROMENT, Daniel; CHUM-Hop Notre-Dame, 1560 rue Sherbrooke E, Montreal QC H2L 4M1; Mon'80; ABIM; LMCC; FRCPC; IntMed; Nephrol (P.Q.). Staff Nephrol, Centre Hospitalier l'Université de Montréal (CHUM) - Hôpital Notre-Dame; adj Prof, Universite de Montreal; Langs: Bilingual(French/English); (514)890-8000 x26616; Fax. (514)412-7831.

FROMENT, Marie-Anne; CHUQ-Hotel-Dieu de Quebec, 11 Cote de Palais, Quebec QC G1R 2J6; Laval'07; FRCPC; RadOncol. Staff, Centre Hospitalier Universitaire de Québec (CHUQ) - Siege Social; (418)525-4444

FRONGILLO, Robert; Clinique du Dr R Frongillo, 108-7240 boul Maurice-Duplessi, Montreal QC H1E 4A7; Laval'79; Langs: English; French; (514)881-2033; Fax. (514)881-2034.

FRONTEDDU, Mavi; Clinique Med Pierre-Boucher, 110-1615 boul Jacques-Cartier, Longueuil QC J4M 2X1; Mon'84; (450)468-6223; Fax. (450)468-5041.

FROST, Craig C; Campbell River & Dist Gen Hosp, 375 2nd Ave, Campbell River BC V9W 3V1; McG'93; CCFP; Staff, Campbell River & District General Hospital; (250)287-7111

FROST, David; Univ Hlth Network-Toronto Western Hosp, 8E 424-399 Bathurst St, Toronto ON M5T 2S8; Tor'06; FRCPC; IntMed. Staff, Toronto Western Hospital - University Health Network; (416)603-5800

FROST, Ian M; The Ottawa Hosp-Riverside, 1967 Riverside Dr, Ottawa ON K1H 7W9; Ott'73; FRCPC; Anes. Staff, The Ottawa Hospital - Riverside Campus; Langs: Bilingual(English/French); (613)738-7100 x88237; Fax. (613)738-8380.

FROST, Peter G; 3 Ovida Blvd, Markham ON L3P 7N8; Birmingham (England)'68; MB ChB; FRCSC; GenSurg. (905)471-2337

FROTTEN, Erin M; McMaster Family Practice, 690 Main St W, Hamilton ON L8S 1A4; Tor'09; CCFP; (905)521-5016

FROUD, Peter J; Queen's University, RR 1 3764 Maple Crest Court, Inverary ON K0H 1X0; Bristol (England)'62; MB ChB; DMRT; FRCR; FRCPC; RadOncol (Breast Cancer). Staff, Kingston General Hospital; Staff, Hotel-Dieu Hospital; Assoc Prof Oncol, Queen's University; (613)653-1937; peter.froud@kingston.net.

FRUCHTERMANN, Lucien-P; Polyclinique Masson, 200-3425 rue Masson, Montreal QC H1X 1R6; Liege (Belgium)'79; Langs: English; French; (514)376-9961; Fax. (514)376-8100.

FRUETEL, Karen; Rockyview Gen Hosp, 5A 150-7007 14 St SW, Calgary AB T2V 1P9; Wes'85; FRCPC; IntMed; GeriatricMed. Staff, Rockyview General Hospital; (403)943-3945; Fax. (403)943-3946.

FRUITMAN, Deborah S; Alberta Children's Hosp, A3 936-2888 Shaganappi Trail N, Calgary AB T3B 6A8; Dal'00; FRCPC; Peds (Pediatric Cardiology); Cardiol. Staff, Alberta Children's Hospital; (403)955-7858; Fax. (403)955-7621.

FRUITMAN, Mark A; St Joseph's Health Centre, 30 The Queensway, Toronto ON M6R 1B5; Wes'96; FRCPC; DiagRad. Staff, St Joseph's Health Centre; (416)530-6010

FRUITMAN, Sheldon; Scarborough North Med Arts, 401-4040 Finch Ave E, Scarborough ON M1S 4V5; Tor'66; FRCSC; ObstGyn. Ac Staff, The Scarborough Hospital - Birchmount Campus; (416)291-9793; Fax. (416)291-8698.

FRUTEAU-DE-LACLOS, Bernard; Ctr Hosp Affilie-St-Sacrement, 1050 ch Sainte-Foy, Quebec QC G1S 4L8; Montpellier (France)'81; FRCPC; MedBiochem. Ac Staff, Centre Hospitalier Affilié Universitaire de Québec - Hôpital du St-Sacrement; (418)682-7558; Fax. (418)682-7965; bernard.fruteau-de-laclos@bcx.ulaval.ca.

FRUTH, Irmgard; Medistat Med Familiale, 4965 rue Saint-Pierre, Pierrefonds QC H9H 5M9; Ulm Univ (Germany)'97; CCFP; (514)624-4774

FRY, Jessica; Royal Jubilee Hosp, 1952 Bay St, Victoria BC V8R 1J8; UBC'10; CCFP; Staff, Royal Jubilee Hospital; (250)370-8000

FRY, Joanne; The Hugh Allen Clinic, PO Box 489 Stn Main, Sioux Lookout ON P8T 1A8; Dal'99; CCFP; Staff, Sioux Lookout Meno-Ya-Win Health Centre; Staff, The Hugh Allen Clinic; (807)737-3803; Fax. (807)737-1771; jfry@slmhc.on.ca.

FRY, Karen J; Keary Med Centre, 105-245 Columbia St E, New Westminster BC V3L 3W4; UBC'90; Staff, Royal Columbian Hospital; (604)522-6800; Fax. (604)540-8126.

FRY, Margaret A; Southlake Reg Health Centre, 596 Davis Dr, Newmarket ON L3Y 2P9; Ott'75; CCFP; Ac Staff, Southlake Regional Health Centre; (905)895-4521; Fax. (905)952-3050.

FRY, Nicholas J; 3100-910 10 Ave W, Vancouver BC V5Z 4E3; Ott'06.

FRY, Peter D; 303-5171 221A St, Langley BC V2Y 0A2; RCS (Ireland)'68; FRCSC; GenSurg; VascSurg (Thoracic). Staff VascSurg, UBC Hospital - Koerner Pavillion; Consultant, Vancouver General Hospital - Centennial Pavillion; Prof, University of British Columbia; (604)534-7515; Fax. (604)534-7501.

FRYATT, Kenneth D; Columbia Health Centre, 2121 29 St NE, Calgary AB T1Y 7H8; Man'95; FRCPC; CommunMed. Med Advisor, Atco Gas; Med Examiner, NRCS Alberta; Med Examiner, Workers' Comp Board of AB; (403)219-5735; Fax. (403)219-5340; ken.fryatt@shaw.ca.

FRYDMAN, Rita B; 145-6000 ch de la Cote-des-Nei, Montreal QC H3S 1Z8; McG'75; FRCOG; FACOG; DAB; FRSOG; FRCSC; ObstGyn (Infertility). Ac Staff, Sir Mortimer B Davis Jewish General; Teacher, McGill University; (514)731-2755; Fax. (514)731-7096.

FRYDRYCH, Seymour; Mount Dennis Med Group, 98 Guestville Ave, Toronto ON M6N 4N6; Tor'77; CCFP; FCFP; Ac Staff Family Pract, Humber River Regional Hospital - Church Street Site; Langs: Yiddish; (416)763-1171; Fax. (416)763-0573.

FRYE, Helen; Alexandra Med Centre, 29 Noxon St, Ingersoll ON N5C 3V6; McM'76; CCFP; FCFP; (519)485-9617

FRYE, June C O; 312-1717 3rd Ave, Prince George BC V2L 3G7; Indiana (USA)'69; FRCPC; Psy. Staff Psy, University Hospital of Northern British Columbia; Asst Prof, University of British Columbia; (250)564-4747

FRYER, Christopher J H; Children's & Women's HC Of BC, A119-4480 Oak St, Vancouver BC V6H 3V4; London (England)'65; LRCP; MRCS; FRCPC; Peds (Pediatric Oncology); RadOncol. Consultant Ped Oncol, BC Children's Hospital; Clin Prof Peds, University of British Columbia; (604)875-2345 x6884

FRYER, Karen E; Von Sakura House Res Hospice, RR 5 715180 Oxford Road 4, Woodstock ON N4S 7V9; Tor'88; CCFP; CCFP(E.M.); FCFP; Ac Staff, Woodstock General Hospital; Med Dir, Von Sakura House Hospice; (519)537-8515; Fax. (519)421-1057.

FRYER, Sonia; Centre Med Familiale de Granby, 48 rue Denison E, Granby QC J2G 4C6; Sher'05; (450)372-3996

FRYER, Veronique; CSSS des Sources, 475 3e av, Asbestos QC J1T 1X6; Sher'07; CCFP; Staff, CSSS des Sources d'Asbestos; (819)879-7158; Fax. (819)879-0075.

FRYKODA, Amy H; PO Box 2119, Minnedosa MB R0J 1E0; Man'04; CCFP.

FU, Anita; 245-809 41st Ave W, Vancouver BC V5Z 2N6; (Philippines)'75; (604)873-3965

FU, Anna; Markham Stouffville Health Ctr, 212-377 Church St, Markham ON L6B 1A1; Tor'97; FRCPC; IntMed (Endoscopy); Gastroent. Staff, Markham Stouffville Hospital; (905)471-6200; Fax. (905)471-6103.

FU, Joseph S L; Lifesource Med Centre, 2130 Robertson Rd, Nepean ON K2H 5Z1; Qns'92; BSc(Hon.); Langs: Cantonese; (613)828-3122; Fax. (613)828-2010.

FU, Lili; MUHC-Montreal Gen Hosp, 1650 av Cedar, Montreal QC H3G 1A4; McG'04; AnatPath. Staff, McGill University Health Centre - Montreal General Campus; (514)934-1934 x43835

FU, Ping; Mackenzie Richmond Hill Hosp, 10 Trench St, Richmond Hill ON L4C 4Z3; Tor'92; FRCPC; CCFP; Neur;CCFP(E.M.); FCFP; Staff, Mackenzie Richmond Hill Hospital; Lecturer DFCM, University of Toronto; (905)883-2041; Fax. (905)883-2138.

FU, Remedios T; Medical Bldg, 201-745 Broadway W, Vancouver BC V5Z 1J6; (Philippines)'70; (604)872-0444; Fax. (604)872-8742.

FU, Stanley; West Winds Med Clinic, 2110-4818 Westwinds Dr NE, Calgary AB T3J 3Z5; Alb'98; CCFP; (403)568-2295; Fax. (403)568-2247.

FUCA, Roland P J; Bank Med Centre, 1935 Bank St, Ottawa ON K1V 8A3; Wes'80; Med Dir Interim Federal Health Prog, Citizenship & Immigration Canada; Langs: French; (613)521-2391; roland.fuca@cic.gc.ca.

FUCHS, Aaron; Lakeshore Gen Hosp, 160 av Stillview, Pointe-Claire QC H9R 2Y2; McG'77; Staff, Lakeshore General Hospital - Pointe Claire; (514)630-2225; Fax. (514)630-4708; afuchs@sympatico.ca.

FUCHS, C Christian; 5423 48 St, Stony Plain AB T7Z 1E3; Alb'78; (780)963-6545; Fax. (780)963-2740.

FUCHS, Graham R; Selkirk & District Gen Hosp, PO Box 5000 Stn Main 100 Easton Dr, Selkirk MB R1A 2M2; Man'69; Staff, Selkirk & District General Hospital; Lecturer Family Pract, University of Manitoba; (204)482-5800

FUCHS, Joachim; 201-2763 Beverly St, Duncan BC V9L 6X2; (Germany)'92; Langs: German; (250)597-3390

FUCHS, Marnie R; Trillium Hlth Ctr-Mississauga, 100 Queensway W, Mississauga ON L5B 1B8; Tor'95; FRCPC; Anes. Staff, Trillium Health Centre - Mississauga; (905)848-7100 x7628

FUCHS-GARCIA, Sigrid; Pitt Street Med Centre, 1335 Pitt St, Cornwall ON K6J 3T7; Mon'69; Langs: German; Spanish; (613)932-6163

FUCHSMAN, Bertha; GMF Cote-des-Neiges, 324-5700 ch de la Cote-des-Neiges, Montreal QC H3T 2A8; Rochester(NY) (USA)'77; CCFP; FCFP; Staff Privil Emerg, McGill University Health Centre - Montreal General Campus; pers Médecin, Sir Mortimer B Davis Jewish General; adj Prof Family Med, McGill University; Langs: English; (514)731-8531; Fax. (514)731-0563.

FUDA, Giuseppe; SMBD Jewish Gen Hosp, A335-3755 ch Cote-Sainte-Cathe, Montreal QC H3T 1E2; Laval'04; FRCPC; Anes. Staff, Sir Mortimer B Davis Jewish General; (514)340-8222 x5701; Fax. (514)340-8108.

FUGER, Jason J; Royal Alexandra Hosp, 10240 Kingsway NW, Edmonton AB T5H 3V9; Alb'04; FRCPC; Anes., Royal Alexandra Hospital; (780)735-4010; Fax. (780)435-4386.

FUGERE, Christina; Stonechurch Family Health Ctre, 1475 Upper Ottawa St, Hamilton ON L8W 3J6; McM'97; CCFP; FCFP; Physician, Stonechurch Family Health Centre; (905)575-7757; Fax. (905)575-7831.

FUGERE, Daniel; Hotel-Dieu d'Arthabaska, 5 rue des Hospitalieres, Victoriaville QC G6P 6N2; Sher'84; CSPQ; Anes. Staff, Hotel-Dieu d'Arthabaska; (819)357-2030; Fax. (819)357-9314.

FUGERE, Francois; Hop Maisonneuve-Rosemont, 5415 boul de l'Assomption, Montreal QC H1T 2M4; Laval'85; CSPQ; FRCPC; Anes. Staff, Hopital Maisonneuve-Rosemont; Clin Teach Staff Anes, Universite de Montreal; (514)252-3426; Fax. (514)252-3542.

FUGERE, Louise; Hop Maisonneuve-Rosemont, 5415 boul de L'Assimption, Montreal QC H1T 2M4; Laval'87; Staff, Institut Universitaire de Gériatrie de Montréal; Staff, Hopital Maisonneuve-Rosemont; Staff, Centre Hospitalier l'Université de Montréal (CHUM) - Hôtel-Dieu; Physician, Clin. Med. Mediclub Sanctuaire(Outremont); (514)252-3869

FUGERE, Pierre; 100-235 boul Rene-Levesque E, Montreal QC H2X 1N8; Mon'59; FRCSC; ObstGyn (Gynecology). ObstGyn, Centre Hospitalier l'Université De Montréal (CHUM) - Hôpital Saint-luc; Prof, Universite de Montreal; (514)866-2446; Fax. (514)866-4013.

FUGERE, Renee; 10905 boul Henri-Bourassa E, Montreal QC H1C 1H1; Laval'76; FRCPC; Psy (Forensic Psychiatry - Adult). Sr Staff, Institut Philippe-Pinel de Montreal; adj Prof Psy, Universite de Montreal; Langs: Bilingual(French/English); (514)648-8461 x559; renee.fugere.ippm@ssss.gouv.qc.ca.

FUGLER, Stephen R; PO Box 9148 Stn Main, Sylvan Lake AB T4S 1S8; Cape Town (South Africa)'89; MB ChB; (403)887-4418; Fax. (403)887-4529.

FUHRMANN, Marlene B; 205-220 Main St, Antigonish NS B2G 2C2; UBC'83; Staff, St Martha's Regional Hospital; (902)863-2674; Fax. (902)867-5662.

FUJII, Hisaki; The Hospital for Sick Children, 555 University Ave, Toronto ON M5G 1X8; (Japan)'96; Staff, The Hospital For Sick Children; (416)813-7654

FUJIOKA, Robert; Clin de Med Fam Cowansville, 499 rue du Sud, Cowansville QC J2K 2X9; McG'80; Staff, Hôpital Brome-Missisquoi-Perkins; (450)263-8890; Fax. (450)263-9737.

FUJIWARA, Joan R; Surrey Mem Hosp, 13750 96 Ave, Surrey BC V3V 1Z2; Tor'76; Staff Youth Clinic & HEAL Team, Surrey Memorial Hospital; (604)585-5999; Fax. (604)585-5929.

FUKS, Abraham; McGill University, 105-3647 Peel St, Montreal QC H3A 1X1; McG'70; AB; FRCPC; ClinImmunol&Allergy. Prof Med, McGill University; Langs: Yiddish; (514)398-4400 x0279; Fax. (514)398-3595; abraham.fuks@mcgill.ca.

FUKS, Maria; CLSC Rene Cassin, 500-5800 boul Cavendish, Cote Saint-Luc QC H4W 2T5; Kazan (Russia (Federation))'58; Langs: Russian; French; (514)488-9163; Fax. (514)485-2978.

FULFORD, Jennifer; The Northwood Park Hlth Ctr, 504N Edward St, Thunder Bay ON P7C 4P9; McM'75; Asst Prof Med, Northwest Medical School; (807)286-2005; Fax. (807)286-2685.

FULGOSI, Don Z; 502-123 Edward St, Toronto ON M5G 1E2; Zagreb (Croatia)'68; FRCPC; Psy. Langs: Croatian; (416)595-2714

FULICEA, Laurentiu; CHUM-Hop Notre-Dame, 1560 rue Sherbrooke E, Montreal QC H2L 4M1; Mon'05; FRCPC; Psy. Staff, Centre Hospitalier l'Université de Montréal (CHUM) - Hôpital Notre-Dame; (514)890-8000

FULLAGAR, Ernest W; 2995 12th Ave W, Vancouver BC V6K 2R2; Cape Town (South Africa)'79; MB ChB; FFPsy(S.A.); FRCPC; Psy. Langs: Afrikaans; (604)559-7729

FULLARD, Ginevra A M H; 101-1516 Fairview Rd, Penticton BC V2A 6A3; Witwatersrand (South Africa)'01; BS; (250)493-7141

FULLER, Barbara E; Queens Family Health Team, 2F-115 Clarence St, Kingston ON K7L 5N6; Qns'84; CCFP; FCFP; Staff, Hotel-Dieu Hospital; Staff, Kingston General Hospital; Staff Clincian/Resd Supvr, Queen's Family Health Team - Corporate Office; Langs: English; French; (613)533-9303; Fax. (613)533-9308.

FULLER, Benjamin R; Bowmanville Professional Bldg, 206-222 King St E, Bowmanville ON L1C 1P6; Dal'88; CCFP; CCFP(E.M.); FCFP; (905)623-5679; Fax. (905)623-1345.

FULLER, Donald; 46 Dundas St, Woodstock ON N4S 1C2; Wes'89; CCFP; FCFP; Physician Designated Medical Practitioner, Citizenship & Immigration Canada; (519)421-9557; Fax. (519)421-9561.

FULLER, Hugh D; St Joseph's Healthcare, 50 Charlton Ave E, Hamilton ON L8N 4A6; London (England)'73; MB BS; MSc; LRCP; MRCS; FRCPC; IntMed. Chief IntMed, St Joseph's Healthcare - Charlton Campus; Assoc Prof Med, McMaster University; (905)540-6560; Fax. (905)521-6068; fullerh@mcmaster.ca.

FULLERTON, Gary M; 103-527 Admiral St, Woodstock ON N4S 5B2; Wes'78; FRCPC; IntMed. Chief IntMed, Woodstock General Hospital; (519)539-1261; Fax. (519)539-9593.

FULLERTON, James E D; 68 Bridge St, Carleton Place ON K7C 2V3; Ott'95; CCFP; FCFP; Staff, Carleton Place & District Memorial Hospital; Langs: Bilingual(English/French); (613)257-4793; Fax. (613)257-4794.

FULLERTON, Merrilee K; Kanata Prof Centre, 103-99 Kakulu Rd, Kanata ON K2L 3C8; Ott'86; (613)592-1448; Fax. (613)591-3778.

FULOP, John C; Ottawa Cardiovascular Centre, 502-1355 Bank St, Ottawa ON K1H 8K7; Tor'79; FACC; FRCPC; Cardiol. Staff, The Ottawa Hospital - General Campus; Langs: Hungarian; (613)738-1584; Fax. (613)738-9097.

FULOP, Katalin; Hop Charles LeMoyne, 3120 boul Taschereau, Longueuil QC J4V 2H1; Sher'06; DiagRad. Staff, Hopital Charles LeMoyne; (450)466-5000

FULOP, Tamas; Inst U Geriatrie Sherbrooke, 1036 rue Belvedere S, Sherbrooke QC J1H 4C4; Geneva (Switzerland)'80; PhD; DSc; IntMed; GeriatricMed. Staff Research Centre, Institut Universitaire de Geriatrie de Sherbrooke-Pavillon Argyll; Prof IntMed, Centre Hospitalier Universitaire de Sherbrooke-Hopital Fleurimont; Staff, CSSS Institut universitaire de gériatrie de Sherbrooke; Langs: Hungarian; (819)780-2220 x46254; Fax. (819)829-7145; tamas.fulop@usherbrooke.ca.

FULTHORPE, Gordon H; Wentworth Limeridge Med Ctre, 405-849 Upper Wentworth St, Hamilton ON L9A 5H4; London (England)'63; MB BS; Staff, Hamilton Health Sciences Centre - McMaster Children's Hospital; (905)387-4508; Fax. (905)387-6093.

FULTON, Dorcas S; Cross Cancer Institute, 11560 University Ave NW, Edmonton AB T6G 1Z2; Tor'72; FRCPC; IntMed (Neuro Oncology); Neur. Staff, Cross Cancer Institute; Staff, University of Alberta Hospital; Prof Oncol & Neur, University of Alberta; (780)432-8517; Fax. (780)432-8380.

FULTON, Gerald A; 17 Richard St, St Catharines ON L2T 2E1; Wes'63; FRCPC; PhysMed&Rehab (Hypnotherapy). (905)684-5681; Fax. (905)684-2556.

FULTON, Jessica; Women's College Hosp, 76 Grenville St, Toronto ON M5S 1B2; Tor'08; CCFP; Staff, Women's College Hospital; Physician, Women's College Family Health Team; (416)323-6060; Fax. (416)323-6351.

FULTON, Lynne A; Sunnybrook Hlth Sciences Ctre, 2075 Bayview Ave, Toronto ON M4N 3M5; McM'73; FRCPC; EmergMed. Staff EmergMed, Sunnybrook Health Sciences Centre; Teach Staff, University of Toronto; (416)480-4037; Fax. (416)480-4704.

FUNARO, Deana; CHUM-Hop St-Luc, 1058 rue Saint-Denis, Montreal QC H2X 3J4; Mon'94; FRCPC; Derm (Vulvar Disease). Staff, Centre Hospitalier l'Université de Montréal (CHUM) - Hôpital Notre-Dame; Staff, Centre Hospitalier l'Université De Montréal (CHUM) - Hôpital Saint-luc; Staff, Hôpital Ste-Justine; Langs: English; French; (514)890-8000; rouleaufunaro@videotron.ca.

FUNDAMENSKI, Marta A; Medica One, 1275 Rymal Rd E, Hamilton ON L8W 3N1; Ott'05; CCFP; (905)387-0005; Fax. (905)387-0010.

FUNDYTUS, Dennis E; Cochrane Primary Care Centre, 103-100 Grande Blvd W, Cochrane AB T4C 0S4; Alb'75; CCFP; FCFP; Staff, Foothills Medical Centre; (403)932-2089; Fax. (403)932-1820.

FUNG, Ambrose Y T; Albany Med Clinic, 807 Broadview Ave, Toronto ON M4K 2P8; Sask'79; CCFP; FCFP; Langs: Chinese; Cantonese; (416)461-9471

FUNG, Anthony Y F; Diamond Hlth Care Centre, 9/F-2775 Laurel St, Vancouver BC V5Z 1M9; (Hong Kong)'77; ABNM; ABCD; ABIM; MB BS; FRCPC; Cardiol; IntMed. Ac Staff, Vancouver General Hospital - Centennial Pavillion; Clin Assoc Prof, University of British Columbia; (604)875-4755; funga@interchange.ubc.ca.

FUNG, Carl A; 206-282 Linwell Rd, St Catharines ON L2N 6N5; National (Ireland)'67; Court Staff, Niagara Health System - St Catharines General Site; Court Staff, Niagara Health System - Ontario Street Site; (905)934-9432; Fax. (905)934-9694.

FUNG, Celeste; St Patricks Home, 2865 Riverside Dr, Ottawa ON K1V 8N5; McG'06; MDCM; CCFP; Langs: Bilingual(English/French); (613)731-4660; Fax. (613)731-4056.

FUNG, Clement; Burnaby Hospital, 3935 Kincaid St, Burnaby BC V5G 2X6; UBC'01; CCFP; Staff, Burnaby Hospital; (604)434-4211

FUNG, Daisy; Westgrove Clinic, 201-505 Queen St, Spruce Grove AB T7X 2V2; Alb'09; CCFP; (780)962-9888; Fax. (780)960-5298.

FUNG, Daniel Y W; Chinatown Centre, 165-288 Georgia St E, Vancouver BC V6A 4H8; Alb'90; (604)605-3382

FUNG, David A; 4420 10th Ave W, Vancouver BC V6R 2H9; Cambridge (England)'78; MB BCh; FRCPC; Psy. Assoc Staff, Providence Health Care - St Paul's Hospital; (604)222-1353

FUNG, Donald E M Y; North Bay Reg Health Centre, 50 College Dr, North Bay ON P1B 0A4; Cal'81; FRCPC; Anes. Staff, North Bay Regional Health Centre - Regional Mental Health; (705)474-8600

FUNG, F Siu-Yue; Sunnybrook Hlth Sciences Ctre, H186-2075 Bayview Ave, Toronto ON M4N 3M5; Mem'05; GenSurg. Staff, Sunnybrook Health Sciences Centre; (416)436-4639

FUNG, Frank; 300 Taunton Rd E, Oshawa ON L1G 7T4; Man'83; Langs: Chinese; (905)725-1131; Fax. (905)725-1132.

FUNG, Gary W T; Riverbend Medicentre, 600 Riverbend Sq NW, Edmonton AB T6R 2E3; Alb'90; Langs: Chinese; (780)434-7234; Fax. (780)988-8903.

FUNG, Gerald; Parkdale Comm Health Centre, 1229 Queen St W, Toronto ON M6K 1L2; Fam Med, Parkdale Community Health Centre; (416)537-2455; Fax. (416)537-3526; gerald.fung@pchc.on.ca.

FUNG, Gordon C; Westview Med Clinic, 9757 90 St, Fort Saskatchewan AB T8L 1K5; National (Ireland)'62; MB ChB; BAO; FRCS; Staff, Fort Saskatchewan Health Centre; (780)998-9290; Fax. (780)998-1616.

FUNG, Harold M Y; Brandon Reg Health Centre, 150 Mctavish Ave E, Brandon MB R7A 2B3; Alb'83; FRCPC; DiagRad. Staff, Brandon Regional Health Centre; (204)727-3513

FUNG, Irving C; 55B-1673 Richmond St, London ON N6G 2N3; McG'70; DABOT; FRCSC; Otol. Langs: Chinese; (519)672-1375; Fax. (519)667-0307.

FUNG, Jason; Corporate Med Centre, 10-78 Corporate Dr, Scarborough ON M1H 3G4; Tor'96; FRCPC; IntMed; Nephrol. Staff, The Scarborough Hospital - General Campus; (416)279-0855; Fax. (416)279-0857.

FUNG, Jonathan; Richmond Mental Hlth Team, 200-6061 No. 3 Rd, Richmond BC V6Y 2B2; UBC'02; FRCPC; Psy. (604)675-3975; Fax. (604)270-6507.

FUNG, Julian; Richmond Public Market, 2270-8260 Westminster Hwy, Richmond BC V6X 3Y2; UBC'95; CCFP; (604)821-1112

FUNG, Kan Ying; 405-3461 Dixie Rd, Mississauga ON L4Y 3X4; Tor'79; Consultant, Trillium Health Centre - Mississauga; Langs: Cantonese; Chinese; Mandarin; (905)624-7225; Fax. (905)624-7225; kfung@thc.on.ca.

FUNG, Kathryn C; The Richmond Hosp, 7000 Westminster Hwy, Richmond BC V6X 1A2; Alb'02; FRCPC; Psy. Staff, Richmond Hospital; (604)278-9711

FUNG, Kee-Wai; 303-89 Humber College Blvd, Etobicoke ON M9V 4B8; National (Taiwan)'60; FAAP; FRCPC; Peds (General Pediatrics). Langs: Chinese; Cantonese; (416)743-6063; Fax. (416)743-0101.

FUNG, Kenneth K; School of Public & Population, 277-2206 East Mall, Vancouver BC V6T 1Z3; Man'78; (604)822-4994

FUNG, Kenneth P L; Univ Hlth Network-Toronto Western Hosp, 9E-399 Bathurst St, Toronto ON M5T 2S8; Tor'95; FRCPC; Psy. Clin Dir, Toronto Western Hospital - University Health Network; Asst Prof, University of Toronto; Langs: Mandarin; Cantonese; Chinese; (416)603-5349; Fax. (416)603-5661; kenneth.fung@utoronto.ca.

FUNG, Kevin; London HSC-Victoria Hosp, PO Box 5010 Stn B B3 427-800 Commissioners Rd E, London ON N6A 5W9; Qns'97; FACS; BA; FRCSC; Otol (Head & Neck Surgery). Staff, London Health Sciences Centre - Victoria Campus; (519)685-8599; Fax. (519)685-8562.

FUNG, Leslie C; Albany Med Clinic, 807 Broadview Ave, Toronto ON M4K 2P8; Tor'00; CCFP; Staff, Sunnybrook Health Sciences Centre; (416)461-9471; Fax. (416)461-2710.

FUNG, Michael E; Kawartha Diagnostic Imaging, 555 George St N, Peterborough ON K9H 3S1; National (Ireland)'70; FRCPC; DiagRad (Interventional Radiology). Div Dir Diag Imaging, Peterborough Regional Health Centre - Hospital Drive; Dir Diag Imaging, Peterborough Regional Health Centre - Rogers St Site; (705)745-1058

FUNG, Michael G; 304-1650 Elgin Mills Rd E, Richmond Hill ON L4S 0B2; Dundee (United Kingdom)'01; MB ChB; CCFP; (905)237-9166

FUNG, Michelle A; Gordon & Leslie Diamond Hlth C, 4117-2775 Laurel St, Vancouver BC V5Z 1M9; McM'98; MHSc; FRCPC; IntMed; Endocrin&Metab. Staff, Vancouver General Hospital - Centennial Pavillion; (604)875-5926; Fax. (604)875-5925.

FUNG, Nancy M; 166 Main St, St Catharines ON L2N 4V5; Ott'88; CCFP; Court Staff, Niagara Health System - St Catharines General Site; (905)935-6880; Fax. (289)206-0641.

FUNG, Peter S M; Parkland Med Associates, 205-505 Queen St, Spruce Grove AB T7X 2V2; Alb'75; BSc; CCFP; FCFP; Langs: Mandarin; Cantonese; (780)962-2001; Fax. (780)962-8176.

FUNG, Raymond C; K 302-650 Sammon Ave, East York ON M4C 5M5; Tor'01; FRCPC; IntMed; Endocrin&Metab. Langs: Cantonese; (416)915-5460

FUNG, Sarah; BCC-St Vincent Hospital, 3F-60 Cambridge St N, Ottawa ON K1R 7A5; UBC'08; CCFP; Staff, Bruyère Continuing Care - Saint-Vincent Hospital; (613)562-6262

FUNG, Scott; Univ Hlth Network-Toronto Gen, 9N 981-200 Elizabeth St, Toronto ON M5G 2C4; Tor'98; BSc; DABIM; FRCPC; IntMed (Hepatology); Gastroent. Staff, Mount Sinai Hospital; Staff, Toronto General Hospital - UHN; Asst Prof, University of Toronto; Langs: Cantonese; Mandarin; (416)340-3893; Fax. (416)340-3258.

FUNG, Shek Hong; St Mary's Hosp Centre, 5N-3830 av Lacombe, Montreal QC H3T 1M5; McG'93; FRCPC; IntMed; GeriatricMed. Staff, St Mary's Hospital Centre; adj Prof, McGill University; Langs: English; French; (514)345-3511 x3453

FUNG, Susanna W S; 1-2060 Ellesmere Rd, Scarborough ON M1H 2V6; Tor'06; CCFP; (416)439-2273

FUNG, Thomas K H; PO Box 73012 Rpo Woodbine, Calgary AB T2W 6E4; Qns'05; CCFP; (403)467-1457

FUNG, Vincent W H; Care Point Med Centres-Joyce, 5138 Joyce St, Vancouver BC V5R 4H1; UBC'06; FRCPC; MedBiochem. Staff, Vancouver General Hospital - Centennial Pavillion; (604)436-0800

FUNG, W L Alan; North York Gen Hosp-Branson, 555 Finch Ave W, North York ON M2R 1N5; Tor'04; FRCPC; Psy (Neuro Psychiatry). Staff, North York General Hospital - Branson Division; Langs: Cantonese; Mandarin; (416)632-8701; Fax. (416)632-8718.

FUNG, Wayne A; Wellington Ortho & Rehab, 3-86 Dawson Rd, Guelph ON N1H 1A8; (Jamaica)'96; FRCSC; OrthSurg. (519)837-2020; Fax. (519)837-2022.

FUNG, Wing-Tai; 113-385 Silver Star Blvd, Scarborough ON M1V 0E3; (Taiwan)'59; Langs: Chinese; Cantonese; Mandarin; (416)551-2888

FUNG KEE FUNG, Karen M C; The Ottawa Hosp-Gen Campus, 8420-501 Smyth Rd Box 804, Ottawa ON K1H 8L6; Mem'83; BMedSci; BSc; FRCSC; ObstGyn (Maternal Fetal Medicine). Prog Dir Maternal Fetal Medicine, The Ottawa Hospital - General Campus; Assoc Prof, University of Ottawa; (613)737-8551; Fax. (613)737-8070; kfung@toh.on.ca.

FUNG KEE FUNG, Michael; The Ottawa Hosp-Gen Campus, 501 Smyth Rd, Ottawa ON K1H 8L6; (Jamaica)'83; MB; BS; FRCSC; ObstGyn (Gynecologic Oncology). Staff Gyn Oncol, The Ottawa Hospital - General Campus; Head Div of Surg Oncol/Prof Dept ObstGyn & Surgery, University of Ottawa; (613)737-8560; Fax. (613)737-8828.

FUNK, Duane J; Health Sciences Centre, 2F-671 William Ave, Winnipeg MB R3E 0Z2; Man'00; FRCPC; Anes; Critical Care Medicine.

FUNK, Kathryn M; Eden Mental Health Centre, 1500 Pembina Ave, Winkler MB R6W 1T4; Man'80; BSc; FRCPC; Psy. Psychiatrist, Eden Mental Health Centre; (204)325-4325; Fax. (204)325-8429.

FUNK, Sandi; Meadow Lake Associate Clinic, PO Box 1510, Meadow Lake SK S9X 1Z1; Sask'07; CCFP; (306)236-5661; Fax. (306)236-4355.

FUOCO, Angelo; Centre Med Brunswick, 955 boul St-Jean, Pointe-Claire QC H9R 5K3; McG'89; CCFP; Staff, St Mary's Hospital Centre; assoc Prof, McGill University; (514)426-6677; Fax. (514)426-3323.

FUOCO, Gabriel G C; The Medical Centre, PO Box 4200 Stn Main 707 Charlotte St, Peterborough ON K9J 7B3; Tor'99; MSc; FRCSC; Otol. Langs: French; Italian; (705)876-4559; Fax. (705)876-4558.

FURER, Basheva; Norfinch Med Centre, 313-2100 Finch Ave W, North York ON M3N 2Z9; Latvia (Russia (Federation))'61; Staff, Humber River Regional Hospital - Finch Avenue Site; Langs: Russian; (416)661-7566; Fax. (416)661-7567; sonya12@rogers.ca.

FURESZ, Eva B; Access Medical Centre, 1395 Bank St, Ottawa ON K1H 8N1; Budapest (Hungary)'51; Hon Staff, The Ottawa Hospital - Riverside Campus; Langs: Hungarian; German; (613)731-1114; Fax. (613)731-1116.

FUREY, Beth; NCSB1C 571-585 University Ave, Toronto ON M5G 2N2; Dal'07; DiagRad.

FUREY, Michael U G; Cardiology Consultants, 101-99 Airport Rd, St. John's NL A1A 4Y3; Mem'79; FACC; FRCPC; IntMed (Interventional Cardiology); Cardiol. Ac Staff, Health Sciences Centre; (709)726-5311; Fax. (709)726-1028; cardiologyconsultants@nfld.net.

FUREY, William; South Shore Reg Hosp, 90 Glen Allan Dr, Bridgewater NS B4V 3S6; Dal'04; FRCPC; Anes. Staff, South Shore Regional Hospital; (902)527-5215

FURLAN, Andrea D; Toronto Rehab University Ctr, 550 University Ave, Toronto ON M5G 2A2; Sao Paulo (Brazil)'92; Staff, Toronto Rehabilitation Institute - University Centre; (416)597-3422; Fax. (416)516-6373.

FURLANI, Aldo A; Red Deer Reg Hosp Ctr, 3942 50A Ave, Red Deer AB T4N 4E7; Buenos Aires (Argentina)'96; Staff, Red Deer Regional Hospital Centre; Langs: Spanish; (403)356-4201; Fax. (403)358-4342.

FURLONG, Brian G; Homewood Health Centre, 150 Delhi St, Guelph ON N1E 6K9; McM'84; FRCPC; Psy. Consultant psy, Guelph General Hospital; Asst Prof Psy & Behavioural Neurosciences, McMaster University; (519)824-1010; Fax. (519)767-3532.

FURLONG, Dennis J; 1-396 William St, Dalhousie NB E8C 2X2; Mem'76; (506)684-6800; Fax. (506)684-6802.

FURLONG, F Wayne; 401-5799 Yonge St, North York ON M2M 3V3; Tor'64; DABPN; FRCPC; Psy (Anxiety Disorder). (416)224-9665; Fax. (416)224-9665.

FURLONG, Michael B; St Clare's Mercy Hosp, 154 Le Marchant Rd, St. John's NL A1C 5B8; Mem'76; FRCPC; IntMed. Staff, St Clare's Mercy Hospital; Clin Asst Prof Med, Memorial University Of Newfoundland; (709)726-7187; Fax. (709)726-8699.

FURLONG, Stephen B; Paradise Health Complex, 203-1386 Topsail Rd, Paradise NL A1L 1P6; Mem'92; CCFP.

FURLONG, Susan M; Paradise Health Complex, 203-1386 Topsail Rd, Paradise NL A1L 1P6; Mem'87; (709)782-4445

FURNESS, Alexander; Georgetown Med Associates, 199 Princess Anne Dr, Georgetown ON L7G 0E3; Tor'65; Staff, Halton Healthcare Services Corporation - Georgetown Hospital; (905)873-3000; Fax. (905)873-3035.

FURNESS, Robert A H; Red Deer Med Centre, 210-3947 50a Ave, Red Deer AB T4N 6V7; Man'83; FRCSC; PlasSurg. Staff, Red Deer Regional Hospital Centre; (403)343-2666; Fax. (403)340-1221.

FURQAN, Naila; New Best Care Med Centre, 4-790 Burnhamthorpe Rd W, Mississauga ON L5C 4G3; Karachi (Pakistan)'89; MB BS; CCFP; Physician, New Best Care Medical Centre; Langs: Hindi; Urdu; (905)848-8686; Fax. (905)848-8796; nfurqan@sasktel.net.

FURST, Katherine A; Mental Health Services, 525 Montreal St, Kingston ON K7K 3H9; Ott'91; FRCPC; Psy. Staff, Providence Care - Mental Health Services; (613)540-6165 x4314

FURSTENBERG, Josias; Supermed Walk in Clinic, 591 15th St E, Prince Albert SK S6V 1G3; MB ChB; CAFCI; Physician, Northern Medical Clinic; (306)922-9444; Fax. (306)922-5505; dutwa@shaw.ca.

FURSTENBURG, Dietrich; 32-665 Front St, Quesnel BC V2J 5J5; Pretoria (South Africa)'10; MB ChB; (250)983-2190

FURTADO, J C Sarah; Dept of Clinical Neurosciences, 3 UCMC-3350 Hospital Dr NW, Calgary AB T2N 4Z5; Cal'95; MD; PhD; FRCPC; Neur (Movement Disorders). Staff Clinical Neurosciences, Foothills Medical Centre; (403)944-4364; Fax. (403)283-2907.

FURTADO, Norman; Alisa Craig Family Clinic, PO Box 340 147 Main St, Ailsa Craig ON N0M 1A0; Wes'07; BHSc; BSc; CCFP; Staff, Strathroy Middlesex General Hospital - Middlesex Hospital Alliance; (519)293-3981; Fax. (519)518-2258.

FURTADO, Richard J; Collingwood Gen & Marine Hosp, 459 Hume St, Collingwood ON L9Y 1W9; Wes'02; Staff, Collingwood General & Marine Hospital; (705)444-8601

FURUE, Koto; Hôpital Ste-Justine, 3175 ch Cote-Sainte-Catherine, Montreal QC H3T 1C5; Dal'99; CSPQ; FRCPC; Anes. Staff, Hôpital Ste-Justine; (514)345-4733

FUSCH, Christoph; McMaster University, HSC 4F5-1280 Main St W, Hamilton ON L8S 4K1; (Germany)'84; FRCPC; Peds. Staff, Hamilton Health Sciences Centre - McMaster University Medical Centre; Teach Staff, McMaster University; Langs: German; French; (905)521-2100

FUSS, Carolyn; Centre for Family Medicine, 10B Victoria St S, Kitchener ON N2G 1C5; Tor'07; CCFP; Associate Clin Prof, McMaster University; (519)783-0021; Fax. (519)783-0031.

FUSS, Jeffrey W; London HSC-Victoria Hosp, PO Box 5010 Stn B 800 Commissioners Rd E, London ON N6A 5W9; Wes'86; FRCPC; EmergMed. Staff, London Health Sciences Centre - Victoria Campus; (519)685-8500

FUTERMAN, David H; 5016-3080 Yonge St, Toronto ON M4N 3N1; Tor'82; FRCPC; Psy. Ac Staff, Centre for Addiction & Mental Health (CAMH) - College Street Site; Lecturer, University of Toronto; (416)789-3012; Fax. (416)789-3012.

FUZESI, Gabor; Campbellton Reg Hosp, PO Box 880 Stn Main 189 Lily Lake Rd, Campbellton NB E3N 3H3; Szeged (Hungary)'93; Staff, Hôpital Régional Campbellton; (506)753-6433; Fax. (506)753-7920; fuzesi@nb.sympatico.ca.

FYFE, Jennifer M; Able-Care Med Clinic, 56-2991 Lougheed Hwy, Coquitlam BC V3B 6J6; McG'82; CCFP; (604)945-7819; Fax. (604)945-2884.

FYFE, Mary-Lyn R; 601A Discovery St, Victoria BC V8T 5G4; UBC'86; (250)386-0023

FYFE, Murray W; Vancouver Island Health, 430-1900 Richmond Rd, Victoria BC V8R 4R2; UBC'85; MSc(Epidemiol); FRCPC; CommunMed (Infectious Diseases). Physician, BC Centre For Disease Control; Teach Staff, University of British Columbia; (250)519-7066; murray.fyfe@bccdc.ca.

FYHN, Melissa A; South Calgary Med Clinic, 118-40 Sunpark Plaza SE, Calgary AB T2X 3X7; Cal'06; CCFP; (403)254-4000; Fax. (403)254-1282.

FYLES, Anthony W; Univ Hlth Network-Princess M, 610 University Ave, Toronto ON M5G 2M9; Tor'79; FRCPC; RadOncol., Princess Margaret Hospital - University Health Network; Prof RadOncol & ObstGyn, University of Toronto; (416)946-6522; Fax. (416)946-2111; anthony.fyles@rmp.uhn.on.ca.

FYLES, Gillian M; BC Cancer Ctre-Southern Interi, 399 Royal Ave, Kelowna BC V1Y 5L3; Man'81; Staff, BC Cancer Agency Sindi Ahluwalia Hawkins Centre for the Southern Interior; (250)712-3994; Fax. (250)712-3911.

FYNN, Joanne P C; South Hill Med Clinic, 890A Lillooet St W, Moose Jaw SK S6H 8B4; (South Africa) MB ChB; Staff Emerg Room Phys, Moose Jaw Union Hospital; Langs: Afrikaans; (306)691-0030; Fax. (306)694-5666.

FYNN, John K; Cumberland Reg Hlth Care Centr, 19428 Hwy 2, Amherst NS B4H 1N6; (Ghana)'92; MRCOG; BSc(Hon); MB ChB; (902)667-5124; Fax. (902)667-4060; john.fynn@cha.nshealth.ca.

GAAL, Judit M; Dundas Med Centre, 404-220 Dundas St W, Whitby ON L1N 8M7; Tor'77; BSc; MSc; Langs: Hungarian.

GAAS, Masoud Ali; M7-9509 156 St NW, Edmonton AB T5P 4J5; (Libya)'98; Gen Physician, Fogo Island Health Centre; (780)756-3300; Fax. (780)756-3301.

GABA, Priya; Bruyere Family Med Centre, 75 Bruyere St, Ottawa ON K1N 5C7; (Russia (Federation))'97; CCFP; Langs: Hindi; Russian; (613)241-3344

GABA IDIAMEY, Francine; CHUM-Hop Notre-Dame, F2117-1560 rue Sherbrooke E, Montreal QC H2L 4M1; Laval'04; FRCPC; IntMed; GeriatricMed. Staff, Centre Hospitalier l'Université de Montréal (CHUM) - Hôpital Notre-Dame; (514)890-8000; Fax. (514)412-7506.

GABANA, Cori-Ann; Royal Columbian Hosp, 330 Columbia St E, New Westminster BC V3L 3W7; UBC'05; FRCPC; IntMed. Staff, Royal Columbian Hospital; (604)520-4253

GABAY, Betty; Hop du Sacre-Coeur de Mtl, 5400 boul Gouin O, Montreal QC H4J 1C5; Mon'96; FRCPC; Derm. Staff, Hôpital du Sacre-Coeur de Montréal; (514)338-3008

GABAY, Jose; Jane Medical Clinic, L6-2780 Jane St, North York ON M3N 2J2; Madrid (Spain)'62; Staff Fam & CommunMed, Mount Sinai Hospital; Assoc Staff Fam & CommunMed, Humber River Regional Hospital - Finch Avenue Site; (416)749-2084; Fax. (416)741-3464.

GABBAY, Moshe; Clinique Mediplex, 15610 boul Gouin O, Sainte-Genevieve QC H9H 1C4; McG'98; FRCPC; IntMed. Staff, Lakeshore General Hospital - Pointe Claire; (514)675-4554

GABEL, Jesse D; CFB Wainwright, 12 CFHS Wainwright, Denwood AB T0B 1B0; Cal'10; CCFP; (780)842-1363; Fax. (780)842-1809.

GABEL, Kevin D; The Hincks Dellcrest Centre, 114 Maitland St, Toronto ON M4Y 1E1; Wes'06; FRCPC; Psy. (416)972-1935

GABEL, Nancy A; Norfolk Gen Hosp, 365 West St, Simcoe ON N3Y 1T7; Sask'83; Staff, Norfolk General Hospital; (519)426-0750

GABER, Mohamed I; Quinte HC Corp-Belleville Gen, 265 Dundas St E, Belleville ON K8N 5A9; Ain Shams (Egypt)'65; MB ChB; LRCP; MRCS; FRCS; FRCPC; AnatPath., QHC Belleville General; Langs: Arabic; (613)969-5511; drgaber@hotmail.com.

GABOR, Alexander; 17866 Leslie St, Newmarket ON L3Y 3E6; Bratislava (Slovakia)'83; Staff, Southlake Regional Health Centre; Langs: Slovak; (905)836-0899; Fax. (905)836-5988.

GABOR, Jonathan; Concordia Gen Hosp, 1095 Concordia Ave, Winnipeg MB R2K 3S8; Tor'06; FRCPC; IntMed. Staff, Concordia General Hospital; (204)667-1560

GABOR, Robert Z; Royal Victoria Hosp, 201 Georgian Dr, Barrie ON L4M 6M2; Semmelweis (Hungary)'01; CCFP; Staff, Royal Victoria Regional Health Centre; Langs: Hungarian; (705)728-9090

GABOR, Zsuzsanna; Doctor's Office, 325 Bamburgh Cir, Scarborough ON M1W 3Y1; Tor'87; Med Dir, MCI the Doctors Office; Langs: Hungarian; (416)492-8068; Fax. (416)497-7796.

GABOS, Zsolt; Cross Cancer Institute, 11560 University Ave NW, Edmonton AB T6G 1Z2; Alb'02; FRCPC; RadOncol. Staff, Cross Cancer Institute; (780)432-8783; Fax. (780)432-8380.

GABOURY, Jean; Centre Hosp Honore-Mercier, 2750 boul Laframboise, Saint-Hyacinthe QC J2S 4Y8; Mon'66; FRCPC; IntMed; Gastroent (P.Q.). Consultant Gastroent, Centre Hospitalier Honore-Mercier; (450)771-3333

GABOURY, Jeffrey P; Queen Street Surgical Assoc, 202-610 Queen St, Saskatoon SK S7K 0M8; Cal'99; BASc; PhD; FRCSC; GenSurg (Trauma). Clinical Asst Prof, University of Saskatchewan; (306)244-6818; Fax. (306)664-3462.

GABOURY, Louis; CHUM-Hotel-Dieu, 3840 rue Saint-Urbain, Montreal QC H2W 1T8; Mon'78; CSPQ; AB; PhD; FCAP; FRCPC; AnatPath (Research). Attending Pathologist, Centre Hospitalier l'Université de Montréal (CHUM) - Hôtel-Dieu; Prof Path & Biology, Universite de Montreal; Langs: Bilingual(French/English); (514)890-8000 x14262; louis.gaboury@umontreal.ca.

GABRA, Genevieve; Richmond Hosp, 7000 Westminster Hwy, Richmond BC V6X 1A2; Laval'02; FRCPC; IntMed. Staff, Richmond Hospital; (604)244-5470

GABRAIL, Yousry; Bronte Med Group, 78 Jones St, Oakville ON L6L 6C5; Cairo (Egypt)'79; CCFP; Langs: Arabic; (905)827-9865; Fax. (905)827-3583.

GABRIEL, Adel A R; Airport Business Centre, 2000 Pegasus Rd NE, Calgary AB T2E 8K7; Cairo (Egypt)'71; MB ChB; DPM(Ire); DTMH(UK); FRCPC; Psy (Adult General Psychiatry). Staff, Peter Lougheed Centre; Asst Prof, University of Calgary; (403)291-9122; Fax. (403)717-2899.

GABRIEL, Alexandra; 8F-311 Coloumbia St, Kamloops BC V2C 2T1; Washington(WA) (USA)'00; Staff, BC Cancer Agency Sindi Ahluwalia Hawkins Centre for the Southern Interior; (250)314-2734

GABRIEL, Anthony M; Gander Med Clinic, 177 Elizabeth Dr, Gander NL A1V 1H6; Mem'90; CCFP; FCFP; (709)256-7101; Fax. (709)256-7109; sherry.gabriel@nf.sympatico.ca.

GABRIEL, Maila J; St Boniface Clinic, 343 Tache Ave, Winnipeg MB R2H 2A5; Man'96; CCFP.

GABRIEL, Patricia S; 212-3001 Gordon Ave, New Westminster BC V3C 2K7; UBC'08; CCFP; (604)944-4077

GABRIEL, Robert P; Oakville Med Arts Bldg, 18-358 Reynolds St, Oakville ON L6J 3L9; Sher'85; Staff Family Pract, Halton Healthcare Services Corporation - Oakville Site; Langs: Bilingual(English/French); (905)844-4383; Fax. (905)844-9135.

GABRIEL, Vincent; Foothills Medical Centre, 1403 29 St NW, Calgary AB T2N 2T9; Sask'00; FRCPC; PhysMed&Rehab. Staff, Foothills Medical Centre; (403)944-1260

GABRIL, Manal Y; London HSC-University Hosp, PO Box 5339 Stn B 339 Windermere Rd, London ON N6A 5A5; Minya (Egypt)'92; FRCPC; AnatPath. Staff, London Health Sciences Centre - University Hospital; Langs: Arabic; (519)685-8500 x36353

GABRUCH, Thomas K; City Centre Fam Physicians, 100-514 Queen St, Saskatoon SK S7K 0M5; Sask'92; CCFP; FCFP; (306)244-3016; Fax. (306)244-4737.

GAD, Nadia; Harwood Med Centre, 2-320 Harwood Ave S, Ajax ON L1S 2J1; Tanta (Egypt)'88; MB ChB; CCFP; (905)231-1122

GADACZ, Ihor; Ivan Franko Home for Aged, 767 Royal York Rd, Etobicoke ON M8Y 2T3; Tor'66; Court Staff, St Joseph's Health Centre; Med Dir, Ivan Franko Ukranian Home for the Aged; Langs: Polish; Ukrainian; (416)767-5352; Fax. (416)239-2771.

GADHAFI, Fathi A; 5546 Portage Rd PO Box 1018, Niagara Falls ON L2E 6X2; Al-Fateh (Libya)'99; MB ChB; CCFP; Staff, Green Bay Community Health Centre; Langs: Arabic; (905)358-0171; fathi2007@hotmail.com.

GADIR, Yousif; 207 Willow St, Truro NS B2N 4Z9; Mosul (Iraq)'86; MB ChB; CCFP; Staff, Colchester East Hants Health Centre.

GADSDEN, Lori J; Rocky Mountain Hlth Centre, PO Box 2019, Fernie BC V0B 1M0; UBC'96; (250)423-4718

GAEDE, Lisa A; 306-125 13th St E, North Vancouver BC V7L 2L3; Alb'94; BSc; CCFP; (604)985-2712; Fax. (604)988-8191.

GAERBER, Shari J; 60 3rd Ave W, Vancouver BC V5Y 1E4; Wes'92; (604)961-5020

GAERTNER, Paul H; St Paul's Hosp, 1702 20th St W, Saskatoon SK S7M 0Z9; Sask'91; CCFP; CCFP(E.M.); FCFP; Staff, St Paul's Hospital (Grey Nuns) of Saskatoon; Teach Staff Family Med, University of Saskatchewan; (306)655-5113; Fax. (306)655-5963.

GAFFIERO, Patricia; CSSS de Saint-Jerome, 290 rue de Montigny, Saint-Jerome QC J7Z 5T3; Mon'86; CSPQ; FRCSC; GenSurg; VascSurg. Staff, Hôtel-Dieu de Saint-Jérôme; (450)431-8200 x2418; Fax. (450)431-8303.

GAFFNEY, Gregory M; 5 Beck Blvd, Penetanguishene ON L9M 1C1; Ott'81; (705)549-3433

GAFNI, Inbal; Women's College Hosp, 76 Grenville St, Toronto ON M5S 1B2; McM'04; FRCPC; Psy. Staff, Women's College Hospital; (416)323-6400

GAFOOR, Farah; Willowgrove Med Group, 2-527 Nelson Rd, Saskatoon SK S7S 1P4; Natal (South Africa)'02; DCH; MB ChB; DObst; CCFP; Staff, St Paul's Hospital (Grey Nuns) of Saskatoon; Staff, Royal University Hospital; Staff, Rosthern Hospital; (306)653-1543; fgafoor@sasktel.net.

GAFOOR, Mohamed M; Oakville Med Arts Bldg, 5-358 Reynolds St, Oakville ON L6J 3L9; RCS (Ireland)'72; FRCSC; GenSurg; Cardiovasc&ThorSurg. Ac Staff Surg, Joseph Brant Memorial Hospital; Ac Staff Surg, Halton Healthcare Services Corporation - Oakville Site; (905)842-4918; Fax. (905)842-4118.

GAFOOR, Tamara A; MUHC-Montreal Children Hosp, 2300 rue Tupper, Montreal QC H3H 1P3; McG'08; Peds. Staff, McGill University Health Centre - Montreal Children's Hospital; (514)412-4400

GAFOOR, Tasnim; Erindale Health Centre, 2-50 Kenderdine Rd, Saskatoon SK S7N 3A1; '05; MB ChB; (306)934-6601; Fax. (306)934-6615.

GAFSI, Aicha; CSSS de Rimouski-Neigette, CP 3150 succ A 150 av Rouleau, Rimouski QC G5L 5T1; Laval'03; FRCPC; IntMed; Nephrol. Staff, Hôpital Regional Rimouski; Langs: Spanish; English; (418)724-3000 x8159; Fax. (418)724-8757.

GAGARIN, Ruben; 2877A Ellesmere Rd, Scarborough ON M1E 4C1; (Russia (Federation))'96; ABPN; Psy (Child & Adolescent Psychiatry). Langs: Russian; (416)281-7301; Fax. (416)281-7465.

GAGE, Laura E; Toronto East Gen Hosp Inc, 825 Coxwell Ave, Toronto ON M4C 3E7; McM'99; FRCPC; Psy. Staff, Ontario Shores Centre for Mental Health Sciences; Staff, Toronto East General Hospital Inc; (416)461-8272

GAGIC, Nenad; Wentworth Limeridge Med Ctre, 402-849 Upper Wentworth St, Hamilton ON L9A 5H4; Belgrade (Serbia)'66; FACS; FRCSC; GenSurg. Associate Clin Prof, McMaster University; Langs: Serbian; (905)387-6460; Fax. (905)387-7470.

GAGLIARDI, Menuccia; Ocean Pier Med Centre, 207-2537 Beacon Ave, Sidney BC V8L 1Y3; Dal'89; CCFP; Staff, Saanich Peninsula Hospital; Staff, Vancouver Island Health Authority; Langs: Italian; (250)656-4114; Fax. (250)656-7118; menuccia@shaw.ca.

GAGNE, Alexandra; CSSS de Lac-Saint Jean-Est, CP 1300 Succ Bureau-Chef 300 boul Champlain S, Alma QC G8B 5W3; Laval'02; ObstGyn. Staff, CSSS de Lac-Saint Jean-Est; Langs: Bilingual(French/English); (418)669-2000

GAGNE, Alexandra; CSSS de Jonquiere, 2230 rue de l'Hopital, Jonquiere QC G7X 4H6; Laval'09; Staff, Centre Hospitalier Jonquiere; (418)695-7700

GAGNE, Ann A; Cita Health, 700-890 Pender St W, Vancouver BC V6C 1J9; McG'75; Assoc Staff, Providence Health Care - St Paul's Hospital; (604)647-2236

GAGNE, Annie-Claude; CSSS Drummond-Hop Sainte-Croix, 570 rue Heriot, Drummondville QC J2B 1C1; Sher'05; CCFP; Staff, Hôpital Sainte-croix; (819)478-6464; Fax. (819)478-6453.

GAGNE, Carl E; Groupe Med de Trois-Rivieres, 305-1900 boul des Recollets, Trois-Rivieres QC G8Z 4K4; Laval'93; CSPQ; Cardiol (P.Q.). Staff, CSSS de Trois-Rivières; Cardiology, Centre Hospitalier Regional de Trois-Rivieres; (819)375-4313

GAGNE, Caroline; Clinique de Med Familiale Jonq, 3835 boul Harvey, Jonquiere QC G7X 2Z5; Laval'99; Staff, Centre Hospitalier Jonquiere; (418)542-7519; Fax. (418)542-6541.

GAGNE, Chantal; CSSSG-Hop de Gatineau, CP 2000 Succ Bureau-Chef 909 boul de la Verendrye O, Gatineau QC J8P 7H2; Sher'88; FRCPC; Peds. Staff, Hôpital de Gatineau; (819)561-8565; Fax. (819)561-8103.

GAGNE, Christian J M; Trillium Med Clinic, 305-1062 Ghislain St, Hawkesbury ON K6A 3B2; Mem'95; BMedSci; Dip SportMed; LMCC; CCFP; FCFP; Langs: French; (613)632-2779; Fax. (613)632-4011.

GAGNE, Christine; CSST, CP 1200 Succ Terminus 280-524 rue Bourdages, Quebec QC G1K 7E2; Laval'76; Physician, Commission de la Sante Securite du Travail; (418)266-4670 x5917; Fax. (418)266-4672; christine.gagne@csst.qc.ca.

GAGNE, Claire; Dir de la Sante Publique-Mtl, 1301 rue Sherbrooke E, Montreal QC H2L 1M3; Mon'86; (514)528-2400 x3270; Fax. (514)528-2598; cgagne@santepub-mtl.qc.ca.

GAGNE, Claude; Clin des Maladies Lipidiques, 225-2590 boul Laurier, Quebec QC G1V 4M6; Laval'72; Ac Staff, Centre Hospitalier Universitaire de Quebec-CHUL; Clin Prof Med, Université Laval; (418)780-1376

GAGNE, Colombe; CSSS de Rimouski-Neigette, CP 3150 Succ A 150 av Rouleau, Rimouski QC G5L 5T1; Laval'89; Staff, Hôpital Regional Rimouski; (418)724-4672

GAGNE, Denise; Direction de Sante Publique, 2400 av D'Estimauville, Quebec QC G1E 7G9; Laval'70; FRCPC; CommunMed (Geriatric Medicine). Ac Staff, Centre Hospitalier Universitaire de Quebec-CHUL; Associate, Centre Hospitalier Universitaire De Québec - Pavillon De St-françois-d'assise; Acad Membre Med & Ambulatory Team, CSSS Vieille-Capitale; (418)666-7000; Fax. (418)666-2776; denise_gagne@ssss.gouv.qc.ca.

GAGNE, Dominique; Hôpital Laval, 2725 ch Sainte-Foy, Quebec QC G1V 4G5; Laval'01; Respir; IntMed (Intensive Care). Staff Pneumologue Intensiviste (IUCPQ), Hôpital Laval; Langs: Bilingual(French/English); (418)656-8711 x5504; Fax. (418)656-4762; dominique.gagne@criucpq.ulaval.ca.

GAGNE, Elaine; CLSC Laurier-Station, 135 rue de la Station SS 1, Laurier-Station QC G0S 1N0; Laval'92; (418)728-3435; Fax. (418)728-2233.

GAGNE, Eric; 345 rue St-Laurent CP 100, Saint-Simeon QC G0T 1X0; Laval'77; Staff, CSSS de Rivière-du-Loup - Centre d'hebergement St-Joseph; (418)638-2404

GAGNE, Eric J; CHUQ-Hotel-Dieu de Quebec, 11 Cote du Palais, Quebec QC G1R 2J6; Laval'86; CSPQ; AnatPath (Dermatological Pathology). Staff, Centre Hospitalier Universitaire de Québec (CHUQ) - Siege Social; Université Laval; (418)691-5233

GAGNE, Eve-Marie; CLSC Paul-Gilbert, 200-1205 boul de la Rive-Sud, Saint-Romuald QC G6W 0J6; Laval'95; Physician, CRC Appalaches & CLSC St-Romuald; Clin Prof, Université Laval; (418)380-8991; Fax. (418)839-5750.

GAGNE, Eve-Reine; CHUS-Hop Fleurimont, 6212 13-3001 12e av N, Sherbrooke QC J1H 5N4; Sher'84; Nephrol; IntMed. Staff, Centre Hospitalier Universitaire de Sherbrooke-Hopital Fleurimont; vice Doyen Predoctoral Med Studies, Universite de Sherbrooke; (819)346-1110; Fax. (819)820-6420.

GAGNE, Eveline; Ctr Hosp Laurentien, 234 rue Saint-Vincent, Ste-Agathe-Des-Mts QC J8C 2B8; Sher'03; Staff, Centre Hospitalier Laurentien; (819)324-4000

GAGNE, Gaston; Hop Louis-H Lafontaine, 7401 rue Hochelaga, Montreal QC H1N 3M5; Laval'82; Staff, Hopital Louis-H Lafontaine; (514)251-4000 x2082

GAGNE, Genevieve; Centre de Sante Valcartier, CP 1000 Bdp Succ Forces, Courcelette QC G0A 4Z0; Sher'07; CCFP; (418)844-5000; Fax. (418)844-6671.

GAGNE, Gilbert; Clinique Med Mirabel, 200-13714 boul du Cure-Labelle, Mirabel QC J7J 2K8; Mon'89; LMCC; CCFP; FCFP; Langs: Spanish; English; (450)435-7666; Fax. (450)435-1716.

GAGNE, Ginette; CLSC Verdun, 6161 rue Laurendeau, Montreal QC H4E 3X6; Mon'89; (514)766-0546

GAGNE, Guy; Centre Med Montcalm, B10-165 Grande Allee E, Quebec QC G1R 2L1; Laval'82; Pres, Clinique Rajeunissement Esthetique; Langs: English; Spanish; (418)524-0585; Fax. (418)524-8817.

GAGNE, Guy-Paul; GPG Consultant MD, 444 rue Beatty, Verdun QC H4H 1X6; Sher'77; FRCS; FSOGC; FRCSC; ObstGyn (Colposcopy). Langs: English; (514)449-8487

GAGNE, Guylaine; Inst Albert Prevost, 6555 boul Gouin O, Montreal QC H4K 1B3; Laval'88; Psy (P.Q.) (Pedology Psychiatry). Staff Psy, Hôpital du Sacre-Coeur de Montréal; Staff Psy, Hôpital Riviere des Prairies; Clin Teacher, Universite de Montreal; (514)338-4280; Fax. (514)338-4223.

GAGNE, Helene; CHUQ-Ctr Hosp Univ Laval, 2705 boul Laurier, Quebec QC G1V 4G2; Mon'99; Staff, Centre Hospitalier Universitaire de Quebec-CHUL; (418)656-4141

GAGNE, Helene; 444 rue Beatty, Verdun QC H4H 1X6; Sher'77; (514)761-1487

GAGNE, Helene M; Harmony Med Centre, 110-152 Cleopatra Dr, Nepean ON K2G 5X2; Qns'00; BSc(McGill); FRCPC; ObstGyn (Colposcopy). Assoc Staff, The Ottawa Hospital - Civic Campus; Assoc Staff, The Ottawa Hospital - Riverside Campus; Langs: Bilingual(English/French); (613)725-1870

GAGNE, Isabelle; Univ Hlth Network-Toronto Gen, 11F EW-200 Elizabeth St, Toronto ON M5G 2C4; Mon'07; AnatPath.

GAGNE, Jacques; CSSS de Rimouski-Neigette, CP 3150 Succ A 150 av Rouleau, Rimouski QC G5L 5T1; Mon'85; Staff, Hôpital Regional Rimouski; (418)723-7851

GAGNE, Jacques; 767 boul des Mille-Iles O, Sainte-Therese QC J7E 4E7; Mon'78; (450)430-7520; Fax. (450)437-5839.

GAGNE, Jean-Pierre; CHUQ-St-Francois D'Assise, B1 520-10 rue de l'Espinay, Quebec QC G1L 3L5; Laval'92; CSPQ; FRCSC; GenSurg (Laparoscopic Surgery). Staff, Centre Hospitalier Universitaire De Québec - Pavillon De St-françois-d'assise; (418)525-4160

GAGNE, Jeannine; Clinique Med Deux-Montagnes, 201 9e av, Deux-Montagnes QC J7R 3M1; Mon'89; BSc; Geriatric Med, CSSS de Thérèse de Blainville; Staff, Hôpital de Saint-Eustache; Langs: Bilingual(French/English); (450)472-7520

GAGNE, Johanne; Centre Med Christ-Roi, 40 du President-Kennedy Rte, Levis QC G6V 6C4; Laval'97; CCFP; (418)833-4977; Fax. (418)833-9557.

GAGNE, Julie; CHUQ-Ctr Hosp Univ Laval, 2705 boul Laurier, Quebec QC G1V 4G2; Mon'00; FRCPC; Peds; Endocrin&Metab. Staff, Centre Hospitalier Universitaire de Quebec-CHUL; (418)654-2282; Fax. (418)654-2137.

GAGNE, Kevin R; North Bay Reg Health Centre, 50 College Dr, North Bay ON P1B 0A4; McM'01; BSc; MSc; FRCPC; Anes (Critical Care Medicine). Staff, North Bay Regional Health Centre - Regional Mental Health; Langs: Bilingual(English/French); (705)474-8600 x2139

GAGNE, Louise E M; Saskatoon Community Clinic, 455 2nd Ave N, Saskatoon SK S7K 2C2; Sask'83; LMCC; Clinical Asst Prof, University of Saskatchewan; (306)652-0300; Fax. (306)652-5692.

GAGNE, Louise; CSSS de la Region de Thetford, 1717 rue Notre-Dame E, Thetford Mines QC G6G 2V4; Mon'88; FRCPC; Peds. Staff, Hopital du CSS de la Region de Thetford; (418)338-7777

GAGNE, Marc; Centre Hospitalier de Verdun, 4000 boul Lasalle, Verdun QC H4G 2A3; Mon'95; Staff, Centre Hospitalier de Verdun; (514)362-1000

GAGNE, Marc; Hop Jean-Talon, 1385 rue Jean-Talon E, Montreal QC H2E 1S6; McG'86; Staff, CSSS du Coeur de l'Isle Hôpital Jean-Talon; (514)495-6767

GAGNE, Marc-Andre; CSSS du Nord de Lanaudière, 1000 boul Sainte-Anne, St-Charles-Brromee QC J6E 6J2; Sher'98; Gastroent; IntMed. Staff, Centre Hospitalier Régional de Lanaudière; (450)759-8222

GAGNE, Marcel C; CSSS Haut-Richelieu-Rouville, 920 boul du Seminaire N, St-Jean-Sur-Richel QC J3A 1B7; Mon'77; CSPQ; FRCPC; Anes. Staff, Hôpital du Haut-Richelieu; (450)359-5000

GAGNE, Marie; CSSS de Lac-Saint Jean-Est, CP 1300 Succ Bureau-Chef 300 boul Champlain S, Alma QC G8B 5W3; Sher'05; FRCPC; DiagRad. Staff, CSSS de Lac-Saint Jean-Est; (418)669-2000

GAGNE, Michel; Polyclinique St-Eustache, 75 rue Grignon, St-Eustache QC J7P 4J2; Mon'73; Rheum; IntMed (P.Q.) (Osteoporosis). Langs: Bilingual(French/English); (450)473-6777; Fax. (450)473-1916; mi.gagne@videotron.ca.

GAGNE, Michelle; 301-1062 rue Charcot, Boucherville QC J4B 0C1; Mon'81; (450)655-4383

GAGNE, Monique; 3F-575 rue Saint-Amable, Quebec QC G1R 2G4; Laval'76; Med Evaluator, Ministry of Social Solidarity; (418)646-3361; Fax. (418)644-9319.

GAGNE, Nancy; CHUS-Hop Fleurimont, 3001 12e av N, Sherbrooke QC J1H 5N4; Sher'92; FRCPC; Peds (Endocrinology); Endocrin&Metab. Staff, Centre Hospitalier Universitaire de Sherbrooke-Hopital Fleurimont; Langs: English; (819)346-1110 x13147

GAGNE, Nathalie; CSSS de Temiscouata, CP 310 58 rue de l'Eglise, Notre-Dame-du-Lac QC G0L 1X0; Laval'91; FRCPC; IntMed (Cardiology). Staff, Centre Hospitalier Notre-Dame-du-Lac; (418)899-6751; Fax. (418)899-1180.

GAGNE, Pierre; 300-234 rue Dufferin, Sherbrooke QC J1H 4M2; Laval'69; FRCPC; Psy (Forensic Psychiatry). Consultant Dept of Justice & Solicitor General, Province of Quebec; Aj Prof Psy, McGill University; assoc Prof Med, Universite de Sherbrooke; (819)821-2297; Fax. (819)821-9917; pierre_gagne@ssss.gouv.qc.ca.

GAGNE, Pierre; Institut de Cardiologie de Mtl, 5000 rue Belanger, Montreal QC H1T 1C8; Mon'65; CSPQ; Cardiol (P.Q.). Staff, Institut de Cardiologie de Montréal; Teach Staff, Universite de Montreal; (514)376-3330; Fax. (514)593-2540.

GAGNE, Pierre; Clinique Med Chaudiere, 102 18e rue, Saint-Georges QC G5Y 4T9; Laval'83; (418)228-6820; Fax. (418)226-0358.

GAGNE, Pierre; CSSS de Trois-Rivières, 1991 boul du Carmel, Trois-Rivieres QC G8Z 3R9; Sher'88; FRCPC; NuclearMed (Academic Medicine). Staff, CSSS de Trois-Rivières; vice Doyen Campus Mauricie, Universite de Montreal; (819)697-3333 x63375; pierre_gagne_chrtr@sss.gouv.qc.ca.

GAGNE, Pierre-Thomas; CSSS Des Iles, 430 ch Principal, Cap-aux-Meules QC G4T 1R9; Laval'08; Staff, Hôpital de l'Archipel; (418)986-2121

GAGNE, Richard; CHUQ-Ctr Hosp Univ Laval, 2705 boul Laurier, Quebec QC G1V 4G2; Laval'67; MSc; PhD; CSPQ; MedGenetics (P.Q.). Staff, Centre Hospitalier Universitaire de Quebec-CHUL; Staff Teacher, Université Laval; (418)654-2103; Fax. (418)654-2780.

GAGNE, Richard; Hop Regional Rimouski, CP 3150 succ Bureau Chef 150 av Rouleau, Rimouski QC G5L 5T1; Mon'68; MCPS; GenSurg. Staff, Hôpital Regional Rimouski; Langs: English; (418)723-7851; gagner@globetrotter.net.

GAGNE, Sandrine; Clinique Med Centre Ville, 95 av Rousseau, Rimouski QC G5L 5S4; Laval'01; CCFP; (418)722-6816; sandrinegagne@hotmail.com.

GAGNE, Sebastien; CHUM-Hop Notre-Dame, 1560 rue Sherbrooke E, Montreal QC H2L 4M1; Sher'01; FRCSC; Ophth. Staff, Centre Hospitalier l'Université de Montréal (CHUM) - Hôpital Notre-Dame; (514)890-8000; sebastien.gagne@mail.mcgill.ca.

GAGNE, Serge; Hop Du Sacre-Coeur De Montreal, 5400 boul Gouin O, Montreal QC H4J 1C5; Mon'85; FRCPC; Psy. Staff, Hôpital du Sacre-Coeur de Montréal; (514)338-4390

GAGNE, Stephen; Clinique Medi-Val, 100-408 rue Jeanne-Mance, Salaber-de-Valleyf QC J6T 4G1; Sher'89; Staff, Centre Hospitalier Régional du Suroît; (450)370-3387; Fax. (450)370-3595.

GAGNE, Suzanne; Clin Medicale De Roberval, 714 boul Marcotte, Roberval QC G8H 1Z6; Laval'82; LMCC; Staff, Hotel-Dieu de Roberval; (418)275-3833; Fax. (418)275-6747.

GAGNE, Sylvain; The Ottawa Hosp-Gen Campus, 501 Smyth Rd, Ottawa ON K1H 8L6; Ott'00; FRCPC; Anes. Staff, The Ottawa Hospital - General Campus; Langs: Bilingual(English/French); (613)737-8187

GAGNE, Thierry; CSSS de la Baie-des-Chaleurs, RR 2 419 boul Perron, Maria QC G0C 1Y0; Laval'03; FRCSC; GenSurg. Staff, CSSS de la Baie-des-Chaleurs; (418)759-3443

GAGNER, Michel; Clinique Michel Gagner MD Inc, 191-315 Pl d'Youville, Montreal QC H2Y 0A4; Sher'82; CSPQ; FRCSC; GenSurg (Laparoscopic Surgery). (514)757-9199

GAGNEUR, Arnaud; CHUS-Hop Fleurimont, 3001 12e av N, Sherbrooke QC J1H 5N4; Brest (France)'99; Staff, Centre Hospitalier Universitaire de Sherbrooke-Hopital Fleurimont; (819)346-1110

GAGNIER, Rachel M; London HSC-Victoria Hosp, PO Box 5010 Stn B 800 Commissioners Rd E, London ON N6A 5W9; McM'09; CCFP; CCFP(E.M.); Staff, London Health Sciences Centre - Victoria Campus; Langs: Bilingual(English/French); (519)667-6538

GAGNIER, Stephane; Inst de Readaptation de Mtl, 6300 av de Darlington, Montreal QC H3S 2J4; Mon'81; FRCPC; Psy (Consultant Liaison Psychiatry). Staff, Institut de Réadaptation Gingras-Lindsay de Montréal; Universite de Montreal; (514)340-2770; Fax. (514)340-2775.

GAGNON, Alain; BC Women's Hosp & Health Ctre, B241-4500 Oak St, Vancouver BC V6H 3N1; Sher'89; FRCSC; ObstGyn (Prenatal Care). Sr Med Dir, BC Women's Hospital & Health Centre; Clin Prof, University of British Columbia; Langs: French; (604)875-3174; Fax. (604)875-3099; agagnon@cw.bc.ca.

GAGNON, Alain; Clinique Med D'Esthetique, 200-1050 boul Cure-Poirier O, Longueuil QC J4K 2E4; Sher'78; CCBOM; Media Dir, QIT-Sorel; Medical Officer, IOC-Sept Isles & Labrador City; Langs: Bilingual(French/English); (450)651-3000; Fax. (450)651-3335; clin.med.a.gagnon@videotron.ca.

GAGNON, Alain; CHUM-Hop Notre-Dame, 1560 rue Sherbrooke E, Montreal QC H2L 4M1; McG'99; FRCSC; PlasSurg. Staff, Centre Hospitalier l'Université de Montréal (CHUM) - Hôpital Notre-Dame; (514)890-8000 x23757; Fax. (514)412-7575.

GAGNON, Alexandre; CSSS de Beauce-Etchemin, 1515 17e rue, Saint-Georges QC G5Y 4T8; Laval'03; FRCPC; DiagRad. Staff, Centre Hospitalier Beauce-Etchemin; (418)228-2031

GAGNON, Alexis; CSSSG-Hop de Hull, 116 boul Lionel-Emond, Gatineau QC J8Y 1W7; Laval'98; FRCPC; Neur. Staff, Hull Hospital; Langs: English; (819)595-6212; Fax. (819)595-6213.

GAGNON, Andre; Ctr Hosp Pierre-Janet, 20 rue Pharand, Gatineau QC J9A 1K7; Laval'75; FRCPC; Psy (Suicide Risk). Staff, CSSS de Gatineau; Staff, Centre Hospitalier Pierre-Janet; Physician, Clinique de Psyhotherapie de L'Outaouais; Teach Staff, University of Ottawa; Langs: Bilingual(French/English); (819)776-8093; Fax. (819)771-7195; andre_gagnon@sssss.gouv.qc.ca.

GAGNON, Andre; Clinique Med Jean-Talon Pie IX, 4679 rue Jean-Talon E, Saint-Leonard QC H1S 1K3; Mon'81; CSPQ; FRCPC; IntMed; Cardiol. Staff, Hopital Maisonneuve-Rosemont; (514)374-5901; Fax. (514)374-1668.

GAGNON, Andre F; Polyclinique de Trois-Rivieres, 320-1900 boul des Recollets, Trois-Rivieres QC G8Z 4K4; Laval'70; FRCPC; Electroenceph (P.Q.) (Electromyography); Neur. Staff Neurol, CSSS de Trois-Rivières; Langs: English; (819)373-3733; Fax. (819)373-8137.

GAGNON, Andree; Clinique Med St-Antoine, 609 9e rue, Saint-Jerome QC J7Z 2Z2; Mon'89; CCFP; Staff, Hôtel-Dieu de Saint-Jérôme; (450)432-3308; Fax. (450)432-1004.

GAGNON, Andree-Anne; Ctr Hosp Laurentien, 234 rue Saint-Vincent, Ste-Agathe-des-Mts QC J8C 2B8; Laval'07; CCFP; Staff, Centre Hospitalier Laurentien; Staff, Centre de L'Annonciation; (819)324-4000

GAGNON, Annie; 105-185 av Acadie, Dieppe NB E1A 1G6; Sher'00; CCFP; (506)862-4182; Fax. (506)862-4179.

GAGNON, Annie; Clin Perinatalitie Trois-Rivie, 100-4900 boul des Forges, Trois-Rivieres QC G8Y 1X1; Laval'96; CCFP; (819)373-2303; Fax. (819)373-0765.

GAGNON, Antoine; Orillia Soldiers' Mem Hosp, 170 Colborne St W, Orillia ON L3V 2Z3; Ott'03; CCFP; Staff, Orillia Soldiers' Memorial Hospital; (705)331-1666

GAGNON, Antoine; Clin De Med Family D'Embrun, PO BOX 1259 869 Notre-Dame St, Embrun ON K0A 1W0; Ott'04; CCFP; (613)443-3311

GAGNON, Bernard; 2615 av Laporte, Saint-Hyacinthe QC J2S 7T1; Laval'67; Urol. Staff, Centre Hospitalier Honore-Mercier; (450)773-3000; Fax. (450)773-4953; bernard.gagnon2@hy.cgocable.ca.

GAGNON, Bernard P; Tower Prof Centre, 5520 50 Ave, Wetaskiwin AB T9A 0T3; Alb'85; VP Med Staff, Wetaskiwin Hospital & Care Centre; (780)352-9700

GAGNON, Bruno; CHUQ-Hotel-Dieu de Quebec, 11 Cote du Palais, Quebec QC G1R 2J6; Laval'85; MSc; Staff, McGill University Health Centre - Royal Victoria Hospital; Staff, Centre Hospitalier Universitaire de Québec (CHUQ) - Siege Social; Asst Prof Med & Oncol, McGill University; Langs: Spanish; English; (418)525-4444

GAGNON, Caroline; CSSS des Îles, CP 730 430 ch Principal, Cap-aux-Meules QC G4T 1R9; Laval'00; CSPQ; FRCPC; Anes. Staff, Hôpital de l'Archipel; (418)986-2121 x8118

GAGNON, Caroline; Hotel-Dieu de Levis, 143 rue Wolfe, Levis QC G6V 3Z1; Laval'99; FRCPC; Psy. Staff, Hôtel-Dieu de Lévis; (418)835-7155; Fax. (418)838-8873.

GAGNON, Caroline; Clinique Bloui-Valois, 299 boul Sir Wilfrid Laurier, Longueuil QC J4R 2L1; Sher'81; Ac Staff, Centre Hospitalier Universitaire de Sherbrooke-Hôpital Hôtel-Dieu; (450)465-7358

GAGNON, Catherine; CSSS Kamouraska-Hop-Notre Dame, CP 460 1201 6e av, La Pocatiere QC G0R 1Z0; Laval'08; CCFP; Staff, CSSS de Kamouraska; (418)856-7000

GAGNON, Catherine; Reseau de Sante du Temiscouata, 45 rue du Foyer S RR 1, Riviere-Bleue QC G0L 2B0; Laval'77; (418)893-5549; Fax. (418)893-1084.

GAGNON, Catherine; Hop Jeffery Hale, 1250 ch Sainte-Foy, Quebec QC G1S 2M6; Laval'86; CCFP; Staff, Jeffery Hale Hospital-Saint Brigid's; (418)683-4471

GAGNON, Christiane; Hop Maisonneuve-Rosemont, 160-5415 boul de l'Assomption, Montreal QC H1T 2M4; Mon'85; FRCPC; Peds. Staff, Hopital Maisonneuve-Rosemont; (514)252-3400; Fax. (514)252-3548.

GAGNON, Christine; Clinique Med Fleur de Lys, 8 rue Du Terminus E, Rouyn-Noranda QC J9X 3B4; Mon'01; Staff, Centre Hospitalier Rouyn-Noranda; Langs: English; (819)764-6185

GAGNON, Claire; CLSC St-Leonard, 5540 rue Jarry E, Saint-Leonard QC H1P 1T9; Sher'86; (514)328-3460; Fax. (514)328-1468.

GAGNON, Claude; Rio Tinto Alcan, 1-1955 boul Mellon, Jonquiere QC G7S 3H2; Laval'81; Chef Gen Med, Centre Hospitalier Jonquiere; (418)699-2111 x3598; Fax. (418)695-8698.

GAGNON, Claude-Francois; CLSC Jardin du Quebec, 2 rue Ste-Famille, Saint-Remi QC J0L 2L0; Sher'95; (450)454-4671; Fax. (450)454-4538.

GAGNON, Claudia; CHUQ-Ctr Hosp Univ Laval, B0027-2705 boul Laurier, Quebec QC G1V 4G2; Sher'01; FRCPC; IntMed; Endocrin&Metab. Staff, Centre Hospitalier Universitaire de Quebec-CHUL; Langs: Bilingual(French/English); (418)525-4444; Fax. (418)654-2792.

GAGNON, D'Arcy W; Downtown Doctors, 418-720 Spadina Ave, Toronto ON M5S 2T9; Ott'90; Langs: Spanish; English; (416)929-1530; Fax. (416)929-7398.

GAGNON, Daniel; CHUS-Hop Fleurimont, 3001 12e av N, Sherbrooke QC J1H 5N4; Sher'89; LMCC; CSPQ; FRCPC; Anes (Intensive Care). Staff, Centre Hospitalier Universitaire de Sherbrooke-Hopital Fleurimont; Clin Prof, Universite de Sherbrooke; (819)346-1110 x14403; Fax. (819)820-6420.

GAGNON, Daniel; Centre Med & Chir Rockland, 110-100 ch Rockland, Mont-Royal QC H3P 2V9; Mon'93; (514)667-3833; Fax. (514)667-3834.

GAGNON, Dominique; Centre Cleophas-Claveau, 1000 rue Du Docteur-desgagne, La Baie QC G7B 2Y6; Laval'99; Staff, Centre Maria-Chapdelaine - CH de Dolbeau-Mistassini; (418)544-3381

GAGNON, Elaine; Centre Medical de l'Hetriere, 201-3520 rue de l'Hetriere, St-Augustin-D-Desm QC G3A 0B4; Laval'88; Langs: Bilingual(French/English); (418)651-3933; Fax. (418)651-0256.

GAGNON, Elisabeth; CSSS de Chicoutimi, 305 rue Saint-Vallier, Chicoutimi QC G7H 5H6; Laval'98; GeriatricMed; IntMed. Staff, Complexe hospitalier de la Sagamie; (418)541-1000

GAGNON, Elyse; CSSS Haut-Richelieu-Rouville, 920 boul du Seminaire N, St-Jean-Sur-Richel QC J3A 1B7; Mon'90; Staff, Hôpital du Haut-Richelieu; (450)359-5000; Fax. (450)359-5251.

GAGNON, Emilie C; CSSS Haute Gaspesie, 50 rue du Belvedere, Ste-Anne-des-Monts QC G4V 1X4; Laval'07; CCFP; Staff, Centre Hospitalier des Monts; (418)763-2261

GAGNON, Emilie; CSSS de Manicouagan, 635 boul Jolliet, Baie-Comeau QC G5C 1P1; Mon'06; CCFP; Staff, Centre Hospitalier Régional Baie-Comeau; (418)589-3701

GAGNON, Eric; Hosp Maisonneuve-Rosemont, 5415 boul de l'Assomption, Montreal QC H1T 2M4; Mon'88; Staff, Hopital Maisonneuve-Rosemont; (514)252-3523

GAGNON, Fabien; Direction de la Sante Publique, 800 boul Chomedey, Laval QC H7V 3Y4; Laval'89; MSc; FRCPC; CommunMed. Médecin, Direction de la Sante Publique de Laval; (450)978-2121; Fax. (450)978-2100; fabien_gagnon@ssss.gouv.qc.ca.

GAGNON, Fabien; CHUQ-Ctr Hosp Univ Laval, 2705 boul Laurier, Quebec QC G1V 4G2; Laval'81; DFAPA; DPsychol; FRCPC; CCFP; FCFP; Psy (Anxiety Disorder). Staff, Centre Hospitalier Universitaire de Quebec-CHUL; Teach Staff, Université Laval; (418)654-2121; Fax. (418)654-2132; fgagnon.psy@fmed.ulaval.ca.

GAGNON, Fabienne; Clinique Med St-Etienne, 2-965 Rte Lagueux, St-Etienne-De-Lauz QC G6J 1T5; Laval'87; Associate, Centre Hospitalier Universitaire de Quebec-CHUL; (418)831-9538; Fax. (418)831-8552.

GAGNON, Francois; 75 rue Saint-Henri, Riviere-Du-Loup QC G5R 2A4; Laval'90; FRCPC; IntMed (Hospital Consultation). Staff, CSSS de Kamouraska; Staff, Centre Hospitalier Regional du Grand-Portage; Langs: English; (418)868-1000; Fax. (418)868-1059; fgportage@gmail.com.

GAGNON, Francois; Clinique Med Val-Belair, 202-1147 boul Pie-XI N, Quebec QC G3K 2P8; Sher'80; (418)843-2473; Fax. (418)843-0224.

GAGNON, Francois; 160 rue Principale, Saint-Jacques NB E7B 1W4; Laval'82; Staff, Hôpital regional d'Edmundston; Physician, Travail Securitaire NB; adj Prof, Universite de Sherbrooke; Langs: Bilingual(French/English); (506)739-7708; Fax. (506)739-5839.

GAGNON, Gabrielle; CSSS de Rimouski-Neigette, CP 3150 Succ A 150 av Rouleau, Rimouski QC G5L 5T1; Laval'98; FRCPC; IntMed; MedOncol; Hem. Staff, Hôpital Regional Rimouski; (418)723-7851

GAGNON, Genevieve; CSSS-Hopital De Hull, 116 boul Lionel-Emond, Gatineau QC J8Y 1W7; Sher'07; CCFP; Staff, Hull Hospital; (819)966-6222

GAGNON, Genevieve; Centre de Obst/Gyn de la Cite, 4250 1re av, Quebec QC G1H 2S5; Laval'03; FRCSC; ObstGyn (Echography Obstetrics & Gynecology). Obst/Gyne, CH St-Francois Inc; Langs: Bilingual(French/English); (418)654-0810; Fax. (418)654-1898.

GAGNON, Genevieve; CHUQ-St-Francois D'Assise, 10 rue du l'Espinay, Quebec QC G1L 3L5; Laval'08; Staff, Centre Hospitalier Universitaire De Québec - Pavillon De St-françois-d'assise; (418)525-4444

GAGNON, Ginette; Cite de la Sante de Laval, 2012 boul Rene-Laennec, Laval QC H7M 4J8; Laval'85; Staff, Hopital de la Cite de la santé; (450)662-3665; Fax. (450)662-9124; ginette_gagnon_csssl@ssss.gouv.qc.ca.

GAGNON, Helene; Centre Med Pour Enfants, 1791 av Dollard, LaSalle QC H8N 1T9; Mon'93; (514)368-0444; Fax. (514)368-0445.

GAGNON, Helene; CLSC du Grand Chicoutimi, 411 rue de l'Hotel-Dieu, Chicoutimi QC G7H 7Z5; Laval'76; (418)543-2221; Fax. (418)543-9512.

GAGNON, Isabelle; Clinique du Coteau, 100-440 boul Saint-Luc, St-Jean-sur-Richel QC J2W 0E2; Mon'98; Staff, Hôpital de Gatineau; Langs: Bilingual(English/French); (450)359-6819; Fax. (450)359-3247; isabelle_gagnon@ssss.gouv.qc.ca.

GAGNON, Isabelle; Clin Chir Plastique Grande-All, 425 Grande Allee E, Quebec QC G1R 2J5; Laval'97; FRCSC; PlasSurg (Breast Reconstruction). Staff PlasSurg, Centre Hospitalier Affilié Universitaire de Québec - Hôpital De L'Enfant Jésus; Staff PlasSurg, Centre Hospitalier Affilié Universitaire de Québec - Hôpital du St-Sacrement; Langs: English; (418)682-2182; Fax. (418)681-2930.

GAGNON, Isabelle; Klondyke Med Clinic, 2-3089 3rd Ave, Whitehorse YT Y1A 5B3; Laval'97; Staff, Whitehorse General Hospital; Staff, Klondyke Medical Clinic; Langs: Bilingual(English/French); (867)668-4046; Fax. (867)668-4078.

GAGNON, Isabelle; CSSSG-Hop de Gatineau, CP 2000 Succ Bureau-Chef 909 boul la Verendrye O, Gatineau QC J8P 7H2; Sher'98; Staff, Hôpital de Gatineau; (819)561-8100; isabelle_gagnon@sss.gouv.qc.ca.

GAGNON, Jacques; Clinique Med de levis, 100-4975 boul de la Rive-Sud, Levis QC G6V 4Z5; Laval'79; Ac Staff, Hôtel-Dieu de Lévis; (418)833-5810; Fax. (418)833-2720.

GAGNON, Jacques R; 205-6070 rue Sherbrooke E, Montreal QC H1N 1C1; Mon'65; FRCPC; Psy (Forensic Psychiatry). Langs: English; French; (514)251-4790; Fax. (514)251-4792; gagnonja@videotron.ca.

GAGNON, Jacques-Eric; Ctr Hosp de Verdun, 4000 boul Lasalle, Verdun QC H4G 2A3; Mon'78; ABIM; FCCP; CSPQ; FRCPC; IntMed (Electrophysiology); Cardiol (P.Q.). Cardiology, Centre Hospitalier de Verdun; Staff Cardiol, Hôpital du Haut-Richelieu; Langs: Bilingual(French/English); (514)362-1000 x2449; Fax. (514)765-7314.

GAGNON, Jean; Bureau Reg CSST Laval, 200-1700 boul Laval, Laval QC H7S 2G6; Mon'66; Ac Staff, Hôpital du Sacre-Coeur de Montréal; Physician, CSST de Laval; (450)967-3200 x3294

GAGNON, Jean; Clinique Med Saint-Gabriel, 85 rue Saint-Gabriel CP 599, St-Gabriel-D-Brand QC J0K 2N0; Sher'75; (450)835-3431

GAGNON, Jean; 102-5495 boul Jean-XXIII, Trois-Rivieres QC G8Z 4A8; Laval'74; Derm. Langs: English; French; (819)376-1144 x0; Fax. (819)376-1147.

GAGNON, Jean-Guy R; Dr Jean-Guy Gagnon Med Prof Co, 102-109 Elm St, Sudbury ON P3C 1T4; Sher'91; BSc(Hon); FRCPC; Psy (Brain Injury Psychiatry). Med Dir, North Bay Regional Health Centre - Kirkwood; Langs: Bilingual(English/French); (705)670-2000

GAGNON, Jean-Paul; Centre Medical Familial, 189 av Damase-Potvin, Baie-Comeau QC G4Z 2Y9; Laval'74; (418)296-4499; Fax. (418)296-9446.

GAGNON, Joel; 4219-2775 Laurel St, Vancouver BC V5Z 1M9; Sher'99; CSPQ; FRCSC; GenSurg; VascSurg. Staff, Vancouver General Hospital - Centennial Pavillion; Staff, Richmond Hospital; (604)875-5819; Fax. (604)875-5542.

GAGNON, Johanne; Commission des Lesions Prof, 250-1200 boul Alphonse-desjard, Levis QC G6V 6Y8; Laval'79; (418)835-0852; Fax. (418)835-4443; johanne.gagnon.md@clp.gouv.qc.ca.

GAGNON, Josee A; CHUQ-Ctr Hosp Univ Laval, 2705 boul Laurier, Quebec QC G1V 4G2; Laval'86; CSPQ; FRCPC; Peds; Critical Care Medicine. Staff, Centre Hospitalier Universitaire de Quebec-CHUL; (418)525-4444; Fax. (418)656-4141.

GAGNON, Josee; Clinique Med St-Antoine, 609 9e rue, Saint-Jerome QC J7Z 2Z2; Sher'85; Staff, Hôtel-Dieu de Saint-Jérôme; (450)432-3308; Fax. (450)432-1004.

GAGNON, Josee; Ctr Hosp Affilie-Enfant-Jesus, 1401 18e rue, Quebec QC G1J 1Z4; Laval'88; LMCC; CSPQ; FRCSC; GenSurg (Intensive Care); Critical Care Medicine (P.Q.). Chef chir gén, Centre Hospitalier Affilié Universitaire de Québec - Hôpital De L'Enfant Jésus; Langs: Bilingual(English/French); (418)649-0252; Fax. (418)649-5579.

GAGNON, Judith; CLSC de Villeray, 1425 rue Jarry E, Montreal QC H2E 1A7; Mon'82; (514)376-4141

GAGNON, Julie; CLSC Saint-Leonard, 5540 rue Jarry E, Saint-Leonard QC H1P 1T9; Mon'04; Staff, Hopital Maisonneuve-Rosemont; (514)328-3460

GAGNON, Julie; Centre Med Fusion, 200-2035 av Sainte-Anne, Saint-Hyacinthe QC J2S 5H3; Mon'96; CCFP; (450)773-9554

GAGNON, Linda; Dartmouth Med Centre, 310-46 Portland St, Dartmouth NS B2Y 1H4; Dal'82; BSc; CCFP; FCFP; Langs: American Sign Language; (902)465-4533; Fax. (902)464-4906.

GAGNON, Linda; CSSS de Jonquiere, 2230 rue de l'Hopital, Jonquiere QC G7X 4H6; Sher'83; CSPQ; FRCPC; Anes. Staff, Centre Hospitalier Jonquiere; (418)695-7707

GAGNON, Lisa M; Foothills Medical Centre, 1403 29 St NW, Calgary AB T2N 2T9; Alb'01; FRCPC; Psy (Perinatal Psychiatry). Staff, Foothills Medical Centre; (403)944-5872; Fax. (403)944-2409.

GAGNON, Louis; 5055 rue Saint-Zotique E, Montreal QC H1T 1N6; Mon'72; (514)844-7818; Fax. (514)844-0786.

GAGNON, Louis; Hotel-Dieu de Levis, 143 rue Wolfe, Levis QC G6V 3Z1; Laval'99; DiagRad (Angiography/Interventional). Staff, Hôtel-Dieu de Lévis; (418)835-7101

GAGNON, Louis; CSSS de Chicoutimi, 305 rue Saint-Vallier, Chicoutimi QC G7H 5H6; Laval'91; FRCPC; EmergMed (P.Q.);CCFP; CCFP(E.M.); Staff, Centre de Sante et de Services Sociaux; Staff, Complexe hospitalier de la Sagamie; Langs: English; (418)541-1010

GAGNON, Louis-Olivier; Hotel-Dieu de Levis, 143 rue Wolfe, Levis QC G6V 3Z1; Laval'06; Urol. Staff, Hôtel-Dieu de Lévis; (418)835-7121

GAGNON, Louis-Simon; Centre Med Berger, 116-1000 ch Sainte-Foy, Quebec QC G1S 2L6; Laval'73; Ac Staff, Centre Hospitalier Affilié Universitaire de Québec - Hôpital du St-Sacrement; (418)688-1385; Fax. (418)688-3249.

GAGNON, Louise; CHUM-Hop Notre-Dame, 1560 rue Sherbrooke E, Montreal QC H2L 4M1; Laval'76; Staff, Centre Hospitalier l'Université de Montréal (CHUM) - Hôpital Notre-Dame; (514)890-8000 x26727

GAGNON, Luc; CSSS de Rimouski-Neigette, CP 3150 Succ A 150 av Rouleau, Rimouski QC G5L 5T1; Sher'86; CSPQ; AnatPath. Staff, Hôpital Regional Rimouski; (418)723-7851; Fax. (418)724-8637.

GAGNON, Luc; Centre Med Chambly, 205-1101 boul Brassard, Chambly QC J3L 5R4; Laval'98; (450)658-6601; Fax. (450)658-7849.

GAGNON, Lucie; Ctr des Service de Sante FC, 6560 rue Hochelaga, Montreal QC H1N 1X9; Mon'83; (514)252-2777

GAGNON, Patricia; 101-210 Centrum Blvd, Orleans ON K1E 3V7; McG'87; Langs: French; (613)837-5454; Fax. (613)837-3781.

GAGNON, Madeleine; Polyclinique de la Sante, 102-1688 boul des Laurentides, Vimont QC H7M 2P4; Mon'77; LMCC; FAAD; CSPQ; FRCPC; Derm (Esthetic Dermatology). Langs: English; (450)668-4812; Fax. (450)668-4547; msgagnon@dermato.ca.

GAGNON, Marianne; Clinique de Med Fam Le Norois, 201-641 4e rue O, Amos QC J9T 2S1; Sher'79; Staff Obst & Lab, CH Hôtel-Dieu d'Amos; Langs: Bilingual(English/French); (819)732-3368; Fax. (819)732-3442.

GAGNON, Marie-Anne; CHUS-Hop Fleurimont, 3001 12e av N, Sherbrooke QC J1H 5N4; Mon'08; CCFP; CCFP(E.M.); Staff, Centre Hospitalier Universitaire de Sherbrooke-Hopital Fleurimont; (819)346-1110

GAGNON, Marie-Anne; CRSSS Baie-James-Chibougamau, 51 3e rue, Chibougamau QC G8P 1N1; Mon'79; Staff, CRSSS de la Baie-James; (418)748-2676; Fax. (418)748-2549.

GAGNON, Marie-Claude; CSSS de Lac-Saint Jean-Est, CP 1300 Succ Bureau-Chef 300 boul Champlain S, Alma QC G8B 5W3; Mon'05; GenSurg. Staff, CSSS de Lac-Saint Jean-Est; (416)669-2000

GAGNON, Marie-Claude; Family Practice 535, 535 Montreal Rd, Ottawa ON K1K 0V1; Mon'03; CCFP; Staff, Montfort Hospital; Langs: Bilingual(French/English); (613)746-5350; Fax. (613)746-5340.

GAGNON, Marie-Elaine; Clin Medicale des 21, 101-171 6e rue, La Baie QC G7B 0A3; Laval'91; CCFP; FCFP; Staff Emerg, CSSS de Lac-Saint Jean-Est; VP-Expl, Université Laval; (418)544-3331; Fax. (418)544-7571.

GAGNON, Marie-Eve; Clinique Med de Saint-Jovite, CP 19069 Csp Place Ouimet 992 rue St-Jovite, Mont-Tremblant QC J8E 3C1; Mon'10; (819)425-2728

GAGNON, Marie-Eve; Hotel-dieu De Levis, 143 rue Wolfe, Levis QC G6V 3Z1; Laval'02; FRCPC; Neur. Staff, Hôtel-Dieu de Lévis; (418)835-7121

GAGNON, Marie-Josee; Ctr Hosp St-Joseph La Malbaie, CP 340 Succ Bureau-Chef 303 rue St-Etienne, La Malbaie QC G5A 1T8; Laval'92; CCFP; FCFP; Staff, Hôpital de la Malbaie; Langs: English; (418)665-1700

GAGNON, Marie-Therese; CHUQ-St-Francois D'Assise, 10 rue de l'Espinay, Quebec QC G1L 3L5; Laval'79; Ac Staff, Centre Hospitalier Universitaire De Québec - Pavillon De St-françois-d'assise; Langs: Bilingual(French/English); (418)525-4397; Fax. (418)525-4424.

GAGNON, Marjolaine M; Ctr d'Ophtalmologie Gagnon-Men, 240-214 boul de la Cite-des-Je, Gatineau QC J8Y 6S8; Mon'90; FRCSC; Ophth. ac Membre, Hôpital de Gatineau; Langs: English; (819)775-2900; Fax. (819)775-2557; les2yeux@videotron.ca.

GAGNON, Martine; 1394 rue Notre-Dame, Repentigny QC J5Y 3X1; Mon'73; ObstGyn. (450)585-1422

GAGNON, Maude; 944 6e av, Grand-Mere QC G9T 2J1; Laval'84; (819)533-5783; Fax. (819)533-5759.

GAGNON, Maurice; Cite de la Sante de Laval, 1755 boul Rene-Laennec, Laval QC H7M 3L9; Mon'63; (450)668-1010 x23488

GAGNON, Melanie; Ctr Medi Soleil St-Jean-Sur-Ri, 120-383 boul du Seminaire N, St-Jean-sur-Richel QC J3B 8C5; Mon'02; CCFP; Staff, Hôpital Anna-Laberge; (450)347-7557; Fax. (450)347-3099.

GAGNON, Melanie; CHUS-Hop Hotel-Dieu, 580 rue Bowen S, Sherbrooke QC J1G 2E8; Sher'95; FRCPC; IntMed. Staff, Centre Hospitalier Universitaire de Sherbrooke-Hôpital Hôtel-Dieu; (819)346-1110 x28303

GAGNON, Michael P; Goodfellow Prof Bldg, 209-170 McEwan Dr E, Bolton ON L7E 4C8; (Ireland)'04; BAO; MB BCh; CCFP; Court Staff Privil, Headwaters Health Care Centre - Orangeville Site; (905)951-7525; Fax. (905)951-3419.

GAGNON, Michel B; Clin Med, 6-39 rue Laurier E, Victoriaville QC G6P 6P6; Laval'64; FRCP; CSPQ; DiagRad (Radiology). Langs: Bilingual(French/English); (819)357-2323; Fax. (819)357-2323; miuic@videotron.ca.

GAGNON, Michel P; Clin Med Du Plateau, 300-195 rue de l'Atmosphere, Gatineau QC J9A 0A3; Mon'83; Prod Mgr, Hull Hospital; (819)776-0001; Fax. (819)776-2171.

GAGNON, Michel; Clinique Millenia, CP 62 Succ Pl-desjardins 303-4 Complexe desjardins, Montreal QC H5B 1B2; Mon'60; Gastroent (P.Q.); IntMed. ac Staff, Centre Hospitalier l'Université De Montréal (CHUM) - Hôpital Saint-luc; (514)861-9686

GAGNON, Michel P; CSSS de Lac-Saint Jean-Est, CP 1300 Succ Bureau-Chef 300 boul Champlain S, Alma QC G8B 5W3; Laval'88; Respir; IntMed. Staff, CSSS de Lac-Saint Jean-Est; Staff, Hôpital Laval; (418)669-2000; Fax. (418)662-6823.

GAGNON, Micheline D M; St Joseph's Healthcare F401-50 Charlton Ave E, Hamilton ON L8N 4A6; McM'88; ABIM; FACP; FRCPC; IntMed; GeriatricMed. Staff Geriatrics, St Joseph's Healthcare - Charlton Campus; Staff, Norfolk General Hospital; Prof Med/Head Geriatric Services, McMaster University; (905)521-6124; Fax. (905)521-6103; gagnonm@mcmaster.ca.

GAGNON, Mylene; Ctr Med Saint-Leonard, 360 rue Beliveau, St-Leonard-d'Aston QC J0C 1M0; Laval'05; (819)399-2030; Fax. (819)399-2343; mylene_gagnon@gmf.gouv.qc.ca.

GAGNON, Nadine; Inst U en Sante Mentale de QC, 2601 ch de la Canardiere, Quebec QC G1J 2G3; Laval'96; FRCPC; Psy. Staff, Institut Universitaire Sante; (418)663-5020; Fax. (418)663-5758.

GAGNON, Nadya; Ctr de Med Familiale de Granby, 48 rue Denison E, Granby QC J2G 4C6; Sher'93; Staff, Centre Hospitalier de Granby; (450)372-3996

GAGNON, Nathalie; CHUS-Hop Fleurimont, 3001 12e av N, Sherbrooke QC J1H 5N4; Sher'89; CSPQ; CCFP; CCFP(E.M.); FCFP; EmergMed. Staff, Centre Hospitalier Universitaire de Sherbrooke-Hopital Fleurimont; Langs: Bilingual(French/English); (819)346-1110 x14274; Fax. (819)564-5386.

GAGNON, Nathalie; Clinique Med Ahuntsic, 241 rue Fleury O, Montreal QC H3L 1V2; Laval'91; Staff, Centre Hospitalier Régional Baie-Comeau; (514)382-0062; Fax. (514)384-1422.

GAGNON, Nathalie; Chuq-St-Francois D'assise, 10 rue de l'Espinay, Quebec QC G1L 3L5; Laval'03; FRCPC; IntMed. (418)525-4444; Fax. (418)525-4467.

GAGNON, Nathalie; CSSS de Rivière-de-Loup, 75 rue Saint-Henri, Riviere-Du-Loup QC G5R 2A4; Mon'88; Urol. Staff Urol, Centre Hospitalier Regional du Grand-Portage; Staff, Denseignement Clinique University Laval; Langs: Bilingual(French/English); (418)868-1000; Fax. (418)868-3337.

GAGNON, Olivier; Clinique de Med Fam Montcalm, 309 rue Montcalm, Chicoutimi QC G7J 2V1; Sher'99; (418)545-4211; Fax. (418)545-2920.

GAGNON, Pauline R; CSSS Drummond-Hop Sainte-Croix, 570 rue Heriot, Drummondville QC J2B 1C1; Sher'85; FRCSC; Ophth (P.Q.). Staff, Hôpital Sainte-croix; (819)478-6464

GAGNON, Pierre; Ctr Hosp Anna-Laberge, 200 boul Brisebois, Chateauguay QC J6K 4W8; Laval'65; FRCPC; Psy. Staff, Hôpital Anna-Laberge; (450)692-0002

GAGNON, Pierre; CHUQ-Ctr Hosp Univ Laval, 580-2705 boul Laurier, Quebec QC G1V 4G2; Laval'82; FRCPC; IntMed (Therapeutic Endoscopy); Gastroent. Ac Staff, Centre Hospitalier Universitaire de Quebec-CHUL; Teach Staff Med, Université Laval; Langs: English; (418)654-2168; Fax. (418)654-2164.

GAGNON, Pierre R; CHUQ-Hotel-Dieu de Quebec, 11 Cote du Palais, Quebec QC G1R 2J6; Laval'86; NBME; AB; LMCC; ABPN; FRCPC; Psy (Psychiatric Oncology). Staff Psy, Centre Hospitalier Universitaire de Québec (CHUQ) - Siege Social; Psychiatre, Maison Michel Sarrazin; Prof Pharmacology, Université Laval; Langs: Bilingual(French/English); (418)691-5151 x15808; Fax. (418)691-5019; pierre.gagnon@crhdq.ulaval.ca.

GAGNON, Raymonde F; MUHC-Montreal Gen Hosp, L4 516-1650 av Cedar, Montreal QC H3G 1A4; Laval'66; FRCPC; IntMed (Urology); Nephrol (P.Q.). Staff Nephrol, McGill University Health Centre - Montreal General Campus; (514)934-1934 x44051; Fax. (514)934-8248; raymonde.gagnon@muhc.mcgill.ca.

GAGNON, Rebecca; CSSS de Beauce-Etchemin, 1515 17e rue, Saint-Georges QC G5Y 4T8; Laval'02; Staff, Centre Hospitalier Beauce-Etchemin; (418)228-2031

GAGNON, Remi; CHUQ-Ctr Hosp Univ Laval, 1355-2705 boul Laurier, Quebec QC G1V 4G2; Laval'98; FRCPC; IntMed; ClinImmunol&Allergy. Staff, Centre Hospitalier Universitaire de Quebec-CHUL; Langs: English; (418)654-2240

GAGNON, Rene; Centre Med Berger, 116-1000 ch Sainte-Foy, Quebec QC G1S 2L6; Laval'68; ac Staff, Centre Hospitalier Affilié Universitaire de Québec - Hôpital du St-Sacrement; (418)688-1385; Fax. (418)688-3249; rene_gagnon@ssss.gouv.qc.ca.

GAGNON, Renee; Ctr Hosp de Matane, 333 rue Thibault, Matane QC G4W 2W5; Laval'01; CCFP; CCFP(E.M.); Staff, Centre Hospitalier de Matane; (418)562-3135

GAGNON, Robert; Clinique Med Familiale Clermon, 500-106 boul Notre-Dame, Clermont QC G4A 1G3; Laval'77; Prés, Hôpital de la Malbaie; (418)439-3935; Fax. (418)439-4548.

GAGNON, Robert; MUHC-Royal Victoria Hosp, F4 34-687 av des Pins O, Montreal QC H3A 1A1; Mon'80; FRCSC; ObstGyn (Obstetrics). Staff, McGill University Health Centre - Royal Victoria Hospital; (514)934-1934 x31385

GAGNON, Roger; Clinique Med Cartier, 804-1851 rue Sherbrooke E, Montreal QC H2K 4L5; Mon'66; CSPQ; Cardiol. Chef Services/ac Staff, Centre Hospitalier l'Université de Montréal (CHUM) - Hôpital Notre-Dame; (514)522-9102

GAGNON, Roger; Clin Med R Gagnon et G Fortier, 2231 rue de l'Hopital, Jonquiere QC G7X 9Y4; Mon'71; (418)542-8153; Fax. (418)542-8151.

GAGNON, Serge R; Les Obst & Gyn de l'Amiante, 102-718 boul Frontenac E, Thetford Mines QC G6G 6H1; Laval'72; ObstGyn. (418)338-2161; Fax. (418)338-2162.

GAGNON, Serge; CHUQ-Hotel-Dieu de Quebec, 11 Cote du Palais, Quebec QC G1R 2J6; Laval'84; CSPQ; Anes. Staff, Centre Hospitalier Universitaire de Québec (CHUQ) - Siege Social; (418)691-5323; Fax. (418)691-5097.

GAGNON, Serge; 10445 av 1Re, Saint-Georges QC G5Y 6X8; Laval'70; CSPQ; FRCSC; OrthSurg (Trauma). Ac Staff, Centre Hospitalier Beauce-Etchemin; Langs: Bilingual(French/English); (418)228-2899; Fax. (418)228-2875; serge@cliniqueiena.com.

GAGNON, Serge; Anciens Combattants Canada, 85 rue Bellehumeur, Gatineau QC J8T 8B7; Mon'78; Langs: English; French; (819)934-3974

GAGNON, Simon; Clin Orl Quebec Metropolition, 110-2880 ch des Quatre-Bourgeo, Quebec QC G1V 4X7; Laval'90; ABOtol; CSPQ; FRCSC; Otol (Laryngology). assoc Membre, Hôpital Laval; ac Membre, Centre Hospitalier Affilié Universitaire de Québec - Hôpital De L'Enfant Jésus; assoc Membre, Centre Hospitalier Chauveau; Langs: English; (418)653-8717; Fax. (418)653-7199; gagnon.si@videotron.ca.

GAGNON, Sonia I; Centre de Sante des Femmes, 5180 boul Gouin O, Montreal QC H4J 1C3; Mon'98; FRCPC; ObstGyn. Chief Service Obs, Hôpital du Sacre-Coeur de Montréal; Langs: Bilingual(French/English); (514)333-8105; Fax. (514)333-8150.

GAGNON, Sonny; Centre Cleophas-Claveau, 1000 rue du Docteur-Desgagne, La Baie QC G7B 2Y6; Laval'90; (418)544-3381 x355

GAGNON, Sonia; CSSS Les Eskers de l'Abitibi, 622 4e rue O, Amos QC J9T 2S2; Sher'92; CCFP; Ac Member, CH Hôtel-Dieu d'Amos; (819)732-3341; Fax. (819)732-4646.

GAGNON, Sophie; CSSSG-Hop de Hull, 116 boul Lionel-Emond, Gatineau QC J8Y 1W7; Mon'95; FRCPC; Neur. Staff, Hull Hospital; Langs: Spanish; English; (819)595-6000 x6244; Fax. (819)595-6213.

GAGNON, Sophie; CHUQ-Ctr Hosp Univ Laval, 2705 boul Laurier, Quebec QC G1L 3L5; Laval'95; CSPQ; FRCPC; Anes. Staff, Centre Hospitalier Universitaire de Quebec-CHUL; (418)656-4141

GAGNON, Sophie-Genevieve; CSSS de la Baie-des-Chaleurs, RR 2 419 boul Perron, Maria QC G0C 1Y0; Mon'98; Staff, CSSS de la Baie-des-Chaleurs; (418)759-3443

GAGNON, Steeve; CSSS Becancour-Nicolet-Yamaska, 216 rue Principale, Fortierville QC G0S 1J0; Laval'88; LMCC; (819)287-4442 x300; Fax. (819)287-4017; steeve_gagnon@ssss.gouv.qc.ca.

GAGNON, Stephan; CHUM-Hop Notre-Dame, 1560 rue Sherbrooke E, Montreal QC H2L 4M1; Mon'84; Neur (P.Q.). Staff, Centre Hospitalier l'Université de Montréal (CHUM) - Hôpital Notre-Dame; (514)890-8123; Fax. (514)412-7373.

GAGNON, Stephane; CHUS-Hop Hotel-Dieu, 580 rue Bowen S, Sherbrooke QC J1G 2E8; Sher'98; FRCPC; Psy. Staff, Centre Hospitalier Universitaire de Sherbrooke-Hôpital Hôtel-Dieu; (819)346-1110 x26535

GAGNON, Stephanie; Ctr Hosp Affilie-Enfant-Jesus, 1401 18e rue, Quebec QC G1J 1Z4; Laval'97; FRCPC; Psy. Staff, Centre Hospitalier Affilié Universitaire de Québec - Hôpital De L'Enfant Jésus; (418)649-5769

GAGNON, Suzanne; Polyclinique de la Sante, 102-1688 boul des Laurentides, Vimont QC H7M 2P4; Mon'72; LMCC; FAAD; CSPQ; FRCPC; Derm (Cosmetic & Laser Surgery). Langs: English; (450)668-4812; msgagnon@dermato.ca.

GAGNON, Suzanne; Ministere de la Sante, 7E-1075 ch Sainte-Foy, Quebec QC G1S 2M1; Laval'82; (418)266-7533

GAGNON, Suzanne; Dir de Sante Publique National, 2400 av D'Estimauville, Quebec QC G1E 7G9; Laval'77; CCFP; FCFP; Ac Staff, Centre Hospitalier Universitaire de Québec (CHUQ) - Siege Social; Prof Family Med, Université Laval; (418)666-7000 x286; Fax. (418)666-2776; suzanne.gagnon@ssss.gouv.qc.ca.

GAGNON, Sylvain; 200-394 rue Saint-Vallier, Chicoutimi QC G7H 4J1; Laval'73; FRCSC; ObstGyn. Chief ObstGyn, Complexe hospitalier de la Sagamie; (418)545-2666; Fax. (418)545-3924; femina@clinique-femina.com.

GAGNON, Sylvain; Hop du Sacre-Coeur de Mtl, 5400 boul Gouin O, Montreal QC H4J 1C5; McG'81; DABOS; CSPQ; FRCSC; OrthSurg (Hand Surgery). Staff, Hôpital du Sacre-Coeur de Montréal; Staff, Hôpital de Saint-Eustache; assoc Prof, Universite de Montreal; Langs: English; (514)661-2166; Fax. (514)661-2833; sgagnon@videotron.ca.

GAGNON, Sylvie; CSSS Pierre Boucher, 1333 boul Jacques-Cartier E, Longueuil QC J4M 2A5; Mon'88; Staff, Centre Hospitalier Pierre Boucher; (450)468-8111

GAGNON, Sylvie; CSSS de Rivière-de-Loup, 75 rue Saint-Henri, Riviere-Du-Loup QC G5R 2A4; Laval'85; CSPQ; AnatPath. Staff AnatPath, Centre Hospitalier Regional du Grand-Portage; Langs: English; (418)868-1010 x2474

GAGNON, Sylvie; CHUS-Hop Fleurimont, 3001 12e av N, Sherbrooke QC J1H 5N4; Sher'89; CSPQ; FRCPC; IntMed (Echocardiography); Cardiol (P.Q.). Staff, Centre Hospitalier Universitaire de Sherbrooke-Hopital Fleurimont; (819)346-1110 x14947; Fax. (819)820-6897; sylvie.gagnon@usherbrooke.ca.

GAGNON, Violaine; CSSS de Montmagny-l'Islet, RR 1 430 rue Jean-Leclerc, St-Jean-Port-Joli QC G0R 3G0; Laval'85; Staff, CSSS de Montmagny-l'Islet; (418)598-3355; Fax. (418)598-9794.

GAGNON, Yves; CSSS de Chicoutimi, 305 rue Saint-Vallier, Chicoutimi QC G7H 5H6; Laval'87; CSPQ; AnatPath. Staff, Complexe hospitalier de la Sagamie; (418)541-1000 x2288; Fax. (418)541-1143.

GAGNON, Yves; CSSS du Suroît, 150 rue Saint-Thomas, Salaber-de-Valleyf QC J6T 6C1; Laval'98; CCFP; Staff, Centre Hospitalier Régional du Suroît; (450)371-9920

GAGNON, Yves; CSSS de la Matapedia, 135 Gaetan-Archambeault, Amqui QC G5J 2K5; Laval'08; CCFP; CCFP(E.M.); Staff, CSSS de la Matapedia; (418)629-2211

GAGNON, Yves-David; Clinique Med du Boise Langevin, 130-288 rue Pierre-Saindon, Rimouski QC G5L 9A8; Laval'84; Staff, Hôpital Regional Rimouski; (418)724-4672; Fax. (418)724-4753.

GAGNON, Yvon-Rene; PO Box 250, Vermilion Bay ON P0V 2V0; Man'90; CCFP; FCFP; Langs: Bilingual(English/French); (807)227-2675

GAGNON-OUELLET, Caroline; Clin Med Frontenac, 24 rue Frontenac, Riviere-du-Loup QC G5R 1S5; Laval'06; CCFP; (418)862-0333; Fax. (418)863-0505.

GAGNON-PERREAULT, Annabelle; CSSS de Sept-Iles, 45 rue du Pere-Divet, Sept-Iles QC G4R 3N7; Laval'05; CCFP; Staff, Centre Hospitalier Regional de Sept-Iles; (418)962-9761

GAGNON-TROTTIER, Ariane; CSSS De Sept-Iles, 45 rue du Père-Divet, Sept-iles QC G4R 3N7; Laval'07; FamilyMed. Staff, Centre Hospitalier Regional de Sept-Iles; (418)962-9761

GAGOVSKI, Vlade M; 511-18 Wynford Dr, North York ON M3C 3S2; (Bulgaria)'84; Langs: Bulgarian; Macedonian; Russian; Serbian; (416)385-9900; Fax. (416)385-9907.

GAHIDE, Gerald; CHUS-Hop Fleurimont, 3001 12e av N, Sherbrooke QC J1H 5N4; (France)'04; DiagRad (P.Q.). Staff, Centre Hospitalier Universitaire de Sherbrooke-Hopital Fleurimont; (819)346-1110

GAI, Luis; Health Sciences Centre, 300 Prince Phillip Dr, St. John's NL A1B 3V6; Buenos Aires (Argentina)'86; FRCPC; AnatPath. Staff, Health Sciences Centre.

GAI, Tina D; West Lincoln Mem Hosp, 169 Main St E, Grimsby ON L3M 1P3; Bombay (India)'85; MRCOG; MB BS; FRCSC; ObstGyn. Staff, West Lincoln Memorial Hospital; Langs: Gujarati; Hindi; Marathi; (905)309-8723; Fax. (905)309-8724.

GAIARDO, Robert R; Guelph Emerg Med Services, 103-73 Delhi St, Guelph ON N1E 6L9; Tor'81; Staff, Guelph General Hospital; (519)837-1401

GAID, Magdi M A; Rouge Valley-Ajax & Pickering, 580 Harwood Ave S, Ajax ON L1S 2J4; Alexandria (Egypt)'75; MB ChB; FRCPC; Anes (Intensive Care). Chief Anes, Rouge Valley Health System - Ajax & Pickering Health Centre Site; Langs: Arabic; (905)683-2320 x1288; Fax. (905)683-8542.

GAID, Nahed; Rouge Valley-Ajax & Pickering, 580 Harwood Ave S, Ajax ON L1S 2J4; Alexandria (Egypt)'75; FRCPC; AnatPath. Dir Labs, Rouge Valley Health System - Ajax & Pickering Health Centre Site; (905)683-2320 x1412; Fax. (905)683-9329.

GAILEY, Carol B; Keary Med Centre, 110-245 Columbia St E, New Westminster BC V3L 3W4; McG'90; BSc; FRCPC; IntMed (Critical Care Medicine); Cardiol. Staff Cardiol, Royal Columbian Hospital; Langs: French; Spanish; (604)522-5727; Fax. (604)522-5578; c_gailey_med@hotmail.com.

GAILLARD, Felix; CSSS Les Eskers de l'Abitibi, 622 4e rue O, Amos QC J9T 2S2; Laval'92; CSPQ; FRCSC; GenSurg (Thoracic). Staff, CH Hôtel-Dieu d'Amos; Physician, Commission Sante Securite Travail; (819)732-3341; Fax. (819)732-0549.

GAILLARDETZ, Eveline; CSSS Hôpital De Verdun, 4000 boul Lasalle, LaSalle QC H4G 2A3; Laval'09; Staff, CSSS Hôpital De Verdun; (514)362-1000

GAILLOUX, Benoit; CSSS Hôpital De Verdun, 4000 boul Lasalle, LaSalle QC H4G 2A3; Mon'08; Staff, CSSS Hôpital De Verdun; (514)362-1000 x2141

GAILLOUX, Pierre; 460 2e av, Weedon QC J0B 3J0; Sher'75; Langs: Bilingual(English/French); (819)877-3434; piega@bellnet.ca.

GAILLOUX, Tom; GMF Centre medical AJC, 110 rue Saint-Jean, Drummondville QC J2B 7T1; Sher'03; CCFP; (819)477-1800

GAIN, Robert H; CBI Health Centre, 1F-4915 54 St, Red Deer AB T4N 2G7; Alb'75; Staff, Red Deer Regional Hospital Centre; (403)341-4983; Fax. (403)346-0498; robgain@hotmail.com.

GAIND, Gagan S; St Joseph's Healthcare, T10 157-50 Charlton Ave E, Hamilton ON L8N 4A6; McM'85; FRCPC; Psy (Inpatient Psychiatry). Ac Staff, St Joseph's Healthcare - Charlton Campus; Court Staff, Hamilton Health Sciences Centre - Hamilton General Hospital; Clin Prof, McMaster University; (905)522-1155 x34370

GAIND, Karandeep S; Univ Hlth Network-Princess M, 16 718-610 University Ave, Toronto ON M5G 2M9; Tor'92; FRCPC; Psy. Assoc Staff Psychosocial Oncol, Princess Margaret Hospital - University Health Network; Assoc Staff, Toronto General Hospital - UHN; Lecturer, University of Toronto; (416)946-4518; Fax. (416)946-2047.

GAINER, Anita L; Abbottsfield Shoppers Mall, 214-3210 118 Ave NW, Edmonton AB T5W 4W1; Alb'86; (780)471-2071

GAINER, C Jane; PO Box 1058, Hanna AB T0J 1P0; Dundee (Scotland)'75; MB ChB; (780)445-6543; jgainer@dthr.ab.ca.

GAIPTMAN, Jack H; Clinique Med Ville-Emard, 5824 boul Monk, Montreal QC H4E 3H3; Sher'76; (514)767-5307; Fax. (514)767-0214.

GAIR, Graeme A; Cottage Country Fam Hlth Team, 1-5 Pineridge Gate, Gravenhurst ON P1P 1Z3; Wes'70; Staff, South Muskoka Memorial Hospital - Muskoka Algonquin Healthcare; Med Examiner, Canadian Aviation; Staff, Northern Ontario School of Medicine; (705)687-2271; Fax. (705)687-7575.

GAISANO, Herbert Y; Univ Hlth Network-Toronto Western Hosp, 8MP 327-399 Bathurst St, Toronto ON M5T 2S8; (Philippines)'81; FACP(IntMed); FACP(Gastroent); FRCPC; IntMed; Gastroent. Staff, Toronto Western Hospital - University Health Network; Langs: Chinese; Tagalog; (416)603-5949; Fax. (416)603-6204; herbert.gaisano@utoronto.ca.

GAISBICHLER, Wolfgang H; Northern Lights Health Region, 7 Hospital St, Fort McMurray AB T9H 1P2; (Germany)'88; Staff, Northern Lights Regional Health Centre; (780)714-5622

GAISINSKY, Igor; Windsor Radiological Assoc, 1568 Ouellette Ave, Windsor ON N8X 1K7; Tor'97; FRCPC; DiagRad. (519)256-4914

GAJARDO, Paz A; Davenport Perth Community Hlth, 1900 Davenport Rd, Toronto ON M6N 1B7; McM'06; CCFP; Langs: Spanish; (416)658-6812; Fax. (416)658-4611.

GAJECKI, Peter; Lions Gate Hosp, 231 15th Ave E, North Vancouver BC V7L 2L7; Warsaw (Poland)'03; FRCPC; Anes. Staff, Lions Gate Hospital; (604)984-5720

GAJEWSKI, Jerzy; Urology Consultants, 620-5991 Spring Garden Rd, Halifax NS B3H 1Y6; Poznan (Poland)'73; Urol; FRCSC; Urol. Att Staff, Queen Elizabeth II Health Sciences Centre - Halifax Infirmary Site; Prof Urol, Dalhousie University; Langs: German; Polish; (902)425-3940; Fax. (902)422-0033; jgajew@dal.ca.

GAJEWSKI, Martin; 520 University Ave W, Waterloo ON N2T 2Z6; Wes'97; CCFP; FCFP; Langs: Polish; (519)743-3641; Fax. (519)743-1042.

GAJIC, Desanka; High Park Health Centre, 406-2333 Dundas St W, Toronto ON M6R 3A6; Tor'78; BSc; AB(Family Pract.); Langs: Croatian; Macedonian; Serbian; (416)534-1030; Fax. (416)534-1024.

GAKHAL, Natasha K; 604-790 Bay St, Toronto ON M5G 1N8; Wes'06; FRCPC; IntMed; Rheum. (416)323-0630

GALAN, Neville E; Grace Women's Health Centre, 4F-1441 29 St NW, Calgary AB T2N 4J8; (West Indies) (Jamaica)'77; FRCSC; ObstGyn. Staff, Foothills Medical Centre; Staff, Tom Baker Cancer Centre; (403)944-1438; Fax. (403)270-4249; neville.galan@calgaryhealthregion.ca.

GALANIS, Eleni; BC Centre for Disease Control, 655 12th Ave W, Vancouver BC V5Z 4R4; Sher'95; MPH; FRCPC; CommunMed. Langs: Greek; Spanish; Bilingual(French/English); (604)707-2558; Fax. (604)707-2516; eleni.galanis@bccdc.ca.

GALANOS, Christopher J; Lansdowne Professional Ctr Ii, 135-3066 Shelbourne St, Victoria BC V8R 6T9; Witwatersrand (South Africa)'86; MB ChB; (250)598-1889; Fax. (250)592-6386.

GALANTE, Samy; Baker Clinic, 220-10405 Jasper Ave NW, Edmonton AB T5J 1G5; (Zimbabwe)'79; MB ChB; FRCPC; Peds. Asst/Clin Prof Med, University of Alberta; (780)421-1990; Fax. (780)944-9599.

GALANTER, Elizabeth; 455 Trafalgar Rd, Oakville ON L6J 3H8; Gdansk (Poland)'80; FRCPC; Peds. Staff, Toronto General Hospital - UHN; Staff, The Hospital For Sick Children; Staff, Mount Sinai Hospital; Langs: German; Polish; Russian; (905)338-9594; Fax. (905)338-8611.

GALARNEAU, France; UMF Shawinigan, 80 rue 118e, Shawinigan-Sud QC G9P 3E4; Laval'84; LMCC; Staff Family Med UMF Shawinigan, Centre Hospitalier du Centre la Mauricie; Langs: Bilingual(French/English); (819)536-7511; Fax. (819)537-3489.

GALARNEAU, Lise-Andree; CSSS de Trois-Rivières, 1991 boul du Carmel, Trois-Rivieres QC G8Z 3R9; Laval'90; Microbio & Infect Dis (P.Q.); MedMicrobiol. Staff, CSSS de Trois-Rivières; (819)697-3333

GALARNEAU, Louise; Tribunal Admin du Quebec, 21e-500 boul Rene-Levesque O, Montreal QC H2Z 1W7; Sher'71; MD(TropMed); CommunMed (P.Q.) (Environmental Health). Med Consultant, Direction de la Sante Publique; Langs: Bilingual(English/French); (514)873-7154; lgalarneau.agence05@ssss.gouv.qc.ca.

GALARNEAU, Pierre; 991 ch des Iles, Entrelacs QC J0T 2E0; Mon'66; CSPQ; FRCSC; GenSurg (Administration). Ac Staff, Centre Hospitalier Honore-Mercier; Langs: Bilingual(French/English); (450)228-2660

GALARNEAU, Sophie; CLSC des Faubourgs, 2260 rue Parthenais, Montreal QC H2K 3T5; Sher'91; CCFP; (514)527-2361; Fax. (514)527-6016; sophie_galarneau@ssss.gouv.qc.ca.

GALARNEAU, Yolaine; Agence SSS GIM, 144 boul de Gaspe, Gaspe QC G4X 1A9; Mon'79; Staff, CSSS de la Baie-des-Chaleurs; (418)368-2349; yolaine.galarneau@msss.gouv.qc.ca.

GALARNEAU-GIRARDIN, Justine; CLSC de Paspebiac, CP 7000 273 boul Gerard-D-Levesque, Paspebiac QC G0C 2K0; Sher'10; CCFP; Staff, CLSC de Paspebiac; (418)752-2572

GALARRAGA, Willy; KW Sleep Laboratory, 290-180 King St S, Waterloo ON N2J 1P8; Los Andes (Venezuela)'78; FRCPC; Psy. (519)745-2621; Fax. (519)745-7174.

GALBAUD DU FORT, Guillaume; MUHC-Montreal Gen Hosp, B6 253-1650 av Cedar, Montreal QC H3G 1A4; (France)'87; Psy (P.Q.). Staff, McGill University Health Centre - Montreal General Campus; (514)934-8010; Fax. (514)934-8237.

GALBRAITH, Beverley D; The U of Toronto-Mississauga, 3359 Mississauga Rd, Mississauga ON L5L 1C6; Man'77; (905)828-5255; Fax. (905)828-3852.

GALBRAITH, Donald A; 9698 Tobias Lane, Lambton Shores ON N0N 1J2; Wes'61; FRCPC; Psy (Forensic Psychiatry). Member, Ontario Review Board; Member, Ontario Consent and Capacity Board; (519)786-6095; dgalbrai@xcelco.on.ca.

GALBRAITH, Jack W; Chatham-Kent Family Health Team, 109-20 Emma St, Chatham ON N7L 5K5; Wes'84; Staff, Chatham-Kent Health Alliance; (519)355-0382; Fax. (519)355-1567; jgalbraith@ckha.on.ca.

GALBRAITH, John C T; Royal Jubilee Hosp, DT 1215-1952 Bay St, Victoria BC V8R 1J8; Alb'83; ABIM; FRCPC; IntMed; InfectDis; MedMicrobiol. Staff, Royal Jubilee Hospital; Staff, Victoria General Hospital; Asst Clin Prof, University of British Columbia; (250)370-8755; Fax. (250)519-1628.

GALBRAITH, L Dawn; Mill Bay Med Centre, 230-2720 Mill Bay Rd RR 1, Mill Bay BC V0R 2P1; Cal'84; CCFP; FCFP; (250)743-3211; Fax. (250)743-2800.

GALBRAITH, Lorri J; 178-11215 Jasper Ave NW, Edmonton AB T5K 0L5; UBC'87; Dir, Healthcare Services, Workplace Health Safety & Compensation Comm.; (780)498-4313

GALBRAITH, Paul F; Abbotsford Reg Hosp & Cancer C, 32900 Marshall Rd, Abbotsford BC V2S 0C2; Man'87; FRCPC; IntMed; Hem. Staff, Providence Health Care - St Paul's Hospital; Staff Med Oncol, Abbotsford Regional Hospital & Cancer Centre; (604)851-4710

GALBRAITH, Robert M; Bigelow-Fowler Clinic, 1605 9 Ave S, Lethbridge AB T1J 1W2; Midwestern University (USA)'06; Dip Ortho; CCFP; (403)327-3121; Fax. (403)327-3905.

GALBRAITH, Roger; Alberta Children's Hosp, 2888 Shaganappi Trail NW, Calgary AB T3B 6A8; McG'89; FRCPC; Peds. Staff Emerg Dept, Alberta Children's Hospital; Med Dir, Health Link Alberta; Clin Assoc Prof Peds, University of Calgary; (403)935-7070; roger.galbraith@calgaryhealthregion.ca.

GALE, George D; Rothbart Centre for Pain Care, 9-4646 Dufferin St, North York ON M3H 5S4; Durham (England)'58; MB BS; FRCA; FAADEP(EP); DAAPM; FRCPC; Anes (Pain Management). (416)512-6407; Fax. (416)512-6375; drgdgale@rothbart.com.

GALE, Jeffrey S; Hotel-Dieu Hosp, 225B-166 Brock St, Kingston ON K7L 5G2; Ott'98; FRCSC; Ophth. Staff, Hotel-Dieu Hospital; (613)544-3310 x3391; Fax. (613)544-3641.

GALE, Mark C; Alberta Children's Hosp, 2888 Shaganappi Trail NW, Calgary AB T3B 6A8; UBC'00; FRCPC; Anes;CCFP; Staff, Alberta Children's Hospital; (403)955-7810

GALE-ROWE, Margaret; Public Hlth Agency of Canada, 2375-100 Eglantine Dr, Ottawa ON K1A 0K9; Ott'87; (613)946-5706; Fax. (613)941-9813.

GALEA, Anthony M; I S M Health & Wellness Cente, 230 Browns Line, Etobicoke ON M8W 3T4; McM'86; MD; BSc; Teach Staff, University of Toronto; Langs: Maltese; (416)620-6861; Fax. (416)620-9774; anthonygalea@mac.com.

GALEMA, Chris J; 307-1950 Algonquin Ave, North Bay ON P1B 4Z2; Qns'92; (705)840-5351

GALESSIERE, Paul F; Steinbach Family Med Centre, 10-333 Loewen Blvd, Steinbach MB R5G 0C3; Tor'87; FRCSC; GenSurg. General Surgery, Bethesda Hospital Steinbach; (204)326-3401; Fax. (204)326-3899; pgalessiere@sehealth.mb.ca.

GALGAY, Susan M; Western Memorial Reg Hosp, PO Box 2005 Stn Main 1 Brookfield Ave, Corner Brook NL A2H 6J7; Mem'06; FRCPC; Anes. Staff, Western Memorial Regional Hospital; (709)637-5000

GALIC, John I; Montreal Retina Institute, 2F-4120 rue Sainte-Catherine O, Westmount QC H3Z 1P4; Qns'97; FRCSC; Ophth. (514)285-8838

GALIK, Marika Y; Valley Care Med, E-310 8th St, Courtenay BC V9N 1N3; Mem'05; CCFP; (250)331-0500

GALIMOVA, Lena; Rehabilitation Centre, RR 135-800 Sherbrook St, Winnipeg MB R3A 1M4; Russia (Ukraine)'83; FRCPC; PhysMed&Rehab (Musculoskeletal). Dir of the Traumatic Brain Injury Rehabilitation Unit/Att Physician, Riverview Health Centre; Asst Prof, University of Manitoba; Langs: Russian; Ukrainian; (204)787-2206; Fax. (204)787-1476.

GALINSKI, Saramin E; Brant Community HC-Brantford, 200 Terrace Hill St, Brantford ON N3R 1G9; McM'99; FRCPC; Anes. Staff, The Brant Community Healthcare System - Brantford General Hospital Site; (519)752-5508

GALIPEAU, Anne V; U of Ottawa Health Services, 302-1 Nicholas St, Ottawa ON K1N 7B7; Tor'91; FCPA; BSc(Hon); CRCP; DCPsy; Psy (Adult Psychiatry & Psychotherapy). Chief Psy, University of Ottawa; (613)564-3950 x225; Fax. (613)564-6627; agalipea@uohs.uottawa.ca.

GALIPEAU, Daniel; Clinique Med Brien, 102-223 boul Brien, Repentigny QC J6A 6M4; Mon'81; (450)585-9810

GALIPEAU, Jean-Luc; 2-867 boul Saint-René O, Gatineau QC J8T 7X6; Guadalajara (Mexico)'82; Ac Staff, Hôpital de Gatineau; (819)243-3221; Fax. (819)243-9684.

GALIPEAU, Jocelyn F; Lakeshore Med Centre, 156 Lakeshore Dr, North Bay ON P1A 2A8; Ott'80; Langs: French; (705)476-7802; Fax. (705)476-3185; jfgalipeau@lakeshoremedicalcentre.com.

GALIPEAU, Louise; Clin De Med Fam Cowansville, 499 rue du Sud, Cowansville QC J2K 2X9; Sher'88; Staff Obst, Hôpital Brome-Missisquoi-Perkins; Langs: English; (450)263-8890

GALIPEAU, M Lynne; York Medical, 3-17215 Leslie St, Newmarket ON L3Y 8E4; Tor'91; Staff Family Pract, Southlake Regional Health Centre; Langs: English; French; (905)853-7107; Fax. (905)853-3702.

GALIWANGO, Joseph; Pediatric Associates, 200-630 Tecumseh Rd E, Windsor ON N8X 4W2; Bristol (England)'72; FAAP; FRCPC; Peds (Consultant Pediatrics). Staff, Windsor Regional Hospital - Metropolitan Site; (519)254-8667; Fax. (519)254-4616.

GALIWANGO, Paul J; Corcare Inc, 410-325 Milner Ave, Scarborough ON M1B 5N1; Tor'01; Cardiol; IntMed. (416)284-4744; Fax. (416)284-0141.

GALL, Brent D; Eagle Ridge Hosp & Health C C, 475 Guildfprd Way, New Westminster BC V3H 3W9; UBC'08; CCFP; Staff, Eagle Ridge Hospital & Health Care Centre; (604)461-2022

GALL, James M; 6038 Empress St, Windsor ON N8T 1B5; Wes'73; CCFP; FCFP; Asst Clin Prof, University of Western Ontario; (519)974-7100 x2229; Fax. (519)974-7672.

GALL, Perry; Northern Med Unit, T162-770 Bannatyne Ave, Winnipeg MB R3E 0W3; Man'87; CCFP; FCFP; (204)789-3711

GALL, Richard M; Sterling Lyon Health Centre, 201-1020 Lorimer Blvd, Winnipeg MB R3P 1C7; Man'94; BSc(Med); FRCSC; Otol (Rhinology). Staff, Health Sciences Centre; Staff, St Boniface General Hospital; Staff, Victoria General Hospital; University of Manitoba; (204)943-0629

GALLAB, Nagy F A E; 1D-570 King St, Welland ON L3B 3L2; Cairo (Egypt)'84; FRCPC; IntMed. Langs: Arabic; (905)735-9672; Fax. (905)735-5597.

GALLACCIO, Alicia A; Caroline Family Hlth Team-CMG, 15-3305 Harvester Rd, Burlington ON L7N 3N2; McM'05; BSc; CCFP; (905)632-8007; Fax. (905)681-6341.

GALLACHER, William; Queen Elizabeth II HSC-Halifax, 1796 Summer St, Halifax NS B3H 2Y9; Glasgow (Scotland)'73; MB ChB; FRCPC; Anes (Intensive Care). Staff, Queen Elizabeth II Health Sciences Centre - Halifax Infirmary Site; (902)473-3606; Fax. (902)473-3610.

GALLAGHER, Clare N; Foothills Med Centre, 1403 29 St NW, Calgary AB T2N 2T9; Alb'00; PhD; FRCSC; Neursurg. Staff, Foothills Medical Centre; (403)944-2230; Fax. (403)283-2270.

GALLAGHER, Finbar P G; James Paton Mem Hosp, 125 Trans-Canada Hwy, Gander NL A1V 1P7; National (Ireland)'82; MB ChB; BAO; MMedSci(Path); FRCPC; AnatPath. Staff, James Paton Memorial Hospital.

GALLAGHER, Genevieve; Ctr Hosp Affilie-Enfant-Jesus, 1401 18e rue, Quebec QC G1J 1Z4; Laval'99; FRCPC; IntMed (Stem Cell Transplantation); Hem. Staff, Centre Hospitalier Affilié Universitaire de Québec - Hôpital De L'Enfant Jésus; Langs: Bilingual(French/English); (418)649-0252

GALLAGHER, Julie A; Couchiching Family Health Team, 103-119 Memorial Ave, Orillia ON L3V 5X1; Tor'92; CCFP; Assoc Staff, Orillia Soldiers' Memorial Hospital; (705)326-3549; Fax. (705)326-9529.

GALLAGHER, Karen; CLSC La Region-Sherbrookoise, 1200 rue King E, Sherbrooke QC J1G 1E4; Mon'91; (819)780-2222; Fax. (819)563-5521.

GALLAGHER, Katherine L; St Boniface Gen Hosp, M 4-409 Tache Ave, Winnipeg MB R2H 2A6; Sask'82; FRCPC; Psy. Staff, St Boniface General Hospital; (204)233-8563

GALLAGHER, Kathleen M; Bedford Waterfront Hlth Clin, 207-967 Bedford Hwy, Bedford NS B4A 1A9; Dal'89; BSc; (902)835-6444; Fax. (902)832-1193.

GALLAGHER, Lawrence P; Cowichan Dist Hosp, 3045 Gibbins Rd, Duncan BC V9L 1E5; UBC'78; BSc; CCFP; CCFP(E.M.); FCFP; Ac Staff, Cowichan District Hospital; Clinical Asst Prof, University of British Columbia; (250)746-4141; millmed@shaw.ca.

GALLAGHER, Michael C J; Niagara H System-G Niagara, PO Box 1018 Stn Main 5546 Portage Rd, Niagara Falls ON L2E 6X2; Liverpool (England)'83; MB ChB; DA(UK); FRCPC; Anes. Staff Anes, Niagara Health System - Greater Niagara General Site; (905)358-0171; Fax. (905)732-6111.

GALLAGHER, Patrick F; Fenelon Falls Med Centre, PO Box 849 205 Francis St E, Fenelon Falls ON K0M 1N0; Tor'82; CAFCI; Ac Staff, Ross Memorial Hospital; (705)887-1310; Fax. (705)887-1326.

GALLAGHER, Pierre; CHUQ-Ctr Hosp Univ Laval, 2705 boul Laurier, Quebec QC G1V 4G2; Laval'71; CSPQ; Cardiol (P.Q.) (Clinical Research). Staff, Centre Hospitalier Universitaire de Quebec-CHUL; (418)654-4141; Fax. (418)691-5717.

GALLAGHER, Romayne; St Paul's Hosp, 1081 Burrard St, Vancouver BC V6Z 1Y6; UBC'84; CCFP; Staff/Head Residential Care Family & Comm Med, Providence Health Care - St Paul's Hospital; Clin Prof Family Pract, University of British Columbia; (604)682-2344 x63734; rgallagher@providencehealth.bc.ca.

GALLANT, Catherine A; The Ottawa Hosp-Gen Campus, 501 Smyth Rd, Ottawa ON K1H 8L6; Mem'90; FRCPC; Anes (Obstetrics Anesthesia). Staff Anes, The Ottawa Hospital - General Campus; Asst Prof, University of Ottawa; (613)737-8187; Fax. (613)737-8189; catherinegallant@rogers.com.

GALLANT, Christopher J; Dartmouth Med Centre, 301-46 Portland St, Dartmouth NS B2Y 1H4; Dal'81; MSc; FRCPC; Derm. Consultant, Dartmouth General Hospital; Consultant Derm, Queen Elizabeth II Health Sciences Centre - Victoria General Site; Assoc Prof Med, Dalhousie University; (902)465-8720; Fax. (902)465-8712.

GALLANT, Christopher R; Moncton Med Clinic, 302-860 Mountain Rd, Moncton NB E1C 2N7; Mem'09; BSc; MHSA; CCFP; Ac Staff, Horizon Health Network; (506)853-5155; Fax. (506)853-5123.

GALLANT, Denise L; 48-650 Champlain St, Dieppe NB E1A 1P5; Laval'89; CCFP; Langs: English; French; (506)204-3313; Fax. (506)204-8340.

GALLANT, Joanne; New Brunswick College of FM, 614 rue Dysart, Dieppe NB E1A 4T9; (506)852-1086; Fax. (506)855-7134; jg@cfpc.ca.

GALLANT, Lee Ann; Gallent Med Clinic, 302-2797 Bathurst St, North York ON M6B 4B9; Tel Aviv (Israel)'81; FRCPC; Peds (Alternative Medicine). Assoc Staff, The Hospital For Sick Children; Court Staff, Women's College Hospital; Lecturer, University of Toronto; Langs: Hebrew; Italian; (416)789-4376; Fax. (416)789-5321.

GALLANT, Marc; Centre Med Acton, CP 550 967 rue Boulay, Acton Vale QC J0H 1A0; Sher'84; (450)546-3245; Fax. (450)546-4720.

GALLANT, Marco; 581 rue Heriot, Drummondville QC J2B 1B8; Laval'92; IntMed (P.Q.). Staff, Hôpital Sainte-croix; (819)478-6464; Fax. (819)472-3105.

GALLANT, Marie-Josee; Ctr D'Hebergement Maison, 134 rue Jean-Rene-Monette, Gatineau QC J8P 7C3; Sher'95; (819)966-6450; Fax. (819)966-6453.

GALLANT, Michel; 200-343 Preston Street, Ottawa ON K1S 1N4; Sher'00; FRCP; FRCSC; PlasSurg (Aesthetic Medicine). Langs: French; (613)729-1616 x3; Fax. (613)567-0148.

GALLANT, Paula M; Valley Prof Centre, 70 Exhibition St, Kentville NS B4N 4K9; Dal'86; BScPharm; FRCSC; GenSurg (Breasts). Staff GenSurg, Valley Regional Hospital; (902)679-2323; Fax. (902)678-1080.

GALLANT, Stephen E; 256-2155 Leanne Blvd, Mississauga ON L5K 2K8; Wes'96; FRCPC; Psy. (905)823-8156

GALLANT, Steven J; 133 Church St, Antigonish NS B2G 2E3; Dal'89; CCFP; Staff, St Martha's Regional Hospital; Teach Staff, Dalhousie University; (902)863-4497; Fax. (902)863-2207; sgallant@ns.sympatico.ca.

GALLANT, Tania M; West Main Plaza, 108C-1600 Main St, Moncton NB E1E 1G5; Dal'03; FRCPC; IntMed; Endocrin&Metab. (506)857-5758; Fax. (506)857-5086; dr.tania.gallant@horizonnb.ca.

GALLANT, Tsvi; North York Health Centre, 207-1262 Don Mills Rd, North York ON M3B 2W7; (Israel)'81; Staff, Humber River Regional Hospital - Finch Avenue Site; Langs: Hebrew; Italian; (416)741-7412; Fax. (416)741-9131.

GALLARDO, Rodolfo C; Lakeshore Med & Prof Bldg, 306-3170 Lake Shore Blvd W, Etobicoke ON M8V 3X8; Santo Tomas (Philippines)'72; BSc; Langs: Ilican; Tagalog; (416)252-6451; Fax. (416)252-1783.

GALLAY, Henry M; Sheppard Associates, 649 Sheppard Ave W, North York ON M3H 2S4; McG'65; FRCPC; Psy (Adult & Geriatric Psychiatry). Ac Staff, North York General Hospital; Ac Staff, North York General Hospital - Branson Division; Langs: Yiddish; (416)630-0610; Fax. (416)398-5712.

GALLAY, Stephen H; Ajax Med Arts Bldg, 200-601 Harwood Ave S, Ajax ON L1S 2J5; McG'89; FRCSC; OrthSurg (Reconstructive Surgery). Staff, Rouge Valley Health System - Ajax & Pickering Health Centre Site; Langs: Portuguese; French; (905)426-3098; Fax. (905)426-6667.

GALLER, Pamela H; PO Box 1003, Yellowknife NT X1A 2N7; Ott'09; CCFP; (250)808-0338

GALLER, Shelly; 1105-180 Bloor St W, Toronto ON M5S 2V6; McG'79; FRCPC; Psy. Langs: Hebrew; French; Fax. (416)297-6031.

GALLEY, Anik; CSSS du Nord de Lanaudière, 1000 boul Sainte-Anne, St-Charles-Brromee QC J6E 6J2; Sher'03; Staff, Centre Hospitalier Régional de Lanaudière; Langs: English; (450)759-8222

GALLEY, Daniel J; Cornwall Comm Hosp-McConnell, PO Box 100 Stn Main 840 McConnell Ave, Cornwall ON K6H 5S5; McG'88; FRCPC; DiagRad. Staff, Cornwall Community Hospital; Langs: Bilingual(English/French); (613)938-4240 x2274; Fax. (613)938-4066.

GALLEY, Peter W; Lakeside Med Clinic, 203-227 Lake St, Pembroke ON K8A 5M2; McG'81; BSc; Langs: English; French; (613)735-2597; Fax. (613)735-5158.

GALLICK, David; Dr Everett Chalmers Reg Hosp, PO Box 9000 Stn A 700 Priestman St, Fredericton NB E3B 5N5; Staff, Dr Everett Chalmers Regional Hospital; (506)452-5400

GALLIE, Brenda L; The Hosp For Sick Children, 555 University Ave, Toronto ON M5G 1X8; Qns'69; MD; FRCSC; Ophth (Medical Genetics). Staff, Toronto Western Hospital - University Health Network; Ac Staff, The Hospital For Sick Children; Sr Scientist Research Institute, Princess Margaret Hospital - University Health Network; Researcher Research Institute, Ontario Cancer Institute; Teacher Med Genetics & Biophysics, University of Toronto; (416)946-2324; Fax. (416)946-4619.

GALLIEN, Annelise; The Moncton Hosp, 135 MacBeath Ave, Moncton NB E1C 6Z8; Dal'07; FRCPC; IntMed. Staff, The Moncton Hospital; (506)857-5111

GALLIEN, Roger; Orthopedie Pediatrique, 297-2600 boul Laurier, Quebec QC G1V 4T3; Laval'65; LMCC; CSPQ; FRCSC; OrthSurg (Pediatric Orthopedics). Staff Ped, Centre Hospitalier Universitaire de Quebec-CHUL; Clin Prof Surg, Université Laval; (418)623-1864; Fax. (418)623-8926.

GALLIFORD, Brian W; Victoria Med Bldg, 315-1669 Victoria St, Prince George BC V2L 2L5; UBC'64; FRCSC; ObstGyn. (250)562-3151; Fax. (250)562-1660.

GALLIMORE, Christopher H; Toronto East Gen Hosp Inc, 825 Coxwell Ave, Toronto ON M4C 3E7; Tor'00; FRCSC; OrthSurg. Staff, Toronto East General Hospital Inc; (416)330-0825

GALLIMORE, Ian C G; Davisville Med & Dental Centre, 210-1849 Yonge St, Toronto ON M4S 1Y2; Tor'70; Court Staff, St Michael's Hospital; (416)964-7621; Fax. (416)964-2564.

GALLINARO, Brian J; St Thomas-Elgin Gen Hosp, PO Box 2007 Stn Main 189 Elm St, St Thomas ON N5P 3W2; Wes'96; CCFP; FCFP; Staff, St Thomas Elgin General Hospital; (519)631-2030

GALLINGER, Steven; Univ Hlth Network-Toronto Gen, 10EN 206-200 Elizabeth St, Toronto ON M5G 2C4; Tor'81; MSc; FRCSC; GenSurg (Hepatobiliary Surgical Oncology). Staff, Toronto General Hospital - UHN; Staff, Princess Margaret Hospital - University Health Network; Prof Institute of Med Sciences, University of Toronto; (416)340-4412; Fax. (416)340-3808; steven.gallinger@uhn.ca.

GALLINS, Colin; Victoria Hosp, PO Box 3000 Stn Main 1200 24th St W, Prince Albert SK S6V 5T4; CCFP; Staff, Victoria Hospital; (306)765-6200; Fax. (306)765-6224.

GALLINS, Kelly; PO Box 52007 Rpo Beacon Ave, Sidney BC V8L 5V9; UBC'02; CCFP; CCFP(E.M.); Staff, Stanton Territorial Health Authority; (250)656-4904

GALLINS, Shannon; PO Box 52007 Rpo Beacon Ave, Sidney BC V8L 5V9; UBC'05; CCFP; CCFP(E.M.).

GALLIVAN, Glenn G; Antigonish Mall, 133 Church St, Antigonish NS B2G 2E3; Dal'90; (902)863-2455; Fax. (902)867-6336.

GALLIVAN, Michael P J; Glace Bay Healthcare Complex, PO Box 131 Stn Main, Glace Bay NS B1A 5V2; Dublin (Ireland)'78; MB BS; DObst; MB BCh; BAO; (902)849-0300; Fax. (902)849-1409; mgallivan@ns.sympatico.ca.

GALLIVER, Robert; Brantford Med Centre, 40 Shellington Place, Brantford ON N3S 0C5; Cardiff (Wales)'67; MB ChB; AB; MRCS(Eng); LRCP(Lond); (519)753-9581; Fax. (519)753-9547.

GALLO, Richard; Institut de Cardiologie de Mtl, 5000 rue Belanger, Montreal QC H1T 1C8; Laval'87; CSPQ; FRCPC; IntMed; Cardiol. Staff, Institut de Cardiologie de Montréal; assoc Prof Med, Universite de Montreal; (514)376-3330 x3616; Fax. (514)376-1076.

GALLOW, Mark D; Lasalle Community Health Care, 2125 Front Rd, Windsor ON N9J 2C1; Caribbean (Montserrat)'95.

GALLOWAY, Emma; Lions Gate Hosp, 3F-231 15th St E, North Vancouver BC V7L 2L7; UBC'10; CCFP; Staff, Lions Gate Hospital; (604)985-6408

GALLOWAY, Lyle D; Foothills Med Centre, 47-1403 29 St NW, Calgary AB T2N 2T9; Alb'92; CCFP; Staff, Foothills Medical Centre; (403)944-2304; Fax. (403)270-9652; lgallowa@telusplanet.net.

GALLOWAY, Meriel A; The Rainbow Med Group, 202-5511 West Boulevard, Vancouver BC V6M 3W6; UBC'91; CCFP; (604)266-3453; Fax. (604)266-3276.

GALLOWAY, Victoria A; Waterview Med & Chiro Centre, 464 Locust St, Burlington ON L7S 1V1; Tor'02; BSc; MSc; CCFP; Ac Staff, Joseph Brant Memorial Hospital; (289)245-1071

GALPERIN, Ilana; Groupe Sante Medisys, 1100-500 rue Sherbrooke O, Montreal QC H3A 3C6; McG'03; CCFP; (514)499-2777; Fax. (514)845-4842.

GALT, Elaine L; Lions Gate Maternity Clinic, 302-231 13th St E, North Vancouver BC V7L 2L7; UBC'92; BSc; Staff Privil, Lions Gate Hospital; (604)985-6408

GALTER, Meri K; 11-398 Steeles Ave W, Thornhill ON L4J 6X3; Yerevan (Armenia (Republic))'93; DABIM; (905)881-0334; Fax. (905)881-1721; merimd70@yahoo.com.

GALVIN, Imelda M; Kingston Gen Hosp, 76 Stuart St, Kingston ON K7L 2V7; (Ireland)'92; Staff, Kingston General Hospital; (613)533-2952

GALVIN, Patti A; Wellington Ortho & Rehab, 3-86 Dawson Rd, Guelph ON N1H 1A8; McM'89; Dip SportMed(Hon); ABIME; DABPMR; CASM; FRCPC; PhysMed&Rehab (Sports Medicine). (519)837-2020 x1; Fax. (519)763-9871.

GALWA, Ram; Dr Everett Chalmers Reg Hosp, PO Box 9000 Stn A 700 Priestman St, Fredericton NB E3B 5N5; (India)'02; Staff, Dr Everett Chalmers Regional Hospital; (506)474-4548

GALWAY, A Brenda; Health Sciences Centre, 300 Prince Philip Dr, St. John's NL A1B 3V6; Mem'81; FRCPC; IntMed (Endocrinology); Endocrin&Metab. Staff, Health Sciences Centre; Assoc Prof Med, Memorial University Of Newfoundland; (709)777-7069

GALWAY, Carol S; Highland Family Practice, 107C-1966 Guthrie Rd, Comox BC V9M 3X7; UBC'95; BSc; CCFP; Ac Staff, St Joseph's General Hospital; (250)890-0919; Fax. (250)890-0929.

GAMACHE, Andre; CHUM-Hop Notre-Dame, 2E-1560 rue Sherbrooke E, Montreal QC H2L 4M1; Laval'81; CSPQ; Psy (P.Q.). Staff, Centre Hospitalier l'Université de Montréal (CHUM) - Hôpital Notre-Dame; (514)890-8000

GAMACHE, Claire; CSSS de Laval, 1755 boul Rene-Laennec, Laval QC H7M 3L9; Mon'92; FRCPC; Psy. Staff, Hopital de la Cite de la santé; (450)668-1010 x23707; Fax. (450)662-9124.

GAMACHE, Germain; 185A rue Grande-Allee E CP 187, Grande-Riviere QC G0C 1V0; Laval'74; Staff, Centre Hospitalier de Chandler; (418)385-2626; Fax. (418)385-4527.

GAMACHE, Ghislaine; Ctr Hosp Anna-Laberge, 200 boul Brisebois, Chateauguay QC J6K 4W8; Mon'81; FRCPC; IntMed (Cardiology). Staff, Hôpital Anna-Laberge; (450)699-2425

GAMACHE, Jean; Clinique Maisonneuve-Rosemont, 60-5345 boul de l'Assomption, Montreal QC H1T 4B3; Mon'80; (514)257-7000

GAMACHE, Louis; CLSC de Chertsey, 485 rue Dupuis, Chertsey QC J0K 3K0; Laval'70; Langs: English; (450)882-2488; Fax. (450)882-3072; louis.gamache@ssss.gouv.qc.ca.

GAMACHE, Nathalie; Clinique Med du Plateau, 106-195 rue de l'Atmosphere, Gatineau QC J9A 0A3; Man'99; FRCSC; ObstGyn. Staff, The Ottawa Hospital - Riverside Campus; Langs: French; (819)770-4664; Fax. (819)770-8108; ngamache@ottawahospital.on.ca.

GAMACHE, Stephan; CLSC et CHSLD Pommeraie, 660 rue Saint-Paul, Farnham QC J2N 3B9; Laval'90; (450)293-3622; Fax. (450)293-3974.

GAMACHE, Suzanne; Clinique Med St-Vallier, 201-205 rue Montmagny, Quebec QC G1N 4V3; Laval'77; Staff, CSSS de Quebec-Sud; (418)688-0872

GAMACHE, Sylvie; Clinique de Ped de Rimouski, 301-161 av Rouleau, Rimouski QC G5L 5T3; Mon'83; FRCPC; Peds. Staff, Hôpital Regional Rimouski; Langs: English; (418)724-4221; Fax. (418)725-3025.

GAMBAROTTA, Nicola; Quinte HC Corp-Belleville Gen, 265 Dundas St E, Belleville ON K8N 5A9; Ott'06; FRCPC; DiagRad. Staff, Quinte Healthcare Pharmacy-Belleville General; (613)969-7400; Fax. (800)483-2811.

GAMBAROTTO, Kathryn R; 12-1300 Garth St, Hamilton ON L9C 4L7; McM'95; FRCPC; Peds. (905)575-0611; Fax. (905)575-7737.

GAMBETTI, Andrea; St Paul's Hosp, 1081 Burrard St, Vancouver BC V6Z 1Y6; Qns'91; FRCPC; Psy. Staff, Providence Health Care - St Paul's Hospital; (604)682-2344

GAMBHIR, Indu B; 300-24 Selkirk Ave, Ottawa ON K1L 0A4; Punjab (India)'69; Langs: Hindi; Punjabi; (613)740-0999; Fax. (613)740-0991.

GAMBHIR, Puneeta; Brampton Urgent Care Centre, 8-51 Mountain Ash Rd, Hamilton ON L8R 1W4; (India)'00; CCFP; Langs: Hindi; Punjabi; (905)799-2722; Fax. (905)709-6727.

GAMBLE, Brian; Thamesview Family Health Team, 465 Grand Ave W, Chatham ON N7L 1C5; Wes'67; CCFP; FCFP; Staff, Chatham-Kent Health Alliance; (519)354-5540; Fax. (519)354-6120.

GAMBLE, Carmen; Royal Univ Hosp, 103 Hospital Dr, Saskatoon SK S7N 0W8; Sask'02; FRCPC; Peds. Staff, Royal University Hospital; (306)655-6900; Fax. (306)655-2897.

GAMBLE, D Gregory; 206-1205 Amber Dr, Thunder Bay ON P7B 6M4; McG'93; FRCPC; IntMed; InfectDis. Staff, Thunder Bay Regional Health Sciences Centre; (807)622-3848; Fax. (807)622-4268.

GAMBLE, Eamon N; Hogans Bldg, 457 London Rd, Sarnia ON N7T 4W9; Cork (Ireland)'73; DCH; Ac Staff, Bluewater Health - Norman Site; Ac Staff, Bluewater Health - Mitton Site; (519)337-0606; Fax. (519)337-4567.

GAMBLE, Jonathan; Royal University Hosp, 103 Hospital Dr, Saskatoon SK S7N 0W8; Sask'02; Critical Care Medicine; Anes. Staff, Royal University Hospital; (306)655-1183; Fax. (306)655-1279.

GAMBLE, Kenneth; International Med Services, 4000 Leslie St, North York ON M2K 2R9; Sask'77; Ac Staff, North York General Hospital; Missionary Health Institute; (416)494-7512; Fax. (416)492-3740.

GAMBLE, Mardelle H; Foothills Med Centre, 1403 29 St NW, Calgary AB T2N 2T9; Alb'95; FRCPC; CCFP; EmergMed. Staff Emerg Med, Foothills Medical Centre; Staff, Peter Lougheed Centre; (403)944-1596; Fax. (403)944-2419.

GAMBLE, Patrick; Gamble James Med Prof Inc, 304-679 Davis Dr, Newmarket ON L3Y 5G8; McM'02; BSc; FRCSC; OrthSurg (Hip & Knee Replacement). Staff, Southlake Regional Health Centre; Aj Clinical Asst Prof, McMaster University; (905)895-4445; Fax. (905)895-8596.

GAMBREL, Jason; Brockville Gen Hosp, 75 Charles St, Brockville ON K6V 1S8; Man'02; FRCSC; OrthSurg (Sports Medicine). Staff, Brockville General Hospital - Charles Street; (613)345-8341; Fax. (613)345-8353.

GAMBU, Helene; CSSS de Chicoutimi, 305 rue Saint-Vallier, Chicoutimi QC G7H 5H6; Sher'98; CCFP; CCFP(E.M.); Staff, Complexe hospitalier de la Sagamie; (418)541-1000

GAME, Kathleen E; Rocky Med Clinic, PO Box 99 Stn Main 5127 49 St, Rocky-Mtn-House AB T4T 1A1; UBC'90; CCFP; (403)845-2815; Fax. (403)845-2177.

GAME, Melaku M; Hys Med Centre, 302-11010 101 St NW, Edmonton AB T5H 4B9; Leipzig (Germany)'91; Staff, Royal Alexandra Hospital; (780)496-1390; Fax. (780)496-1387.

GAMELIN, Adrian; Royal University Hosp, 4544-103 Hospital Dr, Saskatoon SK S7N 0W8; Sask'01; FRCSC; ObstGyn (Reproductive Endocrinology & Infertility). Staff, Royal University Hospital; (306)966-1953; Fax. (306)966-8040.

GAMELIN, Sylvain D; Clinique Med de Nicolet, 1691 boul Louis-Frechette, Nicolet QC J3T 1Z6; Sher'86; Staff, Hôpital de Christ-Roi; (819)293-2022; Fax. (819)293-2024.

GAMER, Meghan; Royal Univ Hosp, 103 Hospital Dr, Saskatoon SK S7N 0W8; Sask'08; Peds. Staff, Royal University Hospital; (306)966-2922; Fax. (306)966-8640.

GAMMAL, Amir S; Health Sciences Centre, 300 Prince Philip Dr, St. John's NL A1B 3V6; Alb'01; FRCPC; Anes. Staff, Health Sciences Centre; (709)777-6300

GAMMAL, Nadia T; Quinte HC Corp-Bellville Gen, 265 Dundas St E, Belleville ON K8N 5A9; Wes'96; FRCPC; DiagRad. Staff, QHC Belleville General; (613)969-5511; Fax. (613)969-5561.

GAMMELL, Lisa; 208-45 Weatherbee Rd, Sydney NS B1M 0A1; Dal'03; CCFP; Staff, Cape Breton Healthcare Complex; (902)539-8566

GAMMON, Braden; St Joseph's Health Care, PO Box 5777 Stn B D209-268 Grosvenor St, London ON N6A 4V2; Tor'06; FRSCS; OrthSurg. Staff, St Joseph's Hospital - St Joseph's Health Care; (519)646-6100

GAMMON, Jessica; Children's Aid Society, 1680 Oxford St E, London ON N5Y 5R8; Tor'06; FRCPC; Peds. Staff, Kingston General Hospital; (519)455-9000

GAMMON, Kristy L; Haliburton Family Med Centre, PO Box 870 7217 Gelert Rd, Haliburton ON K0M 1S0; Wes'87; CCFP; FCFP; Ac Staff, Haliburton Highlands Health Services - Haliburton Site; (705)457-1212; Fax. (705)457-3955.

GAMRA, Tarek A R; 205-505 Queen St, Spruce Grove AB T7X 2V2; (Libya)'98; MB BCh; (780)962-2001; Fax. (780)905-2191.

GAMULKA, Beth D; Scarborough Hosp-General Div, 3050 Lawrence Ave E, Scarborough ON M1P 2V5; McG'93; FRCPC; Peds. Staff, The Scarborough Hospital - General Campus; Staff Peds, The Hospital For Sick Children; Asst Prof Peds, University of Toronto; Langs: Hebrew; (416)431-8200 x6671; gamulka@rogers.com.

GAN, Bing Siang; St Joseph's Health Care, PO Box 5777 Stn B D0 215-268 Grosvenor St, London ON N6A 4V2; Rotterdam (Netherlands)'88; MD; PhD; FACS; FRCSC; PlasSurg (Hand & Reconstructive Microvascular Surgery). Staff Plastic Surg, St Joseph's Hospital - St Joseph's Health Care; Prof Surg, University of Western Ontario; Langs: Dutch; German; (519)646-6097; Fax. (519)646-6049.

GAN, S W Helen; 370-5740 Cambie St, Vancouver BC V5Z 3A6; Alb'98; CCFP; Langs: Cantonese; Mandarin; (604)322-6658; Fax. (604)321-8771.

GAN-GAISANO, Margaret C; The Court Clinic, 315-2863 Ellesmere Rd, Scarborough ON M1E 5E9; (Philippines)'81; FAAP(Peds&PedEndocrin); FRCPC; Peds (Clinical Nutrition). Staff, Rouge Valley Health System - Centenary Health Centre Site; Langs: Tagalog; Mandarin; Fookien; (416)724-8290; Fax. (416)724-1985.

GANAME, Javier; St Joseph's Healthcare, F506 2-50 Charlton Ave, Hamilton ON L8N 4A6; (Argentina)'95; Staff, St Joseph's Healthcare - Charlton Campus; Staff, McMaster University; (905)522-1155; Fax. (905)521-6068.

GANAPATHY, Anusoumya; Guelph Gen Hosp, 115 Delhi St, Guelph ON N1E 4J4; (India)'03; Staff, Guelph General Hospital; (519)837-6440; anusoumya.ganapathy@gghorg.ca.

GANAPATHY, Gobi R; London Medical-Dental Bldg, 308-450 Central Ave, London ON N6B 2E8; Sambalpur (India)'66; MB BS; FRCPC; Neur (Epilepsy). Langs: Hindi; Tamil; (519)642-1911; Fax. (519)642-3487.

GANAPATHY, Sugantha; London HSC-University Hosp, PO Box 5339 Stn B 339 Windermere Rd, London ON N6A 5A5; Madras (India)'71; FRC(Eng); FFARCS(Ire); FRCPC; Anes (Regional Anesthesia). Staff, London Health Sciences Centre - University Hospital; Staff, St Joseph's Hospital - St Joseph's Health Care; Langs: Tamil; (519)685-8500 x35115

GANDELL, Dov; Sunnybrook Hlth Sciences Ctr, HG 69-2075 Bayview Ave, Toronto ON M4N 3M5; McG'02; FRCPC; IntMed; GeriatricMed. Staff, Sunnybrook Health Sciences Centre; (416)480-4076

GANDER, Sarah L G; 160-600 Main St, Saint John NB E2K 1J5; Mem'04; FRCPC; Peds. Staff, Saint John Regional Hospital; Asst Prof, Dalhousie University; Asst Prof, Memorial University Of Newfoundland; (506)648-6554; Fax. (506)648-7620.

GANDHAM, Prem; Rosthern Med Clinic, PO Box 1089, Rosthern SK S0K 3R0; BSc; Physician Emerg Med, Rosthern Hospital; Langs: Punjabi; English; (306)232-4894; Fax. (306)232-4970; pgandham@sasktel.net.

GANDHAM, Satnam S; Dr S Gandham Inc, 135-8291 Ackroyd Rd, Richmond BC V6X 3K5; UBC'83; Langs: Punjabi; Hindi; (604)270-3121; Fax. (604)270-3931.

GANDHI, Amita; Gandhi Med Clinic, 101-6935 120 St, Delta BC V4E 2A8; Rohtak (India)'80; MB BS; FRCPC; Psy (Adult Psychiatry). Langs: Punjabi; Hindi; (604)599-4373; Fax. (604)599-4374.

GANDHI, Harjeet S; Hamilton HSC-McMaster Site, PO Box 2000 Stn Lcd 1200 Main St W, Hamilton ON L8N 3Z5; Punjab (India)'79; FRCSC; OrthSurg. Staff, Hamilton Health Sciences Centre - McMaster Children's Hospital; (905)521-2100

GANDHI, Jasmine; Children's Hosp Eastern Ontari, 4F-401 Smyth Rd, Ottawa ON K1H 8L1; Man'99; FRCPC; Psy. Staff, Children's Hospital of Eastern Ontario (CHEO); (613)722-7000

GANDHI, Karamchand J; Gandhi Med Practice Inc, PO Box 189 Stn Main 172 Jubilee Rd, Bridgewater NS B4V 2W8; Bombay (India)'59; MB BS; DA(Eng.); DObstRCOG; FFARCSI; Ac Staff Fam Med, South Shore Regional Hospital; Langs: Hindi; Gujarati; Marathi; (902)543-5314; Fax. (902)543-4002.

GANDHI, M Suhail; Stayner Med Centre, PO Box 220, Stayner ON L0M 1S0; Tor'90; Staff, Collingwood General & Marine Hospital; (705)428-3246

GANDHI, Rajiv; Univ Hlth Network-Toronto Western Hosp, EW1 439-399 Bathurst St, Toronto ON M5T 2S8; McM'01; FRCSC; OrthSurg. Staff, Toronto Western Hospital - University Health Network; (416)603-5642; Fax. (416)603-3437.

GANDHI, Sanjiv; Children's & Women's HC of BC, AB307-4480 Oak St, Vancouver BC V6H 3V4; McG'93; FRCSC; GenSurg; CardSurg. Staff, BC Children's Hospital; (604)875-3165

GANDHI, Shital; Mount Sinai Hosp, 431-600 University Ave, Toronto ON M5G 1X5; McG'95; MPH; FRCPC; IntMed (Obstetric Medicine). Staff, Mount Sinai Hospital; Asst Prof, University of Toronto; Langs: Bilingual(English/French); (416)586-4857; Fax. (416)586-5377; sgandhi@mtsinai.on.ca.

GANDHI, Shruti; Westend Ctr Assisted Reproduct, 201-101 Westmore Dr, Etobicoke ON M9V 3Y6; (India)'75; MB BS; FRCPC; MedBiochem (Infertility). Staff Family Med, William Osler Health System - Etobicoke General Hospital; Consultant Satellite IVF & Create IVF Program, Westend Centre for Assisted Reproduction; Langs: Hindi; Punjabi; Urdu; (416)748-2800; Fax. (416)748-8865.

GANDHI, Sonal; Sunnybrook Hlth Sciences Ctre, TW 2F-2075 Bayview Ave, Toronto ON M4N 3M5; Qns'05; BSc; MSc; FRCPC; IntMed; MedOncol. Staff Med Oncol, Sunnybrook Health Sciences Centre; Langs: Hindi; (416)480-4617; Fax. (416)480-6002.

GANDHI, Vinod K; Gandhi Med Clinic, 101-6935 120 St, Delta BC V4E 2A8; Punjab (India)'75; MB BS; CCFP; FCFP; Langs: Punjabi; Hindi; (604)599-4373; Fax. (604)599-4374; vinodagandhi@hotmail.com.

GANDILO, Sargon B; Nepean Imaging Centre, 1 Centrepointe Dr, Nepean ON K2G 6E2; Baghdad (Iraq)'68; MD; BAP; FRCPC; DiagRad (Diagnostic Ultrasound). Langs: Assyrian; Arabic; (613)723-6924; Fax. (613)723-5216.

GANDY, Alan C; Summerside Med Centre, 1-475 Granville St, Summerside PE C1N 3N9; McM'88; PhD; MSc; BPHE; FRCPC; Peds. Consultant Peds, Prince County Hospital; (902)432-8124

GANDY, Hazen M; Children's Hosp Eastern Ont, 401 Smyth Rd, Ottawa ON K1H 8L1; Mem'86; FRCPC; Psy. Staff, Children's Hospital of Eastern Ontario (CHEO); Div Chief, Hospital Based Psychiatry; Med Dir, Mental Health Patient Service Unit; Asst Prof, University of Ottawa; (613)737-2703; Fax. (613)738-4202; gandy@cheo.on.ca.

GANESAN, Arun; Kliniek on Main, 351 Main St N, Moose Jaw SK S6H 0W2; (306)694-1440; Fax. (306)693-9990.

GANESAN, Ramakrishnan; Cedar Springs Prof Centre, G-960 Cumberland Ave, Burlington ON L7N 3J6; McM'91; FRCPC; Neur. Staff, Joseph Brant Memorial Hospital; Physician, Cedar Springs Professional Centre; (905)639-8566; Fax. (905)639-7966; rganesan@cogeco.ca.

GANESAN, Soma; Vancouver Health Centre, 715 12th Ave W, Vancouver BC V5Z 1M9; Saigon (Vietnam)'75; FRCP; FRCPC; Psy (Emergency Psychiatry). Med Dir Psy, Vancouver General Hospital - Centennial Pavillion; Med Dir Psy UBC Hosp-Detwiller Pavilion, UBC Hospital - Koerner Pavillion; Commissioner/Med Dir VCH Mental Health/Exec Member Forensic Serv Comm, Ministry of Health-British Columbia; Med Dir, Vancouver Community Mental Health Services; Clin Prof Psy/Dir Cross Cultural Program, University of British Columbia; Langs: French; Vietnamese; (604)875-4023; Fax. (604)875-4987; soma.ganesan@vch.ca.

GANESHRAM, Tharini; Appletree Med Group, 15-1 Rossland Rd, Ajax ON L1Z 1Z2; (India)'90; MB BS; CCFP; (647)722-2370; Fax. (647)426-3196.

GANGAM, Nirupama; Fontbonne Bldg, 2F-301 James St S, Hamilton ON L8P 3B6; Qns'02; BSc; FRCSC; ObstGyn., St Joseph's Healthcare - Charlton Campus; Asst Prof, McMaster University; (905)521-6041; Fax. (905)521-6089.

GANGANI, Asmitha; Magna Hlth Centre, 375 Magna Dr, Aurora ON L4G 7L6; (Kazakhstan)'03; CCFP; Langs: Hindi; Gujarati; Tamil; Russian; (905)726-7470; Fax. (905)726-7471.

GANGBAR, Eric W; York Medical Bldg, 208-250 Harding Blvd W, Richmond Hill ON L4C 9M7; McM'87; MA; FAHA; FRCPC; FRCPC; Cardiol; IntMed (Cardiac Catheterization). Staff, Mackenzie Richmond Hill Hospital; Court Staff, Southlake Regional Health Centre; Teacher, University of Toronto; Langs: Yiddish; French; (905)737-6641; Fax. (905)737-8285; egangbar@rogers.com.

GANGBAR, Randy A; 8-421 Eglinton Ave W, Toronto ON M5N 1A4; Tor'79; FRCPC; Psy. Staff, Centre for Addiction & Mental Health (CAMH) - Queen Site; Staff, Centre for Addiction & Mental Health (CAMH) - College Street Site; Consultant Psy, Jewish Family & Child Service; Asst Prof, University of Toronto; (416)544-9884

GANGDEV, Prakash S; 232 Oxford St W, London ON N6H 1S7; Bombay (India)'84; Langs: Gujarati; Hindi; Marathi; (519)933-3067; Fax. (519)672-6886.

GANGJI, Alnoor; Medical Arts Centre, 314-770 6 St SW, Medicine Hat AB T1A 8M7; Russia (Russia (Federation))'81; FAAP; Staff, Medicine Hat Regional Hospital; Physician Georgia(USA), Rockdale Conyer; (403)527-2281; Fax. (403)502-8934.

GANGJI, Azim; St Joseph's Healthcare, 450-50 Charlton Ave E, Hamilton ON L8N 4A6; McM'99; FRCPC; IntMed (Transplant Nephrology); Nephrol. Staff, St Joseph's Healthcare - Charlton Campus; (905)522-1155 x33261; Fax. (905)308-7222.

GANGODAWILA, Shantha; Upper River Valley Hosp, 11300 130 Rte, Waterville NB E7P 0A4; CCFP; Staff, Upper River Valley Hospital - Waterville; (506)375-5900

GANGOLLI, Vinod K; Grand River Hosp-KW Hlth Ctre, PO Box 9056 Stn C 835 King St W, Kitchener ON N2G 1G3; Karnatak (India)'71; MB BS; MRCPsy; FRCPC; Psy (Psycho Geriatrics). Staff, Grand River Hospital - Kitchener/Waterloo Health Centre; Langs: Hindi; Marathi; (519)749-4300; Fax. (519)749-4261.

GANGULI, Rohan; 500-901 King St W, Toronto ON M5V 3H5; (India)'73; FRCPC; Psy. Staff, Centre for Addiction & Mental Health (CAMH) - Queen Site; Langs: Hindi; (416)535-8501; Fax. (416)583-3485.

GANGULI, Satyajit N; William Osler HC-Brampton, 2100 Bovaird Dr E, Brampton ON L6R 3J7; Tor'94; FRCPC; DiagRad (Nuclear Cardiology); NuclearMed. Locum Tenens, Headwaters Health Care Centre - Orangeville Site; Staff, William Osler Health System - Brampton Civic Hospital; Lecturer Diagnostic Imaging, University of Toronto; Langs: Italian; French; Bengali; (905)494-2120

GANGULI, Subhas C; St Joseph's Healthcare, 50 Charlton Ave E, Hamilton ON L8N 4A6; Sask'90; MSc; ABIM; FRCPC; IntMed (Functional Bowel Disorder); Gastroent. Staff Gastroent, Hamilton Health Sciences Centre - McMaster Children's Hospital; Staff, St Joseph's Healthcare - Charlton Campus; Asst Prof Gastroent, McMaster University; (905)522-1155 x35109; Fax. (905)521-6064.

GANJAVI, Hooman; London HSC-Victoria Hosp, PO Box 5010 Stn B ZB E8 122-800 Commissioners Rd, London ON N6A 5W9; Tor'06; FRCPC; Psy. Staff, London Health Sciences Centre - Victoria Campus.

GANJIZADEH ZAVAREH, Farahnaz; Synergy Wellness Centre, 221-501 Bethel Dr, Sherwood Park AB T8H 0N2; (Iran)'90; (780)464-0123; Fax. (780)449-5609.

GANNAGE, Christopher; Southlake Reg Health Centre, 596 Davis Dr, Newmarket ON L3Y 2P9; McM'88; CCFP; CCFP(E.M.); FCFP; Staff, Southlake Regional Health Centre; (905)895-4521 x7032; Fax. (905)853-2251.

GANNAGE, John M; GF-300 Main St N, Markham ON L3P 1Y8; Tor'90; CCFP; (905)294-2335 x2335; Fax. (905)294-6498.

GANNON, Anne B; Huronia Med Centre, PO Box 790 Stn Main 103-1070 Hugel Ave, Midland ON L4R 4P4; Galway (Ireland)'89; MB ChB; MRCGPract; CCFP; (705)526-8482; Fax. (705)526-8789; aga@cablelan.net.

GANNON, Brian; Queensway-Carleton Hosp, 3045 Baseline Rd, Nepean ON K2H 8P4; Ott'02; FRCPC; AnatPath. Staff, Queensway Carleton Hospital; (613)721-2000

GANNON, Celine M; Salvus Family Med Clinic, 62-143 Liberton Dr, St. Albert AB T8N 6A7; Alb'03; CCFP; (780)460-4562

GANNON, Kathleen; 440 Central Ave, London ON N6B 2E5; Dublin (Ireland)'07; CCFP; (519)601-7577; Fax. (519)601-7737.

GANNON, William; London Road Diagnostic Clinic, 481 London Rd, Sarnia ON N7T 4X3; Dublin (Ireland)'69; Med Dir, Vision Nursing Home; Med Dir, Sumac Lodge Nursing Home; (519)344-8849; Fax. (519)344-8840.

GANS, Maja G; 505-18 Wynford Dr, North York ON M3C 3S2; Tor'91; BSc; FRCSC; ObstGyn. Staff, Toronto East General Hospital Inc; (416)385-3431; Fax. (416)385-1945.

GANS, Mark S; MUHC-Montreal Gen Hosp, L4 211-1650 av Cedar, Montreal QC H3G 1A4; McG'81; AB; FRCSC; Ophth (Medical & Surgical Ophthalmology). Staff, Sir Mortimer B Davis Jewish General; Staff, McGill University Health Centre - Montreal General Campus; assoc Prof, McGill University; Langs: English; French; (514)934-1934 x44081; Fax. (514)934-8223.

GANS, Marvin H; North Toronto Med Bldg, 314-250 Lawrence Ave W, Toronto ON M5M 1B2; Tor'63; FRCPC; Peds. Staff, The Hospital For Sick Children; Assoc Prof, University of Toronto; (416)783-5411; Fax. (416)783-0080.

GANSHORN, Keren D; Regina Community Clinic, 1106 Winnipeg St, Regina SK S4R 1J6; Sask'89; CCFP; FCFP; Staff Family Med, Regina General Hospital; Asst Prof Family Med, University of Saskatchewan; (306)543-7880; Fax. (306)543-6888.

GANT, Peter T; Foothills Medical Centre, C231-1403 29 St NW, Calgary AB T2N 2T9; Cal'79; FRCPC; EmergMed. Staff, Foothills Medical Centre; (403)478-6157

GANTOUS, Andres; St Joseph's Health Centre, 230-30 The Queensway, Toronto ON M6R 1B5; Guadalajara (Mexico)'84; FRCS; FAAFPRS; ABFPS; FRCSC; Otol (Facial Plastic Surgery). Staff, St Joseph's Health Centre; Staff, St Michael's Hospital; Staff Surg, Toronto Facial Plastic Surgery; Teach Staff Otol, University of Toronto; Langs: Italian; Spanish; French; (416)530-6659; Fax. (416)530-6742; drgantous@torontofacialplastic.com.

GANUGAPATI, Usharani; St Paul's Hosp, 1702 20th St W, Saskatoon SK S7M 0Z9; Andhra (India)'80; FRCPC; AnatPath. Staff, St Paul's Hospital (Grey Nuns) of Saskatoon; (306)655-5162

GANZ, Gregory M F; Medical Bldg, 203-1990 Fort St, Victoria BC V8R 6V4; McG'91; FRCPC; IntMed; Nephrol. (250)370-5257; Fax. (250)592-1599.

GAO, Dongsheng; Queen Elizabeth II HSC-Halifax, 2501-1796 Summe St, Halifax NS B3H 3A7; (Chile)'94; Staff, Queen Elizabeth II Health Sciences Centre - Halifax Infirmary Site; (902)473-4272

GAO, Zu-Hua; Duff Med Bldg, B6-3775 rue Universite, Montreal QC H3A 2B4; Peking (China)'92; MSc; PhD; FRCPC; AnatPath (Gastroenterology Pathology). Chef Pathology, McGill University; Langs: Mandarin; (514)398-5599

GAOUETTE, Christian; CSSS de Memphremagog, 50 rue Saint-Patrice E, Magog QC J1X 3X3; Laval'99; CCFP; Staff, Centre Hospitalier et CLSC de Memphremagog; (819)843-3381

GAPSKI, John A P; 505-3025 Hurontario St, Mississauga ON L5A 2H1; Ott'74; FRCPC; IntMed (Medical Oncology). Staff Consultant, Trillium Health Centre - Mississauga; Langs: Polish; (905)270-3842; Fax. (905)270-3843.

GARACH, Anil; 101-130 Mitton St N, Sarnia ON N7T 6G6; Bombay (India)'83; FRCSC; OrthSurg. Langs: Gujarati; Hindi; (519)332-3330

GARADY, Cherif Issa; Royal Alexandra Hosp, DTC 5002-10240 Kingsway NW, Edmonton AB T5H 3V9; Khartoum (Sudan)'95; FRCPC; AnatPath. Staff, Royal Alexandra Hospital; (780)735-5281

GARAND, Lise J; Clinique Ophth Lebourgneuf, 200-777 boul Lebourgneuf, Quebec QC G2J 1C3; Laval'73; Ophth. ac Membre, Centre Hospitalier Affilié Universitaire de Québec - Hôpital du St-Sacrement; (418)628-1417; Fax. (418)623-4517.

GARAND, M T Linda; Edifice Pierre Lemoyne d'Iberv, 193-6560 rue Hochelaga, Montreal QC H1N 1X9; Mon'83; CCFP; Physician, National Defence Montreal Detachment Services Group; (514)252-2777 x4682

GARAND, Marie-Josee; Clinique Notre-Dame, 147 rue Notre-Dame E, Victoriaville QC G6P 3Z8; CCFP; (819)758-3664; Fax. (819)758-0745.

GARAND, Mark; Polyclinique de Trois-Rivieres, 305-1900 boul des Recollets, Trois-Rivieres QC G8Z 4K4; Mon'88; CSPQ; FRCPC; IntMed; Cardiol. Staff, CSSS de Trois-Rivières; (819)375-4313; Fax. (819)378-7897.

GARANT, Dominique; CSSS Les Eskers de l'Abitibi, 622 4e rue O, Amos QC J9T 2S2; Mon'98; Staff, CH Hôtel-Dieu d'Amos; (819)732-3341

GARANT, Dorothee; CSSS de Memphremagog, 50 rue Saint-Patrice E, Magog QC J1X 3X3; Sher'99; Staff, Centre Hospitalier et CLSC de Memphremagog; (819)843-3381

GARANT, Jacques; 337 av Victoria, Saint-Lambert QC J4P 2H7; Laval'68; CSPQ; FRCPC; Psy (Medico Legal Issues). Consultant, Standard Life; Langs: English; (450)465-1993; jacques@standardlife.ca.

GARANT, Jean-Philippe; Centre Medical de Cowanville, 101-370 rue de la Riviere, Cowansville QC J2K 1N3; Sher'06; Staff, Centre Maria-Chapdelaine - CH de Dolbeau-Mistassini; (450)263-0774

GARANT, Marie-Claude; Clinique Med Mirabel, CP 1059 Succ St-Janvier 200-13714 boul du Cure-Labelle, Mirabel QC J7J 2K8; Mon'85; (450)435-7666; Fax. (450)435-1716.

GARANT, Philippe; CHUQ-Hotel-Dieu de Quebec, 11 Cote du Palais, Quebec QC G1R 2J6; Laval'95; Staff, Centre Hospitalier Universitaire de Québec (CHUQ) - Siege Social; (418)691-5042; Fax. (418)691-5024.

GARAVAGLIA, Marco M; St Michael's Hosp, 1 026 SW-30 Bond St, Toronto ON M5B 1W8; (Italy)'00; Staff, St Michael's Hospital; (416)864-5032

GARAY, Michael E; Queen Square Doctors FHT, 201-366 Main St N, Brampton ON L6V 1P8; Wes'98; CCFP; CCFP(E.M.); FCFP; Staff, William Osler Health System - Brampton Civic Hospital; (905)455-1455; Fax. (905)455-5498.

GARBA, Sule; Steinbach Family Med Centre, 10-333 Loewen Blvd, Steinbach MB R5G 0C3; Ahmadu Bello (Nigeria)'78; FRCSC; GenSurg. General Surgery, Bethesda Hospital Steinbach; (204)326-3401; Fax. (204)326-3899; sgarba@sehealth.mb.ca.

GARBE, George J; Regina Cardiology Assoc, 701-2125 11th Ave, Regina SK S4P 3X3; Sask'69; ABIM; FRCPC; IntMed (Interventional Cardiology); Cardiol. Ac Staff, Regina General Hospital; Clin Prof Med Cardiol, University of Saskatchewan; Langs: English; French; (306)781-7944; Fax. (306)781-6997.

GARBEDIAN, Shawn; Mount Sinai Hosp, 600 University Ave, Toronto ON M5G 1X5; Ott'05; FRCSC; OrthSurg. Staff, Mount Sinai Hospital; (416)586-4200

GARBER, Bryan; Canadian Forces Supp Unit HCC, 210-1745 Alta Vista Dr, Ottawa ON K1A 0K6; Mem'86; FRCSC; GenSurg; Critical Care Medicine. Staff, Canadian Forces Health Services Centre (Atlantic); Langs: Bilingual(English/French); (613)949-6339

GARBER, Cheryl; Lakeshore Gen Hosp, 160 av Stillview, Pointe-Claire QC H9R 2Y2; Ott'87; Staff, Lakeshore General Hospital - Pointe Claire; (514)630-2225; Fax. (514)630-2080.

GARBER, Gary E; Public Health Ontario, 1406-751 Parkdale Ave, Ottawa ON K1J 1J7; Cal'80; FACP; FRCPC; IntMed (Infection Control); InfectDis. Staff, The Ottawa Hospital-Research Institute; Prof Med & Cross-appt, University of Ottawa; Langs: French; (613)737-8173; ggarber@ottawahospital.on.ca.

GARBER, Gayle D; Kelligrews Med Clinic, PO Box 17160 Stn Main, Conception Bay S NL A1X 3H1; Dal'79; BSc; BA; MLS; (709)834-2171; Fax. (709)834-1241; gayle_garber@yahoo.ca.

GARBER, Lesley Z; Health Sciences Centre, GB421-820 Sherbrook St, Winnipeg MB R3A 1R9; Man'85; FRCSC; Otol (Neuro Otolaryngology). Staff, Health Sciences Centre; Asst Prof Orol/Prog Dir Residency, University of Manitoba; (204)787-3349; Fax. (204)787-1727.

GARBER, Peter N; 202-4700 Jane St, North York ON M3N 2L3; McG'80; CCFP; (416)661-0004; Fax. (416)661-0810.

GARBER, Philip J; St Boniface Gen Hosp, Y3027-409 Tache Ave, Winnipeg MB R2H 2A6; Man'87; ABIM; FRCPC; IntMed; Cardiol. Staff Med, Health Sciences Centre; Staff, Victoria General Hospital; Staff Bergen Cardiac Centre, St Boniface General Hospital; Asst Prof, University of Manitoba; (204)258-1275; Fax. (204)233-2157.

GARBER, Stanley I; Campbell River & Dist Gen Hosp, 375 2nd Ave, Campbell River BC V9W 3V1; McG'74; FRCPC; DiagRad. Ac Staff DiagImaging, Campbell River & District General Hospital; (250)286-7044; Fax. (250)286-7081.

GARBER, Susan E; 226-1982 Kensington Rd NW, Calgary AB T2N 3R5; Cal'87; CCFP; (403)283-3370

GARBETT, Sally E; Dawson Creek & Dist Hosp, 11100 13 St, Dawson Creek BC V1G 3W8; London (England)'81; MB BS; MRCPsy; MMedSci; FRCPC; Psy. Staff, Dawson Creek & District Hospital; (250)782-8501; sally.garbett@northernhealth.ca.

GARBHARRAN, Hari N; 10C-50 Bur Oak Ave, Markham ON L6C 0A2; Natal (South Africa)'79; MB ChB; FFPsy(SA); MMed(Psy); DPM; FRCPC; Psy. Langs: Hindi; (416)823-4078

GARBOLL, G Michael; Waterloo Sports Med Centre, 4-65 University Ave E, Waterloo ON N2J 2V9; Tor'74; Ad Staff Privil, Grand River Hospital - Kitchener/Waterloo Health Centre; Ad Staff Privil, St Mary's General Hospital; (519)886-2241; Fax. (519)886-3260.

GARBUTT, Allan S; PO Box 370, Bellevue AB T0K 0C0; Wes'91; PhD; MSc; CCFP; FCFP; Staff, Crowsnest Pass Health Centre; Clin Lecturer Family Med, University of Calgary; (403)562-8804; Fax. (403)562-2905; allan@crowsnestpass.com.

GARBUZ, Donald S; Orthopaedic Reconstruction Cli, 3F-2775 Laurel St, Vancouver BC V5Z 1M9; McG'86; FRCSC; OrthSurg. (604)875-5767 x2

GARCEA, Cristina; Royal Alexandra Hosp, 10240 Kingsway NW, Edmonton AB T5H 3V9; Alb'08; CCFP; CCFP(E.M.); Staff, Royal Alexandra Hospital; (780)735-4111

GARCEAU, Audrey; CSSS de Trois-Rivières, 1991 boul du Carmel, Trois-Rivieres QC G8Z 3R9; Sher'06; Staff, CSSS de Trois-Rivières; (819)697-3333

GARCEAU, Claude; Hôpital Laval, 2725 ch Sainte-Foy, Quebec QC G1V 4G5; Laval'80; FRCPC; IntMed (Diabetes). Staff, Hôpital Laval; Langs: Bilingual(English/French); (418)656-4511; claudegarceau@videotron.ca.

GARCEAU, Daniel; Hôpital Laval, 2725 ch Sainte-Foy, Quebec QC G1V 4G5; Laval'83; FRCPC; IntMed (Hypertension); Nephrol. Staff Internist, Hôpital Laval; Clin Teach Staff, Université Laval; (418)656-8711; Fax. (418)656-4587.

GARCEAU, Nicole; Ctr Hosp Anna-Laberge, 200 boul Brisebois, Chateauguay QC J6K 4W8; McG'85; FRCPC; IntMed. Staff, Hôpital Anna-Laberge; (450)699-2425; Fax. (450)699-2525.

GARCEAU, Patrick; Institut de Cardiologie de Mtl, 5000 rue Belanger, Montreal QC H1T 1C8; Laval'01; FRCPC; IntMed (Echocardiography); Cardiol. Staff, Institut de Cardiologie de Montréal; Langs: Spanish; English; (514)376-3330; Fax. (514)293-2557.

GARCEAU, Richard; Dr Georges-L Dumont Reg Hosp, 330 av Universite, Moncton NB E1C 2Z3; Laval'85; FRCPC; MedMicrobiol (AIDS/HIV); Microbio & Infect Dis (P.Q.). Staff Med Microbiol, Dr Georges-L-Dumont University Hospital Centre; Associé Clin Prof, Universite de Sherbrooke; Langs: English; (506)862-4140; Fax. (506)862-4827.

GARCEAU, Sylvie; 324 boul Notre-Dame-des-Champs, Repentigny QC J6A 3B6; Sher'87; Derm. (450)654-9124

GARCES, Luis M; Upper Thornhill Med Clinic, 112-955 Major Mackenzie Dr, Vaughan ON L6A 4P9; Tor'97; BSc; MBA; CCFP; FCFP; (905)417-8880; Fax. (905)417-5803.

GARCES, Patricio B; 4002 Sheppard Ave E, Scarborough ON M1S 4R5; Cal'90; FRCPC; DiagRad. Staff Radiol, Timmins & District Hospital; Langs: Tagalog; (416)299-9895

GARCIA, Andrea; 79 Dundas St W, Mississauga ON L5B 1H7; (Uruguay)'05; CCFP; Langs: Spanish; (905)275-1309

GARCIA, Bertha; London HSC-University Hosp, PO Box 5339 Stn B 339 Windermere Rd, London ON N6A 5A5; (Peru)'72; ABACPath; FACPath; LMCC; FRCP; FRCPC; AnatPath. Chief Path/Chair, London Health Sciences Centre - University Hospital; Vice Dean Education, Schulich School of Medicine & Dentistry; Vice Dean Education/Prof, University of Western Ontario; Langs: Italian; Spanish; (519)663-2954; Fax. (519)663-2930; bertha.garcia@lhsc.on.ca.

GARCIA, Carla S; London HSC-University Hosp, PO Box 5339 Stn B A10 220-339 Windermer Rd, London ON N6A 5A5; Wes'00; FRCPC; Psy. Staff, London Health Sciences Centre - University Hospital; (519)685-8500 x75136

GARCIA, Cesar P; Dixon Med Centre, 202-531 Davis Dr, Newmarket ON L3Y 6P5; Santo Tomas (Philippines)'84; MB BS; FRCPC; Psy (Geriatric Psychiatry). Staff Psy, Southlake Regional Health Centre; Consultant Geriatric Psy, Arbor Living Centre Nursing Homes; Physician, Park Place Manor Retirement Residence; Physician, Aurora Rest Haven; Physician, Versa Care Centre; Langs: Tagalog; (905)895-5199; Fax. (905)895-4033; cgarcia@extendicare.com.

GARCIA, Elio D; CSSSG-Hop de Gatineau, CP 2000 Succ Bureau-Chef 909 boul de la Verendrye O, Gatineau QC J8P 7H2; Cuyo (Argentina)'94; ObstGyn (P.Q.). Staff, Hôpital de Gatineau; (819)561-8100

GARCIA, Javier; Hôpital de Christ-Roi, 675 rue Saint-Jean-Baptiste, Nicolet QC J3T 1S4; Staff, Hôpital de Christ-Roi; (819)293-2071

GARCIA, Michel; Clinique Medicale des Monts, 20 boul Sainte-Anne O, Ste-Anne-des-Monts QC G4V 1P6; Mon'69; MSc(Harvard); Staff, Centre Hospitalier des Monts; VP, CIM & Management Inc; Langs: Spanish; English; (418)763-5731; Fax. (418)763-7401.

GARCIA, Sebasian; CSSS d'Antoine-Labelle-Mt Laur, RR 1 2561 ch de la Lievre S, Mont-Laurier QC J9L 3G3; IntMed (P.Q.). Staff, CSSS d'Antoine-Labelle; (819)623-1234; Fax. (819)440-4606.

GARCIA, Yasmin M A; Community First Med Clinic, 105-518 Lake St, Nelson BC V1L 4C6; (Other Foreign)'04; CCFP; Staff, Fort Nelson General Hospital; Langs: Tagalog; (250)352-5259; yasmin.garcia@northernhealth.ca.

GARCIA, Yelian; 105-126 Wellington St W, Aurora ON L4G 2N9; Saba (Netherlands Antilles)'08; CCFP; (905)841-1633

GARCIA, Angeles; Providence CCC-St Mary's, PO Box 3600 Stn Main 1 157-340 Union St, Kingston ON K7L 5A2; Barcelona (Spain)'75; PhD; FRCPC; IntMed (Dementia); GeriatricMed. Staff, Providence Care - St Mary's of the Lake Hospital Site; Staff, Kingston General Hospital; Staff, Hotel-Dieu Hospital; Assoc Prof, Queen's University; Langs: French; Spanish; Catalan; (613)544-5220 x2229; Fax. (613)544-4017.

GARCIA DEL BUSTO CANO, Elena; Victoria County Mem Hosp, PO Box 220 30 Old Margaree Rd, Baddeck NS B0E 1B0; Dal'08; CCFP; Staff, Victoria County Memorial Hospital; (902)295-3701; Fax. (902)295-3704.

GARCIA DEL SOL, Idania; 280 boul Du Roi-Du-Nord, Laval QC H7L 4L2; Havana (Cuba)'90; Staff, Hopital de la Cite de la santé; Langs: Spanish; (450)622-5110; Fax. (450)622-4150.

GARCIA-ERDELJAN, Meivys; Markham Fertility Center, 5F-379 Church St, Markham ON L6B 0T1; Wes'04; FRCPC; ObstGyn (Infertility). (905)472-4484; Fax. (905)472-3219.

GARCIA GONTHIER, Maite; Clinique Med 3000, 3000 rue Belanger, Montreal QC H1Y 1A9; Mon'07; Médecin, CLSC De Hochelaga-Maisonneuve; (514)376-7702; Fax. (514)376-2639.

GARCIA GUERRA, Gonzalo; University of Alberta Hosp, 3A3 03-8440 112 St NW, Edmonton AB T6G 2B7; (Argentina)'99; Staff, University of Alberta Hospital; (780)407-1673; Fax. (780)407-3214.

GARCIA-RODRIGUEZ, Juan A; Sunridge Family Med Teaching C, 2685 36 St NE, Calgary AB T1Y 5S3; Pontifical (Colombia)'87; CCFP; CommunMed. Staff Emerg, Strathmore District Health Services; Langs: Spanish; (403)943-5000

GARCIA-SALINAS, Raul; Medical Centre Pasqua Hosp, 1-4101 Dewdney Ave, Regina SK S4T 1A5; Monterrey (Mexico)'80; MSc; FACS; FRCSC; Ophth (Retina). Ophthalmology, Pasqua Hospital; Ac Staff, Regina General Hospital; Ophthalmology, Wascana Rehabilitation Centre; Clinical Asst Prof, University of Saskatchewan; Langs: Spanish; (306)522-3937; Fax. (306)522-8252.

GARD, Sherry L; AE231-671 William Ave, Winnipeg MB R3E 0Z2; Man'98; FRCPC; Anes. Staff, Health Sciences Centre.

GARDAM, Michael A; Univ Hlth Network-Toronto Gen, 9 CSB-200 Elizabeth St, Toronto ON M5G 2C4; McG'92; MSc; FRCPC; IntMed; InfectDis. Staff, Toronto General Hospital - UHN; Dir. Inf. Ctrl., University of Toronto; Langs: English; French; (416)340-4800 x3758

GARDEE, Suliman; Appletree Med Centre, 150 Katimavik Rd, Kanata ON K2L 2N2; Dublin (Ireland)'69; LRCPSI(Irish); LMCC; Langs: Swedish; (613)592-1539; Fax. (613)592-1024.

GARDEN, Dana L; Chinook Reg Hosp, 960 19 St S, Lethbridge AB T1J 1W5; Alb'89; CCFP; FCFP; Staff, Chinook Regional Hospital; (403)388-6524; Fax. (403)388-6708.

GARDENER, Kenneth J; Telus Plaza South, 2700-10020 100 St NW, Edmonton AB T5J 0N3; Alb'76; CCFP; FCFP; Staff, Covenant Health - Misericordia Community Hospital; Asst Registrar, College of Physicians & Surgeons of Alberta; Clin Prof Family Med, University of Alberta; (780)392-3110; Fax. (780)420-0651; kgardener@cpso.ob.ca.

GARDIE, Juan; Sir Mortimer B Davis Jewish Ge, 3755 ch Cote-sainte-Catherine, Montreal QC H3T 1E2; CCFP; Staff, Sir Mortimer B Davis Jewish General; (514)340-8253

GARDIN, Letizia L; Children's Hosp Eastern Ont, 401 Smyth Rd, Ottawa ON K1H 8L1; Dal'96; FAB; FRCPC; Peds; Cardiol. Staff, Children's Hospital of Eastern Ontario (CHEO); (613)737-7600; Fax. (613)738-4835.

GARDINER, Dennis; 35B-2121 Carling Ave, Ottawa ON K2A 1H2; Glasgow (Scotland)'75; BSc(Hons); MB ChB; MRCP(UK); Lecturer Family Med, University of Ottawa; (613)761-6777; Fax. (613)761-7744; dennis.gardiner@hrsdc-rhdcc.gc.ca.

GARDINER, Donald B; Saskatoon Cancer Centre, 20 Campus Dr, Saskatoon SK S7N 4H4; Alb'87; MSc; BSc; FRCPC; RadOncol. Staff, Saskatoon Cancer Centre; Staff, Royal University Hospital; Asst Prof Med, University of Saskatchewan; (306)655-2743; Fax. (306)655-2910.

GARDINER, Donald I; Huronia Med Centre, PO Box 790, Midland ON L4R 4P4; Ott'94; CCFP; Ac Staff Oak Ridge Div, Waypoint Centre for Mental Health Care; Ac Staff, Georgian Bay General Hospital - Midland; Langs: Bilingual(English/French); (705)526-8482; Fax. (705)526-8789.

GARDINER, Edward M; P/T CPM Pain Clinic, 110-300 Earl Grey Dr, Ottawa ON K2T 1B8; Ott'74; CCFP; CCFP(E.M.); FCFP; Consultant Occup Med, Renfrew Victoria Hospital; Langs: English; French; (613)302-1669; Fax. (613)622-5606; dr.gardiner@ergomed.ca.

GARDINER, Fritz A; Clinique Med de Vimont, 1768B boul des Laurentides, Laval QC H7M 2P6; (Haiti)'64; (450)668-1221; Fax. (450)661-1224.

GARDINER, Geoffrey W; Gamma Dynacare Laboratories, 115 Midlair Court, Brampton ON L6T 5M3; Alb'68; FRCPC; AnatPath. Ac Staff Pathologist, St Michael's Hospital; Asst Prof, University of Toronto; (905)790-3000

GARDINER, Ian C; 45 St Thomas St, St. Albert AB T8N 6Z1; UBC'89; FRCPC; DiagRad. (780)470-5551; Fax. (780)458-0104.

GARDINER, J Paul; St Clare's Mercy Hosp, SM330-154 Lemarchant Rd, St. John's NL A1C 5B8; Dal'74; BSc; FRCSC; GenSurg; ThorSurg. Gen Surgeon, St Clare's Mercy Hospital; (709)777-5422; Fax. (709)777-5849.

GARDINER, Jane A; BC Women's Hosp & Health Ctre, A139B-4500 Oak St, Vancouver BC V6H 3N1; Mem'86; BMedSci; FRCSC; Ophth (Pediatric Ophthalmology). Staff Ophth, Providence Health Care - St Paul's Hospital; Staff, BC Women's Hospital & Health Centre; Clin Assoc Prof, University of British Columbia; (604)875-3079; Fax. (604)875-3142.

GARDINER, Richard R; Royal Columbian Hosp, 104-330 Columbia St E, New Westminster BC V3L 3W7; UBC'07; Anes. Staff, Royal Columbian Hospital; (604)528-5002

GARDNER, Angus J; Cape Breton Hlthcare Complex, 1482 George St, Sydney NS B1P 1P3; Dal'73; BSc; FRCSC; ObstGyn. Med Dir, Cape Breton Healthcare Complex; Consultant, Northside General Hospital; Clin Instructor, Dalhousie University; (902)567-8118; Fax. (902)567-8116; gardnera@cbdha.nshealth.ca.

GARDNER, Charles; Simcoe Muskoka Dist Health, 15 Sperling Dr, Barrie ON L4M 6K9; Qns'88; MHSc; FRCPC; CommunMed (Public Health);CCFP; Med Officer of Hlth, Simcoe Muskoka District Health Unit Corporate Office; Aj Teach Staff, University of Toronto; (705)721-7520; charles.gardner@smdhu.org.

GARDNER, Douglas; Athlete's Care, C100-11 King St W, Toronto ON M5H 4C7; Mem'84; FRCPC; DiagRad. (416)864-1814; 2brats@wincom.net.

GARDNER, Jillian; Stein Med Clinic, 887 Dunsmuir St, Vancouver BC V6C 1N9; Adelaide (Australia)'04; MB BS; CCFP; (604)688-5924

GARDNER, Marieke; Ctre Hosp de Lasalle, 8585 Terrasse Champlain, LaSalle QC H8P 1C1; Tor'08; CCFP; Staff, Centre Hospitalier de LaSalle; (514)362-8000

GARDNER, Martin J; Queen Elizabeth II HSC-Halifax, 2501A-1796 Summer St, Halifax NS B3H 3A7; Dal'76; FACC; FRCPC; Cardiol. Dir EPS Lab, Queen Elizabeth II Health Sciences Centre - Halifax Infirmary Site; (902)473-2187; martin.gardner@dal.ca.

GARDNER-MAHER, Bertha; SGH Medical Mall, 401-3030 Lawrence Ave E, Scarborough ON M1P 2T7; Sher'70; Neur. Staff, The Scarborough Hospital - General Campus; Langs: Bilingual(English/French); (416)431-5656; Fax. (416)431-4469.

GARDNER-NIX, Jacqueline S; St Michael's Hosp, 30 Bond St, Toronto ON M5B 1W8; London (England)'79; MB BS; PhD(Biochem); MRC; Consultant Chronic Pain, Sunnybrook Health Sciences Centre; Consultant Chronic Pain, St Michael's Hospital; Founder, Scarborough Pact; Asst Prof, University of Toronto; (416)264-2424; Fax. (416)864-5854.

GARE, Douglas J; 601-123 Edward St, Toronto ON M5G 1E2; Tor'60; BSc(Med); FRCSC; ObstGyn (Office Gynecology). Staff, Mount Sinai Hospital; Prof ObstGyn, University of Toronto; (416)813-2288; Fax. (416)813-4179.

GAREAU, Annie; Whister Health Care Centre, 4380 Lorimer Rd, Whistler BC V0N 1B4; Mon'85; FACEP; FRCPC; EmergMed. Att Staff Emerg, Vancouver General Hospital - Centennial Pavillion; Med Consultant, British Columbia Ambulance Services; Instructor Surg, University of British Columbia; (604)932-4911; annie.gareau@gov.bc.ca.

GAREAU, Jacques Y; CSSS de Saint-Jerome, 290 rue de Montigny, Saint-Jerome QC J7Z 5T3; Mon'57; BSc; Staff Psy, Hôtel-Dieu de Saint-Jérôme; Langs: English; French; (450)431-8200 x2501; Fax. (450)227-7490; caron-garo@sympatico.ca.

GAREAU, Julie; Hop Charles Lemoyne, 3120 boul Taschereau, Greenfield Park QC J4V 2H1; Mon'02; CCFP; Staff, Hopital Charles LeMoyne; (450)466-5000

GAREAU, Marilyn; Ctr Hosp Laurentien, 234 rue Saint-Vincent, Ste-Agathe-des-Mts QC J8C 2B8; McG'07; MDCM; CCFP; Staff, Centre Hospitalier Laurentien; (819)324-4000

GAREAU, Pierre; Clinique Medicale du Faubourg, 145-1160 boul Saint-Joseph, Gatineau QC J8Z 1T3; McG'92; Staff, Centre Hospitalier Pierre-Janet; (819)595-1991

GAREAU, Rejean; Thunder Bay Reg HSC-T-Bay, 980 Oliver Rd, Thunder Bay ON P7B 6V4; Alb'05; FRCPC; Anes. Staff, Thunder Bay Regional Health Sciences Centre; (807)684-6000

GAREIW, Salah H; Hamilton HS-General Site, 237 Barton St E, Hamilton ON L8L 2X2; Al Fateh (Libya)'87; Staff, Hamilton Health Sciences Centre - Hamilton General Hospital; Langs: Arabic; (905)527-0271

GAREL, Laurent; Hôpital Ste-Justine, 3175 ch Cote-Ste-Catherine, Montreal QC H3T 1C5; Paris (France)'74; FRCPC; DiagRad (P.Q.). Ac Staff, Hôpital Ste-Justine; Prof, Universite de Montreal; (514)345-4931; Fax. (514)345-4816; laurent_garel@ssss.gouv.qc.ca.

GAREL, Patricia; Hôpital Ste-Justine, 3175 ch Cote-Sainte-Catherine, Montreal QC H3T 1C5; Paris (France)'84; Psy (P.Q.). Ac Staff, Hôpital Ste-Justine; (514)345-4931

GARFAT, Ronald E; 2-316 Wharncliffe Rd N, London ON N6G 1E2; Wes'68; Court Staff, London Health Sciences Centre - Victoria Campus; Court Staff, St Joseph's Health Centre; (519)673-0101; Fax. (519)673-0637.

GARFIELD, Bruce; Rheumatic Disease Ctr of Mtl, 740-4060 rue Sainte-Catherine, Montreal QC H3Z 2Z3; (Grenada)'97; ABIM; FRCPC; Rheum (P.Q.). Langs: Bilingual(French/English); (514)932-7438; Fax. (514)932-1469; doctorgarfield@hotmail.com.

GARFIELD, Hartley; Create Fertility Centre, 540-790 Bay St, Toronto ON M5G 1N8; Tor'68; FAAP; FRCPC; Peds (Neonatology). Court Staff, Mount Sinai Hospital; Court Staff, Sunnybrook Health Sciences Centre; Sr Staff, The Hospital For Sick Children; Court Staff, Toronto General Hospital - UHN; Assoc Prof Dept of Med, University of Toronto; Aj Associate Prof Dept of Med, Queen's University; Langs: Danish; (416)960-5883; Fax. (416)960-9877; hartley.garfield@gmail.com.

GARFIELD, Natasha; MUHC-Royal Victoria Hosp, 687 av des Pins O, Montreal QC H3A 1A1; McG'95; FRCPC; IntMed; Endocrin&Metab. Staff, McGill University Health Centre - Montreal General Campus; Staff, McGill University Health Centre - Royal Victoria Hospital; Langs: French; (514)934-1934; natasha.garfield@muhc.mcgill.ca.

GARFINKEL, Paul; Addiction & Mental Hlth-Clarke, 250 College St, Toronto ON M5T 1R8; Man'69; FRCPC; Psy. Staff, Centre for Addiction & Mental Health (CAMH) - College Street Site; Prof Psy, University of Toronto; (416)535-8501; Fax. (416)583-1288; paul_garfinkel@camh.net.

GARG, Amit; London HSC-Victoria Hosp, PO Box 5010 Stn B ELL 101-800 Commissioners Rd E, London ON N6A 5W9; Tor'95; MEd; PhD; FACP; FRCPC; IntMed (Dialysis); Nephrol. Staff Kidney Clinical Research Unit, London Health Sciences Centre - Victoria Campus; (519)685-8502; Fax. (519)685-8072.

GARG, Arun K; Royal Columbian Hosp, 330 Columbia St E, New Westminster BC V3L 3W7; UBC'77; PhD; FRCPC; MedBiochem. Dir Lab & Med Biochem Serv Fraser Health Authority, Royal Columbian Hospital; Consultant Med Biochem, C J Coady Associates; Programmer Med, Fraser Health Authority; Consultant Med Biochem, BC Biomedical Laboratories Ltd; Clin Prof Path, University of British Columbia; Langs: Hindi; (604)520-4330

GARG, Avinash; Four Corners Med Bldg, 307-2009 Long Lake Rd, Sudbury ON P3E 6C3; Ott'85; DAB; FACS; FRCSC; GenSurg (Cardiac Surgery); CardiothorSurg. Staff Cardio Thoracic Surg, Health Sciences North - Memorial Site; (705)523-4400; Fax. (705)523-4050.

GARG, Divya; Central Comm Hlth Ctr, 359 Talbot St, St Thomas ON N5P 1B7; McM'09; CCFP; Langs: Hindi; (519)633-7989

GARG, Narinder K; Karolbagh Plaza, 104-1090 Peter Robertson Blvd, Brampton ON L6R 3B3; Madagh (India)'80; MB BS; CCFP; FCFP; Langs: Urdu; Hindi; Punjabi; (905)799-0000; Fax. (905)799-1966.

GARG, Naveen; Centre Medical Brunswick, 401-955 boul Saint-Jean, Pointe-Claire QC H9R 5K3; (Netherlands Antilles)'08; CCFP; Langs: Hindi; Punjabi; English; (514)426-6677

GARG, Pallav; London HSC-University Hosp, PO Box 5339 Stn B 399 Windermere Rd, London ON N6A 5A5; Staff, London Health Sciences Centre - University Hospital; (519)663-3627; Fax. (519)663-2997.

GARG, Sunil; Ctr Hosp de lachine, 650 16e av, Lachine QC H8S 3N5; McG'04; FRCPC; IntMed; Cardiol. Staff, Centre Hospitalier de Lachine; Langs: Bilingual(English/French); (514)934-1934 x77250

GARGOUM, Hassan A M; 2275 Broad St, Regina SK S4P 1Y7; Garyunis (Libya)'79; ABIM; FACP; FACC; FRCP; ABCD; CRCP; FRCPC; IntMed (Adult Cardiology); Cardiol. Staff Coronary Care Unit & Invasive Cardiol, Regina General Hospital; Prof Med, University of Saskatchewan; Langs: Arabic; Bilingual(English/French); (306)757-2478; Fax. (306)585-3993; h.gargoum@usask.ca.

GARIC, Mirjana; Medica One, 2019 Caroline St, Burlington ON L7R 1L1; (Croatia)'82; CCFP; Langs: Croatian; Serbian; (905)333-0911 x803; Fax. (905)333-0311.

GARIEPY, Celine; CLSC Saint-Hubert, 6800 boul Cousineau, Saint-Hubert QC J3Y 8Z4; Laval'91; (450)443-7400 x7425; Fax. (450)676-3488; c.gariepy@rrsss16.gouv.qc.ca.

GARIEPY, Daniel; CLSC Jardin du Quebec, 2 rue Ste-Famille, Saint-Remi QC J0L 2L0; Mon'92; (450)454-4671; Fax. (450)454-4538.

GARIEPY, Elizabeth L; Mediclub du Sanctuaire, 6100 av du Boise, Montreal QC H3S 2W1; Mon'85; Ophth. Staff, CSSS du Coeur de l'Isle Hôpital Jean-Talon; Staff, Institut Universitaire de Gériatrie de Montréal; (514)739-6515; Fax. (514)739-6773.

GARIEPY, Gaetan; Polyclinique St-Eustache, 75 rue Grignon, St-Eustache QC J7P 4J2; Mon'81; (450)473-5782; Fax. (450)473-1916.

GARIEPY, Gilles; CHUM-Hop St-Luc, 1058 rue Saint-Denis, Montreal QC H2X 3J4; Mon'65; CSPQ; FRCPC; AnatPath. Pathology, Centre Hospitalier l'Université De Montréal (CHUM) - Hôpital Saint-luc; assoc Prof, Universite de Montreal; (514)890-8000 x36216

GARIEPY, Jacques; Clinique Solumed, 8230 boul Taschereau, Brossard QC J4X 1C2; Mon'64; FRCSC; Neursurg. Langs: Bilingual(French/English); (450)671-2891; Fax. (450)621-1853; jjgariepy@videotron.ca.

GARIEPY, Jean-Luc; Ctr Hosp Affilie-Enfant-Jesus, 1401 18e rue, Quebec QC G1J 1Z4; Mon'92; FRCPC; DiagRad (Neuro Radiology). Staff, Centre Hospitalier Affilié Universitaire de Québec - Hôpital De L'Enfant Jésus; (418)649-5782; Fax. (418)649-5903.

GARIEPY, Linda; CSSS de Trois-Rivières, 1991 boul du Carmel, Trois-Rivieres QC G8Z 3R9; Laval'85; FRCPC; IntMed; Gastroent. Staff, CSSS de Trois-Rivières; (819)697-3333 x63473; Fax. (819)372-3516.

GARIEPY, Philippe; CSSS de la Haute-Yamaska, 205 boul Leclerc O, Granby QC J2G 1T7; Mon'95; CCFP; Staff, Centre Hospitalier de Granby; (450)372-5491; Fax. (450)372-7197.

GARIEPY, Ursule; CSST-Direction Regionale Montr, CP 3 Succ Pl-desjardins 35e-1 Complexe Desjardins, Montreal QC H5B 1H1; Laval'74; Médecin, CSST-Direction Regionale Montreal; (514)906-3484; Fax. (514)906-3430.

GARINTHER, Ross; Appletree Medical Group, 150 Katimavik Rd, Ottawa ON K2L 4A2; Ott'88; (613)592-1539; Fax. (613)592-1024.

GARISA, Padma L; Nolin Center, LL-435 Notre Dame Ave, Sudbury ON P3C 5K6; Venkateswara (India)'85; MB BS; FRCSC; ObstGyn. Staff, Health Sciences North-Laurentian Site; (705)523-7100

GARLAND, Allan B; Health Sciences Centre, GF222-820 Sherbrook St, Winnipeg MB R3A 1R9; Chicago (USA)'86; Staff, Health Sciences Centre.

GARLAND, Allan R; Massey Med Clinic, PO Box 119 260 Cameron St, Massey ON P0P 1P0; Qns'70; (705)865-2300; allan.garland@personainternet.com.

GARLAND, Andrea D; 201-1 Magazine St, Saint John NB E2K 5S9; Mem'85; FRCSC; Otol. Staff, Saint John Regional Hospital; Staff, St Joseph's Hospital; Langs: Bilingual(English/French); (506)658-1379; Fax. (506)632-6955.

GARLAND, Brian E; 206-107 Catherwood St, Saint John NB E2M 5J7; Dal'69; Assoc Staff, Saint John Regional Hospital; Assoc Staff, St Joseph's Hospital; (506)635-8881

GARLAND, E Jane; BC Women's Hosp & Health Ctre, Box 141 P4 215-4500 Oak St, Vancouver BC V6H 3N1; Qns'77; FRCPC; Psy (Child Psychiatry). Staff, BC Women's Hospital & Health Centre; Clin Prof, University of British Columbia; (604)875-2737; Fax. (604)875-2099; jgarland@cw.bc.ca.

GARLAND, Jocelyn S; Queen's Univ-Etherington Hall, 2043-115 Barrack St, Kingston ON K7L 3N6; Mem'97; FRCPC; IntMed; Nephrol. (613)533-3207; Fax. (613)533-2306.

GARLAND, Leslie A; Crowsnest Medl Clinic, PO Box 370, Bellevue AB T0K 0C0; Alb'92; (403)562-8804; Fax. (403)562-2905.

GARLAND, Marie S; Joseph Brant Mem Hosp, 1230 North Shore Blvd, Burlington ON L7S 1W7; Wes'95; CCFP; FCFP; Staff, Joseph Brant Memorial Hospital; (905)632-3730

GARLAND, Paul A; London Road Diagnostic Clinic, 481 London Rd, Sarnia ON N7T 4X3; Liverpool (England)'64; MB ChB; DMRD; FRCPC; DiagRad. (519)332-3434; Fax. (519)332-8214.

GARLICH, Fiona M; Foothills Med Centre, 1403 29 St NW, Calgary AB T2N 2T9; (USA)'07; Staff, Foothills Medical Centre; (403)944-6900; Fax. (403)944-1472.

GARNEAU, Daniel; CSSS de Montmagny-L'Islet, 350 boul Tache O RR 1, Montmagny QC G5V 3R8; Laval'00; CSPQ; FRCSC; OrthSurg. Staff, CSSS de Montmagny-L'Islet; (418)248-0630

GARNEAU, Francois X; Hop du Sacre-Coeur de Mtl, 5400 boul Gouin O, Montreal QC H4J 1C5; Mon'84; FRCPC; EmergMed (P.Q.). Staff, Hôpital du Sacre-Coeur de Montréal; (514)338-2222 x2002

GARNEAU, Genevieve; Centre Hosp Honore-Mercier, 2750 boul Laframboise, Saint-Hyacinthe QC J2S 4Y8; Mon'99; CCFP; CCFP(E.M.); Staff, Centre Hospitalier Honore-Mercier; Langs: Spanish; English; (450)771-3333 x3322; gingembreg@hotmail.com.

GARNEAU, Genevieve; CSSS du Lac-des-Deux-Montagnes, 520 boul Arthur-Sauve, Saint-Eustache QC J7R 5B1; Mon'00; Staff, Hôpital de Saint-Eustache; (450)473-6811

GARNEAU, Guillaume; CHUQ-St-Francois D'Assise, 10 rue de l'Espinay, Quebec QC G1L 3L5; Laval'02; FRCPC; DiagRad. Staff, Centre Hospitalier Universitaire De Québec - Pavillon De St-françois-d'assise; (418)525-4444

GARNEAU, Jacques; Polyclinique de la Capitale, 7-4225 4e av O, Quebec QC G1H 6P3; Laval'79; CSPQ; OrthSurg. Ac Staff, Centre Hospitalier Universitaire De Québec - Pavillon De St-françois-d'assise; (418)623-9871; Fax. (418)623-9873.

GARNEAU, Jessica; Ctr Hosp Trois-Riv-St-Joseph, 2F-731 rue Sainte-Julie, Trois-Rivieres QC G9A 1Y1; Mon'10; CCFP; Staff, Centre Hospitalier Regional de Trois-Rivieres; (819)372-3536

GARNEAU, Jocelyn; CRSSS Baie-James-Chibougamau, 51 3e rue, Chibougamau QC G8P 1N1; Laval'02; CCFP; Staff, CRSSS de la Baie-James; (418)748-2676; Fax. (418)748-2549.

GARNEAU, Melanie; CSSS de Manicouagan, 635 boul Jolliet, Baie-Comeau QC G5C 1P1; Laval'09; Staff, Centre Hospitalier Régional Baie-Comeau; (418)589-3701

GARNEAU, Pascale; Hop Maisonneuve-Rosemont, 5415 boul de l'Assomption, Montreal QC H1T 2M4; Sher'93; IntMed. Staff, Hopital Maisonneuve-Rosemont; (514)252-3400 x4558

GARNEAU, Pierre; Ctr Hosp Affilie-Enfant-Jesus, 1401 18e rue, Quebec QC G1J 1Z4; Laval'75; CSPQ; FRCSC; GenSurg (Digestive Endoscopy). Ac Staff, Centre Hospitalier Affilié Universitaire de Québec - Hôpital De L'Enfant Jésus; (418)649-5882

GARNEAU, Pierre Y; Centre Med & Chir Rockland, 100-100 ch Rockland, Mont-Royal QC H3P 2V9; Laval'91; CSPQ; FRCSC; GenSurg. Staff, Hôpital du Sacre-Coeur de Montréal; (514)334-1499; Fax. (514)331-8683.

GARNEAU, Sara; CSSS de Manicouagan, 635 boul Jolliet, Baie-Comeau QC G5C 1P1; Sher'10; CCFP; Staff, Centre Hospitalier Régional Baie-Comeau; (418)589-3701

GARNEAU, Sebastien; CHUM-Hop Notre-Dame, 1560 rue Sherbrooke E, Montreal QC H2L 4M1; Mon'03; FRCPC; Anes. Staff, Centre Hospitalier l'Université de Montréal (CHUM) - Hôpital Notre-Dame; (514)890-8000 x26876

GARNEAU, Sebastien; Centre Hosp Honore-Mercier, 2750 boul Laframboise, Saint-Hyacinthe QC J2S 4Y8; Laval'02; FRCPC; Anes. Staff, Centre Hospitalier Honore-Mercier; (450)771-3333

GARNEAU, Suzanne; CSSS de Trois-Rivières, 110-1991 boul du Carmel, Trois-Rivieres QC G8Z 3R9; Mon'91; FRCPC; Peds. Staff, CSSS de Trois-Rivières; (819)697-3333; Fax. (819)375-0686.

GARNEAU, Valerie; Centre Medical Fusey, 200 rue Fusey, Trois-Rivieres QC G8T 2V8; Laval'96; Chef Emerg, Centre de santé Cloutier-du-Rivage; Langs: Bilingual(French/English); (819)378-7211; Fax. (819)378-5625.

GARNEAU, Yvon; CHUQ-Ctr Hosp Univ Laval, RC 157-2705 boul Laurier, Quebec QC G1V 4G2; Laval'70; Psy (Adult Psychiatry). Ac Staff, Centre Hospitalier Universitaire de Quebec-CHUL; Clin Assoc Prof, Université Laval; Langs: Bilingual(French/English); (418)654-2121; Fax. (418)654-2132.

GARNER, Michel; Hop du Sacre-Coeur de Mtl, 5400 boul Gouin O, Montreal QC H4J 1C5; Mon'80; EmergMed (P.Q.). Chief Emerg Service, Hôpital du Sacre-Coeur de Montréal; Clin Asst Prof, Universite de Montreal; (514)335-1252; Fax. (514)335-1753.

GARNER, Scott H; Med Works Assessments, 855 Harrington Crt, Burlington ON L7N 3P3; Man'79; BSc; FRCPC; PhysMed&Rehab (Electromyography). Staff Phys, Joseph Brant Memorial Hospital; (905)681-7577; Fax. (905)681-0855.

GARNETT, Robert L; The Ottawa Hosp-Civic Campus, 1053 Carling Ave, Ottawa ON K1Y 4E9; Ott'70; DAB; Anes. Dir Vascular Anes, The Ottawa Hospital - Civic Campus; Staff Teacher, University of Ottawa; (613)761-4169; Fax. (613)761-5209.

GARNETT, Ronald T; South Health Campus, 4448 Front St SE, Calgary AB T3M 1M4; Alb'82; CASM(CASM); CCFP; CCFP(E.M.); FCFP; (403)956-2300

GARNEYS, Glenn G; Peterborough Reg Hlth Centre, 1 Hospital Dr, Peterborough ON K9J 7C6; Man'89; MSc; FRCPC; DiagRad. Staff, Ross Memorial Hospital; Chief Radiol, Peterborough Regional Health Centre - Hospital Drive; Staff, Peterborough Regional Health Centre - Rogers St Site; (705)743-2121; Fax. (705)745-6106; ggarneys1@cogeco.ca.

GARNHAM, Jennifer A; Ottawa Integrative Cancer Ctre, 29 Bayswater Ave, Ottawa ON K1Y 2E5; McM'81; BSc; MSc; FRCPC; Psy (Psychotherapy). (613)792-1222; Fax. (613)792-1620.

GARNIER, Marie-Lise; CSSS Pierre Boucher, 1333 Boul Jacques-Cartier E, Longueuil QC J4M 2A5; Sher'83; FRCPC; Psy. Staff, Centre Hospitalier Pierre Boucher; (450)468-8111

GARNIER, Pascale; CLSC des Patriotes, 300 boul Serge-Pepin, Beloeil QC J3G 0B8; Sher'91; (450)536-2572 x6704

GARNIS-JONES, Sylvia G; Northtown Med Centre, 325 Thorold Rd, Welland ON L3C 3W4; McG'80; FRCPC; Derm. Langs: Latvian; French; (905)732-4777

GARNISS, Derek; Sault Area Hosp, 750 Great Northern Rd, Sault Ste. Marie ON P6B 0A8; Ott'02; CCFP; CCFP(E.M.); Staff, Sault Area Hospital - Sault Ste Marie; (705)759-3434

GARON, Andre; Ctr Hosp Affilie-Enfant-Jesus, 1401 rue 18E, Quebec QC G1J 1Z4; Laval'76; Staff, Centre Hospitalier Affilié Universitaire de Québec - Hôpital De L'Enfant Jésus; (418)649-5604

GARON, Claire; CLSC De Dorval-Lachine, 1900 rue Notre-Dame, Lachine QC H8S 2G2; Laval'81; (514)639-0650; Fax. (514)639-8593.

GARON, Jean; Clin D'Endocrin de l'Outaouais, 3E-520 Boul de l'Hopital, Gatineau QC J8V 2P5; Sher'87; FRCPC; IntMed (Diabetes); Endocrin&Metab. Langs: English; (819)771-8778

GAROUFALIS, Evgenia; MUHC-Royal Victoria Hosp, 204-687 av des Pins O, Montreal QC H3A 1A1; West Indies (Jamaica)'99; CCFP; Staff, McGill University Health Centre - Royal Victoria Hospital; (514)934-1934

GARRARD, Michael J; Cariboo Mem Hosp, 517 Sixth Ave N, Williams Lake BC V2G 2G8; Witwatersand (South Africa)'04; MB ChB; CCFP; Staff, Cariboo Memorial Hospital and Health Centre; (250)392-4411; michael_garrard@telus.net.

GARRAWAY, Naisan; Vancouver Gen Hosp, 855 12th Ave W, Vancouver BC V5Z 1M9; Alb'95; FRCSC; GenSurg;CCFP; Staff, Vancouver General Hospital - Centennial Pavillion; (604)875-5094

GARREL, Dominique; 3840 rue Saint-Urbain, Montreal QC H2W 1T8; Lyon (France)'80; Endocrin (P.Q.) (Nutrition). Staff, Centre Hospitalier l'Université de Montréal (CHUM) - Hôtel-Dieu; Teach Staff, Universite de Montreal; Langs: English; (514)890-8444; dominique.garrel@umontreal.ca.

GARRETT, Cynthia A; Vancouver Native Hlth Society, 449 Hastings St E, Vancouver BC V6A 1P5; UBC'88; (604)255-9766; Fax. (604)254-5750.

GARRETT, Gerry; PO Box 20166 Rpo Towne Centre, Kelowna BC V1Y 9H2; Alb'96; (250)859-1362

GARRETT, J Daniel; Victoria Westmount Med Centre, B106-751 Victoria St S, Kitchener ON N2M 5N4; Qns'72; Coroner, Province of Ontario; (519)748-8510; Fax. (519)742-9717.

GARRETT, Kyle J; Rocky Med Clinic, PO Box 99 Stn Main 5127 49 St, Rocky-Mtn-House AB T4T 1A1; Cal'05; CCFP; Staff, Rocky Mountain House Health Centre; (403)845-2815; Fax. (403)845-2177.

GARRETT, Rex M; 105-704 Mara St, Point Edward ON N7V 1X4; Wes'72; Staff, Bluewater Health - Mitton Site; Staff, Bluewater Health - Norman Site; (519)337-3201

GARREY, Matthew M; Business Bldg, 406-1200 Burrard St, Vancouver BC V6Z 2C7; Glasgow (Scotland)'72; MB ChB; FRCSC; ObstGyn. Ac Staff, BC Women's Hospital & Health Centre; Ac Staff, Providence Health Care - St Paul's Hospital; Consultant, Vancouver General Hospital - Centennial Pavillion; (604)683-8416

GARRIDO-RUSSO, Maria; 15 rue de Moncel, Quebec QC G1E 5M8; (Mexico)'69; FRCPC; IntMed; Endocrin (P.Q.). Staff Teacher, Centre Hospitalier Universitaire De Québec - Pavillon De St-françois-d'assise; Langs: Spanish; garrido@sympatico.ca.

GARRIOCH, Gregory; 1935 Paris St, Sudbury ON P3E 3C6; Tor'81; BSc(Chemistry); Med Dir/Ac Staff Cardiac Rehab/Staff Health Sciences North, Health Sciences North - Memorial Site; Med Dir, Vale Canada; (705)522-1018; Fax. (705)522-0930; drgreg@bellnet.ca.

GARRISON, Scott R; Medical Bldg, 120-6180 Blundell Rd, Richmond BC V7C 4W7; UBC'91; (604)271-1822; Fax. (604)241-8815.

GARROS, Daniel; Edmonton Clinic Health Academy, 4 537-11405 87 Ave NW, Edmonton AB T6G 1C9; Passo Fundo (Brazil)'85; Staff Pediatric Intensive Care, University of Alberta Hospital; Staff, Edmonton Clinic Health Academy; Asst/Clin Prof Peds, University of Alberta; Langs: Portuguese; Spanish; (780)248-5444; Fax. (780)248-5627.

GARRY, Benedict M; Surrey Mem Hosp, 13750 96 Ave, Surrey BC V3V 1Z2; Georgetown (USA)'94; CCFP; Staff, Surrey Memorial Hospital; (604)581-2211

GARRY, Steven C; Radiology Consultants Assoc, 120A-6707 Elbow Dr SW, Calgary AB T2V 0E3; Alb'99; FRCPC; DiagRad. (403)777-3003; Fax. (403)777-3006.

GARSIDE, Kevin; CFB Esquimalt, PO Box 17000 Stn Forces 1200 Colville Rd, Victoria BC V9A 7N2; Leicensed (United Kingdom)'05; CCFP; (250)363-4416

GARSIDE, Sarah L; Hamilton HS-McMaster Site, PO Box 2000 Stn Lcd 1 1200 Main St W, Hamilton ON L8N 3Z5; McM'95; FRCPC; Psy. Staff, Hamilton Health Sciences Centre - McMaster Children's Hospital; (905)521-2100

GARSTON, Ronald G; Albert County Hlth & Wellness, 8 Forestdale Rd, Riverside-Albert NB E4H 3Y7; Ott'71; Urol (Family Medicine). Staff Family Med, The Moncton Hospital; Langs: English; French; (506)882-3100; Fax. (506)882-3101; woof@nbnet.nb.ca.

GARTKE, Kathleen; Parkdale Med Tower, 301-1919 Riverside Dr, Ottawa ON K1H 1A2; Ott'77; FRCS; FRCSC; OrthSurg (Foot Problems). Ac Staff, The Ottawa Hospital - General Campus; (613)722-0210

GARTNER, John G; Univ Of Manitoba, P234-770 Bannatyne Ave, Winnipeg MB R3E 0W3; McG'76; LMCC; FRCPC; AnatPath. Dept Head Path/Prof, University of Manitoba; Langs: English; French; (204)789-3382; gartner@cc.umanitoba.ca.

GARTNER, Sean; 2-453 Park St, Kitchener ON N2G 1N5; Wes'94; CCFP; Staff, Stratford General Hospital - Huron Perth Healthcare Alliance; Staff, Grand River Hospital - Kitchener/Waterloo Health Centre; Staff, St Mary's General Hospital; (519)576-1630; Fax. (519)576-4461.

GARVEY, Brian M; 9878 Main St PO Box 339 Stn Main, Canning NS B0P 1H0; Cork (Ireland)'60; DPM(Eng); MRCPsy(Lond); MB BCh; BAO; FRCPC; Psy (Affective Disorders). Consultant Psy, Valley Regional Hospital; Consultant Psy, Soldiers Memorial Hospital; Consultant Telehealth, South Shore Regional Hospital; Teacher Pt-Time Psy, Dalhousie University; (902)582-7535; Fax. (902)582-7576.

GARVEY, M Bernadette; St Michael's Hosp, 2 085Q-30 Bond St, Toronto ON M5B 1W8; Ott'60; BSc; FRCPC; IntMed (Hematology). Staff Hem, St Michael's Hospital; Prof, University of Toronto; (416)864-5119; Fax. (416)864-5693.

GARVIN, Gregory J; St Joseph's Health Care, PO Box 5777 Stn B 286 Grosvenor St, London ON N6A 4V2; Wes'88; FRCPC; DiagRad. Staff, St Joseph's Hospital - St Joseph's Health Care; (519)646-6035; Fax. (519)646-6204.

GARVIN, Robin W; 103-7110 120 St, Surrey BC V3W 3M8; UBC'70; (604)591-8008

GARZON, Jacob; SMBD Jewish Gen Hosp, 3755 ch Cote-Sainte-Catherine, Montreal QC H3T 1E2; Paris (France)'64; CSPQ; FRCSC; GenSurg. Asst Staff Surg, Sir Mortimer B Davis Jewish General; (514)342-4848; Fax. (514)933-1442.

GARZON, Philippe M; Trillium Cardiovascular Assoc, 500-89 Queensway W, Mississauga ON L5B 2V2; McG'03; FRCSC; GenSurg. Langs: Bilingual(English/French); (905)848-6613; Fax. (905)848-6363.

GASCON, Bernard; Commission des Lesions Prof, 249-500 boul des Laurentides, Saint-Jerome QC J7Z 4M2; Mon'60; CCBOM; FCBOM; Assesseur, Commission des Lesions Professionelles; Langs: English; (450)569-7665; Fax. (450)569-7626.

GASCON, Chantal; CSSS du Nord de Lanaudière, 1000 boul Sainte-Anne, Joliette QC J6E 6J2; Mon'90; FRCSC; ObstGyn. Staff Gynecology, Centre Hospitalier Régional de Lanaudière; (450)759-8222; gynécologue.visitation@bellnet.ca.

GASCON, Georges; CSSS du Nord de Lanaudière, 1000 boul Sainte-Anne, St-Charles-Brromee QC J6E 6J2; Mon'71; Nephrol (P.Q.). Staff Nephrology, Centre Hospitalier Régional de Lanaudière; (450)759-8222; Fax. (450)759-1389.

GASCON, Louis; Groupe Sante Medisys Inc, 500-500 rue Sherbrooke O, Montreal QC H3A 3C6; Laval'67; FRCPC; Psy (Administration). Consultant, Medisys Group; (514)845-1211; Fax. (514)845-4842.

GASCON, Michel; CHUM-Hop St-Luc, 1058 rue Saint-Denis, Montreal QC H2X 3J4; Mon'80; FRCPC; IntMed; Nephrol. Staff, Centre Hospitalier l'Université De Montréal (CHUM) - Hôpital Saint-luc.

GASCON, Suzy; Centre Obst & Gyn, 203-1361 av Beaumont, Mont-Royal QC H3P 2W3; Mon'84; FRCSC; ObstGyn (Pediatric & Adolescent Gynecology). Ac Staff, Hôpital Ste-Justine; (514)344-4411; Fax. (514)344-1991.

GASCOYNE, Randy D; BC Cancer Agency Research Ctr, 5 113-675 10th Ave W, Vancouver BC V5Z 1L3; UBC'82; FRCPC; HemPath (General Pathology). Staff, BC Cancer Agency Vancouver Centre; (604)675-8025; rgascoyn@bccancer.bc.ca.

GASEWICZ, Wilson R J; Waypoint Centre for Mental H C, 500 Church St, Penetanguishene ON L9M 1G3; Tor'68; FRCPC; Psy. Court Staff, Royal Victoria Regional Health Centre; Staff Admissions & Assessment Prog, Waypoint Centre for Mental Health Care; (705)549-3181 x2313; Fax. (705)549-1812.

GASH, Todd G; Advanced Spinal Care Centre, 201-2000 Veteran's Pl NW, Calgary AB T2N 4N2; Mem'93; (403)210-9969; tgash@starpoint.ca.

GASIOROWSKA, Paulina; CSSS d'Argenteuil, 145 av de la Providence, Lachute QC J8H 4C7; UBC'08; CCFP; CCFP(E.M.); Staff, Centre Hospitalier d'Argenteuil; (450)562-3761

GASKIN, Anne M; 182 Bagot St, Kingston ON K7L 3G1; Ott'92; CCFP; FCFP; Assoc Staff Family Med, Hotel-Dieu Hospital; Assoc Staff Family Med & Privileges in Med, Kingston General Hospital; Att Staff, Fairmount Home For The Aged; Langs: Bilingual(English/French); (613)542-8783; Fax. (613)546-1321; cdmin@bagot.com.

GASKIN, David Allan; IWK Health Centre, PO Box 9700 Rpo CSC K3610-5850 University Ave, Halifax NS B3K 6R8; Mem'88; BSc; BMedSci; LMCC; CSPQ; MD; GenPath (P.Q.) (Pediatric Pathology). Staff Pediatric Pathologist, IWK Health Centre; Assoc Prof, Dalhousie University; (902)470-8181; Fax. (902)470-7215; david.gaskin@iwk.nshealth.ca.

GASPARD, Antoine; Clinique Med Havre Sante, 521 boul du Havre, Salaber-de-Valleyf QC J6S 4Z5; Beyrouth (Lebanon)'69; LMCC; CSPQ; FRCSC; OrthSurg (Orthopedic Consultant). Med Vérificateur, Centre Hospitalier Régional du Suroît; Med Vérificateur, Barrie Memorial Hospital; Langs: Bilingual(French/English); (450)371-6444; Fax. (450)371-8512; antoine.gaspard@sftl.ca.

GASPARD, Henry S; CSSG-Hop de Hull, 116 boul Lionel-Emond, Gatineau QC J8Y 1W7; Laval'93; CSPQ; FRCSC; OrthSurg (Shoulder). Staff, Hull Hospital; (819)595-6022; Fax. (819)595-6326; henrygaspard@hotmail.com.

GASPARELLI, Rudolph E; 1965 Chiefswood Rd PO Box 9, Ohsweken ON N0A 1M0; Tor'72; CCFP; FCFP; Ac Staff, Sault Area Hospital - Sault Ste Marie; Ac Staff, Lady Dunn Health Centre; Langs: Italian; Bilingual(French/English); (519)445-4590; wawadoc@hotmail.com.

GASS, David A; Dept of Health and Wellness, PO Box 488 Stn Central 1894 Barrington St, Halifax NS B3J 2R8; Dal'73; MD; CCFP; FCFP; Ac Staff, Queen Elizabeth II Health Sciences Centre - Victoria General Site; Chief Staff, Cumberland Health Authority; Prof, Dalhousie University; (902)424-2900

GASSAS, Adam; The Hosp for Sick Children, 555 University Ave, Toronto ON M5G 1X8; Baghdad (Iraq)'86; MB ChB; MSc; FRCP; DCH; Assoc Prof/Staff, The Hospital For Sick Children; Assoc Prof, University of Toronto; (416)813-8227; Fax. (416)813-5327; adam.gassas@sickkids.ca.

GASSE, Tiffany; Sir Mortimer B Davis Jewish Ge, 3755 ch cote-Sainte-Catherine, Montreal QC H3T 1E2; McG'08; CCFP; CCFP(E.M.); Staff, Sir Mortimer B Davis Jewish General; (514)340-8222

GASSER, Joseph; 28 Bartley Dr, Toronto ON M4A 1B8; Tor'85; FACS; FRCSC; Ophth. Ac Staff, Toronto East General Hospital Inc; Langs: Slovak; French; (416)750-8149; Fax. (416)750-8150.

GASTALDO, Fernando; Hamilton HS-General Site, 237 Barton St E, Hamilton ON L8L 2X2; (Brazil)'92; Staff, Hamilton Health Sciences Centre - Hamilton General Hospital; (905)527-4322; Fax. (905)527-5761.

GASTON, Isabelle; CSSS de Saint-Jerome, 290 rue de Montigny, Saint-Jerome QC J7Z 5T3; Laval'00; Staff, Hôtel-Dieu de Saint-Jérôme; (450)431-8200

GASTONGUAY, Johanne I; Foothills Med Centre, C231-1403 29 St NW, Calgary AB T2N 2T9; McG'87; EmergMed. Staff, Foothills Medical Centre; (403)944-1820; Fax. (403)944-2419.

GAT, E Douglas; 405-304 Stone Rd W, Guelph ON N1G 4W4; Wes'78; Med Dir, Group Disability/Manulife Financial & Med. Dir., Clarica; Teacher Family Practice & Psy, University of Toronto.

GATCHEV, Margarita; North Bay Reg Health Centre, 50 College St, North Bay ON P1B 0A4; Ott'93; CCFP; Staff, North Bay Regional Health Centre - Regional Mental Health; Langs: Bulgarian; French; (705)474-1200; Fax. (705)495-7892.

GATENBY, Allan D; Penticton Reg Hosp, 550 Carmi Ave, Penticton BC V2A 3G6; UBC'06; CCFP; CCFP(E.M.); Staff, Penticton Regional Hospital; (250)492-4000

GATES, Allan B; Abbotsford Reg Hosp & Cancer C, 32900 Marshall Rd, Abbotsford BC V2S 0C2; Dal'86; FCAP; FRCPC; GenPath (Anatomical Pathology). Staff, Abbotsford Regional Hospital & Cancer Centre; (604)851-4700 x64656

GATES, C Bronwen; Women's College Hosp, 43 Wellesley St E, Toronto ON M4Y 1H1; Tor'70; FRCPC; Anes. Ac Staff, Sunnybrook Health Sciences Centre - Holland Orthopaedic & Arthritic Centre; Court Staff, Women's College Hospital; (416)967-8500

GATFIELD, Charles T; Happy Valley Family Hlth Team, PO Box 1120 Stn Main 268 Maiden Lane, St Marys ON N4X 1B7; Ott'92; Ac Staff, St Marys Memorial Hospital - Huron Perth Healthcare Alliance; (519)284-3450; Fax. (519)284-4471; cgatfield@stmmc.ca.

GATHA, Mark; 3114-910 10th Ave W, Vancouver BC V5Z 1M9; Cal'06; OrthSurg. Physician, University of Calgary; (604)875-4111

GATIEN, John G; 30 Farnham Gate Rd, Halifax NS B3M 3W8; Dal'69; FRCPC; Peds (Clinical Immunology & Allergy). Ac Staff, IWK Health Centre; Asst Prof Peds, Dalhousie University; (902)422-4057

GATIEN, Mathieu M; The Ottawa Hosp-Gen Campus, 501 Smyth Rd, Ottawa ON K1H 8L6; Ott'97; CCFP; CCFP(E.M.); Staff Emerg, The Ottawa Hospital - General Campus; Staff Emerg, Cornwall Community Hospital; Langs: English; French; (613)737-8000

GATTO, Joan; Mount St Joseph Hosp, 3080 Prince Edward St, Vancouver BC V5T 3N4; UBC'82; Staff, Providence Health Care - Mount Saint Joseph Hospital; (604)877-8167

GATZKE, Jason B; Associate Family Phys Clinic, 262 2nd Ave NE, Swift Current SK S9H 2C8; Sask'96; CCFP; CCFP(E.M.); (306)773-1555; Fax. (306)773-6817.

GAUCHER, Anita L; Surrey Prenatal Clinic, 2F-9655 137 St, Surrey BC V3T 4G8; UBC'90; (778)395-0085

GAUCHER, Christine; CSSS Haut-Richelieu-Rouville, 920 boul du Seminaire N, St-Jean-sur-Richel QC J3A 1B7; Laval'82; Staff Emerg, Hôpital du Haut-Richelieu; Langs: English; (450)359-5000 x2222

GAUCHER, Nathalie; Hôpital Ste-Justine, 3175 ch Cote-Ste-Catherine, Montreal QC H3T 1C5; Mon'05; PedEmergMed; Peds. Staff, Hôpital Ste-Justine; (514)345-4931

GAUDELLI, Cinzia A; Hop du Sacre-Coeur de Mtl, 5400 boul Gouin O, Montreal QC H4J 1C5; McG'07; MDCM; OrthSurg. Staff, Hôpital du Sacre-Coeur de Montréal; (514)338-2222

GAUDET, Adrienne; Prog Daide aux Medecins du Que, 200-1 boul Rene-Levesque E, Montreal QC H2X 3Z5; Laval'91; FRCPC; Psy. Staff, Hôpital du Sacre-Coeur de Montréal; (514)397-0888; Fax. (514)397-0654.

GAUDET, Celine; 6130 Route 335, Saint-Calixte QC J0K 1Z0; Mon'77; Staff, Hôtel-Dieu de Saint-Jérôme; (450)222-2233; Fax. (450)222-3900; dr_c_gaudet@hotmail.com.

GAUDET, Cynthia; CLSC de la Region-Sherbrooke, 50 rue Camirand, Sherbrooke QC J1H 4J5; (819)780-2220 x48394; Fax. (819)823-0238.

GAUDET, Daniel; CSSS de Chicoutimi, 305 rue Saint-Vallier, Chicoutimi QC G7H 5H6; Laval'86; PhD; MSc; Dir recherche Group, Complexe hospitalier de la Sagamie; Staff, Chaire de Recherche du Canada en Genetique Preventive et genomique; Prof, Universite de Montreal; Langs: English; (418)541-1077; Fax. (418)541-1116; daniel.gaudet@umontreal.ca.

GAUDET, Guylaine P; Hop du Sacre-Coeur de Mtl, 5400 boul Gouin O, Montreal QC H4J 1C5; Mon'94; ABIM; FRCPC; IntMed; MedOncol; Hem (Lymphoma). Staff, Hôpital du Sacre-Coeur de Montréal; Langs: English; (514)338-2150; Fax. (514)338-2631.

GAUDET, Jonathan E C; Peter Lougheed Centre, 3500 26 Ave NE, Calgary AB T1Y 6J4; Dal'05; FRCPC; EmergMed; Critical Care Medicine. Staff, Peter Lougheed Centre; (403)943-4221

GAUDET, Laura; The Moncton Hosp, 135 MacBeath Ave, Moncton NB E1C 6Z8; Qns'02; FRCSC; ObstGyn (Maternal Fetal Medicine). Staff, The Moncton Hospital; (506)857-5111

GAUDET, Louise; GMF Montee de la Baie, 3942 ch Oka, St-Joseph-Du-Lac QC J0N 1M0; Sher'82; Langs: English; (450)473-7225; Fax. (450)473-2160.

GAUDET, Lyne; 1F-6 rue McMahon, Quebec QC G1R 3S1; Laval'87; FRCPC; Psy. Staff, Hôtel-Dieu de Lévis; (418)525-4444

GAUDET, Marc; CSSSG-Hop de Gatineau, CP 2000 Succ Bureau-Chef 909 boul de la Verendrye O, Gatineau QC J8P 7H2; Laval'06; FRCPC; RadOncol (Clinician Investigator Program). Staff, Hôpital de Gatineau; (819)966-6130; Fax. (819)966-6284.

GAUDET, Matthieu; 247 av Universite, Moncton NB E1C 5K4; Sher'03; FRCPC; IntMed (Sleep Medicine); Respir. Staff, Dr Georges-L-Dumont University Hospital Centre; Langs: Bilingual(French/English); (506)858-8985; Fax. (506)383-4492.

GAUDET, Michael E; 211-99 Kakulu Rd, Kanata ON K2L 3C8; Qns'86; FRCPC; Psy (Depression & Anxiety). (613)591-0606; Fax. (613)591-0612.

GAUDET, Olivier P; 30 rue des Trembles RR 1, Ste-Marg-Esterel QC J0T 1L0; Laval'55; Hon Member, Centre Hospitalier Laurentien; (450)228-3301

GAUDET, Pascale; CSSS Les Eskers de l'Abitibi, 622 4e rue O, Amos QC J9T 2S2; Sher'91; FRCSC; ObstGyn. Staff, CH Hôtel-Dieu d'Amos; Langs: English; (819)732-3341; Fax. (819)732-6484.

GAUDET, Rachel; CLSC Samuel de Champlain, 100-5811 boul Taschereau, Brossard QC J4Z 1A5; Sher'85; Clin Prof, Universite de Montreal; (450)445-4452; Fax. (450)445-5535.

GAUDET, Sylvie; CSSSG-Hop de Hull, 116 boul Lionel-Emond, Gatineau QC J8Y 1W7; Laval'91; MedOncol; Hem; IntMed. Staff HemOncol, Hull Hospital; (819)595-6000

GAUDETTE, Emilie; CHUS-Hopital Fleurimont, 3001 12e av N, Sherbrooke QC J1H 5N4; Sher'04; Respir; IntMed. Staff, Centre Hospitalier Universitaire de Sherbrooke-Hopital Fleurimont; (819)346-1110 x14252; Fax. (819)822-6763.

GAUDREAU, Andre; CSST Dir Reg de la Yamaska, 2710 rue Bachand, Saint-Hyacinthe QC J2S 8B6; Mon'71; IntMed; Rheum. (450)771-3900 x3996

GAUDREAU, Annie; Ctr Hosp Anna-Laberge, 200 boul Brisebois, Chateauguay QC J6K 4W8; Sher'07; Anes. Staff, Hôpital Anna-Laberge; (450)699-2425

GAUDREAU, Christiane; CHUM-Hop St-Luc, 1058 rue Saint-Denis, Montreal QC H2X 3J4; Mon'74; FRCPC; MedMicrobiol; Microbio & Infect Dis (P.Q.). Staff, Centre Hospitalier l'Université De Montréal (CHUM) - Hôpital Saint-luc; (514)890-8305 x36209; Fax. (514)412-7311; christiane.gaudreau.chum@ssss.gouv.qc.ca.

GAUDREAU, Eric; Clinique familiale de Thetford, 1001-926 rue Labbe, Thetford Mines QC G6G 2A8; Laval'91; Staff Hospitalistic, Hopital du CSS de la Region de Thetford; (418)338-3521; Fax. (418)338-4580.

GAUDREAU, Genevieve; Ctr Hosp Fleury, 2180 rue Fleury E, Montreal QC H2B 1K3; Laval'06; FRCSC; PlasSurg. Staff, Centre Hospitalier Fleury; (514)381-2000

GAUDREAU, Jean-Marc; CSSS du Nord de Lanaudière, 1000 boul Sainte-Anne, St-Charles-Brromee QC J6E 6J2; Mon'83; Staff, Centre Hospitalier Régional de Lanaudière; (450)834-5407; Fax. (450)834-5400.

GAUDREAU, Jules; Ministere Emploi et Solidarite, 1e-575 rue Saint-Amable, Quebec QC G1R 2G4; Laval'77; LMCC; Med Advisor, Ministere de l'Emploi et Solidarite Sociale; Langs: English; (418)528-6710

GAUDREAU, Marie-Josee; 430-1265 rue Berri, Montreal QC H2L 4X4; Mon'81; (514)483-7904; Fax. (514)843-6706.

GAUDREAU, Mario; Clinique Med-Dent de Montmagny, 104-63 boul Tache O, Montmagny QC G5V 3A3; Laval'83; Staff, CSSS de Montmagny-L'Islet; (418)248-9755; Fax. (418)248-9755; mgmf@globetrotter.qc.ca.

GAUDREAU, Pierre J; 79 rue Leblanc O, Longueuil QC J4J 1K1; Mon'68; Derm. (450)463-3881; Fax. (450)463-0908.

GAUDREAU, Vincent; Hôpital Laval, 2725 ch Sainte-Foy, Quebec QC G1V 4G5; Laval'02; FRCPC; IntMed; Critical Care Medicine (P.Q.); Respir. Staff, Hôpital Laval; (418)656-4747

GAUDREAULT, Claire; Clinique Horizon Sante Enr, 8 boul des Iles, Port-Cartier QC G5B 2J4; Sher'83; CCFP; FCFP; Staff, CLSC-CSSS de Port-Cartier; (418)766-4647; Fax. (418)766-4374.

GAUDREAULT, Gaetan; Poluclinique, 220-874 boul de l'Universite E, Chicoutimi QC G7H 6B9; Laval'75; ac Staff, Complexe hospitalier de la Sagamie; (418)545-1217; Fax. (418)545-4782.

GAUDREAULT, Gertie; Hop Charles Lemoyne, 3120 boul Taschereau, Greenfield Park QC J4V 2H1; Sher'84; CSPQ; FRCPC; IntMed; Cardiol. Staff, Hopital Charles LeMoyne; Staff, Centre Hospitalier Universitaire de Sherbrooke-Hopital Fleurimont; (450)466-5000; Fax. (450)466-5003.

GAUDREAULT, Gilles; Clinique Med Barrette, 150 boul Barette, Chicoutimi QC G7H 7W8; Laval'67; Ophth (P.Q.). Staff, CSSS de Lac-Saint Jean-Est; (418)545-2972

GAUDREAULT, Judith; CSSS de Rivière-de-Loup, 75 rue Saint-Henri, Riviere-Du-Loup QC G5R 2A4; Mon'88; CSPQ; FRCSC; GenSurg. Staff, Centre Hospitalier Regional du Grand-Portage; (418)868-1000; Fax. (418)868-1032.

GAUDREAULT, Lynn; Clin Med Fleury, 2157 rue Fleury E, Montreal QC H2B 1K1; McG'90; ABOtol; FRCSC; Otol (Laser Surgery). Ac Member, CSSS du Coeur de l'Isle Hôpital Jean-Talon; Langs: Spanish; (514)858-6110; Fax. (514)381-9872.

GAUDREAULT, Lynn; CHUS-Hop Hotel-Dieu, 580 rue Bowen S, Sherbrooke QC J1G 2E8; Sher'87; FRCPC; Psy (In-Patient Hospital Psychiatry). Staff, Centre Hospitalier Universitaire de Sherbrooke-Hôpital Hôtel-Dieu; Universite de Sherbrooke; (819)346-1110 x25545

GAUDREAULT, Marc; Clinique Med Caron, 721 rue Caron, Chicoutimi QC G7J 2Z9; Laval'90; (418)690-9395; Fax. (418)690-9412; marc.gaud@videotron.ca.

GAUDREAULT, Mauril D; CSSS de Chicoutimi, 305 rue Saint-Vallier, Chicoutimi QC G7H 5H6; Laval'72; Dir, Complexe hospitalier de la Sagamie; Assoc Dean, Universite de Sherbrooke; (418)541-1079; Fax. (418)541-1159.

GAUDREAULT, Melina; CSSS Maria-Chapdelaine, 2000 boul du Sacre-Coeur, Dolbeau-Mistassini QC G8L 2R5; Laval'09; CCFP; Staff, Centre Maria-Chapdelaine - CH de Dolbeau-Mistassini; (418)276-1234

GAUDREAULT, Nancy; CHUQ-Hotel-Dieu du Quebec, 11 Cote du Palais, Quebec QC G1R 2J6; Laval'97; Staff, Centre Hospitalier Universitaire de Québec (CHUQ) - Siege Social; (418)691-5151

GAUDREAULT, Nicolas; Polyclinique St-Jerome, 204-200 rue Durand, Saint-Jerome QC J7Z 7E2; Sher'01; CSPQ; FRCSC; GenSurg. Staff, Complexe hospitalier de la Sagamie; (450)438-5922; Fax. (450)438-1717.

GAUDREAULT, Pierre; Hôpital Ste-Justine, 3175 ch Cote-Ste-Catherine, Montreal QC H3T 1C5; Laval'76; FRCPC; Peds. Dir Section of Pharmacol & Toxicol, Hôpital Ste-Justine; Treas, Association des Pediatres de Quebec; Clin Adj Prof, Universite de Montreal; Langs: English; (514)345-4675; Fax. (514)345-4744; pierre_gaudreault@ssss.gouv.qc.ca.

GAUDREAULT, Valerie; CHUQ-Hotel-Dieu de Quebec, 11 Cote du Palais, Quebec QC G1R 2J6; Laval'03; FRCPC; IntMed (Clinician Investigator Program); Cardiol. Staff, Centre Hospitalier Universitaire de Québec (CHUQ) - Siege Social; (418)525-4444

GAUDRY, Stefane; CSSS de la Cote-de-Gaspe, 215 boul de York O, Gaspe QC G4X 2W2; Laval'04; CCFP; Staff, Centre Hospitalier de Gaspe; Clin Teach Staff, Université Laval; (418)368-3301

GAUL, H Penney; Gulf Canada Square, 300-401 9 Ave SW, Calgary AB T2P 3C5; Ott'85; FRCPC; DiagRad. (403)284-0230; Fax. (403)726-9883.

GAUL, Karine; CSSS de la Cote-De-Gaspe, 215 boul de York O, Gaspe QC G4X 2W2; Mon'99; CSPQ; FRCSC; GenSurg. Staff, Centre Hospitalier de Gaspe; (418)368-3301

GAUL, Martine; Clinique familiale des Hauts-B, 99 boul des Hauts-Bois, Sainte-Julie QC J3E 3J9; Sher'92; CCFP; Langs: Bilingual(French/English); (450)649-2490

GAUL, Neil; Pavillon Rosemont, 5689 boul Rosemont, Montreal QC H1T 2H1; Mon'81; CCFP; (514)252-3814; Fax. (514)252-3854.

GAULIN, Christian; CLSC-CHSLD du Haut St-Francois, 840 rue Papineau, Sherbrooke QC J1E 1Z2; Laval'91; (819)829-9772 x1616; Fax. (819)829-1789.

GAULIN, Colette; Ministere de la Sante, 1075 ch Sainte-Foy, Quebec QC G1S 2M1; Laval'84; MPH; Ac Staff, Centre Hospitalier Affilié Universitaire de Québec - Hôpital du St-Sacrement; Langs: English; French; (418)266-6733; Fax. (418)266-6708.

GAULIN, Francois; CSSS de Trois-Rivières, 1991 boul du Carmel, Trois-Rivieres QC G8Z 3R9; Mon'07; Anes. Staff, CSSS de Trois-Rivières; (819)697-3333

GAULT, Michael H; LA Medical Clinic, 30-5201 50 St, Leduc AB T9E 6T4; National (Ireland)'78; MB ChB; DObstRCOG; (780)986-9600; Fax. (780)986-9732.

GAUMOND, Marjolaine; CSSS de la Haute-Cote-Nord, RR 1 4 rue de l'Hopital CP 1000, Les Escoumins QC G0T 1K0; Sher'96; CCFP; Staff, Centre de santé des Côté-Nord; (418)233-2931

GAUMOND, Sylvie; CSSS de la Haute-Yamaska, 205 boul Leclerc O, Granby QC J2G 1T7; Laval'83; CSPQ; Anes. Staff Anes, Centre Hospitalier de Granby; (450)372-5491; Fax. (450)372-2478.

GAUMONT, J R Francois; 220-1575 boul de l'Avenir, Laval QC H7S 2N5; Laval'97; FRCPC; EmergMed. Staff, Hopital de la Cite de la santé; (450)696-1025

GAUMONT, Yves A; Centre Med Laennec, 400-1750 av de Vitre, Quebec QC G1J 1Z6; Laval'65; FRCPC; Peds. Assoc Staff, Centre Hospitalier Affilié Universitaire de Québec - Hôpital De L'Enfant Jésus; Ac Staff, Centre Hospitalier Universitaire De Québec - Pavillon De St-françois-d'assise; (418)522-4741; Fax. (418)522-7179.

GAUR, Shiva K; 112-885 Progress Ave, Scarborough ON M1H 3G3; Delhi (India)'77; Staff, Rouge Valley Health System - Centenary Health Centre Site; Langs: Hindi; Urdu; Gujarati; Punjabi; (416)289-0944; Fax. (416)439-3990.

GAURI, Mohammed A; Fort Walk in Clinic, 104-9425 94 Ave, Fort Saskatchewan AB T8L 1N6; (India)'75; MB BS; DCH; Staff Psy Fort Saskatchewan Correction Ctre, Fort Saskatchewan Health Centre; Langs: Hindi; Urdu; Punjabi; (780)997-0888; Fax. (780)997-0858; magauri@hotmail.com.

GAUSVIK, Amy L; Vulcan Clinic, PO Box 419 610 Elizabeth St S, Vulcan AB T0L 2B0; Cal'04; CCFP; (403)485-2216; Fax. (403)485-2218.

GAUTAM, Mamta; 1-72 Queen Elizabeth Dr, Ottawa ON K2P 1E4; Ott'85; FRCPC; Psy (Child & Adolescent Psychiatry). Asst Prof Psy, University of Ottawa; (613)729-3794; Fax. (613)739-5842; mgautam@rogers.com.

GAUTAMA, Sadhana K; 201-300 Veterans Blvd NE, Airdrie AB T4B 3P2; UBC'91; BSc; CCFP; (403)945-2461; Fax. (403)945-2471; mmnhand@shaw.ca.

GAUTHIER, Alain; Perth Family Med, 39 Drummond St W, Perth ON K7H 2J9; Tor'98; PhD; CCFP; Staff, Perth & Smiths Falls District Hospital - Perth Site (Great War Memorial Site); Langs: English; French; (613)264-2686; Fax. (613)264-0454.

GAUTHIER, Alain; CHUM-Hop Notre-Dame, 1560 rue Sherbrooke E, Montreal QC H2L 4M1; McG'97; CSPQ; FRCPC; Anes (Cardio & Thoracic Surgery). Staff, Centre Hospitalier l'Université de Montréal (CHUM) - Hôpital Notre-Dame; Langs: English; (514)890-8000 x26876; Fax. (514)412-7653.

GAUTHIER, Alain; Clinique Camu, 100-2984 boul Taschereau, Greenfield Park QC J4V 2G9; Mon'70; Staff, Hopital Charles LeMoyne; (450)466-4333

GAUTHIER, Aline; Dir de la Sante Publique, 930 rue Jacques-Cartier E, Chicoutimi QC G7H 7K9; Laval'75; Staff, Complexe hospitalier de la Sagamie; (418)545-4980 x429; Fax. (418)549-9710; aline.gauthier@ssss.gouv.qc.ca.

GAUTHIER, Andre L; McArthur Med Centre, 390 McArthur Ave, Vanier ON K1L 6N6; Ott'75; CCFP; (613)741-1134; Fax. (613)741-4276.

GAUTHIER, Andreanne; CHUM-Hotel-Dieu, 3840 rue Saint-Urbain, Montreal QC H2W 1T8; Mon'06; Respir; IntMed. Staff, Centre Hospitalier l'Université de Montréal (CHUM) - Hôtel-Dieu; (514)890-8000

GAUTHIER, Anne-Genevieve; CSSS de Memphremagog, 50 rue Saint-Patrice E, Magog QC J1X 3X3; Laval'00; Staff, Centre Hospitalier et CLSC de Memphremagog; (819)843-3381

GAUTHIER, Ariane; CLSC Haute-Ville-des Rivieres, 55 ch Sainte-Foy, Quebec QC G1R 1S9; Mon'01; CCFP; Staff, CH-CHSLD de Papineau - Pavillon du centre hospitalier; (418)641-2572; Fax. (418)641-0282.

GAUTHIER, Beauregard; Centre Med St-Bruno, 1435 rue Roberval, Saint-Bruno QC J3V 3P7; Mon'71; (450)653-3041; Fax. (450)653-5518.

GAUTHIER, Benoit; Hotel-Dieu du Sacre-Coeur, 1 av du Sacre-Coeur, Quebec QC G1N 2W1; Laval'79; BSc(Med); FRCPC; Psy (Child & Adolescent Psychiatry). Staff Adolescent Psy, Hotel-Dieu du Sacre-Coeur de Jesus de Quebec; Prof, Université Laval; (418)529-6851 x20364; Fax. (418)691-0750.

GAUTHIER, Benoit; CSSS de Memphremagog, 50 rue Saint-Patrice E, Magog QC J1X 3X3; Sher'93; Staff, Centre Hospitalier et CLSC de Memphremagog; (819)843-2572; Fax. (819)843-2786.

GAUTHIER, Bernard; Clinique Med Jean Talon-Pie IX, 4679 rue Jean-Talon E, Saint-Leonard QC H1S 1K3; Mon'83; (514)374-5901; Fax. (514)374-1668.

GAUTHIER, Bernard G A; Inst Albert Prevost, 6555 boul Gouin O, Montreal QC H4K 1B3; Mon'73; FRCPC; Psy. Ac Staff, Hôpital du Sacre-Coeur de Montréal; (514)338-4300

GAUTHIER, Cajetan M; Regie l'Assurance Maladie QC, 44-1125 Grande Allee O, Quebec QC G1S 1E7; Laval'67; ObstGyn (P.Q.) (Echography). Langs: English; (418)682-5144 x4022; Fax. (418)643-3858.

GAUTHIER, Carole; 305-5835 boul Leger, Montreal-Nord QC H1G 6E1; Mon'82; Langs: English; (514)324-3818; Fax. (514)324-4108.

GAUTHIER, Celine; UMF CHRTR-Pavillon St-Joseph, 2e-731 rue Sainte-Julie, Trois-Rivieres QC G9A 1Y1; Sher'81; Staff Gen Med & Obst, Centre Hospitalier Rouyn-Noranda; Staff Med, Centre de Sante et de Services Sociaux; Staff Med, CLSC Malauze; Staff Med, Centre Hospitalier de Soins de Longue Duree; Langs: English; (819)372-3536; Fax. (819)372-3509.

GAUTHIER, Chantal; Clinique Med Pierre-Boucher, 1615 boul Jacques-Cartier E, Longueuil QC J4M 2X1; Mon'93; (450)468-6223

GAUTHIER, Charles E; PO Box 2548 Stn Main, Banff AB T1L 1C3; Cal'89; BSc; CCFP; CCFP(E.M.); FCFP; Med Staff, Covenant Health - Banff Mineral Springs Hospital; Med Staff, Foothills Medical Centre; (403)609-5075; Fax. (403)762-4193; cegauthier@telusplanet.net.

GAUTHIER, Christine; CSSS de Memphremagog, 50 rue Saint-Patrice E, Magog QC J1X 3X3; Sher'87; FRCPC; IntMed. Staff, Centre Hospitalier et CLSC de Memphremagog; (819)843-3381

GAUTHIER, Claude; 7732 rte Marie-Victorin, Contrecoeur QC J0L 1C0; Laval'82; (450)587-2133; Fax. (450)401-0695.

GAUTHIER, Claude; 855-76 rue Dalhousie, Quebec QC G1K 8W6; Mon'78; Staff, Centre Hospitalier Affilié Universitaire de Québec - Hôpital De L'Enfant Jésus; (418)649-5604

GAUTHIER, Claude P; CSSS de Rimouski-Neigette, CP 3150 Succ A 150 av Rouleau, Rimouski QC G5L 5T1; Sher'76; Assoc Staff Commun Health, Hôpital Regional Rimouski; (418)724-8464; Fax. (418)723-3103.

GAUTHIER, Claudie; Clin Med Privee-Rendez-Vous Sa, 101-3195 boul de la Piniere, Terrebonne QC J6X 4P7; Sher'98; CCFP; CCFP(E.M.); Staff Emerg, Hopital de la Cite de la santé; (450)824-1515

GAUTHIER, Daniel; Clinique Med Sainte-Rosalie, 4700 boul Laurier E, Saint-Hyacinthe QC J2R 2C2; Mon'79; Staff, Centre Hospitalier Honore-Mercier; (450)799-5511; Fax. (450)799-5517.

GAUTHIER, Daniel; Clin Ophtalmologie Drummondvil, 103-4534 boul Saint-Joseph, Saint-Nicephore QC J2A 1B5; Mon'78; FRCSC; Ophth. Ac Staff, Hôpital Sainte-croix; Langs: English; (819)475-4200; Fax. (819)475-4246.

GAUTHIER, Danielle; UMF Laurier, 2875 boul Laurier, Quebec QC G1V 2M2; Sher'75; (418)654-2701

GAUTHIER, Danny; 1300 rue Sherbrooke E, Montreal QC H2L 1M2; Mon'94; FRCSC; Ophth. (514)521-4488; Fax. (514)521-8517.

GAUTHIER, Dominic; Clinique Med St-Eugene, 397 rue Jacques-Cartier S, St-Jean-Sur-Richel QC J3B 7T1; Sher'00; LMCC; CCFP; Staff, Hôpital du Haut-Richelieu; Langs: English; (450)347-3748; Fax. (450)347-4287.

GAUTHIER, Dominic; CSSS des Aurores Boreales, CP 6000 679 2e rue E, La Sarre QC J9Z 2X7; Sher'09; CCFP; Staff, Centre Hospitalier La Sarre; (819)333-2311

GAUTHIER, Emmanuelle; CSSS de Haut Saint-Maurice, 885 boul Ducharme, La Tuque QC G9X 3C1; Laval'93; LMCC; Staff EmergMed, Centre Hospitalier Saint-Joseph de la Turque; (819)523-3084; Fax. (819)523-5019; emmanuelle_gauthier@ssss.gouv.qc.ca.

GAUTHIER, Francois; College des Med du Quebec, 2170 boul Rene-Levesque O, Montreal QC H3H 2T8; Mon'70; MBA; FamilyMed. Prof, College des Medecins du Quebec; Langs: English; French; (514)933-4441 x5213; Fax. (514)933-2291.

GAUTHIER, Gilles; Inst U en Sante Mentale de QC, 2601 ch de la Canardiere, Quebec QC G1J 2G3; Laval'97; Ministry of Social Services; Staff, Hema-Quebec; Médecin, Institut Universitaire Sante; Médecin, Anapharm Inc; Langs: English; (418)663-5321; gillesrgauthier@hotmail.com.

GAUTHIER, Gilles; Clinique du Havre, 79A rue Jacques-Cartier, Gaspe QC G4X 1M5; Mon'80; (418)368-5609; Fax. (418)368-6498.

GAUTHIER, Guylaine; Clinique Med de Nicolet, 1691 boul Louis-Frechette, Nicolet QC J3T 1Z6; Laval'91; Staff, Hôpital de Christ-Roi; (819)293-2022

GAUTHIER, Helene; Clinique Medicale Optimum, 158-1 Pl Laval, Laval QC H7N 1A1; Sher'98; Staff, Hopital de la Cite de la santé; (450)668-7400

GAUTHIER, Isabelle; CHUS-Hop Fleurimont, 3001 12e av N, Sherbrooke QC J1H 5N4; Mon'05; FRCPC; RadOncol. Staff, Centre Hospitalier Universitaire de Sherbrooke-Hopital Fleurimont; (819)346-1110

GAUTHIER, Jacques; Clinique Med Rock Forest, 1-4870 boul Bourque, Sherbrooke QC J1N 3S5; Mon'78; Consultant, Centre Hospitalier Universitaire de Sherbrooke-Hôpital Hôtel-Dieu; (819)820-2673; Fax. (819)820-2112.

GAUTHIER, Jacques; CHUM-Hop St-Luc, 6120-1058 rue Saint-Denis, Montreal QC H2X 3J4; Laval'74; FRCSC; Psy. Staff, Centre Hospitalier l'Université De Montréal (CHUM) - Hôpital Saint-luc; (514)890-8000 x36155

GAUTHIER, Jean; Base Militaire Valcartier, CP 1000 Bdp Succ Forces, Courcelette QC G0A 4Z0; Mon'10; CCFP; (418)844-5000

GAUTHIER, Jean; CSSS de Saint-Jerome, 290 rue de Montigny, Saint-Jerome QC J7Z 5T3; Sher'82; CSPQ; FRCPC; AnatPath. Staff, Hôtel-Dieu de Saint-Jérôme; (450)431-8200 x2135; Fax. (450)431-8206.

GAUTHIER, Jean-Claude; The Ottawa Hosp-Civic Campus, 326-1053 Carling Ave, Ottawa ON K1Y 4E9; Ott'07; GenSurg. Staff, The Ottawa Hospital - Civic Campus; (613)798-5555; Fax. (613)761-4124.

GAUTHIER, Jean-Elzear; CSSS de la Haute-Yamaska, 205 boul Leclerc O, Granby QC J2G 1T7; Mon'89; CSPQ; Anes. Staff, Centre Hospitalier de Granby; (450)375-8000 x2219

GAUTHIER, Jean-Guy; Carrefour Med Vallee Richelieu, 665 boul Sir-Wilfrid-Laurier, Beloeil QC J3G 4J1; Laval'78; (450)467-0088; Fax. (450)467-4936.

GAUTHIER, Jeannot; Centre Med de la Vallee, 1-22 rue du Pont, Amqui QC G5J 3T5; Laval'68; Langs: Bilingual(French/English); (418)629-6611; Fax. (418)629-4484.

GAUTHIER, Johanne; Ctr Hosp Trois-Riv-St-Joseph, 2E-731 rue Sainte-Julie, Trois-Rivieres QC G9A 1Y1; Mon'92; Staff, Centre Hospitalier Regional de Trois-Rivieres; Staff Clin de Med Familiale UMF 6MF, CSSS de Trois-Rivières; Langs: English; (819)372-3536; Fax. (819)372-3509.

GAUTHIER, Josee; CRSSS Baie-James-Chibougamau, 51 3e rue, Chibougamau QC G8P 1N1; Laval'99; CCFP; Staff, CRSSS de la Baie-James; (418)748-2676; Fax. (418)748-2549.

GAUTHIER, Jules; Dr Jules Gauthier, 201-425 boul Cure-Poirier O, Longueuil QC J4J 2H3; Laval'79; Langs: English; (450)651-8888; Fax. (450)651-5586; ipa@bellnet.ca.

GAUTHIER, Julie; Clinique Med Familliale Chandl, CP 788 60B boul Rene Levesque E, Chandler QC G0C 1K0; Laval'92; Staff, Centre Hospitalier de Chandler; (418)689-3344

GAUTHIER, Julie; Hop Santa Cabrini Ospedale, 5655 rue Saint-Zotique E, Montreal QC H1T 1P7; Mon'03; CCFP; Staff, Hôpital Santa Cabrini Ospedale; (514)252-6546; Fax. (514)252-6453.

GAUTHIER, Karine; CLSC Jardin Du Quebec, 509 rue Saint-Jacques, Napierville QC J0J 1L0; Mon'05; CCFP; (450)245-3336; Fax. (450)245-0278.

GAUTHIER, Kathryn; Family Med Associates, 306-267 O'Connor St, Ottawa ON K2P 1V3; McM'80; BA; CCFP; Ac Staff Maternal & Newborn Care, The Ottawa Hospital - Civic Campus; Asst Prof Dept of Fam Med, University of Ottawa; (613)233-6652

GAUTHIER, Louis-Marie; 134 8e rue, Shippagan NB E8S 1B7; Laval'73; (506)336-4666

GAUTHIER, Louise F; The Ottawa Hosp-Gen Campus, 1401 CCW-501 Smyth Rd, Ottawa ON K1H 8L6; Ott'79; FRCPC; Anes. Staff Anes, The Ottawa Hospital - General Campus; Langs: English; French; (613)737-8187; Fax. (613)737-8189.

GAUTHIER, Louise F; Le Carrefour Medical, 200-3030 boul Le carrefour, Laval QC H7T 2P5; Mon'79; (450)686-8899; Fax. (450)686-7466.

GAUTHIER, Louise; CLSC des Seigneuries, 203-160 boul de Montarville, Boucherville QC J4B 6S2; Mon'89; CSPQ; FRCSC; GenSurg. Staff General Surg, Centre Hospitalier de Chandler; Langs: English; (450)449-1119

GAUTHIER, Luke E; IWK Health Centre, PO Box 9700 Rpo CSC 5850-5980 University Ave, Halifax NS B3K 6R8; Mem'07; FRCSC; OrthSurg. Staff, IWK Health Centre; (902)473-7015; Fax. (902)473-4442.

GAUTHIER, M Todd; North Hastings Famuly Hlth Tea, 1P Manor Lane, Bancroft ON K0C 1C0; NOSM'10; CCFP; (613)332-5692

GAUTHIER, Marcel; Clinique Med Des 21, 101-171 6e rue, La Baie QC G7B 0A3; Laval'78; Staff, CHSLD-CLSC Cleophas-Claveau; (418)544-3331; Fax. (514)544-7571.

GAUTHIER, Marie-Sophie; Clinique D'ORL du Littoral, 111-822 boul Sainte-Anne, Rimouski QC G5M 1J5; Mon'98; FRCSC; Otol. Staff, Hôpital Regional Rimouski; Staff, CSSS de la Matapedia; Staff, Centre Hospitalier de Matane; Staff, Centre Hospitalier de Gaspe; Langs: Bilingual(French/English); (418)724-0042; Fax. (418)723-0180.

GAUTHIER, Marlene; MUHC-Royal Victoria Hosp, 687 av des Pins O, Montreal QC H3A 1A1; Laval'75; CSPQ; FRCPC; Anes. Staff, McGill University Health Centre - Royal Victoria Hospital; Teach Staff, McGill University; (514)934-1934 x34880

GAUTHIER, Martin G; 4000 av Marcil, Montreal QC H4A 2Z6; Mon'79; Psy. Staff, McGill University Health Centre - Montreal Children's Hospital; (514)485-6747; Fax. (514)412-4346; martin.gauthier3@sympatico.ca.

GAUTHIER, Michel D J; Northeastern Ontario Med Offic, B1-2009 Long Lake Rd, Sudbury ON P3E 6C3; Wes'78; CCFP; (705)586-3601

GAUTHIER, Michel J; CMS-CMI Monteregie, 260-1215 ch du Tremblay, Longueuil QC J4N 1R4; Sher'85; ACLS; (450)442-1018; Fax. (450)442-1967.

GAUTHIER, Michel; 201-835 boul des Recollets, Trois-Rivieres QC G8Z 3W5; Laval'85; Staff, Centre de santé Cloutier-du-Rivage; (819)375-6666; Fax. (819)375-3423.

GAUTHIER, Michel; Clinique Place du Marche, 3490 boul des Sources, Dollard-D-Ormeaux QC H9B 1Z9; Sher'83; (514)421-3762; Fax. (514)683-4540.

GAUTHIER, Michel; SAAQ, CP 266 CSP Magog, Magog QC J1X 3W8; Mon'74; (819)679-0957

GAUTHIER, Nadia; Clinique Med de la Cite, 101-3801 rue de Montcalm, Jonquiere QC G7X 1W1; Sher'97; (418)542-1510; Fax. (418)542-1512.

GAUTHIER, Nadine; The Ottawa Hosp-Gen Campus, CCW 1682-501 Smyth Rd, Ottawa ON K1H 8L6; Ott'03; FRCPC; IntMed; Cardiol. Staff, The Ottawa Hospital - General Campus; (613)737-8165; Fax. (613)739-6727.

GAUTHIER, Nathalie; Hop Charles-Lemoyne, 3120 boul Taschereau, Greenfield Park QC J4V 2H1; Mon'88; FRCSC; Neursurg (P.Q.). Staff, Hopital Charles LeMoyne; (450)466-5053

GAUTHIER, Nicolas; Clin Medicale Privee, 102-17 boul de la Salette, Saint-Jerome QC J5L 2H8; Laval'89; (450)569-4777; Fax. (450)569-4688.

GAUTHIER, Normand; CHUS-Hop Hotel-Dieu, 580 rue Bowen S, Sherbrooke QC J1G 2E8; Mon'87; FRCPC; DiagRad. Staff, Centre Hospitalier Universitaire de Sherbrooke-Hôpital Hôtel-Dieu; (819)346-1110

GAUTHIER, Patrice; CSSS de Trois-Rivières, 1991 boul du Carmel, Trois-Rivieres QC G8Z 3R9; Sher'98; FRCPC; IntMed; Respir. Staff, CSSS de Trois-Rivières; (819)697-3333; Fax. (819)372-3528.

GAUTHIER, Philippe; CHUM-Hop Notre-Dame, 1560 rue Sherbrooke E, Montreal QC H2L 4M1; Mon'76; AB(Gyn/Oncol); FRCSC; ObstGyn (Gynecologic Oncology). Staff Gyn/Oncol, Centre Hospitalier l'Université de Montréal (CHUM) - Hôpital Notre-Dame; assoc Prof, Universite de Montreal; (514)890-8000 x27244; Fax. (514)412-7605; philippe.gauthier.chum@ssss.gouv.qc.ca.

GAUTHIER, Pierre A; 200-3030 boul Le carrefour, Laval QC H7T 2P5; McG'76; CCFP; Staff, St Mary's Hospital Centre; adj Prof, McGill University; Langs: English; German; (450)686-8899; Fax. (450)686-7466.

GAUTHIER, Pierre; CSSS de Sept-Iles, 45 rue du Piere-Divet, Sept-Iles QC G4R 3N7; Mon'64; FRCPC; Peds. Staff, Centre Hospitalier Regional de Sept-Iles; (418)962-1216; Fax. (418)968-2111.

GAUTHIER, Pierre; Clinique ORL, 203-222 rue de la Visitation, St-Charles-Brromee QC J6E 4N5; Laval'78; FRCSC; Otol (Skin Cancer). Staff, Centre Hospitalier Régional de Lanaudière; Langs: English; (450)759-1241; Fax. (450)759-3737.

GAUTHIER, Raphaelle; CSSS de Trois-Rivières, 1991 boul du Carmel, Trois-Rivieres QC G8Z 3R9; Mon'09; CCFP; CCFP(E.M.); Staff, CSSS de Trois-Rivières; (819)697-3333

GAUTHIER, Remi; La Cite Medicale, 295-2600 boul Laurier, Quebec QC G1V 4T3; Laval'70; (418)781-0480; Fax. (418)659-7072.

GAUTHIER, Richard; Hop Maisonneuve-Rosemont, 5415 boul de l'Assomption, Montreal QC H1T 2M4; Mon'80; FRCPC; Respir. Staff, Hopital Maisonneuve-Rosemont; (514)252-3400; Fax. (514)252-3848.

GAUTHIER, Robert J; Hôpital Ste-Justine, 3175 ch Cote-Ste-Catherine, Montreal QC H3T 1C5; Mon'70; FACOG; FRCSC; ObstGyn (Fetal & Maternal Medicine). Chief ObstGyn, Hôpital Ste-Justine; Prof ObstGyn, Universite de Montreal; (514)345-4706; Fax. (514)345-4648; robert_gauthier@ssss.gouv.qc.ca.

GAUTHIER, Serge G; McGill Centre, 6825 boul Lasalle, Verdun QC H4H 1R3; Mon'73; AB; FRCPC; Neur (Geriatric Medicine). Consultant, Douglas Mental Health University Institute; Consultant, McGill University Health Centre - Montreal Neurological Hospital; Prof Psy Neurology, McGill University; Langs: Bilingual(French/English); (514)766-2010; Fax. (514)888-4050; serge.gauthier@mcgill.ca.

GAUTHIER, Serge; Clin de Pedopsy de l'Est de La, 485-2 Place Laval, Laval QC H7N 5N6; Mon'73; FRCPC; Psy (Pediatric Psychiatry). Staff Pedopsychiatry Serv, Hôpital du Sacre-Coeur de Montréal; Asst Clin Prof, Universite de Montreal; Langs: Bilingual(French/English); (450)669-5600; Fax. (450)669-0997; serge051@sympatico.ca.

GAUTHIER, Shaun W; Brandon Reg Hlth Ctr, 150 McTavish Ave E, Brandon MB R7A 2B3; Man'00; CCFP; CCFP(E.M.); Staff, Brandon Regional Health Centre; (204)726-1122

GAUTHIER, Steve; CSSS du Nord de Lanaudière, 1000 boul Sainte-Anne, St-Charles-Boromee QC J6E 6J2; Sher'00; DiagRad. Staff, Centre Hospitalier Régional de Lanaudière; (450)759-8222 x2845

GAUTHIER, Sylvianne; Clin Fam des Basses Laurentide, 2100 boul Labelle, Saint-Jerome QC J7Y 1S8; Sher'89; (450)565-6493; Fax. (450)565-1099.

GAUTHIER, Sylvie; CSSS Pierre Boucher, 1333 boul Jacques-Cartier E, Longueuil QC J4M 2A5; Mon'89; FRCPC; IntMed. Staff, Centre Hospitalier Pierre Boucher; (450)468-8111

GAUTHIER, Valere; 1-206 ch de la Beauce, Beauharnois QC J6N 2N1; Laval'75; Physician, Ministere Affaires Sociales(Quebec); Langs: English; (450)225-1900; Fax. (450)225-1900; gauthiervalere@yahoo.ca.

GAUTHIER, Veronique; CSSS De Saint-Jerome, 290 rue de Montigny, Saint-Jerome QC J7Z 5T3; Mon'08; CCFP; CCFP(E.M.); Staff, Hôtel-Dieu de Saint-Jérôme; (450)431-8200

GAUTHIER, Yvan; CHU De Quebec, D3000-1401 18e rue, Quebec QC G1J 1Z4; Laval'86; LMCC; FRCPC; Psy (Psycho Pharmacology). Staff, Centre Hospitalier Affilié Universitaire de Québec - Hôpital De L'Enfant Jésus; Psychiatre, Institut Universitaire Sante; Staff Emerg Psy Services, CHU De Quebec; Prof, Université Laval; (418)649-5769; Fax. (418)649-5934; citadin@videotron.ca.

GAUTHIER-BIZIER, Sabrina; Clinique Med Cadillac, 3435 rue Bossuet, Montreal QC H1M 2M1; Mon'10; CCFP; (514)253-1211

GAUTHIER-CHOUINARD, Marie; Hôpital Ste-Justine, 3175 ch Cote-Sainte-Catherine, Montreal QC H3T 1C5; Laval'73; FRCPC; Peds. ac Staff, Hôpital Ste-Justine; (514)345-4931 x5353; Fax. (514)345-4822.

GAUTHIER-PARE, Anne-Sophie; CSSS de Laval, 1755 boul Rene-Laennec, Laval QC H7M 3L9; Mon'04; FRCPC; RadOncol. Staff, Hopital de la Cite de la santé; (450)668-1010

GAUTIER, Jean-Joseph; CSSS de Saint-Jerome, 290 rue de Montigny, Saint-Jerome QC J7Z 5T3; Montpellier (France)'71; CSPQ; Cardiol (P.Q.). ac Staff, Hôtel-Dieu de Saint-Jérôme; (450)431-8495

GAUTREAU, Renelle; 208-600 boul Dieppe, Dieppe NB E1A 9J8; Sher'09; CCFP; (506)857-1680; Fax. (506)857-1669.

GAUVIN, Constance; Centre Med St Redempteur, 210-600 Rte 116, Saint-Nicolas QC G7A 4X8; Laval'78; (418)831-4455; Fax. (418)831-7967.

GAUVIN, France; Hôpital Ste-Justine, 3175 ch Cote-Sainte-Catherine, Montreal QC H3T 1C5; Mon'93; ABPeds; FRCPC; Peds (Emergency Medicine). Staff Peds, Hôpital Ste-Justine; (514)345-4931 x6812; Fax. (514)345-7731; france_gauvin@ssss.gouv.qc.ca.

GAUVIN, Michel; CSSS du Rocher-Perce, CP 3300 451 rue Mgr Ross, Chandler QC G0C 1K0; Laval'68; CSPQ; Anes. Staff, Centre Hospitalier de Chandler; (418)689-2261

GAUVIN, Micheline; 275 av Brittany, Mont-Royal QC H3P 3C2; Mon'87; Ac Member, CHSLD Vigi Reine Elizabeth; Ac Member, CHSLD Vigi Dollard des Ormeaux; Ac Member, CHSLD Vigi Mont-Royal; Ac Member, CHSLD Vigi L'Orchidée Blanche; Med Staff, CHSLD Vigi Marie-Claret; Langs: English; French; (514)739-5593 x301; Fax. (514)733-7973; mgauvin@vigisante.com.

GAUVIN, Nathalie; UMF CHRTR-Pavillon St-Joseph, 2F-731 rue Sainte-Julie, Trois-Rivieres QC G9A 1Y1; McG'94; CCFP; Staff, Centre Hospitalier Regional de Trois-Rivieres; (819)372-3536

GAUVREAU, Alain; Clinique Med des Monts, 20 boul Sainte-Anne O, Ste-Anne-des-Monts QC G4V 1P6; Mon'82; Staff, Centre Hospitalier des Monts; Chief Medical Services, Centre d'Accueil de Cap-Chat; Langs: Bilingual(French/English); (418)763-5731; Fax. (418)763-7401.

GAUVREAU, Frederic; Hop Charles LeMoyne, 3120 boul Taschereau, Greenfield Park QC J4V 2H1; Laval'01; CSPQ; FRCSC; GenSurg (Surgical Oncology); General Surgical Oncology (P.Q.). Staff, Hopital Charles LeMoyne; (450)466-5000

GAUVREAU, Lyette; Clinique Med Acces-Sante, 3-8 rue du Terminus E, Rouyn-Noranda QC J9X 3B4; Sher'94; Staff, Centre Hospitalier Rouyn-Noranda; (819)764-6185; Fax. (819)762-6079.

GAUVREAU, Michel; Clinique Med Fam Mailloux, 130-1900 av Mailloux, Quebec QC G1J 5B9; Laval'71; Langs: Bilingual(French/English); (418)667-7014; Fax. (418)667-5808.

GAUVREAU, Robert; Barrhaven Sport Medicine, 3-3570 Strandherd Dr, Nepean ON K2J 5L4; Ott'80; Dip(SportsMed); Staff Surgical Assistant, The Ottawa Hospital - General Campus; (613)823-4991; Fax. (613)823-6221.

GAUVREAU-GADOUA, Louise; Polyclinique Masson, 200-3425 rue Masson, Montreal QC H1X 1R6; Mon'74; (514)376-9961; Fax. (514)376-8100.

GAUZE, Joseph; Westmount Med Bldg, 550-5025 rue Sherbrooke O, Montreal QC H4A 1S9; Sask'64; LMCC; FRCSC; Otol. Hon Staff, Sir Mortimer B Davis Jewish General; Ac Staff, St Mary's Hospital Centre; Langs: English; French; (514)482-6320; Fax. (514)482-6009.

GAVLAS, Shirley J; Medicentre Pincourt, 88 5e Av, Pincourt QC J7V 5K7; McG'85; (514)425-1000; Fax. (514)425-1288.

GAVSIE, Adam; Centre De Medecine Familiale, 1141 boul St Joseph E, Montreal QC H2J 1L3; McG'96; CCFP; Langs: Spanish; French; (514)908-6246; Fax. (514)908-6247.

GAWEL, Marek J; 806-1849 Yonge St, Toronto ON M4S 1Y2; Cambridge (England)'71; FRCP; FRCPC; Neur. Staff, Rouge Valley Health System - Centenary Health Centre Site; Staff, Sunnybrook Health Sciences Centre; Assoc Prof, University of Toronto; Langs: Polish; (416)485-7749; marek.gawel@wchospital.ca.

GAWLEY, Emily; Misericordia Community Hlth, PO Box 1998 16940 87 Ave NW, Edmonton AB T5R 4H5; (Other Foreign)'07; MB BCh; BAO; CCFP; CCFP(E.M.); (780)735-2000

GAWLEY, William F; 201-37979 Cleveland Ave PO Box 198, Squamish BC V8B 0A2; Dublin (Ireland)'76; FRCS(Ed); MB BCh; BAO; FRCSC; GenSurg. Staff Gen Surg, Squamish General Hospital / Hilltop House; (604)815-4552

GAWLIK, Janusz D; 301 Metcalfe St, Ottawa ON K2P 1R9; Lodz (Poland)'71; FRCPC; Psy (Adult Psychiatry). Langs: Polish; (613)569-2300; jgawlik@gmail.com.

GAWLINSKI, Mary J; Richmond Square Med Ctr, 70-3915 51 St SW, Calgary AB T3E 6N1; Cal'78; CCFP; FCFP; (403)229-2273

GAWMAN, William G; True North Imaging, 751 Victoria St S, Kitchener ON N2M 5N4; Tor'55; DABR; FRCPC; DiagRad (Bone Radiol).

GAWRON, Stephen J; Guelph Family Health Team, 101-83 Dawson Rd, Guelph ON N1H 1B1; Tor'87; BSc; Med Constable Health & Performance Centre, University Of Guelph; (519)766-1360

GAY, Brian C; Minor Surgery Clinic, 207-194 Main St, Ottawa ON K1S 1C2; Ott'51; FACS; DABS; FRCSC; GenSurg (Aviation). Ac Associate Surg, The Ottawa Hospital - Riverside Campus; (613)232-0658; Fax. (613)232-3606.

GAY, Raymond B; 205-39 Robertson Rd, Ottawa ON K2H 8R2; Ott'93; FRCSC; GenSurg. Langs: Bilingual(English/French); (613)828-0896; Fax. (613)828-4807.

GAY, Raymond J; 7-1848 Paris St, Sudbury ON P3E 3C7; Dublin (Ireland)'66; MB ChB; BAO; FRCS(Lond & Ire); FRCSC; GenSurg. Hon Staff Dept of Surg, Health Sciences North-St Joseph's Health Centre; Asst Prof Surg, Northern Ontario School of Medicine-Laurentian University; (705)522-4477; Fax. (705)674-2504; raymondguy@hotmail.com.

GAYAPERSHAD, Thasvir K; Carbonear Gen Hosp, 86 Highroad South, Carbonear NL A1Y 1A4; Southern Africa (South Africa)'99; MB ChB; CCFP; Staff, Carbonear General Hospital; (709)945-5111; thasvir@hotmail.com.

GAYDA, Edward X; Northern Mental Health Unit, 300 3rd Ave W, Prince Rupert BC V8J 1L4; Seattle (USA)'79; (250)622-6310

GAYED, Alaa M M; Newport Med Clinic, 100-205 Newport Dr, New Westminster BC V3H 5C9; Ain Shams (Egypt)'94; MB BCh; CCFP; (604)461-0013

GAYLE, Barrington A; Leslie Medical Centre, 407-4800 Leslie St, North York ON M2J 2K9; Tor'66; FRCPC; IntMed. Teacher, University of Toronto; Langs: Spanish; (416)491-8159; Fax. (416)491-0022.

GAYTAN-GRAHAM, Silvia R M; Sudbury Reg Hosp-Laurentian Si, 41 Ramsey Lake Rd, Sudbury ON P3E 5J1; (Mexico)'79; MSc; FRCPC; NeurPath; AnatPath. Staff, Health Sciences North-Laurentian Site; Langs: Spanish; (705)675-4779; Fax. (705)675-4780; sgraham@hrsrh.on.ca.

GAYTON, David C; Peace Arch Hosp, 15521 Russell Ave, White Rock BC V4B 2R4; UBC'76; FRCPC; IntMed; GeriatricMed. Staff Geriatric Med, Peace Arch Hospital; (604)535-4577; Fax. (604)535-4587; david.gayton@fraserhealth.ca.

GAZALA, Khalid; Halton HS Corp-Oakville, 327 Reynolds St, Oakville ON L6J 3L7; Baghdad (Iraq)'98; FRCPC; Neur. Staff, Halton Healthcare Services Corporation - Oakville Site; Langs: Arabic; (905)845-2571 x6765

GAZALA, Sayf; University of Alberta Hosp, 8440 112 St NW, Edmonton AB T6G 2B7; (Iraq)'04; MB ChB; Staff, University of Alberta Hospital; (780)407-8822

GAZELEY, Sharon G; Regent Park Comm Health Centre, 465 Dundas St E, Toronto ON M5A 2B2; McM'95; BSc; CCFP; CCFP; Langs: Bilingual(English/French); (416)203-4507; Fax. (416)364-0822.

GAZENDAM, Mary Kate; Amherstview Med Centre, 18 Manitou Cres W, Amherstview ON K7N 1S3; Qns'87; CCFP; FCFP; Assoc Staff, Kingston General Hospital; Assoc Staff Family Med, Hotel-Dieu Hospital; (613)634-9898; Fax. (613)634-3555.

GAZIT, Vered; IWK Health Centre, PO Box 9700 Rpo CSC 5850-5980 University Ave, Halifax NS B3K 6R8; Hadassah (Israel)'99; Staff, IWK Health Centre; (902)470-8823; Fax. (902)470-7248.

GAZZOLA, Steve; Rouge Valley-Ajax & Pickering, 580 Harwood Ave S, Ajax ON L1S 2J4; Tor'92; FRCPC; DiagRad. Staff, Grey Bruce Health Services - Owen Sound; Staff, Rouge Valley Health System - Ajax & Pickering Health Centre Site; (905)683-2320

GBINIGIE, Nosakhare I; Regina Qu'Appelle HR-Pasqua, 4101 Dewdney Ave, Regina SK S4T 1A5; Lagos University (Other Foreign)'87; FRCPC; Anes. Staff, Pasqua Hospital; (306)766-2222

GBINIGIE, Victoria A; Regina First Consultant Physic, 3125F E Woodhams Dr, Regina SK S4V 2R5; lagos (Nigeria)'94; FRCPC; Psy. (306)522-3043; Fax. (306)522-3044.

GDALEVITCH, Marie; Shriners Hosp for Children, 1529 av Cedar, Montreal QC H3G 1A6; McG'04; FRCSC; OrthSurg. Staff, Shriners Hospitals For Children - Canada; (514)282-7150

GDALEVITCH, Perry; Vancouver Gen Hosp, 855 12th Ave W, Vancouver BC V5Z 1M9; McG'04; FRCSC; PlasSurg. Staff, Vancouver General Hospital - Centennial Pavillion; (604)875-4084

GDIH, Gdih Abulgasem M; Winnipeg Clinic, 425 St Mary Ave, Winnipeg MB R3C 0N2; (Libya)'98; FRCSC; Ophth. (204)957-3274

GE, Hong; Markham Heritage Hlth Clinic, 218-5970 16th Ave, Markham ON L3P 7R1; Shanghai (China)'95; FRCPC; Public Health & Preventive Med;CCFP; (905)471-2967; Fax. (905)471-0476.

GEADAH, Christian; Centre Med Robinson Inc, 4 rue Robinson N, Granby QC J2G 8Z9; Mon'97; CCFP; Staff, Centre Hospitalier Regional de Sept-Iles; (450)378-8435

GEAGEA, Justin; Addiction & Mental Hlth Clarke, 1001 Queen St W, Toronto ON M6J 1H4; McG'00; FRCPC; Psy. Staff, Centre for Addiction & Mental Health (CAMH) - College Street Site; (416)535-8501 x1133; Fax. (416)583-4355.

GEAGEA, Khalil; SMBD Jewish Gen Hosp, A 545-3755 ch Cote-Sainte-Cath, Montreal QC H3T 1E2; St. Joseph (Lebanon)'68; MD; Psy (P.Q.) (Administration). Staff, Sir Mortimer B Davis Jewish General; (514)340-8222 x5896; Fax. (514)340-8126; geagea@canada.com.

GEAR, Marie; PO Box 119, Teeswater ON N0G 2S0; Wes'78; Ac Staff/Chief Medical Staff, Wingham & District Hospital - Listowel Wingham Hospitals Alliance; (519)392-6813; Fax. (519)392-6597.

GEARY, Denis F; The Hosp for Sick Children, 5265-555 University Ave, Toronto ON M5G 1X8; Dublin (Ireland)'73; MB ChB; BAO; MRC(UK); FAAP; FRCPC; Peds. Chief Nephrol, The Hospital For Sick Children; Assoc Prof, University of Toronto; (416)813-6283; Fax. (416)813-6271; denis.geary@sickkids.on.ca.

GEATES, Barry; Mainstreet Med Services, 4929 50 Ave, Lacombe AB T4L 1K3; Alb'85; BSc; Physician, Lacombe Community Health Centre; Staff Hospitalist, Centennial Centre for Mental Health & Brain Injury; (403)782-3732; Fax. (403)782-4240; msms@telusplanet.net.

GEBARA, Nadine; Univ Hlth Network-Toronto Western Hosp, MCL8 431-399 Bathurst St, Toronto ON M5T 2S8; McM'08; CCFP; Staff, St Joseph's Health Centre; (416)603-5800; Fax. (416)603-5315.

GEBEYEHU, Yidersal; New Vision Family Health Team, 421 Greenbrook Dr, Kitchener ON N2M 4K1; Jimma (Ethiopia)'97; CCFP; Langs: Amharic; (519)578-3570; Fax. (519)578-6040.

GEBHARDT, Ian N; Crescent Heights Med Clinic, 49 8 St NW, Medicine Hat AB T1A 6N9; McM'05; BA(Computer Science); CCFP; Staff, Medicine Hat Regional Hospital; (403)526-7422; Fax. (403)526-3349.

GEBHARDT, Vernon A; Regina Internal Med Specialist, 1821 Rose St, Regina SK S4P 1Z7; Sask'76; FRCPC; IntMed (Cardiology). Dir CSU, Pasqua Hospital; (306)525-5769; Fax. (306)525-6025.

GEBIEN, Darryl; Royal Victoria Hosp, 201 Georgian Dr, Barrie ON L4M 6M2; Queensland (Australia)'00; Staff, Royal Victoria Regional Health Centre; (705)728-9802

GEBRE-HEYWOT, Tsedale; TGH Med Inc, 205-159 Cobequid Rd, Lower Sackville NS B4C 2N1; Addis Ababa (Ethiopia)'82; MSc(GenPath); CCFP; FCFP; (902)252-3332; Fax. (902)252-3334.

GEBRECHRISTOS, Ephrem; Westlaw Bldg, 210-1920 Weston Rd, York ON M9N 1W4; Addis Abba (Ethiopia)'83; FRCSC; GenSurg. Langs: Amharic; Tigrigna; (416)241-2441

GEBREMICAEL, Eyob; North Oshawa Med Centre, 1400 Ritson Rd N, Oshawa ON L1G 7W4; (Ethiopia)'89; Langs: Amharic; (905)433-4284

GEDDES, Carol A; Avon Med Centre, 2781 Avonhurst Dr, Regina SK S4R 3J3; Sask'77; DTMH; CCFP; Ac Staff, Regina General Hospital; Ac Staff, Pasqua Hospital; (306)543-4955; Fax. (306)545-7006.

GEDDES, Jay; Health Link Med Clinic, 10-350 Conestoga Blvd, Cambridge ON N1R 7L7; Saba University School of Medicine (Netherlands Antilles)'03; CCFP; (519)740-5010

GEDDES, John A; 404-85 Ontario St, Kingston ON K7L 5V7; Wes'74; CCFP; Assoc Staff, Kingston General Hospital; Assoc Staff, Hotel-Dieu Hospital; Dir, Kingston/Frontenac/Lennox & Addington STD Clinic; Teach Staff Family Med, Queen's University; (613)384-7318

GEDDES, Michael; Foothills Medical Centre, 1403 29 St NW, Calgary AB T2N 2T9; Alb'05; FRCPC; EmergMed. Staff, Foothills Medical Centre; (403)944-1110

GEDDES, Michelle N; Foothills Med Centre, 601-1403 29 St NW, Calgary AB T2N 2T9; Alb'00; FRCPC; IntMed; Hem. Hematologist, Foothills Medical Centre; (403)944-8047

GEDDES, Murray; The Moncton Hosp, 135 MacBeath Ave, Moncton NB E1C 6Z8; Stellenbosch (South Africa)'93; Staff, The Moncton Hospital.

GEDDES, Ross; Lions Gate Hosp, 231 15th St E, North Vancouver BC V7L 2L7; Monash (Australia)'71; AB; MB BS; CCFP; CCFP(E. M.); Staff, Lions Gate Hospital; (604)925-6281

GEDDES, Scott A; Medical Arts Bldg, 2-715 Coronation Blvd, Cambridge ON N1R 7R1; Wes'73; FRCSC; GenSurg. Staff Consultant, Cambridge Memorial Hospital; (519)740-1715; Fax. (519)740-9371.

GEDDES, Valerie; BC Cancer Agency-Fraser Valley, 600 10 Ave W, Vancouver BC V5Z 4E6; UBC'91; CCFP; FCFP; Staff, BC Cancer Agency Vancouver Centre; (604)877-6000

GEDDIE, William R; 11E219-200 Elizabeth St, Toronto ON M5G 2C4; Tor'78; FRCPC; AnatPath (Cytopath). Staff, Toronto General Hospital - UHN; (416)340-3722; william.geddie@uhn.ca.

GEDDIS, Rodney H; Sparling East Med Centre, PO Box 820, Fernie BC V0B 1M0; Cal'76; Ac Staff, Elk Valley Hospital; (250)423-4442; Fax. (250)423-3424; rodney.geddis@interiorhealth.ca.

GEDMINTAS, Audra; Saint John Reg Hosp Facility, PO Box 2100 Stn Main 400 University Ave, Saint John NB E2L 4L2; London (England)'00; Staff, Saint John Regional Hospital; (506)648-6000

GEE, Andrew S; The Ottawa Hosp-Civic Campus, 1053 Carling Ave, Ottawa ON K1Y 4E9; McG'92; FRCPC; EmergMed. Staff, The Ottawa Hospital - Civic Campus; Langs: Bilingual(English/French); (613)761-4000

GEE, Brian; Pacific Med Clinic, 6176 Fraser St, Vancouver BC V5W 3A1; Saba (Netherlands Antilles)'07; CCFP; (604)434-2222

GEE, David; Lakeridge Hlth Corp-Oshawa, 1 Hospital Court, Oshawa ON L1G 2B9; McG'91; CCFP; Staff, Lakeridge Health - Oshawa Site; Langs: Bilingual(English/French); (905)576-8711 x4579

GEE, Douglas F; Chemainus Med Clinic, 9892 Esplanade St RR 1, Chemainus BC V0R 1K1; Alb'77; Staff, Cowichan District Hospital; Staff, Chemainus Health Care Centre; (250)246-3261; Fax. (250)246-9144.

GEE, Edward; Village Park Med Clinic, 110-937 Fir St, Sherwood Park AB T8A 4N6; Alb'78; (780)467-8886; Fax. (780)467-6763; ed.gee54@gmail.com.

GEE, Peter; Courtenay Med Associates, 201-1350 England Ave, Courtenay BC V9N 8X6; Birmingham (United Kingdom)'86; BS; CCFP; (250)334-4411

GEE, Shirl A D; Queen Elizabeth II HSC, 049 7N-1276 South Park St, Halifax NS B3H 2Y9; Alb'95; BSc; FRCPC; IntMed (Endocrinology); Endocrin&Metab. Staff, Queen Elizabeth II Health Sciences Centre - Victoria General Site; (902)473-3740; Fax. (902)473-3726.

GEE, Sydney R; Joseph Brant Mem Hosp, 1230 North Shore Blvd E, Burlington ON L7S 1W7; McM'83; PhD; MSc; FRCPC; IntMed; Hem. Court Staff Privil, Hamilton Health Sciences Centre - McMaster Children's Hospital; Ac Staff, Joseph Brant Memorial Hospital; (905)336-4103; Fax. (905)336-6492.

GEENEN, Caroline L; Markham Stouffville Health Ctr, 206-377 Church St, Markham ON L6B 1A1; Tor'89; FRCPC; Neur (Multiple Sclerosis). Ac Staff, Markham Stouffville Hospital; Ac Staff, St Michael's Hospital; (905)472-6551; Fax. (905)472-5490.

GEERS, Johannes A S M; 1910 20 Ave PO Box 1359 Stn Main, Coaldale AB T1M 1N2; Alb'80; CCFP; FCFP; (403)345-5500; Fax. (403)345-5507.

GEERTS, William H; Sunnybrook Hlth Sciences Ctre, A459-2075 Bayview Ave, Toronto ON M4N 3M5; Mem'79; FRCPC; IntMed (Thromboembolism); Respir. Ac Staff, Sunnybrook Health Sciences Centre; Prof Med, University of Toronto; (416)480-5953; Fax. (416)480-5153.

GEFFEN, Allison S; Hampton Med Centre, 216-1419 Carling Ave, Ottawa ON K1Z 7L6; Wes'93; CCFP; FCFP; Supvr Residency Program, University of Ottawa; (613)728-8880

GEFT, Colin H; Glenhurst Medical Centre, 102-2797 Bathurst St, North York ON M6B 4B9; Cape Town (South Africa)'73; MB ChB; DCH; FRCPC; Peds. Langs: Hebrew; (416)789-4593; Fax. (416)781-6399.

GEHA, Sameh; CHUS-Hop Fleurimont, 3001 12e av N, Sherbrooke QC J1H 5N4; Saint Joseph (Lebanon)'98; Staff, Centre Hospitalier Universitaire de Sherbrooke-Hopital Fleurimont; (819)346-1110 x15331

GEHMAN, Kenneth E; Kenneth Gehman Med Prof Corp, 306-984 Oliver Rd, Thunder Bay ON P7B 7C7; UBC'87; FRCSC; GenSurg (Surgical Oncology); ThorSurg. Staff, Thunder Bay Regional Health Sciences Centre; (807)345-4337; Fax. (807)345-4319.

GEHRELS, Corrine M; Parry Sound Family Health Team, 75 Bowes St, Parry Sound ON P2A 2L6; Wes'89; CCFP; FCFP; Staff, West Parry Sound Health Centre; (705)746-5595; Fax. (705)746-6576.

GEIER, Pavel; Children's Hosp of Eastern Ont, 401 Smyth Rd, Ottawa ON K1H 8L1; Prague (Czech Republic)'87; Staff, Children's Hospital of Eastern Ontario (CHEO); Langs: Czech; (613)737-7600

GEIGER, Glen W; The Ottawa Hosp-Gen Campus, PO Box 124 501 Smyth Rd, Ottawa ON K1H 8L6; McG'88; BASc; MASc; FRCPC; IntMed. Staff, The Ottawa Hospital - General Campus; (613)722-7000 x79362

GEISLER, Arthur E M; 290-1175 Johnson St, New Westminster BC V3B 7K1; Tor'70; BSc; DOHS; CCFP; FCFP; (604)472-1005

GEISLER, William O; 109 Park Rd, Toronto ON M4W 2N8; Tor'48; FRCPC; IntMed (Neuro Rehabilitation); PhysMed&Rehab. Consultant Rehab Med, St Michael's Hospital; Staff, Toronto General Hospital - UHN; Internal Med, Toronto Rehabilitation Institute - Lyndhurst Centre; Emeritus Prof Med Rehab, University of Toronto; Langs: German; English; French; (416)921-4392; Fax. (416)922-0374.

GEIST, Rose; The Hosp for Sick Children, 555 University Ave, Toronto ON M5G 1X8; Tor'75; BSc; FRCPC; Psy (Child Psychiatry). Staff Psy, The Hospital For Sick Children; Dir Child & Adolescent Med Psy Prog, University of Toronto; (416)813-7533; Fax. (416)813-5326.

GEIZER, Marie; Mount St Joseph Hosp, 3080 Prince Edward St, Vancouver BC V5T 3N4; Karlova (Czech Republic)'84; FRCPC; Psy (Geriatric Psychiatry). Staff, Providence Health Care - Mount Saint Joseph Hospital; Asst Prof, University of British Columbia; Langs: Czech; (604)874-1141 x78430

GEKAS, Jean; CHUQ-Ctr Hosp Univ Laval, RC 9300-2705 boul Laurier, Quebec QC G1V 4G2; Amiens (France)'97; AddicMed; ObstGyn (P.Q.). Staff MedGenetics, Centre Hospitalier Universitaire de Quebec-CHUL; Staff MedGenetics, Centre Hospitalier Universitaire De Québec - Pavillon De St-françois-d'assise; adj Prof, Université Laval; (418)656-4141 x48114; Fax. (418)654-2748; jean.gekas@mail.chuq.qc.ca.

GELBER, Herman; Medical Bldg, B 1104-3000 Lawrence Ave E, Scarborough ON M1P 2V1; McG'60; AB; FRCPC; Psy. Consultant Psy, The Scarborough Hospital - General Campus; Associate Psy, St Michael's Hospital; Teacher Psy, University of Toronto; Langs: Bilingual(English/French); (416)430-0661 x6283; Fax. (416)430-0352.

GELBER, Stephen G; North York Gen Hosp-Branson, 103-555 Finch Ave W, North York ON M2R 1N5; Qns'00; MSc; FRCPC; Psy. Staff Psy, North York General Hospital - Branson Division; Langs: French; (416)633-9420 x6788; Fax. (416)635-2428; sgelber@nygh.on.ca.

GELBER, Tobias N M; Associate Med Clinic, PO Box 549, Pincher Creek AB T0K 1W0; Cal'99; CCFP; (403)627-3321; Fax. (403)627-2280; tgelber@panchermedical.ca.

GELBERG, Jacob; Foothills Medical Centre, 1403 29 St NW, Calgary AB T2N 2T9; Qns'07; Respir; IntMed. Staff, Foothills Medical Centre; (905)522-4241

GELDENHUYS, Laurette; DJ Mackenzie Bldg, 742-5788 University Ave, Halifax NS B3H 1V8; Witwatersrand (South Africa)'87; FIAC; MB BCh; MMed; MAED; FRCPC; AnatPath (Cytopath). Sec Head Cytopathology/Service Chief Anatomical Pathology, Queen Elizabeth II Health Sciences Centre - Victoria General Site; Prof, Dalhousie University; Langs: Afrikaans; (902)473-7334; Fax. (902)473-1049.

GELEFF, John S; 1840 Eglinton Ave W, Toronto ON M6E 2J4; RCS (Ireland)'86; (416)789-6100; Fax. (416)789-3735.

GELEIDI, Aladdin; Apple Wellness Clinic, 229 1 St SW, Airdrie AB T4B 3L8; Al Fateh (Libya)'01; MB ChB; CCFP; (403)948-3342; Fax. (403)945-1783.

GELFAND, Gary A J; Foothills Med Centre, G33-1403 29 St NW, Calgary AB T2N 2T9; Alb'84; MSc; MHSc; FRCSC; GenSurg; ThorSurg. Staff, Foothills Medical Centre; Asst Clin Prof, University of Calgary; (403)944-4268; Fax. (403)270-8431; gelfand@ucalgary.ca.

GELFANT, Benjamin M; 100-1333 Broadway W, Vancouver BC V6H 4C1; UBC'78; FRCSC; PlasSurg. Staff, Delta Hospital; Staff, Richmond Hospital; Clin Instructor, University of British Columbia; (604)874-2078; Fax. (604)876-6354.

GELHORN, Donald G; Hudson Bay Med Group, PO Box 1170 607 Albert St, Hudson Bay SK S0E 0Y0; Sask'79; CCFP; FCFP; Staff, Hudson Bay Health Care Facility; Preceptor Family Med, University of Saskatchewan; (306)865-2238; Fax. (306)865-2074; dgelhorn@kthr.sk.ca.

GELINAS, Bernard; Coop Sante des Collines, 393 montee de la Source, Gatineau QC J8V 0J2; Laval'69; Langs: English; (819)607-0650

GELINAS, Bernard; Clinique Medicale le Frontenac, 202-5200 rue Frontenac, Lac-Megantic QC G6B 1H3; Mon'84; Staff, CSSS du Témiscamingue; (819)583-0157; bernard_gelinas@ssss.gouv.qc.ca.

GELINAS, Catherine; Hotel-Dieu D'Arthabaska, 5 rue des Hospitalieres, Victoriaville QC G6P 6N2; Laval'06; Staff, Hotel-Dieu d'Arthabaska; (819)357-2030

GELINAS, Catherine; CSSS Kamouraska-Hop Notre-Dame, CP 460 1201 6e av, La Pocatiere QC G0R 1Z0; Laval'04; CCFP; Staff, CSSS de Kamouraska; (418)856-7000

GELINAS, Christian; CSSS de Saint-Jerome, 290 rue de Montigny, Saint-Jerome QC J7Z 5T3; Mon'88; Staff, Hôtel-Dieu de Saint-Jérôme; (450)431-8200

GELINAS, Claude; Clin Radiologie Boucherville, 202-600 boul du Fort-St-Louis, Boucherville QC J4B 1S7; Laval'70; DiagRad (Echocardiography). Langs: English; (450)655-2430; Fax. (450)655-8308.

GELINAS, Daniel; Polyclinique Les Gres, 104-190 rue St Honore, St-Etienne-Ds-Gres QC G0X 2P0; Laval'90; Ac Member Gen Med, Centre Hospitalier du Centre la Mauricie; (819)535-6512; Fax. (819)535-1627.

GELINAS, Danielle; Clinique Med Vieux Aylmer, 101-204 ch d'Aylmer, Gatineau QC J9H 1A1; Laval'84; Medical Staff, Maison Mathieu-Froment-Savoie Centre de Soins Palliatifs; Langs: English; (819)682-5464

GELINAS, Denis; CRSSS Baie-James-Chibougamau, 51 3e rue, Chibougamau QC G8P 1N1; Mon'87; CSPQ; GenSurg. Staff, CRSSS de la Baie-James; (418)748-2676

GELINAS, France; Hop Jean-Talon, 1385 rue Jean-Talon E, Montreal QC H2E 1S6; Sher'89; Staff, CSSS du Coeur de l'Isle Hôpital Jean-Talon; (514)495-6767

GELINAS, Ginette; Clinique Medicale GMF-1851, 1100-1851 rue Sherbrooke E, Montreal QC H2K 4L5; Mon'74; (514)526-3351; Fax. (514)526-4594.

GELINAS, Guy; Clinique Ophtal de la Cite, 10-2600 boul Laurier, Quebec QC G1V 4T3; Laval'74; FRCSC; Ophth. (418)650-5065; Fax. (418)654-1580.

GELINAS, Jean; Campbell River & Dist Gen Hosp, 375 2nd Ave, Campbell River BC V9W 3V1; Laval'88; CSPQ; Critical Care Medicine (P.Q.); Anes. Staff, Campbell River & District General Hospital; (250)287-7111

GELINAS, Jean-Pierre; 610 boul du Seminaire N, St-Jean-Sur-Richel QC J3B 7B4; Mon'80; (450)348-9218; Fax. (450)348-0377.

GELINAS, Jill M J; Trillium Cardiovascular Assoc, 609-89 Queensway W, Mississauga ON L5B 2V2; Wes'95; FRCSC; OrthSurg. (905)848-7580 x3113

GELINAS, Leonce; 147 A boul E, Maskinonge QC J0K 1N0; Laval'73; (819)626-0080

GELINAS, Louise; Centre Med St-Stanislas, 1380 rue Principale, St-Stanislas-D-Cha QC G0X 3E0; Laval'83; Physician, CHSLD Valee de la Batiscan; Langs: Bilingual(French/English); (418)328-8417; Fax. (418)328-8446.

GELINAS, Lucie M; Clinique Med St-Pierre, 200-85 rue Saint-Pierre, Saint-Constant QC J5A 1G8; Mon'72; LMCC; Langs: Bilingual(French/English); (450)845-4646; Fax. (450)845-4104.

GELINAS, Manon; Clinique Med de l'Est Inc, 100-30 boul Saint-Joseph E, Montreal QC H2T 1G9; Mon'92; (514)845-4240; Fax. (514)845-5493.

GELINAS, Marcien; Clinique de Radiologie, 185-1900 boul des Recollets, Trois-Rivieres QC G8Z 4K4; Mon'66; DiagRad. (819)379-5506; Fax. (819)379-9710.

GELINAS, Marie-Christine; Clin Med Sainte-Julie, 286 rue de Normandie, Sainte-Julie QC J3E 1A7; Mon'02; Langs: English; (450)649-1593; Fax. (450)649-0361.

GELINAS, Melanie; Centre Med Familiale de Granby, 48 rue Denison E, Granby QC J2G 4C6; Mon'00; Staff, Centre Hospitalier de Granby; (450)372-3996

GELINAS, Michel; Hop Santa Cabrini Ospedale, 5655 rue Saint-Zotique E, Montreal QC H1T 1P7; Laval'60; CSPQ; Cardiol (P.Q.). Staff, Hôpital Santa Cabrini Ospedale; (514)252-6000

GELINAS, Paul R; 200-1055 boul des Forges, Trois-Rivieres QC G8Z 4J9; Laval'74; Staff, Governement de Quebec CSST; (819)372-3400 x3455

GELINAS, Pierre; Clinique Med St-Villier, 201-205 rue Montmagny, Quebec QC G1N 4V3; Laval'74; Ac Staff, CSSS de Quebec-Sud; (418)688-0872; Fax. (418)688-4951.

GELINAS, Renee-Claude; Ctr Hosp Laurentien, 234 rue Saint-Vincent, Ste-Agathe-Des-Mts QC J8C 2B8; Mon'95; Staff, Centre Hospitalier Laurentien; (819)324-4000

GELINAS CHAINE, Karine; CSSS de Trois-Rivières, 1991 boul du Carmel, Trois-Rivieres QC G8Z 3R9; McG'06; MDCM; OrthSurg. Staff, CSSS de Trois-Rivières; (819)697-3333

GELKOPF, Marvin A; Doctor's Office, 101-491 Lawrence Ave W, North York ON M5M 1C7; Tor'89; CCFP; FCFP; Asst Prof, University of Toronto; Langs: Yiddish; Hebrew; (416)787-5693; Fax. (416)787-8094.

GELLER, Brian E; Saskatchewan Med Assoc, 402-321A 21st St E, Saskatoon SK S7K 0C1; Sask'92; CCFP; FCFP; Asst Clin Prof, University of Saskatchewan; (306)244-2196; Fax. (306)653-1631.

GELLER, Carol A; Centretown Comm Health Centre, 420 Cooper St, Ottawa ON K2P 2N6; Tor'91; CCFP; FCFP; (613)233-4697; Fax. (613)233-4541.

GELLNER, Darcie L; Red Deer Reg Hosp Centre, 5030-3942 50A Ave, Red Deer AB T4N 4E7; Sask'92; CCFP; CCFP(E.M.); FCFP; Staff Emerg Med, Red Deer Regional Hospital Centre; (403)343-4444; dargel@telusplanet.net.

GELLY, Andre L; 7715 boul Newman, LaSalle QC H8N 1X7; Laval'74; CSPQ; FRCP; LMCC; FRCPC; IntMed; Gastroent. Staff, Centre Hospitalier de LaSalle; Staff, Hôpital Anna-Laberge; Staff, McGill University Health Centre - Montreal General Campus; Langs: English; (514)363-6638; Fax. (514)363-0492.

GELMAN, Gregory D; North York Med Group, 704-240 Duncan Mill Rd, North York ON M3B 3S6; Tor'99; CCFP; FCFP; Staff, North York General Hospital; Teacher, University of Toronto; (416)497-0880; Fax. (416)497-2650.

GELMAN, Marc L; Scarborough Hosp-General Div, 3050 Lawrence Ave E, Scarborough ON M1P 2V5; Buffalo (USA)'91; Staff, The Scarborough Hospital - General Campus; (416)431-8200

GELMAN, Tara D; Medical & Dental Bldg, 404-586 Eglinton Ave E, Toronto ON M4P 1P2; Tor'01; FRCPC; Peds. (416)489-3273; Fax. (416)489-1510.

GELMON, Karen A; BC Cancer Agency-Vancouver CC, 600 10th Ave W, Vancouver BC V5Z 4E6; Sask'79; FRCPC; IntMed; MedOncol. Staff, BC Cancer Agency Vancouver Centre; Staff, Vancouver General Hospital - Centennial Pavillion; Clin Prof, University of British Columbia; (604)877-6000; Fax. (604)877-0585; kgelmon@bccancer.bc.ca.

GELOSO, Angela; Hop Louis-H Lafontaine, 7401 rue Hochelaga, Montreal QC H1N 3M5; Sher'96; Psy. Staff, Hopital Louis-H Lafontaine; (514)251-4000 x3060; Fax. (514)251-1604.

GELOSO, Corrado G; Peterborough Reg Hlth Centre, 1 Hospital Dr, Peterborough ON K9J 7C6; Wes'89; FRCPC; Anes. Staff, Peterborough Regional Health Centre - Hospital Drive; (705)876-5038

GELSTON, Arthur L; Jewish Rehab Hosp, 3205 Pl alton-Goldbloom, Laval QC H7V 1R2; Cornell (USA)'77; FRCPC; IntMed. Staff, Jewish Rehabilitation Hospital; (450)688-5728

GEMAYEL, Kange P; Clinique Med Jean-Talon Pie IX, 4679 rue Jean-Talon E, Saint-Leonard QC H1S 1K3; Alexandria (Egypt)'69; MB ChB; FRCSC; ObstGyn (Colposcopy). Staff, St Mary's Hospital Centre; Staff, Hôpital Santa Cabrini Ospedale; (514)374-5901; Fax. (514)374-1668.

GEMEINHARDT, Christine E; Ladner Centre Med, 5132 Ladner Trunk Rd, Delta BC V4K 1W3; McM'82; MSc; CCFP; Langs: French; German; (604)940-0917

GEMME, Emilie; CLSC Vallee-des-Forts, 978 boul du Seminaire, St-Jean-sur-Richel QC J3A 1E5; Mon'08; Médecin, CLSC Haute-Ville des Rivieres; (450)299-2828; Fax. (450)299-9779.

GEMME, Michel; Centre Med Fusion, 200-2035 av Sainte-Anne, Saint-Hyacinthe QC J2S 5H3; Laval'87; Staff, Centre Hospitalier Honore-Mercier; Langs: English; (450)773-6023

GEMME, Nathalie; Ctr Hosp Affilie-St-Sacrement, 1050 ch Sainte-Foy, Quebec QC G1S 4L8; Mon'06; CCFP; Staff, Centre Hospitalier Affilié Universitaire de Québec - Hôpital du St-Sacrement; (418)682-7511; Fax. (418)682-7977.

GEMMILL, H Ian M; KFLA Public Health, 221 Portsmouth Ave, Kingston ON K7M 1V5; Qns'76; FRCPC; CommunMed (Public Health);CCFP; FCFP; Med Officer of Hlth, KFL & A Public Health Unit; Assoc Prof Community Hth & Family/Dir Community Med Residency Prog, Queen's University; (613)549-1232 x1234; Fax. (613)549-1209.

GENDEMANN, Klaus D; University of Alberta Hosp, 1E7 27WCM-8440 112 St NW, Edmonton AB T6G 2B7; Alb'80; FRCPC; Psy. Chief Site Dept of Psy/Staff, University of Alberta Hospital; Coord Phase III, University of Alberta; (780)407-6574; Fax. (780)407-6672.

GENDREAU, Raymond; Institut de Med Specialisee de, 101-1875 rue Maurice-Gauvin, Laval QC H7S 2M5; Mon'91; CSPQ; FRCPC; IntMed (Cardiology); Cardiol. Staff, Hopital de la Cite de la santé; (450)902-9990; Fax. (450)902-9989.

GENDREAU-REID, M F Liliane; Landsowne Prof Bldg, 260-1641 Hillside Ave, Victoria BC V8T 5G1; Laval'78; ABAI; ABPeds; FRCPC; Peds (Allergy & Immunology); ClinImmunol&Allergy. Consultant, Victoria General Hospital; Langs: Spanish; Bilingual(French/English); (250)595-7844; allergyvictoria@yahoo.ca.

GENDRON, Cathy; CSSS de Trois-Rivières, 1991 boul du Carmel, Trois-Rivieres QC G8Z 3R9; Sher'01; FRCSC; Neursurg. Staff, CSSS de Trois-Rivières; (819)697-3333

GENDRON, Claudie; Polyclinique St-Eustache, 75 rue Grignon, Saint-Eustache QC J7P 4J2; Laval'92; ObstGyn. Staff, Hôpital Santa Cabrini Ospedale; (450)491-1150; Fax. (450)491-7470.

GENDRON, Daniel; MUHC-Montreal Neurology Inst, 3801 rue University, Montreal QC H3A 2B4; Laval'76; FRCPC; Neur; Electroenceph (P.Q.). Staff, McGill University Health Centre - Montreal Neurological Hospital; (514)398-1920; Fax. (514)398-1285.

GENDRON, Francoise; Dir Sante Pub L'Estrie, 300-300 rue King E, Sherbrooke QC J1G 1B1; Mon'88; Staff Clin Planning, Centre Hospitalier Universitaire de Sherbrooke-Hopital Fleurimont; (819)829-3400; Fax. (819)569-8894.

GENDRON, Gilles; Hotel-Dieu de Levis, 143 rue Wolfe, Levis QC G6V 3Z1; Laval'82; CSPQ; FRCPC; Anes. Ac Member, Hôtel-Dieu de Lévis; (418)835-7121; Fax. (418)835-3969.

GENDRON, Guy; CSSS du Sud de Lanaudière, 911 montee des Pionniers, Terrebonne QC J6V 2H2; Sher'82; CSPQ; Anes (P.Q.). Staff, Centre Hospitalier Pierre le Gardeur; (450)654-7525 x32214

GENDRON, Jean-Paul; CLSC-CHSLD La Source, 190 76e rue E, Quebec QC G1H 7K4; Laval'79; Ac Staff, Centre Hospitalier Universitaire De Québec - Pavillon De St-françois-d'assise; (418)628-2572; Fax. (418)628-8668.

GENDRON, Jean-Sebastien; CHUS-Hop Hotel-Dieu, 580 rue Bowen S, Sherbrooke QC J1G 2E8; Sher'96; Staff, Centre Hospitalier Universitaire de Sherbrooke-Hôpital Hôtel-Dieu; (819)346-1110 x21000

GENDRON, Louise; CSSS d'Argenteuil, 145 av de la Providence, Lachute QC J8H 4C7; Mon'80; FRCPC; Psy. Staff, Centre Hospitalier d'Argenteuil; Physician, CLSC d'Argenteuil; (450)562-3761 x7106

GENDRON, Marie-Danielle; Clinique méd Brome-Missiquoi, 280 rue Victoria, Knowlton QC J0E 1V0; Sher'07; CCFP; (450)243-5043; Fax. (450)243-0537.

GENDRON, Olivier-M; 810 rue Montcalm RR 2, Berthierville QC J0K 1A0; Mon'56; (514)836-4224; Fax. (514)836-8135.

GENDRON, Robert; CLSC Grande Riviere, 425 rue Leguerrier, Gatineau QC J9H 6N8; Mon'84; (819)684-2251

GENDRON, Sebastien; Ctr Hosp Soins Psychiatriques, CP 800 1141 rue Royale, Malartic QC J0Y 1Z0; Sher'03; FRCPC; Psy. Staff, Hôpital psychiatrique de Malartic; (819)825-6711; sebastien_gendron@ssss.gouv.qc.ca.

GENDRON, Stephane; CSSS de Laval, 1755 boul Rene-Laennec, Laval QC H7M 3L9; Mon'85; Staff, Hopital de la Cite de la santé; (450)668-1010

GENDRON, Tina-Louise; Clin de Chirurgie du Littoral, 111-822 boul Sainte-Anne, Rimouski QC G5M 1J5; Sher'97; CSPQ; FRCSC; OrthSurg (Sports Medicine). Staff OrthSurg, Hôpital Regional Rimouski; Langs: English; (418)723-0194

GENEREUX, Alexandre; Ctr Hosp Affilie-Enfant-Jesus, 1401 18e rue, Quebec QC G1J 1Z4; Mon'01; FRCPC; IntMed; Gastroent. Staff, Centre Hospitalier Affilié Universitaire de Québec - Hôpital De L'Enfant Jésus; (418)649-0252; Fax. (418)649-5570.

GENEREUX, Mélissa; 300 rue King E, Sherbrooke QC J1G 1B1; Mon'04; FRCPC; CommunMed. (819)829-3400 x42547

GENEREUX, Philippe; Hop Du Sacre-Coeur De Montreal, 5400 boul Gouin O, Montreal QC H4J 1C5; Mon'01; Cardiol; IntMed. Staff, Hôpital du Sacre-Coeur de Montréal; (514)338-2222; philgen36@hotmail.com.

GENESOVE, Leon J; Susan Giangioppo-ON Mol Div, 19th Flr-505 University Ave, Toronto ON M7A 1T7; Tor'79; DIH; CCBOM; FRCPC; OccupMed;CCFP; Chief Physician Gage Occup & Environmental Health Unit, Ontario Ministry of Labour; Occupational Medicine, University of Toronto; (416)326-2913; Fax. (416)326-2988; leon.genesove@ontario.ca.

GENESSE, Dany; Clinique Med de l'Ouest, 2200 6e av, Saint-Georges QC G5Y 3X3; Laval'83; (418)228-2024; Fax. (418)228-7715.

GENEST, Herve; Clin de Chirurgie Plastique Ha, 300-34 Cote de la Fabrique, Quebec QC G1R 3V7; Laval'82; FRCSC; PlasSurg. Ac Staff, Centre Hospitalier Affilié Universitaire de Québec - Hôpital De L'Enfant Jésus; Consultant, Centre Hospitalier Universitaire de Quebec-CHUL; (418)692-3843

GENEST, Isabelle; CHUQ-Ctr Hosp Univ Laval, 2705 boul laurier, Quebec QC G1V 4G2; Laval'01; FRCPC; EmergMed. Staff, Centre Hospitalier Universitaire de Quebec-CHUL; Langs: German; English; (418)525-4444

GENEST, Jacques A P R; The Ottawa Hosp-Gen Campus, 501 Smyth Rd, Ottawa ON K1H 8L6; Laval'79; FACR; CSPQ; FRCPC; RadOncol. Staff, The Ottawa Hospital - General Campus; Prof RadOncol, University of Ottawa; Langs: English; (613)737-7700 x70204; Fax. (613)247-3511.

GENEST, Jocelyne; Hop Santa Cabrini Ospedale, 5655 rue Saint-Zotique E, Montreal QC H1T 1P7; Mon'77; FRCSC; GenSurg (Endoscopic Surgery). Staff, Hôpital Santa Cabrini Ospedale; (514)252-6000

GENEST, Marcel; Central Park Med Centre, 104-3965 Kingsway, Burnaby BC V5H 1Y8; Laval'75; Court Staff, Burnaby Hospital; Langs: Bilingual(English/French); (604)434-8781; Fax. (604)434-8699.

GENEST, Marie-Josee; Centre Medical St-Jean, 202-1018 rue de la Prairie O, St-J-Chrysostome QC G6Z 0A7; Laval'85; Gen Practice, CSSS du Grand Littoral; (418)839-4433; Fax. (418)839-3574.

GENEST, Mathieu; Clin de Chirurgie du Littoral, 111-822 boul Ste-Anne, Rimouski QC G5M 1J5; Laval'00; CSPQ; FRCSC; OrthSurg (Arthroplasty). Langs: English; (418)723-0194; Fax. (418)723-0180.

GENEST, Pierre; Polyclinique Med des Ponts, 140-1100 boul de la Rive-Sud, Saint-Romuald QC G6W 5M6; Laval'59; Physician, Multi Gite Med Industrielle; (418)834-1177; Fax. (418)834-9275.

GENEST, Rene; Clinique Med St-Louis, 220-3165 ch Saint-Louis, Quebec QC G1W 4R4; Laval'89; Staff, Hôtel-Dieu de Lévis; Langs: Bilingual(English/French); (418)653-1970

GENEST, Sylvain; Polyclinique St-Jerome, 204-200 rue Durand, Saint-Jerome QC J7Z 7E2; Mon'80; CSPQ; FRCSC; GenSurg. Staff, Hôtel-Dieu de Saint-Jérôme; Langs: Bilingual(English/French); (450)438-5922; genests@citenet.net.

GENEST JR., Jacques J G; MUHC-Royal Victoria Hosp, 687 av des Pins O, Montreal QC H3A 1A1; McG'80; CSPQ; FRCPC; IntMed (Cardiovascular Disease); Cardiol. Dir Div of Cardiol, McGill University Health Centre - Royal Victoria Hospital; assoc Prof Med, McGill University; (514)934-1934 x34642; Fax. (514)843-2813; jacques.genest@muhc.mcgill.ca.

GENEVE, Mustafa M; Gateway Primacy Med Clinic, 1035 Gateway Rd, Winnipeg MB R2K 4C1; MB ChB; CCFP; Staff, St. Anthony General Hospital; Staff, AMC Clinic; Langs: Arabic; (204)667-5227; Fax. (204)667-5242; drgeneve@yahoo.ca.

GENGE, A Gaylene; Westgrove Med Clinic, 201-505 Queen St, Spruce Grove AB T7X 2V2; Alb'08; CCFP; (780)962-9888; Fax. (780)960-5298.

GENGE, Angela L; MUHC-Montreal Neurology Inst, 3801 rue University, Montreal QC H3A 2B4; Mem'86; FRCPC; IntMed (AIDS/HIV); Neur. Neurology, McGill University Health Centre - Montreal Neurological Hospital; adj Prof, McGill University; Langs: English; French; (514)398-5262; Fax. (514)398-2745.

GENGE, Leah M; 1001 10th Ave SW, Calgary AB T2R 0B7; Dal'10; CCFP; (403)221-8780

GENGE, Margot M; Detwiller Pavillion, 2255 Wesbrook Mall, Vancouver BC V6T 2A1; Mem'88; FRCPC; Psy (Geriatric Psychiatry). Staff, UBC Hospital - Koerner Pavillion; University of British Columbia; (604)822-7298; Fax. (604)822-7887; mgenge@interchange.ubc.ca.

GENGE, Roland J; Baddeck Med Clinic, PO Box 130, Baddeck NS B0E 1B0; Dal'71; Staff, Victoria County Memorial Hospital; Teacher, Dalhousie University; (902)295-2443; Fax. (902)295-1775.

GENGE, Stephanie I; 8 Maypark Place, St. John's NL A1B 2E3; Mem'90; FRCPC; IntMed. Langs: Bilingual(English/French); (709)754-6317

GENNAOUI, Jean-Pierre; Hotel-Dieu de Levis, 143 rue Wolfe, Levis QC G6V 3Z1; Mon'98; FRCSC; ObstGyn. Staff, Hôtel-Dieu de Lévis; (418)835-7121

GENOT, Roxane; 2032 Kingsway, Vancouver BC V5N 2T3; Ott'06; CCFP; (604)874-5555

GENOT, Veronique; Hop Charles Lemoyne, 3120 boul Taschereau, Greenfield Park QC J4V 2H1; Sher'95; Staff, Hopital Charles LeMoyne; (450)466-5000

GENTILI, Fred; Univ Hlth Network-Toronto Western Hosp, WW4 445-399 Bathurst St, Toronto ON M5T 2S8; Tor'72; FACS; FRCSC; Neursurg. Staff, Toronto Western Hospital - University Health Network; Langs: Italian; (416)603-5250; Fax. (416)603-5298; fred.gentili@uhn.on.ca.

GENTIS, Edward F H; Medical Bldg, 1605-805 Broadway W, Vancouver BC V5Z 1K1; Leiden (Netherlands)'72; DABS; FRCSC; GenSurg. Langs: Dutch; Spanish; (604)872-4281; Fax. (604)876-4202.

GENUIS, Stephen J; Family Med Centre, 2935 66 St NW, Edmonton AB T6K 4C1; Tor'79; DAB; FRCSC; ObstGyn (Environmental Health). Clin Prof, University of Alberta; (780)450-3504; Fax. (780)490-1803.

GEOFFRION, Genevieve; Seaforth Med Bldg, 770-3550 ch de la Cote-des-Nei, Montreal QC H3H 1V4; McG'95; FRCPC; Derm. Langs: English; (514)935-9955; Fax. (514)935-7838.

GEOFFRION, Paul C; PO Box 1693, Raymond AB T0K 2S0; McG'03; CCFP; CCFP(E.M.); Staff, Northern Lights Regional Health Centre; Langs: Bilingual(English/French).

GEOFFRION, Roxana; 4F-1190 Hornby St, Vancouver BC V6Z 2K5; McG'01; FRCSC; ObstGyn (Urogynecology). Staff, Providence Health Care - St Paul's Hospital; (604)806-9835

GEOFFROY, Louis; Hôpital Ste-Justine, 3175 ch Cote-Ste-Catherine, Montreal QC H3T 1C5; Sher'74; Peds (Diabetology). Chef méd urgence, Hôpital Ste-Justine; Asst Clin Prof, Universite de Montreal; (514)345-4980; Fax. (514)345-4604.

GEOFFROY, Marie-Helene; UMF Charles Lemoyne, 100B-299 boul Sir-Wilfrid-Laur, Longueuil QC J4R 2L1; Sher'04; CCFP; Staff, Centre Hospitalier Universitaire de Québec (CHUQ) - Siege Social; (450)465-5541

GEOFFROY, Normand; Clinique Med Laurier, 1814 boul Saint-Joseph E, Montreal QC H2H 1C7; Mon'74; (514)527-8228; Fax. (514)527-6364.

GEOFFROY, Pierre; Enhanced Care Clinic, 14872 Yonge St, Aurora ON L4G 1N2; McG'89; MSc(Nutrition); MSc(Epidemiol); CCFP; FCFP; Dir Clinical Research & Development, Wyeth-Ayerst Canada Inc; Langs: Bilingual(English/French); (905)505-0905; Fax. (905)841-9404.

GEOGHEGAN, Michael A; The Doctor's Office, 104-4935 40 Ave NW, Calgary AB T3A 2N1; Dundee (Scotland)'77; MB ChB; FFARCS; DA(Eng.); Staff, Foothills Medical Centre; Langs: German; French; (403)247-2253; Fax. (403)247-0669; mag911@hotmail.com.

GEONZON, Radzfel A; 311-2675 36 St NE, Calgary AB T1Y 6H6; (Philippines)'03; BSc; MSc; CCFP; Langs: Cebuano; Tagalog; (403)291-3801; Fax. (403)291-3795.

GEONZON, Rose Marie E; Sunridge Prof Centre, 311-2675 36 St NE, Calgary AB T1Y 6H6; Cebu (Philippines)'71; AB; CCFP; FCFP; Staff, Peter Lougheed Centre; Langs: Tagalog; (403)291-3801; Fax. (403)291-3795.

GEORGE, Anthony G; Univ Hlth Network-Toronto Gen, 200 Elizabeth St, Toronto ON M5G 2C4; Cape Town (South Africa)'00; Clin Fellow Anes, Toronto General Hospital - UHN; (416)340-3000

GEORGE, Charles F P; London HSC-South Street Hosp, 375 South St, London ON N6A 4G5; Dal'79; ABIM; AB; FRCPC; IntMed (Sleep Medicine); Respir. Staff, London Health Sciences Centre - South Street; Ac Staff, London Health Sciences Centre - Victoria Campus; Prof Med, University of Western Ontario; (519)667-6860

GEORGE, David H; Foothills Med Centre, 1403 29 St NW, Calgary AB T2N 2T9; Man'79; FRCPC; AnatPath. Staff, Foothills Medical Centre; (403)944-8198; Fax. (403)944-4748.

GEORGE, Deepu J; Simon Fraser Health Region, 600-22470 Dewdney Trunk Rd, Maple Ridge BC V2X 5Z6; Transkei (South Africa)'98; MB ChB; FRCPC; IntMed. Staff, Cowichan District Hospital; (604)436-0321

GEORGE, Elizabeth; Medical Centre, 4-1939 Kennedy Rd, Scarborough ON M1P 2L9; (India)'70; Affil Staff, The Scarborough Hospital - Birchmount Campus; Langs: Malayalam; Tamil; (416)754-3335; Fax. (416)754-9518.

GEORGE, Eric J; 201-9775 Fourth St, Sidney BC V8L 2Z8; UBC'91; CCFP; (250)656-4011; Fax. (250)656-4014.

GEORGE, Lillian K F; Family First Family Health Team, 4270 Innes Rd, Orleans ON K4A 5E6; Cairo (Egypt)'90; MB ChB; CCFP; Langs: Arabic; (613)841-7009; Fax. (613)841-0106.

GEORGE, Lindsey J; 3F-10 George St, Hamilton ON L8P 1C8; McM'95; FRCPC; Psy. (905)667-4848

GEORGE, M Catherine; Wortley Village Med Centre, 208-190 Wortley Rd, London ON N6C 4Y7; Dal'78; (519)438-5101; Fax. (519)438-0369.

GEORGE, Mini; Beddington Med Clinic, 207-8120 Beddington Blvd NW, Calgary AB T3K 2A8; (India)'84; MB BS; CCFP; (403)275-4611; Fax. (403)275-4613.

GEORGE, Philip; Thunder Bay Reg HSC-T-Bay, 980 Oliver Rd, Thunder Bay ON P7B 6V4; (India)'94; FRCPC; IntMed (Critical Care Medicine). Staff, Thunder Bay Regional Health Sciences Centre; (807)684-6027; Fax. (807)684-5864.

GEORGE, Puthenkalathil P; 3 Duncan Ave, Kentville NS B4N 1N3; Kerala (India)'60; MB BS; MSc(Psy.); AB; FRCPC; Psy (Adult Psychiatry). Staff Psy, Valley Regional Hospital; Teach Staff, Dalhousie University; Langs: Malayalam; (902)678-6685; Fax. (902)678-6685.

GEORGE, Ralph L; St Michael's Hosp, 30 Bond St, Toronto ON M5B 1W8; Qns'84; FRCSC; GenSurg (Surgical Oncology). Staff, St Michael's Hospital; Med Dir, CIBC Breast Centre; Assoc Prof, University of Toronto; (416)864-6060; Fax. (416)864-5965.

GEORGE, Ron; IWK Health Centre, PO Box 9700 Rpo CSC 5850-5980 University Ave, Halifax NS B3K 6R8; Dal'01; FRCPC; Anes. Staff, IWK Health Centre; (902)470-6627; Fax. (902)470-6626.

GEORGE, Ronald; Salvation Army Grace Gen Hosp, 300 Booth Dr, Winnipeg MB R3J 3M7; Sask'89; CCFP; CCFP(E.M.); FCFP; Physician Emerg, The Salvation Army Grace Hospital; (204)837-8311; Fax. (204)831-0029.

GEORGE, Rosamma; Trillium Hlth Ctr-Mississauga, 100 Queensway W, Mississauga ON L5B 1B8; Kerala (India)'87; FRCPC; AnatPath. Staff, Trillium Health Centre - Mississauga; Langs: Malayalam; (905)848-7580

GEORGE, Sabine R; Queensway Prof Centre, 313-190 Sherway Dr, Etobicoke ON M9C 5N2; Justus-Liebig (Germany)'83; FRCPC; Peds (Emergency Medicine). Assoc Staff, The Hospital For Sick Children; Asst Prof, University of Toronto; Langs: German; (416)626-2193; Fax. (416)626-8992.

GEORGE, Shaun R; 121 Orchard St RR 3, Berwick NS B0P 1E0; Ott'90; Dep Head Physiotherapy, Western Kings Memorial Health Centre; (902)538-0163; Fax. (902)538-1803.

GEORGE, Shawn S; Fairmont Med Bldg, 1314-750 Broadway W, Vancouver BC V5Z 1J3; UBC'02; FAAP; FRCPC; Peds. Staff, BC Women's Hospital & Health Centre; Clin Lecturer, University of British Columbia; (604)879-4564

GEORGE, Stanley P; 800-5991 Spring Garden Rd, Halifax NS B3H 1Y6; Dal'83; FRCSC; Ophth (Cataract). (902)429-2760; Fax. (902)425-0666.

GEORGE, Susan R; Univ Hlth Network-Toronto Gen, EN12 215-200 Elizabeth St, Toronto ON M5G 2C4; Tor'75; ABIM; FACP; FRCPC; IntMed (Endocrinology). Sr Scientist, Centre for Addiction & Mental Health (CAMH) - Russell Street Site; Staff, Toronto General Hospital - UHN; Prof, University of Toronto; Langs: Hindi; Malayalam; (416)340-4360; Fax. (416)340-3314.

GEORGE, Susan; Cambridge Med Place, 5-695 Coronation Blvd, Cambridge ON N1R 7J9; Delhi (India)'69; CCFP; Staff Privil, Cambridge Memorial Hospital; Langs: Hindi; (519)623-2830; Fax. (519)623-9569.

GEORGE, Tony P; Addiction & Mental Hlth-Clarke, 732-250 College St, Toronto ON M5T 1R8; Dal'92; FRCPC; Psy. Staff, Centre for Addiction & Mental Health (CAMH) - College Street Site.

GEORGE, W Derek M; The Wright Clinic, 57 James St, Parry Sound ON P2A 1T6; Tor'74; CCFP; FCFP; Staff, West Parry Sound Health Centre; Med Examiner Civil Aviation/Coroner Inquest, City of Parry Sound; (705)746-2181; Fax. (705)746-4753.

GEORGE, William S; Perry Street Med Centre, 101-12 Perry St, Woodstock ON N4S 3C2; Sofia (Bulgaria)'86; BSc; Assoc Staff, Woodstock General Hospital; Langs: Bulgarian; German; (519)539-1526; Fax. (519)539-7508; wgeorge4001@rogers.com.

GEORGESCU, Leonida-Mihai; Hop Maisonneuve-Rosemont, 5415 boul de l'Assomption, Montreal QC H1T 2M4; Mon'05; Anes. Staff, Hopital Maisonneuve-Rosemont; (514)252-3100

GEORGEVICH, Lila L; The Court, 408-2863 Ellesmere Rd, Scarborough ON M1E 5E9; Wes'88; DipEEG; CSCN; FRCPC; IntMed (Epilepsy); Neur. Staff Neurol, Rouge Valley Health System - Centenary Health Centre Site; Langs: English; French; (416)281-3533; Fax. (416)281-3671.

GEORGIADIS, Nina J; 108 Sterling St, Hamilton ON L8S 4J4; McM'88; Staff, Hamilton Health Sciences Centre - McMaster Children's Hospital; Langs: Polish; French; (905)529-0990

GEORGIEFF, Nancy; CSSS de Portneuf, 700 rue Saint-Cyrille, Saint-Raymond QC G3L 1W1; Laval'95; Staff, Centre Hospitalier Portneuf; (418)337-4611 x2518; Fax. (418)337-6703; nancygeorgieff@videotron.ca.

GEORGIEVSKI, Aleksander; Shouldice Hosp, 7750 Bayview Ave, Thornhill ON L3T 4A3; Zagreb (Croatia)'53; Staff, Shouldice Hospital; Langs: Bulgarian; Croatian; Macedonian; Serbian; (905)889-1125; Fax. (905)889-4216.

GEORGILAS, Mary; Vancouver Gen Hosp, 6F-855 12th Ave W, Vancouver BC V5Z 1M9; UBC'95; Staff, Vancouver General Hospital - Centennial Pavillion; (604)875-4073

GEPRAEGS, Tobi; Lakeridge Hlth Corp-Oshawa, 1 Hospital Crt, Oshawa ON L1G 2B9; McM'04; CCFP; Staff, Lakeridge Health - Oshawa Site; (905)576-8711

GERA, Rakesh M; Light House Med Clinic, PO Box 40 41 Centre St, Gimli MB R0C 1B0; Gujarat (India)'83; (204)642-9616; Fax. (204)642-9624.

GERACE, Rocco V; College of Phys & Surgs of ON, 80 College St, Toronto ON M5G 2E2; Wes'72; MD; FRCPC; EmergMed (Clinical Toxicology). Registrar, College of Physicians & Surgeons of Ontario; Aj Prof, University of Toronto; Prof, University of Western Ontario; (416)967-2600 x400; Fax. (416)967-2618.

GERANMAYEGAN, Amir A; Albion-Kipling Med Centre, 301-1525 Albion Rd, Etobicoke ON M9V 5G5; Mem'88; FRCPC; IntMed; Cardiol. (416)740-0956; Fax. (416)740-0958.

GERARD, Lauren M; Sunnybrook Hlth Sciences Ctre, 2075 Bayview Ave, Toronto ON M4N 3M5; Tor'08; FRCPC; IntMed. Staff, Sunnybrook Health Sciences Centre; (416)480-4662

GERARD, Marisa A; South Urgent Care Center, 31 Sunpark Plaza SE, Calgary AB T2X 3W5; Dal'02; CCFP; CCFP(E.M.); (403)943-9476; Fax. (403)943-9482.

GERBER, Christiaan J F; Lloydminster Clinic, 5120 46 St, Lloydminster AB T9V 2P7; Stellenbosch (South Africa)'89; MB ChB; Langs: Afrikaans; (780)875-2221; Fax. (780)875-0605.

GERBER, David; Meridia Med Group, 501-1881 Yonge St, Toronto ON M4S 3C4; Stellenbosch (South Africa)'87; ObstGyn (Colposcopy). Langs: Afrikaans; Dutch; (416)484-8383; Fax. (416)481-4963.

GERBER, Dorothy I; Grande Cache Med Centre, PO Box 540 1600A Acorn Mall, Grande Cache AB T0E 0Y0; (South Africa)'05; CCFP; Staff, Grande Cache Community Health Complex; Langs: Afrikaans; (780)827-2540; Fax. (780)827-5698.

GERBER, John D W; Santa Maria Clinic, 1123 St Mary's Rd, Winnipeg MB R2M 3T7; Orange Free State (South Africa)'80.

GERBER, Laura K; Beech Tree Med Centre, 4-700 Guelph Line, Burlington ON L7R 3M8; McM'99; BSc; FRCPC; Peds. Staff, Joseph Brant Memorial Hospital; (289)288-0061; Fax. (289)288-0473.

GERBER, Lionel; Sunnybrook Hlth Sciences Ctre, FG 52-2075 Bayview Ave, Toronto ON M4N 3M5; Pretoria (South Africa)'85; FRCPC; Psy. Staff Psy, Sunnybrook Health Sciences Centre; (416)480-4070; Fax. (416)480-6878.

GERBER, Michelle R; Panorama Place, 103-15240 56 Ave, Surrey BC V3S 5K7; Cape Town (South Africa)'85; MB ChB; Staff, Cloverdale Crossing Medical Clinic; Langs: Afrikaans; (604)372-2203

GERBER FINN, Lianne; Sioux Lookout First Nations HA, 61 Queen St, Sioux Lookout ON P8T 1B8; McM'07; CCFP; Dryden Regional Health Centre; Staff, Sioux Lookout First Nations Health Authority; (807)737-5160

GERBIS, Christine; Pembroke Reg Hosp, 705 Mackay St, Pembroke ON K8A 1G8; Wes'75; CCFP; Staff, Pembroke Regional Hospital Inc; (613)735-2811 x8108

GERBRANDS, Bea; Regina Qu'Appelle HR-Regina, 1440 14th Ave, Regina SK S4P 0W5; Pretoria (South Africa)'96; MB ChB; DA; CCFP; Associate Critical Care, Pasqua Hospital; Staff, Regina General Hospital; Langs: Afrikaans; (306)766-4444

GEREIN, Richard B; Children's Hosp Eastern Ont, 401 Smyth Rd, Ottawa ON K1H 8L1; Sask'99; FRCPC; Peds; PedEmergMed. Staff, Children's Hospital of Eastern Ontario (CHEO); (613)767-7600

GEREMIA, Brian; Foothills Med Centre, 1403 29 St NW, Calgary AB T2N 2T9; Sask'78; Staff, Peter Lougheed Centre; Staff, Foothills Medical Centre; (403)944-2800; Fax. (403)283-7365.

GERGELY, Anna E; Courtice Health Centre, 1450 Highway 2, Courtice ON L1E 3C3; Timosoara (Romania)'93; PhD; MD; CCFP; Court Staff, Lakeridge Health - Bowmanville Site; Langs: Hungarian; Romanian; (905)721-4956; Fax. (905)721-6176.

GERGES, Ayman; Mississauga Urgent Care, 1201 Britannia Rd W, Mississauga ON L5V 1N2; Zagazig (Egypt)'86; MB BCh; LMCC; CCFP; Staff, Conestoga Medical Centre; Langs: Arabic; (905)826-2273; Fax. (905)826-4010; ayman_gerges@yahoo.com.

GERGES, Hanan; Riverton Comm Hlth Office, PO Box 724 79 Main St, Riverton MB R0C 2R0.

GERGES, Maged; Ravines Med Center, 535 Larry Uteck Blvd, Halifax NS B3M 0E3; Zagazig (Egypt)'92; MB BCh; CCFP; Staff, Queen Elizabeth II Health Sciences Centre - Halifax Infirmary Site; (902)407-4382; Fax. (902)407-4381; maged.gerges@cdha.nshealth.ca.

GERGES, Maha F G; 820 Main St E, Milton ON L9T 0J4; Alexandria (Egypt)'95; CCFP; Langs: Arabic; (905)864-9393

GERGES, Michael M M; Interlake Med Centre, PO Box 430, Arborg MB R0C 0A0; (Egypt)'87; CCFP; (204)376-2781; Fax. (204)376-5356.

GERGES, Nasim K S; 6-2200 Martin Grove Rd, Etobicoke ON M9V 5H9; Tanta (Egypt)'75; MB ChB; CCFP; Langs: Arabic; (416)740-0900; Fax. (416)740-9010.

GERGOVICH, Richard M; Upper Grand Family Health Team, 753 Tower St S, Fergus ON N1M 2R2; McG'77; Assoc Staff, North Wellington Health Care - Louise Marshall Hospital; Ac Staff, Groves Memorial Community Hospital; (519)843-4380; Fax. (519)843-3211; drnovember@sympatico.ca.

GERHART, Stanley; 101-5796 Glover Rd, Langley BC V3A 4H9; Cal'84; (604)530-3233

GERICKE, Werner; Lakewood Common Cardiology, 411C Herold Crt, Saskatoon SK S7V 0A7; Stellenbosch (South Africa)'93; MB ChB; LMCC; Langs: Afrikaans; (306)933-2868; Fax. (306)933-2865.

GERIN, Camille; Clin Communataire Pointe-St-Ch, 500 av Ash, Montreal QC H3K 2R4; Mon'05; CCFP; (514)937-9251; Fax. (514)937-3492.

GERIN-LAJOIE, Annie; CSSS de Trois-Rivières, 1991 boul du Carmel, Trois-Rivieres QC G8Z 3R9; Sher'99; LMCC; Staff, CSSS de Trois-Rivières; (819)697-3333; Fax. (819)372-3535.

GERIN-LAJOIE, Caroline M A; The Ottawa Hosp-Gen Campus, 4306-501 Smyth Rd, Ottawa ON K1H 8L6; Ott'95; MD; FRCPC; Psy (Psycho Oncology). Staff Psy/Med Head Psychosocial Oncology Prog TOH Cancer Centre, The Ottawa Hospital - General Campus; Asst Prof, University of Ottawa; Langs: Bilingual(English/French); (613)737-8899 x70516; Fax. (613)737-8115.

GERIN-LAJOIE, Jean; Smyth Med Centre, 302-1929 Russell Rd, Ottawa ON K1G 4G3; Laval'66; Otol. (613)526-5737

GERIN-LAJOIE, Michele; Clin Pointe St-Charles, 500 av Ash, Montreal QC H3K 2R4; U. of Vermont (USA)'88; (514)937-9251; Fax. (514)937-3492.

GERLACH, Rebecca M; Kingston Orthopaedic & Pain Cl, 500-797 Princess St, Kingston ON K7L 1G1; Qns'08; (613)507-7246

GERMA, Fikre A; Brant Community HS-Brantford, 200 Terrace Hill St, Brantford ON N3R 1G9; Lagos (Nigeria)'86; CCFP; CCFP(E.M.); FCFP; Staff, The Brant Community Healthcare System - Brantford General Hospital Site; Langs: Amharic; (519)752-7871

GERMAIN, Carlie; PO Box 52045 Rpo Garneau, Edmonton AB T6G 2T5; Cal'10; CCFP.

GERMAIN, Caroline; CSSS de la Haute-Yamaska, 205 boul Leclerc O, Granby QC J2G 1T7; Sher'87; FRCPC; IntMed. Staff, Centre Hospitalier de Granby; (450)372-5491; Fax. (450)375-8042.

GERMAIN, Caroline; CSSS Maria-Chapdelaine, 2000 boul du Sacre-Coeur, Dolbeau-Mistassini QC G8L 2R5; Laval'04; CCFP; Staff, Centre Maria-Chapdelaine - CH de Dolbeau-Mistassini; (418)276-1234

GERMAIN, David; CSSS Pierre Boucher, 1333 boul Jacques-Cartier E, Longueuil QC J4M 2A5; Sher'01; FRCPC; IntMed; Respir. Staff, Centre Hospitalier Pierre Boucher; (450)468-8111; Fax. (450)468-8269.

GERMAIN, Elizabeth; CLSC Vallee de la Batiscan, 90 Riviere-A-Veillette RR 4, Ste-Genev-d-Batisc QC G0X 2R0; Laval'04; (418)362-2728

GERMAIN, Estelle; CSSS de Rouyn-Noranda, 1 9e rue, Rouyn-Noranda QC J9X 2A9; Laval'72; ac Staff, Centre Hospitalier Rouyn-Noranda; (819)762-5599 x45159

GERMAIN, Francois; BC Cancer Ctre-Southern Interi, 399 Royal Ave, Kelowna BC V1Y 5L3; Laval'01; FRCPC; RadOncol. Staff, BC Cancer Agency Sindi Ahluwalia Hawkins Centre for the Southern Interior; Langs: Bilingual(French/English); (250)712-3900

GERMAIN, Gilles; Dr Gilles Germain, 15380 av Bourdages S, Saint-Hyacinthe QC J2T 3P7; Mon'74; Assoc Staff, Centre Hospitalier Honore-Mercier; (450)773-7770; Fax. (450)773-2731.

GERMAIN, Guy; 2065 rue Alexandre-deseve, Montreal QC H2L 2W5; Mon'52; CSPQ; FRCPC; IntMed; Rheum (P.Q.). principale Staff Med, Centre Hospitalier l'Université de Montréal (CHUM) - Hôpital Notre-Dame; Hon Staff Rheum Program, Universite de Montreal; Langs: English; (514)890-8211; Fax. (514)412-7672.

GERMAIN, Hughes; Hop Jean-Talon, 1385 rue Jean-Talon E, Montreal QC H2E 1S6; Mon'77; CSPQ; FRCPC; Anes. Staff, CSSS du Coeur de l'Isle Hôpital Jean-Talon; (514)495-6767; Fax. (514)495-6662.

GERMAIN, Isabelle; CHUQ-Hotel-Dieu de Quebec, 11 Cote du Palais, Quebec QC G1R 2J6; Laval'96; RadOncol; LMCC; MMedSci; FRCP; FRCPC; RadOncol (Breast Cancer). Staff, Centre Hospitalier Universitaire de Québec (CHUQ) - Siege Social; (418)691-5264; Fax. (418)691-5268.

GERMAIN, Isabelle; CLSC La Region-Sherbrookoise, 1200 rue King E, Sherbrooke QC J1G 1E4; Sher'91; CCFP; FCFP; (819)563-2572; Fax. (819)563-8502.

GERMAIN, Jean-Francois; CSSS Haut-Richelieu-Rouville, 920 boul du Seminaire N, St-Jean-Sur-Richel QC J3A 1B7; Laval'95; CCFP; Staff, Hôpital du Haut-Richelieu; (450)359-5000; Fax. (450)359-5251.

GERMAIN, Jennifer M; 202-2401 Yonge St, Toronto ON M4P 3H1; Tor'08; CCFP; (416)322-3700; Fax. (416)322-3707.

GERMAIN, Judith; CSSS de Quebec-Sud, 900 boul Wilfrid-Hamel, Quebec QC G1M 2R9; Laval'92; CCFP; Staff, CSSS de Quebec-Sud; (418)682-1762; Fax. (418)682-1763.

GERMAIN, Julie; Hotel-Dieu de levis, 143 rue Wolfe, Levis QC G6V 3Z1; Sher'97; CSPQ; FRCPC; Anes. Staff, Hôtel-Dieu de Lévis; (418)835-7121 x3218

GERMAIN, Louis; Ctr Hosp de lachine, 650 16e av, Lachine QC H8S 3N5; Sher'79; MSc(Physiol.); FRCPC; Psy (P.Q.) (External Clinic). Staff, CSSS de Dorval-Lachine-Lasalle; Langs: Bilingual(French/English); (514)637-2351 x5130

GERMAIN, Louis-Philippe; Clin du Chirurgie Esthetique G, 3A-520 boul de l'Hopital, Gatineau QC J8V 2P5; Ott'00; FRCSC; GenSurg (Cosmetic Surgery); PlasSurg. Staff, Hôpital de Gatineau; Langs: Bilingual(English/French); (819)561-8739; Fax. (819)561-6929.

GERMAIN, Marc; Hema-Quebec, 1070 av Des Sciences-de-la-Vie, Quebec QC G1V 5C3; Laval'85; PhD; FRCPC; MedMicrobiol (Epidemiology); Microbio & Infect Dis (P.Q.). Vice Pres Human Tissues, Hema-Quebec; Assoc Prof Dept of Social Med & Preventive, Université Laval; (418)780-4362 x2209

GERMAIN, Michel M; 200-2984 boul Taschereau, Greenfield Park QC J4V 2G9; Laval'73; CSPQ; OrthSurg. (450)465-9789; Fax. (450)672-4578.

GERMAIN, Mitchel; CSSS de Vaudreuil-Soulanges, 490 boul Harwood, Vaudreuil-Dorion QC J7V 7H4; (Other Foreign)'03; CCFP; Staff, CSSS de Vaudreuil-Soulanges; (450)455-9301; mitchel_germain@rrsss16.gouv.qc.ca.

GERMAIN, R Michel; MUHC-Royal Victoria Hosp, 687 av des Pins O, Montreal QC H3A 1A1; Mon'77; CSPQ; FRCPC; Anes (Echocardiography). Staff, McGill University Health Centre - Royal Victoria Hospital; adj Prof, McGill University; (514)934-1934 x34880

GERMAIN, Richard D; CLSC Lac Saint-Louis, 180 av Cartier, Pointe-Claire QC H9S 4S1; McG'92; Chief Dept of General Medicine-CLSC, CSSS de l'Ouest de l'Île; Langs: Bilingual(French/English); (514)697-4110; Fax. (514)697-4117; rickgermain@rocketmail.com.

GERMAIN, Richard; Clinique Med de Coaticook, 206-18 rue du Manege, Coaticook QC J1A 3B3; Laval'76; Sec Med Council, Centre Hospitalier de Coaticook; Physician, Centre D'Accueil Dixville Home Inc.; Dir, Clinique Familiale de Coaticook; Langs: English; (819)849-4808; Fax. (819)849-7400; rickgermain@rocketmail.com.

GERMAIN, Sophie; Clin Pediatrique Laurentienne, 106-200 rue Durand, Saint-Jerome QC J7Z 7E2; Mon'90; FRCPC; Peds. Staff, Hôtel-Dieu de Saint-Jérôme; (450)438-1241; Fax. (450)438-3501.

GERMAIN, Susan T; Burnaby Hosp, 2D-3935 Kincaid St, Burnaby BC V5G 2X6; McG'92; Staff, Providence Health Care - St Paul's Hospital; Staff, Burnaby Hospital; (604)412-6298

GERMAIN, Veronique; Ctr Hosp de Verdun, 4000 boul LaSalle, Verdun QC H4G 2A3; Mon'99; FRCPC; DiagRad. Staff, Centre Hospitalier de Verdun; (514)362-1000 x2172

GERMAIN, Violaine; Inst U en Sante Mentale de QC, 2525 ch de la Canardiere, Quebec QC G1J 2G3; Laval'98; Staff, Institut Universitaire Sante; Langs: Bilingual(French/English); (418)663-5008; Fax. (418)687-3585; viloaine.germain@ssss.gouv.qc.ca.

GERMAIN-LACROIX, Nicolas; CSSS de la Vallée de l'Or, 725 6e rue, Val-d'Or QC J9P 3Y1; Mon'06; FRCPC; IntMed; Respir. Staff, Centre Hospitalier de Val d'Or; (819)825-5858

GERMAN, Gregory; Queen Elizabeth Hosp, PO Box 6600 Stn Ctrl 60 Riverside Dr, Charlottetown PE C1A 8T5; Ott'07; FRCPC; MedMicrobiol. Staff, Queen Elizabeth Hospital; (902)894-2111

GERMANUS, Faten; Community Health Centre, PO Box 27 111-3640 Hwy 3, Barrington Passage NS B0W 1G0; Cairo (Egypt)'79.

GERNTHOLTZ, Werner E; Surrey Mem Hosp, 13750 96 Ave, Surrey BC V3V 1Z2; Bloemfontein (South Africa)'98; MB ChB; CCFP; CCFP(E.M.); Staff, Surrey Memorial Hospital; Langs: Afrikaans.

GERRARD, Jon M; Legislative Bldg, 169-450 Broadway, Winnipeg MB R3C 0V8; McG'71; ABPeds; FRCPC; Peds (Pediatric Hematology Oncology). Langs: Bilingual(French/English); (204)945-5194; Fax. (204)948-3220; jon.gerrard@leg.gov.mb.ca.

GERRED, R Kent; 64 Ontario St, Trenton ON K8V 6H9; Qns'73; (613)392-6597; Fax. (613)392-5646.

GERRETSEN, Martin; Sea Courses CME, 715-402 Pender St W, Vancouver BC V6B 1T6; UBC'85; Dir CME, Sea Courses Cruises & Tours; (604)684-7327; Fax. (604)684-7337; martin@seacourses.com.

GERRETSEN, Philip M; Addiction & Mental Hlth-Clarke, 250 College St, Toronto ON M5T 1R8; McM'07; FRCPC; Psy. Staff, Centre for Addiction & Mental Health (CAMH) - College Street Site; (416)535-8501

GERRIDZEN, Ronald; B327-1053 Carling Ave, Ottawa ON K1Y 4E9; Ott'78; MD; FACS; FRCSC; Urol (Neuro Urology). Chief Div of Urol, The Ottawa Hospital - Civic Campus; Consultant, Children's Hospital of Eastern Ontario (CHEO); Chair Div of Urology/Prof Surg, University of Ottawa; (613)761-4500; Fax. (613)761-5305.

GERRIE, Alexandra; UWO Student Health Services, 11 UCC-1151 Richmond St, London ON N6A 5B8; Tor'90; CCFP; FCFP; Staff Health Services, University of Western Ontario; (519)661-3771; Fax. (519)661-3380.

GERRING, David R; Care Point Med Centre, 1175 Denman St, Vancouver BC V6G 2N1; Bristol (England)'66; DObstRCOG; DCH; MB ChB; (604)681-5338; Fax. (604)681-0425; dgerring@gmail.com.

GERRITSEN, Jennifer A; PO Box 34123 Rpo Westbrook, Calgary AB T3C 3W2; Cal'96; FRCPC; MedGenetics.

GERSCHMAN, Tommy D; Alberta Children's Hosp, 2888 Shaganappi Trail NW, Calgary AB T3B 6A8; UBC'06; Rheum; Peds. Staff, Alberta Children's Hospital; (403)955-2721; Fax. (403)955-2215.

GERSHATER, Elize; St Joseph's Health Centre, 30 The Queensway, Toronto ON M6R 1B5; McG'98; FRCPC; DiagRad. Staff, St Joseph's Health Centre; (416)530-6010; Fax. (416)530-6025.

GERSHMAN, Stuart M; Univ of Victoria Health Serv, PO Box 1700 Stn CSC, Victoria BC V8W 2Y2; Man'88; Dip SportMed; Staff, Vancouver Island Health Authority; (250)721-8492; Fax. (250)721-6224; sgershman@sumhab.com.

GERSHON, Andrea S; G1 06-2075 Bayview Ave, Toronto ON M4N 3M5; Tor'96; MSc; MD; FRCPC; IntMed (Respiratory Disease); Respir. Physician, Sunnybrook Health Sciences Centre; (416)480-4758; Fax. (416)480-5153.

GERSHON, Sydney L; 504-55 Queen St E, Toronto ON M5C 1R6; Ott'66; FRCPC; IntMed (Rheumatology). Assoc Staff, St Michael's Hospital; Asst Prof, University of Toronto; (416)361-1784

GERSON, Marvin; York-Finch Med Centre, 216C-2115 Finch Ave W, North York ON M3N 2V6; McG'76; FRCPC; MedMicrobiol (Infectious Diseases). Staff, Humber River Regional Hospital - Finch Avenue Site; (416)744-8386; Fax. (416)747-7105.

GERSTEIN, Betty F; Sheppard Beecroft Med Clinic, 48 Sheppard Ave W, North York ON M2N 1M2; Tor'90; CCFP; FCFP; Staff, North York General Hospital; (416)222-1477; Fax. (416)222-5707.

GERSTEIN, Francine H; CMH Med Centre, 111-1315 Finch Ave W, North York ON M3J 2G6; Tor'97; CCFP; (416)631-6888

GERSTEIN, Hertzel; McMaster University Med Centre, PO Box 2000 Stn Lcd 1 1200 Main St W, Hamilton ON L8N 3Z5; Tor'81; MSc(Clin.Epidemiol.); FRCPC; IntMed; Endocrin&Metab. Staff, Hamilton Health Sciences Centre - McMaster Children's Hospital; Staff, Hamilton Health Sciences Centre-Juravinski Site; Dir Endocrinology & Metab/Prof, McMaster University; gerstein@mcmaster.ca.

GERSTEIN, Samuel M; 5016-3080 Yonge St, Toronto ON M4N 3N1; Tor'82; Staff, Humber River Regional Hospital - Church Street Site; Physician Psychotherapist, Yonge-Lawrence Centre for Counselling & Consulting; (416)480-1471; Fax. (416)221-5089; samgerstein@rogers.com.

GERSTEIN, William; MUHC-Montreal Gen Hosp, L8 148-1650 av Cedar, Montreal QC H3G 1A4; Baylor(Texas) (USA)'56; DABD; FRCPC; Derm. Chief Derm, McGill University Health Centre - Montreal General Campus; assoc Prof Med, McGill University; (514)934-1934; Fax. (514)934-8520.

GERSTLE JR, Justin T; The Hosp for Sick Children, 1526-555 University Ave, Toronto ON M5G 1X8; Dartmouth(NH) (USA)'88; FRCSC; GenSurg. Staff, The Hospital For Sick Children; (416)813-6401; Fax. (416)813-7477.

GERSTNER, Thomas V; Meadowood Med Centre, 1555 St Mary's Rd, Winnipeg MB R2M 5L9; Man'90; FRCPC; Peds; ClinImmunol&Allergy. Teacher Peds & Child Hlth, University of Manitoba; (204)255-7650

GERTENSTEIN, Robyn J; Manitoba Clinic, 790 Sherbrook St, Winnipeg MB R3A 1M3; Man'91; FRCSC; ObstGyn. Fax. (204)786-8092.

GERTH, Sjaan C; Harbourfront Med Centre, 4-8 York St, Toronto ON M5J 2Y2; Tor'08; CCFP; (416)366-2273; Fax. (416)366-5665.

GERTLER, Michael M; Dundas Med Centre, 405-220 Dundas St W, Whitby ON L1N 8M7; McG'83; Langs: Bilingual(English/French); (905)668-2778; Fax. (905)668-2919.

GERTLER, Stanley Z; The Ottawa Hosp-Reg Cancer Ctr, 913-501 Smyth Rd, Ottawa ON K1H 1C4; Ott'83; BSc; BMedSci; FRCPC; MedBiochem; MedOncol; IntMed. Staff Consultant/Staff MedOncol Cancer Centre, The Ottawa Hospital - General Campus; Asst Prof, University of Ottawa; Langs: Czech; French; (613)737-7700 x70179

GERTSMAN, Cynthia M; 305-1100 Sheppard Ave E, North York ON M2K 2W1; Ott'68; FRCPC; Psy. Asst Prof Psy, University of Toronto; (416)223-4802

GERULATH, Alan H; Women's Health Care Ctr, 5F-61 Queen St E, Toronto ON M5C 2T2; Tor'63; MS(BioMed.); FACOG; FRCSC; ObstGyn (Colposcopy). Ac Staff, St Michael's Hospital; Assoc Prof ObstGyn, University of Toronto; Langs: German; (416)867-7480; Fax. (416)867-7478.

GERULL, Brenda; Foothills Medical Centre, 1403 29 St NW, Calgary AB T2N 2T9; (Germany)'97; Staff, Foothills Medical Centre; (403)944-1110

GERUS, Lorraine R; Pembroke Reg Hosp, 705 Mackay St, Pembroke ON K8A 1G8; Tor'84; FRCPC; Anes. Staff, Pembroke Regional Hospital Inc; (613)732-2811; Fax. (613)732-9986.

GERVAIS, Andre; CHUS-Hop Fleurimont, 3001 12e av N, Sherbrooke QC J1H 5N4; Mon'68; CSPQ; Cardiol (P.Q.) (Hemodynamics). Staff, Centre Hospitalier Universitaire de Sherbrooke-Hopital Fleurimont; (819)346-1110; Fax. (819)820-6897.

GERVAIS, Andre; CLSC de la Jacques-Cartier, 62 boul Valcartier, Quebec QC G2A 2M5; Laval'75; (418)843-3001

GERVAIS, Andre J G; Dir de la Sante Publique-Mtl, 1301 rue Sherbrooke E, Montreal QC H2L 1M3; McG'75; Respir; IntMed. ac Staff Resp Med, Centre Hospitalier l'Université de Montréal (CHUM) - Hôpital Notre-Dame; adj Prof Med, Universite de Montreal; (514)528-2400 x3497; Fax. (514)528-2425; agervais@santepub-mtl.qc.ca.

GERVAIS, Anne; CSSSG-Hop de Hull, 116 boul Lionel-Emond, Gatineau QC J8Y 1W7; Sher'95; CCFP; Staff, Hull Hospital; (819)561-8100

GERVAIS, Annie; CLSC-CHSLD Champagnat, 978 boul du Seminaire N, St-Jean-sur-Richel QC J3A 1E5; Mon'04; Staff, CLSC-CHLSD Champagnat Vallee des Forts; (450)358-2572; Fax. (450)349-0724.

GERVAIS, Benoit; GMF Centre medical AJC, 110 rue Saint-Jean, Drummondville QC J2B 7T1; Sher'85; ac Staff, Hôpital Sainte-croix; Prof Med, Universite de Sherbrooke; (819)477-1800; Fax. (819)477-9865.

GERVAIS, Carole; 458 Maclaren St, Ottawa ON K1R 5K6; Laval'84; FRCPC; Psy (Pharmacotherapy). Clin Teacher Faculty Med, University of Ottawa; (613)230-0838

GERVAIS, Carolyne; Ctr Hosp du Centre la Mauricie, 50 119e rue, Shawinigan-Sud QC G9P 5K1; Sher'02; FRCSC; ObstGyn. Staff, Centre Hospitalier du Centre la Mauricie; (819)536-7575 x2168

GERVAIS, Chantal; CLSC des Faubourgs, 1705 rue de la Visitation, Montreal QC H2L 3C3; Mon'90; CCFP; Aj Prof, Universite de Montreal; (514)527-2361

GERVAIS, Coralie; Centre Hosp de LaSalle, 8585 Terrasse Champlain, LaSalle QC H8P 1C1; CCFP; Staff, Centre Hospitalier de LaSalle; (514)362-8000

GERVAIS, Daniel; Centre Hosp Honore-Mercier, 2750 boul Laframboise, Saint-Hyacinthe QC J2S 4Y8; Sher'96; CSPQ; AnatPath; GenPath (P.Q.). Anatomical Pathol/Gen Pathol, Centre Hospitalier Honore-Mercier; (450)771-3333; daniel.gervais@rrsss16.gouv.qc.ca.

GERVAIS, Daniel; Clinique Med du Sud-Ouest, 4475 rue Bannantyne, Verdun QC H4G 1E2; Mon'82; Staff, Centre Hospitalier de Verdun; Universite de Montreal; (514)765-3600; Fax. (514)765-9625.

GERVAIS, Hugues; CSSS du Nord de Lanaudière, 1000 boul Sainte-Anne, Joliette QC J6E 6J2; Sher'98; FRCSC; ObstGyn. Staff, Centre Hospitalier Régional de Lanaudière; (450)759-8222

GERVAIS, Jean-Dominique; Ctr Hosp de Verdun, 4000 boul Lasalle, Verdun QC H4G 2A3; Mon'93; FRCPC; DiagRad. Staff, Centre Hospitalier de Verdun; (514)362-1000 x2171

GERVAIS, Jean-Guy; CLSC-CHSLD de L'Erable, 105-1500 av Saint-Louis, Plessisville QC G6L 2M8; Laval'60; Langs: English; (819)362-6301; jggervais@videotron.ca.

GERVAIS, Jocelyn; Ctr Hosp du Centre la Mauricie, 50 119e rue, Shawinigan-Sud QC G9P 5K1; Sher'94; IntMed. Staff, Centre Hospitalier du Centre la Mauricie; (819)536-7500; jocelyn.gervais@sh.cgocable.ca.

GERVAIS, Marc H; CSSS de la Montagne, 7085 rue Hutchison, Montreal QC H3N 1Y9; Mon'61; MSc; Nephrol (P.Q.); Peds (P.Q.). Langs: English; (514)273-3800 x6436; Fax. (514)380-8138.

GERVAIS, Marie; Clinique Med St-Louis, 220-3165 ch St-Louis, Quebec QC G1W 4R4; Mon'90; Staff, Hotel-Dieu d'Arthabaska; (418)653-1970

GERVAIS, Maryse; Hop Louis-H Lafontaine, 7401 rue Hochelaga, Montreal QC H1N 3M5; Mon'00; FRCPC; Psy. Staff, Hopital Louis-H Lafontaine; (514)251-4000; Fax. (514)251-4083.

GERVAIS, Michel; CSSS de l'Energie-Ste-Therese, 1705 av Georges, Shawinigan QC G9N 2N1; Laval'81; FRCPC; Psy. Staff, CH du Centre-de-la-Mauricie (Ste-Thérèse de Shawinigan); Staff, Centre Hospitalier du Centre la Mauricie; (819)536-2299; Fax. (819)537-1827; michel_gervais@ssss.gouv.qc.ca.

GERVAIS, Mireille; CHUS-Hop Hotel-Dieu, 580 rue Bowen S, Sherbrooke QC J1G 2E8; Sher'96; FRCSC; Otol. Staff, Centre Hospitalier Universitaire de Sherbrooke-Hôpital Hôtel-Dieu; (819)346-1110; Fax. (819)566-5244.

GERVAIS, Normand; CSSS de Rivière-de-Loup, 75 rue Saint-Henri, Riviere-Du-Loup QC G5R 2A4; Mon'81; CSPQ; FRCSC; GenSurg. Staff, Centre Hospitalier Regional du Grand-Portage; (418)868-1000; Fax. (418)868-3336.

GERVAIS, Pascale; CHUQ du CHUL, 1740-2705 boul Laurier, Quebec QC G1V 4G2; Mon'97; FRCPC; Peds. Staff, Centre Hospitalier Universitaire de Quebec-CHUL; (418)656-4141

GERVAIS, Philippe; Hôpital Laval, 2725 ch Sainte-Foy, Quebec QC G1V 4G5; Laval'07; FRCPC; MedBiochem. Staff, Hôpital Laval; (418)656-8711

GERVAIS, Pierre B; Polyclinique de Trois-Rivieres, 305-1900 boul des Recollets, Trois-Rivieres QC G8Z 4K4; Laval'64; CSPQ; FRCPC; Cardiol (P.Q.). (819)378-8028; Fax. (819)378-7897.

GERVAIS, Robert; Centre Med Saint-Francois, 200-2125 boul Lemire, Drummondville QC J2B 8N8; Sher'88; Ac Staff, Hôpital Sainte-croix; Langs: English; (819)477-6793; Fax. (819)477-6962; robert_gervais@gmf.gouv.qc.ca.

GERVAIS, Robert; CSSS de Sept-Iles, 45 rue du Pere-Divet, Sept-Iles QC G4R 3N7; Mon'92; DiagRad. Staff, Centre Hospitalier Regional de Sept-Iles; (418)962-9761 x2510; Fax. (418)962-2816.

GERVAIS, Robert-Paul; Agence de Sante Pub du Canada, 0601E2-100 Eglantine Tunney's, Ottawa ON K1A 0K9; Sher'79; FRCPC; CommunMed (Public Health);CCFP; Med Advisor Public Health, Public Health Agency of Canada; Langs: English; (613)946-0360; Fax. (613)952-6668; robert.gervais@phac-aspc.gc.ca.

GERVAIS, Sophie; CSSS de la Matapedia, 135 av Gaetan-Archambault, Amqui QC G5J 2K5; Mon'93; CCFP; Staff, CSSS de la Matapedia; Langs: Bilingual(French/English); (418)629-2211

GERVAIS, Vanessa; Ctr Hosp Reg Chisasibi, PO Box 250, Chisasibi QC J0M 1E0; McG'09; CCFP; Staff, Cree Board of Health & Social Services James Bay; (819)855-9001; Fax. (819)855-2867.

GERVAIS, Yves; College des medecins du Quebec, 2170 boul Rene-Levesque O, Montreal QC H3H 2T8; Laval'99; CCFP; Prof, College des Medecins du Quebec; (514)933-4441 x5239; Fax. (514)933-4668.

GERVAIS-FAGNOU, Danielle D; U of Ottawa Health Services, 300-100 Marie Curie Pvt, Ottawa ON K1N 1A2; Tor'00; CCFP; (613)564-3950; Fax. (613)564-6627.

GERVAISE, Amelie; CSSSG-Hop de Gatineau, CP 2000 Succ Bureau-Chef 909 boul de la Verendrye O, Gatineau QC J8P 7H2; (France)'98; Staff, Hôpital de Gatineau; (819)966-6100

GESSNER, Alessandra; University of Alberta Hosp, 8440 112 St NW, Edmonton AB T6G 2B7; (Brazil)'97; Staff, University of Alberta Hospital; (780)407-8822

GETAHUN, Tajedin Y; King Street Med Arts Centre, 406-71 King St W, Mississauga ON L5B 4A2; Wes'00; FRCSC; OrthSurg. Staff, The Ottawa Hospital - General Campus; (905)897-1119

GETTING, Philip R; Properties Med Clinic, 5102 Rundlehorn Dr NE, Calgary AB T1Y 1C1; London (England)'80; MB; BSc; DRCOG; MRC; DA; Staff, Properties Medical Clinic; (403)280-2700

GETU, Haregua; 102-2009 Danforth Ave, Toronto ON M4C 1J7; McM'85; BSc; Langs: Amharic; Hungarian; (416)690-7269; Fax. (416)690-1864.

GETZ, Corina; Broadway Family Physicians, 1801 Broadway Ave, Saskatoon SK S7H 2B6; Sask'02; BSc; CCFP; (306)652-2632; Fax. (306)652-2637.

GEUKJIAN, S K Gregory; Centre Med Ormstown, GD 24 rue Gale, Ormstown QC J0S 1K0; McG'74; Ac Staff, Barrie Memorial Hospital; Affil Staff, McGill University Health Centre - Montreal General Campus; Prog Dir Ormstown Site, McGill Family Medicine Rural Program; (450)829-2331; Fax. (450)829-3636.

GEUMEI, Ahmed; Hop Santa Cabrini Ospedale, 5655 rue Saint-Zotique E, Montreal QC H1T 1P7; Ain Shams (Egypt)'94; FRCPC; ObstGyn. Staff, Hôpital Santa Cabrini Ospedale; Chef obst & gynécol, Clinique Medical Mile End; (514)252-6000

GEURTS, Jill M; Salvation Army Grace Gen Hosp, 300 Booth Dr, Winnipeg MB R3J 3M7; Man'07; EmergMed. Staff, The Salvation Army Grace Hospital; (204)837-0391

GEVORGYA, Artur; Univ Hlth Network-the Toronto, RFE 32 438-190 Elizabeth St, Toronto ON M5G 2N2; Yerevan (Armenia (Republic))'01.

GEVORGYAN, Artur; Univ Hlth Network-Toronto Gen, 200 Elizabeth St, Toronto ON M5G 2C4; Yerevan (Armenia (Republic))'01; FRCSC; Otol. Staff, Toronto General Hospital - UHN; (416)946-8743

GEVORKYAN, Rafael; Cambridge Mem Hosp, 700 Coronation Bllvd, Cambridge ON N1R 3G2; Kharkov Medical University (Other Foreign)'95; CCFP; Staff, Cambridge Memorial Hospital; (519)621-2330; Fax. (519)740-4938.

GEWURZ, Lauren A; Albany Clinic, 807 Broadview Ave, Toronto ON M4K 2P8; McG'09; CCFP; Langs: Bilingual(English/French); (416)461-9471

GEYER, Willem J; 819 Main St N, Moose Jaw SK S6H 0W8; Orange Free State (South Africa)'87; (306)693-5955; Fax. (306)693-5954.

GFELLER, Kenneth F; The Ottawa Hosp-Civic Campus, 1053 Carling Ave, Ottawa ON K1Y 4E9; Qns'69; FRCPC; Peds. Staff, Children's Hospital of Eastern Ontario (CHEO); Staff, The Ottawa Hospital - Civic Campus; University of Ottawa; (613)796-4073; Fax. (613)825-8966.

GFELLER, Pierre; CSSS d'Antoine-Labelle-Mt Laur, 2561 ch Lievre S, Mont-Laurier QC J9L 3G3; McG'80; Staff, CSSS d'Antoine-Labelle; Staff, Centre Hospitalier Régional de Lanaudière; Langs: French; (819)623-1234 x4202

GHABBOUR, Nagi N R; St Joseph's Health Centre, 30 The Queensway, Toronto ON M6R 1B5; Ain-Shams (Egypt)'84; MB BS; FRCP; FRCPC; Psy (Child & Adolescent Psychiatry). Staff, The Hospital For Sick Children; Staff Child & Adolescent Mental Hlth Prog, St Joseph's Health Centre; Lecturer Psy, University of Toronto; Langs: Arabic; (416)530-6000 x4061; Fax. (416)530-6393.

GHADAI, Talha I; Southlake Reg Health Centre, 596 Davis Dr, Newmarket ON L3Y 2P9; Universidad Iberoamericana(UNIBE) (Dominican Republic)'03; CCFP; Staff, Southlake Regional Health Centre; Langs: Spanish; Urdu; (905)895-4521; Fax. (905)853-2202.

GHADERI, Bahareh; 806-250 ch de la Pointe-Sud, Verdun QC H3E 0A8; Sher'10.

GHADIRIAN, A Missagh; 1025 av des Pins O, Montreal QC H3A 1A1; Tabriz (Iran)'62; MSc; DPsy; FRCPC; Psy (Mood Disorders). Prof, McGill University; (514)934-1934

GHADIRIAN, Gissou S; 204-1436 Royal York Rd, Etobicoke ON M9P 3A9; McG'94; CCFP; Langs: Spanish; Persian; French; (416)614-9134

GHAEMMAGHAMI, Toghra; 134 Banbury Rd, North York ON M3B 2L3; Tehran (Iran)'69; FRCPC; Psy. Langs: Farsi; (416)449-6699; Fax. (416)449-6699.

GHAFFAR, Abdul; Great Lakes Medical Centre, 25 Great Lakes Dr, Brampton ON L6R 2S5; Karachi (Pakistan)'58; AB; DCH; FRCPC; Peds (Asthma & Allergy). Langs: Urdu; Punjabi; (905)494-0302; Fax. (905)494-0754.

GHAFFAR, Hasan; St Michael's Hosp, 30 Bond St, Toronto ON M5B 1W8; Saba University (Netherlands Antilles)'03; FRCPC; AnatPath. Staff, St Michael's Hospital; (416)360-4000 x2368

GHAFFAR, Omar; Sunnybrook Hlth Sciences Ctr, FG 08-2075 Bayview Ave, Toronto ON M4N 3M5; Tor'02; FRCPC; Psy. Staff, Sunnybrook Health Sciences Centre; (416)480-4216; Fax. (416)480-4613.

GHAFFAR-SEDEH, Maryam; Pickering Holistic Hlth Ctr, 220-1101 Kingston Rd, Pickering ON L1V 1B5; Tehran (Iran)'98; CCFP; Langs: Farsi; Persian; (905)831-9797; Fax. (905)839-9984.

GHAFFARI, Mojgan; 12620 132 Ave NW, Edmonton AB T5L 3P9; (Iran)'93; (780)990-1820; Fax. (780)488-0988.

GHAFFARI, Seyed R; South Shore Reg Hosp, 90 Glen Allan Dr, Bridgewater NS B4V 3S6; Tehran (Iran)'98; Staff, South Shore Regional Hospital; (902)543-4603

GHAFOOR, Akmal; Windsor Reg Cancer Centre, 2220 Kildare Rd, Windsor ON N8W 2X3; Karachi (Pakistan)'87; DABIM(IntMed); Staff, Windsor Regional Hospital - Windsor Regional Cancer Centre; (519)253-5253; gakmal@hotmail.com.

GHAFOURI, Seyed M; Humber River Reg Hosp, 2111 Finch Ave W, North York ON M3N 1N1; Teheran (Iran)'89; FRCPC; IntMed. Staff, Humber River Regional Hospital - Finch Avenue Site; Langs: Farsi; (416)744-2500

GHAHARY, Ali; 984 Broadway W PO Box 53565 Rpo West Broadway, Vancouver BC V5Z 4M6; Alb'03; (604)960-3098

GHAHREMANI, Mandana; 3F-507 Broadway W, Vancouver BC V5Z 1E6; Tor'02; FRCPC; ObstGyn.

GHAI, Sandeep; Women's College Hosp, 76 Grenville St, Toronto ON M5S 1B2; Guru Nanak (India)'93; Staff, Women's College Hospital; Langs: Hindi; Punjabi; (416)340-4800 x6558

GHAI, Sangeet; N C S B -1C544, 585 University Ave, Toronto ON M5G 2N2; Dibrugarh (India)'91; Staff, Toronto General Hospital - UHN; Langs: Hindi; (416)340-4800; Fax. (416)593-0502.

GHAIS, Ahmad; CSSS du Nord de Lanaudière, 1000 boul Sainte-Anne, St-Charles-Brromee QC J6E 6J2; Staff, Centre Hospitalier Régional de Lanaudière; (450)759-8222

GHALI, Ashraf M; 201-906 Brant St, Burlington ON L7R 2J5; Ain Shams (Egypt)'87; CCFP; Langs: Arabic; (905)637-5885; Fax. (905)637-0372.

GHALI, Atef M S; The Ottawa Hosp-Civic Campus, 1053 Carling Ave, Ottawa ON K1Y 4E9; Zagazig Faculty of Medicine (Other Foreign)'88; CCFP; Staff, The Ottawa Hospital - Civic Campus; (613)722-7000

GHALI, Kamil; Devon Med Clinic, 5-106 Erie St S, Devon AB T9G 1A7; Alb'78; BSc(Med); CCFP; FCFP; Staff, Devon General Hospital; Asst Clin Prof, University of Alberta; (780)987-3315; Fax. (780)987-4009; kamilghali@gmail.com.

GHALI, Maged; MUHC-Royal Victoria Hosp, R2 28-687 av des Pins O, Montreal QC H3A 1A1; McG'98; FRCPC; IntMed (Hepatology); Gastroent. Staff, McGill University Health Centre - Royal Victoria Hospital; Langs: Bilingual(English/French); (514)934-1934 x31616; Fax. (514)843-1421.

GHALI, Rafik; Hop Maisonneuve-Rosemont, 5415 boul de l'Assomption, Montreal QC H1T 2M4; Laval'88; CSPQ; FRCSC; GenSurg. VascSurg. Staff, Hopital Maisonneuve-Rosemont; (514)252-3822

GHALI, Robert J; 203-749 King St W, Kitchener ON N2G 1E4; Wes'96; CCFP; (519)744-5221; Fax. (519)742-8133.

GHALI, Saad; Clinique Medicale le Trait-d'U, 38 boul Marie-Victorin, Delson QC J5B 1A9; Mon'76; Langs: Arabic; English; (450)633-0123

GHALI, Samia S K; Windsor Reg Hosp-Metropolitan, 1995 Lens Ave, Windsor ON N8W 1L9; Cairo (Egypt)'74; MB BCh; FRCPC; NuclearMed. Ac Staff, Windsor Regional Hospital - Metropolitan Site; Langs: Arabic; (519)254-5577 x52374; Fax. (519)254-4759; samia_sk@yahoo.ca.

GHALI, William A; HSC-Faculty of Med, 3330 Hospital Dr NW, Calgary AB T2N 4N1; Cal'90; FRCPC; IntMed. (403)210-9317; Fax. (403)210-3818.

GHALI, Zineb; Centre Hosp Honore-Mercier, 2750 boul Laframboise, Saint-Hyacinthe QC J2S 4Y8; Mon'06; FRCSC; Ophth. Staff, Centre Hospitalier Honore-Mercier; (450)771-3333

GHALLY, Gehan R; Westheights Med Clinic, 201-10 Westheights Dr, Kitchener ON N2N 2A8; (Egypt)'91; CCFP; Langs: Arabic; (519)578-5555; Fax. (519)578-5551.

GHALY, Ezzat G; McConnell Med Centre, 111-820 McConnell Ave, Cornwall ON K6H 4M4; Cairo (Egypt)'86; FRCPC; IntMed. Staff, Cornwall Community Hospital; Staff, Cornwall Community Hospital - Second Street Site; Langs: Arabic; French; (613)937-0164; Fax. (613)937-4839.

GHANDEHARI, Hournaz; Sunnybrook Hlth Sciences Ctre, 2075 Bayview Ave, Toronto ON M4N 3M5; Tehran (Iran)'95; FRCPC; DiagRad. Staff, Sunnybrook Health Sciences Centre; Langs: Persian; (416)480-6100

GHANEKAR, Anand; Clinical Sciences Bldg, 11C 1227-585 University Ave, Toronto ON M5G 2N2; Tor'98; PhD; FRCSC; GenSurg (Clinician Investigator Program). Staff, Toronto General Hospital - UHN; Staff, The Hospital For Sick Children; (416)340-4606; Fax. (416)340-4767.

GHANEM, Sara; Courtyard Med Clinic, 12-380 Main St, Hartland NB E7P 2N2; Mem'91; (506)375-4250; Fax. (506)375-1992.

GHANEM, Yazan; Pictou West Clinic, PO Box 1060 222 Halliburton Rd, Pictou NS B0K 1H0; (Jordan)'04; MB BS; CCFP; (902)485-6231; Fax. (902)485-6217.

GHANI, Afshan Y; University of Alberta Hosp, 2F1 12-8440 112 St NW, Edmonton AB T6G 2B7; Islamic International Medical College (Other Foreign)'02; FRCPC; IntMed. Staff, University of Alberta Hospital; (780)407-7020; Fax. (780)407-3132.

GHANI, Ikram; The Credit Valley Hosp, 2200 Eglinton Ave W, Mississauga ON L5M 2N1; Karachi (Pakistan)'86; Staff, The Credit Valley Hospital; Langs: Hindi; Punjabi; Urdu; (905)813-2200; Fax. (905)813-4036.

GHANI, Sayeeda S; Lymburn Med Centre, 7526 178 St NW, Edmonton AB T5T 2Y5; Hyderabad (India)'73; (780)481-2076; Fax. (780)481-1380.

GHANIPOUR FARAHANI, Ali; Cedar Med Centre, 106-9648 128 St, Surrey BC V3T 2X9; UBC'10; CCFP; (604)584-5242

GHANNADI, Fatemeh; Seawall Med Center, 102-1590 Bellevue Ave, West Vancouver BC V7V 3R5; Debrecen (Hungary)'94; CCFP; Staff, Seawall Medical Centre; Langs: Arabic; Farsi; Hungarian; (604)281-2444

GHANNOUM, Marc; Ctr Hosp de Verdun, 4000 boul Lasalle, Verdun QC H4G 2A3; McG'97; Nephrol; IntMed. Staff, Centre Hospitalier de Verdun; (514)362-1000

GHANNY, Shari; St Joseph's Healthcare, L208-50 Charlton Ave E, Hamilton ON L8N 4A6; McM'07; FRCPC; IntMed; Hem. Staff, St Joseph's Healthcare - Charlton Campus; (905)521-2100

GHANTOUS, Youssef; McConnell Med Centre, 210-820 McConnell Ave, Cornwall ON K6H 4M4; Sher'95; CCFP; FCFP; Langs: Arabic; French; (613)933-1441; Fax. (613)933-1977.

GHARAGOZLOO, Mehrdad; Red River Valley H D-Morris, PO Box 519 215 Railroad Ave E, Morris MB R0G 1K0; Staff, Morris General Hospital; (204)746-2301

GHARAPETIAN, Angineh; Vancouver Gen Hosp, 855 12th Ave W, Vancouver BC V5Z 1M9; UBC'08; Staff, Vancouver General Hospital - Centennial Pavillion; (604)875-4575

GHAREDAGHI, Mahshid; 1884 Maine Dr, West Vancouver BC V7V 1J6; (Iran)'03; CCFP; Staff, Ocean Walk Medical Centre; Langs: Farsi; Turkish; (604)925-1884

GHARGOUM, Abdussalam M H; PO Box 2489, La Crete AB T0H 2H0; (Libya)'03; (780)928-2030

GHARIB, Rami; CSSS De La Haute-Yamaska, 205 boul Leclerc O, Granby QC J2G 1T7; St Joseph (Lebanon)'89; CSPQ; FRCSC; GenSurg. Staff, Centre Hospitalier de Granby; (450)375-8000

GHARIB, Shler; Brantford Health Clinic, 40 Shellington Pl, Brantford ON N3S 0C5; (Iraq)'93; CCFP; Langs: Kurdish; Arabic.

GHARSAA, Osama; Taunton Surgical Centre, SS 201 1F-1290 Keith Rd Dr, Oshawa ON L1H 7K4; Al-Fateh (Libya)'00; FRCSC; OrthSurg. Staff, Lakeridge Health - Oshawa Site; Langs: Arabic; (905)721-6156

GHATAGE, Prafull; Tom Baker Cancer Centre, 1331 29 St NW, Calgary AB T2N 4N2; RCS (Ireland)'81; MB ChB; BSc(Hons); BAO; LRCPSI; FRCSC; ObstGyn (Gynecologic Oncology). Staff, Tom Baker Cancer Centre; Assoc Prof, University of Calgary; (403)521-3721; Fax. (403)521-3573; prafull.ghatage@albertahealthservices.ca.

GHATAK, Sasanka S; 7550 Cumberland St, Burnaby BC V3N 3X5; Calcutta (India)'55; MRCS(Eng); DPM(Eng); DCH(Eng); MB BS; FRCPC; IntMed. Staff, Richmond Hospital; Media Coord, George Desby Centre; (604)527-4495

GHATALIA, Samir; Montfort Hosp, 713 Montreal Rd, Ottawa ON K1K 0T2; Tor'01; FRCPC; Anes. Staff, Montfort Hospital; Langs: Arabic; (613)746-4621

GHATAVI, Kayhan R; Peterborough Reg HC-Hospital, 1 Hospital Dr, Peterborough ON K9J 7C6; Tor'97; FRCPC; Psy (Consultation-Liaison). Staff, Peterborough Regional Health Centre - Hospital Drive; Teacher, Dalhousie University; (705)876-5028; Fax. (705)876-5013.

GHATE, Hemant B; Hotel-Dieu Grace Hosp, 1030 Ouellette Ave, Windsor ON N9A 1E1; Poona (India)'78; FRCPC; Anes. Staff, Hôtel-Dieu Grace Hospital; Langs: Marathi; Hindi; (519)973-4421; Fax. (519)255-2130; hghate@hotmail.com.

GHATTAS, Aiman Y; CSSS de la Vallée de l'Or, 725 6e rue, Val-d'Or QC J9P 3Y1; Staff, Centre Hospitalier de Val d'Or; (819)825-5858

GHATTAS, Georges; MUHC Royal Victoria Hosp, 687 av des Pins O, Montreal QC H3A 1A1; Mon'84; Gastroent (P.Q.); IntMed (P.Q.) (Therapeutic Endoscopy). Staff, McGill University Health Centre - Royal Victoria Hospital; adj Prof, McGill University; Aj Prof, Universite de Montreal; Langs: Bilingual(French/English); (514)934-1934; Fax. (514)843-1421.

GHATTAS, Paul B; Appletree Med Group, 205-2948 Baseline Rd, Nepean ON K2H 8T5; Ott'80; Staff, Queensway Carleton Hospital; Langs: Arabic; (613)596-6603

GHAURI, Imran K; Riverside Med Complex, PO Box 628, Turtleford SK S0M 2Y0; CCFP; (306)845-2277; Fax. (306)845-4434.

GHAURI, Sabira; Campbellton Reg Hosp, PO Box 880 Stn Main 189 Lily Lake Rd, Campbellton NB E3N 3H3; Punjab (India)'80; Staff, Hôpital Régional Campbellton; (506)789-5000

GHAVAM-RASSOUL, Abbas; St James Town Health Centre, 1F-410 Sherbourne St, Toronto ON M4X 1K2; Tor'97; MHSc; CCFP; FCFP; Staff, St Michael's Hospital; Langs: Farsi; French; (416)864-3096; Fax. (416)864-6035.

GHAVAMI, Ali; CSSSG-Hop de Hull, 116 boul Lionel-Emond, Gatineau QC J8Y 1W7; Liege (Belgium)'94; FRCPC; Cardiol. Staff, Hull Hospital; (819)595-6200

GHAZAL, Zaid; Labrador South Health Centre, PO Box 70 1 Main St, Forteau NL A0K 2P0; Baghdad (Iraq)'02; MB ChB; Staff, Labrador South Health Centre; (709)931-2450; zaid.ghazal@lghealth.ca.

GHAZALA, Khalida K; 206-3885 Duke of York Blvd, Mississauga ON L5B 0E4; Baghdad (Iraq)'86; MB ChB; CCFP; FCFP; Langs: Arabic; (905)848-2119

GHAZALI, Jufri; 158A-19653 Willowbrook Dr, Langley BC V2Y 1A5; (Australia)'01; MB BS; CCFP; (604)530-1333

GHAZALI, Susan M N; Greencrest Clinic, B-2750 Pembina Hwy, Winnipeg MB R3T 2H8; King Abdul Aziz (Saudi Arabia)'91; FRCS; FRCSC; GenSurg (Surgical Oncology). sghazali@brha.mb.ca.

GHAZAN-SHAHI, Sassan; Kingston Gen Hosp, 76 Stuart St, Kingston ON K7L 2V7; Tehran (Iran)'05; IntMed. Staff, Kingston General Hospital; (613)533-2623

GHAZAR, Nancy J; Alberta Children's Hosp, 2888 Shaganappi Trail NW, Calgary AB T3B 6A8; Cal'00; FRCPC; Anes. Staff, Alberta Children's Hospital; (403)955-7810

GHAZARIAN, Boulos A; Blue Water Health, 108-704 Mara St, Point Edward ON N7V 1X4; Ain Shams (Egypt)'82; FRCSC; ObstGyn. Langs: Arabic; (519)383-0003; Fax. (519)383-6499.

GHAZARIAN, Danny M D; Univ Hlth Network-Toronto Gen, 11F 205-200 Elizabeth St, Toronto ON M5G 2C4; Baghdad (Iraq)'81; MB ChB; PhD; FRCPC; AnatPath. Staff, Toronto General Hospital - UHN; Langs: Armenian; Arabic; (416)340-3839; danny.ghazarian@uhn.on.ca.

GHAZAVI, Mohammed T; Scarborough Hosp-Birchmount, 3030 Birchmount Rd, Scarborough ON M1W 3W3; Tehran (Iran)'84; FRCSC; OrthSurg. Staff, The Scarborough Hospital - Birchmount Campus; Langs: Farsi; (416)495-2600; Fax. (416)495-2530.

GHAZI-MIRSAEED, Sayedeh-Bahareh; Brookfield Bonnews HC Centre, PO Box 209 57 Main St, Brookfield NL A0G 1J0; Tehran (Iran)'01; Staff, Brookfield Bonnews Health Care Centre; (709)536-2405; Fax. (709)536-3189.

GHAZIGIAN, Taline; Family Med Centre, 202-3400 rue du Marche, Dollard-D-Ormeaux QC H9B 2Y1; McG'98; CCFP; (514)683-0414; Fax. (514)683-5528.

GHAZNAVI, Sameera; Royal Oak Clinic, C2-2524 Third Line, Oakville ON L6M 0G8; Alb'87; BMedSci; FCFP; CCFP; FCFP; Physician, Dr Bernstein Health & Diet Clinic; Langs: Urdu; Hindi; (905)827-7000; Fax. (905)827-7755; sameera.ghaznavi@shaw.ca.

GHEBRAY, Tesfay M; Steinbach Family Med Centre, 10-333 Loewen Blvd, Steinbach MB R5G 0C3; Addis Ababa (Ethiopia)'85; CCFP; (204)326-8877; Fax. (204)326-4618.

GHEBRIAL, Maged S N; Wheat City Med Clinic, C1-1711 Kirkcaldy Dr, Brandon MB R7A 0B9; (Other Foreign)'79; CCFP; (204)727-1711

GHEDIRA, Monia; Dr Georges-L Dumont Reg Hosp, 330 av Universite, Moncton NB E1C 2Z3; Monastir (Tunisia)'03; Staff, Dr Georges-L-Dumont University Hospital Centre; (506)862-4000

GHEISSARI, Saeid; University of Alberta Hosp, OR L3-8440 112 St NW, Edmonton AB T6G 2B7; (Iran)'88; Staff, University of Alberta Hospital; (780)407-8822

GHEMLAS, Ibrahim A M; Children's Hosp of Eastern Ont, 401 Smyth Rd, Ottawa ON K1H 8L1; King Saud University (Saudi Arabia)'03; Clin Fellow Ped Hem, Children's Hospital of Eastern Ontario (CHEO); (613)737-7600

GHENEA, Irina; Northside Harbor View Hosp, PO Box 399 Stn Main, North Sydney NS B2A 3M4; McG'96; CCFP; Staff, Northside General Hospital; (902)794-7250; Fax. (902)794-7259.

GHEORGHE, Camelia M; A103-11685 Yonge St, Richmond Hill ON L4E 0K7; (Romania)'99; CCFP; Langs: Romanian; (905)770-9057; Fax. (905)917-0215.

GHEORGHE, Rodica C; Health Sciences Centre, MS459-820 Sherbrook St, Winnipeg MB R3A 1R9; (Romania)'86; FRCPC; AnatPath. Staff, Health Sciences Centre.

GHERIANI, Heitham A A; Park Ave Med Centre ENT Clinic, 500-4634 Park Ave, Terrace BC V8G 1V7; (Libya)'94; MB ChB; FRCSC; Otol. Langs: Arabic; (250)615-5070

GHERT, Michelle A; Hamilton HS-Henderson Site, B3-711 Concession St, Hamilton ON L8V 1C3; Vanderbilt(TN) (USA)'96; FRCSC; OrthSurg (Orthopedic Oncology). Staff, Hamilton Health Sciences Centre-Juravinski Site; Physician, The Juravinski Cancer Centre; (905)387-9495; Fax. (905)381-7071.

GHESQUIERE, Mark H; West Street Health Centre, 201-216 West St, Simcoe ON N3Y 1S8; Wes'90; CCFP; (519)428-0442; Fax. (519)428-4144.

GHESQUIERE, Wayne; Foul Bay Prof Centre, 206-1964 Fort St, Victoria BC V8R 6R3; McM'83; BSc; FRCPC; IntMed (Tropical & Travel Medicine); InfectDis. Staff, Vancouver Island Health Authority; Staff, Royal Jubilee Hospital; Staff, Victoria General Hospital; Clin Assoc Prof Medicine, University of Victoria; Clin Assoc Prof Med, University of British Columbia; (250)370-7717

GHIASSI-RAZAVI, Rezvan; Tudor Glen Medicentre, 2520 Tudor Glen Market, St. Albert AB T8N 3V3; (South Africa)'04; MB ChB; (780)458-5776

GHINEA, Mircea D; Ctr Hosp Fleury, 2180 rue Fleury E, Montreal QC H2B 1K3; Carol Davila (Romania)'96; Staff, Centre Hospitalier Fleury; (514)384-2000

GHITTER-MANNES, Sandra; Forest Heights Med Clinic, 7461 101 Ave NW, Edmonton AB T6A 3Z5; Alb'81; Clin Lecturer, University of Alberta; (780)463-2323; Fax. (780)463-5514.

GHITULESCU, Gabriela; SMBD Jewish Gen Hosp, A500-3755 ch Cote-Sainte-Cathe, Montreal QC H3T 1E2; McG'92; CSPQ; FRCSC; GenSurg (Colon & Rectal Surgery). Staff, Sir Mortimer B Davis Jewish General; Langs: Romanian; Spanish; French; (514)340-8222 x3937; Fax. (514)340-8132; gabriela.ghitulescu@mcgill.ca.

GHOBADIAN, M Reza; Whitby Med Arts Centre, 18-1615 Dundas St E, Whitby ON L1N 2L1; Tehran (Iran)'92; CCFP; Physician, Avicenna Health Centre; Langs: Farsi; Persian; (905)240-2880; Fax. (905)240-3880; medicalhealthcentre2@hotmail.com.

GHOBASSY, Bahar; 6060 Minoru Blvd PO Box 43160 Rpo Richmond Ctr, Richmond BC V6Y 3Y3; UBC'08; CCFP; (604)754-0648

GHOBRIAL, M; Parkdale Med Tower, 502-1081 Carling Ave, Ottawa ON K1Y 4G2; Cairo (Egypt)'64; MB ChB; DAB; FRCPC; Peds (Newborn Medicine). Ac Staff, Children's Hospital of Eastern Ontario (CHEO); Ac Staff, The Ottawa Hospital - Civic Campus; Staff, Queensway Carleton Hospital; University of Ottawa; Langs: Arabic; French; (613)728-0608; Fax. (613)728-4286.

GHOBRIAL, Mohab; Acadia & Buena Vista Drive Cli, 100-739 Lake Bonavista Dr SE, Calgary AB T2J 0N2; Assiut (Egypt)'84; CCFP; (403)271-7763; Fax. (403)271-7715.

GHOBRIL, Victor P; CSSS du Nord de Lanaudière, 1000 boul Sainte-Anne, St-Charles-Brromee QC J6E 6J2; Ein Shams (Egypt)'69; FRCPC; HemPath; MedOncol. Staff Hematology, Centre Hospitalier Régional de Lanaudière; (450)759-8222; Fax. (450)759-7861.

GHOCHE, Roger; Univ Hlth Network-Toronto Western Hosp, 8MCL 433-399 Bathurst St, Toronto ON M5T 2S8; McG'07; MDCM; CCFP; Staff, Sunnybrook Health Sciences Centre; Langs: Bilingual(French/English); (416)603-5800; Fax. (416)603-5315.

GHOHARI, Foroozan; Willoughby Med Centre, B1A-20202 66 Ave, Langley BC V2Y 1P3; (Iran)'92; CCFP; Staff, Willoughby Medical Centre; (604)514-8800

GHOLAM, Bassam I A; Norfolk Gen Hosp, 365 West St, Simcoe ON N3Y 1T7; King Faisal University (Saudi Arabia)'93; CCFP; CCFP(E.M.); Staff, Norfolk General Hospital; Langs: Arabic; (519)426-0750; Fax. (519)429-6998.

GHOLAMABBAS JAVAN, Asef; Municipal Med Centre, PO Box 70, Wakaw SK S0K 4P0; (306)233-4443; Fax. (306)233-4433.

GHOLAMI, Amir S; The Hosp for Sick Children, 555 University Ave, Toronto ON M5G 1X8; Saba University School of Medicine (Other Foreign)'04; Staff, The Hospital For Sick Children; (416)813-7445

GHONEIM, Mostafa S A F; Portage Clinic, 140 9th St SE, Portage La Prairie MB R1N 3V5; Alexandria (Egypt)'75; CCFP; (204)239-2211

GHOOKAL, Dharmendra M; Guelph Gen Hosp, 115 Delhi St, Guelph ON N1E 4J4; Witwatersrand (South Africa)'93; MB ChB; FRCPC; DiagRad. Staff, Guelph General Hospital; (519)837-6440

GHOORAH, Sanyukta K; 21st Medical Clinic, 502-402 21st St E, Saskatoon SK S7K 0C3; (United Kingdom)'90; MB ChB; MRCP(UK); FRCPC; IntMed. Langs: Bilingual(English/French); (306)956-3444; Fax. (306)956-3577.

GHOPRIAL-GHALI, Marcelle; Clinique Metro Papineau, 1900 rue Sainte-Catherine E, Montreal QC H2K 2H5; Ain Shams (Egypt)'78; (514)525-4555; Fax. (514)525-3338.

GHORAB, Zeina; Sunnybrook Hlth Sciences Ctre, E4 37-2075 Bayview Ave, Toronto ON M4N 3M5; Tichreen (Syria)'84; Staff, Sunnybrook Health Sciences Centre; Langs: Arabic; French; (416)480-6100

GHORAYEB, Sahar H; 3-45 Grist Mill Rd, Holland Landing ON L9N 1M7; Wes'05; CCFP; (905)853-8966

GHORBANI, Farnaz; A204-11685 Yonge St, Richmond Hill ON L4E 0K7; Shahid Beheshti (Iran)'92; CCFP; FCFP; Langs: Farsi; (905)237-7474; Fax. (905)237-7476.

GHORI, Aqeel; 6-1061 Central Ave N, Swift Current SK S9H 4Y9; (306)773-5855; Fax. (306)778-3799.

GHORPADE, Nitin; University of Alberta Hosp, 3H2 14-8440 112 St NW, Edmonton AB T6G 2B7; Bombay (India)'89; FRCSC; CardSurg. Staff Cardiac Surg, University of Alberta Hospital; (780)407-8822; Fax. (780)407-7657.

GHOSE, Abhijit; Chinook Reg Hosp, 1A122-960 19 St S, Lethbridge AB T1J 1W5; McM'06; FRCPC; RadOncol. Staff, Chinook Regional Hospital; (403)388-6871

GHOSH, Debasish; Medical Specialists Clinic, 101-901 Island Hwy, Campbell River BC V9W 2C2; Calcutta (India)'83; Staff, Campbell River & District General Hospital; (250)287-8764

GHOSH, Indraneel; BP Health Clinics, 554 John St N, Hamilton ON L8L 4S1; Qns'00; CCFP; CCFP(E.M.); Staff, Hamilton Health Sciences Centre - McMaster University Medical Centre; Staff, Mackenzie Richmond Hill Hospital; Langs: Bengali; Hindi; (905)318-0911; Fax. (905)318-7219; clinics@bphealth.ca.

GHOSH, Mahua; Heritage Med Research Ctr, 362-107 University Campus NW, Edmonton AB T6G 2S2; (India)'96; FRCPC; IntMed; Endocrin&Metab. Langs: Bengali; Hindi; (780)407-3636; Fax. (780)407-6702.

GHOSH, Nina; Health Sciences North, 41 Ramsey Lake Rd, Sudbury ON P3E 5J1; Wes'05; FRCPC; IntMed; Cardiol. (705)523-7100; Fax. (705)671-5358.

GHOSH, Rishi K; 750 Great Northern Rd, Sault Ste. Marie ON P6B 0A8; Ott'02; FRCPC; EmergMed; Critical Care Medicine. Staff, Sunnybrook Health Sciences Centre; Staff, Sault Area Hospital - Sault Ste Marie; Langs: Bilingual(English/French); (705)759-3434

GHOSH, Shuvo; MUHC-Montreal Children Hosp, D 280-2300 rue Tupper, Montreal QC H3H 1P3; Illinois(MI) (USA)'98; Staff, McGill University Health Centre - Montreal Children's Hospital; (514)412-4314; Fax. (514)412-4280.

GHOSH, Subrata; Foothills Med Centre, NT930-1403 29 St NW, Calgary AB T2N 2T9; (India)'82; FRCP(Edin); FRCP(London); MB BS(Calcutta); FRCPC; Gastroent (Inflammatory Bowel Disease). Staff, Foothills Medical Centre; Prof Med/Head Div of Gastroenterology/Dept Head Med, University of Calgary; (403)944-6555; ghosh@ucalgary.ca.

GHOSH, Surajit; Associated Med Specialists, 1555 Second Ave, Trail BC V1R 1M3; Calcutta (India)'59; LRCP(Lond); MRCS(Eng); MRCP; FCCP; MB BS; FRCPC; IntMed. Staff, Kootenay Boundary Regional Hospital; (250)368-3301; Fax. (250)368-5053; imed@shawcable.com.

GHOSN, Pierre B; Hôpital St-Luc, 8302-1058 rue Saint-Denis, Montreal QC H2X 3J4; Beyrouth (Lebanon)'77; CSPQ; FRCSC; GenSurg; Cardiovasc&ThorSurg; VascSurg. Thoracic & Cardiovasc Surg, Centre Hospitalier l'Université de Montréal (CHUM) - Hôpital Saint-luc; Prof Surg, Universite de Montreal; (514)890-8000 x15980; Fax. (514)412-7332.

GHOSSI-MARAGHEH, Nazanine; 3945 17 Ave SW, Calgary AB T3E 0C3; (Other Foreign)'10; CCFP; (403)242-8633

GHOSTINE, Jimmy; CHUM-Hop Notre-Dame, 1560 rue Sherbrooke E, Montreal QC H2L 4M1; McG'03; FRCPC; DiagRad. Staff, Centre Hospitalier l'Université de Montréal (CHUM) - Hôpital Notre-Dame; (514)890-8000

GHOTRA, Harpreet S; Danforth Med Centre, 880 Danforthh Rd, Scarborough ON M1K 1H8; (India)'03; (416)264-4848

GHOUBRIL, Suzette; Clinique Domus Medica, 5601 rue Belanger, Montreal QC H1T 1G3; Mon'81; Staff, Hôpital Santa Cabrini Ospedale; Physician, Centre d'Accueil Elorie Lepage; (514)256-5011 x223

GHOUSE, Ali T; 4-688 Concession St, Hamilton ON L8V 4T1; Osmania (India)'75; FRCPC; PhysMed&Rehab (Electromyography). Staff, Hamilton Health Sciences Centre-Juravinski Site; Clinical Asst Prof, McMaster University; Langs: Hindi; Persian; Urdu; (905)389-4099; Fax. (905)389-4906.

GHREDISH, Tareg; 15345 97 ST NW, Edmonton AB T5X 5V3; (Libya)'99; MB BCh; (780)457-6060; Fax. (780)457-6111.

GHREMIDA, Shukri A M; Cornwall Prof Bldg, 706-2125 11th Ave, Regina SK S4P 3X3; Tripoli (Libya)'90; MB ChB; FRCSC; PlasSurg. Staff, Pasqua Hospital; (306)546-4460; Fax. (306)546-4461.

GHUFRAN, Shazia; 5132 Lander Trunk Rd, Delta BC V4K 1W3; Peshawar (Pakistan)'94; FRCPC; Peds. (604)940-0917

GHUMAN, Harleen K; Grand River Hosp-KW Hlth Ctre, PO Box 9056 835 King St W, Kitchener ON N2G 1G3; Baba Farid (India)'03; FRCPC; Psy. Staff, Grand River Regional Cancer Centre; (519)749-4300

GHUMAN, Jaspinder; Surrey Mem Hosp, 13750 96 Ave, Surrey BC V3V 1Z2; Sask'00; CCFP; CCFP(E.M.); Staff, Surrey Memorial Hospital; Langs: Hindi; Punjabi; (604)581-2211

GHUMMAN, Ejaz A; Leamington District Mem Hosp, 1F-194 Talbot St W, Leamington ON N8H 1N9; Punjab (Pakistan)'82; MB BS; FRCSC; GenSurg. Chief Gen Surg/Chief of Staff, Leamington District Memorial Hospital; Langs: Punjabi; Persian; Urdu; (519)326-2830; Fax. (519)326-4461.

GHURA, Parminder S; Ocean Park Med Clinic, 12894 16th Ave, Surrey BC V4A 1N7; Newcastle (England)'97; MB BS; (604)531-1626

GIACCONE, Roberto A; Nepean Med Centre, 306-1 Centrepointe Dr, Nepean ON K2G 6E2; Ott'87; FRCPC; Neur (Parkinson's Disease). Staff, The Ottawa Hospital - Civic Campus; Staff, Kemptville District Hospital; Langs: Italian; French; (613)723-8733; Fax. (613)723-2925; roberto.giaccone@sympatico.ca.

GIACHINO, A Alan; Smyth Med Centre, 206-1929 Russell Rd, Ottawa ON K1G 4G3; Tor'71; FRCSC; OrthSurg (Rheumatology). Staff, The Ottawa Hospital - Riverside Campus; Ac Staff, The Ottawa Hospital - General Campus; Assoc Prof OrthSurg, University of Ottawa; Langs: Bilingual(English/French); (613)738-0965; Fax. (613)738-1197.

GIACOBBE, Peter; Univ Hlth Network-Toronto Gen, 8EN 225-200 Elizabeth St, Toronto ON M5G 2C4; Wes'01; FRCPC; Psy. Staff, Toronto General Hospital - UHN; (416)340-4672; Fax. (416)340-4198.

GIACOMANTONIO, Carman A; Queen Elizabeth II HSC, 509-1276 South Park St, Halifax NS B3H 2Y9; Mem'91; MSc(Path); FRCSC; GenSurg (Surgical Oncology). Staff, Queen Elizabeth II Health Sciences Centre - Victoria General Site; Staff, IWK Health Centre; (902)473-6177; Fax. (902)473-6178; carman.giacomantonio@dal.ca.

GIACOMANTONIO, J Michael; IWK Health Centre, PO Box 9700 rpo CSC 5850-5980 University Ave, Halifax NS B3K 6R8; Dal'76; FRCSC; GenSurg; PedGenSurg. Div Chief Ped GenSurg/Ac Staff, IWK Health Centre; Assoc Prof Div of Ped & GenSurg, Dalhousie University; (902)470-8114; Fax. (902)470-7260; michael.giacomantonio@iwk.nshealth.ca.

GIACOMANTONIO, Nicholas B; Queen Elizabeth II HSC-Halifax, 2132-1796 Summer St, Halifax NS B3H 3A7; Mem'92; BSc(Hon); FRCPC; IntMed (Preventive Cardiology); Cardiol. Assoc Prof/Cardio Rehabilitation Prog/ Undergraduet Med Educ for Cardiology/Assoc Assoc Dir Clerkship Dept Med, Queen Elizabeth II Health Sciences Centre - Victoria General Site; Assoc Prof Med, Dalhousie University; (902)473-3815; Fax. (902)473-2434; domnbg@cdha.nshealth.ca.

GIACOMINI, Paul S; MUHC-Montreal Neurology Inst, RM 365A-3801 rue University, Montreal QC H3A 2B4; Tor'01; FRCPC; Neur. Staff, McGill University Health Centre - Montreal Neurological Hospital; (514)398-1931; Fax. (514)398-2975.

GIAMMARCO, Rosella; Charlton Med Centre, 808-25 Charlton Ave E, Hamilton ON L8N 1Y2; McM'82; FRCPC; Neur (Headache). Staff, St Joseph's Healthcare - Charlton Campus; Physician, Charlton Medical Centre; Staff Pt-Time, McMaster University; Langs: Italian; (905)523-5788; Fax. (905)523-7880.

GIANCOLA, Lina; Yonge-Eglinton Med Centre, 210-2401 Yonge St, Toronto ON M4P 3H1; McM'91; MSW; CCFP; Langs: Italian; (416)485-9044; Fax. (416)485-8525.

GIANFELICE, David C; Radiologie Laennec Inc, 1100 av Beaumont, Mont-Royal QC H3P 3H5; McG'82; FRCPC; DiagRad. (514)738-6866

GIANG, Clarence; PO Box 4123 Stn South CRO, Edmonton AB T6E 4T2; Alb'07; CCFP.

GIANG, Hudson K H; Ross Mem Hosp, 10 Angeline St N, Lindsay ON K9V 4M8; Ho Chi Minh (Vietnam)'79; FRCPC; GenPath. Staff/Med Dir Laboratory, Ross Memorial Hospital; Langs: Chinese; Vietnamese; Fax. (705)328-6129.

GIANNAKIS, Andreas; 303-7200 rue Hutchison, Montreal QC H3N 1Z2; McG'77; (514)278-8877; Fax. (514)278-8205.

GIANNANGELO, Dominique; Clinique méd Brome-Missiquoi, 280 rue Victoria, Knowlton QC J0E 1V0; McM'99; CCFP; (450)243-5043; Fax. (450)243-0537.

GIANNELIS, Taxiarhoula; Clinique Med l'Envolee, 5025 rue de Salaberry, Montreal QC H4J 1J1; Mon'06; Staff, Centre Hospitalier de LaSalle; (514)331-2323

GIANNETTI, Nadia S; MUHC-Royal Victoria Hosp, A401-687 av des Pins O, Montreal QC H3A 1A1; McG'91; CSPQ; FRCPC; IntMed; Cardiol. Staff, McGill University Health Centre - Royal Victoria Hospital; (514)934-1934 x32850; nadia.giannetti@muhc.mcgill.ca.

GIANNOCCARO, John P; Cardiology Consultants, 103-803 1 Ave NE, Calgary AB T2E 7C5; Tor'85; FRCPC; IntMed; Cardiol. Staff, Peter Lougheed Centre; Staff, Rockyview General Hospital; Staff, Foothills Medical Centre; (403)571-8642; Fax. (403)215-2213.

GIANNOULI, Eleni; RS311-810 Sherbrook St, Winnipeg MB R3A 1R8; Thessaloniki (Greece)'87; FRCPC; IntMed; Respir. Staff, Health Sciences Centre; egiannouli@hsc.mb.ca.

GIANNOULIAS, Dimitrios; 203-421 Bloor St E, Toronto ON M4W 3T1; Athens (Greece)'73; FRCSC; ObstGyn (Prenatal Care). Staff, Mount Sinai Hospital; Med Associate/VP, Hippocrates Hellenic Canadian; Lecturer ObstGyn, University of Toronto; Langs: Greek; (416)975-2549; Fax. (416)975-2568.

GIANOULIS, Mary E; Burnaby Hosp, 3935 Kincaid St, Burnaby BC V5G 2X6; Sask'86; FRCPC; GenPath. Staff Lab, Burnaby Hospital; (604)412-6245; Fax. (604)431-2806.

GIANTOMASO, Tony; Caleo Health, 340-600 Crowfoot Cres NW, Calgary AB T3G 0B4; Sask'03; BSc; DC; FRCPC; PhysMed&Rehab (Pain Management). Clin Assoc Prof, University of Calgary; Langs: Italian; French; (403)452-0999; Fax. (403)452-0995.

GIARD, Alain; Ctr Hosp Laurentien, 234 rue Saint-Vincent, Ste-Agathe-des-Mts QC J8C 2B8; Mon'72; CSPQ; FRCSC; GenSurg (Vasculities). Chef chir gén, Centre Hospitalier Laurentien; Langs: Bilingual(French/English); (819)324-4000

GIARD, Annie; Hop du Sacre-Coeur de Mtl, 5400 boul Gouin O, Montreal QC H4J 1C5; Mon'06; FRCPC; EmergMed. Staff, Hôpital du Sacre-Coeur de Montréal; (514)338-2222

GIARD, Chantale; Ctr Hosp de LaSalle, 8585 Tsse Champlain, LaSalle QC H8P 1C1; Mon'00; CCFP; Staff, Centre Hospitalier de LaSalle; (514)362-8000; chantale_giard@hotmail.com.

GIARD, Francoise; Clinique de Dermatologie, 110-500 boul Greber, Gatineau QC J8T 7W3; Sher'86; FRCPC; Derm. Staff Derm, Hull Hospital; (819)561-5553; Fax. (819)561-5554.

GIARD, Marie-Claude; Ctr Hosp De Verdun, 4000 boul Lasalle, Verdun QC H4G 2A3; Mon'06; Rheum; IntMed. Staff, Centre Hospitalier de Verdun; (514)362-1000

GIASSON, Marc; Hop du Sacre-Coeur de Mtl, 5400 boul Gouin O, Montreal QC H4J 1C5; Mon'87; Critical Care Medicine (P.Q.); IntMed. Staff, Hôpital du Sacre-Coeur de Montréal; (514)338-2050

GIASSON JR., Carl; Groupe Sante Medisys Inc, 550-500 rue Sherbrooke O, Montreal QC H3A 3C6; Mon'68; (514)845-1211; Fax. (514)845-4842.

GIAVEDONI, Louis R; St Michael's Health Centre, 801-61 Queen St E, Toronto ON M5C 2T2; Tor'82; DAB(USA); FRCSC; Ophth (Vitreo Retina). Staff, St Michael's Hospital; Asst Prof, University of Toronto; Langs: Italian; (416)867-7400; Fax. (416)864-0600; giavedonil@smh.toronto.on.ca.

GIBARA, Magdy R B; Postmaster Med Clinic, 2540 Postmaster Dr, Oakville ON L6M 0N2; Tanta (Egypt)'83; CCFP; FCFP; Langs: Arabic; (905)845-4039; Fax. (905)845-6795.

GIBB, Donald R; Bigelow Fowler Clinic West, 30 Jerry Potts Blvd W, Lethbridge AB T1K 5M5; Alb'90; CCFP; FCFP; (403)381-8444; Fax. (403)381-8166.

GIBB, Graham K; The Peterborough Clinic, 301-26 Hospital Dr, Peterborough ON K9J 7C3; Tor'93; BSc; FRCSC; GenSurg (Colon & Rectal Surgery). Staff, Peterborough Regional Health Centre - Hospital Drive; (705)740-6890; Fax. (705)740-6899; ggibb@ptboclinic.com.

GIBB, Paul S; City of Lakes Family Hlth Team, C-960 Notre Dame Ave, Sudbury ON P3A 2T4; Qns'96; BScPharm; CCFP; FCFP; Staff, Health Sciences North-Laurentian Site; Asst Prof Section of Family Med, Northern Ontario School of Medicine; (705)560-1018; Fax. (705)566-7617.

GIBB, Robert A; 4411 Tecumseh Rd E, Windsor ON N8W 1K6; Wes'79; Assoc Staff, Hôtel-Dieu Grace Hospital; (519)944-7811; Fax. (519)944-6105.

GIBBARD, W Benton; Alberta Children's Hosp, 2888 Shaganappi Trail NW, Calgary AB T3B 6A8; UBC'97; FRCPC; Peds (Developmental Pediatrics). Staff, Alberta Children's Hospital; (403)955-7815; Fax. (403)955-7649; ben.gibbard@albertahealthservices.ca.

GIBBINGS, Grant W J; Hilltop Medical, 12894 16 Ave, Surrey BC V4A 1N7; Sask'67; CCFP; (604)531-7712; Fax. (604)542-2559.

GIBBON, Stephen B; Family Practice Associates, 6155 North St, Halifax NS B3K 5R3; Dal'77; BSc; Physician, IWK Health Centre; (902)453-3511; Fax. (902)454-9010.

GIBBONS, Amber; Clinique Med Deux-Montagnes, 201 9e Avenue, Saint-Eustache QC J7R 3M1; Mon'07; CCFP; Staff, Hôpital de Saint-Eustache; (450)472-7545

GIBBONS, Jeannette M; Upstream Family Med, RR 1 108-4330 Sunshine Coast Hwy, Sechelt BC V0N 3A1; Cal'83; CCFP; Staff, St Mary's Hospital; (604)885-6400; Fax. (604)885-6411.

GIBBONS, Maria K; Owen Sound Med Associates, 2000-1415 1st Ave W, Owen Sound ON N4K 4K8; Tor'03; CCFP; CCFP(E.M.); (519)470-3030

GIBBONS, Maria T; Major's Path Family Practice, 301-35 Major's Path, St. John's NL A1A 4Z9; (Ireland)'79.

GIBBONS, Patrick J; Fillmore Union Hlth Centre, PO Box 246, Fillmore SK S0G 1N0; Galway (Ireland)'71; MB ChB; BAO; (306)722-2308; Fax. (306)722-3877.

GIBBONS, Sherri; Maternity Care Clinic, 201-178 96 Ave NE, Calgary AB T3K 6G4; Cal'98; FRCSC; ObstGyn. Staff, Maternity Care Clinic; (403)806-2496; Fax. (403)806-2497.

GIBBONS GOMEZ, Paul; Niagara H System-Welland Site, 65 Third St, Welland ON L3B 4W6; Dal'08; CCFP; Staff, Niagara Health System - Welland Hospital Site; (905)378-4647

GIBBS, David J; Sheldon M Chumir Health Centre, M-1213 4 St SW, Calgary AB T2R 0X7; Man'96; FRCPC; Psy. Staff, Peter Lougheed Centre; Consultant Psy, Calgary Consulting Centre; (403)955-6566; Fax. (403)955-6585; david.gibbs@albertahealthservices.ca.

GIBBS, Gaetan; Hop Regional D'Edmundston, 275 Hebert Blvd, Edmundston NB E3V 4E4; Mon'00; CCFP; Staff, Hôpital regional d'Edmundston; (506)739-2200

GIBBS, Laurence H S; 125 King St PO Box 329 Stn Main, Thedford ON N0M 2N0; Birmingham (England)'78; MRCP(UK); MB ChB; (519)296-5807; Fax. (519)296-4887; la.ha@hotmail.com.

GIBEAULT, Audrey; Hôpital Anna-Laberge, 200 boul Brisebois, Chateauguay QC J6K 4W8; Sher'08; CCFP; Staff, Hôpital Anna-Laberge; (450)699-2425

GIBEAULT, Robert; 37 av de la Moselle, Saint-Lambert QC J4S 1W6; Mon'65; Hopital Charles LeMoyne; Langs: English.

GIBERSON, Warren G; Professional Arts Bldg, 625-100 Arden St, Moncton NB E1C 4B7; Mem'86; DAB; FRCSC; Otol. Consultant, Dr Georges-L-Dumont University Hospital Centre; (506)383-2992; Fax. (506)854-4869.

GIBNEY, Eugene; Viking Health Centre, PO Box 60 5110 57 Ave, Viking AB T0B 4N0; Dublin (Ireland)'80; MB ChB; BAO; FRCS; MSc; Staff, Viking Health Centre; (780)336-4786

GIBNEY, Patrick F; Portage Med FHT-Morrison St Si, 102-6453 Morrison St, Niagara Falls ON L2E 7H1; Dublin (Ireland)'74; MB ChB; BAO; MBA; CCFP; Ac Staff General Pract & EmergMed, Niagara Health System - Greater Niagara General Site; (905)357-6636

GIBNEY, R T Noel; University of Alberta Hosp, 3C1 12-8440 112 St NW, Edmonton AB T6G 2B7; Dublin (Ireland)'75; MB ChB; FRCPI(Ire); FRCPC; Respir (Critical Care Medicine). Ac Staff, University of Alberta Hospital; Div Dir & Prof Critical Care Med/Prof, University of Alberta; (780)407-6755; Fax. (780)407-1228.

GIBSON, Brian L; LAMP Community Health Centre, 185 Fifth St, Etobicoke ON M8V 2Z5; Tor'74; FRCPC; CommunMed (Occupational Health);CCFP; FCFP; Assoc Prof Public Health Serv, University of Toronto; (416)252-6471 x272; Fax. (416)252-5100; brian.gibson@utoronto.ca.

GIBSON, Bruce A; Vancouver Gen Hosp, CP5-855 12th Ave W, Vancouver BC V5Z 1M9; Alb'90; CCFP; Staff, Vancouver General Hospital - Centennial Pavillion; (604)875-4754

GIBSON, Christine L; PO Box 61202 Rpo Kensington, Calgary AB T2N 4S6; Tor'99; BSc; MD; CCFP; Staff, Peter Lougheed Centre; (403)943-5461

GIBSON, Craig R; The Hosp for Sick Children, 555 University Ave, Toronto ON M5G 1X8; University of Western Australia (Australia)'02; Clin Fellow Medical Imaging, The Hospital For Sick Children; (416)813-6025

GIBSON, Douglas S; 4C-256 Jarvis St, Toronto ON M5B 2J4; Qns'72; BSc; Ac Staff, The Brant Community Healthcare System - Brantford General Hospital Site; (416)977-0281

GIBSON, G Thomas C; 8675 Granville St, Vancouver BC V6P 5A3; Tor'62; LMCC; CCFP; FCFP; Ac Staff, Vancouver General Hospital - Centennial Pavillion; Att Staff, UBC Hospital - Koerner Pavillion; (604)263-2646; Fax. (604)263-2649.

GIBSON, Gillian M; Diamond Hlth Care Centre, 8F-2775 Laurel St, Vancouver BC V5Z 1M9; Cal'78; BSc(Biol.); FRCPC; Neur (Peripheral Neuropathology). Ac Staff, Vancouver General Hospital - Centennial Pavillion; Clin Assoc Prof, University of British Columbia; (604)875-4247

GIBSON, Glenn; Campbellford Mem Hosp, 146 Oliver Rd, Campbellford ON K0L 1L0; Wes'70; CCFP; Chief Anes & Family Med, Campbellford Memorial Hospital; Aj Asst Prof Dept Family Med, Queen's University; (705)653-1140; gibson_gc@hotmail.com.

GIBSON, Ian; Health Sciences Centre, MS 435T-820 Sherbrook St, Winnipeg MB R3A 1R9; Staff, Health Sciences Centre.

GIBSON, J Malcolm S; Quinte HC Corp-Belleville Gen, PO Box 428 265 Dundas St E, Belleville ON K8N 5A9; Qns'67; FRCPC; Anes. Ac Staff, QHC Belleville General; (613)969-5511

GIBSON, James; St Joseph's Healthcare, F536-50 Charlton Ave E, Hamilton ON L8N 4A6; Tor'75; BSc; FRCPC; IntMed. Staff, St Joseph's Healthcare - Charlton Campus; Associate Clin Prof, McMaster University; (905)521-6061; Fax. (905)521-6176.

GIBSON, John W; Four Villages Comm Health Ctr, 1700 Bloor St W, Toronto ON M6P 4C3; Tor'75; CCFP; FCFP; Court Staff, Trillium Health Centre - West Toronto; Court Staff, St Joseph's Health Centre; (416)604-3361; Fax. (416)604-3367.

GIBSON, Julia; Annapolis Colaborative Practic, PO Box 573 821 St George St, Annapolis Royal NS B0S 1A0; Seba (Northern Ireland)'10; CCFP; (902)532-2324; Fax. (902)532-5424.

GIBSON, Kara J; St Josep's Healthcare, 50 Charlton Ave E, Hamilton ON L8N 4A6; Cal'04; FRCPC; Anes. Staff, St Joseph's Healthcare - Charlton Campus; Langs: Creole; (905)522-1155 x33853

GIBSON, Keith K; 123-11910 111 Ave NW, Edmonton AB T5G 0E5; Cal'85; FRCPC; Psy (Brain Injury Rehabilitation). (780)453-8985

GIBSON, Kevin F; The Med Centre FHT, PO Box 4200 Stn Main 707 Charlotte St, Peterborough ON K9J 7B3; Qns'77; CCFP; FCFP; Ac Staff, Peterborough Regional Health Centre - Rogers St Site; Ac Staff, Peterborough Regional Health Centre - Hospital Drive; (705)743-6222; Fax. (705)741-1264.

GIBSON, Leila; Taylor Street Med Clinic, 3020 Taylor St E, Saskatoon SK S7H 4J2; Staff Psy, Royal University Hospital; Langs: Russian; Ukrainian; (306)374-8082; Fax. (306)374-0047.

GIBSON, Malcolm A S; Guelph Family Health Team, 109-83 Dawson Rd, Guelph ON N1H 1B1; Qns'03; CCFP; (519)766-1360; Fax. (519)766-0469.

GIBSON, Michael; Weeneebayko Gen Hosp, PO Box 34 19 Hospital Dr, Moose Factory ON P0L 1W0; Qns'90; CCFP; Staff Privil, Pembroke Regional Hospital Inc; Staff, Weeneebayko General Hospital; (705)658-4544

GIBSON, Michelle C; Providence CCC-St Mary's, PO Box 3600 Stn Main 340 Union St, Kingston ON K7L 5A2; Mem'99; BEng; CCFP; Att Physician, Providence Care - St Mary's of the Lake Hospital Site; Lecturer Geriatric Med., Queen's University; Langs: French; (613)544-5220 x2242; Fax. (613)544-4017; gibsonm1@providencecare.ca.

GIBSON, Neil E; Sturgeon Community Hosp, 201 Boudreau Rd, St. Albert AB T8N 6C4; McM'89; BSc; MSc; DOHS; DTMH; FRCPC; IntMed. Staff, Sturgeon Community Hospital; Clin Prof, University of Alberta; (780)418-8200; Fax. (780)459-9704; neil.gibson@ualberta.ca.

GIBSON, Paul J; London HSC-Victoria Hosp, PO Box 5010 Stn B 800 Commissioners Rd E, London ON N6A 5W9; Qns'04; FRCPC; Peds; PedHemaOncol. Staff, London Health Sciences Centre - Victoria Campus; (519)685-8494

GIBSON, Paul S; HSC-Faculty Of Med, 1476-3330 Hospital Dr NW, Calgary AB T2N 4N1; Man'93; FRCPC; IntMed (Pregnancy Medical Complications). Assoc Prof Med & Ob/Gyn, University of Calgary; (403)220-6376; Fax. (403)283-6151.

GIBSON, Peter F; Glenmore Landing, D273-1600 90 Ave SW, Calgary AB T2V 5A8; Edinburgh (Scotland)'59; FRCS(Ed); FRCS(Glas); Dip Ortho(Eng.); FRCSC; Ophth. Staff, Alberta Children's Hospital; Asst Prof, University of Calgary; (403)253-7060; Fax. (403)253-2477.

GIBSON, Peter; Richmond Hosp, 2F-7000 Westminster Hwy, Richmond BC V6X 1A2; Alb'85; FRCPC; Psy (Community Psychiatry). Staff, Richmond Hospital; Clinical Asst Prof Psy, University of British Columbia; (604)244-5241

GIBSON, R John; London HSC-Victoria Hosp, PO Box 5010 Stn B E1 102-800 Commissioners Rd E, London ON N6A 5W9; Wes'82; FRCPC; EmergMed. Staff, London Health Sciences Centre - Victoria Campus; Asst Prof Med, University of Western Ontario; (519)667-6538

GIBSON, Rebecca D; Findlay Creek Med Centre, 3-4744 Bank St, Ottawa ON K1T 3W7; Ott'05; CCFP; (613)317-2584; Fax. (613)822-2775.

GIBSON, Richard J; Cole Harbour Family Med, 203A-240 Baker Dr, Dartmouth NS B2W 6L4; Cal'80; CCFP; FCFP; Staff, Dartmouth General Hospital; (902)435-6312; Fax. (902)434-7920.

GIBSON, Ronald E; PO Box 18012 Rpo Kerrisdale, Vancouver BC V6M 4L3; Sask'70; DTMH; FRCPC; Psy. Clin Assoc Prof, University of British Columbia.

GIBSON, Sean; Oshawa Clinic, 117 King St E, Oshawa ON L1H 1B9; Louvain (Belgium)'76; BSc; FRCSC; Urol (Trans Rectal Prostate). Consultant, Lakeridge Health - Bowmanville Site; Staff, Lakeridge Health - Oshawa Site; Consultant, Lakeridge Health - Whitby Site; Langs: Bilingual(English/French); (905)721-4324; Fax. (905)721-6612.

GIBSON, William T; BC Women's Hosp & Health Ctre, C234-4500 Oak St, Vancouver BC V6H 3N1; Wes'95; FRCPC; MedGenetics (Obesity Genetics). Staff Med Genetics, BC Women's Hospital & Health Centre; Langs: Spanish; French; (604)875-2157; Fax. (604)875-2376.

GICK, Susan V; 119 Royal York St PO Box 746, Richmond ON K0A 2Z0; McG'79; BSc; CCFP; Staff Palliative Care Unit, SCO Health Service - Élisabeth Bruyère Hospital; Langs: English; French.

GIDDENS, J David; 202-1635 Lawrence Ave W, Toronto ON M6L 3C9; Tor'74; FACEP; CCFP; CCFP(E.M.); FCFP; Sr Staff, Humber River Regional Hospital - Church Street Site; Sr Staff, Humber River Regional Hospital - Finch Avenue Site; Staff Physician, Leisure World Nursing Home; City Of Toronto; Staff Physician, Village of Humber Heights; (416)243-3300; Fax. (416)244-1252.

GIDDENS, Jonathan L; 101-18 Kensington Rd, Brampton ON L6T 4S5; Tor'94; FRCSC; Urol. (905)874-0092; Fax. (905)874-0703; jgiddens.md@gmail.com.

GIDDINGS, C Raymond; 2F-400 Queen St W, Brampton ON L6X 1B3; Wes'65; FRCPC; DiagRad.

GIDDINGS, Gordon R; Windsor Reg Cancer Centre, G018-2220 Kildare Rd, Windsor ON N8W 2X3; Birmingham(AL) (USA)'00; CCFP; Staff, Windsor Regional Hospital - Windsor Regional Cancer Centre; Langs: French; (613)562-6262; Fax. (519)255-8676.

GIDEON, Salva; 200-201 Lloyd Manor Rd, Etobicoke ON M9B 6H6; Tor'83; BSc(Hon); BEd; CCFP; Staff, William Osler Health System - Etobicoke General Hospital; (416)239-1138; Fax. (416)239-1944.

GIDON, Martie S; Davisville Med & Dental Centre, 307-1849 Yonge St, Toronto ON M4S 1Y2; McM'77; FAAD; FRCPC; Derm. Staff, Toronto General Hospital - UHN; Staff, Women's College Hospital; Lecturer Med, University of Toronto; (416)483-4541

GIDWANI, Andy J; Royal Health Care Centre, 130 Adelaide St W, Toronto ON M5H 3P5; Wes'02; (416)361-6142; Fax. (416)361-1200.

GIDWANI, Ram; Bluewater Health-Norman Site, 89 Norman St, Sarnia ON N7T 6S3; Bombay (India)'63; MB BS; ABP; ABFP; FRCPC; GenPath (Forensic Pathology). Chief Lab Med, Bluewater Health - Mitton Site; Staff, Bluewater Health - Norman Site; Dir-Lab Serv, Bluewater Health - Charlotte Eleanor Englehart Hospital; University of Western Ontario; (519)464-4400

GIEDE, Johannes A; Univ Hosp of Northern BC, 1475 Edmonton St, Prince George BC V2M 1S2; UBC'88; FRCPC; Psy. Staff, University Hospital of Northern British Columbia; (250)565-7426; Fax. (250)565-2343.

GIEDE, K Christopher; Royal University Hosp, 4515-103 Hospital Dr, Saskatoon SK S7N 0W8; UBC'88; FRCSC; ObstGyn; GynOnco. Staff, Royal University Hospital; Assoc Prof ObstGyn, University of Saskatchewan; Langs: German; (306)966-8693; Fax. (306)966-8040; christopher.giede@usask.ca.

GIEN, Lilian T; Sunnybrook Hlth Sciences Ctre, T2 104-2075 Bayview Ave, Toronto ON M4N 3M5; Wes'01; FRCSC; ObstGyn; GynOnco. Staff, Sunnybrook Health Sciences Centre; (416)480-4026; Fax. (416)480-6002.

GIENI, Melissa E; Spesmed Med Specialist Ctre, 2591 99th St, North Battleford SK S9A 3W1; Sask'07; BSc; FRCSC; GenSurg (Community General Surgeon). (306)446-5543; Fax. (306)446-1661.

GIENI, Rose-Marie A L; Algoma District Med Group, 240 McNabb St, Sault Ste. Marie ON P6B 1Y5; Man'86; Staff, Sault Area Hospital - Sault Ste Marie; Langs: Bilingual(English/French); (705)759-1234; Fax. (705)541-2231; rose.gieni@sympatico.ca.

GIERL, Paul; Beddington Medical Clinic, Box 248 300-8120 Beddington Blvd NW, Calgary AB T3K 2A8; (USA)'83; Staff, Medicine Hat Regional Hospital; Staff, Peter Lougheed Centre; (403)827-9539

GIESBRECHT, Ellen M; 330-507 Broadway W, Vancouver BC V5Z 1E6; Cal'93; FRCSC; ObstGyn. (604)872-5484; Fax. (604)708-0748.

GIESBRECHT, J Elizabeth; Tuxedo Fam Med Centre, 981 Corydon Ave, Winnipeg MB R3M 0X1; Man'88; CCFP; FCFP; (204)988-6040; Fax. (204)989-6047.

GIESBRECHT, Janice L; 201-112 Queenston St, St Catharines ON L2R 2Z4; McM'83; FRCPC; IntMed; MedOncol. Staff Med, Hotel-Dieu Hospital; Staff, Niagara Health System - St Catharines General Site; Court Staff, Niagara Health System - Welland Hospital Site; (905)685-8082; Fax. (905)988-5776.

GIESBRECHT, Sunshine J; PO Box 80150 Rpo Tower Lane, Airdrie AB T4B 2V8; Tor'07; CCFP.

GIESINGER, Carolyn L A; Regina Qu'Appelle HR-Pasqua, 100-4101 Dewdney Ave, Regina SK S4T 1A5; Sask'91; BSc; FRCPC; Anes. Staff, Pasqua Hospital; (306)766-2295; Fax. (306)949-7018.

GIESINGER, Regan E; PG Medical Education Office, 602-500 University Ave, Toronto ON M5G 1V7; Qns'08; Peds.

GIFFARD, Eric; CSSSG-Hop de Gatineau, CP 2000 Succ Bureau-Chef 909 boul de la Verendry O, Gatineau QC J8P 7H2; Sher'97; CSPQ; Anes. Staff, Hôpital de Gatineau; (819)561-8100

GIFFIN, Barry D; PO Box 11, Md Musquodbt NS B0N 1X0; Mem'86; CCFP; (902)384-2834; Fax. (902)384-2719.

GIFFIN, D Mitch; UBC-Dept Of Med, 2449-910 10th Ave W, Vancouver BC V5Z 1M9; Man'88; FRCPC; Anes. (604)875-4304; Fax. (604)875-5209.

GIFFIN, J Robert; Fowler-Kennedy Sports Med Clin, 3M-1151 Richmond St, London ON N6A 3K7; Dal'94; FRCSC; OrthSurg. (519)661-3454; Fax. (519)850-2496.

GIFFIN, Scott C; Public Health Services, PO Box 93 Stn Main, Saint John NB E2L 3X1; Dal'80; ABIM; (506)643-2807; Fax. (506)643-7894.

GIFTOCHRISTOS, Nick T; Woodbine Med Centre, B9-76 Arlington Dr, Keswick ON L4P 0A9; Tor'93; LMCC; CCFP; Langs: Greek; (905)476-0308; Fax. (905)476-1079.

GIGG, Anthony C; Claro Family Practice, 107-4930 55 Ave, Drayton Valley AB T7A 1W2; Wales (United Kingdom)'82; MB ChB; BSc(Hons Biochem); CCFP; (780)621-0202; Fax. (780)621-0213.

GIGLIA, Lucia G; Hamilton HS-McMaster Site, PO Box 2000 Stn Lcd 1 1200 Main St W, Hamilton ON L8N 3Z5; McM'98; FRCPC; Peds. Staff, Hamilton Health Sciences Centre - McMaster Children's Hospital; Langs: Italian; French; (905)523-6766

GIGNAC, Julie; C M F Chicoutimi-Nord, 2185 boul de Tadoussac, Chicoutimi QC G7G 4X2; Sher'03; Staff Gen Med & Obstetrics, Complexe hospitalier de la Sagamie; Staff Gen Med Obstetrics, Clinique Medecine Fam de Chicoutimi; Clin Prof Chicoutimi Campus, Universite de Sherbrooke; Langs: Bilingual(French/English); (418)698-2414

GIGNAC, Martin; Inst Philippe Pinel de Mtl, 10905 boul Henri-Bourassa E, Montreal QC H1C 1H1; McG'98; FRCPC; Psy. Staff, Institut Philippe-Pinel de Montreal; (514)648-8461; Fax. (514)494-4406.

GIGOUX, Celine; Clinique Med Havre Sante, 521 boul du Havre, Salaber-de-Valleyf QC J6S 4Z5; Mon'76; Staff, Centre Hospitalier Régional du Suroît; Langs: English; (450)371-6444; Fax. (450)371-5315.

GIGUERE, Anick; Clin Med Visuelle Notre-Dame, 504 rue Notre-Dame, Repentigny QC J6A 2T8; Sher'91; Staff, Centre Hospitalier Pierre le Gardeur; (450)841-3318

GIGUERE, Brigitte; CLSC des Pres-Bleus, CP 10 Succ Bureau-Chef 1209 boul Sacre-Coeur, Saint-Felicien QC G8K 2P8; Laval'85; (418)679-5270; Fax. (418)679-4748.

GIGUERE, Caroline; Ctr Hosp Affilie-Enfant-Jesus, 1401 rue 18E, Quebec QC G1J 1Z4; Laval'93; FRCPC; DiagRad (Angiography/Interventional). Staff, Centre Hospitalier Affilié Universitaire de Québec - Hôpital De L'Enfant Jésus; (418)649-0252

GIGUERE, Caroline S; CHUS-Hop Fleurimont, 3001 12e av N, Sherbrooke QC J1H 5N4; Sher'93; FRCPC; DiagRad. Staff, Centre Hospitalier Universitaire de Sherbrooke-Hopital Fleurimont; (819)346-1110; caroline.s.giguere@usherbrooke.ca.

GIGUERE, Catherine; Douglas Mental Hlth Univ Inst, 6875 boul LaSalle, Verdun QC H4H 1R3; Sher'84; Psy (Adult Psychiatry). Staff, Douglas Mental Health University Institute; (514)761-6131; Fax. (514)762-3025.

GIGUERE, Chantal M; Hôpital Ste-Justine, 3175 ch Cote-Sainte-Catherine, Montreal QC H3T 1C5; McG'95; MSc; CSPQ; FRCSC; Otol (Pediatric Otolaryngology). Staff, Inuulitsivik Health Centre; Staff, Hôpital Ste-Justine; Staff, Le Medi-Club; Langs: Spanish; French; Italian; (514)345-4857; Fax. (514)345-4791.

GIGUERE, Dominic; Clin Perinatalitie Trois-Rivie, 100-4900 boul des Forges, Trois-Rivieres QC G8Y 1X1; Laval'01; CCFP; (819)373-2303

GIGUERE, Eliane; Clinique Med Asclepios, 2-750 Taylor Creek Dr, Orleans ON K1C 1T1; Mon'06; CCFP; Langs: Bilingual(French/English); (613)830-8388

GIGUERE, Eric; Ctr Med Giguere Pronovost, 1465 rue Roberval, Saint-Bruno QC J3V 3P8; Sher'87; FRCPC; Psy. (450)441-5222; Fax. (450)441-0938.

GIGUERE, Gaetan; Hop Santa Cabrini Ospedale, 5655 rue Saint-Zotique E, Montreal QC H1T 1P7; Mon'76; Ac Staff, Hôpital Santa Cabrini Ospedale; (514)252-6000; Fax. (514)252-6501.

GIGUERE, Isabelle; Polyclinique St-Eustache, 75 rue Grignon, Saint-Eustache QC J7P 4J2; Mon'92; Asst Operator Obstetic Nursery, Hôpital de Saint-Eustache; (450)623-6635

GIGUERE, Jean-Francois; Hop du Sacre-Coeur de Mtl, 5400 boul Gouin O, Montreal QC H4J 1C5; Mon'91; Neursurg. Staff, Hôpital du Sacre-Coeur de Montréal; (514)338-2222; Fax. (514)338-3113.

GIGUERE, Marie-Chantal; Clin Med Du Coteau, 100-440 boul Saint-Luc, St-Jean-sur-Richel QC J2W 0E2; Sher'93; Staff, Hôpital du Haut-Richelieu; Langs: Bilingual(French/English); (450)359-6819; Fax. (450)359-3247.

GIGUERE, Michel; Hotel-Dieu de Levis, 143 rue Wolfe, Levis QC G6V 3Z1; Laval'77; CSPQ; FRCSC; OrthSurg. Staff, Hôtel-Dieu de Lévis; (418)835-7121; migiguere@hotmail.com.

GIGUERE, Michel; ASSS-Chaudiere Appalaches, 363 Rte Cameron, Sainte-Marie QC G6E 3E2; Laval'85; Pub Hlth, Centre d'hébergement de Beauceville; (418)389-1510

GIGUERE, Nicole; Centre Med Drummond, 60 rue Loring, Drummondville QC J2C 7Y9; Laval'90; ac Staff, Hôpital Sainte-croix.

GIGUERE, Paul; Centre Med Beauport, 737 av Royale, Quebec QC G1E 1Z1; Laval'67; FRCSC; Otol. (418)667-7114; Fax. (418)667-5843.

GIGUERE, Richard; Hotel-Dieu de levis, 143 rue Wolfe, Levis QC G6V 3Z1; Mon'85; IntMed (P.Q.). Staff, Hôtel-Dieu de Lévis; (418)835-7121

GIGUERE, Sylvie; Clinique Sante de Thetford, 2000-926 rue Labbe, Thetford Mines QC G6G 2A8; Laval'93; Staff, Hopital du CSS de la Region de Thetford; (418)338-4581; Fax. (418)338-4584.

GIGUERE, Yves; CHUQ-Ctr Hosp Univ Laval, S 220-2705 boul Laurier, Quebec QC G1V 4G2; McG'91; BSc(BioChem); CSPQ; FRCP; DPhil; FRCPC; MedBiochem (Inborn Errors of Metabolism). Staff, Centre Hospitalier Universitaire de Quebec-CHUL; Langs: Czech; (418)654-2103; Fax. (418)654-2748; yves.giguere@crsfa.ulaval.ca.

GIGUERRE, Genevieve; CSSS Vieille Capital, 55 ch Sainte-Foy, Quebec QC G1R 1S9; Laval'05; CCFP; Staff, CSSS Haute-Ville; (418)641-2572; Fax. (418)641-0282; genevieve.giguerre@irdpq.qc.ca.

GIL, Lucas; Winchester Dist Mem Hosp, 566 Louise St, Winchester ON K0C 2K0; Ott'07; CCFP; Staff, Winchester District Memorial Hospital; (613)774-2420

GIL, Michel R; CSSSNL-Psychiatrie, 2-465 rue Notre-Dame, Repentigny QC J6A 2T3; Paris (France)'88; FRCPC; Psy (P.Q.) (Pediatric Psychiatry). Head Psy & Child and Adolescent Psy, Centre Hospitalier Régional de Lanaudière; Langs: English; (450)581-5100; Fax. (450)581-2302; michel.gil@ssss.gouv.qc.ca.

GILAD, Elyahu E; Alberta Children's Hosp, 2888 Shaganappi Trail NW, Calgary AB T3B 6A8; (Israel)'86; Staff Pediatric Intensivist, Alberta Children's Hospital; Langs: Hebrew; (403)955-7931; Fax. (403)955-7081; eli.gilad@albertahealthservices.ca.

GILANI, Ammar; Hamilton HS-Henderson Site, 70W GF24-711 Concession St, Hamilton ON L8V 1C3; Punjab (Pakistan)'91; Staff, Hamilton Health Sciences Centre-Juravinski Site; Assoc Prof Neurology, McMaster University; (905)389-4411 x42760; Fax. (905)381-7042; georgeh@hhsg.ca.

GILANI, Hamid J; Norfolk Med Centre, 206-85 Norfolk St, Guelph ON N1H 4J4; Wes'80; Court Staff, Homewood Health Centre; Court Staff, Guelph General Hospital; Ac Staff, St Joseph's Health Centre; Langs: Urdu; Hindi; (519)837-3900; Fax. (519)837-3632.

GILANI, Sadia; 688 Concession St, Hamilton ON L8V 4T9; Punjab (Pakistan)'93; FRCPC; Psy. Langs: Punjabi; Urdu; (905)538-4146; Fax. (905)538-4147.

GILARDINO, Miroslav; MUHC-Montreal Children Hosp, C11 35-2300 rue Tupper, Montreal QC H3H 1P3; McG'01; FACS; FRCSC; PlasSurg (Cranio Facial Surgery). Staff Plastic/Craniofacial Surg, McGill University Health Centre - Montreal Children's Hospital; Prof Div of Platic Surg/Dir Plastic Surg Residency Program, McGill University; (514)934-1934 x23472; Fax. (514)412-4341; gelsy.mastrangelo@muhc.mcfill.ca.

GILAS, Thomas; 402 KW-650 Sammon Ave, East York ON M4C 5M5; Tor'78; FRCSC; GenSurg (Laparoscopic Surgery). Ac Staff Surg, Toronto East General Hospital Inc; Teacher, University of Toronto; (416)778-5522; tgilas@sympatico.ca.

GILBART, Michael K; UBC Hosp, 2C-2211 Wesbrook Mall, Vancouver BC V6T 2B5; Tor'95; OrthSurg (Clinical & Investigative Medicine). Staff, UBC Hospital - Koerner Pavillion; (604)822-5699

GILBERG, Steven M; The Ottawa Hosp-Gen Campus, 3107-501 Smyth Rd, Ottawa ON K1H 8L6; Ott'84; FRCSC; Ophth (Ophthalmic Plastic & Reconstructive Surgery). Staff Eye Institute, The Ottawa Hospital - General Campus; Dept Chair Ophth, University of Ottawa; Langs: Bilingual(English/French); (613)737-8834; Fax. (613)739-6139.

GILBERT, Alain; CHUQ-Hotel-Dieu de Quebec, 11 Cote du Palais, Quebec QC G1R 2J6; Laval'80; CSPQ; FRCSC; GenSurg. Staff, Centre Hospitalier Universitaire de Québec (CHUQ) - Siege Social; (418)691-5151; Fax. (418)691-5020.

GILBERT, Andree; Direction de la Sante Publique, 1301 rue Sherbrooke E, Montreal QC H2L 1M3; Sher'81; (514)528-2400 x3013; Fax. (514)528-2426.

GILBERT, Barry L R; 1104-170 Bloor St W, Toronto ON M5S 1T9; McM'78; FRCPC; CCFP; Psy (Post Traumatic Stress Disorder). Staff Mood & Anxiety Disorders, Centre for Addiction & Mental Health (CAMH) - College Street Site; Staff Psy, Toronto General Hospital - UHN; Asst Prof Psy, University of Toronto; (416)925-0804

GILBERT, Bernard; CLSC des Pres-Bleus, CP 10 Succ Bureau-Chef 1209 boul Sacre-Coeur, Saint-Felicien QC G8K 2P8; Laval'85; Physician, CSSS Domaine-Du-Roy; (418)679-5270; Fax. (418)679-1748; bernard@leblond.com.

GILBERT, Brian W; Sunnybrook Hlth Sciences Ctre, E205-2075 Bayview Ave, Toronto ON M4N 3M5; Tor'71; FRCPC; Cardiol. VP Cardiovasc Serv, Sunnybrook Health Sciences Centre; Prof, University of Toronto; (416)480-6771; Fax. (416)480-4072.

GILBERT, Christine; CLSC du Richelieu, 300 ch de Marieville, Richelieu QC J3L 3V8; Mon'88; (450)658-7561; Fax. (450)658-4390.

GILBERT, Danielle; Hop du Sacre-Coeur de Mtl, 5400 boul Gouin O, Montreal QC H4J 1C5; Sher'87; FRCPC; DiagRad. Staff, Hôpital du Sacre-Coeur de Montréal; (514)338-2130; Fax. (514)338-3164.

GILBERT, Elise; CSSS du Suroît, 150 rue Saint-Thomas, Salaber-de-Valleyf QC J6T 6C1; Laval'01; FRCPC; IntMed; Critical Care Medicine (P.Q.). Staff, Centre Hospitalier Régional du Suroît; (450)371-9920

GILBERT, France; CSSS de Jonquiere, 2230 rue de l'Hopital, Jonquiere QC G7X 4H6; Mon'93; Staff, Centre Hospitalier Jonquiere; (418)695-7700

GILBERT, Francois; Lakeshore Gen Hosp, 160 av Stillview, Pointe-Claire QC H9R 2Y2; McG'90; FRCPC; EmergMed (Endocrinology). Staff, Lakeshore General Hospital - Pointe Claire; Langs: English; Italian; (514)630-2225

GILBERT, François; 200-17001 Route Trans-Canada, Kirkland QC H9H 5J1; Laval'78; BSc; MSc; FRCPC; IntMed (Diabetology); Endocrin (P.Q.). Medical Staff Endoc, Centre Multi-Medic; Medical Staff Endoc, Medisys Health Group; Med Staff Endocrinology, Clinique Access Med; Langs: German; English; (514)694-4644; Fax. (514)694-4646; fgilbert@accessmed.ca.

GILBERT, Roy; Coleman Clinic, 186 Kenneth St, Duncan BC V9L 1N4; UBC'81; CCFP; FCFP; (250)746-4102; Fax. (250)746-5960.

GILBERT, Jane C; The Bear Clinic, 243 North Service Rd W, Oakville ON L6M 3E5; Tor'89; BSc; FRCPC; Psy. (905)844-4673

GILBERT, Jasmine; Centre Med Fafard Enr, 201-975 boul Monseigneur-de La, Baie-Saint-Paul QC G3Z 2W3; Laval'86; Staff, CSSS de Charlevoix; (418)435-6310; Fax. (418)435-3203.

GILBERT, Jean; 7589 rue Saint-Denis, Montreal QC H2R 2E7; Mon'87; Langs: Spanish; English; (514)273-6111; Fax. (514)273-7770; info@cliniquejeangilbert.com.

GILBERT, Jeremy D; Sunnybrook Hlth Sciences Ctre, H166-2075 Bayview Ave, Toronto ON M4N 3M5; Tor'02; FRCPC; IntMed; Endocrin&Metab. Staff, Sunnybrook Health Sciences Centre; (416)480-6717; Fax. (416)480-4744.

GILBERT, Kenneth; St Joseph's Health Care, PO Box 5777 Stn B A2 519-268 Grosvenor St, London ON N6A 4V2; McG'89; MPH; FRCPC; IntMed. Staff Teacher, St Joseph's Hospital - St Joseph's Health Care; Asst Prof Med, University of Western Ontario; Langs: Bilingual(English/French); (519)646-6000

GILBERT, Linda; CSSS Pierre Boucher, 1333 boul Jacques-Cartier E, Longueuil QC J4M 2A5; Mon'95; Staff, Centre Hospitalier Pierre Boucher; (450)468-8111

GILBERT, Linda; CSSS Deux-Montagne, 111 rue Saint-Laurent, St-Eustache QC J7P 3Z5; Mon'97; FRCPC; Psy. Staff Psy, CSSS du Lac Des Deux; (450)473-1720; Fax. (450)473-6369; linda.gilbert.hse@ssss.gouv.qc.ca.

GILBERT, Luc; CSSS Drummond-Hop Sainte-Croix, 570 rue Heriot, Drummondville QC J2B 1C1; Sher'88; FRCPC; Psy. Dir gén, Hôpital Sainte-croix; (819)478-6464 x3402; Fax. (819)478-6490.

GILBERT, Lucie; CSSS de Beauce-Etchemin, 1515 17e rue, Saint-Georges QC G5Y 4T8; Laval'91; LMCC; CCFP; Staff Emerg & Family Clinic, Centre Hospitalier Beauce-Etchemin; Physician Palliative Care, Catherine de Longpre; Médecin Family Med, Clinique Familiale; (418)228-2031

GILBERT, Lucy; F9.26-687 av des Pins O, Montreal QC H3A 1A1; Mysore (India)'78; MSc; FRCOG; ObstGyn (P.Q.) (Gynecologic Oncology). Chef Div of Gyn & Oncol, McGill University Health Centre - Royal Victoria Hospital; assoc Prof ObstGyn, McGill University; Langs: Bilingual(English/French); (514)843-2833; Fax. (514)843-2830; lucy.gilbert@mcgill.ca.

GILBERT, Marcel; Hôpital Laval, 2725 ch Sainte-Foy, Quebec QC G1V 4G5; Laval'66; CSPQ; Cardiol (P.Q.) (Electrophysiology). Staff, Hôpital Laval; Université Laval; (418)656-4598; Fax. (418)656-4581.

GILBERT, Marie-Eve; CSSS de la Region de Thetford, 1717 rue Notre-Dame E, Thetford Mines QC G6G 2V4; Laval'08; Staff, Hopital du CSS de la Region de Thetford; (418)338-7715; Fax. (418)335-7676.

GILBERT, Marie-Odile; CSSS de la Vallée de l'Or, 725 6e rue, Val-d'Or QC J9P 3Y1; Laval'01; Staff, Centre Hospitalier de Val d'Or; (819)875-6711

GILBERT, Mark P J; BC Centre for Disease Control, 655 12th Ave W, Vancouver BC V5Z 4R4; Ott'00; FRCPC; CommunMed. (604)707-5615

GILBERT, Martin; CSSS de Chicoutimi, 305 rue Saint-Vallier, Chicoutimi QC G7H 5H6; Sher'96; CSPQ; FRCPC; Anes. Staff, Complexe hospitalier de la Sagamie; (418)541-1000

GILBERT, Martin; Ctr Hosp Affilie-Enfant-Jesus, 1401 18e rue, Quebec QC G1J 1Z4; Laval'80; FRCPC; Derm. Ac Staff, Centre Hospitalier Affilié Universitaire de Québec - Hôpital De L'Enfant Jésus; Staff, Hôtel-Dieu de Lévis; Staff, Centre Hospitalier Universitaire de Québec (CHUQ) - Siege Social; Clin Prof, Université Laval; (418)649-5520; Fax. (418)649-5527.

GILBERT, Michael R; Kelso Lake Medl Centre, 112-330 Bronte St S, Milton ON L9T 7X1; Wes'99; CCFP; Staff, Kelso Lake Medical Centre.

GILBERT, Monica; CLSC Desjardins, 15 rue de l'Arsenal, Levis QC G6V 4P6; Laval'81; Staff, Hôtel-Dieu de Lévis; (418)835-3400 x3244; Fax. (418)835-6413; monica_gilbert@ssss.gouv.qc.ca.

GILBERT, Nathalie; CHUQ-St-Francois D'Assise, 10 rue de l'Espinay, Quebec QC G1L 3L5; Laval'95; CSPQ; FRCSC; GenSurg; VascSurg. Staff, Centre Hospitalier Universitaire De Québec - Pavillon De St-françois-d'assise; Clin Prof, Université Laval; Langs: English; (418)525-4444; Fax. (418)525-2264.

GILBERT, Patrick; CHUM-Hosp Notre Dame, 1560 rue Sherbrooke E, Montreal QC H2L 4M1; Laval'03; FRCPC; DiagRad. Staff, Centre Hospitalier l'Université de Montréal (CHUM) - Hôpital Notre-Dame; (514)890-8000; patrick.gilbert@mail.mcgill.ca.

GILBERT, Philippe; Ctr Hosp Affilie-Enfant-Jesus, 1401 18e rue, Quebec QC G1J 1Z4; Laval'03; FRCPC; IntMed; Cardiol. Staff, Centre Hospitalier Affilié Universitaire de Québec - Hôpital De L'Enfant Jésus; (418)649-0252

GILBERT, Philippe; 4302 Pl Guillet, Montreal QC H1X 3H5; Laval'96; FRCPC; IntMed (Cardiology). Langs: English; (514)679-8454

GILBERT, Ralph W; Univ Hlth Network-Princess M, 3 955-610 University Ave, Toronto ON M5G 2M9; Tor'80; FRCSC; Otol (Reconstructive Micro Surgery). Ac Staff, Princess Margaret Hospital - University Health Network; Assoc Staff, Sunnybrook Health Sciences Centre; Prof Otolaryngology Head & Neck Surg, University of Toronto; (416)946-2822; Fax. (416)946-2300; ralph.gilbert@uhn.on.ca.

GILBERT, Rebekah; Royal Alexandra Hosp, 3228 ATC-10240 Kingsway NW, Edmonton AB T5H 3V9; (United Kingdom)'97; MB BS; Staff, Royal Alexandra Hospital; (780)735-4038; Fax. (780)735-5880.

GILBERT, Reynald; CSSS des Etchemins, 331 rue du Sanatorium RR 1, Lac-Etchemin QC G0R 1S0; Laval'78; Staff, CSSS des Etchemins; Staff, Centre d'hébergement de Beauceville; Staff, Centre Hospitalier Beauce-Etchemin; (418)625-8001

GILBERT, Richard E; St Michael's Hosp Health Centr, 6 138-61 Queen St E, Toronto ON M5C 2T2; (Australia)'81; FRCPC; IntMed; Endocrin&Metab. Staff, St Michael's Hospital; (416)867-3747

GILBERT, Rosemarie G; PO Box 1043 Stn Main, Pembroke ON K8A 6Y6; London (England)'64; MB BS; LRCP; MRCS; DObstRCOG; (613)735-8137; rjgilbert@sympatico.ca.

GILBERT, Sebastien; The Ottawa Hosp-Gen Campus, 6363-501 Smyth Rd, Ottawa ON K1H 8L6; McG'96; CSPQ; ABTS; ABS; FRCSC; GenSurg (Surgical Oncology); ThorSurg. Staff/Dir Minimally Intesive & Aerodigestive Surg, The Ottawa Hospital - General Campus; Langs: Bilingual(French/English); (613)737-8899 x74033; Fax. (613)737-8668.

GILBERT, Serge W; Clinique D'Anesthesie 5540, 145-100 ch Rockland, Mont-Royal QC H3P 2V9; Mon'76; CSPQ; FRCPC; Anes. Staff, Hôpital Santa Cabrini Ospedale; (514)955-6787

GILBERT, Valerie; Unite de Med Familiale, 100-1205 boul de la Rive-Sud, Saint-Romuald QC G6W 0J4; Laval'02; Staff, CSSS de Montmagny-L'Islet; (418)380-8597; Fax. (418)380-8596.

GILBERT, Vanessa; Clinique Med Familiale, 2185 boul Tadoussac, Chicoutimi QC G7G 4X2; McG'10; MDCM; CCFP; (418)698-2414

GILBRIDE, Patrick; CFB Gagetown, PO Box 17000 Stn Forces, Oromocto NB E2V 4J5; Dal'09; CCFP.

GILCA, Rodica; INSPQ, 2400 av D'Estimauville, Quebec QC G1E 7G9; Chisinau (Moldova)'87; PhD; Langs: Romanian; French; Russian; (418)666-7000 x278; rodica.gilca@ssss.gouv.qc.ca.

GILCHRIST, Andrew D; Royal Victoria Hosp, 201 Georgian Dr, Barrie ON L4M 6M2; Tor'01; FRCPC; Anes. Staff, Royal Victoria Regional Health Centre; (705)728-9802

GILCHRIST, Angus; Delta Hosp, 5800 Mountain View Blvd, Delta BC V4K 3V6; UBC'98; MSc; BSc; CCFP; CCFP(E.M.); Staff Emerg Phys, Delta Hospital; (604)946-1121 x78322; Fax. (604)946-3086.

GILCHRIST, Dawna M; Medical Sciences Bldg, 8 53 MSB-131 University Campus, Edmonton AB T6G 2H7; Alb'83; FCCMG; FRCPC; IntMed (Medical Genetics). Staff, University of Alberta Hospital; Prof Med, University of Alberta; (780)407-7333; Fax. (780)407-6845.

GILCHRIST, James A; London Reg Cancer Centre, 3021-790 Commissioners Rd E, London ON N6A 4L6; London (England)'65; MB BS; DMRT; FRCPC; RadOncol. Staff RadOncol, London Health Sciences Centre - Victoria Campus; Staff, London Regional Cancer Center; Associate Clin Prof, University of Western Ontario; (519)685-8650 x5361; Fax. (519)685-8627.

GILCHRIST, Lawrence I; Service d'Urologie Rive-Sud, 304-3234 boul Taschereau, Greenfield Park QC J4V 2H3; Qns'74; FRCSC; Urol. Chef Urology, Centre Hospitalier Pierre Boucher; (450)671-2945; Fax. (450)671-8045.

GILDAY, David L; Toronto Nuclear Med Services, 210-123 Edward St, Toronto ON M5G 1E2; McG'66; FRCPC; DiagRad; NuclearMed. Chief Nuclear Med, The Hospital For Sick Children; Prof Radiol, University of Toronto; (416)597-1016 x3060; david.gilday@sickkids.on.ca.

GILDINER, Michael; Humber River Reg Hosp-Finch, 2111 Finch Ave W, North York ON M3N 1N1; Tor'76; FRCPC; DiagRad. Staff, Humber River Regional Hospital - Finch Avenue Site; (416)744-2500

GILE, David S; Orillia Soldiers Mem Hosp, 170 Colborne St W, Orillia ON L3V 2Z3; McM'89; CCFP; CCFP(E.M.); Staff, Orillia Soldiers' Memorial Hospital; (705)325-2201

GILES, Ann M W; Workers' Compensation Board, PO Box 4700 Stn Terminal, Vancouver BC V6B 1J1; UBC'86; CCFP; (250)881-7297

GILES, Brenda-Louise; Children's Hosp, CS516-840 Sherbrook St, Winnipeg MB R3A 1S1; Wes'91; FRCPC; Peds (Critical Care Medicine). Assoc Staff, Health Sciences Centre; Asst Prof, University of Manitoba.

GILES, Catherine E; Crescent Beach Med Arts, 2781 Gordon Ave, Surrey BC V4A 3J5; UBC'91; (604)535-2520

GILES, Christopher A; Sioux Lookout Zone Fam Phys, PO Box 4000, Sioux Lookout ON P8T 1K2; McM'85; CCFP; FCFP; (807)737-6080; Fax. (807)737-4866; gilesc@mcmaster.ca.

GILES, Kathryn A; Cambridge Place Business Bldg, 603-73 Water St N, Cambridge ON N1R 7L6; Tor'86; FRCPC; Neur. Staff, Cambridge Memorial Hospital; (519)624-0129; Fax. (519)624-4928.

GILES, Sarah M; 1403 Edward St PO Box 8000, Hearst ON P0L 1N0; Dal'05; CCFP; (705)362-8262

GILET, Danielle; Hotel-Dieu de Sorel, 400 av de l'Hotel-Dieu, Sorel-Tracy QC J3P 1N5; Mon'09; Staff, Hôtel-Dieu de Sorel; (450)746-6000

GILFIX, Brian M; MUHC-Royal Victoria Hosp, 687 av des Pins O, Montreal QC H3A 1A1; McG'89; PhD; DABCC; CSPQ; FRCPC; MedBiochem. Staff Div of Med Biochem, McGill University Health Centre - Royal Victoria Hospital; assoc Prof, McGill University; (514)934-1934 x34409; brian.gilfix@mcgill.ca.

GILFOYLE, Elaine; Alberta Children's Hosp, 2888 Shaganappi Trail NW, Calgary AB T3B 6A8; Wes'99; FRCPC; Peds (Critical Care Medicine). Staff Critical Care & PICU, Alberta Children's Hospital; (403)955-7931

GILHOOLY, Timothy R; Med Clinic Associates, 200-3207 30 Ave, Vernon BC V1T 2C6; UBC'91; CCFP; (250)542-5909; Fax. (250)545-8260.

GILI, Adrian F; South Calgary Med Clinic, 326-40 Sunpark Plaza SE, Calgary AB T2X 3X7; Tor'88; BEng; FRCPC; Derm. (403)278-1997; Fax. (403)278-2052.

GILIC, Filip; 242 King St, Trenton ON K8V 3X1; Tor'05; CCFP; CCFP(E.M.); Langs: Serbian; (613)392-2541

GILIGSON, Ari; 403-11861 88 Ave, Delta BC V4C 3C6; UBC'95; FRCSC; Ophth. Staff, Delta Hospital; (604)572-4407; Fax. (604)572-4417; dr@giligson.com.

GILKINSON, Trevor L; London HSC-Victoria Hosp, PO Box 5010 Stn B 800 Commissioners Rd E, London ON N6A 5W9; Ott'78; FRCPC; EmergMed. Staff, London Health Sciences Centre - Victoria Campus; Staff, London Health Sciences Centre - South Street; (519)667-6538 x77572; Fax. (519)667-6769; tgilkins@uwo.ca.

GILKS, C Blake; Vancouver Gen Hosp, 1457-855 12th Ave W, Vancouver BC V5Z 1M9; Dal'82; FRCPC; AnatPath. Staff, Vancouver General Hospital - Centennial Pavillion; A-Dept Head Pathology & Laboratory Med, University of British Columbia; (604)875-4901; Fax. (604)875-4797; blake.gilks@supportvgh.ca.

GILL, Andrew J; Lahey Med Centre, 2204-120 5 Ave W, Cochrane AB T4C 0A4; (United Kingdom)'02; BSc; MB ChB; MRCGPract(UK); (403)981-6000; Fax. (403)981-6001.

GILL, Aneeqa A; West London Family Hlth Clinic, 2F-785 Wonderland Rd S, London ON N6K 1M6; Peshawar (Pakistan)'00; CCFP; Langs: Punjabi; Urdu; (519)649-6712; Fax. (519)641-6189.

GILL, Anne-Marie; Whitemud Crossing Med Clinic, 127-4211 106 St NW, Edmonton AB T6J 6L7; Alb'86; BSc; CCFP; FCFP; (780)435-7555; Fax. (780)436-0582.

GILL, Atamjit; Health Sciences Centre, 300 Prince Philip Dr, St. John's NL A1B 3V6; Ranchi (India)'82; MB BS; FRCSC; ObstGyn. Staff, Health Sciences Centre; Chair Clinical Disciplines ObstGyn, Memorial Univ of Newfoundland; (709)777-7445

GILL, Balbinder S; Richmond Health Science Ctre, 440-6091 Gilbert Rd, Richmond BC V7C 5L9; Punjab (India)'85; MB BS; FRCPC; Peds. (604)270-4456; Fax. (604)273-6146.

GILL, Balwinder S; Teulon Med Clinic, PO Box 89, Teulon MB R0C 3B0; (Other Foreign)'78.

GILL, C A; Carmi Clinic, 716-650 Duncan Ave W, Penticton BC V2A 7N1; UBC'71; Ac Staff, Penticton Regional Hospital; (250)490-7256

GILL, Curtis R; Willowbrook Oral Surgery, 301-6351 197 St, Langley BC V2Y 1X8; Sask'94; Otol (Oral Surgery). (604)532-9686; Fax. (604)532-9687.

GILL, Daljit S; Manitoba Clinic, 790 Sherbrook St, Winnipeg MB R3A 1M3; Man'08.

GILL, David A; 26-8180 Macleod Trail SE, Calgary AB T2H 2B8; Alb'73; (403)531-0585; Fax. (403)259-6110.

GILL, Davinder S; Windsor Reg Hosp-Metropolitan, 1995 Lens Ave, Windsor ON N8W 1L9; Sask'01; FRCPC; DiagRad. Staff, Windsor Regional Hospital - Metropolitan Site; Langs: Punjabi; (519)254-5577

GILL, Eunice C; Psychealth Centre, PZ420-771 Bannatyne Ave, Winnipeg MB R3E 3N4; Man'84; FRCPC; Psy. Att Staff Psy, Health Sciences Centre; Assoc Prof Med, University of Manitoba; (204)787-7098; Fax. (204)787-4879; egill@hsc.mb.ca.

GILL, Francis; Ctr Hosp Affilie Enfant-Jesus, 1401 18e rue, Quebec QC G1J 1Z4; Laval'93; CCFP; CCFP(E.M.); Staff, Centre Hospitalier Affilié Universitaire de Québec - Hôpital De L'Enfant Jésus; (418)649-5632

GILL, Ginjeet K; Vancouver Gen Hosp, 855 12th Ave W, Vancouver BC V5Z 1M9; UBC'07; EmergMed. Staff, Vancouver General Hospital - Centennial Pavillion; (604)875-4995

GILL, Glenn H; Cariboo Mem Hosp, 401-517 Sixth Ave N, Williams Lake BC V2G 2G8; Dal'85; BSc; FRCSC; ObstGyn (Colonoscopy). Staff Specialist Phy, Cariboo Memorial Hospital and Health Centre; Clin Assoc Prof ObstGyn, University of British Columbia; (250)398-8280; Fax. (250)398-8287.

GILL, Gurpreet S; 404-5400 Portage Rd, Niagara Falls ON L2G 5X7; Punjab (India)'91; ABIM; FRCPC; IntMed. Langs: Hindi; Punjabi; (905)356-2044; Fax. (905)356-4344; docggill@yahoo.com.

GILL, Gursharan; Chase Medical Clinic, 826 Thompson Ave Box 410, Chase BC V0E 1M0; Punjabi (India)'89; MB BS; CCFP; (250)679-1420

GILL, Harmander S; Star Med Centre, 124-2980 Drew Rd, Richmond Hill ON L4C 0A5; Tor'08; CCFP; Staff, The Credit Valley Hospital; (905)405-9900; Fax. (905)405-9901.

GILL, Harmeet; Kensington Eye Institute, 600-340 College St, Toronto ON M5T 3A9; McM'05; FRCSC; Ophth. (416)928-2132; Fax. (416)928-5075.

GILL, Harpreet; 385-5780 Cambie St, Vancouver BC V5Z 3A7; UBC'99; FRCSC; Ophth. (604)327-5014 x3

GILL, Jagbir; 602-1160 Burrard St, Vancouver BC V6Z 2E8; UBC'01; FRCPC; IntMed; Nephrol. (604)681-7191

GILL, Jasbir; Waterford Hospital, 306 Waterford Bridge Rd, St. John's NL A1E 4J8; Mem'00; FRCPC; Psy. Staff, Waterford Hospital; (709)777-3300

GILL, Jasdeep S; Etobicoke Walk in & Family Phy, 100 Humber College Blvd, Etobicoke ON M9V 4E4; American University of Antigua (Antigua & Barbuda)'09; CCFP; (416)742-9449; Fax. (416)742-6963.

GILL, Jasdildar; 429 4th Ave NE, Swift Current SK S9H 2J9; (Other Foreign)'08; CCFP.

GILL, Joginder S; 101-4383 Portage Rd, Niagara Falls ON L2E 6A6; Magadh (India)'81; MB BS; CCFP; Assoc Staff, Niagara Health System - Greater Niagara General Site; Langs: Hindi; Punjabi; Urdu; (905)356-5945; Fax. (905)356-7206.

GILL, John S; Burrard Health Bldg, 602-1160 Burrard St, Vancouver BC V6Z 2E8; UBC'95; MS; FRCPC; IntMed (Transplantation); Nephrol. Staff, Providence Health Care - St Paul's Hospital; Pres, Canadian Society of Nephrology; Assoc Prof Med, University of British Columbia; (604)681-7191; Fax. (604)681-4482.

GILL, Julie; Hop Brome-Missisquoi-Perkins, 950 rue Principale, Cowansville QC J2K 1K3; Mon'99; CCFP; Staff, Hôpital Brome-Missisquoi-Perkins; (450)266-4342

GILL, K Kevin S; Eagle Ridge Med Clinc Inc, 102-1173 The High St, Coquitlam BC V3B 0B1; UBC'91; Ac Staff, Eagle Ridge Hospital & Health Care Centre; (604)945-0032; Fax. (604)945-4739.

GILL, Karamjit K; BC Cancer Agency-Fraser Valley, 13750 96 Ave, Surrey BC V3V 1Z2; Wes'96; MRCP; ABIM; MD; BSc; FRCPC; IntMed (Hematological Oncology); MedOncol; Hem. Staff, BC Cancer Agency Fraser Valley Centre; Staff, Surrey Memorial Hospital; Clinical Asst Prof, University of British Columbia; Langs: Punjabi; (604)930-2098

GILL, Kimberlee D; 202-10 Unionville Gate, Unionville ON L3R 0W7; Tor'80; BSc; CCFP; FCFP; Staff, Markham Stouffville Hospital; (905)305-7655; Fax. (905)305-8571.

GILL, Kulvinder K; 517-2250 Boivard Dr E, Brampton ON L6R 0W3; Man'06; FRCPC; Peds. (905)452-0015

GILL, Kulwant S; 1380 Regent St, Sudbury ON P3E 3Z4; Punjab (India)'81; FRCPC; HemPath (Cardiology); Hem; IntMed. Dir, Health Sciences North-Laurentian Site; Langs: Punjabi; Hindi; (705)523-1550

GILL, M John; HSC-Faculty of Med, 3330 Hospital Dr NW, Calgary AB T2N 4N1; Birmingham (England)'76; MB ChB; ABIM; FACP; FRCPC; IntMed (AIDS); InfectDis. Staff, Foothills Medical Centre; Prof Med, University of Calgary; (403)220-6032; john.gill@albertahealthservices.ca.

GILL, Manmohanjit S; 300-2845 Cruickshank St, Abbotsford BC V2T 6X1; UBC'89; Langs: Punjabi; (604)852-6659; Fax. (604)852-6708.

GILL, Navdip S; 13719 72 Ave, Surrey BC V3W 2P2; UBC'98; CCFP; Langs: Punjabi; (604)572-5551

GILL, Paramjit; Credit Valley Med Arts Centre, 414-2000 Credit Valley Rd, Mississauga ON L5M 4N4; Jabalpur (India)'76; MS; Court Staff, The Credit Valley Hospital; Langs: Hindi; Punjabi; Urdu; (905)820-2121

GILL, Paramjit; William Osler HC-Brampton, N2 880-2100 Bovaird Dr E, Brampton ON L6R 3J7; Tor'96; FRCPC; IntMed; Critical Care Medicine. Staff, William Osler Health System - Brampton Civic Hospital; Langs: Punjabi; (905)494-2120

GILL, Prabhjot; 303-22112 52 Ave, Langley BC V2Y 2M6; (India)'01; MB BS; CCFP; (604)530-5656

GILL, Rajinder S; John Street Clinic, 14 John St N, Hamilton ON L8R 1G9; Man'97; CCFP; Staff, Hamilton Health Sciences Centre - Hamilton General Hospital; (905)546-0050

GILL, Randeep S; Medreach Med Centre, 400-1642 Merivale Rd, Nepean ON K2G 4A1; Ravi Shankar University (India)'99; Langs: Hindi; Punjabi; (613)228-2020; Fax. (613)228-2737.

GILL, Richdeep; University of Alberta Hosp, 8440 112 St NW, Edmonton AB T6G 2B7; Alb'06; Staff, University of Alberta Hospital; (780)407-8822

GILL, Sabrina; St Paul's Hosp, 470-1081 Burrard St, Vancouver BC V6Z 1Y6; UBC'94; BScPharm(Pharm); MPH; FRCPC; IntMed; Endocrin&Metab. Staff, Providence Health Care - St Paul's Hospital; Consultant, BC Women's Hospital & Health Centre; Clin Associate Prof, University of British Columbia; (604)806-9156; Fax. (604)806-8594.

GILL, Sarbjit S; Brockville Gen Hosp, 75 Charles St, Brockville ON K6V 1S8; Tor'91; Staff, Brockville General Hospital - Charles Street; (613)345-5645

GILL, Satinderpal S; Toronto East Gen Hosp Inc, 825 Coxwell Ave, Toronto ON M4C 3E7; McM'10; CCFP; Staff, Toronto East General Hospital Inc; (416)461-8272

GILL, Satvir; Meadowbrook Med Clinic, 3905 34 St NW, Edmonton AB T6T 1L5; (England)'94; MB ChB; CCFP; Physician, Meadowbrook Medical Clinic; Langs: Punjabi; (780)448-1166; Fax. (780)448-2830.

GILL, Sharlene; BC Cancer Agency-Vancouver CC, 600 10th Ave W, Vancouver BC V5Z 4E6; UBC'96; FRCPC; IntMed; MedOncol. Staff, BC Cancer Agency Vancouver Centre; (604)877-6000; Fax. (604)877-0585.

GILL, Shawn; Campbell River & Dist Gen Hosp, 375 2nd Ave, Campbell River BC V9W 3V1; UBC'99; CCFP; Staff, Campbell River & District General Hospital; (250)287-7111

GILL, Sudeep S; Providence CCC-St Mary's, PO Box 3600 Stn Main 1 152-340 Union St, Kingston ON K7L 5A2; Wes'97; FRCPC; IntMed; GeriatricMed. Staff, Providence Care - St Mary's of the Lake Hospital Site; (613)544-5220 x2242; Fax. (613)544-4017.

GILL, Sukhdev; 27514A Fraser Hwy, Aldergrove BC V4W 3N5; Birmingham (England)'77; MB ChB; Ac Staff, Abbotsford Regional Hospital & Cancer Centre; (604)856-3134

GILL, Sylvie; Clinique de médecine familiale, 300 rue Paradis, Sorel-Tracy QC J3P 3G6; Mon'82; LMCC; ac Staff, Hôtel-Dieu de Sorel; ac Staff, CHSLD du Bas-Richelieu; (450)742-0485; Fax. (450)742-6965; sylvie@medecinefamiliale.com.

GILL, T Michael D; 21 McGivern St PO Box 1328, Walkerton ON N0G 2V0; Dublin (Ireland)'80; (519)881-1278; Fax. (519)881-3968.

GILL, Tara M; Kootenay-Boundary Reg Hosp, 1200 Hospital Bench, Trail BC V1R 4M1; Tor'01; CCFP; CCFP(E.M.); Staff, Kootenay Boundary Regional Hospital; (250)368-3311

GILL, Vikramjit S; Trillium Hlth Ctr-Mississauga, 100 Queensway W, Mississauga ON L5B 1B8; Punjabi (India)'96; Langs: Hindi; Punjabi; Urdu.

GILLANDERS, Brian S; Weinlos Clinic, 15508 87 Ave NW, Edmonton AB T5R 4G5; Alb'80; CCFP; Ac Staff, Covenant Health - Misericordia Community Hospital; Ac Staff, Capital Care - Lynwood; (780)484-8151; Fax. (780)483-1435.

GILLANDERS, David A; 2756 1st Ave W, Vancouver BC V6K 1H3; UBC'57; Otol. Staff, Vancouver General Hospital - Centennial Pavillion; Staff, BC Children's Hospital; (604)733-4857; Fax. (604)742-2070.

GILLELAND, Jonathan C; McMaster University, 3A 74-1280 Main St W, Hamilton ON L8S 4K1; McM'00; FRCPC; Peds; Critical Care Medicine. Staff, Hamilton Health Sciences Centre - McMaster Children's Hospital; Teach Staff, McMaster University; (905)521-2100; Fax. (905)570-8973.

GILLEN, Lorna E R; Bay & Algoma Health Centre, 153 Algoma St S, Thunder Bay ON P7B 3B7; McM'81; BSc; DrMedCh; Staff, Thunder Bay Regional Health Sciences Centre; Asst Prof, Northern Ontario School of Medicine-Lakehead University; (807)344-2527; Fax. (807)344-2614.

GILLEN, Rael T; Burnaby Hosp, 3935 Kincaid St, Burnaby BC V5G 2X6; Alb'91; FRCPC; GenPath. General Pathology, Burnaby Hospital; (604)434-6353; Fax. (604)431-2806.

GILLESE, J Timothy; PO Box 78083 Rpo Callingwood, Edmonton AB T5T 6A1; Alb'80; FRCPC; Psy. Physician, Alberta Mental Health Board; (780)444-2776; Fax. (780)481-8545; gillese@telusplanet.net.

GILLESPIE, Brian G; 710 Pembina Hwy, Winnipeg MB R3M 2M6; Man'83; FRCSC; Ophth. Staff, Misericordia Health Centre; Assoc Prof, University of Manitoba; (204)943-9248; Fax. (204)949-1143.

GILLESPIE, Ian A; PO Box 48210, Victoria BC V8Z 7H6; UBC'71; DABPN; FRCPC; Psy. (250)595-4222

GILLESPIE, Jamie L; 203-900 Harrow St E, Winnipeg MB R3M 3Y7; Man'84; FRCSC; GenSurg (Breasts). Staff, Victoria General Hospital.

GILLESPIE, John D N; Gillespie Clinic, 5116 Elbow Dr SW, Calgary AB T2V 1H1; Alb'70; Ac Staff, Rockyview General Hospital; (403)259-6798; Fax. (403)255-6547; john@gillespieclinic.com.

GILLESPIE, Kenneth E; Professional Arts Bldg, 223-100 Arden St, Moncton NB E1C 4B7; Dal'94; FRCSC; ObstGyn. (506)382-2162; Fax. (506)854-9738.

GILLESPIE, Laurie; South West Health, 315-50 Vancouver St, Yarmouth NS B5A 2P5; Georgia (USA)'99; (902)742-1068; Fax. (902)742-2513.

GILLETT, Dennis G; Internal Medicine Consultant, 4514 Chatterton Way, Victoria BC V8X 5H2; Alb'73; FRCPC; IntMed. (250)881-7268

GILLETT, John A; PO Box 540, Grande Cache AB T0E 0Y0; (South Africa)'86; (780)827-2540; Fax. (780)827-5698.

GILLETT, Michael K; 19 Grange St, Stratford ON N5A 3P7; London (England)'77; MB BS; MRC; FRCPC; IntMed (Cardiology). Ac Staff IntMed, Stratford General Hospital - Huron Perth Healthcare Alliance; Consultant, Listowel Memorial Hospital - Listowel Wingham Hospitals Alliance; (519)273-0095; Fax. (519)273-1720.

GILLETT, Peter G; MUHC-Royal Victoria Hosp, F9 26-687 av des Pins O, Montreal QC H3A 1A1; McG'63; FRCOG; ObstGyn. Chief Obs/Gyn, McGill University Health Centre - Montreal General Campus; Consultant, McGill University Health Centre - Royal Victoria Hospital; Prof Div of Gyn, McGill University; (514)934-1934 x44287

GILLEY, Heather J; St Michael's Hosp, 4S-30 Bond St, Toronto ON M5B 1W8; Cal'84; FRCPC; IntMed; GeriatricMed. Staff Regional Geriatric Program, St Michael's Hospital; Asst Prof, University of Toronto; (416)864-5015

GILLIES, Anne M W; Smyth Med Centre, 204-1929 Russell Rd, Ottawa ON K1G 4G3; McM'98; FRCPC; Peds. Staff, Children's Hospital of Eastern Ontario (CHEO); Langs: Bilingual(English/French); (613)736-9976; Fax. (613)288-1467.

GILLIES, Jean H; Van Prolo & MSK Diag Clinic, 340-1144 Burrard St, Vancouver BC V6Z 2A5; UBC'82; FRCPC; IntMed (Orthopedic Medicine); Rheum. Clin Instructor, University of British Columbia; (604)685-6114; Fax. (604)685-6142.

GILLIES, Judy R M; Timmins Family Health Team, 208-38 Pine St N, Timmins ON P4N 6K6; McM'98; CCFP; FCFP; Staff, Timmins & District Hospital; Staff, White Pines Health Network; Langs: Bilingual(English/French); (705)267-3272; Fax. (705)267-4212.

GILLIES, Liesel; Glenmore Landing, A301-1600 90 Ave SW, Calgary AB T2V 5A8; Stellenbosch (South Africa)'90; MB ChB; CCFP; Langs: Afrikaans; (403)246-0200; Fax. (403)301-0046.

GILLIES, Pamela M; 6-505 23rd St E, Saskatoon SK S7K 4K7; Sask'86; FRCPC; Psy (Anxiety & Mood Disorders). Asst Prof College of Medicine, University of Saskatchewan; (306)652-4687; Fax. (306)652-4685; pgillies@sasktel.net.

GILLILAND, G Barry; Pacific Avenue Med Centre, 300-149 Pacific Ave, Saskatoon SK S7K 1N8; Sask'72; FACOG; FRCSC; ObstGyn (Endoscopic Gynecology). Ac Staff ObstGyn, Saskatoon District Health Board; Clin Prof ObstGyn, University of Saskatchewan; (306)653-5970; Fax. (306)653-5383.

GILLIS, Amy E; Cape Breton Hlthcare Complex, 1482 George St, Sydney NS B1P 1P3; Tor'04; FRCSC; GenSurg (Surgical Oncology). Staff, Cape Breton Healthcare Complex; (902)567-8000

GILLIS, Amy E; Dalhousie Fam Med Mumford Clin, 265-6960 Mumford Rd, Halifax NS B3L 4P1; Dal'02; BSc(Hon); CCFP; (902)473-4700

GILLIS, Anne M; Calgary Heart Centre, GAC 72-3280 Hospital Dr NW, Calgary AB T2N 4Z6; Dal'79; FRCPC; Cardiol (Cardiac Electrophysiology). Media Dir Pacing & Electrophysiol., Foothills Medical Centre; Med Dir Pacing & Electrophysiol, Calgary Health Region; Prof Med, University of Calgary; (403)220-6841; Fax. (403)270-0313; amgillis@ucalgary.ca.

GILLIS, Cory F; C205-600 Main St, Saint John NB E2K 1J5; Mem'03; FRCPC; IntMed; Gastroent. (506)635-0420; Fax. (506)635-0430.

GILLIS, Gregory F; Spingbank Med Centre, 301-460 Springbank Dr, London ON N6J 0A8; Wes'77; CCFP; FCFP; Staff Family Med, St Joseph's Hospital - St Joseph's Health Care; Aj Prof Family Med/Dir CME Development Disabilities Div Dept of Psy, University of Western Ontario; (519)438-7026; Fax. (519)438-7027.

GILLIS, John M; Woodside Hlth Ctr for Pain Man, 18 Acadia St, Dartmouth NS B2Y 4H3; Wes'99; CCFP; CCFP(E.M.); Staff, Dartmouth General Hospital; (902)463-7857; Fax. (902)463-7564.

GILLIS, Judith L; Crowfoot West Business Ctre, 210-600 Crowfoot Cres NW, Calgary AB T3G 0B4; Cal'10; (403)239-9733

GILLIS, Katharine A; The Ottawa Hosp-Civic Campus, 1053 Carling Ave, Ottawa ON K1Y 4E9; Mem'82; FRCPC; Psy. Staff Psy, The Ottawa Hospital - Civic Campus; Dept Chair Psy, University of Ottawa; (613)761-4581; Fax. (613)761-5328.

GILLIS, L Jane; IWK Health Centre, PO Box 9700 Rpo CSC 5850-5980 University Ave, Halifax NS B3K 6R8; Dal'03; FCCMG; FRCPC; MedGenetics. Staff, IWK Health Centre; Asst Prof Peds, Dalhousie University; (902)470-2630; Fax. (902)470-8709.

GILLIS, Lisa A; Chinook Reg Hosp, 960 19 St S, Lethbridge AB T1J 1W5; Mem'98; CCFP; Staff, Chinook Regional Hospital; (403)388-6135; Fax. (403)388-6708.

GILLIS, Melissa C; PO Box 953 Stn A, Prince George BC V2L 4V1; Dal'03; CCFP; CCFP(E.M.); (250)613-2053

GILLIS, Thomas M; 300-1011 Glenmore Trail SW, Calgary AB T2V 4R6; Dal'74; BSc; ABOtol; FACS; FRCSC; Otol (Endoscopy). Ac Staff, Tom Baker Cancer Centre; Ac Staff, Rockyview General Hospital; Ac Staff, Alberta Children's Hospital; Assoc Prof, University of Calgary; (403)571-5205; Fax. (403)571-5206; tgillis@arczone.com.

GILLIS-DOYLE, Jennifer A; 203-170 Simcoe St, Peterborough ON K9H 2H7; Dal'03; CCFP; (705)876-4523

GILLMAN, Lawrence; St Boniface Gen Hosp, Z3053-409 Tache Ave, Winnipeg MB R2H 2A6; Man'02; FRCSC; GenSurg; Critical Care Medicine. Staff, St Boniface General Hospital; (204)233-8563

GILLMAN, Marcia L; SMBD Jewish Gen Hosp, 3755 ch Cote-Sainte-Catherine, Montreal QC H3T 1E2; Man'88; CCFP; FCFP; Ac Member Family Med, Sir Mortimer B Davis Jewish General; Staff, Jewish Rehabilitation Hospital; (514)340-8232

GILLMAN, Ross G; The Doctors Walk-In Med Clinic, 105-641 Commissioners Rd E, London ON N6C 2T9; Wes'59; PhD; FRCSC; GenSurg (Proctology). Staff, Four Counties Health Services - Middlesex Hospital Alliance; (519)963-0233; Fax. (519)963-0232.

GILLMORE, Trevor A; 2316 Major Mackenzie Dr, Maple ON L6A 1W6; McM'88; (905)832-2010; Fax. (905)832-2782.

GILLOT, Nicolas P M; CSSSG-Hop de Hull, 116 boul Lionel-Emond, Gatineau QC J8Y 1W7; Staff, Hull Hospital; (819)966-6200

GILLOTEAUX, Laurent C; Scarborough Hosp-General Div, 3050 Lawrence Ave E, Scarborough ON M1P 2V5; Ohio(OH) (USA)'98; FRCPC; DiagRad. Staff, The Scarborough Hospital - General Campus; Langs: Bilingual(English/French); (416)431-8107

GILLSON, Ashley; Royal Alexandra Hosp, CSC 419-10240 Kingsway Ave, Edmonton AB T5H 3V9; Ott'06; FRCPC; IntMed; Respir. Staff, Royal Alexandra Hospital; (780)735-4243; Fax. (780)735-4245.

GILMAN, Cara E; Assossiate Clinic, 340-401 9 Ave SW, Calgary AB T2P 3C5; Man'92; BA; FRCP; FRCPC; Peds (Community Pediatrics). (403)221-4434; Fax. (403)221-4466.

GILMAN, Michael L; 301-2797 Bathurst St, North York ON M6B 4B9; Tor'71; Staff, Humber River Regional Hospital - Keele Street Site; Staff, Baycrest Centre for Geriatric Care; Staff, Mount Sinai Hospital; (416)787-1297; Fax. (416)781-9580.

GILMAN, Sean A; Centre Hospitalier de Verdun, 4000 boul Lasalle, LaSalle QC H4G 2A2; McG'97; FRCPC; IntMed; Respir. (514)362-1000

GILMER, Deborah; BC Women's Hosp & Health Ctre, 1N22-4500 Oak St, Vancouver BC V6H 3N1; Richmond(VA) (USA)'83; FRCPC; Peds. Staff, BC Women's Hospital & Health Centre; (604)875-2424

GILMORE, Andrew; Westcoast Family Practice Ctre, 2775 Laurel St, Vancouver BC V5Z 1M9; (United Kingdom)'89; (604)875-5691

GILMORE, Kendra; 14-654 Main St, Sussex NB E4E 7H9; Dal'09; CCFP; (506)434-4081

GILMORE, Norbert; MUHC-Montreal Chest Institute, J8 02-3650 rue Saint-Urbain, Montreal QC H2X 2P4; (USA)'70; PhD(Pharm); Sr Physician Clin Immurol, McGill University Health Centre - Royal Victoria Hospital; Dir Chronic Viral Dis Servs, McGill University Health Centre - Montreal Chest Institute; Dir Chronic Viral Diseases Serv, McGill University Health Centre - Montreal General Campus; Langs: French; (514)843-2090; Fax. (514)843-2092; norbert.gilmore@muhc.mcgill.ca.

GILMOUR, Donna T; IWK Health Centre, PO Box 9700 Rpo CSC 5850-5980 Univesity Ave, Halifax NS B3K 6R8; Alb'92; FRCSC; ObstGyn (Gynecological Surgery) (Urogynecology). Court Staff, Queen Elizabeth II Health Sciences Centre - Victoria General Site; Ac Staff ObstGyn, IWK Health Centre; Court Staff, New Halifax Infirmary Sites; Asst Prof, Dalhousie University; (902)470-7491; Fax. (902)425-1125.

GILMOUR, Janet G; HSC-Faculty of Med, 3330 Hospital Dr NW, Calgary AB T2N 4N1; Tor'83; FRCPC; IntMed (AIDS/HIV). Staff, Foothills Medical Centre; Clin Assoc Prof, University of Calgary; (403)220-4506; Fax. (403)283-6151.

GILMOUR, Jeffrey L; 3-96 Cornell Park Ave, Markham ON L6B 1B6; Tor'83; FRCSC; ObstGyn. Ac Staff, Markham Stouffville Hospital; (905)294-1934; Fax. (905)294-7843.

GILMOUR, Kimberly E; Happy Valley Family Hlth Team, PO Box 1120 Stn Main 268 Maiden Ave, St Marys ON N4X 1B7; Wes'03; CCFP; CCFP(E.M.); Staff, Kingston General Hospital; (519)284-3450; kgilmour@stmmc.ca.

GILMOUR, Michael M; Medl Assoc Of Port Perry, 462 Paxton St, Port Perry ON L9L 1L9; Tor'88; CCFP; FCFP; Ac Staff, Lakeridge Health - Port Perry Site; Lecturer, University of Toronto; (905)985-9738; Fax. (905)985-8378.

GILMOUR, Susan; Edmonton Clinic Health Academy, 3 468-11405 87 Ave NW, Edmonton AB T6G 1C9; Sask'90; MSc; FRCPC; Peds (Hepatology). Staff Stollery Children's Health Centre, University of Alberta Hospital; Staff, Edmonton Clinic Health Academy; Assoc Prof Peds/Dept Chair Ped, University of Alberta; (780)407-3339

GILPIN, Sharon D; 307-140 Oxford St E, London ON N6A 5R9; Tor'86; (519)642-7131; Fax. (519)642-7786.

GILRON, Ian; Kingston Gen Hosp, V2-76 Stuart St, Kingston ON K7L 2V7; Ott'90; FRCPC; Anes. Staff, Kingston General Hospital; Clin Dir-Research, Queen's University; (613)549-6666 x3963; Fax. (613)548-1375.

GIMAEL, Jean-Francois; 1055 av du Pont S, Alma QC G8B 2V7; Sher'99; CSPQ; FRCSC; OrthSurg. Staff, CSSS de Lac-Saint Jean-Est; (418)662-7813; Fax. (514)843-2092.

GIMBARZEVSKY, Boris P; Summit Med Clinic, 4-1380 Summit Dr, Kamloops BC V2C 1T8; Cal'90; BSc(Hon.); MSc; Staff Family Pract, Providence Health Care - St Paul's Hospital; Langs: Ukrainian; Croatian; (250)374-9800; borisg@unixg.ubc.ca.

GIMBEL, Howard V; Gimbel Eye Centre, 450-4935 40 Ave NW, Calgary AB T3A 2N1; Loma Linda(CA) (USA)'60; MPH; FAAOO; FRCSC; Ophth (Cataract Surgery). Associate/Clin Prof Surg, University of Calgary; Prof/Chairman Dept of Ophth Loma Linda Univ, University of California-San Francisco(USA); (403)286-3022; Fax. (403)286-2943; hvgimbel@gimbel.com.

GIMON, Eglee; St Paul's Hosp, 1702 20th St W, Saskatoon SK S7M 0Z9; CCFP; Staff, St Paul's Hospital (Grey Nuns) of Saskatoon; Asst Prof Academic Family Med, University of Saskatchewan; (306)655-5530; Fax. (306)655-5918.

GIN, Christopher S W; Castlemore Family Med Centre, 2-9960 Airport Rd, Brampton ON L6S 0C5; Qns'08; CCFP; (905)799-2273

GIN, Davey Y M; Guildford Med Dental Centre, 10-15300 105 Ave, Surrey BC V3R 6A7; UBC'88; CCFP; FCFP; Langs: Nepali; (604)581-6711; Fax. (604)583-2818.

GIN, Kenneth G; Cardiac Ultrasound, 9117-2775 Laurel St, Vancouver BC V5Z 1M9; UBC'85; MCPS; NBEchoTestamur; FRCPC; IntMed; Cardiol. Head Div of Cardiol, Vancouver General Hospital - Centennial Pavillion; Clin Prof/Head Div of Card Vancouver Acute/Med Mgr Vancouver Acute, University of British Columbia; (604)875-5898; Fax. (604)875-5361; kenneth.gin@vch.ca.

GINDI, Gimiana N; Credit Valley Med Arts Centre, 215-2000 Credit Valley Rd, Mississauga ON L5M 4N4; Mansourah (Egypt)'83; MB ChB; CPH; CCFP; Staff, The Credit Valley Hospital; Langs: Arabic; (905)828-9008; Fax. (905)828-9372.

GINDI, Medhat F; Credit Valley Med Arts Centre, 201-2000 Credit Valley Rd, Mississauga ON L5M 4N4; Assiut (Egypt)'83; MB ChB; FRCPC; CommunMed (Travel Medicine). Langs: Arabic; (905)828-6000

GINDI, Raafat F; 206-1366 Yonge St, Toronto ON M4T 3A7; Assuit (Egypt)'75; Staff, St Joseph's Health Centre; Staff, North York General Hospital - Branson Division; Langs: Arabic; (416)654-6779; Fax. (416)654-4894.

GINGELL-POTTS, Ruth; Greenbrook Family Med Centre, 421 Greenbrook Dr, Kitchener ON N2M 4K1; McM'86; CCFP; FCFP; Assoc Staff, Grand River Hospital - Kitchener/Waterloo Health Centre; Assoc Staff, St Mary's General Hospital; Physician, Greenbrook Family Med Centre; (519)570-1655; Fax. (519)570-3477.

GINGERICH, Joel R; St Boniface Gen Hosp, L1 101-409 Tache Ave, Winnipeg MB R2H 2A6; Indiana(PA) (USA)'01; FRCPC; IntMed (Palliative Care); MedOncol. Staff, St Boniface General Hospital; (204)233-8563; joel.gingerich@cancercare.mb.ca.

GINGERICH, Roger L; Steinbach Family Med Centre, 10-333 Loewen Blvd, Steinbach MB R5G 0C3; Man'85; (204)326-8872; Fax. (204)326-3899.

GINGLES, Carmen R; Heritage Med Clinic, 105-2841 109 St NW, Edmonton AB T6J 6B7; Alb'96; CCFP; FCFP; (780)436-3790; Fax. (780)434-8378.

GINGRAS, Alain; Clin Med Saint-Martin, 91 1e Av E RR 1, Saint-Martin QC G0M 1B0; Mon'85; (418)382-5570; Fax. (418)382-3828.

GINGRAS, Andre; 111 12e av, Drummondville QC J2B 2Y6; Laval'77; (819)477-7555; Fax. (819)477-7582.

GINGRAS, Anne-Isabelle; Clinique D'Ophtalmologie, 2e-2875 boul Laurier, Quebec QC G1V 2M2; Laval'02; CCFP; CCFP(E.M.); Staff, CSSS de Trois-Rivières; Staff, Centre Hospitalier Universitaire De Québec - Pavillon De St-françois-d'assise; (418)654-2701

GINGRAS, Benoit; ASSS-Chaudiere Appalaches, 363 Rte Cameron, Sainte-Marie QC G6E 3E2; Laval'71; MSc; Physician, Public Health & Welfare; (418)389-1526; Fax. (418)389-1525; benoit.gingras@ssss.gouv.qc.ca.

GINGRAS, Caroline; CSSS du Lac-des-Deux-Montagnes, 520 boul Arthur-Sauve, Saint-Eustache QC J7R 5B1; Mon'02; Staff, Hôpital de Saint-Eustache; Langs: English; French; (450)473-6811

GINGRAS, Claude R; Clinique Med St-David, 4497 boul de la Rive-Sud, Levis QC G6W 6M9; Laval'75; Ac Staff, Hôtel-Dieu de Lévis; (418)833-4791; Fax. (418)837-0254.

GINGRAS, France; CSSS de Trois-Rivières, 1991 boul du Carmel, Trois-Rivieres QC G8Z 3R9; Laval'00; CSPQ; FRCPC; Anes. Staff, CSSS de Trois-Rivières; (819)697-3333

GINGRAS, Guy; CSSS de Haut Saint-Maurice, 885 boul Ducharme, La Tuque QC G9X 3C1; Laval'80; Staff, Centre Hospitalier Saint-Joseph de la Turque; (819)523-3084; Fax. (819)523-5019; guy_gingras@ssss.gouv.qc.ca.

GINGRAS, Isabelle; CSSS de Sept-Iles, 45 rue du Pere-Divet, Sept-Iles QC G4R 3N7; Mon'99; FRCPC; Psy. Staff, Centre Hospitalier Regional de Sept-Iles; (418)962-9761

GINGRAS, Manon; Regie Cote Nord, 691 rue Jalbert, Baie-Comeau QC G5C 2A1; Mon'89; (418)589-9845

GINGRAS, Marc; CSSS d'Argenteuil, 145 av de la Providence, Lachute QC J8H 4C7; Sher'85; ACLS; ATLS; CSPQ; GenSurg (P.Q.) (C-Section(Caesarean)). Staff, Centre Hospitalier d'Argenteuil; Instructeur (AILS), Hôpital du Sacre-Coeur de Montréal; Staff, CSSS d'Antoine-Labelle; Langs: English; French; (450)562-3761

GINGRAS, Michel; Hôpital Laval, 2725 ch Sainte-Foy, Quebec QC G1V 4G5; Laval'90; LMCC; FRCPC; DiagRad (Abdominal). Staff, Hôpital Laval; Prof, Universite de Sherbrooke; (418)656-4512

GINGRAS, Michele S; North Okanagan Paediatric Clin, 3-2802 34 St, Vernon BC V1T 5X1; Tor'00; FRCPC; Peds. Staff Ped, Vernon Jubilee Hospital; (250)558-5506; Fax. (250)558-5108; nopc@shawcable.ca.

GINGRAS, Nathalie; Hotel-Dieu du Sacre-Coeur, 1 av du Sacre-Coeur, Quebec QC G1N 2W1; Laval'90; FRCPC; Psy. Staff, Hotel-Dieu du Sacre-Coeur de Jesus de Quebec; Chef Psy & Neurosciences, Université Laval; (418)529-6851 x20281

GINGRAS, Pascale; Ctr Hosp Trois-Riv-St-Joseph, 2F-731 rue Sainte-Julie, Trois-Rivieres QC G9A 1Y1; Laval'89; Staff, Centre Hospitalier Regional de Trois-Rivieres; Staff, CLSC Les Forges Soutien a Domicile; (819)372-3536; Fax. (819)372-3509.

GINGRAS, Pierre; Clinique Med Soleil des Tanner, 3767 rue Notre-Dame O, Montreal QC H4C 1P8; Mon'79; (514)932-8912; Fax. (514)932-8944; pierre.gingras@ssss.gouv.qc.ca.

GINGRAS, Rene; CSSS Kamouraska-Hop Notre-Dame, 1201 6e Av CP 460, La Pocatiere QC G0R 1Z0; Laval'68; CSPQ; FRCPC; Anes. Staff, CSSS de Kamouraska; (418)856-7000

GINGRAS, Serge; Hop Ste-Anne, 305 boul des Anciens-Combattan, Ste-Anne-de-Bellev QC H9X 1Y9; Mon'76; Staff, Hopital Ste-Anne; (514)457-3440 x2545; Fax. (514)457-8410.

GINGRAS, Stefanie; MUHC-Montreal Gen Hosp, E10 128 2-1650 av Cedar, Montreal QC H3G 1A4; Mon'97; CCFP; FCFP; Staff Family Phy & Palliative Care, McGill University Health Centre - Montreal General Campus; Teacher, McGill University; Langs: Bilingual(French/English); (514)934-1934 x46000

GINGRICH, Emerson; Richmond Square Med Centre, 70-3915 51 St SW, Calgary AB T3E 6N1; Wes'67; CCFP; (403)229-2273; Fax. (403)246-9688.

GINGRICH, Ruth A; City Pharmacy, 12 West Ave, Corner Brook NL A2H 4K2; Wes'69; CCFP; FCFP; Staff, Western Memorial Regional Hospital; Staff Teacher, Memorial University Of Newfoundland; (709)634-6841; Fax. (709)639-3265.

GINN, Jeffery; Grand River Hosp-KW Hlth Ctre, PO Box 9056 Stn C 835 King St W, Kitchener ON N2G 1G3; Dal'00; CCFP; CCFP(E.M.); Staff, Grand River Hospital - Kitchener/Waterloo Health Centre; (519)749-4300

GINN, John L; 1802-45 Alderney Dr, Dartmouth NS B2Y 2N6; Mem'88; (902)452-7726; Fax. (902)435-0914.

GINNISH, Amanda; Colchester East Hants Hlth Ctr, 600 Abenaki Rd, Truro NS B2N 5A1; Dal'07; Psy. Staff, Colchester East Hants Health Centre; (902)893-4321; Fax. (902)893-5551.

GINSBERG, Donald; MUHC-Montreal Gen Hosp, L10 212-1650 av Cedar, Montreal QC H3G 1A4; McG'02; CCFP; Staff, McGill University Health Centre - Montreal General Campus; Langs: French; (514)934-1934 x43938

GINSBERG, Howard J; St Michael's Hosp, 30 Bond St, Toronto ON M5B 1W8; Tor'93; FRCSC; Neursurg (Spine). Staff, St Michael's Hospital; (416)864-5703

GINSBERG, Jeffrey; St Joseph's Healthcare, H319-50 Charlton Ave E, Hamilton ON L8N 4A6; Ott'78; FRCPC; IntMed (Thromboembolism); Hem. Staff, St Joseph's Healthcare - Charlton Campus; Prof, McMaster University; (905)522-1155

GINSBERG, Leonard S; Addiction & Mental Hlth-Queen, 2-1001 Queen St W, Toronto ON M6J 1H4; Tor'81; FRCPC; Psy. Ac Staff, Centre for Addiction & Mental Health (CAMH) - Queen Site; Asst Prof, University of Toronto; (416)535-8501 x2622; Fax. (416)583-4352.

GINSBURG, Jonathan C; West Lincoln Mem Hosp, 169 Main St E, Grimsby ON L3M 1P3; Cape Town (South Africa)'72; MB ChB; FACP; FRCPC; IntMed (Cardiology). Ac Staff, West Lincoln Memorial Hospital; (905)945-6655; Fax. (905)945-8235.

GINSBURG, M Neale; Lakeridge Hlth Corp-Oshawa, 1 Hospital Crt, Oshawa ON L1G 2B9; Tor'92; CCFP; Staff, Lakeridge Health - Oshawa Site; (905)576-8711 x4579; Fax. (905)721-7763.

GINSBURG, Shiphra R; Mount Sinai Hosp, 433-600 University Ave, Toronto ON M5G 1X5; McG'90; MD; MEd; FRCPC; IntMed; Critical Care Medicine; Respir. Asst Prof, Mount Sinai Hospital; Staff, Princess Margaret Hospital - University Health Network; Asst Prof, University of Toronto; (416)586-8671; Fax. (416)586-8864; sginsburg@mtsinai.on.ca.

GINSON, Deborah; High Point Health Centre, 1-283 New Maryland Hwy, New Maryland NB E3C 2H3; Dal'86; BSc(Hon); Physician, Dr Everett Chalmers Regional Hospital; (506)458-2004; Fax. (506)458-2006.

GINTER, Douglas; Le Marchand Mansion, 408-11523 100 Ave NW, Edmonton AB T5K 0J8; Alb'80; FRCPC; Psy. Clin Instructor, University of Alberta; (780)488-8209; Fax. (780)453-1219.

GINTHER, D Glen; 2654A-5955 Veterans Memorial L, Halifax NS B3H 2E1; Man'82; FRCPC; IntMed; GeriatricMed. (902)473-2495; Fax. (902)473-7133.

GINTING, Nadra; The Langley Business Ctre, 180-8700 200 St, Langley BC V2Y 0G4; Tor'05; VascSurg; GenSurg. (604)888-7505

GINTY, Alexandra C; Dorval Med Assoc Fam Hlth Team, 465 Morden Rd, Oakville ON L6K 3W6; McM'90; CCFP; CCFP(E.M.); FCFP; (905)842-7154; Fax. (905)845-2439; aginty@cogeco.ca.

GINTY, Mark R; Argus Med Centre, 201-581 Argus Rd, Oakville ON L6J 3J4; McM'89; FRCSC; OrthSurg (Sports Medicine). (905)339-0707; Fax. (905)339-1886.

GINZBERG, Hedy H; 5A-5230 Dundas St W, Etobicoke ON M9B 1A8; McG'90; PhD; FRCPC; Peds. (416)234-5442; Fax. (416)234-1483; hginzberg@on.lung.ca.

GINZBURG, Amir; Trillium Hlth Centre-Missiauga, 100 Queensway W, Mississauga ON L5B 1B8; Tor'01; FRCPC; IntMed. Staff, Trillium Health Centre - Mississauga; (905)848-7100

GINZBURG, Brian M; North York Gen Hosp, 4001 Leslie St, North York ON M2K 1E1; Witwatersrand (South Africa)'82; FRCPC; DiagRad. Staff, North York General Hospital; Lecturer, University of Toronto; (416)756-6186

GINZBURG, Val E; Oak Ridge Med Centre, 400-13291 Yonge St, Richmond Hill ON L4E 4L6; McM'05; CCFP; Staff, Stevenson Memorial Hospital; (905)751-2930; val.ginzburg@gmail.com.

GINZER, Matthew E; South Calgary Med Clinic, 118-40 Sunpark Plaza SE, Calgary AB T2X 3X7; Cal'92; BSc(H); CCFP; FCFP; (403)254-4000; Fax. (403)254-1282.

GIOBBE, Stefania; East Kootenay Reg Hosp, 13 24th Ave N, Cranbrook BC V1C 3H9; St George's (Grenada)'03; Staff, East Kootenay Regional Hospital; (250)489-6435

GIONET, Dominique; CSSS de Sept-Iles, 45 rue du Pere-Divet, Sept-Iles QC G4R 3N7; Mon'99; FRCPC; IntMed. Staff, Centre Hospitalier Regional de Sept-Iles; (418)962-9761

GIONET, Edmonde; 1057 St. Peter Ave, Bathurst NB E2A 2Z6; Mon'81; CCFP; FCFP; Staff, Hôpital Général de Grand-Falls; Langs: English; (506)546-1300; Fax. (506)547-1916.

GIONET, Larry R; Merivale Medical Imaging, 1370 Clyde Ave, Nepean ON K2G 3H8; Ott'75; FRCPC; DiagRad. (613)727-1072

GIONET, Melanie; CSSS de Rimouski-Neigette, CP 3150 succ A Bureau Chef 150 av Rouleau, Rimouski QC G5L 5T1; Mon'01; FRCPC; RadOncol. Staff, Hôpital Regional Rimouski; (418)724-8362

GIORDANO, Isabelle; West End Family Care Hlth Team, 80 Michael Cowpland Dr, Kanata ON K2M 1P6; McG'05; CCFP; Staff, Westend Family Care Clinic Family Health Team; Langs: Bilingual(English/French); (613)596-3321; Fax. (613)599-3366.

GIORGI, Conrado; Clinique Med de Montreal, 101-8415 rue Saint-Denis, Montreal QC H2P 2H1; Buenos Aires (Argentina)'73; (514)388-5723

GIORNO, Andrew; Cape Breton Hlthcare Complex, 1482 George St, Sydney NS B1P 1P3; Dal'09; MB ChB; BAO; CCFP; Staff, Cape Breton Healthcare Complex; (902)567-8000

GIORSHEV, Chris; The Simcoe Clinic, 2-279 Yonge ST, Barrie ON L4N 7T9; Tor'91; CCFP; CCFP(E.M.); FCFP; Staff, Royal Victoria Regional Health Centre; (705)728-8869

GIOVANNETTI, Brian L; 26-1917 4th Ave W, Vancouver BC V6J 1M7; Dal'74; (604)816-8142

GIOVANNONI, Aldo; Dr Everett Chalmers Reg Hosp, PO Box 9000 Stn A 700 Priestman St, Fredericton NB E3B 5N5; Pretoria (South Africa)'93; CCFP; Staff, Dr Everett Chalmers Regional Hospital; Langs: Afrikaans.

GIOVINAZZO, George A; 276 Island Park Dr, Ottawa ON K1Y 0A4; Alb'77; Physician, Citizenship & Immigration Canada; (613)698-7870

GIRALDEAU-BELANGER, Sarah-Emilie; CHUM-Hotel-Dieu, 3840 rue Saint-Urbain, Montreal QC H2W 1T8; Mon'05; CCFP; Staff, Centre Hospitalier l'Université de Montréal (CHUM) - Hôtel-Dieu; (514)890-8000 x14996

GIRALDO, Hernan; Ctr Hosp Anna-Laberge, 200 boul Brisebois, Chateauguay QC J6K 4W8; Valle (Colombia)'75; MSc; Peds (P.Q.). Staff, Hôpital Anna-Laberge; Staff, McGill University Health Centre - Montreal Children's Hospital; Associate, McGill University; Langs: Spanish; French; (450)699-2436; Fax. (450)699-2525.

GIRARD, Alain; Clinique Med du Phare, 101-822 boul Sainte-Anne, Rimouski QC G5M 1J5; Laval'96; CCFP; Chef gériatrie, Hôpital Regional Rimouski; (418)723-5135

GIRARD, Andre; 610 boul du Seminaire N, St-Jean-Sur-Richel QC J3B 7B4; Sher'86; (450)348-9218; Fax. (450)348-0377.

GIRARD, Anne-Marie; Polyclinique St-Jerome, 206-200 rue Durand, Saint-Jerome QC J7Z 7E2; Mon'86; FRCSC; ObstGyn. Staff, Hôtel-Dieu de Saint-Jérôme; (450)565-6332; Fax. (450)436-5488.

GIRARD, Benoit; 2500 rue Einstein, Quebec QC G1P 0A2; Laval'71; Médecin, Anapharm Inc; (418)527-3067; Fax. (418)527-3456.

GIRARD, Brigitte; Hop Charles Lemoyne, 3120 boul Taschereau, Greenfield Park QC J4V 2H1; Sher'82; CSPQ; Anes. Ac Staff, Hopital Charles LeMoyne; (450)466-5474

GIRARD, Bruno; CSSS du Sud de Lanaudière, 911 montee des Pionniers, Terrebonne QC J6V 2H2; Laval'99; CSPQ; FRCSC; OrthSurg. Staff, Centre Hospitalier Pierre le Gardeur; (450)654-7525

GIRARD, Claude; CSSS de la Baie-des-Chaleurs, RR 2 419 boul Perron, Maria QC G0C 1Y0; Mon'97; IntMed (P.Q.). Staff, CSSS de la Baie-des-Chaleurs; (418)759-3443 x2421

GIRARD, Claude; 201-1656 rue Sherbrooke E, Montreal QC H2L 1M5; Mon'64; FAB; FRCPC; Derm. ac Staff Derm, Centre Hospitalier l'Université de Montréal (CHUM) - Hôpital Notre-Dame; assoc Prof, Universite de Montreal; (514)526-3783; Fax. (514)412-7620.

GIRARD, Claude; Hotel-Dieu de Levis, 143 rue Wolfe, Levis QC G6V 3Z1; Sher'90; FRCPC; Psy. Staff, Hôtel-Dieu de Lévis; (418)835-7155; Fax. (418)835-7199.

GIRARD, Dominique; CHUM-Hop Notre-Dame, AS1115 3-1560 rue Sherbrooke E, Montreal QC H2L 4M1; Mon'81; CSPQ; FRCPC; Anes. Chef anesth, Centre Hospitalier l'Université de Montréal (CHUM) - Hôpital Notre-Dame; (514)890-8000 x26876; Fax. (514)876-6874.

GIRARD, Drew; Portage Med FHT-Morrison St Si, 303-6453 Morrison St, Niagara Falls ON L2E 7H1; Wes'84; CCFP; (905)356-8500; Fax. (905)356-1367.

GIRARD, Francois; CHUM-Hop Notre-Dame, AS1115 3-1560 rue Sherbrooke E, Montreal QC H2L 4M1; Mon'92; CSPQ; FRCPC; Anes. Staff, Centre Hospitalier l'Université de Montréal (CHUM) - Hôpital Notre-Dame; (514)890-8000 x26876

GIRARD, Gilles; CSSS Pierre Boucher, 1333 boul Jacques-Cartier E, Longueuil QC J4M 2A5; Mon'83; CSPQ; Anes (Family Medicine). Staff, Centre Hospitalier Pierre Boucher; (450)468-8111

GIRARD, Ginette; Clin Med Plateau Marquette, 200-731 rue Galt O, Sherbrooke QC J1H 1Z1; Sher'79; Ac Staff, Centre Hospitalier Universitaire de Sherbrooke-Hôpital Hôtel-Dieu; (819)564-8662

GIRARD, Guy; 120-504 rue Notre-Dame, Repentigny QC J6A 2T8; Mon'77; ObstGyn (P.Q.). Staff, Centre Hospitalier Pierre le Gardeur; (514)582-3999

GIRARD, Guy; Hop du Sacre-Coeur de Mtl, 5400 boul Gouin O, Montreal QC H4J 1C5; Sher'82; FRCSC; Urol. Staff, Hôpital du Sacre-Coeur de Montréal; (514)338-2050

GIRARD, Guylaine; CSSS de la Region de Thetford, 1717 rue Notre-Dame E, Thetford Mines QC G6G 2V4; Laval'86; LMCC; Staff, Hopital du CSS de la Region de Thetford; (418)338-7763; Fax. (418)338-7762.

GIRARD, Guylaine; Clinique Fam Notre Dame, 6F-2120 rue Sherbrooke E, Montreal QC H2K 1C3; Mon'95; Staff Obst, Centre Hospitalier l'Université de Montréal (CHUM) - Hôpital Notre-Dame; Clin Teach Staff, Universite de Montreal; Langs: Bilingual(French/English); (514)527-1958; Fax. (514)527-1649.

GIRARD, Isabelle; CHUS-Hop Fleurimont, 3001 12e av N, Sherbrooke QC J1H 5N4; Laval'03; FRCSC; ObstGyn. Staff, Centre Hospitalier Universitaire de Sherbrooke-Hopital Fleurimont; (819)346-1110

GIRARD, Isabelle; 500-5300 ch de la Cote-des-Nei, Montreal QC H3T 1Y6; Mon'91; FRCSC; ObstGyn. (514)343-0636; Fax. (514)343-0530; i_girard@yahoo.com.

GIRARD, Isabelle M; Foothills Medical Centre, 1403 29 St NW, Calgary AB T2N 2T9; Sher'03; Fellow Ulogynecologie, Foothills Medical Centre; Langs: Bilingual(French/English); (403)944-1437; Fax. (403)283-7136.

GIRARD, J Marc; CHUM-Hop Notre-Dame, 1560 rue Sherbrooke E, Montreal QC H2L 4M1; Mon'83; NBME; LMCC; FRCPC; Neur (Electromyography); Electroenceph (P.Q.). Staff, Centre Hospitalier l'Université de Montréal (CHUM) - Hôpital Notre-Dame; adj Prof, Universite de Montreal; Langs: English; (514)890-8212; Fax. (514)412-7668.

GIRARD, Jacques E; Comm à la santé et au bien-êtr, 700-1020 Rte de l'Eglise, Quebec QC G1V 3V9; Laval'76; MPH; FRCPC; CommunMed (International Health). Langs: Spanish; (418)643-3040

GIRARD, Jean-Baptiste; Clinique Fam D'Hebertville, 9 rue Commerciale, Hebertville QC G8N 1N3; Laval'74; (418)344-1018; Fax. (418)344-1688.

GIRARD, Jean-Francois; CSSS de Saint-Jérôme, 290 rue de Montigny, Saint-Jerome QC J7Z 5T3; Mon'91; Staff, Hôtel-Dieu de Saint-Jérôme; (450)431-8200

GIRARD, Jean-Francois; 9469 rue Lajeunesse, Montreal QC H2M 1S5; Mon'83; Staff Fam Med, Hôpital du Sacre-Coeur de Montréal; (514)381-7192; Fax. (514)387-4293.

GIRARD, Jean-Guy; CSSS de la Region de Thetford, 1717 rue Notre-Dame E, Thetford Mines QC G6G 2V4; Laval'73; Urol (P.Q.) (Palliative Care). Staff, Hopital du CSS de la Region de Thetford; (418)338-7777

GIRARD, Jean-Marc; Clinique familiale d'Arthabask, 2-39 rue Laurier E, Victoriaville QC G6P 6P6; Laval'76; (819)357-9322

GIRARD, John V J; Health Sciences Centre, GH611-820 Sherbrook St, Winnipeg MB R3A 1R9; Man'86; FRCPC; Anes. Staff, Health Sciences Centre; (204)774-6511

GIRARD, Karine; Ctr Obstetrique et Gynecologie, 01D-4250 1re av, Quebec QC G1H 2S5; Laval'03; FRCSC; ObstGyn. (418)654-0555

GIRARD, Kevin; CSSS Domaine du Roy, 450 rue Brassard, Roberval QC G8H 1B9; Sher'08; Staff, Hotel-Dieu de Roberval; (418)275-0110

GIRARD, Liliane; Derma Centre Dr Liliane Girard, 2995 boul de la Piniere, Terrebonne QC J6X 4V5; Sher'88; Derm. (450)312-6151; Fax. (450)326-1004.

GIRARD, Linda; Centre Med Donnacona, 420 Rte 138, Donnacona QC G3M 1C2; Laval'88; Chef psychiatrie, Centre Hospitalier Portneuf; (418)285-1122; Fax. (418)285-0006.

GIRARD, Louis C; The Med Clinic, 265 Yorkland Blvd, North York ON M2J 1S5; Mon'82; CCFP; FCFP; Langs: Italian; English; French; (416)229-2399; Fax. (416)229-9771.

GIRARD, Louis-Phillipe; Foothills Medical Centre, 721-1403 29 St NW, Calgary AB T2N 2T9; Cal'05; BSc; FRCPC; IntMed (Plasmaphaeresis); Nephrol. Staff, Foothills Medical Centre; Clinical Asst Prof, University of Calgary; (403)944-3590; Fax. (403)283-4657; louis.girard@albertahealthservices.ca.

GIRARD, Louise; GMF des Seigneuries, 2220 boul Rene-Gaultier, Varennes QC J3X 1E3; Mon'89; CCFP; FCFP; (450)652-2917; Fax. (450)652-9902.

GIRARD, Luc; Polyclinique 55, 4825 av Bouvet, Becancour QC G9H 1X5; Laval'84; Staff, Centre de santé Cloutier-du-Rivage; (819)233-3123; Fax. (819)233-3124.

GIRARD, Lynne; Kilborn Med Centre, 215-1385 rue Bank, Ottawa ON K1H 8N4; Sher'82; FRCSC; Otol. (613)562-9000; Fax. (613)562-9001.

GIRARD, Marc; Hop Maisonneuve-Rosemont, 5415 boul de l'Assomption, Montreal QC H1T 2M4; Laval'78; DABR; DiagRad (Abdominal Imaging). Dir Radiol Services, Hopital Maisonneuve-Rosemont; Clin Coord, Universite de Montreal; (514)252-3546; Fax. (514)252-3537.

GIRARD, Marc-A; Hôpital Ste-Justine, 3175 ch Cote-Sainte-Catherine, Montreal QC H3T 1C5; Laval'78; IntMed (Adolescent Medicine). ac Staff, Hôpital Ste-Justine; Head Peds, Universite de Montreal; (514)345-4673; Fax. (514)345-2361; marc_girard@ssss.gouv.qc.ca.

GIRARD, Marie; INESSS, 60-1195 av Lavigerie, Quebec QC G1V 4N3; Laval'76; MBA; Gen Dir, Centre Hospitalier Affilié Universitaire de Québec - Hôpital De L'Enfant Jésus; (418)644-8342

GIRARD, Marie-Andree; Hôpital Ste-Justine, 3175 ch Cote-Sainte-Catherine, Montreal QC H3T 1C5; Sher'04; FRCPC; Anes. Staff, Hôpital Ste-Justine; (514)345-4931

GIRARD, Marie-Eve; CSSSG-Hop de Gatineau, 909 boul de la Verendrye O, Gatineau QC J8P 7H2; Mon'09; CCFP; Staff, Hôpital de Gatineau; (819)966-6100

GIRARD, Marie-Eve; CSSS de Saint-Jerome, 290 rue de Montigny, Saint-Jerome QC J7Z 5T3; Sher'05; Neur. Staff, Hôtel-Dieu de Saint-Jérôme; (450)432-2777

GIRARD, Mario; Hotel-Dieu de levis, 143 rue Wolfe, Levis QC G6V 3Z1; Laval'78; CSPQ; FRCPC; Anes. Staff, Hôtel-Dieu de Lévis; (418)835-7121 x3218; Fax. (418)835-3969.

GIRARD, Martin; CHUM-Hosp Notre Dame, 1560 rue Sherbrooke E, Montreal QC H2L 4M1; McG'00; CSPQ; FRCPC; Anes; Critical Care Medicine (P.Q.). Staff, Centre Hospitalier l'Université de Montréal (CHUM) - Hôpital Notre-Dame; (514)890-8000 x26876; Fax. (514)412-7653.

GIRARD, Michel; Hop Maisonneuve-Rosemont, 5415 boul de l'Assomption, Montreal QC H1T 2M4; Mon'74; CSPQ; FRCPC; Anes. Staff, Hopital Maisonneuve-Rosemont; (514)252-3426

GIRARD, Michel; Clinique du Mont-Carmel, 933 rue Rene-Levesque E, Montreal QC H2L 4S4; Mon'84; Ac Staff, Centre Hospitalier de LaSalle; Staff Emerg, CSSS du Coeur de l'Isle Hôpital Jean-Talon; (514)282-9197

GIRARD, Michel; Clinique Med Ahuntsic, 116-241 rue Fleury O, Montreal QC H3L 1V2; Mon'82; Langs: Bilingual(French/English); (514)381-5387; Fax. (514)381-5388.

GIRARD, Philippe; Clin de Physiotherapie des Nei, RR 2 201-10516 boul Sainte-Anne, Ste-Anne-d-Beaupre QC G0A 3C0; Laval'02; (418)827-8331; Fax. (418)827-8332.

GIRARD, Philippe; Polyclinique Saint-Jerome, 102-200 rue Durand, Saint-Jerome QC J7Z 7E2; Sher'97; CCFP; CCFP(E.M.); Staff, Centre Hospitalier Laurentien; (450)431-7666; Fax. (450)431-1275.

GIRARD, Pierrette; Mcdermott Med Clinic, 37 av Donegani, Pointe-Claire QC H9R 2V7; Mon'85; CSPQ; FRCSC; OrthSurg. (514)697-1410; Fax. (514)697-1411.

GIRARD, Procter R M; PO Box 757, Breton AB T0C 0P0; Sask'76; (780)396-3533; Fax. (780)542-3778.

GIRARD, Ronald; Clinique Med des Cantons, 1474 rue King O, Sherbrooke QC J1J 2C2; Mon'83; Langs: Bilingual(French/English); (819)565-1955; Fax. (819)565-5516.

GIRARD, Stephanie M; Joseph Brant Mem Hosp, 1230 North Shore Blvd E, Burlington ON L7S 1W7; Ott'95; FRCPC; DiagRad. Staff, Joseph Brant Memorial Hospital; Langs: Bilingual(English/French); (905)632-3730 x5667

GIRARD, Sylvie; Westmount Med Bldg, 630-5025 rue Sherbrooke O, Montreal QC H4A 1S9; Sher'80; FRCPC; Psy. Ac Staff, Douglas Mental Health University Institute; (514)939-2631

GIRARD, Yvan M; Clinique Fertilite Ovo, 8000 boul Decarie, Montreal QC H4P 2S4; Mon'58; FACS; FACOG; ObstGyn. Staff, Centre Hospitalier l'Université De Montréal (CHUM) - Hôpital Saint-luc; (514)798-2000

GIRARD, Yves; CSSS de Manicouagan, 635 boul Jolliet, Baie-Comeau QC G5C 1P1; Laval'93; FRCPC; IntMed. Staff, Centre Hospitalier Régional Baie-Comeau; (418)589-3701; Fax. (418)589-3099.

GIRARD-DESBIENS, Catherine; Centre Hosp Honore-Mercier, 2750 boul Laframboise, Saint-Hyacinthe QC J2S 4Y8; Mon'07; Hem; IntMed. Staff, Centre Hospitalier Honore-Mercier; (450)771-3333

GIRARDIN, Catherine; CHUM-Hop Notre-Dame, 1560 rue Sherbrooke E, Montreal QC H2L 4M1; Mon'92; FRCPC; IntMed; Nephrol. Staff, Centre Hospitalier l'Université de Montréal (CHUM) - Hôpital Notre-Dame; (514)890-8000 x26616; Fax. (514)412-7831.

GIRARDIN, Colette; CHUS-Hop Fleurimont, 3001 12e av N, Sherbrooke QC J1H 5N4; Sher'87; FRCPC; Peds (Pediatric Nephrology). Staff, Centre Hospitalier Universitaire de Sherbrooke-Hopital Fleurimont; (819)346-1110; Fax. (819)564-5398.

GIRARDIN, Joel-Roger; Le 444 Parent, 444 rue Parent, Saint-Jerome QC J7Z 2A2; Mon'85; Staff, Hôtel-Dieu de Saint-Jérôme; (450)436-9944 x22

GIRDHARI, Rajesh P; Lakeridge Health-Oshawa Site, 1 Hospital Crt, Oshawa ON L1G 2B9; McG'08; CCFP; (905)576-8711

GIRGENTI, Kaylene M; McKenzie Towne Medical, 102-620 McKenzie Towne Dr SE, Calgary AB T2Z 0Y6; (Australia)'05; MB BS; CCFP; (403)262-6311; Fax. (403)262-5911.

GIRGIS, Adel; MCI The Doctor Office, 203-300 John St, Thornhill ON L3T 5W4; Ain Shams (Egypt)'79; CCFP; Langs: Arabic; French; (905)764-0188; Fax. (905)764-0189.

GIRGIS, Ehab S S; Centennial CMH & Brain Injury, PO Box 1000 Stn Main, Ponoka AB T4J 1R8; Assiut (Egypt)'90; MB BCh; Staff, Centennial Centre for Mental Health & Brain Injury; (403)783-7661; Fax. (403)783-7790.

GIRGIS, Emile F; Centre Med Lacordaire, 201-5650 rue Jean-Talon E, Saint-Leonard QC H1S 1M1; Alexandria (Egypt)'70; MB ChB; FRCSC; ObstGyn (P.Q.). (514)255-5595; Fax. (514)255-8550.

GIRGIS, Hossam; Cartier Health Centre, PO Box 447 7 Main St E, Elie MB R0H 0H0; CCFP.

GIRGIS, Ireen; Chinguacousy & Sandalwood Med, 6-10671 Chinguacousy Rd, Brampton ON L7A 0N5; Cairo (Egypt)'95; MB ChB; CCFP; (905)840-4343

GIRGIS, Magdy; Sheppard Med Bldg, 303-701 Sheppard Ave E, North York ON M2K 2Z3; Assiut (Egypt)'67; CCFP; Assoc Staff, North York General Hospital; Langs: Arabic; (416)250-7778; Fax. (416)250-7111.

GIRGIS, Mona; 418-220 Duncan Mill Rd, North York ON M3B 3J5; Ein Shams (Egypt)'65; FRCPC; Psy. Staff, North York General Hospital; Langs: Arabic; (416)447-8053

GIRGIS, Safwat A M; University of Alberta Hosp, 5B2 36WCM-8440 112 St NW, Edmonton AB T6G 2B7; (Egypt)'81; MB ChB; FRCPC; GenPath. Staff Pathologist, University of Alberta Hospital; (780)407-3061; sgirgis@cha.ab.ca.

GIRGIS, Samira W A; 6-3050 Artesian Dr, Mississauga ON L5M 7P5; Alexandria (Egypt)'78; CCFP; Langs: Arabic; (905)607-6495; Fax. (905)607-0881.

GIRGIS, Siham; Dream Crest Med Centre, 6-1010 Dream Crest Rd, Mississauga ON L5V 3A4; CCFP; Langs: Arabic; (905)813-9674

GIRGLA, Satpal S; 35-1495 Cornwall Rd, Oakville ON L6J 0B2; Delhi (India)'79; MB BS; DPM; MRCPsy; FRCPC; Psy (General Adult Psychiatry). Ac Staff, Halton Healthcare Services Corporation - Oakville Site; Langs: Punjabi; Urdu; Hindi; (905)339-3211; Fax. (416)339-3246.

GIRLAN, Larisa; Whitby Med Clinic, 200 Brock St N, Whitby ON L1N 4H5; (Romania)'91; LMCC; CCFP; (905)668-3378; Fax. (905)668-3807.

GIRODIAS, Jean-Bernard; Hôpital Ste-Justine, 3175 ch Cote-Ste-Catherine, Montreal QC H3T 1C5; Lyon (France)'70; Peds. Staff Emerg Peds, Hôpital Ste-Justine; Asst Clin Prof, Universite de Montreal; (514)345-4611

GIRON, Marie-France; CLSC Lac Saint-Louis, 500-1405 Rte Trans-Canada, Dorval QC H9P 2V9; Mon'79; MSc; DIMOH; Med Assessor, Commission des Lesions Professionelles; Staff, CLSC Lac St-Louis; Langs: English; French; (514)421-5756; Fax. (514)421-5779; mfgiron@ssss.gouv.qc.ca.

GIRONNE, Claude; CRSSS Baie-James-Chibougamau, 51 3e rue, Chibougamau QC G8P 1N1; Mon'85; CCFP; FCFP; Staff, CRSSS de la Baie-James; (418)748-2676; Fax. (418)748-6983.

GIROUARD, Caroline; Hop Du Sacre-Coeur De Mtl, 5400 boul Gouin O, Montreal QC H4J 1C5; Mon'88; ABIM; FRCPC; IntMed (Auto Transplantation); MedOncol (P.Q.); Hem. Staff, Hôpital du Sacre-Coeur de Montréal; Universite de Montreal; Langs: Italian; (514)338-2150; beauchampmarc@sympatico.ca.

GIROUARD, France; Clinique Ped des Mille-Iles, 203-233 rue Turgeon, Sainte-Therese QC J7E 3J8; Sher'94; Peds. Staff Peds, Hôpital de Saint-Eustache; (450)434-8006

GIROUARD, Gabriel; Dr Georges-L Dumont Reg Hosp, 330 av Université, Moncton NB E1C 2Z3; Laval'01; FRCPC; InfectDis; IntMed; MedMicrobiol., Dr Georges-L-Dumont University Hospital Centre; Langs: Bilingual(French/English); (506)862-4140; Fax. (506)862-4827; gabriel.girouard@vitalitenb.ca.

GIROUARD, Gilles R; Hôpital Ste-Justine, 3175 ch Cote-Ste-Catherine, Montreal QC H3T 1C5; Mon'79; CSPQ; FRCPC; Anes. Ac Staff, Hôpital Ste-Justine; (514)345-4733

GIROUARD, Joel; CHUQ-Ctr Hosp Univ Laval, S 228-2705 boul Laurier, Quebec QC G1V 4G2; Laval'96; CSPQ; FRCPC; MedBiochem. Staff, Centre Hospitalier Universitaire de Quebec-CHUL; (418)656-4141 x48504

GIROUARD, Marie-Helene; CSSS de Trois-Rivières, 1991 boul Du Carmel, Trois-Rivieres QC G8Z 3R9; Mon'88; CSPQ; FRCSC; GenSurg. Staff, CSSS de Trois-Rivières; Staff, CSSS de Maskinongé; Langs: English; (819)697-3333

GIROUARD, Michele; 200-84 rue Dumas, Gatineau QC J8Y 2N3; Sher'78; DAB; FRCPC; Derm. Ac Staff, Hull Hospital; (819)778-6597; Fax. (819)778-0709.

GIROUARD, Nathalie; Clinique Med du Sud-Ouest, 4475 rue Bannantyne, LaSalle QC H4G 1E2; Mon'87; Staff, Centre Hospitalier de Verdun; Staff, Centre Hospitalier de LaSalle; Universite de Montreal; Langs: Bilingual(French/English); (514)765-3600; Fax. (514)765-9625.

GIROUARD, Yves; Hop du Sacre-Coeur de Mtl, 5400 boul Gouin O, Montreal QC H4J 1C5; Mon'74; FRCPC; MedMicrobiol (Medical Microbiology & Infectious Diseases); InfectDis (P.Q.). Staff, Hôpital du Sacre-Coeur de Montréal; (514)333-2222 x2913; Fax. (514)338-2909.

GIROUX, Anne-Marie; Centre Med Sillery, 1270 av William, Quebec QC G1S 4G1; Laval'92; Staff, Jeffery Hale Hospital-Saint Brigid's; (418)688-0664

GIROUX, Charles; MUHC-Montreal Gen Hosp, 1650 av Cedar, Montreal QC H3G 1A4; Mon'10; CCFP; Staff, McGill University Health Centre - Montreal General Campus; (514)934-1934

GIROUX, Charlotte; 406-2984 boul Taschereau, Greenfield Park QC J4V 2G9; Sher'76; Nephrol (P.Q.). (450)671-4512

GIROUX, Cynthia; CSSS du Rocher-Perce, CP 3300 451 rue Mgr Ross E, Chandler QC G0C 1K0; Laval'00; FRCSC; ObstGyn. Staff, Centre Hospitalier de Chandler; (418)689-2261

GIROUX, Diane; Centre de Read Lucie-Bruneau, 2275 av Laurier E, Montreal QC H2H 2N8; Laval'93; Langs: Bilingual(French/English); (514)527-4527; Fax. (514)527-6637; dgiroux@total.net.

GIROUX, Dominique; CHUQ-Hotel-Dieu de Quebec, 11 Cote du Palais, Quebec QC G1R 2J6; Laval'88; FRCPC; DiagRad. Staff, Centre Hospitalier Universitaire de Québec (CHUQ) - Siege Social; (418)691-5453; Fax. (418)691-5394; dominique.giroux@chuq.qc.ca.

GIROUX, Geraldine; Clin Medicale le Frontenac, 202-5200 rue Frontenac, Lac-Megantic QC G6B 1H3; Laval'07; Staff, Carrefour Sante Granit; (819)583-0157

GIROUX, Jason P; 1-677 Great Northern Rd, Sault Ste. Marie ON P6B 5A1; Sask'97; FRCSC; Ophth;CCFP; (705)949-5182; Fax. (705)251-9969.

GIROUX, Josee; Ctr Hosp de Verdun, 4000 boul Lasalle, Verdun QC H4G 2A3; Sher'87; Staff, Centre Hospitalier de Verdun; Staff, CLSC La Salle; Langs: Bilingual(French/English); (514)765-7325; Fax. (514)362-2823.

GIROUX, Julie; Mediclub, 6100 av du Boise, Montreal QC H3S 2W1; Mon'00; Staff, Hopital de la Cite de la santé; (514)739-5646

GIROUX, Lina; Clinique Med Donnacona, 420 rte 138, Donnacona QC G3M 1C2; Laval'92; (418)285-1122; Fax. (418)285-0006.

GIROUX, Linda; CSSS Becancour-Nicolet-Yamaska, 216 rue Principale QC, Fortierville QC G0S 1J0; Laval'89; Médecin, CLSC Les Bles d'Or; Langs: Spanish; (819)287-4442; Fax. (819)287-4017.

GIROUX, Louise; 509 rue Adoncour, Longueuil QC J4G 2M6; Mon'76; Ophth. (450)646-7788

GIROUX, Louise-Marie; CSSS de Rimouski-Neigette, CP 3150 succ Bureau Chef 150 av Rouleau, Rimouski QC G5L 5T1; Mon'03; FRCPC; AnatPath. Staff, Hôpital Regional Rimouski; (418)724-3000

GIROUX, Manon; CSSS du Sud de Lanaudière, 911 montee des Pionniers, Terrebonne QC J6V 2H2; Laval'95; CSPQ; FRCSC; GenSurg (Breast Cancer). Staff, Centre Hospitalier Pierre le Gardeur; (450)654-7525; manon_giroux@videotron.ca.

GIROUX, Marc F; 101-1800 boul le Corbusier, Laval QC H7S 2K1; Sher'86; Neursurg (Tumor). Staff Neurosurgery, Hôpital du Sacre-Coeur de Montréal; Langs: English; (450)686-9847; Fax. (450)686-0252.

GIROUX, Marc; Regie l'Assurance Maladie QC, 1125 Grande Allee O, Quebec QC G1S 1E7; Laval'69; Prés/gén Dir, Regie de l'Assurance Maladie du Quebec; Langs: English; (418)682-5162; Fax. (418)644-3767; marc.giroux@ramq.gouv.qc.ca.

GIROUX, Marie; CLSC La Region-Sherbrookoise, 1200 rue King E, Sherbrooke QC J1G 1E4; Sher'88; CCFP; FCFP; Staff, Centre Hospitalier Universitaire de Sherbrooke-Hopital Fleurimont; Chef Family Med, Universite de Sherbrooke; (819)563-0913; Fax. (819)563-9912.

GIROUX, Marie-France; CHUM-Hop Notre-Dame, 1560 rue Sherbrooke E, Montreal QC H2L 4M1; Sher'95; FRCPC; DiagRad (Interventional Radiology). Staff, Centre Hospitalier l'Université de Montréal (CHUM) - Hôtel-Dieu; Staff, Centre Hospitalier l'Université de Montréal (CHUM) - Hôpital Notre-Dame; Staff Cardiologie, Institut de Cardiologie de Montréal; Langs: Spanish; English; (514)412-7547; Fax. (514)412-7547.

GIROUX, Mario; 210-7175 rue Marion, Trois-Rivieres QC G9A 5Z9; Laval'87; CSPQ; FRCSC; OrthSurg (P.Q.) (Industrial Occupational Medicine). Staff, CSSS du Coeur de l'Isle Hôpital Jean-Talon; Langs: English; (819)379-0008; Fax. (819)379-4640; drmariogiroux@bellnet.ca.

GIROUX, Michel; CSSS du Suroît, 150 rue Saint-Thomas, Salaber-de-Valleyf QC J6T 6C1; Mon'76; FRCPC; DiagRad. Staff, Centre Hospitalier Régional du Suroît; (450)371-9920 x2032; Fax. (450)377-2800.

GIROUX, Monique; Clinique Med Pierre Boucher, 1615 boul Jacques-Cartier E, Longueuil QC J4M 2X1; Mon'88; (450)468-6223; Fax. (450)468-5041.

GIROUX, Patrick; Dr Georges-L Dumont Reg Hosp, 330 av Universite, Moncton NB E1C 2Z3; Mon'94; FRCPC; PhysMed&Rehab. Staff, Dr Georges-L-Dumont University Hospital Centre; (506)869-2126; Fax. (506)869-2130; cliphysiatrie@health.nb.ca.

GIROUX, Pierre F; Sanagex, 115-5345 boul de l'Assomption, Montreal QC H1T 4B3; Mon'66; (514)251-9331; Fax. (514)251-0511.

GIROUX, Renald; Clinique de Cardiologie de Lev, 4975 boul de la Rive-Sud, Levis QC G6V 4Z5; Laval'67; CSPQ; FRCPC; Cardiol. Staff Cardiol, Hôtel-Dieu de Lévis; (418)833-5750

GIROUX, Richard P; Oshawa Clinic, 117 King St E, Oshawa ON L1H 1B9; Qns'70; (905)723-8551; Fax. (905)721-4329.

GIROUX, Roger; Clinique Ped Ste-Foy, 295-2600 boul Laurier, Quebec QC G1V 4T3; Laval'87; FRCPC; Peds (Neonatology). Ac Staff, Centre Hospitalier Universitaire De Québec - Pavillon De St-françois-d'assise; Ac Staff, Centre Hospitalier Universitaire de Quebec-CHUL; (418)658-0906; Fax. (418)652-7094.

GIROUX, Rosaire; Hop Brome-Missisquoi-Perkins, 950 rue Principale, Cowansville QC J2K 1K3; Laval'81; Staff, Hôpital Brome-Missisquoi-Perkins; Langs: English; (450)266-4342 x55546

GIROUX, Sylvie; CSSS de Beauce-Etchemin, 1515 17e rue, Saint-Georges QC G5Y 4T8; Laval'99; FRCPC; IntMed. Staff, Centre Hospitalier Beauce-Etchemin; (418)228-2031

GIROUX, Yvon; Complexe Med Selection, 1-3 boul Samson, Laval QC H7X 3S5; Mon'68; FRCPC; IntMed; Gastroent. Staff, Hopital de la Cite de la santé; Langs: Bilingual(French/English); (450)969-9911

GIRSCHEK, Peter K; 212-2238 Dundas St W, Toronto ON M6R 3A9; McG'78; DAB; FRCSC; Ophth. Staff, Women's College Hospital; Langs: German; French; (416)536-3658; Fax. (416)536-5282.

GIRVAN, Andrew; Nepean Med Centre, 303-1 Centrepointe Dr, Nepean ON K2G 6E2; Qns'00; FRCSC; Urol. Staff, Queensway Carleton Hospital; (613)228-6929; Fax. (613)228-0191.

GIRVIN, Theresa C; CFB Edmonton-Health Services, PO Box 10500 Stn Forces, Edmonton AB T5J 4J5; UBC'89; FRCPC; Psy. (780)973-4011 x5332; Fax. (780)973-1496; maxifreudbird@yahoo.ca.

GIRVITZ, Sheldon C; Peel Med Arts Bldg, 305-145 Queen St E, Brampton ON L6W 3P8; McM'84; FRCSC; ObstGyn. Staff, William Osler Health System - Brampton Civic Hospital; (905)459-1881; Fax. (905)459-8571.

GISBERT, Ramon; CSSS de Trois-Rivières, 1991 boul du Carmel, Trois-Rivieres QC G8Z 3R9; Cuyo (Argentina)'97; Cardiol (P.Q.). Staff, CSSS de Trois-Rivières; (819)384-8850

GISH, George J; Claresholm Med Centre, PO Box 730, Claresholm AB T0L 0T0; Cal'77; CCFP; FCFP; (403)625-4484; Fax. (403)625-3969.

GISLADOTTIR, Kristin; Bloor-Jane Med Bldg, 203-2425 Bloor St W, Toronto ON M6S 4W4; Reykjavik (Iceland)'63; FRCPC; Psy. Hon Staff, St Joseph's Health Centre; Langs: Danish; Icelandic; (416)762-1119; Fax. (416)762-1600.

GISLASON, Rachel T P; William Osler HC-Brampton, 2100 Bovaird Dr E, Brampton ON L6R 3J7; Man'01; FRCPC; Anes. Staff, William Osler Health System - Brampton Civic Hospital; (905)494-2120

GISSLOW, Mary T; UBC Hospital, M334-2211 Wesbrook Mall, Vancouver BC V6T 2B5; UBC'85; Staff Student Health Services, UBC Hospital - Koerner Pavillion; (604)822-7011; Fax. (604)822-7889.

GITEV, Margarita; Rosedale Med Centre, 503-600 Sherbourne St, Toronto ON M4X 1W4; Sofia (Bulgaria)'67; FRCPC; Psy (Child Psychiatry). Langs: Bulgarian; (416)443-1169; Fax. (416)443-1169; mgitev@gmail.com.

GITLAN, Dan Liviu; CSSS de Manicouagan, 635 boul Jolliet, Baie-Comeau QC G5C 1P1; (Romania)'94; GenSurg (P.Q.). Staff, Centre Hospitalier Régional Baie-Comeau; (418)589-3701

GITLAN, Iulia; CSSS de Manicouagan, 635 boul Jolliet, Baie-Comeau QC G5C 1P1; Staff, Centre Hospitalier Régional Baie-Comeau; (418)589-3701

GITTENS, Rudolph; Riverside Professional Bldg, 312-1919 Riverside Dr, Ottawa ON K1H 1A2; Ott'66; CSPQ; BSP; FRCSC; OrthSurg (Independent Medical Evaluations). Hon Staff, The Ottawa Hospital - General Campus; Langs: French; Spanish; (613)731-3642; Fax. (613)731-6873; rgittensn232@rogers.com.

GITTENS, Winston O; Keary Med Centre, 207-245 Columbia St E, New Westminster BC V3L 3W4; (Jamaica)'70; MB BS; BSc(Anatomy); FRCSC; Neursurg. Consultant, Burnaby Hospital; Ac Staff, Royal Columbian Hospital; Consultant, Surrey Memorial Hospital; (604)520-1120; Fax. (604)524-4447; drwinstongittens@telus.net.

GITTERMAN, Allan; Nepean Med Centre, 106-1 Centrepointe Dr, Nepean ON K2G 6E2; Ott'69; FRCPC; DiagRad. (613)723-5215; Fax. (613)725-5216.

GITTERMAN, J Lawrence; St Lawrence Dist Med Centre, PO Box 39 1012A Prince St, Lansdowne ON K0E 1L0; McG'73; (613)659-2525

GITTERMAN, Michael M; Apple Hills Medical Associates, 1221 Bloor St, Mississauga ON L4Y 2N8; Man'70; CCFP; CCFP(E.M.); Staff, Trillium Health Centre - Mississauga; (905)625-1241; Fax. (905)625-9514; mgitterman@summervillefht.com.

GIUFFRE, Jennifer L; Pan Am Clinic, 3F-75 Poseidon Bay, Winnipeg MB R3M 3E4; Alb'04; FRCSC; PlasSurg. (204)927-2772

GIUFFRE, Martin J; Meadowlark Health Centre, 176 Meadowlark Shopping Ctr NW, Edmonton AB T5R 5W9; Alb'77; FRCSC; PlasSurg. Staff, Royal Alexandra Hospital; Staff, Covenant Health - Grey Nuns Community Hospital; Staff, Covenant Health - Misericordia Community Hospital; (780)428-7739; Fax. (780)428-7737.

GIUFFRE, R Michael; Providence Children Hlth Ctr, 5232 4 St SW, Calgary AB T2V 0Z4; Cal'84; FACC; MBA; FRCPC; Peds (Pediatric Cardiology); Cardiol. Staff, Peter Lougheed Centre; Staff, Alberta Children's Hospital; Staff, Foothills Medical Centre; Clin Prof, University of Calgary; (403)255-2737; giuffrecardiology@live.com.

GIUGOVAZ, Sophie; Clin de Med Fam Cowansville, 499 rue du Sud, Cowansville QC J2K 2X9; Mon'96; (450)263-8890

GIULIANI, Fabrizio; Glen Sather Sports Med Clinic, 4D-11400 University Ave NW, Edmonton AB T6G 1Z1; (Italy)'95; (780)407-5515; Fax. (780)407-1507.

GIULIVI, Antonio; Active Care, 35B-2121 Carling Ave, Ottawa ON K2A 1H2; Pavia (Italy)'84; FRCPC; HemPath (Transfusion Medicine). Consultant, Montfort Hospital; Staff HemPath, The Ottawa Hospital - Civic Campus; Consultant Hem Lab, Queensway Carleton Hospital; Staff, The Ottawa Hospital - General Campus; Asst Prof Path, University of Ottawa; Langs: Italian; French; (613)761-6777; agiulivi@ottawahospital.on.ca.

GIUNTA, Michel; Go Giunta Ophtalmology, 200-1335 rue King O, Sherbrooke QC J1J 2B8; Mon'87; AB; FRCSC; Ophth (Vitreo Retinal Surgery). Staff Ophth/Conférencier, Centre Hospitalier Universitaire de Sherbrooke-Hôpital Hôtel-Dieu; Teacher, Universite de Sherbrooke; (819)563-6889; Fax. (819)563-4558; cliniquemichelgiunta@gmail.com.

GIURISTANTE, Frank A; Polyclinique Cabrini, 214-5700 rue Saint-Zotique E, Montreal QC H1T 3Y7; Mon'76; MCFP(EM); Staff, Hopital Maisonneuve-Rosemont; (514)257-4848

GIUSTINO, Giuseppe; Parklane Surgical Clinic, 210-13710 94A Ave, Surrey BC V3V 1N1; Tor'93; BSc; FRCPC; IntMed; Respir. Staff, Surrey Memorial Hospital; Langs: Italian; (604)582-2100; Fax. (604)582-2199.

GIVELAS, Danny; 303-2175 Sheppard Ave E, North York ON M2J 1W8; Tor'62; FRCPC; Peds. Langs: Macedonian; (416)492-7700; Fax. (416)492-5776.

GIVELICHIAN, Laurentiu M; Royal University Hosp, 103 Hospital Dr, Saskatoon SK S7N 0W8; (Romania)'85; FRCPC; Peds (Neonatology). Staff, Royal University Hospital; Assoc Prof Med/A-Dept Head Ped, University of Saskatchewan; (306)966-8123; Fax. (306)966-8640; dr.givelichian@usask.ca.

GIVEN, John P; Workplace Hlth & Public Safety, Pl 3712M 12F-171 Slater St, Ottawa ON K1A 0K9; Ott'86; (613)946-6583; Fax. (613)990-9397.

GJEVRE JR., John A; Royal University Hosp, 5F-103 Hospital Dr, Saskatoon SK S7N 0W8; Mayo(MN) (USA)'91; ABIM; FRCPC; IntMed (Critical Care Medicine); Respir. Staff, Royal University Hospital; (306)966-8274; Fax. (306)966-8694.

GLACKEN, Robert P; Pan Am Sports Med Centre, 75 Poseidon Bay, Winnipeg MB R3M 3E4; Man'99; CCFP; (204)925-1550; Fax. (204)452-5362.

GLADDY, Rebecca A; Mount Sinai Hosp, 1225-600 University Ave, Toronto ON M5G 1X5; Qns'96; FRCSC; GenSurg (Clinical & Investigative Medicine). Staff, Mount Sinai Hospital; (416)586-4800 x3812; Fax. (416)586-8392.

GLADMAN, Aviv S; Mackenzie Richmond Hill Hosp, 10 Trench St, Richmond Hill ON L4C 4Z3; Tor'03; FRCPC; IntMed; Critical Care Medicine. Staff, Mackenzie Richmond Hill Hospital; (905)883-1212

GLADMAN, Dafna D; Univ Hlth Network-Toronto Western Hosp, EW1 410B-399 Bathurst St, Toronto ON M5T 2S8; Tor'71; FRCPC; IntMed; Rheum. Ac Staff, Toronto Western Hospital - University Health Network; Consultant, Women's College Hospital; (416)603-5753; Fax. (416)603-9387; dgladman@uhnres.utoronto.ca.

GLADMAN, Donald J; PO Box 34274 Rpo Westbrook, Calgary AB T3C 3W2; UBC'62.

GLADMAN, Paul D; PO Box 34274 Rpo Westbrook, Calgary AB T3C 3W2; Cal'89; CCFP; Med Staff, Royal Inland Hospital.

GLADSTONE, David J; Sunnybrook Hlth Sciences Ctre, A442-2075 Bayview Ave, Toronto ON M4N 3M5; Tor'96; BSc; PhD; FRCPC; FRCPC; Neur (Stroke). Dir Stroke Prevention Clinic, Sunnybrook Health Sciences Centre; (416)480-4866; Fax. (416)480-5753.

GLADSTONE, Joan S; North York Med Arts Bldg, 122-1333 Sheppard Ave E, North York ON M2J 1V1; Tor'69; Hon Staff Family Practice, North York General Hospital; (416)494-8811; Fax. (416)494-0756.

GLADSTONE, Jonathan P; Gladstone Headache Clinic, 122-1333 Sheppard Ave E, North York ON M2J 1V1; Tor'00; BSc; FRCPC; Neur (Head Injury). Staff Headache Specialist, Sunnybrook Health Sciences Centre; Co-Dir Headache Clinic, The Hospital For Sick Children; Specialist Headache & Head Injury, Toronto Rehabilitation Institute - University Centre; Dir Neuology & Headache Medicine, Cleveland Clinic Canada; Consultant Neurologist and Headache Specialist/Dir, Gladstone Headache Clinic; (416)492-4144; Fax. (416)492-9864; jon.gladstone@sunnybrook.ca.

GLADSTONE, Julie A; St Joseph's Life Care Centre, 99 Wayne Gretzky Parkway, Brantford ON N3S 6T6; Qns'07; CCFP; (519)756-6400; Fax. (519)756-7343.

GLADSTONE, Peter S J; Scarborough Prof Centre, 406-1371 Neilson Rd, Scarborough ON M1B 4Z8; Tor'79; FRCPC; IntMed; Cardiol. Staff, Rouge Valley Health System - Centenary Health Centre Site; Asst Prof, University of Toronto; (416)281-9499; Fax. (416)283-5705; psjgladstone@rogers.com.

GLADSTONE, Richard M; North York Med Arts Bldg, 122-1333 Sheppard Ave E, Toronto ON M2J 1V1; Tor'64; BSc(Med); Cert Geront(Gerontology); FRCPC; Neur (Electroencephalography). Consultant, North York General Hospital; Court Staff, Humber River Regional Hospital - Finch Avenue Site; Court Staff, Sunnybrook Health Sciences Centre; Asst Prof Med Neurology, University of Toronto; (416)494-8811; Fax. (416)494-0756.

GLADU, Francois-Pierre; Inst U Geriatrie de Montreal, 4565 ch Queen-Mary, Montreal QC H3W 1W5; Mon'97; CCFP; Ac Staff, Institut Universitaire de Gériatrie de Montréal; Universite de Montreal; (514)340-2800

GLADU, Yvan; Clinique Med Ste-Adele, 1150 rue du Bourg-Joli, Sainte-Adele QC J8B 1W8; Mon'78; (450)229-6633; Fax. (450)229-5765.

GLADWELL, Heather E; London HSC-Victoria Hosp, PO Box 5010 Stn B 800 Commissioners Rd E, London ON N6A 5W9; Wes'09; CCFP; CCFP(E.M.); Staff, London Health Sciences Centre - Victoria Campus; (519)685-8500

GLADY, Christine A; Red Deer Reg Hosp Centre, PO Box 5030 Stn Postal Box Ctr 3942 50A Ave, Red Deer AB T4N 6R2; Dal'98; FRCPC; IntMed; Respir. Staff, Red Deer Regional Hospital Centre; (403)343-4422; c_glady@hotmail.com.

GLAESKE, Daniel M; South Country Med Clinic, PO Box 2106 131 3rd Ave W, Assiniboia SK S0H 0B0; Alb'93; Staff, Assiniboia Union Hospital; (306)642-4454; dglaeske@fhr.ca.

GLANC, Phyllis; Sunnybrook Hlth Sciences Ctre, MG104-2075 Bayview Ave, Toronto ON M4N 3M5; McG'83; FRCPC; DiagRad. Staff, Sunnybrook Health Sciences Centre; Asst Prof, University of Toronto; (416)480-6100; Fax. (416)480-5855.

GLANCY, Graham D; 303-720 Spadina Ave, Toronto ON M5S 2T9; Manchester (England)'76; MB ChB; FRCPsy; FRCPC; Psy (Forensic Psychiatry). Asst Prof, McMaster University; Asst Prof, University of Toronto; (416)236-5602; Fax. (416)323-3166; graham.glancy@utoronto.ca.

GLANVILLE, Brook W; Mount IDA Med Centre, PO Box 1870 Stn Main, Salmon Arm BC V1E 4P9; UBC'07; CCFP; Staff, Queen Victoria Hospital; Staff, Shuswap Lake General Hospital; Langs: Spanish; French; (250)833-1990

GLANZ, Anthony E; Windsor Health Clinic, 267-1720 Howard Ave, Windsor ON N8X 5A6; Tor'86; FRCPC; IntMed; Cardiol. Att Staff, Hôtel-Dieu Grace Hospital; Att Staff, Windsor Regional Hospital - Metropolitan Site; Langs: Bilingual(English/French); (519)254-5726; Fax. (519)977-0792.

GLANZBERG, Monte M; 110-3540 41st Ave W, Vancouver BC V6N 3E6; UBC'72; CCFP; Ac Staff, Vancouver General Hospital - Centennial Pavillion; Court Staff, BC Women's Hospital & Health Centre; Teach Staff Family Pract, University of British Columbia; (604)261-6361; Fax. (604)261-1656.

GLAS, Mario R; 3-2020 Strachan Rd SE, Medicine Hat AB T1B 0M9; Pretoria (South Africa)'91; MB ChB; CCFP; Langs: Afrikaans; (403)580-1882

GLASER, Stuart R; 385-1255 boul Laird, Mont-Royal QC H3P 2T1; McG'74; CCFP; FCFP; Assoc Prof Family Med, McGill University; (514)735-4634; Fax. (514)735-4635.

GLASGOW, Daniel F G; Cape Breton Hlthcare Complex, 1482 George St, Sydney NS B1P 1P3; Dal'75; AB; Staff Path Lab Serv, Cape Breton Healthcare Complex; (902)567-7784; Fax. (902)567-7947.

GLASGOW, Donald L M; 11202 76 Ave NW, Edmonton AB T6G 0K1; Alb'04; FRCSC; OrthSurg. (780)439-4945; Fax. (780)439-0396.

GLASGOW, Kevin; Crohns & Colitis Foundation, 600-60 St Clair Ave E, Toronto ON M4T 1N5; Wes'88; FAB(PM); DTMH; MHSc; MBA; FRCPC; CommunMed (Public Health);CCFP; FCFP; CEO, Crohn's Colitis Foundation of Canada; Teach Staff Public Health Services, University of Toronto; (416)920-5035

GLASGOW, Michael J; 34 Maple Ave PO Box 100, Tatamagouche NS B0K 1V0; Dal'86; (902)657-2910

GLASGOW, Robert M; Northgate Centre, 2068-9499 137 Ave NW, Edmonton AB T5E 5R8; Alb'64; FRCSC; OrthSurg. Ac Staff, Covenant Health - Grey Nuns Community Hospital; Staff, Glenrose Rehabilitation Hospital; (780)433-3155; Fax. (780)432-6395.

GLASGOW, Robert R M; 10150 121 St NW, Edmonton AB T5N 1K4; Cal'96; BSc; FRCSC; OrthSurg (Arthroscopic Knee & Shoulder Surgery). Langs: English; French; (780)434-3668; Fax. (780)434-4859.

GLASNER, Carly S; Southland Medical, 110-3540 41st Ave W, Vancouver BC V6N 3E6; Alb'10; CCFP.

GLASS, David H; Grey Bruce HS-Southampton, PO Box 310 340 High St, Southampton ON N0H 2L0; Tor'85; CCFP; FCFP; Staff, Grey Bruce Health Services - Southampton Site; (519)797-3230 x3237; glassd@bmts.com.

GLASS, Judy E; Inst of Commun & Family Psy, 4333 ch Cote-Sainte-Catherine, Montreal QC H3T 1E4; McG'80; FRCPC; Psy. Staff, Sir Mortimer B Davis Jewish General; McGill University; (514)340-8210; Fax. (514)340-7507.

GLASS, Karen B; Create Fertility Centre, 1100-790 Bay St, Toronto ON M5G 1N8; Ott'91; FRCSC; ObstGyn (Infertility). Staff, Women's College Hospital; Staff, Sunnybrook Health Sciences Centre; Teach Staff, University of Toronto; (416)323-7727; Fax. (416)323-7334.

GLASS, Lisa B; Castlemore Health Centre, 3-65 Braydon Blvd, Brampton ON L6P 2S4; Wes'87; (905)794-7649; Fax. (905)794-7650.

GLASSCO, M Jane; Amherstview Med Centre, 18 Manitou Cres W, Amherstview ON K7N 1S3; McM'78; BSc; CCFP; (613)384-4888; Fax. (613)384-0889.

GLASSMAN, Steven J; The Ottawa Hosp-Civic Campus, 13-737 Parkdale Ave, Ottawa ON K1Y 1J8; Witwatersrand (West Africa)'88; Staff, The Ottawa Hospital - Civic Campus; (613)761-4689; Fax. (613)761-4087.

GLAUDE, Simon-Pierre; Cape Breton Hlthcare Complex, 1482 George St, Sydney NS B1P 1P3; Ott'06; CCFP; Staff, Cape Breton Healthcare Complex; (902)567-8000

GLAUDE, Yvon; CSSS Domaine du Roy, 450 rue Brassard, Roberval QC G8H 1B9; Mon'84; DiagRad. Staff, Hotel-Dieu de Roberval; Langs: English; (418)275-0110 x2296; Fax. (418)275-1115; yvonglaude@hotmail.com.

GLAVAS, Panagiotis; Hôpital Ste-Justine, 3175 ch cote-Sainte-Catherine, Montreal QC H3T 1C5; Mon'04; FRCSC; OrthSurg. Staff, Hôpital Ste-Justine; (514)345-4931

GLAVIN, Verne J; Cambridge Mem Hosp, 700 Coronation Blvd, Cambridge ON N1R 3G2; Ott'88; FRCPC; Peds; InfectDis. Staff, Cambridge Memorial Hospital; Langs: Bilingual(English/French); (519)621-2330; vglavin@cmh.org.

GLAY, Jack D; 600-5300 ch de la Cote-des-Nei, Montreal QC H3T 1Y3; McG'75; FRCPC; DiagRad. (514)738-5306; Fax. (514)738-2741.

GLAZE, Sarah J; Tom Baker Cancer Centre, 1331 29 St NW, Calgary AB T2N 4N2; Sask'04; FRCSC; ObstGyn; GynOnco. Staff, Tom Baker Cancer Centre; Staff, Foothills Medical Centre; (403)521-3721; Fax. (403)521-3573.

GLAZEBROOK, Katherine M; Gladstone Professional Ctr, 201-6155 North St, Halifax NS B3K 5R3; Dal'94; BScChemEng; MSc; CCFP; Clin Associate, Queen Elizabeth II Health Sciences Centre - Victoria General Site; Court Staff, IWK Health Centre; (902)453-3511; Fax. (902)454-9010.

GLAZEBROOK, Mark A; Queen Elizabeth II HSC-Halifax, 4867-1796 Summer St, Halifax NS B3H 3A7; Dal'94; FRCSC; OrthSurg. Asst Prof, Queen Elizabeth II Health Sciences Centre - Victoria General Site; (902)473-7137; Fax. (902)473-7201.

GLAZER, Peter R; Univ Hlth Network-the Toronto, 200 Elizabeth St, Toronto ON M5G 2C4; McG'97; CCFP; CCFP(E.M.); Staff, Toronto General Hospital - UHN; Langs: English; French; (416)340-3856

GLAZER, Sheldon; Royal Columbian Hosp, 330 Columbia St E, New Westminster BC V3L 3W7; McG'74; AB; FRCPC; EmergMed. Staff, Royal Columbian Hospital; Staff, Eagle Ridge Hospital & Health Care Centre; Asst Prof Surg, University of British Columbia; (604)520-4283; Fax. (604)520-4722.

GLAZER, Stephen A; York Finch Med Centre, 203A-2115 Finch Ave W, North York ON M3N 2V6; Tor'89; FRCPC; IntMed; Critical Care Medicine. Staff, Humber River Regional Hospital - Church Street Site; Langs: Hebrew; (416)749-2600; Fax. (416)749-2602.

GLAZIER, Lee; PO Box 23052 Rpo Cook Street, Victoria BC V8V 4Z8; UBC'08; (250)858-8410

GLAZIER, Richard H; SMH Health Centre, 4F-410 Sherbourne St, Toronto ON M4X 1K2; Wes'79; CCFP; FCFP; Ac Staff, St Michael's Hospital; Assoc Prof Family & Commun Med, University of Toronto; (416)867-3728; Fax. (416)867-3726.

GLAZMAN, Bernard G; 546 Palmerston Blvd, Toronto ON M6G 2P5; Tor'56; (416)531-5673; Fax. (416)489-5262.

GLAZMAN, Trevor N; 314 Russell Hill Rd, Toronto ON M4V 2T8; Wes'94.

GLAZNER, Kathryn; Pritchard Family Hlth Centre, 5-3014 Henderson Hwy, East St Paul MB R2E 0H9; Man'10; CCFP.

GLEASON, Thomas P; 192-17010 90 Ave NW, Edmonton AB T5T 1L6; Alb'86; FRCSC; ObstGyn. Ac Staff, Covenant Health - Misericordia Community Hospital; (780)483-2901; Fax. (780)483-2910.

GLEAVE, Danica A; Cool Aid Community Health Ctre, 713 Johnson St, Victoria BC V8W 1M8; UBC'93; Physician, Cool Aid Community Health Centre; (250)385-1466; Fax. (250)383-1327.

GLEAVE, Martin E; 6-2775 Laurel St, Vancouver BC V5Z 1M9; UBC'84; Urol (Urological Oncology). Ac Staff Urol/Dir Clin Research The Prostate Centre, Vancouver General Hospital - Centennial Pavillion; Consultant, BC Cancer Agency Vancouver Centre; Prof Surg/Dir Vancouver Prostate Centre, University of British Columbia; (604)875-5603; Fax. (604)875-5604; gleave@interchange.ubc.ca.

GLEDHILL, N Scott; Univ Hlth Network-Toronto Gen, 200 Elizabeth St, Toronto ON M5G 2C4; Wes'94; CCFP; Staff, Toronto General Hospital - UHN; Staff, Medcan Health Management Inc; (416)340-3111

GLEESON, Joseph T; Dragonfly Medical, PO Box 970 Stn Main, Gravenhurst ON P1P 1V3; (Montserrat)'96; BA(Hons); MSc; LMCC; CCFP; Staff, South Muskoka Memorial Hospital - Muskoka Algonquin Healthcare; (705)687-0558; Fax. (705)687-5742; jgleeson5@cogeco.ca.

GLEESON, Peter F; 137 Catherine St, Fort Erie ON L2A 2H9; Wes'79; BSc; Staff, Niagara Health System - Douglas Memorial Hospital Site; (905)871-1333; Fax. (905)871-0163.

GLEESON, Susan E; Burnham Med Services, 370B Burnham St, Peterborough ON K9H 1T6; Qns'79; MSc; CCFP; FCFP; Court Staff, Peterborough Regional Health Centre - Rogers St Site; (705)740-1966; Fax. (705)740-9621.

GLEETON, Dave; 522 rte 132 GD, Cloridorme QC G0E 1G0; Laval'07; FRCPC; Anes.

GLEETON, Onil; Hôpital Laval, 2725 ch Sainte-Foy, Quebec QC G1V 4G5; Laval'80; CSPQ; FRCPC; IntMed; Cardiol. Staff, Hôpital Laval; (418)656-8711 x4862; Fax. (418)656-4544.

GLEISNER, George R; Hawthorne Village Med Clinic, 205-10220 Derry Rd, Milton ON L9T 7J3; Wisconsin (USA)'92; Langs: Spanish; (905)878-0676; Fax. (905)878-0521.

GLEIZE-EMPHOUX, Sandrine; CHSLD de la MRC de Champlain, 831 av Notre-Dame, Longueuil QC J4R 1S1; Aix-Marseille (France)'94; Staff, CHSLD de la MRC de Champlain-Centre Saint-Lambert; (450)672-3328; sandrine.gleize-emphoux@rrsss16.gouv.qc.ca.

GLEN, David R; Royal Jubilee Hosp, 1952 Bay St, Victoria BC V8R 1J8; Cal'87; Staff, Royal Jubilee Hospital; (250)413-6261

GLEN, Silvia P; 106-4360 Lorimer Rd PO Box 654, Whistler BC V0N 1B4; London (England)'66; MB BS; LRCP; MRCS; DObstRCOG; (604)789-0222

GLENDINNING, Karan R; South Calgary Med Clinic, 118-40 Sunpark Plaza SE, Calgary AB T2X 3X7; London (England)'89; MB BS; (403)254-4000; Fax. (403)254-1472.

GLENN, David M; Newmount Med Clinic, 624 18th St, Brandon MB R7A 5B4; Man'93.

GLENN, Joan; Pavillon Ferdinand-Landry, 1050 av de la Medecine, Quebec QC G1V 0A6; Laval'89; DPhil; Staff, Centre Hospitalier Affilié Universitaire de Québec - Hôpital De L'Enfant Jésus; Prof, Université Laval; Langs: English; (418)656-2131 x5439; Fax. (418)656-2733; joan.glenn@fmed.ulaval.ca.

GLENN, John J; Queen Elizabeth II HSC, 314 10S-1276 South Park St, Halifax NS B3H 2Y9; St. Andrews (Scotland)'70; MB ChB; FRCPC; Anes. Staff, Queen Elizabeth II Health Sciences Centre - Victoria General Site; Dalhousie University; (902)473-1393

GLENN, John W; Nepean Sports Med & Phy Ctr, 1701 Woodroffe Ave, Ottawa ON K2G 1W2; Ott'07; CCFP; (613)727-5755

GLENNS, Vivian P; North York Med Arts Bldg, 335-1333 Sheppard Ave E, North York ON M2J 1V1; McG'93; ABIM; FRCPC; IntMed; MedOncol. Ac Staff, North York General Hospital; Langs: English; French; (416)498-4888; Fax. (416)498-6770.

GLETSU, Stephen K; Chatham-Kent Health Alliance, PO Box 2030 Stn Main 80 Grand Ave W, Chatham ON N7M 5L9; Sask'96; CCFP; CCFP(E.M.); Staff, Chatham-Kent Health Alliance; (519)352-6400

GLEW, Wade B; Prairie Trail Med Centre, 100-1345 Taylor Ave, Winnipeg MB R3M 3Y9; Cal'83; CCFP; Ac Staff, Victoria General Hospital; Assoc Prof Family Med, University of Manitoba; (204)475-0088

GLEZOS, James D; New Westminster TB Clinic, 100-237 Columbia St E, New Westminster BC V3L 3W4; Ott'69; FRCPC; IntMed; Respir. Staff Med Resp, Royal Columbian Hospital; Physician TB Control New West Chest Clinic, BCCDC Public Health; Langs: French; (604)707-2698; Fax. (604)808-2694.

GLICK, Naomi H G; 20-1521 Dufferin Cres, Nanaimo BC V9S 5H6; UBC'02; FRCPC; IntMed (Rural Health); Nephrol. Staff, University of Alberta Hospital; (250)591-1898

GLICKMAN, Aaron; Toronto East Gen & Orth Hosp, 825 Coxwell Ave, Toronto ON M4C 3E7; Wes'00; BA; MSc; FRCPC; DiagRad (Radiology). Staff, Toronto East General Hospital Inc; (416)461-8272

GLIKLICH, Ian; 1A-1152 Morningside Ave, Scarborough ON M1B 3A4; Tor'93; BSc; CCFP; Assoc Staff, The Scarborough Hospital - Birchmount Campus; Court Staff, The Credit Valley Hospital; (416)284-2853; Fax. (416)284-4951.

GLIKSTEIN, Rafael S; The Ottawa Hosp-Civic Campus, 1053 Carling Ave, Ottawa ON K1Y 4E9; Buenos Aires (Argentina)'82; DiagRad (P.Q.). Staff, The Ottawa Hospital - Civic Campus; Langs: Spanish; French; (613)761-4476

GLIMPEL, Perry B; 2897 17 Ave SE, Calgary AB T2A 0P7; Cal'92; LMCC; CCFP; (403)272-3384; Fax. (403)272-5671.

GLINSKI, Robert G; Cambridge Family Med Centre, 551 Cambridge St S, Ottawa ON K1S 4J4; Ott'76; CCFP; CCFP(E.M.); Assoc Staff, Children's Hospital of Eastern Ontario (CHEO); Staff Privil, The Ottawa Hospital - Civic Campus; University of Ottawa; (613)236-8132; Fax. (613)236-7482.

GLINSKI-OOMEN, Margaret B; 5-17250 Highway 27, Schomberg ON L0G 1T0; Ott'86; PhD; Staff, Stevenson Memorial Hospital; (905)939-1025; Fax. (905)939-1057.

GLOBERMAN, Daniel J; 218-2025 Corydon Ave, Winnipeg MB R3P 0N5; Man'78; FRCPC; Psy (Forensic Psychiatry). (204)415-5377; Fax. (204)415-3142.

GLODJO, Armansa; Sunny Hill Hlth Ctr for Childr, 3644 Slocan St, Vancouver BC V5M 3E8; Qns'02; FRCPC; Peds (Developmental Pediatrics). Staff, Sunny Hill Health Centre for Children; (604)453-8300

GLOFCHESKIE, B A Ron; 28 Crowfoot Terr NW PO Box 68206 Rpo Crowfoot, Calgary AB T3G 3N8; Tor'87.

GLOOR, Jane; Spingbank Med Centre, 206-460 Springbank Dr, London ON N6J 0A8; Wes'86; FRCPC; Peds (Pediatric Emergency Medicine). Staff, London Health Sciences Centre - Victoria Campus; Asst Prof Med, University of Western Ontario; (519)641-8687; Fax. (519)641-6518; jane.gloor@lhsc.on.ca.

GLORIEUX, Francis; Shriners Hosp for Children, 1529 av Cedar, Montreal QC H3G 1A6; Louvain (Belgium)'63; PhD(McG); FCCMG; Pediatrics, Hôpital Ste-Justine; Associé Peds, McGill University Health Centre - Montreal Children's Hospital; Prof, McGill University; Aj Prof, Universite de Montreal; Langs: Bilingual(English/French); (514)849-7685; Fax. (514)842-5581; glorieux@shriners.mcgill.ca.

GLORION, Antoine; Ctr Hosp Laurentien, 234 rue Saint-Vincent, Ste-Agathe-des-Mts QC J8C 2B8; Staff, Centre Hospitalier Laurentien; (819)324-4000

GLOTMAN, C Stephanie; Immunodeficiency Clinic (IDC), W 10C-1081 Burrard St, Vancouver BC V6Z 1Y6; UBC'89; (604)682-2344

GLOUTNEY, Kim; Centre Med Nazareth, 1771 av Dollard, LaSalle QC H8N 1T9; Laval'04; Langs: Bilingual(French/English); (514)368-5500; Fax. (514)368-0056.

GLOVER, Christopher A; Univ of Ottawa Heart Institute, 3406-40 Ruskin Ave, Ottawa ON K1Y 4W7; Qns'94; FRCPC; IntMed (Interventional Cardiology); Cardiol. Staff, University of Ottawa Heart Institute; Assoc Prof Med, University of Ottawa; (613)761-4119; Fax. (613)761-5332; cglover@ottawaheart.ca.

GLOVER, Janice A; 216 Stewart Green SW PO Box 75094, Calgary AB T3H 3C8; Sask'71; CCFP; Fax. (403)532-6007.

GLOVER, John; Queen Square Doctors FHT, 201-366 Main St N, Brampton ON L6V 1P8; London (England)'67; Med Dir, Grace Manor; Med Dir, Faith Manor; (905)455-1331; Fax. (905)455-5498.

GLOVER, Rodger M; Oakville Health Centre, 210-1060 Speers Rd, Oakville ON L6L 2X4; Tor'80; BSc; PhD; CCFP; Court Staff, Halton Healthcare Services Corporation - Oakville Site; (905)844-0311; Fax. (905)844-0836.

GLOWACKI, Adam R; South Walkerville Med Centre, 131-2224 Walker Rd, Windsor ON N8W 5L7; Warsaw (Poland)'74; FRCSC; ObstGyn. Ac Staff, Windsor Regional Hospital - Metropolitan Site; Langs: Polish; (519)971-7733; Fax. (519)971-0854.

GLOWCZEWSKI-PARK, Elizabeth Y H; The Doctor's Office, 2251 Lawrence Ave E, Scarborough ON M1P 2P5; Wes'05; CCFP; Langs: Korean; Spanish; (416)759-5251; Fax. (416)759-1253.

GLUBE, Mark L; Scarborough Hosp-General Div, 3050 Lawrence Ave E, Scarborough ON M1P 2V5; Wes'95; FRCPC; Anes. Staff, The Scarborough Hospital - General Campus; (416)320-9080

GLUMAC, George; 1 Pheasant Run Dr, Guelph ON N1C 1A3; Qns'77; MSc; FRCPC; Psy (Child Psychiatry). (519)763-6036; Fax. (519)763-8005.

GLUSZYNSKI, Malgorzata; The Ottawa Hosp-Riverside Camp, 1967 Riverside Dr, Ottawa ON K1H 7W9; Ott'04; CCFP; Staff, The Ottawa Hospital - Riverside Campus; Langs: Polish; (613)738-8219

GLYNN-MORRIS, Rodney; Royal Oak Med Clinic, 103-1638 Broadway E, Vancouver BC V5N 1W1; Liverpool (England)'70; AddicMed; MRCS; LRCP; DObstRCOG; CCFP; Langs: German; (604)438-6184

GMORA, Scott B; St Joseph's Healthcare, 836-50 Charlton Ave E, Hamilton ON L8N 4A6; Qns'02; FRCSC; GenSurg. Staff, St Joseph's Healthcare - Charlton Campus; (905)522-1155

GMORA, Shawn W; Ctre Francophone de Toronto, 280-5 Fairview Mall Dr, North York ON M2J 2Z1; McG'92; CCFP; FCFP; Langs: English; French; (416)492-2672; Fax. (416)492-3157.

GNAM, William H; CAMH Psychological Trauma Prog, 200-455 Spadina Ave, Toronto ON M5S 2G8; Cal'85; MSc(Physiol.); FRCPC; Psy (Eating Disorders). Consultant, Princess Margaret Hospital - University Health Network; Staff Psy, Centre for Addiction & Mental Health (CAMH) - Russell Street Site; Teacher Psy, University of Toronto; (416)535-8501; Fax. (416)971-7172; william_gnam@camh.net.

GNANABASKARAN, Ajantha; Dawson Creek Med Clinic, 816 103 Ave, Dawson Creek BC V1G 2G1; (Sri Lanka)'97; MB BS; CCFP; Langs: Sinhalese; Tamil; (250)782-5271

GNANABASKARAN, Sangarapillai; Dawson Creek Med Clinic, 816 103 Ave, Dawson Creek BC V1G 2G1; (Sri Lanka)'88; MB BS; Langs: Sinhalese; Tamil; (250)782-5271; Fax. (250)782-6360.

GNANAPANDITHEN, Kumudini; Markham Stouffville Hosp, PO Box 1800 Stn Main 381 Church St, Markham ON L3P 7P3; Tor'03; FRCPC; IntMed. Staff, Markham Stouffville Hospital; (905)472-7000

GNANATISSA, Asha S; Heathplex Med Centre, 100-150 West Dr, Brampton ON L6T 4P9; Colombo (Sri Lanka)'90; CCFP; (905)454-7410

GNANENDRAN, Kandiah P; Windsor Reg Hosp-Metropolitan, 1995 Lens Ave, Windsor ON N8W 1L9; Colombo (Sri Lanka)'84; MB BS; FFARCS; FRCPC; Anes (Pain Management). Staff, Windsor Regional Hospital - Metropolitan Site; Langs: Tamil; Sinhalese; (519)254-1661

GNANESWARAN, Aiyathurai; Lakeridge Hlth Corp-Oshawa, 1 Hospital Crt, Oshawa ON L1G 2B9; Ceylon (Sri Lanka)'74; MB BS; MRCPsy(UK); FRCPC; Psy. Staff, Lakeridge Health - Oshawa Site; Langs: Sinhalese; Tamil; (905)576-8711; Fax. (905)721-4784.

GNAWALI, Meghraj; Alder Med Center, 277 Evergreen Rd, Campbell River BC V9W 5Y4; Tribhuvan (Nepal)'91; (250)287-7454

GO, Cristina; The Hosp For Sick Children, 555 University Ave, Toronto ON M5G 1X8; Santo Tomas (Philippines)'94; Staff, The Hospital For Sick Children; (416)813-6295

GO, May L; 3750 Lawrence Ave E, Scarborough ON M1G 1R1; Tor'81; Staff, The Scarborough Hospital - General Campus; Langs: Italian; (416)439-3400

GOAD, Ralph F; Chatham-Kent Health Alliance, PO Box 2030 Stn Main 80 Grand Ave W, Chatham ON N7M 5L9; Wes'75; Staff, Chatham-Kent Health Alliance; (519)352-6401 x6081; rgoad@bigfoot.com.

GOB, Alan; London HSC-Victoria Hosp, PO Box 5010 Stn B A2 401-800 Commissioners Rd E, London ON N6A 5W9; Wes'07; FRCPC; IntMed; Hem. Staff, London Health Sciences Centre - Victoria Campus; (519)685-8500

GOBBI, Gabriella; Institut Allan Memorial, 220-1033 av des pins O, Montreal QC H3A 1A1; Rome (Italy)'91; Psy (P.Q.) (Depression). Staff Psy, Institut Philippe-Pinel de Montreal; Staff Psy, Allan Memorial Institute; assoc Prof, McGill University; Langs: Italian; English; (514)398-1290; gabriella.gobbi@mcgill.ca.

GOBBURU, Ram M; Stratford Gen Hosp, 45 General Hosp Dr, Stratford ON N5A 2Y6; Kakatiya (India)'94; Staff, Stratford General Hospital - Huron Perth Healthcare Alliance; (519)271-2120

GOBEIL, Annie-Emmanuelle; Centre Med Laval, 1110 boul Vanier, Laval QC H7C 2R8; Sher'96; (450)661-2521; Fax. (450)661-7193.

GOBEIL, Francois; CSSS Pierre Boucher, 1333 boul Jacques-Cartier E, Longueuil QC J4M 2A5; Mon'88; CSPQ; FRCPC; Anes (Hospitalist). Staff, Centre Hospitalier Pierre Boucher; Chief Dept of Anes, Hopital Charles LeMoyne; Universite de Sherbrooke; (450)468-8225; Fax. (450)466-5007.

GOBEIL, Francois; CHUM-Hotel-Dieu, 3840 rue Saint-Urbain, Montreal QC H2W 1T8; Sher'93; CSPQ; FRCPC; IntMed; Cardiol. Staff, Centre Hospitalier l'Université de Montréal (CHUM) - Hôpital Notre-Dame; Staff, Centre Hospitalier l'Université de Montréal (CHUM) - Hôtel-Dieu; (514)890-8000

GOBEIL, Gerald; CSSS de Chicoutimi, 305 rue Saint-Vallier, Chicoutimi QC G7H 5H6; Laval'79; CSPQ; FRCPC; Anes. Staff, Complexe hospitalier de la Sagamie; (418)541-1000 x2217; Fax. (418)545-3455.

GOBEIL, Marie-Helene; Ilnst Albert Prevost, 6555 boul Gouin O, Montreal QC H4K 1B3; Laval'06; FRCPC; Psy. (514)338-4280

GOBEIL, Martine; CLSC Verdun, 6161 rue Laurendeau, Montreal QC H4E 3X6; Mon'94; Staff, CSSS du Sud-Ouest Verdun; Staff, Centre Hospitalier de LaSalle; Langs: Spanish; English; (514)766-0546 x3228; Fax. (514)765-3265.

GOBEIL, Nicole; La Cite Medicale, 295-2600 boul Laurier, Quebec QC G1V 4T3; Laval'86; (418)781-0480; Fax. (418)659-7072.

GOBESSI, Linda; Geriatric Psy Commun Services, 129Y-75 Bruyere St, Ottawa ON K1N 5C7; Tor'90; FRCPC; Psy (Geriatric Psychiatry). Langs: Bilingual(English/French); (613)562-0283; Fax. (613)562-0497; lgobessi@bruyere.org.

GOBRAN, Gehad G M; Duffus Health Center, 208-7071 Bayers Rd, Halifax NS B3L 2C2; Ain Shams (Egypt)'86; MB BCh; CCFP; Langs: Arabic; Fax. (902)453-5657; gehadgobran@yahoo.ca.

GOBRIAL, Marcos; M & D Med Center, 1-872 Sheppard Ave W, North York ON M3H 5V5; Ain Shams (Egypt)'93; MB ChB; MB BCh; CCFP; FCFP; Staff FD, Bayviewhills Clinic; Langs: Arabic; (416)633-1600; Fax. (416)633-1608.

GOCKER, Marianne; 875 Manning Ave, Toronto ON M6G 2X3; Georgetown DC(Washington) (USA)'78; FRCPC; Psy. Staff, The Hincks-Dellcrest Centre - Toronto; (416)516-9988; Fax. (416)535-6068.

GODBOUT, Ariane; CHUM-Hop St-Luc, 1058 rue Saint-Denis, Montreal QC H2X 3J4; Mon'03; FRCPC; IntMed; Endocrin&Metab. Staff, Centre Hospitalier l'Université De Montréal (CHUM) - Hôpital Saint-luc; (514)890-8000 x32597; Fax. (514)412-7365.

GODBOUT, Bruno; Ctr Hosp Affilie-Enfant-Jesus, 1401 18e rue, Quebec QC G1J 1Z4; Laval'82; CSPQ; FRCPC; Anes. Staff, Centre Hospitalier Affilié Universitaire de Québec - Hôpital De L'Enfant Jésus; (418)649-5803

GODBOUT, Caroline; Centre Hosp Honore-Mercier, 2750 boul Laframboise, Saint-Hyacinthe QC J2S 4Y8; Sher'91; Staff, Centre Hospitalier Honore-Mercier; (450)771-3333; Fax. (450)771-3652.

GODBOUT, Cynthia; 201-6624 av Somerled, Montreal QC H4V 1T2; McG'94; CCFP; Staff Privil Obst & Peds, St Mary's Hospital Centre; Teacher, McGill University; Langs: English; French; (514)486-6656; Fax. (514)486-0309.

GODBOUT, Francois; Hotel-Dieu de Sorel, 400 av de l'Hotel-Dieu, Sorel-Tracy QC J3P 1N5; Mon'91; CCFP; Staff, Hôtel-Dieu de Sorel; (450)746-6000; francois.godbout@sympatico.ca.

GODBOUT, Jacques-Andre; Dr Georges-L Dumont Reg Hosp, 330 av Universite, Moncton NB E1C 2Z3; Mon'03; Staff, Dr Georges-L-Dumont University Hospital Centre; (506)862-4000

GODBOUT, Jean; Clin Med Dr Jean Godbout, 201-28 boul du Mont-Bleu, Gatineau QC J8Z 1J1; Ott'72; Staff, Hull Hospital; (819)770-7304; Fax. (819)770-5502.

GODBOUT, Manon; CSSS Drummond-Hop Sainte-Croix, 570 rue Heriot, Drummondville QC J2B 1C1; Laval'00; FRCSC; Urol. Staff, Hôpital Sainte-croix; (819)478-6464 x2351; Fax. (819)478-6418.

GODBOUT, Marie-Josee; Hotel-Dieu de levis, 143 rue Wolfe, Levis QC G6V 3Z1; Laval'97; FRCPC; DiagRad. Staff, Hôtel-Dieu de Lévis; (418)835-7121; Fax. (418)835-7204.

GODBOUT, Richard; Radiologie CLM, 2984 boul Taschereau, Greenfield Park QC J4V 2G9; Dal'64; DiagRad (Interventional Radiology). Staff Radiologie Diagnost, Hopital Charles LeMoyne; Langs: Bilingual(French/English); (450)671-6173; Fax. (450)671-9284; richard.godbout@videotron.ca.

GODBOUT, Sylvie; CHUS-Hop Hotel-Dieu, 580 rue Bowen S, Sherbrooke QC J1G 2E8; Sher'82; FRCPC; Psy. Staff, Centre Hospitalier Universitaire de Sherbrooke-Hôpital Hôtel-Dieu; Universite de Sherbrooke; (819)346-1110; Fax. (819)829-6284.

GODBOUT, Veronique; CHUM-Hosp Notre Dame, 1560 rue Sherbrooke E, Montreal QC H2L 4M1; Mon'02; FRCSC; OrthSurg (Sports Medicine). Staff, Centre Hospitalier l'Université de Montréal (CHUM) - Hôpital Notre-Dame; Langs: Bilingual(French/English); (514)890-8000 x25900; Fax. (514)412-7619.

GODBOUT, Yves-Laurent; Clinique Med Pointe-Du-Lac, CP 4099 Succ A 10300 ch Sainte-Marguerite, Trois-Rivieres QC G9B 7Y6; Laval'72; Langs: Bilingual(French/English); (819)377-5015; Fax. (819)377-5550.

GODDARD, Christopher M; 103-5631 Inlet Ave, Sechelt BC V0N 3A3; Alb'91; FRCSC; GenSurg. Staff, St Mary's Hospital; (604)741-0590

GODDARD, Gwyllyn; PO Box 363 Stn Main, Chilliwack BC V2P 6J4; Sask'03; BSc; CCFP; (604)858-5300; Fax. (604)858-5264.

GODDARD, Karen J; BC Cancer Agency-Vancouver CC, 600 10th Ave W, Vancouver BC V5Z 4E6; Manchester (England)'79; MB ChB; MRC(UK); FRCPC; RadOncol. Staff, BC Cancer Agency Vancouver Centre; Ac Staff, Vancouver General Hospital - Centennial Pavillion; (604)877-6000; Fax. (604)708-2000.

GODDARD, Karin G; McGill Mental Health Service, 3600 rue McTavish, Montreal QC H3A 1X9; Man'87; FRCPC; Psy (Crisis Intervention). Staff, Centre Hospitalier l'Université de Montréal (CHUM) - Hôpital Notre-Dame; Langs: Dutch; French; (514)398-6019

GODDARD, Michele D; Meadpoint Health Care Centre, 233-355 Wellington St, London ON N6A 3N7; Otago (New Zealand)'60; MB ChB; FRACP; FRCPC; IntMed (Cardiology). (519)432-1919; Fax. (519)432-2566.

GODDARD, Peter; PO Box 118, Aylesford NS B0P 1C0; Dal'67; Staff, Valley Regional Hospital; Med Dir, Grandview Manor Nursing Home; Physician, Berwick Community Health Centre; (902)847-3446; Fax. (902)847-1527.

GODDARD, Shannon L; Sunnybrook Health Sciences Ctr, D108c-2075 Bayview Ave, Toronto ON M4N 3M5; Tor'06; FRCPC; IntMed; Critical Care Medicine. Staff, Sunnybrook Health Sciences Centre; (416)480-6100

GODDARD, Stephen P T; 421 Shepherdson Rd, Temagami ON P0H 2H0; Wes'93; BSc; CCFP; Ac Staff, Temiskaming Hospital; (705)647-8121

GODDARD, Thomas A; PO Box 14, Grand Pre NS B0P 1M0; Dal'97; CCFP; CCFP(E.M.); FCFP; Staff, Valley Regional Hospital; (902)542-0375; Fax. (902)542-7315.

GODDARD, Yvette N; The Ottawa Hosp-Gen Campus, 1401 CCW-501 Smyth Rd, Ottawa ON K1H 8L6; Qns'03; FRCPC; Anes. Staff, The Ottawa Hospital - General Campus; (613)737-8187; Fax. (613)727-8189.

GODDARD-HILL, Alban C; 306-210 Dundas St E, Belleville ON K8N 5G8; Qns'78; BSc; CCFP; Ac Staff, QHC Belleville General; (613)968-8692; Fax. (613)968-5009; alban.goddardhill@ontariomd.ca.

GODEL, J Mark; Lakeland Med Clinic, 206-314 25 St, Cold Lake AB T9M 1G6; Alb'85; CCFP; FCFP; Staff, Cold Lake Healthcare Centre; Clin Teacher Family Med, University of Alberta; Langs: Bilingual(French/English); (780)639-3001; Fax. (780)639-3009; mgodel@yahoo.com.

GODENIR, Victor J B; Radiology Consultants Assoc, 120-6707 Elbow Dr SW, Calgary AB T2V 0E3; Sask'99; FRCPC; DiagRad. (403)777-3007; Fax. (403)777-3008.

GODET, Patrick; Ctr Hosp de Lasalle, 8585 Tss Champlain, LaSalle QC H8P 1C1; Mon'82; ABIM; FRCPC; IntMed (Inflammatory Bowel Disease); Gastroent. Staff, Centre Hospitalier de LaSalle; Staff, Centre Hospitalier de Verdun; (514)362-8000; Fax. (514)367-8624.

GODFREY, Charles M; Rosedale Med Centre, 308-600 Sherbrourne St, Toronto ON M4X 1W4; Tor'53; FRCPC; PhysMed&Rehab (Electromyography). Langs: French; German; Spanish; (416)923-7127; Fax. (416)923-8639.

GODFREY, Sean E; 1058-200 Taunton Rd W, Whitby ON L1R 3H8; Edinburgh (Scotland)'91; MB ChB; FAAP; FRCPC; Peds (Consultant Pediatrics). Ac Staff Peds, Lakeridge Health - Oshawa Site; (905)444-9636; Fax. (905)444-9853; babydocs@rogers.com.

GODIN, Anick; Glenmore Med Bldg, 1605 Gordon Dr, Kelowna BC V1Y 3G8; Sher'05; FRCPC; IntMed; Rheum. (250)762-3808

GODIN, Bernard; Dr Georges-L Dumont Reg Hosp, 330 av Universite, Moncton NB E1C 2Z3; Mon'97; CCFP; Staff, Dr Georges-L-Dumont University Hospital Centre; Langs: English; (506)862-4000

GODIN, Chantal; 200-620 rue King E CP 21501 Csp Ste-Famille, Sherbrooke QC J1G 5K2; Sher'86; CSPQ; FRCPC; IntMed; Endocrin&Metab. Staff Endocrin, Centre Hospitalier Universitaire de Sherbrooke-Hôpital Hôtel-Dieu; Endocrin/Metabolism, Carrefour Sante Granit; Clin Prof, Universite de Sherbrooke; (819)563-2734; Fax. (819)563-0260; endomdcg@sympatico.ca.

GODIN, Christian; CHUQ-Ctr Hosp Univ Laval, 2705 boul Laurier, Quebec QC G1V 4G2; McG'93; Staff, Centre Hospitalier Universitaire de Quebec-CHUL; (418)656-4141 x70554

GODIN, Claude; Centre Med St-Urbain, 209-3875 rue Saint-Urbain, Montreal QC H2W 1V1; Mon'72; FRCSC; OrthSurg. Staff OrthSurg, Centre Hospitalier l'Université de Montréal (CHUM) - Hôtel-Dieu; Associate Clin Prof, Universite de Montreal; (514)849-8391; Fax. (514)849-9313; godin.claude@sympatico.ca.

GODIN, Daniel; Clin Cardio, 103-130 rue Saint-Nicolas, Sorel-Tracy QC J3P 6X9; Mon'80; CSPQ; FRCPC; IntMed (P.Q.); Cardiol (P.Q.). (450)730-0020

GODIN, Danny; Dr Georges-L Dumont Reg Hosp, 330 av Universite, Moncton NB E1C 2Z3; Mon'01; CCFP; CCFP(E.M.); Staff, Dr Georges-L-Dumont University Hospital Centre; (506)862-4000

GODIN, Dominique; Clinique Medicine Nepisiguit, 950 Picot Ave, Bathurst NB E2A 4Z9; Sher'06; CCFP; (506)546-6696

GODIN, Isabelle; CSSS Drummond-Hop Sainte-Croix, 570 rue Heriot, Drummondville QC J2B 1C1; Mon'94; LMCC; Staff, Hôpital Sainte-croix; (819)477-2231; Fax. (819)478-6464.

GODIN, Jacques; Hotel-Dieu de Sorel, 400 av de l'Hotel-Dieu, Sorel-Tracy QC J3P 1N5; Mon'75; Respir (P.Q.). Staff, Hôtel-Dieu de Sorel; (450)746-6000

GODIN, Jean; Groupe Sante Medisys Inc, 1110-500 rue Sherbrooke O, Montreal QC H3A 3C6; Mon'88; Dir gén, Teva Canada Innovation; (514)845-1211; Fax. (514)433-9536; jean.godin@tevapharm.com.

GODIN, Johanne; Clinique Medical Riel, 455 boul Riel, Gatineau QC J8Z 2J8; Laval'89; CCFP; (819)777-7416; Fax. (819)777-5061.

GODIN, Johanne; CSSS du Nord de Lanaudière, 1000 boul Sainte-Anne, St-Charles-Brommee QC J6E 6J2; Sher'94; Staff, Centre Hospitalier Régional de Lanaudière; (450)759-8222

GODIN, Louis; FMOQ, 1000-1440 rue Sainte-Catherine, Montreal QC H3G 1R8; Laval'77; Prés/Dir gén, Federation des Medecins Omnipracticiens du Quebec; (514)878-1911; Fax. (514)878-4455; lgodin@fmoq.org.

GODIN, Marie-Christine; Centre Med & Prof de Dorval, 667 ch Bord-Du-Lac Lakeshore, Dorval QC H9S 2B7; Mon'99; CCFP; (514)633-1510; Fax. (514)633-8299.

GODIN, Marie-Eve; Clin De La Cite, 3801 rue De Montcalm, Jonquiere QC G7X 1W1; Sher'04; CCFP; Staff, Centre Hospitalier Jonquiere; (418)542-1510

GODIN, Marie-Eve; CLSC-CHSLD de la Petite-Nation, 14 rie Saint-Andre, St-Andre-Avellin QC J0V 1W0; Mon'06; (819)983-7341; Fax. (819)983-1315.

GODIN, Maurice; MUHC-Montreal Gen Hosp, L6-211-1650 av Cedar, Montreal QC H3G 1A4; Laval'69; CSPQ; FRCPC; IntMed; Cardiol (P.Q.). Sr Physician, McGill University Health Centre - Montreal General Campus; assoc Prof, McGill University; Langs: Bilingual(French/English); (514)934-1934 x42308; maurice.godin@mcgill.ca.

GODIN, Paul-Emile; 1060 av Royale, Quebec QC G1E 2A6; Laval'60; Ac Staff, Centre Hospitalier Affilié Universitaire de Québec - Hôpital De L'Enfant Jésus; (418)661-3669; Fax. (418)661-2995.

GODIN, Pierre; Centre Med Fusion, 200-2035 av Sainte-Anne, Saint-Hyacinthe QC J2S 5H3; Mon'87; (450)773-6023

GODIN, Stephane; Hôpital régional Chaleur, 1750 Sunset Dr, Bathurst NB E2A 4L7; Sher'05; FRCPC; Psy. Staff, Hopital Regional Chaleur; (506)544-3000

GODINEZ-LUNA, Tomas; McCaig Tower, 3134 Hospital Dr NW, Calgary AB T2N 5A1; (Mexico)'77; IntMed (Critical Care Medicine). Staff, Foothills Medical Centre; (403)944-2586; tomas.godinez@crha-health.ab.ca.

GODINHO, Derek V; Eyewest Vision Inc, 300-1343 Lonsdale Ave, North Vancouver BC V7M 2H7; UBC'85; DABOph; FRCSC; Ophth (Cataract). Staff Ophth, Lions Gate Hospital; Staff Consultant, Vancouver General Hospital - Centennial Pavillion; Clin Assoc Prof Opht, University of British Columbia; (604)985-0405; Fax. (604)985-1271.

GODKIN, Timothy; Queen Elizabeth II HSC-Halifax, 1796 Summer St, Halifax NS B3H 2Y9; Dal'90; Anes. Staff, Queen Elizabeth II Health Sciences Centre - Halifax Infirmary Site; (902)473-2331

GODLEWSKI, Bartosz; Grey Nuns Community Hosp, 1100 Youville Drive West NW, Edmonton AB T6L 5X8; Mem'07; FRCPC; Anes. Staff, Covenant Health - Grey Nuns Community Hospital; (780)735-7020

GODLEWSKI, Marek; Saint John Reg Hosp, PO Box 2100 Stn Main, Saint John NB E2L 4L2; Bialystok (Poland)'82; FRCPC; AnatPath. Pathologist, Saint John Regional Hospital.

GODLEWSKI, Wojciech; Clinical Sciences Bldg, 152 University Campus NW, Edmonton AB T6G 2G3; Warsaw (Poland)'76; FRCPC; Anes. (780)407-8887

GODLEY, Mark B; 6F-555 8th Ave W, Vancouver BC V5Z 1C6; (South Africa)'87; MB ChB; FRCPC; Anes. (604)739-9695

GODON, Patricia; Polyclinique D'Argenteuil, 201-551 rue Berry, Lachute QC J8H 1S4; Liege (Belgium)'98; Staff, Centre Hospitalier d'Argenteuil; Langs: Bilingual(French/English); (450)562-3751; Fax. (450)562-1852; tita222@hotmail.com.

GODOY DALBONI DE LIMA, Renato; CSSS Pierre Boucher, 1333 boul Jacques-Cartier E, Longueuil QC J4M 2A5; Staff, Centre Hospitalier Pierre Boucher; (450)468-8111

GODOY PIMENTA, Newton J; CSSS de Chicoutimi, 305 rue Saint-Vallier, Chicoutimi QC G7H 5H6; Staff, Complexe hospitalier de la Sagamie; (418)541-1000

GODSALVE, Valerie M; Saskatoon City Hops, 701 Queen St, Saskatoon SK S7K 0M7; Sask'75; LMCC; FRCPC; AnatPath (General Pathology). Staff, Saskatoon City Hospital; (306)655-8315; Fax. (306)655-8399.

GODSELL, Sally J; Okanagan Clinical Trials, 204-1353 Ellis St, Kelowna BC V1Y 1Z9; Ott'78; Physician, Kelowna General Hospital; Physician, Okanagan Clinical Trials; (250)862-8141; Fax. (250)862-8130; sjg@oktrials.ca.

GODSOE, Deborah E; 5F-189 Prince William St, Saint John NB E2L 2B9; Dal'77; Staff, Saint John Regional Hospital; (506)636-4075; Fax. (506)636-4788.

GODSOE, Suzanne; Queensway-Carleton Hosp, 3045 Baseline Rd, Nepean ON K2H 8P4; Dal'04; FRCPC; EmergMed. Staff, Queensway Carleton Hospital; Langs: Bilingual(English/French); (613)721-2000

GODUE, Francois; GMF Concorde, 300 boul de la Concorde E, Laval QC H7G 2E6; Sher'83; ATLS; ACLS; (450)667-5310

GODWIN, Elaine I; 1510 9 Ave S, Lethbridge AB T1J 1V8; Sask'94; BSc; CCFP; (403)942-0555; Fax. (403)942-3373; dgodwin@telusplanet.net.

GODWIN, N Marshall S; Health Sciences Centre, 1776-300 Prince Philip Dr, St. John's NL A1B 3V6; Mem'77; BMedSci; CCFP; FCFP; Staff, Health Sciences Centre; Prof, Memorial University Of Newfoundland; (709)777-8373; Fax. (709)777-6118; godwinm@mun.ca.

GOEBEL, Cindy R; 205-323 Wilson St E, Ancaster ON L9G 4A8; McM'95; CCFP; FCFP; (905)648-8786; Fax. (905)648-7730.

GOEBEL, Gary R; 11140 109 St NW, Edmonton AB T5G 2T4; Alb'81; BSc; (780)412-5150

GOEBEL, Pamela J; One World Med Ctr, 3575 20 Ave NE, Calgary AB T1Y 6R3; Tor'81; FRCSC; GenSurg. Med Examiner, Civil Aviation Canada; (403)248-7955; pamela.goebel@tc.gc.ca.

GOECKE, Michelle E; Keary Med Centre, 210-245 Columbia St E, New Westminster BC V3L 3W4; Qns'02; FRCSC; GenSurg. Staff Trauma Services, Vancouver General Hospital - Centennial Pavillion; (604)522-7737

GOEKE, Fredrick J; Seven Oaks Gen Hosp, 2300 Mcphillips St, Winnipeg MB R2V 3M3; Man'90; CCFP; CCFP(E.M.); FCFP; Staff, Seven Oaks General Hospital; (204)632-3113

GOEL, Danny P; 106-3825 Sunset St, Burnaby BC V5G 1T4; Man'03; FRCSC; OrthSurg. (604)437-9600

GOEL, Devendra P; 106-3825 Sunset St, Burnaby BC V5G 1T4; Lucknow (India)'50; MSc(Exp.Surg.); MB BS; FRCSC; GenSurg. Vis Staff, BC Women's Hospital & Health Centre; Vis Staff, BC Children's Hospital; Langs: Hindi; Punjabi; (604)437-9600

GOEL, Nand K; Sunridge Prof Centre, 416-2675 36 St NE, Calgary AB T1Y 6H6; Cal'89; FRCSC; Ophth. Med Staff, Foothills Medical Centre; Med Staff, Peter Lougheed Centre; Med Staff, Alberta Children's Hospital; Asst Prof, University of Calgary; (403)543-5000; Fax. (403)543-5002.

GOEL, Raj K; Windsor Reg Hosp-Metropolitan, 1330-1995 Lens Ave, Windsor ON N8W 1L9; Man'02; FRCSC; Urol (Nephrology). Staff, Windsor Regional Hospital - Metropolitan Site; Staff, Leamington District Memorial Hospital; (519)254-5577 x52020; Fax. (519)985-2650.

GOEL, Rakesh; The Ottawa Hosp-Gen Camp, 501 Smyth Rd, Ottawa ON K1H 8L6; UBC'80; ABIM; FRCPC; IntMed (Medical Oncology); MedOncol. Ac Staff, The Ottawa Hospital - Civic Campus; Consultant, Cornwall Community Hospital; Consultant, Pembroke Regional Hospital Inc; Staff, The Ottawa Hospital - General Campus; Asst Prof Med, University of Ottawa; (613)737-7777

GOEL, Reena; Mclaughin Village Med Clinic, 85 Steeles Ave W, Brampton ON L6Y 0K3; Tor'92; CCFP; Langs: Hindi; (905)455-9374; Fax. (905)455-9505.

GOEL, Ritika; Inner City Family Health Team, 4F-69 Queen St E, Toronto ON M5C 1R8; McM'08; CCFP; (416)368-5666

GOEL, Sadan K; Main Street Med Centre, 9-10886 Hurontario St, Brampton ON L7A 3R9; Vikram (India)'61; MB BS; DCH; FRCSC; GenSurg (Gen Endoscopic CVT). Ac Staff, Headwaters Health Care Centre - Orangeville Site; Langs: Hindi; (905)846-9911

GOEL, Sanjeev; Wise Elephant Family Hlth Team, 247 Main St N, Brampton ON L6X 1N3; Tor'95; CCFP; FCFP; Staff, William Osler Health System - Brampton Civic Hospital; Langs: Hindi; French; (905)459-4385; Fax. (905)459-6373; sgoel@ahealingplace.ca.

GOEL, Seema; Sunridge Prof Centre, 416-2675 36 St NE, Calgary AB T1Y 6H6; Dal'95; CCFP; (403)543-5000; Fax. (403)543-5002.

GOEL, Sunita; Cedar Springs Prof Centre, E-960 Cumberland Ave, Burlington ON L7N 3J6; McM'90; CCFP; Ac Staff, Hamilton Health Sciences Centre - McMaster Children's Hospital; Langs: Hindi; (905)333-9799

GOEL, Vivek; Simcoe Hall, 300-480 University Avenue, Toronto ON M5G 1V2; McG'84; MSc; SM(Harvard); FRCPC; CommunMed (Breast Cancer). Pres/CEO, Ontario Agency for Health; Prof Dalla Lana School of Public Hlth Univ of Toronto, University of Toronto; Langs: French; (647)260-7111; Fax. (647)260-7600; president@oahpp.ca.

GOELA, Aashish; London HSC-University Hosp, PO Box 5339 Stn B 339 Windermere Rd, London ON N6A 5A5; Ott'00; FRCPC; DiagRad. Staff, London Health Sciences Centre - University Hospital; Langs: Hindi; French; (519)685-8500 x33648

GOERTZEN, James; Fort William Clinic, 117 Mckellar St S, Thunder Bay ON P7E 1H5; Man'81; MClSc; CCFP; FCFP; Ac Staff, Thunder Bay Regional Health Sciences Centre; Assoc Prof, Northern Ontario School of Medicine; (807)626-1234; Fax. (807)622-1257.

GOERTZEN, Peter J; PO Box 967 Lcd 1, Medicine Hat AB T1A 7G8; Man'74; FRCPC; Anes. Staff, Medicine Hat Regional Hospital; (403)529-8839; Fax. (403)528-8101.

GOETZ, Catherine J; Quinte HC Corp-Belleville Gen, 265 Dundas St E, Belleville ON K8N 5A9; Ott'86; FRCPC; AnatPath. Staff, QHC Belleville General; (613)969-7400 x2354; Fax. (613)968-9912.

GOETZ, Thomas J; 590-1144 Burrard St, Vancouver BC V6Z 2A5; Qns'91; FRCSC; OrthSurg (Hand & Upper Extremity Surgery). Staff Eagle Ridge Hand & Orthopedic Centre, Eagle Ridge Hospital & Health Care Centre; Clin Asst Med, University of British Columbia; (604)689-5101; Fax. (604)689-5144.

GOETZE, Andre; 11301 13 St, Dawson Creek BC V1G 3X1; Stellenbosch (South Africa)'81; MB ChB; MMed; Staff, Dawson Creek & District Hospital; Langs: Afrikaans; (250)782-5834

GOEZ, Rachel H; Edmonton Clinic Health Academy, 4 588-11405 87 Ave NW, Edmonton AB T6G 1C9; (Israel)'87; (780)248-5630

GOFF, Valerie M; Providence Continuing Care Ctr, 525 Montreal St, Kingston ON K7K 3H9; National (Ireland)'71; MB ChB; MRCPsy(Eng); FRCPC; Psy (Critical Care Medicine). Staff, Providence Care - Mental Health Services; (613)540-6165 x4202; Fax. (613)540-6169.

GOFFIN, John; The Juravinski Cancer Centre, 699 Concession St, Hamilton ON L8V 5C2; Wes'96; FRCPC; IntMed; MedOncol. Physician, The Juravinski Cancer Centre; (905)387-9495

GOFINE, Timothy; 1003-2 Carlton St, Toronto ON M5B 1J3; Sask'81; FRCPC; Psy (Adult & Child Psychiatry). Sr Consultant Psy Dual Diagnosis Service, Ontario Shores Centre for Mental Health Sciences; Consultant, Toronto Western Hospital - University Health Network; Asst Prof, University of Toronto; (416)966-1767; Fax. (416)966-3018.

GOFMAN, Frina; Bathurst-Drewry Med Centre, 201-5927 Bathurst St, North York ON M2R 3T5; Leningrad (Russia (Federation))'63; Langs: Russian; (416)223-9066; Fax. (416)223-9108.

GOFTON, Emma N; Carling-Broadview Med Bldg, 309-770 Broadview Ave, Ottawa ON K2A 3Z3; Qns'98; FRCSC; ObstGyn. Staff, Queensway Carleton Hospital; (613)274-7831; Fax. (613)274-3271.

GOFTON, Jeffery; Office of the Chief Med Examin, 4070 Bowness Rd NW, Calgary AB T3B 3R7; (Grenada)'96; (403)297-8123; Fax. (403)297-3429.

GOFTON, Wade T; The Ottawa Hospital-Civic Camp, J153-1053 Carling Ave, Ottawa ON K1Y 4E9; Wes'99; BSc(Hon); FRCSC; OrthSurg (Trauma). Staff, The Ottawa Hospital - Civic Campus; (613)798-5555 x18779; Fax. (613)761-4015.

GOGAN, Nessa R; Saint John Reg Hosp, PO Box 2100 Stn Main, Saint John NB E2L 4L2; Mem'91; FRCPC; IntMed; Nephrol. Staff, Saint John Regional Hospital; (506)648-6843; Fax. (506)648-6841.

GOGELA-SPEHAR, Marketa; 390-1144 Burrard St, Vancouver BC V6Z 2A5; Alb'03; FRCSC; ObstGyn (High Risk Obstetrics). Staff, Providence Health Care - St Paul's Hospital; Langs: Czech; Polish; (604)568-8155; Fax. (604)568-8145.

GOGGIN, Patricia; Inst Nat'L de Sante Publique, 100-190 boul Crémazie E, Montreal QC H2P 1E2; Mon'76; MHSA; Membre Dept of Preventive Med & Public Health, Centre Hospitalier l'Université de Montréal (CHUM) - Hôpital Notre-Dame; Langs: English; Spanish; (514)864-1600 x3214; Fax. (514)864-7646; patricia.goggin@inspq.qc.ca.

GOGIA, Rupinder K; Medmart Med Centre, 68A Centennial Pky N, Hamilton ON L8E 1H6; Maharshi Dayanand University (Other Foreign)'95; CCFP; Langs: Hindi; Punjabi; (905)560-5800; Fax. (905)560-5801.

GOGUEN, Frederic; Hôpital régional Chaleur, 1750 Sunset Dr, Bathurst NB E2A 4L7; Sher'02; CCFP; Staff, Hopital Regional Chaleur; (506)544-3000

GOGUEN, Jeannette M; St Michael's Health Centre, 6F-61 Queen St E, Toronto ON M5C 2T2; Tor'87; FRCPC; IntMed; Endocrin&Metab. Ac Staff, St Michael's Hospital; Teacher, University of Toronto; (416)867-3714; Fax. (416)867-3714.

GOH, Chor; CHUM-Hosp Notre Dame, T2379 1-1560 rue Sherbrooke E, Montreal QC H2L 4M1; McG'03; FRCPC; IntMed; Nephrol. Staff, Centre Hospitalier l'Université de Montréal (CHUM) - Hôpital Notre-Dame; (514)890-8000 x26616; Fax. (514)412-7831.

GOH, Elaine S; The Credit Valley Hosp, 2G500-2200 Eglinton Ave W, Mississauga ON L5M 2N1; Wes'06; FRCPC; MedGenetics. Staff, The Credit Valley Hospital; (905)813-4104; Fax. (905)813-4347.

GOH, Raymond H T; Rouge Valley-Centenary HC, 2867 Ellesmere Rd, Scarborough ON M1E 4B9; Qns'90; FRCPC; DiagRad. Staff Diagnostic Imaging, Rouge Valley Health System - Centenary Health Centre Site; (416)281-7021; Fax. (416)284-1780.

GOHEEN, Mary Susan L B; The Ottawa Hosp-Civic Campus, 1053 Carling Ave, Ottawa ON K1Y 4E9; Dal'91; BPHE; FRCPC; Anes. Staff Anes, Royal Victoria Regional Health Centre; Staff, The Ottawa Hospital - Civic Campus; Langs: English; French; (613)761-4940; Fax. (613)761-5032.

GOHEL, Bhavini; South Hlth Campus, 4448 Front St SE, Calgary AB T3M 1M4; (Other Foreign)'06; (403)956-1111

GOHIL, J Girishdhai; MD Health, 188 Main St S, Brampton ON L6W 2E2; Baroda (India)'83; (905)456-7774

GOHIL, Jyotsna; Valley Creek Med Clinic, 3938 Cottrelle Blvd, Brampton ON L6P 2R1; Baroda (India)'83; (905)794-6065; Fax. (905)794-6067; jgohil58@yahoo.com.

GOHILL, Jitendra; 101-49 Richard Way SW, Calgary AB T3E 7M8; Cal'90; BSc; PhD; FRCSC; Ophth (Cataract Surgery). (403)264-0141; Fax. (403)265-9279.

GOHILL, Lalji R; Deer Valley Walk-In Med Clinic, 50-1221 Canyon Meadows Dr SE, Calgary AB T2J 6G2; Birmingham (England)'61; MB ChB; Langs: Hindi; Gujarati; (403)278-2164; Fax. (403)278-3192.

GOHILL, Lori B; 206-1717 10 St NW, Calgary AB T2M 4S2; Dal'96; CCFP; (403)282-9865; Fax. (403)282-9893.

GOHLA, Gabriela; St Joseph's Healthcare, L222 3-50 Charlton Ave E, Hamilton ON L8N 4A6; Hamburg (Germany)'88; FRCPC; AnatPath. Staff, St Joseph's Healthcare - Charlton Campus; Langs: German; (905)522-1155 x35009; Fax. (905)521-6192.

GOICEA, Daniela; Bigelow Fowler Clinic, 1605 9 Ave S, Lethbridge AB T1J 1W2; (Romania)'00; (403)327-3121; Fax. (403)320-5593.

GOINDI, Reena; Ottawa Reg Cancer Centre, 503 Smyth Rd, Ottawa ON K1H 1C4; Ott'09; CCFP; (613)737-7700

GOINEAU, Jacques; Clinique Externe Jean-Talon, 7345 rue Garnier, Montreal QC H2E 2A1; Mon'77; FRCPC; Psy. Chef, Hopital Louis-H Lafontaine; Clin Teach Staff Psy, Universite de Montreal; (514)729-3036

GOJER, Julian A C; 303-720 Spadina Ave, Toronto ON M5S 2T9; Mysore (India)'81; DPM(Bangalore,India); MRCPsy(U.K.); FRCPC; Psy (Forensic Psychiatry). Staff Psy, Centre for Addiction & Mental Health (CAMH) - College Street Site; Staff Forensic Psy, Ontario Shores Centre for Mental Health Sciences; Asst Prof, University of Toronto; (416)323-9939; Fax. (416)323-3166; julian_gojer@camh.net.

GOJMERAC, Frederic; Diagnostic Imaging, 8407 112 Ave, Fort St. John BC V1J 0J5; Alb'76; DABR; FRCPC; DiagRad (Nuclear Medicine). Staff, Fort Nelson General Hospital; Staff, Fort St John Hospital & Health Centre; (250)261-7429; frederic.gojmerac@northernhealth.ca.

GOKCEN, M Ilhami; Shoniker Clinic, 2877A Ellesmere Rd, Scarborough ON M1E 4C1; Istanbul (Turkey)'54; DPsy; Psy (Child & Adolescent Psychiatry). Staff Shoniker Clinic, Rouge Valley Health System - Centenary Health Centre Site; Langs: Turkish; French; (416)281-7301; Fax. (416)281-7465.

GOKHALE, Sandhya; 302-310 King St E, Kitchener ON N2G 2L3; (India)'88; CCFP; Langs: Gujarati; Hindi; Marathi; (519)743-2142; Fax. (519)743-2405.

GOKUL, Adhikar B; Callingwood Crossing Med Clini, 6905 172 St NW, Edmonton AB T5T 5Y1; (South Africa)'01; CCFP; (780)444-0350; adhikar_gokul@yahoo.com.

GOLAN, Eyal; Univ Hlth Network-Toronto Western Hosp, 2M 411P-399 Bathurst St, Toronto ON M5T 2S8; McG'03; FRCPC; IntMed; Critical Care Medicine. Staff, Toronto Western Hospital - University Health Network; (647)401-4936

GOLAN, Jeff D; SMBD Jewish Gen Hosp, 3755 ch Cote-Sainte-Catherine, Montreal QC H3T 1E2; McG'01; FRCSC; Neursurg. Staff, Sir Mortimer B Davis Jewish General; (514)340-8222

GOLBABAEI, Mehdi; Royal Alexandra Hosp, 10240 Kingsway NW, Edmonton AB T5H 3V9; (Iran)'93; Staff, Royal Alexandra Hospital; (780)735-4111

GOLBERG, Deborah; 3755 ch Cote-Sainte-Catherine, Montreal QC H3T 1E2; Wes'99; CCFP; Prés assem of The CPDP, Kateri Memorial Hospital Centre; Staff, Sir Mortimer B Davis Jewish General; Langs: English; French; (514)340-8222 x8234; Fax. (514)340-8298.

GOLBEY, Michael J; 5-4520 Gallaghers Lkout, Kelowna BC V1W 3Z8; UBC'80; Ac Staff Family Med, Kelowna General Hospital; (250)765-2996; Fax. (250)765-9015.

GOLD, Beverly L; Heritage Pointe Family Med, RR 3 330-412 Pine Creek Rd, De Winton AB T0L 0X0; Cal'86; CCFP; (403)279-4944; Fax. (403)720-3321.

GOLD, David I; Centre de Med Fam de Wakefield, CP 400 777 ch Riverside, Wakefield QC J0X 3G0; Mon'91; CCFP; FCFP; Ac Member, Centre Hospitalier Gatineau Mémorial; Langs: English; Spanish; (819)459-2363; Fax. (819)459-2997.

GOLD, Elisabeth; 201-6009 Quinpool Rd, Halifax NS B3K 5J7; Tor'77; MHSc; MEd; CCFP; FCFP; Assoc Prof, Dalhousie University; (902)478-2266; Fax. (902)425-2266.

GOLD, Ileana-Maria; William Osler HC-Brampton, 2100 Bovaird Dr E, Brampton ON L6R 3J7; Bucharest (Romania)'84; FRCPC; Anes. Staff, William Osler Health System - Brampton Civic Hospital; Langs: Romanian; Hebrew; French; (905)494-2120

GOLD, Jewel; Mount Sinai Hosp, 1604-600 University Ave, Toronto ON M5G 1X5; McG'82; FRCPC; IntMed; Cardiol. Staff, Mount Sinai Hospital; Langs: French; Hebrew; (416)586-4800 x5275; Fax. (416)586-5980; jgold@mtsinai.on.ca.

GOLD, Pamela D; Hanover Med Associates, 118 7th Ave, Hanover ON N4N 2G9; UBC'99; CCFP; FCFP; Langs: English; French; (519)364-2820

GOLD, Phil; MUHC-Montreal Gen Hosp, D13 173-1650 av Cedar, Montreal QC H3G 1A4; McG'61; MSc; PhD; MACP; FRCPC; IntMed; ClinImmunol&Allergy (P.Q.). Staff Research Institute, McGill University Health Centre - Montreal General Campus; Prof Med Oncol & Phys, McGill University; Langs: French; Yiddish; Bilingual(English/French); (514)934-1934 x43061; Fax. (514)934-8338; phil.gold@mcgill.ca.

GOLD, Susan L; SMBD Jewish Gen Hosp, 3755 ch Cote-Sainte-Catherine, Montreal QC H3T 1E2; Man'83; FRCPC; GeriatricMed (P.Q.). Staff, Sir Mortimer B Davis Jewish General; (514)340-7501; Fax. (514)340-7547.

GOLD, Wayne L; Univ Hlth Network-Toronto Gen, EN13 213-200 Elizabeth St, Toronto ON M5G 2C4; Tor'88; FRCPC; IntMed (AIDS/HIV); InfectDis. Staff, Toronto General Hospital - UHN; (416)340-4800 x4410; Fax. (416)340-3357.

GOLDA, Bronislaw L; 204-1051 Upper James St, Hamilton ON L9C 3A6; Wroclaw (Poland)'77; Langs: Polish; (905)527-7000; Fax. (905)527-7006.

GOLDADE, Roxanne M; Southport Pediatrics, 109-10333 Southport Rd SW, Calgary AB T2W 3X6; Cal'90; BSc(BioChem.); FRCPC; Peds (Developmental Medicine). Ac Staff Privil, Alberta Children's Hospital; Clinical Asst Prof Peds, University of Calgary; (403)253-2288; Fax. (403)255-9322; southportspeds@telus.net.

GOLDBACH, Martin M; London Health Science Centre, PO Box 5339 Stn B B6-116-339 Windermere Rd, London ON N6A 5A5; Wes'69; MD; FRCSC; Cardiovasc&ThorSurg (Cardiac Surgery). Ac Staff, London Health Sciences Centre - Victoria Campus; Staff, London Health Sciences Centre - South Street; Ac Staff, London Health Sciences Centre - University Hospital; Assoc Prof Surg, University of Western Ontario; (519)672-3300; Fax. (519)663-2915; goldbach@uwo.ca.

GOLDBACH, Morton; 103-90 Warren Rd, Toronto ON M4V 2S2; Tor'72; FRCPC; Peds. Ac Staff, The Hospital For Sick Children; Asst Prof, University of Toronto; (416)924-7171; Fax. (416)923-9015.

GOLDBERG, Aron; 102-1111 Lonsdale Ave, North Vancouver BC V7M 2H4; Tor'74; DABOph; Dip Ortho; FACS; FRCSC; Ophth. Att Staff, Lions Gate Hospital; (604)988-1166; Fax. (604)988-0166.

GOLDBERG, Aviva M; Children's Hosp, FE009-840 Sherbrook St, Winnipeg MB R3A 1S1; Cal'99; FRCPC; Peds; Nephrol. Fax. (204)787-1075.

GOLDBERG, Benjamin; 33-30 Doon Dr, London ON N5X 3P1; Dal'55; BSc; FRCPC; Psy (Mental Retardation). Emeritus Prof, University of Western Ontario; Langs: Yiddish; (519)858-2700; Fax. (519)434-0842; bengoldberg@rogers.com.

GOLDBERG, Bernard; Dalecliff Med Centre, 1-209 Ellesmere Rd, Scarborough ON M1R 4E2; Tor'84; Ac Staff, The Scarborough Hospital - General Campus; Court Staff, Rouge Valley Health System - Centenary Health Centre Site; Ac Staff, The Scarborough Hospital - Birchmount Campus; (416)444-8900

GOLDBERG, Chaim J; 2235 Kennedy Rd, Scarborough ON M1T 3G8; Tor'76; FRCSC; Ophth (Refractive Surgery). Ac Staff, Rouge Valley Health System - Centenary Health Centre Site; Member, International Institute of Sportsvision; Member, Contact Lens Association of Ophtalmology; Member, Academy of Ophthalmology; Langs: Hebrew; Italian; Yiddish; French; (416)754-3937; Fax. (416)754-7975.

GOLDBERG, Cory S; Queensway Professional Ctr, 401-190 Sherway Dr, Etobicoke ON M9C 5N2; Qns'99; FRCSC; PlasSurg (Clinician Investigator Program). (416)907-5810

GOLDBERG, David J; Lakeshore Med Centre, 3970 Lakeshore Rd, Kelowna BC V1W 1V5; Man'87; (250)764-8878; Fax. (250)764-0889.

GOLDBERG, Deborah R; St Michael's Hosp, 30 Bond St, Toronto ON M5B 1W8; Tor'07; DiagRad.

GOLDBERG, Erwin H; 023-3545 ch de la Cote-des-Nei, Montreal QC H3H 1V1; Dal'60; Staff, McGill University Health Centre - Montreal General Campus; (514)935-1197; Fax. (514)935-1310.

GOLDBERG, Eudice; The Hosp for Sick Children, 555 University Ave, Toronto ON M5G 1X8; McM'75; FRCPC; Peds (Adolescent Medicine). Staff Adolescent Med, The Hospital For Sick Children; Assoc Prof, University of Toronto; Langs: English; French; (416)813-5825; Fax. (416)813-5392; eudice.goldberg@sickkids.ca.

GOLDBERG, Franklin; St Michael's Hosp, 30 Bond St, Toronto ON M5B 1W8; Tor'82; AB; AB; FRCPC; AnatPath (Breast Imaging); DiagRad. Staff, St Michael's Hospital; (416)864-6060 x6474; goldbergf@yahoo.com.

GOLDBERG, Grant M; Winnipeg Reg Health Authority, 102-1001 Corydon Ave, Winnipeg MB R3M 0B6; Wes'93; CCFP; FCFP; Staff Family Pract, Health Sciences Centre; (204)940-2000

GOLDBERG, Jeremy; St Joseph's Mountain H Serv, PO Box 585 Stn Lcd 1 100 West 5th St, Hamilton ON L8N 3K7; Cape Town (South Africa)'80; FRCPC; Psy. Staff, St Joseph's Healthcare Hamilton - West 5th Campus; (905)522-1155 x6250

GOLDBERG, Kevin M; Maple Tree Med Clinic, 1181B 6 Ave NE, Salmon Arm BC V1E 2S5; Cape Town (South Africa)'99; MB ChB; BSc(Zoo); BSc(Hon)(Med); Langs: Afrikaans; (250)832-9361

GOLDBERG, Laurie D; Peterborough Reg HC-Hospital, 1 Hospital Dr, Peterborough ON K9J 7C6; Man'85; FRCPC; Anes. Staff, Peterborough Regional Health Centre - Hospital Drive; (705)743-2121; Fax. (705)876-5105.

GOLDBERG, Mark A; 202-219 St Clair Ave W, Toronto ON M4V 1R3; Tor'72; FRCPC; Psy (Psychoanalysis). (416)920-2861

GOLDBERG, Michael R; 503-85 Skymark Dr, North York ON M2H 3P2; Tor'65; FACS; FRCSC; GenSurg (Pacemaker Surgery); VascSurg. Staff, Mount Sinai Hospital; Staff, Toronto General Hospital - UHN; Assoc Prof, University of Toronto; (416)499-0009

GOLDBERG, Norman A; Manitoba Clinic, 790 Sherbrook St, Winnipeg MB R3A 1M3; Man'72; BSc(Med); FRCPC; Peds (Insurance Medicine). Staff, Health Sciences Centre; Assoc Prof, University of Manitoba; (204)788-5748; Fax. (204)772-2537.

GOLDBERG, Norman V; Bramalea Med Centre, 300-18 Kensington Rd, Brampton ON L6T 4S5; McG'75; Staff, William Osler Health System - Brampton Civic Hospital; (905)791-3133; Fax. (905)791-8441; norm@norcol.com.

GOLDBERG, Orli D; Forest Hill Family Hlth Ctr, 200-491 Eglinton Ave W, Toronto ON M5N 1A8; McM'04; CCFP; (416)782-6111 x119; Fax. (416)782-5515.

GOLDBERG, Pamela R; North York Gen Hosp, 4001 Leslie St, North York ON M2K 1E1; Cape Town (South Africa)'84; FRCPC; Anes. Staff, North York General Hospital; Langs: Afrikaans; (416)756-6265; Fax. (416)756-6384.

GOLDBERG, Peter; MUHC-Royal Victoria Hosp, L3 06-687 av des Pins O, Montreal QC H3A 1A1; McG'78; Critical Care Medicine (P.Q.); Respir; IntMed. Asst Physician, McGill University Health Centre - Royal Victoria Hospital; Dir ICU, McGill University Health Centre - Montreal Chest Institute; adj Prof, McGill University; (514)934-1934; Fax. (514)843-1686; peter.goldberg@muhc.mcgill.ca.

GOLDBERG, Robert J; St Michael's Hosp, CCW 14 077-30 Bond St, Toronto ON M5B 1W8; Tor'10; Staff, St Michael's Hospital; (416)864-5431

GOLDBERG, Ronn E A; North York Gen Hosp, 4001 Leslie St, North York ON M2K 1E1; Tor'81; FRCPC; DiagRad (Oncology Imaging). Staff, North York General Hospital; (416)756-7289

GOLDBERG, Yigal Paul; BC Women's Hosp & Health Ctre, 4500 Oak St, Vancouver BC V6H 3N1; Cape Town (South Africa)'83; MB ChB; FRCPC; MedGenetics. Staff, BC Women's Hospital & Health Centre; (604)875-2157; Fax. (604)875-2825.

GOLDBERG JACOB, Nesya F F; 206-2900 Steeles Ave E, Thornhill ON L3T 4X1; Tor'03; CCFP; (905)881-6667; Fax. (905)731-1298.

GOLDBERGER, Michael H; 206-3825 Sunset St, Burnaby BC V5G 1T4; Belfast (Ireland)'71; MB ChB; BAO; MRCP(UK); (604)433-1248; Fax. (604)433-1203.

GOLDBLOOM, David S; Addiction & Mental Hlth-Clarke, 250 College St, Toronto ON M5T 1R8; McG'81; DPsy; FRCPC; Psy. Med Advisor Sr Educ & Pub Affairs/Chief Physician, Centre for Addiction & Mental Health (CAMH) - College Street Site; Prof Psy, University of Toronto; Langs: Bilingual(English/French); (416)979-6915; Fax. (416)979-6834.

GOLDBLOOM, Ellen B; Children's Hosp Eastern Ont, 5109C-401 Smyth Rd, Ottawa ON K1H 8L1; Dal'04; FRCPC; Peds; Endocrin&Metab. Staff, Children's Hospital of Eastern Ontario (CHEO); (613)737-7600

GOLDBLOOM, Richard B; Parkland at the Gardens, 817-5732 College St, Halifax NS B3H 1X3; McG'49; FAAP; FRCPC; Peds (Consultation). Med Staff, IWK Health Centre; Emeritus Chancellor/Prof Peds, Dalhousie University; Langs: English; French; (902)429-2901; richardgoldbloom@gmail.com.

GOLDCHTAUB, Valeri; Aberdeen Hosp, 835 East River Rd, New Glasgow NS B2H 3S6; Semipalatinsk (Kazakhstan)'89; Staff, Aberdeen Regional Hospital; (902)752-7600

GOLDEN, Jonathan G; Surrey Mem Hosp, 13750 96 Ave, Surrey BC V3V 1Z2; Man'92; CCFP; CCFP(E.M.); Staff, Surrey Memorial Hospital; (604)588-3369

GOLDEN, Ross S; 2F-223 St Clair Ave W, Toronto ON M4V 1R3; Man'80; FRCPC; Psy. Staff Pt-Time, Humber River Regional Hospital - Keele Street Site; (416)920-7355

GOLDEN, Susan J; 106-3195 Granville St, Vancouver BC V6H 3K2; Man'81; FRCPC; Psy (Child & Adolescent Psychiatry). (604)873-6755; Fax. (604)873-4933.

GOLDENBERG, Barry S; Westmount Square Med Centre, C 180-1 Car Westmount, Westmount QC H3Z 2P9; McG'92; GP/Emerg/Fam Med, Centre Hospitalier de LaSalle; Teacher Faculty, McGill University; (514)934-2334; Fax. (514)934-5559.

GOLDENBERG, David J; St Boniface Clinic, 343 Tache Ave, Winnipeg MB R2H 2A5; Man'72; BSc(Med); FRCPC; IntMed (Gastroenterology). Ac Staff, Victoria General Hospital; Ac Staff, St Boniface General Hospital; Assoc Prof Med, University of Manitoba.

GOLDENBERG, Donna A; The Southcom Bldg, 301-2227 South Millway, Mississauga ON L5L 3R6; McG'87; BSc; MDCM; FRCPC; Peds. Assoc Staff Emerg, The Hospital For Sick Children; Ac Staff, The Credit Valley Hospital; Asst Prof, University of Toronto; (905)569-9798; Fax. (905)569-8630.

GOLDENBERG, Jay C; William Osler HC-Etobicoke, 101 Humber College Blvd, Etobicoke ON M9V 1R8; Wes'81; FRCPC; DiagRad. Staff, William Osler Health System - Etobicoke General Hospital; (416)747-3400 x33543; Fax. (416)747-3610.

GOLDENBERG, Lesley P; 400-200 St Clair Ave W, Toronto ON M4V 1R1; Man'83; DABPN; FRCPC; Psy. Consultant, The Canadian Hearing Society; Teacher, University of Toronto; Langs: Hebrew; (416)928-6599; lgoldenberg@chs.ca.

GOLDENBERG, Leslie; Walking Mobility Clinic, U11-750 Dundas St W, Toronto ON M6J 3S3; Tor'75; BSc; ABIM; FAGS; FRCPC; IntMed (Podologic Medicine); GeriatricMed. Assoc Staff Centenary, Mount Sinai Hospital; Consultant, Toronto Western Hospital - University Health Network; Staff, Baycrest Centre for Geriatric Care; Med Dir, Walking Mobility Clinics; Asst Prof Med, University of Toronto; Langs: Hebrew; (416)929-1015; Fax. (416)929-9918.

GOLDENBERG, Ronald M; 17-531 Atkinson Ave, Thornhill ON L4J 8L7; Tor'84; FACE; FRCPC; IntMed (Diabetes Mellitus); Endocrin&Metab. Consultant, North York General Hospital; (905)763-8660; ronald.goldenberg@lmc.ca.

GOLDENBERG, S Larry; G & L Diamond Hlth Care Centre, 6F-2775 Laurel St, Vancouver BC V5Z 1M9; Tor'78; FACS; FRCSC; Urol (Prostate Cancer). Head Urol/Dir, Vancouver General Hospital - Centennial Pavillion; Staff, BC Cancer Agency Vancouver Centre; Physician, Univ. of Washington; Prof/Dept Head & School dir Urol Sciences, University of British Columbia; (604)875-5003; Fax. (604)875-5604.

GOLDENBERG, Teresa; North York Family Health Team, 701-240 Duncan Mill Rd, North York ON M3B 3S6; McG'84; BSc; CCFP; FCFP; Staff, North York General Hospital; (416)229-6300; Fax. (416)229-6283; tgoldenberg@sympatico.ca.

GOLDENSON, Gordon L; Sunnybrook Hlth Sciences Ctre, M3 200-2075 Bayview Ave, Toronto ON M4N 3M5; Tor'72; BSc; Anes. Staff Anes, Sunnybrook Health Sciences Centre; (416)480-4864

GOLDFARB, Bernard; Canada Place Bldg, 206-107 Shirreff Ave, North Bay ON P1B 7K8; McM'88; FRCSC; Urol. Staff, North Bay Regional Health Centre - Regional Mental Health; Staff, West Nipissing General Hospital; (705)474-0992; Fax. (705)474-1148.

GOLDFARB, Cynthia E; North York Gen Hosp-Branson, 555 Finch Ave W, North York ON M2R 1N5; McM'89; FRCPC; Peds (Developmental Pediatrics). Staff, North York General Hospital - Branson Division; Staff, North York General Hospital; (416)632-8730; Fax. (416)632-8704.

GOLDFARB, David M; McMaster Univ, 1280 Main St W, Hamilton ON L8S 4K1; Dal'03; FRCPC; Peds; MedMicrobiol; InfectDis.

GOLDFARB, David R; Leslie Medical Centre, 303-4800 Leslie St, North York ON M2J 2K9; Tor'85; BSc; FRCSC; Otol (Pediatric Otolaryngology). Staff, Toronto East General Hospital Inc; Chief, North York General Hospital; Staff, Mount Sinai Hospital; Asst Prof, University of Toronto; (416)499-5558; Fax. (416)499-9392.

GOLDFARB, Janice; 3650-6900 boul Decarie, Cote Saint-Luc QC H3X 2T8; Laval'90; (514)733-3668

GOLDFARB, Ludmilla; North York Gen Hosp-Branson, 555 Finch Ave W, North York ON M2R 1N5; Odessa (Ukraine)'48; Ac Staff, North York General Hospital - Branson Division; (416)633-9420; Fax. (416)226-5545.

GOLDFARB, Peter; Etobicoke Med Centre, 400 The East Mall, Etobicoke ON M9B 3Z9; Tor'75; Staff, Trillium Health Centre - West Toronto; (416)621-2220; Fax. (416)621-2357.

GOLDFINGER, Morris; 601-155 St Clair Ave W, Toronto ON M4V 0A1; McG'75; FRCPC; DiagRad. (416)400-8007; morrisgoldfinger@gmail.com.

GOLDHAAR, Haviva; Allan Memorial Institute, 1025 av des Pins O, Montreal QC H3A 1A1; Brooklyn(NY) (USA)'79; Psy. Staff, Allan Memorial Institute; (514)934-1934 x35504

GOLDHAMER, Paul M; 510-164 Eglinton Ave E, Toronto ON M4P 1G4; McG'73; FRCPC; Psy. Staff Psy, Mount Sinai Hospital; Consultant Psy, Centre for Addiction & Mental Health (CAMH) - Queen Site; Asst Prof, University of Toronto; (416)926-0799

GOLDHAR, John N H; Cosmedix Md, 105-150 York St, Toronto ON M5H 3S5; Tor'72; DAB; FRCPC; Derm (Cosmetic Dermatology). Staff, Baycrest Centre for Geriatric Care; Staff, Jewish Home for the Aged; Dir, Cosmedix MD Inc; Langs: English; French; (416)977-6502; Fax. (416)977-6915; info@cosmedixmd.com.

GOLDHAR, Sheldon W; 303-3850 Finch Ave E, Scarborough ON M1T 3T6; Tor'83; FRCSC; Ophth. Ac Staff, The Scarborough Hospital - General Campus; Langs: Hebrew; (416)297-7188; Fax. (416)297-7189.

GOLDHAR, Steven M; Canhealth Med Clinic, PO Box 52 595 Bay St, Toronto ON M7A 2C7; Tor'86; (416)598-1703; Fax. (416)598-1778.

GOLDIE, Craig; PO Box 98037 Rpo Yaletown, Vancouver BC V6Z 2Z7; Qns'08; CCFP; (604)283-5586

GOLDIE, Morag E; 103-15157 Hwy 10, Surrey BC V3S 9A5; Edinburgh (Scotland)'73; (604)574-1805

GOLDIE, Sheena; Peace Arch Maternity Clinic, 1713-15521 Russell Ave, White Rock BC V4B 2R4; UBC'04; (604)542-0248

GOLDING, Ian F; The Hosp for Sick Children, 1725G-555 University Ave, Toronto ON M5G 1X8; Qns'95; FRCPC; Peds (Pediatric Cardiology); Cardiol. Staff Cardiol, The Hospital For Sick Children; Asst Prof Peds, University of Toronto; (416)813-6140; Fax. (416)813-7547.

GOLDLIST, Barry J; Mount Sinai Hosp, 422-600 University Ave, Toronto ON M5G 1X5; Tor'74; FACP; FRCPC; IntMed; GeriatricMed. Ac Staff, Toronto General Hospital - UHN; Ac Staff, Mount Sinai Hospital; Ac Staff, Toronto Western Hospital - University Health Network; Prof, University of Toronto; (416)586-4800 x6641; Fax. (416)586-8327; bgoldlist@mtsinai.on.ca.

GOLDLIST, Gerald I; 7 Elmwood Ave, North York ON M2N 6R6; Tor'72; DOphth; DAB; FRCSC; Ophth. Consultant, North York General Hospital; (416)226-6560; Fax. (416)226-6562.

GOLDMAN, Barbara L; Women's Health Clinic, 3F-419 Graham Ave, Winnipeg MB R3C 0M3; Man'80; CCFP; (204)947-1517; Fax. (204)943-3844.

GOLDMAN, David; Regional Mental HC-St Thomas, PO Box 2004 Stn Main 467 Sunset Dr, St Thomas ON N5P 3V9; Madison(WI) (USA)'74; FRCPC; Psy. Staff, Regional Mental Health Care-St Joseph's Health Care; Staff, Regional Mental Health Care-St Joseph's Health Care; Langs: Bilingual(French/English); (519)631-8510; Fax. (519)631-7348.

GOLDMAN, Faye A; Carling-Broadview Med Bldg, 305-770 Broadview Ave, Ottawa ON K2A 3Z3; Tor'91; CCFP; FCFP; Langs: Hebrew; (613)728-7700; Fax. (613)728-5848.

GOLDMAN, Gail; St Mary's Hosp Centre, 3830 av Lacombe, Montreal QC H3T 1M5; Mon'93; FRCPC; IntMed. Staff, St Mary's Hospital Centre; Langs: English; French; (514)345-3511; goldmangail@hotmail.com.

GOLDMAN, Gerald N; Bridlewood Mall, 231-2900 Warden Ave, Scarborough ON M1W 2S8; Tor'68; Staff, The Scarborough Hospital - General Campus; (416)499-1617; Fax. (416)499-2453.

GOLDMAN, H Brian; Mount Sinai Hosp, 206-600 University Ave, Toronto ON M5G 1X5; Tor'80; FACEP; MCFP(EM); Hd EmergMed, Mount Sinai Hospital; Writer/Host, CBC Toronto; Asst Prof, University of Toronto; Langs: Spanish; (416)586-5058; Fax. (416)586-4719; drhbg@rogers.com.

GOLDMAN, Howard H; Weston Road Med Clinic, 2549 Weston Rd, Toronto ON M9N 2A7; Qns'82; AAFPhys; CCFP; FCFP; (416)240-8282; Fax. (416)240-8870; hhgoldman@doctor.com.

GOLDMAN, Hyman; Tiny Tots Med Center, 203-3400 rue du Marche, Roxboro QC H9B 2Y1; Basel (Switzerland)'58; FRCPC; Peds. Staff, McGill University Health Centre - Montreal Children's Hospital; Assoc Prof Peds, McGill University; (514)685-3531

GOLDMAN, Lorne E; 602-581 Davis Dr, Newmarket ON L3Y 2P6; McG'94; FRCPC; IntMed; Cardiol. Staff, Southlake Regional Health Centre; (905)953-7917

GOLDMAN, Marvin B; Albany Clinic, 807 Broadview Ave, Toronto ON M4K 2P8; Tor'62; FRCPC; Neur. Court Staff, The Scarborough Hospital - General Campus.

GOLDMAN, Mindy R; Canadian Blood Services, 1800 Alta Vista Dr, Ottawa ON K1G 4J5; Mon'84; FRCP; IntMed; FRCPC; IntMed (Transfusion Medicine); Hem. Exec Med Dir Donor & Transplantation Services, Canadian Blood Services; Langs: French; Bilingual(English/French); (613)739-2577; Fax. (613)739-2002; mindy.goldman@blood.ca.

GOLDMAN, Ran D; BC Women's & Children's Hosp, K4 226-4480 Oak St, Vancouver BC V6H 3V4; Jerusalem (Israel)'95; FRCPC; Peds. Staff, BC Children's Hospital; (604)875-2345

GOLDMAN, Russell; Temmy Latner Ctr for Palliativ, Box 13 L4-000-60 Murray St, Toronto ON M5T 3L9; Tor'93; CCFP; FCFP; Staff, Mount Sinai Hospital; Dir, Temmy Latner Centre for Palliative Care; Asst Prof, University of Toronto; (416)586-4800 x6149; Fax. (416)586-4804.

GOLDMAN, Ruth A; 1490 Danforth Ave, Toronto ON M4J 1N4; Tor'84; CCFP; FCFP; Med Dir, Heritage Nursing Home; (416)463-4878; Fax. (416)463-4904.

GOLDNER, Elliot M; Simon Fraser University, 2400-515 Hastings St W, Vancouver BC V6B 0B2; Cal'80; FRCPC; Psy. Langs: English; French; (604)291-5148

GOLDNER, Sarah; Children's Hosp, 840 Sherbrook St, Winnipeg MB R3A 1S1; Qns'05; Peds (Pediatric Emergency Medicine).

GOLDSAND, John I; Toronto Rehab Inst-Hillcrest, 47 Austin Terr, Toronto ON M5R 1Y8; Alb'88; Dip SportMed; CCFP; FCFP; Staff, Toronto Rehabilitation Institute - University Centre; Staff, Bridgepoint Health Centre; Langs: Hebrew; (416)597-3422; goldsand.john@torontorehab.on.ca.

GOLDSMAN, Barry; Montreal Sleep Clinic, 4427 rue Sherbrooke O, Westmount QC H3Z 1E5; McG'85; Langs: English; French.

GOLDSMITH, Lindsay; Inst U Geriatrie de Montreal, 4565 ch Queen-Mary, Montreal QC H3W 1W5; Mon'09; CCFP; Staff, Institut Universitaire de Gériatrie de Montréal; (514)340-2800

GOLDSMITH, Robert; Guelph Family Health Team, 19-35 Harvard Rd, Guelph ON N1G 3A2; Wes'80; CCFP; FCFP; Staff, Guelph General Hospital; (519)837-8137; Fax. (519)822-8240; rgoldsmith@in.on.ca.

GOLDSMITH, William J; Westmount Med Bldg, 510-5025 rue Sherbrooke O, Montreal QC H4A 1S9; McG'71; DAB; FACOG; FRCSC; ObstGyn (Aboriginal Health). Associate ObstGyn, McGill University Health Centre - Royal Victoria Hospital; Associate, McGill University Health Centre - Montreal General Campus; Associate, St Mary's Hospital Centre; Asst Prof ObstGyn, McGill University; Langs: French; German; (514)489-5588; Fax. (514)489-6317.

GOLDSMITH, William O; Guelph Family Health Team, 19B-35 Harvard Rd, Guelph ON N1G 3A2; McM'75; CCFP; FCFP; Staff, Guelph General Hospital; Asst Prof Family Med, McMaster University; (519)837-8137; Fax. (519)822-8240; wgoldsmith@in.on.ca.

GOLDSTEIN, Aubrey; BCC-St Vincent Hospital, 60 Cambridge St N, Ottawa ON K1R 7A5; McM'82; Staff Bruyere Continuing Care, Bruyère Continuing Care - Saint-Vincent Hospital; Med Officer, Bureau of Human Prescription Drugs/Office of Clinical Trials; (613)562-6262; Fax. (613)782-2704; vanngold@rogers.com.

GOLDSTEIN, Benjamin I; Sunnybrook Hlth Sciences Ctr, FG53-2075 Bayview Ave, Toronto ON M4N 3M5; Cal'01; FRCPC; Psy. Staff, Sunnybrook Health Sciences Centre; Langs: Hebrew; (416)480-4089

GOLDSTEIN, Cheryl E; Univ of Alberta Hosp-SCC/WCM, 2F1 36 WCM-8440 112 St, Edmonton AB T6G 2B7; (Israel)'97; MPH; BA; ABIM; FRCPC; IntMed. Staff, University of Alberta Hospital; (780)407-3856; Fax. (780)407-3132.

GOLDSTEIN, Christina; Univ Hlth Network-Toronto Western Hosp, 399 Bathurst St, Toronto ON M5T 2S8; McM'06; FRCSC; OrthSurg. Staff, Toronto Western Hospital - University Health Network; (403)944-1110

GOLDSTEIN, David; Kingston Gen Hosp, 76 Stuart St, Kingston ON K7L 2V7; Dublin (Ireland)'87; LRCPSI; FRCPC; Anes (Acute & Chronic Pain). Staff, Kingston General Hospital; Pres, Medical Staff Association; Staff Teacher, Queen's University; (613)549-6666 x3399; Fax. (613)548-1375; goldsted@kgh.kari.net.

GOLDSTEIN, David I; Centric Health Atria 1, W300-2255 Sheppard Ave E, North York ON M2J 4Y1; Tor'82; CCFP; FCFP; (416)495-1988; Fax. (416)495-9215.

GOLDSTEIN, David P; Univ Hlth Network-Princess M, 3 952-610 University Ave, Toronto ON M5G 2M9; Tor'98; MSc; FRCSC; Otol (Head & Neck Oncology). Staff, Women's College Hospital; Staff, Princess Margaret Hospital - University Health Network; (416)946-2301; Fax. (416)946-2300.

GOLDSTEIN, Eric; The Dermatology Clinic, 255-340 College St, Toronto ON M5T 3A9; Wes'87; FRCPC; Derm. Staff Consultant Derm, Toronto Western Hospital - University Health Network; Staff Derm, University of Toronto; Langs: Bilingual(English/French); (416)925-6349; Fax. (416)925-4120.

GOLDSTEIN, Howard; Groupe Sante Medisys, 11F-500 rue Sherbrooke O, Montreal QC H3A 3C6; McG'86; CCFP; FCFP; ac Staff, Sir Mortimer B Davis Jewish General; (514)845-1211; Fax. (514)340-7579.

GOLDSTEIN, Howard J; Oakdale Med Bldg, 306-2065 Finch Ave W, North York ON M3N 2V7; Ott'70; Ac Staff Family & CommunMed, Humber River Regional Hospital - Finch Avenue Site; (416)745-6435

GOLDSTEIN, Irwin H; Chartwell Prof Centre, 202-2331 Brimley Rd, Scarborough ON M1S 3L6; Tor'72; Staff, The Scarborough Hospital - General Campus; Staff, Rouge Valley Health System - Centenary Health Centre Site; (416)291-7919; Fax. (416)291-8663.

GOLDSTEIN, Jeffrey L; 308-435 Reynolds St, Oakville ON L6J 3M5; Wes'04; Nephrol; IntMed. Staff, Toronto General Hospital - UHN; (905)815-8910; Fax. (905)815-8911.

GOLDSTEIN, Mara S; St Michael's Hosp, 17F-30 Bond St, Toronto ON M5B 1W8; McG'97; FRCPC; Psy. Staff, St Michael's Hospital; (416)864-3090

GOLDSTEIN, Marc B; 3060 Shuter-30 Bond St, Toronto ON M5B 1W8; McG'64; BSc; MSc; MDCM; FRCPC; IntMed (Dialysis). Staff Nephrol, St Michael's Hospital; Prof Emeritus, University of Toronto; Langs: Bilingual(English/French); (416)864-5290; Fax. (416)864-3042; goldsteinma@smh.ca.

GOLDSTEIN, Mark L; 401-960 Lawrence Ave W, North York ON M6A 3B5; Tor'87; CCFP; FCFP; (416)256-1150; Fax. (416)256-0742.

GOLDSTEIN, Mark; Markham Stouffville Urgent Car, 100-110 Copper Creek Dr, Markham ON L6B 0P9; Cal'05; CCFP; Physician, Markham Stouffville Urgent Care; (905)472-8911; Fax. (905)472-6081.

GOLDSTEIN, Martin E; Statcare Clinic, 104-175 av Stillview, Pointe-Claire QC H9R 4S3; Mon'83; (514)694-9282

GOLDSTEIN, Roger S; West Park Healthcare Centre, 82 Buttonwood Ave, Toronto ON M6M 2J5; Manchester (England)'72; MB ChB; FRCP; DABIM; FACCP; FRCPC; IntMed (Sleep Medicine); Respir. Staff RespMed, Toronto General Hospital - UHN; Staff, Mount Sinai Hospital; Prof Med & Physical Therapy, University of Toronto; (416)243-3631; Fax. (416)243-8947; rgoldstein@westpark.org.

GOLDSTEIN, Ronald; Amherstview Med Centre, 18 Manitou Cres W, Amherstview ON K7N 1S3; Tor'94; BSc; MScA; CCFP; (613)389-1619; Fax. (613)507-1619.

GOLDSTEIN, Sheldon H; Medical Clinic Bldg, 202-89 Humber College Blvd, Etobicoke ON M9V 4B8; Tor'67; DABIM; FRCPC; IntMed (Cardiology). Staff, William Osler Health System - Etobicoke General Hospital; (416)743-2784; Fax. (416)743-2788.

GOLDSTEIN, Simon G; Alberta Children's Hosp, 2888 Shaganappi Trail NW, Calgary AB T3B 6A8; Cal'89; FRCSC; OrthSurg (Pediatric Surgery). Staff, Alberta Children's Hospital; Clinical Asst Prof, University of Calgary; (403)955-7392

GOLDSTEIN, Sol J; Dr Sol J Goldstein, 254 Viewmount Ave, North York ON M6B 1V2; Dal'63; FRSH; DL(FAPA); FRCPC; Psy (Divorce). Hon Staff Psy, The Hospital For Sick Children; Asst Prof, University of Toronto; Langs: Yiddish; Hebrew; Spanish; Italian; (416)929-3287; ruchamagoldstein@gmail.com.

GOLDSTEIN, Stanley E; Medical Centre, 39 Drummond St W, Perth ON K7H 2J9; McG'60; DPsy; FRCPC; Psy. (613)264-0340; Fax. (613)264-9671.

GOLDSTEIN, Susan R; Yonge-Eglinton Med Centre, 204-2401 Yonge St, Toronto ON M4P 3H1; Tor'83; CCFP; FCFP; Assoc Staff, Mount Sinai Hospital; Asst Prof Faculty of Med, University of Toronto; (416)485-2222; Fax. (416)485-2276.

GOLDSTEIN, Warren C; York Med Medical Arts Centre, 411-250 Harding Blvd W, Richmond Hill ON L4C 9M7; Tor'80; BSc; Neur (Headache). Staff, Mackenzie Richmond Hill Hospital; Staff, Sunnybrook Health Sciences Centre; Lecturer, University of Toronto; Langs: Hebrew; (905)737-9677; Fax. (905)737-3030.

GOLDSTEIN, William; Univ of Ottawa Heart Institute, 40 Ruskin St, Ottawa ON K1Y 4W7; McG'69; FRCSC; GenSurg (Cardiac Surgery); Cardiovasc&ThorSurg. Att Staff, University of Ottawa Heart Institute; Asst Prof, University of Ottawa; Langs: English; French; (613)761-4253; Fax. (613)761-4388.

GOLDSTEIN-COLMAN, Lisa J; 412-250 Harding Blvd W, Richmond Hill ON L4C 9M7; McM'78; CCFP; FCFP; (905)737-7699; Fax. (905)737-5773.

GOLDSTINE, Ian J; Workers' Comp Board Of MB, 2F-333 Broadway, Winnipeg MB R3C 4W3; Man'79; CCFP; FCFP; Staff, Workers' Comp Board of MB.

GOLDSTUCK, Norman D; Dickinsfield Med Clinic, 22-9228 144 Ave NW, Edmonton AB T5E 6A3; Witwatersrand (South Africa)'72; (780)457-0797

GOLDSZMIDT, Eric; Mount Sinai Hosp, 1514-600 University Ave, Toronto ON M5G 1X5; McG'96; FRCPC; Anes. Staff, Mount Sinai Hospital; (416)586-5270; Fax. (416)586-8664; e.goldszmidt@utoronto.ca.

GOLDSZMIDT, Mark; London HSC-University Hosp, PO Box 5339 Stn B 339 Windermere Rd, London ON N6A 5A5; McG'96; FRCPC; IntMed. Staff, London Health Sciences Centre - University Hospital; Langs: Bilingual(English/French); (519)685-8500

GOLESIC, George F; Doctors Bldg, 200-955 Queen St E, Sault Ste. Marie ON P6A 2C3; Ott'80; FACS; FRCSC; Ophth (Oculo Plastic Surgery). Staff, Sault Area Hospital - Sault Ste Marie; (705)759-8387; Fax. (705)759-0562.

GOLEV, Dmitry S; McMaster Univ, MDCL 3101A-1280 Main St W, Hamilton ON L8S 4K1; (Russia (Federation))'99; DiagRad. Teach Staff, McMaster University.

GOLGER, Alexander; 1802 Avenue Rd, North York ON M5M 3Z1; McM'03; FRCSC; PlasSurg. (416)789-9979

GOLGOON, Michael S; Lakeshore Gen Hosp, 160 av Stillview, Pointe-Claire QC H9R 2Y2; Dominican Rep. (Dominican Republic)'96; Staff, Lakeshore General Hospital - Pointe Claire; (514)630-2225

GOLI, Harish; Hôpital régional Chaleur, 1750 Sunset Dr, Bathurst NB E2A 4L7; Osmania (India)'79; Staff, Hopital Regional Chaleur; (506)544-2412

GOLIGHER, Ewan C; Univ Hlth Network-Toronto Western Hosp, 2MCL 411Q-399 Bathurst St, Toronto ON M5T 2S8; UBC'07; FRCPC; IntMed; Critical Care Medicine. Staff, Toronto Western Hospital - University Health Network; (416)603-5800

GOLIN, Peter D; Collingwood Medical, 350-3150 54th Ave E, Vancouver BC V5S 1Z1; UBC'86; BSc; Staff, Burnaby Hospital; Langs: Russian; (604)435-3388; Fax. (604)433-2323.

GOLISKY, Bruno J; Huronia Med Centre, PO Box 790 Stn Main 103-240 Old Penetang Rd, Midland ON L4R 4P4; Tor'76; CCFP; FCFP; Family Medicine, Georgian Bay General Hospital - Midland; (705)526-7956

GOLISKY, Jeffrey M; Huronia Med Centre, PO Box 790 Stn Main 103-240 Old Penetang Rd, Midland ON L4R 4P4; Tor'04; CCFP; CCFP(E.M.); (705)526-7956

GOLLANT, Jerod; Mackenzie Richmond Hill Hosp, 10 Trench St, Richmond Hill ON L4C 4Z3; Tor'05; FRCPC; Anes. Staff, Mackenzie Richmond Hill Hospital; (905)883-1212

GOLLAPUDI, Shreyasi R; Villa Caritas, 16515 88 Ave NW, Edmonton AB T5R 0A4; Alb'07; FRCPC; Psy. Staff, University of Alberta Hospital; (780)342-6552

GOLLISH, Jeffrey D; Sunnybrook Holland Ortho Arthr, 315-43 Wellesley St E, Toronto ON M4Y 1H1; Tor'78; FRCSC; OrthSurg (Arthroplasty). Dir, Sunnybrook Health Sciences Centre - Holland Orthopaedic & Arthritic Centre; Asst Prof, University of Toronto; (416)967-8730; Fax. (416)967-8731.

GOLLOB, Michael H; Univ of Ottawa Heart Institute, H1285-40 Ruskin St, Ottawa ON K1Y 4W7; Tor'94; FRCPC; IntMed. Staff, University of Ottawa Heart Institute; (613)761-5016; Fax. (613)761-5060.

GOLOGAN, Adrian; SMBD Jewish Gen Hosp, G123-3755 ch Cote-Sainte-Cathe, Montreal QC H3T 1E2; Carol Davila (Romania)'96; Staff, Sir Mortimer B Davis Jewish General; (514)340-8222 x3767

GOLOGAN, Olguta-Ecaterina; CHUM-Hop Notre-Dame, 1560 rue Sherbrooke E, Montreal QC H2L 4M1; Carol Davila (Romania)'96; AnatPath (P.Q.). Staff, Centre Hospitalier l'Université de Montréal (CHUM) - Hôpital Notre-Dame; (514)890-8000 x23828

GOLOMBEK, Harvey; West Parry Sound Health Ctre, 6 Albert St, Parry Sound ON P2A 3A4; Tor'60; FRCPC; Psy. Staff, The Hospital For Sick Children; Staff, West Parry Sound Health Centre; Prof, University of Toronto; (705)746-4540

GOLONKA, Naomi R; PO Box 5604 Stn B, Victoria BC V8R 6S4; UBC'91; FRCSC; GenSurg; PedGenSurg. (250)590-9657

GOLOSINSKI, Agata A; 205-3301 24 Ave, Vernon BC V1T 9S8; Alb'95; BSc; FRCSC; ObstGyn. Ac Staff Privil, Vernon Jubilee Hospital; Langs: Polish; (250)542-0353; Fax. (250)558-9986.

GOLSHAN, Ashkan; Abbotsford Reg Hosp & Cancer C, 14-32900 Marshall Rd, Abbotsford BC V2S 0C2; Tor'01; CCFP; CCFP(E.M.); Staff, Abbotsford Regional Hospital & Cancer Centre; (604)851-4700

GOLTS, Marianna; Mount Sinai Hosp, 600 University Ave, Toronto ON M5G 1X5; Qns'03; FRCPC; Psy. Staff, Mount Sinai Hospital; (416)586-4800

GOLTZMAN, David; MUHC-Royal Victoria Hosp, H467-687 av des Pins O, Montreal QC H3A 1A1; McG'68; DABIM; CSPQ; BSc; FRCPC; IntMed (Endocrinology). principale Médecin, McGill University Health Centre - Royal Victoria Hospital; Chef Centre for Bone & Periodontal Research/Prof Med & Physiol, McGill University; Langs: Bilingual(French/English); (514)843-1632; Fax. (514)843-1712; david.goltzman@mcgill.ca.

GOLU, Tatiana; Guelph Gen Hosp, 115 Delhi St, Guelph ON N1E 4J4; Timisoara (Romania)'97; CCFP; Staff, Guelph General Hospital; Langs: Romanian; (519)837-6440

GOLUBOFF, Lanny; Humber River Reg Hosp-Church S, 200 Church St, Toronto ON M9N 1N8; Sask'66; FRCPC; IntMed (Endocrinology). Staff, Humber River Regional Hospital - Church Street Site; Ac Staff/Med Dir Nuclear Med, Humber River Regional Hospital - Finch Avenue Site; Staff Nuclear Med, Humber River Regional Hospital - Keele Street Site; (416)658-2162; Fax. (416)658-2178.

GOLUBOFF, Steven S; City Centre Fam Physicians, 100-514 Queen St, Saskatoon SK S7K 0M5; Sask'73; AB; CCFP; FCFP; Ac Staff, Saskatoon City Hospital; Ac Staff, Royal University Hospital; Associate Clin Prof, University of Saskatchewan; (306)244-3016; Fax. (306)244-4737; sgoluboff@ccfp.ca.

GOLUBOV, Jordan; Queen South Med Centre, 203-585 Queen St S, Kitchener ON N2G 4S4; Tor'85; ABIM; FRCPC; IntMed; Gastroent. Med Staff, St Mary's General Hospital; Med Staff, Grand River Hospital - Kitchener/Waterloo Health Centre; (519)744-9389; Fax. (519)744-8976.

GOLUBOVIC, Dragan; Harbour Landing Med Clinic, 4500 Gordon Rd, Regina SK S4W 0B7; (Other Foreign)'82; (306)545-2888; Fax. (306)545-2844.

GOLUCH, Richard J; Sudbury Reg Hosp-Laurentian S, 41 Ramsey Lake Rd, Sudbury ON P3E 5J1; McM'83; FRCPC; IntMed (Dialysis); Nephrol. Ac Staff, Health Sciences North-Laurentian Site; Court Staff, Health Sciences North - Memorial Site; (705)523-7007; Fax. (705)523-7161.

GOMBERG, Charles L; 604-5858 ch de la Cote-des-Nei, Montreal QC H3S 1Z1; Tulane(LA) (USA)'52; FRCPC; IntMed. Clin Physician, Sir Mortimer B Davis Jewish General; McGill University; Langs: Bilingual(English/French); (514)733-8072; Fax. (514)273-4045.

GOMEL, Victor; Women's Health Centre, D415-4500 Oak St, Vancouver BC V6H 3N1; Istanbul (Turkey)'58; FACOG; FRCSC; ObstGyn (Endoscopy). Ac Staff, BC Women's Hospital & Health Centre; Prof ObstGyn, University of British Columbia; Langs: French; Italian; Spanish; Turkish; (604)875-2588; Fax. (604)224-5015; victorgomel@cs.com.

GOMES, Anthony J; 1921 10 Ave S, Lethbridge AB T1K 0B8; Alb'88; FRCSC; GenSurg (Gastroenterology). Staff, Chinook Regional Hospital; (403)380-4777; Fax. (403)380-3416.

GOMES, David R; Strathroy Middlesex Gen Hosp, 318A-395 Carrie St, Strathroy ON N7G 3C9; Wes'86; FRCPC; IntMed (Cardiology). Staff, Strathroy Middlesex General Hospital - Middlesex Hospital Alliance; Langs: Portuguese; (519)245-5180; Fax. (519)245-3391.

GOMEZ, E G Enrique; 301 Mitchell St, Port Colborne ON L3K 1Y7; Granada (Spain)'57; Court Staff, Niagara Health System - Port Colborne General Site; Med Dir, Northland Pointe Home for the Aged; Langs: Spanish; (905)835-1189; Fax. (905)835-1180.

GOMEZ, Eva; Active Care Med Group, 1108 Klondike Rd, Kanata ON K2K 0G1; Palacky (Czech Republic)'68; Langs: Czech; French; (613)254-9777

GOMEZ, Jose-Daniel; St Baniface Gen Hosp, 409 Tache Ave, Winnipeg MB R2H 2A6; Pontificia (Colombia)'88; FRCPC; AnatPath. Staff, St Boniface General Hospital; Langs: Spanish; (204)233-8563

GOMEZ, Jose-Luis; CHUQ-Ctr Hosp Univ Laval, 2705 boul Laurier, Quebec QC G1V 4G2; Cuyo (Argentina)'79; Ac Staff Med & Clin Research Staff, Centre Hospitalier Universitaire de Quebec-CHUL; (418)654-2291; Fax. (418)654-2732; jose.gomez@crchul.ulaval.ca.

GOMEZ-CASTANO, Nathali; Clinique Med Quyon, A-1111 rue de Clarendon, Quyon QC J0X 2V0; (Colombia)'02; CCFP; Staff, CSSS du Pontiac; Staff, Pontiac Hospital Centre; (819)458-2397

GOMEZ-JIMENEZ, Alfonso; 201-275 rue Main, Bathurst NB E2A 1A9; Cartagena (Colombia)'84; FRCSC; PlasSurg (Micro Surgery). Staff, Hopital Regional Chaleur; Langs: Spanish; English; (506)547-0899; Fax. (506)547-0182.

GOMEZ LEMUS, Jose A; London HSC-University Hosp, PO Box 5339 Stn B 399 Windermere Rd, London ON N6A 5A5; Pontificia (Colombia)'91; FRCPC; AnatPath. Staff, London Health Sciences Centre - University Hospital; Langs: Spanish; (519)685-8500 x32956; Fax. (519)663-2930.

GOMIDE, Jose G S; Brock Comm Hlth Centre, PO Box 69 64 Camreon St E, Cannington ON L0E 1E0; 80Niterol (Brazil)'78; Langs: Portuguese; (705)432-3388; Fax. (705)432-3389.

GOMOLIN, Julius E S; SMBD Jewish Gen Hosp, 3755 ch Cote-Ste-Catherine, Montreal QC H3T 1E2; McG'77; DABOph; FRCSC; Ophth (Retinal Disease). Ac Staff, Sir Mortimer B Davis Jewish General; Assoc Prof Retina Teaching, McGill University; Langs: French; Yiddish; Hebrew; (514)340-8280; Fax. (514)340-8215.

GOMORI, Andrew J; Medical Arts Bldg, 1516-233 Kennedy St, Winnipeg MB R3C 3J5; Man'68; MD; FAAN; BSc; FRCPC; Neur (Multiple Sclerosis). Ac Staff, Health Sciences Centre; Consultant, St Boniface General Hospital; Assoc Prof, University of Manitoba; Langs: Hungarian; (204)942-7815; Fax. (204)942-5329; agomori@cc.umanitoba.ca.

GOMPERTS, Natalie R; Cardiomatters, 11-398 Steeles Ave W, Thornhill ON L4J 6X3; Wes'02; FRCPC; IntMed; Cardiol. Staff, Sunnybrook Health Sciences Centre; (905)881-0334

GONABADY NAMADON, Mojdeh; Ocean Walk Med Centre, 1884 Marine Dr, West Vancouver BC V7V 1J6; Shahid Beheshti (Iran)'96; Staff, Ocean Walk Medical Centre; Langs: Farsi; (604)925-1884; Fax. (604)922-3591.

GONCALVES, Jose L; 146 Dawson Ave, Penticton BC V2A 6Y9; UBC'92; FRCSC; ObstGyn (Urogynecology). (250)492-4015; drjgoncalves@gmail.com.

GONCALVES, M Joana; 308-622 College St, Toronto ON M6G 1B6; Lisbon (Portugal)'75; Langs: Portuguese; Spanish; (416)533-8486; Fax. (416)533-0114.

GONDER, John R; St Joseph's Hlth Care, PO Box 5777 Stn B 268 Grosvenor St, London ON N6A 4V2; Wes'75; FRCSC; Ophth (Vitreo Retina). Staff, London Health Sciences Centre - Victoria Campus; Staff, St Joseph's Hospital - St Joseph's Health Care; Associate Clin Prof, University of Western Ontario; (519)685-8206

GONOR, Saul E; Medical Arts Bldg, 537-750 Spadina Cres E, Saskatoon SK S7K 3H3; Sask'78; FRCSC; Urol. Staff, Royal University Hospital; Staff, St Paul's Hospital (Grey Nuns) of Saskatoon; (306)653-3255; Fax. (306)653-4386.

GONSALVES, Carol; Civic Parkdale Clinic, 467-737 Parkdale Ave, Ottawa ON K1Y 1J8; Ott'00; FRCPC; IntMed (Thromboembolism); Hem. (613)798-5555 x16992

GONSALVES, Charles G; One Med Place, 102-20 Wynford Dr, North York ON M3C 1J4; Tor'59; FRCPC; DiagRad. (416)441-3344; Fax. (416)441-1471.

GONSALVES, Patrick M; Patient Networks, 157 Yonge St, Toronto ON M5C 1X7; Tor'06; CCFP; Staff, Toronto Western Hospital - University Health Network; (416)362-8822

GONSALVES, Violet; 34 Kimberwick Cres, Ottawa ON K1V 0W6; Madras (India)'70; CCFP; FCFP; (613)737-4801

GONSALVEZ, Antony K; Campbell Clinic, 430 Mayor Magrath Dr S, Lethbridge AB T1J 3M1; (India)'99; (403)328-8101; Fax. (403)328-8150.

GONSER, Randal J; 589 West Gore St, Stratford ON N5A 1L4; Wes'83; FRCSC; GenSurg; VascSurg. Ac Staff, Stratford General Hospital - Huron Perth Healthcare Alliance; Staff Consultant, St Marys Memorial Hospital - Huron Perth Healthcare Alliance; (519)273-4100; Fax. (519)273-3208.

GONSKA, Tanja Y; The Hosp for Sick Children, 555 University Ave, Toronto ON M5G 1X8; (Germany)'99; Staff, The Hospital For Sick Children; (416)813-1500

GONTHIER, Danielle; Clin de Med Fam de la Malbaie, 515 rue Saint-Etienne, La Malbaie QC G5A 1W7; Laval'92; (418)665-2533; Fax. (418)665-7766.

GONTHIER, Genevieve; Hotel-Dieu de Levis, 143 rue Wolfe, Levis QC G6V 3Z1; Laval'05; IntMed. Staff, Hôtel-Dieu de Lévis; (418)835-7121; Fax. (418)835-7104.

GONTHIER, Pierre; Clinique de Med Familiale, 101 rue Lavoie, Rimouski QC G5L 5Y2; Laval'77; LMCC; Langs: Bilingual(French/English); (418)723-5272; Fax. (418)725-2030.

GONU, Crystal J; Lennox & Addington Gen Hosp, 8 Richmond Dr, Napanee ON K7R 2Z4; Saba (Netherlands Antilles)'10; Staff, Lennox & Addington County General Hospital.

GONZALES, Sean; Hys Med Centre, 710-11010 101 St NW, Edmonton AB T5H 4B9; McM'06; PhysMed&Rehab. (780)453-5255; Fax. (780)453-9099.

GONZALEZ, Anne V; MUHC-Montreal Chest Institute, K1 09-3650 rue Saint-Urbain, Montreal QC H2X 2P4; McG'98; FRCPC; IntMed; Critical Care Medicine; Respir. Staff, McGill University Health Centre - Montreal Chest Institute; (514)934-1934 x32150; Fax. (514)843-2083.

GONZALEZ, Armando; Markham College Med Clinic, 205-474 College St, Toronto ON M6G 1A4; Yucatan (Mexico)'67; Langs: Italian; Portuguese; Spanish; (416)961-8186

GONZALEZ, Hernan; Ellerslie Medicentre, 102-9404 Ellerslie Rd SW, Edmonton AB T6X 0K6; Casilla University (Chile)'66; FRCPC; Peds (Neonatology). Langs: Spanish; French; (780)466-8064; Fax. (780)466-8095; hgonzl@gmail.com.

GONZALEZ, Mariel; Centre Med Jolibourg, 1271 boul Jolibourg, Laval QC H7Y 1Z8; Mon'89; MSc(Physiol.); Médecin Centre EPIC, Institut de Cardiologie de Montréal; Physician, Family-Programmes, CLSC des Mille-Iles; Langs: Spanish; English; (450)689-2424

GONZALEZ, Yolanda; GMF de Grand-Mere, 200-1050 8e rue, Grand-Mere QC G9T 4L4; San Carlos (Guatemala)'82; CCFP; Staff, Centre Lafleche Grand-Mere; Staff, URFI Centre Lafteche; Langs: Spanish; English; (819)538-5068; Fax. (819)538-7257.

GONZALEZ-ALMEYDA, Roberto; Family Med Village, 206-197 Talbot St W, Leamington ON N8H 1N8; Havana (Cuba)'94; CCFP; Staff, Leamington District Memorial Hospital; Langs: Spanish; (519)322-1300

GONZALEZ-AMAYA, Gonzalo; Clinique Sante Jacques-Cartier, 200-1815 rue King O, Sherbrooke QC J1J 2E3; (Mexico)'70; CSPQ; AB; FRCSC; GenSurg (Breast Surgery). Ac Staff, Centre Hospitalier Universitaire de Sherbrooke-Hôpital Hôtel-Dieu; Consultant, Institute of Geriatric de l'Estrie; Clin Prof Surg, Universite de Sherbrooke; Langs: Spanish; French; (819)569-2715; Fax. (819)565-7780.

GONZALEZ HERNANDEZ, Roberto L; Capt William Jackman Mem Hosp, 410 Booth Ave, Labrador City NL A2V 2K1; Habana (Cuba)'90; Staff, Captain William Jackman Memorial Hospital; (709)944-2632

GONZALEZ HERRERA, Luis A; CSSS de Rimouski-Neigette, CP 3150 Succ A 150 av Rouleau, Rimouski QC G5L 5T1; Colombia (USA)'88; Neur (P.Q.). Staff Neur, Hôpital Regional Rimouski; Langs: Spanish; English; (418)723-7851 x7492; calimachula@yahoo.com.

GONZALEZ LEJARZA, Rogelio; Cambridge Mem Hosp, 700 Coronation Blvd, Cambridge ON N1R 3G2; Guadalajara (Mexico)'97; Staff, Cambridge Memorial Hospital; (519)621-2330

GONZALEZ LORENZO, Anabel; Clin Med Mirabel, CP 1059 Succ Saint-Janvier 13714 boul Cure-Labelle, Mirabel QC J7J 1A1; (Cuba)'95; CCFP; Staff, Centre Hospitalier d'Argenteuil; (450)435-7666; Fax. (450)435-1716.

GONZALEZ-PINO, Fernando; Victoria Gen Hosp, 6-2340 Pembina Hwy, Winnipeg MB R3T 2E8; Buenos Aires (Argentina)'82; FRCPC; Psy. Staff, Victoria General Hospital; (204)269-3570

GONZALEZ-PORRAS, Maria C; Niagara H System-Welland Site, 65 Third St, Welland ON L3B 4W6; Bogota (Colombia)'91; FRCPC; Anes. Staff, Niagara Health System - Welland Hospital Site; Langs: Spanish; (905)732-6111

GONZALEZ PUPO, Rafael; St Michael's Hosp, 30 Bond St, Toronto ON M5B 1W8; (Cuba)'94; Staff, The Hospital For Sick Children; (416)813-6420

GONZALEZ-ROMERO, Luis M; Links Clinic, 104-11910 111 Ave NW, Edmonton AB T5G 3G6; National (Mexico)'71; Staff, Royal Alexandra Hospital; (780)454-0351; Fax. (780)452-6767.

GONZALEZ-ROMULUS, Marie-Christina; 510-1200 Burrard St, Vancouver BC V6Z 2C7; Laval'09; CCFP.

GOO, Sharon; Valley Med Imaging, 102-32475 Simon Ave, Abbotsford BC V2T 5E3; Alb'05; FRCPC; DiagRad. (604)859-8998

GOOBIE, Paul W A; Professional Arts Bldg, 526-100 Arden St, Moncton NB E1C 4B7; Tor'90; BSc; FRCSC; GenSurg (Trauma). Chief Surg, The Moncton Hospital; Clin Instructor, Dalhousie University; (506)383-6083; Fax. (506)383-6042; dr.paul.goobie@horizonnb.ca.

GOOBIE, Sharan L; London HSC-Victoria Hosp, PO Box 5010 Stn B 800 Commissioners Rd E, London ON N6A 5W9; Dal'03; FRCPC; MedGenetics. Staff, London Health Sciences Centre - Victoria Campus; (519)685-8140

GOOCH, Christopher E; Chisel Peak Med Clinic, PO Box 2769 417 10 Ave, Invermere BC V0A 1K0; Qns'99; (250)341-6900; Fax. (250)341-3226.

GOOCH, Peter A; 200-55 Victoria Rd, Nanaimo BC V9R 5N9; Cape Town (South Africa)'75; MB ChB; (250)716-9911

GOOD, Angela M; St Mary's Gen Hosp, 911 Queens Blvd, Kitchener ON N2M 1B2; Qns'04; CCFP; CCFP(E.M.); Staff, St Mary's General Hospital; (519)744-3311

GOOD, David J; Richardson Laboratory, 201C-88 Stuart St, Kingston ON K7L 3N6; Alb'03; FRCPC; HemPath. Chief Hematopathology Dept Pathology & Molecular Med, Kingston General Hospital; (613)533-2823; Fax. (613)533-2907.

GOOD, H Scott; Royal Victoria Hosp, 201 Georgian Dr, Barrie ON L4M 6M2; Sask'93; FRCPC; DiagRad. Staff, Royal Victoria Regional Health Centre; (705)728-9090; Fax. (705)739-5629.

GOOD, Richard I S; Queen Elizabeth II HSC-Halifax, 1796 Summer St, Halifax NS B3H 3A7; (Other Foreign)'00; MB BS; Staff, Queen Elizabeth II Health Sciences Centre - Halifax Infirmary Site.

GOODACRE, Margaret E; 280 Queenston Rd, Hamilton ON L8K 1H1; Wes'05; CCFP; (905)547-0508; Fax. (905)547-6865.

GOODALE, Natalie N; City of Lakes Family Hlth Team, C-960 Notre Dame Ave, Sudbury ON P3A 2T4; Ott'01; CCFP; Langs: Bilingual(English/French); (705)560-1018; Fax. (705)566-7617.

GOODALL, Douglas J; 541 Eglinton Ave E, Toronto ON M4P 1N7; Tor'73; BSc; CCFP; FCFP; Consultant, Bloorview Hugh McMillan Rehabilitation; Consultant, Owens-Corning Fiberglass; (416)487-2442; Fax. (416)487-2508.

GOODALL, John C; Smyth Med Centre, 216-1929 Russell Rd, Ottawa ON K1G 4G3; Qns'70; DABD; FRCPC; IntMed (Pediatric Dermatology); Derm. Staff, The Ottawa Hospital - Civic Campus; Asst Prof Canadian Armed Forces, Montfort Hospital; Staff, Children's Hospital of Eastern Ontario (CHEO); Staff Rehabliliitaion Centre, The Ottawa Hospital - General Campus; Asst Prof, University of Ottawa; Langs: Bilingual(English/French); (613)731-2226; Fax. (613)731-5163.

GOODALL, R Lorne; Townsite Med Clinic, 512 Campbell St, Nanaimo BC V9R 3H1; UBC'88; Dip SportMed(SportMed); CCFP; Staff, Nanaimo Regional General Hospital; (250)753-5665; Fax. (250)755-1408.

GOODALL, Robert J; 161 Bridge St W, Belleville ON K8P 1K2; McM'74; Ac Staff, QHC Belleville General; (613)962-6000

GOODALL, Simon C P; 170 Elgin N PO Box 898 Stn Main, Mount Forest ON N0G 2L0; Oxford (England)'73; Staff, North Wellington Health Care - Louise Marshall Hospital; (519)323-1422; Fax. (519)323-3603.

GOODARZI, Masoud; Niagara H System-G Niagara, 5546 Portage Rd, Niagara Falls ON L2E 6X2; (Russia (Federation))'96; FRCPC; IntMed. Staff, Niagara Health System - Greater Niagara General Site; Langs: Farsi; Tagalog; (905)378-4647

GOODBAUM, Mark; North Med Centre, 201-7131 Bathurst St, Thornhill ON L4J 7Z1; Tor'80; Ac Staff, North York General Hospital; (905)771-1778; Fax. (905)771-9833.

GOODCHILD, Steven R; Medical-Dental Bldg, 304-1120 Yates St, Victoria BC V8V 3M9; UBC'87; (250)383-3473; Fax. (250)383-3713.

GOODE, J Eric; 300-393 First St, Collingwood ON L9Y 1B3; Tor'77; FRCPC; IntMed; Cardiol. Staff Med & Cardiology, Collingwood General & Marine Hospital; Ac Staff, Rouge Valley Health System - Centenary Health Centre Site; Staff Cardiologist, Southlake Regional Health Centre; (705)444-1648; collingwoodcardiology@rogers.com.

GOODEN, Everton A; Leslie Med Centre, 303-4800 Leslie St, North York ON M2J 2K9; Tor'96; BSc; FRCSC; Otol (Otolaryngology). Ac Staff, North York General Hospital; Ac Staff, Sunnybrook Health Sciences Centre; Court Staff, Toronto East General Hospital Inc; Instructor Otol, University of Toronto; (416)499-5558; Fax. (416)499-9392; evertongooden@hotmail.com.

GOODEN, Heather M; Crystal Ridge Family Med Clin, 4-55 Wheatland Trail, Strathmore AB T1P 1R7; Man'06; CCFP; (403)934-5911; Fax. (403)934-6672.

GOODERHAM, Melinda J; Skin Centre for Dermatology, 743 Lansdowne St W, Peterborough ON K9J 1Z2; Wes'99; FRCPC; Derm. (705)775-7546; Fax. (705)775-3376.

GOODERHAM, Virginia A; Victoria Community Hlth Co, 547 Michigan St, Victoria BC V8V 1S5; McM'99; BHScPT; CCFP; (205)388-6811

GOODFELLOW, A Frank; Parrtown Place, 6A-28 King St, Saint John NB E2L 1G3; Dal'71; ABOph; FRCSC; Ophth. Ac Staff, St Joseph's Hospital; Ac Staff, Saint John Regional Hospital; (506)634-1812; Fax. (506)633-0577.

GOODFELLOW, Alfred; Dr Hugh Twomey Hlth Care Ctr, PO Box 250 25 Twomey Dr, Botwood NL A0H 1E0; Mem'09; CCFP; Staff, Dr Hugh Twomey Health Care Centre; (709)257-2999; Fax. (709)257-4687.

GOODFELLOW, Anne F; Lynde Centre for Dermatology, 3 Ovida Blvd, Markham ON L3P 7N8; Tor'04; CCFP; (905)471-5063; Fax. (905)472-6343; agoodfellow@rogers.com.

GOODFELLOW, Mary E; Parrtown Place, 3B-28 King St, Saint John NB E2L 1G3; Dal'71; CCFP; FCFP; Ac Staff, St Joseph's Hospital; Ac Staff, Saint John Regional Hospital; Lecturer, Dalhousie University; (506)634-7772; Fax. (506)634-7101.

GOODGE, John; Brookdale Family Clinic, 304 Bellevue St, Peterborough ON K9H 5G1; Wes'74; (705)743-7101; Fax. (705)743-7104.

GOODHART, David M; Foothills Med Centre, C849-1403 29 St NW, Calgary AB T2N 2T9; Alb'87; FRCPC; IntMed; Cardiol. Staff, Foothills Medical Centre; (403)944-8491; Fax. (403)283-0744.

GOODHART, Joseph M; 6604 131 St NW, Edmonton AB T6H 3Y5; Durham (England)'61; MB BS; MRC; DObstRCOG; FRCPC; IntMed (Gastroenterology). Ac Staff, Royal Alexandra Hospital; Assoc Prof, University of Alberta.

GOODHEW, John E; 2F-491 Church St, Toronto ON M4Y 2C6; Dal'90; BSc; (416)463-6929; Fax. (416)463-6577.

GOODHEW, Rick T; Talbot Med Centre, 50-1063 Talbot St, St Thomas ON N5P 1G4; Tor'93; CCFP; FCFP; Ac Staff, St Thomas Elgin General Hospital; (519)631-8460; Fax. (519)631-2633.

GOODHUE, Angelique; Mental Health & Addictions, 526 Wentworth St, Nanaimo BC V9R 3E4; Texas((USA)'95; FRCPC; Psy. Staff, Nanaimo Regional General Hospital; (250)740-6998

GOODINE, C William; 1-11300 130 Rte, Waterville Carleton Co NB E7P 0A4; Dal'81; FRCSC; Ophth. Staff, Upper River Valley Hospital - Waterville; (506)375-4181; Fax. (506)375-4183.

GOODINE, Frederick S; Woodstock Med Clinic, 5-110 Chapel St, Woodstock NB E7M 1H1; Dal'59; CCFP; FCFP; Preceptor, Dalhousie University; (506)328-3154; Fax. (506)328-8400.

GOODINE, Grant A D; 491 Main St PO Box 40, Lawrencetown NS B0S 1M0; Dal'84; (902)584-3445; Fax. (902)584-3432.

GOODING, Geoffrey T; Port Arthur Health Centre Inc, 194 Court St N, Thunder Bay ON P7A 4V7; London (England)'58; MRCS; LRCP; MRCP(London); MB BS(London); FRCPC; IntMed (Diagnostic Ultrasound). Ac Staff, Thunder Bay Regional Health Sciences Centre; Langs: Creole; (807)346-1000; Fax. (807)346-6206.

GOODING, John T; Port Arthur Health Centre Inc, 194 Court St N, Thunder Bay ON P7A 4V7; McG'54; FACS; BSc; GenSurg (Vascular Surgery). Court Staff, Thunder Bay Regional Health Sciences Centre Port-Arthur; (807)346-1000; Fax. (807)346-6206.

GOODING, Vivian J; 4A-505 23rd St E, Saskatoon SK S7K 4K7; Sask'76; CCFP; FCFP; Ac Staff Family Med, Saskatoon City Hospital; (306)242-5808; Fax. (306)242-5919.

GOODIS, Leslie; The Two Hundred, 302-200 St Clair Ave W, Toronto ON M4V 1R1; McG'83; FRCPC; Peds. (416)925-7890; Fax. (416)925-1655.

GOODISON, Karin L; PO Box 2155, Rossland BC V0G 1Y0; Alb'94; Staff, Forensic Psychiatric Hospital; (250)362-5999; kgoodison@forensic.bc.ca.

GOODMAN, Daniel N F; MRI/CT Imaging Centre, 300 Harwood Ave S, Ajax ON L1S 2J1; Wes'89; FRCPC; DiagRad. (905)426-8976; Fax. (905)426-7843.

GOODMAN, Earl L; 205-7031 Westminster Hwy, Richmond BC V6X 1A3; Man'69; Staff/Member, Richmond Hospital; (604)273-0538; Fax. (604)273-5817.

GOODMAN, Jesse B; Summerville Family Health Team, 5F-101 Queensway W, Mississauga ON L5B 2P7; Cal'78; Ac Staff, St Joseph's Health Centre; Ac Staff, Trillium Health Centre - Mississauga; (905)272-9700

GOODMAN, Joseph; Lonsdale Med Dental Bldg, 108-1940 Lonsdale Ave, North Vancouver BC V7M 2K2; Cal'87; (604)987-0917; Fax. (604)987-7624.

GOODMAN, Marni A; Birchwood Prof Centre, 24 Kentucky Crt, New Minas NS B4N 4N2; Tor'01; BSc; CCFP; Langs: English; French; (902)681-1080; Fax. (902)681-0600.

GOODMAN, Melvin P; North Toronto Med Bldg, 112-250 Lawrence Ave W, Toronto ON M5M 1B2; Tor'74; CCFP; FCFP; Att Staff, Toronto Rehabilitation Institute - University Centre; Court Staff, Sunnybrook Health Sciences Centre; (416)789-5331; Fax. (416)789-4014; mel.goodman@sympatico.ca.

GOODMAN, Robert L; London HSC-University Hosp, PO Box 5339 Stn B B6 118-339 Winderemere Rd, London ON N6A 5A5; Sask'81; FRCSC; GenSurg; Cardiovasc&ThorSurg. Staff, London Health Sciences Centre - University Hospital; Langs: Bilingual(English/French); (519)685-8300

GOODMAN, Rusty C J; Markham Stouffville Health Ctr, 403-377 Church St, Markham ON L6B 1A1; McG'84; BSc; MDCM; FRCPC; IntMed; Rheum. Staff, Markham Stouffville Hospital; (905)472-7147; Fax. (905)472-6943.

GOODMAN, Saul H; 304-9200 Mary St, Chilliwack BC V2P 4H6; Dal'92; FRCSC; Urol. (604)792-6512; Fax. (604)792-6156.

GOODMAN, Shaun G; St Michael's Hosp, 6 034Q-30 Bond St, Toronto ON M5B 1W8; McM'87; FRCPC; IntMed; Cardiol. Assoc Head Cardiol/Prof Med, St Michael's Hospital; Consultant, Canadian Heart Research Centre; Prof, University of Toronto; (416)864-5722; Fax. (416)864-5407; goodmans@smh.ca.

GOODMAN, Trisha A; Phoenix Med Centre, 106-2155 10th Ave, Prince George BC V2M 5J6; UBC'09; CCFP; (250)563-5111

GOODRIDGE, Alan E; Health Sciences Centre, 300 Prince Philip Dr, St. John's NL A1B 3V6; Mem'79; FRCPC; Neur (Electromyography). Neurologist, Health Sciences Centre; Assoc Prof Med(Neurol)/Chair Clinical Disciplines Med (Acting), Memorial University Of Newfoundland; (709)777-6737; Fax. (709)777-6656; agoodrid@mun.ca.

GOODROW, Gwendolyn J; Isis Regional Fertility Centre, 2180 Meadowvale Blvd, Mississauga ON L5N 5S3; Tor'96; FACOG; FRCSC; ObstGyn (Reproductive Endocrinology & Infertility). Staff, Hamilton Health Sciences Centre - McMaster University Medical Centre; (905)816-9822; Fax. (905)816-9833.

GOODWIN, Beverly J; Lanark Country Mental Health, A2-88 Cornelia St W, Smiths Falls ON K7A 5K9; Qns'87; FRCPC; Psy;CCFP; Court Staff, Almonte General Hospital; Court Staff, Carleton Place & District Memorial Hospital; Court Staff, Perth & Smiths Falls District Hospital - Smiths Falls Site; Assoc Staff, Royal Ottawa Mental Health Centre - Royal Ottawa Health Care Group; Asst Prof Adjunct Dept of Psy, Queen's University; (613)283-2170; Fax. (613)283-9018.

GOODWIN, D Michael; Stamford Med Centre, 201-4256 Portage Rd, Niagara Falls ON L2E 6A4; Belfast (Ireland)'70; Ac Staff, Niagara Health System - Greater Niagara General Site; (905)357-1661

GOODWIN, Grainne M; 1-315 Avenue Rd, Toronto ON M4V 2H2; Dublin (Ireland)'78; FRCPC; Psy. Staff, St Michael's Hospital; Teacher, University of Toronto; (416)921-1094

GOODWIN, Janice R; Woodlawn Med Clinic, 92 Main St, Dartmouth NS B2X 1R5; McM'91; (902)434-1500

GOODWIN, Jodi L; Postgraduate Med Education, MDCL 3101A-1280 Main St W, Hamilton ON L8S 4K1; Wes'06; IntMed.

GOODWIN, John L; Queen Elizabeth Hosp, PO Box 6600 Stn Central 60 Riverside Dr, Charlottetown PE C1A 8T5; Dal'80; FRCPC; DiagRad. Staff, Queen Elizabeth Hospital; (902)894-2111; Fax. (902)894-2276.

GOODWIN, Michael; 984 Broadway Ave W PO Box 53598 Rpo West Broadway, Vancouver BC V5Z 4M6; UBC'04; FRCSC; GenSurg. General Surgery, Fort St John Hospital & Health Centre; (778)228-2722

GOODWIN, Pamela J; Mount Sinai Hosp, 1284-600 University Ave, Toronto ON M5G 1X5; Ott'79; ABIM; FRCPC; IntMed; MedOncol. Dir Marvelle Koffler Breast Centre, Mount Sinai Hospital; Prof Med, University of Toronto; (416)586-8605; Fax. (416)586-8659; pgoodwin@mtsinai.on.ca.

GOODWIN, Rachel; The Ottawa Hosp-Gen Campus, 501 Smyth Rd, Ottawa ON K1H 8L6; Ott'03; FRCPC; IntMed; MedOncol. Staff, The Ottawa Hospital - General Campus; (613)737-7700; Fax. (613)247-3532.

GOODWIN, Susan E B; Henderson Prof Arts Bldg, 662 Concession St, Hamilton ON L8V 1B8; Tor'75; FRCP; FRCPC; IntMed; Neur. Ac Staff, St Joseph's Healthcare - Charlton Campus; Asst Prof, McMaster University; (905)387-1178; Fax. (905)387-6115.

GOODYEAR, Christopher P; Priestman Centre, 207-565 Priestman St, Fredericton NB E3B 5X8; Mem'93; FRCSC; GenSurg. (506)458-0270; Fax. (506)457-4705.

GOODYEAR, Emilie; Hôpital Ste-Justine, 3175 ch cote-Sainte-Catherine, Montreal QC H3T 1C5; McG'05; FRCSC; Ophth. Staff, Hôpital Ste-Justine; (514)345-4931

GOODYEAR, Jillian D; UNB Student Services Center, 26 Bailey Dr, Fredericton NB E3B 5A3; Mem'96; CCFP; (506)453-4837

GOODYEAR, Lisa; Dr Charles A Janeway Child Hc, 300 Prince Philip Dr, St. John's NL A1B 3V6; Mem'01; FRCPC; Peds; PedHemaOncol. Staff, Janeway Children's Health & Rehabilitation Centre; (709)777-4303

GOODYEAR, M Dawn; Foothills Medical Centre, 603 ST-1403 29 St NW, Calgary AB T2N 2T9; Mem'05; FRCPC; IntMed; Hem. Staff, Foothills Medical Centre; (403)944-3265; Fax. (403)944-8352.

GOODYER, Paul R; MUHC-Montreal Children's Hosp, 2300 rue Tupper, Montreal QC H3H 1P3; Rochester(NY) (USA)'72; Nephrol (P.Q.) (Pediatric Nephrology). Staff, McGill University Health Centre - Montreal Children's Hospital; Prof, McGill University; (514)934-4461; Fax. (514)934-4359.

GOOI, Adrian C C; Manitoba Clinic, 790 Sherbrook St, Winnipeg MB R3A 1M3; Wes'04; FRCSC; Otol. Staff, Health Sciences Centre.

GOOI, Patrick C H; Credit Valley Eyecare, 3200 Erin Mills Parkway, Mississauga ON L5L 1W8; Tor'06; Ophth. (905)820-3937

GOOI, Teong Hean; Westwood Clinic, 3320 Portage Ave, Winnipeg MB R3K 0Z1; Manchester (England)'77; MB ChB; (204)832-1363; Fax. (204)896-3445.

GOOI, Teong Lam; Manitoba Clinic, 790 Sherbrook St, Winnipeg MB R3A 1M3; Manchester (England)'78; MB ChB; FRCSC; Ophth (Cataract Surgery). Staff Ophth, Misericordia Health Centre; Asst Prof, University of Manitoba; (204)788-5766; Fax. (204)774-5772.

GOOJHA, Ciaran; Northmount Med Centre, 203-145 13th St E, North Vancouver BC V7L 2L4; (Ireland)'04; MB BCh; BAO; FRCSC; ObstGyn (Endoscopy). (604)982-9139

GOOJHA, Devdass; Westgate Med Clinic, 18-2410 22nd St W, Saskatoon SK S7M 5S6; RCS (Ireland)'75; LRCP; LRCPSI; Medical Staff, Moose Jaw Union Hospital; Med Staff Assoc, Spiritwood & District Health Complex; Med Staff, Saskatoon Health Region; Langs: French; (306)384-7800; Fax. (306)384-7550.

GOOLAM HUSSAIN, M Rashid; The Collonde Bldg, 208-3024 Hurontario St, Mississauga ON L5B 4M4; Witwatersrand (South Africa)'77; MB ChB; DABSM; CCFP; FCFP; Ac Staff, The Credit Valley Hospital; Teacher, Toronto General Hospital - UHN; Med Dir, TRI Hospital Sleep Lab. West; Lecturer, University of Toronto; (905)566-1010; Fax. (905)566-0440.

GOONETILLAKE, Piyanthi; 120-330 Bronte St S, Milton ON L9T 7X1; Ceykon (Sri Lanka)'00; CCFP; (905)693-1314; Fax. (905)693-8892.

GOORAH, Berenice; Hop du Sacre-Coeur de Mtl, G2010-5400 boul Gouin O, Montreal QC H4J 1C5; McG'05; FRCSC; ObstGyn. Staff, Hôpital du Sacre-Coeur de Montréal; (514)338-2222

GOOSEN, Hilgard; Family Health Clinic, PO Box 4127 Stn Main, Ponoka AB T4J 1R5; Orange Free (South Africa)'96; MB ChB; (403)783-5305; Fax. (403)783-8722.

GOOSSEN, Christine; Anaesthesia Associates, 439 Park St, Kitchener ON N2G 1N4; Qns'88; FRCPC; Anes. Staff, Health Sciences North-Laurentian Site; (519)744-7361

GOOSSEN, Marvin J H; The Brandon Clinic, 620 Dennis St, Brandon MB R7A 5E7; Man'84; FRCSC; GenSurg. (204)728-4440

GOOSSEN, Randolph B; Dr Randolph Goossen Med Corp, 212 Kingston Row, Winnipeg MB R2M 0T4; Man'81; FRCPC; Psy;CCFP; Med Dir of WRHA, Community Mental Health; Asst Prof Psy/Med Dir Community Mental Hlth, University of Manitoba; (204)940-2421; Fax. (204)940-6620.

GOPAL, Vanita; 629 Markham Rd, Scarborough ON M1H 2A4; Ott'01; CCFP; Staff, Toronto Rehabilitation Institute - University Centre; (416)642-9445

GOPALAN, Bhaskar S; Queensway-Carleton Hosp, 3045 Baseline Rd, Nepean ON K2H 8P4; Wes'01; CCFP; CCFP(E.M.); Staff, Queensway Carleton Hospital; (613)721-2000

GOPAUL, Darindra D; Grand River Reg Cancer Ctr, PO Box 9056 Stn C 835 King St W, Kitchener ON N2G 1G3; Tor'96; FRCPC; RadOncol. (519)749-4380; Fax. (519)749-4378; darin.gopaul@grhosp.on.ca.

GOPIDASAN, Balaji; Niagara H System-G Niagara, 5546 Portage Rd, Niagara Falls ON L2E 6X2; Tamil (India)'94; FRCPC; Psy. Staff, Niagara Health System - Greater Niagara General Site; Langs: Tamil; (905)378-4647

GOPINATH, Hirekatur V; Haney Health Associates, 22338 Selkirk Ave, Maple Ridge BC V2X 2X5; Mysore (India)'81; MB BS; DPM; MRCPsy; DABPN; FRCPC; Psy (General Psychiatry). Staff, Ridge Meadows Hospital & Health Care Centre; Langs: Hindi; (604)477-7202

GOPINATH, Malar; 2-510 Charolais Blvd, Brampton ON L6Y 0R5; Madras (India)'87; CCFP; (905)455-0500

GOPINATH, Nanda; Medical Office, 211-840 Coxwell Ave, Toronto ON M4C 5T2; Tor'84; FRCPC; IntMed; Gastroent. Staff, Toronto East General Hospital Inc; (416)463-6053; Fax. (416)463-6052.

GOPINATHAN, Asha; Niagara H System-Welland Site, 65 Third St, Welland ON L3B 4W6; Kerala (India)'84; FRCPC; Anes. Staff, Niagara Health System - Welland Hospital Site; (905)732-6111

GOPLEN, Gary B; 303-3320 Richter St, Kelowna BC V1W 4V5; Sask'86; FRCSC; Neursurg (Cerebrovascular Surgery). Staff, Kelowna General Hospital; (250)763-7241; Fax. (250)763-2912; lefk@telus.net.

GOPLEN, Gordon R; Orthopaedic Associates, 11202 76 Ave NW, Edmonton AB T6G 0K1; Sask'95; BA; BSc; FRCSC; OrthSurg (Foot & Ankle Surgery). (780)439-4945; Fax. (780)439-0396.

GORA, Irving; St Lawrence Health Centre, 3-140 The Esplanade, Toronto ON M5A 4P5; McM'74; CCFP; FCFP; Staff, St Michael's Hospital; Asst Prof, University of Toronto; (416)864-6000; Fax. (416)360-4902; gorai@smh.toronto.on.ca.

GORA, Michael; Kingston Comm Med Clinic, 44 Queen St, Kincardine ON N2Z 3C1; McM'07; FRCSC; GenSurg.

GORANSON, Blair D; Red Deer Reg Hosp Centre, PO Box 5030 Stn Postal Box Ctr 3942 50A Ave, Red Deer AB T4N 6R2; Sask'88; FRCPC; Anes. Staff/Chief Anesthetist, Red Deer Regional Hospital Centre; (403)343-4768; Fax. (403)309-2800.

GORANSON, David C; Saddle Mountain Med Clinic, PO Box 159, Nakusp BC V0G 1R0; Sask'79; CCFP; CCFP(E.M.); FCFP; Emergency Family Med, Arrow Lakes Hospital; (250)265-3694; Fax. (250)265-3050.

GORANSON, Sandra L; 200-110 Point Mckay Cres NW, Calgary AB T3B 5B4; Cal'89; CCFP; FCFP; (403)221-9331; Fax. (403)210-0098.

GORCSI, Mary Ann; St Paul Family Health Network, 4F-99 Wayne Gretzky Parkway, Brantford ON N3S 6T6; Wes'96; CCFP; FCFP; Asst Clin Prof Family Med, McMaster University; (519)756-6400; Fax. (519)756-7343.

GORCZYCA, Wojciech; Centre Med St-Bruno, 1435 rue Roberval, Saint-Bruno QC J3V 3P7; Cracow (Poland)'79; (450)653-3631; Fax. (450)653-5518.

GORDILLO, Andres E; Baywood Med Centre, 403-95 Bayly St W, Ajax ON L1S 7K8; Bogota (Colombia)'82; FRCPC; ObstGyn. Langs: Spanish; (905)428-6837; Fax. (905)428-3169.

GORDILLO, Chris G; Grove Med Centre, PO Box 3850 Stn Main 115-187 Hwy 16A, Spruce Grove AB T7X 4P9; Man'01; CCFP; (780)962-4455; Fax. (780)962-4461.

GORDNER, Stuart; Norfinch Med Centre, 202-2100 Finch Ave W, North York ON M3N 2Z9; Tor'74; FACP(Ped); FRCPC; Peds. Ac Staff, The Hospital For Sick Children; Asst Prof, University of Toronto; (416)665-8515; Fax. (416)661-9848.

GORDON, Aida R; MUHC-Montreal Gen Hosp, D10-1650 av Cedar, Montreal QC H3G 1A4; McG'85; CSPQ; FRCPC; Anes. Ac Staff, McGill University Health Centre - Montreal General Campus; assoc Prof, McGill University; (514)934-1934 x43267; Fax. (514)934-8249.

GORDON, Alan; Edmonton Mental Health Clinic, 5F-9942 108 St NW, Edmonton AB T5K 2J5; Cambridge (England)'75; MB ChB; FRCPsy; FRCPC; Psy. Sr Staff Psy, Alberta Hospital Edmonton; Clin Prof, University of Alberta; Fax. (780)427-0424.

GORDON, Alfred; 200-33 Ochterloney St PO Box 135 Stn Main, Dartmouth NS B2Y 4P5; Dal'53; FAGS; Court Staff, Queen Elizabeth II Health Sciences Centre - Victoria General Site; (902)469-3511; Fax. (902)469-3513.

GORDON, Allan S; Mount Sinai Hosp, 1170-600 University Ave, Toronto ON M5G 1X5; Tor'68; FRCPC; Neur. Assoc Staff, Baycrest Centre for Geriatric Care; Dir Wasser Pain Mgmt Centre, Mount Sinai Hospital; Staff, Toronto General Hospital - UHN; Teach Staff, University of Toronto; (416)586-5181; Fax. (416)586-8430; allan.gordon@utoronto.ca.

GORDON, Ann K; Valley Reg Hosp, 150 Exhibition St, Kentville NS B4N 5E3; McG'84; BSc; MDCM; FRCPC; IntMed; Respir. Staff, Valley Regional Hospital; Langs: French; (902)678-1411

GORDON, Benjamin; Medistat Med Familiale, 4965 rue Saint-Pierre, Pierrefonds QC H9H 5M9; McG'87; MSc; CCFP; ac Staff Family Med, St Mary's Hospital Centre; adj Prof Family Med, McGill University; (514)624-4774

GORDON, Danielle M; Aquarius Medical, 179 Davie St, Vancouver BC V6Z 2Y1; Wes'09; CCFP; (604)669-7772

GORDON, Edward G; The Nova Scotia Hosp, PO Box 1004 Stn Main 300 Pleasant St, Dartmouth NS B2Y 3Z9; (Ireland)'85; MB BCh; BAO; FRCPC; Psy. Staff, The Nova Scotia Hospital; (902)464-3049; Fax. (902)464-6172.

GORDON, Elaine; McMaster University HSC, PO Box 2000 Stn Lcd 1 846-1200 Main St W, Hamilton ON L8N 3Z5; McM'77; BSc; FRCPC; Cardiol (Congenital Heart Disease); IntMed. Dir, Adult Congenital Cardiac Clinic; Assoc Prof Med Cardiol/Staff Cardiol, Hamilton Health Sciences Centre; (905)521-2100 x76645; Fax. (905)521-5053; gordone@hhsc.ca.

GORDON, Gayle S; 2F-333 Eglinton Ave E, Toronto ON M4P 1L7; Dal'81; Ac Staff, Rouge Valley Health System - Centenary Health Centre Site; (416)785-5185

GORDON, Heather; Wall Street Med Bldg, 300-140 Wall St, Saskatoon SK S7K 1N4; Sask'01; FRCPC; DiagRad. (306)244-1167

GORDON, Hester A; 4713 48 Ave SS 3, St Paul AB T0A 3A3; (South Africa)'07; MB ChB; (780)645-3331

GORDON, J David; Colchester East Hants Hlth Ctr, 600 Abenaki Rd, Truro NS B2N 5A1; Dal'74; DiagRad. Staff, Colchester East Hants Health Centre; (902)893-5509

GORDON, Janet E; Abbie J Lane Mem Bldg, 1308-5955 Veterans Memorial La, Halifax NS B3H 2E1; Mem'92; FRCPC; IntMed; GeriatricMed. Assoc Prof, Dalhousie University; (902)473-3888; Fax. (902)473-7133.

GORDON, Jeremy; 1500-444 St Mary Ave, Winnipeg MB R3C 3T1; London (England)'62; MB BS; FRCPC; Psy (Psychotherapy).

GORDON, John A; Carling-Broadview Med Bldg, 202-770 Broadview Ave, Ottawa ON K2A 3Z3; Qns'69; FRCSC; OrthSurg (Hip & Knee Arthroplasty). Staff, Queensway Carleton Hospital; Staff, The Ottawa Hospital - Civic Campus; (613)729-3310; Fax. (613)729-3321; john.gordon4@sympatico.ca.

GORDON, Kevin E; IWK Health Centre, PO Box 9700 Rpo CSC 5850-5980 Unviesity Ave, Halifax NS B3K 6R8; Qns'82; MS; FRCPC; Neur (Clinical Research). Consultant, IWK Health Centre; Assoc Prof Peds, Dalhousie University; (902)470-8475; Fax. (902)470-8486.

GORDON, Lloyd P; Humber River Reg Hosp-Church, 200 Church St, Toronto ON M9N 1N8; Tor'76; Staff, Humber River Regional Hospital - Church Street Site; Court Staff, Toronto Western Hospital - University Health Network; (416)243-4191

GORDON, Marla; Mariners Clinic, 505-1160 Burrard St, Vancouver BC V6Z 2E8; UBC'92; CCFP; Staff, Providence Health Care - St Paul's Hospital; Fam Med, Providence Health Care - St Vincent's Hospital-Heather Site; (604)683-0206; Fax. (604)683-0203.

GORDON, Mary E; Sexual Health Centre, 179 Clarence St, Ottawa ON K1N 5P7; Qns'74; FRCPC; CommunMed (Sexually Transmitted Diseases). (613)580-2424 x22556; Fax. (613)560-6069.

GORDON, Michael; Baycrest Ctre/Geriatric Care, 3560 Bathurst St, North York ON M6A 2E1; St Andrews (Scotland)'66; MB ChB; MSc; FRCPC; IntMed; GeriatricMed. Med Prog Dir Palliative Care, Baycrest Centre for Geriatric Care; Head Geriatric Med, Mount Sinai Hospital; Prof, University of Toronto; Langs: Hebrew; (416)785-2500 x3460; Fax. (416)785-2863; m.gordon@baycrest.org.

GORDON, Michelle; Medical Arts Bldg, 17 Dunedin St, Orillia ON L3V 5T3; Tor'96; FRCPC; Peds. Staff, Orillia Soldiers' Memorial Hospital; Assoc Prof, Northern Ontario School of Medicine; Assoc Prof, McMaster University; Assoc Prof Med, Northern Ontario School of Medicine-Laurentian University; Assoc Prof, University of Toronto; Langs: Bilingual(English/French); (705)327-9188; Fax. (705)327-9189.

GORDON, Morris; 310-6411 Buswell St, Richmond BC V6Y 2G5; UBC'77; Ac Staff, Richmond Hospital; Vis Staff, Vancouver General Hospital - Centennial Pavillion; (604)278-6838; Fax. (604)278-8826.

GORDON, Neil; London HSC-Victoria Hosp, PO Box 5010 Stn B 800 Commissioners Rd E, London ON N6A 5W9; McG'86; FRCPC; Anes (Pediatric Anesthesia). Staff, London Health Sciences Centre - Victoria Campus; (519)685-8525

GORDON, Paula B; Vancouver Breast Centre, 505-750 Broadway W, Vancouver BC V5Z 1H4; Tor'78; FRCPC; DiagRad (Bone Densitometry) (Breast Imaging). Consultant, BC Cancer Agency Fraser Valley Centre; Consultant Screening Mammography Prog of BC-Sceener, BC Children's Hospital; Clin Prof Radiol, University of British Columbia; (604)879-4177; Fax. (604)879-4147.

GORDON, Philip H; SMBD Jewish Gen Hosp, 3755 ch Cote-Sainte-Catherine, Montreal QC H3T 1E2; Sask'66; DAB; FACS; FASCRS; FRSM; CSPQ; FRCSC; GenSurg (Colon & Rectal Surgery). Dir Colon & Rectal Surg, Sir Mortimer B Davis Jewish General; Dir Colon & Rectal Surg/Prof, McGill University; (514)342-1772; Fax. (514)340-7560; philip.gordon@mcgill.ca.

GORDON, Philip; 555 University Ave, Toronto ON M5G 1X8; Cape Town (South Africa)'65; MB ChB; MRCP(UK); FRCPath; FRCPC; HemPath. Chief Paediatric Lab Med, The Hospital For Sick Children; Prof Lab Med & Pathbiol, University of Toronto; (416)358-4464; philip.gordon@sickkids.ca.

GORDON, Randy D; 203-3910 Bathurst St, North York ON M3H 5Z3; Dal'82; BSc; Court Staff, North York General Hospital - Branson Division; Court Staff, North York General Hospital; Assoc Staff, Mount Sinai Hospital; Langs: French; Italian; (416)636-6313; Fax. (416)636-3347.

GORDON, Rhona M; 203-1448 Commercial Dr, Vancouver BC V5L 3X9; UBC'84; (604)255-6565; Fax. (604)255-6559.

GORDON, Robert G; Medical Clinic Bldg, 106-89 Humber College Blvd, Etobicoke ON M9V 4B8; Cal'88; FRCSC; OrthSurg (Sports Medicine). Staff, William Osler Health System - Etobicoke General Hospital; Staff, Toronto Western Hospital - University Health Network; Langs: Spanish; French; (416)545-1166; Fax. (416)741-8424.

GORDON, Robert; 102-2210 2 St SW, Calgary AB T2S 3C3; Glasgow (Scotland)'58; MB ChB; FRCS; FRCSC; Ophth (Cataract). Asst Prof, University of Calgary; (403)209-1810; Fax. (403)209-0201.

GORDON, Sherif A A E; Glen Derry Clinic, 3-2760 Derry Rd W, Mississauga ON L5N 3N5; Cairo (Egypt)'89; CCFP; Langs: Arabic; (289)997-3220; Fax. (289)997-3205.

GORDON, Steven C; 200-1075 Pendergast St, Victoria BC V8V 0A1; Cape Town (South Africa)'90; MB ChB; LMCC; (250)477-5433

GORDON, Terrance M; Southwest Med-Centre, SS 2 500-1 Springs Dr, Swift Current SK S9H 3X6; Alb'78; BEd; BA; Physician, Cypress Regional Hospital; (306)773-4681; Fax. (306)778-3449.

GORDON, Tracey A; Mokala Medical, 161-31 Southridge Dr, Okotoks AB T1S 2N3; (Scotland)'98; MB ChB; BSc(Hon); LMCC; (403)995-5740; Fax. (403)995-5743.

GORDON, Vallerie L; Cancer Care Manitoba, ON2006-675 McDermot Ave, Winnipeg MB R3E 0V9; Man'05; FRCPC; IntMed; MedOncol. Staff, Health Sciences Centre; (204)787-2197; Fax. (204)786-0185.

GORDON, W Earl; Primary Health Care Centre, 346 John St N, Arnprior ON K7S 2P6; Wes'72; Ac Staff, Arnprior & District Memorial Hospital; (613)623-7939; Fax. (613)623-8334; rpm59@sympatico.ca.

GORE, Bing Quon; 3185 Grandview Hwy, Vancouver BC V5M 2E9; Cal'77; Court Staff, Providence Health Care - St Vincent's Hospital-Heather Site; Vis Staff, BC Women's Hospital & Health Centre; Vis Staff, Burnaby Hospital; (604)434-2222

GORE, Brian; Sainte Catherine medical Group, 660-5025 rue Sherbrooke O, Montreal QC H4A 1S9; Toulouse (France)'77; Dir-svcs prof, Donald Berman Maimonides Geriatric Centre; Prof Dept of Family Med, McGill University; (514)932-6122; Fax. (514)933-8739; brian.gore@videotron.ca.

GORE, Ron; 101-4600 Lakeshore Rd, Kelowna BC V1W 1X4; Alb'83; (250)764-5211

GORE, Stanley; 10 Silver Birch Ave, Toronto ON M4E 3K9; McM'73; LLB; Ac Staff, Rouge Valley Health System - Centenary Health Centre Site; Court Staff, St Michael's Hospital; Court Staff, The Scarborough Hospital - General Campus; (416)690-2160; Fax. (416)698-0337.

GORE-HICKMAN, Patrick O; Wall Street Med Bldg, 230-140 Wall St, Saskatoon SK S7K 1N4; Sask'80; FRCSC; Otol. (306)244-7865; Fax. (306)244-8864.

GORE-HICKMAN, Wendy L; 105 Red River Rd, Saskatoon SK S7K 1G4; Sask'85; FRCPC; Anes (Cardiovascular Anesthesia). Staff, St Paul's Hospital (Grey Nuns) of Saskatoon; Clin Asst Prof, University of Saskatchewan; (306)668-1879; Fax. (306)655-5964.

GORECKI, Margaret A; Calgary Lab Services, 9-3535 Research Rd NW, Calgary AB T2L 2K8; Warsaw (Poland)'71; PhD; FRCPC; AnatPath (Cytopath). Staff, Calgary Laboratory Services; Langs: Polish; (403)770-3752

GORESKY, Gerald V; Children's & Women's HC of BC, B321-4480 Oak St, Vancouver BC V6H 3V4; McG'72; FRCPC; Anes. Staff, BC Children's Hospital; Prof Anes & Peds, University of Calgary; (604)875-2711; gerald.goresky@calgaryhealthregion.ca.

GORFINKEL, Iris; Medical & Dental Bldg, 516-1849 Yonge St, Toronto ON M4S 1Y2; McG'89; Prin Investigator, Prime Health Clinical Research; (416)486-8444; Fax. (416)486-2193; iris.gorfinkel@primehealthresearch.com.

GORFINKEL, John A; Doctors Hosp Phase 1, 310-340 College St, Toronto ON M5T 3A9; McG'82; FRCSC; Ophth. Staff, Toronto General Hospital - UHN; Instructor, University of Toronto; Langs: Bilingual(English/French); (416)924-2766; Fax. (416)924-0329.

GORGOS, Andreea-Bogdana; MUHC-Montreal Children's Hosp, 2300 rue Tupper, Montreal QC H3H 1P3; McG'05; FRCPC; Peds. Staff, McGill University Health Centre - Montreal Children's Hospital; (514)412-4400

GORGOS, Andrei-Bogdan; CHUM-Hosp Notre Dame, 1560 rue Sherbrooke E, Montreal QC H2L 4M1; McG'02; FRCPC; DiagRad. Staff, Centre Hospitalier l'Université de Montréal (CHUM) - Hôpital Notre-Dame; (514)890-8000

GORGUY, Nermine; Alexandra Marine & Gen Hosp, 120 Napier St, Goderich ON N7A 1W5; Dal'09; CCFP; Staff, Alexandra Marine & General Hospital; (519)524-8689

GORGUY, Verkeen S; Rouge Valley-Centenary HC, 600-2867 Ellesmere Rd, Scarborough ON M1E 4B9; Cairo (Egypt)'72; FRCPC; Psy. Staff, Rouge Valley Health System - Centenary Health Centre Site; Langs: Arabic; (416)281-7318; Fax. (416)281-7320.

GORI-NACHNANI, Maya D; St Mary's Hosp, 4607 53 St, Camrose AB T4V 1Y5; (Pakistan)'92; MB BS; Staff, Covenant Health - St Mary's Hospital; (780)679-6100; Fax. (780)679-6196.

GORIN, Ian C; Westside Med Clinic, 240-4260 av Girouard, Montreal QC H4A 3C9; Sher'72; MSc; Ac Staff Polyclinic, Hopital Maisonneuve-Rosemont; Langs: English; French; (514)489-5753; Fax. (514)489-1616.

GORJA, Juliana; Whitby Urgent Care Clinic, 1615 Dundas St E, Whitby ON L1N 2L1; (Albania)'01; CCFP; Langs: Albanian; Italian; (905)436-2273; Fax. (905)436-2263; gentiga@yahoo.com.

GORLICK, Steven Z; 190 Wilson Ave, North York ON M5M 4N7; Tor'86; Staff, North York General Hospital; Staff, Toronto Western Hospital - University Health Network; (416)482-2111; Fax. (416)482-2174.

GORMAN, Christopher; St Paul's Hosp, 250-1081 Burrard St, Vancouver BC V6Z 1Y6; Alb'80; DABPN; FRCPC; Psy (Inpatient Psychiatry). Staff, Providence Health Care - St Paul's Hospital; Teach Staff, University of Calgary; (604)806-8004

GORMAN, Daniel A; The Hosp for Sick Children, EW 1146-555 University Ave, Toronto ON M5G 1X8; Tor'98; DABPN; FRCPC; Psy (Attention Deficit Hyperactivity Disorder). Staff Psy, The Hospital For Sick Children; (416)813-6936; Fax. (416)813-5326.

GORMAN, Howard E; 9-315 Avenue Rd, Toronto ON M4V 2H2; Tor'75; Psy. Associate Psy, Centre for Addiction & Mental Health (CAMH) - College Street Site; Lecturer, University of Toronto; (416)964-6932; Fax. (416)962-8719.

GORMAN, James A; Markham Med Clinic, 200 Bullock Dr, Markham ON L3P 1W2; Sask'87; Staff, Markham Stouffville Hospital; (905)294-7111; Fax. (905)294-0750.

GORMAN, Kyle; Regina Gen Hosp, 1440 14th Ave, Regina SK S4P 0W5; Sask'07; FRCPC; Anes. Staff, Regina General Hospital; (306)766-4444

GORMAN, Mary C; 206-220 Main St, Antigonish NS B2G 2C2; Dal'82; CCFP; Med Dir/Consultant Geriatrics & Family Pract, St Martha's Regional Hospital; (902)863-3737; Fax. (902)863-5956.

GORMAN, Peter B C; Professional Arts Bldg, 504-100 Arden St, Moncton NB E1C 4B7; Ott'69; BA; FRCSC; Neursurg. Langs: French; (506)857-5376; Fax. (506)857-5378.

GORMAN, Peter; Thompson Rivers Med Clinic, 851 Seymour St, Kamloops BC V2C 2H6; Cal'80; BSc; CCFP; FCFP; Clinical Asst Prof, University of British Columbia; (250)562-5166

GORMAN, Peter R; Regina Qu'Appelle HR-Pasqua, 4F 9-4101 Dewdney Ave, Regina SK S4T 1A5; Sask'80; FRCSC; GenSurg. Staff, Pasqua Hospital; Asst Prof, University of Saskatchewan; (306)757-0171; Fax. (306)757-3866.

GORMAN, Richard F; 554 Spadina Cres, Toronto ON M5S 2J9; Tor'69; Psy (Psychoanalysis). Ac Staff, Toronto East General Hospital Inc; (416)964-8713; Fax. (416)964-6351.

GORMAN, Todd E; CHUQ-Hotel-Dieu de Quebec, 11 Cote-du-Palais, Quebec QC G1R 2J6; Cornell(New York) (USA)'96; Critical Care Medicine; IntMed (P.Q.). Staff, Centre Hospitalier Universitaire de Québec (CHUQ) - Siege Social; Langs: French; (418)691-5151; tgorman@ccapcable.com.

GORMANDY, Winston D; Grey Bruce HS-Owen Sound, PO Box 1800 Stn Main 1800 8th St E, Owen Sound ON N4K 6M9; (Jamaica)'72; MB BS; FRCPC; Psy. Staff, Grey Bruce Health Services - Owen Sound; (519)376-2121

GORMLEY, Lynda; CHUM-Hop St-Luc, 1058 rue Saint-Denis, Montreal QC H2X 3J4; Laval'89; CCFP; Staff, Centre Hospitalier l'Université De Montréal (CHUM) - Hôpital Saint-luc; (514)890-8000

GORNALL, Annie; Selkirk Medical Group, 201-101 First St W, Revelstoke BC V0E 2S0; UBC'10; CCFP; (250)837-9321

GORNALL, Wayne R; PO Box 1232 Stn A, Comox BC V9M 7Z8; Ott'76; FRCPC; Anes. Staff, St Joseph's General Hospital.

GORODETSKY, Olga; Southlake Family Health Team, 201-581 Davis Dr, Newmarket ON L3Y 2P6; Minskij (Russia (Federation))'82; MHSc; CCFP; Langs: Russian; Hebrew; (905)853-3103; Fax. (905)853-2533.

GORODZINSKY, Fabian P; 610 Colborne St, London ON N6B 2V2; National Autonomous (Mexico)'73; CAB; FRCPC; Peds (Community Pediatrics). Ac Staff, London Health Sciences Centre - Victoria Campus; Ac Staff, St Joseph's Hospital - St Joseph's Health Care; Consultant, Clinton Public Hospital - Huron Perth Healthcare Alliance; Assoc Prof Peds, University of Western Ontario; Langs: Hebrew; Spanish; Yiddish; (519)672-4051; Fax. (519)672-4394.

GOROMBEY, Steve J; Calgary Lab Services, 9-3535 Research Rd NW, Calgary AB T2L 2K8; Debrecen (Hungary)'93; FRCPC; AnatPath. Staff, Calgary Laboratory Services; (403)770-3201; Fax. (403)770-3295.

GORRELL, Gerald J; Four Oaks Family Care, 418 Seacliff Dr W, Leamington ON N8H 4E1; Birmingham (England)'69; DObstRCOG; BSc(Hon); MB ChB; Staff, Leamington District Memorial Hospital; (519)326-0344; Fax. (519)326-3285.

GORRIE, Christopher J; Strathcona Health Care Centre, 200-555 Strathcona Blvd SW, Calgary AB T3H 2Z9; Cal'88; BSc; CCFP; FCFP; Ac Staff, Rockyview General Hospital; (403)686-3062; Fax. (403)686-3063; cgorrie@telus.net.

GORSCHE, Ronald G; 117 Macleod Trail PO Box 5580 Stn Main, High River AB T1V 1M6; Alb'69; CCFP; FCFP; Fam Med, High River General Hospital; (403)652-2929; Fax. (403)652-1510.

GORTLER, Judith R; All About Health, E-1070 Major Mackenzie Dr E, Richmond Hill ON L4S 1P3; Wes'98; CCFP; Fam Med, Kateri Memorial Hospital Centre; (905)884-0666

GORWILL, Susan M; Creditview Medical, B14-1240 Eglinton Ave W, Mississauga ON L5V 1N3; Tor'91; Ac Staff, The Credit Valley Hospital; (905)567-4622; Fax. (905)567-7545.

GORZALKA, Frances; 203-3400 rue du Marche, Dollard-D-Ormeaux QC H9B 2Y1; Ott'83; (514)683-0414

GOSAL, Kaviraj; Mistissini Clinic, 395 boul Mistissini, Mistissini QC G0W 1C0; UBC'97; CCFP; (418)923-3376

GOSAL, Manjit; 300-2845 Cruickshank St, Abbotsford BC V2T 6X1; Manchester (England)'92; MB ChB; Staff, Abbotsford Regional Hospital & Cancer Centre; Langs: Punjabi; (604)852-6659; Fax. (604)852-6708.

GOSCIMSKI, Jacqueline; Brant Community HC-Brantford, 200 Terrace Hill St, Brantford ON N3R 1G9; (Other Foreign)'08; CCFP; Staff, The Brant Community Healthcare System - Brantford General Hospital Site; (519)752-7871

GOSEVITZ, J Bernard; Rogers Communication Inc, 3F-333 Bloor St E, Toronto ON M4W 1G9; Ott'71; CCFP; Court Staff, Toronto General Hospital - UHN; Court Staff, Sunnybrook Health Sciences Centre; Court Staff, St Michael's Hospital; Med Advisor, Sun Media Corporation; VP/Chief Medical Officer, Rogers Communications Inc; Med Advisor, Canwest; Med Advisor, Global Television; Med Advisor, Bell Globemedia Inc; Med Advisor, Barrick Gold; Teach Staff, University of Toronto; (416)935-4210; Fax. (416)935-4211; bernie.gosevitz@rci.rogers.com.

GOSHKO, Victor G; Victoria Emerg Phys Mgmt Ltd, 325-1627 Fort St, Victoria BC V8R 1H8; Alb'78; FACEP; FRCPC; EmergMed. Staff, Royal Jubilee Hospital; (250)479-1442

GOSO, T Joseph; 10620 104 Ave, Grande Prairie AB T8V 8J8; Medunsa (South Africa)'85; MB ChB; Langs: Xhosa; Afrikaans; (780)814-5800; Fax. (780)538-4400; jgoso@prha.mb.ca.

GOSPODAROWICZ, Maria K; Univ Hlth Network-Princess M, 5 975-610 University Ave, Toronto ON M5G 2M9; Tor'71; AB(MedOncol); FRCPC; IntMed; RadOncol. Med Dir, Princess Margaret Hospital - University Health Network; Prof, University of Toronto; (416)946-4421; Fax. (416)946-2038.

GOSS, Glenwood D; The Ottawa Hosp-Gen Campus, 501 Smyth Rd, Ottawa ON K1H 8L6; Witwatersrand (South Africa)'75; MB ChB; FRCPC; IntMed; MedOncol. Ac Staff OCF Gen Div, The Ottawa Hospital - General Campus; Consultant, The Ottawa Hospital - Civic Campus; Staff, Ontario Cancer Treatment Fdn.; Assoc Prof, University of Ottawa; Langs: Afrikaans; (613)737-7700

GOSSARD, Denis; CSSS Haut-Richelieu-Rouville, 920 boul du Seminaire N, St-Jean-Sur-Richel QC J3A 1B7; Mon'78; CSPQ; FRCPC; Cardiol (P.Q.) (Clinical Cardiology). Staff, Hôpital du Haut-Richelieu; Clin Prof, Universite de Montreal; (450)359-5000; Fax. (450)359-5254.

GOSSARD, Francis; Clin Med de Saint-Hippolyte, 201-780 ch des Hauteurs, Saint-Hippolyte QC J8A 1H1; Mon'96; CCFP; (450)224-8271; Fax. (450)224-1985.

GOSSE, G Craig; 207-967 Bedford Hwy, Bedford NS B4A 1A9; Mem'83; BSc; BMedSci; FRCPC; Psy. (902)452-8357; Fax. (902)835-1512.

GOSSE, Gordon D; 4 Pine St, Belleville ON K8N 2L8; Qns'66; FRCPC; Peds (Developmental/Behavioural Pediatrics). Consultant Privil, Northumberland Hills Hospital; (613)962-0707; Fax. (613)962-0425.

GOSSELIN, Caroline; Vancouver Gen Hosp, 5D-855 12th Ave W, Vancouver BC V5Z 1M9; Sask'82; FRCPC; Psy (Geriatric Psychiatry). Staff Centennial Pavilon, Vancouver General Hospital - Centennial Pavilion; (604)875-4728

GOSSELIN, Christine; Clin Med de Lauzon, 213 rue Saint-Joseph, Levis QC G6V 1C8; Laval'85; Staff Geriatrics, Hôtel-Dieu de Lévis; Staff, Centre Hospitalier Paul-Gilbert; (418)833-5040; Fax. (418)833-6954.

GOSSELIN, Claire; Ctr Hosp Anna-Laberge, 200 boul Brisebois, Chateauguay QC J6K 4W8; Laval'94; CSPQ; AnatPath. Staff, Hôpital Anna-Laberge; (450)699-2425; Fax. (450)699-4393; c.gosselin@rrsss16.gouv.qc.ca.

GOSSELIN, Claire; CSST Chaudiere-Appalaches, 835 rue de la Concorde, Saint-Romuald QC G6W 7P7; Laval'88; CSPQ; VascSurg; GenSurg. (418)839-2340; Fax. (418)839-1262; claire.gosselin@csst.qc.ca.

GOSSELIN, Emile; Carrefour Med Vallee Richelieu, 665 boul Sir-Wilfrid-Laurier, Beloeil QC J3G 4J1; Laval'72; ac Staff, Centre Hospitalier Honore-Mercier; Physician, CLSC Vallee des Patriotes; Physician, Centre d'Accueil Marguerite-Adam; (450)467-0088; Fax. (450)467-4936.

GOSSELIN, Eve; CSSS de Saint-Jerome, 290 rue de Montigny, Saint-Jerome QC J7Z 5T3; Sher'08; IntMed. Staff, Hôtel-Dieu de Saint-Jérôme; (450)432-2777

GOSSELIN, Francois; Ctr Hosp Laurentien, 234 rue Saint-Vincent, Ste-Agathe-des-Mts QC J8C 2B8; Mon'01; Staff, Centre Hospitalier Laurentien; Langs: English; Spanish; (819)324-4000; francoisgosselin@yahoo.fr.

GOSSELIN, Gabriel; Centre de Sante Valcartier, CP 1000 Bdp Succ Forces, Courcelette QC G0A 4Z0; Laval'63; FRCSC; Urol. Ac Staff, Jeffery Hale Hospital-Saint Brigid's; Consultant, Centre Hospitalier Chauveau; (418)844-5000 x5888

GOSSELIN, Genevieve; Centre Med Saint-Hubert, 206-5125 boul Cousineau, Longueuil QC J3Y 3K7; Mon'04; Staff, Hopital Charles LeMoyne; (450)678-3500

GOSSELIN, Gilbert; Institut de Cardiologie de Mtl, 5000 rue Belanger, Montreal QC H1T 1C8; McG'77; FACC; CSPQ; FRCPC; Cardiol (Interventional Cardiology). Staff, Institut de Cardiologie de Montréal; Chef Dept of Specialized Med, Centre Hospitalier Pierre le Gardeur; adj Prof, Universite de Montreal; Langs: Bilingual(French/English); (514)376-3330 x4060; Fax. (514)593-2155.

GOSSELIN, Gino; CSSS de Laval, 1755 boul Rene-Laennec, Laval QC H7M 3L9; Mon'83; DiagRad. Staff, Hopital de la Cite de la santé; (450)975-5406; Fax. (450)975-5350.

GOSSELIN, Guylaine; CLSC des Etchemins, 331 rue du Sanatorium GD, Lac-Etchemin QC G0R 1S0; Laval'92; Staff, CSSS des Etchemins; (418)625-8001; Fax. (418)625-3109.

GOSSELIN, Isabelle I; CLSC St-Hubert, 6800 boul Cousineau, Saint-Hubert QC J3Y 8Z4; Sher'96; CCFP; FCFP; Staff, CLSC-CHSLD La Pommeraie - Centre hospitalier de Bedford; (450)443-7407; isabelle_gosselin@rrsss16.gouv.qc.ca.

GOSSELIN, Jean; CSSS de Trois-Rivières, 1991 boul du Carmel, Trois-Rivieres QC G8Z 3R9; Sher'92; CSPQ; FRCPC; AnatPath. Staff, CSSS de Trois-Rivières; (819)697-3333 x63494

GOSSELIN, Johanne; Clin Med Vallee-Jonction, 315B rue Principale, Vallee-Jonction QC G0S 3J0; Mon'81; Langs: Bilingual(French/English); (418)253-5481; Fax. (418)253-5157.

GOSSELIN, Johanne; Clinique Med Mellon, 303-2075 boul Mellon, Jonquiere QC G7S 5Z8; Mon'95; LMCC; Médecin, Centre Hospitalier Jonquiere; Physical Med & Rehab, Centre Réadaptation en Déficience Intellectualle du Saguenay-Lac-St-Jean; (418)542-1121; Fax. (418)548-5345.

GOSSELIN, Kim; COOP Sante Gatineau, 370-200 boul Greber, Gatineau QC J8T 6K2; Laval'06; Staff, Centre Hospitalier Portneuf; (819)568-0444

GOSSELIN, Marc; Ctr Hosp Laurentien, 234 rue Saint-Vincent, Ste-Agathe-des-Mts QC J8C 2B8; Mon'95; CCFP; CCFP(E.M.); Staff, Centre Hospitalier Laurentien; (819)324-4000

GOSSELIN, Marc-Andre; Clinique Med Monteuil, 200-4650 boul des Laurentides, Laval QC H7K 2J4; Mon'84; Staff, Hopital Maisonneuve-Rosemont; (450)628-8717

GOSSELIN, Michel; Hop Charles LeMoyne, 3120 boul Taschereau, Longueuil QC J4V 2H1; Mon'97; CSPQ; FRCSC; GenSurg. Staff, Centre Hospitalier l'Université de Montréal (CHUM) - Hôtel-Dieu; Staff, Hopital Charles LeMoyne; Prof, Universite de Sherbrooke; Langs: Bilingual(French/English); (450)466-5000

GOSSELIN, Michel P; 215 rue du Sud, Cowansville QC J2K 2X5; Sher'74; FRCSC; Ophth. Staff, McGill University Health Centre - Montreal General Campus; (450)263-8551; Fax. (450)263-8937.

GOSSELIN, Patrice; Clinique Med St-Damase, 192 rue Principale, St-Damase QC J0H 1J0; Laval'83; ac Membre, Centre Hospitalier Honore-Mercier; (450)797-3385; Fax. (450)797-1062.

GOSSELIN, Pierre; Clin Med Horizon Sante Enr, 8 boul des Iles, Port-Cartier QC G5B 2J4; Sher'83; CCFP; FCFP; Staff, CLSC-CSSS de Port-Cartier; (418)766-4643

GOSSELIN, Pierre; Inst Nat'L de Sante Publique, 945 av Wolfe, Quebec QC G1V 5B3; Laval'76; MPH; Pres Environmental Health Committee, Centre Hospitalier Universitaire de Quebec-CHUL; Coord Institute Climatic Changes, National of Public Health of Quebec; Physician, Health Professionals Task Force International Joint Commission; adj Prof, Université Laval; Langs: Bilingual(English/French); Spanish; (418)650-5115 x5205; Fax. (418)654-3134; pierre-l.gosselin@crchul.ulaval.ca.

GOSSELIN, Richard; Ctr de Med Familiale de Granby, 48 rue Denison E, Granby QC J2G 4C6; Sher'70; Chef, Centre Hospitalier de Granby; Prof, Universite de Sherbrooke; (450)372-3996; Fax. (450)372-0430.

GOSSELIN, Richard; MUHC-Montreal Children's Hosp, C 920-2300 rue Tupper, Montreal QC H3H 1P3; Laval'91; FRCPC; Peds (Neonatal & Perinatal Medicine). Staff, McGill University Health Centre - Montreal Children's Hospital; (514)412-4452; Fax. (514)412-4356; richard.gosselin@muhc.mcgill.ca.

GOSSELIN, Sophie; MUHC-Royal Victoria Hosp, C4 18-687 av des Pins O, Montreal QC H3A 1A1; Laval'97; FRCPC; EmergMed (Toxicology). Staff, McGill University Health Centre - Royal Victoria Hospital; (514)843-2852

GOSSELIN, Sophie; Clinique Med Saint-Vincent, 250 rue King E, Sherbrooke QC J1G 1A9; Sher'96; CCFP; Langs: English; (819)563-0510; Fax. (819)564-6889.

GOSSELIN, Suzanne; Inst U Geriatrie Sherbrooke, 1036 rue Belvedere S, Sherbrooke QC J1H 4C4; Sher'82; CCFP; FCFP; Staff, CSSS Institut universitaire de gériatrie de Sherbrooke; assoc Prof, Universite de Sherbrooke; (819)821-1150 x2089; Fax. (819)829-7153; suzanne.gosselin@usherbrooke.ca.

GOSSELIN, Sylvie; CHUS-Hop Fleurimont, 3001 12e av N, Sherbrooke QC J1H 5N4; Sher'81; FRCPC; Neur; Electroenceph (P.Q.). Consultant, Centre Hospitalier Universitaire de Sherbrooke-Hopital Fleurimont; Langs: English; (819)346-1110 x14586; Fax. (819)564-5395.

GOSSELIN-BRISSON, Anne; Clin Fam des Basses-Laurentide, 2100 boul Labelle, Saint-Jerome QC J7Y 1S8; Mon'06; (450)565-4320; Fax. (450)565-1099.

GOSSELIN-HUNTER, Anne-Marie; MUHC-Montreal Children's Hosp, 2300 rue Tupper, Montreal QC H3H 1P3; Ott'93; FRCPC; Peds. Staff, McGill University Health Centre - Montreal Children's Hospital; (514)412-4400 x22309; Fax. (514)412-4399.

GOSSET, Brian D; Manulife Affinity, 2 Queen St E, Toronto ON M5C 3G7; Tor'82; Med Dir, Manulife Affinity; (416)687-3373; brian_gosset@manulife.com.

GOSSIER, Suzanne M; Vintage View Med, 107-3500 Carrington Rd, Westbank BC V4T 3C1; Tor'95; (250)452-6742; Fax. (250)452-9328.

GOSSMANN, Antoinette; Claro Family Practice, 107-4930 55 Ave, Drayton Valley AB T7A 1W2; (South Africa)'96; MB ChB; (780)621-0202

GOSTIMIROVIC, Milka; University of Ottawa Hlth Serv, 300-100 Marie Curie Pvt, Ottawa ON K1N 1A2; Rijeka (Croatia)'85; CCFP.

GOSWAMI, Anurag; 407 Marlborough Way NE, Calgary AB T2A 7E7; (India)'92; MB BS; (403)272-2211; Fax. (403)248-4906.

GOSWAMI, Duna D; PO Box 2540 Stn A, Abbotsford BC V2T 6R3; UBC'00; FRCSC; ObstGyn. (778)549-8220

GOSWAMI, Rupashi; Medical Arts Bldg, 165 Plymouth Rd, Welland ON L3B 3E1; (Jamaica)'06; CCFP; Langs: Hindi; Punjabi.

GOTESMAN, Galina; 402-4430 Bathurst St, North York ON M3H 3S3; Ott'90; BSc; FRCPC; IntMed; GeriatricMed. Consultant, Baycrest Centre for Geriatric Care; Instructor, University of Toronto; Langs: Russian.

GOTH, Alexis; 2-105 Progress Cres, Kapuskasing ON P5N 3J4; Dal'04; CCFP; Langs: Bilingual(English/French); (705)335-8866; Fax. (705)337-1233.

GOTH, Gary L; PO Box 2348, Cardston AB T0K 0K0; Alb'71; FRCPC; DiagRad. Head Radiol, Chinook Regional Hospital; (403)915-3211

GOTLIB, David A; St Joseph's Health Centre, 30 The Queensway, Toronto ON M6R 1B5; Ott'85; FRCPC; Psy. Staff, St Joseph's Health Centre; (416)530-6000 x3663; Fax. (416)530-6076; gotlid@stjoe.on.ca.

GOTLIEB, Avrum I; Medical Services Bldg, 2113B-1 King's College Circle, Toronto ON M5S 1A8; McG'71; CSPQ; FRCPC; AnatPath. Staff, Toronto General Hospital - UHN; Vice DeanGraduate Affairs(Interim) Sr Academic Advisor & Prf, University of Toronto; (416)978-4635; avrum.gotlieb@utoronto.ca.

GOTLIEB, Stephanie; Medistat Med Familiale, 4965 rue Saint-Pierre, Roxboro QC H9H 5M9; Laval'09; CCFP; (514)624-4774

GOTLIEB, Walter H; SMBD Jewish Gen Hosp, 3755 ch Cote-Sainte-Catherine, Montreal QC H3T 1E2; Bruxelles (Belgium)'84; PhD; ObstGyn (P.Q.) (Gynecologic Oncology). Dir Gyn-Oncology, Sir Mortimer B Davis Jewish General; Prof Gyn-Oncology, McGill University; Langs: English; German; Hebrew; Yiddish; Dutch; (514)340-8222 x3114; Fax. (514)340-8619.

GOTOWIEC, Andrew P; St Joseph's Health Centre, 30 The Queensway, Toronto ON M6R 1B5; McM'03; FRCPC; Psy. Staff Psy, St Joseph's Health Centre; (416)530-6000; Fax. (416)530-6076.

GOTTESMAN, Irving S; Credit Valley Prof Bldg, 506-2300 Eglinton Ave W, Mississauga ON L5M 2V8; Tor'76; FACP; ABIM; ABIM(Endocrin); FRCPC; IntMed; Endocrin&Metab. Assoc Staff, Mount Sinai Hospital; Staff, The Credit Valley Hospital; Asst Prof, University of Toronto; (905)820-2311

GOTTESMAN, Maureen C; North York Gen Hosp, 4S-4001 Leslie St, North York ON M2K 1E1; Wes'98; CCFP; Staff, North York General Hospital; (416)756-6980; Fax. (416)756-6979.

GOTTESMAN, Ronald D; MUHC-Montreal Children's Hosp, C808-2300 rue Tupper, Montreal QC H3H 1P3; McG'82; ABPeds(Peds); ABPeds(Critical Care); FRCPC; Peds (Pediatric Critical Care); Critical Care Medicine (P.Q.). Dir Ped Intensive Care & Geog, McGill University Health Centre - Montreal General Campus; Prog Dir, McGill University; (514)412-4400 x22696; Fax. (514)412-4205; ronald.gottesman@muhc.mcgill.ca.

GOTTESMAN, Steven P; Doctor's Office, 101-491 Lawrence Ave W, North York ON M5M 1C7; Tor'86; CCFP; FCFP; Lecturer, Mount Sinai Hospital; Lecturer, University of Toronto; (416)787-0117; Fax. (416)787-8094.

GOTTFRIED, Stewart B; MUHC-Royal Victoria Hosp, L 411-687 av des Pins O, Montreal QC H3A 1A1; Pennsylvania (USA)'76; ABIM; Respir (P.Q.) (Critical Care Medicine). Staff, McGill University Health Centre - Montreal Chest Institute; Staff, McGill University Health Centre - Royal Victoria Hospital; Staff, Meakins-Christie Laboratories; assoc Prof Med, McGill University; (514)934-1934 x36117; Fax. (514)843-1695; stewart.gottfried@muhc.mcgill.ca.

GOTTKE, Markus U; Hop Brome-Missisquoi-Perkins, 950 rue Principale, Cowansville QC J2K 1K3; Berlin (Germany)'90; IntMed (P.Q.) (Cardiology). Staff, Hôpital Brome-Missisquoi-Perkins; (450)266-4342 x4193

GOTTLIEB, Chloe; The Ottawa Hosp-Gen Campus, Box 307 501 Smyth Rd, Ottawa ON K1H 8L6; McM'03; ABD; FRCSC; Ophth (Uveitis). Staff, The Ottawa Hospital - General Campus; Asst Prof, University of Ottawa Eye Institute; Langs: Bilingual(English/French); (613)739-6845; Fax. (613)739-6635; chloe@fishermansmarket.com.

GOTTLIEB, Sidney O; Collingwood Cardiol & IntMed, 300-393 First St, Collingwood ON L9Y 1B3; Georgia(GA) (USA)'79; Langs: Spanish; (705)444-1648

GOTTMAN, Elizabeth; Montfort Hosp, 713 Montreal Rd, Ottawa ON K1K 0T2; Ott'08; CCFP; Staff, Montfort Hospital; Langs: Bilingual(English/French); (613)983-1628

GOTTNER, Michael J; 105-20644 Eastleigh Cres, Langley BC V3A 4C4; Los Angeles(CA) (USA)'79; FRCSC; Ophth (Retina). (604)530-2323

GOTTO, Geoffrey T; Rockyview Gen Hosp, 6638-7007 14 St SW, Calgary AB T2V 1P9; UBC'04; FRCSC; Urol. Staff, Rockyview General Hospital; (403)943-3000

GOTTSCHALK, Raymond; The Sleep Disorders Clinic, 7-55 Frid St, Hamilton ON L8P 4M3; Cape Town (South Africa)'81; MB ChB; DAB; FRCPC; IntMed (Sleep Medicine); Respir. Staff Respiro, Hamilton Health Sciences Centre - McMaster Children's Hospital; Asst Clin Prof Med, McMaster University; Langs: Afrikaans; (905)529-2259; Fax. (905)529-2262.

GOUACHE, Alain; CLSC Montreal-Nord, 11441 boul Lacordaire, Montreal-Nord QC H1G 4J9; Mon'80; Staff Family Planning Clin, Hopital Maisonneuve-Rosemont; Physician, Clinique Medical Femina; Médecin, CLSC Montreal Nord; (514)389-2000; Fax. (514)788-1262.

GOUBRAN, Ashraf W H; St Boniface Gen Hosp, 409 Tache Ave, Winnipeg MB R2H 2A6; Ain Shams (Egypt)'93; FRCPC; DiagRad., Thompson General Hospital; Staff, St Boniface General Hospital.

GOUBRAN, Mona R; Parkdale Med Tower, 401-1081 Carling Ave, Ottawa ON K1Y 4G2; Cairo (Egypt)'79; MB ChB; CCFP; Langs: Bilingual(English/French); (613)728-5554; Fax. (613)728-7078.

GOUBRAN MESSIHA, Hadi; Royal University Hosp, 103 Hospital Dr, Saskatoon SK S7N 0W8; Staff, Royal University Hospital; (306)655-1483; Fax. (306)655-1809.

GOUDA, Amira F B; Leduc Med Arts Clinic, 7-5204 50 St, Leduc AB T9E 6Z6; (Egypt)'85; MB ChB; CCFP; (780)986-1400; Fax. (780)986-9759.

GOUDA, Zinab; Clinique Medicale, 6185 boul Taschereau, Brossard QC J4Z 1A6; Ain Shams (Egypt)'79; CCFP; Staff, McGill University Health Centre - Montreal General Campus; (450)462-8080

GOUDEZEUNE, Lynne; 101-254 boul Cure-Labelle, Sainte-Rose QC H7L 3A2; Sher'84; Staff, Hopital Maisonneuve-Rosemont; (450)622-3603; Fax. (450)622-3605.

GOUDIE, Richard; Royal Victoria Hosp, 201 Georgian Dr, Barrie ON L4M 6M2; Ott'91; BSc; Dip SportMed(CASM); CCFP; Ac Staff Emerg, Royal Victoria Regional Health Centre; Langs: English; French; (705)728-9802

GOUDREAU, Alain; CSSS de Laval, 1755 boul Rene-Laennec, Laval QC H7M 3L9; Mon'75; MHA; Staff, Hopital de la Cite de la santé; (450)975-5588; Fax. (450)975-5029.

GOUDREAU, Daniel; Clinique Med de Cacouna, 535 rue du Patrimoine, St-Georges-Cacouna QC G0L 1G0; Mon'77; Staff, Centre Hospitalier Regional du Grand-Portage; (418)862-2170; Fax. (418)862-2506.

GOUDREAU, Guy; Hop du Sacre-Coeur de Mtl, 5400 boul Gouin O, Montreal QC H4J 1C5; Mon'83; FRCPC; Neur. Staff, Hôpital du Sacre-Coeur de Montréal; (514)338-2014

GOUDREAU, Stephane; CSSS de Saint-Jerome, 290 rue de Montigny, Saint-Jerome QC J7Z 5T3; Laval'95; Staff, Hôtel-Dieu de Saint-Jérôme; (450)431-8200

GOUDREAU, Veronique; CSSS de la Vallée de l'Or, 725 6e rue, Val-d'Or QC J9P 3Y1; Sher'06; CCFP; CCFP(E.M.); Staff, Centre Hospitalier de Val d'Or; (819)825-5858

GOUDREAU-MICHEL, Joanie; CSSS de Rimouski-Neigette, CP 3150 succ Bureau Chef 150 av Rouleau, Rimouski QC G5L 5T1; Sher'09; Staff, Hôpital Regional Rimouski; (418)724-3000

GOUGEON, Alexandre; CHUQ-Ctr Hosp Univ Laval, 2705 boul Laurier, Quebec QC G1V 4G2; Mon'03; Gastroent; IntMed. Staff, Centre Hospitalier Universitaire de Quebec-CHUL; (418)525-4444

GOUGEON, Francois W; High River Gen Hosp, 560 9 Ave SW, High River AB T1V 1B3; McG'70; SAGES; FRCSC; GenSurg. Gen Surgery, High River General Hospital; Langs: Spanish; French; (403)652-0133; Fax. (403)652-0198; fwgougeon@yahoo.ca.

GOUGEON, Nathalie; Hop Charles Lemoyne, 3120 boul Taschereau, Greenfield Park QC J4V 2H1; Sher'93; FRCPC; Psy. Staff, Hopital Charles LeMoyne; (450)466-5020; Fax. (450)466-5015.

GOUGEON, Nicole; Hop Maisonneuve-Rosemont, 5415 boul de l'Assomption, Montreal QC H1T 2M4; Mon'85; FRCPC; DiagRad. Staff, Hopital Maisonneuve-Rosemont; (514)252-3535; Fax. (514)252-3537.

GOUGH, David W; Cornwall Clinic, 325 Hamilton Ave, St. John's NL A1E 1K1; Dal'63; (709)579-0055; Fax. (709)579-0766.

GOUGH, Ellen R; PO Box 5091 Stn B, Victoria BC V8R 6N3; Tor'84; FRCPC; IntMed; Respir. Staff, Vancouver Island Health Authority.

GOUGH, James; Foothills Med Centre, 11F-1403 29 St NW, Calgary AB T2N 2T9; Dublin (Ireland)'75; FRCPath; MB ChB; BSc; AnatPath (Kidney Pathology). Staff Path., Foothills Medical Centre; Clin Prof, University of Calgary; (403)944-1326; Fax. (403)944-4748; gough@ucalgary.ca.

GOUGH, Kevin A; St Michael's Hosp, 4 179-30 Bond St, Toronto ON M5B 1W8; McM'91; MEd; FRCPC; IntMed (HIV); InfectDis. Head InfectDis, St Michael's Hospital; Asst Prof, University of Toronto; (416)864-5568; Fax. (416)864-5310; kevin.gough@utoronto.ca.

GOUGH, Lisa S; Cook Medical Bldg, 107-1175 Cook St, Victoria BC V8V 4A1; Alb'84; (250)383-3311; Fax. (250)383-1117.

GOUGOUX, Andre; CHUM-Hop Notre-Dame, 1560 rue Sherbrooke E, Montreal QC H2L 4M1; Mon'65; ABIM(Nephrol); Nephrol; IntMed. Staff Nephrol, Centre Hospitalier l'Université de Montréal (CHUM) - Hôpital Notre-Dame; Prof, Universite de Montreal; Langs: Bilingual(French/English); (514)343-5754; Fax. (514)343-2111.

GOUGOUX, David; CSSS de Rivière-de-Loup, 75 rue Saint-Henri, Riviere-Du-Loup QC G5R 2A4; Sher'94; FRCPC; Psy. Staff, Centre Hospitalier Regional du Grand-Portage; (418)868-1020 x4; Fax. (418)868-0530.

GOUGOUX, Fanny; CSSS de Rivière-de-Loup, 75 rue Saint-Henri, Riviere-du-Loup QC G5R 2A4; Laval'99; Staff, Centre Hospitalier Regional du Grand-Portage; (418)868-1000

GOUGOUX, Francois; Clinique Med de Cacouna, RR 1 535 rue du Patrimoine, Cacouna QC G0L 1G0; Mon'67; Langs: Bilingual(French/English); (418)862-2170; Fax. (418)862-2506.

GOUGOUX-TREMBLAY, Stephanie; Institut de Cardiologie de Mon, 5055 rue Saint-Zotique E, Montreal QC H1T 1N6; Mon'94; (514)374-1480

GOUIN, Emilie; CSSS de Trois-Rivieres, 1991 boul du Carmel, Trois-Rivieres QC G8Z 3R9; Sher'06; CCFP; Staff, CSSS de Trois-Rivières; (819)697-3333

GOUIN, Jean-Pierre; UMF Charles-Lemoyne, 215-1144 rue Saint Laurent O, Longueuil QC J4K 1E2; Sher'94; (450)677-4238; Fax. (450)651-4271.

GOUIN, Katy; CHUQ-Ctr Hosp Univ Laval, 2321-2705 boul Laurier, Quebec QC G1V 4G2; Sher'02; FRCSC; ObstGyn (Maternal Fetal Medicine). Staff, Centre Hospitalier Universitaire de Quebec-CHUL; (418)525-4444

GOUIN, Serge; Hôpital Ste-Justine, 3175 ch Cote-Sainte-Catherine, Montreal QC H3T 1C5; McG'90; FAAP; AB; FRCPC; Peds; PedEmergMed (P.Q.). adj Prof, Hôpital Ste-Justine; (514)345-4931 x3498; Fax. (514)345-2358.

GOULARD, Ginette; Ctr Hosp Pierre-Janet, 20 rue Pharand, Gatineau QC J9A 1K7; Ott'91; FRCPC; Psy. Staff, Centre Hospitalier Pierre-Janet; Langs: Bilingual(English/French); (819)776-8085; Fax. (819)771-4727.

GOULARD, Jean-Francois; Vanier Med Centre, 1-325 boul Vanier, Bathurst NB E2A 3N1; Angers (France)'69; LMCC; Ac Staff, Hopital Regional Chaleur; Langs: Bilingual(French/English); (506)548-8951; Fax. (506)548-2011.

GOULART, Jennifer M; Vancouver Island Cancer Center, 2410 Lee Ave, Victoria BC V8R 6V5; Mem'05; FRCPC; RadOncol. Staff, BC Cancer Agency Vancouver Island Centre; (250)519-5500

GOULD, Brent; Royal Jubilee Hosp, 1952 Bay St, Victoria BC V8R 1J8; Man'97; FRCPC; Psy. Staff, Royal Jubilee Hospital; (250)661-6887

GOULD, Glenn D; Foothills Prof Bldg, 350-1620 29 St NW, Calgary AB T2N 4L7; Alb'78; CCFP; FCFP; Staff, Foothills Medical Centre; (403)282-1247; Fax. (403)282-9545.

GOULD, H Marion F; Children's Hosp Eastern Ont, 401 Smyth Rd, Ottawa ON K1H 8L1; Sask'75; FRCP; Anes. Staff, Children's Hospital of Eastern Ontario (CHEO); Asst Prof, University of Ottawa; (613)737-2431; Fax. (613)738-4815.

GOULD, John R; Public Health Services, 7 Mellor Ave, Dartmouth NS B3B 0E8; Tor'77; BSc; MHSc; FRCPC; MedMicrobiol; CommunMed. Staff, Capital Health IWK Health Centre Public Health Dartmouth; Med Officer of Hlth, Western Health Region-Nova Scotia; (902)481-5834

GOULD, Lisa F; Winnipeg Clinic, 425 St Mary Ave, Winnipeg MB R3C 0N2; Man'86; FRCSC; Ophth (Glaucoma). Staff, Misericordia Health Centre; Assoc Prof, University of Manitoba; (204)957-1900; Fax. (204)942-0677.

GOULD, Michael I; Medical Clinic Bldg, 222-89 Humber College Blvd, Etobicoke ON M9V 4B8; Tor'85; FRCPC; IntMed (Hepatology); Gastroent. Court Staff, Women's College Hospital; Vice Pres, Toronto Digestive Disease Associates; Pres/Med Dir, Vaughan Endoscopy Clinic Inc; Asst Prof Med, University of Toronto; (416)745-9994; Fax. (416)745-3653.

GOULD, Peter V; Ctr Hosp Affilie-Enfant-Jesus, 1401 18e rue, Quebec QC G1J 1Z4; McG'86; CSPQ; FRCPC; AnatPath. Staff, Centre Hospitalier Affilié Universitaire de Québec - Hôpital De L'Enfant Jésus; (418)649-5725; Fax. (418)649-5856.

GOULD, Wendy M; 202 St Clair Ave W, Toronto ON M4V 1R2; (Grenada)'06; (416)944-8333; Fax. (416)944-1582.

GOULDEN, Keith J; Glenrose Rehab Hosp, 6-10230 111 Ave NW, Edmonton AB T5G 0B7; Wes'80; FRCPC; Peds (Emotional Injury). Clin Dir Preschool Assessment Serv, Glenrose Rehabilitation Hospital; Assoc Prof Peds, University of Alberta; (780)735-8235; Fax. (780)735-7977.

GOULDING, James F; Victoria Emerg Phys Mgmt Ltd, 325-1627 Fort St, Victoria BC V8R 1H8; Dal'80; MCFP(EM); (250)479-1442; Fax. (250)479-1472.

GOULDING, Krista A; The Ottawa Hosp-Gen Campus, 501 Smyth Rd, Ottawa ON K1H 8L6; McM'07; FRCSC; OrthSurg. Staff, The Ottawa Hospital - General Campus; (613)798-5555 x78213

GOULDING, Thomas H; St Stephen Med Clinic, 33 Wall St, St Stephen NB E3L 2L5; Dal'78; FACS; FRCSC; GenSurg. (506)466-2125; Fax. (506)466-6685.

GOULET, Alain; Clinique Med Havre Sante, 521 boul du Havre, Salaber-de-Valleyf QC J6S 4Z5; Laval'86; Med Dir, Canadian BOAT Federation; (450)371-6444; Fax. (450)371-5315.

GOULET, Audrey-Anne; Clinique Med Champlain, 103-195 rue de l'Atmosphere, Gatineau QC J9A 0A3; Sher'08; Staff Emerg, CSSS de Papineau; Langs: Bilingual(French/English); (819)777-7270; Fax. (819)777-4361; audrey-anne_goulet@ssss.gouv.qc.ca.

GOULET, Benoit; MUHC-Montreal Neurology Inst, 122D-3801 rue University, Montreal QC H3A 2B4; Laval'89; FRCSC; Neursurg (Spinal Neuro Surg). Staff, McGill University Health Centre - Montreal Neurological Hospital; Asst Prof Neurosurg, McGill University; (514)398-5738; Fax. (514)398-8540.

GOULET, Conrad A; Great Leg Clinique, 220-1595 McKenzie Ave, Victoria BC V8N 1A4; Laval'75; Langs: Bilingual(French/English); (250)477-9100; Fax. (250)477-9121; drgouletveinclinic@gmail.com.

GOULET, Constance; CRSS-Sociaux de la Baie James, 199 rue Joliet CP 340, Radisson QC J0Y 2X0; Mon'76; Staff, Centre De Sante Radisson; Langs: English; (819)638-8991; Fax. (819)638-7496; gouletconstance@hotmail.com.

GOULET, David J; Dingwall Med Group, PO Box 3011 Stn Main 40 Goodall St, Dryden ON P8N 2Z6; Ott'07; CCFP; (807)223-6683; Fax. (807)223-4733.

GOULET, Francois; College des Med du Quebec, 2170 boul Rene-Levesque O, Montreal QC H3H 2T8; Mon'80; CCFP; CCFP(E.M.); FCFP; Staff, Centre Hospitalier de Verdun; (514)933-4441 x5237; Fax. (514)933-4668.

GOULET, Genevieve; CHUM-Hotel-Dieu, 3840 rue Saint-Urbain, Montreal QC H2W 1T8; Sher'05; CCFP; CCFP(E.M.); Staff, Centre Hospitalier l'Université de Montréal (CHUM) - Hôtel-Dieu; (514)890-8000

GOULET, Gilles; CHUM-Hotel-Dieu, 3840 rue Saint-Urbain, Montreal QC H2W 1T8; Sher'87; FRCPC; IntMed (Hemodynamics); Cardiol. Staff, Centre Hospitalier l'Université de Montréal (CHUM) - Hôtel-Dieu; Staff, Cardiol, Centre Hospitalier l'Université De Montréal (CHUM) - Hôpital Saint-luc; (514)412-7212

GOULET, Jean; CSSS de Laval, 1755 boul Rene-Laennec, Laval QC H7M 3L9; Mon'85; MSc; FRCPC; Psy (Anxiety Disorder). Staff, Hopital de la Cite de la santé; Clin Teacher, Universite de Montreal; (450)975-5589; Fax. (450)975-5090.

GOULET, Karine; CSSS de l'Energie-Ste-Therese, 1705 av Georges, Shawinigan QC G9N 2N1; Sher'03; FRCPC; Psy. Staff, CH du Centre-de-la-Mauricie (Ste-Thérèse de Shawinigan); (819)536-7575 x4276; karine_goulet@ssss.gouv.qc.ca.

GOULET, Kristian B; Active Care Clinic, 1108 Klondike Rd, Kanata ON K2K 0G1; (Ireland)'07; (613)254-9777

GOULET, Lise; Univ de Montreal, CP 6128 Succ Centre Ville, Montreal QC H3C 3J7; Laval'75; CommunMed. Consultant, Hopital Maisonneuve-Rosemont; (514)343-2442; Fax. (514)343-5645.

GOULET, Marc; Groupe Sante Medisys Inc, 1100-500 rue Sherbrooke O, Montreal QC H3A 3C6; Mon'62; OrthSurg. Ac Staff, Centre Hospitalier Régional de Lanaudière; Med Consultant, Medicolegal CSST; (514)845-1211; Fax. (514)845-4842; marcgoulet@videotron.ca.

GOULET, Marie; Health Protection Bldg, 1117-200 Tunney's Pasture Drwy, Ottawa ON K1A 0K9; Ott'83; FRCSC; ObstGyn (Colposcopy). Staff, Montfort Hospital; Consultant, The Ottawa Hospital - General Campus.

GOULET, Marie-Claude; CHUM-Hop St-Luc, 1058 rue Saint-Denis, Montreal QC H2X 3J4; Mon'05; CCFP; Staff, Centre Hospitalier l'Université De Montréal (CHUM) - Hôpital Saint-luc; (514)890-8000; mariegoulet@hotmail.com.

GOULET, Marie-Helene; Clin de Med Familiale Wakefiel, CP 400 777 rue Riverside, Wakefield QC J0X 3G0; McG'99; CCFP; FCFP; Staff, Hôpital de Gatineau; (819)459-2363; Fax. (819)459-2997.

GOULET, Michelle; Hop Du Sacre-Coeur De Montreal, 5400 boul Gouin O, Montreal QC H4J 1C5; Mon'04; FRCPC; IntMed. Staff, Hôpital du Sacre-Coeur de Montréal; (514)338-2050

GOULET, Richard; Centre Med Laennec, 400-1750 av de Vitre, Quebec QC G1J 1Z6; Laval'71; FRCPC; Peds. Staff, Centre Hospitalier Affilié Universitaire de Québec - Hôpital De L'Enfant Jésus; Ac Staff, Centre Hospitalier Universitaire De Québec - Pavillon De St-françois-d'assise; (418)522-4741; Fax. (418)522-7179.

GOULET, Ronald; CHUS-Hop Hotel-Dieu, 580 rue Bowen S, Sherbrooke QC J1G 2E8; Mon'76; FRCPC; Psy. Staff, Centre Hospitalier Universitaire de Sherbrooke-Hôpital Hôtel-Dieu; (819)346-1110 x24512

GOULET, Sara; University of Manitoba, T162-770 Bannatyne Ave, Winnipeg MB R3E 0W3; Man'05; CCFP; (204)789-3711

GOULET, Serge; UMF Charles Lemoyne, 201-299 boul Sir-Wilfrid-Lauri, Saint-Lambert QC J4R 2L1; Mon'75; Langs: Bilingual(French/English); (450)466-5630

GOULET, Steeve; CSSS de Rimouski-Neigette, CP 3150 Succ A 150 av Rouleau, Rimouski QC G5L 5T1; Laval'92; FRCPC; IntMed (Pneumology); Respir. Chief Pneumol Service, Hôpital Regional Rimouski; Université Laval; (418)724-8122; Fax. (418)724-8596.

GOULET, Stephen C; Victoria Gen Hosp, 2340 Pembina Hwy, Winnipeg MB R3T 2E8; Man'05; FRCPC; IntMed. Staff, Victoria General Hospital; (204)269-3570

GOULET-DION, Sophie; CSSS de Trois-Rivieres, 1991 boul du Carmel, Trois-Rivieres QC G8Z 3R9; Mon'06; FRCPC; IntMed; Respir. Staff, CSSS de Trois-Rivières; (819)697-3333

GOULET-PAGE, Suzanne; Centre Med Brunswick, 401-955 boul Saint-Jean, Pointe-Claire QC H9R 5K3; Mon'78; (514)459-3428

GOUMENIOUK, Alexander D; Dept Of Pharmacology-UBC, C225-2176 Health Sciences Mall, Vancouver BC V6T 1Z3; UBC'87; FRCPC; Psy. Pres, CINEDOCS Consulting Corp; Consultant Psy, University of British Columbia; (604)822-7366

GOUNDEN, Kandasamy; 402-20395 Lougheed Hwy, Maple Ridge BC V2X 2P9; Natal (South Africa)'88; MB ChB; CCFP; (604)465-3900

GOUNDEN, Ranjeeta; ALCA Health Centre, 4821 Calgary Trail NW, Edmonton AB T6H 5W8; (Fiji)'01; MB BS; CCFP; Staff, University of Alberta Hospital; (780)437-1711; Fax. (780)437-1727.

GOUNDREY, Shirley J; Langley Mem Hosp, 22051 Fraser Hwy, Langley BC V3A 4H4; Mem'82; FRCPC; Anes. Staff, Langley Memorial Hospital; (604)534-4121

GOUPIL, Jean-Noel; Dsc St-Luc, 1001 rue Saint-Denis, Montreal QC H2X 3H9; Mon'73; CommunMed. Staff, Hôpital Ste-Justine; (514)277-2660; Fax. (514)873-3239.

GOUPIL-SORMANY, Isabelle; Centre de Sante Publique, 2400 av d'Estimauville, Quebec QC G1E 7G9; Laval'98; FRCPC; CommunMed (Public Health & Preventive Medicine);CCFP; Staff, Hotel-Dieu de Roberval; Langs: Bilingual(French/English); (418)666-7000; isabelle.goupil.sormany@ssss.gouv.qc.ca.

GOURDE, Marjolaine; CLSC-CHSLD Pat Montreal Est, 13926 rue Notre-Dame E, Pte-aux-Trembles QC H1A 1T5; Mon'91; CCFP; FCFP; (514)642-4050

GOURDEAU, Alain; Ctr Hosp Affilie-Enfant-Jesus, 1401 18e rue, Quebec QC G1J 1Z4; Laval'74; Ophth. Ac Staff, Centre Hospitalier Affilié Universitaire de Québec - Hôpital De L'Enfant Jésus; Consultant, Centre Hospitalier Universitaire De Québec - Pavillon De St-françois-d'assise; Associate, Centre Hospitalier Affilié Universitaire de Québec - Hôpital du St-Sacrement; (418)649-0252; Fax. (418)649-5557.

GOURDEAU, Marie; Ctr Hosp Affilie-Enfant-Jesus, 1401 18e rue, Quebec QC G1J 1Z4; Laval'78; FRCPC; MedMicrobiol (Medical Microbiology & Infectious Diseases); InfectDis. Staff, Centre Hospitalier Affilié Universitaire de Québec - Hôpital De L'Enfant Jésus; (418)649-0252 x3033

GOURDEAU, Martin; CHUQ-Ctr Hosp Univ Laval, 2705 boul Laurier, Quebec QC G1V 4G2; Laval'81; CSPQ; Anes. Staff, Centre Hospitalier Universitaire de Quebec-CHUL; (418)656-4141

GOURDEAU, Pierre; CSSS Vieille-Capitale, 2400 av D'Estimauville, Quebec QC G1E 7G9; Laval'77; MSc; Médecin Industrial Med, CSSS Vieille-Capitale; (418)623-1010; Fax. (418)623-7513; pierre.gourdeau@csssvc.qc.ca.

GOURDEAU, Sophie; CSSS de Quebec-Sud, 900 boul Wilfrid-Hamel, Quebec QC G1M 2R9; Laval'90; CCFP; Staff, CSSS de Quebec-Sud; (418)682-1711 x2377; Fax. (418)682-6628.

GOURDES, Denis; Clinique familiale de Thetford, 1001-926 rue Labbe, Thetford Mines QC G6G 2A8; Laval'79; Affil Prof, Centre Hospitalier Universitaire de Sherbrooke-Hopital Fleurimont; Staff, Hopital du CSS de la Region de Thetford; (418)338-3521; Fax. (418)338-4580.

GOURE, Camille A J; Montfort Hosp, 713 Montreal Rd, Ottawa ON K1K 0T2; Ott'06; FRCPC; Anes. Staff, Montfort Hospital; (613)746-4621

GOURGARIS, Adriana; Regina Radiology Associates, 6-2727 Parliament Ave, Regina SK S4S 6X5; Sask'02; FRCP; FRCPC; DiagRad (Radiology). Staff, Radiology Associates of Regina; (306)352-7653

GOURGUE, Martin; Ctr Hosp Affilie-St-Sacrement, 1050 ch Sainte-Foy, Quebec QC G1S 4L8; Laval'82; Psy. Staff, Centre Hospitalier Affilié Universitaire de Québec - Hôpital du St-Sacrement; (418)682-7898

GOURGUES, Alain; Clinique Med Saint-Etienne, 2-965 Rte Lagueux, St-Etienne-de Lauz QC G6J 1T5; McG'90; (418)831-9538; Fax. (418)831-8552.

GOURIOU, Dominique; CSSS de Papineau, 155 rue MacLaren E, Gatineau QC J8L 0C2; Brest (France)'76; Staff, Hôpital de Papineau; Staff, CH-CHSLD de Papineau - Pavillon du centre hospitalier; (819)986-4115

GOURIOU, Louis; Ctr Hosp Pierre-Janet, 20 rue Pharand, Gatineau QC J9A 1K7; Brest (France)'82; FRCPC; Psy (P.Q.). Staff, Centre Hospitalier Pierre-Janet; (819)776-8060; Fax. (819)771-7800.

GOURISHANKAR, Sita; Clinical Sciences Bldg, 11 107-8440 112 St, Edmonton AB T6G 2G3; Alb'95; BSc; MSc(Epidem.); ABIM; FRCPC; IntMed (Renal Transplant); Nephrol. Clin Prof, University of Alberta Hospital; Asst Prof Med Div of Nephrol, University of Alberta; Langs: Tamil; (780)407-3218; Fax. (780)407-7878.

GOURLAY, Douglas L; Wentworth Limeridge Med Ctre, 203-849 Upper Wentworth St, Hamilton ON L9A 5H4; McM'86; MSc; ASAM; Anes (Pain & Chemical Dependence). Staff, Centre for Addiction & Mental Health (CAMH) - Russell Street Site; Staff, Mount Sinai Hospital; Med Consultant, Addiction Research Foundation Pharmacy; Teach Staff, University of Toronto; (905)387-6897

GOURLAY, William A; St Paul's Hosp, 6001-1081 Burrard St, Vancouver BC V6Z 1Y6; McG'88; FRCSC; Urol. Staff Transplant Services Office, Providence Health Care - St Paul's Hospital; (604)806-9610

GOUS, Roelof; Edson Med Centre, PO Box 6660 Stn Main 616 50th St, Edson AB T7E 1V1; (South Africa)'05; MB ChB; Staff, Edson Healthcare Centre; Langs: Afrikaans; (780)723-3366; Fax. (780)723-3437.

GOUSSE-MATTE, Olivier; CSSS Drummond-Hop Sainte-Croix, 570 rue Heriot, Drummondville QC J2B 1C1; Sher'09; Staff, Hôpital Sainte-croix; (819)478-6464

GOUSSEAU, Helene; Quinte HC Corp-Trenton Mem, PO Box 1600 Stn Main 242 King St, Trenton ON K8V 5S6; Cal'96; BSc(Hons.); PhD; CCFP; FCFP; Staff, Deep River & District Hospital; Staff, QHC Trenton Memorial; Langs: English; French; (613)392-2540

GOUSSEV, Igor; Baywood Med Centre, 206-95 Bayly St W, Ajax ON L1S 7K8; Moscow (Russia (Federation))'95; FRCSC; GenSurg (Trauma). Langs: Russian; (905)231-2989; Fax. (905)231-2987.

GOUWS, Daniel R; Ultima Health Assessments, PO Box 49324 Stn Bentall Ctre 410-1055 Dunsmuir St, Vancouver BC V7X 1L4; Stellenbosch (South Africa)'84; MB ChB; Consultant, CBI Occupational Rehab Program & Back-In-Motion; Med Dir, Ultima Health Assessments Corp; Langs: Afrikaans; (604)678-3363; Fax. (604)683-8128.

GOUWS, Willem J; Bonnyville Med Clinic, PO Box 1007 Stn Main, Bonnyville AB T9N 2J7; (South Africa)'07; MB ChB; (780)826-3346; Fax. (780)826-6362.

GOVAN, Jairaj J; 405-5 Fairview Mall Dr, North York ON M2J 2Z1; Witwatersrand (South Africa)'78; FRCPC; Peds (Neonatal & Perinatal Medicine). Ac Staff, North York General Hospital; Staff, North York General Hospital - Branson Division; Teach Staff, University of Toronto; Langs: Gujarati; (416)499-6161; Fax. (416)499-6301; jgovan@nygh.on.ca.

GOVE, Anne E; Ajax Med Arts Bldg, 211-601 Harwood Ave S, Ajax ON L1S 2J5; Wes'76; (905)683-6310; Fax. (905)683-3645.

GOVENDER, Bhagwathee; Weinlos Clinic, 15508 87 Ave NW, Edmonton AB T5R 4G5; RCS (Ireland)'70; LRCPSI; Physician, Weinlos Clinic; (780)484-8151 x3315; Fax. (780)483-1435.

GOVENDER, Indhri; Athabascan Place, 210-80 Chippewa Rd, Sherwood Park AB T8A 4W6; Alb'96; BSc; CCFP; (780)464-6300; Fax. (780)464-2120.

GOVENDER, Kevin; Alta-Sask Wellness Inc, 3-5202 12th St, Lloydminster AB T9V 0W1; Witwatersrand (South Africa)'03; BSc(Hons); MB BCh; (306)825-8877

GOVENDER, Krishnasamy; 2152 Robinson St, Regina SK S4T 2P7; Dublin (Ireland)'71; Ac Staff, Pasqua Hospital; Ac Staff, Regina General Hospital; Dir CME-& MS Health Centre, Regina Qu'Appelle Health Region; (306)569-8544; Fax. (306)522-1598; kgovender@sasktel.net.

GOVENDER, Prakashen; Health Sciences Centre, 820 Sherbrook St, Winnipeg MB R3A 1R9; Durban (South Africa)'87; FRCPC; Anes. Staff, Health Sciences Centre; (204)774-8511

GOVENDER, Preneshlin V; 303-3320 Richter St, Kelowna BC V1W 4V5; Natal (South Africa)'91; MB ChB; FRCSC; Neursurg (Spine Surgery). Staff, Kelowna General Hospital; (250)763-2999; Fax. (250)763-2912.

GOVENDER, Priya; Pacific Med Clinic, 3185 Grandview Hwy, Vancouver BC V5M 2E9; (Other Foreign)'06; MB ChB; (604)434-2222

GOVENDER, Rajan; Maple Creek Primary Hlth Care, PO Box 517 36A Pacific Ave, Maple Creek SK S0N 1N0; (306)662-2829; Fax. (306)662-2332.

GOVENDER, Sivalingum J; Meadowlark Place Prof Centre, 103-8708 155 St NW, Edmonton AB T5R 1W2; RCS (Ireland)'66; Ac Staff, Covenant Health - Misericordia Community Hospital.

GOVENDER, Sundren; Jubilee Centre, 1823 Fort St, Victoria BC V8R 1J6; (South Africa)'97; MB ChB; LMCC; CCFP; Langs: Afrikaans; Zulu; (250)592-6667; Fax. (250)592-2248.

GOVENDER, Tinesha; Prairie North Hlth Centre, 4806 50 St, Lloydminster SK S9V 0M9; (306)820-5997

GOVERNO, Nelson J; Interlake Surgical Assoc, 210D Clandeboye Ave, Selkirk MB R1A 0X1; Man'03; FRCSC; GenSurg.

GOVIG, Bert A; CSSS Les Eskers de l'Abitibi, 622 4e rue O, Amos QC J9T 2S2; McG'88; FRCPC; IntMed. Staff, CH Hôtel-Dieu d'Amos; (819)732-3341 x444; Fax. (819)732-6484.

GOVINDARAJAN, Anand; Mount Sinai Hosp, 1220-600 University Ave, Toronto ON M5G 1X5; Tor'03; FRCSC; GenSurg (Clinician Investigator Program). Staff, Mount Sinai Hospital; (416)586-4800; Fax. (416)586-8392.

GOVINDARAJULU, Arun P; Univ Hlth Network-Toronto Western Hosp, 2 405-399 Bathurst St, Toronto ON M5T 2S8; (India)'99; FRCPC; Anes. Staff, Toronto Western Hospital - University Health Network; (416)603-5118

GOW, Alan L; 700 11th St NE PO Box 1990 Stn Main, Salmon Arm BC V1E 4P9; Glasgow (Scotland)'71; MB ChB; (250)804-3565; Fax. (250)833-3605; allangow@telus.net.

GOW, Barbara L; Peterborough Family Health, 302-170 Simcoe St, Peterborough ON K9H 2H7; Wes'82; CCFP; Staff, Peterborough Regional Health Centre - Hospital Drive; (705)741-1191; Fax. (705)741-1192.

GOW, Janet S; PO Box 308, Deep River ON K0J 1P0; Qns'75; FRCPC; Anes. Ac Staff/Chief Anes, Pembroke Regional Hospital Inc; (613)584-3596; jandabeav@hotmail.com.

GOW, Nina M; Fenwick Med Centre, 311-5595 Fenwick St, Halifax NS B3H 4M2; Dal'88; Dip SportMed; Lecturer Surg, Dalhousie University; (902)421-7512; Fax. (902)429-7138; ngow1@hotmail.com.

GOW, Robert M; Children's Hosp Eastern Ont, 401 Smyth Rd, Ottawa ON K1H 8L1; Queensland (Australia)'76; MB BS; FRACP; FRCPC; Cardiol (Pediatrics). Staff Cardiologist, Children's Hospital of Eastern Ontario (CHEO); Assoc Prof Med, University of Ottawa; (613)737-7600 x2390; Fax. (613)738-4835.

GOWAN, Amy J; Saugeen Shores Med Bldg, 36 Grey St N, Southampton ON N0H 2L0; Tor'05; CCFP; (519)797-9940; Fax. (519)797-1225.

GOWAN, Debra; Dr Everett Chalmers Reg Hosp, 700 Priestman St., Fredericton NB E3B 5N5; Qns'85; MCFP; Staff Palliative Care, Dr Everett Chalmers Regional Hospital; Staff Palliative Care, Cape Breton Healthcare Complex; (506)452-5700; Fax. (506)443-2638; Dr.Debra.Gowan@HorizonNB.ca.

GOWAN, Russell T; 507A-1015 Regent St, Fredericton NB E3B 6H5; Dal'87; FRCSC; GenSurg; Critical Care Medicine; ThorSurg. Staff, Cape Breton Healthcare Complex; (902)562-6409; Fax. (902)562-5796.

GOWAN, Susan E; Dalhousie Univ Health Services, PO Box 15000 Lcd 2 6230 Cobourg Rd, Halifax NS B3H 4R2; Ott'82; CCFP; FCFP; (902)494-2171; Fax. (902)494-2727.

GOWDA, Kempe; 207 2nd Ave N, Saskatoon SK S7K 3P2; Mysore (India)'74; FACP; ABIM; FRCPC; IntMed (Respirology). Clin Prof Med, Royal University Hospital; Clin Prof Med, Saskatoon City Hospital; Staff IntMed, Saskatoon District Health Board; Clin Prof Med, University of Saskatchewan; Langs: Kanarese; Hindi; (306)664-8833; Fax. (306)653-3166; specintmed@sasktel.net.

GOWDA, Shruthi; 105B-10220 Derry Rd, Milton ON L9T 7J3; Bangalore (India)'00; CCFP; (905)875-3369

GOWDA, Sweta; Victoria Gen Hosp, 2340 Pembina Hwy, Winnipeg MB R3T 2E8; Dublin (Ireland)'08; CCFP; Staff, Victoria General Hospital; (204)269-3570

GOWER, Sarah K; Upper Grand Family Health Team, 753 Tower St S, Fergus ON N1M 2R2; Qns'00; CCFP; (519)843-4380; Fax. (519)843-3211.

GOWING, Robert N; 50 Alliance Blvd, Barrie ON L4M 5K3; Qns'05; FRCSC; GenSurg; VascSurg. Staff, Hamilton Health Sciences Centre - McMaster Children's Hospital; (705)728-8778; Fax. (705)728-3053.

GOWRISHANKAR, Manjula; Edmonton Clinic Health Academy, 4 518-11405 87 Ave NW, Edmonton AB T6G 1C9; Ceylon (Sri Lanka)'80; FRCPC; Peds; Nephrol. Staff, Edmonton Clinic Health Academy; (780)248-5470; Fax. (780)248-5627.

GOYAL, Kimmy; Sandalwood Med Clinic, 1-170 Sandalwood Pky E, Brampton ON L6Z 1Y5; Windsor U School of Med (Saint Kitts-Nevis)'07; ABFM; CCFP; Langs: Hindi; Punjabi; (905)846-8282

GOYAL, Kunal; Radiology Associates of Regina, 6-2727 Parliament Ave, Regina SK S4S 6X5; Tamil Nadu (India)'00; MRCP(UK); FRCR(UK); FRCPC; DiagRad (Interventional Cardiology). Staff, Radiology Associates of Regina; Staff DiagRad, Regina Qu'Appelle Health Region; (306)352-7653; Fax. (306)522-4311.

GOYAL, Mayank; Foothills Med Centre, 1403 29 St NW, Calgary AB T2N 2T9; Delhi (India)'90; FRCPC; DiagRad. Staff, Foothills Medical Centre; (403)944-3379

GOYAL, Michelle S; Queen Elizabeth Health Complex, 2111 av Northcliffe, Montreal QC H4A 3K6; McG'94; CCFP; (514)481-4343; michellegoyal@hotmail.com.

GOYAL, Seema; Albert Park Family Ctr, 3992 Albert St, Regina SK S4S 3R1; MRCGPract; DRCOG(UK); CCFP; (306)584-3833; Fax. (306)585-3833.

GOYAL, Sohal V; West Mississauga Medical, 3050 Argentia Rd, Mississauga ON L5N 8E1; Tor'00; BSc; CCFP; Associate Clin Prof Adjuct, McMaster University; (905)785-3627; Fax. (905)785-3628.

GOYAL, Supriya M; 220-339 Aspen Glen Landng SW, Calgary AB T3H 0N6; (India)'90; CCFP; Langs: Hindi; Punjabi; (403)263-7997

GOYEAU, Francis; Harrow H C Inc-A Family Hlth Team, PO Box 430 1480 Erie Rd S, Harrow ON N0R 1G0; Ott'61; (519)738-2000; Fax. (519)738-9944.

GOYER, Caroline; MUHC-Royal Victoria Hosp, S5 05-687 av des Pins O, Montreal QC H3A 1A1; McG'95; CSPQ; FRCPC; Anes. Staff, McGill University Health Centre - Royal Victoria Hospital; (514)934-1934; Fax. (514)843-1723.

GOYER, Eric; Direction de la Sante Publique, 210-1000 rue Labelle, Saint-Jerome QC J7Z 5N6; Laval'95; FRCPC; CommunMed (P.Q.); Public Health & Preventive Med. Langs: Bilingual(English/French); (450)436-8622; eric_goyer@ssss.gouv.qc.ca.

GOYER, Marie-Eve; CSSS Pierre Boucher, 1333 boul Jacques-Cartier E, Longueuil QC J4M 2A5; Laval'03; Staff, Centre Hospitalier Pierre Boucher; (450)468-8111

GOYER, Normand; Polyclinique St-Eustache, 75 rue Grignon, St-Eustache QC J7P 4J2; Mon'74; Staff, Hôpital de Saint-Eustache; (450)472-0552; Fax. (450)473-1916.

GOYER, Pierre; Centre Med Jolibourg, 649-1271 boul Jolibourg, Laval QC H7Y 1Z8; Mon'73; Langs: Bilingual(French/English); (450)689-2424

GOYER, Ronald; Polyclinique St-Eustache, 75 rue Grignon, St-Eustache QC J7P 4J2; Mon'70; (450)472-2474; Fax. (450)473-1916.

GOYET, Martine; Ctr Hosp de LaSalle, 8585 Tsse Champlain, LaSalle QC H8P 1C1; Mon'01; FRCSC; ObstGyn. Staff, Centre Hospitalier de LaSalle; (514)362-8000

GOYETTE, Anne-Marie; CSSS Les Eskers de l'Abitibi, 622 4e rue O, Amos QC J9T 2S2; Laval'05; FRCPC; Anes. Staff, CH Hôtel-Dieu d'Amos; (819)732-3341

GOYETTE, Anne-Marie; MUHC-Montreal Children Hosp, D280-2300 rue Tupper, Montreal QC H3H 1P3; Mon'06; FRCPC; Peds (Developmental Pediatrics). Staff, McGill University Health Centre - Montreal Children's Hospital; (514)412-4314

GOYETTE, Annie; Ctr Hosp Affilie-St-Sacrement, 1050 ch Sainte-Foy, Quebec QC G1S 4L8; Laval'94; FRCSC; Ophth. Staff, Centre Hospitalier Affilié Universitaire de Québec - Hôpital du St-Sacrement; (418)682-7680; Fax. (418)682-7534.

GOYETTE, Claude; Clinique Med St-Antoine, 609 9e rue, Saint-Jerome QC J7Z 2Z2; Mon'77; (450)432-3308

GOYETTE, Maxime; Clinique de Varices, 200-10690 av Peloquin, Montreal QC H2C 2K3; Laval'04; (514)384-0861; Fax. (514)384-3300.

GOYETTE, Monique; CSSS de Trois-Rivières, 1991 boul du Carmel, Trois-Rivieres QC G8Z 3R9; Mon'83; Microbio & Infect Dis (P.Q.); MedMicrobiol (Clinical Research). Staff, CSSS de Trois-Rivières; Langs: Bilingual(French/English); (819)697-3333 x68363; Fax. (819)371-5007; monique_goyette@ssss.gouv.qc.ca.

GOYETTE, Raphael; CLSC Saint-Hubert, 6800 boul Cousineau, Saint-Hubert QC J3Y 8Z4; McG'10; MDCM; CCFP; (450)443-7400

GOYETTE, Roger; Centre Med Chambly, 205-1101 boul Brassard, Chambly QC J3L 5R4; Mon'70; Langs: Bilingual(French/English); (450)658-6601; Fax. (450)658-7849.

GOYTAN, Michael J; AD4-820 Sherbrook St, Winnipeg MB R3A 1R9; Man'89; BSc; FRCSC; OrthSurg (Spine). Staff Surg, St Boniface General Hospital; Med Staff/Staff Surgeon Children's Hosp, Health Sciences Centre; Head, Winnipeg Spine Program; Asst Prof OrthSurg, University of Manitoba; spayette@hsc.mb.ca.

GRABE, Willem A; Village Mall Med Clinic, 22-6320 50 Ave, Red Deer AB T4N 4C6; Orange Free (South Africa)'97; CCFP; (403)314-5357

GRABEC, Jaroslav; 201-180 James St S, Hamilton ON L8P 3A7; Purkyne (Czech Republic)'63; Otol. Physician, Charlton Medical Centre; (905)521-6379; Fax. (905)521-6345.

GRABEC, Marie; Charlton Med Centre, 201-180 James St S, Hamilton ON L8P 4V1; Palacky (Czech Republic)'66; Physician, Charlton Medical Centre; Langs: Czech; Slovak; (905)521-6379; Fax. (905)521-6345.

GRABENSTETTER, Christine L; Inglewood Family Health Centre, 1217 10 Ave SE, Calgary AB T2G 0W6; Tor'83; (403)237-5855; Fax. (403)269-8513.

GRABHER, John J; Nanaimo Reg Gen Hosp, 1200 Dufferin Cres, Nanaimo BC V9S 2B7; Wes'91; CCFP; CCFP(E.M.); Staff, Nanaimo Regional General Hospital; (250)754-2141

GRABIEC, Joseph T; Royal Columbian Hosp, 330 Columbia St E, New Westminster BC V3L 3W7; Man'78; FRCPC; GenPath; AnatPath. Staff, Royal Columbian Hospital; (604)520-4306

GRABNER, Claudia J; Brant Community HC-Brantford, 200 Terrace Hill St, Brantford ON N3R 1G9; Ott'02; Staff, The Brant Community Healthcare System - Brantford General Hospital Site; Langs: French; Spanish; German; (519)752-7871

GRABOSKI, Corrie L; 301-9775 Fourth St, Sidney BC V8L 2Z8; Wes'02; FRCPC; PhysMed&Rehab. Staff, Royal Jubilee Hospital; (250)665-7972

GRABOVAC, Andrea D; BC Cancer Agency-Vancouver CC, 552-600 10th Ave W, Vancouver BC V5Z 4E6; UBC'97; FRCPC; Psy (Mindfulness-Based Stress Reduction). Staff, BC Cancer Agency Vancouver Centre; Staff, Vancouver General Hospital - Centennial Pavillion; (604)877-6000 x2194; Fax. (604)877-6249.

GRABOVE, Matthew A; Saint John Reg Hosp, PO Box 2100 Stn Main 400 Unviersity Ave, Saint John NB E2L 4L2; Mem'04; CCFP; CCFP(E.M.); Staff, Saint John Regional Hospital; (506)648-6000

GRABOWSKA, Kirsten M; Jim Pattison Outpatient & Surg, 9750 140 St, Vancouver BC V5T 0G9; Wes'03; FRCSC; ObstGyn (Maternal Fetal Medicine). (604)582-4588

GRABOWSKI, Arthur; Baywood Med Centre, 300-95 Bayly St W, Ajax ON L1S 7K8; Tor'98; FRCSC; Urol (Urological Oncology). Ac Staff, Rouge Valley Health System - Ajax & Pickering Health Centre Site; Court Staff, Lakeridge Health - Oshawa Site; Langs: Polish; (905)426-9426; Fax. (905)426-9322.

GRABOWSKI, Janet L; Manitoba Clinic, 790 Sherbrook St, Winnipeg MB R3A 1M3; Man'89; BSc(Med); FRCPC; Peds. Ac Staff Children's Hosp, Health Sciences Centre; Ac Staff, Victoria General Hospital; Ac Staff, The Salvation Army Grace Hospital; Asst Prof, University of Manitoba; (204)788-5750; Fax. (204)783-7163.

GRACE, Archie N; Carling Heights Med Centre, 124 Barker St, London ON N5Y 1Y1; Wes'74; BSc; CCFP; FCFP; Ac Staff, St Joseph's Hospital - St Joseph's Health Care; Coroner, Province of Ontario; Asst Prof, University of Western Ontario; (519)451-1363; Fax. (519)451-1162.

GRACE, Donald A; 210-9764 Fifth St, Sidney BC V8L 2X2; Alb'60; FACS; FRCSC; Urol. Staff, Saanich Peninsula Hospital; (250)655-4428; Fax. (250)655-0151.

GRACE, Douglas E; 200-481 John St, Burlington ON L7R 2K8; Tor'97; FRCSC; PlasSurg. Staff, Toronto General Hospital - UHN; (905)336-9636; Fax. (905)336-9651.

GRACE, Francine S; 7025 Myron Rd, Lantzville BC V0R 2H0; Des Moines(IA) (USA)'86; (250)390-8008; Fax. (250)390-8009.

GRACE, James C A; River City Med Clinic, PO Box 369 Stn A, Campbell River BC V9W 5B6; UBC'78; (250)287-2111; Fax. (250)287-2444.

GRACE, Jennifer E; 130-520 D 2nd Ave, Campbell River BC V9W 6G2; UBC'96; FRCPC; IntMed. Staff, Campbell River & District General Hospital; Clin Instructor, University of British Columbia; (250)286-4061

GRACE, Kevin J; Transcona Med Clinic, 200-701 Regent Ave W, Winnipeg MB R2C 1S3; Man'91; CCFP; FCFP; (204)222-5221; Fax. (204)224-2053.

GRACE, S Maureen; Merivale Med Imaging Inc, 1370 Clyde Ave, Nepean ON K2G 3H8; Wes'89; CCFP; (613)727-2745

GRACEY, Janel L; Thomas St Treatment Centre, 813 Richmond St, London ON N6A 3H6; (Dominica)'05; AddicMed; CCFP; Physician Addiction Med, Methadone Clinic; Staff Pain Managment, InMedic; (519)205-0152; Fax. (519)205-0473.

GRACIA, Mark E; Cariboo Mem Hosp, 517 Sixth Ave N, Williams Lake BC V2G 2G8; McG'97; CCFP; CCFP(E.M.); Staff, Cariboo Memorial Hospital and Health Centre; Langs: Bilingual(English/French); (250)392-4411; Fax. (250)398-5712; mark_gracia@telus.net.

GRACIAS, Gavin; Burnaby Hosp, 3935 Kincaid St, Burnaby BC V5G 2X6; Ott'02; FRCPC; Anes. Staff, Burnaby Hospital; (604)412-6311

GRACIE, Glenn A; Sydney Family Practice, 196 Kings Rd, Sydney NS B1S 1A1; Dal'73; CCFP; (902)567-0040; Fax. (902)539-9250.

GRACZYK, Joanna; Sunnybrook Hlth Sciences Ctre, T2033-2075 Bayview Ave, Toronto ON M4N 3M5; Tor'08; IntMed.

GRAD, Elliott; Medical Clinic Bldg, 319-89 Humber College Blvd, Etobicoke ON M9V 4B8; Tor'67; FAAP; FRCPC; Peds (Allergy). Ac Staff, William Osler Health System - Etobicoke General Hospital; (416)743-5652; Fax. (416)743-5491.

GRAD, Roland; SMBD Jewish Gen Hosp, E 0010-3755 ch Cote-Sainte-Cat, Montreal QC H3T 1E2; McG'84; MSc; CCFP; FCFP; Dir recherche Family Med, Sir Mortimer B Davis Jewish General; Med Scientifique Clinical Epidemiology, McGill University Health Centre - Royal Victoria Hospital; assoc Prof Family Med, McGill University; (514)340-8234; Fax. (514)340-8298.

GRAD, Sharon; Regional Rehabilitation Centre, 300 Wellington St N, Hamilton ON L8L 0A4; McM'93; LMCC; FRCP; FRCPC; PhysMed&Rehab (Multiple Sclerosis). Staff, Hamilton Health Sciences Centre - Regional Rehabilitation Centre; Staff, Hamilton Health Sciences Centre - Hamilton General Hospital; Clin Team Dir Prosthetics & Orthotics Reg Rehab Centre, Hamilton Health Sciences Centre - McMaster University Medical Centre; Clinical Asst Prof Med, McMaster University; (905)527-0271 x40819; Fax. (905)577-8233.

GRAD, Willis B; SMBD Jewish Gen Hosp, 3755 ch Cote-Sainte-Catherine, Montreal QC H3T 1E2; McG'88; FRCPC; EmergMed (P.Q.);CCFP; CCFP(E.M.); FCFP; Staff Emerg Dept, Sir Mortimer B Davis Jewish General; Aj Prof Family Med, McGill University; (514)340-8222 x5568; Fax. (514)340-7917.

GRADA, Atef; Scotia Square Med Clinic, 270-5201 Duke St, Halifax NS B3J 1N9; Al Fateh (Libya)'01; MB BCh; (902)431-1800; Fax. (902)431-1818.

GRADE, A C Roxane; PO Box 40056 Rpo Baker Centre, Edmonton AB T5J 4M9; Utrecht (Netherlands)'85; CCBOM; CCFP; FCFP.

GRADER, Joseph; Keele-Ingram Prof Centre, 206-2221 Keele St, North York ON M6M 3Z5; Tor'59; FRCSC; Ophth (Contact Lenses). Senior Active Staff, Humber River Regional Hospital - Keele Street Site; (416)249-7661; Fax. (416)249-5839.

GRADINGER, Charles; 104-4351 boul Notre-Dame, Laval QC H7W 1T3; Geneva (Switzerland)'64; FRCPC; Peds (P.Q.). Staff, McGill University Health Centre - Montreal Children's Hospital; Staff, Sir Mortimer B Davis Jewish General; Staff, Hôpital Ste-Justine; (450)681-7388

GRADINGER, Harvey; 104-4351 boul Notre-Dame, Laval QC H7W 1T3; Geneva (Switzerland)'66; ABPeds; FRCPC; Peds (P.Q.). Att Staff, Hôpital Ste-Justine; Att Staff, McGill University Health Centre - Montreal Children's Hospital; Att Staff, Sir Mortimer B Davis Jewish General; (450)681-7388

GRADSTEIN, Janneke S; Amherst Family Health Clinic, 200-158 Robert Angus Dr, Amherst NS B4H 4R7; Dal'04; CCFP; (902)667-3330; Fax. (902)667-4176.

GRADSTEIN, Roetka; Ravines Med Centre, 2-535 Larry Uteck Blvd, Halifax NS B3M 0E3; Dal'07; CCFP; (902)407-4382; Fax. (902)407-4381.

GRAEB, Douglas A; Vancouver Gen Hosp, 855 12th Ave W, Vancouver BC V5Z 1M9; Tor'71; FRCPC; DiagRad (Neuro Radiology). Ac Staff, Vancouver General Hospital - Centennial Pavillion; Consultant, BC Cancer Agency Vancouver Centre; Consultant, BC Children's Hospital; Assoc Prof Diag Rad, University of British Columbia; (604)875-4111 x63757; Fax. (604)875-4723.

GRAETZ, Michael A; Burns Lake Med Clinic, PO Box 6000, Burns Lake BC V0J 1E0; Stellenbosch (South Africa)'84; MB ChB; CCFP; Staff/Chief of Staff, Lakes District Hospital & Health Centre; (250)692-3111; Fax. (250)692-7477.

GRAF, Rose; Humboldt Med Clinic, PO Box 220, Humboldt SK S0K 2A0; CCFP; (306)682-2618; Fax. (306)682-4499.

GRAFF, Michael; 5966 Mullen Way NW, Edmonton AB T6R 0S9; UBC'10; CCFP; (780)801-1220; Fax. (780)801-1225.

GRAFF, Peter; 1110-160 14th St E, North Vancouver BC V7L 2N3; Witwatersrand (South Africa)'80; MB BS; FRCPC; IntMed. Staff, Lions Gate Hospital; (604)904-0810

GRAFF GUERRERO, Ariel; Addiction & Mental Hlth-Clarke, 250 College St, Toronto ON M5T 1R8; Michoacan (Mexico)'96; Staff, Centre for Addiction & Mental Health (CAMH) - College Street Site; (416)535-8501

GRAFHAM, Mark R G; King West Med Associates, 505 King St W, Hamilton ON L8P 1B9; Qns'90; (905)525-3501; Fax. (905)528-5468; mgrafham@cogeco.ca.

GRAFSTEIN, Eric J; St Paul's Hosp, 1081 Burrard St, Vancouver BC V6Z 1Y6; Tor'85; EmergMed. Staff, Providence Health Care - St Paul's Hospital; (604)806-8982; Fax. (604)806-8488.

GRAGASIN, Ferrante S; Clinical Sciences Bldg, 8 120-152 University Campus NW, Edmonton AB T6G 2G3; Alb'05; FRCPC; Anes. (780)407-8861; Fax. (780)407-3200.

GRAHAM, Alistair D; Kelowna Gen Hosp, 2268 Pandosy St, Kelowna BC V1Y 1T2; Edinburgh (Scotland)'94; MB ChB; BSc; FRCPC; Anes. Staff, Kelowna General Hospital; (250)682-4022

GRAHAM, Andrew J; Foothills Med Centre, G33-1403 29 St NW, Calgary AB T2N 2T9; Tor'87; FRCSC; GenSurg; ThorSurg. Staff, Foothills Medical Centre; (403)944-8258; Fax. (403)270-8431.

GRAHAM, Anthony D; Sudbury Reg Hosp-Laurentian, 1F-41 Ramsey Lake Rd, Sudbury ON P3E 5J1; Qns'83; FRCPC; PhysMed&Rehab (Electromyography). Med Dir Rehab Serv/Staff Physiatrist, Health Sciences North-Laurentian Site; (705)523-7006; Fax. (705)523-7051; agrahama@hrsh.on.ca.

GRAHAM, Anthony F; St Michael's Hosp, 7056 QW-30 Bond St, Toronto ON M5B 1W8; Qns'66; FACC; FRCPC; Cardiol (Cardiovascular Disease). Dir Robert McRae Heart Health Unit/Ambulatory Care/Prof Med, St Michael's Hospital; Leader Volunteer, Heart & Stroke Foundation; Prof Med, University of Toronto; (416)864-5602; Fax. (416)864-6072; agraham@smh.ca.

GRAHAM, Brent A; UHN -Toronto Western Hosp, EW2 425-399 Bathurst St, Toronto ON M5T 2S8; McG'81; FRCSC; OrthSurg (Hand Microsurgery). Staff, Toronto Western Hospital - University Health Network; Asst Prof Surg, University of Toronto; (416)603-5647; Fax. (416)603-5716.

GRAHAM, Candida R; Univ Hosp of Northern BC, 1475 Edmonton St, Prince George BC V2M 1S2; (United Kingdom)'89; MB ChB; MMedSci; Staff, University Hospital of Northern British Columbia; (250)565-2000; Fax. (250)565-2343.

GRAHAM, Caroline H; 400-3910 Bathurst St, North York ON M3H 5Z3; Tor'89; FRCPC; IntMed. (416)638-6107; Fax. (416)638-9484.

GRAHAM, Christopher; Health Sciences Centre, AD401-820 Sherbrook St, Winnipeg MB R3A 1R9; Sask'99; FRCSC; OrthSurg. Staff, Health Sciences Centre.

GRAHAM, Christopher; Trillium Hlth Ctr-Mississauga, 100 Queensway W, Mississauga ON L5B 1B8; Tor'00; FRCPC; IntMed; InfectDis. Staff, Trillium Health Centre - Mississauga; (905)848-7100; Fax. (416)521-4082.

GRAHAM, Christopher H D; Rockingham Ridge Plaza, 30 Farnham Gate Rd, Halifax NS B3M 3W8; Dal'83; (902)457-2222; Fax. (902)443-7800.

GRAHAM, Christopher S; Lorraine Wing Tower C, 201 Deacon St, Pembroke ON K8A 2J6; Qns'93; FRCSC; GenSurg. Staff/Chief GenSurg, Pembroke Regional Hospital Inc; (613)732-9381; Fax. (613)732-6347.

GRAHAM, David J; Aberdeen Hosp, 835 East River Rd, New Glasgow NS B2H 3S6; Tor'75; Staff, Aberdeen Regional Hospital; (902)752-8311

GRAHAM, David M; 1-418 Talbot St W, Aylmer ON N5H 1K9; Wes'82; CCFP; FCFP; Staff, St Thomas Elgin General Hospital; (519)765-1208; Fax. (519)765-1279.

GRAHAM, Debra G; Churchill Med Clinic, 6750 Winston Churchill Blvd, Mississauga ON L5N 4C4; Tor'84; Ac Staff, The Credit Valley Hospital; (905)824-3700; Fax. (905)824-9956.

GRAHAM, Dianne; 1605 Gordon Dr, Kelowna BC V1Y 3G8; Sask'76; CCFP; FCFP; Clin Prof, University of British Columbia; (250)762-2729

GRAHAM, Duncan C M; 21 McGivern St PO Box 1300, Walkerton ON N0G 2V0; McM'84; BA; FRCSC; GenSurg. Att Staff, South Bruce Grey Health Centre - Walkerton Site; (519)881-2880; Fax. (519)881-4648; duncan-graham@wightman.ca.

GRAHAM, Gail E; Children's Hosp Eastern Ontari, 401 Smyth Rd, Ottawa ON K1H 8L1; Qns'92; MSc; FCCMG; FRCPC; MedGenetics. Staff Genetics, Children's Hospital of Eastern Ontario (CHEO); Langs: French; (613)737-7600 x3218; Fax. (613)738-4420; ggraham@cheo.on.ca.

GRAHAM, Heather R; Alberta Children's Hosp, 2888 Shaganappi Trail NW, Calgary AB T3B 6A8; McG'83; FRCPC; Peds (Emergency Pediatrics). Staff, Alberta Children's Hospital; (403)955-7211

GRAHAM, Ian Davidson; 2-206 St Clair Ave W, Toronto ON M4V 1R2; Wes'58; FIPA; FRCPC; Psy (Psychoanalysis). (416)920-5546; Fax. (416)920-5151.

GRAHAM, James A; Chrysalis Obst & Gyn Clinic, 21-10 Richard Way SW, Calgary AB T3E 7M9; Mem'96; BSc; BMedSci; FRCSC; ObstGyn (Gynecology). (403)242-0770; Fax. (403)242-0711; reproendo@gmail.com.

GRAHAM, Jamie; Medical Consultents of West NL, 304-2 Herald Ave, Corner Brook NL A2H 4B5; Tor'63; FRCPC; IntMed (Cardiology). Staff Consulting, Western Memorial Regional Hospital; (709)639-9181; Fax. (709)639-1210.

GRAHAM, Janet E; 250 Dundas St E SS 2, Waterdown ON L0R 2H4; McM'84; CCFP; FCFP; Asst Clin Prof Family Med, McMaster University; (905)690-6748; Fax. (905)690-6750.

GRAHAM, Janice S; 809-123 Edward St, Toronto ON M5G 1E2; Cape Town (South Africa)'82; MB ChB; FRCOG; FRCSC; ObstGyn (Colposcopy). Court Staff Lyndhurst Clinic, University Health Network; (416)962-7777

GRAHAM, Jennifer M; BC Children's Hosp, 4480 Oak St, Vancouver BC V6H 3V4; Cal'06; FRCPC; Peds; PedEmergMed. Staff, BC Children's Hospital; (604)875-2000

GRAHAM, Johanna H; 629-5991 Spring Garden Rd, Halifax NS B3H 1Y6; Dal'92; (902)422-8488; Fax. (902)422-8494.

GRAHAM, John D; Queen Square Doctors FHT, 201-366 Main St N, Brampton ON L6V 1P8; Ott'92; CCFP; CCFP(E.M.); FCFP; (905)455-1455; Fax. (905)455-5498.

GRAHAM, John; St Michael's Hosp, 30 Bond St, Toronto ON M5B 1W8; Glasgow (Scotland)'95; Staff Interventional Cardiol/Asst Prof Med, St Michael's Hospital; Asst Prof, University of Toronto; (416)864-5918

GRAHAM, John S; Gulf Canada Square, 320-401 9 Ave SW, Calgary AB T2P 3C5; Alb'91; FRCSC; GenSurg. Staff, Rockyview General Hospital; (403)221-4489; Fax. (403)221-4420.

GRAHAM, John W; 7010-105 Allen St W, Waterloo ON N2L 1E6; Tor'65; Peds (Child & Adolescent Psychiatry). Court Staff, St Mary's General Hospital; Court Staff, Grand River Hospital - Kitchener/Waterloo Health Centre; Consultant, Kids Link; Consultant, Lutherwood; Consultant, Hope Manor; johngraham@execulink.com.

GRAHAM, Karen L; Kingston Gen Hosp, 76 Stuart St, Kingston ON K7L 2V7; Qns'86; CCFP; CCFP(E.M.); FCFP; Staff Emerg, Kingston General Hospital; (613)549-6666; Fax. (613)548-1374.

GRAHAM, Keith; PO Box 340, Quathiaski Cove BC V0P 1N0; UBC'92; BSc; Member Manpower Utilization Committee, Campbell River & District General Hospital; Staff Interviewer Admissions, University of British Columbia; (250)285-3540

GRAHAM, Kerr; Interlake Medical Clinic, PO Box 70 2-330 3rd Ave S, Stonewall MB R0C 2Z0; Glasgow (Scotland)'75; MB ChB; (204)467-9707; Fax. (204)467-9767.

GRAHAM, Kevin P; 3-2650 Lawrence Ave E, Scarborough ON M1P 2S1; Cal'86; (416)289-0593

GRAHAM, Lawrie J; 43-3075 Ridgeway Dr, Mississauga ON L5L 5M6; Tor'89; CCFP; FCFP; (905)828-6061; Fax. (905)820-9468.

GRAHAM, Lindsay A; 301A-117 Murray St, Ottawa ON K1N 5M5; McG'51; MDCM; (613)238-7729

GRAHAM, Lois E; Oak Grove Clinic, 1872 Kingsway, Vancouver BC V5N 2S7; (Jamaica)'66; EmergMed. Ac Staff Emerg Dept, Vancouver General Hospital - Centennial Pavillion; (604)876-6257

GRAHAM, Louise; 202-285 Aurora Cres, Kelowna BC V1X 7N6; Wes'83; MA; CCFP; FCFP; (250)765-7756; Fax. (250)765-9015.

GRAHAM, Lyla M; St Paticks Home, 2865 Riverside Dr, Ottawa ON K1V 8N5; McM'82; CCFP; FCFP; Ac Staff, SCO Health Service - Élisabeth Bruyère Hospital; Staff, The Ottawa Hospital - General Campus; Assoc Prof Family Med, University of Ottawa; Langs: French; (613)731-4660; Fax. (613)731-4056; lgraham@bruyere.org.

GRAHAM, M Ruth; Health Sciences Ctr Gen Hosp, 700 William Ave, Winnipeg MB R3E 0Z3; Man'83; FRCPC; Anes. Ac Staff Anes, Health Sciences Centre; Asst Prof, University of Manitoba; (204)774-6511

GRAHAM, Marianne D; Sunnybrook Hlth Sciences Ctre, 200MW-2075 Bayview Ave, Toronto ON M4N 3M5; Tor'89; FRCPC; Anes. Staff, Sunnybrook Health Sciences Centre; Asst Prof, University of Toronto; (416)480-6100 x6087; Fax. (416)480-6039.

GRAHAM, Martha B; 28-1495 Cornwall Rd, Oakville ON L6J 0B2; McM'98; CCFP; FCFP; (289)291-0440; Fax. (289)291-0442.

GRAHAM, Melissa; Credit Valley Family Hlth Team, 105-2300 Eglinton Ave W, Mississauga ON L5M 2V8; Ott'08; CCFP; (905)813-3850

GRAHAM, Michelle M; University of Alberta Hosp, 2C2 WCM-8440 112 St NW, Edmonton AB T6G 2B7; Ott'93; FRCPC; IntMed (Interventional Cardiology); Cardiol. Att Staff, University of Alberta Hospital; Asst Prof, University of Alberta; (780)407-1590; Fax. (780)407-1496; mmgraham@cha.ab.ca.

GRAHAM, Nancy J; Kingsway Plaza Phase III, 100-4980 Kingsway, Burnaby BC V5H 4K7; UBC'86; FRCPC; DiagRad. Staff, Langley Memorial Hospital; (604)434-1345

GRAHAM, Nicholas R; Coast Med Clinic, 1018 Seymour St, Vancouver BC V6B 3M6; Alb'08; CCFP; (604)569-3632

GRAHAM, Paul A; 204-45625 Hodgins Ave, Chilliwack BC V2P 1P2; Cal'06; CCFP; (604)792-1908

GRAHAM, Robert D; Fundy Trail Med Centre, 68 Robie St, Truro NS B2N 1L2; Dal'78; CCFP; (902)895-3001; Fax. (902)895-3185; dr.rob_graham@hotmail.com.

GRAHAM, Robert E; Drumheller Assoc Physicians, PO Box 5600 140 Riverside Dr E, Drumheller AB T0J 0Y0; Sask'79; Staff, Drumheller Health Centre; (403)823-3345; Fax. (403)823-7823; rgraham@dthr.ab.ca.

GRAHAM, Robert T; 3-125 Pedersen DR, Aurora ON L4G 0E3; Wes'78; FRCPC; DiagRad. Staff, Southlake Regional Health Centre; (416)996-5824

GRAHAM, Roger C; Selkirk Mental Health Centre, PO Box 9600 Stn Main 825 Manitoba Ave, Selkirk MB R1A 2B5; Man'84; FRCPC; Psy. Staff Psy, Selkirk Mental Health Centre; (204)482-3810; Fax. (204)785-8936.

GRAHAM, Sandra; Clinique Privee Enfant Sante, 206-75 boul des Chateaux, Sainte-Therese QC J7B 2A4; Mon'98; Langs: Spanish; English; (514)738-4445; Fax. (514)738-8284.

GRAHAM, Shelley M; North Hill Prof Centre, 258-1632 14 Ave NW, Calgary AB T2N 1M7; McG'80; CCFP; FCFP; (403)291-3001; Fax. (403)291-3139.

GRAHAM, Steve; Centre Medical Montreal-Est, 201-11370 rue Notre-Dame E, Montreal-Est QC H1B 2W6; Mon'73; Langs: Bilingual(French/English); (514)645-7426; Fax. (514)645-7420.

GRAHAM, Susan F B; Delhi Family Health Team, 105 Main Street of Delhi, Delhi ON N4B 2L8; Tor'88; BSc(Hon); CCFP; Med Staff, Norfolk General Hospital; (519)582-2323; Fax. (519)582-1513.

GRAHAM, Timothy A D; University of Alberta Hosp, 1A7 19-8440 112 St NW, Edmonton AB T6G 2B7; Man'97; CCFP; CCFP(E.M.); Staff, University of Alberta Hospital; (780)407-7047; Fax. (780)407-3314.

GRAHAM, Tracy-Jean M; University of Alberta Hosp, 8440 112 St NW, Edmonton AB T6G 2B7; Man'99; CCFP; Staff, University of Alberta Hospital; (780)407-8822

GRAHAM, Wendy; Main Street, PO Box 10, Port-aux-Basques NL A0M 1C0; Mem'97; CCFP; Staff, Dr Charles L Legrow Health Centre; Co-Principal Investigator, Memorial University Of Newfoundland; (709)695-7775; Fax. (709)695-5757; drwgraham@nf.aibn.com.

GRAHAM, Wendy; 304-111 Main St W, North Bay ON P1B 2T6; Tor'80; CCFP; FCFP; Staff, North Bay Regional Health Centre - Regional Mental Health; (705)476-7747; Fax. (705)476-9373.

GRAHAM-ROWE, Sydney G; L Gervais Memorial Health Cent, PO Box 100 First Ave N, Goodsoil SK S0M 1A0; (Jamaica)'66; Staff, L Gervais Memorial Health Centre; (306)238-2100; Fax. (306)238-4449.

GRAHOVAC, Stephen Z; Kingston Gen Hosp, 76 Stuart St, Kingston ON K7L 2V7; Ott'84; FRCPC; DiagRad (Neuro Radiology). Staff, Kingston General Hospital; (613)549-6666

GRAICE, Renee A M F; Killarney Med Clinic, PO Box 1690, Killarney MB R0K 1G0.

GRAILLON, Ann; CHUS-Hop Fleurimont, 3001 12e av N, Sherbrooke QC J1H 5N4; Sher'88; FRCPC; Peds (Developmental Pediatrics). Staff, Centre Hospitalier Universitaire de Sherbrooke-Hopital Fleurimont; Assoc Prof Peds, Universite de Sherbrooke; (819)346-1110 x14644; Fax. (819)564-5398; ann.graillon@usherbrooke.ca.

GRAINGER, Diana; Foothills Med Centre, 1403 29 St NW, Calgary AB T2N 2T9; Cal'06; CCFP; Staff, Foothills Medical Centre; (403)944-1110

GRAINGER, Fredric R; Queen Square Doctors FHT, 201-366 Main St N, Brampton ON L6V 1P8; Tor'76; CCFP; FCFP; Court Staff, William Osler Health System - Brampton Civic Hospital; (905)455-1455; Fax. (905)455-5498.

GRAINGER, Mark R; Bonavista Med Clinic, 739 Lake Bonavista Dr SE, Calgary AB T2J 0N2; Alb'82; Staff, Rockyview General Hospital; (403)278-1440

GRAINGER, Sharon L; 104A-1803 St. Joseph Blvd, Orleans ON K1C 6E7; Mem'83; BSc; BMedSci; (613)841-1158; Fax. (613)841-1158.

GRAMLICH, Leah M; Royal Alexandra Hosp, 323-10240 Kingsway NW, Edmonton AB T5H 3V9; Alb'87; FRCPC; IntMed (Nutrition); Gastroent. Chief Gastroent., Royal Alexandra Hospital; Dir, Nutrition Support Capital Health Edmonton; Clin Assoc Prof, University of Alberta; (780)735-6839; Fax. (780)735-5650; leah.gramlich@ualberta.ca.

GRAMMATICO, Dino J; Regina Qu'appelle Hr-Pasqua, 4101 Dewdney Ave, Regina SK S4T 1A5; (Grenada)'84; FRCPC; AnatPath. Staff, Pasqua Hospital; (306)766-2134; Fax. (306)766-2752.

GRAMMOND, Pierre; Hotel-Dieu de Levis, 143 rue Wolfe, Levis QC G6V 3Z1; Laval'92; FRCPC; Neur; Electroenceph (P.Q.). Staff, Hôtel-Dieu de Lévis; (418)835-7158; Fax. (418)835-7122.

GRANBERG, Karl-Erik; Thunder Bay Reg HSC-T-Bay, 980 Oliver Rd, Thunder Bay ON P7B 6V4; Man'97; FRCPC; DiagRad. Staff, Thunder Bay Regional Health Sciences Centre; (807)684-6300

GRAND, Laurence; CSSS De La Haute-Yamaska, 205 boul Leclerc O, Granby QC J2G 1T7; Lausanne (Other Foreign)'02; DiagRad. Staff, Centre Hospitalier de Granby; (450)375-8000

GRAND'MAISON, Anne; Juravinski Cancer Centre, 699 Concession St, Hamilton ON L8V 5C2; Sher'88; FRCPC; IntMed; Hem. Staff, Mount Sinai Hospital; (905)387-9711

GRAND'MAISON, Francois; Neuro Rive-Sud, 250-4896 boul Taschereau, Greenfield Park QC J4V 2J2; Sher'83; FRCPC; Neur (Electromyography); Electroenceph (P.Q.). Chief Service Neurologie, Hopital Charles LeMoyne; assoc Prof, Universite de Sherbrooke; Langs: Spanish; English; (450)672-1931; Fax. (450)672-3308.

GRAND'MAISON, Genevieve; Hop Brome-Missisquoi-Perkins, 950 rue Principale, Cowansville QC J2K 1K3; Sher'01; CCFP; Staff, Hôpital Brome-Missisquoi-Perkins; (450)266-4342 x5; ggrandmaison@hotmail.com.

GRAND'MAISON, Nicole; CLSC Champagnat Vallee des For, 2-275 boul Saint-Luc, St-Jean-sur-Richel QC J2W 0B7; Sher'85; LMCC; (450)348-1061 x202

GRANDE, Maria S; Brock University, 500 Glenridge Ave, St. Catharines ON L2S 3A1; Tor'80; CCFP; Teach Staff, Brock University; Langs: English; French; Italian; (905)688-5550

GRANDISSON, Remi; Clinique Med de Saint-Tite, 264 rue du Moulin GD, Saint-Tite QC G0X 3H0; Laval'81; CCFP; FCFP; (418)365-5122; Fax. (418)365-3932.

GRANDMONT, Brigitte; CSSS Drummond-Hop Sainte-Croix, 570 rue Heriot, Drummondville QC J2B 1C1; Sher'91; DiagRad. Staff, Hôpital Sainte-croix; (819)478-6464; Fax. (819)478-6480.

GRANDMONT, Danielle; Hop Du Sacre-Coeur De Montreal, 5400 boul Gouin O, Montreal QC H4J 1C5; Mon'95; Staff, Hôpital du Sacre-Coeur de Montréal; (514)338-2050

GRANDMONT, Dominique; Centre Hosp Honore-Mercier, 2750 boul Laframboise, Saint-Hyacinthe QC J2S 4Y8; Mon'86; CSPQ; Cardiol; IntMed. Staff, Centre Hospitalier Honore-Mercier; (450)771-3333

GRANDMONT, Julie; CSSS du Sud de Lanaudière, 911 montee des Pionniers, Terrebonne QC J6V 2H2; Laval'03; FRCPC; Psy. Staff, Centre Hospitalier Pierre le Gardeur; (450)654-7525

GRANDWILEWSKI, Waldemar; Hamilton Comm Health Ctr, M1B-414 Victoria Ave N, Hamilton ON L8L 5G8; Warsaw (Poland)'78; PhD; Staff Emerg, Niagara Health System - St Catharines General Site; Staff Emerg, The Brant Community Healthcare System - Brantford General Hospital Site; Consultant Environmental, Inline Enterprises International; Clinical Asst Prof OrthSurg, McMaster University; Langs: Polish; German; (905)529-5221; Fax. (905)667-1082.

GRANDY, Barbara; Health Sciences Centre, 300 Prince Philip Dr, St. John's NL A1B 3V6; Mem'87; CCFP; FCFP; Asst Registrar, Health Sciences Centre; College of Physicians & Surgeons of Newfoundland & Labrador; (709)777-6300

GRANDY, Elwood C; 59 Payzant Dr PO Box 2820, Windsor NS B0N 2T0; Dal'82; (902)798-8600; Fax. (902)798-9550.

GRANER, Jerry L; The Doctor's Office, 245 Eglinton Ave E, Toronto ON M4P 3B7; Tor'68; BScPharm; Court Staff, Sunnybrook Health Sciences Centre; (416)488-1455; Fax. (416)488-8846.

GRANGER, Beatrice; CHUM-Hosp Notre Dame, 1560 rue Sherbrooke E, Montreal QC H2L 4M1; Mon'73; CSPQ; FRCSC; GenSurg; Psy. Staff, Centre Hospitalier l'Université de Montréal (CHUM) - Hôpital Notre-Dame; (514)890-8242; Fax. (514)412-7236.

GRANGER, Jean; Clin Medico Familiale Aylmer, C12-181 rue Principale, Gatineau QC J9H 6A6; Mon'77; LMCC; Staff, Hull Hospital; Langs: English; (819)684-7171; Fax. (819)685-0406; grangerjean@msn.com.

GRANGER, Jean; Polyclinique St-Jerome, 305-200 rue Durand, Saint-Jerome QC J7Z 7E2; Mon'82; FRCSC; Otol. (450)565-9898; Fax. (450)565-2702.

GRANGER, Louis R; 4577 rue Beaubien E, Montreal QC H1T 1T5; Mon'74; ObstGyn. Assoc Staff, Hôpital Ste-Justine; (514)725-9136; Fax. (514)725-9138.

GRANGER, Micheline; Polyclinique Med Beaubien-Sant, 107-6494 rue Beaubien E, Montreal QC H1M 1A9; Mon'75; (514)353-7161; Fax. (514)353-0081.

GRANGER, Nathalie; Ctr Hosp Anna-Laberge, 200 boul Brisebois, Chateauguay QC J6K 4W8; McG'99; FRCPC; IntMed. Staff, Hôpital Anna-Laberge; Langs: French; (450)699-2425

GRANGER, Perrine; CHUS-Hop Fleurimont, 3001 12e av N, Sherbrooke QC J1H 5N4; Staff, Centre Hospitalier Universitaire de Sherbrooke-Hopital Fleurimont; (819)346-1110 x14422

GRANGER, Pierre; CSSS Bordeaux-Cartierville-St-, 555 boul Gouin O, Montreal QC H3L 1K5; Mon'65; PhD; Staff, Pavillon Notre-Dame de la Merci; Clinical Asst Prof Family Med, Universite de Montreal; Langs: German; Bilingual(English/French); (514)331-3025; Fax. (514)331-0781.

GRANGER, Robert D C; Villa Caritas, 1411-16515 88 Ave NW, Edmonton AB T5R 0A4; Cal'03; FRCPC; Psy. Staff, Alberta Hospital Edmonton; (780)342-6552; Fax. (780)342-6579.

GRANGER, Robert; Royal City Med Bldg, 208-250 Keary St, New Westminster BC V3L 5E7; UBC'89; FACS; FRCSC; GenSurg. Staff, Royal Columbian Hospital; Clin Instructor Surg, University of British Columbia; (604)526-3721; Fax. (604)526-3811.

GRANGER-JUNEAU, Eugenie; CHUQ-Hotel-Dieu de Quebec, 11 Cote du Palais, Quebec QC G1R 2J6; Laval'01; Staff, Centre Hospitalier Universitaire de Québec (CHUQ) - Siege Social; Langs: English; Spanish; (418)691-5042

GRANGER VALLEE, Alexandre; CHUM-Hop Notre-Dame, 1560 rue Sherbrooke E, Montreal QC H2L 4M1; Mon'04; FRCPC; IntMed; Nephrol. Staff, Centre Hospitalier l'Université de Montréal (CHUM) - Hôpital Notre-Dame; (514)890-8000 x26616

GRANICH, Annette; Allan Mem Institute, P2 037-1025 av des Pins O, Montreal QC H3A 1A1; McG'75; FACP; FRCPC; Psy. Staff Outpatient Dept, McGill University Health Centre - Royal Victoria Hospital; Asst Prof Psy, McGill University; (514)934-1934 x35502

GRANOVSKY, Shawna; North York Gen Hosp, 4001 Leslie St, North York ON M2K 1E1; Wes'92; FRCPC; Peds. Staff, North York General Hospital; (416)756-6002; Fax. (416)638-5286.

GRANT, Leigh; Medical & Dental Bldg, 211-250 Lawrence Ave W, Toronto ON M5M 1B2; Qns'98; CCFP; (416)787-3771; Fax. (416)782-3030.

GRANT, Andrew A; Rouge Valley-Centenary HC, 2867 Ellesmere Rd, Scarborough ON M1E 4B9; Tor'03; CCFP; Staff, Rouge Valley Health System - Centenary Health Centre Site; (416)284-8131; Fax. (416)281-7038.

GRANT, Andrew D M; South Health Campus, 4448 Front St SE, Calgary AB T3M 1M4; Tor'04; FRCPC; IntMed; Cardiol. (403)956-3769; Fax. (403)956-1482.

GRANT, Andrew M; CHUS-Hop Fleurimont, 3001 12e av N, Sherbrooke QC J1H 5N4; Birmingham (England)'70; MRC; PhD(Oxon); FACMI; FRCPC; MedBiochem (Medical Informatics). Dir Collaborative Research for Effective Diag, Centre Hospitalier Universitaire de Sherbrooke-Hopital Fleurimont; Prof, Universite de Sherbrooke; Langs: German; Bilingual(French/English); (819)346-1110 x74158; andrew.grant@usherbrooke.ca.

GRANT, Andrew N; Royal Victoria Hosp, 201 Georgian Dr, Barrie ON L4M 6M2; Tor'93; CCFP; CCFP(E.M.); Staff, Royal Victoria Regional Health Centre; (705)728-9090

GRANT, Anna; Maple Key Clinic Fam Hlth Team, D2-1036 Princess St, Kingston ON K7L 1H2; Man'06; CCFP; (613)546-9721; Fax. (613)546-2799.

GRANT, Carol M R; The Hosp for Sick Children, 555 University Ave, Toronto ON M5G 1X8; Tor'78; FRCPC; Anes. Staff, The Hospital For Sick Children; (416)813-7445; carol.grant@sickkids.ca.

GRANT, Christina; McMaster University, HSC 3A-1280 Main St W, Hamilton ON L8S 4K1; McM'94; FRCPC; Peds (Adolescent Medicine). Asst Prof Dept Ped, Hamilton Health Sciences Centre - McMaster Children's Hospital; Teach Staff, McMaster University; (905)521-2100 x75644; Fax. (905)308-7548.

GRANT, D Augustus; Public Gardens Med, 200-5675 Spring Garden Rd, Halifax NS B3J 1H1; Dal'97; CCFP; (902)425-5440

GRANT, Darrell W; Brock University, 500 Glenridge Ave, St Catharines ON L2S 3A1; Cal'88; CCFP; CCFP(E.M.); FCFP; Staff, Niagara Health System - St Catharines General Site; (905)688-5550

GRANT, David A; Centennial Prof Centre, 81 Exhibition St, Kentville NS B4N 1C2; Dal'82; (902)678-3466; Fax. (902)678-1977.

GRANT, David R; 11C 1248-585 University Ave, Toronto ON M5G 2N2; Wes'78; FRCSC; GenSurg (Hepatobiliary Surgery)., Toronto General Hospital - UHN; Prof Surg, University of Toronto; (416)340-4800; david.grant@uhn.ca.

GRANT, David R; 201-520 University Ave W, Waterloo ON N2T 2Z6; McM'80; BSc; MSc; Med Dir, Parkwood Manor Home for the Aged; (519)744-7200; Fax. (519)745-3684.

GRANT, Dennis R; Surrey Mem Hosp, 13750 96 Ave, Surrey BC V3V 1Z2; Alb'78; FRCPC; GenPath; AnatPath. Consultant, Vancouver General Hospital - Centennial Pavillion; Staff Lab Med, Surrey Memorial Hospital; Clin Assoc Prof Path, University of British Columbia; (604)585-5614; Fax. (604)585-5562.

GRANT, Doris J; Brockville Gen Hosp, 75 Charles St, Brockville ON K6V 1S8; Tor'66; FRCPC; DiagRad (Diagnostic Imaging). Staff, Brockville General Hospital - Charles Street; (613)345-5645 x1157; Fax. (613)345-8324.

GRANT, Elizabeth L; 1862 Oak Bay Ave, Victoria BC V8R 1C5; Cal'81; Staff, Vancouver Island Health Authority South Island Region; (250)592-3220; Fax. (250)592-3225.

GRANT, Elizabeth R L; BC Women's & Children's Hosp, NICU-4480 Oak St, Vancouver BC V6H 3V4; UBC'02; FRCPC; Peds. Staff, BC Children's Hospital; (604)875-2136

GRANT, Eric N; Saint John Reg Hosp, PO Box 2100 Stn Main 400 University Ave, Saint John NB E2L 4L2; Dal'74; FRCPC; IntMed; Rheum. Staff, Saint John Regional Hospital; (506)648-6804; Fax. (506)648-7349.

GRANT, Estee C; Alberta Children's Hosp, 2888 Shaganappi Trail NW, Calgary AB T3B 6A8; Ott'00; FRCPC; Peds; Critical Care Medicine. Staff Pediatric Intensivist, Alberta Children's Hospital; (403)955-7931; Fax. (403)955-7081; estee.grantl@albertahealthservices.ca.

GRANT, F Curry; 204-265 Dundas St E, Belleville ON K8N 5A9; Qns'71; FACC; FACP; DABIM(Cardiol.); MSc(Epidemiol.); FRCPC; IntMed (Stroke Prevention); Cardiol. Staff, QHC Belleville General; Asst Prof, Queen's University; (613)969-7400; Fax. (613)961-2544; cgrant@qhc.on.ca.

GRANT, Heather A; Foothills Med Centre, 4F-1403 29 St NW, Calgary AB T2N 2T9; UBC'05; FRCSC; ObstGyn. Staff, Foothills Medical Centre; (403)944-1110

GRANT, Ian; Halifax Infirmary, 3822-1796 Summer St, Halifax NS B3H 3A7; Dal'89; FRCPC; Neur (Neuromuscular Diseases). Staff, Queen Elizabeth II Health Sciences Centre - Halifax Infirmary Site; (902)473-3731; Fax. (902)473-4438; ian.grant@cdha.nshealth.ca.

GRANT, Ian M; Crown St Med Clinic, 110 Crown St, Saint John NB E2L 2X7; Dal'85.

GRANT, Ian R; Kootenay-Boundary Reg Hosp, 1200 Hospital Bench, Trail BC V1R 4M1; Ott'91; FRCPC; Anes. Staff, Kootenay Boundary Regional Hospital; (250)368-3311; Fax. (250)364-3419.

GRANT, James M; 4565 Wallace St, Port Alberni BC V9Y 3Y3; Dal'83; (250)723-7391; Fax. (250)724-6086.

GRANT, James R; 636 Kennedy Rd, Scarborough ON M1K 2B3; UBC'10; CCFP; (647)247-2600; Fax. (647)247-2601.

GRANT, Jeffry M; Foothills Med Centre, C231-1403 29 St NW, Calgary AB T2N 2T9; Dal'83; FRCPC; EmergMed. Staff, Foothills Medical Centre; (403)670-1635

GRANT, Jennifer M; Vancouver Gen Hosp, 1110 JPPN-855 12th Ave W, Vancouver BC V5Z 1M9; McG'00; FRCPC; IntMed; MedMicrobiol; InfectDis. Staff, Vancouver General Hospital - Centennial Pavillion; (604)875-4111

GRANT, John A; Saint John Reg Hosp, PO Box 2100 Stn Main 400 University Ave, Saint John NB E2L 4L2; Cal'05; FRCSC; OrthSurg. Staff, Saint John Regional Hospital; (506)648-7725; Fax. (506)648-7726.

GRANT, K Gordon J; Health & Wellness Centre, 125-589 South Pelham Rd, Welland ON L3C 3C7; Wes'91; CCFP; CCFP(E.M.); FCFP; Staff, Niagara Health System - Ontario Street Site; (905)788-1500

GRANT, Kelly E; Flemingdon Health Centre, 10 Gateway Blvd, North York ON M3C 3A1; Tor'00; CCFP; Staff, Toronto East General Hospital Inc; Lecturer, University of Toronto; (416)429-4991; Fax. (416)422-3573.

GRANT, Kevin; 606-18 Wynford Dr, North York ON M3C 3S2; Ott'97; FRCSC; OrthSurg (Spine). Staff, The Scarborough Hospital - General Campus; (647)352-8100; Fax. (647)352-8200.

GRANT, Margaret H; The Credit Valley Hosp, 2200 Eglinton Ave W, Mississauga ON L5M 2N1; Tor'95; FRCPC; IntMed; GeriatricMed. Staff, The Credit Valley Hospital; (905)813-1100 x5415; Fax. (905)813-3855.

GRANT, Martin; Clin Serv Sante Rosemere, 400 ch de la Grande-Cote, Rosemere QC J7A 1K7; Mon'04; CCFP; (450)621-9776; Fax. (450)621-1296.

GRANT, Mary M; Postgraduate Med Education, MDCL 3101A-1280 Main St W, Hamilton ON L8S 4K1; McM'07; DiagRad.

GRANT, Nasha E; Medical Dental South Bldg, 312-650 41st Ave W, Vancouver BC V5Z 2M9; Wes'05; CCFP; (604)261-8177

GRANT, Nathalie; 204-387 Main St, Shediac NB E4P 2B5; Mon'98; CCFP; Staff, Dr Georges-L-Dumont University Hospital Centre; (506)533-8366

GRANT, Paul H H; 6383 Main St, Stouffville ON L4A 1G4; Tor'83; (905)591-2626; Fax. (905)591-2627.

GRANT, Peter A; Radiology Consultants Assoc, 120A-6707 Elbow Dr SW, Calgary AB T2V 0E5; Tor'91; FRCPC; DiagRad. Ac Staff, Rockyview General Hospital; Ac Staff, Peter Lougheed Centre; (403)777-3009; Fax. (403)777-3008.

GRANT, Peter; 706-5863 Leslie St, North York ON M2H 1J8; Otago (New Zealand)'60; MB BS; DABPN(P); FRANZCP; FRCPC; Psy. Consultant Staff, North York General Hospital; Court Staff, St Michael's Hospital; Fax. (416)492-7999.

GRANT, Raymer P; 2449 JP2-899 12th Ave W, Vancouver BC V5Z 1M9; UBC'76; FRCPC; Anes. Ac Staff Anes, Vancouver General Hospital - Centennial Pavillion; (604)875-4304

GRANT, Ronald M; The Hosp for Sick Children, 555 University Ave, Toronto ON M5G 1X8; Cal'77; FRCPC; Peds (Pediatric Oncology). Staff, The Hospital For Sick Children; (416)813-5188; Fax. (416)813-5327.

GRANT, Vincent J; 2888 Shaganappi Trail NW, Calgary AB T3B 6A8; Cal'96; FRCPC; Peds (Pediatric Emergency Medicine). Staff, Alberta Children's Hospital; Asst Prof, University of Calgary; Langs: English; French; (403)955-7093; Fax. (403)955-7552; vincent.grant@albertahealthservices.ca.

GRANT, William F; Wedgewood Med Centre, 202-12 Gleneyre St, St. John's NL A1A 2M7; Mem'77; (709)722-9000

GRANT-HALL, Susan C; Grey Bruce Health Unit, 101 17th St E, Owen Sound ON N4K 0A5; Ott'83; CCFP; (519)376-9420

GRANT-OYEYE, Lind; University Hosp of Northern BC, 1475 Edmonton St, Prince George BC V2M 1S2; Benin (Nigeria)'99; Psy. Staff, University Hospital of Northern British Columbia; (250)645-6045

GRANTCHAROV, Teodor P; St Michael's Hosp, 16 CC56-30 Bond St, Toronto ON M5B 1W8; (Bulgaria)'96; Staff, St Michael's Hospital; (416)864-5110

GRANTMYRE, John E; Urology Consultants, 332-5991 Spring Garden Rd, Halifax NS B3H 1Y6; Dal'82; FRCSC; Urol. Prof, Dalhousie University; (902)420-0044; Fax. (902)420-0240.

GRANTNER, Eric W; Nanaimo Reg Gen Hosp, 1200 Dufferin Cres, Nanaimo BC V9S 2B7; Qns'76; Ac Staff, Nanaimo Regional General Hospital; (250)755-7691

GRANTON, Jeffrey T; London HSC-University Hosp, PO Box 5339 Stn B B3 218-339 Windermere Rd, London ON N6A 5A5; Wes'98; FRCPC; Anes; Critical Care Medicine. Staff, London Health Sciences Centre - University Hospital; (519)685-8500

GRANTON, John T; Univ Hlth Network-Toronto Gen, 11UCSB1170-200 Elizabeth St, Toronto ON M5G 2C4; McM'87; FRCPC; IntMed (Critical Care Medicine); Respir. Staff, Toronto General Hospital - UHN; Consultant, Princess Margaret Hospital - University Health Network; Asst Prof, University of Toronto; (416)340-4485; Fax. (416)340-3359; john.granton@uhn.on.ca.

GRAPES, Gavin P; Holley Clinic, 348 Front St, Quesnel BC V2J 2K3; Cape Town (South Africa)'85; MB ChB; Ac Staff, G R Baker Memorial Hospital; (250)992-2158; Fax. (250)992-9391.

GRAPKO-MYSAK, Deborah A; Chamber of Commerce Bldg, 502-345 Lakeshore Rd E, Oakville ON L6J 1J5; Tor'79; CCFP; FCFP; Court Staff, Halton Healthcare Services Corporation - Oakville Site; (905)845-4511; Fax. (905)845-8133.

GRASEMAN, Hartmut; The Hosp for Sick Children, 555 University Ave, Toronto ON M5G 1X8; Essen (Germany)'92; Staff, The Hospital For Sick Children; Langs: German; (416)813-6346; Fax. (416)813-6246; hartmut.grasemann@sickkids.ca.

GRASS, Stephen B; Assiniboine Clinic, 633 Lodge Ave, Winnipeg MB R3J 0S9; Man'02; CCFP.

GRASSWICK, Linda; PO Box 547 Stn A, Abbotsford BC V2T 6Z8; UBC'95; FRCPC; Psy (Forensic Psychiatry). (604)217-2174

GRATTON, Adele; Royal Bank Plaza South Tower, PO Box 83 Stn Royal Bank 2975-200 Bay St, Toronto ON M5J 2J2; Ott'78; Physician Occup Health & Safety, St John's Rehabilitation Hospital; Med Consultant, BMO Life of Canada; Langs: English; French; (416)601-9990; Fax. (416)363-9466.

GRATTON, Celine; Inst U Geriatrie de Montreal, 4565 ch Queen-Mary, Montreal QC H3W 1W5; Mon'81; Staff, Institut Universitaire de Gériatrie de Montréal; (514)340-3514

GRATTON, Jacques; Centre Med St-Urbain, 411-3875 rue Saint-Urbain, Montreal QC H2W 1V1; Mon'73; FRCPC; Gastroent; IntMed. Staff, Centre Hospitalier l'Université de Montréal (CHUM) - Hôtel-Dieu; (514)842-3865; Fax. (514)842-4981.

GRATTON, Madeleine; Clinique Med Lanaudiere, 222 rue Bernard, St-Charles-Brromee QC J6E 2C5; Sher'85; Staff, Centre Hospitalier Régional de Lanaudière; (450)755-1033; Fax. (450)753-5558.

GRATTON, Nicole; CLSC-CHSLD du Marigot, 250 boul Cartier O, Laval QC H7N 5S5; Mon'94; (450)668-1803

GRATTON, Robert; London HSC-Victoria Hosp, PO Box 5010 Stn B B2 412-800 Commissioners Rd E, London ON N6A 5W9; Wes'89; FRCSC; ObstGyn. Staff, London Health Sciences Centre - Victoria Campus; (519)685-8500

GRATTON, Valerie; Montfort Hosp, 713 Montreal Rd, Ottawa ON K1K 0T2; Ott'05; Staff, Montfort Hospital; Langs: Bilingual(English/French); (613)748-4621

GRATZER, David; Scarborough Hosp-Birchmount, 3030 Birchmount Rd, Scarborough ON M1W 3W3; Man'00; FRCPC; Psy. Staff, The Scarborough Hospital - Birchmount Campus; (416)495-2701; Fax. (416)495-2426.

GRAVA-GUBINS, Inese; College of Family Physicians, 1F-2630 Skymark Ave, Mississauga ON L4W 5A4; Staff, College Of Family Physicians Of Canada-Ontario; (905)629-0900; igrava-gubins@cfpc.ca.

GRAVEL, Alain; Hotel-Dieu de Levis, 143 rue Wolfe, Levis QC G6V 3Z1; Sher'96; DiagRad. Staff, Hôtel-Dieu de Lévis; (418)835-7121

GRAVEL, Andre; CLSC Kateri, 90 boul Marie-Victorin, Candiac QC J5R 1C1; Laval'80; (450)659-7661; Fax. (450)444-6276.

GRAVEL, Anne-Marie; Westmount Med Bldg, 225-5025 rue Sherbrooke O, Montreal QC H4A 1S9; McG'91; DDerm; FRCPC; Derm. Langs: Bilingual(English/French); (514)482-6465; Fax. (514)482-3380.

GRAVEL, Caroline; Medi-Club du Sanctuaire, 106-6100 av du Boise, Montreal QC H3S 2W1; Sher'91; FRCPC; Peds. Staff, Hôpital du Haut-Richelieu; (514)739-5646; Fax. (514)739-2368.

GRAVEL, Celine; CSSS de Rivière-de-Loup, 75 rue Saint-Henri, Riviere-Du-Loup QC G5R 2A4; Laval'76; Ophth. Staff, Centre Hospitalier Regional du Grand-Portage; (418)868-1000 x2397; Fax. (418)868-0166.

GRAVEL, Charles A; Clinique Chir Ortho C-Lemoyne, 126 rue Saint-Louis, Lemoyne QC J4R 2L5; Ott'86; FRCSC; OrthSurg (Spine). Staff Surg, Hopital Charles LeMoyne; Langs: English; French; (450)672-1212; Fax. (450)672-9834.

GRAVEL, Christine; CSSS de Chicoutimi, CP 5006 305 rue Saint-Vallier, Chicoutimi QC G7H 5H6; Laval'01; FRCPC; Psy. Staff, Complexe hospitalier de la Sagamie; (418)541-1000

GRAVEL, Claude; Clinique medicale du Luc, 33 rue Saint-Patrice E, Magog QC J1X 5B7; Laval'67; (819)843-3353; Fax. (819)843-7217.

GRAVEL, Denis; CSSS de Laval, 1755 boul Rene-Laennec, Laval QC H7M 3L9; Mon'77; CSPQ; FRCSC; GenSurg. Staff, Hopital de la Cite de la santé; (450)668-1010; Fax. (450)975-5545.

GRAVEL, Denis; Societe Ass Automobile du QC, CP 19600 Succ Terminus 333 boul Jean Lesage, Quebec QC G1K 8J6; Laval'67; (418)528-4043

GRAVEL, Denis H; The Ottawa Hosp-Gen Campus, 501 Smyth Rd, Ottawa ON K1H 8L6; Ott'92; CSPQ; FRCPC; AnatPath. Staff Path, The Ottawa Hospital - General Campus; Asst Prof, University of Ottawa; Langs: English; French; (613)737-8289; Fax. (613)737-8853.

GRAVEL, Diane; CLSC Norman-Bethune, 200-800 boul Chomedey, Laval QC H7V 3Y4; Mon'76; (450)682-2952; Fax. (450)973-1689.

GRAVEL, Evelyne; Hop Du Sacre-Coeur De Montreal, 5400 boul Gouin O, Montreal QC H4J 1C5; Mon'07; CCFP; CCFP(E.M.); Staff, Hôpital du Sacre-Coeur de Montréal; (514)338-2222

GRAVEL, Jacques; CLSC Hochelaga-Maisonneuve, 4201 rue Ontario E, Montreal QC H1V 1K2; Laval'72; (514)253-2181; Fax. (514)253-4550.

GRAVEL, Jean; 101-783 rue Notre-Dame, Repentigny QC J5Y 1B4; Mon'81; Staff Emerg, Centre Hospitalier Pierre le Gardeur; (450)582-1260; Fax. (450)582-0677; graj82@hotmail.com.

GRAVEL, Jean-Pierre; 1601 boul Laurier, Quebec QC G1S 1M5; Laval'65; DABOph; FRCSC; Ophth. Langs: English; Spanish; (418)688-1480; Fax. (418)688-4143; drgravel@videotron.ca.

GRAVEL, Jocelyn; Hôpital Ste-Justine, 3175 ch Cote-Sainte-Catherine, Montreal QC H3T 1C5; Mon'97; FRCPC; Peds; PedEmergMed (P.Q.). Staff, Hôpital Ste-Justine; (514)345-4931

GRAVEL, Julie; Clinique medicale Notre-Dame, 120-504 rue Notre-Dame, Repentigny QC J6A 2T8; Sher'96; (450)585-3232; Fax. (450)582-9763.

GRAVEL, Louis; Clin Medicale Chateauguay, 120 boul Saint-Jean-Baptiste, Chateauguay QC J6K 3A9; Mon'89; Staff, Hôpital Anna-Laberge; (450)691-8191

GRAVEL, Marie-Pascale; CSSS du Lac-des-Deux-Montagnes, 520 boul Arthur-Sauve, Saint-Eustache QC J7R 5B1; Sher'99; Staff, Hôpital de Saint-Eustache; Langs: English; (450)473-6811

GRAVEL, Maxime; CSSS de Rimouski-Neigette, CP 3150 Succ A 150 av Rouleau, Rimouski QC G5L 5T1; Laval'07; NuclearMed (P.Q.). Staff, Hôpital Regional Rimouski; (418)724-3000 x8692

GRAVEL, Michel; Clinique Ophtalmovision, 308-5995 boul Gouin O, Montreal QC H4J 2P8; Mon'86; FRCSC; Ophth. Staff, Hôpital du Sacre-Coeur de Montréal; (514)335-4492

GRAVEL, Normand; Ctr Hosp de Verdun, 4000 boul Lasalle, Verdun QC H4G 2A3; Mon'79; CSPQ; FRCPC; Anes. chef Staff, Centre Hospitalier de Verdun; Langs: Bilingual(French/English); (514)362-1000 x2829

GRAVEL, Robert; Clinique Med Duberger, 2810 boul Pere-Lelievre, Quebec QC G1P 2Y1; Laval'78; (418)688-8414; Fax. (418)688-4273.

GRAVEL, Serge; CLSC de Pohenegamook, 1922 rue Saint-Vallier, Pohenegamook QC G0L 1J0; Mon'92; Staff, Centre Hospitalier Trois-Pistoles; (418)859-2450

GRAVEL, Stephane; CSSS de Saint-Jerome, 290 rue de Montigny, Saint-Jerome QC J7Z 5T3; Sher'84; CSPQ; FRCSC; GenSurg. Staff, Hôtel-Dieu de Saint-Jérôme; (450)431-8200

GRAVELINE, Ronald; CSSS de Laval, 1755 boul Rene-Laennec, Laval QC H7M 3L9; Mon'84; FRCPC; NuclearMed. Chief Nuclear Med, Hopital de la Cite de la santé; (450)975-5546; Fax. (450)975-5548.

GRAVELLE, Catherine; 200B-745 Montreal Rd, Ottawa ON K1K 0T1; Ott'98; FRCSC; ObstGyn. Staff, Montfort Hospital; (613)741-6767; Fax. (613)741-4147.

GRAVELLE, M R Joan; Smyth Med Centre, 220-1929 Russell Rd, Ottawa ON K1G 4G3; Ott'82; FRCPC; Peds. (613)737-7707; Fax. (613)737-4867.

GRAVEN, Michael A; IWK Health Centre, PO Box 9700 Rpo CSC 5850-5980 University Ave, Halifax NS B3K 6R8; Florida(FL) (USA)'91; Staff, IWK Health Centre; (902)470-8888

GRAVES, Carl O; St Joseph's Gen Hosp, 2137 Comox Ave, Comox BC V9M 1P2; McG'87; CCFP; FCFP; Staff, St Joseph's General Hospital; (250)339-2242

GRAVES, Darren F; Health Sciences Centre, 820 Sherbrook St, Winnipeg MB R3A 1R9; Man'89; CCFP; Staff Emerg, Health Sciences Centre; (204)774-6511

GRAVES, Gillian R; IWK Health Centre, PO Box 9700 Rpo CSC 5850-5980 University Ave, Halifax NS B3K 6R8; UBC'78; FRCSC; ObstGyn (Reproductive Endocrinology & Infertility). Obst/Gynec, Queen Elizabeth II Health Sciences Centre - Victoria General Site; Ac Staff ObstGyn, IWK Health Centre; Prof, Dalhousie University; Langs: Bilingual(English/French); (902)470-6726; Fax. (902)425-1125.

GRAVES, Lisa; Northern Ont School of Med, 935 Ramsey Lake Rd, Sudbury ON P3E 2C6; Ott'91; CCFP; FCFP; Assoc Dean Undergraduate Med Education/Assoc Prof, Northern Ontario School of Medicine; Langs: Bilingual(English/French); (705)662-7165; Fax. (705)662-7192.

GRAVES, Nana; Clinique Enfant-Medic, 3221 boul des Sources, Dollard-D-Ormeaux QC H9B 1Z6; McG'74; FRCP; FRCPC; Peds (Ambulatory Pediatrics). Langs: Fanti; Akan; Twi; (514)685-0880; Fax. (514)685-6162.

GRAVES, Peter S; Queensway-Carleton Hosp, 3045 Baseline Rd, Nepean ON K2H 8P4; Ott'91; CCFP; CCFP(E.M.); FCFP; Staff, Queensway Carleton Hospital; Langs: Bilingual(English/French); (613)721-4710

GRAY, Aileen A; Kingston Family Health Team, 202-275 Bagot St, Kingston ON K7L 3G4; Qns'97; CCFP; Asst Prof Family Med, Queen's University; (613)549-7477; Fax. (613)549-4920.

GRAY, Allison J; IWK Health Centre, PO Box 9700 Rpo CSC 5850-5980 University Ave, Halifax NS B3K 6R8; Mem'87; FRCPC; Anes. Staff, IWK Health Centre; (902)470-8888

GRAY, Bruce G; St Michael's Hosp, 3 084-30 Bond St, Toronto ON M5B 1W8; Tor'87; ABR; ABNM; FRCPC; DiagRad (Neuro Radiology); NuclearMed. Staff NeuroRadiologist & Nuclear Phys, St Michael's Hospital; Teacher Med Imaging, University of Toronto; (416)864-5792; Fax. (416)864-5380.

GRAY, Catharina A; 3130 Weald Rd, Victoria BC V8R 6E1; Alb'98; BSc; CCFP; (250)595-5195

GRAY, Catharina; Brandon Reg Health Centre, 150 McTavish Ave E, Brandon MB R7A 2B3; Pretoria (South Africa)'93; CCFP; Staff, Brandon Regional Health Centre; (204)578-4166

GRAY, Catherine; Civic Parkdale Clinic, 408-737 Parkdale Ave, Ottawa ON K1H 8L6; UBC'05; IntMed. Staff, The Ottawa Hospital - Civic Campus; (613)761-4473; Fax. (613)761-4036.

GRAY, Christine E; Bonaventure Med Clinic, 101-12427 Bonaventure Dr SE, Calgary AB T2J 3N8; Cal'94; CCFP; (403)225-9499; Fax. (403)225-2572.

GRAY, Christopher; Queen Elizabeth II HSC-Halivax, 2501C-1796 Summer St, Halifax NS B3H 3A7; Dal'01; FRCPC; IntMed; Cardiol. Staff, Queen Elizabeth II Health Sciences Centre - Halifax Infirmary Site; (902)473-4907; Fax. (902)473-3158.

GRAY, Clare E; Children's Hosp Eastern Ont, 401 Smyth Rd, Ottawa ON K1H 8L1; Qns'88; FRCPC; Psy (Child Psychiatry). Staff Outpatient Psy, Children's Hospital of Eastern Ontario (CHEO); (613)737-7600 x2714; Fax. (613)737-2257; gray_c@cheo.on.ca.

GRAY, D Shaun; Centennial CMH & Brain Injury, PO Box 1000 Stn Main, Ponoka AB T4J 1R8; Cal'85; PhD; FRCPC; PhysMed&Rehab;CCFP; FCFP; Ac Staff, Centennial Centre for Mental Health & Brain Injury; Assoc Prof/Div Dir Phys Med & Rehab, University of Alberta; (403)783-7810

GRAY, Dale E H; North York Med Arts Bldg, 343-1333 Sheppard Ave E, North York ON M2J 1V1; Qns'82; BSc; MSc(Tor.); DABOph; FRCSC; Ophth (Medical Ophthalmology). Court Staff, North York General Hospital; Ac Staff, St Michael's Hospital; Assoc Prof Ophth, University of Toronto; (416)494-6155; Fax. (416)494-0010.

GRAY, Dan P; University of Alberta Hosp, 120-8440 112 St NW, Edmonton AB T6G 2B7; Cal'82; FRCPC; Anes. Staff, University of Alberta Hospital; (780)407-8861; Fax. (780)407-3200.

GRAY, Danielle R; Downey Family Med Centre, 2-115 Downey Rd, Guelph ON N1C 1A2; McM'01; CCFP; (519)827-9779; Fax. (519)827-0162.

GRAY, Daryl K; London HSC-Victoria Hosp, PO Box 5010 Stn B E2 217-800 Commissioners Rd E, London ON N6A 5W9; Wes'92; FRCSC; GenSurg. Staff, London Health Sciences Centre - Victoria Campus; (519)667-6583; Fax. (519)667-6546.

GRAY, Donovan O N; Victoria Gen Hosp, 2340 Pembina Hwy, Winnipeg MB R3T 2E8; Man'87; BSc(Med); CCFP; CCFP(E.M.); FCFP; Physician ER, Victoria General Hospital; (204)477-3121

GRAY, Gail L; The U of Toronto-Mississauga, 3359 Mississauga Rd, Mississauga ON L5L 1C6; Tor'83; BSc; MSc; CCFP; FCFP; Court Staff, The Credit Valley Hospital; Clin Educator, University of Toronto; (905)828-5255; gail_gray@hotmail.com.

GRAY, Gary J; Hys Med Centre, 400-11010 101 St NW, Edmonton AB T5H 4B9; Cal'93; MSc; FRCSC; Urol (Female Urology). Staff, Royal Alexandra Hospital; Staff, Covenant Health - Misericordia Community Hospital; Clinical Asst Prof Urol, University of Alberta; (780)425-5598

GRAY, Gary W; Defence Research & Dev Canada, PO Box 2000 Stn Downsview A 1133 Sheppard Ave W, North York ON M3M 3B9; McG'68; PhD(Tor); FRCPC; IntMed. Court Staff, Mount Sinai Hospital; Med Dir, MDS Executive Health Services; (416)635-2015

GRAY, Gerald; IWK Health Centre, PO Box 9700 Rpo CSC 5850-5980 University Ave, Halifax NS B3K 6R8; Dal'75; FRCPC; Psy (Child & Adolescent Psychiatry). Staff, IWK Health Centre; (902)456-8515; Fax. (902)470-8382.

GRAY, Ian A; Alliston Family Physicians, 40-180 Parsons Rd, Alliston ON L9R 1E8; Aberdeen (Scotland)'70; MB ChB; Ac Staff, Stevenson Memorial Hospital; (705)435-5633; Fax. (705)435-2860.

GRAY, James R; 5153-2775 Laurel St, Vancouver BC V5Z 1M9; UBC'77; ABIM; FRCPC; IntMed; Gastroent. Ac Staff Gastroent, Vancouver General Hospital - Centennial Pavillion; Clin Prof, University of British Columbia; (604)875-5618; Fax. (604)875-5373.

GRAY, Janice; Carleton Place, 44 Lansdowne Ave, Carleton Place ON K7C 2T8; Wes'90; CCFP; FCFP; Ac Staff, Carleton Place & District Memorial Hospital; (613)257-7002; Fax. (613)257-8177.

GRAY, Jason H; Lansdowne Prof Bldg, 380-1641 Hillside Ave, Victoria BC V8T 5G1; UBC'84; FRCSC; PlasSurg. Ac Staff, Royal Jubilee Hospital; Ac Staff, Victoria General Hospital; (250)592-8668; Fax. (250)592-8625.

GRAY, Jonathan D; Royal Ottawa Hlth Care Group, 1145 Carling Ave, Ottawa ON K1Z 7K4; Qns'01; FRCPC; Psy. Staff, Royal Ottawa Mental Health Centre - Royal Ottawa Health Care Group; Langs: Bilingual(English/French); (613)722-6521

GRAY, Katherine A; Oakville Health Centre, 115-1060 Speers Rd, Oakville ON L6L 2X4; Wes'82; (905)842-9735; Fax. (905)842-9731.

GRAY, Michael G; Portage Clinic Inc, 140 9th St SE, Portage La Prairie MB R1N 3V5; Manchester (England)'83; (204)857-3445; Fax. (204)239-1278.

GRAY, P Ainslie; Springboard Clinic, 301-1055 Yonge St, Toronto ON M4W 2L2; McM'75; (416)901-3077; Fax. (416)901-3079.

GRAY, Perry R; Health Sciences Centre, JBRC709-820 Sherbrook St, Winnipeg MB R3A 1R9; Man'84; FRCSC; GenSurg (Critical Care Medicine). Assoc Prof, University of Manitoba; (204)787-1872

GRAY, Peter; Bay View Mall Med Offices, 50-470 Dundas St E, Belleville ON K8N 1G1; Manchester (England)'83; MB ChB; MRCGPract; CCFP; (613)966-4045; Fax. (613)966-0072.

GRAY, Phebe; The Wright Clinic, 57 James St, Parry Sound ON P2A 1T6; Wes'03; CCFP; Staff Family Med, West Parry Sound Health Centre; (705)746-2181

GRAY, Robin R; Foothills Med Centre, 1403 29 St NW, Calgary AB T2N 2T9; McG'72; ABR; FRCPC; DiagRad (Interventional Radiology). Staff Radiol, Foothills Medical Centre; Prof Radiol, University of Calgary; (403)944-1969; Fax. (403)944-2549; robin.gray@crha-health.ab.ca.

GRAY, Robin S; 1408-750 Broadway W, Vancouver BC V5Z 1H8; Wes'94; Derm. (604)876-3333

GRAY, Samantha; Saint John Reg Hosp, PO Box 2100 Stn Main 400 University Ave, Saint John NB E2L 4L2; Dal'07; FRCPC; IntMed; MedOncol. Staff, Saint John Regional Hospital.

GRAY, Sara H; St Michael's Hosp, 30 Bond St, Toronto ON M5B 1W8; Wes'99; FRCPC; EmergMed; Critical Care Medicine. Staff, St Michael's Hospital; (416)864-5095

GRAY, Stanley W; Penticton Reg Hosp, 550 Carmi Ave, Penticton BC V2A 3G6; Alb'71; Staff, Penticton Regional Hospital; (250)492-4000

GRAY, Stephen J; Rocky Mountain Hlth Ctr, PO Box 2019, Fernie BC V0B 1M0; Wes'92; LMCC; (250)423-4718; Fax. (250)423-6463.

GRAY, Stephen J; Provincial Health Authority, 301-931 Fort St, Victoria BC V8V 3K3; Ott'80; MHSc(UBC); CCFP; (250)519-5728; Fax. (250)384-0447.

GRAY, Susan J; 723 Millidge Ave, Saint John NB E2K 2N7; Dal'81; Staff, Saint John Regional Hospital; (506)634-6869; Fax. (506)634-6851.

GRAY, W Alexander; 550 Lakeshore Rd, Sarnia ON N7V 2S5; Wes'52; DAB; FACS; FRCSC; GenSurg. Consultant, Bluewater Health - Charlotte Eleanor Englehart Hospital; Ac Staff Surg, Bluewater Health - Mitton Site; Ac Staff Surg, Bluewater Health - Norman Site; (519)344-8941; Fax. (519)344-8822.

GRBAC, Leonard; Workplace Safety & Insurance B, 4F-200 Front St W, Toronto ON M5V 3J1; Tor'85; CCFP; CCFP(E.M.); FCFP; (416)344-4508; leonard_grbac@wsib.on.ca.

GRBIC, Dusanka; CHUS-Hop Hotel-Dieu, 580 rue Bowen, Sherbrooke QC J1G 2E8; Sher'07; Gastroent; IntMed. Staff, Centre Hospitalier Universitaire de Sherbrooke-Hôpital Hôtel-Dieu; (819)346-1110

GREAVES, Francis W; Grey Bruce HS-Owen Sound, PO Box 1800 Stn Main 1800 8th St E, Owen Sound ON N4K 6M9; Qns'79; FRCPC; DiagRad. Ac Staff, Grey Bruce Health Services - Meaford Site; Ac Staff Diagnostic Imaging, Grey Bruce Health Services - Owen Sound; (519)376-2121 x2202; Fax. (519)372-3954.

GREAVETTE, Thomas; 8-118 Lake St, St. Catharines ON L2R 5Y1; McM'04; CCFP; Ad Staff Privil, Niagara Health System - St Catharines General Site; (905)685-6555; Fax. (905)685-6558.

GREBEN, Daniel H; Addiction & Mental Hlth-Clarke, G5-250 College St, Toronto ON M5T 1R8; Tor'86; FRCPC; Psy. Staff Psy, Centre for Addiction & Mental Health (CAMH) - College Street Site; Staff Psy, Mount Sinai Hospital; Asst Prof, University of Toronto; (416)410-4151; Fax. (416)979-6815; daniel_greben@camh.net.

GREBENYUK, Julia; Med-Scan Xray & Ultrasound, 2810 Major MacKenzie Dr, Vaughan ON L6A 1R8; Tor'04; FRCPC; DiagRad. Staff, St Joseph's Hospital - St Joseph's Health Care; Langs: Russian; (905)832-8984

GREBENYUK, Liliya; Guelph Gen Hosp, 115 Delhi St, Guelph ON N1E 4J4; (Kazakhstan)'98; FRCPC; IntMed. Staff, Guelph General Hospital; (519)837-6440; Fax. (519)822-2170.

GRECO, Robert A; Sudbury Reg Hosp-Laurentian, 41 Ramsey Lake Rd, Sudbury ON P3E 5J1; Tor'76; FRCPC; DiagRad. Staff, Health Sciences North-Laurentian Site; Langs: Italian; French; (705)522-2200

GREEFF, Herman; PO Box 2250 Rpo Banks Centre, Kelowna BC V1X 4K6; Orange Free State (South Africa)'91; MB ChB; CCFP; FCFP; Med Dir Long Term Care, Northern Health Authority; (250)763-5152

GREEFF, Leon L; 208-803 Chaparral Dr SE, Calgary AB T2X 0E5; (South Africa)'02; (403)873-7734; Fax. (403)873-7735.

GREEFF, Michael P; Chinook Reg Hosp, 960 19 St S, Lethbridge AB T1J 1W5; Stellenbosch (South Africa)'78; MB ChB; FRCPath; FRCPC; AnatPath. Staff, Chinook Regional Hospital; (403)388-6158

GREEFF, Wessel; 3-2020 Strachan Rd SE, Medicine Hat AB T1B 0M9; (South Africa)'05; MB BCh; Staff, Medicine Hat Regional Hospital; (403)580-1882; Fax. (403)504-5799.

GREEK, L Shane; Royal Jubilee Hosp, 1952 Bay St, Victoria BC V8R 1J8; UBC'01; FRCPC; DiagRad. Staff, Royal Jubilee Hospital; (250)370-8272

GREEN, Albert H; Valleyview Nursing Home, 541 Finch Ave W, North York ON M2R 3Y3; Wes'57; Vis Court Staff, North York General Hospital - Branson Division; Vis Court Staff, Sunnybrook Health Sciences Centre; Langs: Yiddish; (416)398-0555

GREEN, Andrew F D; Trillium Hlth Ctr-Mississauga, 100 Queensway W, Mississauga ON L5B 1B8; Tor'00; CSPQ; FRCPC; Anes. Staff, Trillium Health Centre - Mississauga; (416)689-2810

GREEN, Bernard M; 209-4430 Bathurst St, North York ON M3H 3S3; Tor'68; Staff, North York General Hospital; Langs: Hebrew; (416)636-4815; Fax. (416)636-0471.

GREEN, Cheryl L; Islington Med Clinic, 702-1243 Islington Ave, Etobicoke ON M8X 1Y9; RCS (Ireland)'82; MB ChB; BAO; LRCS; Ac Staff, St Joseph's Health Centre; (416)766-5888; Fax. (416)766-5885.

GREEN, Daniel M; Oshawa Clinic, 117 King St E, Oshawa ON L1H 1B9; Tor'02; FRCPC; IntMed; Gastroent (Therapeutic Endoscopy). (905)721-4964; Fax. (905)721-6614.

GREEN, Daphne E; Group One Medical, 1111 Springfield Rd, Kelowna BC V1Y 8R7; London (England)'84; MB BS; CCFP; (250)762-4006; Fax. (250)762-4290.

GREEN, David J M; Charlotte County Hosp, 4 Garden St, St Stephen NB E3L 2L9; London (England)'64; MB BS; DABFP; FRCS(Ed); LRCP; Ac Staff Anes & Emerg Med, Charlotte County Hospital; Staff, Horizon Health Network St. Stephen Public Health; Langs: French; (506)465-4444; Fax. (506)465-4410; davidjm.green@horizonnb.ca.

GREEN, Douglas S; The Ottawa Hosp-Gen Campus, 501 Smyth Rd, Ottawa ON K1H 8L6; Ott'90; FRCPC; Psy. Staff, The Ottawa Hospital - General Campus; (613)737-8010; Fax. (613)739-9980.

GREEN, Francis; HSC-Faculty of Med, 3330 Hospital Dr NW, Calgary AB T2N 4N1; Manchester (England)'68; Staff Path, Foothills Medical Centre; Prof, University of Calgary; (403)220-4514; Fax. (403)270-8928; fgreen@ucalgary.ca.

GREEN, James S E; University of Alberta Hosp, 8440 112 St NW, Edmonton AB T6G 2B7; (United Kingdom)'98; MB BS; Staff, University of Alberta Hospital; (780)407-8887

GREEN, Janet E; Courtenay Med Associates, 201-1350 England Ave, Courtenay BC V9N 8X6; Qns'78; CCFP; Staff Family Practice & Obst, St Joseph's General Hospital; (250)334-4411; Fax. (250)338-1245.

GREEN, Jason P; Grand River Hosp-KW Hlth Ctre, 835 King St W, Kitchener ON N2G 1G3; Wes'06; FRCPC; EmergMed. Staff, Grand River Hospital - Kitchener/Waterloo Health Centre; (519)742-3611

GREEN, Jennifer A; Vernon Jubilee Hosp, 2101 32 St, Vernon BC V1T 5L2; UBC'00; FRCPC; Anes (Pain Management). Staff, Vernon Jubilee Hospital; (250)545-2211 x1426

GREEN, Jennifer; Sexual Health Clinic, 2340 Dundas St W, Toronto ON M6P 4A9; Wes'95; ACLS; CCFP; Staff, Women's College Hospital; Langs: Bilingual(English/French); (416)338-7088; jenny.green@wchospital.ca.

GREEN, Jeremy A; B1-350 Conestoga Blvd, Cambridge ON N1R 7L7; Wes'98; FRCSC; ObstGyn. Staff, Cambridge Memorial Hospital; (519)624-8820; Fax. (888)389-9273.

GREEN, Jerome A; Bayview Business Centre, 218-16700 Bayview Ave, Newmarket ON L3X 1W1; Mem'99; FRCSC; Urol. Staff, Southlake Regional Health Centre; (905)836-5561; Fax. (905)836-0038.

GREEN, Kevin H I; 17-600 King St E, Oshawa ON L1H 1G6; Ott'96; CCFP; (905)432-1017; Fax. (905)432-0070.

GREEN, Kevin W; 304C-101 Queensway W, Mississauga ON L5B 2P7; Tor'94; FRCPC; IntMed; Respir. Ac Consultant, Trillium Health Centre - Mississauga; (905)848-5599; Fax. (905)848-8606.

GREEN, Kristy-Jill; 310 Juliana Dr, Woodstock ON N4V 0A4; Alb'03; CCFP; CCFP(E.M.); (519)421-4211

GREEN, Larry T; 103-2245 James White Blvd, Sidney BC V8L 1Z5; Wes'72; DABOph; FRCSC; Ophth. Staff, Royal Jubilee Hospital; Staff, Saanich Peninsula Hospital; (250)656-1813; Fax. (250)656-2551.

GREEN, Laurence D; MUHC-Montreal Gen Hosp, B2 118-1650 av Cedar, Montreal QC H3G 1A4; Tor'74; FRCPC; IntMed. Staff, McGill University Health Centre - Montreal General Campus; (514)934-8054; Fax. (514)937-7298.

GREEN, Laurie K; St Lawrence Health Services, 3-140 The Esplanade, Toronto ON M5A 4P5; Tor'84; CCFP; CCFP(E.M.); FCFP; Court Staff, St Michael's Hospital; (416)864-6000; Fax. (416)360-4902.

GREEN, Lawrence; Canamera Med Centre, B7B-350 Conestpga Blvd, Cambridge ON N1R 7L7; Ott'98; MSc; BSc; FRCSC; GenSurg (Surgical Oncology). Staff, Cambridge Memorial Hospital; Aj Clin Assoc Prof, McMaster University; Langs: French; (519)623-1114; Fax. (519)623-1814.

GREEN, Lee; Glen Sather Sports Med Clinic, 11400 University Ave NW, Edmonton AB T6G 1Z1; (USA)'83; DABFP; Staff, University of Alberta Hospital; (780)433-4211

GREEN, Mark C; Cedar Med Centre, 106-9648 128 St, Surrey BC V3T 2X9; UBC'85; Staff Hospitalist, Surrey Memorial Hospital; Staff, Boundary Park Medical Centre; (604)584-5242; Fax. (604)589-1242.

GREEN, Martin S; Univ of Ottawa Heart Institute, H1285-40 Ruskin St, Ottawa ON K1Y 4W7; Tor'75; FRCP; FRCPC; IntMed (Arrhythmias); Cardiol. Staff, University of Ottawa Heart Institute; Staff, The Ottawa Hospital - Civic Campus; Prof Med Cardiol, University of Ottawa; (613)761-4820; Fax. (613)761-4549.

GREEN, Michael E; Family Med Centre, PO Box 8888 Stn Main 220 Bagot St, Kingston ON K7L 5E9; UBC'93; BSc; MPH; CCFP; FCFP; Ac Staff, Kingston General Hospital; Ac Staff, Hotel-Dieu Hospital; Asst Prof Family Med, Queen's University; Langs: Spanish; (613)533-9303; Fax. (613)549-5403; mg13@queensu.ca.

GREEN, Michael; Port Hope Med Centre, 205-249 Ontario St, Port Hope ON L1A 3Y9; Tor'71; FSOGC; FRCSC; ObstGyn (Gynecology). Consultant, Northumberland Hills Hospital; Asst Prof Family Practice, Queen's University; (905)885-1774; Fax. (905)885-7309.

GREEN, Nicole; Collingwood Gen & Marine Hosp, 459 Hume St, Collingwood ON L9Y 1W9; Tor'08; BMedSci(H); CCFP; Staff, Collingwood General & Marine Hospital; (705)445-2550

GREEN, Peter; 4198-5820 University Ave, Halifax NS B3H 1V7; Dal'95; FRCPC; IntMed; Derm. Assoc Prof, Dalhousie University; (902)473-2814; Fax. (902)473-2655; peter.green@cdha.nshealth.ca.

GREEN, Raymond; Murakami Med Clinic, PO Box 1000 735 4th Ave, Hope BC V0X 1L0; UBC'84; CCFP; Langs: English; French; (604)869-5648

GREEN, Robert S; Queen Elizabeth II HSC, 377-1276 South Park St, Halifax NS B3H 2Y9; Dal'96; FRCPC; EmergMed; Critical Care Medicine. Att Physician, Queen Elizabeth II Health Sciences Centre - Victoria General Site; Prof, Dalhousie University; (902)473-3486

GREEN, Ruth-Ann F; Montfort Hosp, 713 Montreal Rd, Ottawa ON K1K 0T2; Ott'05; FRCPC; Anes. Staff, Montfort Hospital; (613)746-4621

GREEN, Stefanie L; 326-1964 Fort St, Victoria BC V8R 6R3; McG'93; MDCM; CCFP; Staff, Victoria General Hospital; Staff Clinical Faculty, University of British Columbia; Clinical Faculty, University of Victoria; Langs: French; (250)592-4710; Fax. (250)592-4712.

GREEN, Stephen C; Kipling Heights Med Centre, 2291 Kipling Ave, Etobicoke ON M9W 4L6; Tor'73; Staff, William Osler Health System - Etobicoke General Hospital; (416)741-4545; Fax. (416)744-1484.

GREEN, Steven A; Thunder Bay Reg HSC-T-Bay, 980 Oliver Rd, Thunder Bay ON P7B 6V4; Wes'07; CCFP; CCFP(E.M.); Fam Med, Northwestern Ontario Regional Cancer Centre - Cancer Care Ontario; greens@tbh.net.

GREEN, Thomas J; Royal Columbian Hosp, 330 Columbia St E, New Westminster BC V3L 3W7; Qns'06; FRCPC; EmergMed. Staff, Royal Columbian Hospital; (604)520-4000

GREEN, W Scott; Health Services Complex, 3-20 Kennedy Dr, Sussex NB E4E 2P1; Dal'84; Staff, Sussex Health Centre; (506)433-6060; Fax. (506)432-3701.

GREEN-STARR, Iris R; Drs I Green Starr & S Starr In, 1520 Fort St, Victoria BC V8S 5J2; Tor'88; BSc; (250)598-1621

GREENAWAY, Christina A; SMBD Jewish Gen Hosp, G143-3755 ch Cote-Sainte-Cathe, Montreal QC H3T 1E2; Man'86; FRCPC; IntMed (Medical Microbiology & Infectious Diseases); MedMicrobiol; InfectDis. Att Staff, Sir Mortimer B Davis Jewish General; adj Prof, McGill University; (514)340-8222 x2933

GREENAWAY, John R; 1881 Cabana Rd W, Windsor ON N9G 1C7; Qns'65; CCFP; FCFP; (519)566-5664; Fax. (519)253-8599.

GREENAWAY, Masa'il; BC Women's Hosp & Health Ctre, P2 213-4500 Oak St, Vancouver BC V6H 3N1; Alb'97; FRCPC; Psy. Staff, BC Women's Hospital & Health Centre; (604)875-2000 x5599; mgreenaway@cw.bc.ca.

GREENBAUM, Joseph; Charlton Med Ctr, 805-25 Charlton Ave E, Hamilton ON L8N 1Y2; Tor'71; BSc; FRCPC; IntMed (Allergy); ClinImmunol&Allergy. Affil Staff, Hamilton Health Sciences Centre - McMaster Children's Hospital; Ac Staff, St Joseph's Healthcare - Charlton Campus; Physician, Charlton Medical Centre; Asst Clin Prof Med, McMaster University; Langs: Hebrew; Yiddish; (905)522-7703

GREENBERG, David E; 619 Bathurst St, Toronto ON M5S 2P8; Wes'89; Langs: Hebrew; (416)964-1131; Fax. (416)964-8898.

GREENBERG, Gary H; The Ottawa Hosp-Gen Campus, 501 Smyth Rd, Ottawa ON K1H 8L6; Ott'77; FRCPC; EmergMed (Sports Medicine). Ac Staff EmergMed, The Ottawa Hospital - General Campus; Dir Sports Med Centre/Clin Asst Prof, University of Ottawa; Langs: English; French; (613)737-8899; Fax. (613)737-8967.

GREENBERG, Gordon R; Mount Sinai Hosp, 445-600 University Ave, Toronto ON M5G 1X5; Alb'70; FRCPC; IntMed; Gastroent. Staff Gastoent, Mount Sinai Hospital; Prof, University of Toronto; (416)586-4800 x4727; Fax. (416)586-4802.

GREENBERG, H Joseph; 619 Bathurst St, Toronto ON M5S 2P8; Tor'52; (416)964-3307; Fax. (416)964-8898.

GREENBERG, Howard M; Medical Arts Bldg, 202-233 Kennedy St, Winnipeg MB R3C 3J5; Man'74; FACP; FRCPC; DiagRad (Abdominal Imaging). Assoc Staff, Health Sciences Centre; Asst Prof, University of Manitoba; (204)942-6453; Fax. (204)944-8101; hgreenbe5@shaw.ca.

GREENBERG, I David; Health Sciences Centre, F GD157-820 Sherbrook St, Winnipeg MB R3A 1R9; McG'71; FRCPC; DiagRad; NuclearMed. Physician Sect of Nuclear Med, Health Sciences Centre; Assoc Prof Radiol, University of Manitoba; (204)787-3375; Fax. (204)787-3090; dgreenberg@hsc.mb.ca.

GREENBERG, Manuel S; North Med Centre, 206-7131 Bathurst St, Thornhill ON L4J 7Z1; Cal'83; FRCPC; Peds. Staff, Mount Sinai Hospital; Staff, Mackenzie Richmond Hill Hospital; Staff Pt-Time Er, The Hospital For Sick Children; Teacher, University of Toronto; Langs: Hebrew; (905)731-7596; Fax. (905)731-4975.

GREENBERG, Mark A; 202-4700 Jane St, Toronto ON M3N 2L3; Tor'88; BSc; ASAM; CCFP; FCFP; Ac Staff, Humber River Regional Hospital - Finch Avenue Site; Court Staff, Sunnybrook Health Sciences Centre; Langs: Hebrew; (416)661-0004; Fax. (416)661-0810.

GREENBERG, Mark L; The Hosp for Sick Children, 555 University Ave, Toronto ON M5G 1X8; Witwatersrand (South Africa)'66; DABPed; MB ChB; FRCPC; Peds (Pediatric Oncology). Staff Hem/Oncol, The Hospital For Sick Children; Prof POGO Chair, University of Toronto; (416)813-5886; Fax. (416)813-5327; mark.greenberg@sickkids.ca.

GREENBERG, Michael; Groupe Medical Ste-Catherine, 5025 rue Sherbrooke O, Montreal QC H4A 1S9; Mon'10; (514)932-6122

GREENBERG, Ronald B; 212-2678 Broadway W, Vancouver BC V6K 2G3; Tor'76; (604)733-1055

GREENBERG, Saul; Farber Robert & Greenberg Saul, 206-2401 Yonge St, Toronto ON M4P 3H1; Tor'70; FRCP; FRCPC; Peds (Dermatology). Court Staff Newborn Sunnybrook Health Sciences Ctr, Sunnybrook Health Sciences Centre; Staff Major Pt-time Peds, The Hospital For Sick Children; Assoc Prof, University of Toronto; (416)485-4419; Fax. (416)485-2936.

GREENBERG, Stephen H; 1540-800 boul René-Lévesque O, Montreal QC H3B 1X9; McG'82; Staff Family Med, McGill University Health Centre - Royal Victoria Hospital; (514)874-0483; Fax. (514)874-0947.

GREENBLATT, Ellen M; Ctr for Fertility & Reproducti, 700-250 Dundas St W, Toronto ON M5T 2Z5; McG'82; ABOG; ABOG(REI); FRCSC; ObstGyn (Fertility). Staff, Mount Sinai Hospital; Assoc Prof, University of Toronto; Langs: Bilingual(English/French); (416)586-4748; Fax. (416)586-5386.

GREENBLOOM, Susan L; Medical Clinic Bldg, 322-89 Humber College Blvd, Etobicoke ON M9V 4B8; Tor'89; FRCPC; IntMed (Hepatology); Gastroent. Staff, William Osler Health System - Etobicoke General Hospital; (416)740-4113; Fax. (416)740-4816.

GREENE, Calvin A; Regional Fertility Prog, 400-2000 Place Veteran's NW, Calgary AB T3B 4N2; Alb'80; BSc; FRCSC; ObstGyn (Gynecology). Div Chief REI, Foothills Medical Centre; Dir, Regional Fertility Programme; Clin Prof ObstGyn/Div Chief Reproductive Endocrinology & Infertility, University of Calgary.

GREENE, Mabel T; Midtown Medical Clinic, 35 Campbell Ave, St. John's NL A1E 2Z3; Dal'70; (709)579-0703; Fax. (709)579-1477.

GREENE, Marian E; Blackmarsh Med Clinic, 205-496 Topsail Rd, St. John's NL A1E 2C3; Mem'77; (709)579-3725

GREENE, Richard E; Salvation Army Grace Gen Hosp, 300 Booth Dr, Winnipeg MB R3J 3M7; Man'91; CCFP; CCFP(E.M.); FCFP; Staff Emerg, The Salvation Army Grace Hospital; Teacher Family Practice, University of Manitoba; (204)837-0117; Fax. (204)837-5421.

GREENFIELD, Brian J; MUHC-Montreal Children's Hosp, D567-2300 rue Tupper, Montreal QC H3H 1P3; Seattle(WA) (USA)'80; AB; FRCPC; Psy (Child Psychiatry). Dir Outpatient Crisis Team, McGill University Health Centre - Montreal Children's Hospital; Member, McGill University; Langs: English; French; (514)412-4400; Fax. (514)412-4250; brian.greenfield@muhc.mcgill.ca.

GREENFIELD, Garry; CSSS du Lac-des-Deux-Montagnes, 520 boul Arthur-Sauve, Saint-Eustache QC J7R 5B1; McG'87; FRCSC; OrthSurg. Staff, Hôpital de Saint-Eustache; (450)473-7222

GREENFIELD, Gavin J; Foothills Med Centre, C231-1403 29 St NW, Calgary AB T2N 2T9; Wes'98; CCFP; CCFP(E.M.); Asst Prof, University of Calgary; (403)944-8178; Fax. (403)944-2419.

GREENFIELD, Thomas; 3-109 Banting Dr PO Box 1630, Deep River ON K0J 1P0; Qns'89; (613)584-1912; Fax. (613)584-1912; tom.greenfield@drdh.org.

GREENHILL, Alexandra; Crossroads Clinics, 3F-507 Broadway W, Vancouver BC V5Z 1E6; Mon'99; CCFP; Physician, British Columbia Medical Association; Langs: Spanish; German; (604)347-7338

GREENHILL, Brian J; Western Med Assessments, 17204 106A Ave NW, Edmonton AB T5S 1E6; (England)'57; FRCSC; OrthSurg (Medico Legal Assessments). (780)433-1191; Fax. (780)433-1127.

GREENLAND, Jonathan; Dr H Bliss Murphy Cancer Ctr, 300 Prince Philip Dr, St. John's NL A1B 3V6; Mem'95; FRCPC; RadOncol (Lung Cancer). Staff, Dr H Bliss Murphy Cancer Centre; Clinical Asst Prof Med, Memorial University Of Newfoundland; (709)777-7805; Fax. (709)777-8756; Jonathan.Greenland@easternhealth.ca.

GREENOUGH, M Catherine; Primary Health Care Centre, 60-346 John St N, Arnprior ON K7S 2P6; Qns'85; MSc; BSc; MBA; FRCPC; IntMed. Staff, Arnprior & District Memorial Hospital; (613)623-8090; Fax. (613)623-9631.

GREENSMITH, Christopher T; St Clair Corporate Centre, 401-265 Front St N, Sarnia ON N7T 7X1; Dundee (Scotland)'74; MB ChB; FRCPC; CommunMed. Med Officer of Hlth, Sarnia-Lambton Health Unit; (519)336-6039; Fax. (519)336-4943.

GREENSPAN, Lorne; Medcan Health Mgmt Inc, 1500-150 York St, Toronto ON M5H 3S5; Tor'73; FRCPC; EmergMed (Corporate Consultant). Staff, Medcan Health Management Inc; Teach Staff Family & Commun Med, University of Toronto; (416)350-5963; Fax. (416)350-5981; lornegreenspan@medcan.com.

GREENSPAN, Michael; Hamilton Comm Health Centre, M11-414 Victoria Ave N, Hamilton ON L8L 5G8; Tor'74; FRCS; FRCSC; Urol (Sexual Dysfunction). Ac Staff, Hamilton Health Sciences Centre - Hamilton General Hospital; Court Staff, St Joseph's Healthcare - Charlton Campus; Teach Staff, McMaster University; (905)529-0988; Fax. (905)529-0296; ppdoc99@hotmail.com.

GREENSPAN, Stanley; Hys Med Centre, 202-11010 101 St NW, Edmonton AB T5H 4B9; (South Africa)'79; MB ChB; (780)426-1121; Fax. (780)425-5979.

GREENSPOON, Allen; Hamilton Comm Health Ctre, M1-414 Victoria Ave N, Hamilton ON L8L 5G8; Tor'77; Physician, Hamilton Community Health Centre; (905)529-5221; Fax. (905)546-0361; hchc@cogeco.net.

GREENSPOON, Jeffrey N; Hamilton Reg Cancer Ctr, 699 Concession St, Hamilton ON L8V 5C2; Ott'05; FRCPC; RadOncol. (905)387-9495; Fax. (905)575-6323.

GREENSPOON, Mark; 110-164 Queen St E, Brampton ON L6V 1B4; McG'85; (905)456-9600; Fax. (905)456-9606.

GREENSPOON, Todd T; Hamilton Comm Health Centre, 414 Victoria Ave N, Hamilton ON L8L 5G8; Wes'10; CCFP; (905)529-5221

GREENSTONE, Gerrard C; Careplace Med Centre, 7154 120 St, Surrey BC V3W 3M8; McG'70; Peds. Consultant, Surrey Memorial Hospital; (604)590-5811

GREENSTONE, Ilana R; Montreal Children's Hosp, 2300 Tupper St, Montreal QC H3H 1P3; McG'97; FRCPC; Peds; PedEmergMed. Staff, McGill University Health Centre - Montreal Children's Hospital; (514)412-4400 x23039

GREENTREE, David M; CHUS-Hop Fleurimont, 3001 12e av N, Sherbrooke QC J1H 5N4; Alb'88; MSc; CSPQ; FRCSC; GenSurg;CCFP; Cardiovasc&ThorSurg (P.Q.); CardSurg. Staff, Centre Hospitalier Universitaire de Sherbrooke-Hopital Fleurimont; (819)346-1110 x14356; Fax. (819)820-6871; david.greentree@usherbrooke.ca.

GREENWALD, Eric R; Health Sciences Centre, 2F55-1280 Main St W, Hamilton ON L8S 4K1; Qns'02; FRCPC; IntMed; Gastroent. (905)521-2100; Fax. (905)523-6048.

GREENWALD, Ilana; Markham Stouffville Hosp, PO Box 1800 Stn Main 381 Church St, Markham ON L3P 7P3; Tor'06; CCFP; CCFP(E.M.); Staff, Markham Stouffville Hospital; (905)472-5342

GREENWALD, Iris C; Oak Ridge Med Centre, 403-13291 Yonge St, Richmond Hill ON L4E 4L6; Tor'95; CCFP; (905)773-4444

GREENWALD, Joseph A; Hamilton HS-General Site, 237 Barton St E, Hamilton ON L8L 2X2; Tor'07; FRCPC; EmergMed. Staff, Hamilton Health Sciences Centre - Hamilton General Hospital; (905)527-4322

GREENWALD, Kenneth J; Mount Dennis Med Group, 98 Guestville Ave, Toronto ON M6N 4N6; Tor'76; CCFP; Ac Staff, Humber River Regional Hospital - Church Street Site; Langs: Hebrew; (416)763-1171; Fax. (416)763-0573.

GREENWALD, Marci R; Bay Centre for Birth Control, 8F-790 Bay St, Toronto ON M5G 1N8; Tor'05; CCFP; Staff, Women's College Hospital.

GREENWALD, Mark; NorFinch Med Centre, 312-2100 Finch Ave W, North York ON M3N 2Z9; Tel Aviv (Israel)'79; PhD; FRCPC; Peds (Allergy); Rheum. Staff, North York General Hospital; Staff, Humber River Regional Hospital - Church Street Site; Dir, Asthma Society of Canada; Assoc Prof, University of Toronto; Langs: Hebrew; French; (416)748-0008; Fax. (416)748-9957.

GREENWAY, Keith T; Joseph Brant Mem Hosp, 1230 North Shore Blvd E, Burlington ON L7S 1W7; Tor'76; FRCPC; EmergMed. Staff, Joseph Brant Memorial Hospital; Clin Assoc Prof Dept of Med, McMaster University; (905)632-3730

GREENWAY, Matthew; Montebello Med Centre, 8-118 Lake St, St Catharines ON L2R 5Y1; (Ireland)'02; FamilyMed. (289)668-0324

GREENWAY, Steven; Alberta Children's Hosp, 2888 Shaganappi Treail NW, Calgary AB T3B 6A8; Man'00; FRCPC; Peds; Cardiol. Staff, Alberta Children's Hospital; (403)955-7858

GREENWOOD, Eric D; William Osler HC-Brampton, 2100 Bovaird Dr E, Brampton ON L6R 3J7; Cincinnati (OH) (USA)'03; Staff, William Osler Health System - Brampton Civic Hospital; (416)494-2120

GREENWOOD, I Ronald; Scarborough Prof Centre, 210-1371 Neilson Rd, Scarborough ON M1B 4Z8; Tor'72; CCFP; FCFP; Ac Staff, Rouge Valley Health System - Centenary Health Centre Site; Consultant, Complain(CCM) Legal Services; (416)282-5749; Fax. (416)282-9144.

GREENWOOD, Julian D; Julian Greenwood Med Prof Corp, 90 Joanne Crt, Leamington ON N8H 5N5; Qns'83; CCFP; FCFP; Staff, Leamington District Memorial Hospital; (519)326-2373; Fax. (519)322-0041.

GREENWOOD, Michael T; 100-230 Menzies St, Victoria BC V8V 2G7; Cambridge (England)'74; MB BCh; CAFCI; CCFP; FCFP; Assoc Staff, Royal Jubilee Hospital; Assoc Staff, Victoria General Hospital; Med Dir, Victoria Pain Clinic; (250)388-9934

GREER, Mary-Louise C; The Hosp For Sick Children, 555 University Ave, Toronto ON M5G 1X8; Brisbane (Australia)'89; Staff, The Hospital For Sick Children; (416)813-5823; mary-louise.gree@sickkids.ca.

GREER, Matthew; Saint John Reg Hosp, PO Box 2100 Stn Main 400 University Ave, Saint John NB E2L 4L2; Dal'08; CCFP; CCFP(E.M.); Staff, Saint John Regional Hospital; (506)648-6000

GREF, Pauline; College des Med Du Quebec, 2170 boul Rene-Levesque O, Montreal QC H3H 2T8; Sher'82; FRCPC; Peds. Insp, College des Medecins du Quebec; (514)933-4441

GREGAN, Ida-Lynn; Nine Circles Comm Hlth Centre, 705 Broadway Ave, Winnipeg MB R3G 0X2; Man'93; CCFP; (204)940-6001; Fax. (204)940-6003.

GREGG, John S; Niagara HS-St Catharines, 142 Queenston St, St. Catharines ON L2R 7C6; Wes'70; Court Staff, Niagara Health System - St Catharines General Site; (905)684-7271

GREGG, Randall J; Edmonton Sport Institute, 11828 111 Ave NW, Edmonton AB T5G 0E1; Alb'79; (780)451-1234; Fax. (780)452-9303.

GREGG, Richard W; Kingston Reg Cancer Centre, 25 King St W, Kingston ON K7L 5P9; West Indies (Barbados)'83; MB BS; FRCPC; IntMed; MedOncol. Staff, Kingston General Hospital; Asst Prof Med, Queen's University; (613)544-2631 x4502; Fax. (613)544-9708; richard.gregg@krcc.on.ca.

GREGG, Sean M T; Medical & Dental Bldg, 3939 50A Ave, Red Deer AB T4N 4E6; Cal'04; FRCSC; GenSurg. (403)347-9037; Fax. (403)347-9038.

GREGGAIN, Joshua; Murakami Med Clinic, PO Box 1000 735 4th Ave, Hope BC V0X 1L0; Cal'03; CCFP; (604)869-5648; Fax. (604)793-9804.

GREGOIRE, Alain D; CHUS-Hop Hotel-Dieu, 580 rue Bowen S, Sherbrooke QC J1G 2E8; Laval'94; FRCSC; Ophth. Staff, Centre Hospitalier Universitaire de Sherbrooke-Hôpital Hôtel-Dieu; (819)346-1110

GREGOIRE, Caroline; CSSS des Îles, 430 ch Principal, Cap-aux-Meules QC G4T 1R9; Mon'07; Staff, Hôpital de l'Archipel; (418)986-2121; Fax. (418)986-6845.

GREGOIRE, Danielle; CSSS de Montmagny-L'Islet, 350 boul Tache O RR 1, Montmagny QC G5V 3R8; Laval'87; FRCSC; Otol (P.Q.) (Head & Neck Surgery). Staff, CSSS de Montmagny-L'Islet; (418)248-0630; Fax. (418)248-0947.

GREGOIRE, Edith; CSSS des Iles, 430 ch Principal, Cap-aux-Meules QC G4T 1R9; Laval'86; Staff, Hôpital de l'Archipel; Langs: English; (418)986-2121; Fax. (418)986-7010.

GREGOIRE, Elyse; CLSC de Sherbrooke, 8 rue Speid, Sherbrooke QC J1M 1R6; Sher'01; (819)563-2572; Fax. (819)566-8059.

GREGOIRE, Gabrielle; CSSS du Suroît, 150 rue Saint-Thomas, Salaber-de-Valleyf QC J6T 6C1; Mon'07; CCFP; Staff, Centre Hospitalier Régional du Suroît; (450)371-9920; Fax. (450)371-7454.

GREGOIRE, Genevieve; Hop du Sacre-Coeur de Mtl, 5400 boul Gouin O, Montreal QC H4J 1C5; Mon'91; FRCPC; IntMed (Critical Care Medicine). Staff Intensive Care & IntMed, Hôpital du Sacre-Coeur de Montréal; adj Prof, Universite de Montreal; Langs: English; (514)338-2050; Fax. (514)338-2424; margen@videotron.ca.

GREGOIRE, Ginette; 10345 av Papineau, Montreal QC H2B 2A3; Mon'72; LMCC; Psy (Geriatric Psychiatry)., Universite de Montreal; Langs: Italian; English; (514)384-2000 x5080; Fax. (514)383-1462; ginette.gregoirecsssamn@ssss.gouv.qc.ca.

GREGOIRE, Jacques C; 1-321 rue Woodward, Sherbrooke QC J1G 1V7; Laval'65; Ophth. (819)565-8647

GREGOIRE, Jean; Clinique Familiale, 13555 boul Lacroix, Saint-Georges QC G5Y 1P1; Laval'80; CCFP; FCFP; Staff, Centre Hospitalier Beauce-Etchemin; (418)228-8001; Fax. (418)228-5583.

GREGOIRE, Jean; CHUQ-Hotel-Dieu de Quebec, 11 Cote du Palais, Quebec QC G1R 2J6; Mon'98; FRCSC; ObstGyn (Gynecologic Oncology). Staff, Centre Hospitalier Universitaire de Québec (CHUQ) - Siege Social; Langs: Bilingual(French/English); (418)691-5392; Fax. (418)691-5720.

GREGOIRE, Jean; Institut de Cardiologie de Mtl, 5000 rue Belanger, Montreal QC H1T 1C8; Mon'82; ABNM; FRCPC; NuclearMed. Staff, Institut de Cardiologie de Montréal; adj Prof Radiol, Universite de Montreal; (514)376-3330; Fax. (514)376-0936.

GREGOIRE, Jean; Institut de Cardiologie de Mtl, 5000 rue Belanger, Montreal QC H1T 1C8; Mon'85; CSPQ; FRCPC; IntMed; Cardiol. Staff, Institut de Cardiologie de Montréal; (514)376-3330 x3612; Fax. (514)376-6299.

GREGOIRE, Jocelyn; Hôpital Laval, 2725 ch Sainte-Foy, Quebec QC G1V 4G5; Sher'82; CSPQ; Cardiovasc&ThorSurg; GenSurg (Pulmonary Diseases). Staff, Hôpital Laval; adj Prof, Université Laval; Langs: English; (418)656-8711; Fax. (418)656-4762.

GREGOIRE, Julie; Ctr Hosp de Verdun, 4000 boul Lasalle, Verdun QC H4G 2A3; Mon'95; CCFP; Staff, Centre Hospitalier de Verdun; (514)362-1000

GREGOIRE, Keith R; 107-121 Dundas St E, Belleville ON K8N 1C3; Qns'94; FRCPC; Peds. Staff, Kingston General Hospital; QHC Belleville General; Assoc Prof, Queen's University; (613)968-8288; Fax. (613)968-6433.

GREGOIRE, Louise; Clinique Med de Nutrition, 360-979 av de Bourgogne, Quebec QC G1W 2L4; Sher'88; (418)652-1121; Fax. (418)652-0055.

GREGOIRE, Lucie H; Brant Community HC-Brantford, 200 Terrace Hill St, Brantford ON N3R 1G9; Ott'80; Ac Staff, The Brant Community Healthcare System - Brantford General Hospital Site; (519)752-7871

GREGOIRE, Marie-Claude; CSSS de la Haute-Yamaska, 205 boul Leclerc O, Granby QC J2G 1T7; Sher'90; Affil Staff Family Med, Centre Hospitalier de Granby; Langs: Bilingual(French/English); (450)372-5491; Fax. (450)375-8042.

GREGOIRE, Marie-Claude; IWK Health Centre, PO Box 7900 Rpo CSC 5850-5980 University Ave, Halifax NS B3K 6R8; Mon'99; FRCPC; Peds. Staff, IWK Health Centre; (902)470-7707

GREGOIRE, Michel F; Clinique Maisonneuve-Rosemont, 230-5345 boul de l'Assomption, Montreal QC H1T 4B3; Mon'68; FRCPC; Psy. Staff, Hopital Maisonneuve-Rosemont; (514)256-3165; Fax. (514)256-9385.

GREGOIRE, Mireille; Clinique D'Urologie Berger, 416-1000 ch Sainte-Foy, Quebec QC G1S 2L6; McG'86; FRCSC; Urol. Staff, Centre Hospitalier Universitaire de Québec (CHUQ) - Siege Social; Université Laval; Langs: Bilingual(French/English); (418)266-2876; Fax. (418)266-2879.

GREGOIRE, Pascale; Hop Riviere-des-Prairies, 7070 boul Perras, Montreal QC H1E 1A4; Laval'94; LMCC; FRCPC; Psy (Pediatric Psychiatry). Staff, Hôpital Riviere des Prairies; (514)323-7260; Fax. (514)323-3286.

GREGOIRE, Philippe; CHUQ-St-Francois D'Assise, 10 rue de l'Espinay, Quebec QC G1L 3L5; Sher'97; FRCPC; IntMed; Gastroent. Staff, Centre Hospitalier Universitaire De Québec - Pavillon De St-françois-d'assise; (418)525-4444; Fax. (418)525-4331.

GREGOIRE, Pierre; Hop Maisonneuve-Rosemont, 5415 boul de l'Assomption, Montreal QC H1T 2M4; Sher'74; Respir; IntMed. Staff, Hopital Maisonneuve-Rosemont; (514)369-3654; Fax. (514)252-3434.

GREGOIRE, Roger C; CHUQ-St-Francois D'Assise, B1 520-10 rue de l'Espinay, Quebec QC G1L 3L5; Laval'81; CSPQ; FRCSC; GenSurg. Ac Staff, Centre Hospitalier Universitaire De Québec - Pavillon De St-françois-d'assise; (418)525-4160; Fax. (418)525-4162.

GREGOIRE, Scott A; 172-17010 90 Ave NW, Edmonton AB T5T 1L6; Man'07; FRCPC; DiagRad. (780)484-1672

GREGOIRE, Serge; GMF Boreal, 668 rue de Parfondeval, Baie-Comeau QC G5C 3R3; Mon'91; BSc; MSc; CCFP; FCFP; Médecin, Centre de santé des Côté-Nord; Langs: Bilingual(French/English); (418)589-2222; Fax. (418)589-8302.

GREGOIRE, Sylvie; 203-311 McArthur Ave, Vanier ON K1L 8M3; Mon'81; FRCPC; IntMed; Gastroent. Staff The Ottawa Hosp, The Ottawa Hospital - Riverside Campus; Langs: Bilingual(English/French); (613)744-8180; Fax. (613)744-7982.

GREGOIRE, Trixie L; Parkland Med Cl, 203-998 Parkland Dr, Halifax NS B3M 0A6; Wes'00; CCFP; (902)457-4499

GREGOIRE CHAMPAGNE, Samuel; CSSS de la Maskinonge, 420 2e rue, Louiseville QC J5V 1V3; Laval'09; CCFP; Staff, CSSS de Maskinongé; (819)228-2731

GREGOR, James C; London HSC-Victoria Campus, PO Box 5010 Stn B E1 319-800 Commissioners Rd E, London ON N6A 5W9; Wes'88; FRCPC; IntMed; Gastroent. Chief IntMed, London Health Sciences Centre - Victoria Campus; Asst Prof/Prog Dir Gastroent, University of Western Ontario; (519)667-6582; Fax. (519)667-6620; jamie.gregor@lhsc.on.ca.

GREGOR, Laura H; Grand River Hosp-KW Hlth Ctre, PO Box 9056 Stn C 835 King St E, Kitchener ON N2G 1G3; Dal'99; FRCPC; IntMed; Nephrol. Staff, Grand River Hospital - Kitchener/Waterloo Health Centre; (519)749-4300 x2189

GREGOR, Paul; Victoria Med Centre, 405-304 Victoria Ave N, Hamilton ON L8L 5G4; Komensky (Slovakia)'67; FACS; FRCSC; GenSurg. Ac Staff, Hamilton Health Sciences Centre - Hamilton General Hospital; Langs: Czech; Slovak; (905)527-5121

GREGORET-QUINN, Michael G; Royal Alexandra Hosp, 10240 Kingsway NW, Edmonton AB T5H 3V9; Alb'94; FRCPC; Anes. Staff Anes, Royal Alexandra Hospital; (780)735-4111; Fax. (780)735-4386.

GREGORY, Alexander J; Foothills Medical Centre, 1403 29 St NW, Calgary AB T2N 2T9; Cal'07; Anes. Staff, Foothills Medical Centre; (403)944-1403

GREGORY, Alfred J; 223 rue des Draveurs, Gatineau QC J9J 1T4; Mon'59.

GREGORY, Brian W; Fairmont Med Bldg, 1010-750 Broadway W, Vancouver BC V5Z 1H9; Ott'86; Derm. Member Council of Specialist, British Columbia Medical Association; Dir Undergraduate Derm Education, University of British Columbia; (604)876-7222; Fax. (604)876-7216.

GREGORY, David A; 108-230 First Ave, St Thomas ON N5R 4P5; Wes'79; (519)631-1101

GREGORY, Erin L; Town Circle Med Clinic, 101B-1771 Comox Ave, Comox BC V9M 3L9; Cal'00; BSc; CCFP; Staff, St Joseph's General Hospital; (250)339-5780

GREGORY, Walter; MUHC-Royal Victoria Hosp, M 928-687 av des Pins O, Montreal QC H3A 1A1; Qns'66; FRCPC; IntMed (Endocrinology). Sr Physician Med, McGill University Health Centre - Royal Victoria Hospital; assoc Prof, McGill University; (514)843-1455; Fax. (514)843-2838.

GREGORY, Wayne D; The Medical Place, 202-178 John St, Brampton ON L6W 2A4; Tor'79; FACS; FRCSC; GenSurg (Thoracic Surgery). Staff, William Osler Health System - Brampton Civic Hospital; (905)456-1260; Fax. (905)456-1260.

GREGORY-EVANS, Kevin; UBC Eye Care Centre, 2550 Willow St, Vancouver BC V5Z 3N9; (United Kingdom)'85; MB BS; FRCSC; Ophth. (604)875-5275

GREGORYANZ, Tatiana; Edgeland Clinic, 218-2025 Corydon Ave, Winnipeg MB R3P 0N5; Moscow (Russia (Federation))'89; FRCPC; Psy. Asst Prof Psy, University of Manitoba.

GREGSON, Alison N; Psychiatric Assessment Unit, 910 10th Ave W, Vancouver BC V5Z 1M9; Alb'07; Psy. Staff, Abbotsford Regional Hospital & Cancer Centre; (604)875-4018

GREGSON, Daniel B; Calgary Lab Services, 9-3535 Research Rd NW, Calgary AB T2L 2K8; Tor'83; FRCPC; IntMed; MedMicrobiol; InfectDis. Staff, Calgary Laboratory Services; Assoc Prof Path/LabMed & Med, University of Calgary; (403)770-3338; dan.gregson@cls.ab.ca.

GREGSON, John C; Lakeside Clinic, 202-15379 Castle Downs Rd NW, Edmonton AB T5X 3Y7; Alb'84; CCFP; (780)472-7575; Fax. (780)472-7404.

GREGUS, Vojtech; Dartmouth Med Centre, 44 Portland St, Dartmouth NS B2Y 1H3; Bratislava (Slovakia)'75; (902)465-4546; Fax. (902)465-4530.

GREIDANUS, Marc; Chilliwack Gen Hosp, 45600 Menholm Rd, Chilliwack BC V2P 1P7; Alb'04; CCFP; CCFP(E.M.); Staff, Chilliwack General Hospital; (604)795-4141

GREIDANUS, Margriet; Foothills Med Centre, C231-1403 29 St NW, Calgary AB T2N 2T9; Cal'03; CCFP; CCFP(E.M.); Staff, Foothills Medical Centre; (403)944-1635

GREIDANUS, Nelson V; 3F-2775 Laurel St, Vancouver BC V5Z 1M9; Alb'93; MPH; OrthSurg (Hip & Knee Reconstruction). Staff, Vancouver General Hospital - Centennial Pavillion; Asst Prof OrthSurg, University of British Columbia; (604)875-5767; Fax. (604)875-5768.

GREIDANUS, Peter G; Bigelow Fowler Clinic, 1605 9 Ave S, Lethbridge AB T1J 1W2; Alb'73; BSc; Ac Staff, Chinook Regional Hospital; Ac Staff, Covenant Health - St Michael's Health Centre; Langs: Dutch; (403)327-3121; Fax. (403)327-3905.

GREIDANUS, Robert I; PO Box 7435 Stn Main, Peace River AB T8S 1T1; Alb'93; CCFP; (780)624-2581; Fax. (780)624-4015.

GREIDANUS, Thomas H; Meadowlark Health Centre, 212 Meadowlark Shopping Ctr NW, Edmonton AB T5R 5W9; Alb'64; FAAOS; FACS; FRCSC; OrthSurg (Hips Surgery). Ac Staff, Covenant Health - Misericordia Community Hospital; Ac Staff, Glenrose Rehabilitation Hospital; Ac Staff, Royal Alexandra Hospital; Clin Instructor, University of Alberta; (780)484-8051; Fax. (780)484-2194.

GREIG, Anita R A; 303-343 Wilson Ave, North York ON M3H 1T1; Tor'88; FCFP; MD; CCFP; FCFP; Ac Staff, Mount Sinai Hospital; Asst Prof, University of Toronto; (416)785-8412; Fax. (416)785-8324; a.greig@utoronto.ca.

GREIG, Bradley; Associate Med Group, 4705 48 Ave, Red Deer AB T4N 3T1; Alb'92; Staff, Red Deer Regional Hospital Centre; Physician, Associate Medical Group; (403)346-2057; Fax. (403)347-2989.

GREIG, Jean M M; Vaughan Med Centre, H 26-9200 Weston Rd, Woodbridge ON L4H 2P8; Glasgow (Scotland)'64; MB ChB; Court Staff, Humber River Regional Hospital - Finch Avenue Site; (905)417-2273; Fax. (905)417-7088.

GREIG, Paul D; NCSB 11C-1230, 585 University Ave, Toronto ON M5G 2N2; Tor'76; FACS; FRCSC; GenSurg (Hepatobiliary & Pancreatic Surgery). Staff, The Hospital For Sick Children; Staff, Mount Sinai Hospital; Dir GI Transplantation, Toronto General Hospital - UHN; Prof Surg, University of Toronto; (416)340-4252; Fax. (416)340-4039; paul.greig@uhn.on.ca.

GREINER, Karin; Peterborough Reg HC-Hospital, 1 Hospital Dr, Peterborough ON K9J 7C6; Qns'98; CCFP; Staff, Peterborough Regional Health Centre - Hospital Drive; (705)743-2121; Fax. (705)876-5120.

GREINER, Violetta; 12 Streathroy Cres, Waterdown ON L0R 2H5; McM'75; CCFP; FCFP.

GREISMAN, Bernard; West Mississauga Medical, 3050 Argentina Rd, Mississauga ON L5N 8E1; Ott'67; FACOG; FRCSC; ObstGyn (Gynecology). Surg Asst, Shouldice Hospital; Staff Gynecologist-Office Practice, MCI the Doctors Office; Staff Gynecology-Office Practice, Dr E Medical & Travel Clinic; (905)785-3627; pappadok@yahoo.com.

GREISS, Isabelle; CHUM-Hotel-Dieu, 3840 rue Saint-Urbain, Montreal QC H2W 1T8; Mon'97; CSPQ; FRCPC; IntMed (Electrophysiology); Cardiol. Staff ElectroPhysiol, Institut de Cardiologie de Montréal; Staff, Centre Hospitalier l'Université de Montréal (CHUM) - Hôtel-Dieu; (514)890-8000 x1444

GREIVER, Michelle; North York Med Group, 705-240 Duncan Mill Rd, North York ON M3B 3S6; Tor'84; MSc; CCFP; FCFP; Staff, North York General Hospital; Asst Prof Family & CommunMed, University of Toronto; Langs: English; French; (416)222-3011; Fax. (416)221-3097; nyfht705@rogers.com.

GREK, Adrian; Mount Sinai Hosp, L1 012-60 Murray St, Toronto ON M5T 3L9; Witwatersrand (South Africa)'74; MB BS; MRCP(UK); FRCPC; Neur; Psy. Staff Psy, Centre for Addiction & Mental Health (CAMH) - College Street Site; Staff Psychiatrist, Mount Sinai Hospital; Assoc Prof Psy, University of Toronto; (416)586-4800; Fax. (416)586-8654; agrek@mtsinai.on.ca.

GRELL, Natashia G K; 101-2200 Yonge St, Toronto ON M4S 2C6; (Jamaica)'96; MB BS; CCFP.

GRENIER, Alain; Clinique Med Familiale Dolbeau, 1521 rue des Erables, Dolbeau-Mistassini QC G8L 1C4; Sher'89; (418)276-0041; Fax. (418)276-7170.

GRENIER, Andre; CHUQ-St Francois d'Assise, 10 rue de l'Espinay, Quebec QC G1L 3L5; Laval'81; CSPQ; Anes. Staff, Centre Hospitalier Universitaire De Québec - Pavillon De St-françois-d'assise; (418)525-4340; Fax. (418)525-4434.

GRENIER, Anne-Marie; Direction de la Sante Publique, 550 rue Bonaventure, Trois-Rivieres QC G9A 2B5; Laval'90; FRCPC; CommunMed. Staff, CSSS de Trois-Rivières; (819)693-3915; Fax. (819)373-1627.

GRENIER, Benoit; CHUS-Hop Hotel-Dieu, 580 rue Bowen S, Sherbrooke QC J1G 2E8; Mon'78; FRCSC; Ophth. Staff, Centre Hospitalier Universitaire de Sherbrooke-Hôpital Hôtel-Dieu; (819)346-1110; Fax. (819)822-6795.

GRENIER, Benoit; Centre Medical de l'Hetriere, 201-3520 rue de l'Hetriere, St-Augustin-D-Desm QC G3A 0B4; Laval'90; (418)651-3933; Fax. (418)651-0256.

GRENIER, Chantal; CLSC du Grand Chicoutimi, 411 rue de l'Hotel-Dieu, Chicoutimi QC G7H 7Z5; Laval'99; CCFP; (418)543-2221; Fax. (418)543-9512.

GRENIER, Claude; 2924 boul Taschereau, Greenfield Park QC J4V 2G8; Laval'70; DPsy; FRCPC; Psy (Child Psychiatry). Staff, Hopital Charles LeMoyne; Langs: English; French; (450)466-5496 x6114; Fax. (450)466-8789.

GRENIER, Danielle; Clinique de Pediatrie, 105 av Gatineau, Gatineau QC J8T 4J4; Ott'73; FRCPC; Peds (Internal Medicine). (819)561-4412

GRENIER, Debjani; St Boniface Gen Hosp, L1 102-409 Tache Ave, Winnipeg MB R2H 2A6; Sask'93; FRCPC; IntMed; MedOncol. Staff MedOncol, St Boniface General Hospital; Asst Prof, University of Manitoba; (204)235-3141; Fax. (204)237-6048; debjani.grenier@cancercare.mb.ca.

GRENIER, Gilles; CSSS de l'Energie, 1265 rue Trudel, Shawinigan QC G9N 8T3; Laval'69; (819)539-8371; Fax. (819)533-3193.

GRENIER, Gilles; Clinique Medisoleil, 120-383 boul du Seminaire N, St-Jean-sur-Richel QC J3B 8C5; Mon'74; Staff, Hôpital du Haut-Richelieu; Staff, Canadian Armed Forces; Langs: English; (450)347-7557; Fax. (450)347-3099.

GRENIER, Gilles W; Direction Rég Sante Publique, 550 rue Bonaventure, Trois-Rivieres QC G9A 2B5; Laval'77; Staff, CSSS de Trois-Rivières; (819)693-3938

GRENIER, Guy; GMF Clin Med Saint-Laurent, 201-200 av Saint-Laurent, Louiseville QC J5V 1J9; Sher'87; (819)228-4964; Fax. (819)228-1480.

GRENIER, Hugo; CSSS de la Region de Thetford, 1717 rue Notre-Dame E, Thetford Mines QC G6G 2V4; Laval'99; Staff, Hopital du CSS de la Region de Thetford; (418)338-7777

GRENIER, Isabelle; Centre Hospitalier Fleury, 2180 rue Fleury E, Montreal QC H2B 1K3; Mon'05; CCFP; Staff, Centre Hospitalier Fleury; (514)381-9311

GRENIER, Jean-Luc; Direction de la Sante Publique, 210-1000 rue Labelle, Saint-Jerome QC J7Z 5N6; Mon'83; MSc(CommunHealth); Med Consultant Dept of Public Health, Hôtel-Dieu de Saint-Jérôme; (450)436-8622 x2288; Fax. (450)569-6305; jean-luc_grenier@ssss.gouv.qc.ca.

GRENIER, Jean-Paul; Centre Auditif King, 1435 rue King O, Sherbrooke QC J1J 2C1; Sher'83; FRCSC; Otol (Allergy). Consultant Privil, Centre Hospitalier Universitaire de Sherbrooke-Hopital Fleurimont; Consultant, Centre Hospitalier Universitaire de Sherbrooke-Hôpital Hôtel-Dieu; Otolaryngol Consultant, Centre Hospitalier et CLSC de Memphremagog; Otolaryngology, CSSS Institut universitaire de gériatrie de Sherbrooke; Langs: Bilingual(French/English); (819)562-5722; Fax. (819)564-6911; jean.p.grenier@videotron.ca.

GRENIER, Julie; CLSC Vallee de la Batiscan, RR 4 90 ch Rivere-A-Veillet, Ste-Genev-d-Batisc QC G0X 2R0; Laval'04; (418)362-2727; Fax. (418)632-3125.

GRENIER, Julie; Clin D'Obstetrique Gynecologie, 102-222 rue de la Visitation, St-Charles-Boromee QC J6E 4N5; Sher'98; FRCPC; ObstGyn. (450)759-1665; Fax. (450)759-3919.

GRENIER, Lise; Carefour Vallee Ricelieu, 665 boul Sir-Wilfrid-Laurier, Beloeil QC J3G 4J1; Sher'89; (450)467-0088

GRENIER, Lise; Polyclinique Ancienne-Lorette, 204-6385 boul Wilfrid-Hamel, L'Ancienne-Lorette QC G2E 5W2; Sher'78; (418)872-2012; Fax. (418)872-2349.

GRENIER, Louis; Clinique Med St-Agapit, 105-1125 rue Principale RR 1, Saint-Agapit QC G0S 1Z0; Laval'73; Staff Health Services, Hôpital Regional Rimouski; Staff Health Services, Hopital du CSS de la Region de Thetford; (418)888-3951; Fax. (418)888-3952.

GRENIER, Louis-Philippe; CLSC des Mille Iles, 4731 boul Levesque E, Laval QC H7C 1M9; Mon'03; (450)661-2572

GRENIER, Louis-Pierre; Hop Maisonneuve-Rosemont, 5415 boul de l'Assomption, Montreal QC H1T 2M4; McG'08; IntMed. Staff, Hopital Maisonneuve-Rosemont; (514)252-3400

GRENIER, Louis-Simon; Carrefour Sante de Jonquiere, CP 1200 Stn Pdf Jonquiere 2230 rue De l'Hopital, Jonquiere QC G7X 7X2; Sher'02; CCFP; Staff EmergMed, Centre Hospitalier Jonquiere; Clin Prof, Universite de Sherbrooke; Langs: Bilingual(French/English); (418)695-7700; Fax. (418)695-7729.

GRENIER, Louise; Clinique de Med Familiale, 442 boul Sainte-Anne RR 3, Ste-Anne-Plai QC J0N 1H0; Mon'89; Staff, Hôtel-Dieu de Saint-Jérôme; (450)478-4737; Fax. (450)478-7508.

GRENIER, Lucie; Clinique Grande-Allee, 425 Grande Allee E, Quebec QC G1R 2J5; Laval'73; CSPQ; Anes. Staff, Centre Hospitalier Universitaire De Québec - Pavillon De St-françois-d'assise; (418)682-0182

GRENIER, Lucien; Bureau d'Administration, RR 2 477 av Saint-Joseph, East Broughton QC G0N 1G0; Laval'59; (418)427-3630; Fax. (418)427-4929.

GRENIER, M M Catherine; Trillium Hlth Ctr-Mississauga, 100 Queensway W, Mississauga ON L5B 1B8; McG'00; FRCPC; EmergMed. Staff, Trillium Health Centre - Mississauga; Langs: Bilingual(English/French); (905)848-7100

GRENIER, Marie-Andree; Clinique medicale Havre-Sante, 521 boul du Havre, Salaber-de-Valleyf QC J6S 4Z5; Mon'83; Staff CHSLD, Centre Hospitalier Régional du Suroît; Langs: Bilingual(French/English); (450)371-6444; Fax. (450)371-5315.

GRENIER, Mathieu; CSSS de Chicoutimi, CP 5006 305 rue Saint-Vallier, Chicoutimi QC G7H 5H6; Laval'00; FRCPC; Psy. Staff, Complexe hospitalier de la Sagamie; (418)549-5477; Fax. (418)549-7604.

GRENIER, Paule; CHUQ-St-Francois D'Assise, 10 rue de l'Espinay, Quebec QC G1L 3L5; Laval'97; Staff, Centre Hospitalier Universitaire De Québec - Pavillon De St-françois-d'assise; (418)525-4425; Fax. (418)525-4322.

GRENIER, Raynald; CHUQ-St-Francois D'Assise, 10 rue de l'Espinay, Quebec QC G1L 3L5; Laval'65; DABD; LMCC; FASLMS; Derm (Laser Surgery). Staff Derm, Centre Hospitalier Universitaire De Québec - Pavillon De St-françois-d'assise; Langs: Bilingual(French/English); (418)525-4444; Fax. (418)525-4464.

GRENIER, Rejean; CSSS de Rivière-de-Loup, 75 rue Saint-Henri, Riviere-Du-Loup QC G5R 2A4; Laval'76; Ophth (P.Q.). Staff, Centre Hospitalier Regional du Grand-Portage; (418)868-1000 x2496; Fax. (418)868-1032.

GRENIER, Robert; CSSS de Manicouagan, 635 boul Jolliet, Baie-Comeau QC G5C 1P1; Mon'85; Staff, Centre Hospitalier Régional Baie-Comeau; (418)589-3701

GRENIER, Solene; Hotel-Dieu d'Arthabaska, 5 rue Hospitalieres, Victoriaville QC G6P 6N2; Sher'09; Staff, Hotel-Dieu d'Arthabaska; (819)363-3030; Fax. (819)363-3030.

GRENIER, Stefanie; CSSS du Sud de Lanaudière, 911 montee des Pionniers, Terrebonne QC J6V 2H2; Laval'07; OrthSurg. Staff, Centre Hospitalier Pierre le Gardeur; (450)654-7525 x23000

GRENIER, Valerie; Ctr Hosp Laurentien, 234 rue Saint-Vincent, Ste-Agathe-Des-Mts QC J8C 2B8; Laval'01; CCFP; Staff, Centre Hospitalier Laurentien; (819)324-4006; Fax. (819)324-4058.

GRENIER, Yvan; Hop Maisonneuve-Rosemont, 5415 boul de l'Assomption, Montreal QC H1T 2M4; Sher'82; CSPQ; Anes. Staff, Hopital Maisonneuve-Rosemont; Langs: English; (514)252-3400; Fax. (514)252-3542.

GRENIER CLICHE, Catherine; Clinique Urologie Saguenay, 475 boul Talbot, Chicoutimi QC G7H 4A3; Laval'04; Peds. Staff, Complexe hospitalier de la Sagamie; (418)549-1034

GRENNAN, J Troy; Maple Leaf Med Arts, 501-14 College St, Toronto ON M5G 1K2; McM'05; FRCPC; IntMed; InfectDis; MedMicrobiol. Staff, St Joseph's Healthcare - Charlton Campus; Staff, Maple Leaf Medical Clinic; (416)465-0756; Fax. (416)465-8344.

GRENON, Denis; Centre Med Dorion Vaudreuil, 600 boul Harwood, Vaudreuil-Dorion QC J7V 6A3; Mon'77; (450)455-9301; Fax. (450)455-9549.

GRENON, Hugues; Ctr Hosp Affilie-Enfan, 1401 18e rue, Quebec QC G1J 1Z4; Laval'88; FRCPC; DiagRad. Staff, Centre Hospitalier Affilié Universitaire de Québec - Hôpital De L'Enfant Jésus; (418)649-5782; Fax. (418)649-5972.

GRENON, Jean-Francois; Clinique medicale des Erables, 120-578 Rte 138, Neuville QC G0A 2R0; Laval'87; BSc; PhD; LMCC; (418)876-2895; Fax. (418)876-2894; gresim@globetrotter.net.

GRENON, Lisa; Clinique de Carrefour, 1005 Rte Lagueux, St-Etienne-De-Lauz QC G6J 1J8; Laval'91; Staff, CHSLD St-Apollinaire; (418)836-2002; Fax. (418)836-2070.

GRENON, Lorraine; Clin Med Metro St-Michel, 7281 boul Shaughnessy, Montreal QC H2A 1J6; Mon'81; (514)374-0991; Fax. (514)374-0991.

GRENON, Louise; Centre médicale des Carrières, 800-1000 boul Bona-Dussault RR, St-Mar-Des-Carr QC G0A 4B0; Laval'83; Staff, Centre D'Accueil; (418)268-5596; Fax. (418)268-5729.

GRENON, Marie; CHUQ-St-Francois D'Assise, 10 rue de l'Espinay, Quebec QC G1L 3L5; Mon'00; Staff, Centre Hospitalier Universitaire De Québec - Pavillon De St-françois-d'assise; (418)525-4444

GRESCHNER, Michael; The Moncton Hosp, 135 Macbeath Ave, Moncton NB E1C 6Z8; McG'84; FRCPC; Anes. Ac Staff, The Moncton Hospital; Consultant, Dr Georges-L-Dumont University Hospital Centre; Asst Prof Anes, Dalhousie University; Langs: English; French; (506)857-5111; Fax. (506)857-5261.

GRESKO, Peter A; 2650 Tecumseh Rd E, Windsor ON N8W 1G2; Komensky (Slovakia)'65; Court Staff, Windsor Regional Hospital - Metropolitan Site; Langs: Czech; Ukrainian; Slovak; Polish; French; (519)974-6000; Fax. (519)251-0317.

GRETSINGER, Paula C C; Lawrence Warden Med Centre, 2050A Lawrence Ave E, Scarborough ON M1R 2Z5; Man'80; Staff, Rouge Valley Health System - Centenary Health Centre Site; (416)752-2207; Fax. (416)752-0636.

GRETTON, Adrian R; Westbrook Prof Bldg, 211-1610 37 St SW, Calgary AB T3C 3P1; Cal'84; CCFP; FCFP; Att Physician, Foothills Medical Centre; Clinical Asst Prof, University of Calgary; (403)246-2052; Fax. (403)246-2219.

GREVE, Mark D J; Alberta Retina Consultants, 400-10924 107 Ave NW, Edmonton AB T5H 0X5; Sask'88; FRCSC; Ophth (Retina). Clin Assoc Prof Ophth, Royal Alexandra Hospital; Teach Staff, University of Alberta; (780)448-1801; Fax. (780)448-1809.

GREVILLOT, Marie-Helene; CSSS De La Haute-Yamaska, 205 boul Leclerc O, Granby QC J2G 1T7; Sher'01; DiagRad. Staff, Centre Hospitalier de Granby; (450)375-8000 x2180

GREVLER, Joanne M; 1001-2200 Yonge St, Toronto ON M4S 2C6; McG'98; CCFP; Langs: English; French; (416)481-1173; Fax. (416)481-7431.

GREWAL, Anita; 170 Rebecca St, Oakville ON L6K 1J6; McM'00; BSc; CCFP; Langs: Punjabi; (905)845-9293; Fax. (905)845-0981.

GREWAL, Damanpreet S; Family Care Med Centre, 112-55 Castleridge Blvd NE, Calgary AB T3J 3J8; (India)'97; CCFP; (403)280-5500

GREWAL, Deepa; Markham Stouffville Hosp, PO Box 1800 Stn Main 381 Church St, Markham ON L3P 7P3; (Jamaica)'00; FRCPC; Peds. Staff, Markham Stouffville Hospital; (905)472-7000

GREWAL, Jasmine; St Paul's Hosp, B478-1081 Burrard St, Vancouver BC V6Z 1Y6; Man'01; FRCPC; IntMed; Cardiol. Staff, Providence Health Care - St Paul's Hospital; (604)682-2344

GREWAL, Jaspreet S; 307-1017 Wilson Ave, North York ON M3K 1Z1; Man'99; CCFP; (416)636-3800; Fax. (416)636-3840.

GREWAL, Jasvir K; Trillium Hlth Ctr-Mississauga, 100 Queensway W, Mississauga ON L5B 1B8; Tor'03; FRCPC; Anes. Staff, Trillium Health Centre - Mississauga; (905)848-7100

GREWAL, Jeevan K; 4349 Hastings St, Burnaby BC V5C 2J8; UBC'05; CCFP; (604)299-4388

GREWAL, Kamal P; Family Hlth Med Centre, 11-10035 Hurontario St, Brampton ON L6Z 0E6; Rajasthan University (India)'02; CCFP; Langs: Hindi; Urdu; Punjabi; (905)453-2441; Fax. (905)453-4624.

GREWAL, Kharak S; Bramalea Med Centre, 505-18 Kensington Rd, Brampton ON L6T 4S5; Punjab (India)'75; Staff, William Osler Health System - Brampton Civic Hospital; Langs: Hindi; Punjabi; Urdu; (905)458-0177; Fax. (905)458-0178.

GREWAL, Kuljit S; Health Sciences Centre, 300 Prince Philip Dr, St. John's NL A1B 3V6; Mem'83; FRCPC; IntMed (Hematological Oncology); Hem. Ac Staff Med, Health Sciences Centre; Assoc Prof Med, Memorial University Of Newfoundland; (709)777-7061; kgrewal@mun.ca.

GREWAL, Manavdeep; 505-18 Kensington Rd, Brampton ON L6T 4S5; McM'06; CCFP; Langs: Hindi; Punjabi; (905)458-0177

GREWAL, Navdeep K; Mount St Joseph Hosp, 3080 Prince Edward St, Vancouver BC V5R 3N4; UBC'93; CCFP; CCFP(E.M.); Staff, Providence Health Care - Mount Saint Joseph Hospital; (604)877-8341

GREWAL, Parbeer; Stratica Med Clinic, 200-10140 117 St NW, Edmonton AB T5K 1X3; Alb'06; FRCPC; Derm. (780)428-5554; Fax. (780)428-5556.

GREWAL, Puneet; Burlington Prof Centre, 206-3155 Harvester Rd, Burlington ON L7N 3V2; Punjabi (India)'03; CCFP; Langs: Hindi; Punjabi; Urdu; (905)335-4616

GREWAL, Rajdeep; Hamilton HS-General Site, 237 Barton St E, Hamilton ON L8L 2X2; McM'03; CCFP; CCFP(E.M.); Staff, Hamilton Health Sciences Centre - Hamilton General Hospital; Langs: Hindi; Punjabi; (905)527-4322

GREWAL, Rajwant K; 6 Queen St S, Mississauga ON L5M 1K1; Bombay (India)'79; Staff Emerg, William Osler Health System - Etobicoke General Hospital; Langs: Hindi; Punjabi; (905)826-0808; Fax. (905)826-2385.

GREWAL, Rasveg S; 201-1370 Clyde Ave, Nepean ON K2G 3H8; St George (Grenada)'02; FRCPC; IntMed; Cardiol. Langs: Punjabi; (613)722-8086

GREWAL, Ruby; St Joseph's Health Care, PO Box 5777 Stn B 268 Grosvenor St, London ON N6A 4V2; UBC'99; FRCSC; OrthSurg (Hand & Limb Surgery). Staff, St Joseph's Hospital - St Joseph's Health Care; (519)646-6286; Fax. (519)646-6049.

GREWAL, S Tony; Oak Bay Med Clinic, 101-1640 Oak Bay Ave, Victoria BC V8R 1B2; Alb'84; CCFP; Staff, Vancouver Island Health Authority; (250)598-6744; Fax. (250)598-6778.

GREWAL, Sarbjit S; Preventous Collaborative Healt, 1635 17 Ave SW, Calgary AB T2T 0E5; Dublin (Ireland)'84; MB ChB; BAO; DA; LRCP; Langs: Punjabi; (403)229-0129; Fax. (403)398-0193; sarb@shaw.ca.

GREWAL, Seena; Hosp for Sick Children, 555 University Ave, Toronto ON M5G 1X8; UBC'01; FRCPC; Psy. Staff, North York General Hospital; Staff, The Hospital For Sick Children; (416)813-7195

GREWAL, Shiv Pal; Grey Bruce HS-Wiarton, PO Box 310 203-369 Mary St, Wiarton ON N0H 2T0; Man'96; MPH(Harvard); CCFP; FCFP; Assoc Prof, University of Toronto; Assoc Prof, McMaster University; (519)534-5220; Fax. (519)534-1024.

GREWAL, Simarjot K; Leaside Health Centre, 795 Eglinton Ave E, East York ON M4G 4E4; Saba University (Other Foreign)'05; CCFP; Langs: Hindi; (416)424-3145; Fax. (416)424-2611.

GREWAL, Simran; Edmonton Clinic Health Academy, 3 512-11405 87 Ave NW, Edmonton AB T6G 1C9; UBC'99; FRCPC; Peds; PedEmergMed. Staff, Edmonton Clinic Health Academy; (780)248-5575

GREWAL, T Paul S; Pleasantview Med Clinic, 11028 51 Ave NW, Edmonton AB T6H 0L4; Alb'82; (780)434-5129; Fax. (780)434-9992.

GREY, Jane; Rossland Castlegar & Trail, PO Box 1825 2038 Washington St, Rossland BC V0G 1Y0; London (England)'73; MB BS; (250)362-7009; Fax. (250)362-7091; info@rmaads.ca.

GREY, Robert G; 305-1101 Dewdney Ave, Trail BC V1R 4T1; Cape Town (South Africa)'66; MB ChB; FRCS; Staff OrthSurg, Kootenay Boundary Regional Hospital.

GREYLING, Gertie; 480-3033 Immel St, Abbotsford BC V2S 6S2; Orange Free State (South Africa)'86; MB ChB; Staff, Menno Extended Care Hospital; Staff, Abbotsford Regional Hospital & Cancer Centre; Langs: Afrikaans; Zulu; (604)852-6781; Fax. (604)852-0869.

GREYLING, Johannes C; Ramblewood Med Clinic, 101-14 Ramblewood Dr, Wasaga Beach ON L9Z 0C4; MB ChB; Langs: Afrikaans; (705)429-8270

GREYLING, Louw De Lange; Dr C W Wuebe Med Centre, 385 Main St, Winkler MB R6W 1J2; (Other Foreign)'06; (204)325-4312

GREYLING, Schalk J; Family Health Clinic, PO Box 4127 Stn Main 5111 51 Ave, Ponoka AB T4J 1R5; (South Africa)'02; MB ChB; (403)783-5305; Fax. (403)783-8722.

GREYSON, N David; Toronto Nuclear Med Services, 210-123 Edward St, Toronto ON M5G 1E2; Tor'65; BSc(Tor); DMRD; DAB; FRCPC; DiagRad (Diagnostic Imaging); NuclearMed. Consultant, The Hospital For Sick Children; Consultant, Toronto General Hospital - UHN; Assoc Prof, University of Toronto; (416)593-5458; greyson@smh.toronto.on.ca.

GREYVENSTEIN, Ernst L; 123-15566 McIvor Blvd SE, Calgary AB T2Z 4Y2; Pretoria (South Africa)'97; MB ChB; CCFP; Langs: Afrikaans; (403)726-0524; Fax. (403)726-0579.

GRIEF, Cindy J; Baycrest Ctre/Geriatric Care, 3560 Bathurst St, North York ON M6A 2E1; Tor'95; BSc; MSc; FRCPC; Psy (Geriatric Psychiatry). Staff, Baycrest Centre for Geriatric Care; (416)785-2500 x3070; Fax. (416)785-2450.

GRIER, Elizabeth; 309 Alfred St, Kingston ON K7L 3S4; Cal'05; CCFP; (613)344-2090; Fax. (613)531-5956.

GRIERSON, Robert A; Health Sciences Centre, 820 Sherbrook St, Winnipeg MB R3A 1R9; Man'94; BSc; FRCPC; EmergMed. Staff Emerg, Health Sciences Centre; (204)774-6511

GRIESDALE, Donald E; Vancouver Gen Hosp, 2449-855 12th Ave W, Vancouver BC V5Z 1M9; Tor'69; FRCSC; Neursurg (Spine Surgery). Ac Staff, Vancouver General Hospital - Centennial Pavillion; Assoc Prof Surg, University of British Columbia; (604)875-4304

GRIESMAN, Helene C; North Med Centre, 201-7131 Bathurst St, Thornhill ON L4J 7Z1; Tor'88; BSc; Assoc Staff, North York General Hospital; (905)771-1778; Fax. (905)771-9833.

GRIESMAN, Jordan A; Healthwise Diagnostic, 100-12 Morgan Ave, Thornhill ON L3T 1R1; Tor'86; FRCPC; DiagRad; NuclearMed. Dir Nuclear Med, Toronto East General Hospital Inc; (905)695-5665; Fax. (905)695-5666.

GRIEVE, Catharine D; 9912 107 St NW PO Box 2415 Stn Main, Edmonton AB T5J 2S5; Alb'96; CCFP; FCFP; (780)498-4502; Fax. (780)498-7807.

GRIEVE, Geoff; The Med Centre FHT, PO Box 4200 Stn Main 707 Charlotte St, Peterborough ON K9J 7B3; (Ireland)'04; MB; BAO; BCh; BSc; CCFP; Langs: Bilingual(English/French); (705)876-4507

GRIEVE, Kimberley A; Montebello Med Clinic Ltd, PO Box 32 Stn Main 302-320 Alexander St, Salmon Arm BC V1E 4N2; Man'91; CCFP; (250)833-4677; Fax. (250)833-4765.

GRIEVE-EGLIN, Leandra H; Quinte HC Corp-Belleville Gen, 265 Dundas St E, Belleville ON K8N 5A9; Basle (Switzerland)'01; IntMed. Staff, QHC Belleville General; (613)969-7400

GRIFFIN, Ann P; CPM London, 458 Central Ave, London ON N6B 2E5; Tor'85; FRCPC; Anes. Staff, Stratford General Hospital - Huron Perth Healthcare Alliance; (905)576-3444

GRIFFIN, Barbara S; St Vincent's Langara, 255 62nd Ave W, Vancouver BC V5X 4V4; UBC'95; MD; BSc(Hon); CCFP; FCFP; Staff, Providence Health Care - St Vincent's Hospital-Langara Site; Med Staff Med, Providence Health Care - St Paul's Hospital; Clinical Asst Prof, University of British Columbia; (604)325-4116 x64642

GRIFFIN, Desmond J; 200-2099 152 St, Surrey BC V4A 4N7; National (Ireland)'64; MB ChB; BAO; FRAM; FRCPC; Psy (General). (604)542-1161; Fax. (604)541-1625.

GRIFFIN, Glenn H; Quinte West Medical Ctr, 80 Catherine St, Trenton ON K8V 6N8; Tor'80; MSc; MEd; CCFP; FCFP; Ac Staff, QHC Trenton Memorial; (613)394-0770; Fax. (613)394-7079.

GRIFFIN, Griselda K; Humber River Reg Hosp-Church, 200 Church St, Toronto ON M9N 1N8; Dublin (Ireland)'65; LRCPSI; FRCPC; Anes. Staff, Humber River Regional Hospital - Church Street Site; (416)249-8111 x4154

GRIFFIN, Jennifer A; Children's Hosp, 840 Sherbrook St, Winnipeg MB R3A 1A1; Man'06; FRCPC; Peds.

GRIFFIN, Jonathan P M; Jonathan Griffin Inc, 341 Festubert St, Duncan BC V9L 3T1; Cal'85; (250)746-3677; Fax. (250)746-3679.

GRIFFIN, Leslie B; Northwest Med Group, 30 Farnham Gate Rd, Halifax NS B3M 3W8; Dal'94; BSc; CCFP; Langs: French; (902)443-8388; Fax. (902)443-9887.

GRIFFIN, Lisa J; Scotia Med Clinic, 961 Bedford Hwy, Bedford NS B4A 1A9; Dal'02; BSc; CCFP; Physician, Scotia Medical Clinic; (902)832-2360; Fax. (902)444-3074.

GRIFFIN, Patrick M G; Adult Med Clinic, 2735 Pembina Hwy, Winnipeg MB R3T 2H5; Dublin (Ireland)'77; FRCPC; IntMed. Staff, St Boniface General Hospital; Med Staff Assoc, Victoria General Hospital.

GRIFFIN, Steven R; Bancroft Family Health Team, PO Box 578 2F-16 Billa St, Bancroft ON K0L 1C0; Tor'05; CCFP; Assoc Staff, QHC North Hastings; (613)332-1565; Fax. (613)332-0526.

GRIFFIN, Timohty; Broadway Family Hlth Clinic, PO Box 900 Stn Main 3 Herald Ave, Corner Brook NL A2H 6J2; McM'05; CCFP; (709)639-5920; Fax. (709)639-5920.

GRIFFIN, Virginia M; North Toronto Med Bldg, 216-250 Lawrence Ave W, Toronto ON M5M 1B2; Tor'80; CCFP; FCFP; Ac Staff, North York General Hospital; Assoc Prof Family Med, University of Toronto; (416)785-5001; Fax. (416)785-6539; ginny.griffin@rogers.com.

GRIFFIN, Wendy A; Credit Valley Prof Bldg, 205-2300 Eglinton Ave W, Mississauga ON L5M 2V8; Tor'89; BScPharm; CCFP; Ac Staff, The Credit Valley Hospital; (905)820-8144; Fax. (905)820-1631.

GRIFFIN, William; Northern Lights Health Region, 7 Hospital St, Fort McMurray AB T9H 1P2; Galway (Ireland)'81; MB; Staff, Fort Chipewyan Nursing Station; Staff, Northern Lights Regional Health Centre; Staff Chief, Mayerthorpe Health Care Centre; (780)791-6161; williamg@mayerthorpe.ca.

GRIFFIOEN, John P H; Family Practice Associates, PO Box 2010 223 16th Ave, Creston BC V0B 1G0; Qns'92; CCFP; FCFP; (250)428-9371; Fax. (250)428-9350.

GRIFFIOEN, Timothy; 2-125 Muskoka Rd 118 W, Bracebridge ON P1L 1T2; Wes'90.

GRIFFITH, Philip S; Univ of Alberta Hosp, 8440 112 St NW, Edmonton AB T6G 2B7; (Jamaica)'00; MB BS; Staff, University of Alberta Hospital; (780)407-8822

GRIFFITHS, Anne-Marie; The Hosp for Sick Children, 8417-555 University Ave, Toronto ON M5G 1X8; Tor'77; FRCPC; Peds (Pediatric Gastroenterology). Ac Staff Ped Gastroent, The Hospital For Sick Children; Prof Peds, University of Toronto; (416)813-8757; Fax. (416)813-6531; anne.griffiths@sickkids.ca.

GRIFFITHS, Gregory B; 104-532 Lake St, St Catharines ON L2N 4H4; McG'86; ABIM(Rheum.); FRCPC; IntMed; Rheum., Niagara Health System-St Catharines General Site, Rheum.; Consultant Rheum, Hotel-Dieu Hospital; Consultant, Rheumatol., Niagara Rehab; Langs: Bilingual(English/French); (905)935-4949; Fax. (905)937-4242.

GRIFFITHS, Jane M; Family Med Centre, PO Box 8888 Stn Main 220 Bagot St, Kingston ON K7L 5E9; Qns'85; CCFP; FCFP; Clin Assoc Staff, Providence Care - St Mary's of the Lake Hospital Site; Att Staff, Kingston General Hospital; Att Staff, Hotel-Dieu Hospital; Asst Prof, Queen's University; (613)533-9303; Fax. (613)544-9899; jg4@queensu.ca.

GRIFFITHS, Jill C; Southside Women's Health Centr, 120-3017 66 St NW, Edmonton AB T6K 4B2; Alb'01; FRCSC; ObstGyn. Staff, Covenant Health - Grey Nuns Community Hospital; (780)461-6220; Fax. (780)461-4197.

GRIFFITHS, Lesley A; Timmins & District Hosp, 700 Ross Ave E, Timmins ON P4N 8P2; McM'02; MD; BSc; CCFP; Staff ER Family Practice, Timmins & District Hospital; (705)267-2131

GRIFFITHS, Melanie; Hamilton HS-Henderson Site, 711 Concession St, Hamilton ON L8V 1C3; London (England)'88; Staff, Hamilton Health Sciences Centre-Juravinski Site; (905)521-2100

GRIFFITHS, Nancy; CSSS de Sept-Iles, 45 rue du Pere-Divet, Sept-Iles QC G4R 3N7; Mon'97; FRCSC; OrthSurg. Staff, Centre Hospitalier Regional de Sept-Iles; (418)962-9761

GRIFFITHS, Patricia E; Family Med Associates, 500-267 O'Connor St, Ottawa ON K2P 1V3; Ott'77; CCFP; FCFP; Langs: Bilingual(English/French); (613)232-3333; Fax. (613)232-4818.

GRIFFITHS, Robert A; The Richmond Hosp, 7000 Westminster Hwy, Richmond BC V6X 1A2; UBC'77; Staff EmergMed, Richmond Hospital; (604)244-5151; Fax. (604)434-2161.

GRIGG, Megan J; Grey Bruce Health Services, 204-369 Mary St, Wiarton ON N0H 2T0; Mem'06; CCFP; Staff, Grey Bruce Health Services - Wiarton Site; (519)534-1260; Fax. (519)534-1744.

GRIGGS, Gordon Bruce; Deer Lodge Centre Inc, 2109 Portage Ave, Winnipeg MB R3J 0L3; Man'58; CCFP; FCFP; Fam Med, WRHA - Deer Lodge Centre; (204)293-9230; Fax. (204)831-6685.

GRIGNANO, Maria C; Thistlewood Prof Centre, 306-8077 Islington Ave, Woodbridge ON L4L 7X7; Tor'95; CCFP; Langs: Italian; (905)856-8714

GRIGNON, Andree; Hôpital Ste-Justine, 3175 ch Cote-Sainte-Catherine, Montreal QC H3T 1C5; Mon'73; DiagRad (Echography). Ac Staff, Hôpital Ste-Justine; (514)345-4633; Fax. (514)345-4816.

GRIGNON, Michel; 3210 The Boulevard, Westmount QC H3Y 1S3; McG'78; Psy. Staff, McGill University Health Centre - Montreal Children's Hospital; (514)933-5834

GRIGNON, Sylvain; CHUS-Hop Hotel-Dieu, 580 rue Bowen S, Sherbrooke QC J1G 2E8; Aix-Marseille (France)'90; assoc Prof, Centre Hospitalier Universitaire de Sherbrooke-Hôpital Hôtel-Dieu; Langs: English; (819)346-1110; Fax. (819)829-6263; sylvain.grignon@usherbrooke.ca.

GRIGORE, Emil-Vasile; West Elgin Medical Ctr, PO Box 763 171 Main St, West Lorne ON N0L 2P0; (Romania)'75; Asst Surg, London Health Sciences Centre - Victoria Campus; Langs: Romanian; (519)768-1326; Fax. (519)768-2953.

GRIGOREVA, Diana; Southlake Reg Health Centre, W5-596 Davis Dr, Newmarket ON L3Y 2P9; (Belarus)'93; FRCPC; Psy. Staff, Southlake Regional Health Centre; (905)895-4521; Fax. (905)830-5977.

GRIGORIADIS, Elizabeth; Women's College Hosp, 1001-76 Grenville St, Toronto ON M5S 1B2; Tor'95; FRCPC; Rheum; IntMed. Physician, Women's College Hospital; (416)323-6344; Fax. (416)323-6115.

GRIGORIADIS, Sophie; Sunnybrook Hlth Sciences Ctre, FG29-2075 Bayview Ave, Toronto ON M4N 3M5; McM'97; FRCPC; Psy (Hematology). Psychiatrist, Women's College Hospital; Psychiatrist, Toronto General Hospital - UHN; Staff, Sunnybrook Health Sciences Centre; Asst Prof Psy, University of Toronto; (416)480-6100

GRIGORIAN, Anahid; 112-1600 boul Henri-Bourassa O, Montreal QC H3M 3E2; Russia (Russia (Federation))'70; (514)383-5804; Fax. (514)383-8120.

GRIGORIU, Ariadna; MUHC-Royal Victoria Hosp, 687 av des Pins O, Montreal QC H3A 1A2; McG'03; FRCSC; ObstGyn (Maternal Fetal Medicine). Staff, McGill University Health Centre - Royal Victoria Hospital; (514)934-1934

GRILL, Allan K; Markham Family Health Team, 101-377 Church St, Markham ON L6B 1A1; Tor'00; MPH; CCFP; Staff, Markham Stouffville Hospital; Staff, Sunnybrook Health Sciences Centre; Asst Prof, University of Toronto; (905)471-9999; Fax. (905)471-3627.

GRILLAS, Haralambos B; Ctr Hosp de Lachine, 650 16e av, Lachine QC H8S 3N5; McG'90; CSPQ; BSc; DrMedCh; LMCC; FRCPC; Anes (P.Q.) (Cardiac Anesthesia). Staff, Lakeshore General Hospital - Pointe Claire; Staff, Centre Hospitalier de Lachine; Staff, Sir Mortimer B Davis Jewish General; Langs: French; Greek; (514)637-2351; grillbobca@yahoo.ca.

GRILLS, Gordon R; 45974 Yale Rd, Chilliwack BC V2P 2M3; Qns'77; FRCPC; IntMed; Endocrin&Metab. (604)795-3530; Fax. (604)795-3590.

GRIMARD, Doria; CSSS de chicoutimi, 305 rue Saint-Vallier, Chicoutimi QC G7H 5H6; Sher'74; FRCPC; MedMicrobiol; Microbio & Infect Dis (P.Q.). Chef Biologie Med, Complexe hospitalier de la Sagamie; Pres, Intermed Groupe Sante; (418)541-1046; doria.grimard@ssss.gouv.qc.ca.

GRIMARD, Guy; Hôpital Ste-Justine, 3175 ch Cote-Sainte-Catherine, Montreal QC H3T 1C5; Sher'83; FRCSC; OrthSurg (Orthopedics). Ac Staff, Hôpital Ste-Justine; assoc Prof, Universite de Montreal; Langs: Bilingual(French/English); (514)345-4876; Fax. (514)345-4755.

GRIMARD, Laval J; Ottawa Reg Cancer Centre, 501 Smyth Rd, Ottawa ON K1H 8L6; Mon'76; ABR; FRCP; FRCPC; RadOncol. Ac Staff, The Ottawa Hospital - General Campus; Ac Staff, The Ottawa Hospital - Civic Campus; Consultant, Children's Hospital of Eastern Ontario (CHEO); Langs: Bilingual(French/English); (613)737-7700 x70194; Fax. (613)247-3511; lgrimard@toh.on.ca.

GRIMARD, Marlene; Centre Med Le Mesnil, 300-1300 boul Lebourgneuf, Quebec QC G2K 2N1; Laval'91; BSc; MSc; Emergency Med, Centre Hospitalier Portneuf; Physician CSP Quebec/Health Travel & Clin. Externe, CLSC La Source; (418)624-1800; Fax. (418)624-1820.

GRIMARD, Nicole; Clin Med Plateau Marquette, 200-731 rue Galt O, Sherbrooke QC J1H 1Z1; Sher'80; (819)761-6131; Fax. (819)762-3041.

GRIMBEEK, Francois N; 3410 50 Ave, Red Deer AB T4N 3Y4; Orange Free State (South Africa)'00; Staff, Carberry Plains Health Centre; (403)342-9444

GRIMES, David A; The Ottawa Hosp-Civic Campus, C2-1053 Carling Ave, Ottawa ON K1Y 4E9; Ott'92; FRCPC; Neur (Movement Disorders). Assoc Scientist, The Ottawa Hospital - Civic Campus; (613)761-5353; Fax. (613)761-5360.

GRIMES, Gil; Queen Elizabeth Hosp, PO Box 6600 Stn Ctrl 60 Riverside Dr, Charlottetown PE C1A 8T5; Dallas (TX) (USA)'95; AAFP; Staff, Community Hospital Inc; Staff, Queen Elizabeth Hospital; Lecturer, Dalhousie University; (902)894-2111

GRIMES, Richard; Valley Med Clinic, 335 Jubilee St, Duncan BC V9L 1W9; Dublin (Ireland)'72; MB BCh; (250)748-8151; Fax. (250)748-8157.

GRIMES, Ruth B; 401-1020 Lorimar Blvd, Winnipeg MB R3P 1C7; Sask'87; FRCPC; Hem; Peds (Pediatric Hematology Oncology). Consultant Privil Peds & Hem/Associate Provisional, Health Sciences Centre; Associate Admission Treatment/Consultant Privil, St Boniface General Hospital; Asst Prof Peds, University of Manitoba.

GRIMMER, Joanne; London HSC-Victoria Hosp, PO Box 5010 Stn B 800 Commissioners Rd E, London ON N6A 5W9; Qns'97; BSc; FRCPC; Peds (Pediatric Nephrology); Nephrol. Consultant Admitting, London Health Sciences Centre - Victoria Campus; Consultant, Parkwood Hospital - St Joseph's Health Care; Teach Staff Med, University of Western Ontario; (519)685-8500

GRIMSHAW, Robert; Queen Elizabeth II HSC, 5004-1278 South Park St, Halifax NS B3H 2Y9; Wes'84; FRCSC; ObstGyn. Head Gyn Oncol, Queen Elizabeth II Health Sciences Centre - Victoria General Site; Asst Prof ObstGyn, Dalhousie University; (902)473-4029; Fax. (902)473-7765.

GRIMSRUD, Karen; Transport Canada, 815-9700 Jasper Ave NW, Edmonton AB T5J 4C3; Alb'78; FAB; MHSc; Staff, Transport Canada; (780)495-5303; karen.grimsrud@gov.ab.ca.

GRIMWOOD, H Russell; 303C-1830 Oak Bay Ave, Victoria BC V8R 6R2; UBC'73; (250)598-4561

GRIN, Andrea; St Michael's Hosp, 30 Bond St, Toronto ON M5B 1W8; Tor'05; FRCPC; AnatPath. Staff, St Michael's Hospital; Langs: Bilingual(English/French); (416)360-4000 x5858

GRINBERG, Ralph; Grinberg Med Prof Corp, SS 6 57 Misty River Dr, Conestogo ON N0B 1N0; Wes'78; FRCPC; Anes (Obstetrics Anesthesia). Staff, Grand River Hospital - Kitchener/Waterloo Health Centre; Staff, St Mary's General Hospital; Langs: Latvian; (519)664-3018; grinberg@golden.net.

GRINBLAT, Leonard; North York Gen Hosp, 4001 Leslie St, North York ON M2K 1E1; McM'02; FRCPC; DiagRad; NuclearMed. Staff, North York General Hospital; (416)756-6000

GRINGORTEN, Natalie A; 110 Queen's Plate Dr, Etobicoke ON M9W 0B4; (Grenada)'00; FRCSC; ObstGyn. Staff, William Osler Health System - Etobicoke General Hospital; (416)741-2552; Fax. (416)741-9729.

GRINMAN, Michelle; Univ Hlth Network-Toronto Gen, 200 Elizabeth St, Toronto ON M5G 2C4; Cal'05; FRCPC; IntMed. Staff, Toronto General Hospital - UHN; Langs: Italian; Spanish; (416)340-4800

GRINMAN, Susana E Z; Rockyview Gen Hosp, 7007 14 St SW, Calgary AB T2V 1P9; Buenos Aires (Argentina)'70; FRCPC; IntMed. Ac Staff Privil, Rockyview General Hospital; Clinical Asst Prof, University of Calgary; (403)943-3000; Fax. (403)244-8635.

GRIPP, Karen E; Children's Hosp, 840 Sherbrook St, Winnipeg MB R3A 1S1; Baltimore (USA)'96.

GRIPP, Mark J; Medicine Hat Reg Hosp, 666 5 St SW, Medicine Hat AB T1A 4H6; (Netherlands)'01; Staff, Medicine Hat Regional Hospital; (403)529-8804; Fax. (403)529-8078.

GRISARU, Silviu; Alberta Children's Hosp, 2888 Shaganappi Trail NW, Calgary AB T3B 6A8; (Israel)'93; Staff, Alberta Children's Hospital; (403)955-7950

GRISDALE, Noel W; Foothills Family Med Centre, PO Box 460, Black Diamond AB T0L 0H0; Cal'92; CCFP; Board Member, Canadian Medical Association; (403)933-4368; Fax. (403)933-2026.

GRISDALE, William R; 880 16 Ave SW PO Box 15, Calgary AB T2R 1J9; Alb'63; FRCPC; IntMed. (403)216-6120

GRISE, Ann D; Univ Hlth Network-Toronto Gen, 200 Elizabeth St, Toronto ON M5G 2C4; Tor'76; MBA; FRCPC; Anes. Staff Ctr for Addiction & Mental Hlth Kingston Eye Inst, Toronto General Hospital - UHN; Asst Prof, University of Toronto; (416)340-3242; Fax. (416)340-3698.

GRISE, Mary E; One Kids Place, 400 McKeown Ave, North Bay ON P1B 0B2; Qns'97; FRCPC; Peds. Staff, North Bay Regional Health Centre - Regional Mental Health; (705)495-8115; Fax. (705)495-8114.

GRIST, Robert D; 25393 112 Ave, Maple Ridge BC V2W 1G9; Man'71; (604)818-5445

GRISWOLD, Dean A; Glenmore Clinic, 1605 Gordon Dr, Kelowna BC V1Y 3G8; Alb'77; CCFP; FCFP; (250)762-2729

GRISWOLD, Deborah J; St Paul's Hosp, 1081 Burrard St, Vancouver BC V6Z 1Y6; UBC'75; FRCPC; HemPath. Staff, Providence Health Care - St Paul's Hospital; (604)806-9905

GRITTER, Hilda L; Dynacare Kasper Med Labs, 200-10150 102 St NW, Edmonton AB T5J 5E2; Wes'78; FRCPC; AnatPath. Staff, Royal Alexandra Hospital; (780)451-3702 x8155

GRITTER, Roy A; Westgrove Medicentre, 10232 142 St NW, Edmonton AB T5N 2N8; Alb'90; (780)452-0281; Fax. (780)452-1381.

GRIZENKO, Natalie; Douglas Mental Hlth Univ Inst, 6875 boul LaSalle, Verdun QC H4H 1R3; Sher'84; FRCPC; Psy (Child Psychiatry). Med Dir Child Psy, Douglas Mental Health University Institute; Assoc Prof Psy, McGill University; Langs: Russian; Bilingual(French/English); (514)761-6131 x2053; Fax. (514)762-3041; grinat@douglas.mcgill.ca.

GROARKE, Marie-Therese; Ctr Hosp du Centre la Mauricie, 50 rue 119E, Shawinigan QC G9P 5K1; Sher'05; FRCSC; OrthSurg. Staff, Centre Hospitalier du Centre la Mauricie; (819)536-7500

GROBB, Jacie; Brandon Reg Hlth Ctr, 150 McTavish Ave E, Brandon MB R7A 2B3; (Other Foreign)'09; CCFP; Staff, Brandon Regional Health Centre; (204)578-4000

GROBBELAAR, Barend; Airora Hlth Clinic, 202-1302 7th Ave, Prince George BC V2L 3P1; Royal College of Surgeons (Ireland)'79; MB BCh; LRCPSI; CCFP; Physician, Medical Clinic; Clin Instructor Family Med, University of British Columbia; (250)563-2622; Fax. (250)563-2621; barend.grobbelaar@northernhealth.ca.

GROBBELAAR, Jacobus P D; Newell Associate Clinic, PO Box 280 Stn Main 220 4th St W, Brooks AB T1R 1B3; (South Africa)'98; Langs: Afrikaans; (403)362-5501; Fax. (403)362-8426.

GROBER, Ethan; Murray Koffler Urologic Wellne, 6F-60 Murray St, Toronto ON M5T 3L9; McM'99; FRCSC; Urol (Male Infertility)., Mount Sinai Hospital; Staff, Women's College Hospital; (416)586-5374; Fax. (416)586-4823.

GROBLER, Andre; Estevan Med Clinic, 110-1175 Nicholson Rd, Estevan SK S4A 2S7; CCFP; (306)634-2661; Fax. (306)634-8821.

GROBLER, Gert J; 3-2020 Strachan Rd SE, Medicine Hat AB T1B 0M9; (South Africa)'94; MB ChB; (403)580-1882; Fax. (403)504-5799.

GROBLER, Josias M; Central Alberta Prof Centre, 182-5201 43 St, Red Deer AB T4N 1C7; Pretoria (South Africa)'78; MB ChB; Staff, Red Deer Regional Hospital Centre; Langs: Afrikaans; (403)343-6404; Fax. (403)343-6215.

GROBLER, Wilhelmus P; South Sherbrook Health Centre, B-88 Sherbrook St, Winnipeg MB R3C 2B3; Pretoria (South Africa)'80.

GROCHOWSKI, James; Bluewater Health-Norman Site, 89 Norman St, Sarnia ON N7T 6S3; Wes'00; CCFP; CCFP(E.M.); Staff, Bluewater Health - Norman Site; (519)464-4400

GROCOTT, Hilary P T; St Boniface Gen Hosp, 409 Tache Ave, Winnipeg MB R2H 2A6; Sask'90; FRCPC; Anes (Cardiac Surgery). Staff, St Boniface General Hospital; (204)233-8563

GRODECKI, Richard G; Defence Research & Dev Canada, PO Box 2000 Stn Downsview A 1133 Sheppard Ave W, North York ON M3M 3B9; Tor'93; CCFP; (416)635-2021

GRODINSKY, Stephen H; Appletree Med Group, 201-2948 Baseline Rd, Nepean ON K2H 8T5; McG'85; FAAP; FRCPC; Peds (Neonatology). Att Staff, Children's Hospital of Eastern Ontario (CHEO); Att Staff, The Ottawa Hospital - Civic Campus; Chief Peds, Queensway Carleton Hospital; Langs: English; French; (613)828-3310

GRODZICKY, Roman V; Centre de Read Lucie-Bruneau, 2275 rue Laurier E, Montreal QC H2H 2N8; Mon'86; (514)527-4527

GRODZICKY, Tamara C; CHUM-Hop Notre-Dame, 1560 rue Sherbrooke E, Montreal QC H2L 4M1; Mon'92; FRCPC; IntMed (External Clinic); Rheum. adj Prof, Centre Hospitalier l'Université de Montréal (CHUM) - Hôpital Notre-Dame; adj Prof Med, Universite de Montreal; Langs: Ukrainian; English; (514)890-8000 x28800; Fax. (514)412-7630; grodzicky@yahoo.com.

GROENENBOOM JANKUNIS, Marion B; Chinook Reg Hosp, 960 19 St S, Lethbridge AB T1J 1W5; Alb'95; FRCPC; AnatPath. Staff, Chinook Regional Hospital; (403)388-6093

GROENEWALD, Ettiene; St Mary's Hosp, 4607 53 St, Camrose AB T4V 1Y5; (South Africa)'89; MB ChB; Staff, Covenant Health - St Mary's Hospital; Staff, Covenant Health - St Joseph's General Hospital; Langs: Afrikaans; (780)679-6100

GROENEWALD, L Henriette; Dakota Med Centre, 17-845 Dakota St, Winnipeg MB R2M 5M3; Orange Free State (South Africa)'92; CCFP; Langs: Afrikaans; (204)254-2087; Fax. (204)254-0822.

GROENEWALD, Leon C; Queen Elizabeth II Hosp, 10409 98 St, Grande Prairie AB T8V 2E8; (South Africa)'76; MB ChB; Staff, Queen Elizabeth II Hospital; Langs: Afrikaans; German; Norwegian; (780)538-7618; Fax. (780)538-7600.

GROENEWALD, Petrus J; Broadway Med Clinic, 200-41 Broadway St W, Yorkton SK S3N 0L6; Pretoria (South Africa)'89; MB ChB; CCFP; (306)783-2555

GROENEWALD, Wendy C; Associated Medical Clinica, PO BOX 510 10017 101 Ave, Lac La Biche AB T0A 2C0; (780)623-4421; Fax. (780)623-3442.

GROENEWEGE, Donald R; MUHC-Montreal Gen Hosp, A2 230-1650 av Cedar, Montreal QC H3G 1A4; McG'82; FRCPC; Psy. Staff, McGill University Health Centre - Montreal General Campus; Langs: English; French; (514)934-1934; Fax. (514)934-8237.

GROENEWOUD, Yolanda A; 407-474 College St, Toronto ON M6G 1A4; Cal'87; BSc; FRCPC; IntMed; Endocrin&Metab. Consultant Privil, Toronto General Hospital - UHN; Lecturer, University of Toronto; (416)920-3933; Fax. (416)920-4814.

GROF, Paul; Mood Disorders Centre, 202-1929 Russell Rd, Ottawa ON K1G 4G3; Karlova (Czech Republic)'59; PhD; Psy. Staff, Royal Ottawa Mental Health Centre - Royal Ottawa Health Care Group; Langs: Czech; (613)262-8770

GROGAN, J Anthony; Leila Med Clinic, 630 Leila Ave, Winnipeg MB R2V 3N7; Glasgow (Scotland)'59; MB ChB; Med Examiner Teulon Area, MB Gov't Procurement Services; (204)632-0024; Fax. (204)697-2047; anthony.grogan@gov.mb.ca.

GROGAN, Johanne; 118 rue Saint-Jacques, St-Jean-Sur-Richel QC J3B 2K1; Laval'79; (450)346-5885

GROH, Catherine D; Elliot Lake Family Health Team, 2F-31 Nova Scotia Walk, Elliot Lake ON P5A 1Y9; McM'96; CCFP; (705)461-8882; Fax. (705)848-3449.

GROLEAU, Isabelle; CHUQ-St-Francois D'assise, 10 rue de l'Espinay, Quebec QC G1L 3L5; Laval'02; CCFP; Staff, Centre Hospitalier Universitaire de Québec - Pavillon De St-françois-d'assise; (418)525-4351

GROLEAU, Jean-Paul; Centre Med Pierrefonds, 12774 boul Gouin O, Pierrefonds QC H8Z 1W5; Mon'77; Ac Staff, Hôpital du Sacre-Coeur de Montréal; Ac Staff, Lakeshore General Hospital - Pointe Claire; (514)684-8987; Fax. (514)684-5063.

GROLEAU, Maroussia; Clinique Med L'Envolee, 5025 rue De Salaberry, Montreal QC H4J 1J1; Mon'00; (514)331-2323

GROLEAU, Nathalie; Service de L'Evaluation Med, CP 7777 Succ Terminus, Quebec QC G1K 7T4; Laval'95; (418)657-8709 x4153

GROLEAU, Sylvie; Hop Charles Lemoyne, 3120 boul Taschereau, Greenfield Park QC J4V 2H1; Sher'81; DiagRad. Staff, Hopital Charles LeMoyne; Ac Staff Rad, Centre Hospitalier Universitaire de Sherbrooke-Hopital Fleurimont; (450)466-5000 x2327; Fax. (450)466-5072.

GROLL, Ryan J; 303-855 Broadview Ave, Toronto ON M4K 3Z1; Tor'02; FRCSC; Urol. Staff, Toronto East General Hospital Inc; (416)461-7170

GRONAS, Rolf; North York Gen Hosp, 4001 Leslie St, North York ON M2K 1E1; Tor'97; FRCPC; Anes. Staff, St Joseph's Health Centre; Staff, North York General Hospital; Langs: Bilingual(English/French); (416)756-6000

GRONAU, Karen A; 233-2130 North Park Dr, Brampton ON L6S 0C9; Tor'98; BSc; MSc; FRCSC; ObstGyn. Langs: Italian; Aklanon; (905)789-8966

GRONDIN, Anne; Clinique de Pediatrie de St-Je, 218-383 boul du Seminaire N, St-Jean-sur-Richel QC J3B 8C5; Mon'96; Peds. (450)348-4911; Fax. (450)348-6401.

GRONDIN, Charlotte; CHUQ-Ctr Hosp Univ Laval, H3165-2705 boul Laurier, Quebec QC G1V 4G2; Laval'81; FRCPC; IntMed; Rheum. ac Staff, Centre Hospitalier Universitaire de Quebec-CHUL; Clin Prof, Université Laval; (418)654-2242; Fax. (418)654-2798.

GRONDIN, Danielle; Citizenship & Immigration Cda, C357-219 Laurier Ave W, Ottawa ON K1A 1L1; Laval'74; FRCPC; Peds (Public Health). Physician, Citizenship & Immigration Canada; Dep Minister Assistant Interimaire, Public Health Agency of Canada; Langs: Bilingual(French/English); (613)946-5597; Fax. (613)954-8653.

GRONDIN, Fernande M H; Royal Ottawa Health Care Group, 5457-1145 Carling Ave, Ottawa ON K1Z 7K4; Ott'77; FRCPC; Psy (Geriatric Psychiatry). Staff, Royal Ottawa Mental Health Centre - Royal Ottawa Health Care Group; Consultant, Children's Hospital of Eastern Ontario (CHEO); Consultant, Timmins & District Hospital; (613)715-5827; Fax. (613)715-5839.

GRONDIN, Francois R; Clin de Cardiologie de Levis, 600-4975 boul de la Rive-Sud, Levis QC G6V 4Z5; McG'88; CSPQ; FRCPC; IntMed; Cardiol. Staff, Hôtel-Dieu de Lévis; Langs: English; (418)833-5750; Fax. (418)833-5837.

GRONDIN, Gaetan; Centre Bois de Boulogne, 505-1575 boul Henri-Bourassa O, Montreal QC H3M 3A9; Laval'66; CSPQ; LMCC; FRCPC; Psy (Mood Disorders). Staff Psy, Hôpital du Sacre-Coeur de Montréal; Member, Canadian Psychoanalytic Society; Aj Prof Psy Clinic, Universite de Montreal; (514)338-4300; Fax. (514)338-4493.

GRONDIN, Jerome; 103-2984 boul Taschereau, Longueuil QC J4V 2G9; Sher'88; (450)466-4333

GRONDIN, Katherine; CHUQ-Hotel-Dieu de Quebec, 11 Cote du Palais, Quebec QC G1R 2J6; Laval'01; AnatPath. Staff, Centre Hospitalier Universitaire de Québec (CHUQ) - Siege Social; (418)691-5233

GRONDIN, Louis; Cosmetic & Laser Vein Centre, 3F-1504 15 Ave SW, Calgary AB T3C 0X9; Laval'79; MD; MBA; ACLS; FACPh; Langs: Spanish; French; (403)245-8008; Fax. (403)245-5212; grondin@telusplanet.net.

GRONDIN, Louis; Clinique Med du Grand L'Islet, 82 10e rue, L'Isletville QC G0R 2C0; Laval'74; (418)247-5065; Fax. (418)247-3140.

GRONDIN, Louis; Centre Med Mont-Bleu, 719 boul Saint-Joseph, Gatineau QC J8Y 4B6; Laval'76; ACLS; LMCC; Assoc Member, Montfort Hospital; Médecin, Centre Med Mont-Bleu; Langs: Bilingual(French/English); (819)771-6345; Fax. (819)771-4148; lmgrondin@sympatico.ca.

GRONDIN, Luc; CSSS de Trois-Rivières, 1991 boul du Carmel, Trois-Rivieres QC G8Z 3R9; Laval'91; DiagRad. Staff, CSSS de Trois-Rivières; (819)697-3333

GRONDIN, Philippe P; CHUM-Hop Notre-Dame, 1560 rue Sherbrooke E, Montreal QC H2L 4M1; McG'01; FRCSC; OrthSurg. Staff, Centre Hospitalier l'Université de Montréal (CHUM) - Hôpital Notre-Dame; (514)890-8000 x26106

GRONDIN, Pierre; CSSS de Manicouagan, 635 boul Jolliet, Baie-Comeau QC G5C 1P1; Sher'83; FRCPC; DiagRad. Staff, Centre Hospitalier Régional Baie-Comeau; Langs: English; (418)589-3701

GRONDIN, Renee J; CHUQ-Ctr Hosp Univ Laval, 2705 boul Laurier, Quebec QC G1V 4G2; Laval'81; Assoc Dir Prof Services, Centre Hospitalier Universitaire de Quebec-CHUL; (418)654-2287; Fax. (418)577-4661; renee.grondin@chuq.qc.ca.

GRONDIN, Sean C; Foothills Med Centre, G33 D-1403 29 St NW, Calgary AB T2N 2T9; Dal'90; MPH; BSc; FRCSC; GenSurg; ThorSurg. Staff, Foothills Medical Centre; Assoc Prof Surg, University of Calgary; Langs: French; (403)944-8798; Fax. (403)270-8431; sean.grondin@albertahealthservices.ca.

GRONDIN, Valerie; Centre Oculaire de Victorialle, 340 rue Notre-Dame E, Victoriaville QC G6P 4A6; Laval'06; Ophth. Staff, Hotel-Dieu d'Arthabaska; (819)751-5595

GRONDIN BEAUDOIN, Brian; CSSS de Chicoutimi, CP 5006 305 rue Saint-Vallier, Chicoutimi QC G7H 5H6; Sher'08; IntMed. Staff, Complexe hospitalier de la Sagamie; (418)541-1000

GRONSKA, Margaret A; Jane Medical Clinic, 101-2780 Jane St, North York ON M3N 2J2; Ott'03; CCFP; Langs: Polish; (416)745-8500; Fax. (416)748-8730.

GROOT, Donald W; Groot Dermasurgery Centre, 200-9670 142 St NW, Edmonton AB T5N 4B2; Alb'73; FACP; FRCPC; Derm (Laser Surgery). Clin Prof Med, University of Alberta; (780)482-1414; Fax. (780)482-7097; dg@grootdermasurgery.com.

GROOT, Gary; Surgical Associates, 222-750 Spadina Cres E, Saskatoon SK S7K 3H3; Sask'82; FRCSC; GenSurg (Surgical Oncology). (306)653-3366; Fax. (306)653-8832.

GROOT, Marcel C; Northern Health Authority, 410-299 Victoria St, Prince George BC V2L 5B8; Pretoria (South Africa)'01; MB ChB; (250)564-8869

GROOTENDORST, Martin W J; North Road Med Centre, 435 North Rd, Coquitlam BC V3K 3V9; UBC'07; CCFP; (604)936-0411

GROPPER, Peter T; 121-555 12th Ave W, Vancouver BC V5Z 3X7; Sask'69; FRCSC; OrthSurg. Ac Staff, Vancouver General Hospital - Centennial Pavillion; (604)733-4222

GROS, Michelle L; London HSC-Victoria Hosp, PO Box 5010 Stn B D2 315-800 Commissioners Rd E, London ON N6A 5W9; Tor'01; FRCPC; Anes. Staff, London Health Sciences Centre - Victoria Campus; Staff, London Health Sciences Centre - University Hospital; (519)685-8500

GROSCH, Richard D; 210-560 Nicola St NW, Vancouver BC V6G 3J7; Tor'67; BA; FRCPC; Neur. Staff Neurol, Royal Columbian Hospital; Examiner, Licentiate of the Medical Council of Canada; (604)420-6181; grosch@myreflex.com.

GROSETT, Oswald W; 324 College St, Toronto ON M5T 1S3; North Dakota (USA)'65; MB BS; (416)960-3229; Fax. (416)960-9253.

GROSHAUS, Horacio; Rockyview Gen Hosp, 7007 14 St SW, Calgary AB T2V 1P9; (Argentina)'85; FRCPC; IntMed. Staff, Rockyview General Hospital; (403)943-3000

GROSJEAN-NICLOUX, Francine; Clinique Privamed, 203-1052 rue Lionel-Daunais, Boucherville QC J4B 0B2; Nancy (France)'80; CCFP; Staff, Centre Hospitalier de Val d'Or; (450)262-6222

GROSLOUIS, Lise; CSSS de Quebec Nord, 3666 ch Royal, Quebec QC G1E 1X5; Laval'79; Staff, Hôpital de l'Archipel; (418)663-3099

GROSMAN, Harvey; Scarborough Hosp-Birchmount, 3030 Birchmount Rd, Scarborough ON M1W 3W3; Tor'70; DMRD; AB; FRCPC; DiagRad (Neuro Radiology). Chief Diag Imaging, The Scarborough Hospital - Birchmount Campus; Staff, Rouge Valley Health System - Centenary Health Centre Site; Asst Prof, University of Toronto; (416)495-2614; Fax. (416)495-2619.

GROSS, Allan E; Mount Sinai Hosp, 476A-600 University Ave, Toronto ON M5G 1X5; Tor'62; FRCSC; OrthSurg (Lower Extremity Reconstruction). Staff, Mount Sinai Hospital; Teach Staff OrthSurg, University of Toronto; (416)586-4653; Fax. (416)586-8673.

GROSS, Donald W; University of Alberta Hosp, 2E319WCM-8440 112 St NW, Edmonton AB T6G 2B7; Sask'92; BSc; FRCPC; Neur (Epilepsy). Staff, University of Alberta Hospital; Asst Prof Med, University of Alberta; (780)407-3616; Fax. (780)407-1325.

GROSS, Gil; The Hosp for Sick Chilren, 555 University Ave, Toronto ON M5G 1X8; Qns'84; FRCPC; Peds (Electrophysiology); PedCardiol. Staff, The Hospital For Sick Children; Langs: Hebrew; French; (416)813-7326

GROSS, Ian G; Monfort Hosp, 713 Montreal Rd, Ottawa ON K1K 0T2; McG'71; MDCM; FRCSC; PlasSurg (Hand Surgery). Ac Staff, Montfort Hospital; Court Staff, Children's Hospital of Eastern Ontario (CHEO); Staff, The Ottawa Hospital - Civic Campus; Staff, The Ottawa Hospital - General Campus; Langs: English; French; (613)745-6879; Fax. (613)745-6879.

GROSS, Katherine R; 22-88 Duncan Ave W, Penticton BC V2A 7J7; Monash (Australia)'76; MB BS; FRCPC; Peds (Pediatric Rheumatology); Rheum. Asst Staff Consultant Ped, Penticton Regional Hospital; Ac Staff, Vancouver General Hospital - Centennial Pavillion; Consultant, Canadian Arthritis Society; (250)492-2944; Fax. (250)492-2920.

GROSS, M Shirley; Misericordia Community Hosp, 16940 87 Ave NW, Edmonton AB T5R 4H5; Staff, Covenant Health - Misericordia Community Hospital; (780)735-2577; Fax. (780)735-2794.

GROSS, Marie M S; Misericordia Comm Hosp, 2F-16940 87 Ave NW, Edmonton AB T5R 4H5; McG'83; CCFP; Dir The Edmonton Breastfeeding Clinic, Covenant Health - Misericordia Community Hospital; Asst Prof, University of Alberta; Langs: German; French; (780)735-2577; Fax. (780)735-2794.

GROSS, Melissa L; Alberta Children's Hosp, 2888 Shaganappi Trail NW, Calgary AB T3B 6A8; Wes'02; FRCPC; Peds. Staff, Alberta Children's Hospital; (403)955-2953; Fax. (403)933-3055.

GROSS, Michael; Queen Elizabeth II HSC-Halifax, 4879-1796 Summer St, Halifax NS B3H 3A7; Newcastle (England)'75; FRCS; OrthSurg. Staff, Queen Elizabeth II Health Sciences Centre - Victoria General Site; Prof, Dalhousie University; (902)473-6811; Fax. (902)473-2042.

GROSS, Paul; Spectrum Health, 702-1080 Howe St, Vancouver BC V6Z 2T1; McG'07; MDCM; CCFP; (604)681-1080

GROSS, Peter L; Hamilton HS-Henderson Site, G-711 Concession Rd, Hamilton ON L8V 1C3; Tor'94; BSc; MSc; ABIM; FRCPC; IntMed. Staff, Hamilton Health Sciences Centre-Juravinski Site; Asst Prof, University of Toronto; (905)527-6322

GROSS, Veronica A; Ontario Telemdicine Network, 1100-105 Moatfield Dr, North York ON M3B 0A2; Cape Town (South Africa)'75; Langs: Afrikaans; (416)446-4110; Fax. (416)446-4139.

GROSS, Zeev Zvi; 20-10458 Mayfield Rd NW, Edmonton AB T5P 4P4; (Israel)'88; (780)483-7115; Fax. (780)484-6531.

GROSS, Zuzana; Bathurst Med Centre, 207-7117 Bathurst St, Thornhill ON L4J 2J6; Safarika (Slovakia)'81; Langs: Slovak; Hungarian; Russian; (905)764-0333

GROSSE-WORTMANN, Lars; The Hosp for Sick Children, 555 University Ave, Toronto ON M5G 1X8; Wurzburg (Germany)'99; Staff, The Hospital For Sick Children; Langs: German; (416)813-7326; Fax. (416)813-5857; lars.grosse-wortmann@sickkids.ca.

GROSSER, Elana; North York Gen Hosp, 4001 Leslie St, North York ON M2K 1E1; Qns'02; FRCPC; Peds. Staff, North York General Hospital; (416)756-6479

GROSSER, Norman; Medisys Health Group Inc, 12F-95 St Clair Ave W, Toronto ON M4V 1N6; Tor'69; (416)926-6464 x2722; Fax. (416)324-7905.

GROSSMAN, Daphna L; Baycrest Ctre/Geriatric Care, W6-3560 Bathurst St, North York ON M6A 2E1; Tor'92; CCFP; CCFP(E.M.); FCFP; Staff, Sunnybrook Health Sciences Centre; Staff, Baycrest Centre for Geriatric Care; Staff, Halton Healthcare Services Corporation - Georgetown Hospital; (416)785-2500

GROSSMAN, David W; 202-40 Wellesley St E, Toronto ON M4Y 1G4; Tor'95; BSc; FRCPC; CommunMed (AIDS/HIV);CCFP; Public Health & Preventive Med. Staff Family & CommunMed, St Michael's Hospital; Asst Prof Family & CommunMed, University of Toronto; (416)968-6437

GROSSMAN, Harold A; 215-9019 Bayview Ave, Richmond Hill ON L4B 3M6; Qns'71; FRCPC; Psy. Staff, Mackenzie Richmond Hill Hospital; (905)731-9766; Fax. (905)731-1711.

GROSSMAN, Jennifer K; Foothills Med Centre, 1403 29 St NW, Calgary AB T2N 2T9; Cal'06; FRCPC; IntMed; Hem. Staff, Foothills Medical Centre; (403)944-4451

GROSSMAN, Lawrence; Mackenzie Richmond Hill Hosp, 10 Trench St, Richmond Hill ON L4C 4Z3; Tor'67; FRCPC; IntMed (Palliative Care); Hem. Chief of Staff, Mackenzie Richmond Hill Hospital; The Scarborough Hospital - Birchmount Campus; (905)883-1212 x7455

GROSSMAN, Liuba; 5-4646 Dufferin St, North York ON M3H 5S4; Tel Aviv (Israel)'77; Staff, North York General Hospital - Branson Division; Langs: Hebrew; Russian; Lithuanian; Yiddish; (416)736-3505

GROSSMAN, Loren D; LMC Diabetes & Endo Centre, 107-1929 Bayview Ave, Toronto ON M4G 3E8; Tor'82; FACP; FRCPC; IntMed (Diabetology); Endocrin&Metab. Court Staff, The Scarborough Hospital - Birchmount Campus; Att Staff Outpatient, St Michael's Hospital; Staff, LMC Diabetes & Endocrinology Centres-Bayview; VP Research & Development, Eli Lilly Canada Inc; Lecturer Med, University of Toronto; Langs: Bilingual(English/French); (416)645-2929

GROSSMAN, Robert; 205-1735 Kipling Ave, Etobicoke ON M9R 2Y8; Tor'76; Ac Staff Family Practice, William Osler Health System - Etobicoke General Hospital; Consultant, Desjardins Financial Security; Med Consultant, Ontario Teachers Insurance Plan; Med Consultant Disability Division, The Great-West Life Assurance; (416)244-5601; Fax. (416)244-5054.

GROSSMAN, Ronald F; Credit Valley Prog Bldg, 201-2300 Eglinton Ave W, Mississauga ON L5M 2V8; Tor'73; FACP; FCCP; FRCPC; IntMed (Respirology). Staff, Women's College Hospital; Staff Respirologist, The Credit Valley Hospital; Staff, Mount Sinai Hospital; Prof, University of Toronto; (905)828-5168; Fax. (905)828-0113; rgrossman@cvh.on.ca.

GROSSMAN, Stacey; 214-7330 Yonge St, Thornhill ON L4J 7Y7; Tor'03; FRCSC; ObstGyn. Staff, Sunnybrook Health Sciences Centre; (905)707-9900

GROSSMAN, Steven M; 17 Bedford Park Ave, Richmond Hill ON L4C 2N9; Tor'88; Staff, Mackenzie Richmond Hill Hospital; (905)883-1100; Fax. (905)884-1195.

GROSSO, Paul M; 115-675 Queen St S, Kitchener ON N2M 1A1; Tor'96; FRCSC; OrthSurg. (519)603-0623

GROSSO, William T; The Group Health Centre, 240 Mcnabb St, Sault Ste. Marie ON P6B 1Y5; Ott'77; Ac Staff, Sault Area Hospital - Sault Ste Marie; (705)759-1234; Fax. (705)759-7487.

GROTHE, Anne-Marie; Hop du Sacre-Coeur de Mtl, 5400 boul Gouin O, Montreal QC H4J 1C5; Mon'79; CSPQ; Endocrin&Metab; IntMed (Diabetes). Staff Endocrinology, Hôpital du Sacre-Coeur de Montréal; Langs: Bilingual(French/English); (514)338-2050; Fax. (514)338-3549.

GROU, Evelyne; GMF Centre Med du Parc, 101-84 rue Court, Granby QC J2G 4Y5; Laval'92; Staff, Hôpital Regional Rimouski; (450)375-1161; Fax. (450)375-7740.

GROU, Fabienne; CLSC du Marigot, 1351 boul des Laurentides, Vimont QC H7M 2Y2; Mon'78; CCFP; FCFP; Staff, Hôpital du Sacre-Coeur de Montréal; (450)668-1803; Fax. (418)668-1503.

GROU-LECLERC, Etienne; CSSS du Grand Littoral, 1205 boul de la Rive-Sud, Levis QC G6W 0J6; Laval'04; CCFP; Staff, Centre Hospitalier Regional du Grand-Portage; (418)380-8597

GROUHI, Masoud; 9981 Yonge St, Richmond Hill ON L4C 1T9; Tehran (Iran)'82; MD; FRCP; ABPeds; LRCP; FRCPC; Peds (Clinical Immunology & Allergy). Ac Staff, Mackenzie Richmond Hill Hospital; (905)884-5638

GROUHI, Shahpar; 9981 Yonge St, Richmond Hill ON L4C 1T9; (Iran)'87; Langs: Persian; Turkish.

GROULX, Antoine; Ctr de Sante SS Cote-De-Gaspe, 215 boul de York O, Gaspe QC G4X 2W2; Laval'02; MCFP; CCFP; Staff, Centre Hospitalier de Gaspe; Clin Prof, Université Laval; Langs: English; (418)368-6663; Fax. (418)368-5358.

GROULX, Daniel; CSSSG-Hop de Hull, 116 boul Lionel-Emond, Gatineau QC J8Y 1W7; Mon'83; CSPQ; FRCPC; Anes. Ac Staff, Hull Hospital; (819)595-6033; Fax. (819)595-6039.

GROULX, Olivier; CSSS de Rimouski-Neigette, CP 3150 succ A 150 av Rouleau, Rimouski QC G5L 5T1; Laval'06; CCFP; Staff, Hôpital Regional Rimouski; (418)723-7851

GROULX, Pierre-Claude; Clinique Med Jean-Talon Pie IX, 4679 rue Jean-Talon E, Saint-Leonard QC H1S 1K3; Mon'83; (514)374-5901; Fax. (514)374-1668.

GROULX, Stephane; Clin Medicale Pierre-Boucher, 1615 boul Jacques-Cartier E, Longueuil QC J4M 2X1; Mon'78; CCFP; FCFP; (450)468-6223; Fax. (450)468-5041.

GROVER, Arvinder; 2075 Hadwen Rd, Mississauga ON L5K 2L4; Tor'90; FACC; FRCP; FRCPC; IntMed (Adult Cardiology); Cardiol. Dir, The International Heart Institute; Langs: Punjabi; Hindi; Urdu; (905)855-1320

GROVER, Deepak; 102-9123 Mary St, Chilliwack BC V2P 4H7; Delhi (India)'85; FRCS(UK); FRCS(Ortho); MB BS; FRCSC; OrthSurg (Trauma). Staff, Delta Hospital; Staff, Chilliwack General Hospital; Physician, South Fraser Surgigal Ctr Abbotsford; Physician, Fraser Health Authority; Langs: Hindi; Punjabi; (604)795-5122; Fax. (604)792-9175.

GROVER, Gagan C; 111-2580 Cedar Park Pl, Abbotsford BC V2T 3S5; Punjab (India)'84; MB BS; CCFP; (604)853-2120; Fax. (604)853-2116.

GROVER, Harpreet S; St Joseph's Health Care, T2141-50 Charlton Ave E, Hamilton ON L8N 4A6; Wes'06; FRCSC; GenSurg. Staff, St Joseph's Healthcare - Charlton Campus; (905)522-4941

GROVER, Leonard F L; Oakdale Med Bldg, 307-2065 Finch Ave W, North York ON M3N 2V7; Tor'66; FCFP; FAAFP; CCFP; FCFP; Ac Staff, Humber River Regional Hospital - Finch Avenue Site; Ac Staff, St Joseph's Health Centre; Inspector, College of Physicians & Surgeons of Ontario; Asst Prof, University of Toronto; (416)745-7455; len.grover@utoronto.ca.

GROVER, Maya; Preventous Collaborative Healt, 1635 17 Ave SW, Calgary AB T2T 0E5; UBC'09; CCFP; Staff, Foothills Medical Centre.

GROVER, Raj Pal S; Royal Victoria Reg Hlth Ctr, 201 Georgian Dr, Barrie ON L4M 6M2; Ott'01; FRCPC; DiagRad. Staff, Royal Victoria Regional Health Centre; (705)728-9802

GROVER, Ramon S; 101-515 7 St S, Lethbridge AB T1J 2G8; Sask'97; MD; FRCS; FRCSC; PlasSurg (Cranio Maxillofacial Surgery). Clin Lecturer, University of Alberta; (403)320-7181

GROVER, Samir C; St Michael's Hosp, 16 036CCW-30 Bond St, Toronto ON M5B 1W8; Tor'01; BSc; MEDes; FRCPC; IntMed; Gastroent. Staff, St Michael's Hospital; (416)864-6060; Fax. (416)864-5882.

GROVER, Steven A; MUHC-Montreal Gen Hosp, 1650 av Cedar, Montreal QC H3G 1A4; McG'79; IntMed. Staff, McGill University Health Centre - Montreal General Campus; Prof Med, McGill University; (514)934-8292; Fax. (514)934-8293.

GROVES, Lawrence E; The Brandon Clinic, 620 Dennis St, Brandon MB R7A 5E7; Man'74; Staff, Brandon Regional Health Centre; (204)728-4440; Fax. (204)728-1765.

GROVES, Sean; La Ronge Med Clinic, PO Box 240, La Ronge SK S0J 1L0; Sask'03; BSc; CCFP; (306)425-2174; Fax. (306)425-4199.

GROVES, Terence; Cardiometabolic Evaluation Ris, 210-1016 68 Ave SW, Calgary AB T2V 4J2; Alb'65; FRCPC; IntMed (Cardiology). Staff, Rockyview General Hospital; Staff, Cardiometabolic Evaluation & Risk Assessment Centre; (403)541-0033; Fax. (403)541-0032.

GROWE, Gershon H; Canadian Blood Services, 4750 Oak St, Vancouver BC V6H 2N9; Tor'63; FRCPC; IntMed (Transfusion Medicine). Med Dir, Canadian Blood Services; (604)707-3480; Fax. (604)875-8004; gershon.growe@blood.ca.

GRUBER, Dinah C; 307 Sheppard Ave W, North York ON M2N 1N6; Tor'60; FRCPC; Peds. Court Staff Nursery, North York General Hospital; Langs: Yiddish; Hebrew; (416)221-1177

GRUBER, James M; MUHC-Montreal Gen Hosp, D7 201-1650 av Cedar, Montreal QC H3G 1A4; Albert Einstein(NY) (USA)'78; FRCP; FRCPC; IntMed; Respir. Sr Physician, McGill University Health Centre - Montreal General Campus; Sr Physician, McGill University Health Centre - Montreal Chest Institute; assoc Prof, McGill University; Langs: Spanish; French; (514)934-1934 x43881; Fax. (514)934-8226; jim.gruber@muhc.mcgill.ca.

GRUBER, Wayne M; Wayne M Gruber Med Prof Corp, 115 Queen St, St Catharines ON L2R 5H4; Ott'68; BSc; FRCPC; IntMed (Cardiology). Staff, Niagara Health System - St Catharines General Site; (905)984-3400; Fax. (905)984-3370.

GRUBNER, Karin H; 206A-1011 Dufferin St, Toronto ON M6H 4B5; Tor'73; Langs: German; Portuguese; Spanish; (416)534-6331

GRUCHY, Steven E; Queen Elizabeth II HSC, 911-1276 South Park St, Halifax NS B3H 2Y9; Mem'02; FRCPC; IntMed; Gastroent. Staff, Queen Elizabeth II Health Sciences Centre - Victoria General Site; (902)473-4979; Fax. (902)473-4406.

GRUDER, Alicja N; North Lanark Country Comm Hlth, 207 Robertson Rd, Lanark ON K0G 1K0; (Poland)'99; CCFP; Langs: Polish; (613)259-2182

GRUEGER, Barbara; Pediatric Consult Clinic, 9010 Quartz Rd, Whitehorse YT Y1A 2Z5; McM'98; FRCPC; Peds. Staff, Alberta Children's Hospital.

GRUJICH, Nikola; Sunnybrook Hlth Sciences Ctre, 2075 Bayview Ave, Toronto ON M4N 3M5; Tor'06; Psy. Staff, Sunnybrook Health Sciences Centre; (416)480-6100

GRUNAU, Brian; St Paul's Hosp, 1081 Burrard St, Vancouver BC V6Z 1Y6; Man'08; CCFP; CCFP(E.M.); Staff, Providence Health Care - St Paul's Hospital; (604)806-8877

GRUNAU, Esther S; Peace Arch Hosp, 15521 Russell Ave, White Rock BC V4B 2R4; UBC'02; MA; MA; CCFP; CCFP(E.M.); Staff, Peace Arch Hospital; (604)541-7133

GRUNBAUM, Beatrice; Centre medical Metro Monk, 2376 rue Allard, Montreal QC H4E 2K9; (France)'01; Staff, Centre Hospitalier de LaSalle; (514)769-9999

GRUNBAUM, David; Hop Maisonneuve-Rosemont, 5415 boul de l'Assomption, Montreal QC H1T 2M4; Tel Aviv (Israel)'76; CSPQ; FRCPC; IntMed (Diabetes); Endocrin (P.Q.). Staff, Hopital Maisonneuve-Rosemont; Staff, McGill University Health Centre - Royal Victoria Hospital; McGill University; Prof Adjoint de Clinique, Dept of Med, Universite de Montreal; (514)252-3400 x3723; davidgrunbaum@yahoo.com.

GRUNBERG, Sabetai; 203-1711 4 St SW, Calgary AB T2S 1V8; Cuyo (Argentina)'63; Med Dir Age Care, Age Care Beverly; (403)248-5555; Fax. (403)255-3534; sasha.g@shaw.ca.

GRUNDLAND, Batya N; 76 Grenville St, Toronto ON M5S 1B2; Wes'03; CCFP; Physician, Women's College Hospital; Physician, Sunnybrook Health Sciences Centre; Langs: Hebrew; (416)323-6065 x1; Fax. (416)323-6351.

GRUNDLING, Christiaan J; Easthill Med Walk-In Clinic, 610-3020 22 St, Red Deer AB T4R 3J5; Pretoria (South Africa)'78; MB ChB; Langs: Afrikaans; (403)343-0115; Fax. (403)343-8551; cjgrundling@shaw.ca.

GRUNDMANIS, Mark A; Huronia Med Cnetre, PO Box 790 Stn Main 240 Penetanguishene Rd, Midland ON L4R 4P4; Tor'86; CCFP; Staff Privil, Georgian Bay General Hospital - Midland.

GRUNDY, Paul E; University of Alberta Hosp, 4E2 WMC-8440 112 St NW, Edmonton AB T6G 2B7; Alb'79; ABP(HemOncol); FRCPC; Peds (Pediatric Hematology Oncology). Staff, University of Alberta Hospital; Prof, University of Alberta; (780)407-8829; Fax. (780)407-7476; pgrundy@cha.ab.ca.

GRUNDY, Peter D; Gult Canada Square, 352-401 9 Ave SW, Calgary AB T2P 3C5; Cal'88; FRCPC; IntMed; Endocrin&Metab. (403)221-4476; Fax. (403)221-4418.

GRUNEBAUM, Eyal; The Hosp For Sick Children, 7283-555 University Ave, Toronto ON M5G 1X8; Jerusalem (Israel)'88; Head Div of Immunology & Allergy, The Hospital For Sick Children; Langs: Hebrew; (416)813-7654 x1320; Fax. (416)813-8624; eyal.grunebaum@sickkids.ca.

GRUNEBAUM, Margaret J; Bayview-Finch Med Clinic, 301-3292 Bayview Ave, North York ON M2M 4J5; Cape Town (South Africa)'69; MB ChB; Court Staff, North York General Hospital; Langs: Afrikaans; (416)733-9991; Fax. (416)224-9880.

GRUNEIR, Richard K; Princess Centre, 505-33 Princess St, Leamington ON N8H 5C5; Tor'73; FRCSC; ObstGyn. Staff ObstGyn, Leamington District Memorial Hospital; (519)322-1944; Fax. (519)326-8899.

GRUNER, Carole; Inst de Readaptation de Mtl, 6300 av Darlington, Montreal QC H3S 2J4; Staff, Institut de Réadaptation Gingras-Lindsay de Montréal; (514)340-2085

GRUNER, Douglas; Bruyere Academic Fam Hlth Team, 75 Bruyere St, Ottawa ON K1N 5C7; McM'93; CCFP; FCFP; Langs: Bilingual(English/French); (613)241-3344

GRUNFELD, Anton F; Eagle Ridge Hosp & Hlth CC, 475 Guildford Way, Port Moody BC V3H 3W9; Tor'77; FRCPC; EmergMed. Staff, Eagle Ridge Hospital & Health Care Centre; (604)461-2022

GRUNFELD, Eva; 1502-62 Wellesley St W, Toronto ON M5S 2X3; McM'86; MSc; PhD; CCFP; FCFP; Staff Clinician Scientist, Ontario Institute for Cancer Research; Dir Research Prog, University of Toronto; (647)345-3641; eva.grunfeld@utoronto.ca.

GRUNOW, Michael D; Hollyburn Med Bldg, 207C-575 16 St, West Vancouver BC V7V 4Y1; Cape Town (South Africa)'95; MB ChB; CCFP; Langs: Afrikaans; (604)926-3516

GRUSCHENKO, Pavlo; College Avenue East Med, 233 College Ave, Regina SK S4N 0V7; (306)522-3327; Fax. (306)522-3349.

GRUSHKA, Daniel H; Strathroy Middlesex Gen Hosp, 395 Carrie St, Strathroy ON N7G 3C9; Wes'05; CCFP; CCFP(E.M.); Staff, Strathroy Middlesex General Hospital - Middlesex Hospital Alliance; (519)245-1550

GRUSLIN, Andree M R; The Ottawa Hosp-Gen Campus, 8480-501 Smyth Rd, Ottawa ON K1H 8L6; Ott'89; FRCSC; ObstGyn (Maternal Fetal Medicine). Assoc Scientist, The Ottawa Hospital - General Campus; Dept Chair ObstGyn(interim), University of Ottawa; Langs: English; French; (613)737-8797; Fax. (613)737-8070; agruslin@ottawahospital.on.ca.

GRUSON, Valerie J; Vancouver Gen Hosp, 855 12th Ave W, Vancouver BC V5Z 1M9; Cal'78; MD; FRCPC; Psy. Ac Staff, Vancouver General Hospital - Centennial Pavillion; Clin Assoc Prof Psy, University of British Columbia; (604)875-4018; gruson@interchange.ubc.ca.

GRUSZCZYNSKI, Adam; Academic Family Med, 172-1621 Albert St, Regina SK S4P 2S5; Alb'85; CCFP; FCFP; Staff, Regina General Hospital; Asst Prof, University of Saskatchewan; (306)766-0444; Fax. (306)766-0471.

GRYFE, Robert; Mount Sinai Hosp, 455-600 University Ave, Toronto ON M5G 1X5; Tor'93; FRCSC; GenSurg (Colon & Rectal Surgery). Staff, Princess Margaret Hospital - University Health Network; Staff, Mount Sinai Hospital; (416)586-4800 x5088; Fax. (416)586-1586; rgryfe@mtsinai.on.ca.

GRYGOWSKI, Beata K; 203-3101 Bloor St W, Etobicoke ON M8X 2W2; Qns'93; FRCSC; ObstGyn. Langs: Polish; (416)232-1687; Fax. (416)232-1928.

GRYMALA, John P; Royal Ottawa Hlth Care Group, 1145 Carling Ave, Ottawa ON K1Z 7K4; Ott'78; Staff GP, Royal Ottawa Mental Health Centre - Royal Ottawa Health Care Group; (613)722-6508

GRYMALOSKI, Kim; Mill Bay Med Centre, RR 1 230-2720 Mill Bay Rd, Mill Bay BC V0R 2P1; Sask'97; CCFP; (250)743-3211

GRYMONPRE, Ilona M A; Kootenay Lake Med Clinic, 1140 Lakeside Dr, Nelson BC V1L 5Z3; Man'79; (250)352-4666; Fax. (250)352-4696.

GRYN, David M; Mackenzie Richmond Hill Hosp, 10 Trench St, Richmond Hill ON L4C 4Z3; Tor'03; FRCPC; Peds (Neonatal & Perinatal Medicine). Staff, Mackenzie Richmond Hill Hospital; (905)883-1212

GRYNOCH, A Robert; Tawa Centre, 210-3017 66 St NW, Edmonton AB T6K 4B2; Qns'78; FRCPC; IntMed. Ac Staff, Covenant Health - Grey Nuns Community Hospital; (780)465-2716; Fax. (780)465-2825.

GRYNOCH, J Richard; Univ of Alberta Hosp-SCC/WCM, 11 107CSB-8440 112 St NW, Edmonton AB T6G 2B7; Tor'73; FRCPC; IntMed (Nephrology). Asst Prof Nephrol., University of Alberta Hospital; (780)407-8822; Fax. (780)407-7771; richard.grynoch@ualberta.ca.

GRYNOCH, Roberta E; 245-10405 Jasper Ave NW, Edmonton AB T5J 3N4; Alb'83; CCFP; Med Staff, Royal Alexandra Hospital; Med Staff, The Good Samaritan Society; Med Staff Continuing Care Group, Capital Care - Grandview; (780)424-7990; Fax. (780)423-7004; roberta.grynoch@capitalhealth.ca.

GRYNSPAN, David; Children's Hosp of Eastern Ont, 401 Smyth Rd, Ottawa ON K1H 8L1; Tor'00; FRCPC; AnatPath. Staff, Children's Hospital of Eastern Ontario (CHEO); (613)737-7600 x2427

GRYNSPAN, Jonathan; Sudbury Reg Hosp-Laurentian, 41 Ramsey Lake Rd, Sudbury ON P3E 5J1; Tor'00; FRCPC; DiagRad. Staff, Health Sciences North-Laurentian Site; (705)523-7100

GRYNSPAN, Shlomo S; 409-4430 Bathurst St, North York ON M3H 3S3; (Mexico)'71; FRCSC; ObstGyn. Ac Staff, Mount Sinai Hospital; (416)638-9944

GRYPINICH, Michel; 90 rue Bernard, St-Charles-Brromee QC J6E 2C3; Mon'81; FRCPC; IntMed; Gastroent. Ac Staff Gastroenterology, Centre Hospitalier Régional de Lanaudière; (450)752-6667; Fax. (450)752-5507.

GRYPMA, Martin P; 101-20230 64 Ave, Langley BC V2Y 1N3; Wes'84; FRCSC; OrthSurg. Langs: Dutch; (604)996-4066

GRZESLO, Adam G Z; Caroline Family Hlth Team-BFMG, 208-3155 Harvester Rd, Burlington ON L7N 3V2; Tor'76; CCFP; FCFP; Staff, Joseph Brant Memorial Hospital; Teacher Pt-Time Family Med, McMaster University; (905)333-8222; Fax. (905)333-9343.

GRZYBOWSKI, Michelle M; St Boniface Gen Hosp, D1048-409 Tache Ave, Winnipeg MB R2H 2A6; Ott'05; CCFP; Staff, St Boniface General Hospital; (204)233-8563

GRZYBOWSKI, Stefan C W; 530-1501 Broadway W, Vancouver BC V6J 4Z6; UBC'79; MClSc; CCFP; FCFP; Staff, BC Women's Hospital & Health Centre; Co-Dir, Centre for Rural Health Research; Prof, University of British Columbia; Langs: Polish; Bilingual(French/English); (604)742-1794; Fax. (604)742-1798; sgrzybow@interchange.ubc.ca.

GRZYWACZ, Kelly; Centre Med Tiny Tots, 6900 boul Décarie, Cote Saint-Luc QC H3X 2T8; Mon'07; FRCPC; Peds; Gastroent. (514)342-9911

GU, Shian; Burnaby Med Centre, M37-4277 Kingsway, Burnaby BC V5H 3Z2; Tianjin (China)'80; Langs: Mandarin; (604)438-9991; Fax. (604)438-9960.

GUAIANA, Giuseppe; Regional Mental HC-St Thomas, PO Box 2004 Stn Main 467 Sunset Dr, St Thomas ON N5P 3V9; Milan (Italy)'98; Staff, Regional Mental Health Care-St Joseph's Health Care; Langs: Italian; (519)631-8510; Fax. (519)631-9224.

GUAN, Brian; Psychiatry Sherbrooke Centre, 4F-260 Sherbrooke St, New Westminster BC V3L 3M2; UBC'00; FRCPC; Psy (Forensic Psychiatry). (604)524-7171

GUAN, Meng; 203-274 Dundas St E, Belleville ON K8N 1E6; McG'04; FRCSC; Urol. (613)779-6805

GUASPARINI, Roland; Fraser Health Authority, C200-9801 King George Blvd, Surrey BC V3T 5H5; UBC'79; FRCPC; CommunMed. Med Officer of Hlth, Fraser Health Authority; Clin Prof, University of British Columbia; (604)587-7620; Fax. (604)587-7625.

GUAY, Alain; Centre de Sante Carillon, 20 rue de Carillon, Sherbrooke QC J1J 2K8; Sher'77; Consultant, Centre Hospitalier Universitaire de Sherbrooke-Hôpital Hôtel-Dieu; (819)564-1022

GUAY, Andree A; Clinique Med St-Cesaire, 1245 rue Plamondon GD, Saint-Cesaire QC J0L 1T0; Sher'83; (514)469-5551; Fax. (514)469-1521.

GUAY, Benoit; The Ottawa Hosp-gen Campus, 501 Smyth Rd, Ottawa ON K1H 8L6; Sher'05; FRCSC; Otol. Staff, The Ottawa Hospital - General Campus; Langs: Bilingual(English/French); (613)562-5400

GUAY, Bernard; Inst U en Sante Mentale de QC, 2601 ch de la Canardiere, Quebec QC G1J 2G3; Laval'78; Staff, Institut Universitaire Sante; (418)663-5020; Fax. (418)661-6841.

GUAY, Caroline; CSSS du Suroît, 150 rue Saint-Thomas, Salaber-de-Valleyf QC J6T 6C1; Mon'07; CCFP; Staff, Centre Hospitalier Régional du Suroît; (450)371-9920; Fax. (450)377-1372.

GUAY, Celine; Clinique Med Renault, D-595 9e av, Beauceville QC G5X 1J3; Laval'78; Geriatric Med, CHSLD de l'Assomption; Physician, CHSLD de Beauceville; (418)774-2080; Fax. (418)774-2090.

GUAY, Christian; CSSS de Beauce-Etchemin, 1515 17e rue, Saint-Georges QC G5Y 4T8; Laval'98; NuclearMed. Staff, Centre Hospitalier Beauce-Etchemin; (418)228-2031 x7483; Fax. (418)868-1032.

GUAY, Elizabeth; Clin Dermatologique de Lachena, 345-950 Montee de Pionniers, Terrebonne QC J6V 1S8; Mon'96; FRCPC; Derm. Staff, Centre Hospitalier de Granby; Langs: Bilingual(French/English); (450)470-1221; Fax. (450)470-1586.

GUAY, Francine; Hotel-Dieu de Levis, 143 rue Wolfe, Levis QC G6V 3Z1; Laval'78; FRCSC; Ophth. Ac Staff, Hôtel-Dieu de Lévis; Langs: English; Spanish; (418)835-7121

GUAY, Genevieve; Unite de Med Familiale, 100-500 boul de l'Hopital, Gatineau QC J8V 2P5; Laval'99; Supvr Med, Hôpital de Gatineau; (819)561-8107

GUAY, Ghislaine; Clinique Medicale St-Joseph, 841 av Sainte-Therese RR 1, St-Joseph-D-Beauce QC G0S 2V0; Laval'77; (418)397-6891; Fax. (418)397-4170.

GUAY, Helene; Clinique Med D'Amos, 641 4e rue O, Amos QC J9T 2S1; Mon'80; Staff, CH Hôtel-Dieu d'Amos; Langs: Bilingual(English/French); (819)732-1244; Fax. (819)732-4646; lnguay@mac.com.

GUAY, J Michel; 411-420 rue du Charron, St-Augustin-D-Desm QC G3A 0M1; Laval'60; CSPQ; FRCPC; Peds; Cardiol (P.Q.). (418)878-5496; michelguay@videotron.ca.

GUAY, J A Michel; Carrefour Sante Le St-Laurent, 140-5300 boul Saint-Laurent, Sainte-Catherine QC J5C 1A8; Mon'90; (450)638-6383; Fax. (450)635-6359.

GUAY, Jean-Pierre; Clin Med La Cite Place du Parc, 900-300 rue Leo Pariseau, Montreal QC H2X 4B3; Mon'72; ac Staff, Centre Hospitalier l'Université de Montréal (CHUM) - Hôtel-Dieu; Physician, Clinique Medicale de la Cite; (514)281-1722; Fax. (514)281-6697.

GUAY, Jean-Pierre; CHUM-Hop Notre-Dame, AR1001A-1560 rue Sherbrooke E, Montreal QC H2L 4M1; Mon'68; FRCPC; RadOncol. Staff, Centre Hospitalier l'Université de Montréal (CHUM) - Hôpital Notre-Dame; assoc Prof, Universite de Montreal; (514)890-8000 x25726; Fax. (514)890-8254.

GUAY, Joanie; Hotel-Dieu de Roberval, 450 rue Brassard, Roberval QC G8H 1B9; Sher'10; CCFP; Staff, Hotel-Dieu de Roberval; (418)275-0110

GUAY, Joanne M; Hop Maisonneuve-Rosemont, 5415 boul de l'Assomption, Montreal QC H1T 2M4; Mon'77; CSPQ; FRCPC; Peds; Anes. Staff, Hopital Maisonneuve-Rosemont; (514)252-3426; Fax. (514)252-3542.

GUAY, Louise; CHUM-Hop St-Luc, 1058 rue Saint-Denis, Montreal QC H2X 3J4; Mon'75; Psy (P.Q.) (Consultation-Liaison). Staff, Centre Hospitalier l'Université De Montréal (CHUM) - Hôpital Saint-luc; adj Prof, Universite de Montreal; (514)890-8000 x36155; Fax. (514)412-7358; louise.guay.chum@ssss.gouv.qc.ca.

GUAY, Louise; Unite de Med Familiale, 500 boul de l'Hopital, Gatineau QC J8V 2P5; Laval'91; CCFP; Staff, Hôpital de Gatineau; Resd Supvr, McGill University; Langs: Bilingual(French/English); (819)966-6380; Fax. (819)966-6175.

GUAY, Louise; CSSS Les Eskers de l'Abitibi, 622 4e rue O, Amos QC J9T 2S2; McG'88; FRCPC; DiagRad. Staff, CH Hôtel-Dieu d'Amos; (819)732-3341; Fax. (819)732-6484.

GUAY, Marcel; Centre Hosp Honore-Mercier, 2750 boul Laframboise, Saint-Hyacinthe QC J2S 4Y8; Mon'93; CSPQ; FRCPC; Anes (P.Q.). Staff, Centre Hospitalier Honore-Mercier; (450)771-3333 x3353

GUAY, Martine; CSSS Jeanne-Mance, 100-15 av du Mont-Royal O, Montreal QC H2T 2R9; Mon'86; AddicMed; Prof Faculty Pt-Time, McGill University; (514)286-9657; Fax. (514)940-3621.

GUAY, Maryse; Direction de la Sante Publique, 1255 rue Beauregard, Longueuil QC J4K 2M3; Sher'79; FRCPC; CommunMed; Public Health & Preventive Med. Staff, Hopital Charles LeMoyne; Physician, Institut National de Sante Publique; dép Chef/Prof Commun Health Sciences, Universite de Sherbrooke; (450)928-6777 x3070; Fax. (450)928-3295; m.guay@rrsss16.gouv.qc.ca.

GUAY, Michel A; Clinique de Pediatrie SENCRL, 218-383 boul du Seminaire N, St-Jean-sur-Richel QC J3B 8C5; Mon'68; Peds. (450)348-4911; Fax. (450)348-6401.

GUAY, Michel; Clinique Medicale Du Manoir, 1441 av du Manoir, Alma QC G8B 4X3; Laval'91; LMCC; CCFP; (418)662-3944; Fax. (418)662-2607.

GUAY, Micheline; Clinique Med de levis, 100-4975 boul de la Rive-Sud, Levis QC G6V 4Z5; Laval'75; Staff, Hôtel-Dieu de Lévis; (418)833-5810; Fax. (418)833-2720.

GUAY, Nicolas A; The Ottawa Hosp- Civic Campus, 1053 Carling Ave, Ottawa ON K1Y 4E9; Mon'94; FRCSC; PlasSurg. Staff, The Ottawa Hospital - Civic Campus; (613)798-5555; Fax. (613)361-4827.

GUAY, Patrice; Centre Med Robinson Inc, 4 rue Robinson N, Granby QC J2G 8Z9; Mon'94; FRCPC; Peds. (450)387-8435; Fax. (450)375-8832.

GUAY, Pierre; Serv Externe De Psychiatrie, 230-383 boul du Seminaire N, St-Jean-sur-Richel QC J3B 8C5; Mon'80; FRCPC; Psy. Staff, Hôpital du Haut-Richelieu; (450)346-2222; Fax. (450)346-2311.

GUAY, Raynald; Medi-Centre Chomedey, 610 boul Cure-Labelle, Laval QC H7V 2T7; Mon'75; (450)687-6452; Fax. (450)687-3243.

GUAY, Sebastien; CSSS Haut-Richelieu-Rouville, 920 boul du Seminaire N, St-Jean-sur-Richel QC J3A 1B7; Laval'07; CCFP; Staff, Hôpital du Haut-Richelieu; (450)359-5000 x5175

GUAY, Serge; Clinique Med du Carrefour, 1221 boul Marcotte, Roberval QC G8H 3B8; Laval'73; ac Staff, Hotel-Dieu de Roberval; (418)275-5333; Fax. (418)275-5334.

GUAY, Stephane; CSSS de Sept-Iles, 45 rue du Pere-Divet, Sept-Iles QC G4R 3N7; Sher'94; FRCSC; OrthSurg. Staff, Centre Hospitalier Regional de Sept-Iles; (418)962-9761

GUAY LANGEVIN, Vincent; Ctr Hosp Anna-Laberge, 200 boul Brisebois, Chateauguay QC J6K 4W8; Sher'07; Anes. Staff, Hôpital Anna-Laberge.

GUAY-PELLETIER, Louise; Clin Med du Vieux-Terrebonne, 883 rue Saint-Pierre, Terrebonne QC J6W 1E6; Laval'76; Staff, Hopital de la Cite de la santé; (450)964-9111; Fax. (450)964-1450.

GUBANOV, Alexander; Maples Adolescent Treatment, 3405 Willingdon Ave, Burnaby BC V5G 3H4; Tor'01; FRCPC; Psy. (604)660-5800; Fax. (604)660-5814.

GUBBAY, Jonathan B; Public Health Lab Toronto, 81 Resources Rd, Toronto ON M9P 3T1; Sydney (Australia)'92; FRCPC; MedMicrobiol. (416)235-6258

GUBBINS, Beresford G; 1B-219 Fern Rd W PO Box 550, Qualicum Beach BC V9K 1T1; Queen's (Ireland)'70; MB ChB; BAO; Med Dir, Langley Memorial Hospital; (250)752-6568

GUBERMAN, Alan; The Ottawa Hosp-Civic Campus, 2178-1053 Carling Ave, Ottawa ON K1Y 4E9; McG'70; FRCPC; Neur (Epilepsy). Staff, The Ottawa Hospital - Civic Campus; Prof Med Neurol, University of Ottawa; Langs: English; French; (613)761-5353; Fax. (613)761-5360.

GUBERMAN, Daniel S; Hop Jean-Talon, 1385 rue Jean-Talon E, Montreal QC H2E 1S6; Ott'05; FRCSC; PlasSurg. Staff, CSSS du Coeur de l'Isle Hôpital Jean-Talon; (514)495-6767; Fax. (514)495-6734.

GUBITZ, Gordon J; Halifax Infirmary, 3833-1796 Summer St, Halifax NS B3H 3A7; McM'90; FRCP(Edin); FRCPC; Neur. (902)473-6330; Fax. (902)473-4438; ggubitz@dal.ca.

GUCCIARDI, Enza-Josie; Highlands Health Network, 140 Rolling Hills Dr, Orangeville ON L9W 4X8; Ott'04; CCFP; CCFP(E.M.); Ac Staff, Halton Healthcare Services Corporation - Oakville Site; Langs: Italian; French; (519)941-7575; Fax. (519)941-7060; egucciardi@haltonhealthcare.on.ca.

GUDAPATI, Sumathi; Whitehorse Med Services Ltd, 406 Lambert St, Whitehorse YT Y1A 1Z7; (India)'93; Staff Family Phy, Whitehorse General Hospital; Staff, Whitehorse Medical Services Ltd; (867)393-6600; Fax. (867)393-6601.

GUDAS, Virginia M; St Paul's Hosp, 494-1081 Burrard St, Vancouver BC V6Z 1Y6; Mem'78; FRCSC; GenSurg (Cardio Thoracic Transplant); Cardiovasc&ThorSurg. Staff, Providence Health Care - St Paul's Hospital; (604)806-9914; virginia.gudas@vch.ca.

GUDELIS, Susan; The Juravinski Cancer Centre, 699 Concession St, Hamilton ON L8V 5C2; McM'97; CCFP; Staff, Cambridge Memorial Hospital; Physician, The Juravinski Cancer Centre; (905)387-9495

GUDEON, Nina; Alberta Children's Hosp, 2888 Shaganappi Trail NW, Calgary AB T3B 6A8; Mem'02; Staff, Alberta Children's Hospital; (403)955-2226; Fax. (403)955-3105.

GUDERIAN, Angela; 401-111 Main St W, North Bay ON P1B 2T6; McM'89; CCFP; FCFP; Med Staff, North Bay Regional Health Centre - Regional Mental Health; (705)495-6066; Fax. (705)495-6195.

GUDGEON, Avery M; 15-555 12 Ave W, Vancouver BC V5Z 3X7; Wes'09; CCFP; (604)450-2050

GUDGEON, Patrick; Mount Sinai Hosp, 427-600 University Ave, Toronto ON M5G 1X5; Tor'07; FRCPC; IntMed. Staff, Mount Sinai Hospital; (416)585-4800

GUDMUNDSON, Catherine A; East Parkland Med Group, PO Box 310, Ste Rose du Lac MB R0L 1S0; Man'99; CCFP.

GUEDES-MARCHAND, Cecile; CLSC Saint-Tite, 750 rue du Couvent, Saint-Tite QC G0X 3H0; Paris (France)'08; Staff, CLSC Saint-Tite; (418)365-7555

GUENARD, Dominique; Hotel-Dieu de Levis, 143 rue Wolfe, Levis QC G6V 3Z1; Mon'94; BACC(Psych); Staff, Hôtel-Dieu de Lévis; Langs: Bilingual(English/French); (418)835-7121; doguenard@hotmail.com.

GUENETTE, Claudine; Clinique Med 201, 104 rue Sainte-Agathe, Ste-Agathe-Des-Mts QC J8C 2K3; Mon'81; (819)326-1505; Fax. (819)326-8801.

GUENETTE-LEMIEUX, Marie; CSSS de la Baie-des-Chaleurs, RR 2 419 boul Perron, Maria QC G0C 1Y0; Sher'07; CCFP; Staff, CSSS de la Baie-des-Chaleurs; (418)759-3443

GUENTER, C Dale; McMaster Family Practice, A-690 Main St W, Hamilton ON L8S 1A4; Cal'87; MPH; CCFP; FCFP; Staff, Hamilton Health Sciences Centre - McMaster Children's Hospital; Assoc Prof Family Med, McMaster University; (905)521-5015; Fax. (905)521-5010.

GUENTHER, Craig R; Univ of Alberta Hosp-SCC/WCM, 3B232W-8440 112 St NW, Edmonton AB T6G 2B7; Alb'82; FRCPC; Anes (Cardiac Anesthesia). Staff, University of Alberta Hospital; (780)407-8861; Fax. (780)407-3200.

GUENTHER, Lyn C C; The Guenther Derm Research Ctr, 835 Richmond St, London ON N6A 3H7; Wes'79; FAAD; FRCPC; Derm (Research). Prof, University of Western Ontario; Langs: Spanish; French; (519)435-1738; Fax. (519)435-1740.

GUENTHER, Neil V; Darke Creek Acupuncture, 1124 Fish Lake Rd, Summerland BC V0H 1Z8; UBC'85; Ac Staff, Penticton Regional Hospital; (250)404-0454

GUEORDJEV, Svetoslav A; Kootenay Lake Hosp, 3 View St, Nelson BC V1L 2V1; Plovdiv (Bulgaria)'91; Staff, Kootenay Lake General Hospital; Langs: Russian; Bulgarian; (250)352-6611

GUERETTE, Pierre; CHUS-Hop Fleurimont, 3001 12e av N, Sherbrooke QC J1H 5N4; Mon'92; CSPQ; EmergMed. Staff, Centre Hospitalier Universitaire de Sherbrooke-Hopital Fleurimont; Langs: English; (819)346-1110 x14314; Fax. (819)564-5386.

GUERETTE, Pierre-Jean; Clinique Sante Jacques-Cartier, 200-1815 rue King O, Sherbrooke QC J1J 2E3; Laval'78; (819)565-7446; Fax. (819)565-7780.

GUERGUERIAN, Anne-Marie; The Hosp for Sick Children, 555 University Ave, Toronto ON M5G 1X8; Mon'93; PhD; FAAP; FRCPC; Peds (Critical Care Medicine). Staff/Asst Prof, The Hospital For Sick Children; Langs: Bilingual(French/English); (416)813-6477; Fax. (416)813-7299.

GUERIN, Caroline; Centre Hosp Honore-Mercier, 2750 boul Laframboise, Saint-Hyacinthe QC J2S 4Y8; Mon'09; CCFP; CCFP(E.M.); Staff, Centre Hospitalier Honore-Mercier; (450)771-3333

GUERIN, Danielle; CSSSG-Hop de Gatineau, CP 2000 Succ Bureau-Chef 909 boul de la Verendrey O, Gatineau QC J8P 7H2; Mon'92; Staff, Hôpital de Gatineau; Langs: English; (819)561-8265; Fax. (819)561-8394.

GUERIN, Helene; CSSS de Memphremagog, 50 rue Saint-Patrice E, Magog QC J1X 3X3; Sher'81; Staff, Centre Hospitalier et CLSC de Memphremagog; (819)843-3381

GUERIN, John M; Queen Elizabeth II HSC, 1276 South Park St, Halifax NS B3H 2Y9; (Ireland)'00; MB ChB; BAO; Staff, Queen Elizabeth II Health Sciences Centre - Victoria General Site; (902)473-7015; Fax. (902)473-4442.

GUERIN, Linda; CLSC Basse-Ville-Limoilou, 50 rue Saint-Joseph E, Quebec QC G1K 3A5; Sher'82; (418)529-2572; Fax. (418)529-1515.

GUERIN, Lucie C; Ctr Hosp de Verdun, 4000 boul Lasalle, Verdun QC H4G 2A3; Sher'79; FRCPC; IntMed (Hypertension). Staff, Centre Hospitalier de Verdun; Langs: English; (514)362-1000; Fax. (514)765-7306.

GUERIN, Marc; 22-41 rue de l'Eglise, Verdun QC H4G 2L8; Laval'72; Psy. (514)769-2943; Fax. (514)769-0602.

GUERIN, Ronald; Imagix Radiologie St-Eustache, 75 rue Grignon, Saint-Eustache QC J7P 4J2; Laval'65; DiagRad. ac Staff, Hôpital Ste-Justine; (450)473-4250; Fax. (450)473-0240.

GUERN, Claude; Mini-Urgence Chicoutimi, 715 boul Sainte-Genevieve, Chicoutimi QC G7G 4Z4; Poitiers (France)'79; Staff Emerg, Complexe hospitalier de la Sagamie; (418)696-2330

GUERRA, Enrique C; Leamington Dist Mem Hosp, 167-194 Talbot St W, Leamington ON N8H 1N9; (Mexico)'77; FRCPC; IntMed. Chief Med, Leamington District Memorial Hospital; Langs: Spanish; (519)326-3330; Fax. (519)326-0104; eguerra22@hotmail.com.

GUERRA, Luis A; Children's Hosp Eastern Ont, 401 Smyth Rd, Ottawa ON K1H 8L1; Pernambuco (Brazil)'84; Staff Urology, Children's Hospital of Eastern Ontario (CHEO); (613)737-7600 x1353; Fax. (613)738-4271.

GUERRA, Peter G; Institut de Cardiologie de Mtl, 5000 rue Belanger, Montreal QC H1T 1C8; McG'91; CSPQ; FRCPC; IntMed; Cardiol. Staff, Institut de Cardiologie de Montréal; (514)376-3330; Fax. (514)593-2581.

GUERRA PAEZ, Jose G; Scarborough Hosp-Birchmount, 3030 Birchmount Rd, Scarborough ON M1W 3W3; Oklahoma(U.S.A.) (USA)'87; FRCSC; OrthSurg. Staff, The Scarborough Hospital - Birchmount Campus; (416)495-2400; jguerrapaez@hotmail.com.

GUERRIERE, Michael; 21F-25 York St, Toronto ON M5J 2V5; Tor'86; MBA; Asst Prof Med, University of Toronto; (647)837-4286; michael.guerriere@telus.com.

GUERTIN, Benoit; Polyclinique Med Concorde, 300 boul de la Concorde E, Laval QC H7G 2E6; Mon'80; FRCSC; Urol. (450)667-5310; Fax. (450)667-5248.

GUERTIN, Benoit-Jean; GMF Centre Med du Parc, 101-84 rue Court, Granby QC J2G 4Y5; Sher'79; Ophth. Staff, Centre Hospitalier de Granby; (450)375-2074; Fax. (450)375-8719.

GUERTIN, Catherine; Ctr Hosp du Centre la Mauricie, 50 119e rue, Shawinigan-Sud QC G9P 5K1; Laval'01; CCFP; Staff, Centre Hospitalier du Centre la Mauricie; (819)536-7575

GUERTIN, Charles; 5270 rue de Bellechasse, Montreal QC H1T 2A9; Mon'96; FRCS; CSPQ; ACLS; ATLS; LMCC; BBA; DS; LRCPS; MBA; MCPS; FRCSC; PlasSurg (Aesthetic Surgery). Staff, Centre Hospitalier l'Université de Montréal (CHUM) - Hôpital Notre-Dame; Staff, Hôtel-Dieu de Saint-Jérôme; Chief Plastic Surg, Hopital Maisonneuve-Rosemont; Staff, Institut de Cardiologie de Montréal; Langs: Bilingual(English/French); (514)257-1860; drguertin@bellnet.ca.

GUERTIN, Ghislaine O; Clinique Cadillac, 3435 rue Bossuet, Montreal QC H1M 2M1; Mon'79; ac Staff, Centre Hospitalier l'Université de Montréal (CHUM) - Hôpital Notre-Dame; (514)253-1211

GUERTIN, Louis; Polyclinique de l'Oreille, 252-1111 rue Saint-Charles O, Longueuil QC J4K 5G4; Sher'86; FRCSC; Otol. Staff, Centre Hospitalier l'Université de Montréal (CHUM) - Hôpital Notre-Dame; (450)651-9000; Fax. (450)679-1651.

GUERTIN, Paul; GMF Centre Med du Parc, 101-84 rue Court, Granby QC J2G 4Y5; Sher'82; Staff, Centre Hospitalier de Granby; (450)375-1161; Fax. (450)375-7740.

GUEST, Cameron B; Sunnybrook Hlth Sciences Ctre, D108-2075 Bayview Ave, Toronto ON M4N 3M5; Tor'91; FRCPC; Anes; Critical Care Medicine. Staff Anes, Sunnybrook Health Sciences Centre; (416)480-4522; Fax. (416)480-4999.

GUEST, Christopher L; Georgian Radiology Consultants, 114-121 Wellington St W, Barrie ON L4N 1L2; Tor'96; DiagRad (Interventional Radiology). Staff, Royal Victoria Regional Health Centre.

GUEST, Joan E; 10 Lower Jarvis St, Toronto ON M5E 1Z2; Tor'60; Att Staff, Centre for Addiction & Mental Health (CAMH) - Queen Site; (416)304-1118; Fax. (416)304-1119.

GUEST, R Gerald; O'Connor Doctors, B1 20-1450 O'Connor Dr, East York ON M4B 2T8; Tor'59; Med Dir, CIHS Ltd; (416)285-4075; Fax. (416)285-4076.

GUEST, William A; Rouge Valley-Centenary HC, 2867 Ellesmere Rd, Scarborough ON M1E 4B9; Tor'60; DPsy; FRCPC; Psy. Staff Psy, Rouge Valley Health System - Centenary Health Centre Site; (416)281-7318; Fax. (416)281-7320.

GUEVIN, Raymond; Polyclinique Med Populaire, 1988 rue Sainte-Catherine E, Montreal QC H2K 2H7; Mon'58; MedOncol (P.Q.); Hem (P.Q.); IntMed. Langs: Bilingual(French/English); (514)524-3637; Fax. (514)524-3638.

GUEVREMONT, Mylene; CSSS du Nord de Lanaudière, 1000 boul Sainte-Anne, St-Charles-Brromee QC J6E 6J2; McG'01; Neur. Staff, Centre Hospitalier Régional de Lanaudière; (450)759-8222; Fax. (450)759-0077.

GUEVREMONT, Pierre; CSSS de Sept-Iles, 45 rue du Pere-Divet, Sept-Iles QC G4R 3N7; Mon'65; FRCSC; Otol. Staff, Centre Hospitalier Regional de Sept-Iles; (418)962-9761; pierre.guevremont@cgocable.ca.

GUGGISBERG, Kelly A; Rockyview Gen Hosp, 4N43-7007 14 St SW, Calgary AB T2V 1P9; UBC'96; FRCPC; AnatPath. Staff, Rockyview General Hospital; Staff, Foothills Medical Centre; Staff, Calgary Laboratory Services; (403)943-3438; Fax. (403)943-3333.

GUGLIELMIN, Darryl R; Foothills Medical Centre, 1403 29 St NW, Calgary AB T2N 2T9; Alb'99; BSc; FRCPC; Anes (Chronic Pain Management). Staff, Foothills Medical Centre; Staff, Calgary Health Region Chronic Pain Centre; (403)944-1430

GUGLIOTTA, Donato; 105-30 King St, Trenton ON K8V 6B1; Tor'85; Staff Anes, QHC Trenton Memorial; (613)392-3887; Fax. (613)392-1700.

GUHLE, Mark E; Synergy Med Clinic, 221-501 Bethel Dr, Sherwood Park AB T8H 0N2; Alb'93; CCFP; FCFP; (780)464-0123; Fax. (780)449-5138; familymedicinegp@telus.net.

GUI, Xianyong; Foothills Medical Centre, 11F-1403 29 St NW, Calgary AB T2N 2T9; (China)'84; Staff, Foothills Medical Centre; (403)944-1363; Fax. (403)944-4748.

GUIANG, Charlie B; Health Centre at 410 St Michae, 4F-410 Sherbourne St, Toronto ON M4X 1K2; Man'97; BSc; CCFP; Staff Physician, St Michael's Hospital; Asst Prof Family & Commun Med, University of Toronto; (416)867-3728; Fax. (416)867-3726; guiangc@smh.ca.

GUIBERT, Remi; Clinique Medicale Sainte-Adele, 1150 rue du Bourg-Joli, Sainte-Adele QC J8B 1W8; Mon'72; MSc; (450)229-6633

GUICHAOUA, Yves; Clin de Med Fam Cowansville, 499 rue du Sud, Cowansville QC J2K 2X9; Mon'81; (450)263-8890; Fax. (450)263-9737.

GUICHON, Donald M P; Parklane Surgical Clinic, 319-13710 94A Ave, Surrey BC V3V 1N1; UBC'72; FRCSC; PlasSurg (Cosmetic Surgery). Ac Staff, Royal Columbian Hospital; Ac Staff, Eagle Ridge Hospital & Health Care Centre; Staff, Surrey Memorial Hospital; (604)589-6021; Fax. (604)589-6841.

GUIGNARD, Jimmy; 2-1 av de L'Eglise, Saint-Antoine NB E4V 1L6; Laval'02; CCFP; Staff Family Med/Emerg Med, Dr Georges-L-Dumont University Hospital Centre; Langs: Bilingual(French/English); (506)525-2409; Fax. (506)525-2240.

GUIGUI, Jean-Yves; CHSLD Emilie-Gamelin, 1440 rue Dufresne, Montreal QC H2K 3J3; Mon'79; Prés, CHSLD Emilie-Gamelin; (514)527-8921; Fax. (514)523-4820; jean.guigui@ssss.gouv.qc.ca.

GUIJON, Fernando B; 317-456 Moberly Rd, Vancouver BC V5Z 4L7; Santiago (Chile)'67; FACOG; FSOGC; FRCSC; ObstGyn (Colposcopy). guijon@cc.umanitoba.ca.

GUIJON, Juan-Carlos; 100-5791 No. 3 Rd, Richmond BC V6X 2C9; Man'94; FRCPC; NuclearMed; DiagRad. (604)278-9151; Fax. (604)278-9291.

GUILBAULT, Francois; CSSS de Montmagny-L'Islet, 350 boul Tache O RR 1, Montmagny QC G5V 3R8; Laval'01; CSPQ; FRCPC; AnatPath. Staff, CSSS de Montmagny-L'Islet; (418)248-0630 x4435; Fax. (418)248-9791.

GUILBAULT, Marcel; Centre de Med Fam de Gatineau, 201-908 boul Maloney E, Gatineau QC J8P 1H5; Mon'84; Staff, Hôpital de Gatineau; (819)663-7711; Fax. (819)663-9326.

GUILBAULT, Mathieu; Centre Medical St-Jovite, 992 rue de Saint-Jovite, Mont-Tremblant QC J8E 3J8; Mon'10; (819)425-2728

GUILBAULT, Nathalie; CSSS du Sud de Lanaudière, 911 montee des Pionniers, Terrebonne QC J6V 2H2; McG'95; Peds. Staff, Centre Hospitalier Pierre le Gardeur; (450)654-7525; Fax. (450)582-7688.

GUILBAULT, Normand; Ctr Hosp Laurentien, 234 rue Saint-Vincent, Ste-Agathe-des-Mts QC J8C 2B8; Mon'64; Ophth. Staff, Centre Hospitalier Laurentien; (819)324-4000

GUILBAULT, Paul; IRDPQ-Site Boulevard-Hamel, 525 boul Wilfrid-Hamel, Quebec QC G1M 2S8; Sher'84; Langs: English; (418)529-9141 x6737; Fax. (418)529-3197.

GUILBEAULT, Helene; St Mary's Hosp Centre, 3830 av Lacombe, Montreal QC H3T 1M5; McG'85; DiagRad (P.Q.). Staff, St Mary's Hospital Centre; Langs: Bilingual(French/English); (514)734-2620; Fax. (514)734-2659.

GUILBEAULT, Julie; CSSS du Suroît, 150 rue Saint-Thomas, Salaber-de-Valleyf QC J6T 6C1; Sher'98; FRCSC; Otol. Staff, Centre Hospitalier Régional du Suroît; (450)371-9920

GUILBEAULT, Nathalie; Csss de la Cote-De-Gaspe, 215 boul de York O, Gaspe QC G4X 2W2; Laval'90; FRCSC; ObstGyn. Staff, Centre Hospitalier de Gaspe; (418)368-3301; Fax. (418)368-8772.

GUILBEAULT, Valerie; CSSS de Papineau, 155 rue MacLaren E, Gatineau QC J8L 0C2; Mon'97; Staff, Hôpital de Papineau; Staff, CH-CHSLD de Papineau - Pavillon du centre hospitalier; Langs: Bilingual(French/English); (819)986-3341; Fax. (819)986-1616.

GUILBERT, Edith; Inst Nat'l de Sante Publique, 945 av Wolfe, Quebec QC G1V 5B3; Laval'77; LMCC; MSc; Staff Med Clinique in Family Planning, Centre Hospitalier Universitaire de Quebec-CHUL; Med Consultant, Institut National de Santé Publique du Québec; Clin Prof ObstGyn, Université Laval; Langs: English; (418)650-5115; edith.guilbert@inspq.qc.ca.

GUILBERT, Francois; CHUM-Hop Notre-Dame, 1560 rue Sherbrooke E, Montreal QC H2L 4M1; Sher'95; DiagRad. Staff, Centre Hospitalier l'Université de Montréal (CHUM) - Hôpital Notre-Dame; (514)890-8000 x26579

GUILBERT, Jacques; Canadian Med Protective Assn, PO Box 8225 Stn T CSC, Ottawa ON K1G 3H7; Mon'65; MSc; FACS; CSPQ; GenSurg. Staff, Centre Hospitalier l'Université de Montréal (CHUM) - Hôpital Notre-Dame; (613)725-2000

GUILCHER, Gregory M T; Alberta Children's Hosp, 2888 Shaganappi Trail NW, Calgary AB T3B 6A8; Mem'01; FRCPC; Peds (Pediatric Oncology); PedHemaOncol; Hem. Staff PedOncol, Alberta Children's Hospital; Langs: Bilingual(English/French); (403)955-7272; greg.guilcher@albertahealthservices.ca.

GUILE, Jean M; Douglas Mental Hlth Univ Inst, 6875 boul LaSalle, Verdun QC H4H 1R3; Paris (France)'85; FRCPC; Psy (P.Q.). Dir Div Child & Adolescent Psy, Douglas Mental Health University Institute; (514)761-6131; Fax. (514)762-3041.

GUILFOYLE, F John; 90 Queen St PO Box 35 Stn Main, Sioux Lookout ON P8T 1A1; Dublin (Ireland)'80; MB ChB; CCFP; FCFP; Langs: Irish; French; (604)898-1740

GUILFOYLE, F Jonathan; Alberta Children's Hosp, 2888 Shaganappi Trail NW, Calgary AB T3B 6A8; Man'03; FRCPC; Peds; PedEmergMed. Staff, Alberta Children's Hospital; (403)955-7070; Fax. (403)955-7398.

GUILFOYLE, Shoshauna E; 100-820 59 Ave SE, Calgary AB T2H 2G5; Man'04; CCFP; (403)531-3250; Fax. (403)531-3255.

GUILLAUME, Eddy; Clinique Maisonneuve-Rosemont, RC60-5345 boul de l'Assomption, Montreal QC H1T 4B3; (Haiti)'63; (514)257-7000

GUILLEMETTE, Annie; CHUQ-St-Francois D'Assise, 10 rue de l'Espinay, Quebec QC G1L 3L5; Sher'04; FRCPC; Neur. Staff, Centre Hospitalier Universitaire De Québec - Pavillon De St-françois-d'assise; (418)525-4444

GUILLEMETTE, Chantal; CSSS de la Minganie, 1035 Prom des Anciens CP 190, Havre-Saint-Pierre QC G0G 1P0; Laval'02; CCFP; Fam Med, CSSS de la Minganie; Langs: English; Spanish; (418)538-2212; Fax. (418)538-2254.

GUILLEMETTE, Fernand; Direction de Sante Publique, 550 rue Bonaventure, Trois-Rivieres QC G9A 2B5; McG'73; Peds (P.Q.) (Public Health). Med Consultant, Direction de la Sante Publique Trois Rivieres; Langs: Bilingual(French/English); (819)693-3959; Fax. (819)373-1627; Fernand.Guillemette.Agence04@ssss.gouv.qc.ca.

GUILLEMETTE, Gaetan; Clinique Med Richelieu, 200-500 Rte Marie-Victorin, Sorel-Tracy QC J3R 1K7; Sher'71; Ac Staff, Hôtel-Dieu de Sorel; (450)742-5638; Fax. (450)742-0995.

GUILLEMETTE, Gilles; 690 av Roberval CP 338 Succ Bureau-Chef, Roberval QC G8H 2N7; Laval'75; Ac Staff, Hotel-Dieu de Roberval; (418)275-4141; Fax. (418)275-9119.

GUILLEMETTE, Helene; CRSSS Baie-James-Chibougamau, 51 3e rue, Chibougamau QC G8P 1N1; Sher'05; CCFP; Staff, CRSSS de la Baie-James; (418)748-6435; Fax. (418)748-4208.

GUILLEMETTE, Jeanne; 824 av Myrand, Quebec QC G1V 2V5; Laval'79; (418)688-8399; Fax. (418)688-2136.

GUILLEMETTE, Julie; Ctr Obstetrique et Gynecologie, 4250 1re av, Quebec QC G1H 2S5; Laval'94; FRCSC; ObstGyn. Langs: English; (418)654-0555; Fax. (418)654-1898.

GUILLEMETTE-GRIGNET, Helene; Clinique de Pediatrie SENCRL, 218-383 boul du Seminaire N, St-Jean-sur-Richel QC J3B 8C5; Sher'81; Peds. Staff, Hôpital du Haut-Richelieu; Clin Prof Ped, Universite de Sherbrooke; (450)348-4911; Fax. (450)348-6401.

GUILLEMI, Silvia; St Paul's Hosp, PO Box 23608 1081 Burrard St, Vancouver BC V6Z 1Y6; La Plata (Argentina)'79; Staff, Providence Health Care - St Paul's Hospital; (604)682-2344

GUILLEMOT, Yolande; Clin Med Guillemot, 6804 rue du Fusain, Quebec QC G1G 6L7; Mon'85; (418)626-0495; Fax. (418)626-0678.

GUILLET, France; Clin Med Pierre-Boucher, 1615 boul Jacques-Cartier E, Longueuil QC J4M 2X1; Mon'87; (450)468-6223

GUILLET, Mario A; 220A-2944 boul Taschereau, Greenfield Park QC J4V 2G8; Buenos Aires (Argentina)'54; IntMed. Staff, Hopital Charles LeMoyne; (514)256-5011; Fax. (514)342-1519.

GUILLET, Suzanne; Centre de Med Sportive de Lava, 3095 Autoroute Laval O, Laval QC H7P 4W5; Mon'85; Physician, Centre de Med. Sportive de Laval; (450)688-5134 x200; Fax. (450)688-8566.

GUILLETTE, Lyne; Clinique Med du Coteau, 100-440 boul Saint-Luc, St-Jean-sur-Richel QC J2W 0E2; Sher'93; CCFP; Staff, Hôpital du Haut-Richelieu; (450)359-6819; Fax. (450)359-3247.

GUILLON, Simone; GMF de Verdun au 55, 3e-55 av de l'Eglise, Verdun QC H4G 3E7; McG'80; DPH; CCFP; FCFP; ac Staff Family Med, Centre Hospitalier de Verdun; Teach Staff Univ de Montreal Ecole d'Arch, Universite de Montreal; (514)737-2496; Fax. (514)733-2759.

GUILLOT-HARDY, Denise; CLSC des Etchemins, RR 1 331 rue du Sanatorium, Lac-Etchemin QC G0R 1S0; Laval'95; BSc; Staff, CSSS des Etchemins; (418)625-8001

GUILLOTTE, Eve; CSSS du Pontiac, CP 430 160 ch de la Chute, Fort-Coulonge QC J0X 1V0; Mon'05; CCFP; Staff, CSSS du Pontiac; (514)683-3000; Fax. (514)683-2008.

GUILMAIN-MAURICE, Micheline; Ctr Medico Prof de Brossard, 101-2424 boul Lapiniere, Brossard QC J4Z 2K9; Mon'77; (450)678-9033 x105

GUILMETTE, Constance; CLSC La Source, 190 76e rue E, Quebec QC G1H 7K4; Laval'81; (418)628-2572

GUILMETTE, Pierre; Clinique Med du Carrefour, 8585 boul Lacroix, Saint-Georges QC G5Y 5L6; Sher'85; (418)227-1271; Fax. (418)227-2781.

GUIMARAES, Daniel B S; CHUS-Hop Hotel-Dieu, 580 rue Bowen S, Sherbrooke QC J1G 2E8; Bahia (Brazil)'93; Psy (P.Q.). Staff, Centre Hospitalier Universitaire de Sherbrooke-Hôpital Hôtel-Dieu; Langs: English; Spanish; Portuguese; (819)346-1110 x25541; Fax. (819)829-6263.

GUIMOND, Claude; Medi-Centre Lasalle, 206-1500 av Dollard, LaSalle QC H8N 1T5; Mon'68; CSPQ; Cardiol (P.Q.) (Electrocardiology). hon Membre, Centre Hospitalier l'Université de Montréal (CHUM) - Hôpital Notre-Dame; Med Consultant, Centre de Sante Newman; Langs: English; (514)363-8955; Fax. (514)685-0013; guimondc@videotron.ca.

GUIMOND, Claude; FMOQ, 2000-3500 boul de Maisonneuve, Montreal QC H3Z 3C1; Mon'86; Dir Adjoint DFP, Federation des Medecins Omnipracticiens du Quebec; (514)878-1911; Fax. (514)878-4455; cguimond@fmoq.org.

GUIMOND, Gaston; Centre Med des Carrieres, 800-1000 boul Bona-Dussault RR, St-Mar-Des-Carr QC G0A 4B0; Laval'80; ac Staff, Centre Hospitalier Universitaire de Quebec-CHUL; Physician, CLSC de Portneuf; (418)268-5596; Fax. (418)268-5729.

GUIMOND, Gerard; Clinique de l'Alternative, 2034 rue Saint-Hubert, Montreal QC H2L 3Z5; Mon'71; (514)281-9848

GUIMOND, Isabelle; CSSS Pierre Boucher, 1333 boul Jacques-Cartier E, Longueuil QC J4M 2A5; Mon'09; Staff, Centre Hospitalier Pierre Boucher; (450)468-8111

GUIMOND, Jean C; Hôpital Laval, 2725 ch Sainte-Foy, Quebec QC G1V 4G5; Laval'82; FRCPC; NuclearMed. Head Med Imaging Dept, Hôpital Laval; (418)656-4580; Fax. (418)656-4857.

GUIMOND, Jean-Gilles; CHUM-Hop Notre-Dame, 1560 rue Sherbrooke E, Montreal QC H2L 4M1; Sher'78; FCCP; ABIMCCM; FRCPC; IntMed; Critical Care Medicine (P.Q.). Staff, Centre Hospitalier l'Université de Montréal (CHUM) - Hôpital Notre-Dame; assoc Prof Med, Universite de Montreal; Langs: English; (514)890-8000 x27120; Fax. (514)412-7623; jean-gilles.guimond.chum@ssss.gouv.qc.ca.

GUIMOND, Jean-Pierre; Mediclub, 6100 av Du Boise, Montreal QC H3S 2W1; Mon'89; CCFP; Staff, Centre Hospitalier Laurentien; (514)739-5646

GUIMOND, Jean-Victor; Clinique des Jeunes St-Denis, 1250 rue Sanguinet, Montreal QC H2X 3E7; Laval'72; (514)527-2361 x3674

GUIMOND, Joanne; Ctr Hosp Rouyn-Noranda, 4 9e rue, Rouyn-Noranda QC J9X 2B2; Mon'78; ObstGyn. Staff, Centre Hospitalier Rouyn-Noranda; (819)764-5131

GUIMOND, Julie; CPFM, 4577 rue Beaubien E, Montreal QC H1T 1T5; Mon'93; LMCC; ObstGyn. Staff, Hopital Maisonneuve-Rosemont; (514)722-1162; Fax. (514)725-9138.

GUIMOND, Marie-Claude; North York Gen Hosp, 8F-4001 Leslie St, North York ON M2K 1E1; McG'96; FRCPC; Psy. Staff, North York General Hospital; Langs: Bilingual(English/French); (416)756-6676; Fax. (416)756-6671.

GUIMOND, Marie-France; CHUQ-St-Francois D'Assise, 10 rue de l'Espinay, Quebec QC G1L 3L5; Mon'95; CSPQ; FRCSC; GenSurg; VascSurg. Staff, Centre Hospitalier Universitaire De Québec - Pavillon De St-françois-d'assise; (418)525-4422

GUIMOND, Mauril; SAAQ, 333 boul Jean-Lesage, Quebec QC G1K 8J6; Laval'71; Langs: English; (418)528-3920

GUIMOND, Nathalie; CSSS de la Mitis, 800 av du Sanatorium, Mont-Joli QC G5H 3L6; Laval'91; LMCC; PhysMed&Rehab. Staff, CSSS de la Mitis; (418)775-7261; Fax. (418)775-1686.

GUIMOND, Richard; Clin de Gynecologie du Saguena, 200-394 rue Saint-Vallier, Chicoutimi QC G7H 4J1; Laval'67; FACOG; FICS; DAB; CSPQ; FRCSC; ObstGyn. ac Staff, Complexe hospitalier de la Sagamie; ac Staff, CRSSS de la Baie-James; Clin Prof Med, Universite de Sherbrooke; Clin Prof Med, Universite de Montreal; Langs: English; (418)545-2666; Fax. (418)545-3924; guimondr@videotron.ca.

GUIMOND, Timothy H; St Michael's Hosp, CCW 17 047-30 Bond St, Toronto ON M5B 1W8; Baltimore(MD) (USA)'03; FRCPC; Psy. Staff, St Michael's Hospital; (416)360-4000

GUIMOND HEMMINGS, Jessica; Saint John Reg Hosp, PO Box 2100 400 University Ave, Saint John NB E2L 4L2; Mem'05; CCFP; Staff, Saint John Regional Hospital; (506)648-6000; Fax. (506)649-2634.

GUIMOND-SIMARD, Sebastien; Centre Med Sport Laval, 3095 Autoroute Laval O, Laval QC H7P 4W5; Sher'96; FRCSC; OrthSurg. Staff, Hôpital de Saint-Eustache; (450)688-5132; Fax. (450)688-8566.

GUIMONT, Marie-Christine; CSSS de Montmagny-L'Islet, 350 boul Tache O RR 1, Montmagny QC G5V 3R8; Mon'08; Staff, CSSS de Montmagny-L'Islet; (418)248-0630; Fax. (418)248-6838.

GUINARD, Francois; 60 av Bateman, Edmundston NB E3V 4X6; McG'89; FRCSC; Ophth. Ophthalmology, Hôpital regional d'Edmundston; Staff, Hôtel-Dieu St-Joseph de Saint-Quentin; Ophthalmology, Hôpital Général de Grand-Falls; (506)735-5033; Fax. (506)739-9050.

GUINDI, Nizar S; St George Med Centre, 15-2727 Portage Ave, Winnipeg MB R3J 0R2; Ain Shams (Egypt)'86; CCFP; Staff, Thompson General Hospital.

GUINDO, Fatouma S; Med Privee Notre-Dame, 597 av Notre-Dame, Saint-Lambert QC J4P 2K8; Sher'00; Staff, Centre Hospitalier Regional de Sept-Iles; (450)766-0766; Fax. (450)766-0767.

GUINDON, Benoit; 130 2nd St W PO Box 1266 Stn Main, Cornwall ON K6H 5V3; Ott'77; FRCSC; Ophth. Langs: Bilingual(English/French); (613)938-9742; Fax. (613)938-0388.

GUINDON, Karine; CSSS du Lac-des-Deux-Montagnes, 11-520 boul Arthur-Sauve, Saint-Eustache QC J7R 5B1; Sher'03; FRCSC; GenSurg. Staff, Hôpital de Saint-Eustache; (450)473-6811; Fax. (450)473-6966.

GUINDON, Myriam; Polyclinique Med de La Lievre, 536 rue de la Madone, Mont-Laurier QC J9L 1S7; Laval'09; (819)440-2345

GUINDON, Noemi; 1598 Ouellette Ave, Windsor ON N8X 1K7; Ott'58; Langs: English; French; (519)258-6923; Fax. (519)254-2765.

GUINDY, Sherine M; Assiniboine Clinic, 633 Lodge Ave, Winnipeg MB R3J 0S9; Ain Shams (Egypt)'86; CCFP; Staff, Percy E Moore Hospital.

GUINHAWA, Dante R; Regional Mental Health Service, 5F-9942 108 St NW, Edmonton AB T5K 2J5; Santo Tomas (Philippines)'74; FRCPC; Psy (Consultant Liaison Psychiatry). Consultant Psy & Clin Coord, Royal Alexandra Hospital; Consultant Psy, Sturgeon Community Hospital; Consultant Psy, University of Alberta Hospital; Clin Assoc Prof, University of Alberta; (780)342-7727; Fax. (780)342-7602.

GUIOT, Marie-Christine; MUHC-Montreal Neurology Inst, 3801 rue University, Montreal QC H3A 2B4; Bordeaux (France)'83; AnatPath (P.Q.). Staff, McGill University Health Centre - Montreal Neurological Hospital; (514)398-5319; Fax. (514)398-5825.

GUIRAUDON, Gerard M; London HSC-University Hosp, PO Box 5339 Stn B 339 Windermere Rd, London ON N6A 5A5; Paris (France)'65; FACC; FRCSC; Cardiovasc&ThorSurg (Arrhythmia Surgery). Staff, London Health Sciences Centre - University Hospital; (519)685-8500

GUIRGIS, Hany; 101-7117 Bathurst St, Thornhill ON L4J 2J6; Ain Shams (Egypt)'76; MB ChB; FRCSC; Otol (Sleep Medicine). Chief ENT Division/Ac Staff, The Scarborough Hospital - Birchmount Campus; Pres, Scarborough North Sleep Disorder Clinic; Langs: Arabic; French; (905)597-6222

GUIRGUIS, Adel F; AIM Health Group, B22-550 Terminal Ave, Ottawa ON K1G 0Z3; Cairo (Egypt)'58; FRCS(Eng); Langs: French; Arabic; (613)731-4770

GUIRGUIS, Dina; Credit Valley Med Arts Centre, 311-2000 Credit Valley Rd, Mississauga ON L5M 4N4; Ain Shams (Egypt)'91; CCFP; Langs: Arabic; (905)828-6525; Fax. (905)828-4208.

GUIRGUIS, Emad F T; 153-1880 Eglinton Ave E, Scarborough ON M1L 2L1; Ain Shams (Egypt)'87; MB BCh; CCFP; Staff, Western Memorial Regional Hospital; (416)285-7575; Fax. (416)285-7574.

GUIRGUIS, Emad M; Lakeview Surgery Centre, 1 Kempenfelt Dr, Barrie ON L4M 1B8; McM'85; BA; FRCSC; GenSurg (Dermatology). Staff, Stevenson Memorial Hospital; (705)737-3933; Fax. (705)737-1176; info@lakeviewsurgery.com.

GUIRGUIS, Emad S L; Oakville Med Clinic, 2501 Prince Michael Dr, Oakville ON L6H 0E9; Asyut (Egypt)'87; CCFP; Langs: Arabic; (905)257-4943; Fax. (905)257-2582.

GUIRGUIS, Ezzat F; Orillia Soldiers' Mem Hosp, 170 Colborne St W, Orillia ON L3V 2Z3; Alexandria (Egypt)'62; FRCPC; Psy. Staff, Orillia Soldiers' Memorial Hospital; Langs: Arabic; French; Italian; (705)325-2201; Fax. (705)325-7953.

GUIRGUIS, Hany R Y; Sunnybrook Hlth Sciences Ctre, 2075 Bayview Ave, Toronto ON M4N 3M5; Cairo (Egypt)'95; Hem; IntMed. Staff, Sunnybrook Health Sciences Centre; (416)480-6100

GUIRGUIS, Hesham S R; 400 av de L'Hotel-Dieu, Sorel-Tracy QC J3P 1N5; Ain Shams (Egypt)'86; MSc; PhD; CSPQ; IntMed (P.Q.) (Nephrology). Staff, Hôtel-Dieu de Sorel; Langs: Arabic; English; French; (450)746-6000 x6027; Fax. (450)746-6227; hguirguis@hotmail.com.

GUIRGUIS, Isis K; Alpha-One Med Centre, 12-1891 Rathburn Rd E, Mississauga ON L4W 3Z3; Ain Shams (Egypt)'79; CCFP; (905)212-9955

GUIRGUIS, Nancy; Clin Med Du Vieux Aylmer, 101-204 ch d'Aylmer, Gatineau QC J9H 1A1; Alexandria (Egypt)'02; MB ChB; (819)682-5464

GUIRGUIS, Samir S; Akron Med Centre, 302-2318 Lake Shore Blvd W, Etobicoke ON M8V 1B5; Ain Shams (Egypt)'64; FCBOM; DIMOH; Ac Staff, St Joseph's Health Centre; Langs: Arabic; French; (416)252-5921; Fax. (416)252-9343; drguirguis@aol.com.

GUIRGUIS, Suzette K; CSSS de Laval, 1755 boul Rene-Laennec, Laval QC H7M 3L9; McG'91; CCFP; FCFP; Staff Family Med, Hopital Marie Clarac; Fam Med, Hopital de la Cite de la santé; Consultant, McGill University Health Centre - Montreal Chest Institute; (450)668-1010

GUIRGUIS, Suzy; 201-1131 Nottinghil Gate, Oakville ON L6M 1K5; Alexandria (Egypt)'80; CCFP; (905)815-9090; Fax. (905)815-1834.

GUIRGUIS, Wael; South Country Med Clinic, PO Box 2106 131 3rd Ave W, Assiniboia SK S0H 0B0; (306)642-4454; Fax. (306)642-5949.

GUISE, Roxan M; Niagara Med Group Fam Hlth Team, 4421 Queen St, Niagara Falls ON L2E 2L2; Tor'91; CCFP; FCFP; Langs: French; (905)356-2236; Fax. (905)356-2568.

GUITARD, Sylvianne; CHUS-Hop Hotel-Dieu, 580 rue Bowen S, Sherbrooke QC J1G 2E8; Mon'00; CCFP; CCFP(E.M.); Staff, Centre Hospitalier Universitaire de Sherbrooke-Hôpital Hôtel-Dieu; (819)346-1110 x21000

GUITE, Charles; CSSS de Trois-Rivières, 1991 boul du Carmel, Trois-Rivieres QC G8Z 3R9; Sher'91; FRCPC; Neur; Electroenceph (P.Q.). Staff, CSSS de Trois-Rivières; (819)379-7336; Fax. (819)370-6681.

GUITE, Christian; Centre Med Berger, 116-1000 ch Sainte-Foy, Quebec QC G1S 2L6; Laval'86; ac Staff, Centre Hospitalier Affilié Universitaire de Québec - Hôpital du St-Sacrement; (418)688-1385; Fax. (418)688-3249; christian_guite@ssss.gouv.qc.ca.

GUIZANI, Sinda; Institut de Cardiologie de Mtl, 5000 rue Belanger, Montreal QC H1T 1C8; Mon'09; CCFP; CCFP(E.M.); Staff, Institut de Cardiologie de Montréal; (514)376-3330

GUJRAL, Paramjeet; Four Rivers Med Clinic, 647 Broadway, Winnipeg MB R3C 0X2; Man'05; CCFP.

GUL, Shahid M; 405-125 13th St E, North Vancouver BC V7L 2L3; UBC'99; FRCSC; Neursurg. (604)904-2484

GULA, Lorne J; London HSC-University Hosp, PO Box 5339 Stn B C6 110-339 Windermere Rd, London ON N6A 5A5; Ott'97; FRCPC; IntMed; Cardiol. Staff, London Health Sciences Centre - University Hospital; (519)663-3746; Fax. (519)663-3782.

GULAMHUSEIN, Sajadhussein S; Cedars Prof Park, 2937 66 St NW, Edmonton AB T6K 4C1; Wes'74; ABIM; FRCPC; IntMed (Cardiac Electrophysiology); Cardiol. Dir Cardiac Device Clinic, Covenant Health - Grey Nuns Community Hospital; Dir Arrhythmia Serv, University of Alberta Hospital; Clin Prof, University of Alberta; Langs: Urdu; Gujarati; (780)461-6856; Fax. (780)461-6908; sajadgulamhusein@gmail.com.

GULAMHUSSEIN, Murtaza; West Lincoln Mem Hosp, 169 Main St E, Grimsby ON L3M 1P3; Tor'90; Staff, West Lincoln Memorial Hospital; Langs: Gujarati; Kacchi; (905)945-2253 x202; Fax. (905)945-0504; mg@pathcom.com.

GULAN, Mirjana; 10-100 Highland Rd W, Kitchener ON N2M 3B5; Tor'78; FRCPC; IntMed (Endocrinology). Staff, Grand River Hospital - Kitchener/Waterloo Health Centre; Staff, St Mary's General Hospital; (519)745-1014; Fax. (519)745-1015.

GULAN-VUJNOVIC, Ljubica; Bloor-Jane Med Bldg, 512-2425 Bloor St W, Toronto ON M6S 4W4; Belgrade (Serbia)'66; Ac Staff, St Joseph's Health Centre; Langs: Serbian; Yugoslavian; (416)763-3816

GULATI, Brahm B; Dept of Veteran's Affairs, PO Box 7700 Stn Central, Charlottetown PE C1A 8M9; Agra (India)'56; MB BS; FRCS(Ed & Ire); FFARCS(Eng); MSc(McG); FRCSC; GenSurg. Physician, Veterans Affairs Canada; (902)566-8858; Fax. (902)566-8525; brahm.gulati@vac-acc.gc.ca.

GULATI, Brij B; Ross Mem Hosp, 10 Angeline St N, Lindsay ON K9V 4M8; Nagpur (India)'76; Staff, Ross Memorial Hospital; Langs: Hindi; Punjabi; (705)324-6111

GULATI, Harleena; Harry Medovy House, 2F-671 William Ave, Winnipeg MB R3E 0Z2; Man'05; FRCPC; Anes.

GULATI, Meena; Peterborough Reg Hlth Centre, 1 Hospital Dr, Peterborough ON K9J 7C6; (India)'81; Staff, Peterborough Regional Health Centre - Hospital Drive; (705)743-2121

GULATI, Sanjiv K; Brockville Mental Health Ctre, PO Box 1050 Stn Main 1804 Highway 2 E, Brockville ON K6V 5W7; Himachal Pradesh (India)'96; Staff, Brockville Mental Health Centre - Royal Ottawa Health Care Group; Langs: Hindi; Punjabi; (613)803-4860; Fax. (613)341-2882.

GULAVITA, Sunil; Thunder Bay Reg HSC-T-Bay, 980 Oliver Rd, Thunder Bay ON P7B 6V4; Colombo (Sri Lanka)'71; DMRT; FRCR(UK); FRCPC; RadOncol (Genito Urinary Oncology). Ac Staff Reg Cancer Care, Thunder Bay Regional Health Sciences Centre; Radiation Oncology, Northwestern Ontario Regional Cancer Centre - Cancer Care Ontario; (807)684-7211; Fax. (807)684-5801; gulavitas@tbh.net.

GULENCHYN, Karen Y; Hamilton HS-McMaster Site, HSC 1P15-1200 Main St W, Hamilton ON L8N 3Z5; Wes'76; FRCPC; IntMed; NuclearMed. Staff, Hamilton Health Sciences Centre - McMaster Children's Hospital; Chief Nuclear Med, St Joseph's Hospital - St Joseph's Health Care; Assoc Prof, McMaster University; (905)521-2100 x75667; Fax. (905)546-1125.

GULENS, Voldemars; 19 Oaklands Ave, Toronto ON M4V 2E4; Tor'63; Dip; Psy (Family Psychiatry). Langs: Latvian; (416)920-5861; Fax. (416)920-2680.

GULKA, Irene B; London HSC-University Hosp, PO Box 5339 Stn B 339 Windermere Rd, London ON N6A 5A5; Sask'78; FRCPC; DiagRad (Neuro Radiology). Ac Staff, London Health Sciences Centre - University Hospital; Asst Prof DiagRad & Clin Neurological Sciences, University of Western Ontario; (519)663-3203; Fax. (519)663-8803; ibgulka@uwo.ca.

GULKA, Mark O; Langley Mem Hosp, 22051 Fraser Hwy, Langley BC V3A 4H4; Sask'92; Staff, Langley Memorial Hospital; (604)534-4121

GULLANE, Patrick J; Univ Hlth Network-Toronto Gen, 8N4 877-200 University Ave, Toronto ON M5G 2C4; Galway (Ireland)'70; FRACS(Hon); FRCS(Hon); FRCSI(Hon); FACS; FRCSC; Otol (Head & Neck Surgery). Chair Head & Neck Surgery, Princess Margaret Hospital - University Health Network; Chief Otol Head & Neck Surg, Toronto General Hospital - UHN; Teach Staff, University of Toronto; (416)946-2143; Fax. (416)946-2300.

GULLER, Dmitry; Orillia Soldiers Mem Hosp, 170 Colborne St W, Orillia ON L3V 2Z3; Wes'05; FRCPC; Psy. Staff, Orillia Soldiers' Memorial Hospital; (705)325-2201

GULLIPALLI, Ravindra; St Clare's Mercy Hosp, 154 LeMarchant Rd, St. John's NL A1C 5B8; (India)'96; MB BS.

GULLIVER, Wayne P; 187 Lemarchant Rd, St. John's NL A1C 2H5; Mem'82; BMedSci; FRCPC; Derm. Med Dir/Pres NewLab Clinical Research Inc/Chief Derm, St. John's Health Care Corporation; Assoc Prof Med Derm, Memorial University Of Newfoundland; (709)753-5520; wgulliver@newlab-cro.com.

GULLY, Robert M; Royal Inland Hosp, 311 Columbia St, Kamloops BC V2C 2T1; Alb'76; BMedSci; FRCPC; Anes. Ac Staff, Royal Inland Hospital; Hon Staff, Vancouver General Hospital - Centennial Pavillion; Clinical Asst Prof, University of British Columbia; (250)314-2620; rgully@mail.ocis.net.

GUMBER, Rhythmpal S; Steinbach Med Centre, 10-333 Loewen Blvd, Steinbach MB R5G 0C3; (Other Foreign)'07; CCFP; (204)899-4613

GUMBS, Darren G; St Michael's Health Centre, 1400 9 Ave S, Lethbridge AB T1J 4V5; Alb'04; FRCPC; PhysMed&Rehab. Staff, Covenant Health - St Michael's Health Centre; (403)382-6466; Fax. (403)382-6451.

GUMMESON, Ian D; 101-164 Kings Lane SE, Salt Spring Island BC V8K 2P7; Cal'79; CCFP; (250)537-1828

GUNARATNAM, Lakshman; Univ Hlth Network-Toronto Western Hosp, PO Box 5339 Stn B ALL 139-339 Windermere Rd, London ON N6A 5A5; Ott'02; Staff, London Health Sciences Centre - University Hospital; (519)663-3632; Fax. (519)663-3449.

GUNARATNAM, Selvaratnam; Halton HCS Corp-Georgetown, 1 Princess Anne Dr, Georgetown ON L7G 2B8; Ceylon (Sri Lanka)'74; MB BS; LRCP(Lond); MRC(UK); MRCS(Eng); FRCSC; ObstGyn (Laparoscopic Surgery). Staff, Halton Healthcare Services Corporation - Georgetown Hospital; Langs: Tamil; Sinhalese; (905)873-0111 x228; Fax. (905)702-8738.

GUNASEKERA, Shiny D; St Joseph's Healthcare, FB 639-50 Charlton Ave E, Hamilton ON L8N 4A6; Man'97; FRCPC; Psy. Asst Clin Prof, St Joseph's Healthcare - Charlton Campus; (905)522-1155 x3179; Fax. (905)521-6098.

GUNASINGAM, Padumanithi; Strathroy Middlesex Gen Hosp, 395 Carrie St, Strathroy ON N7G 3J4; Colombo (Sri Lanka)'85; CCFP; Staff, Strathroy Middlesex General Hospital - Middlesex Hospital Alliance; (519)245-5295

GUNATILAKE, K Deepthi; Community Mental Hlth, 200 King St, Woodstock NB E7M 1Z7; Vinnitsa (Ukraine)'86.

GUNAWARDENA, Dishani; 100-1 Belton Blvd, St. Catharines ON L2T 3Y4; (Other Foreign)'09; (905)688-6460

GUNAWARDENA, S Yamuna; North Richmond Hill Kids Clini, 412-1650 Elgin Mills Rd E, Richmond Hill ON L4C 7B5; Havana (Cuba)'93; FRCPC; Peds (Asthma). Consultant Peds, Mackenzie Richmond Hill Hospital; Consultant Peds, Kenswick Family Medicine; Langs: Spanish; Sinhalese; drg@northrichmondhillkidsclinic.ca.

GUNDOGAN, Munire; IWK Health Centre, PO Box 9700 Rpo CSC 5850-5980 University Ave, Halifax NS B3K 6R8; Istanbul (Turkey)'91; FRCPC; DiagRad. Staff, IWK Health Centre; (902)470-7832

GUNDRUM, Susan; 786 Goderich St, Port Elgin ON N0H 2C3; McM'92; CCFP; FCFP; Ac Staff, Grey Bruce Health Services - Southampton Site; (519)389-5501; Fax. (519)389-5509; sgundrum@bmts.com.

GUNKA, Vit B; BC Women's Hosp & Health Ctre, 1Q72-4500 Oak St, Vancouver BC V6H 3N1; Palacky (Czech Republic)'90; DAB; FRCPC; Anes. Staff, BC Women's Hospital & Health Centre; Langs: Czech; (604)875-2158; Fax. (604)875-2733.

GUNN, Adam M; Lansdowne Professional Ctr II, 265-3066 Shelbourne St, Victoria BC V8R 6T9; Man'94; FRCPC; Psy. Staff, Royal Jubilee Hospital; (250)370-7731

GUNN, Beth M; 18F-655 Bay St, Toronto ON M5G 2K4; Alb'04; FRCSC; ObstGyn. (416)217-3974

GUNN, C Robin; Concordia Health Serv, GM200-1550 boul de Maisonneuve, Montreal QC H3G 1M8; Alb'78; MHSc; CCFP; (514)848-2424 x3573; Fax. (514)848-2834.

GUNN, Chit-Chan; 828 Broadway W, Vancouver BC V5Z 1J8; Cambridge (England)'57; MB BCh; FRCP; Pres/Med Dir, Institute for the Study & Treatment of Pain; Clin Prof Multidisciplinary Pain Centre, University of Washington(Seattle-USA); (604)873-4866; Fax. (604)872-4481; c.changunn@gmail.com.

GUNN, David E; 202-255 Main St PO Box 1059, Liverpool NS B0T 1K0; Saba (Netherlands Antilles)'03; BA; CCFP; Staff, Queens General Hospital; (902)356-3044; Fax. (902)354-3626.

GUNN, Harold D; Centre for Integrated Healing, 200-1330 8th Ave W, Vancouver BC V6H 4A6; UBC'81; Teach Staff, University of British Columbia; (604)734-7125 x226; Fax. (604)734-7105.

GUNN, Robert F; Valley Prof Centre, 70 Exhibition St, Kentville NS B4N 4K9; Dal'76; CCFP; FCFP; Ac Staff, Valley Regional Hospital; (902)678-6845; Fax. (902)678-4550.

GUNNARSSON, Thorsteinn; Hamilton HS-General Site, 237 Barton St E, Hamilton ON L8L 2X2; Reykjavik (Iceland)'95; Staff, Hamilton Health Sciences Centre - McMaster Children's Hospital; Staff, Hamilton Health Sciences Centre - Hamilton General Hospital; (905)521-2100

GUNNING, Alan L; 3-245 Argyle St S, Caledonia ON N3W 1K7; McM'87; CCFP; FCFP; (905)765-5245; Fax. (905)765-1090.

GUNNING, Derek J R; 105-245 Columbia St E, New Westminster BC V3L 3W4; UBC'00; FRCSC; CardSurg; Critical Care Medicine. (604)522-6800

GUNNINK, Sara E; Meadowlands Family Hlth Clinic, 888 Meadowlands Dr, Ottawa ON K2C 3R2; Wes'05; CCFP; (613)228-2882; Fax. (613)228-2856.

GUNSON, Kimberly A; Broadway Family Hlth Clinic, 3F-3 Herald Ave, Corner Brook NL A2H 6J2; Mem'07; CCFP; Staff, Western Memorial Regional Hospital; (709)639-5920

GUNTAMUKKALA, Padmavathy; Dr Charles S Curtis Mem Hosp, 178-200 West St, St Anthony NL A0K 4S0; Nagarjuna (India)'80; MB BS; DCH; FAAP; FRCPC; Peds., Charles S Curtis Memorial Hospital; (709)454-3333; mgmukkala@hotmail.com.

GUNTER, Heinz J; Mills Memorial Hosp, 4720 Haugland Ave, Terrace BC V8G 2W7; Cape Town (South Africa)'86; MB ChB; LMCC; FRCPC; Anes. Chief Staff Anes, Mills Memorial Hospital; (250)635-2211; Fax. (250)638-4015.

GUNTLEY-LORIMER, Edith M; Rosedale Med Centre, 412-600 Sherbourne St, Toronto ON M4X 1W4; McM'74; BSc(Hon); MSc; Physician, Shout Clinic CTCHS; Langs: French; Creole; (416)929-6453; Fax. (416)929-6281.

GUNZ, Anna C; Children's Hosp Eastern Ont, 401 Smyth Rd, Ottawa ON K1H 8L1; McM'08; FRCPC; Peds. Staff, Children's Hospital of Eastern Ontario (CHEO); (613)737-7600

GUO, Hans C T; The Doctor's Office, 2251 Lawrence Ave E, Scarborough ON M1P 2P5; Tor'96; BSc; MSc; CCFP; Staff, Markham Stouffville Hospital - Uxbridge Site; Langs: Taiwanese; (416)759-5251; Fax. (416)759-1253.

GUO, Lin Rui; London HSC-University Hosp, Po Box 5339 Stn B B6 112-339 Windermere Rd, London ON N6A 5A5; Shanxi (China)'83; FRCSC; Cardiovasc&ThorSurg. Staff, London Health Sciences Centre - University Hospital; Langs: Chinese; (519)663-3468; Fax. (519)663-3477.

GUO, Peter Y; Misericordia Community Hosp, 1N86-16940 87 Ave NW, Edmonton AB T5R 4H5; Alb'02; FRCPC; IntMed; Nephrol. Staff, Covenant Health - Misericordia Community Hospital; (780)735-2512; Fax. (780)735-2298.

GUO, Ray; Sunnybrook Health Sciences Ctr, 2075 Bayview Ave, Toronto ON M4N 3M5; Tor'10; Staff, Sunnybrook Health Sciences Centre; (416)480-6100

GUPPY, Barry R; Lakeridge Health-Oshawa Site, 1 Hospital Crt, Oshawa ON L1G 2B9; McM'91; BSc; FRCPC; Neur (Neuromuscular Diseases). Ac Staff, QHC Belleville General; Staff, Lakeridge Health - Oshawa Site; Instructor Neurol, Queen's University; (905)576-8711; Fax. (905)721-4784.

GUPTA, Abha A; The Hosp for Sick Children, 9215-555 University Ave, Toronto ON M5G 1X8; Tor'00; FRCPC; Peds (Pediatric Oncology). Staff, The Hospital For Sick Children; Staff, Princess Margaret Hospital - University Health Network; Langs: Hindi; (416)813-8795; Fax. (416)813-5327; abha.gupta@sickkids.ca.

GUPTA, Aditya K; 645 Windermere Rd, London ON N5X 2P1; Southampton (England)'81; FAAD; PhD; MBA; MA; FRCPC; Derm. Prof Derm, University of Toronto; Langs: Hindi; (519)657-4222; Fax. (519)657-4233; agupta@execulink.com.

GUPTA, Anil; The Collonde Bldg, 307-3024 Hurontario St, Mississauga ON L5B 4M4; Dal'96; BSc; Cardiol; IntMed. Staff, Trillium Health Centre - Mississauga; Langs: Hindi; (905)276-4535

GUPTA, Anil K; Albion Finch Med Centre, 106-1620 Albion Rd, Etobicoke ON M9V 4B4; Tor'92; CCFP; FCFP; Langs: Punjabi; (416)741-1500; Fax. (416)741-1506.

GUPTA, Anjalee; Peel Med Arts Bldg, 247-2130 North Park Dr, Brampton ON L6S 0C9; McM'06; CCFP; (905)595-1586

GUPTA, Anjali; Manitoba Clinic, 203-790 Sherbrook St, Winnipeg MB R3A 1M3; Alb'03; FRCSC; ObstGyn;CCFP; (204)788-5745

GUPTA, Anjali; Joseph Brant Mem Hosp, 1230 North Shore Blvd E, Burlington ON L7S 1W7; Tor'84; Staff, Joseph Brant Memorial Hospital; (905)336-4116; Fax. (905)336-6484.

GUPTA, Anup K; Pape Med Centre, 215-751 Pape Ave, Toronto ON M4K 3T1; Meerut (India)'79; ABIM(Cardiol); FRCPC; IntMed; Cardiol. Ac Staff Cardiol, Toronto East General Hospital Inc; (416)462-3884; Fax. (416)462-3895; agupta@outer-net.com.

GUPTA, Aparna; Rouge Valley HS-Ajax/Pickering, 580 Harwood Ave S, Ajax ON L1S 2J4; Kasturba (India)'02; Neur. Staff, Rouge Valley Health System - Ajax & Pickering Health Centre Site; (905)683-2320

GUPTA, Arun T; Crowfoot West Business Ctre, 340-600 Crowfoot Cres NW, Calgary AB T3G 0B4; Alb'04; FRCPC; PhysMed&Rehab. Staff, Foothills Medical Centre; (403)547-9135; Fax. (403)452-0995.

GUPTA, Asha; The Credit Valley Hosp, 4F-2200 Eglinton Ave W, Mississauga ON L5M 2N1; McM'04; CCFP; Staff, The Credit Valley Hospital; Langs: Hindi; (905)813-1100 x5125; Fax. (905)813-4024.

GUPTA, Ashish; The Ottawa Hos-Gen Campus, 501 Smyth Rd, Ottawa ON K1H 8L6; Rajashtan (India)'02; Staff, The Ottawa Hospital - General Campus; (613)737-8571

GUPTA, Chander; Lakeland Medical Clinic, 203-314 25 St, Cold Lake AB T9M 1G6; (India)'92; MB BS; Staff, Foothills Medical Centre; (780)639-3322 x820

GUPTA, Chander K; Boyd Med Centre, 202-388 Portage Ave, Winnipeg MB R3C 0C8; Punjab (India)'64; MB BS; FRCSC; ObstGyn (Urological Gynecology). Ac Staff, Victoria General Hospital; Ac Staff, Seven Oaks General Hospital; Ac Staff Women's Hosp, Winnipeg Regional Health Authority; Assoc Prof, University of Manitoba; Langs: Hindi; Punjabi; chandergupta@shaw.ca.

GUPTA, Chantal R; Cachet Family Physicians, 2-9255 Woodbine Ave, Markham ON L6C 1Y9; Tor'83; BSc; Court Staff, Markham Stouffville Hospital; Court Staff, The Scarborough Hospital - Birchmount Campus; Court Staff, Rouge Valley Health System - Centenary Health Centre Site; (905)887-2222; Fax. (905)887-3655.

GUPTA, Daya K; Boyd Med Centre, 202-388 Portage Ave, Winnipeg MB R3C 0C8; Punjab (India)'62; MS(Ophth.); Dip Ortho(Lond.); FACS; DAB; FRCSC; Ophth (Cataract). Ac Staff, St Boniface General Hospital; Ac Staff, Misericordia Health Centre; Staff, Health Sciences Centre; Asst Prof, University of Manitoba; Langs: Hindi; Punjabi; (204)956-2222; Fax. (204)942-6651; info@ultravision.ca.

GUPTA, Deepak; Bayview Business Centre, 101-16700 Bayview Ave, Newmarket ON L3X 1W1; Tor'87; FRCSC; GenSurg; VascSurg. Ac Staff, Southlake Regional Health Centre; (905)953-0637; Fax. (905)953-0943.

GUPTA, Gaurav; MUHC-Montreal Gen Hosp, E19-1650 av Cedar, Montreal QC H3G 1A4; Tor'05; FRCPC; PhysMed&Rehab. Staff, McGill University Health Centre - Montreal General Campus; (514)934-8223

GUPTA, Geeta; Clinic Cardiogenix, 100-8250 boul Decarie, Montreal QC H4P 2P5; Calcutta (India)'66; MRCOG(Lond); CCFP; Ac Staff, St Mary's Hospital Centre; Asst Prof Family Med, McGill University; (514)731-7717

GUPTA, Geetha; 303-22112 52 Ave, Langley BC V2Y 2M6; Karnataka (India)'78; MB BS; CCFP; Clin Instructor, University of British Columbia; Langs: Hindi; (604)530-1040; Fax. (604)530-4718; guptagita@hotmail.com.

GUPTA, Hansa M; 10 Parkside Dr PO Box 37010, St Jacobs ON N0B 2N0; Tor'02; CCFP; (519)664-3794; Fax. (519)664-2182.

GUPTA, Hemi; The Group Health Centre, 240 McNabb St, Sault Ste. Marie ON P6B 1Y5; Karnatak (India)'92; FRCSC; ObstGyn;CCFP; Langs: Hindi; Punjabi.

GUPTA, Inder P; 3-683 Great Northern Rd, Sault Ste. Marie ON P6B 5A1; Rohtak (India)'83; FRCPC; IntMed (Adult Cardiology); Cardiol. Langs: Hindi; (705)254-7009; Fax. (705)254-7856.

GUPTA, Indra R; MUHC-Montreal Children's Hosp, 2300 rue Tupper, Montreal QC H3H 1P3; Alb'88; FRCPC; Peds; Nephrol. Staff, McGill University Health Centre - Montreal Children's Hospital; (514)934-4400; Fax. (514)934-4359.

GUPTA, Jacqueline P; Newmarket Med Centre, 6-17725 Yonge St, Newmarket ON L3Y 7C1; Delhi (India)'87; CCFP; (905)853-7600

GUPTA, Jagdeep S; Toronto Poly Clinic, 204-5460 Yonge St, North York ON M2N 6K7; UBC'05; CCFP; Physician, Toronto Poly Clinic; Langs: Punjabi; (416)250-7171; Fax. (416)250-0323.

GUPTA, K Kashyap; AMS Toronto, 439 King St E, Toronto ON M5A 1L5; Man'94; CCFP; (416)368-6304

GUPTA, Kapil; Village Park Med, 210A-6640 Vedder Rd, Chilliwack BC V2R 0J2; (Russia (Federation))'03; (604)858-2246

GUPTA, Kaveri; Winchester Dist Mem Hosp, RR 4 566 Louise St, Winchester ON K0C 2K0; Dal'04; IntMed. Staff, Winchester District Memorial Hospital; (613)774-2420; Fax. (613)482-5110.

GUPTA, Madhu; 230-5780 Cambie St, Vancouver BC V5Z 3A7; Kanpur (India)'74; MB BS; FRCSC; ObstGyn. Ac Staff, BC Women's Hospital & Health Centre; Langs: Hindi; Punjabi; Urdu; (604)873-3336

GUPTA, Madhulika A; 101-585 Springbank Dr, London ON N6J 1H3; Tor'78; MD; DABPN; DABSM; FRCPC; Psy;CCFP; Prof Psy, University of Western Ontario; Langs: Bengali; Hindi; (519)641-1001; Fax. (519)641-1033; magupta@uwo.ca.

GUPTA, Malati; Addiction & Mental Hlth-Queen, 1001 Queen St W, Toronto ON M6J 1H4; Bihar (India)'72; FRCPC; Psy. Staff Psy, Centre for Addiction & Mental Health (CAMH) - Queen Site; Langs: Bengali; Hindi; (416)535-8501 x2673; Fax. (416)583-4352.

GUPTA, Meera; Westmount Square Med Centre, 300-1 Car Westmount, Montreal QC H3Z 2P9; Dal'07; Neur. (514)934-2334 x242

GUPTA, Melanie; Mount Carmel Clinic, 886 Main St, Winnipeg MB R2W 5L4; Man'05; CCFP.

GUPTA, Michael; St Joseph's Healthcare, G836-50 Charlton Ave E, Hamilton ON L8N 4A6; Alb'03; FRCSC; Otol (Cancer Head & Neck). Staff, St Joseph's Healthcare - Charlton Campus; Asst Prof, McMaster University; (905)522-1155; Fax. (905)521-6077.

GUPTA, Milan; Osler Cardiology Associates, 200-3 Conestoga Dr, Brampton ON L6Z 4N5; Tor'88; FACC; FRCPC; IntMed (Adult Cardiology); Cardiol. Staff, William Osler Health System - Brampton Civic Hospital; Aj Scientist Div of CU Surg, St Michael's Hospital; Clinical Asst Prof, McMaster University; Langs: Urdu; Hindi; Punjabi; (905)495-4278; Fax. (905)452-1052.

GUPTA, Milli; South Hlth Campus, 4448 Front St SE, Calgary AB T3M 1M4; Wes'06; FRCPC; IntMed; Gastroent. Staff, Foothills Medical Centre; Physician, South Health Campus; (403)956-3804

GUPTA, Mona; CHUM-Hop St-Luc, 1058 rue Saint-Denis, Montreal QC H2X 3J4; McG'95; PhD; FRCPC; Psy. Staff, Centre Hospitalier l'Université De Montréal (CHUM) - Hôpital Saint-luc; (514)890-8000; mona.gupta@wchospital.ca.

GUPTA, Namta; GMF Côté-des-Neiges, 5700 ch Cote des Neiges, Montreal QC H3T 2A8; Man'93; CCFP; FCFP; Staff, CSSS de la Montagne; adj Doyen Student Affairs, McGill University; Langs: Hindi; French; (514)731-1386 x2263; namtagupta@videotron.ca.

GUPTA, Neelam K; Meadowlark Health Centre, 162 Meadowlark Shopping Ctr NW, Edmonton AB T5R 5W9; Alb'06; FRCSC; ObstGyn. (780)428-9516; Fax. (780)428-0629.

GUPTA, Neeru; St Michael's Hosp, CCW8 072-30 Bond St, Toronto ON M5B 1W8; Man'86; PhD; MBA; FRCSC; Ophth (Glaucoma). Dir Glaucoma Unit, St Michael's Hospital; Dir Pitts Chair, Li Ka Shing Knowledge Institute; Prof Ophth & Vision Sciences, University of Toronto; Langs: English; French; (416)864-5444; Fax. (416)864-5208.

GUPTA, Nikhil; LMC Brampton, 238-2130 North Park Dr, Brampton ON L6S 0C9; (India)'05; (905)595-0560

GUPTA, Priya; Alberta Children's Hosp, 2888 Shaganappi Trail NW, Calgary AB T3B 6A8; Delhi (India)'02; Staff, Alberta Children's Hospital; (403)955-7211; Fax. (403)955-7214.

GUPTA, Rahul K; Gibsons Med Clinic, 211-1100 Sunshine Goast Hwy, Gibsons BC V0N 1V7; Qns'93; CCFP; (604)886-2868

GUPTA, Rajeev; Peel Med Arts Bldg, 202-2120 North Park Dr, Brampton ON L6S 0C9; Ross (Dominica)'98; BSc; FAAP; FRCPCH; Peds (Oncology). Staff, William Osler Health System - Brampton Civic Hospital; (905)799-1399; Fax. (905)799-5950.

GUPTA, Rajesh; St Michael's Hosp, 4 150-30 Bond St, Toronto ON M5B 1W8; Tor'94; FRCPC; IntMed (Addiction Medicine). Staff, St Michael's Hospital; (416)864-5361; Fax. (416)864-5714.

GUPTA, Rajiv; 207-100 Humber College Blvd, Etobicoke ON M9V 5G4; Tor'93; FRCSC; Urol. Staff, William Osler Health System - Etobicoke General Hospital; (416)745-2038; Fax. (416)742-2139.

GUPTA, Ram; Shoppers World Med Centre, 106-499 Main St S, Brampton ON L6Y 1N7; Ranchi (India)'78; CCFP; Langs: Hindi; Punjabi; Urdu; (905)796-6570; drramgupta@gmail.com.

GUPTA, Rasna; WIndsor Reg Cancer Centre, 220 Kildare Rd, Windsor ON N8W 2X3; (India)'11; Langs: Hindi; Punjabi; (519)253-5253

GUPTA, Ravi; 23 HSC Canadian Forces Base, PO Box 17000 Stn Forces, Winnipeg MB R3J 3Y5; Man'05; (204)833-2500; Fax. (204)833-2836.

GUPTA, Rekha; 725-5790 University Ave, Halifax NS B3H 1V7; Gujarat (India)'69; MB BS; FRCPC; AnatPath. Asst Path, Queen Elizabeth II Health Sciences Centre - Victoria General Site; Assoc Prof Path, Dalhousie University; Langs: Hindi; Punjabi; Gujarati; (902)473-6895; Fax. (902)473-1049.

GUPTA, Renu; 801-30 Eglinton Ave W, Mississauga ON L5R 3E7; Ross (USA)'05; (416)535-8501

GUPTA, Rohit; South Muskoka Mem Hosp, 75 Ann St, Bracebridge ON P1L 2E4; Punjab (India)'96; GenSurg (Surgical Oncology). Staff, South Muskoka Memorial Hospital - Muskoka Algonquin Healthcare; Langs: Hindi; Punjabi; (705)645-7749; Fax. (705)646-1473.

GUPTA, Salil Kumar; 344 Riverside Dr, Sudbury ON P3E 1H7; Rajasthan (India)'79; Neur. (705)586-3101; Fax. (705)586-3103.

GUPTA, Samir; St Michael's Hosp, 6045 BW-30 Bond St, Toronto ON M5B 1W8; McG'00; FRCPC; IntMed; Respir. Staff, St Michael's Hospital; Langs: Hindi; (416)864-6026; Fax. (416)864-5649.

GUPTA, Samir; 100-1333 Neilson Rd, Scarborough ON M1B 4Y9; Tor'95; BSc; FRCPC; Derm (Cosmetic Dermatology). (416)291-7719; Fax. (416)287-3775.

GUPTA, Sanjay K; Canada Diagnostic Centres, 6020 1A St SW, Calgary AB T2H 0G3; Dal'94; BSc; Dip SportMed; FRCPC; DiagRad;CCFP; CCFP(E.M.); Staff, Toronto General Hospital - UHN; Staff, The Brant Community Healthcare System - Brantford General Hospital Site; Lecturer, University of Toronto; (403)253-4666

GUPTA, Sanjeev; 3429 Fieldgate Dr, Mississauga ON L4X 2J4; Delhi (India)'81; Langs: Punjabi; Hindi; Urdu; (905)602-8448; Fax. (905)602-8448.

GUPTA, Sanjiv; The Ottawa Hosp-Civic Campus, 1053 Carling Ave, Ottawa ON K1Y 4E9; Ott'03; FRCPC; Anes. Staff, The Ottawa Hospital - Civic Campus; (613)761-4940

GUPTA, Sanjoy; 601-1265 East Arthur St, Thunder Bay ON P7E 6E7; Dal'97; MSc; PhD; FRCSC; Ophth. Ac Medical Staff (All Sites), Thunder Bay Regional Health Sciences Centre; Langs: French; Hindi; Bengali; (807)623-3937; Fax. (807)623-3946.

GUPTA, Seema; Mango Tree Family Health Team, 16-35 Harvard Rd, Guelph ON N1G 3A2; McG'95; CCFP; Langs: Hindi; French; (519)837-5410; Fax. (519)837-4853.

GUPTA, Shivani; 404-2151A McCallum Rd, Abbotsford BC V2S 3N8; (Ireland)'06; FRCPC; DiagRad. (604)859-8998

GUPTA, Sumit; The Hosp For Sick Children, 555 Unviersity Ave, Toronto ON M5G 1X8; Tor'05; FRCPC; Peds; PedHemaOncol; OrthSurg. Staff, The Hospital For Sick Children; (416)813-1500

GUPTA, Sunil N; Royal Alexandra Hosp, 10240 Kingsway NW, Edmonton AB T5H 3V9; Alb'89; FRCPC; Anes. Staff, Royal Alexandra Hospital; (780)735-4010

GUPTA, Sunjay; Grandview Med Ctr Fam Hlth Team, 167 Hespeler Rd, Cambridge ON N1R 3H7; (Other Foreign)'08; (519)623-4200

GUPTA, Vikas; Univ Hlth Network-Princess M, 5 217-610 University Ave, Toronto ON M5G 2M9; Guru Nanak (India)'88; FRCP; Staff, Princess Margaret Hospital - University Health Network; Asst Prof Med, University of Toronto; Langs: Hindi; Punjabi; Urdu; (416)946-4521; Fax. (416)946-6546.

GUPTA, Vinesh; Alberta Hosp Edmonton, PO Box 307 Stn Main 17480 Fort Rd, Edmonton AB T5J 2J7; (India)'93; MB BCh; Staff, Alberta Hospital Edmonton; (780)472-5337; Fax. (780)472-5595.

GUPTA, Vishal; 203-3825 Sunset St, Burnaby BC V5G 1T4; (Ireland)'07; MB BCh; BAO; (604)434-9515

GUPTILL, Elizabeth; South Shore Reg Hosp, 90 Glen Allan Dr, Bridgewater NS B4V 3S6; Dal'78; CCFP; Ac Staff Family Med & Obst, South Shore Regional Hospital; Preceptor Family Med., Dalhousie University; (902)543-9151

GURALNICK, Marla S; Kensington Children's Clinic, 6548 Hastings St, Burnaby BC V5B 1S2; New York(NY) (USA)'96; FRCPC; Peds. (604)299-9769

GURALNICK, Melvin S; Westmount Med Centre, 550-1 Car Westmount, Westmount QC H3Z 2P9; McG'65; ObstGyn (Gynecology). Staff, Sir Mortimer B Davis Jewish General; McGill University; (514)934-2334; Fax. (514)731-8824.

GURAM, Karmdeep; The Credit Valley Hosp, 2200 Eglinton Ave W, Mississauga ON L5M 2N1; Wes'03; FRCPC; DiagRad. Staff, The Credit Valley Hospital; Langs: Punjabi; (905)522-1155

GURBIN, Gary M; Kincardine Family Health Team, 44 Queen St, Kincardine ON N2Z 3C1; Wes'65; Staff, South Bruce Grey Health Centre - Kincardine Site; (519)396-6751; Fax. (519)396-3199; gurbin@bmts.com.

GUREKAS, Vydas; Ctr de Sante de Temiscaming, 180 rue Anvik CP 760, Temiscaming QC J0Z 3R0; McG'75; Coroner Investigator, Province of Quebec; pers Prof, McGill University; Langs: Bilingual(English/French); (819)627-3385; Fax. (819)627-9932.

GUREVICH, Lev; PrimeCare Health, 120-109 Quarry Park Blvd SE, Calgary AB T2C 5E7; CCFP; (403)930-7111; Fax. (403)930-7114.

GURGES, Ramy; Barrhead Healthcare Centre, 4815 51 Ave, Barrhead AB T7N 1M1; (Egypt)'94; MB ChB; Staff, Barrhead Healthcare Centre; (780)674-2221

GURJAL, Anagha; Abbotsford Reg Hosp & Cancer C, 32900 Marshall Rd, Abbotsford BC V2S 0C2; Karnatak (India)'85; MB BS; Staff, Abbotsford Regional Hospital & Cancer Centre; (604)851-4710

GURKE, Richard A; Cabrini Centre, 4F-16811 88 Ave NW, Edmonton AB T5R 5Y6; Alb'82; FRCPC; Psy. Ac Staff, Covenant Health - Misericordia Community Hospital; Consultant Psy, Alberta Mental Health Services; Clin Teacher, University of Alberta; (780)735-2934; Fax. (780)735-2973.

GURLAND, Paul R; Credit Valley Med Arts Centre, 502-2000 Credit Valley Rd, Mississauga ON L5M 4N4; Tor'78; FRCSC; ObstGyn (Coloscopy). Ac Staff, The Credit Valley Hospital; (905)820-8748; Fax. (905)820-0255.

GURR, Kevin R; London HSC-Victoria Hosp, PO Box 5010 Stn B 800 Commissioners Rd E, London ON N6A 5W9; Wes'80; FRCSC; OrthSurg (Spine). Staff, London Health Sciences Centre - Victoria Campus; Assoc Prof, University of Western Ontario; (519)685-8500; Fax. (519)685-8059.

GURSAHANEY, Ashvini H; MUHC-Montreal Gen Hosp, E6 188-1650 av Cedar, Montreal QC H3G 1A4; McG'87; MDCM; FRCPC; IntMed (Intensive Care); Critical Care Medicine (P.Q.); Respir. Dir Critical Care Services, McGill University Health Centre - Montreal General Campus; Dir Pulmonary & Critical Care & Ass't Prof, McGill University; Langs: English; French; (514)934-1934 x43255; Fax. (514)934-8244.

GURTU, Rachita; 106B - 100 Humber College Blvd, Toronto ON M9V 5G4; Cal'04; CCFP; (416)742-9449.

GURU, Kiran; 5B-1474 Pickwick Dr, Mississauga ON L5V 2G2; Tor'87; Langs: Hindi; (905)812-0700; Fax. (905)812-7501.

GURWITZ, E Dennis; Scarborough Prof Centre, 302-1371 Neilson Rd, Scarborough ON M1B 4Z8; Witwatersrand (South Africa)'72; MB ChB; DCH; FRCPC; Peds (Pediatric Respirology). Ac Staff, Rouge Valley Health System - Centenary Health Centre Site; Consultant, The Hospital For Sick Children; Lecturer, University of Toronto; (416)281-1100; Fax. (416)281-1105.

GUSCOTT, Jesse R; Collingwood Gen & Marine Hosp, 459 Hume St, Collingwood ON L9Y 1W9; McM'03; CCFP; Staff, Collingwood General & Marine Hospital; (705)444-8606

GUSCOTT, Richard G; Mood Disorders Clinic, 400-723 Rymal Rd W, Hamilton ON L9B 2W2; McM'83; MA; FRCPC; Psy (Anxiety Disorder). (905)522-1384; Fax. (905)522-2738.

GUSDAL, Jeffrey D; Justik Med Clinic, 8225 105 St NW, Edmonton AB T6E 4H2; Alb'95; BSc; CCFP; (780)432-0211; Fax. (780)439-9349.

GUSELLE, Tracey L; Lakeside Med Clinic, 3919 8th St E, Saskatoon SK S7H 5M7; Sask'93; BSc(Biol); CCFP; (306)374-6884

GUSHATY, Leonard N; Justik Med Clinic, 8225 105 St NW, Edmonton AB T6E 4H2; Alb'75; CCFP; Ac Staff Family Med, Covenant Health - Edmonton General Continuing Care Centre; (780)432-0211; Fax. (780)439-9349.

GUSHE, Leonard D; 310 7th St PO Box 599 Stn Main, Mattawa ON P0H 1V0; Tor'89; (705)744-5541

GUSHULAK, Brian D; PO Box 463, Qualicum Beach BC V9K 1S9; Sask'81.

GUSPIE, Brian D; Hys Med Centre, MF-11010 101 St NW, Edmonton AB T5H 4B9; Alb'80; FRCPC; DiagRad (Angiography). (780)426-1121; Fax. (780)425-5979.

GUSTAFSON, Kerstin D; Grandview Business Centre, 300-2626 Croydon Cres, Surrey BC V3S 0C5; UBC'00; FRCSC; ObstGyn. (604)531-3915; Fax. (604)531-3924.

GUSTAFSON, Larry O J; 400-13450 102 Ave, Surrey BC V3T 0H1; UBC'79; BSc; MHSc; LTh; Langs: Urdu; (604)587-4483

GUSTAFSON, Reka Z; Vanc Coastal Hlth Authority, 800-601 Broadway W, Vancouver BC V5Z 4C2; UBC'98; FCFP; FRCPC; CommunMed (Public Health); FamilyMed. Langs: Hungarian; (604)675-3925; Fax. (604)731-2756.

GUSTAFSON, Robert L; Workers Compensation Board, 333 Broadway, Winnipeg MB R3C 4W3; UBC'74; Staff, Workers' Comp Board of MB.

GUSTAFSSON, Jan C; Med Assoc Of Port Credit, 2F-333 Lakeshore Rd W, Mississauga ON L5H 1G9; Tor'72; Court Staff, The Credit Valley Hospital; (905)274-7044; Fax. (905)274-0227.

GUSTAVSSON, Eric S; 105-2231 Louie Dr, Kelowna BC V4T 3K3; UBC'92; (250)768-6985; Fax. (250)768-5490.

GUSZTAK, Leo W; Lloydminster Health District, 3820 43 Ave, Lloydminster SK S9V 1Y5; Man'79; Staff Radiology, Lloydminster Hospital; Staff, Prairie North Health Region; (306)820-6045; Fax. (306)820-6054.

GUT, Roman; Windsor Med Clinic, 101-4465 boul des Sources, Roxboro QC H8Y 3C1; McG'72; CCFP; Ac Staff, Lakeshore General Hospital - Pointe Claire; (514)684-7440

GUTAUSKAS, Andrea; Carling Broadview Med Bldg, 107-770 Broadview Ave, Ottawa ON K2A 3Z3; Ott'04; GenSurg. Staff, Arnprior & District Memorial Hospital; Staff, Queensway Carleton Hospital; Langs: Bilingual(English/French); Spanish; (613)725-9180; Fax. (613)725-1852.

GUTAUSKAS, Jose; 107-770 Broadview Ave, Ottawa ON K2A 3Z3; Ott'68; FRCSC; GenSurg (Cosmetic Surgery). Staff, Arnprior & District Memorial Hospital; Staff, Queensway Carleton Hospital; Langs: Spanish; Lithuanian; French; (613)725-9180; Fax. (613)725-1852.

GUTFREUND, Klaus S; Zeidler Ledcor Centre, 130 University Campus NW, Edmonton AB T6G 2X8; (Germany)'84; FRCPC; IntMed (Hepatology); Gastroent. Staff, University of Alberta Hospital; Assoc Prof Med, University of Alberta; Langs: English; French; (780)492-0388; Fax. (780)492-8143.

GUTGUTIA, Kanan; St Joseph's Health Centre, 30 The Queensway, Toronto ON M6R 1B5; Punjab (India)'94; Staff, St Joseph's Health Centre; Langs: Punjabi; (416)530-6695

GUTHRIE, Bing D; Stanton Terr Health Authority, PO Box 10 Stn Main, Yellowknife NT X1A 2N1; Auckland (New Zealand)'87; MB ChB; FRCSC; ObstGyn. Staff, Stanton Territorial Health Authority; (867)669-4151; Fax. (867)669-4139; bing_guthrie@gov.nt.ca.

GUTHRIE, John B; Glenrose Rehab Hosp, 1238-10230 111 Ave NW, Edmonton AB T5G 0B7; Alb'81; FRCPC; PhysMed&Rehab. Asst Clin Prof, University of Alberta; (780)735-8213; Fax. (780)735-7976.

GUTHRIE, Tara E; 319 15 Ave N PO Box 969, Creston BC V0B 1G0; UBC'90; (250)428-8873; Fax. (250)428-3346.

GUTIERREZ, Carlos A; North York Gen Hosp, 4001 Leslie St, North York ON M2K 1E1; Bogota (Colombia)'77; Staff, North York General Hospital; (416)756-6000

GUTIERREZ, Marinett R; Hôpital régional Chaleur, 1750 Sunset Dr, Bathurst NB E2A 4L7; (Philippines)'88; Staff, Hopital Regional Chaleur; Acadie Bathurst Health Authority; Physician, Vitalite Network; Langs: Tagalog; (506)544-2416 x2417

GUTKIN, Calvin L; College of Fam Phys of Canada, 2630 Skymark Ave, Mississauga ON L4W 5A4; Man'69; CCFP; CCFP(E.M.); FCFP; Exec Dir/CEO, College Of Family Physicians Of Canada-Ontario; (905)629-0900 x237; Fax. (905)629-0893; cgutkin@cfpc.ca.

GUTMAN, I Edward; St Joseph's Health Centre, 30 The Queensway, Toronto ON M6R 1B5; Tor'82; CCFP; FCFP; Hamilton Health Sciences Centre - Hamilton General Hospital; Ac Staff, St Joseph's Health Centre; Ac Staff, Baycrest Centre for Geriatric Care; Teacher Family & CommunMed, University of Toronto; (416)530-6174; Fax. (416)530-8598.

GUTMAN, Jimmy; Groupe Sante Physimed, 121-6363 route Transcanadienne, Saint-Laurent QC H4T 1Z9; Cal'82; Staff, Sir Mortimer B Davis Jewish General; adj Prof, McGill University; (514)747-8888; Fax. (514)747-0655.

GUTMAN, Mory M; Gen Hlthcare Males of All Ages, 201-2318 Lakeshore Blvd W, Etobicoke ON M8X 1B5; Tor'75; (416)259-8898

GUTMAN, Samuel J; 110-916 Broadway W, Vancouver BC V5Z 1K7; Wes'91; CCFP; FamilyMed(EM). Staff, Lions Gate Hospital; Clin Asst Staff ICU/Emerg, Providence Health Care - St Paul's Hospital; (604)718-6990; Fax. (604)324-1706.

GUTMANIS, Peter; Harbour City Health Centre, 202-1125 Dufferin Cres, Nanaimo BC V9S 2B5; Wes'73; FRCSC; OrthSurg. Ac Staff, Nanaimo Regional General Hospital; Ac Staff, University of British Columbia; Langs: English; French; Latvian; (250)714-1983; Fax. (250)714-1951.

GUTOSKI, Donald R; St Joseph's Health Care, PO Box 5777 Stn B 268 Grosvenor St, London ON N6A 4V2; Wes'79; Physician Emerg, St Joseph's Hospital - St Joseph's Health Care; Asst Prof, University of Western Ontario; (519)646-6000 x64233

GUTTERIDGE, Tim J; Surrey Mem Hosp, 13750 96 Ave, Surrey BC V3V 1Z2; Alb'09; CCFP; Staff, Surrey Memorial Hospital; (604)581-2211

GUTTERIDGE, Ursula; Vancouver Coastal/Burnaby Offi, L50-4946 Canada Way, Burnaby BC V5G 4H7; UBC'02; FRCPC; Psy. (604)918-7540; Fax. (604)918-7550.

GUTTMAN, Alex; SMBD Jewish Gen Hosp, D 010-3755 ch Cote-Sainte-Cath, Montreal QC H3T 1E2; McG'84; EmergMed (P. Q.). Clin Asst Emerg Rm, Sir Mortimer B Davis Jewish General; (514)340-8222 x5568; Fax. (514)340-7519.

GUTTMAN, Mark; Centre for Movement Disorders, 2780 Bur Oak Ave, Markham ON L6B 1C9; McM'80; FRCPC; Neur (Movement Disorders). Staff, Markham Stouffville Hospital; (905)472-7082; Fax. (905)472-6270.

GUTTMAN, Orlee R; Children's & Women's HC of BC, 4480 Oak St, Vancouver BC V6H 3V4; Tor'02; FRCPC; Peds; Gastroent. Staff, BC Children's Hospital; (604)875-4111

GUTTMANN, Astrid; The Hosp for Sick Children, 555 University Ave, Toronto ON M5G 1X8; McG'94; MHSc; FRCPC; Peds. Staff, The Hospital For Sick Children; Langs: English; French; German; (416)480-4055 x3783; astrid.guttmann@ices.on.ca.

GUTU, Liana E; CSSS de Laval, 1755 boul Rene-Laennec, Laval QC H7M 3L9; (Romania)'92; AnatPath. Staff, Hopital de la Cite de la santé; (450)668-1010

GUTZIN, Sheryl J; North York Gen Hosp, 4001 Leslie St, North York ON M2K 1E1; Ott'97; FRCPC; IntMed. Staff, North York General Hospital; (416)756-6000

GUY, David J; Central City Med Clinic, PO Box 1138 3110-10153 King George Blvd, Surrey BC V3T 2W1; Mem'74; (604)951-0885; Fax. (604)951-0689.

GUY, Donald A; Nepean Med Centre, 409-1 Centrepointe Dr, Nepean ON K2G 6E2; McM'80; (613)228-8860

GUY, John; Royal Inland Hosp, 311 Columbia St, Kamloops BC V2C 2T1; McG'89; FRCPC; Anes. Staff, Royal Inland Hospital; (250)374-5111

GUY, John R; MUHC-Royal Victoria Hosp, 687 av des Pins O, Montreal QC H3A 1A1; Cal'85; BSc; FRCPC; EmergMed. Staff, McGill University Health Centre - Royal Victoria Hospital; (514)934-1934

GUY, John R F; Health Sciences Centre, 1355-300 Prince Philip Dr, St. John's NL A1B 3V6; Dal'71; FACS; FCCP; FRCSC; GenSurg; ThorSurg. Staff, Health Sciences Centre; (709)777-1378

GUY, K James; 104-386 Cambria St, Stratford ON N5A 1J4; Ott'98; FRCSC; OrthSurg. (519)272-1811; Fax. (519)272-1822.

GUY, Meghan L; Golden Med Clinic, PO Box 1170, Golden BC V0A 1H0; Cal'09; CCFP; (250)575-8255

GUY, Pierre; Ortho Trauma Office, 3F-2775 Laurel St, Vancouver BC V5Z 1M9; McG'89; FRCSC; OrthSurg (Trauma). Langs: Bilingual(English/French); (604)875-5809

GUY, Roger G; Clinique Metro Medic, 100-1538 rue Sherbrooke O, Montreal QC H3G 1L5; Mem'75; BSc; MMedSci; Langs: French; (514)932-2122

GUY, Trevor; Pier Medical, 788 Victoria Rd, Sydney NS B1N 1J7; Dal'05; BSc; BEd; CCFP; CCFP(E.M.); Lecturer Family Med, Dalhousie University; (902)564-8185; Fax. (902)567-6161.

GUYATT, Gordon H; McMaster University HSC, 2C12-1200 Main St W, Hamilton ON L8N 3Z5; McM'77; FRCPC; IntMed. Ac Staff Clin Epidemiol & Biostat, Hamilton Health Sciences Centre - McMaster Children's Hospital; Prof Clin Epidemiol, McMaster University; (905)525-9140; Fax. (905)524-3841; guyatt@mcmaster.ca.

GUYON, Akingabe; DSP du Bas Saint-Laurent, 225-288 rue Pierre-Saindon, Rimouski QC G5L 9A8; McG'04; FRCPC; CommunMed;CCFP; (418)724-5231 x6036

GUYOT, Catherine; CSSS du Suroit, 150 rue Saint-Thomas, Salaber-de-Valleyf QC J6T 6C1; Mon'05; FRCSC; GenSurg. Staff, Centre Hospitalier Régional du Suroît; (450)371-9920

GUZAR, Rebecca L; University Down Fam Practice, 425 University Ave E, Waterloo ON N2K 4C9; McM'00; CCFP; (519)569-8821; Fax. (519)569-8823.

GUZDER, Jaswant; Centre for Child Dev Ment Hlth, 4335 ch Cote-Sainte-Catherine, Montreal QC H3T 1E4; McG'73; DPsy; FRCPC; Psy (Child Psychiatry). Ac Staff Psy, Sir Mortimer B Davis Jewish General; Assoc Prof Psy, McGill University; Langs: Punjabi; Hindi; (514)340-8226; Fax. (514)340-7903; jaswant@videotron.ca.

GUZDER, Rustom N; 1165 Dufferin Cres, Nanaimo BC V9S 2B5; Bangalore (India)'94; (250)591-3200

GUZIK, Elaine C; 9368 Southfort Dr, Fort Saskatchewan AB T8L 0C5; Wes'01; CCFP; (780)997-0177

GUZMAN, D Antonio; Elizabeth Bruyere Pavilion, 261Y-75 Bruyere St, Ottawa ON K1N 5C7; McG'60; FRCPC; Neur (Dementia); Electroenceph (P.Q.). Ac Staff Neurol, SCO Health Service - Élisabeth Bruyère Hospital; Consultant Neurol, The Ottawa Hospital - General Campus; Asst Prof, University of Ottawa; Langs: Spanish; (613)562-6322; Fax. (613)562-6013; dguzman@bruyere.org.

GUZMAN, Jaime; BC Women's Hosp & Health Ctre, K4 115-4500 Oak St, Vancouver BC V6H 3N1; Guanajuato (Mexico)'85; MSc; FRCPC; PhysMed&Rehab (Rheumatology). Staff, BC Women's Hospital & Health Centre; Langs: Spanish; (604)875-2437

GUZMAN, Randolph P; St Boniface Gen Hosp, Z3021-409 Tache Ave, Winnipeg MB R2H 2A6; Man'83; FRCSC; GenSurg; VascSurg. Dept Head Surgery, St Boniface General Hospital; Prof, University of Manitoba; Langs: English; French; (204)235-3349; Fax. (204)237-3429; rguzman@sbgh.mb.ca.

GUZMAN, Venus B; 1765 Eglinton Ave W, Toronto ON M6E 2H7; Manila (Philippines)'61; Ac Staff, St Joseph's Health Centre; Ac Staff, Trillium Health Centre - West Toronto; Langs: Spanish; Tagalog; (416)782-2327; Fax. (416)782-2469.

GUZMAN BUSTAMANTE, Juan; Ctr Hosp de Val-d'Or, 725 6e rue, Val-d'Or QC J9P 3Y1; (Colombia)'94; Anes (P.Q.). Staff, Centre Hospitalier de Val d'Or; (819)825-5858 x2280; Fax. (819)825-7909.

GUZMAN ORDUZ, Juan; Hamilton HS-General Site, 237 Barton St E, Hamilton ON L8L 2X2; Santander (Mexico)'00; FRCPC; IntMed. Staff, Hamilton Health Sciences Centre - Hamilton General Hospital; Langs: Spanish; (905)527-4322

GUZOWSKI, Ann V; Niagara H System-Welland Site, 65 Third St, Welland ON L3B 4W6; Tor'86; BSc; FRCPC; GenPath (Anatomical Pathology). Staff, Hamilton Health Sciences Centre-Juravinski Site; Assoc Staff, St Joseph's Healthcare - Charlton Campus; Staff, Niagara Health System - Welland Hospital Site; Niagara Health System - St Catharines General Site; McMaster University; (905)378-4647; Fax. (905)984-5578.

GUZZO, Angelina; MUHC-Montreal Gen Hosp, D10 144-1650 av Cedar, Montreal QC H3G 1A4; McG'01; FRCPC; Anes. Staff, McGill University Health Centre - Montreal General Campus; (514)934-1934 x43261; Fax. (514)934-8249.

GVERZDYS, Sharunas A; London HSC-Victoria Hosp, PO Box 5010 Stn B 800 Commissioners Rd E, London ON N6A 5W9; Wes'85; FRCPC; Anes. Staff, London Health Sciences Centre - Victoria Campus; (519)685-8300; Fax. (519)685-8275.

GWARDJAN, Andrzej J; 240 James St S, Hamilton ON L8P 3B3; Warsaw (Poland)'83; FRCPC; PhysMed&Rehab (Electromyography). Langs: Polish; (905)521-6376; Fax. (905)777-9399.

GWARDJAN, Ewa; 101-460 Main St E, Hamilton ON L8N 1K4; Warsaw (Poland)'83; Langs: Polish; (905)521-1622; Fax. (905)521-1874; e.gward@sympatico.ca.

GWIAZDA, Katarzyna M; Trillium Health Centre-Mississ, 100 Queensway W, Mississauga ON L5B 1B8; Lodz (Poland)'99; FRCPC; Peds. Staff, Trillium Health Centre - Mississauga; Langs: Polish; (905)848-7100

GWIAZDA, Zbigniew; Municipal Med Centre, PO Box 70, Wakaw SK S0K 4P0; (306)233-4443; Fax. (306)233-4433.

GWIZDAL, Mary; 41 Front St S, Belleville ON K8N 2Y5; Wes'64; BSc(Med); FACOG; FRCSC; ObstGyn. Court Staff, QHC Belleville General; Langs: Polish; (613)962-8211; Fax. (613)968-2051.

GWOZDECKI, Taras M; Lakewood Med Centre, 30 Lakewood Blvd, Winnipeg MB R2J 2M6; Man'88; Staff, Health Sciences Centre; (204)257-3395; Fax. (204)257-6843.

GWYN, Alice; Bonne Bay Health Centre, PO Box 70, Norris Point NL A0K 3V0; Belfast (Ireland)'03; MB BCh; CCFP; Staff, Bonne Bay Health Centre; Langs: Spanish; French; (709)458-2201

GYE, Emmanuel A; Associate Med Clinic, 201-836 1 Ave NW, Airdrie AB T4B 0V2; (Nigeria)'95; (403)948-6422; Fax. (403)948-4492.

GYENES, Gabor T; University of Alberta Hosp, 2C2WCM-8440 112 St NW, Edmonton AB T6G 2B7; Semmelweis (Hungary)'84; PhD; Staff, University of Alberta Hospital; Assoc Prof Cardiol, University of Alberta; Langs: Hungarian; (780)407-2704; Fax. (780)407-6452; gabor.gyenes@albertahealthservices.ca.

GYENES, Tal Ora; Bathurst-Drewry Med Centre, 202-5927 Bathurst St, North York ON M2R 3T5; Tel-Aviv (Israel)'82; FRCPC; PhysMed&Rehab. Teacher Med, University of Toronto; (416)225-0095; Fax. (416)225-0099.

GYETVAI, Kristen M; F-300 Giles Boulevard E, Windsor ON N9A 4C4; Tor'00; FRCSC; GenSurg. (519)252-6538; Fax. (519)252-3389.

GYGER, Genevieve; Sir Mortimer B Davis Jewish Ge, 3755 ch cote-Sainte-Catherine, Montreal QC H3T 1E2; Laval'03; Rheum; IntMed. Staff, Sir Mortimer B Davis Jewish General; (514)340-8222 x4840; Fax. (514)340-7906.

GYGER, Martin; SMBD Jewish Gen Hosp, 3755 ch Cote-Sainte-Catherine, Montreal QC H3T 1E2; Mon'71; FRCPC; HemPath (Bone Marrow Transplant); Hem (P.Q.)., Sir Mortimer B Davis Jewish General Hospital, Stem Cell Transplant Prog.; Dir Stem Cell Transplant Prog, Sir Mortimer B Davis Jewish General; Langs: English; French; (514)340-8207

GYIMAH, Albert; William Osler HC-Brampton, 2100 Bovaird Dr E, Brampton ON L6R 3J7; (Ghana)'79; MB ChB; FRCPC; Psy (General Adult Psychiatry). Staff, William Osler Health System - Brampton Civic Hospital; Langs: Ghanaian; Akan; (905)494-2120; Fax. (905)494-6710.

GYOMOREY, Katalin; Thunder Bay Reg HSC-T-Bay, 980 Oliver Rd, Thunder Bay ON P7B 6V4; McM'03; FRCPC; Psy. Staff, Thunder Bay Regional Health Sciences Centre; Langs: German; Hungarian; French; (807)684-6000

GYOMOREY, Sandor; 206-89 Humber College Blvd, Etobicoke ON M9V 4B8; Tor'03; FRCSC; OrthSurg. Staff, Mount Sinai Hospital; Staff, William Osler Health System - Etobicoke General Hospital; Langs: German; Hungarian; (416)774-3199

GYONGYOSSY, Edward A; Healthcare, 3163 Winston Churchill Blvd, Mississauga ON L5L 2W1; Qns'89; (905)607-2001; Fax. (905)607-1553.

GYOPAR, Andrew F; Ctr Hosp Anna-Laberge, 200 boul Brisebois, Chateauguay QC J6K 4W8; McG'88; CSPQ; FRCSC; GenSurg. Staff, Hôpital Anna-Laberge; Langs: Hungarian; French; (450)699-2425

GYSLER, Mathias; Credit Valley Med Arts Centre, 2180 Meadowvale Blvd, Mississauga ON L5N 5S3; Wes'73; FRCSC; ObstGyn. Chief/Medical Staff, The Credit Valley Hospital; Ac Staff, The Hospital For Sick Children; Langs: German; (905)816-9822; Fax. (905)816-9833.

GZIK, Danusia J; 141 Roe Rd RR 4, Huntsville ON P1H 0A5; McM'94; CCFP; (705)788-9352

HA, Andrew; Hamilton HS-General Site, NW8N 01-237 Barton St E, Hamilton ON L8L 2X2; Qns'06; Cardiol; IntMed. Staff, Hamilton Health Sciences Centre - Hamilton General Hospital; Langs: Korean; (905)521-2100

HA, Andrew C T; Univ Hlth Network-Toronto Gen, 200 Elizabeth St, Toronto ON M5G 2C4; Ott'02; FRCPC; IntMed; Cardiol. Staff, Toronto General Hospital - UHN; Langs: Cantonese; (416)340-5206

HA, David J; University of Alberta Hosp, 1A7 19WCM-8440 112 St NW, Edmonton AB T6G 2B7; UBC'01; FRCPC; EmergMed. Staff Emerg, University of Alberta Hospital; (780)407-8432

HA, Duc Vinh; Foothills Med Centre, 1403 29 St NW, Calgary AB T2N 2T9; Sask'99; FRCPC; Anes. Staff, Foothills Medical Centre; (403)944-1430

HA, Hang Chu; St Paul's Hosp, 1702 20th St W, Saskatoon SK S7M 0Z9; Saigon (Vietnam)'72; FRCPC; Anes. Staff, St Paul's Hospital (Grey Nuns) of Saskatoon; (306)655-5240; Fax. (306)655-5964.

HA, Michael; St Joseph's Healthcare, 50 Charlton Ave E, Hamilton ON L8N 4A6; Man'98; FRCPC; EmergMed. Staff, St Joseph's Healthcare - Charlton Campus; Langs: Cantonese; (905)522-1155

HA, Valerie; Danforth Medical Arts, 105-235 Danforth Ave, Toronto ON M4K 1N2; Tor'00; CCFP; Court Staff, Humber River Regional Hospital - Church Street Site; (416)462-1777; Fax. (416)462-1775; danforthmedicalartsclinic@gmail.com.

HAAF, Dana J; 306-125 13th St E, North Vancouver BC V7L 2L3; UBC'03; CCFP; (604)988-0727

HAAGER, Moritz B; Royal Alexandra Hosp, 541 CSC-10240 Kingsway NW, Edmonton AB T5H 3V9; Alb'01; FRCPC; EmergMed. Staff, Royal Alexandra Hospital; (780)735-4449

HAAK, Diane S; Orillia Soldiers Mem Hosp, 170 Colborne St W, Orillia ON L3V 2Z3; Ott'99; BSc; CCFP; Staff, Orillia Soldiers' Memorial Hospital; (705)325-2201; dhaak@gbhs.on.ca.

HAALAND, Derek A; Georgian Prof Centre, 001-125 Bell Farm Rd, Barrie ON L4M 6L2; Dal'03; FRCPC; IntMed; ClinImmunol&Allergy; Rheum. (905)734-9343; Fax. (905)734-0007.

HAALBOOM, Erijka W; Sheldon Chumuik Centre, 1213 4 St SW, Calgary AB T2R 0X7; Ott'06; FRCPC; Psy. (403)955-6155

HAAPALA, Eric M; Central Algoma Med Group, PO Box 398, Bruce Mines ON P0R 1C0; McM'01; CCFP; Langs: Bilingual(English/French); (705)785-3495; Fax. (705)785-3672.

HAAS, Yvonne M; St Joseph's Hlth Ctr Urban FHT, 306-27 Roncesvalles Ave, Toronto ON M6R 3B2; Tor'93; CCFP; Staff, St Joseph's Health Centre; (416)761-0133; Fax. (416)761-1915; yvonne.haas@sickkids.ca.

HAASE, David A; Queen Elizabeth II HSC, 5014-1278 Tower Rd, Halifax NS B3H 2Y9; (Jamaica)'73; MB BS; FRCPC; IntMed (Infectious Diseases); InfectDis. Staff IntMed, Queen Elizabeth II Health Sciences Centre - Victoria General Site; Assoc Prof IntMed, Dalhousie University; (902)473-8477; Fax. (902)473-7394; david.haase@dal.ca.

HAASE, Erika; 205-3017 66 St NW, Edmonton AB T6K 4B2; McG'99; MDCM; MSc; GenSurg (Surgical Oncology). Gen Surgeon & Surgical Oncologist, Covenant Health - Grey Nuns Community Hospital; Gen Surgeon & Surgical Oncologist/Asst Prof, University of Alberta; Langs: German; French; (780)461-6012; Fax. (780)461-5442.

HAASZ, Maya; The Hosp for Sick Children, 555 University Ave, Toronto ON M5G 1X8; McG'06; MDCM; FRCPC; Peds (Pediatric Emergency Medicine). Staff, The Hospital For Sick Children; (416)813-7832

HABAL, Flavio; Univ Hlth Network-Toronto Gen, 9EN 229-200 Elizabeth St, Toronto ON M5G 2C4; Tor'77; PhD; FRCPC; Gastroent (Hepatology); IntMed. Ac Staff, Toronto General Hospital - UHN; Assoc Prof Med, University of Toronto; Langs: Italian; French; (416)340-5023; Fax. (416)595-5251; flavio.habal@uhn.on.ca.

HABASHY, Suzane F; Stadium Med Centre, 21-1941 Uxbridge Dr NW, Calgary AB T2N 2V2; Ain Shams (Egypt)'81; LRCP; LRCS(Edin); LRCPS(Glas); CCFP; (403)248-8807

HABAZ, Yehuda; Campelton Reg Hosp, PO Box 880 189 Lily Lake Rd, Campbellton NB E3N 3H3; Tel Aviv (Israel)'88; FRCSC; ObstGyn. Staff, Hôpital Régional Campbellton; (506)789-5000

HABBAB, Fadi; MUHC-Royal Victoria Hosp, 687 av des Pins O, Montreal QC H3A 1A1; McG'03; FRCPC; DiagRad. Staff, McGill University Health Centre - Royal Victoria Hospital; (514)934-1934 x48084

HABDANK-KOSSOWSKI, Katherine; Niagara H System-Welland Site, 65 Third St, Welland ON L3B 4W6; Qns'03; FRCPC; IntMed; Respir. Staff, Niagara Health System - Welland Hospital Site; (905)378-6111

HABDANK-KOSSOWSKI, Krzysztof; Niagara H System-Welland Site, 65 Third St, Welland ON L3B 4W6; Qns'03; DiagRad. Staff, Niagara Health System - Welland Hospital Site; Langs: Polish; (905)732-6111

HABEL, Jean-Paul; Clinique Med East Angus, 1A-150 rue Angus S, East Angus QC J0B 1R0; Laval'68; (819)832-2438; Fax. (819)832-2104.

HABEL, Maryline; Clinique Medicale Lacroix, 210-880 rue Commerciale, Levis QC G6Z 2E3; Laval'00; CCFP; Staff, Centre Hospitalier La Sarre; (418)834-9911

HABEL, Michel; 4255 av Papineau, Montreal QC H2H 2P6; Mon'76; (514)526-4981

HABEL, Pierre-David; CSSS du Haut Saint-Maurice, 885 boul Ducharme, La Tuque QC G9X 3C1; Mon'10; Staff, Centre Hospitalier Saint-Joseph de la Turque; (819)523-4581

HABER, George D; Clinique Med En Route, F5-895 rue de la Gauchetiere O, Montreal QC H3B 4G1; Wayne State (USA)'66; AB; ObstGyn. (514)954-1444

HABER, Julia A; Rockyview Gen Hosp, 7007 14 St SW, Calgary AB T2V 1P9; Qns'05; Anes. Staff, Rockyview General Hospital; (403)943-3000

HABER, L Richard; Plaza Baie D'Urfe, 14-90 Morgan Rd, Ste-Anne-de-Bellev QC H9X 3A8; McM'72; FAAP; MPhil; MTS; FRCPC; Peds. Dir Ped Consultation Center, McGill University Health Centre - Montreal Children's Hospital; assoc Prof Ped, McGill University; Langs: Bilingual(English/French); (514)695-6345; richard.haber@mcgill.ca.

HABER, Richard M; Richmond Road Diag & Trmt Ctre, 1153-1820 Richmond Rd SW, Calgary AB T2T 5C7; Tor'76; FRCPC; Derm. Staff, Foothills Medical Centre; (403)955-8659

HABERER, Marie-Pierre; Campbellton Reg Hosp, PO Box 880 189 Lily Lake Rd, Campbellton NB E3N 3H3; Montpellier (France)'94; Staff, Hôpital Régional Campbellton; Staff, Centre de santé Communitaire - St-Joseph.

HABERMAN, Craig J; Harry Medovy House, 2F-671 William Ave, Winnipeg MB R3E 0Z2; Man'98; FRCPC; Anes. Staff, Health Sciences Centre.

HABERMAN, Herbert F; Univ Hlth Network-Toronto Western Hosp, EW8-399 Bathurst St, Toronto ON M5T 2S8; Tor'59; FRCPC; Derm. Court Staff, Toronto Western Hospital - University Health Network; (416)603-5721; Fax. (416)603-2782.

HABERMAN, John J R; Campbell Clinic, 430 Mayor Magrath Dr S, Lethbridge AB T1J 3M1; Alb'70; Assoc Staff, Chinook Regional Hospital; Assoc Staff, Covenant Health - St Michael's Health Centre; Med Advisor, Victorian Order of Nurses; (403)328-8101; Fax. (403)328-8150.

HABERMEHL, Lisa M; Kenora Med Centre, 45 Wolsley St, Kenora ON P9N 3W7; Wes'00; CCFP; (807)468-3021; lhabermehl@redlakehospital.ca.

HABERT, Jeffrey S; Shops on Steeles Med Centre, 206-2900 Steeles Ave E, Thornhill ON L3T 4X1; Tor'87; CCFP; FCFP; Ac Staff, The Scarborough Hospital - Birchmount Campus; Court Staff, North York General Hospital; (905)881-6667; Fax. (905)731-1298; jhabert@rogers.com.

HABIB, Adel F; Hotel-Dieu de Sorel, 400 av de l'Hotel-Dieu, Sorel-Tracy QC J3P 1N5; Cairo (Egypt)'87; Psy (P.Q.). Staff Psy, Hôtel-Dieu de Sorel; Langs: Arabic; English; (450)746-6150; Fax. (450)746-6225.

HABIB, Adnan; West Main Plaza, 175-1273 Main St, Moncton NB E1E 0P4; Aga Khan (Pakistan)'98; ABIM; Staff Respirologist, The Moncton Hospital; (506)857-5748; Fax. (506)857-5728; dr.adnan.habib@horizon.nb.ca.

HABIB, Bahaa S; Bathurst Med Centre, LL56-7117 Bathurst St, Thornhill ON L4J 2J6; Ain Shams (Egypt)'86; MB BCh; CCFP; Langs: Arabic; (905)731-5662; Fax. (905)731-6841.

HABIB, Emad A; Ottawa Reg Cancer Centre, 503 Smyth Rd, Ottawa ON K1H 1C4; Assiut (Egypt)'74; MSc(Orth); CCFP; Physician, Ottawa Regional Cancer Centre; Langs: Arabic; (613)737-7700 x8469

HABIB, Khawaja; Athabasca Health Authority, PO Box 124, Black Lake SK S0J 0H0; Punjab (Pakistan)'86; CCFP; (306)439-2200

HABIB, Nader H; Centre Med Samson, 202-4599 boul Samson, Laval QC H7W 2H2; Mon'73; Staff, Hôpital du Sacre-Coeur de Montréal; Langs: English; Arabic; (450)688-7170; Fax. (450)688-3335; n.habib@videotron.ca.

HABIB, Naiyer; 1225 Sumas Way PO Box 4106, Abbotsford BC V2S 8H0; Patna (India)'64; MB BS; FACC; FACP; FRCPC; IntMed (Cardiology). Clin Prof Med Cardiology, University of Saskatchewan; Langs: Urdu; Hindi; (604)556-9213; drnhabib@yahoo.ca.

HABIB, Rami; U of Ottawa Health Services, 300-100 Marie Curie Pvt, Ottawa ON K1N 6N5; McM'93; FRCPC; Psy. Staff, Royal Ottawa Mental Health Centre - Royal Ottawa Health Care Group; (613)564-3950

HABIB, Samir; Clinique du Dr Ivy Matouk, 116-1600 boul Henri-Bourassa o, Montreal QC H3M 3E2; Sofia (Bulgaria)'86; CCFP; Langs: Bulgarian; French; Arabic; (514)832-0333; Fax. (514)832-3742.

HABIB, Syed W; Clinical Sciences Bldg, 11 107-152 University Campus N, Edmonton AB T6G 2G3; Karachi (Pakistan)'87; MB BS; Asst Prof, University of Alberta Hospital; Clinical Asst Prof, University of Alberta; Langs: Urdu; (780)407-3604; Fax. (780)407-7771; syed.habib@ualberta.ca.

HABIBA, Ayman A; Cape Breton Healthcare Complex, 1482 George St, Sydney NS B1P 1P3; Cairo (Egypt)'81; MB BCh; Staff, Cape Breton Healthcare Complex; (902)567-8000

HABIBI, Hamid R; Bridgeland Med Bldg, 306-803 1 Ave NE, Calgary AB T2E 7C5; (Iran)'89; Staff, Foothills Medical Centre; (403)571-8600; Fax. (403)571-8659.

HABIBI, Mehri; 1502-101 Humber College Blvd, York ON M9N 1R8; Shahid Beheshti (Iran)'90; Anes. Staff, William Osler Health System - Brampton Civic Hospital; Langs: Farsi; (416)747-3400

HABIBIAN, Sonia; Ocean Walk Med Centre, 1884 Marine Dr, West Vancouver BC V7V 1J6; Shahid Beheshti (Iran)'86; CCFP; Staff, Ocean Walk Medical Centre; Langs: Farsi; (604)925-1884

HABING, David K; Lincoln Med Centre, 4413 Ontario St, Beamsville ON L0R 1B5; Dal'94; CCFP; Staff, West Lincoln Memorial Hospital; (905)563-1212; Fax. (905)563-4404.

HABJAN, Andrej J; Thunder Bay Med Centre, 330-63 Algoma St N, Thunder Bay ON P7A 4Z6; Ljubljana (Slovenia)'77; BSc; Staff, St Joseph's Care Group; Staff, Thunder Bay Regional Health Sciences Centre; Langs: Croatian; Slovenian; (807)343-0070; Fax. (807)343-0101.

HABOT, Juda; 602-581 Davis Dr, Newmarket ON L3Y 2P6; Cal'92; BSc; FRCPC; IntMed (Echocardiography); Cardiol. Staff, Southlake Regional Health Centre; Langs: Hebrew; Yiddish; (905)953-7917

HABRA, Magdi; GMF Chapleau, 87 montee Gagnon, Bois-des-Filion QC J6Z 4C4; Ain Shams (Egypt)'77; assoc Staff, Hopital de la Cite de la santé; Langs: French; Arabic; (450)621-7420; Fax. (450)621-5007.

HABRA, Munir; 300-3234 boul Taschereau, Greenfield Park QC J4V 2H3; St. Joseph (Lebanon)'74; Staff Emerg & Outpatient Clin, Hopital Charles LeMoyne; Langs: Arabic; English; (450)466-1125; Fax. (450)466-9646; munir.h@videotron.ca.

HABRA, Natalie; Inst de Readaptation de Mtl, 6300 av de Darlington, Montreal QC H3S 2J4; Mon'05; FRCPC; PhysMed&Rehab. Staff, Institut de Réadaptation Gingras-Lindsay de Montréal; (514)340-2088

HABTESELASSIE, Biruk Y; York Med Green Lane, RR 1 Lcd 1 18120 Yonge St, Newmarket ON L3Y 4V8; Addis Ababa University (Ethiopia)'97; CCFP; Langs: Amharic; (905)868-9243

HACCOUN, Charles; Clin Pedia Laurentienne, 106-200 rue Durand, Saint-Jerome QC J7Z 7E2; McG'96; FRCPC; Peds. (450)438-1241; Fax. (450)438-3501.

HACHACHENA, Fatima; Ctr Hosp de Lachine, 650 16e av, Lachine QC H8S 3N5; Alger (Algeria)'87; Staff, CSSS de Dorval-Lachine-Lasalle; (514)637-2351

HACHE, Chantal; Hotel-Dieu de Levis, 143 rue Wolfe, Levis QC G6V 3Z1; Sher'00; FRCPC; IntMed (Hepatology); Gastroent. Staff, Hôtel-Dieu de Lévis; Langs: Bilingual(French/English); (418)835-7121

HACHE, Louise; Clinique Med De Tracadie, PO Box 3634 Stn Main, Tracadie-Sheila NB E1X 1G5; Laval'93; CCFP; (506)395-1140; Fax. (506)395-1150.

HACHE, M K Nanette D; Health Sciences Centre, 300 Prince Philip Dr, St. John's NL A1B 3V6; Mem'95; FRCPC; DiagRad. Staff, Health Sciences Centre; (709)777-7810

HACHE, Marilene; Clinique Med Nepisiquit, 950 av Picot, Bathurst NB E2A 4Z9; Sher'02; CCFP; Staff, Hopital Regional Chaleur; Langs: Bilingual(French/English); (506)546-6696; cmni@nbnet.nb.ca.

HACHE, Mireille C; Hôpital régional Chaleur, 1750 Sunset Dr, Bathurst NB E2A 4L7; Sher'96; LMCC; FRCPC; Psy. Staff, Hopital Regional Chaleur; Langs: Bilingual(French/English); (506)544-2316; Fax. (506)544-2326; mireille.hache@vitalitenb.ca.

HACHE, Nathalie; Regie des Rentes du Quebec, 348-2600 boul Laurier, Quebec QC G1V 4T3; Laval'97; Staff, Hôtel-Dieu de Lévis; (418)657-8709 x3305

HACHE, Rachelle; 4-1116 Mountain Rd, Moncton NB E1C 2T3; Sher'01; CCFP; (506)857-5011; Fax. (506)857-5013.

HACHED BAITICHE, Leila; CSSS de Laval, 1755 boul Rene-Laennec, Laval QC H7M 3L9; (Algeria)'87; Staff, Hopital de la Cite de la santé; (450)668-1010

HACHEMI, Latifa; CSSS de Papineau, 155 rue MacLaren E, Gatineau QC J8L 0C2; CCFP; Staff, Hôpital de Papineau; (819)986-4115 x4006; Fax. (819)961-8018.

HACHINSKI, Vladimir; London Hlth Sciences Ctr, PO Box 5339 Stn B B7 003-339 Windermere Rd, London ON N6A 5A5; Tor'66; MSc(DME); DSc(Med); FRCPC; Neur (Stroke). Staff Dept of Neurological Sciences, London Health Sciences Centre - University Hospital; Staff, Schulich School of Medicine & Dentistry; Prof Neurol, University of Western Ontario; Langs: Spanish; (519)663-3624; Fax. (519)663-3910; rebecca.clarke@lhsc.on.ca.

HACK, Anna T; Appletree Med Center, 1309 Carling Ave, Ottawa ON K1Z 7L3; Tor'10; CCFP; (613)482-0118

HACK, Arshad; Fairview Med Arts Centre, 208-2200 Fairview St, Burlington ON L7R 4H9; (USA)'07; BSc(Hon); MHSA; CCFP; Chief Family Med, Joseph Brant Memorial Hospital; Asst Clin Prof, McMaster University; (905)632-2542; Fax. (905)632-2617.

HACK, Kalesha; Sunnybrook Hlth Sciences Ctre, 2075 Bayview Ave, Toronto ON M4N 3M5; Wes'04; FRCPC; DiagRad. Staff, Sunnybrook Health Sciences Centre; (416)480-6100

HACK, M Imran; Aberdeen Hosp, 835 East River Rd, New Glasgow NS B2H 3S6; Mem'79; BSc(Biol.); IntMed (Cardiology). Staff IntMed, Aberdeen Regional Hospital; (902)752-1965; Fax. (902)752-6330.

HACK, Muhammad U; 215-1315 Finch Ave W, North York ON M3J 2G6; Tor'76; CCFP; Chief Family Pract, North York General Hospital - Branson Division; Ac Staff, Humber River Regional Hospital - Finch Avenue Site; (416)630-3301; Fax. (416)630-3303; unus_hack@hotmail.com.

HACKAM, Daniel G; 1400 Weston Rd, London ON N6G 2V2; Wes'00; FRCPC; IntMed (Clinical Pharmacology). (519)663-3838

HACKENBERG, Libusa; Northern alberta Eye Institute, 10115 99 Ave, Grande Prairie AB T8V 0S1; (Slovakia)'96; (780)538-9997; Fax. (780)538-9788.

HACKER, David C; 560-135 Queen's Plate Dr, Etobicoke ON M9W 6V1; Tor'92; FRCSC; Otol (Pediatric Otolaryngology). (416)745-1661; Fax. (416)745-4496.

HACKER, Paul L; 320-1861 Robertson Rd, Nepean ON K2H 1B9; Tor'89; Staff, Queensway Carleton Hospital; (613)801-0035

HACKER, Paul M; Boxgrove Med Arts Centre, 205-110 Copper Creek Dr, Markham ON L6B 0P9; Tor'86; FRCPC; IntMed; Cardiol. Court Staff Cardiol, Sunnybrook Health Sciences Centre; Staff Cardiol, Markham Stouffville Hospital; (905)472-8228; Fax. (905)472-8548.

HACKER, Peter; Seaforth Med Bldg, 770-3550 ch de la Cote-des-Nei, Montreal QC H3H 1V4; Ott'63; DAA; FRCPC; Derm. Court Staff, St Michael's Hospital; Asst Prof Adjunt Med, University of Toronto; Langs: Hungarian; (416)233-3340; Fax. (416)233-0488.

HACKETT, Michael A; The Group Health Centre, 240 Mcnabb St, Sault Ste. Marie ON P6B 1Y5; Ott'81; Ac Staff, Sault Area Hospital - Sault Ste Marie; Med Dir, Algoma District Cancer Program; (705)759-1234

HACKETT, R Andrew; Senior Mental Health Program, 200-1164 Devonshire Ave, North Bay ON P1B 6X7; Tor'73; DipCE; FRCPC; Psy (Geriatric Psychiatry);CCFP; FCFP; Staff, North Bay Regional Health Centre - Regional Mental Health; (705)474-5885

HACKETT, Richard J; PO Box 360, Tofield AB T0B 4J0; National U (Ireland)'82; MB ChB; DObstRCOG; DCH; DA; Fam Med, Tofield Health Centre; (780)662-2080; Fax. (780)662-2140; richard.hackett@albertahealthservices.ca.

HACKETT, Sharon L; The Dermatology Centre, 124 42 Ave SW, Calgary AB T2S 3B3; McM'79; FRCPC; Derm. Langs: Bilingual(English/French); (403)299-5800; Fax. (403)299-5844.

HACKING, Frederick J; Kenogami Clinic, PO Box 528 RR 2, Swastika ON P0K 1T0; Bristol (England)'69; DRCOG; (705)642-3317

HACKING, Jennifer J; Greenwood Med Centre, 10-496 Discovery Ave, Kingston ON K7K 7E9; Man'99; CCFP; (613)507-7003

HACKING, Susan M; Hinton Healthcare Centre, 1280 Switzer Dr, Hinton AB T7V 1V2; Cape Town (South Africa)'75; MB ChB; FRCR; FRCPC; DiagRad. Staff, Hinton Healthcare Centre; (780)865-3333; Fax. (780)865-3581.

HACKMANN, Thomas; IWK Health Centre, PO Box 9700 Rpo CSC 5850-5980 University Ave, Halifax NS B3K 6R8; Dusseldorf (Germany)'80; FRCPC; Anes. Staff, IWK Health Centre; (902)470-8251

HACQUEBARD, Simone M A; Wilson Centre Family Practice, 1-2185 Wilson Ave, Port Coquitlam BC V3C 6C1; Ott'74; Court Staff Privil, Royal Columbian Hospital; Court Staff Privil, Eagle Ridge Hospital & Health Care Centre; (604)942-7227; Fax. (604)942-7058.

HADAD, Keyvan; Pediatric & Newborn Care, 303-1750 10th Ave E, Vancouver BC V5N 5K4; Wes'95; FRCPC; Peds. Langs: Farsi; French; (604)602-0931; keyvan@telus.net.

HADCOCK, Steven J; 160 Dundurn St S, Hamilton ON L8P 4K3; Tor'95; CCFP; Ac Staff, St Joseph's Healthcare - Charlton Campus; (905)528-5480; Fax. (905)528-2884.

HADDAD, Alain; CSSSG-Hop De Gatineau, 909 boul de la Verendrye O, Gatineau QC J8P 7H2; Ott'05; FRCPC; RadOncol. Staff, Hôpital de Gatineau; (819)966-6130; Fax. (819)966-6284.

HADDAD, Camille; Pleasant Street Med Clinic, 4-250 Pleasant St, Miramichi NB E1V 1Y5; Dal'90; (506)622-6140; Fax. (506)627-0484.

HADDAD, Dimitri E; Grand River Sports Med, 40 George St N, Cambridge ON N1S 2M8; Qns'01; FRCSC; OrthSurg. Langs: Bilingual(English/French); (519)624-5999; Fax. (519)624-1917; info@grsm.ca.

HADDAD, Elie; Hôpital Ste-Justine, 3175 ch Cote-Sainte-Catherine, Montreal QC H3T 1C5; Paris (France)'93; ClinImmunol&Allergy (P.Q.). Staff, Hôpital Ste-Justine; Langs: Bilingual(French/English); (514)345-4713; Fax. (514)345-4897; elie.haddad@umontreal.ca.

HADDAD, Elizabeth M; Chatham Kent Health Alliance, 65 Thames St, Chatham ON N7L 1S4; Ott'00; BSc(Hon); FRCSC; GenSurg. (519)354-7676; Fax. (519)358-1361.

HADDAD, Georges; Pavillon Rosemont, 5F-5689 boul Rosemont, Montreal QC H1T 2H1; Paris (France)'71; Psy (P.Q.). Staff, Hopital Maisonneuve-Rosemont; (514)252-3400 x4770

HADDAD, Georges; 203-369 boul Fiset, Sorel-Tracy QC J3P 3R3; Beyrouth (Lebanon)'69; ABPeds; Peds. (450)742-3755; Fax. (450)746-3756.

HADDAD, Haissam A; Univ of Ottawa Heart Institute, 1289C-40 Ruskin St, Ottawa ON K1Y 4W7; Tishneen (Syria)'83; BSc; ABIM; FRCP; FRCPC; IntMed (Heart Transplantation); Cardiol. Staff, University of Ottawa Heart Institute; Langs: Arabic; French; (613)761-5165; Fax. (613)761-5212.

HADDAD, Henri K; CSSS de Laval, 1755 boul Rene-Laennec, Laval QC H7M 3L9; Mon'07; FRCPC; IntMed. Staff, Hopital de la Cite de la santé; (450)668-1010

HADDAD, Henry; CHUS, 555 rue Murray, Sherbrooke QC J1G 2K8; Ott'63; FRCPC; IntMed; Gastroent (P.Q.). Staff, Centre Hospitalier Universitaire de Sherbrooke-Hôpital Hôtel-Dieu; (819)346-1110

HADDAD, Jacob P; Polyclinique de Trois-Rivieres, 110-1900 boul des Recollets, Trois-Rivieres QC G8Z 4K4; Sher'73; PlasSurg (P.Q.). (819)376-1552; Fax. (819)373-9563.

HADDAD, Jacques; CHUS Hotel-Dieu, 580 rue Bowen S, Sherbrooke QC J1G 2E8; Sher'98; FRCSC; PlasSurg. Staff, Centre Hospitalier Universitaire de Sherbrooke-Hôpital Hôtel-Dieu; (819)346-1110

HADDAD, Margaret M; Albany Med Clinic, 807 Broadview Ave, Toronto ON M4K 2P8; McM'84; (416)461-9471; Fax. (416)461-2710.

HADDAD, Michel; Bluewater Health-Norman Site, 89 Norman St, Sarnia ON N7T 6S3; Ott'99; FRCSC; CardSurg; Critical Care Medicine. Staff, Bluewater Health - Norman Site; (519)464-4400

HADDAD, Richard G; London HSC-Victoria Hosp, PO Box 5010 Stn B 800 Commissioners Rd E, London ON N6A 5W9; Wes'74; DiagRad. Staff Radiol, London Health Sciences Centre - Victoria Campus; Assoc Prof, University of Western Ontario; (519)685-8500 x51388

HADDAD, Susan J P; 204-967 Bedford Hwy, Bedford NS B4A 1A9; Dal'07; CCFP; (902)835-6200; Fax. (902)832-7100.

HADDARA, Wael M; London HSC-University Hosp, PO Box 5339 Stn B 339 Windermere Rd E, London ON N6A 4G5; Qns'99; FRCPC; IntMed; Critical Care Medicine; Endocrin&Metab. Staff, London Health Sciences Centre - University Hospital; Asst Prof, University of Western Ontario; Langs: Arabic; (519)646-6082

HADDON, Roger W T; 2-809 Brant St, Burlington ON L7R 2J4; Durham (England)'62; MB BS; MRC; FCCP; FRCPC; IntMed (Respirology). (905)632-9015

HADDUD, Ahmed; US Memorial Hlth Ctr, PO Box 398, St Lawrence NL A0E 2V0; Al Fath (Libya)'04; MB BCh; Staff, US Memorial Health Centre; (709)873-2807

HADE-HETU, Sebastien; CSSS de la Baie-des-Chaleurs, RR 2 419 boul Perron, Maria QC G0C 1Y0; Mon'01; CCFP; Staff, CSSS de la Baie-des-Chaleurs; (418)759-3443

HADER, Walter J; Foothills Med Centre, 1403 29 St NW, Calgary AB T2N 2T9; Sask'94; FRCSC; Neursurg (Pediatrics). Staff, Alberta Children's Hospital; Staff, Foothills Medical Centre; (403)944-3498

HADER, Walter; Saskatoon City Hosp, 701 Queen St, Saskatoon SK S7K 0M7; Ott'58; MD; FRCPC; PhysMed&Rehab (Neuro Rehabilitation). Staff, Saskatoon City Hospital; (306)655-7742; Fax. (306)655-8404.

HADI, Ali; 2079 Lakeshore Rd, Burlington ON L7R 1E2; Baghdad (Iraq)'01; MB BS; CCFP; Langs: Arabic; (905)634-1625; Fax. (905)634-5332.

HADI, Ghassan M; 205-3017 66 St NW, Edmonton AB T6K 4B2; Baghdad (Iraq)'95; MB ChB; FRCSC; GenSurg (Minimal Invasive Surgery). Langs: Arabic; (780)461-6012; Fax. (780)461-5442.

HADI, Haidar M; Phoenix Med Centre, 209-2155 10th Ave, Prince George BC V2M 5J6; (Iraq)'94; MB ChB; (250)561-0666

HADI, Hani; Alberta Children's Hosp, 2888 Shaganappi Trail NW, Calgary AB T3B 6A8; Tor'00; FRCPC; Peds. Staff, Alberta Children's Hospital; (403)943-2953

HADI, Mohammed; Port Dover Med Centre, PO Box 728 807 St George St, Port Dover ON N0A 1N0; Ott'06; CCFP; (519)583-0893; Fax. (519)583-0010.

HADIAN, Abbas H; 310-1110 Sheppard Ave E, North York ON M2K 2W2; Tehran (Iran)'60; Staff, North York General Hospital; Staff, North York General Hospital - Branson Division; Staff Physician, North York After Hours Clinic; Langs: Farsi; (416)223-6929; Fax. (416)223-6820; dr.hadlan@rogers.com.

HADID, David; Royal Columbian Hosp, 330 Columbia St E, New Westminster BC V3L 3W7; McG'06; MDCM; Staff, Royal Columbian Hospital; (604)520-4253

HADJ KACEM, Chiraz; Hop Maisonneuve-Rosemont, 5415 boul de l'Assomption, Montreal QC H1T 2M4; (Tunisia)'03; FRCPC; AnatPath. Staff, Hopital Maisonneuve-Rosemont; (514)252-3400

HADJ TAHAR, Abdallah; Clinique Neuro Outaouais, 200-147 boul d'Europe, Gatineau QC J9J 0N3; Monastir (Tunisia)'95; FRCPC; Neur. (819)777-2500; Fax. (819)777-2502.

HADJERES, Rachid; CHUM-Hop Notre-Dame, 1560 rue Sherbrooke E, Montreal QC H2L 4M1; Alger (Algeria)'83; AnatPath (P.Q.). Staff, Centre Hospitalier l'Université de Montréal (CHUM) - Hôpital Notre-Dame; (514)890-8000 x26972

HADJIPAVLOU, George A; UBC-Dept Of Psychiatry, 2C7-2255 Wesbrook Mall, Vancouver BC V6T 2A1; Dal'03; FRCPC; Psy. Staff, UBC Hospital Pharmacy - Koerner Pavillion; Teach Staff, University of British Columbia; (604)822-7707; ghadjipavlou@psych.ubc.ca.

HADJIS, Tomy A; MUHC-Montreal Gen Hosp, E5 200-1650 av Cedar, Montreal QC H3G 1A4; Laval'87; CSPQ; FRCPC; IntMed; Cardiol. Staff, McGill University Health Centre - Montreal General Campus; (514)934-1934 x2654; Fax. (514)934-8344.

HADJIYANNAKIS, Anastasia; Children's Hosp Eastern Ont, 401 Smyth Rd, Ottawa ON K1H 8L1; Tor'96; BSc; FRCPCH; FRCPC; Peds (Pediatric Endocrinology); Endocrin&Metab. Staff, Children's Hospital of Eastern Ontario (CHEO); Langs: Greek; (613)737-2393 x3939; Fax. (613)738-4236; shadjiyannakis@cheo.on.ca.

HADJOUDJ, Hachemi; 1755 boul Rene-Laennec, Laval QC H7M 3L9; Alger (Algeria)'72; IntMed (P.Q.). Staff, Hopital de la Cite de la santé; Langs: English; Arabic; (450)668-1010; hachemih@gmail.com.

HADLAW, Violetta A; 1437 Belcher St PO Box 300, Port Williams NS B0P 1T0; Krakow (Poland)'89; FRCPC; IntMed. Langs: Polish; (902)542-0990; Fax. (902)542-1759.

HADLEY, Brian P; Napanee MMT Clinic, 104 John St, Napanee ON K7R 1R2; Qns'76; (613)354-9993

HADLEY, David L; Foothills Med Centre, C231-1403 29 St NW, Calgary AB T2N 2T9; UBC'96; BSc; MBA; CCFP; CCFP(E.M.); Staff, Foothills Medical Centre; (403)944-1820

HADLEY, John D; St Paul Family Health Network, Box 119 4F-99 Wayne Gretzky Pky, Brantford ON N3S 6T6; McM'91; CCFP; FCFP; (519)756-6400; Fax. (519)756-7343; john.hadley@sympatico.ca.

HADLEY, Katherine E; 116 Lansdowne St, Fredericton NB E3B 1T4; Mem'11.

HADLEY, Linda D; Sault Area Hosp, 750 Great Northern Rd, Sault Ste. Marie ON P6B 0A8; Tor'69; BSc; FRCPC; Anes. Staff Anesthetist, Sault Area Hospital - Sault Ste Marie; (705)759-3630

HADZIMUREZIC, Dzenita; Queen Elizabeth II HSC, 1276 South Park St, Halifax NS B3H 2Y9; Staff, Queen Elizabeth II Health Sciences Centre - Victoria General Site; (902)473-2700

HADZIOMEROVIC, Adnan; The Ottawa Hosp-Civic Campus, 1053 Carling Ave, Ottawa ON K1Y 4E9; Ott'93; FRCPC; DiagRad. Staff, The Ottawa Hospital - Civic Campus; (613)761-4054

HAEBE, James R; Soundcare Med Centre, 560-1145 Hunt Club Rd, Ottawa ON K1V 0Y3; Tor'86; FRCSC; ObstGyn. Staff, The Ottawa Hospital - General Campus; Asst Prof, University of Ottawa; (613)738-2378

HAEBE, Jeffrey J; Ottawa Fertility Centre, 955 Green Valley Cres, Ottawa ON K2C 3V4; Tor'94; FRCSC; ObstGyn (Gynecological Reproductive Endocrinology). (613)686-3378 x430

HAECK, Olivier; CSSS de Laval, 1755 boul Rene-Laennec, Laval QC H7M 3L9; Mon'02; FRCPC; MedMicrobiol; Microbio & Infect Dis (P.Q.). Staff, Hopital de la Cite de la santé; (450)975-5558; Fax. (450)975-5095.

HAEGERT, David; Duff Med Bldg, 3775 University St, Montreal QC H3A 2B4; UBC'68; CSPQ; FRCPC; AnatPath. Prof, McGill University; Fax. (514)398-5599; david.haegert@muhc.mcgill.ca.

HAENE, Roger; Dr Everett Chalmers Reg Hosp, PO Box 9000 Stn A 700 Priestman St, Fredericton NB E3B 5N5; (South Africa)'97; Staff, Dr Everett Chalmers Regional Hospital; (506)452-5400

HAENSEL, Heidi M; London HSC-Victoria Hosp, PO Box 5010 Stn B 800 Commissioners Rd E, London ON N6A 5W9; Mem'03; FRCPC; Psy. Staff, London Health Sciences Centre - Victoria Campus; (519)685-8500

HAF GAGNE, Valerie; CLSC des Faubourgs, 1250 rue Sanguinet, Montreal QC H2X 3E7; Mon'08; CCFP; (514)527-2361

HAFAZALLA, Basem K; 1F-75 Charles St, Brockville ON K6V 1S8; Assiut (Egypt)'85; FRCOG(UK); FRCSC; ObstGyn (Minimal Invasive Surgery). Staff, Yarmouth Regional Hospital; Langs: Arabic; (613)498-0740; Fax. (613)345-3036; bkhafazalla@hotmail.com.

HAFEZ, Ali; Hop du Sacre-Coeur de Mtl, 5400 boul Gouin O, Montreal QC H4J 1C5; Cairo (Egypt)'81; Ophth (P.Q.). Staff, Hôpital du Sacre-Coeur de Montréal; (514)338-2222; Fax. (514)338-3515.

HAFEZ, Kevin; Sunridge Family Med Teaching C, 2685 36th St NE, Calgary AB T1Y 5S3; Debrecen (Hungary)'94; MHSA; MA; CCFP; FCFP; Staff, Sunridge Family Medicine Teaching Centre; Langs: Hungarian; Finnish; Arabic; (403)943-5000

HAFEZ, Mohammed N; Ottawa Cardiovascular Centre, 502-1355 Bank St, Ottawa ON K1H 8K7; Damascus (Syria)'94; FRCPC; IntMed; Cardiol. Staff, University of Ottawa Heart Institute; (613)738-1584; Fax. (613)738-9097.

HAFEZ, Shahira O; Trillium Hlth Ctr-Queensway, 150 Sherway Dr, Etobicoke ON M9C 1A5; Ain Shams (Egypt)'74; FRCPC; Anes. Staff, Trillium Health Centre - West Toronto; (416)259-6671; Fax. (905)602-5674.

HAFEZI, Rod; Bose & Hafezi Med Specialists, 140B Idylwyld Dr N, Saskatoon SK S7L 0Y7; Saba (Netherlands Antilles)'99; FACP; FRCPC; IntMed (Sleep Medicine); Respir. Staff, Saskatoon City Hospital; Clin Assoc Prof, Royal University Hospital; Langs: Farsi; Spanish; (306)933-3004; rhafezi@yahoo.com.

HAFEZI BAKHTIARI, Sara; Univ Hlth Network-Toronto Gen, 200 Elizabeth St, Toronto ON M5G 2C4; Isfahan (Iran)'01; AnatPath. Staff, Toronto General Hospital - UHN; Langs: Farsi; (416)340-4800

HAFFNER, Thomas D; Jenny trouit Centre, 110-342 Erie St, Stratford ON N5A 2N4; Wes'08; FRCPC; IntMed. (519)273-1990

HAFIDH, Maky; Eastside Orthopedics Inc, LL-1481 George St, Sydney NS B1P 1P2; Baghdad (Iraq)'90; FRCSI; FRCSC; Otol (Head & Neck). Staff, Cape Breton Healthcare Complex; (902)270-3356; Fax. (902)270-3357.

HAFIZ, Hasan; 2070-11300 Tuscany Blvd NW, Calgary AB T3L 2V7; Ain Shams (Egypt)'82; Langs: Turkish; Arabic; German; (403)263-0091; Fax. (403)263-0082; hasan.hafiz@shaw.ca.

HAFIZ, Shujauddin F; The Southcom Bldg, 301-2227 South Millway, Mississauga ON L5L 3R6; Karnatak (India)'80; MB BS; MRCP; FRCPC; Peds (Neonatology). Langs: Urdu; (905)569-9798; Fax. (905)569-8630.

HAFUTH, Falih M; Guelph Gen Hosp, 115 Delhi St, Guelph ON N1E 4J4; Mosil (Iraq)'83; MB ChB; CCFP; FCFP; Staff, Woodstock General Hospital; Langs: Arabic; Farsi; (519)837-6440

HAGE, Bechir; CSSS de Laval, 1755 boul Rene-Laennec, Laval QC H7M 3L9; Sher'05; Urol. Staff, Hopital de la Cite de la santé; (450)668-1010

HAGEL, Jeffrey A; Peace Arch Hosp, 15521 Russell Ave, White Rock BC V4B 2R4; UBC'02; FRCPC; DiagRad. Staff, Peace Arch Hospital; (604)531-5512

HAGEN, Arlene D; 4018 rue Sainte-Catherine O, Westmount QC H3Z 1P2; Mayo Minnesota (USA)'89; Psy (P.Q.). (514)412-4449 x22401; Fax. (514)412-4346.

HAGEN, Barry A; Phoenix Med Centre, 307-2155 10th Ave, Prince George BC V2M 5J6; UBC'65; Ac Staff, University Hospital of Northern British Columbia; (250)563-8013; Fax. (250)563-7105.

HAGEN, Catherine A; Univ Hosp of Northern BC, 1475 Edmonton St, Prince George BC V2M 1S2; Cal'86; CCFP; CCFP(E.M.); FCFP; Staff, University Hospital of Northern British Columbia; Aj Prof, University of Northern British Columbia; Clin Instructor, University of British Columbia; (250)565-2000

HAGEN, John A; 504-960 Lawrence Ave W, North York ON M6A 3B5; Alb'79; FRCSC; GenSurg (Laparoscopy). Staff/Head Gen Surg, Humber River Regional Hospital - Keele Street Site; Lecturer, University of Toronto; (416)782-2616; Fax. (416)782-5899.

HAGEN, Margarietha J; Viking Med Clinic, PO BOX 868 5301 51 St, Viking AB T0B 4N0; (780)336-4780; Fax. (780)336-2020.

HAGEN, Neil A; Tom Baker Cancer Centre, 1331 29 St NW, Calgary AB T2N 4N2; Alb'82; FRCPC; Neur (Cancer Pain Management). Staff, Tom Baker Cancer Centre; Prof, Foothills Medical Centre; Assoc Prof/Dir Palliative Med Residency Prog, University of Calgary; (403)521-3446

HAGEN, Paul; Cowichan Dist Hosp, 3045 Gibbins Rd, Duncan BC V9L 1E5; UBC'95; FRCPC; DiagRad. Staff, Campbell River & District General Hospital; (250)709-3000

HAGENS, John E; Dr J Hagens & J Norheim Partne, PO Box 5219 Stn Main 117 Macleod Trail, High River AB T1V 1M4; Cal'96; CCFP; Med Staff, High River General Hospital; Med Examiner, Alberta Department of Justice; Associate Clin Prof of Med Dept of Family Med, University of Calgary; (403)652-5333; Fax. (403)652-5375.

HAGERMAN, R Neil; Acadia Med Centre, 202-8330 Fairmount Dr SE, Calgary AB T2H 0Y8; Alb'83; FRCSC; GenSurg. Ac Staff, Rockyview General Hospital; (403)252-5674; Fax. (403)252-3938.

HAGGAR, Carine; MUHC-Royal Victoria Hosp, 687 av des Pins O, Montreal QC H3A 1A1; McG'96; MD; FRCPC; EmergMed. Staff, McGill University Health Centre - Montreal Children's Hospital; Staff Emerg, McGill University Health Centre - Royal Victoria Hospital; Staff Emerg, McGill University Health Centre - Montreal General Campus; adj Prof, McGill University; Langs: Bilingual(French/English); (514)934-1934 x32557; carine71@yahoo.com.

HAGGARD, Gian; Dakota Med Centre, 17-845 Dakota St, Winnipeg MB R2M 5M3; Orange Free State (South Africa)'95; CCFP; (204)254-2087; Fax. (204)254-0822.

HAGGARTY, John M; St Joseph's Health Centre, 710 Victoria Ave E, Thunder Bay ON P7C 5P7; McM'88; BSc(Hon); FRCPC; Psy. Staff, Lakehead Psychiatric Hospital - St. Joseph's Care Group; Prof Clerkship Lead, Northern Ontario School of Medicine-Laurentian University; (807)624-3400; Fax. (807)624-3401.

HAGGBLAD, John S; Gulf Canada Square, 362-401 9 Ave SW, Calgary AB T2P 3C5; Cal'84; CCFP; FCFP; Staff, Rockyview General Hospital; (403)221-4424; Fax. (403)221-4426.

HAGGERTY, Mary E; Family Med Associates, 7004 98 Ave NW, Edmonton AB T6A 0A5; Alb'72; MSc; (780)468-6035; Fax. (780)466-9132.

HAGHIGHAT, Kasra; 2-10660 Yonge St, Richmond Hill ON L4C 3C9; Sask'04; (905)770-9096; Fax. (905)770-4703.

HAGHIGHAT TALAB, Amir Tinouch; CSSSG-Hop de Hull, 116 boul Lionel-Emond, Gatineau QC J8Y 1W7; Paris (France)'99; FRCPC; Cardiol. Staff, Hull Hospital; Langs: Persian; Bilingual(English/French); Farsi; (819)966-6200; hagh@rogers.com.

HAGOPIAN, Salpi; 301-1600 boul Cure-Labelle, Laval QC H7V 2W2; Aleppo (Syria)'79; CCFP; Ac Staff, CSSS du Coeur de l'Isle Hôpital Jean-Talon; (450)978-9173; Fax. (450)978-0782; salpih@sympatico.ca.

HAGSHI, Judy L; Clinique Med VMS, 201-6260 av Victoria, Montreal QC H3W 2S3; Tor'96; CCFP; Staff, Sir Mortimer B Davis Jewish General; (514)344-0098; Fax. (514)344-0061.

HAGUE, Cameron J; St Paul's Hosp, 1081 Burrard St, Vancouver BC V6Z 1Y6; UBC'03; FRCPC; DiagRad. Staff, Providence Health Care - St Paul's Hospital; (604)682-2344

HAGUE, Jayne L A; Kingsland Med Clinic, 7712 Elbow Dr SW, Calgary AB T2V 1K2; Sask'84; CCFP; FCFP; Staff, Rockyview General Hospital; (403)252-6681; Fax. (403)252-9741.

HAHLWEG, Kenneth A; J A Hildes Northern Medical, T162-770 Bannatyne Ave, Winnipeg MB R3E 0W3; Man'93; BSc; CCFP; FCFP; Staff, Health Sciences Centre; Dir, University Health Services; University of Manitoba; Langs: German; (204)789-3711

HAHN, Angelika F G; London HSC-University Hosp, PO Box 5339 Stn B 339 Windermere Rd, London ON N6A 5A5; Munich (Germany)'65; FRCPC; Neur (Neuromuscular Diseases). Dir Neuromuscular Clinic, London Health Sciences Centre - University Hospital; Prof, University of Western Ontario; (519)663-3110; Fax. (519)663-3328; angelika.hahn@lhsc.on.ca.

HAHN, Cecil D A; 555 University Ave, Toronto ON M5G 1X8; Tor'98; MPH; CSCN; FRCPC; Neur (Clinical Neurophysiology). Staff, The Hospital For Sick Children; Langs: French; German; (416)813-6659; Fax. (416)813-6334.

HAHN, Ernest M; Huron Business Centre, 8B-31 Mcbrine Dr, Kitchener ON N2R 1J1; McM'82; BSc; MD; CCFP; CCFP(E.M.); Staff Family Med, St Mary's General Hospital; Staff Family Med, Grand River Hospital - Kitchener/Waterloo Health Centre; Langs: Spanish; (519)893-5568; Fax. (519)893-5795.

HAHN, Johann A; Yorkton Reg Hlth Centre, 270 Bradbrooke Dr, Yorkton SK S3N 2K6; Cape Town (South Africa)'72; Staff, Yorkton Regional Health Centre; (306)786-0427; Fax. (306)786-0424.

HAHN, Karin M E; London Reg Cancer Centre, 790 Commissioners Rd E, London ON N6A 4L6; Tor'94; FRCPC; MedOncol; IntMed. Staff, London Health Sciences Centre - London Regional Cancer Centre; (519)685-8600; karin.hahn@lhsc.on.ca.

HAHN, Margaret K; Addiction & Mental Hlth-Clark, 250 College St, Toronto ON M5T 1R8; Cal'04; FRCPC; Psy. Staff, Centre for Addiction & Mental Health (CAMH) - College Street Site; Langs: Polish; French; (416)535-8501

HAHN, Miah; The Court, 101-2863 Ellesmere Rd, Scarborough ON M1E 5E9; Tor'88; FRCSC; OrthSurg (Pediatric Orthopedic Surgery). Ac Staff OrthSurg, Rouge Valley Health System - Ajax & Pickering Health Centre Site; Ac Staff OrthSurg, Rouge Valley Health System - Centenary Health Centre Site; (416)283-2311; Fax. (416)284-1218.

HAHN, Michael E J; 204-135 15th St E, North Vancouver BC V7L 2P7; Wes'79; BSc; FRCPC; IntMed (Gastrointestinal & Hepatic Disease); Gastroent. Staff, Lions Gate Hospital; (604)984-4138; Fax. (604)984-6606.

HAHN, Peter J; 535 Broadway E, Vancouver BC V5T 1X4; Alb'03; CCFP; Staff, Eagle Ridge Hospital & Health Care Centre; (778)229-0502

HAHN-LEE, June H; Windsor Health Unit, 254-1720 Howard Ave, Windsor ON N8X 5A6; Seoul (Korea)'66; Peds. Ac Staff, Windsor Regional Hospital - Metropolitan Site; Ac Staff, Hôtel-Dieu Grace Hospital; Langs: Korean; (519)252-9445; Fax. (519)252-8080.

HAIART, Dominique C; Thompson Gen Hosp, 871 Thompson Dr S, Thompson MB R8N 0C8; London (England)'76; FRCSC; GenSurg. Staff, Thompson General Hospital; (204)677-2381

HAICHIN, Richard N; MUHC-Royal Victoria Hosp, M4 76-687 av des Pins O, Montreal QC H3A 1A1; McG'79; CSPQ; FRCPC; IntMed (Echocardiography); Cardiol (P.Q.). Staff, McGill University Health Centre - Royal Victoria Hospital; Staff, St Mary's Hospital Centre; Staff, McGill University Health Centre - Montreal General Campus; Langs: English; French; (514)934-1934 x35737; Fax. (514)843-2813; richard.haichin@muhc.mcgill.ca.

HAIDAR, Mukhtar; Associate Clinic, 5215 49 Ave, Wetaskiwin AB T9A 0R1; Punjab (Pakistan)'65; CCFP; Langs: Urdu; (780)352-7157; Fax. (780)352-2273.

HAIDAR, Nadim; 335-955 Queen St E, Sault Ste. Marie ON P6A 2C3; Wes'05; Urol. Staff, Sault Area Hospital - Sault Ste Marie; (705)254-4364

HAIDAR, Rafid; Ctr de Sante Vallee-Gatineau, 309 boul Desjardins, Maniwaki QC J9E 2E7; McG'94; FRCPC; IntMed. Staff, CSSS de la Vallée de la Gatineau; (819)449-2300

HAIDASH, Serhii; Eastside Med Clinic, 82 Great Plains Rd, Emerald Park SK S4L 1C3; (Ukraine)'87; (306)871-7077

HAIDER, Aamir; Chamber of Commerce Bldg, 302-345 Lakeshore Rd E, Oakville ON L6J 1J5; Sask'97; PharmD; BScPharm; FRCPC; Derm;CCFP; Langs: Urdu; (905)842-8500; Fax. (905)842-8502.

HAIDER, Ehsan A H; St Joseph's Healthcare, T0733-50 Charlton Ave E, Hamilton ON L8N 3Z5; Cairo (Egypt)'98; FRCPC; DiagRad. Staff, St Joseph's Healthcare - Charlton Campus; (905)522-1155 x37326

HAIDER, Erum; Medical Health Centre, 18-1615 Dundas St E, Whitby ON L1N 2L1; (Pakistan)'96; CCFP; Langs: Urdu; (905)240-2880

HAIDER, Esam M S; Grey Bruce HS-Owen Sound, PO Box 1800 Stn Main 7219-1800 8th St E, Owen Sound ON N4K 6M9; Al-Fateh (Libya)'92; FRCSC; OrthSurg. Staff, Grey Bruce Health Services - Owen Sound; Langs: Arabic; (519)376-2121; Fax. (519)372-3358.

HAIDER, Kamal-Uddin; Saskatoon Cancer Centre, 20 Campus Dr, Saskatoon SK S7N 4H4; Karachi (Pakistan)'91; MB BS; Clin Assoc Prof, Royal University Hospital; Staff, Saskatoon Cancer Centre; (306)655-2710; Fax. (306)655-2910.

HAIDER, Kamil; William Osler HC-Etobicoke, 101 Humber College Blvd, Etobicoke ON M9V 1R8; Sask'00; BSc; CCFP; Chief EmergMed Etobicoke Gen Hosp, William Osler Health System - Etobicoke General Hospital; Asst Clin Prof (Adjunct), McMaster University; Langs: Urdu; Hindi; (416)747-3400

HAIDER, Masoom A; Sunnybrook Hlth Sciences Ctre, 2075 Bayview Ave, Toronto ON M4N 3M5; Ott'86; FRCPC; DiagRad. Staff, Princess Margaret Hospital - University Health Network; Staff, Sunnybrook Health Sciences Centre; (416)480-6100

HAIDER, Seemab; Alberta Children's Hosp, 2888 Shaganappi Trail NW, Calgary AB T3B 6A8; (Turkey)'95; Staff, Alberta Children's Hospital; (403)955-7985; seemab.haider@calgaryhealthregion.ca.

HAIDER, Shariq; Hamilton HS-Juravinski Site, A3 79-711 Concession St, Hamilton ON L8V 1C3; Sask'95; FRCPC; IntMed; InfectDis. Staff, Hamilton Health Sciences Centre - McMaster Children's Hospital; Staff, Hamilton Health Sciences Centre-Juravinski Site; (905)389-4411

HAIDER, Syed N; Ridge Meadows Hosp & Hlth CC, 11666 Laity St, Maple Ridge BC V2X 5A3; Rawalpindi (Pakistan)'96; MB BS; Staff, Ridge Meadows Hospital & Health Care Centre; (604)463-1870

HAIDER, Syed Y A; Markham Stouffville Health Ctr, 406-377 Church St, Markham ON L6B 1A1; Punjab (Pakistan)'89; MB BS; FRCSOrth; FRCSC; OrthSurg (Sports Medicine). Staff, Markham Stouffville Hospital; Langs: Punjabi; Urdu; (905)472-2755; Fax. (905)472-3455.

HAIDER, Umar; Clayton Park Med Centre, 101C-278 Lacewood Dr, Halifax NS B3M 3N8; Punjab, Pakistan (Pakistan)'84; MB BS; CCFP; Langs: Urdu; (902)445-9600; Fax. (902)445-4270.

HAIDUK, Michael J; Kimberley Med Clinic, PO Box 160, Kimberley BC V1A 2Y6; Tor'78; BSc(Hon); CCFP; FCFP; Staff, East Kootenay Regional Hospital; (250)427-4861; Fax. (250)427-2082.

HAIEK, Laura N; Roper Clinic, 4500 rue Sherbrooke O, Westmount QC H3Z 1E6; Buenos Aires (Argentina)'84; MSc(Epidem&Biostats); MSc(Nutrition); CCFP; Langs: Spanish; French; (514)937-8000; Fax. (514)937-8884; l.haiek@rrsss16.gouv.qc.ca.

HAIG, Aaron R; London HSC-University Hosp, PO Box 5339 Stn B 339 Windermere Rd, London ON N6A 5A5; Wes'03; FRCPC; AnatPath. Staff, London Health Sciences Centre - University Hospital; (519)685-8500

HAIG, Charlotte E; Haig Clinic, 601 6 Ave S, Lethbridge AB T1J 0Z2; Alb'98; BSc; CCFP; FCFP; (403)328-6641; Fax. (403)328-6118.

HAIG, Cynthia L; Atrium Prof Centre, 203-190 Cundles Rd E, Barrie ON L4M 4S5; McM'83; CCFP; FCFP; Staff, Royal Victoria Regional Health Centre; (705)726-8393; Fax. (705)726-8398.

HAIG, Margaret J; Hôpital Ste-Justine, 3175 ch Cote-Sainte-Catherine, Montreal QC H3T 1C5; McM'76; CSPQ; FRCPC; Anes. Staff, Hôpital Ste-Justine; (514)345-4931

HAIG, Sara L; St Joseph's Health Care, PO Box 5777 Stn B 268 Grosvenor St, London ON N6A 4V2; Wes'04; FRCPC; IntMed; Rheum. Staff, St Joseph's Hospital - St Joseph's Health Care; (519)646-6330

HAIGH, Donald; Praxes Emerg Specialists, 6030 Almon St, Halifax NS B3K 1T8; McG'71; MSc; Asst Prof, School of Epidemiology & Community Medicine; Langs: French; (902)420-9725; Fax. (902)420-9987.

HAIGH, Kim D; 4-389 Main St E PO Box 2200, Picton ON K0K 2T0; Alb'98; CCFP; FCFP; (613)476-3103; Fax. (613)476-1604.

HAIGH, Susan E; 1102-160 14th St E, North Vancouver BC V7L 2N3; Cal'78; FRCPC; IntMed (Diabetology); Endocrin&Metab. Ac Staff, Lions Gate Hospital; Clin Instructor, University of British Columbia; (604)987-0480; Fax. (604)987-3699.

HAIGHT, James S J; North Toronto Med Bldg, 308-250 Lawrence Ave W, Toronto ON M5M 1B2; Oxford (England)'73; PhD; FACS; FRCSC; Otol (Nasal & Sinus Surgery). Staff, North York General Hospital - Branson Division; Staff, Humber River Regional Hospital - Keele Street Site; Staff, St Michael's Hospital; Assoc Prof, University of Toronto; Langs: Italian; German; French; (416)787-5511; Fax. (416)787-1592.

HAIKAL, Youssef; Polyclinique de l'Oreille, 252-1111 rue Saint-Charles O, Longueuil QC J4K 5G4; St. Joseph (Lebanon)'84; ABOtol; FRCSC; Otol (Head & Neck Surgery). Staff, Hopital Charles LeMoyne; Staff, Centre ORL de Montreal; Staff, Institut ORL de Montreal; Langs: Arabic; English; (450)651-9000; Fax. (450)679-1651.

HAILE MESKEL, Helena; Centenary Health Centre, 2867 Ellesmere Rd, Scarborough ON M1E 4B9; Addis Ababa (Ethiopia)'73; FCAP; FRCPC; AnatPath (Hematology Pathology). Staff, Rouge Valley Health System - Centenary Health Centre Site; Langs: Amharic; (416)284-8131; Fax. (416)281-7486; hmeskel@rougevalley.ca.

HAILEMESKEL, Yemisrach; 206B-1011 Dufferin St, Toronto ON M6H 4B5; Komensky (Slovakia)'83; CCFP; Ac Staff Family Med, St Joseph's Health Centre; Langs: Amharic; Slovak; (416)537-2438; Fax. (416)537-9056.

HAILEY, Jane; Fairmont Med Bldg, 1314-750 Broadway W, Vancouver BC V5Z 1J3; Cambridge (England)'85; MB ChB; FRCPC; Peds. Staff, BC Children's Hospital; Staff, BC Women's Hospital & Health Centre; (604)879-4564; Fax. (604)879-5191.

HAILU, Maru E; North Oshawa Med Centre, 101-1400 Ritson Rd N, Oshawa ON L1G 7W4; (Ethiopia)'93; CCFP; Langs: Amharic; (905)433-0001; Fax. (905)721-1366.

HAILU, Tadesse; Caswell Med Clinic, 511H 33rd St W, Saskatoon SK S7L 0V7; Medunsa (South Africa)'78; (306)244-5529

HAILU, Tesfu; Dynacare Kasper Med Lab, 200-10150 102 St NW, Edmonton AB T5J 5E2; Addis Ababa (Ethiopia)'94.

HAINC, Milan; 3-1767 152 St, Surrey BC V4A 4N3; Giessen (Germany)'87; (604)535-3388; Fax. (604)542-2667.

HAINEAULT, Caroline; Ctr Hosp Anna-Laberge, 200 boul Brisebois, Chateauguay QC J6K 4W8; Laval'08; CCFP; Staff, Hôpital Anna-Laberge; Médecin, Clinique Medicale Napierville; Langs: Bilingual(French/English); (450)699-2424; Fax. (450)699-2525; chaineault@hotmail.com.

HAINEAULT, Rejean; CLSC des Mille-Iles, 4731 boul Levesque E, Laval QC H7C 1M9; Mon'68; (450)661-2572; Fax. (450)661-5322.

HAINER, Steven C; 87 Adelaide St N, Lindsay ON K9V 4L4; Ott'94; CCFP; FCFP; (705)324-2561; Fax. (705)328-1816.

HAINER, Tammy L; Tillsonburg Med Centre, 200 Broadway St, Tillsonburg ON N4G 5A7; McM'07; CCFP; (519)842-4231; Fax. (519)842-3793.

HAINES, A Theodore S; McMaster University, 125-1280 Main St W, Hamilton ON L8S 4K1; Tor'78; DOHS; MSc; FRCPC; CommunMed; OccupMed. Staff, Hamilton Health Sciences Centre - McMaster Children's Hospital; Physician, Lakeshore Multiservice Project Occup Health Program; Teach Staff Clin Epidemiol, McMaster University; hainest@mcmaster.ca.

HAINES, Alexander M; Barrie Family Medicine, 18 Cundles Rd E, Barrie ON L4M 2Z5; Wes'88; Ac Staff, Royal Victoria Regional Health Centre; (705)737-1887; Fax. (705)735-6949.

HAINES, Barbara J; 101-1032 Austin Ave, Coquitlam BC V3K 3P3; UBC'89; (604)939-2441; Fax. (604)939-2420.

HAINES, Gregory C; Gagetown Med Clinic, 209 Ross Terrace, Fredericton NB E3A 8E5; Dal'81; CCFP; Ac Staff Privil, Oromocto Public Hospital; Court Staff Privil, Dr Everett Chalmers Regional Hospital; (506)488-2312; Fax. (506)488-1091.

HAINS, Melanie; Ctr Hosp Affilie-Enfant-Jesus, 1401 18e rue, Quebec QC G1J 1Z4; Laval'99; FRCPC; IntMed; GeriatricMed. Staff, Centre Hospitalier Affilié Universitaire de Québec - Hôpital De L'Enfant Jésus; (418)649-0252

HAIR, Amarjit S; 103-7130 120 St, Surrey BC V3W 3M8; UBC'88; (604)572-4437

HAISLIP, Heidi L; Family Practice Associates, 6155 North St, Halifax NS B3K 5R3; Dal'94; (902)453-3511; Fax. (902)454-9010.

HAIST, David W; 389 Greenwood Ave, North Bay ON P1B 5G3; Tor'71; Staff, North Bay Regional Health Centre - Regional Mental Health; (705)494-9643

HAJAR, Khaled; 235-9450 137 Ave NW, Edmonton AB T5E 6C2; (Cayman Islands)'09; (780)475-0934; Fax. (780)475-0732.

HAJAS, Adriana; James Snow Med & Walk-In Clini, C2-51 James Snow Pky, Milton ON L9T 0R3; Washington (WA)'90; CCFP; (905)636-1050; Fax. (905)636-1090.

HAJCSAR, Elizabeth M; 526 Guelph Line, Burlington ON L7R 3M4; Qns'91; CCFP; FCFP; (289)337-9628

HAJCSAR, Ernest E; EH2 Med Assoc/Aesthetica MD, B6-645 Plains Rd E, Burlington ON L7T 4J5; Qns'99; PhD; BSc; BEd; CCFP; FCFP; (905)681-3430; Fax. (905)681-7525.

HAJEK, David M; 230-1333 Sheppard Ave E, North York ON M2J 1V1; Minneapolis(MN) (USA)'01; FRCSC; Urol. Staff, Mount Sinai Hospital; (416)494-7900

HAJEK, Jan J; Heather Pavilion, 452 D-2733 Heather St, Vancouver BC V5Z 3J5; Qns'01; FRCPC; IntMed; InfectDis. Staff, The Ottawa Hospital - General Campus; (604)875-4588

HAJEK, Tomas; Abbie J Lane Mem Bldg, 3093-5909 Veterans Memorial La, Halifax NS B3H 2E2; Czech.Rep. (Czech Republic)'99; Staff, Queen Elizabeth II Health Sciences Centre - Victoria General Site; (902)473-8299; Fax. (902)473-4877.

HAJELA, Raju; 305-320 23 Ave SW, Calgary AB T2S 0J2; Dal'82; MPH(Harvard); CCFP; FCFP; Consultant Addiction Med & Chronic Pain, Alberta Health Services Calgary; Langs: Hindi; Urdu; (403)536-2480; Fax. (403)536-2482; rajuhajela@hotmail.com.

HAJI, Salah A; Leaf Rapids Health Centre, PO Box 370, Leaf Rapids MB R0B 1W0; (Somalia)'85; Staff, Percy E Moore Hospital; (204)376-2781; salah_haji@hc-sc.gc.ca.

HAJI PAVLOU, Christopher; Mainland Medical Clinic, 1061 Hamilton St, Vancouver BC V6B 5T4; Pretoria (South Africa)'04; MB ChB; (604)683-3973

HAJIDIACOS, Nicholas P; St Boniface Gen Hosp, C5104-409 Tache Ave, Winnipeg MB R2H 2A6; Man'00; FRCPC; IntMed. Staff, St Boniface General Hospital; (204)233-8563

HAJJAR, Edward; Ctr Hosp de Verdun, 4000 boul Lasalle, LaSalle QC H4G 2A3; Mon'08; CCFP; Staff, Centre Hospitalier de Verdun; (514)362-1000

HAJJAR, Eliane; Hydro Quebec, 101-75 boul Rene-Levesque O, Montreal QC H2Z 1A4; Mon'89; CCFP; (514)289-2211 x4291

HAJJAR, Georges E; The Ottawa Hosp-Civic Campus, A2 80-1053 Carling Ave, Ottawa ON K1Y 4E9; Ott'84; FRCSC; GenSurg; VascSurg. Prog Dir Div of Vasc Surg, The Ottawa Hospital - Civic Campus; Staff, The Ottawa Hospital - General Campus; Assoc Prof Surg, University of Ottawa; (613)761-4766; Fax. (613)761-5362; ghajjar@ottawahospital.on.ca.

HAJRA, Leena; Markham Stouffville Health Ctr, 407-377 Church St, Markham ON L6B 1A1; Tor'05; FRCPC; IntMed; MedOncol. Staff, Sunnybrook Health Sciences Centre; (905)472-7072; Fax. (905)472-0529.

HAJY AGHAEI, Roya; Bayview-Finch Med Clinic, 202-3292 Bayview Ave, North York ON M2M 4J5; (Iran)'92; CCFP; Langs: Farsi; Persian; (416)222-9955; Fax. (416)222-8088.

HAK, Hendrik C; Medical Arts Centre, 770 6 St SW, Medicine Hat AB T1A 8M7; Utrecht (Netherlands)'78; FRCPC; Peds. (403)502-8931

HAKA-IKSE, Katerina K; 908-123 Edward St, Toronto ON M5G 1E2; Athens (Greece)'52; FAAP; FRCPC; Peds (Developmental/Behavioural Pediatrics). Sr Physician, The Hospital For Sick Children; Emeritus Prof Peds, University of Toronto; Langs: French; Greek; (416)596-8918; Fax. (416)596-1041; haka-Ikse@bellnet.ca.

HAKAMI, M Taghi; CSSS de Chicoutimi, 305 rue Saint-Vallier, Chicoutimi QC G7H 5H6; Toulouse (France)'64; Staff, Complexe hospitalier de la Sagamie; Langs: Farsi; English; (418)541-1000; t.hakami@sympatico.ca.

HAKES, Jacqueline J; Peter Lougheed Centre, 3500 26 Ave NE, Calgary AB T1Y 6J4; Tor'98; CCFP; Staff, Peter Lougheed Centre; (403)943-5461; Fax. (403)943-5438.

HAKES, John A A; Greenestone Clinic, 300-5734 Yonge St, North York ON M2M 4E7; Bristol (England)'59; MB ChB; FRCA; FRCPC; Anes. Assoc Staff Anes, Markham Stouffville Hospital.

HAKIM, Antoine M; Univ of Ottawa, 2413-451 Smyth Rd, Ottawa ON K1H 8M5; Albany(NY) (USA)'75; PhD; FRCPC; Neur. Ac Staff, The Ottawa Hospital - General Campus; Staff, University of Ottawa; (613)562-5462; Fax. (613)562-5403; ahakim@ohri.ca.

HAKIM, David; CSSS de Trois-Rivières, 1991 boul du Carmel, Trois-Rivieres QC G8Z 3R9; Mon'07; Anes. Staff, CSSS de Trois-Rivières; (819)697-3333

HAKIM, Hassan R; Royal Victoria Hosp, 201 Georgian Dr, Barrie ON L4M 6M2; Dacca (Bangladesh)'76; MRCPsy; DTMH; DCH; DPM; FRCPC; Psy. Staff, Royal Victoria Regional Health Centre; Langs: Bengali; (705)728-9090 x47210; Fax. (705)739-5631.

HAKIM, M Omar; Windsor Reg Hosp-Metropolitan, 1995 Lens Ave, Windsor ON N8W 1L9; Aga Khan (Pakistan)'90; MB BS; FRCPC; AnatPath. Staff, Hôtel-Dieu Grace Hospital; Staff, Windsor Regional Hospital - Metropolitan Site; (519)254-5577

HAKIM, Miriam; Medistat Med Familiale, 4965 rue Saint-Pierre, Pierrefonds QC H9H 5M9; Cincinnati(OH) (USA)'98; FRCPC; Derm (Pediatric Dermatology). Att Staff, McGill University Health Centre - Montreal Children's Hospital; Consultant Derm, Lakeshore General Hospital - Pointe Claire; adj Prof, McGill University; (514)624-4774

HAKIM, Omar; 316-1235 Trafalgar Rd, Oakville ON L6H 3P1; Wes'87; FRCSC; Ophth. Ac Consultant, Halton Healthcare Services Corporation - Oakville Site; Affil Consultant, Joseph Brant Memorial Hospital; Affil Consultant, Halton Healthcare Services Corporation - Georgetown Hospital; (905)338-6786

HAKIM, Ronnie; First Med Place, 205-170 Queensway W, Mississauga ON L5B 3A8; Sher'80; FRCSC; ObstGyn. Ac Staff, Trillium Health Centre - Mississauga; (905)896-3443; Fax. (905)896-4848.

HAKIM, Samira; Clinique Medicale, 205-1850 boul Le Corbusier, Laval QC H7S 2K1; Alger (Algeria)'75; (450)686-6661; Fax. (450)686-4811.

HAKIM, Sania; Northumberland Hills Hosp, 1000 DePalma Dr, Cobourg ON K9A 5W6; (Pakistan)'89; Staff, Northumberland Hills Hospital; (905)372-6811

HAKOUN, Jack; 105-5 Broadway Ave, Toronto ON M4P 1T7; Tor'83; Staff Family Practice, North York General Hospital; Langs: French; Hebrew; (416)480-1460

HALAC, Ugur; Hôpital Ste-Justine, 3175 ch Cote-Ste-Catherine, Montreal QC H3T 1C5; (Belgium)'02; Gastroent (P.Q.). Staff, Hôpital Ste-Justine; Langs: Bilingual(French/English); (514)345-4931; Fax. (514)345-4741; ugur_halac@yahoo.fr.

HALASA, L Nicole; Bridgeland Prof Centre, 306-1010 1 Ave NE, Calgary AB T2E 7W7; Cal'84; CCFP; FCFP; (403)263-5760; Fax. (403)263-9493.

HALASA, M Christine; Bridgeland Prof Centre, 306-1010 1 Ave NE, Calgary AB T2E 7W7; Cal'86; CCFP; FCFP; (403)263-5760

HALBERT, Cyril; 41 Frederick St, Orillia ON L3V 5W6; Washington (USA)'84; Staff, Orillia Soldiers' Memorial Hospital; (705)325-3645; Fax. (705)325-9004.

HALDANE, David J M; 326-5788 University Ave, Halifax NS B3H 2Y9; Dundee (Scotland)'80; MB ChB; FRCPC; MedMicrobiol. Staff, Queen Elizabeth II Health Sciences Centre - Victoria General Site; Dir, Bacteriology Special Pathogens, N.S.; Clin Dir, Provincial Public Health Laboratory Network; Assoc Prof Microbiol & Pathology, Dalhousie University; (902)473-2392; david.haldane@cdha.nshealth.ca.

HALDER, Smita L S; McMaster Univ, 1280 Main St W, Hamilton ON L8S 4K1; Edinburgh (United Kingdom)'94; Teach Staff, McMaster University; (905)521-2100; Fax. (905)521-4958.

HALE, Ilona; 622 5th Ave, Kimberley BC V1A 2T2; Ott'93; CCFP; Staff, East Kootenay Regional Hospital; Langs: German; French; (250)427-4861; Fax. (250)427-2082.

HALE, Kathryn B; 203-1199 Bay Ave, Trail BC V1R 4A4; Alb'94; FRCSC; ObstGyn. (250)368-6663; Fax. (250)368-6681.

HALE, Nicole; Queensway-Carleton Hosp, 3045 Baseline Rd, Nepean ON K2H 8P4; Tor'05; FRCPC; Anes. Staff, Queensway Carleton Hospital; (613)721-4700

HALEEM, Saima; Health Park, 206-45 Weatherbee Rd, Sydney NS B1M 0A1; (Pakistan)'98; MB BS; CCFP; Staff, Cape Breton Healthcare Complex; Langs: Punjabi; Urdu; (902)270-3340; Fax. (905)270-3339.

HALEIS, Ahmed R; St James Street Med Clinic, 1600 Portage Ave, Winnipeg MB R3J 0C6; (Libya)'98.

HALENAR, Mario A; PO Box 92031, West Vancouver BC V7V 4X4; Alb'84; BSc; BMedSci; Staff, Dawson Creek & District Hospital; Langs: Slovak; mahalenar@yahoo.ca.

HALES, Kristine E; 572 Arthur St PO Box 32063, Thunder Bay ON P7E 5H0; Wes'08; CCFP; (613)878-3638

HALES, Sarah; Princess Margret Hosp, 16747-610 University Ave, Toronto ON M5G 2M9; Qns'00; FRCPC; Psy. Staff Psy, Princess Margaret Hospital - University Health Network; (416)946-4501; Fax. (416)946-2047.

HALEY, George F; Northern Interior Health Unit, 3F-1444 Edmonton St, Prince George BC V2M 6W5; Dal'73; (250)565-7406

HALEY, Lawrence P; Royal Columbian Hosp, 330 Columbia St E, New Westminster BC V3L 3W7; UBC'77; FRCPC; HemPath. Staff, Royal Columbian Hospital; (604)520-4318; Fax. (604)520-4769; lawrence.haley@fraserhealth.ca.

HALEY, Nancy; Dir de la Sante Publique-Mtl, H2-1301 rue Sherbrooke E, Montreal QC H2L 1M3; McM'76; Peds. ac Staff, Hôpital Ste-Justine; (514)528-2400 x3893; Fax. (514)528-2452; nhaley@santepub-mtl.qc.ca.

HALEY, Susan L; Kingston Gen Hosp, 76 Stuart St, Kingston ON K7L 2V7; Tor'81; FRCPC; Anes. Staff Anes, Kingston General Hospital; (613)548-3232; Fax. (613)548-6042.

HALF, Nicholas P; 402-3210 25th Ave, Vernon BC V1T 1P1; UBC'04; FRCSC; ObstGyn. (250)503-3913; nhalf@me.com.

HALIGOWSKI, David J; Rivergrove Med Clinic, 2-2605 Main St, Winnipeg MB R2V 4W3; Man'85; Pres Med Staff, Seven Oaks General Hospital; Med Examiner, Province of Manitoba; (204)632-0024; Fax. (204)697-2047.

HALIK, Jerry J; Markham Stouffville Health Ctr, 202-377 Church St, Markham ON L6B 1A1; Tor'80; DAB; FRCSC; Otol. Ac Staff, Markham Stouffville Hospital; Asst Prof, University of Toronto; (905)472-7123; Fax. (905)472-2003.

HALIKOWSKI, Marvin J; Sunnybrook Hlth Sciences Ctre, 2075 Bayview Ave, Toronto ON M4N 3M5; Tor'91; Staff, Sunnybrook Health Sciences Centre; (416)480-5248; Fax. (416)480-6002.

HALIL, Alexander; Queensway-Carleton Hosp, 3045 Baseline Rd, Nepean ON K2H 8P4; Ott'94; FRCPC; GenPath. Staff, Queensway Carleton Hospital; (613)721-4700 x1008; Fax. (613)721-4747.

HALINEN, Lea I; 405-10030 107 St NW, Edmonton AB T5J 3E4; Alb'69; (780)735-0012; Fax. (780)735-0015.

HALIOTIS, Photini; SMBD Jewish Gen Hosp, 3755 ch Cote-Sainte-Catherine, Montreal QC H3T 1E2; Athens (Greece)'77; FRCPC; GenPath; HemPath (P.Q.). Staff, Sir Mortimer B Davis Jewish General; (514)340-8222 x5472; tina.haliotis@mcgill.ca.

HALISCHUK, Grant F; Eric Martin Pavilion, 2334 Trent St, Victoria BC V8R 4Z3; McG'83; FRCPC; Psy. (250)370-8408

HALJAN, Gregory; Richmond Hosp, 7000 Westminster Hwy, Richmond BC V6X 1A2; Alb'99; Critical Care Medicine; IntMed. Staff, Richmond Hospital; (604)244-5153

HALKA, Hany H I; Wheat City Med Clinic, C1-1711 Kirkcaldy Dr, Brandon MB R7A 0B9; Assiut (Egypt)'92; MB BCh; CCFP.

HALKIER, Bradley K; Royal Columbian Hosp, 330 Columbia St E, New Westminster BC V3L 3W7; Alb'78; BSc; DABR; FRCPC; DiagRad (Interventional Radiology). Staff, Eagle Ridge Hospital & Health Care Centre; Staff Med Imaging, Royal Columbian Hospital; (604)520-4648; Fax. (604)520-4801.

HALL, Aaron; Radiology Consultants Assoc, 120-6707 Elbow Dr SW, Calgary AB T2V 0E3; Sask'99; FRCPC; DiagRad. (403)777-3003; Fax. (403)777-3008.

HALL, Andrew; Manitoba Adolescent Trmt Ctre, 120 Tecumseh St, Winnipeg MB R3E 2A9; Man'94; FRCPC; Psy (Child & Adolescent Psychiatry). Staff, Man.Adolescent Treatment Ctr; (204)477-6391

HALL, Ann Mary; Brant Community HC-Brantford, 200 Terrace Hill St, Brantford ON N3R 1G9; Wes'93; FRCPC; GenPath. Staff, The Brant Community Healthcare System - Brantford General Hospital Site; Langs: English; French; (519)751-5544; Fax. (519)740-4916.

HALL, Barbara; 4-408 Main St, Stonewall MB R0C 2Z0; Brown(RI) (USA)'85; ABIM; (204)467-7782

HALL, Carolyn M; PO Box 56043 Rpo 1st Ave Marke, Vancouver BC V5L 5E2; Dal'97; CCFP.

HALL, Christine A; Victoria Gen Hosp, 1 Hospital Way, Victoria BC V8Z 6R5; Cal'96; FRCPC; EmergMed. Staff, Victoria General Hospital; (250)727-4212

HALL, Christopher; Foothills Medical Centre, C231-1403 29 St NW, Calgary AB T2N 2T9; Tor'03; FRCPC; EmergMed. Staff, Foothills Medical Centre; (403)944-1110

HALL, Christopher W; Glazier Med Centre, 11 Gibb St, Oshawa ON L1H 2J9; McG'73; BSc; CCFP; FCFP; Staff, Lakeridge Health - Oshawa Site; Lecturer, University of Toronto; Langs: Bilingual(English/French); (905)579-1212; Fax. (905)579-1583.

HALL, David A; St Michael's Hosp, 6B 045-30 Bond St, Toronto ON M5B 1W8; Tor'00; FRCPC; IntMed; Critical Care Medicine; Respir. Staff, St Michael's Hospital; (416)864-5516; Fax. (416)864-5649.

HALL, David F; Peterborough Reg Hlth Ctr, 1 Hospital Dr, Peterborough ON K9J 7C6; Mem'92; FRCPC; Anes. Staff, Peterborough Regional Health Centre - Hospital Drive; (705)743-2121

HALL, David R A; Vancouver Comm UrbanPrimary, 200-520 6 Ave W, Vancouver BC V5Z 4H5; UBC'02; CCFP; Staff Immunodeficiency Clinic, Providence Health Care - St Paul's Hospital; (604)731-3792

HALL, Dennis K; Southlands Med Clinic, 110-7 Strachan Bay SE, Medicine Hat AB T1B 4Y2; Wes'70; CCFP; FCFP; (403)528-4490; Fax. (403)528-4481.

HALL, Elaine J; Algonquin College Hlth Serv, C141-1385 Woodroffe Ave, Ottawa ON K2G 1V8; Ott'93; CCFP; (613)727-4723

HALL, Gordon W; Ontario Power Generation, 1675 Montgomery Park Rd, Pickering ON L1V 2R5; Qns'71; Court Staff, Timmins & District Hospital; (905)839-1151 x3541

HALL, Gregory S; Brantford Gen Hosp, 200 Terrace Hill St, Brantford ON N3R 1G9; Wes'93; BSc; CCFP; CCFP(E.M.); FCFP; Staff, The Brant Community Healthcare System - Brantford General Hospital Site; (519)752-7871

HALL, Gwendolen C E; Rockyview Gen Hosp, 7007 14 St SW, Calgary AB T2V 1P9; Sask'98; FRCPC; Anes. Staff, Rockyview General Hospital; (403)943-8720

HALL, Hamilton; PO Box 434, Markdale ON N0C 1H0; Tor'63; FRCSC; OrthSurg (Spine). Court Staff, Grey Bruce Health Services - Markdale; Staff, Sunnybrook Health Sciences Centre; Staff, Orthopaedic & Arthritic Institute; Prof Surg, University of Toronto; (519)986-4444; Fax. (519)986-2579.

HALL, Henry J E; Orillia Soldiers' Mem Hosp, 170 Colborne St W, Orillia ON L3V 2Z3; Tor'59; CCFP; FCFP; Ac Staff, Orillia Soldiers' Memorial Hospital; Asst Prof Med, University of Toronto; (705)325-2201

HALL, J Douglas; 204-599 Main St, Hampton NB E5N 6C2; Qns'07; CCFP; (506)832-0528; Fax. (506)832-3037.

HALL, Jeffery A; MUHC-Montreal Neurology Inst, 122C-3801 rue University, Montreal QC H3A 2B4; Tor'98; FRCSC; Neursurg. Staff, McGill University Health Centre - Montreal Neurological Hospital; (514)398-8871; Fax. (514)398-2811.

HALL, Jennifer L; Whitemud Crossing Med Clinic, 127-4211 106 St NW, Edmonton AB T6J 6L7; UBC'99; CCFP; (780)435-7555; Fax. (780)436-0582.

HALL, Jennifer L; St Joseph's Hosp, 130 Bayard Dr, Saint John NB E2L 3L6; Mem'92; CCFP; FCFP; Staff, St Joseph's Hospital; (506)632-5483; Fax. (506)632-5447.

HALL, Jeremy A; St Michael's Orthopaedic Assoc, 800-55 Queen St E, Toronto ON M5C 1R6; Tor'99; BSc(Hon); MEd; FRCSC; OrthSurg (Trauma & Reconstructive Surgery). Staff Ortho, St Michael's Hospital; (416)864-6006; Fax. (416)359-1601.

HALL, Jeremy; Chilliwack Gen Hosp, 45600 Menholm Rd, Chilliwack BC V2P 1P7; UBC'04; CCFP; Staff, Chilliwack General Hospital; (604)795-4141

HALL, John D; Port Dover Med Centre, 807 St George St, Port Dover ON N0A 1N0; Tor'71; (519)583-0891; Fax. (519)583-2814.

HALL, John S; 103-152 High St PO Box 1108, Sutton West ON L0E 1R0; Tor'80; CCFP; FCFP; Ac Staff, Southlake Regional Health Centre; (905)722-9011; Fax. (905)722-9376.

HALL, Lacresha L; St Paul's Hosp, 1081 Burrard St, Vancouver BC V6Z 1Y6; Galveson (USA)'99; Staff, Providence Health Care - St Paul's Hospital; (604)682-2344

HALL, Leslie E; Children's Hosp Eastern Ont, 401 Smyth Rd, Ottawa ON K1H 8L1; Man'77; FRCPC; Anes (Pediatric Anesthesia). Staff, Children's Hospital of Eastern Ontario (CHEO); Court Staff, The Ottawa Hospital - General Campus; Asst Prof Med, University of Ottawa; (613)737-2431; Fax. (613)737-4815.

HALL, M Jeremy; Southlake Reg Health Centre, 596 Davis Dr, Newmarket ON L3Y 2P9; London (England)'72; MB BS; Staff, Southlake Regional Health Centre; (905)895-4521

HALL, Matthew; Rockyview Gen Hosp, ER-7007 14 St SW, Calgary AB T2V 1P9; Qns'94; CCFP; CCFP(E.M.); Staff, Rockyview General Hospital; (403)943-3449

HALL, Melinda H; 304-5450 ch de la Cote-des-Nei, Montreal QC H3T 1Y6; McG'00; FRCSC; ObstGyn. (514)739-6943

HALL, Michael S; 201-193 LeMarchant Rd, St. John's NL A1C 2H5; Mem'88; FRCPC; Peds (Asthma & Allergy). (709)738-2200; Fax. (709)738-2204.

HALL, Patricia; London HSC-Victoria Hosp, PO Box 5010 Stn B 800 Commissioners Rd E, London ON N6A 5W9; Ott'04; FRCPC; Psy. Staff, London Health Sciences Centre - Victoria Campus; (519)685-8500; Fax. (519)685-8590.

HALL, Philippa; Univ of Ottawa, 451 Smyth Rd, Ottawa ON K1H 8M5; Sask'83; CCFP; FCFP; Dir Portfolio on core competencies, University of Ottawa; (613)562-5800

HALL, Renee N; Aquarius Med Clinic, 202-179 Davie St, Vancouver BC V6Z 2Y1; Tor'99; CCFP; (604)669-7772

HALL, Richard I; Queen Elizabeth II HSC-Halifax, 5452-1796 Summer St, Halifax NS B3H 3A7; Dal'81; FRCPC; Anes (Critical Care Medicine). Staff, Queen Elizabeth II Health Sciences Centre - Victoria General Site; Prof Anes/Pharmacology & Med, Dalhousie University; (902)473-2328; Fax. (902)473-4828; rihall@dal.ca.

HALL, Robert E; Foothills Medical Centre, C231-1403 29 St NW, Calgary AB T2N 2T9; Sask'00; FRCPC; EmergMed. Staff Emerg, Foothills Medical Centre; (403)944-8430

HALL, Robert O M; Ashgrove Med Centre, 305-6633 Highway 7, Markham ON L3P 7P2; (Jamaica)'79; MB BS(Hons); FRCSC; ObstGyn (Colposcopy). Staff, Markham Stouffville Hospital; (905)294-4405; Fax. (905)294-2334.

HALL, Ronald L; Kanata Prof Centre, 215-99 Kakulu Rd, Kanata ON K2L 3C8; Ott'86; (613)592-5096; Fax. (613)592-4493.

HALL, Sarah A; Alberta Children's Hosp, 2888 Shaganappi Trail NW, Calgary AB T3B 6A8; Tor'03; FRCPC; Peds. Staff Peds, Alberta Children's Hospital; (403)955-2953; Fax. (403)955-3055.

HALL, Sarah C; Nanaimo Reg Gen Hosp, 1200 Dufferin Cres, Nanaimo BC V9S 2B7; McM'91; BSc; FRCPC; Anes. Staff, Nanaimo Regional General Hospital; (250)755-7605

HALL, Stephanie; Cole Harbor Family Medicine, 920 Cole Harbour Rd, Dartmouth NS B2V 2J5; Dal'01; CCFP; (902)435-6312; Fax. (902)434-7920.

HALL, Stephen F; Hotel Dieu Hosp, 166 Brock St, Kingston ON K7L 5G2; Qns'73; MSc; FRCSC; Otol (Head & Neck Surgery). Staff, Kingston General Hospital; Staff Otol, Hotel-Dieu Hospital; Prof Otol, Queen's University; (613)544-3400 x3618; Fax. (613)547-5654.

HALL, Susan E H; 1882 Niagara Stone Rd PO Box 10, Niagara-on-the-Lke ON L0S 1T0; McM'86; PhD; DAB(Derm.); BSc(Hons); FRCP; FRCPC; Derm. Consultant Privil, Niagara Health System - Ontario Street Site; Asst Prof Med, McMaster University; (905)468-3275; Fax. (905)468-7960.

HALL, Thomas A; Torbay Med Clinic, B-1345 Torbay Rd, Torbay NL A1K 1B2; Mem'06; CCFP; Staff, Carbonear General Hospital; (709)437-6301

HALL, Trevor L; Grand River Sports Med, 40 George St N, Cambridge ON N1S 2M8; Tor'94; CCFP; Asst Prof, University of Waterloo; Langs: English; French; (519)622-4529; Fax. (519)622-3563.

HALL, Trudy M; Bayshore Med Bldg, 101-3029 Carling Ave, Ottawa ON K2B 8E8; Tor'83; MSc; CCFP; FCFP; Staff, The Ottawa Hospital - Civic Campus; Staff, Children's Hospital of Eastern Ontario (CHEO); (613)820-1123

HALL, William A; Park Towers, 134-400 Walmer Rd, Toronto ON M5P 2X7; Glasgow (Scotland)'53; DPM; MRCPsy; Member, Canadian Psychoanalytic Society; (416)920-3702

HALL, William G; 171-1402 8 Ave NW, Calgary AB T2N 1B9; Tor'73; CCFP; FCFP; Assoc Staff, Alberta Children's Hospital; Ac Staff, Foothills Medical Centre; Clin Associate Prof, University of Calgary; (403)777-5760; Fax. (403)777-5764; wmghall@shaw.ca.

HALL BARBER, Karen; Queen's FHT-Corporate Office, PO Box 8888 319-220 Bagot St, Kingston ON K7L 3G2; Ott'96; CCFP; (613)533-9303

HALL-FINDLAY, Elizabeth J; 340-317 Banff Ave PO Box 2009 Stn Main, Banff AB T1L 1B7; Wes'76; BSc; AB; FRCSC; PlasSurg (Cosmetic Surgery). Ac Staff, Covenant Health - Banff Mineral Springs Hospital; (403)762-2055; Fax. (403)762-8297; info@banffplasticsurgery.ca.

HALL-LOSIER, Suzanne M; Moncton Med Clinic, 203-860 Mountain Rd, Moncton NB E1C 2N7; Dal'90; CCFP; FCFP; (506)853-5135; Fax. (506)389-2425.

HALLAGE, Marie G; CSSS du Suroît, 150 rue Saint-Thomas, Salaber-de-Valleyf QC J6T 6C1; Mon'09; Staff, Centre Hospitalier Régional du Suroît; (450)371-9920

HALLAK, Jean J; Hop Sainta Cabrini Ospedal, 5655 rue Saint-Zotique E, Montreal QC H1T 1P7; Istanbul (Turkey)'61; AB; FACOG; FRCSC; ObstGyn (P.Q.). Chef, Hôpital Santa Cabrini Ospedale; Langs: Armenian; Turkish; Arabic; English; (514)252-6000

HALLDORSON, Heather G; Herold Road Family Physicians, 1-325 Herold Rd, Saskatoon SK S7V 1J7; Sask'99; CCFP; FCFP; (306)374-2404; Fax. (306)477-0300.

HALLE, Amelie; CSSS de Trois-Rivières, 1991 boul du Carmel, Trois-Rivieres QC G8Z 3R9; Laval'06; FRCPC; DiagRad. Staff, CSSS de Trois-Rivières; (819)697-3333

HALLE, Denis; Clinique Neuro-Outaouais, 200-147 boul d'Europe, Gatineau QC J9J 0N3; Laval'80; CSPQ; FRCPC; IntMed (Adult Neurology); Neur (P.Q.). Ac Staff, Hull Hospital; Consultant, Hôpital de Gatineau; Langs: English; (819)777-2500; Fax. (819)777-2502.

HALLE, Jean-Pierre; Hop Maisonneuve-Rosemont, 5415 boul de l'Assomption, Montreal QC H1T 2M4; Mon'68; CSPQ; FRCPC; IntMed (Diabetology); Endocrin (P.Q.). Staff Endocrinol, Hopital Maisonneuve-Rosemont; Prof, Universite de Montreal; Langs: English; (514)252-3400 x3305; hallejp@videotron.ca.

HALLE, Pierre; Ctr Hosp Affilie-St-Sacrement, 1050 ch Sainte-Foy, Quebec QC G1S 4L8; Laval'73; FRCPC; IntMed; Gastroent. Ac Staff Gastroent, Centre Hospitalier Affilié Universitaire de Québec - Hôpital du St-Sacrement; (418)682-7623; Fax. (418)682-7588; pierre.halle.cha@ssss.gouv.qc.ca.

HALLE, Suzanne; CSSS Montmagny-l'Islet, 214-848 rue Commerciale, St-J-Chrysostome QC G6Z 2T6; Laval'73; (418)839-2070 x2307; Fax. (418)839-9161.

HALLERAN, Sarah; Hys Med Centre, 604-11010 101 St NW, Edmonton AB T5H 4B9; Alb'00; FRCSC; ObstGyn (Pediatric & Adolescent Gynecology). (780)421-4728; Fax. (780)426-6698.

HALLETT, Kristen M; Health Sciences Bldg, 201-15 Mountain Ave S, Stoney Creek ON L8G 2V6; McM'95; BScPharm; MD; Peds; FRCPC; Peds. Staff, St Joseph's Healthcare - Charlton Campus; Assoc Prof, McMaster University; (905)664-9992; Fax. (905)664-9910; kristen.hallett@sympatico.ca.

HALLEY, Kathleen M; Family Wellness Place, 48 Commonwealth Ave, Mount Pearl NL A1N 5B6; Mem'80; (709)364-6650; kmh@cruisejunkie.com.

HALLIDAY, April; Westgate Family Med Clinic, 172-17010 90 Ave NW, Edmonton AB T5T 1L6; UBC'04; FRCPC; DiagRad. Staff, Cross Cancer Institute; (780)484-1672

HALLIDAY, David M; Family Med Associates, 607-267 O'Connor St, Ottawa ON K2P 1V3; Ott'80; (613)235-8146; Fax. (613)235-8146.

HALLIDAY, Fiona; 201-4256 Portage Rd, Niagara Falls ON L2E 6A4; Belfast (Ireland)'94; BSc; (905)354-9822; Fax. (905)354-9823.

HALLIDAY, Frederick; Niagara H System-G Niagara, 5546 Portage Rd, Niagara Falls ON L2E 6X2; Belfast (Ireland)'62; MB ChB; FFARCSI(I); FRCPC; Anes. Staff, Niagara Health System - Greater Niagara General Site; (905)358-0171

HALLIDAY, Kelly; William Osler HC-Etobicoke, 101 Humber College Blvd, Etobicoke ON M9V 1R8; Ott'06; CCFP; Staff, William Osler Health System - Etobicoke General Hospital; Langs: Bilingual(English/French); (416)747-3400

HALLIDAY, Sarah M F; Royal Ottawa Hlth Care Group, 1145 Carling Ave, Ottawa ON K1Z 7K4; Ott'01; FRCPC; Psy (Geriatric Psychiatry). Staff, Royal Ottawa Mental Health Centre - Royal Ottawa Health Care Group; Langs: Bilingual(English/French); (613)722-6521; Fax. (613)798-2999.

HALLIDAY, William R S; Copeman Health Care Centre, 400-628 12 Ave SW, Calgary AB T2R 0H6; Cal'91; CCFP; FCFP; Med Staff, Foothills Medical Centre; (403)270-2273; Fax. (403)521-2250.

HALLIGAN, Rachael; Cambridge Mem Hosp, 700 Coronation Blvd, Cambridge ON N1R 3G2; McM'98; CCFP; Staff, Grand River Hospital - Kitchener/Waterloo Health Centre; Staff, Cambridge Memorial Hospital; (519)621-2330

HALLIWELL, Oliver T; Radiology Consultants Assoc, 120-6707 Elbow Dr SW, Calgary AB T2V 0E3; (United Kingdom)'95; BSc(Lond); MRCS(Eng); FRCR; MB BS(Lond); (403)777-3007; Fax. (403)777-3008.

HALLMAN, Melissa J; GM-200-1455 boul de Maisonneuv, Montreal QC H3G 1M8; Ott'95; CCFP; (514)848-2424 x3565

HALLORAN, Brendan P; Ziedler Ledcor Centre, 1 59-130 University Campus NW, Edmonton AB T6G 2X8; Alb'05; Gastroent; IntMed. (780)492-8691; Fax. (780)492-8121.

HALLORAN, Kieran; University of Alberta Hospital, 8440 112 St NW, Edmonton AB T6G 2B7; Alb'07; FRCPC; IntMed; Respir. Staff, University of Alberta Hospital; (780)407-8822

HALLORAN, Philip F; Heritage Med Research Centre, 250-107 University Campus NW, Edmonton AB T6G 2S2; Tor'68; PhD; FRCPC; IntMed (Nephrology). Dir Div of Nephrol & Immunol/Med, University of Alberta Hospital; Prof, University of Alberta; (780)492-6160; Fax. (780)492-0145; phil.halloran@ualberta.ca.

HALLS, Steven B; St Mary's Hosp, 4607 53 St, Camrose AB T4V 1Y5; Alb'85; FRCPC; DiagRad. Staff, Cross Cancer Institute; Staff Oncology Imaging, Covenant Health - St Mary's Hospital; (780)679-6113; Fax. (780)679-2815.

HALMAN, Mark H; St Michael's Hosp, 17033-30 Bond St, Toronto ON M5B 1W8; Tor'87; FRCPC; Psy (Gay Affirmative Psychiatry). Dir HIV Psychiatry Prgm, St Michael's Hospital; Asst Prof Psy, University of Toronto; (416)864-3082; Fax. (416)864-3091; halmanm@smh.toronto.on.ca.

HALMAN, Samantha; The Ottawa Hosp-Gen Campus, 501 Smyth Rd, Ottawa ON K1H 8L6; Ott'08; FRCPC; IntMed. Staff, The Ottawa Hospital - General Campus; (613)737-8726

HALMAN, Stephen I; Oakdale Med Bldg, 424-2065 Finch Ave W, North York ON M3N 2V7; McG'93; BASc; FRCSC; OrthSurg (Upper Extremity Surgery). Staff, Humber River Regional Hospital - Finch Avenue Site; (416)745-9195; Fax. (416)745-9175.

HALMARSON, Erica B; River East Health Access Ctre, 975 Henderson Hwy, Winnipeg MB R2K 4L7; Man'06; CCFP; (204)938-5000

HALMO, Stephen D; 1-737 Belmont Ave W, Kitchener ON N2M 1P3; Wes'79; FRCSC; ObstGyn. Staff, Grand River Hospital - Kitchener/Waterloo Health Centre; (519)741-8710; Fax. (519)741-1359.

HALONEN, Mark A; Windsor Essex Community HC, 1585 Ouellette Ave, Windsor ON N8X 1K5; Michigan State Univ (USA)'80; (519)253-8481

HALPARIN, Elliot; Georgetown Med Associates, 199 Princess Anne Dr, Georgetown ON L7G 0E3; Man'74; CCFP; FCFP; Ac Staff, Halton Healthcare Services Corporation - Georgetown Hospital; (905)873-3000; Fax. (905)873-0800.

HALPARIN, Lawrence S; Pacific Gastroenterology Assoc, 770-1190 Hornby St, Vancouver BC V6Z 2K5; Man'69; FRCPC; IntMed; Gastroent. Ac Staff, Providence Health Care - St Paul's Hospital; (604)688-6332 x223

HALPENNY, David G; Peter Lougheed Centre, 3500 26 Ave NE, Calgary AB T1Y 6J4; McG'77; FRCPC; EmergMed; Anes. Staff, Peter Lougheed Centre; (403)943-5554; Fax. (403)219-3574.

HALPENNY, Robert; Interior Health Authority, 220-1815 Kirschner Rd, Kelowna BC V1Y 4N7; Sask'80; Pres/CEO, Interior Health Authority Corpoate Office; (250)862-4205

HALPERIN, Frank A; Cardiology Associates, 2606 Pandosy St, Kelowna BC V1Y 1V6; Tor'89; FRCPC; IntMed; Cardiol. (250)762-9211; frankhalperin@yahoo.com.

HALPERIN, Harvey I; Fairmont Med Bldg, 1109-750 Broadway W, Vancouver BC V5Z 1J1; McG'74; BSc(Hon)Geriatrics; Assoc Staff, BC Children's Hospital; Assoc Staff, Vancouver General Hospital - Centennial Pavillion; Assoc Staff, Women's & Children's Health Centre; Langs: Bilingual(French/English); Yiddish; (604)873-0557; Fax. (604)873-5819.

HALPERIN, Michael; 202-3461 Dixie Rd, Mississauga ON L4Y 3X4; Tor'73; Staff, Trillium Health Centre - Mississauga; (905)624-2558; Fax. (905)602-6481.

HALPERIN, Ross M; BC Cancer Agency-Southern Int, 399 Royal Ave, Kelowna BC V1Y 5L3; Alb'93; BSc; FRCPC; RadOncol. Staff PPL Radiation Oncology, BC Cancer Agency Sindi Ahluwalia Hawkins Centre for the Southern Interior; (250)979-6645; Fax. (250)712-3911; rhalperin@bccancer.bc.ca.

HALPERIN, Scott; IWK Health Centre, PO Box 9700 rpo CSC 5850-5980 University Ave, Halifax NS B3J 3G8; New York(NY) (USA)'77; FRCPC; Peds. Ac Staff, IWK Health Centre; (902)470-8141; Fax. (902)470-7232.

HALPERN, Janice R; 244 Dupont St, Toronto ON M5R 1V7; Tor'78; FRCPC; Psy (Psychoanalysis). (416)962-0228; Fax. (416)787-6741.

HALPERN, Stephen H; Sunnybrook Hlth Sciences Ctre, M5 318-2075 Bayview Ave, Toronto ON M4N 3M5; Tor'77; FRCPC; Anes. Staff, Women's College Hospital; Staff, Sunnybrook Health Sciences Centre; (416)480-6100; Fax. (416)323-2666.

HALSE, Robert A; Family Health Clinic, 10-5011 48 Ave, Ponoka AB T4J 1J3; London (England)'83; Ac Staff, Centennial Centre for Mental Health & Brain Injury; Staff Anes, Ponoka Hospital & Care Centre; Anesthetist, Lacombe Hospital & Care Centre; (403)783-5305; Fax. (403)783-8722; robert.halse@gov.ab.ca.

HALSTEAD, A Catherine; Children's & Women's HC of BC, 4480 Oak St, Vancouver BC V6H 3V4; Tor'78; FRCPC; MedBiochem (General Pathology). Ac Staff Path & Lab Med, BC Children's Hospital; Clin Assoc Prof, University of British Columbia; (604)875-2918; chalstead@cw.bc.ca.

HALTON, Jacqueline M L; Children's Hosp Eastern Ont, 2636-401 Smyth Rd, Ottawa ON K1H 8L1; Detroit(MI) (USA)'84; FRCPC; Peds (Hematological Oncology). Staff HemOncol, Children's Hospital of Eastern Ontario (CHEO); Prof, University of Ottawa; (613)737-2370; Fax. (613)738-4828; halton@cheo.on.ca.

HALUK, Myron; Trillium Hlth Ctr-Mississauga, 100 Queensway W, Mississauga ON L5B 1B8; Tor'92; BSc; CCFP; CCFP(E.M.); Assoc Staff Family Med., The Credit Valley Hospital; Assoc Staff Emerg, Trillium Health Centre - West Toronto; Staff, Trillium Health Centre - Mississauga; Langs: Ukrainian; (905)848-7100

HALVORSON, James; Cowichan District Hosp, 3045 Gibbins Rd, Duncan BC V9L 1E5; McG'85; CCFP; CCFP(E.M.); Staff, Cowichan District Hospital; Langs: English; French; (250)746-4141

HALWANI, Fawaz; The Ottawa Hosp- Gen Campus, 501 Smyth Rd, Ottawa ON K1H 8L6; Shiraz (Iran)'81; PhD; FRCPC; AnatPath (Breasts). Staff, Peterborough Regional Health Centre - Hospital Drive; Staff, The Ottawa Hospital - General Campus; Langs: English; French; Arabic; Persian; (613)737-8899

HALYK, Mark A; Crescent Heights Fam Med Ctr, 114-2805 6th Ave E, Prince Albert SK S6V 6Z6; Sask'86; Ac Staff, Victoria Hospital; (306)763-2681; Fax. (306)953-1024.

HAM, Clayton L; Namgis Health Centre, PO Box 49, Alert Bay BC V0N 1A0; Sask'70; (250)974-5520; Fax. (250)974-5952.

HAM, Kevin; 4438 10th Ave W PO Box 802, Vancouver BC V6R 4R8; UBC'98; (604)351-4156

HAM, Sharon A; Royal Jubilee Hosp, 1952 Bay St, Victoria BC V8R 1J8; McM'07; CCFP; Staff, Royal Jubilee Hospital; (250)370-8000

HAM, Trevor J; Bay Street Clinic, 960 3rd Ave E, Owen Sound ON N4K 2K9; McG'63; FRCPC; Peds (Attention Deficit Hyperactivity Disorder). Langs: Spanish; French; (519)376-4865; Fax. (519)376-4409.

HAM PONG, Antony J; Smyth Medical Centre, 208-1929 Russell Rd, Ottawa ON K1G 4G3; (Jamaica)'78; MB BS; AB; FRCPC; Peds; ClinImmunol&Allergy (Allergy & Immunology). Consultant Chest Clinic, Children's Hospital of Eastern Ontario (CHEO); Clin Lecturer School of Med & Faculty, University of Ottawa; (613)526-3501; Fax. (613)741-4325.

HAMAD, Fatin; Parkway Forest Med Centre, 40-105 Parkway Forest Dr, North York ON M2J 1L8; Baghdad (Iraq)'79; MB BS; CCFP; Langs: Arabic; (416)502-3404; Fax. (416)502-3017.

HAMADAH, Abdulaziz A; Civic Parkdale Clinic, 465-737 Parkdale Ave, Ottawa ON K1Y 1J8; (Kuwait)'00; FRCPC; IntMed; Hem. (613)798-5555

HAMADEH, Mohamad; University of Alberta Hosp, 4G1 12-8440 112 St NW, Edmonton AB T6G 2B7; Syria (Syria)'94; Staff, University of Alberta Hospital; (780)407-7018; Fax. (780)407-3839.

HAMAM, Al-Walid; Sunnybrook Hlth Sciences Ctre, 2075 Bayview Ave, Toronto ON M4N 3M5; Ott'07; FRCSC; OrthSurg. Staff, Sunnybrook Health Sciences Centre.

HAMANDI, Husein Z; Rebecca Med Associates, 170A Rebecca St, Oakville ON L6K 1J6; Al-Mustansiriyah (Iraq)'86; CCFP; FCFP; Staff Emerg, Halton Healthcare Services Corporation - Milton District Hospital; Langs: Arabic; (905)845-9293; Fax. (905)845-0981.

HAMANI, Clement; Univ Hlth Network-Toronto Western Hosp, WW4 437-399 Bathurst St, Toronto ON M5T 2S8; Sao Paolo (Brazil)'93; Staff, Toronto Western Hospital - University Health Network; (416)603-2581

HAMANN, Adolf; Western Memorial Clinic, 347 O'Connell Dr, Corner Brook NL A2H 7E4; Montevideo (Uruguay)'85; MRC(U.K.); MRCOG; LMCC; Chief ObstGyn, Western Memorial Regional Hospital; Langs: Spanish; German; (709)634-2355; Fax. (709)634-4177.

HAMANN, Richard; Clinique Med Courcelles, 137 rue Principale RR 1, Courcelles QC G0M 1C0; Laval'83; (418)483-5346; Fax. (418)483-5846.

HAMANN, Steven; Clin Medicale de Pintendre, 5-792 Rte Du President-Kennedy, Levis QC G6C 1C8; Laval'93; Staff Emerg Med, CSSS de Montmagny-L'Islet; (418)837-6943; Fax. (418)837-0487.

HAMAOUI, Charles; Hop Maisonneuve-Rosemont, 5415 boul de l'Assomption, Montreal QC H1T 2M4; Mon'83; FRCPC; Peds. Staff, Hopital Maisonneuve-Rosemont; (514)252-3400; Fax. (514)252-3548.

HAMAT, Richard B; Vaughan Pediatric Clinic, 310-8333 Weston Rd, Woodbridge ON L4L 8E2; Tor'84; FRCPC; Peds. Assoc Staff, Humber River Regional Hospital - Church Street Site; Assoc Staff, Humber River Regional Hospital - Keele Street Site; (905)850-3250; Fax. (905)850-5607.

HAMAWY, Nabil N; St Mary's Hosp Centre, 3830 av Lacombe, Montreal QC H3T 1M5; Alexandria (Egypt)'63; CSPQ; FRCPC; Anes (Pain Management). Staff, St Mary's Hospital Centre; Asst Prof Anes, McGill University; (514)345-3511 x3344; Fax. (514)342-1376; nhamawy@hotmail.com.

HAMBLETON, Corey R; Living Health, 103-6033 London Rd, Richmond BC V7E 0A7; Alb'96; CCFP; (604)277-0307

HAMBLY, David; Kings County Med Centre, PO Box 817, Montague PE C0A 1R0; Mem'76; Court Staff, Queen Elizabeth Hospital; Ac Staff, Kings County Memorial Hospital; (902)838-3680; Fax. (902)838-2758; kcmc@pei.aibn.com.

HAMBOYAN, Herag; Sheridan College Davis Campus, B202-7899 McLaughlin Rd S, Brampton ON L6V 1G6; Dal'94; BSc(Hons); CCFP; FCFP; Langs: Spanish; French; Armenian; (905)459-7533 x5153

HAMBURGER, Jaap N; Gordon & Leslie Diamond HCC, 9121-2775 Laurel St, Vancouver BC V5Z 1M9; Amsterdam (Netherlands)'86; PhD; FRCPC; Cardiol (Interventional Cardiology). Ac Staff Cardiol, Vancouver General Hospital - Centennial Pavillion; Ac Staff, Providence Health Care - St Paul's Hospital; Staff, Gordon & Leslie Diamond Health Care Centre; Dir Interventional Cardiol Research Prog, University of British Columbia; Langs: Dutch; (604)875-5523; Fax. (604)875-5544.

HAMDAD-VITRE, Nadia; Groupe Sante Physimed, 121-6363 rte Transcanadienne, Saint-Laurent QC H4T 1Z9; Mon'02; CCFP; (514)747-8888; Fax. (514)747-4705.

HAMDAN, Helena; Family Health Centre, 200-2462 Howard Ave, Windsor ON N8X 3V6; Wes'05; CCFP; (519)258-5837; Fax. (519)258-4456.

HAMDAN, Loai M K; Slave Lake Family Clinic, SS 3 608 6 St SE, Slave Lake AB T0G 2A3; (Libya)'08; MB BCh; (780)849-2860

HAMDANI, Aziza; Serv Externe De Psychiatrie, 230-383 boul du Seminaire N, St-Jean-sur-Richel QC J3B 8C5; (Algeria)'93; Psy (P.Q.). (450)346-2222

HAMDI, Amre; Health Science Centre, 3330 Hospital Dr NW, Calgary AB T2N 4N1; Jeddah (Saudi Arabia)'03; FRCSC; OrthSurg. Staff, Foothills Medical Centre; (403)220-2724

HAMDY, Ahmed; St Michael's Hosp, 30 Bond St, Toronto ON M5B 1W8; Ain Shams (Egypt)'01; FRCPC; Anes. Staff, St Michael's Hospital; Langs: Arabic; (416)864-5071

HAMDY, Hazem A; 58 James St, Ottawa ON K2P 0T6; Cairo (Egypt)'68; CCFP; Staff, The Ottawa Hospital - Civic Campus; Langs: Arabic; (613)233-6240; Fax. (613)233-8205.

HAMDY, Nermeen R I; 201-1448 Lawrence Ave E, North York ON M4A 2V6; Cairo (Egypt)'86; CCFP; Staff, Rouge Valley Health System - Centenary Health Centre Site; Langs: Arabic; (416)759-0184; Fax. (416)759-4583.

HAMDY, Reggie C A; Shriners Hosp for Children, 1529 av Cedar, Montreal QC H3G 1A6; Alexandria (Egypt)'76; MSc; FRCSC; OrthSurg (Pediatrics). adj Chef Surg, Shriners Hospitals For Children - Canada; Consultant, Centre de Réadaptation Marie Enfant du CHU Sainte-Justine; Consultant, McGill University Health Centre - Montreal Children's Hospital; assoc Prof, McGill University; Langs: Arabic; English; (514)842-4464; Fax. (514)842-8664; rhamdy@shriners.mcgill.ca.

HAMED, Azza A W M; 300-2338 Hurontario St, Mississauga ON L5B 1N1; Cairo (Egypt)'81; MB BCh; FRCPC; Peds (Pediatric Allergy). Langs: Arabic; (905)268-0385; Fax. (905)268-0567.

HAMED ABDELAZIM, Hala M F; Niagara H System-Welland Site, 65 Third St, Welland ON L3B 4W6; Cairo (Egypt)'92; FRCPC; Anes. Staff, Niagara Health System - Welland Hospital Site; Langs: Arabic.

HAMEDANCHI, Reza; MCI The Doctors Office, PO Box 52 595 Bay St, Toronto ON M5G 2C2; (Other Foreign)'00; CCFP; (416)598-1703; Fax. (416)598-1778.

HAMEED, Adnan K; 205-589 Lake St, St. Catharines ON L2N 7L6; Man'05; FRCPC; IntMed; Cardiol. (905)646-2525

HAMEED, Asiya; NHH Cobourg, RR 4 8542 Majestic Hills Dr, Cobourg ON K9A 4J7; Aligarh (India)'77; MB BS; (905)342-5726; Fax. (905)373-6996.

HAMEED, Babar; Beechwood Comm Hlth Centre, PO Box 550, O'Leary PE C0B 1V0; Punjab (India)'89; MB BS; Physician, O'Leary Health Centre; (902)859-3929

HAMEED, Faiza; Peterborough Reg HC-Hospital, 1 Hospital Dr, Peterborough ON K9J 7C6; Kilpauk (India)'87; Staff, Peterborough Regional Health Centre - Hospital Drive; (705)743-2121; Fax. (705)876-5120.

HAMEED, Kazi A; 210-2200 McPhillips St, Winnipeg MB R2V 3P4; Peshawar (Pakistan)'63; MB BS; FRCPC; IntMed (Cardiology). Ac Staff, Seven Oaks General Hospital; Langs: Urdu; Pashtu; Punjabi; (204)633-3664; Fax. (204)633-3664.

HAMEED, Nageen; Oakville Med Clinic, 307-331 Sheddon Ave, Oakville ON L6J 1X8; Man'96; FRCPC; IntMed. Langs: Pashtu; Urdu; (905)338-0550; Fax. (905)338-3187.

HAMEED, S Morad; Vancouver Gen Hosp, 855 12th Ave W, Vancouver BC V5Z 1M9; Alb'93; FRCSC; GenSurg. Staff Trauma Services, Vancouver General Hospital - Centennial Pavillion; (604)875-4111

HAMEED, Saadia; St Joseph's Family Med Centre, 346 Platt's Lane, London ON N6G 1J1; Punjab (Pakistan)'01; CCFP; Asst Prof, University of Western Ontario; Langs: Punjabi; Urdu; (519)672-9660; Fax. (519)672-7727.

HAMEER, Taslim; University Village Med Clinic, 228-2155 Allison Rd, Vancouver BC V6T 1T5; UBC'00; (604)222-2273

HAMEL, Alexandra; Hôp de Saint-Eustache, 520 boul Arthur-Sauve, Saint-Eustache QC J7R 5B1; Mon'09; CCFP; Staff, Hôpital de Saint-Eustache; (450)473-6811

HAMEL, Annick; Horizon Feminin, 206-200 rue Durand, Saint-Jerome QC J7Z 7E2; Mon'97; FRCSC; ObstGyn. (450)436-4228; Fax. (450)436-5488.

HAMEL, Bernard; Clinique Med Chaudiere, 102 18e rue, Saint-Georges QC G5Y 4T9; Laval'92; Staff, Centre Hospitalier Beauce-Etchemin; (418)228-6820

HAMEL, Bruno; CSSS de Chicoutimi, 305 rue Saint-Vallier, Chicoutimi QC G7H 5H6; Sher'86; CCFP; CCFP(E.M.); FCFP; EmergMed (P.Q.). Affil Member, Universite de Sherbrooke; (418)541-1000; brunohamel1@videotron.ca.

HAMEL, Caroline; Hotel-Dieu de Sorel, 400 av de l'Hôtel-Dieu, Sorel-Tracy QC J3P 1N5; Mon'09; CCFP; Staff, Hôtel-Dieu de Sorel.

HAMEL, Catherine; CLSC Chateauguay, 95 av de la Verdure, Chateauguay QC J6K 0E8; Laval'07; CCFP; (450)699-3333; Fax. (450)699-2325.

HAMEL, Emilie; CLSC Montreal Nord, 11441 boul Lacordaire, Montreal-Nord QC H1G 4J9; Laval'06; (514)384-2000 x7225

HAMEL, Erick; Clinique Med Saint-Vincent, 250 rue King E, Sherbrooke QC J1G 1A9; Sher'83; FRCPC; DiagRad. (819)563-1443

HAMEL, Gilles; Centre Med Saint-Raymond, 220 rue Saint-Joseph, Saint-Raymond QC G3L 1J1; Laval'80; Staff, Hôtel-Dieu de Lévis; (418)337-2214; Fax. (418)337-3749.

HAMEL, Jean; CSSS de Rimouski-Neigette, 150 av Rouleau, Rimouski QC G5L 5S9; Laval'85; CSPQ; Cardiol; IntMed. Staff, Hôpital Regional Rimouski; (418)723-7851

HAMEL, Jean-Francois; Clinique Familiale, 13555 boul Lacroix, Saint-Georges QC G5Y 1P1; Laval'86; (418)228-8001; Fax. (418)228-5583.

HAMEL, Jean-Pierre; Centre de Sante Newman, 7715 boul Newman, LaSalle QC H8N 1X7; Mon'81; (514)365-3142; Fax. (514)365-2074.

HAMEL, Jean-Rene; CSSS de la Cote-de-Gaspe, 215 boul de York O, Gaspe QC G4X 2W2; Laval'93; CSPQ; FRCPC; Anes. Staff, Centre Hospitalier de Gaspe; (418)368-3301 x3204; Fax. (418)368-6850; carojr@globetrotter.net.

HAMEL, Jean-Yves; Clinique Med Saint-Vincent, 318-250 rue King E, Sherbrooke QC J1G 1A9; Laval'66; CSPQ; GenSurg. (819)566-8336; Fax. (819)566-1646.

HAMEL, Joanne; Hop du Sacre-Coeur de Mtl, 5400 boul Gouin O, Montreal QC H4J 1C5; Laval'81; FRCPC; IntMed; Gastroent (P.Q.). Staff, Hôpital du Sacre-Coeur de Montréal; Staff, Jeffery Hale Hospital-Saint Brigid's; Assoc Member, Centre Hospitalier Beauce-Etchemin; Université Laval; (514)338-2794

HAMEL, Louise; Tribunal Administratif du Qc, 500 boul Rene-Levesque O, Montreal QC H2Z 1W7; Mon'77; (514)873-8030; Fax. (514)873-4137.

HAMEL, Lysianne; CSSS de Trois-Rivieres, 1191 boul du Carmel, Trois-Rivieres QC G8Z 3R9; Sher'07; CCFP; CCFP(E.M.); Staff, CSSS de Trois-Rivières; (819)697-3333

HAMEL, Melanie; CSSS de Laval, 1755 boul Rene-Laennec, Laval QC H7M 3L9; Sher'01; Nephrol; IntMed. Staff, Hopital de la Cite de la santé; (450)668-1010

HAMEL, Nathalie; Polyclinique Med Concorde, 225-300 boul de la Concorde E, Laval QC H7G 2E6; Mon'88; FRCSC; OrthSurg. (450)668-3840; Fax. (450)667-5248.

HAMEL, Pascale; Place Val des Arbres, 175-1600A boul Saint-Martin E, Laval QC H7G 4R8; Mon'89; FRCPC; Peds. (450)669-6666; Fax. (450)669-5412.

HAMEL, Patrick; Hôpital Ste-Justine, 3175 ch Cote-Sainte-Catherine, Montreal QC H3T 1C5; Laval'93; FRCSC; Ophth. Staff, Hôpital Ste-Justine; Universite de Montreal; Langs: Bilingual(English/French); (514)345-4715; Fax. (514)345-4880; patrick_hamel@ssss.gouv.qc.ca.

HAMEL, Pierre; CHUQ-Ctr Hosp Univ Laval, 2705 boul Laurier, Quebec QC G1V 4G2; Laval'88; CCFP; CCFP(E.M.); FCFP; EmergMed (P.Q.). Staff, Centre Hospitalier Universitaire de Quebec-CHUL; (418)656-4141 x70553; Fax. (418)688-2089.

HAMEL, Robert; Clinique Med Monk, 6023 boul Monk, Montreal QC H4E 3H5; Mon'74; GP/Family Med & Obst, Centre Hospitalier de LaSalle; Physician, Unite Familiale Des Naissances; Langs: Italian; (514)761-5527; Fax. (514)761-0790.

HAMEL-BREAULT, Daphné; Centre de Peri-Maternite, 575 rue Saint-Charles E, Longueuil QC J4H 1B8; Mon'06; Staff, Centre Hospitalier Pierre Boucher; Staff, Clinique Adoncour Longueuil; Langs: Bilingual(French/English); (450)332-9833

HAMELIN, Bernard; CLSC Rivieres Et Marees, 22 rue Saint-Laurent, Riviere-du-Loup QC G5R 4W5; Laval'94; Staff General Med, Centre Hospitalier Regional du Grand-Portage; (418)867-2642 x309; Fax. (418)867-4713.

HAMELIN, Christine; CLSC-CHSLD Pat Montreal Est, 13926 rue Notre-Dame E, Pte-aux-Trembles QC H1A 1T5; Mon'93; (514)642-4050; Fax. (514)642-5438.

HAMELIN, Claude; 310-369 boul Fiset, Sorel-Tracy QC J3P 3R3; Mon'76; Hôtel-Dieu de Sorel; (450)743-7133

HAMELIN, Lucie; CHUQ-St-Francois d'Assise, 10 rue de l'Espinay, Quebec QC G1L 3L5; Laval'81; CCFP; Staff, Centre Hospitalier Universitaire De Québec - Pavillon De St-françois-d'assise; (418)525-4444

HAMEON, Brigitte; CLSC du Richelieu, 300 ch de Marieville, Richelieu QC J3L 3V8; Mon'86; (450)658-7561; Fax. (450)658-4390.

HAMER, Edward S; 405-360 Bloor St W, Toronto ON M5S 1X1; Tor'73; FRCPC; Psy (Psychotherapy & Psychoanalysis). Asst Prof, University of Toronto; (416)921-1820; edward.hamer@sympatico.ca.

HAMES, Heather; London HSC-Victoria Hosp, 800 Commissioners Rd E, London ON N6A 5W9; Wes'06; FRCPC; EmergMed. Staff, London Health Sciences Centre - Victoria Campus; (519)685-8500

HAMES, J Danelle; Tom Baker Cancer Centre, 1331 29 St NW, Calgary AB T2N 4N2; Qns'73; CCFP; FCFP; Staff, Tom Baker Cancer Centre; (403)521-3740; Fax. (403)270-8407; danellehames@albertahealthservices.ca.

HAMES, Linda; Cardiometabolic Evaluation Ris, 210-1016 68 Ave SW, Calgary AB T2V 4J2; Cal'75; BScPharm; FRCPC; IntMed. Staff, Foothills Medical Centre; Staff Physician, Southern Alberta (HIV) Clinic; Staff, Cardiometabolic Evaluation & Risk Assessment Centre; Teacher, University of Calgary; (403)541-0033; Fax. (403)541-0032.

HAMET, Pavel; CHUM-Hotel-Dieu, 3840 rus Saint-Urbain, Montreal QC H2W 1T8; Prague (Czech Republic)'67; PhD(McG); FRCPC; Endocrin (P.Q.); MedScient(Med). Staff, Centre Hospitalier l'Université de Montréal (CHUM) - Hôtel-Dieu; Langs: Czech; English; Russian; (514)890-8000

HAMID, Haroon; 1050 91 St SW, Edmonton AB T6X 0P2; CCFP; Staff, Royal Alexandra Hospital; (780)463-7050; Fax. (780)463-7551.

HAMID, Muhammad A; Rouge Valley-Centenary HC, 2867 Ellesmere Rd, Scarborough ON M1E 4B9; Karachi (Pakistan)'92; Staff, Rouge Valley Health System - Centenary Health Centre Site; (416)284-8131

HAMID, Salim; Campana Place, 204-609 14 St NW, Calgary AB T2N 2A1; Karachi (Pakistan)'84; MB BS; DPM(Ire); FRCPC; Psy. Asst Prof/Staff, University of Calgary; (403)457-1953; Fax. (403)457-1727.

HAMID, Samina; 6176 Fraser St, Vancouver BC V5W 3A1; Punjab (Pakistan)'89; MB BS; (604)301-9955

HAMID, Zinia; Charlotte County Hosp, 4 Garden St, St Stephen NB E3L 2L9; (Bangladesh)'97; Staff, Charlotte County Hospital; (506)465-4586

HAMIDEH, Fayad; The Doctor's Office, 1011 Upper Middle Rd E, Oakville ON L6H 4L1; (Syria)'87; ABIM; Med Staff, Bluewater Health - Norman Site; Langs: Arabic; French; (905)849-7007; Fax. (905)849-7883.

HAMIDI, Bijan; Crowfoot Corner Medicentre, 217-150 Crowfoot Cres NW, Calgary AB T3G 3T2; (Iran)'98; (403)241-8900; Fax. (403)241-8909.

HAMIDI, Jinous; East Tower, 123-400 Walmer Rd, Toronto ON M5P 2X7; Wes'01; FRCPC; Psy. Staff, Centre for Addiction & Mental Health (CAMH) - Queen Site; (647)401-6116

HAMIELEC, Cindy M; Hamilton HS-General Site, 436-237 Barton St E, Hamilton ON L8L 2X2; McM'80; FRCPC; IntMed (Intensive Care); Respir. Ac Staff, Hamilton Health Sciences Centre - Hamilton General Hospital; Staff, St Joseph's Healthcare - Charlton Campus; Pres., Canadian Intensive Care Fdn; Assoc Prof, McMaster University; (905)522-9017; Fax. (905)577-1466.

HAMILTON, A Mark; PO Box 1708, Oliver BC V0H 1T0; Alb'79; (250)498-3488; Fax. (250)498-3566.

HAMILTON, Anderw A D; Penticton Reg Hosp, 550 Carmi Ave, Penticton BC V2A 3G6; Manchester (England)'79; MB ChB; FFARCS; FRCPC; Anes (Cardiovascular Anesthesia). Hd Anes, Penticton Regional Hospital; (250)492-4000

HAMILTON, Andrew W; Geraldton Med Clinic, 510 Hogarth St W, Geraldton ON P0T 1M0; Dal'04; CCFP; (807)854-0224; ahamilton@geraldtondh.com.

HAMILTON, Anne; Perley & Rideau Veterans HC, 1750 Russell Rd, Ottawa ON K1G 5Z6; Ott'84; CCFP; FCFP; Staff, The Perley & Rideau Veterans' Health Centre; Langs: Bilingual(English/French); (613)526-7171

HAMILTON, Anthony C; Beechy Hlth Centre, PO Box 158, Beechy SK S0L 0C0; Witwatersrand (South Africa)'70; (306)859-2113

HAMILTON, Brian T; 89 Kingswood Dr, Fredericton NB E3B 6Z8; Mem'75; FRCPC; Anes. Ac Staff Anes, Dr Everett Chalmers Regional Hospital; (506)452-5400

HAMILTON, Danielle; 104-1220 D'Orleans Dr, Orleans ON K1C 7K3; NOSM'09; CCFP; (613)841-5397

HAMILTON, David M P; Queensway-Carleton Hosp, 3045 Baseline Rd, Nepean ON K2H 8P4; Dublin (Ireland)'97; FRCPC; Psy. Staff Psy, Queensway Carleton Hospital; (613)721-2000

HAMILTON, Donald J; Central Alberta Prof Centre, 167-5201 43 St, Red Deer AB T4N 1C7; Alb'80; FRCSC; GenSurg; VascSurg. Staff GenSurg & Vascular Surg, Red Deer Regional Hospital Centre; Langs: Bilingual(English/French); (403)347-5200; Fax. (403)347-6215.

HAMILTON, Dorothy J; Doctors Med Clinic, 215-3066 Shelbourne St, Victoria BC V8R 6T9; Alb'88; CCFP; FCFP; (250)388-4211

HAMILTON, Douglas B; 204-595 Columbia St W, Kamloops BC V2C 1K7; UBC'85; Staff, Royal Inland Hospital; (250)377-8182; Fax. (250)377-8183.

HAMILTON, Douglas R; Research & Inovation Centre, W21C-3280 Hospital Dr NW, Calgary AB T2N 4Z6; Cal'91; FRCPC; IntMed. (403)210-7541; Fax. (403)210-9850.

HAMILTON, Emily F; Perigen Canada Ltd, 314-5252 boul de Maisonneuve O, Montreal QC H4A 3S5; McG'75; FRCSC; ObstGyn (Research). Staff, McGill University Health Centre - Royal Victoria Hospital; Principale Vp Clinical Research, Perigen Canada Ltd; Aj Prof, McGill University.

HAMILTON, Erin; Mount Royal Family Physicians, 701 Avenue P N, Saskatoon SK S7L 2W1; Sask'10; CCFP; (306)382-5854; Fax. (306)382-7477.

HAMILTON, G Andrew; Kingston Gen Hosp, 76 Stuart St, Kingston ON K7L 2V7; Dal'84; FRCSC; GenSurg; CardiothorSurg. Chief CardiacSurg, Kingston General Hospital; Lecturer, Queen's University; (613)548-2422 x4939; Fax. (613)548-2406.

HAMILTON, George D; 22-14 Richard Way SW, Calgary AB T3E 7M9; Cal'79; BSc; FRCSC; PlasSurg (Cosmetic Surgery). Site Chief PlasSurg, Peter Lougheed Centre; Asst Prof Clinical Surg, University of Calgary; (587)353-0244; Fax. (587)352-7448.

HAMILTON, Gillian R; Duffus Health Ctr, 208-7071 Bayers Rd, Halifax NS B3L 2C2; Dal'00; CCFP; (902)453-4585; Fax. (902)453-5657.

HAMILTON, Holly D M; Notre Dame Lourdes Fam Practic, PO Box 393 44 Rogers St, Notre-Dame-Lourdes MB R0G 1M0; Man'06; CCFP; (204)248-2252; Fax. (204)248-2781.

HAMILTON, J Douglas; Holly Street Endoscopy Clinic, 301-40 Holly St, Toronto ON M4S 3C3; Wes'56; FRCSC; GenSurg (Colon & Rectal Surgery). Physician, Holly Street Endoscopy Clinic; (416)486-8088; Fax. (416)486-7888.

HAMILTON, James J A; Woodstock & Area Commn HC, 35 Metcalf St, Woodstock ON M4S 3E6; Tor'08; (519)539-1111; Fax. (519)539-9111.

HAMILTON, Janet; Nanaimo Reg Gen Hosp, 1200 Dufferin Cres, Nanaimo BC V9S 2B7; Manchester (England)'83; MB ChB; BSc; FRCSC; ObstGyn (Surgical Assistant). Staff, Nanaimo Regional General Hospital; (250)755-7605

HAMILTON, Jeanette M; Smiths Falls Comm Hlth Ctr, 2 Gould St, Smiths Falls ON K7A 2S5; McM'83; BSc(Pharm); CCFP; FCFP; (613)283-1952; Fax. (613)283-6322.

HAMILTON, Jill K; The Hosp for Sick Children, 555 University Ave, Toronto ON M5G 1X8; Ott'92; MSc; FRCPC; Peds (Pediatric Endocrinology); Endocrin&Metab. Staff, The Hospital For Sick Children; Assoc Prof, University of Toronto; (416)813-5115; Fax. (416)813-6304; jill.hamilton@sickkids.ca.

HAMILTON, Joan; Regina Community Clinic, 1106 Winnipeg St, Regina SK S4R 1J6; Sask'07; CCFP; (306)543-7880; Fax. (306)543-6888.

HAMILTON, Joanne M; Children's Hosp, AE 305-671 William Ave, Winnipeg MB R3E 0Z2; Wes'05; FRCPC; Peds.

HAMILTON, John A; Dr John A Hamilton Inc, 9146 Mary St, Chilliwack BC V2P 4J1; UBC'94; CCFP; Med Dir Part-Time/Staff, Chilliwack General Hospital; Clin Associate Prof, University of British Columbia; (604)792-5966; Fax. (604)792-5961.

HAMILTON, John G; 2B-150 Sidney St, Belleville ON K8P 5E2; Wes'86; BSc; CCFP; FCFP; Staff, QHC Belleville General; (613)969-5217; Fax. (613)969-5218.

HAMILTON, John R; St Martha's Reg Hosp, 25 Bay St, Antigonish NS B2G 2G5; Dal'77; BSc(Hons.); FRCSC; Ophth. Staff Chief Ophth, St Martha's Regional Hospital; Assoc Consultant, Aberdeen Regional Hospital; Assoc Consultant, Inverness Consolidated Memorial Hospital; Assoc Consultant, St. Anne Centre(Arichat); Langs: English; French; (902)863-2830

HAMILTON, Julia E; Sports Med Specialists, 5F-150 Eglinton Ave E, Toronto ON M4P 1E8; Tor'06; CCFP; (416)481-1601; Fax. (416)481-1267.

HAMILTON, Kirk; 406-746 Base Line Rd E, London ON N6C 5Z2; Wes'92; CCFP; FCFP; Ac Staff Fam Med & Obst, London Health Sciences Centre - Victoria Campus; (519)472-2920

HAMILTON, Kristin; AE 305-671 William Ave, Winnipeg MB R3E 0Z2; Man'06; FRCPC; Peds.

HAMILTON, Linda D; 213-1535 Dresden Row, Halifax NS B3J 3T1; Cal'96; FRCSC; ObstGyn (Infertility). Staff, IWK Health Centre; (902)404-8600; Fax. (902)404-8601; linda.hamilton23@gmail.com.

HAMILTON, M Lynn; Rosedale Med Centre, 502-600 Sherbourne St, Toronto ON M4X 1W4; Ott'81; FRCPC; IntMed (Osteoporosis); Rheum. Ac Staff, Sunnybrook Health Sciences Centre - Holland Orthopaedic & Arthritic Centre; Lecturer, University of Toronto; Langs: Polish; (416)963-9292; Fax. (416)963-8057.

HAMILTON, Mark G; Foothills Medical Centre, 12F-1403 29 St NW, Calgary AB T2N 2T9; McG'83; FRCSC; Neursurg (Neuro Oncology). Staff, Alberta Children's Hospital; Staff, Foothills Medical Centre; Staff, Tom Baker Cancer Centre; (403)944-1626; Fax. (403)283-2270; mark-hamilton@shaw.ca.

HAMILTON, Marlene A; Clinical Sciences Bldg, 13 109-152 University Campus N, Edmonton AB T6G 2G3; Alb'95; BSc; FRCPC; IntMed; MedOncol; Hem. Staff, University of Alberta Hospital; (780)407-1584 x8; Fax. (780)407-2680.

HAMILTON, Matthew J; Kilborn Med Centre, 316-1385 Bank St, Ottawa ON K1H 8N4; Ott'62; FRCPC; Psy. (613)733-7372; Fax. (613)733-2093.

HAMILTON, Michael J; 8808 92 St NW, Edmonton AB T6C 3R1; Alb'91; CCFP; FCFP; (780)469-7147; Fax. (780)469-3871.

HAMILTON, Michael J A; 15900 Bayview Ave, Aurora ON L4G 7Y3; Qns'00; CCFP; (905)726-9755

HAMILTON, Nicolas; Chinook Reg Hosp, 960 19 St S, Lethbridge AB T1J 1W5; Laval'08; CCFP; CCFP(E.M.); Staff, Chinook Regional Hospital; (403)388-6300

HAMILTON, Paul A; Sunnybrook Hlth Sciences Ctre, 2075 Bayview Ave, Toronto ON M4N 3M5; Mem'78; FRCPC; DiagRad. Staff Med Imaging, Sunnybrook Health Sciences Centre; Asst Prof, University of Toronto; (416)480-4336; Fax. (416)480-5228.

HAMILTON, Peter G; University of Alberta Hosp, 22-8440 112 St NW, Edmonton AB T6G 2B7; Witwatersrand (South Africa)'79; MB ChB; FRCPC; IntMed (Nephrology). Asst Prof, University of Alberta Hospital; Asst Prof, University of Alberta; (780)407-8153; Fax. (780)407-3132.

HAMILTON, Philip P; CSSSG Hop de Hull, 116 boul Lionel-Emond, Gatineau QC J8Y 1W7; Qns'77; BA; BPHE; MSc; CSPQ; FRCPC; Anes (Hyperbaric Medicine). Ac Staff, Hull Hospital; Court Staff Anes, University of Ottawa; Langs: French; (819)595-6033; pphamilton@hotmail.com.

HAMILTON, Robert J; 70 Meredith St PO Box 219, Gore Bay ON P0P 1H0; Alb'79; DCH(NZ); Staff, Manitoulin Health Centre - Little Current; Med Dir, Manitoulin Lodge; Asst Prof Family Medicine, Northern Ontario School of Medicine; (705)282-2262; Fax. (705)282-2370.

HAMILTON, Robert M; The Hosp for Sick Children, 555 University Ave, Toronto ON M5G 1X8; Dal'82; Cardiol; Peds (Electrophysiology). Ac Staff Cardiol, The Hospital For Sick Children; Asst Prof Peds, University of Toronto; (416)813-6142; Fax. (416)813-7547; robert.hamilton@sickkids.ca.

HAMILTON, Roger D; Wolfville Prof Centre, PO Box 2016 6-4 Little Rd, Wolfville NS B4P 1P4; Qns'85; Staff, Valley Regional Hospital; (902)542-7016; rh@eastlink.ca.

HAMILTON, Ronald W; 205-751 King St W, Kitchener ON N2G 1E5; Cambridge (England)'59; FRCS(Eng); FRCSC; GenSurg; Urol. Ac Staff, Grand River Hospital - Kitchener/Waterloo Health Centre; Ac Staff, St Mary's General Hospital; (519)744-3503; Fax. (519)744-7372.

HAMILTON, Scott; 103-361 George St N, Peterborough ON K9H 3R2; Wes'04; FRCSC; Otol (Head & Neck Surgery). Staff, Peterborough Regional Health Centre - Hospital Drive; (705)743-8221; Fax. (705)743-4416.

HAMILTON, Sean F; St Clare's Mercy Hosp, 154 Lemarchant Rd, St. John's NL A1C 5B8; Mem'80; FRCPC; IntMed; Rheum. Staff, St Clare's Mercy Hospital; Assoc Prof Med, Memorial University Of Newfoundland; (709)777-5582; Fax. (709)722-5526.

HAMILTON, Stewart M; University of Alberta Hosp, 2D447WCM-8440 112 St NW, Edmonton AB T6G 2B7; McG'77; FRCSC; GenSurg (Breast Aesthetic Surgery). Staff, University of Alberta Hospital; (780)407-6306; Fax. (780)407-1422; stewart.hamilton@albertahealthservices.ca.

HAMILTON, Trevor; Foothills Medical Centre, 1403 29 St NW, Calgary AB T2N 2T9; Dal'08; Staff, Foothills Medical Centre; (403)944-1110

HAMILTON, W Keith; Medical Arts Bldg, 208-750 Spadina Cres E, Saskatoon SK S7K 3H3; Sask'85; FRCSC; Ophth (Cataract Surgery). Ac Staff, Royal University Hospital; Ac Staff, Saskatoon City Hospital; Assoc Prof, University of Saskatchewan; (306)242-9990; Fax. (306)244-1909.

HAMILTON, Wendy; The Westend Family Care Clinic, 80 Michael Cowpland Dr, Kanata ON K2M 1P6; Ott'90; CCFP; FCFP; Staff, Westend Family Care Clinic Family Health Team; (613)599-3321; Fax. (613)599-3366.

HAMILTON-IRVING, Jonathan; Quinte HC Corp-Belleville Gen, 265 Dundas St E, Belleville ON K8N 5A9; Dal'06; CCFP; CCFP(E.M.); Staff, QHC Belleville General; (613)969-7400

HAMIWKA, Lorraine A; Alberta Children's Hosp, C4 604-2888 Shaganappi Trail N, Calgary AB T3B 6A8; Man'96; BSc; FRCPC; Peds (Transplantation); Nephrol. Staff PedsNephrol, Alberta Children's Hospital; (403)955-7821; Fax. (403)955-2203.

HAMLET, Bevin; 322 Silverthorn Ave, Toronto ON M6N 3K6; Tor'85; CCFP; FCFP; Staff, St Joseph's Health Centre; Staff, Humber River Regional Hospital - Keele Street Site; (416)656-8777; Fax. (416)656-5489.

HAMLYN, Margaret O; Pearlgate Med Clinic, 18 Gibson Dr, Mount Pearl NL A1N 5K8; Mem'06; CCFP; (709)364-3909

HAMM, Caroline M; Windsor Reg Cancer Centre, 2220 Kildare Rd, Windsor ON N8W 2X3; Dal'92; FRCPC; IntMed; MedOncol. (519)253-5253; Fax. (519)253-4204; lend@wincom.net.

HAMM, Charles; Valley Women's & Children's Ce, 60 Aberdeen St, Kentville NS B4N 2N3; Massachusetts (USA)'02; FRCSC; ObstGyn. Physician, Valley Women's & Children's Centre; (902)678-4626; Fax. (902)678-6338.

HAMM, Darrell A; Capri Med Centre, 132-1835 Gordon Dr, Kelowna BC V1Y 3H5; Sask'98; LMCC; CCFP; (250)717-3211; Fax. (250)717-3233.

HAMM, Jason S; Glen Sather Sports Med Clinic, 1A 102-11400 University Ave NW, Edmonton AB T6G 1Z1; Alb'06; CCFP; Staff, University of Alberta Hospital; Clin Lecturer Family Med Dept, University of Alberta.

HAMMAD, Nazik H M; Kingston Reg Cancer Ctr, 25 King St W, Kingston ON K7L 5P9; Khartoum (Sudan)'89; Staff, Cancer Centre of Southeastern Ontario; (613)544-2631 x4505; Fax. (613)546-8209.

HAMMAMI, Hachmi; 58 rue du Marche, Salaber-de-Valleyf QC J6T 1P4; Lausanne (Switzerland)'67; LMCC; FRCSC; Ophth (Neuro Ophthalmology). Langs: Italian; Arabic; English; (450)747-0851; Fax. (450)747-0855.

HAMMAMJI, Karim; 301-5340 1 St SW, Calgary AB T2H 0C8; McG'06; MDCM; FRCSC; Ophth. (403)252-3937

HAMMAN, Wessel; Humboldt Med Clinic, PO Box 3841, Humboldt SK S0K 2A0; (306)682-4405; Fax. (306)682-4405.

HAMMEL, Kenneth H; Aberdeen Prof Centre, 835 East River Rd, New Glasgow NS B2H 3S6; Alb'83; BMedSci; FRCSC; Ophth (Cataract Surgery). Ac Staff, Aberdeen Regional Hospital; (902)752-2216; Fax. (902)752-4593.

HAMMELL, Darlene M S; Med Sciences Bldg, PO Box 1700 Stc Csc, Victoria BC V8W 2Y2; Tor'73; CCFP; FCFP; Ac Staff, Vancouver Island Health Authority; Clin Prof Family Med/Asst Dean Student Affairs Island Med Prog, University of British Columbia; (250)472-5500; Fax. (250)472-5505; dhammell@uvic.ca.

HAMMELL, Jennifier; Virden Associate Med Clinic, PO Box 730, Virden MB R0M 2C0; NOSM'09; CCFP.

HAMMER, Antony; 3019 Tecumseh Rd E, Windsor ON N8W 1G8; London (England)'73; MB BS; MRCS; LRCP; CISAM; Ac Staff, Windsor Regional Hospital - Metropolitan Site; Staff Addiction Medicine, Erie-St Clair Clinic; (519)945-4503

HAMMER, Debra M; University of Alberta Hosp, 2C2WCM-8440 112 St NW, Edmonton AB T6G 2B7; Sask'84; ABIM; FACC; FRCPC; IntMed (Cardiology). Clin Teacher/Staff, University of Alberta Hospital; (780)407-2176; Fax. (780)407-6452.

HAMMERBERG, Ole; 2-520 Sarnia Rd, London ON N6G 5A3; UBC'75; BSc; MSc; FRCPC; Peds (Infectious Diseases); MedMicrobiol. Consultant, St Joseph's Hospital - St Joseph's Health Care; Consultant, London Health Sciences Centre - University Hospital; Assoc Prof, University of Western Ontario; Langs: Danish; (519)432-5508; Fax. (519)433-3394.

HAMMERLINDL, Donna M A; Seventh Street Plaza, 405-10030 107 St NW, Edmonton AB T5J 3E4; Alb'79; Staff, Birth Control Centre; Staff, After Hours Clinic; (780)735-0010

HAMMETT, D Clayton; Peterson Med Centre, RR 1 Stn Main 45 Wolosley St, Kenora ON P9N 3W7; Qns'98; FRACGP; CCFP; (807)468-3021

HAMMETT, John; Paterson Med Centre, 45 Wolsley St, Kenora ON P9N 3W7; Tor'68; MHSc; CCFP; FCFP; Staff, Lake of the Woods District Hospital; Coroner, District of Kenora; (807)468-3021; Fax. (807)468-8145.

HAMMETT, Tess; Health Point Care Center, 1454 Hillside Ave, Victoria BC V8T 2B7; Qns'09; CCFP; (250)370-5637

HAMMING, Jeremy A D; Foothills Med Centre, 1403 29 St NW, Calgary AB T2N 2T9; UBC'01; FRCPC; Anes. Staff, Foothills Medical Centre; (403)944-1430; Fax. (403)944-2425.

HAMMOND, Allan; Health Sciences Centre, 820 Sherbrook St, Winnipeg MB R3A 1R9; Man'03; FRCSC; OrthSurg. Staff, Health Sciences Centre; (204)774-8511

HAMMOND, Cecil M; Prince Albert Med Clinic, 681 15th St W, Prince Albert SK S6V 7H9; Physician, Prince Albert Medical Clinic; (306)764-1505; Fax. (306)764-7775.

HAMMOND, D Ian; 501 Smyth Rd, Ottawa ON K1H 8L6; McG'72; FACR; FRCPC; DiagRad. Consultant, Arnprior & District Memorial Hospital; Consultant, Winchester District Memorial Hospital; Consultant, Almonte General Hospital; Staff, The Ottawa Hospital - General Campus; Langs: French; (613)788-8965; Fax. (613)737-8957; ihammond@ottawahospital.on.ca.

HAMMOND, Diana R; 101-230 Cook St PO Box 23074, Victoria BC V8V 4Z9; Alb'08; CCFP; (403)617-2244

HAMMOND, Gregory W; 730 William Ave, Winnipeg MB R3E 0W3; McG'72; FRCPC; IntMed (Public Health); InfectDis; MedMicrobiol. Staff Med Microbiol & InfectDis, Health Sciences Centre; Teach Staff Med Microbiol, University of Manitoba.

HAMMOND, J Alex; London Reg Cancer Centre, 790 Commissioners Rd E, London ON N6A 4L6; Witwatersrand (South Africa)'69; MB ChB; AB; BSc(Med); FRCPC; RadOncol (Head Neck & Gynecology). Consultant, London Health Sciences Centre - Victoria Campus; Prof, University of Western Ontario; (519)685-8650; Fax. (519)685-8627.

HAMMOND, Jo-Anne S; Thames Valley FHT-Victoria Fam, 60 Chesley Ave, London ON N5Z 2C1; Wes'84; MClSc; CCFP; FCFP; Ac Staff, London Health Sciences Centre - Victoria Campus; Ac Staff, St Joseph's Hospital - St Joseph's Health Care; Asst Prof Family Med, University of Western Ontario; (519)433-8424; Fax. (519)433-2244; joanne.hammond@lhsc.on.ca.

HAMMOND, Karsten M; 206-1964 Fort St, Victoria BC V8R 6R3; Alb'07; FRCPC; IntMed; InfectDis. (250)370-7717

HAMMOND, Lynda C; 3335 Dougall Ave, Windsor ON N9E 1S8; Tor'91; CCFP; FCFP; (519)948-8000

HAMMOND, Michael; Grand Bend Area CHC, 69 Main St, Grand Bend ON N0M 1T0; Qns'05; CCFP; Staff Physician, South Huron Hospital Association; (519)238-2362; Fax. (519)238-6478.

HAMMOND, Robert R; London HSC-University Hosp, PO Box 5339 Stn B B3 148-339 Windermere Rd, London ON N6A 5A5; Wes'87; FRCPC; NeurPath. Med Staff, London Health Sciences Centre - Victoria Campus; Med Staff, London Health Sciences Centre - University Hospital; Med Staff, St Joseph's Hospital - St Joseph's Health Care; Prof Path & Clin Neurological Sciences/Assoc Dean Admissions, University of Western Ontario; (519)685-8500 x36367; Fax. (519)663-2930; rhammond@uwo.ca.

HAMMOUD, Souhaila; Erindale Med Centre, 1101 McBride Ave, Mississauga ON L5C 1M6; (Syria)'82; CCFP; Langs: Arabic; (905)270-4020; Fax. (905)270-6374.

HAMMOUDA, M Wahbi; Chinguacousy & Sandalwood Med, 6-10671 Chinguacousy Rd, Brampton ON L7A 0N5; McG'80; FRCPC; IntMed (Benign Hematology); Hem. Court Staff, Clin Path, Sunnybrook Health Sciences Centre; Consultant Hematologist, Royal Health Care Centre; Consultant Hematologist, MCI-Royal Bank Plaza; Langs: Arabic; French; Italian; (905)840-4343; Fax. (905)840-4303.

HAMMOUDI, Dena; 401-7900 Hurontario St, Brampton ON L6Y 0P6; Tor'06; FRCSC; Ophth. (905)456-9500; Fax. (905)456-9508.

HAMODAT, Mowafak; Health Sciences Centre, 1547-300 Prince Philip Dr, St. John's NL A1B 3V6; (Iraq)'84; FRCPC; AnatPath. Staff, Health Sciences Centre; (709)777-6300

HAMOUDI, Aseel; McMaster University, 2F-1280 Main St W, Hamilton ON L8S 4K1; Baghdad (Iraq)'94; FRCSC; ObstGyn. Teach Staff, McMaster University; Langs: Arabic; (905)521-2100; Fax. (905)577-0471.

HAMOUR, Abuobeida; Phoenix Med Centre, 303-2155 10th Ave, Prince George BC V2M 5J6; Khartoum (Sudan)'81; MB BS; MSc; MRCP(UK); FRCP(Edin); DTM&H(Lond); CCST(UK); FRCPC; IntMed (Travel Medicine); InfectDis. Staff, University Hospital of Northern British Columbia; Clinical Asst Prof, University of British Columbia; Langs: Arabic; (250)563-8284; abu.hamour@northernhealth.ca.

HAMOUR, Faisal A; Professional Bldg, 3101-222 King St E, Bowmanville ON L1C 1P6; Alexandria (Egypt)'85; MB ChB; FRCSC; GenSurg. (905)697-4499; Fax. (905)623-1835.

HAMPE, Kyle; Dryden Reg Hlth Centre, PO Box 3003 Stn Main 58 Goodall St, Dryden ON P8N 2Z6; McM'94; FRCPC; Psy. Staff, Dryden Regional Health Centre; (807)223-6678; Fax. (807)223-7183.

HAMPEL, Elizabeth; Reddendale Family Hlth Centre, 125 Lakeview Ave, Kingston ON K7M 3T6; (Poland)'86; FRCPC; Psy. Staff, Providence Care - Mental Health Services; (613)384-4664; Fax. (613)384-4182.

HAMPOLE, Rahul K; 502-550 Victoria St, Prince George BC V2L 2K1; Qns'91; FRCSC; Urol. Staff Urol, University Hospital of Northern British Columbia; (250)561-3007; Fax. (250)561-2990.

HAMRAHI, Hormoz; Toronto Grace Hosp, 6F-650 Church St, Toronto ON M4Y 2G5; Tor'02; CCFP; Staff Family Med, The Salvation Army Toronto Grace Health Centre; Langs: Persian; (416)925-2251; Fax. (416)925-9136.

HAMSON, Andrew C; Thompson Gen Hosp, 871 Thompson Dr, Thompson MB R8N 0C8; Liverpool (England)'70; MB ChB; FRCPC; Peds. Staff, Thompson General Hospital; (204)677-2381

HAMSTRA, Joel M; St Joseph's Healthcare, 50 Charlton Ave E, Hamilton ON L8N 4A6; McM'03; FRCPC; Anes. Staff Anes, St Joseph's Healthcare - Charlton Campus; (905)522-1155 x33853

HAMZA, Essam; Cambie Plaza Med Clinic, 180-11700 Cambie Rd, Richmond BC V6X 1L5; Alb'97; CCFP; (604)270-9833

HAMZA, Sate; Health Sciences Centre, MS477K-820 Sherbrook St, Winnipeg MB R3A 1R9; Aleppo (Syria)'95; FRCPC; AnatPath. Staff, Health Sciences Centre; (204)774-6511

HAN, Christina E; Westminster Med Bldg, 606-625 Fifth Ave, New Westminster BC V3M 1X4; UBC'07; FRCPC; Derm. (604)528-3961

HAN, Guangming; Sunnybrook Hlth Sciences Ctre, 2075 Bayview Ave, Toronto ON M4N 3M5; Tor'04; FRCPC; AnatPath. Staff, Sunnybrook Health Sciences Centre; (416)480-6100

HAN, John; South Hlth Campus, 260180-4448 Front St SE, Calgary AB T3M 1M4; UBC'10; CCFP; Staff, Rockyview General Hospital; (403)462-0225

HAN, Lily; Unite de Med Familiale, 100-500 Boul de l'Hopital, Gatineau QC J8V 2P5; McG'10; MDCM; CCFP; (819)966-6171

HAN, Ra Kyung; 2F-61 Queen St E, Toronto ON M5C 2T2; Tor'00; BSc; FRCPC; Peds (Pediatric Cardiology); Cardiol. Staff Pediatric Cardiology Clinic, St Michael's Hospital; Staff, The Hospital For Sick Children; Staff, Women's College Hospital; Staff, Sunnybrook Health Sciences Centre; (416)867-3655; Fax. (416)867-3736; hanra@smh.ca.

HAN, Thomas M K; Oakdale Med Bldg, 402-2065 Finch Ave W, North York ON M3N 2V7; UBC'96; FRCPC; PhysMed&Rehab. (416)745-2314; Fax. (416)745-9336.

HAN, Victor; London HSC-Victoria Hosp, PO Box 5010 Stn B D4 215-800 Commissioner's Rd E, London ON N6A 5W9; Rangoon (Burma)'73; FRCP(Lond); DAB; FRCPC; Peds (Neonatal & Perinatal Medicine). Staff Neonatol, St Joseph's Hospital - St Joseph's Health Care; Staff, London Health Sciences Centre - Victoria Campus; Chair, Canada Research; Prof, University of Western Ontario; Langs: Burmese; (519)685-8500

HAN, Yung; St Mary's Hosp Centre, 3830 av Lacombe, Montreal QC H3T 1M5; Chicago (USA)'06; OrthSurg. Staff, St Mary's Hospital Centre; (514)345-3511

HANADA, Edwin Y; Nova Scotia Rehab Centre, 209-1341 Summer St, Halifax NS B3H 4K4; UBC'96; FRCPC; PhysMed&Rehab. Staff, Nova Scotia Rehabilitation Centre; (902)473-2612

HANADA, Philip M; Grand River Hosp-KW Hlth Ctre, PO Box 9056 Stn C 835 King St W, Kitchener ON N2G 1G3; Qns'88; FRCPC; Anes. Staff Anes, Grand River Hospital - Kitchener/Waterloo Health Centre; Staff, St Mary's General Hospital; (519)749-4300

HANAM, Philip J; Royal Oak Med Centre, 204-6440 Royal Oak Ave, Burnaby BC V5H 3P2; Alb'91; CCFP; (604)482-6100; Fax. (604)482-6102.

HANBIDGE, Anthony E; Univ Hlth Network-Toronto Western Hosp, EW 3MC 426-399 Bathurst St, Toronto ON M5T 2S8; Dublin (Ireland)'82; MB ChB; BAO; FRCPC; DiagRad (Body Imaging). Staff, Toronto Western Hospital - University Health Network; Staff, Toronto General Hospital - UHN; Asst Prof, University of Toronto; (416)603-5800 x3761; anthony.hanbidge@uhn.on.ca.

HANCKE, Petrus; 219B 3 St W, Brooks AB T1R 0S3; (South Africa)'76; MB ChB; (403)362-3040

HANCOCK, B J; Children's Hosp, AE401-840 Sherbrook St, Winnipeg MB R3A 1S1; Man'84; MSc(Surg.); FACS; BSc(Hon); FRCSC; GenSurg (Pediatric Surgery); Critical Care Medicine; PedGenSurg. Staff, Health Sciences Centre; Assoc Prof, University of Manitoba; Langs: French; (204)787-1246; Fax. (204)787-4618; bjhancock@hsc.mb.ca.

HANCOCK, Caroline A; Annapolis Family Med Group, PO Box 573 821 St George St, Annapolis Royal NS B0S 1A0; Cardiff (Wales)'87; MB ChB; MSc; CCFP; (902)532-2324

HANCOCK, David J; Rouge Valley-Ajax & Pickering, 580 Harwood Ave S, Ajax ON L1S 2J4; Edinburgh (Scotland)'69; Chief Emerg, Rouge Valley Health System - Ajax & Pickering Health Centre Site; Dir Medical & Health Services, Toronto Police Services; (905)683-2320

HANCOCK, E Jolene; Complete Medical, 573 Torbay Rd, St. John's NL A1A 5G9; Mem'02; FRCPC; Psy. (709)754-3787

HANCOCK, Gregg W; The Jenny Trout Centre, 203-342 Erie St, Stratford ON N5A 2N4; Wes'93; BSc(Hon); FRCSC; ObstGyn. Staff Consultant, Alexandra Hospital; Staff Consultant, Listowel Memorial Hospital - Listowel Wingham Hospitals Alliance; Chief Dept of ObstGyn, Stratford General Hospital - Huron Perth Healthcare Alliance; Aj Prof, University of Western Ontario; (519)271-1912; Fax. (519)271-5772; gregghancock@sympatico.ca.

HANCOCK, Jennifer; Queen Elizabeth II HSC, 348-1276 South Park St, Halifax NS B3H 2Y9; Mem'00; FRCPC; IntMed; Critical Care Medicine. Staff, Queen Elizabeth II Health Sciences Centre - Victoria General Site; (902)473-2700

HANCOCK, Julian A; Dr Skinlaser Clinics, 214-911 Yates St, Victoria BC V8V 4X3; London (England)'78; MB BS; DCH; DRCOG; DA; FRCPC; Derm (Laser Surgery). Fellow, American Society of Lasers Medicine & Surgery; (250)384-3202; Fax. (250)383-0612.

HANCOCK, Larry G; 283-4035 Gellatly Rd S, Kelowna BC V4T 1R7; Tor'73; Staff, Kelowna General Hospital; Teach. Assoc., University of British Columbia; (250)768-3846; Fax. (250)768-8684.

HANCOCK, Lindsay E; Sioux Lookout Zone Family Phys, PO Box 4000, Sioux Lookout ON P8T 1K2; Tor'05; CCFP; (807)737-5166; Fax. (807)737-4364.

HANCOCK, Michael; Victoria Med Centre, 6915 109 St NW, Edmonton AB T6H 3B7; London (England)'74; MB BS; MRCS; LRCP; FRCS(Eng); Surg Asst Dept of Cardiovascular Surgery, University of Alberta Hospital; Langs: French; (780)433-7211; Fax. (780)433-7758.

HANCOCK, Ronald J; 135 Jensen Ave E PO Box 1141 Stn Main, Parksville BC V9P 2H2; Cal'92; (250)248-6969; Fax. (250)248-4275.

HANCOCK, Sherri R M; 275 Island Hwy, Victoria BC V9B 1G4; UBC'94; FRCSC; ObstGyn. Staff, Cowichan District Hospital; Locum Tenens, Victoria General Hospital; (250)380-9002

HANCOCK, Trevor G; 3800 Finnerty Rd, Victoria BC V8W 2Y2; London (England)'73; MHSc; MB BS; (250)472-5374

HANCOCK FRIESEN, Camille L; IWK Health Centre, PO Box 9700 Rpo CSC 5850-5980 University Ave, Halifax NS B3K 6R8; Alb'92; MSc; FACS; FRCSC; GenSurg (Pediatric Cardiac Surgery); CardSurg. Staff, IWK Health Centre; Assoc Prof Surg, Dalhousie University; (902)473-7597; Fax. (902)473-4448; camillehf@hotmail.com.

HANCU, Dan J; 403-1017 Wilson Ave, North York ON M3K 1Z1; Tor'76; CCFP; FCFP; Ac Staff, Humber River Regional Hospital - Keele Street Site; Langs: Italian; Spanish; French; Romanian; (416)636-5500; Fax. (416)636-5501; danhancu10@yahoo.ca.

HAND, Gregory R F; Kootenay Lake Hosp, 3 View St, Nelson BC V1L 2V1; Qns'99; Staff, Kootenay Lake General Hospital; (250)352-3111

HAND, Karen M; Consent and Capacity Board, 10F-151 Bloor St W, Toronto ON M5S 2T5; Mem'81; FRCPC; Psy. Staff Consultant, Regional Mental Health Care-St Joseph's Health Care.

HANDA, Pooja; 10660 Yonge St, Richmond Hill ON L4C 3C9; Windsor (England)'08; (905)770-9096

HANDANOS, Daphne; Ctr Hosp de Verdun, 4000 boul Lasalle, Verdun QC H4G 2A3; Mon'89; CCFP; Staff Med/Supvr, Centre Hospitalier de Verdun; Physician, CLSC Verdun; Universite de Montreal; (514)765-7310

HANDELMAN, Kenneth L; Halton Hlth Care Oakville Corp, 6F-700 Dorval Dr, Oakville ON L6K 3V3; Tor'95; DABPN; FRCPC; Psy (Child & Adolescent Psychiatry). Aj Prof Psy, University of Western Ontario; (905)815-5140 x4826; Fax. (905)815-5076.

HANDELSMAN, Sam; Keele-Ingram Prof Centre, 315-2221 Keele St, North York ON M6M 3Z5; Tor'77; FRCPC; Rheum; IntMed. Staff, Humber River Regional Hospital - Finch Avenue Site; (416)235-0814; Fax. (416)245-1166; handelsman@rogers.com.

HANDFIELD-JONES, Richard S; Cdn Forces Hlth Services Ctre, 101 Colonel By Dr, Ottawa ON K1A 0K2; Ott'81; CCFP; FCFP; Langs: French; (613)945-1340

HANDFORD, Curtis D; Wellesley Health Centre, 4F-410 Sherbourne St, Toronto ON M4X 1K2; Man'01; BSc; MHSc; CCFP; Staff, Centre for Addiction & Mental Health (CAMH) - Russell Street Site; (416)867-3728; Fax. (416)867-3726.

HANDFORD, Robert G; Health Sciences Ctr Gen Hosp, GC 423-700 William Ave, Winnipeg MB R3E 0Z3; Man'55; BA; FRCPC; IntMed.

HANDLER, Jeffrey D; William Osler HC-Brampton, 2100 Bovaird Dr E, Brampton ON L6R 3J7; Tor'92; MSc; Dip SportMed; CCFP; CCFP(E.M.); FCFP; Staff, William Osler Health System - Brampton Civic Hospital; (905)494-2120

HANDLEY, David; 302-125 Bell Farm Rd, Barrie ON L4M 6L2; Tor'68; Assoc Staff, Royal Victoria Regional Health Centre; (705)737-1532; Fax. (705)737-3703.

HANDLEY-DERRY, Mark H; 210-658 Danforth Ave, Toronto ON M4J 5B9; London (England)'78; MB BS; DCH; FRCPC; Peds (Developmental Pediatrics). Staff, The Hospital For Sick Children; Court Staff, Toronto East General Hospital Inc; Asst Prof, University of Toronto; (416)461-3937; Fax. (416)461-7425; mark.handley.derry@utoronto.ca.

HANDS, Brian W; The Two Hundred, 406-200 St Clair Ave W, Toronto ON M4V 1R1; Tor'68; FRCSC; Otol (Ears). Associate Scientific, Mount Sinai Hospital; (416)922-0070; Fax. (416)922-0071.

HANDSCOMB, Arthur; Windsor Reg Hosp-Metropolitan, 1995 Lens Ave, Windsor ON N8W 1L9; Glasgow (Scotland)'60; MRCOG; ObstGyn. Staff, Windsor Regional Hospital - Metropolitan Site; (519)254-5577

HANDSCOMB, Sheina E W; Harrow Hlth Clinic Incorporate, PO Box 430 1480 County Rd 13, Harrow ON N0R 1G0; Glasgow (Scotland)'60; MB ChB; Court Staff, Hôtel-Dieu Grace Hospital; (519)738-2000

HANDY, Shaheda; Southlake Reg Health Centre, 596 Davis Dr, Newmarket ON L3Y 2P9; Poona (India)'73; MB BS; FRCPC; GenPath. Staff Path, Southlake Regional Health Centre; (905)895-4521 x2493; Fax. (905)952-2824.

HANEKOM, Pierre; Family Physicians Group, PO Box 2170, Melfort SK S0E 1A0; Stellenbosch (South Africa)'82; MB ChB; LMCC; (306)752-3253; Fax. (306)752-5099.

HANEL, Erich; Hamilton HS-General Site, 237 Barton St E, Hamilton ON L8L 2X2; MB; BAO; BCh; MSc; CCFP; CCFP(E.M.); Staff, Hamilton Health Sciences Centre - Hamilton General Hospital; (905)521-2100; e.hanel@ontariomd.ca.

HANEL, Robert; CSSS des Iles, 430 ch Principal, Cap-aux-Meules QC G4T 1R9; Sher'95; FRCPC; IntMed. Staff, Hôpital de l'Archipel; Langs: English; (418)986-2121

HANELT, Richard R; 9534 87 St NW, Edmonton AB T6C 3J1; UBC'02; CCFP; Physician, Meadowbrook Medical Clinic; (780)440-8274

HANET, Stephen H; Bloor Med Clinic, 844 Bathurst St, Toronto ON M5R 3G1; Tor'71; CCFP; FCFP; Assoc Staff, Mount Sinai Hospital; (416)534-4214; Fax. (416)534-4582.

HANEY, Colleen M; 201 Deacon St, Pembroke ON K8A 2J6; Ott'06; FRCSC; GenSurg. (613)732-3675; Fax. (613)732-6347.

HANEY, Elizabeth; St Thomas-Elgin Gen Hosp, PO Box 2007 Stn Main 189 Elm St, St Thomas ON N5P 3W2; Dal'04; CCFP; CCFP(E.M.); Staff, London Health Sciences Centre - South Street; Staff, St Thomas Elgin General Hospital; (519)631-2020; Fax. (519)631-1083.

HANEY, Isabel M M; 105-3950 14th Ave, Markham ON L3R 0A9; McG'90; FRCPC; Peds. (905)305-1700; Fax. (905)305-1706.

HANI, Antoine; Clinique Med Viau, 4750 rue Jarry E, Saint-Leonard QC H1R 1X8; Mon'75; Staff Gen Med, Hôpital Santa Cabrini Ospedale; (514)326-7203; Fax. (514)326-3656.

HANIAK, William A; 209-125 13th St E, North Vancouver BC V7L 2L3; UBC'89; BSc(Pharm); FRCPC; IntMed; Gastroent. (604)988-2855; Fax. (604)988-2846.

HANICK, Adrian N; 702-120 Eglinton Ave E, Toronto ON M4P 1E2; Tor'74; FACP; FRCPC; Psy (Pain Medicine). (416)322-3522; Fax. (416)322-6448; schiap1@sympatico.ca.

HANKEY, Arthur V; Stroud Med Centre, 1-7869 Yonge St, Innisfil ON L9S 1K8; Tor'75; Staff, Royal Victoria Regional Health Centre; (705)436-2251; Fax. (705)436-7991.

HANKINS, Jennifer E; Alberni Med Bldg, 4-3855 9th Ave, Port Alberni BC V9Y 4T9; Wes'99; FRCSC; GenSurg. Staff, West Coast General Hospital; (250)736-1900

HANKINSON, James J; Hamilton HS-GenSite, 237 Barton St E, Hamilton ON L8L 2X2; Alb'91; Anes. Staff, Hamilton Health Sciences Centre - Hamilton General Hospital; (905)527-0271

HANKINSON, Jeffrey J; The Med Centre, PO Box 4010 Stn Main, Barrhead AB T7N 1A1; Alb'80; CCFP; Staff, Barrhead Healthcare Centre; (780)674-2246; Fax. (780)674-6164.

HANKINSON, Keith; Two Rivers FHT-Hespeler Med Cl, B12-350 Conestoga Blvd, Cambridge ON N1R 7L7; Tor'87; CCFP; Staff, Cambridge Memorial Hospital; (519)629-4615 x224; Fax. (519)629-4630.

HANKS, David G; 204-300 Columbia St, Kamloops BC V2C 6L1; UBC'91; FRCSC; GenSurg. Staff Privil, Royal Inland Hospital; (250)374-0028; Fax. (250)374-0328.

HANLEY, Brendan E; Mental Health Services, 4 Hospital Rd, Whitehorse YT Y1A 3H8; Alb'82; CCFP; CCFP(E.M.); Staff, Whitehorse Medical Services Ltd.

HANLEY, Catherine L; Brant Community HC-Brantford, 200 Terrace Hill St, Brantford ON N3R 1G9; McM'04; Staff, The Brant Community Healthcare System - Brantford General Hospital Site; (519)752-7871

HANLEY, David A; Richmond Road Diag & Tremt Ctr, 1820 Richmond Rd SW, Calgary AB T2T 5C7; Tor'70; FRCPC; IntMed (Endocrinology & Metabolism). Staff Med Endocrin & Metab, Foothills Medical Centre; Staff Med Endocrin & Metab, Tom Baker Cancer Centre; Prof of Med Community Hlth Sciences & Oncology, University of Calgary; (403)955-8327; Fax. (403)955-8249; dahanley@ucalgary.ca.

HANLEY, S Anne; MDS Laboratory Services, 100 International Blvd, Etobicoke ON M9W 6J6; Galway (Ireland)'73; FRCPC; GenPath (Anatomical Pathology).

HANLEY, William B; 660 Eglinton Ave E PO Box 50030 Rpo Sunnybrook, East York ON M4G 4G1; Tor'54; FRCPC; Peds (Newborn Screening). Hon Physician, St Michael's Hospital; Hon Physician, North York General Hospital; Hon Physician, The Hospital For Sick Children; (416)781-1805; Fax. (416)781-8515.

HANLON, Brian A; East York Med Health Centre, 27E-45 Overlea Blvd, Toronto ON M4H 1C3; Dublin (Ireland)'68; DRCOG; (416)696-9836 x222; Fax. (416)696-7881.

HANLON, John G; St Michael's Hosp, 30 Bond St, Toronto ON M5B 1W8; Tor'05; FRCPC; Anes. Staff, St Michael's Hospital; (416)864-5071

HANLON, William M; Cochrane Primary Care Centre, 103-100 Grande Blvd W, Cochrane AB T4C 0S4; Cork (Ireland)'81; BAO; MRCGPract; CCFP; Staff Family Med & Obst, Foothills Medical Centre; (403)932-2089; Fax. (403)932-1820.

HANLON-DEARMAN, Ana C; Children's Hosp, CK253-840 Sherbrook St, Winnipeg MB R3A 1S1; Man'94; FRCPC; Peds (Developmental Pediatrics). Staff Developmental Peds Children's Hosp, Health Sciences Centre; Assoc Prof Peds & Child Health, University of Manitoba; (204)787-2424; Fax. (204)787-1138.

HANLY, John G; Nova Scotia Rehab Centre, 245-1341 Summer St, Halifax NS B3H 4K4; National (Ireland)'78; MRC; FRCPC; IntMed; Rheum. Staff Rheumatologist, Nova Scotia Rehabilitation Centre; Att Staff, Queen Elizabeth II Hospital; Teach Staff, Dalhousie University; (902)473-3818; Fax. (902)473-7019; john.hanly@cdha.nshealth.ca.

HANLY, Patrick J; HSC-Faculty of Med, 1421-3330 Hospital Dr NW, Calgary AB T2N 4N1; National (Ireland)'78; MB ChB; BAO; FRCPC; IntMed (Critical Care Medicine); Respir. (403)210-8694; hanlyp@smh.toronto.on.ca.

HANMIAH, Rajendar; St Joseph's Healthcare, F533-50 Charlton Ave E, Hamilton ON L8N 4A6; Man'92; FRCPC; IntMed. Staff, St Joseph's Healthcare - Charlton Campus; (905)521-6146

HANNA, Adala; Family Focus Med Clinic, 3601 Joseph Howe Dr, Halifax NS B3L 4H8; (Other Foreign)'86; MB BCh; CCFP; (902)443-2038; Fax. (902)443-2110.

HANNA, Albert H H; Glazier Med Centre, 11 Gibb St, Oshawa ON L1H 2J9; Cairo (Egypt)'91; CCFP; (905)579-1228

HANNA, Amir K; 6F-61 Queen St E, Toronto ON M5C 2T2; Ain Shams (Egypt)'63; MB BCh; ABIM; FACP; FRCPC; IntMed (Diabetes Mellitus); Endocrin&Metab. Hd Dir Div of Endocrinology & Metabolism, St Michael's Hospital; Langs: Arabic; (416)867-3721

HANNA, Basma; Justik Med Clinic, 8225 105 St NW, Edmonton AB T6E 4H2; (Iraq)'93; MB ChB; CCFP; Langs: Arabic; (780)432-0211; Fax. (780)439-9349.

HANNA, Brian D; Briand D Hanna Medicine, 1145 Concession Rd, Cambridge ON N3H 4L5; Belfast (Ireland)'67; MRCP; MB; FRCPC; IntMed (Rheumatology). Dir Rheumatology Clinic, St Mary's General Hospital; Assoc Staff, Grand River Hospital - Kitchener/Waterloo Health Centre; Assoc Staff, Cambridge Memorial Hospital; Clin Assoc Prof, McMaster University; (519)743-4351

HANNA, Claudine; Clin Pediatrique Aux Petits So, 201-6624 av Somerled, Montreal QC H4V 1T2; McG'04; (514)486-6656

HANNA, Dominique; CHUS-Hop Fleurimont, 3001 12e av N, Sherbrooke QC J1H 5N4; Mon'01; ABD; FRCPC; Derm. Staff, Centre Hospitalier Universitaire de Sherbrooke-Hopital Fleurimont; Langs: Bilingual(English/French); (819)346-1110 x13774; dominique.hanna@usherbrooke.ca.

HANNA, Emad S A; Hanna Med Clinic, PO Box 700, Hanna AB T0J 1P0; Mansura (Egypt)'76; CCFP; (403)854-3351; Fax. (403)854-4116.

HANNA, Enas; Gander Med Clinic, 177 Elizabeth Dr, Gander NL A1V 1H6; Staff, Brookfield Bonnews Health Care Centre.

HANNA, Glen R; Southlake Reg Health Centre, 596 Davis Dr, Newmarket ON L3Y 2P9; McM'99; FRCPC; Anes. Staff, Southlake Regional Health Centre; (905)895-4521

HANNA, Hala; CSSS de Temiscouata, CP 310 58 rue de l'Eglise, Notre-Dame-du-Lac QC G0L 1X0; (Lebanon)'94; GenSurg (P.Q.). Staff, Centre Hospitalier Notre-Dame-du-Lac; (418)899-0214; Fax. (418)899-2809.

HANNA, Hany S H; 1-6 Clairmont St, Thorold ON L2V 1R1; Cairo (Egypt)'80; CCFP; Langs: Arabic; (905)680-9703; Fax. (905)680-9705; hany_amelhann5@hotmail.com.

HANNA, Irin S F; Lasalle Med Clinic, 3-49 rue Principale, La Salle MB R0G 1B0; Ain Shams (Egypt)'92; CCFP; (204)736-2416; Fax. (204)736-2418.

HANNA, Ivan W; Finchgate Med Centre, 221-40 Finchgate Blvd, Brampton ON L6T 3J1; Belfast (Ireland)'65; DRCOG; Court Staff, William Osler Health System - Brampton Civic Hospital; (905)792-2247; Fax. (905)792-9661.

HANNA, Jean T; CLSC de la Petite-Nation, 14 rue St-Andre RR 1, St-Andre-Avellin QC J0V 1W0; 80Besancon (France)'80; (819)983-7341; Fax. (819)983-7708.

HANNA, Linda; Yonge-Eglinton Med Centre, 210-2401 Yonge St, Toronto ON M4P 3H1; McM'99; CCFP; Langs: Arabic; (416)485-9044; Fax. (416)485-8525.

HANNA, Magda W; 3-305 Baldwin Ave, Cornwall ON K6H 4J6; Ain Shams (Egypt)'81; MB ChB; FRCPC; Psy. Staff The Cornwall Community Hospital 2nd Street Site, Cornwall Community Hospital; Langs: Arabic; (613)938-6167; Fax. (613)938-0720.

HANNA, Magdy M; Finch-Midland Med Centre, 308-4190 Finch Ave E, Scarborough ON M1S 4T7; Alexandria (Egypt)'61; CCFP; FCFP; Langs: Arabic; (416)299-5260

HANNA, Marni K; Manitoba Clinic, 790 Sherbrook St, Winnipeg MB R3A 1M3; Man'04; FRCPC; Peds.

HANNA, Mary H G; Lacewood Med Center, 200-366 Lacewood Dr, Halifax NS B3S 1M7; Ain Shams (Egypt)'87; MB ChB; (902)445-9400; Fax. (902)445-7108.

HANNA, Mary M; 4788 Rosebush Rd, Mississauga ON L5M 5N1; (Australia)'59; CCFP.

HANNA, Mary; St Mary Ancaster Med Clinic, 201-1144 Wilson St W, Ancaster ON L9G 3K9; (Egypt)'79; CCFP; Langs: Arabic; (905)648-2666; Fax. (905)648-7793; dr_hanna@hotmail.ca.

HANNA, Michael H; Mccreary/Alonsa Health Centre, PO Box 250, McCreary MB R0J 1B0; Ain Shams (Egypt)'77; (204)835-2586; Fax. (204)835-2713.

HANNA, Michael Y G; Wheat City Med Centre, 920 Victoria Ave, Brandon MB R7A 1A7.

HANNA, Nader; CSSS de Temiscouata, CP 310 58 rue de L'eglise, Notre-Dame-du-Lac QC G0L 1X0; Staff, Centre Hospitalier Notre-Dame-du-Lac; (418)899-0214

HANNA, Nermeen S; Pinawa Primary Hlth Care Ctr, PO Box 400 30 Vanier Dr, Pinawa MB R0E 1L0; Ain Shams (Egypt)'95; CCFP.

HANNA, Neveen M; Martin Grove Med Centre, 6-2200 Martin Grove Rd, Etobicoke ON M9V 5H9; Ain Shams (Egypt)'91; CCFP; Langs: Arabic; (416)740-0900

HANNA, Nevin-Wadie N; Huron Square Med Centre, 2500 Hurontario St, Mississauga ON L5B 1N4; (Egypt)'89; CCFP; Langs: Arabic; (905)897-6160

HANNA, Noha; Oak Park Family Care Centre, 201 Oak Walk Dr, Oakville ON L6H 6M3; Alexandra (Egypt)'95; MB ChB; CCFP; (905)257-3297; Fax. (905)257-8621.

HANNA, Phebe; 3-5283 Rutherford Rd, Woodbridge ON L4H 2T2; (Egypt)'87; CCFP; Langs: Arabic; (905)264-8311; Fax. (905)264-0801.

HANNA, Rafik B A M; Queenston Walk in Clinic, 631 Queenston Rd, Hamilton ON L8K 6R5; Ain Shams (Egypt)'89; CCFP; Langs: Arabic; (905)578-5738

HANNA, Rania; Deerfoot Meadows Med Clinic, 7979 11 St SE, Calgary AB T2H 0B8; Ain Shams (Egypt)'02; MB BCh; (403)251-2690; Fax. (403)251-2695.

HANNA, Rose K F A; Britannia Med Clinic, 3-5980 Churchill Meadows Blvd, Mississauga ON L5M 7M5; Mansura (Egypt)'75; CCFP; Langs: Arabic; (905)814-1342; Fax. (905)814-8724.

HANNA, Sameh K; Oak Park Family Care Centre, 201 Oak Walk Dr, Oakville ON L6H 6M3; Ain Shams (Egypt)'85; MB ChB; CCFP; Langs: Arabic; French; (905)257-3297; Fax. (905)257-8621.

HANNA, Sameh; The Dermatology Centre, 403-208 Bloor St W, Toronto ON M5S 3B4; Pennsylvania (USA)'96; (416)922-9620; Fax. (416)922-4358.

HANNA, Samer K F; 48-2140 North Park Dr, Brampton ON L6S 0C9; Ain Shams (Egypt)'94; FRCSC; OrthSurg (Trauma). Langs: Arabic; (905)595-4970; Fax. (905)595-4980.

HANNA, Samer; Polyclinique Concorde, 300 boul de la Concorde E, Laval QC H7G 2E6; Sher'02; FRCSC; Urol (Laparoscopy). Staff Urol, Hopital de la Cite de la santé; Staff Urol, Hôpital de Saint-Eustache; Langs: Arabic; English; (450)667-5310; Fax. (450)667-2163.

HANNA, Samia; Providence Care-Mental Health, PO Box 603 Stn Main 752 King St W, Kingston ON K7L 4X3; (Egypt)'78; FRCPC; Psy. Staff, Providence Care - Mental Health Services; (613)546-1101

HANNA, Samim Y; The Dr G B Cross Mem Hosp, 67 Manitoba Dr, Clarenville NL A5A 1K3; Baghdad (Iraq)'96; MB ChB; CCFP; Staff, The Dr G B Cross Memorial Hospital; (709)466-3411

HANNA, Sherif S; Odette Cancer Centre, T2011-2075 Bayview Ave, Toronto ON M4N 3M5; Cairo (Egypt)'70; MB ChB; AB; FACS; FICS; FRCSC; GenSurg (Surgical Oncology). Staff Surg Oncol, Sunnybrook Health Sciences Centre; Physician, Odette Cancer Centre; Assoc Prof, University of Toronto; (416)480-4774; Fax. (416)480-6002.

HANNA, Shoukry; Medical Bldg, 202-250 Harding Blvd W, Richmond Hill ON L4C 9M7; Alexandria (Egypt)'83; MB ChB; CCFP; Langs: Arabic; (905)737-8402; shoukry@hotmail.com.

HANNA, Viola; 13718 113A ST NW, Edmonton AB T5X 4H7; (Egypt)'90; MB BCh.

HANNA, Wedad M; Sunnybrook Hlth Sciences Ctre, E432-2075 Bayview Ave, Toronto ON M4N 3M5; Alexandria (Egypt)'68; FRCPC; AnatPath. Chief Anatomic Path, Sunnybrook Health Sciences Centre; Prof Div of Path, University of Toronto; Langs: French; Arabic; (416)480-6100 x4012; Fax. (416)480-4271.

HANNA, Yousri; 6-8525 av des Ponts-de-Ce, Anjou QC H1J 1X3; Mon'74; Chief Palliative Care, Hôpital Santa Cabrini Ospedale; Langs: Arabic; English; (514)353-4160; Fax. (514)353-3284.

HANNA DIEF, Sarwat K; Rouge Valley-Centenary HC, 2867 Ellesmere Rd, Scarborough ON M1E 4B9; Cairo (Egypt)'79; FRCPC; Psy. Staff, Rouge Valley Health System - Centenary Health Centre Site; Langs: Arabic; (416)496-0359

HANNA SARSAM, Haithem S; 234-1821 Walker's Line, Burlington ON L7M 0H6; Baghdad (Iraq)'82; CCFP; (905)335-5959; Fax. (905)335-4757; hsarsam@hotmail.com.

HANNACH, Barbara R; Canadian Blood Services, 67 College St, Toronto ON M5G 2M1; McG'78; FRCPC; IntMed (Administration); Hem. Langs: Bilingual(French/English); (416)313-4431; Fax. (416)974-9757.

HANNAFORD, Maureen C; Medical Consultants Group, 193 Lemarchant Rd, St. John's NL A1C 2H5; Mem'76; FRCPC; IntMed (Nephrology). Ac Staff, Waterford Hospital; Ac Staff Health Care Corp of St John's, Health Sciences Centre; Chief Div of Nephrol/Clinical Asst Prof Med, Memorial University Of Newfoundland; (709)579-4191; Fax. (709)579-1302; drmchannaford@medicalconsultants.nf.net.

HANNAM, Paul D; Toronto East Gen Hosp Inc, 825 Coxwell Ave, Toronto ON M4C 3E7; UBC'99; CCFP; CCFP(E.M.); FCFP; A-Chief Dept of EmergMed, Toronto East General Hospital Inc; (416)461-8272

HANNAM, Thomas G; Hannam Fertility Centre, 1103-655 Bay St, Toronto ON M5G 2K4; UBC'95; FRCSC; ObstGyn (Reproductive Endocrinology & Infertility). (416)595-1521; Fax. (416)506-0680; info@fertility.ca.

HANNIGAN, Jay; Saint John Reg Hosp, PO Box 2100 Stn Main 400 University Ave, Saint John NB E2L 4L2; Dal'01; CCFP; CCFP(E.M.); Staff, Saint John Regional Hospital; (506)648-6000

HANNIGAN, Jennifer; Saint John Reg Hosp, PO Box 2100 Stn Main 400 University Ave, Saint John NB E2L 4L2; Cal'05; CCFP; Staff, Saint John Regional Hospital; (506)648-6000

HANNINEN, Mikael V W; London HSC-University Hosp, PO Box 5339 Stn B 339 Windermere Rd, London ON N6A 5A5; Alb'06; Cardiol; IntMed. Staff, London Health Sciences Centre - University Hospital.

HANNON, Judith L; Canadian Blood Services, 8249 114 St NW, Edmonton AB T6G 2R8; Alb'71; FRCPC; HemPath (Transfusion Medicine). Staff, University of Alberta Hospital; Consultant, Cross Cancer Institute; Medical Officer, Canadian Blood Services; Clin Prof, University of Alberta; (780)431-8714; Fax. (780)431-8770; judy.hannon@blood.ca.

HANNON, Patricia J; Upper Appleby Med Assoc, 36-1960 Appleby Line, Burlington ON L7L 0B7; McM'88; (905)315-9929; Fax. (905)315-9314.

HANNOUCHE, Fadi; Lakeridge Hlth Corp-Oshawa, 1 Hospital Crt, Oshawa ON L1G 2B9; Saba (Netherlands Antilles)'02; FRCPC; Anes. Staff, Lakeridge Health - Oshawa Site; Langs: Arabic; (905)576-8711

HANNOUCHE, M Georges; Clinique Domus Medica, 302-5601 rue Belanger, Montreal QC H1T 1G3; Beyrouth (Lebanon)'69; ac Staff, St Mary's Hospital Centre; ac Staff ObstGyn, Hôpital Santa Cabrini Ospedale; Langs: Arabic; English; (514)256-5011 x247; Fax. (514)342-1227.

HANNOUCHE, Nabil; Hop Santa Cabrini Ospedale, 5655 rue Saint-Zotique E, Montreal QC H1T 1P7; Beirut (Lebanon)'76; DiagRad. Staff, Hôpital Santa Cabrini Ospedale; Langs: Arabic; Bilingual(French/English); (514)252-6567; nhannouche@hotmail.com.

HANOMAN, Marguerite B C; 185 Oxford St, Ingersoll ON N5C 2V8; Ireland (Ireland)'79; MB ChB; BAO; ABIM; FRCPC; IntMed. Staff, Alexandra Hospital; (519)485-5829

HANON, Neil H; Outreach Urban Health, 455 Leon St, Kelowna BC V1Y 1J4; Alb'83; DABPN; FRCPC; Psy (Adult General Psychiatry). Med Staff, Kelowna General Hospital; (250)868-2230

HANRAHAN, Kevin M; Foothills Med Centre, C231-1403 29 St NW, Calgary AB T2N 2T9; Cal'87; CCFP; CCFP(E.M.); FCFP; Staff, Foothills Medical Centre; (403)944-1820

HANRAHAN, Renee; 1B-560 Bryne Dr, Barrie ON L4N 9P6; Mem'02; FRCSC; GenSurg (Surgical Oncology). Staff, Royal Victoria Regional Health Centre; (705)735-9300; Fax. (705)735-9391.

HANS, Harninder P; Capt William Jackman Mem Hosp, 410 Booth St, Labrador City NL A2V 2K1; Punjabi (India)'98; MB BS; Staff, Captain William Jackman Memorial Hospital; (709)944-2632

HANS, Jeffrey P; Pleasant Street Med Clinic, 2-250 Pleasant St, Miramichi NB E1V 1Y5; Dal'82; Staff, Miramichi Regional Hospital; (506)622-1971; Fax. (506)622-6888.

HANS, Laura M; St Michael's Hosp, 30 Bond St, Toronto ON M5B 1W8; Tor'95; CCFP; CCFP(E.M.); Staff, St Michael's Hospital; (416)864-5094

HANS, Narpinder; Meadowbrook Med Clinic, 3905 34 St NW, Edmonton AB T6T 1L5; Alb'95; MSc; CCFP; Member College of Family Physician, Alberta Medical Association; Board Member, Southside Primary Care Network; Clin Assoc Prof, University of Alberta; Langs: Punjabi; (780)448-1166; Fax. (780)448-2830.

HANSEN, Frederick M; Red Deer Med Centre, 202-3947 50A Ave, Red Deer AB T4N 6V7; Alb'86; FRCPC; Psy (Adult Psychiatry). Ac Staff, Centennial Centre for Mental Health & Brain Injury; Consultant, Red Deer Regional Hospital Centre; (403)341-4303; Fax. (403)341-4322.

HANSEN, Gregory; New West Ortho & Sports, 102-65 Richmond St, New Westminster BC V3L 5P5; Dal'07; OrthSurg. (604)526-7885

HANSEN, James L; Bridgeland Med Bldg, 306-803 1 Ave NE, Calgary AB T2E 7C5; Cal'76; BSc; FRCPC; IntMed (Interventional Cardiology); Cardiol. Att Staff, Foothills Medical Centre; Att Staff, Peter Lougheed Centre; Att Staff, Rockyview General Hospital; Clin Assoc Prof, University of Calgary; (403)215-2212; Fax. (403)215-2208.

HANSEN, Mark G; Montfort Hosp, 713 Montreal Rd, Ottawa ON K1K 0T2; Sask'10; CCFP; Staff, Montfort Hospital; (613)746-4621

HANSEN, Mark S; Sunnybrook Hlth Sciences Ctre, A253-2075 Bayview Ave, Toronto ON M4N 3M5; Tor'99; FRCPC; IntMed (Echocardiography); Cardiol. Staff, Sunnybrook Health Sciences Centre; (416)480-5505; Fax. (416)480-4745.

HANSEN, Maxim T T; 204-300 Columbia St, Kamloops BC V2C 6L1; Alb'99; FRCSC; GenSurg (Intensive Care). Staff Gen Surg & Intensive Care Spec, Royal Inland Hospital; (250)374-0028

HANSEN, Miriam; Royal Court Med Centre, 208-1 Quarry Ridge Rd, Barrie ON L4M 7G1; McM'01; FRCPC; Peds. Staff, Royal Victoria Regional Health Centre; (705)728-3766

HANSEN, Philip R; 479 Main St PO Box 399, Alberton PE C0B 1B0; Alb'82; CCFP; FCFP; Staff, Western Hospital - Health PEI; Preceptor, Dalhousie University; (902)853-3197; Fax. (902)853-3309.

HANSEN, Ruben G; Royal Alexandra Hosp, 5F CSC-10240 Kingsway NW, Edmonton AB T5H 3V9; Alb'92; FRCPC; EmergMed. Staff, Royal Alexandra Hospital; (780)735-4442; Fax. (780)735-4916.

HANSEN, Shandi M; Univ Hlth Network-Toronto Gen, 480-200 Elizabeth St, Toronto ON M5G 2C4; (USA)'06; Staff, Toronto General Hospital - UHN.

HANSEN, Steven G; 302-22112 52 Ave, Langley BC V2Y 2M6; Alb'86; Staff, Langley Memorial Hospital; (604)533-0551

HANSIA, Mohammed R; Stapleford Med Clinic, 327 McCarthy Blvd N, Regina SK S4R 7M2; (306)545-3000; Fax. (306)545-5584.

HANSON, Alexandra J; Foothills Med Centre, 12F-1403 29 St NW, Calgary AB T2N 2T9; Ott'95; BSc; FRCPC; Neur (Epilepsy). Staff, Foothills Medical Centre; Clin Prof, University of Calgary; (403)944-8087; Fax. (403)283-2270.

HANSON, Amanda E; Royal Alexandra Hosp, 10240 Kingsway NW, Edmonton AB T5H 3V9; Alb'00; FRCPC; EmergMed. Staff, Royal Alexandra Hospital; (780)735-4447

HANSON, B Margaret; South Walkerville Med Centre, 260-2224 Walker Rd, Windsor ON N8W 5L7; Jagiellonian (Poland)'85; (519)971-8242; Fax. (519)971-8827.

HANSON, Dana W; Fredericton Med Clinic, 302-1015 Regent St, Fredericton NB E3B 6H5; Dal'74; FRCPC; Derm (Family Medicine). Consultant, Dr Everett Chalmers Regional Hospital; Lecturer, Dalhousie University; (506)458-0206; Fax. (506)458-0222.

HANSON, Everette M; Oromocto Public Hosp, 103 Winnebago St, Oromocto NB E2V 1C6; Dal'82; Staff, Oromocto Public Hospital; (506)357-4700

HANSON, Garth J; Peterborough Reg Nephrology, 239 Charlotte St, Peterborough ON K9J 2V2; Qns'00; FRCPC; IntMed; Nephrol (Critical Care Medicine). (705)750-1786

HANSON, Jacelyn; Natawihin/Natasuwenik Med Clin, GD, Ile-a-la-Crosse SK S0M 1C0; Sask'08; CCFP; Teach Staff, University of British Columbia; (306)833-2044; Fax. (306)833-2401.

HANSON, Johnathon; Regina Qu'Appelle Hr-Pasqua, 4101 Dewdney Ave, Regina SK S4T 1A5; Sask'07; CCFP; CCFP(E.M.); Staff, Pasqua Hospital; (306)766-2979; Fax. (306)766-2751.

HANSON, Mark D; 102-272 Lawrence Ave E, North York ON M4N 1T4; Tor'81; FRCPC; Psy (Child Psychiatry). Assoc Prof Psy/Assoc Dean Undergraduate Admissions & Student Finance, University of Toronto; (416)787-9055

HANSON, Mary K; 504-49 St Clair Ave W, Toronto ON M4V 1K6; Tor'77; FRCPC; Psy. (416)588-7084

HANSON, Paul R; 101-2475 McDougall Ave, Windsor ON N8X 3N9; Jagiellonian (Poland)'85; (519)966-0089; Fax. (519)966-5622.

HANSON, Peter G; Royal Bank Plaza, PO Box 134 Stn Royal Bank LR8-200 Bay St, Toronto ON M5J 2J3; Tor'71; Langs: Bilingual(English/French); (416)368-6787

HANSON, Robert E; MUHC-Royal Victoria Hosp, 687 av des Pins O, Montreal QC H3A 1A1; McG'65; FRCPC; DiagRad. Staff, McGill University Health Centre - Royal Victoria Hospital; (514)842-1231

HANSON, Sonya; Saint John Reg Hosp, PO Box 2100 Stn Main 400 University Ave, Saint John NB E2L 4L2; McG'98; CCFP; CCFP(E.M.); Staff, Saint John Regional Hospital; (506)648-6900

HANSON, Wayne G; 205-230 First Ave, St Thomas ON N5R 4P5; Wes'88; FRCSC; Otol. (519)631-6391; whanson@stegh.on.ca.

HANSPAL, Rajvinder; New Waterford Consolidated Hos, 716 King St, New Waterford NS B1H 3Z5; Guru Nanak (India)'89; MB BS; FamilyMed. Staff, New Waterford Consolidated Hospital; (902)862-6411; Fax. (902)592-3308.

HANSSON, Ann M; Vancouver Gen Hosp, JPP16-855 12th Ave W, Vancouver BC V5Z 1M9; Qns'91; CCFP; Staff Palliative Care Unit, Vancouver General Hospital - Centennial Pavillion; (604)875-4715; Fax. (604)875-4967.

HANTHO, Janet E; Rockyview Gen Hosp, 7007 14 St SW, Calgary AB T2V 1P9; Alb'86; Ac Staff, Rockyview General Hospital; Langs: English; French; (403)943-3558; Fax. (403)253-5895.

HANTON, David A; 5118 48 St PO Box 150, Castor AB T0C 0X0; (Scotland)'92; MB ChB; CCFP; Chief EmergMed, Covenant Health - Our Lady of the Rosary Hospital; (403)882-2665; Fax. (403)882-3525.

HANTON, Timothy E; PO Box 729, Killam AB T0B 2L0; (Scotland)'96; CCFP; (780)385-3741; Fax. (780)385-3007.

HANY, Richard W; Mackenzie Richmond Hill Hosp, 10 Trench St, Richmond Hill ON L4C 4Z3; Wes'84; FRCPC; DiagRad. Staff, Mackenzie Richmond Hill Hospital; (905)883-2004

HANZAL, Djilali; 3-276 rue Marie, Beresford NB E8K 1P8; Alger (Algeria)'89; Staff, Hopital Regional Chaleur.

HAOUARA, Fatiha; CLSC Cote-des-Neiges, 6600 ch de la cote-des-Neiges, Montreal QC H3T 2A8; (Algeria)'83; (514)731-1386; Fax. (514)739-8132.

HAPCHYN, Carole A; Child & Adolesc Serv Assoc, 10645 63 Ave NW, Edmonton AB T6H 1P7; Alb'82; FRCPC; Psy (Child Psychiatry). Consultant Privil, University of Alberta Hospital; Consultant Privil, Glenrose Rehabilitation Hospital; Consultant, Child & Adolescent Services Association; Clin Prof Psy, University of Alberta; (780)438-0011; Fax. (780)437-6133.

HAPGOOD, Conamara A; St Clare's Mercy Hosp, 154 Lemarchant Rd, St. John's NL A1C 5B8; Mem'03; FRCPC; DiagRad. Staff, St Clare's Mercy Hospital; (709)777-5000

HAPONIUK, Adrienne D; University of Alberta Hosp, 1A7 19WCM-8440 112 St NW, Edmonton AB T6G 2B7; UBC'01; FRCPC; EmergMed. Staff, University of Alberta Hospital; (780)407-8822

HAPUARACHCHI, Milanthi; Urgentcare Med Clinic, 1-6941 Derry Rd, Milton ON L9T 7H5; (Sri Lanka)'98; MB BS; CCFP; Langs: Sinhalese; (905)875-9999; Fax. (905)875-9940.

HAQ, Aamir; St Joseph's Hlth Centre, 30 The Queensway, Toronto ON M6R 1B5; NOSM'10; CCFP; Staff, St Joseph's Health Centre; (416)530-6860; Fax. (416)530-6160.

HAQ, Anwar U; Apple Tree Med Group, 2016 Ogilve Rd, Ottawa ON K1J 7B3; Punjab (Pakistan)'59; MRC(Lond); DABIM; FRCPC; IntMed (Hematological Oncology). (613)749-5549

HAQ, Farhan; Langley Mem Hosp, 22051 Fraser Hwy, Langley BC V3A 4H4; Islamia (Pakistan)'97; Staff, Langley Memorial Hospital; (604)534-4121

HAQ, Farzana; Emkiro Hlth Services, 70 University Ave, Toronto ON M5J 2M4; Tor'07; CCFP; (416)977-7474; Fax. (416)977-7464.

HAQ, Iftikhar U; Medical Centre, 102-984 Oliver Rd, Thunder Bay ON P7B 7C7; Nishtar (Pakistan)'87; FRCS; FRCSC; Neursurg (Spine Surgery). Staff, Thunder Bay Regional Health Sciences Centre Port-Arthur; Staff, Thunder Bay Regional Health Sciences Centre; Asst Prof Surg, Lakehead University / Library; Asst Prof Surg, Northern Ontario School of Medicine-Lakehead University; Langs: Urdu; Punjabi; (807)766-3590

HAQ, M Mansoor; Allan Blair Cancer Centre, 300-4101 Dewdney Ave, Regina SK S4T 7T1; Karachi (Pakistan)'85; MB BS; (306)766-2498; Fax. (306)766-2688.

HAQ, Rashida; 2085Q-30 Bond St, Toronto ON M5B 1W8; Punjab (Pakistan)'76; MB BS; FACP; FRCPC; IntMed (Breast Cancer); MedOncol. Consultant MedOncol, St Michael's Hospital; Teacher Med, University of Toronto; Langs: Urdu; (416)864-5912; haqr@smh.ca.

HAQ, Sheira; 762 King St, New Waterford NS B1H 3Z5; Dhaka (Bangladesh)'93; MB BS; CCFP; (902)862-6792; Fax. (902)862-7963.

HAQ, Syed M S; 102-5990 Fraser St, Vancouver BC V5W 2Z7; Chittagong (Bangladesh)'88; MB BS; CCFP; Langs: Bengali; (604)322-3366

HAQ CHOUDHURI, Akm Ziaul; Hop Regional D'Edmundston, 275 Hebert Blvd, Edmundston NB E3V 4E4; Chittagong (Bangladesh)'75; Staff Diagnostic Imaging, Hôpital regional d'Edmundston; (506)739-2847; Fax. (506)739-2745; hagchoudhuri@health.nb.ca.

HAQQ, Andrea M; University of Alberta Hosp, WMC 1C4-8440 112 St NW, Edmonton AB T6G 2B7; Cal'94; FAAP; FRCPC; Peds; Endocrin&Metab. Staff, University of Alberta Hospital; (780)407-1568

HAQUE, Farah N; St. Boniface Hosp, 409 Tache Ave, Winnipeg MB R2H 2A6; (Pakistan)'89; Staff, St Boniface General Hospital.

HAQUE, Khurshid; Restigouche Health Centre, PO Box 10 Stn Main 63 Prom Gallant, Campbellton NB E3N 3G2; Santo Domingo (Dominican Republic)'85; Asst Head Dept of Psy, Centre Hospitalier Restigouche; Langs: Urdu; Bengali; (506)789-7014; Fax. (506)789-6726.

HAQUE, M Samiul; Child & Youth Services, 1680 Albert St, Regina SK S4P 2S6; Sask'91; FRCPC; Psy. (306)766-6700

HAQUE, Nargis; IWK Health Centre, PO Box 9700 Rpo CSC 5850-5980 University Ave, Halifax NS B3K 6R8; Punjab (Pakistan)'80; MB BS; Staff, IWK Health Centre; (902)470-7426; Fax. (902)470-6469.

HAQUE, Shelby; PO Box 4477 Stn South Cro, Edmonton AB T6E 4T5; Alb'04; CCFP; CCFP(E.M.); Staff, University of Alberta Hospital; (780)407-8432

HAQUE, Zia-Ul; Abbotsford Mental Health Ctre, 11-32700 George Ferguson Way, Abbotsford BC V2T 4V6; Punjab (Pakistan)'92; (604)870-7800

HAR, Bryan J N; Foothills Med Centre, C807-1403 29 St NW, Calgary AB T2N 2T9; Cal'05; FRCPC; IntMed; Cardiol. Staff, Foothills Medical Centre; (403)944-4243; Fax. (403)944-1592.

HARABOR, Andrei; Foothills Med Centre, C211-1403 29 St NW, Calgary AB T2N 2T9; (Romania)'91; FRCPC; Peds. Staff Neonatologist, Calgary Health Region; Langs: French; Romanian; (403)944-1615

HARADA, Glenn K; 122 Buckigham Lane PO Box 97, Annan ON N0H 1B0; Tor'71; Staff, Grey Bruce Health Services - Owen Sound; (519)371-3963

HARAOUI, Boulos; Inst de Rhumatologie de Montré, 1551 rue Ontario E, Montreal QC H2L 1S6; Beyrouth (Lebanon)'77; ABIM(IntMed,Rheum); FRCPC; IntMed (Anti-Rheumatic Medicine); Rheum. Dir Clin Research, Centre Hospitalier l'Université de Montréal (CHUM) - Hôpital Notre-Dame; assoc Prof, Universite de Montreal; (514)523-3305; boulos.haraoui@ssss.gouv.qc.ca.

HARAOUI, Louis-Patrick; Hop Charles Lemoyne, AN302-3120 boul Taschereau, Longueuil QC J4V 2H1; McG'05; FRCPC; IntMed; MedMicrobiol. Staff, Hopital Charles LeMoyne; (450)466-5000

HARAPHONGSE, Mant; University of Alberta Hosp, 2C2 38WCM-8440 112 St NW, Edmonton AB T6G 2B7; Bangkok (Thailand)'64; FRCPC; IntMed (Cardiology). Staff, University of Alberta Hospital; Emeritus Prof, University of Alberta; (780)407-7206; Fax. (780)407-6452.

HARAPHONGSE, Yada; 301-2377 111 St NW, Edmonton AB T6J 5E5; Alb'94; CCFP; (780)436-8731

HARARI, Maya V; Rockyview Gen Hosp, 7007 14 St SW, Calgary AB T2V 1P9; Tor'86; FRCPC; EmergMed (Sports Medicine). Staff, Rockyview General Hospital; (403)943-3449

HARASYMOWYCZ, Paul J; Hop Maisonneuve-Rosemont, 5415 boul de l'Assomption, Montreal QC H1T 2M4; McG'95; FRCSC; Ophth (Glaucoma). Staff, Hopital Maisonneuve-Rosemont; (514)252-3878; Fax. (514)252-3905.

HARATI, Osama; Salvation Army Grace Gen Hosp, 300 Booth Dr, Winnipeg MB R3J 3M7; Al Fateh (Libya)'97; CCFP; Staff, The Salvation Army Grace Hospital; (204)837-0391

HARB, Mohammed; The Moncton Hosp, 135 MacBeath Ave, Moncton NB E1C 6Z8; Staff, The Moncton Hospital; (506)867-5267

HARB, Raymond T; Garden City Family Health Team, 121 Oakdale Ave, St Catharines ON L2P 2L3; Ott'79; CCFP; Ac Staff, Niagara Health System - Ontario Street Site; Ac Staff, Niagara Health System - St Catharines General Site; Sec, Lincoln County Academy of Medicine; Langs: Arabic; French; (905)685-8700; Fax. (905)988-1616.

HARBOUR, Jacques; CSSS de la Vieille Capitale, 900 boul Wilfrid-Hamel, Quebec QC G1M 2R9; Laval'74; Otol (P.Q.). Ac Staff, CSSS de Quebec-Sud; Associate, CHSLD St-Jude-de-Laval Ltée; (418)682-1711 x2251

HARCZY, Martha; Centrepointe Med Consultants, 106 Centrepointe Dr, Nepean ON K2G 6B1; Semmelweis (Hungary)'79; MSc; FRCPC; IntMed (Lung); MedOncol. Court Staff Oncology, The Ottawa Hospital - General Campus; Langs: Hungarian; French; (613)224-6151; Fax. (613)224-7228; martha.harczy@sympatico.ca.

HARDER, Arthur; Cannon Clinic, 4-2151 McCallum Rd, Abbotsford BC V2S 3N9; UBC'89; (604)853-3314; Fax. (604)853-2171.

HARDER, Carroll D; St Thomas-Elgin Gen Hosp, PO Box 2007 Stn Main 189 Elm St, St Thomas ON N5P 3W2; McM'06; CCFP; CCFP(E.M.); Staff, St Thomas Elgin General Hospital; Langs: German; (519)631-2020

HARDER, James A; Alberta Children's Hosp, 2888 Shaganappi Trail NW, Calgary AB T3B 6A8; Alb'74; BSc; MD; FRCS; FRCSC; OrthSurg (Limb Defiency). Ac Staff, Alberta Children's Hospital; Ac Staff, Foothills Medical Centre; Assoc Prof, University of Calgary; (403)955-7633; jharder@ucalgary.ca.

HARDER, Joyce A R; Alberta Children's Hosp, 2888 Shaganappi Trail NW, Calgary AB T3B 6A8; Alb'74; FRCPC; Peds; PedCardiol. Ac Staff PedCardiol, Alberta Children's Hospital; Ac Staff, Foothills Medical Centre; Associate Clin Prof, University of Calgary; (403)955-7858; Fax. (403)955-7621; joyce.harder@albertahealthservices.ca.

HARDER, Kenneth K; Gaetz Family Practice, 104-45744 Gaetz St, Chilliwack BC V2R 3P1; Sask'92; CCFP; FCFP; Site Dir Chillwack, UBC Family Practice; Clin Assoc Prof, University of British Columbia; (604)824-1588; Fax. (604)824-8743; ken.harder@fraserheatlh.ca.

HARDIAL, Janine L; PO Box 78055 Rpo Grandview, Vancouver BC V5N 5W1; UBC'06; CCFP; (778)840-8044

HARDIE, Brenda J; Latchford Med Centre, PO Box 100 66 Main St, Latchford ON P0J 1N0; Tor'91; BPHE; CCFP; FCFP; Med Advisor Cardiopulmonary Rehab & CME Coordinator, Temiskaming Hospital; (705)676-2200; Fax. (705)676-2111.

HARDIE, David P; West Parry Sound Health Ctre, 6 Albert St, Parry Sound ON P2A 3A4; Mem'74; BSc; DA; BMedSci; Court Staff Part-Time, Huntsville District Memorial Hospital - Muskoka Algonquin Healthcare; Court Staff Part-Time, Burks Falls Hosp; Staff, West Parry Sound Health Centre; (705)746-9321; Fax. (705)746-7364.

HARDIN, Barry E; Dr B E Hardin Prof Corp, 33-240 Midpark Way SE, Calgary AB T2X 1N4; Alb'77; BMedSci; CCFP; FCFP; (403)256-2355; Fax. (403)256-4852; bhardin@telus.net.

HARDIN, Earl D; Broadway Med Centre, 902-601 Broadway W, Vancouver BC V5Z 4C2; Alb'58; FRCPC; Psy. (604)734-0511; Fax. (604)731-7764.

HARDIN, Evelyn; Haig Clinic, 601 6 Ave S, Lethbridge AB T1J 0Z2; Alb'71; Staff, Chinook Regional Hospital; Staff, Covenant Health - St Michael's Health Centre; (403)328-6641; Fax. (403)328-6118.

HARDIN, Philip A; Links Clinic Office, 104-11910 111 Ave NW, Edmonton AB T5G 3G6; Alb'78; FACP; FRCPC; IntMed (Diabetology). Dir, West Edmonton Diabetes Centre; Associate Clinical Prof Div of Endocrin Dept of Med, University of Alberta; (780)452-1999; Fax. (780)451-6384.

HARDING, Anita; Pacific Avenue Med Centre, 300-149 Pacific Ave, Saskatoon SK S7K 1N8; Pretoria (South Africa)'94; MB ChB; FRCSC; ObstGyn (Urogynecology). Staff, Foothills Medical Centre; Langs: Afrikaans; (306)653-5970; Fax. (306)653-5383.

HARDING, David M; Timmins & Dist Hosp, 700 Ross Ave E, Timmins ON P4N 8P2; Tor'81; FRCSC; OrthSurg. Staff, Timmins & District Hospital; (705)267-2131

HARDING, Gary A J; ON 2074-675 McDermot Ave, Winnipeg MB R3E 0V9; Man'00; FRCPC; IntMed; MedOncol.

HARDING, Gregory E J; Health Sciences Centre, GF547-820 Sherbrook St, Winnipeg MB R3A 1R9; Man'98; FRCPC; GenSurg; VascSurg. Staff, Health Sciences Centre; (204)774-8511

HARDING, Kevin P; St Thomas-Elgin Gen Hosp, PO Box 2007 Stn Main 189 Elm St, St Thomas ON N5P 3W2; Wes'79; FRCPC; DiagRad. Chief Radiol, St Thomas Elgin General Hospital; (519)631-2030

HARDING, Peter W; Medical-Surgical Eye Bldg, 879 Shefford Rd, Gloucester ON K1J 8H9; Ott'86; Ophth (Retina). Staff, The Ottawa Hospital - General Campus; Staff, Montfort Hospital; Langs: Slovak; French; (613)741-6904; Fax. (613)741-7338.

HARDING, Roy A; 653 Hwy 1 PO Box 42 Mount Uniacke, Mount Uniacke NS B0N 1Z0; Dal'77; (902)256-3300; Fax. (902)256-3301.

HARDING, Sheila M R; U Of Saskatchewan, A204-107 Wiggins Rd, Saskatoon SK S7N 5E5; Wes'81; FRCPC; IntMed (Clinical Hematology); Hem. Staff, Royal University Hospital; Assoc Staff, Saskatchewan Cancer Commission; Staff, Saskatoon Health Region; Assoc Dean Undergraduate Med Education, University of Saskatchewan; (306)966-6150; sheila.harding@usask.ca.

HARDT, Barbara J; Bowness Family Med Centre, 52-7930 Bowness Rd NW, Calgary AB T3B 0H3; McG'85; MSc; BSc; CCFP; Langs: English; French; (403)247-1303; Fax. (403)288-6670.

HARDWICK, David F; Dean's Office Faculty of Med, 317-2194 Health Sciences Mall, Vancouver BC V6T 1Z3; UBC'57; AB; FCAP; FRCP; LLD; FRCPC; GenPath (Administration). Ac Staff, BC Children's Hospital; Prof Path & Peds, University of British Columbia; (604)822-4305; david.f.hardwick@ubc.ca.

HARDWICK, James M; 150 Huron St, Stratford ON N5A 5S8; London (England)'69; MB BS; LRCP; MRCS; FRCS(Glas); FRCSC; GenSurg. Consultant, Listowel Memorial Hospital - Listowel Wingham Hospitals Alliance; Staff, Stratford General Hospital - Huron Perth Healthcare Alliance; (519)273-2223; Fax. (519)273-2262.

HARDY, Brian W; Medical Arts Bldg, 202-233 Kennedy St, Winnipeg MB R3C 3J5; Man'83; FRCPC; DiagRad. (204)942-6453; Fax. (204)944-8101.

HARDY, C David; Rockyview Gen Hosp, 7007 14 St SW, Calgary AB T2V 1P9; Cal'89; FRCPC; Anes. Staff, Rockyview General Hospital; (403)541-3410

HARDY, Christine; Clinique Med Sainte-Dorothee, 102-1 boul Samson, Laval QC H7X 3S5; Mon'89; Staff, EmergMed, Hopital de la Cite de la santé; Universite de Montreal; (450)689-6334; Fax. (450)689-6339.

HARDY, Christopher D; Beddington Med Clinic, 207-8120 Beddington Blvd NW, Calgary AB T3K 2A8; Leeds (England)'82; MB ChB; MRC(Eng); (403)275-4611; Fax. (403)275-4613.

HARDY, Dean W; Jasper Avenue Med Centre, 11464 Jasper Ave NW, Edmonton AB T5K 0M1; Cal'78; BSc; BEd; (780)756-9212; Fax. (780)756-9211.

HARDY, Dorothy A; Misericordia Community Hosp, 16940 87 Ave NW, Edmonton AB T5R 4H5; Cal'81; Anes. Staff, Covenant Health - Misericordia Community Hospital; (780)484-8811; Fax. (780)930-5967.

HARDY, Douglas A; Vernon Jubilee Hosp, 2101 32 St, Vernon BC V1T 5L2; Sask'84; FRCPC; GenPath (Clinical Pathology). Staff, Vernon Jubilee Hospital; (250)558-1350; Fax. (250)558-1368.

HARDY, Edward L G; Vernon Jubilee Hosp, 2101 32 St, Vernon BC V1T 5L2; Sask'92; FRCPC; IntMed; MedOncol. Pres/Medical Staff, Vernon Jubilee Hospital; Staff, BC Cancer Agency Sindi Ahluwalia Hawkins Centre for the Southern Interior; (250)558-1235; Fax. (250)558-4113; ehardy@bccancer.bc.ca.

HARDY, Guillaume; CLSC-CHSLD Mrc Denis-Riverin, 50 rue du Belvedere, Ste-Anne-des-Monts QC G4V 1X4; Laval'10; CCFP; Staff, Centre Hospitalier des Monts; (418)763-2261

HARDY, Isabelle; Hop Maisonneuve-Rosemont, 5415 boul de l'Assomption, Montreal QC H1T 2M4; Mon'88; AB; FRCSC; Ophth (Oculo Plastic Surgery). Staff, Hopital Maisonneuve-Rosemont; (514)252-3878; Fax. (514)252-3905.

HARDY, Jean-Francois; CHUM-Hop Notre-Dame, 1115 3-1560 Sherbrooke E, Montreal QC H2L 4M1; Mon'74; FRCP; DABA; CSPQ; FRCPC; Anes (Cardiac Anesthesia). Chef Anes, Centre Hospitalier l'Université de Montréal (CHUM) - Hôpital Notre-Dame; Langs: English; (514)890-8000 x26876; Fax. (514)412-7653; jean-francois.hardy.chum@ssss.gouv.qc.ca.

HARDY, John J; Kelligrews Medical Clinic, PO Box 17160 Stn Main, Conception Bay S NL A1X 3H1; Mem'73; (709)834-2171; Fax. (709)834-1241.

HARDY, Jules J; CHUM-Hop Notre-Dame, 1560 rue Sherbrooke E, Montreal QC H2L 4M1; Mon'56; FRCSC; Neursurg. Consultant, Centre Hospitalier l'Université de Montréal (CHUM) - Hôtel-Dieu; Staff NeuroSurg, Centre Hospitalier l'Université de Montréal (CHUM) - Hôpital Notre-Dame; Consultant, McGill University Health Centre - Montreal General Campus; Prof, Universite de Montreal; Aj Prof, McGill University; (514)526-0419; Fax. (514)412-7816; juleshardy@yahoo.com.

HARDY, Krista; St Boniface Gen Hosp, 409 Tache Ave, Winnipeg MB R2H 2A6; Tor'02; FRCSC; GenSurg. Staff, St Boniface General Hospital; (204)233-8563

HARDY, Mark; Sir Mortimer B Davis Jewish Ge, 3755 ch cote-Sainte-Catherine, Montreal QC H3T 1E2; London (England)'79; MB BS; MSc(Epidem.); FRCSC; GenSurg (Surgical Oncology). Staff, Sir Mortimer B Davis Jewish General; Langs: English; French; Fax. (514)340-7510.

HARDY, Paul E; City View Surgical Associates, 400-3939 50A Ave, Red Deer AB T4N 4E6; Wes'86; FRCSC; GenSurg. Staff, Red Deer Regional Hospital Centre; (403)347-9037; Fax. (403)347-9038.

HARDY, Pierre; Hôpital Ste-Justine, 3175 ch Cote-Sainte-Catherine, Montreal QC H3T 1C5; Laval'83; FRCPC; Peds (Neonatal & Perinatal Medicine). Staff Peds & Neonatologist, Hôpital Ste-Justine; Universite de Montreal; (514)345-4931 x6700; Fax. (514)345-4801.

HARDY-BROWN, Karolyn W; The Peterborough Clinic, 26 Hospital Dr, Peterborough ON K9J 7C3; Qns'05; FRCPC; Peds. (705)740-6841; Fax. (705)740-6891.

HARE, Gregory M T; St Michael's Hosp, 30 Bond St, Toronto ON M5B 1W8; Tor'90; FRCPC; Anes. Staff, St Michael's Hospital; (416)864-5259; Fax. (416)864-6014.

HAREBOTTLE, Ronald R; Miramichi Med Arts Centre, Box 8 7-679 King George Hwy, Miramichi NB E1V 1N9; Stellenbosch (South Africa)'83; MB ChB; (506)778-4140; Fax. (506)778-2585.

HAREL, Francois; Institut de Cardiologie de Mtl, 5000 rue Belanger, Montreal QC H1T 1C8; Laval'94; FRCPC; NuclearMed. Staff, Institut de Cardiologie de Montréal; (514)376-3330 x3656; Fax. (514)376-0936.

HAREL, Shai; Misericordia Health Centre, 99 Cornish Ave, Winnipeg MB R3C 1A2; CCFP; CCFP(E.M.); Staff, Misericordia Health Centre; (204)788-8364

HAREL, Simon-Pierre; Chus-Hop Hotel-Dieu, 580 rue Bowen S, Sherbrooke QC J1G 2E8; Mon'85; Staff, Centre Hospitalier Universitaire de Sherbrooke-Hôpital Hôtel-Dieu; (819)346-1110 x23599; Fax. (819)820-6899.

HAREL, Ziv; 61 Queen St, Toronto ON M5C 2T2; Wes'04; FRCPC; IntMed; Nephrol. (416)360-4000; Fax. (416)363-9338.

HARES, Mark; Algonquin Med Centre, 201-227 Algonquin Blvd W, Timmins ON P4N 2R8; London (England)'67; MB BS; FRCS(Edinburgh); FRCSC; Urol. Staff, Timmins & District Hospital; Physician Urologist, Algonquin Medical Centre; Asst Prof Surg, Northern Ontario School of Medicine; (705)268-1600; Fax. (705)268-1616.

HARESHA, Abdullatif; Red River Clinic, 139 Carmen Ave, Winnipeg MB R2L 0E5; Al Fateh (Libya)'92; FRCPC; Peds;CCFP.

HARETH, Rezkallah; CSSS de la Region de Thetford, 1717 rue Notre-Dame E, Quebec QC G2G 2V4; Damascus (Syria)'96; GenSurg (P.Q.). (418)338-7715

HARFA, Leah; Markham Endoscopy Diag Inc, 130-100 Renfrew Dr, Markham ON L3R 9R6; Victoria (Australia)'88; MB BS; FRCPC; Anes. Staff, The Scarborough Hospital - General Campus.

HARGADON, John M; St Joseph's Hosp, PO Box 3251 Stn P 35 Algoma St N, Thunder Bay ON P7B 5G7; Qns'79; DABPMR; FAANEM; FRCPC; PhysMed&Rehab. Physician Advisor-Rehab, St Joseph's Care Group - St Joseph's Hospital; Asst Prof Div of Clin Sciences, Northern Ontario School of Medicine-Lakehead University; (807)345-0510; Fax. (807)344-3891; hargadoj@tbh.net.

HARGASSNER, Edward; Geraldston Dist Hosp, 510 Hogarth Ave W, Geraldton ON P0T 1M0; Wes'98; General Practice, Geraldton District Hospital; (807)854-1862; Fax. (807)854-1568; ehargassner@geraldtondh.com.

HARGOT, Leonard; R2-581 Plains Rd E, Burlington ON L7T 2E6; Ott'67; (905)631-0911; Fax. (905)631-0912.

HARGREAVES, James A; 1113 103 Ave, Dawson Creek BC V1G 2G8; Alb'90; CCFP; Staff, Dawson Creek & District Hospital; (250)782-2827; Fax. (250)782-2867.

HARGROVE, Andrea L; Associate Med Centre, 5016 48 Ave, Taber AB T1G 1R8; Alb'08; CCFP; (403)223-3525; Fax. (403)223-9020.

HARGROVE, Gaylene M; 201-1990 Fort St, Victoria BC V8R 6V4; Cal'93; FRCPC; IntMed (Peritonial Dialysis); Nephrol. Staff, Royal Jubilee Hospital; Asst Clin Prof, University of British Columbia; (250)598-9395; Fax. (250)598-5469.

HARI, Krishna S P; Guildford Town Ctr Med Clinic, 100-15170 104 Ave, Surrey BC V3R 1N3; Kerala (India)'73; MB BS; (604)583-8482

HARI SINGH, Manjeet; Canora Med Clinic, PO Box 2040, Canora SK S0A 0L0; Gen Practice, Yorkton Mental Health & Addiction Centre; (306)563-5557; Fax. (306)563-4175.

HARIBHAI, Jayshree C; Cedar Hills Med Clinic, 12860 96 Ave, Surrey BC V3V 6A8; Natal (South Africa)'83; MB ChB.

HARIKUMAR, Usha; 304-1200 Markham Rd, Scarborough ON M1H 3C3; Kerala (India)'96; FRCSC; ObstGyn. Staff, Women's College Hospital; Langs: Hindi; Malayalam; Tamil; (647)345-8627

HARILAL, Mayadevi; 1619 9 Ave S, Lethbridge AB T1J 1W1; S. Africa (South Africa)'78; MMed(Peds.); FRCPC; Peds. (403)320-2236; Fax. (403)331-2268.

HARILD, Laura D; The Credit Valley Hosp, 2200 Eglinton Ave W, Mississauga ON L5M 2N1; McM'08; CCFP; Staff, The Credit Valley Hospital; (905)813-2200

HARINGTON, Michael B; Medical Arts Bldg, 222-750 Spadina Cres E, Saskatoon SK S7K 3H3; Salisbury (Zimbabwe)'81; MB ChB; FRCS(Edin); LRCPS; LMCC; FRCSC; GenSurg (Breasts). Staff, St Paul's Hospital (Grey Nuns) of Saskatoon; Clin Associate Prof, University of Saskatchewan; (306)653-3366; Fax. (306)653-8832.

HARIRI, Farzad; William Osler HC-Etobicoke, 101 Humber College Blvd, Etobicoke ON M9V 1R8; (Iran)'94; FRCSC; GenSurg. Staff, William Osler Health System - Etobicoke General Hospital; Langs: Farsi; (416)747-3400

HARISH, Srinivasan; St Joseph's Health Care, 50 Charlton Ave E, Hamilton ON L8N 4A6; Tamil Nadu (India)'96; FRCPC; DiagRad. Staff, St Joseph's Healthcare - Charlton Campus; Langs: Tamil; (905)522-1155

HARISSI DAGHER, Jehan; Inst Readaptation de Montréal, 6300 av de Darlington, Montreal QC H3S 2J4; Mon'00; ABPMR; CMQ; BScPT; FRCPC; PhysMed&Rehab (Electromyography). Staff, McGill University Health Centre - Montreal General Campus; Staff, Institut de Réadaptation Gingras-Lindsay de Montréal; Langs: Bilingual(French/English); (514)340-2085

HARISSI DAGHER, Mona; CHUM-Hop Notre-Dame, 1560 rue Sherbrooke E, Montreal QC H2L 4M1; Mon'00; FRCSC; Ophth. Staff, Centre Hospitalier l'Université de Montréal (CHUM) - Hôpital Notre-Dame; (514)890-8000 x23122

HARITON, Gregory B; C P M Hamilton, 1605 Main St W, Hamilton ON L8S 1E6; Arizona (USA)'89; Staff, CPM Health Centres Inc; Langs: Spanish; French; (905)574-4911; Fax. (905)574-8290; ghariton@med-emerg.com.

HARITON, Nicolas C; 200-101 16th St W, North Vancouver BC V7M 1T3; Tor'03; FRCPC; IntMed. Staff, Lions Gate Hospital; (604)904-0810; Fax. (604)904-0812.

HARIZANOV, Velizar A; Rosedale Med Centre, 204-600 Sherbourne St, Toronto ON M4X 1W4; Sofia (Bulgaria)'63; Langs: Serbian; Bulgarian; Serbo-Croatian; Russian; (416)927-8346; Fax. (416)927-0709.

HARJI, Fayaz G; Rockyview Gen Hosp, 7007 14 St SW, Calgary AB T2V 1P9; Wes'01; CCFP; CCFP(E.M.); Staff, Rockyview General Hospital; (403)943-3449

HARKER, Lynda A; Stratford Gen Hosp, 46 General Hospital Dr, Stratford ON N5A 2Y6; Wes'81; DiagRad. Med Prog Dir Med Imag, Stratford General Hospital - Huron Perth Healthcare Alliance; Aj Prof, University of Western Ontario; (519)272-8210 x2668

HARKNESS, Debra L; Townsite Med Clinic, 512 Campbell St, Nanaimo BC V9R 3H1; UBC'88; CCFP; Ac Staff, Nanaimo Regional General Hospital; (250)753-5665; Fax. (250)755-1408.

HARLE, Christopher; London HSC-University Hosp, PO Box 5339 Stn B 339 Windermere Rd, London ON N6A 5A5; Stellenbosch (South Africa)'89; FRCPC; Anes. Staff, London Health Sciences Centre - University Hospital; (519)663-3270

HARLE, Ingrid A; Queen's Palliative Care Med, 34 Barrie St, Kingston ON K7L 3J7; Wes'81; BSc; FRCSC; GenSurg;CCFP; Asst Prof Med & Oncology, Queen's University; Langs: Norwegian; (613)548-2485; Fax. (613)548-2436.

HARLESS, William; Cape Breton Healthcare Hosp, 1482 George St, Sydney NS B1P 1P3; (USA)'96; Staff, Cape Breton Healthcare Complex.

HARLEY, Charles H; Glenrose Rehab Hosp, 2319-10230 111 Ave NW, Edmonton AB T5G 0B7; Alb'65; MSc; FRCPC; IntMed. Staff Faculty Medical Disorder, Glenrose Rehabilitation Hospital; (780)735-7982; charles.harley@albertahealthservices.ca.

HARLEY, Frances L; Edmonton Clinic Health Academy, 4 555-11405 87 Ave, Edmonton AB T6G 1C9; Wes'65; DABPed; DABPed; FRCPC; Peds; Nephrol. Staff, University of Alberta Hospital; (780)248-5560

HARLEY, Stephen L; Dartmouth Med Centre, 203-46 Portland St, Dartmouth NS B2Y 1H4; Dal'96; CCFP; (902)465-4547; Fax. (902)469-2400.

HARLOCK, John A; Hamilton HS-General Site, 1200 Main St W, Hamilton ON L8N 3Z5; McM'05; FRCSC; GenSurg; VascSurg. Staff, Hamilton Health Sciences Centre - Hamilton General Hospital; (905)521-2100

HARLOS, Hans E; B-40 Yonge St S, Elmvale ON L0L 1P0; Man'79; Langs: German; (705)322-6330; Fax. (705)322-6320.

HARLOS, Michael S; St Boniface Gen Hosp, A8024-409 Tache Ave, Winnipeg MB R2H 2A6; UBC'84; CCFP; FCFP; Med Dir WRHA Palliative Care Sub-Program, St Boniface General Hospital; (204)235-3912; Fax. (204)231-3671.

HARLOS, Sandra C; Winnipeg Reg Health Authority, 490 Hargrave St, Winnipeg MB R3A 0X7; UBC'84; FRCPC; CommunMed. (204)940-3610

HARMAN, Jeremy J; 407-421 Bloor St E, Toronto ON M4W 3T1; National (Ireland)'68; MB ChB; FRCPC; Psy. Staff Psy, The Hospital For Sick Children; Staff, West End Creche; Teacher Psy, University of Toronto; (416)963-4363

HARMAN, John K; Medical Arts Bldg, 211-121 Wellington St W, Barrie ON L4N 1L2; National (Ireland)'80; MB ChB; CCFP; (705)792-1222

HARMAN, Karen E; Hamilton HS-Chedoke Site, PO Box 2000 Stn Lcd 1 1200 Main St W, Hamilton ON L8N 3Z5; McM'94; BSc; FRCPC; Peds (Developmental Pediatrics). Assoc Prof Peds, Hamilton Health Sciences Centre - McMaster University Medical Centre; (905)521-2100 x77212; Fax. (905)521-7953; harmank@mcmaster.ca.

HARMAN, Lisa M; The Ottawa Hosp - Civic Campus, 1053 Carling Ave, Ottawa ON K1Y 4E9; Qns'09; CCFP; Staff, The Ottawa Hospital - Civic Campus; (613)798-5555

HARMAN, Stuart; Children's Hosp of Eastern Ont, 401 Smyth Rd, Ottawa ON K1H 8L1; Qns'05; PedEmergMed; Peds. Staff, Children's Hospital of Eastern Ontario (CHEO); (613)737-7600

HARMANTAS, Athanasios; St Joseph's Health Centre, 230-30 The Queensway, Toronto ON M6R 1B5; McM'89; MSc; FRCSC; GenSurg (Head & Neck Surgery). Court Staff, Toronto General Hospital - UHN; Ac Staff Surg, St Joseph's Health Centre; Asst Prof Surg, University of Toronto; Langs: Greek; (416)530-6694; Fax. (416)530-6742.

HARMANTAS, Nikolaos; Cargill Meat Solutions, 165 Dunlop Dr, Guelph ON N1L 1P4; Wes'98; CCFP; (905)856-2100

HARMAR, Heather C; 40 Empire St, London ON N5Y 1G7; UBC'80; (204)747-2461

HARMATHY, Tibor A; 125-210 Memorial Ave, Orillia ON L3V 7V1; Ott'82; CAFCI; CCFP; FCFP; Ac Staff, Orillia Soldiers' Memorial Hospital; Langs: Hungarian; (705)326-5565; Fax. (705)329-2582.

HARMER, Andrea L; Kensington Med Clinic, 6548 Hastings St, Burnaby BC V5B 1S2; UBC'02; CCFP; (604)299-9769

HARMON, Christopher G; Bracebridge Med Arts Centre, 253 James St, Bracebridge ON P1L 2C2; Qns'76; CCFP; Staff, South Muskoka Memorial Hospital - Muskoka Algonquin Healthcare; (705)645-2281; Fax. (705)645-0057.

HARMON, Heather C; Admirals Walk, PO Box 56007 1511 Admirals Rd, Victoria BC V9A 2P0; UBC'10; CCFP; (250)380-3039

HARMON, Thomas P; 1100-1090 Pender St W, Vancouver BC V6E 2N7; UBC'63; (604)669-8188

HARMS, Sheila C; Hamilton HSC-McMaster Site, PO Box 2000 Stn Lcd 1 1200 Main St W, Hamilton ON L8N 3Z5; McM'03; FRCPC; Psy. Staff Child & Youth Mental Health, Hamilton Health Sciences Centre - McMaster Children's Hospital; (905)521-2100; Fax. (905)521-7978.

HARMS, Stefan; St Boniface Gen Hosp, 409 Tache Ave, Winnipeg MB R2H 2A6; Orange Free State (South Africa)'86; MB ChB; FRCPC; Anes. Staff, St Boniface General Hospital; Staff, Health Sciences Centre; (204)233-8563

HARMSE, Albert C; Associated Med Centre, PO Box 219 4909 50 Ave, St Paul AB T0A 3A0; (South Africa)'78; MB ChB; CCFP; (780)645-4411; Fax. (780)645-4566.

HARMSEN, Merril A; Canadian Med Protective Assn, 875 Carling Ave, Ottawa ON K1S 5P1; Qns'79; Med Advisor, Ministry of Health & Long Term Care.

HARNOIS, Bryan D; Prince County Hosp, PO Box 3000 Stn Main 65 Roy Boates Ave, Summerside PE C1N 2A9; McG'78; CCFP; Ac Staff, Prince County Hospital; (902)888-2212

HARNOIS, Carmen; CSSS de Quebec-Sud, 900 boul Wilfrid-Hamel, Quebec QC G1M 2R9; Laval'94; Staff, CSSS de la Vieille-Capitale; Langs: Bilingual(French/English); (418)682-1762; Fax. (418)682-1763.

HARNOIS, Dominic; CHUS-Hop Fleurimont, 3001 12e av N, Sherbrooke QC J1H 5N4; Sher'90; CCFP; CCFP(E.M.); FCFP; Staff, Centre Hospitalier Universitaire de Sherbrooke-Hopital Fleurimont; (819)346-1110

HARNOIS, Pierre A; Clinique Med Manseau, 584 boul Manseau, Joliette QC J6E 3E4; Mon'82; (450)753-9234; Fax. (450)755-1157.

HARNOIS, Yves; CSSS de Lac-Saint Jean-Est, CP 1300 Succ Bureau-Chef 300 boul Champlain S, Alma QC G8B 5W3; Sher'87; CSPQ; GenSurg. Staff, CSSS de Lac-Saint Jean-Est; (418)669-2000; Fax. (418)668-9697.

HAROLD, S Brent; South Albert Med Centre, 5-4150 Albert St, Regina SK S4S 3R8; Sask'92; FRCPC; Psy. (306)584-6230; Fax. (306)352-5395.

HAROON, Aroosa; 903-8210 111 St NW, Edmonton AB T6G 2C7; (Pakistan)'88; CCFP; (780)834-7124

HAROON, Nigil; Univ Hlth Network-Toronto Western Hosp, IE 423-399 Bathurst St, Toronto ON M5T 2S8; Kerala (India)'00; Staff, Toronto Western Hospital - University Health Network; (416)603-5634; Fax. (416)603-4348.

HAROUN, Gamal W; Bramalea Med Centre, 206-18 Kensington Rd, Brampton ON L6T 4S5; Cairo (Egypt)'65; MB ChB; FRCPC; DiagRad. Langs: Arabic; (905)793-5858; Fax. (905)278-2535.

HARPER, Byrne D J; West Main Plaza, 220-1600 Main St, Moncton NB E1E 1G5; Dal'84; FRCPC; Neur. Chief Neurosciences, The Moncton Hospital; (506)383-4472; Fax. (506)383-4267.

HARPER, Debra L; White Rock Medical Assoc, 101-15451 Russell Ave, White Rock BC V4B 2R5; UBC'82; Med Staff, Peace Arch Hospital; (604)531-5595; Fax. (604)531-9818; dh@wrma.ca.

HARPER, Jon A; Associated Anaes Services, M2A-601 Broadway W, Vancouver BC V5Z 4C2; UBC'76; FRCPC; Anes. Ac Staff, Vancouver General Hospital - Centennial Pavillion; (604)874-5291; Fax. (604)874-6852.

HARPER, Kelly M; Ajax Family Care Centre, 30 Kingston Rd W, Ajax ON L1T 4K8; Tor'92; Langs: French; (905)426-2501; Fax. (905)426-4852.

HARPER, Richard; 3310 32 Ave, Vernon BC V1T 2M6; (United Kingdom)'88; MB ChB; (250)545-5321

HARPER, Robert I; Glenmore Landing, D261-1600 90 Ave SW, Calgary AB T2V 5A8; Wes'81; CCFP; FCFP; (403)252-8855

HARPER, Samuel A; Clinique des Jeunes St-Denis, 1250 rue Sanguinet, Montreal QC H2X 3E7; Mon'02; CCFP.

HARPER, Telen T; 204-1931 Mount Newton Cross Rd, Saanichton BC V8M 2A9; UBC'88; Ac Staff, Saanich Peninsula Hospital; Ac Staff, Vancouver Island Health Authority; (250)652-9227; Fax. (250)652-9224.

HARPER, William B; Moncton Med Clinic, 308-860 Mountain Rd, Moncton NB E1C 2N7; Dal'78; CCFP; FCFP; (506)853-5145; Fax. (506)853-5177.

HARPER, William L; Hamilton HS-General Site, 627-237 Barton St E, Hamilton ON L8L 2X2; Tor'96; FRCPC; IntMed; Endocrin&Metab. Staff, Hamilton Health Sciences Centre - Hamilton General Hospital; (905)540-3560; Fax. (905)577-1404.

HARPIN, Chantal; Clinique médicale de Fleurimon, 210-2140 rue King E, Sherbrooke QC J1G 5G6; Sher'95; FRCPC; Peds. (819)563-4462; Fax. (819)563-4464.

HARPUR, George D; Tobermory Med Clinic, PO Box 220, Tobermory ON N0H 2R0; Tor'64; CCFP; FCFP; Ac Staff Lion's Head Unit, Grey Bruce Health Services - Owen Sound; Med Dir, Tobermory Hyperbaric Facility & Coroner, Prov. of Ontario & Med. Examiner Civil Aviation; Asst Prof Family Med, University of Western Ontario; Asst Clin Prof Family Med, McMaster University; Asst Prof Family Med, University of Toronto; (519)596-2305; Fax. (519)596-2979; pma@amtelecom.net.

HARPUR, George E; Allied Health Bldg, 300-5673 North St, Niagara Falls ON L2G 1J4; McM'91; BSc(H.K.); FRCSC; GenSurg. Chief Surg, Niagara Health System - Greater Niagara General Site; Clinical Asst Prof GenSurg, McMaster University; (905)357-5333; Fax. (905)357-0668.

HARPUR, Lisa L; Rockyview Gen Hosp, 7007 14 St SW, Calgary AB T2V 1P9; Cal'06; FRCPC; Psy. Staff, Rockyview General Hospital; (403)943-8704; Fax. (403)259-6289.

HARPUR, R Arthur; Laurel Family Practice Clinic, 2775 Laurel St, Vancouver BC V5Z 1M9; McG'77; MHSc; Ac Staff, Vancouver General Hospital - Centennial Pavillion; (604)875-5691; Fax. (604)875-5694.

HARRAD, Upninderjit S; Windsor Square Shopp Centre, 141-1959 152 St, Surrey BC V4A 9E3; Punjabi (India)'85; MB BS; FRCPC; Psy (General Psychiatry). Langs: Punjabi; Hindi; Urdu; (604)542-1190; Fax. (604)542-1191.

HARRICHARAN, Rajendra; London HSC-Victoria Hosp, PO Box 5010 Stn B 800 Commissioners Rd E, London ON N6A 5W9; Utkal (India)'84; FRCPC; Psy (Psychosis). Ac Staff, London Health Sciences Centre - Victoria Campus; Assoc Prof, University of Western Ontario; (519)667-6604; Fax. (519)667-6689.

HARRICHARAN, Tanujaa; 18-1960 Appleby Line, Burlington ON L7L 0B7; Academy of Medicine (USA)'01; CCFP; (905)319-2000

HARRIES, Jeffrey K; Medical Services Inc, 465 Ellis St, Penticton BC V2A 4M1; Cal'89; (250)492-6700; Fax. (250)492-6060.

HARRIES, Leona T; Dr's J & L Harries Med Service, 465 Ellis St, Penticton BC V2A 4M1; Cal'88; (250)492-6700; Fax. (250)492-6060; jeffharries@shaw.ca.

HARRIES, Didi V; Chilliwack Gen Hosp, 45600 Menholm Rd, Chilliwack BC V2P 1P7; Palacky (Czech Republic)'83; FRCPC; Peds (Neonatology). Staff, Chilliwack General Hospital; Langs: Czech; German; English; (604)795-4141

HARRIGAN, Erin K; Base Hosptal-CFB Petawawa, PO Box 9999 Stn Main, Petawawa ON K8H 2X3; McM'07; BEd; BScH; CCFP; Staff, Base Hospital-CFB Petawawa; (613)687-5511; familyht@drdh.org.

HARRIGAN, Gordon R; Joseph Brant Mem Hosp, 1230 North Shore Blvd E, Burlington ON L7S 1W7; Tor'74; FAB; FRCPC; Anes. Staff, Joseph Brant Memorial Hospital; (905)632-3730 x4135

HARRIGAN, Lynne A; AVH Corprate Office, 15 Chipman Dr, Kentville NS B4N 3V7; Dal'83; FRCPC; IntMed. (902)538-3424; Fax. (902)538-3432.

HARRIMAN, Maureen M A; 222-601 Sixth St, New Westminster BC V3L 3C1; McM'89; FRCSC; Otol. Staff, Burnaby Hospital; Staff, Surrey Memorial Hospital; Staff, Squamish General Hospital / Hilltop House; Staff, Royal Columbian Hospital; Staff, Eagle Ridge Hospital & Health Care Centre; Clin Instructor, University of British Columbia; (604)521-5301; Fax. (604)521-5311.

HARRINGTON, Andrew J; Wall Street Med Bldg, 220-140 Wall St, Saskatoon SK S7K 1N4; Sask'68; BA; Ac Staff, St Paul's Hospital (Grey Nuns) of Saskatoon; Ac Staff, Saskatoon City Hospital; (306)653-5522; Fax. (306)653-1723.

HARRINGTON, Brian D; The Peterborough Clinic, 302-26 Hospital Dr, Peterborough ON K9J 7C3; Wes'01; BSc; FRCSC; ObstGyn. (705)740-6507; Fax. (705)740-6891.

HARRINGTON, David M; 206 Lemarchant Rd, St. John's NL A1C 5B8; Mem'04; FRCSC; GenSurg; VascSurg. (709)739-8700

HARRINGTON, Gregory D R; Haney Prof Bldg, 206-11743 224 St, Maple Ridge BC V2X 6A4; UBC'79; FRCSC; Urol. (604)463-5433; Fax. (604)466-1622; gharr@telus.net.

HARRINGTON, Ian; One Med Place, 317-20 Wynford Dr, North York ON M3C 1J4; Wes'65; BASc; MSc; FRCSC; OrthSurg. Staff, Providence Healthcare; Court Staff, Toronto East General Hospital Inc; Aj Prof Surg, University of Toronto; (416)441-3656; Fax. (416)441-3604.

HARRINGTON, John P; 48-2140 North Park Dr, Brampton ON L6S 0C9; Tor'93; FRCSC; OrthSurg (Arthroplasty). Ac Staff, Halton Healthcare Services Corporation - Georgetown Hospital; Ac Staff, Headwaters Health Care Centre - Orangeville Site; Staff, William Osler Health System - Brampton Civic Hospital; (905)455-7987; Fax. (905)455-7486; jpharrington@rogers.com.

HARRINGTON, Karen P; Hôpital Ste-Justine, 3175 ch Cote-Sainte-Catherine, Montreal QC H3T 1C5; McG'96; FRCPC; Peds; Critical Care Medicine (P.Q.). Staff, Hôpital Ste-Justine; (514)345-4931 x5549

HARRINGTON, Leah D; Westway Med Clinic, 4-1723 Kipling Ave, Etobicoke ON M9R 4E1; McM'90; FRCPC; Peds. Staff, The Hospital For Sick Children; (416)244-8404; Fax. (416)244-7916; leah.harrington@sickkids.ca.

HARRINGTON, Michael; Psychealth Centre, PZ 202-771 Bannatyne Ave, Winnipeg MB R3E 3N4; Qns'06; FRCSC; Psy. (204)787-5151

HARRIS, Alison C; Vancouver Gen Hosp, 855 12th Ave W, Vancouver BC V5Z 1M9; Leicester (England)'90; BSc; LMCC; MB ChB; FRCPC; DiagRad. Staff Radiol, Vancouver General Hospital - Centennial Pavillion; (604)875-4340; Fax. (604)875-4225; alison.harris@vch.ca.

HARRIS, Andrew S; Abbie J Lane Mem Bldg, 7509-5909 Veterans Memorial La, Halifax NS B3H 2E2; Dal'96; FRCPC; Psy (Consultant Liaison Psychiatry). Staff, Queen Elizabeth II Health Sciences Centre - Victoria General Site; Dir Psy/Asst Prof, Dalhousie University; (902)473-2508; Fax. (902)473-4545.

HARRIS, Bradley J; Comox Med Clinic, 100-1695 Comox Ave, Comox BC V9M 3M1; UBC'99; CCFP; (250)339-2266

HARRIS, Colin J; Valley Reg Hosp, 150 Exhibition St, Kentville NS B4N 5E3; Dal'04; FRCPC; DiagRad. Staff, Valley Regional Hospital; (902)678-7381

HARRIS, David; Endocrine Fellow's Office, 4F-2775 Laurel St, Vancouver BC V5Z 1M9; UBC'08; FRCPC; IntMed. (604)875-4552

HARRIS, David J; 1381 Sprucedale Ave, London ON N5X 2N7; Leeds (England)'68; MRCPsy; LRCP; MRCS; FRCPC; Psy (Geriatric Psychiatry). Consultant Psy, St Thomas Elgin General Hospital; Consultant Psy, Parkwood Hospital - St Joseph's Health Care; Emeritus Prof Psy, University of Western Ontario; (519)433-1777; Fax. (519)433-1747.

HARRIS, David P; Royal Jubilee Hosp, 1952 Bay St, Victoria BC V8R 1J8; Cal'87; Staff, Royal Jubilee Hospital; (250)370-8000

HARRIS, Denis; Centre Med Laval, 1110 boul Vanier, Laval QC H7C 2R8; Mon'67; Staff, Hopital de la Cite de la santé; (450)661-2521; Fax. (450)661-7193; harrisdenis@yahoo.com.

HARRIS, Devin R; St Paul's Hosp, 128-1081 Burrard St, Vancouver BC V6Z 1Y6; UBC'98; MHSc; CCFP; CCFP(E.M.); FCFP; Staff Emerg Med, Providence Health Care - St Paul's Hospital; Clin Instructor Family Pract, University of British Columbia; (604)806-8480; Fax. (604)806-8488.

HARRIS, Donald J F; London Intercommunity Hlth Ctr, 659 Dundas St, London ON N5W 2Z1; Wes'75; Staff, London Intercommunity Health Centre - Dundas Street; (519)660-0874; Fax. (519)642-1532.

HARRIS, Donald R H; Queensway-Carleton Hosp, 3045 Baseline Rd, Nepean ON K2H 8P4; Ott'93; Staff, Queensway Carleton Hospital; Langs: Spanish; (613)721-2000

HARRIS, Elaine M; 258-1011 Glenmore Trail SW, Calgary AB T2V 4R6; Cal'83; (403)640-0600; Fax. (403)253-0124.

HARRIS, Eleanor J; PO Box 43015 Rpo Deer Valley, Calgary AB T2J 7A7; Mem'78; Ac Staff, Rockyview General Hospital.

HARRIS, Evan W; Walter Mackenzie HSC, 1D1-132 Meadowlark Shopping Ct, Edmonton AB T6G 2R7; Alb'85; FRCPC; Peds. Staff, University of Alberta Hospital; (780)407-6370; Fax. (780)407-6414.

HARRIS, Howard M; Credit Valley Prof Bldg, 202-2300 Eglinton Ave W, Mississauga ON L5M 2V8; McG'73; FRCPC; Derm. Ac Staff, The Credit Valley Hospital; Lecturer, University of Toronto; (905)828-0770; Fax. (905)828-4130.

HARRIS, J Kent; Arbutas Med Clinic, 203-149 Ingram St, Duncan BC V9L 1N8; Alb'76; BSc; MD; CCFP; FCFP; Assoc Staff, Cowichan District Hospital; Clin Prof Family Practice, University of British Columbia; (250)715-0049

HARRIS, James G; 303-8055 Anderson Rd, Richmond BC V6Y 1S2; UBC'72; FRCPC; Psy. (604)276-9339; Fax. (604)276-9345.

HARRIS, James M; Crescent Heights Fam Med Ctr, 114-2805 6th Ave E, Prince Albert SK S6V 6Z6; Sask'80; (306)763-2681; Fax. (306)953-1024.

HARRIS, Jeffrey R; University of Alberta Hosp, 1E429-8440 112 St NW, Edmonton AB T6G 2B7; Alb'95; FRCSC; Otol. Staff, University of Alberta Hospital; (780)407-7958; Fax. (780)407-3885.

HARRIS, Jennifer M I; Dr Charles A Janeway Child HC, 300 Prince Philip Dr, St. John's NL A1B 3V6; Mem'89; FRCPC; Anes. Staff, Janeway Children's Health & Rehabilitation Centre; (709)777-4381

HARRIS, Jeremy R; London HSC-University Hosp, PO Box 5010 Stn B E2 117-800 Commissioners Rd E, London ON N6A 5W9; Wes'02; FRCSC; GenSurg; VascSurg. Staff, London Health Sciences Centre - Victoria Campus; (519)685-8500

HARRIS, Kenneth; PO Box 5010, London ON N6A 5W9; Qns'77; FRCSC; GenSurg; VascSurg. Consultant Surg, Winchester District Memorial Hospital; Dir Office of Education, Royal College Of Physicians &; Emeritus Prof, University of Western Ontario; Aj Prof, University of Ottawa.

HARRIS, Kevin C; Children's & Women's HC of BC, 1F-4480 Oak St, Vancouver BC V6H 3V4; UBC'05; FRCPC; Peds; Cardiol. Staff, BC Children's Hospital; (604)875-2345 x2120

HARRIS, Kevin J; Misericordia Community Hosp, 16940 87 Ave NW, Edmonton AB T5R 4H5; Tor'95; CCFP; CCFP(E.M.); Staff, Covenant Health - Misericordia Community Hospital; (780)735-2627; Fax. (780)735-2966.

HARRIS, Kristin R; Lake of the Woods Dist Hosp, 21 Sylvan St, Kenora ON P9N 3W7; Alb'09; BSc(Hon); CCFP; Staff, Lake of the Woods District Hospital; (807)468-9861; Fax. (807)468-3939.

HARRIS, Leonard; 3532 Commerce Court, Burlington ON L7N 3L7; Tor'89; MSc; FRCSC; PlasSurg. Court Staff, Halton Healthcare Services Corporation - Oakville Site; Head Plastic Surg/Staff Plastic Surg, Joseph Brant Memorial Hospital; (905)333-9402; Fax. (905)333-0872.

HARRIS, Lia C; North Okanagan Paediatric Clin, 3-2802 34 St, Vernon BC V1T 5X1; UBC'97; FRCPC; Peds. (250)558-5506

HARRIS, Louise; Univ Hlth Network-Toronto Gen, GW3 562-200 Elizabeth St, Toronto ON M5G 2C4; Cape Town (South Africa)'75; FRCPC; Cardiol. Ac Staff, Toronto General Hospital - UHN; (416)340-3324; Fax. (416)340-3352.

HARRIS, Marianne; St Paul's Hosp, B 518-1081 Burrard St, Vancouver BC V6Z 1Y6; Alb'81; BMedSci; CCFP; Staff, Providence Health Care - St Paul's Hospital; Clinical Asst Prof Family Practice, University of British Columbia; (604)806-8771; Fax. (604)806-8412; mharris@cfenet.ubc.ca.

HARRIS, Nancy L; Orillia Solders' Mem Hosp, 170 Colborne St W, Orillia ON L3V 2Z3; Mem'79; BSc; BEd; CCFP; FCFP; Staff, Orillia Soldiers' Memorial Hospital; Langs: English; French; (705)325-2201

HARRIS, Neil S; 175 6 St SE, Medicine Hat AB T1A 1G7; Alb'81; Otol. Staff, Medicine Hat Regional Hospital; (403)527-2626; Fax. (403)529-5510.

HARRIS, Patricia E; Manitoba Clinic, 790 Sherbrook St, Winnipeg MB R3A 1M3; Tor'72; FRCPC; Hem (Medical Oncology); IntMed. Ac Staff, Health Sciences Centre; Ac Staff, The Salvation Army Grace Hospital; Ac Staff, Concordia General Hospital; Asst Prof, University of Manitoba.

HARRIS, Patrick G; CHUM-Hop Notre-Dame, G 3132-1560 rue Sherbrooke E, Montreal QC H2L 4M1; McG'88; FRCS; FRCSC; PlasSurg (Hand Surgery). Staff, Centre Hospitalier l'Université de Montréal (CHUM) - Hôpital Notre-Dame; Teacher Staff, Universite de Montreal; Langs: Bilingual(English/French); (514)890-8000 x23757; Fax. (514)412-7575; patrick.harris.chum@ssss.gouv.qc.ca.

HARRIS, Paul M; 2210 Broad St, Regina SK S4P 4V6; Witwatersrand (South Africa)'89; MB BCh; BSc; LMCC; CCFP; Langs: Afrikaans; (306)781-8080; Fax. (306)781-5644; pharris_physn@sasktel.net.

HARRIS, Robert W; Cornwall Comm Hosp-Second St, 510 Second St E, Cornwall ON K6H 1Z6; UBC'57; MSc(Exp.Surg.); PlasSurg (Hand Surgery). Ac Staff, Cornwall Community Hospital - Second Street Site; Ac Staff, Cornwall Community Hospital; Staff, Massena Gen. & Canton-Potsdam Hospitals(NY,USA); Langs: English; French; (613)534-8330

HARRIS, Russell B; 11-88 Duncan Ave W, Penticton BC V2A 7J7; UBC'70; Derm. Staff, Penticton Regional Hospital; (250)492-6565; Fax. (250)492-5103.

HARRIS, Scott Rodney; Health Sciences Centre, 300 Prince Philip Dr, St. John's NL A1B 3V6; Mem'02; FRCPC; DiagRad. Staff, Health Sciences Centre; (709)777-6300

HARRIS, Stewart B; St Joseph's Family Med Centre, 346 Platt's Lane, London ON N6G 1J1; Cal'82; MPH; FACPrevMed; CCFP; FCFP; Ac Staff, St Joseph's Hospital - St Joseph's Health Care; Prof Family Med, University of Western Ontario; Langs: Hebrew; (519)672-9660; Fax. (519)672-7727; sharris1@uwo.ca.

HARRIS, Thomas R; Central Alberta Med Imaging, 4312 54 Ave, Red Deer AB T4N 4M1; Tor'01; FRCPC; DiagRad. (403)343-6172

HARRIS, Wendy M; Barrie Community Health Centre, 490 Huronia Rd, Barrie ON L4N 6M2; McM'85; (705)734-9690; Fax. (705)734-0239.

HARRIS, William A; 103-1205 Amber Dr, Thunder Bay ON P7B 6M4; Tor'97; GenSurg (Endoscopy). Staff, Thunder Bay Regional Health Sciences Centre; (807)346-1440; Fax. (807)346-1445.

HARRIS-EZE, Ayodeji; Queen Elizabeth Hosp, PO Box 6600 Stn Central 60 Riverside Dr, Charlottetown PE C1A 8T5; FRCPC; IntMed. Staff, Queen Elizabeth Hospital; (902)894-2111; Fax. (902)894-0346.

HARRISON, Adele M; Victoria Gen Hosp, 1 Hospital Way, Victoria BC V8Z 6R5; Edinburgh (Scotland)'90; MB ChB; FRCPC; Peds (Neonatology). Staff, Victoria General Hospital; (250)727-4151

HARRISON, Alan W; Woodbridge Vascular Lab, 200-4600 Hwy 7, Woodbridge ON L4L 4Y7; Tor'49; FRCSC; GenSurg. Vis Staff Vascular Surg/Med Dir Univ of Toronto Clinic, Sunnybrook Health Sciences Centre; Prof Surg, University of Toronto; (905)850-2991

HARRISON, Christine E; Family Med Associates, 500-267 O'connor St, Ottawa ON K2P 1V3; Sask'74; MEd; CCFP; FCFP; Asst Prof Community, University of Ottawa; (613)760-3707; Fax. (613)232-4818.

HARRISON, David A; 206-101 Queensway W, Mississauga ON L5B 2P7; Qns'87; BSc; MSc; FRCPC; IntMed; Cardiol. Staff, Trillium Health Centre - Mississauga; (905)615-1441; Fax. (905)615-8537.

HARRISON, David W; Vancouver Gen Hosp, 855 12th Ave W, Vancouver BC V5Z 1M9; Wes'83; FRCPC; CCFP; EmergMed;CCFP(E.M.); Ac Staff EmergMed, Vancouver General Hospital - Centennial Pavillion; (604)875-4033; Fax. (604)875-4872.

HARRISON, Dean R; 126 Albion St S, Amherst NS B4H 2X3; Dal'02; CCFP; Staff, Miramichi Regional Hospital; Staff, Cumberland Regional Health Care Center; Locum Tenens ER, Saint John Regional Hospital; (902)661-7618; Fax. (902)661-7428.

HARRISON, Dorothy A; BC Cancer Agency-Vancouver CC, 600 10th Ave W, Vancouver BC V5Z 4E6; Cal'76; FRCPC; DiagRad. Ac Staff, BC Cancer Agency Vancouver Centre; (604)877-6098

HARRISON, Edmund R; Queen Elizabeth Hosp, PO Box 6600 Stn Central 60 Riverside Dr, Charlottetown PE C1A 8T5; Ott'78; FRCPC; PhysMed&Rehab (Electrodiagnosis). Staff, Queen Elizabeth Hospital; (902)894-2062; Fax. (902)894-2416; canoehed@dal.ca.

HARRISON, Kenneth F; Dow Chemical Canada ULC, PO Box 16 Stn Main, Fort Saskatchewan AB T8L 2P4; Alb'73; Med Dir Canadian Region, DOW Chemical Canada ULC; (780)998-8107; Fax. (780)998-8422.

HARRISON, Kenneth J; Addiction & Mental Hlth-Queen, 2 4-1001 Queen St W, Toronto ON M6J 1H4; Tor'90; Staff, Centre for Addiction & Mental Health (CAMH) - Queen Site; (416)535-8501 x2620

HARRISON, Linda M; Lions Gate Hosp, 3F-231 15th St E, North Vancouver BC V7L 2L7; UBC'74; Staff, Lions Gate Hospital; (604)985-6406

HARRISON, Lloyd W; The Medical Dental Centre, 300-16 O'Brien St, Orillia ON L3V 5S2; Tor'73; BSc(Hons.); FRCSC; GenSurg (Endoscopy). Staff, Orillia Soldiers' Memorial Hospital; (705)325-6197; Fax. (705)325-6198.

HARRISON, Mariam N; Kingston Gen Hosp, 76 Stuart St, Kingston ON K7L 2V7; Tor'06; FRCPC; IntMed; Respir. Staff, Kingston General Hospital; (613)548-3232

HARRISON, Mark M; Kingston Gen Hosp, N3-76 Stuart St, Kingston ON K7L 2V7; Qns'89; FRCSC; OrthSurg (Lower Extremity Joint Surgery). Staff Orthopedics, Kingston General Hospital; Staff Orthopedics, Hotel-Dieu Hospital; (613)549-6666 x4537; Fax. (613)548-2526; harrison@kgh.kart.net.

HARRISON, Megan E; Children's Hosp of Eastern Ont, 401 Smyth Rd, Ottawa ON K1H 8L1; McM'02; FRCPC; Peds. Staff, Children's Hospital of Eastern Ontario (CHEO); (613)737-7600

HARRISON, Philip B; St Paul's Hosp, 1081 Burrard St, Vancouver BC V6Z 1Y6; Cal'74; FACR; DiagRad. Ac Staff, Providence Health Care - St Paul's Hospital; Asst Prof, University of British Columbia; (604)806-8006

HARRISON, R Joseph; 208-565 Priestman St, Fredericton NB E3B 5X8; Dal'72; DAA; FRCSC; Ophth. Ac Staff, Dr Everett Chalmers Regional Hospital; (506)458-8875; Fax. (506)459-7458; jh@nbnet.nb.ca.

HARRISON, Robert G; Selkirk Medical, 22313 Selkirk Ave, Maple Ridge BC V2X 2X6; Alb'75; BSc; Staff, Ridge Meadows Hospital & Health Care Centre; (604)463-8814; Fax. (604)463-9927.

HARRISON, Robyn A; Grey Nuns Community Hosp, 0639-1100 Youville Drive West, Edmonton AB T6L 5X8; Dal'03; FRCPC; IntMed; InfectDis. Staff, Covenant Health - Grey Nuns Community Hospital; (780)735-7236; Fax. (780)735-9760.

HARRISON, Sarah D; Associate Family Phys Clinic, 262 2nd Ave NE, Swift Current SK S9H 2C8; Sask'08; CCFP; (306)773-1555; Fax. (306)773-6817.

HARRISON, Sidney W; 502 7 Ave SW, Medicine Hat AB T1A 5B9; Alb'90; CCFP; FCFP; (403)527-3200; Fax. (403)527-8695; docsid@telusplanet.net.

HARRISON, Stephen D; Medicentre Saint-Angelique, 1811 ch Sainte-Angelique, Saint-Lazare QC J7T 2X9; Ott'95; (450)424-7030

HARRISON, Susan A L; U of Toronto-Health Services, 214 College St, Toronto ON M5T 2Z9; Wes'84; CCFP; FCFP; (416)978-8030; Fax. (416)971-2089.

HARRISON, Warren E; 560-1145 Hunt Club Rd, Ottawa ON K1V 0Y3; Wes'71; FACOG; FRCSC; ObstGyn. Staff, The Ottawa Hospital - General Campus; Asst Prof, University of Ottawa; (613)738-2378; Fax. (613)738-2653.

HARRISON, Wayne D; Brandon Reg Health Centre, G 149-150 Mctavish Ave E, Brandon MB R7A 2B3; Man'85; FRCPC; DiagRad. Staff, Brandon Regional Health Centre; (204)726-2155; Fax. (204)726-2448.

HARRISON, Yasmin; 206-815 College St, Toronto ON M6G 1C9; McG'97; CCFP; Staff, Glengarry Memorial Hospital; Langs: Hindi; (416)923-5500

HARROLD, A John; Vendome Centre, 100-5175 boul de Maisonneuve W, Montreal QC H4A 1Z3; McG'61; BSc; CM; CCFP; (514)484-4711; Fax. (514)484-9828.

HARROLD, Brent D; Penticton Reg Hosp, 550 Carmi Ave, Penticton BC V2A 3G6; UBC'95; CCFP; CCFP(E.M.); FCFP; Staff, Penticton Regional Hospital; (250)492-4000; Fax. (250)492-9068.

HARROLD, Catherine G; 13214 Kelly Ave PO Box 1620, Summerland BC V0H 1Z0; UBC'95; BSc; CCFP; Staff, Penticton Regional Hospital; (250)494-3432; Fax. (250)494-4392.

HARROLD, Deborah L; Huntsville Prof Bldg, 202-348 Muskoka Rd 3 N, Huntsville ON P1H 1H8; McM'99; CCFP; (705)788-3623; Fax. (705)788-3624.

HARROLD, JoAnn E; Children's Hosp Eastern Ont, 8231-401 Smyth Rd, Ottawa ON K1H 8L1; McM'97; FRCPC; Peds (Neonatal & Perinatal Medicine). Staff, Children's Hospital of Eastern Ontario (CHEO); Staff, The Ottawa Hospital - General Campus; Asst Prof, University of Ottawa; Langs: Bilingual(French/English); (613)737-7600 x2415; Fax. (613)738-4847; jharrold@cheo.on.ca.

HARROP, A Robertson; Alberta Children's Hosp, 2888 Shaganappi Trail NW, Calgary AB T3B 6A8; Qns'86; FRCSC; PlasSurg (Plastic & Reconstructive Surgery). Staff, Foothills Medical Centre; Staff, Alberta Children's Hospital; (403)955-2840; Fax. (403)955-7634.

HARRY, Gervais A; Rathburn Med Centre, 600 The East Mall, Etobicoke ON M9B 4B1; London (England)'64; MB BS; LMCC; FRCSC; Urol. Langs: Spanish; Portuguese; Italian; (416)626-9222; Fax. (416)626-9205; gervaisharry@rogers.com.

HART, Brian; Stone's Mill Family Hlth Ctre, 25 Mill St, Gananoque ON K7G 2L5; Qns'90; CCFP; Med Examiner, Civil Aviation Canada; (613)382-3974; Fax. (613)382-4417; bhart@smartchartsmd.com.

HART, Claire; 827-10 Discovery Ridge Hill SW, Calgary AB T3H 5X2; Cal'07; Psy. Staff, Foothills Medical Centre; (403)452-6272; Fax. (403)452-6242.

HART, David G; Cowan Avenue Med Clinic, 201-496 Topsail Rd, St. John's NL A1E 2C2; Mem'75; (709)368-2115; Fax. (709)368-2120.

HART, Greg C; Abbotsford Village Med Clinic, 302-2050 Sumas Way, Abbotsford BC V2S 2C7; UBC'94; CCFP; (604)504-7145

HART, Jason J; BC Cancer Agency-Vanc Isl Ctr, 2410 Lee Ave, Victoria BC V8R 6V5; Alb'99; BSc; FRCPC; IntMed; MedOncol; Hem. Staff, BC Cancer Agency Vancouver Island Centre; (250)519-5570; Fax. (250)519-5595.

HART, Julian G; Joseph Brant Mem Hosp, 1230 North Shore Blvd E, Burlington ON L7S 1W7; Tor'83; BSc; MSc; FASCP; ABPath; FRCPC; AnatPath (Laboratory Medicine). Chief Path & Laboratory Med Dir, Joseph Brant Memorial Hospital; (905)681-4826; jhart@jbmh.com.

HART, Lawrence; Charlton Med Centre, 608-25 Charlton Ave E, Hamilton ON L8N 1Y2; Witwatersrand (South Africa)'76; MB BCh; MSc(ClinEpid); FACP; FRCPC; IntMed (Rheumatology). Ac Staff, St Joseph's Healthcare - Charlton Campus; Physician, Charlton Medical Centre; Prof, McMaster University; (905)529-9749; Fax. (905)521-0098.

HART, Meryl E; Red Deer Reg Hosp Centre, 3942 50A Ave, Red Deer AB T4N 4E7; (Jamaica)'74; FRCPC; IntMed. Staff, Red Deer Regional Hospital Centre; (403)343-4422; Fax. (403)358-4324.

HART, Michelle; Glenwood Med Clinic, 3945 17 Ave SW, Calgary AB T3E 0B3; (South Africa)'00; MB ChB; Langs: Afrikaans; (403)242-8633; Fax. (403)242-8884; michelle.hart@shaw.ca.

HART, Michelle; Baycrest Ctre/Geriatric Care, 5W26-3560 Bathurst St, North York ON M6A 2E1; Tor'06; CCFP; Staff, Baycrest Centre for Geriatric Care; (416)785-2500

HART, Paul J; 204-3140 Lakeshore Rd, Kelowna BC V1W 3T1; Glasgow (Scotland)'79; MB ChB; DRCOG; (250)763-1131; Fax. (250)763-3455.

HART, Paul L; Kirkland & District Hosp, PO Box 3000 Stn Main 145 Goverment Rd E, Kirkland Lake ON P2N 3P4; Mem'73; Staff, Kirkland & District Hospital; (705)567-5251

HART, Paul M; King West Med Associates, 505 King St W, Hamilton ON L8P 1B9; Wes'92; Ac Staff, St Joseph's Healthcare - Charlton Campus; (905)525-3501; Fax. (905)528-5468.

HART, R Allan; Digestive Health Clinic, 510-330 Highway 7 E, Richmond Hill ON L4B 3P8; Tor'61; FACG; FRCPC; IntMed (Gastroenterology). Ac Staff, North York General Hospital; (905)707-5007; Fax. (905)707-5008.

HART, Randy; White Hills Med Clinic, 262 Newfoundland Dr, St. John's NL A1A 3R5; Mem'75; (709)753-1091; Fax. (709)753-3790; rhart@nl.rogers.com.

HART, Renee S; Woodlawn Med Centre, 92 Main St, Dartmouth NS B2X 1R5; Dal'99; CCFP; (902)434-1500; Fax. (902)434-4368.

HART, Richard S; St Joseph's Health Centre, 215-30 The Queensway, Toronto ON M6R 1B5; Wes'93; FRCSC; GenSurg (Hepatobiliary & Pancreatic Surgery). Staff, St Joseph's Health Centre; Lecturer, University of Toronto; (416)530-6841; Fax. (416)530-6844.

HART, Robert D; Queen Elizabeth II HSC, 1276 South Park St, Halifax NS B3H 2Y9; Dal'00; FRCSC; Otol. Asst Prof, Queen Elizabeth II Health Sciences Centre - Victoria General Site; (902)473-7002; Fax. (902)473-5667.

HART, Stephanie E; Foothills Family Practice, 102-30 Crystalridge Dr, Okotoks AB T1S 2C3; Cal'03; BSc; CCFP; Fam Med, High River General Hospital; (403)938-5455

HARTE, Susannah E; Univ of Toronto, 112-150 College St, Toronto ON M5S 3E2; Dublin (Ireland)'01.

HARTERRE, Trevor D; Timmins & Dist Hosp, 700 Ross Ave E, Timmins ON P4N 8P2; Ott'95; CCFP; CCFP(E.M.); FCFP; Staff, Timmins & District Hospital; Langs: English; French; (705)267-6340

HARTFIELD, Dawn; Edmonton Clinic Hlth Academy, 3 597-11405 87 Ave NW, Edmonton AB T6G 1C9; Sask'94; FRCPC; Peds (Hospitalist). Staff, University of Alberta Hospital; Staff, Edmonton Clinic Health Academy; (780)407-8822; Fax. (780)248-5625.

HARTFORD, Brian; The Spence Clinic, 500-1265 Arthur St E, Thunder Bay ON P7E 5H7; Tor'83; (807)626-1123; Fax. (807)626-1142.

HARTFORD, James A; 24 Gerrard St, London ON N6C 4C5; Wes'79; FRCPC; Psy. (519)432-1430; Fax. (519)432-1430.

HARTFORD, Lesley A; Mill Bay Med Centre, 230-2720 Mill Bay Rd RR 1, Mill Bay BC V0R 2P1; UBC'90; CCFP; (250)743-3211

HARTFORD, Samuel D; 150-3200 Shelbourne St, Victoria BC V8P 5G8; UBC'90; (250)595-1121

HARTH, Manfred M; AIM Healthcare Group, 458 Central Ave, London ON N6B 2E5; Tor'60; FRCPC; IntMed (Rheumatology). Consultant, St Joseph's Hospital - St Joseph's Health Care; Emeritus Prof Cons, University of Western Ontario; manfred.harth@sjhc.london.on.ca.

HARTLEIB, Michael C; Kawartha Cardiology Clinic, 402-327 Charlotte St, Peterborough ON K9J 0B2; Tor'98; FRCPC; IntMed (Critical Care Medicine); Cardiol. Staff, Peterborough Regional Health Centre - Hospital Drive; Physician, Kawartha Cardiology Clinic; (705)775-0320; Fax. (705)775-0128.

HARTLEY, Duane M; Charleswood Med Clinic, 3360 Roblin Blvd, Winnipeg MB R3R 0C5; Man'95; CCFP; FCFP; Staff, The Salvation Army Grace Hospital; (204)889-7200

HARTLEY, Elizabeth J; Rouge Valley-Centenary HC, 2867 Ellesmere Rd, Scarborough ON M1E 4B9; Tor'82; BSc; MSc; FRCPC; Anes. Staff Anes, Rouge Valley Health System - Centenary Health Centre Site; Asst Prof, University of Toronto; (416)284-8131 x4054; Fax. (416)281-7453.

HARTMAN, Alexander; True North Imaging, 120-7330 Yonge St, Thornhill ON L4J 7Y7; Tor'82; FRCPC; DiagRad. Langs: Hebrew; Hungarian; (905)707-1777; ahartman@truenorthimaging.com.

HARTMAN, Darrell J; Town Centre Family Clinic, 320-6203 28 Ave NW, Edmonton AB T6L 6K3; Alb'88; Staff, Covenant Health - Grey Nuns Community Hospital; (780)462-8120; Fax. (780)461-9437.

HARTMAN, Dennis L; 101-1757 Beaufort Ave, Comox BC V9M 1R8; Sask'88; BSc; FRCSC; ObstGyn. (250)339-3114; Fax. (250)339-4186.

HARTON, Elisabeth; CLSC du Richelieu, 1394 rue Notre-Dane, Saint-Cesaire QC J0L 1T0; Mon'94; (514)469-0269

HARTON, Jacques; CLSC Mer Et Montagnes, 600 av William-May, Murdochville QC G0E 1W0; Laval'73; Membre Active, Centre Hospitalier de Gaspe; Member Active, CLSC Mont-Louis-CSSS Haute-Gaspesie; Langs: Portuguese; (418)784-2572; Fax. (418)784-3629.

HARTRICK, Terrance R; 103-9710 Second St, Sidney BC V8L 3C4; UBC'81; CCFP; Ac Staff, Saanich Peninsula Hospital; (250)656-7261; Fax. (250)655-1219.

HARTRIDGE, Allan D; Wall Street Med Bldg, 300-140 Wall St, Saskatoon SK S7K 1N4; Sask'67; DiagRad. Ac Staff, St Paul's Hospital (Grey Nuns) of Saskatoon; Ac Staff, Saskatoon City Hospital; University of Saskatchewan; (306)244-1167; Fax. (306)244-2911.

HARTRY, A Shane; Seven Oaks Gen Hosp, 2300 McPhillips St, Winnipeg MB R2V 3M3; Man'04; CCFP; CCFP(E.M.); Staff, Seven Oaks General Hospital.

HARTRY, Zoa; Lakewood Med Centre, 30 Lakewood Blvd, Winnipeg MB R2J 2M6; Man'02; CCFP; (204)257-4900; Fax. (204)257-6843.

HARTSBURG, Cory J; Royal Court Med Centre, 206-1 Quarry Ridge Rd, Barrie ON L4M 7G1; Qns'97; BSc; FRCSC; Urol. Staff, Royal Victoria Regional Health Centre; (705)728-4501; Fax. (705)728-8332.

HARTT, Donald J; Terwillegar Med Clinic, 101-121 Haddow Close NW, Edmonton AB T6R 3W3; Alb'99; CCFP; (780)989-5300

HARTT, Marcia R; Grey Nuns Community Hosp, 1100 Youville Drive West NW, Edmonton AB T6L 5X8; Alb'05; CCFP; Staff, Covenant Health - Grey Nuns Community Hospital; (780)735-7000

HARTWICK, Karl; The Ottawa Hosp-Gen Campus, Box 206 LM 12-501 Smyth Rd, Ottawa ON K1H 8L6; Cal'04; FRCPC; IntMed; Critical Care Medicine. Staff, The Ottawa Hospital - General Campus; (613)737-8755; Fax. (613)737-8851.

HARTWICK, Karl R; Haliburton Family Med Centre, PO Box 870 7217 Gelert Rd, Haliburton ON K0M 1S0; Wes'72; CCFP; FCFP; Staff, Haliburton Highlands Health Services - Haliburton Site; Asst Prof Family & Commun Med, University of Toronto; (705)457-1212; Fax. (705)457-3955.

HARTWIG, Karen S; 508 15 Ave SW, Calgary AB T2R 0R2; Alb'85; (403)398-5449; Fax. (403)229-1759.

HARTWIG, Michael C; Health First Med Centre, 100-15129 100 Ave, Surrey BC V3R 9P4; Alb'86; Langs: German; (604)583-3550

HARVEY, Adrian M; Foothills Med Centre, 1403 29 St NW, Calgary AB T2N 2T9; Tor'01; FRCSC; GenSurg. Staff, Foothills Medical Centre; (403)944-0966; Fax. (403)944-1277.

HARVEY, Amelie; CSSS de Lac-Saint Jean-Est, CP 1300 Succ Bureau-Chef 300 boul Champlain S, Alma QC G8B 5W3; Sher'09; Staff, CSSS de Lac-Saint Jean-Est; (418)668-2477; amelie.harvey@ssss.gouv.qc.ca.

HARVEY, Anne; CHUS-Hop Fleurimont, 3001 12e av N, Sherbrooke QC J1H 5N4; Laval'77; FRCPC; PhysMed&Rehab. Staff, Centre Hospitalier Universitaire de Sherbrooke-Hopital Fleurimont; Consultant, Centre Hospitalier Universitaire de Sherbrooke-Hôpital Hôtel-Dieu; (819)346-1110; Fax. (819)820-6420.

HARVEY, Annie; Clinique Med Des 21, 101-171 6e rue, La Baie QC G7B 0A3; Laval'88; Staff Family Med & Emerg, CSSS de Charlevoix; (418)544-3073; Fax. (418)544-7571.

HARVEY, Bartholomew J; Dalla Lana School of Public Hl, 688-155 College St, Toronto ON M5T 1P8; Tor'81; MSc(BiomedEng); MEd; PhD(Epidemiol); FACPrevMed; FRCPC; CommunMed (Public Health). Coroner, Ministry of Public Safety & Corrections; Assoc Prof Dalla Lana School of Public Health, University of Toronto; (416)946-5793; Fax. (416)978-8299; bart.harvey@utoronto.ca.

HARVEY, Berthold; Clinique Med Notre-Dame Inc, 147 rue Notre-Dame E, Victoriaville QC G6P 3Z8; Laval'71; Staff, Hotel-Dieu d'Arthabaska; (819)758-3165; Fax. (819)758-0745.

HARVEY, Catherine A; 400-1128 Hornby St, Vancouver BC V6Z 2L4; UBC'82; CCFP; FCFP; Vis Staff, Providence Health Care - St Paul's Hospital; Vis Staff, BC Children's Hospital; Ac Staff, Vancouver General Hospital - Centennial Pavillion; Staff, West Coast Family Practice Centre; Clinical Asst Prof, University of British Columbia; (604)707-2273; Fax. (604)707-2250.

HARVEY, Claude; 102-739 rue Notre-Dame, Repentigny QC J5Y 1N1; Mon'79; Staff, Residence de la Rive Nord; Staff, Residence de la Rive; Staff, Residence la Belle Epoque; (450)581-6294

HARVEY, Claudette; CSSS des Iles, 430 ch Principal CP 730, Cap-aux-Meules QC G4T 1R9; Sher'86; Staff, Hôpital de l'Archipel; (418)986-2121; Fax. (418)986-7001; claudette.harvey.archipel@ssss.gouv.qc.ca.

HARVEY, Daniel G; Clinique Med Mont St-Hilaire, 261 boul Laurier, Mont-Saint-Hilaire QC J3H 3N8; Sher'87; (450)464-5151; Fax. (450)464-3703.

HARVEY, Dany; CSSS de Lac-Saint Jean-Est, CP 1300 Succ Bureau-Chef 300 boul Champlain S, Alma QC G8B 5W3; Sher'88; Peds (Allergy). Staff, CSSS de Lac-Saint Jean-Est; (418)669-2000; Fax. (418)662-8003.

HARVEY, David; Univ of Ottawa, 2044-451 Smyth Rd, Ottawa ON K1H 8M5; Mem'08.

HARVEY, David T; Hamilton HS-Henderson Site, 711 Concession St, Hamilton ON L8V 1C3; Wes'79; FRCPC; PhysMed&Rehab. Ac Staff, Hamilton Health Sciences Centre-Juravinski Site; Staff, Joseph Brant Memorial Hospital; Assoc Prof, McMaster University; (905)574-8515; Fax. (905)575-2598; dharvey@hhsc.ca.

HARVEY, Edward J; MUHC-Montreal Gen Hosp, B51595-1650 av Cedar, Montreal QC H3G 1A4; McG'89; FRCSC; OrthSurg. Staff, McGill University Health Centre - Montreal General Campus; Teach Staff, McGill University; (514)934-1934 x42734; Fax. (514)934-8453.

HARVEY, Elizabeth A; The Hosp for Sick Children, 555 University Ave, Toronto ON M5G 1X8; Mem'82; FRCPC; Peds (Pediatric Nephrology). Staff Nephrol, The Hospital For Sick Children; Assoc Prof Peds, University of Toronto; (416)813-5082; Fax. (416)813-6271; elizabeth.harvey@sickkids.ca.

HARVEY, Guy; 1055 av du Pont S, Alma QC G8B 2V7; Laval'87; OrthSurg (Arthroscopy). (418)662-4997; Fax. (418)662-2660.

HARVEY, Isabelle; CHUQ-Hotel-Dieu de Quebec, 11 Cote du Palais, Quebec QC G1R 2J6; Mon'99; CSPQ; FRCPC; AnatPath. Staff, Centre Hospitalier Universitaire de Québec (CHUQ) - Siege Social; (418)691-5233; Fax. (418)691-5226.

HARVEY, Janice A; Campus Hlth Centre-Musc, B101-1280 Main St W, Hamilton ON L8S 4K1; McM'86; Dip SportMed; CCFP; FCFP; Clin Prof Pt-Time, McMaster University; (905)525-9140 x24578; Fax. (905)546-0805; jaharvey@mcmaster.ca.

HARVEY, Janice; 203-542 7 St S, Lethbridge AB T1J 2H1; Alb'74; Dip SportMed; BMedSci; MD; (403)320-1540; Fax. (403)329-3778.

HARVEY, Janique; Douglas Mental Hlth Univ Inst, 6875 boul LaSalle, Verdun QC H4H 1R3; Laval'02; Psy (Transcultural Med). Staff, Douglas Mental Health University Institute; Langs: Bilingual(French/English); (514)761-6131; Fax. (514)888-4460; janique.harvey@douglas.mcgill.ca.

HARVEY, Johanne; CSSS de Chicoutimi, CP 5006 305 rue Saint-Vallier, Chicoutimi QC G7H 5H6; Laval'92; FAAP; MPH; FRCPC; Peds (Adolescent Medicine). Clin Staff Peds/Med Coord Adolesent Med Speciolist, Complexe hospitalier de la Sagamie; Consultant, Direction de Sante Publique du Saguenay-Lac St-Jean; Langs: English; (418)541-1059; Fax. (418)541-1157; johanne.harvey.chs@ssss.gouv.qc.ca.

HARVEY, John T; Hamilton Reg Eye institute, 2112-2757 King St E, Hamilton ON L8G 5E4; Wes'75; DAB; FRCSC; Ophth (Oculo Plastic Surgery). Ac Staff, Hamilton Health Sciences Centre - McMaster Children's Hospital; Ac Staff, St Joseph's Healthcare - Charlton Campus; Prof, McMaster University; (905)573-7777 x3809; Fax. (905)573-4826; jtharvey@mcmaster.ca.

HARVEY, Julie; CSSS de Trois-Rivières, 1991 boul du Carmel, Trois-Rivieres QC G8Z 3R9; Laval'01; FRCPC; RadOncol. Staff, CSSS de Trois-Rivières; (819)697-3333 x63900; Fax. (819)378-9712.

HARVEY, Kathleen; Dr Everett Chalmers Reg Hosp, PO Box 9000 Stn A 700 Priestman St, Fredericton NB E3B 5N5; Staff, Dr Everett Chalmers Regional Hospital; (506)452-5400

HARVEY, Marianne; COOP Solidarite-sante-Hubert R, 1 rue Masse, St-Hubert-Riv-Du-L QC G0L 2L0; Mon'93; Staff, Centre Hospitalier Regional du Grand-Portage; (418)497-3903; Fax. (418)497-3905.

HARVEY, Marie-Andree; Kingston Gen Hosp, V4-76 Stuart St, Kingston ON K7L 2V7; Laval'92; MSc; FRCOG; LMCC; FRCSC; ObstGyn (Urological Gynecology). Staff, Kingston General Hospital; Assoc Prof, Queen's University; (613)548-6115; Fax. (613)548-1330; harveym@queensu.ca.

HARVEY, Martin C; Mission Med Clinic, 201-2303 4 St SW, Calgary AB T2S 2S7; Nottingham (England)'85; MRCGPract; BMedSci; (403)640-4320; Fax. (403)640-4397.

HARVEY, Michel; Clin Orl Du Saguenay, 1577 boul Talbot, Chicoutimi QC G7H 4C3; Laval'86; FRCSC; Otol. Staff, Complexe hospitalier de la Sagamie; Langs: Bilingual(French/English); (418)545-9989; Fax. (418)545-1766; orldoc@videotron.ca.

HARVEY, Normand; Clin Med Fam de la Malbaie, 515 rue Saint-Etienne, La Malbaie QC G5A 1W7; Laval'73; Langs: Bilingual(French/English); (418)665-2366 x13; Fax. (418)665-7766.

HARVEY, Robert C; 408-73 Water St N, Cambridge ON N1R 7L6; Tor'81; (519)740-2020; Fax. (519)740-6658.

HARVEY, Patricia T; 310-750 Dundas St W, Toronto ON M6J 3S3; McM'78; DAA; FRCSC; Ophth (Retina). Ac Staff, Toronto Western Hospital - University Health Network; Court Staff, Hamilton Health Sciences Centre - McMaster Children's Hospital; Asst Prof, University of Toronto; Associate Clin Prof Surg, McMaster University; (416)603-1116; Fax. (416)603-1118.

HARVEY, Paula; Women's College Hosp, 766-76 Grenville St, Toronto ON M5S 1B2; Adelaide (Australia)'86; PhD; MB BS; FRACP; Staff Cardiol, Mount Sinai Hospital; Staff Cardiol, Toronto Western Hospital - University Health Network; Staff, Women's College Hospital; Asst Prof, University of Toronto; (416)323-7703; Fax. (416)323-6304; paula.harvey@ewhospital.ca.

HARVEY, Pierre; Clinique de Med Fam Montcalm, 309 rue Montcalm, Chicoutimi QC G7J 2V1; Laval'74; assoc Staff, Complexe hospitalier de la Sagamie; Langs: Bilingual(English/French); (418)545-4211; Fax. (418)545-2920; pharvey@royaume.com.

HARVEY, Pierre; CSSS de Rivière-de-Loup, 75 rue Saint-Henri, Riviere-du-Loup QC G5R 2A4; Mon'88; FRCP; Microbio & Infect Dis (P.Q.); MedMicrobiol (Infectiology). Staff, Centre Hospitalier Regional du Grand-Portage; (418)868-1010 x2624

HARVEY, Pierre-Claude; Clinique Med de l'Anse, 78 rue Lemaire, Sept-Iles QC G4S 1A3; Mon'78; Chef Dept of Med, Centre Hospitalier Regional de Sept-Iles; (418)962-1212; pcharvey49@hotmail.com.

HARVEY, Richard D; Fredericton Med Clinic, 302-1015 Regent St, Fredericton NB E3B 6H5; Dal'90; FRCPC; IntMed. (506)458-0213

HARVEY, Richard; CHUS-Hop Fleurimont, 3001 12e av N, Sherbrooke QC J1H 5N4; Sher'76; FACC; CSPQ; Cardiol. Ac Staff, Centre Hospitalier Universitaire de Sherbrooke-Hopital Fleurimont; Langs: Bilingual(French/English); (819)346-1110 x14947; Fax. (819)820-6897.

HARVEY, Sylvie; CSSS de Rivière-de-Loup, 75 rue Saint-Henri, Riviere-Du-Loup QC G5R 2A4; Mon'82; FRCPC; DiagRad. Staff, Centre Hospitalier Regional du Grand-Portage; (418)868-1010 x2386; Fax. (418)868-1035.

HARVEY, William L G; Elmsdale Med Centre, 106 Elmsdale Rd, Elmsdale NS B2S 1K6; Mem'97; CCFP; FCFP; Clin Preceptor, Dalhousie University; (902)883-2216; Fax. (902)883-1734; wharvey@accesswave.ca.

HARVEY-BLANKENSHIP, Michele; Royal Alexandra Hosp, 10240 Kingsway NW, Edmonton AB T5H 3V9; Tor'04; FRCPC; Peds. Staff, Royal Alexandra Hospital; (780)735-4605; Fax. (780)735-4071.

HARVIE, Christopher J; Maples Surgical Centre, 9-1291 Jefferson Ave, Winnipeg MB R2P 1S7; Dal'82; BSc(Hons); FRCPC; Anes.

HARVIE, Sarah; Peterborough Reg Health Centre, 1 Hospital Dr, Peterborough ON K9J 7C6; Dal'01; FRCPC; DiagRad. Staff, Peterborough Regional Health Centre - Hospital Drive; (705)743-2121

HARWOOD, Robin; Sault Area Hosp, 750 Great Northern Rd, Sault Ste. Marie ON P6B 0A8; Sask'05; Anes. Staff, Sault Area Hospital - Sault Ste Marie; (705)759-3434

HARWOOD, Roger A E; Rouge Valley-Centenary HC, 2867 Ellesmere Rd, Scarborough ON M1E 4B9; London (England)'68; MB BS; LRCP; MRCS; FFARCS; FRCPC; Anes. Staff, Rouge Valley Health System - Centenary Health Centre Site; (416)284-8131 x4054; Fax. (416)281-7453.

HASAL, Simona; University of Alberta Hosp, 8440 112 St NW, Edmonton AB T6G 2B7; (Czech Republic)'95; Staff, University of Alberta Hospital; (780)407-8822

HASAN, Anwar A A; Windsor Reg Hosp- Metropolitan, 1995 Lens Ave, Windsor ON N8W 1L9; Bahrain (Saudi Arabia)'94; FRCPC; EmergMed. Staff, Windsor Regional Hospital - Metropolitan Site; (519)254-1661; Fax. (519)254-3150.

HASAN, Azra; Medical Arts Bldg, 102-336 Kings Rd, Sydney NS B1S 1A9; Karachi (Pakistan)'94; MB BS; Associate, Cape Breton District Health Authority; (902)562-8222; Fax. (902)564-4783.

HASAN, Bushra F; Justik Med Clinic, 8225 105 St NW, Edmonton AB T6E 4H2; (Iraq)'89; MB ChB; CCFP; (780)432-0211; Fax. (780)439-9349.

HASAN, Fauzia; The Credit Valley Hosp, 2200 Eglinton Ave W, Mississauga ON L5M 2N1; Karachi (Pakistan)'98; AnatPath. Staff, The Credit Valley Hospital; (905)813-2200

HASAN, Fyeza; The Hosp for Sick Children, 555 University Ave, Toronto ON M5G 1X8; Bristol (United Kingdom)'03; Peds.

HASAN, Khalid H A; 10538 124 St NW, Edmonton AB T5N 1R9; (Libya)'02; (780)756-3090; Fax. (780)756-3089.

HASAN, Omar N; CSSS de la Matapedia, 135 av Gaetan-Archambault, Amqui QC G5J 2K5; Moscow (Russia (Federation))'88; DGS; DPhil; LMCC; ATLS; CSPQ; LRCPS; CRCP; FRCSC; GenSurg (P.Q.) (Endoscopy). Chef de Chirurgie, CSSS de la Matapedia; Langs: Russian; Arabic; Kurdish; Persian; Bilingual(English/French); Farsi; (418)629-2211 x2138; Fax. (418)629-4498; omar.n.hasan@gmail.com.

HASAN, Osama; Grand River Hosp-KW Hlth Ctre, PO Box 9056 Stn C 835 King St W, Kitchener ON N2G 1G3; Saddam (Iraq)'93; CCFP; CCFP(E.M.); Staff, Grand River Hospital - Kitchener/Waterloo Health Centre; Langs: Arabic; (519)742-3611

HASAN, S K Mahmud; University Health Centre, 104-65 Chancellers Cr, Winnipeg MB R3T 2N2; Dhaka (Bangladesh)'76; Langs: Bengali; (204)474-8411; Fax. (204)474-7573.

HASAN, Sadiq; Ontario Shores Ctr Mental HS, 700 Gordon St, Whitby ON L1N 5S9; Karachi (Pakistan)'80; MB; BSc; DPM; FRCPC; Psy (Adult Psychiatry). Staff, Ontario Shores Centre for Mental Health Sciences; Langs: Urdu; Punjabi; Hindi; (905)668-5881; Fax. (905)430-4032.

HASAN, Shabih U; HSC-Faculty of Med, 211-3330 Hospital Dr NW, Calgary AB T2N 4N1; Karachi (Pakistan)'76; MB BS; DCH; FRCPC; Peds (Neonatal). Ac Staff Neonatol/Prof Dept of Ped, Alberta Health Services; Langs: Urdu; (403)220-3741; Fax. (403)270-8928; hasans@ucalgary.ca.

HASAN, Shaukat; Lakeridge Hlth Corp-Oshawa, 2F-1 Hospital Crt, Oshawa ON L1G 2B9; Jiwaji (India)'82; CCFP; Staff, Lakeridge Health - Oshawa Site; Langs: Hindi; Urdu; Gujarati; (905)576-8711 x4579; Fax. (905)721-7763.

HASANEE, Khalid; 826 Main St E, Hamilton ON L8M 1L6; McM'00; FRCSC; Ophth. (905)549-3002; Fax. (905)548-0770.

HASANNI, Sameer A H; Victoria Hospital, PO Box 3000 Stn Main 1200 24th St W, Prince Albert SK S6V 5T4; Aziz (Saudi Arabia)'01; FRCPC; Anes. Staff, Victoria Hospital; (306)765-6200; Fax. (306)765-6224.

HASDAN, Galit; St Boniface Gen Hosp, E4003-409 Tache Ave, Winnipeg MB R2H 2A6; Kalinin (Israel)'89; CCFP; Staff, St Boniface General Hospital; (204)233-8563

HASEEB, Sabiha; Riverview Helath Centre, 1 Morley Ave, Winnipeg MB R3L 2P4; Osmania (India)'78; Staff, Riverview Health Centre.

HASEGAWA, Brian J; The Hasegawa Clinic, 156 Waterloo St S, Stratford ON N5A 4B4; McG'87; FACS; FRCSC; PlasSurg. Ac Staff, Stratford General Hospital - Huron Perth Healthcare Alliance; (519)271-6711; Fax. (519)271-8533.

HASEGAWA, Naomi A; 240-315 boul Brunswick, Pointe-Claire QC H9R 5M7; McG'91; FRCSC; Ophth (Comprehensive Ophthalmology). Ac Member Ophth, Lakeshore General Hospital - Pointe Claire; Assoc Member Ophth, Sir Mortimer B Davis Jewish General; Assoc Member Ophth, McGill University Health Centre - Royal Victoria Hospital; Langs: English; French; (514)694-2010; Fax. (514)694-0772.

HASEGAWA, Wanda; Queen Elizabeth II HSC, 1276 South Park St, Halifax NS B3H 2Y9; Qns'94; FRCPC; IntMed; Hem. Staff, Queen Elizabeth II Health Sciences Centre - Victoria General Site; (902)473-7006; wanda.hasegawa@cdha.ns.health.ca.

HASEL, Raymond; Lakeshore Gen Hosp, 160 av Stillview, Pointe-Claire QC H9R 2Y2; McG'89; CSPQ; FRCPC; Anes. Langs: English; French; (514)630-2225 x2699; Fax. (514)630-3097.

HASELL, John S; 301-410 7 St S, Lethbridge AB T1J 2G6; Sask'86; FRCSC; PlasSurg (Cosmetic Surgery). Assoc Staff, Chinook Regional Hospital; Consultant, Covenant Health - St Michael's Health Centre; (403)328-1300; Fax. (403)327-7471.

HASEMZADEH-BALOUCHI, Maliheh; York Health Centre, 302-1650 Elgin Mills E, Richmond Hill ON L4S 0B2; (Kuwait)'90; CCFP; Langs: Arabic; Farsi; (289)809-3131; Fax. (289)809-3132.

HASEN, Gregory A; 204-2425 Tecumseh Rd E, Windsor ON N8W 1E6; Wes'80; FSOGC; FACOG; MD; BSc(Hon); AddicMed; FRCSC; ObstGyn (Infertility). Staff, Windsor Regional Hospital - Metropolitan Site; Pres., Academy of ObstGyn., Windsor; Acad Dir ObstGyn, University of Western Ontario; (519)254-6461; Fax. (519)254-1349; ghasen@sympatico.ca.

HASEY, Gary M; St Joseph's Mountain H Serv, PO Box 585 Stn Lcd 1 100 West 5th St, Hamilton ON L8N 3K7; Alb'77; MSc; FRCPC; Psy (Affective Disorders). Clin Dir Mood Disorders Prog, St Joseph's Healthcare Hamilton - West 5th Campus; Asst Prof, McMaster University; (905)388-2511 x5444; Fax. (905)575-6054.

HASHAM, Aliya; Civic Family Med Centre, 210 Melrose Ave, Ottawa ON K1Y 4K7; Chicago (USA)'10; CCFP; (613)761-4334

HASHAM, Amin M; Elgin Med Centre, 101-2255 Elgin Ave, Port Coquitlam BC V3C 2B4; UBC'88; Staff, Royal Columbian Hospital; Clin Instructor, University of British Columbia; (604)942-7292; Fax. (604)942-9698; elginmedical@telus.net.

HASHAM, Parviz M; Conestoga Med Centre, 26-380 Bovaird Dr E, Brampton ON L6Z 2S8; Makerere (Uganda)'72; MB BS; Langs: Kacchi; Gujarati; (905)791-2230; Fax. (905)840-3912.

HASHEM, Fathi; Pine Falls Hlth Complex, PO Box 2000, Pine Falls MB R0E 1M0; Al Fateh (Libya)'95.

HASHIM, Ezat; Plastic Surgery Clinic of Mont, 2381 boul Gouin O, Montreal QC H3M 1B5; McG'91; MSc; BSc; FACS; FRCSC; PlasSurg. Langs: French; Spanish; (514)277-6644; Fax. (514)277-2774; info@ccpmtl.com.

HASHIM, Shahzad; The Credit Valley Hosp, 2200 Eglinton Ave W, Mississauga ON L5M 2N1; Aga Khan (Pakistan)'99; Staff, The Credit Valley Hospital; (905)813-2200

HASHIMOTO, Mariko M; 203-16 Green St, Nepean ON K2J 3R2; Sask'88; (613)825-7710

HASHIMOTO, Stanley A; Clinical Professor Emeritus, PO Box 38049 968 King Edward Ave W, Vancouver BC V5Z 2E0; Alb'62; FRCPC; Neur (Multiple Sclerosis). Staff Vancouver Coastal Health MS Clinic, UBC Hospital - Koerner Pavillion; Clin Prof Emeritus, University of British Columbia; (604)822-7131

HASHMAN, Kenneth; Southern Alberta Forensic Psy, 11333 85 St NW, Calgary AB T3R 1J3; Alb'87; DABPN; BMedSci; FRCPC; Psy (Administrative Psychiatry). Site Coord Dept of Psy, Peter Lougheed Centre; Med Dir Program/Chief Academic Div & Psy Div of Forensic, Alberta Health Services-Calgary Zone; Med Dir Program/Chief Academic Div & Psy Div of Forensic, University of Calgary; (403)944-6810; Fax. (403)944-6852; ken.hashman@albertahealthservices.ca.

HASHMI, Sajjad; Health Plus Med Centre, 1075 Autumnwood Dr, Winnipeg MB R2J 1C6; Man'03; CCFP; (204)594-2100; Fax. (204)594-2101.

HASIC, Aida; 200-1735 Kipling Ave, Etobicoke ON M9R 2Y8; Sarajevo (Bosnia-Herzegovina)'85; MD; CCFP; Court Staff, Humber River Regional Hospital - Church Street Site; (416)247-2196 x4162; Fax. (416)247-0402.

HASIMJA SARAQINI, Delvina; The Ottawa Hosp-Gen Campus, Box 209 501 Smyth Rd, Ottawa ON K1H 8L6; Pristina (Albania)'00; FRCPC; IntMed. Staff, The Ottawa Hospital - General Campus; Langs: Albanian; (613)737-8899; Fax. (613)739-6833.

HASINOFF, David A; Allin Clinic, 10155 120 St NW, Edmonton AB T5K 2A2; Alb'95; CCFP; Physician Long Term Care, Capital Care - Grandview; (780)482-7551; Fax. (780)701-5397; david.hasinoff@capitalhealth.ca.

HASINOFF, Erin A; 306-125 13th St E, North Vancouver BC V7L 2L3; UBC'99; CCFP; (604)988-8133

HASKINS, Catherine A; CLSC Lac Saint-Louis, 180 av Cartier, Pointe-Claire QC H9S 4S1; Qns'90; CCFP; FCFP; (514)697-4110 x1316; Fax. (514)697-4117.

HASKINS, Marlowe; PO Box 3760, Smithers BC V0J 2N0; Cal'90; CCFP; FCFP; (250)847-8761; Fax. (250)847-2814; drhaskinsoffice@telus.net.

HASLAH, Maja; West Park Healthcare Centre, 82 Buttonwood Ave, Toronto ON M6M 2J5; Zagreb (Croatia)'79; CCFP; Staff, West Park Healthcare Centre; Langs: Croatian; (416)243-3600 x4020

HASLAM, David R S; St Joseph's HC-Parkwood Hosp, 801 Commissioners Rd E, London ON N6C 5J1; McM'94; FRCPC; Psy. Staff, Parkwood Hospital - St Joseph's Health Care; (519)685-4292; Fax. (519)685-4585.

HASLETT, Michael; Sussex Health Centre, 2-20 Kennedy Dr, Sussex NB E4E 2P1; Dal'07; (506)433-2406; Fax. (506)433-2347.

HASLETT, Peter J; 173 Fern Rd W, Qualicum Beach BC V9K 1S4; (United Kingdom)'87; BCh; (250)752-6907

HASNAIN, Haider; Tecumseh Comm Hlth Care Ctr, 101-13278 Tecumseh Rd E, Tecumseh ON N8N 5E1; Wes'92; DOHS; CCFP; FCFP; Med Dir, Caesars Windsor; Prog Dir Schulich Med, University Of Windsor; Langs: Urdu; (519)979-5260; Fax. (519)979-8085.

HASNAIN, Mehrul; Waterford Hosp, 306 Waterford Bridge Rd, St. John's NL A1E 4J8; Rawalpindi (Pakistan)'89; Staff, Waterford Hospital; (709)777-3300

HASON, Yaniv; The Credit Valley Hosp, 2200 Eglinton Ave W, Mississauga ON L5M 2N1; McM'04; Staff, The Credit Valley Hospital; Langs: Hebrew; (905)813-1100

HASS, Ian; Medical Bldg, 1401-805 Broadway W, Vancouver BC V5Z 1K1; Otago (New Zealand)'69; MB ChB; FAAO; FRCSC; Ophth. Ac Staff, Richmond Hospital; Vis Staff, Vancouver General Hospital - Centennial Pavillion; Asst Prof, University of British Columbia; (604)879-4277

HASSA, Agnieszka; Royal Victoria Hosp, 201 Georgian Dr, Barrie ON L4M 6M2; Wes'06; FRCSC; PlasSurg. Staff, Royal Victoria Regional Health Centre; (705)728-9802

HASSAINE, Assia; Polyclinique Coeur de 'Ile, 529 rue Jarry E, Montreal QC H2P 1V5; McG'07; MDCM; ClinImmunol&Allergy; Peds. (514)270-1555

HASSALL, Eric; BC Women's Hosp & Health Ctre, K4 182-4500 Oak St, Vancouver BC V6H 3N1; Cape Town (South Africa)'73; MB ChB; FACG; DCH; AB(Gastroent); FRCPCH; FRCPC; Peds (Gastroesophageal Reflux Dis). Staff, BC Women's Hospital & Health Centre; Staff Member, BC Children's Hospital; Prof Pediatrics, University of British Columbia; (604)875-2332

HASSAM, Imtiaz K; Yaletown Med Clinic, 1296 Pacific Blvd, Vancouver BC V6Z 2V1; Alb'96; BSc; MSc; Dip SportMed; Staff Family & Commun Med, Providence Health Care - St Paul's Hospital; Clinical Asst Prof Family Pract, University of British Columbia; (604)633-2474; Fax. (604)633-2475.

HASSAN, Abdalla A; 209-129 Aberdeen Rd, Bridgewater NS B4V 2S7; Khartoum (Sudan)'75; MB BS; LMCC; FACS; FRCSC; GenSurg. Ac Staff Surg, South Shore Regional Hospital; Langs: Arabic; (902)543-6535; Fax. (902)543-1383.

HASSAN, Abubaker M M; St Paul's Hosp, 1702 20th St W, Saskatoon SK S7M 0Z9; Al-Arab (Libya)'91; FRCPC; IntMed; Nephrol. Staff Nephrology/Transplant Prog, St Paul's Hospital (Grey Nuns) of Saskatoon; (306)655-5930

HASSAN, Ahmed; William Osler HC-Etobicoke, 101 Humber College Blvd, Etobicoke ON M9V 1R8; Alb'00; CCFP; CCFP(E.M.); Staff, William Osler Health System - Etobicoke General Hospital; (416)747-3400

HASSAN, Ali; 001-525 Park Rd N, Brantford ON N3R 7K8; Ott'93; Ac Staff Family Med, The Brant Community Healthcare System - Brantford General Hospital Site; Assoc Prof Family Med, McMaster University; Langs: Punjabi; Urdu; (519)756-2512

HASSAN, Amal; Medicine Professional Corp, 302-3024 Hurontario St, Mississauga ON L5B 4M4; Khartoum (Sudan)'81; MB BS; CCFP; Staff, Trillium Health Centre - West Toronto; Langs: Arabic; (905)272-6776; Fax. (905)272-1566.

HASSAN, Ansar; Saint John Reg Hosp, PO Box 2100 Stn Main 400 University Ave, Saint John NB E2L 4L2; McG'98; FRCSC; CardSurg (Clinician Investigator Program). Staff, Saint John Regional Hospital; (506)648-6000

HASSAN, Ayman; Medical Center, 201-984 Oliver Rd, Thunder Bay ON P7B 7C7; Ain Shams (Egypt)'85; (807)684-6707

HASSAN, Durreshahwar; Medi-Centre des Sources, 4465 boul des Sources, Roxboro QC H8Y 3C1; Lahore (Pakistan)'80; MB BS; FRCSC; ObstGyn (P.Q.) (Infertility). Langs: Urdu; French; Arabic; (514)683-1089; Fax. (514)683-0058.

HASSAN, Fathi T B; PO Box 4010 Stn Main, Barrhead AB T7N 1A1; (Libya)'96; MB BCh; (780)674-2246; Fax. (780)674-6164.

HASSAN, Hanadi; Alliston Family Hlth Team, PO Box 280 36 Victoria St W, Alliston ON L9R 1S8; Khartoum (Sudan)'91; CCFP; Staff, Toronto Western Hospital - University Health Network.

HASSAN, Haron; Chand Med Clinic, 104-15122 72 Ave, Surrey BC V3S 2G2; University of South Pacific (Fiji)'99; MB BS; CCFP; Fam Med, Lillooet District Hospital; Langs: Hindi; Urdu; (604)593-5156

HASSAN, Paul; Halton HCS Corp-Milton, 7030 Derry Rd, Milton ON L9T 7H6; Qns'04; CCFP; CCFP(E.M.); Staff, Halton Healthcare Services Corporation - Milton District Hospital; (905)878-2383

HASSAN, Saima; Univ Hlth Network-Princess M, 3 130-610 University Ave, Toronto ON M5G 2M9; McG'02; FRCSC; GenSurg. Staff, Princess Margaret Hospital - University Health Network; (416)946-6583

HASSAN, Sameh A; 201-3300 Yonge St, Toronto ON M4N 2L6; Aleppo (Syria)'78; FRCPC; Psy (Child Psychiatry). Langs: Arabic; (416)481-2280; Fax. (416)481-2280.

HASSAN, Sameh; The Nova Scotia Hosp, 1115-300 Pleasant St, Dartmouth NS B2Y 3Z9; Cairo (Egypt)'91; MB BCh; Staff, The Nova Scotia Hospital; (902)464-6064; Fax. (902)464-3002.

HASSAN, Sarah; Polyclinique Med Concorde, 300 boul de la Concorde E, Laval QC H7G 2E6; Sher'10; CCFP; (450)667-5310

HASSAN, Shabbir; Trans Canada Mall, 1440 52 ST NE, Calgary AB T2A 4T8; (Pakistan)'89; MB BS; CCFP; (403)273-6471; Fax. (403)272-3647.

HASSAN, Tariq; Providence Care-Mental Health, PO Box 603 Stn Main 1076-752 King St W, Kingston ON K7L 4X3; Nishtar (Pakistan)'98; Staff, Providence Care - Mental Health Services; Langs: Hindi; (613)548-5567; Fax. (613)540-6113.

HASSAN, Waseem; PO Box 690, Two Hills AB T0B 4K0; (South Africa)'06; MB ChB; (780)657-3337; Fax. (780)657-3382.

HASSAN, Youssef; Clinique Medicentre, 5050 boul des Forges, Trois-Rivieres QC G8Y 1X2; Picardie (France)'76; (819)376-4444; Fax. (819)372-0260.

HASSAN, Ziauddin; Moose Jaw Union Hosp, 455 Fairford St E, Moose Jaw SK S6H 1H3; Staff, Moose Jaw Union Hospital; (306)694-0200; Fax. (306)694-0329.

HASSAN ABDELMOTLEB, Hassa A; Golf Links Community Clinic, 5-1077 Golf Links Rd, Thunder Bay ON P7B 7A3; Cairo (Egypt)'87; (807)622-3995; Fax. (807)622-3430.

HASSANAIN, Mazen; MUHC-Royal Victoria Hosp, S10 30-687 av des Pins O, Montreal QC H3A 1A1; Riyadh (Saudi Arabia)'99; FRCSC; GenSurg. Staff, McGill University Health Centre - Royal Victoria Hospital; (514)843-1600; Fax. (514)843-1503.

HASSANALIZADEH, Hamid; CSSS d'Argenteuil, 145 av de la Providence, Lachute QC J8H 4C7; Liege (Belgium)'83; Staff, Centre Hospitalier d'Argenteuil; (450)562-3761; Fax. (450)683-5850.

HASSARD, Frank A; 565 King St, Welland ON L3B 3L3; Dal'96; FRCSC; Ophth. (905)735-4600; Fax. (905)735-6031.

HASSARD, Mary K; EFW Radiology, 401 9 Ave SW, Calgary AB T2P 4Z4; Tor'99; FRCPC; DiagRad. (403)284-0228

HASSARD, Philip V; 307-595 Montreal Rd, Ottawa ON K1K 4L2; Tor'93; FRCPC; IntMed (Crohn's Disease); Gastroent. Staff, Montfort Hospital; Assoc Prof, University of Ottawa; (613)746-5393; Fax. (613)746-4840.

HASSEIN BEY, Leila; Ctr Hosp du Centre la Mauricie, 50 119E rue, Shawinigan-Sud QC G9P 5K1; Sher'07; Staff, Centre Hospitalier du Centre la Mauricie; (819)536-7500

HASSELBACK, Paul D; Interior Health Authority, 3F-6475 Mentral Dr, Nanaimo BC V9T 2L9; Ott'81; MSc(Epidem.); FRCPC; CommunMed. Chair, BC Health Officers Council; Clinical Asst Prof, University of British Columbia; (205)755-7944; paul.hasselbackdr@interiorhealth.ca.

HASSELL, Patricia R; BC Cancer Agency-Vancouver CC, 600 10th Ave W, Vancouver BC V5Z 4E6; McG'71; DABR; FRCPC; DiagRad. Ac Staff, BC Cancer Agency Vancouver Centre; (604)877-6000 x2267

HASSEN, Riyaan; PO Box 690, Wabasca AB T0G 2K0; Witwatersrand (South Africa)'04; MB BCh; Langs: Afrikaans; (780)891-3839; Fax. (780)891-2926.

HASSON, Paul K; Queens Park Hlth, 899 Bay St, Toronto ON M5S 3K6; Dal'91; (416)927-8462; Fax. (416)927-9431.

HASSON, Victor; The Doctor's Office, 600-1001 Broadway W, Vancouver BC V6H 4B1; Cape Town (South Africa)'84; MB ChB; (604)739-4247

HASSOUN, Joelle; CHUS Hotel-Dieu, 585 rue Bowen S, Sherbrooke QC J1G 2E8; Nice (France)'82; Psy (P.Q.) (Biomedical Ethics). Staff, Centre Hospitalier Universitaire de Sherbrooke-Hôpital Hôtel-Dieu; Langs: English; (819)346-1110; Fax. (819)829-6263.

HASSOUNA, Magdy; Univ Hlth Network-Toronto Western Hosp, MP8 306-399 Bathurst St, Toronto ON M5T 2S8; Alexandria (Egypt)'75; PhD; AB; FACS; FRCSC; Urol (Incontinence). Staff, Toronto Western Hospital - University Health Network; Urology, Toronto Rehabilitation Institute - Lyndhurst Centre; Staff, Lyndhurst Hospital; Assoc Prof, University of Toronto; Langs: Arabic; French; (416)603-5018; mhassouna@yahoo.com.

HASSWANI, Samer; Ctre de Sante Psychologique, 2101 boul Edouard-Montpetit, Montreal QC H3T 1J3; Mon'97; CCFP; (514)343-6452; Fax. (514)343-7236.

HASTIE, Ian G; Huntsville District Mem Hosp, 100 Frank Miller Dr, Huntsville ON P1H 1H7; Tor'69; FRCPC; EmergMed. Staff, Huntsville District Memorial Hospital - Muskoka Algonquin Healthcare; (705)789-2311

HASTINGS, Deborah M; Hamilton HS-Henderson Site, 711 Concession St, Hamilton ON L8V 1C3; Tor'79; FRCPC; IntMed; Cardiol. Ac Staff, Hamilton Health Sciences Centre-Juravinski Site; Asst Prof Med, McMaster University; (905)547-3708; Fax. (905)547-9878.

HASTINGS, Donald; Chatham-Kent Family Health Team, 20 Emma St, Chatham ON N7L 5K5; Ott'80; Staff, Chatham-Kent Health Alliance; (519)354-2172; dhastings@ckha.on.ca.

HASTINGS, Donna; Edmonton Gen Cont Care Centre, 11111 Jasper Ave NW, Edmonton AB T5K 0L4; Alb'95; DipCE; CCFP; Site Leader, Covenant Health - Edmonton General Continuing Care Centre; Att Physician, Youville Home; Att Physician, University of Alberta; (866)334-1211; Fax. (780)634-2699; donna.hastings@covenanthealth.ca.

HASTINGS, Peter C; 3461 Cook St, Victoria BC V8X 1B3; Dal'87; (250)386-6161

HASTINGS, Thomas J E K; Halton HSC Corp-Oakville, 327 Reynolds St, Oakville ON L6J 3L7; McM'98; FRCPC; Psy. Med Staff, Halton Healthcare Services Corporation - Oakville Site; (905)845-2571 x5631; Fax. (905)815-5096.

HASULO, Lori A; U of Guelph Student Hlth Servi, 1-176 Wyndham St N, Guelph ON N1H 8N9; Tor'95; BSc; CCFP; Assoc Staff Family Pract, Guelph General Hospital; (519)821-6638; Fax. (519)821-5834; lhasulo@guelphchc.ca.

HASWELL, W Timothy F; 750 Brunswick St, Fredericton NB E3B 1H9; Dal'87; FRCSC; PlasSurg. Ac Staff, Dr Everett Chalmers Regional Hospital; (506)455-7311; Fax. (506)443-4351; wtfhaswell@nb.aibn.com.

HATALA, Rosemarie A; St Paul's Hosp, 5907-1081 Burrard St, Vancouver BC V6Z 1Y6; McM'90; FRCPC; IntMed. Staff, Providence Health Care - St Paul's Hospital; (604)682-2344

HATALEY, Joy M; Frontenac Med Associates, 201-791 Princess St, Kingston ON K7L 1E9; Man'93; BSc; CCFP; FCFP; Staff Family Med & Obst, Kingston General Hospital; Staff Emerg Phys, Lennox & Addington County General Hospital; (613)542-7002 x239; hataley@frontenacmedical.ca.

HATAMI, Afshin; Hôpital Ste-Justine, 3175 ch Cote-Sainte-Catherine, Montreal QC H3T 1C5; Mon'95; FRCPC; Derm. Staff, Hôpital Ste-Justine; (514)345-4931; Fax. (514)345-2134.

HATAMI, Shahin; All In One Med Clinic, 100-10083 Keele St, Maple ON L6A 3Y8; Utesa (Dominican Republic)'98; CCFP; Langs: Farsi; (905)832-4644; Fax. (905)832-7717.

HATASHITA, Eric; 1106-123 Edward St, Toronto ON M5G 1E2; Tor'79; CCFP; FCFP; (416)340-0700; Fax. (416)340-0400.

HATCHER, David S; Grey Bruce HS-Owen Sound, PO Box 1800 Stn Main 1800 8th St E, Owen Sound ON N4K 6M9; Wes'93; FRCPC; Anes. Staff, Grey Bruce Health Services - Owen Sound; (519)376-2121

HATCHER, Lydia B; Family Wellness Place, 48 Commonwealth Ave, Mount Pearl NL A1N 5B6; Mem'82; CCFP; FCFP; Clin Assoc Prof, Memorial University Of Newfoundland; (709)364-6650; Fax. (709)364-6040.

HATCHER, Michael C E; 142 Queenston St, St. Catharines ON L2R 2Z7; Mem'93; BSc; EmergMed. Staff, St Joseph's Healthcare - Charlton Campus; (905)378-4647

HATCHER, Ronagh J; Grace Maternal Child Clinic, 130-1402 8 Ave NW, Calgary AB T2N 1B9; Cal'02; CCFP; Staff, Foothills Medical Centre; (403)289-9051

HATCHER, Sharon N; CSSS de Chicoutimi, 305 rue Saint-Vallier, Chicoutimi QC G7H 5H6; Ott'84; CCFP; FCFP; Ac Staff, Complexe hospitalier de la Sagamie; Assoc Prof Full-Time, Universite de Sherbrooke; Langs: English; French; (418)541-1088; Fax. (418)541-1129; sharon.hatcher@usherbrooke.ca.

HATCHER, Simon; Royal Ottawa Hlth Care Group, 5458-1145 Carling Ave, Ottawa ON K1Z 7K4; London (England)'85; FRCPC; Psy. Staff, Royal Ottawa Mental Health Centre - Royal Ottawa Health Care Group.

HATCHETTE, Todd F; DJ Mackenzie Bldg, 315-5788 University Ave, Halifax NS B3H 1V8; Mem'95; FRCPC; IntMed; InfectDis; MedMicrobiol. (902)473-6885; Fax. (902)473-7971.

HATCHWELL, Anthony R; Nanaimo Reg Gen Hosp, 1200 Dufferin Cres, Nanaimo BC V9S 2B7; (Zimbabwe)'83; MB ChB; Staff, Nanaimo Regional General Hospital; (250)755-7691

HATEGAN, Ana; St Joseph's Mountain H Service, PO Box 585 Lcd 1 E116A-100 West 5th St, Hamilton ON L8N 3K7; Timisoara (Romania)'95; FRCPC; Psy. Psychiatrist, Regional Mental Health Care-St Joseph's Health Care; Staff, St Joseph's Healthcare Hamilton - West 5th Campus; (905)388-2511

HATFIELD, M Christine; North Okanagan Women's Health, 303-3210 25 Ave, Vernon BC V1T 1P1; Wes'94; ABAAM; FRCSC; ObstGyn (Hormone Replacement). (250)542-4490; Fax. (250)558-9986.

HATFIELD, Peter W; Canadian Forces Hlth Serv Ctr, PO Box 99000 Stn Forces, Halifax NS B3K 5X5; Alb'88; CCFP; FCFP; Fam Med, Canadian Forces Health Services Centre (Atlantic); (902)721-7881

HATFIELD, Richard H; 2-140 Athabascan Ave, Sherwood Park AB T8A 4E3; Witwatersrand (South Africa)'94; MB ChB; CCFP; (780)467-3244; Fax. (780)464-9044.

HATHEWAY, Ronald J; South Shore Med Arts, 302-42 Glen Allan Dr, Bridgewater NS B4V 3N2; Dal'75; FRCPC; IntMed (Echocardiography); Cardiol. Ac Staff, South Shore Regional Hospital; (902)543-1866; Fax. (902)543-6028.

HATHORN, John F; 8675 Granville St, Vancouver BC V6P 5A3; Edinburgh (Scotland)'68; MB ChB; (604)266-9408; Fax. (604)263-1093; jfh@shaw.ca.

HATHOUT, Deana; Trillium Hlth Ctr-Mississauga, 100 Queensway W, Mississauga ON L5B 1B8; Tor'08; CCFP; CCFP(E. M.); Staff, Trillium Health Centre - Mississauga; (905)848-7100

HATLAPA, Karolina; Etobicoke Med Centre, 400 The East Mall, Etobicoke ON M9B 3Z9; (Other Foreign)'05.

HATLELID, Keith; 2480 Heather St, Vancouver BC V5Z 3H9; Cal'80; Ac Staff, BC Women's Hospital & Health Centre; Vis Staff, Vancouver General Hospital - Centennial Pavillion; Ac Staff, Providence Health Care - St Paul's Hospital; Clin Assoc Prof Family Pract, University of British Columbia; (604)879-3900; Fax. (604)879-3969.

HATLELID, Leonard W; B-22195 Dewdney Trunk Rd, Maple Ridge BC V2X 3H7; Cal'86; Ac Staff, Ridge Meadows Hospital & Health Care Centre; (604)463-4102

HATTERSLEY, Beverly A; St Peter's Hosp, 88 Maplewood Ave, Hamilton ON L8M 1W9; McM'91; BSc; CCFP; FCFP; Fam Med, Hamilton Health Sciences Centre - St Peter's Hospital; (905)777-3837; Fax. (905)549-6829.

HATTINGH, Evert; Life Medical Clinic, PO Box 1406 Stn Main 4740 50 Ave, Whitecourt AB T7S 1P3; Stellenbosch (South Africa)'01; Langs: Afrikaans; (780)706-7080; Fax. (780)706-7064.

HATTINGH, H Suzanne; Saskatoon City Hosp, 701 Queen St, Saskatoon SK S7K 0M7; Orange Free State (South Africa)'81; MB ChB; Staff, Saskatoon City Hospital; Langs: Afrikaans; (306)655-7434

HATTINGH, Jacolette; 102-9814 97 St, Grande Prairie AB T8V 8H5; (South Africa)'98; MB ChB; (780)539-4770; Fax. (780)532-6997.

HATTINGH, Jozua F; 9820 101 Ave, Fort St. John BC V1J 2B2; Orange Free State (South Africa)'79; MB ChB; (250)787-1123; Fax. (250)787-1221.

HATZAKORZIAN, Roupen; MUHC-Royal Victoria Hosp, P9 16-687 av des Pins O, Montreal QC H3A 1A1; Sher'97; CSPQ; FRCPC; Anes. Staff, McGill University Health Centre - Royal Victoria Hospital; (514)842-1231

HATZIDIAKOS, Peter; Southlake Reg Hlth Ctr, 596 Davis Dr, Newmarket ON L3Y 2P9; Tor'95; FRCPC; Anes. Staff, Rouge Valley Health System - Centenary Health Centre Site; (905)895-4521

HAU, Cheryl S; Crestwood Med Dental, 208-6051 Gilbert Rd, Richmond BC V7C 3V3; UBC'06; CCFP; (604)278-0090

HAU, Monica; Peel Public Health, 7120 Hurontario St, Mississauga ON L5M 2C1; McM'06; FRCPC; Public Health & Preventive Med;CCFP.

HAUBRICH, Jay M; Ermineskin Med Clinic, 301-2377 111 St NW, Edmonton AB T6J 5E5; Alb'03; CCFP; (780)436-8731

HAUCH, Susan G; Family Med Centre, 500-400 Tache Ave, Winnipeg MB R2H 3E1; Man'77; CCFP; Ac Staff, St Boniface General Hospital; Assoc Prof, University of Manitoba; (204)237-2863; Fax. (204)231-2648; shauch@sbgh.mb.ca.

HAUCK, Brian A; Foothills Prof Bldg, 210-1620 29 St NW, Calgary AB T2N 4L7; Alb'82; FRCSC; ObstGyn. Staff, Foothills Medical Centre; (403)289-1940; Fax. (403)210-3331.

HAUG, Delmer O; Mediclinic, 101-3333 8th St E, Saskatoon SK S7H 4K1; Sask'69; CCFP; Staff, Royal University Hospital; (306)955-1530

HAUGEN, Richard D; University of Alberta Hosp, 3B232WCM-8440 112 St NW, Edmonton AB T6G 2B7; Alb'89; FRCPC; Anes. Staff, University of Alberta Hospital; (780)407-8887; Fax. (780)407-3200.

HAUGHTON, David A; Children's & Women's HC of BC, B321-4480 Oak St, Vancouver BC V6H 3V4; Cornell(NY) (USA)'84; FRCPC; Peds. Staff, BC Children's Hospital; (604)875-2045

HAUGRUD, Mark J; Bow River Prof Centre, 218-4411 16 Ave NW, Calgary AB T3B 0M3; Alb'78; FRCSC; PlasSurg. (403)234-8008; Fax. (403)264-6214.

HAUKIOJA, Ari H O; Cobourg Clinic, PO Box 86 Stn Main 44 University Ave, Cobourg ON K9A 4K4; Tor'74; Ac Staff, Northumberland Hills Hospital; (905)372-3323; Fax. (905)372-3692.

HAUMAN, Helena; Frederiction Family Med Clinic, 302-1015 Regent St, Fredericton NB E3B 6H5; Orange Free State (South Africa)'93; MB ChB; CCFP; FCFP; (506)458-9445; Fax. (506)458-8118.

HAUNTS, Kirk; Coborag Hlth Centre, 203-316 King St E, Cobourg ON K9A 5R8; Leicester (United Kingdom)'07; CCFP; Physician, Cobourg Health Centre; (905)373-1282; Fax. (905)373-9335.

HAUPTMAN, Robert S; Salvus Family Med Clinic, 62-143 Liberton Dr, St. Albert AB T8N 6A7; Alb'87; Chief Dep Family Med, Sturgeon Community Hospital; Med Dir Med Managment Program, Healthpointe Pain Clinic; Clin Assoc Prof, University of Alberta; (780)460-4562; Fax. (780)460-4550.

HAUSEN, Doris M; 5-1310 Don Mills Rd, North York ON M3B 2W6; Tor'80; FRCPC; DiagRad; NuclearMed. (416)444-6999; Fax. (416)444-0896.

HAUSER, Jo; 28 Osborne Street, Ottawa ON K2H 8P4; Ott'66; BSc; MD; CCFP; Ac Staff (All Sites), The Ottawa Hospital - Riverside Campus; Ac Staff, St Francis Memorial Hospital; Staff, Queensway Carleton Hospital; Langs: French; (613)730-2646

HAUSER, Ronda J; Tillicum Med Clinic, 14-3170 Tillicum Rd, Victoria BC V9A 7C5; McG'83; (250)381-8112

HAUSMANIS, Larisa I; Sherbourne Hlth Centre, 333 Sherbourne St, Toronto ON M5A 2S5; Tor'08; CCFP; Langs: Latvian; Spanish; (416)324-4180 x5275; Fax. (416)324-4181.

HAUSSER, Christian; Polyclinique St-Martin, 301-1435 boul Saint-Martin O, Laval QC H7S 2C6; Mon'76; Peds. ac Staff, Hôpital Ste-Justine; ac Staff, Hopital de la Cite de la santé; (450)629-3405

HAUSSER, Jean-Louis; Ctr Hosp Fleury, 2180 rue Fleury E, Montreal QC H2B 1K3; Mon'79; Staff, Centre Hospitalier Fleury; Langs: Bilingual(English/French); (514)381-9311; Fax. (514)858-2435.

HAUSSMANN, Jessica; 351-4411 16 Ave NW, Calgary AB T3B 0M3; UBC'02; FRCPC; IntMed; Gastroent. Clin Teach Staff Gastroent, University of Calgary; Langs: Bilingual(English/French); (403)984-4240; Fax. (403)984-4339.

HAUTALA, Bronwyn R; Maternity Care Westside, 853 Anders Rd, West Kelowna BC V1Z 1K2; Adelaide (Australia)'86; MB BS; (778)755-5720

HAVELOCK, Jon C; Pacific Ctre for Reproductive, 500-4601 Canada Way, Burnaby BC V5G 4X7; Man'98; BSc; FACOG; FRCSC; ObstGyn (Infertility). Staff, Vancouver General Hospital - Centennial Pavillion; (604)422-7276; jhavelock@pacificfertility.ca.

HAVENS, John R; 434 Tatchell Rd, Quesnel BC V2J 6N7; Wes'62; CCFP; FCFP; (250)983-6828

HAVER, William J; Lakeside Med Clinic, 3919 8th St E, Saskatoon SK S7H 5M7; Sask'78; BSc; Staff Chief Family Med, Saskatoon City Hospital; (306)374-6884; Fax. (306)374-2552.

HAVERS, Melanie; Hamilton HS-McMaster Site, 2U8-1200 Main St W, Hamilton ON L8N 3Z5; McM'05; FRCPC; Anes. Staff, Hamilton Health Sciences Centre - McMaster Children's Hospital; Staff, Hamilton Health Sciences Centre - Hamilton General Hospital; (905)521-2100

HAVRANKOVA, Jana B; Clinique Familiale St-Lambert, 209 rue de Woodstock, Saint-Lambert QC J4P 1W7; Mon'72; Endocrin (P.Q.); IntMed (Diabetology). Langs: English; (450)466-8583; Fax. (450)466-4072; janahavrankova@videotron.ca.

HAW, Charles S; Gordon & Leslie Diamond HCC, 8121-2775 Laurel St, Vancouver BC V5Z 1M9; UBC'92; MEd; FRCSC; Neursurg. Staff, Vancouver General Hospital - Centennial Pavillion; Staff, Gordon & Leslie Diamond Health Care Centre; (604)875-4391

HAW, Peter M; Markham Family Health Team, 1-122 Cornell Park Ave, Markham ON L6B 1B6; Tor'82; CCFP; Fax. (905)209-1501; phaw@msh.on.ca.

HAW FOR CHIN, Oliver R; Rockyview Gen Hosp, 7007 14 St SW, Calgary AB T2V 1P9; Laval'02; FRCPC; IntMed; Nephrol. Staff, Rockyview General Hospital; Langs: Bilingual(English/French); (403)943-3000; Fax. (403)210-8723.

HAWA, Raed J; Univ Hlth Network-Toronto Western Hosp, 7F-399 Bathurst St, Toronto ON M5T 2S8; Alb'94; DABSM(SleepMed.); DABPN; FRCPC; Psy (Consultation-Liaison). Psychiatrist, Toronto Western Hospital - University Health Network; Teacher Psy, University of Toronto; (416)603-5847; Fax. (416)603-5292; raed.hawa@uhn.ca.

HAWALESHKA, Adrian; Health Sciences Centre, GH 611-820 Sherbrook St, Winnipeg MB R3A 1R9; Man'94; FRCPC; Anes. Staff, Health Sciences Centre; (204)787-3796

HAWASH-MOSTAFA, Fatma E; 1234 Richmond St, London ON N6A 3M3; Cairo (Egypt)'72; AddicMed; Langs: Arabic; (519)439-0318; Fax. (519)439-5216; fhawash@hotmail.com.

HAWASS, Ammar N; William Osler HC-Brampton, 2100 Bovaird Dr E, Brampton ON L6R 3J7; Punjab (India)'96; MB BS; Staff, William Osler Health System - Brampton Civic Hospital; (905)494-2120

HAWASS, Oubada; William Osler HC-Etobicoke, 101 Humber College Blvd, Etobicoke ON M9V 1R8; Punjab (Pakistan)'97; CCFP; Staff, William Osler Health System - Etobicoke General Hospital; (416)494-2120

HAWBOLDT, Geoffrey S; Chronic Pain Centre, 160-2210 2 St SW, Calgary AB T2S 3C3; Dal'94; Anes (Pain Management). Att Staff Anes., Foothills Medical Centre; Asst Prof Anes, University of Calgary; (403)943-9900; Fax. (403)209-2954.

HAWE, Richard; St Boniface Genl Hosp, M4-409 Tache Ave, Winnipeg MB R2H 2A6; UBC'05; FRCPC; Psy. Staff, St Boniface General Hospital; (204)233-8563

HAWEGI, Tarek H; Shawnessy Village Shopping Ctr, 70 Shawville Blvd SE, Calgary AB T2Y 2Z3; (Libya)'97; CCFP; (403)984-3193

HAWES, Violet C; Dr Violet Hawes Inc, PO Box 93, Md Musquodbt NS B0N 1X0; Dal'83; (902)384-2834; Fax. (902)384-2719.

HAWKE, W Michael; Medical & Dental Bldg, LF 10-1849 Yonge St, Toronto ON M4S 1Y2; Tor'65; DAB; BSc(Med.); Otol (Sinusitis). Ac Staff, St Joseph's Health Centre; Ac Staff, Toronto General Hospital - UHN; Prof, University of Toronto; (416)487-1525; m.hawke@utoronto.ca.

HAWKEN, Katherine A S; 103-460 Wellington St, St Thomas ON N5R 6H9; Tor'75; ABIM; FRCPC; IntMed (Gastroenterology). Consultant IntMed, St Thomas Elgin General Hospital; (519)631-1380; Fax. (519)631-6143.

HAWKER, Gillian; Women's College Hosp, 815-76 Grenville St, Toronto ON M5S 1B2; Tor'84; FRCPC; IntMed (Osteoarthritis & Osteoporosis); Rheum. Chief Med, Women's College Hospital; Prof, University of Toronto; (416)323-7722; Fax. (416)323-7513; g.hawker@utoronto.ca.

HAWKER, Linda J; 18-1710 Ellis St, Kelowna BC V1Y 2B5; Alb'77; CCFP; (250)763-5427; Fax. (250)763-2922; lhawker@shaw.ca.

HAWKES, Christopher A; The Moncton Hosp, 135 MacBeath Ave, Moncton NB E1C 6Z8; Mem'91; FRCPC; Anes. Ac Staff Anes, The Moncton Hospital; (506)857-5520; chawk@nb.sympatico.ca.

HAWKES, Robert P; Grey Bruce HS-Owen Sound, PO Box 1800 Stn Main 1800 8th St E, Owen Sound ON N4K 6M9; Tor'02; FRCPC; DiagRad. Staff, Grey Bruce Health Services - Owen Sound; (519)376-2121; Fax. (519)372-3954.

HAWKES, Toni P; South Calgary Urgent Care Clin, 31 Sunpark Plaza SE, Calgary AB T2X 3W5; Ott'75; BA; CCFP; Staff, South Calgary Urgent Care Centre; Langs: English; French; (403)943-9476

HAWKESWOOD, Jonathan P; Seafield Med Bldg, 3-1179 Seafield Cres, Nanaimo BC V9S 4S1; UBC'06; FRCPC; PhysMed&Rehab. Staff, G F Strong Rehabilitation Centre; (250)741-0755

HAWKESWOOD, Michael L; Dr Michael Hawkeswood & Assoc, 3893 Dougall Ave, Windsor ON N9G 1X3; McM'78; (519)258-1154; Fax. (519)258-2056.

HAWKINS, Ann E; IWK Health Centre, PO Box 9700 Rpo CSC 5850-5980 University Ave, Halifax NS B3K 6R8; Mem'77; ABPeds; FAAP; FRCPC; Peds (Developmental/Behavioural Pediatrics). Staff, IWK Health Centre; Assoc Prof Peds, Dalhousie University; (902)470-8951; Fax. (902)470-7284; ahawkins@dal.ca.

HAWKINS, Cynthia E; The Hosp for Sick Children, 555 University Ave, Toronto ON M5G 1X8; Wes'97; FRCPC; NeurPath. Staff, The Hospital For Sick Children; (416)813-5938; Fax. (416)813-5974; cynthia.hawkins@sickkids.ca.

HAWKINS, David F; Towne Centre Med, 19-2475 Dobbin Rd, Westbank BC V4T 2E9; Tor'82; (250)768-8315

HAWKINS, Lindsay; 547 Michigan St, Victoria BC V8V 1S5; Tor'08; CCFP; Staff, North York General Hospital; (250)388-6811

HAWKINS, Mark G; Canmore Associate Med Clinic, 124-1151 Sidney St, Canmore AB T1W 3G1; Cal'98; CCFP; (403)678-5585; Fax. (403)678-6262.

HAWKINS, Paul; Sunnybrook Hlth Sciences Ctre, C753-2075 Bayview Ave, Toronto ON M4N 3M5; Man'81; MCFP(EM); DAB; FACEP; Staff, Sunnybrook Health Sciences Centre; Teach Staff, University of Toronto; (416)480-4037; Fax. (416)480-4704.

HAWKINS, Ralph G; HSC-Faculty Of Med, 1444-3330 Hospital Dr NW, Calgary AB T2N 4N1; Sask'81; DABIM; FRCPC; IntMed; Nephrol. Staff Int Med, Foothills Medical Centre; (403)220-8382; Fax. (403)283-6151.

HAWKINS, Robert H; Regent Med Bldg, 550-2184 Broadway W, Vancouver BC V6K 2E1; Qns'69; FRCSC; OrthSurg (Shoulder). Ac Staff, UBC Hospital - Koerner Pavillion; Clin Prof OrthSurg, University of British Columbia; (604)739-2029; Fax. (888)467-4045.

HAWKINS, T Lee-Ann; HSC-Faculty Of Med, 1432-3330 Hospital Dr NW, Calgary AB T2N 4N1; Cal'03; FRCPC; IntMed.

HAWKWOOD, Joseph N H; 102 Allen Cove, Hinton AB T7V 2A6; Alb'07; CCFP; (780)865-3338; Fax. (780)865-7024.

HAWLEY, Kristopher S; Hamilton HS-McMaster Site, PO Box 2000 Stn Lcd 1 1200 Main St W, Hamilton ON L8N 3Z5; Qns'98; FRCPC; EmergMed. Staff, Hamilton Health Sciences Centre - McMaster Children's Hospital; (905)521-2100

HAWLEY, Philippa H; BC Cancer Agency-Vancouver CC, 600 10th Ave W, Vancouver BC V5Z 4E6; Southampton (England)'85; FRCPC; IntMed (Palliative Medicine). Staff Palliative Care, BC Cancer Agency Vancouver Island Centre; Staff, BC Cancer Agency Vancouver Centre; Asst Prof, University of British Columbia; (604)877-6000 x2445; Fax. (604)877-0585.

HAWLING, Christopher A; Scarborough Hosp-General Div, 3050 Lawrence Ave E, Toronto ON M1P 2V5; Tor'87; FRCPC; Anes. Staff, The Scarborough Hospital - General Campus; Langs: Polish; (416)431-8133

HAWORTH, Angela C; Joseph Brant Mem Hosp, 1230 North Shore Blvd E, Burlington ON L7S 1W7; Ott'80; FRCPC; GenPath. Staff, Joseph Brant Memorial Hospital; (905)632-3730

HAWRYLUCK, Laura A; 11F 1176-585 University Ave, Toronto ON M5G 2N2; Wes'92; FRCPC; IntMed (Critical Care Medicine). (416)340-4605

HAWRYLYSHYN, Peter A; Ontario Hydro, 3F-700 University Ave, Toronto ON M5G 1Z5; Tor'79; PhD; MSc; FACOG; FRCSC; ObstGyn (Infertility). Staff, Mount Sinai Hospital; Teach Staff ObstGyn, University of Toronto; Langs: German; (416)586-4534; Fax. (416)586-4512; phawrylyshyn@mtsinai.on.ca.

HAWTHORNE, Diane W; Real Canadian Super Store, UL-1205 Oxford St W, London ON N6H 1V8; Wes'82; CCFP; FCFP; Ac Staff, St Joseph's Hospital - St Joseph's Health Care; Aj Prof, University of Western Ontario; (519)672-8460; Fax. (519)672-4947.

HAXUAN, Sandra; CLSC Saint-Michel, 3355 rue Jarry E, Montreal QC H1Z 2E5; Mon'01; CCFP; (514)374-8223

HAY, Elizabeth J; 201-1650 Terminal Ave N, Nanaimo BC V9S 0A3; UBC'81; BSc; FAAO; FRCSC; Ophth (Retina). Staff, Nanaimo Regional General Hospital; (250)753-3230; Fax. (250)753-1881.

HAY, Gregory J; 6217-2850 Shaughnessy St, Port Coquitlam BC V3C 6K5; Qns'75; DAB; FRCSC; Ophth. Staff, Royal Columbian Hospital; Consultant, Vancouver General Hospital - Centennial Pavillion; University of British Columbia; (604)552-0991; Fax. (604)552-0992; gjhay62@shaw.ca.

HAY, J Keith; 105 Shipley St PO Box 1030, Clinton ON N0M 1L0; McG'83; CCFP; FCFP; Ac Staff/Member, Clinton Public Hospital - Huron Perth Healthcare Alliance; Aj Prof, University of Western Ontario; (519)482-5512; Fax. (519)482-7648; jkhay@tcc.on.ca.

HAY, John H; BC Cancer Agency-Vancouver CC, 4515-600 10th Ave W, Vancouver BC V5Z 4E6; Cambridge (England)'74; FRCR; FRCPC; RadOncol (Oncology). Staff, BC Cancer Agency Vancouver Centre; Clin Prof Surg, University of British Columbia; (604)877-6000 x2660; Fax. (604)708-2000.

HAY, Kevin M; KM Hay Prof Corp, 901 22 St, Wainwright AB T9W 1T8; Dublin (Ireland)'80; MRC; DCH; CCFP; FCFP; Staff, Wainwright Health Centre; (780)842-4920; Fax. (780)842-4983; khay@telusplanet.net.

HAY, Marie D; Trinity Med Centre, 101-1668 Tamarack St, Prince George BC V2L 2T3; Dublin (Ireland)'76; MB ChB; MRC(UK); DCH; DRCOG; BAO; FRCPC; Peds (Child Abuse). Consultant Peds, University Hospital of Northern British Columbia; Clinical Asst Prof Med, University of British Columbia; (250)564-8999; Fax. (250)564-8966.

HAY, Marshall A; Create Fertility Centre, PO Box 11 322-790 Bay St, Toronto ON M5G 1N8; Tor'01; FRCSC; Otol. (416)598-5665; Fax. (416)591-1162.

HAY, Peter J; 875 4th Ave A W, Owen Sound ON N4K 6L5; Dublin (Ireland)'76; CCFP; (519)371-6400

HAY, Richard C; East Van Med Bldg, M01-1750 10th Ave E, Vancouver BC V5N 5K4; UBC'74; Court Staff, BC Women's Hospital & Health Centre; Vis Staff, Vancouver General Hospital - Centennial Pavillion; (604)874-0424; Fax. (604)879-5411.

HAY, W John; Hawkesbury Dist Gen Hosp, 2F-1111 Ghislain St, Hawkesbury ON K6A 3G5; Qns'78; FRCPC; IntMed. Staff, Hawkesbury & District General Hospital; (613)632-1111; Fax. (613)632-3720.

HAY, William L; 350-425 Carrall St, Vancouver BC V6B 6E3; Man'79; CSAM; FRCPC; Psy (Addiction Medicine). (604)708-1117; Fax. (604)708-1145.

HAYAKAWA, Thomas E J; Health Sciences Centre, GF547-820 Sherbrook St, Winnipeg MB R3A 1R9; Man'95; FRCSC; PlasSurg. Staff, Health Sciences Centre; Asst Prof Surg, University of Manitoba; (204)787-7147

HAYAMI, Douglas A; Institut de Cardiologie de Mtl, 5040-5000 rue Belanger, Montreal QC H1T 1C8; McG'06; MDCM; FRCPC; IntMed; Cardiol. Staff, Institut de Cardiologie de Montréal; (514)376-3330 x2192

HAYAMI, John A; 25 Centre St W, Richmond Hill ON L4C 3P3; Tor'69; Ac Staff, Mackenzie Richmond Hill Hospital; (905)884-1156; Fax. (905)884-2409.

HAYANI, Omar; William Osler HC-Brampton, 2100 Bovaird Dr E, Brampton ON L6R 3J7; Tor'07; Critical Care Medicine; IntMed. Staff, William Osler Health System - Brampton Civic Hospital; (416)417-8284

HAYASHI, Allen H; Richmond Med Bldg, 302-2020 Richmond Rd, Victoria BC V8R 6R5; Wes'81; DAB; FRCSC; GenSurg (Surgical Oncology); PedGenSurg. Consultant, Vancouver Island Health Authority; Clin Asst Prof, University of British Columbia; (250)592-4313; Fax. (250)592-5020.

HAYASHIDA, Peter J K; Baywood Med Centre, 504-95 Bayly St W, Ajax ON L1S 7K8; Tor'81; BSc; FRCSC; GenSurg; PlasSurg. Ac Staff, Rouge Valley Health System - Ajax & Pickering Health Centre Site; (905)426-9928; Fax. (905)426-6857.

HAYAT, Sikandar; Sir Thomas Roddick Hosp, PO Box 5000 Stn Main 142 Minnesota Dr, Stephenville NL A2N 2V6; (Pakistan)'88; FRCSC; Staff, Sir Thomas Roddick Hospital; (709)643-5111

HAYDEN, Brian C; Liberton Med Centre, 212-31 Liberton Dr, St. Albert AB T8N 3X6; Alb'84; CCFP; FCFP; (780)459-7760

HAYDEN, David S; Medical Arts Bldg, 308-42 Glen Allan Dr, Bridgewater NS B4V 3N2; McG'94; FRCSC; PlasSurg. Langs: English; French; (902)543-5900; Fax. (902)543-5900.

HAYDEN, Huguette S; 107-22190 48 Ave, Langley BC V3A 3N5; Bordeaux (France)'69; FRCPC; Psy (Child & Adolescent Psychiatry). Staff Child & Adolescent Psy, Child & Adolescent Mental Health; Staff Child & Adolescent Psy, Children Foundation; Staff Child & Adolescent Psy, Toronto North Support Services; Staff Child & Adolescent Psy, Non Promotion Organization; Asst Prof, University of British Columbia; Langs: French; (604)534-2989; huguetteh@tnss.ca.

HAYDEN, Michael R; 3026-950 28th Ave W, Vancouver BC V5Z 4H4; Cape Town (South Africa)'75; MB ChB; FRSC; FRCPC; IntMed (Medical Genetics). Chair Research, Canada Medical Genetics; Sr Scientist/Dir Centre for Molecular Med & Therapeutics, University of British Columbia; (604)875-3535; Fax. (604)875-3819.

HAYDEN, Robert I; Keary Med Centre, 105-245 Columbia St E, New Westminster BC V3L 3W4; McG'70; FRCSC; GenSurg; Cardiovasc&ThorSurg; ThorSurg. Ac Staff, Royal Columbian Hospital; Consultant, Vancouver General Hospital - Centennial Pavillion; Clin Prof Surg, University of British Columbia; (604)522-6800; Fax. (604)540-8126; erh@telus.net.

HAYDEY, Richard P; Winnipeg Clinic, 425 St Mary Ave, Winnipeg MB R3C 0N2; Man'76; BSc(Med.); DABD; FRCPC; Derm. Staff, St Boniface General Hospital; Staff Children's Hosp, Health Sciences Centre; Assoc Prof Med, University of Manitoba; (204)957-3226; Fax. (204)943-2614.

HAYEEMS, Eran B Z; William Osler HC-Etobicoke, 101 Humber College Blvd, Etobicoke ON M9V 1R8; Tor'95; FRCPC; DiagRad. Staff, William Osler Health System - Etobicoke General Hospital; (416)747-3400

HAYER, Kuldip S; 4-135 Whitefield Dr NE, Calgary AB T1Y 5X1; Alb'95; CCFP; FCFP; (403)590-9992; Fax. (403)590-9994.

HAYES, Aubrey C; Rideau Med & Dental Centre, 210-1711 4 St SW, Calgary AB T2S 1V8; Dublin (Ireland)'52; MCh; Dip Ortho; (403)228-3948; Fax. (403)228-5068; dr.hayes@telus.net; Semi-Retired.

HAYES, Christopher W; St Michael's Hosp, QW4 036-30 Bond St, Toronto ON M5B 1W8; Tor'00; FRCPC; IntMed; Critical Care Medicine. Staff, St Michael's Hospital; (416)340-6000

HAYES, Claire L; Clinique Duvernay, 765 rue Roland-Forget, Laval QC H7E 4C1; Laval'81; FRCPC; Psy. Staff Psy, Hopital de la Cite de la santé; (450)668-2620 x1; Fax. (450)668-1077.

HAYES, Dennis W; Cochrane Primary Care Centre, 103-100 Grande Blvd W, Cochrane AB T4C 0S4; Cal'97; (403)932-2089 x7; Fax. (403)932-1820; MyFamilyDoc@gmail.com.

HAYES, Evelyn A; 35 Providence St, Moncton NB E1C 8X3; Laval'86; FRCPC; Derm. Dermatology, Dr Georges-L-Dumont University Hospital Centre; (506)857-1422; Fax. (506)857-1430.

HAYES, Gary W; Westwood Mall, 142-3000 Lougheed Hwy, Coquitlam BC V3B 1C5; Man'78; (604)945-0100; Fax. (604)945-0171.

HAYES, Jason A; The Hosp for Sick Children, 555 University Ave, Toronto ON M5G 1X8; Tor'95; FRCPC; Anes (Pediatric Anesthesia). Clin Associate Anes, The Hospital For Sick Children; (416)813-8963; jason.hayes@sickkids.ca.

HAYES, K Oona; Univ of Victoria Health Serv, PO Box 1700 Stn CSC, Victoria BC V8W 2Y2; McM'99; CCFP; (250)721-8492; Fax. (250)721-6224.

HAYES, Malcolm M M; BC Cancer Agency-Vancouver CC, 600 10th Ave W, Vancouver BC V5Z 4E6; Rhodesia (Zimbabwe)'76; MB ChB; MRCS(Eng); LRCP(Lond); MRCPath; FRCPC; AnatPath. Staff, BC Cancer Agency Vancouver Centre; (604)877-6098 x2050; Fax. (604)873-5384.

HAYES, Marie; Clinique Sante Jacques-Cartier, 200-1815 rue King O, Sherbrooke QC J1J 2E3; Ott'85; CCFP; ac Staff, Centre Hospitalier Universitaire de Sherbrooke-Hopital Fleurimont; Clin Prof, Universite de Sherbrooke; Langs: Bilingual(French/English); (819)565-7446; Fax. (819)565-7780; mjh06@sympatico.ca.

HAYES, Megan; Shea Heights Comm Hlth Ctr, PO Box 13122 Stn A 57B Linegar Ave, St. John's NL A1B 4A4; Mem'07; CCFP; (709)752-4300

HAYES, Paul R; Queen Street Surgical Assoc, 202-610 Queen St, Saskatoon SK S7K 0M8; Sask'94; BSc(Hon.); FACS; FRCSC; GenSurg (Critical Care Medicine). Clinical Asst Prof Surg/Asst Prog Dir Dept of Surg Div of Gen Surg, University of Saskatchewan; Langs: French; (306)244-6818; Fax. (306)664-3462.

HAYES, Robert C; 175 Hampton Rd PO Box 21008, Rothesay NB E2E 4Y7; Dal'00; FRCPC; Derm (Mohs Micrographic Surgery). Dir Mohs Surgery Clinic, Horizon Health Network Saint John Public Health; (506)847-8330; Fax. (506)847-8392.

HAYES, Tracy; 9-2120 Regent Rd S, Sudbury ON P3E 3Z9; Ott'03; CCFP; CCFP(E.M.); Staff, Health Sciences North-St Joseph's Health Centre; Assoc Prof, Northern Ontario School of Medicine; Langs: Bilingual(English/French); (705)523-9199; Fax. (705)523-9197.

HAYES, Vonda; Abbie J Lane Mem Bldg, 8F-5909 Veterans Memorial Lane, Halifax NS B3H 2E2; Dal'71; CCFP; FCFP; Court Staff, Queen Elizabeth II Health Sciences Centre - Halifax Infirmary Site; Teach Staff, Dalhousie University; (902)473-4748; Fax. (902)473-4760; vonda.hayes@dal.ca.

HAYES, William A; 65 Dundas St E, Belleville ON K8N 1B9; Galway (Ireland)'70; MB ChB; BAO; (613)966-7144; Fax. (613)966-3878.

HAYFRON-BENJAMIN, Jonathan; Appletree Medical Group, 1A-1595 Merivale Rd, Ottawa ON K2G 3J4; Aberdeen (Scotland)'66; MB ChB; Staff Family Med, Appletree Medical Group; (613)224-2880; Fax. (613)224-2804.

HAYLEY, John H; Nanaimo Reg Gen Hosp, 1200 Dufferin Cres, Nanaimo BC V9S 2B7; Wes'74; FRCPC; EmergMed. Staff, Burnaby Hospital; Staff, Nanaimo Regional General Hospital; (250)755-7691

HAYMAN, Christopher; Quinte HC Corp-Trenton Mem, PO Box 1600 Stn Main 242 King St, Trenton ON K8V 5S6; Man'02; CCFP; Staff, QHC Trenton Memorial; Medical Officer, Canadian Forces Base; (613)392-2541; Fax. (613)961-5503.

HAYMAN, Coryn; Addiction & Mental Hlth-Queen, 1001 Queen St W, Toronto ON M6J 1H4; Wes'01; CCFP; Weeneebayko General Hospital; Staff, Centre for Addiction & Mental Health (CAMH) - Queen Site; Staff, West Nipissing General Hospital; Fax. (416)535-8501; corynhayman@yahoo.com.

HAYMAN, Kellie; Ross Mem Hosp, 10 Angeline St N, Lindsay ON K9V 4M8; McM'02; CCFP; CCFP(E.M.); Staff, Ross Memorial Hospital; (705)324-6111

HAYNES, Alison; The Hosp for Sick Children, 555 University Ave, Toronto ON M5G 1X8; Mem'08; Peds.

HAYNES, Gordon R; 1-107 Main St, Minto NB E4B 3L6; Dal'67; Staff, Queens North Community Health Centre; Court Staff, Dr Everett Chalmers Regional Hospital; Court Staff, Oromocto Public Hospital; (506)327-3347; Fax. (506)327-4519.

HAYNES, R Brian; McMaster Campus Health Centre, CRL 133-1280 Main St W, Hamilton ON L8S 4K1; Alb'71; PhD; OC; MACP; FRCPC; IntMed (Clinical Epidemiology). Ac Staff, Hamilton Health Sciences Centre - McMaster Children's Hospital; Prof Clin Epidemiology & Med Health Information Research Unit, McMaster University; (905)525-9140 x20152; Fax. (905)526-8447.

HAYS, Luke; Pemberton Med Clinic, PO Box 69 1403 Portage Rd, Pemberton BC V0N 2L0; UBC'08; CCFP; Staff, Haliburton Highlands Health Services - Haliburton Site; (604)894-6633; Fax. (604)894-6918.

HAYTER, Charles; The Credit Valley Hosp, 2200 Eglinton Ave W, Mississauga ON L5M 2N1; Qns'84; FRCPC; RadOncol. Staff, The Credit Valley Hospital; (905)813-1100 x5000

HAYTER, Megan; St Michaels Hosp, 30 Bond St, Toronto ON M5B 1W8; UBC'05; FRCPC; Anes. Staff, St Michael's Hospital; (416)864-5071

HAYTER, Michael; Dr Everett Chalmers Reg Hosp, PO Box 9000 Stn A 700 Priestman St, Fredericton NB E3B 5N5; Dal'95; CCFP; Staff, Dr Everett Chalmers Regional Hospital; (506)452-5400

HAYTON, Barbara C; Inst of Commun & Family Psy, 4333 ch Cote-Sainte-Catherine, Montreal QC H3T 1E4; McG'83; CCFP; FCFP; Clin Asst Psy, Sir Mortimer B Davis Jewish General; Asst Prof Psy & Family Med, McGill University; (514)340-8210

HAYTON, Peter M; Lonsdale Place, 403-1200 Lonsdale Ave, North Vancouver BC V7M 3H6; Sask'90; (604)984-8788

HAYTON, Susan; Royal University Hosp, 103 Hospital Dr, Saskatoon SK S7N 0W8; Sask'85; FRCSC; GenSurg (Family Medicine). Staff, Royal University Hospital; (306)655-1000

HAYWARD, Andrew C; Toronto East Gen Hosp Inc, 825 Coxwell Ave, Toronto ON M4C 3E7; Tor'07; FRCSC; OrthSurg. Staff, Toronto East General Hospital Inc; (416)469-6580

HAYWARD, Catherine P M; 2N29A-1200 Main St W, Hamilton ON L8N 3Z5; Wes'84; MB; FRCPC; IntMed; Hem. Staff, Hamilton Health Sciences Centre - McMaster Children's Hospital; Staff, St Joseph's Hospital - St Joseph's Health Care; Staff, Hamilton Regional Laboratory Medicine Program; Assoc Prof Path, McMaster University; (905)521-2100 x76274; Fax. (905)521-2338.

HAYWARD, Clyde; Medi-Kel Family Prac & Walk in, PO Box 2100 Rpo Banks Centre, Kelowna BC V1X 4K5; (South Africa)'06; MB ChB; (250)862-4996

HAYWARD, Diana; Lakeridge Hlth Corp-Oshawa, 1 Hospital Crt, Oshawa ON L1G 2B9; Wes'06; FRCPC; Anes. Staff, Lakeridge Health - Oshawa Site; (905)576-8711

HAYWARD, James M; Northmount Med Centre, 501-145 13th St E, North Vancouver BC V7L 2L4; Ott'78; CCFP; Court Staff, Lions Gate Hospital; Clinical Asst Prof Family Med, University of British Columbia; (604)988-1211; Fax. (604)980-3707; drjameshayward@telus.net.

HAYWARD, Judith E; Pine Clinic, 1985 4th Ave W, Vancouver BC V6J 1M7; Cal'77; (604)733-3525; Fax. (604)731-9479.

HAYWARD, Lindsey; Three Lakes Med Ctr, 202-3005 30 St, Vernon BC V1T 2M1; Manchester (England)'97; MB ChB; (250)542-1353

HAYWARD, Lori; Dr H Bliss Murphy Cancer Ctr, 300 Prince Philip Dr, St. John's NL A1B 3V6; Mem'01; BSc(Hons); CCFP; Staff, Dr H Bliss Murphy Cancer Centre; (709)737-6300; dlhayward@nl.rogers.com.

HAYWARD, Melissa L; St Joseph's Healthcare, 50 Charlton Ave E, Hamilton ON L8N 4A6; Tor'07; FRCPC; EmergMed. Staff, St Joseph's Healthcare - Charlton Campus; (905)522-1155

HAYWARD, Robert S A; 2105 RTF-8308 114 St NW, Edmonton AB T6G 2V2; Qns'84; MPH; FRCPC; IntMed (Medical Informatics). Staff, Capital Health Authority; Staff, Research Transition Facility; Teach Staff, University of Alberta; (780)492-6633; Fax. (780)492-1748.

HAYWARD, Rowland J; Pembina Village Walk-In Clinic, 2-2077 Pembina Hwy, Winnipeg MB R3T 5J9; Man'83; BSc(Hons); PhD; CCFP; Ac Staff, Victoria General Hospital; Staff, Misericordia Health Centre; (204)261-5743; Fax. (204)489-5680.

HAYWARD, Susan L; Queen Square FHT, 201-366 Main St N, Brampton ON L6V 1P8; Ott'91; BSc(Hon); CCFP; FCFP; Staff, William Osler Health System - Brampton Civic Hospital; Lecturer, University of Toronto; Asst Prof, McMaster University; (905)455-1455; Fax. (905)455-5498.

HAYWARD-STEWART, Amber; 7-389 Main St, Picton ON K0K 2T0; McM'95; Dip SportMed; CASM; CCFP; Chief Emerg, QHC Trenton Memorial; Coroner, Province of Ontario; Clin Associate Part Time Family Med, Queen's University; (613)476-5744; Fax. (613)476-8773.

HAYWOOD, Catherine T; 219-284 Queen St E, Brampton ON L6V 1C2; McG'95; BSc; MDCM; FRCSC; PlasSurg. Langs: Bilingual(English/French); (905)451-2285

HAYWOOD-FARMER, Eric; Brockville Gen Hosp, 75 Charles St, Brockville ON K6V 1S8; Ott'06; CCFP; CCFP(E.M.); Staff, Brockville General Hospital - Charles Street; (613)345-5645

HAZAN, Ariel; Clinique Med Joliette, 3841 rue Ontario E, Montreal QC H1W 1S5; Sher'87; (514)524-3731; Fax. (514)524-0675.

HAZAN, Joelle; 201-6164 ch de la Cote-Saint-L, Montreal QC H3X 2H1; Mon'84; FRCPC; Peds. Staff, Centre Hospitalier l'Université De Montréal (CHUM) - Hôpital Saint-luc; (514)369-9999; Fax. (514)369-6016.

HAZAN, Sandra J; 608-10 St Mary St, Toronto ON M4Y 1P9; McM'88; DPsy; AB; FRCPC; Psy. (416)483-3144

HAZEL, Elizabeth; MUHC-Montreal Gen Hosp, A6 123-1650 av Cedar, Montreal QC H3G 1A4; McG'00; FRCPC; IntMed; Rheum. Staff, McGill University Health Centre - Montreal General Campus; (514)934-1934

HAZELL, Paul M; Port Hope Med Centre, 204-249 Ontario St, Port Hope ON L1A 3Y9; Tor'72; (905)885-5770; Fax. (905)885-2568.

HAZELTINE, Mark; Ctr de Rhumatlogie de Laval, 3095 Autoroute Laval O, Laval QC H7P 4W5; Mon'80; FRCPC; IntMed; Rheum. (450)988-1026; Fax. (450)688-8566.

HAZELTON, Lara D K; The Nova Scotia Hosp, PO Box 1004 Stn Main 300 Pleasant St, Dartmouth NS B2Y 3Z9; Dal'94; FRCPC; Psy. Staff, The Nova Scotia Hospital; (902)464-3039; Fax. (902)464-3002.

HAZIZA, Muriel; Clinique Med St-Jacques, 201-5515 rue St-Jacques O, Montreal QC H4A 2E3; Mon'00; FRCPC; PhysMed&Rehab (Botox Injection). Staff, Institut de Réadaptation Gingras-Lindsay de Montréal; (514)735-5547; Fax. (514)735-5722.

HAZIZA, Philippe; PO Box 74212 Rpo Beechwood, Ottawa ON K1M 2H9; Mon'90.

HAZLETT, David L; Northmount Med Centre, 704-145 13th St E, North Vancouver BC V7L 2L4; UBC'97; BSc; MSc; CCFP; (604)988-0677; Fax. (604)987-9607.

HAZLETT, Melinda M; Wellington Med Arts Bldg, 216-121 Wellington St W, Barrie ON L4N 1L2; McM'91; BSc(Hon); FAAP; FRCPC; Peds (Diabetes). Staff, Royal Victoria Regional Health Centre; Court Consultant, Orillia Soldiers' Memorial Hospital; Asst Clin Prof, McMaster University; (705)721-1113; Fax. (705)721-7815.

HAZLEWOOD, Glen S; Health Science Ctr Faculty of, 3330-3330 Hospital Dr NW, Calgary AB T2N 4N1; Cal'05; FRCPC; IntMed; Rheum. (403)220-5903; Fax. (403)210-9717.

HAZRA, Sachin K; Niagara Health Centre, 107-180 Vine St S, St Catharines ON L2R 7P3; Calcutta (India)'56; FRCP(Edin); MB BS; DCH(Lond); FRCPC; IntMed (Diabetology)., Niagara Health System - St Catharines General Site; Langs: Bengali; Hindi; (905)685-1444; Fax. (905)685-6109.

HAZRA, Samir K; Univ of Ottawa Heart Institute, 40 Ruskin St, Ottawa ON K1Y 4W7; Ott'08; FRCPC; IntMed. Staff, University of Ottawa Heart Institute; (613)761-5000

HAZRATI, Ali; Greenstone Clinic, 300-5734 Yonge St, North York ON M2M 4E7; Tehran (Iran)'95; FRCSC; GenSurg;CCFP; Langs: Farsi; Persian; (416)222-5501; Fax. (416)222-1932.

HAZRATI, Lili-Naz; Univ Hlth Network-The Toronto, 11F-200 Elizabeth St, Toronto ON M5G 2C4; Mon'02; FRCPC; NeurPath. Staff, Toronto General Hospital - UHN; (416)340-4800

HAZZI, Cherine; Centre de Sante Valcartier, CP 1000 Bdp Succ Forces, Courcelette QC G0A 4Z0; Laval'80; Ac Staff, Institut Universitaire Sante; (418)844-5000 x3186

HEAD, Donald R; Trillium Hlth Ctr-Mississauga, 100 Queensway W, Mississauga ON L5B 1B8; Man'88; FRCPC; Psy (Hospital Consultation). Consultant Liason Psy, Trillium Health Centre - Mississauga; (905)848-7585

HEAD, James A; 103-107 Edward St, St Thomas ON N5P 1Y8; Mem'76; Staff, St Thomas Elgin General Hospital; (519)631-6147; Fax. (519)631-6149.

HEAD, Pauline W; Rockyview Gen Hosp, 7007 14 St SW, Calgary AB T2V 1P9; Sask'80; FRCPC; EmergMed. Staff, Rockyview General Hospital; University of Calgary; (403)943-3449; Fax. (403)943-3220.

HEAD, Robert B; Powell River Gen Hosp, 5000 Joyce Ave, Powell River BC V8A 5R3; UBC'93; CCFP; CCFP(E.M.); Staff, Powell River General Hospital; (604)485-3211

HEAD, Stephen J; St Paul's Hosp, 1081 Burrard St, Vancouver BC V6Z 1Y6; Cal'99; FRCPC; Anes. Staff, Providence Health Care - St Paul's Hospital; (604)682-2344

HEALE, V Robert; Health Sciences Centre, 300 Prince Philip Dr, St. John's NL A1B 3V6; Mem'99; FRCPC; DiagRad. Staff, Health Sciences Centre; (709)777-8844

HEALEY, Andrew J; St Joseph's Healthcare, 50 Charlton Ave E, Hamilton ON L8N 4A6; Mem'04; FRCPC; EmergMed; Critical Care Medicine. Staff, St Joseph's Healthcare - Charlton Campus; (905)522-4941

HEALEY, Ara A; Dr Charles A Janeway Child HC, 300 Prince Philip Dr, St. John's NL A1B 3V6; Mem'02; FRCPC; Peds; Endocrin&Metab. Staff, Janeway Children's Health & Rehabilitation Centre; (709)777-6300

HEALEY, Christopher J; Western Mem Reg Hosp, PO Box 2005 Stn Main 1 Brookfield Ave, Corner Brook NL A2H 6J7; London (England)'69; MB BS; FRCOG; FRCSC; ObstGyn. Chief ObstGyn/Staff, Western Memorial Regional Hospital; Clinical Asst Prof, Memorial University Of Newfoundland; (709)637-5000

HEALEY, David C; South Hlth & Life Managment Ct, 2-2120 Regent St, Sudbury ON P3E 3Z9; Mem'95; FRCSC; OrthSurg (Adult Reconstructive Surgery). (705)522-9101; Fax. (705)522-5744.

HEALEY, Francis B; 3411 32 Ave, Vernon BC V1T 2M9; London (England)'76; MB BS; MRCGPract; LMCC; Physician Emerg, South Okanagan General Hospital; Langs: English; French; (250)545-3233; healeyf@shaw.ca.

HEALEY, Jane; The Credit Valley Hosp, 2200 Eglinton Ave W, Mississauga ON L5M 2N1; Tor'01; BSc; FRCPC; Peds. Clin Asst, Hamilton Health Sciences Centre - McMaster Children's Hospital; Staff, The Credit Valley Hospital; Langs: Czech; (905)813-4466

HEALEY, Jeffrey S; Hamilton HS-General Site, 237 Barton St E, Hamilton ON L8L 2X2; Ott'95; BSc; MSc; FRCPC; IntMed (Electrophysiology); Cardiol. Staff, Hamilton Health Sciences Centre - Hamilton General Hospital; Asst Prof, McMaster University; Langs: French; (905)577-8004; Fax. (905)523-9165; healeyj@hhsc.ca.

HEALEY, Kathryn L; 543 Eglinton Ave E, Toronto ON M4P 1N7; Tor'84; CCFP; (416)487-7721

HEALEY, Linda M; Correction Serv of Canada, PO Box 4500 Stn Del Ctr 3391 Gladys Ave, Abbotsford BC V2S 2E8; Mem'93; FRCPC; Psy. Staff, Regional Treatment Centre & Pacific Institution; (604)870-2752; lhealey@forensic.bc.ca.

HEALEY, Paul D; Halton HSC Corp-Oakville, 327 Reynolds St, Oakville ON L6J 3L7; Wes'01; CCFP; CCFP(E.M.); Staff, Halton Healthcare Services Corporation - Oakville Site; Staff, St Joseph's Health Centre; Staff, The Credit Valley Hospital; (905)338-4605

HEALEY, Sarah; 103-35 Major's Path, St. John's NL A1A 4Z9; Mem'96; FRCOG; FSOGC; FRCSC; ObstGyn (Reproductive Endocrinology & Infertility). Staff OB/Gyn REI, Eastern Health Authoriy; Asst Prof, Memorial University Of Newfoundland; (709)777-7444; Fax. (709)752-3648.

HEALLEY, William M; Midpark Family Med Centre, 100-290 Midpark Way SE, Calgary AB T2X 1P1; Pretoria (South Africa)'76; MB ChB; Langs: Afrikaans; (403)254-8405

HEALY, Conor M; Quinte HC Corp-Trenton Mem, PO Box 1600 Stn Main, Trenton ON K8V 5S6; Galway (Ireland)'68; Staff, QHC Trenton Memorial; (613)392-2541; Fax. (613)392-3749.

HEALY, Jane; Burnside Medical Clinic, 101 Burnside Rd W, Victoria BC V9A 1B7; (Australia)'01; (250)381-4353

HEANEY, Michael J P; Ministry Of Health, 1515 Blanshard St, Victoria BC V8W 3C8; Sask'69; (250)952-3032

HEAPES, Mary B; Lakehead Psychiatric Hosp, PO Box 2930 Stn P 580 Algoma St, Thunder Bay ON P7B 5G4; Dublin (Ireland)'83; FRCPC; Psy. Staff, Lakehead Psychiatric Hospital - St. Joseph's Care Group; (807)343-4300

HEARD, Janice; HSC-Faculty of Med, G740E-3330 Hospital Dr NW, Calgary AB T2N 4N1; Cal'84; BSc(Hon); BPHE; FRCPC; Peds. Staff, Alberta Children's Hospital; Consultant Ped, Cope Community Outreach Ped Psy & Education; Staff, Cups Health Centre; Physician, Calgary Urban Project Society; Clin Asst Prof, University of Calgary; (403)210-8935; Fax. (403)255-6744.

HEARD, Neil M; PO Box 3182 Stn Main, Sherwood Park AB T8H 2T2; (Zimbabwe)'81; MB ChB; CCFP; FCFP; (780)998-2231; Fax. (780)998-4399.

HEARD, Patricia M; South Calgary Hlth Clinic, 113-31 Sunpark Plaza SE, Calgary AB T2X 3W5; McM'82; CCFP; FCFP; University of Calgary; (403)254-2030; Fax. (403)254-2929.

HEARD, S Mark A; Dr Mark Heard Banff Sport Med, PO Box 1300 Stn Main 207-303 Lynx St, Banff AB T1L 1B3; Cal'86; CASM; FRCSC; OrthSurg (Arthroscopic Surgery). Staff Consultant OrthSurg, Golden & District General Hospital; Ac Staff, Covenant Health - Banff Mineral Springs Hospital; Staff Consultant, Canmore General Hospital; (403)760-2897; Fax. (403)760-8234.

HEARN, Taryn L; Waterford Hosp, 306 Waterford Bridge Rd, St. John's NL A1E 4J8; Mem'02; FRCPC; Psy. Staff, Waterford Hospital; (709)777-3082

HEARNDEN, Trevor A; 91 King St E PO Box 209, Colborne ON K0K 1S0; Qns'81; (905)355-2075; Fax. (905)355-3366.

HEARTWELL, Barbara J E; 101-1106 Ouellette Ave, Windsor ON N9A 1C9; Tor'72; FRCSC; GenSurg. Ac Staff, Hôtel-Dieu Grace Hospital; (519)258-4433; Fax. (519)258-8793.

HEASMAN, Kaaren Z; 501-131 Bloor St W, Toronto ON M5S 1R1; Tor'86; FRCPC; Psy (Psychotherapy- Individual & Couple). (416)928-0361

HEATH, Andrea M; 2-32904 Ventura Ave, Abbotsford BC V2S 6J3; UBC'08; CCFP; Staff, Chilliwack General Hospital; (604)859-1211

HEATH, David S; New Vision Family Hlth Team, 421 Greenbrook Dr, Kitchener ON N2M 4K1; Liverpool (England)'67; MB ChB; FRCPC; Psy. Staff, Cambridge Memorial Hospital; (519)578-3510; Fax. (519)578-6040.

HEATH, Diana S; International Med Services, 4000 Leslie St, North York ON M2K 2R9; Tor'77; CCFP; (416)494-7512; Fax. (416)492-3740.

HEATH, Jennifer; Alberta Children's Hosp, 2888 Shaganappi Trail NW, Calgary AB T3B 6A8; Columbia (USA)'90; Staff, Alberta Children's Hospital; Aj Asst Prof, University of Calgary; (403)955-7326

HEATH, John W; Alder Med Centre, 277 Evergreen Rd, Campbell River BC V9W 5Y4; McG'76; FRCPC; IntMed (Respirology). (250)287-7454; Fax. (250)287-4384.

HEATH, V Ann; Alder Med Centre, 277 Evergreen Rd, Campbell River BC V9W 5Y4; McG'76; (250)287-7454; Fax. (250)286-3628.

HEATHCOTE, Jenny L; Univ Hlth Network-Toronto Western Hosp, 6BFW156-399 Bathurst St, Toronto ON M5T 2S8; London (England)'68; MB BS; FRCP; MD; FRCPC; IntMed (Hepatology); Gastroent. Head, Toronto Western Hospital - University Health Network; Head Patient Based Clin Research Div, Toronto Western Research Institute; Prof Med, University of Toronto; (416)603-5914; Fax. (416)603-6281; jenny.heathcote@utoronto.ca.

HEATHCOTE, J Godfrey; DJ Mackenzie Bldg, 702A-5788 University Ave, Halifax NS B3H 1V8; Cambridge (England)'74; MB ChB; PhD; FRCPC; AnatPath (Head & Neck). Head Dept of Path, Dalhousie University; (902)473-3734; Fax. (902)473-7161; godfrey.heathcote@cdha.nshealth.ca.

HEATHCOTE, John C; BC Biomedical Laboratories, 7455 130 St, Surrey BC V3W 1H8; Qns'79; FRCPC; MedBiochem. (604)507-5000; Fax. (604)507-5215; jheathcote@bcbio.com.

HEATHCOTE, Karen; Red Deer Reg Hosp Centre, PO Box 5030 Stn Postal Box Ctr 3942 50A Ave, Red Deer AB T4N 6R2; Sask'05; FRCPC; IntMed; Respir. Staff, Central Alberta Cancer Centre; Staff, Red Deer Regional Hospital Centre; (403)356-4201; Fax. (403)358-4342; heathcote@telusplanet.net.

HEATON, Catherine J; 4712 Bowness Rd NW, Calgary AB T3B 0B4; Cal'76; CCFP; (403)247-1616; Fax. (403)247-0310.

HEATON, Kenneth; 301-423 Devonshire Ave, Woodstock ON N4S 0B2; McM'83; DDS; CME Advisory Commitee, Woodstock General Hospital; Aj Prof Family Med, University of Western Ontario; (519)537-8303; Fax. (519)539-3838; ken@khmd.ca.

HEAVEN, Charles G; Stettler Med Clinic, PO Box 1210 B4-4710 50 St, Stettler AB T0C 2L0; Alb'70; Ac Staff, Stettler Hospital and Care Centre; Med Examiner Civial Aviation, Employment & Immigration; (403)742-3441; Fax. (403)742-3299; cheaven@dthr.ab.ca.

HEBB, A Michael O; Woodlawn Med Clinic, 92 Main St, Dartmouth NS B2X 1R5; Dal'67; DAB; CCFP; CCFP(E.M.); Physician Emerg/Ac Staff, Dartmouth General Hospital; (902)434-1500; Fax. (902)434-4058.

HEBB, Jonathan P O; Abbotsford Reg Hosp & Cancer C, 32900 Marshall Rd, Abbotsford BC V2S 0C2; Dal'01; FRCPC; IntMed; Critical Care Medicine; Hem. Staff, Abbotsford Regional Hospital & Cancer Centre; (604)851-4700

HEBB, Linda M; Dr Everett Chalmers Reg Hosp, PO Box 9000 Stn A 700 Priestman St, Fredericton NB E3B 5N5; McG'84; CCFP; CCFP(E.M.); FCFP; Ac Staff, Dr Everett Chalmers Regional Hospital; Dalhousie University; (506)452-5058

HEBB, Matthew O; London HSC-University Hosp, PO Box 5339 Stn B 339 Windermere Rd, London ON N6A 5A5; Tor'02; FRCSC; Neursurg. Staff, London Health Sciences Centre - University Hospital; (519)663-2981

HEBBARD, Pamela; Health Sciences Centre, GF434-820 Sherbrook St, Winnipeg MB R3A 1R9; Mem'04; FRCSC; GenSurg; General Surgical Oncology. Staff, Health Sciences Centre; (204)774-8511

HEBER, Alexandra S; Montfort Hosp, 713 Montreal Rd, Ottawa ON K1K 0T2; Man'89; FRCPC; Psy. Staff, Montfort Hospital; (613)746-4621

HEBERT, Amelie; Centre de Peri-Maternite, 575 rue Saint-Charles E, Longueuil QC J4H 1B8; Laval'02; (450)332-9833

HEBERT, Annie; CHUS-Hop Fleurimont, 3001 12e av N, Sherbrooke QC J1H 5N4; Sher'99; CCFP; CCFP(E.M.); Staff, Centre Hospitalier Universitaire de Sherbrooke-Hopital Fleurimont; (819)346-1110

HEBERT, Annie; CLSC Beauce-Sartigan, RR 1 763 av 14E, La Guadeloupe QC G0M 1G0; Sher'02; (418)459-3441; Fax. (418)459-3142; annielhebert@hotmail.com.

HEBERT, Benedict; CSSS Haut-Richelieu-Rouville, 920 boul du Seminaire N, St-Jean-sur-Richel QC J3A 1B7; Sher'10; CCFP; Staff, Hôpital du Haut-Richelieu; (450)359-5000

HEBERT, Christian-Rene; Hôpital Laval, 2725 ch Sainte-Foy, Quebec QC G1V 4G5; Laval'94; BSc; MSc; CCFP; Staff, Hôpital Laval; Langs: Bilingual(English/French); (418)656-4550; Fax. (418)658-1448; c.r.hebert@sympatico.ca.

HEBERT, Denis L; 143-175 av Stillview, Pointe-Claire QC H9R 4S3; Mon'82; FRCPC; Derm. (514)695-9646

HEBERT, Diane; The Hosp for Sick Children, 555 University Ave, Toronto ON M5G 1X8; Sher'76; FRCPC; Peds. Staff, The Hospital For Sick Children; (416)813-6287; Fax. (416)813-6271; diane.hebert@sickkids.ca.

HEBERT, Diane; CLSC Haute-Ville, 55 ch Sainte-Foy, Quebec QC G1R 1S9; Laval'99; Staff Palliative Care, Centre Hospitalier Affilié Universitaire de Québec - Hôpital du St-Sacrement; (418)641-2572; Fax. (418)522-5437; dihebert@yahoo.com.

HEBERT, France; Clinique Med Sorel-Tracy, 330 av de l'Hotel-Dieu, Sorel-Tracy QC J3P 1N4; Mon'94; CCFP; FCFP; (450)742-9459; Fax. (450)742-9450.

HEBERT, Francois; Centre Med Robinson Inc, 4 rue Robinson N, Granby QC J2G 8Z9; Mon'90; (450)378-8435; Fax. (450)375-8832.

HEBERT, Guy J; The Ottawa Hosp-Civic Campus, 1053 Carling Ave, Ottawa ON K1Y 4E9; Ott'90; FRCPC; IntMed; EmergMed. Staff, The Ottawa Hospital - Civic Campus; Langs: Bilingual(English/French); (613)761-4347

HEBERT, Helene; Hop Louis-H Lafontaine, 406-7401 rue Hochelaga, Montreal QC H1N 3M5; Mon'85; Staff, Hopital Louis-H Lafontaine; Staff, Centre Hospitalier Pierre Boucher; (514)251-4050

HEBERT, Hugo; CLSC Olivier-Guimond, 5810 rue Sherbrooke E, Montreal QC H1N 1B2; Sher'02; (514)255-2365

HEBERT, Isabelle; Hop du Sacre-Coeur de Mtl, 5400 boul Gouin O, Montreal QC H4J 1C5; Mon'08; CCFP; Staff, Hôpital du Sacre-Coeur de Montréal; (514)338-2222; Fax. (514)338-3155.

HEBERT, Isabelle; CSSS de Beauce-Etchemin, 1515 17e rue, Saint-Georges QC G5Y 4T8; Laval'06; Staff, Centre Hospitalier Beauce-Etchemin; (418)228-2031; Fax. (418)228-3825.

HEBERT, Isabelle; CSSS du Rocher-Perce, CP 3300 451 rue Mgr Ross, Chandler QC G0C 1K0; Sher'94; FRCPC; IntMed (Diabetes). Staff, Centre Hospitalier de Chandler; Langs: English; (418)689-2261; Fax. (418)689-4620.

HEBERT, Jacqueline S; Glenrose Rehab Hosp, 10230 111 Ave NW, Edmonton AB T5G 0B7; Cal'95; BSc; FRCPC; PhysMed&Rehab (Amputee Rehabilitation). Staff, Glenrose Rehabilitation Hospital; Clin Dir, Glenrose Adult Amputee Program; Assoc Prof, University of Alberta; (780)735-8218; Fax. (780)735-6018.

HEBERT, Jacques R; CHUQ-Ctr Hosp Univ Laval, 2705 boul Laurier, Quebec QC G1V 4G2; Laval'71; ClinImmunol&Allergy (P. Q.). Ac Staff, Centre Hospitalier Universitaire de Quebec-CHUL; Teacher, Université Laval; (418)654-2240; Fax. (418)780-1583; hebert.j@videotron.ca.

HEBERT, Jean; CSSS de la Vallée de l'Or, 725 6e rue, Val-d'Or QC J9P 3Y1; Sher'04; NuclearMed. Staff, Centre Hospitalier de Val d'Or; (819)825-6711

HEBERT, Jean; Serv Correctionel du Canada, RR 1 242 montee Gagnon, Ste-Anne-d-Plaines QC J0N 1H0; Mon'86; Psy. Dir Prof Services, Hôpital Riviere des Prairies; Dir Psy, Universite de Montreal; (450)478-5960

HEBERT, Jean-Marc; GMF de Saint-Donat, 377 rue du Foyer, St-Donat-De-Mtcalm QC J0T 2C0; McG'82; VP, AMCCSQ; (819)424-1511; Fax. (819)424-4682.

HEBERT, Jean-Pierre; Centre Medical de Huntington, RR 3 72A rue Chateauguay, Huntingdon QC J0S 1H0; Mon'75; Gen Practice, Huntingdon County Hospital Centre; Staff, Barrie Memorial Hospital; Langs: Bilingual(French/English); (450)264-6101

HEBERT, Jocelyn; Polyclinique 55, 4825 av Bouvet, Becancour QC G9H 1X5; Laval'80; Staff, Hôpital de Christ-Roi; (819)233-3123; Fax. (819)233-3124.

HEBERT, Jocelyne; 110-667 rue Champlain, Dieppe NB E1A 1P6; Sher'96; FRCSC; GenSurg (Endoscopy). General Surgery, Dr Georges-L-Dumont University Hospital Centre; Langs: Bilingual(French/English); (506)854-6293; Fax. (506)858-9012.

HEBERT, Josee; Clinique Med du Sud-Ouest, 300-185 boul Saint-Jean-Baptis, Chateauguay QC J6K 3B4; Mon'93; ObstGyn. Staff, Hôpital Anna-Laberge; Langs: Bilingual(French/English); (450)692-3232; Fax. (450)692-3535.

HEBERT, Josee; Hop Maisonneuve-Rosemont, 5415 boul de l'Assomption, Montreal QC H1T 2M4; Mon'84; FRCPC; IntMed (Leukemia); Hem. Staff, Hopital Maisonneuve-Rosemont; Assoc Researcher IRIC, University of Montana; Langs: English; (514)252-3404; jhebert.hmr@ssss.gouv.qc.ca.

HEBERT, Julie; GMF Centre De Sante, 3745 rue Georges-Couture, Drummondville QC J2B 7P4; Sher'95; (819)477-2231

HEBERT, Julien; Inst U en Sante Mentale de QC, 2601 ch de la Canardiere, Quebec QC G1J 2G3; Laval'04; FRCPC; Psy. (418)663-5000

HEBERT, Louis P; Le Centre Medicale, 427-4 rue Taschereau, Gatineau QC J8Y 2V5; Laval'61; Peds (P.Q.). Staff, Hull Hospital; (819)771-8367

HEBERT, Marie-Josee; CHUM-Hop Notre-Dame, 1560 rue Sherbrooke E, Montreal QC H2L 4M1; Mon'89; FRCPC; IntMed; Nephrol. Staff, Centre Hospitalier l'Université de Montréal (CHUM) - Hôpital Notre-Dame; (514)890-8000 x25017; Fax. (514)412-7804; marie-josee.hebert.chum@ssss.gouv.qc.ca.

HEBERT, Mario; Ctr Hosp Affilie-St-Sacrement, 1050 ch Sainte-Foy, Quebec QC G1S 4L8; Laval'81; FRCPC; DiagRad. Staff, Centre Hospitalier Affilié Universitaire de Québec - Hôpital du St-Sacrement; (418)682-7700

HEBERT, Michel; La Cite Medicale, 295-2600 boul Laurier, Quebec QC G1V 4T3; Laval'81; (418)781-0480; Fax. (418)659-7072.

HEBERT, Michel; Ctr Hosp de Verdun, 4000 boul Lasalle, Verdun QC H4G 2A3; Mon'08; CCFP; Staff, Centre Hospitalier de Verdun; (514)362-1000

HEBERT, Michele; CSSSG-CLSC de Gatineau, 777 boul de la Gappe, Gatineau QC J8T 8R2; Ott'75; Langs: English; (819)561-2001 x1129

HEBERT, Mireille; Clinique Med D'Alma, 935 av du Pont S, Alma QC G8B 2V5; Mon'88; Staff, CSSS de Lac-Saint Jean-Est; (418)668-6121; Fax. (418)668-5298.

HEBERT, Nancy; CSSS de Beauce-Etchemin, 1515 17E rue, Saint-Georges QC G5Y 4T8; Laval'01; CCFP; CCFP(E.M.); Staff, Centre Hospitalier Beauce-Etchemin; (418)228-2031 x7800

HEBERT, Natacha; 105A-667 rue Cjamplain, Dieppe NB E1A 1P6; Sher'03; FRCPC; Peds. Staff, Dr Georges-L-Dumont University Hospital Centre; (506)869-2150; Fax. (506)869-2147.

HEBERT, Nathalie; 105-2160 ch du Tremblay, Longueuil QC J4N 1A8; Laval'94; FRCPC; Peds. (450)448-4440; Fax. (450)448-5403.

HEBERT, Nathalie; Ctr Hosp de LaSalle, 8585 Terrasse Champlain, LaSalle QC H8P 1C1; Mon'93; Staff, Centre Hospitalier de LaSalle; (514)362-8000

HEBERT, Odette; CSSS Domaine du Roy, 450 rue Brassard, Roberval QC G8H 1B9; Sher'86; FRCPC; IntMed (Rheumatology). Staff, Hotel-Dieu de Roberval; (418)275-0110 x2355; Fax. (418)275-2109; odette.hebert@cgocable.ca.

HEBERT, Paul C; The Ottawa Hosp- Civic Campus, 1053 Carling Ave, Ottawa ON K1Y 4E9; Ott'86; MHSc; FRCPC; IntMed; Critical Care Medicine. Sr Scientist, The Ottawa Hospital - General Campus; Staff, The Ottawa Hospital - Civic Campus; Prof Med Critical Care, Anesthesiology, Surgery Epidemiol/Chair, University of Ottawa; Langs: English; French; (613)798-5555; Fax. (613)761-5402; phebert@ohri.ca.

HEBERT, Paulin; CSSS de Maskinonge, 450 2e rue, Louiseville QC J5V 1V3; Laval'60; Staff, CSSS de Maskinongé; (819)228-2731

HEBERT, Philip C; Sunnybrook Hlth Sciences Ctre, A100-2075 Bayview Ave, Toronto ON M4N 3M5; Tor'84; PhD; CCFP; FCFP; Staff, Sunnybrook Health Sciences Centre; Assoc Prof Family & Commun Med, University of Toronto; (416)480-4963; Fax. (416)480-6038; philip.hebert@sunnybrook.ca.

HEBERT, Pierre A; Centre Med St-Charles, 357 rue de la Visitation, St-Charles-Brromee QC J6E 4N8; Mon'72; Staff, Centre Hospitalier Régional de Lanaudière; (450)759-5421; Fax. (450)759-5424.

HEBERT, Real; Centre de Sante Valcartier, CP 1000 Bdp Succ Forces, Courcelette QC G0A 4Z0; Mon'90; PhD; MSc; CCFP; (418)844-5000 x8243

HEBERT, Rejean; Inst U Geriatrie Sherbrooke, 1036 rue Belvedere S, Sherbrooke QC J1H 4C4; Sher'79; FRCPC; GeriatricMed (P.Q.). Staff, CSSS Institut universitaire de gériatrie de Sherbrooke; Scientist Inst of Aging/Dir, Canadian Institute of Health Research; Dir succ, Universite de Sherbrooke; (819)821-1150; Fax. (819)829-7141.

HEBERT, Richard J; 1921 10 Ave S, Lethbridge AB T1K 0B8; Alb'71; FRCSC; GenSurg. Ac Staff, Chinook Regional Hospital; (403)380-4777; Fax. (403)380-3416.

HEBERT, Yves; Institut de Cardiologie de Mtl, 5000 rue Belanger, Montreal QC H1T 1C8; Mon'72; CSPQ; Cardiovasc&ThorSurg; GenSurg. Staff, Institut de Cardiologie de Montréal; (514)376-3330; Fax. (514)593-2540.

HEBERT, Yves; Medecine Esthetique Dr Hebert, 2e-1832 rue Sherbrooke O, Montreal QC H3H 1E4; Mon'78; (514)935-6616; Fax. (514)933-2104.

HEBERT-BLOUIN, Marie-Noelle; MUHC-Montreal Neurology Inst, 109-3801 rue University, Montreal QC H3A 2B4; McG'02; FRCSC; Neursurg. Staff, McGill University Health Centre - Montreal Neurological Hospital; (514)398-2591

HEBERT CROTEAU, Nicolas; Brockville Gen Hosp, 75 Charles St, Brockville ON K6V 1S8; Sher'86; FRCPC; IntMed. Staff, Brockville General Hospital - Charles Street; Langs: Bilingual(French/English); (613)498-0365; Fax. (613)498-1479.

HEBERT-CROTEAU, Nicole; 1706-60 rue Berlioz, Verdun QC H3E 1M4; Mon'77; Staff, Centre Hospitalier l'Université de Montréal (CHUM) - Hôpital Notre-Dame; (514)751-2434; nicole.hebert-croteau@inspq.qc.ca.

HEBERT-SEMCO, Genevieve; CSSS Drummond-Hop Sainte-Croix, 570 rue Heriot, Drummondville QC J2B 1C1; Laval'08; CCFP; Staff, Hôpital Sainte-croix; (819)478-6464

HECHLER, Peter; Rosser Med Group, 841 Rosser Ave, Brandon MB R7A 0L1; Frankfurt (Germany)'87; CCFP.

HECHT, Kristian K; Foothills Medical Centre, C231-1403 29 St NW, Calgary AB T2N 2T9; UBC'06; CCFP; CCFP(E.M.); Staff, Foothills Medical Centre; (403)944-1635

HECHTENTHAL, Norman; Oakfield Med Clinic, 106-1021 Court Ave, Winnipeg MB R2P 1V7; Man'78; FRCPC; IntMed. Staff, Seven Oaks General Hospital; University of Manitoba; (204)334-4368; Fax. (204)339-3971.

HECHTMAN, Lily T; 4018 rue Sainte-Catherine O, Westmount QC H3Z 1P2; McG'67; AB; DPsy; FRCPC; Psy (Adult Psychiatry). Chief ADHD Psy Servs, McGill University Health Centre - Montreal General Campus; Dir Research Div Child Psy, McGill University; Langs: English; French; (514)412-4449; Fax. (514)412-4346.

HECKMAN, George A W; Grand River Hosp-KW Hlth Ctre, PO Box 9056 Stn C 835 King Street W, Kitchener ON N2G 1G3; Tor'95; FRCPC; IntMed (Heart Failure); GeriatricMed. Staff, St Joseph's Hospital - St Joseph's Health Care; Ac Staff, St Mary's General Hospital; Ac Staff, Grand River Hospital - Kitchener/Waterloo Health Centre; Asst Prof, Hamilton Health Sciences Centre - Hamilton General Hospital; Asst Prof Med, McMaster University; Assoc Prof Hlth Sciences & Gerontology, University of Waterloo; Langs: French; (519)749-4300 x7068; ggheckma@uwaterloo.ca.

HECTOR, R Ian; Canadian Mental Hlth Assoc, 21 Bradford St, Barrie ON L4N 1W2; Tor'57; DPsy; MRC(Lond); MRCPsy; FRCPC; Psy (Adult Psychiatry). (705)726-5033 x284; Fax. (705)726-4887.

HECTOR, Yanick; CLSC Saint-Michel, 3355 rue Jarry E, Montreal QC H1Z 2E5; Monterrey (Mexico)'87; Langs: English; Spanish; (514)374-0776; Fax. (514)374-5931.

HEDDEN, David; Concordia Joint Replacement Gr, 301-1155 Concordia Ave, Winnipeg MB R2K 2M9; Cape Town (South Africa)'84; BSc; MB ChB; FRCSC; OrthSurg (Arthroplasty). Staff/Dir Orth Surg, Concordia General Hospital; Asst Prof Section of OrthSurg., University of Manitoba; (204)926-1230; Fax. (204)940-2263.

HEDDEN, Douglas M; University of Alberta Hosp, 2D2 23WMC-8440 112 St NW, Edmonton AB T6G 2B7; Qns'78; FRCSC; OrthSurg (Pediatric Orthopedics). Chair Surg, University of Alberta Hospital; Clin Dept Head, Alberta Health Services; Dept Chair Surg, University of Alberta; (780)407-6605; Fax. (780)407-6606; dhedden@ualberta.ca.

HEDDEN, John R; Portage Clinic Inc, 140 9th St SE, Portage La Prairie MB R1N 3V5; Cape Town (South Africa)'80; Att Physician, Portage District General Hospital; Langs: Afrikaans; (204)857-3445; Fax. (204)239-1278; jhedden@shaw.ca.

HEDGCOCK, Malcolm A; Maple Leaf Med Arts, 501-14 College St, Toronto ON M5G 1K2; Tor'03; CCFP; Physician, Maple Leaf Medical Clinic; (416)465-0756

HEDGES, Bruce M; Richmond Rd. Family Med Centre, 290-5255 Richmond Rd, Calgary AB T3E 7C4; Qns'77; Med Staff, Penticton Regional Hospital; (403)532-1631

HEDGES, Donald G; Columia Med Bldg, 208-301 Columbia St E, New Westminster BC V3L 3W5; UBC'83; Assoc Staff, Burnaby Hospital; Instructor, Simon Fraser University; (604)525-5211; Fax. (604)525-2475.

HEDGES, James D; 250 German School Rd PO Box 790, St George Brant ON N0E 1N0; McM'80.

HEDIGER, Marcel; Forensic Psychiatric Hosp, 70 Colony Farm Rd, Coquitlam BC V3C 5X9; Orange Free State (South Africa)'92; MB ChB; Staff, Forensic Psychiatric Hospital; (604)524-7700; mhediger@forensic.bc.ca.

HEDLEY, David W; Univ Hlth Network-Princess M, 610 University Ave, Toronto ON M5G 2M9; Leeds (England)'70; Sr Scientist, Princess Margaret Hospital - University Health Network; Prof Med & Med Biophysics, University of Toronto; (416)946-4501 x3428; Fax. (416)946-6546; dhedley@uhnres.utoronto.ca.

HEDREI, Philip; Children's & Women's HC of BC, 4480 Oak St, Vancouver BC V6H 3V4; McG'00; FRCPC; Peds; PedEmergMed. Staff, BC Children's Hospital; (604)875-2345

HEED, Marni R; Simon Fraser Health Region, 600-22470 Dewdney Trunk Rd, Maple Ridge BC V2X 5Z6; UBC'96; FRCSC; GenSurg. (604)476-1855; Fax. (604)476-1850.

HEEDE, Santa; IWK Health Centre, PO Box 9700 Rpo CSC 5850-5980 University Ave, Halifax NS B3K 6R8; (Germany)'00; Staff, IWK Health Centre; (902)470-8731

HEEG, J Christopher; South Macleod Family Med, 100-15915 Macleod Trail SE, Calgary AB T2Y 3R9; Sask'90; CCFP; (403)457-2457; Fax. (403)457-2458.

HEELAN, John A; Queen Elizabeth II HSC, 1276 South Park St, Halifax NS B3H 2Y9; National (Ireland)'83; MB ChB; BAO; MRC; FFR; FRCPC; DiagRad (Interventional Radiology). Ac Staff, Queen Elizabeth II Health Sciences Centre - Victoria General Site; Dalhousie University; (902)473-7770; Fax. (902)473-3482.

HEELEY-RAY, Timothy; Cornwall Comm Hosp-Second St, 510 Second St E, Cornwall ON K6H 1Z6; McG'06; MDCM; FRCPC; EmergMed. Staff, Cornwall Community Hospital - Second Street Site; (613)932-3300

HEEREMA, Timothy; Hanover Med Associates, 118 7th Ave, Hanover ON N4N 2G9; Wes'05; BSc; CCFP; CCFP(E.M.); Chief FamilyMed(EM), Hanover & District Hospital; Aj Prof, University of Western Ontario; (519)364-2820; Fax. (519)364-3965.

HEESE, Heinz B; St James Street Med Clinic, 1600 Portage Ave, Winnipeg MB R3J 0C6; Sask'62; Dist Coroner, Winnipeg Area; Langs: German; (204)774-1868; Fax. (204)774-7303.

HEFFER, Matthew; St Joseph's Hlth Centre, 30 The Queensway, Toronto ON M6R 1B5; Tor'05; FRCPC; IntMed; Respir. Staff, St Joseph's Health Centre; (416)530-6043

HEFFERNAN, Mary C; Reach Community Health Centre, 1145 Commercial Dr, Vancouver BC V5L 3X3; McM'74; Ac Staff, Queen Charlotte Islands General Hospital - Queen Charlotte Site; Clin Instructor, University of British Columbia; (604)254-1354; cheffernan@reachcentre.bc.ca.

HEFFERNAN, Michael L; M Heffernan Med Prof Corp, 300-690 Dorval Dr, Oakville ON L6K 3W7; Tor'95; PhD; FRCPC; IntMed; Cardiol. Staff Cardiol, Halton Healthcare Services Corporation - Oakville Site; (905)849-4567 x3; Fax. (905)815-0299.

HEFFERNAN, Patrick A T; Brameast Family Health Org, 38-2130 North Park Dr, Brampton ON L6S 0C9; Tor'78; CCFP; FCFP; Staff, William Osler Health System - Brampton Civic Hospital; (905)792-2211; Fax. (905)792-2901.

HEFFERNAN, Paul; Quinte HC Corp-Belleville Gen, PO Box 428 Stn Main 265 Dundas St E, Belleville ON K8N 5A9; Mem'04; FRCPC; IntMed; Critical Care Medicine; Respir. Staff, QHC Belleville General; (613)969-7400

HEFFERON, Michael D; 305-275 Bagot St, Kingston ON K7L 3G4; Dublin (Ireland)'76; FRCPC; Peds (Consultant Pediatrics). Att Staff, Hotel-Dieu Hospital; Att Staff Neonatology Unit, Kingston General Hospital; Asst Prof, Queen's University; Langs: Gaelic; French; (613)549-4403; Fax. (613)549-4409.

HEFFNER, Gary I; West Oaks Med Centre, 310-32700 South Fraser Way, Abbotsford BC V2T 4M5; UBC'75; (604)557-9938; Fax. (604)557-9948.

HEFFORD, Brenda C; George Street Family Practice, 1-1400 George St, White Rock BC V4B 4A3; Mem'86; Ac Staff, Peace Arch Hospital; (604)536-1686; Fax. (604)536-6440.

HEGARTY, C Colette; Toronto Grace Hosp, 650 Church St, Toronto ON M4Y 2G5; National (Ireland)'68; FRCPC; Anes. Staff, The Salvation Army Toronto Grace Health Centre; Langs: Bilingual(English/French); (416)925-2251 x261; Fax. (416)925-9136.

HEGARTY, Raymond; St Martha's Reg Hosp, 25 Bay St, Antigonish NS B2G 2G5; National (Ireland)'60; MB ChB; MAO; MRCOG; FRCSI; ObstGyn. Staff, St Martha's Regional Hospital; (902)863-2830

HEGAZY, Nasr A E; William Osler HC-Etobicoke, 101 Humber College Blvd, Etobicoke ON M9V 1R8; Ain Shams (Egypt)'90; MB ChB; FRCPC; Anes. Staff, William Osler Health System - Etobicoke General Hospital; Langs: Arabic; (416)494-2120

HEGDE, Hardally R; Temple Med Clinic, 210-5401 Temple Dr NE, Calgary AB T1Y 3R7; Mysore (India)'70; FRCPC; Peds. (403)293-5705; Fax. (403)293-5372.

HEGDEKAR, Mona; St Boniface Gen Hosp, 409 Tache Ave, Winnipeg MB R2H 2A6; Man'93; CCFP; CCFP(E.M.); Staff, St Boniface General Hospital; (204)233-8563

HEGEDUS, Csaba; Chinook Reg Hosp, 960 19 St S, Lethbridge AB T1J 1W5; Szeged (Hungary)'75; FRCPC; AnatPath. Staff, Chinook Regional Hospital; (403)388-6628; Fax. (403)388-6067; csaba.hegedus@albertahealthservices.ca.

HEGELE, Richard G; The Hosp for Sick Children, 555 University Ave, Toronto ON M5G 1X8; Tor'84; PhD; DABPath; FRCPC; AnatPath. Staff, The Hospital For Sick Children; Chair Laboratory Med & Pathobiology, University of Toronto; (416)813-1500

HEGELE, Robert A; Robarts Research Institute, PO Box 5015 Stn B 4288-100 Perth Dr, London ON N6A 5K8; Tor'81; FACP; FRCPC; IntMed (Lipidology); Endocrin&Metab. Staff, London Health Sciences Centre - University Hospital; Teach Staff, University of Western Ontario; (519)931-5774; Fax. (519)931-5218; hegele@robarts.ca.

HEGGE, Susan G; 201-1221 Algonquin Ave, North Bay ON P1B 4Y3; Tor'94; FRCSC; GenSurg. Staff, North Bay Regional Health Centre - Regional Mental Health; (705)494-1076; Fax. (705)494-9827.

HEGGIE, Jane E; Univ Hlth Network-Toronto Gen, 200 Elizabeth St, Toronto ON M5G 2C4; Tor'86; FRCPC; Anes (Adult Congenital Heart Disease). Staff Anes, Toronto General Hospital - UHN; Lecturer Anes, University of Toronto; (416)340-3242; Fax. (416)340-3698; jane.heggie@uhn.on.ca.

HEGMANN, Erik J; Kanata Med Arts Bldg, 200-99 Kakulu Rd, Kanata ON K2L 3C8; Tor'96; MSc; BSc; CCFP; (613)592-3202; Fax. (613)592-9225; erikhegmann@hotmail.com.

HEIBER, Michael J; The Scarborough Hosp-General, 3050 Lawrence Ave E, Scarborough ON M1P 2V5; Tor'98; BSc; MSc; CCFP; CCFP(E.M.); Staff, The Scarborough Hospital - General Campus; Staff, The Scarborough Hospital - Birchmount Campus; Langs: Swedish; French; (416)431-8200

HEIBESH, Suzy G F; Princess Med Clinic, 1239A Princess Ave, Brandon MB R7A 0R2.

HEID, Robert D; Pererborough Reg HC-Hospital, 1 Hospital Dr, Peterborough ON K9J 7C6; Tor'91; FRCPC; Anes. Staff, Peterborough Regional Health Centre - Hospital Drive; (705)743-2121 x5038

HEIDARPOUR MEYMEH, Reza; Royal Victoria Hosp, 201 Georgian Dr, Barrie ON L4M 6M2; (Iran)'92; CCFP; Staff, Royal Victoria Regional Health Centre; Langs: Farsi; Fax. (705)728-9090.

HEIDENREICH, Wolfgang W F; Meadowood Med Centre, 1555 St Mary's Rd, Winnipeg MB R2M 5L9; Freiburg (Germany)'72; Langs: German; (204)255-5577; Fax. (204)254-0730.

HEIDT, Lisa K; Vernon Jubilee Hosp, 2101 32 St, Vernon BC V1T 5L2; UBC'04; CCFP; CCFP(E.M.); Staff, Vernon Jubilee Hospital; (250)558-1200

HEIER, Krista J; Stevenson Mem Hosp, PO Box 4000 Stn Main 200 Fletcher Cres, Alliston ON L9R 1W7; Wes'95; FRCPC; Anes;CCFP; Court Staff, Stevenson Memorial Hospital; (705)435-6281; Fax. (705)434-5138.

HEIKAL, Ruby S; 6-3420 Rebecca St, Oakville ON L6L 6W2; Alexandrea (Egypt)'95; MB ChB; CCFP; Langs: Arabic; (905)847-2525

HEIKKILA, Andew J; Hamilton HS-McMaster Site, PO Box 2000 Stn Lcd 1 1200 Main St W, Hamilton ON L8N 3Z5; McM'09; Staff, Hamilton Health Sciences Centre.

HEILBRON, Brett G; Burrard Med Bldg, 350-1144 Burrard St, Vancouver BC V6Z 2A5; Cape Town (South Africa)'84; MB ChB; FRCPC; IntMed (General Cardiology); Cardiol. Staff, Providence Health Care - St Paul's Hospital; University of British Columbia; (604)688-5215; Fax. (604)688-5229.

HEILBRUNN, David L; Surrey Mem Hosp, 13750 96 Ave, Surrey BC V3V 1Z2; Cape Town (South Africa)'70; MB ChB; DAB; FRCPC; Psy (Acupuncture). Staff Psy, Surrey Memorial Hospital; (604)585-5666 x2967; Fax. (604)587-3943; david.heilbrunn@fraserhealth.ca.

HEILBUT, Michele D; 41 Alvin Ave, Toronto ON M4T 2A7; Cape Town (South Africa)'75; MB ChB; DABPed; FRCPC; Cardiol (Pediatric Cardiology); Peds. Consultant, Sunnybrook Health Sciences Centre; (416)960-8012; Fax. (416)782-7965.

HEILMAN, James; East Kootenay Reg Hosp, 13 24th Ave N, Cranbrook BC V1C 3H9; Sask'03; CCFP; CCFP(E.M.); Staff, Moose Jaw Union Hospital; Staff, East Kootenay Regional Hospital; (250)426-5281

HEILPERN, Paul L; SMBD Jewish Gen Hosp, 3755 ch Cote-Sainte-Catherine, Montreal QC H3T 1E2; McG'72; DABIM; IntMed (Geriatric Medicine). Staff Geriatrics, Sir Mortimer B Davis Jewish General; adj Prof, McGill University; Langs: English; French; (514)340-7501; Fax. (514)340-7547.

HEIMANN, G Allen; Windsor-Essex County Hlth Unit, 1005 Ouellette Ave, Windsor ON N9A 4J8; Iowa(IA) (USA)'76; MHSc; (519)258-2146 x1402; Fax. (519)258-6003.

HEIMBACH, Catherine E; Southport Family Practice, 110-10333 Southport Rd SW, Calgary AB T2W 3X6; Alb'82; CCFP; FCFP; Assoc Staff, Rockyview General Hospital; (403)258-1960; Fax. (403)253-5735.

HEIN, Kent S; 1819 9 Ave S, Lethbridge AB T1J 1W6; Cal'75; FRCSC; PlasSurg (Breasts). Staff, Chinook Regional Hospital; (403)329-0600; Fax. (403)329-4686.

HEINE, John A; Suitor House, 1004 8 Ave SE, Calgary AB T2G 0M4; Ott'83; FACS; FASCRS; FRCSC; GenSurg (Colon & Rectal Surgery). Chief Division GenSurg, Peter Lougheed Centre; Clin Asst Prof of Surg, University of Calgary; Langs: French; (403)264-6720; Fax. (403)237-6646.

HEINECK, Katja; Senior People's Res in North T, 2F-140 Merton St, Toronto ON M4S 1A1; McM'09; CCFP; Staff, Women's College Hospital; Langs: German; Spanish; French; (416)481-5099; Fax. (416)481-2590.

HEINEGG, Jennifer; Ctr Hosp de Verdun, 4000 boul Lasalle, LaSalle QC H4G 2A3; Mon'06; Staff, Centre Hospitalier de Verdun; (514)362-1000

HEINRICH, Lee E; Southlake Reg Health Centre, 596 Davis Dr, Newmarket ON L3Y 2P9; Sask'93; Anes. Staff, Southlake Regional Health Centre; (905)895-4521

HEINRICHS, David A; 209-9123 Mary St, Chilliwack BC V2P 4H7; UBC'83; MSc(Biostat&Epidemiol); FRCSC; Ophth. Ac Staff, Chilliwack General Hospital; (604)792-4600; Fax. (604)792-0045.

HEINRICHS, Irvin H; Central Alberta Prof Centre, 171-5201 43 St, Red Deer AB T4N 1C7; Man'72; FRACP; FRCPC; IntMed; Neur. Staff, Red Deer Regional Hospital Centre; (403)343-7731; Fax. (403)343-7856.

HEINRICHS, Kristin; Prairie Trails at The Oaks, 2300 McPhillips St, Winnipeg MB R2V 3M3; Man'10; CCFP.

HEINTZMAN, John D; Grand River Hosp-Kw Hlth Ctre, PO Box 9056 Stn C 835 King St W, Kitchener ON N2G 1G3; Qns'93; BSc(Hon); FRCPC; Psy (Child & Adolescent Psychiatry). Staff, Grand River Hospital - Kitchener/Waterloo Health Centre; (519)749-4300 x5950

HEIR, Jatinder; Grand Manan Hosp, 196 Route 776, Grand Manan NB E5G 1A3; (India)'93; Staff, Grand Manan Hospital; (506)662-4060

HEISEY, Ruth E; Family Practice Health Centre, 77 Grenville St, Toronto ON M5S 1B3; Qns'86; CCFP; FCFP; Staff, Women's College Hospital; Clin Associate, Princess Margaret Hospital - University Health Network; Asst Prof, University of Toronto; (416)323-6060; Fax. (416)323-6345; r.heisey@utoronto.ca.

HEISLER, Benjamin E; Valley Prof Centre, 70 Exhibition St, Kentville NS B4N 4K9; Dal'95; BSc(Med); FRCSC; GenSurg; VascSurg. Consultant, Fishermen's Memorial Hospital; Staff Surg, Valley Regional Hospital; Consultant, Yarmouth Regional Hospital; (902)678-2821; Fax. (902)678-2945.

HEISLER, Owen R; Telus Plaza South, 2700-10020 100 St NW, Edmonton AB T5J 0N3; Alb'82; MD; MSc; MBA; FRCSC; GenSurg. Staff, University of Alberta Hospital; (780)969-4905; Fax. (780)424-9619; oheisler@dthr.ab.ca.

HEISLER, Ryan L; Medical Clinic Bldg, 221-89 Humber College Blvd, Etobicoke ON M9V 4B8; Qns'94; MSc; FACS; BSc(Hon); FRCSC; GenSurg. Ac Staff GenSurg, William Osler Health System - Etobicoke General Hospital; Lecturer Faculty of Med, University of Toronto; (416)746-3944; Fax. (416)746-9329.

HEISLER, Stanley H; 420-245 av Victoria, Westmount QC H3Z 2M6; McG'72; CCFP; Ac Staff, Sir Mortimer B Davis Jewish General; (514)939-9633; Fax. (514)939-7382.

HEISLER, Terry L; 10010 102A Ave NW, Edmonton AB T5J 0G5; Alb'75; CCFP; FCFP; (780)422-1302; Fax. (780)427-0777.

HEISZ, Erin M; Avon Family Med Centre, 511 Huron St, Stratford ON N5A 5T8; Wes'05; CCFP; (519)508-1212; Fax. (519)508-1240.

HEITMAN, Steven J; Peter Lougheed Centre, 3500 26 Ave NE, Calgary AB T1Y 6J4; Cal'00; MSc; FRCPC; IntMed (Therapeutic Endoscopy); Gastroent. Staff, Peter Lougheed Centre; Teach Staff Gastroenterology/Assoc Prof, University of Calgary; (403)943-2502; Fax. (403)943-4017.

HEITZNER, John D; Belmont Professional Building, 402-564 Belmont Ave W, Kitchener ON N2M 5N6; Tor'93; BSc; FRCPC; PhysMed&Rehab (Chronic Pain). (519)749-7911; Fax. (519)749-5644.

HEITZNER, Maureen C; Aurora-Newmarket Fam Hlth, 405-531 Davis Dr, Newmarket ON L3Y 6P5; Tor'89; BSc; Staff, Southlake Regional Health Centre; (905)898-2240; Fax. (905)898-2253.

HEJAZI, Banafcheh; Clin Med Avicenne, 23 rue Rachel O, Montreal QC H2W 2T1; Mon'94; CCFP; Staff, Hopital Maisonneuve-Rosemont; (514)849-7373; Fax. (514)288-4682.

HEJDANKOVA, Barbara; 400-2609 Westview Dr, North Vancouver BC V7N 4M2; Prague (Czech Republic)'86; CCFP; Clin Asst, University of British Columbia; Langs: Czech; (604)980-0012; Fax. (604)980-0063.

HEJEILY, Antoine; Hotel-Dieu de Sorel, 400 av de l'Hotel-Dieu, Sorel-Tracy QC J3P 1N5; Laval'98; FRCSC; Urol (Andrology). Staff, Hôtel-Dieu de Sorel; Langs: English; Lebanese; (450)746-6000; tonymd26@hotmail.com.

HEJJAJI, Hanna E; Trillium Hlth Ctr-Mississauga, 100 Queensway W, Mississauga ON L5B 1B8; Al Fateh (Libya)'87; FRCPC; DiagRad. Staff, Trillium Health Centre - Mississauga; Langs: Arabic; (905)848-7100 x3284; Fax. (905)848-7676.

HEKKENBERG, Rob J; Georgian Prof Centre, 203-125 Bell Farm Rd, Barrie ON L4M 6L2; Tor'92; FRCSC; Otol. Langs: Dutch; (705)726-6900; Fax. (705)725-7330.

HELDE, Michael; Hotel Dieu Grace Hosp, 1030 Ouellette Ave, Windsor ON N9A 1E1; Wes'63; FRCPC; GenPath. Staff, Hôtel-Dieu Grace Hospital; (519)973-4444; mhelde@hdgh.org.

HELDZINGER, Derek; Horizon Square Med Centre, 401-3508 32 Ave NE, Calgary AB T1Y 6J2; Stellenbosch (South Africa)'87; MB ChB; CCFP; (403)291-5599

HELEWA, Michael E; St Boniface Gen Hosp, D 2051-409 Tache Ave, Winnipeg MB R2H 2A6; American Univ of Beirut (Lebanon)'80; FACOG; FRCSC; ObstGyn (High Risk Obstetrics). Staff/Head Clin Obst Section/Med Dir Woman & Child Program, St Boniface General Hospital; Prof ObstGyn, University of Manitoba; Langs: French; Arabic; (204)237-2549; Fax. (204)233-1751; helewam@cc.umanitoba.ca.

HELFRICH, Leanne C; Lakeside Med Clinic, 3919 8th St E, Saskatoon SK S7H 5M7; Sask'94; LMCC; CCFP; (306)374-6884

HELIE, Frederic; Polyclinique St-Jerome, 305-200 rue Durand, Saint-Jerome QC J7Z 7E2; Laval'92; FRCSC; Otol. ac Membre, Hôpital de Saint-Eustache; Langs: Bilingual(English/French); (450)473-6811

HELIE, Genevieve; Centre Med Fontainebleau, 102-10 boul des Chateaux, Blainville QC J7B 1Z5; Mon'89; Staff, Hopital de la Cite de la santé; Médecin, Centre Medicale Fontainebleau; (450)419-8811; Fax. (450)419-7758.

HELLEMAN, Krista; London HSC-Victoria Hosp, PO Box 5010 Stn B 800 Commissioners Rd E, London ON N6A 5W9; Wes'98; BScN; FRCPC; Peds; PedEmergMed. Staff, London Health Sciences Centre - Victoria Campus; (519)685-8500 x13617; Fax. (519)685-8347.

HELLER, Barbara; Southwest Family Health Ctre, 307-200 James St S, Hamilton ON L8P 3A9; Wes'91; BSc(Hon); FRCSC; GenSurg (Surgical Oncology). Staff, St Joseph's Healthcare - Charlton Campus; Staff Surgical Oncologist, The Juravinski Cancer Centre; Asst Clin Prof, McMaster University; (905)526-6829; Fax. (905)526-6230.

HELLER, Brian W; 110-20611 Fraser Hwy, Langley BC V3A 4G4; Alb'75; Ac Staff, Langley Memorial Hospital; (604)534-2922; Fax. (604)534-2919.

HELLER, Martin; York-Finch Med Centre, 400-2115 Finch Ave W, North York ON M3N 2V6; McG'78; FRCSC; OrthSurg. Dep Chief Med, Humber River Regional Hospital - Finch Avenue Site; Langs: Bilingual(English/French); (416)746-7442; Fax. (416)746-3311.

HELLEUR, Katherine A; The Airfield Clinic YYC, 105A-5621 11 St NE, Calgary AB T2E 6Z7; Cal'87; CCFP; FCFP; (403)275-7705; Fax. (403)275-7701.

HELLIAR, Stephen G; Saskatoon Community Clinic, 455 2nd Ave N, Saskatoon SK S7K 2C2; Wes'75; Ac Staff, Saskatoon City Hospital; Ac Staff, St Paul's Hospital (Grey Nuns) of Saskatoon; Ac Staff, Royal University Hospital; Staff Teacher, University of Saskatchewan; (306)652-0300; Fax. (306)652-5692.

HELLIWELL, James A; St Paul's Hosp, 1081 Burrard St, Vancouver BC V6Z 1Y6; UBC'01; FRCPC; Anes. Staff, Providence Health Care - St Paul's Hospital; (604)682-2344

HELLMAN, David; PO Box 4050 Stn Yarrow Main, Chilliwack BC V2R 5H8; Man'85; FRCPC; Anes. Staff, Abbotsford Regional Hospital & Cancer Centre; (604)823-7299

HELLMAN, Karyn J; Midpark Family Med Centre, 100-290 Midpark Way SE, Calgary AB T2X 1P1; Man'92; BSc; CCFP; (403)258-2290

HELLMANN, Jonathan; The Hosp for Sick Children, 38102-555 University Ave, Toronto ON M5G 1X8; Witwatersrand (South Africa)'70; MHSc; DCH; FAAP; FRCPC; Peds (Neonatology). Clin Dir Neonatal ICU, The Hospital For Sick Children; Prof, University of Toronto; (416)813-6341; Fax. (416)813-5245; jonathan.hellmann@sickkids.ca.

HELLOU, Gisele; CHUS-Hop Fleurimont, 3001 12e av N, Sherbrooke QC J1H 5N4; Mon'79; CSPQ; FRCSC; GenSurg. Staff, Hôpital du Sacre-Coeur de Montréal; Centre Hospitalier Universitaire de Sherbrooke-Hôpital Hôtel-Dieu; Staff, Centre Hospitalier Universitaire de Sherbrooke-Hopital Fleurimont; (819)346-1110

HELLYAR, Andrew G; Dawson Creek Med Clinic, 816 103 Ave, Dawson Creek BC V1G 2G1; London (United Kingdom)'76; MB BS; (250)782-5271

HELLYER, Deborah J; Windsor Reg Hosp-Western Camp, AC 3417-1453 Prince Rd, Windsor ON N9C 3Z4; Wes'78; FRCPC; IntMed (Occupational Lung Disease); Respir. Staff, Windsor Regional Hospital - Tayfour Site; Physician, Occupational Health Clinic; (519)254-5577 x72344; dhellyer@ohcow.on.ca.

HELM, Charles W; Tumbler Ridge Med Clinic, PO Box 1690, Tumbler Ridge BC V0C 2W0; Cape Town (South Africa)'81; MB ChB; CCFP; FCFP; (250)242-4251; Fax. (250)242-4076.

HELMAN, Anton D; North York Gen Hosp, 4001 Leslie St, North York ON M2K 1E1; Ott'99; CCFP; CCFP(E.M.); FCFP; Staff, North York General Hospital; (416)756-6000

HELMER, Richard P; Valley Care Med Clinic, E-310 8th St, Courtenay BC V9N 1N3; UBC'72; (250)331-0500

HELMERSEN, Douglas S; Peter Lougheed Centre, 3500 26 Ave NE, Calgary AB T1Y 6J4; Cal'96; BSc; FRCPC; IntMed (Pulmonary Hypertention); Respir. Staff Respirol., Peter Lougheed Centre; Staff Respirol., Foothills Medical Centre; Clinical Asst Prof Med, University of Calgary; (403)943-4833; Fax. (403)943-4017; doug.helmersen@albertahealthservices.ca.

HELMI, Sanaa T H A; Grand River Hosp-KW Hlth Ctre, PO Box 9056 Stn C 835 King St W, Kitchener ON N2G 1G3; Ain Shams (Egypt)'88; FRCPC; Psy. Staff, Grand River Hospital - Kitchener/Waterloo Health Centre; Langs: Arabic; (519)749-4300; Fax. (519)749-4289.

HELMS, Johan B; The Brandon Clinic, 620 Dennis St, Brandon MB R7A 5E7; Orange Free State (South Africa)'83; FRCSC; ObstGyn. (204)728-4440

HELMS, Nelly W; Radville Marian Health Centre, PO Box 310, Radville SK S0C 2G0; Orange Free State (South Africa)'89; MB ChB; (306)869-3111; Fax. (306)869-3256.

HELOU, Hussam A; Lakeshore Gen Hosp, 160 av Stillview, Pointe-Claire QC H9R 2Y2; McG'94; BSc; CCFP; Staff, Lakeshore General Hospital - Pointe Claire; Langs: Arabic; French; (514)967-3888

HELOU, Joe; CHUM-Hotel-Dieu, 2 402-3840 Saint-Urbain, Montreal QC H2W 1T8; Ott'91; CSPQ; FRCSC; CardSurg. Staff, Centre Hospitalier l'Université de Montréal (CHUM) - Hôtel-Dieu; (514)890-8000 x15808; Fax. (514)412-7694; joe.helou.chum@ssss.gouv.qc.ca.

HELOU, Maggy; Hop du Sacre-Coeur de Mtl, 5400 boul Gouin O, Montreal QC H4J 1C5; St. Joseph (Lebanon)'75; FRCPC; IntMed. Staff, Hôpital du Sacre-Coeur de Montréal; (514)338-2050

HELOU, Tarek M; Hinton Healthcare Centre, 1280 Switzer Dr, Hinton AB T7V 1V2; UBC'02; FRCPC; DiagRad. (780)865-3333; Fax. (780)865-3134.

HELPER, Steven R M; False Creek Surgical Centre, 6F-555 8th Ave W, Vancouver BC V5Z 1C6; Man'01; FRCPC; PhysMed&Rehab (Back Pain). Physician, False Creek Surgical Centre; Clin Instructor, University of British Columbia; (604)739-9695; Fax. (604)709-9676; stevenhelper@mac.com.

HELSON, Kenneth G; Courtice Medical Imaging, 1450 Highway 2, Courtice ON L1E 3C3; Wes'56; FRCPC; DiagRad (Diagnostic Imaging). (905)721-4932

HELSZAJN, Judith; GMF de Mascouche, 100-880 Montee Masson, Mascouche QC J7K 2L7; Brussels (Belgium)'85; Staff Observation & Hospitalisation, Hopital de la Cite de la santé; Langs: English; (450)966-0324; Fax. (450)966-0156.

HELT, Bruno R; Haliburton High Hlth Serv-Mide, PO Box 30 6 McPherson St, Minden ON K0M 2K0; McM'92; CCFP; Staff, Haliburton Highlands Health Services - Miden Site; Staff, Ross Memorial Hospital; (705)286-2288; bruno@hhfht.com.

HELT, Robert P; Huronia Med Centre, PO Box 790 Stn Main 240 Old Penetang Rd, Midland ON L4R 4P4; Amsterdam (Netherlands)'84; Ac Staff, Georgian Bay General Hospital - Midland; Langs: Dutch; (705)526-4033; Fax. (705)526-5565.

HELYAR, Richard G; 306-77 Westmount Rd, Guelph ON N1H 5J1; McM'96; CCFP; FCFP; Staff, Guelph General Hospital; Asst Prof, McMaster University; (519)827-1399; Fax. (519)827-1858.

HELYER, Lucy K; Queen Elizabeth II HSC, 809 CB-1276 South Park St, Halifax NS B3H 2Y9; Dal'98; FRCSC; GenSurg; General Surgical Oncology. Staff, Queen Elizabeth II Health Sciences Centre - Victoria General Site; (902)473-1887; Fax. (902)429-3313.

HEMA, Karumpuzha; Western Memorial Health Clinic, 3 Herald Ave, Corner Brook NL A2H 4B8; Madras (India)'82; MB BS; FRCSC; ObstGyn. Staff, Western Memorial Regional Hospital; Staff, Sir Thomas Roddick Hospital; (709)637-3900 x3900; Fax. (709)634-9572.

HEMANI, Razi; Yarmouth Reg Hosp, 60 Vancouver St, Yarmouth NS B5A 2P5; (Pakistan)'92; MB BS; Staff, Yarmouth Regional Hospital; (902)742-3541

HEMANS, Clover A; Halton HSC Corp-Oakville, 327 Reynolds St, Oakville ON L6J 3L7; McM'88; CCFP; FCFP; Staff, Halton Healthcare Services Corporation - Oakville Site; (905)845-2571

HEMBROFF, Tristan; Foothills Family Med Centre, PO Box 460 114 1 St SW, Black Diamond AB T0L 0H0; Sask'06; BSc; CCFP; Staff, Oilfields General Hospital; (403)933-4368; Fax. (403)933-2026; tristan.hembroff@albertahealthservices.ca.

HEMENS, William D; South Muskoka Mem Hosp, 75 Ann St, Bracebridge ON P1L 2E4; Mon'84; CCFP; FCFP; Staff Emerg Med, South Muskoka Memorial Hospital - Muskoka Algonquin Healthcare; (705)645-4400 x121

HEMINGS, David J; Riverside South Med Centre, 665C Earl Armstrong Rd, Gloucester ON K1V 2G2; St. Andrews (Scotland)'64; MB ChB; (613)822-0411; hemings@kingston.net.

HEMMELGARN, Brenda; Foothills Med Centre, 1403 29 St NW, Calgary AB T2N 2T9; McM'98; FRCPC; IntMed; Nephrol. Staff, Foothills Medical Centre; (403)944-2745; Fax. (403)944-2876.

HEMMERICH, David; CFB Comox, PO Box 1000 Stn Main 19 Wing Comox, Lazo BC V0R 2K0; Cal'89; Staff Flight Surgeon, CFB Comox; (250)339-8267

HEMMERICH, Eva E; Sea Cove Med Clinic, 201-1757 Beaufort Ave, Comox BC V9M 1R8; Mem'89; CCFP; Langs: Swedish; (250)339-5335; Fax. (250)339-1898.

HEMMERLING, Thomas M; MUHC-Montreal Gen Hosp, 1650 av Cedar, Montreal QC H3G 1A4; Saarland (Germany)'91; Anes (P.Q.). Staff, McGill University Health Centre - Montreal General Campus; (514)934-1934

HEMMING, Anthony R; Peace Arch Hosp, 15521 Russell Ave, White Rock BC V4B 2R4; UBC'86; FRCPC; Anes. Staff, Peace Arch Hospital; (604)531-5512 x7910

HEMMINGS, Christian; Comm des lesions Professionnel, 17401-500 boul Rene-Levesque O, Montreal QC H2Z 1W7; Mon'81; Langs: English; (514)873-1593; christian.hemmings@clp.gouv.qc.ca.

HEMMINGS, Robert; Clin Med La Cite, 500-300 rue Leo Pariseau, Montreal QC H2X 4B3; Sher'77; FRCSC; ObstGyn. Ac Staff, St Mary's Hospital Centre; Langs: English; French; (514)343-0636; Fax. (514)343-0530.

HEMOND, Claude; Clin Medicale de Bromptonville, 201-103 rue Saint-Lambert, Sherbrooke QC J1C 0N8; Sher'80; CCFP; FCFP; Ac Staff, Centre Hospitalier Universitaire de Sherbrooke-Hôpital Hôtel-Dieu; (819)846-2811; Fax. (819)846-0594.

HEMPHILL, Douglas J; Barrie GI Associates, 301-5 Quarry Ridge Rd, Barrie ON L4M 7G1; McM'89; BSc(Hon); FRCPC; IntMed; Gastroent. Med Staff, Royal Victoria Regional Health Centre; Clin Dir, Barrie GI Associates; (705)721-3344; Fax. (705)721-5522.

HEMY, Melissa D; Group Health Centre, 240 McNabb St, Sault Ste. Marie ON P6B 1Y5; Tor'07; CCFP; (705)759-1234

HENBEST, Ronald; Souris Hosp Inc, PO Box 640, Souris PE C0A 2B0; Alb'78; MClSc; CCFP; FCFP; Staff, Souris Hospital Inc; (902)687-7150

HENDEL, Mary-Jane; Queen Street Diagnostic Imagin, 200-514 Queen St, Saskatoon SK S7K 0M5; Cardiff (Wales)'82; MB ChB; FRCPC; DiagRad (Diagnostic Imaging). Staff, Royal University Hospital; Clin Asst, University of Saskatchewan; (306)664-3200; Fax. (306)664-0032.

HENDEL, Raymond; 257 Larch St, Sudbury ON P3B 1M2; UBC'79; GenSurg; PlasSurg. Staff, Health Sciences North-St Joseph's Health Centre; Staff, Northeastern Ontario Regional Cancer Centre; Langs: English; French; (705)674-9677; Fax. (705)674-6353.

HENDER, Kimberley J; Queen Elizabeth Hosp, PO Box 6600 Stn Central 60 Riverside Dr, Charlottetown PE C1A 8T5; Dal'89; FRCPC; DiagRad. Staff, Queen Elizabeth Hospital; (902)894-2111

HENDERSON, Allison M; 350-2755 Lougheed Hwy, Port Coquitlam BC V3B 5Y9; Wes'10; CCFP; (604)941-8366

HENDERSON, Ann E; 2F-117 Cedar St, Sudbury ON P3E 1A9; McG'81; CCFP; FCFP; (705)673-6353; Fax. (705)673-7935.

HENDERSON, Blair T; Medical Arts Bldg, 202-233 Kennedy St, Winnipeg MB R3C 3J5; Man'99; FRCPC; DiagRad.

HENDERSON, Cynthia L; 2922 3rd Ave W, Vancouver BC V6K 1M7; Wes'86; FRCPC; Anes (Hyperbaric Medicine). Staff Anes, Vancouver General Hospital - Centennial Pavillion; Clin Assoc Prof, University of British Columbia; (604)737-1883; Fax. (604)875-5209; cynthia.henderson@vch.ca.

HENDERSON, David L; Victoria Gen Hosp, 1 Hospital Way, Victoria BC V8Z 6R5; Dal'73; MPH; FAB(Occ); Staff, Victoria General Hospital; (250)727-4212

HENDERSON, David M; Surrey North Comm Hlth Centre, PO Box 500 Stn Main, Surrey BC V3T 5B7; UBC'90; Staff, Vancouver Native Health Society.

HENDERSON, Donald R; Port Arthur Health Centre Inc, 194 Court St N, Thunder Bay ON P7A 4V7; Tor'63; BSc; DMRD; FRCPC; DiagRad (Diagnostic Imaging). Staff, Thunder Bay Regional Health Sciences Centre; (807)345-5728; donhend@tbaytel.net.

HENDERSON, Douglas M; Chelsea House Fam Med Group, 33623 Wildwood Dr, Abbotsford BC V2S 1S2; Edinburgh (Scotland)'70; (604)853-4377; Fax. (604)853-2626.

HENDERSON, Garry; Wellpoint Health, 103-2025 Broadway W, Vancouver BC V6J 1Z6; Glasgow (Scotland)'81; MB ChB; DRCOG(UK); MRCGPract(UK); Physician Emerg Room, Mission Memorial Hospital; (604)730-9769; Fax. (604)730-0110.

HENDERSON, Gordon T; 1-2379 Bevan Ave, Sidney BC V8L 4M9; Qns'90; (250)656-4143; Fax. (250)656-9285.

HENDERSON, J David; Colchester East Hants Hlth Ctr, 601 Abenaki Rd, Truro NS B2N 5A1; Mem'91; CCFP; FCFP; Staff/Med Dir Palliative Care, Colchester East Hants Health Centre; (902)893-5554; Fax. (902)893-7781.

HENDERSON, James M; Fredericton Med Clinic, 407-1015 Regent St, Fredericton NB E3B 6H5; Ott'75; Rheum. Pres, Canadian Rheumatology Associatioin; Lecturer, Dalhousie University; Langs: Bilingual(English/French); (506)458-0324; Fax. (506)457-4754.

HENDERSON, Jane M; Queen Elizabeth II HSC-Halifax, 1796 Summer St, Halifax NS B3H 2Y9; Dal'82; FRCPC; Anes. Staff, Queen Elizabeth II Health Sciences Centre - Victoria General Site; (902)473-4326

HENDERSON, John E S; Allin Clinic, 10155 120 St NW, Edmonton AB T5K 2A2; Alb'75; (780)482-7551; Fax. (780)482-3533; jeshenderson@shaw.ca.

HENDERSON, John; Pleasant Street Med Clinic, PO Box 11 6-250 Pleasant St, Miramichi NB E1V 1Y5; Mem'97; CCFP; FCFP; Member, Horizon Health Network Corporate Office; (506)622-8908; Fax. (506)622-6566.

HENDERSON, Julie L; 60 White Squirrel Way, Toronto ON M6J 1H4; Dal'05; FRCPC; Psy. Staff, Centre for Addiction & Mental Health (CAMH) - Queen Site; (416)535-8501

HENDERSON, K Muriel; 802-1243 Islington Ave, Etobicoke ON M8X 1Y9; Tor'68; Court Staff, Women's College Hospital; Court Staff, St Michael's Hospital; (416)767-9289; Fax. (416)767-5276.

HENDERSON, Kenneth J; Dr Charles A Janeway Child HC, 300 Prince Philip Dr, St. John's NL A1B 3V6; Dal'72; FRCPC; Peds. Ac Staff, Dr Everett Chalmers Regional Hospital; Staff, Janeway Children's Health & Rehabilitation Centre; Langs: English; French; (709)777-4222

HENDERSON, Laura J W; 1424 Commercial Dr PO Box 21565 Rpo Little Italy, Vancouver BC V5L 5G2; Tor'08; CCFP; (604)255-6565

HENDERSON, Lemay E; 125A Mind Longevity Ctr Inc, 557-1030 Denman St, Vancouver BC V6G 2M6; Cal'92; CCFP; (604)685-2469

HENDERSON, M Melanie; 27-1020 av des Pins O, Montreal QC H3A 1A2; McG'99; FRCPC; Peds; Endocrin&Metab. Staff, Hôpital Ste-Justine.

HENDERSON, Mark; Curans Health Centre, 384 Fort William Rd, Thunder Bay ON P7B 2Z3; London (England)'75; MB BS; FRCPC; Cardiol. Staff, Thunder Bay Regional Health Sciences Centre; (807)345-3355; Fax. (807)345-0099.

HENDERSON, Nadene D; Kirkland & District Hosp, 145 Government Rd W, Kirkland Lake ON P2N 2E8; UBC'97; CCFP; FCFP; Staff, Kirkland & District Hospital; (705)568-2138

HENDERSON, Richard J; Jensen Med Clinic, PO Box 1141 Stn Main 135 Jensen Ave E, Parksville BC V9P 2H2; Queensland (Australia)'79; MB BS; (250)248-6969; Fax. (250)248-4275.

HENDERSON, Robert J; 700 Main St E, Hamilton ON L8M 1K7; Tor'76; CCFP; FCFP; (905)547-3901; Fax. (905)547-4051.

HENDERSON, Robert W; Trent Hills Family Health Team, 119 Isabella St, Campbellford ON K0L 1L0; Man'73; CCFP; FCFP; Staff, Campbellford Memorial Hospital; Asst Prof Family Med, University of Toronto; (705)653-1801; Fax. (705)653-5483.

HENDERSON, Ronald L; Meadowlark Health Centre, 166 Meadowlark Shopping Ctr NW, Edmonton AB T5R 5W9; Alb'83; FRCSC; OrthSurg (Spine). Staff, Covenant Health - Misericordia Community Hospital; University of Alberta; (780)483-0283; Fax. (780)486-1739.

HENDERSON, Rosemary; Queen Elizabeth Hosp, PO Box 6600 Stn Central 60 Riverside Dr, Charlottetown PE C1A 8T5; Dal'82; FRCPC; GenPath., Queen Elizabeth Hospital; (902)894-2411; Fax. (902)894-2385.

HENDERSON, Sylvia; Delta Health Sciences Centre, 202-4515 Harvest Dr, Delta BC V4K 4L1; UBC'81; BSc(Hons); MSc(Math); CCFP; FCFP; Med Staff, Vancouver General Hospital - Centennial Pavillion; Med Staff, Richmond Hospital; Med Staff, Delta Hospital; Physician, Delta Health Sciences Centre; Fellow, Canadian College of Family Practice; Clin Assoc Prof Family Pract, University of British Columbia; (604)946-6411; Fax. (604)946-0372.

HENDERSON, Tamara A; Kingston Gen Hosp, 76 Stuart St, Kingston ON K7L 2V7; Qns'04; FRCPC; Anes. Staff, Kingston General Hospital; Langs: Bilingual(English/French); (613)549-6666

HENDERSON, William R; Dr W R Henderson Prof Corp, 503-1015 Regent St, Fredericton NB E3B 6H5; Dal'75; DABOT; CCFP; Staff, Dr Everett Chalmers Regional Hospital; (506)459-4898; Fax. (506)452-0814.

HENDERSON, William R; Vancouver Gen Hosp, 2438-855 12th Ave W, Vancouver BC V5Z 1M9; UBC'97; Critical Care Medicine; EmergMed. Staff, Vancouver General Hospital - Centennial Pavillion; (604)875-5949

HENDERSON, Winston B; 300-4309 52 Ave, Red Deer AB T4N 6S4; Man'99; FRCSC; OrthSurg (Foot & Ankle Surgery). Staff, Central Zone David Thompson Health Region; (403)309-2001

HENDLER, Aaron L; Univ Hlth Network-Toronto Gen, ES1 416-200 Elizabeth St, Toronto ON M5G 2C4; McG'84; FRCPC; IntMed; NuclearMed; DiagRad. Staff, Toronto General Hospital - UHN; (416)340-4489; Fax. (416)340-4198.

HENDRICK, A Corbin; Alliston Family Physicians, 40-180 Parsons Rd, Alliston ON L9R 1E8; Tor'78; CCFP; FCFP; Ac Staff, Stevenson Memorial Hospital; (705)435-5633; Fax. (705)435-2860; corbin.hendrick@sympatico.ca.

HENDRICK-HALLET, Julie; 2801-10 Yonge St, Toronto ON M5E 1R4; Laval'06; FRCPC; GenSurg. Sec-trés, Centre Hospitalier Universitaire De Québec - Pavillon De St-françois-d'assise; (416)737-6679

HENDRICKSON, Donna V; Knox Manse, 505 4th Ave N, Saskatoon SK S7K 2M5; Sask'86; FRCPC; Psy (Psychological Sexual Disorders). (306)665-0505; Fax. (306)668-0507.

HENDRIE, Douglas S; 353 St Paul Ave, Brantford ON N3R 4N3; Wes'78; FRCPC; DiagRad. Ac Staff Radiol, The Brant Community Healthcare System - Brantford General Hospital Site; (519)759-6089

HENDRIE, Peter M; Guelph Family Health Team, 207-55 Wyndham St N, Guelph ON N1H 7T8; Wes'75; CCFP; FCFP; Ac Staff, Guelph General Hospital; (519)836-1455; Fax. (519)836-1321.

HENDRIKS, J A Edouard; Horizan Health Network, B-155 Pleasant St, Miramichi NB E1V 1Y3; Laval'78; MHA; CCFP; CCFP(E.M.); FCFP; Vice Pres Medical Academic Affairs, Horizon Health Network Corporate Office; Langs: Bilingual(French/English); (506)623-5527; Fax. (506)623-5534; edouard.hendricks@horizonnb.ca.

HENDRIKS, Johannes; 316 8th Ave PO Box 700 Stn Main, Brooks AB T1R 1B6; Stellenbosch (South Africa)'01; Staff Family ER & Obst, Brooks Health Centre; (403)793-8883

HENDRIKS, Rene; Centre Med Racine Sainte-Foy, 102-2880 ch des Quatre-Bourgeo, Quebec QC G1V 4X7; Laval'87; Langs: English; (418)657-6363; Fax. (418)657-6898.

HENDRIKS, William L J; Wetaskiwin Fam Med Practice, 5107 50 St, Wetaskiwin AB T9A 1K1; Ott'87; CCFP; FCFP; (780)352-3010; Fax. (780)352-7413.

HENDRY, Graeme A; 91 Cornelia St W, Smiths Falls ON K7A 5L3; McG'90; CCFP; FCFP; Staff, Perth & Smiths Falls District Hospital - Smiths Falls Site; Langs: Bilingual(English/French); (613)283-1149; Fax. (613)283-9730.

HENDRY, James N; Canmore Gen Hosp, 1100 Hospital Pl, Canmore AB T1W 1N2; Qns'90; CCFP; CCFP(E.M.); Staff, Canmore General Hospital; (403)678-7214

HENDRY, Jerrod; Peace Arch Hosp, 15521 Russell Ave, White Rock BC V4B 2R4; UBC'01; BSc; MSc; MD; CCFP; CCFP(E.M.); Staff, Peace Arch Hospital; Staff, UBC Hospital - Koerner Pavillion; (604)531-5512

HENDRY, Khati L; Rosedale Med Associates, PO Box 460 13009 Rosedale Ave, Summerland BC V0H 1Z0; San Francisco(CA) (USA)'77; CCFP; Langs: Spanish; (250)404-4242

HENDRY, Paul J; Univ of Ottawa Heart Institute, 3404 B-40 Ruskin St, Ottawa ON K1Y 4W7; Ott'81; AB; MSc; FRCSC; GenSurg (Cardiac Surgery); Cardiovasc&ThorSurg. Staff, University of Ottawa Heart Institute; Ac Staff, The Ottawa Hospital - General Campus; Vice Dean Continuing Med Educ, University of Ottawa; (613)761-5001; Fax. (613)761-4388.

HENDSON, Glenda; BC Women's Hosp & Health Ctre, 4500 Oak St, Vancouver BC V6H 3N1; Witwatersrand (South Africa)'86; MB BCh; FRCPC; AnatPath (General Pathology). Staff, BC Women's Hospital & Health Centre; (604)875-3554; Fax. (604)875-3529.

HENDSON, Leonora; Royal Alexandra Hosp, DTC 5027-10240 Kingsway NW, Edmonton AB T5H 3V9; Witwatersrand (South Africa)'92; FRCPC; Peds (Neurology). Staff, Royal Alexandra Hospital; (780)735-4670; Fax. (780)735-4072.

HENDY, Ayman; Queen Elizabeth II HSC-Halifax, 5452-1796 Summer St, Halifax NS B3H 3A7; Cairo (Egypt)'93; MB BCh; FRCPC; Anes. Staff, Queen Elizabeth II Health Sciences Centre - Halifax Infirmary Site; (902)473-2700

HENDY, Ramez H M; Univ of Ottawa, 2115-451 Smyth Rd, Ottawa ON K1H 8M5; Ain Shams (Egypt)'96; Anes. Staff, University of Ottawa.

HENEGAN, Charles P; 3945 17 Ave SW, Calgary AB T3E 0C3; (South Africa)'01; MB ChB; (403)242-8633; chenegan50@hotmail.com.

HENEGHAN, Paul D; 206 LeMarchant Rd, St. John's NL A1C 2H6; Mem'89; FRCSC; GenSurg; VascSurg. Staff, Health Sciences Centre.

HENEIN, Emad; AIM Health Group, 320 Adelaide St S, London ON N5Z 3L2; Alexandria (Egypt)'91; CCFP; Langs: Arabic; (519)668-3969

HENEIN, John; River Oaks Med Clinic, A3-2163 Sixth Line, Oakville ON L6H 3N7; Ain Shams (Egypt)'99; MB ChB; CCFP; Ac Staff, Halton Healthcare Services Corporation - Oakville Site; Langs: Arabic; (905)582-5030; Fax. (905)582-5133.

HENEIN, Sam; York Prof Bldg, 221-679 Davis Dr, Newmarket ON L3Y 5G8; Tor'80; Asst Prof Fam Med, Queen's University; Asst Prof Fam Med, McMaster University; (905)898-2931; Fax. (905)898-0983.

HENEMAN, Anaïs; Clinique Med du Sud-Ouest, 4475 rue Bannantyne, LaSalle QC H4G 1E2; Mon'08; (514)765-3600

HENEN, Manal F Y; McKnight Village Medical, 5486 Falsbridge Dr NE, Calgary AB T3J 5H4; (Egypt)'84; MB BCh; (403)280-2272; Fax. (403)280-2268.

HENEN, Raafat; 203-1585 Markham Rd, Scarborough ON M1B 2W1; Ain Shams (Egypt)'91; FRCSC; Ophth. Langs: Arabic; French; (416)284-0289; Fax. (416)284-7594.

HENG, Daniel Y C; Tom Baker Cancer Centre, 1331 29 St NW, Calgary AB T2N 4N2; Cal'02; FRCPC; IntMed (Genito Urinary Cancers); MedOncol. Staff, Tom Baker Cancer Centre; (403)521-3166; Fax. (403)283-1651.

HENG, Marilyn M; Mount Sinai Hosp, 4761-600 University Ave, Toronto ON M5G 1X5; Tor'07; FRCSC; OrthSurg. Staff, Mount Sinai Hospital; (416)586-4800

HENIN, Catherine Y; MUHC-Montreal Children's Hosp, F134 4-2300 rue Tupper, Montreal QC H3H 1P3; Qns'00; FRCPC; Peds. Staff, McGill University Health Centre - Montreal Children's Hospital; (514)412-4400

HENIS, Mohsen; Bonis-Birchmount Med Clinic, 5 Bonis Ave, Scarborough ON M1T 2T9; Asiyut (Egypt)'81; CCFP; Langs: Arabic; (416)335-0077; Fax. (416)335-9277.

HENLEY, Jeanette L; 202-3005 30 St, Vernon BC V1T 9J5; Manchester (United Kingdom)'85; MB ChB; (250)542-1353

HENLEY, Peter A; 202-3005 30 St, Vernon BC V1T 9J5; Manchester (United Kingdom)'94; MB ChB; (250)542-1353

HENNEBERRY, Ryan; Queen Elizabeth II HSC-Halifax, 355-1796 Summer St, Halifax NS B3H 3A7; Dal'01; CCFP; CCFP(E.M.); Staff, Queen Elizabeth II Health Sciences Centre - Halifax Infirmary Site; (902)473-8769; Fax. (902)473-3617.

HENNEN, Brian K E; Abbie J Lane Mem Bldg, 5909 Veterans Memorial Lane, Halifax NS B3H 2E2; Qns'62; CCFP; FCFP; (902)473-8548

HENNENFENT, Brett W; 78 Masons Beach Rd PO Box 1617, Lunenburg NS B0J 2C0; Cal'92; (902)634-1951; Fax. (902)634-3522.

HENNES, Claire Sadek; Dr Noor's Medical Centre, 14-10088 Mclaughlin Rd, Brampton ON L7A 2X6; Ain Shams (Egypt)'82; MB ChB; CCFP; Langs: Arabic; French; (905)495-9040

HENNESSEY, Katherine K; 650-6091 Gilbert Rd, Richmond BC V7C 5L9; UBC'06; FRCSC; Urol. (604)273-4320

HENNESSEY, Trevor; CSSSG-Hop de Gatineau, CP 2000 Succ Bureau-Chef 909 boul de la Verendrye O, Gatineau QC J8P 7H2; UBC'04; FRCPC; Anes. Staff, Hôpital de Gatineau; (819)966-6100

HENNESSY, Anne D M; Medical Expertise Division CPP, 333 North River Rd, Ottawa ON K1A 0L1; Dublin (Ireland)'79; FRCPC; Psy (Geriatric Psychiatry). (613)952-3622

HENNESSY, Colleen; Victoria Med Bldg, 303-1669 Victoria St, Prince George BC V2L 2L5; Dal'86; DABIM; BSc(Hon)(Hon); FRCPC; IntMed (Cardiology). Staff, UBC Hospital - Koerner Pavillion; Clinical Asst Prof, University of British Columbia; Assoc Prof, University of Northern British Columbia; (250)563-9995

HENNIG, Kevin R; Oliver Eye Centre, 11652 104 Ave NW, Edmonton AB T5K 2T7; Alb'89; FRCSC; Ophth. Staff, Royal Alexandra Hospital; Asst Clin Prof, University of Alberta; (780)488-5600; Fax. (780)488-5682.

HENNIG, Ronald C; Cross Cancer Institute, 11560 University Ave NW, Edmonton AB T6G 1Z2; Alb'79; BMedSci; ABR; FRCPC; DiagRad. Staff Radiol., Cross Cancer Institute; Clin Prof, University of Alberta; (780)432-8771; Fax. (780)451-2891.

HENNING, Beth M; London Medical-Dental Bldg, 102-450 Central Ave, London ON N6B 2E8; Cal'81; MPH; AB; CCFP; Med Officer of Hlth, Huron Country Health Unit; (519)672-1421; bhenning@quadro.net.

HENNING, Christopher; First Care Med Centre, 2590 Commercial Dr, Vancouver BC V5N 4C2; Wes'93; CCFP; Staff, Grey Bruce Health Services - Owen Sound; (604)871-1535

HENNING, Hartmut; Gordon & Leslie Diamond HCC, 9F-2775 Laurel St, Vancouver BC V5Z 1M9; Munich (Germany)'64; CRCP; FACC; PhD; IntMed (Cardiology). Assoc Prof Med, Vancouver General Hospital - Centennial Pavillion; Assoc Prof Med, University of British Columbia; Langs: German; (604)875-4540; Fax. (604)875-4642; hhenning@mail.ubc.ca.

HENNING, Jan L; Grey Bruce HS-Owen Sound, PO Box 1800 Stn Main 5116-1800 8th St E, Owen Sound ON N4K 6M9; Pretoria (South Africa)'83; MB ChB; MMed(Ortho); FRCSC; OrthSurg (Orthopedics). Staff, Grey Bruce Health Services - Owen Sound; Langs: Afrikaans; (519)376-6066; Fax. (519)376-3446.

HENNING, Jan-Willem; Tom Baker Cancer Centre, 1331 29 St NW, Calgary AB T2N 4N2; Orange Free State (South Africa)'99; MB ChB; FRCPC; IntMed; MedOncol. Staff, Tom Baker Cancer Centre; Langs: Afrikaans; (403)944-1110

HENNING, Slavica; 10211 149 Ave, Edmonton AB T5E 2M4; (Other Foreign)'87.

HENNINK, Maurice H J; Regina Mental Health Clinic, 2110 Hamilton St, Regina SK S4P 2E3; Stellenbosch (South Africa)'81; MB ChB; MMed(ComHealth); Langs: Afrikaans; Dutch; (306)766-7772; Fax. (306)766-7607.

HENRI, Manon; Hotel-Dieu D'Arthabaska, 5 rue des Hospitalieres, Victoriaville QC G6P 6N2; Laval'99; Staff, Hotel-Dieu d'Arthabaska; (819)357-2030 x2059

HENRI, Marcel; CRSSS Baie-James-Chibougamau, 51 3e rue, Chibougamau QC G8P 1N1; Mon'79; ac Staff, CRSSS de la Baie-James; (418)748-2676

HENRI, Margaret; Hop Maisonneuve-Rosemont, 5415 boul de l'Assomption, Montreal QC H1T 2M4; Mon'96; CSPQ; FRCSC; GenSurg. Staff, Hopital Maisonneuve-Rosemont; (514)252-3400

HENRI, Richard; Hop du Sacre-Coeur de Mtl, 5400 boul Gouin O, Montreal QC H4J 1C5; Mon'74; CSPQ; FRCPC; Anes (Pain Control). Staff Anes, CRSSS de la Baie-James; Staff, Hôpital du Sacre-Coeur de Montréal; Langs: English; Spanish; (514)338-2222 x2680; Fax. (514)338-2009.

HENRI-BHARGAVA, Alexandre R; Baycrest Ctre/Geriatric Care, 644-3560 Bathurst St, North York ON M6A 2E1; McG'04; FRCPC; Neur (Behavioural Neurology). Staff, Baycrest Centre for Geriatric Care; Staff, Toronto East General Hospital Inc; Langs: Spanish; French; (416)785-4294; Fax. (416)785-2484.

HENRIKSON, Donna G; Albany Med Clinic, 807 Broadview Ave, Toronto ON M4K 2P8; Man'85; Langs: English; French; (416)461-9471; Fax. (416)461-2710.

HENRIQUES, Tania R; H-960 Cumberland Ave, Burlington ON L7N 3J6; McM'06; FRCPC; PhysMed&Rehab. (905)681-7577; Fax. (905)681-0855.

HENRY, Alison; 45779 Luckackuck Way, Chilliwack BC V2R 0G8; Ott'07; CCFP; Staff, Chilliwack General Hospital; (604)858-5544

HENRY, Alison; Workers' Comp Board, 110-2045 Enterprise Way, Kelowna BC V1Y 9T5; Cape Town (South Africa)'89; MB ChB; CCFP; (250)979-4161

HENRY, Bonnie J F; BC Centre for Disease Control, 2104-655 12th Ave W, Vancouver BC V5Z 4R4; Dal'90; FACPrevMed; MPH; FRCPC; CommunMed (Infectious Diseases). Asst Prof, University of British Columbia; (604)660-1823

HENRY, Caroline; Ctr Hosp de Verdun, 4000 boul Lasalle, Verdun QC H4G 2A3; Mon'07; CCFP; Staff, Centre Hospitalier de Verdun; (514)362-1000

HENRY, David A; Glenridge Med Bldg, 203-1 Belton Blvd, St Catharines ON L2T 3Y4; (Jamaica)'67; (905)682-7776; Fax. (905)682-9908.

HENRY, David G; Niagara HS-Douglas Mem Site, 238 Bertie St, Fort Erie ON L2A 1Z3; Wes'69; Ac Staff, Niagara Health System - Douglas Memorial Hospital Site; (905)871-6622; Fax. (905)871-1221.

HENRY, Douglas; Parkview Professional Centre, 102-2110 Main St, Winnipeg MB R2V 2C2; Man'02; CCFP.

HENRY, Elizabeth A; North Vancouver Med Clinic, 115 16th St, North Vancouver BC V7M 1T3; UBC'90; BSc; MSc; CCFP; (604)904-8804

HENRY, Eric L; Kilborn Med Centre, 215-1385 Bank St, Ottawa ON K1H 8N4; Ott'02; FRCSC; Otol. (613)562-9000; Fax. (613)562-9898.

HENRY, J Paul; Health Care VIRCC, 4216 Wilkinson Rd, Victoria BC V8Z 5B2; Wes'72; Assoc Staff, Royal Jubilee Hospital; Assoc Staff, Victoria General Hospital; (250)953-4409

HENRY, James A C; 204-245 Pelham Rd, St Catharines ON L2S 1X8; Tor'84; (905)688-1224; Fax. (905)688-9249.

HENRY, Louise; Regie des Rentes du Quebec, CP 5200 Succ Terminus, Quebec QC G1K 7S9; Mon'89; Médecin, Regie des Rentes du Quebec; (418)657-8709 x4716

HENRY, Mary A; 910-515 St Laurent Blvd, Ottawa ON K1K 3X5; McM'82; CCFP; CCFP(E.M.); (613)234-4683; Fax. (613)842-8188.

HENRY, Michael M; North Toronto Med Bldg, 203-250 Lawrence Ave W, Toronto ON M5M 1B2; Tor'71; DABOph; FAAO; FRCSC; Ophth. Chief Ophth, North York General Hospital; (416)787-1121; Fax. (416)787-4778; mm.henry@rogers.com.

HENRY, Monica M; Misericordia Comm Hosp & H C, 16940 87 Ave NW, Edmonton AB T5R 4H5; Dal'95; FRCPC; IntMed; Critical Care Medicine. Staff Neurosurgical ICU, University of Alberta Hospital; Staff Intensive Care Unit, Covenant Health - Misericordia Community Hospital; (780)735-2858; Fax. (780)735-2953.

HENRY, Patrick D G; 800-55 Queen St E, Toronto ON M5C 1R6; Sydney (Australia)'04.

HENRY, Pauline C L; Toronto East Gen & Orth Hosp, 825 Coxwell Ave, Toronto ON M4C 3E7; Tor'05; FRCPC; AnatPath. Staff, Toronto East General Hospital Inc; (416)469-6580

HENRY, Rachel; Forensic Outreach Prog, 200-1164 devonshire Ave, North Bay ON P1B 6X7; Cal'02; FRCPC; Psy. Staff, North Bay Regional Health Centre - Regional Mental Health; (705)474-5885; Fax. (705)495-7823.

HENRY, Richard; Kingston Gen Hosp, 76 Stuart St, Kingston ON K7L 2V7; Cape Town (South Africa)'81; MB ChB; FRCPC; Anes (Pain Management). Staff Anes, Hotel-Dieu Hospital; Staff Anes, Kingston General Hospital; Med Dir, Richard Henry Pain Managment; Asst Prof Anes, Queen's University; (613)548-7827; Fax. (613)548-1375.

HENRY, Sean; Royal Jubilee Hosp, 1900 Fort St, Victoria BC V8R 1J8; Wes'90; CCFP; CCFP(E.M.); Staff, Royal Jubilee Hospital; (250)370-8000

HENRY, Stephen F; Concordia Gen Hosp, 1095 Concordia Ave, Winnipeg MB R2K 3S8; Man'87; BSc; FRCPC; IntMed; Nephrol., Concordia General Hospital; Asst Prof, University of Manitoba; (204)667-1560

HENRY, Tracy; Sudbury Reg Hosp-Laurentian, 41 Ramsey Lake Rd, Sudbury ON P3E 5J1; Tor'95; CCFP; Staff, Health Sciences North-Laurentian Site; (705)523-7100

HENRY, Willa J; UBC Family Med Clinic, 300-5950 University Blvd, Vancouver BC V6T 1Z3; McM'83; CCFP; FCFP; Teach Staff, University of British Columbia; (604)822-6811

HENRY EBEID, Jacqueline; Centre Medical Samson, 202-4599 boul Samson, Laval QC H7W 2H2; Alexandria (Egypt)'77; CCFP; (450)688-7170

HENRY-GANESH, Brenda P; Guelph Family Health Team, 207-55 Wyndham St N, Guelph ON N1H 7T8; Tor'81; CCFP; Staff, Guelph General Hospital; (519)836-1455; Fax. (519)836-1321.

HENSON, John; 105-348 Bagot St, Kingston ON K7K 3B7; Qns'80; FRCSC; GenSurg (Surgical Oncology). Ac Staff Surg, Hotel-Dieu Hospital; Ac Staff Surg, Kingston General Hospital; Assoc Lecturer, Queen's University; (613)544-9797; Fax. (613)544-8590.

HENSTOCK, Hendrik D; Golden Ears Fam Pract & Walk-I, 140-20395 Lougheed Hwy, Maple Ridge BC V2X 2P9; Stellenbosch (South Africa)'82; MB ChB; Langs: Afrikaans; (604)465-1066; Fax. (604)465-7776.

HENSTRIDGE, David G; West Nipissing Gen Hosp, 725 Coursol Rd, Sturgeon Falls ON P2B 2Y6; Mem'77; BMedSci; CCFP; CCFP(E.M.); Staff EmergMed, North Bay Regional Health Centre - Regional Mental Health; Staff, West Nipissing General Hospital; Med Advisor, Base Hosp. Program; (705)753-3110

HENTELEFF, Harry J A; Queen Elizabeth II HSC, 7 010-1276 South Park St, Halifax NS B3H 2Y9; Man'86; BSc(Med); MSc; FRCSC; GenSurg; Critical Care Medicine; ThorSurg. Staff, Queen Elizabeth II Health Sciences Centre - Victoria General Site; Asst Prof, Dalhousie University; (902)473-5685; Fax. (902)473-5851; hhenteleff@tupdean2.med.dal.ca.

HENTELEFF, Sybil M; 404-11861 88 Ave, Delta BC V4C 3C6; Man'82; Langs: Bilingual(English/French); (604)599-0077; Fax. (604)599-8531.

HENTSCHEL, Eric P; Medical Bldg, 306-18 Pine St, Kitchener ON N2H 5Z8; Qns'83; FRCPC; IntMed (Chronic Osturctive); Respir. Consultant Staff, North Wellington Health Care - Louise Marshall Hospital; Staff, Grand River Hospital - Kitchener/Waterloo Health Centre; Med Dir, St Mary's General Hospital; Med Dir, Freeport Pulmonary Rehabilitation Program; Asst Prof Adjunct, McMaster University; (519)570-0062; Fax. (519)570-9551.

HENTSCHEL, Stephen J; CBI Health Centre, 605 Discovery St, Victoria BC V8T 5G4; UBC'96; BSc; FRCSC; Neursurg (Oncology). (250)383-3638

HENWICK, Scott; BC Biomedical Laboratories, 7455 130 St, Surrey BC V3W 1H8; UBC'85; FRCPC; Peds; InfectDis; MedMicrobiol. Staff Lab Med, Surrey Memorial Hospital; Staff, Chilliwack General Hospital; Staff, Royal Columbian Hospital; Assoc., Dr. C. J. Coady; (604)507-5000

HENZLER, Dietrich; Queen Elizabeth II HSC, 10 W-1276 South Park St, Halifax NS B3H 2Y9; Hannover (Germany)'93; FRCPC; Anes. Staff, Queen Elizabeth II Health Sciences Centre - Victoria General Site; (902)473-2700

HEON, Elise; The Hosp for Sick Children, 555 University Ave, Toronto ON M5G 1X8; Sher'87; FRCSC; Ophth (Ocular Genetics). Staff Ophth & Vision Sciences, The Hospital For Sick Children; Prof Ophth, University of Toronto; Langs: English; French; (416)813-8606; Fax. (416)813-6261; eheon@attglobal.net.

HEPBURN, Andrew; 5525 West Boulevard Box 437, Vancouver BC V6M 3W6; Glasgow (Scotland)'66; MB ChB; FRCS(Ed); LMCC; FRCSC; OrthSurg. Ac Staff, Royal Columbian Hospital; Ac Staff, Eagle Ridge Hospital & Health Care Centre; Asst Prof, University of British Columbia; (604)263-4038; Fax. (604)263-4028.

HEPBURN, Beth; Caledonian Med Clinic, 340 Campbell St, Nanaimo BC V9R 3G7; Aberdeen (Scotland)'85; (250)753-3202

HEPBURN, David F; 105-911 Yates St, Victoria BC V8V 4X3; Ott'86; Langs: Bislama; (250)388-3080

HEPBURN, Douglas S; Durham Fertility Center, 117 King St E, Oshawa ON L1H 1B9; Wes'86; DABOG; FRCSC; ObstGyn (Infertility). Staff, Lakeridge Health - Oshawa Site; Queen's University; (905)721-3543; Fax. (905)721-3558.

HEPBURN, Keith G; Shuswap Fam Practice, 102-571 6 St NE, Salmon Arm BC V1E 1R6; UBC'95; CCFP; CCFP(E.M.); FCFP; (250)832-2151; Fax. (250)832-3669.

HEPBURN, Laura D; Shuswap Family Practice, 102-571 6 St NE, Salmon Arm BC V1E 1R6; UBC'95; BSc; CCFP; FCFP; Staff, Shuswap Lake General Hospital; (250)832-2151; Fax. (250)832-3669.

HEPBURN, Robert W A; 106-9648 128 St, Surrey BC V3T 2X9; Oxford (England)'71; BMus; BCh; MRCGPract; CCFP; FCFP; Ac Staff, Surrey Memorial Hospital; (604)584-2233; Fax. (604)589-1242.

HEPPELL, Josee; CSSS du Sud de Lanaudière, 911 montee des Pionniers, Terrebonne QC J6V 2H2; Sher'06; CCFP; Staff, Centre Hospitalier Pierre le Gardeur; (450)654-7525

HEPTING, Kristin L; Sudbury Reg Hosp-Laurentian, 41 Ramsey Lake, Sudbury ON P3E 5J1; NOSM'10; CCFP; Staff, Health Sciences North-Laurentian Site; (705)523-7100

HERAN, Manraj K S; Children's & Women's HC of BC, 4480 Oak St, Vancouver BC V6H 3V4; UBC'96; FRCPC; DiagRad (Neuro Radiology). Staff, BC Children's Hospital; Staff Neurorodiologist, Vancouver General Hospital - Centennial Pavillion; Langs: Punjabi; (604)875-2131; manraj.heran@vch.ca.

HERAN, Navraj S; 207-245 Columbia St E, New Westminster BC V3L 3W4; UBC'98; FRCSC; Neursurg. Langs: Punjabi; (604)520-1120

HERAR, Daljit S; Cedar Hills Med Clinic, 12860 96 Ave, Surrey BC V3V 6A8; UBC'86; GenPath. Staff, Surrey Memorial Hospital; Langs: Punjabi; Hindi; Urdu; (604)584-3531

HERARD, Genevieve; Clinique Medicale Desy, 5636 boul Henri-Bourassa E, Montreal-Nord QC H1G 2T2; Mon'10; CCFP; (514)326-9060

HERARD, Jean-Francois; CSSS de Rivière-de-Loup, 75 rue Saint-Henri, Riviere-du-Loup QC G5R 2A4; Laval'02; Staff, Centre Hospitalier Regional du Grand-Portage; Langs: English; (418)868-1010; jeffherard@hotmail.com.

HERATH, Jayantha; Ontario Forensic Pathology Ser, 26 Grenville St, Toronto ON M7A 2G9; Varna (Bulgaria)'93; FRCPC; AnatPath (Forensic Pathology). Staff, Health Sciences Centre; (416)314-4040

HERATH, Subarathna M; Lakeridge Hlth Corp-Oshawa, 1 Hospital Crt, Oshawa ON L1G 2B9; (Sri Lanka)'75; MB BS; FFARCS(Eng); FRCPC; Anes. Staff Anes, Lakeridge Health - Oshawa Site; (905)576-8711 x3237; Fax. (905)721-4848.

HERBA, Karl; Hop Maisonneuve-Rosemont, 5415 boul de l'Assomption, Montreal QC H1T 2M4; McG'04; FRCPC; IntMed; Gastroent. Staff, Hopital Maisonneuve-Rosemont; (514)252-3400

HERBERT, Carol P; Ctre for Studies in Family Med, 245-100 Collip Circle, London ON N6G 4X8; UBC'69; CCFP; FCFP; (519)858-5028; carol.herbert@schulich.uwo.ca.

HERBERT, John W; Carrot River Med Clinic, PO Box 160, Carrot River SK S0E 0L0; Qns'89; LMCC; Staff, Carrot River Medical Clinic; (306)768-2000; Fax. (306)768-2001.

HERBERT, Linda T; Bigelow Fowler Clinic West, 30 Jerry Potts Blvd W, Lethbridge AB T1K 5M5; Mon'86; Ac Staff, Chinook Regional Hospital; (403)381-8444; Fax. (403)381-8166.

HERBERT, Melodie; BC Cancer Agency-Fraser Valley, 13750 96 Ave, Surrey BC V3V 1Z2; UBC'93; BScN; CCFP; Clin Associate Radiation Oncology, BC Cancer Agency Fraser Valley Centre; (604)930-2098; Fax. (604)930-4065.

HERCIG, Dragan; The Two Hundred, 416-200 St Clair Ave W, Toronto ON M4V 1R1; Zagreb (Croatia)'80; FRCPC; Psy. Langs: Croatian; (416)934-0098; Fax. (416)444-0452.

HERCZ, Amos R; Hop Santa Cabrini Ospedale, 5655 rue Saint-Zotique E, Montreal QC H1T 1P7; Cal'02; FRCPC; IntMed. Staff, Hôpital Santa Cabrini Ospedale; (514)252-6000; Fax. (514)252-6453.

HERCZ, Gavril; 2175 Keele St, Toronto ON M6M 3Z4; McG'78; FRCP; ABIM; FACP; FRCPC; IntMed; Nephrol. Staff, Humber River Regional Hospital - Keele Street Site; Staff Nephrol Kidney Care Clinic, Humber River Regional Hospital - Church Street Site; Assoc Prof, University of Toronto; Langs: English; French; Hungarian; (416)658-2241; Fax. (416)658-2242.

HERD, Anthony; Salvation Army Grace Gen Hosp, 300 Booth Dr, Winnipeg MB R3J 3M7; Man'86; CCFP; CCFP(E.M.); FCFP; Staff, The Salvation Army Grace Hospital; (204)837-0391

HERD, Stuart W; Vancouver Gen Hosp, 855 12th Ave W, Vancouver BC V5Z 1M9; Wes'80; FRCPC; Anes (Echocardiography). Staff, Vancouver General Hospital - Centennial Pavillion; (604)875-4111

HEREDIA, Armando; Taiga Medical Clinics, 210 Elliott St, Whitehorse YT Y1A 2A2; (Mexico)'92; Consultant, Whitehorse General Hospital; Dir, Taiga Medical Clinics Inc; Langs: Spanish; (867)456-4362; Fax. (867)393-4362.

HEREDIA, Cesar; 300-4135 rue de Rouen, Montreal QC H1V 1G5; Lausanne (Switzerland)'72; Ophth (P.Q.). (514)256-0007; Fax. (514)256-4966.

HEREDIA, Maria; CSSS de Beauce-Etchemin, 1515 17e rue, Saint-Georges QC G5Y 4T8; (Other Foreign)'04; CCFP; Staff, Centre Hospitalier Beauce-Etchemin; (418)228-2031

HEREISH, Jean-Pierre; Clinique Med St-Sulpice, 12-1420 rue Legendre E, Montreal QC H2M 1H5; Mon'84; Staff, Hôpital du Sacre-Coeur de Montréal; Staff, Centre Hospitalier Fleury; Pres, ABH Informatique; Staff Clin Formation, Universite de Montreal; (514)382-0552

HEREISH, Michel; College des Med du Quebec, 2170 boul Rene Levesque O, Montreal QC H3H 2T8; Laval'88; Staff, Centre Hospitalier de Chandler; Staff, CLSC Perce; Clin Teacher, Université Laval; Langs: Arabic; (514)933-4441; mhereish@globetrotter.net.

HERER, Elaine R; Sunnybrook Hlth Sciences Ctr, B722-2075 Bayview Ave, Toronto ON M4N 3M5; Cal'82; BSc; FRCS; FSOGC; FRCSC; ObstGyn. Staff, Women's College Hospital; Ac Staff, Sunnybrook Health Sciences Centre; Assoc Prof, University of Toronto; (416)480-4680; Fax. (416)480-4751.

HERGET, Robert J; Gulf Canada Square, 366-401 9 Ave SW, Calgary AB T2P 3C5; Alb'74; (403)266-3353; Fax. (403)266-4828.

HERGETT, Susan C; Wolfville Prof Centre, 2-4 Little Rd, Wolfville NS B4P 1P4; Dal'91; (902)542-7016; Fax. (902)542-1544.

HERGOTT, Christopher A; Royal University Hosp, 544-103 Hospital Dr, Saskatoon SK S7N 0W8; Tor'03; FRCPC; IntMed; Respir. Staff, Royal University Hospital; (306)655-1000

HERGOTT, Paul A; 208-974 Queen St E, Sault Ste. Marie ON P6A 2C5; Wes'76; FRCSC; ObstGyn (Obstetrics & Gynecology). Consultant, Sault Area Hospital - Sault Ste Marie; (705)942-6845; Fax. (705)942-6880.

HERING, Ramm; Northend Community Hlth Ctr, 2165 Gottingen St, Halifax NS B3K 3B5; Cal'07; CCFP; (902)420-0303; Fax. (902)422-0859.

HERITZ, Dianne M; Urology Clinic, 202-180 Vine St S, St Catharines ON L2R 7P3; McM'87; BScN; FACS; FRCSC; Urol (Female Urology). Staff, Niagara Health System - Ontario Street Site; Staff, Niagara Health System - St Catharines General Site; Asst Prof, McMaster University; (905)688-2761; Fax. (905)688-6638.

HERMA, Messaoud; CSSS De Sept-Iles, 45 rue du Pere-Divet, Sept-Iles QC G4R 3N7; (Other Foreign)'98; Staff, Centre Hospitalier Regional de Sept-Iles; (418)962-9761

HERMAN, Bruce A; North Bramalea Med Centre, 202-9780 Bramalea Rd, Brampton ON L6S 2P1; Tor'83; CCFP; FCFP; Staff, William Osler Health System - Brampton Civic Hospital; (905)791-2390; Fax. (905)791-8476.

HERMAN, Dorli; Spingbank Med Centre, 303-460 Springbank Dr, London ON N6J 0A8; Qns'86; BSc; MSc; CCFP; CCFP(E.M.); FCFP; (519)439-0200; Fax. (519)439-0205.

HERMAN, Jaclyn; William Osler HC-Etobicoke, 101 Humber College Blvd, Etobicoke ON M9V 1R8; Tor'06; CCFP; CCFP(E.M.); Staff, Lakeridge Health - Oshawa Site; William Osler Health System - Etobicoke General Hospital; (416)747-3400

HERMAN, Leon; 103-333 Wilson Ave, North York ON M3H 1T2; Tor'72; (416)636-1279; Fax. (416)636-2975.

HERMAN, Rebecca C; Medical Dental Bldg, 516-1849 Yonge St, Toronto ON M4S 1Y2; Wes'04; CCFP; (416)486-8444; Fax. (416)486-2193.

HERMAN, Robert J; HSC-Faculty of Med, 1474-3330 Hospital Dr NW, Calgary AB T2N 4N1; Sask'77; FRCPC; IntMed (Clinical Pharmacology). Staff, Foothills Medical Centre; Prof, University of Calgary; (403)220-5926; herman@ucalgary.ca.

HERMAN, Shauna P; Crossroads Famly Practice, 201-5110 St Margarets Bay Rd, Upper Tantallon NS B3Z 1E2; Dal'06; CCFP; (902)826-9096; Fax. (902)820-9399.

HERMAN, Stanley L; Mackenzie Richmond Hill Hosp, 10 Trench St, Richmond Hill ON L4C 4Z3; McM'94; BSc; MSc; FRCPC; Anes (Chronic Pain). Staff, Mackenzie Richmond Hill Hospital; (905)883-2110

HERMAN, Stephen J; NCSB-1C 566, 585 Unviersity Ave, Toronto ON M5G 2N2; Tor'75; AB; FRCPC; DiagRad. Staff Radiol, Toronto General Hospital - UHN; Assoc Prof, University of Toronto; (416)340-4800 x4522; Fax. (416)340-3900.

HERMAN-KIDECKEL, Sari M; North York Med Group, 704-240 Duncan Mill Rd, North York ON M3B 3S6; McM'04; FRCPC; IntMed; ClinImmunol&Allergy. (416)497-0880; Fax. (416)497-2650.

HERMAN-LEMELIN, Antoine; CSSS de Chicoutimi, CP 5006 305 rue Saint-Vallier, Chicoutimi QC G7H 5H6; Mon'07; CCFP; CCFP(E.M.); Staff, Complexe hospitalier de la Sagamie; (418)541-1000

HERMANN, Laura L; Dartmouth Gen Hosp, 325 Pleasant St, Dartmouth NS B2Y 4G8; Man'05; FRCPC; IntMed; InfectDis. Staff, Dartmouth General Hospital; (902)465-8300

HERMANS, Pierre; Ctr Hosp de Verdun, 4000 boul Lasalle, Verdun QC H4G 2A3; Sher'84; CSPQ; FRCSC; GenSurg (Thoracic Surgery). Staff, Centre Hospitalier de Verdun; Langs: Bilingual(English/French); (514)362-1000; pierrehermans@mac.com.

HERMANT, Tammy G; 702-110 Eglinton Ave E, Toronto ON M4P 2Y1; Wes'94; BSc(Hon); CCFP; FCFP; (416)486-3300; Fax. (416)486-9433.

HERMANUTZ, Katie E; 160-6900 Taylor Dr, Red Deer AB T4P 1K4; Cal'10; CCFP; (403)342-2234; Fax. (403)342-2655.

HERMIZ, Fadia; Andy's Pharm & Walkin Clinic, 1500-2055 Sandwich West Pky, Windsor ON N9H 2S4; (Iraq)'83; MB ChB; CCFP; Staff, Hôtel-Dieu Grace Hospital; Staff, Windsor Regional Hospital - Metropolitan Site; Langs: Arabic; French; (519)915-5516; Fax. (519)915-5718.

HERMON, Orly; Medistat Med Familiale, 4965 rue Saint-Pierre, Pierrefonds QC H9H 5M9; McG'92; CCFP; Conférencier Faculty of Herzl Family Med Unit, Sir Mortimer B Davis Jewish General; assoc Staff, Lakeshore General Hospital - Pointe Claire; Langs: French; Romanian; (514)624-4774; Fax. (514)624-4704.

HERNANDEZ, Maria D R; Cumberland Reg Hlth Care Centr, 19428 Hwy 2, Amherst NS B4H 3Y4; Havana (Cuba)'87; FRCPC; Anes. Staff, Cumberland Regional Health Care Center; (902)667-3361

HERNANDEZ, Paul; Queen Elizabeth II HSC-Halifax, 4458-1796 Summer St, Halifax NS B3H 3A7; McG'87; BSc; MDCM; FRCPC; IntMed (Pulmonary Hypertention); Respir. Staff Respirologist, Queen Elizabeth II Health Sciences Centre - Victoria General Site; Ac Staff Respirologist, Capital District Health Authority; Med Dir, Pulmonary Rehabilitation Prog; Assoc Prof, Dalhousie University; Langs: French; (902)473-3698; Fax. (902)473-6202; paul.hernandez@cdha.nshealth.ca.

HERNANDEZ ALEJANDRO, Roberto; London HSC-University Hosp, PO Box 5339 Stn B C4 211B-339 Windermere Rd, London ON N6A 5A5; La Salle (Mexico)'95; Staff, London Health Sciences Centre - University Hospital; (519)663-2920; Fax. (519)663-3858.

HERNANDEZ MURCIA, Lizeth A; Hamilton HS-McMaster Site, PO Box 2000 Stn Lcd 1 1200 Main St W, Hamilton ON L8N 3Z5; (Australia)'94; Staff, Hamilton Health Sciences Centre - McMaster Children's Hospital; (905)521-2100; Fax. (905)521-5092.

HERNANDEZ-SANCHEZ, Olivia; Direction de la Sante Publique, 1 9e rue, Rouyn-Noranda QC J9X 2A9; Guadalajara (Mexico)'77; Staff, CSSS de Rouyn-Noranda; Langs: Spanish; English; (819)764-3264 x49418; Fax. (819)797-1947.

HERNBERGER, Julie A; 101-190 Pelican Pl, Sylvan Lake AB T4S 1K2; Alb'04; CCFP; Staff Phy, Red Deer Regional Hospital Centre; Physician, Wolf Creek Primary Care Network; (403)887-2224

HERON, Timothy A; Clin Ortho Saint-Urbain, 209-3875 rue Saint-Urbain, Montreal QC H2W 1V1; McG'86; BSc; MDCM; DAB; FRCSC; OrthSurg (Sports Medicine). Staff, Centre Hospitalier l'Université de Montréal (CHUM) - Hôtel-Dieu; adj Prof, Universite de Montreal; Langs: English; French; (514)849-8391; Fax. (514)849-9313.

HEROUX, Isabelle; CSSS Becancour-Nicolet-Yamaska, 216 rue Principale, Fortierville QC G0S 1J0; Mon'05; CCFP; (819)287-4442

HEROUX, Josee; Centre Med Robinson Inc, 4 rue Robinson N, Granby QC J2G 8Z9; Sher'92; FRCPC; Derm (Psoriasis). Staff Derm, Centre Hospitalier de Granby; Langs: Bilingual(French/English); (450)378-1000; Fax. (450)770-8567.

HEROUX, Julie; Ctr Hosp Rouyn-Noranda, 4 9e rue, Rouyn-Noranda QC J9X 2B2; Mon'90; FRCPC; IntMed. Staff Internal Med, Centre Hospitalier Rouyn-Noranda; Langs: Bilingual(French/English); (819)764-5131; Fax. (819)764-2946.

HEROUX, Martin; Regina Qu'Appelle Hr-Pasqua, 4A-4101 Dewdney Ave, Regina SK S4T 1A5; Sask'01; CCFP; CCFP(E.M.); Staff, Pasqua Hospital; Staff, Regina General Hospital; (306)766-2222; Fax. (306)766-2669.

HEROUX, Micheline; PAMQ, 200-1 boul Rene-Levesque E, Montreal QC H2X 3Z5; Laval'72; CSPQ; FRCPC; Anes. Staff, Centre Hospitalier Paul-Gilbert; Staff Anes, Hôtel-Dieu de Lévis; (514)397-0888; Fax. (514)397-0654.

HEROUX, Michelle; Clinique Med Centre-Ville, 5-167 rue de la Reine, Gaspe QC G4X 2W6; Laval'82; CCFP; FCFP; Université Laval; (418)368-1811; Fax. (418)368-2616.

HERR, Steven J; Huntsville Prof Bldg, 102-348 Muskoka Rd 3 N, Huntsville ON P1H 1H8; Wes'97; BScChemEng; CCFP; CCFP(E.M.); FCFP; (705)789-4377; Fax. (705)789-1640.

HERRERA, Pedro; Ctr Hosp Anna-Laberge, 200 boul Brisebois, Chateauguay QC J6K 4W8; Mon'03; Staff, Hôpital Anna-Laberge; (450)699-2425; Fax. (450)699-2525.

HERRERA-CORREA, Jose R; Ctr Hosp de Verdun, 4000 boul Lasalle, LaSalle QC H4G 2A3; (Chile)'71; Endocrin (P.Q.). Assoc Staff, McGill University Health Centre - Royal Victoria Hospital; Consultant, CSSS de Dorval-Lachine-Lasalle; Staff, Centre Hospitalier de Verdun; (514)362-1000

HERRICK, Ian A; London HSC-University Hosp, PO Box 5339 Stn B B3 216-339 Windermere Rd, London ON N6A 5A5; Cal'82; MPA; FRCPC; Anes (Neuro Anesthesia).; Staff, London Health Sciences Centre - University Hospital; Staff Anesthetist, St Joseph's Hospital - St Joseph's Health Care; Assoc Prof, University of Western Ontario; (519)663-3283; Fax. (519)663-3079; iherrick@uwo.ca.

HERRIDGE, M Margaret S; NCSB 11C-1170, 585 University Ave, Toronto ON M5G 2N2; Qns'90; MSc; ABIM; FRCPC; IntMed (Critical Care Medicine); Respir. Staff Physician, Toronto General Hospital - UHN; Asst Prof Med, University of Toronto; (416)340-3057; Fax. (416)340-3109.

HERRMANN, Nathan; Sunnybrook Hlth Sciences Ctre, 2075 Bayview Ave, Toronto ON M4N 3M5; Tor'83; FRCPC; Psy. Staff, Sunnybrook Health Sciences Centre; (416)480-6133

HERRMANN, Trevor J H; Anaesthetic Services, 213-2186 Oak Bay Ave, Victoria BC V8R 1G3; Cape Town (South Africa)'86; MB ChB; FRCPC; Anes. Staff, Victoria General Hospital; (250)595-7211

HERSCH, Edwin L; Medical & Dental Bldg, 707-586 Eglinton Ave E, Toronto ON M4P 1P2; Tor'83; MA(Psychol); FRCPC; Psy (Psychotherapy). (416)480-0042

HERSCHMAN, Peter L; 4-208 St Clair Ave W, Toronto ON M4V 1R2; McG'67; DABPN; FRCPC; Psy (Psychoanalysis). (416)922-7279

HERSCHORN, Andrea; Omega Med Associates, 304-2 Lansing Sq, North York ON M2J 4P8; Tor'09; CCFP; (416)489-0711; Fax. (416)489-7009.

HERSCHORN, Sender; Sunnybrook Hth Sciences Ctr, MG408-2075 Bayview Ave, Toronto ON M4N 3M5; McG'72; FRCSC; Urol. Consultant, Toronto Western Hospital - University Health Network; Staff Urol, Sunnybrook Health Sciences Centre; Staff Lithotripsy, St Michael's Hospital; (416)480-4733; Fax. (416)480-6121; s.herschorn@utoronto.ca.

HERSELMAN, Paul J; 19-1599 Cliffe Ave, Courtenay BC V9N 2K6; S.Africa (South Africa)'92; MB ChB; CCFP; CCFP(E.M.); (250)334-1512

HERSHBERG, Dane M; 201-55 Nassau St N, Winnipeg MB R3L 2G8; Man'72; BSc; FRCPC; Psy (Anxiety Disorder). Staff Psy, Victoria General Hospital.

HERSHBERG, Melissa B; 6F-55 St Clair Ave W, Toronto ON M4V 2Y7; McM'04; CCFP; (416)435-6650; Fax. (416)435-7807.

HERSHENFELD, Seymour; 240-30 Disera Dr, Thornhill ON L4J 0A7; McG'76; FRCSC; Ophth. Ac Staff, North York General Hospital - Branson Division; (905)881-8050; Fax. (905)881-8050.

HERSHENFIELD, Karen R; 501-1110 Sheppard Ave E, North York ON M2K 2W2; Tor'07; CCFP; (416)223-0555; Fax. (416)223-0540.

HERSHFIELD, Earl S; Eaton Place Med Centre, 81-333 St Mary Ave, Winnipeg MB R3C 4A5; Man'58; FRCP; BSc(Med.); DABIM; FCCP; FRCPC; IntMed (Respirology). (204)942-0933; Fax. (204)942-2491; samuel17@shaw.ca.

HERSHFIELD, Melvyn; Royal City Med Bldg, 301-250 Keary St, New Westminster BC V3L 5E7; Man'63; FICS; FRCSC; Urol. Ac Staff, Royal Columbian Hospital; Court Staff, Burnaby Hospital; Ac Staff, Eagle Ridge Hospital & Health Care Centre; (604)524-6735; Fax. (604)525-2956.

HERSHFIELD, Noel B; Richmond Road Fam Med Ctre, 5255 Richmond Rd SW, Calgary AB T3E 7C4; Dublin (Ireland)'59; LRCPSI; FACP; FRCPC; IntMed (Gastroenterology). Ac Staff, Foothills Medical Centre; Clin Prof Gastro, University of Calgary; (403)249-3165

HERSHKOP, Marlon S; 201-300 King St W, Oshawa ON L1J 2K1; Tor'86; AB; FRCPC; NuclearMed. Staff Nuclear Med, Toronto General Hospital - UHN; Staff, Princess Margaret Hospital - University Health Network; Staff, Mount Sinai Hospital; Asst Prof Med Imaging, University of Toronto; (905)723-1653; marlon.hershkop@uhn.on.ca.

HERSHKOP, Sheldon; Mississauga Treatment Ctr, 3047A Hurontario St, Mississauga ON L5A 2G9; Tor'85; CCFP; FCFP; Langs: English; French; (905)279-4848

HERSHKOP, Susan K; Sunnybrook Hlth Sciences Ctre, 2075 Bayview Ave, Toronto ON M4N 3M5; Tor'96; FRCPC; Psy. Staff, Sunnybrook Health Sciences Centre; (416)480-4693; Fax. (416)480-6878.

HERSHLER, Abby; Women's College Hosp, W948-76 Grenville St, Toronto ON M5S 1B2; McM'04; FRCPC; Psy. Staff, Women's College Hospital; (416)323-6400; Fax. (416)323-6356.

HERSHLER, Cecil; MacDonald Med Centre, 104-2786 16th Ave W, Vancouver BC V6K 4M1; McM'80; PhD; MSc; FRCPC; PhysMed&Rehab. (604)732-7060; Fax. (604)732-5913; chershler@gmail.com.

HERSI, Ali I; Hamilton HS-General Site, 237 Barton St E, Hamilton ON L8L 2X2; McG'00; FRCPC; EmergMed. Staff, Hamilton Health Sciences Centre - Hamilton General Hospital; Langs: Somali; (905)527-4322

HERSKOVITZ, Mariana L N; Carlington Comm Hlth Services, 900 Merivale Rd, Ottawa ON K1Z 5Z8; Man'89; BSc(Med); Clin Associate Heart Check Centre, University of Ottawa; Langs: Spanish; (613)722-2161; Fax. (613)722-8471.

HERSKOVITZ, Steven; St Mary's Hosp Centre, 3830 av Lacombe, Montreal QC H3T 1M5; McG'99; CCFP; CCFP(E.M.); Staff, St Mary's Hospital Centre; (514)345-3511; hersste@hotmail.com.

HERSSON-EDERY, Fanny; La Maison Bleue, 3735 av Plamondon, Montreal QC H3S 1L8; McG'97; (514)509-0833

HERST, Jordan A; Sudbury Reg Hosp-Laurentian, 41 Ramsey Lake Rd, Sudbury ON P3E 5J1; Tor'86; ABIM; FRCPC; IntMed; Hem. Staff, Health Sciences North-Laurentian Site; Asst Prof, University of Ottawa; (705)522-6237; jherst@hsnsudbury.ca.

HERTWIG, Brian K; First Avenue Fam Med Centre, 6 First Ave, St Thomas ON N5R 4M2; Wes'81; CCFP; Court Staff, St Thomas Elgin General Hospital; (519)633-6050

HERTZMAN, Clyde; Univ of British Columbia, 462-2206 East Mall, Vancouver BC V6T 1Z8; McM'79; MSc; FRCPC; CommunMed. Asst Prof Health Care & Epidemiol, University of British Columbia; (604)822-3002

HERTZMAN-CHALOUH, Daniel; London HSC-Victoria Hosp, PO Box 5010 800 Commissioners Rd E, London ON N6A 4G5; Mon'05; FRCPC; Psy. Psychiatrist, London Health Sciences Centre - Victoria Campus; (519)685-8500; Fax. (519)667-6539; hertzman-chalouhd@lhsc.on.ca.

HERVIEUX, David; Clinique Med Lavaltrie, 1400 rue Notre-Dame, Lavaltrie QC J5T 1M6; Mon'01; Staff, Centre Hospitalier Pierre le Gardeur; (450)586-1033

HERVIEUX, Matyas; Sioux Lookout Zone Fam Phys, PO Box 4000, Sioux Lookout ON P8T 1K2; McM'05; CCFP; (807)737-3030

HERVOUET-ZEIBER, Catherine; Hôpital Ste-Justine, 3175 ch Cote-Ste-Catherine, Montreal QC H3T 1C5; McG'00; FRCPC; Peds. Staff, Hôpital Ste-Justine; (514)345-4931

HERZENBERG, Martin A; 7885 Wyandotte St E, Windsor ON N8S 1S8; Witwatersrand (South Africa)'64; Langs: Afrikaans; (519)944-3144; Fax. (519)944-7660.

HERZIG, Sheldon; Herzig Eye Institute, 210-131 Bloor St W, Toronto ON M5S 1R1; Tor'73; FRCSC; Ophth (Cataract & Refractive). Ac Staff, North York General Hospital; Med Dir, Herzig Eye Institute; Lecturer, University of Toronto; (416)929-2020; Fax. (416)929-0232; eyes@herzig-eye.com.

HERZOG, Melvin; 1750 Jane St, York ON M9N 2T1; Wes'65; (416)244-4845

HESELTINE, N Geoffrey; Cornwall Comm Hosp-Second St, PO Box 100 Stn Main 840 McConnell Ave, Cornwall ON K6H 5S5; RCS (Ireland)'85; MBA; CCFP; Staff, Cornwall Community Hospital; (613)938-4240

HESHKA, Jodi; Ottawa Cardiovasculer Centre, 502-1355 Bank St, Ottawa ON K1H 8K7; Ott'07; FRCPC; IntMed. (613)738-1584

HESLIP, Laura A M; 200-7031 Westminster Hwy, Richmond BC V6X 1A3; Alb'97; FRCSC; ObstGyn. Staff, Richmond Hospital; (604)207-2500; Fax. (604)207-2550.

HESLOP, Winston L; Dundas Med Centre, 301-220 Dundas St W, Whitby ON L1N 8M7; (Jamaica)'78; MB BS; ABIM; FRCPC; IntMed (Cardiology). Consultant, Lakeridge Health - Bowmanville Site; (905)668-7899; Fax. (905)668-3156.

HESOM, Margaret S; Dr CW Wiebe Med Centre, 385 Main St, Winkler MB R6W 1J2; Cape Town (South Africa)'90; MB ChB; (204)325-4312; Fax. (204)325-4594; info@winklerclinic.com.

HESS, Allan R; Allan R Hess Med Prof Corp, 100-637 Davis Dr, Newmarket ON L3Y 2R2; Tor'79; FACC; FRCPC; Cardiol; IntMed. Ac Staff, Southlake Regional Health Centre; Langs: Estonian; (905)898-7924

HESS, Lembi M; Dixon Med Clinic, 405-531 Davis Dr, Newmarket ON L3Y 6P5; Wes'09; CCFP; (905)898-2240; Fax. (905)898-2253.

HESS, Talvi M; Postgraduate Med education, MDCL 3101A-1280 Main St W, Hamilton ON L8S 4K1; Wes'06; IntMed.

HESSAMI-BOOSHEHRI, Morvarid; SGH Medical Mall, 3030 Lawrence Ave E, Scarborough ON M1P 2T7; Tehran (Iran)'92; FRCPC; Derm;CCFP; (416)438-6442

HESSE, Stephen R; Students Union Bldg, 2 200-66 University Campus NW, Edmonton AB T6G 2J7; Alb'95; FRCPC; Psy. (780)492-5205; Fax. (780)492-0013.

HESSELSON, Jeffrey P; 1225B 100th St, North Battleford SK S9A 0V6; Witwatersrand (South Africa)'76; CCFP; Staff Anes & Family Med, Battlefords Union Hospital; (306)445-0233; Fax. (306)445-0235.

HESSENTHALER, Doris M; 225-45 Edenwold Dr NW, Calgary AB T3A 3S8; Wes'85; CCFP; FCFP; (403)241-2888; Fax. (403)241-3505.

HESSIAN, Renee C; Univ of Ottawa Heart Institute, H 145A-40 Ruskin St, Ottawa ON K1Y 4W7; Qns'86; FRCPC; IntMed; Cardiol. Staff, The Ottawa Hospital - General Campus; Langs: Bilingual(English/French); (613)761-4377; Fax. (613)761-5022; rhessian@ottawaheart.ca.

HESTER, Valerie L; Meadowvale Prof Centre, 224-6855 Meadowvale Town Ctre, Mississauga ON L5N 2Y1; Wes'78; (905)814-5884; Fax. (905)814-4841.

HESTON, Jonathan P A; Landmark Prof Centre, 101-2731 Hewes Way NW, Edmonton AB T6L 6W6; Cal'78; MSc; FRCSC; Ophth. (780)450-3200; Fax. (780)450-9861.

HETAIMISH, Bandar; Postgraduate Med Education, MDCL 3101A-1280 Main St W, Hamilton ON L8S 4K1; King Abdul Aziz (Saudi Arabia)'04; OrthSurg.

HETHERINGTON, D Maxine; Smyth Associate Clinic, 4904 48 St, Leduc AB T9E 6X4; Alb'96; CCFP; (780)986-2715; Fax. (780)986-0356.

HETHERINGTON, Gabrielle S E; Grey Nuns Community Hosp & HC, 1100 Youville Drive West NW, Edmonton AB T6L 5X8; (Ireland)'66; FRCPC; Psy. Staff, Covenant Health - Grey Nuns Community Hospital; (780)735-7292; Fax. (780)735-7496.

HETHERINGTON, Kerri; Kliniek on Main, 351 Main St N, Moose Jaw SK S6H 0W2; Sask'06; CCFP; Staff, Regina General Hospital; (306)694-1440; Fax. (306)693-9990.

HETLAND, Ray K D; Grey Nuns Community Hosp, 1100 Youville Drive West NW, Edmonton AB T6L 5X8; Loma Linda(CA) (USA)'82; MPH; Staff, Covenant Health - Grey Nuns Community Hospital; (780)735-7000

HETU, Jessika; CHUS Hotel-Dieu, 580 rue Bowen S, Sherbrooke QC J1G 2E8; Mon'07; GenSurg. Staff, Centre Hospitalier Universitaire de Sherbrooke-Hôpital Hôtel-Dieu; (819)346-1110

HETU, Marc A; 22 rue Michel CP 130, St-Chrysostome QC J0S 1R0; Mon'65; Staff, Barrie Memorial Hospital; (450)826-3110; Fax. (450)826-1177; marc_hetu@hotmail.com.

HETU, Valerie; CSSS du Nord de Lanaudière, 1000 boul Sainte-Anne, St-Charles-Brromee QC J6E 6J2; Mon'04; FRCSC; ObstGyn. Staff, Centre Hospitalier Régional de Lanaudière; Langs: French; (450)759-8222

HEUGHAN, Caroline E; Parkdale Med Tower, 308-1081 Carling Ave, Ottawa ON K1Y 4G2; Dal'06; FRCPC; Derm. (613)722-8532

HEUGHAN, David; Victoria County Mem Hosp, PO Box 220 30 Old Margaree Rd, Baddeck NS B0E 1B0; Dal'08; CCFP; Staff, Victoria County Memorial Hospital; (902)794-8521

HEULE, Mark K; Misericordia Comm Hosp & H C, 16940 87 Ave NW, Edmonton AB T5R 4H5; Alb'75; FCCP; FRCPC; IntMed (Respirology). Ac Staff, University of Alberta Hospital; Ac Staff ICU, Covenant Health - Misericordia Community Hospital; Clin Assoc Prof, University of Alberta; (780)735-2880; Fax. (780)735-2953; mheule@cha.ab.ca.

HEUNIS, Adriaan; 200 Trans Canada Hwy W PO Box 1870 Stn Main, Salmon Arm BC V1E 4P9; (South Africa)'82; MB ChB; Langs: Afrikaans; Dutch; German; Zulu; (250)833-1990; Fax. (250)833-1988.

HEVENOR, Robert D; Tillsonburg Medical Clinic, PO Box 516 Stn Main 154 Rolph St, Tillsonburg ON N4G 4J1; Tor'84; (519)842-3682; Fax. (519)842-8711.

HEVEY, Simon; Clinique Medicale de Roberval, 714 boul Marcotte, Roberval QC G8H 1Z6; Sher'99; Staff, Hotel-Dieu de Roberval; (418)275-3833; Fax. (418)275-6747.

HEW, Amy; Norfinch Med Centre, 201-2100 Finch Ave W, North York ON M3N 2Z9; (Jamaica)'62; MB BS; Staff, Humber River Regional Hospital - Finch Avenue Site; (416)739-7225; Fax. (416)739-7226.

HEW, Eleanor; Clinique Med Roper, 4500 rue Sherbrooke O, Westmount QC H3Z 1E6; Tor'92; CCFP; FCFP; Staff Family Med Centre, McGill University Health Centre - Montreal General Campus; Langs: English; French; (514)937-8000; Fax. (514)937-8884.

HEW, Ernest M; Greenstone Clinic, 300-5734 Yonge St, North York ON M2M 4E7; (Trinidad & Tobago)'64; FFARCSI; FRCPC; Anes. Staff, North York General Hospital; (416)222-5501

HEW, Jeremy O; Scarborough Hosp-Birchmount, 3030 Birchmount Rd, Scarborough ON M1W 3W3; Qns'99; Anes (Family Medicine). Staff, The Scarborough Hospital - Birchmount Campus; (416)495-2561

HEW, Karen E; Scarborough North Med Arts, LL1C-4040 Finch Ave E, Scarborough ON M1S 4V5; McM'91; FRCSC; ObstGyn (Prenatal Care). Ac Staff, The Scarborough Hospital - Birchmount Campus; (416)298-2757; Fax. (416)298-2757.

HEW, Lincoln R; Norfinch Med Centre, 201-2100 Finch Ave W, North York ON M3N 2Z9; London (England)'62; MB BS; ABOG; FRCOG; FRCSC; ObstGyn. Staff ObstGyn, Humber River Regional Hospital - Finch Avenue Site; (416)739-7225; Fax. (416)739-7226.

HEW, Sheila L; 1A-3585 Lawrence Ave E, Scarborough ON M1G 1P4; McM'05; CCFP; Langs: Cantonese; Malay; Mandarin; (416)431-0756; Fax. (416)431-0648.

HEW-WING, Philip; Scarborough Hosp-General Div, 3050 Lawrence Ave E, Scarborough ON M1P 2V5; Tor'83; FRCPC; Anes. Staff, The Scarborough Hospital - General Campus; (416)431-8133

HEWAK, James C; Surrey G I Clinic, 105-21 Surrey St W, Guelph ON N1H 3R3; Wes'91; FRCPC; IntMed; Gastroent. (519)836-8201; Fax. (519)836-1341.

HEWES, Deborah K M; Windermere Clinic, 104B-32450 Simon Ave, Abbotsford BC V2T 4J2; London (England)'85; MB BS; FRCPC; Peds. (604)853-4323

HEWETT, Fraser G; Trilake Health Centre, PO Box 1690, Killarney MB R0K 1G0; (Other Foreign)'04; CCFP.

HEWGILL, Randolph T; Lions Gate Hosp, 231 15th St, North Vancouver BC V7L 2L7; UBC'01; FRCPC; Anes. Staff, Providence Health Care - St Paul's Hospital; Staff, Lions Gate Hospital; (604)987-5938

HEWINS, Edward A; 108-10 Webster St, Kentville NS B4N 1H7; Alb'89; FRCSC; OrthSurg. (902)679-3399; Fax. (902)679-3350.

HEWITT, Cheryl A W; Summerville Family Health Team, 5F-101 Queensway W, Mississauga ON L5B 2P7; McM'84; CCFP; FCFP; Staff, Trillium Health Centre - Mississauga; (905)272-9700; Fax. (905)272-1416.

HEWITT, Daniel C; New World Island Clinic, PO Box 240, Summerford NL A0G 4E0; Wes'84; CCFP; FCFP; (709)629-3681

HEWITT, Mathew; Vernon Jubilee Hosp, 2101 32 St, Vernon BC V1T 5L2; Qns'06; CCFP; CCFP(E.M.); Staff, Vernon Jubilee Hospital; (250)558-1200

HEWITT, Morgan; Royal Univ Hosp, 103 Hospital Dr, Saskatoon SK S7N 0W8; Sask'08; FRCPC; Peds. Staff, Royal University Hospital; (306)966-2922; Fax. (306)966-8640.

HEWITT, Richard J; Health Sciences Centre, 300 Prince Philip Dr, St. John's NL A1B 3V6; Mem'90; FRCSC; Urol. Staff, Health Sciences Centre; Physician, St. John's Health Care Corp.; (709)722-4050; Fax. (709)722-4082.

HEWKO, Robert A; 8191-2775 Laurel St, Vancouver BC V5Z 1M9; Alb'80; FRCPC; Psy (Consultation-Liaison). Ac Staff Psy, Vancouver General Hospital - Centennial Pavillion; Asst Prof, University of British Columbia; (604)875-4809; rahewko@shaw.ca.

HEWLETT, Patrick T; LuCliff Place, PO Box 206 604-700 Bay St, Toronto ON M7A 2B1; London (England)'64; MB BS; LRCP; MRCS; DRCOG; FRCSC; ObstGyn (Infertility). (416)591-3992; Fax. (416)591-3992.

HEWLETT, Thomas J C; Cape Breton Hlthcare Complex, 3651 1-1482 George St, Sydney NS B1P 1P3; McG'90; MDCM; FRCPC; IntMed; Nephrol. Staff, Cape Breton Healthcare Complex; (902)567-8035; Fax. (902)567-8037.

HEWTON-BACKFAT, Latisha; Siksika Health Services, PO Box 1130, Siksika AB T0J 3W0; Alb'10; CCFP; Staff, Victoria General Hospital; (403)734-5690

HEY, Amanda J; Sudbury Reg Hosp-Mem Site, 865 Regent St, Sudbury ON P3E 3Y9; Cal'83; CCFP; FCFP; Staff, Health Sciences North - Memorial Site; (705)523-7100

HEY, Jonathan D; Lakeside Med Clinic, 3919 8th St E, Saskatoon SK S7H 5M7; Stellenbosch (South Africa)'80; CCFP; FCFP; (306)374-6884; Fax. (306)374-2552.

HEY, Norman T P; Sudbury Reg Hosp-Laurentian, 41 Ramsey Lake Rd, Sudbury ON P3E 5J1; Qns'80; DAB; FRCPC; Anes (Critical Care Medicine). Staff Anes, Health Sciences North-Laurentian Site; (705)522-2200; normandy.hey@sympatico.ca.

HEYDARZADEH-AZAR, Kamran; Fort St John Hosp & Health Cen, 9636 100 Ave, Fort St. John BC V1J 1Y3; Mem'94; CSPQ; FRCPC; AnatPath (Surgical Pathology). Staff, Fort St John Hospital & Health Centre; Langs: Spanish; Persian; French; (250)262-5240; Fax. (250)785-1323; kheyda@yahoo.ca.

HEYDENRYCH, Siegfriedt L; Cold Lake Health Centre, 206-314 25 St, Cold Lake AB T9M 1G6; Stellenbosch (South Africa)'89; MB ChB; LMCC; CCFP; (780)639-3001; Fax. (780)639-3009.

HEYDING, Robert K; Leaside Health Centre, 795 Eglinton Ave E, East York ON M4G 4E4; Tor'81; (416)424-3145; Fax. (416)424-2611.

HEYEN, Francoise; Hop Maisonneuve-Rosemont, 5415 boul de l'Assomption, Montreal QC H1T 2M4; Mon'81; CSPQ; FRCSC; GenSurg (Colon & Rectal Surgery). Staff, Hopital Maisonneuve-Rosemont; adj Prof, Universite de Montreal; (514)252-3822; Fax. (514)252-3894.

HEYES, Robert H; Haliburton Family Med Centre, PO Box 870 7217 Gelert Rd, Haliburton ON K0M 1S0; Wes'71; CCFP; FCFP; Ac Staff/Chief Med Staff, Haliburton Highlands Health Services - Haliburton Site; (705)457-1212; Fax. (705)457-3955.

HEYLAND, Daren K; Kingston Gen Hosp, 76 Stuart St, Kingston ON K7L 2V7; Alb'89; MSc; FRCPC; IntMed (Critical Care Medicine). Staff, Kingston General Hospital; Prof, Queen's University; (613)549-6666 x3339; Fax. (613)548-1351.

HEYLBROECK, Christophe; Hop Du Sacre-Coeur De Montreal, 5400 boul Gouin O, Montreal QC H4J 1C5; Mon'03; FRCPC; Anes; Critical Care Medicine (P.Q.). Staff, Hôpital du Sacre-Coeur de Montréal; (514)338-2222

HEYMAN, Marsha R; Inst of Commun & Family Psy, 4333 ch Cote-Sainte-Catherine, Montreal QC H3T 1E4; McG'86; FRCPC; Psy. Staff, Sir Mortimer B Davis Jewish General; McGill University; Langs: French; (514)340-8226; heyman@videotron.ca.

HEYMANS, Gerry A; Russell Med Centre, PO Box 610 Stn Main 110 Craig St, Russell ON K4R 1E7; Tor'78; CCFP; FCFP; Ac Staff, Winchester District Memorial Hospital; (613)445-5333; Fax. (613)445-3659.

HEYN, Sujiva; Health Sciences Centre, 300 Prince Philip Dr, St. John's NL A1B 3V6; Wes'06; CCFP; CCFP(E.M.); Staff, Health Sciences Centre; (709)777-6300

HEYNS, Daniel B; 419 5 St S, Lethbridge AB T1J 2B6; (South Africa)'84; FRCSC; Ophth. Staff, University of Alberta Hospital; (403)320-8200

HEYS, Luther; Leamington Dist Mem Hosp, 194 Talbot St W, Leamington ON N8H 1N9; (South Africa)'93; MB ChB; CCFP; Staff, Leamington District Memorial Hospital; (519)326-2373

HEYWOOD, Mark; BC Cancer Agency, 600 10th Ave W, Vancouver BC V5Z 4E6; Dundee (Scotland)'83; MB ChB; FRCSC; ObstGyn (Gynecologic Oncology). Staff, BC Cancer Agency Vancouver Centre; Staff, Gordon & Leslie Diamond Health Care Centre; (604)877-6000 x2367

HEZAM, Wael; 10620 104 Ave, Grande Prairie AB T8V 8J8; (Libya)'01; Langs: Arabic; (780)814-5800; Fax. (780)538-4400; waelhezam@yahoo.com.

HIBBARD, Jennifer; Foothills Med Centre, 1403 29 St NW, Calgary AB T2N 2T9; Alb'98; BSc; FRCPC; Psy (Child & Adolescent Psychiatry). Staff, Foothills Medical Centre; Clin Lecturer, University of Alberta; (403)944-1298

HIBBARD, Kate; Students Union Bldg, 2 200-66 University Campus NW, Edmonton AB T6G 2J7; Alb'04; FRCPC; Psy. (780)492-5205; Fax. (780)492-0172.

HIBBARD, Richard E; Royal Alexandra Hosp, 6F-10240 Kingsway NW, Edmonton AB T5H 3V9; Tor'71; FRCPC; Psy. Staff Outpatient Psy, Royal Alexandra Hospital; Clin Prof, University of Alberta; (780)735-4564; Fax. (780)735-4797.

HIBBERT, Nadira D; Kingston Gen Hosp, 76 Stuart St, Kingston ON K7L 2V7; West Indies (Jamaica)'02; IntMed.

HIBBERT, Rebecca; The Ottawa Hosp-Civic Campus, 1053 Carling Ave, Ottawa ON K1Y 4E9; McM'05; FRCPC; DiagRad. Staff, Sault Area Hospital - Sault Ste Marie; Staff, The Ottawa Hospital - Civic Campus; (613)798-5555

HIBBITTS, Erin D; 1B-200 Thickwood Blvd, Fort McMurray AB T9K 1X9; UBC'08; CCFP; (780)790-9342; Fax. (780)791-0221.

HICK, Anthony; Sudbury Reg Hosp-Laurentian, 41 Ramsey Lake Rd, Sudbury ON P3E 5J1; Tor'88; FRCPC; Anes. Staff, Health Sciences North-Laurentian Site; Staff, QHC Trenton Memorial; (705)675-4733

HICK, Katherine M; The Hosp For Sick Children, 555 University Ave, Toronto ON M5G 1X8; Tor'89; FRCPC; Peds (Adolescent Medicine). Staff, The Hospital For Sick Children; (416)813-5825; khick@sympatico.ca.

HICKCOX, Samuel E; Dalhousie Univ Hlth Services, 1459 Oxford St, Halifax NS B3H 4R2; McM'05; BA; CCFP; Staff Physician GP Rhumatology, Capital District Health Authority; (902)494-2171; Fax. (902)494-6872; sam-hickcox@yahoo.ca.

HICKEN, W Blair; Centennial CMH & Brain Injury, PO Box 1000 Stn Main, Ponoka AB T4J 1R8; Dal'80; FRCPC; Psy (Emergency Psychiatry). Staff, Centennial Centre for Mental Health & Brain Injury; (403)783-7600

HICKESON, Marc P; MUHC-Royal Victoria Hosp, M2 11-687 av des Pins O, Montreal QC H3A 1A1; Ott'96; FRCPC; NuclearMed. Staff, McGill University Health Centre - Royal Victoria Hospital; Langs: French; (514)843-1501; Fax. (514)843-1469.

HICKEY, Andrea E; 102-435 Regent St, Fredericton NB E3B 3X6; Dal'87; BSc; (506)458-0273; Fax. (506)458-0090.

HICKEY, Bruce M; First Med Place, 105-170 Queensway W, Mississauga ON L5B 3A8; RCS (Ireland)'85; Staff, Trillium Health Centre - Mississauga; (905)848-4454

HICKEY, Catherine; Dr L A Miller Centre, 100 Forest Rd, St. John's NL A1A 3Z9; Mem'99; FRCPC; Psy (Clinical Psychiatry). Physician, Dr Leonard A Miller Centre; (709)777-3300; drcatherinehickey@gmail.com.

HICKEY, Chantal; Hôpital Ste-Justine, 3175 ch Cote-Sainte-Catherine, Montreal QC H3T 1C5; Mon'97; CSPQ; FRCPC; Anes. Staff, Hôpital Ste-Justine; (514)345-4931

HICKEY, D Paul; Northside Family Practice, 145 King St, North Sydney NS B2A 3S1; Dal'72; BSc; Ac Staff, Northside General Hospital; (902)794-7242; Fax. (902)794-8429.

HICKEY, Dean; Hôpital régional Chaleur, 1750 Sunset Dr, Bathurst NB E2A 4L7; Dal'01; FRCPC; IntMed; Nephrol. Staff, Hopital Regional Chaleur; Langs: Bilingual(English/French); (506)544-2501; Fax. (506)544-2041.

HICKEY, Denise M; Dr Charles A Janeway Child HC, 300 Prince Philip Dr, St. John's NL A1B 3V6; Mem'97; FRCPC; Peds. Staff, Janeway Children's Health & Rehabilitation Centre; (709)777-4126; Fax. (709)777-4726.

HICKEY, Donald R; SMBD Jewish Gen Hosp, 3755 ch Cote-Sainte-Catherine, Montreal QC H3T 1E2; Mem'78; CSPQ; FRCPC; Anes. Staff, Sir Mortimer B Davis Jewish General; Assoc Prof Anes, McGill University; (514)340-8222 x5701; Fax. (514)340-8108.

HICKEY, James P; Elizabeth Avenue Fam Practice, 116-100 Elizabeth Ave, St. John's NL A1B 1S1; Mem'92; CCFP; FCFP; (709)579-5006

HICKEY, Joanne; Health Sciences Centre, 300 Prince Philip Dr, St. John's NL A1B 3V6; Mem'03; FRCPC; IntMed; Hem. Staff, Health Sciences Centre; (709)777-8967

HICKEY, John S; A-26 Market St, Antigonish NS B2G 3B4; Dal'74; CCFP; Staff, St Martha's Regional Hospital; (902)863-1775; Fax. (902)863-0572.

HICKEY, Kristin M; Univ of Western Ontario, UCC 25-1151 Richmond St, London ON N6A 3K7; Dal'00; CCFP; (519)661-2047; Fax. (519)661-3824.

HICKEY, Liam; Fredericton Med Clinic, 402-1015 Regent St, Fredericton NB E3B 6H5; Dal'00; FRCSC; Urol. Staff, Dr Everett Chalmers Regional Hospital; (506)457-4783; Fax. (506)457-4757; lhickey@dul.ca.

HICKEY, Michael C; North Lambton CHC, PO Box 1120 59 King St W, Forest ON N0N 1J0; Wes'65; CCFP; FCFP; (519)786-4545; Fax. (519)786-6318.

HICKEY, Michael; 41 Frederick St, Orillia ON L3V 5W6; McM'06; FRCSC; OrthSurg. Staff, Queen Elizabeth II Health Sciences Centre - Halifax Infirmary Site; (705)242-0447

HICKEY SOMERVILLE, Julia M; Parksville Med Clinic, PO Box 250 Stn Main 154 Memorial Ave W, Parksville BC V9P 2G4; Dal'87; Ac Staff, Nanaimo Regional General Hospital; (250)248-5757; Fax. (250)248-2128.

HICKIE, John P; Crowchild Square, 130-5403 Crowchild Trail NW, Calgary AB T3B 4Z1; Cal'91; CCFP; FCFP; University of Calgary.

HICKMAN, Donald N; New Vision Family Health Team, 206-525 Belmont Ave W, Kitchener ON N2M 5E2; Wes'78; CCFP; Staff, St Mary's General Hospital; Staff, Grand River Hospital - Kitchener/Waterloo Health Centre; (519)576-4070

HICKMAN, Robert S; Workplace Safety & Ins Board, WSIB-30 Cedar St, Sudbury ON P3E 1A4; Alb'72; Anes. (705)675-9301

HICKS, Christopher; St Michael's Hosp, 30 Bond St, Toronto ON M5B 1W8; Qns'04; FRCPC; EmergMed. Staff, St Michael's Hospital; (416)864-5095

HICKS, Cynthia D A; Winnipeg Clinic, 425 St Mary Ave, Winnipeg MB R3C 0N2; Man'93; MSc; ABIM; ABAI; (204)957-3204; Fax. (204)943-7921.

HICKS, Frank S; Green Bay Med Centre, PO Box 820 292 Main St, Springdale NL A0J 1T0; Mem'75; CCFP; FCFP; Staff, Green Bay Community Health Centre; (709)673-3867; Fax. (709)673-2803.

HICKS, Heather A; 10-5268 Memorial Dr NE, Calgary AB T2A 2R1; McM'81; BScN; Ac Staff, Tom Baker Cancer Centre; Ac Staff, Foothills Medical Centre; Clin Assoc Prof Med, University of Calgary; (403)235-6333; Fax. (403)235-6349.

HICKS, Lisa K; St Michael's Hosp, 2084-30 Bond St, Toronto ON M5B 1W8; Tor'99; FRCPC; IntMed (Hematological Oncology); Hem. Staff, St Michael's Hospital; (416)864-5632; Fax. (416)864-3055.

HICKS, Lisa K; Burnham Med Services, 105-380 Burnham St, Peterborough ON K9H 1T6; McM'91; CCFP; FCFP; (705)741-3489; Fax. (705)741-3715.

HICKS, Roger A G; 201-143 Fourth Ave S, Williams Lake BC V2G 1J8; UBC'73; (250)398-8242

HICKS, Susan B; Conroy Med Centre, 100-2 Lorry Greenberg Dr, Ottawa ON K1G 5H6; Ott'82; CCFP; FCFP; (613)737-0654; Fax. (613)737-3265.

HICKS, Todd D; Aurora Med Dental Prof Bldg, 102-372 Hollandview Trail, Aurora ON L4G 0A5; Tor'92; CCFP; FCFP; Surg Asst, Southlake Regional Health Centre; (905)727-1711; Fax. (905)727-1411.

HICKS, Tracy E; Orthopedics & Surgery Inc, 5515 208 St, Langley BC V3A 2K4; Sask'70; FRCSC; OrthSurg (Hand & Wrist Surgery). Ac Staff, Langley Memorial Hospital; Vis Staff, Peace Arch Hospital; Langs: French; (604)534-9218; Fax. (604)534-9810.

HIDVEGI, Robert I S; MUHC-Montreal Chest Institute, 3650 rue Saint-Urbain, Montreal QC H2X 2P4; Budapest (Hungary)'52; FRCPC; DiagRad (Chest Radiology). Diagnostic-Radiology, McGill University Health Centre - Royal Victoria Hospital; Staff, McGill University Health Centre - Montreal General Campus; Chief Dept of Radiol, McGill University Health Centre - Montreal Chest Institute; adj Prof, McGill University; (514)934-1934 x32341; Fax. (514)873-2088.

HIDVEGI, Sylvia; 408-600 Sherbourne St, Toronto ON M4X 1W4; McG'87; FRCPC; Psy (Psychiatric Disorders/Elderly). Staff, Toronto East General Hospital Inc; Lecturer, University of Toronto; (416)551-1900

HIEBERT, Gayle D; Ermineskin Med Clinic, 301-2377 111 St NW, Edmonton AB T6J 5E5; Alb'72; Staff, Covenant Health - Edmonton General Continuing Care Centre; (780)436-8731

HIEBERT, Mervin P J; Chinook Reg Hosp, 960 19 St S, Lethbridge AB T1J 1W5; Man'91; CCFP; CCFP(E.M.); Staff Emerg Med, Chinook Regional Hospital; (403)388-6304

HIEBERT, Ron M; Royal Jubilee Hosp, HW 118-1952 Bay St, Victoria BC V8R 1J8; Alb'94; CCFP; Staff, Royal Jubilee Hospital; (250)519-1539

HIEBERT, Tim; St. Boniface Hosp, 409 Tache Ave, Winnipeg MB R2H 2A6; Man'05; FRCPC; IntMed. Staff, St Boniface General Hospital; (204)233-8563

HIEMSTRA, Laurie A; Banff Sport Medicine, PO Box 1300 Stn Main, Banff AB T1L 1B3; Mem'95; PhD; PhC; BMedSci; FRCS; FRCSC; OrthSurg (Sports Medicine). Staff, Covenant Health - Banff Mineral Springs Hospital; (403)760-2897; Fax. (403)760-8234; hiemstra@banffsportmed.ca.

HIEMSTRA, Robert; Alexandra Hosp, 29 Noxon St, Ingersoll ON N5C 1B8; Mem'96; BSc; CCFP; Staff, Alexandra Hospital; Staff Emerg Phys, South Huron Hospital Association; Staff Emerg Phys, West Haldimand General Hospital; (519)485-1732 x256; Fax. (519)453-4306.

HIER, Michael; SMBD Jewish Gen Hosp, 3755 ch Cote-Sainte-Catherine, Montreal QC H3T 1E2; McG'90; FRCSC; Otol (Head & Neck Surgery & Oncology). Staff, Sir Mortimer B Davis Jewish General; Assoc Prof Otolaryngology & Oncolgy, McGill University; Langs: Bilingual(English/French); (514)340-8222; Fax. (514)340-7581.

HIERLIHY, Lynn E; Halton HSC Corp-Oakville, 327 Reynolds St, Oakville ON L6J 3L7; Qns'94; BSc(Hon); PhD; FRCPC; Peds. Court Staff, Halton Healthcare Services Corporation - Oakville Site; (905)845-2571

HIERLIHY, Phyllis J; 202-100 Marie Curie Pvt, Ottawa ON K1N 1A2; Tor'69; FRCPC; IntMed (Endocrinology). Ac Staff Med, The Ottawa Hospital - General Campus; Assoc Prof Med, University of Ottawa; (613)860-3632; Fax. (613)569-0889; phierlihy@sympatico.ca.

HIEW, Moo-Khon; Foothills Med Centre, 1403 29 St NW, Calgary AB T2N 2T9; Alb'91; FRCPC; Anes. Staff, Foothills Medical Centre; (403)944-1430; Fax. (403)944-2425.

HIGA, Thomas E; DynaLIFEdx Med Labs, 200-10150 102 St NW, Edmonton AB T5J 5E2; Alb'77; BMedSci; FRCPC; AnatPath (Laboratory Medicine). Consultant, Sturgeon Community Hospital; Consultant, DynaLIFE Diagnostics; Clin Prof, University of Alberta; (780)451-3702; Fax. (780)454-2845.

HIGGIN, Douglas M; Cochrane Comm Hlth Centre, 60 Grande Blvd W, Cochrane AB T4C 0S4; Cal'97; CCFP; CCFP(E.M.); (403)851-6261; Fax. (403)851-6279; dhiggin@mdh.ab.ca.

HIGGINS, Brian P; The Credit Valley Hosp, 2200 Eglinton Ave W, Mississauga ON L5M 2N1; Tor'87; DABIM; FRCPC; IntMed; MedOncol. Court Staff, Headwaters Health Care Centre - Orangeville Site; Staff, The Credit Valley Hospital; (905)813-2200 x5135; bhiggins@cvh.on.ca.

HIGGINS, Darren S; 201-720 Spadina Ave, Toronto ON M5S 2T9; Dal'90; FRCPC; Psy. Staff, Mount Sinai Hospital; Staff Mood & Anxiety Prog, Centre for Addiction & Mental Health (CAMH) - Queen Site; Teach Staff Psy, University of Toronto; (416)972-6019

HIGGINS, David A; St Joseph's Healthcare, 50 Charlton Ave E, Hamilton ON L8N 4A6; National (Ireland)'79; MB ChB; MRC(PI); BSc; DABSM; FRCPC; IntMed (Sleep Disorders); Respir. Pres, St Joseph's Healthcare - Charlton Campus; Clin Prof Med, McMaster University; (905)522-1155 x33960; Fax. (905)521-6184; dhiggins@stjosham.on.ca.

HIGGINS, Derek A; Sparwood Primary Health Centre, PO Box 1120 570 Pine Ave, Sparwood BC V0B 2G0; Aberdeen (Scotland)'91; MB ChB; CCFP; Staff, Sparwood Healthcare Centre; (250)425-4501; Fax. (250)425-4549.

HIGGINS, Eric J; CSSS de Saint-Jerome, 290 rue de Montigny, Saint-Jerome QC J7Z 5T3; Mon'95; Staff, Hôtel-Dieu de Saint-Jérôme; (450)431-8400

HIGGINS, Ethel; Centre Med St Redempteur, 210-600 rte 116, Saint-Nicolas QC G7A 4X8; Laval'81; CCFP; FCFP; assoc Membre, Centre Hospitalier Universitaire de Quebec-CHUL; Université Laval; (418)831-3677; Fax. (418)831-7967; ethel.higgins@gmf.gouv.qc.ca.

HIGGINS, Geoffrey C; St Clare's Mercy Hosp, 154 Lemarchant Rd, St. John's NL A1C 5B8; Dal'73; DABR; FRCPC; DiagRad (Body Computed Tomography). Chief Dept of Diagnostic Imaging, St Clare's Mercy Hospital; Ac Staff, Health Care Corporation Of St John's; Clin Assoc Prof Radiol, Memorial University Of Newfoundland; (709)777-5362; Fax. (709)777-5793.

HIGGINS, Gina; Killick Health Centre, 54 Union St, Grnd-Falls-Windsor NL A2A 2E2; Mem'08; CCFP; (709)292-3000

HIGGINS, Gordon A; The Wellness Centre, 98 Bonaventure Ave, St. John's NL A1B 2X4; Mem'75; CCFP; FCFP; Court Staff, Health Sciences Centre; Dist Med Officer of Hlth, Newfoundland & Labrador-Veterans Affairs Canada; (709)753-8883; Fax. (709)726-9571.

HIGGINS, Greg; Prince Edward Family Hlth Team, GD 2-35 Bridge St, Picton ON K0K 2T0; Qns'87; CCFP; Staff, QHC Prince Edward County Memorial; Instructor Family Med, Queen's University; (613)476-0400

HIGGINS, Kevin; Sunnybrook Hlth Sciences Ctre, M1 102-2075 Bayview Ave, Toronto ON M4N 3M5; Tor'97; BSc; MSc; FRCSC; Otol (Endocrinology Surgery). Court Staff, Women's College Hospital; Court Staff, North York General Hospital; Court Staff, Toronto East General Hospital Inc; Staff, Sunnybrook Health Sciences Centre; (416)480-5104; Fax. (416)480-5761.

HIGGINS, Louise J; Saugeen Shores Med Bldg, 36 Grey St N, Southampton ON N0H 2L0; Mem'00; CCFP; (519)797-9940; Fax. (519)797-1225.

HIGGINS, Richard J; Children's Hosp, 840 Sherbrook St, Winnipeg MB R3A 1S1; Man'83; FRCPC; DiagRad. Staff, Health Sciences Centre.

HIGGINS, Terrance F; Spryfield Med Centre, 205 Herring Cove Rd, Halifax NS B3P 1L1; Dal'70; (902)477-5693; Fax. (902)477-0502.

HIGGINS, Thomas J; Parry Sound Family Health Team, 15 James St, Parry Sound ON P2A 1T4; Qns'80; CCFP; Ac Staff, West Parry Sound Health Centre; (705)746-9382; Fax. (705)746-7758.

HIGGINS, Liam; Hoy Med Clinic, 402-2155 10th Ave, Prince George BC V2M 5J6; Dublin (Ireland)'78; MB ChB; BAO; DObst; DCH; (250)563-8878; Fax. (250)564-9847.

HIGGINSON, Judy J; Langley Mem Hosp, 22051 Fraser Hwy, Langley BC V3A 4H4; McM'82; CCFP; CCFP(E.M.); Staff, Langley Memorial Hospital; (604)534-4121 x5265; Fax. (604)533-6467.

HIGGINSON, Lyall A J; Univ Of Ottawa Heart Institute, H3412A-40 Ruskin St, Ottawa ON K1Y 4W7; McG'71; FRCPC; IntMed; Cardiol. Staff, Royal Jubilee Hospital; (613)761-4039; Fax. (613)761-4170.

HIGGS, Jillian; Oromocto Family Physicans, 66 Broad Rd, Oromocto NB E2V 1C2; Dal'05; BSc; MSc; CCFP; (506)357-1813; Fax. (506)357-3712.

HIGGS, Stewart I L; Iroquois Ridge Med Centre, B5-360 Dundas St E, Oakville ON L6H 6Z9; (United Kingdom)'79; MB BS; CCFP; (905)257-8777

HIGH, Sasha M; The Credit Valley Hosp, 2200 Eglinton Ave W, Mississauga ON L5M 2N1; Tor'08; FRCPC; IntMed. Staff, The Credit Valley Hospital; (905)813-2200

HIGHAM, M Scott; Centennial Med Centre, 299 Lake Ave E, Carleton Place ON K7C 1J3; McG'78; CCFP; FCFP; Chief Medical Staff, Carleton Place & District Memorial Hospital; Court Staff, Almonte General Hospital; Asst Prof Family Med, University of Ottawa; (613)257-2311; Fax. (613)257-4435.

HIGHMORE, Kerri A; Children's Hosp Eastern Ont, 401 Smyth Rd, Ottawa ON K1H 8L1; Mem'06; DiagRad. Staff, Children's Hospital of Eastern Ontario (CHEO); (613)737-7600

HIGNELL, Allen B; Guisachan Family Medicine, 105-2395 Gordon Dr, Kelowna BC V1W 3X7; UBC'69; CCFP; Staff, Kelowna General Hospital; Assoc Prof Family Pract, University of British Columbia; (250)860-5888; Fax. (250)860-5880.

HII, Anthony Y P; 105-1971 Queen St E, Toronto ON M4L 1H9; Tor'70; Langs: Chinese; (416)699-9219; Fax. (416)691-8383.

HII, James F K; East Van Med Bldg, 401-1750 10th Ave E, Vancouver BC V5N 5K4; UBC'68; DAB; Staff Board of Directors, American Board of Anti-Aging Medicine; Langs: Mandarin; Foochow; Fookien; (604)873-2688; Fax. (604)873-2680; jameshii@telus.net.

HII, John; 401-372 Bay St, Toronto ON M5H 2W9; McG'84; FRCPC; MedMicrobiol (Infectious Diseases). Court Staff, St Joseph's Health Centre; Langs: Malay; Hokkin; English; French; Chinese; (416)350-3555; Fax. (416)350-3167.

HII, Ting H; Columbia Family Med, 302-1101 Dewdney Ave, Trail BC V1R 4T1; Alb'87; Ac Staff, Kootenay Boundary Regional Hospital; Langs: Mandarin; (250)368-9394; Fax. (250)368-8281.

HIJAL, Tarek; MUHC-Montreal Gen Hosp, D5 400-1650 av Cedar, Montreal QC H3G 1A4; McG'03; FRCPC; RadOncol. Staff, McGill University Health Centre - Montreal General Campus; (514)934-8040

HILAL, Ali Abbas M; 129-2224 Walker Rd, Windsor ON N8W 5L7; Baghdad (Iraq)'92; FRCSI; FRCSC; Otol (Laryngology). Langs: Arabic; French; (519)946-0230

HILAREGUY, Natacha; CSSS Haut-Richelieu-Rouville, 300-920 boul du Seminaire N, St-Jean-sur-Richel QC J3A 1B7; Sher'06; Otol. Staff, Hôpital du Haut-Richelieu; (450)376-1300

HILBORN, David J; South Bank Med Centre, 3-2430 Bank St, Ottawa ON K1V 0T7; Qns'60; Staff, The Ottawa Hospital - Riverside Campus; Med Examiner, Canadian & American Civil Aviation; Clin Instructor, University of Ottawa; (613)736-6946; Fax. (613)736-6938.

HILDAHL, Craig R; Bison Primacy Med Clinic, 1-80 Bison Dr, Winnipeg MB R3T 4Z7; Man'78; CCFP; FCFP; (204)275-1500; Fax. (204)269-9938.

HILDAHL, V Keith; Manitoba Adolescent Trmt Ctr, 120 Tecumseh St, Winnipeg MB R3E 2A9; Man'81; FRCPC; Psy (Child & Adolescent Psychiatry). CEO, Manitoba Adolescent Treatment Centre; Asst Prof, University of Manitoba; (204)477-6391; Fax. (204)783-8948; khildahl@matc.ca.

HILDAHL, Wayne; Pan Am Clinic, 75 Poseidon Bay, Winnipeg MB R3M 3E4; Man'74; COO, Pan Am Sports Med Centre; (204)927-2772; Fax. (204)925-4878; whildahl@panamclinic.com.

HILDEBRAND, Ainslie M; London HSC-Victoria Hosp, PO Box 5010 800 Commissioners Rd E, London ON N6A 4G5; Man'07; FRCPC; IntMed; Nephrol. Staff, London Health Sciences Centre - Children's Hospital; (519)685-8500

HILDEBRAND, B Mark; 101-532 Lake St, St Catharines ON L2N 4H4; Man'87; CCFP; (905)646-0015

HILDEBRAND, Brenda; St Boniface Gen Hosp, Z3012-409 Tache Ave, Winnipeg MB R2H 2A6; Man'05; FRCSC; Urol. Staff, St Boniface General Hospital; (204)233-8863

HILDEBRAND, Kevin A; Health Research Innovation Ctr, 3280 Hospital Dr NW, Calgary AB T2N 4Z6; Cal'89; FRCSC; OrthSurg (Elbow & Wrist Surgery). Physician, Health Research Innovation Centre; Prof, University of Calgary; (403)220-7282; Fax. (403)270-3679.

HILDEBRAND, Kyla J; St Joseph's Health Care, B3 110-268 Grosvenor St, London ON N6A 4V2; Man'05; FRCPC; Peds; ClinImmunol&Allergy. Staff, St Joseph's Hospital - St Joseph's Health Care; (519)685-8167

HILDEBRAND, Mary M; Wilson Centre Family Practice, 1-2185 Wilson Ave, Port Coquitlam BC V3C 6C1; McM'90; (604)942-7227; Fax. (604)942-7058.

HILDEBRANDT, Walter H; Highland Park Med Clinic, 2B-6315 Horn St, Red Deer AB T4N 6H5; (South Africa)'90; MB ChB; (403)342-2040; Fax. (403)342-7390.

HILDERMAN, Ernest D; Smith Clinic, 1-6601 48 Ave, Camrose AB T4V 3G8; Cal'78; Ac Staff, Covenant Health - St Mary's Hospital; (780)672-2424; Fax. (780)608-5895.

HILDERMAN, Lorraine; Markham Med Centre, 200-2265 Pembina Hwy, Winnipeg MB R3T 5J3; Man'89; Staff, Victoria General Hospital; Staff Breast Screening Program, Manitoba Cancer Treatment & Research Foundation; lorraine.hilderman@cancercare.mb.ca.

HILDERMAN, Timothy E; Stonewall & District Hlth Cent, 589 3rd Ave S, Stonewall MB R0C 2Z0; Man'91; FRCPC; CommunMed (Public Health). Staff, Stonewall & District Health Centre; (204)467-5514

HILDES-RIPSTEIN, G Elizabeth E; Children's Hosp, CH 102-840 Sherbrook St, Winnipeg MB R3A 1S1; Man'88; FRCPC; Peds. Staff Children's Hosp Ambulatory Group, Health Sciences Centre; University of Manitoba.

HILL, Alan; Children's & Women's HC Of BC, K3 145-4480 Oak St, Vancouver BC V6H 3V4; Sask'75; PhD; BSc; FRCPC; Peds (Child Neurology); Neur. Vis Staff, Providence Health Care - St Paul's Hospital; Hd Neurol & Child Ambulatory Care, BC Children's Hospital; Prof, University of British Columbia; (604)875-2121; Fax. (604)875-2285; ahill@cw.bc.ca.

HILL, Alan M; 744 Centre St PO Box 6000, Burns Lake BC V0J 1E0; (United Kingdom)'70; MB BS; (250)692-3111; Fax. (250)692-7477.

HILL, Amanda J; St Paul's Hosp, 9F-1081 Burrard St, Vancouver BC V6Z 1Y6; Witwatersrand (South Africa)'78; MB BCh; FRCPC; IntMed (Dementia); GeriatricMed. Staff, Providence Health Care - St Paul's Hospital; Staff, Vancouver General Hospital - Centennial Pavillion; Consultant, Geriatric Consultation Team; Clin Assoc Prof, University of British Columbia; (778)389-8793; amanda.hill@vch.ca.

HILL, Andrew B; The Ottawa Hosp-Civic Campus, A280 014-1053 Carling Ave, Ottawa ON K1Y 4E9; McG'86; CSPQ; BSc; MSc; FRCSC; GenSurg; VascSurg. Staff, The Ottawa Hospital - Civic Campus; Assoc Prof Surg, University of Ottawa; Langs: French; (613)798-5555 x16043; Fax. (613)761-5362; ahill@ottawahospital.on.ca.

HILL, Christine; CLSC de la Haute Yamaska, 294 rue Deragon, Granby QC J2G 5J5; Laval'91; LMCC; (450)375-1442 x6279; Fax. (450)375-9345.

HILL, Danny G; Sault Area Hosp, 750 Great Northern Rd, Sault Ste. Marie ON P6B 0A8; Alb'07; Hem; IntMed. Staff, Sault Area Hospital - Sault Ste Marie; (705)759-3434

HILL, David J; 202-1017 Wilson Ave, North York ON M3K 1Z1; Dublin (Ireland)'71; MSc; MRC(Lond); Langs: Gaelic; Spanish; Italian; French; (416)633-5880; Fax. (416)633-6278.

HILL, Denise C; Foothills Med Centre, SSB AC144A-1403 29 St NW, Calgary AB T2N 2T9; McM'97; FRCPC; PhysMed&Rehab (Spinal Cord Injury). Staff, Foothills Medical Centre; Clinical Asst Prof, University of Calgary; (403)944-4475; Fax. (403)283-2526.

HILL, Douglas A; 207-2004 14 St NW, Calgary AB T2M 3N3; Cal'86; MSW; BA(Hons); DAB(Phlebology); CCFP; FCFP; (403)220-9353; Fax. (403)210-0593; vtcentre@telus.net.

HILL, Gary V; Peterborough Reg HC-Hospital, 1 Hospital Dr, Peterborough ON K9J 7C6; Tor'83; AB; Staff, Peterborough Regional Health Centre - Hospital Drive; (705)876-5022

HILL, Jeanne; CSSS La Pommeraie, 200 rue Principale, Cowansville QC J2K 1J2; Mon'87; Physician, CSSS la Pommeraie; Langs: English; (450)263-5142 x3300; Fax. (450)263-5218; jeanne_hill@yahoo.com.

HILL, Joanna E; Valley Park Lodge Nursing Home, 6400 Valley Way, Niagara Falls ON L2E 7E3; Wes'78; BSc; Court Staff, Niagara Health System - Greater Niagara General Site; (905)358-3277; Fax. (905)358-3012.

HILL, Karen; Six Nations Family Hlth Team, PO Box 5000 1745 Chiefswood Rd, Ohsweken ON N0A 1M0; McM'03; CCFP; Associate Clin Prof, McMaster University; (519)445-4019

HILL, Kenneth C; Kingsway Plaza Phase III, 601-4980 Kingsway, Burnaby BC V5H 4K7; Man'56; FRCSC; OrthSurg. Staff, Burnaby Hospital; (604)435-7822; Fax. (604)435-1498; ken_hill@telus.net.

HILL, Laurie L; Brampton Cardio-Pulmonary Serv, 31 Centre St S, Brampton ON L6W 2X7; West Indies (Jamaica)'77; MB BS; FACP; FACC; FACCP; FRCPC; IntMed (Sleep Medicine); Cardiol. (905)455-3010; Fax. (905)455-3011; info@bramptoncardio.com.

HILL, Mariana G; Keele-Ingram Prof Centre, 103-2221 Keele St, North York ON M6M 3Z5; Bucharest (Romania)'61; FRCPC; Psy (General Psychiatry). Staff, North York General Hospital; Langs: Romanian; French; (416)614-9696; Fax. (416)614-9696.

HILL, Mark K; Gordon & Leslie Diamond HCC, 3L-2775 Laurel St, Vancouver BC V5Z 1M9; Sask'82; FRCSC; PlasSurg. (604)875-5866

HILL, Michael; Foothills Med Centre, 1242A-1403 29 St NW, Calgary AB T2N 2T9; Ott'93; BSc; MSc; FRCPC; IntMed (Stroke); Neur. Ad Staff Privil, Foothills Medical Centre; Assoc Dean Clinical Research, University of Calgary; Langs: English; French; (403)944-8065; Fax. (403)283-2270.

HILL, Monica L; 51 Riverside Gate PO Box 376 Stn Main, Okotoks AB T1S 1A6; Sask'90; CCFP; FCFP; Assessment Physician, Alberta Medical Association Physician & Family Support Prog; (403)995-4409

HILL, N Grant; PO Box 430 Stn Main, Okotoks AB T1S 1A6; Alb'68; (403)938-1424; Fax. (403)938-4184.

HILL, Norman S; Queensway Prof Centre, 412-190 Sherway Dr, Etobicoke ON M9C 5N2; Tor'76; FRCSC; GenSurg. VP-Med Affairs, Trillium Health Centre - Mississauga; Ac Staff, Trillium Health Centre - West Toronto; (416)621-3551; Fax. (416)621-3335.

HILL, Robert W; The Two Hundred, 401W E-200 St Clair Ave W, Toronto ON M4V 1R1; Tor'70; FRCPC; Psy (Forensic Medicine). (416)944-0186

HILL, Samantha; St Michael's Hosp, 30 Bond St, Toronto ON M5B 1W8; McG'03; FRCSC; CardSurg. Staff, St Michael's Hospital; Langs: Bilingual(English/French); (416)360-4000

HILL, Stephen D; Huntsville District Mem Hosp, 8-100 Frank Miller Dr, Huntsville ON P1H 1H7; Wes'83; CCFP; Ac Staff, Huntsville District Memorial Hospital - Muskoka Algonquin Healthcare; (705)789-0022 x372

HILL, Vivian E; 344-933 17 Ave SW, Calgary AB T2T 5R6; Ott'96; BSc(Hon); FRCSC; Ophth (Pediatric Ophthalmology). Staff, Alberta Children's Hospital; Staff, Rockyview General Hospital; Staff, Peter Lougheed Centre; University of Calgary; Langs: German; French; (403)245-3171; Fax. (403)245-3080.

HILL-ELIAS, Rachel; 3700 Westfield Rd, Saint John NB E2M 5Z4; Dal'89; Staff, Saint John Regional Hospital; (506)738-4727

HILLARY, Edward W; 1301-1255 Main St, Vancouver BC V6A 4G5; Cape Town (South Africa)'85; MB ChB; CCFP; Langs: Afrikaans.

HILLEN, James; Regional Treatment Centre, PO Box 22 Stn Main 560 King St W, Kingston ON K7L 4V7; McM'83; MSc; FRCPC; ObstGyn; Psy. Staff Forensic Services, Providence Care - Mental Health Services; Consultant Psy, Correctional Services of Canada; Aj Asst Prof, Queen's University; (613)545-8476

HILLER, Bruce; Burnaby Hosp, 3935 Kincaid St, Burnaby BC V5G 2X6; UBC'95; BSc(Microbiol); DTMH; FRCPC; IntMed. Staff, Burnaby Hospital; (604)434-4211

HILLER, Stella; CSSS Lac-des-Deux Montagnes, 201-1 Place de la Gare, Saint-Eustache QC J7R 0B4; Mon'75; (450)473-6811 x7474; Fax. (450)491-5408; stella.hiller@ssss.gouv.qc.ca.

HILLHOUSE, Brian; 2-1230 Alward St, Prince George BC V2M 7B1; UBC'08; CCFP; Staff, University Hospital of Northern British Columbia; (250)563-0414

HILLIARD, Jennifer; 202-60 Aberdeen St, Kentville NS B4N 2N3; Dal'07; FRCPC; Peds. (902)678-1221; Fax. (902)678-2331.

HILLIARD, Neil K; 100-2296 McCallum Rd, Abbotsford BC V2S 3P4; Tor'77; Ac Staff, Chilliwack General Hospital; Staff, Abbotsford Regional Hospital & Cancer Centre; Staff, Mission Memorial Hospital; (604)851-4700; Fax. (604)859-2929.

HILLIARD, Robert I; The Hosp for Sick Children, 555 University Ave, Toronto ON M5G 1X8; Tor'67; ABPeds; FAAP; EdD; FRCPC; Peds (Medical Education). Staff Peds, The Hospital For Sick Children; Prof Peds, University of Toronto; (416)813-5795; Fax. (416)813-5663; robert.hilliard@sickkids.ca.

HILLIER, Linda G; Children Hosp of Eastern Ont, 401 Smyth Rd, Ottawa ON K1H 8L1; Mem'82; FRCPC; Peds (General Pediatrics). Staff, Children's Hospital of Eastern Ontario (CHEO); (613)737-7600 x2571; Fax. (613)738-4878.

HILLIER, Mark R; 3935 Kincaid St, Burnaby BC V5G 2X6; UBC'87; Staff, Burnaby Hospital; (604)431-2811

HILLIER, Stephen F; Burnaby Hosp, 3935 Kincaid St, Burnaby BC V5G 2X6; McM'74; BSc(Med); Staff, Burnaby Hospital; (604)412-6311

HILLIER, Tracey L B; Meadowlark Hlth Ctr, 200 Meadowlark Shopping Ctr NW, Edmonton AB T5R 5W9; McM'97; FRCPC; DiagRad. Staff, University of Alberta Hospital; (780)489-5313

HILLIS, Joanne; Radiology Associates Of Regina, 6-2727 Parliament Ave, Regina SK S4S 6X5; Sask'83; FRCPC; DiagRad (Mammography). Staff, Pasqua Hospital; Staff, Regina General Hospital; Staff, Radiology Associates of Regina; (306)352-7653; Fax. (306)522-4311.

HILLIS, Michael T; Valley Reg Hosp, 150 Exhibition St, Kentville NS B4N 5E3; Dal'92; FRCPC; Anes. Staff, Valley Regional Hospital; (902)678-7381; Fax. (902)679-1904.

HILLIS, Robert A; PO Box 1329 Stn Main, Vernon BC V1T 6N6; Alb'81; FCBOM; (250)542-6485; Fax. (250)549-4165.

HILLMAN, Alison J; North Plaza Med Bidgood's Plaz, PO Box 1060 Stn C, Goulds NL A1S 1H2; Mem'90.

HILLMER, Melinda; Toronto East Gen & Orth Hosp, 825 Coxwell Ave, Toronto ON M4C 3E7; Tor'04; FRCPC; IntMed; Critical Care Medicine. Staff, Toronto East General Hospital Inc; (416)461-8272

HILLSON, Tim R; 2-384 West St N, Orillia ON L3V 5E6; McM'96; MA; FRCSC; Ophth (Cataract). Staff, Orillia Soldiers' Memorial Hospital; (705)325-6591; Fax. (705)325-9309.

HILLYARD, David; Cottage Country Fam Hlth Team, 1-5 Pineridge Gate, Gravenhurst ON P1P 1Z3; Wes'73; CCFP; Ac Staff Family Pract, South Muskoka Memorial Hospital - Muskoka Algonquin Healthcare; (705)687-2795; Fax. (705)687-8652.

HILLYARD, Jeremy W; Guysborough Antigonish Hlth Au, 25 Bay St, Antigonish NS B2G 2G5; Liverpool (England)'74; MB ChB; FRCS; (902)867-4500 x4170; Fax. (902)867-1059; jeremy.hillyard@gasha.nshealth.ca.

HILLYER, Cheryl; 150 Huron St, Stratford ON N5A 5S8; Leicester (England)'90; MB ChB; BSc(Hon.); FRCSC; ObstGyn. Staff, Stratford General Hospital - Huron Perth Healthcare Alliance; (519)271-2822; Fax. (519)271-2266.

HILNER, Jon S; Grandin Med Clinic, 1 St Anne St, St. Albert AB T8N 2E8; Alb'10; CCFP; (780)459-5581; Fax. (780)458-7515.

HILSDEN, Richard; London HSC-University Hosp, PO Box 5339 Stn B 339 Windermere Rd, London ON N6A 5A5; McM'06; CCFP; Staff, London Health Sciences Centre - University Hospital; (519)663-3269

HILSDEN, Robert J; University of Calgary, 3330 Hospital Dr NW, Calgary AB T2N 4N1; Sask'88; PhD; MSc; MD; FRCPC; FRCPC; Gastroent; IntMed. Ac Staff, Peter Lougheed Centre; Health Research Innovation Centre; Asst Prof, University of Calgary; (403)943-2502; Fax. (403)943-4017; rhilsden@ucalgary.ca.

HILSDEN, Shannon; Grand River Comm Hlth Centre, 347 Colborne St, Brantford ON N3S 3N2; McM'07; CCFP; (519)754-0777; Fax. (519)754-0757.

HILTON, J David; Richmond Med Bldg, 202-2020 Richmond Rd, Victoria BC V8R 6R5; Tor'75; FRCPC; Cardiol (Interventional Cardiology). Staff Interventional Cardiol, Royal Jubilee Hospital; Co-Dir, Victoria Heart Institute Foundation; (250)595-3111; Fax. (250)595-4278; dhilton@westheart.net.

HILTON, Jack G; 100 Division St, Trenton ON K8V 4W8; McG'83; FRCPC; IntMed (Oncology). (613)394-8540; Fax. (613)394-8538.

HILTON, James D; North Toronto Med Bldg, 202-250 Lawrence Ave W, Toronto ON M5M 1B2; McG'69; BSc; MDCM; FRCPC; Peds. Staff Physician, The Hospital For Sick Children; Court Staff Sunnybrook Health Ctr, Sunnybrook Health Sciences Centre; Asst Prof Peds, University of Toronto; (416)789-4818

HILTON, Jennifer; Queen City Obst & Gyn, 3271 Quance St E, Regina SK S4V 3B7; Sask'03; MSc; BSc; FRCSC; ObstGyn. Staff, Regina General Hospital; Physician, Queen City Obstetrics & Gynecology; (306)585-9565; Fax. (306)585-9209.

HILTZ, David W; Riverview Shopping Mall, 102-720 Coverdale Rd, Riverview NB E1B 3L8; Dal'72; CCFP; FCFP; (506)387-4402; Fax. (506)387-4037.

HILZENRAT, Nir; SMBD Jewish Gen Hosp, 3755 ch Cote-Ste-Catherine, Montreal QC H3T 1E2; Technion (Israel)'89; FRCPC; Gastroent. Staff, Sir Mortimer B Davis Jewish General; (514)340-8286; Fax. (514)340-8282.

HIMAL, Harry S; St Michal's Hosp Academic-FHT, 935-790 Bay St, Toronto ON M5G 1N8; Ott'63; FACS; FRCSC; GenSurg. Langs: English; French; (416)613-5050; Fax. (416)513-5051.

HIMANN, Joan E; 202-170 Simcoe St, Peterborough ON K9H 2H7; McM'90; PhD; Dip SportMed; CCFP; FCFP; Staff, Peterborough Regional Health Centre - Hospital Drive; (705)743-3804; Fax. (705)872-4357; jhimann@prhc.on.ca.

HIMAYA, Eric; Clinique Ovo, 100-8000 boul Decarie, Montreal QC H4P 2S4; Mon'06; FRCSC; ObstGyn. (514)798-2000

HIMEL, Naomi; 245 Eglinton Ave E, Toronto ON M4P 3B7; Tor'84; CCFP; FCFP; Langs: Hebrew; (416)485-7663; Fax. (416)488-8846.

HIMELFARB, Erite; Kerrisdale Station Med Clinic, 2077 42nd Ave W, Vancouver BC V6M 2B4; Tor'78; Court Staff, BC Women's Hospital & Health Centre; Vis Staff, Vancouver General Hospital - Centennial Pavillion; Vis Staff, Providence Health Care - St Paul's Hospital; (604)261-9494

HIMIDAN, Sharifa A; The Hosp For Sick Children, 555 University Ave, Toronto ON M5G 1X8; Abdul Aziz (Saudi Arabia)'90; MB BS; FRCSC; GenSurg (Neonatal); PedGenSurg. Staff, The Hospital For Sick Children; Staff PedSurg, North York General Hospital; Langs: Arabic; (416)813-7654; Fax. (416)813-7181; sharifa.himidan@sickkids.ca.

HIMMEL, Susan; Ashgrove Med Centre, 103-6633 Highway 7, Markham ON L3P 7P2; Tor'80; (905)472-3322; Fax. (905)472-4323.

HIMMEL, Walter M; North York Gen Hosp, 4001 Leslie St, North York ON M2K 1E1; Tor'76; CCFP; CCFP(E.M.); FCFP; Ac Staff, North York General Hospital; Staff, The Scarborough Hospital - General Campus; Staff, Toronto East General Hospital Inc; (416)756-6002; Fax. (416)346-9049; wmhim@sympatico.ca.

HIMMELMAN, Donald W; South Shore Med Arts Bldg, 307-42 Glen Allan Dr, Bridgewater NS B4V 3N2; Dal'71; Ophth (Medical & Surgical Ophthalmology). Ac Staff, South Shore Regional Hospital; (902)543-6819; Fax. (902)543-9273; dwhimmelman@eastlink.ca.

HIMMELSBACH, Sherillynne; Whitehorse Med Services Ltd, 406 Lambert St, Whitehorse YT Y1A 1Z7; UBC'84; CCFP; FCFP; Staff, Whitehorse Medical Services Ltd; (867)393-6640; Fax. (867)393-6601.

HINCHLIFFE, Mary J; Hycroft Med Bldg, 115-3195 Granville St, Vancouver BC V6H 3K2; UBC'89; CCFP; FCFP; (604)732-0525

HIND, Sharon A; 110-200 St Clair Ave W, Toronto ON M4V 1R1; Ott'05; CCFP; Staff, Women's College Hospital; Staff, William Osler Health System - Etobicoke General Hospital; (416)928-9343

HINDLE, Hugh R; Red Deer Reg Hosp Centre, 3942 50A Ave, Red Deer AB T4N 4E7; London (England)'78; DRCOG; MRCGPract; MB BS; CCFP; CCFP(E.M.); FCFP; Staff, Red Deer Regional Hospital Centre; Ac Staff, Hinton Healthcare Centre; Med Dir Cardiac Rehab Program, Westview Regional Health Authority; Clin Assoc Prof Med. & Unit Dir., University of Alberta; (403)343-4444; hugh.hindle@arfmn.ab.ca.

HINDLE, Peter R; Port Arthur Health Centre Inc, 194 Court St N, Thunder Bay ON P7A 4V7; McM'76; (807)346-1000

HINDLE, Valerie; 3F-219 Laurier Ave W, Ottawa ON K1A 1L1; Man'85; BSc(Med); Dip SportMed; CCFP; Med Officer of Hlth, Citizenship & Immigration Canada; Staff Occuptional Health, Health Canada; Physician Community Med, University of Ottawa; Langs: Spanish; French; Fax. (613)941-2179; valerie.hindle@gmail.com.

HINDLER, Lionel R; Shubenacadie Med Centre, PO Box 304 2815 Main St, Shubenacadie NS B0N 2H0; Witwatersrand (South Africa)'84; MB ChB; (902)758-2296

HINDOCHA, Sandeep P; 1 Henderson Dr, Aurora ON L4G 4J7; Ott'93; CCFP; (905)713-6800; Fax. (905)713-6539.

HINDOOSH, Raghad A N A; Hurontario Clinic, C7-4555 Hurontario St, Mississauga ON L4Z 3M1; (Iraq)'00; CCFP; (416)992-3957

HINDS, Catharine A; Canmore Associate Med Clinic, 124-1151 Sidney St, Canmore AB T1W 3G1; Tor'77; BSc; CCFP; FCFP; Ac Staff, Canmore General Hospital; Vis Staff, Covenant Health - Banff Mineral Springs Hospital; (403)678-5585; Fax. (403)678-6262.

HINDS, Philip R; Seawatch Med Clinic, 203-2276 Island Hwy S, Campbell River BC V9W 1C3; Belfast (United Kingdom)'87; MB BCh; BAO; (250)923-1189

HINDSON, Judith M; King West Med Associates, 505 King St W, Hamilton ON L8P 1B9; Wes'92; CCFP; FCFP; Asst Prof Family Med, McMaster University; (905)525-3501; Fax. (905)528-5468.

HINEK, Anna; Credit Valley Prof Bldg, 202-2300 Eglinton Ave W, Mississauga ON L5M 2V8; Tor'07; Derm. (905)828-0770; Fax. (905)828-4130.

HINGS, Ingrid M; MUHC-Montreal Gen Hosp, B7 119-1650 av Cedar, Montreal QC H3G 1A4; McG'86; BSc; ABIM; AB(Hem/MedOncol.); FRCPC; IntMed; Hem; MedOncol. Assoc Physician Oncol & IntMed, McGill University Health Centre - Montreal General Campus; Assoc Prof Oncol & IntMed, McGill University; Langs: English; French; German; (514)934-8007; Fax. (514)934-8379; ingrid.hings@muhc.mcgill.ca.

HINGWALA, Jay P; 602-500 University Ave, Toronto ON M5G 1V7; Man'08; FRCPC; IntMed.

HINKEWICH, Christopher; Queen Elizabeth II HSC, 1276 South Park St, Halifax NS B3H 2Y9; Dal'07; FRCSC; Anes. Staff, Queen Elizabeth II Health Sciences Centre - Victoria General Site; (902)473-3608

HINKKALA, Kaarlo S; London HSC-University Hosp, ALL 139-339 Windermere Rd, London ON N6A 5A5; Wes'08; FRCPC; IntMed. Staff, London Health Sciences Centre - University Hospital; (519)685-8500

HINKLE, Molli E; Queen Alexandra Ctre Children, 2400 Arbutus Rd, Victoria BC V8N 1V7; (USA)'97; Staff, Queen Alexandra Centre for Children's Health; (250)217-0054

HINNAWI, Hanna M; The Westway Plaza, 208-1735 Kipling Ave, Etobicoke ON M9R 2Y8; (Jordan)'80; Ac Staff, St Joseph's Health Centre; Ac Staff, William Osler Health System - Etobicoke General Hospital; Langs: Arabic; (416)235-2655; Fax. (416)235-0886.

HINNELL, Claire J; Jim Pattison Out patient Centr, 9750 140 St, Surrey BC V3T 0G9; UBC'06; FRCPC; Neur. (604)582-4550

HINSE, Michel; Centre Med de Dolbeau, 1530 rue des Erables, Dolbeau-Mistassini QC G8L 2W7; Mon'70; (418)276-0111; Fax. (418)276-6298.

HINSHAW, Deena L; 4703 53 St, Camrose AB T4V 1Y8; Alb'04; FRCPC; CommunMed;CCFP; (780)608-8805; Fax. (780)608-8600.

HINTON, Joan M; Edmonton Mental Health Clinic, 3F-9942 108 St NW, Edmonton AB T5K 2J5; London (England)'58; Clinical Asst Prof Psy, Edmonton Mental Health Clinic; Clinical Asst Prof Psy, University of Alberta; (780)428-1776; Fax. (780)425-9317.

HINTON, Patricia V; York-Finch Med Centre, 407-2115 Finch Ave W, North York ON M3N 2V6; Wes'80; FRCSC; Ophth. Consultant Canadian Forces, DRDC Toronto; (416)482-3311; Fax. (416)482-0831.

HINTON, Stephen W; Frontenac Med Associates, 201-791 Princess St, Kingston ON K7L 1E9; Qns'85; CCFP; FCFP; Staff, Kingston General Hospital; Staff, Hotel-Dieu Hospital; (613)544-2727; Fax. (613)544-7247.

HINZ, Bradley J; Brad J Hinz Prof Corp, 400-10924 107 Ave NW, Edmonton AB T5H 0X5; Alb'92; DABOph; FRCSC; Ophth (Retina Vitreous Surgery). Staff, Royal Alexandra Hospital; Asst Prof Ophth, University of Alberta; (780)448-1801; Fax. (780)448-1809; bhinz@alberta-retina.com.

HIPPOLA, Dimithra N; Evergreen Community Health Ctr, 3425 Crowley Dr, Vancouver BC V5R 6G3; Alb'96; BSc; CCFP; FCFP; Staff Admitling-Obstetnical, BC Women's Hospital & Health Centre; Langs: Sinhalese; (604)707-3639; Fax. (604)432-6632.

HIPWELL, Alexander E; Mental Health Services, 4-51 Forest Hills Pky, Dartmouth NS B2W 6C6; Dublin (Ireland)'74; MB BCh; BAO; FRCPC; Psy. Staff, The Nova Scotia Hospital; Asst Prof, Dalhousie University; (902)434-3263; Fax. (902)434-0181.

HIRALAL, Rajesh; Surrey Med Arts Bldg, 117-13798 94A Ave, Surrey BC V3V 1N1; UBC'03; FRCPC; IntMed; Cardiol. (604)588-5598

HIRAM-KARASMANIS, Rania; Royal Court Med Centre, 211-5 Quarry Ridge Rd, Barrie ON L4M 7G1; Ott'02; FRCPC; Peds. Staff, Royal Victoria Regional Health Centre; (705)797-0800

HIRANI, Naushad; Peter Lougheed Centre, 3500 26 Ave NE, Calgary AB T1Y 6J4; Tor'99; BSc; ABIM; FRCPC; IntMed (Pulmonary Hypertention); Respir. Staff, Peter Lougheed Centre; Langs: Hindi; Urdu; (403)943-4833; Fax. (403)943-4017; nhirani@ucalgary.ca.

HIRANO, David Y; Mackenzie Richmond Hill Hosp, 10 Trench St, Richmond Hill ON L4C 4Z3; Wes'78; Staff, Mackenzie Richmond Hill Hospital; (905)883-2320

HIRANO, Gail M; The Credit Valley Hosp, 2200 Eglinton Ave W, Mississauga ON L5M 2N1; Tor'82; FRCPC; Anes. Staff, The Credit Valley Hospital; (905)813-2200

HIRAWAN, Natasha; Associate Med Clinic, PO Box 510, Slave Lake AB T0G 2A0; (South Africa)'05; MB ChB; (780)849-4155; Fax. (780)849-4574; n_hirawan@yahoo.com.

HIREMATH, Swapnil; The Ottawa Hosp-Riverside, 1967 Riverside Dr, Ottawa ON K1H 7W9; Bombay (India)'97; Staff, The Ottawa Hospital - Riverside Campus; (613)738-8400; Fax. (613)738-8337.

HIRJI, Alim; 1624 7th Ave, Prince George BC V2L 3P6; McM'07; Respir; IntMed. Staff, Gordon & Leslie Diamond Health Care Centre; Langs: Kacchi; (250)596-9180

HIRJI, Jamil; Allin Clinic, 10155 120 St NW, Edmonton AB T5K 2A2; UBC'08; CCFP; Staff, Sturgeon Community Hospital; (780)482-7551

HIRJI, Rahim; Richmond Hill After Hours Clin, 301 High Tech Rd, Richmond Hill ON L4B 4R2; Tor'04; CCFP; (905)709-4274; Fax. (905)709-4985.

HIRMIZ, Khalid J; Windsor Reg Cancer Centre, 2220 Kildare Rd, Windsor ON N8W 2X3; Baghdad (Iraq)'94; MB ChB; FRCPC; RadOncol. Staff, Windsor Regional Hospital - Windsor Regional Cancer Centre; Langs: Arabic; French; (519)253-5253; Fax. (519)255-8670; khalid_hirmiz@wrh.on.ca.

HIRON, Peter; Sault Area Hosp, 750 Great Northern Rd, Sault Ste. Marie ON P6B 0A8; McG'70; BSc; MDCM; Staff, Sault Area Hospital - Sault Ste Marie; (705)759-3434; Fax. (705)759-3616; peterhiron@rogers.com.

HIROWATARI, Sandra; PO Box 1300, Aldergrove BC V4W 2V1; Wes'90; CCFP; FCFP; (604)514-2340

HIRSCH, Andrei E; B-2900 Eglinton Ave E, Scarborough ON M1J 2E4; Bucharest (Romania)'79; Staff, The Scarborough Hospital - General Campus; Langs: German; Hungarian; Romanian; (416)289-6777; Fax. (416)289-6778.

HIRSCH, Andrew M; SMBD Jewish Gen Hosp, G203-3755 ch Cote-Sainte-Cathe, Montreal QC H3T 1E2; McG'89; FRCPC; IntMed (Pulmonary Hypertention); Respir. Staff, Sir Mortimer B Davis Jewish General; adj Prof Med, McGill University; (514)340-8275; Fax. (514)340-7555.

HIRSCH, Byron D; 725-3271 Dunmore Rd SE, Medicine Hat AB T1B 3R2; Alb'81; CCFP; Staff, Medicine Hat Regional Hospital; (403)526-1092; Fax. (403)526-0188.

HIRSCH, David J; 5081-5820 University Ave, Halifax NS B3H 1V7; Dal'78; FRCPC; IntMed; Nephrol. Staff, Queen Elizabeth II Health Sciences Centre - Victoria General Site; Prof Med, Dalhousie University; (902)473-7764; Fax. (902)473-2675.

HIRSCH, Gabriel H; Pacific Rehab Medicine, 140-943 Broadway W, Vancouver BC V5Z 4E1; Hamburg (Germany)'83; BSc; FRCPC; PhysMed&Rehab (Acquired Brain Injury). Staff, G F Strong Rehabilitation Centre; Consultant, Vancouver General Hospital - Centennial Pavillion; Consultant, George Pearson Centre, Rehab.; Clin Asst Prof, University of British Columbia; Langs: German; (604)733-2222; Fax. (604)733-2202; rehabmd@pacificrehab.net.

HIRSCH, Gregory M; Queen Elizabeth II HSC-Halifax, 2006-1796 Summer St, Halifax NS B3H 3A7; New York(NY) (USA)'84; ABS; AB; BA; FRCSC; CardiothorSurg (Cardiac Surgery). Staff, Queen Elizabeth II Health Sciences Centre - Victoria General Site; Prof Surg/Div Head Cardiac Surg, Dalhousie University; (902)473-7890; Fax. (902)473-7149.

HIRSCH, Kristine J; Queen Elizabeth II HSC-Halifax, 1796 Summer St, Halifax NS B3H 3A7; Seattle(WA) (USA)'90; FRCPC; Anes. Staff Anes, Queen Elizabeth II Health Sciences Centre - Victoria General Site; (902)473-4326; Fax. (902)473-3820.

HIRSCH, Steven L; Winston Park Family Physicians, 104-2315 Bristol Cir, Oakville ON L6H 6P8; Dal'81; CCFP; FCFP; Ac Staff, The Credit Valley Hospital; (905)829-2826

HIRSCHEIMER, Andrea; Spingbank Med Centre, 202-460 Springbank Dr, London ON N6J 0A8; McG'91; CCFP; FCFP; Langs: English; French; (519)672-0060; Fax. (519)661-0597; ahirscheimer@rogers.com.

HIRSH, Denton; Surrey Mem Hosp, 13750 96 Ave, Surrey BC V3V 1Z2; UBC'99; FRCPC; Peds. Staff, Surrey Memorial Hospital; Langs: French; (778)868-1365

HIRSH, Jack; Hamilton HS-Hamilton Site, C2 116-237 Barton St E, Hamilton ON L8L 2X2; Melbourne (Australia)'59; MB BS; MRACP; FRACP; FRCPC; IntMed; MedScient(Med). Staff, Hamilton Health Sciences Centre - Hamilton General Hospital; (905)527-4322; Fax. (905)297-3781.

HIRSH, Michael S; Parkdale Med Tower, 507-1081 Carling Ave, Ottawa ON K1Y 4G2; McG'80; CCFP; FCFP; Court Staff, The Ottawa Hospital - Civic Campus; Asst Prof/Dept Chair Family Med(interim), University of Ottawa; Langs: Bilingual(English/French); (613)728-4605; Fax. (613)728-3083.

HIRSH, Vera; Hop Santa Cabrini Ospedale, 5655 rue Saint-Zotique E, Montreal QC H1T 1P7; Karlova (Czech Republic)'71; FRCPC; Hem; MedOncol. ac Staff, Hôpital Santa Cabrini Ospedale; Staff, McGill University Health Centre - Royal Victoria Hospital; Staff, McGill University Health Centre - Montreal General Campus; assoc Prof Med & Oncol, McGill University; (514)252-6000 x7157; vera.hirsh@sunnybrook.ca.

HIRSHBERG, Eric D; Guelph Urology Associates, 205-77 Westmount Rd, Guelph ON N1H 5J1; Tor'90; BSc; FRCSC; Urol (Incontinence). Ac Staff, Guelph General Hospital; Ac Staff, South Bruce Grey Health Centre - Walkerton Site; Court Staff, Cambridge Memorial Hospital; (519)824-7272; Fax. (519)824-0833.

HIRSHFELD, Steven M; Sarbroro Centre for Hlth Comm, 3545 Kingston Rd, Scarborough ON M1M 1R6; Tor'76; Court Staff Privil, St Joseph's Health Centre; Staff, West Hill Community Health Centre; Teacher Health Service, University of Toronto; (416)284-6439

HIRST, Clinton G; 300-2580 32 St NE, Calgary AB T1Y 7M8; UBC'97; FRCPC; Psy. Staff, Peter Lougheed Centre; (403)944-9800; Fax. (403)944-9850.

HIRST, Georgia C; Nanaimo Reg Gen Hosp, 1200 Dufferin Cres, Nanaimo BC V9S 2B7; Witwatersrand (South Africa)'85; MB ChB; FRCPC; Anes. Staff, Nanaimo Regional General Hospital; (250)755-7605; Fax. (250)755-7633.

HIRST, Jason O; Bluewater Health-Norman Site, 89 Norman St, Sarnia ON N7T 6S3; Wes'00; CCFP; CCFP(E.M.); Staff, Bluewater Health - Mitton Site; Staff, Bluewater Health - Norman Site; (519)464-4400

HIRST, Kenneth R; 203-9123 Mary St, Chilliwack BC V2P 4H7; UBC'75; Staff, Chilliwack General Hospital; (604)795-9161; Fax. (604)795-9937.

HIRSZ, Abraham I; Taddle Creek Fam Hlth Team, Box 58/59 522-790 Bay St, Toronto ON M5G 1N8; Man'74; CCFP; FCFP; Court Staff, Mount Sinai Hospital; Instructor Family & Commun Med, University of Toronto; Langs: Yiddish; (416)591-1222; Fax. (416)591-1227; abehirsz@gmail.com.

HIRTE, Holger; The Juravinski Cancer Centre, 699 Concession St, Hamilton ON L8V 5C2; Tor'80; FRCPC; IntMed (Gynecologic Oncology); MedOncol. Court Staff, Hamilton Health Sciences Centre - McMaster Children's Hospital; Court Staff, St Joseph's Healthcare - Charlton Campus; Court Staff, Joseph Brant Memorial Hospital; Assoc Staff Med, Hamilton Health Sciences Centre-Juravinski Site; Physician, The Juravinski Cancer Centre; Assoc Prof Oncology & ObstGyn, McMaster University; Langs: German; French; (905)387-9495 x64603; Fax. (905)575-6326.

HIRTENFELD, Adi; 13311 Yonge St PO Box 2838 Stn B, Richmond Hill ON L4E 1A7; Tor'82; MSc; Med Staff, Mackenzie Richmond Hill Hospital; (905)773-1210; Fax. (905)773-1978.

HIRTLE, Ann; MUHC-Montreal Gen Hosp, 1650 av Cedar, Montreal QC H3G 1A4; Mem'91; CCFP; FCFP; Staff, McGill University Health Centre - Montreal Children's Hospital; (514)934-1934

HIRUKI, Tadaaki; 3225-600 10th Ave W, Vancouver BC V5Z 4E6; Alb'86; FRCPC; AnatPath. Staff Path, BC Cancer Agency Vancouver Centre; (604)877-6000 x2133

HIRVI, Edward; Group Health Centre, 240 McNabb St, Sault Ste. Marie ON P6B 1Y5; McM'06; CCFP; (705)759-1234; Fax. (705)579-7469.

HIRZER, Robert; Northside Med Group, 102-1015 Austin Ave, Coquitlam BC V3K 3N9; Wes'77; CCFP; FCFP; Ac Staff, Royal Columbian Hospital; (604)939-9251; Fax. (604)939-2592.

HISCOCK, Carrie; Foothills Med Centre, C231-1403 29 St NW, Calgary AB T2N 2T9; Cal'93; CCFP; CCFP(E.M.); FCFP; Staff Emerg Med, Foothills Medical Centre; (403)944-1635

HISCOCK, Jeffery G; 215 LeMarchant Rd, St. John's NL A1C 2H5; Mem'79; FRCPC; IntMed. (709)738-3113

HISCOCK, Stephen M; PO Box 852 Stn Main, Salmon Arm BC V1E 4N9; Mem'92; FRCSC; GenSurg. Staff, Shuswap Lake General Hospital; (250)832-1052

HISCOCK, Susan L; 268 Maiden Lane PO Box 160 Stn Main, St Marys ON N4X 1B1; Qns'86; CCFP; FCFP; (519)284-1280; Fax. (519)284-4816.

HISCOX, Christina M; Kingston Gen Hosp, 76 Stuart St, Kingston ON K7L 2V7; Man'06; FRCSC; OrthSurg. Staff, Kingston General Hospital; (613)548-3232

HISCOX, Michael; Toronto East Gen & Orth Hosp, 825 Coxwell Ave, Toronto ON M4C 3E7; UBC'05; FRCPC; Anes. Staff, Toronto East General Hospital Inc; (416)461-8272

HISLOP, Alan John; 120-2797 Main St SW, Airdrie AB T4B 3S6; Sint Eustatius (Netherlands Antilles)'05; BSc; BMedSci; MD; (403)948-4168

HISLOP, Jonathan A; Ambleside Med Clinic, 250 16th St, West Vancouver BC V7V 3R5; McG'06; MDCM; CCFP; (604)926-1510

HISLOP, Lois; PO Box 7111 Stn Main, Saskatoon SK S7K 4J1; (306)665-7714; Fax. (306)665-7714.

HISLOP, Robert I; Bluewater Health - Norman Site, 89 Norman St, Sarnia ON N7T 6S3; Wes'88; CCFP; CCFP(E.M.); Staff EmergMed, Bluewater Health - Mitton Site; Staff Family Pract, Bluewater Health - Norman Site; (519)464-4400

HITCHCOCK, Deborah J; Richmond Square Med Centre, 70-3915 51 St SW, Calgary AB T3E 6N1; Alb'80; BMedSci; CCFP; FCFP; Ac Staff, Rockyview General Hospital; (403)229-2273; Fax. (403)246-9688.

HITCHCOCK, William G; Victoria Gen Hosp, 2340 Pembina Hwy, Winnipeg MB R3T 2E8; Man'98; CCFP; Staff, Victoria General Hospital; (204)269-3570

HITCHMAN, Derek W; Trinity Western University, 7600 Glover Rd, Langley BC V2Y 1Y1; UBC'89; Physician-in-Charge Student Health Services, Trinity Western U.; (604)513-2024; Fax. (604)513-2041.

HITCHON, Carol A; Health Sciences Centre, RR149-820 Sherbrook St, Winnipeg MB R3A 1R9; Alb'92; FRCPC; IntMed; Rheum. Staff, Health Sciences Centre; (204)774-6511

HITKARI, Jason A; Genesis Fertility Center, 300-1367 Broadway Ave W, Vancouver BC V6H 4A7; UBC'00; FRCSC; ObstGyn. (604)879-3032

HITZLER, Johann K; The Hosp for Sick Children, 9402-555 University Ave, Toronto ON M5G 1X8; ULM (Germany)'87; FRCPC; Peds (Pediatric Oncology); Hem. Staff, The Hospital For Sick Children; Langs: German; (416)813-8887; johann.hitzler@sickkids.ca.

HIVERT, Marie-France; CHUS-Hop Fleurimont, 580 rue Bowen S, Sherbrooke QC J1G 2E8; Sher'01; FRCPC; IntMed; Endocrin&Metab. Staff, Centre Hospitalier Universitaire de Sherbrooke-Hôpital Hôtel-Dieu; (819)346-1110 x23599; Fax. (819)820-6899.

HIVON, Jacinthe; CLSC de la Jacques-Cartier, 11999A rue de L'Hopital, Quebec QC G2A 2T7; Laval'79; (418)843-2572; Fax. (418)843-3880.

HIVON, Marilene; Clinique Med la Providence, 16405 av Bourdages S, Saint-Hyacinthe QC J2T 4G9; Mon'85; Staff, Centre de Sante et de Services Sociaux; (450)773-1322; Fax. (450)773-9909.

HIVON, Pierre; CHUQ-St-Francois D'Assise, 10 rue de l'Espinay, Quebec QC G1L 3L5; Laval'84; Microbio & Infect Dis (P.Q.); MedMicrobiol. Ac Staff, Centre Hospitalier Universitaire De Québec - Pavillon De St-françois-d'assise; (418)525-4444 x53380

HJELKREM, Michel; Riverside Med Clinic, 305-1101 Dewdney Ave, Trail BC V1R 4T1; Dal'89; FACS; FRCSC; OrthSurg. Langs: English; French; (250)364-1599; Fax. (250)368-8886.

HJERTAAS, Kenneth R; Red Deer Reg Hosp Centre, 3942 50A Ave, Red Deer AB T4N 4E7; Alb'73; Staff, Red Deer Regional Hospital Centre; (403)343-4442

HJERTAAS, Richard J; Woodland Hills, 119-27475 Township Road 380, Red Deer County AB T4S 2B7; Sask'74; FRCSC; Otol. Ac Staff, Red Deer Regional Hospital Centre; (403)343-1372

HLA, Nan Htwe; Rockyview Gen Hosp, 7007 14 St SW, Calgary AB T2V 1P9; (Malaysia)'02; Staff, Rockyview General Hospital; (403)944-3700

HLADKOWICZ, Richard B; The Ottawa Hosp-Civic Campus, B3-1053 Carling Ave, Ottawa ON K1Y 4E9; Ott'76; FRCPC; Anes. Staff Anes, The Ottawa Hospital - Civic Campus; Langs: Polish; (613)761-4169; Fax. (613)761-5209.

HLADKY, Eugene N; Clin Sante Visuelle de Montrea, 200-7355 boul Saint-Michel, Montreal QC H2A 2Z9; Mon'93; DABOph; CSPQ; FRCSC; Ophth (P.Q.) (Cataract). Staff, CSSS du Coeur de l'Isle Hôpital Jean-Talon; Staff, Centre Hospitalier Fleury; Langs: Ukrainian; Polish; English; (514)593-6161; Fax. (514)593-3937; dr_eugene_hladky@mac.com.

HLADUNEWICH, Michelle A; Sunnybrook Hlth Sciences Ctre, 139-2075 Bayview Ave, Toronto ON M4N 3M5; Alb'94; FRCPC; IntMed; Nephrol. Staff, Sunnybrook Health Sciences Centre; (416)480-4773; Fax. (416)480-5755.

HLADY, Lois J; Children's & Women's Hc Of Bc, H201-4480 Oak St, Vancouver BC V6H 3V4; UBC'74; BSc; FRCPC; Peds (Addiction Issues). Dir Child Protective Serv Unit, BC Children's Hospital; Clin Prof Peds, University of British Columbia; (604)875-3270

HLAS, Lucie; Northwest Coop Comm Health Ctr, 103-61 Tyndall Ave, Winnipeg MB R2X 2T4; Prague (Czech Republic)'85; Att Staff Family Med, Seven Oaks General Hospital; (204)633-5955; Fax. (204)632-4666.

HLOUSEK, Daniela B; Whitby Mental Hlth Ctr, 700 Gordon St, Whitby ON L1N 5S9; Tor'00; FRCPC; Psy. (905)668-5881; Fax. (905)430-4470.

HLUSEK, Emilia; North Bay Reg Health Centre, 50 College Dr, North Bay ON P1B 0A4; Safarika (Slovakia)'63; FRCPC; Psy. Staff, North Bay Regional Health Centre - Regional Mental Health; Langs: Slovak; (705)474-1200; Fax. (705)495-7835; ehusek@nemhe.on.ca.

HLUSHAK, Curtis R; Hys Med Centre, 710-11010 101 St NW, Edmonton AB T5H 4B9; (Australia)'06; MB BS; FRCPC; PhysMed&Rehab. (780)453-5255; Fax. (780)453-9099.

HLYNKA, Anthony; Eaton Place Med Centre, 81-333 St Mary Ave, Winnipeg MB R3C 4A5; Man'03; CCFP.

HLYNSKY, Julia A; Elaho Med Clinic, 1337 Pemberton Ave, Squamish BC V8B 0J8; UBC'09; CCFP; (604)892-5688

HNATIUK, Bradley; Hys Med Centre, 11010 101 St NW, Edmonton AB T5H 4B9; Alb'06; FRCPC; DiagRad. (780)426-1121

HNATIUK, Melanie L; South Health Campus, 4448 Front St SE, Calgary AB T3M 1M4; Wes'04; CCFP; (403)956-2300; Fax. (403)476-9624.

HNATOWICH, Rachel; Alberta Children's Hosp, 2888 Shaganappi Trail NW, Calgary AB T3B 6A8; McG'06; MDCM; FRCPC; Psy. Staff, Alberta Children's Hospital; (403)955-7211

HNYDYK, William S; Alberta Med Association, 12230 106 Ave NW, Edmonton AB T5N 3Z1; Alb'74; Staff, Alberta Medical Association; (780)482-2626; Fax. (780)482-5445.

HO, Adrian W J; William Osler HC-Brampton, 2100 Brovaird Dr E, Brampton ON L6R 3J7; Qns'89; (905)494-2120

HO, Alexander S; St Michael's Hosp, 30 Bond St, Toronto ON M5B 1W8; Tor'98; FRCPC; Anes. Staff, St Michael's Hospital; Langs: Cantonese; (416)864-5071; Fax. (416)864-6014.

HO, Alice; Oakridge Ctre Med/Dental Bldg, 226-650 41st Ave W, Vancouver BC V5Z 2M9; UBC'84; CCFP; FCFP; Vis Staff, Vancouver General Hospital - Centennial Pavillion; (604)267-3333; Fax. (604)267-3360.

HO, Alice W; Alberta Children's Hosp, 2888 Shaganappi Trail NW, Calgary AB T3B 6A8; UBC'99; FRCPC; Neur. Staff, Alberta Children's Hospital; (403)955-7816; Fax. (403)955-7609.

HO, Allan; Synergy Wellness Centre, 137-501 Bethel Dr, Sherwood Park AB T8H 0N2; (United Kingdom)'97; MB BS; Staff, Covenant Health - Grey Nuns Community Hospital; (780)735-7113; Fax. (780)570-5493.

HO, Angela L H; Toronto East Gen Hosp Inc, 825 Coxwell Ave, Toronto ON M4C 3E7; Tor'99; FRCPC; DiagRad. Staff, Toronto East General Hospital Inc; (416)469-6580 x6073

HO, Ben; Nanaimo Reg Gen Hosp, 1200 Dufferin Cres, Nanaimo BC V9S 2B7; Alb'91; CCFP; CCFP(E.M.); Med Staff, Nanaimo Regional General Hospital; (250)755-7627; Fax. (250)755-7660.

HO, Benjamin G M; 1-1101 Brock St S, Whitby ON L1N 4M1; Tor'88; FRCPC; IntMed; Gastroent. Staff, Lakeridge Health - Oshawa Site; (905)668-1676; Fax. (905)668-5053; bengiho@rogers.com.

HO, C John; Athlete's Care, C120-11 King St W, Toronto ON M5H 4C7; Wes'00; BSc(Hon); BPHE; Dip SportMed; CCFP; (416)368-9990

HO, Catherine K Y; North York Gen Hosp, 4001 Leslie St, North York ON M2K 1E1; Wes'05; CCFP; CCFP(E.M.); Staff, North York General Hospital; (416)756-6882

HO, Cedric D S W; Royal Columbian Hosp, 330 Columbia St E, New Westminster BC V3L 3W7; UBC'94; FRCPC; Anes. Staff Anes, Royal Columbian Hospital; (604)520-4602

HO, Charmaine S; East York Med Hlth Ctr, 27E-45 Overlea Blvd, Toronto ON M4H 1C3; Tor'97; BSc; MSc; CCFP; (416)696-9836 x222; charmaine.ho@utoronto.ca.

HO, Cheryl C; BC Cancer Agency-Vancouver CC, 600 10th Ave W, Vancouver BC V5Z 4E6; Wes'00; FRCPC; IntMed; MedOncol. Staff, BC Cancer Agency Vancouver Centre; (604)877-6000

HO, Chester; Foothills Med Centre, 1195-1403 29 ST NW, Calgary AB T2N 2T9; Staff, Foothills Medical Centre; (403)944-2061; Fax. (403)270-7878.

HO, Chia-Sing; Univ Hlth Network-Toronto Gen, 200 Elizabeth St, Toronto ON M5G 2C4; (Hong Kong)'65; FRCPC; DiagRad. Chief Radiology, Toronto General Hospital - UHN; Prof Radiol, University of Toronto; Langs: Chinese; (416)340-3371; Fax. (416)593-0502.

HO, Christopher T M; Family Health Centre, 3003 Danforth Ave, Toronto ON M4C 1M9; Tor'90; (416)694-4343; Fax. (416)694-4241.

HO, Clinton; Life Labs, 3680 Gilmore Way, Burnaby BC V5G 4V8; Cal'94; FRCPC; GenPath; HemPath. Staff, University of Alberta Hospital; Langs: Chinese; (604)431-5005

HO, Cosmas V J; 35 Hallett Cres, St. John's NL A1B 4C4; National (Taiwan)'61; Med Staff, St Clare's Mercy Hospital; (709)368-9300; Fax. (709)364-8759.

HO, Daniel T; 1-6219 Centre St NW, Calgary AB T2K 0V2; (Taiwan)'87; Staff GP, Olive Medical Clinic; (403)275-5300; Fax. (403)275-5301.

HO, Darius M S; 206-230 First Ave, St Thomas ON N5R 4P5; Wes'76; FRCPC; MedBiochem. (519)633-6020; Fax. (519)633-6025.

HO, Della S W; Gulf Canada Square, 340-401 9 Ave SW, Calgary AB T2P 3C5; (Hong Kong)'71; MB BS; FRCPC; Peds. Ac Staff, Alberta Children's Hospital; Ac Staff, Rockyview General Hospital; Clin Assoc Prof, University of Calgary; Langs: Chinese; (403)221-4434; Fax. (403)221-4466.

HO, Derek C; London HSC-Victoria Hosp, PO Box 5010 Stn B 800 Commissioners Rd E, London ON N6A 5W9; Wes'02; FRCPC; DiagRad. Staff, London Health Sciences Centre - Victoria Campus; (519)685-8500 x56176; derek.ho@lhsc.on.ca.

HO, Doris S C; 225-279 Wharncliffe Rd N, London ON N6H 2C2; Wes'76; Court Staff Family Med, St Joseph's Hospital - St Joseph's Health Care; Langs: Cantonese; (519)673-3836; Fax. (519)673-3837.

HO, Duncan T H; Clareview Family Med Clinic, 4950-137 Ave NW, Edmonton AB T5Y 2V4; UBC'00; CCFP; (780)478-1999; Fax. (780)478-1166.

HO, Edward S; 225 Fairview Dr PO Box 28017 Rpo N Park Plaza, Brantford ON N3R 7X5; Tor'77; Staff, The Brant Community Healthcare System - Brantford General Hospital Site; Langs: Cantonese; (519)759-4060; Fax. (519)759-8807; siusunho2000@yahoo.com.

HO, Elaine P L; Bowmanville Prof Bldg, 1100-222 King St E, Bowmanville ON L1C 1P6; Tor'94; CCFP; FCFP; Ac Staff, Lakeridge Health - Bowmanville Site; Langs: Cantonese; (905)623-6458

HO, Elinda P L; QE Park Med Clinic, 4060 Cambie St, Vancouver BC V5Z 2X8; UBC'92; Langs: Cantonese; (604)874-4060

HO, Esther C Y; Chinook Reg Hosp, 960 19 St S, Lethbridge AB T1J 1W5; Alb'04; FRCPC; Anes. Staff, Medicine Hat Regional Hospital; Staff, Chinook Regional Hospital; (403)388-6111

HO, Gerald C L; Chalmers Gate Med Bldg, 306-328 Highway 7 E, Richmond Hill ON L4B 3P7; (Hong Kong)'83; MB BS; MRCP(UK); FRCPC; Peds (Consultation). Att Staff Peds, Mackenzie Richmond Hill Hospital; Langs: Chinese; (905)731-5092; Fax. (905)731-5106.

HO, Gilian C; Rural Palliative Care Consulta, 11 Cimarron Common, Okotoks AB T1S 2E9; Alb'04; CCFP; Consultant Palliative Care, Regional Palliative & Hospice Care; (403)995-2714; Fax. (403)995-2619.

HO, Grant K C; 125-210 Memorial Ave, Orillia ON L3V 7V1; Tor'97; CCFP; FCFP; Staff, Orillia Soldiers' Memorial Hospital; Langs: Cantonese; (705)329-1223; Fax. (705)329-3255; g.ho@utoronto.ca.

HO, H Henry; 705-5799 Yonge St, North York ON M2M 3V3; Tor'94; CCFP; Langs: Mandarin; Spanish; (416)221-8612; Fax. (416)221-8784.

HO, Harmony A; 303-600 Sherbourne St, Toronto ON M4X 1W4; Cal'05; FRCSC; ObstGyn (Gynecological Reproductive Endocrinology). (416)922-0840

HO, Helen H Y; 1113-123 Edward St, Toronto ON M5G 1E2; (Hong Kong)'65; FRCSC; ObstGyn (Gynecology). Assoc Staff, Toronto Western Hospital - University Health Network; Assoc Staff, Mount Sinai Hospital; Langs: Chinese; (416)596-1089; Fax. (416)596-7491.

HO, Herbert K K; 103 Parkway Forest Dr, North York ON M2J 1L8; Man'71; Staff, The Scarborough Hospital - General Campus; (416)491-7451; Fax. (416)491-8008.

HO, Hip Wah; Guildford Med Dental Centre, 27-15300 105 Ave, Surrey BC V3R 6A7; Sheffield (England)'68; MB ChB; FRCPC; IntMed (Clinical Immunology & Allergy). Consultant, Surrey Memorial Hospital; Langs: Chinese; (604)585-1391; Fax. (604)585-8833.

HO, Hoi Shing; 3-3039 Kingsway, Vancouver BC V5R 5J6; Alb'73; Ac Staff, Burnaby Hospital; Langs: Chinese; (604)430-1438; Fax. (604)430-1438.

HO, Hon-Fai; Quality Med Imaging, 306-280 Spadina Ave, Toronto ON M5T 3A5; (Taiwan)'67; AB; FRCPC; DiagRad (Diagnostic Imaging). Court Staff, Stevenson Memorial Hospital; Locum Tenens, North York General Hospital - Branson Division; Langs: Chinese; (416)603-1197; Fax. (416)603-1199.

HO, Hon-Lau; Pacific Med Centre, F33-4300 Steeles Ave E, Markham ON L3R 0Y5; (Hong Kong)'68; MB BS; FRACS; FRCS(E); CCFP; FCFP; Court Staff, Rouge Valley Health System - Centenary Health Centre Site; Court Staff, The Scarborough Hospital - Birchmount Campus; Court Staff, The Scarborough Hospital - General Campus; Langs: Mandarin; Cantonese; (905)604-7889; Fax. (905)604-7890.

HO, Jenny M; Civic Parkdale Clinic, 737 Parkdale Ave, Ottawa ON K1Y 1J8; Ott'05; Hem; IntMed. (613)737-8899

HO, Jeremy J; Richmond Hosp, 7000 Westminster Hwy, Richmond BC V6X 1A2; Qns'06; FRCPC; IntMed; MedOncol. Staff, Richmond Hospital; Staff, BC Cancer Agency Vancouver Centre; (604)278-9711

HO, Jin K; Northmount Med Centre, 602-145 13th St E, North Vancouver BC V7L 2L4; Dublin (Ireland)'99; MRCP; FRCPC; IntMed; Gastroent. Staff, Lions Gate Hospital; Clin Instructor Gastroent, University of British Columbia; (604)770-4478

HO, Joanne M; Sunnybrook Hlth Sciences Ctre, L1 01D-2075 Bayview Ave, Toronto ON M4N 3M5; UBC'05; FRCPC; IntMed (Clinical Pharmacology & Toxicology); GeriatricMed. Staff, Sunnybrook Health Sciences Centre; Langs: Cantonese; (416)480-4076

HO, Josephine; Alberta Children's Hosp, 2888 Shaganappi Trail NW, Calgary AB T3B 6A8; Wes'99; FRCPC; Peds; Endocrin&Metab. Staff, Alberta Children's Hospital; (403)955-7819

HO, Juliet; Health Sciences Centre, GE421-820 Sherbrook St, Winnipeg MB R3A 1R9; Wes'01; FRCPC; IntMed; Nephrol. Staff IntMed, Health Sciences Centre.

HO, Karen C T; Toronto East Gen Hosp Inc, 825 Coxwell Ave, Toronto ON M4C 3E7; Wes'08; CCFP; CCFP(E.M.); Staff, Toronto East General Hospital Inc; (416)469-6580

HO, Kay; 106-9181 Main St, Chilliwack BC V2P 4M9; (Hong Kong)'74; MB BS; Ac Staff, Chilliwack General Hospital; Langs: Chinese; Cantonese; (604)792-7361; Fax. (604)792-7362.

HO, Kendall; Vancouver Gen Hosp, 855 12th Ave W, Vancouver BC V5Z 1M9; UBC'86; FRCPC; EmergMed. A-Staff Emerg, Vancouver General Hospital - Centennial Pavillion; Teach Staff, University of British Columbia; Langs: Cantonese; Mandarin; (604)875-4111; Fax. (604)875-4872.

HO, Kennely J; Keary Med Centre, 207-245 Columbia St E, New Westminster BC V3L 3W4; Alb'77; FRCPC; Neur. (604)526-1848; Fax. (604)526-1847; ho@myreflex.com.

HO, Kenneth S W; William Osler HC-Brampton, 2100 Bovaird Dr E, Brampton ON L6R 3J7; (Hong Kong)'73; FRCPC; Anes. Staff, William Osler Health System - Brampton Civic Hospital; Langs: Chinese; (905)494-2120

HO, Kwok Fan; Credit Valley Med Arts Centre, 124-2000 Credit Valley Rd, Mississauga ON L5M 4N4; Tor'77; Langs: Chinese; (905)569-1744; Fax. (905)569-9620.

HO, Man Fan; 212-701 Sheppard Ave E, North York ON M2K 2Z3; Tor'77; FRCSC; ObstGyn. Ac Staff, North York General Hospital; Asst Prof ObstGyn, University of Toronto; (416)221-1661

HO, Maria Y; Cross Cancer Institute, 11560 University Ave NW, Edmonton AB T6G 1Z2; Man'06; FRCPC; IntMed; MedOncol. (780)432-8771

HO, Michael S C; 312-280 Spadina Ave, Toronto ON M5T 3A5; Ott'75; BSc; Court Staff, Toronto General Hospital - UHN; Court Staff, Mount Sinai Hospital; Langs: Chinese; Mandarin; (416)977-4111; Fax. (416)977-4495.

HO, Minnie M W; Southwood Med Clinic, 1700-2751 Cliffe Ave, Courtenay BC V9N 2L8; UBC'93; CCFP; FCFP; Court Staff, St Joseph's General Hospital; (250)334-2212

HO, Nancy S K; Chalmers Med Office, 8-360 Highway 7 E, Richmond Hill ON L4B 3Y7; Tor'89; Langs: Cantonese; (905)881-0900; Fax. (905)881-0906.

HO, Nhung T C; 201-1017 Wilson Ave, North York ON M3K 1Z1; Sher'83; FAAD; CSPQ; FRCP; FRCPC; Peds (Pediatric Dermatology); Derm. Assoc Staff Derm, The Hospital For Sick Children; Court Staff Derm, Humber River Regional Hospital - Finch Avenue Site; Asst Prof, University of Toronto; Aj Prof Schulich School of Medicine, University of Western Ontario; Langs: Vietnamese; Bilingual(French/English); (416)398-0292; Fax. (416)398-8389; nhung.ho@utoronto.ca.

HO, Peter H T; Mount Sinai Hosp, 600 University Ave, Toronto ON M5G 1X5; Man'95; Anes. Staff Anes, Mount Sinai Hospital; (416)586-5270

HO, Peter S C; Surrey Med Bldg, 304-9656 King George Blvd, Surrey BC V3T 2V5; Tor'75; FACOG; BSc; FRCSC; ObstGyn. Ac Staff, Surrey Memorial Hospital; (604)584-7677; Fax. (604)584-3902.

HO, Philip C; 2983 Bloor St W, Etobicoke ON M8X 1C1; (Hong Kong)'73; DABPed; FRCPC; Peds (Allergy). Court Staff, Trillium Health Centre - West Toronto; Langs: Cantonese; Mandarin; (416)232-2118; Fax. (416)232-9494.

HO, Quang Nhan; Clin Med Rosemont, 1969 boul Rosemont, Montreal QC H2G 1S9; Saigon (Vietnam)'71; FACS; CSPQ; FRCSC; GenSurg (Oncology). Ac Staff, Hôpital Santa Cabrini Ospedale; Assoc Staff, CSSS du Coeur de l'Isle Hôpital Jean-Talon; Langs: Vietnamese; French; (514)274-7344; Fax. (514)274-1165.

HO, Ru-Chie; Glazier Med Centre, 11 Gibb St, Oshawa ON L1H 2J9; (Taiwan)'66; FRCSC; Otol. Langs: Mandarin; (905)579-1212; Fax. (905)579-2021.

HO, Shen-Pang E; Ross Memorial Hosp, 10 Angeline St N, Lindsay ON K9V 4M8; Montpellier (France)'70; FRCPC; GenPath. Staff, Ross Memorial Hospital; Langs: Mandarin; Cantonese; Fukinese; (705)324-6100

HO, Shu Fung; 3255 Hospital Rd RR 2, Vanderhoof BC V0J 3A2; UBC'10; CCFP; Staff, University Hospital of Northern British Columbia; (250)567-6211

HO, Stephen G F; Vancouver Gen Hosp, 899 12th Ave W, Vancouver BC V5Z 1M9; UBC'89; FRCPC; DiagRad. Assoc Staff, Vancouver General Hospital - Centennial Pavillion; Dir Residency Prog/Asst Prof Radiol, University of British Columbia; (604)875-5253; Fax. (604)875-4806; Stephen.Ho@vch.ca.

HO, Suzanne; Clin Med Rosemont, 1969 boul Rosemont, Montreal QC H2G 1S9; Laval'99; FRCPC; Otol. (514)274-7344; Fax. (514)274-1165.

HO, Terrence T L; Ultima Med Services Inc, PO Box 32301 Rpo Yvr Terminal, Richmond BC V7B 1W2; UBC'07; (604)207-6900

HO, Thi Kim; CLSC Saint-Henri, 3833 rue Notre-Dame O, Montreal QC H4C 1P8; Sher'87; CCFP; Médecin, CLSC Chateauguay; (514)933-7541; Fax. (514)933-2411.

HO, Thi Nguyet; CLSC Saint-Henri, 3833 rue Notre-Dame O, Montreal QC H4C 1P8; Mon'86; (514)933-7541; Fax. (514)937-7052.

HO, Thi Nhu M; CSSS Pierre Boucher, 1333 boul Jacques-Cartier E, Longueuil QC J4M 2A5; Mon'91; Staff, Centre Hospitalier Pierre Boucher; (450)468-8111

HO, Thomas M W; 3484 Main St, Vancouver BC V5V 3N2; UBC'80; CCFP; Ac Medical Staff, Providence Health Care - Mount Saint Joseph Hospital; Ac Medical Staff, Providence Health Care - St Paul's Hospital; Assoc Staff, Vancouver General Hospital - Centennial Pavillion; Clin Assoc Prof Family Med, University of British Columbia; Langs: Cantonese; Mandarin; (604)877-2233; Fax. (604)877-0802.

HO, Tommy K L; 402-700 Bay St, Toronto ON M5G 1Z6; Qns'94; MSc; FRCPC; Peds (Clinical). Staff Peds, The Scarborough Hospital - Birchmount Campus; Clin Asst, The Hospital For Sick Children; Lecturer, University of Toronto; Langs: Mandarin; Cantonese; (416)596-1155

HO, Tze May; HSC-Faculty Of Med, 3330 Hospital Dr NW, Calgary AB T2N 4N1; Tor'71; FRCPC; IntMed; InfectDis. Consultant Med, Foothills Medical Centre; Assoc Prof Med, University of Calgary; (403)220-8516; Fax. (403)210-8862.

HO, Victoria Y W; Belmont Prof Centre, 403-564 Belmont Ave W, Kitchener ON N2M 5N6; Tor'78; DABIM; FCCP; FRCPC; IntMed; Respir. Ac Staff, Grand River Hospital - Kitchener/Waterloo Health Centre; Ac Staff, St Mary's General Hospital; Langs: Cantonese; (519)742-2900; Fax. (519)742-3140.

HO, Vincent C Y; Skin Care Centre, 835 10th Ave W, Vancouver BC V5Z 4E8; UBC'81; FRCPC; Derm (Skin Cancer). Staff, BC Cancer Agency Vancouver Centre; Ac Staff Derm, Vancouver General Hospital - Centennial Pavillion; Prof, University of British Columbia; Langs: Cantonese; Mandarin; (604)875-5151; Fax. (604)873-9919; vho@interchange.ubc.ca.

HO, Vincent W G; Royal Victoria Hosp, 201 Georgian Dr, Barrie ON L4M 6M2; Qns'92; FRCPC; Peds (Neonatology). Staff Neonatal Intensive Care Unit, Royal Victoria Regional Health Centre; (705)728-9802

HO, Vincent W K; Professional Bldg, 3100-222 King St E, Bowmanville ON L1C 1P6; Tor'95; CCFP; FCFP; Court Staff, The Scarborough Hospital - General Campus; Staff, Lakeridge Health - Bowmanville Site; Lecturer, University of Toronto; (905)623-2355; Fax. (905)623-9607.

HO, Vincent W S; Trillium Health Centre, 7F-101 Queensway W, Mississauga ON L5B 2P7; Tor'10; CCFP; (905)272-9900

HO, W Steve; The Ottawa Hosp-Gen Campus, LM 10-501 Smyth Rd, Ottawa ON K1Y 4E9; National University of Ireland (Ireland)'07; IntMed (Gastroenterology). Staff, The Ottawa Hospital - Civic Campus; (613)737-8899

HO, W M Amy; 406-1110 Sheppard Ave E, North York ON M2K 2W2; Tor'91; Langs: Cantonese; (416)733-4151; Fax. (416)221-4047.

HO, Wei-Ning; 3695 10 Ave W PO Box 39218 Rpo Point Grey, Vancouver BC V6R 4P1; UBC'92; BSc; Langs: Cantonese; Mandarin; (604)738-1793

HO, Yvonne; Credit Valley Prof Bldg, 209-2300 Eglinton Ave W, Mississauga ON L5M 2V8; Tor'97; FRCPC; DiagRad;CCFP; Staff, The Credit Valley Hospital; Langs: Cantonese; (905)607-8334; Fax. (905)607-8184; hoyeewan@yahoo.com.

HO-A-SHOO, Deanne P; Aberfoyle Health Centre, 102-304 The East Mall, Etobicoke ON M9B 6E2; Loma Linda(CA) (USA)'84; BSc; MD; CGPP; CCFP; FCFP; (416)231-7968; Fax. (416)231-7982.

HO-ASJOE, Marianne P K; 6681 Victoria Dr, Vancouver BC V5P 3Y2; Tor'90; CCFP; (604)321-8712; Fax. (604)321-2446.

HO CHEN, Anthony; 1353 Aster Rd PO Box 134, Pemberton BC V0N 2L0; Witwatersrand (South Africa)'79; MB ChB; (604)894-6365; Fax. (604)894-6365.

HO-KIM, Thu-Lan; Dr Poon's Metabolic Clinic, 6-375 Kingston Rd, Pickering ON L1V 1A3; McG'93; CCFP; (905)509-6888

HO NGOC HAP, Annie; Ctr Hosp Affilie-St-Sacrement, 1050 ch Sainte-Foy, Quebec QC G1S 4L8; Laval'88; Staff, Centre Hospitalier Affilié Universitaire de Québec - Hôpital du St-Sacrement; (418)682-7515; Fax. (418)682-7956.

HO PING KONG, Barbara S; Balmoral Med Arts Facility, 209-1366 Yonge St, Toronto ON M4T 3A7; West Indies (Jamaica)'69; MB BS; ABD; FRCPC; Derm. Staff, Toronto Western Hospital - University Health Network; Asst Prof, University of Toronto; (416)963-5955; Fax. (416)963-5612; b.hopingkong@sympatico.ca.

HO PING KONG, Wayne; Scarborough North Med Arts, 404-4040 Finch Ave E, Scarborough ON M1S 4V5; Tor'93; FRCPC; IntMed; Cardiol. Ac Staff, The Scarborough Hospital - Birchmount Campus; Staff, Rouge Valley Health System - Centenary Health Centre Site; (416)297-7277; Fax. (416)299-4842.

HO-TAI, Lily M; Rouge Valley-Centenary HC, 2867 Ellesmere Rd, Scarborough ON M1E 4B9; Tor'88; FRCPC; Anes. Court Staff, Thunder Bay Regional Health Sciences Centre; Staff Anes, Rouge Valley Health System - Centenary Health Centre Site; Langs: Cantonese; (416)284-8131 x4054; Fax. (416)281-7453.

HO-TAI, Paul; KMH Cardiol & Diagnostic Ctr, 108-751 Victoria St S, Kitchener ON N2M 5N4; Tor'81; FRCPC; DiagRad (Diagnostic Imaging). Staff, Grand River Hospital - Freeport Site; Staff, Guelph General Hospital; Staff, Groves Memorial Community Hospital; Langs: Cantonese; (519)570-2198

HO YUEN, Diana E; 104-1061 Ridgeway Ave, Coquitlam BC V3J 1S6; Witwatersrand (South Africa)'74; MB BS; (604)931-7596; Fax. (604)937-8841.

HO YUEN, Vernon; 101-111 Kootenay St N, Cranbrook BC V1C 3T5; Tor'94; DAB; FRCSC; Ophth (Cataract Surgery). (250)426-7997

HOAG, Christopher C; 102-123 15th St E, North Vancouver BC V7L 2P7; Ott'03; FRCSC; Urol. (604)987-8171

HOAG, Gordon N; Vancouver Island Hlth Authorit, 5902-1952 Bay St, Victoria BC V8R 1J8; Sask'82; MSc; PhD; FRCPC; GenPath. (250)370-8437; Fax. (250)370-8873.

HOANG, Antoine; Lakeshore Gen Hosp, 160 av Stillview, Pointe-Claire QC H9R 2Y2; Mon'03; Staff, Lakeshore General Hospital - Pointe Claire; Langs: English; Vietnamese; (514)630-2225; hoang_antoine@hotmail.com.

HOANG, Diem-Quan; Hop du Sacre-Coeur de Mtl, 5400 boul Gouin O, Montreal QC H4J 1C5; Laval'03; FRCPC; DiagRad. Staff, Hôpital du Sacre-Coeur de Montréal; (514)338-2222

HOANG, Dinh Le; CSSS de Laval, 1755 boul Rene-Laennec, Laval QC H7M 3L9; Sher'95; CCFP; CCFP(E.M.); Staff, Hopital de la Cite de la santé; (514)323-7435

HOANG, Duc Hieu N; Clinique Med Desy, 5636 boul Henri-Bourassa E, Montreal-Nord QC H1G 2T2; Sher'93; (514)326-9060; Fax. (514)326-0919.

HOANG, Holly; Grey Nuns Community Hosp & HC, 640-1100 Youville Drive West N, Edmonton AB T6L 5X8; Alb'07; FRCPC; IntMed; InfectDis. Staff, Covenant Health - Grey Nuns Community Hospital; (780)735-7236; Fax. (780)735-9760.

HOANG, Le Uyen; CSSS de Laval, 1755 boul Rene-Laennec, Laval QC H7M 3L9; Mon'97; Staff, Hopital de la Cite de la santé; Staff Clin Formation, Universite de Montreal; (450)668-1010; anh_hoang50@hotmail.com.

HOANG, Minh Chau; Clin Medicale 8260, 212-8260 boul Maurice-Duplessi, Montreal QC H1E 3A3; Mon'87; Langs: Vietnamese; English; (514)643-1113; Fax. (514)643-1767.

HOANG, Ngoc Bich; Hotel-Dieu D'arthabaska, 5 rue des Hospitalieres, Victoriaville QC G6P 6N2; Sher'02; FRCPC; Psy. Staff, Hotel-Dieu d'Arthabaska; (819)357-2030

HOANG, Ngoc Vinh; Clin Med du Haut-Anjou, 45-7500 boul Les Galeries d'An, Anjou QC H1M 3M4; Hue (Vietnam)'74; (514)493-1999; Fax. (514)493-4428.

HOANG, Ngoc-Khoi; Bathurst Medical Centre, 204-800 Bathurst St, Toronto ON M5R 3M8; Saigon (Vietnam)'60; Assoc Staff, Toronto Western Hospital - University Health Network; Langs: English; French; (416)533-5882

HOANG, Que Chi; GMF Saint-Laurent, 1605 boul Marcel-Laurin, Saint-Laurent QC H4R 0B7; Mon'08; CCFP; Médecin, Centre De Sante De Rigaud; (514)747-2555

HOANG, T Boi-Ngoc; 53 Augusta St, Hamilton ON L8N 1P8; Saigon (Vietnam)'63; FRCSC; ObstGyn. Court Staff, St Joseph's Healthcare - Charlton Campus; Ac Staff, Hamilton Health Sciences Centre - McMaster Children's Hospital; Teach Staff Pt-Time, McMaster University; Langs: French; Vietnamese; (905)523-8484; Fax. (905)523-6075.

HOANG, Tina Y H; 225-45 Edenwold Dr NW, Calgary AB T3A 3S8; Cal'03; CCFP; (403)241-2888

HOANG, Tuan Van; Hop Santa Cabrini Ospedale, 5655 rue Saint-Zotique E, Montreal QC H1T 1P7; Saigon (Vietnam)'73; Staff Medical Imaging, Hôpital Santa Cabrini Ospedale; Langs: Bilingual(English/French); (514)252-6567

HOANG, Tuan-Khai; Clin Med D'Urgence Mediz, 200-5900 boul Leger, Montreal-Nord QC H1G 1K9; Hue (Vietnam)'73; (514)323-2072

HOAR, Glen G; 201-1771 Comox Ave, Comox BC V9M 3L9; Mem'97; FRCSC; Ophth. (250)890-0089; Fax. (250)890-0090; ghoar@shawbiz.ca.

HOAR, Karen; 203-300 Brae Rd, Duncan BC V9L 3T8; UBC'98; FRCSC; Ophth. (250)748-2922

HOAR, Stephanie E; The Ottawa Hosp-Riverside, 5 26-1967 Riverside Dr, Ottawa ON K1H 7W9; Mem'95; FRCPC; IntMed; Nephrol. Staff, The Ottawa Hospital - Riverside Campus; Asst Prof Med, University of Ottawa; (613)738-7100; Fax. (613)738-8337; shoar@ottawahospital.on.ca.

HOARE, Connie; Summerside Med Centre, 101-475 Granville St, Summerside PE C1N 4P7; Ott'85; FRCPC; IntMed (Gastroenterology). Staff, Prince County Hospital; (902)432-8181

HOBART, Michael G; Hys Med Centre, 400-11010 101 St NW, Edmonton AB T5H 4B9; Alb'90; FRCSC; Urol (Laparoscopic Urology). Staff, Royal Alexandra Hospital; Staff, Covenant Health - Misericordia Community Hospital; Clin Assoc Prof, University of Alberta; (780)425-5892; Fax. (780)441-2596.

HOBBS, Barry B; London X-Ray Associates, 104-450 Central Ave, London ON N6B 2E8; Wes'66; DMRD(Tor); FRCPC; DiagRad. Staff, St Joseph's Hospital - St Joseph's Health Care; Prof Radiol & Nuclear Med, University of Western Ontario; (519)672-5270

HOBBS, Cheryl L; St James Street Med Clinic, 1600 Portage Ave, Winnipeg MB R3J 0C6; Man'82; Staff, St Boniface General Hospital; (204)774-1868; Fax. (204)774-7303.

HOBBS, Cynthia A; St Joseph's Hosp, 130 Bayard Dr, Saint John NB E2L 3L6; McM'94; FRCPC; IntMed; GeriatricMed. Staff, St Joseph's Hospital; (506)632-5555

HOBBS, R Neil; Tamworth Med Centre, RR 1, Tamworth ON K0K 3G0; Cambridge (England)'72; MB ChB; DRCOG; CCFP; FCFP; Physician, Sehtu HSS, North West Terrories; (613)379-2946; Fax. (613)379-5138.

HOBBS, Sandra E; Grandview Heights Med Clinic, 12313 63 Ave NW, Edmonton AB T6H 1R4; Alb'72; CCFP; FCFP; Staff, Glenrose Rehabilitation Hospital; (780)437-1968; Fax. (780)438-4395.

HOBDARI, Ilda; Columbus Med Arts Bldg, 300-8333 Weston Rd, Woodbridge ON L4L 8E2; Bucharest (Romania)'99; CCFP; (905)264-9859; Fax. (905)264-9311.

HOBDEN, Alexandra; CSSS du Sud de Lanaudière, 911 montee des Pionniers, Terrebonne QC J6V 2H2; Mon'85; FRCPC; Psy. Staff, Centre Hospitalier Pierre le Gardeur; (450)654-7525

HOBDEN, Christian; Centre Medical des Boises, 4670 boul Saint-Martin O, Laval QC H7T 2Y2; Mon'89; Staff, Centre Hospitalier d'Argenteuil; (450)687-8585

HOBDEN, Elisabeth J; The Ottawa Hosp-Civic Campus, 1053 Carling Ave, Ottawa ON K1Y 4E9; Mon'01; FRCPC; EmergMed. Staff, The Ottawa Hospital - Civic Campus; Langs: Bilingual(English/French); (613)798-5555

HOBDEN, Roger; CLSC des Faubourg, 1705 rue de la Visitation, Montreal QC H2L 3C3; Mon'77; Physician, CLSC Centre-Sud; (514)527-2361; Fax. (514)527-3074.

HOBDEN, Susan D; Brockville Gen Hosp, 75 Charles St, Brockville ON K6V 1S8; Qns'97; FRCSC; GenSurg. Staff, Brockville General Hospital - Charles Street; (613)345-8345; Fax. (613)345-8318.

HOBEIKA, Chaker A; Dr Charles A Janeway Child HC, 300 Prince Philip Dr, St. John's NL A1B 3V6; Alexandria (Egypt)'60; MB ChB; FRCPC; Peds. Staff, Janeway Children's Health & Rehabilitation Centre; Langs: Bilingual(English/French); (709)777-4766; Fax. (709)777-4343.

HOBEIKA, Sharon L; 200-2550 12th Ave, Regina SK S4P 3X1; Mem'97; FRCPCH; ABPeds; FRCPC; Peds. (306)566-1010; Fax. (306)566-4158.

HOBEN, Lionel E; 140-339 Wellington Rd, London ON N6C 5Z9; Wes'87; BSc(Biochem.Concordia); (519)668-7566; Fax. (519)668-7567.

HOBSON, Bruce C; A1-6935 Harvie Ave, Powell River BC V8A 5H9; UBC'81; Ac Staff, Powell River General Hospital; (604)485-0136; Fax. (604)485-0130; docbruce@telus.net.

HOBSON, Douglas; Deer Lodge Centre, 200 Woodlawn St, Winnipeg MB R3J 2H7; Man'81; FRCPC; Neur (Movement Disorders). Asst Prof Med/Dir Movement Disorder Clinic, University of Manitoba; (204)940-8400; Fax. (204)940-8414.

HOBSON, John W; 203-300 Willow Rd, Guelph ON N1H 7C6; Wes'83; BSc; FRCSC; GenSurg; VascSurg. Staff, Guelph General Hospital; Staff, Grand River Hospital - Kitchener/Waterloo Health Centre; Staff, St Mary's General Hospital; (519)822-4521; Fax. (519)822-0030.

HOBSON, Steven G; Cedar Care Clinic, 104-32423 Lougheed Hwy, Mission BC V2V 7B8; Lund (Sweden)'88; Langs: Swedish; (604)820-7676; Fax. (604)820-7726.

HOCA, Asim; Connaigre Peninsula Hlth Centr, PO Box 70 1 Alexander Ave, Hermitage NL A0H 1S0; Staff, James Paton Memorial Hospital.

HOCH, N Charles W; Ilderton Med Clinic, Main St, Ilderton ON N0M 2A0; McG'74; (519)666-1610

HOCHART, Laurent; 102-1617 Baker St, Cranbrook BC V1C 1B4; (Belgium)'91; (250)426-7500

HOCHBAN, Ty J; Albert Park Family Med Ctr, 3992 Albert St, Regina SK S4S 3R1; Sask'90; (306)584-3833; Fax. (306)585-3833.

HOCHMAN, David J; St Boniface Clinic, 343 Tache Ave, Winnipeg MB R2H 2A5; Man'00; FRCSC; GenSurg.

HOCHMAN, Gary P; Mackenzie Richmond Hill Hosp, 10 Trench St, Richmond Hill ON L4C 4Z3; Man'81; FRCPC; DiagRad. Staff Radiol, Southlake Regional Health Centre; Staff Radiol, Mackenzie Richmond Hill Hospital; (905)883-2004

HOCHMAN, Jacqueline R; Women's College Hosp, 1001-76 Grenville St, Toronto ON M5S 1B2; Qns'01; FRCPC; IntMed (Clinician Investigator Program); Rheum. Staff, Women's College Hospital; (416)323-6400

HOCHMAN, Jay; Heartline Medical, 110-2504 Skaha Lake Rd, Penticton BC V2A 6G1; Man'05; FRCPC; IntMed; Nephrol. Staff, Penticton Regional Hospital; (250)492-3511

HOCHMAN, Jordan; Health Sciences Centre, GB4-820 Sherbrook St, Winnipeg MB R3A 1R9; Man'02; FRCSC; Otol. Staff, Health Sciences Centre; (204)787-7773

HOCHMAN, Michael; Eaton Place Med Centre, 81-333 St Mary Ave, Winnipeg MB R3C 4A5; (Other Foreign)'07; CCFP.

HOCHMAN, Mitchel I; Radiology Consultants Assoc, 120-6707 Elbow Dr SW, Calgary AB T2V 0E3; Man'00; FRCPC; DiagRad. (403)777-3007

HOCKE, Volker S; London HSC-Victoria Campus, PO Box 5010 Stn B 800 Commissioners Rd E, London ON N6A 5W9; FRCPC; Psy (Forensic Pathology). Staff, London Health Sciences Centre - Victoria Campus; Langs: German; (519)667-6861

HOCKIN, James C; Centre for Surveillance Coord, AI 6503A-130 Colonnade Rd, Nepean ON K2E 1B6; Tor'80; MSc(Epidem); Aj Prof Epidemiol & Community Health, University of Ottawa; (613)957-1764; Fax. (613)952-3196; james.hockin@hc-sc.gc.ca.

HOCKING, Deborah A; 3317 Wesbrook Mall, Vancouver BC V6S 0B1; UBC'90; Med Staff, Powell River General Hospital; (604)259-7744

HOCKMANN, Edgar R; Sunnybrook Hlth Sciences Ctre, D1 08-2075 Bayview Ave, Toronto ON M4N 3M5; Qns'02; FRCPC; Anes. Staff, Sunnybrook Health Sciences Centre; (416)480-4522

HOCKMANN, Guido I; 48-2140 North Park Dr, Brampton ON L6S 0C9; Wes'03; FRCSC; OrthSurg (Shoulder). (905)595-4971; Fax. (905)595-0515.

HODAIE, Mojgan; Univ Hlth Network-Toronto Western Hosp, 4WW 443-399 Bathurst St, Toronto ON M5T 2S8; Qns'96; FRCSC; Neursurg. Staff, Toronto Western Hospital - University Health Network; Langs: Spanish; Farsi; (416)603-5800

HODBY, Elizabeth D; Markham Ellesmere X-Ray & Ultr, 112-1200 Markham Rd, Scarborough ON M1H 3C3; London (England)'68; MB BS; FRCPC; DiagRad. (416)439-4866

HODDER, Andre; Dr Charles A Janeway Child HC, 300 Prince Philip Dr, St. John's NL A1B 3V6; Mem'02; FRCPC; GenSurg; PedGenSurg. Staff, Janeway Children's Health & Rehabilitation Centre; (709)777-6300

HODDER, David M; 105-645 Commissioners Rd E, London ON N6C 2T9; Mem'86; Staff, South Huron Hospital Association; (519)963-0232

HODDER, Donald G; Grand Falls Med Clinic, 164 Goodyear Ave, Grnd-Falls-Wi NL A2A 1M4; Dal'69; Staff, Central Newfoundland Regional Health Centre; (709)489-3744; Fax. (709)489-0081.

HODELET, Nicola; Vernon Mental Health Centre, 1440 14 Ave, Vernon BC V1B 2T1; Aberdeen (Scotland)'91; Staff, Vernon Jubilee Hospital; (250)549-5737

HODES, Peter K; 101-50 William St, Milverton ON N0K 1M0; Tor'82; Ac Staff, Stratford General Hospital - Huron Perth Healthcare Alliance; (519)595-8548; Fax. (519)595-8856.

HODGE, Eleanor A; Centretown Comm Health Centre, 420 Cooper St, Ottawa ON K2P 2N6; Alb'81; (613)233-4697; Fax. (613)233-4541; ehodge@centretownchc.org.

HODGE, Matthew J; Mount Sinai Hosp, 206-600 University Ave, Toronto ON M5G 1X5; McG'96; PhD; FRCPC; CommunMed;CCFP; CCFP(E.M.); Staff, Toronto General Hospital - UHN; Langs: English; French; (416)586-4800; Fax. (416)586-4719.

HODGE, Steven A; Cardiology Associates, 2606 Pandosy St, Kelowna BC V1Y 1V6; Man'97; FRCPC; IntMed (Interventional Cardiology); Cardiol. Staff, Kelowna General Hospital; (250)762-9211

HODGE, William G; Ivey Eye Institute, 268 Grosvenor St, London ON N6A 4V2; McG'88; MPH; PhD; FRCSC; Ophth (Cornea). Dept Chair Ophth, University of Western Ontario; Langs: English; French; (519)646-6210; Fax. (519)646-6136.

HODGE, William R; North Bay Reg Health Centre, 50 College Dr, North Bay ON P1B 0A4; Tor'75; FRCPC; DiagRad. Staff, North Bay Regional Health Centre - Regional Mental Health; (705)474-8600 x2038

HODGES, Brian D; R Fraser Elliott Bldg, 1 410-190 Elizabeth St, Toronto ON M5G 2C4; Qns'89; FRCPC; Psy (Education). Staff, Toronto General Hospital - UHN; Langs: Bilingual(English/French); (416)340-3079; Fax. (416)340-3792; brian.hodge@utoronto.ca.

HODGES, Daniel J; 245-10405 Jasper Ave NW, Edmonton AB T5J 3N4; Cal'82; FACOG; FRCSC; ObstGyn (Colposcopy). Med Staff Assoc/Dir Colposcopy Clinic, Royal Alexandra Hospital; Asst Clin Prof, University of Alberta; (780)423-1840; Fax. (780)423-7004.

HODGES, David C; Gordon Professional Ctr, 100-3001 Gordon Ave, Coquitlam BC V3C 2K7; Tor'88; FRCPC; DiagRad. Staff, Royal Columbian Hospital; (604)941-7611; Fax. (604)924-4612; david.hodges@fraserhealth.ca.

HODGES, Ernest J; 400-10216 124 St NW, Edmonton AB T5N 4A3; Alb'80; BSc; DAB; FRCSC; Ophth (Cataract Surgery). Staff Surg., Royal Alexandra Hospital; Clin Assoc Prof, University of Alberta; (780)482-6770; Fax. (780)482-4410; ejhodges@telusplanet.net.

HODGETTS, P Geoffrey; Queen's FHT-Corporate Office, PO Box 8888 220 Bagot St, Kingston ON K7L 3G2; Tor'71; CCFP; FCFP; Att Staff, Kingston General Hospital; Att Staff, Hotel-Dieu Hospital; Assoc Prof, Queen's University; (613)549-4480 x3906; Fax. (613)544-9899; hodgetts@post.queensu.ca.

HODGINS, G Walter; Royal Jubilee Hosp, 1952 Bay St, Victoria BC V8R 1J8; Tor'69; FRCPC; DiagRad. Ac Staff DiagRad, Royal Jubilee Hospital; (250)370-8272; Fax. (250)370-8594.

HODGINS, Michael B; The Ottawa Hosp-Gen Campus, 501 Smyth Rd Box 508, Ottawa ON K1H 8L6; Qns'87; CCFP; FCFP; Staff, The Ottawa Hospital - General Campus; (613)737-8899

HODGKISS, David R; SGH Medical Mall, 411-3030 Lawrence Ave E, Scarborough ON M1P 2T7; Tor'74; FACS; FRCSC; GenSurg (Laparoscopic Surgery). Staff, The Scarborough Hospital - General Campus; (416)439-4873; Fax. (416)439-7077; drhodgkiss@rogers.com.

HODGSON, Alyssa L; Royal Columbian Hosp, 330 Columbia St E, New Westminster BC V3L 3W7; UBC'00; FRCPC; Anes. Staff, Royal Columbian Hospital; (778)230-2882

HODGSON, Christopher J; University Village Med Clinic, 228-2155 Allison Rd, Vancouver BC V6T 1T5; UBC'81; (604)222-2273; Fax. (604)222-3403.

HODGSON, Craig D; Whitecourt Med Clinic, PO Box 1076 Stn Main, Whitecourt AB T7S 1P9; Alb'96; CCFP; FCFP; Chief Clinical Offices/Residency Coord & Med Staff, Whitecourt Healthcare Centre; (780)778-2224; Fax. (780)778-2127.

HODGSON, Darlene; Royal University Hosp, 103 Hospital Dr, Saskatoon SK S7N 0W8; Mem'03; FRCPC; Anes. Staff, Royal University Hospital; (306)655-1183; Fax. (306)655-1279.

HODGSON, David C; Univ Hlth Network-Princess M, 610 University Ave, Toronto ON M5G 2M9; Tor'93; FRCPC; RadOncol (Leukemia & Lymphoma). Prof, Princess Margaret Hospital - University Health Network; Asst Prof RadOncol, University of Toronto; (416)946-2919; Fax. (416)946-4586.

HODGSON, Nicole C; Hamilton HS-Henderson Site, B3-711 Concession St, Hamilton ON L8V 1C3; Ott'97; MSc; FRCSC; GenSurg (Surgical Oncology). Staff, Hamilton Health Sciences Centre-Juravinski Site; Physician, The Juravinski Cancer Centre; (905)575-6365; Fax. (905)381-7071.

HODGSON, Therese M M; 1-2530 St. Joseph Blvd, Orleans ON K1C 1G1; Ott'86; CCFP; FCFP; Langs: Bilingual(English/French); (613)830-5888; Fax. (613)830-1791.

HODGSON, Todd R; Brockville Gen Hosp, 75 Charles St, Brockville ON K6V 1S8; Qns'07; CCFP; Staff, Brockville General Hospital - Charles Street; (613)345-5077

HODGSON-VIDEN, Heather; Royal University Hosp, 103 Hospital Dr, Saskatoon SK S7N 0W8; Alb'04; FRCPC; Peds. Staff, Royal University Hospital; (306)966-8144; Fax. (306)966-8640.

HODKINSON, Roger G; Western Med Assessments, 17204 106A Ave NW, Edmonton AB T5S 1E6; Cambridge (England)'68; MB BCh; MA; FRCPC; GenPath. Staff, Bio-Id Diagnostics Inc; (780)433-1191; rhodkinson@westernmedicalassessments.com.

HODLEVSKYY, Oleksandr; Glenrose Rehab Hosp, 327-10230 111 Ave NW, Edmonton AB T5G 0B7; Ukraine (Russia (Federation))'84; Staff, Glenrose Rehabilitation Hospital; (780)735-7939; Fax. (780)735-8246.

HODSMAN, Anthony B; St Joseph's Health Care, PO Box 5777 Stn B A2 105-268 Grosvenor St, London ON N6A 4V2; London (England)'71; MB BS; FRCP(UK); MRCP(UK); FRCPC; IntMed (Metabolic Bone Disease). Consultant, London Health Sciences Centre - University Hospital; Consultant, St Joseph's Hospital - St Joseph's Health Care; Member Scientific Advisory Counsel, Osteoporosis Canada; Prof, University of Western Ontario; (519)646-6100 x64316; Fax. (519)646-6074.

HODSON, D Ian; The Juravinski Cancer Centre, 699 Concession St, Hamilton ON L8V 5C2; Oxford (England)'74; MA(Physiol); BMus; BCh; FRCPC; RadOncol (Therapeutic Radiology). Staff, Hamilton Health Sciences Centre - McMaster University Medical Centre; Staff, The Juravinski Cancer Centre; Head Div of RadOncol, McMaster University; (905)387-9495; Fax. (905)575-6326.

HODUC, Viviane; CLSC Pat-Mtl-Est, 13926 rue Notre-Dame E, Pte-Aux-Trembles QC H1A 1T5; Mon'87; LMCC; CCFP; FCFP; Staff, Hopital Maisonneuve-Rosemont; (514)642-4050; Fax. (514)642-5438.

HOE, Walter; The Ottawa Hosp-Gen Campus, Box 400 501 Smyth Rd, Ottawa ON K1H 8L6; Tor'86; FRCPC; Psy. Staff, The Ottawa Hospital - General Campus; (613)737-8010

HOEBERG, Debbie J; Business Bldg, 200-1200 Burrard St, Vancouver BC V6Z 2C7; UBC'80; Ac Staff, Providence Health Care - St Paul's Hospital; (604)685-4398; Fax. (604)685-7110.

HOEGLER, David; BC Cancer Ctre-Southern Interi, 399 Royal Ave, Kelowna BC V1Y 5L3; McM'90; FRCPC; RadOncol. Staff, BC Cancer Agency Sindi Ahluwalia Hawkins Centre for the Southern Interior; (250)712-3900; Fax. (250)712-3911.

HOEGLER, Kathy A; 303-21 Surrey St W, Guelph ON N1H 3R3; McM'90; FRCPC; Peds (Neonatology). Asst Clin Prof, Hamilton Health Sciences Centre; Staff, Grand River Hospital - Kitchener/Waterloo Health Centre; (519)836-3020; Fax. (519)836-5377.

HOEPPNER, Vernon H; Royal University Hosp, 3544-103 Hospital Dr, Saskatoon SK S7N 0W8; Man'68; FRCPC; IntMed; Respir. Staff Tuberculosis Control, Royal University Hospital; Dir, Tuberculosis Control Program, Saskatchewan Health; Prof/Dept Head Med, University of Saskatchewan; (306)966-8000; Fax. (306)966-8021.

HOESCHEN, Lawrence; 2F-7000 Westminster Hwy, Richmond BC V6X 1A2; Man'73; PhD(Pharm); FRCPC; IntMed (Addiction Medicine). Staff, Richmond Hospital; (604)244-5579; Fax. (604)244-5366; lawrence.hoeschen@vch.ca.

HOEVE, Allan J; 4607 50 Ave PO Box 3955 Stn Main, Olds AB T4H 1P6; Cal'94; CCFP; (403)556-7130; Fax. (403)556-1944.

HOEY, John R; Medical Assoc of Port Perry, 462 Paxton St, Port Perry ON L9L 1L9; McG'67; ABIM; FACP; FAB; FRCPC; IntMed (P.Q.); CommunMed. Langs: Bilingual(English/French); (905)985-5572; Fax. (905)985-8378.

HOEY, Steven A; 204-49 Emma St, Guelph ON N1E 6X1; Wes'90; FRCSC; OrthSurg. (519)763-5345; Fax. (519)821-8872.

HOFER, Michael; Dr Russell M Hall Fam Hlth Ctr, PO Box 550 32 South Court St E, Norwich ON N0J 1P0; (Czech Republic)'01; CCFP; (519)863-2338; Fax. (519)863-2073.

HOFER, Stefan O P; Univ Hlth Network-The Toronto, 8N 865-200 Elizabeth St, Toronto ON M5G 2C4; Amsterdam (Netherlands)'92; PhD; FRCSC; PlasSurg (Oncology Reconstruction). Staff, Princess Margaret Hospital - University Health Network; Staff, Toronto General Hospital - UHN; Langs: Dutch; (416)340-3449; Fax. (416)340-4403.

HOFF, Mark; Bethesda Hosp Steinbach, PO Box 939 Stn Main 316 Henry St, Steinbach MB R5G 1A3; Alb'98; CCFP; Staff, Bethesda Hospital Steinbach; (204)326-6411; mhoff@sehealth.mb.ca.

HOFFE, Charles D; Lytton Med Clinic, PO Box 39, Lytton BC V0K 1Z0; Witwatersrand (South Africa)'87; MB BCh; BSc; Chief Med Staff, St Bartholomew's Health Centre; (250)455-2202; Fax. (250)455-2237.

HOFFER, L John; SMBD Jewish Gen Hosp, 3755 ch Cote-Sainte-Catherine, Montreal QC H3T 1E2; McG'75; BSc; PhD; FRCPC; IntMed (Clinical Nutrition). Sr Physician, Sir Mortimer B Davis Jewish General; Prof Med, McGill University; (514)340-8222; Fax. (514)340-7502.

HOFFER, Mayer; 223 St Clair Ave W, Toronto ON M4V 1R3; Man'78; BSc(Med); DCH; DCHPsy; DABPN; FRCPC; Psy (Child & Adolescent Psychiatry). (416)967-1890; Fax. (416)482-8971.

HOFFERT, Blake M; 4474 Joyce Ave, Powell River BC V8A 3A6; Tor'78; FRCPC; IntMed (Cardiology)., Powell River General Hospital; (604)485-5340; Fax. (604)485-5341.

HOFFMAN, Alan S; 19-279 Kingston Rd E, Ajax ON L1Z 0K5; Guadalajara (Mexico)'77; Ac Staff, Rouge Valley Health System - Ajax & Pickering Health Centre Site; Court Staff, Rouge Valley Health System - Centenary Health Centre Site; (905)686-3811; Fax. (905)686-1295.

HOFFMAN, Bertrand; 2239 rue du Parc de Lotbiniere, Quebec QC G1T 1G5; Laval'72; FRCSC; Ophth (P.Q.). Ac Staff, Jeffery Hale Hospital-Saint Brigid's; Consultant, CSSS de Quebec-Sud; (418)658-2010; Fax. (418)658-8310.

HOFFMAN, Brian F; North York Gen Hosp-Branson, 262-555 Finch Ave W, North York ON M2R 1N5; Tor'66; FRCPC; Psy (Post Traumatic Stress Disorder). Staff Psy, North York General Hospital - Branson Division; Assoc Prof Psy, University of Toronto; (416)635-2583; Fax. (416)632-8718; brianhoffman@nygh.on.ca.

HOFFMAN, Bruce O; Hoffman Ctr for Integrative Me, 1133 17 Ave NW, Calgary AB T2M 0P7; Cape Town (South Africa)'81; (403)206-2333; Fax. (403)206-2334; info@hoffmancentre.com.

HOFFMAN, Christine; Linden Prof Centre, 101-24 Linden Ave, Charlottetown PE C1A 5Y8; Tor'91; CCFP; (902)367-3285; Fax. (902)569-8661.

HOFFMAN, Dale H M; 11336 Sheffield Place, Delta BC V4E 2H8; UBC'78; (604)809-8360

HOFFMAN, Daniel B; Aberdeen Hosp, 835 East River Rd, New Glasgow NS B2H 3S6; Dal'89; FRCPC; DiagRad. Staff, Aberdeen Regional Hospital; (902)752-8311

HOFFMAN, David V; Port Arthur Health Centre Inc, 194 Court St N, Thunder Bay ON P7A 4V7; Tor'65; FRCSC; OrthSurg. Ac Staff, Thunder Bay Regional Health Sciences Centre Port-Arthur; Ac Staff, St Joseph's Care Group - St Joseph's Hospital; (807)346-1000 x6225; Fax. (807)346-6251.

HOFFMAN, Harold E; Meadowlark Place Prof Centre, 410-8708 155 St NW, Edmonton AB T5R 1W2; Alb'73; FRCPC; OccupMed;CCFP; FCFP; Staff, University of Alberta Hospital; Staff, Covenant Health - Misericordia Community Hospital; Adjunct Assoc. Prof., University of Alberta; (780)439-9491; Fax. (780)433-9091.

HOFFMAN, Jaco; PO Box 3955 Stn Main, Olds AB T4H 1P7; (South Africa)'02; MB ChB; (403)556-7130

HOFFMAN, Joanne M; 107-22190 48 Ave, Langley BC V3A 3N5; McM'85; FRCPC; Psy. (604)534-2989

HOFFMAN, Kerri-Lyn; Kingston Laser & Cosmetic Clin, 863 Norwest Rd, Kingston ON K7P 2N2; Ott'95; CCFP; (613)384-4200

HOFFMAN, Lawrence H; Allan Memorial Institute, 1025 av des Pins O, Montreal QC H3A 1A1; McG'79; FRCPC; Psy. Staff, McGill University Health Centre - Royal Victoria Hospital; (514)842-1231

HOFFMAN, Maria E; Wild Rose Med Centre, 4607 50 Ave, Olds AB T4H 1W1; (South Africa)'02; MB ChB; (403)556-7130; Fax. (403)556-1944.

HOFFMAN, Norman; Norman Hoffman Med Serv Inc, 250-2015 rue Drummond, Montreal QC H3G 1W7; McG'79; FRCPC; Psy. Staff, Sir Mortimer B Davis Jewish General; (514)448-2800; Fax. (514)800-0782.

HOFFMAN, Shawn; SMBD Jewish Gen Hosp, 3755 ch Cote-Sainte-Catherine, Montreal QC H3T 1E2; McG'06; MDCM; FRCPC; Anes. Staff, Sir Mortimer B Davis Jewish General; (514)340-8222

HOFFMAN, Shayna E; Thunder Bay Reg HSC-T-Bay, 980 Oliver Rd, Thunder Bay ON P7B 6V4; McM'07; CCFP; CCFP(E.M.); Staff, Thunder Bay Regional Health Sciences Centre; (807)684-6000

HOFFMAN, Thomas M; Windsor Prof Centre, 124-2462 Howard Ave, Windsor ON N8X 3V6; Tor'90; CCFP; (519)258-7335; Fax. (519)971-9120.

HOFFMANN, Daile R; 124 14 Ave N PO Box 698, Creston BC V0B 1G0; Alb'97; CCFP; (250)428-5381

HOFFMANN, Kristin M I; 107-770 6 St SW, Medicine Hat AB T1A 4J6; (Belgium)'98; (403)487-5109; Fax. (403)487-5260.

HOFFMANN, Renee A; Springborough Prof Centre, 108-30 Springborough Blvd SW, Calgary AB T3H 0N9; Witwatersrand (South Africa)'89; MB ChB; DA(SA); (403)240-2221; Fax. (403)240-4670.

HOFFMANN, Susan M; East End Commun Health Centre, 1619 Queen St E, Toronto ON M4L 1G4; Alb'91; CCFP; (416)778-5858; Fax. (416)778-5855.

HOFFSTEIN, Victor; St Michael's Hosp, 30 Bond St, Toronto ON M5B 1W8; Miami(FL) (USA)'75; FRCPC; Respir. Ac Staff, St Michael's Hospital; Langs: Russian; Polish; French; Italian; (416)864-5516; Fax. (416)864-5649; victor.hoffstein@utoronto.ca.

HOFHUIS, John A; 285 Bridge St, Port Stanley ON N5L 1J5; Wes'78; CCFP; Langs: Dutch; (519)782-4195; Fax. (519)782-3743.

HOFMANN, Adam; CSSS de Saint-Jerome, 290 rue De Montigny, Saint-Jerome QC J7Z 5T3; McG'05; FRCPC; IntMed. Staff, CSSS St-Jerôme; (450)432-2777

HOFMANN, Karen H; Athabascan Place, 114-80 Chippewa Rd, Sherwood Park AB T8A 4W6; Qns'72; FRCPC; DiagRad (Diagnostic Imaging)., University of Alberta; Langs: German; (780)467-2773; Fax. (780)467-2982; karenhof@cancerboard.ab.ca.

HOFNER, Anne Marie; Dr Charles A Janeway Child HC, 300 Prince Philip Dr, St. John's NL A1B 3V6; Warsaw (Poland)'07; Psy. Staff, Health Sciences Centre; (709)737-6300

HOFNER, Grazyna W; Colchester East Hants Hlth Ctr, 600 Abenaki Rd, Truro NS B2N 5A1; Warsaw (Poland)'81; FRCPC; Psy. Staff, Colchester East Hants Health Centre; Langs: Polish; Czech; Russian; (902)897-4357; Fax. (902)895-5829.

HOFSTADER, Sophie L R; SGH Medical Mall, 201-3030 Lawrence Ave E, Scarborough ON M1P 2T7; Dal'56; MDCM; FRCPC; Derm (Psoriasis). Staff, Women's College Hospital; Ac Staff, The Scarborough Hospital - General Campus; Asst Prof Med, University of Toronto; Langs: Polish; Russian; (416)438-6442; Fax. (416)438-8227; sophiehofstader@hotmail.com.

HOGAN, Angela; Hopital Montfort, 713 Montreal Rd, Ottawa ON K1K 0T2; Ott'05; FRCPC; Anes. Staff, Montfort Hospital; Langs: Bilingual(English/French); (613)746-4621

HOGAN, Darryl R; Commonwealth Med Clinic, 77 Commonwealth Ave, Mount Pearl NL A1N 1W7; Mem'98; CCFP; Staff, The Dr G B Cross Memorial Hospital; (709)364-7555

HOGAN, David B; HSC-Faculty Of Med, 3330 Hospital Dr NW, Calgary AB T2N 4N1; Dal'77; FACP; FRCPC; IntMed; GeriatricMed. Ac Staff, Foothills Medical Centre; Chair Geriatric Med, The Brenda Strafford Foundation; Prof/Chair Geriatric Med Faculty of Med, University of Calgary; (403)220-4578; Fax. (403)283-6151; dhogan@ucalgary.ca.

HOGAN, Gillian M M; Erinoakkids Ctr for Treatment, 2277 South Millway, Mississauga ON L5L 2M5; National (Ireland)'80; FRCPC; Peds (Developmental Pediatrics). VP Med Services, Erinoakkids Centre for Treatment & Development; Clin Associate Part-Time, McMaster University; (905)828-3217

HOGAN, Kevin P; Waterford Hosp, 306 Waterford Bridge Rd, St. John's NL A1E 4J8; Mem'75; FRCPC; Psy. Staff, Waterford Hospital; Clinical Asst Prof Commun Med, Memorial University Of Newfoundland; (709)777-3614; Fax. (709)777-3553.

HOGAN, Marie-Pier; CSSS De Sept-Iles, 45 rue du Pere-Divet, Sept-Iles QC G4R 3N7; Mon'06; Respir; IntMed. Staff, Centre Hospitalier Regional de Sept-Iles; (418)962-9761

HOGAN, Matthew J; The Ottawa Hosp-Civic Campus, 1053 Carling Ave, Ottawa ON K1Y 4E9; Qns'79; FRCPC; Neur. Staff, The Ottawa Hospital - Civic Campus; (613)798-5555; mhogan@uottawa.ca.

HOGAN, Maureen; Health Sciences Centre, 300 Prince Phillip Dr, St. John's NL A1B 3V6; McM'04; FRCPC; DiagRad. Staff, Health Sciences Centre; (709)737-6300

HOGAN, Megan R; 445 Inglehart St N, Oakville ON L6J 3J5; McM'06; CCFP; Derm. Staff, The Credit Valley Hospital; Langs: Bilingual(English/French); (905)844-8800; Fax. (905)844-8200.

HOGAN, Michael P; Health Sciences Centre, 300 Prince Philip Dr, St. John's NL A1B 3V6; Mem'00; FRCSC; GenSurg. Staff, Health Sciences Centre; (709)777-6439

HOGAN, Michael S N; University of Alberta Hosp, 8440 112 St NW, Edmonton AB T6G 2B7; (Ireland)'03; MB BCh; BAO; Staff, University of Alberta Hospital; (780)407-8887; Fax. (780)407-3200; mhogan@ualberta.ca.

HOGAN, W Patrick D; Queensway-Carleton Hosp, 3045 Baseline Rd, Nepean ON K2H 8P4; Ott'77; FRCPC; Anes. Staff, Queensway Carleton Hospital; (613)721-4700

HOGARTH, Margaret T; Burlington After Hours Clinic, 183-2025 Guelph Line, Burlington ON L7P 4M8; Dayton(OH) (USA)'95; CCFP; (905)681-7755

HOGARTH, Teresa K; Keary Med Centre, 105-245 Columbia St E, New Westminster BC V3L 3W4; UBC'84; Staff, Royal Columbian Hospital; Staff, Surrey Memorial Hospital; (604)522-6800

HOGARTH, Walter D; Red Deer Reg Hosp Centre, 3942 50A Ave, Red Deer AB T4N 4E7; Wes'86; CCFP; CCFP(E.M.); FCFP; Staff Emerg Med, Red Deer Regional Hospital Centre; (403)343-4448; Fax. (403)343-4459.

HOGBEN, Reed M; 315-401 9 Ave SW, Calgary AB T2P 3C5; Alb'83; (403)263-0661; Fax. (403)233-9026.

HOGENBIRK, Barbara F; Brunswick Med Centre, 401-955 boul Saint-Jean, Pointe-Claire QC H9R 5K3; Ott'88; CCFP; FCFP; (514)426-6677; Fax. (514)426-3323.

HOGG, David H; Univ Hlth Network-Princess M, 5 108-610 University Ave, Toronto ON M5G 2M9; Tor'80; ABIM; FRCPC; IntMed (Melanoma); Hem. Staff/Prof Med, Princess Margaret Hospital - University Health Network; (416)946-4521; david.hogg@uhn.on.ca.

HOGG, Donald W; Hunt Club Med Centre, 104-3328 McCarthy Rd, Ottawa ON K1V 0H9; Tor'69; (613)526-5515; Fax. (613)526-0740.

HOGG, L Craig; Niagara H System-Welland Site, 65 Third St, Welland ON L3B 4W6; Tor'85; Staff, Niagara Health System - Port Colborne General Site; (905)732-6111

HOGG, Lori M; 303-6707 Elbow Dr SW, Calgary AB T2V 0E5; Cal'89; FRCPC; Psy. Staff, Foothills Medical Centre; (403)571-2480; Fax. (403)571-2499.

HOGG, Susan C; MCI The Doctors Office, PO Box 134 Royal Bank Plaza 220 Bay St, Toronto ON M5J 2J3; Tor'90; (416)368-6787; Fax. (416)368-7632.

HOGGE, Donna E; Gordon & Leslie Diamond Hlth C, 10F-2775 Laurel St, Vancouver BC V5Z 1M9; Alb'73; MD; FRCPC; IntMed (Hematological Oncology); Hem. Ac Staff, Vancouver General Hospital - Centennial Pavillion; Staff Hem, BC Cancer Agency Vancouver Centre; Clin Prof Med, University of British Columbia; (604)875-4662; Fax. (604)875-4763.

HOGUE, Dominique; Ctr Hosp Anna-Laberge, 200 boul Brisebois, Chateauguay QC J6K 4W8; Mon'88; CSPQ; FRCSC; GenSurg. Staff, Hôpital Anna-Laberge; (450)699-2425; Fax. (450)699-2525.

HOGUE, Nadia; CSSS du Lac-des-Deux-Montagnes, 520 boul Arthur-Sauve, Saint-Eustache QC J7R 5B1; Mon'99; Staff, Hôpital de Saint-Eustache; (450)473-6811

HOH, Erin S Y; Region of Waterloo Public Hlth, 99 Regina St W, Waterloo ON N2J 4V3; McM'08; CCFP; Physician, Region of Waterloo Public Health Corporate Office; (519)883-2000

HOH, Lydia O K; North York Gen Hosp, 4001 Leslie St, North York ON M2K 1E1; Tor'87; Ac Staff Family Med, North York General Hospital; (416)756-6265

HOHL, Christopher M; St Boniface Gen Hosp, A8024-409 Tache Ave, Winnipeg MB R2H 2A6; Man'04; FRCPC; Peds (Palliative Medicine). Staff, St Boniface General Hospital; (204)233-8563

HOHL, Corinne M; Vancouver Gen Hosp, 855 12th Ave W, Vancouver BC V5Z 1M9; McG'99; FRCPC; EmergMed. Staff, Vancouver General Hospital - Centennial Pavillion; Langs: German; French; (604)875-4995

HOHOL, Maria J; 943-55 Queen St E, Toronto ON M5C 1R6; Tor'85; BSc; FRCPC; Neur (Multiple Sclerosis). Staff Neurol, St Michael's Hospital; Assoc Prof Div of Neurol, University of Toronto; Langs: Ukrainian; (416)864-5533; Fax. (416)864-5610.

HOIRCH, Adam R; Near North Med Clinic, 202-66 Josephine St, North Bay ON P1B 0A7; Saba (United Kingdom)'09; CCFP; (705)476-1512; Fax. (705)495-4500.

HOJYO TOMOKA, Margarita K; Royal York Med Arts Bldg, 311-1436 Royal York Rd, Etobicoke ON M9P 3A9; (Mexico)'69; Court Staff, St Joseph's Health Centre; Langs: Spanish; Japanese; (416)241-4689; Fax. (416)241-4680.

HOKANSON, Michelle R M; Peter Lougheed Centre, 3500 26 Ave NE, Calgary AB T1Y 6J4; Sask'96; FRCPC; Anes. Staff, Peter Lougheed Centre; (403)943-5721

HOLAN, Jan; 4950 Heather St, Vancouver BC V5Z 3L9; Purkyne (Czech Republic)'80; Staff, BC Mental Health & Addiction Service; (604)806-9565

HOLBROOK, Anne M; St Joseph's Healthcare, G623A-50 Charlton Ave E, Hamilton ON L8N 4A6; McM'83; MSc; PharmD; FRCPC; IntMed (Clinical Pharmacology). Staff, St Joseph's Healthcare - Charlton Campus; Staff Med, Hamilton Health Sciences Centre - McMaster Children's Hospital; Dir Div of Clin Pharmacol & Assoc of Prof, McMaster University; (905)522-1155 x35269; Fax. (905)528-7386.

HOLDEN, Dean A; Queensway Carleton Hosp, 3045 Baseline Rd, Nepean ON K2H 8P4; Ott'03; FRCPC; DiagRad. Staff, Queensway Carleton Hospital; (613)721-4700

HOLDEN, Jana P; Griffiths Med Clinic, 28-5201 50 St, Leduc AB T9E 6T4; Cal'95; CCFP; CCFP(E.M.); (780)986-6200; Fax. (780)986-5200.

HOLDEN, Janet K; St Paul's Hosp, 1081 Burrard St, Vancouver BC V6Z 1Y6; Sask'80; FRCPC; AnatPath. Ac Staff Path, Providence Health Care - St Paul's Hospital; (604)806-8204; Fax. (604)806-8158.

HOLDEN, Rachel M; Queen's Univ-Etherington Hall, 3048C-115 Barrack St, Kingston ON K7L 3N6; Ott'96; FRCPC; IntMed; Nephrol. (613)533-3134

HOLDEN, Timothy J; Royal Jubilee Hosp, 1952 Bay St, Victoria BC V8R 1J8; Cape Town (South Africa)'77; MMed(Psych); FRCPC; Psy (Consultation). Staff, Royal Jubilee Hospital; (250)519-1554; Fax. (250)370-8814.

HOLDER, Chanse L; QHC Belleville Gen Hosp, 265 Dundas St E, Belleville ON K8N 5A9; Dal'98; CCFP; Staff, QHC Belleville General; (613)969-7400

HOLDER, Douglas A; Hamilton HS-General Site, 514-237 Barton St E, Hamilton ON L8L 2X2; Wes'69; FRCPC; IntMed (Interventional Cardiology); Cardiol. Member Cardiol, Hamilton Health Sciences Centre - Hamilton General Hospital; Prof Med, McMaster University; (905)523-1241; Fax. (905)523-8352; holderd@hhsc.ca.

HOLDER, Fryderyk; Norwood Walk-In & Fam Med Ctr, 43A Marion St, Winnipeg MB R2H 0S8; Silesian (Poland)'65; (204)233-9477

HOLDSWORTH, Judith A; CFB Kingston, PO Box 17000 Stn Forces, Kingston ON K7K 7B4; Tor'79; BASc; Staff, Guelph General Hospital; (613)541-5010 x5522

HOLDSWORTH, Rosalynd E; Community Psych Service, 1350 St. Andrews Ave, North Vancouver BC V7L 3L4; Cal'90; FRCPC; Psy. Staff, Providence Health Care - St Paul's Hospital; (604)983-6020

HOLDWAY, Geoffrey M; Rosedale Med Group, 280 Queenston Rd, Hamilton ON L8K 1H1; Cardiff (Wales)'74; MB ChB; MRCGPract; DObstRCOG; Staff Women's Health Clinic, Hamilton Health Sciences Centre-Juravinski Site; (905)547-0508; Fax. (905)547-6865.

HOLEK, Arlene R; 574A Upper James St, Hamilton ON L9C 2Y6; Wes'86; Ac Staff, Hamilton Health Sciences Centre - McMaster Children's Hospital; Court Staff, St Joseph's Healthcare - Charlton Campus; (905)574-2668; Fax. (905)318-1115.

HOLFELD, Karen I; Victoria East Med Clinic, 2F-2068 Prince of Wales Dr, Regina SK S4V 3A6; Sask'83; FRCPC; Derm. (306)789-4677; Fax. (306)789-0945.

HOLINATY, Carla; Kenderdine Med Clinic, 110-1804 McOrmond Dr, Saskatoon SK S7S 0A6; Sask'10; CCFP; (306)934-6606; Fax. (306)242-4171.

HOLLAAR, Gwendolyn L; Peter Lougheed Centre, 3500 26 Ave NE, Calgary AB T1Y 6J4; Alb'89; FRCSC; GenSurg. Staff, Peter Lougheed Centre; (403)943-4843; Fax. (403)219-3574.

HOLLAND, Anthony J C; West Coast Gen Hosp, 3949 Port Alberni Hwy, Port Alberni BC V9Y 4S1; Adelaide (Australia)'63; DCH; FRCA; CSPQ; MB BS; Anes (P.Q.) (Pain Management). Staff Anes, West Coast General Hospital; Langs: Swedish; French; (250)723-2135; Fax. (250)724-8805.

HOLLAND, Bernard; Montague Health Centre, PO Box 877, Montague PE C0A 1R0; Dal'91; BSc; MCFP; Ac Staff, Kings County Memorial Hospital; (902)838-0830; Fax. (902)838-0834; bjholland@ihis.org.

HOLLAND, David C; Queen's Univ Etherington Hall, 2058-115 Barrack St, Kingston ON K7L 3N6; McM'88; LMCC; FRCPC; IntMed (Renal Transplant); Nephrol. Staff, Kingston General Hospital; Teach Staff, Queen's University; (613)533-6983

HOLLAND, David R; 1903 9 Ave S, Lethbridge AB T1J 1W8; Alb'84; FACP; ABMO; FRCPC; IntMed; MedOncol. Med Dir, Lethbridge Cancer Centre; Ac Staff, Covenant Health - St Michael's Health Centre; Ac Staff, Chinook Regional Hospital; Clinical Asst Prof Med, University of Calgary; (403)320-0633; Fax. (403)320-0353.

HOLLAND, F John; Ont Cancer Research Ethics Boa, 401-790 Bay St, Toronto ON M5G 1N8; Queen's (Ireland)'69; MB ChB; BAO; FRCP; FRCPC; Peds; Endocrin&Metab. Staff, Toronto General Hospital - UHN; (416)673-6662

HOLLAND, Joanna; IWK Health Centre, PO Box 9700 Rpo CSC 5850-5980 University Ave, Halifax NS B3K 6R8; Tor'01; FRCPC; Peds. Staff, IWK Health Centre; (902)470-6866; Fax. (902)470-6913.

HOLLAND, John E; Chinook Paediatric Clinic, 951 19 St S, Lethbridge AB T1J 3H5; Pretoria (South Africa)'81; MB BS; MMed(Ped); FRCPCH; FRFPS; FRCPC; Peds. Sr Med Dir, Chinook Regional Hospital; (403)320-7825; Fax. (403)320-8613.

HOLLAND, Lind G; Strabane Medical Office, RR 4 1436 Brock Rd, Dundas ON L9H 5E4; McM'84; CCFP; (905)659-1663; Fax. (905)659-0681; lholland2@cogeco.ca.

HOLLAND, Roy V; Maples Adolescent Centre, 250-3405 Willingdon Ave, Burnaby BC V5G 3H4; McM'78; FRCPC; Psy (Forensic Psychiatry). Staff/Clin Dir, Maples Adolescent Treatment Centre; (604)986-3667

HOLLAND, Sharon A; Quinte HC Corp-Belleville Gen, 265 Dundas St E, Belleville ON K8N 5A9; Mem'77; BSc; BMedSci; FRCPC; DiagRad. Staff, QHC Trenton Memorial; Staff, Lennox & Addington County General Hospital; Staff Radiol, QHC Belleville General; (613)969-7400

HOLLAND, Simon P; UBC Eye Care Centre, 2550 Willow St, Vancouver BC V5Z 3N9; Salisbury (Zimbabwe)'75; MRC(UK); DAB; FRCS; FRC; MB ChB; FRCSC; Ophth (Cataract). Staff, Providence Health Care - Mount Saint Joseph Hospital; Staff, Vancouver General Hospital - Centennial Pavillion; Staff, Dawson Creek & District Hospital; Pacific Laser Eye Centre; Clin Prof, University of British Columbia; (604)875-5850; Fax. (604)875-5860; simon_holland@telus.net.

HOLLAND, Stephen G; Yarrow Med Bldg, 305-645 Fort St, Victoria BC V8W 1G2; Cal'73; BSc; FRCP; FRCPC; Gastroent (Gastrointestinal & Hepatic Disease); IntMed. Asst Prof Med, University of British Columbia; (250)384-1544; gioffice@telus.net.

HOLLAND, Stewart H; Woodlawn Med Clinic, 92 Main St, Dartmouth NS B2X 1R5; McG'73; MDCM; Ac Staff, Dartmouth General Hospital; (902)434-1500; Fax. (902)434-4368.

HOLLAND-MUTER, Elizabeth M; Dr C W Wiebe Med Centre, 385 Main St, Winkler MB R6W 1J2; Pretoria (South Africa)'84; (204)325-4312

HOLLANDER, Andree L; Professional Bldg, 2100-222 King St E, Bowmanville ON L1C 1P6; Tor'88; CCFP; CCFP(E.M.); FCFP; Ac Staff, Lakeridge Health - Bowmanville Site; (905)623-0323; Fax. (905)697-0230.

HOLLANDS, Hussein; 3105 27 St, Vernon BC V1T 4W4; UBC'05; Ophth. (250)549-4362

HOLLANDS, Laurence S; 8840 210 St E PO Box 505, Langley BC V1M 2Y2; Cal'84; FRCPC; IntMed (Rheumatology). Staff Clinical Instructor, Royal Columbian Hospital; Consultant, Langley Memorial Hospital; Staff, Fraser Arthritis Centre; Clin Instructor, University of British Columbia; (604)469-0028

HOLLANDS, Ralph T; 43 Aylmer Ave, Ottawa ON K1S 5R4; McM'76; CCFP; FCFP; Ac Staff, The Ottawa Hospital - Riverside Campus.

HOLLENBERG, Robert D; McMaster University HSC, 4E-1200 Main St W, Hamilton ON L8S 4J9; Harvard(MA) (USA)'65; FACS; FRCSC; Neursurg (Pediatric Neuro Surgery); Electroenceph (P.Q.). Ac Staff Ped Neurosurg, Hamilton Health Sciences Centre - McMaster Children's Hospital; Affil Staff, St Joseph's Healthcare - Charlton Campus; Clin Assoc Prof Surg & Peds, McMaster University; (905)521-2100 x75237; Fax. (905)521-9992.

HOLLENBERG, Susan L; UBC Health Clinic, 310-5950 University Blvd, Vancouver BC V6T 1Z3; UBC'88; DSc; Staff, Travel Medicine & Vaccination Centre; Clinical Asst Prof, University of British Columbia; (604)822-5431

HOLLENHORST, Helmut; 5820 University Ave, Halifax NS B3H 1V7; Munich (Germany)'95; FRCPC; RadOncol. Staff Rad Oncol, Queen Elizabeth II Health Sciences Centre - Victoria General Site; Asst Prof, Dalhousie University; Langs: German; (902)473-6185; Fax. (902)473-7205.

HOLLER, Theresa A M; St Michael's Hosp, 8CCWN-30 Bond St, Toronto ON M5B 1W8; McM'06; FRCSC; Otol. Staff, St Michael's Hospital; (416)864-5276

HOLLETT, Bruce; Waterford Hosp, 306 Waterford Bridge Rd, St. John's NL A1E 4J8; Mem'87; CCFP; Staff, Waterford Hospital; (709)777-3300; bruceh@nl.rogers.com.

HOLLETT, Peter D; Health Sciences Centre, 300 Prince Philip Dr, St. John's NL A1B 3V6; Mem'82; FRCPC; NuclearMed. Consultant/Staff Nuclear Med, St Clare's Mercy Hospital; Consultant, Janeway Children's Health & Rehabilitation Centre; Clinical Asst Prof Radiol, Memorial University Of Newfoundland; (709)777-7159; Fax. (709)777-8267.

HOLLETT, Peter M; 303-274 Dundas St E, Belleville ON K8N 1E6; Mem'99; FRCPC; IntMed; Cardiol. Staff, QHC Belleville General.

HOLLETT-CAINES, Jackie R; St Joseph's Health Care, PO Box 5777 Stn B 268 Grosvenor St, London ON N6A 4V2; Mem'99; FRCSC; ObstGyn (Reproductive Endocrinology & Infertility). Staff, London Health Sciences Centre - University Hospital; Staff, London Health Sciences Centre - Victoria Campus; Staff, St Joseph's Hospital - St Joseph's Health Care; Teach Staff Obst/Gyn, University of Western Ontario; (519)646-6000

HOLLIDAY, Ronald L; Galleria London, 355 Wellington St, London ON N6A 3N7; Wes'66; FACS; FRCSC; GenSurg (Breasts). Staff GenSurg, London Health Sciences Centre - Victoria Campus; Prof, University of Western Ontario; (519)432-1919

HOLLIDGE, Melanie G; Hamilton HS-General Site, 237 Barton St E, Hamilton ON L8L 2X2; McM'02; FRCPC; Anes; Critical Care Medicine. Staff, Hamilton Health Sciences Centre - Hamilton General Hospital; (905)525-9140

HOLLING, Tamara L; 3-715 Coronation Blvd, Cambridge ON N1R 7R1; Wes'10; (519)740-1700

HOLLINGER, C Gerald; Old Quebec Street Mall, 203-55 Wyndham St N, Guelph ON N1H 7T8; McG'77; BSc; MSc(Mon.); ABIM(IntMed&Resp.); FCCP; MDCM; FRCPC; IntMed. Staff, Guelph General Hospital; Staff, Groves Memorial Community Hospital; (519)837-1011; Fax. (519)837-3352.

HOLLINGER, Horst; Tsawwassen Fam Health Centre, 101-5461 12 Ave, Delta BC V4M 2B2; UBC'96; (604)943-1148; Fax. (604)943-1140.

HOLLINGER, Shawn M; Children's Hosp of Eastern Ont, 401 Smyth Rd, Ottawa ON K1H 8L1; Saba (Netherlands Antilles)'08; Peds.

HOLLINGSWORTH, Christopher W; Medicine Prof Corp, 12 Lakeview Cir, St Thomas ON N5P 4B2; Wes'03; CCFP; CCFP(E.M.); Staff, St Thomas Elgin General Hospital; (519)633-4364

HOLLINGSWORTH, W John; PO Box 1299, Cardston AB T0K 0K0; Alb'64; FACS; FRCSC; GenSurg (Obesity Surgery). (403)653-4884; Fax. (403)653-1912.

HOLLINGWORTH, Gary R; Univ of Ottawa, 2045A-451 Smyth Rd, Ottawa ON K1H 8M5; Ott'73; CCFP; FCFP; Ac Staff, The Ottawa Hospital - General Campus; Asst Dean Admissions/Assoc Prof, University of Ottawa; Langs: French; (613)562-5800; Fax. (613)562-5651.

HOLLINGWORTH, James L; Goderich Med Centre, 181 Cambria Rd N, Goderich ON N7A 2R2; London (England)'69; DCH; DRCOG; CCFP; FCFP; Staff, Alexandra Marine & General Hospital; (519)524-5385; Fax. (519)524-8926.

HOLLINGWORTH, Roger W; Credit Valley Prof Bldg, 509-2300 Eglinton Ave W, Mississauga ON L5M 2V8; McM'78; BSc; FRCPC; IntMed; Gastroent. Ac Staff, The Credit Valley Hospital; (905)820-7877; Fax. (905)820-4887.

HOLLINGWORTH, Sean; Medicine Hat Reg Hosp, 666 5 St SW, Medicine Hat AB T1A 4H6; (South Africa)'94; FRCPC; Anes. Staff Anes, Medicine Hat Regional Hospital; (403)529-8024; Fax. (403)529-8998.

HOLLINS, Russell J; 144 Brock St, Kingston ON K7L 5G2; Ott'95; FRCSC; Otol. Staff, Hotel-Dieu Hospital; Staff, Kingston General Hospital; Asst Prof, Queen's University; Langs: French; (613)544-3400; Fax. (613)547-5654.

HOLLINSHEAD, Robert M; Sports Med Centre, 2500 University Dr NW, Calgary AB T2N 1N4; Man'71; FRCSC; OrthSurg (Shoulder). Clin Prof Med, University of Calgary; (403)220-5077; Fax. (403)282-6170; rholl@shaw.ca.

HOLLIS, Brian A; Ernest Walk-In Med Clinic, 1101 Jalna Blvd, London ON N6E 3B3; Tor'92; (519)668-2208

HOLLIS, Harlow R; Derma Spa Clinic, 101-1830 Oak Bay Ave, Victoria BC V8R 6R2; Dal'69; FRCSC; PlasSurg (Cosmetic Surgery). Assoc Staff, Vancouver Island Health Authority; Med Dir, Derma Spa; (250)598-6968; Fax. (250)592-8998; hollismd@dermaspa.ca.

HOLLOHAN, Brendan T; Healey's Pharmacy Bldg, 132 Casey St, St. John's NL A1C 4X7; Mem'92; (709)753-4011; Fax. (709)753-3130.

HOLLOHAN, Kirk G; 786 Goderich St, Port Elgin ON N0H 2C3; Mem'93; BMedSci; CCFP; CCFP(E.M.); Staff Emerg, Providence Health Care - St Paul's Hospital; (519)832-4997; Fax. (519)832-4999.

HOLLOMBY, David J; LHSC-University Hosp, PO Box 5339 Stn B ALL 135-339 Windermere Rd, London ON N6A 5A5; McG'71; DABIM; FACP; BSc; FRCP(Glasg); FRCPC; IntMed (Transplant Nephrology); Nephrol (P.Q.). Staff, London Health Sciences Centre - University Hospital; Staff, St Joseph's Hospital - St Joseph's Health Care; (519)663-3239; Fax. (519)663-8619; dj.hollomby@lhsc.on.ca.

HOLLOWAY, Caroline L; BC Cancer Agency-Vanc Isl Ctr, 2410 Lee Ave, Victoria BC V8R 6V5; UBC'00; FRCPC; RadOncol. Staff, BC Cancer Agency Vancouver Island Centre; (250)519-5500

HOLLOWAY, Claire M B; Sunnybrook Health Science Ctre, T2 015-2075 Bayview Ave, Toronto ON M4N 3M5; Wes'84; PhD; MRCS; FRCSC; GenSurg (Breast Surgery) (Breast Disease). Staff Breast Surg & Oncologic Reconstruction, Sunnybrook Health Sciences Centre - Edmond Odette Cancer Centre; Asst Prof, University of Toronto; (416)480-4210; Fax. (416)480-6002; claire.holloway@sunnybrook.ca.

HOLLOWAY, Erica; Dr Everett Chalmers Reg Hosp, PO Box 9000 Stn A 700 Priestman St, Fredericton NB E3B 5N5; Mem'01; FRCSC; ObstGyn (Fetal & Maternal Medicine). Staff, Dr Everett Chalmers Regional Hospital; (506)452-5286; Fax. (506)447-4421.

HOLLOWAY, Michael A; 1950 Broadway W PO Box 29101 Rpo South Granvil, Vancouver BC V6J 5C2; Cal'95; CCFP; CCFP(E.M.); Staff, Peace Arch Hospital.

HOLLOWAY, Peter J; 2-30 45th St S, Wasaga Beach ON L9Z 0A6; McM'03; CCFP; (705)429-9445

HOLLOWAY, Randy W; Leamington Dist Mem Hosp, 194 Talbot St W, Leamington ON N8H 1N9; Mem'89; Staff, Leamington District Memorial Hospital; (519)322-2501 x4242

HOLLOWELL, Jill S; Preston Med Centre, 506 King St E, Cambridge ON N3H 3N2; Nova Southeastern University (USA)'03; CCFP; (519)653-3321; Fax. (519)653-3498.

HOLLWAY, Gordon; Rothesay Med Clinic, 11 Gondola Point Rd, Rothesay NB E2E 5J6; Dal'85; CCFP; FCFP; Staff, Horizon Health Network Saint John Public Health; Lecturer, Dalhousie University; (506)847-7592; Fax. (506)847-7509.

HOLLY, Ralph; Campbellton Reg Hosp, PO Box 880 Stn Main 189 Lily Lake Rd, Campbellton NB E3N 3H3; (Haiti)'92; Staff, Hôpital Régional Campbellton; (506)789-5000

HOLLY, Tania M; Campbellton Reg Hosp, PO Box 880 Stn Main 189 Lily Lake Rd, Campbellton NB E3N 3H3; (Haiti)'92; Staff, Hôpital Régional Campbellton; (506)789-5000

HOLM JHASS, Jacqueline L; Grandin Med Clinic, 1 St Anne St, St. Albert AB T8N 2E8; Alb'05; CCFP; Langs: Bilingual(English/French); (780)459-5581; Fax. (780)458-7515.

HOLMAN, Joan L; 101-4695 Hastings St, Burnaby BC V5C 2K6; UBC'86; CCFP; Staff, Burnaby Hospital; (604)298-7201; Fax. (604)291-6176.

HOLMAN, Terry G; South Muskoka Med Centre, 230 Manitoba St, Bracebridge ON P1L 2E1; Tor'92; (705)646-7634; Fax. (705)646-0476.

HOLMEN, Carol D; Mineral Spring Hosp, PO Box 1050 Stn Main 301 Lynx St, Banff AB T1L 1H7; Alb'96; FRCPC; EmergMed. Physician Emerg, Foothills Medical Centre; Staff, Covenant Health - Banff Mineral Springs Hospital; (403)762-2222

HOLMES, Alan R; Brantford Med Centre, 40 Shellington Place, Brantford ON N3S 0C5; Mem'82; CCFP; FCFP; (519)753-9581

HOLMES, Allan E; 1644 3rd Ave W, Vancouver BC V6J 1K2; UBC'87; FRCPC; EmergMed. (604)685-4747 x430; Fax. (604)685-4748; aholmes@global-medical.ca.

HOLMES, Andrew I; PO Box 167, Baddeck NS B0E 1B0; Dal'87; CCFP; (902)295-2443; Fax. (902)295-1775.

HOLMES, Candice N; Family Practice Unit, 3F-61 Queen St E, Toronto ON M5C 2T2; Tor'99; CCFP; Staff, St Michael's Hospital; (416)867-7428; Fax. (416)867-7498.

HOLMES, Carol D; Agassiz Med Clinic, 130-30 Stephen St, Morden MB R6M 2G3; Man'81; CCFP; FCFP; (204)822-4474; Fax. (204)822-6886.

HOLMES, Colin L; Piper Creek Med Clinic, 200-3215 49 Ave, Red Deer AB T4N 0M8; Alb'73; Staff, Red Deer Regional Hospital Centre; (403)986-7265; Fax. (403)986-7604.

HOLMES, Daniel T; St Paul's Hosp, 1081 Burrard St, Vancouver BC V6Z 1Y6; UBC'01; BSc; FRCPC; MedBiochem (Laboratory Medicine). Staff Med Biochemist, Providence Health Care - St Paul's Hospital; Prof, University of British Columbia; (604)806-8919; dtholmes@interchange.ubc.ca.

HOLMES, David N P; Chelsea Court Health Centre, 779 Chelsea St, Brockville ON K6V 6J8; Dal'76; Staff, Brockville General Hospital - Charles Street; Staff, Providence Continuing Care Centre (PCCC) - St Vincent de Paul Hospital; (613)342-1199; Fax. (613)342-2900.

HOLMES, Donald H; Central Alberta Med Imaging, 4312 54 Ave, Red Deer AB T4N 4M1; Cal'74; FRCPC; DiagRad. Ac Staff, Red Deer Regional Hospital Centre; (403)343-6172; Fax. (403)309-3063.

HOLMES, Edward S; Abbottsfield Shoppers Mall, 214-3210 118 Ave NW, Edmonton AB T5W 4W1; Alb'71; (780)471-2071; Fax. (780)474-8001.

HOLMES, John E; Medical & Dental Bldg, 207-1221 Algonquin Ave, North Bay ON P1B 4Y3; Wes'70; FRCSC; OrthSurg. Staff, North Bay Regional Health Centre - Regional Mental Health; (705)476-0165; Fax. (705)476-5243.

HOLMES, John J; Fairview Med Bldg, 208-2200 Fairview St, Burlington ON L7R 4H9; McM'86; Head Family Med/Staff, Joseph Brant Memorial Hospital; Member Information Standards Committee, Ministry of Health; McMaster University; (905)333-5245; Fax. (905)632-2617; john.holmes@uhn.on.ca.

HOLMES, Kathryn J; Lynn Valley Med & Travel Clin, 102-1200 Lynn Valley Rd, North Vancouver BC V7J 2A2; UBC'79; Court Staff, Lions Gate Hospital; (604)988-3747; Fax. (604)988-5339; holmes@istar.ca.

HOLMES, Matthew C; 300A-984 Oliver Rd, Thunder Bay ON P7B 7C7; Ott'02; FRCSC; GenSurg. (807)346-9747; Fax. (807)346-4312.

HOLMES, Roger G; Roger Holmes Med Corp, 283 Aylmer St N, Peterborough ON K9J 7M4; Qns'72; BSc; MSc; Ac Staff, Peterborough Regional Health Centre - Hospital Drive; (705)743-8006; Fax. (705)743-8022.

HOLMES, S Bruce; Cornwall Prof Bldg, 705-2125 11th Ave, Regina SK S4P 3X3; Man'80; BSc(Med); FRCPC; Peds. Med Dir, Regina Cystic Fibrosis Clinic; Clin Assoc Prof, University of Saskatchewan; (306)352-4900; Fax. (306)352-6500.

HOLMES, Stewart E; Eston Clinic, PO Box 9, Eston SK S0L 1A0; Man'55; (306)962-3616

HOLMES, Thomas S; St Joseph's Gen Hosp, 2137 Comox Ave, Comox BC V9M 1P2; UBC'99; FRCPC; Anes. Staff, St Joseph's General Hospital; (250)339-2242

HOLMES, Vicki R; City Centre Family Physicians, 100-514 Queen St, Saskatoon SK S7K 0M5; Sask'73; Ac Staff, St Paul's Hospital (Grey Nuns) of Saskatoon; Ac Staff, Royal University Hospital; Ac Staff, Saskatoon City Hospital; (306)244-3016; Fax. (306)244-4737.

HOLMES BOULTON, Cheryl L; B9 400-3151 Lakeshore Rd, Kelowna BC V1W 3S9; UBC'84; FRCPC; IntMed; Critical Care Medicine. Dir Critical Care Unit, Kelowna General Hospital; Clinical Asst Prof IntMed, University of British Columbia; (250)212-9450

HOLMVANG, Annette M; Crestwood Medical Dental, 207-6051 Gilbert Rd, Richmond BC V7C 3V3; UBC'79; FRCSC; GenSurg; VascSurg. (604)276-0952; Fax. (604)231-0583.

HOLNESS, D Linn; 4082A-30 Bond St, Toronto ON M5B 1W8; Tor'77; MHSc; FFOM(Hon.); FRCPC; OccupMed (Occupational Skin Diseases). Chief Occup & Environmental Health, St Michael's Hospital; Dir Gage Occup & Environmental Health Unit & Occup Med, University of Toronto; (416)864-5074; Fax. (416)864-5421; holnessl@smh.ca.

HOLODY, Erik A J; Ctr Hosp Reg Chisasibi, PO Box 250, Chisasibi QC J0M 1E0; Wes'08; CCFP; CCFP(E.M.); Staff, Cree Board of Health & Social Services James Bay; (819)855-9001

HOLOWACHUK, Brian M; Tillsonburg Fam Physicians, 4-594 Broadway St, Tillsonburg ON N4G 5K9; Tor'94; CCFP; (519)842-3636; Fax. (519)842-9522.

HOLOWATY, Eric J; Cancer Care Ontario, 1500-620 University Ave, Toronto ON M5G 2L7; UBC'75; MSc; FRCPC; CommunMed. Sr Consultant Div of Preventive Oncology, Cancer Care Ontario - Provincial Office; Assoc Prof Public Health Services, University of Toronto; (416)971-9800 x1125; Fax. (416)971-6888; eric.holowaty@cancercare.on.ca.

HOLOWATY, Melissa N; 1 Madoc St PO Box 520, Marmora ON K0K 2M0; Tor'08; CCFP; (613)472-6131; Fax. (613)472-6135.

HOLOWENKO, Dedeshya S; Tuxedo Fam Med Centre, 981 Corydon Ave, Winnipeg MB R3M 0X1; Man'94; CCFP; CCFP(E.M.); FCFP; Staff, Misericordia Health Centre; (204)788-8364

HOLROYD, Brian R; University of Alberta Hosp, 1G1 62 WCM-8440 112 St NW, Edmonton AB T6G 2B7; Alb'81; FACEP; FRCPC; EmergMed;CCFP; FCFP; Chair Dept. of EmergMed., University of Alberta Hospital; Prof, University of Alberta; (780)407-7047; Fax. (780)407-3314; bholroyd@ualberta.ca.

HOLROYD-LEDUC, Jayna M; Foothills Med Centre, 105-1403 29 St NW, Calgary AB T2N 2T9; Tor'96; FRCPC; IntMed (Geriatric Medicine). Staff, Foothills Medical Centre; Staff, Peter Lougheed Centre; Assoc Prof, University of Calgary; (403)944-1771; Fax. (403)944-1095; jayna-holroyd-leduc@calgaryhealthregion.ca.

HOLT, Alana; Royal University Hosp, H170-103 Hosptial Dr, Saskatoon SK S7N 0W8; Sask'00; BSc; FRCPC; Psy (Adult & Child Psychiatry). Staff Psy, Royal University Hospital; Consultant Psy, Mental Health & Addiction Services; Asst Prof/Consultant Psy, University of Saskatchewan; (306)655-0264; Fax. (306)655-0186.

HOLT, David J; St Michaels Hosp, 30 Bond St, Toronto ON M5B 1W8; Tor'07; Anes. Staff, St Michael's Hospital; (416)360-4000

HOLT, Martha; Bruyere Family Med Centre, 75 Bruyere St, Ottawa ON K1N 5C7; Ott'06; CCFP; (613)241-3344

HOLT, Susan C; Health Sciences Centre, E3-820 Sherbrook St, Winnipeg MB R3A 1R9; Man'79; FRCPC; DiagRad. Staff, Health Sciences Centre; Asst Prof Radiol, University of Manitoba; (204)774-6511

HOLT, Tanya; Royal University Hosp, 103 Hospital Dr, Saskatoon SK S7N 0W8; Sask'01; FRCPC; Peds; Critical Care Medicine. Staff, Royal University Hospital; (306)966-8125

HOLTBY, Helen M K; The Hosp for Sick Children, 555 University Ave, Toronto ON M5G 1X8; London (England)'79; MB BS; FRCPC; Anes (Pediatric Anesthesia). Staff Anes, The Hospital For Sick Children; Asst Prof Anes, University of Toronto; (416)813-7445; Fax. (416)813-7543; helen.holtby@sickkids.ca.

HOLTBY, Joanne L; North Bay Reg Health Centre, 50 College Dr, North Bay ON P1B 0A4; Mem'89; BSc; BMedSci; FRCPC; Psy. Staff, North Bay Regional Health Centre - Regional Mental Health; (705)474-1205 x2285

HOLTBY, Richard M; 634-43 Wellesley St E, Toronto ON M4Y 1H1; London (England)'77; FRCSC; OrthSurg (Shoulder). Staff, Sunnybrook Health Sciences Centre - Holland Orthopaedic & Arthritic Centre; Staff, Women's College Hospital; Asst Prof, University of Toronto; (416)967-8701; Fax. (416)967-8704; richard.holtby@sunnybrook.ca.

HOLTBY, Stuart G; 820 Red River Rd, Thunder Bay ON P7B 1K2; Wes'78; FCCP; AB; FRCPC; IntMed (Sleep Medicine); Respir. (807)683-4415; Fax. (807)683-4420.

HOLTON, Donna L; Peter Lougheed Centre, 3500 26 Ave NE, Calgary AB T1Y 6J4; Alb'80; FRCPC; IntMed (AIDS/HIV); InfectDis. Consultant Infection Diseases, Peter Lougheed Centre; Chief Div of Infectious Diseases, Alberta Health Services; Chief Div of Infectious Diseases, University of Calgary; (403)943-5681; Fax. (403)943-4017.

HOLTON, Gordon R; 5529 Hwy 62 RR 7, Belleville ON K8N 4Z7; Cal'90; CCFP; FCFP; (613)967-8000; Fax. (613)967-8007.

HOLTON, Peggy J; Crescent Heights Fam Med Ctr, 114-2805 6th Ave E, Prince Albert SK S6V 6Z6; Sask'87; (306)763-2681; Fax. (306)953-1024.

HOLTZHAUSEN, Peter J; 1292 99th St, North Battleford SK S9A 0P5; Cape Town (South Africa)'86; MB ChB; CCFP; (306)445-5070; Fax. (306)445-4224.

HOLUB, Darren J; 6F-700 Dorval Dr, Oakville ON L6K 3V3; Tor'01; FRCPC; Psy. (905)338-4630 x4811; Fax. (905)845-6419.

HOLUB, Jacob A; 1935 Paris St, Sudbury ON P3E 3C6; Tor'79; Ac Staff, Health Sciences North-Laurentian Site; (705)522-8300; Fax. (705)522-0930.

HOLUB, Roger V; Meadowlak Health Centre, 200 Meadowlark Shopping Ctr NW, Edmonton AB T5R 5W9; Alb'85; FRCPC; DiagRad. (780)489-7851; Fax. (780)486-5160.

HOLWELL, James P; E & D Physicians Services, PO Box 1110, Englehart ON P0J 1H0; Mem'99; CCFP; (705)544-2321; Fax. (705)544-5224; jholwell@edhospital.on.ca.

HOLZAPFEL, G Stephen; Women's College Hosp, 76 Grenville St, Toronto ON M5S 1B2; Tor'82; CCFP; FCFP; Staff, Sunnybrook Health Sciences Centre; Ac Staff Family Practice Health Centre, Women's College Hospital; Assoc Staff, Mount Sinai Hospital; Assoc Prof Family & CommunMed., University of Toronto; Langs: German; (416)323-6060 x17; Fax. (416)323-6402; s.holzapfel@utoronto.ca.

HOLZER, Gideon; MUHC-Royal Victoria Hosp, 687 av des Pins O, Montreal QC H3A 1A1; Jerusalem (Israel)'92; Staff, McGill University Health Centre - Royal Victoria Hospital; Dir, MUHC Reproductive Centre; adj Prof, McGill University; (514)843-1650

HOMAYOUNFAR, Freydoun; Pontiac Health Centre, 200 rue Argue, Shawville QC J0X 2Y0; Santiago (Dominican Republic)'85; Gen Practice, Pontiac Hospital Centre; Langs: Farsi; French; (819)647-3851; Fax. (819)647-3275.

HOMER, Ivy M; Medical Assoc of Port Perry, 462 Paxton St, Port Perry ON L9L 1L9; Wes'09; CCFP; (905)985-2895

HOMIER, Valerie; MUHC-Royal Victoria Hosp, 687 av des Pins O, Montreal QC H3A 1A1; Sher'05; FRCPC; EmergMed. Staff, McGill University Health Centre - Royal Victoria Hospital; (514)934-1934

HOMIK, Joanne E; Heritage Med Research Centre, 562 HMRC-107 University Campus, Edmonton AB T6G 2S2; Man'86; MSc; FRCP; FRCPC; IntMed (Osteoporosis); Rheum. Assoc Prof Med, University of Alberta; (780)407-8070; Fax. (780)407-6055; jhomik@gpu.srv.ualberta.ca.

HOMIK, Lawrence A; Winnipeg Clinic, 425 St Mary Ave, Winnipeg MB R3C 0N2; Man'81; FRCPC; IntMed; Respir. (204)957-3231; Fax. (204)957-7410.

HOMSY, Alfred A; Ctr Hosp de Lasalle, 8585 Tsse Champlain, LaSalle QC H8P 1C1; Lyon (France)'78; FRCPC; Anes. Assoc Member, Centre Hospitalier de Verdun; Assoc Member, Centre Hospitalier de LaSalle; adj Prof, Universite de Montreal; (514)362-8000

HONDUBRATA, Linda; Coronation Health Centre, 203-725 Coronation Blvd, Cambridge ON N1R 7S9; (Indonesia)'89; CCFP; Langs: Indonesian; (519)624-2262; Fax. (519)624-2263.

HONEIN, Charles F; Medical Clinic Person-Ctred Ps, 403-265 Yorkland Blvd, North York ON M2J 1S5; Cairo (Egypt)'58; Staff, The Medical Clinic for Person-Centred Psychotherapy; (416)229-2399; Fax. (416)229-9771.

HONER, William G; Centre for Complex Disorders, A3 127-938 28th Ave W, Vancouver BC V5Z 4H4; Qns'84; FRCPC; Psy (Schizophrenia). Dept Head & School Dir Psy, University of British Columbia; (604)875-3664

HONEY, Christopher R; Gordon & Leslie Diamond HCC, 8105-2775 Laurel St, Vancouver BC V5Z 1M9; Tor'86; FRCSC; Neursurg. Staff, Vancouver General Hospital - Centennial Pavillion; Staff, Gordon & Leslie Diamond Health Care Centre; (604)875-5894; Fax. (604)875-4882.

HONEY, Liisa L; Nepean Med Centre, 308-1 Centrepointe Dr, Nepean ON K2G 6E2; Wes'94; BSc(Hon); FRCSC; ObstGyn. Staff, Queensway Carleton Hospital; (613)274-7282

HONEY, R John D'A; St Michael's Hospital Health C, 9103Q-61 Queen St E, Toronto ON M5C 2T2; Cambridge (England)'70; MB ChB; FRCSC; Urol (Endoscopy Urology) (Minimal Invasive Surgery) (Stone Disorders) (Endourology). Chief Div of Urol, St Michael's Hospital; Dir Kidney Stone Centre/Assoc Prof, University of Toronto; (416)867-3705; Fax. (416)867-7433; honeyj@smh.toronto.on.ca.

HONEYWOOD, Kallie; Vernon Jubilee Hosp, 2101 32 St, Vernon BC V1T 5L2; McM'01; FRCPC; Anes. Staff, Royal Columbian Hospital; Staff, Kootenay Boundary Regional Hospital; Staff, Vernon Jubilee Hospital; (778)887-6627

HONG, Aaron P; St Michael's Hosp, 30 Bond St, Toronto ON M5B 1W8; Tor'96; FRCPC; Anes. Staff, St Michael's Hospital; (416)360-4000

HONG, Angie S; Bayview-Finch Med Clinic, 301-3292 Bayview Ave, North York ON M2M 4J5; Tor'01; CCFP; (416)224-9333; Fax. (416)224-9880.

HONG, Collin; 3-302 Sheppard Ave W, North York ON M2N 1N5; Tor'84; FRCSC; PlasSurg. Staff, Rouge Valley Health System - Centenary Health Centre Site; Staff, Mackenzie Richmond Hill Hospital; Langs: Chinese; (416)222-6986; Fax. (416)222-0955.

HONG, Dennis; St Joseph's Healthcare, G814-50 Charlton Ave E, Hamilton ON L8N 4A6; Tor'96; FRCSC; GenSurg. Staff, St Joseph's Healthcare - Charlton Campus; (905)522-1155 x32938; Fax. (905)521-6123; dennis.hong@nygh.on.ca.

HONG, Diana; Palisades Med Clinic, 12808 137 Ave NW, Edmonton AB T5L 4Y8; Cal'08; CCFP; (780)457-1100; Fax. (780)457-0033.

HONG, Harry H L; 210-13710 94A Ave, Surrey BC V3V 1N1; Tor'93; FRCPC; IntMed (Critical Care Medicine); Respir. Staff Palmonologist & Intensivist, Surrey Memorial Hospital; (604)582-2100

HONG, Hilary C; Guildford Med Dental Centre, 20-15300 105 Ave, Surrey BC V3R 6A7; Tor'97; FRCPC; Derm (Psoriasis). Staff Rapid Access Clinic, Providence Health Care - St Paul's Hospital; Langs: Cantonese; (604)585-1110; Fax. (604)585-1170.

HONG, Julie; Rockyview Gen Hosp, 6625-7007 14 St SW, Calgary AB T2V 1P9; Qns'02; CCFP; Staff, Rockyview General Hospital; (403)943-8994; Fax. (403)943-8996.

HONG, Paul; IWK Health Centre, PO Box 9700 Rpo CSC 5850-5980 University Ave, Halifax NS B3K 6R8; Ott'04; FRCSC; Otol (Pediatric Otolaryngology). Staff, IWK Health Centre; Asst Prof, Dalhousie University; (902)470-8641; Fax. (902)470-8929.

HONG, Tommy; 142 Nahani Way, Mississauga ON L4Z 3J1; Tor'87; CCFP; Ac Staff Hospitalist, The Credit Valley Hospital; Langs: Cantonese; (905)568-0355; Fax. (905)568-0307; tommyhong@sympatico.ca.

HONIBALL, James; Dakota Med Centre, 17-845 Dakota St, Winnipeg MB R2M 5M3; Pretoria (South Africa)'98; CCFP; Fam Med, Russell Health Centre; (204)773-2125

HONICKMAN, Debbie F; Queen West Commun Health Ctre, 168 Bathurst St, Toronto ON M5V 2R4; McM'81; DOHS; CCFP; FCFP; Langs: Bilingual(English/French); (416)703-8480; Fax. (416)703-8479.

HONISH, Colin; St Paul's Hosp, 1702 20th St W, Saskatoon SK S7M 0Z9; Sask'04; CCFP; Staff, St Paul's Hospital (Grey Nuns) of Saskatoon; (306)655-5000

HONJO, Osami; The Hosp for sick Children, 555 University Ave, Toronto ON M5G 1X8; (Japan)'97; Staff, The Hospital For Sick Children; (416)813-8977; Fax. (416)813-7984.

HONOS, George N; CHUM-Hotel-Dieu, 3840 rue Saint-Urbain, Montreal QC H2W 1T8; McG'82; AB; FACC; ABIM; CSPQ; FRCPC; IntMed; Cardiol. Staff, Centre Hospitalier l'Université de Montréal (CHUM) - Hôtel-Dieu; Pres, Quebec Echo Society; assoc Prof Med, McGill University; Langs: Hungarian; English; (514)890-8000 x15447; Fax. (514)412-7830.

HONS, Ronald B; Foothills Med Centre, C210B-1403 29 St NW, Calgary AB T2N 2T9; Qns'67; FACP; FRCPC; IntMed (Nephrology). Staff Nephrology, Foothills Medical Centre; Associate Clin Prof/Dir Nephrology Training Prog, University of Calgary; (403)944-1169; Fax. (403)270-0055.

HONSINGER, Philip; West Parry Sound Health Ctre, 6 Albert St, Parry Sound ON P2A 3A4; Tor'07; CCFP; Staff, West Parry Sound Health Centre; (705)746-9321

HONSL, Evelyn M; Carling-Broadview Med Bldg, 301-770 Broadview Ave, Ottawa ON K2A 3Z3; Karlova (Czech Republic)'65; Ac Staff, Queensway Carleton Hospital; Langs: Czech; Slovak; (613)233-0625; Fax. (613)233-5143.

HOOD, David T; 304-73 Delhi St, Guelph ON N1E 6L9; Wes'81; CCFP; FCFP; Ac Staff Family Pract, Guelph General Hospital; (519)837-2321; Fax. (519)837-9534.

HOOD, Eric; 210-200 St Clair Ave W, Toronto ON M4V 1R1; Glasgow (Scotland)'64; MB ChB; FRCPC; Psy (Child & Adolescent Psychiatry). Consultant, Centre for Addiction & Mental Health (CAMH) - College Street Site; Consultant, Childrens Aid Society of Tor; Asst Prof, University of Toronto; (416)966-5466

HOOD, Nancy A; North York Gen Hosp, 4001 Leslie St, North York ON M2K 1E1; Tor'80; Staff, North York General Hospital; Med Dir Family Practice, Combined Insurance Co of America; (416)756-6000

HOOD, Roberta; Markham Stouffville Hosp, PO Box 1800 Stn Main 381 Church St, Markham ON L3P 7P3; Tor'06; CCFP; Staff, Markham Stouffville Hospital; (905)472-7000

HOOGE, John P; 555 12 Ave W PO Box 47058 Rpo City Square, Vancouver BC V5Z 4L6; Sask'69; MD; FRCPC; Neur (Multiple Sclerosis). Clin Assoc Prof, University of British Columbia; (604)822-7131; Fax. (604)879-7443.

HOOGERBOORD, C Marius; Queen Elizabeth II HSC-VG Site, 821-1276 South Park St, Halifax NS B3H 2Y9; Orange Free State (South Africa)'00; MB ChB; FRCSC; GenSurg (Minimal Invasive Surgery). Staff, Queen Elizabeth II Health Sciences Centre - Victoria General Site; Assoc Prof Surg, Dalhousie University; (902)473-7272; Fax. (902)473-5147.

HOOGEVEEN, Larry G; 99 Park Meadows Crt SE, Medicine Hat AB T1B 4C3; Sask'69; (403)502-2624

HOOGEVEEN, Paul; The Simcoe Clinic, 279 Yonge St, Barrie ON L4N 7T9; Tor'93; CCFP; CCFP(E.M.); FCFP; Staff, Royal Victoria Regional Health Centre; (705)728-8860

HOOGEWERF, Simon E C; Victoria Emerg Phys Mgmt Ltd, 325-1627 Fort St, Victoria BC V8R 1H8; UBC'96; BSc(Hon); CCFP; CCFP(E.M.); FCFP; Fax. (250)479-1442.

HOOGSTRA, Jason A; Children's Hosp of Western Ont, 800 Commissioners Rd E, London ON N6C 2V5; Tor'96; BSc; FRCPC; Anes. Staff, Children's Hospital of Western Ontario; Staff, Victoria Hospital; Asst Prof, University of Western Ontario; (519)685-8525; Fax. (519)685-8275.

HOOK, Kenneth; Star FHT-Tavistock Comm Hlth I, PO Box 310 80 Maria St, Tavistock ON N0B 2R0; McG'71; BSc; MDCM; CCFP; FCFP; Ac Staff, Stratford General Hospital - Huron Perth Healthcare Alliance; Asst Prof Family Med, University of Western Ontario; Langs: Bilingual(English/French); (519)655-2322; Fax. (519)655-3073.

HOOKENSON, Brenda J; 1521 6th Ave W, Prince Albert SK S6V 5K1; Sask'74; brendahookenson@hotmail.com.

HOOKER, Ross W; Victoria Gen Hosp, 1 Hospital Way, Victoria BC V8Z 6R5; (Ireland)'07; FRCPC; EmergMed. Staff, Victoria General Hospital; (250)727-4212

HOOKEY, Lawrence C; Hôtel-Dieu Hosp, S4-166 Brock St, Kingston ON K7L 5G2; Mem'98; FRCPC; IntMed; Gastroent. Staff, Hotel-Dieu Hospital; Langs: Bilingual(English/French); (613)544-3310; Fax. (613)544-3114.

HOOKS, Rosalie J; Flemingdon Health Centre, 10 Gateway Blvd, North York ON M3C 3A1; Wes'80; CCFP; FCFP; Staff, Sunnybrook Health Sciences Centre; Staff Obst, Toronto East General Hospital Inc; Teach Staff, University of Toronto; (416)429-4991; Fax. (416)422-3573.

HOOLEY, Peter J D; 30 Linden Ave, Charlottetown PE C1A 5Y9; Dal'04; CCFP; (902)628-6660; Fax. (902)367-3760.

HOONJAN, Malvinder S; 301-550 West Ave, Kelowna BC V1Y 4Z4; Piscataway (USA)'03; Ophth. (250)860-3937

HOOPER, Davyd R; Riverview Health Centre, PE319-1 Morley Ave, Winnipeg MB R3L 2P4; Man'02; FRCPC; PhysMed&Rehab.

HOOPER, Elizabeth D; Leamington District Mem Hosp, 194 Talbot St W, Leamington ON N8H 1N9; Ott'81; FRCPC; DiagRad. Staff, Leamington District Memorial Hospital; (519)326-2373

HOOPER, Jonathan G V; The Ottawa Hosp-Civic Campus, 1053 Carling Ave, Ottawa ON K1Y 4E9; Ott'82; FRCPC; Anes; Critical Care Medicine. Staff, Royal Ottawa Mental Health Centre - Royal Ottawa Health Care Group; Staff Anes, The Ottawa Hospital - Civic Campus; Asst Prof, University of Ottawa; (613)761-4169

HOOPER, Monika; Royal University Hosp, 103 Hospital Dr, Saskatoon SK S7N 0W8; FRCPC; Psy. Staff, Royal University Hospital; (306)655-1000

HOOPER, Philip L; St Joseph's Health Care, 268 Grosvenor St, London ON N6A 4V2; Wes'82; ABOph; FRCSC; Ophth (Ocular Inflamation). Staff, St Joseph's Hospital - St Joseph's Health Care; Staff, London Health Sciences Centre - Victoria Campus; Assoc Prof/Dept Chair Ophthalmology, University of Western Ontario; (519)685-8312; Fax. (519)646-6160; phil.hooper@lhsc.on.ca.

HOOPER, R Allen; Sports Med Clinic, 325 Power St, Penticton BC V2A 7K9; Cal'87; CCFP; FCFP; Clin Asst Prof Family Med, University of Calgary; (250)487-1455

HOOPER, Richard O; Hooper Cardiology, 1002-1708 Dolphin Ave, Kelowna BC V1Y 9S4; UBC'68; CSPQ; FRCPC; IntMed; Cardiol. (250)763-6118; Fax. (250)860-0992; richard@hoopercardiology.com.

HOOPER, Wendy M; 305-400 Tache Ave, Winnipeg MB R2H 3C3; Man'95; FRCSC; ObstGyn. Assoc Staff, St Boniface General Hospital; University of Manitoba; (204)233-4224; Fax. (204)233-6636.

HOORNWEG, Karen L; Brameast Family Health Org, 38-2130 North Park Dr, Brampton ON L6S 0C9; McM'96; CCFP; FCFP; Staff, William Osler Health System - Brampton Civic Hospital; (905)792-2211; Fax. (905)792-2901.

HOOSEN, Naushad; Fourth Avenue Med Clinic, 411 Louth St, St Catharines ON L2S 4A2; Durban (South Africa)'88; MB ChB; CCFP; Physician Emerg, Niagara Health System - St Catharines General Site; (905)682-3692

HOOSHANGI, Hedieh; Rouge Valley-Centenary HC, 2867 Ellesmere Rd, Scarborough ON M1E 4B9; Tehran (Iran)'92; FRCPC; Anes. (416)284-8131

HOPE, Andrew; Univ Hlth Network-Princess M, 5 606-610 University Ave, Toronto ON M5G 2M9; Wisconsin (USA)'02; FRCPC; RadOncol. Staff, Princess Margaret Hospital - University Health Network; (416)946-2124

HOPE, Kim; 214-9181 Main St, Chilliwack BC V2P 4M9; UBC'97; FRCPC; Psy. (604)795-0084

HOPE, L Anna; 132 Parkdale Ave S, Hamilton ON L8K 3P3; McG'69; CCFP; FCFP; Court Staff, St Joseph's Healthcare - Charlton Campus; Ac Staff, Hamilton Health Sciences Centre - Hamilton General Hospital; McMaster University; (905)544-6599; Fax. (905)544-9094.

HOPE, Paula; CSSS Jeanne-Mance, 100-15 av du Mont-Royal O, Montreal QC H2T 2R9; Alb'98; CCFP; (514)286-9657; Fax. (514)940-3621.

HOPE, Sarah J; 765 Canboro Rd PO Box 128, Fenwick ON L0S 1C0; London (England)'73; MRCS; LRCP; DRCOG; (905)892-8722; Fax. (905)892-8220.

HOPFNER, Joseph; Associate Med Group, 4705 48 Ave, Red Deer AB T4N 3T1; Man'68; Physician, Associate Medical Group; (403)346-2057; Fax. (403)347-2989; jhopfner@telusplanet.net.

HOPGOOD, Derek C; 201-747 Queen St E, Sault Ste. Marie ON P6A 2A8; London (England)'71; MB BS; LRCP; MRCS; DRCOG; FRCPC; Psy. Dir Commun Mental Health Prog, Sault Area Hospital - Sault Ste Marie; (705)253-9671; Fax. (705)254-1840.

HOPKINS, Gary W; Forest Hills Med Clinic, 4 Forest Hills Pky, Dartmouth NS B2W 5G7; Mem'77; CCFP; (902)435-5530; Fax. (902)462-6398.

HOPKINS, Howard; 404 Parliment Place, 2631 28th Ave, Regina SK S4S 6X3; Cardiff(Wales) (United Kingdom)'59; MB ChB; FRCP(Edin); LMCC; FRCPC; IntMed (Respirology). Ac Staff, Regina General Hospital; Consultant, Pasqua Hospital; Consultant, Regina Health District; Clin Assoc Prof, University of Saskatchewan; (306)352-8626; Fax. (306)347-3020.

HOPKINS, Ian A; Meadowlark Health Centre, 178 Meadowlark Shopping Ctr NW, Edmonton AB T5R 5W9; Glasgow (Scotland)'62; FRCPC; Anes. (780)424-6520

HOPKINS, Jessica P; Niagara Reg Public Health Unit, PO Box 1052 2201 St David's Rd, Thorold ON L2V 4T7; Wes'04; FRCPC; CommunMed;CCFP; Public Health & Preventive Med.

HOPKINS, John G; Health Sciences Centre, 300 Prince Philip Dr, St. John's NL A1B 3V6; Mem'97; FRCPC; DiagRad. Staff Radiol, Health Sciences Centre; (709)777-8378

HOPKINS, John P; Medical & Dental Bldg, 502-1849 Yonge St, Toronto ON M4S 1Y2; Tor'74; BScPharm; Assoc Staff, Toronto Rehabilitation Institute - University Centre; Assoc Staff Family Pract Unit, Sunnybrook Health Sciences Centre; (416)485-9111; Fax. (416)485-3232.

HOPKINS, Kathleen D; Heritage Med Research Centre, 362-107 University Campus NW, Edmonton AB T6G 2S2; Alb'82; Staff, Royal Alexandra Hospital; (780)407-3636

HOPKINS, M Laura; The Ottawa Hosp-Gen Campus, 8130-501 Smyth Rd, Ottawa ON K1H 8L6; Tor'95; FRCSC; ObstGyn (Gynecologic Oncology). Staff, The Ottawa Hospital - General Campus; (613)737-8560; Fax. (613)737-8828.

HOPKINS, Peter D; 506-2425 Bloor St W, Toronto ON M6S 4W4; Tor'56; CCFP; FCFP; Consultant Occupational Health, Air Canada Medical Clinic; (416)763-3425; Fax. (416)763-3312; brown.hopkins@sympatico.ca.

HOPKINS, Suzanne E; Osprey Med Clinic, 12-1000 Northwest Blvd, Creston BC V0B 1G6; (Other Foreign)'93; CCFP; (250)428-7887

HOPKINS, Tammy M H; White Pines Health Network, 208-38 Pine St N, Timmins ON P4N 6K6; Ott'04; BSc(Hon); CCFP; Med Staff, Timmins & District Hospital; Staff, White Pines Health Network; (705)267-3272; Fax. (705)267-4212; thopkins@pht.ca.

HOPKINS, Thomas M; 45637 Lark Rd, Chilliwack BC V2R 3N5; UBC'72; Staff, Chilliwack General Hospital; (604)858-7111; Fax. (604)858-6897.

HOPMAN, Michael; Mission Park, PO Box 25075 Rpo Mission Park, Kelowna BC V1W 3Y7; Alb'06; CCFP; (250)717-3211

HOPP, Marilyn H; Lakeshore Med Centre, 3970 Lakeshore Rd, Kelowna BC V1W 1V5; Wes'72; CAFCI; (250)764-8878; Fax. (250)764-0889.

HOPP, Peter M; Nicola Med Dental Bldg, 207-321 Nicola St, Kamloops BC V2C 6G6; Witwatersrand (South Africa)'81; MB ChB; FRCSC; Ophth (Cataract Surgery). Staff, Royal Inland Hospital; (250)314-1073; Fax. (250)374-5375.

HOPPE, Barbara J; Health Sciences Centre, 300 Prince Philip Dr, St. John's NL A1B 3V6; Warsaw (Poland)'64; PhD; Staff Neurol, Health Sciences Centre; Asst Prof Neurol, Memorial University Of Newfoundland; Langs: Polish; (709)777-6554; Fax. (709)777-6656.

HOPPER, Gordon H I; Rockyview Gen Hosp, 7007 14 St SW, Calgary AB T2V 1P9; Aberdeen (Scotland)'73; FRCPC; Anes. Staff Anes, Rockyview General Hospital; (403)943-3410; Fax. (403)943-3360.

HOPWOOD, Marie-Clare; Dunsmuir Med Clinic, PO Box 719 2765A Dunsmuir Ave, Cumberland BC V0R 1S0; Sheffield (United Kingdom)'04; MB ChB; (250)336-2208

HOPYAN, Julia J; Sunnybrook Hlth Sciences Ctre, A233-2075 Bayview Ave, Toronto ON M4N 3M5; New South Wales (Australia)'00; FRCPC; Neur. Staff, Sunnybrook Health Sciences Centre; (416)480-4473; Fax. (416)480-4833.

HOPYAN, Sevan; The Hosp for Sick Children, S107-555 University Ave, Toronto ON M5G 1X8; Tor'95; PhD; FRCSC; OrthSurg (Pediatric Orthopedics). Staff, The Hospital For Sick Children; Langs: Armenian; (416)813-7654 x1277; Fax. (416)813-6414; sevan.hopyan@sickkids.ca.

HOQUE, Asadul; Health Sciences Centre, 300 Prince Philip Dr, St. John's NL A1B 3V6; Dacca (Pakistan)'60; MB BS; FRCPC; DiagRad. Staff Radiol, Health Sciences Centre; (709)777-7721

HOQUE, M Zahirul; Fort Saskatchewan Med Clinic, 9421 94 Ave, Fort Saskatchewan AB T8L 1N6; Dacca (Bangladesh)'61; MB BS; LRCP(Ed); LRCS(Ed); LRCPS(Glas); Staff, Fort Saskatchewan Health Centre; Staff, Lamont Health Care Centre; Langs: Bengali; (780)998-2231; Fax. (780)998-4399.

HOQUE, Mohamed N; Sturgeon Community Hosp, 201 Boudreau Rd, St. Albert AB T8N 6C4; Alb'04; FRCPC; IntMed (Gastroenterology). Staff, Sturgeon Community Hospital; (780)418-8587; Fax. (780)418-8584.

HOQUE, Mohd E; Leader Med Clinic, PO Box 638, Leader SK S0N 1H0; (306)628-4584; Fax. (306)628-3998.

HOQUET, France; CLSC St Jerome, 1000 rue Labelle, Saint-Jerome QC J7Z 5N6; Mon'91; Langs: Bilingual(French/English); (450)431-8001 x26489; Fax. (450)436-8478.

HORAK, Ladislav; Rothbart Centre for Pain Care, 9-4646 Dufferin St, North York ON M3H 5S4; Kosice (Slovakia)'60; Langs: Slovak; Hungarian; (416)512-6407; Fax. (416)512-6375.

HORAK, Martin J; St Michael's Hosp, 30 Bond St, Toronto ON M5B 1W8; UBC'94; FRCPC; EmergMed (Trauma). Staff EmergMed, St Michael's Hospital; (416)864-5095; Fax. (416)864-5341.

HORAK, Stuart Z; Lions Gate Hosp, 231 15th St E, North Vancouver BC V7L 2L7; UBC'96; CCFP; CCFP(E.M.); Staff, Lions Gate Hospital; Clin Instructor, University of British Columbia; Langs: Czech; (604)984-5982; shorak@telus.net.

HORAN, P Frank; Belleville Medical Arts Buildi, 204-210 Dundas St E, Belleville ON K8N 5G8; Ott'72; FRCPC; Derm. Staff, QHC Belleville General; Langs: English; French; (613)966-4989; Fax. (613)966-6419.

HORAN, Vanessa T; 250-333 Aspen Glen Landing SW, Calgary AB T3H 0N6; Wes'01; CCFP; Staff, University of Alberta Hospital; (403)984-9025; Fax. (403)984-9029.

HORANI, Maria A; Rothbart Centre, 9-4646 Dufferin St, North York ON M3H 5S4; Prague (Czech Republic)'66; Langs: Czech; (416)512-6407; Fax. (416)512-6375.

HOREN, Sheila A; Leamington & Area Fam Hlth Team, 197 Talbot St W, Leamington ON N8H 1N8; Qns'96; CCFP; FCFP; Ac Staff Hospitalist, Leamington District Memorial Hospital; (519)322-1100; Fax. (519)322-0324; shoren@ldmh.org.

HORGAN, Kevin P; 201-1990 Fort St, Victoria BC V8R 6V4; McM'96; BSc; MSc; FRCPC; IntMed; Nephrol. (250)598-1021; Fax. (250)598-5469; khorgan@shaw.ca.

HORGAN-BELL, Caroline B; Wellington Dermatology Assoc, 272 Oxford St W, London ON N6H 1S9; Tor'86; BSc(Hon); MSc; FRCPC; Derm (Skin Cancer). (519)434-2193; Fax. (519)434-9676.

HORII, Allan H; Medical Bldg, 120-6180 Blundell Rd, Richmond BC V7C 4W7; UBC'89; Asst Clinical Prof Dept of Family Practice, University of British Columbia; (604)275-4111; Fax. (604)241-8615.

HORLICK, Eric M; Univ Hlth Network-Toronto Gen, 6E-249-200 Elizabeth St, Toronto ON M5G 2C4; McG'96; FRCPC; IntMed (Interventional Cardiology); Cardiol. Staff, Toronto General Hospital - UHN; Langs: French; (416)340-3835; Fax. (416)340-3000; eric.horlick@uhn.on.ca.

HORLICK, Simon G D; Burrard Med Bldg, 500-1144 Burrard St, Vancouver BC V6Z 2A5; Qns'87; FRCSC; OrthSurg. (604)683-3585; Fax. (604)683-3531.

HORMOZDI, Homa; Quality Care Clinic, 414-250 Harding Blvd W, Richmond Hill ON L4C 9M7; Tehran (Iran)'99; CCFP; (905)237-7723; Fax. (905)291-0768.

HORN, Marilyn J; Business Bldg, 410-1200 Burrard St, Vancouver BC V6Z 2C7; Wes'77; Ac Staff, Providence Health Care - St Paul's Hospital; Staff, Bentall 4 Clinic; Clin Instructor, University of British Columbia; (604)681-7561; Fax. (604)681-6995.

HORN, Ojistoh; Kateri Memorial Hosp Ctr, PO Box 10, Kahnawake QC J0L 1B0; UBC'05; MSc; BSc; CCFP; Staff, Barrie Memorial Hospital; Staff, Hôpital Anna-Laberge; Staff, Kateri Memorial Hospital Centre; (450)638-3930; Fax. (450)638-4634.

HORN, Pieter W; Smith Clinic, 1-6601 48 Ave, Camrose AB T4V 3G8; Stellenbosch (South Africa)'82; MB ChB; (780)672-2425; Fax. (780)608-5895.

HORN, Ruth; MUHC-Royal Victoria Hosp, L502-687 av des Pins O, Montreal QC H3A 1A1; McG'79; FRCPC; IntMed (Medical Microbiology & Infectious Diseases); MedMicrobiol; InfectDis. Att Physician Microbiol, McGill University Health Centre - Royal Victoria Hospital; adj Prof, McGill University; Langs: Bilingual(English/French); (514)543-1611; Fax. (514)844-7526; hornruth@hotmail.com.

HORNBECK, Tiffany K; Royal Inland Hosp, 311 Columbia St, Kamloops BC V2C 2T1; Alb'99; CCFP; Staff Family Med, Royal Inland Hospital; (250)374-5111

HORNBERGER, Lisa; University of Alberta Hosp, 4C2 WCMC-8440 112 St NW, Edmonton AB T6G 2B7; San Diego (USA)'89; Peds (Pediatric Cardiology). Staff Ped/Cardiol, University of Alberta Hospital; Dir Fetal & Neonatal Cardiology Prog Section Head Ped Echocardiology, University of Alberta; (780)407-3355; Fax. (780)407-3954.

HORNE, Bruce D; 101-3825 Sunset St, Burnaby BC V5G 1T4; Cal'75; BSc; MSc; ABIM; FACC; FRCPC; IntMed (Cardiology). Ac Staff, Burnaby Hospital; Asst Clin Prof, University of British Columbia; (604)430-4577; Fax. (604)430-5022.

HORNE, Duff D; Crowfoot Corner Medicentre, 217-150 Crowfoot Cres NW, Calgary AB T3G 3T2; Alb'82; FRCPC; IntMed (Clinical Virology); InfectDis. (403)241-8900; Fax. (403)241-8109.

HORNE, Garnet J; Red Deer Reg Hosp Centre, PO Box 5030 Stn Postal Box Ctr 3942 50A Ave, Red Deer AB T4N 6R2; Alb'03; FRCPC; AnatPath. Staff, Red Deer Regional Hospital Centre; (403)343-4717; Fax. (403)343-4877.

HORNE, J Digby; Johnstone Crossing Comm Hlth C, 300 Jordan Pky, Red Deer AB T4P 0G8; Alb'85; FRCPC; CommunMed. (403)356-6425

HORNE, Jonathan B; 825 Oxford St E, London ON N5Y 3J8; Wes'85; Staff, St Joseph's Health Centre; (519)673-0159; Fax. (519)673-5384.

HORNE, Mark R; Bigelow Fowler Clinic East, 3515 Mayor Magrath Dr S, Lethbridge AB T1K 8A8; (South Africa)'08; MB ChB; (403)327-3977

HORNE, Pamela E; Vanier Children's Services, 871 Trafalgar St, London ON N5Z 1E6; National University of Ireland (Ireland)'04; (519)433-3101

HORNE, S Gabrielle; Queen Elizabeth II HSC-Halifax, 2102-1796 Summer St, Halifax NS B3H 3A7; London (England)'86; MB BS; PhD; FRCPC; IntMed (Congenital Heart Disease); Cardiol. Staff Cardiol, Queen Elizabeth II Health Sciences Centre - Victoria General Site; Assoc Prof Med & Biomedical Eng, Dalhousie University; (902)473-6815; Fax. (902)473-2434.

HORNER, Gordon; Queen Charlotte Med Clinic, PO Box 9, Queen Charlotte BC V0T 1S0; UBC'96; CCFP; Staff, Queen Charlotte Islands General Hospital - Queen Charlotte Site.

HORNER, Richard H; 430-943 Broadway W, Vancouver BC V5Z 4E1; UBC'76; Ac Staff, Vancouver General Hospital - Centennial Pavillion; (604)731-5559

HORNER, Robert; Regina Qu'Appelle HR-Regina, 1440 14th Ave, Regina SK S4P 0W5; Saba (Netherlands)'85; CCFP; CCFP(E.M.); Staff, Regina General Hospital; (306)766-4444

HORNICH, Adrian A; Rosedale Med Group, 280 Queenston Rd, Hamilton ON L8K 1H1; McM'76; CCFP; FCFP; Court Staff, St Joseph's Healthcare - Charlton Campus; Ac Staff, Hamilton Health Sciences Centre - McMaster University Medical Centre; Med Dir, Arbour Creek Long Term Care; Langs: Ukrainian; (905)547-0508; Fax. (905)547-6865.

HORNING, C E Maxwell; Primary Health Care Clinic, PO Box 355 176 Wellington St, Niagara-Lk ON L0S 1J0; Tor'63; Ac Staff, Niagara Health System - Niagara-on-the-Lake Hospital Site; Instructor Family & Commun Med, University of Toronto; (905)468-0742; Fax. (905)468-1998.

HORNSTEIN, David; MUHC-Montreal Gen Hosp, 1650 Cedar Ave, Montreal QC H3G 1A4; McG'86; FRCPC; IntMed. Staff, McGill University Health Centre - Montreal General Campus; (514)934-1934 x43255; Fax. (514)340-8133.

HORNSTEIN, Stanley J; Delta Hosp, 5800 Mountain View Blvd, Delta BC V4K 3V6; Man'80; FRCPC; Anes. Staff, Delta Hospital; (604)946-1121; Fax. (604)946-3086.

HORNY, Stefan; Institut Canadien-Polonais, 5655 rue Belanger, Montreal QC H1T 1G2; Prague (Czech Republic)'66; Staff, Centre Hospitalier Régional du Suroît; Langs: Polish; Czech; Slovak; French; Russian; German; (514)259-2551

HORODEZKY, L Sandford; 201-73 Warren Rd, Toronto ON M4V 2R9; McG'71; FRCPC; Psy. Staff, Mount Sinai Hospital; Member, Toronto Psychoanalytic Society; Asst Prof, University of Toronto; (416)960-5812; Fax. (416)961-7081.

HOROWITZ, Glenda A; Addiction & Mental Health-Quee, 2 4-1001 Queen St W, Toronto ON M6J 1H4; Ott'04; FRCPC; Psy. Staff Schizophrenia Program, Centre for Addiction & Mental Health (CAMH) - Queen Site; Staff, North York General Hospital; (416)535-8501; Fax. (416)583-1208.

HORREY, Kathleen A; Cowie Family Med Centre, PO Box 27 16 Dentith Rd, Halifax NS B3R 2H9; Cal'99; CCFP; Asst Prof, Dalhousie University; (902)473-1234; Fax. (902)473-4353.

HORRICKS, Colin H; Hycroft Med Bldg, 205-3195 Granville St, Vancouver BC V6H 3K2; Sask'74; CCFP; FCFP; Vis Staff, Providence Health Care - St Paul's Hospital; (604)731-6212; Fax. (604)731-9703.

HORSEY, Mary E; 235-400 Bayfield St, Barrie ON L4M 5A1; Qns'63; MRCPsy(UK); FRCPC; Psy (Adult Psychiatry). Court Staff Psy, Royal Victoria Regional Health Centre; (705)726-5453; Fax. (705)726-2707.

HORSEY, Michael W; Perth & Smiths Falls Dist Hosp, 60 Cornelia St W, Smiths Falls ON K7A 2H9; Wes'96; CCFP; Ac Staff, Perth & Smiths Falls District Hospital - Smiths Falls Site; (613)283-2330 x1102; Fax. (613)283-9342.

HORSFALL, Susan J; A1-6935 Harvie Ave, Powell River BC V8A 5H9; McM'05; CCFP; (604)485-0136

HORSHAM, Patricia A M; 111-21 Queensway W, Mississauga ON L5B 1B6; Newcastle (England)'73; MB BS; FRCPC; Peds. Physician Emerg, Children's Hospital of Eastern Ontario (CHEO); Langs: Bilingual(English/French); (905)897-0788; Fax. (905)897-9229.

HORSMAN, Catherine A; Carry Drive Med Centre, 101-116 Carry Dr SE, Medicine Hat AB T1B 3Z8; Alb'90; BScDistinction; CCFP; FCFP; Vis Staff, Medicine Hat Regional Hospital; (403)580-4212; Fax. (403)504-1164.

HORSMAN, Douglas E; BC Cancer Agency-Vancouver CC, 600 10th Ave W, Vancouver BC V5Z 4E6; Sask'73; GenPath (Cancer Genetics). Staff, BC Cancer Agency Vancouver Centre; Clin Prof Path, University of British Columbia; (604)877-6000

HORSMAN, Gregory B; Saskatchewan Disease Control L, 5 Research Dr, Regina SK S4S 0A4; Man'72; FRCPC; MedMicrobiol (Public Health). Assoc Staff, Regina General Hospital; Teacher Adjunct Biology, University Of Regina; (306)787-8316; Fax. (306)787-1525; ghorsman@health.gov.sk.ca.

HORTH, Caroline; CSSS de Trois-Rivières, 1991 boul du Carmel, Trois-Rivieres QC G8Z 3R9; Laval'06; FRCSC; OrthSurg. Staff, CSSS de Trois-Rivières; (819)697-3333

HORTH, Marie-Christine; Ctr Hosp de Granby, 205 boul Leclerc O, Granby QC J2G 1T7; Sher'03; FRCSC; Otol. Staff, Centre Hospitalier de Granby; (450)375-8000

HORTON, Jillian J; Health Sciences Centre, GC 419-820 Sherbrook St, Winnipeg MB R3A 1R9; McM'00; FRCPC; IntMed.

HORTON, Joan M; Westbrook Prof Bldg, PO Box 34076 P55-1610 37 St SW, Calgary AB T3C 3P1; Cal'85; BSc; CCFP; FCFP; Staff, Foothills Medical Centre; Member, College of Family Physicians of Canada-Alberta; Clin Assoc Prof Family Med, University of Calgary; (403)246-2052; Fax. (403)246-2219; horton@ucalgary.ca.

HORTON, Lesley; Student Health Services, 100 49th Ave W, Vancouver BC V5Y 2Z6; Wes'94; CCFP; Staff Student Health Services, Langara College; (604)323-5256

HORTON, Robert P; Queen Elizabeth II HSC, 308-1276 South Park St, Halifax NS B3H 2Y9; Dal'92; CCFP; Staff, Queen Elizabeth II Health Sciences Centre - Victoria General Site; (902)473-2700

HORTON, Ross C; Metrotown Surgery Centre, 505-4885 Kingsway, Burnaby BC V5H 4T2; UBC'82; FRCSC; PlasSurg (Cosmetic Surgery). (604)435-8483; Fax. (604)435-8409; doctorhorton@shawcable.com.

HORTON, Sheryl; 220 Stewart Green SW, Calgary AB T3H 3C8; (USA)'05; (403)240-0090; Fax. (403)240-0579.

HORTOP, John; Centre Med D'ormstown, CP 2001 24 rue Gale, Ormstown QC J0S 1K0; Tor'74; ABPeds; Cardiol; Peds. Staff, Barrie Memorial Hospital; McGill University; Langs: Bilingual(English/French); (450)829-2321; Fax. (450)829-3636.

HORVAT, Amy M K; Highlands Health Network, 140 Rolling Hills Dr, Orangeville ON L9W 4X8; Ott'02; CCFP; Ac Physician, Headwaters Health Care Centre - Orangeville Site; Assoc Prof, University of Toronto; (519)941-7575

HORVAT, Daniel; 2-1230 Alward St, Prince George BC V2M 7B1; UBC'92; BSc; Staff Family Physician, University Hospital of Northern British Columbia; Asst Prof Family Practice, University of British Columbia; (250)563-0414

HORVATH, Anna M B; North York Gen Hosp, 3S 376-4001 Leslie St, North York ON M2K 1E1; Tor'72; CCFP; FCFP; Staff Consultant Palliative Care Initiative, Sunnybrook Health Sciences Centre; Staff, North York General Hospital; Asst Prof Commun & Family Med, University of Toronto; (416)756-6468; nina.horvath@utoronto.ca.

HORVATH, Gabriela A; Children's & Women's HC of BC, K3 207-4480 Oak St, Vancouver BC V6H 3V4; Tirgu-Mures (Romania)'86; FRCPC; Peds (Biochemical Genetics). Staff Clin Instructor, BC Children's Hospital; Clin Fellow Biochemical Genetics, UBC Hospital - Koerner Pavilion; Locum Tenens Peds, Peace Arch Hospital; Locum Tenens Peds, Ridge Meadows Hospital & Health Care Centre; Langs: Romanian; (604)875-2880

HORVATH, Gary P; Doc-Side Medical, 125 Main St, Vancouver BC V6A 2S5; UBC'91; CASAM; MSc; Dip SportMed; ABAM; CCFP; (604)633-1234; Fax. (604)633-1233.

HORVATH, Jeffrey F; Victoria Gen Hosp, 2340 Pembina Hwy, Winnipeg MB R3T 2E8; Man'89; BSc(Med); CCFP; Physician, Victoria General Hospital; Lecturer Family Practice, University of Manitoba; (204)269-3570

HORVATH, Robert D; North York Gen Hosp, 4001 Leslie St, North York ON M2K 1E1; Tor'80; CCFP; FCFP; Ac Staff/Physician Emerg, North York General Hospital; Asst Prof Family & Commun Med, University of Toronto; (416)756-6000

HORVATH, Zoltan; 104-22112 52 Ave, Langley BC V2Y 2M6; Ott'95; FAAP; FRCPC; Peds. Consultant Peds, Langley Memorial Hospital; Consultant Peds, Abbotsford Regional Hospital & Cancer Centre; (604)539-2222; Fax. (604)534-8016.

HORWITZ, Trevor A; Medical Imaging Consultants, 202-11010 101 St NW, Edmonton AB T5H 4B9; Witwatersrand (South Africa)'80; MB ChB; FRCPC; DiagRad. (780)426-1121; Fax. (780)425-5979.

HORWOOD, John C; Peterborough Reg HC-Hosp, 1 Hospital Dr, Peterborough ON K9J 7C6; Ott'73; FRCPC; GenPath. Staff Path, Peterborough Regional Health Centre - Hospital Drive; (705)743-2121; Fax. (705)876-5008.

HORWOOD, Karen L; Labrador Grenfell Health, PO Box 7000 Stn C 227 Hamilton River Rd, Goose Bay NL A0P 1C0; Mem'95; BSc; BMedSci; MCFP; CCFP; FCFP; Staff, Labrador Health Centre; Memorial University Of Newfoundland; Fax. (709)897-2372; kalourie@hotmail.com.

HORWOOD, Paula L; Primary Med Centre, 150 Old Placentia Rd, Mount Pearl NL A1N 4Y9; Mem'87.

HORWOOD, Sargent P; 948A King St W, Hamilton ON L8S 1K8; Western Reserve(Ohio) (USA)'60; FRCPC; Peds (Psychotherapy). (905)528-1815; Fax. (905)529-7279.

HOSAIN, Jason; West Winds Health Centre, 3311 Fairlight Dr, Saskatoon SK S7M 3Y5; Sask'03; CCFP; (306)655-4200

HOSAIN, Shahid; Manitoba Adolescent Trmt Ctre, 165 St Mary's Rd, Winnipeg MB R2H 1J1; Man'98; FRCPC; Psy. Staff, Manitoba Adolescent Treatment Centre; (204)958-9660; shosain@matc.ca.

HOSDIL, Jane M J; East Wellington Family Hlth Team, PO Box 340 A-175 Alma St, Rockwood ON N0B 2K0; Tor'69; BSc; Court Staff, Guelph General Hospital; Court Staff, Homewood Health Centre; Media Dir, Eden House Long Term Care Facility; Court Staff, St Joseph's Health Centre; Langs: Dutch; (519)856-4611; Fax. (519)856-4612; jhosdil@ewfht.ca.

HOSE, Patricia M; Davisville Fam Practice, 600-1881 Yonge St, Toronto ON M4S 3C4; Tor'85; CCFP; FCFP; Staff, Toronto General Hospital - UHN; Court Staff, Toronto Western Hospital - University Health Network; (416)932-3172; Fax. (416)440-0238.

HOSEIN, Alana N; WOHC-Brampton Civic Hosp, 2100 Bovaird Dr E, Brampton ON L6R 3J7; McM'05; FRCSC; GenSurg. Staff, William Osler Health System - Brampton Civic Hospital; (905)494-2120

HOSEIN, Jalal; Fenwick Med Centre, 5595 Fenwick St, Halifax NS B3H 4M2; Dal'73; (902)422-5595; Fax. (902)429-8125.

HOSEIN, Rasheed A; Meadowlark Health Centre, 224 Meadowlark Shopping Ctr NW, Edmonton AB T5R 5W9; Alb'92; FRCPC; IntMed. Staff, University of Alberta Hospital; (780)484-8474; Fax. (780)489-3836.

HOSEK, Paul; Grand River Hosp-KW Hlth Ctre, PO Box 9056 Stn C 835 King St W, Kitchener ON N2G 1G3; McM'96; FRCPC; EmergMed; Critical Care Medicine. Staff, Grand River Hospital - Kitchener/Waterloo Health Centre; (519)749-4300

HOSENBOCUS, Sheik N; 782 Seymour St, Kamloops BC V2C 2H3; RCS (Ireland)'76; LRCP; LRCS; DPsy; DABPN; FRCPC; Psy (Child & Adolescent Psychiatry). Dir Child & Adolesc Psy Program/Ac Staff, Royal Inland Hospital; Clin Dir, Parkview Child & Adolescent Mental Hlth Centre; Clinical Asst Prof Psy, University of British Columbia; Langs: Bilingual(English/French); (250)314-2122; Fax. (250)314-2281; drsheik.hosenbocus@interiorhealth.ca.

HOSHIZAKI, Dale K; Peace Arch Hosp, 15521 Russell Ave, White Rock BC V4B 2R4; UBC'88; CCFP; CCFP(E.M.); Staff, Peace Arch Hospital; (604)541-7133

HOSHIZAKI, David K; University of Alberta Hosp, 1G162WCM-8440 112 St NW, Edmonton AB T6G 2B7; Alb'92; Staff, University of Alberta Hospital; (780)407-8433

HOSHOWSKY, B; Acadia Med Centre, 101-8330 Fairmount Dr SE, Calgary AB T2H 0Y8; Cal'87; FRCSC; Otol (Otolaryngology). Staff, Calgary Health & Headwaters Health Regions; University of Calgary; Langs: Ukrainian; (403)640-1199; Fax. (403)640-1582; drborys@shaw.ca.

HOSIE, Andrew D; 2425A Bevan Ave, Sidney BC V8L 4R5; Sask'84; (250)656-1164; Fax. (250)656-7870.

HOSKIN, Robert W; Royal Columbian Hosp, 330 Columbia St E, New Westminster BC V3L 3W7; Cal'90; FRCPC; Anes. Staff, Royal Columbian Hospital; (604)520-4602

HOSKIN-MOTT, Ann E D; Queen Elizabeth II HSC, 2035-1276 South Park St, Halifax NS B3H 2Y9; Qns'73; FRCS; FRCSC; Ophth (Retina Vitreous Ophthalmology). Staff, Queen Elizabeth II Health Sciences Centre - Victoria General Site; Asst Prof Ophth, Dalhousie University; (902)473-4302; Fax. (902)473-2839; ann.hoskin-mott@dal.ca.

HOSKING, Denis H; Health Sciences Centre, AD203-820 Sherbrook St, Winnipeg MB R3A 1R9; Cape Town (South Africa)'72; MB ChB; FRCS(Ed); AB; FRCSC; Urol (Endoscopy Urology). Spec Staff Privil, St Boniface General Hospital; Prof Surg Urol, University of Manitoba; (204)787-3677; Fax. (204)787-3040.

HOSKING, Martin C K; Children's & Women's HC of BC, 1F20-4480 Oak St, Vancouver BC V6H 3V4; Cal'80; FRCPC; Peds (Pediatric Intervention); Cardiol. Staff Heart Centre, BC Children's Hospital; Clin Assoc Prof, University of British Columbia; (604)875-2296; Fax. (604)875-3463; mhosking@chs.bc.ca.

HOSKINS, Christopher F; Hys Med Centre, 604-11010 101 St NW, Edmonton AB T5H 4B9; Otago (New Zealand)'74; MB ChB; DObst; FRCSC; ObstGyn. Ac Staff/Chief Ob/Gyn, Royal Alexandra Hospital; Clin Prof, University of Alberta; (780)421-4728; Fax. (780)426-6698.

HOSKINS, Eric W; 2009 Danforth Ave, Toronto ON M4C 1J7; McM'85; MPH; PhD(PublicHealth&Epidem; FRCPC; CommunMed (International Health). (416)690-7269

HOSKINS, Paul J; BC Cancer Agency-Vancouver CC, 600 10th Ave W, Vancouver BC V5Z 4E6; Cambridge (England)'78; MB ChB; MRCP(UK); FRCPC; IntMed; MedOncol. Staff MedOncol, BC Cancer Agency Vancouver Centre; Staff, Vancouver General Hospital - Centennial Pavillion; Assoc Prof, University of British Columbia; (604)877-6000; Fax. (604)877-6179.

HOSKINSON, Michael E; 202-11010 101 St NW, Edmonton AB T5H 4B9; McG'76; FRCPC; NuclearMed. Staff Rad, University of Alberta Hospital; (780)426-1121

HOSOKAWA, Akiko N; North York Med Group, 705-240 Duncan Mill Rd, North York ON M3B 3S6; Tor'01; CCFP; Langs: Japanese; (416)222-3011; Fax. (416)221-3097.

HOSSACK, Karen J; 1153 56 St PO Box 19074, Delta BC V4L 2P8; UBC'84; CCFP; Staff, Pender Community Health Centre; (604)839-6582

HOSSAIN, Mohammad M; Saint John Reg Hosp, PO Box 2100 Stn Main 400 University Ave, Saint John NB E2L 4L2; Dhaka (Bangladesh)'93; FRCPC; GenPath. Staff, Saint John Regional Hospital; (506)648-6025

HOSSAIN, Muhammad; Miramichi Reg Hosp, 500 Water St, Miramichi NB E1V 3G5; Staff, Miramichi Regional Hospital; (506)623-3000

HOSSAIN, Rana Md Iftekhar; 9312 137 Ave NW, Edmonton AB T5E 6C2; (Bangladesh)'90; MB BS; (780)456-0658; Fax. (780)456-3015.

HOSSEINI, Mona; Queen Elizabeth II HSC-Halifax, 1796 Summer St, Halifax NS B3H 3A7; Shiraz (Iran)'91; Staff, Queen Elizabeth II Health Sciences Centre - Halifax Infirmary Site; (902)473-6540; Fax. (902)473-2434.

HOSSEINI, Seyed H; Hamilton HS-Juravinski Site, 711 Concession St, Hamilton ON L8V 1C3; Babol University of Health Sciences (Iran)'95; Staff, Hamilton Health Sciences Centre-Juravinski Site.

HOSSEINI MOGHADDAM, Syed M; London HSC-University Hosp, PO Box 5339 Stn B 339 Winderemere Rd, London ON N6A 5A5; Babol University of Health Sciences (Iran)'96; Staff, London Health Sciences Centre - University Hospital; (519)670-2647

HOSSEININEJAD, Mir M; PO Box 818 Stn B, Happy-Valley-Goose NL A0P 1E0; (Iran)'94.

HOSSENBUX, Farook; 339 Churchill Ave N, Ottawa ON K1Z 5B8; Sheffield (England)'64; MB ChB; MRCP; ABIM; FRCPC; IntMed. Langs: Creole; (613)722-2959; Fax. (613)722-3547; farook@virtualwave.com.

HOSSIE, Helen L; Waypoint Centre for Mental HC, 500 Church St, Penetanguishene ON L9M 1G3; Qns'91; FRCPC; Psy. Staff, Waypoint Centre for Mental Health Care; (705)549-3181

HOSTETLER, Jason L; 207-440 Boler Rd, London ON N6K 4L2; Man'92; CCFP; (519)472-1846

HOSTETLER, John C; 2054 Sooke Rd, Victoria BC V9B 1W3; Qns'90; Neur. Langs: English; French; (250)474-1664; Fax. (250)474-1683.

HOSTLAND, Sara; Bruyere Family Med Centre, 75 Bruyere St, Ottawa ON K1N 5C8; Ott'09; CCFP; CCFP(E.M.); Staff, Bruyère Continuing Care - Elisabeth Bruyere Hospital; (613)241-1154; sara@bruyere.org.

HOTA, Susy S; Univ Hlth Network-Toronto Gen, 9CSB 804-200 Elizabeth St, Toronto ON M5G 2C4; Tor'02; FRCPC; IntMed; InfectDis. Staff, Toronto General Hospital - UHN; (416)340-4800; Fax. (416)340-5047.

HOTA, Valli L B; Richmond Med Clinic, 307 Bridge St W, Napanee ON K7R 2G3; India (India)'78; CCFP; FCFP; (613)354-6409; Fax. (613)354-3801.

HOTA, Venkata S V B; Lennox & Addington Gen Hosp, 8 Richmond Park Dr, Napanee ON K7R 2Z4; Andra (India)'73; MB BS; FRCS(ENG); FRCSC; GenSurg. Staff, Lennox & Addington County General Hospital; Langs: Telugu; (613)354-3301; Fax. (613)354-3985.

HOTSON, Kenneth E; Bracebridge Med Arts Ctr, 253 James St, Bracebridge ON P1L 2C2; Man'01; CCFP; (705)645-2281; Fax. (705)645-0057.

HOTTE, Dominique; CLSC des Faubourgs, 2260 rue Parthenais, Montreal QC H2K 3T5; Sher'04; CCFP; (514)527-2361; Fax. (514)527-6016; dominique_hotte@ssss.gouv.qc.ca.

HOTTE, Marie-Josee; Inst U Geriatric Sherbrooke, 1036 rue Belvedere S, Sherbrooke QC J1H 4C4; Sher'94; CCFP; Staff, CSSS Institut universitaire de gériatrie de Sherbrooke; (819)821-1150; Fax. (819)829-7153.

HOTTE, Marie-Josee; Clin Le Medical, 285-1750 boul Marie-Victorin, Longueuil QC J4G 1A5; Mon'95; (450)442-9531; Fax. (450)442-1553.

HOTTE, Sebastien J; The Juravinski Cencer Centre, 699 Concession St, Hamilton ON L8V 5C2; Ott'96; FRCPC; IntMed; MedOncol. Physician, The Juravinski Cancer Centre; Asst Prof Med, McMaster University; Langs: English; French; (905)387-9495; Fax. (905)575-6326; sebastien.hotte@hrcc.on.ca.

HOTTE, Simon L; Clinique de Pediatrie, 105 av Gatineau, Gatineau QC J8T 4J4; Ott'02; FRCPC; Peds; ClinImmunol&Allergy. Staff, McGill University Health Centre - Montreal Children's Hospital; (819)561-4412

HOTTIN, Paule; Inst U Geriatrie Sherbrooke, 375 rue Argyll, Sherbrooke QC J1J 3H5; Sher'82; FRCPC; Psy (Geriatric Psychiatry). Staff, Institut Universitaire de Geriatrie de Sherbrooke-Pavillon Argyll; Consultant, Centre Hospitalier Universitaire de Sherbrooke-Hôpital Hôtel-Dieu; Prof, Universite de Sherbrooke; (819)569-3661 x413; Fax. (819)569-5502.

HOTTLET, Helene; CSSS des Aurores Boreales, CP 6000 Succ Bureau-Chef 679 2e rue E, La Sarre QC J9Z 2X7; Mon'94; Staff, Centre Hospitalier La Sarre; Langs: Bilingual(French/English); (819)333-2311

HOTZ, Aaron; Doctor's Office, 101-491 Lawrence Ave W, North York ON M5M 1C7; McM'94; CCFP; Assoc Lecturer, Mount Sinai Hospital; (416)787-5693; Fax. (416)787-8094.

HOTZ, Harry; Wilson Med Centre, 130 Wilson St, Hamilton ON L8R 1E2; Tor'44; FAAP; FRCPC; Peds. (905)526-6250; Fax. (905)526-9745.

HOU, Daniel J; Laurel Med Centre, 215-888 8th Ave W, Vancouver BC V5Z 3Y1; UBC'08; (604)872-0345

HOU, Frank L; Laurel Med Centre Ltd, 215-888 8th Ave W, Vancouver BC V5Z 3Y1; UBC'75; BSc; PhD; Ac Staff, Vancouver General Hospital - Centennial Pavillion; Court Staff, BC Women's Hospital & Health Centre; Court Staff, Providence Health Care - Mount Saint Joseph Hospital; Clin Assoc Prof, University of British Columbia; Langs: Chinese; (604)872-0345

HOUBE, Jill S; Sunny Hill Hlth Centre for Chi, 3644 Slocan St, Vancouver BC V5M 3E8; Boston(MA) (USA)'88; FRCPC; Peds. Staff, BC Children's Hospital; Langs: Spanish; French; (604)875-2345

HOUBI, Yasin; Aspen Health Clinic, 221-339 Aspen Glen Landng SW, Calgary AB T3H 0N6; ABFM; CCFP; (403)263-7997; Fax. (403)263-7996.

HOUCK, Leslie V H; 205-316 Willow St, Truro NS B2N 5A1; Dal'83; FRCSC; ObstGyn. (902)895-4477

HOUDE, Bryan; CSSS Pierre Boucher, 1333 boul Jacques-Cartier E, Longueuil QC J4M 2A5; Mon'04; FRCPC; Anes. Staff, Centre Hospitalier Pierre Boucher; (450)468-8111

HOUDE, Catherine; CSSS de Jonquiere, CP 1200 Stn Pdf Jonquiere 2230 rue de l'Hopital, Jonquiere QC G7X 7X2; Mon'97; CCFP; Staff, Centre Hospitalier Jonquiere; (418)695-7700; Fax. (418)695-7715.

HOUDE, Christine; CHUQ-Ctr Hosp Univ Laval, 2705 boul Laurier, Quebec QC G1V 4G2; Laval'85; CSPQ; FRCPC; Peds (Interventional Cardiology); Cardiol. Ac Staff, Centre Hospitalier Universitaire de Quebec-CHUL; Ac Staff, Hôpital Laval; adj Prof, Université Laval; Langs: Bilingual(French/English); (418)656-4141 x48347; Fax. (418)654-2710; christine.houde@chuq.qc.ca.

HOUDE, Danielle; Clin Med Valcartier, SS 481 118-190 rue Dube, Courcelette QC G0A 1R1; Laval'88; Assoc Member, Centre Hospitalier Chauveau; Langs: English; (418)844-3721; Fax. (418)844-3318; d.houde@videotron.ca.

HOUDE, Dominique; Ctr Hosp Anna-Laberge, 200 boul Brisebois, Chateauguay QC J6K 4W8; Mon'88; CSPQ; AnatPath. Staff, Hôpital Anna-Laberge; (450)699-2425 x4276; dominique.houde@rrsss16.gouv.qc.ca.

HOUDE, Gaetan; Centre Med Laennec, 200-1750 av de Vitre, Quebec QC G1J 1Z6; Laval'78; CSPQ; FRCPC; Cardiol (P.Q.). Cardiology, Centre Hospitalier Affilié Universitaire de Québec - Hôpital De L'Enfant Jésus; Langs: English; (418)663-2858; Fax. (418)663-2352.

HOUDE, Ghislaine; CHUS-Hop Fleurimont, 3001 12e av N, Sherbrooke QC J1H 5N4; Sher'86; FRCP; FRCPC; IntMed; Endocrin&Metab. Staff, Centre Hospitalier Universitaire de Sherbrooke-Hopital Fleurimont; (819)564-5244

HOUDE, Isabelle; CHUQ-Hotel-Dieu de Quebec, 11 Cote du Palais, Quebec QC G1R 2J6; Laval'83; FRCPC; IntMed (Transplantation); Nephrol. Dir, Centre Hospitalier Universitaire de Québec (CHUQ) - Siege Social; (418)691-5464; Fax. (418)691-5253.

HOUDE, Jacques; Regie l'Assurance Maladie QC, Q044-1125 Grande Allee O, Quebec QC G1S 1E7; Laval'66; Med Assessor, Regie de l'Assurance Maladie du Quebec; (418)682-5144 x3159; Fax. (418)643-3858; jacques.houde@ramq.gouv.qc.ca.

HOUDE, Jean; Ctr Hosp Rouyn-Noranda, 4 9e rue, Rouyn-Noranda QC J9X 2B2; Mon'79; Staff, Centre Hospitalier Rouyn-Noranda; (819)764-5131

HOUDE, Jean-Luc; CSSS de Chicoutimi, 305 rue Saint-Vallier, Chicoutimi QC G7H 5H6; Mon'00; CSPQ; FRCSC; GenSurg. Staff Gen Surg, Complexe hospitalier de la Sagamie; Langs: Spanish; English; (418)541-1234

HOUDE, Josee; CSSS de Laval, 1755 boul Rene-Laennec, Laval QC H7M 3L9; Mon'91; Staff, Hopital de la Cite de la santé; (450)668-1010

HOUDE, Julie; Carrefour Med Vallee Richelieu, 665 boul Sir-Wilfrid-Laurier, Beloeil QC J3G 4J1; Mon'01; CCFP; Staff, Centre Hospitalier Honore-Mercier; (450)467-0088

HOUDE, Lucien; CHUQ-Hotel-Dieu de Quebec, 11 Cote du Palais, Quebec QC G1R 2J6; Laval'86; Staff, Centre Hospitalier Universitaire de Québec (CHUQ) - Siege Social; (418)691-5042; Fax. (418)691-5024.

HOUDE, Madeleine; Clin Med Pasteur, 770 1re av, Quebec QC G1L 3K2; Laval'76; Ac Staff, Centre Hospitalier Universitaire De Québec - Pavillon De St-françois-d'assise; Ac Staff, CSSS de Quebec-Sud; (418)529-0042; Fax. (418)529-4924.

HOUDE, Marc; Hop Maisonneuve-Rosemont, 5415 boul de l'Assomption, Montreal QC H1T 2M4; Mon'69; Nephrol (P.Q.) (Hypertension). Staff, Hopital Maisonneuve-Rosemont; Prof Adjoint De Clinique, Universite de Montreal; Langs: English; (514)252-3489; Fax. (514)255-3026.

HOUDE, Marie-Christine; CSSS de Saint-Jerome, 290 rue de Montigny, Saint-Jerome QC J7Z 5T3; Mon'06; Staff, Hôtel-Dieu de Saint-Jérôme; (450)431-8200; Fax. (450)431-8302.

HOUDE, Michele; CHUQ-Ctr Hosp Univ Laval, 2705 boul Laurier, Quebec QC G1V 4G2; Laval'97; FRCPC; Psy. Staff, Centre Hospitalier Universitaire de Quebec-CHUL; (418)654-2177

HOUDE, Michelle; CHUM-Hop Notre-Dame, 1560 rue Sherbrooke E, Montreal QC H2L 4M1; Mon'81; CSPQ; FRCPC; AnatPath (P.Q.) (Legal Pathology). Staff, Centre Hospitalier l'Université de Montréal (CHUM) - Hôpital Notre-Dame; Staff, Legal Sciences Lab. & Med.; (514)890-8000 x28759

HOUDE, Rene; Polyclinique du Cap, 110-700 boul Thibeau, Trois-Rivieres QC G8T 7A1; Laval'77; (819)373-4551; Fax. (819)373-6516.

HOUDE, Robert; Clin Med du Quartier, 1191 av Cartier, Quebec QC G1R 2S9; Sher'74; (418)522-1911; Fax. (418)522-1789.

HOUDE, Stefaine; Moonashee Med Clinic, PO Box 700 2067 Columbia Ave, Rossland BC V0G 1Y0; Mon'00; MSc; CCFP; Langs: Bilingual(English/French); (250)362-9070

HOUDE, Sylvie; Inst de Readaptation de Mtl, 6300 av de Darlington, Montreal QC H3S 2J4; Sher'86; FRCPC; Neur (P.Q.) (Cranio Encephalic); PhysMed&Rehab. Staff, Institut de Réadaptation Gingras-Lindsay de Montréal; Universite de Montreal; Langs: Bilingual(French/English); (514)340-2065; Fax. (514)340-2775; sylvie.houde.irglm@ssss.gouv.qc.ca.

HOUDE-SAUVE, Mathieu; Clinique Psychiatrie, 190 rue Labonte, Longueuil QC J4H 2P7; Mon'97; FRCPC; Psy. Staff, Hopital Charles LeMoyne; (450)466-5453; Fax. (450)466-5473.

HOUETO, Sohoueto; Ctr Hosp Laurentien, 234 rue Saint-Vincent, Ste-Agathe-des-Mts QC J8C 2B8; Staff, Centre Hospitalier Laurentien; (819)324-4000

HOUGESEN, Bent; 2485 62 Hwy PO Box 215, Hazelton BC V0J 1Y0; Tor'75; MPH; FRCPC; CommunMed (International Health);CCFP; CCFP(E.M.); FCFP; Public Health & Preventive Med. Hon Staff, Wrinch Memorial Hospital; Staff, Hazelton Family & Community Clinic; Clin Prof, University of British Columbia; Langs: Danish; (250)842-4060

HOUGH, Henry; Sir Thomas Roddick Hosp, PO Box 5000 Stn Main 142 Minnesota Dr, Stephenville NL A2N 2V6; (South Africa)'89; Staff, Sir Thomas Roddick Hospital; (709)643-5111

HOUGHTON, Kelvin T; Gracemed Clinic, 102-1629 Townsite Rd, Nanaimo BC V9S 1N3; Natal (South Africa)'93; MB ChB; (250)755-4031

HOUGHTON, Peter G H; 135-5325 Cordova Bay Rd, Victoria BC V8Y 2L3; Cape Town (South Africa)'76; MB ChB; (250)658-5228; Fax. (250)658-5241.

HOUGHTON, Scott D; Pawassan & Area Med Centre, PO Box 39 8 King St, Powassan ON P0H 1Z0; Wes'89; (705)724-5511; Fax. (705)724-5499.

HOULACHI, Jean-Pascal; Clinique d'Urgence Forcemedic, 1021 rue Jean-Talon E, Montreal QC H2R 1V6; Mon'95; Staff, Centre Hospitalier Régional du Suroît; (514)787-1818

HOULD, Frederic S; UMF Laval, 2725 ch Sainte-Foy, Quebec QC G1V 4G5; McG'84; CSPQ; FRCSC; GenSurg (Bariatric Surgery). Staff GenSurg, Institut Universitaire Cardiologie & Pneumologie de Quebec; Assoc Prof Surg Part Time, Université Laval; Langs: Bilingual(English/French); (418)656-4810; Fax. (418)656-4825.

HOULD, Melanie; Hawkesbury & Dist Gen Hosp, 1111 Ghislain St, Hawkesbury ON K6A 3G5; Mon'08; CCFP; Staff, Hawkesbury & District General Hospital; Langs: Bilingual(French/English); (613)632-1111

HOULD, Nathalie; Hotel-Dieu d'Arthabaska, 5 rue des Hospitalieres, Victoriaville QC G6P 6N2; Sher'04; CCFP; CCFP(E.M.); Staff, Hotel-Dieu d'Arthabaska; (819)357-2030

HOULD, Raymond; Clin Orth des Bois-Francs, 5-39 rue Laurier E, Victoriaville QC G6P 6P6; Laval'75; OrthSurg. Ac Staff, Hotel-Dieu d'Arthabaska; (819)357-8683; Fax. (819)357-2331.

HOULDEN, Robyn L; Kingston Gen Hosp, 4 330-76 Stuart St, Kingston ON K7L 2V7; Ott'83; FRCPC; IntMed (Diabetes); Endocrin&Metab. Ac Staff, Hotel-Dieu Hospital; Ac Staff, Kingston General Hospital; Prof, Queen's University; (613)548-1379; Fax. (613)548-6105; houldenr@queensu.ca.

HOULE, Andreane; Dir de la Sante Publique-Mtl, 200-300 rue King E, Sherbrooke QC J1G 1B1; Sher'06; Staff, Carrefour Sante Granit; (819)346-8411

HOULE, Anne-Marie; Hôpital Ste-Justine, 3175 ch Cote-Sainte-Catherine, Montreal QC H3T 1C5; Laval'83; FRCSC; Urol (Pediatric Urology). Chef PedUrol Service, Hôpital Ste-Justine; (514)345-4716 x4; Fax. (514)345-4824.

HOULE, Annie; CSSS de Laval, 1755 boul Rene-Laennec, Laval QC H7M 3L9; Mon'06; FRCPC; RadOncol. Staff, Hopital Charles LeMoyne; (450)668-1010

HOULE, Claude; CSSS Pierre Boucher, 1333 boul Jacques-Cartier E, Longueuil QC J4M 2A5; Laval'88; Staff, Centre Hospitalier Pierre Boucher; (450)468-8111

HOULE, Claudia; CSSS de Trois-Rivières, 1991 boul du Carmel, Trois-Rivieres QC G8Z 3R9; Laval'03; MedMicrobiol. Staff, CSSS de Trois-Rivières; Langs: Bilingual(French/English); (819)697-3333; claudia-houle-chrtr@ssss.gouv.qc.ca.

HOULE, Cynthia; Ctr Hosp du Centre la Mauricie, 50 119e rue, Shawinigan-Sud QC G9P 5K1; Mon'06; CCFP; Staff, Centre Hospitalier du Centre la Mauricie; (819)536-7500

HOULE, Francois; Bathurst Shopping Mall, 212-1300 St. Peter Ave, Bathurst NB E2A 3A6; Sher'93; CSPQ; FRCSC; GenSurg. Staff, Hôpital de Gatineau; (506)548-2727; Fax. (506)546-3943.

HOULE, Gabriel; Clin Med Saint-Fabien, 115 1re rue CP 310, Saint-Fabien QC G0L 2Z0; Sher'78; Langs: Bilingual(French/English); (418)869-2142; Fax. (418)869-3632.

HOULE, Gaetan; Clinique Med Ahuntsic, 116-241 rue Fleury O, Montreal QC H3L 1V2; Mon'74; Chef Geriatric, Centre Hospitalier Fleury; (514)381-5387; Fax. (514)381-5388.

HOULE, Gregory A; 201-3301 24 Ave, Vernon BC V1T 9S8; Sask'94; BSc(Hons); FRCSC; Urol. (250)542-8715; Fax. (250)542-2798.

HOULE, Jean-Rene; CSSS de Laval, 1755 boul Rene-Laennec, Laval QC H7M 3L9; Mon'94; CSPQ; FRCSC; GenSurg; VascSurg. Staff, Hopital de la Cite de la santé; (450)668-1010 x3986; Fax. (450)975-5031.

HOULE, Marie-Andree; CSSS de Chicoutimi, CP 5006 305 rue Saint-Vallier, Chicoutimi QC G7H 5H6; Sher'07; FRCPC; IntMed; Respir. Staff, Complexe hospitalier de la Sagamie; (418)541-1000

HOULE, Marie-Claude; CHUQ-Hotel-Dieu de Quebec, 11 Cote du Palais, Quebec QC G1R 2J6; McG'05; FRCPC; Derm. Staff, Centre Hospitalier Universitaire de Québec (CHUQ) - Siege Social; (418)691-5200

HOULE, Michele; CLSC Villeray, 1425 rue Jarry E, Montreal QC H2E 1A7; Mon'85; LMCC; (514)376-4141; Fax. (514)722-3752.

HOULE, Noemi; Ctr Hosp le Gardeur, 911 montee des Pionniers, Terrebonne QC J6V 2H2; Mon'08; CCFP; Staff, Centre Hospitalier Pierre le Gardeur; (450)654-7525

HOULE, Normand; 425 Grande Allée est, Quebec QC G1R 2J5; Laval'75; FRCS; FRCSC; PlasSurg (Cosmetic Surgery). Langs: Bilingual(French/English); (418)682-4182; Fax. (418)681-2930; doctornormandhoule@cliniquegrandeallee.com.

HOULE, Patrick; Polyclinique Les Gres, 104-190 rue St Honore, St-Etienne-Ds-Gres QC G0X 2P0; Sher'91; (819)535-6512 x5701; Fax. (819)535-1627.

HOULE, Pierre-Alain; Polyclinique du Cap, 110-700 boul Thibeau, Trois-Rivieres QC G8T 7A1; Laval'79; (819)373-4551; Fax. (819)373-6516.

HOULE, Raymond; Comm de la Sante du Travail, 280-524 rue Bourdages, Quebec QC G1K 7E2; Sher'75; Staff, Hôpital de l'Archipel; (418)266-4670

HOULE, Serge; Clin Medicale, 100-1226 boul Sainte-Foy, Longueuil QC J4K 1X3; Mon'77; (450)646-4364; Fax. (450)646-6412.

HOULE, Stephanie; CSSS de Rimouski-Neigette, CP 3150 Succ A 150 av Rouleau, Rimouski QC G5L 5T1; Laval'01; Staff, Hôpital Regional Rimouski; (418)723-7851

HOULE, Sylvain; Addiction & Mental Hlth-Clarke, 250 College St, Toronto ON M5T 1R8; Tor'79; FRCPC; NuclearMed. Dir Research Imaging Centre PET, Centre for Addiction & Mental Health (CAMH) - College Street Site; Langs: Bilingual(English/French); (416)979-4651; Fax. (416)979-4656.

HOULE, Virginie; Ctr Hosp Affilie-St-Sacrement, 1050 ch Sainte-Foy, Quebec QC G1S 4L8; Mon'06; DiagRad. Staff, Centre Hospitalier Affilié Universitaire de Québec - Hôpital du St-Sacrement; (418)682-7511

HOULE, Yves E; Clin Medicale St-Louis, 220-3165 ch Saint-Louis, Quebec QC G1W 4R4; Laval'81; Staff, Centre Hospitalier Universitaire de Québec (CHUQ) - Siege Social; (418)653-1970; Fax. (418)653-9956.

HOULGRAVE, Albert W; St Joseph's Gen Hosp, 2137 Comox Ave, Comox BC V9M 1P2; UBC'01; CCFP; CCFP(E.M.); Staff, St Joseph's General Hospital.

HOUPT, Daniel R; Peterborough Reg HC-Hospital, 1 Hospital Dr, Peterborough ON K9J 7C6; McM'93; CCFP; Staff Family Practice, Peterborough Regional Health Centre - Hospital Drive; Fam Med, Peterborough Regional Health Centre - Rogers St Site; (705)876-5014

HOURIGAN, John F; Gibsons Med Clinic, 211-1100 Sunshine Coast Hwy, Gibsons BC V0N 1V7; UBC'85; (604)886-2870; Fax. (604)886-9716.

HOURTOVENKO, Clyde D; Riverside Cardiac Clinic, 2147 Armstrong St, Sudbury ON P3E 4W2; Wes'87; FRCPC; IntMed; Cardiol. (705)670-0654; Fax. (705)670-9348.

HOUSE, A Maxwell; Health Sciences Centre, 300 Prince Philip Dr, St. John's NL A1B 3V6; Dal'52; FRCPC; Neur. Staff, Health Sciences Centre; (709)777-8837

HOUSE, Andrew A; London HSC-University Hosp, PO Box 5339 Stn B 339 Windermere Rd, London ON N6A 5A5; Ott'92; MSc(Epidemiol&Biostats); FRCPC; IntMed (Transplant Nephrology); Nephrol. Prof Med, London Health Sciences Centre - University Hospital; (519)663-3167; Fax. (519)663-3449; andrew.house@lhsc.on.ca.

HOUSE, Ronald A; St Michael's Hosp, 30 Bond St, Toronto ON M5B 1W8; McG'74; MSc(ClinEpidem); DIH; CCBOM; FRCPC; OccupMed. Ac Staff Occup & Environ Health, St Michael's Hospital; Asst Prof Public Hlth Sciences, University of Toronto; Langs: Bilingual(English/French); (416)867-7470; Fax. (416)867-3673.

HOUSE, Sheilagh J; Sheddon Avenue Med Assoc, 308-331 Sheddon Ave, Oakville ON L6J 1X8; Mem'83; Assoc Staff, Halton Healthcare Services Corporation - Oakville Site; (905)845-8771; Fax. (905)845-8379.

HOUSE, W Peter; The Copeman Health Care Ctr, 400-1128 Hornby St, Vancouver BC V6Z 2L4; Dal'68; Med Dir, The Copeman Healthcare Centre; (604)707-2273; Fax. (604)707-2250; phouse@copemanhealthcare.com.

HOUSEFATHER, Leslie S; Polyclinic Family & Specialty, 5-4646 Dufferin St, North York ON M3H 5S4; McG'98; CCFP; Langs: Hebrew; French; (416)222-6160; Fax. (416)222-9604.

HOUSHMAND, Henry; Hotel-Dieu de Saint-Joseph, 10 Woodland Hill, Perth-Andover NB E7H 5H5; (Iran)'81; Staff, Hôtel-Dieu of St Joseph Hospital; (506)273-7100

HOUSLEY, Richard J; 301-5673 North St, Niagara Falls ON L2G 1J4; McG'85; DABIM(IntMed&Gastroent); FRCPC; IntMed; Gastroent. Court Staff, Niagara Health System - St Catharines General Site; Ac Staff, Niagara Health System - Greater Niagara General Site; Aj Prof, University of Western Ontario; Langs: English; French; (905)354-3242; Fax. (905)354-3830.

HOUSTON, David M; East End Family Health Team, PO Box 3211 4715 Hwy 101 E, South Porcupine ON P0N 1H0; Tor'93; MD; BMath; CCFP; CCFP(E.M.); FCFP; (705)235-6900; Fax. (705)235-6901.

HOUSTON, Donald S; CancerCare Manitoba, 675 Mcdermot Ave, Winnipeg MB R3E 0V9; Sask'82; PhD; MD; FRCPC; FRCPC; Hem; IntMed. Att Physician, Health Sciences Centre; Staff, CancerCare Manitoba; Assoc Prof IntMed, University of Manitoba; (204)787-2108

HOUSTON, Gordon T M; 307-7031 Westminster Hwy, Richmond BC V6X 1A3; Man'86; FRCSC; GenSurg; VascSurg. (604)270-2726; Fax. (604)270-3431.

HOUSTON, James G; Yates Quadra Integreted Hlth C, 105-911 Yates St, Victoria BC V8V 4X3; London (England)'77; MB BS.

HOUSTON, Patricia L; St Michael's Hosp, 30 Bond St, Toronto ON M5B 1W8; Tor'78; FRCPC; Anes (Administration). Staff/Chief, St Michael's Hospital; Assoc Prof, University of Toronto; (416)864-5071; Fax. (416)864-6014; houstonp@smh.toronto.on.ca.

HOUSTON, Scott A W; Creemore Med Centre, GD 1-15 Elizabeth St E, Creemore ON L0M 1G0; Tor'79; CCFP; FCFP; Staff, Collingwood General & Marine Hospital; (705)466-3077; Fax. (705)466-2587.

HOUSTON, Stanley C; University of Alberta Hosp, 2E412WCM-8440 112 St NW, Edmonton AB T6G 2B7; Sask'75; FRCPC; IntMed (HIV); InfectDis. Ad Staff, University of Alberta Hospital; Consultant, Royal Alexandra Hospital; Prof Med & Public Health Sciences, University of Alberta; Langs: Spanish; (780)407-8035; Fax. (780)407-7137; shouston@ualberta.ca.

HOUSTOUN, Anne L; North End Comm Health Centre, 2165 Gottingen St, Halifax NS B3K 3B5; McG'85; MDCM; (902)420-0303; Fax. (902)422-0859.

HOVAN, Shirley; Associate Med Group, 4705 48 Ave, Red Deer AB T4N 3T1; Alb'72; BSc; Dir Community Med, Red Deer Regional Hospital Centre; Physician, Associate Medical Group; Dir Community Med, Central Zone David Thompson Health Region; (403)346-2057; Fax. (403)347-2989; sahovan@shaw.ca.

HOVEY, Jeffrey T; Manotick Family Health Org, PO Box 580 Stn Main 5230 Mitch Owens Rd, Manotick ON K4M 1A5; Mem'88; CCFP; FCFP; Asst Prof, University of Ottawa; (613)692-2571; Fax. (613)692-0271.

HOW, Angela R; 102B-6440 Royal Oak Ave, Burnaby BC V5H 3P2; Cal'74; FRCPC; Peds; Rheum. Ac Staff, Burnaby Hospital; Staff Consultant, Vancouver General Hospital - Centennial Pavillion; Member Medical Advisory Board, Arthritis Society of British Columbia; (604)436-3323; Fax. (604)436-5590.

HOW, Benjamin K; Oak Bay Family Phys Ltd, 101-1640 Oak Bay Ave, Victoria BC V8R 1B2; Alb'82; Ac Staff, Vancouver Island Health Authority; (250)598-6744; Fax. (250)598-6778.

HOW, Jacques S; MUHC-Montreal Gen Hosp, C6 252-1650 av Cedar, Montreal QC H3G 1A4; Glasgow (Scotland)'71; MRCP(UK); FRCPC; Endocrin (P.Q.) (Thyroid Diseases); Endocrin&Metab. Assoc Dir Endocrin, McGill University Health Centre - Montreal General Campus; assoc Prof Med, McGill University; Langs: Hakka; (514)934-8362; Fax. (514)934-8361; jacques.how@muhc.mcgill.ca.

HOW, Jonathan; MUHC-Royal Victoria Hosp, 687 av des Pins O, Montreal QC H3A 1A1; McG'05; FRCPC; IntMed; Hem. Staff Hematol, McGill University Health Centre - Royal Victoria Hospital; (514)934-1934

HOW, Richard K; Tillicum Mall Med Centre, 14-3170 Tillicum Rd, Victoria BC V9A 7C5; Wes'65; (250)381-8112; Fax. (250)381-8252.

HOWARD, Andrew K; Detwiller Pavilion, 0007-2255 Wesbrook Mall, Vancouver BC V6T 2A1; Qns'98; FRCPC; Psy (Neuro Psychiatry). Staff BC Neuropsychiatry Prog, UBC Hospital - Koerner Pavillion; Clinical Asst Prof Psy, University of British Columbia; (604)822-7921; Fax. (604)822-7921.

HOWARD, Andrew W; The Hosp for Sick Children, S107-555 University Ave, Toronto ON M5G 1X8; Qns'90; MSc; FRCSC; OrthSurg (Cerebral Palsy). Staff, The Hospital For Sick Children; Consultant, Erinoak Children's Treatment Centre; Asst Prof, University of Toronto; Langs: Bilingual(English/French); (416)813-6430; Fax. (416)813-6414; andrew.howard@sickkids.ca.

HOWARD, Craig R; Trillium Cardiovascular Assoc, 608-89 Queensway W, Mississauga ON L5B 2V2; Tor'79; Staff, Trillium Health Centre - Mississauga; (905)848-3113; Fax. (905)848-7513.

HOWARD, Douglas J; Royal Victoria Hosp, 201 Georgian Dr, Barrie ON L4M 6M2; Sask'91; CCFP; CCFP(E.M.); FCFP; Staff, Royal Victoria Regional Health Centre; (705)728-9802

HOWARD, Edward W; Comox Med Clinic, 100-1695 Comox Ave, Comox BC V9M 3M1; Sask'97; BSc; CCFP; Ac Staff, St Joseph's General Hospital; (250)339-2266; edcorrie@shaw.ca.

HOWARD, James L; London Hsc-Univ Campus Site, PO Box 5339 Stn B 339 Windermere Rd, London ON N6A 5A5; Cal'00; FRCSC; OrthSurg. Staff, London Health Sciences Centre - University Hospital; (519)663-3551

HOWARD, Jane A; Antigonish Medical Assoc, 40 Church St, Antigonish NS B2G 2C7; Dal'06; CCFP; CCFP(E.M.); (902)863-4558; Fax. (902)867-5665.

HOWARD, Jane M; Senior's Mental Hlth Clinic, 200-1164 Devonshire Ave, North Bay ON P1B 6X7; Qns'78; FRCPC; Psy (Geriatric Psychiatry). Langs: Bilingual(English/French); (705)494-3054

HOWARD, Janet L; Albro Lake Med Centre, 6 Primrose St, Dartmouth NS B3A 4C5; Dal'83; (902)465-4444

HOWARD, Jason J; IWK Health Centre, PO Box 9700 Rpo CSC 5850-5980 University Ave, Halifax NS B3K 6R8; Mem'98; BMedSci; FRCPC; OrthSurg (Pediatrics). Staff, IWK Health Centre; (902)470-7238; jason.howard@calgryhealthregion.ca.

HOWARD, Jessica C; Middlesex Centre Reg Clinic, PO Box 160 36 Heritage Dr, Ilderton ON N0M 2A0; Wes'07; CCFP; (519)666-1610

HOWARD, John M; London HSC-Victoria Hosp, PO Box 5010 Stn B B1 162-800 Commissioners Rd E, London ON N6A 5W9; Qns'77; FRCP; ABIM; FRCPC; IntMed (Pediatric Gastroenterology); Gastroent. Att Staff, London Health Sciences Centre - Victoria Campus; Prof Med & Peds, University of Western Ontario; (519)685-8048; Fax. (519)685-8062.

HOWARD, Kathleen G; Espanola Family Health Team, 801 McKinnon Dr, Espanola ON P5E 1T2; Ott'74; Langs: German; French; (705)862-7991

HOWARD, Paisley G; 408-125 13th St E, North Vancouver BC V7L 2L3; Tor'96; BSc; MSc; CCFP; (604)980-3411

HOWARD, Paul L; Complete Med of Barrie, 103-1 Quarry Ridge Rd, Barrie ON L4M 7G1; Wes'95; BSc; CCFP; CCFP(E.M.); FCFP; Staff, Royal Victoria Regional Health Centre; (705)725-1862

HOWARD, Peter R S; Sunnybrook Hlth Sciences Ctre, 8G31-2075 Bayview Ave, Toronto ON M4N 3M5; Wes'00; FRCPC; DiagRad (Neuro Radiology). Staff, Sunnybrook Health Sciences Centre; (416)480-6100 x89323

HOWARD, Raymond; Telus Plaza North, PO Box 1360 Stn Main 13F-10025 Jasper Ave NW, Edmonton AB T5J 2N3; Edinburgh (Scotland)'65; MB ChB; FRCS(Ed); FRCS(Lond); Med Consultant, Alberta Health & Wellness; (780)415-1551; Fax. (780)415-0963.

HOWARD, Richard J; Canadian Forces Hlth Serv Ctr, PO Box 99000 Stn Forces, Halifax NS B3K 5X5; Dublin (Ireland)'68; DPM; DCH; DRCOG; MRCPsy; MB BCh; BAO; FRCPC; Psy (Clinical Psychiatry). Consultant, Queen Elizabeth II Health Sciences Centre - Victoria General Site; Consultant, Canadian Forces Health Services Centre (Atlantic); Asst Prof Psy, Dalhousie University; (902)721-8054; Fax. (902)721-0326.

HOWARD, Robert J; 1 028BW-30 Bond St, Toronto ON M5B 1W8; McM'75; MD; MBA; FRCPC; Cardiol; IntMed. Exec VP/Prof Med, St Michael's Hospital; Prof, University of Toronto; (416)864-5617; Fax. (416)864-5669; howardr@smh.ca.

HOWARD, Robert S; Mental Hlth & Addictions, 5000 Joyce Ave, Powell River BC V8A 5R3; Cape Town (South Africa)'78; MB ChB; FRCPC; Psy. Staff, East Kootenay Regional Hospital; (604)485-3300

HOWARD, Sheldon; 234-475 Main St, Vancouver BC V6A 2T7; Tor'69; Ac Staff, Vancouver General Hospital - Centennial Pavillion; (604)681-0248

HOWARD-TRIPP, Micheal E; Telus Plaza South, 2700-10020 100 St NW, Edmonton AB T5J 0N3; Cape Town (South Africa)'93; MB ChB; BSc(Med) (Hons.); CCFP; Senior Med Advisor, College of Physicians & Surgeons of Alberta; Langs: Afrikaans; (780)969-4954; Fax. (780)424-9617; micheal.howard-tripp@cpsa.ab.ca.

HOWARTH, Andrew G; Foothills Med Centre, 700-1403 29 St NW, Calgary AB T2N 2T9; UBC'99; FRCPC; IntMed; Cardiol. Staff, Foothills Medical Centre; (403)944-8806; Fax. (403)944-8510.

HOWARTH, Barbara J; Market Mall Prof Ctr, 301-4935 40 Ave NW, Calgary AB T3A 2N1; London (England)'76; MB BS; LMCC; CCFP; FCFP; (403)286-4924; Fax. (403)247-2644.

HOWARTH, David J C; Mount Sinai Hosp, 6F-600 University Ave, Toronto ON M5G 1X5; Tor'86; FRCPC; AnatPath. Staff Path, Mount Sinai Hospital; Assoc Prof, University of Toronto; (416)586-4670

HOWARTH, Erik; 354 Read St PO Box 550, Merrickville ON K0G 1N0; Ott'97; CCFP; Langs: English; French; (613)269-3400; Fax. (613)269-4958.

HOWARTH, Paul A; Hamilton Health Sciences, 217 Barton St E, Hamilton ON L8L 2W7; McM'75; EmergMed (Surgical Assistant). (905)527-0271 x46277

HOWATT, Alison L; Montobello Med Clinic, PO Box 32 Stn Main 302-320 Alexander St NE, Salmon Arm BC V1E 4N2; McM'96; BSc; CCFP; FCFP; Staff, Shuswap Lake General Hospital; (250)833-4677; Fax. (250)833-4765; alisonhowatt@telus.net.

HOWATT, Eric B; Valley Prof Centre, 125-70 Exhibition St, Kentville NS B4N 4K9; Mem'81; BMedSci; Dip SportMed; FRCSC; OrthSurg (Personal Injury). Ac Staff, Valley Regional Hospital; (902)678-4404; Fax. (902)678-1177; ebhortho@eastlink.ca.

HOWATT, Jesse; J A Hides Northern Med, T162-770 Bannatyne Ave, Winnipeg MB R3E 0W3; Man'10; CCFP.

HOWE, B Anne; 2-418 Talbot St W, Aylmer ON N5H 1K9; Tor'80; CCFP; FCFP; Court Staff, St Thomas Elgin General Hospital; (519)765-1280; Fax. (519)765-1283.

HOWE, David; Parrsboro & Area Professional, PO Box 638 76 Jenks Ave, Parrsboro NS B0M 1S0; London (England)'66; MB BS; CCFP; FCFP; (902)254-3760; davidhowe282@gmail.com.

HOWE, Marnie L; Temmy Latner Centre, 60 Murray St Box 13, Toronto ON M5T 3L9; Wes'08; CCFP; Staff, Mount Sinai Hospital; (416)586-4800; Fax. (416)586-4804.

HOWE, William A; Women Walk in Clinic, 106-6453 Morrison St, Niagara Falls ON L2E 7H1; Wes'62; BSc; (905)374-3344

HOWELL, Brandon G; Guelph Medical Place 2, 107-89 Dawson Rd, Guelph ON N1H 1B1; Tor'06; FRCPC; Derm. (519)836-7326; Fax. (519)763-5440.

HOWELL, Jane C; Mount Dennis Med Group, 98 Guestville Ave, Toronto ON M6N 4N6; Tor'80; CCFP; FCFP; Ac Staff, Humber River Regional Hospital - Church Street Site; (416)763-1171; Fax. (416)763-0573.

HOWELL, Kathleen; Royal Ottawa Hlth Care Group, 1145 Carling Ave, Ottawa ON K1Z 7K4; McM'05; FRCPC; Psy. Staff, Royal Ottawa Mental Health Centre - Royal Ottawa Health Care Group; Teach Staff, University of Ottawa; (613)722-6521

HOWELL, Oscar J; Health Sciences Centre, 300 Prince Philip Dr, St. John's NL A1B 3V6; Mem'75; BMedSci; MSc; CCBOM; Staff, Health Sciences Centre; Pres, Medserv Solutions Inc; Ac Staff Ambulatory Care, Health Care Corporation Of St John's; Clin Asst Prof Family Med, Memorial University Of Newfoundland; (709)777-1308; ohowell@nf.sympatico.ca.

HOWELLS, Steven R; Health Sciences Centre, 300 Prince Philip Dr, St. John's NL A1B 3V6; Dal'90; FRCPC; Anes. Staff, Health Sciences Centre; (709)777-6300

HOWES, Daniel W; Kingston Gen Hosp, 20 202-76 Stuart St, Kingston ON K7L 2V7; Dal'94; FRCPC; EmergMed (Hypothermia); Critical Care Medicine. Staff, Kingston General Hospital; Dir, Regional Trauma Program; (613)549-6666 x3637

HOWEY, Jeannine I; Primary Westside Med Clinic, 835 Langford Pky, Victoria BC V9B 4V5; Alb'84; (250)391-0300

HOWIE, Graham M; PO Box 438, Shawnigan Lake BC V0R 2W0; Aberdeen (Scotland)'80; MB ChB; MRCGPract; DA(UK); DRCOG; (250)952-1104

HOWIE, James F; Aspen Med Centre, 21-429 Tranquille Rd, Kamloops BC V2B 3G9; UBC'81; (250)376-7242

HOWIE, Sebastian; 204-3811 Chatham St, Richmond BC V7E 2Z4; UBC'00; CCFP; (604)277-7166

HOWITT, Patricia A; Reach Community Health Ctre, 1145 Commercial Dr, Vancouver BC V5L 3X3; McM'88; BScN; BA; Clin Consultant, University of British Columbia; (604)254-1354; Fax. (604)258-9190.

HOWK, Shelley D; Cochrane Primary Care, 103-100 Grande Blvd W, Cochrane AB T4C 0S4; Man'90; BSc; CCFP; (403)932-2089; Fax. (403)932-1820.

HOWLETT, Alexandra A; Alberta Children's Hosp, 2888 Shaganappi Trail NW, Calgary AB T3B 6A8; Tor'89; FAAP; FRCPC; Peds (Neonatology). Staff, Foothills Medical Centre; Staff, Alberta Children's Hospital; (403)955-3171; Fax. (403)955-2203; alixe.howlett@dal.ca.

HOWLETT, Andrew L; St Josephs Health Centre, 3L 234-30 The Queensway, Toronto ON M6R 1B5; Dal'07; FRCPC; Psy. Staff Our Lady of Mercy Wing, St Joseph's Health Centre; (416)530-6486; Fax. (416)530-6393.

HOWLETT, Christopher J; London HSC-University Hosp, PO Box 5339 Stn B 339 Windermere Rd, London ON N6A 5A5; Cal'04; FRCPC; AnatPath. Staff, London Health Sciences Centre - University Hospital; (519)685-8500 x36338

HOWLETT, Evan J; Lenore Centre Med Clinic, 4-123 Lenore Dr, Saskatoon SK S7K 7H9; Sask'85; (306)242-6700; Fax. (306)242-1168.

HOWLETT, Jonathan; Foothills Medical Centre, C838-1403 29 St NW, Calgary AB T2N 2T9; Tor'89; FACC; FRCPC; IntMed (Invasive Cardiology); Cardiol. Prof of Med, Foothills Medical Centre; (403)944-3232; Fax. (403)944-3262; howlettjonathan@gmail.com.

HOWLETT, Laura A; Grey Bruce HS-Owen Sound, PO Box 1800 Stn Main 1800 8th St E, Owen Sound ON N4K 6M9; Dal'94; FRCPC; DiagRad. Staff, Grey Bruce Health Services - Owen Sound; (519)376-2121 x2279; Fax. (519)372-3954.

HOWLETT, Michael K; Saint John Reg Hosp, PO Box 2100 Stn Main 400 University Ave, Saint John NB E2L 4L2; Dal'86; CCFP; CCFP(E.M.); Staff, Emerg Fam Med, Saint John Regional Hospital; (506)648-6092

HOWLETT, Todd C; Dartmouth Gen Hosp, 325 Pleasant St, Dartmouth NS B2Y 4G8; Ott'92; CCFP; CCFP(E.M.); FCFP; Staff, Dartmouth General Hospital; Langs: English; French; (902)465-8525; Fax. (902)460-4142.

HOWLEY, D Brent; 100-585 Mapleton Rd, Moncton NB E1G 2K5; Dal'01; BSc(Hon); FRCSC; PlasSurg. Ac Staff Plastic Surg, Sackville Memorial Hospital; Ac Staff Plastic Surg, Dr Georges-L-Dumont University Hospital Centre; Ac Staff Plastic Surg, The Moncton Hospital; (506)853-5164; Fax. (506)853-4104; info@drhowley.com.

HOWSE, David C N; Thunder Bay Reg Hlth Sciences, 201-984 Oliver Rd, Thunder Bay ON P7B 7C7; Tor'62; FRCPC; Neur (Stroke). Med Dir Regional Stroke Prog, Thunder Bay Regional Health Sciences Centre; (807)684-6707; Fax. (807)684-5883.

HOWSE, G Dawn; Carbonear Gen Hosp, 86 Highroad South, Carbonear NL A1Y 1A4; Mem'78; Staff, Carbonear General Hospital; (709)945-5111

HOWSE, Kelly L; Queen's Family Hlth Team, 115 Clarence St, Kingston ON K7L 5N6; Ott'07; CCFP; (613)533-9303; Fax. (613)533-9308.

HOWSON-JAN, Kang; London Hlth Sciences Centre, PO Box 5375 Stn B A2 401-800 Commissioners Rd E, London ON N6C 6B5; Qns'81; FRCPC; IntMed (Bone Marrow Transplant). Staff Hematology, London Health Sciences Centre - Victoria Campus; Consultant, London Regional Cancer Centre; Assoc Prof, University of Western Ontario; (519)685-8500 x52169; Fax. (519)685-8477.

HOY, Conrad S G; Assoc Rehab Consultants Canada, 1850 Main St, Winnipeg MB R2V 3J4; Man'91; BSc(Med); FRCPC; PhysMed&Rehab (Pain & Disability Evaluation). (204)942-3128; Fax. (204)942-3172.

HOY, Gerald J F; Turtle Mountain Med Clinic, 968 Main St, Winnipeg MB R2W 3P5; Man'03; CCFP; (204)589-3999; Fax. (204)589-8467.

HOY, Monica; Foothills Medical Centre, 1403 29 St NW, Calgary AB T2N 2T9; Alb'08; Staff, Foothills Medical Centre; (403)944-1110

HOY, Paul J; Professional Bldg, 304-222 King St E, Bowmanville ON L1C 1P6; Ott'74; CCFP; FCFP; Staff, Lakeridge Health - Bowmanville Site; (905)623-1161; Fax. (905)623-6397.

HOY, Peter; Park Avenue Med Centre, 3F-4634 Park Ave, Terrace BC V8G 1V7; UBC'76; BSc; Langs: Chinese; (250)615-5025; Fax. (250)615-5035.

HOY, Wayne K F; Beddington Co-Op Mall, 110-8220 Centre St NE, Calgary AB T3K 1J7; Alb'80; CCFP; FCFP; (403)275-1141; Fax. (403)275-1143.

HOYECK, Antoine; Flin Flon Gen Hosp Inc, PO Box 340, Flin Flon MB R8A 1N2; Laval'85; CSPQ; FRCSC; GenSurg (Biliary Surgery). Staff, Flin Flon General Hospital Inc; (204)687-7591

HOYER, Emelie M L; 920 Kennedy Ave, North Vancouver BC V7R 1L3; UBC'84; BSc; FRCSC; ObstGyn (Colposcopy). Ac Staff, Lions Gate Hospital; (604)319-5055

HOYER, Irene; Westglen Med Clinic, 108-30 Springborough Blvd SW, Calgary AB T3H 0N9; Karlova (Czech Republic)'72; Langs: Czech; (403)240-2221; Fax. (403)240-4670.

HOYER, Vaclav R; Westglen Med Clinic, 108-30 Springborough Blvd SW, Calgary AB T3H 0N9; Prague (Czech Republic)'73; Staff, CRHA Extendicare; Langs: Czech; Slovak; (403)240-2221; Fax. (403)240-4670; hoyermed@hughes.net.

HOYT, Benjamin J A; 340 Brunswick St, Fredericton NB E3B 1H1; Dal'03; FRCSC; Otol.

HOYT, Linda C; Fredericton Mental Hlth Clinic, 65 Brunswick St, Fredericton NB E3B 1G5; Dal'02; FRCPC; Psy. (506)453-2132; Fax. (506)453-8766.

HOYTE, Keith M; Peter Lougheed Centre, 3500 26 Ave NE, Calgary AB T1Y 6J4; Qns'72; ABIM; FRCPC; IntMed (Stroke); Neur. Staff, Peter Lougheed Centre; Clin Assoc Prof Neuroscience, University of Calgary; (403)943-5477; Fax. (403)219-3296; hoyte@ucalgary.ca.

HRABAR, Zenona M I; Orion Health Centre, 120-16555 Fraser Hwy, Surrey BC V4N 0E9; Alb'68; Langs: Polish; Ukrainian; (604)575-2325

HRABARCHUK, Blair E; Dauphin Med Clinic, 622 3rd St SW, Dauphin MB R7N 1R5; Man'88; FRCPC; IntMed. (204)638-6445; Fax. (204)638-5670.

HRADECKY, Cyril M; Queensway-Carleton Hosp, 3045 Baseline Rd, Ottawa ON K2H 8P4; Ott'70; FRCSC; OrthSurg. Staff, Queensway Carleton Hospital; (613)721-4700

HRADSKY, Nadine S; The Doctors Bldg, 804-208 Bloor St W, Toronto ON M5S 3B4; Tor'63; FRCPC; Derm. Asst Prof, University of Toronto; Langs: Czech; Italian; (416)961-9881; Fax. (416)961-0708.

HRAMIAK, O M Irene; St Joseph's Health Care, PO Box 5777 Stn B 268 Grosvenor St, London ON N6A 4V2; Wes'76; MD; FRCPC; IntMed (Diabetes); Endocrin&Metab. Staff, St Joseph's Hospital - St Joseph's Health Care; Staff, London Health Sciences Centre - University Hospital; Prof Med, University of Western Ontario; Langs: Ukrainian; (519)646-6353; Fax. (519)646-6059.

HRAZDIL, Chantelle T; VGH Epilepsy Clinic, 8257-2775 Laurel St, Vancouver BC V5Z 1M9; Alb'06; FRCPC; Neur (Epilepsy). Staff Neurologist, Vancouver General Hospital - Centennial Pavillion; Physician, Vancouver Gen Hosp Epilepsy Clinic; Asst Clin Prof, University of British Columbia; (604)875-4403; Fax. (604)875-4786; chantallehrazdil@vch.ca.

HRAZDIL, Jiri; Primrose Med Centre, 8436 182 St NW, Edmonton AB T5T 1Y7; Karlova (Czech Republic)'80; FRCPC; Anes (Pain Management). Staff Anes., Royal Alexandra Hospital; Lecturer, University of Alberta; (780)487-7532; Fax. (780)487-8862.

HRDINA, Josef; St Joseph's Health Centre, 30 The Queensway, Toronto ON M6R 1B5; Prague (Czech Republic)'93; FRCPC; Anes. Staff Anes, St Joseph's Health Centre; (416)530-6090

HRDLICKA, Adam J; Medical Clinic, 5031 49 St, Innisfail AB T4G 1A4; Alb'09; CCFP; (403)227-3356

HRDLICKA, Ash T; Medical Centre, 1-1036 7 St SW, Medicine Hat AB T1A 8V7; Alb'10; CCFP; (403)528-4141; Fax. (403)528-2162.

HREBICEK, Olinka K; 208-1964 Fort St, Victoria BC V8R 6R3; McM'94; FRCPC; Neur. Staff, Victoria General Hospital; (250)592-5115

HRIMIUC, Ramona; Royal Alexandra Hosp, 10240 Kingsway NW, Edmonton AB T5H 3V9; Alb'06; FRCPC; IntMed. Staff, Royal Alexandra Hospital; (780)735-5312

HRISTOV, Hristo N; Paterson Med Centre, RR 1 45 Wolsley St, Kenora ON P9N 3W7; Sofia (Bulgaria)'94; FRCSC; GenSurg. Staff, Lake of the Woods District Hospital; (807)468-5410

HRNCIRIK, Joseph; Miramichi East Med Clinic, 4 Johnson Ave, Miramichi NB E1N 3B7; Purkyne (Czech Republic)'71; Ac Staff, Miramichi Regional Hospital; Langs: Czech; Slovak; French; (506)773-6281; Fax. (506)773-3568; jhrncirik@rogers.com.

HRUBY, Lorna E; Burnaby Youth Clinic, 4734 Imperial St, Burnaby BC V5J 1C2; UBC'84; CCFP; (604)293-1764

HRUCZKOWSKI, Tomasz W; University of Alberta Hosp, 8440 112 St NW, Edmonton AB T6G 2B7; McM'98; MScE; FRCPC; IntMed; Cardiol (Cardiac Electrophysiology). Staff, University of Alberta Hospital; Langs: Polish; (780)407-3146; Fax. (780)407-6452.

HRYCIUK, Daniel J; Sturgeon Community Hosp, 201 Boudreau Rd, St. Albert AB T8N 6C4; Alb'76; Staff, Sturgeon Community Hospital; (780)418-8228; Fax. (780)418-8376.

HRYCIUK, Laura E; East Edmonton Mental Hlth Serv, 7910 112 Ave NW, Edmonton AB T5B 0C2; Alb'76; Staff, Sturgeon Community Hospital; (780)342-4926

HRYCKO, Sophia; Children's Hosp Eastern Ont, 401 Smyth Rd, Ottawa ON K1H 8L1; Ott'93; CSPQ; FRCPC; Psy. Staff Child Psy, Children's Hospital of Eastern Ontario (CHEO); Langs: English; French; (613)737-7600 x3476; Fax. (613)738-3233; hrycko@cheo.on.ca.

HRYNCHAK, Monica; Royal Columbia Hosp, B180-330 Columbia St E, New Westminster BC V3L 3W7; Sask'83; FCCMG; FRCPC; GenPath (Anatomical Pathology). Staff, BC Children's Hospital; Dir Cytogenetic Lab & Path, Royal Columbian Hospital; (604)520-4486; monica.hrynchak@fraserhealth.ca.

HRYNCHYSHYN, Gregory J; 205-9148 23 Ave NW, Edmonton AB T6N 1H9; Alb'94; FRCPC; IntMed. (780)462-3010; Fax. (780)440-2911.

HRYNIOWSKI, Ronald G; 465 rue Main CP 788, Hudson QC J0P 1H0; McG'76; CCFP; (450)458-5393; Fax. (450)458-4464.

HRYNIUK, William M; 502-123 Edward St, Toronto ON M5G 1E2; Man'61; FRCP(Scientist); FRCPC; MedScient(Med) (Administration). Med Dir, Carepath Inc; Langs: Ukrainian; (416)595-2720 x2822; Fax. (416)595-2710.

HSIA, Cyrus C; London HSC-Victoria Hosp, PO Box 5010 Stn B A2 401-800 Commissioners Rd E, London ON N6A 5W9; Wes'03; BSc(Hon); FRCPC; IntMed; Hem. Staff Hem, London Health Sciences Centre - Victoria Campus; (519)685-8500 x5606; cyrus.hsia@lhsc.on.ca.

HSIA, David; Delta Health Sciences Centre, 204-4515 Harvest Dr, Delta BC V4K 4L1; UBC'74; Physician, Delta Health Sciences Centre; (604)946-0665; Fax. (604)946-0494.

HSIA, Ivan K; Hotel-Dieu Grace Hosp, 1030 Ouellette Ave, Windsor ON N9A 1E1; McM'04; FRCPC; Anes. Staff, Hôtel-Dieu Grace Hospital; (519)973-4421; Fax. (519)255-2130.

HSIANG, Diana; Family Practice Health Centre, 3F-77 Grenville St, Toronto ON M5S 1B3; McG'10; MDCM; CCFP; (416)323-6060

HSIANG, York N H; 510-943 Broadway W, Vancouver BC V5Z 1K3; Otago (New Zealand)'79; MB; MHSc; FRCSC; GenSurg; VascSurg. Prof Surg, UBC Hospital - Koerner Pavillion; Staff, Vancouver General Hospital - Centennial Pavillion; Asst Prof, University of British Columbia; (604)876-5882; Fax. (604)876-8085; yhsiang@vanhosp.bc.ca.

HSIAO, Janey S C; Women's College Hosp, 5F-76 Grenville St, Toronto ON M5S 1B2; McG'00; FRCPC; IntMed; Hem. Staff, Women's College Hospital; (416)323-6118; Fax. (416)323-6403.

HSIAO, Jerry L C; Terrace Hill Med Clinic, 217 Terrace Hill St, Brantford ON N3R 1G8; UBC'91; Court Staff, The Brant Community Healthcare System - Brantford General Hospital Site; (519)756-4240; Fax. (519)756-0840.

HSIAO, Marvin M; Sunnybrook Hlth Sciences Ctre, 2075 Bayview Ave, Toronto ON M4N 3M5; Tor'08; Staff, Sunnybrook Health Sciences Centre; (416)810-6100

HSIAO, Yann J; 17-2949 Main St, Vancouver BC V5T 3G4; Man'85; Langs: Cantonese; Mandarin; Taiwanese; (604)879-1168; Fax. (604)872-5668.

HSIEH, Daniel T T; Dundas Med Centre, 401-220 Dundas St W, Whitby ON L1N 8M7; Kaohsiung (Taiwan)'79; Ac Staff, Lakeridge Health - Oshawa Site; Ac Staff, Lakeridge Health - Whitby Site; (905)666-1777; Fax. (905)666-1922.

HSIEH, Eugene T K; Sunnybrook Hlth Sciences Ctre, 4 35-2075 Bayview Ave, Toronto ON M4N 3M5; McG'93; FRCPC; AnatPath. Staff, Sunnybrook Health Sciences Centre; (416)480-6100 x7894; eugene.hsieh@sunnybrook.ca.

HSIEH, Tauyee; Scarborough Prof Centre, 302-1371 Neilson Rd, Scarborough ON M1B 4Z8; Qns'01; FRCPC; Peds; Respir. (416)281-1100; Fax. (416)281-1105.

HSIEH, Wayne W Y; Lapsley Family Doctors, 13 Lapsley Rd, Scarborough ON M1B 1K1; Wes'95; CCFP; Langs: Mandarin; (416)754-9595; Fax. (416)754-3946; kaarway@sympatico.ca.

HSIN, Mabel; 6-52 Holland St E PO Box 1209 Stn Main, Bradford ON L3Z 2B6; Tor'88; Ac Staff, Southlake Regional Health Centre; Langs: Mandarin; Cantonese; (905)775-0081; Fax. (905)775-9290.

HSIUNG, G Y Robin; UBC Hospital-Koerner Pavillion, S162-2211 Wesbrook Mall, Vancouver BC V6T 2B5; Qns'92; MHSc; FACP; FRCPC; Neur (Dementia). Staff Neurol, Providence Health Care - St Paul's Hospital; Staff Neurol, UBC Hospital - Koerner Pavillion; Staff Neurol, Vancouver General Hospital - Centennial Pavillion; Asst Prof, University of British Columbia; Langs: Chinese; (604)822-3610; Fax. (604)822-7177.

HSU, Chia-Wen; Peterborough Clinic, 26 Hospital Dr, Peterborough ON K9J 7C3; Mem'90; CCFP; FCFP; (705)740-6886

HSU, David H; Vancouver Gen Hosp, 855 12th Ave W, Vancouver BC V5Z 1M9; UBC'77; Staff Palliative Care Unit, Vancouver General Hospital - Centennial Pavillion; (604)875-4715

HSU, David H J; Thunderbird Family Practice, D114-20159 88 Ave, Langley BC V1M 0A4; Wes'93; CCFP; (604)888-6220; Fax. (604)882-1383.

HSU, David M; 404-1100 Sheppard Ave E, North York ON M2K 2W1; Qns'05; CCFP; (416)222-0660; Fax. (416)222-9238.

HSU, Fred H C; Abbotsford Reg Hosp & Cancer C, 32900 Marshall Rd, Abbotsford BC V2S 0C2; Ott'03; FRCPC; RadOncol. Staff, Abbotsford Regional Hospital & Cancer Centre; (604)851-4710

HSU, Howard C; 100-739 Lake Bonavista Dr SE, Calgary AB T2J 0N2; Alb'10; (403)271-7763

HSU, Justin W; PO Box 32589 Rpo Aberdeen Cent, Richmond BC V6X 3S1; Man'09; CCFP; (604)629-6655

HSU, Katherine; 107-3825 Sunset St, Burnaby BC V5G 1T4; Wes'00; FRCSC; GenSurg (Laparoscopic Surgery). Staff, Burnaby Hospital; Langs: Mandarin; (604)568-5026; Fax. (604)568-5027.

HSU, Pei-Ti; Crossroads Med Clinic, 350-507 Broadway Ave W, Vancouver BC V5Z 1E6; Vienna (Austria)'97; CCFP; (604)568-7229

HSU, Richard C; Thunderbird Family Practice, D114-20159 88 Ave, Langley BC V1M 0A4; UBC'90; CCFP; CCFP(E.M.); (604)888-6220; Fax. (604)882-1383.

HSU, Tina Y; BC Cancer Agency, 600 10th Ave W, Vancouver BC V5Z 4E6; McM'06; FRCPC; IntMed; MedOncol. Staff, BC Cancer Agency Vancouver Centre; (604)877-6000

HSU, Vivienne; Scarborough Hosp-Birchmount, 3030 Birchmount Rd, Scarborough ON M1W 3W3; Tor'93; FRCPC; Anes. Staff, The Scarborough Hospital - Birchmount Campus; (416)495-2400

HSUEN, John S C; 67 Churchill Ave, North York ON M2N 1Y8; Madras (India)'63; MB BS; ABPeds; FRCPC; Peds. Ac Staff, North York General Hospital - Branson Division; Asst Prof, University of Toronto; Langs: Chinese; Cantonese; Mandarin; Japanese; (416)222-7358; Fax. (416)221-5624.

HTUN, Ye; 203-2825 Clearbrook Rd, Abbotsford BC V2T 6S3; Myanmar (Burma)'82; MB BS; (604)852-1567; Fax. (604)852-8949.

HU, Fang; South Simcoe Medical, 239 Holland St W, Bradford ON L3Z 1H9; Zhong Shan (China)'84; CCFP; Langs: Chinese; (905)775-4863; Fax. (905)775-8351.

HU, John H W; 118-10151 No. 3 Rd, Richmond BC V7A 4R6; UBC'01; CCFP; (604)273-9920

HU, Lin Aung (Rex); Albany Med Clinic, 807 Broadview Ave, Toronto ON M4K 2P8; Inst of Medicine II (Burma)'00; CCFP; (416)461-9471; Fax. (416)461-2710.

HU, Richard W; Foothills Med Centre, MT 0492-1403 29 St NW, Calgary AB T2N 2T9; Mem'84; FRCSC; OrthSurg (Spine Surgery). Staff, Foothills Medical Centre; University of Calgary; (403)944-2036; Fax. (403)270-8004.

HU, Weimin; Trillium Hlth Ctr-Mississauga, 100 Queensway W, Mississauga ON L5B 1B8; Hebei (China)'83; PhD; FRCPC; AnatPath. Staff Lab Med, Trillium Health Centre - Mississauga; Lecturer, University of Toronto; Langs: Chinese; (905)848-7580 x2011

HU, William; Scarborough Hosp-Birchmount, 3030 Birchmount Rd, Scarborough ON M1W 3W3; Tor'85; ATLS; ACLS; Staff, The Scarborough Hospital - Birchmount Campus; (416)495-2600

HU, William Y; Foothills Med Centre, 1403 29 St NW, Calgary AB T2N 2T9; Alb'87; FRCPC; DiagRad (Neuro Radiology). Staff Diag Imaging, Foothills Medical Centre; (403)944-2520; Fax. (403)670-1687.

HU, Xiao W; MUHC-Royal Victoria Hosp, M9 05-687 av des Pins O, Montreal QC H3A 1A1; McG'03; FRCPC; IntMed; Endocrin&Metab. Staff, McGill University Health Centre - Royal Victoria Hospital; (514)843-1659

HUA, Johnson T S; 663 Coronation Blvd, Cambridge ON N1R 3G4; National (Taiwan)'61; FAAP; FRCPC; Peds. Staff, Cambridge Memorial Hospital; (519)623-6010

HUAN, Susan D; 3330 Hospital Dr NW, Calgary AB T2N 4N1; Cebu (Philippines)'80; FRCPC; IntMed; MedOncol. Staff, Rockyview General Hospital.

HUANG, Alice; Nicola Med Dental Bldg, 200-321 Nicola St, Kamloops BC V2C 6G6; Tor'88; (250)372-5522; Fax. (250)372-8412.

HUANG, Allen R; The Ottawa Hosp-Civic Campus, 678-1053 Carling Ave, Ottawa ON K1Y 4E9; McG'84; ABIM; BSc; FRC; FACP; FRCPC; IntMed; GeriatricMed. Staff, The Ottawa Hospital - Civic Campus; Langs: French; (613)761-4795

HUANG, Amy Y; Burnaby Med Centre, M37-4277 Kingsway, Burnaby BC V5H 3Z2; UBC'02; Langs: Mandarin; (604)438-9991; Fax. (604)438-9960.

HUANG, Ann C; North Burlington Med Centre, 18-1960 Appleby Line, Burlington ON L7L 0B7; Wes'83; CCFP; CCFP(E.M.); (905)319-2000; Fax. (905)319-6292; ann@pol.net.

HUANG, Anne A; Academic Family Medicine, 3311 Fairlight Dr, Saskatoon SK S7M 3Y5; UBC'07; CCFP; (306)655-4200

HUANG, Annie A; The Hosp for Sick Children, 555 University Ave, Toronto ON M5G 1X8; Tor'95; FRCPC; Peds (Hematology). Staff Hematol Oncol, The Hospital For Sick Children; Asst Prof Peds, University of Toronto; (416)813-7360; annie.huang@sickkids.ca.

HUANG, Brian C; Rockyview Gen Hosp, 7007 14 St SW, Calgary AB T2V 1P9; Dal'03; BSc; CCFP; Staff, Rockyview General Hospital; Langs: Mandarin; (403)281-2020; Fax. (403)943-8411.

HUANG, Carol T L; Alberta Children's Hosp, 2888 Shaganappi Trail NW, Calgary AB T3B 6A8; Tor'96; BSc; PhD; FRCPC; Peds; Endocrin&Metab. Staff, Alberta Children's Hospital; (403)955-7819

HUANG, David J T; St Michael's Hosp, 30 Bond St, Toronto ON M5B 1W8; Qns'08; IntMed. Staff, St Michael's Hospital; (416)360-4000

HUANG, Eileen Y; Trillium Hlth Ctr-Mississauga, 100 Queensway W, Mississauga ON L5B 1B8; Tor'76; FRCPC; Anes; IntMed. Staff, Trillium Health Centre - Mississauga; (905)848-7628; Fax. (905)848-0348.

HUANG, Eleanor C Y; AIM Clinic North, 302-235 North Centre Rd, London ON N5X 4E7; Cal'78; CCFP; FCFP; Langs: Chinese; (519)645-2444; Fax. (519)645-2545.

HUANG, Eric M; HSC-Faculty of Medicine, 3330-3330 Hospital Dr NW, Calgary AB T2N 4N1; Alb'06; FRCSC; OrthSurg. (403)402-5991

HUANG, Felicia; Whitehorse Gen Hosp, 5 Hospital Rd, Whitehorse YT Y1A 3H7; Ott'95; MSc; FRCSC; GenSurg. Staff, Whitehorse General Hospital; Langs: French; (867)393-8907

HUANG, Fleur; Cross Cancer Institute, 11560 University Ave NW, Edmonton AB T6G 1Z2; McG'03; FRCPC; RadOncol. Staff, Cross Cancer Institute; (780)432-8516; Fax. (780)432-8380.

HUANG, Gloria W S; 460-5525 West Boulevard, Vancouver BC V6M 3W6; Tor'85; Ac Staff, Vancouver General Hospital - Centennial Pavillion; Vis Staff, BC Women's Hospital & Health Centre; Asst Prof, University of British Columbia; (604)263-3589; Fax. (604)263-3589.

HUANG, Harvey Y; Rouge Valley-Ajax & Pickering, 580 Harwood Ave S, Ajax ON L1S 2J4; Tor'95; FRCPC; Anes. Staff, Rouge Valley Health System - Ajax & Pickering Health Centre Site; Langs: Taiwanese; (905)683-2320 x1288; harvey.huang@hotmail.com.

HUANG, Henry Y; Ajax Med Arts Bldg, 106-601 Harwood Ave S, Ajax ON L1S 2J5; Tor'93; BA; MD; FRCS; FRCSC; Otol (Facial Plastic Surgery). Staff Surg, Rouge Valley Health System - Centenary Health Centre Site; Staff Surg, The Scarborough Hospital - General Campus; Langs: Taiwanese; French; (905)428-8862; Fax. (905)427-9174.

HUANG, Ian T; 102-2210 2 St SW, Calgary AB T2S 3C3; Alb'82; BMedSci; AB; FRCSC; Otol (Allergy). Staff, Foothills Medical Centre; Staff, Alberta Children's Hospital; University of Calgary; (403)244-6700; Ian.Huang@playstarmusic.com.

HUANG, Jane; Sunnybrook Hlth Sciences Ctre, 2075 Bayview Ave, Toronto ON M4N 3M5; Tor'89; FRCPC; Anes; Critical Care Medicine. Staff, Sunnybrook Health Sciences Centre; (416)480-4864

HUANG, John T; PO Box 67035 Rpo Northland Vlg, Calgary AB T2L 2L2; Alb'87; DAB; FRCSC; Ophth. Clin Prof Ophth/Dir Undergraduate Medical Eductaion Dept of Ophth, University Of Calgary; (403)286-3335; Fax. (403)273-3668.

HUANG, Lennox; McMaster University, HSC 3A-1280 Main St W, Hamilton ON L8S 4K1; Tor'97; FAAP; Dep Chief Peds, Hamilton Health Sciences Centre - McMaster Children's Hospital; Dept Head Peds, McMaster University; (905)521-2100 x75697; Fax. (905)570-8967.

HUANG, Li Ming; 570 Mountainview Sq, Kitimat BC V8C 2N2; Alb'94; Staff/Chief of Staff, Kitimat Hospital & Health Centre; (250)632-2118; Fax. (250)632-5578.

HUANG, Ling Ling; King Street Med Arts Centre, 401-71 King St W, Mississauga ON L5B 4A2; Cal'81; CCFP; Staff, Trillium Health Centre - Mississauga; Med Dir, Cawthra Garden Long Term Care; Med Dir, Westoak Village Long Term Care; Physician, Chelsey Park Nursing Home; Langs: Mandarin; Cantonese; Taiwanese; (905)273-9793; Fax. (905)273-7054.

HUANG, Louis; Rouge Valley-Centenary HC, 2867 Ellesmere Rd, Scarborough ON M1E 4B9; Tor'94; FRCPC; Anes. Staff, Rouge Valley Health System - Centenary Health Centre Site; Langs: Mandarin; Taiwanese; Cantonese; (416)281-7454; Fax. (416)281-7453; sleepydr@yahoo.com.

HUANG, Madeline W C; 100-5 Fairview Mall Dr, North York ON M2J 2Z1; Tor'90; FRCPC; DiagRad. (416)499-3559; Fax. (416)499-4631.

HUANG, Max; 402-100 Humber College Blvd, Etobicoke ON M9V 5G4; Qns'00; FRCPC; IntMed (Sleep Medicine); Respir. Staff, William Osler Health System - Etobicoke General Hospital; (416)640-1755

HUANG, Patrick O; 1550-4380 No 3 Rd, Richmond BC V6X 3V7; (Hong Kong)'71; MB BS; ABPeds; Langs: Cantonese; (604)273-9899

HUANG, Paul B T; Vancouver Gen Hosp, 899 12th Ave W, Vancouver BC V5Z 1M9; UBC'82; FRCPC; EmergMed. Staff, Royal Columbian Hospital; Staff, Vancouver General Hospital - Centennial Pavillion; Langs: Cantonese; (604)875-4111

HUANG, Pein-Pein; Montfort Hosp, 713 Montreal Rd, Ottawa ON K1K 0T2; Manchester (England)'80; MB ChB; FRCPC; Peds (Neonatology). Staff, Montfort Hospital; Langs: Cantonese; Chinese; Fookien; (613)748-4950

HUANG, Peter T S; Bow River Prof Centre, 313-4411 16 Ave NW, Calgary AB T3B 0M3; Alb'82; FRCSC; Ophth (Cornea/External Disease). Staff, Calgary Health Region; Clin Prof, University of Calgary; (403)286-3335; Fax. (403)286-3316.

HUANG, Qingli L; Oakville Med Clinic, 307-331 Sheddon Ave, Oakville ON L6J 1X8; McG'96; BSc; FRCPC; IntMed (Diabetes); Endocrin&Metab. Staff, Halton Healthcare Services Corporation - Oakville Site; Langs: Mandarin; (905)338-0550; Fax. (905)338-3187.

HUANG, Shih-Han S; London HSC-South St, PO Box 5375 Stn B 800 Commissioners Rd E, London ON N6A 4G5; Ott'05; FRCPC; IntMed; Nephrol. Staff, London Health Sciences Centre - South Street; (519)685-8361

HUANG, Shirley C; The Ottawa Hosp-Civic Campus, 1053 Carling Ave, Ottawa ON K1Y 4E9; UBC'07; IntMed. Staff Geriatric Med, The Ottawa Hospital - Civic Campus; (613)761-4195

HUANG, Simon H K; Burrard Health Bldg, 501-1160 Burrard St, Vancouver BC V6Z 2E8; Sask'71; FRCPC; IntMed. Ac Staff, Providence Health Care - St Paul's Hospital; (604)684-4551

HUANG, Virgil Y F; Cassandra Clinic, 2044-2048 Victoria Park Ave, North York ON M1R 1V2; Chicago (USA)'03; ABPeds; Langs: Chinese; Mandarin; (416)331-9111; Fax. (416)331-9050.

HUANG, Vivian W; Univ Hlth Network-Toronto Western Hosp, 326-399 Bathurst St, Toronto ON M5T 2S8; Qns'07; FRCPC; IntMed; Gastroent. Staff, Toronto Western Hospital - University Health Network; (416)603-5724

HUANG, Weei-Yuarn; DJ MacKenzie Bldg, 5788 University Ave, Halifax NS B3H 1V8; Taipei (Taiwan)'89; ABPath; FRCPC; AnatPath. Langs: Chinese; (902)473-7665; Fax. (902)473-1049.

HUANG, Yu Lun; York Medical Green Lane, 18120 Yonge St, East Gwillimbury ON L9N 0J3; Tor'95; CCFP; (905)868-9243; Fax. (905)836-1597; yulun0110@yahoo.ca.

HUARD, Genevieve; CHUM-Hop St-Luc, 1058 rue Saint-Denis, Montreal QC H2X 3J4; Mon'06; Gastroent; IntMed. Staff, Centre Hospitalier l'Université De Montréal (CHUM) - Hôpital Saint-luc; (514)890-8000

HUARD, Joseph; Clinique Med Loretteville, 250-11000 boul de l'Ormiere, Quebec QC G2B 5S1; Laval'67; CSPQ; FRCPC; Derm. ac Staff, Centre Hospitalier Universitaire De Québec - Pavillon De St-françois-d'assise; Conférencier, Université Laval; (418)842-6556

HUARD, Pierre J; Harmony Med Centre, 106-152 Cleopatra Dr, Nepean ON K2G 5X2; Ott'75; FRCSC; ObstGyn (Perinatology). Att Staff, The Ottawa Hospital - Civic Campus; Asst Prof, University of Ottawa; (613)729-9178; Fax. (613)729-4633.

HUARD, Verilibe; Hop du Sacre-Coeur de Mtl, 5400 boul Gouin O, Montreal QC H4J 1C5; Mon'99; CCFP; CCFP(E.M.); Staff, Hôpital du Sacre-Coeur de Montréal; (514)335-1252; Fax. (514)335-1753.

HUBACEK, Jaroslav; Saint John Reg Hosp, PO Box 2100 400 University Ave, Saint John NB E2L 4L2; Comenius (Slovakia)'97; FRCPC; IntMed; Cardiol. Staff, Saint John Regional Hospital; (506)648-6000

HUBAND, Donald M; Guelph Gen Hosp, 115 Delhi St, Guelph ON N1E 4J4; Wes'68; FSOGC; FRCSC; ObstGyn. Staff, Guelph General Hospital; (519)837-6440

HUBAND, Louisa A; Medical Office, 105-840 Coxwell Ave, East York ON M4C 5T2; Man'02; CCFP; Staff Obst Privileges/Dir Residency Prog Family Practice, Toronto East General Hospital Inc; (416)469-6464

HUBAY, Stacey A; Grand River Hosp-KW Hlth Ctre, PO Box 9056 Stn C 835 King St W, Kitchener ON N2G 1G3; Tor'97; FRCPC; IntMed; MedOncol. Staff, Grand River Hospital - Kitchener/Waterloo Health Centre; (519)749-4300

HUBBES, Claudia H; 100-11 Rosemount Ave, Ottawa ON K1Y 4R8; McM'92; CCFP; FCFP; Asst Prof Med, University of Ottawa; Langs: English; French; German; (613)724-5852; Fax. (613)724-9965.

HUBER, Adam M; IWK Health Centre, PO Box 9700 Rpo CSC 5850 University Ave, Halifax NS B3K 6R8; UBC'93; FRCPC; Peds (Pediatric Rheumatology); Rheum. Staff, IWK Health Centre; (902)470-8827; Fax. (902)470-7217; adam.huber@iwk.nshealth.ca.

HUBER, Alan G; The Richmond Hosp, 7000 Westminster Hwy, Richmond BC V6X 1A2; Otago (New Zealand)'83; MB ChB; FRCPC; EmergMed. Staff, Richmond Hospital; (604)278-9711; Fax. (604)244-5194.

HUBER, Christopher J; The Richmond Hosp, 7000 Westminster Hwy, Richmond BC V6X 1A2; Cal'77; FFARCS; FRCPC; Anes. Staff, Richmond Hospital; (604)278-9711

HUBER, Douglas R; RCMP Health Services, 11140 109 St NW, Edmonton AB T5G 2T4; Sask'87; CCFP; FCFP; Staff Health Services, Royal Canadian Mounted Police; (780)412-5150; Fax. (780)412-5174.

HUBER, Joelene F H; Paediatric Ambulatory Clinic, 2F-61 Queen St E, Toronto ON M5C 2T2; McM'05; FRCPC; Peds (Developmental Pediatrics). (416)867-3655

HUBER, Jonathan D; Kingston Gen Hosp, 76 Stuart St, Kingston ON K7L 2V7; Qns'06; FRCSC; ObstGyn. Staff Obst & Gyn, Kingston General Hospital; (613)548-1372

HUBER, Keith D; Royal Alexandra Hosp, 10240 Kingsway NW, Edmonton AB T5H 3V9; Alb'10; LMCC; CCFP; Staff, Royal Alexandra Hospital; (780)735-4201

HUBER, Warren N; Humboldt Med Clinic, PO Box 220, Humboldt SK S0K 2A0; Sask'70; Chief Medical Staff, Humboldt District Hospital; (306)682-2618; Fax. (306)682-4499; humboldtclinic@sasktel.net.

HUBERMAN, Marvin; Gain Med Centre, 1199 Austin Ave, Coquitlam BC V3K 3P4; McG'72; Langs: English; French; (604)939-7345; Fax. (604)939-7781; mrhub2001@shaw.ca.

HUBERT, Amelie; CSSS des Iles, 430 ch Principal, Cap-aux-Meules QC G4T 1R9; Sher'04; CCFP; Staff, Hôpital de l'Archipel; (418)986-2121

HUBERT, Christophe; Hop Jean-Talon, 1385 rue Jean-Talon E, Montreal QC H2E 1S6; Paris (France)'95; Staff, CSSS du Coeur de l'Isle Hôpital Jean-Talon; (514)495-6767

HUBINETTE, Maria M; Ctre for Hlth Educ Scholarship, 910 10th Ave W, Vancouver BC V5Z 1M9; UBC'03; CCFP; Staff Centre for Health Education Scholarship, Vancouver General Hospital - Centennial Pavillion; (604)875-4111 x68718

HUBLALL, Ronald V; South West Health, 60 Vancouver St, Yarmouth NS B5A 2P5; Matamoros (Mexico)'98; (902)742-3541; Fax. (902)742-0369.

HUBLER, Dana G; Port Alice Health Centre, PO Box 188 1090 Marine Dr, Port Alice BC V0N 2N0; Cal'02; CCFP; (250)636-2221

HUBNER, Rurik; Dunsmuir Med Clinic, PO Box 719 2765A Dunsmuir Ave, Cumberland BC V0R 1S0; Munich (Germany)'93; CCFP; (250)336-2208

HUCAL, Sandie G; 126 3 Ave W PO Box 1913 Stn Main, Cochrane AB T4C 1B7; McG'93; BSc; CCFP; (403)889-9059; Fax. (403)206-7357.

HUCHET, Emmanuelle; Clinique Med l'Actuel, 1001 boul de Maisonneuve E, Montreal QC H2L 4P9; Sher'96; (514)524-1001

HUCKELL, Caitlin L; Surrey Med Arts Bldg, 116-13798 94A Ave, Surrey BC V3V 1N1; UBC'97; FRCSC; ObstGyn. (604)580-1210; Fax. (604)580-1230.

HUCKELL, Victor F; Gordon & Leslie Diamond HCC, 9F-2775 Laurel St, Vancouver BC V5Z 1M9; UBC'69; BSc; DABIM; FACC; FESC; FRCPC; IntMed; Cardiol. Consultant, BC Children's Hospital; Consultant, BC Women's Hospital & Health Centre; Ac Staff Cardiol, Vancouver General Hospital - Centennial Pavillion; Staff, Gordon & Leslie Diamond Health Care Centre; Clin Prof Med, University of British Columbia; (604)875-5483; Fax. (604)875-4358; huckell@uniserve.com.

HUCKER, Stephen J C; 101-427 Princess St, Kingston ON K7L 5S9; Newcastle (England)'70; MB BS; MRCPsy; FRCPsy; FRCPC; Psy (Forensic Psychiatry). Staff, Centre for Addiction & Mental Health (CAMH) - College Street Site; Prof, University of Toronto; (416)533-6455; Fax. (416)533-6455.

HUCULAK, George E; Byron Street Med Centre, 200-320 Byron St S, Whitby ON L1N 4P8; RCS (Ireland)'90; Langs: Ukrainian; French; (905)668-5835; Fax. (905)668-8942.

HUDA, Noureen; London HSC-University Hosp, PO Box 5339 Stn B 339 Windermere Rd, London ON N6A 5A5; Ajman (United Arab Emirates)'06; FRCPC; IntMed. Staff Internal Med, London Health Sciences Centre - University Hospital; (519)685-8500 x19283

HUDAK, Alan P; Medical Arts Bldg, 17 Dunedin St, Orillia ON L3V 5T3; McM'78; FRCPC; Peds. (705)327-9188; Fax. (705)327-9189.

HUDANI, Sayeeda A; Royal Columbian Hosp, 330 Columbia St E, New Westminster BC V3L 3W7; Dal'90; Staff, Royal Columbian Hospital; (604)506-5965

HUDEC, Mary-Ann; 7504-5909 Veterans Memorial La, Halifax NS B3H 2E2; Wes'84; FRCPC; Psy. (902)473-4409; Fax. (902)473-1422.

HUDES, Elliot T; The Credit Valley Hosp, 2200 Eglinton Ave W, Mississauga ON L5M 2N1; Tor'82; FRCPC; Anes. Staff, The Credit Valley Hospital; (905)813-4466

HUDGEL, David W; Misericordia Health Centre, 370-99 Cornish Ave, Winnipeg MB R3C 1A2; Iowa City (USA)'67; Staff Sleep Disorder Centre, Misericordia Health Centre; (204)788-8364

HUDICOURT, Martine; CSSS du Nord de Lanaudière, 1000 boul Sainte-Anne, St-Charles-Brromee QC J6E 6J2; Port-au-Prince (Haiti)'91; CCFP; Staff, Centre Hospitalier Régional de Lanaudière; Langs: Creole; English; (450)759-8222

HUDLICKY, Ivo J; Lower Mainland Drug Freedom, 25 Blackwood St, New Westminster BC V3L 2T3; Qns'73; CCFP; Staff, Royal Columbian Hospital; Staff, Lower Mainland Drug Freedom Clinic; (604)520-1068

HUDOBA DE BADYN, Monika; Vancouver Gen Hosp, 1505-855 12th Ave W, Vancouver BC V5Z 1M9; Bratislava (Slovakia)'87; FRCPC; HemPath. Staff, Vancouver General Hospital - Centennial Pavillion; (604)875-4381

HUDOBA DE BADYN, Peter; 160-5172 Kingsway, Burnaby BC V5H 2E8; Komensky (Slovakia)'82; FRCSC; Neursurg. (604)435-9151

HUDON, Andre; Clinique Med Saint-Rodrigue, 5000 3e av O, Quebec QC G1H 7J1; Laval'69; Staff, Centre Hospitalier Universitaire de Québec (CHUQ) - Siege Social; Université Laval; (418)623-9172

HUDON, Catherine; CSSS de Chicoutimi, 305 rue Saint-Vallier, Chicoutimi QC G7H 5H6; Laval'96; MSc; CCFP; Staff, Complexe hospitalier de la Sagamie; Prof, Universite de Sherbrooke; (418)541-1079; Fax. (418)541-1129.

HUDON, Claire; CHUQ-Ctr Hosp Univ Laval, R1742-2705 boul Laurier, Quebec QC G1V 4G2; Laval'82; FRCPC; Peds. ac Staff, Centre Hospitalier Universitaire de Quebec-CHUL; Langs: English; (418)654-2282; Fax. (418)654-2771.

HUDON, Claude; Centre de Sante du Littoral, 110-822 boul Sainte-Anne, Rimouski QC G5M 1J5; Laval'71; OrthSurg (P.Q.). (418)723-8680

HUDON, Eveline; Ctr Hosp de Verdun, 4000 boul Lasalle, Verdun QC H4G 2A3; Mon'85; CCFP; FCFP; Staff, Centre Hospitalier de Verdun; (514)765-7325

HUDON, Francois; Plyclinique Med Concorde, 300 boul de la Concorde E, Laval QC H7G 2E6; Mon'87; FRCPC; DiagRad. Staff, Hopital de la Cite de la santé; (450)668-7376; Fax. (450)668-8300.

HUDON, J J Gilles; 112 av de Charente, Saint-Lambert QC J4S 1K3; Laval'67; DABR; FRCPC; DiagRad (Administration). (450)671-6632

HUDON, Jean; 209 rue de la Montagne CP 1767, La Pocatiere QC G0R 1Z0; Mon'80; (418)856-4292

HUDON, Lynda; Hôpital Ste-Justine, 3175 ch Cote-Sainte-Catherine, Montreal QC H3T 1C5; Mon'91; FRCSC; ObstGyn (Maternal Fetal Medicine). Staff, Hôpital Ste-Justine; (514)345-4705

HUDON, Marcel; Pavillon Rosemont, 5689 boul Rosemont, Montreal QC H1T 2H1; Laval'66; Psy. Staff, Hopital Maisonneuve-Rosemont; (514)252-3400 x4780; Fax. (514)252-3810.

HUDON, Marck P J; 502-1150 Marine Dr, North Vancouver BC V7P 1S8; UBC'95; BSc; MSc; Langs: Bilingual(English/French); (604)971-5153

HUDON, Mark E; Foothills Med Centre, 1403 29 St NW, Calgary AB T2N 2T9; McG'87; FRCPC; DiagRad. Staff Diag Imaging, Foothills Medical Centre; (403)944-1969

HUDON, Martin; Clinique Med Elysee, 451 rue des Champs-Elysees, Chicoutimi QC G7H 2W3; Laval'83; ac Staff, Complexe hospitalier de la Sagamie; (418)545-2323; Fax. (418)545-2756.

HUDON, Nathalie; Clinique Med Elysees, 451 rue des Champs-Elysees, Chicoutimi QC G7H 2W3; Laval'87; Langs: English; (418)545-2323

HUDON, Pascale; Centre Hosp Honore-Mercier, 2750 boul Laframboise, Saint-Hyacinthe QC J2S 4Y8; Sher'01; CCFP; Staff, Centre Hospitalier Honore-Mercier; (450)771-3333; Fax. (450)771-3246.

HUDON, Paul-Andre; Clinique Med Deux-Montagnes, 201 9e av, Deux-Montagnes QC J7R 3M1; Mon'77; Staff, Hôpital de Saint-Eustache; (450)472-7520 x6; Fax. (450)472-0886.

HUDON, Sylvie R; 4F-347 Preston St, Ottawa ON K1S 3J4; Ott'93; CCFP; Langs: Spanish; English; (613)727-2816

HUDSON, Carl R; Miramichi Med Arts Centre, 679 King George Hwy, Miramichi NB E1V 1N9; Mem'75; CCFP; FCFP; (506)627-2729; Fax. (506)627-2728.

HUDSON, Christopher C C; Univ of Ottawa Heart Institute, 40 Ruskin St, Ottawa ON K1Y 4W7; Dal'03; FRCPC; Anes. Staff, University of Ottawa Heart Institute; (613)761-4379

HUDSON, Craig J; Alexandra Marine & Gen Hosp, 120 Napier St, Goderich ON N7A 1W5; Tor'88; FRCPC; Psy. Staff, Alexandra Marine & General Hospital; (905)668-5881

HUDSON, Darren A; University of Alberta Hosp, 12-8440 112 St NW, Edmonton AB T6G 2B7; Cal'96; FRCPC; IntMed; Critical Care Medicine. Staff, University of Alberta Hospital; (780)407-6755

HUDSON, Emmanuel W; Cross Cancer Institute, 11560 University Ave NW, Edmonton AB T6G 1Z2; Mem'78; FRCPC; DiagRad; NuclearMed. Staff, Cross Cancer Institute; (780)432-8220

HUDSON, Gregory N; Hudson Med Centre, 11-605 K.L.O. Rd, Kelowna BC V1Y 8E7; Man'89; (250)763-0999

HUDSON, Jacqueline T; Dr Jacqueline Hudson Inc, 2212 Kitchener St, Vancouver BC V5L 2X2; UBC'06; FRCPC; Anes. Staff, Vancouver General Hospital - Centennial Pavillion.

HUDSON, Jean E; Credit Valley Prof Bldg, 205-2300 Eglinton Ave W, Mississauga ON L5M 2V8; Qns'88; CCFP; FCFP; Ac Staff, The Credit Valley Hospital; (905)820-8144; Fax. (905)820-1631.

HUDSON, Jordan K; The Ottawa Hosp-Civic Campus, 1053 Carling Ave, Ottawa ON K1Y 4E9; Wes'03; FRCPC; Anes. Staff, The Ottawa Hospital - Civic Campus; (613)722-7000

HUDSON, Linda G; Miramichi Med Arts Centre, 679 King George Hwy, Miramichi NB E1V 1N9; Mem'76; (506)627-2729; Fax. (506)627-2728.

HUDSON, Marie; SMBD Jewish Gen Hosp, 3755 ch Cote-Sainte-Catherine, Montreal QC H3T 1E2; McG'96; FRCPC; IntMed; Rheum. Staff, Sir Mortimer B Davis Jewish General; (514)340-8222 x3476; Fax. (514)340-7906; marie.hudson@mcgill.ca.

HUDSON, Nancy; Nicola Med Dental Bldg, 201-321 Nicola St, Kamloops BC V2C 6G6; McG'89; FRCPC; IntMed; Rheum. (250)377-3892; Fax. (250)377-3896.

HUDSON, Neil C; The Medical Centre, PO Box 4200 Stn Main 707 Charlotte St, Peterborough ON K9J 7B3; Cape Town (South Africa)'85; MB ChB; CCFP; (705)876-4517; Fax. (705)742-7076.

HUDSON, Patricia; Direction de la Sante Publique, 1255 rue Beauregard, Longueuil QC J4K 2M3; Mon'85; FRCPC; CommunMed. (450)928-6777 x3148

HUDSON, Richard E K; James Bay Med Centre, 547 Michigan St, Victoria BC V8V 1S5; Alb'74; CCFP; (250)388-6811

HUDSON, Robert J; Clinical Sciences Building, 8-120-152 University Campus NW, Edmonton AB T6G 2G3; Man'77; DABA; LMCC; FRCPC; Anes (Cardiac Anesthesia). Staff Anes & Pain Med, University of Alberta Hospital; Clin Prof Anes & Pain Med, University of Alberta; (780)407-8861; Fax. (780)407-3200.

HUDSON, Robert W; Kingston Gen Hosp, 76 Stuart St, Kingston ON K7L 2V7; Tor'66; PhD; FRCPC; IntMed (Andrology)., Kingston General Hospital; Consultant, Hotel-Dieu Hospital; Prof, Queen's University; (613)533-2973; Fax. (613)533-6574; hudsonr@queensu.ca.

HUDSON, Sharlene M; Vulcan Med Clinic, PO Box 419, Vulcan AB T0L 2B0; Alb'03; CCFP; (403)485-2216; sharlenehudson@hotmail.com.

HUDSON, Shauna G; Sun Country Health Region, PO Box 2003 Stn Main, Weyburn SK S4H 2Z9; Sask'86; FRCPC; CommunMed (Public Health);CCFP; FCFP; (306)842-8659

HUDSON, Stephen P; Victoria Fertility Centre, 207-4400 Chatterton Way, Victoria BC V8X 5J2; Cape Town (South Africa)'78; FRCSC; ObstGyn (Infertility). Staff, Victoria General Hospital; Staff, Royal Jubilee Hospital; Asst Prof ObstGyn, University of British Columbia; (250)704-0024; Fax. (250)704-0034.

HUDSPITH, Elizabeth; 3423 Normandy St, Saskatoon SK S7M 3R1; Birmingham (England)'62; MB ChB; (306)384-1140; Fax. (306)384-1209.

HUDY, Simon M P; Properties Med Clinic, 5102 Rundlehorn Dr NE, Calgary AB T1Y 1C1; Cal'83; CCFP; Staff, Properties Medical Clinic; (403)280-2700; Fax. (403)285-2641.

HUEBEL, Stephen C; Rouge Valley-Centenary HC, 2867 Ellesmere Rd, Scarborough ON M1E 4B9; Tor'88; Staff, Rouge Valley Health System - Centenary Health Centre Site; (416)898-0061

HUEBERT, David M; Pan Am Sports Med Centre, 75 Poseidon Bay, Winnipeg MB R3M 3E4; Man'89; FRCSC; OrthSurg. Staff, Health Sciences Centre; (204)925-1550

HUEBERT, Helmut T; Winnipeg Clinic, 425 St Mary Ave, Winnipeg MB R3C 0N2; Man'58; FRCSC; OrthSurg (Bone Tumour). Staff, Health Sciences Centre; Staff, Concordia General Hospital; Langs: German; (204)957-3261; Fax. (204)947-2671.

HUEBSCH, Lothar B; The Ottawa Hosp-Gen Campus, 7208-501 Smyth Rd, Ottawa ON K1H 8L6; Ott'75; Hem; IntMed. Assoc Staff, Children's Hospital of Eastern Ontario (CHEO); Assoc Staff, Canadian Forces Health Services Centre; Ac Staff Med, The Ottawa Hospital - General Campus; Prof Med, University of Ottawa; (613)737-8158; Fax. (613)737-8861; lhuebsch@ottawahospital.on.ca.

HUEHN, Linda L; Ground Floor, 458 MacLaren St, Ottawa ON K1R 5K6; Tor'82; FRCPC; Psy (Psychotherapy). Staff Consulting, The Ottawa Hospital - General Campus; (613)233-8271

HUEN, K M Nicoletta; Citygate Med Centre, 107C-3939 Duke of York Blvd, Mississauga ON L5B 4N2; McG'95; CCFP; Langs: Chinese; (905)361-0970; Fax. (905)361-0971.

HUET, Madeleine; Clinique Med Saint-Luc, 264 boul Saint-Luc, St-Jean-Sur-Richel QC J2W 1C3; Mon'77; (450)348-6126; Fax. (450)348-4163.

HUET, Marc-Andre; CLSC Frontenac, 17 rue Notre-Dame O, Thetford Mines QC G6G 1J1; Mon'75; (418)338-3511; Fax. (418)338-1668; marcandrehuet@ssss.gouv.qc.ca.

HUEY, Henry H L; 100-5791 No. 3 Rd, Richmond BC V6X 2C9; UBC'80; FRCPC; DiagRad. (604)278-9152; Fax. (604)278-9291.

HUFF, Lynn; Vancouver Family Health Centre, 100-2732 Hastings St E, Vancouver BC V5K 1Z9; UBC'93; CCFP; (604)253-3166; Fax. (604)253-2048.

HUFF, Hildegard R; 2000-1415 1st Ave W, Owen Sound ON N4K 4K8; McM'78; CCFP; Dir Palliative Care, Grey Bruce Health Services - Owen Sound; (519)470-3030; Fax. (519)370-4052.

HUFFMAN, David A W; Thamesview Family Health Team, 465 Grand Ave E, Chatham ON N7L 1C5; Wes'00; CCFP; (519)352-2686; Fax. (519)352-2176.

HUFFMAN, James L; Foothills Med Centre, 1403 29 St NW, Calgary AB T2N 2T9; Cal'06; FRCPC; EmergMed. Staff, Foothills Medical Centre; (403)944-1405

HUG, Martin B; St Thomas-Elgin Gen Hosp, PO Box 2007 Stn Main 189 Elm St, St Thomas ON N5P 3W2; Tor'95; CCFP; CCFP(E.M.); FCFP; Staff, St Thomas Elgin General Hospital; (519)631-2020; Fax. (519)631-1825.

HUGGETT, Philip M; Lansdowne Prof Bldg, 270-1641 Hillside Ave, Victoria BC V8T 5G1; UBC'79; (250)595-5644; Fax. (250)592-3897.

HUGGINS, David G; 2 Broomhead Rd PO Box 757, Chapleau ON P0M 1K0; Qns'70; Staff, Chapleau General Hospital - Division of Services de santé de Chapleau Health Services; (705)864-0210; hugssrt6@msn.com.

HUGGINS, Joseph E; Don Mills Family Health Team, 200-20 Wynford Dr, North York ON M3C 1J4; Tor'72; Staff, North York General Hospital; (416)444-6161; Fax. (416)444-5792.

HUGGINS, Mary-Anne; Dorothy Ley Hospice, 220 Sherway Dr, Etobicoke ON M9C 0A7; McG'82; BSc; MHSc; CCFP; Lecturer, University of Toronto; (416)626-0116

HUGH, Judith C; University of Alberta Hosp, 5B4 21-8440 112 St NW, Edmonton AB T6G 2B7; McG'83; FRCPC; AnatPath. Staff Lab Med & Path, University of Alberta Hospital; (780)407-2872; Fax. (780)407-3009; judith.hugh@capitalhealth.ca.

HUGHAN, Isabelle C; Upstream Family Medicine, 108-4330 Sunshine Coast Hwy, Sechelt BC V0N 3A1; London (England)'96; MB BS; (604)885-6400; Fax. (604)885-6411.

HUGHES, Adrian M; Lakeshore Med Centre, 3970 Lakeshore Rd, Kelowna BC V1W 1V5; Dal'92; (250)764-8878; Fax. (250)764-0889.

HUGHES, Ariana; PO Box 138, Forest Grove BC V0K 1M0; UBC'99; FRCPC; IntMed.

HUGHES, Barbara L; Haney Prof Bldg, 207-11743 224 St, Maple Ridge BC V2X 6A4; UBC'95; FRCPC; PhysMed&Rehab; IntMed. (604)466-5822

HUGHES, Bevan G; UBC-Dept of Anes, 2449 JPP-910 10th Ave W, Vancouver BC V5Z 1M9; Cal'99; FRCPC; Anes. Langs: Bilingual(English/French).

HUGHES, Brendan J; 1-150 Strickland Rd, Lakefield ON K0L 2H0; Mem'97; BSc; BMedSci; CCFP; FCFP; (705)651-0502; Fax. (705)651-0503.

HUGHES, Brian D; 289 Huron St, Stratford ON N5A 5T3; Wes'00; FRCSC; Otol (Head & Neck Surgery). (519)273-7400; Fax. (519)273-2899.

HUGHES, Carol M E; St Joseph's Health Centre, 30 The Queensway, Toronto ON M6R 1B5; Wes'83; FCFP; MCFP; AddicMed; CGPP; MB; MCPS; CCFP; FCFP; Staff, St Joseph's Health Centre; (416)530-6162; cmehughes@hotmail.com.

HUGHES, Daniel M; IWK Health Centre, PO Box 9700 Rpo CSC 5980 University Ave, Halifax NS B3K 6R8; Dal'73; FRCPC; Peds (Pediatric Respiratory Medicine). Staff, IWK Health Centre; (902)470-8218; Fax. (902)470-7223; dan.hughes@iwk.nshealth.ca.

HUGHES, David A; Whites Road Med Clinic, 5A-750 Oklahoma Dr, Pickering ON L1W 3G9; Tor'77; Court Staff, The Scarborough Hospital - Birchmount Campus; Court Staff, The Scarborough Hospital - General Campus; Court Staff, Rouge Valley Health System - Centenary Health Centre Site; (905)831-8666; Fax. (905)831-8749.

HUGHES, David R; Saint John Reg Hosp, PO Box 2100 Stn Main, Saint John NB E2L 4L2; Tor'82; FRCPC; Anes (Intensive Care). Staff, Saint John Regional Hospital; (506)648-6861

HUGHES, Edward G; One Fertility, 3210 Harvester Rd, Burlington ON L7N 3T1; Liverpool (England)'79; MB ChB; MSc; FRCSC; ObstGyn (Infertility). Langs: English; French; (905)634-4440; Fax. (905)639-3810.

HUGHES, Frances J; Burlington Prof Centre, 409-3155 Harvester Rd, Burlington ON L7N 3V2; Leicester (England)'82; MB ChB; FRCPC; Peds. Staff, St Joseph's Healthcare - Charlton Campus; (905)333-5437; Fax. (905)333-5352.

HUGHES, Jeffrey R; Associate Med Centre, 5016 48 Ave, Taber AB T1G 1R8; Alb'08; CCFP; (403)223-3525; Fax. (403)223-9020.

HUGHES, Jennifer G; Foothills Med Centre, C231-1403 29 St NW, Calgary AB T2N 2T9; McM'03; CCFP; CCFP(E.M.); Staff Emerg Med, Foothills Medical Centre; (403)944-1820; Fax. (403)944-2419.

HUGHES, John B; 210-1255 av Greene, Westmount QC H3Z 2A4; McG'76; Langs: French; (514)488-3697; Fax. (514)488-1790; john.hughes@mcgill.ca.

HUGHES, John M; 601 Martin St, Penticton BC V2A 5L5; McM'78; (250)493-7700; Fax. (250)490-9079.

HUGHES, Kenneth F; Richmond Health Sciences Ctre, 310-6091 Gilbert Rd, Richmond BC V7C 5L9; Cal'77; FRCSC; OrthSurg (Arthroplasty). Staff, Richmond Hospital; Teach Staff, University of British Columbia; (604)273-6148; Fax. (604)273-3421; khrichmondortho@telus.net.

HUGHES, Margaret H; St Mary's Hosp Centre, 3830 av Lacombe, Montreal QC H3T 1M5; Man'86; CCFP; Staff, St Mary's Hospital Centre; (514)345-3511 x3460

HUGHES, Miranda C; New Denver Med Clinic, PO Box 9, New Denver BC V0G 1S0; Wes'88; Ac Staff, Slocan Community Health Centre; (250)358-7211; mhughes@cw.bc.ca.

HUGHES, Owen P; 204-474 Holland Ave, Ottawa ON K1Y 0Z5; Mem'77; MBA; MB; BSc; BMedSci; CCFP; FCFP; Chief Maternal & Newborn Care, Ottawa Health Research Institute; (613)725-1523; Fax. (613)691-0620.

HUGHES, Patricia-Lynn M; Pine Seven Med Centre, 165-4600 Highway 7, Woodbridge ON L4L 4Y7; Tor'78; CCFP; FCFP; (905)856-5757

HUGHES, Peter L; Peterborough Clinic, 103-26 Hospital Dr, Peterborough ON K9J 7C3; Tor'89; FRCPC; Peds. (705)740-6844; Fax. (705)740-6897.

HUGHES, P; 201-112 Queenston St, St Catharines ON L2R 2Z4; Qns'80; FRCPC; IntMed (Medical Oncology). Staff, Niagara Health System - Ontario Street Site; Staff, Niagara Health System - St Catharines General Site; (905)685-8082; Fax. (905)988-5776.

HUGHES, Philip M; Southdale Med Centre, 45 Vermillion Rd, Winnipeg MB R2J 4A1; London (England)'85; DRCOG; LMCC; (204)253-6762; Fax. (204)256-1384.

HUGHES, Rhiannon M; 3-4565 Wallace St, Port Alberni BC V9Y 3Y3; Tor'86; FRCPC; Peds; MedGenetics. Ac Staff, West Coast General Hospital; (250)724-3233; Fax. (250)724-3238; pediatricsgenetics@telus.net.

HUGHES, Robin J; Regina Qu'Appelle Hr-Pasqua, 4101 Dewdney Ave, Regina SK S4T 1A5; Sask'96; CCFP; CCFP(E.M.); FCFP; Staff, Pasqua Hospital; (306)766-2238

HUGHES, Shannon M; Foothills Med Centre, C231-1403 29 St NW, Calgary AB T2N 2T9; Cal'99; CCFP; CCFP(E.M.); Staff, Foothills Medical Centre; (403)944-1820; shannonhughes@telus.net.

HUGHES, Sheila L; College Plaza, 205-8215 112 St NW, Edmonton AB T6G 2C8; Alb'76; BMedSci; Ac Staff, Royal Alexandra Hospital; Assoc Prof Family Med, University of Alberta; (780)492-3622; Fax. (780)492-8191.

HUGHES, Tracy; Two Rivers FHT-Hespeler Med Cl, B12-350 Conestoga Blvd, Cambridge ON N1R 7L7; McM'96; CCFP; FCFP; (519)629-4615 x224

HUGHES, William G; Kawartha Cardiology Clinic, 327 Charlotte St, Peterborough ON K9J 0B2; McM'79; FRCPC; IntMed; Cardiol. Physician, Kawartha Cardiology Clinic; (705)743-3555; Fax. (705)775-3555.

HUGIE, Tammy R; Mental Health & Addiction Serv, 14007 50 St NW, Edmonton AB T5A 5E4; Sask'93; BSc; FRCPC; Psy (Personality Disorders). Staff, Mental Health & Addiction Services; (780)492-2612; Fax. (780)492-0172.

HUGLO, Evelyne; Complexe Sante Reine-Elizabeth, 2100 av de Marlowe, Montreal QC H4A 3L5; Mon'73; (514)486-4980

HUGO, Andre; 107-3500 Carrington Rd, Westbank BC V4T 3C1; Orange Free State (South Africa)'97; MB ChB; (250)452-6762

HUGO, Daniel; Cranbrook OB/GYN Med Clinic, 225-1629 Baker St, Cranbrook BC V1C 1B4; Stellenbosch (South Africa)'90; MB ChB; FRCSC; ObstGyn. (250)426-1124; Fax. (250)426-1164.

HUGO, Pierre M; Union Family Med Centre, 278 4th Ave NE, Moose Jaw SK S6H 0C6; Pretoria (South Africa)'85; MB ChB; (306)694-1717

HUGO, Wouter L; Smith Clinic, 1-6601 48 Ave, Camrose AB T4V 3G8; Stellenbosch (South Africa)'80; MRCOG(Eng); MB ChB; FRCSC; ObstGyn. Staff, Covenant Health - St Mary's Hospital; Langs: Afrikaans; (780)608-5877

HUH, Caroline C; The Court, 410-2863 Ellesmere Rd, Scarborough ON M1E 5E9; Tor'92; FRCSC; ObstGyn. Ac Staff ObstGyn, Rouge Valley Health System - Centenary Health Centre Site; Langs: Korean; (416)286-3743

HUH, Linda L; BC Children's Hosp, B321-4480 Oak St, Vancouver BC V6H 3V4; Ott'99; Neur; Peds. Staff, BC Children's Hospital; (604)875-2121

HUHLEWYCH, Roman; SGH Medical Mall, 502-3030 Lawrence Ave E, Scarborough ON M1P 2T7; Alb'81; FRCSC; GenSurg; VascSurg. Staff Surg, The Scarborough Hospital - General Campus; Court Staff, Southlake Regional Health Centre; (416)439-1504; Fax. (416)439-7807.

HUHN, Karen M M; 201-2139 4 Ave NW, Calgary AB T2N 0N6; Cal'91; (403)270-8081; Fax. (403)270-8087.

HUHN, Otto H; Mineral Spring Hosp, PO Box 1050 Stn Main 301 Lynx St, Banff AB T1L 1H7; Alb'63; FRCPC; GenPath (Hematology Pathology). Dir Lab & Emeritus Kasper Med Labs/Staff, Covenant Health - Banff Mineral Springs Hospital; Langs: French; German; (403)226-0068; Fax. (403)226-0068.

HUI, Adrian W Y; Family Care Med Centre, 30-747 Don Mills Rd, North York ON M3C 1T2; Tor'79; (416)421-8372; Fax. (416)421-8379.

HUI, Alphonsus Z; Oakridge Centre South Tower, 203-650 41st Ave W, Vancouver BC V5Z 2M9; Tor'73; Langs: Cantonese; Mandarin; (604)263-0828

HUI, Anita K W; 4626 Bowness Rd NW, Calgary AB T3B 0B3; Cal'96; AB; AAFPRS; FRCSC; Otol (Head & Neck Surgery). (403)452-8816; Fax. (403)452-8817.

HUI, Anthony Y T; The Doctors Bldg, 602-208 Bloor St W, Toronto ON M5S 3B4; Tor'76; FAAP; FRCPC; Peds. Staff Nursery, Sunnybrook Health Sciences Centre; Hon Staff, The Hospital For Sick Children; Asst Prof, University of Toronto; (416)968-3777; Fax. (416)968-3780.

HUI, Carolyn M W; Royal Alexandra Hosp, 10240 Kingsway NW, Edmonton AB T5H 3V9; Cal'06; FRCPC; Anes. Staff, Royal Alexandra Hospital; (780)708-1688

HUI, Catherine C M; 370-5740 Cambie St, Vancouver BC V5Z 3A6; UBC'99; CCFP; Langs: Cantonese; (604)322-6658

HUI, Catherine M T; Strathcona Med Dental Bldg, 200-8225 105 St NW, Edmonton AB T6E 4H2; Cal'04; FRCSC; OrthSurg. (780)439-5858

HUI, Charles P S; Children's Hosp Eastern Ont, 401 Smyth Rd, Ottawa ON K1H 8L1; Ott'96; FRCPC; Peds (Pediatric Infectious Diseases); InfectDis. Staff, Children's Hospital of Eastern Ontario (CHEO); (613)737-7600 x2651; Fax. (613)738-4878; chui@cheo.on.ca.

HUI, Creighton; Rockyview Gen Hosp, 7007 14 St SW, Calgary AB T2V 1P9; UBC'08; CCFP; CCFP(E.M.); Staff, Rockyview General Hospital; (403)943-3000

HUI, Dini; Sunnybrook Hlth Sciences Ctr, M4 168-2075 Bayview Ave, Toronto ON M4N 3M5; Tor'02; FRCSC; ObstGyn (Maternal Fetal Medicine). Staff, Sunnybrook Health Sciences Centre; (416)480-4920; Fax. (416)480-4933.

HUI, Edith W Y; Don Mills Med Clinic, 825 Don Mills Rd, North York ON M3C 1V4; Saba (Netherlands Antilles)'09; CCFP; (416)383-1251

HUI, Frederick; 313-18 Wynford Dr, North York ON M3C 3S2; Tor'79; CCFP; Court Staff, St Michael's Hospital; Teach Staff Family Med, University of Toronto; Langs: Chinese; (416)443-0811; Fax. (416)443-0482; drhui@drhui.com.

HUI, Gavin; 202-6990 Derry Rd, Milton ON L9T 7H3; Wes'90; FRCPC; IntMed. (905)878-4556; Fax. (905)878-4296.

HUI, Gladwin C W; Canada Diagnostic Centres, 1-6020 1A St SW, Calgary AB T2H 0G3; Tor'05; FRCPC; DiagRad. (403)253-4666

HUI, Hilary K; Dr Hilary Hui Inc, 115-8120 Cook Rd, Richmond BC V6Y 1T9; Tor'73; Ac Staff, Richmond Hospital; Langs: Cantonese; Mandarin; (604)278-5192; Fax. (604)278-5127.

HUI, Ivy Y C; 4060-8171 Ackroyd Rd, Richmond BC V6X 3K1; Tor'89; CCFP; FCFP; Assoc Member Family Pract, Richmond Hospital; Langs: Cantonese; Mandarin; (604)232-1099; Fax. (604)232-1098; ivyhui@shaw.ca.

HUI, Jacqueline C W; Northeast Mental Health Team, 222-2750 Hastings St E, Vancouver BC V5K 1Z9; UBC'97; FRCPC; Psy. Staff, Vancouver Adult Mental Health Intake; Langs: Cantonese; (604)675-3890

HUI, Jacqueline Y; Mount Sinai Hosp, 1001B-600 University Ave, Toronto ON M5G 1X5; Tor'01; CCFP; Staff, Mount Sinai Hospital; (416)586-4800; Fax. (416)586-4804.

HUI, Melody; McMaster Innovation Park, 201A-175 Longwood Rd S, Hamilton ON L8P 0A1; McM'10; CCFP; (905)525-9140 x20501

HUI, Philip L Y; UBC Faculty of Medicine, 7F-2775 Laurel St, Vancouver BC V5Z 1M9; UBC'08; FRCPC; IntMed.

HUI, William K; Hys Med Centre, 350-11010 101 St NW, Edmonton AB T5H 4B9; (Hong Kong)'77; MB BS; FRCP(Edin); DABIM(CardioVasDis); FRCPC; IntMed; Cardiol. Consultant, Covenant Health - Edmonton General Continuing Care Centre; Consultant, Covenant Health - Grey Nuns Community Hospital; Chief Div. of Cardiol., Royal Alexandra Hospital; Clin Prof, University of Alberta; (780)428-3246; Fax. (780)425-0487.

HUIDOVICI, Elia; 202-3335 Dougall Ave, Windsor ON N9E 1S8; Bucharest (Romania)'93; CCFP; Aj Prof, Schulich School of Medicine-Windsor Campus; Langs: Romanian; Bulgarian; French; (519)258-3478; elia.huidovici@yahoo.ca.

HUIKESHOVEN, Menno; Gordon & Leslie Diamond HCC, 3F-2775 Laurel St, Vancouver BC V5Z 1M9; Amsterdam (Netherlands)'04; Staff, Vancouver General Hospital - Centennial Pavillion; Staff, Gordon & Leslie Diamond Health Care Centre; Langs: Dutch; (604)857-5866

HUISAMEN, Charles C; St Joseph's Gen Hosp, 2137 Comox Ave, Comox BC V9M 1P2; Stellenbosch (South Africa)'91; MB ChB; CCFP; CCFP(E.M.); Staff, St Joseph's General Hospital; Langs: Afrikaans; (250)339-2242

HUJIC, Nirvana; Albany Med Clinic, 807 Broadview Ave, Toronto ON M4K 2P8; Banja Luka (Bosnia-Herzegovina)'94; CCFP; (416)461-9471

HUK, Michael; Victoria Gen Hosp, 1 Hospital Way, Victoria BC V8Z 6R5; Alb'94; FRCPC; DiagRad. Staff, Victoria General Hospital; (250)727-4208

HUK, Olga L; SMBD Jewish Gen Hosp, 3755 ch Cote-Sainte-Catherine, Montreal QC H3T 1E2; McG'84; BSc; MDCM; MSc; FRCSC; OrthSurg (Adult Hip & Knee Reconstruction). Att Staff OrthSurg, Sir Mortimer B Davis Jewish General; Asst Prof Surg, McGill University; (514)340-7532; Fax. (514)340-7595; ohuk@ldi.jgh.mcgill.ca.

HUKIN, Juliette; Children's & Women's HC of BC, B321-4480 Oak St, Vancouver BC V6H 3V4; Sydney (Australia)'87; MB BS; FRCPC; Peds (Pediatric Neurology); Neur. Staff, BC Children's Hospital; (604)875-3684

HULL, Christopher M; Four Counties Med Clinic, RR 3 1824 Concessions Dr, Newbury ON N0L 1Z0; Cal'05; BSc(UBC); MSc(UC); CCFP; (519)693-0350

HULL, Constance L; UBC Faculty of Medicine, 3333 University Way, Kelowna BC V1V 1V7; Mem'80; DTMH; CCFP; FCFP; Staff, Vernon Jubilee Hospital; Staff, Kelowna General Hospital; (250)807-8789

HULL, M Louise; The Core Family Health Centre, 825 Richmond St, London ON N6A 3H7; Cal'86.

HULL, Mark; St Paul's Hosp, 667B-1081 Burrard St, Vancouver BC V6Z 1Y6; Sask'00; FRCPC; IntMed (AIDS/HIV); InfectDis. Staff, Providence Health Care - St Paul's Hospital; (604)682-2344 x69051; Fax. (604)806-8527.

HULL, Peter R; Royal University Hosp, 103 Hospital Dr, Saskatoon SK S7N 0W8; Witwatersrand (South Africa)'70; MB ChB; PhD; FRCPC; Derm. Staff Derm, Royal University Hospital; (306)966-5157

HULL, Russell D; Foothills Med Centre, ST 906-1403 29 St NW, Calgary AB T2N 2T9; Sydney (Australia)'69; MB BS; FRACP; FACP; FCCP; FRCPC; IntMed. Staff, Foothills Medical Centre; Prof Med. & Hd., University Of Calgary; (403)944-8052; Fax. (403)944-3266.

HULL, Stephen; Saint John Reg Hosp, PO Box 2100 400 University Ave, Saint John NB E2L 4L2; Belfast (United Kingdom)'95; Staff, Saint John Regional Hospital; (506)648-7412; Fax. (506)653-2939.

HULME, W Terrance; Rockyview Gen Hosp, 7007 14 St SW, Calgary AB T2V 1P9; Ott'82; FRCPC; IntMed; Critical Care Medicine; Respir. Ac Staff, Rockyview General Hospital; (403)943-3788; Fax. (403)212-1241; terry.hulme@calgaryhealthregion.ca.

HULSBOSCH, Hanna; Northern Medical Unit, T162-770 Bannatyne Ave, Winnipeg MB R3E 0W3; Man'96; CCFP; (204)789-3711; Fax. (204)774-8919.

HULT, Keith W; Professional Med Clinic, 202-9425 94 Ave, Fort Saskatchewan AB T8L 1N6; Alb'82; CCFP; (780)998-4434; Fax. (780)998-3634.

HULTZER, Michele V; Trillium Hlth Ctr-Mississauga, 100 Queensway W, Mississauga ON L5B 1B8; Witwatersrand (South Africa)'87; MB ChB; FRCPC; Anes;CCFP; Consultant, Trillium Health Centre - Mississauga; (905)848-7628

HULYK, Raymond; Associate Med Group, 4705 48 Ave, Red Deer AB T4N 3T1; Alb'64; CCFP; FCFP; Physician, Associate Medical Group; (403)346-2057; Fax. (403)347-2989.

HUM, Annie; Canadian Ctre Integrative Med, 12 Main St N, Markham ON L3P 1X2; Tor'90; CAFCI; LMCC; Staff Family Med, The Scarborough Hospital - Birchmount Campus; Langs: English; French; Chinese; (905)471-9355; Fax. (905)471-4348.

HUM, Betty M; Medical Office, 105-840 Coxwell Ave, Toronto ON M4C 5T2; Tor'01; CCFP; Ac Staff, Toronto East General Hospital Inc; Langs: Cantonese; (416)469-6464; Fax. (416)469-6164.

HUM, Hing-Sang; Ellendale Med Bldg, 690-5845 ch de la Cote-des-Nei, Montreal QC H3S 1Z4; McG'82; ObstGyn (Endoscopic Surgery). Staff, McGill University Health Centre - Montreal General Campus; Staff, Sir Mortimer B Davis Jewish General; Clin Staff Part-Time, McGill University; (514)738-5621

HUM, Peter C M; Belmead Med Centre, 18220 89 Ave NW, Edmonton AB T5T 2K6; Alb'81; CCFP; FCFP; (780)481-8812; Fax. (780)489-7853.

HUM, Teresa Y K; A202-3000 Highway 7, Markham ON L3R 6E1; Tor'99; CCFP; (905)480-1050; Fax. (905)480-0898.

HUMAN, Anthony P; 520 Nicola St, Kamloops BC V2C 2R1; Cape Town (South Africa)'79; MB ChB; FRCSC; ObstGyn. (250)372-0126; Fax. (250)372-8026.

HUMAN, David S; 4802 Highway St E GD, Valleyview AB T0H 3N0; Pretoria (South Africa)'05; MB ChB; (780)524-3365

HUMAN, Derek G; BC Women's Hosp & Health Ctre, 1F22-4500 Oak St, Vancouver BC V6H 3N1; Oxford (England)'71; FRCPC; Peds; Cardiol. Staff, BC Women's Hospital & Health Centre; (604)875-2296; dhuman@cw.bc.ca.

HUMAR, Atul; Katz-Rexall Centre, 6 030-1A University Campus NW, Edmonton AB T6G 2E1; Ott'92; MSc; FRCPC; IntMed; InfectDis. Staff, University of Alberta Hospital; Staff, Research Transition Facility; (780)492-3885; atul.humar@ualberta.ca.

HUMAYUN, Kiran; Harbour Landing Med Clinic, 4500 Gordon Rd, Regina SK S4W 0B7; (Other Foreign)'09; CCFP; Langs: Urdu; (306)545-2888; Fax. (306)545-2844.

HUMAYUN, Muhammad; Dartmouth Med Centre, 311-46 Portland St, Dartmouth NS B2Y 1H4; Nishtar (Pakistan)'67; MB BS; FRCSC; Ophth. Staff, Queen Elizabeth II Health Sciences Centre - Victoria General Site; Consultant, Dartmouth General Hospital; (902)465-8724; Fax. (902)461-9997.

HUMBER, Nancy L; Lillooet Med Clinic PO Box 850, Lillooet BC V0K 1V0; Mem'93; CCFP; (250)256-7505; Fax. (250)256-7591; saffron2@telus.net.

HUMBER, Robert E; Humber Med Clinic, PO Box 670 51-53 Conception Bay Hwy, Bay Roberts NL A0A 1G0; Dal'74; Pentecostal Senior Citizen's Home; (709)786-7144

HUMBLE, Richard G; Cottage Country Fam Hlth Team, 1-5 Pineridge Gate, Gravenhurst ON P1P 1Z3; McM'79; Staff, South Muskoka Memorial Hospital - Muskoka Algonquin Healthcare; (705)687-2794

HUME, Cheryl A; Riverside Med Clinic, 304-1101 Dewdney Ave, Trail BC V1R 4T1; Cal'85; CCFP; (250)368-5656; Fax. (250)368-8811.

HUME, Heather; Hôpital Ste-Justine, 3175 ch Cote-Sainte-Catherine, Montreal QC H3T 1C5; Qns'78; FRCPC; Peds (Pediatric Hematology Oncology); MedOncol (P.Q.); Hem. Staff, Hôpital Ste-Justine; Prof Clinical Med, Universite de Montreal; (514)345-4931; heather.hume@umontreal.ca.

HUME, Laura J; Wilson Centre Family Practice, 1-2185 Wilson Ave, Port Coquitlam BC V3C 6C1; Southampton (England)'05; MB BS; (604)942-7227

HUMEN, Dennis P; London HSC-University Hosp, PO Box 5339 Stn B C6 127-339 Windermere Rd, London ON N6A 5A5; Alb'75; FRCPC; IntMed; Cardiol. Staff, London Health Sciences Centre - University Hospital; (519)663-3505; Fax. (519)663-3506; dennishumen@gmail.com.

HUMER, Michael F; 201-2903 Pandosy St, Kelowna BC V1Y 1W1; UBC'87; FRCSC; GenSurg; ThorSurg. Staff, Kelowna General Hospital; (250)763-7660; Fax. (250)763-7685; info@thoracicsurgery.bc.ca.

HUMES, R Trevor; Health Sciences Centre, 300 Prince Philip Dr, St. John's NL A1B 3V6; Mem'00; CCFP; CCFP(E.M.); Staff, Health Sciences Centre; (709)737-6300

HUMMEL, David B; Bayview-Finch Med Clinic, 301-3292 Bayview Ave, North York ON M2M 4J5; Pretoria (South Africa)'77; MB ChB; FRCPC; Peds; ClinImmunol&Allergy (Allergy). Court Staff, Markham Stouffville Hospital; Court Staff, Rouge Valley Health System - Centenary Health Centre Site; Staff Pt-time Allergy & Immunol, The Hospital For Sick Children; (416)733-7772; Fax. (416)224-9880.

HUMMEL, Jonathan S; The Court, 101-2863 Ellesmere Rd, Scarborough ON M1E 5E9; Witwatersrand (South Africa)'81; MB ChB; FRCSC; OrthSurg. Staff, Rouge Valley Health System - Centenary Health Centre Site; (416)284-0488; Fax. (416)284-1218.

HUMNICKA-SZOTT, Malgorzata; Saskatoon Community Clinic, 455 2nd Ave N, Saskatoon SK S7K 2C2; Silesian (Poland)'79; CCFP; FCFP; Assoc Staff, Saskatoon City Hospital; Assoc Staff, Royal University Hospital; Assoc Staff, St Paul's Hospital (Grey Nuns) of Saskatoon; Langs: Polish; (306)652-0300; Fax. (306)664-4120; szott.md@shaw.ca.

HUMNISKI, Anne-Marie P; The Credit Valley Hosp, 2200 Eglinton Ave W, Mississauga ON L5M 2N1; Tor'96; BSc; CCFP; CCFP(E.M.); FCFP; Staff Emerg, The Credit Valley Hospital; (905)813-4141

HUMPHREY, Andrew B; Family Practice Associates, 200-6155 North St, Halifax NS B3K 5R3; Dal'91; BSc; (902)453-3511; Fax. (902)454-9010.

HUMPHREY, Diane B; 203-20 Hobson St, Cambridge ON N1S 2M6; Wes'94; CCFP; (519)621-7831

HUMPHREY, Robert J; 302-600 Princess St, Woodstock ON N4S 4H4; Wes'05; FRCSC; GenSurg. Staff, London Health Sciences Centre - University Hospital; (519)539-6622; Fax. (519)539-7954.

HUMPHREY, Shannon D; Skin Care Centre, 3F-835 10th Ave W, Vancouver BC V5Z 4E8; Dal'04; FRCPC; Derm. (604)875-5151

HUMPHREY, Susan M; The Ottawa Hosp-Riverside, 1967 Riverside Dr, Ottawa ON K1H 7W9; Ott'89; MEd; FRCPC; IntMed; Rheum. Ad Staff Privil, The Ottawa Hospital - Riverside Campus; Dep Registrar, Medical Council of Canada Examination Board; Assoc Dir AIME/Assoc Prof, University of Ottawa; Langs: English; French; (613)737-8899; Fax. (613)738-8228.

HUMPHREY, Wayne A; Thunder Bay Reg HSC-T-Bay, 980 Oliver Rd, Thunder Bay ON P7B 6V4; McM'85; MSc; CCFP; CCFP(E.M.); FCFP; Staff, Thunder Bay Regional Health Sciences Centre; (807)684-6100

HUMPHREYS, Douglas B; MacLeod Trail Plastic Surgery, 7425 MacLeod Trail SW, Calgary AB T2H 0L8; Sask'97; FRCSC; PlasSurg. (403)242-5080; Fax. (403)242-5090.

HUMPHREYS, Karen M; 1822B Comox Ave, Comox BC V9M 3M7; Man'95; FRCPC; IntMed. (250)339-1110

HUMPHREYS, Michael R; Vernon Jubilee Hosp, 2101 32 St, Vernon BC V1T 5L2; Tor'06; FRCPC; IntMed; MedOncol. Staff, Vernon Jubilee Hospital; (250)558-1235

HUMPHREYS, Peter; Children's Hosp Eastern Ont, 401 Smyth Rd, Ottawa ON K1H 8L1; McG'66; FRCP; BSc; FRCPC; Neur (Pediatric Neurology). Staff Consultant Neurol, The Ottawa Hospital - General Campus; Staff Neurol, Children's Hospital of Eastern Ontario (CHEO); Ac Staff Neurol, Ottawa Children's Treatment Centre; Prof Peds, University of Ottawa; Langs: French; (613)737-7600 x2605; Fax. (613)738-4886; phumphreys@cheo.on.ca.

HUMPHREYS, Robert A; Surrey Pediatric Associates, 103-13710 94A Ave, Surrey BC V3V 1N1; Mem'02; FRCPC; Peds; Nephrol. Staff, BC Children's Hospital; Staff, Surrey Memorial Hospital; (604)583-7070

HUMPHREYS, Shaun W; 315-1105 Pandora Ave, Victoria BC V8V 3P9; (Wales)'84; MB BCh; (250)598-2231

HUMPHRIES, Alexander; Island Emerald Med Centre, 3-1273 Island Hwy S, Nanaimo BC V9R 7A4; London (England)'92; MB BS; CCFP; (250)754-3218

HUMPHRIES, Paul W A; Royal Alexandra Hosp, 10240 Kingsway NW, Edmonton AB T5H 3V9; McM'77; CCFP; FCFP; Staff, Royal Alexandra Hospital; Prof Family Med, University of Alberta; (780)735-4201; Fax. (780)735-4978.

HUMPHRIES, R Keith; BC Cancer Agency Research Ctre, 675 10th Ave W, Vancouver BC V5Z 1L3; UBC'75; Staff, BC Cancer Agency Research Centre; (604)675-8140

HUMPL, Tilman F; The Hosp for Sick Children, 555 University Ave, Toronto ON M5G 1X8; Mainz (Germany)'90; Staff Critical Care Med & Cardiol, The Hospital For Sick Children; Assoc Prof Peds, University of Toronto; Langs: German; (416)813-6477; Fax. (416)813-7299; tilman.humpl@sickkids.ca.

HUNCHAK, Cheryl L; Mount Sinai Hosp, 600 University Ave, Toronto ON M5G 1X5; Wes'05; CCFP; CCFP(E.M.); Staff, Mount Sinai Hospital; (416)586-5058

HUNCHAK, John F; Lakeridge Hlth Corp-Oshawa, 1 Hospital Crt, Oshawa ON L1G 2B9; Man'70; Ac Staff, Lakeridge Health - Oshawa Site; (905)576-8711; Fax. (905)721-4742.

HUNDAL, Prabhjot; University Hosp of Northern BC, 3333 University Way, Prince George BC V2N 4Z9; Flinders (Australia)'08; (250)960-5555

HUNEAULT, David R; Sudbury Med Centre, 300A-65 Larch St, Sudbury ON P3E 1B8; Tor'95; FRCSC; ObstGyn. Langs: French; (705)673-8778; Fax. (705)675-8245.

HUNEAULT, J Gaetan O; Rayside Med Office, PO Box 549 93 Notre Dame St, Azilda ON P0M 1B0; Laval'65; (705)983-4222; Fax. (705)983-2019.

HUNEAULT, Pierre; Clinique Med Notre-Dame Inc, 147 rue Notre-Dame E, Victoriaville QC G6P 3Z8; Mon'90; (819)758-3165; Fax. (819)758-0745.

HUNG, Anthony R T; Trillium Hlth Ctr-Mississauga, 100 Queensway W, Mississauga ON L5B 1B8; Tor'03; FRCPC; IntMed (Palliative Medicine). Staff, Trillium Health Centre - Mississauga; (905)848-7641

HUNG, C Francis; CML Health Care Inc, 5-5801 Yonge St, North York ON M2M 3T9; (Hong Kong)'64; DABR; FRCPC; DiagRad. Langs: Cantonese; Mandarin; (416)222-6989; Fax. (416)222-4278.

HUNG, Frederico A; 9-1425 Dundas St E, Mississauga ON L4X 2W4; Tor'77; BSc; Staff, Trillium Health Centre - Mississauga; Langs: Cantonese; (905)624-0688; Fax. (905)624-9262.

HUNG, Geoffrey R; Children's & Women's HC of BC, K4 164-4480 Oak St, Vancouver BC V6H 3V4; Qns'00; FRCPC; Peds; PedEmergMed. Staff, BC Children's Hospital; (604)875-2345

HUNG, James; 2270-3700 No. 3 Rd, Richmond BC V6X 3X2; UBC'83; (604)273-0990 x2596; Fax. (604)974-0999.

HUNG, Lick San; St Joseph's Health Centre, 30 The Queensway, Toronto ON M6R 1B5; (Hong Kong)'76; MB BS; FRCPC; AnatPath. Staff Path, St Joseph's Health Centre; Langs: Cantonese; Mandarin; (416)530-6000 x3344

HUNG, Orlando; Queen Elizabeth II HSC, 1276 South Park St, Halifax NS B3H 2Y9; Dal'83; FRCPC; Anes. Staff, Queen Elizabeth II Health Sciences Centre - Victoria General Site; Prof Anes, Surg & Pharmacology, Dalhousie University; Langs: Cantonese; (902)473-7767; Fax. (902)473-4493; hungorla@dal.ca.

HUNG, Peggy; PO Box 19174 Rpo Fourth Ave, Vancouver BC V6K 4R8; Man'95; CCFP.

HUNG, Richard H; 6014 Yonge St, North York ON M2M 3V9; Witwatersrand (South Africa)'65; FRCPC; Peds. Ac Staff, North York General Hospital; (416)221-8255; Fax. (416)221-8255.

HUNG, Ryan M T; Holland Bloorview Kids Rehab, 150 Kilgour Rd, Toronto ON M4G 1R8; Qns'03; MSc; FRCP; FRCPC; Peds (Acquired Brain Injury); Neur. Staff, Holland Bloorview Kids Rehabilitation Hospital; Assoc Staff, The Hospital For Sick Children; (416)425-6220; Fax. (416)494-6621; rhung@hollandbloorview.ca.

HUNG, Ryan W Y; University of Alberta Hosp, 8440 112 St NW, Edmonton AB T6G 2B7; UBC'05; DiagRad. Staff, University of Alberta Hospital; (780)407-6810

HUNG, Tawny W; 1501-899 12th Ave W, Vancouver BC V5Z 1M9; UBC'08; Staff, Vancouver General Hospital - Centennial Pavillion; Langs: Cantonese; (604)875-4759

HUNG, Violet W T; The Richmond Hosp, 7000 Westminster Hwy, Richmond BC V6X 1A2; UBC'08; CCFP; CCFP(E.M.); Staff Emerg, Richmond Hospital; (604)278-9711

HUNI, Gerard E; Hop Brome-Missisquoi-Perkins, 950 rue Principale, Cowansville QC J2K 1K3; McG'00; FRCPC; Anes. Staff, Hôpital Brome-Missisquoi-Perkins; Langs: Armenian; English; (450)266-4342

HUNKA, Larry E; Meadowlark Health Centre, 166 Meadowlark Shopping Ctr NW, Edmonton AB T5R 5W9; Alb'73; FRCSC; OrthSurg. Ac Staff, University of Alberta Hospital; Ac Staff, Covenant Health - Misericordia Community Hospital; Clin Assoc Prof, University of Alberta; (780)483-0283; Fax. (780)486-1739.

HUNKIN, John B; Parry Sound Family Health Team, 15 James St, Parry Sound ON P2A 1T4; Wes'74; Staff Physician, West Parry Sound Health Centre; (705)746-9382; Fax. (705)746-7758.

HUNSINGER, Leigh A; University Hosp of Northern BC, 1475 Edmonton St, Prince George BC V2M 1S2; McM'07; CCFP; CCFP(E.M.); Staff, University Hospital of Northern British Columbia; (250)565-2000

HUNT, Alan P; 1165 Dufferin Cres, Nanaimo BC V9S 2B5; Orange Free State (South Africa)'82; MB ChB; FRCSC; ObstGyn. Staff, Nanaimo Regional General Hospital; Clin Instructor, University of British Columbia; (250)754-6323; Fax. (250)754-6354.

HUNT, Allan J A; Centenary Site, 2867 Ellesmere Rd, Scarborough ON M1E 4B9; (Jamaica)'78; MB BS; DMJ; FASCP; FRCPath; FRCPC; AnatPath (Forensic Pathology); GenPath. Ac Staff Pathology Dept, Rouge Valley Health System - Centenary Health Centre Site; Staff Office of the Coroner, Forensic Pathology Unit; (416)281-7388; jhunt@rougevalley.ca.

HUNT, Andrew J; Notre Dame Bay Mem Hlth Ctr, GD Hospital Lane, Twillingate NL A0G 4M0; Mem'09; CCFP; Staff, Notre Dame Bay Memorial Health Centre; (709)884-2131

HUNT, Anita S; Credit Valley Med Arts Centre, 206-2000 Credit Valley Rd, Mississauga ON L5M 4N4; Tor'84; CCFP; FCFP; Langs: Tamil; (905)820-1046; Fax. (905)820-1899.

HUNT, Barry H; Linden Prof Centre, 203-24 Linden Ave, Charlottetown PE C1A 5Y8; Cal'83; FRCPC; IntMed; Respir. Ac Staff, Queen Elizabeth Hospital; (902)367-4130; Fax. (902)367-4132.

HUNT, Brian M; 460 16th St E, North Vancouver BC V7L 2T5; UBC'64; FACS; FRCSC; Neursurg (Spinal Injury). Ac Staff, Lions Gate Hospital; (604)988-2715; brian.hunt@telus.net.

HUNT, Carolyn P; Grandview Treatment Centre, RR 4 600 Townline Rd S, Oshawa ON L1H 7K6; McM'96; FRCPC; Peds (Developmental Pediatrics). (905)728-1673 x2562; Fax. (905)728-2961; carolyn.hunt@grtc.ca.

HUNT, Christopher G E; 810-777 Hornby St, Vancouver BC V6Z 1S4; London (England)'70; LRCP; MRCS; DObstRCOG; Ac Staff, Providence Health Care - St Paul's Hospital; Physician, Vancouver School Board Employee Health Service & Three Bridges Drop-In Clinic; (604)669-6099; Fax. (604)669-2912.

HUNT, Daniel; Carman Commun Health Centre, 360 4th St SW, Carman MB R0G 0J0; Alb'90; CCFP.

HUNT, David G; St Paul's Hosp, 4B 432-1081 Burrard St, Vancouver BC V6Z 1Y6; UBC'69; FRCPC; EmergMed (Chronic Pain). Staff, Vancouver General Hospital - Centennial Pavillion; Consultant Pain Management Centre, Providence Health Care - St Paul's Hospital; Member Chronic Pain Committee, College of Physicians & Surgeons of British Columbia; (604)806-9381; Fax. (604)806-8782.

HUNT, Dereck L; Hamilton HS-Henderson Site, 711 Concession St, Hamilton ON L8V 1C3; Wes'92; FRCPC; IntMed (Diabetology). Staff, Hamilton Health Sciences Centre-Juravinski Site; Assoc Prof Med, McMaster University; (905)318-9084; Fax. (905)575-7320; huntdl@mcmaster.ca.

HUNT, Edgar W; Kirkland & District Hosp, PO Box 3000 Stn Main 145 Government Rd E, Kirkland Lake ON P2N 3P4; Mem'76; Staff, Kirkland & District Hospital; (705)567-5251

HUNT, George D; West Parry Sound Health Ctr, 6 Albert St, Parry Sound ON P2A 3A4; Manchester (England)'56; MB ChB; FRCS; FACS; FRCSC; GenSurg. Consultant, West Parry Sound Health Centre; (705)746-2240; Fax. (705)746-2282; drhunt@wpshc.com.

HUNT, Georgia C; Sheway Maternity Services, 533 Hastings St E, Vancouver BC V6A 1P9; McM'75; CCFP; Consultant Perinatal Addictions, BC Women's Hospital & Health Centre; Clin Assoc Prof Family Practice, University of British Columbia; Langs: French; (604)216-1684; Fax. (604)216-1683.

HUNT, Gordon S; 1923 9 Ave S, Lethbridge AB T1J 1W8; Alb'83; BSc; FRCPC; IntMed. (403)394-7100; Fax. (403)380-4024.

HUNT, Harold G; 101-1964 Fort St, Victoria BC V8R 6R3; Wes'94; BSc; FRCSC; ObstGyn. Staff, Victoria General Hospital; Assoc Consultant, BC Cancer Agency Vancouver Island Centre; Discipline Specific Site Leader, Island Medical Program; Clin Assoc Prof, University of British Columbia; (250)386-1964; Fax. (250)386-1994; h.hunt@shaw.ca.

HUNT, Jennifer; St Boniface Gen Hosp, 409 Tache Ave, Winnipeg MB R2H 2A6; Ott'04; FRCSC; ObstGyn (Maternal Fetal Medicine). Staff, St Boniface General Hospital; (204)233-8563

HUNT, Richard H; Hamilton HS-McMaster Site, PO Box 2000 Stn Lcd 1 1200 Main St W, Hamilton ON L8N 3Z5; Edinburgh (Scotland)'66; FRCP; FACG; FRCPC; IntMed (Gastroenterology). Staff, St Joseph's Healthcare - Charlton Campus; Prof Med, Hamilton Health Sciences Centre - McMaster Children's Hospital; Prof Med, McMaster University; (905)521-2100 x73219; Fax. (905)521-5072.

HUNT, Ryan D; CLSC Metro, 300-1801 boul de Maisonneuve O, Montreal QC H3H 1J9; McG'91; CCFP; CCFP(E.M.); FCFP; Staff, Centre Hospitalier de LaSalle; Physician, CLSC de Metro; Langs: French; Spanish; German; (514)934-0354; Fax. (514)934-6155; rhunt@ssss.gouv.qc.ca.

HUNT, Stephen B; Foothills Med Centre, 1403 29 St NW, Calgary AB T2N 2T9; Mem'07; OrthSurg. Staff, Foothills Medical Centre; (403)944-1110

HUNT, Travis L; Selkirk Medical Group, PO Box 590 101 First St W, Revelstoke BC V0E 2S0; Detroit(MI) (USA)'96; CCFP; (250)837-9321

HUNTER, Alasdair G W; Children's Hosp Eastern Ont, 401 Smyth Rd, Ottawa ON K1H 8L1; McG'71; MSc; FRCPC; Peds; MedGenetics. Consultant Staff Genetics, Children's Hospital of Eastern Ontario (CHEO); Langs: French; (613)737-2275; Fax. (613)738-4822; heddalasdair@aol.com.

HUNTER, Andrea J; 12-1300 Garth St, Hamilton ON L9C 4L7; McM'03; FRCPC; Peds. Staff, Hamilton Health Sciences Centre - McMaster Children's Hospital; (905)575-0611

HUNTER, Brad C; 275-1555 McKenzie Ave, Victoria BC V8N 1A4; Cal'85; (250)477-7221; Fax. (250)477-2853.

HUNTER, Cameron M; 27 Cherry Point Crt, North Bay ON P1A 4E4; Tor'79; FRCPC; NuclearMed; DiagRad. Staff, North Bay Regional Health Centre - Regional Mental Health; (705)476-1690

HUNTER, Charlene A; Calgary Lab Services, 9-3535 Research Rd NW, Calgary AB T2L 2K8; Alb'02; FRCPC; AnatPath. Staff, University of Alberta Hospital; (403)770-3514

HUNTER, Christopher; Portage Med Clinic, 140 9th St SE, Portage la Prairie MB R1N 3V5; Man'10; CCFP; (204)857-3445

HUNTER, Christopher D; Dr Christopher Hunter Inc, 718-333 Brooksbank Ave, North Vancouver BC V7J 3V8; UBC'81; FRCPC; Psy. Staff, Regional Treatment Centre & Pacific Institution; (604)836-9549; chunter@forensic.bc.ca.

HUNTER, Gary R W; 112-3502 Taylor St E, Saskatoon SK S7H 5H9; Sask'04; FRCPC; Neur. Clinical Asst Prof, University Of Saskatchewan; (306)244-8002; Fax. (306)244-8012.

HUNTER, Glen A; Commercial Street Med Centre, 208-311 Commercial St, Milton ON L9T 3Z9; Wes'89; FRCSC; ObstGyn. (905)875-2280; Fax. (905)875-9172.

HUNTER, Gordon A; 6 Saint Aubyn's Cres, Toronto ON M4N 3K2; London (England)'60; MB BS(Hons); MRCS; LRCP; FRCS; OrthSurg. Hon Consultant OrthSurg, Sunnybrook Health Sciences Centre; Emeritus Prof Orth, University of Toronto; (416)482-2975; Fax. (416)482-9597.

HUNTER, Graham N; 3-3525 26 Ave SE, Calgary AB T2B 2M9; Cal'75; (403)273-7076; Fax. (403)235-3018.

HUNTER, Ivan A; Hunter Med Centre, 200 Mill St, Milton ON L9T 1S2; Wes'65; Court Staff, Joseph Brant Memorial Hospital; Ac Staff, Halton Healthcare Services Corporation - Milton District Hospital; Med Dir, Allendale L T C Halton; Coroner Area 8, City of Milton; (905)878-3575; Fax. (905)876-1205.

HUNTER, J Barry; 1391 Ontario St, Burlington ON L7S 1G2; Wes'74; MSc(Physiol.); FRCSC; ObstGyn. Ac Staff, Joseph Brant Memorial Hospital; Assoc Prof, McMaster University; (905)639-7732; Fax. (905)639-9612; jbob@cogeco.ca.

HUNTER, J Brad; Foothills Hosp South Tower, 710-3031 Hospital Dr NW, Calgary AB T2N 2T8; Alb'98; BSc; MSc; Staff, Foothills Medical Centre; (403)944-2304; Fax. (403)270-9652.

HUNTER, James M; 202-168 13th St E, North Vancouver BC V7L 4W8; UBC'85; BSc; FRCSC; GenSurg; VascSurg. Staff, Lions Gate Hospital; (604)986-4772; Fax. (604)986-4701.

HUNTER, Jennifer M; North York Family Health Team, 5179 Yonge St, North York ON M2N 5P5; Man'80; Ac Staff Family Med, North York General Hospital; (416)733-0555; Fax. (416)733-0830.

HUNTER, John M; Royal Oak Clinic, 103-1638 Broadway E, Vancouver BC V5N 1W1; UBC'91; (604)438-6184

HUNTER, John R; Beaverlodge Med Clinic, PO Box 209 1030 1st Ave, Beaverlodge AB T0H 0C0; Alb'76; CCFP; FCFP; Medical Staff, Beaverlodge Municipal Hospital; Assoc Medical Staff, Queen Elizabeth II Hospital; (780)354-8993; Fax. (780)354-8181.

HUNTER, Jonathan J; Mount Sinai Hosp, 1285B-600 University Ave, Toronto ON M5G 1X5; Tor'84; FRCPC; Psy (Psychosomatic Medicine). Staff, Mount Sinai Hospital; Asst Prof, University of Toronto; (416)586-4800 x4557; Fax. (416)586-8654.

HUNTER, Julia D; 600-1285 Broadway W, Vancouver BC V6H 3X8; UBC'00; Psy (Child & Adolescent Psychiatry). (778)371-3435

HUNTER, Kathryn L; Garden City Family Health Team, 145 Carlton St, St Catharines ON L2R 1R5; Dal'91; FRCPC; Psy (Child & Adolescent Psychiatry).

HUNTER, Kenneth C; Oak Grove Clinic, 1872 Kingsway, Vancouver BC V5N 2S7; Queen's (Northern Ireland)'72; MB BCh; BAO; (604)876-6257

HUNTER, Meredith D; Ctr for the North Prince Georg, 1215 Lethbridge St, Prince George BC V2M 7E9; Wes'02; CCFP; (250)645-7335

HUNTER, Natalie; BC Women's Hosp & Health Centr, F2-4500 Oak St, Vancouver BC V6H 3N1; UBC'04; FRCPC; DiagRad. Staff Breast Health Program, BC Women's Hospital & Health Centre; (604)775-0026

HUNTER, Robert R T; Grand River Hosp-KW Hlth Ctre, PO Box 9056 Stn C 835 King St W, Kitchener ON N2G 1G3; Wes'70; Staff, Grand River Hospital - Kitchener/Waterloo Health Centre; (519)742-3611

HUNTER, Susan J; Cottage Medical, 559 6th St, Courtenay BC V9N 1M5; Ott'87; BSc; CCFP; FCFP; Staff, St Joseph's General Hospital; Staff, Clacier View Lodge; (250)338-1391; Fax. (250)338-2385.

HUNTER-ORANGE, Jessica M; London Skin Disorders Clinic, 611 Wonderland Rd N, London ON N6H 4V6; McM'05; CCFP; (519)471-5815; Fax. (519)471-2801.

HUNTING, Erika A; Le Marchand Mansion, 407-11523 100 Ave NW, Edmonton AB T5K 0J8; Alb'98; FRCPC; Psy. (780)452-4505; Fax. (780)453-1219.

HUNTINGTON, Katrina D; The Ottawa Hosp-Gen Campus, 4327-501 Smyth Rd, Ottawa ON K1H 8L6; Ott'98; FRCPC; Psy. Staff Psy, The Ottawa Hospital - General Campus; (613)737-8010

HUNTLEY, Margaret E; 301-1407 Yonge St, Toronto ON M4T 1Y7; London (England)'55; MB BS; LRCP; MRCS; DCH; FRCPC; Psy (Psychoanalysis). Asst Prof, University of Toronto; (416)944-2904

HUNTSMAN, David G; BC Cancer Agency-Vancouver CC, 3427-600 10th Ave W, Vancouver BC V5Z 4E6; Mem'88; FCCMG; FRCPC; GenPath (Cancer Genetics). Staff Genetic Pathol, Vancouver General Hospital - Centennial Pavillion; Staff Genetic Pathol/Med Dir CTAG Lab, BC Cancer Agency Vancouver Centre; Assoc Prof, University of British Columbia; (604)877-6000 x2148; Fax. (604)877-6089.

HUNTSMAN, Jennifer C; 1633 Mountain Rd PO Box 29109 Rpo North End, Moncton NB E1G 4R3; Mem'81; CCFP; CCFP(E.M.); FCFP; (506)855-6030; Fax. (506)855-6003.

HUNTSMAN, Richard J; Royal University Hosp, 103 Hospital Dr, Saskatoon SK S7N 0W8; Mem'98; FRCPC; Peds; Neur. Assoc Prof Ped & Neur, Royal University Hospital; Langs: Bilingual(English/French); (306)966-8115; Fax. (306)975-3767.

HUOT, Ann; Cross Cancer Institute, 2001-11560 University Ave NW, Edmonton AB T6G 1Z2; Laval'93; CCFP; Staff, Cross Cancer Institute; (780)432-8318

HUOT, Caroline; Centre de Read Lucie-Bruneau, 2275 av Laurier E, Montreal QC H2H 2N8; Mon'86; (514)527-4521; Fax. (514)527-7968.

HUOT, Caroline; Dir Reg de Sante Publique, 2400 av d'Estimauville, Quebec QC G1E 7G9; Sher'04; FRCPC; CommunMed; Public Health & Preventive Med. (418)666-7000; Fax. (418)666-2776.

HUOT, Celine; CHUQ-Ctr Hosp Univ Laval, 2705 boul Laurier, Quebec QC G1V 4G2; Laval'72; FRCSC; ObstGyn. Staff, Centre Hospitalier Universitaire de Quebec-CHUL; (418)525-4444; Fax. (418)577-2058.

HUOT, Celine; 3175 ch de la Côte-Sainte-Cath, Montreal QC H3T 1C5; McG'83; FRCPC; Peds (Diabetes); Endocrin&Metab. ac Staff, Hôpital Ste-Justine; assoc Prof, Universite de Montreal; (514)345-4735; Fax. (514)345-4988.

HUOT, David J; Carrefour Vanier Med Centre, 108-355 Montreal Rd, Vanier ON K1L 8H3; Ott'72; FRCPC; Peds. Langs: English; French; (613)744-2786; Fax. (613)744-0711.

HUOT, Denis; Clinique Med de Shawingian-Sud, 200-2355 5e av, Shawinigan-Sud QC G9P 1P4; Laval'80; Staff, Centre Hospitalier du Centre la Mauricie; (819)537-6205; Fax. (819)537-5596.

HUOT, Denys; CSSS de la Region de Thetford, 1717 rue Notre-Dame E, Thetford Mines QC G6G 2V4; Sher'80; NBME; FRCPC; NuclearMed. Chef Dept of Nuclear Med, Hopital du CSS de la Region de Thetford; (418)338-7777; Fax. (418)338-7757.

HUOT, Denyse; CHUQ-Ctr Hosp Univ Laval, 2705 boul Laurier, Quebec QC G1V 4G2; Laval'94; CSPQ; Anes. Staff, Centre Hospitalier Universitaire de Quebec-CHUL; (418)656-4141 x47565

HUOT, Helene; Ctr Medi Soleil St-Jean-Sur-Ri, 120-383 boul du Semaire N, St-Jean-sur-Richel QC J3B 8C5; Laval'79; Physician, Ministry of National Defense; (450)349-5555; Fax. (450)347-7557.

HUOT, Marie-Pierre; CSSS de Laval, 1755 boul Rene-Laennec, Laval QC H7M 3L9; Laval'02; Anes. Staff, Hopital de la Cite de la santé; (450)668-1010

HUOT, Michele; Centre Med Iberville, 101-235 2e av, St-Jean-sur-Richel QC J2X 2B2; Mon'80; (450)347-5548

HUOT, Philippe; Baycrest Ctre/Geriatric Care, 3560 Bathurst St, Toronto ON M6A 2E1; Laval'03; FRCPC; Neur (Movement Disorders). Staff, Baycrest Centre for Geriatric Care; (416)758-2500

HUOT, Pierre; Cliniqu Med Ste-Catherine, 4570 rte de Fossambault, Ste-Cath-d-I-J-Car QC G3N 2T6; Laval'70; Ac Staff, Centre Hospitalier Universitaire De Québec - Pavillon De St-françois-d'assise; Ac Staff, Centre Hospitalier Chauveau; Ac Staff, Centre Hospitalier Universitaire de Quebec-CHUL; Langs: English; (418)875-4356; Fax. (418)875-1446; cliniquestc@hotmail.com.

HUOT, Richard; Polyclinique Med Fabreville, 207-380 boul Curé-Labelle, Laval QC H7P 5L3; Mon'77; Staff, Hopital de la Cite de la santé; (450)628-5800 x314; Fax. (450)628-0217.

HUOT, Roger; Institut de Cardiologie de Mtl, 5000 rue Belanger, Montreal QC H1T 1C8; Mon'65; Cardiol (P.Q.). Staff, Institut de Cardiologie de Montréal; (514)376-3330; Fax. (514)593-2540.

HUPE, Anne; CSSS de la Mitis, 800 av du Sanatorium, Mont-Joli QC G5H 3L6; Sher'90; CCFP; FCFP; Staff Emerg, CSSS de la Mitis; Teach Staff, Université Laval; Langs: English; (418)775-7261 x3100; Fax. (418)775-6487.

HUPEL, Thomas M; 115-657 Queen St S, Kitchener ON N2M 1A1; Tor'93; MSc; FRCSC; OrthSurg. Staff, St Mary's General Hospital; Staff, Palmerston & District Hospital; Staff, Grand River Hospital - Kitchener/Waterloo Health Centre; (519)603-0630

HUPPE, Alain; CLSC Bois-Francs, 339 boul des Bois-Francs N, Victoriaville QC G6P 7B7; Laval'76; Staff, Hotel-Dieu d'Arthabaska; Dir exéc, CLSC Suzor-Cote-Victoriaville; (819)758-7281; Fax. (819)758-2706; alain_huppe@ssss.gouv.qc.ca.

HUPPE, Chantal; Clinique Med du Plateau, 300-195 rue de l'Atmosphere, Gatineau QC J9A 0A3; Laval'97; CCFP; FCFP; Ac Staff, CHSLD Vigi de l'Outaouais; Langs: English; (819)776-0001; Fax. (819)776-2171.

HUPPE, Diane; CSSS de la Haute-Yamaska, 205 boul Leclerc O, Granby QC J2G 1T7; Sher'91; FRCPC; Psy (Hospitalist). Staff, Centre Hospitalier de Granby; (450)375-8000

HUPPE, Rene; Ctr Hosp Affilie-Enfant-Jesus, 1401 18e rue, Quebec QC G1J 1Z4; Laval'07; Psy. Staff, Centre Hospitalier Affilié Universitaire de Québec - Hôpital De L'Enfant Jésus; (418)649-5769

HUPPE, Rivard; Clinique Med St-Bernard, CP 100 1629 rue St-Georges, Saint-Bernard QC G0S 2G0; Mon'75; (418)475-6615; Fax. (418)475-4369.

HUPPE, Xavier; Hop de la Malbaie, 303 rue Saint-Etienne, La Malbaie QC G5A 1T1; Laval'08; CCFP; Staff, Hôpital de la Malbaie; (418)665-1713

HUQ, M Momenul; Sunnybrook Hlth Sciences Ctre, H4 10-2075 Bayview Ave, Toronto ON M4N 3M5; Chittagong (Bangladesh)'85; MB BS; CardSurg. Staff, Sunnybrook Health Sciences Centre; (416)480-6073

HUQ, Nasimul S; Niagara Plastic Surgery Centre, 1-5668 Main St, Niagara Falls ON L2G 5Z4; Wes'93; MSc; FACS; DAB; CAQSH; FRCS; FRCSC; PlasSurg (Adult Reconstructive Surgery). Court Staff PlasSurg & Clin Ass't, Hamilton Health Sciences Centre - Hamilton General Hospital; Ac Staff PlasSurg, Niagara Health System - Greater Niagara General Site; Clinical Asst Prof Dept of Surg, McMaster University; Langs: French; (905)357-2360; Fax. (905)357-4714.

HUQ, Nisarul M; 101-1368 Ouellette Ave, Windsor ON N8X 1J9; Wes'91; ABIM; FRCPC; IntMed; Cardiol. Langs: English; French; (519)977-6643

HUQ, Rokaiya; Queensway-Carleton Hosp, 3045 Baseline Rd, Ottawa ON K2H 8P4; Ott'04; CCFP; Staff, Queensway Carleton Hospital; (613)721-2000; Fax. (613)721-4757.

HURD, Carmen A; Health Sciences Centre, 820 Sherbrook St, Winnipeg MB R3A 1R9; Man'06; FRCPC; IntMed; Endocrin&Metab. Staff, Health Sciences Centre; (204)774-8511

HURDALEK, Jiri T; The Doctors Bldg, 501-208 Bloor St W, Toronto ON M5S 3B4; Purkyne (Czech Republic)'67; DABPN; FRCPC; Psy. Staff, Centre for Addiction & Mental Health (CAMH) - Queen Site; Lecturer Psy, University of Toronto; (416)971-6666

HURDLE, Ian B; PO Box 370, Bellevue AB T0K 0C0; Cal'76; FRCSC; OrthSurg;CCFP; Staff Ortho., Chinook Regional Hospital; Staff Ortho, Crowsnest Pass Health Centre; (403)562-8804; Fax. (403)562-2905; ian@crowsnestpass.com.

HURDLE, Maureen; Main Street Med Centre, 9-10886 Hurontario St, Brampton ON L7A 3R9; McM'99; CCFP; (905)846-9911

HURENS, Cindy; Clinique Med de Lavaltrie, 89C ch Lavaltrie, Lavaltrie QC J5T 2H5; Laval'07; CCFP; Staff, Centre Hospitalier Pierre le Gardeur; (450)586-1033; Fax. (450)586-4498.

HURIK, Ilona; CSSS de Papineau, 155 rue MacLaren E, Gatineau QC J8L 0C2; Mon'02; Staff, CH-CHSLD de Papineau - Pavillon du centre hospitalier; Staff, Winchester District Memorial Hospital; (819)986-4115; Fax. (819)961-8018.

HURLBERT, R John; Foothills Med Centre, 1403 29 St NW, Calgary AB T2N 2T9; Sask'85; PhD; FACS; FRCSC; Neursurg (Spine Surgery). Staff Clin Neurosci, Foothills Medical Centre; Assoc Prof, University of Calgary; (403)283-4449; Fax. (403)283-5559; jhurlber@ucalgary.ca.

HURLBURT, Mary E; 404-10216 124 St NW, Edmonton AB T5N 4A3; Alb'83; CCFP; FCFP; Staff, University of Alberta Hospital; (780)735-3757

HURLBUT, David J; Kingston Gen Hosp, 76 Stuart St, Kingston ON K7L 2V7; Wes'85; FRCPC; AnatPath. Staff, Kingston General Hospital; Staff, Hotel-Dieu Hospital; Assoc Prof Path, Queen's University; (613)549-6666 x6035; hurlbutd@kgh.kari.net.

HURLEY, Bernard R; The Ottawa Hosp-Gen Campus, 501 Smyth Rd, Ottawa ON K1H 8L6; Wes'99; FRCPC; Ophth. Staff, The Ottawa Hospital - General Campus; (613)737-8174

HURLEY, Janette A; PO Box 61046 Rpo Kensington, Calgary AB T2N 4S6; Dal'81; FPIM; CCFP; Ac Staff, Foothills Medical Centre; (403)650-1004; Fax. (403)283-5531.

HURLEY, Katrina F; IWK Health Centre, PO Box 9700 Rpo CSC, Halifax NS B3K 6R8; Mem'01; FRCPC; EmergMed. Staff, IWK Health Centre; (902)470-8823

HURLEY, Michael; Bluewater Area Family Hlth Tea, PO Box 98 43 Main St, Zurich ON N0M 2T0; National (Ireland)'68; BCh; BAO; MB; (519)236-4314; Fax. (519)236-7508; michael@womenshealthclinic.co.uk.

HURLEY, Thomas C; Pembroke Reg Hosp, 705 Mackay St, Pembroke ON K8A 1G8; Wes'95; CCFP; CCFP(E.M.); FCFP; Staff/Chief EmergMed, Pembroke Regional Hospital Inc; (613)732-2811; Fax. (613)732-6351.

HURMATOV, Tetyana Y; Dr Hurmatov Med Clinic, 3-448 Welland Ave, St Catharines ON L2N 7V3; (Ukraine)'00; Langs: Russian; Ukrainian; (905)688-2000; Fax. (905)688-2008.

HUROWITZ, Eric E; Scarborough North Med Arts, 406-4040 Finch Ave E, Scarborough ON M1S 4V5; Tor'80; FRCPC; IntMed; Gastroent. Staff, The Scarborough Hospital - Birchmount Campus; Teacher, Sunnybrook Health Sciences Centre; Teacher, University of Toronto; (416)335-4669; Fax. (416)335-4672.

HURST, David E; North Shore FHT-Schreiber Site, PO Box 760 415 Scotia St, Schreiber ON P0T 2S0; Man'86; The McCausland Hospital; (807)824-2934; Fax. (807)824-2758.

HURST, David W; Kingston Family Health Team, 200-2437 Princess St, Kingston ON K7M 3G1; Qns'79; (613)546-6652; Fax. (613)546-5292; dhurst@kfhn.net.

HURST, Jody L; Jackson Park Health Centre, 230-2475 McDougall Ave, Windsor ON N8X 3N9; Ott'88; CCFP; (519)258-2230; Fax. (519)258-5883; sljhwin@cogeco.ca.

HURST, Lorne D C; Medical Arts Bldg, 1602-233 Kennedy St, Winnipeg MB R3C 3J5; National (Ireland)'88; MB ChB; FRCPC; Derm (Cutaneous Laser Surgery). (204)942-4808

HURST, Margaret M; 4B-119 Queen St N PO Box 449, Tottenham ON L0G 1W0; New England(ME) (USA)'94; ABPeds; (905)406-0171; Fax. (905)406-0172.

HURST, Randall R; 101-860 Tecumseh Rd E, Windsor ON N8X 2S5; Tor'75; (519)255-7118

HURTEAU, Julie M; Children's Hosp Eastern Ont, 401 Smyth Rd, Ottawa ON K1H 8L1; Sher'91; FRCPC; DiagRad (Pediatric Radiology). Staff Radiol, Children's Hospital of Eastern Ontario (CHEO); Langs: English; (613)737-7600 x2810; Fax. (613)737-2306; hurteau@cheo.on.ca.

HURTELOUP, Valerie; Institut de Cardiologie de Mtl, 5000 rue Belanger, Montreal QC H1T 1C8; Mon'96; Staff, Institut de Cardiologie de Montréal; (514)376-3330

HURTIG, Avery I; 200-200 St Clair Ave W, Toronto ON M4V 1R1; Man'83; Psy. (416)932-1333

HURTUBISE, Andre; Clinique Med des Laurentides, 1950 boul du Cure-Labelle, Saint-Jerome QC J7Y 1S1; Mon'76; (450)432-1442; Fax. (450)432-6814.

HURTUBISE, Andre L; Temiskaming Hosp, PO Box 4040 538-421 Shepherdson Rd, New Liskeard ON P0J 1P0; Ott'68; BSc; CCFP; FCFP; Staff, Centre de Sante Communautaire; Staff, Temiskaming Hospital; Langs: French; (705)647-8121; Fax. (705)647-0182.

HURTUBISE, Johann; CHUQ-Ctr Hosp Univ Laval, 2705 boul Laurier, Quebec QC G1V 4G2; Laval'79; FRCSC; ObstGyn. Staff, Centre Hospitalier Universitaire de Quebec-CHUL; (418)577-2057

HURTUBISE, Michel G; MGH Consultant Inc, 1979 rue Montarville, Saint-Bruno QC J3V 3V8; Mon'70; Staff, Hopital Charles LeMoyne; Physician, Pratt & Whitney Canada; Langs: Bilingual(French/English); (514)891-5083; mgh.consultant@bell.net.

HURTUBISE, Severine; Ctr Hosp de Verdun, 4000 boul Lasalle, Verdun QC H4G 2A3; Mon'99; Staff, Centre Hospitalier de Verdun; (514)362-1000 x2141

HURTUBISE, Suzanne; Groupe Med de Trois-Rivieres, 225-1900 boul des Recollets, Trois-Rivieres QC G8Z 4K4; Sher'83; Staff Dept of Public Health, CSSS de Trois-Rivières; (819)375-6666; Fax. (819)375-3423.

HURWITZ, Gilbert A; St Michael's Hosp, 30 Bond St, Toronto ON M5B 1W8; Tor'70; FRCPC; IntMed; NuclearMed. Staff, St Michael's Hospital; (416)864-5115

HURWITZ, Jeffrey J; The Joseph & Wolf Lebovic Bldg, 1 001-60 Murray St, Toronto ON M5T 3L9; Tor'67; FRCSC; Ophth (Eyelid Lacrimal Orbital). Ac Staff, The Hospital For Sick Children; Staff, The Scarborough Hospital - General Campus; Teach Staff, University of Toronto; (416)586-4800 x8385; Fax. (416)586-5915; jhurwitz@mtsinai.on.ca.

HURWITZ, Joel S; St Joseph's Health Care, PO Box 5777 Stn B A3 120-268 Grosvenor St, London ON N6A 4V2; Belfast (Ireland)'71; MB ChB; BAO; FRCP(Lond); FRCPC; IntMed (Geriatric Medicine). Ac Staff Med, St Joseph's Hospital - St Joseph's Health Care; Ac Staff Med, London Health Sciences Centre - South Street; (519)646-6188; Fax. (519)646-6260.

HURWITZ, Stanley D; Medical Bldg, 170-6180 Blundell Rd, Richmond BC V7C 4W7; Pretoria (South Africa)'78; MB ChB; CCFP; Langs: Afrikaans; (604)275-8228; Fax. (604)271-4900.

HURWITZ, Trevor A; UBC-Dept Of Psychiatry, 7-2255 Wesbrook Mall, Vancouver BC V6T 2A1; Pretoria (South Africa)'74; MB ChB; MRCP(UK); FRCPC; Psy; Neur (Neuro Psychiatry). Ac Staff Psy/Assoc Member Neurology, UBC Hospital - Koerner Pavillion; Med Dir BC Neuropsychiatry Program/Clin Prof, University of British Columbia; (604)822-7066; Fax. (604)822-7105; t.hurwitz@ubc.ca.

HURYN, Mark J; 2F-11 King St W, Toronto ON M5H 4C7; Tor'81; CCFP; FCFP; Court Staff, North York General Hospital; Court Staff, St Michael's Hospital; (416)864-0728; Fax. (416)864-0729.

HUSA, Regina; SMBD Jewish Gen Hosp, 3755 ch Cote-Sainte-Catherine, Montreal QC H3T 1E2; Mem'97; FRCPC; IntMed (Echocardiography); Cardiol. Staff Cardiologist, Sir Mortimer B Davis Jewish General; Staff Cardiologist, McGill University Health Centre - Montreal General Campus; Langs: French; (514)340-8232; Fax. (514)340-7510.

HUSAIN, Aisha T; Uxbridge Family Health Clinic, B-2 Elgin Park Dr, Uxbridge ON L9P 0B1; (Grenada)'04; CCFP; (905)852-1009

HUSAIN, Ali M A; 270-200 rue Champlain, Dieppe NB E1A 1P1; Arabian Gulf (Bahrain)'91; MD; FRCSC; PlasSurg (Breast Reconstruction). Staff, The Moncton Hospital; Staff Pt-Time, Dr Georges-L-Dumont University Hospital Centre; Langs: French; (506)853-5154; Fax. (506)854-2520; info@alluraclinics.ca.

HUSAIN, Almas S; The Moncton Hosp, 135 MacBeath Ave, Moncton NB E1C 6Z8; Osmania (India)'78; MB BS; FRCPC; AnatPath. Staff, The Moncton Hospital; (506)857-5321

HUSAIN, Amna F; Temmy Latner Centre, L4 000-60 Murray St, Toronto ON M5T 3L9; Alb'87; BMedSci; CCFP; Staff The Temmy Latner Centre for Palliative Care, Mount Sinai Hospital; (416)586-4800 x6777; Fax. (416)586-4804.

HUSAIN, Juhi; William Osler HC-Brampton, 2100 Bovaird Sr E, Brampton ON L6R 3J7; (India)'00; Staff, William Osler Health System - Brampton Civic Hospital; (905)494-6542; Fax. (905)494-6416.

HUSAIN, Mansoor; Univ Hlth Network-Toronto Gen, EN6 236-200 Elizabeth St, Toronto ON M5G 2C4; Alb'86; BMedSci; FRCPC; IntMed (Cardiovascular Imaging); Cardiol. Sr Scientist, Toronto General Hospital - UHN; Dir, Heart & Stroke Richard Lewar Centre for Excellence; Prof, University of Toronto; Langs: Urdu; (416)340-3188; Fax. (416)340-4021.

HUSAIN, Navaid; PO Box 1149, Three Hills AB T0M 2A0; (India)'95; MB BS; MRCGPract; (403)443-5522; Fax. (403)443-5535.

HUSAIN, Rafi A; Heritage Lane Med Clinic, 10835 23 Ave NW, Edmonton AB T6J 7B5; Alb'88; (780)424-6490; Fax. (780)425-4920.

HUSAIN, S Baqir; Prince Albert Mental Hlth Ctre, PO Box 3003 Stn Main, Prince Albert SK S6V 6G1; Karachi (Pakistan)'62; MB BS; DPM(Eng); MRCPsy(Eng.); Psy. Consultant Psy, Victoria Hospital; Consultant Psy, Prince Albert Parkland Health Region; Langs: Urdu; Hindi; (306)765-6055; Fax. (306)765-6349; bhusain@paphr.sk.ca.

HUSAIN, Saima F; St Joseph's Healthcare, 50 Charlton St E, Hamilton ON L8N 4A6; Dal'07; FRCPC; IntMed. Staff, St Joseph's Healthcare - Charlton Campus; (905)521-5070

HUSAIN, Shahid; Univ Hlth Network-Toronto Gen, 11C 1206-200 Elizabeth St, Toronto ON M5G 2C4; Karachi (Pakistan)'89; Staff, Toronto General Hospital - UHN; (416)340-4800; Fax. (416)340-5442.

HUSAIN, Siraj M; Tom Baker Cancer Centre, 1331 29 St NW, Calgary AB T2N 4N2; Dal'79; FRCPC; RadOncol. Staff, Tom Baker Cancer Centre; (403)521-3164; Fax. (403)283-1651.

HUSAREWYCZ, Stephen; Parkview Prof Centre, 107-2110 Main St, Winnipeg MB R2V 2C2; Russia (Russia (Federation))'70.

HUSBAND, Carol A; 33 Somerset St W, Ottawa ON K2P 0H3; Ott'79; DPsy; FRCPC; Psy (Individual Psychotherapy). (613)233-2269

HUSBAND, Daniel M; 203-2051 McCallum Rd, Abbotsford BC V2S 3N5; Sask'89; (604)855-0677; Fax. (604)855-0722.

HUSEIN, Murad; London HSC-Victoria Hosp, PO Box 5010 Stn B B3 440-800 Commissioners Rd E, London ON N6A 5W9; Wes'96; MSc; FRCSC; Otol (Pediatric Otolaryngology). Staff, London Health Sciences Centre - Victoria Campus; Staff, Thames Valley Children's Centre; (519)685-8184; Fax. (519)685-8185.

HUSEIN, Nadira; Northfield Med Centre, 201-99 Northfield Dr E, Waterloo ON N2K 3P9; Wes'93; BSc; FRCPC; IntMed; Endocrin&Metab. Assoc Staff Privil, Grand River Hospital - Kitchener/Waterloo Health Centre; Assoc Staff Privil, St Mary's General Hospital; Aj Prof Endocrin&Metab, University of Western Ontario; (519)744-2592; Fax. (519)585-7528.

HUSEYNOV, Khumar; Univ Hlth Network-Toronto Gen, 6F-200 Elizabeth St, Toronto ON M5G 2C4; (Azerbaijan)'97; VascSurg; GenSurg. Staff, Toronto General Hospital - UHN; (416)340-3303

HUSIEN, Mohamed E M; 453 Park St, Kitchener ON N2G 1N5; Al Fateh (Libya)'91; MB ChB; FRCSC; GenSurg (Surgical Oncology). (519)742-3341; mehusien@hotmail.com.

HUSKA, Linda A; Harbour City Health Centre, 102-1125 Dufferin Cres, Nanaimo BC V9S 2B5; Man'86; CCFP; FCFP; (250)753-2500

HUSNI, Mariwan H; Thunder Bay Reg HSC-T-Bay, 3049-980 Oliver Rd, Thunder Bay ON P7B 6V4; Mosul (Iraq)'86; MB ChB; FRCPC; Psy. Staff, Thunder Bay Regional Health Sciences Centre; (807)684-6029; Fax. (807)684-5893.

HUSNI, Tawfik; Port Aux Basques Med Centre, PO Box 1329 11 Water St W, Port-aux-Basques NL A0M 1C0; Ain Shams (Egypt)'69; MB BCh; CCFP.

HUSSAIN, Amna; Finch-Weston Med Centre, 2367B Finch Ave W, North York ON M9M 2W8; Aligarh Muslim (India)'71; (416)741-6062

HUSSAIN, Asmaa S; London HSC-Victoria Hosp, PO Box 5010 Stn B 800 Commissioners Rd E, London ON N6A 5W9; Basra (Iraq)'03; Peds. Staff, London Health Sciences Centre - Victoria Campus; (519)685-8500

HUSSAIN, Ayesha; Summerville Family Health Team, 211-190 Sherway Dr, Etobicoke ON M9C 5N2; McM'02; CCFP; (416)621-9700; Fax. (416)621-4438.

HUSSAIN, Chaudry L; Child & Family Services, 782 Seymour St, Kamloops BC V2C 2H3; Punjabi (India) MB BS; Staff, Royal Inland Hospital; (250)374-5111

HUSSAIN, Farha; Royal Health Care Centre, 130 Adelaide St W, Toronto ON M5H 3P5; Sask'96; CCFP; (416)361-6142

HUSSAIN, Farida K; Tillsonburg Dist Mem Hosp, 167 Rolph St, Tillsonburg ON N4G 3Y9; Peshawar (Pakistan)'63; MB BS; FRCPC; Psy. Staff, Tillsonburg District Memorial Hospital; (519)688-0960; Fax. (519)842-3134.

HUSSAIN, Farrukh; St Boniface Gen Hosp, Y3533-409 Tache Ave, Winnipeg MB R2H 2A6; Tor'98; FRCPC; IntMed; Cardiol. Staff, St Boniface General Hospital; (204)237-2023; Fax. (204)233-2157; fhussain@sbgh.mb.ca.

HUSSAIN, Fatima M; William Osler HC-Brampton, 2100 Bovaird Dr E, Brampton ON L6R 3J7; (Ireland)'03; FRCPC; IntMed; GeriatricMed. Staff Geriatric Med, William Osler Health System - Brampton Civic Hospital; (905)494-2120

HUSSAIN, Ijaz; Surrey Mem Hosp, 13750 96 Ave, Surrey BC V3V 1Z2; Peshawar (Pakistan)'99; Staff, Surrey Memorial Hospital; (604)581-2211

HUSSAIN, Kamal S; Women's College Hosp, 76 Grenville St, Toronto ON M5S 1B2; Punjab (Pakistan)'87; FRCPC; Anes. Staff, Women's College Hospital.

HUSSAIN, Khalid M; Cape Breton Hlthcare Complex, 1482 George St, Sydney NS B1P 1P3; Karachi (Pakistan)'96; MB BS; FRCPC; DiagRad. Staff, Cape Breton Healthcare Complex; (902)567-7778

HUSSAIN, M Zulfiquar; 2727 2nd Ave W, Prince Albert SK S6V 5E5; Punjab (Pakistan)'63; MB BS; DPM; MRCPsy; FRCPC; Psy (Adult Psychiatry). Staff Psy, Victoria Hospital; Chief Psy., Prince Albert Mental Health Centre; (306)922-6676; Fax. (306)922-5574; dianehus@sasktel.net.

HUSSAIN, Mahjabeen; Salveo Family Med Clinic, B8-6455 MacLeod Trail SW, Calgary AB T2H 0K8; (Pakistan)'90; MB BS; LMCC; CCFP; Staff, Calgary Sexual Responce Team; Physician, Calgary Sexual & Reproductive Health; Langs: Urdu; Hindi; Gujarati; Punjabi; (403)444-0428; Fax. (403)537-0029.

HUSSAIN, Maria; Hotel Dieu Hosp, 166 Brock St, Kingston ON K7L 5G2; Aga Khan (Pakistan)'05; Psy. Staff, Hotel-Dieu Hospital; (613)544-3310

HUSSAIN, Mohammad A; Trillium Hlth Ctr-Mississauga, 100 Queensway W, Mississauga ON L5B 1B8; Karachi (Pakistan)'90; MB BS; ABMO; ABIM; FRCPC; IntMed. Staff, Trillium Health Centre - Mississauga; (905)848-7160; Fax. (905)848-7161.

HUSSAIN, Mohammed F I; William Osler HC-Etobicoke, 5F-101 Humber College Blvd, Etobicoke ON M9V 1R8; Karachi (Pakistan)'94; Staff, William Osler Health System - Etobicoke General Hospital; (905)747-4300; Fax. (905)747-3350.

HUSSAIN, Mohammed T; 1400 Windsor Ave, Windsor ON N8X 3L9; Tor'02; BSc; CCFP; Ac Staff, Windsor Regional Hospital - Metropolitan Site; Langs: Urdu; (519)971-0116

HUSSAIN, Munawar; Clareview Medical Office, 3504 137 Ave NW, Edmonton AB T5Y 1Y7; (Pakistan)'92; MB BS; LMCC; CCFP; (780)456-8552; Fax. (780)456-8505.

HUSSAIN, Nabil; Family Med Centre, 611 Wonderland Rd N, London ON N6H 4V6; Ott'03; BSc(Hon); MSc; CCFP; (519)471-6686

HUSSAIN, Nadeem A; St Joseph's Health Centre, PO Box 5777 Stn B E 4 113-268 Grosvenor St, London ON N6A 4V2; McG'92; ERCP; EUS; FRCPC; Gastroent (Endoscopic Ultrasound). Staff, London Health Sciences Centre - South Street; Staff, St Joseph's Hospital - St Joseph's Health Care; Langs: English; French; Urdu; (519)646-6100 x64312; Fax. (519)646-6130; nadeem.hussain@sjhc.london.on.ca.

HUSSAIN, Nusrat; Halton HCS Corp-Oakville, 327 Reynolds St, Oakville ON L6J 3L7; Punjab (Pakistan)'96; FRCPC; GenPath. Staff, Halton Healthcare Services Corporation - Oakville Site; (905)338-4690 x6489; Fax. (905)845-3376.

HUSSAIN, R; Charolais Med Clinic, 12-305 Charolais Blvd, Brampton ON L6Y 2R2; RCS (Ireland)'86; CCFP; (905)456-8099; Fax. (905)456-1888.

HUSSAIN, Saad A; Minnedosa Med Group, PO Box 810, Minnedosa MB R0J 1E0; Mosul (Iraq)'77.

HUSSAIN, Saba; Glenashton Med Clinic, 2-333 Glenashton Dr, Oakville ON L6H 7P6; (Grenada)'01; (905)582-4929

HUSSAIN, Safdar; R J A Medicentres Cnd Inc, 204-10458 Mayfield Rd NW, Edmonton AB T5P 4P4; (Pakistan)'82; MB BS; (780)483-7115; Fax. (780)484-6531.

HUSSAIN, Sajida S; Centre Med Brunswick, 955 boul Saint-Jean, Pointe-Claire QC H9R 5K3; Osmania (India)'66; CSPQ; AnatPath; GenPath (P.Q.). (514)426-6677; sajidashariff@hotmail.com.

HUSSAIN, Samiruddin S; MUHC-Montreal Children's Hosp, T 131-2300 rue Tupper, Montreal QC H3H 1P3; McG'03; FRCPC; Peds. Staff, McGill University Health Centre - Montreal Children's Hospital; (514)412-4400 x23039; Fax. (514)412-4397.

HUSSAIN, Seema; Foothills Med Centre, 1403 29 St NW, Calgary AB T2N 2T9; Sask'94; FRCPC; Psy (Consultant Liaison Psychiatry). Staff, Foothills Medical Centre; (403)944-3369; Fax. (403)944-8340.

HUSSAIN, Shabnam; Smyth Med Centre, 200-1929 Russell Rd, Ottawa ON K1G 4G3; Karachi (Pakistan)'82; MB BS; CCFP; Prof/Teacher Dept of Medicine, University of Ottawa; Langs: Urdu; Hindi; Gujarati; (613)249-0803; Fax. (613)249-0804.

HUSSAIN, Syed S; Westgate Med Clinic, 18-2410 22nd St W, Saskatoon SK S7M 5S6; (Other Foreign)'96; MB BS; CCFP; Staff, Saskatoon Cancer Centre; Langs: Urdu; Punjabi; (306)384-7800; Fax. (306)384-7550.

HUSSAIN, Tabassum M; 2810 Major MacKenzie Dr, Maple ON L6A 1R8; Universidad Iberoamericana (Dominican Republic)'99; CCFP; (905)832-3838

HUSSAIN, Tasneem; Credit Valley Med & Cosmetic C, 229A-5100 Erin Mills Pky, Mississauga ON L5M 4Z5; Punjab (Pakistan)'80; CCFP; Staff, The Credit Valley Hospital; (905)607-2600; Fax. (905)607-9292.

HUSSAIN, Tousief; Royal University Hosp, 103 Hospital Dr, Saskatoon SK S7N 0W8; Sask'94; FRCSC; OrthSurg. Staff, Royal University Hospital; (306)655-6323; Fax. (306)384-2179.

HUSSAIN, Yasmine E; 117-1060 Speers Rd, Oakville ON L6L 2X4; McM'05; CCFP; (905)845-8884

HUSSAIN-AUTENRIED, Irene; 404-3101 Bloor St W, Etobicoke ON M8X 2W2; Berne (Switzerland)'71; Ac Staff Family Pract., St Joseph's Health Centre; Langs: French; German; Italian; (416)231-4708

HUSSAINI, Syed M; South Walkerville Med Centre, 179-2224 Walker Rd, Windsor ON N8W 5L7; Osmania (India)'78; MB BS; FRCPC; IntMed. (519)977-6768; Fax. (519)977-7690.

HUSSAN, Naila N; Wal Mart Canada, 1212 37 St SW, Calgary AB T3C 1S3; (Pakistan)'91; MB BS; (403)451-5788; Fax. (403)451-5789.

HUSSEIN, Abir H; 306C-60 Vancouver St, Yarmouth NS B5A 2P5; Ain Shams (Egypt)'02; MB BCh; (902)742-4365; Fax. (902)742-9234.

HUSSEIN, Ahmed; Sturgeon Community Hosp, 201 Boudreau St, St. Albert AB T8N 6C4; Alb'93; FRCPC; IntMed; InfectDis. Staff, Sturgeon Community Hospital; Staff, Leduc Community Hospital; Langs: Arabic; (780)418-8200

HUSSEIN, Elhadi F; Markham Stouffville Hosp, PO Box 1800 Stn Main 381 Church St, Markham ON L3P 7P3; Al-Fateh (Libya)'90; FRCPC; Anes. Staff, Markham Stouffville Hospital; (905)472-7000

HUSSEIN, Elysha; Albany Med Clinic, 807 Broadview Ave, Toronto ON M4K 2P8; Wes'08; CCFP; Staff, North York General Hospital.

HUSSEIN, Mahmoud R; Saint John Reg Hosp, PO Box 2100 Stn Main, Saint John NB E2L 4L2; Assuit (Egypt)'90; FRCPC; AnatPath. Staff, Saint John Regional Hospital; (506)648-6000

HUSSEIN, Mohamed R; Cape Breton Hlthcare Complex, Level 3-1482 George St, Sydney NS B1P 1P3; Ain Shams (Egypt)'85; MB ChB; Staff, Cape Breton Healthcare Complex; (902)567-7205; Fax. (902)567-7207.

HUSSEIN, Mohammed H; Ross Mem Hosp, 10 Angeline St N, Lindsay ON K9V 4M8; Baghdad (Iraq)'93; MB ChB; CCFP; Staff, Ross Memorial Hospital; (705)324-6111

HUSSEIN, Naushad; 127-8787 Woodbine Ave, Markham ON L3R 9S2; McG'82; FRCSC; Ophth. Ac Staff, Markham Stouffville Hospital; (905)474-3937; Fax. (905)415-3937.

HUSSEIN, Shaukat N; 506 Trethewey Dr, Toronto ON M6M 4C2; London (England)'64; MB BS; LRCP; MRCS; LMCC; (416)244-5210; Fax. (416)244-5208; shaukat.hussein@sympatico.ca.

HUSSEIN, Sohaileh; 506 Trethewey Dr, Toronto ON M6M 4C2; Sask'91; (416)244-5210; Fax. (416)244-5208.

HUSSEIN, Wissam M; Appletree Med Centre, 2016 Ogilvie Rd, Gloucester ON K1J 7N9; Mosul (Iraq)'89; CCFP.

HUSSEY, Andrew A; The Jenny Trout Centre, 201-342 Erie St, Stratford ON N5A 2N4; West Indies (Jamaica)'70; MB BS; FRCSC; Urol (Minimal Invasive Urology). Chief GenSurg, Stratford General Hospital - Huron Perth Healthcare Alliance; Chief GenSurg, Seaforth Community Hospital - Huron Perth Healthcare Alliance; St Marys Memorial Hospital - Huron Perth Healthcare Alliance; (519)271-7900; Fax. (519)271-2830; ahussey@rogers.com.

HUSSEY, Danielle M; James Paton Mem Hosp, 125 Trans Canada Hwy, Gander NL A1V 1P7; Mem'01; FRCPC; Neur. Staff, James Paton Memorial Hospital; (709)256-2500

HUSSEY, Jeffrey A; Kootenay-Boundary Reg Hosp, 1200 Hospital Bench, Trail BC V1R 4M1; Tor'00; CCFP; CCFP(E.M.); Staff, Kootenay Boundary Regional Hospital; (250)368-3311; jeffhussey@hotmail.com.

HUSSEY, Linda S; Bluewater Health-Norman Site, 89 Norman St, Sarnia ON N7T 6S3; Dal'83; FRCPC; Psy. Staff, Bluewater Health - Norman Site; University of Western Ontario; (519)464-4500

HUSSMAN, Edward A; Bloor Park Med Centre, 208-726 Bloor St W, Toronto ON M6G 4A1; Tor'77; Staff Family & CommunMed, Mount Sinai Hospital; (416)535-3164; Fax. (416)532-4453.

HUSSMAN, M Ruth; 402-235 Danforth Ave, Toronto ON M4K 1N2; McM'88; CCFP; FCFP; (416)466-4290; Fax. (416)466-4393.

HUSTON, Marcy A; 210-688 Coxwell Ave, Toronto ON M4C 3B7; Alb'81; (416)406-5088; Fax. (416)406-1319.

HUTCHEON, Michael A; NCSB 11C 1196, 200 Elizabeth St, Toronto ON M5G 2C4; Tor'70; FRCPC; IntMed (Transplantation); Respir. Prof Med, University of Toronto; (416)340-4019; Fax. (416)598-1819.

HUTCHINGS, Leslie A; Stayner Med & Dental Clinic, PO Box 220, Stayner ON L0M 1S0; McM'96; CCFP; (705)428-3246; Fax. (705)428-5652.

HUTCHINGS, Reg S; Linden Avenue Med Centre, 24 Linden Ave, Charlottetown PE C1A 5Y8; Dal'71; FRCPC; Neur (Adult Neurology). Ac Staff, Queen Elizabeth Hospital; (902)368-1084; Fax. (902)569-5293; rsh@pei.aibn.com.

HUTCHINGS, Robyn J; Edmonton Clinic Health Academy, 11405 87 Ave NW, Edmonton AB T6G 1C9; Mem'06; FRCPC; Peds. (780)248-5539

HUTCHINSON, Angela; North Road Med Centre, S-435 North Rd, Coquitlam BC V3K 3V9; UBC'93; CCFP; (604)936-0411

HUTCHINSON, Clare M; North York Gen Hosp, 4001 Leslie St, North York ON M2K 1E1; McG'04; FRCPC; Peds; Rheum. Staff, North York General Hospital; (416)756-6300

HUTCHINSON, Debra L; Hamilton HS-Hamilton Gen Site, 320-237 Barton St N, Hamilton ON L8L 2X2; Ott'86; CCFP; CCFP(E.M.); FCFP; Ac Staff Physician Education Specialist Clinical Practice & Education, Hamilton Health Sciences Centre - Hamilton General Hospital; Court Staff, St Joseph's Healthcare - Charlton Campus; Clinical Asst Prof EmergMed, McMaster University; (905)527-4322 x75465

HUTCHINSON, Gordon B; 5040 Block Dr PO Box 506, 108 Mile Ranch BC V0K 2Z0; McG'81; CCFP; CCFP(E.M.); (250)791-6584

HUTCHINSON, James M; Royal Jubilee Hosp, 1952 Bay St, Victoria BC V8R 1J8; Alb'85; FRCPC; MedMicrobiol. Staff, Royal Jubilee Hospital; (250)519-1941

HUTCHINSON, Janine M; Montebelle Med Centre, 8-118 Lake St, St Catharines ON L2R 5Y1; Qns'03; CCFP; (905)685-6555; Fax. (905)685-6558.

HUTCHINSON, Lisa G; Southlake Reg Health Centre, 596 Davis Dr, Newmarket ON L3Y 2P9; Tor'87; FRCPC; IntMed; Anes. Staff, Southlake Regional Health Centre; University of Toronto; (905)895-4521; Fax. (905)830-5972.

HUTCHINSON, Lois J; Lakenhead Psychiatric Hosp, PO Box 2930 Stn P, Thunder Bay ON P7B 5G4; Qns'74; FRCPC; Psy (Geriatric Medicine). Staff, Thunder Bay Regional Health Sciences Centre; Staff, Lakehead Psychiatric Hospital - St. Joseph's Care Group; (807)343-4300; Fax. (807)343-4373.

HUTCHINSON, Neil T; Port Hope Med Centre, 204-249 Ontario St, Port Hope ON L1A 3Y9; Tor'79; FRCSC; PlasSurg (Breast Surgery). Ac Staff, Lakeridge Health - Oshawa Site; (905)432-2419

HUTCHINSON, Tom A; MUHC-Royal Victoria Hosp, R409-687 av des Pins O, Montreal QC H3A 1A1; Dublin (Ireland)'71; MB ChB; FRCPC; IntMed (Palliative Care); Nephrol (P.Q.). Staff, McGill University Health Centre - Royal Victoria Hospital; Prof, McGill University; (514)934-1934

HUTCHINSON, Vivien; South Muskoka Med Centre, 230 Manitoba St, Bracebridge ON P1L 2E1; Sheffield (England)'64; (705)646-7634; Fax. (705)646-0476.

HUTCHINSON-JAFFE, Adam B; Univ of Toronto, 602-500 University Ave, Toronto ON M5G 1V7; Wes'08; FRCPC; IntMed.

HUTCHISON, Carolyn; 3330 Hospital Dr NW, Calgary AB T2N 4N1; McM'86; BSc; FRCSC; OrthSurg (Joint Replacement). Staff, Foothills Medical Centre; Assoc Prof, University of Calgary; (403)220-8737; Fax. (403)210-8165; cmantei@ucalgary.ca.

HUTCHISON, Mary E; 176 Commercial St PO Box 146 Stn Main, North Sydney NS B2A 3M1; Dal'75; (902)794-3494; Fax. (902)794-3702.

HUTCHISON, Robert J; 1309 Main St W, Hamilton ON L8S 1C5; McG'74; MDCM; FRCSC; ObstGyn. Court Staff, St Joseph's Healthcare - Charlton Campus; Ac Staff ObstGyn, Hamilton Health Sciences Centre - McMaster Children's Hospital; Clin Assoc Prof ObstGyn, McMaster University; (905)529-6571; Fax. (905)529-6573.

HUTCHISON, S Keith; Royal Inland Hosp, 311 Columbia St, Kamloops BC V2C 2T1; Alb'87; Staff, Royal Inland Hospital; (250)374-5111

HUTCHISON, Stuart J; Foothills Med Centre, C852A-1403 29 St NW, Calgary AB T2N 2T9; McG'86; FRCPC; IntMed; Cardiol. Staff, Foothills Medical Centre; (403)944-3258

HUTCHISON, Susan J; Worker's Comp Board, PO Box 2415 Stn Main, Edmonton AB T5J 2S5; Dal'87; (780)498-7942; Fax. (780)498-7807.

HUTCHISON, Trevor; Health Sciences Centre, GC419-820 Sherbrook St, Winnipeg MB R3A 1R9; Man'06; FRCPC; IntMed. Staff, Health Sciences Centre; (204)774-8511

HUTFLUSS, George J; Waverley Surgical Assoc, 4-871 Waverley St, Winnipeg MB R3T 5P4; Tor'81; BSc(Hons); FRCSC; GenSurg. Ac Staff, Victoria General Hospital; Ac Staff, The Salvation Army Grace Hospital; (204)488-3996; Fax. (204)888-0705.

HUTFLUSS, Richard M; St Mary's Gen Hosp, 911 Queens Blvd, Kitchener ON N2M 1B2; Tor'83; FRCPC; Anes. Staff Anes, St Mary's General Hospital; (519)744-3311

HUTH, Brian J; 204-10 Westheights Dr, Kitchener ON N2N 2A8; Tor'95; CCFP; FCFP; (905)745-7950; Fax. (905)885-8862.

HUTNIK, Cindy M; St Joseph's Health Centre, PO Box 5777 Stn B 268 Grosvenor St, London ON N6A 4V2; Ott'94; DAB; PhD; FRCSC; Ophth (Cataract & Glaucoma). Staff, London Health Sciences Centre - University Hospital; Staff, Clinton Public Hospital - Huron Perth Healthcare Alliance; Staff Eye Clinic, St Joseph's Hospital - St Joseph's Health Care; Aj Prof, University of Windsor; Asst Prof, University of Western Ontario; (519)646-6272; Fax. (519)646-6410.

HUTNYK, David J; Brief Intervention Unit, 715 12th Ave W, Vancouver BC V5Z 1M9; Cal'94; FRCPC; Psy. Staff, Vancouver General Hospital - Centennial Pavillion; Clinical Asst Prof, University of British Columbia; (604)875-5720; Fax. (604)875-5721; hutnyk@telus.net.

HUTSON, Maureen L; Hys Med Centre, 202-11010 101 St NW, Edmonton AB T5H 4B9; Sask'78; FRCPC; DiagRad. Ac Staff, Royal Alexandra Hospital; University of Alberta; (780)426-1121; Fax. (780)425-5979.

HUTTEN-CZAPSKI, Peter A; Family Health Clinic, PO Box 3000 293 Meridian Ave, Haileybury ON P0J 1K0; Qns'86; CCFP; FCFP; Staff, Temiskaming Hospital; (705)672-2442; Fax. (705)672-2384.

HUTTNER, Istvan; CSSS du Suroît, 150 rue Saint-Thomas, Salaber-de-Valleyf QC J6T 6C1; Budapest (Hungary)'61; PhD(McG); ABPath; CSPQ; FRCPC; AnatPath. Staff, Centre Hospitalier Régional du Suroît; (450)371-9920

HUTTON, Andrew S; Shoppers Drug Mart Bldg, 250 LeMarchant Rd, St. John's NL A1E 1P7; Mem'83; CCFP; (709)739-7444

HUTTON, Linda C; London HSC-University Hosp, PO Box 5339 Stn B 339 Windermere Rd, London ON N6A 5A5; McG'68; FACR; FRCPC; DiagRad. Staff, London Health Sciences Centre - University Hospital; Emeritus Prof, University of Western Ontario; (519)685-8500 x33648; Fax. (519)663-8803; linda.hutton@lhsc.on.ca.

HUTTON, Shannon K; Downey Family Med Centre, 2-115 Downey Rd, Guelph ON N1C 1A2; Qns'01; CCFP; Staff, Guelph General Hospital; (519)827-9779

HUTTON, Stewart A; 350-1620 29 St NW, Calgary AB T2N 4L7; (Ireland)'05; CCFP; (403)282-1269

HUTTON, Timothy; Prima Care Comm FHT-St George, 2 Sunnyside Dr, St George Brant ON N0E 1N0; Rochester(NY) (USA)'83; FAAFP; CCFP; Staff, The Brant Community Healthcare System - Brantford General Hospital Site; Clin Assoc Prof Family Med, McMaster University; (519)448-3331; Fax. (519)448-3334.

HUTTUNEN, K T Henrik; 2449-910 10th Ave W, Vancouver BC V5Z 1M9; UBC'01; FRCPC; Anes. Staff, Vancouver General Hospital - Centennial Pavillion; (604)875-4304

HUTZAL, Carolyn E; Andrew Street Family Hlth Ctre, 16 Andrew St, Kitchener ON N2H 5R2; Wes'07; Peds. (519)804-9234

HUWAIT, Hassan; Vancouver Gen Hosp, 855 12th Ave W, Vancouver BC V5Z 1M9; King Abdul Aziz (Saudi Arabia)'01; MB BS; FRCPC; AnatPath. Staff, Vancouver General Hospital - Centennial Pavillion; (604)875-4111 x54892

HUXTABLE, Leslie J; Medi-Kel CLinic, 105-330 Highway 33 W, Kelowna BC V1X 6A8; (Other Foreign)'02; MB ChB; (250)862-5915

HUYER, Dirk W; 1F-1 Stone Rd W, Guelph ON N1G 4Y2; Tor'86; Asst Prof Peds, University of Toronto; (519)837-6330

HUYNH, Chau Cong; 67-3175 Rutherford Rd, Concord ON L4K 5Y6; (Vietnam)'82; CCFP; Staff, Sunnybrook Health Sciences Centre; Langs: Vietnamese; (905)761-6082; Fax. (905)761-2144; chau.huynh@sunnybrook.ca.

HUYNH, Hien; Edmonton Clinic Health Academy, 4 579-11405 87 Ave NW, Edmonton AB T6G 1C9; Monash (Australia)'90; FRACP; MB BS; FRCPC; Peds (Pediatric Gastroenterology). Staff Gastroent, University of Alberta Hospital; Staff, Edmonton Clinic Health Academy; Assoc Prof, University of Alberta; Langs: Cantonese; Vietnamese; (780)248-5420; hien.huynh@ualberta.ca.

HUYNH, Huu Hung; CSSS Pierre Boucher, 1333 boul Jacques-Cartier E, Longueuil QC J4M 2A5; Sher'93; FRCPC; IntMed. Internal Med, Centre Hospitalier Pierre Boucher; Langs: Vietnamese; (450)468-8111 x2223

HUYNH, Khanh-Cong; Ctr Hosp de Verdun, 4000 boul Lasalle, Verdun QC H4G 2A3; Sher'88; CSPQ; AnatPath. Staff, Centre Hospitalier de Verdun; (514)362-1000 x2217

HUYNH, Nam Phuong T; Hop Santa Cabrini Ospedale, 5655 rue Saint-Zotique E, Montreal QC H1T 1P7; Mon'09; CCFP; Staff, Hôpital Santa Cabrini Ospedale; (514)252-6000

HUYNH, Nhu Nguyet; Providence Healthcare, C207-3276 St Clair Ave E, Scarborough ON M1L 1W1; Tor'08; CCFP; (416)285-3666 x4514

HUYNH, Phuoc Hai; Hop du Sacre-Coeur de Mtl, 5400 boul Gouin O, Montreal QC H4J 1C5; Sher'03; FRCSC; GenSurg. Staff, Hôpital du Sacre-Coeur de Montréal; (514)338-2222; Fax. (514)338-3515.

HUYNH, Quoc Hung P; 504-960 Lawrence Ave W, North York ON M6A 3B5; Tor'01; BSc; FRCSC; GenSurg (Bariatric Surgery). Langs: Vietnamese; (416)782-2616

HUYNH, Suong Ngoc; 10904B 107 Ave NW, Edmonton AB T5H 0X5; Saigon (Vietnam)'78; (780)429-1813; Fax. (780)424-0195.

HUYNH, Thi Phuong T; Centre Medical Alexandre, 8100 boul Taschereau, Longueuil QC J4X 1C2; Sher'96; (450)465-5589; Fax. (450)465-0092.

HUYNH, Xinh; Creditview Medical, 14B-1240 Eglinton Ave W, Mississauga ON L5V 1N3; Tor'94; Assoc Staff Family Pract, The Credit Valley Hospital; (905)567-4622

HUYNH BAO, Giang Thanh; CSSS de Saint-Jerome, 290 rue de Montigny, Saint-Jerome QC J7Z 5T3; Sher'95; GenSurg. Staff, Hôtel-Dieu de Saint-Jérôme; (450)431-8200

HUYNH THANH, Thao; MUHC-Montreal Gen Hosp, L6 200-1650 av Cedar, Montreal QC H3G 1A4; Mon'86; CSPQ; FRCPC; IntMed; Cardiol. Staff, McGill University Health Centre - Montreal General Campus; (514)934-1934; Fax. (514)934-8569; thao.huynh@muhc.mcgill.ca.

HUYSER, Charles A; East Kootenay Reg Hosp, 13 24th Ave N, Cranbrook BC V1C 3H9; Pretoria (South Africa)'90; MB ChB; FRCSC; ObstGyn. Staff, East Kootenay Regional Hospital; (250)426-5281

HUZEL, Leah N; Trainor Laboratory, 306-233 Kennedy St, Winnipeg MB R3C 0L7; Man'95; FRCPC; GenPath. (204)944-9707; Fax. (204)943-4797.

HUZEL, Lisa L; Lakeridge Hlth Corp-Oshawa, 1 Hospital Crt, Oshawa ON L1G 2B9; Man'94; FRCPC; IntMed (Asthma); Critical Care Medicine; Respir. Staff, Lakeridge Health - Oshawa Site; (905)576-8711 x3353

HWANG, Angela; Hillside Med Centre, 2867 Lawrence Ave E, Scarborough ON M1P 2T2; London (England)'81; MB BS; CCFP; FCFP; Staff, The Scarborough Hospital - General Campus; Lecturer, University of Toronto; Langs: Cantonese; Mandarin; (416)261-7223; Fax. (416)261-6374.

HWANG, Christine; Crossway Sexual Health Clinic, 2340 Dundas St W, Toronto ON M6P 4A9; McG'92; MSc; Langs: Cantonese; French; (416)338-7088

HWANG, David M; Univ Hlth Network-Toronto Gen, E11444-200 Elizabeth St, Toronto ON M5G 2C4; Tor'00; FRCPC; AnatPath. Pathologist, Toronto General Hospital - UHN; (416)340-4988; Fax. (416)586-9901; david.hwang@uhn.ca.

HWANG, Hamish S; Medical Clinic Associates, 200-3207 30 Ave, Vernon BC V1T 2C6; UBC'00; FRCSC; GenSurg (Endoscopic Surgery). Clin Instructor Med, University of British Columbia; (250)545-2288; Fax. (250)545-2781.

HWANG, Irene I L; 210-31 Disera Dr, Thornhill ON L4J 0A7; Cal'09; CCFP; (905)771-7755

HWANG, John M; Windsor Square Shopp Centre, 201-1959 152 St, Surrey BC V4A 9E3; Tor'00; FRCSC; GenSurg. (604)535-0525

HWANG, June H K; Royal Alexandra Hosp, 10240 Kingsway NW, Edmonton AB T5H 3V9; Tor'04; FRCPC; AnatPath. Staff, Royal Alexandra Hospital; (780)735-5133

HWANG, Liana L A; PO Box 65128 Rpo North Hill, Calgary AB T2N 4T6; Cal'06; CCFP; (403)284-3711; Fax. (403)284-3719.

HWANG, Mei L; Hillside Med Centre, 2867 Lawrence Ave E, Scarborough ON M1P 2T2; Ott'86; BMedSci; Staff, The Scarborough Hospital - General Campus; Staff, The Scarborough Hospital - Birchmount Campus; Langs: Mandarin; Cantonese; (416)261-7223; Fax. (416)261-6374.

HWANG, Naomi; VISTA/Elderly Outreach Service, 2828 Nanaimo St, Victoria BC V8T 4W9; Wes'98; CCFP; FCFP; (250)953-3966

HWANG, Norman H; Metrotown Med Centre, 303-6411 Nelson Ave, Burnaby BC V5H 4H3; Sask'94; FRCSC; Ophth. (604)433-1258

HWANG, Paul A L S; 402-1110 Sheppard Ave E, Toronto ON M2K 2W2; McG'74; BSc; MSc; FRCP; FRCPC; Neur (Clinical Neurophysiology). Staff Ped Neurol Dept of Peds, North York General Hospital; Associate, Toronto Western Hospital - University Health Network; Staff, Holland Bloorview Kids Rehabilitation Hospital; Consultant, Youthdale Centre; Assoc Prof Neurol/Co-Dir Epilepsy Research Program, University of Toronto; Langs: Chinese; Mandarin; Cantonese; Bilingual(French/English); (416)224-1922; Fax. (416)224-0056; phwang@nygh.on.ca.

HWANG, Peter M; University of Alberta Hosp, 8440 112 St NW, Edmonton AB T6G 2B7; Tor'07; FRCPC; IntMed. Staff, University of Alberta Hospital; (780)407-8822

HWANG, Stephen W; St Michael's Hosp, 30 Bond St, Toronto ON M5B 1W8; Johns Hopkins(MD) (USA)'88; MPH; FRCPC; IntMed. Staff, St Michael's Hospital; Assoc Prof, University of Toronto; (416)864-5991; Fax. (416)864-5485; hwangs@smh.toronto.on.ca.

HWANG, Theng G; 3107 35 Ave, Vernon BC V1T 2T2; Glasgow (Scotland)'74; MB ChB; DAB; FRCSC; GenSurg. Ac Staff/Chief GenSurg, Vernon Jubilee Hospital; (250)545-6443

HWEE, Peter T; 303-310 King St E, Kitchener ON N2G 2L3; Rangoon (Burma)'71; Staff, Grand River Hospital - Kitchener/Waterloo Health Centre; Staff, St Mary's General Hospital; Langs: Chinese; Burmese; (519)894-8800

HYACINTHE, Jean M F; Dr Jean-Michel Hyacinthe, 1904 rue Sherbrooke E, Montreal QC H2K 1B5; Port-au-Prince (Haiti)'73; CSPQ; FRCSC; PlasSurg (Maxillo Facial Surgery). Langs: Spanish; English; (514)509-9945

HYAKUTAKE, Momoe T; 11F-1190 Hornby St, Vancouver BC V6Z 2K5; Alb'07; ObstGyn. (604)806-9090

HYAMS, Ian A; Golden Ears Family Practice, 140-20395 Lougheed Hwy, Maple Ridge BC V2X 2P9; Pretoria (South Africa)'87; MB ChB; (604)465-1066

HYATT, H John; 4095 Pear Tree Crt SS 2, Vineland ON L0R 2C0; Wes'64; FRCSC; GenSurg (Vascular Surgery). Ac Staff, Niagara Health System - St Catharines General Site; (905)380-3127; Fax. (289)567-0762.

HYATT, Peter J; 211-282 Linwell Rd, St Catharines ON L2N 6N5; Wes'86; BSc; CCFP; FCFP; Staff, Niagara Health System - St Catharines General Site; (905)934-6165; Fax. (905)934-2251.

HYDE, Byron M; 121 Iona St, Ottawa ON K1Y 3M1; Ott'66; Chairman, Nightingale Research Foundation; Langs: Bilingual(English/French); (613)722-5555; Fax. (613)729-0148; office@nightingale.ca.

HYDE, J Patrick; Meadowlark Health Centre, 200 Meadowlark Shopping Ctr NW, Edmonton AB T5R 5W9; Witwatersrand (South Africa)'78; MB ChB; DTMH; FRCPC; DiagRad. (780)489-7851; Fax. (780)486-5160.

HYDE, Mandy M; Horizons Family Medicine, A-5016 51Ave, Red Deer AB T4N 4H5; Alb'02; BSc; CCFP; Staff, Red Deer Regional Hospital Centre; Physician, Associate Medical Group.

HYDERI, Abbas; Grey Nuns Community Hosp, 3301-1100 Youville Drive West, Edmonton AB T6L 5X8; (India)'00; MB BS; Staff, Covenant Health - Grey Nuns Community Hospital; (780)735-7037

HYDORN, Thomas G; 204-2 Lawrence St, Amherst NS B4H 3G5; Dal'86; Staff, Cumberland Regional Health Care Center; (902)667-2331; Fax. (902)667-4638.

HYDRI, Muneeb S; 9213 Lakeshore Dr, Grande Prairie AB T8X 8C9; (Pakistan)'87; MB BS; DiagRad. (780)814-9972; Fax. (780)814-9967.

HYLAND, G M Denise; East End Health Children's Centre, 2 Mount Cashel Rd, St. John's NL A1A 1X7; Dublin (Ireland)'82; MB ChB; BAO; Langs: Spanish; (709)579-5297

HYLAND, Robert H; St Michael's Hosp, 30 Bond St, Toronto ON M5B 1W8; Tor'73; FCCP; FACP; FRCPC; IntMed; Respir. Staff, St Michael's Hospital; (416)864-5811; Fax. (416)864-5649; hylandb@smh.ca.

HYLES, Rudolph S; 1758 Wedmore Way, Mississauga ON L5J 2J9; Dal'72; Ac Staff Family Pract, Halton Healthcare Services Corporation - Oakville Site; (905)823-1555; Fax. (905)822-2432.

HYMAN, Andrew R; Appletreee Med Group, 1-275 Dundas St W, Toronto ON M5T 1G1; Tor'95; FRCPC; IntMed; Nephrol. (647)722-2370

HYMAN, David I; Oxbow Med Clinic, PO Box 780, Oxbow SK S0C 2B0; Pretoria (South Africa)'96; MB ChB; CCFP; (306)483-2332

HYMAN, Jeffrey R; Children's Hosp, CH102-840 Sherbrook St, Winnipeg MB R3A 1S1; Man'00; FRCPC; Peds (Sports Medicine). Staff, Children's Hospital of Winnipeg; jhyman@hsc.mb.ca.

HYND, Jamie W H; 7-7748 Kent Blvd, Brockville ON K6V 7J9; Wes'83; FRCPC; IntMed; Cardiol. Head, Brockville General Hospital - Charles Street; Head Dept of Med, Bruyère Continuing Care - Saint-Vincent Hospital; Clin Asst, Queen's University; (613)345-1236; Fax. (613)345-4285.

HYNDMAN, C William; Alberta Children's Hosp, 2888 Shaganappi Trail NW, Calgary AB T2V 1P9; Alb'67; FAAP; FRCSC; Urol (Pediatrics). Staff, Alberta Children's Hospital; (403)955-2266; Fax. (403)955-7634.

HYNDMAN, John C; IWK Health Centre, PO Box 9700 Rpo CSC 5980 University Ave, Halifax NS B3K 6R8; Dal'69; DABOS; OrthSurg (Pediatric Orthopedics). Ac Staff, IWK Health Centre; Prof Surg, Dalhousie University; (902)470-7245; Fax. (902)470-7341; jc.hyndman@iwk.nshealth.ca.

HYNDMAN, Lucy T; Foothills Med Centre, 1403 29 St NW, Calgary AB T2N 2T9; Cal'98; CCFP; Staff, Foothills Medical Centre; (403)944-2800; Fax. (403)283-7365; lucy.hyndman@calgaryhealthregion.ca.

HYNDMAN, Matthew E; Rockyview Gen Hosp, 7007 14 St SW, Calgary AB T2V 1P9; Cal'04; FRCSC; Urol. Staff, Rockyview General Hospital; (403)943-8910

HYNES, Adrian F M; PsycHealth Centre, PZ202-771 Bannatyne Ave, Winnipeg MB R3E 3N4; Dublin (Ireland)'76; MB ChB; MRC; DCH; DRCOG; FRCPC; Psy (Addiction Medicine). Staff, Psychealth Centre; (204)787-5005

HYNES, Brian P; 2-110 Water St, Sarnia ON N7T 5T3; McM'83; FRCSC; Otol (Head & Neck Surgery). (519)332-5707; Fax. (519)332-0638.

HYNES, David M; Haldimand War Mem Hosp, 206 John St, Dunnville ON N1A 2P7; Cambridge (England)'61; MB ChB; DMRD; FRCP; FRCR; FRCPC; DiagRad. Staff, Haldimand War Memorial Hospital; (905)774-7431; Fax. (905)774-6776.

HYNES, Mark S; Univ of Ottawa Heart Institute, H 24-40 Ruskin St, Ottawa ON K1Y 4W7; McG'85; FRCPC; Anes. Staff, University of Ottawa Heart Institute; Staff, The Ottawa Hospital - Civic Campus; (613)761-4379; Fax. (613)761-4925.

HYNES, Nicolas M; Lotus Cosmetic Surg Ctr/Medisp, 199 MacNab St S, Hamilton ON L8P 3C8; McM'91; MSc; FRCSC; PlasSurg (Cosmetic Surgery). Staff Surgeon, St Joseph's Healthcare - Charlton Campus; Staff, Hamilton Health Sciences Centre - McMaster Children's Hospital; Med Dir, Lotus Cosmetic Surgery Centre & Medispa; Clinical Asst Prof, McMaster University; (905)645-5640; Fax. (905)645-5643; hynesplasticsurgery@sympatico.ca.

HYNES, Sally L; The Hosp for Sick Children, 5425-555 University Ave, Toronto ON M5G 1X8; Qns'05; PlasSurg. Staff Plastic & Reconstructive Surg, The Hospital For Sick Children; (416)813-6448

HYNES, William; Polyclinique Isabell-sur-Mer, 8224 rue St-Paul, Bas-Caraquet NB E1W 6E2; Sher'09; CCFP; (506)727-7549

HYNIE, Vera; 601-333 Preston St, Ottawa ON K1S 5N4; Prague (Czech Republic)'66; Langs: Czech; (613)234-7777; Fax. (613)235-5421.

HYNSCHT, Harold G; Dover Shores Family Practice, GD 410 Main St, Port Dover ON N0A 1N0; Tor'85; Staff, Norfolk General Hospital; Langs: German; (519)583-0892; Fax. (519)583-3981.

HYPPOLITE, Renaud; Centre de Cardiologie Rive-Sud, 303-3234 boul Taschereau, Greenfield Park QC J4V 2H3; Port-Au-Prince (Haiti)'58; Cardiol (P.Q.). (450)671-4182; Fax. (450)671-2249.

HYPPOLITE, Shirley-Rose; Centre de Sante Publique, 2400 av D'Estimauville, Quebec QC G1E 7G9; Laval'92; FRCPC; CommunMed. (418)666-7000

HYRMAN, Vaclav; 201-3701 Hastings St, Burnaby BC V5C 2H6; Karlova (Czech Republic)'65; LMCC; FRCPC; Psy (Electroconvulsive Therapy). Court Staff, Burnaby Hospital; Consultant Psy, Surrey Mental Health & Addictions; (604)299-6191; Fax. (604)299-6190; vhyrman@shaw.ca.

HYSHKA, Sandra A; Medical Assoc of Port Perry, 462 Paxton St, Port Perry ON L9L 1L9; Ott'94; Staff, Lakeridge Health - Port Perry Site; (905)985-2895; Fax. (905)985-8931.

HYSLOP, Douglas R; Georgian Bay Gen Hosp, PO Box 760 Stn Main 1112 St Andrews Dr, Midland ON L4R 4P4; McM'77; Staff, Georgian Bay General Hospital - Midland; (705)526-3751; Fax. (705)526-3448.

HYSON, H Christopher; 105-396 Queens Ave, London ON N6B 1X8; Dal'96; BScPharm; FRCPC; Neur (Movement Disorders). Staff, London Health Sciences Centre - University Hospital; Asst Prof, University of Western Ontario; (519)663-3404; Fax. (519)663-3416.

IABONI, Andrea; Univ Hlth Network-Toronto Gen, 8E 216-200 Elizabeth St, Toronto ON M5G 2C4; Tor'06; FRCPC; Psy. Staff, Toronto General Hospital - UHN; (416)340-3814

IACUCCI, Marietta; Health Research Innovation Ctr, 3280 Hospital Dr NW, Calgary AB T2N 4Z6; (Italy)'94; (403)592-5034; Fax. (403)592-5080.

IAKOUB, Elena; Aylmer-Lucerne Med Centre, 67 rue du Couvent, Gatineau QC J9H 6A2; Moscow (Russia (Federation))'95; CCFP; (819)684-1234; Fax. (819)684-1240.

IAKOVLEV, Vladimir V; St Michael's Hosp, CC 2 093-30 Bond St, Toronto ON M5B 1W8; Tjumen State (Russia (Federation))'94; FRCPC; AnatPath. Staff, St Michael's Hospital; (416)864-6060 x3176

IAKOVLEVA, Gaiane K; Markham Stouffville Hosp, PO Box 1800 Stn Main 381 Church St, Markham ON L3P 7P3; Tyumen State (Russia (Federation))'92; FRCPC; AnatPath. Staff, Markham Stouffville Hospital; (905)472-7000

IAMPEN, Corrina; Elle Ambiance Spa Vein/Skin, 302 Crowchild Trail NW, Calgary AB T2N 2R5; Sask'98; CCFP; (403)313-7546

IANCU, Andreea; CSSS de Vaudreuil-Soulanges, 490 boul Harwood, Vaudreuil-Dorion QC J7V 7H4; Cluj (Romania)'88; CCFP; Staff, CSSS de Vaudreuil-Soulanges; (450)455-6171; Fax. (450)455-6145; andreea_iancu@rrsss16.gouv.qc.ca.

IANCU, Daniela-Elena; The Ottawa Hosp-Civic Campus, 1053 Carling Ave, Ottawa ON K1Y 4E9; Bucharest (Romania)'97; Staff, The Ottawa Hospital - Civic Campus; (613)722-7000

IANKOVA, Vesselina; All Med Health, 1-16880 Yonge St, Newmarket ON L3Y 0A3; Sofia (Bulgaria)'85; CCFP; (905)895-9777; Fax. (905)895-9720.

IANNANTUONO, Biagio; South Muskoka Mem Hosp, 75 Ann St, Bracebridge ON P1L 2E4; Wes'92; FRCSC; GenSurg. Ac Staff, South Muskoka Memorial Hospital - Muskoka Algonquin Healthcare; Court Staff, Huntsville District Memorial Hospital - Muskoka Algonquin Healthcare; Langs: Italian; (705)646-1043; Fax. (705)646-1473.

IANNI, Floriana; Inst of Commun & Family Psy, 4333 ch Cote-Sainte-Catherine, Montreal QC H3T 1E4; Mon'90; FRCPC; Psy. Staff, Sir Mortimer B Davis Jewish General; Lecturer Psy, McGill University; (514)340-8210

IANNI, Frank A; The Group Health Centre, 320-955 Queen St E, Sault Ste. Marie ON P6A 2C3; Tor'75; CCFP; FCFP; Ac Staff, Sault Area Hospital - Sault Ste Marie; (705)759-1234 x7474; frank.ianni@sympatico.ca.

IANNICELLO, Carman M; Windsor Vein Centre, 300-880 North Service Rd E, Windsor ON N8X 3J5; Padova (Italy)'80; FRCSC; VascSurg. (519)250-4284

IBACH, Deborah M; 200-156 Meadowlark Shopping Ct, Edmonton AB T5R 5W9; Alb'88; BMedSci; FRCPC; DiagRad. (780)489-5313

IBACH, Richard J; Northern Lights Health Region, 7 Hospital St, Fort McMurray AB T9H 1P2; Alb'96; BSc; CCFP; CCFP(E.M.); (780)791-6161

IBARRETA, Nelson Y; Battlefords Union Hosp, 1092 107th St, North Battleford SK S9A 1Z1; Santo Tomas (Philippines)'60; Staff, Battlefords Union Hospital; (306)446-6500; Fax. (306)446-6546.

IBBITT, Christopher J; Medical Arts Bldg, 1611-233 Kennedy St, Winnipeg MB R3C 3J5; London (England)'68; DObst(Obs); (204)942-7339

IBBOTSON, Geoffrey C; 214 Med Place, 928-9909 102 St, Grande Prairie AB T8V 2V4; Tor'94; FRCSC; GenSurg. (780)539-4545

IBEY, Christopher C; Parry Sound Family Health Team, 57 James St, Parry Sound ON P2A 1T6; Tor'73; Staff, West Parry Sound Health Centre; (705)746-2181; Fax. (705)746-4753.

IBEY, Margaret M; Parry Sound Family Health Team, 57 James St, Parry Sound ON P2A 1T6; Tor'73; Assoc Staff, West Parry Sound Health Centre; (705)746-2181; Fax. (705)746-4753; mmibey@hotmail.com.

IBRAHIEM, Kawa M A; Cambridge Mem Hosp, 700 Coronation Blvd, Cambridge ON N1R 3G2; Mustansyriah (Iraq)'85; MB BS; CCFP; Clin Associate, University Health Network; Staff Psy, Cambridge Memorial Hospital; Langs: Kurdish; (519)621-2330 x3331; Fax. (519)740-4936; kawani_98@yahoo.com.

IBRAHIM, Abdulmajid S; Taunton Surgical Centre, SS 201 1F-1290 Keith Ross Dr, Oshawa ON L1H 7K4; Tripoli (Libya)'87; FRCSC; OrthSurg. (905)721-4922

IBRAHIM, Adel F A; Meadowood Gardens, 303-566 St Anne's Rd, Winnipeg MB R2M 1G5; Cairo (Egypt)'85; MB BCh; CCFP; Langs: French; Arabic; (204)415-6562; Fax. (204)255-5290; aibrahim@brha.mb.ca.

IBRAHIM, Amir A; 3101-222 King St E, Bowmanville ON L1C 1P6; Vinnitsa (Ukraine)'91; FRCSC; GenSurg.

IBRAHIM, Edgar; 301-164 rue des Tresors-de-l'i, Repentigny QC J5Z 4P7; Mon'76; Langs: Italian; English.

IBRAHIM, Evelin; 100-205 Newport Dr, Port Moody BC V3H 5C9; Cairo (Egypt)'86; MB ChB; CCFP; Langs: Arabic; (604)461-0016; Fax. (604)461-0013.

IBRAHIM, Fahim K F; 115-704 Mara St, Point Edward ON N7V 1X4; Ain Shams (Egypt)'74; FRCSC; Ophth. (519)336-9988; Fax. (519)336-8069.

IBRAHIM, Hany S H; Bridletowne Med Centre, 5-3245 Finch Ave E, Scarborough ON M1W 4C1; Ain Shams (Egypt)'92; CCFP; FCFP; Langs: Arabic; (416)490-0544; Fax. (416)490-0644; bridletownemedical@yahoo.ca.

IBRAHIM, Hisham G E M; Fitzgerald Bldg, 121-150 College St, Toronto ON M5S 3E2; Cairo (Egypt)'95; (416)978-4306

IBRAHIM, Hisham; 180-17010 90 Ave NW, Edmonton AB T5T 1L6; (Libya)'03; MB ChB; (780)487-4260; Fax. (780)481-6776.

IBRAHIM, Ihab I S; 100-205 Newport Dr, Port Moody BC V3H 5C9; Cairo (Egypt)'80; MB ChB; (604)461-0016; Fax. (604)461-0013.

IBRAHIM, Imran; Shellbrook Primary Hlth Care C, PO Box 1030, Shellbrook SK S0J 2E0; (Other Foreign)'99; CCFP; (306)747-2552

IBRAHIM, Jawahir I A; McConnell Med Centre, 207-820 McConnell Ave, Cornwall ON K6H 4M4; Ain Shams (Egypt)'96; CCFP; (613)935-6414; Fax. (613)935-8560.

IBRAHIM, Julie; Hop Sante Cabrini Ospedale, 5655 rue Saint-Zotique E, Montreal QC H1T 1P7; Mon'03; CCFP; Staff, Hôpital Santa Cabrini Ospedale; (514)252-6000

IBRAHIM, Khaled M O; Niagara Health Centre, 308-180 Vine St S, St Catharines ON L2R 7P3; Al Fateh (Libya)'95; FRCPC; IntMed; Gastroent. (905)682-8693

IBRAHIM, Magdy L A; Steinbach Family Med Centre, 10-333 Loewen Blvd, Steinbach MB R5G 0C3; Mansoura (Egypt)'83; (204)326-3401; Fax. (204)326-3899.

IBRAHIM, Magdy; 41 Edgewood Cres, Markham ON L6C 2K7; (Other Foreign)'83; CCFP.

IBRAHIM, Maged S H; Bridle Towne Med Centre, 5-3245 Finch Ave E, Scarborough ON M1W 4C1; Ain Shams (Egypt)'91; CCFP; (416)490-0544

IBRAHIM, Mahdi K; Bonavista Peninsula Health Ctr, Postal Service 1 1 Hospital Rd, Bonavista NL A0C 1B0; Baghdad (Iraq)'92; MB ChB; Staff, Bonavista Peninsula Health Centre; Langs: Kurdish; Arabic; (709)468-7881; Fax. (709)468-7690; madi.jaff@gmail.com.

IBRAHIM, Mohammed A; 216-2120 North Park Dr, Brampton ON L6S 0C9; Glasgow (Scotland)'72; MB ChB; FACS; DABU; FRCSC; Urol (Oncology). Associate, Headwaters Health Care Centre - Orangeville Site; Ac Staff, William Osler Health System - Brampton Civic Hospital; Langs: Urdu; Punjabi; (905)453-3251; Fax. (905)453-9623.

IBRAHIM, Mohammud S; Valley Med Clinic, 335 Jubilee St, Duncan BC V9L 1W9; Cape Town (South Africa)'01; MB ChB; (250)748-8151

IBRAHIM, Moheb S; St Mary's Gen Hosp, 911 Queens Blvd, Kitchener ON N2M 1B2; Asyut (Egypt)'81; MB ChB; FRCS(Ed); FRCSC; CardSurg. Staff, Southlake Regional Health Centre; (519)744-3311

IBRAHIM, Nancy; Ctr Hosp Anna-Laberge, 200 boul Brisebois, Chateauguay QC J6K 4W8; Alexandria (Egypt)'05; CCFP; FCFP; Staff, Hôpital Anna-Laberge; (450)699-2425

IBRAHIM, Narmin; Community Clinic, 455 2nd Ave N, Saskatoon SK S7K 2C2; (Iraq)'86; CCFP; Langs: Kurdish; Arabic; (306)652-0300; Fax. (306)652-0682.

IBRAHIM, Nathalie; Hop Santa Cabrini Ospedale, 5655 rue Saint-Zotique E, Montreal QC H1T 1P7; McG'05; FRCPC; DiagRad. Staff, Hôpital Santa Cabrini Ospedale; (514)252-6000

IBRAHIM, Nurain; Medical Associates, 100-155 Main St E, Grimsby ON L3M 1P2; Karachi (Pakistan)'98; CCFP.

IBRAHIM, Ragui A B; Institut de Cardiologie de Mtl, 5000 rue Belanger, Montreal QC H1T 1C8; Cairo (Egypt)'95; IntMed. Staff, Institut de Cardiologie de Montréal; (514)376-3330

IBRAHIM, Reda; Institut de Cardiologie de Mtl, 5000 rue Bélanger, Montreal QC H1T 1C8; Mon'94; FRSM; Cardiol; IntMed (Hemodynamics). Dir Medical Intensive Care, Institut de Cardiologie de Montréal; assoc Prof, Universite de Montreal; Langs: Bilingual(French/English); (514)376-3330 x3800; Fax. (514)593-2158; reda.ibrahim@icm-mhi.org.

IBRAHIM, Rizqi N; Associate Family Phys Clinic, 262 2nd Ave NE, Swift Current SK S9H 2C8; Cairo (Egypt)'70; MB ChB; Ac Staff, Cypress Regional Hospital; Ac Staff, Palliser Regional Care Centre; Ac Staff, Swift Current Care Centre; (306)773-1555; Fax. (306)773-6817; rdjib@shaw.ca.

IBRAHIM, Salwa N K; 209-3410 Sheppard Ave E, Scarborough ON M1T 3K4; (Egypt)'83; CCFP; (416)293-4942

IBRAHIM, Samia M R; St Mary Clinic, 2010 Trim Rd, Orleans ON K4A 0G4; Cairo (Egypt)'82; Langs: Arabic; French; (613)590-1433

IBRAHIM, Sarwat; Brampton Multidisciplinary Cli, 180 Sandalwood Pky E, Brampton ON L6Z 1Y4; Cairo (Egypt)'82; CCFP; (905)846-5271; Fax. (905)846-2525; sarwatri@hotmail.com.

IBRAHIM, Wael F; Stellarton Med Centre, PO Box 2550 10 Jubilee Ave, Stellarton NS B0K 1S0; Cairo (Egypt)'90; MB BCh; (902)695-3246; Fax. (902)695-3247.

IBSEN, David G B; 200 Brock St N, Whitby ON L1N 4H5; Tor'86; CCFP; (905)668-3378; Fax. (905)668-3807.

IBUDE, Bose E; Dr Charles S Curtis Mem Hosp, 178-200 West St, St Anthony NL A0K 4S0; (Nigeria)'01; MB BS; Staff, Charles S Curtis Memorial Hospital.

ICKOWICZ, Abel; The Hosp for Sick Children, 555 University Ave, Toronto ON M5G 1X8; (Costa Rica)'78; FRCPC; Psy (Child & Adolescent Psychiatry). Staff Psychiatrist, The Hospital For Sick Children; Assoc Prof Psy, University of Toronto; (416)813-7524; Fax. (416)813-5326.

ICTON, Carolyn D; 106-15252 32 Ave, Surrey BC V3S 0R7; UBC'05; CCFP; (604)542-4885

IDAMI, Wilson O; Hollidge Med Centre, B6-130 Hollidge Blvd, Aurora ON L4G 8A3; Benin (Nigeria)'91; CCFP; (905)841-5554

IDANWEKHAI, Evaristus; Princeton Gen Hosp, PO Box 610 98 Ridgewood Dr, Princeton BC V0X 1W0; Benin (Nigeria)'95; MB BS; CCFP; Staff, Princeton General Hospital; (250)295-4482

IDESTRUP, Christopher; Sunnybrook Hlth Sciences Ctre, 2075 Bayview Ave, Toronto ON M4N 3M5; Tor'00; MSc; BSc; FRCPC; Anes (Regional Anesthesia). Staff, Sunnybrook Health Sciences Centre; (416)480-6100 x3230

IDIONG, N Daniel; Women's Hosp, WS012-735 Notre Dame Ave, Winnipeg MB R3E 0L8; Enugu (Nigeria)'76.

IDZIOR, Janusz M; Stephenville Comm Med Clinic, 1 Washington Dr, Stephenville NL A2N 2V5; Wroclaw (Poland)'68; DrMedCh; Staff, Sir Thomas Roddick Hospital; Langs: Polish; (709)643-5656; Fax. (709)643-5543; jidzior@nf.sympatico.ca.

IFABIYI, Godwin O; Hamilton Comm Health Centre, M6-414 Victoria Ave N, Hamilton ON L8L 5G8; Ibadan (Nigeria)'87; MB BS; CCFP; (905)525-1741

IFERGAN, Nathalie; Pavillon Rosemont, 5689 boul Rosemont, Montreal QC H1T 2H1; Mon'94; CCFP; Staff, Hopital Maisonneuve-Rosemont; (514)252-3400

IFTENE, Felicia; Providence Care-Mental Health, PO Box 603 Stn Main 752 King St W, Kingston ON K7L 4X3; Cluj (Romania)'84; FRCPC; Psy. Staff, Providence Care - Mental Health Services; (613)548-6164; Fax. (613)540-6196.

IFTIKHAR, Asma; Park Royal Med Centre, 2425 Truscott Dr, Mississauga ON L5J 2B4; Punjab (India)'86; CCFP; (905)823-5020

IGARTUA, Karine J; MUHC-Montreal Gen Hosp, A2 224-1650 av Cedar, Montreal QC H3G 1A4; McG'94; DPsy; FRCPC; Psy (Emergency Psychiatry). Staff Psy, McGill University Health Centre - Montreal General Campus; adj Prof Psy/Co-Dir Sexual Identity Centre, McGill University; (514)934-1934 x42365; Fax. (514)934-8471.

IGBEKOYI, Olawale F; Rosetown & Dist Primary Care C, PO Box 1810, Rosetown SK S0L 2V0; (306)882-1212

IGBINOSA, Christine; Ladysmith Comm Health Centre, PO Box 10 1111 4th Ave, Ladysmith BC V9G 1A1; Benin (Nigeria)'93; MB BS; (250)739-5738

IGBINOSA, Osayuwame; 3-1273 Island Hwy S, Nanaimo BC V9R 7A4; Benin (Nigeria)'93; MB BS; (250)754-3822

IGE, Olabode A; Family Physicians Group, PO Box 2170, Melfort SK S0E 1A0; (Other Foreign)'98; CCFP; (306)752-5505; Fax. (306)752-5508; olabodeigea@gmail.com.

IGHEMA, Mohamed R; 12620A 132 Ave NW, Edmonton AB T5L 3P9; Tripoli (Libya)'99; MB BCh; (780)990-1820

IGIDBASHIAN, Levon; Hop de la Cite-de-la-Sante, 1755 boul Rene-Laennec, Laval QC H7M 3L9; Mon'04; FRCPC; RadOncol. Staff, Hopital de la Cite de la santé; (450)668-1010

IGLAR, Karl T; St Michael's Hosp, 30 Bond St, Toronto ON M5B 1W8; Tor'91; CCFP; Staff, St Michael's Hospital; (416)867-7428; Fax. (416)867-7498.

IGLESIAS, Ivan R; London HSC-University Hosp, PO Box 5339 Stn B 339 Windermere Rd, London ON N6A 5A5; Santander (Colombia)'84; FRCPC; Anes. Staff, London Health Sciences Centre - University Hospital; (519)685-8300

IGLESIAS, Juan R; INESSS, 60-1195 av Lavigne, Quebec QC G1V 4N3; Sher'72; MSc; (418)644-8120

IGLESIAS, Marie-Helene; Hôpital Ste-Justine, 3175 ch Cote-Sainte-Catherine, Montreal QC H3T 1C5; Mon'03; FRCSC; ObstGyn (Maternal Fetal Medicine). Staff, Hôpital Ste-Justine; (514)345-4706; Fax. (514)345-4648.

IGLESIAS, Stuart J; R W Large Mem Hosp, 88 Waglisla St, Bella Bella BC V0T 1Z0; Tor'79; Staff, R W Large Memorial Hospital; Clinical Asst Prof Family Med, University of British Columbia; Langs: Bilingual(French/English); (250)957-2332; Fax. (250)957-2360; drsiglesias@gmail.com.

IGNACIO, Bayani S; 750 Main St PO Box 208 Stn Sydney Mines, Sydney Mines NS B1V 2Y5; Santo Tomas (Philippines)'58; FACS; FRCSC; GenSurg (Endoscopy). Staff, Cape Breton Healthcare Complex; Chief Surg, Northside General Hospital; (902)544-0210; Fax. (902)736-8882.

IGNACIO, Eugene E; 750 Main St PO Box 208 Stn Sydney Mines, Sydney Mines NS B1V 2Y5; Dal'84; CCFP; (902)544-0210; Fax. (902)736-8882.

IGNASZEWSKI, Andrew P; St Paul's Hosp, 180-1081 Burrard St, Vancouver BC V6Z 1Y6; Lublin (Poland)'83; FRCPC; IntMed (Nuclear Medicine); Cardiol. Staff, Providence Health Care - St Paul's Hospital; Staff, Vancouver General Hospital - Centennial Pavillion; Langs: Polish; (604)806-8605; Fax. (604)806-8596.

IGNASZEWSKI, Wojciech M; Carbonear Gen Hosp, 86 Highroad South, Carbonear NL A1Y 1A4; Lublin (Poland)'87; Staff, Carbonear General Hospital; (709)945-5111

IGOE, Michael P; Northside Harbor View Hosp, PO Box 399 Stn Main, North Sydney NS B2A 3M4; Galway (Ireland)'67; MB BCh; BAO; MRC; FRCPC; IntMed (Rheumatology). Staff Internist, Northside General Hospital; (902)794-7704; Fax. (902)794-7801.

IGRAS-KULACH, Dorothy; Sunridge Prof Centre, 308-2675 36 St NE, Calgary AB T1Y 6H6; Cal'92; FRCSC; ObstGyn. Staff ObstGyn, Peter Lougheed Centre; Langs: Polish; (403)215-4070; Fax. (403)215-4071.

IHSAN, Novin; South Health Campus, 4448 Front St SE, Calgary AB T3M 1M4; UBC'07; Psy. (403)889-6321

IIZUKA, Megumi; St Joseph's Health Centre, 30 The Queensway, Toronto ON M6R 1B5; Cal'01; BASc; MSc; FRCSC; Ophth. Staff Eye Clinic, St Joseph's Health Centre; Lecturer, University of Toronto; (416)530-6118

IJAZ, Mohammad S; Broad Med Specialists, 2275 Broad St, Regina SK S4P 1Y7; (Pakistan)'88; Langs: Urdu; Punjabi; (306)352-4441; Fax. (306)352-4446.

IJAZ, Sabina P; George M Guimond Care Ctr Inc, PO Box 308, Pine Falls MB R0E 1M0; McM'00; CCFP; Physician Emerg & Admitting Privil, Pine Falls Health Complex; Physician, Fort Alexander Health Centre; Physician, George M Guimond Care Centre; Langs: Bilingual(French/English); German; isabina@hotmail.com.

IKARI, Michael Y; Second Avenue Med Clinic, 330 2nd Ave W, Prince Rupert BC V8J 1G6; UBC'97; CCFP; Staff, Prince Rupert Regional Hospital; (250)624-5500

IKEJI, Ngozi; Aurora Clinic, 5 Hospital Rd, Whitehorse YT Y1A 3H7; Lagos (Nigeria)'78; MB BS; Langs: Ibo; (867)393-8923

IKEJIANI, Charles E; Royal Court Med Centre, 209-5 Quarry Ridge Rd, Barrie ON L4M 7G1; Dal'95; FRCSC; OrthSurg. (705)727-4050; Fax. (705)727-4055.

IKEMURA, Maki; Bella Bella Med Clinic, 88 Waglisla St, Bella Bella BC V0T 1Z0; Alb'95; CCFP; FCFP; (250)957-2332

IKIZLER, Yasemin; St Joseph's Hlth Ctre, 306-27 Roncesvalles Ave, Toronto ON M6R 3B2; Tor'93; CCFP; (416)761-0133; Fax. (416)761-1915; yasemin.ikizler@sickkids.ca.

IKUTA, Roland M; Chinook Reg Hosp, 960 19 St S, Lethbridge AB T1J 1W5; Alb'86; FRCPC; IntMed; GeriatricMed. Sr Med Dir, Chinook Regional Hospital; Langs: Japanese; (403)388-6600; rolikuta@shaw.ca.

ILAGAN-NYAME, Matilde; Lloydminster Hosp, 3820 43rd Ave, Lloydminster SK S9V 1Y5; Staff, Lloydminster Hospital; (306)820-6000

ILAN, Roy; Queen's Univ-Etherington Hall, 1005-94 Stuart St, Kingston ON K7L 2V6; Haifa (Israel)'98; MSc; Staff, Kingston General Hospital; Asst Prof, Queen's University; (613)533-2131; Fax. (613)533-6654; ilanr@kgh.kari.net.

ILANGO, Sumathy; Dr Charles A Janeway Child HC, 300 Prince Philip Dr, St. John's NL A1B 3V6; Jaffna (Sri Lanka)'91; MB BS; Clin Associate, Janeway Children's Health & Rehabilitation Centre; (709)777-4222

ILCEWICZ-KLIMEK, Magdalena I; Neuropsychiatry Dept, 2255 Wesbrook Mall, Vancouver BC V6T 2B5; Warsaw (Poland)'98; FRCPC; Psy. Staff, UBC Hospital - Koerner Pavillion; Langs: Polish; (604)822-7549

ILCHYNA, Daniel C; Steinbach Family Med Centre, 10-333 Loewen Blvd, Steinbach MB R5G 0C3; Man'95; CCFP; FCFP; Staff, Bethesda Hospital Steinbach; (204)326-3401; Fax. (204)326-3899; dilchyna@sehealth.mb.ca.

ILES, David L; Saint John Reg Hosp, PO Box 2100 Stn Main, Saint John NB E2L 4L2; Dal'86; FRCPC; DiagRad (Cardiovascular Imaging). Staff Diagnostic Imaging, Saint John Regional Hospital; Assoc Prof, Dalhousie University; (506)648-6918; Fax. (506)648-6925; diles@health.nb.ca.

ILES, Sian E; Queen Elizabeth II HSC, 3237-1276 South Park St, Halifax NS B3H 2Y9; Dal'82; FRCPC; DiagRad; NuclearMed. Staff, Queen Elizabeth II Health Sciences Centre - Victoria General Site; Asst Prof, Dalhousie University; (902)473-2388; Fax. (902)473-2018.

ILIE-HAYNES, Radu T; 201-20 14th St W, Prince Albert SK S6V 3K8; Timisoara (Romania)'80; FRCPC; IntMed. (306)763-9580; Fax. (306)763-9583.

ILIES, Drigissa A; CSSSNL, 204-465 rue Notre-Dame, Repentigny QC J6A 2T3; Mon'02; FRCPC; Psy. (450)581-5100 x428

ILIESCU, Eduard A; Kingston Gen Hosp, 76 Stuart St, Kingston ON K7L 2V7; Wes'90; FRCPC; IntMed; Nephrol. Staff, Kingston General Hospital; (613)549-6666

ILIVITSKY, Vadim B; Royal Ottawa Hlth Care Group, 1145 Carling Ave, Ottawa ON K1Z 7K4; Donetsk (Russia (Federation))'63; FRCPC; Psy (Schizophrenia). Staff Schizophrenia Serv, Royal Ottawa Mental Health Centre - Royal Ottawa Health Care Group; Asst Prof, University of Ottawa; Langs: Russian; (613)722-6521 x6533; Fax. (613)798-2971; vadiri.ilivitsy@rohcg.on.ca.

ILK, Lisa A; Flemingdon Health Centre, 10 Gateway Blvd, North York ON M3C 3A1; Tor'03; CCFP; (416)429-4991

ILKOV-MOOR, Snezana S; Providence Care-Mental Health, PO Box 603 Stn Main 752 King St W, Kingston ON K7L 4X3; Qns'00; FRCPC; Psy (Geriatric Psychiatry). Staff, Providence Care - Mental Health Services; (613)546-1101

ILLAMPERUMA, Chamani; Promenade Med Centre, 129 Church St S, Richmond Hill ON L4C 1W4; Colombo (Sri Lanka)'00; FRCPC; IntMed. (905)884-0977; Fax. (905)884-6454.

ILLAMPERUMA ARACHCHIGE, Dilum C; Promenade Med Centre, 46-7700 Bathurst St, Thornhill ON L4J 7Y3; Ross(Edison,NJ) (USA)'02; CCFP; (905)707-0977

ILLAMPERUMA ARACHCHIGE, Lasith R; Promenade Med Centre, 46-7700 Bathurst St, Thornhill ON L4J 7Y3; Ross(Edison,NJ) (USA)'02; CCFP; (905)707-0977

ILLESCAS, Alfred W; 1-227 boul Saint-Joseph E, Montreal QC H2T 1H9; McG'79; Att Physician, McGill University Health Centre - Royal Victoria Hospital; Langs: French; Spanish; Italian; (514)288-2488; Fax. (514)288-2022.

ILLICAL, Emmanuel M; The Ottawa Hosp-Gen Campus, W1650-501 Smyth Rd, Ottawa ON K1H 8L6; Alb'06; FRCSC; OrthSurg. Staff, The Ottawa Hospital - General Campus; (613)737-8774

ILLING, Leigh H G; Foothills Med Centre, 1403 29 St NW, Calgary AB T2N 2T9; Cape Town (South Africa)'84; FRCPC; Anes. Staff Anes, Foothills Medical Centre; (403)944-1430

ILLING, Martin A J; Mount St Joseph Hosp, 3080 Prince Edward St, Vancouver BC V5T 3N4; Ott'88; FRCPC; Psy (Geriatric Psychiatry). Staff, Providence Health Care - Mount Saint Joseph Hospital; (604)877-8163

ILLING, V Kim; Foothills Med Centre, 1403 29 St NW, Calgary AB T2N 2T9; Sask'86; FRCPC; Anes. Staff Anes, Foothills Medical Centre; (403)944-1430

ILLINGWORTH, Meghan; Elaho Med Clinic, PO Box 10003 Rpo The Chieftain 1337 Pemberton Ave, Squamish BC V8B 0R1; UBC'03; CCFP; (604)892-5618

ILLMAN, Jeffery E; Sudbury Reg Hosp-Laurentian, 41 Ramsey Lake Rd, Sudbury ON P3E 5J1; Tor'96; DiagRad (Neuro Radiology). Staff, Health Sciences North-Laurentian Site; (705)523-7100 x580

ILNICKI, Teresa M; Alberta Children's Hosp, 2888 Shaganappi Trail NW, Calgary AB T3B 6A8; Cal'92; CCFP; CCFP(E.M.); FCFP; Staff, Alberta Children's Hospital; (403)955-7862

ILNYCKYJ, Alexandra; St Boniface Gen Hosp, 409 Tache Ave, Winnipeg MB R2H 2A6; Man'87; FRCPC; IntMed. Staff, St Boniface General Hospital; (204)237-2796; Fax. (204)233-7154.

ILO, Mary P; Brant Community HC-Brantford, 200 Terrace Hill St, Brantford ON N3R 1G9; (Italy)'94; CCFP; CCFP(E.M.); Staff, The Brant Community Healthcare System - Brantford General Hospital Site; (519)751-5544 x5507

ILORETA, Aileen; Hye Park Express, 15-555 12 Ave W, Vancouver BC V5Z 3X7; Cal'09; CCFP; (778)918-5963

ILSE, Werner K; Health Sciences Centre, GE 248-820 Sherbrook St, Winnipeg MB R3A 1R9; Wes'83; BSc; MSc; FRCPC; IntMed (Neuromuscular Diseases); Neur. Att Staff Neurol, Health Sciences Centre; Att Staff, St Boniface General Hospital; Asst Prof Neurol, University of Manitoba; Langs: Afrikaans; French; (204)787-7252; Fax. (204)787-5158.

ILYAS, Amir; 306-1669 Victoria St, Prince George BC V2L 2L5; Karachi (Pakistan)'95; MB BS; FRCPC; Neur. (250)612-0221; Fax. (250)612-0228.

IM, Stephen S; 404-55 Queen St E, Toronto ON M5C 1R6; Tor'78; FACOG; FRCSC; ObstGyn (Micro Surgery). Ac Staff, St Michael's Hospital; Consultant Gyn, Centre for Addiction & Mental Health (CAMH) - College Street Site; Asst Prof, University of Toronto; Langs: Korean; (416)864-5913; Fax. (416)864-5572.

IM, Tae-Bin T; Terrace Hill Med Centre, 217 Terrace Hill St, Brantford ON N3R 1G8; Tor'82; Langs: Korean; (519)752-7863; Fax. (519)752-7824.

IMAM, Isam E D B; Healthway/Four Seasons Clinic, 713 Portage Ave, Winnipeg MB R3G 0M8; (Romania)'83; CCFP.

IMANA, Mohammed M; Brookfield Bonnews HC Centre, PO Box 209 57 Main St, Brookfield NL A0G 1J0; Ibadan (Nigeria)'91; MB BS; Staff, Brookfield Bonnews Health Care Centre; (709)536-9440; Fax. (709)536-1344.

IMASOGIE, Ngozi; Leamington Dist Mem Hosp, 194 Talbot St W, Leamington ON N8H 1N9; Ibadan (Nigeria)'84; Staff, Leamington District Memorial Hospital; (519)326-2373

IMBEAU, Eric; Hotel-Dieu de Levis, 143 rue Wolfe, Levis QC G6V 3Z1; Laval'92; FRCSC; GenSurg. Staff, Hôtel-Dieu de Lévis; (418)835-7121

IMBEAULT, Annie; Clinique d'urologie Berger, 416-1000 ch Sainte-Foy, Quebec QC G1S 2L6; Laval'07; Urol. (418)266-2876

IMBEAULT, Bruno; CSSS de Sept-Iles, 45 rue du Pere-Divet, Sept-Iles QC G4R 3N7; Mon'84; FRCPC; IntMed; Respir. Staff, Centre Hospitalier Regional de Sept-Iles; (418)962-9761

IMBEAULT, Carrol; Ctr Hosp Affilie-Enfant-Jesus, 1401 18e rue, Quebec QC G1J 1Z4; Laval'81; Ac Staff, Centre Hospitalier Affilié Universitaire de Québec - Hôpital De L'Enfant Jésus; (418)649-5882; carol.imbeault@cha.quebec.qc.ca.

IMBEAULT, Jean; CHUM-Hop Notre-Dame, 1560 rue Sherbrooke E, Montreal QC H2L 4M1; Laval'70; FRCPC; Psy. Staff, Centre Hospitalier l'Université de Montréal (CHUM) - Hôpital Notre-Dame; (514)890-8000 x25665

IMBEAULT, Sarto; Clinique de Readap de l'Avenir, 210-1150 boul de l'Avenir, Laval QC H7N 6L2; Mon'75; FRCPC; PhysMed&Rehab (Industrial Occupational Medicine). Staff, Clinique de Physiatrie; (450)973-9280; Fax. (450)973-8100.

IMBEAULT, Stephanie; CSSS de Lac-Saint Jean-Est, CP 1300 Succ Bureau-Chef 300 boul Champlain, Alma QC G8B 5W3; Sher'05; Psy. Staff, CSSS de Lac-Saint Jean-Est; (418)669-2000

IMBULGODA, Manel R; 25-255 Dundas St E, Waterdown ON L0R 2H4; Colombo (Sri Lanka)'82; MB BS; CCFP; Associate, Dr Everett Chalmers Regional Hospital; Langs: Sinhalese; (905)689-8242

IMLAH, Shona M; 12230 106 Ave NW, Edmonton AB T5N 3Z1; UBC'08; CCFP; (780)482-2626

IMMELMAN, Lynleigh J; Lansdowne Professional Ctr II, 265-3066 Shelbourne St, Victoria BC V8R 6T9; Witwatersrand (South Africa)'75; FRCPC; Psy.

IMMELMAN, Philip L; Associate Med Clinic, PO Box 510, Slave Lake AB T0G 2A0; Stellenbosch (South Africa)'74; MB ChB; Langs: Afrikaans; German; (780)849-4155; Fax. (780)849-4574.

IMOUKHUEDE, Unuigboje; Rockyview Gen Hosp, 7007 14 St SW, Calgary AB T2V 1P9; (Nigeria)'98; MB BS; Staff Neurol, Rockyview General Hospital; (403)943-3579

IMPERIAL, Miguel; Station Square Med Clinic, 146-6200 McKay Ave, Burnaby BC V5H 4L7; UBC'05; FRCPC; MedMicrobiol. Staff, Station Square Medical Clinic; (604)438-8288

IMRAN, Aatika; 499 Oxford St E, London ON N5Y 3H8; Islamabad (Pakistan)'05; CCFP.

IMRAN, Ayesha; 510-1110 Panatella Blvd NW, Calgary AB T3K 0S6; (Pakistan)'88; MB BS; CCFP; (403)274-9712

IMRAN, Syed A; Queen Elizabeth II HSC, 47-1276 South Park St, Halifax NS B3H 2Y9; Punjab (Pakistan)'87; MB BS; FRCPC; IntMed; Endocrin&Metab. Staff, Queen Elizabeth II Health Sciences Centre - Victoria General Site; (902)473-2952; Fax. (902)473-3726.

IMRIE, Diana M G; Group One Med Associates, 1111 Springfield Rd, Kelowna BC V1Y 8R7; Dal'84; Physician, Outreach Urban Health; (250)762-4286; Fax. (250)762-4213; dmgimrie@shaw.ca.

IMRIE, John R; 100-123 15th St E, North Vancouver BC V7L 2P7; National (Ireland)'82; MB ChB; FRCPC; IntMed (Adult Cardiology); Cardiol. Staff Cardiol, Lions Gate Hospital; (604)980-1031; Fax. (604)980-1032; johnimrie@telus.net.

IMRIE, Kevin R; Odette Cancer Centre, 2075 Bayview Ave, Toronto ON M4N 3M5; Ott'88; FRCPC; IntMed (Malignant Lymphoma); Hem., Sunnybrook Health Sciences Centre; Prof Med, University of Toronto; (416)480-5145

INACIO, Joao M S R; The Ottawa Hosp-Gen Campus, 501 Smyth Rd, Ottawa ON K1H 8L6; Lisboa (Portugal)'99; Staff Radiol, The Ottawa Hospital - General Campus; (613)737-8571

INAMDAR, Mangesh; Halton HCS Corp-Oakville, 327 Reynolds St, Oakville ON L6J 3L7; McG'95; CCFP; CCFP(E.M.); FCFP; Staff, Halton Healthcare Services Corporation - Oakville Site; (905)338-4618; Fax. (905)338-4616.

INANDAN, Elnora S; Bathurst Med Centre, 307-4256 Bathurst St, North York ON M3H 5Y8; Manila (Philippines)'73; Physician Health Serv, North York General Hospital - Branson Division; (416)630-1010; Fax. (416)916-6703.

INCARDONA, Nadia K; Univ Hlth Network-Toronto Western Hosp, 2F WW-399 Bathurst St, Toronto ON M5T 2S8; Qns'06; CCFP; Staff, Toronto Western Hospital - University Health Network; (416)603-5397; nadia.incardona@uhn.on.ca.

INCE-CUSHMAN, Daniel; CLSC Cote-des-Neiges, 500-5700 ch Cote-des-Neiges, Montreal QC H3T 2A8; Wes'02; CCFP; Médecin, CLSC Cote-des-Neiges; (514)731-8531

INCH, Cam J; Front-Frederick Health Service, 14F-365 Bloor St E, Toronto ON M4W 3L4; Wes'97; CCFP; CCFP(E.M.); Langs: Bilingual(English/French); (416)362-8777; Fax. (416)362-7879.

INCH, Nicole G; Medical & Dental Bldg, 602-586 Eglinton Ave E, Toronto ON M4P 1P2; Tor'89; Peds (Oncology). Staff, Mount Sinai Hospital; Staff, The Hospital For Sick Children; Staff, Women's College Hospital; University of Toronto; (416)489-3263; Fax. (416)489-7808.

INCITTI, Filomena; Geddes Medical Group, 143 Metcalfe St, Elora ON N0B 1S0; McM'98; BSc; MD; CCFP; FCFP; Staff, Groves Memorial Community Hospital; (519)846-2224; Fax. (519)846-2005; fincitti@cogeco.ca.

INCULET, Richard; London HSC-Victoria Hosp, PO Box 5010 Stn B E2 122-800 Commissioners Rd E, London ON N6A 5W9; Wes'78; AB; FACS; FRCSC; GenSurg (Thoracic Oncology); ThorSurg. Consultant, London Health Sciences Centre - University Hospital; Consultant, St Joseph's Hospital - St Joseph's Health Care; Staff, London Health Sciences Centre - Victoria Campus; Consultant, London Regional Cancer Centre; Assoc Prof Surg, University of Western Ontario; (519)667-6679; Fax. (519)667-6762; rinculet@lhsc.on.ca.

INCZE, Peter F; Trafalgar Prof Centre, 407-1235 Trafalgar Rd, Oakville ON L6H 3P1; McM'91; FRCSC; Urol. Staff Urol, Halton Healthcare Services Corporation - Oakville Site; (905)842-1393; Fax. (905)338-3150.

INDECH, Michael; 902-5799 Yonge St, North York ON M2M 3V3; London (England)'61; MRCS; LRCP; FRCS; FRCSC; OrthSurg (Tort Cases). Sr Consultant Honorary Staff, North York General Hospital - Branson Division; (416)630-9992; Fax. (416)630-9992.

INFANTE-RIVARD, Claire; 1110 Av des Pins O, Montreal QC H3A 1A3; Mon'70; PhD(McG); MPH(UCLA); CommunMed; PH (P.Q.) (Research). Staff, Hôpital Ste-Justine; Prof, McGill University; Langs: English; Spanish; (514)398-4231; Fax. (514)398-7435.

ING, Alan F M; Markham Stouffville Health Ctr, 402-377 Church St, Markham ON L6B 1A1; Tor'78; FRCSC; GenSurg. Staff Surg, Markham Stouffville Hospital; (905)472-7122; Fax. (905)472-2290.

ING, Douglas J; Univ Hlth Network-Toronto Gen, 3PMCC 526-200 Elizabeth St, Toronto ON M5G 2C4; Tor'91; ABIM(CardiovascDis); FRCPC; IntMed (Cardiology). Staff Interventional Cardiol & Electrophysiol, Toronto General Hospital - UHN; Assoc Prof Med, University of Toronto; (416)340-5237; Fax. (416)340-4710.

ING, Edsel B; Toronto Eyelid Strabismus, 306 KW-650 Sammon Ave, Toronto ON M4C 5M5; Tor'88; DABOph; FRCSC; Ophth (Oculo Plastic Surgery). Staff, Toronto East General Hospital Inc; Staff, Sunnybrook Health Sciences Centre; Assoc Prof, University of Toronto; Langs: Cantonese; (416)465-7900; Fax. (416)465-2035.

ING, Gary; 6020 Malden Rd, Windsor ON N9H 1S8; Wes'77; FCFP; Chief of Staff, Windsor Regional Hospital - Metropolitan Site; (519)258-9313; Fax. (519)258-9312.

ING, Horne D; Scarborough Extendicare, 3830 Lawrence Ave E, Scarborough ON M1G 1R6; Tor'79; BSc; Ac Staff, Rouge Valley Health System - Centenary Health Centre Site; Ac Staff, The Scarborough Hospital - General Campus; (416)439-1243; Fax. (416)484-1651; ingjeu@sympatico.ca.

ING, Sabrina Y; Oak Park Med Clinic, 2530 Sixth Line, Oakville ON L6H 6W5; Tor'00; CCFP; (905)257-1006; Fax. (905)257-0661.

ING, Tom G E; 1617 Ouellette Ave, Windsor ON N8X 1K9; Wes'61; AB; FRCSC; Ophth. Staff I O D E Unit, Windsor Regional Hospital - Tayfour Site; Staff, Hôtel-Dieu Grace Hospital; (519)252-4494

ING, Vincent W; Montebello Med Clinic, 1-249 Waverley Rd, Dartmouth NS B2X 2C5; Tor'60; FACP; FRCPC; IntMed (Hematology). Att Staff, Queen Elizabeth II Health Sciences Centre - Victoria General Site; Asst Prof, Dalhousie University; (902)406-4444

INGBER, Linda G; Malvern Med Arts Bldg, 100-1333 Neilson Rd, Scarborough ON M1B 4Y9; Tor'78; (416)291-7719; Fax. (416)287-3775; malvernmedical@rogers.com.

INGBER, Neil J; Jane-Finch Family Health Team, 136A-1 Yorkgate Blvd, North York ON M3N 3A1; Tor'10; CCFP; (416)745-4555; Fax. (416)745-0786.

INGBER, Sarah A; 335-1333 Sheppard Ave E, North York ON M2J 1V1; Tor'06; FRCPC; IntMed; Hem. (416)498-4888; Fax. (416)498-6770.

INGELS, Anne; CSSS de Beauce-Etchemin, 1515 17e rue, Saint-Georges QC G5Y 4T8; Laval'80; Staff, Centre Hospitalier Beauce-Etchemin; (418)228-2031 x7864

INGERSOLL, Ruth E; 14 King Square S, Saint John NB E2L 1E5; Dal'91; (506)658-1667; Fax. (506)648-0706.

INGHAM, Andrew B; Dartmouth Gen Hosp, 325 Pleasant St, Dartmouth NS B2Y 4G8; Dal'93; FRCPC; DiagRad. Staff, Dartmouth General Hospital; Staff, The Nova Scotia Hospital; Staff, Eastern Shore Memorial Hospital; (902)465-8320; Fax. (902)465-8360; aingham@ns.sympatico.ca.

INGIMUNDSON, Janice C; 603-1661 Portage Ave, Winnipeg MB R3J 3T7; Man'67; FRCPC; Psy (Intensive Psychotherapy).

INGLEDEW, Paris-Ann; BC Cancer Agency-Fraser Valley, 13750 96 Ave, Surrey BC V3V 1Z2; UBC'02; FRCPC; RadOncol. Staff, BC Cancer Agency Fraser Valley Centre; (604)930-4033

INGLES, Julia; 200-16 O'Brien St, Orillia ON L3V 5S2; Dal'01; FRCSC; ObstGyn. (705)330-4060

INGLES, Martha G C; Wild Rose Med Centre, PO Box 3955 Stn Main, Olds AB T4H 1P6; Alb'08; CCFP; (403)556-7130; Fax. (403)556-5976.

INGLIS, Douglas S; 149 Church St, Moncton NB E1C 4Z8; Dal'66; DAB; PlasSurg. Staff Plastic Surg, The Moncton Hospital; Staff Plastic Surg, Dr Georges-L-Dumont University Hospital Centre; Consultant, Sackville Memorial Hospital; (506)855-4644; Fax. (506)853-8291.

INGLIS, Duncan L; Assiniboine Clinic, 633 Lodge Ave, Winnipeg MB R3J 0S9; Man'89; FRCSC; GenSurg.

INGLIS, Edward K; Family Med Centre, 2931 20 Ave S, Lethbridge AB T1K 3M5; Manchester (England)'72; (403)328-2326; Fax. (403)327-0123.

INGLIS, Gary; MUHC-Montreal Gen Hosp, 1650 av Cedar, Montreal QC H3G 1A4; Laval'92; FRCPC; IntMed; GeriatricMed. Staff, McGill University Health Centre - Montreal General Campus; (514)934-8015

INGO, Steven K; 2876 Campbell St PO Box 270, Sydenham ON K0H 2T0; Tor'92; (613)376-3327; Fax. (613)376-9868.

INGRAM, Alistair J; St Joseph's Healthcare, M342-50 Charlton Ave E, Hamilton ON L8N 4A6; Wes'90; BSc; FRCPC; IntMed; Nephrol. Court Staff, Hamilton Health Sciences Centre - Hamilton General Hospital; Ac Staff, St Joseph's Healthcare - Charlton Campus; Assoc Prof Med, McMaster University; Langs: English; French; (905)521-6151; Fax. (905)521-6153; ingrama@mcmaster.ca.

INGRAM, Andrea D; F W Green Med Centre, 1629 Baker St, Cranbrook BC V1C 1B4; Ott'95; BSc; MSc; (250)426-6601; Fax. (250)426-6470.

INGRAM, David W; St Clare's Mercy Hosp, 154 Lemarchant Rd, St. John's NL A1C 5B8; Queen's Univ-Belfast (Ireland)'50; MB ChB; BAO; MSMed; FACP; MCFPHon; FRCPC; IntMed (Thyroid Diseases). Ac Staff, St Clare's Mercy Hospital; Consultant, Health Sciences Centre; Prof Pt-Time Gen Med & Therapeutics, Memorial University Of Newfoundland; (709)777-5575; Fax. (709)777-5290; david.ingram@easternhealth.ca.

INGRAM, Diana R; Victoria Gen Hosp, 1 Hospital Way, Victoria BC V8Z 6R5; McM'76; FRCPC; ObstGyn (Mood Disorders); Psy. Staff, Victoria General Hospital; (250)272-4266

INGRAM, Heidi M; Carmi Clinic, 114-725 Carmi Ave, Penticton BC V2A 3G8; Witwatersrand (South Africa)'98; MB ChB; CCFP; (250)492-4274

INGRAM, K Jennifer; Kawartha Reg Memory Clinic, 168 Brock St, Peterborough ON K9H 2P4; Qns'74; FRCP; FRCPC; IntMed; GeriatricMed (Clinical Trials). Consultant Memory Clinic, Ontario Shores Centre for Mental Health Sciences; Staff, Peterborough Regional Health Centre - Hospital Drive; Board Member, Osteoporosis Society; I-Leader GAIN Program, Geriatric Assesstment & Intervention Network; Principal Investigator, Kawartha Regional Memory Clinic & Research Group; (705)749-3906; Fax. (705)749-2778; ingrams@bellnet.ca.

INGRAM, Peter F; 1500-444 St Mary Ave, Winnipeg MB R3C 3T1; Man'79; FRCPC; Psy (General Psychiatry). Asst Prof, University of Manitoba.

INGRAM, Wessel J; 3103 36 Ave, Vernon BC V1T 2V7; Orange Free State (South Africa)'84; MB ChB; MMed(SA); FRCSC; Ophth (Cataract & Refractive). Head Ophth, Vernon Jubilee Hospital; Langs: Afrikaans; (250)542-8345; Fax. (250)542-8398.

INGRAM-CROOKS, Jennifer L; St Lawrence Med Clinic, PO Box 772, Morrisburg ON K0C 1X0; Ott'04; CCFP; (613)543-2963; Fax. (613)543-4171.

INGREY, James R; 331C 6th St, Courtenay BC V9N 1M2; Glasgow (Scotland)'99; MB ChB; CCFP; (250)338-1333

INJOYAN, Rita; 158-1 Place Laval, Laval QC H7N 1A1; Mon'95; CCFP; (450)668-7400; Fax. (450)668-5855.

INKPEN, Linda L; Memorial U-Student Health Serv, PO Box 4200 Stn C, St. John's NL A1C 5S7; Mem'74; BSc(Biol.); BMedSci; (709)737-7595

INKPEN, Peter C; 3203 34 St, Vernon BC V1T 5X7; Mem'06; FRCPC; PhysMed&Rehab. (778)475-5919

INKSTER, John R; Trafalgar Med Clinic, 200-1235 Trafalgar Rd, Oakville ON L6H 3P1; Wes'72; Ac Staff, Halton Healthcare Services Corporation - Oakville Site; (905)844-3281; Fax. (905)849-1076.

INMAN, Geoffrey A B; Jubilee Centre, 1823 Fort St, Victoria BC V8R 1J6; UBC'94; CCFP; (250)370-0024

INMAN, Richard J; Credit Valley Prof Bldg, 405-2300 Eglinton Ave W, Mississauga ON L5M 2V8; Tor'78; FRCSC; PlasSurg. Assoc Staff, The Credit Valley Hospital; Court Staff, Trillium Health Centre - Mississauga; (905)820-8077; Fax. (905)820-2520.

INMAN, Robert D; Univ Hlth Network-Toronto Western Hosp, IE 423-399 Bathurst St, Toronto ON M5T 2S8; McM'74; FACP; FRCPC; IntMed; Rheum. Staff Rheum, Toronto Western Hospital - University Health Network; (416)603-5869; robert.inman@uhn.on.ca.

INNES, A Micheil; Alberta Children's Hosp, 2888 Shaganappi Trail NW, Calgary AB T3B 6A8; Alb'95; BSc(McG); FRCPC; MedGenetics (Dysmorphology). Staff Clinical Geneticist, Alberta Children's Hospital; Associate, University of Calgary; Langs: Bilingual(French/English); (403)955-7373; micheil.innes@albertahealthservices.ca.

INNES, C Peter; 1902 Richmond Rd, Victoria BC V8R 4R2; Sheffield (England)'68; DObstRCOG; Chief Family Practice/Pres Medical Staff Association, Vancouver Island Health Authority South Island Region; (250)385-3622; drinnes@telus.net.

INNES, Duncan M; Valley Medical Laboratories, 105-537 Leon Ave, Kelowna BC V1Y 6J5; Bristol (England)'57; MB ChB; GenPath. (250)763-4813; Fax. (250)862-2843.

INNES, Grant D; North Hill Centre, 1633-1632 14 Ave NW, Calgary AB T2N 1M7; Alb'80; FRCPC; EmergMed. Staff Emerg Med, Foothills Medical Centre; (403)944-8430

INNES, Marilyn E; London HSC-Victoria Hosp, PO Box 5010 Stn B 800 Commissioners Rd E, London ON N6A 5W9; Qns'02; FRCPC; EmergMed. Staff, London Health Sciences Centre - Victoria Campus; (519)685-8500

INNISS, Michael W; Salmo Wellness Centre, PO Box 730 423 Davies St, Salmo BC V0G 1Z0; Tor'89; (250)357-2627; Fax. (250)357-2687.

INOUYE, Phillip K; 250-2039 Robertson Rd, Nepean ON K2H 8R2; Cal'00; FRCPC; IntMed; Gastroent. (613)726-3263

INOUYE, Tetsuo; Credit Valley Prof Bldg, 512-2300 Eglinton Ave W, Mississauga ON L5M 2V8; UBC'71; FRCPC; IntMed; Respir. Court Staff, The Credit Valley Hospital; (905)828-0226; Fax. (905)828-4703; tinouye@rogers.com.

INSANALLY, S S A Reza; Village Park Med, 210A-6640 Vedder Rd, Chilliwack BC V2R 0J2; RCS (Ireland)'94; (604)858-2246

INSLEY, Kristyn J; Medical & Cosmetic Clinic, 1-601 8th St E, Saskatoon SK S7H 0R1; Sask'06; CCFP; (306)974-3939; kji804@mail.usask.ca.

INTERNOSCIA, Karine; Clinique Med La Rose des Vents, 3498 boul Sainte-Rose, Laval QC H7P 4K7; Mon'08; CCFP; (450)624-1844

INTRATER, Howard M; Harry Medovy House, 2F-671 William Ave, Winnipeg MB R3E 0Z2; Man'85; FRCPC; Anes. Staff, Health Sciences Centre.

INTWALA, Chaitasi R; Flin Flon Gen Hosp Inc, PO Box 340, Flin Flon MB R8A 1N2; Staff, Flin Flon General Hospital Inc; (204)687-7591

INWOOD, Matthew J; University of Alberta Hosp, 1A7 19WCM-8440 112 St NW, Edmonton AB T6G 2B7; (Ireland)'04; CCFP; CCFP(E.M.); Staff, University of Alberta Hospital; (780)407-8433

INY, Alan I; 480 Metcalfe St, Ottawa ON K1S 3N6; McG'89; CCFP; Physician, Aim Health Group; Langs: French; Hebrew; (613)369-7812; Fax. (613)565-8902.

INY, Karen; Hop Brome-Missisquoi-Perkins, 950 rue Principale, Cowansville QC J2K 1K3; McG'06; MDCM; CCFP; Staff, Hôpital Brome-Missisquoi-Perkins; (450)266-4342

INY, Robert; QHC Trenton Mem Hosp, PO Box 1600 Stn Main 242 King St, Trenton ON K8V 5S6; McG'06; CCFP; Staff, QHC Trenton Memorial; (613)392-2540; robbieiny@yahoo.com.

IOANNOU, K Panagiotis; Gordon & Leslie Diamond HCC, 9F-2775 Laurel St, Vancouver BC V5Z 1M9; McM'07; IntMed. Staff, Gordon & Leslie Diamond Health Care Centre; (604)875-4111

IOCCA, Angelo J; Royal Court Med Centre, 206-1 Quarry Ridge Rd, Barrie ON L4M 7G1; Tor'93; BSc; MD; FRCSC; Urol (Prostrate Cancer). Ac Staff/Chief Urology, Royal Victoria Regional Health Centre; (705)792-6796; Fax. (705)728-8332.

IONESCU, Adriana; Lakeshore Gen Hosp, 4N-160 av Stillview, Pointe-Claire QC H9R 2Y2; Bucharest (Romania)'85; CCFP; Staff, Lakeshore General Hospital - Pointe Claire; Langs: Romanian; English; (514)630-2225

IONESCU, Diana; BC Cancer Agency-Vancouver CC, 600 10th Ave W, Vancouver BC V5Z 4E6; Cluj-Napaco (Romania)'95; FRCPC; AnatPath. Staff, BC Cancer Agency Vancouver Centre; Langs: Romanian; (604)877-6000 x2117

IONESCU, Loretta V; Centre Med Hochelaga, 9080 rue Hochelaga, Montreal QC H1L 2N9; Bucarest (Romania)'88; CCFP; (514)353-8742

IONITA, Mihaela; Cite de la sante Laval, 255-1755 boul Rene-Laennec, Laval QC H7M 3L9; Carol Davila (Romania)'01; CCFP; Staff, Hopital de la Cite de la santé; Langs: Bilingual(English/French); (450)668-1010; Fax. (450)975-5497.

IORDACHE, Claudiu; Lamont Health Care Centre, PO Box 10 5216 53rd St, Lamont AB T0B 2R0; (Romania)'89; MSc; PhD; Staff, Lamont Health Care Centre; Langs: Romanian; (780)579-1333; Fax. (780)579-1334.

IORDACHE, Irina-Liliana; Kipling Heights Med Centre, 2291 Kipling Ave, Etobicoke ON M9W 4L6; (Romania)'96; CCFP; (416)741-4545; Fax. (416)744-1484.

IORDACHESCU, Andrei; CLSC Bordeaux-Cartierville, 11822 av du Bois-de-Boulogne, Montreal QC H3M 2X6; Mon'10; CCFP; (514)331-2572

IORDANESCU, Vlad; Clinique Med du Sud-Ouest, 103-4475 rue Bannatyne, Verdun QC H4G 1E2; Laval'93; FRCSC; Otol (Head & Neck Surgery). (514)765-3600 x214

IORDANOV, Kolio; Quinte HC Corp-Belleville Gen, 265 Dundas St E, Belleville ON K8N 5A9; Sofia (Bulgaria)'75; FRCPC; Anes. Staff, QHC Belleville General; (613)969-7400

IORIO, Alfonso; Hemophilia Program, 1200 Main St W, Hamilton ON L8N 3Z5; University of Perugia (Italy)'91; FRCPC; IntMed.

IOSIF, Alina R; Addiction & Mental Hlth-Queen, 1001 Queen St W, Toronto ON M6J 1H4; Cal'01; FRCPC; Psy. Staff, Centre for Addiction & Mental Health (CAMH) - Queen Site; (416)535-8501

IP, Andrew P; Sault Area Hosp, 750 Great Northern Rd, Sault Ste. Marie ON P6B 0A8; Qns'99; CCFP; CCFP(E.M.); Staff, Sault Area Hospital - Sault Ste Marie; (705)759-3434

IP, Angel H; Healthway Medical, 865 Portage Ave, Winnipeg MB R3G 0N8; (Taiwan)'70; (204)783-6464; Fax. (204)772-5554.

IP, Gregory J C; North York Gen Hosp, 4001 Leslie St, North York ON M2K 1E1; Tor'97; FRCPC; Anes. Staff, North York General Hospital; (416)756-6265

IP, Hui Yun V; Clinical Sciences Bldg, 8 120-152 University Campus NW, Edmonton AB T6G 2G3; Birmingham (England)'00; (780)407-8861; Fax. (780)407-3200.

IP, Janet L; 3029 Cambie St, Vancouver BC V5Z 4N2; UBC'03; CCFP; Staff, Pacific Dermaesthetics; (604)875-8999

IP, Joseph K H; Royal Columbia Hosp, 330 Columbia St E, New Westminster BC V3L 3W7; UBC'98; FRCPC; EmergMed. Staff, Royal Columbian Hospital; (604)520-4283

IP, Shannon; Univ of Alberta Hosp, 8440 112 St NW, Edmonton AB T6G 2B7; Cal'07; FRCPC; IntMed. Staff, University of Alberta Hospital; (780)407-8822

IP, Terence K Y; Sunnybrook Hlth Sciences Ctre, D1 08-2075 Bayview Ave, Toronto ON M4N 3M5; McM'06; Anes. Staff, Sunnybrook Health Sciences Centre; (416)480-4522

IP, Vincent K L; Richmond Hosp, 7000 Westminster Hwy, Richmond BC V6X 1A2; Man'67; Staff, Richmond Hospital; (604)725-3229

IP, W William; MDCL 3101A-1280 Main St W, Hamilton ON L8S 4K1; Tor'03; CCFP; IntMed.

IP, Yiu Ban; Surrey Mem Hosp, 13750 96 Ave, Surrey BC V3V 1Z2; Man'82; BSc(Med.); BSc(Microbiol); FACEP; Med Dir, Surrey Memorial Hospital; Chief Medical Officer School of Health Sciences, Justice Institute Of Bc; Langs: Cantonese; Chinese; (604)585-5530; Fax. (604)588-3320; urbain.ip@fraserhealth.ca.

IPP, Moshe M; 103-90 Warren Rd, Toronto ON M4V 2S2; Witwatersrand (South Africa)'70; MB ChB; FAAP; FRCPC; Peds (Consultation). Court Staff, Sunnybrook Health Sciences Centre; Court Staff, Mount Sinai Hospital; Prof Peds, University of Toronto; (416)924-7171; Fax. (416)923-9015.

IPSIROGLU, Osman S; Sunny Hill Hlth Ctr for Child, 3644 Slocan St, Vancouver BC V5M 3E8; Vienna (Austria)'85; Staff, BC Children's Hospital; Staff, Sunny Hill Health Centre for Children; Langs: German; Turkish; (604)875-2345

IQBAL, Bland; Grey Bruce HS-Owen Sound, PO Box 1800 Stn Main 1800 8th St E, Owen Sound ON N4K 6M9; Pakistan (Pakistan)'90; MB BS; Staff, Grey Bruce Health Services - Owen Sound; (519)376-2121

IQBAL, Fawaad O; Lakeridge Hlth Corp-Oshawa, 1 Hospital Crt, Oshawa ON L1G 2B9; Alb'03; FRCPC; RadOncol. Staff, Lakeridge Health - Oshawa Site; (905)576-8711

IQBAL, Irum; Four Rivers Med Clinic, 647 Broadway, Winnipeg MB R3C 0X2; Punjab (Pakistan)'01; CCFP; Staff, Seven Regions Health Centre.

IQBAL, Mirza N; Yarmouth Reg Health Centre, 60 Vancouver St, Yarmouth NS B5A 2P5; Karachi (Pakistan)'91; MB BS; Staff, Yarmouth Regional Hospital.

IQBAL, Mudassir; Royal Inland Hosp, 311 Columbia St, Kamloops BC V2C 2T1; Punjab (India)'99; Staff, Royal Inland Hospital; (250)374-5111

IQBAL, Muhammad; Health Sciences Centre, 2749-300 Prince Philip Dr, St. John's NL A1B 3V6; Punjab (Pakistan)'94; FRCPC; IntMed. Staff, Health Sciences Centre; (709)777-6330

IQBAL, Nayyer; Saskatoon Cancer Centre, 20 Campus Dr, Saskatoon SK S7N 4H4; (306)655-2710; Fax. (306)655-0633.

IQBAL, Sahar J; St Clare's Mercy Hosp, 154 Lemarchant Rd, St. John's NL A1C 5B8; Rawalpindi (Pakistan)'91; MB BS; FRCPC; IntMed. Staff, St Clare's Mercy Hospital; (709)777-5000

IQBAL, Sameena Z; MUHC-Montreal Gen Hosp, L4 512-1650 av Cedar, Montreal QC H3G 1A4; Qns'93; FRCPC; IntMed; Nephrol. Staff, McGill University Health Centre - Montreal General Campus; (514)934-1934 x44035; Fax. (514)934-8248; sameena.iqbal@mcgill.ca.

IQBAL, Tariq; Brockville Med Centre, 108-100 Strowger Blvd, Brockville ON K6V 5J9; Peshawar (Pakistan)'89; FRCPC; IntMed; Rheum. (613)342-5118

IQBAL, Zafar; 102-1669 Victoria St, Prince George BC V2L 2L5; Karachi (Pakistan)'91; MB BS; FRCPC; IntMed. (250)564-3133

IRACE-CIMA, Alejandra; Dir Sante Publique de Laval, Tour A 3E-800 boul Chomedey, Laval QC H7V 3Y4; Cordoba (Argentina)'84; FRCPC; CommunMed. (450)978-2121 x2993

IRACLEOUS, Panayiotis; Rouge Valley-Centenary HC, 2867 Ellesmere Rd, Scarborough ON M1E 4B9; Tor'05; CCFP; Staff, Rouge Valley Health System - Centenary Health Centre Site; (416)281-7270

IRAJI, Mandana; Royal Victoria Hosp, 201 Georgian Dr, Barrie ON L4M 6M2; (Dominican Republic)'02; CCFP; Staff, Royal Victoria Regional Health Centre; (705)728-9802

IRANI, Carla A; College Plaza 3, 404-8215 112 ST NW, Edmonton AB T6G 2C8; (Lebanon)'95; DABACI; (780)433-5891; Fax. (780)439-1061.

IRANI, Farhad; 106-1929 Russell Rd, Ottawa ON K1G 4G3; Ott'89; (613)260-3497; Fax. (613)260-3725.

IRANI, Kaizad S; Lower Mainland Drug Freedom In, 25 Blackwood St, New Westminster BC V3L 2T3; Bombay (India)'95; MB BS; FRCPC; Psy. (604)520-1068

IRANI, Nabil; Hop Jean-Talon, 1385 rue Jean-Talon E, Montreal QC H2E 1S6; (Lebanon)'91; Staff, CSSS du Coeur de l'Isle Hôpital Jean-Talon; (514)495-6767

IRANI, Zeubin; CSSS Jeanne-Mance, 100-15 av du Mont-Royal O, Montreal QC H2T 2R9; Mon'91; (514)286-9657; Fax. (514)940-3621.

IRAZUZTA, Jorge O E; Crown Point Family Hlth Ctre, 67 Kenilworth Ave N, Hamilton ON L8H 4R6; (Argentina)'67; DPH; CCFP; FCFP; (905)577-0667; Fax. (905)577-0259.

IRELAND, Brenda J; Chinook Reg Hosp, 960 19 St S, Lethbridge AB T1J 1W5; UBC'83; CCFP; FCFP; Ac Staff, Covenant Health - St Michael's Health Centre; Ac Staff GenPract, Chinook Regional Hospital; (403)388-6325

IRELAND, Kim L; Burlington Prof Centre, 202-3155 Harvester Rd, Burlington ON L7N 3V2; Ott'90; BSc(Hons.); (905)639-3666; Fax. (905)639-6662.

IRELAND, Laurie F; Nine Circles Med Clinic, 705 Broadway, Winnipeg MB R3G 0X2; Man'05; CCFP; (204)940-6000; Fax. (204)940-6003.

IRELAND, Ronald M; Lincoln Med Centre, 4413 Ontario St, Beamsville ON L0R 1B5; Wes'86; CCFP; FCFP; Staff, West Lincoln Memorial Hospital; (905)563-1212; Fax. (905)563-4404; lkmc@sympatico.ca.

IRFAN, Jeewani; Medical Clinic, PO Box 40, Port au Choix NL A0K 4C0; (Russia (Federation))'92; LMCC; Staff, Rufus Guinchard Health Centre; Langs: Sinhalese; Russian; Tamil; (709)861-4999; Fax. (709)861-2152.

IRFAN, Mohamed H; Medical Clinic, PO Box 40 47 Fisher St, Port au Choix NL A0K 4C0; North Colombo (Sri Lanka)'95; MB BS; MSc; CCFP; FCFP; Chief/Staff, Rufus Guinchard Health Centre; Sr Medical Officer, Port Saunders District; Langs: Malay; Tamil; Sinhalese; (709)861-4999; Fax. (709)861-2152; mohamed.irfan@umontreal.ca.

IRIARTE, Paula L; 103-3195 Granville St, Vancouver BC V6H 3K2; Buenos Aires (Argentina)'95; CCFP; Langs: Spanish; (604)739-8011

IRIOGBE, Itua G; Smith Clinic, 1-6601 48 Ave, Camrose AB T4V 3G8; (Nigeria)'96; (780)672-2425; Fax. (780)672-5607.

IRISH, Craig L; Trillium Hlth Ctr-Mississauga, 100 Queensway W, Mississauga ON L5B 1B8; Tor'83; FRCPC; Anes. Staff, Trillium Health Centre - Mississauga; (905)848-7100

IRISH, Jonathan C; Univ Hlth Network-Princess M, 3 954-610 University Ave, Toronto ON M5G 2M9; Tor'84; MSc(MedSciences); DABOT; FACS; FRCSC; Otol (Head & Neck & Reconstructive Surgery Oncology). Chief Surgical Oncology, Princess Margaret Hospital - University Health Network; Chief Surgical Oncol, Mount Sinai Hospital; Prof, University of Toronto; (416)946-2149; Fax. (416)946-2300; jonathan.irish@uhn.on.ca.

IRISH, Kevin E; East Kootaney Reg Hosp, 13 24th Ave N, Cranbrook BC V1C 3H9; St George's (Grenada)'05; FRCPC; DiagRad. Staff, East Kootenay Regional Hospital; (250)426-5281

IRISH, Leon D; 2100-222 King St E, Bowmanville ON L1C 1P6; Tor'86; BSc; Ac Staff, Lakeridge Health - Bowmanville Site; Ac Staff, Lakeridge Health - Oshawa Site; (905)623-0323; Fax. (905)697-0230.

IRO, Chinedu J; Lions Gate Hosp, 231 15th St E, North Vancouver BC V7L 2L7; (Nigeria)'96; MB BS; Staff, Lions Gate Hospital; (604)988-3131

IROBI, Clara C; Winchester Dist Mem Hosp, RR 4 566 Louise St, Winchester ON K0C 2K0; (Nigeria)'82; FRCPC; IntMed. Staff, Winchester District Memorial Hospital; (613)774-2420

IRONS, Shawna M; St Joseph Health Centre, 30 The Queensway, Toronto ON M6R 1B5; Tor'07; CCFP; Staff, St Joseph's Health Centre; (416)530-6860

IRRINKI, Anand; Fredericton Family Med Clinic, 479 Smythe St, Fredericton NB E3B 3E3; Mem'96; CCFP; (506)458-9446; Fax. (506)458-8118.

IRSHAD, Fauzia; Winston Churchill Med Centre, 1A-6975 Meadowvale Town Ctr Ci, Mississauga ON L5N 2W7; Birmingham (England)'70; MB BS; CCFP; Langs: French; Urdu; Punjabi; (905)812-4874

IRSHAD, Kashif; Springdale Prof Bldg, 315-2250 Bovaird Dr, Brampton ON L6R 0W3; McG'98; FRCSC; GenSurg; ThorSurg. Staff, William Osler Health System - Etobicoke General Hospital; Langs: Hindi; English; Punjabi; Urdu; (905)458-4520

IRVINE, Brendon R; Saanich Peninsula Hosp, 2166 Mount Newton Cross Rd, Saanichton BC V8M 2B2; UBC'93; CCFP; CCFP(E.M.); Staff, Saanich Peninsula Hospital; (250)652-3911

IRVINE, Elizabeth Jan; 16 052-30 Bond St, Toronto ON M5B 1W8; Tor'77; MSc; FRC; FRCPC; IntMed (Gastroenterology). Head Div of Gastroent, St Michael's Hospital; Prof Med, University of Toronto; (416)864-5060; Fax. (416)861-8378.

IRVINE, Harland S; Greenwood Fam Physicians, PO Box 5 709 1 St NE, Sundre AB T0M 1X0; Cal'77; CCFP; FCFP; Vis Staff, Olds Hospital & Care Centre; Ac Staff/Chief FamilyMed, Sundre Hospital & Care Centre; Clin Assoc Prof Family Med, University of Calgary; (403)638-2424; Fax. (403)638-3580; irvineh@airenet.com.

IRVINE, Harley R; Fairview Med Clinic, PO Box 725 10624 110 St, Fairview AB T0H 1L0; (Other Foreign)'09; (780)835-4255

IRVINE, James D; Mamawetan Churchill River RHA, PO Box 6000, La Ronge SK S0J 1L0; Sask'76; MSc; FRCPC; CommunMed;CCFP; FCFP; Public Health & Preventive Med. Staff, Mamawetan Churchill River Health Region Corporate Office; Med Officer of Hlth Population Health Unit, Northern Saskatchewan Health Authorities; Prof Family Med/Assoc Member School of Public Health, University of Saskatchewan; (306)425-8585; Fax. (306)425-8530; james.irvine@mcrrha.sk.ca.

IRVINE, James E; Brant Community HC-Brantford, 200 Terrace Hill St, Brantford ON N3R 1G9; Wes'89; CCFP; CCFP(E.M.); FCFP; Staff Emerg, The Brant Community Healthcare System - Brantford General Hospital Site; (519)751-5507

IRVINE, Jamie J; Hys Med Centre, 710-11010 101 St NW, Edmonton AB T5H 4B9; Man'98; BSc; FRCPC; PhysMed&Rehab (Electrodiagnostic Medicine). Clin Staff, Glenrose Rehabilitation Hospital; Clin Lecturer, University of Alberta; (780)453-5255

IRVINE, Lorne G; Caledonian Med Clinic, 340 Campbell St, Nanaimo BC V9R 3G7; Sask'79; Staff, Nanaimo Regional General Hospital; (250)753-3202; Fax. (250)753-1039.

IRVINE, Michael A; Summerside Med Centre, 101-475 Granville St, Summerside PE C1N 3N9; Alb'85; FRCPC; IntMed. (902)432-8133; Fax. (902)436-3789.

IRVINE, Rebecca E; Brockville Family Health Org, 2-5 Home St, Brockville ON K6V 0A5; (Netherlands Antilles)'09; CCFP; (613)423-1111

IRVINE, Richard A; Nith Valley Family Practice, 1-10 Waterloo St, New Hamburg ON N3A 1V5; Wes'72; (519)662-1551; Fax. (519)662-1402.

IRVINE, Robert A; St Paul's Hosp, 1081 Burrard St, Vancouver BC V6Z 1Y6; Sask'84; ABOtol; FRCSC; Otol (Thyroid Diseases). Ac Staff, Providence Health Care - St Paul's Hospital; Ac Staff, Providence Health Care - Mount Saint Joseph Hospital; Clin Assoc Prof, University of British Columbia; (604)806-9075; Fax. (604)806-9253; rirvine@providencehealth.bc.ca.

IRVINE, Thomas E; Cottage Country Fam Hlth Team, 1-5 Pineridge Gate, Gravenhurst ON P1P 1Z3; Wes'73; CCFP; FCFP; Fam Med, Huronia Regional Centre; Staff Family Pract, South Muskoka Memorial Hospital - Muskoka Algonquin Healthcare; Physician, Leisure World Nursing Home; (705)687-2271; Fax. (705)687-7575.

IRVINE, Thomas R; Belmont Med Centre, 101-535 Belmont Ave W, Kitchener ON N2M 5E9; Tor'09; CCFP; (519)579-0350; Fax. (519)579-7476.

IRVINE CHAMBERLAIN, Leanne B; Scarborough Hosp-Birchmount, 3030 Birchmount Rd, Scarborough ON M1W 3W3; Sask'04; CCFP; CCFP(E.M.); Staff, The Scarborough Hospital - Birchmount Campus; (416)495-2400

IRVING, Antony M; Associate Med Clinic, PO Box 549, Pincher Creek AB T0K 1W0; London (England)'70; MB BS; CCFP; FCFP; Asst Prof, University of Calgary; (403)627-3321; Fax. (403)627-2280.

IRVING, Christopher J; Mineral Springs Hosp, PO Box 1050 Stn Main 301 Lynx St, Banff AB T1L 1H7; Man'01; BSc; BSc(Med); CCFP; Staff Anes, Covenant Health - Banff Mineral Springs Hospital; (403)760-2897; Fax. (403)760-8234.

IRVING, Hugh D; 3-3110 8th St E, Saskatoon SK S7H 0W2; Alb'82; FRCPC; DiagRad. Clinical Asst Prof, Royal University Hospital; (306)477-1000; Fax. (306)477-1071; dr.irving@sasktel.net.

IRVING, James E; Pan Am Clinic, 75 Poseidon Bay, Winnipeg MB R3M 3E4; Man'76; FRCSC; OrthSurg (Knee Surgery). Staff, The Salvation Army Grace Hospital; (204)927-2680; Fax. (204)927-2685; jeirv@mts.net.

IRVING, Julie A; Royal Jubilee Hosp, 1952 Bay St, Victoria BC V8R 1J8; UBC'98; FRCPC; AnatPath. Staff, Royal Jubilee Hospital; (250)370-8938

IRVING, William E; 168 Rothesay Ave, Saint John NB E2J 2B5; Dal'74; (506)674-2080; Fax. (506)674-2086.

IRWIN, D June; 131-175 av Stillview, Pointe-Claire QC H9R 4S3; McG'61; DAA; FRCPC; Derm. Clin Staff, Lakeshore General Hospital - Pointe Claire; (514)697-7980

IRWIN, Darryl J; North York Gen Hosp, 4001 Leslie St, North York ON M2K 1E1; Wes'00; FRCPC; Anes. Staff, North York General Hospital; (416)756-6265 x1

IRWIN, David A J; West End Mental Health Team, 1555 Robson St, Vancouver BC V6G 1C3; UBC'84; FRCPC; Psy. Staff, West End Mental Health Team; Staff, UBC Hospital - Koerner Pavillion; (604)687-7994; dirwin@forensic.bc.ca.

IRWIN, Joanne L; 110-3540 41st Ave W, Vancouver BC V6N 3E6; Qns'89; MSc(Anat.); CCFP; FCFP; Ac Staff, BC Women's Hospital & Health Centre; Asst Prof, University of British Columbia; (604)261-6361; Fax. (604)261-1656.

IRWIN, Mandi R; Dalhousie Fam Med Spryfield MC, 27-16 Dentith Rd, Halifax NS B3R 2H9; Dal'08; CCFP; (902)473-1234

IRWIN, Marsha L A; Calgary Women's Imaging Centre, 20 Richard Way SW, Calgary AB T3E 7M9; UBC'75; FRCPC; DiagRad (Breast Imaging). (403)685-3123; Fax. (403)685-3235.

IRWIN, Meredith S; The Hosp for Sick Children, 555 University Ave, Toronto ON M5G 1X8; Harvard(MA) (USA)'92; FRCPC; Peds. Staff, The Hospital For Sick Children; Assoc Prof, University of Toronto; (416)813-7654 x2912; meredith.irwin@sickkids.ca.

IRWIN, Michael E; Roseville Garden Walk in Clini, 2425 Roseville Garden Dr, Windsor ON N8T 3J8; Tor'63; CCFP; (519)944-3393

IRWIN, S Patrick; 39 Park Rd N, Oshawa ON L1J 4K8; Edinburgh (Scotland)'69; MB ChB; (905)576-6251; Fax. (905)576-0374.

IRWIN, Susan; 20B-385 Frederick St, Kitchener ON N2H 2P2; Wes'97; CCFP; FCFP; (519)747-1200; Fax. (519)747-1560.

IRWIN, William F; 288 Westdale Ave, Kingston ON K7L 4S7; Edinburgh (Scotland)'71; MB ChB; DRCOG; Physician, Carveth Care Nursing Home; (613)382-1334

ISAAC, Carey D; Concordia Health Associates, 102-1155 Concordia Ave, Winnipeg MB R2K 2M9; UBC'87; CCFP; FCFP; Staff, Concordia General Hospital; (204)415-0322; Fax. (204)415-3714.

ISAAC, Debra L; Foothills Med Centre, 1403 29 St NW, Calgary AB T2N 2T9; Cal'87; FRCPC; IntMed (Transplantation); Cardiol. Dir Cardiac Transplant, Foothills Medical Centre; Clin Assoc Prof, University of Calgary; (403)944-2124; Fax. (403)944-1592; dlisaac@ucalgary.ca.

ISAAC, Errol B; 2-760 Brant St, Burlington ON L7R 4B7; Tor'69; FRCPC; DiagRad (Diagnostic Imaging). Consultant, Joseph Brant Memorial Hospital; (905)637-7606

ISAAC, Isaac F; 100-231 Wharncliffe Rd S, London ON N6J 2L3; Alexandria (Egypt)'72; MB ChB; FRCPC; Psy (Addiction Issues). Langs: Arabic; (519)641-5789; Fax. (519)641-3949.

ISAAC, Lisa A; The Hosp for Sick Children, 555 University Ave, Toronto ON M5G 1X8; Wes'93; CSPQ; FRCP; FRCPC; Anes (Pediatric Anesthesia). Staff Anes, The Hospital For Sick Children; Lecturer Anes, University of Toronto; Langs: French; (416)813-7445; Fax. (416)813-7543; lisa.isaac@sickkids.ca.

ISAAC, Neil R A; North York Gen Hosp, 4001 Leslie St, North York ON M2K 1E1; Dal'02; FRCPC; DiagRad. Staff, North York General Hospital; (416)756-6000

ISAAC, Nicole S; Lakeridge Hlth Corp-Oshawa, 1 Hospital Crt, Oshawa ON L1G 2B9; Wes'97; FRCPC; DiagRad. Staff, Lakeridge Health - Oshawa Site; (905)576-8711

ISAAC, Richard G; Queen Elizabeth Centre, 130 Dunn Ave, Toronto ON M6K 2R7; Tor'69; LLB; Coroner, Province of Ontario; Lecturer Family & Commun Med, University of Toronto; (416)597-3422 x2235; Fax. (416)530-2470; isaac.richard@torontorehab.on.ca.

ISAAC, Sandra L; Unison Hlth & Commun Services, 12 Flemington Rd, North York ON M6A 2N4; Tor'88; BSc; CCFP; Court Staff, The Scarborough Hospital - General Campus; Court Staff, Women's College Hospital; (416)787-1661

ISAAC-RENTON, Judith L; BC Centre For Disease Control, 655 12th Ave W, Vancouver BC V5Z 4R4; Tor'72; DPH(Public Health); FRCPC; MedMicrobiol (Infection Control). Consultant Med Microbiol, Ministry of Healthy Living & Sport-British Columbia; Consultant Med Microbiol, Ministry of Health-British Columbia; Prof, University of British Columbia; (604)707-2646; isaacren@interchange.ubc.ca.

ISAACS, Gwenyth F; Cook St Village Med Clinic, 101A-230 Cook St, Victoria BC V8V 3X3; Man'75; (250)220-9999

ISAACS, Theodore R; Haliburton Family Med Centre, PO Box 870 7217 Gelert Rd, Haliburton ON K0M 1S0; Cape Town (South Africa)'59; (705)457-1212

ISAACSON, Steven; Southlake Reg Health Centre, 596 Davis Dr, Newmarket ON L3Y 2P9; Witwatersrand (South Africa)'84; MB ChB; FRCPC; DiagRad (Body Imaging). Staff Diag Imaging, Southlake Regional Health Centre; (905)895-4521 x2251; Fax. (905)830-5986.

ISAAK, Verner H; Sheridan College Health, 1430 Trafalgar Rd, Oakville ON L6H 2L1; Tor'65; Staff, Halton Healthcare Services Corporation - Oakville Site; Staff Health Services, Sheridan Institute of Technology; Staff Phys, Maplehurst Correctional Centre; Staff Phys, Syl Apps Youth Centre; (905)845-9430; Fax. (905)815-4012.

ISABEL, Liette; CSSS de Laval, 1755 boul Rene-Laennec, Laval QC H7M 3L9; Laval'87; CSPQ; Anes. Staff, Hopital de la Cite de la santé; (450)668-1010; Fax. (450)975-5545.

ISAC, George D; UBC-Dept of Anes, 2449-910 10th Ave W, Vancouver BC V5Z 1M9; Dal'99; FRCPC; Anes.

ISAC, Michelle M; Hamilton HS-General Site, 237 Barton St E, Hamilton ON L8L 2X2; Dal'02; FRCPC; Anes. Staff, Hamilton Health Sciences Centre - Hamilton General Hospital; (905)521-2100

ISAIAH, Joel H; 3911 51 Ave, Lloydminster AB T9V 2Z2; (India)'86; MB BS; (780)875-6460

ISAYAMA, Tetsuya; The Hosp for Sick Children, 555 University Ave, Toronto ON M5G 1X8; (Japan)'03.

ISAZA-ZAPATA, Gloria M; Hamilton HS-McMaster Site, PO Box 2000 Stn Lcd 1 4V2-1200 Main St W, Hamilton ON L8N 3Z5; Antioquia (Colombia)'89; Staff, Hamilton Health Sciences Centre - McMaster Children's Hospital; (905)521-2100; Fax. (905)521-2332.

ISBISTER, Carolyn M; 108-575 16th St, West Vancouver BC V7V 4Y1; UBC'03; FRCSC; Ophth. (604)926-5722

ISCOE, Neill A; Odette Cancer Centre, 2075 Bayview Ave, Toronto ON M4N 3M5; McG'75; FRCPC; IntMed; MedOncol. Ac Staff, Sunnybrook Health Sciences Centre; Assoc Prof Med, University of Toronto; (416)480-5248

ISCOVE, Melvyn L; 204-272 Lawrence Ave W, Toronto ON M5M 4M1; Tor'69; FRCPC; Psy. (416)782-6253; Fax. (416)782-3040.

ISEMAN, Wendy E; Markham Stouffville Hosp, PO Box 1800 Stn Main 381 Church St, Markham ON L3P 7P3; Wes'86; CCFP; CCFP(E.M.); Emergency Family Med, Markham Stouffville Hospital; (905)472-7111; Fax. (905)472-7026.

ISEN, Susan J C; 41 Windhaven Terrace, Thornhill ON L4J 7N8; Tor'94; CCFP; FCFP; (905)731-9147; Fax. (905)731-5417.

ISENBERG, Gerald N; 401-294 Main St, Toronto ON M4C 4X5; Tor'66; Assoc Staff, Mount Sinai Hospital; (416)694-3427; Fax. (416)694-3430.

ISENBERG, Joel H; NOAH, 42 Second St, Kirkland Lake ON P2N 1R1; McG'83; FRCPC; IntMed (Addiction Medicine). (705)567-7778; Fax. (705)567-6664.

ISENBERG, Jonathan R; Red Lake Med Associates, PO Box 311, Red Lake ON P0V 2M0; Tor'09; CCFP; Staff, St Joseph's Health Centre; (807)727-2617

ISENBERG, Meyer L; Rouge Valley-Centenary HC, 6F-2867 Ellesmere Rd, Scarborough ON M1E 4B9; Lausanne (Switzerland)'66; FRCPC; Psy. Staff Psy Serv, Rouge Valley Health System - Centenary Health Centre Site; (416)281-7318; Fax. (416)281-7320.

ISENRING, Paul; CHUQ-Hotel-Dieu de Quebec, 11 Cote Du Palais, Quebec QC G1R 2J6; Laval'85; FRCPC; IntMed; Nephrol. Staff, Centre Hospitalier Universitaire de Québec (CHUQ) - Siege Social; (418)691-5464; Fax. (418)691-5757.

ISENSTEIN, Norman G; 201-40 Westmore Dr, Etobicoke ON M9V 4C2; Man'80; Staff, William Osler Health System - Etobicoke General Hospital; (416)744-9758; Fax. (416)746-1071.

ISHAC, Magda; 101-2780 Jane St, North York ON M3N 2J2; Alexandria (Egypt)'76; DOHS; Ac Staff Family Med, Humber River Regional Hospital - Finch Avenue Site; Langs: Arabic; (416)748-6936; Fax. (416)748-8730.

ISHAK, Fadel A; 272 Cedar St, Sudbury ON P3B 1M7; Cairo (Egypt)'77; FACS; FRCSC; Otol (Head & Neck Surgery). (705)673-4415

ISHAK, Magued; Ctr Hosp De Verdun, 4000 boul Lasalle, Verdun QC H4G 2A3; Mon'79; Microbio & Infect Dis (P.Q.); MedMicrobiol. Staff, Centre Hospitalier de Verdun; adj Prof, Universite de Montreal; (514)362-1000 x2246; magued.ishak@videotron.ca.

ISHAK-BOUSHAKI, Fatma-Zohra; Hop Santa Cabrini Ospedale, 5655 rue Saint-Zotique E, Montreal QC H1T 1P7; (Algeria)'94; Staff, Hôpital Santa Cabrini Ospedale; (514)252-6000

ISHAQZAY, Rahmatullah; Milton Urgent Care Clinic, 103-400 Bronte St S, Milton ON L9T 0H7; Punjab (Pakistan)'88; MB BS; LMCC; CCFP; Langs: Urdu; Punjabi; Persian; (905)876-3843; Fax. (905)876-2486.

ISHKANIAN, Adrian S; Sunnybrook Hlth Sciences Ctre, 2075 Bayview Ave, Toronto ON M4N 3M5; UBC'06; RadOncol. Staff RadOncol, Sunnybrook Health Sciences Centre; (416)480-6100

ISHRAT ALI KHAN, Pervez; Cross Cancer Centre, 11560 University Ave NW, Edmonton AB T6G 1Z2; Peshawar (Pakistan)'78; MB BS; MRC(I); Staff, Cross Cancer Institute; Langs: Urdu; Punjabi; Arabic; (780)432-8771; Fax. (780)412-6326.

ISHWARLALL, Sujay; Moose Jaw Union Hosp, 455 Fairford St E, Moose Jaw SK S6H 1J3; Staff, Moose Jaw Union Hospital; (306)694-0200

ISIGUZO, Obinna F; Associate Med Clinic, GD 215 Centre St, McLennan AB T0H 2L0; (Nigeria)'01; MB BS; (780)324-3730

ISKANDAR, Evette; CLSC Notre-Dame-De-Grace, 110-2525 boul Cavendish, Montreal QC H4B 2Y4; Ain Shams (Egypt)'76; (514)485-1670

ISKANDAR, Hani; Douglas Mental Hlth Univ Inst, 6875 boul Lasalle, Verdun QC H4H 1R3; Alexandria (Egypt)'70; DPsy; Staff, Douglas Mental Health University Institute; Asst Prof Psy, McGill University; Langs: French; Arabic; Italian; (514)761-6131; Fax. (514)762-3045; iskhan@douglas.mcgill.ca.

ISKANDER, Alexander W; 303-1017 Wilson Ave, North York ON M3K 1Z1; Gazira (Sudan)'84; MB BS; FRCS(Ed); FRCSC; GenSurg (Colonoscopy). Staff, Humber River Regional Hospital - Church Street Site; Langs: Arabic; (416)782-1016; Fax. (416)782-1742.

ISKANDER, John W; Halton HSC-Georgetown, 203-1A Princess Anne Dr, Georgetown ON L7G 2B8; Khartoum (Sudan)'86; MB BS; FRCSC; GenSurg (Surgical Oncology). Ac Staff General Surgeon, Halton Healthcare Services Corporation - Georgetown Hospital; Langs: Arabic; (905)702-1088; Fax. (905)702-1028.

ISKANDER, Mamdouh A S; 128-8401 Weston Rd, Vaughan ON L4L 1A6; Khartoum (Sudan)'88; MB BS; CCFP; (905)856-6142

ISKANDER, Mariam F G; The Doctor's Office, 203-300 John St, Thornhill ON L3T 5W4; Cairo (Egypt)'77; CCFP; Langs: Arabic; (905)764-0188; Fax. (905)764-0189; m.iskander@rogers.com.

ISKANDER, Nagi M; 379-5 Fairview Mall Dr, North York ON M2J 2Z1; Alexandria (Egypt)'82; MB ChB; CCFP; (416)498-7282

ISKANDER, Salah S G; Lakewood Med Centre, 34 Lakewood Blvd, Winnipeg MB R2J 2M6; Alexandria (Egypt)'86; MB BS; ACLS; ATLS; FCFP; CCFP; Langs: Arabic; (204)257-4900 x242

ISKANDER, Sam; Dept of Psychiatry, 70 Colony Farm Rd, Coquitlam BC V3C 5X9; Tor'04; FRCPC; Psy. (604)524-7700

ISKANDER, Suzan F; Lakewood Med Centre, 34 Lakewood Blvd, Winnipeg MB R2J 2M6; Alexandria (Egypt)'84; CCFP; (204)257-4900; Fax. (204)257-7240.

ISKANDIR, Amal K E; Burnhamthorpe Med Centre, 4-350 Burnhamthorpe Rd E, Mississauga ON L5A 3S5; Asyut (Egypt)'87; CCFP; Langs: Arabic; (905)270-9700; Fax. (905)270-5779.

ISKHAKOVA, Maria A; Geraldton Med Group, PO Box 1240 510 Hogarth Ave W, Geraldton ON P0T 1M0; Kyrgyz State (Kyrgyzstan)'84; CCFP; (807)854-0224; Fax. (807)854-0227; mariaishakova@yahoo.ca.

ISLAM, Ali; St Joseph's Health Care, PO Box 5777 Stn B 268 Grosvenor St, London ON N6A 4V2; Tor'99; FRCPC; DiagRad (Cardiovascular Radiology). Staff Radiol, Tillsonburg District Memorial Hospital; Staff Radiol, Strathroy Middlesex General Hospital - Middlesex Hospital Alliance; Staff Diagnostic Radiol, St Joseph's Hospital - St Joseph's Health Care; (519)646-6035; ali.islam@sjhc.london.on.ca.

ISLAM, Ashiqul; 222 King St E, Bowmanville ON L1C 1P6; Chittagong (Bangladesh)'88; FRCPC; IntMed. (905)697-9770

ISLAM, Bonnieca F; North Edmonton Health Centre, 14007 50 St NW, Edmonton AB T5A 5E4; Alb'02; FRCPC; Peds. Clinical Asst Prof, University of Alberta; Langs: Bengali; (780)342-4169; Fax. (780)342-4196.

ISLAM, Mohammad Z; Golden Mile Centre, 208-3806 Albert St, Regina SK S4S 3R2; (306)569-1565

ISLAM, Muhammad U; Valley Medical Imaging, 404A-2151 McCallum Rd, Abbotsford BC V2S 3N8; Punjab (India)'86; MB BS; FRCPC; DiagRad. Langs: Punjabi; Urdu.

ISLAM, Omar S; Kingston Gen Hosp, 76 Stuart St, Kingston ON K7L 2V7; Tor'95; ABR; LMCC; FRCPC; DiagRad (Neuro Radiology). Staff DiagRad, Kingston General Hospital; Staff, Hotel-Dieu Hospital; Asst Prof DiagRad, Queen's University; Langs: Urdu; (613)548-2301; Fax. (613)548-2413.

ISLAM, Shahidul; The Ottawa Hosp-Gen Campus, 1440-501 Smyth Rd, Ottawa ON K1H 8L6; Dhaka (Bangladesh)'92; FRCPC; AnatPath. Staff, The Ottawa Hospital - General Campus; (613)737-8899 x78297; Fax. (613)737-8853.

ISLER, Marc H; Les Ortho de Maisonneuve, 320-5345 boul de l'Assomption, Montreal QC H1T 4B3; Mon'86; FRCSC; OrthSurg (Orthopedic Oncology). Staff, Hôpital Ste-Justine; Staff, Hopital Maisonneuve-Rosemont; Prof, Universite de Montreal; Langs: Bilingual(English/French); (514)254-6161; Fax. (514)254-1596.

ISLER, Monique; Dir de la Sante Publique-Mtl, 1301 rue Sherbrooke E, Montreal QC H2L 1M3; Mon'77; OccupMed (P.Q.). (514)528-2400 x3202; Fax. (514)528-2459; misler@santepub-mtl.qc.ca.

ISLES, Katherine K; 102-304 The East Mall, Etobicoke ON M9B 6E2; Tor'78; DIH; CCBOM; MASc; FRCPC; OccupMed. Court Staff, Women's College Hospital; Att Staff, St Michael's Hospital; (416)231-7968; Fax. (416)231-7982; kisles@tpclinic.com.

ISLUR, Avinash; St Boniface Gen Hosp, Z3036-409 Tache Ave, Winnipeg MB R2H 2A6; Tor'02; FRCSC; PlasSurg (Plastic & Reconstructive Surgery). Staff, St Boniface General Hospital; Asst Prof/Prog Dir Plastic Surg Residency, University of Manitoba; (204)237-2571; Fax. (204)237-3429; aislur@sbgh.mb.ca.

ISLUR, Jaya M; 1-1033 Pape Ave, Toronto ON M4K 3W1; Mysore (India)'61; MB BS; DABPed; FAAP; FRCPC; Peds (Infectious Diseases). Staff Physician, The Hospital For Sick Children; Asst Prof, University of Toronto; Langs: Hindi; Kanarese; (416)425-0605; Fax. (416)291-1969.

ISMAEIL, Nabeel H A; Univ of Ottawa Heart Institute, 40 Ruskin St, Ottawa ON K1Y 4W7; King Abdul Aziz (Saudi Arabia)'03; FRCPC; IntMed. Staff, University of Ottawa Heart Institute.

ISMAEL, Mahmoud; Northgate Centre, 2074-9499 137 Ave NW, Edmonton AB T5E 5R8; (Libya)'97; MB BCh; (780)479-3318; Fax. (780)479-3810.

ISMAIL, Abdel-Raouf; 750 Brunswick St, Fredericton NB E3B 1H9; Tor'75; DAB; PlasSurg. (506)447-8979; Fax. (506)447-8294.

ISMAIL, Aden A; 210-633 Colborne St, London ON N6B 2V3; (Somalia)'82; FRCPC; Psy (Child & Adolescent Psychiatry). Staff, Woodstock General Hospital; Langs: Somali; Arabic; Italian; (519)936-0810; Fax. (519)936-1169.

ISMAIL, Alnashir; Toronto Centre for Med Imaging, 910-150 York St, Toronto ON M5H 3S5; McG'85; FRCPC; DiagRad. (416)368-8488

ISMAIL, Farooq F; West Park Healthcare Centre, R3 92-82 Buttonwood Ave, Toronto ON M6M 2J5; Wes'99; FRCPC; PhysMed&Rehab. Staff, West Park Healthcare Centre; (416)243-3600 x3680; Fax. (416)243-1177.

ISMAIL, Ibrahim T; Grand Rapids Nursing Station, PO Box 53, Grand Rapids MB R0C 1E0; Mosul (Iraq)'87; CCFP; ibrahim_ismail@hc-sc.gc.ca.

ISMAIL, Laila; CLSC Pierrefonds, 13800 boul Gouin O, Pierrefonds QC H8Z 3H6; Sher'01; FRCPC; Peds. Médecin, CLSC Pierrefonds; Physician, Centre Jeunesse de Montreal; Langs: English; (514)626-2572; Fax. (514)624-7486.

ISMAIL, Michelle M; Valley Med Clinic, 335 Jubilee St, Duncan BC V9L 1W9; Cape Town (South Africa)'95; MB ChB; (250)748-8151; Fax. (250)748-8157.

ISMAIL, Shiraz H; 12 Brandy Court, North York ON M3B 3L3; Makerere (Uganda)'70; Hon Staff, St Joseph's Health Centre; Assoc Staff, Toronto East General Hospital Inc; Physician, Leisureworld Nursing Home-Cheltenham; Physician, Leisureworld Nursing Home; Langs: Urdu; Kacchi; Gujarati; Hindi; Swahili; (416)469-0491; Fax. (416)469-0773.

ISMAIL, Waleed S; Saskatoon Cancer Centre, 20 Campus Dr, Saskatoon SK S7N 4H4; Staff, Saskatoon Cancer Centre; (306)655-2980

ISMAIL, Yahya A; Milbrook Mall, 304-2 Herald Ave, Corner Brook NL A2H 4B5; (Jordan)'80; Staff, Western Memorial Regional Hospital.

ISMAIL, Zahinoor; Foothills Med Centre, C203-1403 29 St NW, Calgary AB T2N 2T9; Alb'94; FRCPC; Psy. Staff, Foothills Medical Centre; (403)944-1321

ISMAILI, Arif M A; 309-751 King St W, Kitchener ON N2G 1E5; Cal'00; FRCPC; IntMed; Gastroent. Staff Physician, St Mary's General Hospital; Staff Physician, Grand River Hospital - Kitchener/Waterloo Health Centre; Langs: Punjabi; Urdu; Hindi; (519)741-5786; Fax. (519)741-0030.

ISMAILY, Nasreen S; 103-3195 Granville St, Vancouver BC V6H 3K2; Ott'97; PhmB; BSc; CCFP; (604)739-8011

ISMAT-RAHEEM, Alia; Carbonear General Hosp, 86 Highroad South, Carbonear NL A1Y 1A4; Punjab (Pakistan)'92; MB BS; Staff, Carbonear General Hospital; (709)945-5035

ISMEAL, Ali K; Bishop Falls Medical Clinic, PO Box 580 2 Helen Tulk Dr, Bishops Falls NL A0H 1C0; Baghdad (Iraq)'92; CCFP; Staff, Connaigre Peninsula Community Health Centre; (709)258-5555; ali.ismeal@easternhealth.ca.

ISMIIL, Nadia D; Sunnybrook Hlth Sciences Ctre, E432-2075 Bayview Ave, Toronto ON M4N 3M5; Basra (Iraq)'81; FRCPC; AnatPath. Staff, Sunnybrook Health Sciences Centre; (416)480-6100; Fax. (416)480-4271.

ISOARD, Lionel A; CSSS du Lac-des-Deux-Montagnes, 520 boul Arthur-Sauve, Saint-Eustache QC J7R 5B1; Lyon (France)'98; Staff, Hôpital de Saint-Eustache; (450)473-6811 x2152; Fax. (450)473-9234.

ISOMURA, M Theresa K; Fraser Health Authority, 4F-260 Sherbrooke St, New Westminster BC V3L 3M2; UBC'79; FRCPC; Psy. (604)520-4662; Fax. (604)520-4871.

ISPAHANY, M Mehdi; 33 2nd Ave SE PO Box 389, Chesley ON N0G 1L0; Saba (Netherlands Antilles)'08; CCFP; (519)363-3220; Fax. (519)363-0385.

ISPAS, Cristina L; Dynacare Kasper Med Lab, 200-10150 102 St NW, Edmonton AB T5J 5E2; (Romania)'93; (780)451-3702; Fax. (780)452-8488.

ISRAEL, Aliza T; Women's College Hosp, 76 Grenville St, Toronto ON M5S 1B2; Tor'04; FRCPC; Psy. Staff, Women's College Hospital; (416)323-6230

ISRAEL, David M; BC Women's & Hosp & Health Ctr, K4 184-4500 Oak St, Vancouver BC V6H 3N1; Tel Aviv (Israel)'84; FRCPC; Peds (Pediatric Gastroenterology). Hd Gastroent, BC Children's Hospital; Clin Prof Peds, University of British Columbia; (604)875-2332

ISRAEL, Koma D; 503 Concession St, Hamilton ON L9A 1C1; Baghdad (Iraq)'79; MB ChB; CCFP; Langs: Hebrew; Arabic; Kurdish; (905)529-8111; Fax. (905)529-6336.

ISRAEL, Mimi; Douglas Mental Hlth Univ Inst, 6875 boul Lasalle, Verdun QC H4H 1R3; McG'83; FRCPC; Psy. Chef Psychiatry/assoc Prof, McGill University; (514)761-6131; isrmim@douglas.mcgill.ca.

ISRAELIAN, Gaspar; Credit Valley Prof Bldg, 503-2300 Eglinton Ave W, Mississauga ON L5M 2V8; London (England)'70; MB BS; FRCPC; Neur. Ac Staff, The Credit Valley Hospital; Court Staff, Toronto General Hospital - UHN; University of Toronto; (905)820-9197; Fax. (905)820-7543.

ISRAELS, Sara J; CancerCare Manitoba, 675 McDermot Ave, Winnipeg MB R3E 0V9; Man'79; FRCPC; Peds (Pediatric Hematology Oncology); Hem. Dir Haemostasis Lab & Hemophilia Prog, Health Sciences Centre; Prof Peds, University of Manitoba; (204)787-4141; israels@cc.umanitoba.ca.

ISSA, Kheirie; 401 Smyth Rd, Ottawa ON K1H 8L1; Tichreen (Syria)'86; FAAP; FRCPC; Peds. Staff Peds, Children's Hospital of Eastern Ontario (CHEO); Langs: Arabic; (613)737-7600

ISSA-CHERGUI, Badia; CSSS du Sud de Lanaudière, 911 montee des Pionniers, Terrebonne QC J6V 2H2; Damascus (Syria)'80; CSPQ; FRCPC; AnatPath. Staff, Centre Hospitalier Pierre le Gardeur; (450)654-7525

ISSAIVANAN, Magimairajan; CancerCare Manitoba, 675 McDermot Ave, Winnipeg MB R3E 0V9.

ISSAKOFF-MELLER, Anna M; Guelph Family Health Team, 311-85 Norfolk St, Guelph ON N1H 4J4; Ott'85; Langs: Italian; Spanish; French; (519)836-7861; Fax. (519)836-8842.

ISSAR, Ajay; Doctor's Office, 150 Yardley Ave, East York ON M4B 2B2; Tor'87; (416)755-2541

ISSEKUTZ, Andrew C; IWK Health Centre, PO Box 9700 Rpo CSC 5850-5980 University Ave, Halifax NS B3K 6R8; Dal'74; FRCPC; Peds (Immunology). Staff, IWK Health Centre; (902)470-8491; andrew.issekutz@iwk.nshealth.ca.

ISSEKUTZ, Thomas B; IWK Health Centre, PO Box 9700 Rpo CSC K8518-5850 University Ave, Halifax NS B3K 6R8; Dal'76; Peds (Pediatric Immunology). Ac Staff, IWK Health Centre; Prof Peds, Dalhousie University; (902)470-6935; thomas.issekutz@iwk.nshealth.ca.

ISSENMAN, Robert; McMaster University, HSC 3A-1280 Main St W, Hamilton ON L8S 4K1; McM'73; FAAP; FRCPC; Peds (Pediatric Gastroenterology). Chief Peds Gastroent, Hamilton Health Sciences Centre - McMaster Children's Hospital; Affil Staff, Joseph Brant Memorial Hospital; Prof Peds, McMaster University; Langs: English; French; (905)521-2100 x75637; Fax. (905)521-2655.

ISSERLIN, Jonathan; Greenbank Med Centre, 106-139 Greenbank Rd, Nepean ON K2H 9A5; London (England)'67; LRCP; MRCS; DA; Ac Staff, Queensway Carleton Hospital; (613)596-1320; Fax. (613)596-3933.

ISSERLIN, Leanna E; Children's Hosp of Western Ont, B8 178-800 Commissioners Rd E, London ON N6C 2V5; Dal'04; FRCPC; Psy. Staff, Children's Hospital of Western Ontario; Staff, London Health Sciences Centre - Victoria Campus; (519)685-8500; Fax. (519)685-8595.

ISSEROW, Saul H; UBC Hospital, S110-2211 Wesbrook Mall, Vancouver BC V6T 2B5; Witwatersrand (South Africa)'86; MB ChB; FRCPC; IntMed; Cardiol. Assoc Dir Cardiol, UBC Hospital - Koerner Pavillion; Assoc Dir Healthy Heart Program, Vancouver General Hospital - Centennial Pavillion; Clin Instructor, University of British Columbia; (604)822-1747; Fax. (604)822-7625.

ISSID, Simon; Centre d'Urgence St-Laurent, 200-1605 boul MArcel-Laurin, Saint-Laurent QC H4R 0B7; St. Joseph (Lebanon)'72; Langs: French; Arabic; (514)747-2555; Fax. (514)747-7624.

ISSLEY, Steven B; Hotel-Dieu Grace Hosp, 1030 Ouellette Ave, Windsor ON N9A 1E1; McG'97; CCFP; EmergMed. Staff, Hôtel-Dieu Grace Hospital; (519)973-4411

ISTASY, Victor F; Children's Hosp, 840 Sherbrook St, Winnipeg MB R3A 1S1; Ain Shams (Egypt)'92; FRCPC; Peds.

ISTEAD, Jannice M; Quinte HC Corp-Belleville Gen, 265 Dundas St E, Belleville ON K8N 5A9; Qns'80; BSc(Biology); Staff, QHC Belleville General; (613)969-7400; Fax. (613)969-0229.

ISTVAN, Jurai; Ctr Hosp De Verdun, 4000 boul Lasalle, Verdun QC H4G 2A3; Mon'06; FRCPC; Anes. Staff, Centre Hospitalier de Verdun; (514)362-1000

ITALIANO, Marc A; 203-100 Colborne St W, Orillia ON L3V 2Y9; Tor'96; CCFP; Staff, Orillia Soldiers' Memorial Hospital; (705)326-3529; Fax. (705)326-8802.

ITCUSH, Laurie L; Surrey Mem Hosp, 13750 96 Ave, Surrey BC V3V 1Z2; UBC'89; Staff, Surrey Memorial Hospital; Langs: Bilingual(English/French); (604)581-2211

ITH, Rinda-Bun H; Clinique Medicale KARE, 104-4415 boul Notre-Dame, Laval QC H7W 1T7; Laval'96; Staff, Jewish Rehabilitation Hospital; Langs: Bilingual(French/English); (450)686-0701; Fax. (450)686-7511.

ITO, Shinya; E 8229-555 University Ave, Toronto ON M5G 1X8; (Japan)'79; FRCPC; Peds. Staff, The Hospital For Sick Children; Prof, University of Toronto; Langs: Japanese; (416)813-5781; Fax. (416)813-7562.

ITOVITCH, Joseph J; CSSS du Suroît, 150 rue Saint-Thomas, Salaber-de-Valleyf QC J6T 6C1; McG'92; FRCSC; Urol. Staff, Centre Hospitalier Régional du Suroît; Langs: English; French; (450)371-9920

IU, Alvin C L; 10-10 Headdon Gate, Richmond Hill ON L4C 8A3; (Hong Kong)'81; FRCPC; Peds. (905)770-5661; Fax. (905)770-3381.

IU, Simon C M; 506-1110 Sheppard Ave E, North York ON M2K 2W2; Tor'82; MSc; FRCSC; GenSurg (Thoracic Surgery). Staff, Toronto East General Hospital Inc; Staff, North York General Hospital; University of Toronto; Langs: Cantonese; (416)221-1233; Fax. (416)221-7873.

IURASCO, Vladislav; 250-8730 Country Hills Blvd NW, Calgary AB T3G 0E2; (Moldova)'03; LMCC; (403)262-7787

IVANANS, Nicholas C; 134-318 21st St E, Saskatoon SK S7K 6C8; UBC'00; BSc; CCFP; CCFP(E.M.); Staff Emerg, Royal University Hospital; Assoc Prof, University of Saskatchewan; (306)881-5660

IVANKOVIC, Maria N; The Credit Valley Hosp, 2200 Eglinton Ave W, Mississauga ON L5M 2N1; McM'03; CCFP; CCFP(E.M.); Staff, The Credit Valley Hospital; (905)813-4530

IVANOV, T N Teodor; 101-12165 Harris Rd, Pitt Meadows BC V3Y 2E9; Sofia (Bulgaria)'91; CCFP; Langs: Bulgarian; Russian; (604)465-3010

IVANOVICH, Den M; 69 Lake Ave W, Carleton Place ON K7C 1L5; Wes'86; Ac Staff, Carleton Place & District Memorial Hospital; (613)257-1818; Fax. (613)257-5890.

IVANTCHEV, Sergei; Upper River Valley Hosp, 11300 130 Rte, Watervil-Carleton NB E7P 0A4; (Moldova)'89; CCFP; Staff, Upper River Valley Hospital - Waterville; (506)375-5900; Fax. (506)325-2772.

IVANY, Linda E; Primary Medical, 150 Old Placentia Rd, Mount Pearl NL A1N 4Y9; Mem'83; Teacher Family Practice, Memorial University Of Newfoundland; (709)368-8883

IVANYI, Katalin E; Stonechurch Family Health Ctre, 1475 Upper Ottawa St, Hamilton ON L8W 3J6; McM'91; CCFP; FCFP; Assoc Staff, St Joseph's Healthcare - Charlton Campus; (905)575-7757

IVERS, Noah; Women's College Hosp, 76 Grenville St, Toronto ON M5S 1B2; Wes'07; CCFP; Staff, Women's College Hospital; (416)323-6060; Fax. (416)323-6255.

IVERSON, Gregory C; Kingston Med Arts Centre, 301-800 Princess St, Kingston ON K7L 5E4; Ott'77; (613)549-8754; Fax. (613)549-2736.

IVERSON, Lance M; Royal University Hosp, 103 Hospital Dr, Saskatoon SK S7N 0W8; Sask'96; CCFP; CCFP(E.M.); FCFP; Staff, Royal University Hospital; (306)655-1398; Fax. (306)655-1011.

IVES, Michael S; Coldwater Med Centre, PO Box 489 45 River St, Coldwater ON L0K 1E0; Qns'85; (705)686-3335; Fax. (705)686-3837.

IVEY, Jeffrey A; Eden Mental Health Centre, 1500 Pembina Ave, Winkler MB R6W 1T4; Man'73; BSc(Med.); FRCPC; Psy (Administration). Consultant, Churchill Regional Health Authority; Staff Psy, Eden Mental Health Centre; (204)325-4325; Fax. (204)325-8429.

IWAMA, Tom T; Guildford Med Dental Centre, 10-15300 105 Ave, Surrey BC V3R 6A7; UBC'82; BSc; CCFP; Staff Palliative Care, Surrey Memorial Hospital; Clin Instructor, University of British Columbia; (604)581-5611; Fax. (604)583-2818.

IWANCHYSHYN, George J; Martinway Plaza, 415 The Westway, Etobicoke ON M9R 1H5; Qns'90; Staff Privil, William Osler Health System - Etobicoke General Hospital; Court Staff Privil, Humber River Regional Hospital - Church Street Site; Court Staff Privil, Humber River Regional Hospital - Keele Street Site; (416)249-0009

IWANICKI, Stanislaw M; Sunridge Prof Centre, 301-2675 36 St NE, Calgary AB T1Y 6H6; Akademia Medyczna (Poland)'73; LRCP(Lond); MRCS(Eng); FRCOG; FRCSC; ObstGyn (Maternal Fetal Medicine). Clin Assoc Prof, University of Calgary; (403)291-0270; Fax. (403)250-3419.

IWANOCHKO, Robert M; Univ Hlth Network-Toronto Western Hosp, EW5 423-399 Bathurst St, Toronto ON M5T 2S8; Tor'87; FACC; FRCPC; IntMed; Cardiol., Trillium Health Centre - West Toronto; Staff Cardiol, Toronto General Hospital - UHN; Med Dir, Toronto Western Hospital - University Health Network; Asst Prof Med, University of Toronto; (416)603-5236; Fax. (416)603-5680; robert.iwanochko@uhn.on.ca.

IWASA, Carolyn T; Guildwood Village Shopping Ctr, 5-123 Guildwood Pky, Scarborough ON M1E 4V2; Tor'85; (416)269-5088; Fax. (416)261-3112.

IWASHKIW, Boris M; 3-4402 37 St, Stony Plain AB T7Z 2A9; Alb'83; BSc; (780)963-7800; Fax. (780)963-0468; iwashkiw@shaw.ca.

IYAYI, Ehinomen A; Park Avenue Med Centre, 4634 Park Ave, Terrace BC V8G 1V7; (South Africa)'04; MB ChB; CCFP; (250)615-5030

IYENGAR, Akshai M; The Ottawa Hosp-Gen Campus, 209-501 Smyth RD, Ottawa ON K1H 8L6; Mem'06; FRCPC; IntMed; Critical Care Medicine. Staff, The Ottawa Hospital - General Campus; (613)737-8222

IYENGAR, Pratibha; The Credit Valley Hosp, 2200 Eglinton Ave W, Mississauga ON L5M 2N1; McG'99; ABP; FRCP; LMCC; FRCPC; AnatPath (Cytology). Staff Path, The Credit Valley Hospital; (905)813-2696; piyengar@cvh.on.ca.

IYER, Hariharan S; London HSC-University Hosp, PO Box 5339 Stn B ALL 135-339 Windermere Rd, London ON N6A 5A5; Pramukhswami (India)'98; Staff, London Health Sciences Centre - University Hospital; (519)663-3892

IYER, L Priya; 515-3030 Lawrence Ave E, Scarborough ON M1P 2T7; Wes'05; FRCPC; IntMed; Respir. (416)431-2300

IYER, Mahalaxmi V; Valley Medical Centre, 11948 227 St, Maple Ridge BC V2X 6J3; Bombay (India)'97; MB BS; FRCPC; Anes.

IYER, Natasha; 518-922 5 Ave SW, Calgary AB T2P 5R4; Natal (South Africa)'95; MB ChB; CCFP; (403)237-2353; Fax. (403)237-9533.

IYER, R Padmanabhan; 596 McNaughton Ave W, Chatham ON N7L 4J6; Banaras Hindu (India)'69; MD; MB BS; FRCP; FACP; FCCP; FRCPC; IntMed. Chief Dept of Med/Med Prog Dir ICU, Chatham-Kent Health Alliance; Aj Prof Med, University of Western Ontario; Langs: Tamil; Malayalam; Telugu; (519)351-0111; Fax. (519)351-0112; piyer@uwo.ca.

IYER, Sriram N; Valley Medical Centre, 11948 227 St, Maple Ridge BC V2X 6J3; Gujarat (India)'94; FRCPC; Peds. (604)477-0165

IYER, Sugantha P; Niagara H System-Welland Site, 65 Third St, Welland ON L3B 4W6; St. Maarten (Netherlands Antilles)'07; Staff, Niagara Health System - Welland Hospital Site; (905)378-4647

IYER, Vikram S; Hamilton HS-General Site, 5N-237 Barton St E, Hamilton ON L8L 2X2; Wes'98; FRCSC; GenSurg; VascSurg. Staff, Hamilton Health Sciences Centre - Hamilton General Hospital; (905)528-1321; iyer@hhsc.ca.

IZAWA, Jonathan I; London HSC-South St, PO Box 5375 Stn B C3 120-800 Commissioners Rd E, London ON N6A 4G5; Wes'94; BSc; FRCSC; Urol (Urological Oncology). Staff, London Health Sciences Centre - South Street; Asst Prof Surg & Oncol Div of Urol, University of Western Ontario; (519)685-8550; Fax. (519)685-8455; jonathan.izawa@lhsc.on.ca.

IZEN, Randi J; 414-750 Broadway W, Vancouver BC V5Z 1H3; Man'96; BSc; CCFP; Staff Privil, BC Women's Hospital & Health Centre; (604)675-9433

IZENBERG, O Samuel; 223A St Clair Ave W, Toronto ON M4V 1R3; Tor'65; FRCPC; Psy. (416)960-1415; Fax. (416)445-2983.

IZEVBAYE, Iyare E; University of Alberta Hosp, 4B4.31-8440 112 St NW, Edmonton AB T6G 2B7; (Nigeria)'98; DABPath; MB BS; Staff, University of Alberta Hospital; (780)407-8025; Fax. (780)407-8599.

IZSO, Peter; 6179 Main St PO Box 1089 Stn Main, Stouffville ON L4A 8A1; Tor'72; BSc; Court Staff, Markham Stouffville Hospital; Court Staff, Markham Stouffville Hospital - Uxbridge Site; (905)640-2300; Fax. (905)640-5256.

IZUKAWA, Dennis M S; 210-101 Queensway W, Mississauga ON L5B 2P7; Tor'83; FRCSC; Neursurg. Staff, Trillium Health Centre - Mississauga; (905)566-9750; Fax. (905)566-9717.

IZUKAWA, Terumi A; Baycrest Ctre/Geriatric Care, 1C13-3560 Bathurst St, Toronto ON M6A 2E1; Tor'85; BSc; FRCPC; IntMed (Geriatric Medicine). Consultant, Mount Sinai Hospital; Consultant, Markham Stouffville Hospital; Hd GeriatricMed/Hd IntMed, Baycrest Centre for Geriatric Care; Asst Prof Geriatric Med & Prog Dir, University of Toronto; (416)785-2500 x2607; Fax. (416)785-2873.

IZZARD, J Brad; Woodlawn Med Clinic, 92 Main St, Dartmouth NS B2X 1R5; Dal'97; BSc; CCFP; Staff, Dartmouth General Hospital; (902)434-1500; Fax. (902)434-4368.

IZZELDIN, Abuelgasim; Westney Heights Med Centre, 2-15 Westney Rd N, Ajax ON L1T 1P4; (Romania)'88; CCFP; FCFP; (905)428-8055

IZZELDIN, Mohamed S; A I M Health Group, 1051 Wonderland Rd S, London ON N6K 3X4; Gezira (Sudan)'86; CCFP; Langs: Arabic; (519)472-2060

JAAKKIMAINEN, R Liisa; Sunnybrook Hlth Sciences Ctre, A103-2075 Bayview Ave, Toronto ON M4N 3M5; McM'95; BSc; MSc; CCFP; Assoc Staff Family & Commun Med, Sunnybrook Health Sciences Centre; Asst Prof, University of Toronto; (416)480-4936; Fax. (416)480-6038.

JAAMOUR, Mohammad; South Walkerville Med Centre, 368-2224 Walker Rd, Windsor ON N8W 5L7; Damascus (Syria)'76; Langs: Arabic; (519)973-1800; Fax. (519)973-1805.

JABADO, Nada; MUHC-Montreal Children's Hosp, B300-2300 rue Tupper, Montreal QC H3H 1P3; Paris (France)'95; Staff, McGill University Health Centre - Montreal Children's Hospital; (514)412-4400 x23270; Fax. (514)412-4331; nada.jabado@mcgill.ca.

JABBAR, Faiza; Northern Interior Health Unit, 3F-1444 Edmonton St, Prince George BC V2M 6W5; Karachi (Pakistan)'96; MB BS; Physician, Northern Interior Health Unit; faiza.jabbar@northernhealth.ca.

JABBAR, Faraz; University Hosp of Northern BC, 1475 Edmonton St, Prince George BC V2M 1S2; Karachi (Pakistan)'00; MB BS; Staff, University Hospital of Northern British Columbia; (250)565-2450

JABBAR, Yasmeen; Georgetown Med Associates, 199 Princess Anne Dr, Georgetown ON L7G 0E3; Karachi (Pakistan)'98; CCFP; (905)873-3000; Fax. (905)873-0800.

JABBARI-ZADEH, Shahram; Millwoods Medicentre, 6426 28 Ave NW, Edmonton AB T6L 6N3; (Iran)'93; CCFP; (780)462-3491

JABBOUR, Mona L; Children's Hosp Eastern Ont, W1401-401 Smyth Rd, Ottawa ON K1H 8L1; McM'87; FRCPC; Peds. Staff EmergMed, Children's Hospital of Eastern Ontario (CHEO); (613)737-7600 x2318; Fax. (613)738-4285.

JABEEN, Shaifta; Scotia Med Family Practice, 961 Bedford Hwy, Bedford NS B4A 1A9; Karachi (Pakistan)'83; MB BS; LMCC; CCFP.

JABER, Wisam M A; Bay St George Med Centre, 129 Montana Dr, Stephenville NL A2N 2T4; Baghdad (Iraq)'96.

JABER, Zaid M A; Grand River Hosp-KW Hlth Ctre, PO Box 9056 Stn Main 835 King St W, Kitchener ON N2G 1G3; Al-Nahrain (Other Foreign)'97; CCFP; CCFP(E.M.); Staff, Grand River Hospital - Kitchener/Waterloo Health Centre; (519)749-4300

JABI, Maha; Gamma-Dynacare Lab, 750 Peter Morand Cres, Ottawa ON K1G 6S4; Damascus (Syria)'71; AnatPath. Staff, The Ottawa Hospital - General Campus; (613)729-0200 x6009; Fax. (613)729-1127.

JABLANCZY, Alexander J N; Doctors Bldg, 105-955 Queen St E, Sault Ste. Marie ON P6A 2C3; Dal'76; Ac Staff, Sault Area Hospital - Sault Ste Marie; (705)949-1216; Fax. (705)949-1241.

JABLONOWSKI, Karin; 3-7700 Bathurst St, Thornhill ON L4J 7Y3; McG'00; FRCPC; Psy (Psycho Geriatrics). Consultant Psy, Canadian Mental Health Associaton; Langs: French; (905)660-9760; Fax. (905)660-9762.

JABLONSKI, Eric V; PO Box 460, Black Diamond AB T0L 0H0; Cal'10; CCFP; (403)933-4368

JABLONSKI, Theodore J; Crowfoot Village Fam Practice, 210-600 Crowfoot Cres NW, Calgary AB T3G 0B4; Man'84; BSc(Med); ACLS; CCFP; FCFP; Ad Staff Privil, Foothills Medical Centre; (403)239-9733; Fax. (403)241-8112.

JABLONSKY, George; London HSC-University Hosp, PO Box 5339 Stn B 339 Windermere Rd, London ON N6A 5A5; Tor'76; FACP; FACC; FCCP; FAHA; FRCPC; Cardiol (Internal Medicine). Cardiologist, London Health Sciences Centre - University Hospital; Assoc Prof Med, University of Western Ontario; (519)663-3266; Fax. (519)434-3278; George.Jablonsky@lhsc.on.ca.

JABOR, Ammar K A; Carbonear Gen Hosp, 86 Highroad South, Carbonear NL A1Y 1A4; Baghdad (Iraq)'02; MB ChB; Staff, Carbonear General Hospital; (709)945-5111

JABOUIN, Serge; 421 Rideau St, Ottawa ON K1N 5Y9; (Haiti)'73; (613)789-7707; Fax. (613)789-2682.

JABS, Corrine F I; Parliament Place, 405-2631 28th Ave, Regina SK S4S 6X3; Sask'93; BSc(Med); FRCSC; ObstGyn (Urological Gynecology). (306)586-3120; Fax. (306)586-3128; corrinejabs@hotmail.com.

JABS, Doris K; Hotel-Dieu Hosp, 166 Brock St, Kingston ON K7L 5G2; Man'96; FRCPC; DiagRad. Staff, Kingston General Hospital; (613)544-3400

JABS, Marlis E; Riverwood Med Centre, 1295 Pembina Hwy, Winnipeg MB R3T 2B3; Man'93; CCFP; Langs: German; (204)452-3345; Fax. (204)452-5339.

JACIW, George A; Byron Street Med Centre, 320 Byron St S, Whitby ON L1N 4P8; Ott'55; Langs: Ukrainian; Polish; German; (905)668-5835; Fax. (905)668-8942.

JACK, Kristin L; University of Western Ontario, M106-1151 Richmond St, London ON N6A 5C1; Sask'07; Neur.

JACK, Zita; Parkland Med Clinic, 203-998 Parkland Dr, Halifax NS B3M 0A6; (Other Foreign)'08; CCFP.

JACKA, Michael J; University of Alberta Hosp, 8 120 CSB-8440 112 St NW, Edmonton AB T6G 2B7; Qns'88; MSc; MBA; FRCPC; Anes; Critical Care Medicine. Staff, University of Alberta Hospital; Staff, Covenant Health - Grey Nuns Community Hospital; Staff, Covenant Health - Misericordia Community Hospital; Clin Prof, University of Alberta; Langs: English; French; (780)407-8861; Fax. (780)407-3200; mjacka@ualberta.ca.

JACKA, Robert M; B-370 Burnham St, Peterborough ON K9H 1T6; Tor'89; CCFP; (705)740-0066; Fax. (705)740-0046.

JACKIEWICZ, Allan W; Stamford Med Centre, 103-4256 Portage Rd, Niagara Falls ON L2E 6A4; Warsaw (Poland)'81; FRCSC; ObstGyn. Ac Staff ObstGyn, Niagara Health System - Greater Niagara General Site; Clinical Asst Prof ObstGyn, McMaster University; Langs: Polish; (905)374-0781; Fax. (905)374-6265.

JACKIEWICZ, Grazyna; 103-4256 Portage Rd, Niagara Falls ON L2E 6A4; Warsaw (Poland)'81; FRCPC; Peds (Consultant Pediatrics). Pediatrics, Niagara Peninsula Children's Centre; Asst Prof Peds, McMaster University; Langs: Polish; (905)374-0781; Fax. (905)374-6265.

JACKMAN, Christopher S; Newfoundland Drive Med Clinic, 201-427 Newfoundland Dr, St. John's NL A1A 4A5; Mem'01; FRCSC; Ophth. (709)576-7676

JACKMAN, Heather R; Dr Charles A Janeway Child Hc, 300 Prince Philip Dr, St. John's NL A1B 3V6; Mem'98; FRCSC; OrthSurg. Staff, Janeway Children's Health & Rehabilitation Centre; (709)777-4046

JACKMAN, Kevin F M; Callingwood Crossing Med Clini, 6905 172 St NW, Edmonton AB T5T 5Y1; (Ireland)'76; BSc(Anatomy); FRCSI; LMCC; Staff, Viking Health Centre; Staff, Viking Medical Clinic; (780)444-0350; kevin.jackman@ech.ab.ca.

JACKMAN, Michelle L; Alberta Children's Hosp, 2888 Shaganappi Trail NW, Calgary AB T3B 6A8; Tor'01; FRCPC; Peds. Staff, Alberta Children's Hospital; (403)955-7211

JACKMAN, Paul D; Quidi Vidi Family Practice, 3F-20 Lake Ave, St. John's NL A1A 1H4; Mem'91; BMedSci; (709)576-7040; Fax. (709)576-7151.

JACKMAN, Stephanie S; Dr Charles A Janeway Child HC, 300 Prince Philip Dr, St. John's NL A1B 3V6; Mem'01; FRCPC; DiagRad. Staff, Janeway Children's Health & Rehabilitation Centre; (709)777-6300

JACKS, Duncan A; Rebalance MD, 104-3551 Blanshard St, Victoria BC V8Z 0B9; McG'04; OrthSurg. (250)940-4444

JACKSON, A Beverley; 207-726 Bloor St W, Toronto ON M6G 4A1; Alb'79; CCFP; FCFP; Ac Staff, Sunnybrook Health Sciences Centre; Ac Staff, Women's College Hospital; Lecturer, University of Toronto; (416)538-3939; Fax. (416)538-2980; bloorparkdocs@gmail.com.

JACKSON, Aaron L; Ottawa Fertility Centre, 200-955 Green Valley Cres, Ottawa ON K2C 3V4; Wes'04; FRCSC; ObstGyn. (613)686-3378

JACKSON, Alan C; Health Sciences Centre, GF 543-820 Sherbrook St, Winnipeg MB R3A 1R9; Qns'78; FRCP; FRCPC; IntMed; Neur. Sec Head Neurol, Winnipeg Regional Health Authority; Prof, University of Manitoba; (204)787-1578; Fax. (204)787-1486; ajackson2@hsc.mb.ca.

JACKSON, Andora T K; The Pas Health Complex, PO Box 240 61 1st ST W, The Pas MB R9A 1K4; Man'07; FRCSC; ObstGyn. Staff, St. Anthony General Hospital.

JACKSON, Andrew D; Silverfern Med Clinic, PO Box 309 1710B 20 St, Didsbury AB T0M 0W0; Dunedin (New Zealand)'95; Physician, Didsbury District Health Services; (403)335-8895

JACKSON, Bernard S; Charlton Med Centre, 810-25 Charlton Ave E, Hamilton ON L8N 1Y2; Witwatersrand (South Africa)'72; MB BCh; ABOtol; FRCSC; Otol (Head & Neck Surgery). Ac Staff, St Joseph's Healthcare - Charlton Campus; McMaster University; (905)528-0109; Fax. (905)528-7176.

JACKSON, Bethany J; Carleton Univ Student Health, 1125 Colonel By Dr, Ottawa ON K1S 5B6; Sask'02; CCFP; Assoc Physician Surgical Asst, Queensway Carleton Hospital; (613)520-6674

JACKSON, Christopher A; 201-86 Angeline St S, Lindsay ON K9V 6C5; Wes'84; Court Staff, Ross Memorial Hospital; (705)324-6255; Fax. (705)324-9046.

JACKSON, Colin M; Surrey Med Arts Bldg, 101-13798 94A Ave, Surrey BC V3V 1N1; UBC'98; BSc; FRCSC; OrthSurg (Hand & Wrist Surgery). Staff, Surrey Memorial Hospital; (604)588-6528; Fax. (604)588-1241.

JACKSON, Craig S; 225-2306 Highway 6, Vernon BC V1T 7E3; UBC'94; (250)260-3800

JACKSON, Elaine E; Guildford Med Dental Centre, 37-15300 105 Ave, Surrey BC V3R 6A7; UBC'90; (604)588-6411

JACKSON, Gary C; Peace Arch Hosp, 15521 Russell Ave, White Rock BC V4B 2R4; UBC'79; FRCSC; ObstGyn. Staff, Peace Arch Hospital; (604)531-5512

JACKSON, John; Clin Med Physergo du Sud-Ouest, 5260 rue de Verdun, Verdun QC H4H 1K1; McG'78; (514)766-1696; Fax. (514)766-3472.

JACKSON, John R; Radiology Consultants Assoc, 120-6707 Elbow Dr SW, Calgary AB T2V 0E3; Alb'77; FRCPC; DiagRad. (403)777-3003; Fax. (403)777-3008.

JACKSON, Lauren E; Alderlea Med Clinic, 101-330 Festubert St, Duncan BC V9L 3S9; UBC'86; CCFP; FCFP; Staff, Cowichan District Hospital; (250)748-9000; Fax. (250)748-1299.

JACKSON, Lori; Dr Everett Chalmers Reg Hosp, PO Box 9000 Stn A, Fredericton NB E3B 5N5; New England (USA)'04; Staff, Dr Everett Chalmers Regional Hospital; (506)452-5400

JACKSON, Louise M; Comox Valley Surgical Centre, PO Box 3477 Stn Main, Courtenay BC V9N 5N5; Amsterdam (Netherlands)'69; FRCPC; Anes (Acute Pain Management). Langs: Dutch.

JACKSON, Martin R; Group One Med Associates, 1111 Springfield Rd, Kelowna BC V1Y 8R7; Edinburgh (Scotland)'69; BSc(Hon); MB ChB; CCFP; (250)762-4286

JACKSON, Mary E; Medical Bldg, 202-18 Pine St, Kitchener ON N2H 5Z8; Qns'82; FRCPC; IntMed; Respir. Ac Staff, Grand River Hospital - Kitchener/Waterloo Health Centre; Ac Staff, St Mary's General Hospital; (519)741-8660; Fax. (519)741-1657.

JACKSON, Mary Lou; Royal Jubilee Hosp, 1952 Bay St, Victoria BC V8R 1J8; McM'80; Ophth. Staff, Royal Jubilee Hospital; (250)370-8677

JACKSON, Mervyn M; North York Family Health Team, PO Box 91130 Rpo Bayview Village 2901 Bayview Ave, North York ON M2K 2Y6; Dublin (Ireland)'75; BAO; LM; CCFP; FCFP; Med Dir Palliative Care Outreach Team, North York General Hospital; Asst Prof Family & CommunMed, University of Toronto; (416)493-3611; Fax. (416)491-6428; mervynjackson@rogers.com.

JACKSON, Michael H; McBride & Dist Hosp, PO Box 669, McBride BC V0J 2E0; Kansas(KS) (USA)'75; Fam Med, McBride & District Hospital; (250)569-2251; Fax. (250)569-3369; michael.jackson@northernhealth.ca.

JACKSON, Paul A; St Joseph's Healthcare, 50 Charlton Ave E, Hamilton ON L8N 4A6; McM'88; FRCPC; Anes. Consultant Anes, St Joseph's Healthcare - Charlton Campus; Ass't Clin Prof, McMaster University; (905)522-4941; Fax. (905)521-6019.

JACKSON, Peter D; 1726 Kings Rd, Sydney NS B1S 1E9; Guy's Hosp. (England)'62; LRCP(Lond); MRCS(Eng); Ac Staff, Cape Breton Healthcare Complex; (902)562-3134; Fax. (902)562-8155.

JACKSON, R Jeffrey D; Brockville Gen Hosp, 75 Charles St, Brockville ON K6V 1S8; Wes'73; FRCPC; Psy (Adult Psychiatry). Staff, Brockville General Hospital - Charles Street; (613)345-5645

JACKSON, Renee N M; Alberta Children's Hosp, 2888 Shaganappi Trail NW, Calgary AB T3B 6A8; Cal'05; FRCPC; Peds. Staff, Alberta Children's Hospital; (403)955-7211

JACKSON, Robert; 82 Viscount Ave, Ottawa ON K1Z 7M9; McG'50; BSc; MDCM; FRCPC; Derm. Emeritus Prof, University of Ottawa; (613)729-2192; Fax. (613)729-8179; robertnonie@rogers.com.

JACKSON, Robin M; Hillcrest Clinic, 7381 Hurd St, Mission BC V2V 3H8; Witwatersrand (South Africa)'02; MB BCh; (604)826-8345

JACKSON, Rose J; 201-86 Angeline St S, Lindsay ON K9V 6C5; Wes'84; Court Staff, Ross Memorial Hospital; (705)324-6255; Fax. (705)324-9046.

JACKSON, Roy P; Southern Health Centre, 15157 Roper Ave, White Rock BC V4B 5C9; Witwatersrand (South Africa)'87; MB ChB; BSc; FRCSC; ObstGyn (Gynecology). Member Dept of ObstGyn, Peace Arch Hospital; Physician, False Creek Surgical Centre; Med Dir, Southern Health Centre; Dir, Gynaecological Services; (604)531-8707; Fax. (604)531-8725; info@southernhealthcentre.com.

JACKSON, Shannon C; Burrard Med Bldg, 490-1144 Burrard St, Vancouver BC V6Z 2A5; Cal'01; FRCPC; IntMed; Hem. (604)684-5794 x2

JACKSON, Simon D; Queen Elizabeth II HSC-Halifax, 2134-1796 Summer St, Halifax NS B3H 3A7; Dal'90; FRCPC; IntMed; Cardiol. Att Staff, Queen Elizabeth II Health Sciences Centre - Victoria General Site; (902)473-6608

JACKSON, Steven J; 208-3030 Lawrence Ave E, Scarborough ON M1P 2T7; McG'87; MBA; FRCSC; GenSurg (Surgical Oncology). Lecturer, University of Toronto; Langs: English; French; (416)438-6824; Fax. (416)438-7006.

JACKSON, Timothy D; Univ Hlth Network-Toronto Western Hosp, 322-399 Bathurst St, Toronto ON M5T 2S8; McM'03; FRCSC; GenSurg. Staff, Toronto Western Hospital - University Health Network; (416)603-5599

JACKSON, W Bruce; The Ottawa Hosp-Gen Campus, W6221A-501 Smyth Rd, Ottawa ON K1H 8L6; Wes'67; DABOph; FRCSC; Ophth (Cornea/External Disease). Dir Refractive Surg/Laser Prog Univ of Ottawa Eye Institute, The Ottawa Hospital - General Campus; Prof, University of Ottawa; (613)737-8759; Fax. (613)737-8374.

JACKSON, Wesley D; Sunridge Fam Med Teaching Ctr, 2685 26 St NE, Calgary AB T1Y 5S3; Cal'82; BSc; CCFP; FCFP; Langs: Italian; (403)943-5000; Fax. (403)347-8784; wjackson@ucalgary.ca.

JACKSON, Zane S; Medical Clinic Bldg, 117-89 Humber College Blvd, Etobicoke ON M9V 4B8; Tor'05; FRCSC; GenSurg. Staff, William Osler Health System - Etobicoke General Hospital; (416)741-8998

JACKSON-HUGHES, John F; Nipigon Health Centre, PO Box 67 125 Hogan Rd, Nipigon ON P0T 2J0; Ott'74; BSc; CCFP; FCFP; Instructor, Northern Ontario Medical Plan; (807)887-2102; Fax. (807)887-2903; jjackson@ndmh.ca.

JACO, Jennifer M; Windsor Reg Hosp-Metropolitan, 1995 Lens Ave, Windsor ON N8W 1L9; Tor'84; CCFP; Staff, Windsor Regional Hospital - Metropolitan Site; (519)254-5577

JACOB, Abraham J; Markham Stouffville Urgent Car, 110 Copper Creek Dr, Markham ON L6B 0P9; Wes'08; CCFP; (905)472-8911

JACOB, Andre M; Unite de Med Familiale, 80 118e rue, Shawinigan-Sud QC G9P 3E4; Laval'76; Teach Staff, Centre Hospitalier du Centre la Mauricie; (819)537-8878; Fax. (819)537-3489.

JACOB, Anu; Medical Care Clinic, 205 Markham Rd, Scarborough ON M1J 3C3; Mysore (India)'96; (416)265-6663

JACOB, Francois-Dominique J R; Edmonton Clinic Health Academy, 4-588 11405 87 Ave NW, Edmonton AB T6G 1C9; Ott'06; Neur. Staff, University of Alberta Hospital; (780)248-5630

JACOB, Gaetan; Centre de Med Familiale, 189 av Damase-Potvin, Baie-Comeau QC G4Z 2Y9; Laval'77; Staff, Centre Hospitalier Régional Baie-Comeau; (418)296-6609

JACOB, Genevieve; Hop du Sacre-Coeur de Mtl, 5400 boul Gouin O, Montreal QC H4J 1C5; McG'97; Staff Geriatric Serv, Hôpital du Sacre-Coeur de Montréal; Prof, Universite de Montreal; Langs: English; French; (514)338-2222 x2763

JACOB, Helene; La Cite Medicale, 295-2600 boul Laurier, Quebec QC G1V 4T3; Laval'94; BSc; MBA; Langs: Bilingual(French/English); (418)781-0480

JACOB, Jacob C; Wedgewood Med Centre, 307-12 Gleneyre St, St. John's NL A1A 2M7; Madras (India)'56; FRCPC; Neur (Adult Neurology). Ac Staff, Health Sciences Centre; Ac Staff, Janeway Children's Health & Rehabilitation Centre; Clin Prof Med Peds Neur, Memorial University Of Newfoundland; (709)753-1051; Fax. (709)753-1883.

JACOB, Laurent; CSSS de Saint-Jerome, 290 rue de Montigny, Saint-Jerome QC J7Z 5T3; Mon'91; Staff, Hôtel-Dieu de Saint-Jérôme; (450)431-8400

JACOB, Mary V; Boundary Trails Health Centre, PO Box 2000 Stn Main, Winkler MB R6W 1H8; Man'94; FRCPC; DiagRad. Staff, Boundary Trails Health Centre; (204)331-8811; Fax. (204)331-8812.

JACOB, Moire S; North Park Med Centre, 1365 Lawrence Ave W, North York ON M6L 1A4; Madras (India)'63; MB BS; FRCPC; IntMed. (416)244-4377

JACOB, Phillip; Hôtel Dieu de Saint-Joseph, 10 Woodland Hill, Perth-Andover NB E7H 5H5; Wisconsin (USA)'99; Staff, Hôtel-Dieu of St Joseph Hospital.

JACOB, Punnaran; Medical Care Clinic, 205 Markham Rd, Scarborough ON M1J 3C3; Mysore (India)'96; CCFP; (416)265-6663

JACOB, Renee; Centre Med De Beauport, 737 av Royale, Quebec QC G1E 1Z1; Laval'75; (418)667-7114; Fax. (418)667-5843.

JACOB, Sanjay M; Regina Qu'Appelle HR-Regina, 1440 14th Ave, Regina SK S4P 0W5; Ott'03; FRCSC; GenSurg; VascSurg. Staff, Regina General Hospital; (306)766-6900

JACOB, Sheila V; Hôpital Ste-Justine, 3175 ch Cote-Sainte-Catherine, Montreal QC H3T 1C5; Tor'87; CSPQ; FRCPC; Peds; Respir (P.Q.). Staff, Hôpital Ste-Justine; adj Prof, Universite de Montreal; Langs: Bilingual(English/French); (514)345-4931 x5409; Fax. (514)345-4804; sheila_jacob@ssss.gouv.qc.ca.

JACOB, Simon; Ctr Hosp Affilie-St-Sacrement, 1050 ch Sainte-Foy, Quebec QC G1S 4L8; Laval'72; CSPQ; AnatPath (Cytogenetics). Ac Staff, Centre Hospitalier Affilié Universitaire de Québec - Hôpital du St-Sacrement; Staff Teacher, Université Laval; (418)682-7813; simon.jacob.cha@ssss.gouv.qc.ca.

JACOB, Thomas K; Health Sciences Centre, GC430-820 Sherbrook St, Winnipeg MB R3A 1R9; Bangalore (India)'97; FRCPC; IntMed (Critical Care Medicine); Rheum. Staff, Health Sciences Centre; (204)774-8511

JACOB, V Chandy; Dr CW Wiebe Med Centre, 385 Main St, Winkler MB R6W 1J2; Kerala (India)'58; GenSurg (Orthopedics). Staff, Boundary Trails Health Centre; Langs: Hindi; (204)325-4312; Fax. (204)325-4594.

JACOB-GOUDREAU, Ariane; CSSS de la Cote-de-Gaspe, 215 boul de York O, Gaspe QC G4X 2W2; Sher'07; Staff, Centre Hospitalier de Gaspe; (418)368-3301

JACOB-GOUDREAU, Philippe; CSSS du Lac-des-Deux-Montagnes, 520 boul Arthur-Sauve, Saint-Eustache QC J7R 5B1; Sher'02; FRCSC; OrthSurg. Staff, Hôpital de Saint-Eustache; (450)473-6811

JACOBI, Nicole; Sudbury Reg Hosp-Laurentian, 41 Ramsey Lake Rd, Sudbury ON P3E 5J1; Mainz (Germany)'93; Staff, Health Sciences North-Laurentian Site; (705)523-7100

JACOBS, David A; Humber River Reg Hosp-Church, 200 Church St, York ON M9N 1N8; Qns'96; FRCPC; DiagRad. Staff, Humber River Regional Hospital - Church Street Site; (416)249-8111

JACOBS, Gerhardus C; Quinsam Med Group, 280-1400 Dogwood St, Campbell River BC V9W 3A6; Stellenbosch (South Africa)'94; MB ChB; CCFP; Staff Emerg, Campbell River & District General Hospital; (250)286-0601; Fax. (250)286-0504.

JACOBS, Howard; The Jacobs Pain Centre, 102-8920 Woodbine Ave, Markham ON L3R 9W9; RCS (Ireland)'77; LRCPSI; DAAPM; Chair Section Chronic Pain, Ontario Medical Association; Pres, Canadian Academy of Pain Management; Langs: Hebrew; (905)305-9484; Fax. (905)305-7381; drjacobs@rogers.com.

JACOBS, Irving G; North York Gen Hosp, 4001 Leslie St, North York ON M2K 1E1; Tor'83; FRCPC; DiagRad. Staff, North York General Hospital; (416)398-4411

JACOBS, Johan J; South Sherbrook Health Centre, 88 Sherbrook St, Winnipeg MB R3C 2B3; Pretoria (South Africa)'89; MB ChB; LMCC; Med Dir, Fast Air Medivac; Physician, Northern Medical Unit; Langs: Afrikaans; (204)774-7196; Fax. (204)774-9260; jjjacobs@mts.net.

JACOBS, Lawrence; 201-2475 McDougall St, Windsor ON N8X 3N9; Wayne (USA)'07; IntMed. (519)915-2241; Fax. (519)915-5225.

JACOBS, Robert J; Highlands Med Clinic, GD, Neils Harbour NS B0C 1N0; Wake Forest (USA)'81; (902)336-2621; Fax. (902)336-2229.

JACOBS, Steve R; 600-123 Edward St, Toronto ON M5G 1E2; Tor'84; FRCPC; DiagRad. (416)597-1016

JACOBS, Susan; Agincourt Mall, 3850 Sheppard Ave E, Scarborough ON M1T 3L4; Tor'87; (416)335-5532

JACOBS, Thomas B; Wilson Centre Family Practice, 1-2185 Wilson Ave, Port Coquitlam BC V3C 6C1; McM'87; BSc; MSc; PhD; Staff, Eagle Ridge Hospital & Health Care Centre; Staff, Royal Columbian Hospital; Langs: German; (604)942-7227; Fax. (604)942-7058.

JACOBS, W Bradley; Foothills Med Centre, 1250-1403 29 St NW, Calgary AB T2N 2T9; Cal'98; FRCSC; Neursurg (Spinal Neuro Surg). Staff Clinical Neurosciences, Foothills Medical Centre; (403)944-3406

JACOBS, Gerhardus W F; Associate Med Clinic, 25 St Michael St, St. Albert AB T8N 1C7; Stellenbosch (South Africa)'96; MB ChB; (780)458-1234; Fax. (780)460-7941.

JACOBSEN, Craig A; QE Park Med Clinic, 4060 Cambie St, Vancouver BC V5Z 2X8; McG'92; (604)874-4060

JACOBSEN, Marnie; Selkirk Family Medicine, 307-1101 Dewdney Ave, Trail BC V1R 4T1; Sask'77; Staff, Kootenay Boundary Regional Hospital; (250)368-8802; Fax. (250)368-8813.

JACOBSEN, Niels-Erik B; Hys Med Centre, 400-11010 101 St NW, Edmonton AB T5H 4B9; Alb'99; FRCSC; Urol. (780)441-2588

JACOBSOHN, Eric; Health Sciences Centre, 2F-671 Wiliam Ave, Winnipeg MB R3E 0Z2; Cape Town (South Africa)'84; MB ChB; FRCPC; Anes; Critical Care Medicine. Staff, Health Sciences Centre; Dept Head Anes, University of Manitoba.

JACOBSOHN, Friedrich G; G R Baker Mem Hosp, 543 Front St, Quesnel BC V2J 2K7; Orange Free State (South Africa)'01; Staff, G R Baker Memorial Hospital; (250)985-5600

JACOBSON, Avrum I; 200-175 av Stillview, Pointe-Claire QC H9R 4S3; McG'96; FRCSC; Urol (Oncology). Staff Urol, Lakeshore General Hospital - Pointe Claire; Langs: Bilingual(French/English); (514)697-5323; Fax. (514)697-6610.

JACOBSON, Bradley A; Thunder Bay Reg HC-T-Bay, 980 Oliver Rd, Thunder Bay ON P7B 6V4; McM'05; CCFP; CCFP(E.M.); Staff, Thunder Bay Regional Health Sciences Centre.

JACOBSON, Edward L; Oakville Health Centre, 212-1060 Speers Rd, Oakville ON L6L 2X4; Tor'78; Langs: Hebrew; (905)582-7777

JACOBSON, Elliot S; Cornwall Comm Hosp-McConnell, PO Box 100 Stn Main 840 McConnell Ave, Cornwall ON K6H 5S5; Alb'99; CCFP; CCFP(E.M.); Staff, Cornwall Community Hospital; (613)938-4240

JACOBSON, Kevan; Children's & Women's HC of BC, K4 184-4480 Oak St, Vancouver BC V6H 3V4; Witwatersrand (South Africa)'83; FRCPC; IntMed (Pediatric Gastroenterology); Gastroent. Div Head/Staff, BC Children's Hospital; (604)875-2332

JACOBSON, Paul D M; 425-1200 Markham Rd, Scarborough ON M1H 3C3; Qns'95; CCFP; CCFP(E.M.); FCFP; Staff, Humber River Regional Hospital - Church Street Site; (416)438-7080

JACOBSON, Perry A; Brampton Hlth & Wellness Ctre, 2 Kennedy Rd S, Brampton ON L6W 3E1; Man'92; (905)796-2270; Fax. (905)796-5241.

JACOBSON, Perry D; Royal University Hosp, 103 Hospital Dr, Saskatoon SK S7N 0W8; Alb'02; FRCPC; Anes. Staff Anes, Royal University Hospital; (306)655-1183; Fax. (306)655-1279.

JACOBSON, Roger S; 15 Wing Canadian Forces Base, PO Box 5000 Stn Main, Moose Jaw SK S6H 7Z8; Sask'71; Ac Staff, Moose Jaw Union Hospital; (306)756-2262; Fax. (306)756-2262.

JACOBSON, Sheila J; Clairhurst Med Centre, 201-1466 Bathurst St, Toronto ON M5R 3S3; Witwatersrand (South Africa)'83; FRCPC; Peds (Clinical Pharmacology). Staff, The Hospital For Sick Children; Asst Prof, University of Toronto; (416)531-3331; Fax. (416)531-1639.

JACOBSON, Stephen A; SMBD Jewish Gen Hosp, 3755 ch Cote-Sainte-Catherine, Montreal QC H3T 1E2; Dal'63; FACS; FRCSC; Urol (Uro Oncology). Staff, Sir Mortimer B Davis Jewish General; Staff, McGill University Health Centre - Royal Victoria Hospital; Staff, McGill University Health Centre - Montreal General Campus; Prof Urol, McGill University; Langs: English; French; (514)340-8222 x3700; Fax. (514)340-7559.

JACOBSZ, Nicolette; Regina Qu'Appelle HR-Regina, 1440 14th Ave, Regina SK S4P 0W5; (Other Foreign)'06; (306)766-2096; Fax. (306)766-2842.

JACOBY, Colin S; Pacific Med Clinic, 3185 Grandview Hwy, Vancouver BC V5M 2E4; (Other Foreign)'02; (604)434-2222

JACOBY, Lynn M; Appletree Med Group, 1582 Bank St, Ottawa ON K1H 7Z5; Michigan (USA)'01; MB BS; (613)731-0259

JACOBY, Michael E; Tudor Village Clock Tower, 105-1315 Summit Dr, Kamloops BC V2C 5R9; Cal'93; FRCSC; PlasSurg (Plastic & Reconstructive Surgery). (250)377-4949; Fax. (250)377-4664; mjacoby@shaw.ca.

JACONELLO, Paul P; Jaconello Health Centre, 6F-615 Yonge St, Toronto ON M4Y 1Z5; London (England)'67; MB BS; DRCOG(Eng); FFARCS(Eng); Dir, Jaconello Centre for Nutritional & Preventive Medicine; (416)463-2911; Fax. (416)469-0538.

JACOT, Francis R M; 50 ch Lacroix RR 3, Danville QC J0A 1A0; McG'72; adj Prof, Universite de Sherbrooke; Langs: English; French; (819)839-3688

JACQMIN, Marc L; Sault Area Hosp, 750 Great Northern Rd, Sault Ste. Marie ON P6B 0A8; Mon'67; FAAOS; FRCSC; OrthSurg. Ac Staff, Sault Area Hospital - Sault Ste Marie; (705)759-3434

JACQUEMIN, Geraldine; Inst De Readaptation De Mtl, 6300 av De Darlington, Montreal QC H3S 2J4; Mon'95; FRCPC; PhysMed&Rehab (Spinal Cord Injury). Assoc Member, Hôpital du Sacre-Coeur de Montréal; Staff, Institut de Réadaptation Gingras-Lindsay de Montréal; Langs: Spanish; English; (514)340-2146

JACQUEMIN, Jean-Pierre; CSSS de la Hauet-Yamaska, 205 boul Leclerc O, Granby QC J2G 1T7; Louvain (Belgium)'66; FRCSC; GenSurg. Staff, Centre Hospitalier de Granby; (450)375-8000

JACQUEMIN, Paul J; Ctr Hosp de Verdun, 4000 boul Lasalle, Verdun QC H4G 2A3; Louvain (Belgium)'72; FRCPC; Respir. Staff, Centre Hospitalier de Verdun; Langs: Belgian; English; (514)362-1000; Fax. (514)767-1766; p.jacquemin@videotron.ca.

JACQUES, Aline; Hotel-Dieu de Sorel, 400 av de l'Hotel-Dieu, Sorel-Tracy QC J3P 1N5; Mon'06; Staff, Hôtel-Dieu de Sorel; (450)746-6000

JACQUES, Andre; GMF de Grand-Mere, 200-1050 8e rue, Grand-Mere QC G9T 4L4; Laval'79; CCFP; Membre, Centre Lafleche Grand-Mere; (819)538-0773; Fax. (819)538-0774.

JACQUES, Andre; Clinique Sante Jacques-Cartier, 200-1815 rue King O, Sherbrooke QC J1J 2E3; Sher'74; LMCC; Ac Staff Family Med & Emerg, Centre Hospitalier Universitaire de Sherbrooke-Hôpital Hôtel-Dieu; Prof, Universite de Sherbrooke; (819)565-7446; Fax. (819)565-7780.

JACQUES, Andre J; College des Med Du Quebec, 2170 boul Rene-Levesque O, Montreal QC H3H 2T8; Mon'74; CCFP; FCFP; Dir, College des Medecins du Quebec; (514)933-4441; Fax. (514)933-4668; jacques.cmq@sympatico.ca.

JACQUES, Christine; CLSC-CHSLD Vallee de la Batisc, 90 Riviere-A-Veillette RR 4, Ste-Genev-D-Batisc QC G0X 2R0; Mon'98; CCFP; (418)362-2727; Fax. (418)362-3125.

JACQUES, Cindi N; The Ottawa Hosp-Gen Campus, 501 Smyth Rd, Ottawa ON K1H 8L6; McM'05; FRCPC; IntMed; Hem. (613)737-8899

JACQUES, Denis; Clinique Med St-Vallier, 201-205 rue Montmagny, Quebec QC G1N 4V3; Laval'75; ac Staff, CSSS de Quebec-Sud; (418)688-0872; Fax. (418)688-4951.

JACQUES, Francois H; Clinique Neuro-Outaouais, 200-147 boul d'Europe, Gatineau QC J9J 0N3; Ott'88; FRCPC; Neur. Staff, Hull Hospital; (819)777-2500; Fax. (819)777-2502; francois.jacques@ssss.gouv.qc.ca.

JACQUES, Frederic; Hôpital Laval, 2725 chemin Sainte-Foy, Quebec QC G1V 4G5; Laval'04; MSc; FRCSC; CardSurg (Pediatric Cardiac Surgery). Staff, Hôpital Laval; Médecin, Institut Universitaire Cardiologie & Pneumologie de Quebec; Langs: English; Spanish; (418)656-4717

JACQUES, Graham A; St Lawrence Med Clinic, PO Box 329, Ingleside ON K0C 1M0; Ott'75; Ac Staff, Winchester District Memorial Hospital; Physician, ROHMAX Canada; (613)543-2963; Fax. (613)543-4171; gjacques@personainternet.com.

JACQUES, Ian R; North Bay Reg Health Centre, 50 College Dr, North Bay ON P1B 0A4; Ott'77; BSc; FRCPC; Psy. Staff Forensic Psy Program, North Bay Regional Health Centre - Regional Mental Health; (705)474-1200 x3436; Fax. (705)495-7814.

JACQUES, John; Dynacare Kasper Med Labs, 200-10150 102 St NW, Edmonton AB T5J 5E2; Queen's (Ireland)'65; MRCPath; FRCPC; AnatPath. (780)451-3702

JACQUES, Line; MUHC-Montreal Neurology Inst, 145-3801 rue University, Montreal QC H3A 2B4; Mon'90; BSc; MSc; FRCSC; Neursurg. Staff, McGill University Health Centre - Montreal Neurological Hospital; assoc Prof, McGill University; (514)398-3081; Fax. (514)398-2037; ljacques@yahoo.com.

JACQUES, Louis; Dir de la Sante Publique-Mtl, 1301 rue Sherbrooke E, Montreal QC H2L 1M3; Sher'77; FRCPC; CommunMed; OccupMed (P.Q.). (514)528-2400 x3305; ljacques@santepub-mtl.qc.ca.

JACQUES, Marc-Andre; Hop de Readaptation Lindsay, 6363 ch Hudson, Montreal QC H3S 1M9; (Haiti)'71; Staff, Institut de Réadaptation Gingras-Lindsay de Montréal; Langs: English; Spanish; (514)737-3661 x4127

JACQUES, Martin; Cite de la Sante de Laval, 1755 boul Rene-Laennec, Laval QC H7M 3L9; Mon'98; Staff, Hopital de la Cite de la santé; (450)668-1010

JACQUES, Martine; CHUQ-St-Francois D'Assise, 10 rue de l'Espinay, Quebec QC G1L 3L5; Laval'95; CCFP; Staff, Centre Hospitalier Universitaire De Québec - Pavillon De St-françois-d'assise; (418)525-4351

JACQUES, Michel; Centre Med Le Mesnil, 300-1300 boul Lebourneuf, Quebec QC G2K 2N1; Laval'03; (418)624-1800

JACQUES, Nicole; Clinique Med Saint-Hippolyte, 201-780 ch des Hauteurs, Saint-Hippolyte QC J8A 1H1; Laval'86; (450)224-8271

JACQUES, Paul; Inst U en Sante Mentale de QC, 2601 ch de la Canardiere, Quebec QC G1J 2G3; Laval'94; FRCPC; Psy. Staff, Institut Universitaire Sante; (418)663-5020; Fax. (418)663-5758.

JACQUES, Pierre; CSSS de la Cote-De-Gaspe, 215 boul De York O, Gaspe QC G4X 2W2; Laval'87; FRCPC; Derm. Staff, Centre Hospitalier de Gaspe; (418)368-3301

JACQUES, Raymond G; 44 First Ave, Coniston ON P0M 1M0; Ott'86; Langs: Bilingual(English/French); (705)694-0999; Fax. (705)694-0444.

JACQUES, Rene; CSSS de Quebec-Nord, 791 rue de Sherwood, Quebec QC G2N 1X7; Laval'87; Langs: English; (418)849-2572; rejacques55@yahoo.ca.

JACQUES, Romeo; 179 av Mercier, Rouyn-Noranda QC J9X 4X8; Laval'74; (819)762-0804; Fax. (819)762-7584.

JACQUES, Stephanie; Centre Hosp Rouyn-Noranda, 4 9e rue, Rouyn-Noranda QC J9X 2B2; Mon'97; FRCPC; Neur (Pediatric Neurology). Staff, Centre Hospitalier Rouyn-Noranda; Langs: Bilingual(French/English); (819)797-8811

JACQUES, Ulrick; Clinique Med Perrier, 10-10794 rue Lajeunesse, Montreal QC H3L 2E8; Port-au-Prince (Haiti)'62; OrthSurg (P.Q.). (514)274-7344; Fax. (514)274-1165.

JACQUES, Valerie; La Cite Medicale, 295-2600 boul Laurier, Quebec QC G1V 4T3; Mon'99; Staff, Centre Hospitalier Affilié Universitaire de Québec - Hôpital du St-Sacrement; Langs: Bilingual(French/English); (418)781-0480; Fax. (418)659-7072.

JACQUES, Yvan D; CSSS Haut-Richelieu-Rouville, 920 boul Du Seminaire N, St-Jean-Sur-Richel QC J3A 1B7; Laval'65; CSPQ; Anes. Staff, Hôpital du Haut-Richelieu; (450)359-5000 x5212; yvanjacques@sympatico.ca.

JACQUIER, Jennifer E; Heritage Med Research Centre, 362-107 University Campus NW, Edmonton AB T6G 2S2; Mem'05; FRCPC; IntMed; Endocrin&Metab. (780)407-3636

JACYK, Peter; Islington Med Clinic, 805-1243 Islington Ave, Etobicoke ON M8X 1Y9; Tor'77; MSc(Pharmacol.); Ac Staff Family & CommunMed, St Joseph's Health Centre; Langs: Ukrainian; (416)644-1890; Fax. (416)644-1892.

JACYK, William R; Greene Stone Muskoka, 3571 Muskoka Road 169, Bala ON P0C 1A0; Man'64; FRCPC; IntMed (Addiction Medicine). (705)762-5501

JACYNA, Stephan M; Rockyview Gen Hosp, 7007 14 St SW, Calgary AB T2V 1P9; Man'83; FRCPC; Anes. Staff Anes, Rockyview General Hospital; (403)943-3410

JADAD BECHARA, Alejandro R; Univ Hlth Network-Toronto Gen, RFE 4-190 Elizabeth St, Toronto ON M5G 2C4; Javeriana (Colombia)'86; Staff, Toronto General Hospital - UHN; Staff Physician, Princess Margaret Hospital - University Health Network; Chair Canada Research/Chief Innovator & Founder, Centre for Global eHealth Innovation; Prof, Dalla Lana School of Public Health; Prof Anes Institute of health policy Management & Evaluation, University of Toronto; Langs: Spanish; (416)340-4800 x6903; Fax. (416)340-3595.

JADAVJI, Nadeem; Royal Inland Hosp, 311 Columbia St, Kamloops BC V2C 2T1; Cal'03; FRCPC; Anes;CCFP; Staff, Royal Inland Hospital; (250)374-5111

JADAVJI, Tajdin P; Alberta Children's Hosp, 2888 Shaganappi Trail NW, Calgary AB T3B 6A8; Sind (Pakistan)'76; FAAP; FRCPC; Peds (AIDS/HIV); InfectDis. Staff, Alberta Children's Hospital; Prof Microbiol InfectDis Peds/Assoc Dean International Health, University of Calgary; (403)955-7813; Fax. (403)955-3045.

JADD, Jerome L; 469 William St S SS 2 Stn Main, Exeter ON N0M 1S2; Wes'85; (519)235-0910

JADI, Mohamed S; Guelph Med Place, 210-83 Dawson Rd, Guelph ON N1H 1B1; Al-Fateh (Libya)'81; FRCSC; ObstGyn (Prenatal Care). Staff, Guelph General Hospital; Langs: Arabic; (519)821-2440; Fax. (519)821-2448.

JADICK, Carmen H C; 206-51 Inglewood Dr, St. Albert AB T8N 4E7; Cal'88; FRCSC; GenSurg. Staff, Medicine Hat Regional Hospital; (780)419-6007; Fax. (780)459-6609.

JADOT, Sabina; CFB Kingston, PO Box 17000 Stn Forces, Kingston ON K7K 7B4; Buenos Aires (Argentina)'78; FRCPC; Psy. Staff, Brockville Mental Health Centre - Royal Ottawa Health Care Group; (613)541-5010 x5776

JADUSINGH, Inderman H; Tower Centre, 415-131 9 Ave SW, Calgary AB T2P 1K1; (Jamaica)'75; DABPath(AP/Cytopath.); FCAP; FRCPC; AnatPath (Fine Needle Aspiration Cytopathology). Specialist, Calgary Regional Health Authority; (403)299-0600; Fax. (403)299-0603.

JAEGER, Claire P; Manitoba Clinic, 790 Sherbrook St, Winnipeg MB R3A 1M3; Man'85; CCFP; FCFP.

JAEGER, Dominique; Clinique Med Du 5e Rang, 1091 rue Principale RR 1, St-Ambroise-D-Kild QC J0K 1C0; (Haiti)'82; (450)755-2555

JAEGER, Hilary F; Veterans Affairs Canada, 606-66 Slater St, Ottawa ON K1A 0P4; Tor'86; Staff, Canadian Forces Health Services Centre; Langs: Bilingual(English/French); (613)992-7424

JAEGER, Melanie T; Kingston Gen Hosp, 76 Stuart St, Kingston ON K7L 2V7; McM'90; FRCPC; Anes. Staff Anes, Kingston General Hospital; (613)548-7827; Fax. (613)548-1375; jaeger@kgh.kari.net.

JAEGER, Valerie A; Niagara Reg Public Health Unit, PO Box 1052 Stn Main 2201 St David's Rd W, Thorold ON L2V 0A2; McG'82; CCFP.

JAEGGI, Edgar T; The Hosp For Sick Children, 555 University Ave, Toronto ON M5G 1X8; Basel (Switzerland)'84; FRCPC; Peds. Staff Cardiol, The Hospital For Sick Children; Prof Peds, University of Toronto; Langs: German; French; (416)813-7467; edgar.jaeggi@sickkids.ca.

JAESCHKE, Roman Z; Fontbonne Bldg, 301 James St S, Hamilton ON L8P 3B6; Krakow (Poland)'81; FRCPC; IntMed (Critical Care Medicine). Staff, St Joseph's Healthcare - Charlton Campus; Clin Prof, McMaster University; (905)521-6077; Fax. (905)521-6068.

JAFARI, Siavash; 20 Hastings St W, Vancouver BC V6B 1J6; Shiraz (Iran)'99; Langs: Farsi; Persian; Turkish; (604)683-0073 x354

JAFARIAN, Fatemeh; MUHC-Montreal Children's Hosp, 2300 rue Tupper, Montreal QC H3H 1P3; Shahid Beheshti (Iran)'95; Staff, McGill University Health Centre - Montreal Children's Hospital; (514)412-4310; Fax. (514)412-4202; fatemeh.jafarian@mcgill.ca.

JAFFER, Ashif S; Jacaranda Med Clinic, 141-3292 Dunmore Rd SE, Medicine Hat AB T1B 2R4; Mem'98; FRACGP; CCFP; Fam Med, St Theresa General Hospital; Staff, Central Zone David Thompson Health Region; Staff, Calgary Health Region; (403)502-1465; Fax. (403)526-6448; didsburymedicalclinic@shaw.ca.

JAFFER, Kassamali M F; 207-2250 Bovaird Dr E, Brampton ON L6R 0W3; McM'74; FRCSC; ObstGyn. (905)457-6389

JAFFER, Naaznin K; 501 Pharmacy Ave, Scarborough ON M1L 3G7; Wes'83; Langs: Gujarati; Hindi; Persian; (416)466-7598; Fax. (416)466-6537; naazjaffer@hotmail.com.

JAFFER, Nasir M; Mount Sinai Hosp, 600 University Ave, Toronto ON M5G 1X5; UBC'75; DACR; FRCPC; DiagRad. Staff Radiol, Mount Sinai Hospital; Asst Prof, University of Toronto; (416)586-4800 x5278

JAFFER, Perhez; 4446 Hastings St, Burnaby BC V5C 2K2; UBC'91; CCFP; (604)298-4491

JAFFER, Salina; The Westend Family Care Clinic, 80 Michael Cowpland Dr, Kanata ON K2M 1P6; Ott'92; BSc; Staff, Westend Family Care Clinic Family Health Team; (613)599-3321; Fax. (613)599-3366.

JAFFER, Shahin; 230-4977 Trenant St, Delta BC V4K 2K5; Mem'86; MHSc; FRCPC; IntMed (Endocrinology). Staff Clinician, Delta Hospital; Clin Asst Prof, University of British Columbia; (604)940-8840

JAFFERJEE, Juzar; Grand River Family Physicians, 753 Tower St S, Fergus ON N1M 2R2; (India)'03; CCFP; (519)843-4380; Fax. (519)843-3211.

JAFFRAY, Fiona K; Glenrose Rehab Hosp, 10230 111 Ave NW, Edmonton AB T5G 0B7; (United Kingdom)'90; MB BS; DRCOG; MRCPsy; Staff, Glenrose Rehabilitation Hospital; (780)735-8845; Fax. (780)735-8846; fionajaffray@cha.ab.ca.

JAFFRI, Syed N; 101-2845 Cruickshank St, Abbotsford BC V2T 6X1; Punjab (Pakistan)'88; MB BS; (604)556-3550

JAFRUDY, Russell H; 105-235 Danforth Ave, Toronto ON M4K 1N2; (Iran)'96; CCFP; (416)462-1777

JAGAN, Gavin S; One Care Med Clinic, 1755 Brimley Rd, Scarborough ON M1P 0A3; Tor'91; CCFP; (416)290-0361; Fax. (416)290-5986.

JAGAN, Nigel N; Whitby Medical Arts Centre, 206-1615 Dundas St E, Whitby ON L1N 2L1; Tor'83; Staff, Lakeridge Health - Oshawa Site; (905)434-8600

JAGAN, Sarva; 101-2001 av Victoria, Saint-Lambert QC J4S 1H1; Ceylon (Sri Lanka)'76; Staff, McGill University Health Centre - Montreal General Campus; (450)465-9927; Fax. (450)465-1781.

JAGAS, Ivan F; 16-385 Frederick St, Kitchener ON N2H 2P2; Tor'91; (519)745-7482; Fax. (519)745-1881.

JAGDEO, Amit; Seven Oaks Gen Hosp, 2300 McPhillips St, Winnipeg MB R2V 3M3; Man'06; FRCPC; Psy. Staff, Seven Oaks General Hospital; (204)632-7133

JAGDEO, Dayanand G; SGH Medical Mall, 409-3030 Lawrence Ave E, Scarborough ON M1P 2T7; Tor'72; FRCPC; Peds (Consultant Pediatrics). Consultant, The Scarborough Hospital - General Campus; Asst Prof Peds, University of Toronto; (416)439-9699; Fax. (416)439-8656.

JAGGA, Michele; Medical Arts Clinic, 780 Central Ave N, Swift Current SK S9H 0M3; (Other Foreign)'01; (306)733-3949

JAGGASSAR, Theo A; Maxville Med Centre, PO Box 350 72 Mechanic St W, Maxville ON K0C 1T0; McG'66; CCFP; FCFP; Court Staff, Cornwall Community Hospital - Second Street Site; Ac Staff, Glengarry Memorial Hospital; Ac Staff, Cornwall Community Hospital; Med Dir, Maxville Manor; (613)527-2030; Fax. (613)527-2030.

JAGGER, Justin; Thunder Bay Paediatrics, 588 Arthur St, Thunder Bay ON P7E 5R7; Wes'04; FRCPC; Peds. Asst Prof, Northern Ontario School of Medicine; (807)766-3370; Fax. (807)766-3374.

JAGIELLO, Lukasz W; 301-2227 South Millway, Toronto ON M5G 1X8; Wes'08; Peds. (905)569-9798

JAGLALSINGH, L Harry; Baker Centre, 709-10025 106 St NW, Edmonton AB T5J 1G4; Alb'65; Physician, Industrial & Psychological Medicine; (780)428-7777; Fax. (780)428-7801; jaglal@telusplanet.net.

JAGODZINSKI, Daniel; Hop Jean-Talon, 1385 rue Jean-Talon E, Montreal QC H2E 1S6; Staff, CSSS du Coeur de l'Isle Hôpital Jean-Talon; (514)495-6767

JAGOE, Robert T; SMBD Jewish Gen Hosp, Suite G 221 3755 ch Cote-Sainte-Catherine, Montreal QC H3T 1E2; Cambridge (England)'89; Staff, Sir Mortimer B Davis Jewish General; (514)340-8222 x8275; Fax. (514)340-7555.

JAGOTA, Ajay; Steeple Hill Med Centre, 205-650 Kingston Rd, Pickering ON L1V 1A6; Tor'90; CCFP; (905)831-4547; Fax. (905)831-5109.

JAHANDAR, Parveen F; Royal Alexandra Hosp, 6408-10240 Kingsway NW, Edmonton AB T5H 3V9; (Iran)'94; FRCPC; Psy. Staff, Royal Alexandra Hospital; Langs: Farsi; (780)735-4564; Fax. (780)735-4797.

JAHANDARDOOST, Mohammad R; Medical Arts Centre, 202-770 6 St SW, Medicine Hat AB T1A 4J6; (Iran)'95; ABIM; FRCPC; IntMed (Geriatric Medicine). Staff Geriatric & IntMed, Medicine Hat Regional Hospital; Langs: Farsi; (403)487-5313; Fax. (403)487-5305; mjahandardoost@palliserhealth.ca.

JAHANGIR, Mubeen; Campbellton Reg Hosp, PO Box 880 Stn Main 189 Lily Lake Rd, Campbellton NB E3N 3H3; Peshawa (Pakistan)'92; Staff, Hôpital Régional Campbellton; (506)789-5000

JAHJAH, Laila; Hotel-Dieu Du Sacre-Coeur, 1 av Du Sacre-Coeur, Quebec QC G1N 2W1; Laval'85; Ac Staff, Hotel-Dieu du Sacre-Coeur de Jesus de Quebec; (418)529-6851 x293; Fax. (418)529-2971.

JAHNKE, Natalie Ann; Valley Med Clinic, 335 Jubilee St, Duncan BC V9L 1W9; (Venezuela)'94; CCFP; (250)748-8151

JAHNS, Krystyna M; Heritage Plaza, 8330 MacLeod Trail SE, Calgary AB T2H 2V2; Silesian Academy (Poland)'59; (403)258-3000

JAHROMI, Afshin; 202-73 Delhi St, Guelph ON N1E 6L9; Tor'99; FRCSC; GenSurg; VascSurg. Staff Vascular & Endovascular surg, Guelph General Hospital; (519)836-9441; drjahromioffice@gmail.com.

JAIDKA, Rajesh; Springdale Prof Bldg, 505-2250 Bovaird Dr E, Brampton ON L6R 0W3; Kurukshetra (India)'76; MB BS; MS(Ophth); Langs: Hindi; Punjabi; Urdu; (905)790-7400; Fax. (905)794-1668.

JAIGOBIN, Cheryl S; Univ Hlth Network-Toronto Gen, 306-200 Elizabeth St, Toronto ON M5G 2C4; Tor'92; MSc; FRCPC; Neur (Stroke). Staff Stroke Neurol, Toronto General Hospital - UHN; Asst Prof Med, University of Toronto; (416)340-3007; Fax. (416)340-3670; cheryl.jaigobin@uhn.on.ca.

JAILALL, Davindra N; Springdale Prof Bldg, 308-2250 Bovaird Dr E, Brampton ON L6R 0W3; New Jersey (USA)'02; (905)595-2870; Fax. (905)595-2869.

JAIN, Anil; 118-1025 Grenon Ave, Ottawa ON K2B 8S5; Ott'85; (613)596-3211; Fax. (613)596-3212.

JAIN, Arsh K; London HSC-University Hosp, PO Box 5010 Stn B 800 Commissioners Rd E, London ON N6A 5W9; Tor'02; FRCPC; IntMed; Nephrol. Staff IntMed, London Health Sciences Centre - University Hospital; (519)665-8500

JAIN, Deepak B; Hop Sante Cabrini Ospedale, 5655 rue Saint-Zotique E, Montreal QC H1T 1P7; Cal'96; FRCPC; IntMed; Cardiol. Staff, Hôpital Santa Cabrini Ospedale; (514)252-6000 x7172

JAIN, Evelyn; 70-3915 51 St SW, Calgary AB T3E 6N1; Cal'87; CCFP; FCFP; Clinical Asst Prof Family Med, University of Calgary; (403)246-7076; Fax. (403)249-0156.

JAIN, Hem C; 302-927 King St E, Cambridge ON N3H 3P4; Cal'79; MSc; FRCPC; Derm. Langs: Hindi; Punjabi; Gujarati; (519)650-0006; Fax. (519)650-6060.

JAIN, Leena; Specialized Geriatric Clinic, 232 Ross Dr, New Westminster BC V3L 0B2; Delhi (India)'90; MB BS; FRCPC; IntMed; GeriatricMed. Staff, Royal Columbian Hospital; Staff Internist-Geriatrician, Queen's Park Geriatric Outpatient Clinic; Langs: Hindi; Urdu; Punjabi; (604)528-5031

JAIN, Madhuri; Jain Med Centre, 83A Sherbrook St, Winnipeg MB R3C 2B2; Allahabad (India)'69; MB BS; Staff, Misericordia Health Centre; Staff, Health Sciences Centre; (204)783-6265; Fax. (204)783-4293.

JAIN, Mahendra K; Danforth Med Centre, 880 Danforth Rd, Scarborough ON M1K 1H8; Rajasthan (India)'81; Langs: Hindi; (416)264-4848; Fax. (416)264-0547.

JAIN, Mukesh K; 246 Matheson Blvd E, Mississauga ON L4Z 1X1; Tor'94; FACR; DiagRad. (905)712-9500

JAIN, Narendra K; Jain Med Centre, 83A Sherbrook St, Winnipeg MB R3C 2B2; Allahabad (India)'69; MB BS; Med Officer, WRHA - Deer Lodge Centre; Langs: Hindi; (204)783-6265; Fax. (204)783-4296.

JAIN, Neelesh K; North York Gen Hosp, 4001 Leslie St, North York ON M2K 1E1; McG'98; FRCSC; GenSurg. Staff Surg, North York General Hospital; Langs: Hindi; French; (416)756-6011

JAIN, Nita; City Square Mall, 495-555 12th Ave W, Vancouver BC V5Z 3X7; UBC'94; BSc; FRCP; MD; FRCPC; Peds (Child Abuse). Staff, BC Children's Hospital; Clinical Asst Prof, University of British Columbia; Langs: Hindi; Punjabi; (604)730-5622; Fax. (604)875-6717; nita.jain@telus.net.

JAIN, Padma; 207-801 York Mills Rd, North York ON M3B 1X7; Jiwaji Gwalior (India)'67; MB BS; Ac Staff, The Scarborough Hospital - Birchmount Campus; (416)495-1919; Fax. (416)495-9525; pjain@fairviewcosmeticsurgery.com.

JAIN, Praveen; University of Alberta Hosp, 8440 112 St NW, Edmonton AB T6G 2B7; Alb'93; FRCPC; EmergMed. Staff Emerg, University of Alberta Hospital; (780)407-7047; Fax. (780)407-3314.

JAIN, Preeti; 306-726 Bloor St W, Toronto ON M6G 4A1; Udaipur (India)'89; FAAP; FRCPC; Peds (Neonatology). Staff Peds, Mount Sinai Hospital; Langs: Hindi; (416)534-1159; Fax. (416)572-0083.

JAIN, Raagini; Children's Hosp of Eastern Ont, 401 Smyth Rd, Ottawa ON K1H 8L1; Sask'05; FRCPC; Peds; PedEmergMed. Staff, Children's Hospital of Eastern Ontario (CHEO); (613)737-7600

JAIN, Rachna; South Bank Med Centre, 3-2430 Bank St, Ottawa ON K1V 0T7; Ott'89; BSchem/Nutri) - (Bio-Ch; Langs: Hindi; (613)736-6946; Fax. (613)736-6948.

JAIN, Sajal; 214-7885 6th St, Burnaby BC V3N 3N4; Bangalore (India)'95; MB BS; FACP; FRCPC; IntMed. Langs: Hindi; Punjabi; Urdu; (778)759-9919

JAIN, Sanjive; 2C-201 King St W, Oshawa ON L1J 2J5; Tor'85; CCFP; Staff, Lakeridge Health - Oshawa Site; (905)436-5335

JAIN, Shailly; Univ of Alberta Hosp, 8440 112 St NW, Edmonton AB T6G 2B7; Wes'05; FRCPC; MedGenetics. Staff, University of Alberta Hospital; (780)492-0874; Fax. (780)492-1998.

JAIN, Shalini; Lakeview Medical, Q-6 Speers Blvd, Amherstview ON K7N 1Z6; Meerut (India)'94; CCFP; Langs: Hindi; Urdu; (613)634-9597; Fax. (613)634-1668.

JAIN, Shauna A; The Hosp For Sick Children, 555 University Ave, Toronto ON M5G 1X8; Qns'97; FRCPC; Peds; PedEmergMed. Staff, The Hospital For Sick Children; (416)813-1500

JAIN, Sherry; Dalhousie Health Services, 6230 Coburg Rd, Halifax NS B3H 4J5; Mem'00; CCFP; (902)494-2171

JAIN, Subhash C; 29-1225 Wonderland Rd N, London ON N6G 2V9; Gwalior (India)'64; FRCPsy(UK); MRCP(London); FRCP(Glas); MRCPsy(UK); FRCPC; Psy (Mood Disorders). Langs: Hindi; (519)690-1001; Fax. (519)690-1309; drjainsubhash@yahoo.com.

JAIN, Trevor; Queen Elizabeth Hosp, PO Box 6600 Stn Central 60 Riverside Dr, Charlottetown PE C1A 8T5; Dal'99; CCFP; CCFP(E. M.); Staff, Queen Elizabeth Hospital; (902)894-2111

JAIN, Umesh; Bloor-Jane Med Bldg, 501-2425 Bloor St W, Toronto ON M6S 4W4; Patiala (India)'83; MB BS; FRCSC; Urol (Endocrinology). Court Staff, Mackenzie Richmond Hill Hospital; Ac Staff/Head Urol, St Joseph's Health Centre; Langs: Hindi; Punjabi; Urdu; (416)767-0995; Fax. (416)767-0992; jainu@stjoe.on.ca.

JAIN, Venu; Royal Alexandra Hosp, 10240 Kingsway NW, Edmonton AB T5H 3V9; Patiula (India)'92; FRCSC; ObstGyn (Maternal Fetal Medicine). Staff, Royal Alexandra Hospital; (780)735-4812; Fax. (780)735-4981.

JAIN, Vikas K; Brant Community HC-Brantford, 200 Terrace Hill St, Brantford ON N3R 1G9; Ott'05; FRCPC; DiagRad. Staff, The Brant Community Healthcare System - Brantford General Hospital Site; (519)752-7871

JAIN, Vipan K; Strathroy Middlesex Gen Hosp, PO Box 5001 Stn Main 395 Carrie St, Strathroy ON N7G 3J4; Ott'06; FRCSC; GenSurg. Staff, Strathroy Middlesex General Hospital - Middlesex Hospital Alliance; (519)246-6321

JAIPARGAS, Charles C; EMR Advantage Software, 400-53 Yonge St, Toronto ON M5E 1J3; McM'92; (647)722-2370; Fax. (647)367-4301.

JAIRATH, Ashok K; Norfinch Med Centre, 104-2100 Finch Ave W, North York ON M3N 2Z9; Punjab (India)'77; Staff, Humber River Regional Hospital - Finch Avenue Site; (416)739-7664; Fax. (416)739-7665.

JAIYESIMI, Olufemi B; PO Box 160, Trochu AB T0M 2C0; (Nigeria)'91; MB BCh; (403)442-3814

JAKDA, Ahmed I; Grand River Hosp-KW Hlth Ctre, PO Box 9056 Stn C 835 King St W, Kitchener ON N2G 1G3; Gardner(MA) (USA)'03; CCFP; Staff, Grand River Hospital - Kitchener/Waterloo Health Centre; (519)742-3611

JAKDA, Almas; Langs Med Clinic, RR 1 2958 Greenfield Rd, Ayr ON N0B 1E0; Saba (Netherlands Antilles)'04; (519)632-1229

JAKELSKI, Klaus D; 2F-117 Cedar St, Sudbury ON P3E 1A9; Tor'78; (705)670-8930; Fax. (705)670-1743.

JAKIBCHUK, Jerry; 7 Welland Ave, St Catharines ON L2R 2L8; Wes'73; Court Staff, Niagara Health System - St Catharines General Site; Langs: Ukrainian; Polish; (905)684-8555; Fax. (905)684-2542.

JAKLIS, Ziad; 106-1353 Ellis St, Kelowna BC V1Y 1Z9; Ott'93; FRCSC; Urol. (250)448-7408

JAKOVCIC, Carmela M; Glen Erin Med-Dental Centre, 11-2318 Dunwin Dr, Mississauga ON L5L 1C7; Tor'85; CCFP; Court Staff, The Credit Valley Hospital; (905)828-1145; Fax. (905)828-1144.

JAKSIC-TOMANOVIC, Ljiljana; Bloor-Jane Med Bldg, 505-2425 Bloor St W, Toronto ON M6S 4W4; Sarajevo (Bosnia-Herzegovina)'83; CCFP; Langs: Serbian; Croatian; (416)604-4400; Fax. (416)604-4100; drljiljana@bellnet.ca.

JAKUBEC, Darren M; Bulkley Valley Dist Hosp, PO Box 370 3950 8th Ave, Smithers BC V0J 2N0; UBC'94; CCFP; Staff, Bulkley Valley District Hospital; (250)847-2611

JAKUBOVIC, Henry R; Glazier Med Centre, 11 Gibb St, Oshawa ON L1H 2J9; Tor'77; FRCPC; Derm (Dermatological Pathology); AnatPath. Staff Derm & Path, St Michael's Hospital; Consultant Derm, Providence Healthcare; Asst Prof Med & Lab Med, University of Toronto; (905)579-1212

JAKUBOVICZ, Difat E; St Joseph's Health Centre, 30 The Queensway, Toronto ON M6R 1B5; Tor'92; CCFP; FCFP; Staff, St Joseph's Health Centre; Asst Prof, University of Toronto; Langs: Hebrew; French; (416)530-6860

JAKUBOW, Andre N; Sioux Lookout Meno-Ya-Win HC, PO Box 909 Stn Main, Sioux Lookout ON P8T 1B4; McM'08; CCFP; Staff, Sioux Lookout Meno-Ya-Win Health Centre; (807)737-3030

JAKUBOWSKI, Andrew T; Richmond Health Sciences Ctre, 750-6091 Gilbert Rd, Richmond BC V7C 5L9; Warsaw (Poland)'78; FRCPC; IntMed (Cardiac Rehabilitation); Cardiol. Ac Staff, Richmond Hospital; Dir, Healthy Heart Program; Langs: Polish; (604)273-1555; Fax. (604)273-2969.

JAKUBOWSKI, Marek J; West Parry Sound Health Ctre, 6 Albert St, Parry Sound ON P2A 3A4; Warsaw (Poland)'86; FRCPC; IntMed. Med Staff, West Parry Sound Health Centre; Langs: Polish; (705)746-4540 x4302; Fax. (705)773-4066.

JALA, Vikram R; Aberdeen Hosp, 835 East River Rd, New Glasgow NS B2H 3S6; Osmania (India)'98; MB BS; Staff, Aberdeen Regional Hospital; (902)752-7600

JALALI, Fereshteh; Peter Lougheed Centre, 3500 26 Ave NE, Calgary AB T1Y 6J4; Cal'06; FRCPC; Psy. Staff, Peter Lougheed Centre; (403)943-4555

JALALI, Subash; Medical Arts Bldg, 413-1 Young St, Hamilton ON L8N 1T8; Kashmir (India)'79; FRCPC; IntMed (Gastroenterology). (905)577-4670; Fax. (905)577-6204.

JALAYER, Massoud; Hamilton HS-General Site, 237 Barton St E, Hamilton ON L8L 2X2; (Iran)'94; EmergMed. Staff Emerg, Hamilton Health Sciences Centre - Hamilton General Hospital; (905)521-2100

JALBERT, Marc; Clinique Med de Lavaltrie, 1400 rue Notre-Dame, Lavaltrie QC J5T 1M6; Mon'10; (450)586-1033

JALBERT, Maya; Hop Charles LeMoyne, 3120 boul Taschereau, Greenfield Park QC J4V 2H1; Mon'97; FRCPC; Psy. Staff, Hopital Charles LeMoyne; Langs: English; (450)466-5020; Fax. (450)466-5015.

JALBERT, Yves; Ministere de la Sante, 9e-1075 ch Sainte-Foy, Quebec QC G1S 2M1; Sher'89; Staff, Centre Hospitalier de Gaspe; Staff, Ministry of Health-Quebec; (418)266-6946; yves.jalbert@msss.gouv.qc.ca.

JALIL, Rabiya; East Calgary Health Centre, 4715 8 Ave SE, Calgary AB T2A 3N4; Sask'09; CCFP; (403)955-1400

JALINK, Diederick W; Kingston Gen Hosp, Burr 2 059-76 Stuart St, Kingston ON K7L 2V7; Cal'89; BSc; FACS; FRCSC; GenSurg (Hepatobiliary & Pancreatic Surgery). Att Staff, Kingston General Hospital; Asst Prof, Queen's University; Langs: Dutch; (613)544-3400 x2415; Fax. (613)546-4854; jalinkd@hdh.kari.net.

JAMAL, Abeed; Burrard Health Bldg, 605-1160 Burrard St, Vancouver BC V6Z 2E8; McG'96; FRCPC; IntMed; Nephrol. (604)639-1177

JAMAL, Abida S; Women's College Hosp, 805-76 Grenville St, Toronto ON M5S 1B2; Tor'91; FRCPC; IntMed; Endocrin&Metab. Staff, Women's College Hospital; (416)323-6400

JAMAL, Aliff; Burnaby Hosp, 526-3935 Kincaid St, Burnaby BC V5G 2X6; UBC'98; BSc(Pharm); CCFP; Staff, Burnaby Hospital; (604)434-4211

JAMAL, Alykhan M; East York Med Health Centre, 27E-45 Overlea Blvd, Toronto ON M4H 1C3; Tor'94; CCFP; (416)696-9836 x222; Fax. (416)696-7881.

JAMAL, Dawood I; East Toronto Health Centre, 1496 Danforth Ave, Toronto ON M4J 1N4; RCS (Ireland)'62; LRCPSI; LM; Ac Staff, North York General Hospital; Langs: Urdu; Gujarati; (416)778-1496

JAMAL, Dried E; Headwaters Health Care Centre, 100 Rolling Hills Dr, Orangeville ON L9W 4X9; (Iraq)'97; MB ChB; CCFP; Staff, Headwaters Health Care Centre - Orangeville Site; (519)941-2410

JAMAL, Hafeez L; 374 Lakeshore Rd E, Mississauga ON L5G 1H5; McM'03; CCFP; (905)271-9000

JAMAL, Hanif N; Halton HS Corp-Oakville, 327 Reynolds St, Oakville ON L6J 3L7; McM'04; CCFP; Staff, Halton Healthcare Services Corporation - Oakville Site; (905)338-4618; Fax. (905)338-4146.

JAMAL, John; Univ Hlth Network-Toronto Gen, 200 Elizabeth St, Toronto ON M5G 2C4; Man'83; CCFP; CCFP(E.M.); Staff, Toronto General Hospital - UHN; (416)340-3856

JAMAL, Kishwar; Glenwood Med Clinic, 16114 100A Ave NW, Edmonton AB T5P 4A1; (Pakistan)'97; MB BS; (780)405-7520; Fax. (587)521-1801.

JAMAL, Laila T; Toronto East Gen Hosp Inc, H5 561-825 Coxwell Ave, Toronto ON M4C 3E7; Tor'99; FRCPC; Psy. Staff, Toronto East General Hospital Inc; (416)461-8272

JAMAL, Munir A; Credit Valley Med Arts Centre, 410-2000 Credit Valley Rd, Mississauga ON L5M 4N4; Tor'95; FRCSC; Urol. Assoc Staff, The Credit Valley Hospital; (905)607-6262; Fax. (905)607-6551; munir.jamal@utoronto.ca.

JAMAL, Parviz A; Parkway Mall, 213-85 Ellesmere Rd, Scarborough ON M1R 4B8; Dar Es Salaam (Tanzania)'73; FRCPC; Psy. (416)425-9322

JAMAL, Rahima; CHUM-Hop Notre-Dame, 1560 rue Sherbrooke E, Montreal QC H2L 4M1; Mon'03; MedOncol; Hem; IntMed. Staff, Centre Hospitalier l'Université de Montréal (CHUM) - Hôpital Notre-Dame; (514)890-8000

JAMAL, Shabana; Cross Lake Nursing Station, PO Box 160, Cross Lake MB R0B 0J0; (Other Foreign)'89; Fam Med, Cross Lake Nursing Station; (204)676-2011

JAMAL, Shahin; Gordon & Leslie Diamond HCC, 8205B-2775 Laurel St, Vancouver BC V5Z 1M9; UBC'99; BScPT; MSc; FRCPC; IntMed; Rheum. Staff, Vancouver General Hospital - Centennial Pavillion; (604)875-8270; Fax. (604)875-5992.

JAMAL, Shamir M; Cosmedix MD, 105-150 York St, Toronto ON M5H 3S5; Tor'91; Staff, Cosmedix MD Inc; (416)977-6502; Fax. (416)977-6915.

JAMAL, Shelina M; BC Children's Hosp, 4480 Oak St, Vancouver BC V6H 3V4; Chicago (USA)'06; FRCPC; Peds. Staff, BC Children's Hospital; (604)875-2161

JAMAL, Wael E; Dr Georges-L Dumont Reg Hosp, 330 University Ave, Moncton NB E1C 2Z3; King Abdulaziz (Saudi Arabia)'99; Staff, Dr Georges-L-Dumont University Hospital Centre; (506)862-4000

JAMAL, Wael H; Clinique OVO, 8000 boul Decarie, Montreal QC H4P 2S4; King Abdul Aziz (Saudi Arabia)'98; FRCSC; ObstGyn. (514)798-2000; Fax. (514)798-2001.

JAMAL, Zahirali; PO Box 1260, Mayerthorpe AB T0E 1N0; Alb'96; BSc; CCFP; (780)786-2412; Fax. (780)786-2249; zjamal9@hotmail.com.

JAMAL, Zahra; Albany Med Clinic, 807 Broadview Ave, Toronto ON M4K 2P8; Southampton (England)'98; CCFP.

JAMAL, Zeeya; 2312 King St PO Box 10, Brechin ON L0K 1B0; Chicago(IL) (USA)'08; CCFP; (705)484-0074

JAMALI, Hossein; CSSS du Sud de Lanaudière, 911 montée des Pionniers, Terrebonne QC J6V 2H2; Tehran (Iran)'96; FRCPC; IntMed; Hem; MedOncol. Staff, Centre Hospitalier Pierre le Gardeur; (450)654-7525

JAMALI, Mina; Sunnybrook Hlth Sciences Ctre, B204-2075 Bayview Ave, Toronto ON M4N 3M5; Ott'06; FRCPC; AnatPath. Staff, Sunnybrook Health Sciences Centre; (416)480-6100

JAMALI, Zainab; Ctr Hosp de Lasalle, 8585 Tsse Champlain, LaSalle QC H8P 1C1; McG'03; FRCPC; Anes. Staff, Centre Hospitalier de LaSalle; (514)362-8000 x1871

JAMANI, Sherally K; B-908 Garth St, Hamilton ON L9C 4L2; Welsh National (Wales)'66; Staff, Hamilton Health Sciences Centre - McMaster University Medical Centre; Langs: Gujarati; (905)383-8026; Fax. (905)383-8446.

JAMATY, Chloe; CSSS de Saint-Jerome, 290 rue de Montigny, Saint-Jerome QC J7Z 5T3; McG'04; EmergMed. Staff, Hôtel-Dieu de Saint-Jérôme; (450)431-8400

JAMATY, Georges F; CSSS d'Argenteuil, 145 av de la Providence, Lachute QC J8H 4C7; Beirut (Lebanon)'75; AB; DiagRad. Staff, Centre Hospitalier d'Argenteuil; (450)562-3761 x5170; Fax. (450)566-3308.

JAMBROSIC, Jadranka A; Kingsway Dermatology, 1000-1243 Islington Ave, Etobicoke ON M8X 1Y9; Tor'77; BSc; MSc; FRCPC; AnatPath (Dermatological Pathology); Derm. Consultant Pigmented Lesion Clinic, Women's College Hospital; Consultant Derm Path, Life Labs; Assoc Prof, University of Toronto; Langs: Croatian; (416)231-0100; Fax. (416)231-0109.

JAMENSKY, Neil T; Scarborough Hosp-General Div, 3050 Lawrence Ave E, Scarborough ON M1P 2V5; Qns'00; FRCPC; Anes. Staff, The Scarborough Hospital - General Campus; Langs: French; (416)431-8208

JAMES, Adrian L; 6130-555 University Ave, Toronto ON M5G 1X8; Oxford (England)'90; Staff, The Hospital For Sick Children; Asst Prof, University of Toronto; (416)813-2191

JAMES, Aisha N P; Unison Hlth & Community Servic, 1541 Jane St, North York ON M9N 2R3; Qns'07; CCFP; (416)645-7575

JAMES, Andrew G; The Hosp For Sick Children, 38100-555 University Ave, Toronto ON M5G 1X8; Auckland (New Zealand)'74; MB ChB; BSc; FRACP; FRCPC; Peds (Medical Informatics). Assoc Dir Clinical, The Hospital For Sick Children; Assoc Prof, University of Toronto; (416)813-7202; Fax. (416)813-5245; andrew.james@sickkids.ca.

JAMES, Christopher M; 2425 Bevan Ave, Sidney BC V8L 4R5; Birmingham (England)'80; MB ChB; DA; DRCOG; MRCGPract; Physician, Corrections Service BC; (250)656-1164; Fax. (250)656-7870.

JAMES, David H C; Boniface Park Medical Centre, 700 Markham Rd, Scarborough ON M1H 2A7; Ott'83; BSc; Staff, Lakeridge Health - Oshawa Site; (416)264-3443

JAMES, David M; Niagara H System-Welland Site, 65 Third St, Welland ON L3B 4W6; Tor'85; CCFP; CCFP(E.M.); FCFP; Staff, Niagara Health System - Welland Hospital Site.

JAMES, David N H; 103-901 Island Hwy, Campbell River BC V9W 2C2; London (England)'82; FRCSC; GenSurg. Staff Surg/Asst Prof, Campbell River & District General Hospital; (250)286-0767; Fax. (250)286-8815; dnhjames@telus.net.

JAMES, Debra J; Courtice Health Centre, 1450 Highway 2, Courtice ON L1E 3C3; Ott'85; BSc; Staff, Lakeridge Health - Oshawa Site; (905)721-4934; Fax. (905)721-4369.

JAMES, Elizabeth D F; Brockville Mental Health Ctre, PO Box 1050 Stn Main 1804 Hwy 2 E, Brockville ON K6V 5W7; Sask'05; Psy. Staff, Brockville Mental Health Centre - Royal Ottawa Health Care Group; (613)345-1461

JAMES, Gerald K; Royal Inland Hosp, 311 Columbia St, Kamloops BC V2C 2T1; UBC'92; FRCPC; GenPath. Staff Path, Royal Inland Hospital; (250)314-2640; Fax. (250)314-2505.

JAMES, Heidi K; Riverview Family Practice, 101-639 Pinewood Rd, Riverview NB E1B 5R6; Dal'04; CCFP; (506)853-5888

JAMES, J Marion E; Winnipeg Clinic, 425 St Mary Ave, Winnipeg MB R3C 0N2; Man'67; BSc(Med); FAAAI; FRCPC; Peds (Asthma); ClinImmunol&Allergy. Consultant Allergy & Immun, Health Sciences Centre; Asst Prof, University of Manitoba; (204)957-3204

JAMES, J Walter; 717 Coxwell Ave, Toronto ON M4C 3C1; Tor'63; FRCPC; Peds (Clinical Immunology & Allergy). Ac Staff, North York General Hospital; Assoc Staff, The Hospital For Sick Children; Langs: Spanish; Italian; French; (416)449-8333; Fax. (416)469-0952.

JAMES, Jacqueline; Mount Sinai Hosp, L5 026-600 University Ave, Toronto ON M5G 1X5; Tor'87; BSc; MEd; FRCPC; IntMed (Diabetology); Endocrin&Metab. Staff, Toronto General Hospital - UHN; Staff Physician, Mount Sinai Hospital; Assoc Prof Med/Dir Wrightman-Berris Academy, University of Toronto; (416)586-8369

JAMES, Keleigh J A; Seine Med Centre, 100-142 Centrale Ave, Ste Anne MB R5H 1C3; Man'06; CCFP; (204)422-8811

JAMES, Kristin D; Gamble James Med Prof Inc, 304-679 Davis Dr, Newmarket ON L3Y 5G8; McM'04; Staff, Southlake Regional Health Centre; (905)895-4445

JAMES, M Ray; Carling-Broadview Med Bldg, 306-770 Broadview Ave, Ottawa ON K2A 3Z3; Qns'68; FRCSC; PlasSurg. Staff, Carleton Place & District Memorial Hospital; Staff, Arnprior & District Memorial Hospital; (613)728-5807; Fax. (613)728-3942; dr.rayjames@ca.inter.net.

JAMES, Mark L; Royal University Hosp, 103 Hospital Dr, Saskatoon SK S7N 0W8; Pretoria (South Africa)'90; MB ChB; FRCPC; Anes. Staff, Royal University Hospital; (306)655-1183; Fax. (306)655-1279.

JAMES, Mary E; South Calgary Med Clinic, 118-40 Sunpark Plaza SE, Calgary AB T2X 3X7; Cal'80; CCFP; FCFP; Ac Staff Community Care, Calgary Health Region; (403)254-4000; Fax. (403)254-1282.

JAMES, Matthew T; Foothills Med Centre, 1403 29 St NW, Calgary AB T2N 2T9; UBC'02; FRCPC; IntMed; Nephrol. Staff Nephrol, Foothills Medical Centre; (403)944-2595

JAMES, Michael J; South Ajax Family Doctors, 969 Westney Rd S, Ajax ON L1S 3K7; London (England)'69; MSc(OccMed); CCBOM; DIH; MFOM; (905)428-6311

JAMES, Michelle; Prince Albert Med Clinic, 681 15th St W, Prince Albert SK S6V 7H9; Transkei (South Africa)'00; MB ChB; (306)764-1505; Fax. (306)764-7775.

JAMES, Neil E; 35 Hatt St, Dundas ON L9H 2G2; McM'94; CCFP; FCFP.

JAMES, Nicola D; 4303 10th Ave W, Vancouver BC V6R 2H6; UBC'81; (604)224-1355; Fax. (604)224-0179.

JAMES, Paul D; Foothills Med Centre, 1403 29 St NW, Calgary AB T2N 2T9; Tor'07; Gastroent; IntMed. Staff, Foothills Medical Centre; (403)592-5020

JAMES, Paula D; 2025-94 Stuart St, Kingston ON K7L 2V6; Sask'96; FRCP; FRCPC; IntMed (Hemostasis); Hem. Staff, Kingston General Hospital; (613)533-2946; Fax. (613)533-6855; sac2@queensu.ca.

JAMES, Philip B; 12 A Absalom St E PO Box 370, Mildmay ON N0G 2J0; McM'84; BEd; BA; BPE; (519)367-2600

JAMES, Richard G G; 403-1100 Sheppard Ave E, North York ON M2K 2W1; Queen's (Ireland)'67; MB ChB; BAO; MRCP(UK); FRCPC; IntMed (Cardiology). Staff Consultant, North York General Hospital; (416)226-5881; Fax. (416)226-4582.

JAMES, Richard H B; Ladner Centre Medical, 5132 Ladner Trunk Rd, Delta BC V4K 1W3; Mysore (India)'83; FCFP; Staff, Delta Hospital; (604)940-0917; Fax. (604)940-9827.

JAMES, Sherry L; Mental H S Bedford-Sackville, 40 Freer Lane, Lower Sackville NS B4C 0A2; McM'05; MEd(Counselling); FRCPC; Psy. Staff Mental Health Services Bedford-Sackville, Cobequid Community Health Centre; Asst Prof Psy, Dalhousie University; (902)865-3663; Fax. (902)865-2072; sherry.james@cdha.nshealth.ca.

JAMES, Simon T; 203-15 McRae St PO Box 546 Stn Main, Okotoks AB T1S 1A7; Cal'79; (403)938-3860

JAMES, Stephen R; Rothbart Ctr for Pain Care Ltd, 9-4646 Dufferin St, North York ON M3H 5S4; UNIBE (Dominican Republic)'01; (416)512-6407; Fax. (416)512-6375.

JAMES, Susan H; Quinte HC Corp-Belleville Gen, 265 Dundas St E, Belleville ON K8N 5A9; Tor'05; FRCPC; DiagRad. Staff, QHC Belleville General; (613)979-7400

JAMES, Thresiamma; Thresiamma James Prof Corp, 600-8600 Franklin Ave, Fort McMurray AB T9H 4G8; Kerala (India)'77; MB BS; FRCPC; Peds. (780)790-0739; Fax. (780)743-1913; jamespc@shaw.ca.

JAMES, William; 403-267 O'Connor St, Ottawa ON K2P 1V3; Qns'63; FRCPC; Peds (Attention Deficit Hyperactivity Disorder). Staff, Children's Hospital of Eastern Ontario (CHEO); Ac Staff, The Ottawa Hospital - Civic Campus; Asst Prof Peds, University of Ottawa; (613)237-4621; Fax. (613)567-3917.

JAMESON, Cathy Ann; Okanagan Health Surgical Ctr, 401-3320 Richter St, Kelowna BC V1W 4V5; UBC'83; (250)868-9799

JAMIESON, Bruce H D; ABC Medical Clinic, 9842 101 Ave, Fort St. John BC V1J 2B2; Pretoria (South Africa)'88; BSc(Hons.); MB ChB; DA; CCFP; (250)785-1220; Fax. (250)785-9750; abcmed@northernhealthcare.ca.

JAMIESON, Christopher G; Queen Elizabeth II HSC, 821-1276 South Park St, Halifax NS B3H 2Y9; London (England)'70; MB BS; MRCS; LRCP; FACS; FRCSC; GenSurg (Colon & Rectal Surgery). Staff, Queen Elizabeth II Health Sciences Centre - Victoria General Site; Prof, Dalhousie University; (902)473-5144; Fax. (902)473-5147; l.bisbee@dal.ca.

JAMIESON, Clark B; Phoenix Med Centre, 407-2155 10th Ave, Prince George BC V2M 5J6; Alb'70; FRCSC; Urol. Staff, University Hospital of Northern British Columbia; Lecturer Surg, University of British Columbia; (250)564-2633; Fax. (250)564-7759.

JAMIESON, Donald M; MD Health Med Centre-Brampton, 186 Main St S, Brampton ON L6W 2E2; Glasgow (Scotland)'73; MB ChB; DObstRCOG; MRCGPract(UK); (905)456-7774

JAMIESON, Douglas H; Children's & Women's HC of BC, IL30-4480 Oak St, Vancouver BC V6H 3V4; Cape Town (South Africa)'80; MB ChB; FRCPC; DiagRad. Staff, BC Children's Hospital; (604)875-2345; Fax. (604)875-2367.

JAMIESON, Erin L; McNeely Med Clinic, 455 McNeely Ave, Carleton Place ON K7C 4S6; Qns'09; CCFP; (613)253-2233

JAMIESON, Frances; Public Health Laboratory, 81 Resources Rd, Toronto ON M9P 3T1; Tor'84; FRCPC; MedMicrobiol. Med Dir/Physician Med Microbiol TB & Mycobacteriology, Public Health Ontario Laboratories; Assoc Prof, University of Toronto; (416)235-5841; Fax. (416)235-5951; frances.jamieson@oahpp.ca.

JAMIESON, Iain C; The Medical Centre, PO Box 4200 Stn Main 707 Charlotte St, Peterborough ON K9J 7B3; Tor'85; FRCPC; Peds. Staff, Peterborough Regional Health Centre - Hospital Drive; (705)743-6222; Fax. (705)740-8392.

JAMIESON, James D; Squamish Med Clinic, PO Box 389 Stn Main, Squamish BC V8B 0A3; (Wales)'80; MB BCh; DA; DRCOG; (604)892-3535; Fax. (604)892-3545; jjsqmed@telus.net.

JAMIESON, Jean L; Gordon & Leslie Diamond HCC, 11F-2775 Laurel St, Vancouver BC V5Z 1M9; UBC'84; DTMH; MHSc(Comm. Med.); Admn Staff, Gordon & Leslie Diamond Health Care Centre; (604)875-4111 x69226

JAMIESON, John W; Dr Charles A Janeway Child HC, 300 Prince Philip Dr, St. John's NL A1B 3V6; Mem'77; FRCPC; Anes. Staff, Janeway Children's Health & Rehabilitation Centre; (709)777-4381

JAMIESON, Lucy H; Univ of Alberta Hosp, 2A2 41-8440 112 St NW, Edmonton AB T6G 2B7; Dal'05; FRCPC; DiagRad. Staff, University of Alberta Hospital; (780)407-6907; Fax. (780)407-6907.

JAMIESON, Mary J; Family Med Centre, 5F-400 Tache Ave, Winnipeg MB R2H 3E1; Man'81; CCFP; FCFP.

JAMIESON, Mary Anne; Kingston Gen Hosp, 76 Stuart St, Kingston ON K7L 2V7; McM'90; FRCSC; ObstGyn (Pediatric & Adolescent Gynecology). Staff ObstGyn, Kingston General Hospital; Staff, Hotel-Dieu Hospital; Teach Staff ObstGyn & Peds, Queen's University; (613)548-6069; Fax. (613)548-1330; maj3@post.queensu.ca.

JAMIESON, Peter C; Foothills Med Centre, 1403 29 St NW, Calgary AB T2N 2T9; Cal'95; CCFP; FCFP; Staff, Foothills Medical Centre; Staff, Calgary Regional Health Authority; Clinical Asst Prof Family Med, University of Calgary; (403)944-2800; Fax. (403)283-7365.

JAMIESON, Robin N; Whitehorse Med Services Ltd, 406 Lambert St, Whitehorse YT Y1A 1Z7; Qns'03; CCFP; CCFP(E.M.).

JAMIESON, W R Eric; St Paul's Hosp, B-486-1081 Burrard St, Vancouver BC V6Z 1Y6; Dal'66; FACC; FACS; Cardiovasc&ThorSurg; GenSurg. Ac Staff Providence Bldg, Providence Health Care - St Paul's Hospital; Consultant, Vancouver General Hospital - Centennial Pavillion; Consultant, BC Cancer Agency Vancouver Centre; Clin Prof, University of British Columbia; (604)806-8383; Fax. (604)806-8384; eric.jamieson@ubc.ca.

JAMIESON, William T; St Michael's Hosp, 30 Bond St, Toronto ON M5B 1W8; Tor'06; FRCPC; IntMed. Staff, St Michael's Hospital; (416)864-5928

JAMIL, Fawaz H; Carbonear Gen Hosp, 86 Highroad South, Carbonear NL A1Y 1A4; Al-Mustansiriyah (Iraq)'97; MB BS; CCFP; Staff, Carbonear General Hospital; (709)945-5111; fawaz.jamil@easternhealth.ca.

JAMIL, Khalid; Campbellton Reg Hosp, PO Box 880 Stn Main 189 Lily Lake Rd, Campbellton NB E3N 3H3; Sindh (Pakistan)'90; Staff, Hôpital Régional Campbellton; kjamilmd@yahoo.com.

JAMIL, Najma; Avalon Med Clinic, 23-2605 Broadway Ave, Saskatoon SK S7J 0Z5; Punjab (Pakistan)'73; MB BS; MSc; (306)652-3496; Fax. (306)652-3493.

JAMISON, Bruce M; The Ottawa Hosp-Gen Campus, 501 Smyth Rd, Ottawa ON K1H 8L6; McG'87; BSc; CSPQ; FRCPC; IntMed (Research); AnatPath. Staff, The Ottawa Hospital - General Campus; Asst Prof, University of Ottawa; Langs: English; French; (613)737-8899 x71521

JAMMAL, Marie-Paule; Polyclinique Med Concorde, 303-300 boul de la Concorde E, Laval QC H7G 2E6; Mon'85; FRCSC; Urol. Ac Member, Hopital de la Cite de la santé; Ac Member, Centre Hospitalier l'Université De Montréal (CHUM) - Hôpital Saint-luc; (450)667-5310; Fax. (450)667-2163; urolaval@videotron.ca.

JAMMAL, Wael H; Clinique OVO, 8000 boul Decarie, Montreal QC H4P 2S4; King Abdulaziz (Saudi Arabia)'98; ObstGyn (P.Q.). (514)798-2000; Fax. (514)798-2001.

JAMOULLE, Olivier; Hôpital Ste-Justine, 3175 ch Cote-Ste-Catherine, Montreal QC H3T 1C5; Liege (Belgium)'95; FRCPC; Peds (Adolescent Medicine). Staff, Hôpital Ste-Justine; (514)345-4931; Fax. (514)345-4778; jamoulle@videotron.ca.

JAMSHAID, Mamoona; Montreal Road Med Centre, 398 Montreal Rd, Ottawa ON K1K 0V4; Punjab (Pakistan)'87; CCFP; (613)244-2005; Fax. (613)244-2004.

JAN, Edgar; Cambridge Mem Hosp, 700 Coronation Blvd, Cambridge ON N1R 3G2; Tor'03; FRCPC; DiagRad. Staff, Cambridge Memorial Hospital; (519)621-2330

JAN, F; 111-2580 Cedar Park Pl, Abbotsford BC V2T 3S5; Punjab (Pakistan)'94; MB BS; (604)853-2125

JAN, James E; Children's & Women's HC of BC, 1B10-4480 Oak St, Vancouver BC V6H 3V4; Alb'63; FRCPC; Peds (Electroencephalography). Staff, BC Children's Hospital; Sr Rsch Scientist Emeritus, Child & Family Research Institute; Clin Prof, University of British Columbia; (604)875-2124; jjan@cw.bc.ca.

JANA, Elizabeth V; Oshawa Clinic, 117 King St E, Oshawa ON L1H 1B9; Wes'81; FRCSC; ObstGyn. Staff, Lakeridge Health - Oshawa Site; (905)721-3561; Fax. (905)721-3558.

JANA, Kunal K; Medical Arts Bldg, 537-750 Spadina Cres E, Saskatoon SK S7K 3H3; Sask'01; FRCSC; Urol. Clin Assoc Prof, University of Saskatchewan; (306)653-3255; Fax. (306)653-4386.

JANAKIRAM, Praseedha; 940-790 Bay St, Toronto ON M5G 1N8; McM'05; CCFP; (416)926-0101; Fax. (416)926-1910.

JANBEY, Ehsan M; 1-25 12th Ave S, Cranbrook BC V1C 2R8; Damascus (Syria)'91; FRCPC; IntMed. (250)426-1995

JANCELEWICZ, Zygmunt; 207-190 Sherway Dr, Etobicoke ON M9C 5N2; Gdansk (Poland)'60; AB; FAAA; FRCPC; IntMed (Clinical Immunology & Allergy). Langs: Polish; (416)532-6837; Fax. (416)532-1544.

JANCEWICZ, Miroslav T; Allan Blair Cancer Centre, 300-4101 Dewdney Ave, Regina SK S4T 7T1; Lodz (Poland)'74; DAB(IntMed); FRCPC; IntMed (Medical Oncology). Ac Staff, Pasqua Hospital; Ac Staff MedOncol, Allan Blair Cancer Centre; Ac Staff MedOncol, Regina Health District; Asst Prof Med, University of Saskatchewan; (306)766-2260; Fax. (306)766-2688.

JANDA, Surinder P; Surrey Med Arts Bldg, 201-13798 94A Ave, Surrey BC V3V 1N1; UBC'04; FRCPC; IntMed;CCFP; Respir. (604)581-6727

JANDO, Linda J; Aquarius Med Centre, 202-179 Davie St, Vancouver BC V6Z 2Y1; UBC'98; BSc(Hons.); CCFP; FCFP; Vis Staff Privil, Lions Gate Hospital; Asst Prof, University of British Columbia; (604)669-7772; Fax. (604)669-7772; aquariusmedical@novuscom.net.

JANDO, Victor T; North Mount Med Centre, 213-145 13th St E, North Vancouver BC V7L 2L4; McG'97; MDCM; FRCSC; OrthSurg. (604)984-0044

JANELLE, Chantal; MUHC-Montreal Children's Hosp, C 532-2300 rue Tupper, Montreal QC H3H 1P3; Mon'88; FRCSC; OrthSurg (Pediatric Orthopedics). Staff, McGill University Health Centre - Montreal Children's Hospital; Ac Member, Shriners Hospitals For Children - Canada; (514)412-4437; Fax. (514)412-4353; chantal.janelle@muhc.mcgill.ca.

JANELLE, Christian; Dr Christian Janelle Inc, 4065 rue De Sabrevois, Trois-Rivieres QC G9B 2B2; Sher'02; CCFP; Staff, Centre Hospitalier Regional de Trois-Rivieres; (819)697-3333

JANELLE, France; Direction de la Sante Publique, 1255 rue Beauregard, Longueuil QC J4K 2M3; Laval'80; Ac Staff, Hôpital Sainte-croix; (450)928-6777

JANELLE, Genevieve; CSSS de Beauce-Etchemin, 1515 17e rue, Saint-Georges QC G5Y 4T8; Laval'06; CCFP; Staff, Centre Hospitalier Beauce-Etchemin; (418)228-2031

JANELLE, Sylvie; Clin Med Saint-Jerome, 450 boul Monseigneur-Dubois, Saint-Jerome QC J7Y 3L8; Laval'79; (450)438-1776; Fax. (450)438-6119.

JANES, John C; Commonwealth Med Clinic, 77 Commonwealth Ave, Mount Pearl NL A1N 1W7; Mem'81; (709)364-7555; Fax. (709)364-7554.

JANES, Shawn P; Royal Columbian Hosp, 330 Columbia St E, New Westminster BC V3L 3W7; Mem'92; FRCPC; EmergMed. Staff, Royal Columbian Hospital; (604)520-4283

JANEVSKI, John; Univ Hlth Network-Toronto Western Hosp, 5 471-399 Bathurst St, Toronto ON M5T 2S8; Tor'98; BSc; MSc; FRCPC; IntMed; Cardiol. Staff, Toronto Western Hospital - University Health Network; (416)603-5516

JANG, Douglas K; Ashgrove Med Centre, 214-6633 Highway 7, Markham ON L3P 7P2; Tor'96; CCFP; Assoc Staff, Markham Stouffville Hospital; (905)294-2290; Fax. (905)294-0029.

JANG, Eddy; Parkway Mall, 208-85 Ellesmere Rd, Scarborough ON M1R 4B8; Tor'92; (416)386-0139; Fax. (416)386-0141.

JANG, Frances L; 3568 41st Ave W, Vancouver BC V6N 3E6; UBC'83; FRCPC; Derm. Consultant, Vancouver General Hospital - Centennial Pavillion; (604)737-7100

JANG, Hyun-Jung; Dept of Medical Imaging, 585 University Ave, Toronto ON M5G 2N2; Seoul (Korea)'93; (416)340-4800; Fax. (416)593-0502.

JANG, Karen Y K; Women's College Hosp, 76 Grenville St, Toronto ON M5S 1B2; Tor'09; CCFP; Staff, Women's College Hospital; (416)323-6400

JANG, Raymond W; Univ Hlth Network-Princess M, 5 110-610 University Ave, Toronto ON M5G 2M9; Tor'06; FRCPC; IntMed; MedOncol. Staff, Princess Margaret Hospital - University Health Network; (416)946-2000

JANGAARD, Krista A L; IWK Health Centre, PO Box 9700 Rpo CSC 5850-5980 University Ave, Halifax NS B3K 6R8; Dal'87; FRCPC; Peds (Neonatal & Perinatal Medicine). Staff, IWK Health Centre; Asst Prof Peds, Dalhousie University; (902)470-6643; Fax. (902)470-6469; krista.jangaard@dal.ca.

JANGRA, Dalbhir; 305-2051 McCallum Rd, Abbotsford BC V2S 3N5; Tor'99; FRCSC; GenSurg. Staff, Abbotsford Regional Hospital & Cancer Centre; (604)504-1911

JANHUNEN, David R; Nipigon Health Centre, 125 Hogan Rd, Nipigon ON P0T 2J0; NOSM'09; CCFP; Staff, Nipigon District Memorial Hospital; Staff, Thunder Bay Regional Health Sciences Centre; (807)887-5250; Fax. (807)887-1645.

JANI, Aarti; Northern Interior Health Unit, 3F-1444 Edmonton St, Prince George BC V2M 6W5; Gujarat (India)'86; MB BS; FRCPC; Psy (Adult Clinical Psychiatry). Staff Psy, University Hospital of Northern British Columbia; Consultant Psy, Northern Health Authority; Clin Instructor, University of British Columbia; Langs: Hindi; Gujarati; (250)565-2666; Fax. (250)565-2016; ajani@northernhealth.ca.

JANI, Prashant A; Thunder Bay Reg HSC-T-Bay, 980 Oliver Rd, Thunder Bay ON P7B 6V4; Pune (India)'92; MB BS; FRCPC; AnatPath (Oncology Pathology). Staff AnatPath, Thunder Bay Regional Health Sciences Centre; (807)684-6591; Fax. (807)684-5878.

JANICKA, Alicja W; Royal Alexandra Hosp, 2F-10240 Kingsway NW, Edmonton AB T5H 3V9; Wroclaw (Poland)'84; FRCPC; Peds. Staff, Royal Alexandra Hospital; Ass't Clin Prof, University of Alberta; Langs: Polish; (780)735-4605; Fax. (780)735-4071.

JANICKI, Robert T; 103-1660 Feltham Rd, Victoria BC V8N 2A1; UBC'88; (250)477-1858; cookquadra@telus.net.

JANICKI, Ryan R; 405-125 13th St E, North Vancouver BC V7L 2L3; UBC'06; Neursurg. (604)904-7467

JANICKI, Tomasz; Centennial CMH & Brain Injury, PO Box 1000 Stn Main, Ponoka AB T4J 1R8; Wroclaw (Poland)'82; Staff, Centennial Centre for Mental Health & Brain Injury; (403)783-7600

JANIKOWSKI, Andrew M; 8 Hill St, Picton ON K0K 2T0; Qns'75; CCFP; CCFP(E.M.); FCFP; Ac Staff, QHC Prince Edward County Memorial; Asst Prof, Queen's University; Langs: Polish; (613)969-6798

JANJUA, Arif S; Gordon & Leslie Diamond HCC, 4F-2775 Laurel St, Vancouver BC V5Z 1M9; Alb'02; FRCSC; Otol (Head & Neck Surgery). Staff, Providence Health Care - St Paul's Hospital; Staff, Gordon & Leslie Diamond Health Care Centre; (604)875-8296

JANJUA, Meer M; Greencrest Pembina Clinic, B-2750 Pembina Hwy, Winnipeg MB R3T 2H8; (Other Foreign)'08; CCFP.

JANJUA, Sadiq A; Dundas Street Walk-In Clinic, 209-3416 Dundas St W, Toronto ON M6S 2S1; Aberdeen (Scotland)'62; MB ChB; DPH(Ed); Assoc Staff, Humber River Regional Hospital - Church Street Site; Assoc Staff, William Osler Health System - Etobicoke General Hospital; (416)763-3111; Fax. (416)763-5665.

JANKE, Edwin M; Yarmouth Reg Hosp, 60 Vancouver St, Yarmouth NS B5A 2P5; Alb'71; FRCSC; GenSurg. Staff, Yarmouth Regional Hospital; Chief of Staff, Southwest District Health Authority; (902)742-3541; Fax. (902)742-0369; ejanke@swndha.nshealth.ca.

JANKE, Fred H; 101-190 Pelican Pl, Sylvan Lake AB T4S 1K2; Cal'82; MSc; BSc; CCFP; FCFP; Assoc Staff, Red Deer Regional Hospital Centre; Assoc Prof, University of Alberta; Langs: German; (403)887-2224; Fax. (403)887-2261.

JANKE, Paul G; The Forensic Group, 305-1245 Broadway W, Vancouver BC V6H 1G7; UBC'82; FRCPC; Psy. Consultant, Vancouver General Hospital - Centennial Pavillion; Psychiatrist, Juvenile Services to Court(Burnaby); (604)733-5722

JANKOV, Robert P; The Hosp for Sick Children, 555 University Ave, Toronto ON M5G 1X8; Melbourne (Australia)'87; Assoc Staff Peds, The Hospital For Sick Children; Staff, Women's College Hospital; Asst Prof Peds, University of Toronto; (416)813-6773; Fax. (416)813-5245.

JANKOWSKA, Agnes; Bathurst Shopping Mall, 212-1300 St. Peter Ave, Bathurst NB E2A 3A6; Mon'92; CSPQ; FRCPC; Anes. (506)548-2727; Fax. (506)546-3943.

JANMOHAMED, Amirali K; Scarborough Prof Centre, 406-1371 Neilson Rd, Scarborough ON M1B 4Z8; Aga Khan (Pakistan)'90; FRCPC; IntMed (Cardiac Electrophysiology); Cardiol. Staff, Rouge Valley Health System - Centenary Health Centre Site; Staff, St Michael's Hospital; (416)281-9499; Fax. (416)283-5705.

JANMOHAMED, Anisa; Balmoral Med Arts Facility, 305-1366 Yonge St, Toronto ON M4T 3A7; UBC'01; CCFP; (416)962-2964; Fax. (416)962-2526.

JANMOHAMED, Jamil; Westgrove Clinic, 201-505 Queen St, Spruce Grove AB T7X 2V2; Qns'09; CCFP; (780)962-9888

JANNA, Peter A; Transport Canada, 330 Sparks St, Ottawa ON K1A 0N8; McG'91; CCFP; FCFP; Fax. (613)993-4935.

JANNELLE, Jean-Pierre; CLSC et CHSLD Pommeraie, 660 rue Saint-Paul, Farnham QC J2N 3B9; Mon'78; CCFP; (450)293-3622; Fax. (450)293-3974.

JANOSKI, Michele M; Cross Cancer Institute, 11560 University Ave NW, Edmonton AB T6G 1Z2; Sask'96; FRCPC; DiagRad. Staff, Cross Cancer Institute; (780)432-8643

JANOVCIK, Juraj E; Peter Lougheed Centre, 3500 26 Ave NE, Calgary AB T1Y 6J4; (Slovakia)'04; FRCPC; IntMed; Respir. Staff, Peter Lougheed Centre; (403)943-4555

JANSCHITZ, Kristien N; Westland Market, 144-70 McLeod Ave, Spruce Grove AB T7X 3C7; Alb'08; CCFP; (780)962-9393

JANSE VAN RENSBERG, Annelie; Victoria Hosp, PO Box 3000 Stn Main 1200 24th St W, Prince Albert SK S6V 5T4; Pretoria (South Africa)'98; MB ChB; CCFP; Staff, Victoria Hospital; Langs: Afrikaans; (306)765-6226; Fax. (306)765-6224; annelievr@hotmail.com.

JANSE VAN RENSBURG, Dawid A; Park Avenue Medical Bldg, 500-4634 Park Ave, Terrace BC V8G 1V7; Pretoria (South Africa)'98; MB ChB; FRCSC; ObstGyn. Langs: Afrikaans; (250)615-5121

JANSE VAN RENSBURG, Renier; Medical Arts Centre, 103-650 Terminal Ave, Nanaimo BC V9R 5E2; Orange Free State (South Africa)'85; MB ChB; CCFP; Med Staff, Nanaimo Regional General Hospital; Langs: Afrikaans; (250)753-3431; Fax. (250)754-6897.

JANSE VAN VUUREN, Christoffel J; Jasper Avenue Med Centre, 11464 Jasper Ave NW, Edmonton AB T5K 0M1; Orange Free State (South Africa)'91; Staff, Covenant Health - St Mary's Hospital; (780)756-5262

JANSEN, Ann P; 103-599 Main St PO Box 1069 Stn Main, Hampton NB E5N 8H1; Witwatersrand (South Africa)'99; MB ChB; CCFP; (506)832-2929

JANSEN, Gerard H; The Ottawa Hosp-Civic Campus, 1053 Carling Ave, Ottawa ON K1Y 4E9; Utrecht (Netherlands)'87; FRCPC; NeurPath. Staff, The Ottawa Hospital - Civic Campus; Mgr, Prions Section Population & Public Health Branch-Health Canada; Asst Prof NeuroPath, University of Ottawa; Langs: Dutch; German; (613)737-8899 x19847; gjansen@toh.on.ca.

JANSEN, Gregory W; Medical Arts Bldg, 201-42 Glen Allan Dr, Bridgewater NS B4V 3N2; UBC'84; Staff, South Shore Regional Hospital; (902)543-4446; Fax. (902)543-4446.

JANSEN, Jan W; Hamilton HS-McMaster Site, PO Box 2000 Stn Lcd 1 2N18-1200 Main St W, Hamilton ON L8N 3Z5; Berlin (Germany)'76; Staff, St Joseph's Healthcare - Charlton Campus; Staff, Hamilton Health Sciences Centre - McMaster University Medical Centre; (905)521-2100; Fax. (905)577-0198.

JANSEN, Kara A; 340-943 Broadway W, Vancouver BC V5Z 4E1; Ott'02; CCFP; (604)738-1912

JANSEN, Kurt A; Queen Elizabeth Urgent Care, 2111 av Northcliffe, Montreal QC H4A 3K6; Man'00; CCFP; Langs: German; French; (514)481-4343

JANSEN, Liesbet M; Stevenson Mem Hosp, PO Box 4000 Stn Main 200 Fletcher Cres, Alliston ON L9R 1W7; McM'96; CCFP; Staff, Stevenson Memorial Hospital; Langs: English; French; (705)435-6281

JANSEN, Lisa E; 145-2475 McDougall St, Windsor ON N8X 3N9; Wes'96; BSc; CCFP; FCFP; (519)258-4142; Fax. (519)985-1084.

JANSEN, Nolan P; La Ronge Med Clinic, PO Box 240, La Ronge SK S0J 1L0; (306)425-2174; Fax. (306)425-4199.

JANSEN, Paul J; Meridian Medical, 3-4402 37 St, Stony Plain AB T7Z 2A9; (South Africa)'96; MB ChB; (780)963-7800; Fax. (780)963-0468.

JANSEN VAN RENSBURG, Leon; Fourth Avenue Med Centre, 278 4th Ave NE, Moose Jaw SK S6H 0C6; (South Africa)'82; MB ChB; BSc(Hon); MMedSci; (306)694-1717

JANSEN VAN RENSBURG, Nicholas A; Beausejour Primary Health CC, PO Box 550 151 First St S, Beausejour MB R0E 0C0; Pretoria (South Africa)'80; MB ChB; CCFP; Physician, Beausejour District Hospital; Staff Family Practitioner, Beausejour Primary Health Care Centre; Site Physician, Millner Ridge Correctional Centre; Langs: Afrikaans; (204)268-4966; Fax. (204)268-4399.

JANSEN VAN RENSBURG, Nicolaas M; Tremont Med Clinic, 2A-2F Tremont Dr, St Catharines ON L2T 3B2; Pretoria (South Africa)'91; CCFP; (905)687-8887; Fax. (905)641-3693.

JANSEN VAN RENSBURG, Petrus; Esterhazy Med District, PO Box 940, Esterhazy SK S0A 0X0; (Other Foreign)'03; MB ChB; (306)745-6682; Fax. (306)745-2995.

JANSEN VAN RENSBURG, Stella-Amore; 88 Elizabeth St PO Box 573 Stn Main, Okotoks AB T1S 1A7; (South Africa)'01; (403)982-7771

JANSEN VAN VUUREN, Cornelius J; Family Med Clinic, 4615 49 Ave, Lloydminster SK S9V 0T1; (South Africa)'90; MB ChB; Langs: Afrikaans; (306)825-8877; Fax. (306)825-5167.

JANSEN VAN VUUREN, Cornelius; Daysland Med Centre, PO Box 160, Daysland AB T0B 1A0; (South Africa)'63; MB ChB; Langs: Afrikaans; (780)374-3944; Fax. (780)374-2433.

JANSEN VAN VUUREN, Stephanus J; Sherwood Park Medicentre, 9-101 Bremner Dr, Sherwood Park AB T8H 0M5; (South Africa)'87; MB ChB; Staff, Two Hills Health Centre; Physician, Two Hills Medical Clinic; (780)467-4717; Fax. (780)467-9316.

JANSMA, L Lee-Anne; Glenora Med Clinic, 310-10230 142 St NW, Edmonton AB T5N 3Y6; Alb'99; CCFP; (780)455-3311; Fax. (780)451-4404.

JANSSEN, Henricus L A; Univ Hlth Network-Toronto Western Hosp, 399 Bathurst St, Toronto ON M5T 2S8; Nijmegen (Netherlands)'89; Staff, Toronto Western Hospital - University Health Network; (416)603-6230

JANSSEN, Lyne; Hôpital de Saint-Eustache, 520 boul Arthur-Sauve, Saint-Eustache QC J7R 5B1; Sher'07; Peds. Staff, Hôpital de Saint-Eustache; (450)473-6811

JANSSEN, Nicolaas J C; Caledonian Med Clinic, 340 Campbell St, Nanaimo BC V9R 3G7; UBC'94; CCFP; (250)753-3202; Fax. (250)753-1039.

JANSSEN, Rebecca S; Omineca Medical Clinic, RR 2 3348 Hospital Rd, Vanderhoof BC V0J 3A2; Wes'09; CCFP; (250)567-2201

JANSZ, G Kenneth; Burlington Prof Centre, 303-3155 Harvester Rd, Burlington ON L7N 3V2; Tor'80; BSc; FRCSC; Urol (Adult & Pediatric Urology). Hd Urol, Joseph Brant Memorial Hospital; (905)681-3030; Fax. (905)681-0132; gkjansz@bellnet.ca.

JANSZ, Gwenderlyn F; St Jamestown Health Centre, 410 Sherbourne St, Toronto ON M4X 1K2; McM'91; BSc; MSc; PhD; CCFP; Staff, St Michael's Hospital; Asst Prof, University of Toronto; (416)864-3096; Fax. (416)864-6035.

JANTCHOU MBAKOP, Prevost; Hôpital Ste-Justine, 3175 ch Cote-Sainte-Catherine, Montreal QC H3T 1C5; (France)'01; (514)345-4675

JANUSZ, Michael T; St Paul's Hosp, 458-1081 Burrard St, Vancouver BC V6Z 1Y6; Man'74; FRCSC; GenSurg (Aortic Surg); Cardiovasc&ThorSurg. Staff, Providence Health Care - St Paul's Hospital; Staff, Vancouver General Hospital - Centennial Pavillion; Clin Prof Surg, University of British Columbia; (604)876-8948

JANUSZEWSKA, Mariola S; 301A-15252 32 Ave, Surrey BC V3S 0R7; Gdansk (Poland)'87; CCFP; Langs: Polish; (604)538-6111

JANVIER, Annie F; Hôpital Ste-Justine, 3175 ch Cote Sainte-Catherine, Montreal QC H3T 1C5; Mon'97; LMCC; FRCPC; Peds (Neonatal & Perinatal Medicine). Staff, Hôpital Ste-Justine; Langs: English; Spanish; (514)345-4931 x4658

JANVIER, Jack A; Peter Lougheed Centre, 3500 26 Ave NE, Calgary AB T1Y 6J4; Sask'01; FRCPC; IntMed; InfectDis. Staff, Peter Lougheed Centre; (403)943-5681; Fax. (403)943-4017.

JANY, Mark J; Bayvalley Med Arts Bldg, 202A-145 Queenston St, St Catharines ON L2R 2Z9; Qns'90; FRCPC; IntMed (Respirology); Respir. Ac Staff, Niagara Health System - St Catharines General Site; Ac Staff, Niagara Health System - Ontario Street Site; (905)984-3349; Fax. (905)984-5110.

JANZ, Christopher B; Royal Inland Hosp, 311 Columbia St, Kamloops BC V2C 2T1; UBC'89; Staff, Royal Inland Hospital; (250)314-2782; Fax. (250)314-2280.

JANZ, Rodica F; Kootenay Lake Hosp, 3 View St, Nelson BC V1L 2V1; UBC'03; CCFP; Staff, Kootenay Lake General Hospital; Langs: Romanian; (250)505-9919

JANZ, Trevor W; Kootenay Lake Hosp, 3 View St, Nelson BC V1L 2V1; Cal'84; Staff, Kootenay Lake General Hospital; (250)352-3111

JANZEN, Dennis L; Surrey Mem Hosp, 13750 96 Ave, Surrey BC V3V 1Z2; Sask'88; FRCPC; DiagRad. Staff, Surrey Memorial Hospital; Staff, Vancouver General Hospital - Centennial Pavillion; (604)588-3308; Fax. (604)588-3359.

JANZEN, Derek S; Kensington Med Clinic, 6548 Hastings St, Burnaby BC V5B 1S2; Man'97; CCFP; (604)299-9769

JANZEN, Dorothy M; 34-1199 Lynn Valley Rd, North Vancouver BC V7J 3H2; UBC'86; Clin Instructor, University of British Columbia; Langs: Dutch; French; (604)988-0707; Fax. (604)988-4729.

JANZEN, Ernest P; Professional Corp, 931 19 St S, Lethbridge AB T1J 3H5; Alb'79; FRCPC; IntMed (Cardiology). Ac Staff, Chinook Regional Hospital; Ac Staff, Covenant Health - St Michael's Health Centre; Consultant, Coaldale Health Centre; Asst Prof, University of Calgary; Langs: German; (403)328-0693

JANZEN, James A; Rockyview Gen Hosp, 7007 14 St SW, Calgary AB T2V 1P9; Sask'84; FRCPC; Anes. Staff, Rockyview General Hospital; (403)943-3410; Fax. (403)943-3360.

JANZEN, Jeannette L; Groupe Medical Stillview, 245-175 av Stillview, Pointe-Claire QC H9R 4S3; Sask'86; CCFP; Ac Staff, Mount Sinai Hospital Center; Hon Member, Lakeshore General Hospital - Pointe Claire; (514)697-6387

JANZEN, Matthew; 106-2155 10th Ave, Prince George BC V2M 5J6; UBC'03; CCFP; CCFP(E.M.); (250)563-4004

JANZEN, Rhonda M; Surrey Med Bldg, 205-9656 King George Hwy, Surrey BC V3T 2V5; UBC'95; FRCSC; GenSurg. (604)582-3004; Fax. (604)582-3080.

JANZEN, Thomas; Regional Mental HC-St Thomas, PO Box 2004 Stn Main 467 Sunset Dr, St Thomas ON N5P 3V9; Wes'87; Staff, Regional Mental Health Care-St Joseph's Health Care; (519)455-5110 x49458

JAO, Kevin; CSSS du Lac-des-Deux-Montagnes, 520 boul Arthur-Sauve, Saint-Eustache QC J7R 5B1; Mon'07; Hem; IntMed. Staff, Hôpital de Saint-Eustache; (450)473-6811

JAQUIER, Catherine; Hop Jean-Talon, 1385 rue Jean-Talon E, Montreal QC H2E 1S6; Lausanne (Switzerland)'92; Staff, Pontiac Hospital Centre; (514)495-6767

JARAND, Julie M; Peter Lougheed Centre, 3500 26 Ave NE, Calgary AB T1Y 6J4; Cal'01; FRCPC; IntMed; Respir. Staff, Peter Lougheed Centre; (403)943-5425

JARDINE, Frederick F; Summerhill Med Clinic, 207-130 Conception Bay Hwy, Conception Bay S NL A1W 3A6; Mem'82; CCFP; FCFP; (709)834-2039; Fax. (709)834-9649.

JARDINE, Ivan; Mills Memorial Hosp, 4720 Haugland Ave, Terrace BC V8G 2W7; Witwatersrand (South Africa)'78; MB ChB; Staff Surg, Mills Memorial Hospital; (250)635-2211

JARDINE, Julie A; Canadian Forces Services Ctre, 101 Colonel By Dr, Ottawa ON K1A 0K2; Ott'95; FRCPC; Psy. Staff, Canadian Forces Health Services Centre; (613)945-1060; Fax. (613)945-1070.

JARDINE, Lawrence F; Children's Hosp, B1 114-800 Commissioners Rd E, London ON N6C 2V5; Mem'87; FRCPC; Peds (Hematological Oncology). Staff, Children's Hospital of Western Ontario; Assoc Prof Peds, University of Western Ontario; (519)685-8494; Fax. (519)685-8384.

JARDON, Kris; MUHC-Royal Victoria Hosp, F9 26-687 av des Pins O, Montreal QC H3A 1A1; Auvergne (France)'02; Staff, McGill University Health Centre - Royal Victoria Hospital; (514)934-1934; Fax. (514)843-2830; kris.jardon@mcgill.ca.

JAREMA, Andrew J; Fort Med Clinic, 101-6603 132 Ave NW, Edmonton AB T5C 2A4; Alb'72; BSc; Staff Extended Care, Capital Care - Dickinsfield; Staff, St Michael's Extended Care; Staff, Venta Care Centre; Clin Instructor, University of Alberta; Langs: Ukrainian; (780)476-1388; Fax. (780)473-3530; andyjarema@shaw.ca.

JAREMKO, Jacob L; Hys Med Centre, 202-11010 101 St NW, Edmonton AB T5H 4B9; Cal'03; FRCPC; DiagRad. (780)428-1121

JARIANI, Marjan; Univ Hlth Network-Toronto Gen, 200 Elizabeth St, Toronto ON M5G 2C4; Tehran (Iran)'90; FRCPC; Anes. Staff, Toronto General Hospital - UHN; (416)340-4800 x3242

JARJOUR, Allan M; Medicentre St-Lazare, D-1811 ch Sainte-Angelique, Saint-Lazare QC J7T 2X9; McG'92; FRCPC; Peds. Langs: English; French; (450)424-7030; Fax. (450)424-7033.

JARJOURA, Samir C; CHUS-Hop Fleurimont, 3001 12e Av N, Sherbrooke QC J1H 5N4; Beirut (Lebanon)'70; ABPeds; AB; FRCPC; Peds; Electroenceph (P.Q.); Neur. Staff, Centre Hospitalier Universitaire de Sherbrooke-Hopital Fleurimont; adj Prof Med, Universite de Sherbrooke; (819)342-1110; Fax. (819)822-6776.

JARMAIN, Sarah H; Regional Mental HC-St Thomas, PO Box 2004 Stn Main 467 Sunset Dr, St Thomas ON N5P 3V9; McM'93; BSc; FRCPC; Psy. Site Chief, Regional Mental Health Care-St Joseph's Health Care; Site Chief, Regional Mental Health Care-St Joseph's Health Care; Vice Chair MPC, St Joseph's Hospital - St Joseph's Health Care; Asst Prof, University of Western Ontario; (519)631-8510 x49429; Fax. (519)631-2512.

JARMAN, David; Workers' Comp Board, 801 30th St, Courtenay BC V9N 8G6; Sher'80; Med Advisor, Worker's Comp Board of BC; Langs: English; French.

JARMULA, Bartosz M; Selkirk Med Group, PO Box 590, Revelstoke BC V0E 2S0; Alb'03; CCFP; (250)837-9321

JARMUSKE, Mario B; The Ottawa Hosp-Gen Campus, S6-501 Smyth Rd, Ottawa ON K1H 8L6; Man'82; FRCSC; GenSurg; PlasSurg. Staff/Chief Div of Plastic Surg, The Ottawa Hospital - General Campus; Chief Div of Plastic Surg, University of Ottawa; (613)737-8899 x73047; Fax. (613)737-8676.

JARONI, Arkadiusz N; St Mary's Hosp, 4607 53 St, Camrose AB T4V 1Y5; Alb'91; BSc; CCFP; FCFP; Staff, Covenant Health - St Mary's Hospital; Langs: Polish; (780)679-6100; artjaroni@shaw.ca.

JAROSZYNSKA, Anna M; 23-1960 Appleby Line, Burlington ON L7L 0B7; (Poland)'89; FACR; FRCPC; IntMed (Osteoporosis); Rheum. Langs: Polish; (905)632-4016; Fax. (289)288-5004; annaj@cogeco.ca.

JAROSZYNSKI, Grzegorz C; 23A-1960 Appleby Line, Burlington ON L7L 0B7; Lodz (Poland)'88; FRCSC; OrthSurg (Hip & Knee Replacement). Ac Staff, Joseph Brant Memorial Hospital; Langs: Polish; (905)333-5020; Fax. (905)333-5018.

JARRATT, Mary E; 202-107 Catherwood St, Saint John NB E2M 5J7; Dal'84; Ac Staff, Saint John Regional Hospital; (506)642-1153; Fax. (506)642-1158.

JARRELL, Eugene G; Brant Community HC-Brantford, 200 Terrace Hill St, Brantford ON N3R 1G9; Qns'81; AB; FACEP; CCFP; CCFP(E.M.); FCFP; Dir EmergMed, The Brant Community Healthcare System - Brantford General Hospital Site; (519)751-5544 x4235; Fax. (519)752-0098.

JARRELL, John F; Foothills Med Centre, 1403 29 St NW, Calgary AB T2N 2T9; Qns'72; MSc; FRCSC; ObstGyn (Chronic Pain Management). Staff ObstGyn, Foothills Medical Centre; Staff, Calgary Regional Health Authority; Staff, Calgary Health Region Chronic Pain Centre; Prof Med, University of Calgary; Langs: Bilingual(French/English); (403)944-1438; Fax. (403)270-4249; john.jarrell@calgaryhealthregion.ca.

JARRETT, Francis J; Hotel-Dieu Hosp, 166 Brock St, Kingston ON K7L 5G2; Liverpool (England)'59; MB ChB; DPM(Eng); MRCPsy; FRCPC; Psy (Anxiety Disorder). Att Staff, Hotel-Dieu Hospital; Att Staff, Kingston General Hospital; Asst Prof, Queen's University; (613)544-3400 x3552; Fax. (613)544-9666.

JARRETT, Pamela G; St Joseph's Hosp, 130 Bayard Dr, Saint John NB E2L 3L6; Dal'89; FRCPC; IntMed; GeriatricMed. Head Clin Dept, St Joseph's Hospital; Head Clin Dept, Saint John Regional Hospital; Asst Prof Med & Div of Geriatric Med, Dalhousie University; (506)632-5556; Fax. (506)632-5512; pam.jarret@horizonnb.ca.

JARRY, Marie-Claude; CLSC Rivieres-des-Prairies, 8655 boul Perras, Montreal QC H1E 4M7; Sher'90; CCFP; (514)494-4924

JARRY, Michel; Centre Cardio Rive-Sud, 200-1615 boul Jacques-Cartier, Longueuil QC J4M 2X1; Mon'79; FACC; FRCP; Cardiol (Adult Cardiology). Ac Member, Centre Hospitalier Pierre Boucher; Assoc Member, Centre Hospitalier Pierre le Gardeur; Pres CSSS Pierre-Boucher, CMDP; (450)674-2345; Fax. (450)674-1622; mjarry@sympatico.ca.

JARVI, Keith A; The Joseph & Wolf Lebovic Bldg, 6F-60 Murray St, Toronto ON M5T 3L9; Ott'82; FRCSC; Urol (Infertility). Staff, Toronto General Hospital - UHN; Staff, Mount Sinai Hospital; Staff, St Michael's Hospital; Prof Surg, University of Toronto; (416)586-8867; Fax. (416)586-8354; kjarvi@mtsinai.on.ca.

JARVIE, Andrew; Queen Elizabeth II HSC, 1276 South Park St, Halifax NS B3H 2Y9; Glasgow (Scotland)'91; MB ChB; Staff, Queen Elizabeth II Health Sciences Centre - Victoria General Site; (902)473-2331; Fax. (902)423-9454.

JARVIS, Carl W; Queen Elizabeth II HSC-Halifax, 355-1796 Summer St, Halifax NS B3H 3A7; Dal'93; CCFP; CCFP(E.M.); Staff, Queen Elizabeth II Health Sciences Centre - Halifax Infirmary Site; Langs: French; (902)473-8769

JARVIS, Catherine A; CLSC Cote des Neiges, 5700 ch de la Cote-des-Nieges, Montreal QC H3T 2A8; Alb'94; CCFP; FCFP; (514)731-8531

JARVIS, G Eric; Inst of Commun & Family Psy, 4333 ch Cote-Sainte-Catherine, Montreal QC H3T 1E4; Alb'94; BSc; MSc; DABPN; FRCPC; Psy (Social Psychiatry). Staff, Sir Mortimer B Davis Jewish General; Médecin, Concordia Univ Student Health Services; McGill University; Langs: English; French; (514)340-8210; eric.jarvis@mcgill.ca.

JARVIS, Ingrid M; Kingsway Med Bldg, 7-2917 Bloor St W, Toronto ON M8X 1B4; Tor'77; FRCPC; Derm. Staff, Toronto General Hospital - UHN; Staff, Princess Margaret Hospital - University Health Network; Staff Dermatologist, SpaMedica; University of Toronto; Langs: French; Hungarian; (416)233-3340; Fax. (416)233-0488.

JARVIS, James G; Children's Hosp Eastern Ont, 401 Smyth Rd, Ottawa ON K1H 8L1; Cal'78; FRCSC; OrthSurg (Pediatric Orthopedics). Ac Staff, Children's Hospital of Eastern Ontario (CHEO); Consultant, The Ottawa Hospital - Civic Campus; Ac Staff, Ottawa Children's Treatment Centre; Assoc Prof Surg, University of Ottawa; (613)737-2586; Fax. (613)738-4840.

JARVIS, Jolene E; 140-11 Highway 329 PO Box 249, Hubbards NS B0J 1T0; Ott'97; LMCC; CCFP; (902)857-1312; Fax. (902)857-1471.

JARVIS, Scott E; Foothills Med Centre, 1403 29 St NW, Calgary AB T2N 2T9; Cal'06; FRCPC; Neur. Staff, Foothills Medical Centre; (403)944-4253; Fax. (403)270-7126.

JARVIS, Tanya J; Carbonear Gen Hosp, 86 Highroad South, Carbonear NL A1Y 1A4; Mem'96; FRCPC; DiagRad. Staff, Carbonear General Hospital; (709)945-5111

JARZEM, Peter F; MUHC-Montreal Gen Hosp, B5 111-1650 av Cedar, Montreal QC H3G 1A4; Qns'84; FRCS; FRCSC; OrthSurg (Spinal Injury). Staff Surg, Sir Mortimer B Davis Jewish General; Langs: German; Italian; French; (514)934-8508

JASCHINSKI, Joerg; The Medical Associates Sechelt, PO Box 638 5531 Inlet Ave, Sechelt BC V0N 3A0; Cape Town (South Africa)'98; MB ChB; (604)885-2257

JASELIUNAS, Odetas; CSST, 5e-750 boul Charest E, Quebec QC G1K 3J7; Laval'76; Dir Med Services, CSST-Chaudiere-Appalaches; (418)266-4200

JASEY, Bradley; South Walkerville Med Ctre, 340-2224 Walker Rd, Windsor ON N8W 5L7; Wes'95; FRCSC; ObstGyn. Staff, Windsor Regional Hospital - Metropolitan Site; (519)972-1346; Fax. (519)258-7350.

JASEY, Gordon M; South Walkerville Med Ctre, 340-2224 Walker Rd, Windsor ON N8W 5L7; Dal'56; FRCSC; ObstGyn. Court Staff, Hôtel-Dieu Grace Hospital; Court Staff, Windsor Regional Hospital - Metropolitan Site; (519)258-1592

JASEY, Greg; North Walkerville Med Centre, 216-2425 Tecumseh Rd E, Windsor ON N8W 1E6; Qns'95; FRCSC; OrthSurg (Arthroplasty). Staff, Hôtel-Dieu Grace Hospital; Staff, Windsor Regional Hospital - Metropolitan Site; (519)254-5763; Fax. (519)254-6356; orthopedic@bellnet.ca.

JASEY, Kathleen A; South Walkerville Med Centre, 340-2224 Walker Rd, Windsor ON N8W 5L7; Wes'00; CCFP; (519)258-1592; Fax. (519)258-7350.

JASKOLKA, Jeffrey D; Mount Sinai Hosp, 564-600 University Ave, Toronto ON M5G 1X5; Wes'01; FRCPC; DiagRad. Staff Medical Imaging, Mount Sinai Hospital; (416)586-4800

JASKOLKA, Kenneth M; North York Med Group, 705-240 Duncan Mill Rd, North York ON M3B 3S6; Tor'84; BSc; Ac Staff, North York General Hospital - Branson Division; Ac Staff, North York General Hospital; (416)222-2688; Fax. (416)221-3097.

JASKOT, Thomas P; 10-987 King St E, Hamilton ON L8M 1C6; Warsaw (Poland)'65; (905)545-8785; Fax. (905)545-8838.

JASMIN, Christiane L; Centre Med Fleury, 2157 rue Fleury E, Montreal QC H2B 1K1; Mon'86; Médecin, CLSC Pierrefonds; (514)858-6110; Fax. (514)381-9872.

JASMIN, Francois; Clin Med La Cite Place Du Parc, 900-300 rue Léo-Pariseau, Montreal QC H2X 4B3; Laval'74; ac Staff, Centre Hospitalier l'Université de Montréal (CHUM) - Hôtel-Dieu; (514)281-1722; Fax. (514)281-6697.

JASMIN, Yvon; Hop Jean-Talon, 1385 rue Jean-Talon E, Montreal QC H2E 1S6; Mon'68; ABOG; FACOG; ObstGyn. Chef cabinet, CSSS du Coeur de l'Isle Hôpital Jean-Talon; (514)495-6767

JASON, Marlowe A; Markham Prof Centre, 108-2265 Pembina Hwy, Winnipeg MB R3T 5J3; Man'72; AB; FRCSC; Urol (Benign Prostatic Hypertrophy). Chief Urol, Seven Oaks General Hospital; Chief Urol, Victoria General Hospital; Pt-Time Staff, University of Manitoba; (204)261-3030; Fax. (204)261-3010.

JASSAL, Davinder S; St Boniface Gen Hosp, Y3531-409 Tache Ave, Winnipeg MB R2H 2A6; Man'98; FRCPC; IntMed; Cardiol. Staff, St Boniface General Hospital; Asst Prof Med, University of Manitoba; (204)237-2023; Fax. (204)233-2157; djassal@sbgh.mb.ca.

JASSAL, Harinder; 12811 96 Ave, Surrey BC V3V 6V9; Man'88; (604)588-7976

JASSAL, Inderjit S; 125-15299 68 Ave, Surrey BC V3S 2C1; Sydney (Australia)'05; MB BS; CCFP; (778)218-4100

JASSAL, Kuldip; 307A-15252 32 Ave, Surrey BC V3S 0R7; Amritsar (India)'88; FRCPC; Psy. (604)560-5556

JASSAL, Rajive; Tawa Centre, 222-3017 66 St NW, Edmonton AB T6K 4B2; Man'02; FRCPC; Neur. (780)735-9626

JASSAL, S Vanita; Univ Hlth Network-Toronto Gen, 8N 857-200 Elizabeth St, Toronto ON M5G 2C4; Queen's (Ireland)'87; MB; MSc; FRCPC; IntMed (Dialysis). Researcher, Sunnybrook Health Sciences Centre; Staff, Toronto General Hospital - UHN; Asst Prof, University of Toronto; Langs: German; Punjabi; (416)340-3196; Fax. (416)340-4999.

JASSAM, Jabir M; Health Treasure Med Centre, 104-10 Green St, Nepean ON K2J 3Z6; Mosul (Iraq)'90; CCFP; (613)825-0544; Fax. (613)825-0543.

JASSAR, Balvinder S; Millbourne Road Med Clinic, 131 Millbourne Road East NW, Edmonton AB T6K 1P6; Alb'00; PhD; CCFP; Langs: Punjabi; Hindi; (780)462-4229; Fax. (780)462-3315.

JASSAT, Zaheera E; Glenrose Rehab Hosp, 10230 111 Ave NW, Edmonton AB T5G 0B7; (South Africa)'99; Staff, Glenrose Rehabilitation Hospital; (780)735-8870

JASSERAND, Francoise; Clinique Med Joliette, 3841 rue Ontario E, Montreal QC H1W 1S5; Grenoble (France)'74; Staff, Sir Mortimer B Davis Jewish General; Langs: English; (514)524-3731; Fax. (514)524-0675.

JAST, Zygmunt M; Centre Medical, 200-2615 av Van Horne, Montreal QC H3S 1P7; UBC'65; Staff, St Mary's Hospital Centre; (514)788-1228; Fax. (514)739-5398.

JASTRZEBSKI, Jacek P; Gordon & Leslie Diamond HCC, 5F-2775 Laurel St, Vancouver BC V5Z 1M9; (Poland)'88; FRCPC; IntMed; Nephrol. Staff, Vancouver General Hospital - Centennial Pavillion; Staff, Gordon & Leslie Diamond Health Care Centre; Asst Prof, University of British Columbia; Langs: Polish; (604)875-5950; Fax. (604)875-5952.

JAT, Khalid M; Waterford Hosp, 306 Waterford Bridge Rd, St. John's NL A1E 4J8; Sind (Pakistan)'92; MB BS; FRCPC; Psy. Staff, Waterford Hospital; (709)777-3300

JATTAN, Sarla; The Doctor's Office, 202-3609 Sheppard Ave E, Scarborough ON M1T 3K8; Tor'84; BSc; CCFP; Staff, Rouge Valley Health System - Centenary Health Centre Site; Staff, The Scarborough Hospital - General Campus; Staff Health Services, University of Toronto; (416)321-2643

JAUHARI, Vinod; North Whitby Med Centre, 3975 Garden St, Whitby ON L1R 3A4; Jodhpur (India)'70; CCFP; (905)430-2400

JAUNKALNS, Robert; Sunnybrook Hlth Sciences Ctre, FG 40-2075 Bayview Ave, Toronto ON M4N 3M5; Tor'81; FRCPC; Psy. Ac Staff, Sunnybrook Health Sciences Centre; Asst Prof Psy, University of Toronto; (416)480-4693; Fax. (416)480-6878.

JAURON, Annie; Clinique familiale des Hauts-B, 99 boul des Hauts-Bois, Sainte-Julie QC J3E 3J9; Mon'06; CCFP; Staff, Centre Hospitalier de Matane; (450)649-2490

JAUVIN, Daniel; Coop Solidarite Shooner-Jauvin, GD 10A rue Georges, Pierreville QC J0G 1J0; Sher'78; LMCC; ac Membre Gen Med, Hôtel-Dieu de Sorel; (450)568-3296; Fax. (450)568-0333; djauvin@sympatico.ca.

JAVAHERI, Erfan; 195-4750 Rutherford St, Nanaimo BC V9T 4K6; (Other Foreign)'01; (250)585-7100

JAVAHERI, Sepehr; CSSS Les Eskers de l'Abitibi, 622 4e rue O, Amos QC J9T 2S2; McG'98; FRCPC; IntMed. Staff, CH Hôtel-Dieu d'Amos; (819)732-3341; Fax. (819)732-6465.

JAVALY, Kedarnath; Niagara H System-G Niagara, PO Box 1018 Stn Main 5546 Portage Rd, Niagara Falls ON L2E 6X2; New York (USA)'90; (905)378-4647

JAVANMARD, Mahan; Humber River Reg Hosp-Church, 200 Church St, Toronto ON M9N 1N8; Tor'02; CCFP; CCFP(E.M.); Staff, Humber River Regional Hospital - Church Street Site; (416)243-4191

JAVANMARD, Mahgol; A 8-1390 Major Mackenzie Dr E, Richmond Hill ON L4S 0A1; Ott'01; CCFP; (905)884-7711

JAVED, Arshad; 305-2155 10th Ave, Prince George BC V2M 5J6; Karachi (Pakistan)'90; MB BS; CCFP; (250)564-5656

JAVED, Farrukh; Dr Charles A Janeway Child Hc, 300 Prince Philip Dr, St. John's NL A1B 3V6; Lahore (Pakistan)'90; Staff, Janeway Children's Health & Rehabilitation Centre; (709)777-4642

JAVED, Khalid; Phoenix Med Centre, 201-2155 10th Ave, Prince George BC V2M 5J6; Bahuddin Zakaria (Pakistan)'89; CCFP; (250)563-1502

JAVER, Akbar K; Columbia Med Bldg, 201-301 Columbia St E, New Westminster BC V3L 3W5; UBC'85; Ac Staff Gen Pract, Royal Columbian Hospital; Clin Instructor Med, University of British Columbia; (604)526-4655; Fax. (604)526-7656.

JAVER, Amin R; St Paul's Hosp, 2619-1081 Burrard St, Vancouver BC V6Z 1Y6; UBC'91; FRCSC; Otol (Nasal & Sinus Surgery). Staff ENT Clinic, Providence Health Care - St Paul's Hospital; Langs: Kacchi; Urdu; Hindi; Gujarati; Swahili; (604)806-9926; sinussurgeon@shaw.ca.

JAVID, Sabiha; McCarthy Park Med Clinic, 1039 Devonshire Drive N, Regina SK S4X 2X4; CCFP; (306)924-2220; Fax. (306)775-2720.

JAVIDAN, Manouchehr; Gordon & Leslie Diamond HCC, 8267-2775 Laurel St, Vancouver BC V5Z 1M9; (Iran)'75; MSc(Neurophysiol.); FRCPC; Neur (Epilepsy). Dir Neurophysiol Lab, Vancouver General Hospital - Centennial Pavillion; Staff Epilepsy Clinic, Gordon & Leslie Diamond Health Care Centre; Physician, Canadian Society of Clinical Neurophysiology; Exec Board Member, Canadian Society of Clinical Neurophysiol; Clin Assoc Prof Med, University of British Columbia; Langs: Farsi; (604)875-4402; Fax. (604)875-4786; mjavidan@vch.ca.

JAVIDI, Robert R; Acadie-Bathurst Ophth Center, 2-939 St. Peter Ave, Bathurst NB E2A 2Z3; Laval'98; FRCSC; Ophth. Staff, Hopital Regional Chaleur; Langs: English; (506)548-2722; Fax. (506)548-5722; ophthalmo@nb.aibn.com.

JAVIER, Joseph J; Health Matters Med Clinic, 102-3215 Dunmore Rd SE, Medicine Hat AB T1B 2H2; Guadalajara (Mexico)'72; BSc(Biol.); FRCPC; IntMed (Rheumatology). Staff, Medicine Hat Regional Hospital; (403)504-0450

JAVIER, Romulo E; 201-2444 Hurontario St, Mississauga ON L5B 2V1; Santo Tomas (Philippines)'73; (905)897-0949

JAWAD, Luma R; Medical Centre, 5-5035 Hurontario St, Mississauga ON L4Z 3Y7; Al-Mustansiriyah (Iraq)'92; MB ChB; CCFP.

JAWAHIR, George A; Arbour Med Centre, 281 Stone Rd E, Guelph ON N1G 5J5; McM'84; BSc; (519)823-5133; Fax. (519)827-0255.

JAWANDA, Madhumeet K; 103-7130 120 St, Surrey BC V3W 3M8; Alb'93; CCFP; (604)572-4437; Fax. (604)572-4438.

JAWANDA, Manindar; MedicalWest, 212-3001 Gordon Ave, Coquitlam BC V3C 2K7; UBC'87; (604)944-4077; Fax. (604)944-0677.

JAWARD, M A Abdul; Thunder Bay Radiology Inc, 150-63 Algoma St N, Thunder Bay ON P7A 4Z6; Sheffield (England)'63; LRCP; MRCS; DMRD; FRCR; FRCPC; DiagRad.

JAWORSKI, Anne-France M; 102-135 Ormond St, Brockville ON K6V 5Y2; Qns'89; BScPharm; Staff, Brockville General Hospital - Charles Street; Staff, Providence Continuing Care Centre (PCCC) - St Vincent de Paul Hospital; Langs: Bilingual(English/French); (613)342-8176; Fax. (613)342-8065.

JAWORSKI, Jerzy S; Surrey Med Arts Bldg, 209-13710 94A Ave, Surrey BC V3V 1N1; Lodz (Poland)'72; PhD; FRCPC; PhysMed&Rehab. Med Dir Rehab, Surrey Memorial Hospital; Consultant, Langley Memorial Hospital; Consultant, Peace Arch Hospital; Langs: Polish; (604)951-2323; Fax. (604)951-2324.

JAWORSKI, Laurence; Hop du Sacre-Coeur de Mtl, 5400 boul Gouin O, Montreal QC H4J 1C5; Sher'05; FRCSC; Ophth. Staff, Hôpital du Sacre-Coeur de Montréal; (514)338-2222

JAWORSKI, Martine A; U of Ottawa Health Services, 302-1 Nicholas St, Ottawa ON K1N 7B7; Johns Hopkins (USA)'74; FRCPC; Peds. Langs: English; French; (613)564-3950

JAY, Howard; The Doctor's Office, 2251 Lawrence Ave E, Scarborough ON M1P 2P5; Cambridge (England)'61; MB ChB; MRCS; LRCP; Ac Staff, Rouge Valley Health System - Centenary Health Centre Site; (416)759-5251; Fax. (416)759-1253.

JAY, Jack C; Burnaby Hosp, 3935 Kincaid St, Burnaby BC V5G 2X6; UBC'89; Staff, Burnaby Hospital; (604)434-4211; Fax. (604)412-6170.

JAY, Richard M; Sunnybrook Hlth Sciences Ctre, A 459-2075 Bayview Ave, Toronto ON M4N 3M5; Tor'75; ABIM; FRCPC; IntMed (Thrombosis & Hemostasis); Hem. Ac Staff, Sunnybrook Health Sciences Centre; Assoc Prof Med, University of Toronto; (416)480-6161; Fax. (416)480-5153.

JAY, Robert L; McGill Centre, PO Box 2000 Stn Central, Charlottetown PE C1A 7N8; Ott'99; FRCPC; Psy. Staff, Hillsborough Hospital & Special Care Centre; (902)368-4911

JAY, Venita; Manulife Financial, 2-200 Bloor St E, Toronto ON M4W 1E5; Delhi (India)'82; AB(AP,NP); FRCPC; NeurPath. Staff, Women's College Hospital; Asst Prof Path & Ophth, University of Toronto; (416)926-3000

JAYABARATHAN, Ajantha; Central Halifax Innovative Hlt, 1584 Robie St, Halifax NS B3H 3E6; Wes'89; CCFP; FCFP; Member, National Institute of Health Informatics; Board Member, Collaborative Family Healthcare Association; Staff, Central Halifax Innovative Health Clinic; Asst Prof Family Med, Dalhousie University; Langs: Hindi; Tamil; (902)420-0033; Fax. (902)420-0707; familymedclinic@eastlink.ca.

JAYAKUMAR, Saumya; 6D61-3280 Hospital Dr NW, Calgary AB T2N 4Z6; Man'04; FRCPC; IntMed; Gastroent. Staff, Foothills Medical Centre; (403)592-5049

JAYALATH, Arachchige D; Acton Med Clinic & Urgent Care, 10 Eastern Ave, Acton ON L7J 0A5; Colombo (Sri Lanka)'86; CCFP; (519)853-4449; Fax. (519)853-5242.

JAYAPRAKASH, Makam S; Regina Mental Health Clinic, 2110 Hamilton St, Regina SK S4P 2E3; Bangalore (India)'89; MB BS; FRCPC; Psy. (306)766-7800; Fax. (306)766-7811.

JAYARAJAH, Francia G; 301-1585 Markham Rd, Scarborough ON M1B 2W1; Jaffna (Sri Lanka)'95; MB BS; CCFP; Langs: Tamil; (416)792-2444

JAYARAJAN, Meera; Humber River Reg Hosp, 2111 Finch Ave W, North York ON M3N 1N1; Ott'07; CCFP; CCFP(E.M.); Staff, Humber River Regional Hospital - Finch Avenue Site; (416)744-2500

JAYARAM, Kadamby P; Fredericton Med Clinic, 208-1015 Regent St, Fredericton NB E3B 6H5; Mysore (India)'65; MB BS; DPM(Eng); FRCPC; Psy (General Adult Psychiatry). Ac Staff, Dr Everett Chalmers Regional Hospital; Consultant Psy, Mental Health Clinic; Clin Instructor Psy, Dalhousie University; (506)458-0466; Fax. (506)459-3302.

JAYARAM, Srinidhi K; The Ottawa Hosp-Civic Campus, 1053 Carling Ave, Ottawa ON K1Y 4E9; Mem'04; FRCSC; GenSurg; VascSurg. Staff, The Ottawa Hospital - Civic Campus; (613)761-4221

JAYARAMAN, Chitra; Com El Med Bldg, 202-2620 Commercial Dr, Vancouver BC V5N 4C4; Kilpauk (India)'85; MB BS; CCFP; (604)842-0509

JAYARAMAN, Dev; MUHC-Montreal Gen Hosp, 1650 av Cedar, Montreal QC H3G 1A4; McG'96; FRCPC; IntMed; Critical Care Medicine (P.Q.). Staff, McGill University Health Centre - Montreal General Campus; (514)934-1934

JAYARAMAN, Jai; Humber River Reg Hosp-Church, 200 Church St, Toronto ON M9N 1N8; Cornell(NY) (USA)'01; Staff, Humber River Regional Hospital - Church Street Site; (416)249-8111

JAYARAMAN, Jyothi; Broadway & Burrard Med Clinic, 1816 Broadway Ave W, Vancouver BC V6J 1Y9; Madras (India)'84; MB BS; CCFP; Langs: Tamil; Kanarese; Hindi; (604)736-1888

JAYARAMAN, Shiva; St Joseph's Health Centre, 221-30 The Queensway, Toronto ON M6R 1B5; Wes'02; FRCSC; GenSurg. Staff, St Joseph's Health Centre; (416)530-6653

JAYARAMAN, Vadula; Parksville Med Clinic, PO Box 250 154 Memorial Ave, Parksville BC V9P 1K7; Nagpur (India)'09; MB BS; (250)248-5757

JAYASHANKAR, Komathy; Bur Oak Med Centre, 5B-20 Bur Oak Ave, Markham ON L6C 0A2; Kilpauk (India)'96; MB BS; CCFP; Langs: Tamil; (905)887-0042; Fax. (905)887-0054.

JAYASINGHE, Hettiarachchige; Yorkton Reg Health Centre, 270 Bradbrooke Dr, Yorkton SK S3N 2K6; Staff, Yorkton Regional Health Centre; (306)782-2401

JAYASURIYA, D Sushila; The Ottawa Hosp-Civic Campus, A620-1053 Carling Ave, Ottawa ON K1Y 4E9; Ceylon (Sri Lanka)'70; MB BS; FRCPC; Psy (Consultation-Liaison). Att Staff, The Ottawa Hospital - Civic Campus; Langs: Sinhalese; (613)761-4581; Fax. (613)761-5328; sjayasuriya@ottawahospital.on.ca.

JAYASURIYA, Joseph C; PO Box 4067 Stn Main, Ponoka AB T4J 1R5; RCS (Ireland)'64; MRCPsy; DPM(Eng); Consultant, Red Deer Regional Hospital Centre; Med Consultant, Lacombe Hospital & Care Centre; (403)783-4803

JAYAWARDENE, Nishan C; Niagara H System-Douglas Mem, 230 Bertie St, Fort Erie ON L2A 1Z2; Tor'98; CCFP; Staff, Niagara Health System - Douglas Memorial Hospital Site; (905)871-6605

JAZRAWI, Bashar; 277B Foord St PO Box 3010, Stellarton NS B0K 1S0; (Iraq)'01; MB ChB; CCFP; (902)695-3441

JAZRAWY, Helen; 57 Thornbank Rd, Thornhill ON L4J 2A1; Baghdad (Iraq)'69; MB ChB; DABR; FRCPC; DiagRad., University of Toronto; Langs: Arabic; (905)881-6929; helenjazrawy@gmail.com.

JBALA, Moulay A; CSSS de Papineau, 155 rue Maclaren E, Gatineau QC J8L 0C2; (Other Foreign)'99; CCFP; Staff, Hôpital de Papineau; (819)986-3341

JEAN, Andrea; Ctr Hosp Affilie-St-Sacrement, 1050 ch Sainte-Foy, Quebec QC G1S 4L8; Laval'94; Staff, Centre Hospitalier Affilié Universitaire de Québec - Hôpital du St-Sacrement; (418)686-7511

JEAN, Bernard; CSSS de la Vieille-Capitale, 1 av du Sacre-Coeur, Quebec QC G1N 2W1; Laval'76; Gen Practice, CSSS de la Vieille-Capitale; (418)691-0743

JEAN, Catherine; Centre de Sante des Femmes, 5180 boul Gouin O, Montreal QC H4J 1C3; McG'98; FRCSC; ObstGyn. Staff, Hôpital du Sacre-Coeur de Montréal; Langs: English; (514)333-8105

JEAN, Catherine; Centre Med du Christ-Roi, 102-40 rte du President-Kenned, Levis QC G6V 6C4; Laval'09; (418)833-4977; Fax. (418)833-9557.

JEAN, Christian; CHUQ-Hotel-Dieu De Quebec, 11 Cote Du Palais, Quebec QC G1R 2J6; Laval'84; FRCSC; ObstGyn. Staff, Centre Hospitalier Universitaire de Québec (CHUQ) - Siege Social; (418)691-5222; Fax. (418)691-5720.

JEAN, Claire; Clinique Medicale Sayabec, RR 1 99A rue de l'Eglise, Sayabec QC G0J 3K0; Laval'80; (418)536-5438; Fax. (418)536-5439.

JEAN, Dominique; Hop Du Sacre-Coeur de Mtl, 5400 boul Gouin O, Montreal QC H4J 1C5; Laval'88; CSPQ; Anes. Staff, Hôpital du Sacre-Coeur de Montréal; (514)338-2222 x2680; Fax. (514)338-2009.

JEAN, Gabriel; CSSS de la Cote-De-Gaspe, 215 boul De York O, Gaspe QC G4X 2W2; Mon'73; FRCSC; OrthSurg (Pediatrics). Staff, Centre Hospitalier de Gaspe; Langs: Bilingual(French/English); (418)368-3301; Fax. (418)368-3650.

JEAN, Isabelle; Dr Georges-L Dumont Reg Hosp, 330 av Universite, Moncton NB E1C 2Z3; Mon'88; Staff, Dr Georges-L-Dumont University Hospital Centre; (506)862-4113; isabellej@rogers.com.

JEAN, Renee; Dr Georges L-Dumont Reg Hosp, 330 av Universite, Moncton NB E1C 2Z3; Mon'94; Staff, Dr Georges-L-Dumont University Hospital Centre; (506)862-4000

JEAN, Sara-Elizabeth; CHUS-Hop Fleurimont, 3001 12e av N, Sherbrooke QC J1H 5N4; McG'06; MDCM; FRCPC; Derm. Staff, Centre Hospitalier Universitaire de Sherbrooke-Hopital Fleurimont; (819)346-1110

JEAN, Suzanne; Clin Med La Cite Place Du Parc, 900-300 rue Léo-Pariseau, Montreal QC H2X 4B3; Mon'81; ac Staff, Centre Hospitalier l'Université de Montréal (CHUM) - Hôtel-Dieu; (514)281-1722; Fax. (514)281-6697.

JEAN-DESTIN, Marie N; Clin Med Maisonneuve-Rosemont, 5345 boul de l'Assomption, Montreal QC H1T 4B3; (Haiti)'77; (514)257-7000

JEAN-FRANCOIS, Herve G; Ctr Hosp Pierre-Janet, 20 rue Pharand, Gatineau QC J9A 1K7; (Haiti)'96; Staff, Centre Hospitalier Pierre-Janet; (819)771-7761; Fax. (819)771-2908.

JEAN-LOUIS, Carlo; Clinique Med Mega-Force, 149 rue Saint-Pierre, Rimouski QC G5L 1T7; Port-Au-Prince (Haiti)'76; LMCC; CCFP; FCFP; Langs: Spanish; English; (418)723-7307

JEAN MARY, Evelyne; Hop Charles LeMoyne, 3120 boul Taschereau, Greenfield Park QC J4V 2H1; (Haiti)'95; FRCPC; RadOncol. Staff, Hopital Charles LeMoyne; (450)466-5000

JEAN-ST-MICHEL, Emilie M; The Hosp for Sick Children, 555 University Ave, Toronto ON M5G 1X8; McG'07; MDCM; Peds. Staff, The Hospital For Sick Children; (416)813-7500

JEANES, C William; 100 Island Lodge Rd, Ottawa ON K1N 0A2; Guy's Hospital (England)'43; Consultant Int'l Health & Tropical Med, Public Health Agency of Canada; (613)749-4227 Semi-Retired.

JEANMART, Cecile; Unite Med Familiale Maizerets, 2480 ch de la Canardiere, Quebec QC G1J 2G1; Laval'96; CCFP; (418)661-2428

JEANMART, Hugues; Hop du Sacre-Coeur de Mtl, 5400 boul Gouin O, Montreal QC H4J 1C5; Laval'97; FRCSC; CardSurg. Staff, Hôpital du Sacre-Coeur de Montréal; (514)338-2222

JEANNEAU, Robert; 1801 av Dollard, Lasalle QC H8N 1T9; Sher'75; FRCPC; Peds. Staff, McGill University Health Centre - Montreal Children's Hospital; (514)364-5229; Fax. (514)364-5221.

JEANNERET-GROSJEAN, Alphonse; CHUM-Hotel-Dieu, 3840 rue Saint-Urbain, Montreal QC H2W 1T8; Lausanne (Switzerland)'72; Respir; IntMed (Cystic Fibrosis). Staff, Centre Hospitalier l'Université de Montréal (CHUM) - Hôtel-Dieu; adj Prof, Universite de Montreal; Langs: German; Italian; Spanish; (514)890-8000 x15639; Fax. (514)412-7178; alph.jeanneret@sympatico.ca.

JEANNOT, Sandra; CSSS de Trois-Rivieres, 1991 boul du Carmel, Trois-Rivieres QC G8Z 3R9; Mon'06; CCFP; Staff, CSSS de Trois-Rivières; (819)697-3333

JEANNOTTE, Jean-Pierre; Clinique medicale du Luc, 33 rue Saint-Patrice E, Magog QC J1X 5B7; Mon'76; (819)843-3353; Fax. (819)843-7217.

JEANNOTTE, Simon; Hop Charles LeMoyne, 3120 boul Taschereau, Greenfield Park QC J4V 2H1; Sher'94; FRCPC; NuclearMed. Staff, Hopital Charles LeMoyne; (450)466-5000 x3413

JEANS, E Rose; Advanced Rejuvenation Med Spa, 425 Locust St, Burlington ON L7S 1T8; Wes'89; MedMicrobiol; InfectDis; IntMed. Med Dir, Advanced Rejuvenation Medical Spa; (905)340-0401; info@restoringnaturalbeauty.com.

JEANS-MINGO, Aulayne; 69 Abercrombie Rd, New Glasgow NS B2H 1K4; Dal'86; (902)752-5122

JEANSON, Pierre; Clinique d'Ophtalmologie, 328 boul Antonio-Barrette, N-D-Des-Prairies QC J6E 1G2; Mon'01; Ophth. (450)752-4141

JEAVONS, Michael M; Business Bldg, 604-94 Cumberland St, Toronto ON M5R 1A3; Birmingham (England)'72; MB ChB; FRCPC; Psy (HIV Psychiatry). Consultant, Meno-Ya-Wen Health Centre; Ac Staff, The Hospital For Sick Children; Pres, Source Line Inc.; University of Toronto; (416)925-8160 x225; Fax. (416)923-0438; mjeavons@sourceline.ca.

JEBAMANI, Samuel; 986B Portage Ave, Winnipeg MB R3G 0R6; Madras (India)'63; MB BS; MRCP(Lond); FRCPC; Peds. Staff, Health Sciences Centre; Staff, St Boniface General Hospital; Asst Prof, University of Manitoba; (204)774-1300; Fax. (204)774-2655.

JECEN, Nikole; Ctr Hosp de Lasalle, 8585 tsse Champlain, LaSalle QC H8P 1C1; New York (USA)'05; FRCPC; Anes. Staff, Centre Hospitalier de LaSalle; (514)362-8000; Fax. (514)367-8612.

JECHEL, Peter; Perth Med Clinic, 14 Isabella St, Perth ON K7H 2W6; Qns'84; CCFP; CCFP(E.M.); FCFP; Ac Staff, Perth & Smiths Falls District Hospital - Smiths Falls Site; Langs: German; (613)267-5556; Fax. (613)267-2641.

JEDNAK, Irene; Westmount Square Med Centre, C 180-1 car Westmount, Westmount QC H3Z 2P9; McG'93; Staff Omnipracticienne, Westmount Square Health Centre; Langs: Bilingual(French/English); (514)934-2334; Fax. (514)934-5559.

JEDNAK, Roman; MUHC-Montreal Children's Hosp, C 527-2300 rue Tupper, Montreal QC H3H 1P3; McG'92; BSc; FRCSC; Urol (Pediatric Urology). adj Chef cabinet, Shriners Hospitals For Children - Canada; Staff, McGill University Health Centre - Montreal Children's Hospital; Langs: French; Polish; Ukrainian; (514)412-4316; Fax. (514)412-4384; roman.jednak@muhc.mcgill.ca.

JEDRZKIEWICZ, Sean J; 300-690 Dorval Dr, Oakville ON L6K 3W7; McM'03; FRCPC; IntMed; Cardiol. (905)849-4567

JEE, Katie H; Centre Med Ste-Anne, 500 Old St. Patrick St, Ottawa ON K1N 9G4; Qns'09; CCFP; (613)789-1552

JEE, Robert M; BC Women's Hosp & Health Ctre, 4500 Oak St, Vancouver BC V6H 3N1; Qns'07; FRCPC; Anes. Staff, BC Women's Hospital & Health Centre; (604)875-2158

JEEJEEBHOY, Farida M; 230-2 County Court Blvd, Brampton ON L6W 3W8; Cal'95; FACC; FRCP; MD; FRCPC; IntMed (Clinical Cardiology); Cardiol. Court Staff Cardiologist, William Osler Health System - Brampton Civic Hospital; (905)451-0185; Fax. (905)451-4743; farida.j@sympatico.ca.

JEEJEEBHOY, Khursheed N; 5-4646 Dufferin St, Toronto ON M3H 5S4; Vellore (India)'59; MB BS; PhD(Lond); MRCP(Lond); FRCP(Eng); FRCPC; IntMed (Gastroenterology). Staff Physician, St Michael's Hospital; Emeritus Prof Med, University of Toronto; (416)645-5145; Fax. (416)645-1401; endoscopy@polyclinic.ca.

JEERAKATHIL, Thomas J; University of Alberta Hosp, 2E3 22WCM-8440 112 St NW, Edmonton AB T6G 2B7; Sask'95; BSc; MSc; Neur (Stroke). Staff, University of Alberta Hospital; Asst Prof, University of Alberta; (780)407-8786; Fax. (780)407-1325; thomasj@ualberta.ca.

JEEVA, Adam M; 103 Macleod Trail PO Box 5488 Stn Main, High River AB T1V 1M6; Dublin (Ireland)'58; LRCS; LRCP; Langs: Gujarati; (403)652-2682; Fax. (403)652-3166.

JEEVA, Ashref; 103 Macleod Trail PO Box 5634 Stn Main, High River AB T1V 1M7; Alb'93; CCFP; (403)652-2682; Fax. (403)652-3166.

JEEVA, Imraan; Addiction & Mental Hlth-Clarke, 250 College St, Toronto ON M5T 1R8; Wes'96; FRCPC; Psy. Staff, Centre for Addiction & Mental Health (CAMH) - College Street Site; (416)535-8501

JEEVANANDAM, Sivagami; Springdale Prof Bldg, 609-2250 Bovaird Dr E, Brampton ON L6R 0W3; Madras (India)'75; Ac Staff, William Osler Health System - Etobicoke General Hospital; (905)595-4963

JEEVES, Nicholas G; Mindemoya Med Clinic, PO Box 150 2120B Hwy 551, Mindemoya ON P0P 1S0; McM'90; Emerg Med, Manitoulin Health Centre - Mindemoya Site; (705)377-5371; Fax. (705)377-5372; ngjeeves@mhc.on.ca.

JEFFERIES, Ann Louise; Mount Sinai Hosp, 775A-600 University Ave, Toronto ON M5G 1X5; Tor'76; DABPed; MEd; FRCPC; Peds (Neonatal & Perinatal Medicine). Staff Neonatol, Mount Sinai Hospital; Assoc Staff, The Hospital For Sick Children; Assoc Prof Peds, University of Toronto; (416)586-8295

JEFFERIES, John W; 40 O'Brien St, Orillia ON L3V 5S3; Qns'70; BSc; FRCPC; IntMed (Gastroenterology). Consultant, Orillia Soldiers' Memorial Hospital; (705)326-8022; Fax. (705)326-5319.

JEFFERSON, Debra L; Newcastle Village Med Assoc, 87 Mill St N, Newcastle ON L1B 1H8; Wes'88; CCFP; FCFP; Ac Staff, Lakeridge Health - Bowmanville Site; (905)987-1896; Fax. (905)987-9894.

JEFFERY, Andrew H; Southlake Reg Health Centre, 596 Davis Dr, Newmarket ON L3Y 2P9; Jagiellonian U (Poland)'02; Staff, Southlake Regional Health Centre; (905)895-4521

JEFFERY, Anthony J; The Peterborough Clinic, 26 Hospital Dr, Peterborough ON K9J 7C3; Tor'86; BSc; Staff, Peterborough Regional Health Centre - Hospital Drive; (705)740-6840

JEFFERY, Deborah A; Associate Clinic, 5215 49 Ave, Wetaskiwin AB T9A 0R1; (South Africa)'93; CCFP; (780)352-7157; Fax. (780)352-2273.

JEFFERY, Deborah L; Univ of Waterloo, 200 University Ave W, Waterloo ON N2L 3G1; Tor'82; EmergMed. Teach Staff, University Of Waterloo; (519)888-4096

JEFFERY, Glenn J; Ermineskin Med Clinic, 301-2377 111 St NW, Edmonton AB T6J 5E5; Alb'85; (780)436-8731; Fax. (780)434-8732.

JEFFERY, Hartley F; Temiskaming Hosp, PO Box 4040 421 Shepherdson Rd, New Liskeard ON P0J 1P0; London (England)'62; MB BS; MRCS; LRCP; FRCS(E); FRCSC; GenSurg. Staff, Temiskaming Hospital; Langs: English; French; (705)647-5388; Fax. (705)647-5405.

JEFFERY, James W; 9-2168 Mccallum Rd, Abbotsford BC V2S 6R6; Sask'84; FRCSC; GenSurg. Consultant GenSurg, Mission Memorial Hospital; Consultant, Abbotsford Regional Hospital & Cancer Centre; (604)854-3955; Fax. (604)854-3965.

JEFFERY, John; Medical Arts Centre, 105-770 6 St SW, Medicine Hat AB T1A 4J6; Cal'82; BSc(Biol.); FRCSC; ObstGyn (Colposcopy). Staff, Medicine Hat Regional Hospital; (403)502-8932; Fax. (403)526-8824; aerobat@telusplanet.net.

JEFFERY, Roy D; Little Current Med Associates, PO Box 549, Little Current ON P0P 1K0; Ott'79; CCFP; FCFP; (705)368-2450; Fax. (705)368-2480; rdjeffery@mhc.on.ca.

JEFFERYS, Stephen G; Kelowna Pain Management Assoc, 2-3039 Pandosy St, Kelowna BC V1Y 1W3; Welsh National (Wales)'74; MB ChB; DRCOG; FFARCS; FRCPC; Anes (Pain Management). (778)478-0960

JEFFORD, Cheryl L; St Clare's Mercy Hosp, 154 Lemarchant Rd, St. John's NL A1C 5B8; Mem'98; FRCPC; DiagRad; NuclearMed. Staff, St Clare's Mercy Hospital; (709)777-5329

JEFFORD, Valerie J; Western Mem Reg Hosp, PO Box 2005 Stn Main 1 Brookfiel Ave, Corner Brook NL A2H 6J7; Mem'99; FRCSC; GenSurg. Staff, Western Memorial Regional Hospital; (709)637-5000

JEFFREY, Cam A; Colchester Surg Incorporated, 67 Dominion St, Truro NS B2N 3P2; Dal'04; BSc; MSc; FRCSC; GenSurg. Staff, Colchester East Hants Health Centre; (902)893-0133; Fax. (902)893-4787; cameron.jeffrey@cehha.nshealth.ca.

JEFFREY, John F; Kingston Gen Hosp, 76 Stuart St, Kingston ON K7L 2V7; Qns'78; LMCC; FRCSC; ObstGyn (Gynecologic Oncology). Ac Staff, Kingston General Hospital; Assoc Prof/Div Chair Div ofGynOncol, Queen's University; (613)548-6071; Fax. (613)548-1330.

JEFFRIES, Gregory A; Halton HSC Corp-Oakville, 327 Reynolds St, Oakville ON L6J 3L7; Tor'07; CCFP; Staff, Halton Healthcare Services Corporation - Oakville Site; (905)845-2571

JEFFRIES, J Joel; Addiction & Mental Hlth-Clarke, 250 College St, Toronto ON M5T 1R8; Dublin (Ireland)'63; MB BCh; BAO; MRCPsy; DFCPA; FRCPC; Psy (Psychosis). Staff, Centre for Addiction & Mental Health (CAMH) - College Street Site; Assoc Prof, University of Toronto; (416)979-6863; Fax. (416)979-6815; joel_jeffries@camh.net.

JEFFRIES, Jennifer F; Norwich Med Centre, P O Box 550 32 South Court St E, Norwich ON N0J 1P0; Boston (USA)'94; (519)863-2338

JEFREMOVA, Ljudmilla; East Whitby Med Centre, 6-1916 Dundas St E, Whitby ON L1N 2L6; Tartu (Estonia)'91; CCFP; (905)434-1662

JEGADESH, Beula S; Alberta Hosp Edmonton, PO Box 307 Stn Main, Edmonton AB T5J 2J7; Tamil Nadu (India)'00; FRCPC; Psy. Staff, Alberta Hospital Edmonton; (780)342-5438; Fax. (780)342-5233.

JEGATHEESWARAN, Dharmavathy; 301-3852 Finch Ave E, Scarborough ON M1T 3T9; (Sri Lanka)'72; MB BS; MD; Staff, The Scarborough Hospital - Birchmount Campus; (416)298-9956

JEGATHEESWARAN, Rajadurai; 301-3420 Finch Ave E, Scarborough ON M1W 2R6; (Sri Lanka)'83; MB BS; MRCOG(UK); MRCS; FRCSC; ObstGyn. Staff, The Scarborough Hospital - General Campus; Langs: Tamil; (416)498-3452

JEGEDE, R Olukayode; D-568 Christina St N, Sarnia ON N7T 5W6; Ibadan (Nigeria)'67; FRCPC; Psy (Child, Adolescent Stress). Staff Psy, Bluewater Health - Mitton Site; (519)344-1700; Fax. (519)344-0157.

JEH, Jusli P; Blue Quill Shopping Centre, 374 Saddleback Rd NW, Edmonton AB T6J 4R7; (Taiwan)'73; (780)437-5914; Fax. (780)448-9457.

JEI ALMDHEM, Mohamed Y; 216 D-245 Pelham Rd, St Catharines ON L2S 1X8; Al Fateh (Libya)'99; CCFP; (905)988-3700; Fax. (905)988-3703.

JEICAN, Brandusa R; Clin Externe de Sante Mentale, 200-237 boul Saint-Jean-Baptis, Chateauguay QC J6K 3C3; (Romania)'97; (450)692-0002

JEJE, Oluyemi M; London Reg Cancer Centre, 790 Commissioners Rd E, London ON N6A 4L6; Ibadan (Nigeria)'74; MB BS; LMCC; (519)685-8640; Fax. (519)685-8611.

JELANI, Anwar D; Royal Alexandra Hosp, 418 4-10240 Kingsway NW, Edmonton AB T5H 3V9; (Saudi Arabia)'95; Staff, Royal Alexandra Hospital; (780)735-5962; Fax. (780)669-7207.

JELENICH, Sandra E; St Michael's Hosp, 30 Bond St, Toronto ON M5B 1W8; Tor'75; BSc; FRCPC; Anes. Staff, St Michael's Hospital; Assoc Prof, University of Toronto; (416)864-5071

JELFIMOW, Peter V; 6-1540 Springhill Dr, Kamloops BC V2E 2H1; Sask'03; FRCSC; Ophth.

JELINEK, Henry J; Akron Pharmacy Ltd, 2318 Lake Shore Blvd W, Etobicoke ON M8V 1B5; Prague (Czech Republic)'60; Ac Staff, Trillium Health Centre - West Toronto; Langs: Czech; (416)252-1414; Fax. (416)252-3314.

JELLEMA, Dick; Pair O'Docs Incorporated, 5832 St Margaret's Bay Rd, Hubbards NS B3Z 2E4; UBC'93; FRCPC; Psy. (902)826-1901; Fax. (902)826-7981.

JELLICOE, Paul A; Health Sciences Centre, AD401-820 Sherbrook St, Winnipeg MB R3A 1R9; Manchester (England)'94; FRCSC; OrthSurg. Staff, Health Sciences Centre; (204)774-6511

JELLIE, Hugh G; Belmont Prof Centre, 306-564 Belmont Ave W, Kitchener ON N2M 5N6; Wes'80; DABOph; FRCSC; Ophth (Cornea). Med Dir, TLC Waterloo; (519)579-2020; Fax. (519)579-0800.

JELLOO, Mazin K A; Dr William H Newhook Comm HC, PO Box 449, Whitbourne NL A0B 3K0; Baghdad (Iraq)'81; MB ChB; LMCC; CCFP; Staff, Dr William H Newhook Health Centre; Langs: Arabic; (709)759-2300; jelloo@mun.ca.

JEN, Ho; University of Alberta Hosp, 41-8440 112 St NW, Edmonton AB T6G 2B7; McG'87; FRCPC; DiagRad; NuclearMed. Staff Diag Imaging, University of Alberta Hospital; (780)407-6907

JEN, Yun; Inst Nat'l De Sante Publique, 190 boul Cremazie E, Montreal QC H2P 1E2; Mon'95; FRCPC; CommunMed (Public Health). Physician, Institut National de Sante Publique du Quebec; (514)864-1600 x3737; yun_jen@ssss.gouv.qc.ca.

JENA, Debakanta; 105-266 4 St SW, Medicine Hat AB T1A 4E5; (India)'94; FRCSOrtho(Galsgow); Dip SportMed; MB BS; FRCSC; OrthSurg (Arthroplasty). Staff, Medicine Hat Regional Hospital; Clinical Asst Prof, University of Calgary; (403)488-6666; Fax. (403)488-6677.

JENEY, Christa M; St Joseph's Health Centre, 30 The Queensway, Toronto ON M6R 1B5; Tor'83; BSc; CCFP; FCFP; Ac Staff Family Med/Med Dir, St Joseph's Health Centre; Langs: Hungarian; (416)530-6860; Fax. (416)530-6139; jeneyc@stjoe.on.ca.

JENEY, Elizabeth V M; 634 Stone Church Rd W, Hamilton ON L9B 1A7; Tor'84; FRCSC; Otol (Ear Nose & Throat Surgery). Clinical Asst Prof, McMaster University; Langs: Hungarian; (905)575-4429; Fax. (905)575-4456.

JENICEK, Milos; McMaster University, 1280 Main St W, Hamilton ON L8S 4K1; Prague (Czech Republic)'59; PhD(Epidemiol); FRCPC; CommunMed (Epidemiology & Clinical Epidemiology). Prof Pt-Time/Staff Clin Epidemiol Biostatistics, McMaster University; Langs: French; Czech; (905)525-9140; Fax. (905)577-0017.

JENKEN, Carol L; 4-101 Burnside Rd W, Victoria BC V9A 1B7; Alb'78; (250)727-9932; Fax. (250)727-9936; edora.jenken@shaw.ca.

JENKEN, Daryl A; 2940 17 Ave SW, Calgary AB T3E 0A9; Cal'82; FRCSC; GenSurg (Colon & Rectal Surgery). (403)244-4844; Fax. (403)244-2268.

JENKIN, Jeffrey K; Sault Area Hosp, 750 Great Northern Rd, Sault Ste. Marie ON P6B 0A8; McM'78; DABR; FRCPC; DiagRad. Staff, Sault Area Hospital - Sault Ste Marie; (705)759-3434

JENKINS, Andrea N; Associate Med Clinic, PO Box 1059 1973 Columbia Ave, Rossland BC V0G 1Y0; Alb'98; CCFP; (250)362-7307

JENKINS, Catherine A; Royal Jubilee Hosp, 1952 Bay St, Victoria BC V8R 1J8; UBC'88; GeriatricMed; IntMed. Staff, Royal Jubilee Hospital; (250)370-8509; Fax. (250)370-8285.

JENKINS, Charles O; The Group Health Centre, 240 McNabb St, Sault Ste. Marie ON P6B 1Y5; Cambridge (England)'63; MB ChB; DRCOG; MRC(Lond); FRCPC; IntMed. Consultant, Sault Area Hospital - Sault Ste Marie; (705)759-1234 x630

JENKINS, David J A; Fitzgerald Bldg, 150 College St, Toronto ON M5S 3E2; Oxford (England)'71; BCh; DSc; FRCP(UK); FRCS; MD; FRCPC; MedScient(Med) (Clinical Nutrition). Assoc Physician, Toronto General Hospital - UHN; Prof Med, University of Toronto; (416)867-7475; cyril.kendall@utoronto.ca.

JENKINS, Deirdre A; Foothills Med Centre, C210-1403 29 St NW, Calgary AB T2N 2T9; Cal'98; BMLSc; FRCPC; IntMed (Hematology); Hem. Staff IntMed & Hem, Foothills Medical Centre; Asst Prof, University of Calgary; (403)944-4451

JENKINS, Donald; 643 6th St, Courtenay BC V9N 1M7; UBC'81; BSc; FRCPC; IntMed; Derm. Staff, St Joseph's General Hospital; Staff, Campbell River & District General Hospital; Staff, West Coast General Hospital; (250)334-4172; Fax. (250)334-4473.

JENKINS, Heather D; Dr Heather D Jenkins Inc, 4186 Dunbar St, Vancouver BC V6S 2E7; UBC'95; CCFP; (604)739-9881; Fax. (604)739-9803.

JENKINS, Huw; Central Alberta Prof Centre, 169-5201 43 St, Red Deer AB T4N 1C7; London (England)'71; MB; BSc; FRCPC; IntMed. Staff, Red Deer Regional Hospital Centre; (403)755-9270

JENKINS, John T; Lunenburg Med Clinic, PO Box 1450 42 High St, Lunenburg NS B0J 2C0; Dal'92; CCFP; Staff, Fishermen's Memorial Hospital; Staff, South Shore Regional Hospital; (902)634-7177; Fax. (902)634-4982.

JENKINS, Keith A; Child & Adolescent Trmt Ctre, 1240 10th St, Brandon MB R7A 7L6; Man'05; FRCPC; Psy.

JENKINS, Kenneth; Western Mem Reg Hosp, PO Box 2005 Stn Main 1 Brookfield Ave, Corner Brook NL A2H 6J7; Mem'84; BMedSci; Western Memorial Regional Hospital; Vice Pres Med Services, Western Health Care Corp; Langs: English; French; (709)637-5000

JENKINS, Mark R; 68 1re av, Verdun QC H4G 2V4; McG'10; MDCM; CCFP.

JENKINS, Martin F; 100-5791 No. 3 Rd, Richmond BC V6X 2C9; Cal'77; FRCPC; DiagRad. (604)278-9152; Fax. (604)278-9291.

JENKINS, Mary E; London HSC-University Hosp, PO Box 5339 Stn B A10 335-339 Windermere Rd, London ON N6A 5A5; Wes'97; FRCPC; Neur. Staff, London Health Sciences Centre - University Hospital; (519)663-3404; Fax. (519)663-3416.

JENKINS, Sarah J; Health Sciences Centre, 300 Prince Philip Dr, St. John's NL A1B 3V6; Mem'04; FRCPC; DiagRad. Staff, Health Sciences Centre; (709)737-6300

JENKINSON, Richard J; MG 321-2075 Bayview Ave, Toronto ON M4N 3M5; Wes'01; FRCSC; OrthSurg (Trauma). Staff Div of OrthSurg, Sunnybrook Health Sciences Centre; (416)480-6160; Fax. (416)480-5886.

JENKS, Lorena L; Fort Frances Clinic, 301 Victoria Ave, Fort Frances ON P9A 2C1; Qns'85; CCFP; FCFP; (807)274-3287; Fax. (807)274-7875.

JENNER, Julie A; Centretown Comm Health Centre, 420 Cooper St, Ottawa ON K2P 2N6; Wes'94; CCFP; Ac Staff, The Ottawa Hospital - Civic Campus; (613)233-4697; Fax. (613)233-4541; jjenner@centretownchc.org.

JENNER, Morris; Children's Aid Society, PO Box 7010 Stn Main 1680 Oxford St E, London ON N5Y 5R8; Sask'63; FRCPC; Peds (Pediatric Endocrinology). Staff, Children's Aid Society of London & Middlesex; (519)455-9000 x455

JENNINGS, Stacey L; Cobourg Health Centre, 203-316 King St E, Cobourg ON K9A 5R8; McM'04; CCFP; (905)373-1280

JENSEN, Brian W; PO Box 5695 Stn Main, High River AB T1V 1M7; Alb'81; CCFP; (403)652-7993; Fax. (403)652-7997.

JENSEN, Bryant J; 110-7 Strachan Bay SE, Medicine Hat AB T1B 4Y2; Alb'08; CCFP; (403)528-4490; Fax. (403)528-4481.

JENSEN, Carlye A; Uxbridge Family Health Clinic, B-2 Elgin Park Dr, Uxbridge ON L9P 0B1; Cal'03; CCFP; CCFP(E.M.); (905)852-1009

JENSEN, Christopher W B; Winnipeg Clinic, 5N-425 St Mary Ave, Winnipeg MB R3C 0N2; Man'78; FASTS; FRCSC; Urol (Organ Transplant). Staff, The Salvation Army Grace Hospital; Langs: English; French; (204)957-3306; Fax. (204)947-0450.

JENSEN, Derrek M; 1050 Leila Ave PO Box 49128 Rpo Garden City, Winnipeg MB R2V 4G8; Man'04; CCFP.

JENSEN, John L; Cape Breton Hlthcare Complex, 1482 George St, Sydney NS B1P 1P3; Alb'72; BSc; MedOncol; IntMed (Palliative Care). Staff, Cape Breton Healthcare Complex.

JENSEN, John M; Alder Medical Centre, 277 Evergreen Rd, Campbell River BC V9W 5Y4; Cape Town (South Africa)'78; MB ChB; (250)287-7441

JENSEN, Laura A; Lougheed Med Clinic, 145-9855 Austin Rd, Burnaby BC V3J 1N4; UBC'75; (604)421-2555

JENSEN, Meghan B; Castlegar Med Associates, 1008 Columbia Ave, Castlegar BC V1N 1H2; Alb'07; CCFP; (250)365-2161; Fax. (250)365-2171.

JENSEN, Paul; 208-3410 Sheppard Ave E, Scarborough ON M1T 3K4; Man'98; FRCPC; Neur. (416)492-6071; Fax. (416)492-9515.

JENSEN, Valerie M; Misericordia Community Hosp, 16940 87 Ave NW, Edmonton AB T5R 4H5; Cal'76; FRCPC; Anes. Staff, Covenant Health - Misericordia Community Hospital; (780)735-2863

JEON, Albert; Radiology Associates of Regina, 6-2727 Parliament Ave, Regina SK S4S 6X5; Mem'94; FRCPC; DiagRad. Staff, Radiology Associates of Regina; (306)352-7653; Fax. (306)522-4311.

JEON, Paul M; Health Sciences Centre, 300 Prince Philip Dr, St. John's NL A1B 3V6; Mem'85; FRCPC; DiagRad. Staff Radiol, Health Sciences Centre; (709)777-7650

JERAJ, Anthony F; Crescent Heights Med Centre, 49 8 St NW, Medicine Hat AB T1A 6N9; Guadalajara (Mexico)'86; CCFP; FCFP; Staff, Medicine Hat Regional Hospital; Langs: Spanish; (403)526-7422; Fax. (403)526-3349.

JEREMIC, Goran; Woodstock Gen Hosp, 310 Juliana Dr, Woodstock ON N4V 0A4; Tor'07; FRCSC; Otol (Head & Neck Surgery). Staff, Woodstock General Hospital; (519)421-4211

JERICHO, Monique C; Alberta Children's Hosp, 2888 Shaganappi Trail NW, Calgary AB T3B 6A8; Wes'02; FRCPC; Psy. Staff, Alberta Children's Hospital; (403)955-3066

JERJIAN, Yacoub; CSSS de Manicouagan, 635 boul Jolliet, Baie-Comeau QC G5C 1P1; Damascus (Syria)'84; Staff Anes, Centre Hospitalier Régional Baie-Comeau; (418)589-3701 x2786

JEROME, Amanda L; 14-2025 William O'Connell Blvd, Burlington ON L7M 4E4; McM'06; CCFP; (905)635-3632

JEROME, Dana C; Women's College Hosp, 1001-76 Grenville St, Toronto ON M5S 1B2; Wes'94; FRCPC; IntMed; Rheum. Staff, Women's College Hospital; (416)323-6344; Fax. (416)323-6115.

JEROME, Laurence; 90 Wharncliffe Rd S, London ON N6J 2K1; Manchester (England)'74; MB ChB; MSc; FRCPsy; FRCPC; Psy (Child Psychiatry). Aj Prof Psy, University of Western Ontario; (519)432-3818; Fax. (519)432-1748; ljerom2416@rogers.com.

JERUDI, Maher; Carbonear Gen Hosp, 86 Highroad South, Carbonear NL A1Y 1A4; Damascus (Syria)'94.

JESCHKE, Marc; Sunnybrook Hlth Sciences Ctre, D704-2075 Bayview Ave, Toronto ON M4N 3M5; Eberhard Karls University (Germany)'94; FRCSC; PlasSurg (Telehealth). Staff, Sunnybrook Health Sciences Centre; (416)480-6703; Fax. (416)480-6763.

JESIN, Aaron; Bathurst Med Centre, 203-4256 Bathurst St, North York ON M3H 5Y8; Wes'77; Ac Staff, North York General Hospital - Branson Division; Langs: Yiddish; Hebrew; (416)635-5012; Fax. (416)635-5018; aaron@drjesin.com.

JESIN, Edward C; City Centre Med Clinic, 130-5 Park Home Ave, North York ON M2N 6L4; Tor'87; Staff, North York General Hospital - Branson Division; (416)730-9588; Fax. (416)590-9371.

JESMIN, Rownak S; Medica One, 1275 Rymal Rd E, Hamilton ON L8W 3N1; Chittagong (Bangladesh)'93; CCFP; (905)387-0005; Fax. (905)387-0010.

JESPERSEN, Bruce W; Oakridge Shopp Centre, 45-2580 Southland Dr SW, Calgary AB T2V 4J8; Alb'74; Staff, Rockyview General Hospital; (403)571-0755; Fax. (403)571-0759.

JESPERSEN, Denise M; Dufferin Vaughan Med Clinic, 2-9200 Dufferin St, Vaughan ON L4K 0C6; Tor'95; CCFP; (905)417-3125; Fax. (905)417-3105.

JESSA, Karim K; Mackenzie Richmond Hill Hosp, 10 Trench St, Richmond Hill ON L4C 4Z3; Tor'91; FRCPC; EmergMed. Staff, Mackenzie Richmond Hill Hospital; (905)883-2241

JESSA, Shamim; Saddletowne Med Clinic, 914 Saddletowne Cir, Calgary AB T3J 0H5; New South Wales (Australia)'74; MB BS; LMCC; Langs: Hindi; Gujarati; (403)590-7710; Fax. (403)590-7113; shamimjessa@aol.com.

JESSAMINE, Peter G; The Ottawa Hosp-Gen Campus, 501 Smyth, Ottawa ON K1H 8L6; Ott'83; FRCPC; IntMed; MedMicrobiol; InfectDis. Staff Microbiol & InfectDis, The Ottawa Hospital - General Campus; (613)798-5555 x79138; jessamine@ottawahospital.on.ca.

JESSAMY, Nalya T; Womens Hlth in Womens Hands, 500-2 Carlton St, Toronto ON M5B 1J3; McM'05; CCFP; (416)593-7655 x230; Fax. (416)848-6255.

JESSOP, Darrell J; Pitt Meadows Med Clinic, 125-19150 Lougheed Hwy, Pitt Meadows BC V3Y 2H6; Alb'93; (604)465-4911

JESSUP, Jennifer L; Mount St Joseph Hosp, 3080 Prince Edward St, Vancouver BC V5T 3N4; UBC'04; DiagRad. Staff, Providence Health Care - Mount Saint Joseph Hospital; (604)874-1141

JETHA, Mary M; University of Alberta Hosp, 8440 112 St NW, Edmonton AB T6G 2B7; Cal'00; BPE; BSc; FRCPC; Peds; Endocrin&Metab. Staff, University of Alberta Hospital; Staff, Edmonton Clinic Health Academy; (780)407-1568; Fax. (780)407-1509.

JETHA, Nasir; 201-718 Broadway W, Vancouver BC V5Z 1G8; Pahlavi (Iran)'78; FRCPC; Peds. Med Dir Children's Centre, Providence Health Care - Mount Saint Joseph Hospital; Staff, BC Women's Hospital & Health Centre; Staff, BC Children's Hospital; Clin Assoc Prof, University of British Columbia; Langs: Farsi; Gujarati; Hindi; Kiswahili; Punjabi; Urdu; (604)325-5201

JETHA, Shamin; 202-718 Broadway W, Vancouver BC V5Z 1G8; Shiraz (Iran)'79; CCFP; Ac Staff, Vancouver General Hospital - Centennial Pavillion; Langs: Farsi; Hindi; Persian; Kacchi; Swahili; Urdu; (604)873-8011; Fax. (604)873-5675.

JETHALAL, Bhiku; 316-1200 Markham Rd, Scarborough ON M1H 3C3; Natal (South Africa)'68; FRCPC; IntMed (Clinical Immunology & Allergy). Court Staff, The Scarborough Hospital - Birchmount Campus; Langs: Hindi; Gujarati; (416)289-3221; Fax. (416)289-3181; jethalal@rogers.com.

JETHWA, Anita; 13175 Yonge St, Richmond Hill ON L4E 0G6; Tor'00; FRCPC; Peds. Staff, Markham Stouffville Hospital; (905)954-4011

JETHWA, Arvind K N; Carling Heights Med Centre, 124 Barker St, London ON N5Y 1Y1; Bristol (England)'66; MB ChB; University of Western Ontario; Langs: Gujarati; (519)451-1363; Fax. (519)451-1162.

JETLY, Rakesh; Canadian Forces Supp Unit HCC, 1745 Alta Vista Dr, Ottawa ON K1A 0K6; Tor'91; FRCPC; Psy. Staff, Canadian Forces Health Services Centre; (613)680-3578; Fax. (613)992-6095.

JETTE, Johanie; CSSS du Nord de Lanaudière, 1000 boul Sainte-Anne, St-Charles-Brromee QC J6E 6J2; Laval'09; CCFP; Staff, Centre Hospitalier Régional de Lanaudière; (450)759-8222

JETTE, Julie; CLSC Chateauguay, 95 av de la Verdure, Chateauguay QC J6K 0E8; Mon'06; (450)699-3333

JETTE, Nathalie; Foothills Med Centre, C1209-1403 29 St NW, Calgary AB T2N 2T9; Ott'98; BSc(Hon)Biology; MSc; FRCP; FRCPC; Neur (Epilepsy). Assoc Prof Clinical Neurosciences, Foothills Medical Centre; Asst Prof, University of Calgary; Langs: Bilingual(English/French); (403)944-2760; Fax. (403)944-0988.

JETTE, Pierre; CSSS Pierre Boucher, 1333 boul Jacques-Cartier E, Longueuil QC J4M 2A5; Mon'79; GenSurg. Staff, Centre Hospitalier Pierre Boucher; (450)468-8111

JETTE-GRENIER, Marie; Clinique Familiale, 102-6955 boul Taschereau, Brossard QC J4Z 1A7; Mon'76; (450)656-2310; Fax. (450)656-2619; benoitgrenier@sympatico.ca.

JETTE-YANIRE, Sylvie; Clinique Med Brien, 102-223 Boul Brien, Repentigny QC J6A 6M4; Mon'81; (450)585-9810; Fax. (450)585-8538.

JETTY, Mandip K; 5230 Mitch Owens Rd RR 1, Manotick ON K4M 1B2; Ott'02; CCFP; (613)692-2571; Fax. (613)692-0271.

JETTY, Prasad; The Ottawa Hosp-Civic Campus, A280-1053 Carling Ave, Ottawa ON K1Y 4E9; McG'97; FRCSC; GenSurg; VascSurg. Staff, The Ottawa Hospital - Civic Campus; (613)761-4766

JETTY, Radha; Children's Hosp Eastern Ont, 401 Smyth Rd, Ottawa ON K1H 8L1; McG'03; FRCPC; Peds. Consultant Pediatrician, Children's Hospital of Eastern Ontario (CHEO); (613)737-7600

JEU, Joan P; Ellesmere Health Care, 1-2060 Ellesmere Rd, Scarborough ON M1H 2V6; Tor'83; BScPharm; CCFP; Court Staff, Rouge Valley Health System - Centenary Health Centre Site; (416)439-2273

JEUN, Bing W; 300-1428 Ouellette Ave, Windsor ON N8X 1K4; Ott'60; FRCPC; IntMed (Neurology). Hon Staff Med, Windsor Regional Hospital - Metropolitan Site; (519)258-4121; Fax. (519)258-2184.

JEVNIKAR, Anthony M; London HSC-University Hosp, PO Box 5339 Stn B 339 Windermere Rd, London ON N6A 5A5; Wes'81; FRCPC; IntMed. Staff Nephrol, London Health Sciences Centre - University Hospital; Prof Med, University of Western Ontario; (519)663-3688; Fax. (519)663-8808; anthony.jevnikar@lhsc.on.ca.

JEVREMOVIC, Alexandra; 10-10 Headdon Gate, Richmond Hill ON L4C 8A3; Qns'98; FRCPC; Peds (Pediatric Cardiology); Cardiol. Staff, Mackenzie Richmond Hill Hospital; Assoc Staff, The Hospital For Sick Children; Regional Affiliate, Royal Victoria Regional Health Centre; Langs: French; Serbian; (905)770-5661; Fax. (905)770-3381.

JEVREMOVIC, Tatiana; Fowler Kennedy Sport Med Clin, 3M-1151 Richmond St, London ON N6A 3K7; McG'99; CCFP; CCFP(E.M.); (519)661-3011

JEWELL, Kristyn S; 204-720 Spadina Ave, Toronto ON M5S 2T9; McM'09; CCFP; (416)928-0920

JEWER, Carolyn M; Family First Medical, 207-496 Topsail Rd, St. John's NL A1E 2C2; Mem'09; CCFP.

JEWER, Craig M; Central Nlfd Reg Hlth Centre, 50 Union St, Grnd-Falls-Wi NL A2A 2E1; Mem'00; FRCPC; DiagRad. Staff, Central Newfoundland Regional Health Centre; (709)292-2500

JEWER, D Lee; Social Development Canada, 333 North River Rd, Ottawa ON K1A 0L1; Mem'78; (613)952-3623

JEWER, David D; Health Sciences Centre, 1842-300 Prince Philip Dr, St. John's NL A1B 3V6; Mem'81; BSc(Hon); BMedSci; FRCSC; PlasSurg (Hand Surgery). Staff Surgeon, Janeway Children's Health & Rehabilitation Centre; Staff Surgeon, Health Sciences Centre; Surgeon Full-Time, Eastern Health Authoriy; Clin Assoc Prof Surg, Memorial University Of Newfoundland; (709)777-6437; Fax. (709)777-6295; d.jewer@nf.sympatico.ca.

JEWERS, Paul C; Central Queens Health Centre, PO Box 9, Hunter River PE C0A 1N0; Dal'89; BSc; Physician Family Med, Queen Elizabeth Hospital; (902)621-3050; Fax. (902)621-3069.

JEWETT, Lawrence C; 800 Baker St, Cranbrook BC V1C 1A2; Dal'74; FRCSC; Otol (Facial Plastic Surgery). Member Executive Council, College of Physicians & Surgeons of British Columbia; (250)489-3323; Fax. (250)489-5233; lcjewett.md@shaw.ca.

JEWETT, Michael A S; Univ Hlth Network-Princess M, 3 130-610 University Ave, Toronto ON M5G 2M9; Qns'68; FRCSC; Urol (Oncology)., Princess Margaret Hospital - University Health Network; Chair Div of Urology/Prof, University of Toronto; (416)946-2909; Fax. (416)598-9997; m.jewett@utoronto.ca.

JEWSON, Frederick A; 29 Sparling Cres PO Box 1648 Stn Main, St Marys ON N4X 1B9; Wes'76; Ac Staff, St Marys Memorial Hospital - Huron Perth Healthcare Alliance; (519)284-2370; fjewson@stmmc.ca.

JEYABALAN, Neera; Lakeridge Hlth Corp-Oshawa, 1 Hospital Crt, Oshawa ON L1G 2B9; McM'01; FRCPC; IntMed; MedOncol. Staff, Lakeridge Health - Oshawa Site; (905)387-9495

JEYAKUMAR, Alwin; Queen Elizabeth II HSC, 465-1276 South Park St, Halifax NS B3H 2Y9; Ibadan (Nigeria)'92; MB BS; FRCPC; IntMed; MedOncol. Staff, Queen Elizabeth II Health Sciences Centre - Victoria General Site; (902)473-8317

JEYALINGAM, Kanapathipillai; Rouge Valley-Ajax & Pickering, 580 Harwood Ave S, Ajax ON L1S 2J4; Colombo (Sri Lanka)'82; FRCPC; IntMed. Staff, Rouge Valley Health System - Ajax & Pickering Health Centre Site; (905)683-2320; kjey91@rogers.com.

JEYAPRAGASAN, Manjula; Rosedale Med Centre, 711-600 Sherbourne St, Toronto ON M4X 1W4; Colombo (Sri Lanka)'85; CCFP; Langs: Tamil; (416)929-0929; Fax. (416)929-8084.

JEYARAJ, Hamilton; Oshawa Health Centre, 1F-247 Simcoe St N, Oshawa ON L1G 4T3; Kasturba (India)'03; CCFP; (905)728-7915

JEYARAJ, Leo; The Ottawa Hosp-Civic Campus, 1053 Carling Ave, Ottawa ON K1Y 4E9; Tamil Nadu (India)'93; Staff, The Ottawa Hospital - Civic Campus; (613)798-5555

JEYARANJAN, A Richard; Sheppard Med Bldg, 309-701 Sheppard Ave E, North York ON M2K 2Z3; Peradeniya (Sri Lanka)'82; PhD; MB BS; FRCPC; IntMed (Cardiology). Langs: Tamil; (416)222-8004; Fax. (416)222-8004.

JEZDIC, Dusanka D; Lakeshore Health Centre, PO Box 670 330 Notre Dame St, Belle River ON N0R 1A0; Wes'92; (519)728-0777

JHA, Muneesh; Toronto East Gen & Orth Hosp, 825 Coxwell Ave, Toronto ON M4C 3E7; (Ireland)'05; CCFP; Staff, Toronto East General Hospital Inc; (416)461-8272

JHA, Naresh; Cross Cancer Institute, 11560 University Ave NW, Edmonton AB T6G 1Z2; Delhi (India)'79; MB BS; FRCPC; RadOncol (Head & Neck). Sr Staff RadOncol, Cross Cancer Institute; Asst Prof, University of Alberta; (780)432-8755; Fax. (780)432-8380.

JHA, Neilank K; 105-901 King St W, Toronto ON M5V 3H5; McM'04; FRCSC; Neursurg. Staff, Toronto Western Hospital - University Health Network; (416)599-6000

JHA, Prabhat K S; St Michael's Hosp, 30 Bond St, Toronto ON M5B 1W8; Man'88; PhD; Staff, St Michael's Hospital; (416)864-6042 x2379; Fax. (416)864-5256.

JHA, Sapna; Family Practice Health Centre, 3F-77 Grenville St, Toronto ON M5S 1B3; Tor'10; CCFP; (416)323-6255

JHA, Umesh C; Halifax Prof Centre, 263-5991 Spring Garden Rd, Halifax NS B3H 1Y6; Lucknow (India)'64; BSc; MB BS; DPM(Lond); FRCPC; Psy (Family Therapy). Physician, Halifax Correctional Centre; Physician, Northwood Care Centre; (902)429-1122; Fax. (902)429-1122.

JHAMANDAS, Jack H; Heritage Med Research Centre, 530-107 University Campus NW, Edmonton AB T6G 2S2; Cal'79; PhD; FRCPC; Neur. Medical Staff Neurol, University of Alberta Hospital; Assoc Dean Research/Assoc Prof Neurol, University of Alberta; (780)407-7153; Fax. (780)407-3410.

JHAMEEL, Rafet; 5720 Glover Rd, Langley BC V3A 4H8; Baghdad (Iraq)'92; (604)530-2374

JHANDIR, Muhammad F M; 3330-3330 Hospital Dr NW, Calgary AB T2N 4N1; (Pakistan)'98; MB BS; MD; FRCPC; IntMed (Vascular Medicine). Staff, Foothills Medical Centre; (403)220-8382

JHAVERI, Faeza; Kitchener Waterloo Travel Clin, 902-570 University Ave E, Waterloo ON N2K 4P2; Natal (South Africa)'88; CCFP; Med Dir, Kitchener Waterloo Travel Clinic; (519)570-1280; Fax. (519)570-2808.

JHAVERI, Kartik S; Univ Hlth Network-Princess M, 3 957-610 University Ave, Toronto ON M5G 2M9; Bombay (India)'95; DMRD; Staff, Princess Margaret Hospital - University Health Network; (416)946-4501 x5635; Fax. (416)946-6564.

JHAWAR, Balraj; 205-1106 Ouellette Ave, Windsor ON N9A 1C9; Wes'94; MSc; FRCSC; Neursurg (Skull Base Surgery). Staff Neurosurg, Hôtel-Dieu Grace Hospital; (519)973-8771; Fax. (519)973-4690.

JHIRAD, Reuven R; Halton Family Health Centre, 2951 Walker's Line, Burlington ON L7M 4Y1; Tor'90; CCFP; FCFP; Teach Staff Med, University of Toronto; (905)336-3437; Fax. (905)639-0608.

JHIRAD, Ronen H; Health Park, 403A-45 Weatherbee Rd, Mira Road NS B1M 0A1; Tor'90; FRCSC; GenSurg; VascSurg. (902)567-5304; Fax. (902)567-5305.

JIA, Xiaoyan; Murrayville Health Care Centre, 104-22112 52 Ave, Langley BC V2Y 2M6; (China)'83; FRCPC; Peds. Staff, City Square Medical Centre; Langs: Japanese; Mandarin; (604)514-7777

JIANG, Chaozhe; Joseph Brant Mem Hosp, 1230 North Shore Blvd E, Burlington ON L7S 1W7; Zhejiang (China)'83; FRCPC; AnatPath (Cytopath). Staff, Joseph Brant Memorial Hospital; (905)632-3737 x1212; Fax. (905)336-6483; cjiang@jbmh.com.

JIANG, Charles C Y; Midtown Med Clinic, 130-8780 Blundell Rd, Richmond BC V6Y 3Y8; Shanghai (China)'93; (604)277-9006

JIANG, Hongxing; Orthopaedic Consultants, 10972 124 St NW, Edmonton AB T5M 0H8; (China)'82; FRCSC; OrthSurg (Spine & Hips). Specialist Orthoped, Royal Alexandra Hospital; Specialist Orthoped, University of Alberta Hospital; Asst Prof, University of Alberta; Langs: Chinese; (780)732-3722; Fax. (780)451-1437.

JIANG, Shelly; Clinique Mistissini, GD 395 boul Mistissini, Mistissini QC G0W 1C0; McG'09; (418)923-3376

JIANG, Xiu Yan; Calgary Lab Services, 9-3535 Research Rd NW, Calgary AB T2L 2K8; (China)'85; FRCPC; AnatPath (Hematology Pathology). Staff, Calgary Laboratory Services; (403)770-3548; Fax. (403)770-3738.

JIARAVUTHISAN, Michael; Caroline Med Group, 8-3305 Harvester Rd, Burlington ON L7N 3N2; McM'05; Derm. (905)336-9624

JIARAVUTHISAN, Somchai; Glazier Med Centre, 11 Gibb St, Oshawa ON L1H 2J9; Mahidol (Thailand)'70; FRCPC; Neur (Headache). Court Staff, Lakeridge Health - Oshawa Site; Langs: Thai; (905)579-1212 x334; Fax. (905)579-5548.

JIBB, Norma E; Sunridge Prof Centre, 412-2675 36 St NE, Calgary AB T1Y 6H6; Qns'72; ABIM; FRCPC; IntMed; Rheum. Asst Prof, University of Calgary; (403)265-9494; Fax. (403)291-9474.

JIBODH, Rawle M; 2-700 Markham Rd, Scarborough ON M1H 2A7; West Indies (Jamaica)'73; FSOGC; FACOG; FACS; FRCSC; ObstGyn. Staff, The Scarborough Hospital - Birchmount Campus; (416)430-0010; Fax. (416)430-0064.

JICHICI, Draga; Norfolk Med Centre, 204-85 Norfolk St, Guelph ON N1H 4J4; McM'89; FRCPC; Neur (Critical Care Medicine). Staff, Hamilton Health Sciences Centre - Hamilton General Hospital; Associate Clin Prof Critical Care Med & Neurol, McMaster University; (519)821-4421; Fax. (519)821-3341.

JIJON, Humberto B; Health Science Centre, 3280-3330 Hospital Dr NW, Calgary AB T2N 4N1; Cal'07; Gastroent; IntMed. (403)592-5020

JILANI, Amer M; Kawartha Reg Memory Clinic, 168 Brock St, Peterborough ON K9H 2P4; Punjab (Pakistan)'88; (705)749-3906; Fax. (705)749-2778.

JILAVEANU PELMUS, Manuela; SMBD Jewish Gen Hosp, 3755 ch Cote-Sainte-Catherine, Montreal QC H3T 1E2; Bucarest (Romania)'87; AnatPath. Staff, Sir Mortimer B Davis Jewish General; (514)349-8274; Fax. (514)340-8102.

JILESEN, Herman C; 9292 Highway 93 Box 1 RR 2, Midland ON L4R 4K4; Qns'73; BSc(Hons); Ac Staff, Georgian Bay General Hospital - Midland; Coroner, Ministry of the Solicitor General; (705)527-6560; Fax. (705)527-1773.

JILKINA, Tatiana A; La Vie Executive Health Centre, 525 Legget Dr, Kanata ON K2K 2W2; (Russia (Federation))'87; CCFP; (613)592-0862

JILLOOD, Ibrahim K; Alberta Mental Health Clinic, 200 5 Ave S, Lethbridge AB T1J 4L1; (Iraq)'67; MB ChB; DPM(UK); MRCPsy(UK); FRCPsy(UK); Consultant Psy, Chinook Regional Hospital; Consultant Psy, Alberta Mental Health Board; Consultant Psy, Lethbridge Mental Health Clinic; Consultant Psy, Fort MacLeod Mental Health Rural Clinic; Langs: Arabic; (403)381-5260; Fax. (403)382-4518.

JILWAN, Antoine R; CHUM-Hop Notre-Dame, 1560 rue Sherbrooke E, Montreal QC H2L 4M1; Angers (France)'72; Staff, Centre Hospitalier l'Université de Montréal (CHUM) - Hôpital Notre-Dame; (514)890-8000 x26558; Fax. (514)866-5261.

JIM, Gung Kyn; Queen Elizabeth II Hosp, 10409 98 St, Grande Prairie AB T8V 2E8; UBC'96; FRCPC; DiagRad. Staff, Queen Elizabeth II Hospital; (780)538-7440; Fax. (780)538-7450.

JIM, Harry; Woodbine Med Centre, 9-76 Arlington Dr, Keswick ON L4P 0A9; Mem'82; MD; Med Staff Assoc, Southlake Regional Health Centre; Langs: Chinese; (905)476-0308; Fax. (905)476-1079.

JIM, Jean S; McKnight Village Medical, 5486 Falsbridge Dr NE, Calgary AB T3J 5H4; Dal'84; BScPharm; MBA; CCFP; (403)280-2272

JIM, King T; The Medical Centre, 7 Pinsent Dr, Grnd-Falls-Wi NL A2A 2S8; Dal'75; Staff, Central Newfoundland Regional Health Centre; (709)489-1200; Fax. (709)489-6724.

JIM, Kym Lee; Central Alberta Med Imaging, 4312 54 Ave, Red Deer AB T4N 4M1; Cal'92; FRCPC; IntMed; Nephrol. (403)314-1435; Fax. (403)314-1437.

JIMENEZ, Edgar M; Peace Arch Hosp, 15521 Russell Ave, White Rock BC V4B 2R4; Man'07; Staff, Peace Arch Hospital; (604)531-5512

JIMENEZ, Elizabeth; Bloorview Kids Rehab, 150 Kilgour Rd, Toronto ON M4G 1R8; Tor'98; FRCPC; Peds (Developmental Pediatrics). Staff, Holland Bloorview Kids Rehabilitation Hospital; (416)425-6220 x6057

JIMENEZ, Tomas Y; London East Med Centre, 295 Saskatoon St, Stratford ON N5A 6A2; Wes'04; CCFP; CCFP(E.M.); Staff, Stratford General Hospital - Huron Perth Healthcare Alliance; (519)659-1122

JIMENEZ, Vania J; CLSC Cote-des-Neiges, 5700 ch de la Cote-des-Neiges, Montreal QC H3T 2A8; McG'71; CCFP; FCFP; Staff, Sir Mortimer B Davis Jewish General; (514)731-8531; Fax. (514)731-0563; vjimenez@ssss.gouv.qc.ca.

JIMENEZ FIEDLER, Waldo G; Juravinski Cancer Centre, 699 Concession St, Hamilton ON L8V 5C2; Conception (Peru)'97; (905)389-5688; Fax. (905)575-6343.

JIMENEZ-GUERRA, Idalberto; Kindersley Med Clinic, PO Box 1390, Kindersley SK S0L 1S0; (306)463-2621

JIMENEZ JUAN, Laura; Sunnybrook Hlth Sciences Ctre, 2075 Bayview Ave, Toronto ON M4N 3M5; (Spain)'02; Staff, Sunnybrook Health Sciences Centre; (416)480-6100; Fax. (416)480-6033.

JIMENEZ RIVERA, Carolina D; Children's Hosp of Eastern Ont, 401 Smyth Rd, Ottawa ON K1H 8L1; (Costa Rica)'94; Staff Peds, Children's Hospital of Eastern Ontario (CHEO); (613)737-2516

JIMENEZ ZEPEDA, Victor H; Univ Hlth Network-Princess M, 5 226-610 University Ave, Toronto ON M5G 2M9; (Mexico)'01; Staff, Princess Margaret Hospital - University Health Network.

JIMOH, Olubukola; Niagara Med Prof Centre, PO Box 10 1882 Niagara Stone Rd, Virgil ON L0S 1T0; Kwazulu-Natal (South Africa)'05; CCFP; (905)468-3275

JIN, Albert Y; Kingston Gen Hosp, 76 Stuart St, Kingston ON K7L 2V7; McM'01; FRCPC; Neur. Staff, Kingston General Hospital; (613)548-2472

JIN, Eddy Y H; North York Gen Hosp, 4001 Leslie St, North York ON M2K 1E1; UBC'99; CCFP; CCFP(E.M.); Staff, North York General Hospital; (416)756-6882

JIN, Edward G J; 205-4800 Leslie St, North York ON M2J 2K9; Tor'77; FAAP; FRCPC; Peds. Staff, The Hospital For Sick Children; Staff, St Michael's Hospital; Staff, North York General Hospital; Lecturer, University of Toronto; (416)494-3122; Fax. (416)494-3120.

JIN, Fengling; Thunder Bay Reg HSC-T-Bay, 980 Oliver Rd, Thunder Bay ON P7B 6V4; Beijing (China)'86; FRCPC; Anes. Staff, Thunder Bay Regional Health Sciences Centre; (807)684-6290

JIN, Jing; Yonge-Eglinton Med Centre, LL01-2401 Yonge St, Toronto ON M4P 3H1; Qns'07; CCFP; (416)544-9065; Fax. (416)544-9063.

JIN, Sheila Y M; North York Health Centre, 209-1262 Don Mills Rd, North York ON M3B 2W7; Tor'91; (416)449-2100; Fax. (416)449-2105.

JINA, Abdul F; 1057 Ouellette Ave, Windsor ON N9A 4J8; McM'74; FRCPC; IntMed. (519)255-9670; Fax. (519)255-7075.

JINAPRIYA, Delan; Hotel-Dieu Hosp, 166 Brock St, Kingston ON K7L 5G2; Qns'03; FRCSC; Ophth. Staff, Hotel-Dieu Hospital; (613)544-3400

JINCHEREAU, Pierre; CHUQ-St-Francois D'Assise, 10 rue de l'Espinay, Quebec QC G1L 3L5; Laval'73; CCFP; Ac Staff, Centre Hospitalier Universitaire De Québec - Pavillon De St-françois-d'assise; (418)525-4351; Fax. (418)525-4322; pierre.jinchereau@chuq.qc.ca.

JINDAL, Catherine M; Huntsville Prof Bldg, 106-348 Muskoka Rd 3 N, Huntsville ON P1H 1H8; Ott'92; (705)789-1977; Fax. (705)789-6330.

JINDAL, Kailash K; Clinical Sciences Bldg, CSB 11 107-152 University Camp, Edmonton AB T6G 2G3; Jammu-Kashmir (India)'75; FRCPC; IntMed; Nephrol. Dir, Northern Alberta Renal Program; Prof, University of Alberta; Langs: Punjabi; Hindi; (780)407-1098; Fax. (780)407-7771; kjindal@ualberta.ca.

JINDAL, Sanjay K; Huntsville Prof Bldg, 106-348 Muskoka Rd 3 N, Huntsville ON P1H 1H8; Ott'90; FRCPC; IntMed. Staff, Huntsville District Memorial Hospital - Muskoka Algonquin Healthcare; Langs: Bilingual(English/French); (705)787-1491; Fax. (705)789-6330.

JINDAL, Vinay K; Danforth Med Centre, 880 Danforth Rd, Scarborough ON M1K 1H8; Tor'95; CCFP; FCFP; (416)264-4848

JING, Nin; South Bridge Med Clinic, 2-2780 Totten St, Windsor ON N9B 0A9; Nanjing (China)'95; CCFP; Langs: Chinese; (519)253-2888; Fax. (519)253-0444.

JINNAH, Inez F; Near North Med Clinic, 201-66 Josephine St, North Bay ON P1B 0A7; Witwatersrand (South Africa)'88; CCFP; FCFP; (705)495-2685; Fax. (705)495-4218.

JINNAH, Rashid A; King Street Med Arts Centre, 505-71 Kings St W, Mississauga ON L5B 4A2; Tor'91; OrthSurg. Staff, Trillium Health Centre - Mississauga; (905)848-4362; Fax. (905)848-6929.

JINOT, Christopher P; Central Algoma Med Group, PO Box 398 9242 Taylor St, Bruce Mines ON P0R 1C0; McM'94; CCFP; FCFP; Langs: French; Spanish; (705)785-3495; Fax. (705)785-3672.

JIONA, Andree; Ctr Hosp Trois-Riv-St-Joseph, 731 rue Sainte-Julie, Trois-Rivieres QC G9A 1Y1; Laval'84; Staff, Centre Hospitalier Regional de Trois-Rivieres; (819)372-3536; Fax. (819)372-3509.

JIPA, George; CLSC Notre-Dame-De-Grace, 110-2525 boul Cavendish, Montreal QC H4B 2Y4; Bucarest (Romania)'80; (514)485-1670

JIPA, Ileana; CLSC Villeray, 1425 rue Jarry E, Montreal QC H2E 1A7; Mon'80; CCFP; FCFP; (514)376-4141; Fax. (514)376-7650.

JIRJIS, Luma M; Kingsridge Med Centre, 2-2015 Kingsridge Dr, Oakville ON L6M 4Y7; Baghdad (Iraq)'90; MB ChB; CCFP; (905)827-3006; Fax. (905)825-9431; lumajirjis@hotmail.com.

JIRSCH, Dennis W; 10221 129 St NW, Edmonton AB T5N 1W8; Alb'67; MSc; PhD(Surg); MBA; FRCSC; GenSurg (Gastroenterology). Ac Staff, Royal Alexandra Hospital; Clin Prof Surg/Aj Prof, University of Alberta; (780)735-6924; djirsch@shaw.ca.

JIRSCH, Jeffrey D; Univ of Alberta Hosp, 2E3 31WCM-8440 112 St NW, Edmonton AB T6G 2B7; Tor'98; FRCPC; Neur. Staff Neurol, University of Alberta Hospital; (780)407-3616

JIVAN, Verandra P; Westbram Family Physicians, 104-100 Pertosa Dr, Brampton ON L6X 0H9; Witwatersrand (South Africa)'88; MB BCh; CCFP; FCFP; Staff, William Osler Health System - Brampton Civic Hospital; Teach Staff, McMaster University; (905)451-1244

JIVANJI, Nisreen; 2444 Hurontario St, Mississauga ON L5B 2V1; Karachi (Pakistan)'89; CCFP; (905)566-1444

JIWA, Abdulkarim M; UBC Hospital, 2211 Wesbrook Mall, Vancouver BC V6T 2B5; Makerere (Uganda)'71; MB ChB; FRCPC; Psy. Chief Consultation Liaison Services, UBC Hospital - Koerner Pavillion; Consultant, Vancouver General Hospital - Centennial Pavillion; Clin Assoc Prof, University of British Columbia; Langs: Gujarati; (604)822-7549

JIWA, Ashifa; Grand River Hosp-KW Hlth Ctre, PO Box 9056 Stn C 835 King St W, Kitchener ON N2G 1G3; Wes'02; CCFP; Staff, Grand River Hospital - Kitchener/Waterloo Health Centre; (519)749-4300

JIWA, Gulnaz B; Hys Med Centre, 604-11010 101 St NW, Edmonton AB T5H 4B9; Wes'94; FRCSC; ObstGyn. Langs: Gujarati; (780)421-4728; Fax. (780)426-6698.

JIWA, Karima; Scott Town Med Centre, 9556 120 St, Surrey BC V3V 4C1; UBC'88; BSc(Biol.); CCFP; FCFP; (604)588-0320

JIWA, Nizar H; 1008-900 Greenbank Rd, Ottawa ON K2J 1S8; Cardiff (Wales)'67; FRCPC; IntMed. (613)825-6161

JIWANI, Almas A; 242-121 Orchard St PO Box 432, Berwick NS B0P 1E0; Mumbai (India)'84; MB BS; CCFP; (902)538-0575; Fax. (902)538-3415.

JIWANI, Azim H; Dr Azim H Jiwani Inc, 2363 Folkestone Way, West Vancouver BC V7S 3E1; Makerere (Uganda)'72; MRCS(Eng); LRCP(Lond); MB ChB; CCFP; FCFP; BC Cancer Agency Vancouver Centre; Langs: Gujarati; Hindi; Kiswahili; Punjabi; Urdu; (778)279-8243

JO, Woo Je; Red Deer Reg Hosp Centre, PO Box 5030 Stn Postal Box Ctr, Red Deer AB T4N 6R2; Ott'99; FRCPC; AnatPath. Staff, Red Deer Regional Hospital Centre; (403)343-4735

JOA, Elisabet A E; Business Bldg, 406-1200 Burrard St, Vancouver BC V6Z 2C7; UBC'97; FRCSC; ObstGyn. (604)683-8416; Fax. (604)683-1904.

JOANES, Joseph F; Port Arthur Health Centre Inc, 194 Court St N, Thunder Bay ON P7A 4V7; Galway (Ireland)'61; FRCPI(Ire); FRCPC; IntMed (Gastroenterology). Ac Staff, Thunder Bay Regional Health Sciences Centre; (807)346-6227 x6268; Fax. (807)346-6206; fjoanes@tbaytel.net.

JOANIS, Norman D J; 21st Medical Clinic, 502-402 21st St E, Saskatoon SK S7K 0C3; Sask'95; FRCPC; IntMed. Staff, St Paul's Hospital (Grey Nuns) of Saskatoon; (306)956-3444

JOANIS, Vincent; Rockyview Gen Hosp, 7007 14 St SW, Calgary AB T2V 1P9; Dal'05; CCFP; CCFP(E.M.); Staff, Rockyview General Hospital; (403)943-8741

JOANISSE, John A; Montfort Hosp, 713 Montreal Rd, Ottawa ON K1K 0T2; Ott'71; Chief FamilyMed/Chief GeriatricMed, Montfort Hospital; (613)746-4621 x6000

JOANNISSE, Valerie; Ctr Hosp Gatienau Memorial, 101 ch Burnside, Wakefield QC J0X 3G0; Sher'03; CCFP; CCFP(E.M.); Staff, Centre Hospitalier Gatineau Mémorial; (819)459-1112

JOANNOU, Jason A J; Addiction & Mental Hlth-Clarke, 536-250 College St, Toronto ON M5T 1R8; Tor'06; FRCPC; Psy. Staff, Centre for Addiction & Mental Health (CAMH) - College Street Site; (416)535-8501

JOANNOU, Manuela H E; 279 Canal Bank Rd PO Box 20107 Rpo Perth Mews, Perth ON K7H 3M6; Ott'90; CCFP; CCFP(E.M.); (613)267-9888; Fax. (613)267-8791.

JOAQUIN, Andrew J; 610 St. Charles St, Victoria BC V8S 3N7; London (Jamaica)'62; FRCSC; Neursurg. (250)598-8181

JOARDER, Mohammad Z H; Univ Hlth Network-Toronto Gen, 8N 840-200 Elizabeth St, Toronto ON M5G 2C4; Dhaka (Bangladesh)'85; Staff, Toronto General Hospital - UHN.

JOASSIN, Alfred M; CHUM-Hop Notre-Dame, 1560 rue Sherbrooke E, Montreal QC H2L 4M1; Louvain (Belgium)'66; FRCSC; Cardiovasc&ThorSurg (Thoracic Surgery). ac Staff, Centre Hospitalier l'Université de Montréal (CHUM) - Hôpital Notre-Dame; Ac Staff, Hôpital Santa Cabrini Ospedale; (514)890-8200

JOBIDON, Denis; Clinique Med Sillery, 1270 av William, Quebec QC G1S 4G1; Laval'83; FRCPC; Psy. Staff, Centre Hospitalier Affilié Universitaire de Québec - Hôpital du St-Sacrement; (418)622-7898

JOBIN, Catherine; CHUQ-Ctr Hosp Univ Laval, 2705 boul Laurier, Quebec QC G1V 4G2; Laval'92; FRCPC; Peds (Pneumology); Respir (P.Q.). Staff, Centre Hospitalier Universitaire de Quebec-CHUL; (418)654-2252

JOBIN, Celine M; Hop du Sacre-Coeur de Mtl, 5400 boul Gouin O, Montreal QC H4J 1C5; Mon'04; FRCPC; Neur. Staff, Hôpital du Sacre-Coeur de Montréal; (514)338-2222 x3877

JOBIN, Genevieve; CLSC Malauze, GD 107 132 Rte O, Saint-Omer QC G0C 2Z0; Laval'93; (418)364-7064; Fax. (418)364-7119.

JOBIN, Gilles; Hop Maisonneuve-Rosemont, 5415 boul de l'Assomption, Montreal QC H1T 2M4; Mon'74; Gastroent. Staff, Hopital Maisonneuve-Rosemont; adj Prof, Universite de Montreal; (514)252-3400 x3367; Fax. (514)252-3486.

JOBIN, Jacques R; Ctr Hosp De Verdun, 4000 boul Lasalle, Verdun QC H4G 2A3; Sher'76; Nephrol (P.Q.). Staff, Centre Hospitalier de Verdun; (514)765-8121

JOBIN, Johanne; Institut De Physiatrie Quebec, 2049 rue Sherbrooke E, Montreal QC H2K 1C1; Mon'90; CSPQ; FRCPC; Anes. (514)527-4155

JOBIN, Monique; Clinique Medicale, 105-1055 12e Av N, Sherbrooke QC J1E 2X4; Mon'90; Staff, CSSS du Témiscamingue; (819)821-2142; Fax. (819)821-0248; monique_jobin@ssss.gouv.qc.ca.

JOBIN, Nicolas; CSSS de Manicouagan, 635 boul Jolliet, Baie-Comeau QC G5C 1P1; Laval'95; CCFP; Staff, Centre Hospitalier Régional Baie-Comeau; Prof adj clin, Université Laval; Langs: Bilingual(French/English); (418)589-3701; Fax. (418)294-2862.

JOBIN, Philippe; CSSS de Chicoutimi, 305 rue Saint-Vallier, Chicoutimi QC G7H 5H6; Laval'06; FRCPC; DiagRad. Staff, Complexe hospitalier de la Sagamie; (418)541-1099

JOBIN, Vincent; CHUM-Hotel-Dieu, 3840 rue Saint-Urbain, Montreal QC H2W 1T8; Mon'95; FRCPC; IntMed; Respir. Staff, Centre Hospitalier l'Université de Montréal (CHUM) - Hôtel-Dieu; (514)890-8000 x14444

JOCELYN, Leslie J; Emerging Minds, 97 Hinton Ave N, Ottawa ON K1Y 0Z7; Man'81; FRCPC; Peds (Child & Adolescent Psychiatry); Psy. Staff, Children's Hospital of Winnipeg; Staff, Manitoba Adolescent Treatment Centre; Assoc Prof Peds & Psy, University of Manitoba; (613)883-3716; Fax. (613)233-9561; ljocelyn@matc.ca.

JOCHEM, Klaus; Dir de la Sante Publique-Mtl, 1301 rue Sherbrooke E, Montreal QC H2L 1M3; McG'85; MPH(Harvard); DTMH; MB BS; Consultant Phys Dept of Med & InfectDis, McGill University Health Centre - Montreal General Campus; Consultant Phys of Biological Environmental & Occupational Risk, Institut National de Sante Publique; Langs: German; Nepali; French; (514)528-2400 x3651; Fax. (514)528-2452; kjochem@santepub-mtl.qc.ca.

JOCIC, D Anna; Brant Community HC-Brantford, 200 Terrace Hill St, Brantford ON N3R 1G9; McM'98; CCFP; CCFP(E.M.); FCFP; Staff, The Brant Community Healthcare System - Brantford General Hospital Site; (519)752-7871

JOCOV, Drago; CSSS de Manicouagan, 635 boul Joliet, Baie-Comeau QC G5C 1P1; Sher'07; DiagRad. Staff, Centre Hospitalier Régional Baie-Comeau; (418)589-3701

JODOIN, Alain; Centre Bois De Boulogne, 480-1575 boul Henri-Bourassa O, Montreal QC H3M 3A9; Mon'72; FRCSC; OrthSurg (Spine). ac Staff, Hôpital du Sacre-Coeur de Montréal; Consultant, Hôpital Ste-Justine; Universite de Montreal; (514)332-6025; Fax. (514)332-4243.

JODOIN, Caroline; 2570 av Vanier, Saint-Hyacinthe QC J2S 6L7; Mon'83; FRCSC; Ophth. (450)774-6224; Fax. (450)774-6224.

JODOIN, Christian; Hop Charles LeMoyne, 3120 boul Taschereau, Greenfield Park QC J4V 2H1; Mon'93; CSPQ; FRCPC; Anes. Staff, Hopital Charles LeMoyne; (450)466-5000; Fax. (450)466-5007.

JODOIN, Gilles; Hôp Brome-Missisquoi-Perkins, 950 rue Principale, Cowansville QC J2K 1K3; Mon'65; LMCC; Respir (Pneumology). Staff, Hôpital Brome-Missisquoi-Perkins; Staff, Centre Hospitalier de Granby; Langs: English; (450)266-4342 x5; mgjodoin@sympatico.ca.

JODOIN, Lyne; Clinique Uniderma, 210-1575 boul de l'Avenir, Laval QC H7S 2N5; Mon'90; CCFP; (450)629-3376; Fax. (450)629-3375.

JODOIN, Marcel R; 202-1760 boul Jacques-Cartier, Longueuil QC J4N 1C2; Mon'78; CSPQ; ObstGyn. Staff, Centre Hospitalier Pierre Boucher; Staff, Hopital Maisonneuve-Rosemont; Langs: Bilingual(French/English); (450)468-2151; Fax. (450)468-3309.

JODOIN, Nicolas; CHUM-Hop Notre-Dame, GR 1178-1560 rue Sherbrooke E, Montreal QC H2L 4M1; Mon'00; FRCPC; Neur. Staff, Centre Hospitalier l'Université de Montréal (CHUM) - Hôpital Notre-Dame; (514)890-8123

JODOIN, Richard R; CSSS Les Eskers de l'Abitibi, 622 4e rue O, Amos QC J9T 2S2; Mon'82; FRCSC; PlasSurg. Staff, CH Hôtel-Dieu d'Amos; (819)732-0760

JODOIN, Steve; Ctr Hosp Affilie-Enfant-Jesus, 1401 18e rue, Quebec QC G1J 1Z4; Mon'96; FRCPC; DiagRad. Diagnostic-Radiology, Centre Hospitalier Affilié Universitaire de Québec - Hôpital De L'Enfant Jésus; (418)649-5789; stevejodoin@yahoo.com.

JODOIN, Valerie; Hop Jean-Talon, 1385 rue Jean-Talon E, Montreal QC H2E 1S6; Mon'07; Staff, CSSS du Coeur de l'Isle Hôpital Jean-Talon; (514)495-6767

JODOIN-FONTAINE, Xavier; CSSS Haut-Richelieu-Rouville, 920 boul du Seminaire N, St-Jean-sur-Richel QC J3A 1B7; Sher'06; OrthSurg. Staff, Hôpital du Haut-Richelieu; (450)359-5000

JOE, Barbara A; Algonquin College Health Serv, 1385 Woodroffe Ave, Nepean ON K2G 1V8; Tor'83; CCFP; FCFP; (613)727-4723 x7222

JOE, Howard A; BC Cancer Agency-Vanc Isl Ctr, 2410 Lee Ave, Victoria BC V8R 6V5; UBC'89; FRCPC; RadOncol. Staff, BC Cancer Agency Vancouver Island Centre; (250)519-5639; Fax. (250)519-2000; hjoe@bccancer.bc.ca.

JOE, Ronald S; Vancouver Coastal Health, 20 Hastings St W, Vancouver BC V6B 1G6; Auckland (New Zealand)'87; MB ChB; Staff, Providence Health Care - St Paul's Hospital; Staff, Vancouver Coastal Health; (604)683-0073 x241; ronald.joe@vch.ca.

JOFFE, A Mark; Royal Alexandra Hosp, 303-10240 Kingsway NW, Edmonton AB T5H 3V9; Cal'82; FRCPC; IntMed; InfectDis. Staff, Royal Alexandra Hospital; (780)735-5678

JOFFE, Ari; Edmonton Clinic Health Academy, 4 546-11405 87 Ave NW, Edmonton AB T6G 1C9; Alb'87; FRCPC; Peds (Critical Care Medicine); InfectDis. Staff, University of Alberta Hospital; Staff, Edmonton Clinic Health Academy; Clinical Asst Prof Peds, University of Alberta; (780)248-5435; ari.joffe@albertahealthservices.ca.

JOFFE, Beth E; Hycroft Med Bldg, 115-3195 Granville St, Vancouver BC V6H 3K2; Tor'91; CCFP; FCFP; (604)732-0525; Fax. (604)732-1064.

JOFFE, Denise; MUHC-Montreal Children's Hosp, 2300 rue Tupper, Montreal QC H3H 1P3; McG'86; Anes. Staff, McGill University Health Centre - Montreal Children's Hospital; (514)412-4400

JOFFE, John B; Seymour Med Clinic, 200-1530 7th Ave W, Vancouver BC V6J 1S3; Witwatersrand (South Africa)'86; MB BCh; (604)739-5623

JOFFE, Kenneth M; Misericordia Community Hosp, 16940 87 Ave NW, Edmonton AB T5R 4H5; Alb'99; FRCPC; Psy. Staff, Covenant Health - Misericordia Community Hospital; (780)735-2594; Fax. (780)735-2595.

JOFFE, Robert; Toronto East Gen & Orth Hosp, 825 Coxwell Ave, Toronto ON M4C 3E7; Tor'07; CCFP; CCFP(E.M.); Staff, Toronto East General Hospital Inc; (416)461-8271

JOG, Mandar S; London HSC-University Hosp, PO Box 5339 Stn B A10 026-339 Windermere Rd, London ON N6A 5A5; Mem'88; BSc; FRCPC; Neur (Movement Disorders). Staff, London Health Sciences Centre - University Hospital; Staff, St Joseph's Hospital - St Joseph's Health Care; University of Western Ontario; (519)663-3814; Fax. (519)663-3174.

JOGLEKAR, Anvita S; Sheppard Associates, 649 Sheppard Ave W, North York ON M3H 2S4; Poona (India)'68; FRCPC; Psy (Adult General Psychiatry). Langs: Marathi; Hindi; (416)630-0610

JOGLEKAR, Shashikant A; CMC Medical Centre, 5995 Steeles Ave E, Scarborough ON M1V 5P7; Bihar (India)'64; MB BS; Staff Physician, Homewood Health Centre; Langs: Hindi; Bengali; (416)297-5330

JOHAL, Balvindar S; BC Cancer Agency-Fraser Valley, 13750 96 Ave, Surrey BC V3V 1Z2; UBC'01; FRCPC; IntMed; MedOncol., BC Cancer Agency Fraser Valley Centre; (604)930-4028

JOHAL, Kashmir S; 200-8120 Cook Rd, Richmond BC V6Y 1T9; UBC'77; Ac Staff, Richmond Hospital; (604)270-8008; Fax. (604)270-9531.

JOHAL, Malkit K; Queen West Commun Health Ctre, 168 Bathurst St, Toronto ON M5V 2R4; Punjab (India)'70; CCFP; FCFP; Court Staff, Toronto Western Hospital - University Health Network; Asst Prof Commun Med, University of Toronto; Langs: Punjabi; Hindi; (416)703-8480; Fax. (416)703-8479; mjohal@ctchc.com.

JOHAL, Manraj S; 1545 Johnston Rd, White Rock BC V4B 3Z6; Sint Eustatius (Netherlands Antilles)'09; CCFP; (604)560-6161

JOHANNES, Christine J; Kingston Gen Hosp, 76 Stuart St, Kingston ON K7L 2V7; Cal'08; FRCPC; Peds. Staff, Kingston General Hospital; (613)549-6666

JOHANNSON, Kerri A M; Foothills Med Centre, 1403 29 St NW, Calgary AB T2N 2T9; Cal'06; FRCPC; IntMed; Respir. Staff, Foothills Medical Centre; (403)943-5634

JOHANNSSON, Peter W; 9-389 Main St RR 2, Picton ON K0K 2T0; Tor'77; (613)476-4482; Fax. (613)476-4617.

JOHANSON, Curtis R; The Juravinski Cancer Centre, 3 22-699 Concession St, Hamilton ON L8V 5C2; Cal'76; FRCPC; IntMed; RadOncol. Staff, Hamilton Health Sciences Centre-Juravinski Site; (905)387-9495; Fax. (905)575-6326; curtis.johanson@hrcc.on.ca.

JOHANSSON, Dawn A; Westmount Med Bldg, 640-5025 rue Sherbrooke O, Montreal QC H4A 1S9; McG'76; BSc; MSc; FRCSC; ObstGyn (Ultrasonography). Att Staff, McGill University Health Centre - Royal Victoria Hospital; Att Staff, McGill University Health Centre - Montreal General Campus; adj Prof, McGill University; Langs: English; French; (514)489-4575

JOHANSSON, Joyce E; Westmount Med Bldg, 640-5025 rue Sherbrooke O, Montreal QC H4A 1S9; McG'73; FACS; FRCSC; OrthSurg (Sports Medicine). Asst Prof Ortho, St Mary's Hospital Centre; Asst Prof Ortho, McGill University; Langs: English; French; (514)486-3741

JOHANSSON, Patricia L; Westmount Med Bldg, 640-5025 rue Sherbrooke O, Montreal QC H4A 1S9; McG'74; Langs: French; (514)486-3741

JOHAR, H Paul; Burnaby Hosp, 3935 Kincaid St, Burnaby BC V5G 2X6; Wes'00; CCFP; CCFP(E.M.); Staff, Burnaby Hospital; (604)434-4211

JOHN, A Roxane; The Westend Family Care Clinic, 80 Michael Cowpland Dr, Kanata ON K2M 1P6; Ott'91; CCFP; FCFP; Staff, Westend Family Care Clinic Family Health Team; (613)599-3321; Fax. (613)599-3366.

JOHN, Cyriac; Western Mem Reg Hosp, PO Box 2005 1 Brookfield Ave, Corner Brook NL A2H 6J7; Louisiana (USA)'93; Staff, Western Memorial Regional Hospital; (709)637-5000

JOHN, Elizabeth; Univ Hlth Network-Toronto Western Hosp, 399 Bathurst St, Toronto ON M5T 2S8; Mysore (India)'68; MB BS; DAB; FRCPC; Anes. Staff, Toronto Western Hospital - University Health Network; (416)603-5118

JOHN, Lal; Fraser Health Authority, 4F-260 Sherbrooke St, New Westminster BC V3L 3M2; Madras (India)'64; MB BS; Staff, Royal Columbian Hospital; (604)520-4662

JOHN, Michael A; London HSC-Victoria Hosp, PO Box 5010 Stn B 800 Commissioners Rd E, London ON N6A 5W9; Cape Town (South Africa)'83; MB ChB; MSc; FRCPC; MedMicrobiol. Staff Med Microbiol, London Health Sciences Centre - Victoria Campus; Asst Prof Microbiol & Immunology, University of Western Ontario; (519)685-8474; Fax. (519)685-8203.

JOHN, Miroslava; Smyth Med Centre, 312-1929 Russell Rd, Ottawa ON K1G 4G3; Charles (Czech Republic)'67; Ac Staff, The Ottawa Hospital - General Campus; University of Ottawa; (613)526-3146

JOHN, Nicholas D; Le Marchand Mansion, 408-11523 100 Ave NW, Edmonton AB T5K 0J8; Alb'83; BMedSci; FRCPC; Psy (Group Therapy). Teach Staff University Health Serv, University of Alberta; (780)488-4412

JOHN, Omana E; 41 Westmount Dr, Saint John NB E2K 5G1; Trivandrum (India)'77; FRCPC; Psy (Consulant Cardiologist). Consultant Psy, Horizon Health Network Saint John Public Health; Teacher Pt-Time, Dalhousie University; (506)633-0716; Fax. (506)658-0898.

JOHN, Philip R; The Hosp For Sick Children, 555 University Ave, Toronto ON M5G 1X8; Liverpool (England)'78; FRCPC; DiagRad. Staff Radiol, The Hospital For Sick Children; Assoc Prof Medical Imaging, University of Toronto; (416)813-7591; philip.john@sickkids.ca.

JOHN, Rohan; Univ Hlth Network-Toronto Gen, 200 Elizabeth St, Toronto ON M5G 2C4; Tamil Nadu (India)'93; Staff, Toronto General Hospital - UHN; (416)340-4560; Fax. (416)340-5517.

JOHN, Susan; Scarborough Hosp-General Div, 3050 Lawrence Ave E, Scarborough ON M1P 2V5; McM'05; FRCPC; IntMed; InfectDis. Staff, The Scarborough Hospital - General Campus; (416)431-8165

JOHN, Thomas; Taunton Surgical Centre, SS 201 1290 Keith Ross Dr, Oshawa ON L1H 7K4; Kerala (India)'78; BSc; MB BS; FRCPC; PhysMed&Rehab (Amputee Rehabilitation). Ac Staff, Lakeridge Health - Oshawa Site; Langs: Malayalam; Tamil; (905)721-6164; drsjohnnewall@on.aibn.com.

JOHN, Usha S; Taunton Health Centre, SS 201 3F-1290 Keith Ross Dr, Oshawa ON L1H 7K4; Kerala (India)'93; CCFP; (905)721-6877; Fax. (905)721-6686.

JOHN, Verghese; CMHA Toronto Branch, 500-1200 Markham Rd, Scarborough ON M1H 3C3; Ranchi (India)'82; LMCC; FRCPC; Psy. Langs: Hindi; Malayalam; (416)289-6285 x315

JOHN, Verity J; 500-89 Queensway W, Mississauga ON L5B 2V2; Wes'02; Neur. (905)848-0001; Fax. (905)848-6360.

JOHNS, Christine R; The Ottawa Hosp-Civic Campus, 1053 Carling Ave, Ottawa ON K1Y 4E9; McM'83; CCFP; CCFP(E.M.); Staff, The Ottawa Hospital - Civic Campus; (613)761-4337

JOHNS, Daniel G; Market Mall, 208-3625 Shaganappi Trail NW, Calgary AB T3A 0E2; Cal'03; CCFP; (403)286-9118

JOHNS, David G; 33 Dundas St, Dundas ON L9H 1A1; McM'89; CCFP; FCFP; Ac Staff, Hamilton Health Sciences Centre - McMaster Children's Hospital; Assoc Staff, St Joseph's Healthcare - Charlton Campus; Lecturer Med, McMaster University; (905)628-6151; Fax. (905)628-1609.

JOHNS, Karen; Finance Bldg-Tunney's Pasture, AL0202D2-123 Slater St, Ottawa ON K1A 1B9; Wes'83; (613)941-2134

JOHNS, Katharine L; Crowfoot Village Fam Practice, 210-600 Crowfoot Cres NW, Calgary AB T3G 0B4; Alb'92; FCFP; BMedSci; MCFP(EM); CCFP; CCFP(E.M.); FCFP; Medical Staff Family Med, Foothills Medical Centre; (403)239-9733; Fax. (403)241-8112.

JOHNS, Peter D; The Ottawa Hosp-Gen Campus, 501 Smyth Rd, Ottawa ON K1H 8L6; Ott'84; FRCPC; EmergMed. Staff, The Ottawa Hospital - General Campus; (613)737-8899 x79002; Fax. (613)737-8967.

JOHNSEN, Bonnie L; Fort William Clinic, 117 Mckellar St S, Thunder Bay ON P7E 1H5; Dal'97; CCFP; FCFP; (807)626-1234

JOHNSEN, Jon H; Fort William Clinic, 117 McKellar St S, Thunder Bay ON P7E 1H5; Dal'97; BSc; CCFP; FCFP; Ac Staff, Thunder Bay Regional Health Sciences Centre; (807)626-1234

JOHNSEN, Wendy A; 9th Avenue Med Centre, 7-3855 9th Ave, Port Alberni BC V9Y 4T9; Cape Town (South Africa)'81; MB ChB; CCFP; (250)723-9424; Fax. (250)723-9321.

JOHNSON, Alphonse J; Queen Elizabeth II HSC, 1276 South Park St, Halifax NS B3H 2Y9; Dal'68; DiagRad. Consultant, Queen Elizabeth II Health Sciences Centre - Victoria General Site; Assoc Prof DiagRad, Dalhousie University; (902)473-7770; Fax. (902)473-3482.

JOHNSON, Amy E; Northern Health Authority, 908-299 Victoria St, Prince George BC V2L 5B8; UBC'09; CCFP; (250)563-4706

JOHNSON, Andrea L; Packham Avenue Med Clinic, 104-335 Packham Ave, Saskatoon SK S7N 4S1; Cal'07; CCFP; (306)651-7091

JOHNSON, Andrew A; Cedar Care Clinic, 104-32423 Lougheed Hwy, Mission BC V2V 7B8; Manchester (England)'72; MB ChB; CCFP; (604)820-7676

JOHNSON, Andrew N; Westbram Family Physicians, 208-100 Pertosa Dr, Brampton ON L6X 0H9; Alb'91; CCFP; Staff, Homewood Health Centre; (905)454-2080

JOHNSON, Andrew S; Foothills Med Centre, 302-1403 29 St NW, Calgary AB T2N 2T9; Wes'93; FRCPC; IntMed; InfectDis; MedMicrobiol. Clin Asst Prof, Peter Lougheed Centre; Staff, Foothills Medical Centre; (403)944-2325; johnsona@ucalgary.ca.

JOHNSON, Beverly A; Nepean Med Centre, 402-1 Centrepointe Dr, Nepean ON K2G 6E2; Tor'85; Staff, Queensway Carleton Hospital; (613)226-2266

JOHNSON, Bijai; Salvation Army Grace Gen Hosp, 300 Booth Dr, Winnipeg MB R3J 3M7; Mahatma Gandhi (India)'95; FRCPC; IntMed. Staff, The Salvation Army Grace Hospital; (204)837-8311

JOHNSON, Bruce B; Invermere Med Centre, PO Box 8000 937 7 Ave, Invermere BC V0A 1K0; Cape Town (South Africa)'83; MB ChB; (250)342-9206

JOHNSON, Carey L; 2227 5 Ave NW, Calgary AB T2N 0S8; Cal'84; FRCPC; Peds; MedGenetics. Staff, Alberta Children's Hospital; (403)686-7200; Fax. (403)686-7244.

JOHNSON, Carmen L; Regina Qu'Appelle HR-Pasqua, 4101 Dewdney Ave, Regina SK S4T 1A5; Sask'91; CCFP; Staff, Pasqua Hospital; (306)766-2222

JOHNSON, Caroline; CLSC Metro, 1801 boul de Maisonneuve O, Montreal QC H3H 1J9; Mon'05; CCFP; (514)934-0354

JOHNSON, Carolyne; Hop Maisonneuve-Rosemont, 5415 boul de l'Assomption, Montreal QC H1T 2M4; Mon'94; FRCSC; ObstGyn. Staff, Hopital Maisonneuve-Rosemont; (514)252-3400

JOHNSON, Charles F; EaglesMed Clinic, 315-12445 Lake Fraser Dr SE, Calgary AB T2J 7A4; (Other Foreign)'06; CCFP; (403)723-2453; Fax. (403)723-2463.

JOHNSON, Charles N; Legacy Sport Clinic, 14-160 Meadowood Dr, Winnipeg MB R2M 5L6; Alb'76; FRCPC; PhysMed&Rehab. Staff, Health Sciences Centre; Staff, The Rehabilitation Centre; cjohnson@cc.umanitoba.ca.

JOHNSON, Christopher B; The Ottawa Hosp-Gen Campus, 501 Smyth Rd, Ottawa ON K1H 8L6; Ott'98; FRCPC; IntMed; Cardiol. (613)737-8582

JOHNSON, Claude; 200-1 boul Rene-Levesque E, Montreal QC H2X 3Z5; Laval'87; CSPQ; FRCPC; Anes. Langs: Bilingual(French/English); (514)397-0888; cjohnson@pamq.org.

JOHNSON, Daniel A; Kindersley Med Clinic, PO Box 1390, Kindersley SK S0L 1S0; Sask'71; CCFP; FCFP; Fam Med, Kindersley & District Health Centre; (306)463-2621; Fax. (306)463-4101; daniel.johnson@hrha.sk.ca.

JOHNSON, Darcy E; Henderson Med Centre, 441 Henderson Hwy, Winnipeg MB R2K 2H5; Man'81; CCFP; FCFP; (204)667-8650; Fax. (204)668-1928.

JOHNSON, David; 221 Edgewood Dr, Thunder Bay ON P7B 6A2; University Coll. (Ireland)'66; MB ChB; BAO; FRCSI; Med Dir, St Joseph's Care Group; Court Staff, Thunder Bay Regional Health Sciences Centre; (807)767-8798; Fax. (807)767-2206.

JOHNSON, David W; Alberta Children's Hosp, 2888 Shaganappi Trail NW, Calgary AB T3B 6A8; Dartmouth(NH) (USA)'84; Staff Child Health Research Unit, Alberta Children's Hospital; (403)955-7551; Fax. (403)955-7552; david.johnson@crha-health.ab.ca.

JOHNSON, David W; 2-695 Canterbury St, Woodstock ON N4S 8W7; McG'89; BSc; FRCSC; Ophth (Cataract & Refractive). Staff, Woodstock General Hospital; Staff, Alexandra Hospital; (519)537-5052; Fax. (519)539-0476.

JOHNSON, Donald H; Sports Med Clinic Carleton U, 1125 Colonel By Dr, Ottawa ON K1S 5B6; Qns'66; FACS; OrthSurg (Arthroscopy). Assoc Staff, The Ottawa Hospital - Civic Campus; Clinical Asst Prof OrthSurg, University of Ottawa; (613)520-3510; Fax. (613)520-3974; donnie@carletonsportsmed.com.

JOHNSON, Douglas R E; Suitor House, 1004 8 Ave SE, Calgary AB T2G 0M4; Cal'87; FRCSC; GenSurg. (403)264-6720; Fax. (403)237-6646.

JOHNSON, Edward S; University of Alberta Hosp, 8440 112 St NW, Edmonton AB T6G 2B7; Alb'71; ABNPath; LMCC; ABACPath; FRC; FRCPC; GenPath; NeurPath. Staff Lab Med & AnatPath, University of Alberta Hospital; Assoc Prof Path, University of Alberta; (780)407-8952; edwardj@ualberta.ca.

JOHNSON, Erik P; Associate Clinic, 5215 49 Ave, Wetaskiwin AB T9A 0R1; Alb'05; CCFP; (780)352-7157; Fax. (780)352-2273.

JOHNSON, Ernest B; Fenwick Med Centre, 5595 Fenwick St, Halifax NS B3H 4M2; Dal'61; Physician, Queen Elizabeth II Health Sciences Centre - Victoria General Site; Medical Staff Air Pilot, Ministry Of Transport; Langs: Bilingual(English/French); (902)422-5595; Fax. (902)429-8125.

JOHNSON, Errol; Winnipegosis Med Clinic, PO Box 128, Winnipegosis MB R0L 2G0; Dublin (Ireland)'76; Chief of Staff, Winnipegosis & District Health Centre; (204)656-4492; Fax. (204)656-4627; ejohnson@prha.mb.ca.

JOHNSON, F Gordon; 1863 Oak Bay Ave, Victoria BC V8R 1C6; London (England)'50; MB BS; MRCPsy; FRCPC; Psy (Motor Vehicle Accident Assessment & Rehabilitation). (250)370-2534

JOHNSON, Fiona; Peace Arch Hosp, 15521 Russell Ave, White Rock BC V4B 2R4; Dublin (Ireland)'88; MB BCh; BAO; Staff, Peace Arch Hospital.

JOHNSON, Garth E; The Ottawa Hosp-Civic Campus, 1053 Carling Ave, Ottawa ON K1Y 4E9; Man'66; FRCSC; OrthSurg (General Orthopedics). Staff Orthopedic Surg, The Ottawa Hospital - Civic Campus; Staff Teacher, University of Ottawa; (613)761-5168; Fax. (613)761-4661; gjohnson@ottawahospital.on.ca.

JOHNSON, Gordon H; Dynacare Kasper Med Labs, 200-10150 102 St NW, Edmonton AB T5J 5E2; Alb'77; FRCPC; GenPath (Cytopath). Staff, Royal Alexandra Hospital; Physician, DynaLIFE Diagnostics; Clin Assoc Prof, University of Alberta; (780)451-3702 x152

JOHNSON, Heather O; 102-26 North St, Bridgewater NS B4V 2V6; Mem'94; CCFP; (902)543-2733; Fax. (902)543-1678.

JOHNSON, Ian L; Ont Agency for Hlth Protection, 300-480 University Ave, Toronto ON M5G 1V2; Dal'79; FRCPC; CommunMed. (647)260-7415; Fax. (647)260-7600.

JOHNSON, John E; Primrose Medical Clinic, PO Box 670 Stn Main 2-152 Primrose St N, Qualicum Beach BC V9K 5T2; Durham (England)'57; MB BS; Hon Staff, Nanaimo Regional General Hospital; (250)752-7100

JOHNSON, J Kenneth; Queen Elizabeth II HSC, 1278 Tower Rd, Halifax NS B3H 2Y9; Man'71; Staff, Queen Elizabeth II Health Sciences Centre - Victoria General Site; (902)473-1486; Fax. (902)473-6602; ken.johnson@ns.sympatico.ca.

JOHNSON, James C; North Battleford Med Clinic, 102-11427 Railway Ave, North Battleford SK S9A 3G8; Sask'76; CCFP; FCFP; Staff, Battlefords Union Hospital; (306)445-4415; Fax. (306)445-5145.

JOHNSON, Jennifer K; Bayside Med Centre, 3 Beck Blvd, Penetanguishene ON L9M 1B9; McM'92; BSc(Eng); CCFP; Staff, Georgian Bay General Hospital - Midland; (705)549-3939; Fax. (705)549-0029.

JOHNSON, Jo-Ann M; Foothills Med Centre, 1403 29 St NW, Calgary AB T2N 2T9; Man'80; FRCSC; ObstGyn (Maternal Fetal Medicine). Staff ObstGyn, Foothills Medical Centre; Prof ObstGyn, University of Calgary; (403)944-1438; Fax. (403)270-4249.

JOHNSON, John F; London HSC-University Hosp, PO Box 5339 Stn B 339 Windermere Rd, London ON N6A 5A5; Ott'96; FRCPC; IntMed; Nephrol. Staff, London Health Sciences Centre - University Hospital; (519)685-8300; Fax. (519)663-3449.

JOHNSON, John K; Queen Elizabeth II HSC-VG Site, 7A-1276 South Park St, Halifax NS B3H 2Y9; Man'71; Staff, Queen Elizabeth II Health Sciences Centre - Victoria General Site; (902)473-1486

JOHNSON, Kassia J; Hamilton HS-McMaster Site, PO Box 2000 Stn Lcd 1 1200 Main St W, Hamilton ON L8N 3Z5; McM'03; FRCPC; Peds. Staff, Hamilton Health Sciences Centre - McMaster University Medical Centre; (905)521-2100; Fax. (905)521-7953.

JOHNSON, Kevin N; 66 Braemar St, Calgary AB T3Z 2T2; Qns'83; CCFP; CCFP(E.M.); FCFP; Staff, Foothills Medical Centre; Staff, Alberta Children's Hospital; (403)246-7425; Fax. (403)246-0398.

JOHNSON, Kevin W; Glen Allan Med Centre, 306-42 Glen Allan Dr, Bridgewater NS B4V 3N2; Mem'94; FRCSC; GenSurg. (902)527-0163

JOHNSON, Kim C; Royal Health Care Centre, 130 Adelaide St W, Toronto ON M5H 3P5; Wes'05; CCFP; (416)361-6142

JOHNSON, Kirsten N; MUHC-Royal Victoria Hosp, C418-687 av des Pins O, Montreal QC H3A 1A1; Cal'01; CCFP; CCFP(E.M.); Staff, McGill University Health Centre - Royal Victoria Hospital; (514)934-1934 x34277

JOHNSON, Krista M; Kerrisdale Station Med Clinic, 2077 42nd Ave W, Vancouver BC V6M 2B4; McG'97; CCFP; (604)261-9494

JOHNSON, Kristen M; Alberta Children's Hosp, 2888 Shaganappi Trail NW, Calgary AB T3B 6A8; Alb'06; FRCPC; Peds; PedEmergMed. Staff, Alberta Children's Hospital; (403)955-7211

JOHNSON, L Stephen; 541 Eglinton Ave E, Toronto ON M4P 1N7; Wes'74; Court Staff, Sunnybrook Health Sciences Centre; Ac Staff, North York General Hospital; Consultant, Hospitals of Ontario Pension Plan; (416)487-2442; Fax. (416)487-2508.

JOHNSON, Laura B; Canadian Forces Health Service, 4050 4th Ave W, Vancouver BC V6R 1P6; UBC'76; Medical Officer, Canadian Forces Health Services; (604)225-2520 x2560

JOHNSON, Liane B; IWK Health Centre, PO Box 9700 Rpo CSC 5850-5980 University Ave, Halifax NS B3K 6R8; McG'95; MDCM; FACS; FRCSC; Otol (Pediatric Otolaryngology). Staff, IWK Health Centre; (902)470-8041; Fax. (902)470-8929.

JOHNSON, Louise M; 500-5300 h de la Cote-des-Neig, Montreal QC H3T 1Y3; McG'85; MDCM; FRCSC; ObstGyn. (514)344-8330

JOHNSON, Manamohan; South Peel Med Arts Bldg, 212-77 Queensway W, Mississauga ON L5B 1B7; Madras (India)'73; DPM; MRCPsy(U.K.); FRCPC; Psy. Consultant Psy, Trillium Health Centre - Mississauga; Langs: Tamil; (905)848-8677; Fax. (905)848-5855.

JOHNSON, Marcia M; Coronation Plaza, 104-14310 111 Ave NW, Edmonton AB T5M 3Z7; Sask'80; FRCPC; CommunMed. (780)342-0195; Fax. (780)342-0248; marcia.johnson@capitalhealth.ca.

JOHNSON, Martine; Centre Medical Louvain, 9469 rue Lajeunesse, Montreal QC H2M 1S5; Mon'83; (514)381-7192; Fax. (514)387-4293.

JOHNSON, Mary A; Cross Cancer Institute, 11560 University Ave NW, Edmonton AB T6G 1Z2; Sask'77; DABR; FRCPC; DiagRad. Staff, Cross Cancer Institute; (780)432-8723

JOHNSON, Melissa A; Hys Med Centre, 310-11010 101 St NW, Edmonton AB T5H 4B9; Alb'03; FRCPC; IntMed; Gastroent. (780)421-1029; Fax. (780)425-5533.

JOHNSON, Melissa A; Elmwood Family Clinic, 3-204 First Ave, St Thomas ON N5R 4P5; McM'06; CCFP; (519)631-3223; Fax. (519)631-8005.

JOHNSON, Mervin L; Meadow Lake Associate Clinic, PO Box 1510, Meadow Lake SK S9X 1Z1; Sask'69; CCFP; FCFP; (306)236-5661; Fax. (306)236-4355; mlacdoctors@sasktel.net.

JOHNSON, Michael C; Royal Alexandra Hosp, 2305-10240 Kingsway NW, Edmonton AB T5H 3V9; Alb'02; FRCSC; Ophth (Neuro Ophthalmology). Staff, Royal Alexandra Hospital; (780)735-4769; Fax. (780)735-5242.

JOHNSON, Michael G; Health Sciences Centre, AD401-820 Sherbrook St, Winnipeg MB R3A 1R9; Man'94; BSc; FRCSC; OrthSurg (Spine). Medical Staff, Health Sciences Centre; Medical Staff, Rehabilitation Centre for Children; Staff, CancerCare Manitoba; Asst Prof, University of Manitoba; (204)787-4415; Fax. (204)787-2460; sbowman4@hsc.mb.ca.

JOHNSON, Michelle D; St Paul's Hosp, 470C-1081 Burrard St, Vancouver BC V6Z 1Y6; Man'96; FRCPC; IntMed (Pituitary & Adrenal Disorders); Endocrin&Metab. Staff, Providence Health Care - St Paul's Hospital; Staff, Vancouver General Hospital - Centennial Pavillion; (604)806-9156; Fax. (604)806-8594; mjohnson@providencehealth.bc.ca.

JOHNSON, Natasha I; Hamilton HS-McMaster Site, PO Box 2000 Stn Lcd 1 3A36-1200 Main St W, Hamilton ON L8N 3Z5; McG'97; FRCPC; Peds (Adolescent Medicine). Staff Adolescent Med & Gen Ped, Hamilton Health Sciences Centre - McMaster University Medical Centre; Teach Staff, McMaster University; (905)521-2100 x75658

JOHNSON, Nathalie; SMBD Jewish Gen Hosp, 3755 ch Cote-Sainte-Catherine, Montreal QC H3T 1E2; Ott'98; PhD; FRCPC; IntMed; Hem. Staff, Sir Mortimer B Davis Jewish General; (514)340-8222

JOHNSON, Nelie C; Lougheed Health Centre, 105-22838 Lougheed Hwy, Maple Ridge BC V2X 2V6; UBC'76; CCFP; Staff, Ridge Meadows Care Clinic Inc(East); Staff, Ridge Meadows Care Clinic Inc(West); Langs: English; French; (604)467-4166; Fax. (604)466-5768.

JOHNSON, Nicole A; Alberta Children's Hosp, 2888 Shaganappi Trail NW, Calgary AB T3B 6A8; McM'98; FRCPC; Peds; Rheum. Staff Ped Rheumatol, Alberta Children's Hospital; (403)955-7771

JOHNSON, Pamela J; St Joseph's Health Centre, 231-710 Victoria Ave E, Thunder Bay ON P7C 5P7; McM'89; BScN(Hon); Psy. Staff, Thunder Bay Regional Health Sciences Centre; Assoc Prof, Northern Ontario School of Medicine; Langs: Spanish; (807)624-3400

JOHNSON, Patricia L; Royal Columbian Hosp, 330 Columbia St E, New Westminster BC V3L 3W7; UBC'88; FRCPC; Anes. Staff Anes, Royal Columbian Hospital; Clin Instructor Anes, University of British Columbia; (604)520-4602; Fax. (604)520-4899.

JOHNSON, Paul M; Synergy Wellness Centre, 221-501 Bethel Dr, Sherwood Park AB T8H 0N2; Alb'01; CCFP; (780)464-0123; Fax. (780)449-1245.

JOHNSON, Paul M; Queen Elizabeth II Hosp, 8 025-1276 South Park St, Halifax NS B3H 2Y9; Dal'96; FRCSC; GenSurg. Staff Surg, Queen Elizabeth II Health Sciences Centre - Victoria General Site; (902)473-2851; Fax. (902)473-1018.

JOHNSON, Phyllis J; James Paton Mem Hosp, 125 Trans Canada Hwy, Gander NL A1V 1P7; Mem'85; Staff, James Paton Memorial Hospital; (709)651-2500 x5552; Fax. (709)256-5588.

JOHNSON, Richard R; Market Mall Prof Bldg, 222-4935 40 Ave NW, Calgary AB T3A 2N1; UBC'77; (403)202-0724; Fax. (403)247-0711.

JOHNSON, Robert D A; Madrona Imaging Westhill Ctre, A-1804 Bowen Rd, Nanaimo BC V9S 5W4; McG'90; FRCPC; DiagRad; NuclearMed. (250)753-4351; Fax. (250)753-0856.

JOHNSON, Robert E; 214-89 Dawson Rd, Guelph ON N1H 1B1; Qns'82; FRCSC; Ophth. Staff, Guelph General Hospital; (519)822-5500; Fax. (519)822-5449.

JOHNSON, Robert E; Cariboo Mem Hosp, 517 Sixth Ave N, Williams Lake BC V2G 2G8; Dal'98; CCFP; CCFP(E.M.); FCFP; Staff, Cariboo Memorial Hospital and Health Centre; (250)392-8225; robert_johnson@telus.net.

JOHNSON, Robert G; 102-1155 Concordia Ave, Winnipeg MB R2K 2M9; Man'06; CCFP; (204)415-0322

JOHNSON, Robin L; Cariboo Mem Hosp, 401-517 Sixth Ave N, Williams Lake BC V2G 2G8; UBC'01; FRCSC; ObstGyn. Staff, Cariboo Memorial Hospital and Health Centre; (250)392-4411; robin_johnson@telus.net.

JOHNSON, Roger J; McKenzie Prof Centre, 211-1595 McKenzie Ave, Victoria BC V8N 1A4; Ott'85; MHSc; BSc; FRCPC; Public Health & Preventive Med. Langs: English; French; (250)598-3932

JOHNSON, Ross W; 99 Shuniah St, Thunder Bay ON P7A 2Z2; McM'84; CCFP; (807)346-9400; Fax. (807)346-9123.

JOHNSON, Royce L C; First Edmonton Place, 1190-10665 Jasper Ave NW, Edmonton AB T5J 3S9; Sask'77; FRCSC; Ophth. Ac Staff, Royal Alexandra Hospital; Clin Assoc Prof, University of Alberta; (780)425-4521; Fax. (780)425-5613.

JOHNSON, Sandra M; Eagle Ridge Prof Complex, 490 Huronia Rd, Barrie ON L4N 6M2; Qns'03; (705)734-9690; Fax. (705)734-0239.

JOHNSON, Scott T; Royal Alexandra Hosp, 417-10240 Kingsway NW, Edmonton AB T5H 3V9; Man'01; FRCSC; GenSurg; ThorSurg. Staff, Royal Alexandra Hospital; (780)735-4111

JOHNSON, Sharon B; Primary Care Clinic, 1300-13401 108 Ave, Surrey BC V3T 5T3; McG'75; Med Dir Youth Clinic, Surrey Memorial Hospital; Staff, Youth Clinic; Staff, Fraser North Child & Youth Eating Disorder Program; (604)953-4940

JOHNSON, Sindhu R; Univ Hlth Network-Toronto Western Hosp, EW GF-399 Bathurst St, Toronto ON M5T 2S8; Mem'98; FRCPC; IntMed; Rheum. Clin Associate Rheum, Toronto Western Hospital - University Health Network; Lecturer, University of Toronto; (416)603-6417; Fax. (416)603-4348.

JOHNSON, Sonia C; MCI The Doctor's Office, PO Box 134 Stn Royal Bank 200 Bay St, Toronto ON M5J 2J3; (Other Foreign)'08; (416)368-6787

JOHNSON, Stephanie; PO Box 77007 Kingsway Knight R, Vancouver BC V5V 5E7; UBC'06; FRCSC; ObstGyn. Staff, Providence Health Care - St Paul's Hospital.

JOHNSON, Steven D W L; Foothills Med Centre, 1403 29 St NW, Calgary AB T2N 2T9; Ott'04; Staff, Foothills Medical Centre; (403)944-1110

JOHNSON, Suni J; Grey Bruce HS-Owen Sound, PO Box 1800 Stn Main 7106-1800 8th St E, Owen Sound ON N4K 6M9; Kerala (India)'92; FACP; ABIM; FRCPC; IntMed. Staff, Grey Bruce Health Services - Owen Sound; Langs: Malayalam; (519)376-2747; Fax. (519)376-2097.

JOHNSON, Sunny V; Credit Valley Med Arts Centre, 513-2000 Credit Valley Rd, Mississauga ON L5M 4N4; Padova (Italy)'84; BSc; DSS; FRCPC; Psy (Mood Disorders). Dir Research, The Credit Valley Hospital; Dir, Medical Research Associates; Langs: Italian; (905)607-9320; Fax. (905)607-9785.

JOHNSON, Terrence R; Royal University Hosp, 103 Hospital Dr, Saskatoon SK S7N 0W8; Johannesburg (South Africa)'91; MB ChB; Staff, Royal University Hospital; (306)655-1915; Fax. (306)655-6604.

JOHNSON, Thomas A; Medicine Hat Reg Hosp, 666 5 St SW, Medicine Hat AB T1A 4H6; Sask'80; BSc; FRCPC; Anes. Staff Anes, Medicine Hat Regional Hospital; (403)529-8839; Fax. (403)528-8101; tajohn@shaw.ca.

JOHNSON, Thomas E; Halton Family Health Centre, 2951 Walker's Line, Burlington ON L7M 4Y1; McM'78; CCFP; FCFP; (905)336-3437 x2076

JOHNSON, Troy G; West Lincoln Mem Hosp, 169 Main St E, Grimsby ON L3M 1P3; Alb'99; CCFP; Staff, West Lincoln Memorial Hospital; (905)945-2253

JOHNSON, Wayne D; Arkona Med Centre, PO Box 119 14 Union St, Arkona ON N0M 1B0; Tor'76; BSc; MSc; Ac Staff, Strathroy Middlesex General Hospital - Middlesex Hospital Alliance; (519)828-3821; Fax. (519)828-3429; jashep@xcelco.on.ca.

JOHNSON, William S; 520-89 Queensway W, Mississauga ON L5B 2V2; Qns'04; VascSurg; GenSurg. (905)848-7777

JOHNSON, Yves; Clinique Med Duberger, 2810 boul Pere-Lelievre, Quebec QC G1P 2Y1; Laval'85; ac Staff, CSSS de Quebec-Sud; (418)688-8414; Fax. (418)688-4273.

JOHNSON MORA, Ben H; Children's Hosp of Eastern Ont, 401 Smyth Rd, Ottawa ON K1H 8L1; Costa Rica (Costa Rica)'91; Staff, Children's Hospital of Eastern Ontario (CHEO); (613)737-7600

JOHNSON-OBASEKI, Stephanie E; Univ Hlth Network-Toronto Gen, 200 Elizabeth St, Toronto ON M5G 2C4; Ott'06; Otol (Head & Neck Surgery). Staff, Toronto General Hospital - UHN; (416)340-3111

JOHNSSON, Karen E; PO Box 35053 Rpo Hillside, Victoria BC V8T 5G2; Alb'90; CCFP.

JOHNSTON, A Catherine; Tantramar Commun Health Centre, D-2 Main St, Sackville NB E4L 4A3; Dal'84; (506)536-3111; Fax. (506)536-3199.

JOHNSTON, Aaron; Rockyview Gen Hosp, 7007 14 St SW, Calgary AB T2V 1P9; Qns'03; CCFP; CCFP(E.M.); Staff, Rockyview General Hospital; (403)943-3000

JOHNSTON, Andrew G; The Landing Bldg C, 405-9811 96A St NW, Edmonton AB T6A 4A4; Birmingham (England)'71; (780)432-0037; ajohnston@medicentres.com.

JOHNSTON, Anita G C; Homewood Health Centre, 150 Delhi St, Guelph ON N1E 6K9; Tor'73; FRCPC; Psy (Psychoanalysis). Court Staff, Centre for Addiction & Mental Health (CAMH) - College Street Site; Staff, Homewood Health Centre; Lecturer Psy, University of Toronto; (519)824-1010; anita.johnston@utoronto.ca.

JOHNSTON, Anna L; Dauphin Comm Health Services, 625 3rd St SW, Dauphin MB R7N 1R7; Man'93; BSc; CCFP; Staff, Dauphin Regional Health Centre; (204)638-2124; Fax. (204)638-8622.

JOHNSTON, B Lynn; 5014 ACC-5780 University Ave, Halifax NS B3H 1V7; Dal'79; LMCC; FRCP; FRCPC; IntMed; InfectDis. Ac Staff, Queen Elizabeth II Health Sciences Centre - Victoria General Site; Ac Staff, Capital District Health Authority; Prof, Dalhousie University; (902)473-5553; Fax. (902)473-7394; ljohnsto@dal.ca.

JOHNSTON, Brenda A; 417-190 Sherway Dr, Etobicoke ON M9C 5N2; McG'85; FRCSC; ObstGyn. (416)913-3746; Fax. (647)436-8371.

JOHNSTON, Brian R; Saint John Reg Hosp, PO Box 2100 Stn Main, Saint John NB E2L 4L2; Dal'92; FRCSC; GenSurg (Thoracic Surgery). Staff, Saint John Regional Hospital; Asst Prof, Dalhousie University; (506)648-6489; Fax. (506)648-6490.

JOHNSTON, C Stuart; Main Street Med Associates, PO Box 489 36005 97th St, Oliver BC V0H 1T0; Cape Town (South Africa)'87; MB ChB; MSc; CCFP; Medical Staff, St John Hospital; Clin Assoc Prof Family Pract, University of British Columbia; (250)498-3411

JOHNSTON, Carolina; Delisle Court Prof Centre, 230-1560 Yonge St, Toronto ON M4T 2S9; McM'77; FRCPC; Psy. Staff, Toronto Western Hospital - University Health Network; (416)920-0930

JOHNSTON, Charlene F; 5881 Malden Rd, Windsor ON N9H 1S5; Tor'99; CCFP; (519)966-2473; Fax. (519)966-8961.

JOHNSTON, Christopher A M; 3070-1554 Dresden Row, Halifax NS B3J 2K2; Qns'98; CCFP; (902)442-5199

JOHNSTON, Colleen G; Town Centre Family Clinic, 320-6203 28 Ave NW, Edmonton AB T6L 6K3; Alb'84; BSc(Med); CCFP; FCFP; Assoc Staff, Covenant Health - Grey Nuns Community Hospital; (780)462-8120; Fax. (780)461-9437.

JOHNSTON, Curtis W; Kingsway Nephrology Assoc, 303-10611 Kingsway NW, Edmonton AB T5G 3C8; Alb'96; BSc; FRCPC; IntMed; Critical Care Medicine; Nephrol. Staff/Site Chief Med & Critical Care, Royal Alexandra Hospital; (780)496-9350; Fax. (780)425-8475; curtis.johnston@ualberta.ca.

JOHNSTON, D William C; 11202 76 Ave NW, Edmonton AB T6G 0K1; Alb'75; FRCSC; OrthSurg. Site Med Dir, University of Alberta Hospital; Staff, Glenrose Rehabilitation Hospital; Clin Prof, University of Alberta; (780)439-4945; Fax. (780)439-0396.

JOHNSTON, David A; Associate Family Phys Clinic, 262 2nd Ave NE, Swift Current SK S9H 2C8; Glasgow (Scotland)'56; (306)773-1555; Fax. (306)773-6817.

JOHNSTON, David G; Fontbonne Bldg, 6F-301 James St S, Hamilton ON L8P 3B6; Qns'69; FRCPC; Psy (Anxiety Disorder). Staff, St Joseph's Healthcare - Charlton Campus; Staff, Anxiety Treatment & Research Clinic; Assoc Prof, McMaster University; (905)522-1155 x33697

JOHNSTON, David G; Queen Elizabeth II HSC-Halifax, 4855-1796 Summer St, Halifax NS B3H 3A7; Dal'84; FRCSC; OrthSurg. Staff Orth, Queen Elizabeth II Health Sciences Centre - Halifax Infirmary Site; (902)473-2085; Fax. (902)473-7239.

JOHNSTON, Dean C C; 202-1160 Burrard St, Vancouver BC V6Z 2E8; UBC'92; BSc; MHSc; DABPN; FRCPC; Neur (Cerebrovascular Disease). Clinical Asst Prof, Vancouver General Hospital - Centennial Pavillion; Dir Stroke Prog & Rapid Access Clinic/Clinical Asst Prof, Providence Health Care - St Paul's Hospital; Clinical Asst Prof Div of Neurol, University of British Columbia; (604)602-8118; Fax. (604)683-8150.

JOHNSTON, Donna L; Children's Hosp Eastern Ont, 401 Smyth Rd, Ottawa ON K1H 8L1; Qns'95; BSc(Hon); FRCPC; Peds (Hematology). Att Staff Hem/Oncol, Children's Hospital of Eastern Ontario (CHEO); Assoc Prof, University of Ottawa; (613)737-2370; Fax. (613)738-4828.

JOHNSTON, Eamon F; 450 West Heights, Kitchener ON N2N 2B9; National (Ireland)'79; MB ChB; (519)743-5196; Fax. (519)743-6477; cornwallmed@citenet.net.

JOHNSTON, Edward E; 202-800 Princess St, Kingston ON K7L 5E4; Tor'60; FRCSC; ObstGyn. Consultant Gyn, Ongwanada Resource Centre; (613)544-5378; Fax. (613)542-6868.

JOHNSTON, Elizabeth L; Yorkview Med Centre, 104-3695 Keele St, North York ON M3J 1N2; Tor'75; Staff, Humber River Regional Hospital - Finch Avenue Site; (416)633-3711; Fax. (416)630-7338.

JOHNSTON, Erin L; Hassle Free Clinic, 2F-66 Gerrard St E, Toronto ON M5B 1G3; McM'89; CCFP; (416)922-0566; Fax. (416)922-2018.

JOHNSTON, Geoffrey H F; Royal University Hosp, 103 Hospital Dr, Saskatoon SK S7N 0W8; Ott'78; BSc; MBA; FACS; CHE; FRCSC; OrthSurg (Upper Extremity Surgery). Staff, Royal University Hospital; Prof Surg, University of Saskatchewan; (306)966-8209; Fax. (306)966-8196.

JOHNSTON, Geraldine; Kings County Med Centre, PO Box 817, Montague PE C0A 1R0; Dal'86; Med Dir, Kings County Memorial Hospital; (902)838-4672

JOHNSTON, H Alan; AIM Health Group, B22-550 Terminal Ave, Ottawa ON K1G 0Z3; Tor'63; CCFP; FCFP; Staff, The Ottawa Hospital - Riverside Campus; Langs: English; French; (613)731-4770; Fax. (613)731-4979; pdomc@magma.ca.

JOHNSTON, Hariclia; Etobicoke Med Centre, 400 The East Mall, Etobicoke ON M9B 3Z9; Tor'99; BSc; MSc; CCFP.

JOHNSTON, Ian G; 100-202 King St W, Chatham ON N7M 1E5; Tor'93; PhD; FRCPC; Peds. Staff, Chatham-Kent Health Alliance; Prof Peds, University of Western Ontario; (519)358-1880; Fax. (519)358-1586; ijohnston@ckha.on.ca.

JOHNSTON, Ian R; Tudor Glen Medicentre, 2520 Tudor Glen Market, St. Albert AB T8N 3V3; Manchester (England)'69; MB ChB; DA; DObstRCOG; Physician, Belvedere Medicentre; Physician, Westend Medicentre; Physician, Belmont Medicentre; Physician, Heritage Medicentre; (780)458-5776; Fax. (780)460-1908.

JOHNSTON, J Mark; Valley Prof Centre, 210-70 Exhibition St, Kentville NS B4N 4K9; Dal'97; FRCPC; Psy (Dementia). (902)679-0536

JOHNSTON, James B; Cancercare Manitoba, 675 McDermot Ave, Winnipeg MB R3E 0V9; Dublin (Ireland)'75; FRCPC; IntMed (Hematological Oncology). (204)787-2197; Fax. (204)783-6875; james.johnston@cancercare.mb.ca.

JOHNSTON, James C; BC Centre for Disease Control, 655 12th Ave W, Vancouver BC V5Z 4R4; Qns'03; FRCPC; IntMed; Respir. Staff, Gordon & Leslie Diamond Health Care Centre; (604)707-5662

JOHNSTON, James D; KMH Cardiology & Diag Centres, 108-751B Victoria St S, Kitchener ON N2M 5N4; (Grenada)'87; (519)658-5893

JOHNSTON, James G; Family Med Centre, 387 Cedar St, Simcoe ON N3Y 2J2; Wes'65; Staff, Norfolk General Hospital; (519)426-4821; Fax. (519)426-5430.

JOHNSTON, James W; Sage Med Clinic, 101-2210 Main St, Penticton BC V2A 5H8; UBC'88; Staff GP, Penticton Regional Hospital; (250)492-0990; Fax. (250)492-0992.

JOHNSTON, Janine L; Thomson House, 1835 Corydon Ave, Winnipeg MB R3N 0K6; Man'81; BScPharm; FRCPC; Neur (Neuro Ophthalmology). Ac Staff, Health Sciences Centre; Assoc Prof, University of Manitoba; (204)947-1766; Fax. (204)947-1804.

JOHNSTON, Jean F; Glenrose Rehab Hosp, 1259-10230 111 Ave NW, Edmonton AB T5G 0B7; Glasgow (Scotland)'77; MB ChB; MRCPsy; FRCPC; Psy. Staff, Glenrose Rehabilitation Hospital; (780)735-8800

JOHNSTON, Jeremy V W; 115-6350 120 St, Surrey BC V3X 1Y7; London (England)'63; MB BS; MRCS; LRCP; DObstRCOG; Staff, Surrey Memorial Hospital; (604)591-6300

JOHNSTON, Joan M; First Edmonton Place, 1270-10665 Jasper Ave NW, Edmonton AB T5J 3S9; Alb'72; BMedSci; CCFP; FCFP; (780)423-5508

JOHNSTON, Julie A; Summerside Med Centre, 101-475 Granville St, Summerside PE C1N 3N9; Tor'96; CCFP; Staff, Prince County Hospital; (902)432-8181

JOHNSTON, K Ross; PO Box 114 Rpo Chestermere, Chestermere AB T1X 1K8; Alb'83; (403)999-2589; Fax. (403)398-0503; krjprof@shaw.ca.

JOHNSTON, K Wayne; 6E 228-200 Elizabeth St, Toronto ON M5G 2C4; Tor'66; FACS; FRCSC; GenSurg; VascSurg. Staff/Head Div of VascSurg, Toronto General Hospital - UHN; Chair R Fraser Elliott/Prof Surg, University of Toronto; (416)340-3552; Fax. (416)340-5029; wayne.johnston@uhn.ca.

JOHNSTON, Karen E; 403-265 Yorkland Blvd, North York ON M2J 5C7; Tor'87; CCFP; FCFP; (416)229-2399; Fax. (416)229-9771.

JOHNSTON, Karen M; Athletic Edge Sports Medicine, 1100-121 King St W, Toronto ON M5H 3T9; Tor'91; DrMedCh; FRCSC; Neursurg (Brain Injury). Consultant Athletic Edge Sports Med/Brain Injury-Div of NeuroSurg, University of Toronto; Langs: English; French; (416)800-0800

JOHNSTON, Kelly D; 335-401 9 Ave SW, Calgary AB T2P 3C5; Alb'01; FRCSC; OrthSurg (Hip & Knee Reconstruction). Clin Lecturer, University of Calgary; (403)221-4322

JOHNSTON, Kristin M; Whistler Health Care Centre, 201-4380 Lorimer Rd RR 4, Whistler BC V0N 1B4; UBC'99; CCFP; Physician, Whistler Health Care Centre; (604)932-3977; Fax. (604)932-0660.

JOHNSTON, Lesley M; Dr Charles A Janeway Child HC, 300 Prince Philip Dr, St. John's NL A1B 3V6; Mem'06; Anes. Staff, Janeway Children's Health & Rehabilitation Centre; (709)777-6300

JOHNSTON, Mary E; Carleton Place & Dist Mem Hosp, 211 Lake Ave E, Carleton Place ON K7C 1J4; McM'93; CCFP; CCFP(E.M.); FCFP; Staff, Carleton Place & District Memorial Hospital; Asst Prof, University of Ottawa; (613)257-2200

JOHNSTON, Mary T; 2350 Blind Bay Rd RR 1, Blind Bay BC V0E 1H1; Dal'74; BSc; MSc; Staff, Queen Victoria Hospital; Resd Teach Staff Family Pract, University of British Columbia; (250)675-0023

JOHNSTON, Maureen R; Children's Hosp of Western Ont, 800 Commissioners Rd E, London ON N6C 2V5; Man'83; FRCPC; Peds. Staff, London Health Sciences Centre - University Hospital; Staff, Children's Hospital of Western Ontario; University of Western Ontario; (519)685-8500 x52460; mrjohns2@sympatico.ca.

JOHNSTON, Michael R; Beatrice Hunter Cancer Res Ins, PO Box 15000 Lcd 2 5850 College St, Halifax NS B3H 4R2; Illinois (USA)'72; FRCSC; ThorSurg (Bronchoscopie). Affiliated Scientist, Queen Elizabeth II Health Sciences Centre - Victoria General Site; (902)494-6318

JOHNSTON, Olwyn; Gordon & Leslie Diamond HCC, 5F-2775 Laurel St, Vancouver BC V5Z 1M9; Dublin (Ireland)'96; BAO; MB BCh; (604)875-5950

JOHNSTON, Paul H; Surgical Associates, 13-391 Empire Ave, St. John's NL A1E 1W6; Qns'05; Urol. Staff, Health Sciences Centre.

JOHNSTON, Peter S; Happy Valley Family Hlth Team, PO Box 1120 Stn Main 268 Maiden Lane, St Marys ON N4X 1B7; Wes'74; Chief Chronic Care, St Marys Memorial Hospital - Huron Perth Healthcare Alliance; (519)284-3450; Fax. (519)284-4471; pjohnston@stmmc.ca.

JOHNSTON, Richard G R; Royal Alexandra Hosp, 4228-10240 Kingsway NW, Edmonton AB T5H 3V9; Alb'77; FAB; MBA; FRCPC; Anes (Critical Care Medicine). Chief Critical Care, Royal Alexandra Hospital; Clin Assoc Prof Anes & Div of Critical Care, University of Alberta; (780)735-5172

JOHNSTON, Richard U; 200-16 O'Brien St, Orillia ON L3V 5S2; Wes'69; DABOG; FSOGC; FRCSC; ObstGyn. (705)326-5561

JOHNSTON, Robert S; The Ottawa Hosp-Gen Campus, 501 Smyth Rd, Ottawa ON K1H 8L6; Tor'99; FRCPC; Anes. Staff, The Ottawa Hospital - General Campus; (613)737-7777

JOHNSTON, Robert V; 96 Edendale Cres NW, Calgary AB T3A 3W6; McG'76; EmergMed.

JOHNSTON, Ronald E; Niagara H System-St Catharines, PO Box 3018 Stn Main 142 Queenston St, St Catharines ON L2R 7C6; Tor'51; DPsy; FRCPC; Psy. Staff Site Chief Psy, Niagara Health System - St Catharines General Site; (905)684-7271

JOHNSTON, Sarah J; Port Rowan Medical Centre, 1035 Bay St, Port Rowan ON N0E 1M0; Qns'07; CCFP; (519)586-3143

JOHNSTON, Sharon E; Primrose Family Med Centre, 35 Primrose Ave, Ottawa ON K1R 0A1; Dartmouth(NH) (USA)'03; CCFP; (613)230-7788

JOHNSTON, Shawna L; Kingston Gen Hosp, 76 Stuart St, Kingston ON K7L 2V7; Qns'90; FRCSC; ObstGyn (Urological Gynecology). Att Staff, Kingston General Hospital; Att Staff, Hotel-Dieu Hospital; Assoc Prof ObstGyn & Urol, Queen's University; (613)548-6115; Fax. (613)548-1330.

JOHNSTON, Susan A; North Bay Reg Health Centre, 50 College Dr, North Bay ON P1B 0A4; Dal'96; BSc; FRCPC; Psy. Staff, North Bay Regional Health Centre - Regional Mental Health; (705)474-8600 x3641; Fax. (705)495-7890.

JOHNSTON, Terry G; Kelowna Flightcraft Hangar #8, 5655 Airport Way, Kelowna BC V1V 1S1; Sask'74; (250)807-5372

JOHNSTON, Wendy S W; University of Alberta Hosp, 2E3 17-8440 112 St NW, Edmonton AB T6G 2B7; Qns'85; BSc; FRCPC; Neur (Amyotrophic Lateral Sclerosis). Staff, University of Alberta Hospital; Assoc Prof, University of Alberta; Langs: Bilingual(English/French); (780)407-3638; Fax. (780)407-1325; wendy.johnston@ualberta.ca.

JOHNSTON, William H; 90 John St S, Stratford ON N5A 2Y8; McM'78; FRCPC; Psy. (519)272-8210

JOHNSTON, William H; Wellington Med Clinic, 1651 Boundary Ave, Nanaimo BC V9S 5R8; UBC'84; DAB; FAAO; FRCSC; Ophth (Cataract). (250)248-2266; info@islandcentreforvision.com.

JOHNSTON, Williard P; 495 40th Ave W, Vancouver BC V5Y 2R5; Cal'80; (604)324-4155; Fax. (604)321-6722.

JOHNSTONE, Brian T; Fort Frances Clinic, 301 Victoria Ave, Fort Frances ON P9A 2C1; London (England)'56; MB BS; MRCS(Eng); LRCP(Lond); CCFP; Staff, La Verendrye Hospital - Riverside Health Care Facility; (807)274-3287

JOHNSTONE, David E; Mazankowski Alberta Heart Inst, 4A7 046-8440 112 St NW, Edmonton AB T6G 2B7; McG'73; FACC; FRCPC; IntMed; Cardiol. Staff, University of Alberta Hospital; Clin Dir, Mazankowski Alberta Heart Institute; (780)407-2892; Fax. (780)407-7834.

JOHNSTONE, David W; Huntsville Prof Bldg, 204-348 Muskoka Rd 3 N, Huntsville ON P1H 1H8; Wes'93; FRCPC; IntMed. Staff, Huntsville District Memorial Hospital - Muskoka Algonquin Healthcare; (705)789-1268; Fax. (705)789-9698.

JOHNSTONE, James E; Mill Cove Plaza, 207-967 Bedford Hwy, Bedford NS B4A 1A9; Saba (Netherlands Antilles)'08; CCFP; (902)835-6444; Fax. (902)832-1193.

JOHNSTONE, Jennie; McMaster University, MDCL 3200-1280 Main St W, Hamilton ON L8S 4K1; Dal'02; FRCPC; IntMed; InfectDis. Teacher, McMaster University.

JOHNSTONE, Jennifer L; Packham Avenue Med Clinic, 104-335 Packham Ave, Saskatoon SK S7N 4S1; Sask'09; CCFP; (306)651-7091; Fax. (306)651-7092.

JOHNSTONE, Julie C; The Hosp for Sick Children, 555 University Ave, Toronto ON M5G 1X8; Wes'07; FRCPC; Peds. Staff, The Hospital For Sick Children; (416)813-7500

JOHNSTONE, Kerri L; Horizons Family Medicine, A-5016 51 Ave, Red Deer AB T4N 4H5; Alb'07; (403)342-7270; Fax. (403)343-2677.

JOHNSTONE, Saralaine S; 3000-181 Bay St, Toronto ON M5J 2T3; McM'99; CCFP; FCFP; (416)507-6607

JOHRI, Amer M; Kingston Gen Hosp, 76 Stuart St, Kingston ON K7L 2V7; Qns'02; FRCPC; IntMed; Cardiol. Staff, Kingston General Hospital; (613)549-6666

JOKAY, Eva M; 204-3269 Bloor St W, Etobicoke ON M8X 1E2; Karlova (Czech Republic)'59; DCP; FRCPC; Psy (Child Psychiatry). Langs: Polish; Czech; Slovak; (416)234-8555; Fax. (416)234-8550.

JOKHAN, Rikash; 23 First Ave N, Yorkton SK S3N 1J3; (South Africa)'05; MB BS; Staff Pediatrician, Yorkton Regional Health Centre; (306)783-3226

JOKHANI, Krishna; 3601-1499 Pender St, Vancouver BC V6G 0A7; Banaras Hindu University (India)'71; MRCPsy; FRCPC; Psy (Custody & Access). Clin Instructor/Head ADHD Clinic, BC Children's Hospital; Langs: Hindi; Punjabi; Gujarati; (604)434-7414; Fax. (604)434-7431; kjokhani@cw.bc.ca.

JOKHIO, Raza M; Endoscopy Clinic, 40 Holly St, Toronto ON M4S 3C3; (Pakistan)'76; FRCPC; Anes. (416)486-8088

JOKIC, Ruzica; Providence Care-Mental Health, PO Box 603 Stn Main 752 King St W, Kingston ON K7L 4X3; Belgrade (Serbia)'83; FRCPC; Psy. Staff, Providence Care - Mental Health Services; (613)546-1101 x5402; Fax. (613)540-6114.

JOKINEN, Donna L; Orleans Urgent Care Centre, 100-1220 Place D'Orleans Dr, Orleans ON K1C 7K3; Qns'80; Staff, Kemptville District Hospital; (613)841-5389

JOLIBOIS, Andree-Ann; Hôpital de Saint-Eustache, 520 boul Arthur-Sauve, Saint-Eustache QC J7R 5B1; Laval'04; Staff, Hôpital de Saint-Eustache; (450)473-6811; Fax. (450)473-6966.

JOLICOEUR, Andre; Clinique Familiale, 13555 boul Lacroix, Saint-Georges QC G5Y 1P1; Mon'73; Langs: Bilingual(French/English); (418)228-8001; Fax. (418)228-5583.

JOLICOEUR, Claude; Douglas Mental Hlth Univ Inst, 6875 boul Lasalle, Verdun QC H4H 1R3; Laval'66; Psy (P.Q.). Staff PedoPsy, Douglas Mental Health University Institute; McGill University; Langs: Bilingual(French/English); (514)761-6131 x2041

JOLICOEUR, Denis; Polyclinique des Ponts, 120-1100 boul de la Rive-Sud, Saint-Romuald QC G6W 5M6; Laval'77; Langs: English; (418)834-1177; Fax. (418)834-9275.

JOLICOEUR, Diane; Dir Sante Publique Montreal, 1301 rue Sherbrooke E, Montreal QC H2L 1M3; Mon'82; Langs: English; (514)528-2400 x3536

JOLICOEUR, Dominique; CLSC Saint-Jerome, 1000 rue Labelle, Saint-Jerome QC J7Z 5N6; Mon'88; MSc(Nutrition); BSc(EducPhysique); Médecin, CLSC Saint-Jerome; (450)431-8001; Fax. (450)436-8478.

JOLICOEUR, Emilie; 304-595 Montreal Rd, Ottawa ON K1K 4L2; Ott'00; FRCPC; IntMed; Gastroent. (613)744-7000; Fax. (613)744-8048.

JOLICOEUR, Gilbert; 765 boul Saint-Joseph, Gatineau QC J8Y 4B7; Ott'54; IntMed. Med Dir Long Term Care, Bruyère Continuing Care - Saint-Vincent Hospital; Consultant, Hull Hospital; (819)770-6477; Fax. (819)770-4358.

JOLICOEUR, Isabelle; CLSC Mercier-Est-Anjou, 9503 rue Sherbrooke E, Montreal QC H1L 6P2; Sher'99; (514)356-2572; Fax. (514)493-0083.

JOLICOEUR, Marc; Institut de Cardiologie de Mtl, 5000 rue Belanger, Montreal QC H1T 1C8; Mon'00; FRCPC; IntMed; Cardiol. Staff, Institut de Cardiologie de Montréal; (514)376-3330; Fax. (514)593-2155.

JOLICOEUR, Marjory; Hop Charles Lemoyne, 3120 boul Taschereau, Greenfield Park QC J4V 2H1; Mon'91; RadOncol. Staff, Hopital Charles LeMoyne; (450)466-5650

JOLICOEUR, Paul; Inst de Recherche Clin de Mtl, 110 av des Pins O, Montreal QC H2W 1R7; Laval'68; PhD; Prop, Institut de Recherche Clin de Montreal; Langs: English; (514)987-5569; Fax. (514)987-5794; jolicop@ircm.qc.ca.

JOLICOEUR, Sylvie; 1000-1075 boul Firestone, Joliette QC J6E 6X6; Mon'78; (450)755-2741; Fax. (450)755-4895.

JOLIN, Cathy; CHUM-Hop St-Luc, 1058 rue Saint-Denis, Montreal QC H2X 3J4; Mon'03; Staff, Centre Hospitalier l'Université De Montréal (CHUM) - Hôpital Saint-luc; (514)890-8000 x2444

JOLIN, Diane; CLSC de Jonquiere, 3667 boul Harvey, Jonquiere QC G7X 3A9; Sher'91; Staff, Centre Hospitalier Jonquiere; (418)695-8275; diane.jolin@ssss.gouv.qc.ca.

JOLIN, Isabelle; Clin de Med Fam Cowansville, 499 rue du Sud, Cowansville QC J2K 2X9; Sher'96; Ac Staff, Hôpital Brome-Missisquoi-Perkins; Langs: Bilingual(French/English); (450)263-8890; Fax. (450)263-9737.

JOLIN, Isabelle-Sophie; Clinique Med de Touraine, 2B-520 boul de l'Hopital, Gatineau QC J8V 2P5; McG'94; CCFP; FCFP; Langs: English; (819)568-0212; Fax. (819)568-6310.

JOLIN, Steeve; CSSSG-Hop de Hull, 116 boul Lionel-Emond, Gatineau QC J8Y 1W7; Sher'95; CSPQ; FRCPC; Anes. Staff, Hull Hospital; (819)595-6033; Fax. (819)246-0314; propof@hotmail.com.

JOLIVET, Jacques; CSSS de Saint-Jerome, 290 rue de Montigny, Saint-Jerome QC J7Z 5T3; Mon'76; ABIM; FRCPC; IntMed; MedOncol. Staff, Hôtel-Dieu de Saint-Jérôme; (450)431-8201

JOLIVET, Marie; Ctr Hosp De Verdun, 4000 boul Lasalle, Verdun QC H4G 2A3; Mon'74; FRCPC; MedMicrobiol; Microbio & Infect Dis (P.Q.). Ac Staff, Centre Hospitalier de Verdun; (514)362-1000 x2211

JOLIVET-TREMBLAY, Martine; CHUM-Hop St-Luc, 1058 rue Saint-Denis, Montreal QC H2X 3J4; Mon'93; FRCSC; Urol. Staff, Centre Hospitalier l'Université De Montréal (CHUM) - Hôpital Saint-luc; (514)890-8000; Fax. (514)861-3021.

JOLLANT, Fabrice B; Douglas Mental Hlth Univ Inst, 6875 boul Lasalle, Verdun QC H4H 1R3; Montpellier (France)'04; Staff, Douglas Mental Health University Institute; (514)761-6131

JOLLER, Petra; Health Sciences Centre, 300 Prince Philip Dr, St. John's NL A1B 3V6; Qns'06; CCFP; Staff, Health Sciences Centre; (709)737-6300

JOLLIMORE, Jason V; Colchester East Hants Hlth Ctr, 600 Abenaki Rd, Truro NS B2N 5A1; Dal'99; BSc(Hon); FRCPC; AnatPath. Staff Pathologist, Colchester East Hants Health Centre; Consultant Pathologist, Aberdeen Regional Hospital; Staff, Cumberland Regional Health Care Center; (902)893-5554; drjvjollimore@hotmail.com.

JOLLY, Donald T; Misericordia Community Hosp, 16940 87 Ave NW, Edmonton AB T5R 4H5; Wes'77; FRCPC; Anes (Acute Pain Management);CCFP; CCFP(E.M.); FCFP; Staff Anes, Covenant Health - Misericordia Community Hospital; Clinical Asst Prof Anes, University of Alberta; (780)735-2863

JOLLY, Elaine E; The Ottawa Hosp-Riverside, 7 236-1967 Riverside Dr, Ottawa ON K1H 7W9; Qns'64; ObstGyn (Menopause). Med Dir Shirley E Greenberg Women's Health Centre, The Ottawa Hospital - Riverside Campus; Prof ObstGyn, University of Ottawa; (613)738-8400; Fax. (613)738-8505.

JOLLY, Elizabeth M; 100-2903 32 Ave, Vernon BC V1T 2L6; Wes'81; BSc; CCFP; FCFP; Staff, Vernon Jubilee Hospital; (250)545-9669; Fax. (250)545-9940.

JOLLY, Kanwaljit S; Boyd Med Centre, 513-388 Portage Ave, Winnipeg MB R3C 0C8; Punjab (India)'69; MB BS; LRCP; MRCS; DRCOG; FRCPC; IntMed (Cardiology). Ac Staff, Victoria General Hospital; Consultant, Concordia General Hospital; Ac Staff, St Boniface General Hospital; Asst Prof, University of Manitoba; (204)943-9162

JOLLY, Patrick; 201-1408 rue Jean-Talon E, Montreal QC H2E 1S2; Mon'68; FRCSC; Urol (Surgical Oncology). Ac Staff, CSSS du Coeur de l'Isle Hôpital Jean-Talon; Langs: Bilingual(French/English); (514)270-8337; Fax. (514)270-6336.

JOLLY, Rajnee K; Kingsridge Med Centre, 2-2015 Kingsridge Dr, Oakville ON L6M 4Y7; Tor'99; CCFP; (905)827-3006; Fax. (905)825-9431.

JOLLY, Sanjit S; Hamilton HS-General Site, C3 118-237 Barton St E, Hamilton ON L8L 2X2; Tor'99; FRCPC; IntMed; Cardiol. Staff, Hamilton Health Sciences Centre - Hamilton General Hospital; (905)524-2712; Fax. (905)297-3785.

JOLLY, Shivinder S; Medical Bldg, 104-18 Pine St, Kitchener ON N2H 5Z8; Ott'94; FRCPC; IntMed (Hypertension); Nephrol. (519)743-2573; Fax. (519)743-2792.

JOLLYMORE, Brian D; Valley Reg Hosp, 150 Exhibition St, Kentville NS B4N 5E3; Dal'86; FRCPC; GenPath. Staff, Valley Regional Hospital; (902)678-7381; bdj.path@ns.sympatico.ca.

JOLLYMORE, Gary E; 554 Main St E, Hamilton ON L8M 1J3; Dal'74; BSc; (905)522-9002; Fax. (905)522-2532; gary.jollymore@hamiltonsteel.ca.

JOLLYMORE, George C; Chester Med Services, PO Box 110 57 King St, Chester NS B0J 1J0; Dal'63; BSc; Staff, Fishermen's Memorial Hospital; Staff, South Shore Regional Hospital; (902)275-3529; Fax. (902)275-2594.

JOLLYMORE, John S; Foul Bay Prof Centre, 212-1964 Fort St, Victoria BC V8R 6R3; Dal'85; (250)592-5255; Fax. (250)592-5201.

JOLLYMORE, Kory G; Dingwall Med Group, PO Box 3011 40 Goodall St, Dryden ON P8N 2Z6; Dal'05; CCFP; (807)223-6683

JOLY, Caroline; Espace Sante Ile-des-Soeurs, 200-8 Place du Commerce, Verdun QC H3E 1N3; Mon'92; CCFP; Staff, CSSS de Dorval-Lachine-Lasalle; (514)798-2228

JOLY, Christine; Clinique Med Laval, 1110 boul Vanier, Laval QC H7C 2R8; Mon'90; Staff, Hopital de la Cite de la santé; (450)661-2521; Fax. (450)661-7193.

JOLY, Dominique E; Centre Med Ste-Anne, 113 rue Sainte-Anne, Ste-Anne-De-Bellev QC H9X 1M2; Sher'84; (514)457-2772; Fax. (514)457-4397.

JOLY, Edith; Clin Med du Plateau Mont-Royal, 103-1374 av du Mont-Royal E, Montreal QC H2J 1Y7; Mon'03; Staff, Centre Hospitalier Pierre le Gardeur; (514)527-3997

JOLY, Jacqueline L; 210-99 Kakulu Rd, Kanata ON K2L 3C8; McM'88; FRCPC; Peds. Court Staff Privil, Children's Hospital of Eastern Ontario (CHEO); Langs: English; French; (613)591-3339

JOLY, Jean R; CSSS de la Haute-Yamaska, 205 boul Leclerc O, Granby QC J2G 1T7; Mon'74; MBA; FRCPC; MedMicrobiol; Microbio & Infect Dis (P.Q.). Staff, Centre Hospitalier de Granby; (450)375-8000

JOLY, Jean-Gil; CSSS de Saint-Jerome, 290 rue de Montigny, Saint-Jerome QC J7Z 5T3; Mon'65; MSc; MedBiochem (P.Q.); IntMed (P.Q.). Chef Biochem, Hôtel-Dieu de Saint-Jérôme; Chief, Clinique de la Migraine des Laurentides; Langs: English; (450)431-8200 x2141; Fax. (450)227-7406; dr.joly@cgocable.ca.

JOLY, Johanne; Douglas Mental Hlth Univ Inst, 6875 boul Lasalle, Verdun QC H4H 1R3; McG'77; FRCPC; Psy. Staff, Douglas Mental Health University Institute; (514)761-6131 x2768

JOLY, Lucie; CSSS de Laval, 1755 boul Rene-Laennec, Laval QC H7M 3L9; Laval'99; FRCPC; IntMed; Gastroent. Staff, Hopital de la Cite de la santé; (450)688-1010

JOLY, Melissa; Hotel-Dieu d'Arthabaska, 5 rue des Hospitalieres, Victoriaville QC G6P 6N2; Sher'02; Staff, Hotel-Dieu d'Arthabaska; (819)357-2030

JOLY, Nikola; CHUM-Hop St-Luc, 1058 rue Saint-Denis, Montreal QC H2X 3J4; Mon'05; FRCPC; Anes. Staff, Centre Hospitalier l'Université De Montréal (CHUM) - Hôpital Saint-luc; (514)890-8000

JOLY, Sylvain; Ctr Hosp Pierre-Janet, 20 rue Pharand, Gatineau QC J9A 1K7; Mon'80; FRCPC; Psy. Staff, Centre Hospitalier Pierre-Janet; Consultant Psy, Hull Hospital; University of Ottawa; (819)771-7761; Fax. (819)771-4727.

JOLY NICKOLET, Sarah; Royal Alexandra Hosp, 10240 Kingsway NW, Edmonton AB T5H 3V9; Alb'05; FRCPC; Anes. Staff, Royal Alexandra Hospital; (780)735-4111

JOMHA, Nadr M; University of Alberta Hosp, 2D2 32-8440 112 St NW, Edmonton AB T6G 2B7; Alb'90; FRCSC; OrthSurg (Foot & Ankle Surgery). Clin Associate, University of Alberta Hospital; Staff, Covenant Health - Misericordia Community Hospital; Asst Prof, University of Alberta; (780)407-2816

JOMPHE, Julie; Clin Externe de Psychiatrie, 203-100 rue Grenier, Charlemagne QC J5Z 4C6; Sher'95; FRCPC; Psy. Staff, Centre Hospitalier Pierre le Gardeur; (450)585-9010; Fax. (450)585-2709.

JOMPHE, Michele; 1403 Edward St PO Box 2530, Hearst ON P0L 1N0; Sher'08; CCFP; (705)362-8262

JONAS, Krista M; Brock University, 500 Glenridge Ave, St Catharines ON L2S 3A1; Wes'93; Teach Staff, Brock University; (905)688-5550

JONAT, Lee M; 405-321 Nicola St, Kamloops BC V2C 6G6; UBC'06; FRCSC; Urol. (778)471-5556

JONATHAN, Ernest R; 1176 St Clair Ave W, Toronto ON M6E 1B4; Tor'83; (416)652-5600; Fax. (416)652-5601.

JONATHAN, Stanley R; York-Finch Med Centre, 311A-2115 Finch Ave W, North York ON M3N 2V6; Cape Town (South Africa)'55; MB ChB; Ac Staff Psy, Humber River Regional Hospital - Finch Avenue Site; (416)745-7989

JONCAS, Henri; Ctr Hosp Affilie-Enfant-Jesus, 1401 18e rue, Quebec QC G1J 1Z4; Laval'77; CSPQ; FRCPC; Anes. Staff, Centre Hospitalier Affilié Universitaire de Québec - Hôpital De L'Enfant Jésus; (418)649-5803

JONCAS, Jean-Francois; CHUS-Hop Hotel-Dieu, 580 rue Bowen S, Sherbrooke QC J1G 2E8; Sher'83; FRCSC; OrthSurg. Ac Staff, Centre Hospitalier Universitaire de Sherbrooke-Hôpital Hôtel-Dieu; (819)346-1110

JONCAS, Paul-Aime; Clinique Med Dr Joncas, CP 10 21 rue Bord-de-L'Eau, Lourdes-D-Bl-Sabl QC G0G 1W0; Laval'84; Langs: English; (418)461-3773; Fax. (418)461-3772.

JONCAS, Sebastien X; CSSS de Chicoutimi, 305 rue Saint-Vallier, Chicoutimi QC G7H 5H6; Sher'07; IntMed. Staff, Complexe hospitalier de la Sagamie; (418)541-1000

JONCAS, Valerie; CHUQ-Ctr Hosp Univ Laval, 1207-2705 boul Laurier, Quebec QC G1V 4G2; Mon'04; FRCPC; Derm. Staff, Centre Hospitalier Universitaire de Quebec-CHUL; (418)654-2160

JONEJA, Anu; U of Toronto-Health Services, 214 College St, Toronto ON M5T 2Z9; Sask'01; CCFP; (416)978-8030; Fax. (416)971-2089.

JONEJA, Mala; Queen's Univ-Etherington Hall, 2004-99 University Ave, Kingston ON K7L 3N5; Qns'94; FRCPC; IntMed; Rheum. Att Staff, Kingston General Hospital; Asst Prof Med, Queen's University; Langs: Hindi; Punjabi; (613)533-3230; Fax. (613)533-3244.

JONES, A Frank; 4005-381 Kent St, Ottawa ON K2P 2A8; McM'73; FRCPC; Psy. Consultant, The Ottawa Hospital - General Campus; University of Ottawa; (613)230-4838; Fax. (613)230-3697.

JONES, Alan P; Hys Med Centre, 350-11010 101 St NW, Edmonton AB T5H 4B9; Dal'82; FRCPC; IntMed; Cardiol. (780)428-3246; Fax. (780)425-0487.

JONES, Alan W R; Regina Qu'Appelle HR-Pasqua, 6-4101 Dewdney Ave, Regina SK S4T 1A5; Sask'91; BEd; BSc; FRCSC; OrthSurg (Arthroplasty). Head Section of Orthoaedics, Pasqua Hospital; (306)766-6964; Fax. (306)766-7025.

JONES, Alexander E; 27 John St, York ON M9N 1J4; Tor'66; Staff, Humber River Regional Hospital - Church Street Site; (416)248-6334

JONES, Allan R; Kelowna Gen Hosp, 2268 Pandosy St, Kelowna BC V1Y 1T2; McG'75; MedOncol; Hem; IntMed. Staff, Kelowna General Hospital; Reg Associate Deans Interior, University of British Columbia; (250)862-4300

JONES, Allen S; John Street Clinic, 14 John St N, Hamilton ON L8R 1G9; UBC'98; CCFP; Staff, St Joseph's Healthcare - Charlton Campus; (905)546-0050; Fax. (905)546-0030.

JONES, Andrea K; Georgian Bay Gen Hosp, PO Box 760 Stn Main 1112 St Andrew's Dr, Midland ON L4R 4P4; Dal'96; CCFP; CCFP(E.M.); Staff, Georgian Bay General Hospital - Midland; (705)526-1300; Fax. (705)526-1338.

JONES, Andrew E; London HSC-Victoria Hosp, PO Box 5010 Stn B 102-800 Commissioners Rd E, London ON N6A 5W9; Wes'97; FRCPC; EmergMed. Staff EmergMed, London Health Sciences Centre - Victoria Campus; (519)667-6538

JONES, Angela M; Waterdown Family Med Clinic, 95 Hamilton St N, Waterdown ON L0R 2H0; McM'99; CCFP; FCFP; Associate, Joseph Brant Memorial Hospital; (905)689-6134; Fax. (905)689-5665.

JONES, Angela M; Royal University Hosp, 103 Hospital Dr, Saskatoon SK S7N 0W8; Cal'03; BSc; FRCPC; Peds. Staff Ped Outpatient Dept, Royal University Hospital; (306)966-2922; Fax. (306)966-8640.

JONES, Ann D; Waypoint Centre for Mental H C, 500 Church St, Penetanguishene ON L9M 1G3; Wes'87; FRCPC; Psy. Staff, Waypoint Centre for Mental Health Care; (705)549-3181

JONES, Anthony H D; Meridian Med Clinic, 3-4402 37 St, Stony Plain AB T7Z 2A9; London (England)'68; MB BS; LRCP; MRCS; (780)963-7800; Fax. (780)963-0468; antonj@xplornett.net.

JONES, Arthur L; The Medical Centre, 403-265 Yorkland Blvd, North York ON M2J 5C7; Dublin (Ireland)'48; FRCP(Ire); DPsy; DABPN; Psy (Adult Psychiatry). (416)229-2399; Fax. (416)229-9771; ajone2139@rogers.com.

JONES, Barbara A; Medicine Professional Corp, 29 Northview Rd, Ottawa ON K2E 6A6; McM'80; FRCPC; Psy (Child & Adolescent Psychiatry). Staff Psychiatrist, Children's Hospital of Eastern Ontario (CHEO); Asst Clin Prof, University of Ottawa.

JONES, Brent D; Canadian Forces Supp Unit HCC, 1745 Alta Vista Dr, Ottawa ON K1A 0K6; Alb'91; CCFP; Staff, Canadian Forces Health Services Centre; (613)945-6533

JONES, Bronwen A; Spryfield Med Clinic, 205 Herring Cove Rd, Halifax NS B3P 1L1; Alb'89; CCFP; Med Dir, Harbour View Haven Nursing Home; (902)477-5693; Fax. (902)477-0502.

JONES, C William; Clarenceville Clinic, GD 100 rue Principale, Clarenceville QC J0J 1B0; McG'68; FRCSC; GenSurg; Cardiovasc&ThorSurg. (450)294-2177

JONES, Carl V; Island Centre for Vision, 1651 Boundary Ave, Nanaimo BC V9S 5R8; Oxford (England)'69; MB; BCh; AB; ABOph; FRCS; FRCSC; Ophth. Staff, Providence Health Care - St Paul's Hospital; Staff, Providence Health Care - Mount Saint Joseph Hospital; Clin Assoc Prof, University of British Columbia; (250)753-6960; jonescv@interchange.ubc.ca.

JONES, Carolyn S S; 200-10504 100 Ave, Fort St. John BC V1J 1Z2; Witwatersrand (South Africa)'89; FRCPC; Psy. Staff, Fort St John Hospital & Health Centre; Staff, Dawson Creek & District Hospital; (250)262-5282; Fax. (250)262-5331.

JONES, Charlotte A; UBC Okanagan-HSC, 321-3333 University Way, Kelowna BC V1V 1V7; Cal'89; FRCPC; IntMed; Endocrin&Metab.

JONES, Christine N; Victoria Hospice Society, 3F-1952 Bay St, Victoria BC V8R 1J8; UBC'93; BSc; CCFP; Staff, Victoria Hospice Society; (250)370-8715

JONES, Christopher M; 203-1990 Fort St, Victoria BC V8R 6V4; UBC'84; FRCPC; IntMed; Nephrol. (250)592-1166; Fax. (250)592-1599.

JONES, Christopher T; Queen Elizabeth II HSC-Halifax, 1796 Summer St, Halifax NS B3H 3A7; Monash (Australia)'00; Staff, Queen Elizabeth II Health Sciences Centre - Halifax Infirmary Site; (902)473-2700

JONES, Claire A; 700-250 Dundas St W, Toronto ON M5T 2Z5; Wes'07; FRCPC; ObstGyn. (416)586-5367

JONES, Colin D; Radiology Consultants Assoc, 120-6707 Elbow Dr SW, Calgary AB T2V 0E3; Alb'03; FRCPC; DiagRad. (403)777-4674; Fax. (403)777-3198.

JONES, Cristen D; Brandon Reg Health Centre, 150 McTavish Ave E, Brandon MB R7A 2B3; Staff, Brandon Regional Health Centre; (204)578-4000

JONES, D Stephen R; Thamesville Med Clinic, 14 Victoria St, Thamesville ON N0P 2K0; McG'89; BSc(Hons); CCFP; Court Staff Privil, Chatham-Kent Health Alliance; Staff, Four Counties Health Services - Middlesex Hospital Alliance; (519)692-9584

JONES, David A R; KDH Health Centre, PO Box 2113 2671 Concession Rd, Kemptville ON K0G 1J0; Ott'02; CCFP; (613)258-0100

JONES, David H D; 106-450 Central Ave, London ON N6B 2E8; Wes'87; Physician, London Health Sciences Centre - Victoria Campus; (519)660-1788

JONES, David M; Foothills Med Centre, 1403 29 St NW, Calgary AB T2N 2T9; Mem'04; Hem; IntMed. Staff, Foothills Medical Centre; (403)944-1110

JONES, David R L; Pemberton Med Clinic, PO Box 69 1403 Portage Rd, Pemberton BC V0N 2L0; London (England)'99; MB BS; CCFP; (604)894-6454; Fax. (604)894-6721.

JONES, David W; Royal Oak Med Centre, 204-6440 Royal Oak Ave, Burnaby BC V5H 3P2; UBC'70; BSc; Coord Med, Burnaby Hospital; Court Staff, Vancouver General Hospital - Centennial Pavillion; Court Staff, BC Women's Hospital & Health Centre; (604)482-6100; Fax. (604)482-6102.

JONES, Dean R; Delta Hosp, 5800 Mountain View Blvd, Delta BC V4K 3V6; Qns'99; FRCPC; Anes. Staff, Delta Hospital; (604)946-1121

JONES, Denis; Regina Qu'Appelle HR-Regina, 1440 14th Ave, Regina SK S4P 0W5; Witwatersrand (South Africa)'89; Staff, Regina General Hospital; (306)766-4444

JONES, Donald P; The Credit Valley Hosp, 2200 Eglinton Ave W, Mississauga ON L5M 2N1; Tor'72; FCCP; FACS; FRCSC; GenSurg; ThorSurg (Thoracic Oncology). Head Oncol, William Osler Health System - Etobicoke General Hospital; Ac Staff, The Credit Valley Hospital; Court Staff, North York General Hospital; Head Surgical Oncol, Peel Regional Cancer Centre; Langs: Italian; French; (905)813-1100 x5070; Fax. (905)813-4024.

JONES, Donna V; 4F-1441 29 St NW, Calgary AB T2N 4J8; Man'98; FRCSC; ObstGyn. Staff ObstGyn, Foothills Medical Centre; (403)944-1438; Fax. (403)270-4249.

JONES, E Shani; 90 Ellesmere Dr, Moncton NB E1C 9L6; Mem'82; FRCPC; AnatPath. (506)857-5308; Fax. (506)857-5632; dr.e.shani.jones@horizonnb.ca.

JONES, Edmund F; Hotel-Dieu Hosp, 166 Brock St, Kingston ON K7L 5G2; McG'84; FRCSC; Otol. Staff, Hotel-Dieu Hospital; Langs: Bilingual(English/French); (613)544-3400 x3610; Fax. (613)547-5654.

JONES, Edward A; Regina Qu'Appelle HR-Pasqua, 100-4101 Dewdney Ave, Regina SK S4T 1A5; Alb'73; BSc; FRCPC; AnatPath (General Pathology). Staff Path, Pasqua Hospital; Staff Path, Regina Health District; Asst Prof, University of Saskatchewan; Langs: English; French; (306)766-2157

JONES, Edward C; Vancouver Gen Hosp, 855 12th Ave W, Vancouver BC V5Z 1M9; UBC'80; FRCPC; AnatPath (Urologic Pathology). Consultant Path, Vancouver General Hospital - Centennial Pavillion; Clin Prof Med/Assoc Member, University of British Columbia; Langs: English; French; (604)875-5564; Fax. (604)875-4797.

JONES, Emmanuel E; Clarke's Beach Clinic, PO Box 220, Clarkes Beach NL A0A 1W0; Mem'89; (709)786-6611; Fax. (709)786-6612.

JONES, Ernest R; Humber River Reg Hosp-Church, 200 Church St, Toronto ON M9N 1N8; Tor'52; Staff, Humber River Regional Hospital - Church Street Site; (416)612-7786

JONES, Gareth W; Elmira Med Centre, 2 Park Ave W, Elmira ON N3B 1L1; Wes'85; (519)669-5493; Fax. (519)669-5901.

JONES, Glenn W; The Credit Valley Hosp, 2200 Eglinton Ave W, Mississauga ON L5M 2N1; Qns'84; BSc; MSc; FRCPC; RadOncol (Medical Oncology). Staff, The Credit Valley Hospital; Assoc Prof Med, McMaster University; (905)813-1100 x5000; Fax. (905)813-3962.

JONES, Glynn C; Kelowna Gen Hosp, 2268 Pandosy St, Kelowna BC V1Y 1T2; Stellenbosch (South Africa)'81; MB ChB; CCFP; Staff, Kelowna General Hospital; (250)862-4000; glynnjones@shaw.ca.

JONES, Gordon R; Kingston Gen Hosp, 76 Stuart St, Kingston ON K7L 2V7; Qns'82; FRCPC; EmergMed. Staff, Kingston General Hospital; Staff, Hotel-Dieu Hospital; (613)548-2368; Fax. (613)548-1374; jonesg@kgh.kari.net.

JONES, Gordon R M; Queen Elizabeth II HSC, 1276 South Park St, Halifax NS B3H 2Y9; Edinburgh (Scotland)'65; MB ChB; DMRD; FRCR(UK); MRC(UK); DiagRad (Diagnostic Imaging). Staff Radiol, Queen Elizabeth II Health Sciences Centre - Victoria General Site; Assoc Prof, Dalhousie University; (902)473-7770; Fax. (902)473-3482; gr_jones@hotmail.com.

JONES, Graham L; McMaster University, 3U7-1280 Main St W, Hamilton ON L8S 4K1; Tor'93; MSc; PhD; FRCPC; IntMed (Pulmonary Medicine); Critical Care Medicine; Respir. Staff, Hamilton Health Sciences Centre - McMaster Children's Hospital; Asst Prof Med, McMaster University; (905)521-2100 x73259; Fax. (905)521-5053.

JONES, Griffith D; The Ottawa Hosp-Gen Campus, 8420-501 Smyth Rd, Ottawa ON K1H 8L6; London (England)'87; FRCSC; ObstGyn. Staff, The Ottawa Hospital - General Campus; (613)737-8571; Fax. (613)737-8070.

JONES, Gwynne; The Ottawa Hosp-Gen Campus, 207-501 Smyth Rd, Ottawa ON K1H 8L6; London (England)'69; MB BS; FRCP(UK); FRCPC; IntMed (Critical Care Medicine). Assoc Prof Med, The Ottawa Hospital - General Campus; Assoc Prof Med, University of Ottawa; Langs: English; French; (613)737-9830; Fax. (613)737-8890.

JONES, H Niall; 124 Street Med Group, 10839 124 St NW, Edmonton AB T5M 0H4; UBC'92; FRCPC; IntMed (Scleroderma & Inflammatory Arthritis); Rheum. Associate Clin Prof, University of Alberta; (780)488-1755; Fax. (780)488-1749.

JONES, J H Lloyd; Lasalle Walk In Clinic, 1813 Lasalle Blvd, Sudbury ON P3A 2A3; Oxford (England)'47; BCh; Staff, Health Sciences North - Memorial Site; (705)560-9422; Fax. (705)560-9482; jhlloyd@gmail.com.

JONES, Jeffery B; 722 Mackay St, Pembroke ON K8A 8J8; Qns'84; FRCSC; Otol. (613)732-1037; Fax. (613)732-1041.

JONES, Jeffrey K; Claresholm Med Centre, PO Box 2050, Claresholm AB T0L 0T0; Alb'90; CCFP; CCFP(E.M.); FCFP; (403)625-4484; Fax. (403)625-3969.

JONES, Jennifer K; Health Sciences Bldg, 310-15 Mountain Ave S, Stoney Creek ON L8G 2V6; Qns'08; CCFP; (905)664-3730; Fax. (905)664-9921.

JONES, Jennifer L; Royal University Hosp, 103 Hospital Dr, Saskatoon SK S7N 0W8; Dal'99; BSc; FRCPC; IntMed (Inflammatory Bowel Disease); Gastroent. Staff, Royal University Hospital; (306)655-1000

JONES, Jeremy C; 104-86 Angeline St S, Lindsay ON K9V 6C5; Ott'01; BSc; FRCPC; IntMed. Associate Privil, Ross Memorial Hospital; (705)878-4004; Fax. (705)878-1822.

JONES, Jodi L P; Health Sciences Centre, GB421-820 Sherbrook St, Winnipeg MB R3A 1R9; Man'02; FRCSC; Otol. Staff, Health Sciences Centre; (204)774-8511

JONES, Judith L; 304-4420 Chatterton Way, Victoria BC V8X 5J2; UBC'91; BSc; CCFP; FCFP; Staff, Vancouver Island Health Authority; (250)727-2663; Fax. (250)727-9445.

JONES, Julia J; Taunton Health Centre, SS 201 1290 Keith Ross Dr, Oshawa ON L1H 7K4; Tor'94; BSc; MSc; FRCSC; GenSurg; General Surgical Oncology. (905)721-4315; Fax. (905)721-6647.

JONES, Julie; Prairie Trail Med Centre, 100-1345 Taylor Ave, Winnipeg MB R3M 3Y9; UBC'93; MSc(Nutrition); BSc(Hons); CCFP; Med Dir, St James Medical Clinic; Med Dir, Great West Life Assurance Company; Langs: English; French; (204)475-0088

JONES, Karen E; Maple Leaf Med Clinic, 6F-14 College St, Toronto ON M5G 1K2; McM'91; BSc(Hon); MHSc; FRCP; MD; FCFP; FRCPC; CommunMed (Cognitive-Behavioral Psychotherapy);CCFP; FCFP; Public Health & Preventive Med. Staff, Toronto General Hospital - UHN; Asst Prof Family Commun Med & Psy, University of Toronto; (416)921-6773; Fax. (416)960-0489.

JONES, Kathryn G; Columbia Med Bldg, 303-301 Columbia St E, New Westminster BC V3L 3W5; McG'85; MDCM; Staff, Royal Columbian Hospital; (604)525-5388; Fax. (604)525-4541.

JONES, Keith W; Sow's Ear Clinic, PO Box 190 7186 Lantzville Rd, Lantzville BC V0R 2H0; Cardiff (Wales)'72; MB ChB; (250)390-4542; Fax. (250)390-4561.

JONES, Kelly O; St Thomas-Elgin Gen Hosp, PO Box 2007 Stn Main, St Thomas ON N5P 3W2; Wes'66; Assoc Staff, St Thomas Elgin General Hospital; (519)631-2020

JONES, Kenneth D; Parkdale Medical Tower, 607-1081 Carling Ave, Ottawa ON K1Y 4G2; London (England)'62; MB BS; LRCP; MRCS; (613)725-3117

JONES, Kirsten E; Cambie Surgery Centre, 2836 Ash St, Vancouver BC V5Z 3C6; Qns'04; FRCSC; GenSurg. Staff, Cambie Surgery Centre; (604)874-1349

JONES, Kristen S; Cottage Country Fam Hlth Team, 1-5 Pineridge Gate, Gravenhurst ON P1P 1Z3; Wes'04; CCFP; (705)687-2271; Fax. (705)687-7575.

JONES, Lanice K; 23 McDougall Crt NE, Calgary AB T2E 8R3; Cal'85; BSc; CCFP; FCFP; Clin Lecturer Family Pract, University of Calgary; (403)265-3410; Fax. (403)265-3411.

JONES, Lee D T; Hinton Med Clinic, 102 Allen Cove, Hinton AB T7V 2A6; Alb'06; CCFP; (780)865-3338

JONES, Lize; Village Mall Med Clinic, 22-6320 50 Ave, Red Deer AB T4N 4C6; Pretoria (South Africa)'99; Langs: Afrikaans; (403)314-5357

JONES, Lori; Crossroads Family Practice, 201-5110 St Margarets Bay Rd, Upper Tantallon NS B3Z 1E2; (Other Foreign)'09; CCFP; (902)826-9096

JONES, Mark B; 2F-353 St Paul Ave, Brantford ON N3R 4N3; Tor'02; FRCPC; IntMed; Gastroent. Staff, The Brant Community Healthcare System - Brantford General Hospital Site; (519)512-0058; Fax. (519)512-0611.

JONES, Megan G C; Nova Medical, 496 Topsail Rd, St. John's NL A1B 1S1; Alb'01.

JONES, Michael B; Cook Medical Bldg, 107-1175 Cook St, Victoria BC V8V 4A1; Cape Town (South Africa)'85; MB ChB; LMCC; (250)383-3311

JONES, Michael W; Cobourg Clinic, PO Box 86 Stn Main, Cobourg ON K9A 4K4; London (England)'68; MB BS; MRCS; LRCP; Ac Staff, Northumberland Hills Hospital; (905)372-3323; Fax. (905)372-3692.

JONES, Michele L; St Anthony's Med Centre, 308-582 Goldstream Ave, Victoria BC V9B 2W7; UBC'96; FRCSC; Ophth (Anterior Segment). (250)391-6062

JONES, Michelle-Lee; London HSC-University Hosp, PO Box 5339 Stn B 339 Windermere Rd, London ON N6A 5A5; McG'07; MDCM; FRCPC; Neur. Staff, London Health Sciences Centre - University Hospital; (519)685-8300

JONES, Nicola L; The Hosp For Sick Children, 8409-555 University Ave, Toronto ON M5G 1X8; Tor'89; FRCPC; Peds. Staff, The Hospital For Sick Children; Prof Peds, University of Toronto; (416)813-7734; Fax. (416)813-6531; nicola.jones@sickkids.ca.

JONES, Nicole A; West Durham Family Health Team, 200B-1105 Kingston Rd, Pickering ON L1V 1B5; McM'05; CCFP; (905)420-9999

JONES, Pamela L; 201-17001 Trans Canada, Kirkland QC H9H 5J1; Tor'85; FRCSC; OrthSurg (Foot & Ankle Surgery). Ac Member, CSSS de Dorval-Lachine-Lasalle; Langs: French; Italian; (514)624-0666

JONES, Philip M G; London HSC-University Hosp, PO Box 5339 Stn B C3 110-339 Windermere Rd, London ON N6A 5A5; Wes'00; FRCPC; Anes. Staff, London Health Sciences Centre - University Hospital; (519)685-8500

JONES, Stephen; Lakeridge Hlth Corp-Oshawa, 1 Hospital Crt, Oshawa ON L1G 2B9; Cardiff (Wales)'71; FRCPC; DiagRad. Staff, Lakeridge Health - Oshawa Site; (905)433-4305; Fax. (905)721-4770.

JONES, Ralph W M; 101-9006 Edward St, Chilliwack BC V2P 4E1; Birmingham (England)'76; MB ChB; MRCGPract; Ac Staff, Chilliwack General Hospital; Consultant, Mental Health Centre; (604)701-6866; ralph.jones@viha.ca.

JONES, Robert A; 426 Talbot St, St Thomas ON N5P 1B9; Wes'72; Staff, St Thomas Elgin General Hospital; (519)633-4410

JONES, Robert G; 206-435 Reynolds St, Oakville ON L6J 3M5; McM'79; Staff, Halton Healthcare Services Corporation - Oakville Site; (905)815-9434; Fax. (905)815-1745.

JONES, Russet L; Child & Adolescent Psy, 4450 Oak St, Vancouver BC V6H 3V5; UBC'99; FRCPC; Psy. Staff, BC Children's Hospital; (604)875-2014

JONES, Sarah A; London HSC-Victoria Hosp, PO Box 5010 Stn B B 1 131-800 Commissioners Rd E, London ON N6A 5W9; McM'95; FRCSC; GenSurg; PedGenSurg. Staff, London Health Sciences Centre - Victoria Campus; Asst Prof, Queen's University; (519)685-8500

JONES, Sarah D; Crossroads Family Practice, 201-5110 St Margarets Bay Rd, Upper Tantallon NS B3Z 1E2; Dal'07; CCFP; (902)826-9096; Fax. (902)820-9399.

JONES, Shannon L; PO Box 1304 Stn A, Comox BC V9M 7Z8; Alb'94; CCFP; FCFP.

JONES, Suzanne; Kateri Mem Hosp Centre, PO Box 10, Kahnawake QC J0L 1B0; McG'82; CCFP; FCFP; Dir Prof Services, Kateri Memorial Hospital Centre; Staff, Sir Mortimer B Davis Jewish General; adj Prof, McGill University; (450)638-3930; Fax. (450)638-4634; suzanne.jones@rrsss16.gouv.qc.ca.

JONES, Sylvie A; Academic Family Medicine, 172-1621 Albert St, Regina SK S4P 2S5; McG'92; CCFP; FCFP; Staff Physician, Regina General Hospital; (306)766-0444; Fax. (306)766-0471.

JONES, Tera; Office of the Chief Med Examin, 4070 Bowness Rd NW, Calgary AB T3B 3R7; (USA)'02; DABPath; (403)297-8123; Fax. (780)422-1265.

JONES, Valerie A; 201-3040 Tutt St, Kelowna BC V1Y 2H5; Man'80; FRCPC; Psy (Adult Psychiatry). Staff Admitting Privil, Kelowna General Hospital; (250)763-7448; Fax. (250)763-7440.

JONES, Victoria J; North York Med Arts Bldg, 141-1333 Sheppard Ave E, North York ON M2J 1V1; Wes'77; FRCPC; Psy. Consultant, North York General Hospital; (416)491-4318; Fax. (416)491-1719.

JONES, Wentworth W; 2 Lyall Ave, Toronto ON M4E 1V8; Tor'56; (416)699-9823; Fax. (416)699-0459.

JONES-HISCOCK, Cherie L; Ongwanada Resource Center, 191 Portsmouth Ave, Kingston ON K7M 8A6; Mem'94; FRCPC; Psy (Child & Adolescent Psychiatry). Staff Psy, Ongwanada Development Services; Asst Prof School of Med, Queen's University; (613)548-4417

JONES-LOCKE, Diana C; Physicians Incorporated, 204-316 Willow St, Truro NS B2N 5A4; Dal'89; Staff, Colchester East Hants Health Centre; (902)893-4999; Fax. (902)893-7669.

JONES-STOKREEF, Nicola J; 1080 Mississaga St W, Orillia ON L3V 3C8; Qns'89; FRCPC; Peds (Developmental Pediatrics). Staff, Orillia Soldiers' Memorial Hospital; Langs: English; French; (705)326-2214 x244; Fax. (705)326-0667; njonesstokreef@osmh.on.ca.

JONG, Anthony K; Westwind Med Clinic, 107-755 Goldstream Ave, Victoria BC V9B 2X4; Dal'73; Ac Staff, Victoria General Hospital; (250)478-1764; Fax. (250)478-1300.

JONG, Michael K K; Labrador Grenfell Health, PO Box 7000 Stn C, Happy-Valley-Goose NL A0P 1C0; (Malaysia)'75; MRCP(UK); CCFP; FCFP; Labrador Health Centre; Prof Family Med, Memorial University Of Newfoundland; (709)897-2268; Fax. (709)896-4032.

JONG, Roberta A; Sunnybrook Hlth Sciences Ctre, MG178-2075 Bayview Ave, Toronto ON M4N 3M5; Tor'69; FRCPC; DiagRad. Staff, Sunnybrook Health Sciences Centre; (416)480-4355

JONG, Roland C K; William Osler HC-Brampton, 2100 Bovaird Dr E, Brampton ON L6R 3J7; Tor'93; FRCPC; AnatPath. Staff, William Osler Health System - Brampton Civic Hospital; (905)494-2120

JONG, Winston M; 2180 Meadowvale Blvd, Mississauga ON L5N 5S3; Tor'68; BSc; FACOG; FSOGC; FRCSC; ObstGyn (Infertility). Staff ObstGyn, The Credit Valley Hospital; Asst Prof, University of Toronto; (905)816-9822; Fax. (905)816-9833; wmjong@isisrfc.com.

JONKER, Derek J; The Ottawa Hosp-Gen Campus, 501 Smyth Rd, Ottawa ON K1H 8L6; Qns'93; FRCPC; IntMed (Gastrointestinal Malignancy); MedOncol. Staff, The Ottawa Hospital - General Campus; Asst Prof, University of Ottawa; (613)737-7700; Fax. (613)247-3511.

JONKER, Franz A; 3-2020 Strachan Rd SE, Medicine Hat AB T1B 0M9; Orange Free (South Africa)'87; MB ChB; DA; CCFP; Langs: Afrikaans; (403)580-1882; Fax. (403)504-5799.

JONKER, Garland P; Campbell Clinic, 430 Mayor Magrath Dr S, Lethbridge AB T1J 3M1; Cal'09; CCFP; (403)328-8101; Fax. (403)328-8150.

JONKER, Jacobus M; North Nanaimo Med Clinic, 195-4750 Rutherford Rd, Nanaimo BC V9T 4K6; Pretoria (South Africa)'97; (250)585-7100

JONY, Louai; Aberdeen Hosp, 835 East River Rd, New Glasgow NS B2H 3S6; Cluj-Napaco (Romania)'84; FRCSC; ObstGyn. Staff, Colchester East Hants Health Centre; Staff, Aberdeen Regional Hospital; Langs: Arabic; Romanian; (902)755-3995

JOO, Daisy T; North York Gen Hosp, 4001 Leslie St, North York ON M2K 1E1; Tor'94; FRCPC; Anes. Staff, North York General Hospital; (416)756-6520

JOO, Daniel A; Lion's Gate Hosp, 231 15 St E, North Vancouver BC V7L 2L7; Cal'08; CCFP; CCFP(E.M.); Staff, Lions Gate Hospital; (604)719-7916

JOO, G Pil; 49 Mill St RR 2, Killaloe ON K0J 2A0; McG'07; MDCM; CCFP; (613)757-0004; Fax. (613)757-0005.

JOO, Hwan Suk; St Michael's Hosp, 30 Bond St, Toronto ON M5B 1W8; Tor'92; FRCPC; Anes. Staff Anes, St Michael's Hospital; (416)864-5071

JOOBER, Ridha; Douglas Mental Hlth Univ Inst, 6875 boul Lasalle, Verdun QC H4H 1R3; Tunis (Tunisia)'92; Staff, Douglas Mental Health University Institute; (514)761-6131 x2404; Fax. (514)888-4064; joorid@douglas.mcgill.ca.

JOOMUN, M K Rashid; Medical Clinic, PO Box 668, Whitewood SK S0G 5C0; RCS (Ireland)'65; LRCPSI; LM; Chief Med Staff, Southeast Integrated Care Centre - Moosomin; Langs: English; French; (306)735-2691; Fax. (306)735-2692; rashid.joomun@rqhealth.ca.

JOORAVAN, Sujeeth J; St Paul's Hosp, 1702 20th St W, Saskatoon SK S7N 0W8; Staff, St Paul's Hospital (Grey Nuns) of Saskatoon; (306)371-9752

JORDAN, Andrew; Von Southeast Leads & Grenvill, PO Box 338 11-333 California Ave, Brockville ON K6V 5V5; Qns'89; (613)345-5077; Fax. (613)345-6024; ajordan@rohcg.on.ca.

JORDAN, David D; Brockville Gen Hosp, 75 Charles St, Brockville ON K6V 1S8; Qns'81; BSc(Hon); MSc(Biochem.); Court Staff OR, Brockville General Hospital - Charles Street; Court Staff, Providence Continuing Care Centre (PCCC) - St Vincent de Paul Hospital; (613)345-5645

JORDAN, David R; 301 O'Connor St, Ottawa ON K2P 1V6; Tor'81; FRCSC; Ophth (Oculo Plastic Surgery). Staff, The Ottawa Hospital - General Campus; Staff, Children's Hospital of Eastern Ontario (CHEO); Staff, Pembroke Regional Hospital Inc; Prof Ophth, University of Ottawa; (613)563-3800; Fax. (613)563-1576.

JORDAN, Dean H; Foothills Med Centre, 1403 29 St NW, Calgary AB T2N 2T9; Cal'06; FRCPC; Anes. Staff, Foothills Medical Centre; (403)670-1110

JORDAN, Edward H; Kirkland Disrict Fam Hlth Team, PO Box 10 Stn Main 2 Water Lane, Kirkland Lake ON P2N 3M6; Mem'88; BMedSci; Staff, Kirkland & District Hospital; (705)567-2224

JORDAN, John M; Thames Valley FHT-Byron Fam Me, 1228 Commissioners Rd W, London ON N6K 1C7; Tor'79; MClSc(FM); CCFP; FCFP; Staff, St Joseph's Hospital - St Joseph's Health Care; Staff, London Health Sciences Centre - Victoria Campus; Assoc Prof Family Med, University of Western Ontario; (519)472-9670; Fax. (519)657-1766; jjordan@uwo.ca.

JORDAN, Laurance T; Medical Clinic Associates, 200-3207 30 Ave, Vernon BC V1T 2C6; McG'52; ObstGyn. Ac Staff, Vernon Jubilee Hospital; (250)542-0343; Fax. (250)542-0343.

JORDAN, Michaela R V; Peter Lougheed Centre, 3500 26 Ave NE, Calgary AB T1Y 6J4; Cal'04; FRCPC; IntMed. Staff, Peter Lougheed Centre; (403)943-5526

JORDAN, Rex W; Drumheller Assoc Physicians, PO Box 5600, Drumheller AB T0J 0Y0; West Indies (Jamaica)'65; FRCSC; GenSurg. (403)823-3345; Fax. (403)823-7823.

JORDAN, Victor L; Campbell River & Dist Gen Hsp, 375 2nd Ave, Campbell River BC V9W 3V1; UBC'95; CCFP; CCFP(E.M.); Staff, Campbell River & District General Hospital; Langs: Spanish; (250)287-7111

JORGENSEN, Gayleen; Maternity Care Clinic, 109-178 96 Ave NE, Calgary AB T3K 6G4; Cal'77; CCFP; FCFP; Physician, Maternity Care Clinic; Clin Lecturer, University of Calgary; (403)735-4922; Fax. (403)735-4901.

JORGENSEN, Ian T; Royal University Hosp, 103 Hospital Dr, Saskatoon SK S7N 0W8; Cal'04; FRCPC; Anes. Staff, Royal University Hospital; (306)655-1183; Fax. (306)655-1279.

JORGENSEN, Sally H; 207-42 Glen Allan Dr, Bridgewater NS B4V 3N2; London (England)'77; MB BS; FRCSC; ObstGyn. Staff, South Shore Regional Hospital; Langs: English; French; (902)543-8788; Fax. (902)543-3334; s.h.jorgensen07@gmail.com.

JORGENSON, Keith F; Properties Med Clinic, 5102 Rundlehorn Dr NE, Calgary AB T1Y 1C1; Cal'84; FRCPC; Peds. Staff, Alberta Children's Hospital; Staff, Properties Medical Clinic; (403)280-2700; Fax. (403)285-2641.

JORON, Chantal; Polyclinique St-Eustache, 75 rue Grignon, St-Eustache QC J7P 4J2; Sher'91; LMCC; Staff Nursery, Hôpital de Saint-Eustache; (450)473-2121; Fax. (450)473-1916.

JORUNDSON, Edward R; Meadowlark Health Centre, 142 Meadowlark Shopping Ctr NW, Edmonton AB T5R 5W9; Man'69; MPH; DABPM(Occ.Med.); CCBOM; Med Officer of Hlth Occupational Health, Health Canada Medical Services Branch; (780)486-7777; Fax. (780)486-7747; ejorundson@shaw.ca.

JOSAN, Kiranbir; Columbus Medical Arts Bldg, 401-8333 Weston Rd, Woodbridge ON L4L 8E2; Wes'05; FRCPC; IntMed; Cardiol. (905)264-0022

JOSE, Aurea S; Bluewater Health-Norman Site, 89 Norman St, Sarnia ON N7T 6S3; (Philippines)'63; FRCPC; IntMed; Derm. Assoc Staff, Bluewater Health - Mitton Site; Assoc Staff, Bluewater Health - Norman Site; Court Staff, Bluewater Health - Charlotte Eleanor Englehart Hospital; (519)464-4400

JOSE, Peter F; Peter F Jose Med Prof Corp, 2273 Kingston Rd, Scarborough ON M1N 1T8; Tor'89; Ac Staff, Rouge Valley Health System - Centenary Health Centre Site; Court Staff, The Scarborough Hospital - General Campus; Medical Staff, Craiglee Long Term Care Facility; (416)269-2121

JOSEFCHAK, Robert G; Niagara Health Centre, 207-180 Vine St S, St Catharines ON L2R 7P3; Wes'81; BSc(Hon); FRCSC; OrthSurg (Upper Extremity Surgery). Staff, Niagara Health System - Ontario Street Site; Staff, Hôtel Dieu Shaver Health & Rehabilitation Centre; Staff, Niagara Health System - St Catharines General Site; Clin Coord Michael DeGroote School of Med/Reg Leader Orthopaedics, McMaster University; (905)641-3423; Fax. (905)641-3713.

JOSEPH, Anil P; 680 Kirkwood Dr, Sudbury ON P3E 1X3; Mysore (India)'86; MB BS; MRCPsy(UK); DPM; FRCPC; Psy. Staff, North Bay Regional Health Centre - Kirkwood; Asst Prof Mental Health, Northern Ontario School of Medicine; Aj Prof, University of Western Ontario; Langs: Malayalam; (705)675-5900; Fax. (705)671-3031; ajoseph@hsnsudbury.ca.

JOSEPH, Anu Bala; Peninsula Village Shopping Ctr, 109-15388 24 Ave, Surrey BC V4A 2J2; Stellenbosch (South Africa)'07; MB ChB; (604)531-4131

JOSEPH, Christy S; Waterford Hosp, 306 Waterford Bridge Rd, St. John's NL A1E 4J8; Jaffna (Sri Lanka)'88; MB BS; Staff, Waterford Hospital; (709)777-3300

JOSEPH, Geena; McMaster Univ Med Centre, 3V39-1280 Main St W, Hamilton ON L8S 4K1; Tor'02; FRCPC; IntMed; Nephrol. (905)521-2100 x76992; Fax. (905)524-5500.

JOSEPH, Jacqueline J; Dr J Joseph Med Office, 2276 Lorne St, Regina SK S4P 2M7; Ludhiana (India)'66; MB BS; LRCP; MRCS(Lond); (306)352-8747

JOSEPH, Javed; Northgate Med Centre, 2711 Avonhurst Dr, Regina SK S4R 3J3; Guadalajara (Mexico)'86; BSc; Ac Staff Member, Regina General Hospital; Ac Staff Member, Pasqua Hospital; Langs: Spanish; Hindi; (306)543-4566; Fax. (306)543-4441.

JOSEPH, Jeffrey T; Foothills Med Centre, C1146-1403 29 St NW, Calgary AB T2N 2T9; (USA)'91; Staff, Foothills Medical Centre; (403)944-8849; Fax. (403)944-1460.

JOSEPH, Kurian J T; Cross Cancer Institute, 11560 University Ave NW, Edmonton AB T6G 1Z2; Calicut (India)'87; MB BS; FRCPC; RadOncol. Staff, Cross Cancer Institute; (780)432-8848

JOSEPH, Llewellyn W; Southlake Reg Health Centre, 596 Davis Dr, Newmarket ON L3Y 2P9; Albert Einstein(NY) (USA)'73; FRCPC; Psy (Child & Adolescent Psychiatry). Staff, Southlake Regional Health Centre; (905)895-4521 x6348

JOSEPH, Marcia; Scarborough Prof Centre, 112-1371 Neilson Rd, Scarborough ON M1B 4Z8; McG'81; Staff, Rouge Valley Health System - Centenary Health Centre Site; Staff, The Scarborough Hospital - General Campus; (416)287-9100; Fax. (416)287-0261.

JOSEPH, Mariamma G; London HSC-University Hosp, PO Box 5339 Stn B 339 Windermere Rd, London ON N6A 5A5; Kerala (India)'75; MB BS(AP,CP,Cythopath); FRCPC; GenPath (Cytopath). Staff, London Health Sciences Centre - University Hospital; Affil Investigator, The Lawson Research Institute; Clin Prof Path, University of Western Ontario; Langs: Malayalam; (519)685-8500 x36379; mariamma.joseph@lhsc.on.ca.

JOSEPH, Marissa O; Women's College Hosp, 8F-76 Grenville St, Toronto ON M5S 1B2; Dal'04; FRCPC; Peds; Derm. Staff, Women's College Hospital; (416)323-7546; Fax. (416)323-6236.

JOSEPH, Mary; Canning Med Clinic, PO Box 100 Stn Main 9816 Main St, Canning NS B0P 1H0; Kerala (India)'73; MB BS; Langs: Malayalam; (902)582-7330; Fax. (902)582-7339.

JOSEPH, Mathew B; AIM Orleans Hlth & Wellness Cl, 3-1605 Orleans Blvd, Orleans ON K1C 7E2; Karnatak (India)'61; DAB; FRCP; FRCPC; Peds. (613)830-6890; Fax. (613)830-6312.

JOSEPH, Paul K; Nova Scotia Cancer Centre, 5820 University Ave, Halifax NS B3H 1V7; Ibadan (Nigeria)'74; MB BS; DABR(T); FRCPC; RadOncol. Head RadOncol, Queen Elizabeth II Health Sciences Centre - Victoria General Site; Head Dept of RadOncol, Dalhousie University; (902)473-6012; Fax. (902)473-7205; paul.joseph@cdha.nshealth.ca.

JOSEPH, Steven R; CFB Edmonton, PO Box 10500 Stn Forces, Edmonton AB T5J 4J5; Cal'09; CCFP; (780)973-4011

JOSEPHSON, Brian R; Carry Drive Med Centre, 114-116 Carry Dr SE, Medicine Hat AB T1B 3Z8; UBC'06; CCFP; (403)487-5140; Fax. (403)487-5408.

JOSEPHSON, David A J; Orangeville Family Med Centre, M1-32 First St, Orangeville ON L9W 2E1; Wes'95; CCFP; (519)938-8000; Fax. (519)938-8080.

JOSEPHSON, Deborah; Hillside Family Practice, 100 av Metcalfe, Westmount QC H3Z 2H4; McG'82; (514)931-2162; Fax. (514)931-8436.

JOSEPHSON, E Bruce; Queen Elizabeth II HSC-Halifax, 2129-1796 Summer St, Halifax NS B3H 3A7; Mem'74; FRCPC; IntMed (Echocardiography); Cardiol. Staff, Queen Elizabeth II Health Sciences Centre - Halifax Infirmary Site; Assoc Prof Med, Dalhousie University; (902)473-2307; Fax. (902)473-2434; bruce.josephson@dal.ca.

JOSEPHSON, Robert L; Medical & Dental Bldg, 10-1849 Yonge St, Toronto ON M4S 1Y2; Mem'77; PhD(Path); MSc(Anat.); DABOT; FRCSC; Otol. Ac Staff, St Joseph's Health Centre; Asst Prof, University of Toronto; (416)487-1525; Fax. (416)487-5490.

JOSEPHSON, Timothy B; Univ Hlth Network-Toronto Gen, 200 Elizabeth St, Toronto ON M5G 2C4; Sask'96; FRCPC; EmergMed. Staff, Toronto General Hospital - UHN; (416)340-3131

JOSHI, Ashwini K; The Moncton Hosp, 135 MacBeath Ave, Moncton NB E1C 6Z8; Punjab (India)'70; MB BS; Staff, The Moncton Hospital; (506)856-5251

JOSHI, Atul; Fifth Avenue Med Centre, 300-14 Fifth Ave, Orangeville ON L9W 1G2; Kanpur (India)'92; MB BS; ABIM; FRCPC; IntMed. Langs: Hindi; (519)940-8496

JOSHI, Changulanda M; Aberdeen Prof Centre, 835 East River Rd, New Glasgow NS B2H 3S6; Madras (India)'84; MB BS; MRCOG; FRCSC; ObstGyn (Pelvic Floor Reconst). Staff, Aberdeen Regional Hospital; Langs: Kanarese; Hindi; Tamil; (902)752-8583; Fax. (902)752-8772.

JOSHI, Harshad P; Windsor Med Clinic, 1608 Tecumseh Rd W, Windsor ON N9B 1T8; Nairobi (Kenya)'78; (519)258-4400

JOSHI, Hemlata S; Outpatient Psychiatry, 415-260 Sherbrooke St, New Westminster BC V3L 3M2; UBC'00; FRCPC; Psy. (604)520-4662

JOSHI, Manish D; Gulf Canada Square, 300-401 9 Ave SW, Calgary AB T2P 3C5; Tor'05; FRCPC; DiagRad (Neuro Radiology). (403)210-9980

JOSHI, Manohar L; Queensway Prof Centre, 415-190 Sherway Dr, Etobicoke ON M9C 5N2; Punjab (India)'68; Staff Privil Dept of Psy, Trillium Health Centre - Mississauga; Court Staff Psy, Trillium Health Centre - West Toronto; Langs: Urdu; Punjabi; Hindi; (416)626-5466

JOSHI, Mital; Mount Sinai Hosp, 19 104-600 University Ave, Toronto ON M5G 1X5; Tor'04; FRCPC; Anes. Staff, Mount Sinai Hospital; (416)586-5270

JOSHI, Pradip J; Regatta Plaza, 80 Elizabeth Ave, St. John's NL A1A 1W7; Manchester (England)'75; FRCPC; IntMed. Staff Gen IntMed, Health Sciences Centre; Assoc Prof Med/Clin Chief Medicine Program, Memorial University Of Newfoundland; (709)726-2610; Fax. (709)726-4803.

JOSHI, Prakash C; 79 Rivershore Dr, Saint John NB E2K 4X4; Bombay (India)'62; MB BS; MSc; FCCP; DABIM; FRCPC; IntMed (Intensive Care); Respir. Ac Staff, Saint John Regional Hospital; Asst Prof, Memorial University Of Newfoundland; Asst Prof, Dalhousie University; (506)672-3206; Fax. (506)648-6637.

JOSHI, Ramona; 105-840 Coxwell Ave, Toronto ON M4C 5T2; McM'04; CCFP; Staff, Toronto East General Hospital Inc; (416)469-6464

JOSHI, Sangeeta S; Niagara H System-G Niagara, PO Box 1018 Stn Main 5546 Portage Rd, Niagara Falls ON L2E 6X2; Bhopal (India)'80; MB BS; DABPath; FRCPC; GenPath. Dir Path, Niagara Health System - Douglas Memorial Hospital Site; Associate Path, Niagara Health System - Greater Niagara General Site; (905)358-0171 x53354

JOSHI, Shelendra; Cherryhill Med Centre, 301 Oxford St W, London ON N6H 1S6; UBC'99; (519)850-3999; Fax. (519)850-3990.

JOSHI, Suhas B; Niagara H System-St Catharines, PO Box 3018 Stn Main 142 Queenston St, St Catharines ON L2R 7C6; Indore (India)'76; DABPath; FCAP; FRCPC; AnatPath. Dir Lab, Niagara Health System - Port Colborne General Site; Dir., Labs., MDS Niagara Reference Laboratories; Langs: Marathi; Hindi; (905)684-7271 x46226; Fax. (905)984-5578; sjoshi@niagarahealth.on.ca.

JOSHI, Supriya; 509-2300 Eglinton Ave W, Mississauga ON L5M 2V8; Wes'98; FRCPC; IntMed (Hepatology); Gastroent. Staff, The Credit Valley Hospital; (905)569-9546; Fax. (905)569-9987.

JOSHI, Sushma; Malton Med Arts Bldg, 202-3530 Derry Rd E, Mississauga ON L4T 4E3; Punjab (India)'70; MB BS; (905)673-6211; Fax. (905)673-9520.

JOSHI, Urvi; Royal Columbian Hosp, 330 Columbia St E, New Westminster BC V3L 3W7; Sask'95; FRCPC; NuclearMed (Positron Emission Tomography). Staff Nuclear Med, Royal Columbian Hospital; Langs: Dutch; French; (604)520-4436

JOSHI, V Raman; Finchgate Med Centre, 314-40 Finchgate Blvd, Brampton ON L6T 3J1; Dal'94; BSc; FRCPC; IntMed; Rheum. Staff, William Osler Health System - Brampton Civic Hospital; (905)453-0766; Fax. (905)799-3129.

JOSHI, Vinod S; Mental Health Services, 55 Union St, Saint John NB E2L 5B7; Bombay (India)'86; FRCPC; Psy. (506)658-3737; Fax. (506)658-3739.

JOSHI, Virat; Humber River Reg Hosp-Finch, 2111 Finch Ave W, North York ON M3N 1N1; Birmingham (England)'94; MB ChB; CCFP; CCFP(E.M.); Staff, Humber River Regional Hospital - Finch Avenue Site; (416)747-3857

JOSHI, Vishal; Rouge Valley-Centenary HC, 2867 Ellesmere St, Scarborough ON M1E 4B9; UNIBE (Mexico)'04; Staff, Rouge Valley Health System - Centenary Health Centre Site; (416)284-5131

JOSHIPURA, Mini G; Trillium Hlth Centre-W Toronto, 150 Sherway Dr, Etobicoke ON M9C 1A5; Baroda (India)'93; MB BS; FRCPC; IntMed; GeriatricMed. Staff, Trillium Health Centre - West Toronto; Langs: Malayalam; Hindi; Gujarati; (416)521-4090; mjoshipura@thc.com.

JOSHUA, Anthony M; Univ Hlth Network-Princess M, 5 122-610 University Ave, Toronto ON M5G 2M9; Sydney (Australia)'98; Staff MedOncol, Princess Margaret Hospital - University Health Network; (416)946-4501 x2520; Fax. (416)946-6546.

JOSHUA, Julian M; Salvation Army Grace Gen Hosp, 300 Booth Dr, Winnipeg MB R3J 3M7; Man'88; Staff, The Salvation Army Grace Hospital; (204)837-8311

JOSHUA, Rodney S; Centuria Medical, 2-1499 Gordon Dr, Kelowna BC V1Y 9R2; Cape Town (South Africa)'90; CCFP; (250)762-3807

JOSIUKAS, Anne N E; Collingwood Gen & Marine Hosp, 459 Hume St, Collingwood ON L9Y 1W9; McM'83; FRCPC; Psy. Staff, Collingwood General & Marine Hospital; Langs: Lithuanian; (705)444-6600; Fax. (705)444-5131.

JOSPITRE, Joseph-Marie L; CSSS Du Haut Saint-Maurice, 885 boul Ducharme, La Tuque QC G9X 3C1; (Haiti)'91; Staff, Centre Hospitalier Saint-Joseph de la Turque; (819)523-4581

JOSS, Kasandra; 3-1230 Alward St, Prince George BC V2M 7B1; McG'99; BSc; CCFP; (250)562-1231; Fax. (250)562-1207.

JOSSE, Robert G; St Michael's Hosp, 30 Bond St, Toronto ON M5B 1W8; London (England)'70; MB BS; FRCP(UK); FACP; FRCPC; IntMed (Diabetes); Endocrin&Metab. Staff Endocrinologist, St Michael's Hospital; Prof Med & Nutritional Sciences, University of Toronto; (416)867-7455; Fax. (416)867-3696; josser@smh.ca.

JOSSEAU, Melanie J C; Queensway-Carleton Hosp, 3045 Baseline Rd, Nepean ON K2H 8P4; Ott'09; CCFP; CCFP(E.M.); Staff, Queensway Carleton Hospital; (613)721-2000

JOTA, Jose M; Westville Med Clinic, PO Box 930 1886 Main St, Westville NS B0K 2A0; UE Quezon City (Philippines)'90; (902)396-4142

JOTHY, Serge P; St Michael's Hosp, 30 Bond St, Toronto ON M5B 1W8; Bordeaux (France)'68; PhD(Exp Med); AnatPath (Renal Pathology). Chief Lab Med, St Michael's Hospital; Prof Lab Med & Path, University of Toronto; Langs: Bilingual(English/French); (416)864-5972; Fax. (416)864-5648; jothys@smh.ca.

JOU, Hsing; Edmonton Clinic Health Academy, 3 582D-11405 87 Ave NW, Edmonton AB T6G 1C9; Alb'92; FRCPC; Peds (Emergency Medicine). Staff Ped Emerg, University of Alberta Hospital; Staff, Edmonton Clinic Health Academy; Ass't Clin Prof Ped Emerg, University of Alberta; (780)248-5575; hjou@cha.ab.ca.

JOUBARNE, Francois; GMF Concorde, 300 boul de la Concorde E, Laval QC H7G 2E6; Sher'91; Langs: English; (450)667-5310; Fax. (450)667-5248.

JOUBERT, Carole; Clinique Med Ste-Adele, 1150 rue Du Bourg-Joli, Sainte-Adele QC J8B 1W8; Mon'81; (450)229-6633; Fax. (450)229-5765.

JOUBERT, Gary I E; London HSC-Victoria Hosp, E1-107-800 Commissioners Rd E, London ON N6A 5W9; McM'83; BSc; FAAP; FRCPCH; FRCPC; Peds. Chief Emerg, St Joseph's Hospital - St Joseph's Health Care; Dir Ped Emerg Med, Children's Hospital of Western Ontario; Chief Emerg, London Health Sciences Centre - Victoria Campus; Assoc Prof Peds, University of Western Ontario; (519)685-8134; Fax. (519)667-6769; gary.joubert@lhsc.on.ca.

JOUBERT, Hendrina J; Kenderdine Med Clinic, 110-1804 McOrmond Dr, Saskatoon SK S7S 0A6; BSc(Hons); MB ChB; (306)934-6606; Fax. (306)955-3180.

JOUBERT, Jan G; Medicine Hat Reg Hosp, 666 5 St SW, Medicine Hat AB T1A 4H6; (South Africa)'84; MB ChB; CCFP; CCFP(E.M.); Staff, Medicine Hat Regional Hospital; (403)808-3732

JOUBERT, Jan J M; Second Avenue Med Clinic, 330 2nd Ave W, Prince Rupert BC V8J 1G6; Stellenbosch (South Africa)'96; MB ChB; Langs: Afrikaans; (250)624-5500; Fax. (250)624-4797.

JOUBERT, Johan L; 1025 103 Ave, Dawson Creek BC V1G 2G6; (Other Foreign)'78; MB BCh; Staff, Dawson Creek & District Hospital; Langs: Afrikaans; Dutch; (250)782-1186

JOUBERT, P Renier; F W Green Med Centre, 1629 Baker St, Cranbrook BC V1C 1B4; Kansas (USA)'00; (250)426-6601

JOUBERT, Pierre; Clinique familiale de Thetford, 1001-926 rue Labbe, Thetford Mines QC G6G 2A8; Sher'76; (418)338-3521; Fax. (418)338-4580.

JOUGHIN, Karen E; PO Box 47003 Rpo City Square, Vancouver BC V5Z 4L6; Dal'84; MSc; FRCSC; PlasSurg (Hand Microsurgery).

JOUGHIN, V Elaine; Alberta Children's Hosp, 2888 Shaganappi Trail NW, Calgary AB T3B 6A8; Sask'82; BSc; FRCSC; OrthSurg (Pediatric Orthopedics). Ac Staff, Alberta Children's Hospital; (403)955-7867; Fax. (403)955-7634; elaine.joughin@albertahealthservices.ca.

JOUNDI, Mohamad G; Boyd Med Centre, 811-388 Portage Ave, Winnipeg MB R3C 0C8; Beirut (Lebanon)'75; ABD; ABPath; Langs: Arabic; Bilingual(French/English); (204)943-1387; Fax. (204)831-8403.

JOURDAIN, Sylvain; Hop Brome-Missisquoi-Perkins, 950 rue Principale, Cowansville QC J2K 1K3; Sher'87; CSPQ; FRCPC; Anes. Staff Anes, Hôpital Brome-Missisquoi-Perkins; (450)266-5546

JOURDENAIS, Emmanuelle; CHUM-Hop Notre-Dame, 1560 rue Sherbrooke E, Montreal QC H2L 4M1; Laval'97; CCFP; CCFP(E.M.); FCFP; Staff, Centre Hospitalier l'Université de Montréal (CHUM) - Hôpital Notre-Dame; (514)890-8000; emmanuelle.jourdenais@sympatico.ca.

JOURNEAU, Janice; 103-571 6 St NE PO Box 247, Salmon Arm BC V1E 1R6; John Hopkins (USA)'91; FRCSC; GenSurg. Langs: Spanish; German; (250)803-4233

JOURNET, Charles; Centre Hosp Honore-Mercier, 2750 boul Laframboise, Saint-Hyacinthe QC J2S 4Y8; Laval'98; FRCPC; DiagRad. Staff, Centre Hospitalier Honore-Mercier; (450)771-3377

JOURNET, Michel; 100 Boul Saint-Joseph O, Montreal QC H2T 2P6; Mon'73; Derm. Clin Staff, Centre Hospitalier l'Université De Montréal (CHUM) - Hôpital Saint-luc; (514)271-2594; Fax. (514)271-8594.

JOURNI, Amein; Lessard Med Clinic, 6633 177 St NW, Edmonton AB T5T 4K3; (Libya)'06; MB BCh; (780)399-4441; Fax. (780)757-7991.

JOUTSI, Pentti A; 404 Medical Clinic, 39-1111 Davis Dr, Newmarket ON L3Y 8X2; Wes'77; FRCSC; ObstGyn (Laparoscopic Surgery). Consultant, Southlake Regional Health Centre; Langs: Finnish; (905)898-7221; Fax. (905)898-2553; pjoutsi@rogers.com.

JOUVET, Philippe; Hôpital Ste-Justine, 3175 ch Cote-Sainte-Catherine, Montreal QC H3T 1C5; Paris (France)'89; Critical Care Medicine (P.Q.). Staff, Hôpital Ste-Justine; (514)345-4931 x4927

JOVAISAS, Algis V; 100-194 Main St, Ottawa ON K1S 1C2; Tor'77; FRCPC; IntMed (Osteoporosis); Rheum. Staff, The Ottawa Hospital - General Campus; Staff, Montfort Hospital; Staff, The Ottawa Hospital - Riverside Campus; Asst Prof Rheum & Med, University of Ottawa; (613)233-7426; Fax. (613)233-9912.

JOVANOVIC, John E; Credit Valley Prof Bldg, 504-2300 Eglinton Ave W, Mississauga ON L5M 2V8; Tor'85; FRCPC; IntMed; Cardiol. Ac Staff, The Credit Valley Hospital; (905)828-7935; Fax. (905)820-6342.

JOVANOVIC, Mile; 203-1656 Martin Dr, Surrey BC V4A 6E7; UBC'79; ABD; ABIM; Derm. Consultant, Fraser Valley Cancer Clinic; (604)531-7733; Fax. (604)531-8300.

JOVANOVIC, Radmila; Children's Hosp Eastern Ont, 401 Smyth Rd, Ottawa ON K1H 8L1; Belgrade (Serbia)'81; Staff, Children's Hospital of Eastern Ontario (CHEO); (613)737-7600 x3090

JOVEL, Ramon Eduardo; Oakfield Med Associates, 106-1021 Court Ave, Winnipeg MB R2P 1V7; (El Salvador)'80; Langs: Spanish; (204)956-1057; Fax. (204)956-1057.

JOVEY, Roman D; 9-6400 Millcreek Dr, Mississauga ON L5N 3E7; Tor'80; Dir Addictions & Concurrent Disorders Centre/Physician, The Credit Valley Hospital; Med Dir, CPM Centres for Pain Management; Langs: Ukrainian; (905)858-1368; Fax. (905)858-2144; rjovey@aimhealthgroup.com.

JOVIC, Draga; 309-2453 Beacon Ave, Sidney BC V8L 1X7; McM'87; CCFP; FCFP; Staff, Vancouver Island Health Authority; Staff, Saanich Peninsula Hospital; (250)656-0856; Fax. (250)656-0816.

JOVIC, Jelena; CLSC Montreal-Nord, 11441 boul Lacordaire, Montreal-Nord QC H1G 4J9; Sher'07; CCFP; (514)327-0400

JOWETT, Andrew G; Charleswood Med Clinic, 3360 Roblin Blvd, Winnipeg MB R3R 0C5; London (England)'77; MB BS; MRCGPract; (204)889-7200; Fax. (204)896-5081.

JOWETT, Jonathan E; Hamilton HS-General Site, 237 Barton St E, Hamilton ON L8L 2X2; Tor'97; CCFP; CCFP(E.M.); Staff, Hamilton Health Sciences Centre - Hamilton General Hospital; (905)527-0271

JOY, Andrea E; Forest Hills Med Clinic, 4 Forest Hill Pky, Dartmouth NS B2W 5G7; Dal'95; BSc; CCFP; (902)475-3705; Fax. (902)462-6398.

JOY, Graham A; Dartmouth Gen Hosp, 325 Pleasant St, Dartmouth NS B2Y 4G8; UBC'94; FRCPC; DiagRad. Staff Radiol, Dartmouth General Hospital; (902)465-8539

JOY, Tisha R; St Joseph's Health Care, PO Box 5777 Stn B B5 107-268 Grosvenor St, London ON N6A 4V2; Wes'01; FRCPC; IntMed (Endocrinology); Endocrin&Metab. Staff, St Joseph's Hospital - St Joseph's Health Care; (519)646-6296; Fax. (519)646-6372.

JOYAL, Claude; Base Militaire de Longue Point, CP 4000 Succ K 6363 rue Notre-Dame E, Montreal QC H1N 3V9; Laval'86; Staff, Hopital Charles LeMoyne; (514)252-2777

JOYAL, Dominique; SMBD Jewish Gen Hosp, 3755 ch Cote-Sainte-Catherine, Montreal QC H3T 1E2; McG'98; FRCPC; IntMed; Cardiol. Staff, Sir Mortimer B Davis Jewish General; (514)340-8222

JOYAL, France; CHUM-Hop Notre-Dame, 1560 rue Sherbrooke E, Montreal QC H2L 4M1; Mon'77; FRCPC; IntMed (Vascular Medicine). Prof adj clin, Centre Hospitalier l'Université de Montréal (CHUM) - Hôpital Notre-Dame; Universite de Montreal; Langs: Spanish; (514)890-8000 x27049; Fax. (514)412-7646.

JOYAL, Helene; CSSS Haut-Richelieu-Rouville, 920 boul du Séminaire N, St-Jean-Sur-Richel QC J3A 1B7; Sher'99; FRCSC; Ophth. Staff, Hôpital du Haut-Richelieu; (514)381-9311

JOYAL, Jean-Sebastien; Hôpital Ste-Justine, 3175 ch Cote-Sainte-Catherine, Montreal QC H3T 1C5; McG'00; FRCPC; Peds (Pediatric Intensive Care); Critical Care Medicine (P.Q.). Staff, Hôpital Ste-Justine; (514)345-4931

JOYAL, Marie; Centre Hospitalier de Verdun, 4000 boul Lasalle, Verdun QC H4G 2A3; Mon'81; Staff, Centre Hospitalier de Verdun; (514)762-2777

JOYAL, Marie-Suzanne; Ctr Hosp De Verdun, 4000 boul Lasalle, Verdun QC H4G 2A3; Mon'92; CCFP; Fam Med/Emerg & Cardiol, Centre Hospitalier de Verdun; Langs: English; Spanish; (514)362-1000

JOYAL, Maryse; Ctr Hosp Affilie-St-Sacrement, 1050 ch Sainte-Foy, Quebec QC G1S 4L8; Mon'86; Staff, Centre Hospitalier Affilié Universitaire de Québec - Hôpital du St-Sacrement; (418)682-7511 x2004; Fax. (418)682-7956.

JOYAL, Michel; Institut de Cardiologie de Mtl, 5000 rue Belanger, Montreal QC H1T 1C8; Sher'77; Cardiol. Staff, Institut de Cardiologie de Montréal; (514)376-3330; Fax. (514)593-2540.

JOYAL, Patricia; CSSS de Trois-Rivières, 1991 boul du Carmel, Trois-Rivieres QC G8Z 3R9; Sher'06; FRCPC; Anes. Staff, CSSS de Trois-Rivières; (819)697-3333

JOYAL, Renee; Hop Brome-Missisquoi-Perkins, 950 rue Principale, Cowansville QC J2K 1K3; Mon'01; Staff, Hôpital Brome-Missisquoi-Perkins; (450)266-5535

JOYCE, Brenda M; Nova Scotia Rehab Centre, 1341 Summer St, Halifax NS B3H 4K4; Sask'78; FRCPC; PhysMed&Rehab. Staff, Nova Scotia Rehabilitation Centre; (902)473-1238; Fax. (902)473-3204.

JOYCE, C Mark; 47 Crowfoot Way NW, Calgary AB T3G 2L4; Alb'80; CCFP; Ac Staff, Foothills Medical Centre; Physician, Calgary Foothills Primary Care Network; Langs: German; French; (403)239-3231; Fax. (403)239-3234; mjoyce@ucalgary.ca.

JOYCE, Carol J; Health Sciences Centre, 300 Prince Philip Dr, St. John's NL A1B 3V6; Dal'79; FRCPC; IntMed (Adult Endocrinology); Endocrin&Metab. Assoc Prof Med, Memorial University Of Newfoundland; (709)777-6309; Fax. (709)777-6273; cjoyce@mun.ca.

JOYCE, David P; Pender Community Health Centre, 59 Pender St W, Vancouver BC V6B 1R3; Tor'97; CCFP; CCFP(E.M.); Staff, Chilliwack General Hospital; Staff, Squamish General Hospital / Hilltop House; Staff, Pender Community Health Centre; Langs: Bilingual(English/French); (604)669-9181

JOYCE, Joan E; The Medical Centre, PO Box 4200 Stn Main 707 Charlotte St, Peterborough ON K9J 7B3; Cal'89; CCFP; (705)740-2093

JOYCE, Susan M; 303-343 Wilson Ave, North York ON M3H 1T1; Dublin (Ireland)'84; MRCGPract; MB BCh; BAO; CCFP; Lecturer Family Med, University of Toronto; (416)785-8412; Fax. (416)785-8324.

JOYEUX, Nathalie; CLSC-CHSLD Petite Nation, 14 rue Saint-Andre, St-Andre-Avellin QC J0V 1W0; Paris (France)'01; (819)983-7341

JOYNER, Campbell D; Sunnybrook Hlth Sciences Ctre, E250-2075 Bayview Ave, Toronto ON M4N 3M5; Tor'76; FRCPC; IntMed; Cardiol. Ac Staff Div of Cardiol, Sunnybrook Health Sciences Centre; Prof, University of Toronto; (416)480-4748; Fax. (416)480-6856; cam.joyner@sunnybrook.ca.

JOYNT, Chloe A; University of Alberta Hosp, 3A3.13-8440 112 St NW, Edmonton AB T6G 2B7; Cal'00; FRCPC; Peds (Neonatology). Staff Neonatologist, University of Alberta Hospital; Asst Prof Peds, University of Alberta; (780)407-8822; cjoynt@ualberta.ca.

JOYNT, Margaret S K; 313 Old Quarry Rd, Kingston ON K7M 3L1; London (England)'62; Ac Staff, Kingston General Hospital; Queen's University; (613)542-6769; Fax. (613)542-6169; mjoynt3@cogeco.ca.

JOYNT, Meileen; 208-189 Kent St W, Lindsay ON K9V 5G6; Wes'08; CCFP; (705)880-2525

JOZA, Eva V; 200-300 Main St N, Brampton ON L6V 4H6; Tor'74; Assoc Staff, William Osler Health System - Brampton Civic Hospital; (905)451-1937; Fax. (905)451-8272.

JOZA, Jacqueline; SMBD Jewish Gen Hosp, 3755 ch Cote-Sainte-Catherine, Montreal QC H3T 1E2; Wes'07; FRCPC; IntMed. Staff, Sir Mortimer B Davis Jewish General; (514)340-8222 x5968

JOZA, Paul; The Medical Place, 305-178 John St, Brampton ON L6W 2A4; Tor'73; FRCPC; IntMed; Cardiol. Ac Staff, William Osler Health System - Brampton Civic Hospital; (905)456-2172; Fax. (905)456-2172.

JU, Hui; Sunnybrook Hlth Sciences Ctre, M3 200-2075 Bayview Ave, Toronto ON M4N 3M5; Beijing (China)'02; Staff, Sunnybrook Health Sciences Centre; (416)480-4864

JUBIN, Donna L; 518 Queen St, Saskatoon SK S7K 0M5; Sask'93; CCFP; (306)652-0553; Fax. (306)652-1649; donnajubin@sasktel.net.

JUBY, Angela G; Clinical Sciences Bldg, 1 110-11350 83 Ave NW, Edmonton AB T6G 2P4; (Zimbabwe)'84; Staff, University of Alberta Hospital; Staff, Caritas Health Group-Edmonton; Assoc Prof Med, University of Alberta; (780)492-2470; Fax. (780)492-2874.

JUCE, Karen L; Hamiota Dist Health Centre, 177 Birch Ave, Hamiota MB R0M 0T0; McG'85; BSc(Brandon); MDCM; CCFP; FCFP; Staff, Hamiota District Health Centre; University of Manitoba; (204)764-4218; Fax. (204)764-2325; kjuce@arha.ca.

JUDA, Tibor; 355-340 College St, Toronto ON M5T 3A9; Qns'61; FRCSC; Urol. Staff Urol, Toronto Western Hospital - University Health Network; Langs: Hungarian; Slovak; German; Yiddish; Hebrew; (416)920-8535; Fax. (416)920-8535.

JUDAH, Eli; 604-180 Bloor St W, Toronto ON M5S 2V6; McG'87; (416)925-4560; Fax. (416)925-3353.

JUDAH, Sybil; 650-56 Aberfoyle Cres, Etobicoke ON M8X 2W4; McG'82; FRCS; FRCSC; ObstGyn. Staff, St Joseph's Health Centre; University of Toronto; (416)237-1455; Fax. (416)237-1389.

JUDD, Andrew S; Saskatchewan Med Association, 402-321A 21st St E, Saskatoon SK S7K 0C1; London (England)'73; MB BS; LRCP; MRCS; (306)244-2196; Fax. (306)657-4587.

JUDD, Lyne; Direction de la Sante Publique, 1-205 boul de York O, Gaspe QC G4X 2W5; Mon'97; Med Consultant, Agence de santé et des services sociaux de la Montérégie; (418)368-2443; Fax. (418)368-1317.

JUDELSON, Jeffrey; 2101 Smith St, Regina SK S4P 2P3; Witwatersrand (South Africa)'80; FRCS(Ed); MMed(Wits); FRCSC; Ophth. Ac Staff Ophth & Surg, Pasqua Hospital; Med Supvr Regina Lab, Lions Eye Bank of Saskatchewan; (306)569-3937; Fax. (306)569-4122.

JUDGES, David P; Queen South Med Centre, 303-585 Queen St S, Kitchener ON N2G 4S4; Tor'80; FRCSC; GenSurg. (519)578-7484; Fax. (519)579-2432.

JUDSON, Martyn; 203-240 Wharncliffe Rd N, London ON N6H 4P2; Manchester (England)'71; MB ChB; DObstRCOG; CISAM; MRCGPract; CCFP; FCFP; Staff Consultant Psy, London Health Sciences Centre - University Hospital; Teach Staff Addiction Med, St Joseph's Hospital - St Joseph's Health Care; Med Dir, Clinic 528 Methadone Clinic; Asst Prof Family Med & Psy, University of Western Ontario; (519)642-7676

JUE, Johnny; Gordon & Leslie Diamond HCC, L9-2775 Laurel St, Vancouver BC V5Z 1M9; UBC'79; FACC; ABIM; ABCD; FRCP; FRCPC; IntMed; Cardiol. Ac Staff, Vancouver General Hospital - Centennial Pavillion; Staff, Gordon & Leslie Diamond Health Care Centre; Clin Assoc Prof, University of British Columbia; (604)875-4833; Fax. (604)875-5361; jjue@unixg.ubc.ca.

JUE, Perpetua; 201-513 Main St, Vancouver BC V6A 2V1; (Hong Kong)'73; Court Staff, BC Women's Hospital & Health Centre; Vis Staff, Providence Health Care - St Paul's Hospital; (604)684-2128

JUERGENS, Rosalyn A; The Juravinski Cancer Centre, 3F-699 Concession St, Hamilton ON L8V 5C2; Georgetown U (USA)'00; Physician, The Juravinski Cancer Centre; (905)387-9495

JUERY, Pierre G; Smyth Med Centre, 314-1929 Russell Rd, Ottawa ON K1G 4G3; Ott'80; CCFP; FCFP; Ac Staff, The Ottawa Hospital - General Campus; Asst Prof, University of Ottawa; Langs: English; (613)738-5000; Fax. (613)738-2298.

JUGDAVE, Yajna; KW Sleep Laboratory, 180 King St S, Waterloo ON N2J 1P8; Witwatersrand (South Africa)'98; MB ChB; Langs: Hindi; (519)745-2621

JUGDUTT, Bodh I; University of Alberta Hosp, 2C2 WMC-8440 112 St NW, Edmonton AB T6G 2B7; Glasgow (Scotland)'70; MB ChB; MSc; FACC; FAHA; FESC; FRCPC; MedScient(Med). Staff, University of Alberta Hospital; Prof, University of Alberta; (780)439-0745; Fax. (780)437-3546; bjugdutt@ualberta.ca.

JUGENBURG, Martin; Fairmont Royal York Hotel, Level B-100 Front St W, Toronto ON M5J 1E3; Tor'01; PlasSurg. Staff, Humber River Regional Hospital - Finch Avenue Site; (416)834-6640

JUGGERNATH, Nivas; Midway Health Care, 2102 11th Ave, Regina SK S4P 3Y6; Teach Staff, University Of Regina; (306)522-3346; Fax. (306)522-3348.

JUGLOFF, Lisa S; Etobicoke Med Centre, 400 The East Mall, Etobicoke ON M9B 3Z9; McM'99; MSc; BSc; CCFP; Staff, Trillium Health Centre - Mississauga; (416)621-2220; Fax. (416)621-2203.

JUGNAUTH, Anand; 201-2903 Pandosy St, Kelowna BC V1Y 1W1; Sask'96; FRCSC; GenSurg; ThorSurg. (250)763-7660

JUGNAUTH, Eleonora M; 202-3001 Tutt St, Kelowna BC V1Y 2H4; Man'96; FRCPC; Peds; Nephrol. (778)478-0835

JUGNUNDAN, Pravesh; Enhanced Care Clinic, 14872 Yonge St, Aurora ON L4G 1N2; Durban (South Africa)'87; MB ChB; CCFP; FCFP; Staff, Southlake Regional Health Centre; Physician, OHCOW & WSIB; Langs: Zulu; (905)505-0950

JUGOVIC, Pieter J; Toronto East Gen & Orth Hosp, 825 Coxwell Ave, Toronto ON M4C 3E7; Tor'01; BSc(Biol.); MSc(Biol.); CCFP; Staff, Toronto East General Hospital Inc; (416)469-6580

JUKIER, Lilian; Kildare Family Med Associates, 8-7005 ch Kildare, Cote Saint-Luc QC H4W 1C1; McG'72; FRCPC; IntMed; Endocrin (P.Q.). adj Prof, McGill University; (514)489-5785; Fax. (514)489-5786.

JULIEN, Caroline; Clinique Med de Mont-Joli, 1385 boul Benoit-Gaboury, Mont-Joli QC G5H 4B1; Laval'03; CCFP; (418)775-5353

JULIEN, Gilles; 1600 rue Aylwin, Montreal QC H1W 3B8; Laval'70; Peds (P.Q.) (Community Pediatrics). Staff, Hôpital Ste-Justine; Assoc Prof Ped & Family Med, McGill University; Teach Staff, Universite de Montreal; Langs: English; (514)528-8488; juliengilles@hotmail.com.

JULIEN, Isabelle; Inst U Geriatrie De Montreal, 4565 ch Queen-Mary, Montreal QC H3W 1W5; Laval'00; Staff, Institut Universitaire de Gériatrie de Montréal; (514)340-3514; Fax. (514)340-2832.

JULIEN, Jean-Francois; Clinique Med De Stoneham, 345A ch du Hibou, Stoneham QC G3C 1R9; Mon'86; Staff, CLSC Antoine-Rivard(St-Fabien-de-Panet); Langs: English; (418)848-1919; Fax. (418)848-4004.

JULIEN, Marcel; Hop du Sacre-Coeur De Mtl, 5E-5400 boul Gouin O, Montreal QC H4J 1C5; Mon'77; FRCPC; Respir. Ac Staff, Hôpital du Sacre-Coeur de Montréal; (514)338-2162; Fax. (514)338-3699.

JULIEN, Marlene; CSSS de Portneuf, 700 rue Saint-Cyrille, Saint-Raymond QC G3L 1W1; Laval'97; Staff, Centre Hospitalier Portneuf; (418)337-4611 x2518

JULIEN, Natalie A; CHVO-Hop de Hull, 116 boul Lionel-Emond, Gatineau QC J8Y 1W7; Qns'01; FRCPC; IntMed; Nephrol. Staff, Hull Hospital; (819)595-6000

JULIEN, Pierre G; 2570 av Vanier, Saint-Hyacinthe QC J2S 6L7; Mon'64; FRCSC; Ophth. (450)774-6224

JULIEN, Pierre; Centre Med des Generations, 200-465 rue Bibeau, Saint-Eustache QC J7R 0C8; Mon'80; Chef Cont Med Educ, Hôpital de Saint-Eustache; (450)472-1955; Fax. (450)472-1905; pjulien@cm25.ca.

JULIEN, Rene; Centre Med Le Mesnil, 300-1300 boul Lebourgneuf, Quebec QC G2K 2N1; Laval'91; Staff, CSSS de Kamouraska; Staff, CLSC les Aboiteaux; Langs: English.

JULIEN, Stephane; CRSSS Baie-James-Sante Lebel, GD 950 boul Quevillon N, Lebel-s-Quevillon QC J0Y 1X0; Laval'91; Staff, Centre de santé Lebel; (819)755-4881; Fax. (819)755-3779; daya2345@yahoo.ca.

JULIEN, Warren R; Rosedale Med Associates, PO Box 460 13009 Rosedale Ave, Summerland BC V0H 1Z0; UBC'81; BSc; Langs: Bilingual(English/French); (250)404-4242

JULL, Laura A; Montfort Hosp, 713 Montreal Rd, Ottawa ON K1K 0T2; Qns'07; CCFP; Staff, Montfort Hospital.

JULYAN-GUDGEON, John; Horizons Family Medicine, 5016 51 Ave, Red Deer AB T4N 4H5; Alb'04; CCFP; Physician, Associate Medical Group; (403)342-7270; Fax. (403)343-2677.

JUMA, Azim F; 501 Pharmacy Ave, Scarborough ON M1L 3G7; Wes'96; MHA; MSc; BSc; CCFP; Asst Prof, University of Toronto; Langs: Gujarati; Swahili; Dari; Farsi; Hindi; Urdu; (416)466-7598; Fax. (416)466-6537.

JUMA, Zulfikar A H; 8-2140 Regent St, Sudbury ON P3E 5S8; Manchester (England)'72; FACC; FCCP; FRCPC; IntMed; Cardiol. Staff Cardiol, Health Sciences North - Memorial Site; (705)522-0444; Fax. (705)522-3308.

JUMAA, M Said; Penticton Health Care Centre, 740 Carmi Ave, Penticton BC V2A 8P9; Damascus (Syria)'93; Langs: Arabic; (250)770-3506

JUN, Martin C; Rouge Valley-Ajax & Pickering, 580 Harwood Ave S, Ajax ON L1S 2J4; Ott'99; CCFP; Staff, Rouge Valley Health System - Ajax & Pickering Health Centre Site; (905)683-2320

JUNAID, Amjad; Wentworth Limeridge Med Ctre, 404-849 Upper Wentworth St, Hamilton ON L9A 5H4; Ott'94; MASc; BSc(Hons.); CCFP; CCFP(E.M.); FCFP; Staff Emerg, St Joseph's Healthcare - Charlton Campus; Asst Prof Health Sciences, McMaster University; (905)388-2233; thejunaids@yahoo.com.

JUNAID, Asad I; 1F-408 Booth Dr, Winnipeg MB R3J 3R7; Man'85; FRCPC; IntMed (Nephrology); Critical Care Medicine. Staff, The Salvation Army Grace Hospital; Asst Prof IntMed, University of Manitoba; (204)837-0793; Fax. (204)837-0791.

JUNCK, Randall; Red Deer Reg Hosp, PO Box 5030 Stn Postal Box Ctr 3942 50A Ave, Red Deer AB T4N 6R2; Alb'72; BSc(Med.); DAB; FRCPC; EmergMed (Occupational Health). Staff, Red Deer Regional Hospital Centre; (403)343-4444; Fax. (403)343-4459.

JUNEAU, Francine; CLSC Rivieres et Marees, GD 2E-197 rue Principale, Saint-Cyprien QC G0L 2P0; Mon'92; Physician, Centre Hospitalier Regional du Grand-Portage; (418)963-2769

JUNEAU, Martin M D; 5055 rue Saint-Zotique E, Montreal QC H1T 1N6; Sher'80; Cardiol (Clinical Research). Chef Dept of Med & Cardiol, Institut de Cardiologie de Montréal; Clin Prof, Universite de Montreal; (514)374-1480; Fax. (514)374-2445; martin.juneau@icm-mhi.org.

JUNEAU, Pierre; Clinique Med Antoine-Labelle, 200-555 boul Saint-Antoine, Saint-Jerome QC J7Z 3B8; Mon'84; Ac Staff, Centre Hospitalier Rouyn-Noranda; (450)438-5150

JUNEAU, Valerie; CSSS de Trois-Rivières, 1991 boul du Carmel, Trois-Rivieres QC G8Z 3R9; Laval'06; CCFP; CCFP(E.M.); Staff, CSSS de Trois-Rivières; (819)697-3333

JUNEJA, Namrata V; Grand River Hosp-KW Hlth Ctre, PO Box 9056 Stn C 835 King St, Kitchener ON N2G 1G3; Ravi Shankar (India)'99; MB BS; FRC; ABP; FASCP; FRCPC; AnatPath. Staff, Grand River Hospital - Kitchener/Waterloo Health Centre; (519)749-4300 x5175

JUNEJA, Ravneet S; 850 King St W, Kitchener ON N2G 1E8; Aligarh Muslim (India)'94; MB; BSc; FRCPC; Psy. Staff, Grand River Hospital - Kitchener/Waterloo Health Centre; (519)749-4300; Fax. (519)749-4307.

JUNEJA, Romi; Main Street Med Centre, 9-10886 Hurontario St N, Brampton ON L7A 3R9; Wes'02; CCFP; (905)846-9911; Fax. (905)846-9299.

JUNEK, R Wade; IWK Health Centre, PO Box 9700 Rpo CSC 5850-5980 University Ave, Halifax NS B3K 6R8; Qns'67; FRCPC; Psy (Administration). Staff, IWK Health Centre; Dalhousie University; (902)491-2352; Fax. (902)491-2355.

JUNG, Beverly; Burrard Health Bldg, 605-1160 Burrard St, Vancouver BC V6Z 2E8; Tor'96; FRCPC; IntMed; Nephrol. (604)639-1177; beverlyjung@hotmail.com.

JUNG, Hans W; Canadian Forces Med Group, 1745 Alta Vista Dr, Ottawa ON K1A 0K6; Tor'84; Langs: English; French; (613)945-6827; Fax. (613)990-1345.

JUNG, Hsiao-Ming; Albany Med Clinic, 807 Broadview Ave, Toronto ON M4K 2P8; McG'81; CCFP; Staff, Mount Sinai Hospital; Langs: Mandarin; Chinese; (416)461-9471

JUNG, Jack H; Children's Hosp Western Ont, PO Box 5010 Stn B 800 Commissioners Rd E, London ON N6A 5W9; Cal'77; FCCMG; BSc; FRCP; FABMG; FRCPC; Peds (Medical Genetics). Staff, St Joseph's Hospital - St Joseph's Health Care; Staff, Children's Hospital of Western Ontario; Staff Reg Cancer Program, London Regional Cancer Center; Prof, University of Western Ontario; (519)685-8140; Fax. (519)685-8214.

JUNG, Jacob D; Sunridge Prof Centre, 516-2675 36 St NE, Calgary AB T1Y 6H6; Cal'92; DABFP; CCFP; (403)285-2500; Fax. (403)285-2501; jdjjung@shaw.ca.

JUNG, Marek A; Rocyview Gen Hosp, 7007 14 St SW, Calgary AB T2V 1P9; Warsaw (Poland)'57; FACC; FRCPC; IntMed (Cardiology). Ac Staff, Foothills Medical Centre; Ac Staff, Rockyview General Hospital; Asst Prof, University of Calgary; Langs: Polish; French; Russian; (403)943-3713

JUNG, Sungmi; MUHC-Montreal Gen Hosp, 1650 av Cedar, Montreal QC H3G 1A4; Pusan National (Korea)'95; Staff, McGill University Health Centre - Montreal General Campus; (514)934-1934; Fax. (514)398-4423.

JUNGEN, David R A; Foothills Med Centre, 1403 29 St NW, Calgary AB T2N 2T9; UBC'03; FRCPC; Anes. Staff, Foothills Medical Centre; (403)944-1430

JUNKER, Anne K; Children's & Women's HC of BC, K4 223-4480 Oak St, Vancouver BC V6H 3V4; Cal'76; Peds. Ac Staff, BC Children's Hospital; (604)875-3591; Fax. (604)875-2414.

JUNKER-ANDERSEN, Lorna R; Hamilton HS-General Site, 237 Barton St E, Hamilton ON L8L 2X2; Man'82; CCFP; CCFP(E.M.); FCFP; Staff EmergMed, Hamilton Health Sciences Centre - Hamilton General Hospital; Court Staff, The Brant Community Healthcare System - Brantford General Hospital Site; Court Staff, St Joseph's Healthcare - Charlton Campus; (905)525-4322

JUNOD, Patrice; Clinique Med l'Actuel, 1130-1001 boul de Maisonneuve, Montreal QC H2L 4P9; Mon'87; (514)524-1001; Fax. (514)524-3831.

JURALOWICZ, Pawel; Seniors and Outreach Mental Hl, PO Box 1949 249 West Hirst Ave, Parksville BC V9P 2H7; Lodz (Poland)'88; FRCPC; Psy (Geriatric Psychiatry). Langs: Polish; (250)947-8225

JURAS, Audrey M; CLSC Metro, 1801 boul de Maisonneuve O, Montreal QC H3H 1J9; McG'96; (514)934-0354

JURAVSKY, Louis I; The Moncton Hosp, 135 MacBeath Ave, Moncton NB E1C 6Z8; Man'84; FRCPC; DiagRad. Staff, The Moncton Hospital; (506)857-5520

JURENCAK, Roman; Children's Hosp of Eastern Ont, 401 Smyth Rd, Ottawa ON K1H 8L1; Brno (Czech Republic)'02; Staff, Children's Hospital of Eastern Ontario (CHEO); (613)737-7600

JURENKA, Blanka; Squamish Nation Clinic, 9A-380 Welch St, North Vancouver BC V7P 0A7; UBC'97; CCFP; Med Dir, BC Women's Hospital & Health Centre; Fax. (604)982-0372.

JURGA, Milan; St Martha's Reg Hosp, 25 Bay St, Antigonish NS B2G 2G5; Czech Republic (Czech Republic)'94; CCFP; CCFP(E.M.); Staff, St Martha's Regional Hospital; (902)863-2830

JURGELEIT, Herbert; Upper River Valley Hosp, 11300 130 Rte, Watervil-Carleton NB E7P 0A4; Harvard (USA)'66; Staff, Upper River Valley Hospital - Waterville; (506)375-5900

JURGENS, Dewald; 125-1620 29 St NW, Calgary AB T2N 4L7; (South Africa)'03; MB ChB; (403)452-5049; Fax. (403)289-7523.

JURGENS, Sabine C; 661 Dever Rd, Saint John NB E2M 4J2; Mem'93; CCFP; FCFP; Staff, Saint John Regional Hospital; Staff Privil, St Joseph's Hospital; (506)635-8727

JURIANSZ, Allan R; The Polyclinic, 5-4646 Dufferin St, North York ON M3H 5S4; Sydney (Australia)'64; MB BS; FRCSC; Urol. (416)222-6160

JURIANSZ, Brian D; Binbrook Med Centre, 3137 Highway 56, Binbrook ON L0R 1C0; Loma Linda(CA) (USA)'85; (905)692-5455; Fax. (905)692-5923.

JURRIAANS, Erik; Hamilton HS-Henderson Site, 711 Concession St, Hamilton ON L8V 1C3; Cape Town (South Africa)'83; MB ChB; FRCPC; DiagRad. Staff, Hamilton Health Sciences Centre-Juravinski Site; Assoc Prof, McMaster University; (905)527-4322 x4225; Fax. (905)575-2660.

JURT, Ursula; Brampton Cardiopulmonary Clini, 7-31 Centre St S, Brampton ON L6W 2X7; Tor'97; FRCPC; IntMed; Cardiol. Staff Cardiologist, Peterborough Regional Health Centre - Hospital Drive; Langs: German; (905)455-3010

JUSSAK-KIELLERMAN, Ewa; 1139 Yates St, Victoria BC V8V 3N2; Krakow (Poland)'83; Langs: Polish; (250)381-8500

JUSSAUME, Richard L; Bathurst Pain & Sports Clinic, 101-800 Bathurst St, Toronto ON M5R 3M8; Sher'80; (416)534-6313

JUST, Jon D; 204-300 Columbia St, Kamloops BC V2C 6L1; Sask'90; FRCSC; GenSurg. Staff Privil, Royal Inland Hospital; (250)374-0028; Fax. (250)374-0328.

JUST, Norman W M; Southlake Reg Health Centre, 596 Davis Dr, Newmarket ON L3Y 2P9; McG'75; FRCPC; DiagRad (Neuro Radiology). Dir MRI, Southlake Regional Health Centre; Staff, Mackenzie Richmond Hill Hospital; (905)895-4521

JUSTINICH, Christopher J; Kingston Gen Hosp, 76 Stuart St, Kingston ON K7L 2V7; Qns'84; FRCPC; Peds; Gastroent. Staff, Kingston General Hospital; Assoc Prof Peds, Queen's University; (613)549-6666 x6375; Fax. (613)548-1368.

JUSZKIEWICZ, Piotr; 103-901 Island Hwy, Campbell River BC V9W 2C2; Gdansk (Poland)'81; MD; PhD; FRCSC; GenSurg. Staff, Powell River General Hospital; Langs: Polish; (250)286-0767

JUTA, Dhanesh; 503 Concession St, Hamilton ON L9A 1C1; (South Africa)'97; MB ChB; CCFP; (905)575-1114

JUTA, Manikant M; 503 Concession St, Hamilton ON L9A 1C1; Bombay (India)'74; MB BS; (905)575-1114

JUTA, Meghna P; Summit Centre, 306-200 Boudreau Rd, St. Albert AB T8N 6B9; (India)'86; MB BS; LMCC; CCFP; Langs: Hindi; Nepali; Zulu; (780)458-3318; Fax. (780)458-3348.

JUTA, Ramesh N; The Family Med Centre, 203-9425 94 Ave, Fort Saskatchewan AB T8L 1N6; Lucknow (India)'88; MB BS; FRCSC; GenSurg. Staff, Barrhead Healthcare Centre; Vis Consultant Surg, Whitecourt Healthcare Centre; Vis Consultant Surg, Mayerthorpe Health Care Centre; (780)998-7757; rameshj@mayerthorpe.ca.

JUTA, Sunil; York Medical Health Centre, G-17215 Leslie St, Newmarket ON L3Y 8E4; Natal (South Africa)'89; MB ChB; LMCC; FRCPC; IntMed; Endocrin&Metab. (905)953-9232; Fax. (905)953-9233.

JUTEAU, Eric; Centre Med des Cascades, 101-3639 rue Queen, Rawdon QC J0K 1S0; Mon'98; (450)834-3708; Fax. (450)834-6202.

JUTEAU, Louis-Christopher; Centre la Maillon de Laval, 2255 rue Bienville, Laval QC H7H 3C9; Laval'09; CCFP; (450)937-5290; Fax. (450)937-5295.

JUTRAS, Claire; Agence De le SSSS Laurentides, 210-1000 rue Labelle, Saint-Jerome QC J7Z 5N6; Mon'88; MPH; Langs: English; Fax. (450)436-1761; claire_jutras@ssss.gouv.qc.ca.

JUTRAS, Jean-Francois; CSSS de Trois-Rivières, 1991 boul du Carmel, Trois-Rivieres QC G8Z 3R9; McG'06; MDCM; FRCSC; GenSurg. Staff, CSSS de Trois-Rivières; (819)697-3333

JUTRAS, Jerome-Oliver; Ctr Hosp Anna-Laberge, 200 boul Brisebois, Chateauguay QC J6K 4W8; Laval'90; CCFP; ac Membre, Hôpital Anna-Laberge; Staff, Clinique Medicale Mercier-Ville-Mercier; Dir Education Unite de Med Familiale, McGill University; Langs: Bilingual(French/English); (450)699-2425

JUTRAS, Luc C; MUHC-Montreal Children's Hosp, C352-2300 rue Tupper, Montreal QC H3H 1P3; McG'88; FRCPC; Peds; Cardiol. Staff Ped Cardiol, McGill University Health Centre - Montreal Children's Hospital; Asst Prof Peds, McGill University; Langs: Bilingual(English/French); Bilingual(French/English); (514)412-4423; Fax. (514)412-4273; luc.jutras@muhc.mcgill.ca.

JUTRAS, Marcel; GMF Centre medical AJC, 110 rue Saint-Jean, Drummondville QC J2B 7T1; Mon'75; ac Staff, Hôpital Sainte-croix; (819)477-1800

JUTRAS, Marie; CLSC Richmond, 110 rue Barlow, Richmond QC J0B 2H0; Sher'91; Staff, Centre de Readaptation de l'Estrie; Langs: English; (819)542-2777 x55400; Fax. (819)826-3867; marie.jutras@ssss.gouv.qc.ca.

JUTRAS, Marie-France; CSSS Pierre Boucher, 1333 boul Jacques-Cartier E, Longueuil QC J4M 2A5; Mon'06; Neur. Staff, Centre Hospitalier Pierre Boucher; (450)468-8111

JUTRAS, Maryse; Polyclinique Ancienne-Lorette, 204-6385 boul Wilfrid-Hamel, L'Ancienne-Lorette QC G2E 5W2; Laval'77; ac Staff, Centre Hospitalier Universitaire De Québec - Pavillon De St-françois-d'assise; (418)872-2012; Fax. (418)872-2349.

JUTRAS, Michel N; Lakeside Med Clinic, 3919 8th St E, Saskatoon SK S7H 5M7; Sask'79; CCFP; FCFP; (306)374-6884; Fax. (306)374-2552.

JUTRAS, Philippe A; CSSS de Rimouski-Neigette, CP 3150 Succ A 150 av Rouleau, Rimouski QC G5L 5T1; Laval'86; FRCPC; IntMed (Infection Control); MedMicrobiol; InfectDis. Staff, Hôpital Regional Rimouski; (418)723-7851 x8335

JUTRAS, Pierre; 203-4534 boul Saint-Joseph, Saint-Nicephore QC J2A 1B5; Laval'68; assoc Staff, Hôpital Sainte-croix; (819)477-5790; Fax. (819)477-6732.

JUTRAS, Serge; Ctr Medi Soleil St-Jean-Sur-Ri, 120-383 boul du Seminaire N, St-Jean-sur-Richel QC J3B 8C5; Laval'70; Staff, Service externe de psychiatrie; Staff Clin Med, GRN St Jean BFC Montreal, D.N.D.; Langs: Bilingual(French/English); (450)347-7557; serge.jutras@videotron.ca.

JUTRAS-ASWAD, Didier; CHUM-Hop St-Luc, 1058 rue Saint-Denis, Montreal QC H2X 3J4; Mon'03; FRCPC; Psy. Staff, Centre Hospitalier l'Université De Montréal (CHUM) - Hôpital Saint-luc; (514)890-8000

JUURLINK, David N; Sunnybrook Hlth Sciences Ctre, G 106-2075 Bayview Ave, Toronto ON M4N 3M5; Dal'94; PhmB(Pharm); PhD; LMCC; FRCP; ABIM; DABMT; FRCPC; IntMed (Clinical Pharmacology). Staff, The Hospital For Sick Children; Staff, Sunnybrook Health Sciences Centre; (416)480-6100 x3039; Fax. (416)480-6048; david.juurlink@ices.on.ca.

JUVET, Stephen C; 9N 945-585 University Ave, Toronto ON M5G 2N2; Tor'02; FRCPC; IntMed; Respir.

JUVSHIK, Alexander K; Thunder Bay Med Centre, 340-63 Algoma St N, Thunder Bay ON P7A 4Z6; Ott'97; CCFP; (807)345-5859; Fax. (807)345-2385.

JWELY, Ahmed M; Canadian Mental Health Assoc, 1400 Windsor Ave, Windsor ON N8X 3L9; Al Fateh (Libya)'98; FRCPC; Psy. (519)255-7440

JYU, Christopher A; 3-501 Pharmacy Ave, Scarborough ON M1L 3G7; Man'80; BSc; MBA; CCFP; CCFP(E.M.); FCFP; (416)757-3237; Fax. (647)776-7763.

KAAL, Nuri I M B; Grey Bruce HS-Owen Sound, PO Box 1800 Stn Main 1800 8th St E, Owen Sound ON N4K 6M9; Cairo (Egypt)'79; MB ChB; ABIM; FRCPC; IntMed (Gastroenterology). Staff, Grey Bruce Health Services - Owen Sound; Langs: Arabic; (519)376-2121; Fax. (519)371-8585; nurikaal@hotmail.com.

KAASA, Benjamin M; North York Gen Hosp, 4001 Leslie St, North York ON M2K 1E1; Cal'07; CCFP; Staff, North York General Hospital; (416)756-6000; Fax. (416)756-6508.

KAASA, Roderick B; Magrath Med Clinic, 308-14127 23 Ave NW, Edmonton AB T6R 0G4; Alb'76; CCFP; (780)430-8788; Fax. (780)435-3134.

KABAN, Allan R; Medical Arts Centre, 103-650 Terminal Ave, Nanaimo BC V9R 5E2; Cal'81; CCFP; FCFP; Staff, Nanaimo Regional General Hospital; Langs: Ukrainian; (250)753-3431

KABAN, Glenda D; Regina Qu'Appelle HR-Pasqua, 4101 Dewdney Ave, Regina SK S4T 1A5; Sask'97; BSc; CCFP; CCFP(E.M.); FCFP; Staff, Pasqua Hospital; (306)766-2238

KABAN, Gordie K; Regina Qu'Appelle HR-Regina, 1440 14th Ave, Regina SK S4P 0W5; Sask'97; FRCSC; GenSurg (Laparoscopic Surgery). Staff, Regina General Hospital; (306)766-6911; Fax. (306)766-6917; dr.kaban@sasktel.net.

KABANGU, Emman-Tshiamang; SMBD Jewish Gen Hosp, 3775 ch Cote-Sainte-Catherine, Montreal QC H3T 1E2; Kinshasa (Congo (Democratic Republic))'94; CCFP; Staff, Sir Mortimer B Davis Jewish General; (514)340-8213

KABANI, Amin M; 1502-155 Carlton St, Winnipeg MB R3C 3H8; Bristol (England)'85; MB BS; FAAP; MBA; MedMicrobiol; InfectDis; Peds. Dir Clin Microbiology, Health Sciences Centre; (204)926-8005; akabani7147@dsmanitoba.ca.

KABAROFF, Alison M; University of Alberta Hosp, 1G1 50-8440 112 St NW, Edmonton AB T6G 2B7; Alb'04; EmergMed. Staff, University of Alberta Hospital; (780)407-7047; Fax. (780)407-3314.

KABER, Asem S; Eastwood Med Clinic, 7919 118 Ave NW, Edmonton AB T5B 0R5; (Libya)'05; MB BCh; (780)756-3666; Fax. (780)756-2598.

KABILA, Mbongani; 235-2335 162 Ave SW, Calgary AB T2Y 4S6; (Congo (Democratic Republic))'89; CCFP; (403)873-1500

KABIR, Atif; Appletree Med Clinic, 1309 Carling Ave, Ottawa ON K1Z 7L3; Ott'98; CCFP; (613)715-9816; Fax. (613)715-9278.

KABIRI-ABYANEH, Shadan; 1065 24th St, West Vancouver BC V7V 4H1; Shahid Beheshti (Iran)'98; CCFP; Teacher/Preceptor IMG Program, University of British Columbia; Langs: French; Farsi; (604)925-1301; Fax. (604)925-1314.

KABISIOS, Theodoros; Women's Health Network, 54 Union St, Grnd-Falls-Windsor NL A2A 2E2; Semmelweis (Hungary)'99; Staff, Central Newfoundland Regional Health Centre; (709)489-5312

KABOLI, Fariba; Dr Bernstein Diet & Health Cli, 1558 Broadway W, Vancouver BC V6J 5K9; (Iran)'97; FRCPC; OccupMed. Staff, Lonsdale & 19th Medical Clinic; Langs: Persian; (604)736-3438

KABONGO, Jean-Pierre; 45 Centennial Dr PO Box 2504, Mackenzie BC V0J 2C0; Kinshasa (Congo (Democratic Republic))'97; Staff, Mackenzie & District Hospital & Health Centre; (250)997-4342; jean-pierre.kabongo@northernhealth.ca.

KABONGO, Tshipita; Preeceville Med Clinic, PO Box 409, Preeceville SK S0A 3B0; (Other Foreign)'04; CCFP; (306)547-2011

KABWE, Kazadi N; Hopital Reg D'Edmundston, 275 Hebert Blvd, Edmundston NB E3V 4E4; Sher'01; Staff, Hôpital regional d'Edmundston; (506)739-2200

KACED, Nadia; Medicentre Mascouche, 880 montee Masson, Mascouche QC J7K 2L7; (Other Foreign)'98; (450)966-0324

KACER, Milan R R; Bolton Med Centre, 202-12295 Highway 50, Bolton ON L7E 1M2; Tor'74; Ac Staff, William Osler Health System - Etobicoke General Hospital; (905)857-2655

KACHAN, Paul S; Lansdowne Prof Bldg, 130-1641 Hillside Ave, Victoria BC V8T 5G1; Sask'90; CCFP; (250)595-7122; Fax. (250)598-7125.

KACHOEI, Babak A; Southlake Reg Health Centre, 596 Davis Dr, Newmarket ON L3Y 2P9; Qns'07; IntMed. Staff, Southlake Regional Health Centre; (905)895-4521

KACHOOIE, Alireza; 200-1911 Kennedy Rd, Scarborough ON M1P 2L9; Isfahan (Iran)'75; FRCPC; PhysMed&Rehab (Musculoskeletal & Neurological). Ac Staff, The Scarborough Hospital - Birchmount Campus; Physician, Worker's Safety & Insurance Board; Assoc Teach Staff, University of Toronto; Langs: Persian; (416)299-3800; Fax. (416)299-6025.

KACHOPE, J Twinomujuni; Misericordia Community Hosp, 16940 87 Ave NW, Edmonton AB T5R 4H5; Makerere (Uganda)'90; FRCPC; IntMed. Staff IntMed, Covenant Health - Misericordia Community Hospital; (780)735-2000

KACHRA, Beheram S; 110-175 av Stillview, Pointe-Claire QC H9R 4S3; East Africa (Mozambique)'69; Cardiol (P.Q.) (Echocardiography). Ac Staff, Lakeshore General Hospital - Pointe Claire; (514)697-8113; Fax. (514)697-1069.

KACHROO, Umang B; Sheppard Med Bldg, 203-701 Sheppard Ave E, North York ON M2K 2Z3; Tor'96; MB BS; CCFP; FCFP; Langs: Hindi; (416)221-0176; Fax. (647)776-7696.

KACHTAN, Mohammed; Ctr Hosp du Centre la Mauricie, 8e-50 119e rue, Shawinigan-Sud QC G9P 5K1; Tours (France)'77; Staff, Centre Hospitalier du Centre la Mauricie; (819)536-7629; Fax. (819)536-7676.

KACHUR, Edward; Hamilton HS-General Site, 237 Barton St E, Hamilton ON L8L 2X2; Wes'96; FRCSC; Neursurg (Spine). Staff, Hamilton Health Sciences Centre - Hamilton General Hospital; Asst Prof, McMaster University; (905)522-9884

KACHURA, John R; NCSB 1C-568, 585 University Ave, Toronto ON M5G 2N2; Tor'89; FRCPC; DiagRad (Angiography & Interventional Radiology). Staff Radiol, Princess Margaret Hospital - University Health Network; Staff Radiol, Mount Sinai Hospital; Radiologist, Toronto General Hospital - UHN; Asst Prof Med Imaging, University of Toronto; (416)340-4800 x3250; Fax. (416)593-0502; john.kachura@uhn.on.ca.

KACZMAREK, Susan E; Misiway Comm Hlth Ctre, 130 Wilson Ave, Timmins ON P4N 2S9; Nottingham (England)'82; BMedSci; MHSc; CCFP; Staff, Timmins & District Hospital; Clin Physician, Misiway Milopemahtesewin Community Health Centre; (705)264-2200; Fax. (705)267-5688; skaczmarek@vianet.ca.

KADAMBI, Desikan R; Eyetech Lasik Clinic, 250 Portage Ave, Winnipeg MB R3C 0B1; Mysore (India)'59; LMSSA(Lond); Dip Ortho(Lond.); FRCS(Ed); DAB; FRCSC; Ophth (Refractive Surgery). Langs: Tamil; Kanarese; Hindi; (204)946-5595; Fax. (204)946-5606; ashvini007@hotmail.com.

KADANKA, Hanna; North York Gen Hosp, 4001 Leslie St, North York ON M2K 1E1; Purkyne (Czech Republic)'63; Ac Staff, North York General Hospital; Langs: Czech; (416)756-6265

KADAOUI, Nabila; Direction de la Sante Publique, 1255 rue Beauregard, Longueuil QC J4K 2M3; (Other Foreign)'88; Public Health & Preventive Med; CommunMed (P.Q.). (450)928-6777

KADAR, Paul-Lewis; The Hosp for Sick Children, 555 University Ave, Toronto ON M5G 1X8; Ott'00; FRCPC; Peds. Staff, The Hospital For Sick Children; (416)813-7564

KADER, Hosam E H A; BC Cancer Agency-Vanc Isl Ctr, 2410 Lee Ave, Victoria BC V8R 6V5; Cairo (Egypt)'76; MB ChB; MRCP; FRCR; FRCPC; RadOncol. Staff RadOncol, BC Cancer Agency Vancouver Island Centre; (250)519-5575; Fax. (250)519-2000.

KADER, Tina; SMBD Jewish Gen Hosp, 3755 ch Cote-Sainte-Catherine, Montreal QC H3T 1E2; McG'86; FRCPC; IntMed; Endocrin&Metab. Staff, Sir Mortimer B Davis Jewish General; adj Prof, McGill University; (514)340-8250; Fax. (514)340-7529; tkader@end.jgh.mcgill.ca.

KADHEM, Rasheed H; Lewisporte Med Clinic, PO Box 1195, Lewisporte NL A0G 3A0; Baghdad (Iraq)'91; (709)535-8617

KADIC-MUCEVIC, Edina; Winston Park Family Physicians, 104-2315 Bristol Circle, Oakville ON L6H 6P8; (Bosnia-Herzegovina)'96; CCFP; (905)829-2826; Fax. (905)829-2846.

KADIRI, Yahaya Z; Southlake Reg Health Centre, 596 Davis Dr, Newmarket ON L3Y 2P9; Ibadan (Nigeria)'71; Anes. Staff Anes, Southlake Regional Health Centre; (905)895-4521

KADIRSAHIB, Sadhak; Lac Du Bonnet Dist Health Cent, PO Box 700 89 McIntosh St, Lac du Bonnet MB R0E 1A0; Physician, Lac du Bonnet District Health Centre; (204)345-8647

KADOCH, Harry; Barrie Mem Hosp, CP 2000 28 rue Gale, Ormstown QC J0S 1K0; McG'08; CCFP; Staff, Barrie Memorial Hospital; ac Membre, CLSC Rene-Cassin; Langs: Hebrew; Arabic; French; (450)829-2331

KADOCH, Isaac-Jacques; Clin de Procreation du CHUM, 200-888 boul de Maisonneuve E, Montreal QC H2L 4S8; Paris (France)'00; DGO; Staff, Centre Hospitalier l'Université De Montréal (CHUM) - Hôpital Saint-luc; Dir Programme Endoc Reprod et Infertilite, Universite de Montreal; Langs: English; French; (514)890-8309; ij.kadoch@umontreal.ca.

KADOCH, Laurence; Quinte HC Corp-Belleville Gen, 265 Dundas St E, Belleville ON K8N 5A9; Sher'00; FRCPC; DiagRad. Staff, QHC Belleville General; (613)969-5511

KADRI, Albert; 104-1106 Ouellette Ave, Windsor ON N9A 1C9; Wes'94; FRCPC; IntMed; Nephrol. Langs: Arabic; (519)946-0103; Fax. (519)977-6690.

KADRI, Nadine; CHUM-Hop Notre-Dame, 1560 rue Sherbrooke E, Montreal QC H2L 4M1; McG'97; FRCPC; MedBiochem. Staff, Centre Hospitalier l'Université de Montréal (CHUM) - Hôpital Notre-Dame; (514)890-8000 x27497; Fax. (514)412-7553; nadine.kadri.chum@ssss.gouv.qc.ca.

KADRI, Nadjla; Ctr Hosp de Matane, 333 rue Thibault, Matane QC G4W 2W5; (Algeria)'98; Staff, Centre Hospitalier de Matane; (418)562-3135

KAEGI, Andrew; Whitehorse Gen Hosp, 5 Hosptial Rd, Whitehorse YT Y1A 3H7; Otago (New Zealand)'66; MB ChB; FRACP; FRCPC; IntMed (Laboratory & Clinical Hematology); Hem. Consultant IntMEd & Hem, Whitehorse General Hospital; Langs: German; French; (867)393-8700; andrewkaegi@gmail.com.

KAETHLER, Frieder; Community Health Clinic, PO Box 484 50 Lorne St, Markdale ON N0C 1H0; Ott'84; Locum Tenens Emerg, Grey Bruce Health Services - Markdale; Langs: German; (519)986-1873; Fax. (519)986-1876; fredkaethler@hotmail.com.

KAETHLER, H Wilfried S; Steinbach Med Centre, 10-333 Loewen Blvd, Steinbach MB R5G 0C3; Asuncion (Paraguay)'78; CCFP; FCFP; Physician Family Med, Bethesda Hospital Steinbach; University of Manitoba; Langs: German; Spanish; French; (204)326-3401; Fax. (204)346-3899; wkaethler@sehealth.mb.ca.

KAETHLER, Yvonne E; Winchester Dist Mem Hosp, 566 Louise St, Winchester ON K0C 2K0; McM'97; CCFP; Staff 1, Winchester District Memorial Hospital; (613)774-2420

KAFI, Ayotunde O; Nordic Court, 600-10014 99 St, Grande Prairie AB T8V 3N4; (Nigeria)'89; MB BS; (780)538-5160

KAFKA, Henryk P; Cardiology Services Group, 303-274 Dundas St E, Belleville ON K8N 1E6; Qns'76; FACP; FACC; FRCPC; Cardiol; IntMed. Med Staff, QHC Belleville General; Att Staff, Kingston General Hospital; Queen's University; Langs: Polish; French; (613)966-4377; Fax. (613)966-4730.

KAFKA, Marcella; Dir de Sante Publique l'Outaou, 104 rue Lois, Gatineau QC J8Y 3R7; McG'91; FRCPC; CommunMed;CCFP; (819)777-3871

KAGAL, Allan D; Vaughan Rheumatology Centre, 7-2200 Rutherford Rd, Concord ON L4K 5V2; Tor'97; BSc(Hons.); FRCPC; IntMed; Rheum. Ac Staff, Mackenzie Richmond Hill Hospital; Langs: Hebrew; (416)849-2250; Fax. (416)849-2252.

KAGAL, Darren R; 301-4430 Bathurst St, North York ON M3H 3S3; Wes'04; FRCPC; IntMed; Cardiol. (416)398-2220; Fax. (416)398-2221.

KAGAN, Hershel H B; Family Med Associates, 500-267 O'Connor St, Ottawa ON K2P 1V3; Man'92; CCFP; FCFP; (613)234-5553

KAGAN, Jennifer L; Univ Hlth Network-Toronto Gen, 9N 927-200 Elizabeth St, Toronto ON M5G 2C4; McM'09; CCFP; Staff, Toronto General Hospital - UHN; (416)340-4800

KAGAN, Leon J; Glenrose Rehab Hosp, 1259-10230 111 Ave NW, Edmonton AB T5G 0B7; Alb'79; FRCPC; Psy;CCFP; Staff, Glenrose Rehabilitation Hospital; (780)735-8802

KAGAN, Mary L; 101-4695 Hastings St, Burnaby BC V5C 2K6; Man'89; CCFP; (604)298-7201

KAGAN, Rhoda S; 310-4800 Leslie St, North York ON M2J 2K9; McG'89; MDCM; FRCPC; Peds; ClinImmunol&Allergy. Staff Peds, North York General Hospital; Assoc Prof Peds, University of Toronto; Langs: English; French; (416)492-5888; Fax. (416)492-6569.

KAGEE, Rafeeq; Cambie Plaza Med Clinic, 180-11700 Cambie Rd, Richmond BC V6X 1L5; (South Africa)'01; MB ChB; LMCC; Staff, Cambie Plaza Medical Clinic; (604)270-9833

KAGOMA, Peter K; Medical Arts Bldg, 353 St Paul Ave, Brantford ON N3R 4N3; Lagos (Nigeria)'80; MB BS; FRCPC; IntMed; Hem. Staff, The Brant Community Healthcare System - Willett Hospital Site; Staff, The Brant Community Healthcare System - Brantford General Hospital Site; (519)751-0131

KAHALE, Justin A; Montfort Hosp, 713 Montreal Rd, Ottawa ON K1K 0T2; Ott'07; CCFP; CCFP(E.M.); Staff, Montfort Hospital; (613)746-4621; Fax. (613)748-4914.

KAHAN, Meldon M; Women's College Hosp, 76 Grenville St, Toronto ON M5S 1B2; Tor'82; CCFP; FCFP; CommunMed (Addiction Medicine). Staff, Women's College Hospital; Assoc Prof Family & Comm Med, University of Toronto; (416)323-6400; kahanm@stjoe.on.ca.

KAHANE, Steven G; 311-4800 Leslie St, North York ON M2J 2K9; Tor'93; BSc; CCFP; FCFP; Ac Staff, North York General Hospital; University of Toronto; (416)222-5439; Fax. (416)229-2513.

KAHANOVITCH, I I David; 203-355 Ellice Ave, Winnipeg MB R3B 1X8; Man'73; FRCPC; IntMed. Staff, Seven Oaks General Hospital; Staff, St Boniface General Hospital; Asst Prof Med, University of Manitoba; (204)943-7861; Fax. (204)943-7861.

KAHANSKY, Leonard M; Weston Med Centre, 1953 Weston Rd, York ON M9N 1W8; Ott'87; CCFP; Court Staff, Humber River Regional Hospital - Church Street Site; Ac Staff, St Bernard's Residence; (416)248-5539; Fax. (416)248-0520.

KAHLON, Amrit; Thunder Bay Reg HSC-T-Bay, 3049-980 Oliver Rd, Thunder Bay ON P7B 6V4; UBC'05; FRCPC; IntMed; Hem. Staff, Thunder Bay Regional Health Sciences Centre; (807)684-6029

KAHLON, Baldev S; Scottsdale Med Centre, 100-6950 Nicholson Rd, Delta BC V4E 1Z7; Punjab (India)'76; MB BS; Staff, Scottsdale Medical Centre; Langs: Punjabi; Hindi; Urdu; (604)596-4211; Fax. (604)596-4257.

KAHLON, Kuldip S; Cannon Clinic, 4-2151 McCallum Rd, Abbotsford BC V2S 3N9; National (Ireland)'96; MB BS; LRCPSI; BAO; (604)853-3314; Fax. (604)853-2171.

KAHLON, Navraj; Royal Columbian Hosp, 104-330 Columbia St E, New Westminster BC V3L 3W7; Queensland (Australia)'05; FRCPC; Anes. Staff, Royal Columbian Hospital; (604)528-5002

KAHN, Alan S; Addiction & Mental Hlth-Clarke, 250 College St, Toronto ON M5T 1R8; Wes'04; FRCPC; Psy. Staff, Centre for Addiction & Mental Health (CAMH) - College Street Site; (416)535-8501

KAHN, Frederick; 1-411 Horner Ave, Etobicoke ON M8W 4W3; Tor'55; DABS; FRCSC; GenSurg. (416)251-1055; fred.kahn.md@meditech-bioflex.com.

KAHN, Harriette J; Sunnybrook Hlth Sciences Ctre, E4 33-2075 Bayview Ave, Toronto ON M4N 3M5; Witwatersrand (South Africa)'61; FRCPC; AnatPath. Staff, Sunnybrook Health Sciences Centre; Prof, University of Toronto; (416)480-6100 x7356

KAHN, Larry; 3825 Cadboro Bay Rd PO Box 55024 Stn Cadboro Bay, Victoria BC V8N 6L8; Cape Town (South Africa)'84; MB ChB; BSc(Med); FRCPC; Anes. Staff, Royal Jubilee Hospital; (250)370-8000

KAHN, Michael K; Saint John Reg Hosp, PO Box 2100 Stn Main, Saint John NB E2L 4L2; Peshawar (Pakistan)'00; FRCPC; Anes;CCFP; CCFP(E.M.); Staff, Saint John Regional Hospital; (506)648-6958

KAHN, Susan R; SMBD Jewish Gen Hosp, 3755 ch Cote-Sainte-Catherine, Montreal QC H3T 1E2; McG'85; BSc; MSc(Ep.); FRCPC; IntMed (Thromboembolism). Att Physician, Sir Mortimer B Davis Jewish General; Prof, McGill University; (514)340-8222 x7587; Fax. (514)340-7564.

KAHNAMOUI, Kamyar; Hamilton HS-General Site, 607-237 Barton St E, Hamilton ON L8L 2X2; Ott'95; FRCSC; GenSurg. Staff, Hamilton Health Sciences Centre - Hamilton General Hospital; (905)527-4322; Fax. (905)577-4105.

KAHR, Walter H A; The Hosp For Sick Children, 555 University Ave, Toronto ON M5G 1X8; Tor'94; DPhil; FRCPC; IntMed; Hem. Staff, The Hospital For Sick Children; (416)813-7977; Fax. (416)813-5327; walter.kahr@sickkids.ca.

KAHWAJI, Daniel; Plateau Med Clinic, F8M-1410 Parkway Blvd, Coquitlam BC V3E 3J7; Brussels (Belgium)'89; (604)468-1500; Fax. (604)468-1501.

KAHWAJI, Raymond N; Children's & Women's HC of BC, B321-4480 Oak St, Vancouver BC V6H 3V4; Brussels (Belgium)'83; FRCPC; Anes. Staff, BC Children's Hospital; Clin Instructor, University of British Columbia; Langs: Arabic; French; (604)875-2711

KAHWAJIAN, Lori; Clinique Metro Medic, 100-1538 rue Sherbrooke O, Montreal QC H3G 1L5; McG'08; CCFP; Staff, Sir Mortimer B Davis Jewish General; (514)340-8253

KAHWASH, Eiad; 1940 Gottigen St PO Box 2085 Stn Central, Halifax NS B3J 3B7; Aleppo (Syria)'91; (902)474-8298

KAHWATI, Abed G; Clinique Med Hochelaga, 9080 rue Hochelaga, Montreal QC H1L 2N9; Beirut (Lebanon)'68; FRCPC; Cardiol. (514)788-0904; Fax. (514)353-8701.

KAI, Brian M; Richmond Hosp, 7000 Westminster Hwy, Richmond BC V6X 1A2; UBC'05; FRCPC; DiagRad. Staff Radiol, Richmond Hospital; (604)273-7378

KAIKOV, Yigal; Oakridge Centre South Tower, 207-650 41st Ave W, Vancouver BC V5Z 2M9; Tel-Aviv (Israel)'78; FRCPC; Peds (Pediatric Hematology Oncology). Clin Asst, BC Women's Hospital & Health Centre; Langs: Italian; Hebrew; (604)266-1874; ykaikov@cw.bc.ca.

KAILA, Brinderjit K; 5-4646 Dufferin St, North York ON M3H 5S4; Man'02; FRCPC; IntMed; Gastroent. (416)645-5145; Fax. (416)645-1401.

KAILA, Kendeep S; University of Alberta Hosp, 2C2-8440 112 St NW, Edmonton AB T6G 2B7; Man'07; IntMed. Staff, University of Alberta Hospital; (780)407-6507

KAILA, Sanjeev; 106-704 Mara St, Point Edward ON N7V 1X4; Wes'97; FRCSC; PlasSurg. (519)336-1555

KAILIA, Joel H; Community First Med Clinic, 105-518 Lake St, Nelson BC V1L 4C6; Tor'02; BSc; MSc; CCFP; Langs: Bilingual(English/French); (250)352-5259; office@firstmedical.ca.

KAIN, Brian F; 2-135 Ontario St, Kingston ON K7L 0A5; Qns'71; CCFP; FCFP; (613)531-8040

KAIN, Danielle A; Queen Elizabeth II HSC-Halifax, 8 4-1796 Summer St, Halifax NS B3H 3A7; Tor'09; CCFP; Staff, Queen Elizabeth II Health Sciences Centre - Halifax Infirmary Site; (902)473-2700

KAIN, Kevin C; MaRS & McLaughlin-Rotman Ctre, 10 358-101 College St, Toronto ON M5G 1L7; Wes'80; FRCPC; MedMicrobiol (Infectious Diseases). Dir Tropical Disease Unit, Toronto General Hospital - UHN; Prof Med, University of Toronto; (416)581-7704; Fax. (416)595-5826; kevin.kain@uhn.ca.

KAIPRATH, Soumini; Aberdeen Prof Centre, 835 East River Rd, New Glasgow NS B2H 3S6; Calicut (India)'77; MB BS; CCFP; Staff, Aberdeen Regional Hospital; Langs: Hindi; Malayalam; Tamil; (902)752-1211; soumini@hotmail.com.

KAISER, Carina; Brandon Reg Health Centre, 150 McTavish Ave E, Brandon MB R7A 2B3; CCFP; Staff, Brandon Regional Health Centre; (204)578-4000

KAISER, Grant A; North West Maternity Clinic, 130-1402 8 Ave NW, Calgary AB T2N 1B9; Cal'09; CCFP; (403)284-3711

KAISER, Stephanie M; Queen Elizabeth II HSC, 048-1276 South Park St, Halifax NS B3H 2Y9; Tor'84; FRCPC; IntMed (Endocrinology); Endocrin&Metab. Staff, Queen Elizabeth II Health Sciences Centre - Victoria General Site; (902)473-3712; Fax. (902)473-3726.

KAISER, William J; William Osler HC-Brampton, 2100 Bovaird Dr E, Brampton ON L6R 3J7; Tor'88; CCFP; Staff, William Osler Health System - Brampton Civic Hospital; (905)494-2120

KAITA, Kelly D E; Liver Disease Unit, 803-715 Mcdermot Ave, Winnipeg MB R3E 3P4; Man'89; FRCPC; IntMed (Hepatology). Staff, Health Sciences Centre; Asst Prof Med, University of Manitoba; kaita@cc.umanitoba.ca.

KAIZER, Leonard; The Credit Valley Hosp, 2200 Eglinton Ave W, Mississauga ON L5M 2N1; McG'80; FRCPC; IntMed; MedOncol. Court Staff, Headwaters Health Care Centre - Orangeville Site; Ac Staff, The Credit Valley Hospital; Teach Staff, University of Toronto; (905)813-2200; lkaizer@cvh.on.ca.

KAJBAF, Sahar; 100-3 Conestoga Blvd, Brampton ON L6Z 4N5; Ott'98; FRCPC; IntMed; Nephrol. Langs: Farsi; (905)497-0114; Fax. (905)497-7114.

KAJETANOWICZ, Andrzej J; Cape Breton Hlthcare Complex, 1482 George St, Sydney NS B1P 1P3; Lodz (Poland)'79; Staff Neonatol, Cape Breton Healthcare Complex; Aj Lecturer Peds, Dalhousie University; Langs: Polish; (902)567-7838; Fax. (902)567-7892.

KAJETANOWICZ, Danuta M; Riverside Prof Centre, 31 Riverside Dr, Sydney NS B1S 3N1; McM'88; Staff, Cape Breton Healthcare Complex; Langs: Polish; (902)562-0988; Fax. (902)562-5848; danka@kajetanowicz.com.

KAKADEKAR, Ashok P; Royal University Hosp, 103 Hospital Dr, Saskatoon SK S7N 0W8; Mysore (India)'79; MB BS; MRCP; FRCP; FRCPC; Peds; Cardiol. Staff Peds, Royal University Hospital; (306)966-8114; Fax. (306)966-8640; kakadekar@hotmail.com.

KAKANI, Nirma K; London HSC-University Hosp, PO Box 5339 Stn B 339 Windermere Rd, London ON N6A 5A5; Tamil Nadu (India)'95; Staff, London Health Sciences Centre - University Hospital; (519)663-3221

KAKAR, Ravi; 4597 14th Ave, Markham ON L3S 3K2; Delhi (India)'82; MB BS; LMCC; FRCPC; Psy (Adult Clinical Psychiatry). (905)604-4452; Fax. (905)604-4205; rvkakar@yahoo.ca.

KAKAVAND, Farid; Georgina Family Med Centre, 201-417 The Queensway S, Keswick ON L4P 2C7; Bangalore (India)'93; MB BS; MD; CCFP; (905)989-7800; Fax. (905)989-7803.

KAKI, Reham M S; 300-25 Charlton Ave E, Hamilton ON L8N 1Y2; King Abdul Aziz (Saudi Arabia)'06; FRCPC; IntMed. (905)522-1155

KAKKAR, Fatima; Hopital Sainte-Justine, 3175 ch Cote-Sainte-Catherine, Montreal QC H3T 1C5; McG'03; FRCPC; Peds; InfectDis. Staff, Hôpital Ste-Justine; (514)345-4931

KAKO, Christian Y; All About Health, E-1040 Major Mackenzie Dr E, Richmond Hill ON L4S 1P3; Ott'91; BSc; Langs: English; French; (905)884-0666; Fax. (905)884-5317.

KAKUMANU, Ankineedu S; Allan Blair Cancer Centre, 300-4101 Dewdney Ave, Regina SK S4T 7T1; (India)'95; FRCPC; RadOncol. (306)766-2691; Fax. (306)766-2688.

KAKZANOV, Vered V; Yorkgate Mall, 136A-1 York Gate Blvd, North York ON M3N 3A1; McM'08; CCFP; (416)745-4555

KALADEEN, Stephen M; 64 Ontario St, Trenton ON K8V 6H9; Qns'88; (613)394-1610

KALAHER, Susan G; Keary Med Centre, 204-245 Columbia St E, New Westminster BC V3L 3W4; McM'92; FRCPC; Peds. (604)521-7705; Fax. (604)521-7706.

KALAICHANDRAN, Sivasamboo; 409-2863 Ellesmere Rd, Scarborough ON M1E 5E9; Mysore (India)'77; MB BS; MRCOG(Eng); FRCOG; FSOGC; FRCS; FRCSC; ObstGyn (Endoscopic Surgery). Staff, Rouge Valley Health System - Centenary Health Centre Site; Lecturer ObstGyn, University of Ottawa; (416)431-5592; Fax. (416)289-6536; kalaichandran@sympatico.ca.

KALALA, Tshimanga W; Meadow Lake Associate Clinic, PO Box 1510, Meadow Lake SK S9X 1Z1; (Other Foreign)'98; (306)236-5661

KALANTARI, Saeed; 212-1110 Sheppard Ave E, North York ON M2K 2W2; Tehran (Iran)'93; CCFP; Staff, North York General Hospital; Langs: Farsi; Persian; (416)730-1300

KALAPARAMBATH, Tef; 104-200 Ronson Dr, Etobicoke ON M9W 5Z9; Ott'95; FRCP; FRCPC; IntMed (Adult Cardiology); Cardiol. Staff Cardiol, Trillium Health Centre - Mississauga; Langs: English; (416)740-7200; Fax. (416)740-6100.

KALASH, Joseph; Cite Sante St-Laurent, 1-1077 rue Decarie, Saint-Laurent QC H4L 3M8; Beirut (Lebanon)'83; Staff, Hôpital Santa Cabrini Ospedale; (514)747-5556; Fax. (514)747-5557.

KALCHMAN, Marc J; Seymour-Hannah Sports Plex, 240 St. Paul St W, St Catharines ON L2S 2E7; Wes'90; FRCSC; OrthSurg. Staff, Niagara Health System - St Catharines General Site; Staff, Niagara Health System - Ontario Street Site; (905)688-9338; Fax. (905)688-2398.

KALD, Anne-Ly; 194 Court St N Port Arthur Health Centre Inc, Thunder Bay ON P7A 4V7; Wes'79; Staff, Thunder Bay Regional Health Sciences Centre Port-Arthur; (807)346-1000; Fax. (807)346-6206.

KALDA, Riho; Guinness Business Centre, 300-1055 Hastings St W, Vancouver BC V6E 2E9; Tor'70; FRCPC; Psy (Aviation Psychiatry). Clin Prof, University of British Columbia; Langs: Estonian; (604)609-6163; kalda@interchange.ubc.ca.

KALDAS, Nahed N R; 210 Clandeboye Ave, Selkirk MB R1A 0X1; (Other Foreign)'94; (204)785-2555; Fax. (204)785-4447.

KALDAS, Rhoda M; PO Box 34066 Rpo Fort Richmond, Winnipeg MB R3T 5T5; Ain Shams (Egypt)'97; CCFP; Medical Officer, Selkirk Mental Health Centre; (204)488-7333

KALE, Karna C; Marketingplace Medical, C7-4555 Hurontario St, Mississauga ON L4Z 3M1; Dal'05; BSc; CCFP; Staff Newborn Care, Trillium Health Centre - Mississauga; Asst Prof, University of Toronto; Langs: Urdu; Marathi; Hindi; (905)507-4300

KALE, Rajendra D; The Ottawa Hosp-Civic Campus, 1053 Carling Ave, Ottawa ON K1Y 4E9; Bombay (India)'77; Staff, The Ottawa Hospital - Civic Campus; (613)798-5555

KALENCHUK, Anna L; BC Women's Hosp & Health Ctre, P2 213-4500 Oak St, Vancouver BC V6H 3N1; Alb'07; Psy. Staff, BC Women's Hospital & Health Centre; (604)875-2345 x5599

KALENGA, Jean-Claude M; Alberta Medical Association, 12230 106 Ave NW, Edmonton AB T5N 3Z1; (Congo (Democratic Republic))'90; FRCPC; IntMed; Nephrol. (780)732-3366; Fax. (780)732-3361.

KALER, Harpreet; Ellwood Med Clinic Inc, 200-31205 Maclure Rd, Abbotsford BC V2T 5E5; (Netherlands Antilles)'06; (604)746-4700; hkaler@prospera.ca.

KALI, Aporna; 201-9815 97 St, Grande Prairie AB T8V 8B9; (India)'89; MB BS; MSc(UK); DGO; CCFP; Staff, Queen Elizabeth II Hospital; Langs: Bengali; Hindi; (780)832-3030; Fax. (780)832-3034.

KALIA, Samir; Burlington Prof Centre, 101-3155 Harvester Rd, Burlington ON L7N 3V2; McM'02; CCFP; (905)639-1142; Fax. (905)632-7501.

KALIA, Suneil K; Univ Hlth Network-Toronto Western Hosp, 399 Bathurst St, Toronto ON M5T 2S8; Tor'06; FRCSC; Neursurg. Staff, Toronto Western Hospital - University Health Network; (416)603-5800

KALIA, Sunil; Skin Care Centre, 3F-835 10th Ave W, Vancouver BC V5Z 4E8; Cal'05; FRCPC; Derm. (604)875-4747

KALIANDASANI, Bina; Heritage Village Medicentre, 2041 111 St NW, Edmonton AB T6J 4V9; Delhi (India)'78; MB BS; (780)438-2306; Fax. (780)461-2632.

KALICHARRAN, Ubendranauth; Humber River Reg Hosp-Finch, 2111 Finch Ave W, North York ON M3N 1N1; Tor'93; BSc; FRCPC; Anes. Staff, Humber River Regional Hospital - Finch Avenue Site; Staff, Toronto General Hospital - UHN; (416)747-3835

KALICINSKY, Chrystyna M; Health Sciences Centre, GC319-820 Sherbrook St, Winnipeg MB R3A 1R9; Man'95; FRCPC; IntMed; ClinImmunol&Allergy. Staff, Health Sciences Centre; (204)787-3366

KALIDINDI, Shiva K R; London HSC-Victoria Hosp, 800 Commissioners Rd E, London ON N6A 5W9; Bangalore (India)'00; FRCPC; Peds; EmergMed. Staff, London Health Sciences Centre - Victoria Campus; (519)685-8134

KALIM, Myrlène; Centre Sante Comm-St Joseph's, 1-280 Victoria St, Dalhousie NB E8C 2R6; (Other Foreign)'95; Staff, Centre de santé Communitaire - St-Joseph; (506)684-7000

KALIN, H David; Central Med Bldg, 305-1105 Carling Ave, Ottawa ON K1Y 4G5; Ott'68; CCFP; FCFP; Ac Staff, The Ottawa Hospital - Civic Campus; Asst Prof, University of Ottawa; (613)728-2770; Fax. (613)728-7134.

KALIN, Michael J; Sante Kildare, 14-7005 ch Kildare, Montreal QC H4W 1C1; Tor'99; CCFP; FCFP; Langs: Bilingual(English/French); (514)397-0777

KALINA, Mathias; MUHC-Royal Victoria Hosp, A1 24-687 av des Pins O, Montreal QC H3A 1A1; Mon'72; CCFP; Staff, McGill University Health Centre - Royal Victoria Hospital; Langs: Bilingual(French/English); (514)934-1934 x31996; Fax. (514)843-1490; mathias.kalina@muhc.mcgill.ca.

KALINOWSKI, Leszek; Burrard Health Bldg, 305-1160 Burrard St, Vancouver BC V6Z 2E8; Gdansk (Poland)'80; Langs: Polish; Russian; (604)681-8735; Fax. (604)608-8740.

KALINS, Lauma A; 105-3292 Bayview Ave, North York ON M2M 4J5; Tor'72; Court Staff, North York General Hospital; Court Staff, The Scarborough Hospital - General Campus; Physician, Scarborough, Dept. of Health, Human Resources; Langs: Latvian; (416)445-4067; Fax. (416)445-0206.

KALIRAI, Baljit S; Grand River Hosp-KW Hlth Ctre, PO Box 9056 Stn C 835 King St W, Kitchener ON N2G 1G3; Tor'02; CCFP; CCFP(E.M.); Staff, Grand River Hospital - Kitchener/Waterloo Health Centre; (519)749-4300

KALIRAY, Jagdeepak; 120-6345 120 St, Delta BC V4E 2A6; Aberdeen (Scotland)'04; MB ChB; (604)599-9401

KALISIAK, Maria T; Sunnyside Med Arts Centre, 303-27 Roncesvalles Ave, Toronto ON M6R 3B2; Gdansk (Poland)'72; Langs: Polish; (416)534-4230; Fax. (416)533-7652.

KALISIAK, Michal S; 3C 101-11400 University Ave NW, Edmonton AB T6G 1Z1; Alb'03; FRCPC; Derm. (780)407-1257; Fax. (780)407-3003.

KALKE, Robyn J; St Paul's Hosp, 1081 Burrard St, Vancouver BC V6Z 1Y6; Alb'06; FRCPC; DiagRad. Staff, Providence Health Care - St Paul's Hospital; (604)806-8006

KALKMAN, Peter H; Valley Med Imaging, 102-32475 Simon Ave, Abbotsford BC V2T 5E3; UBC'88; FRCPC; DiagRad. (604)855-0112

KALLA, Daniel M; St Paul's Hosp, 179-1081 Burrard St, Vancouver BC V6Z 1Y6; UBC'91; CCFP; CCFP(E.M.); Staff, Providence Health Care - St Paul's Hospital; (604)806-8480; Fax. (604)806-8488.

KALLAL, E Timothy; Barrhead Clinic, PO Box 4540 Stn Main, Barrhead AB T7N 1A4; Alb'69; Staff, Barrhead Healthcare Centre; (780)674-2231; Fax. (780)674-2447.

KALLAS, Alari; Medical Bldg, 120-6180 Blundell Rd, Richmond BC V7C 4W7; Tor'70; Chief Staff/Ac Staff, Richmond Hospital; Asst Prof, University of British Columbia; (604)448-0223; Fax. (604)241-8615.

KALLURI, Meena; College Plaza 3, 225D-8215 112 St NW, Edmonton AB T6G 2C8; (India)'00; MB BS; Staff Respirology, University of Alberta Hospital; (780)407-1767; Fax. (780)407-3027.

KALMAN, Peter G; Shouldice Hosp, 7750 Bayview Ave, Thornhill ON L3T 4A3; Wes'78; FRCSC; VascSurg. Staff, Shouldice Hospital.

KALMANOVITCH, William A; Foothills Med Centre, 1403 29 St NW, Calgary AB T2N 2T9; Cal'77; DAB; CCFP; CCFP(E.M.); FCFP; Staff, Foothills Medical Centre; (403)944-1315; Fax. (403)670-1833.

KALNINS, Richard E B; 7-5550 Lawrence Ave E, Scarborough ON M1C 3B2; Tor'89; (416)283-3700; Fax. (416)283-1453.

KALNY, Michele T; 10-8180 MacLeod Trail SE, Calgary AB T2H 2B8; Cal'88; FAAP; FRCPC; Peds (Pediatric Emergency Medicine). Staff Emerg, Alberta Children's Hospital; Asst Prof, University of Calgary; (403)252-6651

KALOMBO, Augustin N; Central Nfld Reg Health Centre, 50 Union St, Grnd-Falls-Windsor NL A2A 2E1; Kinshasa (Congo (Democratic Republic))'85; Staff, Central Newfoundland Regional Health Centre; (709)489-1200

KALONI, Rita; 502-345 Lakeshore Rd E, Oakville ON L6J 1J5; Wes'99; CCFP; (905)845-4511

KALOUL, Ismail; CSSS de la Vallée de l'Or, 725 6e rue, Val-d'Or QC J9P 3Y1; Damascus (Syria)'85; Staff, Centre Hospitalier de Val d'Or; (819)825-5858

KALPIN, Allen O; 27 Arnold Cres, Richmond Hill ON L4C 3R6; Tor'81; Physician, Ontario Centre for Short-Term Dynamic Psychotherapy; (905)770-7503

KALRA, Bharat B; Bridlewood Prof Centre, 404-3443 Finch Ave E, Scarborough ON M1W 2S1; (India)'79; MB BS; DCH; Staff, The Scarborough Hospital - General Campus; Staff, Rouge Valley Health System - Centenary Health Centre Site; Langs: Punjabi; Hindi; Urdu; (416)492-9880; Fax. (416)492-9886.

KALRA, Jawahar; Royal University Hosp, 103 Hospital Dr, Saskatoon SK S7N 0W8; Mem'81; PhD; FRCPC; MedBiochem (Laboratory Medicine). Prof Path, Royal University Hospital; Staff Lab Med, Saskatoon District Health Board; (306)655-2152; jay.kalra@saskatoonhealthregion.ca.

KALRA, Sanjay; University of Alberta Hosp, 2E3 18 WCM-8440 112 St NW, Edmonton AB T6G 2B7; Tor'94; FRCPC; Neur. Staff Neurol, University of Alberta Hospital; Asst Prof, University of Alberta; (780)407-7780; Fax. (780)407-1325.

KALRA, Savita; Timmins & Dist Hosp, 700 Ross Ave E, Timmins ON P4N 8P2; Punjab (India)'97; FRCPC; IntMed. Staff, Timmins & District Hospital; (705)264-6339

KALSI, Gursharan S; Surrey Mem Hosp, 13750 96 Ave, Surrey BC V3V 1Z2; Cork (Ireland)'91; MB ChB; BAO; BSc; MSc; Ac Staff, Surrey Memorial Hospital; (604)581-2211

KALSI, Jarnail; West Winds Med Clinic, 2130-4818 Westwinds Dr NE, Calgary AB T3J 3Z5; (Other Foreign)'97; CCFP; (403)293-5454

KALTURNYK, Blake P; Seven Oaks Gen Hosp, 2300 McPhillips St, Winnipeg MB R2V 3M3; Man'87; Staff Emerg, Seven Oaks General Hospital; (204)632-7133; Fax. (204)694-8276.

KALU, Uduma O; 5-63 Walford Rd PO Box 891 Stn B, Sudbury ON P3E 4S1; Washington(DC) (USA)'74; FRCPC; IntMed (Gastroenterology). Consultant, Health Sciences North-St Joseph's Health Centre; Consultant, Health Sciences North - Memorial Site; Consultant, Health Sciences North-Laurentian Site; Langs: Ibo; (705)523-5589; Fax. (705)523-5414.

KALUZIENSKI, Mark H; The Ottawa Hosp-Gen Campus, 501 Smyth Rd, Ottawa ON K1H 8L6; Ott'03; Psy. Staff, The Ottawa Hospital - General Campus; (613)737-7777

KALYAN, Sangeeta; South Shore Reg Hosp, 90 Glen Allan Dr, Bridgewater NS B4V 3S6; Gauhati (India)'94; MB BS; Staff, South Shore Regional Hospital; (902)527-5227

KALYANPUR, Yamuna; Crossroads Obstetrics & Gyn, 330-507 Broadway W, Vancouver BC V5Z 1E6; Madras (India)'62; MB BS; FRCSC; ObstGyn. Langs: Punjabi; Swahili; (604)708-0788

KALYNIUK, Jo-Anne; Bayview Business Centre, 208-16700 Bayview Ave, Newmarket ON L3X 1W1; Ott'78; Ac Staff, Southlake Regional Health Centre; (905)898-7811; Fax. (905)898-0963.

KALYNIUK, Judith A; Bayview Business Centre, 208-16700 Bayview Ave, Newmarket ON L3X 1W1; Ott'78; Ac Staff, Southlake Regional Health Centre; (905)898-7811; Fax. (905)898-0963.

KALYNIUK, Norman J; Bayview Business Centre, 208-16700 Bayview Ave, Newmarket ON L3X 1W1; Wes'87; Assoc Staff, Southlake Regional Health Centre; (905)898-7811; Fax. (905)898-0963; nkalyniuk@rogers.com.

KALYVAS, Maria; Kingston Reg Cancer Centre, 25 King St W, Kingston ON K7L 5P9; Ott'99; FRCPC; RadOncol. Physician, Kingston Regional Cancer Centre; (613)544-2630; maria.kalyvas@krcc.on.ca.

KAM, April J; McMaster University, HSC 3A-1280 Main St W, Hamilton ON L8S 4K1; McM'03; MScPublicHealth; FRCPC; Peds (Emergency Medicine). Staff Ped Emerg, Hamilton Health Sciences Centre - McMaster Children's Hospital; Teach Staff, McMaster University; (905)521-2100 x75607; Fax. (905)524-5707; kama@mcmaster.ca.

KAM, Cindy L S; Trans canada Mall, 152-1440 52 St NE, Calgary AB T2A 4T8; UBC'09; CCFP; (403)272-3627

KAM, Joan S; 4419 Hastings St, Burnaby BC V5C 2K1; UBC'97; CCFP; FCFP; (604)299-3457; joankam@hotmail.com.

KAM, Karen J; Foothills Med Centre, 1403 29 St NW, Calgary AB T2N 2T9; Alb'07; FRCPC; Peds; Respir. Staff Ped Resp, Foothills Medical Centre; (403)944-1110

KAM, Michael S; Mapleton Health Centre, 11 Andrews Dr W, Drayton ON N0G 1P0; Wes'98; CCFP; Medical Staff, North Wellington Health Care - Palmerston & District Hospital; Teach Staff ROMP, McMaster University; (519)638-3088; Fax. (519)638-3982.

KAM, Sau Shun; 2259 Hastings St E, Vancouver BC V5L 1V3; Alb'98; CCFP; FCFP; (604)216-2525

KAM, Timothy W T; 2366 41st Ave W, Vancouver BC V6M 2A4; Tor'93; BSc; Physician Family Med, Vancouver General Hospital - Centennial Pavillion; Langs: Cantonese; Mandarin; (604)263-2726; Fax. (604)263-2736; dr.timkam@shawbiz.ca.

KAMAL, Fadi A B; The Ottawa Hosp-Gen Campus, 501 Smyth Rd, Ottawa ON K1H 8L6; King Abdul Aziz (Saudi Arabia)'00; FRCSC; Urol. Staff Urol, The Ottawa Hospital - General Campus; (613)798-5555

KAMALIA, Fatima R; North Med Centre, 206-7131 Bathurst St, Thornhill ON L4J 7Z1; Qns'93; FAAP; FRCPC; Peds. Staff Emerg, The Hospital For Sick Children; Ac Staff, Mackenzie Richmond Hill Hospital; (905)731-7596; Fax. (905)731-4975.

KAMALUDDEEN, Majeeda S B; Foothills Med Centre, 780A-1403 29 St NW, Calgary AB T2N 2T9; (India)'87; MRCP; DABPed; Staff, Foothills Medical Centre; (403)944-1615

KAMANI, Allaudin A S; BC Women's Hosp & Health Ctre, 4500 Oak St, Vancouver BC V6H 3N1; Man'76; FACA; DABA; FRCPC; Anes. Staff, BC Women's Hospital & Health Centre; Assoc Prof, University of British Columbia; Langs: Gujarati; Hindi; Kacchi; Kiswahili; (604)875-2158; Fax. (604)875-2733.

KAMANI, Azadali A; 320-6330 Fraser St, Vancouver BC V5W 3A4; Mem'74; Langs: Hindi; Gujarati; Urdu; (604)322-3383; Fax. (604)321-4823.

KAMANI, Rozmin F; 304-2083 Alma St, Vancouver BC V6R 4N6; Man'80; CCFP; FCFP; Vis Staff, UBC Hospital - Koerner Pavillion; Ac Asst Staff Family Pract, Providence Health Care - St Paul's Hospital; Vis Staff Neonatal, BC Women's Hospital & Health Centre; Pres., Federation Med. Womens of Canada; Clin Asst Family Pract, University of British Columbia; Langs: Farsi; Kacchi; Gujarati; (604)222-9998; Fax. (604)222-2111.

KAMARA, Hawa; Oakville Health Centre, 117-1060 Speers Rd, Oakville ON L6L 2X4; London (England)'99; CCFP; (905)845-8884

KAMATH, Amisha T; Forbes Park Med Centre, 26 Forbes St, Cambridge ON N3C 2E2; (Anguilla)'08; (519)658-4615

KAMATH, Vranda S; 203-450 Central Ave, London ON N6B 2E8; Bombay (India)'86; MB BS; CCFP; Court Staff, Alexandra Hospital; (519)432-7350; Fax. (519)432-0949.

KAMATH PATEL, Binita M; The Hosp for Sick Children, 555 University Ave, Toronto ON M5G 1X8; Cambridge (England)'95; MB BCh; MRCP; Staff, The Hospital For Sick Children; Asst Prof Peds, University of Toronto; (416)813-6171; Fax. (416)813-4972; binita.kamath@sickkids.ca.

KAMATOVIC, Ralph J; Fort Erie Group Fam Practice, 7-238 Bertie St, Fort Erie ON L2A 1Z3; Ott'03; BSc; CCFP; Staff ER, Niagara Health System - Port Colborne General Site; Staff ER, Niagara Health System - Douglas Memorial Hospital Site; Staff ER, Niagara Health System - Welland Hospital Site; Staff ER, Niagara Health System - Greater Niagara General Site; (905)871-1220; Fax. (905)871-1221.

KAMAU, Allan G; CSSS du Nord de Lanaudière, 1000 boul Sainte-Anne, St-Charles-Brromee QC J6E 6J2; Tours (France)'71; Gastroent (P.Q.). Staff, Centre Hospitalier Régional de Lanaudière; (450)759-8222

KAMAWI, Malalai; Castlemore Health Centre, 3-65 Braydon Blvd, Brampton ON L6P 2S4; Delhi (India)'96; CCFP; (905)794-7649

KAMBA, E Francine; Hôpital régional Chaleur, 1750 Sunset St, Bathurst NB E2A 4L7; Kinshasa (Other Foreign)'91; Staff, Hopital Regional Chaleur; (506)544-3000

KAMBA, Samuel; Hôpital régional Chaleur, 1750 Sunset Dr, Bathurst NB E2A 4L7; Kinshasa (Congo (Brazzaville))'89; Staff, Hopital Regional Chaleur; (506)544-3000

KAMBLE, Vaibhav A; Toronto East Gen Hosp Inc, 825 Coxwell Ave, Toronto ON M4C 3E7; Tor'92; FRCPC; Anes;CCFP; Staff Anes, Toronto East General Hospital Inc; (416)469-6212; Fax. (416)469-6874.

KAMBLI, Kamini C; Finch Midland Med Centre, 428-4190 Finch Ave E, Scarborough ON M1S 4T7; Nagpur (India)'85; MB BS; CCFP; (416)299-1893; Fax. (416)299-1859.

KAMDAR, Lalit K; Tawa Centre, 221-3017 66 St NW, Edmonton AB T6K 4B2; National (Ireland)'65; LRCPSI; FAAFP; Langs: English; (780)462-1446; Fax. (780)450-2892.

KAMEDIEN, Rabiah; Edson Med Centre, PO Box 6660 Stn Main, Edson AB T7E 1V1; (South Africa)'06; MB ChB; (780)723-3366

KAMEL, Emad H; Gambo Med Clinic, PO Box 430, Gambo NL A0G 1T0; Alexandria (Egypt)'79; MS(SA); MB ChB; CCFP; Physician Family Med, Central East Health Institute Medical Board; Langs: Arabic; (709)674-4403; Fax. (709)674-2000.

KAMEL, Hany M; Medico-Centre Mont Royal, 101-4689 av Papineau, Montreal QC H2H 1V4; Alexandria (Egypt)'78; FACCPhys; CCFP; Staff, Barrie Memorial Hospital; (514)521-5555; hanyk@hotmail.com.

KAMEL, Ibrahim D; The Kamel Eye Centre, 310-220 Duncan Mill Rd, North York ON M3B 3J5; Alexandria (Egypt)'64; DOMS; DS; FRCSC; Ophth (Cataract & Glaucoma). Ac Staff, Rouge Valley Health System - Centenary Health Centre Site; Physician, The Kamel Eye Centre; Langs: Arabic; (416)492-6694; Fax. (416)492-3961.

KAMEL, Jean-Pierre; Mayland Medical, 1905 8 Ave NE, Calgary AB T2E 0T2; Cairo (Egypt)'73; (403)242-1188; Fax. (403)242-1124.

KAMEL, Kamel S; St Michael's Hosp, 30 Bond St, Toronto ON M5B 1W8; Ain Shams (Egypt)'79; FRCPC; IntMed; Nephrol. Head Nephrol, St Michael's Hospital; Asst Prof Med, University of Toronto; (416)867-7479; Fax. (416)867-3709.

KAMEL, Mona K; Trillium Hlth Ctr-Mississauga, 100 Queensway W, Mississauga ON L5B 1B8; Cairo (Egypt)'80; MB ChB; FRCPC; AnatPath. Microbiologist, Trillium Health Centre - Mississauga; Langs: Arabic; (905)848-7580 x2344; Fax. (905)848-8313.

KAMEL, Sahar S F; Sheppard Med Bldg, 215-701 Sheppard Ave E, North York ON M2K 2Z3; Ain Shams (Egypt)'82; Psy. (647)346-8649; Fax. (647)352-8650.

KAMEL, Sherief J; Professional Arts Bldg, 226-100 Arden St, Moncton NB E1C 4B7; Dal'05; FRCPC; IntMed; Cardiol. (506)386-3591; Fax. (506)386-2554.

KAMENCIC, Huse; 100-2631 28th Ave, Regina SK S4S 6X3; Sarajevo (Bosnia-Herzegovina)'90; FRCSC; ObstGyn. (306)586-1800; Fax. (306)586-3511.

KAMENS, Cathy A; 302-790 Bay St, Toronto ON M5G 1N8; Connecticut (USA)'97; CCFP; (416)585-9555

KAMENSKAIA, Vera; 4646 Dufferin St, North York ON M3H 5S4; Novosibirsk (Russia (Federation))'97.

KAMERMANS, Rob J; 2230 Main St, Coe Hill ON K0L 1P0; Albuquerque(NM) (USA)'92; Langs: Dutch; Spanish; (613)337-8984

KAMGA-NGANDE, Carole N; CHUM-Hop St-Luc, 1058 rue Saint-Denis, Montreal QC H2X 3J4; Limoges (France)'04; ObstGyn. Staff, Centre Hospitalier l'Université De Montréal (CHUM) - Hôpital Saint-luc; (514)890-8000

KAMIL, Rifaat; Ahousat Holistic Centre, PO Box 91, Ahousat BC V0R 1A0; McG'85; FRCPC; Psy. (250)670-9558

KAMINKER, Arthur; 303-1200 Lawrence Ave E, North York ON M3A 1C1; Tor'54; ABAI; FRCPC; IntMed (Clinical Immunology & Allergy). Court Staff Med/Consultant, The Scarborough Hospital - General Campus; (416)449-1000; Fax. (416)449-7934.

KAMINKER, Richard S; The Court, 101-2863 Ellesmere Rd, Scarborough ON M1E 5E9; Tor'93; FRCSC; OrthSurg (Lower Extremity Reconstruction). Staff, Rouge Valley Health System - Centenary Health Centre Site; Langs: Hebrew; (416)287-2335; Fax. (416)284-1218; drkaminker@rougevalley.ca.

KAMINSKA, Elzbieta A; Richmond Road Diag & Trmt Ctre, G11147-1820 Richmond Rd SW, Calgary AB T2T 5C2; Szczecin (Poland)'79; FRCPC; IntMed; Rheum. Langs: Polish; (403)955-8732

KAMINSKA, Irena; Professional Corporation, 3-19 Main St, St George NB E5C 3H9; Wroclaw (Poland)'68; Staff, Fundy Health Centre; Langs: Polish; (506)755-6133; Fax. (506)755-2259.

KAMINSKA, Malgorzata E; South Health Campus, 4F-4448 Front St SE, Calgary AB T3M 1M4; Tor'05; CCFP; Staff, Oilfields General Hospital; Teacher Undergraduate Med Education/Asst Prof Fac of Med Dept of Family Med, University of Calgary; Langs: French; Polish; (403)956-2300; malgorzata.kaminska@albertahealthservices.ca.

KAMINSKA, Marta; MUHC-Royal Victoria Hosp, 687 av des Pins O, Montreal QC H3A 1A1; McG'01; FRCPC; IntMed; Respir. Staff, McGill University Health Centre - Royal Victoria Hospital; (514)934-1934

KAMINSKI, Michael; 205-4949 Bathurst St, North York ON M2R 1Y1; Rokitnica-Bytom (Poland)'57; Staff, North York General Hospital - Branson Division; (416)225-8809; Fax. (416)225-8800.

KAMINSKY, Victor M; 207-267 O'Connor St, Ottawa ON K2P 1V3; Cape Town (South Africa)'66; MB ChB; FRCS(Ed); FRCSC; GenSurg. Ac Staff, Queensway Carleton Hospital; (613)567-8000; Fax. (613)567-8022; vickaminsky@hotmail.com.

KAMITAKAHARA, Alan T; Royal City Med Bldg, 305-250 Keary St, New Westminster BC V3L 5E7; Tor'68; FRCSC; GenSurg. (604)522-6020; Fax. (604)526-6705.

KAMITAKAHARA, Holly K; 308-14127 23 Ave NW, Edmonton AB T6R 0G4; Alb'10; CCFP; (780)430-8788

KAMMERER, Hubert; Glenrose Rehab Hosp, 10230 111 Ave NW, Edmonton AB T5G 0B7; Alb'82; CCFP; FCFP; Staff, Glenrose Rehabilitation Hospital; (780)735-7934; Fax. (780)735-8837.

KAMMILA, Srinu; Peterborough Reg Nephrology, 239 Charlotte St, Peterborough ON K9J 2V2; Cal'97; FRCPC; IntMed; Nephrol. (705)750-1786; Fax. (705)750-0591.

KAMMINGA, Amanda M; Riverview Med Group, LL-205 Queen St E, Fergus ON N1M 1T2; McM'08; CCFP; (519)787-1200

KAMOUNA, Ahmed K; Military Urgent Care Clinic, 103-400 Bronte St S, Milton ON L9T 0H7; Baghdad (Iraq)'99; MB ChB; CCFP; Langs: Arabic; (905)876-3843

KAMOUNA, Mustafa K; Milton Urgent Care Clinic Unit, 103-400 Bronte St S, Milton ON L9T 0H7; Baghdad (Iraq)'93; MB BS; CCFP; FCFP; Ac Staff, Halton Healthcare Services Corporation - Milton District Hospital; (905)876-3843; Fax. (905)876-2486.

KAMPF, N Noreen; Leaside Health Centre, 795 Eglinton Ave E, Toronto ON M4G 4E4; McM'91; CCFP; FCFP; (416)424-3145; Fax. (416)424-2611.

KAMRA, Chander P; Health Sciences Centre, 300 Prince Philip Dr, St. John's NL A1B 3V6; Punjab (India)'68; MB BS; FFARCS(Eng); FFARCSI; DA(Lond); FRCPC; Anes (Pain Management). Staff Anes, Health Sciences Centre; Clin Assoc Prof, Memorial University Of Newfoundland; (709)777-6300 x6249; chanderkamra@warp.nfld.net.

KAMRA, Juhu; Royal Victoria Hosp, 201 Georgian Dr, Barrie ON L4M 6M2; Dal'93; FRCPC; RadOncol (Epidemiology). Staff, Royal Victoria Regional Health Centre; (705)728-9802; Fax. (705)728-1122.

KAMRA, Palinder; Paton Med Centre, 219-1 Paton St, St. John's NL A1B 4S8; Guru Nanak (India)'76; MB BS; DABPed; FAAP; FRCPC; Peds (Asthma). Clin Assoc Prof, Janeway Children's Health & Rehabilitation Centre; Clin Assoc Prof, Memorial University Of Newfoundland; Langs: Punjabi; Hindi; (709)579-9400; Fax. (709)579-1708.

KAMRAN, Abdul Q; Evergreen Medical Center, 205-4851 Westwinds Dr NE, Calgary AB T3J 4L4; (Pakistan)'92; MB BS; CCFP; (403)590-5585; Fax. (403)590-7750.

KAMRAN, Asim; Dr H Bliss Murphy Cancer Ctr, 300 Prince Philip Dr, St. John's NL A1B 3V6; Punjab (India)'91; FRCPC; RadOncol. Staff, Dr H Bliss Murphy Cancer Centre; (709)777-2440

KAMRUL, Rejina; Family Medicine Unit, 172-1621 Albert St, Regina SK S4P 2S5; CCFP; Staff Family Med, Regina General Hospital; (306)766-0444; Fax. (306)766-4041.

KAMYAB, Mahshid; Eagle Ridge Plaza, 203-1194 Lansdowne Dr, Coquitlam BC V3E 1J7; Shahid Beheshti (Iran)'91; CCFP; Langs: Farsi; (604)472-1104; Fax. (604)472-1103.

KAMYAR, Mandana; Border City Clinic, 2707 50 Ave, Lloydminster SK S9V 2A8; (306)825-4427

KAN, F Dana; 501-4580 Dufferin St, North York ON M3H 5Y2; Tor'92; (416)739-9123

KAN, John Y C; Mon Sheong Court Clinic, 2020 McNicoll Ave, Scarborough ON M1V 0B5; Dal'77; (416)291-8228

KAN, Julio W H; Markham Stouffville Hosp, PO Box 1800 Stn Main 381 Church St, Markham ON L3P 7P3; McG'84; FRCPC; DiagRad. Ac Staff Diag Imaging, Markham Stouffville Hospital; (905)472-7020; Fax. (905)472-7078.

KAN, Lorna C H; 475-4789 Kingsway, Burnaby BC V5H 0A3; UBC'89; CCFP; (604)433-2733; Fax. (604)436-0224.

KAN, Victor C; 475-4789 Kingsway, Burnaby BC V5H 0A3; UBC'87; (604)433-2733

KAN, Wai-On; 6040-8171 Ackroyd Rd, Richmond BC V6X 3K1; UBC'84; Langs: Chinese; (604)273-5508

KANAAN, Hassan D; Bluewater Health-Norman Site, 89 Norman St, Sarnia ON N7T 6S3; Mosul (Iraq)'90; MB ChB; Staff, Bluewater Health - Norman Site; (519)464-4510

KANACHOWSKI, Danusia A; Whitehorse Med Services Ltd, 406 Lambert St, Whitehorse YT Y1A 1Z7; McM'90; Staff, Whitehorse Medical Services Ltd; (867)393-6620; Fax. (867)393-6601; wmsl@klondiker.com.

KANADJIAN, Maral N; Hop Santa Cabrini, 5655 rue Saint-Zotique E, Montreal QC H1T 1P7; Sher'06; CCFP; CCFP(E.M.); Staff, Hôpital Santa Cabrini Ospedale; (514)252-6000; Fax. (514)252-6453.

KANAGANAYAKAM, Shankary; Argus Med Centre, 300-581 Argus Rd, Oakville ON L6J 3J4; McM'05; BSc; CCFP; (905)338-9900

KANAGARATNAM, Christina N; Crescent Beach Med Arts, 2781 Gordon Ave, Surrey BC V4A 3J5; London (England)'96; CCFP; (604)535-0110

KANAGARATNAM, Sivaruban; St Michael's Hosp, 30 Bond St, Toronto ON M5B 1W8; Moscow (Russia (Federation))'05; Staff, St Michael's Hospital; (416)360-4000

KANAGASABAI, Sivakumar; MKS Medical Clinic, 6637 Highway 7, Kentville NS B4R 1B7; Colombo (Sri Lanka)'03; MB BS; (902)679-6650; Fax. (902)679-1739.

KANAKOS, Michael A; 525 Broadway W PO Box 20004 Rpo Fairview, Vancouver BC V5Z 0C1; Qns'05; Cardiol; IntMed.

KANANI, Amin S; Hycroft Med Bldg, 207-3195 Granville St, Vancouver BC V6H 3K2; McG'94; FRCPC; IntMed; ClinImmunol&Allergy. Staff Allergy & Clin Immunol, Providence Health Care - St Paul's Hospital; Clin Instructor, University of British Columbia; Fax. (604)732-4819.

KANANI, Kunal P; Brant Community HC-Brantford, 200 Terrace Hill St, Brantford ON N3R 1G9; Ott'97; Anes. Staff, The Brant Community Healthcare System - Brantford General Hospital Site; (519)752-7871

KANANI, Nisha; The Credit Valley Hosp, 2200 Eglinton Ave W, Mississauga ON L5M 2N1; Cal'04; FRCPC; Anes. Staff, The Credit Valley Hospital; (905)813-2200

KANANI, Ronak S; Bridgeland Med Bldg, 306-803 1 Ave NE, Calgary AB T2E 7C5; McM'96; FRCPC; IntMed; Cardiol. Staff, Foothills Medical Centre; (403)571-8687

KANANI, Ronik; North York Gen Hosp, 4001 Leslie St, North York ON M2K 1E1; Cal'01; FRCPC; Peds. Staff, North York General Hospital; (416)756-6479; Fax. (416)756-6152.

KANANI, Subodh D; Lakeshore Med & Prof Bldg, 302-3170 Lake Shore Blvd W, Etobicoke ON M8V 3X8; McM'74; CCFP; FCFP; (416)259-3507; Fax. (416)259-3507.

KANANI, Suresh R; Mission Med Clinic, 2303 4 St SW, Calgary AB T2S 2S7; Dublin (Ireland)'66; LRCPSI; (403)229-1700; Fax. (403)229-1875.

KANASHIRO, Jeanie; 3500 26 Ave NE, Calgary AB T1Y 6J4; McM'98; FRCSC; GenSurg. Staff Surg, Peter Lougheed Centre; (403)943-5689; Fax. (403)219-3574.

KANAWATY, David S; North York Med Arts Bldg, 123-1333 Sheppard Ave E, North York ON M2J 1V1; Tor'85; FCCP; FACP; FRCPC; IntMed (Critical Care Medicine); Respir. Ac Staff Respirologist & Internist, North York General Hospital; Instructor Med, University of Toronto.

KANBER, Yonca; Universite McGill, 3775 rue University, Montreal QC H3A 2B4; Marmara (Turkey)'95; (514)398-7446

KANCHERLA, Yasodhara; 3-1401 Plains Rd E, Burlington ON L7R 0C2; Andhra (India)'83; FRCSC; GenSurg (Breast Surgery). Staff, Joseph Brant Memorial Hospital; (905)639-3511; Fax. (905)639-1572.

KANDASAMY, Gengatharan; Fenton Med Centre, 4-2 Fenton Rd, Markham ON L3R 7B4; West Indies (Saint Lucia)'03; (905)948-9455

KANDASAMY, Gerald R; Kandasamy Med Prof Corp, 24 Albert St E, Thorold ON L2V 1P1; Natal (South Africa)'82; BSc; MB ChB; LMCC; CCFP; (905)988-1103; Fax. (905)988-1161.

KANDEL, Gabor P; St Michael's Hosp, 30 Bond St, Toronto ON M5B 1W8; Tor'78; FRCPC; IntMed; Gastroent. Staff, St Michael's Hospital; Assoc Prof Med, University of Toronto; (416)864-3093; Fax. (416)864-5994; kandelg@smh.toronto.on.ca.

KANDEL, Rita A; Mount Sinai Hosp, 600 University Ave, Toronto ON M5G 1X5; Tor'78; FRCPC; AnatPath. Chief-Pathol/Lab Med, Mount Sinai Hospital; Prof, University of Toronto; (416)586-8516; rkandel@mtsinai.on.ca.

KANDIAH, Anushiya; PO Box 1292 Stn Main, Port Alberni BC V9Y 7M2; Colombo (Sri Lanka)'95; MB BS.

KANDOLA, Kami; Dept of Health & Social Serv, PO Box 1320 Stn Main, Yellowknife NT X1A 2L9; McG'92; MPH; ABPM; DTMH; CCFP; FCFP; Med Officer of Hlth, Stanton Territorial Health Authority; Physician, Yellowknife Health & Social Services Authority; Langs: English; French; (867)920-8646; Fax. (867)873-0442; kami_kandola@gov.nt.ca.

KANDOLA, Rajdeep R; East Calgary Health Centre, 4715 8 Ave SE, Calgary AB T2A 3N4; Alb'09; CCFP; Staff, Rockyview General Hospital; (403)955-1400; Fax. (403)955-1414.

KANE, Barbara J; University Hosp of Northern BC, 1475 Edmonton St, Prince George BC V2M 1S2; Wes'80; FRCPC; Psy. Consultant, University Hospital of Northern British Columbia; Consultant, University of Northern British Columbia; Asst Prof, University of British Columbia; (250)564-1152; Fax. (250)612-5176; bkane@netbistro.com.

KANE, Jennifer J; Markham Stouffville Hosp, PO Box 1800 Stn Main 381 Church St, Markham ON L3P 7P3; Wes'07; CCFP; Staff, Markham Stouffville Hospital; (905)472-7373

KANE, Lorraine A; Osoyoos Med Centre, PO Box 330, Osoyoos BC V0H 1V0; Alb'99; CCFP; (250)495-2661

KANE, Martin D; New Vision Family Health Team, 421 Greenbrook Dr, Kitchener ON N2M 4K1; McM'02; CCFP; (519)578-3510; Fax. (519)578-6040.

KANE, Nolan P; Promenade Circle, 50-7700 Bathurst St, Thornhill ON L4J 7Y3; Tor'67; FRCSC; Otol. Assoc Staff, North York General Hospital - Branson Division; Assoc Staff, Humber River Regional Hospital - Keele Street Site.

KANE, Sheri-Lynn; St Joseph's HC-Parkwood Hosp, 801 Commissioners Rd E, London ON N6C 5J1; McM'91; BSc(Hons); FRCPC; IntMed; GeriatricMed. Staff, Guelph General Hospital; Staff, St Joseph's Health Centre; Parkwood Hospital - St Joseph's Health Care; Asst Prof, McMaster University; (519)685-4292

KANE-CORRIVEAU, Sandra P; 33 Dundas St, Dundas ON L9H 1A1; McM'93; CCFP; Staff Privil, Hamilton Health Sciences Centre - McMaster Children's Hospital; Staff Privil, St Joseph's Healthcare - Charlton Campus; (905)628-6151; Fax. (905)628-1609.

KANEE, Allan S; Credit Valley Med Arts Centre, 502-2000 Credit Valley Rd, Mississauga ON L5M 4N4; Tor'90; FRCSC; ObstGyn (Urological Gynecology). Staff, The Credit Valley Hospital; (905)820-8748 x223; Fax. (905)820-0255.

KANELLAKOS, George W; Queen Elizabeth II HSC, 1276 South Park St, Halifax NS B3H 2Y9; Dal'99; BSc; FRCPC; Anes (Thoracic Anesthesia). Staff Anes, Queen Elizabeth II Health Sciences Centre - Victoria General Site; (902)473-2700

KANERVA, Kevin J; 101-1865 Dilworth Dr, Kelowna BC V1Y 9T1; Wes'86; CCFP; CCFP(E.M.); (250)859-5433

KANETOS, Emmanuel; Markham Stouffville Hosp, PO Box 1800 Stn Main 381 Church St, Markham ON L3P 7P3; Tor'04; CCFP; Staff, Markham Stouffville Hospital; (905)472-7000

KANG, Amrit K; St Joseph's Health Centre, 332-30 The Queensway, Toronto ON M6R 1B5; Tor'96; BSc; FRCPC; IntMed (Hypertension); Nephrol. Staff, St Joseph's Health Centre; Langs: Punjabi; Hindi; (416)530-6227; Fax. (416)530-6233; akang00@yahoo.com.

KANG, Angela M; 490-5 Fairview Mall Dr, North York ON M2J 2Z1; Tor'87; FRCSC; ObstGyn. (416)492-2667; Fax. (416)492-6189.

KANG, Anna; Burnaby Hosp, 3935 Kincaid St, Burnaby BC V5G 2X6; Cal'99; FRCPC; IntMed. Staff, Burnaby Hospital; (604)434-4211

KANG, Arvind; Lions Gate Hosp, 231 15th St E, North Vancouver BC V7L 2L7; Punjab (India)'85; MB BS; FRCPC; Psy. Staff Geriatric Psy, Lions Gate Hospital; Staff, CREST Program; Langs: Hindi; Punjabi; (604)984-3860

KANG, G Shimi; BC Women's Hosp & Health Ctre, 3-4500 Oak St, Vancouver BC V6H 3N1; Alb'97; FRCPC; Psy (Addiction Psychiatry). Staff Psy, BC Women's Hospital & Health Centre; Clinical Asst Prof, University of British Columbia; Langs: Punjabi; Hindi; (604)875-2025; skang@cw.bc.ca.

KANG, Harbhajan S; Centre Med Cote-des-Neiges, 200-5300 ch Cote-des-Neiges, Montreal QC H3T 1Y3; UBC'97; FRCPC; IntMed; Rheum. Langs: French; Punjabi; (514)731-3601

KANG, Maria; Coast Med Clinic, 1018 Seymour St, Vancouver BC V6B 3M6; Cal'99; BSc; CCFP; Staff, Granville Medical Clinic; (604)569-3632

KANG, Maria; 302-4420 Chatterton Way, Victoria BC V8X 5J2; Man'04; FRCPC; Peds. (250)727-2156

KANG, Nirmal S; Burnaby Hosp, 3935 Kincaid St, Burnaby BC V5G 2X6; Punjab (India)'84; FRCPC; Psy (Geriatric Psychiatry). Staff Burnaby Mental Health & Addiction Services, Burnaby Hospital; (604)434-4211

KANG, Parmjit S; 216-7110 120 St, Surrey BC V3W 3M8; Jabalpur (India)'79; MB BS; FRCPC; IntMed; Endocrin&Metab. Staff, Surrey Memorial Hospital; Langs: Punjabi; Hindi; Urdu; (604)590-7121; parmjit_kang@yahoo.ca.

KANHAI, Neil A; St Joseph's Health Centre, 30 The Queensway, Toronto ON M6R 1B5; Tor'00; CCFP; CCFP(E.M.); Staff, St Joseph's Health Centre; (416)530-6000

KANHERE, Rujuta A; Southlake Reg Health Centre, 596 Davis Dr, Newmarket ON L3Y 2P9; Pune (India)'98; FRCPC; AnatPath. Staff, Southlake Regional Health Centre; (905)895-4521

KANIA, Jadwiga; Professional Bldg, 106-55 Selkirk Ave, Thompson MB R8N 0M5; Gdansk (Poland)'81.

KANIGAN, Arlene M; Hys Med Centre, 202-11010 101 St NW, Edmonton AB T5H 4B9; Sask'95; FRCPC; DiagRad. (780)426-1121

KANIGSBERG, Nordau D; Riverside Prof Centre, 305-1919 Riverside Dr, Ottawa ON K1H 1A2; Dal'71; AB; FRCPC; Derm. Assoc Staff, The Ottawa Hospital - General Campus; Assoc Staff, Children's Hospital of Eastern Ontario (CHEO); Assoc Prof, University of Ottawa; (613)523-4921; Fax. (613)523-5339.

KANJ, Nada; CSSS de Laval, 1755 boul Rene-Laennec, Laval QC H7M 3L9; (Russia (Federation))'90; MedBiochem. Staff, Hopital de la Cite de la santé; (450)688-1010 x24087

KANJEE, Anjum S; 10171 Yonge St, Richmond Hill ON L4C 1T5; Karachi (Pakistan)'87; CCFP; (905)918-1358

KANJEEKAL, S Rajh; Windsor Med Clinic, 6720 Hawthorne Dr, Windsor ON N8T 1J9; Kerala (India)'69; MB BS; FAAFP; (519)944-2295

KANJEEKAL, Santosh S R; Toronto East Gen Hosp Inc, 825 Coxwell Ave, Toronto ON M4C 3E7; Alb'99; CCFP; CCFP(E.M.); Staff, Toronto East General Hospital Inc; (416)469-6435

KANJEEKAL, Sindu M; Windsor Reg Cancer Centre, 2220 Kildare Rd, Windsor ON N8W 2X3; Wes'97; BSc; FRCPC; IntMed; MedOncol; Hem. (519)253-5253; sindu_kanjeekal@wrh.on.ca.

KANJI, Amirali; Medical Centre Walk-In-Clinic, 1428 Ouellette Ave, Windsor ON N8X 1K4; London (England)'56; FRCSC; GenSurg (Family Practice). (519)419-4294; Fax. (519)419-4267.

KANJI, Diamond M; Medical & Dental Bldg, 407-586 Eglinton Ave E, Toronto ON M4P 1P2; Makerere (Uganda)'71; FRCPC; Psy (Group Psychotherapy). Att Staff OPD, St Michael's Hospital; University of Toronto; (416)489-8150; Fax. (416)489-8231.

KANJI, Dilshad A; 298 Sheppard Ave E, North York ON M2N 3B1; Zambia (Zambia)'77; MB ChB; FRCPC; IntMed; Rheum. (416)223-6500; Fax. (416)223-6502.

KANJI, Hussein D; Vancouver Gen Hosp, 2447 C-855 12th Ave W, Vancouver BC V5Z 1M9; Cal'05; FRCPC; EmergMed. Staff, Vancouver General Hospital - Centennial Pavillion; Langs: Gujarati; French; (604)875-4111

KANJI, Jamil; Misericordia Community Hosp, 16940 87 Ave NW, Edmonton AB T5R 4H5; McM'06; FRCPC; IntMed; MedMicrobiol; InfectDis. Staff, Covenant Health - Misericordia Community Hospital; (780)735-2000

KANJI, Mohammed I; 200-2984 boul Taschereau, Greenfield Park QC J4V 2G9; Ott'80; FRCPC; IntMed; Rheum (P.Q.). Staff, Hopital Charles LeMoyne; Staff, Centre Hospitalier de Verdun; (450)465-9789; Fax. (450)672-4578.

KANJI, Rajandra; Saint John Reg Hosp, PO BOx 2100 Stn Main, Saint John NB E2L 4L2; Natal (South Africa)'79; MB ChB; MSc; Staff, Saint John Regional Hospital; (506)648-6000

KANJI, Zainul A A; Bradley Family Health Care, 2F-595 Bradley Ave, London ON N6E 3Z8; UBC'74; (519)936-0704

KANKARIA, Pratibha; Bolton Med Centre, 207-12295 Highway 50, Bolton ON L7E 1M2; Rajasthan (India)'85; MBA; CCFP; (905)857-8855

KANKE, Lorena J; PO Box 74655 Rpo Kitsilano, Vancouver BC V6K 4P4; UBC'67; FRCSC; ObstGyn (Abortion). Att Staff, Vancouver General Hospital - Centennial Pavillion; Ac Staff, BC Women's Hospital & Health Centre; Staff Consultant, BC Cancer Agency Vancouver Centre; Clin Assoc Prof, University of British Columbia.

KANNAB-AYDA, George; CSSS Haut-Richelieu-Rouville, 920 boul du Seminaire N, St-Jean-sur-Richel QC J3A 1B7; Tichreen Univ (Syria)'98; Staff, Hôpital du Haut-Richelieu; (450)359-5000

KANNAMPUZHA, Paul T; 104-200 Ronson Dr, Etobicoke ON M9W 5Z9; Tor'88; FRCPC; IntMed; Cardiol. Dir Cardiac Care Unit, Trillium Health Centre - Mississauga; Clin Instructor, University of Toronto; (416)740-7600; Fax. (416)740-6100.

KANNU, Peter; The Hosp for Sick Children, 555 University Ave, Toronto ON M5G 1X8; Otago Medical School (New Zealand)'94; MB ChB; DCH; FRACP; PhD; Staff, The Hospital For Sick Children; (416)813-6390; Fax. (416)813-5345; peter.kannu@sickkids.ca.

KANTARDJIEFF, Spiridon; Clinique des Med d'Urgence, 632 rue Bowen S, Sherbrooke QC J1G 2E9; Sofia (Bulgaria)'69; Electroenceph (P.Q.); Neur (P.Q.). Staff, Centre Hospitalier Universitaire de Sherbrooke-Hopital Fleurimont; (819)822-2700

KANTHAN, Rani; Royal University Hosp, 2868 GW-103 Hospital Dr, Saskatoon SK S7N 0W8; (India)'79; MS; FRCS(Edin); FACP; FRCPC; AnatPath (Gastroenterology). Staff, Royal University Hospital; Consultant AnatPath, Saskatoon Health Region; Prof, University of Saskatchewan; Langs: Hindi; Tamil; (306)655-2158

KANTOCH, Michal; University of Alberta Hosp, 4C2-8440 112 St NW, Edmonton AB T6G 2B7; Warsaw (Poland)'81; FRCPC; Peds (Adult Congenital Heart Disease); Cardiol. Staff, Stollery Children's Hospital; Staff, University of Alberta Hospital; Prof Peds, University of Alberta; (780)407-3963

KANTOR, David; 56 Aberfoyle Cres, Etobicoke ON M8X 2W4; Man'79; FRCPC; Psy (Mood Disorders). Staff, Humber River Regional Hospital - Keele Street Site; Langs: Hebrew; (416)248-2050 x235; Fax. (416)248-6557; dkantor@bellnet.ca.

KANTOR, Paul F; The Hosp For Sick Children, 555 University Ave, Toronto ON M5G 1X8; Witwatersrand (South Africa)'84; MB ChB; DCH(UK); FRCPC; FRCPC; Cardiol; Peds (Heart Failure). Staff Crdiol, The Hospital For Sick Children; Assoc Prof Peds, University of Toronto; Langs: Afrikaans; (416)813-7239; Fax. (416)813-7547.

KANUNGO, Nachiketa M; Windsor Radiological Assoc, 1568 Ouellette Ave, Windsor ON N8X 1K7; McG'89; FRCPC; DiagRad. Staff, Hôtel-Dieu Grace Hospital; Langs: English; French; (519)256-4914; Fax. (519)256-4358.

KANUNGO, Tarit K; Niagara Health Centre, 105-180 Vine St S, St Catharines ON L2R 7P3; Calcutta (India)'65; MB BS(Cal); CCFP; CCFP(E.M.); FCFP; (905)682-7555; Fax. (905)682-7446.

KANWAL, Jaswinder S; Grnadview Med Clinic, PO Box 399 644 Mill St, Grandview MB R0L 0Y0; (Other Foreign)'99; (204)546-2774

KANWAL, Tejpreet K; Goodfellow Prof Bldg, 201-170 McEwan Dr E, Bolton ON L7E 4C8; Karnataka (India)'98; FRCPC; Peds. (905)857-2356

KANYA-FORSTNER, Nicholas G; Timmins Family Health Team, 208-38 Pine St N, Timmins ON P4N 6K6; Tor'92; CCFP; FCFP; Staff, White Pines Health Network; (705)267-3272; Fax. (705)267-4212; nkanya-forstner@pht.ca.

KANZA EPUNZA, Rene; CSSS de Chicoutimi, 305 rue Saint-Vallier, Chicoutimi QC G7H 5H6; Kinshasa (Congo (Democratic Republic))'98; Staff, Complexe hospitalier de la Sagamie; (418)541-1031

KAO, Pion; 200-233 16 Ave NW, Calgary AB T2M 0H5; Alb'93; FRCPC; Peds. Clinical Asst Prof, University of Calgary; Langs: Mandarin; Chinese; (403)230-3300; Fax. (403)230-3322.

KAO, Dina H; Zeidler-Ledcor Centre, 130 University Campus NW, Edmonton AB T6G 2X8; Alb'99; FRCPC; IntMed (Endoscopy); Gastroent. Staff, University of Alberta Hospital; (780)492-8307

KAO, Ellen; MUHC-Royal Victoria Hosp, 687 av des Pins O, Montreal QC H3A 1A1; Sask'80; ABR; FRCPC; DiagRad. Staff DiagRad, McGill University Health Centre - Royal Victoria Hospital; adj Prof, McGill University; (514)934-1934 x36008; ellen.kao@muhc.mcgill.ca.

KAO, John T S; Boxgrove Med Arts Centre, 300-110 Copper Creek Dr, Markham ON L6B 0P9; UBC'92; FRCSC; PlasSurg. Langs: Mandarin; (905)471-5633; Fax. (905)471-5634.

KAO, K Jesse; The Family Practice Clinic, 2778 104th St, Nanaimo BC V9T 2E4; McG'07; MDCM; MBA; CCFP; CCFP(E.M.); (250)758-1711

KAO, Raymond L C; London HSC-Victoria Hosp, PO Box 5010 Stn B 800 Commissioners Rd E, London ON N6A 5W9; Tor'90; FRCPC; IntMed (Critical Care Medicine). Staff, London Health Sciences Centre - Victoria Campus; (519)685-8500 x55662; Fax. (519)667-6698; rickao@yahoo.com.

KAO, Shawn S K; Finchgate Med Centre, 102-40 Finchgate Blvd, Brampton ON L6T 3J1; Tor'87; Peds. Staff, William Osler Health System - Etobicoke General Hospital; Staff, William Osler Health System - Brampton Civic Hospital; (905)791-6444; Fax. (905)791-7333.

KAO, Yolanda M; Foothills Prof Bldg, 170-1620 29 St NW, Calgary AB T2N 4L7; Cal'92; BSc; CCFP; Staff, Foothills Medical Centre; (403)237-6404; Fax. (403)266-4746; kao.yolanda@shaw.ca.

KAPALA, Marianna M; 200-101 Queensway W, Mississauga ON L5B 2P7; Tor'01; FRCSC; GenSurg. Staff, Trillium Health Centre - West Toronto; Staff, Trillium Health Centre - Mississauga; Langs: Slovak; Ukrainian; (905)624-4531; Fax. (905)624-6988.

KAPALA, Miroslava A; Trillium Hlth Ctr-Mississauga, 100 Queensway W, Mississauga ON L5B 1B8; Tor'04; FRCPC; Anes. Staff, Trillium Health Centre - Mississauga; (905)848-7100

KAPALANGA, Joachim; Summerside Med Centre, 475 Granville St, Summerside PE C1N 3N9; Staff, Prince County Hospital; (902)432-8181

KAPALANGA, Nyolima J B; Grey Bruce HS-Owen Sound, PO Box 1800 Stn Main 8226-1800 8th St E, Owen Sound ON N4K 6M9; Dar Es Salaam (Tanzania)'80; Staff, Grey Bruce Health Services - Owen Sound; (519)376-2121; Fax. (519)378-1583.

KAPASI, Ali M; University of Alberta Hosp, 2E4 42WMC-8440 112 St NW, Edmonton AB T6G 2B7; Alb'03; Respir; IntMed. Staff, University of Alberta Hospital; (780)407-2659; Fax. (780)407-6384.

KAPASI, Tahera Y; Chantham-Kent Hlth Alliance, PO Box 2030 Stn Main 80 Grand Ave W, Chatham ON N7M 5L9; Bombay (India)'86; FRCPC; Anes. Staff, Chatham-Kent Health Alliance.

KAPELUTO, Daniel; Couchiching Family Health Team, 103-119 Memorial Ave, Orillia ON L3V 5X1; Dublin (Ireland)'09; MB BCh; CCFP; (705)326-3549

KAPHENGST, Karla; Kitchener Downtown CHC, 44 Francis St S, Kitchener ON N2G 2A2; (Other Foreign)'97; (519)745-4404; Fax. (519)745-3709.

KAPIJIMPANGA, Lowesha B; Niagara H System-Welland Site, 65 Third St, Welland ON L3B 4W6; Ott'70; GenSurg. Staff, Niagara Health System - Welland Hospital Site; (905)714-1660; Fax. (905)714-1666.

KAPILA, Varun; Univ Hlth Network-Toronto Gen, 6EN 216-200 Elizabeth St, Toronto ON M5G 2C4; Ott'06; FRCSC; GenSurg. Staff, Toronto General Hospital - UHN; (416)340-4800

KAPILAN, Priyadharsini M; Bedford Central Med Clinic, 2F-1650 Bedford Hwy, Bedford NS B4A 4J7; Colombo (Sri Lanka)'90; MB BS; CCFP; (902)835-4777; Fax. (902)835-5502.

KAPITOULSKI, Boris; Red Deer Reg Hosp Centre, PO Box 5030 Stn Postal Box Ctr 3942 50A Ave, Red Deer AB T4N 6R2; Sverdlovsk State (Russia (Federation))'86; FRCPC; Anes. Staff, Red Deer Regional Hospital Centre; (403)343-4519; Fax. (403)309-2809.

KAPLAN, Alan G; 17 Bedford Park Ave, Richmond Hill ON L4C 2N9; Tor'83; CCFP; CCFP(E.M.); FCFP; Physician Hospitalist, William Osler Health System - Brampton Civic Hospital; Chair, Family Physician Airways Group of Canada; Clin Lecturer, University of Toronto; (905)883-1100; Fax. (905)884-1195.

KAPLAN, Allan S; Addiction & Mental Hlth-Clarke, 832-250 College St, Toronto ON M5T 1R8; Tor'78; MSc; FRCPC; Psy. Sr Staff Psy, Toronto General Hospital - UHN; Chief Clinical Research/Staff, Centre for Addiction & Mental Health (CAMH) - College Street Site; Vice Chair Research/Prof Psy, University of Toronto; (416)535-8501 x4980

KAPLAN, David M; North York Doctors, 703-240 Duncan Mill Rd, North York ON M3B 3S6; Tor'01; MSc; BA; CCFP; Chief Family & Commun Med, North York General Hospital; Asst Prof Family & Commun Med, University of Toronto; Langs: Hebrew; (416)494-7396; Fax. (416)494-0129.

KAPLAN, Gilaad; UCMC Area 2 Clinic, G1-3330 Hospital Dr NW, Calgary AB T2N 4N1; Cal'00; FRCPC; IntMed; Gastroent. (403)944-6551; Fax. (403)944-6548.

KAPLAN, Henry D; Medical Clinic Bldg, 112-89 Humber College Blvd, Etobicoke ON M9V 4B8; McG'87; FRCSC; Ophth. (416)746-1617; Fax. (416)746-1619.

KAPLAN-KRASNY, Wendy; Tiny Tots Med Centre, 203-3400 rue Du Marche, Dollard-D-Ormeaux QC H9B 2Y1; Tor'80; (514)685-3531; Fax. (514)685-7971.

KAPLAN-MYRTH, Nili; 151D Second Ave, Ottawa ON K1S 2H6; Ott'08; CCFP; (613)695-6687; Fax. (613)695-6689.

KAPLANSKY-GOLD, Cathy S; U Of Toronto-Psychiatric Serv, 214 College St, Toronto ON M5T 2Z9; McM'86; FRCPC; Psy. Lecturer Psy/Staff Psy, University of Toronto; (416)978-8070; Fax. (416)978-7341.

KAPLOVITCH, Harvey; Bloor Med Clinic, 844 Bathurst St, Toronto ON M5R 3G1; McM'75; CCFP; FCFP; Assoc Staff, Mount Sinai Hospital; Langs: French; Hebrew; (416)534-4214; Fax. (416)534-4582.

KAPNOUDHIS, Paul C; Vancouver Gen Hosp, 855 12th Ave W, Vancouver BC V5Z 1M9; Cape Town (South Africa)'81; FRCPC; Anes. Staff, Vancouver General Hospital - Centennial Pavillion; (604)875-4855; Fax. (604)875-5209.

KAPOOR, Aarti; Univ Hlth Network-Toronto Western Hosp, 2F WW-399 Bathurst St, Toronto ON M5T 2S8; Ott'09; CCFP; Staff, Toronto Western Hospital - University Health Network; (416)603-5888

KAPOOR, Anil; St Joseph's Healthcare, G340-50 Charlton Ave E, Hamilton ON L8N 4A6; Dal'91; MD; FRCSC; Urol (Renal Oncology). Urology, St Joseph's Healthcare - Charlton Campus; Prof Surg, McMaster University; (905)522-6536; Fax. (905)521-6195; kapoor4@mcmaster.ca.

KAPOOR, Anmol S; Marlborough Mall, 280-433 Marlborough Way NE, Calgary AB T2A 5H5; Russia (Russia (Federation))'00; Cardiol; IntMed.

KAPOOR, Monika; Univ Hlth Network-Toronto Gen, 480-200 Elizabeth St, Toronto ON M5G 2C4; McM'04; CCFP; CCFP(E.M.); Staff, Toronto General Hospital - UHN; (416)340-3111

KAPOOR, Pankaj V; 400-871 Ottawa St, Windsor ON N8Y 2C9; Mysore (India)'97; Langs: Hindi; Punjabi; (519)973-1133; Fax. (519)973-1255.

KAPOOR, Sunil; Toronto East Gen Hosp Inc, 825 Coxwell Ave, Toronto ON M4C 3E7; Dal'93; FRCPC; Anes., Toronto East General Hospital Inc; University of Toronto; (416)469-6580 x6212; Fax. (416)469-6874; skapo@tegh.on.ca.

KAPOOR, Videsh; Vancouver Airport Med Clinic, PO Box 32301 Rpo YVR Terminal, Richmond BC V7B 1W2; UBC'93; BSc; BEd; CCFP; FCFP; Staff, Royal Columbian Hospital; Clinical Asst Prof Family Pract, University of British Columbia; Langs: Hindi; French; (604)738-3755; Fax. (604)207-8400; videsh@telus.net.

KAPOOR, Vikram J; William Osler HC-Brampton, 2100 Bovaird Dr E, Brampton ON L6R 3J7; McM'09; CCFP; Staff, William Osler Health System - Brampton Civic Hospital; (905)494-2120

KAPOOR, Vimal S; Markham Stouffville Hosp, PO Box 1800 Stn Main 381 Church St, Markham ON L3P 7P3; Dal'02; BSc(McG); MPH(PublicHealth); ATLS; LMCC; ACLS; FRS; MRCP; DTM&H; AvMed; FRCPC; CommunMed;CCFP; CCFP(E.M.); Public Health & Preventive Med. Staff, Markham Stouffville Hospital; Langs: French; Hindi; Punjabi; (905)668-4113 x3200; vimal.kapoor@mail.mcgill.ca.

KAPP, Magdalena J; Medical Clinic, 5031 49 St, Innisfail AB T4G 1A4; (South Africa)'82; MB ChB; Langs: Afrikaans; (403)227-3356; Fax. (403)227-2702.

KAPP, Sanet; Prince Albert Med Clinic, 681 15th St W, Prince Albert SK S6V 7H9; (306)764-1505

KAPPAGANTULA, Mythri; All Saints Springhill Hosp, 10 Princess St, Springhill NS B0M 1X0; (Other Foreign)'10; CCFP; Staff, All Saints Springhill Hospital; (902)597-3773

KAPPAGANTULA, Usha R; Sandy Hill Comm Health Centre, 221 Nelson St, Ottawa ON K1N 1C7; Ranchi (India)'68; CCFP; FCFP; Staff Physician, Queensway Carleton Hospital; (613)789-8458; Fax. (613)789-8710.

KAPPEL, Joanne E; Saskatoon Nephrology Group, 434-230 Avenue R S, Saskatoon SK S7M 2Z1; Sask'81; FRCPC; IntMed; Nephrol. Staff, St Paul's Hospital (Grey Nuns) of Saskatoon; Clin Prof Med, University of Saskatchewan; (306)934-3300; Fax. (306)934-3355; jekappel@sasktel.net.

KAPPOS, Stamatina; Bracebridge Med Centre, 2-55 Muskoka Rd 118 W, Bracebridge ON P1L 1T2; Wes'92; CCFP; Ac Staff, South Muskoka Memorial Hospital - Muskoka Algonquin Healthcare; Langs: Greek; (705)645-1028; Fax. (705)646-2543.

KAPRAL, Moira K; Univ Hlth Network-Toronto Gen, 14EN 215-200 Elizabeth St, Toronto ON M5G 2C4; Tor'92; MSc; FRCPC; IntMed. Staff Physician, Toronto General Hospital - UHN; Physician, Institute for Clinical Evaluative Sciences; (416)340-4642; Fax. (416)595-5826; moira.kapral@uhn.on.ca.

KAPRELIAN, Suzan; CHUM-Hotel-Dieu, 3840 rue Saint-Urbain, Montreal QC H2W 1T8; Mon'98; CSPQ; FRCPC; Anes. Staff, Centre Hospitalier l'Université de Montréal (CHUM) - Hôtel-Dieu; (514)890-8000 x14570; Fax. (514)412-7222.

KAPRIELIAN, Anoush A; Queensway Carleton Hosp, 3045 Baseline Rd, Nepean ON K2H 8P4; Qns'04; CCFP; Staff, Queensway Carleton Hospital; (613)721-2000

KAPROWY, Richard R; Medical Arts Bldg, 202-233 Kennedy St, Winnipeg MB R3C 3J5; Man'69; DiagRad.

KAPTEIN, Sylvia; 201-4256 Portage Rd, Niagara Falls ON L2E 6A4; Dal'85; CCFP; FCFP; Staff Court Privil, Niagara Health System - Greater Niagara General Site; (905)357-1662; Fax. (905)356-2227.

KAPUR, Farah; Fall River Family Practice, PO Box 2160 Rpo Fall River 3060 Lake Thomas Dr, Fall River NS B2T 1K6; Man'94; CCFP; FCFP; (902)861-2237; Fax. (902)861-1914.

KAPUR, Kusum; Halton HCS Corp-Oakville, 327 Reynolds St, Oakville ON L6J 3L7; Punjab (India)'69; FRCPC; Anes. Staff, Halton Healthcare Services Corporation - Oakville Site; (905)845-2571

KAPUR, Nishitha; Bridlewood Mall, 241-2900 Warden Ave, Scarborough ON M1W 2S8; Bombay (India)'92; MB BS; CCFP; FCFP; Langs: Hindi; Punjabi; (416)497-7277; Fax. (416)498-7588; nishitha.kapur@sympatico.ca.

KAPUR, Sandeep; Halifax Allergy & Asthma, 503-5657 Spring Garden Rd, Halifax NS B3J 3R4; Dal'91; BSc; FRCPC; Peds (Pediatric Allergy); ClinImmunol&Allergy. Ac Staff, IWK Health Centre; Asst Prof, Dalhousie University; (902)425-3927

KAPUR, Shiv; Hopital Reg D'Edmundston, 275 Hebert Blvd, Edmundston NB E3V 4E4; New Delhi (India)'89; Staff Clin Path, Hôpital regional d'Edmundston; (506)739-2537; Fax. (506)739-2232.

KAPUR, Suneil; Greenbank Med Centre, 203-139 Greenbank Rd, Nepean ON K2H 9A5; Wes'97; FRCPC; IntMed; Rheum. Assoc Staff Rheumatol, The Ottawa Hospital - General Campus; Asst Prof, University of Ottawa; Langs: French; (613)422-3861; Fax. (613)422-7538.

KAPUSCINSKA, Maria M; MUHC-Montreal Children's Hosp, 2300 rue Tupper, Montreal QC H3H 1P3; Warsaw (Poland)'68; FRCPC; Psy (Child Psychiatry). Ac Staff, McGill University Health Centre - Montreal Children's Hospital; Asst Prof Psy, McGill University; (514)412-4449; Fax. (514)412-4346.

KAPUSTA, Donald J; 86 Third St, Etobicoke ON M8V 2X9; Sask'86; (416)251-8571; Fax. (416)251-1193.

KAPUSTA, Linda R; The Credit Valley Hosp, 2200 Eglinton Ave W, Mississauga ON L5M 2N1; Sask'86; FRCPC; AnatPath (Cytology). Assoc Staff, The Credit Valley Hospital; Asst Prof, University of Toronto; Asst Prof, McMaster University; (905)813-4243; lkapusta@cvh.on.ca.

KAPUSTA, Michael A; SMBD Jewish Gen Hosp, 3755 ch Cote-Sainte-Catherine, Montreal QC H3T 1E2; McG'90; Ophth (Vitreo Retinal Surgery). Staff, Sir Mortimer B Davis Jewish General; Staff, McGill University Health Centre - Montreal Children's Hospital; Staff, McGill University Health Centre - Royal Victoria Hospital; McGill University; (514)340-8284; Fax. (514)340-8115.

KAPUSTA, Morton A; 205-5885 ch Cote-des-Neiges, Montreal QC H3S 2T2; McG'59; FRCP; FAB; FRCPC; Rheum; IntMed. Staff, Sir Mortimer B Davis Jewish General; assoc Prof, McGill University; Langs: English; French; (514)735-6978; Fax. (514)735-2072.

KAPUSTA, William M; Oshawa Clinic, 117 King St E, Oshawa ON L1H 1B9; Sask'79; BSc; Staff, Lakeridge Health - Oshawa Site; Langs: Ukrainian; (905)723-8551; Fax. (905)721-4329.

KARA, Alnoor F; 282 Erie St, Stratford ON N5A 2N2; Mem'80; (519)273-4993; Fax. (519)273-7830.

KARA, Mahmud; 101-1614 Dundas St E, Whitby ON L1N 8Y8; Tor'88; FRCSC; PlasSurg. (905)438-9000; Fax. (905)438-9001; drahmed@gmail.com.

KARA, Sukaina; Laurel Place Hospice, 9688 137A St, Surrey BC V3T 4H9; Mem'07; CCFP; (604)930-6808

KARA, Zulfikar S; Bay Coll Med Lockwood Diag, 108-790 Bay St, Toronto ON M5G 1N8; McM'91; CCFP; (416)929-1900; Fax. (416)929-7316.

KARA-SHARIFF, Shain; Markham Mews Med Clinic, 7-4997 Highway 7, Unionville ON L3R 1N1; McM'82; Ac Staff, Markham Stouffville Hospital; (905)475-3995; Fax. (905)475-3581.

KARABATSOS, Athanassios; Pontiac Health Centre, 200 rue Argue, Shawville QC J0X 2Y0; Padova (Italy)'79; IntMed. Staff, Pontiac Hospital Centre; Langs: English; Italian; Greek; (819)647-2211; Fax. (819)647-6814.

KARABATSOS, Charalabos B; 48-2140 North Park Dr, Brampton ON L6S 0C9; Tor'96; FRCSC; OrthSurg (Hip & Knee Replacement). Court Staff, Halton Healthcare Services Corporation - Georgetown Hospital; Staff, William Osler Health System - Brampton Civic Hospital; Court Staff, Headwaters Health Care Centre - Orangeville Site; Langs: Greek; (905)455-6884; Fax. (905)455-2398; b.karabatsos@gmail.com.

KARABEGOVIC, Amna; Univ Hlth Network-Toronto Gen, 480-200 Elizabeth St, Toronto ON M5G 2C4; Tor'09; CCFP; CCFP(E.M.); Staff Emerg, Toronto General Hospital - UHN; (416)340-3131

KARACHI, Timothy A; Hamilton HS-Henderson Site, 711 Concession St, Hamilton ON L8V 1C3; Wes'97; FRCPC; IntMed (Critical Care Medicine). Staff, Hamilton Health Sciences Centre-Juravinski Site; (905)521-2100

KARAGIOZOV, Ilko S; 1-2060 Ellesmere Rd, Scarborough ON M1H 2V6; Pavlov (Bulgaria)'94; CCFP; Langs: Bulgarian; Russian; (416)439-2273

KARAGUESIAN, Gregory J; Haliburton Highlands Health S, PO Box 115 7199 Gelert Rd, Haliburton ON K0M 1S0; Qns'90; Staff, Haliburton Highlands Health Services - Haliburton Site; Langs: English; French; (705)457-1392

KARAH, Munia M A; Commercial Street Med Centre, 208-311 Commercial St, Milton ON L9T 3Z9; Al Fateh (Libya)'00; FRCSC; ObstGyn. (905)875-2280

KARAIVANOV, Yordan S; Labrador Grenfell Health, PO Box 7000 Stn C, Happy-Valley-Goose NL A0P 1C0; Sofia (Bulgaria)'95; CCFP; Staff, Labrador Health Centre; (709)897-2000; Fax. (709)897-6774.

KARAKIEWICZ, Pierre; CHUM-Hop St-Luc, 4205-1058 rue Saint-Denis, Montreal QC H2X 3J4; McG'94; FRCSC; Urol. Staff, Centre Hospitalier l'Université De Montréal (CHUM) - Hôpital Saint-luc; Langs: German; Polish; French; (514)890-8000 x35336

KARALIC, Sanja; 1199 Lynn Valley Rd PO Box 16011 Rpo Lynn Valley, North Vancouver BC V7J 3S9; UBC'05; CCFP; Langs: Serbian; Spanish; Croatian; (604)254-1354

KARALIS, Aspasia; MUHC-Montreal Children's Hosp, A 602-2300 rue Tupper, Montreal QC H3H 1P3; McG'07; MDCM; MedGenetics. Staff, McGill University Health Centre - Montreal Children's Hospital; (514)412-4427

KARALIS, Peter; Pape Med Centre, 210-751 Pape Ave, Toronto ON M4K 3T1; Tor'83; BSc(Hon); Staff, Toronto East General Hospital Inc; Media Dir, Nesbit Lodge; Langs: Greek; (416)461-1311; Fax. (416)778-5534; drkaralis@bellnet.ca.

KARAM, Boutros; Ctr Hosp De Verdun, 4000 boul Lasalle, Verdun QC H4G 2A3; St. Joseph (Lebanon)'82; FRCSC; GenSurg; VascSurg. Staff, Centre Hospitalier de Verdun; (514)362-1000

KARAM, Jacques; 202-895 Boul Du Seminaire N, St-Jean-Sur-Richel QC J3A 1J2; Beirut (Lebanon)'71; Cardiol (P. Q.). Ac Staff, Hôpital du Haut-Richelieu; Langs: English; Arabic; (450)359-8080; Fax. (450)359-7577.

KARAM, Rana; Toronto East Gen Hosp Inc, 825 Coxwell Ave, Toronto ON M4C 3E7; Ott'98; FRCPC; DiagRad. Staff, Toronto East General Hospital Inc; (416)469-6580 x3409

KARAM-DAD, Choudhary K; Martensville Med Clinic, PO Box 210, Martensville SK S0K 2T0; Rajshahi (Bangladesh)'67; LRCP; MRCS; (306)931-8582; Fax. (306)931-8589.

KARAMA, Sherif; Pavillon Frank B Common, 6875 boul Lasalle, Verdun QC H4H 1R3; Mon'02; FRCPC; Psy. (514)761-6131 x2221

KARAMANOS, Stavroula V; Queensway-Carleton Hosp, 3045 Baseline Rd, Nepean ON K2H 8P4; McG'95; FRCPC; DiagRad. Staff Diagnostic Radiol, Queensway Carleton Hospital; (613)721-2000 x2701; Fax. (613)721-4774.

KARAMBOLOVA, Kristi K; Rosedale Med Centre, 212-600 Sherbourne St, Toronto ON M4X 1W4; Warsaw (Poland)'81; MedBiochem (Menopause). (416)546-3487; Fax. (416)546-3657.

KARAMCHANDANI, Jason R P; St Michael's Hosp, 30 Bond St, Toronto ON M5B 1W8; Stanford University (USA)'06; Staff, St Michael's Hospital; (416)864-6060 x6130; Fax. (416)864-5648.

KARAMDAD, Nargis; Temple Family Med Clinic, 5401 Temple Dr NE, Calgary AB T1Y 3R7; Sask'01; (403)293-1698

KARAN, Tulika S; Saddletowne Med Clinic, 914 Saddletowne Circle NE, Calgary AB T3J 5M1; (India)'93; MB BS; CCFP; (403)590-7710; Fax. (403)590-7113.

KARANI, Yasir; William Osler HC-Etobicoke, 101 Humber College Blvd, Etobicoke ON M9V 1R8; West Indies (Saint Kitts-Nevis)'06; FRCPC; IntMed. Staff, William Osler Health System - Etobicoke General Hospital; (905)494-2120

KARANICOLAS, Paul J; Sunnybrook Hlth Sciences Ctre, 2075 Bayview Ave, Toronto ON M4N 3M5; Wes'03; FRCSC; GenSurg. Staff, Sunnybrook Health Sciences Centre; (416)480-6100

KARANICOLAS, Stavros; St Joseph's Health Centre, 339-30 The Queensway, Toronto ON M6R 1B5; Athens (Greece)'68; DAB; FRCPC; IntMed (Nephrology). Head Nephrol, St Joseph's Health Centre; Langs: Greek; (416)530-6239; Fax. (416)530-6722.

KARANOFSKY, Mark; SMBD Jewish Gen Hosp, 3755 ch Cote-Sainte-Catherine, Montreal QC H3T 1E2; McG'02; CCFP; Staff, Sir Mortimer B Davis Jewish General; (514)340-8253

KARANTONIS, Anastassios; Pape Med Centre, 214-757 Pape Ave, Toronto ON M4K 3T1; Innsbruck (Austria)'67; Langs: Greek; (416)463-0879; Fax. (416)463-0026.

KARANWAL, Derek A; Cape Breton Hlthcare Complex, 1482 George St, Sydney NS B1P 1P3; Liverpool (England)'95; MB ChB; Staff, Cape Breton Healthcare Complex; (902)567-8000

KARAPAREDDY, Venugopal R; Markham Stouffville Hosp, PO Box 1800 Stn Main 381 Church St, Markham ON L3P 7P3; Mysore (India)'99; Psy. Staff Psy, Markham Stouffville Hospital.

KARAPLIS, Andy C; SMBD Jewish Gen Hosp, 3755 ch Cote-Sainte-Catherine, Montreal QC H3T 1E2; McG'84; Endocrin&Metab; Endocrin (P.Q.); IntMed. Staff, Sir Mortimer B Davis Jewish General; adj Prof, McGill University; (514)340-7550

KARAS, Maria; Hop Marie Clarac, 3530 boul Gouin E, Montreal-Nord QC H1H 1B7; Cracovie (Poland)'82; CCFP; Staff, Hopital Marie Clarac; (514)321-8800

KARAS, Philip; Smyth Med Centre, 224-1929 Russell Rd, Ottawa ON K1G 4G3; McM'81; CCFP; Staff, The Ottawa Hospital - General Campus; University of Ottawa; (613)738-3327

KARAS, Yair; 10014 Yonge St, Richmond Hill ON L4C 1T8; Hebrew (Israel)'67; FRCSC; Ophth. Ac Staff, Mackenzie Richmond Hill Hospital; (905)884-8733; Fax. (905)884-9187.

KARASIK, Arthur E; 202-190 Sherway Dr, Etobicoke ON M9C 5N2; Tor'77; FRCPC; IntMed (Rheumatology); Rheum. Ac Staff, St Joseph's Health Centre; (416)233-1271; Fax. (416)233-3861.

KARASMANIS, George N; Royal Victoria Hosp, 201 Georgian Dr, Barrie ON L4M 6M2; Qns'03; CCFP; CCFP(E.M.); Staff, Royal Victoria Regional Health Centre; (705)728-9090

KARATELA, Kamran; Chatham-Kent Health Alliance, PO Box 2030 Stn Main 80 Grand Ave W, Chatham ON N7M 5L9; Karachi (Pakistan)'98; Staff, Chatham-Kent Health Alliance; (519)352-6400

KARATZIOS, Christos; MUHC-Montreal Children's Hosp, C 1242-2300 rue Tupper, Montreal QC H3H 1P3; McG'98; FRCPC; Peds (AIDS/HIV); InfectDis. Asst Prof Peds InfectDis, McGill University Health Centre - Montreal Children's Hospital; Assoc Member Special Immunol, Universite de Montreal; Langs: Greek; French; (514)412-4485

KARAVATTATHAYYIL, Sebastian; Toronto East Gen Hosp Inc, 825 Coxwell Ave, Toronto ON M4C 3E7; Kerala (India)'78; MB BS; ABAP/CP; ABHemPath; FRCPC; AnatPath. Staff Lab Med, Toronto East General Hospital Inc; (416)469-6580 x2985; Fax. (416)469-6106; sebkaravatt@hotmail.com.

KARAYAN, Lina; Centre sante Queen Elizabeth, 2100 av de Marlowe, Montreal QC H4A 3L5; Laval'94; CCFP; Staff, McGill University Health Centre - Montreal General Campus; (514)934-8080

KARAZIVAN, Philippe; Clinique de Med Familiale, 6e-2120 rue Sherbrooke E, Montreal QC H2K 1C3; Mon'03; CCFP; Staff, Centre Hospitalier l'Université de Montréal (CHUM) - Hôpital Notre-Dame; (514)527-1958; Fax. (514)527-1649.

KARBI, Oscar A; William Osler HC-Brampton, 2100 Bovaird Dr E, Brampton ON L6R 3J7; Tor'86; FRCPC; EmergMed (Family Practice). Staff, William Osler Health System - Brampton Civic Hospital; (905)796-4492; Fax. (905)451-8439.

KARDAL, Lori J; Kaleidoscope Ped Consultants, 10-8180 MacLeod Trail SE, Calgary AB T2H 2B8; UBC'89; FRCPC; Peds. (403)252-6651; Fax. (403)640-0710.

KARDASH, Kenneth J; SMBD Jewish Gen Hosp, 3755 ch Cote-Sainte-Catherine, Montreal QC H3T 1E2; Man'85; CSPQ; Anes. Dir, Sir Mortimer B Davis Jewish General; adj Prof, McGill University; (514)340-8222 x5701

KARDASH, Sidney; 212-2948 Baseline Rd, Nepean ON K2H 8T5; Ott'63; FRCPC; Peds (Primary Care). Ac Staff, Children's Hospital of Eastern Ontario (CHEO); Ac Staff, The Ottawa Hospital - Civic Campus; University of Ottawa; (613)828-9792; Fax. (613)828-9657; skardash@rogers.com.

KARDERA, Edward P; Cedars at Cobble Hill, PO Box 250 3741 Holland Ave, Cobble Hill BC V0R 1L0; UBC'65; (250)733-2006

KAREEMI, Fauzia K; D261-1600 90 Ave SW, Calgary AB T2V 5A8; Punjab (Pakistan)'87; MB BS; CCFP; Langs: Urdu; (403)252-8855

KAREEMI, Raza K; 148 Vidal St N, Sarnia ON N7T 5X7; London (England)'78; FRCSC; GenSurg. (519)383-1585; Fax. (519)383-7990.

KARELLIS, Nicolas; 3828 boul Notre-Dame, Laval QC H7V 1R9; Mon'84; Langs: French; Greek; (450)682-6688; Fax. (450)682-6689.

KARENKOVA, Natalia; Mackenzie Richmond Hill Hosp, 10 Trench St, Richmond Hill ON L4C 4Z3; (Belarus)'96; Staff, Mackenzie Richmond Hill Hospital; (905)883-1212

KARGBO, John; Sault Area Hosp, 750 Great Northern Rd, Sault Ste. Marie ON P6B 0A8; Russia (Russia (Federation))'94; CCFP; CCFP(E.M.); FCFP; Chief-Inpatient Servs, Dryden Regional Health Centre; Staff, Sault Area Hospital - Sault Ste Marie; Asst Prof Family Med, McMaster University; Asst Prof Family Med, Northern Ontario School of Medicine-Laurentian University; Langs: Russian; (705)759-3710; kargbo@sympatico.ca.

KARGBO, Natalia V; Sault Area Hosp, 750 Great Northern Rd, Sault Ste. Marie ON P6B 0A8; IUHS (Saint Kitts-Nevis)'07; CCFP; Staff, Sault Area Hospital - Sault Ste Marie; (705)759-3434

KARGEL, Caroline S; The Simcoe Clinic, 2-279 Yonge St, Barrie ON L4N 7T9; Qns'97; CCFP; CCFP(E.M.); Staff Emerg, Royal Victoria Regional Health Centre; (705)728-8860; Fax. (705)737-4733.

KARGEL, Marcus J; Toronto East Gen Hosp Inc, 825 Coxwell Ave, Toronto ON M4C 3E7; Tor'99; BSc; FRCPC; IntMed; Critical Care Medicine; Respir. Staff, Toronto East General Hospital Inc; (416)469-6580 x7777

KARIA, Narendra K; Heritage Hill Medicenter, 110-8180 Macleod Trail SE, Calgary AB T2H 2B8; Manchester (England)'66; MB ChB; DObstRCOG; FRCOG; Langs: Gujarati; Hindi; Punjabi; Swahili; (403)259-3256; Fax. (403)253-2673; drkaria@shaw.ca.

KARIM, Mandy; 2201 Broadway W, Vancouver BC V6K 2E4; Dhaka (Bangladesh)'81; MB BS; Langs: Bengali; (604)222-2256; Fax. (604)222-2257.

KARIM, Mohamud A; Surrey Med Arts Bldg, 113-13798 94A Ave, Surrey BC V3V 1N1; UBC'83; FRCPC; IntMed; Nephrol. Att Staff, Royal Columbian Hospital; Staff, Surrey Memorial Hospital; (604)582-6606; Fax. (604)581-0580.

KARIM, Nasim A; 109-747 Lake Bonavista Dr SE, Calgary AB T2J 0N2; London (England)'75; MB BS; Langs: Gujarati; (403)271-5611; Fax. (403)271-5678.

KARIM, Ruhin; O'Connor Doctor's Offices Bldg, 20-1450 O'Connor Dr, Toronto ON M4B 2T8; (United Kingdom)'02.

KARIM, Sadiqa; 202-4383 Portage Rd, Niagara Falls ON L2E 6A6; Sind Med College (Pakistan)'90; (905)354-1111; Fax. (905)354-7902.

KARIM, Shahzad S; Keary Med Centre, 105-245 Columbia St E, New Westminster BC V3L 3W4; UBC'89; FRCSC; GenSurg (Pacemaker); CardSurg. Att Staff Surgeon-Cardiac Surg, Royal Columbian Hospital; Att Staff Surgeon-Cardiac Surg/Leader Extraction Program, Providence Health Care - St Paul's Hospital; Clin Assoc Prof, University of British Columbia; Langs: Urdu; (604)522-6800; Fax. (604)540-8126.

KARIM, Zamil; Surrey Med Arts Bldg, 300-13798 94A Ave, Surrey BC V3V 1N1; Tor'07; FRCPC; IntMed; Gastroent. (604)588-2777

KARIMI ZANDI, Shahram; William Osler HC-Brampton, 2100 Bovaird Dr E, Brampton ON L6R 3J7; Tehran (Iran)'95; FRCPC; Anes. Staff, William Osler Health System - Brampton Civic Hospital; (905)494-2120

KARIMIRAD, Helen; Lonsdale Walk-In Clinic, 108-1940 Lonsdale Ave, North Vancouver BC V7M 2K2; Tehran (Iran)'92; CCFP; (604)987-3357

KARIMU, Ande L; The Pas Health Complex, PO Box 240 Stn Main, The Pas MB R9A 1K4; (Nigeria)'84; Staff, St. Anthony General Hospital; Langs: Yoruba; (204)623-6431

KARIMUDDIN, Ahmer A; St Paul's Hosp, 1081 Burrard St, Vancouver BC V6Z 1Y6; Wes'01; FRCSC; GenSurg. Staff, Providence Health Care - St Paul's Hospital; (604)806-8711

KARIVELIL, Joshy; All Saints Springhill Hosp, 10 Princess St, Springhill NS B0M 1X0; (India)'81; CCFP; Staff, All Saints Springhill Hospital; (902)597-2623; Fax. (902)597-2808.

KARKOUTI, Keyvan; Univ Hlth Network-Toronto Gen, 3EN-200 Elizabeth St, Toronto ON M5G 2C4; Tor'90; FRCPC; Anes (Emergency Medicine). Anesthesiologist, Toronto General Hospital - UHN; University of Toronto; (416)340-4800 x3242; Fax. (416)340-3698; keyvan.karkouti@uhn.ca.

KARL, Paul A; 205-73 Delhi St, Guelph ON N1E 6L9; Wes'85; Assoc Staff, Guelph General Hospital; (519)763-6705; Fax. (519)763-4332.

KARLINSKY, Audrey L; Wellpoint Family Practice, 9F-1240 Bay St, Toronto ON M5R 2A7; Tor'84; CCFP; FCFP; Staff, Mount Sinai Hospital; Assoc Staff, Women's College Hospital; Lecturer Family & Commun Med, University of Toronto; (416)971-7601; Fax. (416)971-7718.

KARLINSKY, Harry J; The Richmond Hosp, 2F-7000 Westminster Hwy, Richmond BC V6X 1A2; Man'80; MSc; FRCPC; Psy. Education Site Leader Psy, Richmond Hospital; Clin Prof, University of British Columbia; (604)278-9711 x4112

KARMALI, Alkarim N K; Fraser Med Clinic, 108-22441 Dewdney Trunk Rd, Maple Ridge BC V2X 7X7; Sheffield (England)'81; MB ChB; DRCOG; MRCGPract; (604)463-1300; Fax. (604)463-1301; frasermedicalclinic@shaw.ca.

KARMALI, Mohamed A; 11F Rm 15-180 Queen St W, Toronto ON M5V 3L7; Glasgow (Scotland)'72; MB ChB; FRCP(Glas); FRCPC; MedMicrobiol. Dir General for Foodborne Zoonoses, Public Health Agency of Canada Lab; Prof Lab Med & Path Biology, University of Toronto; Prof Path & Molecular Med, McMaster University; Langs: Gujarati; (519)822-3300; mohamed_karmali@phac-aspc.gc.ca.

KARMALI, Shahzeer; Royal Alexandra Hosp, 405 CSC-10240 Kingsway NW, Edmonton AB T5H 3V9; Alb'02; FRCSC; GenSurg. Staff, Royal Alexandra Hospital; (780)735-6650

KARMALI-RAWJI, Shameela S F; 4440 44 Ave NE, Calgary AB T1Y 4W5; McM'92; MSc; CCFP; FCFP; Langs: Urdu; Hindi; Gujarati.

KARMY, Grigory; Bathurst-Drewry Med Centre, 204-5927 Bathurst St, North York ON M2R 3T5; Man'92; (416)224-5947; Fax. (416)229-5957.

KARN, Eric B; Western Mem Reg Hosp, PO Box 2005 Stn Main 1 Brookfield Ave, Corner Brook NL A2H 6J7; Tor'93; AnatPath. Staff, Western Memorial Regional Hospital; (709)637-5000

KARN, Heather A; King Street Family Physicians, 2-273 King St E, Kingston ON K7L 3B1; Tor'98; CCFP; (613)546-3650

KARNIK, Nachiket S; Links Clinic, 104-11910 111 Ave NW, Edmonton AB T5G 3G6; Alb'94; BMedSci; CCFP; (780)454-0351; Fax. (780)452-6767.

KARNIK, Vikas V; Windsor Med Clinic, 1608 Tecumseh Rd W, Windsor ON N9B 1T8; Bombay (India)'80; MB BS; MD; DPM; Ac Staff, Windsor Regional Hospital - Metropolitan Site; Court Staff, Hôtel-Dieu Grace Hospital; Langs: Hindi; (519)258-4400

KARNIS, Constantine G; North Burlington Med Centre, 18-1960 Appleby Line, Burlington ON L7L 0B7; McG'93; Langs: English; Greek; (905)319-2000; Fax. (905)319-6292.

KARNIS, Megan M F; ONE Fertility Clinic, 3210 Harvester Rd, Burlington ON L7N 3T1; McM'93; FRCOG; BASc; FRCSC; ObstGyn (Reproductive Endocrinology & Infertility). Staff Reproductive Endocrin & Fertility, Hamilton Health Sciences Centre - McMaster Children's Hospital; Med Dir, ONE Fertility; Assoc Prof ObstGyn, McMaster University; Langs: French; (905)634-4440; Fax. (905)639-3810.

KAROL, Savita; 205-640 Prospect St, Fredericton NB E3B 9M7; Himachal (India)'84; MB BS; DCH; CCFP; Langs: Hindi; Punjabi; Urdu; (506)458-0243

KAROLAK, Marek E; Kelowna Gen Hosp, 2268 Pandosy St, Kelowna BC V1Y 1T2; Warsaw (Poland)'78; Staff, Kelowna General Hospital; Langs: Polish; (250)862-4300

KAROLAK, Michael M; Misericordia Community Hosp, 16940 87 Ave NW, Edmonton AB T5R 4H5; (Poland)'04; FRCPC; IntMed. Staff, Covenant Health - Misericordia Community Hospital; (780)735-2611

KAROLAK, Wojtek; Foothills Med Centre, 1403 29 St NW, Calgary AB T2N 2T9; Pozan (Poland)'04; FRCSC; CardSurg. Staff, Foothills Medical Centre; (403)944-1090

KARON, Stanley F; Mariner's Med Clinic, 505-1160 Burrard St, Vancouver BC V6Z 2E8; Witwatersrand (South Africa)'87; MB ChB; CCFP; Ac Staff, Providence Health Care - Mount Saint Joseph Hospital; Ac Staff/Leader Night Phys Prog, Providence Health Care - St Paul's Hospital; Langs: Afrikaans; Hebrew; (604)683-0206; Fax. (604)683-0203; csms@mannersclinic.com.

KAROVITCH, Alan J; The Ottawa Hosp-Gen Campus, 501 Smyth Rd, Ottawa ON K1H 8L6; McG'91; FRCPC; IntMed. Staff, The Ottawa Hospital - General Campus; Langs: English; French; (613)737-7777; Fax. (613)737-8688.

KARPAKIS, Janine; Bigelow Fowler Clinic West, 30 Jerry Potts Blvd W, Lethbridge AB T1K 5M5; (South Africa)'94; MB ChB.

KARPILOW, Craig; Wilson Med Centre, 130 Wilson St, Hamilton ON L8R 1E2; Dal'74; MPH; FACOEM; CCFP; FCFP; Med Dir OccupMed, Workplace Medical Corporation; Langs: French; Spanish; (905)526-6250

KARPINSKI, Jolanta A M; The Ottawa Hosp-Riverside, 1967 Riverside Dr, Ottawa ON K1H 7W9; Sask'90; FRCPC; IntMed; Nephrol. Staff, The Ottawa Hospital - Riverside Campus; Dir Postgraduate Evaluation & Accreditation/Assoc Prof, University of Ottawa; Langs: Polish; French; (613)738-8400 x82538; Fax. (613)738-8337.

KARPINSKI, Martin E; Health Sciences Centre, GE421-820 Sherbrook St, Winnipeg MB R3A 1R9; Sask'94; FRCPC; IntMed; Nephrol. Staff, Health Sciences Centre; Asst Prof IntMed, University of Manitoba; Langs: French; Polish; (204)774-6511; mkarpinski@exchange.hsc.mb.ca.

KARPIYEVICH, Maryna; Westland Market, 144-70 McLeod Ave, Spruce Grove AB T7X 3C7; (Belarus)'86; CCFP; Langs: Russian; (780)962-9393; Fax. (780)962-4295.

KARPLUK, Philip F; Labour Bldg, 8F-10808 99 Ave NW, Edmonton AB T5K 0G5; Alb'72; FRCPC; OccupMed. Dir-Research Medical Services Human Resouces & Employment, Workplace Safety & Health Divisions; (780)415-0607; Fax. (780)422-0014.

KARPMAN, Shelby N; First Edmonton Place, 350-10665 Jasper Ave NW, Edmonton AB T5J 3S9; Alb'87; MHA; Dip SportMed; CCFP; FCFP; Consultant Family Med, Royal Alexandra Hospital; Consultant Primary Care, University of Alberta; Langs: English; French; Hebrew; (780)421-7711; Fax. (780)421-9744; skarpman@ualberta.ca.

KARR, Suzanne M; Bayview-Finch Med Clinic, 300-3292 Bayview Ave, North York ON M2M 4J5; Ott'85; BSc; CCFP; Ac Staff Family Med, North York General Hospital; (416)646-4455; Fax. (416)222-5722.

KARRAS, Beverley E; West Winds Primary Health Ctr, 3311 Fairlight Dr, Saskatoon SK S7M 3Y5; Sask'78; CCFP; Asst Prof Family Med, University of Saskatchewan; (306)655-4200; Fax. (306)655-4894.

KARREL, Abram I G; Workers' Comp Board, 4980 Wills Rd, Nanaimo BC V9T 6C6; McG'90; CCFP; FCFP; Med Advisor, Worksafe BC; (250)751-8014

KARSAI, Helen; BC Cancer Agency-Vancouver CC, 600 10th Ave W, Vancouver BC V5Z 4E6; Tor'72; Clin Associate, BC Cancer Agency Vancouver Centre; Langs: Czech; Slovak; (604)877-6000; Fax. (604)877-0585.

KARSAN, Aly; BC Cancer Agency-Vancouver CC, 600 10th Ave W, Vancouver BC V5Z 4E6; Qns'86; FRCPC; HemPath. Staff, BC Cancer Agency Vancouver Centre; Staff, Vancouver General Hospital - Centennial Pavillion; Staff, Genome Sciences Centre; Staff Teacher, University of British Columbia; Fax. (604)675-8049; akarsan@bccancer.bc.ca.

KARSH, Jacob; The Ottawa Hosp-Riverside, 1967 Riverside Dr, Ottawa ON K1H 7W9; McG'72; FRCPC; Rheum; IntMed. Staff, The Ottawa Hospital - Riverside Campus; (613)738-8400; Fax. (613)738-8378; jkarsh@ottawahospital.on.ca.

KARSKI, Jacek M; Univ Hlth Network-Toronto Gen, 200 Elizabeth St, Toronto ON M5G 2C4; Cracow (Poland)'73; FRCPC; Anes (Cardiac Anesthesia). Staff Anes, Toronto General Hospital - UHN; Asst Prof Anes, University of Toronto; (416)340-3405; Fax. (416)340-4696; jacek.karski@uhn.on.ca.

KARSLI, Cengiz H; The Hosp For Sick Children, 555 University Ave, Toronto ON M5G 1X8; Tor'93; FRCPC; Anes. Staff Anes, The Hospital For Sick Children; University of Toronto; Langs: French; Turkish; (416)813-7445; Fax. (416)813-7543; ckarsli@hotmail.com.

KARSON, Stanley J; Huronia Med Centre, PO Box 790 Stn Main 204-240 Old Penetanguishene Rd, Midland ON L4R 4P4; Tor'80; CCFP; Ac Staff, Georgian Bay General Hospital - Midland; (705)526-0057; Fax. (705)526-1537.

KARTHIKEYAN, Suba; PO Box 63047 Rpo Stadium, Calgary AB T2N 4S5; (India)'95; MB BS; FRCPC; Peds.

KARUNAKARAN, Kumudhini; Regina Qu'Appelle HR-Regina, 1440 14th Ave, Regina SK S4P 0W5; St George's (Grenada)'95; ABIM; FRCPC; IntMed (Infectious Diseases). Staff Infectious Dis Clinic, Regina General Hospital; Clinical Asst Prof, University of Saskatchewan; Langs: Tamil; (306)766-3915; Fax. (306)766-3995.

KARUNAKARAN, Siva; 1821 Rose St, Regina SK S4P 1Z7; St. George's (Grenada)'95; FRCPC; IntMed; Nephrol. Clin Assoc Prof Med, University of Saskatchewan; (306)525-3675; Fax. (306)359-1068.

KARUNANITHY, Anusha; Trinity Conception Med Centre, PO Box 903 Stn Main 16 Goff Ave, Carbonear NL A1Y 1C4; L'vov Medical Institute (Ukraine)'86; (709)596-5135

KARUTHEDATH, Rajesh; Knox Manse, 505 4th Ave N, Saskatoon SK S7K 2M5; Calcutta (India)'91; FRCPC; Psy.

KARVAT, Anand; BC Cancer Agency-Fraser Valley, 13750 96 Ave, Surrey BC V3V 1Z2; Alb'97; BMedSci; FRCPC; RadOncol (Lung Cancer). Staff, BC Cancer Agency Fraser Valley Centre; Clinical Asst Prof, University of British Columbia; (604)930-4033; Fax. (604)930-4065.

KARVELAS, John P; Markham Prof Centre, 102-2265 Pembina Hwy, Winnipeg MB R3T 5J3; Man'91; BSc(Med); FRCSC; Urol. Staff, Seven Oaks General Hospital; Staff, Victoria General Hospital; Langs: Greek.

KARVELAS, Lisa M; Psychealth Centre, PZ246-771 Bannatyne Ave, Winnipeg MB R3E 3N4; Man'91; BSc; FRCPC; Psy (Mood Disorders). Langs: English; French.

KARVELLAS, Constantine J; Zeidler Ledcor Bldg, 1 40-130 University Campus NW, Edmonton AB T6G 2X8; Alb'01; FRCPC; IntMed; Critical Care Medicine; Gastroent. (780)492-4390

KARWA, Laila; Surrey Mem Hosp, 13750 96 Ave, Surrey BC V3V 1Z2; Bombay (India)'92; MB BS; FRCPC; Anes (Pediatrics). Staff, Surrey Memorial Hospital; Langs: Hindi; (604)588-3367

KARWOWSKA, Anna; Children's Hosp Eastern Ont, 401 Smyth Rd, Ottawa ON K1H 8L1; McG'94; FRCPC; Peds. Staff, Children's Hospital of Eastern Ontario (CHEO); (613)737-2318

KARWOWSKI, Andrzej S; Canadian Forces Hlth Services, PO Box 17000 Stn Forces, Victoria BC V9A 7N2; Dublin (Ireland)'05; MB BCh; CCFP.

KARY, Salah S M; Greig Associates, 5732 Victoria Dr, Vancouver BC V5P 3W6; King Khalid (Saudi Arabia)'97; MB BS; FRCPC; DiagRad. (604)321-6774

KARZAZI, Meryem; CSSS de Beauce-Etchemin, 1515 17e rue, Saint-Georges QC G5Y 4T8; Mohammed V (Morocco)'90; IntMed (Cardiology). Staff, Centre Hospitalier Beauce-Etchemin; Langs: English; Arabic; (418)228-2031; Fax. (418)227-3825; meryemkarzazi@hotmail.com.

KASAMALI, Naureen N; Royal Alexandra Hosp, 6408-10240 Kingsway NW, Edmonton AB T5H 3V9; Alb'06; FRCPC; Psy. Staff, University of Alberta Hospital; (780)735-4564; Fax. (780)735-4797.

KASAPI, Marina S; Northeast Mental Health Team, 222-2750 Hastings St E, Vancouver BC V5K 1Z9; UBC'99; FRCPC; Psy. Staff, Providence Health Care - St Paul's Hospital; (604)675-3890

KASATIYA TREVISANI, Elena; CERB Biologics & Genetics, B7-120 Parkdale Ave, Ottawa ON K1A 0L2; Paris (France)'62; MD; Staff Clin Evaluation Div Centre for Biologics Eval Biologics & Genetic Therapies Directorate, Health Canada; Langs: French; Spanish; Italian; Catalan; (613)941-8568; elena_kasatiya@hc-sc.gc.ca.

KASAVAN, Devan S; 8708 155 St NW, Edmonton AB T5R 1W2; Durban (South Africa)'97; MB ChB; DA(SA); Physician Family Med, Slave Lake Health Care Centre; (780)483-7860; Fax. (780)483-7868.

KASBIA, Sukhvinder S; 101-6501 Campeau Dr, Kanata ON K2K 3E9; Bristol (England)'83; MB ChB; LMCC; CCFP; Lecturer, University of Ottawa; Langs: Punjabi; (613)271-0885; Fax. (613)271-0885.

KASBO, Marie-Rose; Cite Sante St-Laurent, 1-1077 rue Decarie, Saint-Laurent QC H4L 3M8; Aleppo (Syria)'80; Staff, Pavillon Notre-Dame de la Merci; (514)747-5556; Fax. (514)747-5557.

KASHA, Katherine A; 201-5651 Riverbend Rd NW, Edmonton AB T6H 5K4; Alb'04; BScZoology(Hons); CCFP; (780)438-8844

KASHANIA, Behnam; Humber River Reg Hosp-Church, 200 Church St, Toronto ON M9N 1N8; Tehran (Iran)'90; FRCPC; Anes. Staff, Humber River Regional Hospital - Church Street Site; (416)249-8111

KASHGARI, Alia Y A; London HSC-South Street Site, PO Box 5375 Stn B C 531-375 South St, London ON N6A 4G5; King Abdul Aziz (Saudi Arabia)'00; MB BS; FRCPC; IntMed; Respir. Staff, London Health Sciences Centre - South Street; (519)667-6860

KASHGARY, Abdullah Y A; London HSC-University Hosp, PO Box 5339 Stn B 339 Windermere Rd, London ON N6A 5A5; King Abdul Aziz (Saudi Arabia)'04; IntMed. Staff, London Health Sciences Centre - University Hospital; (519)663-3511

KASHIF, Muhammad; Adolescent Day Treatment Prog, 9634 King George Blvd, Surrey BC V3T 0G7; Punjab (Pakistan)'98; Staff, Surrey Memorial Hospital; (604)587-3814

KASHIN, Brian A; North York Gen Hosp, 4001 Leslie St, North York ON M2K 1E1; Tor'85; FRCPC; Anes (Critical Care Medicine). Staff/Med Dir Acute Pain Service, North York General Hospital; Lecturer Anes, University of Toronto; (416)756-6520

KASHMERE, Jodi; 10820 124 St NW, Edmonton AB T5M 0H3; Sask'99; FRCPC; Neur. (780)444-4890; Fax. (780)444-4807.

KASHYAP, Rajendra P; The Court, 208-2863 Ellesmere Rd, Scarborough ON M1E 5E9; New Delhi (India)'61; MB BS; Ac Staff, Rouge Valley Health System - Centenary Health Centre Site; Court Staff, The Scarborough Hospital - General Campus; Court Staff, The Scarborough Hospital - Birchmount Campus; Langs: Hindi; Punjabi; Urdu; (416)281-8630

KASHYAP, Sonya; Genesis Fertility Centre, 300-1367 Broadway W, Vancouver BC V6H 4A7; Ott'95; FRCSC; ObstGyn. (604)879-3032

KASIANIK, Larissa; Kincardine Commun Med Clinic, 44 Queen St, Kincardine ON N2Z 3C1; Khabarovsk (Russia (Federation))'80; CCFP; Langs: Russian; (519)396-6752; Fax. (519)396-6177.

KASIM, Yusuf M; 267 Bradbrooke Dr, Yorkton SK S3N 3L3; (306)782-2332; Fax. (306)782-3360.

KASINA, Rafal A; Hants Community Hosp, 610-89 Payzant Dr, Windsor NS B0N 2T0; Crakow (Poland)'81; FRCPC; IntMed. Staff, Hants Community Hospital; (902)792-2016; Fax. (902)798-4019.

KASK, Jennifer A; Campbell River & Dist Gen Hosp, 375 2nd Ave, Campbell River BC V9W 3V1; UBC'01; CCFP; Staff, Campbell River & District General Hospital; (250)287-7111

KASMAIEFAR, Farzin; 1-601 8th St E, Saskatoon SK S7H 0R1; (Other Foreign)'89; (306)974-3939; Fax. (306)974-3941.

KASNER, Oscar P; SMBD Jewish Gen Hosp, 3755 ch Cote-Sainte-Catherine, Montreal QC H3T 1E2; Sher'82; FRCSC; Ophth (Glaucoma). Staff, Sir Mortimer B Davis Jewish General; adj Prof, McGill University; (514)342-8219; Fax. (514)340-8215.

KASON, David V; Delta Health Sciences Centre, 204-4515 Harvest Dr, Delta BC V4K 4L1; UBC'71; CCFP; FCFP; Physician, Delta Health Sciences Centre; (604)946-0665; Fax. (604)946-0494.

KASON, Deborah A; Delta Health Sciences Centre, 204-4515 Harvest Dr, Delta BC V4K 4L1; UBC'04; CCFP; Staff, Delta Health Sciences Centre; Medical Officer, Health Canada; Downtown Community Health Clinic; (604)946-0665

KASON, Jason S; Delta Health Sciences Centre, 204-4515 Harvest Dr, Delta BC V4K 4L1; UBC'03; CCFP; Physician, Delta Health Sciences Centre; (604)946-0665

KASPER, Kenneth D; Health Sciences Centre, GF 329-820 Sherbrook St, Winnipeg MB R3A 1R9; Man'93; FRCPC; IntMed; InfectDis. Staff, Health Sciences Centre; (204)787-1624; kkasper@exchange.hsc.mb.ca.

KASRAI, Leila; Islington Med Clinic, 707-1243 Islington Ave, Etobicoke ON M8X 1Y9; Wes'94; MPH; FRCSC; PlasSurg (Cosmetic Surgery). Staff, St Joseph's Health Centre; Staff, The Hospital For Sick Children; Asst Prof, University of Toronto; Langs: Farsi; (416)236-5559; Fax. (416)236-4591.

KASRAVI, Neema; 304-1333 Sheppard Ave E, North York ON M2J 1V1; Tor'07; FRCPC; Neur. (647)748-6155

KASS, Malek; St Boniface Gen Hosp, 409 Tache Ave, Winnipeg MB R2H 2A6; Man'02; FRCPC; IntMed; Cardiol. Staff, St Boniface General Hospital; (204)233-8563

KASS, Theodore; Ctr Hosp de Lachine, 650 16e av, Lachine QC H8S 3N5; McG'69; FRCSC; GenSurg. Staff, CSSS de Dorval-Lachine-Lasalle; (514)637-2854

KASSA, A Ayalew; Airport Way Med Clinic, PO Box 2000, Fort Nelson BC V0C 1R0; Birmingham (England)'81; MB ChB; Physician, Airport Way Medical Clinic; (250)774-7838

KASSAB, Francois; 210-900 Boul Du Seminaire N, St-Jean-Sur-Richel QC J3A 1C3; Mon'81; Staff, Hôpital du Haut-Richelieu; (450)348-1118; Fax. (450)348-9998.

KASSAB, Jacinthe; Gimble Eye Centre, 450-4935 40 Ave NW, Calgary AB T3A 2N1; Sher'84; FRCSC; Ophth. Langs: English; French; (403)286-3022; Fax. (403)286-2943; jkassab@gimbel.com.

KASSAM, Alisha; The Hosp for Sick Children, 555 University Ave, Toronto ON M5G 1X8; Ott'06; PedHemaOncol; Peds (Palliative Care). Staff, The Hospital For Sick Children; (416)813-1500

KASSAM, Amin; The Ottawa Hosp-Civic Campus, 1053 Carling Ave, Ottawa ON K1Y 4E9; Tor'91; FRCSC; Neursurg. Staff, The Ottawa Hospital - Civic Campus; (613)798-5555

KASSAM, Azaad; Queensway-Carleton Hosp, 3045 Baseline Rd, Nepean ON K2H 8P4; Alb'99; FRCPC; Psy. Staff, Queensway Carleton Hospital; (613)721-2000

KASSAM, Farrah; Stronach Reg Cancer Centre, 596 Davis Dr, Newmarket ON L3Y 2P9; Wes'03; FRCPC; IntMed; MedOncol. Staff, Southlake Regional Health Centre; Staff, Stronach Regional Cancer Centre; (905)895-4521 x6091

KASSAM, Fatma-Zahra; Southlake Reg Health Centre, 596 Davis Dr, Newmarket ON L3Y 2P9; London (England)'95; FRCPC; RadOncol. Staff, Southlake Regional Health Centre; (905)895-4521; Fax. (905)952-3052.

KASSAM, Hanif; 10-8707 Dufferin St, Thornhill ON L4J 0A6; McM'92; BSc(Math); MHSc; FRCPC; CommunMed. Dir Public Health Programs, York Region Health Services; (905)326-7685; Fax. (905)326-6942.

KASSAM, Hassanali A; Bramalea Med Centre, 402A-18 Kensington Rd, Brampton ON L6T 4S5; Kerala (India)'81; (905)791-9301

KASSAM, Jacqueline C; Summit Centre, 209-200 Boudreau Rd, St. Albert AB T8N 6B9; Alb'99; CCFP; Clin Lecturer Family Med, University of Alberta; (780)458-7000; Fax. (780)458-8484.

KASSAM, Narmin; University of Alberta Hosp, 2F1 16-8440 112 St NW, Edmonton AB T6G 2B7; Alb'91; FRCPC; IntMed. Staff, University of Alberta Hospital; Assoc Prof, University of Alberta; Langs: Gujarati; (780)407-7606; Fax. (780)407-3132.

KASSAM, Nizar I F; Coral Spring Medical, 5070 68 St NE, Calgary AB T3J 4J1; (India)'70; MB BS; CCFP; Staff, Peter Lougheed Centre; (403)568-0171; Fax. (403)568-0157.

KASSAM, Saleem A; The Court, 307-2863 Ellesmere Rd, Scarborough ON M1E 5E9; Tor'93; FRCPC; IntMed; Cardiol. (416)284-9727; Fax. (416)284-0141.

KASSAM, Salma; Gates of Maple Family Practice, 201-955 Major Mackenzie Dr, Maple ON L6A 4P9; Tor'91; CCFP; FCFP; (905)417-7899; Fax. (905)417-8905.

KASSAM, Tasneem M; Victoria Health Centre, 2F-521 Victoria Park Ave, Scarborough ON M4C 5H1; Tor'06; CCFP; (416)694-1400

KASSAM, Zarina K; Trillium Hlth Ctr-West Toronto, 150 Sherway Dr, Etobicoke ON M9C 1A5; Bristol (England)'74; FRCPC; Anes. Staff, Trillium Health Centre - West Toronto; (416)259-6671

KASSAS, Emad; 210-2224 Walker Rd, Windsor ON N8W 3P6; Damascus (Syria)'91; (519)255-9991

KASSEL, Edward E; Univ Hlth Network-Princess M, 3 962-610 University Ave, Toronto ON M5G 2M9; Wes'71; DDS; FRCPC; DiagRad. Staff, Princess Margaret Hospital - University Health Network; Assoc Prof, University of Toronto; (416)946-4501

KASSEL, Robert N; Oshawa Clinic, 117 King St E, Oshawa ON L1H 1B9; Tor'83; AB; FRCSC; Otol. Staff, Lakeridge Health - Oshawa Site; (905)721-3575; Fax. (905)721-6640.

KASSEM, Manal H M; Shamrock Med Clinic, PO Box 89, Ferryland NL A0A 2H0; Damascus (Syria)'98; CCFP.

KASSEM, Wail A; Burntwood Reg Health Authority, 867 Thompson Dr S, Thompson MB R8N 1Z4; Staff, Northern Health Thompson Regional Office.

KASSEN, Barry O; St Paul's Hosp, 5910-1081 Burrard St, Vancouver BC V6Z 1Y6; Sask'70; FACP; FRCPC; IntMed. Staff, Providence Health Care - St Paul's Hospital; Head Div of General IntMed/A-Head Div of CommunIntMed, University of British Columbia; (604)806-8668; Fax. (604)806-8338; bkassen@providencehealth.bc.ca.

KASSEN, David M; St Paul's Hosp, 1081 Burrard St, Vancouver BC V6Z 1Y6; Sask'83; FRCPC; EmergMed. Ac Staff, Providence Health Care - St Paul's Hospital; (604)682-2344

KASSETT, Suresh P; PO Box 490, Herbert SK S0H 2A0; Southampton (England)'81; (306)784-2577; Fax. (306)784-2888.

KASSIER, Karl E; The Brandon Clinic, 620 Dennis St, Brandon MB R7A 5E7; Stellenbosh (South Africa)'83; FRCSC; Urol. (204)728-4440

KASSIM, Ali A K; Waterford Hosp, 306 Waterford Bridge Rd, St. John's NL A1E 4J8; Al-Mustansiriyah (Iraq)'96; MB ChB; Staff, Waterford Hospital; (709)777-3300

KASSIM, Olayiwola A; West Parry Sound Health Ctre, 6 Albert St, Parry Sound ON P2A 3A4; Ibadan (Nigeria)'75; MB BS; DABPath; FCAP; FRCPC; AnatPath (Laboratory Medicine). Dir Labs & Path in Chief, West Parry Sound Health Centre; Consultant, Orillia Soldiers' Memorial Hospital; Lecturer Path, University of Toronto; Langs: Yoruba; (705)746-4540 x3820; laboratory@wpshc.com.

KASSIRER, Aubrey G; Newcastle Village Med Assoc, 87 Mill St N, Newcastle ON L1B 1H8; Qns'97; CCFP; FCFP; Staff, Lakeridge Health - Bowmanville Site; Staff, Lakeridge Health - Oshawa Site; (905)987-1896; Fax. (905)987-9894.

KASSIRI, Janani; University of Alberta Hosp, 8440 112 St NW, Edmonton AB T6G 2B7; Man'07; Staff, University of Alberta Hospital; (780)407-8822

KASSIRI, Kamrouz; 103-2731 Hewes Way NW, Edmonton AB T6L 6W6; Man'05; FRCSC; Ophth. (780)450-3335; Fax. (780)461-9430.

KASSIRIAN, Shima; North York Gen Hosp, GS 70-4001 Leslie St, North York ON M2K 1E1; Tor'02; FRCSC; GenSurg. Staff, North York General Hospital; (416)756-6516

KASSIS, Jeannine; Hop Maisonneuve-Rosemont, 5415 boul de l'Assomption, Montreal QC H1T 2M4; Mon'84; FRCPC; IntMed (Hematological Oncology); Hem. Staff Hem, Hopital Maisonneuve-Rosemont; assoc Prof Med, Universite de Montreal; Langs: English; (514)252-3404; jkassis.hmr@ssss.gouv.qc.ca.

KASSIS, Lorette B; Abbey Med Centre, 1131 Nottinghill Gate, Oakville ON L6M 1K5; (Israel)'92; CCFP; (905)815-9090

KASSISSIA, Ibrahim G Y; Clinique Med La Plein Ciel, 475 boul de la Cote-Vertu, Saint-Laurent QC H4L 1X7; Ein Shams (Egypt)'82; MSc; PhD; (514)337-3171; Fax. (514)337-6023.

KASSNER, Rachel; Polyclinic Prof Centre Inc, 199 Grafton St, Charlottetown PE C1A 1L2; Dal'82; Pres, Medical Society of PEI; (902)629-8842; Fax. (902)629-8827; rakassner04@hotmail.com.

KASSOUF, Wassim; MUHC-Montreal Gen Hosp, L8 315-1650 av Cedar, Montreal QC H3G 1A4; McG'98; FRCSC; Urol. Staff, McGill University Health Centre - Montreal General Campus; (514)934-8246

KASSUM, Diamond A; 300-355 Portage Avenue, Winnipeg MB R3B 0J6; Cambridge (England)'70; MB ChB; FRCSC; GenSurg (Surgical Intensive Care). Pres Associate/Ac Staff, St Boniface General Hospital; (204)926-9002; dkassum@manitoba-ehealth.ca.

KASTEEL, Kelly A; Royal Columbia Hosp, 330 Columbia St E, New Westminster BC V3L 3W7; UBC'05; CCFP; CCFP(E.M.); Staff, Royal Columbian Hospital; (604)520-4253

KASTRUKOFF, Lorne F; UBC Hospital, 2211 Wesbrook Mall, Vancouver BC V6T 2B5; UBC'73; BSc; DABPN; FAAN; FRCP; LMCC; MD; NBME; FRCPC; Neur (Multiple Sclerosis). Med Staff Koerner Pavillon, UBC Hospital - Koerner Pavillion; Staff, Vancouver General Hospital - Centennial Pavillion; Assoc Prof Med, University of British Columbia; (604)822-7147; Fax. (604)822-7488.

KASUMOVIC, Janna M; Terwillegar Med Clinic, 101-121 Haddow Close NW, Edmonton AB T6R 3W3; Alb'07; CCFP; (780)989-5300

KASUMU, Yetunde; Avenida Bonavista Shopp Ctre, 315-12445 Lake Fraser Dr SE, Calgary AB T2J 7A4; Obafemi Awolowo (Nigeria)'99; CCFP; (403)723-2453

KASZA, Leslie A; Cedars Prof Park, 2937 66 St NW, Edmonton AB T6K 4C1; Wes'84; ABIM; AB; FRCPC; IntMed; Cardiol. Staff Cardiol, Covenant Health - Grey Nuns Community Hospital; Staff Consultant, Wetaskiwin Hospital & Care Centre; Staff Consultant, Wainwright Health Centre; Clin Assoc Prof, University of Alberta; (780)461-6802; Fax. (780)450-0621.

KASZAS, Zsuzsanna; Kinmount & Dist Health Centre, PO Box 118 31 County Rd 503, Kinmount ON K0M 2A0; Semmelweis (Hungary)'93; CCFP; Langs: Hungarian; (705)488-1105; Fax. (705)488-1119.

KATAKKAR, Jyoti; Ross Mem Hosp, 10 Angeline St N, Lindsay ON K9V 4M8; McM'99; CCFP; Staff, Ross Memorial Hospital; (705)324-6111

KATAKKAR, Suresh B; Prince George Reg Hosp, 1475 Edmonton St, Prince George BC V2M 1S2; Poona (India)'69; MB BS; FRCPC; IntMed. Staff, University Hospital of Northern British Columbia; (250)565-2535

KATALINIC, Z Branislav; 545 Front St, Quesnel BC V2J 2K7; Zagreb (Croatia)'59; FRCS(Ed & Eng); LRCP(Lond); MRCS(Lond); LMCC; FRCSC; GenSurg. General Surgery, G R Baker Memorial Hospital; Langs: Croatian; (250)991-0655; Fax. (250)991-0656.

KATAOKA, Mark T; St Michael's Hosp, 30 Bond St, Toronto ON M5B 1W8; Tor'92; FRCPC; Anes. Staff Anes, St Michael's Hospital; (416)864-5071

KATAREY, Hement K; The Doctor's Office, 1011 Upper Middle Rd E, Oakville ON L6H 4L1; Mysore (India)'81; MB BS; BSc(Hons Physiol); CCFP; FCFP; Langs: Hindi; Gujarati; Punjabi; (905)849-7007; Fax. (905)849-7883.

KATAREY, Mamta; The Doctor's Office, 1011 Upper Middle Rd E, Oakville ON L6H 4L1; Indore (India)'82; MB BS; CCFP; FCFP; (905)849-7007; Fax. (905)849-7883.

KATARZYNIAK-KUNYSZ, Danuta; CRSSS Baie-James-Sante-Lebel, GD 950 boul Quevillon N, Lebel-s-Quevillon QC J0Y 1X0; Poznan (Poland)'65; Staff, Centre de santé Lebel; Langs: Polish; Russian; (819)755-4881 x251; Fax. (819)755-3779.

KATCHAN, Brian M; North York Gen Hosp, 4001 Leslie St, North York ON M2K 1E1; McG'92; FRCPC; IntMed. Staff, North York General Hospital; Langs: French; Hebrew; Yiddish; (416)756-6002

KATES, David M; 312-3001 Tutt St, Kelowna BC V1Y 2H4; UBC'87; FRCPC; IntMed; Nephrol. (250)861-4847; Fax. (250)861-4831.

KATES, Martin L; Summerville Family Health Team, 211-190 Sherway Dr, Etobicoke ON M9C 5N2; Tor'75; CCFP; FCFP; Ac Staff, Trillium Health Centre - West Toronto; (416)621-9700; Fax. (416)621-4438; mkates@thc.on.ca.

KATES, Michael D; Trillium Summerville Teaching, 7F-101 Queensway W, Mississauga ON L5B 2P7; Tor'81; CCFP; Staff, Trillium Health Centre - West Toronto; Ac Staff, Trillium Health Centre - Mississauga; (905)272-9900; Fax. (905)272-9977.

KATES, Nicholas S; Centre for Mountain Hlth Serv, J218-100 5 Ave W, Hamilton ON L8N 3K7; London (England)'76; MB BS; LRCP; MRCS; FRCPC; Psy. Staff, St Joseph's Healthcare Hamilton - West 5th Campus; Advisor Quality Improvement, St Joseph's Healthcare - Charlton Campus; A-Chair Psy, McMaster University; (905)667-4848; Fax. (905)667-4873; nkates@mcmaster.ca.

KATES, W Bradley; Trafalgar Prof Centre, 304-1235 Trafalgar Rd, Oakville ON L6H 3P1; Tor'90; FRCSC; Ophth (Medical Retina). Ac Staff, Halton Healthcare Services Corporation - Oakville Site; Affil Staff, Joseph Brant Memorial Hospital; Att Staff, St Michael's Hospital; (905)842-3555; Fax. (905)849-6990.

KATHIRAV, Satheesh; Peterborough Reg Health Centre, 1 Hospital Dr, Peterborough ON K9J 7C6; Ross U (Dominica)'02; Staff, Peterborough Regional Health Centre - Hospital Drive; (705)743-2121

KATHIRAVELU, Anusha; City Centre Family Physicians, 500-71 King St W, Mississauga ON L5B 4A2; Ott'08; CCFP; (905)270-0415; Fax. (905)848-1500.

KATHIRGAMANATHAN, Kalaimakal; London HSC-University Hosp, PO Box 5339 Stn B 339 Windermere Rd, London ON N6A 5A5; Saba (USA)'07; FRCPC; IntMed. Staff, London Health Sciences Centre - University Hospital; (519)663-3069

KATHIRGAMANATHAN, Mylvaganam; Crestview Med Clinic, 204 O'Connell Dr, Corner Brook NL A2H 5N4; Peradeniya (Sri Lanka)'74; MB BS; FRCS(Ed); LRCP(Lond); MRCS(Eng); Staff, Labrador Health Centre; (709)634-6954

KATHIRGAMANATHAN, Sarathadev; Trillium Hlth Ctr-Mississauga, 100 Queensway W, Mississauga ON L5B 1B8; Peradeniya (Sri Lanka)'76; MB BS; FRCPC; Anes. Staff, Trillium Health Centre - Mississauga; (905)848-7100

KATHRADA, Yacoob A H; Terrace Hill Med Centre, 224-217 Terrace Hill St, Brantford ON N3R 1G8; (South Africa)'85; LMCC; FRCPC; IntMed (Cardiology). Staff Internist, The Brant Community Healthcare System - Brantford General Hospital Site; (519)750-9966; Fax. (519)750-1650.

KATHURIA, Chanchal; 16-585 Ontario St S, Milton ON L9T 2N2; Gandhi (India)'97; CCFP; (905)693-9500

KATHURIA, Sangeet; Halton HSC Corp-Oakville, 327 Reynolds St, Oakville ON L6J 3L7; Delhi (India)'98; MB BS; FRCPC; Peds (Neonatology). Staff Peds, Halton Healthcare Services Corporation - Oakville Site; (905)845-2571

KATI, Arvind A; Regent Primary Med Clinic, 1578 Regent Ave, Winnipeg MB R2C 3B4; Dublin (Ireland)'63; LRCPSI; LM; Langs: Hindi; Swahili.

KATIS, Peter G; Univ Hlth Network-Toronto Gen, GS 434-200 Elizabeth St, Toronto ON M5G 2C4; Tor'97; CCFP; CCFP(E.M.); Staff, Toronto General Hospital - UHN; (416)340-5066

KATSARKAS, Athanasios; MUHC-Royal Victoria Hosp, E4 48-687 av des Pins O, Montreal QC H3A 1A1; Thessaloniki (Greece)'61; MSc; ABOtol; FRCSC; Otol (Vertigo) (Neuro Otolaryngology). Ac Staff, McGill University Health Centre - Royal Victoria Hospital; Prof, Otology Institute; Prof Otol, McGill University; Langs: German; French; Greek; (514)842-2324; Fax. (514)843-1529; akatsarkas@hotmail.com.

KATSIOS, Zaharo; 200-140 Oxford St E, London ON N6A 5R9; Thessaloniki (Greece)'82; CCFP; (519)858-4476; Fax. (519)858-8199.

KATSIRIS, Sandra E; London HSC-Victoria Hosp, PO Box 5010 Stn B 800 Commissioners Rd E, London ON N6A 5W9; Wes'92; FRCPC; Anes. Staff, London Health Sciences Centre - Victoria Campus; (519)685-8500 x58525; Fax. (519)685-8275.

KATSOUNAKIS, John; Greene Avenue Clinic, 210-1255 av Greene, Westmount QC H3Z 2A4; Mem'93; BSc; BMedSci; CCFP; Langs: French; Greek; (514)938-5535; jkatsounakis@yahoo.com.

KATSUNO, Richard M; 1A-172 Ethel St, Sturgeon Falls ON P2B 1V9; Tor'85; BPHE; (705)753-5352; Fax. (705)753-6729.

KATSUTA, Tsuyoshi Tennessee; Mimico Med Centre, 200-398 Royal York Rd, Etobicoke ON M8Y 2R6; Tor'90; Court Staff, Trillium Health Centre - West Toronto; (416)259-8441; Fax. (416)259-5442.

KATTA, Balaraju B; The Richmond Hosp, 2005-7000 Westminster Hwy, Richmond BC V6X 1A2; Tirupati (India)'82; MB BS; MRCPsy(UK); FRCPC; Psy (Adult Psychiatry). Staff, Richmond Hospital; Langs: Telugu; Hindi; (604)278-9711 x4362; bbkatta@hotmail.com.

KATTAN, Abdullah E; Univ of Toronto, 602-500 University Ave, Toronto ON M5G 1V7; King Saud U (Saudi Arabia)'02; FRCSC; PlasSurg.

KATTAR, Mireille M; University of Alberta Hosp, 4B1 WCM-8440 112 St NW, Edmonton AB T6G 2B7; (Lebanon)'91; Staff, University of Alberta Hospital; (780)407-3000; Fax. (780)407-3009.

KATTLEMAN, Barry S; 107-5775 Ch de la Cote-des-Nei, Montreal QC H3S 2S9; McG'81; FRCSC; Ophth. Clin Asst, Sir Mortimer B Davis Jewish General; Teacher Ophth, McGill University; (514)341-3335

KATTYGNARATH, Tiao; Clinique Procrea, 301-1361 av Beaumont, Mont-Royal QC H3P 2W3; Strasbourg (France)'03; ObstGyn (P.Q.). Staff, Hopital Charles LeMoyne; (514)345-8535

KATYAL, Anil; Oakdale Med Bldg, 426-2065 Finch Ave W, Toronto ON M3N 2V7; Tor'97; FRCSC; Otol. Ac Staff, Humber River Regional Hospital - Finch Avenue Site; Court Staff, William Osler Health System - Etobicoke General Hospital; Court Staff, St Michael's Hospital; Lecturer, University of Toronto; (416)744-1211; Fax. (416)744-2644.

KATYAL, Parul; Lakeridge Hlth Corp-Oshawa, 1 Hospital Crt, Oshawa ON L1G 2B9; Aligarh Muslim (India)'98; FRCPC; Anes. Staff, Lakeridge Health - Oshawa Site; (905)576-8711

KATYAL, Sonia; Planned Parenthood Toronto, 36B Prince Arthur Ave, Toronto ON M5R 1A9; McM'04; CCFP; (416)961-0113; Fax. (416)961-9856.

KATZ, Abraham S; St Michael's Hosp, 30 Bond St, Toronto ON M5B 1W8; McG'64; FRCPC; Anes. Ac Staff Anes, St Michael's Hospital; University of Toronto; (416)864-5071

KATZ, Alan; Family Med Centre, 500-400 Tache Ave, Winnipeg MB R2H 3E1; Cape Town (South Africa)'83; MB ChB; MSc; CCFP; FCFP; Ac Staff, St Boniface General Hospital; Dir Research, University of Manitoba; (204)789-3442; Fax. (204)789-3910.

KATZ, Arnon M; Dixon Med Centre, 304-531 Davis Dr, Newmarket ON L3Y 6P5; Tor'87; FRCPC; Derm. Staff, Sunnybrook Health Sciences Centre; Staff, Southlake Regional Health Centre; Staff, Women's College Hospital; Instructor Med, University of Toronto; (905)836-1454

KATZ, Dan G; Ajax Med Arts Bldg, 208-601 Harwood Ave S, Ajax ON L1S 2J5; Bucharest (Romania)'81; FRCPC; PhysMed&Rehab. Langs: Romanian; Hebrew; (905)686-5502; Fax. (905)686-8776.

KATZ, Edward; CSST-Direction Regionale Montr, CP 3 Succ Pl-desjardins 3027-1 Complexe Desjardins, Montreal QC H5B 1H1; McG'70; MSc(A.); Reg Physician, CSST-Direction Regionale Montreal; Langs: English; French; (514)906-3271; Fax. (514)906-3232; docteur@doctor.com.

KATZ, Guido A; 47 Marion St, Winnipeg MB R2H 0S8; FRCSC; ObstGyn.

KATZ, Ian L; Humber River Reg Hosp-Finch, 2111 Finch Ave W, North York ON M3N 1N1; Witwatersrand (South Africa)'78; FAB; Anes. Ac Staff, Humber River Regional Hospital - Finch Avenue Site; (416)633-7797

KATZ, Jerry C; Synergy Wellness Centre, 113-501 Bethel Dr, Sherwood Park AB T8H 0N2; Man'73; CCFP; (780)416-8999

KATZ, Joel M; CSSSG-Hop de Hull, 116 boul Lionel-Emond, Gatineau QC J8Y 1W7; Ott'80; CSPQ; FRCPC; Anes. Staff, Hull Hospital; (819)966-6033; Fax. (819)966-6323.

KATZ, Kevin C; North York Gen Hosp, GW 33-4001 Leslie St, Toronto ON M2K 1E1; McG'97; FRCPC; IntMed; MedMicrobiol; InfectDis. Staff, North York General Hospital; (416)756-6672

KATZ, Laurence Y; Health Sciences Centre, 820 Sherbrook St, Winnipeg MB R3A 1R9; Man'93; FRCPC; Psy. Staff, Health Sciences Centre; (204)787-7470; Fax. (204)787-4975; lkatz@exchange.hsc.mb.ca.

KATZ, Liliana; Medical Centre, 252-2100 Ellesmere Rd, Scarborough ON M1H 3B7; Bucharest (Romania)'81; Court Staff, The Scarborough Hospital - Birchmount Campus; Court Staff, The Scarborough Hospital - General Campus; (416)438-8000; Fax. (416)289-2520.

KATZ, Mark R; Southlake Reg Health Centre, 596 Davis Dr, Newmarket ON L3Y 2P9; Tor'87; FRCPC; Psy. Staff, Southlake Regional Health Centre; Asst Prof, University of Toronto; (905)713-0015

KATZ, Max G; Lakeshore Gen Hosp, 160 av Stillview, Pointe-Claire QC H9R 2Y2; McG'64; FRCPC; IntMed; MedOncol (P.Q.); Hem. Staff, Lakeshore General Hospital - Pointe Claire; (514)630-2225

KATZ, Miriam; 303-85 Grenville St, Toronto ON M5S 3A2; Man'82; FRCPC; IntMed. Staff, Sunnybrook Health Sciences Centre.

KATZ, Mortimer; 2020 Alta Vista Dr, Ottawa ON K1H 7L1; Tor'50; Langs: Bilingual(French/English); (613)733-7202; Fax. (613)733-9606; drmkatz@rogers.com.

KATZ, Murray S; 203-3400 rue du Marche, Dollard-D-Ormeaux QC H9B 2Y1; McG'69; Consultant Peds, McGill University Health Centre - Montreal Children's Hospital; Consultant, Sir Mortimer B Davis Jewish General; Consultant, Medical-Legal Forensic; Teach Staff Family Practice, McGill University; Teach Staff Family Practice, Universite de Montreal; Langs: English; French; (514)685-0933; Fax. (514)685-3880.

KATZ, Nili R; Pureform Diagnostics, 519-4916 130 Ave SE, Calgary AB T2Z 0G4; Cal'00; FRCPC; DiagRad. (403)291-3315; Fax. (403)291-9308.

KATZ, Pamela; St Boniface Gen Hosp, C5113-409 Tache Ave, Winnipeg MB R2H 2A6; Tor'05; FRCPC; IntMed; Endocrin&Metab. Staff, St Boniface General Hospital; (204)233-8563

KATZ, Paul R; Baycrest Ctr/Geriatric Care, 2M07-3560 Bathurst St, Toronto ON M6A 2E1; Michigan (USA)'77; FRCPC; GeriatricMed. Staff, Baycrest Centre for Geriatric Care; (416)785-2500 x2856

KATZ, Philip; 1602-170 Hargrave St, Winnipeg MB R3C 3H4; Man'55; FRCPC; Psy. Ac Staff, Health Sciences Centre; Prof Psy/Dir, University of Manitoba; (204)943-6242; Fax. (204)787-4879.

KATZ, Ronald; 147A Albert St N, Regina SK S4R 3B8; Padua (Italy)'79; (306)525-6466

KATZ, Saul S; C 200-1 car Westmount, Montreal QC H3Z 2P9; Man'69; FRCPC; IntMed; Gastroent (P.Q.). Ac Staff, McGill University Health Centre - Royal Victoria Hospital; (514)904-0666; Fax. (514)904-0668; saul.katz@muhc.mcgill.ca.

KATZ, Sheldon; 204-2221 Keele St, North York ON M6M 3Z5; Tor'67; Staff, Humber River Regional Hospital - Keele Street Site; (416)651-2444; Fax. (416)651-1991.

KATZ, Sherri L; Children's Hosp Eastern Ont, W1403-401 Smyth Rd, Ottawa ON K1H 8L1; McG'97; MDCM; MMedSci; FRCP; FRCPC; Peds (Pediatric Sleep Medicine); Respir. Staff, Children's Hospital of Eastern Ontario (CHEO); Langs: Bilingual(French/English); (613)737-7600 x2868; Fax. (613)738-4886.

KATZ, Shirley; North Med Centre, 201-7131 Bathurst St, Thornhill ON L4J 7Z1; McG'76; CCFP; (905)771-1779; Fax. (905)771-9833.

KATZ, Steven J; Heritage Med Research Ctr, 562-107 University Campus NW, Edmonton AB T6G 2S2; Man'04; FRCPC; IntMed; Rheum. (780)407-6050

KATZBERG, Hans; Univ Hlth Network-Toronto Gen, 5EC 306-200 Elizabeth St, Toronto ON M5G 2C4; UBC'02; FRCPC; Neur. Staff, Toronto General Hospital - UHN; (416)340-3662; Fax. (416)340-4081.

KATZMAN, Debra K; The Hosp For Sick Children, 555 University Ave, Toronto ON M5G 1X8; McM'83; BSc; FRCPC; Peds (Adolescent Medicine). Med Dir The Eating Disorder Prog/Head Div of Adolescent Med, The Hospital For Sick Children; Prof Peds, University of Toronto; (416)813-5804; Fax. (416)813-5392; debbie.katzman@sickkids.ca.

KATZMAN, Martin A; START Clinic, 32 Park Rd, Toronto ON M4W 2N4; Tor'91; FRCPC; Psy (Anxiety Disorder). Staff Psy, Centre for Addiction & Mental Health (CAMH) - College Street Site; Chair, Scientific Advisory Committee/Anxiety Disorders Assoc. & Clin. Dir., START Clinic for Mood & Anxiety Disorders; Aj Prof Psy, Lakehead University / Library; Asst Prof, Northern Ontario School of Medicine; Asst Prof Psy, University of Toronto; (416)598-9344; Fax. (416)598-8198; mkatzman@startclinic.ca.

KATZNELSON, Rita; Univ Hlth Network-Toronto Gen, EN3 451-200 Elizabeth St, Toronto ON M5G 2C4; Taskent (Russia (Federation))'90; FRCPC; Anes. Staff Anes, Toronto General Hospital - UHN; (416)340-3567

KAUCHALI, Muti-Ullah; 101-190 Pelican Pl, Sylvan Lake AB T4S 1K2; (403)887-2224

KAUD, Robert; 2520 Place Keller, Saint-Laurent QC H4K 2T2; McG'77; CCFP; FCFP; Hon Staff Med, Hôpital du Sacre-Coeur de Montréal; Examiner, Medical Council of Canada; Examiner, College of Family Physicians of Canada-Quebec; Langs: English; French; (514)332-0311; Fax. (514)331-0281.

KAUFFMAN-SCHENKER, Tammy; The Market Place, 1881 Steeles Ave W, North York ON M3H 5Y4; Tor'91; CCFP; (416)665-2900; Fax. (416)665-2021.

KAUFMAN, Adam J; Toronto East Gen Hosp Inc, 825 Coxwell Ave, Toronto ON M4C 3E7; Tor'09; CCFP; CCFP(E.M.); Staff, Toronto East General Hospital Inc; (416)469-6580

KAUFMAN, Ian; MUHC-Royal Victoria Hosp, 687 av des Pins O, Montreal QC H3A 1A1; McG'96; CSPQ; FRCPC; Anes. Staff, McGill University Health Centre - Royal Victoria Hospital; (514)934-1934 x34880

KAUFMAN, Jennifer C; The Toronto GI Clinic, 450-5 Fairview Mall Dr, Toronto ON M5J 2Z1; Boston University (USA)'01; MD; (416)322-7517

KAUFMAN, Miriam E; The Hosp For Sick Children, 555 University Ave, Toronto ON M5G 1X8; Qns'80; BScN; FRCPC; Peds (Adolescent Medicine). Staff Adolescent Med Clinic, The Hospital For Sick Children; Prof, University of Toronto; (416)813-6657; Fax. (416)813-5392.

KAUFMAN, Ruebin; Eaton Place Med Centre, 81-333 St Mary Ave, Winnipeg MB R3C 4A5; Man'53; FRCPC; IntMed. (204)942-0933; Fax. (204)942-2491.

KAUFMAN, Tomas; Lakeshore Gen Hosp, 160 av Stillview, Pointe-Claire QC H9R 2Y2; Dal'87; CCFP; Ac Staff, Lakeshore General Hospital - Pointe Claire; (514)630-2166

KAUFMAN-CLAIN, Sanda; CLSC Jean-Olivier-Chenier, 29 ch d'Oka, Saint-Eustache QC J7R 1K6; Laval'91; Physician, CLSC Jean-Olivier-Chenier; Langs: Romanian; English; (450)491-1233; Fax. (450)491-6898.

KAUFMANN, Anthony M; Health Sciences Centre, GB137-820 Sherbrook St, Winnipeg MB R3A 1R9; Man'87; FRCSC; Neursurg. Staff Neurosurg, Health Sciences Centre; (204)774-6511

KAUFMANN, I Michael; Ontario Med Association, 900-150 Bloor St W, Toronto ON M5S 3C1; Tor'79; BSc; CCFP; FCFP; Dir Physician Health Program, Ontario Medical Association; (416)340-2972; Fax. (416)340-2860.

KAUL, Rupert; Univ of Toronto, 6356-1 Kings College Cir, Toronto ON M5S 1A8; Tor'90; PhD(Immunol); FRCPC; IntMed (AIDS/HIV); InfectDis. Staff, Toronto General Hospital - UHN; Staff, Mount Sinai Hospital; Assoc Prof, University of Toronto; Vis Lecturer, U. Nairobi; (416)978-8607; Fax. (416)340-4890; rupert.kaul@utoronto.ca.

KAUL, Thomas; St Michael's Hosp, 30 Bond St, Toronto ON M5B 1W8; Wes'05; FRCPC; EmergMed. Staff, St Michael's Hospital; (416)360-4000

KAUL, William H; York-Med Medical Arts Centre, 410-250 Harding Blvd W, Richmond Hill ON L4C 9M7; London (England)'65; MB BS; FRCSC; Otol (Sinusitis). Ac Staff Otol, Mackenzie Richmond Hill Hospital; University of Toronto; (905)884-9601; Fax. (905)884-5390.

KAUR, Balvindar; Alberta Children's Hosp, 2888 Shaganappi Trail NW, Calgary AB T3B 6A8; (Austria)'03; MB BS; Staff, Alberta Children's Hospital; (403)955-7810; Fax. (403)955-7606.

KAUR, Harkiran; Hamilton HS-Henderson Site, 711 Concession St, Hamilton ON L8V 1C3; Allahabad (India)'01; FRCPC; AnatPath. Staff, Hamilton Health Sciences Centre-Juravinski Site; (905)389-4411

KAUR, Harmeet; Alberta Children's Hosp, 2888 Shaganappi Trail NW, Calgary AB T3B 6A8; Staff, Alberta Children's Hospital; (403)944-1110

KAUR, Manjit; Idylwyld Med Centre, 1216 Idylwyld Dr N, Saskatoon SK S7L 0Z9; (Other Foreign)'98; Staff, Saskatoon City Hospital; (306)652-0400

KAUR, Navpreet; Castlemore Med Centre, 105-4515 Ebenezer Rd, Brampton ON L6P 2K7; (Dominican Republic)'97; CCFP; (905)794-5900

KAUR, Satinder; Belmont Prof Centre, 205-564 Belmont Ave W, Kitchener ON N2M 5N6; Dal'74; CCFP; Langs: Hindi; Punjabi; (519)578-0480; Fax. (519)578-8493.

KAURA, Amit; Stratford Gen Hosp, 46 Hospital Dr, Stratford ON N5A 2Y6; Medical Univ of the Americas (Saint Kitts-Nevis)'04; Staff, Stratford General Hospital - Huron Perth Healthcare Alliance; (519)271-2120

KAURA, Deepak R; Alberta Children's Hosp, 2888 Shaganappi Trail NW, Calgary AB T3B 6A8; Man'97; FRCPC; DiagRad. Dir Radiology, Alberta Children's Hospital; (403)955-7985; Fax. (403)955-7656.

KAUSHAL, Anu; Uptown Health Centre, 8-9325 Yonge St, Richmond Hill ON L4C 0A8; Tor'95; BScPharm; CCFP; (905)508-8876; Fax. (905)508-1087.

KAUSHAL, Ravi D; McKenzie Family Med Centre, 634 Selkirk Ave, Winnipeg MB R2W 2N1; Mysore (India)'80; MB BS; (204)582-7755; Fax. (204)582-7755.

KAUSHIK, Aneel; Appletree Med Group, 240 Sparks St, Ottawa ON K1P 6C9; Cal'03; CCFP; (613)482-0118

KAUSHIK, Swarsha; 1-106 Silvercreek Pky N, Guelph ON N1H 7B4; Delhi (India)'70; CCFP; Ac Staff, Guelph General Hospital; Langs: Hindi; (519)824-4567

KAUSKY, Karin M; Whistler Med Clinic, RR 4 201-4380 Lorimer Rd, Whistler BC V0N 1B4; Tor'88; Dip SportMed; CCFP; Langs: Czech; (604)932-4911; whistlermc@telus.net.

KAUZMAN, George; CSSS de Trois-Rivieres, 1991 boul du Carmel, Trois-Rivieres QC G8Z 3R9; Staff, CSSS de Trois-Rivières; (819)697-3333

KAVADAS, Fotini D; Alberta Children's Hosp, C4 437-2888 Shaganappi Trail N, Calgary AB T3B 6A8; Alb'03; FRCPC; Peds; ClinImmunol&Allergy. Staff, Alberta Children's Hospital; (403)955-3035

KAVALEC, Conrad; Drummond Med Bldg, 322-1414 rue Drummond, Montreal QC H3G 1W1; McG'86; DAB; FRCSC; Ophth (Oculo Plastic Surgery). Dept Chairman, St Mary's Hospital Centre; Ophthalmology, McGill University Health Centre - Royal Victoria Hospital; Staff, McGill University Health Centre - Montreal Children's Hospital; adj Prof, McGill University; Langs: French; (514)842-2983; Fax. (514)842-0777.

KAVALSKY, Dennis M; Levy Med Clinic, 1390 Main St E, Hamilton ON L8K 1C1; Cape Town (South Africa)'80; MB ChB; CCFP; FCFP; Ac Staff, St Joseph's Healthcare - Charlton Campus; Asst Prof, McMaster University; (905)549-1246; Fax. (905)547-2424.

KAVAN, Petr; SMBD Jewish Gen Hosp, 3755 ch Cote-Sainte-Catherine, Montreal QC H3T 1E2; Prague (Czech Republic)'86; MD; PhD; Staff, Sir Mortimer B Davis Jewish General; Program Dir Adolescent & Young Adult Oncology, McGill University; Langs: Czech; Russian; (514)340-8222

KAVANAGH, Brian P W; The Hosp For Sick Children, 555 University Ave, Toronto ON M5G 1X8; National (Ireland)'85; MB; BScPharm(Pharm); MRC; FRCPC; Anes (Critical Care Medicine). Staff, The Hospital For Sick Children; Chair Anes/Prof, University of Toronto; (416)813-6860; Fax. (416)813-5313; brian.kavanagh@sickkids.ca.

KAVANAGH, James M; 203-20 Hobson St, Cambridge ON N1S 2M6; Tor'75; BSc(Hon.); MSc; Staff, Cambridge Memorial Hospital; (519)621-7831

KAVANAGH, Katherine; Health Research Innovation Ctr, GAC82-3280 Hospital Dr NW, Calgary AB T2N 4Z6; Mem'76; FRCPC; IntMed (Electrophysiology); Cardiol. Staff Libin Cardiovascular Research Inst, University of Calgary; (403)210-6152; Fax. (403)984-0870.

KAVANAGH, Sandra T; 304-9426 51 Ave NW, Edmonton AB T6E 5A6; Alb'81; Ac Staff, Covenant Health - Grey Nuns Community Hospital; Ac Staff, Covenant Health - St. Joseph's Auxilliary Hospital; Ac Staff, South Terrace Continuing Care Ctre; (780)784-0139; Fax. (780)669-5740; kfdrsoffice@shaw.ca.

KAVAZANJIAN, Hratch; 2038 Victoria Park Ave, North York ON M1R 1V2; Beirut (Lebanon)'77; (416)444-1700; Fax. (416)444-1703.

KAVERI SELVAN, Kaveri M; Shoppers World Med Centre, 106-499 Main St, Brampton ON L6Y 1N7; Tamilnadu (India)'00; MB BS; CCFP; (905)796-6570

KAVIANI, Mandana; 200-1530 7th Ave W, Vancouver BC V6J 1S3; Shiraz (Iran)'91; FRCPC; IntMed; ClinImmunol&Allergy. Langs: Farsi; (604)739-5612

KAVOURIS, William; D2-125 The Queensway, Etobicoke ON M8Y 1H6; Tor'89; Langs: Greek; (416)253-0632

KAVULU, Anne L; Academic Family Medicine, 172-1621 Albert St, Regina SK S4P 2S5; (Other Foreign)'04; CCFP; (306)766-0444

KAWAI, Susan H; Dr Langer & Associates, 180 Sandalwood Pky E, Brampton ON L6Z 1Y4; McM'92; BSc; FRCPC; Peds. (905)846-9255; Fax. (905)846-2525.

KAWAKAMI, Jun; Rockyview Gen Hosp, 6625-7007 14 St SW, Calgary AB T2V 1P9; Qns'98; BSc; MSc; FRCSC; Urol (Oncology). Staff, Rockyview General Hospital; (403)943-8994; Fax. (403)943-8996.

KAWAM, Michael P; 201-274 Dundas St E, Belleville ON K8N 1E6; Ott'91; FRCSC; OrthSurg. Staff, QHC Belleville General; (613)969-9742; Fax. (613)969-7166.

KAWAMURA, Anne; Holland Bloorview Kids Rehab, 150 Kilgour Rd, Toronto ON M4G 1R8; Tor'97; FRCPC; Peds. Staff, Holland Bloorview Kids Rehabilitation Hospital; (416)425-6220 x3586; Fax. (416)424-3837.

KAWAMURA, Nao; Sunridge Prof Centre, 3-2675 36 St NE, Calgary AB T1Y 6H6; McG'97; FRCPC; DiagRad. (403)291-3315; Fax. (403)291-9308.

KAWCHUK, Janet; IWK Health Centre, PO Box 9700 Rpo CSC, Halifax NS B3K 6R8; Alb'84; FRCPC; Peds (Developmental Pediatrics). Med Staff Developmental Clinic, IWK Health Centre; Lecturer Med, Dalhousie University; (902)470-8483; Fax. (902)470-7284.

KAWCHUK, Joann M; Royal University Hosp, 103 Hospital Dr, Saskatoon SK S7N 0W8; Sask'01; FRCPC; Anes; Critical Care Medicine. Staff Anes, Royal University Hospital; (306)655-1183

KAWCHUK, Terry P; 750-5991 Spring Garden Rd, Halifax NS B3H 1Y6; Alb'84; Court Staff, IWK Health Centre; Staff Health Phys., Technical U. of Nova Scotia; (902)422-5551

KAWERK, Jacques; CSSS du Suroît, 150 rue Saint-Thomas, Salaber-de-Valleyf QC J6T 6C1; (Lebanon)'95; Staff, Centre Hospitalier Régional du Suroît; (450)371-9920 x2146

KAWERNINSKI, Michael S; Stewart Health Centre, PO Box 8, Stewart BC V0T 1W0; Ott'73; CCFP; FCFP; Staff, Stewart Health Centre; (250)636-2221

KAWUN, Ulana B; The Court, 407-2863 Ellesmere Rd, Scarborough ON M1E 5E9; McM'98; FRCSC; GenSurg. (416)283-7338

KAY, Gary P; The Ottawa Hosp-Civic Campus, 1053 Carling Ave, Ottawa ON K1Y 4E9; Wes'01; FRCPC; Psy. Staff Neurol, The Ottawa Hospital - Civic Campus; (613)798-5555

KAY, John D; Wortley Village Med Centre, 209-190 Wortley Rd, London ON N6C 4Y7; Wes'89; DABPN; FRCPC; IntMed; Neur. Physician, Wortley Village Medical Centre; (519)667-2221; Fax. (519)667-2001.

KAY, Joseph; 327 Reynolds St, Oakville ON L6J 3L7; McG'84; MD; FRCPC; Anes (Pain Management). Staff, Halton Healthcare Services Corporation - Oakville Site; Ac Staff Anes, Sunnybrook Health Sciences Centre; Asst Prof, University of Toronto; Clinical Asst Prof, McMaster University; (905)845-2571

KAY, L Rex K; 240 Glengrove Ave W, Toronto ON M4R 1P3; Man'85; BA; FRCPC; Psy. Staff Psy, Mount Sinai Hospital; Lecturer Psy, University of Toronto; (416)482-4518; rex.kay@utoronto.ca.

KAY, Marvin S; 1414-30 Greenfield Ave, North York ON M2N 6N3; Tor'57; (416)222-7780

KAY, Philip W; Campobello Health Centre, 1-640 Route 774, Welshpool NB E5E 1A5; Alb'87; BSc; CCFP; Ac Staff, Charlotte County Hospital; (506)752-4100; Fax. (506)752-4101; kayphi@sympatico.ca.

KAY, Sabina; Kitimat Gen Hosp & Health Ctr, 920 Lahakas Blvd S, Kitimat BC V8C 2S3; Tuzla (Bosnia-Herzegovina)'93; Staff, Kitimat Hospital & Health Centre; (250)632-8679; Fax. (250)632-8631; drkay.drskully@gmail.com.

KAYA, Ebru; Univ Hlth Network-Toronto Gen, NU9 925-200 Elizabeth St, Toronto ON M5G 2C4; London (England)'98; Staff, Toronto General Hospital - UHN; (416)340-4800; Fax. (416)340-4823.

KAYAL, Dounia; CLSC Cote-des-Neiges, 5700 ch de la Cote-des-Neiges, Montreal QC H3T 2A8; Mon'09; Staff Family Med, Institut Universitaire de Gériatrie de Montréal; Langs: English; Spanish; (514)731-8531; dounia.kayal@mail.mcgill.ca.

KAYAL, Magdi D; Centre Med Pierrefonds, 12774 boul Gouin O, Pierrefonds QC H8Z 1W5; Tor'72; Staff Emerg, Lakeshore General Hospital - Pointe Claire; (514)683-3742

KAYE, Geoffrey B; Gimbel Eye Centre, 140-11910 111 Ave NW, Edmonton AB T5G 0E5; Cape Town (South Africa)'82; MB ChB; FRCSC; Ophth (Cataract). Staff, Royal Alexandra Hospital; Langs: Afrikaans; (780)452-4111; Fax. (780)452-4114; gbkaye@gimbel.com.

KAYE, Kathy L; 211-1135 Adelaide St N, London ON N5Y 5K7; Wes'96; BSc; FRCPC; Neur. (519)438-8586; Fax. (519)438-9237.

KAYE, Stephen H; 103-1221 Lonsdale Ave, North Vancouver BC V7M 2H5; Witwatersrand (South Africa)'83; FRCSC; ObstGyn (Urogynecology). Ac Staff ObstGyn, Lions Gate Hospital; Clin Assoc Prof, University of British Columbia; (604)980-2838; Fax. (604)980-0808.

KAYE, Valerie N; Adult Eating Disorder Program, 509-111 Waterloo St, London ON N6B 2M4; McG'80; FRCPC; Psy (Group Therapy). Staff, London Health Sciences Centre - South Street; (519)685-8500 x74801

KAYILASANATHAN, Suganthan; 1701 Martin Grove Rd, Etobicoke ON M9V 4N4; (Saint Kitts-Nevis)'07; CCFP; (416)744-0461; Fax. (416)744-3356.

KAYLER, Douglas E; 4-871 Waverley St, Winnipeg MB R3T 5P4; Tor'72; FRCSC; OrthSurg. (204)832-6560; Fax. (204)888-0705.

KAYSER, Rebecca J; The Credit Valley Hosp, 2200 Eglinton Ave W, Mississauga ON L5M 2N1; McM'02; CCFP; CCFP(E.M.); Staff, The Credit Valley Hospital; (905)813-4141

KAYSSI, Hassan; Clinique Med Versailles, 2215-7275 rue Sherbrooke E, Montreal QC H1N 1E9; Beyrouth (Lebanon)'71; Langs: English; Arabic; (514)353-1093; Fax. (514)353-0039.

KAYUMI, Adam S; Brittany Glen Med Centre, 102-5602 Tenth Line W, Mississauga ON L5M 7L9; Kabul (Afghanistan)'83; CCFP; Langs: Dari; Hindi; Urdu; (905)858-9393; Fax. (905)858-8960.

KAZANDJI, Dalal; 214-6633 Highway 7, Markham ON L3P 7P2; Saba (Netherlands Antilles)'09; CCFP; (905)294-0029

KAZANOWSKI, Davina A; Medical Arts Centre, 103-650 Terminal Ave, Nanaimo BC V9R 5E2; UBC'89; Staff, Nanaimo Regional General Hospital; (250)753-3431; Fax. (250)754-6897; medicalartscentre@shaw.ca.

KAZARIAN, Nancy; Medical Assoc of Port Perry, 462 Paxton St, Port Perry ON L9L 1L9; Tor'97; CCFP; FCFP; Teacher ROMP, University of Toronto; (905)985-2895 x5416; Fax. (905)985-5402.

KAZATCHENKO, Lioubov N; Oasis Med Centre, 103-1800 Market Street SE, Airdrie AB T4A 0K9; (Russia (Federation))'92; CCFP; (403)980-9926

KAZDAN, David M; 101-157 Queen St E, Brampton ON L6W 3X4; Tor'87; Dip SportMed; CCFP; Staff, William Osler Health System - Brampton Civic Hospital; (905)453-1340; Fax. (905)453-5493.

KAZDAN, Jerome J; 240-30 Disera Dr, Thornhill ON L4J 0A7; Tor'60; FRCSC; Ophth. Ac Staff, North York General Hospital - Branson Division; Assoc Prof, University of Toronto; (905)881-8050; Fax. (905)881-8050.

KAZEMBE, V Gertrude; River City Centre, 610-8600 Franklin Ave, Fort McMurray AB T9H 4G8; Lusaka (Zambia)'84; MB ChB; MRCPPeds; (780)743-0178; Fax. (780)743-0820; vivienne_b@yahoo.com.

KAZEMI, Ali-Reza; 212-168 13th St E, North Vancouver BC V7L 4W8; London (England)'88; MSc; FRCS(Edin & Glas); LRCP; MRCS; Staff, Providence Health Care - St Paul's Hospital; Langs: Farsi; (604)985-8561; Fax. (604)985-9561.

KAZEMI, Kamyar; Royal City Med Bldg, 205-250 Keary St, New Westminster BC V3L 5E7; Wes'94; FRCSC; GenSurg; VascSurg. Staff Vascular Surg, Royal Columbian Hospital; (604)521-3917; Fax. (604)521-3918.

KAZEMI, Reza; 305 Helena St, Dunnville ON N1A 2S9; Tor'87 London (England); Langs: Persian; (905)774-8841

KAZEROUNI, Abdul H; Western Mem Reg Hosp, PO Box 2005 Stn Main 1 Brookfield Ave, Corner Brook NL A2H 6J7; (Iran)'97; Staff, Western Memorial Regional Hospital.

KAZHILA, David G; Lindsay Med Centre, 104-86 Angeline St S, Lindsay ON K9V 6C5; Lusaka (Zambia)'91; MB ChB; FRCPC; IntMed (Cardiology). (705)878-9700; Fax. (705)878-4109.

KAZI, Soofia L; 207-240 Wharncliffe Rd N, London ON N6H 4P2; Karachi (Pakistan)'90; CCFP; Aj Prof, University of Western Ontario; Langs: Urdu; Hindi; (519)432-1522

KAZIMI, Syed N; Southlake Reg Health Centre, 596 Davis Dr, Newmarket ON L3Y 2P9; Dow (Pakistan)'95; MB BS; FRCPC; AnatPath. Staff, Southlake Regional Health Centre; (905)895-4521; snkazmi@yahoo.com.

KAZIMIRSKI, Judith C; Hants Shore Community Hlth Ctr, RR 1 5638 Highway 215, Newport NS B0N 2A0; Ott'69; kazimirski@ns.sympatico.ca.

KAZIMIRSKI, Mark; Windsor Med Clinic, PO Box 490 141 Wentworth Rd, Windsor NS B0N 2T0; Ott'69; CCFP; FCFP; Chair, College of Family Physicians of Canada-Nova Scotia; Preceptor, Dalhousie University; (902)798-2227; Fax. (902)798-4554; windsor.med@ns.sympatico.ca.

KAZIUKA, Eric N; Morningside Crossing Med Ctr, H9-4525 Kingston Rd, Scarborough ON M1E 2P1; McG'82; Staff, The Scarborough Hospital - General Campus; (416)284-0189; Fax. (416)284-1491.

KAZMI, Asif A; Royal Court Med Centre, 211-5 Quarry Ridge Rd, Barrie ON L4M 7G1; Punjab (India)'94; FRCPC; Peds. (705)797-0800

KAZMI, Mustapha H; Bridgeland Med Bldg, 306-803A 1 Ave NE, Calgary AB T2E 7C5; Cal'04; FRCPC; IntMed; Cardiol. (403)571-8600

KAZMI, Najma; Landmark Med Centre, 3-4150 Albert St, Regina SK S4S 3R8; (Other Foreign)'87; (306)775-3311

KAZMI, Samina; Southlake Med Centre, 204A-581 David Dr, Newmarket ON L3Y 2P6; Univ of Karachi (Pakistan)'88.

KAZMIE, Huma; Windsor Health Centre, 205-630 Tecumseh Rd E, Windsor ON N8X 4W2; Aligarh (India)'90; MD; BSc; FRCPC; Peds. Staff Pediatrician, Windsor Regional Hospital - Metropolitan Site; Langs: Hindi; Urdu; (519)253-6112; Fax. (519)253-6335; humakazmie@yahoo.com.

KE, Warren J; Dundas Med Centre, 302-220 Dundas St W, Whitby ON L1N 8M7; Tor'79; BSc; Langs: Chinese; (905)666-2222; Fax. (905)666-2222.

KEABLE, Andre; CHSLD Cote Jardins, 880 av Painchaud, Quebec QC G1S 0A3; Laval'82; (418)621-5355

KEALEY, Alayne; Sunnybrook Hlth Sciences Ctre, 2075 Bayview Ave, Toronto ON M4N 3M5; Ott'01; FRCPC; Anes. Staff, Sunnybrook Health Sciences Centre; (416)480-4864; Fax. (416)480-6039.

KEALEY, Angela J; Foothills Med Centre, 1403 29 St NW, Calgary AB T2N 2T9; Ott'01; FRCPC; IntMed; Cardiol. Fellow Cardiol, Foothills Medical Centre; (403)944-8081; Fax. (403)944-3262.

KEALEY, Miles S; Halton HCS Corp-Oakville, 327 Reynolds St, Oakville ON L6J 3L7; Ott'94; FRCSC; GenSurg. Staff, Halton Healthcare Services Corporation - Oakville Site; (905)845-2571

KEALEY, Lynn S; Smyth Med Centre, 312-1929 Russell Rd, Ottawa ON K1G 4G3; Wisconsin (USA)'71; FRCPC; Psy (Psychotherapy). Asst Prof, University of Ottawa; (613)738-7819; lkealey@sympatico.ca.

KEALY, Ciaran L; Sudbury Med Centre, 209-65 Larch St, Sudbury ON P3E 1B8; Dublin (Ireland)'63; FRCS; FRCSC; GenSurg. (705)673-6215; Fax. (705)673-5195.

KEALY, Walter W; Onaping Falls Med Centre 24 Nickel St PO Box 160, Levack ON P0M 2C0; National (Ireland)'69; MB ChB; DCH; (705)966-5180; Fax. (705)966-5182; wwfkealy@hotmail.com.

KEAN, H R Wade; Burin Peninsula Hlth Care Ctr, PO Box 340, Burin NL A0E 1E0; Mem'83; Staff, Burin Peninsula Health Care Centre; (709)891-1040

KEAN, Walter F; 401-1 Young St, Hamilton ON L8N 1T8; Glasgow (Scotland)'72; MB ChB; MD; FRCPC; IntMed (Rheumatology). Consultant, Hamilton Health Sciences Centre; Clin Prof Med, McMaster University; Langs: French; Italian; (905)521-0514; Fax. (905)528-2385.

KEANE, Eimear J; Anaesthetic Services, 213-2186 Oak Bay Ave, Victoria BC V8R 1G3; Dublin (Ireland)'79; MB ChB; BAO; FRCPC; Anes. (250)595-7211

KEARNEY, Ramona A; Zeidler Ledcor Centre, 2 76-130 University Campus NW, Edmonton AB T6G 2X8; Mem'79; FRCPC; Anes (Adult Anesthesia). Staff Anes, Stollery Children's Hospital; (780)492-9722; Fax. (780)492-4144.

KEARNS, Finnualla; CLSC Ste-Foy-Sillery, 3108 ch Sainte-Foy, Quebec QC G1X 1P8; Laval'87; Staff, Hotel-Dieu du Sacre-Coeur de Jesus de Quebec; (418)651-2572; Fax. (418)651-3133.

KEARNS, Katherine; Prairie Trail Med Centre, 100-1345 Taylor Ave, Winnipeg MB R3M 3Y9; Alb'04; CCFP; (204)475-0088

KEARON, M Clive; Hamilton HS-Henderson Site, 711 Concession St, Hamilton ON L8V 1C3; Dublin (Ireland)'80; MRCP(I); PhD; MB; FRCPC; IntMed (Thromboembolism); Respir. Staff Thrombosis Unit, Hamilton Health Sciences Centre-Juravinski Site; McMaster University; (905)383-2251; Fax. (905)575-7320.

KEASHLY, Dena; Canadian Blood Services, 737 13 Ave SW, Calgary AB T2R 1J1; Cal'90; BSc; CCFP; Staff, Canadian Blood Services; (403)410-2680; Fax. (403)410-2799; dena.keashly@blood.ca.

KEAST, David H; St Joseph's HC-Parkwood Hosp, 801 Commissioners Rd E, London ON N6C 5J1; Qns'85; BSc; MSc; CCFP; FCFP; Staff, Parkwood Hospital - St Joseph's Health Care; (519)695-4027

KEATING, Armand; UHN-Princess Margaret Hosp, 610 University Ave, Toronto ON M5G 2M9; Ott'76; FRCPC; IntMed (Bone Marrow Transplant); Hem. Dir Cell Therapy Program, Princess Margaret Hospital - University Health Network; Dir/Prof Med, University of Toronto; (416)946-4595; armand.keating@uhn.on.ca.

KEATING, Frances M; 240 Main St PO Box 538, Thessalon ON P0R 1L0; Dal'86; CCFP; (705)842-2905; Fax. (705)842-0038.

KEATING, Mary-Margaret; Woodlawn Med Clinic, 92 Main St, Dartmouth NS B2X 1R5; Dal'06; FRCPC; IntMed; Hem. Staff, Dartmouth General Hospital; Assoc Prof Capital Health, Queen Elizabeth II Health Sciences Centre - Halifax Infirmary Site; (902)434-1500 x234; Fax. (902)462-8464; keatingm@dal.ca.

KEATING, Michael P; Millidge Place, 707 Millidge Ave, Saint John NB E2K 2N7; Dal'70; CCFP; FCFP; Asst Consultant, Oromocto Public Hospital; (506)696-6544; Fax. (506)696-0787; dr.m.keating@nb.aibn.com.

KEATING, Michael V; The Group Health Centre, 240 McNabb St, Sault Ste. Marie ON P6B 1Y5; McM'85; Langs: English; French; (705)759-1234; Fax. (705)759-5888.

KEATING, Paula M; Miramichi East Med Clinic, 4 Johnson Ave, Miramichi NB E1N 3B7; Dal'90; CCFP; Ac Staff, Miramichi Regional Hospital; (506)778-8994; Fax. (506)778-8719; savoyg@nb.sympatico.ca.

KEATING, Sarah J; Mount Sinai Hosp, 600 University Ave, Toronto ON M5G 1X5; Tor'79; FRCPC; AnatPath. Staff, Mount Sinai Hospital; (416)586-8748

KEATING-POWER, Dianne; Nova Medical, 204-496 Topsail Rd, St. John's NL A1E 2C2; Mem'07; CCFP; (709)745-6682

KEATS, Karen L; Foothills Med Centre, C231-1403 29 St NW, Calgary AB T2N 2T9; Mem'94; FRCPC; EmergMed (Diving Medicine). Staff EmergMed, Foothills Medical Centre; (403)944-1110; Fax. (403)944-2419.

KEAVENEY, Lynda; Kindersley Med Clinic, PO Box 1390, Kindersley SK S0L 1S0; (Other Foreign)'96; CCFP; (306)463-2621

KEAVENY, John A; Associate Med Clinic, PO Box 510, Slave Lake AB T0G 2A0; University Coll. (Ireland)'83; MB ChB; BAO; CCFP; (780)849-4155; Fax. (780)849-4574.

KEAY, James S; Associate Med Clinic, 203-10030 106 St, Westlock AB T7P 2K4; Alb'05; BSc; CCFP; (780)349-3341; Fax. (780)349-6686.

KEAYS, Gloria E; Coronation Plaza, 101-14310 111 Ave NW, Edmonton AB T5M 3Z7; Qns'88; FRCPC; CommunMed;CCFP; FCFP; Public Health & Preventive Med. (780)342-0251; Fax. (780)342-0316.

KEAYS, Tara N; Bank Respiratory Services, 217-1385 Bank St, Ottawa ON K1H 8N4; Tor'03; FRCPC; IntMed; Respir. (613)523-4444

KEBARLE, Paula J; Solid Organ Transplant Clinic, 5F-2775 Laurel St, Vancouver BC V5Z 1M9; Alb'92; BSc; CCFP; CCFP(E.M.); Clin Associate Renal Transplant, Vancouver General Hospital - Centennial Pavillion; Langs: Bilingual(English/French); (604)875-4439

KEBEDE, Daniel; 303-3024 Hurontario St, Mississauga ON L5B 4M4; Sofia (Bulgaria)'88; DrMedCh; CCFP; (905)272-3131; Fax. (905)272-8284.

KECHAOU, Wassim; CSSS du Sud de Lanaudière, 911 montee des Pionniers, Terrebonne QC J6V 2H2; Staff, Centre Hospitalier Pierre le Gardeur; (450)654-7525

KEDDY, John W; 206-1015 Regent St, Fredericton NB E3B 6H5; Dal'73; CCFP; FCFP; Med Dir DVA Unit/Ac Staff, Dr Everett Chalmers Regional Hospital; Lecturer, Dalhousie University; (506)458-0246; Fax. (506)458-0264.

KEDDY-GRANT, Jill A; Winnipeg Clinic, 425 St Mary Ave, Winnipeg MB R3C 0N2; Man'85; FRCPC; Derm (Pediatric Dermatology). Consultant Children's Hosp, Health Sciences Centre; Clin Lecturer, University of Manitoba; (204)957-3226

KEE, Barbara E; 106-1971 Queen St E, Toronto ON M4L 1H9; Tor'71; Ac Staff, Toronto East General Hospital Inc; (416)691-6661; Fax. (416)691-6665.

KEE, Gordon A; Queensway Carleton Hosp, 3045 Baseline Rd, Nepean ON K2H 8P4; McM'02; CCFP; CCFP(E.M.); Staff, Queensway Carleton Hospital; (613)721-2000

KEE, I Heather; Kensington Med Clinic, 6546 Hastings St, Burnaby BC V5B 1S2; RCS (Ireland)'79; FRCPC; Peds. (604)299-9769; heatherkee123@hotmail.com.

KEE, Norman G; 23A Albert St S, Orillia ON L3V 5K6; Tor'66; CCFP; FCFP; Staff, Orillia Soldiers' Memorial Hospital; (705)325-1965; Fax. (705)325-1011; ngkee@bellnet.ca.

KEEBLE, William; Misericordia Community Hosp, 16940 87 Ave NW, Edmonton AB T5R 4H5; Nottingham U (United Kingdom)'93; BMedSci; MRCP; Staff Cardiol, Covenant Health - Misericordia Community Hospital; (780)735-2255; Fax. (780)735-2257.

KEEBLER, Conrad G; Regent Med Bldg, 425-2184 Broadway W, Vancouver BC V6K 2E1; Qns'70; BSc; DACP; FRCPC; IntMed (Cardiology). (604)736-6441; Fax. (604)736-6442.

KEEFE, Kathrene M A; 12 John St W, Waterloo ON N2L 1A7; Wes'79; (519)744-9756; Fax. (519)744-6827.

KEEFE, Peter H; 36 Madison Ave, Toronto ON M5R 2S1; Tor'76; FRCPC; IntMed; Psy. Staff Psy, Mount Sinai Hospital; Asst Prof Psy, University of Toronto; (416)969-9780; Fax. (416)766-8582.

KEEGAN, David A; Sheldon Chumuik Centre, 8F-1213 4 St SW, Calgary AB T2R 0X7; Mem'95; CCFP; CCFP(E.M.); FCFP; (403)955-9300

KEEGAN, David L; Royal University Hosp, 119-103 Hospital Dr, Saskatoon SK S7N 0W8; Sask'64; AB; FRCPC; Psy. Ac Staff Saskatoon Health Region, Royal University Hospital; Ac Staff, Saskatoon Health Region; Emeritus Prof Psy, University of Saskatchewan; (306)966-8226; Fax. (306)966-8237.

KEEGAN, Philippa A; South Calgary Med Clinic, 118-40 Sunpark Plaza SE, Calgary AB T2X 3X7; Dublin (Ireland)'75; MB ChB; BAO; Staff, Rockyview General Hospital; (403)254-4000; Fax. (403)254-1304.

KEEGAN-HENRY, M Jeanne; Burnaby Hosp, 3935 Kincaid St, Burnaby BC V5G 2X6; Queensland (Australia)'86; MB BS; BSc; CCFP; Staff Hospitalist, Burnaby Hospital; (604)434-4211; Fax. (604)412-6185.

KEELER, H S Grant; Wilson Med Centre, 130 Wilson St, Hamilton ON L8R 1E2; Tor'63; (905)526-6250; Fax. (905)522-0425.

KEELER, John E; Shelburne Med Associates, PO Box 700, Shelburne NS B0T 1W0; Dal'84; (902)875-2321; Fax. (902)875-2323.

KEELER, Steven W; 109-284 Helmcken Rd, Victoria BC V9B 1T2; Mem'92; (250)479-6962; Fax. (250)474-5617.

KEELEY, Paul J; Pelham Med Centre, 205-245 Pelham Rd, St Catharines ON L2S 1X8; Dublin (Ireland)'70; CCFP; Staff, Niagara Health System - St Catharines General Site; (905)682-2600; Fax. (905)682-1769.

KEELING, Christopher P; Keystone Dermatology Institute, 303-2377 111 St NW, Edmonton AB T6J 5E5; Dal'00; BSc; MSc; FRCPC; Derm (Dermatology Surgery). Clin Lecturer, University of Alberta Hospital; (780)439-7546; drkeeling@mac.com.

KEELING, Douglas N; 175 Old Hampton Rd PO Box 21008, Quispamsis NB E2E 4Z4; Dal'79; BSc; FRCPC; Derm. Consultant, St Joseph's Hospital; Staff, Saint John Regional Hospital; Dalhousie University; Langs: Bilingual(English/French); (506)849-8330; Fax. (506)849-8392.

KEELING, Patricia; Weeneebayko Gen Hosp, PO Box 34 19 Hospital Dr, Moose Factory ON P0L 1W0; Wes'64; Staff, Weeneebayko General Hospital; (705)658-4544

KEELING, Stephanie O; Heritage Med Research Centre, 562-107 University Campus NW, Edmonton AB T6G 2S2; UBC'99; FRCPC; IntMed; Rheum. Asst Prof Rheum, University of Alberta Hospital; Langs: Ukrainian; (780)407-7540; Fax. (780)407-6055; sokeeling@med.ualberta.ca.

KEELY, Erin J; The Ottawa Hosp-Riverside, 1967 Riverside Dr, Ottawa ON K1H 7W9; Qns'84; FRCPC; IntMed; Endocrin&Metab. Staff, The Ottawa Hospital - Riverside Campus; Assoc Prof Med, University of Ottawa; (613)738-8400 x81946; ekeely@ottawahospital.on.ca.

KEELY, Kathryn L; 505 O'Connor St, Ottawa ON K1S 3P6; Qns'80; FRCPC; Peds. Ac Staff, Children's Hospital of Eastern Ontario (CHEO); Ac Staff, The Ottawa Hospital - Civic Campus; Staff, The Ottawa Hospital - General Campus; (613)230-5958; Fax. (613)230-1612.

KEEN, Brian D; Red Deer Reg Hosp Centre, PO Box 5030 Stn Postal Box Ctr 3942 50A Ave, Red Deer AB T4N 6R2; Cal'76; BSc; Ac Staff, Red Deer Regional Hospital Centre; (403)391-3665; Fax. (403)314-5307.

KEEN, Sabina L C; St Joseph's Ctr for Ambulatory, 2757 King St E, Hamilton ON L8G 5E4; McM'01; FRCPC; IntMed; GeriatricMed. Court Staff, Niagara Health System - Ontario Street Site; Court Staff, Hamilton Health Sciences Centre; (905)573-4818

KEEN, Susan L; 200-489 College St, Toronto ON M6G 1A5; McM'89; BSc; Staff, Women's College Hospital; (416)323-9986; Fax. (416)323-0447.

KEENAN, Maureen P; Family Practice Centre, F326-4500 Oak St, Vancouver BC V6H 3N1; Dublin (Ireland)'03; MB BCh; BAO; CCFP; (604)875-2029

KEENAN, Robert J; Scotia Square Med Centre, 0270-5201 Duke St, Halifax NS B3J 1N9; Mem'90; (902)431-1800; Fax. (902)431-1818.

KEENAN, Tiffany J; Little Current Med Associates, PO Box 549, Little Current ON P0P 1K0; Mem'98; CCFP; (705)368-1488

KEENAN, William G; Hys Med Centre, 202-11010 101 St NW, Edmonton AB T5H 4B9; Alb'81; FRCPC; DiagRad. (780)426-1121; Fax. (780)425-5979.

KEENE, Daniel L; Children's Hosp of Eastern Ont, 401 Smyth Rd, Ottawa ON K1H 8L1; Sask'75; BSc; MA; FRCPC; Peds (Epilepsy); Neur. Court Staff Privil, The Ottawa Hospital - General Campus; Ad Staff Privil, Children's Hospital of Eastern Ontario (CHEO); Assoc Prof Peds & Med, University of Ottawa; (613)737-7600; dkeene@cheo.on.ca.

KEENLEYSIDE, Joel H; 285 Bridge St, Port Stanley ON N5L 1J5; Wes'79; CCFP; FCFP; (519)782-3667; Fax. (519)782-3743.

KEEPING, Brenda; Regina Gen Hosp, 1440 14th Ave, Regina SK S4P 0W5; Mem'93; FRCPC; Anes. Staff, Regina General Hospital; (306)766-4252; Fax. (306)766-4443.

KEEPING, Virginia A; Mount Pearl Med Centre, 12 St. David's Ave, Mount Pearl NL A1N 1G8; Mem'88; BSc; BMedSci; (709)368-8381

KEESAL, Nancy B; 604-790 Bay St, Toronto ON M5G 1N8; McG'88; FRCPC; IntMed; Rheum. Langs: English; French; Spanish; (416)323-0630; Fax. (416)413-9689; nancykeesal@bellnet.ca.

KEESARI, Manohar; Durham Children's Aid Society, SS 201 1320 Airport Blvd, Oshawa ON L1H 7K4; Osmania (India)'62; MB BS; FRCPC; Psy (Child Psychiatry). Langs: Urdu; Telugu; (905)433-1551

KEETBAAS, Shayne D; Canadian Sport Medicine, 2424 University Dr NW, Calgary AB T2N 3Y9; Cal'06; FRCSC; OrthSurg. (403)284-4526

KEETON, Linda H; 101-100 Main St E, Hamilton ON L8N 3W4; McM'87; Staff, Halton Healthcare Services Corporation - Oakville Site; (905)528-5858; Fax. (905)523-7703.

KEETON, Michael; Argus Med Centre, 300-581 Argus Rd, Oakville ON L6J 3J4; Qns'75; PhD; BSc; Ac Staff, Halton Healthcare Services Corporation - Oakville Site; (905)338-9900; Fax. (905)338-9904.

KEEZER, Mark R; Complexe Sante Reine-Elizabeth, 2100 rue Marlowe, Montreal QC H4A 3L5; McG'07; MDCM; FRCPC; Neur. Staff, Centre de santé Queen Elizabeth; (514)485-5030

KEFFER, Glen W; Niagara H System-Welland Site, 65 Third St, Welland ON L3B 4W6; Wes'61; Staff, Niagara Health System - Welland Hospital Site; (905)732-6111

KEFI, Sameh; CSSS Pierre-De Saurel, 400 av de l'Hotel-Dieu, Sorel-Tracy QC J3P 1N5; (Tunisia)'05; (450)746-6000

KEHINDE, Olasunkanmi; 100-200 James St S, Hamilton ON L8P 3A9; (Nigeria)'90; MB BS; CCFP; (905)523-4114; Fax. (905)523-1533.

KEHLER, Faye E; Dingwall Med Group, PO Box 3011 Stn Main 40 Goodall St, Dryden ON P8N 2Z6; Man'85; BSc(Med.); CCFP; FCFP; Med Pres, Dryden Regional Health Centre; (807)223-2258; Fax. (807)223-4733.

KEHLER, Larry D; PO Box 1103, Hope BC V0X 1L0; Sask'67; CCFP; (604)869-5648; Fax. (604)869-2459; ldkehler@telus.net.

KEHOE, Anne; South-East Ottawa Centre, 600-1355 Bank St, Ottawa ON K1H 8K7; McM'86; CCFP; FCFP; Asst Staff, The Ottawa Hospital - General Campus; Lecturer, University of Ottawa; (613)737-4809; Fax. (613)739-3723.

KEI, Olivia C Y; Copeman Healthcare Centre, 400-1128 Hornby St, Vancouver BC V6Z 2L4; Qns'03; CCFP; (604)638-1077

KEIGHAN, Leslie; CSSS de la Matapedia, 135 av Gaetan-Archambault, Amqui QC G5J 2K5; Laval'66; DiagRad (Echography). Staff, CSSS de la Matapedia; (418)629-2211

KEIJZER, Richard; Children's Hosp, 840 Sherbrook St, Winnipeg MB R3A 1S1.

KEITH, Arthur L; North Bay Reg Health Centre, 50 College Dr, North Bay ON P1B 0A4; U of South Alabama (USA)'79; D(P)ABPN; JD; LLB; Staff, North Bay Regional Health Centre - Regional Mental Health; Asst Prof Mental Health, Northern Ontario School of Medicine; (705)474-1200 x3437; Fax. (705)495-7814; arthur.keith@nbrhc.on.ca.

KEITH, Bruce D; BC Cancer Agency-Abbotsford, 32900 Marshall Rd, Abbotsford BC V2S 0C2; Tor'92; FRCPC; IntMed; MedOncol. Staff, Abbotsford Regional Hospital & Cancer Centre; (604)851-4710

KEITH, Ian C; Saint John Reg Hosp, PO Box 2100 Stn Main 400 University Ave, Saint John NB E2L 4L2; Aberdeen (Scotland)'67; MB ChB; PhD(Leeds); FRCA(Lond); Staff, Saint John Regional Hospital; (506)648-6861; Fax. (506)648-6860.

KEITH, Julia L; Sunnybrook Hlth Sciences Ctre, E4 32-2075 Bayview Ave, Toronto ON M4N 3M5; Dal'03; FRCPC; NeurPath. Staff, Sunnybrook Health Sciences Centre; (416)480-6100 x88055; Fax. (416)480-4271.

KEITH, Nabil T; Wilson Medical Centre, 130 Wilson St, Hamilton ON L8R 1E2; Damascus (Syria)'99; (905)526-6250

KEITH, Paul E; Associated Physicians, 2425 Bevan Ave, Sidney BC V8L 4R5; Trinity Coll. (Ireland)'79; MB ChB; BAO; CCFP; (250)656-1164; Fax. (250)656-7870.

KEITH, Paul K; McMaster University, HSC 3V47-1280 Main St W, Hamilton ON L8S 4K1; Wes'86; ABAI; ABIM; FAAAI; FACAAI; MSc; FRCPC; IntMed; ClinImmunol&Allergy. Staff, Hamilton Health Sciences Centre - McMaster Children's Hospital; Staff, St Joseph's Healthcare - Charlton Campus; Assoc Prof, McMaster University; (905)521-2100 x76374; Fax. (905)521-4971; keithp@mcmaster.ca.

KEITH, Roger G; Royal University Hosp, 103 Hospital Dr, Saskatoon SK S7N 0W8; Alb'64; DABS; FACS; FRCS; FRCSC; GenSurg (Hepatobiliary & Pancreatic Surgery). Staff, Royal University Hospital; Prof Surg, University of Saskatchewan; (306)966-8632; Fax. (306)966-1611; roger.keith@usask.ca.

KEIZER, Heather E; Hillsborough Hosp, PO Box 1929 Stn Central, Charlottetown PE C1A 7N5; Dal'94; BSc; FRCPC; Psy (Adult Psychiatry). Staff, Hillsborough Hospital & Special Care Centre; Langs: English; French; (902)368-5400

KEIZER, W Stirling; Parkdale Med Centre, 20 St. Peters Rd, Charlottetown PE C1A 5N4; Dal'97; MA; MDiv; MHSA; CCFP; Staff, Queen Elizabeth Hospital; (902)566-6682; Fax. (902)566-6681.

KEKOSZ, Veronica N H; Sunnybrook Hlth Sciences Ctre, SCIL UG25-2075 Bayview Ave, Toronto ON M4N 3M5; McM'77; BA; BSc; FRCPC; PhysMed&Rehab. Staff Physiatrist, Sunnybrook Health Sciences Centre; Lecturer, University of Toronto; Langs: Ukrainian; (416)480-4685; Fax. (416)480-6885; v.kekosz.paul@utoronto.ca.

KELADA-SEDRA, Ibtisam P; New Creation MediCosmetic Ctr, 107 Lakeshore Rd, St Catharines ON L2N 2T6; Alexandria (Egypt)'73; LMCC; MB ChB; Court Staff, Niagara Health System - Ontario Street Site; Court Staff/Surgical Assist, Niagara Health System - St Catharines General Site; (905)937-1100; Fax. (905)937-5040; newcreationmedicosmetic@gmail.com.

KELEHER, Stephen T; 298 Lawrence Ave, Kitchener ON N2M 1Y4; Tor'06; CCFP; (519)578-9757; Fax. (519)578-6040.

KELEN, Leslie; 5717 av Wildwood, Cote Saint-Luc QC H4W 1W8; Budapest (Hungary)'38; LRCP; FAGS; Langs: Hungarian; (514)483-2000

KELFORD, Alison M; Sheddon Avenue Med Assoc, 308-331 Sheddon Ave, Oakville ON L6J 1X8; McM'93; BSc; MHSc; CCFP; FCFP; (905)845-8771; Fax. (905)845-8379; akelford@hotmail.com.

KELKAR, Kumar V; Addiction Centre of Toronto, 1288 Danforth Ave, Toronto ON M4J 1M6; (India)'56; MB BS; DA; FACA; Anes (Addiction Medicine). (416)462-0228; Fax. (416)461-7690.

KELL, John S; 302-840 Coxwell Ave, Toronto ON M4C 5T2; Tor'93; FRCSC; Urol. Staff, Toronto East General Hospital Inc; Langs: English; French; (416)421-4499; Fax. (416)421-4466; john.kell@utoronto.ca.

KELLAM, George W; Prescott Family Health Team, 555 King St W, Prescott ON K0E 1T0; Qns'74; CCFP; FCFP; Ac Staff, Brockville General Hospital - Charles Street; (613)925-2839; Fax. (613)925-1238.

KELLAND, Alison A; Hants Community Hosp, 89 Payzant Dr, Windsor NS B0N 2T0; Dal'75; FRCPC; Anes. Staff, Hants Community Hospital; (902)456-0977

KELLAND, Diana M; Saddle Mountain Med Clinic, PO Box 159, Nakusp BC V0G 1R0; Ott'72; DObst(Auckland); CCFP; FCFP; Fam Med, Arrow Lakes Hospital; Court Staff, Slocan Community Health Centre; (250)265-3694; Fax. (250)265-3050; dkelland@cw.bc.ca.

KELLAND, Jeffrey M; Bradley Med Centre, 104-595 Bradley Ave, London ON N6E 3Z8; Mem'98; BSc; CCFP; (519)681-2981; Fax. (519)681-0629.

KELLEHER, Barbara E; LL-339 Princess Ave, Brandon MB R7A 0N7; (Other Foreign)'80; BSc; DACP; Rep, Manitoba Medical Association; r, Canadian Society of Phlebology; Member, Canadian Assoc Aesthetic Medicine; (204)727-1920; Fax. (204)727-1922; info@kellehercosmetic.com.

KELLEHER, Samantha M A; College of Phys & Surg of BC, 300-669 Howe St, Vancouver BC V6C 0B4; Man'96; FRCPC; Psy (Eating Disorders). Staff, College of Physicians & Surgeons of British Columbia; (604)733-7758

KELLEN, Philippa E; Manitoba Clinic, 790 Sherbrook St, Winnipeg MB R3A 1M3; Witwatersrand (South Africa)'79; FRCPC; Derm. Staff Children's Hosp, Health Sciences Centre; Teach Staff, University of Manitoba; (204)788-5741; Fax. (204)783-7163.

KELLEN, Rodney I; Manitoba Clinic, 790 Sherbrook St, Winnipeg MB R3A 1M3; Witwatersrand (South Africa)'77; FRCS(E); FRCOphth; FRCSC; Ophth (Cataract Surgery). Att Staff, Misericordia Health Centre; Asst Prof, University of Manitoba; (204)788-5730; Fax. (204)784-4149.

KELLER, Emily; 666 Upper James St, Hamilton ON L9C 2Z3; Komensky (Slovakia)'77; Staff, Hamilton Health Sciences Centre - McMaster University Medical Centre; (905)574-6766

KELLER, Evelyn-Elizabeth; Inst U en Sante Mentale de QC, 2601 ch de la Canardiere, Quebec QC G1J 2G3; Laval'89; FRCPC; Psy. Staff, Institut Universitaire Sante; (418)663-5781

KELLER, Jeremy H; Four Counties Med Clinic, 1824 Concession Dr, Newbury ON N0L 1Z0; Wes'07; CCFP; Staff, Strathroy Middlesex General Hospital - Middlesex Hospital Alliance; (519)693-0350

KELLER, John R; 303-1033 Bay St, Toronto ON M5S 3A5; Tor'88; MA(Hon); PhD; (416)926-9386; Fax. (416)926-0504; jrkeller@hotmail.com.

KELLER, Oliver R; The Ottawa Hosp-Gen Campus, 501 Smyth Rd, Ottawa ON K1H 1C4; Alb'88; FRCPC; IntMed; MedOncol. Staff, The Ottawa Hospital - General Campus; (613)737-8899 x70169

KELLER, Rhona J; Ctr Radiologique Ville Marie, 1000-1538 rue Sherbrooke O, Montreal QC H3G 1L5; McG'61; DiagRad. (514)933-2778 x285; Fax. (514)788-4809.

KELLER, Robert; Allan Memorial Institute, 1025 av des Pins O, Montreal QC H3A 1A1; Man'64; FRCPC; Psy. Dir, McGill University Health Centre - Royal Victoria Hospital; adj Prof, McGill University; (514)934-1934 x35730

KELLER, Ronald E; Family Med Associates, 5021 51 St, Lacombe AB T4L 2A3; Alb'79; (403)782-3351; Fax. (403)782-5879.

KELLERHALS, Erika; Quadra Island Med Clinic, PO Box 340, Quathiaski Cove BC V0P 1N0; UBC'92; BSc; CCFP; (250)285-3540; Fax. (250)285-3549; tsylos@oberon.ark.com.

KELLERMAN, Adriaan I; Lillooet Med Clinic, PO Box 850, Lillooet BC V0K 1V0; Stellenbosch (South Africa)'74; MB ChB; Staff Family Med, Interior Health Authority Central Okanagan Kelowna Health Unit; Langs: Afrikaans; (250)256-7505

KELLERMAN, Madelene S; Lethbridge Mental Hlth Clinic, 200 5 Ave S, Lethbridge AB T1J 4L1; Stellenbosch (South Africa)'85; MB ChB; BSc(Hons); MMed(Psych); Consultant Psy, Chinook Regional Hospital; Consultant Psy, Alberta Mental Health Board; Staff Taber Mental Health Clinic & Raymond Mental Health, Lethbridge Mental Health Clinic; Preceptor, University of Calgary; Langs: Afrikaans; Dutch; Flemish; German; (403)381-5260; Fax. (403)382-4518.

KELLETT, John G; Thunder Bay Reg HSC-T-Bay, 980 Oliver Rd, Thunder Bay ON P7B 6V4; (Ireland)'70; FRCPC; IntMed. Staff, Thunder Bay Regional Health Sciences Centre; (807)684-6028

KELLETT, Lisa M; 108 Avenue Rd, Toronto ON M5R 2H3; Tor'92; DABD; FRCPC; Derm (Laser Cosmetic Surgery). Langs: Bilingual(English/French); Greek; Spanish; (416)440-2597; Fax. (416)923-2597; info@dlkonavenue.com.

KELLETT, Russell H; Coast Specialists Clinic, PO Box 799 103-5631 Inlet Ave, Sechelt BC V0N 3A0; Sask'88; FRCSC; ObstGyn. Staff, St Mary's Hospital; (604)740-0003; Fax. (604)740-0029.

KELLEY, Catherine L; Don Valley Med Associates Inc, 144-1333 Sheppard Ave E, North York ON M2J 1V1; McM'85; CCFP; CCFP(E.M.); FCFP; Court Staff, Sunnybrook Health Sciences Centre; Ac Staff, North York General Hospital; University of Toronto; (416)491-5900; Fax. (416)491-1149; catherine.kelley@utoronto.ca.

KELLEY, Robert J; Boardwalk Prof Centre, 220 Water St, Charlottetown PE C1A 9M5; Dal'94; CCFP; Staff, Queen Elizabeth Hospital; (902)569-7931; Fax. (902)569-7932; dorkel@pei.eastlink.ca.

KELLEY, Simon P; The Hosp for Sick Children, S107-555 University Ave, Toronto ON M5G 1X8; Birmingham (England)'97; MB ChB; Staff, The Hospital For Sick Children; (416)813-6435

KELLNER, Barbara L; PO Box 15006 Rpo Aspenwoods, Calgary AB T3H 0N8; McM'91; FRCPC; Derm. (403)220-0770

KELLNER, James D; Alberta Children's Hosp, 2888 Shaganappi Trail NW, Calgary AB T3B 6A8; Cal'84; MD; MSc; FRCP; FRCPC; Peds; InfectDis. Reg Hd InfectDis/Reg Hd Peds, Alberta Children's Hospital; Prof/Dept Head Peds, University of Calgary; (403)955-7802; jim.kellner@albertahealthservices.ca.

KELLOW, Zina S; Mount St Joseph Hosp, 3080 Prince Edward St, Vancouver BC V5T 3N4; McG'04; DiagRad. Staff, Providence Health Care - Mount Saint Joseph Hospital; (604)874-1141

KELLS, Catherine M; Queen Elizabeth II HSC-Halifax, 2133-1796 Summer St, Halifax NS B3H 3A7; Dal'84; FACC; FRCPC; IntMed; Cardiol. Staff, Queen Elizabeth II Health Sciences Centre - Halifax Infirmary Site; Staff Cardiol/Chief Service Div of Cardiol, Queen Elizabeth II Health Sciences Centre - Victoria General Site; Consultant, IWK Health Centre; Prof Med, Dalhousie University; (902)473-6540; Fax. (902)473-2434.

KELLY, Adrian P; Tantramar Commun Health Centre, H-2 Main St, Sackville NB E4L 4A3; Dal'00; BSc(Hons); CCFP; Langs: French; (506)536-3847; Fax. (506)536-0287; drkelly@istar.ca.

KELLY, Adrienne M; 3114-910 10th Ave W, Vancouver BC V5Z 1M9; Wes'06; FRCSC; OrthSurg. (604)875-4111 x66276

KELLY, Albert S; 1624 7th Ave, Prince George BC V2L 3P6; Glasgow (Scotland)'70; MB ChB; (250)564-6000; Fax. (250)564-1892.

KELLY, Allan J; Hermitage Medicentre, 12747 50 St NW, Edmonton AB T5A 4L8; Alb'82; BMedSci; Dir Research & Clinical Trials, RJA Medicentres; (780)473-2102; Fax. (780)478-9061; akelly@medicentres.com.

KELLY, Alvin G; Brameast Family Health Org, 38-2130 North Park Dr, Brampton ON L6S 0C9; Tor'66; Ac Staff, William Osler Health System - Brampton Civic Hospital; Physician, Assured Assist; (905)792-2211; Fax. (905)792-2901.

KELLY, Anthea G; CHUS-Hop Fleurimont, 3001 12e Av N, Sherbrooke QC J1H 5N4; Ott'62; DPH; MedBiochem (P.Q.). Staff, Centre Hospitalier Universitaire de Sherbrooke-Hopital Fleurimont; Consultant, CSSS Institut universitaire de gériatrie de Sherbrooke; Langs: English; French; (819)346-1110 x13018; akelly.chus@ssss.gouv.qc.ca.

KELLY, Brian F; St Mary's Gen Hosp, 911 Queens Blvd, Kitchener ON N2M 1B2; Wes'80; Grand River Hospital - Kitchener/Waterloo Health Centre; Staff, St Mary's General Hospital; Langs: French; (519)744-3311

KELLY, Brian R; 109-10333 Southport Rd SW, Calgary AB T2W 3X6; Dundee (Scotland)'78; MB ChB; FRCPC; Peds. Staff, Alberta Children's Hospital; Staff, Rockyview General Hospital; Clinical Asst Prof, University of Calgary; (403)253-2288; Fax. (403)255-9322; briankellypc@yahoo.com.

KELLY, C Maeve; 320 Freshwater Rd, St. John's NL A1B 1C2; Dublin (Ireland)'80; FRCPC; Peds (Emergency Pediatrics). Staff Emerg, Janeway Children's Health & Rehabilitation Centre; Teach Staff Peds, Memorial Univ of Newfoundland; (709)579-1813; mkelly@morgan.ucs.mun.ca.

KELLY, C Patrick; Queensway-Carleton Hosp, 3045 Baseline Rd, Nepean ON K2H 8P4; Dal'77; FRCPC; Anes. Staff, Queensway Carleton Hospital; (613)721-2000 x2900

KELLY, Catherine L; Pelham Med Bldg, PO Box 1388 120 Pelham St, Lunenburg NS B0J 2C0; Mem'82; (902)634-4454; Fax. (902)634-3655.

KELLY, Catherine M K; Women's College Hosp, 76 Grenville St, Toronto ON M5S 1B2; McG'80; BSc; MSc(Physiol.); FRCPC; IntMed (Diabetes) (Thyroid Diseases); Endocrin (P.Q.) (Diabetes). Staff Endocrin, Women's College Hospital; Teach Staff, University of Toronto; Langs: English; French; (416)323-6013; catherine.kelly@wchospital.ca.

KELLY, Colleen M; Parkland Med Clinic, 203-998 Parkland Dr, Halifax NS B3M 0A6; Dal'87; FRCPC; Derm. Ac Staff, Queen Elizabeth II Health Sciences Centre - Victoria General Site; (902)404-7737

KELLY, Daniel M; Timmins & Dist Hosp, 700 Ross Ave E, Timmins ON P4N 8P2; Ott'07; FRCSC; GenSurg. Staff, Timmins & District Hospital.

KELLY, Dominick T; Able-Care Med Clinic, 56-2991 Lougheed Hwy, Coquitlam BC V3B 6J6; UBC'91; (604)945-7819

KELLY, Edmond N; Mount Sinai Hosp, 775-600 University Ave, Toronto ON M5G 1X5; University Coll. (Ireland)'74; DCH(Dublin); DABPed; DABPed(Perinatology&Neonat; Peds (Neonatology). Staff Neonatol & Peds, Mount Sinai Hospital; Staff Neonatol, The Hospital For Sick Children; Assoc Prof Peds, University of Toronto; (416)586-4800 x5310; Fax. (416)586-8745; ekelly@sinai.on.ca.

KELLY, Elizabeth G; Wildrose Med Centre, PO Box 3955 Stn Main 4607 50 St, Olds AB T4H 1P6; Pretoria (South Africa)'96; MB ChB; Langs: Afrikaans; (403)556-7130; Fax. (403)556-1944; kellytt@telus.net.

KELLY, Emily R; South Huron Hosp Assoc, 24 Huron St W, Exeter ON N0M 1S2; Wes'07; CCFP; Staff, South Huron Hospital Association; (519)235-2700

KELLY, Erin M; The Ottawa Hosp-Gen Campus, 501 Smyth Rd, Ottawa ON K1H 8L6; McG'08; IntMed. Staff, The Ottawa Hospital - General Campus; (613)737-8899

KELLY, Frances M; 155 Oxford St E, London ON N6A 1T4; National (Ireland)'69; (519)685-0168; Fax. (519)645-0314.

KELLY, Francis B; Holland Cross Tower B, 5F-120 Parkdale Ave, Ottawa ON K1A 0K9; McG'73; Staff, Bruyère Continuing Care - Saint-Vincent Hospital; (613)948-5882

KELLY, Gordon J; Justik Med Clinic, 8225 105 St NW, Edmonton AB T6E 4H2; Alb'96; FRCPC; Psy;CCFP; (780)432-0211

KELLY, Heather L; The Moncton Hosp, 135 MacBeath Ave, Moncton NB E1C 6Z8; Mem'07; CCFP; Staff, The Moncton Hospital; (506)857-5111

KELLY, J Calvin; Bramalea Med Centre, 203-18 Kensington Rd, Brampton ON L6T 4S5; Dublin (Ireland)'71; (905)791-2436; Fax. (905)791-8256.

KELLY, James K; Royal Jubilee Hosp, 1952 Bay St, Victoria BC V8R 1J8; National (Ireland)'72; MB ChB; BAO; FRCPath; FRCPC; AnatPath (Gastrointestinal & Liver Pathology). Chief AnatPath, Royal Jubilee Hospital; Ac Staff/Consultant, BC Cancer Agency Vancouver Island Centre; (250)370-8434; Fax. (250)370-8069.

KELLY, Janet M; The Med Centre FHT, PO Box 4200 Stn Main 707 Charlotte St, Peterborough ON K9J 7B3; Qns'86; CCFP; FCFP; Staff, Peterborough Regional Health Centre - Hospital Drive; (705)876-4540; Fax. (705)743-3865.

KELLY, John J P; Foothills Med Centre, 1403 29 St NW, Calgary AB T2N 2T9; Alb'01; FRCSC; Neursurg. Staff, Foothills Medical Centre; (403)944-1110

KELLY, John L; 108-1022 Pandora Ave, Victoria BC V8V 3P5; Cal'79; Staff, Victoria General Hospital; Staff, Royal Jubilee Hospital; Staff, St Mary's Hospital; (250)383-4442; Fax. (250)383-6442.

KELLY, Kathleen E; Family First Family Health Team, 4270 Innes Rd, Orleans ON K4A 5E6; McM'98; BSc; CCFP; (613)861-7009

KELLY, Kathleen J; Rideau FHT - Lancaster Site, 11-2450 Lancaster Rd, Ottawa ON K1B 5N3; Ott'81; CCFP; Med Staff Member, The Ottawa Hospital - General Campus; Asst Prof, University of Ottawa; (613)738-9119; Fax. (613)738-2736.

KELLY, Larry J; 263-675 Queen St S, Kitchener ON N2M 1A1; Wes'68; MA; (519)885-1935; Fax. (519)885-1889.

KELLY, Laura J; Emergency Dept, 11666 Laity St, Maple Ridge BC V2X 5A3; McM'90; CCFP; CCFP(E.M.); Pres Medical Staff, Ridge Meadows Hospital & Health Care Centre; Chair Local Med Advisory Committee, Fraser Health Authority Fraser North Service Maple Ridge Health Unit; (604)466-6909

KELLY, Leonard; The Hugh Allen Clinic, PO Box 489 Stn Main, Sioux Lookout ON P8T 1A8; Wes'88; MClSc; CCFP; FCFP; Staff, The Hugh Allen Clinic; Assoc Prof, McMaster University; Assoc Prof, Northern Ontario School of Medicine; (807)737-3803; Fax. (807)737-1771.

KELLY, Margaret M; Health Research Innovation Ctr, 4AC66-3280 Hospital Drive NW, Calgary AB T2N 4Z6; (Zimbabwe)'82; FRCPC; AnatPath. Physician, Health Research Innovation Centre; (403)944-8541

KELLY, Meghan L; PO Box 368 Stn A, Nanaimo BC V9R 5L3; Tor'09; CCFP; Langs: Bilingual(English/French).

KELLY, Michael E; Royal University Hosp, 103 Hospital Dr, Saskatoon SK S7N 0W8; Sask'99; PhD; FACS; FRCSC; Neursurg. Staff Neurosurg, Royal University Hospital; (306)966-8187

KELLY, Michael J; Grand River Hosp-KW Hlth Ctre, PO Box 9056 Stn C 835 King St W, Kitchener ON N2G 1G3; McM'78; FRCPC; Psy (Geriatric Psychiatry). Staff, Grand River Hospital - Kitchener/Waterloo Health Centre; Clinical Asst Prof Health Sciences, McMaster University; (519)749-4300 x7448

KELLY, Michael J A; 1015 Queen St E, Sault Ste. Marie ON P6A 2C2; Oxford (England)'55; MA; MB BCh; FRCOG; FACOG; FRCSC; ObstGyn. (705)253-4845; Fax. (705)253-4845.

KELLY, Michael T; Lifelabs Med Laboratory Serv, 3680 Gilmore Way, Burnaby BC V5G 4V8; Indianapolis(IN) (USA)'73; AB; AB; PhD; FRCPC; MedScient(Med) (Medical Microbiology). Consultant, Vancouver General Hospital - Centennial Pavillion; Head Med & Enteric Section, Provincial Health Laboratory; Head Microbiology Dept, Metro-McNair Clinical Laboratory; Prof, University of British Columbia; (604)412-4435; Fax. (604)412-4446.

KELLY, Mirabelle; Hop Jean-Talon, 1385 rue Jean-Talon E, Montreal QC H2E 1S6; Sher'96; FRCPC; IntMed; InfectDis; MedMicrobiol. Staff, CSSS du Coeur de l'Isle Hôpital Jean-Talon; (514)495-6767; Fax. (514)495-6782; mirabelle.kelly.cdi@ssss.gouv.qc.ca.

KELLY, Patricia E; 26 H-9200 Weston Rd, Woodbridge ON L4H 2P8; Ott'67; (905)417-2273

KELLY, Paul B; Harbourside Family Health Ctr, 243 Harbour Dr, Summerside PE C1N 5R1; Dal'72; DTMH; CCFP; FCFP; Staff, Prince County Hospital; (902)432-2600; Fax. (902)432-2610.

KELLY, Philip; Uptown Med Clinic, 3460 Saanich Rd, Victoria BC V8Z 0B9; Otago (New Zealand)'73; (250)479-2593; Fax. (250)479-2624.

KELLY, Rachel S; Squamish Gen Hosp, 38140 Behrner Dr, Squamish BC V8B 0J3; Ott'09; CCFP; Staff, Squamish General Hospital / Hilltop House; (604)726-6527

KELLY, Richard; 223 Av Saint-Charles, Vaudreuil-Dorion QC J7V 2L6; Sher'74; (450)424-4420; kellyr@videotron.ca.

KELLY, Robert G M; King Street Med Arts Centre, 207-71 King St W, Mississauga ON L5B 4A2; Tor'64; FRCSC; Ophth (Cataract & Glaucoma). Teacher, University of Toronto; (905)270-2056; Fax. (905)270-8669.

KELLY, Sarah A; Foothills Med Centre, 1403 29 St NW, Calgary AB T2N 2T9; UBC'01; FRCPC; DiagRad. Staff, Foothills Medical Centre; (403)944-1110

KELLY, Sheila M; Merivale Med Imaging, 1370 Clyde Ave, Nepean ON K2G 3H8; Ott'69; FRCPC; DiagRad. Ac Staff Radiol, The Ottawa Hospital - Civic Campus; Asst Prof, University of Ottawa; (613)727-1072; Fax. (613)727-5873; skelly@mmimaging.com.

KELLY, Stephen R; Hamilton HS-Henderson Camp, 711 Concession St, Hamilton ON L8V 1C3; Cambridge (England)'92; Staff, Hamilton Health Sciences Centre - McMaster Children's Hospital; Staff, Hamilton Health Sciences Centre-Juravinski Site; Assoc Prof, McMaster University; (905)521-2100; Fax. (905)528-9388.

KELLY-SMITH, Carolyn H; Royal Columbian Hosp, 260 Sherbrooke St, New Westminster BC V3L 3W7; UBC'06; FRCPC; EmergMed. Staff, Royal Columbian Hospital; (604)520-4000

KELPIN, Bryce; 202-520 17th St, West Vancouver BC V7V 3S8; UBC'89; Staff, Lions Gate Hospital; (604)913-8183

KELSALL, John T; Burrard Health Bldg, 202-1160 Burrard St, Vancouver BC V6Z 2E8; McG'91; BSc; FRCPC; IntMed; Rheum. Consultant, Vancouver General Hospital - Centennial Pavillion; Ac Staff, Providence Health Care - St Paul's Hospital; Clinical Asst Prof, University of British Columbia; (604)602-8118; Fax. (604)683-8150; jkelsall@providencehealth.bc.ca.

KELSALL, Rosemary; Sicamous Med Clinic, PO Box 715, Sicamous BC V0E 2V0; UBC'90; BSc; DTMH; (250)836-2817; Fax. (250)836-2867.

KELTON, David; William Osler HC-Brampton, S2 749-2100 Bovaird Dr E, Brampton ON L6R 3J7; Tor'05; DiagRad. Staff, William Osler Health System - Brampton Civic Hospital; (905)494-2120; Fax. (905)494-6614.

KELTON, John G; McMaster University, 2E1-1280 Main St W, Hamilton ON L8S 4K1; Wes'73; FRCPC; IntMed (Blood Transfusion); Hem. Dean/VP Health Sciences/Prof, McMaster University; (905)525-9140; keltonj@mcmaster.ca.

KELTON, Peter M; Leamington & Area FHT-Kingsvil, 273 Main St E, Kingsville ON N9Y 1A7; Wes'81; Staff, Leamington District Memorial Hospital; (519)733-2318; Fax. (519)733-2310.

KELTON, Timothy J; The Complete Traveler's Clinic, 410-4040 Finch Ave E, Scarborough ON M1S 4V5; Ott'90; CCFP; CCFP(E.M.); FCFP; Ac Staff, North York General Hospital; Ac Staff, The Scarborough Hospital - Birchmount Campus; Assoc Prof Family & Commun Med, University of Toronto; (416)335-0126

KELTON, Yasmine S; Centre for Women's Health, 13291 Yonge St, Richmond Hill ON L4E 4L6; Ott'01; CCFP; Langs: Portuguese; French; (905)773-4444

KELTZ, Irwin; 702-5799 Yonge St, North York ON M2M 3V3; Tor'59; BA; CCFP; FCFP; Hon Staff, North York General Hospital; Med Dir, Willowdale Manor; (416)221-5588; Fax. (416)221-5580.

KELTZ, Maurice; 572 Eglinton Ave W, Toronto ON M5N 1B7; Tor'57; Asst Volunteer Newborn Care, Mount Sinai Hospital; (416)481-0661

KEMBHAVIE, Nikhil D; Royal Alexandra Hosp, 10240 Kingsway NW, Edmonton AB T5H 3V9; Alb'01; FRCPC; Anes. Staff Anes, Royal Alexandra Hospital; (780)477-4010

KEMBLE, Frank; Richmond Med Bldg, 304-2020 Richmond Rd, Victoria BC V8R 6R5; Manchester (England)'59; MB ChB; MRCP; FRCPC; Neur (Neuromuscular Diseases). Ac Staff, Royal Jubilee Hospital; Ac Staff, Victoria General Hospital; (250)595-6271; Fax. (250)595-8411.

KEMKARAN, Kenneth P F; Eaton Place Med Centre, 81-333 St Mary Ave, Winnipeg MB R3C 4A5; (Ireland)'95; MB ChB.

KEMP, Cornelius J; West Hill Med Clinic, 1A-2995 2nd Ave W, Prince Albert SK S6V 5V5; (306)765-8500; Fax. (306)765-8501.

KEMP, David R; 203 2nd Ave W PO Box 1101, Wilkie SK S0K 4W0; Manchester (England)'69; MB ChB; Staff, Unity & District Health Centre; Staff Chief, Wilkie Health Centre; (306)843-2888; Fax. (306)843-2456; davidrkemp@yahoo.com.

KEMP, Donald G; 1-270 Argyle St S, Renfrew ON K7V 1T7; McG'70; Staff, Renfrew Victoria Hospital; (613)432-3612; Fax. (613)432-5329.

KEMP, Ilse; James Paton Mem Hosp, 125 Trans Canada Hwy, Gander NL A1V 1P7; Orange Free State (South Africa)'84; MB ChB; FRCPC; Peds. Staff, James Paton Memorial Hospital; Langs: Afrikaans; French; (709)651-2500; Fax. (709)256-5472; ilse.kemp@cenralhealth.nl.ca.

KEMP, Isabelle; Clinique Zina Sante, 300-9250 boul de l'Acadie, Montreal QC H4N 3C5; Sher'83; Psy. Langs: English; Spanish; (514)384-9462

KEMP, Kristina M; 605-100 Arden St, Moncton NB E1C 4B7; Wes'99; FRCPC; IntMed; Respir. Lecturer, Dalhousie University; Clinical Asst Prof, Memorial University Of Newfoundland; (506)870-2917; Fax. (506)857-5548.

KEMP, Robert A; Kingscross Med Group, 408-18 Kensington Rd, Brampton ON L6T 4S5; McM'78; CCFP; FCFP; Ac Staff, William Osler Health System - Brampton Civic Hospital; Langs: English; French; (905)792-2280; Fax. (905)792-9832.

KEMP, Sheelagh M; The Hosp For Sick Children, 555 University Ave, Toronto ON M5G 1X8; American (Montserrat)'83; FRCPC; Anes. Staff, The Hospital For Sick Children; (416)813-7445; Fax. (416)813-7543.

KEMP, Theo; Blackfalds Walk-In Med Clinic, PO Box 1419, Blackfalds AB T0M 0J0; Stellenbosch (South Africa)'81; MB ChB; LMCC; Langs: Afrikaans; (403)885-2237; Fax. (403)885-2705; dockemp1@telus.net.

KEMPENAAR, Jacob W; Rouge Valley-Ajax & Pickering, 580 Harwood Ave S, Ajax ON L1S 2J4; Tor'92; Staff Emerg Med, Rouge Valley Health System - Ajax & Pickering Health Centre Site; (905)683-2320

KEMPF, Christina; CSSS du Suroît, 150 rue Saint-Thomas, Salaber-de-Valleyf QC J6T 6C1; Laval'07; FRCPC; IntMed. Staff, Centre Hospitalier Rouyn-Noranda; (450)371-9920

KEMPINSKA, Anna; The Hosp for Sick Children, 555 University Ave, Toronto ON M5G 1X8; Ott'06; PedEmergMed; Peds. Staff, The Hospital For Sick Children; (416)573-5583

KEMPSTON, John D; Bloor-Jane Med Bldg, 513-2425 Bloor St W, Toronto ON M6S 4W4; Tor'69; FRCPC; IntMed (Gastroenterology). Staff Gastroent, St Joseph's Health Centre; Assoc Prof, University of Toronto; (416)766-3401; Fax. (416)766-5076; kempsj@stjoe.on.ca.

KENDAL, David; Mount Sinai Fam Hlth Team, 4F-60 Murray St, Toronto ON M5T 3L9; Tor'68; Ac Staff, Mount Sinai Hospital; Staff, Temmy Latner Centre for Palliative Care; (416)586-4800 x6761; Fax. (416)586-4804; david.kendal@tkpc.org.

KENDAL, Ian K; Heritage Pointe Fam Medicine, RR 3 330-412 Pine Creek Rd, De Winton AB T0L 0X0; Cal'86; CCFP; Physician, South Calgary Urgent Care Centre; Calgary Health Region; (403)278-4944; Fax. (403)720-3321.

KENDAL, Wayne S; The Ottawa Hosp-Gen Campus, 501 Smyth Rd, Ottawa ON K1H 8L6; Alb'77; PhD; FRCSC; GenSurg; RadOncol. Staff, The Ottawa Hospital - General Campus; (613)737-7700; Fax. (613)247-3511.

KENDAL, Wendy M; Business Bldg, 1055 Dunsmuir St, Vancouver BC V7X 1L4; Alb'74; Ac Staff, Providence Health Care - St Paul's Hospital; (604)683-8138

KENDALL, Chris J; Rocky Med Clinic, PO Box 99 Stn Main 5127 49 St, Rocky-Mtn-Hse AB T4T 1A1; Alb'00; CCFP; Clin Lecturer Family Med, University of Alberta; Clin Lecturer Family Med, University of Calgary; (403)845-2815; Fax. (403)845-2177; drckendall@hotmail.com.

KENDALL, Claire E; The Ottawa Hosp-Riverside, 1967 Riverside Dr, Ottawa ON K1H 7W9; Ott'00; CCFP; Staff, The Ottawa Hospital - Riverside Campus; Asst Prof, University of Ottawa; (613)738-8219; Fax. (613)738-8217.

KENDALL, Hugh E A; Durham Endosurgery Centre, B03-95 Bayly St W, Ajax ON L1S 7K8; McG'90; MDCM; FRCSC; GenSurg (Endoscopy). Dir, Durham Endosurgery Centre; (905)426-2028; Fax. (905)426-2033; kendallsurgery@rogers.com.

KENDALL, Perry R W; Ministry of Health, 4F-1515 Blanshard St, Victoria BC V8W 3C8; London (England)'68; MB BS; MSc; FRCPC; CommunMed (Administration). Staff, Vancouver Island Health Authority; Clin Prof Faculty of Med, University of British Columbia; (250)952-1330; Fax. (250)952-1362; perry.kendall@gov.bc.ca.

KENDALL, Richard W; Richmond Health Science Centre, 280-7031 Westminster Hwy, Richmond BC V6X 1A3; UBC'86; BScPharm; FAAOS; DABOS; FRCSC; OrthSurg (Arthroplasty). Staff, Richmond Hospital; (604)207-9119; Fax. (604)207-9118.

KENDALL, T P Adam; Whistler Health Care Centre, 4380 Lorimer Rd RR 4, Whistler BC V0N 1B4; UBC'94; MSc; BPE; Dip SportMed; CCFP; (604)932-4911; Fax. (604)932-4992.

KENDLER, David L; Broadway Med Centre, 150-943 Broadway W, Vancouver BC V5Z 4E1; Tor'77; ABIM(Endocrin); FRCPC; IntMed (Bone Densitometry); Endocrin&Metab. Ac Staff, BC Women's Hospital & Health Centre; Ac Staff, Providence Health Care - St Paul's Hospital; Asst Prof Med, University of British Columbia; (604)263-3644; Fax. (604)263-3744.

KENDRICK, Victoria L; Alberta Children's Hosp, 2888 Shaganappi Trail NW, Calgary AB T3B 6A8; UBC'87; BSc(Hon); FRCPC; Peds. Staff Peds, Alberta Children's Hospital; Staff Peds, Rockyview General Hospital; (403)955-2525; Fax. (403)955-7799.

KENEFICK, Gerald; 204-7885 6th St, Burnaby BC V3N 3N4; Cork (Ireland)'68; MB ChB; BAO; CCFP; FCFP; Med Dir, CN Rail; Med Dir, International Travel Health & Vaccination Clinic; Langs: English; French; (604)521-5941; workdocs@shawbiz.ca.

KENICK, Scott; 205-269 boul Saint-Jean, Pointe-Claire QC H9R 3J1; Man'78; FRCPC; IntMed; Gastroent. ac Staff, St Mary's Hospital Centre; (514)697-0002

KENNECKE, Hagen F; BC Cancer Agency-Vancouver CC, 600 10th Ave W, Vancouver BC V5Z 4E6; Dal'97; FRCPC; IntMed; MedOncol. Staff, BC Cancer Agency Vancouver Centre; (604)877-6000

KENNEDY, Allison T; Perth Med Clinic, 1-500 East Riverside Dr, Perth-Andover NB E7H 1Z1; Dal'84; CCFP; FCFP; Staff, Hôtel-Dieu of St Joseph Hospital; (506)273-9520; Fax. (506)273-9560.

KENNEDY, Ambrose; Souris Hosp Inc, PO Box 640, Souris PE C0A 2B0; (Other Foreign)'88; Staff, Souris Hospital Inc; (902)687-7150

KENNEDY, Andrea L; BC Women's Hosp & Health Ctre, P1 228-4500 Oak St, Vancouver BC V6H 3N1; Alb'05; FRCPC; Psy. Staff, Richmond Hospital; Staff Reproductive Mental Health Program, BC Women's Hospital & Health Centre; (604)875-2025

KENNEDY, Andrew; 43 Hillcrest Dr, Perth Andover NB E7H 2G7; St Maarten (Netherlands Antilles)'09; CCFP; (506)273-3558

KENNEDY, Brent A; Sudbury Reg Hosp-Laurentian Si, 41 Ramsey Lake Rd, Sudbury ON P3E 5J1; UBC'93; FRCPC; Anes. Staff, Health Sciences North-Laurentian Site; (705)674-3181

KENNEDY, Carl J; James Paton Mem Hosp, 125 Trans Canada Hwy, Gander NL A1V 1P7; Mem'99; FRCSC; OrthSurg. Staff, James Paton Memorial Hospital; (709)256-2500

KENNEDY, Charlene M; South Maternity & Fam Practice, 258-1011 Glenmore Trail SW, Calgary AB T2V 4R6; Alb'99; CCFP; (403)640-0600; Fax. (403)253-0124.

KENNEDY, Christine A S; Western Mem Reg Hosp, PO Box 2005 1 Brookfield Ave, Corner Brook NL A2H 6J7; Cal'04; CCFP; Staff, Western Memorial Regional Hospital; (709)637-5000

KENNEDY, Christine D; Alberta Children's Hosp, 2888 Shaganappi Trail NW, Calgary AB T3B 6A8; Man'06; FRCPC; Peds (Pediatric Emergency Medicine). Staff, Alberta Children's Hospital; (403)955-7070

KENNEDY, David R; 381 Cedar St, Simcoe ON N3Y 2J2; Wes'91; FRCPC; IntMed. Associate IntMed, Norfolk General Hospital; (519)426-1013; Fax. (519)426-2029.

KENNEDY, Dorcas D; Legacy Med Centre, 378 4 Ave S, Lethbridge AB T1J 5E9; Cal'86; CCFP; FCFP; (403)320-1504; Fax. (403)329-3778.

KENNEDY, Erin D; Mount Sinai Hosp, 455-600 University Ave, Toronto ON M5G 1X5; Tor'95; FRCSC; GenSurg (Clinician Investigator Program); General Surgical Oncology. Staff, Mount Sinai Hospital; Affil Scientist, Toronto General Hospital - UHN; (416)586-4800 x2159

KENNEDY, Fergus J; Hillside Med Centre, PO Box 700 Stn Main 541 3 Ave, Ladysmith BC V9G 1A5; University Coll. (Ireland)'77; MB BCh; BAO; DObst; DCH; (250)245-2235; Fax. (250)245-3094.

KENNEDY, Grant C; Foothills Med Centre, C231-1403 29 St NW, Calgary AB T2N 2T9; Man'06; CCFP; CCFP(E.M.); Staff, Foothills Medical Centre; (403)944-1635

KENNEDY, Ian; 301-909 Island Hwy, Campbell River BC V9W 2C2; Glasgow (Scotland)'62; MB ChB; DObstRCOG; DTMH; DA; Staff, Campbell River & District General Hospital; (250)286-0313; Fax. (250)287-2679; drianken@shaw.ca.

KENNEDY, Jacqueline M; 205-3017 66 St NW, Edmonton AB T6K 4B2; Dal'93; FRCSC; GenSurg. Asst Prof Clinical, University of Alberta; (780)461-6012; Fax. (780)461-5442.

KENNEDY, James L; Addiction & Mental Hlth-Clarke, R31-250 College St, Toronto ON M5T 1R8; Cal'84; FRCPC; Psy (General Outpatient Psychiatry). Staff, Centre for Addiction & Mental Health (CAMH) - College Street Site; Prof Psy, University of Toronto; (416)979-4987; Fax. (416)979-4666.

KENNEDY, James M C; South Health Campus, 4448 Front St SE, Calgary AB T3M 1M4; Cal'05; FRCSC; PlasSurg. (403)956-3692

KENNEDY, James R; St Paul's Hosp, 5912B-1081 Burrard St, Vancouver BC V6Z 1Y6; Mem'74; BSc(Hon); FRCPC; IntMed (Clinical Pharmacology). Med Staff, Providence Health Care - St Paul's Hospital; Med Consultant, British Columbia Drug & Poison Information Centre; Clin Assoc Prof Med & Pharm, University of British Columbia; Langs: English; French; (604)806-8397; Fax. (604)806-8546; jkennedy@providencehealth.bc.ca.

KENNEDY, Jennifer R; Haig Clinic, 601 6 Ave S, Lethbridge AB T1J 0Z2; Cal'02; CCFP; (403)328-6641; Fax. (403)328-6118.

KENNEDY, Jessica A; Southgate Med Clinic, 1-45905 Yale Rd, Chilliwack BC V2P 2M6; UBC'08; CCFP; (604)795-7228

KENNEDY, Joel N D; Lakeridge Hlth Corp-Oshawa, 1 Hospital Crt, Oshawa ON L1G 2B9; Dal'08; CCFP; Staff, Lakeridge Health - Oshawa Site; (905)576-8711

KENNEDY, John C; Medical Arts Bldg, 10-626 Main St, Penticton BC V2A 5C8; Cal'84; CCFP; FCFP; Staff, Penticton Regional Hospital; Clinical Asst Prof Family Med, University of British Columbia; (250)492-0470

KENNEDY, John S; Raymond Care Centre, PO Box 260, Raymond AB T0K 2S0; Cal'81; FRCPC; Psy (Cognitive Disorders). Aj Prof Neurosciences, Canadian Centre for Behavioural Neurosciences; Clin Prof Psy, University of Alberta; (403)752-3316; john.kennedy@uleth.ca.

KENNEDY, Joseph D; White Med Clinic, 729 Jane St, Toronto ON M6N 4B3; Tor'04; CCFP; Staff, St Joseph's Health Centre; (416)763-8880

KENNEDY, Josephine A; Don Valley Med Centre, 302-855 Broadview Ave, Toronto ON M4K 3Z1; Dal'77; BSc; (416)461-6383; Fax. (416)461-5985.

KENNEDY, Karen M; 234A Colborne St W, Orillia ON L3V 2Z6; Tor'87; CCFP; FCFP; Staff, Orillia Soldiers' Memorial Hospital; Staff, Orillia After Hours Med Clinic; Langs: German; French; (705)325-2487; Fax. (705)325-1906; karen_kennedy@rogers.com.

KENNEDY, Lindsay C; Peace Arch Hosp, 15521 Russell Ave, White Rock BC V4B 2R4; Man'03; FRCPC; Psy. Staff, Peace Arch Hospital; (604)531-5512

KENNEDY, Louis J; Providence Care-Mental Health, PO Box 603 Stn Main 752 King St W, Kingston ON K7L 4X3; Qns'84; Staff, Providence Care - Mental Health Services; Staff, Providence Care - St Mary's of the Lake Hospital Site; Queen's University; Langs: Bilingual(French/English); (613)546-1101; ljk@queensu.ca.

KENNEDY, M Stewart; Harbour View Med Clinic, 43 Court St N, Thunder Bay ON P7A 4T5; McM'84; CCFP; FCFP; (807)345-3070; Fax. (807)345-3071.

KENNEDY, Maureen F; Sports Med Centre, 145 Pacific Ave, Winnipeg MB R3B 2Z6; Man'94; BSc; MSc; CCFP; FCFP.

KENNEDY, Meagan T; Thunder Bay Reg HSC-T-Bay, 980 Oliver Rd, Thunder Bay ON P7B 6V4; Tor'01; FRCPC; AnatPath. Staff, Thunder Bay Regional Health Sciences Centre; (807)684-6594; Fax. (807)684-5877.

KENNEDY, Michael G; Lakeridge Hlth Corp-Oshawa, 1 Hospital Crt, Oshawa ON L1G 2B9; Galway (Ireland)'72; CCFP; Staff, Lakeridge Health - Oshawa Site; (905)576-8711 x3200; Fax. (905)721-7763.

KENNEDY, Michael J; East End Health Centre, 2 Mount Cashel Rd, St. John's NL A1A 1X7; Mem'89; (709)753-1450

KENNEDY, Norman R; Terrace Clinic, 204-35 Major's Path, St. John's NL A1A 4Z9; Mem'91; FRCPC; Psy.

KENNEDY, Paula M; James Paton Mem Hosp, 125 Trans Canada Hwy, Gander NL A1V 1P7; Mem'00; FRCPC; NuclearMed; DiagRad. Staff, James Paton Memorial Hospital; (709)256-2500

KENNEDY, Renee S; St Paul's Hosp, 1702 20th St W, Saskatoon SK S7M 0Z9; Dal'88; BSc; FRCSC; ThorSurg. Staff, Royal University Hospital; Staff Surg, St Paul's Hospital (Grey Nuns) of Saskatoon; Assoc Prof, University of Saskatchewan; Langs: English; French; (306)655-0533; Fax. (306)655-5771; renee.kennedy@usask.ca.

KENNEDY, Richard J; 310-1011 Glenmore Trail SW, Calgary AB T2V 4R6; Qns'63; BSc; FCCP; FRCPC; Respir (Allergy); IntMed. Ac Staff, Peter Lougheed Centre; Consultant, Alberta Health Services; Asst Prof, University of Calgary; Langs: French; (403)213-3990; Fax. (403)213-3994; rjk@rjkennedymd.com.

KENNEDY, Richard; F-7819 East Saanich Rd, Saanichton BC V8M 2B4; Wes'80; BSc; CCFP; (250)652-9518; Fax. (250)652-1256.

KENNEDY, Richard; CSSS du Suroît, 150 rue Saint-Thomas, Salaber-de-Valleyf QC J6T 6C1; Mon'76; IntMed (P.Q.). Staff, Centre Hospitalier Régional du Suroît; (450)371-9920

KENNEDY, Robert C; Terrace On The Square, 8-10 Rowan St, St. John's NL A1B 2X1; Mem'03; FRCSC; ObstGyn.

KENNEDY, Ross A; Surrey Eye Care Centre, 13490 104 Ave, Surrey BC V3T 1V8; McG'78; FRCSC; Ophth (Strabismus). Ac Staff, Vancouver General Hospital - Centennial Pavillion; Staff, Surrey Memorial Hospital; Staff, Delta Hospital; Clinical Asst Prof, University of British Columbia; (604)951-8543; Fax. (604)951-0812.

KENNEDY, Russell G; Crossroads Med Clinic, 3F-507 Broadway W, Vancouver BC V5Z 1E6; Wes'91; BSc; (604)568-7229; dockennedy@shaw.ca.

KENNEDY, Ryan P; Canadian Forces Health Serv, 713 Montreal Rd, Ottawa ON K1K 0T2; Sask'09; CCFP.

KENNEDY, Shayla L; 21st Medical Clinic, 502-402 21st St E, Saskatoon SK S7K 0C3; Man'07; (306)956-3444

KENNEDY, Sidney H; Univ Hlth Network-Toronto Gen, E8 222-200 Elizabeth St, Toronto ON M5G 2C4; Belfast (Ireland)'75; MB BCh; BAO; MRCPsy; MD; FRCPC; Psy (Mood Disorders). Psychiatrist in Chief University Health Network, Toronto General Hospital - UHN; Prof, University of Toronto; (416)340-3888; Fax. (416)340-4198; sidney.kennedy@uhn.ca.

KENNEDY, Tara J T; Stan Cassidy Centre for Rehab, 800 Priestman St, Fredericton NB E3B 0C7; Wes'95; FRCPC; Peds (Developmental Pediatrics). (506)447-4382

KENNEDY, William E; St Joseph's Healthcare, 50 Charlton Ave E, Hamilton ON L8N 4A6; Qns'70; CCFP; FCFP; Med Staff, St Joseph's Healthcare - Charlton Campus; Court Staff, Hamilton Health Sciences Centre - McMaster University Medical Centre; Asst Prof Family Med, McMaster University; (905)522-1155

KENNEL, E Ross; 207-751 King St W, Kitchener ON N2G 1E5; McM'80; CCFP; Med Dir, Columbia Forest Long Term Care Centre; Med Dir, Forest Heights Long Term Care Centre-Kitchener; (519)578-3500; Fax. (519)741-0286; kennelmd@rogers.com.

KENNEL, Richard L; Heritage Park Shopping Centre, 8-200 Lorraine Ave, Kitchener ON N2B 3R3; McM'82; CCFP; FCFP; (519)745-7521; Fax. (519)745-7524.

KENNEY, France; CSSS Pierre Boucher, 1333 boul Jacques-Cartier E, Longueuil QC J4M 2A5; Sher'92; Staff, Centre Hospitalier Pierre Boucher; (450)468-8111

KENNEY, Gordon W; Burnaby Hosp, 3935 Kincaid St, Burnaby BC V5G 2X6; Alb'82; CCFP; CCFP(E.M.); Staff, Burnaby Hospital; (604)412-6500

KENNEY, Michael P; Foothills Med Centre, 1403 29 St NW, Calgary AB T2N 2T9; Qns'94; CCFP; CCFP(E.M.); Staff, Foothills Medical Centre; (403)944-1820

KENNEY, Stephen W; 204-404 St. George St, Moncton NB E1C 1X6; Dal'92; CCFP; (506)858-9892

KENNIE, Robin C; Perth Family Medicine, 39 Drummond St W, Perth ON K7H 2J9; UBC'99; CCFP; (613)264-2686; Fax. (613)264-0454.

KENNY, Anne; Associated Radiologist, 300-140 Wall St, Saskatoon SK S7K 1N4; Sask'89; FRCPC; DiagRad. (306)244-1167; Fax. (306)244-2911.

KENNY, Brendan G; 504-100 Arden St, Moncton NB E1C 4B7; Dublin (Ireland)'78; FRCS(I); Neursurg (P.Q.) (Stereotactic Radiosurgery). Staff Neuroscience, The Moncton Hospital; Langs: Bilingual(English/French); Gaelic; (506)857-5376; Fax. (506)857-5378; dr.brendan.kenny@horizonnb.ca.

KENNY, David J; Courtenay Med Clinic, 788 Grant Ave, Courtenay BC V9N 2T3; Tor'84; CCFP; FCFP; (250)334-2445

KENNY, Erin K; St Paul's Hosp, 1081 Burrard St, Vancouver BC V6Z 1Y6; McG'05; CCFP; CCFP(E.M.); Staff, Providence Health Care - St Paul's Hospital; (604)682-2344

KENNY, Kathryn; Foothills Med Centre, 1403 29 St NW, Calgary AB T2N 2T9; Cal'07; Staff, Foothills Medical Centre; (403)944-1110

KENNY, Lisa P; Univ Hlth Network-Toronto Western Hosp, MC2 411H-399 Bathurst St, Toronto ON M5T 2S8; Mem'01; FRCPC; IntMed; Critical Care Medicine. Staff, Toronto Western Hospital - University Health Network; (416)603-5800

KENNY, Patrick; Medical Arts Bldg, 400-1105 Pandora Ave, Victoria BC V8V 3P9; Galway (Ireland)'70; DABD; FRCPC; Derm. Staff, Capital Health Region; Clinical Asst Prof, University of British Columbia; (250)592-2422; Fax. (250)381-2422.

KENNY, Paul E; C01-310 Bridge St W, Napanee ON K7R 0A4; Tor'77; CCFP; FCFP; Ac Staff, Lennox & Addington County General Hospital; Clinical Asst Prof Family Med, Queen's University; (613)354-9648; Fax. (613)354-7435.

KENNY, William F; Queen's University, 146 Stuart St, Kingston ON K7L 3N6; McG'61; (613)533-2508

KENNY-SCHERBER, A Claire; Refuge Centre for Newcomer, 183 Hughson St S, Hamilton ON L8N 2B6; McM'08; CCFP; Staff, The Brant Community Healthcare System - Brantford General Hospital Site; (519)751-5544

KENSCOFF, Jean-Michel; Clinique Med Saint-Luc, 264 boul Saint-Luc, St-Jean-Sur-Richel QC J2W 1C3; Sher'88; Staff, Hôpital du Haut-Richelieu; (450)348-6124; Fax. (450)348-4163.

KENSHOLE, Anne B; Royal Health Centre, 130 Adelaide St W, Toronto ON M5H 3P5; London (England)'61; MB BS; FACP; FRCPC; IntMed (Diabetes). Emeritus Prof, University of Toronto; (416)361-6142; Fax. (416)361-1200; annekenshole@gmail.com.

KENT, Blaine A; Queen Elizabeth II HSC-Halifax, 1796 Summer St, Halifax NS B3H 3A7; Dal'97; FRCPC; Anes. Staff, Queen Elizabeth II Health Sciences Centre - Halifax Infirmary Site; (902)473-4326

KENT, David A; 1602-318 26 Ave SW, Calgary AB T2S 2T9; Mem'82; FRCPC; Anes (Clinical). (403)943-3410; dkentmd@shaw.ca.

KENT, David C; Archdekin Med Group, PO Box 660 Stn Main 205 Hiram St, Bracebridge ON P1L 1T9; Glasgow (Scotland)'68; MB ChB; CCFP; FCFP; Ac Staff, South Muskoka Memorial Hospital - Muskoka Algonquin Healthcare; (705)645-2223; Fax. (705)645-2342.

KENT, Jerrod S; 2A-800 Southdown Rd, Mississauga ON L5J 4H8; Sask'07; FRCPC; Ophth. (905)822-2020

KENT, Kimberley; Credit Valley Family Hlth Team, 101-2300 Eglinton Ave W, Mississauga ON L5M 2V8; Tor'07; CCFP; (905)813-3850

KENT, Lara C; Centretown Comm Health Centre, 420 Cooper St, Ottawa ON K2P 2N6; Man'02; CCFP; (613)233-4697

KENT, Lenore J; Manotick Medical Centre, 5492 South River Dr, Manotick ON K4M 1J3; McM'86; CCFP; FCFP; (613)692-2571; Fax. (613)692-0271.

KENT, Nancy E; BC Women's Hosp & Health Ctre, 2H35-4500 Oak St, Vancouver BC V6H 3N1; Tor'81; BSc; FRCSC; ObstGyn (Maternal Fetal Medicine). Staff, BC Women's Hospital & Health Centre; Clin Assoc Prof Med, University of British Columbia; (604)875-2021; nkent@cw.bc.ca.

KENT, Rebecca; Marathon Family Health Team, PO Box 399 22 Peninsula Rd, Marathon ON P0T 2E0; Tor'08; CCFP; (807)229-3243

KENT, Shefalee; A2-800 Southdown Rd, Mississauga ON L5J 2Y4; Sask'05; FRCSC; Ophth. (905)822-2020

KENT, Steven N; 302-4420 Chatterton Way, Victoria BC V8X 5J2; Man'76; BSc; FRCPC; Peds (Cystic Fibrosis). Staff, Victoria General Hospital; Consultant, Tofino General Hospital; Clinical Asst Prof Peds, University of British Columbia; (250)727-2156; Fax. (250)727-2143.

KENTNER, Taryn; Georgian Bay Gen Hosp, PO Box 760 1112 St Andrews Dr, Midland ON L4R 4P4; Wes'08; CCFP; Staff, Georgian Bay General Hospital - Midland; (705)526-1300

KENTS, Ilmar J; Brant Community HC-Brantford, 200 Terrace Hill St, Brantford ON N3R 1G9; Ott'73; Staff, The Brant Community Healthcare System - Brantford General Hospital Site; Med Dir, Tranquility Place; Langs: Spanish; (519)752-7871

KENTS, Kersti; South Muskoka Mem Hosp, 75 Ann St, Bracebridge ON P1L 2E4; McM'03; CCFP; CCFP(E.M.); Staff, South Muskoka Memorial Hospital - Muskoka Algonquin Healthcare; (705)645-4404

KENWORTHY, Christopher P; York Prof Bldg, 206-679 Davis Dr, Newmarket ON L3Y 5G8; Liverpool (England)'71; DObstRCOG; MB ChB; DCH; CCFP; Ac Staff, Southlake Regional Health Centre; (905)898-2211; Fax. (905)830-0224.

KENYON, Christopher R; Royal University Hosp, 103 Hospital Dr, Saskatoon SK S7N 0W8; Dal'97; BSc; FRCSC; GenSurg (Colon & Rectal Surgery). Staff Surg, Royal University Hospital; (306)966-8134

KENYON, Cynthia F; London HSC-Victoria Hosp, PO Box 5010 Stn B D4 204-800 Commissioners Rd E, London ON N6A 5W9; Sask'75; FRCPC; Peds (Neonatology). Staff, St Joseph's Hospital - St Joseph's Health Care; Consultant, London Health Sciences Centre - University Hospital; Staff, London Health Sciences Centre - Victoria Campus; Assoc Prof Peds, University of Western Ontario; (519)685-8500 x64361; ckenyon@uwo.ca.

KENYON, Gregory J; 179 Ontario Rd PO Box 10, Mitchell ON N0K 1N0; Wes'87; CCFP; FCFP; (519)348-8797; Fax. (519)348-8756.

KENYON, Jennifer A; 202-2190 West Railway St, Abbotsford BC V2S 2E2; UBC'02; FRCSC; ObstGyn. (604)859-7725

KENYON, Jolene C; Lloydminster Clinic, 5120 46 St, Lloydminster AB T9V 2P7; Sask'05; BSc(Hon); CCFP; (780)875-2221; Fax. (780)875-0605.

KENYON, Michael R; 500-4634 Park Ave, Terrace BC V8G 1V7; Witwatersrand (South Africa)'82; FRCPC; IntMed (Endocrinology). Med Staff, Nanaimo Regional General Hospital; Langs: Afrikaans; Dutch; Italian; Zulu; (250)615-5088

KEOGH, Brendan G; Norwood Med Clinic, PO Box 370 31 King St, Norwood ON K0L 2V0; Dublin (Ireland)'81; BAO; Court Staff, Campbellford Memorial Hospital; (705)639-2245; Fax. (705)639-2764.

KEOGH, Ciaran F; Brooke Radiology Associates, 5791 No. 3 Rd, Richmond BC V6X 2C9; Dublin (Ireland)'93; FRCPC; DiagRad. Staff, BC Cancer Agency Vancouver Centre; (604)278-9151

KEOGH, J Thomas; 2-100 Peel Centre Dr, Brampton ON L6T 4G8; Tor'74; CCBOM; FCBOM; CCFP; FCFP; Court Staff, The Hospital For Sick Children; Court Staff, Toronto Western Hospital - University Health Network; Court Staff, The Credit Valley Hospital; Court Staff, Cambridge Memorial Hospital; Physician, Air Canada; Physician Occupational Hlth, Enbridge Gas Distribution Inc; Physician, Darlington Nuclear; (416)231-7363; dr.jtkeogh@gmail.com.

KEOGH, Kelly A; The Hosp For Sick Children, 555 University Ave, Toronto ON M5G 1X8; Wes'92; FRCPC; Peds (Emergency Medicine). Staff Ped EmergMed, The Hospital For Sick Children; Asst Prof Peds, University of Toronto; (416)813-8950; Fax. (416)813-5043; kelly.keogh@sickkids.ca.

KEOHANE, John D; 11122 142 St NW, Edmonton AB T5M 4G5; Alb'83; FRCSC; Otol. (780)428-7824; Fax. (780)425-1527.

KEOUGH, Gregory G; Gateway Med Clinic, 950-3803 Calgary Trail NW, Edmonton AB T6J 5M8; Cal'95; (780)436-7240; Fax. (780)436-8142.

KEOUGH, Michael; Notre Dame Bay Mem Hlth Ctre, GD Hospital Lane, Twillingate NL A0G 4M0; Mem'08; CCFP; Staff, Notre Dame Bay Memorial Health Centre; (709)884-2131; keough@mun.ca.

KEOUGH, Valerie J; Queen Elizabeth II HSC, 1276 South Park St, Halifax NS B3H 2Y9; Mem'99; FRCPC; DiagRad. Staff, Queen Elizabeth II Health Sciences Centre - Victoria General Site; (902)473-2700

KEOUGH-RYAN, Tammy M; Dickson Bldg, 5097-5820 University Ave, Halifax NS B3H 1V7; Mem'95; BMedSci; MSc; CSPQ; FRCPC; IntMed (Transplant Nephrology); Nephrol. Prog Dir Nephrol/Assoc Prof, Dalhousie University; (902)473-4612; Fax. (902)473-2675; tammy.keough-ryan@cdha.nshealth.ca.

KEOWN, Paul A; Vancouver Gen Hosp, JP1-855 12th Ave W, Vancouver BC V5Z 1M9; Manchester (England)'70; MB ChB; FRCP(Lond); FACP; MD; MBA; DSc; FASN; FRC; FRCPC; IntMed (Immunology). Dir Immunology, Vancouver General Hospital - Centennial Pavillion; Vis Staff, Providence Health Care - St Paul's Hospital; Prof/Head Nephrology, University of British Columbia; (604)875-4393; keown@interchange.ubc.ca.

KEPRON, Charis A; The Ottawa Hosp-Gen Campus, 501 Smyth Rd, Ottawa ON K1H 8L6; Tor'04; FRCPC; AnatPath (Forensic Pathology). Staff, The Ottawa Hospital - General Campus; (613)737-8860

KEPRON, M Wayne; Respiratory Hosp, RS 319-810 Sherbrook St, Winnipeg MB R3A 1R8; Man'67; BSc(Med); FRCPC; IntMed (Respirology). Consultant Med/Att Staff Manitoba Lung Transplant Prog & Adult Cystic Fibrosis Prog, Health Sciences Centre; Prof Med/Asst Prof, University of Manitoba; (204)787-2338; Fax. (204)787-2420; wkepron@exchange.hsc.mb.ca.

KER, Katherine J; North York Gen Hosp, 4S-4001 Leslie St, North York ON M2K 1E1; Tor'09; CCFP; Staff, North York General Hospital; (416)756-6980; Fax. (416)756-6979.

KERAMETLIAN, Vatche; 403-2299 Dundas St W, Toronto ON M6R 1X7; Yerevan (Russia (Federation))'69; Ac Staff, St Joseph's Health Centre; (416)533-7748

KERBA, Jean-Paul; CSSS du Sud de Lanaudière, 911 montee des Pionniers, Terrebonne QC J6V 2H2; Mon'09; CCFP; Staff, Centre Hospitalier Pierre le Gardeur; (450)654-7525

KERBY, Karmen H; Devon Med Clinic, 5-106 Erie St S, Devon AB T9G 1A7; Alb'06; CCFP; (780)987-3315; Fax. (780)987-4009.

KERBY, Lilli D; 2067 Columbia Ave PO Box 404, Rossland BC V0G 1Y0; UBC'05; CCFP; (250)362-9040

KEREN, Arieh; Univ of Ottawa Heart Institute, H1285-40 Ruskin St, Ottawa ON K1Y 4W7; Melbourne (Australia)'96; Staff, University of Ottawa Heart Institute; (613)761-4059; Fax. (613)761-4877.

KEREN, Ron; Toronto Rehabilitation Institu, 550 University Ave, Toronto ON M5G 2A2; Tel Aviv (Israel)'86; FRCPC; Psy (Geriatric Psychiatry). Consultant, Toronto Rehabilitation Institute - University Centre; Consultant, Ontario Shores Centre for Mental Health Sciences; Asst Prof, University of Toronto; Langs: Hebrew; (416)597-3422; Fax. (416)597-0836.

KERFOOT, Karin E; London HSC-University Hosp, PO Bix 5010 Snt B B8 110 800 Commissioners Rd E, London ON N6A 5W9; Cal'01; FRCPC; Psy. Staff, London Health Sciences Centre - Victoria Campus.

KERGOAT, Marie-Jeanne; Inst U Geriatrie De Montreal, 4565 ch Queen-Mary, Montreal QC H3W 1W5; Sher'78; FRCPC; GeriatricMed;CCFP; FCFP; Chief Dept of Med Spec, Institut Universitaire de Gériatrie de Montréal; assoc Prof Med, Universite de Montreal; (514)340-3515; Fax. (514)340-2832; marie-jeanne.kergoat@umontreal.ca.

KERIN, Noel A; KOHC, 1002-3266 Yonge St, Toronto ON M4N 3P6; National (Ireland)'68; BSc(Hons Physiol); MSc(OccupMed); CCBOM; CBC/PWU Union/Global Round Table on Addictions & Mental Hlth. & Phys., Dept. of Nat'l. Defense-Mohawk College; (416)488-2900; Fax. (416)440-8274.

KERKERIAN, Eric J; Ctr Hosp du Centre la Mauricie, 50 119e rue, Shawinigan-Sud QC G9P 5K1; Mon'82; IntMed. Staff, Centre Hospitalier du Centre la Mauricie; (819)536-7500; Fax. (819)536-7611.

KERKHOFF, Ross V; Moosomin Family Practice Ctre, PO Box 1528, Moosomin SK S0G 3N0; Stellenbosch (South Africa)'91; MB ChB; LMCC; CCFP; (306)435-3838; Fax. (306)435-2176.

KERLEY, Brian K; Garden City Family Health Team, 145 Carlton St, St Catharines ON L2R 1R5; McM'81; CCFP; FCFP; Ac Staff, Niagara Health System - St Catharines General Site; (905)988-1352; Fax. (905)988-1201.

KERLIS, Thomas E; Lloydminster Clinic, 5120 46 St, Lloydminster AB T9V 2P7; Stellenbosch (South Africa)'89; MB ChB; Ac Staff, Lloydminster Hospital; Langs: German; Afrikaans; (780)875-2221; Fax. (780)875-0605; thomaskerlis@excite.com.

KERLOW, Thomas N; Agincourt Med Centre, 2020 Brimley Rd, Scarborough ON M1S 4R7; Tor'84; CCFP; FCFP; Staff, Rouge Valley Health System - Centenary Health Centre Site; Staff, The Scarborough Hospital - General Campus; Staff, The Scarborough Hospital - Birchmount Campus; (416)293-2404

KERNAGHAN, Gillian A J; St Joseph's Health Care, PO Box 5777 Stn B 268 Grosvenor St, London ON N6A 4V2; Wes'82; CCFP; FCFP; (519)646-6100 x64200; Fax. (519)646-6054; gillian.kernaghan@sjhc.london.on.ca.

KERNAHAN, Jill; Family Medicine, 1190 Hornby St, Vancouver BC V6Z 2K5; Man'76; BSc(Med); CCFP; FCFP; Prog Dir Family Residency Prog/Assoc Dean Postgraduate Med Education (Interim), University of British Columbia; (604)806-8444; kernahan@familymed.ubc.ca.

KERNER, Cecilia M; Perth-Smith Falls Dist hosp, 60 Cornelia St W, Smiths Falls ON K7A 2H9; Wes'02; FRCSC; ObstGyn. Staff, Perth & Smiths Falls District Hospital - Smiths Falls Site; (613)283-2330; Fax. (613)283-0048.

KERNER, Sarah N; Greene Family Med Group, 800-1310 av Greene, Montreal QC H3Z 2B2; McG'08; CCFP; (514)780-2222

KEROUAC, Marcel; Ctr Hosp De Verdun, 4000 boul Lasalle, Verdun QC H4G 2A3; Sher'80; NuclearMed (P.Q.). Staff, Centre Hospitalier de Verdun; (514)765-7305

KERR, Charles R; 211-1033 Davie St, Vancouver BC V6E 1M7; UBC'73; FRCPC; IntMed (Electrophysiology); Cardiol. Ac Staff Cardiol, Providence Health Care - St Paul's Hospital; Consultant, Vancouver General Hospital - Centennial Pavillion; Prof Cardiol, University of British Columbia; (604)806-8517; Fax. (604)806-8723; ckerr@providencehealth.bc.ca.

KERR, Clifford G; Forensic Clinic, 300-307 Broadway W, Vancouver BC V5Y 1P8; Queen's (Ireland)'69; MB ChB; DPM(Eng); MRCPsy(Eng); FRCPC; Psy. Staff Psy, Providence Health Care - St Paul's Hospital; Clin Instructor, University of British Columbia; (604)529-3350

KERR, D Robert; Hamilton HS-Gen Site, 237 Barton St E, Hamilton ON L8L 2X2; Ott'93; CCFP; CCFP(E.M.); FCFP; Staff, Hamilton Health Sciences Centre - Hamilton General Hospital; (905)527-0271

KERR, Darren; Saint John Reg Hosp, PO Box 2100 Stn Main, Saint John NB E2L 4L2; Dal'94; FRCSC; OrthSurg (Arthroplasty). Staff, Saint John Regional Hospital; Asst Prof, Memorial University Of Newfoundland; Asst Prof, Dalhousie University; (506)648-7872; Fax. (506)648-7874.

KERR, Ernest; Health Care Unit, 550 Gerrard St E, Toronto ON M4M 1X6; Ott'70; Ac Staff, The Scarborough Hospital - General Campus; Ac Staff, Rouge Valley Health System - Centenary Health Centre Site; Med. officer, Toronto Don Jail; (416)325-4444; Fax. (416)325-3284.

KERR, Jonathan R; Belleville Queen's Univ-FMC, 202-145 Station St, Belleville ON K8N 2S9; Tor'06; CCFP; (613)771-1910; Fax. (613)771-1016.

KERR, Kathleen J; Medical & Dental Bldg, 710-1849 Yonge St, Toronto ON M4S 1Y2; Tor'71; DEH; Staff Physician, Women's College Hospital; Lecturer Family & Commun Med, University of Toronto; (416)489-4445

KERR, Larry C; 815 High St, Peterborough ON K9J 8J9; Wes'73; Staff, Peterborough Regional Health Centre - Hospital Drive; Staff, Peterborough Regional Health Centre - Rogers St Site; (705)749-2391

KERR, Leanne A; The Youth Centre, 5-360 Bayly St W, Ajax ON L1S 1P1; Tor'89; BSc; CCFP; (905)428-1212; Fax. (905)428-9151.

KERR, Lorraine M R; Provencher Pediatrics, 103-147 Provencher Blvd, Winnipeg MB R2H 0G2; Man'87; FRCPC; Peds. Assoc Staff, Health Sciences Centre; Assoc Staff, St Boniface General Hospital; University of Manitoba; Langs: English; French.

KERR, Mary; Sudbury Reg Hosp-Laurentian Si, 41 Ramsey Lake Rd, Sudbury ON P3E 5J1; Wes'03; FRCPC; IntMed; Critical Care Medicine. Staff, Health Sciences North-Laurentian Site; (705)522-2200

KERR, PJK Peter J; 1601 Whiteside Way RR 2, Metcalfe ON K0A 2P0; Glasgow (Scotland)'65; DPsy; DABPN; FRCPC; Psy (Psychoanalysis). Consultant, The Ottawa Hospital - Civic Campus; Member, Canadian Psychoanalytic Society; University of Ottawa; (613)224-3777; Fax. (613)821-0970; pjkerrmd@hotmail.com.

KERR, Paul A; 103-426 Talbot St, St Thomas ON N5P 1B9; Sask'96; FRCPC; Peds. Staff Peds, St Thomas Elgin General Hospital; Prof Peds, University of Western Ontario; paulkerr@hotmail.com.

KERR, Paul B; 203-640 Prospect St, Fredericton NB E3B 9M7; Mem'86; CCFP; FCFP; Assoc Staff Family Med, Dr Everett Chalmers Regional Hospital; (506)459-8580; Fax. (506)450-2946.

KERR, Paul D; Health Sciences Centre, GB421-820 Sherbrook St, Winnipeg MB R3A 1R9; Man'87; BSc; FRCSC; Otol (Head & Neck Surgery & Oncology). Assoc Staff, St Boniface General Hospital; Assoc Prof Residency/Dept Head Otol, University of Manitoba; (204)787-3349; Fax. (204)787-1727; pkerr@exchange.hsc.mb.ca.

KERR, Pauline E; Appletree Clinic, 2573 Baseline Rd, Ottawa ON K2H 7B3; McM'96; BSc(Hon); MSc; ABPeds; ABAAI; FRCPC; Peds; ClinImmunol&Allergy. Consultant, Children's Hospital of Eastern Ontario (CHEO); Physician, Appletree Med Group; Langs: Bilingual(English/French); (613)482-0118; Fax. (613)288-2060.

KERR, Roderick G; 201-1131 Nottinghill Gate, Oakville ON L6M 1K5; Belfast (Ireland)'69; DObstRCOG; FAAFP; CCFP; FCFP; Hd Physician, North Oakville Family Health Group; (905)815-9090; Fax. (905)815-1834; rodhikes@yahoo.ca.

KERR, Sarah K; The Credit Valley Hosp, 2200 Eglinton Ave W, Mississauga ON L5M 2N1; Dal'92; CCFP; CCFP(E.M.); Staff Emerg, The Credit Valley Hospital; (905)813-4530

KERR, Thomas A W; Peterborough Clinic FHT, LL03-26 Hospital Dr, Peterborough ON K9J 7C3; Qns'69; (705)740-6817; Fax. (705)740-6520.

KERRIE, Jeffrey P; Royal Columbian Hosp, 330 Columbia St E, New Westminster BC V3L 3W7; Man'08; FRCPC; IntMed. Staff, Royal Columbian Hospital; (604)520-4253

KERRIGAN, Scott A; North Bay Reg Health Centre, 50 College St, North Bay ON P1B 0A4; Wes'98; FRCPC; GenPath. Staff, North Bay Regional Health Centre - Regional Mental Health; (705)474-8600; kerris@nbgh.on.ca.

KERRY, Marie-Paule; PO Box 2003, Lameque NB E8T 3N3; Laval'88; Langs: Bilingual(French/English); (506)344-2518; Fax. (506)344-8409.

KERS, Albert A; 7-3250 60 St NE, Calgary AB T1Y 3T5; (Other Foreign)'94; (403)293-5600; Fax. (403)285-6478.

KERSWELL, Philip; 46 Stanley Rd PO Box 948, Lake Cowichan BC V0R 2G0; Manchester (England)'75; MB ChB; DRCOG; BSc(St.Andrews,Scot.); (250)749-4114; Fax. (250)749-0120; a.kerswell@shaw.ca.

KERTES, Peter J; Sunnybrook Hlth Sciences Ctre, M1 202A-2075 Bayview Ave, Toronto ON M4N 3M5; McG'91; FRCSC; Ophth (Retina Vitreous Surgery). Staff, Sunnybrook Health Sciences Centre; Staff, The Hospital For Sick Children; Assoc Prof, University of Toronto; Aj Prof, University of Ottawa; Langs: French; Hungarian; (416)480-5280; Fax. (416)480-4481.

KERTESZ, Andrew; 39 Doncaster Ave, London ON N6G 2A1; Qns'60; FRCPC; IntMed (Brain Trauma); Neur. Prof Clin Neurological Sciences, University of Western Ontario; (519)471-6088; Fax. (519)646-6226.

KERWIN, Larkin; Clinique des Med d'Urgence, 632 rue Bowen S, Sherbrooke QC J1G 2E9; Laval'78; Chef méd urgence, Centre Hospitalier Universitaire de Sherbrooke-Hôpital Hôtel-Dieu; Clin Assoc Prof, Universite de Sherbrooke; (819)822-2700; Fax. (819)822-2027; direction@cmu.qc.ca.

KERWIN, Stephanie A; 110-10333 Southport Rd SW, Calgary AB T2W 3X6; Ott'05; CCFP; (403)258-1960

KERYAKES, Hany; Clinique Med Samson, 202-4599 boul Samson, Laval QC H7W 2H2; (Egypt)'80; Staff, Centre de L'Annonciation; (450)688-7170

KESAVAN, Vinod; 203-3030 Lincoln Ave, Coquitlam BC V3B 6B4; Mysore (India)'77; MB BS; DCH; ABPeds; FAAP; AB(Neonatal&Perinatal); FRCPC; Peds (Neonatology). Staff/Chief Peds, Royal Columbian Hospital; (604)942-1119; Fax. (604)942-1129.

KESCHTKAR, Nicholas; Dr Everett Chalmers Reg Hosp, PO Box 9000 Stn A, Fredericton NB E3B 5N5; Giessen (Germany)'94; Staff, Dr Everett Chalmers Regional Hospital; (506)452-5400

KESES, Natalie; Queensway-Carleton Hosp, 3045 Baseline Rd, Nepean ON K2H 8P4; Wes'98; FRCPC; IntMed (Cardiology). Ac Staff, Queensway Carleton Hospital; (613)721-4842; Fax. (613)721-4785.

KESHAV, Dattatri L; Regional Mental HC-St Thomas, PO Box 2004 Stn Main 467 Sunset Dr, St Thomas ON N5P 3V9; Mysore (India)'65; MB BS; DPM(Lond); BSc; FRCPC; Psy (General Adult Psychiatry). Staff, Regional Mental Health Care-St Joseph's Health Care; Langs: Kanarese; (519)455-5110

KESHAVARZI, Gholamreza; Capilano Clinic, 85-935 Marine Dr, North Vancouver BC V7P 1S7; (Other Foreign)'09; CCFP; Staff, Pacific Medical Clinic; Staff, Park Royal Medical Clinic; Langs: Farsi; (604)988-3441

KESHAVJEE, Al-Noor M; Milliken Med Centre, 17-5651 Steeles Ave E, Scarborough ON M1V 5P6; Wes'97; BSc; CCFP; (416)291-6323; Fax. (416)291-0890.

KESHAVJEE, Fatehalli C; Fairview Mall, 344-1800 Sheppard Ave E, North York ON M2J 5A7; Dublin (Ireland)'60; LRCS; LRCP; MD; (416)491-0057; Fax. (416)491-3776.

KESHAVJEE, Hassenali C; Fairview Mall, 344-1800 Sheppard Ave E, North York ON M2J 5A7; Witwatersrand (South Africa)'50; MB ChB; DCH; (416)491-0042; Fax. (416)491-3776.

KESHAVJEE, Karim; Queentario Med Centre, 4B-2325 Hurontario St, Mississauga ON L5A 4C7; Tor'93; MSc; MBA; CCFP; Assoc Member, Centre for Evaluation of Med; (905)270-8307; Fax. (905)270-6861; karim@infoclin.ca.

KESHAVJEE, Shaf; Univ Hlth Network-Toronto Gen, 9N 946-200 Elizabeth St, Toronto ON M5G 2C4; Tor'85; MSc; DABS; DABTS; MRCS; MCPS; FRCSC; FACS; GenSurg (Medical Oncology); CardiothorSurg. Staff Surg, The Hospital For Sick Children; Hd Div of Thoracic Surg, Toronto General Hospital - UHN; Sr Scientist, Princess Margaret Hospital - University Health Network; Dir, Thoracic Surgery Research Laboratory; Prof & Chair, Div of Thoracic Surg, University of Toronto; Dir, Toronto Lung Transplant Program; (416)340-4010; Fax. (416)340-4556.

KESHAVJEE, Yasmin; Erie St Clair Clinic, 1574 Lincoln Rd, Windsor ON N8Y 2J4; McM'92; CCFP; (519)977-9772

KESHEN, Aaron R; Abbie J Lane Mem Bldg, 7F-5909 Veterans Memorial Lane, Halifax NS B3H 2E2; Dal'04; Psy. (902)473-2488

KESHMIRI, Mehdi; 202-2151 Mccallum Rd, Abbotsford BC V2S 3N8; Alb'80; FCCP; FRCPC; IntMed (Respirology). Staff Respirol, Mission Memorial Hospital; (604)853-8810; Fax. (604)853-8820.

KESHMIRIAN, Jalal; 102-140 Oxford St E, London ON N6A 5R9; Wes'93; BSc(Hons); PhD; CCFP; Assoc Staff, London Health Sciences Centre - Victoria Campus; Aj Prof, University of Western Ontario; Aj Prof Fac of Medicine, University of Toronto; Langs: French; (519)433-4999; jay.keshmirian@lhsc.on.ca.

KESHOOFY, Mohammad; Carmen Vanderwater Med Ctr, PO Box 382 Stn Main 33-180 Parsons Rd, Alliston ON L9R 1V6; Tehran (Iran)'90; FACS; MCR; FRCSC; GenSurg. Langs: Farsi; (705)435-0391

KESHVARA, A Muru; Southview Clinic, 2-1364 Southview Dr SE, Medicine Hat AB T1B 4E7; London (England)'76; MRCS; LRCP; DA(Eng.); CCFP; FCFP; Staff Privil, Medicine Hat Regional Hospital; (403)527-1233; Fax. (403)528-9774.

KESKINEN, Helen; Clinique Med Notre-Dame, 138 rue Notre-Dame S, Sainte-Marie QC G6E 4A4; Laval'80; (418)387-5200; Fax. (418)387-5283; helen_keskinen@ssss.gouv.qc.ca.

KESSARAM, Robert A; 75 Golfdale Rd, Brantford ON N3T 5H8; McG'73; BSc; FACS; CAB; FRC; DrMedCh; FRCSC; GenSurg. Consultant, The Brant Community Healthcare System - Brantford General Hospital Site; Vis Staff, Hamilton Health Sciences Centre - McMaster Children's Hospital.

KESSEL, Brian R; The West Mall Health Centre, 1-290 The West Mall, Etobicoke ON M9C 1C6; Tor'80; Ac Staff Family Pract, Trillium Health Centre - West Toronto; Court Staff Family Pract, Humber River Regional Hospital - Keele Street Site; (416)621-4461; Fax. (416)620-7476.

KESSELMAN, Edward W; Seven Oaks Gen Hosp, 2300 Mcphillips St, Winnipeg MB R2V 3M3; Man'75; Staff, Seven Oaks General Hospital; (204)632-7133; Fax. (204)694-8276.

KESSELMAN, Murray S; Children's Hosp, JL369-840 Sherbrook St, Winnipeg MB R3A 1R9; Man'74; AB(Critical Care); FRCPC; Peds (Pediatric Critical Care). Dir Ped ICU, Health Sciences Centre; Staff, Children's Hospital of Winnipeg; Assoc Prof Peds & Child Health, University of Manitoba; (204)787-4239; mkesselman@hsc.mb.ca.

KESSIE, Atiemo; Etobicoke Urgent Care Clinic, 10-25 Woodbine Downs Blvd, Etobicoke ON M9W 6N5; Wes'97; CCFP; CCFP(E.M.); (416)741-2273; Fax. (416)741-3542.

KESTENBAUM, Deborah S; Yonge-Eglinton Med Centre, 204-2401 Yonge St, Toronto ON M4P 3H1; McG'90; CCFP; FCFP; Court Staff, Women's College Hospital; (416)485-2222; Fax. (416)485-2276.

KESTER-GREENE, Nicole; Sunnybrook Hlth Sciences Ctre, 2075 Bayview Ave, Toronto ON M4N 3M5; Ott'98; FRCPC; EmergMed. Staff, Sunnybrook Health Sciences Centre; (416)480-6100; Fax. (416)480-4704.

KESTLE, John R W; 3100-910 10th Ave W, Vancouver BC V5Z 4E3; Wes'84; BSc; MSc; FRCSC; Neursurg (Pediatric Neuro Surgery). (604)875-4136

KESTLER, Andrew M; St Paul's Hosp, 1081 Burrard St, Vancouver BC V6Z 1Y6; Pennsylvania (USA)'99; FRCPC; EmergMed. Staff, Providence Health Care - St Paul's Hospital; (604)806-8480

KESTLER, Mary H; BC Women's Hosp & Health Ctre, 4500 Oak St, Vancouver BC V6H 3N1; (Other Foreign)'01; Staff, BC Women's Hospital & Health Centre; (604)875-2424

KESTY, Kenneth R; Near North Med Clinic, 1-66 Josephine St, North Bay ON P1B 0A7; Rochester(MN) (USA)'80; FRCSC; Ophth. Staff, North Bay Regional Health Centre - Regional Mental Health; (705)472-4782; Fax. (705)472-1848.

KESZTHELYI, Eniko J; Royal Columbia Hosp, 330 Columbia St E, New Westminster BC V3L 3W7; Tor'02; CCFP; CCFP(E.M.); Staff, Royal Columbian Hospital; (604)520-4001; Fax. (604)520-4069.

KETABI, Salma; Surrey Mem Hosp, 13750 96 Ave, Surrey BC V3V 1Z2; (Iran)'97; FRCPC; Anes. Staff, Surrey Memorial Hospital; (604)581-2211

KETCH, James E; Guisachan Family Medicine, 105-2395 Gordon Ave, Kelowna BC V1W 3X7; UBC'90; CCFP; CCFP(E.M.); (250)861-3235; Fax. (250)861-3448.

KETCHIAN, Leon V; Centre Med Lacoraire, 201-5650 rue Jean-Talon E, Saint-Leonard QC H1S 1M1; Cairo (Egypt)'70; CSPQ; FRCSC; ObstGyn. Ac Staff, Hôpital Santa Cabrini Ospedale; (514)255-5595; Fax. (514)255-8550.

KETENE, Atila H; 206-2678 Broadway W, Vancouver BC V6K 2G3; Dal'80; Clin Prof, University of British Columbia; (604)737-2699

KETTLE, Charles A; 1493 Paris St, Sudbury ON P3E 3B7; Ott'89; FRCSC; PlasSurg (Cosmetic Surgery). Assoc Prof, Northern Ontario School of Medicine-Laurentian University; (705)673-5035; Fax. (705)673-5931.

KETTLER, Jack J; St Boniface Gen Hosp, M5-409 Tache Ave, Winnipeg MB R2H 2A6; Man'91; FRCPC; Psy. Staff, St Boniface General Hospital; (204)233-8563

KETTLES, M Jane; Toronto East Gen Hosp Inc, 825 Coxwell Ave, Toronto ON M4C 3E7; McM'75; FRCPC; Anes. Staff, Toronto East General Hospital Inc; Court. Lect., University of Toronto; (416)461-8272 x6212; Fax. (416)469-6874.

KETTNER, Adrian S; Psychealth Centre, PX161-771 Bannatyne Ave, Winnipeg MB R3E 3N4; Man'77; FRCPC; Psy.

KETTNER, Joel D; Manitoba Health, 4004-300 Carlton St, Winnipeg MB R3B 3M9; Man'76; MSc(Epidemiol.,Lond.); CommunMed; GenSurg (Travel Medicine). Att Staff CommunMed, Health Sciences Centre; Med Officer of Hlth, Winnipeg Community & Long Term Care Authority; Chief Med Officer of Hlth, Manitoba Health; Asst Prof Commun Health Sciences, University of Manitoba; (204)788-6766; Fax. (204)948-2204; joel.kettner@gov.mb.ca.

KETTOUCHE, Louiza; Clinique Med Belanger, 300-3871 rue Belanger, Montreal QC H1X 3M7; (Algeria)'75; (514)722-1166; Fax. (514)722-6022.

KEU, Khun Visith; CHUS-Hop Fleurimont, 3001 12e ave N, Sherbrooke QC J1H 5N4; Mon'05; FRCPC; NuclearMed. Staff, Centre Hospitalier Universitaire de Sherbrooke-Hopital Fleurimont; (819)346-1110

KEU, Nita; CLSC Riviere-des-Prairies, 8655 boul Perras, Montreal QC H1E 4M7; Sher'07; CCFP; (514)494-4924

KEUHL, Jonathan R; ADMG Group Hlth Centre, 240 McNabb St, Sault Ste. Marie ON P6B 1Y5; Massachussetts (USA)'05; FRCPC; Peds. (705)759-5540

KEUNEN, Johannes E G M; Ontario Power Generation Bldg, 3267-700 University Ave, Toronto ON M5G 1Z5; Maastricht (Netherlands)'91; (416)586-4800 x8513

KEVORK, Raymond B; Bay Coll Med & Lockwood Diag, 320-790 Bay St, Toronto ON M5G 1N8; Cairo (Egypt)'60; MB ChB; FRCPC; IntMed (Diabetes). Court Staff, Women's College Hospital; University of Toronto; (416)921-2121; Fax. (416)921-0569.

KEVORKIAN, Agavni; Ontario Shores Ctr Mental HS, 700 Gordon St, Whitby ON L1N 5S9; Russia (Russia (Federation))'74; FRCPC; Psy (Psychotherapy). Staff, Ontario Shores Centre for Mental Health Sciences; (905)668-5881 x6146; Fax. (905)430-4480.

KEVU, Joseph E; The Goodhouse Bldg, 300-93 West St, Corner Brook NL A2H 2Y6; (Benin)'81.

KEW, Andrea K; Queen Elizsabeth II HSC, 434-1276 South Park St, Halifax NS B3H 2Y9; Dal'01; FRCPC; IntMed; Hem. Staff, Queen Elizabeth II Health Sciences Centre - Victoria General Site; (902)473-4642

KEY, Fiona M; MUHC-Montreal Children's Hosp, 2300 rue Tupper, Montreal QC H3H 1P3; Glasgow (Scotland)'70; MB ChB; MRCP(UK); FRCPC; Peds (Child & Adolescent Psychiatry); Psy. Staff Outpatient Psy, McGill University Health Centre - Montreal Children's Hospital; adj Prof Psy & Peds, McGill University; Langs: Bilingual(French/English); (514)412-4449

KEY, Siobhan L; 908-299 Victoria St, Prince George BC V2L 5B8; UBC'04; CCFP; CCFP(E.M.); (250)563-4706

KEYES, G Elizabeth; 661 Dever Rd, Saint John NB E2M 4J2; Dal'89; (506)635-8727

KEYES, Mira; BC Cancer Agency-Vancouver CC, 600 10th Ave W, Vancouver BC V5Z 4E6; Novi Sad (Serbia)'86; FRCPC; RadOncol (Genito Urinary Oncology). Staff, BC Cancer Agency Vancouver Centre; Assoc Prof RadOncol, University of British Columbia; (604)877-6000 x2660; Fax. (604)877-0505.

KEYES, Paul D; 661 Dever Rd, Saint John NB E2M 4J2; Mem'95; CCFP; CCFP(E.M.); (506)635-8727; Fax. (506)635-5951.

KEYES, Robert D; St Paul's Hosp, 2367-1081 Burrard St, Vancouver BC V6Z 1Y6; UBC'76; BSc; ABIM; FACP; FAANEM; FRSM; FRCPC; Neur (Clinical Neurophysiology). Dir EEG/ER/EML Laboratories, Providence Health Care - St Paul's Hospital; Associate EEG/Staff Consultant, Vancouver General Hospital - Centennial Pavillion; Associate EMG/Staff Consultant, BC Children's Hospital; Clin Prof Neurol, University of British Columbia; (604)806-8354; Fax. (604)806-8354.

KEYES, Robert E; Royal Alexandra Hosp, 541-10240 Kingsway NW, Edmonton AB T5H 3V9; Alb'02; FRCPC; EmergMed; Critical Care Medicine. Staff, Royal Alexandra Hospital; (780)735-5200

KEYES, Sean A; 661 Dever Rd, Saint John NB E2M 4J2; Dal'60; Ac Staff, St Joseph's Hospital; Ac Staff, Saint John Regional Hospital; Dalhousie University; (506)635-8727; Fax. (506)635-5951.

KEYES, Sean J; 661 Dever Rd, Saint John NB E2M 4J2; Mem'90; (506)635-8727; Fax. (506)635-5951; sjkeyes@nbnet.nb.ca.

KEYHAN, Nicola T; The Hosp for Sick Children, 555 University Ave, Toronto ON M5G 1X8; McM'00; FRCPC; Psy. Staff, Sunnybrook Health Sciences Centre; Staff, The Hospital For Sick Children; (416)813-5760

KEYNAN, Yoav; Basic Medical Sciences, 539-745 Bannatyne Ave, Winnipeg MB R3E 0J9; Beersheba (Israel)'95.

KEYSERLINGK, R. John R; Centre Medical Ville-Marie, 1000-1538 rue Sherbrooke O, Montreal QC H3G 1L5; Mon'72; MSc(Exp.Surg.); FACS; FRCSC; GenSurg (Head & Neck Surgery); Otol (P.Q.). Staff Surg, McGill University Health Centre - Montreal General Campus; Staff Surg, McGill University Health Centre - Royal Victoria Hospital; Dir Div of Gen Surg, St Mary's Hospital Centre; Asst Prof Surg, McGill University; Langs: French; (514)933-2778; Fax. (514)933-9635; info@villemariemed.com.

KEYSTON, Rebecca; Vendome Medical, 200-5175 rue de Maisonneuve O, Montreal QC H4A 1Z3; McG'07; MDCM; CCFP; (514)484-4712

KEYSTONE, Edward C; The Joseph & Wolf Lebovic Bldg, PO Box 4 2-006-60 Murray St, Toronto ON M5T 3L9; Tor'69; FRCPC; IntMed (Adult Rheumatology); Rheum. Rheumatologist, Mount Sinai Hospital; Prof Med, University of Toronto; (416)586-8646; Fax. (416)586-8766.

KEYSTONE, Jay; Univ Hlth Network-Toronto Gen, 13N 1347-200 Elizabeth St, Toronto ON M5G 2C4; Tor'69; MSc(CTM); FRCPC; IntMed (Tropical & Travel Medicine). Staff Physician Tropical Disease Unit, Toronto General Hospital - UHN; Dir, Medisys Travel Health Clinic; Prof Med1, University of Toronto; (416)340-3675; Fax. (416)340-3260.

KEYTER, Herman P; PO Box 704, Valemount BC V0E 2Z0; Pretoria (South Africa)'83; MB ChB; CCFP; (250)566-9138

KEYVANI, Leila; University Hosp of Northern BC, 1475 Edmonton St, Prince George BC V2M 1S2; '99; ABIM; FRCPC; IntMed; Gastroent. Staff, University Hospital of Northern British Columbia; Langs: Persian; Farsi; (604)996-9989

KEYZER, Yvonne J; Kimberley Med Clinic, PO Box 160, Kimberley BC V1A 2Y6; Tor'95; CCFP; FCFP; (250)427-4861; Fax. (250)427-2082.

KGOBISA, Lettie; Redvers Med Clinic, PO Box 30, Redvers SK S0C 2H0; Medunsa Medical University (South Africa)'95; (306)452-6362; Fax. (306)452-6317.

KHABAZEH, Youssef; CSSS du Nord de Lanaudière, 1000 boul Sainte-Anne, St-Charles-Brromee QC J6E 6J2; Aleppo (Syria)'92; Staff, Centre Hospitalier Régional de Lanaudière; (450)759-8222; Fax. (450)752-0651.

KHABBAZ, Samir; West Coast Gen Hosp, 3949 Port Alberni Hwy, Port Alberni BC V9Y 4S1; Tor'92; CCFP; Staff, West Coast General Hospital; (250)723-2135

KHADAROO, Rachel; University of Alberta Hosp, 8440 112 St NW, Edmonton AB T6G 2B7; McM'98; FRCSC; GenSurg (Clinician Investigator Program); Critical Care Medicine. Staff, University of Alberta Hospital; (780)407-7728; Fax. (780)407-7674.

KHADEM, Aliasghar; St Boniface Gen Hosp, Y3008-409 Tache Ave, Winnipeg MB R2H 2A6; Shiraz (Iran)'91; Staff, St Boniface General Hospital; Asst Prof Med, University of Manitoba; Langs: Persian; (204)258-1267; Fax. (204)233-2157; akhadem@sbgh.mb.ca.

KHADILKAR, Madhusudan C; Cavendish Med Centre, 130-2545 boul Cavendish, Montreal QC H4B 2Y9; Bangalore (India)'66; MB BS; (514)483-2424; Fax. (514)483-2359.

KHADIM, Hamid Ahmadzai; Woodbridge Urgent Care Centre, 2-4000 Highway 7, Woodbridge ON L4L 8Z2; Varna (Bulgaria)'08; (905)851-3777

KHADIR, Amir A H; CSSS du Sud de Lanaudière, 911 montee des Pionniers, Terrebonne QC J6V 2H2; Laval'90; Microbio & Infect Dis (P.Q.); MedMicrobiol. Microbiol-Infect, Centre Hospitalier Pierre le Gardeur; Assoc Researcher, McGill University; Langs: Persian; Spanish; (450)654-7525; amir.khadir@ssss.gouv.qc.ca.

KHADIR, Saideh; CHUM-Hop St-Luc, 1058 rue Saint-Denis, Montreal QC H2X 3J4; Mon'95; Staff, Centre Hospitalier l'Université De Montréal (CHUM) - Hôpital Saint-luc; (514)890-8000 x36360

KHADOUR, Fadi; Sturgeon Community Hosp, 201 Boudreau Rd, St. Albert AB T8N 6C4; Baghdad (Iraq)'87; FRCPC; IntMed; Cardiol. Staff, Sturgeon Community Hospital; (780)418-7331; Fax. (780)418-8125; fkhadour@ualberta.ca.

KHADOURY, Adeline; Mount Sinai Hosp Centre, 5690 boul Cavendish, Cote Saint-Luc QC H4W 1S7; Mon'07; CCFP; Staff, Mount Sinai Hospital Center; (514)369-2222

KHAIRALLAH, Nicole; Hop Maisonneuve-Rosemont, 5415 boul de l'Assomption, Montreal QC H1T 2M4; Mon'96; FRCPC; Neur. Ac Member, Hopital Maisonneuve-Rosemont; (514)252-3528; Fax. (514)252-3529.

KHAIRY, May; MUHC-Montreal Children's Hosp, A611-2300 rue Tupper, Montreal QC H3H 1P3; McG'94; FRCPC; Peds. Staff Peds, McGill University Health Centre - Montreal Children's Hospital; adj Prof, McGill University; Langs: Bilingual(English/French); (514)412-4302; Fax. (514)412-4367; may.khairy@muhc.mcgill.ca.

KHAIRY, Paul; Institut de Cardiologie de Mtl, 5000 rue Belanger, Montreal QC H1T 1C8; McG'95; FRCPC; IntMed; Cardiol. Staff, Institut de Cardiologie de Montréal; Chair Electrophysiol & Adult Congenital Heart Dis, Canada Research; (514)376-3330 x2114; paul.khairy@lhsc.on.ca.

KHAIRY, Ramez C; St Mary's Hosp Centre, 3830 av Lacombe, Montreal QC H3T 1M5; Cairo (Egypt)'65; MB BCh; DA; CSPQ; Anes (P.Q.). Staff, St Mary's Hospital Centre; adj Prof, McGill University; (514)345-3511 x3344

KHAJEHDEHI, Ali A; C-17215 Leslie St, Newmarket ON L3Y 8E4; Isfahan U (Iran)'86; CCFP; (905)853-0404

KHAKEE, Shamshuddin G; Centre Med de la Plaza, 125-6700 ch de la Cote-des-Nei, Montreal QC H3S 2B2; New South Wales (Australia)'65; Hem (P.Q.); Peds. (514)341-2941

KHAKETLA, Moliehi; Population Health Unit, PO Box 6000, La Ronge SK S0J 1L0; (Other Foreign)'03; (306)425-8526

KHAKSHAEE, Amir H; Mountain Med Walk-In Clinic, 5A-880 Upper Wentworth St, Hamilton ON L9A 5H2; (Iran)'00; CCFP; (905)575-0808; Fax. (905)574-3003.

KHALADKAR, Sunil V; 300-4010 Pasqua St, Regina SK S4S 7B9; Sask'85; CCFP; FCFP; (306)789-3566; Fax. (306)789-3563.

KHALAF, Khalil; CSSSG-Hop de Hull, 116 boul Lionel-Emond, Gatineau QC J8Y 1W7; St. Joseph (Lebanon)'78; FRCSC; Neursurg. Staff, Hull Hospital; (819)595-6000

KHALAFF-ABOURAWAI, Hussein; Windsor Health Centre, 118-700 Tecumseh Rd E, Windsor ON N8X 4T2; Cairo (Egypt)'78; FRCSC; Urol. (519)971-0083; Fax. (519)971-0659.

KHALED, Abdelmoula; Clinique Med Metro Medic, 5950 ch de la Cote-des-Neiges, Montreal QC H3S 1Z5; Paris (France)'92; Staff, Hopital Charles LeMoyne; (514)731-1186

KHALED, Mohamed B; Roseland Med Centre, 1-433 Guelph Line, Burlington ON L7R 3L7; Tor'88; CCFP; Ac Staff, Joseph Brant Memorial Hospital; (905)333-4936; Fax. (905)333-4131.

KHALEDUZZAMAN, Mohammad; The Moncton Hosp, 135 MacBeath Ave, Moncton NB E1C 6Z8; (Bangladesh)'02; Staff, The Moncton Hospital; (506)857-5111

KHALEFIH, Tarek A; Halton HCS Corp-Milton, 7030 Derry Rd, Milton ON L9T 7H6; Damascus (Syria)'83; FRCPC; Peds. Staff, Halton Healthcare Services Corporation - Milton District Hospital; Langs: Arabic; (905)878-2383

KHALEIFA, Ali O; Niagara HS-St Catharines, 142 Queenston St, St. Catharines ON L2R 7C6; Al Fateh (Libya)'00; CCFP; Staff, Niagara Health System - St Catharines General Site.

KHALFAN, Aniz; Mount St Joseph Hosp, 3080 Prince Edward St, Vancouver BC V5T 3N4; Aberdeen (Scotland)'81; MB ChB; FRCPC; Anes. Staff, Providence Health Care - Mount Saint Joseph Hospital; (604)874-1141

KHALID, Hasan F; Marketplace Medical, C 7-4555 Hurontario St, Mississauga ON L4Z 3M1; Ott'03; CCFP; (905)507-4300

KHALID, Muhammad R; 600-299 Victoria St, Prince George BC V2L 5B8; Aga Khan U (Pakistan)'98; FRCPC; IntMed. (250)565-5580

KHALID, Salman; Halton HCS Corp-Milton, 7030 Derry Rd, Milton ON L9T 7H6; Ott'07; CCFP; CCFP(E.M.); Staff, Halton Healthcare Services Corporation - Milton District Hospital; (905)878-2383

KHALID, Tahir R; 102-32475 Simon Ave, Abbotsford BC V2T 5E3; Punjab (Pakistan)'92; MB BS; FRCPC; DiagRad (Abdominal Radiology). (604)859-8998

KHALID, Zahira; St Joseph's Healthcare, 50 Charlton Ave E, Hamilton ON L8N 4A6; Punjab (Pakistan)'03; FRCPC; IntMed. Staff, St Joseph's Healthcare - Charlton Campus; (905)522-1155

KHALID-KHAN, Sarosh; Hotel-Dieu Hosp, 564-166 Brock St, Kingston ON K7L 5G2; Karachi (Pakistan)'89; Staff, Hotel-Dieu Hospital; (613)544-3310; Fax. (613)544-7623.

KHALIDI, Nader A; 708-25 Charlton Ave E, Hamilton ON L8N 1Y2; Man'90; FRCPC; IntMed; Rheum. Staff, St Joseph's Healthcare - Charlton Campus; (905)521-9034; Fax. (905)521-8099.

KHALIF, Marwan; Burin Peninsula Hlth Care Ctr, PO Box 340, Burin NL A0E 1E0; Al Fateh (Libya)'04; MB BCh; CCFP; Staff, Burin Peninsula Health Care Centre; (709)891-1040

KHALIFA, Amer J; Regina Qu'Appelle HR-Pasqua, 4101 Dewdney Ave, Regina SK S4T 1A5; Baghdad (Iraq)'80; MB ChB; AB; FRCPC; CCFP; AnatPath. Staff Path Lab Dept, Pasqua Hospital; (306)766-2156

KHALIFA, Mahmoud A; Sunnybrook Hlth Sciences Ctre, E400-2075 Bayview Ave, Toronto ON M4N 3M5; (Egypt)'78; MB ChB; PhD; ABPath; FRCPC; AnatPath (Gynecological Pathology). Staff Path & Lab Med, Sunnybrook Health Sciences Centre; Prof, University of Toronto; Langs: Arabic; (416)480-4987; Fax. (416)480-4271; mahmoud.khalifa@sunnybrook.ca.

KHALIFA, Nagib M A; 72 Victoria Ave, Chatham ON N7L 3A1; Al Fateh (Libya)'99; FRCPC; IntMed. (519)397-0790; Fax. (519)397-5535.

KHALIFE, Samir; Seaforth Med Bldg, 700-3550 ch de la Cote-des-Nei, Montreal QC H3H 1V4; St. Joseph (Lebanon)'76; FRCSC; ObstGyn. Ac Staff, McGill University Health Centre - Royal Victoria Hospital; Langs: English; Arabic; (514)933-8877; Fax. (514)933-8338.

KHALIL, Andrew; Ctr Hosp de Lachine, 650 16e av, Lachine QC H8S 3N5; McG'06; MDCM; CCFP; CCFP(E.M.); Staff, Centre Hospitalier de Lachine; (514)637-2351; andrew.khalil@mail.mcgill.ca.

KHALIL, Ayman M R; Islington Med Clinic, 1206-1243 Islington Ave, Etobicoke ON M8X 1Y9; El-Minia (Egypt)'93; MB ChB; CCFP; Langs: Arabic; Hebrew; (416)233-5100

KHALIL, Elene O; MUHC-Montreal Children's Hosp, 2300 rue Tupper, Montreal QC H3H 1P3; McG'93; FRCPC; Peds. Staff Peds, McGill University Health Centre - Montreal Children's Hospital; adj Prof, McGill University; (514)412-4400

KHALIL, Evon W H; Holy Trinity Med Clinic, 6-2 Bloomfield Trail, Richmond Hill ON L4E 2H8; Alexandria (Egypt)'97; CCFP; Langs: Arabic; (905)313-8000; holytrinitymedical@gmail.com.

KHALIL, Hisham A; IWK Health Centre, PO Box 9700 Rpo CSC 5850-5980 University Ave, Halifax NS B3K 6R8; McM'06; FRCSC; ObstGyn. Staff, IWK Health Centre; (902)470-6788

KHALIL, Ihab A B; Alliston Family Health, PO Box 280 36 Victoria St W, Alliston ON L9R 1V5; El Minia (Egypt)'92; BCh; CCFP; (705)435-8887

KHALIL, M Arshad; South Walkerville Med Centre, 120-2224 Walker Rd, Windsor ON N8W 5L7; Mem'80; FRCPC; IntMed; Gastroent. (519)977-7880; Fax. (519)977-0094.

KHALIL, Moosa N G; Foothills Med Centre, 1403 29 St NW, Calgary AB T2N 2T9; Assiut (Egypt)'81; MB ChB; FRCPC; AnatPath. Staff Path, Foothills Medical Centre; (403)944-1363; moosa.khalil@cls.ab.ca.

KHALIL, Nasreen; Leslie Diamond Health Care Ctr, 7F-2775 Laurel St, Vancouver BC V5Z 1M9; Mem'78; BMedSci; FCCP; FRCPC; IntMed; Respir. Staff, Vancouver General Hospital - Centennial Pavillion; Assoc Prof Med, University of British Columbia; (604)875-4122

KHALIL, Raghad; William Osler HC-Brampton, S 2508-2100 Bovaird Dr E, Brampton ON L6R 3J7; Baghdad (Iraq)'99; FRCPC; Anes. Staff, William Osler Health System - Brampton Civic Hospital; (905)494-2120

KHALIL, Riad A; 476 rue King, Granby QC J2G 6V1; Lyon (France)'69; Peds (P.Q.). Staff, Centre Hospitalier de Granby; (450)372-3124

KHALIL, Sylvia; Centre Med Saint-Francois, 2125 boul Lemire, Drummondville QC J2B 8N8; Mon'05; CCFP; (819)477-6793

KHALIL, Tarek H Y; Bedford Central Med Clinic, 1650 Bedford Hwy, Bedford NS B4A 4J7; Cairo (Egypt)'92; MB BCh; (902)835-4777

KHALILI, Korosh; Mount Sinai Hosp, 562-600 University Ave, Toronto ON M5G 1X5; Ott'94; FRCPC; DiagRad. Staff, Mount Sinai Hospital; (416)946-4501

KHALILI, Mark; Viva Care Med Clinic, 2150 Hawkins St, Port Coquitlam BC V3B 0G6; Carribean (Netherlands Antilles)'96; CCFP; Langs: Farsi; (778)216-1822

KHALIQ, Anisa L; Garneau Prof Centre, 407-11044 51 Ave NW, Edmonton AB T6H 5B4; Alb'92; FRCPC; Psy. (780)438-6181; Fax. (780)437-3499.

KHALIQ-KAREEMI, Munaa; 1031 Russet Rd NE, Calgary AB T2E 5L2; Punjab (Pakistan)'87; ABIM; FRCPC; IntMed; Gastroent. Staff Gastroenterologist, Rockyview General Hospital; Clin Assoc Prof, University of Calgary; Langs: Urdu; Punjabi; (403)277-7321; Fax. (403)277-7327; clinic@giinx.ca.

KHALSA, Kesar S; 4-8388 128 St, Surrey BC V3W 4G2; Aberdeen (Scotland)'64; MB ChB; (604)590-0662; Fax. (604)501-0416.

KHALSA, Satwant K; 4-8388 128 St, Surrey BC V3W 4G2; Rajasthan (India)'67; (604)590-0662; Fax. (604)501-0416.

KHAMBALIA, Bashir; 72 King St W, Stoney Creek ON L8G 1H8; Dublin (Ireland)'69; LRCPS; LM; CCFP; Staff, St Joseph's Healthcare - Charlton Campus; (905)662-2501; Fax. (905)662-4100; bkhambalia@hotmail.com.

KHAMBHLA, Arvind D; 303-360 College St, Toronto ON M5T 1S6; Gujarat (India)'62; MB BS; FRCOG; FRCSC; ObstGyn. Consultant, St Joseph's Health Centre; Langs: Gujarati; Hindi; Marathi; (416)961-8238; Fax. (416)961-5732.

KHAMIDBAYEV, Timur; Southdale Med Clinic, 395 Southdale Rd E, London ON N6E 1A2; (Kazakhstan)'96; CCFP; (519)691-0100

KHAMISA, Karima; College Square Med Centre, 1980 Baseline Rd, Ottawa ON K2C 0C6; Wes'02; FRCPC; IntMed; Hem. Staff, Queensway Carleton Hospital; (613)224-6606; karima.khamisa@gmail.com.

KHAMSI, Firouz; Rosedale Med Centre, 610-600 Sherbourne St, Toronto ON M4X 1W4; Birmingham (England)'66; FRCPC; IntMed. Assoc Staff, Toronto General Hospital - UHN; Dir, Advanced Diagnostic Facilities; Dir, Toronto Fertility Sterility Institute; Asst Prof Med, University of Toronto; Langs: Farsi; (416)968-2830; tfsi@aaa-tfsi.com.

KHAN, A Ghaffar; Ghaffar Khan Medicine, 20 Montreal Rd, Cornwall ON K6H 1B1; Karachi (Pakistan)'61; MB BS; DPM(Lond); MRCPsy; FRCPC; Psy (Child Psychiatry). Langs: Urdu; (613)937-0303; Fax. (613)937-0663.

KHAN, Mahmood A H; Markham College Med Clinic, 405-474 College St, Toronto ON M6G 1A4; Dacca (Bangladesh)'58; MB BS; FRCPC; IntMed (Cardiology). Langs: Bengali; Hindi; (416)924-8968; Fax. (416)924-4533.

KHAN, A M Safiqul I; Surrey Med Bldg, 203-9656 King George Hwy, Surrey BC V3T 2V5; Dacca (Bangladesh)'59; MB BS; MRCP(UK); FRCPC; IntMed. Consultant Staff, Surrey Memorial Hospital; (604)588-4858; Fax. (604)588-4123.

KHAN, Ahmar; 3625 Shaganappi Trail NW PO Box 84179 Rpo Market Mall, Calgary AB T3A 5C4; Alb'08; CCFP.

KHAN, Airudin S; 223-279 Wharncliffe Rd N, London ON N6H 2C2; Man'65; BSc; FRCPC; IntMed (Cardiology). Consultant Internal Med, Regional Mental Health Care-St Joseph's Health Care; (519)679-0351; Fax. (519)679-7867.

KHAN, Akbar N; 301-4576 Yonge St, North York ON M2N 6N4; Tor'92; MD; Assoc Staff Family Med, The Scarborough Hospital - Birchmount Campus; (416)227-0037; Fax. (416)227-1915; akhan@medicorcancer.com.

KHAN, Ali H; Seven Oaks Surgery Centre, 2DS12-2300 McPhillips St, Winnipeg MB R2V 3M3; Man'96; FRCSC; GenSurg.

KHAN, Aliya A; Oakville Med Centre, 209-331 Sheddon Ave, Oakville ON L6J 1X8; Ott'82; FACP; FACE; FRCPC; IntMed; GeriatricMed (Metabolic Bone Disease). Consultant IntMed Geriatrics & Endoc, Halton Healthcare Services Corporation - Oakville Site; Dir Calcium Disorder Clinic, St Joseph's Healthcare - Charlton Campus; Clin Prof Med, McMaster University; (905)844-5677; Fax. (905)844-8966.

KHAN, Aneal A; Alberta Children's Hosp, 3F-2888 Shaganappi Trail NW, Calgary AB T3B 6A8; Qns'97; MSc; FCCMG; FRCPC; Peds (Medical Genetics). Staff, Alberta Children's Hospital; (403)955-7587

KHAN, Anwar A; 158A-19653 Willowbrook Dr, Langley BC V2Y 1A5; Karachi (Pakistan)'90; MB BS; CCFP; (604)530-1333

KHAN, Arshad; Victoria Westmount Med Centre, 201-751 Victoria St S, Kitchener ON N2M 5N4; Delhi (India)'69; MB BS; FRCPC; Psy (Eating Disorders). Staff Psy, Grand River Hospital - Kitchener/Waterloo Health Centre; Langs: Urdu; Hindi; (519)741-5567; Fax. (519)741-0947.

KHAN, Arshya F; Killarney Physicians, PO Box 1690 86 Elice Dr, Killarney MB R0K 1G0; (Other Foreign)'98; CCFP; (204)523-4609; Fax. (204)523-7340.

KHAN, Ashraf; 161A-31 Southridge Dr, Okotoks AB T1S 2N3; (South Africa)'88; MB ChB; CCFP; Lecturer, University of Alberta; (403)995-5740

KHAN, Asif A; Tillsonburg Dist Mem Hosp, 167 Rolph St, Tillsonburg ON N4G 3Y9; Karachi (Pakistan)'96; MB BS; Staff Anes, Tillsonburg District Memorial Hospital; (519)842-3611

KHAN, Asifjehan; Royal Ottawa Hlth Care Group, 1145 Carling Ave, Ottawa ON K1Z 7K4; Durban (South Africa)'85; MB ChB; FRCPC; Psy. Staff Psy, Royal Ottawa Mental Health Centre - Royal Ottawa Health Care Group; (613)722-6521 x6617

KHAN, Asra S; Valley Med Imaging, 102-32475 Simon Ave, Abbotsford BC V2T 5E3; Wes'99; FRCPC; DiagRad. (604)859-4888

KHAN, Ayesha; MUHC-Montreal Children's Hosp, D 168-2300 ru Tupper, Montreal QC H3H 1P3; Lahore (Pakistan)'83; Staff, McGill University Health Centre - Montreal Children's Hospital; (514)412-4400 x22891; Fax. (514)412-4443.

KHAN, Azra; Brant Community Hc-Brantford, 200 Terrace Hill St, Brantford ON N3R 1G9; Tor'93; FRCPC; DiagRad. Diagnostic-Radiology, The Brant Community Healthcare System - Brantford General Hospital Site; (519)752-7871

KHAN, Badarunisa; The Ottawa Hosp-Gen Campus, 501 Smyth Rd, Ottawa ON K1H 8L6; Osmania (India)'63; MB BS; FRCPC; Psy (Psycho Geriatrics). Staff Psy & OutpatientPsy, The Ottawa Hospital - General Campus; Asst Prof Psy/Clin Lecturer, University of Ottawa; (613)737-8010 x8043; Fax. (613)739-9980.

KHAN, Baseer U; Clarity Eye Institute, 105-8800 Dufferin St, Vaughan ON L4K 0C5; Tor'00; FRCSC; Ophth (Cataract). Ac Staff, Stevenson Memorial Hospital; Staff, Southlake Regional Health Centre; Langs: Urdu; (416)663-3937; Fax. (416)663-3731.

KHAN, Ehsan U; 104-3737 Major Mackenzie Dr, Woodbridge ON L4H 0A2; (Pakistan)'92; CCFP; (905)417-7771

KHAN, Farah I; Windsor Allergy & Asthma Assoc, 1407 Ottawa St, Windsor ON N8X 2G1; Aga Khan Univ (Pakistan)'00; FRCPC; Peds; ClinImmunol&Allergy. (519)258-4356; Fax. (519)258-9918.

KHAN, Farah Y; 3-9581 Weston Rd, Woodbridge ON L4H 3A5; (Other Foreign)'97; CCFP; (905)417-5777; Fax. (905)417-5774.

KHAN, Faraz; Queen Elizabeth Hosp, PO Box 6600 Stn Central, Charlottetown PE C1A 8T5; Staff, Queen Elizabeth Hospital; (902)894-2111

KHAN, Fareeha S; Eskasoni Community Health Ctr, PO Box 7745 Stn Main 15 Medicine Trali, Eskasoni NS B1W 1B3; Punjab (India)'01; MB BS; CCFP; (902)379-1365

KHAN, Farhan I A; 6038 Currents Dr NW, Edmonton AB T6W 0L7; (Pakistan)'00; MB BS; (780)784-3333; Fax. (780)784-3344.

KHAN, Farhana A; The Medical Care Centre, 6-1 Bartley Bull Pky, Brampton ON L6W 2J3; Punjab (Pakistan)'97; MB BS; CCFP; (905)450-2981

KHAN, Farhana A; 100 Humber College Boulevard, Etobicoke ON M9V 5G4; Illinois (USA)'06; (416)743-4961

KHAN, Fariha S; Goodfellow Prof Bldg, 201-170 McEwan Dr E, Bolton ON L7E 4C8; McM'04; CCFP; (905)857-2356

KHAN, Farrukh A; The Court, 319-2863 Ellesmere Rd, Scarborough ON M1E 5E9; Punjab (Pakistan)'94; ABIM; ABEndocrin; FRCPC; IntMed (Endocrinology). (416)281-5426; Fax. (416)281-3600.

KHAN, Fayyaz; Sir Thomas Roddick Hosp, PO Box 5000 Stn Main 142 Minnesota Dr, Stephenville NL A2N 2V6; Karachi (India)'90; MB BS; Staff, Sir Thomas Roddick Hospital; (709)643-5111

KHAN, Ghulam Z; North Bay Reg Health Centre, 50 College Dr, North Bay ON P1B 0A4; Islamia (Pakistan)'84; MB BS; Staff, North Bay Regional Health Centre - Regional Mental Health; (705)474-8600; Fax. (705)495-7890.

KHAN, Hafshah; 108-22441 Dewdney Trunk Rd, Maple Ridge BC V2X 7X7; London (England)'99; MB BS; CCFP; (604)463-1300

KHAN, Hamza N; Medical-Dental Bldg, 400-1120 Yates St, Victoria BC V8V 3M9; Wes'91; MPH; FRCSC; Ophth. (250)382-3937

KHAN, Haroon; Central Nfld Reg Hlth Centre, 50 Union St, Grnd-Falls-Wi NL A2A 2E1; Punjab (Pakistan)'87; MB BS; Staff, Central Newfoundland Regional Health Centre; (709)292-2500

KHAN, Hashmat U; 2291 Kipling Ave, Etobicoke ON M9W 4L6; Wes'03; CCFP; (416)741-4545; Fax. (416)744-1484.

KHAN, Idan; Royasl Columbian Hosp, 330 Columbia St E, New Westminster BC V3L 3W7; Cal'97; FRCPC; EmergMed. Staff, Royal Columbian Hospital; (604)520-4000

KHAN, Iftkhar H; 314-1669 Victoria St, Prince George BC V2L 2L5; Bahuddin Zakaria (Pakistan)'89; MB BS; (250)564-5535; Fax. (250)562-1481.

KHAN, Imtiaz M S; Credit Valley Med Arts Centre, 403-2000 Credit Valley Rd, Mississauga ON L5M 4N4; McG'91; DABIM; BSc; FRCPC; IntMed; Rheum. (905)828-6464

KHAN, Iqbal A; Medical Arts Bldg, 9-165 Plymouth Rd, Welland ON L3B 3E1; Bahauddin Zakariya (Pakistan)'85; MB BS; FRCSEd(Gyne); FRCSC; GenSurg (Gastroenterology). (905)735-4411; Fax. (905)735-4413.

KHAN, Isfandyar; Univ Hosp of Northern BC, 1475 Edmonton St, Prince George BC V2M 1S2; Peshawar (Pakistan)'95; MB BS; FRCPC; Psy. Staff, University Hospital of Northern British Columbia; (250)645-6045

KHAN, Kamran A; Queen Elizabeth II HSC-Halifax, 8896F-1796 Summer St, Halifax NS B3H 3A7; Karachi (Pakistan)'01; MB BS; Staff, Queen Elizabeth II Health Sciences Centre - Halifax Infirmary Site; (902)473-2184

KHAN, Kamran M; St Michael's Hosp, 30 Bond St, Toronto ON M5B 1W8; Tor'96; MPH; FRCPC; IntMed (Tuberculosis); InfectDis. Staff, St Michael's Hospital; (416)864-6060 x2976; Fax. (416)864-5485; khank@smh.toronto.on.ca.

KHAN, Kamran Z; Carbonear Gen Hosp, 86 Highroad South, Carbonear NL A1Y 1A4; Allama Iqbal Medical College (Pakistan)'98; MB BS; Staff, Carbonear General Hospital; (709)945-5111

KHAN, Karim; Ctre for Hip Health & Mobility, 175-828 10th Ave W, Vancouver BC V5Z 1M9; Melbourne (Australia)'84; MB BS; FAB; Dip SportMed; Staff, BC Women's Hospital & Health Centre; Staff Centre for Hip & Health Mobility, Vancouver General Hospital - Centennial Pavillion; Asst Prof Family Practice, University of British Columbia; (604)875-4111 x69611

KHAN, Karla E; 1022 20 St S, Lethbridge AB T1K 2C9; Sask'95; FRCSC; ObstGyn. (403)381-4410

KHAN, Khurram J; St Joseph's Healthcare, H421-50 Charlton Ave E, Hamilton ON L8N 4A6; Wes'04; FRCPC; IntMed; Gastroent. Staff, St Joseph's Healthcare - Charlton Campus; (905)522-1155; Fax. (905)308-7201.

KHAN, Khurshid A; University of Alberta Hosp, 2E3-8440 112 St NW, Edmonton AB T6G 2B7; (Nigeria)'88; MB ChB; FRCPC; Neur (Cerebrovascular Disease). Staff, University of Alberta Hospital; (780)407-7574; Fax. (780)407-1325.

KHAN, Liaquat H; Evergreen Medl Centre, 8960 152 St, Surrey BC V3R 4E4; Peshawar (Pakistan)'92; MB BS; (604)588-8181

KHAN, M Gabriel; Bank Med Centre, 4-1935 Bank St, Ottawa ON K1V 8A3; Queen's (Ireland)'61; MB ChB; FRCP(Lond); FACP; FACC; FRCPC; IntMed (Cardiology). Ac Staff Cardiol, The Ottawa Hospital - General Campus; Assoc Prof Med, University of Ottawa; (613)521-2391 x111; Fax. (613)521-5443; gabriel@terapia.ca.

KHAN, M Ibrahim; 4F-2045 Broad St, Regina SK S4P 3T7; (Pakistan)'94; MB BS; MPH; PhD; Med Officer of Hlth, City of Regina; Langs: German; (306)780-6561; ikhan@regina.ca.

KHAN, M Naeem; IWK Health Centre, PO Box 9700 Rpo CSC 5850-5980 University Ave, Halifax NS B3K 6R8; Peshawar (Pakistan)'89; MB BS; Staff, IWK Health Centre; (902)428-8888

KHAN, M Viqar; Oakville Health Care Centre, 213-1060 Speers Rd, Oakville ON L6L 2X4; Osmania (India)'79; MB BS; CCFP; Langs: Urdu; Hindi; Telugu; (905)842-5455; Fax. (905)842-7788.

KHAN, Rauf M A; 327 Wellington St, Sarnia ON N7T 1H4; Jabalpur (India)'62; MB BS; MRC; FRCP; FRCPC; IntMed (Gastroenterology). Med Staff/Court Staff, Bluewater Health - Mitton Site; Med Staff, Bluewater Health - Norman Site; Med Staff, Bluewater Health - Charlotte Eleanor Englehart Hospital; (519)344-3692; Fax. (519)344-5933; drkhan@ebtech.net.

KHAN, Mahmuda B; Milliken Med Centre, 17-5671 Steeles Ave E, Scarborough ON M1V 5P6; (Kenya)'73; MB ChB; CCFP; FCFP; Court Staff, Rouge Valley Health System - Centenary Health Centre Site; Langs: Gujarati; Urdu; Swahili; Punjabi; (416)291-7643; Fax. (416)291-0890.

KHAN, Mansoor A; Rouge Valley-Ajax & Pickering, 580 Harwood Ave S, Ajax ON L1S 2J4; Karachi (Pakistan)'82; Staff, Rouge Valley Health System - Ajax & Pickering Health Centre Site; (905)683-2320

KHAN, Mateen A; Chatham-Kent Health Alliance, PO Box 2030 Stn Main 80 Grand Ave W, Chatham ON N7M 5L9; Philadelphia (USA)'04; Staff, Chatham-Kent Health Alliance; (519)352-6400

KHAN, Mohamed K; BC Cancer Agency, 600 10th Ave W, Vancouver BC V5Z 4E6; Chicago (USA)'94; Staff, BC Cancer Agency Vancouver Centre; (604)877-6193

KHAN, Mohammad A; Sherbrooke Centre, 4F-260 Sherbrooke St, New Westminster BC V3L 3M2; Peshawar (Pakistan)'96; MB BS; FRCPC; Psy. Staff, Royal Columbian Hospital; (604)520-4662

KHAN, Mohammad A; Kelsey Trail Health Region, PO Box 6500, Melfort SK S0E 1A0; Peshawar (Pakistan)'89; MB BS; MPH; Med Officer of Hlth, Kelsey Trail Health Region; Langs: Urdu; Pashtu; Punjabi; (306)752-6310

KHAN, Mohammad M; Allan Blair Cancer Centre, 300-4101 Dewdney Ave, Regina SK S4T 7T1; Peshawar (Pakistan)'72; (306)766-2213

KHAN, Mohammed A H; 103-535 Belmont Ave W, Kitchener ON N2M 5E9; Manchester (England)'91; MB ChB; MRCGPract; LMCC; Sub-Investigator, Biopharm Inc; Langs: Urdu; (519)578-8050; mkhan@anapharm.com.

KHAN, Muhammad A; Cape Breton Hlthcare Complex, 1482 George St, Sydney NS B1P 1P3; Punjab (India)'98; MB BS; CCFP; CCFP(E.M.); Staff, Cape Breton Healthcare Complex; Langs: Urdu; Arabic; (902)567-7485; khanm@cbdha.nshealth.ca.

KHAN, Muhammad N; Surrey Mem Hosp, 13750 96 Ave, Surrey BC V3V 1Z2; Punjab (Pakistan)'95; MB BS; Staff, Surrey Memorial Hospital; (604)581-2211

KHAN, Mujtaba A; The Medical Care Centre, 6-1 Bartley Bull Parkway, Brampton ON L6W 2J3; Lahore (Pakistan)'87; MB BS; CCFP; (905)450-2981; Fax. (905)450-2532.

KHAN, Mujtaba A; 214-3806 Albert St, Regina SK S4S 3R2; (Other Foreign)'96; CCFP; (306)205-5430; Fax. (306)205-5431.

KHAN, Muniba M; Langley Mem Hosp, 22051 Fraser Hwy, Langley BC V3A 4H4; Aga Khan (Pakistan)'99; MB BS; CCFP; Staff, Langley Memorial Hospital; (604)450-2913

KHAN, Mustafa Z; Lakeridge Hlth Corp-Oshawa, 1 Hospital Crt, Oshawa ON L1G 2B9; Tor'04; FRCPC; DiagRad. Staff, Lakeridge Health - Oshawa Site; (905)433-4305

KHAN, Nadia A; St Paul's Hosp, 620B-1081 Burrard St, Vancouver BC V6Z 1Y6; Alb'95; FRCPC; IntMed. Staff, Providence Health Care - St Paul's Hospital; (604)682-2344; Fax. (604)806-8005.

KHAN, Nadim A; Glendower Fam Healthcare Ctre, 3-331 Glendower Circt, Scarborough ON M1T 2Z7; Tor'85; (416)298-3339; Fax. (416)298-3475.

KHAN, Nadira S; Wellpoint Family Practice, 9F-1240 Bay St, Toronto ON M5R 2A7; Cal'98; CCFP; Staff, Women's College Hospital; (416)969-3250; Fax. (416)971-7718.

KHAN, Naeem A H; 103-127 Westmore Dr, Etobicoke ON M9V 3Y6; Osmania (India)'60; MB BS; DCH(Eng); DABPN; FRCPC; Psy. Staff, William Osler Health System - Brampton Civic Hospital; Langs: Urdu; Hindi; (416)749-3933; Fax. (416)749-3936.

KHAN, Nayla M; William Osler HC-Brampton, 2100 Bovaird Dr E, Brampton ON L6R 3J7; Punjab (Pakistan)'96; ObstGyn. Staff, William Osler Health System - Brampton Civic Hospital; (905)494-2120

KHAN, Nazir A; MUHC-Montreal Gen Hosp, 1650 av Cedar, Montreal QC H3G 1A4; Man'62; FRCPC; DiagRad. Staff, McGill University Health Centre - Montreal General Campus; (514)934-1934

KHAN, Niaz A; Miramichi Reg Hosp, 500 Water St, Miramichi NB E1V 3G5; Dhaka (Bangladesh)'82; FRCPC; IntMed. Staff, Miramichi Regional Hospital; (506)623-3195

KHAN, Noor M; D-844 McLeod Ave, Winnipeg MB R2G 2T7; Punjab (Pakistan)'68; Staff, Seven Oaks General Hospital; (204)987-3030

KHAN, Nusrat U; 206A-1920 Ellesmere Rd, Scarborough ON M1H 2V6; Wes'99; CCFP; (416)850-4167; Fax. (416)850-4168.

KHAN, Obaid-Ur-Rahman; Kelowna Gen Hosp, 2268 Pandosy St, Kelowna BC V1Y 1T2; Punjab (Pakistan)'86; Staff, Kelowna General Hospital; Clinical Asst Prof Med, University of British Columbia; (250)862-4300 x2437; dr.obaid.khan@interiorhealth.ca.

KHAN, Omar D M; Hotel Dieu Shaver Hlth Rehab C, 541 Glenridge Ave, St Catharines ON L2T 4C2; McM'01; FRCPC; PhysMed&Rehab (Spasticity Management). Associate/Consultant, Hôtel Dieu Shaver Health & Rehabilitation Centre; Langs: Urdu; (905)685-1381 x85306

KHAN, Qasim S; 201-331 Sheddon Ave, Oakville ON L6J 1X8; McM'00; FRCSC; GenSurg. (905)618-0148

KHAN, Rabia N; 175 Alma St, Rockwood ON N0B 2K0; Qns'94; CCFP; (519)856-4681; rkhan@ewfht.ca.

KHAN, Raza M; Lawren S Harris Med Clinic, 150 Brant Ave, Brantford ON N3T 3H7; Tor'95; CCFP; FCFP; (519)720-0983; Fax. (519)720-0282.

KHAN, Razaullah; Burin Peninsula Hlth Care Ctr, PO Box 340, Burin NL A0E 1E0; Dow (Pakistan)'89; MB BS; Staff, Burin Peninsula Health Care Centre; (709)891-1040

KHAN, Razi; London HSC-University Hosp, PO Box 5339 Stn B 339 Windermere Rd, London ON N6A 5A5; McG'06; MDCM; Cardiol; IntMed. Staff, London Health Sciences Centre - University Hospital; (519)685-8500 x19428

KHAN, Razia; Wardenwoods Health Centre Inc, 2361 Warden Ave, Scarborough ON M1T 1V7; Hyderabad (India)'68; MB BS; Staff, Rouge Valley Health System - Centenary Health Centre Site; Court Staff, The Scarborough Hospital - Birchmount Campus; Court Staff, North York General Hospital; Langs: Hindi; Urdu; (416)299-4999; Fax. (416)299-1322.

KHAN, Rita R; 96 Highland Rd W, Kitchener ON N2M 3B5; Delhi (India)'69; Court Staff, Grand River Hospital - Kitchener/Waterloo Health Centre; Court Staff, St Mary's General Hospital; Langs: Hindi; Urdu; Punjabi; (519)571-0925; Fax. (519)571-0731.

KHAN, Ruhe S; Crescent Town Health Centre, 4 The Market Place, Toronto ON M4C 5M1; Zaria (Nigeria)'89; CCFP; (416)690-3412; Fax. (416)691-2543.

KHAN, Ruhi A; Urgent Care Centre, 1500 Dundas St E, Mississauga ON L4X 1L4; Karachi (Pakistan)'95; MB BS; CCFP; (416)741-2273

KHAN, Rukhshanda J; Bay 1-601 8th St E, Saskatoon SK S7H 0R1; Karachi (Pakistan)'89; MB BS; CCFP; Staff, Saskatoon City Hospital; Staff, Royal University Hospital; Staff, St Paul's Hospital (Grey Nuns) of Saskatoon; (306)974-3939; Fax. (306)979-3941.

KHAN, Saad M; Dr G B Cross Mem Hosp, 67 Manitoba Dr, Clarenville NL A5A 1K3; Sind (Pakistan)'82; ABACPath; Staff, The Dr G B Cross Memorial Hospital; (709)466-3411

KHAN, Saadia N; 16-2555 Erin Centre Blvd, Mississauga ON L5M 5H1; Ott'94; CCFP; Staff, The Credit Valley Hospital; Langs: Arabic; Urdu; (905)828-0030; Fax. (905)828-4101.

KHAN, Sadia N; Glenboro Health Dist Hosp, PO Box 310, Glenboro MB R0K 0X0; Staff, Glenboro Health District Hospital; (204)827-2633; Fax. (204)827-2741.

KHAN, Sadiqa J; PO Box 1178, Beausejour MB R0E 0C0; (Other Foreign)'99; Staff, Beausejour District Hospital.

KHAN, Safeer A; Peter Lougheed Centre, 25-3500 26 Ave NE, Calgary AB T1Y 6J4; (Pakistan)'81; DABPN; MB BS; Staff Psy, Peter Lougheed Centre; Clin Lecturer, University of Calgary; Langs: Urdu; Hindi; Punjabi; (403)943-5725

KHAN, Saima W; Chatham-Kent Family Health Team, 20 Emma St, Chatham ON N7L 5K5; Ziauddin (Pakistan)'02; CCFP; (519)354-2174; skhan@ckha.on.ca.

KHAN, Sameena A; Deer Valley Walk-In Med Clinic, 26-1221 Canyon Meadows Dr SE, Calgary AB T2J 6G2; Cal'08; BSc; MSc; CCFP; (403)278-2164

KHAN, Sandra M; The Medical Centre FHT, PO Box 4200 Stn Main 707 Charlotte St, Peterborough ON K9J 7B3; Tor'91; CCFP; FCFP; (705)876-4540

KHAN, Seema N; Smyth Medical Centre, 208-1929 Russell Rd, Ottawa ON K1G 4G3; Wisconsin (USA)'94; (613)526-3501

KHAN, Shagufta U; St Joseph's Health Centre, 310-30 The Queensway, Toronto ON M6R 1B5; Lucknow (India)'93; FRCPC; IntMed; Endocrin&Metab. Staff, St Joseph's Health Centre; Langs: Urdu; Hindi; (416)530-6814; Fax. (416)530-6797.

KHAN, Shah F; Abbotsford Mental Health Ctre, 11-32700 George Ferguson Way, Abbotsford BC V2T 4V6; Peshawar (Pakistan)'99; MB BS; (604)870-7800

KHAN, Shahbaz; Health Sense Medical, 8-2983 Westoak Trails Blvd, Oakville ON L6M 5E4; Nishtar (Pakistan)'95; CCFP; (905)901-1217

KHAN, Shahida R; Health With Care, 501-3621 Highway 7, Markham ON L3R 0G6; King Edward (Pakistan)'67; FRCPC; Peds. Langs: Urdu; (905)474-5754 x1008; Fax. (905)474-7667.

KHAN, Shahida; Halton Family Health Centre, 2951 Walker's Line, Burlington ON L7M 4Y1; (Pakistan)'95; CCFP; (905)336-3437

KHAN, Shahnaz; Mackenzie Richmond Hill Hosp, 10 Trench St, Richmond Hill ON L4C 4Z3; Osmania (India)'73; MB BS; Staff, Mackenzie Richmond Hill Hospital; (905)883-1212

KHAN, Shahzia; The Core Family Health Centre, 825 Richmond St, London ON N6A 3H7; (Other Foreign)'93; CCFP.

KHAN, Shajia; 402-267 O'Connor St, Ottawa ON K2P 1V3; Osmania (India)'65; MB BS; FRCPC; IntMed (Diabetes). Ac Staff, The Ottawa Hospital - Civic Campus; University of Ottawa; Langs: Urdu; Hindi; (613)234-2594

KHAN, Sher B; Royal Victoria Hosp, 201 Georgian Dr, Barrie ON L4M 6M2; Peshawar (Pakistan)'90; MB BS; MRCPsy; FRCPC; Psy. Staff, Royal Victoria Regional Health Centre; (705)728-9090

KHAN, Shereena; Surrey Mem Hosp, 13750 96 Ave, Surrey BC V3V 1Z2; Punjab (Pakistan)'01; CCFP; Staff, Surrey Memorial Hospital; (604)581-2211

KHAN, Swaleha; 206-800 Bathurst St, Toronto ON M5R 3M8; Utkal (India)'70; (416)536-0063; Fax. (416)907-7175.

KHAN, Syma; Rockyview Gen Hosp, 7007 14 St SW, Calgary AB T2V 1P9; UBC'08; CCFP; CCFP(E.M.); Staff EmergMed, Rockyview General Hospital; (403)943-3449

KHAN, T Ali; Manitoba Health, 3071-300 Carlton St, Winnipeg MB R3B 3M9; Karachi (Pakistan)'58; MSc; FRCS(Ed & Eng); FRCSC; GenSurg.

KHAN, Tariq S; Victoria Hosp, PO Box 3000 Stn Main 1200 24th St W, Prince Albert SK S6V 5T4; Staff, Victoria Hospital; (306)765-6267

KHAN, Uzma A Z; Kingsway Garden Mall, 303-1 Kingsway Garden Mall NW, Edmonton AB T5G 3A6; (Pakistan)'92; CCFP; (780)479-3699; Fax. (780)479-3399.

KHAN, Vajid A; McMaster University HSC, MDCL 3101A-1280 Main St W, Hamilton ON L8S 4K1; Wes'07; DiagRad.

KHAN, Waheed; Markham Stouffville Urgent Car, 100-110 Copper Creek Dr, Markham ON L6B 0P9; Peshawar (Pakistan)'05; (905)472-8911

KHAN, Y Aaron; Ear Falls Health Centre, PO Box 520 25 Spruce St, Ear Falls ON P0V 1T0; Man'90; (807)222-3728; Fax. (807)222-2053.

KHAN, Yasir H; Major's Path Family Practice, 301-35 Major's Path, St. John's NL A1A 4Z9; Mem'10; CCFP; (709)579-2324

KHAN, Yasir; Univ Hlth Network-Toronto Gen, 200 Elizabeth St, Toronto ON M5G 2C4; McM'03; FRCPC; Psy. Staff, Toronto General Hospital - UHN; (416)340-4464

KHAN, Yasmin; Univ Hlth Network-Toronto Gen, GS 480-200 Elizabeth St, Toronto ON M5G 2C4; Wes'02; FRCPC; EmergMed. Staff EmergMed, Toronto General Hospital - UHN; (416)340-3856

KHAN, Yasser A; 401-7900 Hurontario St, Brampton ON L6Y 0P6; McM'97; FRCSC; Ophth. (905)456-9500

KHAN, Zarin P; Medicine Hat Reg Hosp, 666 5 St SW, Medicine Hat AB T1A 4H6; Bristol (England)'64; MB ChB; FRCS; FACS; FRCSC; GenSurg (Thoracic Surgery). Staff, Medicine Hat Regional Hospital; Langs: Urdu; Spanish; (403)529-8000; Fax. (403)529-8949.

KHAN AFRIDI, Obaid T; 214 Med Place, 909-9909 102 St, Grande Prairie AB T8V 2V4; (Pakistan)'91; MB BS; (780)814-5225; Fax. (780)402-2858.

KHANAHMADI, Shahab; Winnipeg Clinic, 425 St Mary Ave, Winnipeg MB R3C 0N2; Tehran (Iran)'99; shahabmd@yahoo.com.

KHANAM, Humaira; Queen Elizabeth Hosp, PO Box 6600 Stn Central 60 Riverside Dr, Charlottetown PE C1A 8T5; Sind (Pakistan)'91; DAB; FRCPC; AnatPath (Neuropathology). Staff, Queen Elizabeth Hospital; (902)894-2300 x2304; hkhanam@ihis.org.

KHANBADR, Daryoush; Royal Columbian Hosp, 330 Columbia St E, New Westminster BC V3L 3W7; Shahid Beheshti (Iran)'95; CCFP; Staff, Royal Columbian Hospital; (604)520-4001

KHANBHAI, Irfan A; 855 12th Ave W, Vancouver BC V5Z 1M9; UBC'93; FRCPC; Psy (Personality Disorders). Staff Psy, Vancouver General Hospital - Centennial Pavillion; (604)365-2344; ikhanbhai@providencehealth.bc.ca.

KHANDAKER, Masud H; Ottawa Cardiovascular Centre, 502-1355 Bank St, Ottawa ON K1H 8K7; (Ireland)'04; (613)738-1584

KHANDEKAR, Sayra A; Ermineskin Med Clinic, 303-2377 111 St NW, Edmonton AB T6J 5E5; Tulane University (Other Foreign)'05; FRCPC; IntMed; Cardiol. (780)407-8822

KHANDELWAL, Ajai S; Dr Ajai Khandelwal Med Clinic, PO Box 810 420 4th St NE, Minnedosa MB R0J 1E0; Vikram (India)'61; FRCS(Ed); LRCP(Lond); MRCS(Eng); Chief Medical Staff, Erickson Health Centre; Gen Surgery, Minnedosa Health Centre; (204)867-2722

KHANDELWAL, Mukesh Kumar N; Medical Arts Bldg, C-165 Plymouth Rd, Welland ON L3B 3E1; Nagpur (India)'90; FRCPC; IntMed (Nephrology). Staff, St Joseph's Healthcare - Charlton Campus; (905)735-8131

KHANDELWAL, Sanjay; Surrey Mem Hosp, 13750 96 Ave, Surrey BC V3V 1Z2; Man'98; Staff, Surrey Memorial Hospital; (604)585-2211

KHANDELWAL, Surbhi; Family Med Centre, PO Box 8888 Stn Main 220 Bagot St, Kingston ON K7L 5E9; (India)'97; CCFP; (613)533-9300

KHANDUJA, Purva K; Mount Sinai Hosp, 104-600 University Ave, Toronto ON M5G 1X5; Liverpool (England)'99; FRCPC; Anes. Staff, Mount Sinai Hospital; (416)596-4200

KHANDWALA, Hasnain; LMC Endocrinology Centres, 2 B-1723 Kipling Ave, Etobicoke ON M9R 4E1; Karachi (Pakistan)'93; MB BS; DABIM; DAB(DiabetesEndocrin&Me; FRCPC; IntMed; Endocrin&Metab. Langs: Urdu; (416)645-1035

KHANGURA, Davinder S; Health Plus Med Centre, 1075 Autumnwood Dr, Winnipeg MB R2J 1C6; Man'03; CCFP; (204)594-2100; Fax. (204)594-2101.

KHANGURA, Seema S; 525-2755 Lougheed Hwy, Port Coquitlam BC V3B 5Y9; UBC'94; CCFP; (604)294-8540

KHANGURA, Simi; Children's & Women's HC of BC, B321-4480 Oak St, Vancouver BC V6H 3V4; UBC'99; FRCPC; Peds. Staff, BC Children's Hospital; (604)875-2045

KHANI-HANJANI, Abbas; University of Alberta Hosp, 8440 112 St NW, Edmonton AB T6G 2B7; Cal'04; FRCSC; CardSurg. Staff, University of Alberta Hospital; (780)407-8822

KHANNA, Anuradha; Danforth Med Centre, 880 Danforth Rd, Scarborough ON M1K 1H8; Shivaji (India)'97; CCFP; (416)264-4848

KHANNA, Charu; Family Physicians, 101-610 Queen St, Saskatoon SK S7K 0M8; Sask'92; CCFP; (306)244-0766; Fax. (306)665-8838.

KHANNA, Julie J; Inst of Cosmetic & Laser Surg, 100-1344 Cornwall Rd, Oakville ON L6J 7W5; Ott'90; FAB; FRCSC; PlasSurg (Breast Surgery). Ac Staff, Halton Healthcare Services Corporation - Oakville Site; (905)842-2262; Fax. (905)842-3625; info@icls.ca.

KHANNA, Madhur S; 5966 Mullen Way NW, Edmonton AB T6R 0S9; Tor'10; (780)801-1220; Fax. (780)801-1225.

KHANNA, Manish; SMBD Jewish Gen Hosp, 3755 ch Cote-Sainte-Catherine, Montreal QC H3T 1E2; McG'96; FRCPC; Derm (Skin Cancer). Staff, Sir Mortimer B Davis Jewish General; Staff, McGill University Health Centre - Montreal General Campus; McGill University; Langs: English; French; (514)340-8222 x4247; Fax. (514)340-7510.

KHANNA, Nitin V; St Joseph's Health Care, PO Box 5777 Stn B 268 Grosvenor St, London ON N6A 4V2; Mem'98; FRCPC; IntMed (Therapeutic Endoscopy); Gastroent. Staff, St Joseph's Hospital - St Joseph's Health Care; Assoc Prof, University of Western Ontario; (519)646-6125; Fax. (519)646-6130; nitin.khanna@sjhc.london.on.ca.

KHANNA, Parul; The Credit Valley Hosp, 2200 Eglinton Ave W, Mississauga ON L5M 2N1; Alb'01; FRCPC; IntMed. Staff, The Credit Valley Hospital; (905)813-4466

KHANNA, Rahul; Postmaster Med Clinic, 2540 Postmaster Dr, Oakville ON L6M 0N2; (Other Foreign)'00; CCFP; (905)844-1700; Fax. (905)844-1705.

KHANNA, Rajiv; First Med Place, 111-170 Queensway W, Mississauga ON L5B 3A8; Tor'88; (905)566-0121

KHANNA, Rama J; South Georgetown Med Clinic, 2-333 Mountainview Rd S, Georgetown ON L7G 6E8; (India)'71; CCFP; (905)873-4742

KHANNA, Reena; University of Western Ontario, 106-1151 Richmond St, London ON N6A 5C1; Wes'06; FRCPC; IntMed; Gastroent. (519)685-8500

KHANNA, Rokesh K; Woodstock Gen Hosp, 310 Juliana Dr, Woodstock ON N4V 0A4; Tor'86; Staff, Woodstock General Hospital; (519)421-4211 x2204

KHANNA, Vickas; The Ottawa Hosp-Gen Campus, 5004-501 Smyth Rd, Ottawa ON K1H 8L6; Dal'07; OrthSurg. Staff, The Ottawa Hospital - General Campus; (613)737-8785

KHANNA, Vijay; IWK Health Centre, PO Box 9700 Rpo CSC, Halifax NS B3K 6R8; Bhopal (India)'72; MB BS; Staff, IWK Health Centre; (902)420-6669; Fax. (902)420-6469.

KHAOUAM, Nader; Hop Maisonneuve-Rosemont, 5415 boul de l'Assomption, Montreal QC H1T 2M4; Mon'01; FRCPC; RadOncol. Staff, Hopital Maisonneuve-Rosemont; (514)252-3425

KHARA, Milan; Pacific Spirit Commun Hlth Ctr, 3F-2110 43rd Ave W, Vancouver BC V6M 2E1; Leicester (England)'89; MB ChB; CCFP; (604)261-6366

KHARAL, Aysha; London Medicentres, 611 Wonderland Rd N, London ON N6H 4V6; (Pakistan)'03; CCFP; (519)471-6686

KHARE, Suneeta D; Quinte HC Corp-Belleville Gen, 265 Dundas St E, Belleville ON K8N 5A9; Ott'93; FRCPC; GenPath. Staff, QHC Belleville General; Fax. (613)968-9912.

KHARE, Umesh; Phoenix Med Centre, 404-2155 10th Ave, Prince George BC V2M 5J6; Lucknow (India)'60; (250)563-0701; Fax. (250)563-0701; umeshkanakkhare@telus.net.

KHARONSKY, Rita M; 212-4949 Bathurst St, North York ON M2R 1Y1; Kaunas State (Lithuania)'82; CCFP; Langs: Russian; Hebrew; Lithuanian; (416)225-7482; Fax. (416)225-7455.

KHASIMUDDIN, Syed A; William Osler HC-Brampton, 2100 Bovaird Dr E, Brampton ON L6R 3J7; (Grenada)'01; Staff, William Osler Health System - Brampton Civic Hospital; (905)494-2120

KHATAAN, Somaia A M; Hurontario Med Clinic, 201-2338 Hurontario St, Mississauga ON L5B 1N1; Alexandria (Egypt)'82; CCFP; Ac Staff/Member family Pract, Trillium Health Centre - Mississauga; Langs: Arabic; (905)281-9100; Fax. (905)281-9101.

KHATAMI, Kian; Eagle Ridge Family Health Ctre, 203-480 Huronia Rd, Barrie ON L4N 6M2; Shaheed Beheshti (Iran)'97; CCFP; (705)727-7688; Fax. (705)734-6284.

KHATAMI TOUSSI, Mohammad; 2010-4818 Westwinds Dr NE, Calgary AB T3J 3Z5; Islamic Azad U-Mashhad Branch (Iran)'06; (403)568-2295

KHATCHADOURIAN, Karine; Children's & Women's HC of BC, K4 213-4480 Oak St, Vancouver BC V6H 3V4; Mon'07; FRCPC; Peds; Endocrin&Metab. Staff, BC Children's Hospital; (604)875-2117

KHATCHATOURIAN, Marina; The Toronto GI Clinic, 450-5 Fairview Mall Dr, North York ON M2J 2Z1; Tor'91; FRCPC; IntMed; Gastroent. Langs: Armenian; Persian; (416)322-7517; Fax. (416)489-8053.

KHATIB, Ahmad; Campbellton Med Clinic, 4-10 Village Ave, Campbellton NB E3N 3S8; (United Arab Emirates)'96; Staff, Hôpital Régional Campbellton; (506)753-3722

KHATIB, Aisha N; Devon Gen Hosp, 101 Erie St S, Devon AB T9G 1A6; Alb'09; CCFP; CCFP(E.M.); Staff, Devon General Hospital; (780)342-7000

KHATIWADA, Bikalpa; Queensway Carleton Hosp, 3045 Baseline Rd, Nepean ON K2H 8P4; McG'05; CCFP; CCFP(E.M.); Staff, Queensway Carleton Hospital; (613)721-2000

KHATRI, Prateek; Univ Hlth Network-Toronto Gen, 14 217-200 Elizabeth St, Toronto ON M5G 2C4; Ott'10; Staff, Toronto General Hospital - UHN; (416)340-3155

KHATTABI, Mona; Hop Maisonneuve-Rosemont, 5415 boul de l'Assomption, Montreal QC H1T 2M4; Mon'03; CCFP; Staff, Hopital Maisonneuve-Rosemont; (514)252-3400

KHATTAK, Abid S; Abbotsford Mental Health Ctre, 11-32700 George Ferguson Way, Abbotsford BC V2T 4V6; Peshawar (Pakistan)'94; MB BS; (604)870-7800

KHATTAK, M Sohail; The Kids Clinic, 19-1615 Dundas St W, Whitby ON L1N 2L1; Peshawar (Pakistan)'88; FRCP; FRCPC; Peds (Clinical Pharmacology). Staff Peds, Lakeridge Health - Oshawa Site; Langs: Pashtu; Hindi; Punjabi; Urdu; (905)666-4400; Fax. (905)668-2881; skhattak@kidsclinic.ca.

KHATTER, Kapil; 300-100 Marie Curie Pvt, Ottawa ON K1N 1A2; McG'92; CCFP; Langs: English; French; (613)564-3950

KHATTER, Manishi; Synergy Wellness Centre, 225-501 Bethel Dr, Sherwood Park AB T8H 0N2; Man'92; CCFP; (780)467-4343; Fax. (780)449-4951.

KHAWAJA, Noumaan; Great Lakes Med Centre, 25B Great Lakes Dr, Brampton ON L6R 2S5; (Pakistan)'91; MB BS; CCFP; (905)494-0302

KHAYAT, Kamal; Clin Pediatrique Laurentienne, 106-200 rue Durand, Saint-Jerome QC J7Z 7E2; Beirut (Lebanon)'72; FRCPC; Peds. Langs: Arabic; English; (450)438-1241; Fax. (450)438-3501.

KHAYKIN, Yaariv; 602-581 Davis Dr, Newmarket ON L3Y 2P6; Tor'96; ABC; FACC; ABIM; FRCPC; IntMed (Echography); Cardiol. Staff, Southlake Regional Health Centre; Langs: Russian; (905)953-7917; Fax. (905)953-0046; ykhaykin@pace-cardiology.com.

KHAYYAM, Naiyar; Saskatoon City Hosp, 7601-701 Queen St, Saskatoon SK S7K 0M7; Kashmir (India)'78; MB BS; Staff Geriatrics, Saskatoon City Hospital; (306)655-8925; Fax. (306)655-8929.

KHAZAMIPOUR, Kazem; Dr K Khazamipour Med Clinic, 130-8120 Cook Rd, Richmond BC V6Y 1T9; Santiago (Dominican Republic)'98; (604)231-1942

KHAZANDAR, Fatimah; Ctr Hosp de Lasalle, 8585 tsse Champlain, LaSalle QC H8P 1C1; Mon'07; CCFP; Staff, Centre Hospitalier de LaSalle; (514)362-8000

KHAZEI, Afshin; 855 12th Ave W, Vancouver BC V5Z 1M9; UBC'95; ABPM; AAFPhys; DABEM; ACLS; ATLS; FRC; FRCPC; EmergMed (Hyperbaric Medicine). Staff EmergMed, Vancouver General Hospital - Centennial Pavillion; Langs: Farsi; (604)875-4033

KHAZOOM, Stephane; Imagix Brossard, 2340 boul Lapiniere, Brossard QC J4Z 2K7; Laval'85; FRCPC; DiagRad. Staff, Centre Hospitalier Régional de Lanaudière; (450)656-1220

KHDER, Jabbar A S; 2927 137 Ave NW, Edmonton AB T5A 5G8; (Sweden)'91; (780)488-4575; Fax. (780)488-4501.

KHEDIGUIAN, Varoujan; 430-5300 Ch de la Cote-des-Nei, Montreal QC H3T 1Y3; Alexandria (Egypt)'64; Peds. Staff, Sir Mortimer B Davis Jewish General; Staff, McGill University Health Centre - Montreal Children's Hospital; Staff, St Mary's Hospital Centre; McGill University; (514)735-4932; Fax. (514)739-9348.

KHEFIF, Ghania; CSSS de Rivière-du-Loup, 75 rue Saint-Henri, Riviere-du-Loup QC G5R 2A4; (Algeria)'93; Staff, Centre Hospitalier Regional du Grand-Portage; (418)868-1000

KHELIL, Assil I; Linden Ridge Med Centre, E-123 Scurfield Blvd, Winnipeg MB R3Y 1L6; Baghdad (Iraq)'88; MB BS; CCFP; Langs: Arabic; assilkh@hotmail.com.

KHENISSI, Zeineb; Hop General de Grand-Sault, 625 Everard H Daigle Blvd, Gr-Sault/Gr-Falls NB E3Z 2R9; Tunis (Other Foreign)'06; Staff, Hôpital Général de Grand-Falls; (506)473-7555

KHERA, A Sheny; Misericordia Community Hosp, 16940 87 Ave NW, Edmonton AB T5R 4H5; Alb'01; CCFP; Staff, Covenant Health - Misericordia Community Hospital; (780)735-2800; Fax. (780)735-2857.

KHERA, Joginder S; 10-1423 Upper Ottawa St, Hamilton ON L8W 3J6; Cardiff (Wales)'77; MB ChB; CCFP; FCFP; Med Dir, Village & Wentworth Heights; Med Dir, Macassa Lodge Home for the Aged; Asst Prof, McMaster University; (905)575-0228; Fax. (905)575-0311.

KHERA, Vikas; The Credit Valley Hosp, 2200 Eglinton Ave W, Mississauga ON L5M 2N1; McM'04; FRCPC; IntMed; Critical Care Medicine. Staff, The Credit Valley Hospital; (905)813-2200

KHERANI, Amin; 200-5340 1 St SW, Calgary AB T2H 0C8; Alb'93; FRCSC; Ophth. Staff, Rockyview General Hospital; (403)286-6802; Fax. (403)286-6819.

KHERANI, Femida; 3994 Hastings St, Burnaby BC V5C 6C1; Alb'97; FRCSC; Ophth. (604)299-3936

KHERANI, Raheem B; Richmond Health Science Ctre, 230-6091 Gilbert Rd, Richmond BC V7C 5L9; Alb'00; FRCPC; IntMed; Rheum. (604)273-8085; Fax. (604)273-8043.

KHERANI, Safeena; 302-1929 Russell Rd, Ottawa ON K1G 4G3; Alb'03; FRCSC; Otol. Consultant, The Ottawa Hospital - General Campus; Consultant, Children's Hospital of Eastern Ontario (CHEO); Consultant, Carleton Place & District Memorial Hospital; (613)526-5737; Fax. (613)526-3402.

KHETANI, Justin D; University of Alberta Hosp, 1E4-8440 112 St NW, Edmonton AB T6G 2B7; Tor'07; Otol. Staff, University of Alberta Hospital; (780)407-7656; Fax. (780)407-7658.

KHETANI, Karim; Dynacare Kasper Med Labs, 200-10150 102 St NW, Edmonton AB T5J 5E2; Aga Khan (Pakistan)'91; (780)451-3702; Fax. (780)452-8488.

KHIDER, Mehdi; Hôpital régional Chaleur, 1750 Sunset Dr, Bathurst NB E2A 4L7; Algiers (Algeria)'93; Staff, Hopital Regional Chaleur; (506)544-3000

KHIM, Hong-Ly; GMF de L'Assomption, CP 3406 Succ Bureau-Chef 814 boul l'Ange-Gardien N, L'Assomption QC J5W 4M9; Laval'86; Staff, CSSS de la Matapedia; (450)589-5778; Fax. (450)589-5779.

KHIMA, Chahrazed; CSSS du Rocher-Perce, CP 3300 451 rue Mgr Ross E, Chandler QC G0C 1K0; (Other Foreign)'02; Staff, Centre Hospitalier de Chandler; (418)689-2261

KHINDA, Surinder S; Morrison Centre, 13-9914 Morrison St, Fort McMurray AB T9H 4A4; (India)'89; MB BS; FRCPC; IntMed. Langs: Punjabi; Hindi; (780)742-2268; Fax. (780)742-0023; drkhinda@yahoo.com.

KHITHANI, Anil K; 206-3430 Finch Ave E, Scarborough ON M1W 2R5; Bombay (India)'84; MB BS; DA(Anes); MD(Anes.); CCFP; FCFP; Staff, Toronto East General Hospital Inc; Staff, The Scarborough Hospital - Birchmount Campus; Staff, Providence Healthcare; Langs: Hindi; Sindhi; Marathi; (416)497-3303; Fax. (416)497-5458.

KHLIL, Abderrahim; Barrie Mem Hosp, 28 rue Gale, Ormstown QC J0S 1K0; Hassan II (Morocco)'99; CCFP; Staff, Barrie Memorial Hospital; (450)829-2321

KHO, Julian; OakMed Family Health Team, 110-231 Oak Park Blvd, Oakville ON L6H 7S8; Tor'02; BSc; CCFP; (905)901-5111; Fax. (905)901-5122.

KHODABANDEHLOO, Mohammed R; 304-1221 Algonquin Ave, North Bay ON P1B 4Y3; (Iran)'91; FRCSC; OrthSurg. Staff Peds, North Bay Regional Health Centre - Regional Mental Health; (705)494-0201

KHODADAD, Kian; Cape Breton Hlthcare Complex, 1482 George St, Sydney NS B1P 1P3; Shahid Beheshti U (Iran)'91; Staff, Cape Breton Healthcare Complex; (902)567-8000

KHODAEI, Minoo; St Thomas-Elgin Gen Hosp, PO Box 2007 Stn Main 189 Elm St, St Thomas ON N5R 5C4; McM'10; CCFP; Staff, St Thomas Elgin General Hospital; (519)631-2020

KHODAWANDI, Kurosch A; Brant Med Arts Bldg, 307-672 Brant St, Burlington ON L7R 2H3; McM'91; CCFP; FCFP; Staff, Joseph Brant Memorial Hospital; (905)632-5138; Fax. (905)632-9961.

KHODAY, Shanta S; 416-5450 Ch de la Cote-des-Nei, Montreal QC H3T 1Y6; Mysore (India)'59; FRCSC; ObstGyn. (514)739-7050

KHOJA, Murtuza; Etobicoke Urgent Care Clinic, 10-25 Woodbine Downs Blvd, Etobicoke ON M9W 6N5; Dublin (Ireland)'05; CCFP; (416)741-2273; Fax. (416)741-3542.

KHOKHAR, Jawad B; 207-95 Bayly St W, Ajax ON L1S 7K8; Punjab (Pakistan)'89; MB BS; CCFP; FCFP; Staff, Rouge Valley Health System - Ajax & Pickering Health Centre Site; Langs: Urdu; (289)660-2888

KHOKHOTVA, Vladislav; 1060-2109 Ottawa St, Windsor ON N8Y 1R8; Tor'05; FRCSC; GenSurg. (519)254-4154; Fax. (519)254-4158.

KHOMANI, Abderrahim; Health Sciences North-Laurenti, 41 Ramsey Lake Rd, Sudbury ON P3E 6J1; (Russia (Federation))'99; (705)523-7100; Fax. (705)523-7318.

KHONG, Binh K; Hamilton HSC- Hamilton Gen, 237 Basrton St E, Hamilton ON L8L 2X2; McM'95; FRCPC; Anes. Staff, Hamilton Health Sciences Centre - Hamilton General Hospital; (905)527-4322

KHONJE, Tadeyo T; Central Med Clinic, 6-1061 Central Ave N, Swift Current SK S9H 4Y9; London (England)'69; MB BS; LRCP(Lond); MRCS(Eng); FACP; FRCPC; IntMed. Chief Dept of Med, Cypress Regional Hospital; Clinical Asst Prof Med, University of Saskatchewan; (306)773-5855; Fax. (306)778-3799.

KHOO, Kong E; BC Cancer Ctre-Southern Interi, 399 Royal Ave, Kelowna BC V1Y 5L3; McM'85; BSc; FRCPC; IntMed; MedOncol; Hem. Staff, Royal Inland Hospital; Ac Staff, Kelowna General Hospital; Consultant, East Kootenay Regional Hospital; Clinical Asst Prof, University of British Columbia; kkhoo@bccancer.bc.ca.

KHOO, Nee Scze; University of Alberta Hosp, 8440 112 St NW, Edmonton AB T6G 2B7; (New Zealand)'97; MB ChB; Staff, University of Alberta Hospital; (780)407-8822

KHORASANI, Kasra; 67 Wells Hill Ave, Toronto ON M5R 3A7; Qns'89; BASc; FRCPC; Psy (Brief Psychotherapy). Staff Psy, Mount Sinai Hospital; Staff Pt-Time Psy, St Michael's Hospital; Lecturer Psy, University of Toronto; Langs: Farsi; (416)627-4590; kasra.khorasani@utoronto.ca.

KHOROVETS, Andrei; Queen Elizabeth II HSC, 1276 South Park St, Halifax NS B3H 2Y9; Moscow (Russia (Federation))'82; Staff, Queen Elizabeth II Health Sciences Centre - Victoria General Site; (902)473-2331

KHORRAMI, Katayoun S; 1213 4 St SW, Calgary AB T2R 0X7; Cal'90; CCFP; Langs: Persian; French; (403)955-6011; Fax. (403)955-6022.

KHORRAMI-ARANI, Nivmand; Royal Jubilee Hosp, 1952 Bay St, Victoria BC V8R 1J8; Flinders (Australia)'03; Staff, Royal Jubilee Hospital; (250)370-8318

KHORSHIDI, Amirmohsen; Brookfield Bonnews HC Centre, PO Box 209 57 Main St, Brookfield NL A0G 1J0; Tehran (Iran)'00; Staff, Brookfield Bonnews Health Care Centre; (709)536-2405

KHORSI, Sonia R; CSSS du Nord de Lanaudière, 1000 boul Sainte-Anne, Joliette QC J6E 6J2; (Algeria)'95; Staff, Centre Hospitalier Régional de Lanaudière.

KHOSHKISH, Reza; Royal Alexandra Hosp, 10240 Kingsway NW, Edmonton AB T5H 3V9; (Iran)'93; Staff, Royal Alexandra Hospital; (780)735-4524; Fax. (780)735-5877.

KHOSHNOOD, Narges; Tammy Latner Centre, L4-60 Murray St Box 13, Toronto ON M5T 3L9; McM'08; CCFP; Langs: Farsi; (416)586-4800

KHOSID, Herbert I; 217-7330 Yonge St, Thornhill ON L4J 7Y7; Kaunas (Lithuania)'65; Staff, Mount Sinai Hospital; Langs: Lithuanian; Russian; Yiddish; (905)707-5165; Fax. (905)707-5197.

KHOSLA, Indu; Mayfair Med Clinic, 211-6707 Elbow Dr SW, Calgary AB T2V 0E4; (India)'71; DTMH; (403)571-1235; Fax. (403)255-4941.

KHOSLA, Megan A; Cardiometabolic Evaluation Ris, 210-1016 68 Ave SW, Calgary AB T2V 4J2; (USA); Staff, Cardiometabolic Evaluation & Risk Assessment Centre; (403)541-0033; Fax. (403)541-0032.

KHOSLA, Munish; Cardiometabolic Evaluation Ris, 240-1016 68 Ave SW, Calgary AB T2V 4J2; Cracow (Poland)'00; ABIM; FRCPC; IntMed; Endocrin&Metab. Staff Diabetes in Pregnancy, Peter Lougheed Centre; Staff, Cardiometabolic Evaluation & Risk Assessment Centre; (403)541-0033; Fax. (403)541-0032.

KHOSLA, Rahul; Kootenay Lake Hosp, 3 View St, Nelson BC V1L 2V1; UBC'99; CCFP; CCFP(E.M.); FCFP; Staff, Kootenay Lake General Hospital; (250)352-3111

KHOSRODAD, Nasim; PO Box 21023 Rpo Terwillegar, Edmonton AB T6R 2V4; (Iran)'01; CCFP.

KHOSROSHAHY, Reza; East Kootenay Reg Hosp, 13 24th Ave N, Cranbrook BC V1C 3H9; Teheran (Iran)'92; (250)426-5281 x6499

KHOSROVANEH, Amir K; Wellington Med Arts Bldg, 214-121 Wellington St W, Barrie ON L4N 1L2; Islamic Azad (Iran)'93; FRCPC; IntMed; InfectDis. Staff, Royal Victoria Regional Health Centre; (705)733-4061

KHOTIANOV, Natan L; Bathurst-Drewry Med Centre, 102-5927 Bathurst St, North York ON M2R 3T5; Grodno State (Belarus)'89; FAAFP; CCFP; Langs: Russian; (416)512-2651; Fax. (416)512-2653.

KHOUEIR, Jihad P; 101-1800 boul le Corbusier, Laval QC H7S 2K1; Sher'00; FRCSC; Neursurg. Staff, Hôpital du Sacre-Coeur de Montréal; (450)686-1156; Fax. (450)686-0252.

KHOUMAIS, Nuha A O; Fitzgerald Bldg, 112-150 College St, Toronto ON M5S 3E2; King Abdul Aziz University (Saudi Arabia)'98; (416)978-6801

KHOUR, Hamid; CSSS du Nord de Lanaudière, 920 boul du Seminaire N, St-Jean-sur-Richel QC J3A 1B7; Staff, Hôpital du Haut-Richelieu; (450)359-5000

KHOURI, Lucie M; Clin Ophtalmologique Decarie, 587 boul Decarie, Saint-Laurent QC H4L 3L1; Mon'94; DABOph; LMCC; FRCSC; Ophth (Oculo Plastic Surgery). Staff Ophth OculoPlastic, Centre Hospitalier l'Université de Montréal (CHUM) - Hôpital Notre-Dame; Staff Ophth Oculoplastic, Hôpital Santa Cabrini Ospedale; Clin Prof, Universite de Montreal; Langs: Arabic; English; Armenian; Spanish; (514)747-6111; Fax. (514)956-8628.

KHOURY, Elie G; Clin Ophtalmologique Decarie, 587 boul Decarie, Saint-Laurent QC H4L 3L1; Beyrouth (Lebanon)'68; AB; CSPQ; Ophth (P.Q.). assoc Staff, Hôpital Santa Cabrini Ospedale; Langs: Arabic; Armenian; English; Italian; (514)747-6111; Fax. (514)956-8628; dreliekhouri@hotmail.com.

KHOURY, Elie-Philippe; CHUS-Hop Fleurimont, 3001 12e Av N, Sherbrooke QC J1H 5N4; St. Joseph (Lebanon)'70; AB; FRCSC; Urol. Staff, Centre Hospitalier Universitaire de Sherbrooke-Hopital Fleurimont; (819)346-1110; Fax. (819)566-7916.

KHOURY, Khalil; CHUS-Hop Fleurimont, 3001 12e Av N, Sherbrooke QC J1H 5N4; Damascus (Syria)'65; FRCPC; Endocrin (P.Q.) (Diabetology); Peds. Staff EndocrinPed, Centre Hospitalier Universitaire de Sherbrooke-Hopital Fleurimont; Consultant, Centre Hospitalier Universitaire de Sherbrooke-Hôpital Hôtel-Dieu; assoc Prof Peds & Endocrin, Universite de Sherbrooke; Langs: Arabic; English; (819)346-1110 x13353; Fax. (819)564-5398.

KHOURY, Lara; The Ottawa Hosp-Civic Campus, 1053 Carling Ave, Ottawa ON K1Y 4E9; Ott'99; FRCPC; IntMed; GeriatricMed. Staff, The Ottawa Hospital - Civic Campus; Langs: Arabic; French; (613)798-5555

KHOURY, Marzouk; Rock Lake Health District, PO Box 130 135 Machray Ave, Crystal City MB R0K 0N0; CCFP; Staff, Rock Lake Health District Hospital; (204)873-2132

KHOURY, Michael A; The Hosp for Sick Children, 555 University Ave, Toronto ON M5G 1X8; Wes'10; Staff, The Hospital For Sick Children; (416)813-5320

KHOURY, Nabil M; GMF Chapleau, 87 montee Gagnon, Bois-des-Filion QC J6Z 4C4; Cairo (Egypt)'77; MSc(Montreal); LMCC; MB BCh; Langs: Arabic; English; (450)621-7420; Fax. (450)621-5007.

KHOURY, Nagib; Hop Jean-Talon, 1385 rue Jean-Talon E, Montreal QC H2E 1S6; Beirut (Lebanon)'78; FRCSC; GenSurg; General Surgical Oncology (P.Q.). Staff, CSSS du Coeur de l'Isle Hôpital Jean-Talon; (514)495-6767

KHOURY, Samir; Clinique Med Ahuntsic, 104-241 rue Fleury O, Montreal QC H3L 1V2; Alb'96; ABPeds; FRCPC; Peds. Staff, Hôtel-Dieu de Sorel; Langs: Arabic; Spanish; French; Lebanese; (514)389-4786; Fax. (514)389-4839; sammykhoury@hotmail.com.

KHOURY, Shahira S; 210-4800 Leslie St, North York ON M2J 2K9; Ain Shams (Egypt)'80; MB ChB; FRCPC; PhysMed&Rehab. Ac Staff, The Scarborough Hospital - Birchmount Campus; Court Staff, Sunnybrook Health Sciences Centre; Court Staff, Toronto Rehabilitation Institute - Lyndhurst Centre; Langs: Arabic; (416)221-1061; Fax. (416)221-0534.

KHOURY, Viviane; MUHC-Montreal Gen Hosp, 1650 av Cedar, Montreal QC H3G 1A4; McG'96; FRCP; ABR; BSc; FRCPC; DiagRad (Musculoskeletal Imaging). Staff, McGill University Health Centre - Montreal General Campus; Langs: Bilingual(French/English); (514)934-1934; Fax. (514)934-8263; viviane.khoury@hotmail.com.

KHOURY, Zahi; CLSC de Saint-Jerome, 1000 rue Labelle, Saint-Jerome QC J7Z 5N6; Saint Joseph (Lebanon)'85; CCFP; (450)431-8001

KHOUZAM, Pierre; York Medical, RR 5 Lcd 1 11-1111 Davis Dr, Newmarket ON L3Y 7V1; Ain Shams (Egypt)'60; Langs: English; Italian; Arabic; (905)853-0404

KHOZA, Phumelelo H J; Drumheller Assoc Physicians, PO Box 5600, Drumheller AB T0J 0Y0; (South Africa)'02; BSc; MB ChB; (403)823-3345; Fax. (403)823-7823.

KHRAISHI, Majed M; 101-120 Stavanger Dr, St. John's NL A1A 5E8; Ain Shams (Egypt)'79; FRCPC; IntMed; Rheum. Clin Prof Med Rheaum, Memorial University Of Newfoundland; (709)576-3235

KHULBE, Suman S; Med Team Clinic, 99 Kakulu Rd, Kanata ON K2L 3C8; Ott'99; CCFP; (613)592-1448

KHULLAR, Atul; Northern Alberta Sleep Clinic, 302-8702 Meadowlark Rd NW, Edmonton AB T5R 5W5; Alb'99; MSc; DABPN; DABSM; FRCPC; Psy (Sleep Disorders). Staff Psy, Covenant Health - Grey Nuns Community Hospital; Consultant Psy, Edmonton Zone Edmonton Public Health Services; Consultant Specialist, MedSleep Calgary; (780)487-5333; Fax. (780)487-3045; info@edmontonsleep.com.

KHULLAR, Chander M; Devon Med Clinic, 5-106 Erie St S, Devon AB T9G 1A7; Delhi (India)'70; Staff, Devon General Hospital; (780)987-3315; Fax. (780)987-4009.

KHULLAR, Renu; Sentinelle Health Group, 232 boul Saint-Joseph, Gatineau QC J8Y 3X4; Alb'86; BSc; Langs: Bilingual(English/French); (819)778-1330; Fax. (819)778-3455.

KHULLAR, Sarjiwan; Devon Med Clinic, 5-106 Erie St S, Devon AB T9G 1A7; Rajsthan (India)'65; MB BS; FRCS(Ed & Eng); LRCP(Lond); MRCS(Eng); Med Examiner, Civil Aviation Canada; Langs: Hindi; Punjabi; (780)987-3315; Fax. (780)987-4009; sarjiwan.khullar@tc.gc.ca.

KHUMREE, Altaf; Airdrie Med Centre, 103-1800 Market St SE, Airdrie AB T4A 0K9; (South Africa)'08; MB BCh; (403)980-9929; Fax. (403)980-9925.

KHUNKHUN, J Sevena; 6438 Fraser St, Vancouver BC V5W 3A4; UBC'92; CCFP; Langs: Punjabi; Hindi; (604)327-3330

KHUON, David C; Hunt Club Med Centre, 104-3328 McCarthy Rd, Ottawa ON K1V 0H9; Sher'95; CCFP; Langs: Bilingual(English/French); (613)526-5515; Fax. (613)526-0740.

KHUONG, Helene T; Foothills Med Centre, 1403 29 St NW, Calgary AB T2N 2T9; Laval'04; FRCSC; Neursurg. Staff, Foothills Medical Centre; (403)944-1110

KHURAL, Ajay P S; 86 Highroad South, Carbonear NL A1Y 1A4; Punjab (India)'81; MB BS; Hospitalist, Carbonear General Hospital; Langs: Punjabi; Hindi; (709)945-5035; Fax. (709)945-5212; ajaysimrit@hotmail.com.

KHURAL, Simrit K; Wetern Bay Clinic, PO Box 10, Western Bay NL A0A 4J0; Punjab (India)'87; MB BS; Staff, Carbonear General Hospital.

KHURANA, Mahesh C; 1265 100th St, North Battleford SK S9A 0V6; Agra (India)'70; MB BS; MD; Staff, Battlefords Union Hospital; (306)446-4303; Fax. (306)446-4304.

KHURANA, Mona; Humber River Reg Hosp-Church, 200 Church St, Toronto ON M9N 1N8; UBC'08; CCFP; Staff, Humber River Regional Hospital - Church Street Site; Langs: Hindi; Punjabi; (416)243-4191

KHURANA, Reena; Fraser River Endocrinology, 32-15300 105 Ave, Surrey BC V3R 6A7; UBC'02; FRCPC; IntMed; Endocrin&Metab. (604)584-3669

KHURANA, Rosy; Mistissini Clinic, GD 395 boul Mistissini, Mistissini QC G0W 1C0; McG'97; CCFP; Langs: Hindi; French; (418)923-3376; Fax. (418)923-3240.

KHURANA, Rshmi; Royal Alexandra Hosp, 332CSC-10240 Kingsway NW, Edmonton AB T5H 3V9; Alb'92; FRCPC; IntMed. Staff Community Service Ctr, Royal Alexandra Hospital; (780)735-6827; Fax. (780)735-5313.

KHURRAM, Sabahat; Parkland Med Associates, 205-505 Queen St, Spruce Grove AB T7X 2V2; (Other Foreign)'02; CCFP; (780)962-2001

KHURSHID, Faiza; The Hosp for Sick Children, 555 University Ave, Toronto ON M5G 1X8; Punjab (Pakistan)'02; Staff, The Hospital For Sick Children; (416)813-6927

KHWAJA, Kosar A; MUHC-Montreal Gen Hosp, L9 411-1650 av Cedar, Montreal QC H3G 1A4; McG'99; FRCSC; GenSurg (Clinician Investigator Program); Critical Care Medicine (P.Q.). Staff, McGill University Health Centre - Montreal General Campus; (514)934-1934

KHY, Virachit; CSSSG-Hop De Gatineau, CP 2000 Succ Bureau-Chef 909 boul la Verendrye O, Gatineau QC J8P 7H2; Mon'90; CSPQ; FRCPC; Anes. Staff, Hôpital de Gatineau; (819)561-8299

KI, Vincent; 132-101 Queensway W, Mississauga ON L5B 2P7; McM'07; FRCPC; IntMed; Nephrol. Staff Adult Nephrology Residendy Prog, St Joseph's Healthcare - Charlton Campus; (905)272-1104

KIAHOSSEINI, Shirin; Churchill Falls Clinic, GD, Churchill Falls NL A0R 1A0; (Iran)'95; (709)925-3381

KIAI, Cristina A; Lonsdale Med Dental Bldg, 108-1940 Lonsdale Ave, North Vancouver BC V7M 2K2; Manila (Philippines)'83; BSc; CCFP; Langs: Tagalog; (604)987-3347; Fax. (604)987-7624.

KIAII, Bob B; London HSC-University Hosp, PO Box 5339 Stn B 339 Windermere Rd, London ON N6A 5A5; Wes'92; FRCSC; GenSurg (Minimal Invasive Surgery); CardSurg. Staff, London Health Sciences Centre - University Hospital; Langs: Italian; Persian; (519)663-3153; Fax. (519)663-3044; bob.kiaii@lhsc.on.ca.

KIAII, Mercedeh; Burrard Health Bldg, 602-1160 Burrard St, Vancouver BC V6Z 2E8; UBC'94; FRCPC; IntMed; Nephrol. Staff Nephrologist, Providence Health Care - St Paul's Hospital; Asst Prof, University of British Columbia; (604)681-7191; Fax. (604)681-4482.

KIAIRA, Mary K; 12-75 Main St E, Milton ON L9T 1N4; Nairobi (Kenya)'86; Staff, Halton Healthcare Services Corporation - Milton District Hospital; (905)636-1779

KIANG, Michael W J; St Joseph's Mountain H Serv, PO Box 585 Stn Lcd 1 100 West 5th St, Hamilton ON L8N 3K7; Tor'97; FRCPC; Psy. Staff, St Joseph's Healthcare Hamilton - West 5th Campus; (905)522-1155

KIAPWAY, Mosenza; Wadena Group Med Clinic, PO Box 130, Wadena SK S0A 4J0; (Other Foreign)'85; Physician, Saskatoon Health Region; (306)338-2597; Fax. (306)338-2367.

KIARED, Ahmed; Legacy Med Centre, 378 4 Ave S, Lethbridge AB T1J 5E9; Laval'07; (403)320-1504

KIBBLEWHITE, Douglas J; 802-777 Broadway W, Vancouver BC V5Z 4J7; UBC'80; FRCSC; Otol (Facial Plastic & Reconstructive Surgery). Ac Staff, Vancouver General Hospital - Centennial Pavillion; Asst Prof, University of British Columbia; (604)688-5900; Fax. (604)688-5905.

KIBERD, Bryce A; Queen Elizabeth II HSC, 5082-1276 South Park St, Halifax NS B3H 2Y9; Tor'80; FRCPC; IntMed; Nephrol. Staff, Queen Elizabeth II Health Sciences Centre - Victoria General Site; Dalhousie University; (902)473-5160; Fax. (902)473-2675; bryce.kiberd@dal.ca.

KIBIUK, Laurie A M; 103B-984 Oliver Rd, Thunder Bay ON P7B 7C7; Man'98; CCFP; FCFP; (807)768-1333; Fax. (807)768-1348.

KIBOS TALABUR, Elena; CSSS du Haut-Saint-François, RR 3 460 2e Avenue, Weedon QC J0B 3J0; Carol Davila (Romania)'99; Gen Practice, CSSS du Haut-Saint-François; (819)877-3434

KIBRIA, Shawkat; Parkland Med Associates, 205-505 Queen St, Spruce Grove AB T7X 2V2; Man'99; CCFP; Staff Physician, Westview Health Centre; (780)962-2001; Fax. (780)962-8176.

KIBRITE, Antoine; CHUQ-Hotel-Dieu De Quebec, 11 Cote Du Palais, Quebec QC G1R 2J6; St. Joseph (Lebanon)'69; FRCSC; GenSurg (Colon & Rectal Surgery). Staff, Centre Hospitalier Universitaire de Québec (CHUQ) - Siege Social; Clin Prof Faculte de Med, Université Laval; Langs: Arabic; Bilingual(English/French); (418)691-5370; Fax. (418)691-5020.

KIBSEY, Pamela C; Royal Jubilee Hosp, 1952 Bay St, Victoria BC V8R 1J8; Alb'78; FRCPC; MedMicrobiol (Infection Control). Staff, Victoria General Hospital; Staff, Royal Jubilee Hospital; (250)519-1626; Fax. (250)519-1628; pamela.kibsey@viha.ca.

KICHIAN, Krikor; Bayshore Med Bldg, 302-3029 Carling Ave, Ottawa ON K2B 8E8; Tor'99; FRCPC; IntMed; Gastroent. Langs: Arabic; Armenian; French; (613)728-1795; Fax. (613)728-0091.

KIDD, Arthur D F; 1096 Goyeau St, Windsor ON N9A 1J1; Qns'72; FRCPC; IntMed (Endocrinology & Metabolism). Staff Chief, Hôtel-Dieu Grace Hospital; Ac Staff, Windsor Regional Hospital - Metropolitan Site; (519)258-1335; Fax. (519)258-8936; akidd@hdgh.org.

KIDD, Monica G; South Health Campus, 4448 Front St SE, Calgary AB T3M 1M4; Mem'08; CCFP; (403)956-2300

KIDD, Robert F; 175 Argyle St S, Renfrew ON K7V 1T6; McG'70; Court Staff, Renfrew Victoria Hospital; Langs: Bilingual(English/French); (613)432-6596; Fax. (613)432-6596; rfkidd@on.aibn.com.

KIDD, William T; Foothills Med Centre, C827-1403 29 St NW, Calgary AB T2N 2T9; Alb'84; FRCSC; GenSurg (Cardiac Surgery); Cardiovasc&ThorSurg. Staff, Foothills Medical Centre; (403)944-1671; Fax. (403)944-2906.

KIDDOO, Darcie A; University of Alberta Hosp, 2C3 65 WMC-8440 112 St NW, Edmonton AB T6G 2B7; Alb'98; FRCSC; Urol (Pediatric Urology). Staff, University of Alberta Hospital; Asst Prof, University of Alberta; (780)407-7808; dkiddoo@ualberta.ca.

KIDERCHAH, Rabi; CSSS D'Argenteuil, 145 av de la Providence, Lachute QC J8H 4C7; Mon'98; Staff, Centre Hospitalier d'Argenteuil; (450)562-3761

KIDNEY, Maria R; 100-3001 Gordon Ave, Coquitlam BC V3C 2K7; Trinity Coll. (Ireland)'76; FRCPC; DiagRad. Staff Med Imaging, Royal Columbian Hospital; (604)941-7611

KIDWAI, Bakhtiar J; Queen Elizabeth II HSC-Halifax, 6896-1796 Summer St, Halifax NS B3H 3A7; Karachi (Pakistan)'85; MB BS; MSc; MRC; Att Staff Cardiol, Queen Elizabeth II Health Sciences Centre - Halifax Infirmary Site; Asst Prof Med, Dalhousie University; Langs: Urdu; (902)473-4153; Fax. (902)473-6293.

KIDY, A Razak; Brampton Med Bldg, 210-164 Queen St E, Brampton ON L6V 1B4; Cardiff (Wales)'67; MB ChB; Dip; Ac Staff, William Osler Health System - Brampton Civic Hospital; (905)459-6710; Fax. (905)459-5085.

KIEFER, Gerhard N; Alberta Children's Hosp, 2888 Shaganappi Trail NW, Calgary AB T3B 6A8; Cal'80; FRCSC; OrthSurg (Pediatric Orthopedics). Dir Orthopaedics, Alberta Children's Hospital; Staff, Foothills Medical Centre; Assoc Prof, University of Calgary; Langs: German; (403)955-2268; Fax. (403)943-7634; gkiefer@ucalgary.ca.

KIEFER, Lori A; 16F-25 Grosvenor St, Toronto ON M7A 1Y6; Alb'94; MHSc; FRCPC; CommunMed; Public Health & Preventive Med., University of Toronto; (416)327-2389

KIEFFER, Marilyn A; Village Med Associates, 27-1077 North Service Rd, Mississauga ON L4Y 1A6; Tor'89; CCFP; FCFP; Staff, Trillium Health Centre - Mississauga; (905)949-1700; Fax. (905)949-8625.

KIEHN, Lana; Southlake Med Centre, 201-581 Davis Dr, Newmarket ON L3Y 2P6; Qns'08; CCFP; Staff, North York General Hospital; (905)853-3103

KIELAR, Ania Z; The Ottawa Hosp-Civic Campus, 1053 Carling Ave, Ottawa ON K1Y 4E9; Ott'00; FRCPC; DiagRad. Staff, The Ottawa Hospital - Civic Campus; (613)761-4982

KIELEY, Lisa A; Eleven Elizabeth Fam Practice, 201-11 Elizabeth Ave, St. John's NL A1A 1W6; Mem'99; CCFP; lkieley@nl.rogers.com.

KIELLERMAN, Andrew J; 4-101 Burnside Rd W, Victoria BC V9A 1B7; Cracow (Poland)'83; BSc(Hon); Langs: Polish; (250)360-1194; Fax. (250)381-9257.

KIELLY, G Andrew; PO Box 1955 Stn Main, Swift Current SK S9H 4M7; Sask'01; CCFP.

KIELTY, John P; Deer Lake Clinic, 2-4 Clinic Dr, Deer Lake NL A8A 1E2; Dublin (Ireland)'05; MB BCh; CCFP; (709)635-7200

KIELY, Daniel J; Hop du Sacre-Coeur de Mtl, 5400 boul Gouin O, Montreal QC H4J 1C5; McG'06; MDCM; ObstGyn. Staff, Hôpital du Sacre-Coeur de Montréal; (514)338-2222

KIENITZ, Norman G; Royal Inland Hosp, 311 Columbia St, Kamloops BC V2C 2T1; Ott'94; BSc; CCFP; CCFP(E.M.); Staff, Royal Inland Hospital; Langs: German; (250)314-2100

KIERASZEWICZ, Halina; Strathroy-Middlesex Gen Hosp, 395 Carrie St, Strathroy ON N7G 3C9; Wes'76; FRCPC; Anes. Staff, Strathroy Middlesex General Hospital - Middlesex Hospital Alliance; Ac Staff, London Health Sciences Centre - Victoria Campus; (519)245-1550

KIESER, Katharina E; 5003-5820 University Ave, Halifax NS B3H 1V7; Dal'97; BSc; MSc; FRCSC; ObstGyn (Gynecologic Oncology). Asst Prof, Dalhousie University; Langs: German; (902)473-2366; Fax. (902)473-7765; kkieser@dal.ca.

KIESER, Teresa M; Foothills Med Centre, C816-1403 29 St NW, Calgary AB T2N 2T9; Ott'76; ABS; FACS; FRCSC; GenSurg (Cardiac Surgery); Cardiovasc&ThorSurg. Staff Cardiothoracic Surg, Foothills Medical Centre; Assoc Prof, University of Calgary; Langs: English; French; Italian; (403)944-8449; Fax. (403)944-0489.

KIESS, Marla C; St Paul's Hosp, 2375-1081 Burrard St, Vancouver BC V6Z 1Y6; UBC'77; FACC; FRCPC; Cardiol (Adult Congenital Heart Disease). Dir Noninvasive Cardiol & Pacific Adult Congenital Heart Clinic, Providence Health Care - St Paul's Hospital; Staff, BC Women's Hospital & Health Centre; Clin Prof, University of British Columbia; (604)806-8297; Fax. (604)806-8410.

KIEU, Cong Van; Centre Hosp Honore-Mercier, 2750 boul Laframboise, Saint-Hyacinthe QC J2S 4Y8; Mon'87; Cardiol (P.Q.); IntMed (P.Q.). Staff, Centre Hospitalier Honore-Mercier; (450)771-3333 x3288; Fax. (450)771-3283.

KIEU, Khanh-Giao; Clinique Med Provision, 5428 av Victoria, Montreal QC H3W 2P4; Mon'90; LMCC; Chief Medical Serv., CLSC St-Laurent; (514)748-6400; Fax. (514)748-6323; khanh-giao.kieu@ssss.gouv.qc.ca.

KIEU, Vi-Thuy; 5482 rue Victoria, Montreal QC H3W 2P8; Mon'89; (514)342-1251

KIEZ, Debra A; Mackenzie Richmond Hill Hosp, 10 Trench St, Richmond Hill ON L4C 4Z3; McM'85; CCFP; CCFP(E.M.); Court Staff Urgent Care Clinic, North York General Hospital - Branson Division; Staff, Mackenzie Richmond Hill Hospital; Langs: English; French; (905)883-1212; debra.kiez@sympatico.ca.

KIFY, Omar H; Pembroke Regional Hosp, 705 MacKay St, Pembroke ON K8A 1G8; Al-Mustansiriyah (Iraq)'94; FRCPC; IntMed; Respir. Staff, Pembroke Regional Hospital Inc; (613)732-2811

KIGGUNDU, Fredrick; 8115 160 Ave NW, Edmonton AB T5Z 0G3; Makerere (Uganda)'92; MB ChB; (780)475-9635; Fax. (780)478-9635.

KIJEWSKI, Raegan L; Royal Alexandra Hosp, 10240 Kingsway NW, Edmonton AB T5H 3V9; Alb'06; CCFP; Staff, Royal Alexandra Hospital; (780)735-4201; Fax. (780)735-4978.

KILADA, Baher F N; Seven Regions Health Centre, PO Box 1000 24 Mill St, Gladstone MB R0J 0T0; (Egypt)'88; CCFP; Staff, Seven Regions Health Centre; baherfawzy@hotmail.com.

KILAM, Surendar K; Auxiliary Wing, 3K 219AW-935 17 St S, Lethbridge AB T1J 3E4; Kashmir (India)'65; DABS; FACS; FICS; FRCSC; GenSurg (Endoscopy). Staff, Chinook Regional Hospital; Langs: Kashmiri; (403)388-6515; Fax. (403)388-6516; surendar.kilam@gmail.com.

KILANI, Mehrak M; Royal Court Med Centre, 305-1 Quarry Ridge Rd, Barrie ON L4M 7G1; Tehran (Iran)'93; FRCSC; ObstGyn. (705)728-5311; Fax. (705)728-5601.

KILANY, Ali K A A; Dufferin Subspecialty Clinic, 1664 Dufferin St, Toronto ON M6H 3M1; Garyounis (Libya)'94; FRCPC; IntMed; Cardiol. Langs: Arabic; (416)652-6101

KILBERTUS, Frances T; Bruyere Academic Fam Hlth Team, 75 Bruyere St, Ottawa ON K1N 5C7; McM'84; CCFP; FCFP; Langs: French; Spanish; (613)241-3344; Fax. (613)241-1971.

KILBY, Donald L P; U of Ottawa Health Services, 300-100 Marie Curie Pvt, Ottawa ON K1N 1A2; Ott'77; Dir, University of Ottawa Health Services; (613)564-3950; Fax. (613)564-6627; dkilby@uottawa.ca.

KILCOLLINS, Calvin T; 75 Water St PO Box 417, Windsor NS B0N 2T0; Dal'75; CCFP; Staff, Hants Community Hospital; (902)798-4330; Fax. (902)798-4456.

KILCUP, Michael C; Miramichi Reg Hosp, 500 Water St, Miramichi NB E1V 3G5; Dal'04; FRCPC; DiagRad. Staff, Miramichi Regional Hospital; (506)623-3000

KILFOIL, John E; F W Green Med Centre, 1629 Baker St, Cranbrook BC V1C 1B4; Witwatersrand (South Africa)'97; (250)426-6601

KILGAR, Jennifer L; London HSC-Victoria Campus, E1 105-800 Commissioners Rd E, London ON N6A 4G5; Dal'96; FRCPC; Peds; PedEmergMed. Staff, London Health Sciences Centre - Victoria Campus; Clin Researcher Ped Emerg, University of Western Ontario; (519)685-8500 x58134; Fax. (519)667-6769; jennifer.kilgar@lhsc.on.ca.

KILIAN, Daniel S; 100-2210 Main St, Penticton BC V2A 5C2; Stellenbosch (South Africa)'93; LMCC; Langs: Afrikaans; (250)493-6747; dkilian@telusplanet.net.

KILIAN, Lu-Inge; H2 Medical Centre, 7020 4 St NW, Calgary AB T2K 1C4; Stellenbosch (South Africa)'90; MB ChB; CCFP; FCFP; (403)730-7663

KILIAN, Rochagne; Cariboo Mem Hosp, 517 Sixth Ave N, Williams Lake BC V2G 2G8; Orange Free State (South Africa)'05; CCFP; Staff Emergency dept, Cariboo Memorial Hospital and Health Centre; Langs: Afrikaans; (250)392-4411; rochagne_kilian@telus.net.

KILLEEN, Ronald A; Lockview Med Clinic, 204-159 Cobequid Rd, Lower Sackville NS B4C 2N1; Dal'75; CCFP; FCFP; (902)865-7547; Fax. (902)252-3029.

KILLIAN, Fionnuala M; Victoria Med Rehab Consultants, 402-1245 Esquimalt Rd, Victoria BC V9A 3P2; National (Ireland)'75; MB ChB; BAO; FRCPC; PhysMed&Rehab. Staff, Vancouver Island Health Authority; (250)598-9922

KILLIAN, Kieran J; McMaster University, 3U9-1280 Main St W, Hamilton ON L8S 4K1; National (Ireland)'72; FRCP(Ire); FRCPC; IntMed; Respir. Staff Physician RespMed, Hamilton Health Sciences Centre - McMaster Children's Hospital; Prof Med, McMaster University; (905)521-2100; Fax. (905)521-5053.

KILLICK, David G; Northern Lights Health Region, 7 Hospital St, Fort McMurray AB T9H 1P2; Alb'81; CCFP; CCFP(E.M.); Staff, Northern Lights Regional Health Centre; (780)791-6161; Fax. (780)791-6167; dgkillick@shaw.ca.

KILLICK, Geoffrey W; Central Park Med/Dental, 104-3965 Kingsway, Burnaby BC V5H 1Y8; UBC'80; (604)434-8781; Fax. (604)434-8699.

KILLICK, Lyn M; Fraser Med Clinic, 108-22441 Dewdney Trunk Rd, Maple Ridge BC V2X 7X7; Ott'86; FRCPC; Psy. Staff, Surrey Memorial Hospital; (604)463-1300

KILLINGER, Donald W; Medical Clinic Bldg, 309-89 Humber College Blvd, Etobicoke ON M9V 4B8; Wes'57; MSc; PhD; FRCPC; IntMed (Endocrinology). Emeritus Prof Faculty of Med, University of Western Ontario; (416)740-9663; Fax. (416)740-0827; donkillinger@yahoo.com.

KILLINS, Brian A; PO Box 84, Tofino BC V0R 2Z0; Alb'79; (250)726-4443; Fax. (250)726-7333.

KILLORN, Erin E; London HSC-Victoria Hosp, PO Box 5010 Stn B 800 Commissioners Rd E, London ON N6A 5W9; Dal'02; FRCPC; Peds; PedEmergMed. Staff, London Health Sciences Centre - Victoria Campus; (519)685-8500 x58134

KILLORN, W Patrick; Burlington Prof Centre, 401-3155 Harvester Rd, Burlington ON L7N 3V2; Dal'78; FRCPC; IntMed; Respir. (905)639-3209; Fax. (905)639-3452.

KILMARTIN, Patrick E; 6-14 Victoria St W, Alexandria ON K0C 1A0; National (Ireland)'72; (613)525-4599; Fax. (613)525-4673.

KILMARTIN, Patrick J M; Time Square, 270-380 Armour Rd, Peterborough ON K9H 7L7; Dublin (Ireland)'78; MB ChB; DCH; Ac Staff, Peterborough Regional Health Centre - Rogers St Site; Ac Staff, Peterborough Regional Health Centre - Hospital Drive; (705)743-7592; Fax. (705)743-1935; pkilmartin@prhc.on.ca.

KILMURRY, Matthew R; 201-749 King St W, Kitchener ON N2G 1E4; Tor'96; FRCSC; GenSurg; ThorSurg. (519)742-6696; Fax. (519)742-9520.

KILMURY, Alana J; Pasqua Hosp, 4F-4101 Dewdney Ave, Regina SK S4T 1A5; (Other Foreign)'07; CCFP; Staff Palliative Care, Pasqua Hospital; (306)766-2951; Fax. (306)766-2588.

KILPATRICK, Bruce T; Royal Inland Hosp, 311 Columbia St, Kamloops BC V2C 2T1; Witwatersrand (South Africa)'98; Staff, Royal Inland Hospital; (250)374-5111

KILPATRICK, Katherine L; Health for Life Med Centre, 637 Princess St, Kingston ON K7L 1E2; McM'95; BA; CCFP; FCFP; Med Dir, Health for Life Medical Centre; Asst Prof, Queen's University; (613)546-1600; Fax. (613)546-6806.

KILPATRICK, Nevin; BC Women's Hosp & Health Ctre, 4500 Oak St, Vancouver BC V6H 3N1; Stellenbosch (South Africa)'87; MB ChB; FRCPC; Anes; FamilyMed. Staff, BC Women's Hospital & Health Centre; (604)875-2158

KILSHAW, Margaret W; Lansdowne Professional Ctr II, 325-3066 Shelbourne St, Victoria BC V8R 6T9; London (England)'65; MB BS; DOMS(Eng.); FRCSC; Ophth. Consultant, Vancouver Island Health Authority; (250)595-2443; Fax. (250)598-6237; mkilshaw@telus.net.

KILTY, Shaun J; C-1541 Merivale Rd, Ottawa ON K2G 5W1; Ott'02; FRCSC; Otol. (613)729-2312; Fax. (613)729-2412.

KILTZ, Michael R; West Edmonton Mall Clinic, 2-17303 Stony Plain Rd NW, Edmonton AB T5S 1B5; Alb'86; CCFP; (780)484-0800; Fax. (780)484-0907.

KILVERT, Vivan M; PO Box 1187 Stn Main, Ladysmith BC V9G 1A8; Cal'99; CCFP.

KIM, Alexandra V; Sunnybrook Health Sciences Ctr, A421-2075 Bayview Ave, Toronto ON M4N 3M5; Moscow Medical Stomatology Institute (Russia (Federation))'99; Staff, Sunnybrook Health Sciences Centre; (416)480-6100

KIM, Alice D; Vancouver Gen Hosp, JP2 244-899 12th Ave W, Vancouver BC V5Z 1M9; UBC'99; FRCPC; Anes. Staff, Vancouver General Hospital - Centennial Pavillion; (604)875-4303

KIM, Amanda L; Meadowlark Health Centre, 162 Meadowlark Shopping Ctr NW, Edmonton AB T5R 5W9; Dal'01; FRCSC; ObstGyn. (780)428-9516; Fax. (780)428-0629.

KIM, Anne M; 8630 120 St, Surrey BC V3W 3N6; UBC'00; CCFP; (604)591-5505

KIM, Arnold F; Thunder Bay Reg HSC-T-Bay, 980 Oliver Rd, Thunder Bay ON P7B 6V4; Wes'90; Staff, Thunder Bay Regional Health Sciences Centre; (807)684-6100

KIM, Betty Y S; PG Medical Education Office, 2F-500 University Ave, Toronto ON M5G 1V7; McM'02; FRCSC; Neursurg.

KIM, Brian; Circle Med at Copperfield, 123-15566 McIvor Blvd SE, Calgary AB T2Z 4Y2; Man'10; CCFP; Langs: Korean; (403)726-0524

KIM, Catherine Y; Southlake Reg Health Centre, 596 Davis Dr, Newmarket ON L3Y 2P9; Tor'03; FRCPC; Anes. Staff, Southlake Regional Health Centre; (905)895-4521

KIM, Cei-Whan; 1433 Ontario St, Burlington ON L7S 1G5; Tor'98; GenSurg. (905)333-0622; Fax. (905)632-9308.

KIM, Celine C; The Hosp for Sick Children, 555 University Ave, Toronto ON M5G 1X8; Tor'09; Staff, The Hospital For Sick Children; (416)813-1500

KIM, Christie Y; William Osler HC-Brampton, 2100 Bovaird Dr E, Brampton ON L6R 3J7; McG'05; FRCPC; IntMed; Hem. Staff, William Osler Health System - Brampton Civic Hospital; (905)494-6542

KIM, Christina K; 308-435 Reynolds St, Oakville ON L6J 3M5; McG'06; MDCM; FRCPC; IntMed; Nephrol. (905)815-9283

KIM, Dae Tong; Queen Elizabeth Hosp, PO Box 6600 Stn Central, Charlottetown PE C1A 8T5; UBC'98; FRCPC; AnatPath. Staff, Queen Elizabeth Hospital; (902)894-0126; Fax. (902)894-2385.

KIM, Daniel H; Southlake Reg Health Centre, 596 Davis Dr, Newmarket ON L3Y 2P9; Tor'97; FRCPC; Anes. Staff, Southlake Regional Health Centre; (905)895-4521

KIM, Daniel H J; University of Alberta Hosp, 2C2 39-8440 112 St NW, Edmonton AB T6G 2B7; Cal'95; FRCPC; IntMed (Interventional Cardiology); Cardiol. Staff Div of Cardiol, University of Alberta Hospital; Asst Prof Med, University of Alberta; (780)407-7206; Fax. (780)407-6452.

KIM, Daniel J; Vancouver Gen Hosp, 855 12th Ave W, Vancouver BC V5Z 1M9; Wes'07; FRCPC; EmergMed. Staff, Vancouver General Hospital - Centennial Pavillion; (604)875-4111

KIM, David; Bluewater Health-Norman Site, 89 Norman St, Sarnia ON N7T 6S3; Wes'94; Staff, Bluewater Health - Norman Site; Staff, Bluewater Health - Mitton Site; (519)464-4400

KIM, David; BC Cancer Ctre-Southern Interi, 399 Royal Ave, Kelowna BC V1Y 5L3; Alb'95; BSc; FRCPC; RadOncol. Staff, BC Cancer Agency Sindi Ahluwalia Hawkins Centre for the Southern Interior; Staff, Kelowna General Hospital; (250)712-3979; dakim@bccancer.bc.ca.

KIM, David E; Saskatoon Orth & Sports Med Ct, 104-311 Ludlow St, Saskatoon SK S7S 1N6; UBC'96; FRCSC; OrthSurg. (306)651-0800; Fax. (306)651-5323; davidkim.ortho@shaw.ca.

KIM, David H; Markham Stouffville Health Ctr, 405-377 Church St, Markham ON L6B 1A1; Cal'01; BSc(Hon); CSCN; FRCPC; Neur (Electromyography). Court Staff, West Park Healthcare Centre; Court Staff, Sunnybrook Health Sciences Centre; Ac Staff, Markham Stouffville Hospital; (905)294-8053; Fax. (905)294-5652.

KIM, Dennis D H; Univ Hlth Network-Princess M, 5 126-610 University Ave, Toronto ON M5G 2M9; Kyungpook National University (Korea)'95; Staff, Princess Margaret Hospital - University Health Network; Asst Prof, University of Toronto; Langs: Korean; (416)946-4501 x2464; Fax. (416)946-4563.

KIM, Dennis; 1844 Coronation Blvd, Cambridge ON N3H 3R9; Qns'02; FRCSC; Urol. (519)650-4510

KIM, Dennis; Eaton Placve Med Centre, 81-333 St Mary Ave, Winnipeg MB R3C 4A5; (Other Foreign)'09.

KIM, Do-Hoon; The Juravinski Cancer Centre, 699 Concession St, Hamilton ON L8V 5C2; Qns'01; FRCPC; RadOncol. Physician, The Juravinski Cancer Centre; (905)387-9495

KIM, Don Wook; Ridge Meadows Hosp & Hlth CC, 11666 Laity St, Maple Ridge BC V2X 5A3; Tor'92; CCFP; CCFP(E.M.); Staff Emerg, Ridge Meadows Hospital & Health Care Centre; (604)463-4111; Fax. (604)463-1835.

KIM, Don; Credit Valley Prof Bldg, 501-2300 Eglinton Ave W, Mississauga ON L5M 2V8; Tor'78; FRCPC; IntMed; Nephrol. Staff, The Credit Valley Hospital; Staff, Trillium Health Centre - Mississauga; Staff, Headwaters Health Care Centre - Orangeville Site; Langs: Korean; (905)820-8770; Fax. (905)820-3703; drkimdohun@hotmail.com.

KIM, Donna M; CAMH Geriatric Program, 6F-80 Workman Way, Toronto ON M6J 1H4; Wes'04; FRCPC; Psy. Staff, Centre for Addiction & Mental Health (CAMH) - Queen Site; (416)535-8501; Fax. (416)583-1272.

KIM, Edward; 2775 Laurel St, Vancouver BC V5Z 1M9; Qns'96; FRCPC; IntMed; Gastroent. (604)875-4124

KIM, Florence A; St Michael's Hosp, 30 Bond St, Toronto ON M5B 1W8; Sask'01; CCFP; Staff Family Practice Unit, St Michael's Hospital; (416)864-5110; Fax. (416)867-7498.

KIM, George P; Byron Family Med Centre, 1228 Commissioners Rd W, London ON N6K 1C7; Wes'03; CCFP; Physician, West Elgin Comm Health Centre.

KIM, Godfrey J H; Rouge Valley-Centenary HC, 2867 Ellesmere Rd, Scarborough ON M1E 4B9; Tor'91; FRCPC; DiagRad. Staff, Rouge Valley Health System - Centenary Health Centre Site; (416)284-8131 x3873

KIM, Hyung; 205-589 Lake St, St Catharines ON L2N 7L6; McG'87; FACC; FRCPC; IntMed; Cardiol. Staff, Niagara Health System - Ontario Street Site; Staff, Niagara Health System - St Catharines General Site; (905)646-2525; Fax. (905)646-3251.

KIM, H Kenneth; St Michael's Hosp, 30 Bond St, Toronto ON M5B 1W8; Wes'06; FRCPC; Anes. Staff, St Michael's Hospital; (416)864-5071

KIM, H L Nancy; Canada Diagnostic Centres, 200A Stewart Green SW, Calgary AB T3H 3C8; UBC'99; FRCPC; DiagRad. Langs: Korean; (403)685-6175; Fax. (403)685-6199; nkim@canadadiagnostics.ca.

KIM, Hae Ryong; 84 Finch Ave W, North York ON M2N 2H4; Yonsei (Korea)'78; FRCP; FRCPC; Psy (Psychiatric Assessment). Langs: Korean; (416)224-2685; Fax. (416)224-1736; talfinch@rogers.com.

KIM, Hae-Kwan J; Portage Clinic, 140 9th St SE, Portage la Prairie MB R1N 3V5; Man'10; CCFP; (204)857-3445

KIM, Hahn Hoe; 208-564 Belmont Ave W, Kitchener ON N2M 5N6; McG'96; FRCPC; IntMed; Cardiol. Staff, St Mary's General Hospital; (519)576-3099; Fax. (519)576-3112; hoe.kim@utoronto.ca.

KIM, Harold L; Belgage Med Arts Bldg, 205-525 Belmont Ave W, Kitchener ON N2M 5E2; Wes'91; FRCPC; IntMed; ClinImmunol&Allergy. Asst Prof, McMaster University; Aj Prof, University of Western Ontario; (519)745-9525; grandriverallergy@yahoo.ca.

KIM, Hyon Chung; Sunnybrook Hlth Sciences Ctre, H 356-2075 Bayview Ave, Toronto ON M4N 3M5; Tor'97; CCFP; Staff, Sunnybrook Health Sciences Centre; (416)480-6100 x7091

KIM, J John; Univ Hlth Network-Princess M, 610 University Ave, Toronto ON M5G 2M9; Tor'89; FRCPC; RadOncol (Gastrointestinal Disorders). Staff, Princess Margaret Hospital - University Health Network; Asst Prof, University of Toronto; (416)946-2126; Fax. (416)946-6561.

KIM, Jae K; Thunder Bay Reg HSC, 980 Oliver Rd, Thunder Bay ON P7B 6V4; Tor'97; FRCPC; DiagRad. Staff, Thunder Bay Regional Health Sciences Centre; (807)684-6000

KIM, James K; Lions Gate Hosp, 231 15th St E, North Vancouver BC V7L 2L7; UBC'93; FRCPC; Anes. Staff, Lions Gate Hospital; (604)984-5709

KIM, James S J; 2-2 Kennedy Rd S, Brampton ON L6W 3E1; Tor'89; CAFCI; Staff Privil, Humber River Regional Hospital - Church Street Site; Langs: Korean; (905)458-7477; Fax. (905)458-7477; jkim0309@rogers.com.

KIM, Jarmila; Children's Hosp Eastern Ont, 401 Smyth Rd, Ottawa ON K1H 8L1; Ott'91; FRCPC; Anes. Staff Anes, Children's Hospital of Eastern Ontario (CHEO); (613)737-2431; Fax. (613)738-4815.

KIM, Ji Hyun; Harborn Med Associates, 510-89 Queensway W, Mississauga ON L5B 2V2; Qns'09; CCFP; Staff, Mount Sinai Hospital; (905)273-4380; Fax. (905)273-4335.

KIM, Jin Hee; The Doctor's Office, 245 Eglinton Ave E, Toronto ON M4P 3B7; UBC'07; CCFP; (416)488-1455

KIM, Joe; Belmont Family Medicine, 201-535 Belmont Ave, Kitchener ON N2M 5E9; Wes'96; CCFP; (519)579-4870; Fax. (519)579-7903.

KIM, John; The Ottawa Hosp-Gen Campus, W2284-501 Smyth Rd, Ottawa ON K1H 8L6; Qns'94; FRCPC; IntMed; Critical Care Medicine. Staff, The Ottawa Hospital - General Campus; (613)737-8899 x79830

KIM, Joon-Han J; Headwaters Health Care Centre, 100 Rolling Hills Dr, Orangeville ON L9W 4X9; Tor'91; CCFP; CCFP(E.M.); Staff Emerg, Headwaters Health Care Centre - Orangeville Site; (519)941-2410

KIM, Joseph C; Rothbart Centre for Pain Care, 9-4646 Dufferin St, North York ON M3H 5S4; Wes'03; FRCPC; Anes. (416)512-6407; Fax. (416)512-6375.

KIM, Joseph; Rockyview Gen Hosp, 3A 151-7007 14 St SW, Calgary AB T2V 1P9; Alb'04; FRCPC; IntMed; InfectDis. Staff, Rockyview General Hospital; (403)943-3255; joskim@ucalgary.ca.

KIM, Juan; The Well Medical Clinic, E-1001 Austin Ave, Coquitlam BC V3K 3N9; Ott'05; CCFP; (604)937-2520

KIM, Julie; 2113 boul Casavant O, Saint-Hyacinthe QC J2S 8B8; McG'88; FRCSC; Otol. Staff, Centre Hospitalier Honore-Mercier; (450)773-7824

KIM, Jun-Nyun; 700 Ross Ave E, Timmins ON P4N 8P2; Alb'96; CCFP; CCFP(E.M.); Staff, Timmins & District Hospital; (705)267-6340; junkim6@gmail.com.

KIM, Justin; 10A-30 Eglinton Ave W, Mississauga ON L5R 3E7; Tor'03; MD; CCFP; Court Staff, The Credit Valley Hospital; Ac Staff, William Osler Health System - Brampton Civic Hospital; Langs: Korean; (905)712-2288; Fax. (905)712-8228.

KIM, Ki Sun; 101-7380 Westminster Hwy, Richmond BC V6X 1A1; UBC'89; (604)273-9404; Fax. (604)273-3342.

KIM, Lina B; Ermineskin Med Clinic, 301-2377 111 St NW, Edmonton AB T6J 5E5; Alb'97; CCFP; (780)436-8731; Fax. (780)434-8732.

KIM, Linda; Rouge Valley-Ajax & Pickering, 580 Harwood Ave S, Ajax ON L1S 2J4; Tor'93; FRCPC; Anes. Staff, Rouge Valley Health System - Ajax & Pickering Health Centre Site; (905)683-2320 x1288

KIM, M Marie; Erinoak, 2277 South Millway, Mississauga ON L5L 2M5; Tor'84; MSc; FRCPC; Peds (Developmental Pediatrics). Assoc Prof Peds, McMaster University; Langs: Korean; (905)820-7111 x3223; mkim@erinoakkids.ca.

KIM, Matthew C Y; 203-726 Bloor St W, Toronto ON M6G 4A1; Tor'83; (416)532-3397; Fax. (416)532-3531; kim1265@rogers.com.

KIM, Mi Hwa; Wrinch Mem Hosp, PO Box 999, Hazelton BC V0J 1Y0; Seoul (Korea)'83; CCFP; Staff, Wrinch Memorial Hospital; (250)842-5234

KIM, Myung-Gi; Douglas Med Centre, 238 Bertie St, Fort Erie ON L2A 1Z3; Tor'84; Staff, Niagara Health System - Douglas Memorial Hospital Site; Langs: Korean; (905)871-0364; Fax. (905)871-2204.

KIM, Paul R; The Ottawa Hosp-Gen Campus, W1650-501 Smyth Rd, Ottawa ON K1H 8L6; Sask'89; FRCSC; OrthSurg. Staff OrthSurg, The Ottawa Hospital - General Campus; (613)737-8774; Fax. (613)737-8837.

KIM, Peter T W; NCSB 1244-585 University Ave, Toronto ON M5G 2N2; Wes'02; FRCSC; GenSurg (Clinician Investigator Program). Staff, Toronto General Hospital - UHN; (416)340-4252

KIM, Rak Hay; 617-18 William Carson Cres, North York ON M2P 2G6; (Korea)'55; FRCP; FRCPC; IntMed (Endocrinology); Endocrin&Metab. Hon Staff Endocrin, Toronto General Hospital - UHN; Langs: Korean; (416)512-7887; Fax. (416)921-7369; swkooh@rogers.com.

KIM, Raymond H; PG Medical Education Office, 602-500 University Ave, Toronto ON M5G 1V7; Tor'08; FRCPC; IntMed.

KIM, Richard B; London HSC-University Hosp, PO Box 5339 Stn B 339 Windermere Rd, London ON N6A 5A5; Sask'87; FRCPC; IntMed. Staff, London Health Sciences Centre - University Hospital; (519)685-8300

KIM, Richard S J; St Joseph's Health Centre, 30 The Queensway, Toronto ON M6R 1B5; Tor'91; CCFP; CCFP(E.M.); Ac Staff Emerg, St Joseph's Health Centre; (416)530-6857

KIM, Rozaliya; Vancouver Family Health Centre, 100-2732 Hastings St E, Vancouver BC V5K 1Z9; (Other Foreign)'09; CCFP; (604)253-3166

KIM, S Joseph; CSB 11C-585 University Ave, Toronto ON M5G 2N2; Tor'97; FRCPC; IntMed; Nephrol. Staff, Toronto General Hospital - UHN; (416)340-3228; Fax. (416)340-4701.

KIM, Sandra A; Women's College Hosp, 810-76 Grenville St, Toronto ON M5S 1B2; Ott'01; FRCPC; IntMed; Endocrin&Metab. Staff, Women's College Hospital; (416)323-6373

KIM, Sarah; Toronto East Gen Hosp Inc, 825 Coxwell Ave, Toronto ON M4C 3E7; McM'03; CCFP; Staff, Toronto East General Hospital Inc; Lakeridge Health - Bowmanville Site; (416)469-6580

KIM, Seung; Kingsway Plaza Phase III, 600-4980 Kingsway, Burnaby BC V5H 4K7; Alb'93; FRCPC; IntMed; ClinImmunol&Allergy. Staff, Ridge Meadows Care Clinic Inc(West); Langs: Korean; (604)433-0545; Fax. (604)433-2846.

KIM, Sharon; 228-284 Queen St E, Brampton ON L6V 1C2; Cal'01; FRCSC; PlasSurg (Hand & Wrist Surgery). Court Staff Plastic Surg, Trillium Health Centre - Mississauga; Ac Staff Plastic Surg, William Osler Health System - Brampton Civic Hospital; (905)456-7635

KIM, Simon Y; Niagara H SYstem-St Catharine, PO Box 3018 Stn Main 142 Queenston St, St Catharines ON L2R 7C6; Tor'98; FRCPC; IntMed;CCFP; Staff, Niagara Health System - St Catharines General Site; (905)684-7271

KIM, Steve Y; St Joseph's Health Centre, 30 The Queensway, Toronto ON M6R 1B5; Wes'07; FRCPC; Urol. Staff, St Joseph's Health Centre; (416)530-6000

KIM, Susan; 390-1144 Burrard St, Vancouver BC V6Z 2A5; Cal'03; FRCSC; ObstGyn. (604)568-8155

KIM, Susie; Women's College Hosp, 76 Grenville St, Toronto ON M5S 1B2; Wes'07; CCFP; Staff, Women's College Hospital.

KIM, Tae K; Dept Of Medical Imaging, 585 University Ave, Toronto ON M5G 2N2; Seoul (Korea)'91; FRCPC; DiagRad.

KIM, Vy Hong-Diep N; The Hosp For Sick Children, 555 University Ave, Toronto ON M5G 1X8; McM'04; FRCPC; Peds; ClinImmunol&Allergy. Staff, The Hospital For Sick Children; (416)813-1500; Fax. (416)813-8638.

KIM, W James; Scenic Acres Med Clinic, 8555 Scurfield Dr NW, Calgary AB T3L 1Z6; (South Africa)'06; MB ChB; (403)547-2255

KIM, Willy S; GMF Concorde, 300 boul de la Concorde E, Laval QC H7G 2E6; Mon'08; CCFP; (450)667-5310

KIM, Won Oh; 11664 223 St, Maple Ridge BC V2X 5X5; Qns'04; FRCSC; OrthSurg. Staff, Ridge Meadows Hospital & Health Care Centre; (604)467-0454

KIM, Young-In; St Michael's Hosp, 16CC-038-30 Bond St, Toronto ON M5B 1W8; Tor'87; FRCPC; IntMed; Gastroent. Staff Gastroent, St Michael's Hospital; Assoc Prof Med, University of Toronto; Langs: Korean; (416)864-5848; Fax. (416)864-5994.

KIM SING, Charmaine; BC Cancer Agency-Vancouver CC, 600 10th Ave W, Vancouver BC V5Z 4E6; Cape Town (South Africa)'80; FRCPC; RadOncol. Staff, BC Cancer Agency Vancouver Centre; Clin Assoc Prof, University of British Columbia; (604)877-6000; Fax. (604)708-2000.

KIM SING, Malcolm; 108-3825 Sunset St, Burnaby BC V5G 1T4; Witwatersrand (South Africa)'78; FRCPC; Peds. (604)433-5750 x3646; Fax. (604)431-6228.

KIMACOVICH, Richard G; Niagara H System-St Catherine, PO Box 3018 Stn Main 142 Queenston St, St Catharines ON L2R 7C6; Man'88; BSc; CCFP; CCFP(E.M.); FCFP; Staff, Niagara Health System - St Catharines General Site; (905)684-7271

KIMBALL, Brian P; The Sheppard Heart Centre, 740-100 Sheppard Ave E, North York ON M2N 6N5; Alb'77; BMedSci; ABIM(IntMed&CardioVascDis); FACC; Cardiol; IntMed (Non-Invasive Diagnostics). (416)224-0375; Fax. (416)224-1895.

KIMBALL, Lauren E; Academic Family Medicine, 172-1621 Albert St, Regina SK S4P 2S5; McM'10; BScH; CCFP; Asst Prof, University of Saskatchewan; (306)766-0444; Fax. (306)766-0471.

KIMBER, Shane K M; University of Alberta Hosp, 2C2-8440 112 St NW, Edmonton AB T6G 2B7; Qns'84; FRCPC; IntMed; Cardiol. Staff, University of Alberta Hospital; (780)407-6946; Fax. (780)407-6452.

KIMBERLEY, Nicholas A; 302-1757 Beaufort Ave, Comox BC V9M 1R8; UBC'86; BSc; FRCSC; GenSurg. Staff, St Joseph's General Hospital; (250)890-0632; Fax. (250)890-0637.

KIMEL, Gilad; St Paul's Hosp, 1081 Burrard St, Vancouver BC V6Z 1Y6; UBC'05; FRCPC; IntMed (Palliative Medicine). Staff, Providence Health Care - St Paul's Hospital; (604)682-2344 x62297

KIMELMAN, Allen L; Rougeau Plaza Med Centre, N-1522 Regent Ave W, Winnipeg MB R2C 3B4; Man'85; Fax. (204)663-0827.

KIMELMAN, Harold S; 101-9 Madawaska Ave, North York ON M2M 2R1; Tor'71; Ac Staff, North York General Hospital - Branson Division; (416)226-4363; Fax. (416)226-6482.

KIMIA, Dyan; 65 av Hillside, Westmount QC H3Z 1W1; McG'91; FRCPC; Peds. Clin Asst, McGill University Health Centre - Montreal Children's Hospital; Staff Peds, Sir Mortimer B Davis Jewish General; Langs: French; Hebrew; (514)931-5652; Fax. (514)931-2625.

KIMMONS, Gerard M J; 217 Danforth Ave, Toronto ON M4K 1N2; McM'81; Psy (Oppositional Defiant Disorder). Staff, Pine Seven Medical Centre; (416)236-0133; Fax. (416)236-0135; dr.g.kimmons@gmail.com.

KIMOFF, R John; MUHC-Royal Victoria Hosp, 687 av des Pins O, Montreal QC H3A 1A1; McG'83; ABIM; FRCPC; IntMed (Pulmonary Medicine); Respir. Staff, McGill University Health Centre - Royal Victoria Hospital; assoc Prof, McGill University; Langs: English; French; (514)843-1568; Fax. (514)843-1695.

KIMPINSKI, Kurt; London HSC-University Campus, PO Box 5339 Stn B 339 Windermere Rd, London ON N6A 5A5; Dal'02; Neur. Staff Clinical Neurological, London Health Sciences Centre - University Hospital; (519)663-3337; Fax. (519)663-3328.

KIMPTON, Susan; Clinique De Ped De Rimouski, 301-161 av Rouleau, Rimouski QC G5L 5T3; Laval'73; Peds. Ac Staff, Hôpital Regional Rimouski; Langs: English; (418)724-4221; Fax. (418)725-3025.

KINAHAN, Consuelo A P; Medimax, 2479 McCallum Rd, Abbotsford BC V2S 3P8; UBC'85; (604)852-2279

KINAHAN, John F J D; 101-1503 Hillside Ave, Victoria BC V8T 2C1; UBC'91; FRCSC; Urol. (250)384-8515; Fax. (250)386-9323.

KINAHAN, Michael J; Royal Jubilee Hosp, 1952 Bay St, Victoria BC V8R 1J8; UBC'89; FRCPC; Anes. Staff, Royal Jubilee Hospital; (250)370-8441

KINAHAN, Thomas J; 210-3001 Tutt St, Kelowna BC V1Y 2H4; UBC'84; FAAP(Urol); FRCSC; Urol (Pediatric Urology). (250)763-3842; Fax. (250)763-8220.

KINAIA, Ban M; Windsor Med Centre, 3-130 Ouelette Place, Windsor ON N8X 1L9; Univesity of Al-Mustansiriyah (Other Foreign)'90; CCFP; (519)971-2901

KINASH, Barbara L; Family Med Associates, 5021 51 St, Lacombe AB T4L 2A3; Alb'81; Ac Staff, Lacombe Hospital & Care Centre; (403)782-3351; Fax. (403)782-5879.

KINCADE, David D; Penticton Reg Hosp, 102-550 Carmi St, Penticton BC V2A 3G6; UBC'94; FRCPC; IntMed (Cardiology). Staff, Penticton Regional Hospital; Staff, Royal Inland Hospital; Clin Instructor Med, University of British Columbia; (250)493-0887

KINDEKI-LUZINGU, Pierrette; CSSS-Hopital De Hull, 116 boul Lionel-Emond, Gatineau QC J8Y 1W7; Louvain (Belgium)'01; Staff, Hull Hospital; (819)595-6000

KINDLE, Geoffrey F; Brandon Reg Health Centre, 150 McTavish Ave E, Brandon MB R7A 2B3; Qns'70; FRCPC; DiagRad. Staff Imaging Dept, Brandon Regional Health Centre; (204)726-2155; Fax. (204)726-2396.

KINDLE, Gitta K N; Rideau Family Health Team, 11-2450 Lancaster Rd, Ottawa ON K1B 5N3; Qns'72; Langs: Indonesian; (613)738-9119; Fax. (613)738-2736.

KINDLE, John E; Rideau Valley Health Centre, 1221 Greenbank Rd, Ottawa ON K2J 5V7; Qns'72; (613)258-8710; Fax. (613)440-3238; drjkindle@rogers.com.

KINDOPP, A Shawn; Surrey Mem Hosp, 13750 96 Ave, Surrey BC V3V 1Z2; Sask'96; FRCPC; Anes. Staff Anes, Surrey Memorial Hospital; Clinical Asst Prof, University of British Columbia; (604)588-3367; shawnkindopp@hotmail.com.

KINDRACHUK, Gary W; Kelowna Medical Imaging, 101-3330 Richter St, Kelowna BC V1W 4V5; Alb'81; FRCPC; DiagRad; NuclearMed. (250)762-4420

KINDY, Anna O T; North Island Med Clinic, 1405 Spruce St, Campbell River BC V9W 7K1; Alb'86; Physician, North Island Medical Clinic; (250)286-1334

KINDZIERSKI, Robert; Royal Alexandra Hosp, 10240 Kingsway NW, Edmonton AB T5H 3V9; Sask'07; FRCPC; Anes. Staff, Royal Alexandra Hospital; (780)735-4010

KING, Aaron D; 45 Mill St, Toronto ON M5A 3R6; Ott'03; FRCPC; Derm. Staff, Haldimand War Memorial Hospital.

KING, Amy C; Central Nfld Reg Hlth Centre, 50 Union St, Grnd-Falls-Windsor NL A2A 2E1; Mem'08; FRCPC; IntMed. Staff, Central Newfoundland Regional Health Centre.

KING, Anthony E; Royal University Hosp, 103 Hospital Dr, Saskatoon SK S7N 0W8; Mem'90; FRCSC; OrthSurg (Hip & Knee Reconstruction). Staff Orth Surg, Royal University Hospital; Staff Orth Surg, Saskatoon City Hospital; Prog Dir Orthopedics, University of Saskatchewan; (306)966-8089; Fax. (306)966-8196.

KING, Arlene; Hepburn Block, 11F-80 Grosvenor St, Toronto ON M7A 1R3; McM'81; MHSc; FRCPC; CommunMed (Public Health). Langs: English; French; (416)212-3831; arlene.king@ontario.ca.

KING, Barbara J; Markham Stouffville Hosp, PO Box 1800 Stn Main 381 Church St, Markham ON L3P 7P3; Man'92; CCFP; CCFP(E.M.); Staff, Markham Stouffville Hospital; (905)472-7111

KING, Bertram W; 205A-1635 Lawrence Ave W, Toronto ON M6L 3C9; Cape Town (South Africa)'67; Staff, Humber River Regional Hospital - Keele Street Site; (416)245-3555; Fax. (416)245-8949.

KING, Caroline A; 105-17 King St E, Dundas ON L9H 1B7; Wes'96; FRCPC; Psy (General Adult Psychiatry). (905)628-5656

KING, Charles B; Village Family Health Team, 102-171 East Liberty St, Toronto ON M6K 3P6; Rochester (USA)'87; (416)599-8348 x8348; charles.king@villagefht.ca.

KING, Charles D; Crescent Beach Med Arts, 2781 Gordon Ave, Surrey BC V4A 3J5; Tor'71; (604)535-2520

KING, Christopher R; Royal Jubilee Hosp, 1952 Bay St, Victoria BC V8R 1J8; UBC'01; FRCPC; DiagRad. Staff, Royal Jubilee Hospital; (250)370-8000

KING, David B; Dr David King Incorporated, 208-1535 Dresden Row, Halifax NS B3J 3T1; Dal'71; BSc; FRCPC; Neur (Movement Disorders). Staff, Queen Elizabeth II Health Sciences Centre - Victoria General Site; Consultant, Nova Scotia Rehabilitation Centre; Asst Prof, Dalhousie University; (902)425-7343; Fax. (902)423-0879.

KING, David P; Worker's Comp Board of NS, PO Box 1150 5595 Fenwick St, Halifax NS B3J 2Y2; Dal'81; BSc(H.C.); Chief Medical Officer, Worker's Compensation Board of NS; (902)491-8341; Fax. (902)491-8232.

KING, David S; St Paul's Hosp, 1081 Burrard St, Vancouver BC V6Z 1Y6; McG'10; MDCM; CCFP; Staff, Providence Health Care - St Paul's Hospital; (604)682-2344

KING, Dionne V; CSSSG-Hop de Gatineau, CP 2000 Succ Bureau-Chef 909 boul de la Verandrye O, Gatineau QC J8P 7H2; McG'98; Peds. Staff, Hôpital de Gatineau; (819)561-8565

KING, Dolores; Calgary Trail Medicentre, 1-10407 51 Ave NW, Edmonton AB T6H 0K4; Dublin (Ireland)'58; Staff, Calgary Trail Medicentres; (780)436-8071; Fax. (780)435-6034.

KING, Elizabeth A; 20 Jeffrey St PO Box 598, Bridgetown NS B0S 1C0; Mem'87; (902)665-3075; Fax. (902)665-0005.

KING, Francis G; Health Sciences Centre, 300 Prince Philip Dr, St. John's NL A1B 3V6; Mem'75; FRCPC; Anes (Anesthesia-ICU). Staff, Health Sciences Centre; (709)777-6540; Fax. (709)777-6506; fking@mun.ca.

KING, George W; Hawkesbury Dist Gen Hosp, 1111 Ghislain St, Hawkesbury ON K6A 3G5; Dal'92; CCFP; CCFP(E.M.); Staff, Hawkesbury & District General Hospital; (613)632-1111 x346

KING, Graham J W; St Joseph's Health Care, PO Box 5777 Stn B 268 Grosvenor St, London ON N6A 4V2; UBC'82; FRCSC; OrthSurg (Hand Wrist & Elbow Surgery). Ac Staff Hand & Upper Limb Centre, St Joseph's Hospital - St Joseph's Health Care; Prof, University of Western Ontario; (519)646-6011; Fax. (519)646-6049.

KING, Gregory P; Sunnybrook Health Sciences Ctr, 2075 Bayview Ave, Toronto ON M4N 3M5; South Dakota (USA)'07; DiagRad.

KING, Heidi; Saint John Reg Hosp, PO Box 2100 Stn Main, Saint John NB E2L 4L2; Mem'97; FRCPC; DiagRad. Staff, Saint John Regional Hospital; (506)452-5200

KING, James F; Grand Falls Med Clinic, 164 Goodyear Ave, Grnd-Falls-Wi NL A2A 1M4; Mem'78; CCFP; FCFP; Ac Staff, Central Newfoundland Regional Health Centre; Clin Associate Family Med, Memorial University Of Newfoundland; (709)489-7851; Fax. (709)489-0081.

KING, Jason J; Medical Assoc of Port Colborne, 97 Charlotte St, Port Colborne ON L3K 3E2; (Grenada)'02; (905)834-4546

KING, Jeffrey A; Beechwood Forest Med Centre, 2-890 Glasgow St, Kitchener ON N2N 3G6; Wes'86; (519)744-4293; Fax. (519)744-6424.

KING, John W R; North York Gen Hosp, 4001 Leslie St, North York ON M2K 1E1; Cal'85; FRCPC; EmergMed. Staff, North York General Hospital; (416)756-6165

KING, Joseph W; Clearly Lasik Canada Inc, 303-10060 Jasper Ave NW, Edmonton AB T5J 3R8; UBC'92; FRCSC; Ophth. (780)421-7007; jking@clearlyasik.com.

KING, Karen M; Cross Cancer Institute, 11560 University Ave NW, Edmonton AB T6G 1Z2; Alb'98; FRCPC; IntMed; MedOncol. Staff Med Oncol, Cross Cancer Institute; (780)432-8221; Fax. (780)432-8888; karenkin@cancerboard.ab.ca.

KING, Kathryn A; 1450 Waddington Rd, Nanaimo BC V9S 4V9; UBC'95; PhD; CCFP; FCFP; Ac Staff Privil, Nanaimo Regional General Hospital; (250)754-5545; Fax. (250)754-5954; kaking@shaw.ca.

KING, Kebby F G; Peterborough Reg HC, 1 Hospital Dr, Peterborough ON K9J 7C6; West Indies (Jamaica)'97; FRCPC; DiagRad. Staff, Peterborough Regional Health Centre - Hospital Drive; (705)743-2121

KING, Kim W; Caledonian Med Clinic, 340 Campbell St, Nanaimo BC V9R 3G7; UBC'92; FRCPC; IntMed; GeriatricMed. Staff, Nanaimo Regional General Hospital; (250)753-3202

KING, Laval Kon Kam; Summerside Med Centre, 101-475 Granville St, Summerside PE C1N 3N9; Aberdeen (Scotland)'65; MB ChB; MRC; Staff, Prince County Hospital; Langs: Chinese; French; (902)432-8123; Fax. (902)436-9660.

KING, Marion J; 201-6990 Derry Rd, Milton ON L9T 7H3; Qns'82; CCFP; FCFP; Ac Staff Family Med, Halton Healthcare Services Corporation - Milton District Hospital; Court Staff Family Med, Joseph Brant Memorial Hospital; (905)878-2424; Fax. (905)878-0945.

KING, Meghan A; Dalhousie Fam Med Spryfield MC, 16 Dentith Rd, Halifax NS B3R 2H9; Tor'10; CCFP; (902)473-1234

KING, Michael H; 507-3025 Hurontario St, Mississauga ON L5A 2H1; Tor'65; FRCPC; IntMed (Hematology). Ac Staff, Toronto General Hospital - UHN; Staff, Trillium Health Centre - West Toronto; Ac Staff, Trillium Health Centre - Mississauga; Assoc Prof, University of Toronto; (905)270-8470; Fax. (905)270-8478.

KING, Pamela A; Surrey Mem Hosp, 13750 96 Ave, Surrey BC V3V 1Z2; Dal'88; Staff, Surrey Memorial Hospital; (604)588-3367

KING, Peter A C; 1450 Waddington Rd, Nanaimo BC V9S 4V9; Alb'75; Dip SportMed; BMedSci; Ac Staff, Nanaimo Regional General Hospital; Clinical Asst Prof, University of British Columbia; (250)754-5545; Fax. (250)754-5954; packmd@shaw.ca.

KING, Rebecca R; London HSC-Victoria Hosp, PO Box 5010 Stn B 800 Commissioners Rd E, London ON N6A 5W9; Mem'06; FRCPC; Psy. Staff, London Health Sciences Centre - Victoria Campus.

KING, Rebekah M; North Bay Reg Health Centre, 50 College Dr, North Bay ON P1B 0A4; McM'08; CCFP; Staff, North Bay Regional Health Centre - Regional Mental Health; (705)474-8600

KING, Robert J; Pathways to Independence, 289 Pinnacle St, Belleville ON K8N 3B3; Tor'84; FRCPC; Psy. (613)962-2541; Fax. (613)962-6357.

KING, Roger B; Western Mem Reg Hosp, PO Box 2005 Stn Main 1 Brookfield Ave, Corner Brook NL A2H 6J7; Mem'97; CCFP; Staff, Western Memorial Regional Hospital; (709)637-5000

KING, Russell H T; Fredericton Med Clinic, 501-1015 Regent St, Fredericton NB E3B 6H5; Dal'72; BSc; CCFP; Ac Staff, Dr Everett Chalmers Regional Hospital; (506)458-0238; Fax. (506)458-0301.

KING, Susan M; Eleven Elizabeth Fam Practice, 201-11 Elizabeth Ave, St. John's NL A1A 1W6; Mem'80; Staff Health Care Corp of St John's, St Clare's Mercy Hospital.

KING, Timothy R; Injury Management Solutions, 120-16555 Fraser Hwy, Surrey BC V4N 0E9; Dal'90; BSc; PhD; (604)575-2325; Fax. (604)575-2326; solutions@imsrehab.com.

KING, W James B; Children's Hosp Eastern Ont, 401 Smyth Rd, Ottawa ON K1H 8L1; Mem'85; FRCPC; Peds. Staff, Children's Hospital of Eastern Ontario (CHEO); (613)737-7600 x2664; Fax. (613)737-4878.

KING, W I Nelson; Medical Clinic Bldg, 310-89 Humber College Blvd, Etobicoke ON M9V 4B8; Tor'91; FRCSC; GenSurg (Endoscopy). (416)742-0506; Fax. (416)742-1666.

KING, Wei-Shuen; Anaesthetic Services, 213-2186 Oak Bay Ave, Victoria BC V8R 1G3; Cal'03; FRCPC; Anes. (250)595-7211

KING, William; Canadian Vein Institute, 402-1881 Yonge St, Toronto ON M4S 3C4; Tor'65; FRCS; FRCSC; GenSurg; VascSurg. Staff, Canadian Vein Institute; Lecturer Surg, University of Toronto; (416)966-3886

KING, Yvonne M; Valley Prof Centre, 300-70 Exhibition St, Kentville NS B4N 4K9; Mem'78; (902)678-6495; Fax. (902)678-7431.

KINGDOM, John C P; Mount Sinai Hosp, 3265-600 University Ave, Toronto ON M5G 1X5; Dublin (Ireland)'84; FRCOG; MRC(UK); DCH; FRCSC; ObstGyn (Doppler). Staff ObstGyn, Mount Sinai Hospital; Prog Dir Maternal Fetal Med Fellowship/Prof, University of Toronto; (416)586-4800 x8808; Fax. (416)586-3216.

KINGSBURY, Claude; Polyclinique St-Eustache, 75 rue Grignon, St-Eustache QC J7P 4J2; Mon'91; (450)473-3585; Fax. (450)473-1916.

KINGSLEY, Justin J; Wellington Med Clinic, 84C-3200 Island Hwy N, Nanaimo BC V9T 1W1; Alb'07; CCFP; (250)740-2100

KINGSLEY, Normand; Centre Hosp Honore-Mercier, 2750 boul Laframboise, Saint-Hyacinthe QC J2S 4Y8; Mon'73; Chief Med Staff, Centre Hospitalier Honore-Mercier; (450)771-3333; Fax. (450)771-3283; normand.kingsley@rrsss16.gouv.qc.ca.

KINGSLEY, Simon J; St Michael's Hosp, 30 Bond St, Toronto ON M5B 1W8; Tor'94; BSc; CCFP; CCFP(E.M.); Ac Staff, St Michael's Hospital; University of Toronto; (416)864-5095; Fax. (416)864-5341.

KINGSMAN, Ronald N; Oshawa Clinic, 117 King St E, Oshawa ON L1H 1B9; Ott'74; Court Staff, Lakeridge Health - Oshawa Site; (905)723-8551 x2538; Fax. (905)723-1495.

KINGSTON, Gary W; 104-1629 Townsite Rd, Nanaimo BC V9S 1N3; UBC'86; FRCSC; GenSurg. (250)753-8808; Fax. (250)753-8823.

KINGSTON, June; Summerville Family Health Team, 5F-101 Queensway W, Mississauga ON L5B 2P7; Tor'79; CCFP; FCFP; Trillium Health Centre - Mississauga; (905)272-9700; Fax. (905)272-1416.

KINGSTON, Robert; Campbell Clinic, PO Box 180 Stn Main, Coaldale AB T1M 1M3; Sheffield (England)'66; (403)345-3072; Fax. (403)345-2141.

KINGSTON, Susan J; Maternal Child Clinic, 130-1402 8 Ave NW, Calgary AB T2N 1B9; McG'87; CCFP; FCFP; Med Staff, Foothills Medical Centre; (403)289-9051; Fax. (403)284-3129.

KINGSTON, William G R; 410-299 Victoria St, Prince George BC V2L 5B8; Queen's (Ireland)'81; MB ChB; DRCOG; DCH; FRCS; FRCSC; ObstGyn. Staff, University Hospital of Northern British Columbia; (250)564-8869; Fax. (250)564-8863.

KINGSTONE, Eddie; Rosedale Med Centre, 205-600 Sherbourne St, Toronto ON M4X 1W4; McG'56; Dip; FRCPC; Psy. Prof Psy, University of Toronto; (416)967-6200; kingstone@smh.toronto.on.ca.

KINGSTONE, Michael S; The Ottawa Hosp-Civic Campus, 1053 Carling Ave, Ottawa ON K1Y 4E9; Tor'92; FRCPC; DiagRad. Staff, The Ottawa Hospital - Civic Campus; (613)798-5555

KINGSTONE, Robert A; Forest Hill Family Health Cent, 491 Eglinton Ave W, Toronto ON M5N 1A8; Tor'63; (416)782-6111; Fax. (416)782-5515.

KINGSTONE, Sheldon I; Castleview Wychwood Towers, 351 Christie St, Toronto ON M6G 3C3; Tor'57; (416)392-5700; Fax. (416)392-4157.

KINGWELL, Stephen P; The Ottawa Hosp-Civic Campus, 1053 Carling Ave, Ottawa ON K1Y 4E9; Qns'02; FRCSC; OrthSurg (Spine). Staff, The Ottawa Hospital - Civic Campus; (613)798-5555 x13245; Fax. (613)761-5100.

KINI, Vishwas M; 115-4515 Ebenezer Rd, Brampton ON L6P 2K7; Karnatak University Dharwar (India)'00; CCFP; Langs: Hindi; Punjabi.

KINIGAKIS, Tracey D; 1-1261 Beaverbrook Ave, London ON N6H 0G6; Wes'81; CCFP; FCFP; (519)642-2077; Fax. (519)642-1725.

KINLEY, Cecil E; Parkland Med Clinic, 203-998 Parkland Dr, Halifax NS B3M 0A6; Dal'86; (902)404-7737; Fax. (902)404-7066.

KINLOCH, R David; Richmond Med Bldg, 202-2020 Richmond Rd, Victoria BC V8R 6R5; Alb'74; ABIM(IntMed); ABIM(CV); FRCPC; IntMed (Interventional Cardiology); Cardiol. (250)595-3111; Fax. (250)595-4278; david.kinloch@viha.ca.

KINNARD, Patrick R G; Polyclinique de la Capitale, 7-4225 4e av O, Quebec QC G1H 6P3; Louvain (Belgium)'71; FRCSC; OrthSurg. (418)623-9871; Fax. (418)623-9873.

KINNEAR, David W H P; Portage Clinic Inc, 140 9th St SE, Portage La Prairie MB R1N 3V5; Man'92; CCFP; FCFP; (204)857-3445; Fax. (204)239-1278.

KINNEAR, Hilary A; Cole Harbour Family Med Centre, 203-240 Baker St, Dartmouth NS B2W 5L4; Dal'98; BSc; CCFP; FCFP; Staff Family Med, Dartmouth General Hospital; Staff Family Med, IWK Health Centre; (902)435-6312; hkinnear@accesswave.ca.

KINNEAR, Susan E; Associate Clinic, 352-401 9 Ave SW, Calgary AB T2P 3C5; Man'94; BSc(Med); FRCPC; IntMed; Endocrin&Metab. Clinical Asst Prof, University of Calgary; (403)221-4476; Fax. (403)221-4418.

KINNEY, Gary E J; Business Bldg, 406-1200 Burrard St, Vancouver BC V6Z 2C7; Wes'68; FRCSC; ObstGyn (Colposcopy). Assoc Staff, BC Cancer Agency Vancouver Centre; Ac Staff, Providence Health Care - St Paul's Hospital; Assoc Staff, BC Women's Hospital & Health Centre; Asst Prof, University of British Columbia; (604)683-8416; Fax. (604)683-1904.

KINNIE, Brent R; Deer Valley Family Med Centre, 101-83 Deerpoint Rd SE, Calgary AB T2J 6W5; Cal'92; CCFP; FCFP; (403)271-5124; Fax. (403)225-1276; bkinnie@shaw.ca.

KINNIE, Susan M; Deer Valley Family Med Centre, 101-83 Deerpoint Rd SE, Calgary AB T2J 6W5; Alb'91; CCFP; FCFP; (403)271-5124; Fax. (403)225-1276.

KINSLEY, David C; Interlake Surgical Associates, 210D Clandeboye Ave, Selkirk MB R1A 0X1; Man'01; FRCSC; GenSurg.

KINSNER, Kathleen J; The Hugh Allen Clinic, PO Box 489 79 5th Ave N, Sioux Lookout ON P8T 1A8; Man'09; CCFP; Staff, The Hugh Allen Clinic.

KINTZEN, George M; MUHC-Montreal Gen Hosp, 1650 av Cedar, Montreal QC H3G 1A4; McG'78; FRCPC; DiagRad. Staff, McGill University Health Centre - Montreal General Campus; (514)934-8003; Fax. (514)934-8263.

KINZIE, Sarah C; Stonechurch Family Health Ctre, 1475 Upper Ottawa St, Hamilton ON L8W 3J6; McM'97; CCFP; FCFP; Asst Prof, McMaster University; (905)575-7757; Fax. (905)575-1539.

KIP, Sven; 101-436 Lorne St, Kamloops BC V2C 1W3; Pretoria (South Africa)'95; MB ChB; CCFP; Langs: Afrikaans; (250)373-3828; kipmd@msn.com.

KIPNIS, Christopher; Lakeland Med Clinic, 1715 Ellis St, Kelowna BC V1Y 8M9; Mem'84; Associate, Kelowna General Hospital; (778)478-0277; Fax. (778)478-0279.

KIPPEN, James D; Medical Arts Bldg, 202-233 Kennedy St, Winnipeg MB R3C 3J5; Man'97; DiagRad.

KIPPEN, Robert N; Winnipeg Clinic, 425 St Mary Ave, Winnipeg MB R3C 0N2; Man'71; BSc(Med); FRCPC; IntMed; Gastroent. Ac Staff, Health Sciences Centre; Ac Staff, The Salvation Army Grace Hospital; Asst Prof IntMed, University of Manitoba; (204)957-3333; Fax. (204)942-2671.

KIRALY, Dennis A; Mission Hill Clinic, 100-398 St Albert Trail, St. Albert AB T8N 5J9; Alb'79; Ac Staff, Covenant Health - Grey Nuns Community Hospital; (780)460-0424; Fax. (780)460-0524.

KIRALY, Jane M; Yonge-Eglinton Med Centre, 210-2401 Yonge St, Toronto ON M4P 3H1; Wes'71; Court Staff, Women's College Hospital; (416)485-9044

KIRALY, Leslie T; East Toronto Health Centre, 1496 Danforth Ave, Toronto ON M4J 1N4; Tor'74; FRCPC; Psy (Mood Disorders). Staff Consultant, Toronto East General Hospital Inc; Staff Consultant, Collingwood General & Marine Hospital; Physician, Workplace Safety & Insurance Board; University of Toronto; Langs: Hungarian; (416)778-1496; Fax. (416)778-1400; ethc.1496@rogers.com.

KIRALY, Stephen J; West Community Health Centre, 241-2121 Marine Dr, West Vancouver BC V7V 4Y2; Wes'71; FRCPC; Psy. (604)904-6200

KIRAN, Tara; Health Centre @ 80 Bond, 80 Bond St, Toronto ON M5B 1X2; Tor'02; CCFP; (416)864-3011

KIRBY, Angus D; Regina Qu'Appelle HR-Pasqua, 100-4101 Dewdney Ave, Regina SK S4T 1A5; Sask'88; FRCPC; GenPath (Anatomical Pathology). Staff, Pasqua Hospital; Clinical Asst Prof, University of Saskatchewan; (306)766-2222

KIRBY, Ann S; Rockyview Gen Hosp, 7007 14 St SW, Calgary AB T2V 1P9; Tor'83; BSc; MSc; FRCPC; IntMed (Critical Care Medicine). Staff Critical Care & IntMed, Rockyview General Hospital; Assoc Prof, University of Calgary; (403)943-3706; Fax. (403)212-1241; ann.kirby@albertahealthservices.ca.

KIRBY, Christopher E; Kemptville District Hosp, PO Box 2007 2675 Concession Rd, Kemptville ON K0G 1J0; Ott'09; CCFP; Staff, Kemptville District Hospital; (613)258-6133

KIRBY, Colleen V; Complete Medical, 573 Torbay Rd, St. John's NL A1A 5G9; Mem'02; CCFP.

KIRBY, Emily K; Carleton Univ Health Services, 1125 Colonel By Dr, Ottawa ON K1S 5B6; Ott'07; CCFP; Staff Urgent Care, University of Ottawa Health Services; (613)520-6674; Fax. (613)520-4059; ekirb053@uottawa.ca.

KIRBY, Erle J; Wawa Family Health Team, PO Box 2000 17 Government Rd, Wawa ON P0S 1K0; Tor'73; CCFP; FCFP; Ac Staff, Lady Dunn Health Centre; Assoc Prof, McMaster University; Assoc Prof, Northern Ontario School of Medicine-Laurentian University; Langs: French; Spanish; (705)856-1313; Fax. (705)856-9550; ekirby@wawamedicalcentre.com.

KIRBY, Jeffrey C; Dalhousie Univ Hlth Services, PO Box 15000 Lcd 2 6230 Coburg Rd, Halifax NS B3H 4R2; Dal'76; Physician Univ Health Services Graduate Studies in Philosophy & Bioethics, Dalhousie University; (902)494-2171

KIRBY, Joanne N; London HSC-Victoria Hosp, PO Box 5010 Stn B B2 450-800 Commissioners Rd E, London ON N6A 5W9; Tor'90; FRCSC; ObstGyn. Staff, London Health Sciences Centre - Victoria Campus; (519)685-8394

KIRBY, John G; Oakville Med Centre, 206-331 Sheddon Ave, Oakville ON L6J 1X8; National (Ireland)'77; MB ChB; FRCPC; IntMed; Respir. Staff, Halton Healthcare Services Corporation - Oakville Site; (905)842-3366; Fax. (905)842-1180.

KIRBY, Melanie-Ann; The Hosp For Sick Children, 555 University Ave, Toronto ON M5G 1X8; West Indies (Jamaica)'82; FRCPC; Peds (Pediatric Hematology). Staff, The Hospital For Sick Children; Asst Prof Peds, University of Toronto; (416)813-7606; Fax. (416)813-5327; melanie.kirby@sickkids.ca.

KIRBY, Lee; Nova Scotia Rehab Centre, 209-1341 Summer St, Halifax NS B3H 4K4; Dal'71; FRCPC; PhysMed&Rehab. Staff, Nova Scotia Rehabilitation Centre; Staff, Queen Elizabeth II Health Sciences Centre - Victoria General Site; Pres., Tartan Rehab. Ltd.; Prof, Dalhousie University; (902)473-1278; Fax. (902)473-3204; kirby@dal.ca.

KIRBY, Sandra J; 35 Primrose Lane, Guelph ON N1H 7V9; McM'84; CCFP; Staff, Guelph General Hospital; Asst Clinl Prof Michael & Degroote School of Med, McMaster University; (519)767-5943

KIRBY, Sarah; Queen Elizabeth II HSC-Halifax, 3835-1796 Summer St, Halifax NS B3H 3A7; Dal'88; FRCPC; Neur (Neuro Oncology). Consultant, Queen Elizabeth II Health Sciences Centre - Halifax Infirmary Site; Staff, IWK Health Centre; (902)473-2405; Fax. (902)473-4438.

KIRBY, Shane D; Burnaby Hosp, 3935 Kincaid St, Burnaby BC V5G 2X6; Cal'03; FRCPC; GenPath. Staff, Burnaby Hospital; (604)412-6354

KIRBY, Simon D; Health Sciences Centre, 300 Prince Philip Dr, St. John's NL A1B 3V6; Mem'93; FRCSC; Otol. Staff, Health Sciences Centre; (416)340-3111

KIRCHGESNER, Daniel; Humboldt Med Clinic, PO Box 220, Humboldt SK S0K 2A0; Sask'69; CCFP; FCFP; Fam Med, Humboldt District Hospital; (306)682-8703; Fax. (306)682-4499; humboldtclinic@sasktel.net.

KIRDEIKIS, Katherine L; Cabrini Centre, 3F-16811 88 Ave NW, Edmonton AB T5R 5Y6; Alb'91; FRCPC; Psy. Staff Psy, Covenant Health - Misericordia Community Hospital; Clin Lecturer, University of Alberta; (780)735-2594

KIRIGIN, Mladen J; Queensway Prof Centre, 105-190 Sherway Dr, Etobicoke ON M9C 5N2; Zagreb (Croatia)'85; FRCPC; IntMed; Cardiol. Staff Cardiol, Trillium Health Centre - West Toronto; Assoc Staff, Toronto General Hospital - UHN; Instructor, University of Toronto; (416)622-9453; Fax. (416)622-3684.

KIRK, Allan A G; Port Arthur Health Centre Inc, 194 Court St N, Thunder Bay ON P7A 4V7; McM'82; FRCSC; GenSurg. (807)346-1000; Fax. (807)346-6206.

KIRK, Andrew; Royal University Hosp, 103 Hospital Dr, Saskatoon SK S7N 0W8; Wes'83; FRCPC; Neur (Cognitive Neurol). Staff Neurol, Royal University Hospital; Prof, University of Saskatchewan; (306)966-8372; Fax. (306)966-8008; andrew.kirk@usask.ca.

KIRK, Andrew T; Ridgeview Med Centre, 212-1240 Railway Ave, Canmore AB T1W 1P4; (United Kingdom)'02; MB ChB; (403)609-8333; Fax. (403)609-3666.

KIRK, Angus H; Southcentre Prof Offices, 163-100 Anderson Rd SE, Calgary AB T2J 3V1; Alb'67; MSc; FRCSC; Ophth. Ac Staff, Alberta Children's Hospital; (403)271-2244 x9; Fax. (403)271-1494.

KIRK, Brian C T; Queensway-Carleton Hosp, 3045 Baseline Rd, Nepean ON K2H 8P4; Wes'78; FRCPC; Anes. Ac Staff Anes, Queensway Carleton Hospital; (613)721-2000 x2900; b_kreuk@hotmail.com.

KIRK, D Grant; Stellarton Med Clinic, PO Box 819 Stn Main 10 Jubilee Ave, Stellarton NS B0K 1S0; Dal'74; CCFP; FCFP; Ac Staff, Aberdeen Regional Hospital; Physician, Designated RCMP Examiner & Trenton Work's Inc.; (902)752-3200; Fax. (902)752-7126.

KIRK, Gary M; Windsor Essex County Hlth Unit, 1005 Ouellette Ave, Windsor ON N9A 4J8; McG'84; Staff, Windsor-Essex County Health Unit Corporate Office; (519)258-2146

KIRK, John C; SMBD Jewish Gen Hosp, 3755 ch Cote-Sainte-Catherine, Montreal QC H3T 1E2; Man'79; CCFP; FCFP; Staff, Sir Mortimer B Davis Jewish General; Asst Prof Family Med, McGill University; (514)340-7501

KIRK, Peter J; Dept of Family Practice UBC, 5960 University Blvd, Vancouver BC V6T 1Z3; Aberdeen (Scotland)'72; CCFP; FCFP; (250)419-3645

KIRK, Valerie G; Alberta Children's Hosp, 2888 Shaganappi Trail NW, Calgary AB T3B 6A8; Cal'92; FRCPC; Peds (Pediatric Respirology); Respir. Staff, Alberta Children's Hospital; Clinical Asst Prof, University of Calgary; (403)955-2923; val.kirk@calgaryhealthregion.ca.

KIRKER, Andrew W; Eye Care Centre, 2550 Willow St, Vancouver BC V5Z 3N9; UBC'04; FRCSC; Ophth. (604)875-4656

KIRKER, Jennifer M; False Creek Urgent Care Ctre, 107-555 8th Ave W, Vancouver BC V6Z 1C6; UBC'04; CCFP; CCFP(E.M.); Staff, Lions Gate Hospital; (604)628-2822

KIRKHAM, Colleen M; 200-2475 Bayswater St, Vancouver BC V6K 4N3; Qns'88; CCFP; FCFP; (604)731-0091; Fax. (604)731-0081.

KIRKHAM, Kyle R; Univ Hlth Network-Toronto Western Hosp, 2 405-399 Bathurst St, Toronto ON M5T 2S8; UBC'06; Anes. Staff, Toronto Western Hospital - University Health Network; (416)603-5118

KIRKHAM, Yolanda A; Women's College Hosp, 76 Grenville St, Toronto ON M5S 1B2; UBC'05; FRCSC; ObstGyn (Pediatrics). Staff Gyn, Women's College Hospital; Langs: Mandarin; Cantonese; Chinese; (416)323-7744; Fax. (416)323-6237.

KIRKMAN, Stacey D; Montebello Med Clinic, PO Box 32 Stn Main 302-320 Alexander St NE, Salmon Arm BC V1E 4N2; Cape Town (South Africa)'91; MB ChB; DCH(SA); LMCC; CCFP; (250)833-4677

KIRKPATRICK, Andrew W; Foothills Med Centre, 1403 29 St NW, Calgary AB T2N 2T9; Ott'88; FRCSC; GenSurg (Trauma); Critical Care Medicine. Staff, Foothills Medical Centre; (403)944-4262; andrew.kirkpatrick@calgaryhealthregion.ca.

KIRKPATRICK, David A; Queen Elizabeth II HSC, 838-1276 South Park St, Halifax NS B3H 2Y9; Dal'79; AB; FRCSC; Otol. Staff, Queen Elizabeth II Health Sciences Centre - Victoria General Site; Staff, IWK Health Centre; Asst Prof Otol/A-Head Surgery, Dalhousie University; (902)473-2670; Fax. (902)473-3418.

KIRKPATRICK, David; 302-1497 Marine Dr, West Vancouver BC V7T 1B8; Georgia (USA)'70; FRCPC; Psy. (604)913-9154

KIRKPATRICK, H Roy; Huntsville Prof Bldg, 205-348 Muskoka Rd 3 N, Huntsville ON P1H 1H8; Qns'77; FACS; FRCSC; GenSurg. Consultant, Huntsville District Memorial Hospital - Muskoka Algonquin Healthcare; Consultant, South Muskoka Memorial Hospital - Muskoka Algonquin Healthcare; (705)789-6401; Fax. (705)789-4734.

KIRKPATRICK, Iain D C; St Boniface Gen Hosp, 409 Tache Ave, Winnipeg MB R2H 2A6; Man'98; FRCPC; DiagRad. Staff Radiol, St Boniface General Hospital; (204)233-8563

KIRKPATRICK, J Nicole; Shuswap Lake Gen Hosp, PO Box 520 Stn Main 601 10th St NE, Salmon Arm BC V1E 4N6; Qns'05; CCFP; CCFP(E.M.); Staff, Shuswap Lake General Hospital; (250)833-3600

KIRKPATRICK, James R; 302-2955 Jutland Rd, Victoria BC V8T 5J9; Sask'84; Board Member, Provincial Steering Committee on Eating Disorders & B.C.Eating Disorders Assoc.; (250)387-0000; Fax. (250)387-0002.

KIRKPATRICK, Janice M; Fraser Heights Med Clinic, 106-15966 108 Ave, Surrey BC V4N 5V6; Man'81; (604)582-8820

KIRKPATRICK, John H; 8 Peppett St, North Sydney NS B2A 2M7; Dal'82; CCFP; FCFP; Staff, Northside General Hospital; Preceptor Family Med, Dalhousie University; (902)794-2711

KIRKPATRICK, Marilyn H; Canadian Blood Services, 777 William Ave, Winnipeg MB R3E 3R4; Man'98; FRCPC; GenPath (Transfusion Medicine). (204)789-1075

KIRKPATRICK, Sybil M L; A-63 Albert St, Uxbridge ON L9P 1E5; Tor'69; BSc; FRCPC; Peds (Developmental/Behavioural Pediatrics). Consultant Peds, The Hospital For Sick Children; Asst Prof, University of Toronto; (905)862-0762; Fax. (905)862-0762.

KIRKPATRICK, Xenia R; 200-45 St Clair Ave W, Toronto ON M4V 1K9; McM'78; FRCPC; Psy (Disability Assessment). (416)925-6573; Fax. (416)925-9387; conpsych@bellnet.ca.

KIRKWOOD, Jessica E M; Boyle McCauley Health Ctre, 10628 96 St NW, Edmonton AB T5H 2J2; Alb'09; CCFP; (780)422-7333

KIRLEW, Michael L; Sioux Lookout First Nations H, PO Box 4000, Sioux Lookout ON P8T 1K2; Ott'05; CCFP.

KIRMANI, Saleem; Cumberland Med Hlth Services, 33 Havelock St, Amherst NS B4H 4W1; Karachi (Pakistan)'89; MB BS.

KIRMANI, Waheed-Ud-Din; Niagara H System-St Catharine, PO Box 3018 Stn Main 142 Queenston St, St Catharines ON L2R 7C6; Sind (Pakistan)'72; MB BS; CCFP; Staff, Niagara Health System - St Catharines General Site; (905)731-6111

KIRMAYER, Laurence J; Inst of Commun & Family Psy, 4333 ch Cote-Sainte-Catherine, Montreal QC H3T 1E4; McG'78; FRCPC; Psy. Staff Pay, Sir Mortimer B Davis Jewish General; Dir, Culture & Mental Health Research Unit & Research Assoc., Institute of Comm. & Family Psy.; Prof Div of Social & Transcultural Psy, McGill University; (514)340-7549; Fax. (514)340-7503; laurence.kirmayer@mcgill.ca.

KIROUAC, Isabelle; Unite Med Familiale Maizerets, 2480 ch de la Canardiere, Quebec QC G1J 2G1; Laval'92; (418)661-1413; Fax. (418)661-7504.

KIROUAC, Isabelle; Hôpital Laval, 2725 ch Sainte-Foy, Quebec QC G1V 4G5; Laval'89; FRCPC; IntMed. Staff, Hôpital Laval; (418)656-4511; Fax. (418)656-4587.

KIROUAC, Jacques; CSSS de Trois-Rivières, 1991 boul Du Carmel, Trois-Rivieres QC G8Z 3R9; Laval'87; FRCSC; Otol. Staff, CSSS de Trois-Rivières; (819)697-3333

KIROVA, Juliana S; South Health Campus, 4448 Front St SE, Calgary AB T3M 1M4; Sofia (Bulgaria)'00; Psy. (403)956-1111

KIRPALANI, Anish; St Michael's Hosp, 3F-30 Bond St, Toronto ON M5B 1W8; McM'00; FRCPC; DiagRad. Staff, St Michael's Hospital; (416)864-5692

KIRSCH, Richard; Mount Sinai Hosp, 600 University Ave, Toronto ON M5G 1X5; Cape Town (South Africa)'91; FRCPC; AnatPath. Staff, Mount Sinai Hospital; (416)586-4800 x6187

KIRSCH, Susan E; Richmond Children's Clinic, 404-250 Harding Blvd W, Richmond Hill ON L4C 9M7; Temple (USA)'81; FRCPC; Peds; Endocrin&Metab. Court Staff, Royal Victoria Regional Health Centre; Staff, Markham Stouffville Hospital; Staff, Mackenzie Richmond Hill Hospital; Staff, The Hospital For Sick Children; (905)737-9898

KIRSH, Andrea F; Yonge-Eglinton Med Centre, 202-2401 Yonge St, Toronto ON M4P 3H1; Man'87; BSc; CCFP; FCFP; Ad Staff Privil, Toronto General Hospital - UHN; Lecturer Family & Commun Med, University of Toronto; Langs: Bilingual(English/French); (416)322-3700; Fax. (416)322-3707; rkmappointments@rogers.com.

KIRSH, Brian S; 585-340 College St, Toronto ON M5T 2A9; Tor'79; FRCPC; Psy (Pain Management). Consultant Comprehensive Pain Progarm, Toronto Western Hospital - University Health Network; (416)922-8429; Fax. (416)603-3208.

KIRSH, David M; 203-3410 Sheppard Ave E, Scarborough ON M1T 3K4; Tor'99; CCFP; (416)321-3444; Fax. (416)321-2388.

KIRSH, Gerald L; 203-3410 Sheppard Ave E, Scarborough ON M1T 3K4; Tor'70; Ac Staff, North York General Hospital; Court Staff, The Scarborough Hospital - Birchmount Campus; (416)321-3444; Fax. (416)321-2388.

KIRSH, Jerry J; 986 Bloor St W, Toronto ON M6H 1L8; Tor'57; Court Staff, Toronto General Hospital - UHN; (416)531-1193; Fax. (416)531-9969.

KIRSH, Joel A; The Hosp For Sick Children, 555 University Ave, Toronto ON M5G 1X8; Tor'92; BASc; MSc; FRCPC; Peds (Pediatric Cardiology); Cardiol. Staff Cardiol, The Hospital For Sick Children; (416)813-6140; Fax. (416)813-7547.

KIRSH, Joel C; The Credit Valley Hosp, 2200 Eglinton Ave W, Mississauga ON L5M 2N1; Dal'71; AB; AB; FRCPC; DiagRad; NuclearMed. Staff, The Credit Valley Hospital; Staff, Trillium Health Centre - Mississauga; (905)813-4469; Fax. (905)813-3042; jkirsh@cvh.on.ca.

KIRSH, Shari G; 692 Euclid Ave, Toronto ON M6G 2T9; Man'83; FRCPC; Psy (Psychotherapy).

KIRSHEN, Albert J; The Joseph & Wolf Lebovic Bldg, Box 13 4F-60 Murray St, Toronto ON M5T 3L9; Tor'78; MSc(CommunHealth); FRCPC; IntMed (Palliative Care); GeriatricMed. Staff, Mount Sinai Hospital; Asst Prof Geriatric Med, University of Toronto; Langs: Hebrew; Yiddish; (416)586-4800 x7885; Fax. (416)586-4804.

KIRSHNER, Alla; Edgeland Clinic, 218-2025 Corydon Ave, Winnipeg MB R3P 0N5; Man'99; FRCPC; Psy (Psycho Geriatrics). Asst Prof/Staff Psy, University of Manitoba; Langs: Hebrew; Russian; (204)415-5377; Fax. (204)415-3142.

KIRSHNER, Caroline M; 740-118 Eglinton Ave W, Toronto ON M4R 2G4; Tor'86; FRCPC; Psy. (416)964-2540

KIRSTEIN, Dolen D; Rocky Med Clinic, PO Box 99 Stn Main 5127 49 St, Rocky-Mtn-House AB T4T 1A1; Alb'07; CCFP; (403)845-2815; Fax. (403)845-2177.

KIRSTEIN, Florian P; Bracebridge Med Centre, 2-55 Muskoka Rd 118 W, Bracebridge ON P1L 1T2; Wes'96; CCFP; (705)645-1027

KIRSTEN, Andre R; Ancron Med Centre, 108-402 Baker St, Nelson BC V1L 4H8; Pretoria (South Africa)'89; MB ChB; LMCC; CCFP; Langs: Afrikaans; (250)352-9144

KIRSTINE, Ileana B; 401-3500 Dufferin St, North York ON M3K 1N2; (Guatemala)'80; (416)631-8100; Fax. (416)631-8144.

KIRTON, Christopher A; Alberta Children's Hosp, 2888 Shaganappi Trail NW, Calgary AB T3B 6A8; Qns'00; FRCPC; Neur. Staff Neurol, Alberta Children's Hospital; (403)955-2296; Fax. (403)955-2922.

KIRTSMAN, Irina; 2F-4 Montreal Rd, Cornwall ON K6H 1B1; Rostov (Russia (Federation))'81; FAAP; FRCPC; Peds (Neonatology). Clin Associate, The Ottawa Hospital - Civic Campus; Att Staff, Cornwall Community Hospital; Langs: French; Russian; (613)938-7906; Fax. (613)938-2138.

KIRUBAHARAN, Rajaratnam; Fenton Medical Centre, 4-2 Fenton Rd, Markham ON L3R 7B4; Ceylon (Sri Lanka)'91; CCFP; (905)948-9455; Fax. (905)948-0570.

KIRULUTA, Sheila M; Kingston Med Arts Centre, 201-800 Princess St, Kingston ON K7L 5E4; (Jamaica)'70; FRCPC; Peds. Att Staff, Hotel-Dieu Hospital; Att Staff, Kingston General Hospital; Asst Prof, Queen's University; (613)546-6047; Fax. (613)542-9712.

KIRUPANANTHAN, Coomarasamy; 511-2347 Kennedy Rd, Scarborough ON M1T 3T8; (Sri Lanka)'75; MB BS; FRCOG(UK); FRCSC; ObstGyn. Consultant ObstGyn, The Scarborough Hospital - General Campus; Langs: Sinhalese; Tamil; (416)609-1199; Fax. (416)609-2173; ckirupananthan@hotmail.com.

KIRWAN, Katharine E; 316 Kelly St, Essex ON N8M 1V3; Ott'85; (519)776-8459

KIRWAN, Michael C; Associate Clinic, 5215 49 Ave, Wetaskiwin AB T9A 0R1; Dublin (Ireland)'78; BAO; DCH; DObst; MB BCh; Ac Staff Privil, Wetaskiwin Hospital & Care Centre; (780)352-7157; Fax. (780)352-2273.

KIRWIN, Pierre J; Oakdale Med Bldg, 402-2065 Finch Ave W, North York ON M3N 2V7; Tor'86; DABPMR; FRCPC; PhysMed&Rehab (Physiology). Ac Staff, St John's Rehabilitation Hospital; Langs: Afrikaans; Hebrew; (416)745-2314; Fax. (416)745-9336.

KIRZNER, Michael P; 303-7131 Bathurst St, Thornhill ON L4J 7Z1; Tor'83; CCFP; Ac Staff, Baycrest Centre for Geriatric Care; Clinic Leader, Ontario Addiction Treatment Centre; (905)731-5554; drkirzner@rogers.com.

KIRZNER, Steven L; Coal Harbour Eye Centre, 2788-1177 Hastings St W, Vancouver BC V6E 2K3; Tor'79; DABOph; FRCSC; Ophth (Laser Refractive Surgery). Langs: Japanese; Korean; Farsi; (604)682-4900; Fax. (604)682-0707.

KIS, Joanna K; Halton Healthcare Services, 6F-700 Dorval Dr, Oakville ON L6K 3V3; McM'03; FRCPC; Psy. Staff, Halton Healthcare Services Corporation - Oakville Site; (905)845-2571

KIS, Mihaly; 302-101 Queensway W, Mississauga ON L5B 2P7; Qns'04; FRCSC; Neursurg. (905)273-4449

KISAK-TOMIUK, Jeannette L; Centre Med Notre-Dame, 1515 rue Notre-Dame, Lachine QC H8S 2E4; Mon'65; LMCC; Langs: Bilingual(French/English); (514)634-7146; Fax. (514)634-7147.

KISCHUK, Robert P; 33 Confederation Dr RR 3, Niagara-on-the-Lke ON L0S 1J0; Man'86; BSc; FRCPC; IntMed. (905)520-1254

KISH, Marilyn Y; Sunpark Prof Centre, 118-40 Sunpark Plaza SE, Calgary AB T2X 3X7; Alb'66; CCFP; FCFP; (403)254-4000; Fax. (403)254-1282.

KISH, Scott L; Dauphin Med Clinic, 622 3rd St SW, Dauphin MB R7N 1R5; Cal'97; CCFP; FCFP; (204)638-6445; Fax. (204)638-5670; kishs@cc.umanitoba.ca.

KISHI, Ian G; Hodgins Prof Bldg, 204-45625 Hodgins Ave, Chilliwack BC V2P 1P2; UBC'84; (604)792-1908; Fax. (604)792-3589.

KISHKA, Paul; Clinique Med St-Prosper, 2475 28e rue, St-Prosper-d-Dorch QC G0M 1Y0; Mon'78; (418)594-8218; Fax. (418)584-8294.

KISHTA, Waleed E M; IWK Health Centre, PO Box 9700 Rpo CSC, Halifax NS B3K 6R8; Mansoura (Egypt)'96; MB BCh; Staff, IWK Health Centre; (902)470-7238; Fax. (902)470-7237.

KISIEL, Ursula; Windsor Med Centre, 3-130 Ouellette Place, Windsor ON N8X 1L9; (Other Foreign)'05; (519)971-2901; Fax. (519)971-2902.

KISIL, Kathryn E; Health Action Centre, 640 Main St, Winnipeg MB R3B 0L8; Man'94; CCFP; FCFP; Asst Prof Family Med, University of Manitoba; (204)940-1626

KISKIS, Anthony A; Frederick Mall, 385 Frederick St, Kitchener ON N2H 2P2; Tor'79; FRCSC; Ophth. Ac Staff, Grand River Hospital - Kitchener/Waterloo Health Centre; Ac Staff, St Mary's General Hospital; (519)746-1583; Fax. (519)746-0207.

KISKIS, John; 106 Renfrew St PO Box 160, Pakenham ON K0A 2X0; Ott'71; Ac Staff, Arnprior & District Memorial Hospital; Court Staff, Almonte General Hospital; (613)624-5480; Fax. (613)624-5223.

KISS, Andre L; Clinique Med de Vercheres, CP 879 90 montee Calixa-Lavallee, Vercheres QC J0L 2R0; Mon'81; Chercheur, Centre Hospitalier Pierre Boucher; Langs: English; Spanish; (450)583-6643; Fax. (450)583-6487.

KISS, Erzsebet B; 201-190 Cundles Rd E SS 103, Barrie ON L4M 4S5; Cluj (Romania)'94; CCFP; Langs: Romanian; Hungarian; (705)722-3844

KISS, Sabrina; MUHC-Montreal Gen Hosp, 1650 av Cedar, Montreal QC H3G 1A4; McG'07; MDCM; DiagRad. Staff, McGill University Health Centre - Montreal General Campus; (514)934-1934

KISS, Thomas L; Hop Maisonneuve-Rosemont, 5415 boul de l'Assomption, Montreal QC H1T 2M4; Basel (Switzerland)'87; FRCPC; IntMed; Hem. Staff, Hopital Maisonneuve-Rosemont; (514)252-3404; Fax. (514)254-5094; thomas.kiss@umontreal.ca.

KISS, Zelma H T; Foothills Med Centre, 12F-1403 29 St NW, Calgary AB T2N 2T9; Ott'88; PhD; FRCSC; Neursurg (Stereotactic-Functional Neuro Surgery). Staff Clin Neurosciences, Foothills Medical Centre; Langs: Hungarian; (403)944-8602; Fax. (403)283-2270.

KISSEL, Catherine; CHUM-Hop St-Luc, 1058 rue Saint-Denis, Montreal QC H2X 3J4; Bordeaux (France)'69; GeriatricMed (P.Q.); IntMed (P.Q.). Staff, Centre Hospitalier l'Université De Montréal (CHUM) - Hôpital Saint-luc; (514)890-8000; Fax. (514)412-7376.

KISSELGOFF, Dmitry D; 980 Oliver Rd, Thunder Bay ON P7B 6V4; Chelyabinsk State (Russia (Federation))'94; Staff, Thunder Bay Regional Health Sciences Centre; Langs: Hebrew; Russian; (807)684-6720; Fax. (807)684-5893.

KISSICK, James S; Ottawa Sport Med Centre, 1370 Clyde Ave, Ottawa ON K2G 3H8; Qns'83; Dip SportMed; CCFP; Clin Lecturer Family Med, University of Ottawa; (613)727-2745; jkissick@sympatico.ca.

KISSOON, Niranjan; Children's & Women's HC of BC, B245-4480 Oak St, Vancouver BC V6H 3V4; (Jamaica)'78; FRCPC; Peds. Staff, BC Children's Hospital; (604)875-2507

KITA, Paul M; Providence Healthcare, 3276 St Clair Ave E, Scarborough ON M1L 1W1; McM'91; CCFP; Ac Staff Family Pract, Toronto East General Hospital Inc; Ac Staff Geriatric Rehab & Assesment Unit, Providence Healthcare; Lecturer Family & Commun Med, University of Toronto; (416)285-3604; Fax. (416)285-3804.

KITAGAWA, Eva B; Central Peace Health Centre, PO Box 608, Spirit River AB T0H 3G0; Alb'01; BSc; CCFP; Med Examiner, Alberta Dept of Justice; Langs: Hungarian; (780)864-3962

KITAI, Carol; Women's College Hosp, 76 Grenville St, Toronto ON M5S 1B2; Tor'84; CCFP; FCFP; Staff, Women's College Hospital; University of Toronto; (416)323-6062; Fax. (416)323-6255.

KITAI, Ian C; Baywood Med Centre, 202-95 Bayly St W, Ajax ON L1S 7K8; Witwatersrand (South Africa)'77; FRCPC; Peds; InfectDis. Assoc Staff, The Hospital For Sick Children; Staff, Rouge Valley Health System - Ajax & Pickering Health Centre Site; Assoc Prof, University of Toronto; (905)683-7593 x221; Fax. (905)683-7669.

KITAI, Tessa; Ramblewood Med Clinic, 101-14 Ramblewood Dr, Wasaga Beach ON L9Z 0C4; McM'87; CCFP; Staff, Collingwood General & Marine Hospital; (705)429-8270; Fax. (705)429-7611.

KITAMURA, Kelly M; Gladstone Prof Centre, 6155 North St, Halifax NS B3K 5R3; Wes'90; CCFP; FCFP; (902)453-3511; Fax. (902)454-9010.

KITAY, Stanley; Meadowlark Health Centre, 200 Meadowlark Shopping Ctr NW, Edmonton AB T5R 5W9; Witwatersrand (South Africa)'80; FFR(D)SA; FRCR; FRCPC; DiagRad. Staff Radiol, Covenant Health - Misericordia Community Hospital; (780)481-7961; Fax. (780)486-5160.

KITCHELL, Latiff A; Medical Office, 304-840 Coxwell Ave, Toronto ON M4C 5T2; Sask'67; FRCPC; IntMed. Ac Staff, Toronto East General Hospital Inc; Ac Staff, Sunnybrook Health Sciences Centre - Holland Orthopaedic & Arthritic Centre; (416)466-8313

KITCHENS, James M; Bridgepoint Health Centre, 14 St Matthews Rd, Toronto ON M4M 2B5; North Carolina (USA)'80; FRCPC; IntMed. Staff, Bridgepoint Health Centre; Asst Prof, University of Toronto; (416)461-8252

KITCHING, Allan D; Charlton Med Centre, 500-25 Charlton Ave E, Hamilton ON L8N 1Y2; McM'88; BSc; MSc; ABIM; FRCPC; IntMed; Cardiol. Staff Cardiol, St Joseph's Healthcare - Charlton Campus; Clin Asst Prof Faculty of Health Sciences, McMaster University; (905)528-4111; Fax. (905)528-9181; kitchinga@mcmaster.ca.

KITS, Douwe; Brooks Med Clinic, 219B 3 St W, Brooks AB T1R 0S3; Pretoria (South Africa)'88; Langs: Afrikaans; (403)362-3040; Fax. (403)362-0102; douwe_kits@msn.com.

KITSHOFF, Antoinette; 100-700 Elm St PO Box 1472, Ashcroft BC V0K 1A0; Pretoria (South Africa)'07; (250)453-9353

KITSHOFF, Arno; 8-10010 Lakeshore Rd, Port Alberni BC V9Y 8Z5; Stellenbosch (South Africa)'08; MB ChB; Langs: Afrikaans; (250)731-7849

KITSON, C Neil; West Tenth Med Bldg, 835 10th Ave W, Vancouver BC V5Z 4E8; McM'74; FRCPC; Derm. Staff, Vancouver General Hospital - Centennial Pavillion; (604)875-5151; Fax. (604)873-9919.

KITSON, Hilary F; Oakridge Paediatrics, 207-650 41st Ave W, Vancouver BC V5Z 2M9; Birmingham (England)'72; MB ChB; FRACP; Peds (Pediatric Endocrinology). (604)266-1874

KITTO, Kimberley A; South East Toronto Fam Health, 1871 Danforth Ave, Toronto ON M4C 1J3; Tor'09; CCFP; Staff, Toronto East General Hospital Inc; (416)699-7775

KITTS, John B; The Ottawa Hosp-Civic Campus, 1053 Carling Ave, Ottawa ON K1Y 4E9; Ott'80; FRCPC; Anes. Dir Pre Admission Unit & Research, The Ottawa Hospital - Civic Campus; Asst Prof, University of Ottawa; (613)761-4169; Fax. (613)761-4940.

KITTY, Darlene J; Kirkland & District Hosp, PO Box 3000 Stn Main 145 Government Rd E, Kirkland Lake ON P2N 3P4; Ott'02; CCFP; Staff, Kirkland & District Hospital; Dir Alumni & Student Affairs-Aoriginal Students, University of Ottawa; (705)567-5251; Fax. (705)568-2102.

KITWANDA, Lawrence H; Peter Lougheed Ctr/Calgary GH, 3500 26 Ave NE, Calgary AB T1Y 6J4; Medunsa (South Africa)'96; MB ChB; Staff, Peter Lougheed Centre; (403)943-6628

KITZ, Stacey L; Brandon Reg Health Centre, 150 McTavish Ave E, Brandon MB R7A 2B3; Man'05; CCFP; CCFP(E.M.); Staff, Brandon Regional Health Centre; (204)726-1122

KITZUL, Robert D; Medical Bldg, 201-18 Pine St, Kitchener ON N2H 5Z8; Qns'76; Ac Staff, Grand River Hospital - Freeport Site; Ac Staff, Grand River Hospital - Kitchener/Waterloo Health Centre; Ac Staff, St Mary's General Hospital; (519)579-6920; Fax. (519)579-4890.

KIVES, Sari L; 507-55 Queen St E, Toronto ON M5C 1R6; Tor'95; FRCSC; ObstGyn (Pediatric Gynecology). Staff, The Hospital For Sick Children; Staff, St Michael's Hospital; (416)867-7480; Fax. (416)867-7478.

KIVI, Paul; Misericordia Community Hosp, 16940 87 Ave NW, Edmonton AB T5R 4H5; (Ireland)'05; MB BCh; BAO; CCFP; Staff, Covenant Health - Misericordia Community Hospital; (780)735-2899

KIVINEN, Gary W; Sudbury Reg Hosp-Mem Site, 2F-865 Regent St, Sudbury ON P3E 3Y9; Qns'68; FRCPC; IntMed; Respir. Ac Staff, Health Sciences North-Laurentian Site; Ac Staff, Health Sciences North - Memorial Site; Ac Staff, Health Sciences North-St Joseph's Health Centre; Langs: Finnish; (705)671-5464; Fax. (705)671-5465; gkivinen@hrsrh.on.ca.

KIVLICHAN, Robert M; Queen-Lynch Med Centre, 212-157 Queen St E, Brampton ON L6W 3X4; Glasgow (Scotland)'75; MB ChB; Court Staff, William Osler Health System - Brampton Civic Hospital; (905)451-0994; Fax. (905)451-9260.

KIWAN, Emile; Clinique Med Havre Sante, 521 boul du Havre, Salaber-de-Valleyf QC J6S 4Z5; Beirut (Lebanon)'71; FACS; Otol. (450)371-4158; Fax. (450)694-2370.

KIZILBASH, Kamran; Queen Elizabeth Hosp, PO Box 6600 Stn Central, Charlottetown PE C1A 8T5; Karachi (Pakistan)'91; Staff, Queen Elizabeth Hospital; (902)894-2111

KIZIOR-HAJDUK, Anna J; 281 Stone Rd E, Guelph ON N1G 5J5; Lodz (Poland)'85; CCFP; Langs: Polish; (519)823-5133

KIZIS, Jeffrey J; Guelph Emergency Med Services, 103-73 Delhi St, Guelph ON N1E 6L9; McM'08; CCFP; CCFP(E.M.); (519)837-1401; Fax. (519)837-0133.

KIZIS, Saulius J; South Windsor Med Centre, 2-3840 Howard Ave, Windsor ON N9E 3N9; Wes'71; Staff, Hôtel-Dieu Grace Hospital; (519)969-3744; Fax. (519)969-4478.

KIZOFF, Peter; Atrium Prof Bldg, 201-190 Cundles Rd E, Barrie ON L4M 4S5; Mem'81; Ac Staff, Royal Victoria Regional Health Centre; (705)721-0547; Fax. (705)727-4056.

KJELLAND, Colleen B; Royal Alexandra Hosp, 541CSC-10240 Kingsway NW, Edmonton AB T5H 3V9; Cal'04; FRCPC; EmergMed. Staff, Royal Alexandra Hospital; (780)735-4443; Fax. (780)735-4916.

KJERNISTED, Kevin D; 200-545 Clyde Ave, West Vancouver BC V7T 1C5; Man'83; FRCPC; Psy. (604)669-2273

KLAASSEN, Robert J; 2638-401 Smyth Rd, Ottawa ON K1H 8L1; Sask'90; FRCPC; Peds; Hem. Staff, Children's Hospital of Eastern Ontario (CHEO); Asst Prof, University of Ottawa; Langs: French; (613)737-7600 x2210; rklaassen@cheo.on.ca.

KLAGES, Naomi E; 78 King St E PO Box 280, Thornbury ON N0H 2P0; Ott'08; CCFP; (226)665-7000

KLAHSEN, Andrew J; Cambridge Mem Hosp, 700 Coronation Blvd, Cambridge ON N1R 3G2; McM'91; FRCPC; Anes. Chief Serv-Anaesthesia, Cambridge Memorial Hospital; (519)651-4042; Fax. (519)624-8274; aklahsen@cmh.org.

KLAIR, Rajbir S; Etobicoke Walk-In & Family Phy, 106-100 Humber College Blvd, Etobicoke ON M9V 5G4; (Netherlands Antilles)'08; CCFP; (416)742-9449

KLAJN, Christopher L; 18220 89 Ave NW, Edmonton AB T5T 2K6; Alb'75; Langs: Polish; (780)481-8812; Fax. (780)489-7853.

KLAJNER, Felix; Royal Health Care Centre, 130-130 Adelaide St W, Toronto ON M5H 3P5; Tor'89; PhD(Psychol); CCFP; Assoc Prof Psychology, University of Toronto; (416)361-6142; Fax. (416)361-1200.

KLAM, Stephanie; H-325-5790 ch de la Cote-des-N, Montreal QC H3S 1Y9; McG'95; FRCSC; ObstGyn (Prenatal Care). Staff, Sir Mortimer B Davis Jewish General; Langs: French; (514)340-8222 x3666; Fax. (514)340-7941.

KLAMMER, Gayle M; Capri Medical, 132-1835 Gordon Dr, Kelowna BC V1Y 3H4; Alb'01; CCFP; (250)717-3211

KLAPECKI, Karyn C; Inspired Pathways, 405-517 Wellington St W, Toronto ON M5V 1G1; Man'77; CGPP; CCFP; FCFP; Asst Prof Family & Commun Med, University of Toronto; (416)972-9664; Fax. (416)972-0085; karyn@inspiredpathways.com.

KLAPONSKI, John R; Salvation Army Grace Gen Hosp, 300 Booth Dr, Winnipeg MB R3J 3M7; Belgrade (Serbia)'81; CCFP; CCFP(E.M.); FCFP; Staff, The Salvation Army Grace Hospital; Lecturer Med, University of Manitoba; (204)837-0157; Fax. (204)837-5421.

KLAPONSKI, Stanka; St Boniface Gen Hosp, 409 Tache Ave, Winnipeg MB R2H 2A6; Belgrade (Serbia)'81; FRCPC; Psy. Staff, St Boniface General Hospital; (204)233-8563

KLAPSTEIN, Kim F; Prince Rupert Reg Hosp, 1305 Summit Ave, Prince Rupert BC V8J 2A6; Alb'97; CCFP; FCFP; Staff, Prince Rupert Regional Hospital; (250)624-2171

KLAPWYK, Linda A; High Park Health Centre, 507-2333 Dundas St W, Toronto ON M6R 3A6; McM'99; CCFP; FCFP; (416)766-2718

KLAR, Brian D; Pine Seven Med Centre, 180-4600 Highway 7, Woodbridge ON L4L 4Y7; Tor'83; CCFP; FCFP; Staff, William Osler Health System - Etobicoke General Hospital; (905)856-3330; Fax. (905)856-3331.

KLAR, Michael; Health Care Unit, 550 Gerrard St E, Toronto ON M4M 1X6; Tor'76; (416)325-4444; Fax. (416)325-3284.

KLAR, Michael; St Michael's Hosp, 30 Bond St, Toronto ON M5B 1W8; McG'88; BSc; CCFP; Staff, St Michael's Hospital; (416)864-5689; klarm@smh.toronto.on.ca.

KLARENBACH, Scott; Clinical Sciences Bldg, 11 107-152 University Ave NW, Edmonton AB T6G 2G3; Alb'96; FRCPC; IntMed; Nephrol. Staff Nephrologist, University of Alberta Hospital; Assoc Prof, University of Alberta; (780)407-3627

KLARKE, Dorrit; Keary Med Centre, 107-245 Columbia St E, New Westminster BC V3L 3W4; McM'77; BA(Hon.); PhD; Staff, Royal Columbian Hospital; Staff, Eagle Ridge Hospital & Health Care Centre; Staff Part-Time, Queen's Park Hospital; Examiner M.O.T., Aviation & Marine; Langs: Danish; (604)521-7784; Fax. (604)521-7785.

KLAS, Matthew J; PO Box 581, Lions Bay BC V0N 2E0; Mem'92; FRCPC; Anes (Cardiac Anesthesia). Staff Anes, Providence Health Care - St Paul's Hospital; Clin Instructor Med, University of British Columbia.

KLASA, Marc; 4-135 Whitefield Dr NE, Calgary AB T1Y 5X1; McG'95; CCFP; Staff Med & Peds, Peter Lougheed Centre; Dir Diabetes Services, Siksika First Nation; Langs: English; French; (403)590-9992; Fax. (403)590-9994.

KLASA, Richard J; BC Cancer Agency-Vancouver CC, 600 10th Ave W, Vancouver BC V5Z 4E6; McG'76; FRCPC; IntMed; MedOncol. Staff, BC Cancer Agency Vancouver Centre; Ac Staff, Vancouver General Hospital - Centennial Pavillion; Clin Prof Med, University of British Columbia; Langs: English; French; (604)877-6000; Fax. (604)877-0585; rklasa@bccancer.bc.ca.

KLASS, Darren; 899 12th Ave W, Vancouver BC V5Z 1M9; Pretoria (South Africa)'01; MB ChB; (604)875-4111 x68025

KLASSEN, Brian D; Peter Lougheed Centre, 3500 26 Ave NE, Calgary AB T1Y 6J4; Sask'96; FRCPC; Neur. Staff Neurol, Peter Lougheed Centre; (403)943-5550; Fax. (403)219-3296.

KLASSEN, Dennis R; Queen Elizabeth II HSC, 1276 South Park St, Halifax NS B3H 2Y9; Man'93; FRCSC; GenSurg. Staff, Queen Elizabeth II Health Sciences Centre - Victoria General Site; (902)473-5574; Fax. (902)473-2828.

KLASSEN, Donald H; Dr CW Wiebe Med Centre, 385 Main St, Winkler MB R6W 1J2; Man'76; CCFP; FCFP; Staff, Boundary Trails Health Centre; (204)325-4312; Fax. (204)325-4594.

KLASSEN, Ernest H; Lenore Centre Med Clinic, 4-123 Lenore Dr, Saskatoon SK S7K 7H9; Sask'69; Sec Dept of GP/Ac Staff, Saskatoon City Hospital; Court Staff, St Paul's Hospital (Grey Nuns) of Saskatoon; Court Staff, Royal University Hospital; Clin Instructor Obst, University of Saskatchewan; (306)242-6700; Fax. (306)242-1168.

KLASSEN, Jeffrey M; St Boniface Gen Hosp, L1019-409 Tache Ave, Winnipeg MB R2H 2A6; Man'07; FRCPC; EmergMed. Staff, St Boniface General Hospital; (204)233-8563

KLASSEN, John; Foothills Med Centre, 1403 29 St NW, Calgary AB T2N 2T9; Man'62; IntMed. Dir Plasmapheresis Program, Foothills Medical Centre; Prof, University of Calgary; (403)944-1571; Fax. (403)283-4657; john.klassen@albertahealthservices.ca.

KLASSEN, Judith T; Saskatoon Nephrology Group, 434-230 Avenue R S, Saskatoon SK S7M 2Z1; Sask'88; FRCPC; IntMed; Nephrol. (306)934-3300; Fax. (306)934-3355.

KLASSEN, Julie A; PO Box 19612 Rpo Ctre Point Ma, Vancouver BC V5T 4E7; Wes'96; CCFP.

KLASSEN, Larry J; Eden Mental Health Centre, 1500 Pembina Ave, Winkler MB R6W 1T4; Man'99; FRCPC; Psy. Staff, Eden Mental Health Centre; (204)325-4325

KLASSEN, Lisa A; Doctors on Bayview, 15900 Bayview Ave, Aurora ON L4G 7Y3; Wes'96; BSc; CCFP; (905)726-9755; Fax. (905)726-9631.

KLASSEN, Margaret L; Foothills Med Centre, 1403 29 St NW, Calgary AB T2N 2T9; Cal'93; CCFP; Staff, Foothills Medical Centre; (403)944-1110

KLASSEN, Michelle M B; Crowfoot Village Fam Practice, 210-600 Crowfoot Cres NW, Calgary AB T3G 0B4; Cal'08; (403)208-0722

KLASSEN, Miriam; Perth District Health Unit, 653 West Gore St, Stratford ON N5A 1L4; Tor'88; (519)271-7600; Fax. (519)271-2195; klassen@pdhu.on.ca.

KLASSEN, Neil B; Royal Alexandra Hosp, 10240 Kingsway NW, Edmonton AB T5H 3V9; UBC'91; FRCPC; Anes. Staff, Royal Alexandra Hospital; (780)735-4010

KLASSEN, Norma F; Southwood Med Centre, E-2810 Pembina Hwy, Winnipeg MB R3T 2H8; Man'89; Med Staff Assoc, Victoria General Hospital; (204)261-6080

KLASSEN, Orla; Parkview Prof Centre, 111-2110 Main St, Winnipeg MB R2V 2C2; Man'81; Staff, Seven Oaks General Hospital; (204)338-7853

KLASSEN, Philip E; Ontario Shores Ctr Mental HS, 700 Gordon St, Whitby ON L1N 5S9; Man'87; FRCPC; Psy (Forensic Psychiatry). Staff, Ontario Shores Centre for Mental Health Sciences; Consultant Psy, Correctional Services of Canada; Staff, Metropolitan Toronto Forensic Services; Lecturer Psy, University of Toronto; (905)668-5881

KLASSEN, Reginald A; Windsor Med Clinics, 1608 Tecumseh Rd W, Windsor ON N9B 1T8; Man'90.

KLASSEN, Rodney H; Royal Inland Hosp, 311 Columbia St, Kamloops BC V2C 2T1; Cal'98; BSc; CCFP; CCFP(E.M.); FCFP; Staff, Royal Inland Hospital; (250)374-5111

KLASSEN, Ruby A; West Arthur Place, 303-1265 Arthur St E, Thunder Bay ON P7E 6E7; Sask'94; CCFP; FCFP; Staff, Thunder Bay Regional Health Sciences Centre; (807)622-3737; Fax. (807)623-1969.

KLASSEN, Sheri A; 102-200 Boudreau Rd, St. Albert AB T8N 6B9; Alb'01; CCFP; (780)459-1266

KLASSEN, Steven B; West Arthur Place, 303-1265 Arthur St E, Thunder Bay ON P7E 6E7; Sask'94; CCFP; FCFP; (807)622-3737; Fax. (807)623-1969.

KLASSEN, Terry P; Manitoba Institute of Child He, 513-715 McDermot Ave, Winnipeg MB R3E 3P4; Man'82; FACS; FRCPC; Peds. Assoc Dean Academic, University Of Manitoba.

KLASSEN, Vicki J; Pender Community Health Centre, 59 Pender St W, Vancouver BC V6B 1R3; Alb'02; CCFP; Staff, Pender Community Health Centre; (604)669-9181

KLAUS, E Markus; Nova Scotia Rehab Centre, 245-1341 Summer St, Halifax NS B3H 4K4; Stellenbosch (South Africa)'00; MB ChB; IntMed. Staff, Nova Scotia Rehabilitation Centre; (902)473-3818; Fax. (902)473-7019.

KLAVINA, Ieva; St Martha's Reg Hosp, 25 Bay St, Antigonish NS B2G 2G5; Riga (Latvia)'03; FRCPC; DiagRad. Staff, St Martha's Regional Hospital; (902)473-2700

KLAY, Donna M; Devon Med Clinic, 5-106 Erie St S, Devon AB T9G 1A7; Alb'80; BMedSci; CCFP; Ac Staff, Devon General Hospital; (780)987-3315; Fax. (780)987-4009.

KLEIBER, Niina M; Hôpital Ste-Justine, 3175 ch Cote-Sainte-Catheirne, Montreal QC H3T 1C5; (Switzerland)'02; Peds. Staff, Hôpital Ste-Justine; (514)345-4931

KLEIMAN, J Harry; 410-340 College St, Toronto ON M5T 3A9; Tor'58; FRCPC; DiagRad. Staff, Toronto General Hospital - UHN; (416)962-3202; Fax. (416)962-9653; harry.kleiman@sympatico.ca.

KLEIMAN, James E B; Malvern Med Arts Bldg, 100-1333 Neilson Rd, Scarborough ON M1B 4Y9; Man'87; (416)291-7719; Fax. (416)287-3775.

KLEIMAN, Simcha; SMBD Jewish Gen Hosp, 3755 ch Cote-Sainte-Catherine, Montreal QC H3T 1E2; Man'80; CSPQ; FRCPC; Anes. Dir, Sir Mortimer B Davis Jewish General; adj Prof, McGill University; (514)340-8222

KLEIN, Anna E; Kingston Community Health Ctre, 400 Elliott Ave, Kingston ON K7K 6M9; Ott'08; CCFP.

KLEIN, Benjamin D; 1100-1200 av McGill College, Montreal QC H3B 4G7; Lille (France)'78; Staff, Hopital Ste-Anne; (514)733-2106

KLEIN, Bernie E; 10th Street Medical, 75 Tenth St, New Westminster BC V3M 3X4; Man'91; (604)526-3308; Fax. (604)526-2984.

KLEIN, Cheryl A; St Joseph's Healthcare, 50 Charlton Ave E, Hamilton ON L8N 4A6; Tor'73; FRCPC; IntMed; Hem. Ac Staff Hematol, St Joseph's Healthcare - Charlton Campus; (905)521-6024; Fax. (905)540-6568.

KLEIN, David J; St Michael's Hosp, W 4 054C-30 Bond St, Toronto ON M5B 1W8; Tor'99; FRCPC; IntMed; Critical Care Medicine. Staff, St Michael's Hospital; (416)864-6060 x3566

KLEIN, David W; Lindsay Commun Health Clinic, 108 Angeline St S, Lindsay ON K9V 3L5; Tor'79; (705)879-4100

KLEIN, Douglas J; Royal Alexandra Hosp, 10240 Kingsway NW, Edmonton AB T5H 3V9; Ott'98; BSc; MSc; CCFP; Staff Family Med, Royal Alexandra Hospital; Asst Prof, University of Alberta; (780)735-4201; Fax. (780)735-4978.

KLEIN, Gary M; South Health Campus, 4448 Front St SE, Calgary AB T3M 1M4; London (England)'78; FRCPC; Neur. Staff, Rockyview General Hospital; (403)956-2459; Fax. (403)956-2992.

KLEIN, George J; London Cardiac Institute, 302-256 Pall Mall St, London ON N6A 5P6; Tor'72; FACC; FRCPC; IntMed; Cardiol. Staff Electrophysiology Lab & Prof, London Health Sciences Centre - University Hospital; Investigator, Heart & Stroke Foundation; Prof, University of Western Ontario; (519)645-0146; Fax. (519)645-1548; gklein@uwo.ca.

KLEIN, Gunther; River City Med Clinic, 1424B Island Hwy, Campbell River BC V9W 8C9; Pretoria (South Africa)'94; MB ChB; CCFP; Langs: German; (250)287-2111

KLEIN, H Alexander; 491 Church St, Toronto ON M4Y 2C6; Tor'77; BSc; Staff, Mount Sinai Hospital; Physician, Fairmont Hotels & Resorts; (416)463-6929; Fax. (416)463-6577.

KLEIN, Jack; Kirkland Med Centre, 17000 boul Hymus, Kirkland QC H9J 2W2; Chicago(IL) (USA)'76; Langs: French; (514)694-6459; Fax. (514)694-6470.

KLEIN, Jack; Hampton Park Med Centre, 200-1419 Carling Ave, Ottawa ON K1Z 7L6; Tor'83; FRCPC; Psy. (613)226-9444; Fax. (613)820-7892.

KLEIN, Jean-Marc Y; West Royalty Med Centre, 591 North River Rd, Charlottetown PE C1E 1J7; Paris (France)'67; FAB; FRCPC; Derm. Ac Staff, Queen Elizabeth Hospital; Langs: English; French; (902)628-1360; Fax. (902)672-2855.

KLEIN, Julianne R H; St Boniface Gen Hosp, 409 Tache Ave, Winnipeg MB R2H 2A6; Man'90; FRCPC; AnatPath; GenPath. Staff, St Boniface General Hospital; (204)233-8563

KLEIN, Klara P; Colborne Family Med Centre, 612 Colborne St, London ON N6B 2V2; Tor'72; CCFP; FCFP; (519)673-1962; Fax. (519)673-3758; kklein@uwo.ca.

KLEIN, Lawrence W; Elaho Med Clinic, PO Box 10003 Rpo The Chieftain 1337 Pemberton Ave, Squamish BC V8B 0R1; UBC'91; (604)892-5618

KLEIN, Laz V; 504-960 Lawrence Ave W, North York ON M6A 3B5; Tor'96; FRCSC; GenSurg (Laparoscopic Surgery). Staff, Humber River Regional Hospital - Finch Avenue Site; Langs: Hebrew; (416)782-2616; Fax. (416)782-5899; surgery@misgroup.ca.

KLEIN, Linda; Mount Sinai Hosp Centre, 5690 boul Cavendish, Cote Saint-Luc QC H4W 1S7; McG'83; CCFP; Staff, Mount Sinai Hospital Center; (514)369-2222; Fax. (514)369-2225.

KLEIN, Marina B; MUHC-Montreal Chest Institute, 3650 rue Saint-Urbain, Montreal QC H2X 2P4; McG'91; FRCPC; IntMed (AIDS/HIV); InfectDis. Staff, McGill University Health Centre - Montreal Chest Institute; adj Prof, McGill University; Langs: English; French; (514)843-2090; marina.klein@muhc.mcgill.ca.

KLEIN, Michael C; BC Women's Hosp & Health Ctre, L408-4500 Oak St, Vancouver BC V6H 3N1; Stanford (USA)'66; AB; CCFP; FCFP; Staff, BC Women's Hospital & Health Centre; Head Peds & Family Pract/Prof, University of British Columbia; (604)875-2000

KLEIN, Rael; Associated Anaes Services, M217-601 Broadway W, Vancouver BC V5Z 4C2; Stellenbosch (South Africa)'86; MB ChB; FRCPC; Anes. Staff Anes, Vancouver General Hospital - Centennial Pavillion; (604)875-4304

KLEIN, Stuart W; North York Med Arts Bldg, 220-1333 Sheppard Ave E, North York ON M2J 1V1; Wes'62; DABIM; FACP; FACC; FRCPC; IntMed (Cardiology). Consultant, Sunnybrook Health Sciences Centre; Consultant, North York General Hospital; Asst Prof, University of Toronto; (416)494-7375; Fax. (416)494-7376; stuartklein@hotmail.com.

KLEIN, Thomas B; 210-164 Queen St E, Brampton ON L6V 1B4; Tor'87; FACS; FRCSC; Ophth (Anterior Segment Surgery). Staff, North York General Hospital - Branson Division; Court Staff, The Credit Valley Hospital; Chief Ophth, William Osler Health System - Brampton Civic Hospital; (905)451-4560; Fax. (905)459-5085.

KLEIN-PARKER, Helga; BC Cancer Agency-Vancouver CC, 600 10th Ave W, Vancouver BC V6Z 4E6; Lubeck (Germany)'84; FRCPC; AnatPath. Staff, BC Cancer Agency Vancouver Centre; (604)877-6000 x5351

KLEINER-FISMAN, Galit; Baycrest Ctre/Geriatric Care, 3560 Bathurst St, Toronto ON M6A 2E1; McG'96; FRCPC; Neur. Staff, Baycrest Centre for Geriatric Care; (416)784-3600; Fax. (416)784-5600.

KLEINGELD, Johannes A; La Ronge Med Clinic, PO Box 240, La Ronge SK S0J 1L0; Witwatersrand (South Africa)'76; MB ChB; Staff, La Ronge Health Centre; (306)425-2174; Fax. (306)425-4199; kgeld@sasktel.net.

KLEINHANS, Nerine; Kindersley Med Clinic, PO Box 1390, Kindersley SK S0L 1S0; (Other Foreign)'04; (306)463-2621

KLEINMAN, Irwin; The Two Hundred, 401-200 St Clair Ave W, Toronto ON M4V 1R1; McG'76; FRCPC; Psy. Staff, Mount Sinai Hospital; (416)922-2558; Fax. (416)922-4527.

KLEINMAN, Max; Northwest Rehab Associates, 303-960 Lawrence Ave W, North York ON M6A 3B5; Tor'76; ABPMR; BSc; ABIME; FRCPC; PhysMed&Rehab (Musculoskeletal). Court Staff, Humber River Regional Hospital - Keele Street Site; Langs: French; Hebrew; Italian; (416)785-0844; Fax. (416)785-8030.

KLEMKA, Philip J; Edmonton Gen Cont Care Centre, 3B13-11111 Jasper Ave NW, Edmonton AB T5K 0L4; Alb'77; BMedSci; Staff, Covenant Health - Edmonton General Continuing Care Centre; Langs: Lithuanian; (780)430-8784; Fax. (780)342-8947; klemka@shaw.ca.

KLETT, Marie-Josee; Orleans-Cumberland Comm FHT, 202-3095 St. Joseph Blvd, Orleans ON K1E 3W6; Ott'05; Dip SportMed; CCFP; Staff, Physio Sport Plus; Asst Prof, University of Ottawa; Langs: Bilingual(English/French); (613)590-0533; Fax. (613)590-7351.

KLEVAN, Ariel E; 510-330 Highway 7 E, Richmond Hill ON L4B 3P8; Tor'06; FRCSC; GenSurg. (905)707-5007

KLIEWER, Kenneth L; Altona Clinic, PO Box 999, Altona MB R0G 0B0; Man'73; CCFP; FCFP; Fam Med, Altona Community Memorial Health Centre/Eastview Place; Court Staff, Boundary Trails Health Centre; Asst Prof, University of Manitoba; (204)324-6447; Fax. (204)324-5694.

KLIFFER, A Paul; BC Women's Hosp & Health Ctre, 4500 Oak St, Vancouver BC V6H 3N1; UBC'80; FRCPC; Anes. Staff, BC Women's Hospital & Health Centre; (604)875-2158; Fax. (604)875-2289.

KLIGMAN, David H; 2 Marcus Cres, London ON N6G 4Y9; McG'68; MDCM; FRCPC; Psy (Psychoanalysis).

KLIMAN, Jacob J; Steveston Med Group, 204-3811 Chatham St, Richmond BC V7E 2Z4; UBC'82; Staff, Richmond Hospital; (604)277-7166; Fax. (604)277-3811.

KLIMAN, Lorne D; All About Health, E-1070 Major Mackenzie Dr E, Richmond Hill ON L4S 1P3; Tor'79; (905)884-0666

KLIMAN, Michael E; Dr Michael Kliman Inc, 211-2425 Bloor St W, Toronto ON M6S 4W4; Tor'77; FRCSC; OrthSurg. Staff, Toronto Rehabilitation Institute - University Centre; Ac Staff, St Joseph's Health Centre; University of Toronto; (416)762-9163; Fax. (416)762-3951.

KLIMEK, Alexander T; St Paul's Hosp, 1081 Burrard St, Vancouver BC V6Z 1Y6; Warsaw (Poland)'99; FRCPC; Anes. Staff, Providence Health Care - St Paul's Hospital; (604)682-2344

KLIMEK, Edwin H; Bayvalley Med Arts Bldg, 301-145 Queenston St, St Catharines ON L2R 2Z9; Mem'82; AB; FRCPC; Neur. (905)688-2066; Fax. (905)688-9335.

KLIMEK, Marek G; Queen Elizabeth II HSC-Halifax, 1796 Summer St, Halifax NS B3H 3A7; Jagiellonian University (Poland)'73; DrMedCh; Staff, Queen Elizabeth II Health Sciences Centre - Halifax Infirmary Site; Langs: Polish; (902)473-2220; mklimek@hfx.eastlink.ca.

KLINCK, Jennifer R; Royal Alexandra Hosp, 10240 Kingsway NW, Edmonton AB T5H 3V9; Man'97; FRCPC; Anes. Staff, Royal Alexandra Hospital; (780)735-4010

KLINE, Gregory A; Richmond Road Diag & Trmt Ctr, T-1820 Richmond Rd SW, Calgary AB T2T 5C7; Wes'96; FRCPC; IntMed; Endocrin&Metab. Staff, Foothills Medical Centre; Staff, Richmond Road Diagnostic & Treatment Centre; (403)955-8327; Fax. (403)955-8249; gregory.kline@albertahealthservices.ca.

KLINE, Harvey; Albany Med Clinic, 807 Broadview Ave, Toronto ON M4K 2P8; Tor'58; Staff, Toronto East General Hospital Inc; (416)461-9471; Fax. (416)461-2710.

KLINE, Stephen A; St Paul's Hosp, 1081 Burrard St, Vancouver BC V6Z 1Y6; Alb'69; FRCPC; Psy. Head Med, UBC Hospital - Koerner Pavillion; Head Med & Phys-in-Chief, Vancouver General Hospital - Centennial Pavillion; Ac Staff, Providence Health Care - St Paul's Hospital; Staff Regional Sr. Psy., Vancouver/Richmond Health Board; Prof/Head, University of British Columbia; (604)631-5320

KLINGENBERG, Karen J; Lansdowne Prof Bldg, 310-1641 Hillside Ave, Victoria BC V8T 5G1; Stellenbosch (South Africa)'82; MB ChB; CCFP; FCFP; (250)592-5312

KLINGHOFER, Irvin L; 345-340 College St, Toronto ON M5T 3A9; Tor'73; Assoc Staff Fam & CommunMed, Toronto General Hospital - UHN; Lecturer Family & Commun Med, University of Toronto; (416)921-3580; Fax. (416)921-0676; irvin.klinghofer@utoronto.ca.

KLINGHOFFER, Oded; Parkview Nursing Centre, 545 King St W, Hamilton ON L8P 1C1; McM'77; CCFP; FCFP; Ac Staff, Hamilton Health Sciences Centre - St Peter's Hospital; Ac Staff, Hamilton Health Sciences Centre-Juravinski Site; (905)525-7749

KLINGHOFFER, Zachary D; 216-16700 Bayview Ave, Newmarket ON L3X 1W1; Qns'07; FRCSC; Urol. (905)953-0299; Fax. (905)836-9038.

KLINKE, Jennifer A; 202-250 Keary St, New Westminster BC V3L 5E7; UBC'00; FRCPC; IntMed (Diabetology); Endocrin&Metab. (604)520-1135; Fax. (604)520-1132.

KLINKE, W Peter; 200-1900 Richmond Ave, Victoria BC V8R 4R2; Alb'72; FACC; FACP; FRCPC; IntMed (Interventional Cardiology); Cardiol. Dir, Victoria Heart Institute Foundation; (250)595-1884; Fax. (250)595-5367; peterklinke@vhif.org.

KLINKHOFF, Alice V; Arthritis Research Centre of C, 895 10th Ave W, Vancouver BC V5Z 1L7; McG'77; FRCPC; IntMed; Rheum. Ac Staff, Providence Health Care - St Paul's Hospital; Med Dir, Arthritis Research Centre of Canada; Clinical Asst Prof, University of British Columbia; (604)875-5353

KLIPIN, Louise P; Eastern Health Community Serv, 5 Coish Place, Clarenville NL A5A 0C3; Witwatersrand (South Africa)'95; MB BCh; Staff, The Dr G B Cross Memorial Hospital.

KLIPITCH, Oleg; 1278 The Queensway, Etobicoke ON M8Z 1S3; McM'07; CCFP; Clinical Asst Prof Family Med, McMaster University; Langs: Ukrainian; Polish; Russian; (416)848-9795

KLIPPENSTEIN, Jodine R; Lougheed Plaza, 260-9600 Cameron St, Burnaby BC V3J 7N3; UBC'06; CCFP; (604)420-9252

KLIPPENSTEIN, Norman L; The Brandon Clinic, 620 Dennis St, Brandon MB R7A 5E7; Man'85; FRCSC; OrthSurg. (204)728-4440

KLIPPENSTEIN, Wanda Y L; Elkford Health Care Centre, PO Box 250 212 Alpine Dr, Elkford BC V0B 1H0; Man'00; CCFP; (250)865-2215; Fax. (250)865-7289.

KLJAJIC, Djordje; Doc-Side Medical, 125 Main St, Vancouver BC V6A 2S5; Belgrade (Serbia)'67; Staff, Mills Memorial Hospital; Langs: Serbian; (604)633-1234; georgejk98@hotmail.com.

KLJENAK, Diana; Univ Hlth Network-Toronto Western Hosp, 9E 453-399 Bathurst St, Toronto ON M5T 2S8; Zagreb (Croatia)'87; MD; FRCPC; Psy. Staff Psy, Toronto Western Hospital - University Health Network; University of Toronto; Langs: Croatian; Serbian; Serbo-Croatian; Yugoslavian; (416)603-5459; Fax. (416)603-5490.

KLODAS, Slawomir M; High Park Health Centre, 302-2333 Dundas St W, Toronto ON M6R 3A6; Lodz (Poland)'60; Med Dir, Copernicus Lodge; Langs: Polish; (416)535-6009; Fax. (416)535-9019.

KLOIBER, Reinhard; Foothills Med Centre, 1403 29 St NW, Calgary AB T2N 2T9; McG'72; FRCPC; DiagRad; NuclearMed. Staff Chief Nuclear Med, Foothills Medical Centre; Clin Prof Rad, University of Calgary; (403)944-1252; Fax. (403)944-1687; reinhard.kloiber@calgaryhealthregion.ca.

KLOMFASS, Matthias T; Two Rivers FHT-Hespeler Med Cl, 12-350 Conestoga Blvd, Cambridge ON N1R 7L7; Heidelberg (Germany)'98; CCFP; (519)629-4615 x224; Fax. (519)629-4630.

KLOMPJE, Jan; The Specialist Clinic, 200-10504 100 Ave, Fort St. John BC V1J 1Z2; Stellenbosch (South Africa)'76; MMed(Surg); GenSurg (Gastroenterology). (250)785-7732

KLONOWSKA, Maria-Teresa; Albro Lake Med Centre, 6 Primrose St, Dartmouth NS B3A 4C5; Warsaw (Poland)'73; Langs: Polish; (902)465-4444

KLONOWSKI, Paul W; Calgary Lab Services, 9-3535 Research Rd NW, Calgary AB T2L 2K8; (Poland)'06; DABPath; Staff, Calgary Laboratory Services; (403)770-3430; Fax. (403)770-3292.

KLOPFENSTEIN, Jean-Jacques; Societte Centre Chirug Joliett, 202-222 rue de la Visitation, St-Charles-Brromee QC J6E 4N5; Sher'87; FRCSC; GenSurg (Thoracic Surgery). Staff General Surg, Centre Hospitalier Régional de Lanaudière; Langs: Bilingual(French/English); (450)753-7588; jjk@xilo.org.

KLOPPER, Johanna H; Family Health Centre, 4918 52 St, Athabasca AB T9S 1G9; (South Africa)'93; MB ChB; LMCC; Langs: Afrikaans; (780)675-5018; Fax. (780)675-5028.

KLOPPER, Laurens F; Mill Bay Med Centre, RR 1 230-2720 Mill Bay Rd, Mill Bay BC V0R 2P1; Stellenbosch (South Africa)'98; MB ChB; (250)743-3211

KLOPPER, Leila; PO Box 2278, 100 Mile House BC V0K 2E0; Stellenbosch (South Africa)'97; MB ChB.

KLOPPER, Lukas C; Omineca Med Clinic, 3348 Hospital Rd, Vanderhoof BC V0J 3A2; Orange Free State (South Africa)'81; MB ChB; (250)567-2201; Fax. (250)567-2105.

KLOPPERS, Allan A; Border City Clinic, 2707 50 Ave, Lloydminster SK S9V 2A8; (Other Foreign)'06; MB ChB; (306)825-4427; Fax. (306)825-2028.

KLOPPERS, Amor; Second Avenue Med Clinic, 330 2nd Ave W, Prince Rupert BC V8J 1G6; Pretoria (South Africa)'97; MB ChB; (250)624-5500

KLOPPERS, Anton; Four Rivers Med Clinic, 878 Main St, Winnipeg MB R2W 3P1; Pretoria (South Africa)'74; Physician, Aboriginal Health & Wellness; akloppers@ahwc.ca.

KLOPPERS, Stephanus P; 107-9123 Mary St, Chilliwack BC V2P 4H7; Pretoria (South Africa)'75; MB ChB; Staff Ear Nose & Throat Surg, Chilliwack General Hospital; Langs: Afrikaans; (604)795-2282

KLOSOWSKI, Izabela; Centre Med St-Bruno, 1435 rue Roberval, Saint-Bruno QC J3V 3P7; Cracow (Poland)'82; CCFP; Langs: Polish; French; (450)653-3631; Fax. (450)653-5518.

KLOTH, Debra M; 416 Central Ave, London ON N6B 2E5; Qns'97; BSc; MSc; FRCP; FRCPC; Peds (Asthma); ClinImmunol&Allergy. (519)675-1366; Fax. (519)675-0875.

KLOTZ, Laurence H; Sunnybrook Hlth Sciences Ctre, MG 408-2075 Bayview Ave, Toronto ON M4N 3M5; Tor'77; FRCSC; Urol (Surgical Oncology). Ac Staff, Sunnybrook Health Sciences Centre; Ed in Chief, Canadian Journal of Urology; Prof Surg, University of Toronto; (416)480-4673; Fax. (416)480-6121; laurence.klotz@sunnybrook.ca.

KLOUB, Oxana; Queen Elizabeth II Hosp, 10409 98 St, Grande Prairie AB T8V 2E8; (Ukraine)'86; Staff, Queen Elizabeth II Hospital; (780)538-7423

KLUBIEN, Kristine E; MUHC-Montreal Children's Hosp, 2300 rue Tupper, Montreal QC H3H 1P3; (New Zealand)'83; MB ChB; FRCA; Staff, McGill University Health Centre - Montreal Children's Hospital; Langs: English; French; (514)412-4463; Fax. (514)412-4341; kristine.klubien@muhc.mcgill.ca.

KLUCZYNSKI, Pawel M; Sherwood Park Medicentre, 9-101 Bremner Dr, Sherwood Park AB T8H 0M5; Lodz (Poland)'73; Langs: Polish; (780)467-4717; Fax. (780)467-9316.

KLUFTINGER, Andreas M; 203-3040 Tutt St, Kelowna BC V1Y 2H5; UBC'87; FRCSC; GenSurg (Endocrinology Surgery). Ac Staff, Kelowna General Hospital; (250)763-2226; Fax. (250)861-5937.

KLUG, Andrew P; Humber River Reg Hosp-Church, 200 Church St, York ON M9N 1N8; Cal'01; FRCPC; IntMed; Cardiol. Staff, Humber River Regional Hospital - Church Street Site; (416)249-8111

KLUGE, Hagen F N; Richmond Med Bldg, 405-2020 Richmond Ave, Victoria BC V8R 6R5; McM'10; CCFP; (250)598-7234

KLUKACH, John J; Addiction & Mental Hlth-Queen, 1001 Queen St W, Toronto ON M6J 1H4; McM'95; FRCPC; Psy. Staff, Centre for Addiction & Mental Health (CAMH) - Queen Site; (416)535-8501 x7670

KLURFAN, Paula; Hamilton HS-General Site, 724-237 Barton St E, Hamilton ON L8L 2X2; Buenos Aires (Argentina)'98; Staff, Hamilton Health Sciences Centre - Hamilton General Hospital; Langs: Spanish; (905)527-4322 x44698

KLUZ, Agnieszka M; Huron Commun Family Hlth Team, PO Box 460 32B-1 Centennial Dr, Seaforth ON N0K 1W0; Poznan (Poland)'07; CCFP; (519)600-2273

KLUZ, Andrzej T; Seaforth Community Hosp, PO Box 99 24 Centennial Dr, Seaforth ON N0K 1W0; Poznan (Poland)'07; CCFP; Staff, Seaforth Community Hospital - Huron Perth Healthcare Alliance; (519)527-1650; akluz@rogers.com.

KLVANA, Jacqueline; Clinique Med Solumed, 1-8230 boul Taschereau, Brossard QC J4X 1C2; McG'93; CCFP; Staff, Mount Sinai Hospital Center; Langs: English; Spanish; (450)466-0003; Fax. (450)466-0022.

KLYM, Carol M; Family Physicians, 101-610 Queen St, Saskatoon SK S7K 0M8; UBC'89; (306)244-0766; Fax. (306)665-8838.

KLYM, Karen L; Southwood Med Centre, 3/F-2385 Pembina Hwy, Winnipeg MB R3T 2H4; Man'88; CCFP; FCFP; (204)988-1590

KLYM, Kelleigh K A; Okotoks Hlth & Wellness Ctre, 11 Cimarron Common, Okotoks AB T1S 2E9; Man'95; FAAP; FRCPC; Peds. Clin Associate, University of Calgary; (403)995-2670

KNACKSTEDT, Jeffrey V; Port Hope Med Centre, 211-249 Ontario St, Port Hope ON L1A 3Y9; Tor'90; (905)885-8289; Fax. (905)885-4257.

KNAP, Michel; CSSS de Manicouagan, 635 boul Jolliet, Baie-Comeau QC G5C 1P1; Sher'83; Staff, Centre Hospitalier Régional Baie-Comeau; (418)589-3701

KNAPP, Charles D; North York Gen Hosp, 4001 Leslie St, North York ON M2K 1E1; McM'87; BSc; FRCPC; Anes (Obstetrics Anesthesia). Staff, North York General Hospital; Langs: Hungarian; Bilingual(French/English); (416)756-6520; charles.knapp@utoronto.ca.

KNAPP, Harvey K; Enhanced Care Clinic, 3857 Lake Shore Blvd W, Etobicoke ON M8W 0A2; Tor'77; Court Staff Gen Pract, Trillium Health Centre - West Toronto; (416)259-8441; Fax. (416)259-5442.

KNAPP, Thomas R; Halton HCS Corp-Oakville, 327 Reynolds St, Oakville ON L6J 3L7; Tor'90; FRCPC; DiagRad. Staff, Halton Healthcare Services Corporation - Oakville Site; (905)845-2571 x5614

KNARR, Nadia K; 240 Pinnacle St, Belleville ON K8N 3A6; Tor'03; CCFP; (613)968-9840

KNASH, Michael E; Hys Med Centre, 710-11010 101 St NW, Edmonton AB T5H 4B9; Alb'07; FRCPC; Neur. (780)453-5255; Fax. (780)453-9099.

KNAUS, Russell P; Lumsden Med Clinic, PO Box 418, Lumsden SK S0G 3C0; Sask'85; Clin Associate, University of Saskatchewan; (306)731-3129; Fax. (306)731-2604.

KNEBEL, Laura C; Downtown Commun Health Centre, 569 Powell St, Vancouver BC V6A 1G8; Cal'04; CCFP; Staff, Downtown Community Health Clinic; (604)255-3151

KNECHT, Hans; CHUS-Hop Fleurimont, 4141-3001 12e av N, Sherbrooke QC J1H 5N4; Zurich (Switzerland)'77; FRCPC; Hem (Medical Oncology). Staff, Centre Hospitalier Universitaire de Sherbrooke-Hopital Fleurimont; Langs: English; German; Italian; (819)346-1110 x12709; Fax. (819)564-5434; hans.knecht@usherbrooke.ca.

KNEIFEL, Dorle G; 2209 Broadway W, Vancouver BC V6K 2E4; McG'89; (604)736-4616

KNELL, Eva; St Paul's Hosp, 1081 Burrard St, Vancouver BC V6Z 1Y6; UBC'85; CCFP; FCFP; Staff, Providence Health Care - St Paul's Hospital; Clin Prof Family Med, University of British Columbia; (604)682-2344 x63404

KNETEMAN, Norman M; University of Alberta Hosp, 2D4 44-8440 112 St NW, Edmonton AB T6G 2B7; Alb'78; FRCSC; GenSurg (Hepatobiliary & Pancreatic Surgery). Dir Surg & Transplantation Surg, University of Alberta Hospital; Dir Surg, Human Organ Procurement & Exchange, Central & Northern Alberta; Prof Surg, University of Alberta; (780)407-7072; Fax. (780)407-7374; nkneteman@cha.ab.ca.

KNEZEVICH, Mark P; Royal Alexandra Hosp, 10240 Kingsway NW, Edmonton AB T5H 3V9; Alb'04; FRCPC; Anes. Staff, Royal Alexandra Hospital; (780)735-4010; Fax. (780)735-4386.

KNEZIC, Kathy A; 102-1155 Concordia Ave, Winnipeg MB R2K 2M9; Man'02; CCFP; Langs: Croatian; (204)415-0322; Fax. (204)415-3714.

KNIBUTAT, Darren B; Grand River Hosp-KW Hlth Ctre, PO Box 9056 Stn C 835 King St W, Kitchener ON N2G 1G3; Saba (Netherlands Antilles)'05; Staff, Grand River Hospital - Kitchener/Waterloo Health Centre; (519)749-4300 x2381

KNICKLE, David A; Dept of Veteran's Affairs, PO Box 7700 Stn Central, Charlottetown PE C1A 8M9; Dal'67; FRCSC; ObstGyn. (902)566-8888

KNIGHT, Alison J; Edson Med Centre, PO Box 6660 Stn Main 616 50 St, Edson AB T7E 1V1; Alb'96; CCFP; (780)723-3366; Fax. (780)723-3437.

KNIGHT, Allan; Medical & Dental Bldg, 212-586 Eglinton Ave E, Toronto ON M4P 1P2; McG'50; FAACIA; FACP; FRCPC; IntMed (Clinical Immunology & Allergy). Assoc Prof Med, University of Toronto; Langs: Bilingual(English/French); (416)483-4720; Fax. (416)489-4720.

KNIGHT, Andrew C; Northeastern On Reg Cancer Ctr, 41 Ramsey Lake Rd, Sudbury ON P3E 5J1; Tor'82; Staff, Health Sciences North-Laurentian Site; Staff, Northeastern Ontario Regional Cancer Centre; (705)522-6237 x2320; Fax. (705)523-7329.

KNIGHT, B Joan; 104-6404 Bowness Rd NW, Calgary AB T3B 0E7; Alb'83; (403)288-3733; Fax. (403)288-8081.

KNIGHT, Brian; Misericordia Community Hosp, 16940 87 Ave NW, Edmonton AB T5R 4H5; UBC'82; CMedAcup; FRCPC; Anes (Chronic Pain). Staff, Covenant Health - Misericordia Community Hospital; Clin Assoc Prof, University of Alberta; (780)809-0636; Fax. (780)809-0636; drbknight@gmail.com.

KNIGHT, Burton W; North York Med Arts Bldg, 228-1333 Sheppard Ave E, North York ON M2J 1V1; Dal'75; FRCPC; IntMed; Endocrin&Metab. Ac Staff, North York General Hospital; (416)498-1998; bwknight@rogers.com.

KNIGHT, Caroline A; 309-1580 Merivale Rd, Ottawa ON K2G 4B5; UBC'91; CCFP; FCFP; Asst Prof Family Med, University of Ottawa; (613)226-4030; Fax. (613)225-3891.

KNIGHT, Casey T; York Prof Bldg, 304-679 Davis Dr, Newmarket ON L3Y 5G8; McM'04; FRCSC; PlasSurg. (905)895-4423

KNIGHT, Deborah C; Dartmouth Med Centre, 206-46 Portland St, Dartmouth NS B2Y 1H4; Dal'74; IntMed. (902)465-4550; Fax. (902)461-9967.

KNIGHT, Drew A; Kingston Gen Hosp, 76 Stuart St, Kingston ON K7L 2V7; Queensland (Australia)'08; CCFP; Staff, Kingston General Hospital; (613)549-6666

KNIGHT, Gregory J; Grand River Hosp-KW Hlth Ctre, PO Box 9056 Stn C 835 King St W, Kitchener ON N2G 1G3; Mem'88; FRCPC; IntMed; MedOncol. Staff, Grand River Hospital - Kitchener/Waterloo Health Centre; Clinical Asst Prof, McMaster University; (519)749-4300 x5715; Fax. (519)749-4304; gregory.knight@grhosp.on.ca.

KNIGHT, Jennifer W H; The Family Focus Clinic, 207-667 Sackville Dr, Lower Sackville NS B4C 2S4; Witwatersrand (South Africa)'88; MB BCh; (902)869-2038

KNIGHT, Lawrence; Westmount Square Med Centre, T1 550-1 Car Westmount, Westmount QC H3Z 2P9; McG'67; FCCP; FRCPC; IntMed (Pulmonary Diseases); Respir. assoc Prof, McGill University Health Centre - Royal Victoria Hospital; assoc Prof, McGill University Health Centre - Montreal Chest Institute; assoc Prof Med, McGill University; Langs: French; (514)934-2334 x242; Fax. (514)931-2929; lknight@videotron.ca.

KNIGHT, Mary; PO Box 37, Smithers BC V0J 2N0; Alb'94; BSc(Med.); CCFP; FCFP.

KNIGHT, Michael C; Hollyburn Med Centre, 207B-575 16th St, West Vancouver BC V7V 4Y1; Dal'71; (604)926-4322; Fax. (604)926-0653.

KNIGHT, R William; 38 Stewarts Rd, Emsdale ON P0A 1J0; Wes'77; (705)636-5856

KNIGHT, Richard S; 100-175 av Stillview, Pointe-Claire QC H9R 4S3; McG'83; OrthSurg. Staff, Hopital de la Cite de la santé; Staff, Hôpital de Saint-Eustache; Staff, Lakeshore General Hospital - Pointe Claire; (514)695-6067

KNIPPING, Randolph P; DeerFields Clinic Caledon, 17084 Duffy's Lane, Palgrave ON L7E 3C2; Tor'85; BSc; CCFP; Langs: German; (416)253-9769

KNOEFEL, Frank D; 43 Bruyere St., Ottawa ON K1N 5C8; Mon'89; BSc; MPA; CCFP; FCFP; VP Medical Affairs & Health Informatics, SCO Health Service - Élisabeth Bruyère Hospital; Clin Scientist, Bruyère Continuing Care - Saint-Vincent Hospital; Clin Scientist, Elisabeth Bruyere Research Institute; University of Ottawa; Aj Prof Research Systems & Computer Engineering, Carleton University; Langs: German; French; (613)562-6322; Fax. (613)782-2785; fknoefel@bruyere.org.

KNOLL, Gregory A; The Ottawa Hosp-Riverside, 1967 Riverside Dr, Ottawa ON K1H 7W9; Ott'89; FRCPC; IntMed; Nephrol. Staff, The Ottawa Hospital - Riverside Campus; (613)738-8400 x82536; Fax. (613)738-8337; gknoll@ottawahospital.on.ca.

KNOLL, Susan E; 1-1230 Alward St, Prince George BC V2M 7B1; Sask'82; CCFP; FCFP; (250)563-8151; Fax. (250)563-9211.

KNOTT, David C; Halton HCS Corp-Oakville, 327 Reynolds St, Oakville ON L6J 3L7; Ott'91; CCFP; CCFP(E.M.); Staff, Halton Healthcare Services Corporation - Oakville Site; (905)338-4605

KNOTT, Z Marek; 740 Main St, Sydney Mines NS B1V 2L2; Lublin (Poland)'83; Staff, Northside General Hospital; Langs: Polish; (902)736-2013; Fax. (902)736-2026.

KNOWLES, Holly K E; St Michael's Health Centre, 80 Bond St, Toronto ON M5B 1X2; McM'02; CCFP; (416)864-3011; Fax. (416)864-3099.

KNOWLES, Kathleen F; Hop Sante Cabrini Ospedale, 5655 rue Saint-Zotique E, Montreal QC H1T 1P7; Ott'76; BSc; CSPQ; FRC; FRCPC; MedMicrobiol (Diagnostic Microbiology); InfectDis. Affil Staff Microbiol, McGill University Health Centre - Montreal General Campus; Ac Staff, Hôpital Santa Cabrini Ospedale; Langs: Bilingual(French/English); (514)252-6000 x7203; Fax. (514)252-6592; kfknowles@hotmail.com.

KNOWLES, Louise M B; Port Arthur Health Centre, 194 Court St N, Thunder Bay ON P7A 4V7; McM'06; FRCSC; ObstGyn. (807)346-1000

KNOWLING, Margaret A; BC Cancer Agency-Vancouver CC, 4459-600 West 10th Ave, Vancouver BC V5Z 4E6; Mem'74; ABMO(MedOncol); BMedSci; FRCP; FRCPC; IntMed. Full-Time Medical Oncologist, BC Cancer Agency Vancouver Centre; Clinical Asst Prof, University of British Columbia; (604)877-6000 x2746; Fax. (604)877-0585.

KNOWLTON, Robert J; Oakville Laser Clinic & Spa, A5-2427 Trafalgar Rd, Oakville ON L6H 6K7; Tor'59; PlasSurg. (905)842-8346

KNOX, Corinne E L; Kootenay-Boundary Reg Hosp, 1200 Hospital Bench, Trail BC V1R 4M1; Wes'99; CCFP; Staff, Kootenay Boundary Regional Hospital; (250)368-3311

KNOX, David W; Fifth Avenue Med Centre, 500-14 Fifth Ave, Orangeville ON L9W 1G2; Tor'83; CCFP; FCFP; Staff, Headwaters Health Care Centre - Orangeville Site.

KNOX, Jennifer J; Univ Hlth Network-Princess M, 5 210-610 University Ave, Toronto ON M5G 2M9; Tor'95; MSc; BSc; FRCPC; IntMed (Clinical Oncology); MedOncol. Staff Med Oncol, Princess Margaret Hospital - University Health Network; Staff Physician, Mount Sinai Hospital; Teach Staff Med, University of Toronto; (416)946-2399; Fax. (416)946-6546.

KNOX, John R A; Ross Mem Hosp, 10 Angeline St N, Lindsay ON K9V 4M8; Qns'07; CCFP; Staff, Ross Memorial Hospital; (705)324-6111

KNOX, Katherine B; Saskatoon City Hosp, 701 Queen St, Saskatoon SK S7K 0M7; McM'00; FRCPC; PhysMed&Rehab (Multiple Sclerosis). Staff PhysMed & Rehab, Saskatoon City Hospital; Teach Staff, University of Saskatchewan; (306)655-7742; Fax. (306)655-8813.

KNOX, W F John; Espanola Family Med Centre, 801 McKinnon Dr, Espanola ON P5E 1T2; Ott'85; Staff, Espanola Regional Hospital and Health Centre; (705)869-6100; Fax. (705)869-5095.

KNOX, William H; Kincardine Commun Med Clinic, 44 Queen St, Kincardine ON N2Z 3C1; Tor'76; PhD; BSc; MSc; Staff, South Bruce Grey Health Centre - Kincardine Site; (519)396-6753; Fax. (519)396-3199.

KNUDSON, Gail A; 201-1770 Fort St, Victoria BC V8R 1J5; UBC'96; BSc; FRCPC; Psy. Med Dir Transgender Health Program, Vancouver Coastal Health; Clin Assoc Prof Sexual Med, University of British Columbia; (250)592-6183

KNUDTSON, Merril L; Teaching Research & Wellness, GE 54-3280 Hospital Dr NW, Calgary AB T2N 4Z6; Cal'75; BSc; FRCPC; IntMed (Research); Cardiol. Staff, Foothills Medical Centre; Prof, University of Calgary; (403)210-7385; Fax. (403)210-9837; knudtson@shaw.ca.

KO, Benjamin; Northgate Centre, 1058-9499 137 Ave NW, Edmonton AB T5E 5R8; Alb'98; FRCPC; Psy. Staff, Royal Alexandra Hospital; (780)342-2792

KO, Chung Chun; Valley Medical Imaging, 404A-2151 McCallum Rd, Abbotsford BC V2S 3N8; Monash (Australia)'95; FRCPC; DiagRad. (604)859-8988; koc.canada@gmail.com.

KO, Dennis T; Sunnybrook Health Sciences Ctr, D 380-2075 Bayview Ave, Toronto ON M4N 3M5; Ott'96; FRCPC; FRCPC; Cardiol; IntMed. Staff, Sunnybrook Health Sciences Centre; Langs: Chinese; (416)480-6100 x7835; Fax. (416)480-4657; dennisko_md@yahoo.com.

KO, Evan K Y; 206-22 Richmond St, Richmond Hill ON L4C 3Y1; McG'72; MDCM; DOHS; Ac Staff, Mackenzie Richmond Hill Hospital; (905)884-1154; Fax. (905)883-1298.

KO, Gordon D; Canadian Ctre Integrative Med, 12 Main St N, Markham ON L3P 1X2; Tor'82; DABPMR; DABPainMed; DABAAM; FRCPC; PhysMed&Rehab (Pain Management);CCFP; CCFP(E.M.); Consultant Rehab Med, Sunnybrook Health Sciences Centre; Court Staff, The Scarborough Hospital - Birchmount Campus; Specialist Botox, Mon Sheong Richmond Hill Long Term Care; Assoc Prof School of Health & Human Resources, Rutherford University; Lecturer Med, University of Toronto; Langs: Chinese; (905)471-9355; Fax. (905)471-4348; jean@drkoprp.com.

KO, Hin Hin; Pacific Gastroenterology Assoc, 770-1190 Hornby St, Vancouver BC V6Z 2K5; Tor'04; FRCPC; IntMed; Gastroent. (604)688-6332

KO, Hyang Mi; Univ Hlth Network-Toronto Gen, 11F-200 Elizabeth St, Toronto ON M5G 2C4; Chonnam National (South Korea)'91; Ac Staff AnatPath, Toronto General Hospital - UHN; (416)340-4800

KO, Jevan; Scarborough North Med Arts, 305-4040 Finch Ave E, Scarborough ON M1S 4V5; Tor'96; FRCSC; ObstGyn. Staff, The Scarborough Hospital - General Campus; Langs: Cantonese; (416)321-8875; Fax. (416)321-0166.

KO, Karen; Spadina Health Centre, 404-720 Spadina Ave, Toronto ON M5S 2T9; Qns'05; CCFP; (416)928-0920

KO, Michael A; Toronto Rehab Inst-Univ Ctr, 550 University Ave, Toronto ON M5G 2A2; Wes'00; FRCSC; GenSurg; ThorSurg. Staff, Toronto Rehabilitation Institute - University Centre; (416)897-3422

KO, Peter; Champlain Mall, 3188 54th Ave E, Vancouver BC V5S 1Z1; UBC'76; BSc; LMCC; CCFP; Staff, Providence Health Care - Mount Saint Joseph Hospital; Med Dir, Lakeview Care Centre; Clinical Asst Prof, University of British Columbia; Langs: Cantonese; Mandarin; (604)434-6677; Fax. (604)434-5346.

KO, Raynauld; Univ Hlth Network-Toronto Gen, EN3 464-200 Elizabeth St, Toronto ON M5G 2C4; McG'97; BSc(Hon); CSPQ; FRCPC; Anes (Acute & Chronic Pain). Staff, Toronto General Hospital - UHN; (416)340-4800 x3567; Fax. (416)340-3698; raynauld.ko@uhn.on.ca.

KO, Samuel; 405-2330 Kennedy Rd, Scarborough ON M1T 0A2; Qns'03; FRCSC; ObstGyn. (416)773-0102; Fax. (416)773-0103.

KO, Sang Wook; 100-4700 130 Ave SE, Calgary AB T2Z 4E7; Tor'94; CCFP; FCFP; (403)264-0122

KO, Seung S; Malvern Med Arts Bldg, 100-1333 Neilson Rd, Scarborough ON M1B 4Y9; Tor'90; CCFP; FCFP; Staff, Rouge Valley Health System - Centenary Health Centre Site; Langs: Korean; (416)291-7719; Fax. (416)287-3775.

KO, Simon C C; 110 Keefer St, Vancouver BC V6A 1X4; UBC'84; Staff, Vancouver General Hospital - Centennial Pavillion; Staff, Providence Health Care - Mount Saint Joseph Hospital; (604)688-9795

KO, Yong-Kyong; 101-13025 Yonge St, Richmond Hill ON L4E 1A6; Qns'05; FRCPC; PhysMed&Rehab. (905)773-3342

KO, Yoo Joung; Sunnybrook Hlth Sciences Ctre, 2075 Bayview Ave, Toronto ON M4N 3M5; Tor'93; MMedSci; FRCPC; IntMed. Staff, Sunnybrook Health Sciences Centre; (416)424-4928; Fax. (416)480-6002; yoo-joung.ko@sw.ca.

KOBAH, Saif D; Grand Bank Community Hlth Ctre, PO Box 310, Grand Bank NL A0E 1W0; Baghdad (Iraq)'06; MB ChB; Staff, Grand Bank Health Centre; (709)832-2500

KOBAISY, Omaima; Rabbit Hill Med Clinic, 14030 23 Ave NW, Edmonton AB T6R 3L6; Universidad Iberoamericana (Mexico)'03; CCFP; (780)757-4220

KOBAYASHI, Eliane; MUHC-Montreal Neurology Inst, 3801 rue University, Montreal QC H3A 2B4; Campinas (Brazil)'95; Staff, McGill University Health Centre - Montreal Neurological Hospital; (514)398-6644

KOBAYASHI, Jeffrey S; 6D-555 University Ave, Toronto ON M5G 1X8; Tor'79; FRCPC; Peds (Pediatric Neurology). Staff, The Hospital For Sick Children; Asst Prof Peds, University of Toronto; (416)425-6220 x6276; Fax. (416)753-6046.

KOBAYASHI, Kenneth A; Grand River Reg Cancer Centre, PO Box 9056 Stn C 835 King St W, Kitchener ON N2G 1G3; Wes'84; BSc(Hons.); FRCPC; Derm (Cutaneous Oncology). Staff, Grand River Regional Cancer Centre; VP Research & Development, Leo Pharma Inc; (519)749-4370 x5459; jkobayshi@rogers.com.

KOBAYASHI, Robert B; 201-556 Josephine St, Nelson BC V1L 1W6; McM'88; BSc; CCFP; FCFP; Ac Staff, Kootenay Lake General Hospital; Consultant, Kootenay Boundary Regional Hospital; (250)352-1867; Fax. (250)352-1859.

KOBEL, Martin; Foothills Med Centre, C1150-1403 29 St NW, Calgary AB T2N 2T9; (Germany)'97; Staff, Foothills Medical Centre; (403)944-8504; Fax. (403)944-4748.

KOBELEVA, Sofya; Grand River Hosp-KW Hlth Ctre, PO Box 9056 Stn C, Kitchener ON N2G 1G3; (Uzbekistan)'83; FRCPC; RadOncol. Staff, Grand River Hospital - Kitchener/Waterloo Health Centre; (519)749-4370

KOBELKA, Charlotte R; The Group Health Centre, 240 McNabb St, Sault Ste. Marie ON P6B 1Y5; McM'90; Staff, Sault Area Hospital - Sault Ste Marie; (705)759-1234

KOBETZ, Lawrence E; Wentworth Limeridge Med Ctre, 409-849 Upper Wentworth St, Hamilton ON L9A 5H4; Qns'73; FRCSC; Ophth (Cataract Surgery). Staff, St Joseph's Healthcare - Charlton Campus; Asst Prof Surg, McMaster University; (905)574-4666

KOBEWKA, Carlynne J; FIndlay Creek Med Centre, 3-4744 Bank St, Ottawa ON K1T 3W7; Alb'08; CCFP.

KOBIERSKI, B Lynn; PO Box 53549 Rpo Broadmead, Victoria BC V8X 5K2; UBC'74; CCFP; FCFP.

KOBLENTS, Klara; Kristus Darzs Latvian Home, 11290 Pine Valley Dr RR 2, Woodbridge ON L4L 1A6; Riga (Latvia)'69; Langs: Latvian; Russian; (905)832-3300; harry.koblents@sympatico.ca.

KOBLIC, Paul M; Mount Sinai Hosp, 206-600 University Ave, Toronto ON M5G 1X5; Tor'08; CCFP; CCFP(E.M.); Staff, Mount Sinai Hospital; (416)586-4800

KOBULNIK, Jeremy; 11C 1203-585 University Ave, Toronto ON M5G 2N2; McG'04; FRCPC; IntMed; Cardiol. (416)340-3482

KOBY, Robert D; 1900-666 rue Sherbrooke O, Montreal QC H3A 1E7; McG'69; FACOG; ABOG; FSOGC; BSc; FRCSC; ObstGyn (Laparoscopy). Associate ObstGyn, McGill University Health Centre - Royal Victoria Hospital; Associate ObstGyn, Sir Mortimer B Davis Jewish General; adj Prof, McGill University; (514)842-4497; Fax. (514)842-5837; drrkoby@videotron.ca.

KOBYLECKY, Anna A; Ridley Heights Plaza, 29-100 Fourth Ave, St Catharines ON L2S 3P1; McM'80; FRCSC; GenSurg. Staff, Niagara Health System - St Catharines General Site; (905)641-4511; Fax. (905)641-1321.

KOCAEFE, Burcu; CSSSG-Hop de Hull, 116 boul Lionel-Emond, Gatineau QC J8Y 1W7; Laval'10; CCFP; Staff, Hull Hospital; (819)966-6200

KOCANDRLE, Hana; Edmond Odette Cancer Centre, 2075 Bayview Ave, Toronto ON M4N 3M5; Alb'72; Staff GPO Radiation & Preventive Oncology, Sunnybrook Health Sciences Centre - Edmond Odette Cancer Centre; Langs: Czech; (416)480-4951; Fax. (416)480-6002.

KOCH, Christine A; Univ Hlth Network-Princess M, 5F-610 University Ave, Toronto ON M5G 2M9; Tor'95; FRCPC; RadOncol. Staff Radiation Oncol, Princess Margaret Hospital - University Health Network; (416)946-4662

KOCH, Joan L; Credit Valley Prof Bldg, 306-2300 Eglinton Ave W, Mississauga ON L5M 2V8; Man'84; Staff Family Med, The Credit Valley Hospital; (905)828-2970

KOCH, Marcus Werner; Foothills Med Centre, 1403 29 St NW, Calgary AB T2N 2T9; (Germany)'03; Staff, Foothills Medical Centre; (403)944-1260

KOCH, Marion D; Ctr Hosp Gatineau Memorial, 101 ch Burnside, Wakefield QC J0X 3G0; McM'93; FRCPC; Psy (Adult General Psychiatry). Staff, Hull Hospital; Psychiatre, Centre Hospitalier Gatineau Mémorial; Prof/Coord, McGill University; Langs: English; French; (819)459-1112; Fax. (819)459-1148.

KOCH, Patricia; CSSS du Nord de Lanaudière, 1000 boul Sainte-Anne, St-Charles-Brromee QC J6E 6J2; Mon'01; FRCSC; GenSurg. Staff, Centre Hospitalier Régional de Lanaudière; (450)759-8222

KOCHA, Walter H; London Reg Cancer Centre, 790 Commissioners Rd E, London ON N6A 4L6; Wes'74; BSc(BioChem); FRCPC; Hem (Medical Oncology). Staff London Reg Cancer Centre, London Health Sciences Centre - Victoria Campus; Assoc Prof, University of Western Ontario; (519)685-8640 x58640; neuroendocrine.ca@gmail.com.

KOCHENBURGER-BELANGER, Stephanie; GMF Le Carrefour Medical, 200-3030 boul Le carrefour, Laval QC H7T 2P5; Mon'96; (450)686-8899

KOCHENDORFER, Robert L; Elgin Med Centre, 101-2255 Elgin Ave, Port Coquitlam BC V3C 2B4; Alb'68; (604)942-7292; Fax. (604)942-9698.

KOCHUYT, Caroline P R; Hop Ste-Anne-De-Beaupre, 11000 rue des Montagnards RR 1, Beaupre QC G0A 1E0; Louvain (Belgium)'93; Staff, Hôpital Sainte Anne de Beaupré; (418)827-3738 x3218; Fax. (418)827-3730.

KOCLAS, Louise; MUHC-Montreal Children's Hosp, A618-2300 rue Tupper, Montreal QC H3H 1P3; Mon'78; FRCPC; Peds. Staff, McGill University Health Centre - Montreal Children's Hospital; (514)412-4302; louise.koclas@muhc.mcgill.ca.

KOCMUR, Elizabeth; The Doctor's Office at Six Poi, 5230 Dundas St W, Etobicoke ON M9B 1A8; Tor'68; (416)234-8668

KOCSIS, Pongrac; 201-959 Dundas St, Woodstock ON N4S 1H2; Wes'90; CCFP; Chief FamilyMed, Woodstock General Hospital; (519)539-5621; Fax. (519)539-0628.

KOCUR, Ivana; MUHC-Montreal Children's Hosp, C 1117-2300 rue Tupper, Montreal QC H3H 1P3; Palacky (Czech Republic)'65; Staff, McGill University Health Centre - Montreal Children's Hospital; (514)412-4448; Fax. (514)412-4341.

KOCZANSKI, Roman P; Redwood Med Clinic, 203-1750 Main St, Winnipeg MB R2V 1Z7; Wroclaw (Poland)'85; (204)586-8426; Fax. (204)589-5764.

KOCZAPSKI, Andrzej B A; VGH Health Centre, 715 12th Ave W, Vancouver BC V5Z 1M9; UBC'76; BSc; MB; FRCP; DFAPA; FRCPC; CCFP; Psy. Staff Psy, UBC Hospital - Koerner Pavillion; Clin Assoc Prof Psy, University of British Columbia; (604)875-4139

KOCZERGINSKI, David; William Osler HC-Brampton, 2100 Bovaird Dr E, Brampton ON L6R 3J7; Tor'83; FRCPC; Psy. Chief Psy, William Osler Health System - Brampton Civic Hospital; (905)494-2120; Fax. (905)494-6710.

KOCZOROWSKA, Maria T; The Two Hundred, 416-200 St Clair Ave W, Toronto ON M4V 1R1; Cracow (Poland)'82; FRCPC; Psy (Inpatient Psychiatry). Staff Pt-Time, Toronto Western Hospital - University Health Network; Consultant, Niagara Health System - Douglas Memorial Hospital Site; (416)924-3854; Fax. (416)924-9428.

KODAGODA, Dayananda; Family Medicine, 201-185 Bentinck St, Sydney NS B1P 1G7; Ceylon (Sri Lanka)'73; MB BS; CCFP; Staff, Cape Breton Healthcare Complex; Langs: Sinhalese; Tamil; (902)539-0078; Fax. (902)539-0064.

KODAMA, Ronald T; Sunnybrook Hlth Sciences Ctre, MG 406-2075 Bayview Ave, Toronto ON M4N 3M5; Tor'80; FRCSC; Urol (Urethral Reconstruction). Staff Urol, Sunnybrook Health Sciences Centre; Staff, Toronto General Hospital - UHN; Assoc Prof, University of Toronto; (416)480-5956; Fax. (416)480-6121; ron.kodama@utoronto.ca.

KODEESWARAN, Tanuja; Alberta Children's Hosp, E-2888 Shaganappi Trail NW, Calgary AB T3B 6A8; McM'94; BSc; FAAP; FRCPC; Peds (Pediatric Emergency Medicine). Staff, Alberta Children's Hospital; (403)229-7211

KODSI, Maged S; Kingsway Med Bldg, 11-2917 Bloor St W, Etobicoke ON M8X 1B4; Cairo (Egypt)'73; MB ChB; FRCSC; Psy (Child & Family Psychiatry). Physician Leader/Clin Head Child & Adolescent Mental Health, Humber River Regional Hospital - Keele Street Site; (416)239-0154; Fax. (416)239-0254.

KODSI, Sherif S; St George's Med Centre, 101-650 Sheppard Ave E, North York ON M2K 3E4; Ain Shams (Egypt)'78; Staff, The Scarborough Hospital - Birchmount Campus; Staff, North York General Hospital; Physician, St George's Medical Centre; (416)223-5511; Fax. (416)223-5528.

KOE, Sandy S K; Good Samaritan Seniors' Clinic, 9534 87 St NW, Edmonton AB T6C 3J1; Alb'88; BSc(MedSc); Langs: Mandarin; (780)440-8274; Fax. (780)469-6495.

KOEGLER, David P; Family Med Centre, 2931 20 Ave S, Lethbridge AB T1K 3M5; McM'78; BSc; FRCPC; IntMed (Gastroenterology). Staff, Coaldale Health Centre; Staff, Chinook Regional Hospital; Chairman Endoscopy Committee, Chinook Region; (403)328-2326; Fax. (403)327-0123.

KOEGLER, Peter A; Campbell Clinic, 160 Columbia Blvd W, Lethbridge AB T1K 4J4; Alb'95; CCFP; Staff, Chinook Regional Hospital; (403)381-7000; Fax. (403)381-8250.

KOEHLE, Michael S; Allan McGavin Sports Med Ctr, 3055 Wesbrook Mall, Vancouver BC V6T 1Z3; Tor'99; MSc; CCFP; (604)822-3614; Fax. (604)822-9058.

KOEHLE, Shawna L; Mill Creek Family Medicine, 101-1912 Enterprise Way, Kelowna BC V1Y 9S9; Alb'98; CCFP; (250)868-0700; Fax. (250)868-3003.

KOEHLER, Barry E; Richmond Health Science Ctre, 230-6091 Gilbert Rd, Richmond BC V7C 5L9; Tor'65; FRCP; FRCPC; IntMed; Rheum. Consultant Staff, Richmond Hospital; Clin Prof Emeritus Med, University of British Columbia; (604)273-8085; Fax. (604)273-8043; barry.koehler@gmail.com.

KOEHN, Martha E; St Paul's Hosp, C106-1081 Burarrd St, Vancouver BC V6Z 1Y6; UBC'10; Staff, Providence Health Care - St Paul's Hospital; (604)806-8877

KOEHNCKE, Niels K; Royal University Hosp, 103 Hospital Dr, Saskatoon SK S7N 0W8; Alb'95; MSc; FRCPC; OccupMed. Staff, Royal University Hospital; (306)966-8286; Fax. (306)966-8799; niels.koehncke@usask.ca.

KOELINK, Anthony F C; Kerrisdale Station Med Clinic, 2077 42nd Ave W, Vancouver BC V6M 2B4; UBC'75; CCFP; Ac Staff, Vancouver General Hospital - Centennial Pavillion; Court Staff, BC Women's Hospital & Health Centre; (604)261-9494; Fax. (604)261-9405.

KOELINK, Eric A; Dept of Pediatric, 525 University Ave, Toronto ON M5G 2L3; (Australia)'07; FRCPC; Peds.

KOEN, Johannes C; 130-3410 50 Ave, Red Deer AB T4N 3Y4; (South Africa)'97; MB ChB; (403)342-9444; Fax. (403)340-8847.

KOENEKOOP, Robert K; MUHC-Montreal Children's Hosp, D168 1-2300 rue Tupper, Montreal QC H3H 1P3; McG'89; FRCSC; Ophth (Retina). assoc Prof Ophth Tenure & Human Genetics, McGill University Health Centre - Montreal Children's Hospital; Asst Prof Ophth & Human Genetics, McGill University; Langs: French; Dutch; (514)412-4400 x2891; Fax. (514)412-4443.

KOENIG, James K; St Boniface Gen Hosp, 409 Tache Ave, Winnipeg MB R2H 2A6; Man'05; FRCPC; DiagRad. Staff, St Boniface General Hospital; (204)233-8563

KOENIG, Marie-Charlotte; Ungava Tulattavik Health Ctr, CP 149, Kuujjuaq QC J0M 1C0; Mon'88; CCFP; ac Staff, Hull Hospital; Langs: Spanish; English; (819)964-2905

KOENIG, Martial; CHUM-Hop Notre-Dame, 1560 rue Sherbrooke E, Montreal QC H2L 4M1; Grenoble (France)'02; Staff, Centre Hospitalier l'Université de Montréal (CHUM) - Hôpital Notre-Dame; (514)890-8000 x24444

KOESTER, Catherine; Newburgh Clinic, PO Box 129 5 Earl St, Newburgh ON K0K 2S0; Qns'06; CCFP; (613)378-1754; Fax. (613)378-1776.

KOFF, David A; Hamilton HS-Chedoke Hosp, 559 Sanatorium Rd, Hamilton ON L9C 7W8; Paris V (France)'80; FRCPC; DiagRad. Staff, Hamilton Health Sciences Centre - Chedoke Hospital; Dept Head Radiol, McMaster University; Asst Prof, University of Toronto; Langs: French; (905)521-2100; Fax. (905)577-1443; david.koff@sunnybrook.ca.

KOFFMAN, Allyson E; Earl Bales Walk-In Clinic, 100-4256 Bathurst St, North York ON M3H 5Y8; Wes'97; Staff Phys, University of Toronto; (416)352-7188; Fax. (416)352-7190.

KOFFMAN, Gerald A; Don Valley Med Associates Inc, 144-1333 Sheppard Ave E, North York ON M2J 1V1; Tor'69; Staff, North York General Hospital; Physician, Yamaha; (416)491-5900; Fax. (416)491-1149.

KOGAN, Eva; Markham Stouffville Hosp, PO Box 1800 Stn Main 381 Church St, Markham ON L3P 7P3; Wes'04; FRCPC; IntMed (Diabetes); Endocrin&Metab. Staff, Markham Stouffville Hospital; Langs: Russian; (905)472-7000 x6182; Fax. (905)472-7533.

KOGAN, Izabella; Alliston Family Health Team, 36 Victoria St W, Alliston ON L9R 1S8; Russia (Russia (Federation))'91; PhD; CCFP; Staff, Stevenson Memorial Hospital; Asst Prof, McMaster University; Langs: Russian; (705)435-8887; Fax. (705)435-8867.

KOGAN, Sylvia; 221-2025 Corydon Ave, Winnipeg MB R3P 0N5; Man'01; FRCSC; Ophth.

KOGILWAIMATH, Siddhath; Health Sciences Centre, 2184-300 Prince Philip Dr, St. John's NL A1B 3V6; Dal'09; Staff, Health Sciences Centre; (709)737-6300

KOGON, David P; Professional Arts Bldg, 427-100 Arden St, Moncton NB E1C 4B7; Guadalajara (Mexico)'78; FACOG; FRCSC; ObstGyn. Chief of Staff/Med Dir, The Moncton Hospital; Asst Prof, Dalhousie University; Clinical Asst Prof, Memorial University Of Newfoundland; Langs: Spanish; (506)855-6700; Fax. (506)389-2141.

KOGON, Michael D; Gates of Maple Med Center, 103-2200 Rutherford Rd, Concord ON L4K 5V2; Tor'03; FRCSC; Urol. (905)832-8428; Fax. (905)832-6651.

KOH, Clarissa B K; Riverwood Med Centre, 1295 Pembina Hwy, Winnipeg MB R3T 2B3; Man'92; BSc; CCFP; Langs: Mandarin; (204)452-3345; Fax. (204)452-5339.

KOH, Denise M; Manitoba Health, 100-300 Carlton St, Winnipeg MB R3B 3M9; Sask'96; FRCPC; CommunMed;CCFP.

KOHANEK, Frances L; Beauséjour Clinic, 708 Park Ave E, Beausejour MB R0E 0C0; Man'69.

KOHANSAL VAJARGAH, Ali R; University of Alberta Hosp, 8440 112 St NW, Edmonton AB T6G 2B7; (Australia)'02; IntMed. Staff, University of Alberta Hospital; (780)407-8822

KOHEN, Samuel A; Dr Samuel Kohen Med Corp, PO Box 39038 Rpo Point Grey 3695 10th Ave W, Vancouver BC V6R 4P1; UBC'06; Critical Care Medicine; IntMed. Staff, Vancouver General Hospital - Centennial Pavillion; (604)984-5795

KOHJA, Abbas A; Clearspring Med Clinic, 1-390 Main St, Steinbach MB R5G 1Z3; Punjab (Pakistan)'83; MB BS; Langs: Urdu; Punjabi; Hindi; (204)326-6111; Fax. (204)326-6952.

KOHL, Jack H M; 1006-21 St Clair Ave E, Toronto ON M4T 1L9; Tor'82; AB; FRCPC; Psy (Psychiatric Consultant Liaison). (416)324-9585

KOHLER, Andrew J; Callingwood Crossing Med Clini, 6905 172 St NW, Edmonton AB T5T 5Y1; Alb'86; BMedSci; CCFP; (780)444-0350; Fax. (780)444-0476.

KOHLER, Anneliese M; Allin Clinic, 10155 120 St NW, Edmonton AB T5K 2A2; Alb'08; CCFP; Staff Locum, Royal Alexandra Hospital; (780)482-7551; Fax. (780)488-2056.

KOHLI, Jagdeep; Gulf Canada Square, 360-401 9 Ave SW, Calgary AB T2P 3C5; Cal'95; MSc; BSc; FRCPC; Neur (Electromyography). Staff Neurol, Calgary Health Region; (403)221-4447

KOHLI, Sandeep S S; Halton HCS Corp-Oakville, 327 Reynolds St, Oakville ON L6J 3L7; Wes'01; FRCPC; IntMed (Critical Care Medicine). Staff, Halton Healthcare Services Corporation - Oakville Site; (905)338-4618

KOHLL, David E; Family Physicians, 101-610 Queen St, Saskatoon SK S7K 0M8; Cape Town (South Africa)'86; MB ChB; BSc(Hons); (306)244-0766; Fax. (306)665-8838.

KOHLSMITH, Douglas J; 4 Jacob St, Sydney Mines NS B1V 3M4; Dal'85; Ac Staff, Northside General Hospital; (902)736-2821; Fax. (902)736-0141.

KOHLY, Radha P; Sunnybrook Hlth Sciences Ctre, M1 202B-2075 Bayview Ave, Toronto ON M4N 3M5; McM'04; FRCSC; Ophth. Staff, Sunnybrook Health Sciences Centre; (416)480-5607

KOHN, Magdie L; 216-40 Finchgate Blvd, Brampton ON L6T 3J1; Tor'99; FRCPC; IntMed (Sleep Medicine); Respir. (905)456-3699

KOHN, Thomas; 1600 rue Sherbrooke O, Montreal QC H3H 1C9; Cal'77; FRCPC; Derm (Skin Cancer). (514)933-3366; Fax. (514)933-2525.

KOHNO, Yume; Orillia Soldier's Mem Hosp, 170 Colborne St W, Orillia ON L3V 2Z3; UBC'03; FRCPC; DiagRad. Staff, Orillia Soldiers' Memorial Hospital; (705)325-2201

KOHUT, Ludmila B; Markham College Med Clinic, 308-474 College St, Toronto ON M6G 1A4; Safarika (Slovakia)'67; Assoc Staff, Women's College Hospital; Assoc Staff, Mount Sinai Hospital; (416)923-9401; Fax. (416)923-5001.

KOHUT, Nitsa; 103-1849 Yonge St, Toronto ON M4S 1Y2; Tor'87; MSc; Court Staff, North York General Hospital; Staff Phys, Carefree Lodge; Staff Physician, Meighen Manor; (416)486-8788; Fax. (416)486-4515; nitsak@rogers.com.

KOHUT, Vera M; Healthcare 365, 905-1867 Yonge St, Toronto ON M4S 1Y5; Cal'79; BSc(Pharm); CCFP; FCFP; (416)642-9160; Fax. (416)487-3931.

KOIFMAN, Rod; 1A-6758 Kingston Rd, Scarborough ON M1B 1G8; Tor'81; CCFP; CCFP(E.M.); Assoc Staff, Rouge Valley Health System - Centenary Health Centre Site; (416)286-7890; Fax. (416)286-8600.

KOIFMAN, Rolan; 21 Essa Rd, Barrie ON L4N 3K4; McM'02; CCFP; (705)728-5433

KOILPILLAI, Christiansen J; Queen Elizabeth II HSC-Halifax, 2148-1796 Summer St, Halifax NS B3H 3A7; McM'77; FRCPC; IntMed; Cardiol. Staff, Queen Elizabeth II Health Sciences Centre - Halifax Infirmary Site; Dir Echocardiography, Queen Elizabeth II Health Sciences Centre - Victoria General Site; Assoc Prof, Dalhousie University; (902)473-4127; Fax. (902)473-2434.

KOJORI, Fatemeh; Manitoba Clinic, 790 Sherbrook St, Winnipeg MB R3A 1M3; McM'07.

KOK, Kevin D; 314 Duchess St, Saskatoon SK S7K 0R1; Sask'92; FRCPC; Psy. Assoc Prof Psy, University of Saskatchewan; (306)655-0441; Fax. (306)655-0457.

KOKA, H Pavan K; Sudbury Reg Hosp-Laurentian, 41 Ramsey Lake Rd, Sudbury ON P3E 5J1; Ott'02; CCFP; CCFP(E.M.); Staff, Health Sciences North-Laurentian Site; (705)675-4700

KOKA, Hanumantha R; Northeast Mental Hlth Centre, 680 Kirkwood Dr, Sudbury ON P3E 1X3; Karnatak (India)'72; MB BS; DPM(Eng); FRCPC; Psy. Ac Staff, North Bay Regional Health Centre - Kirkwood; Section Leader Mental Health, Northern Ontario School of Medicine; (705)675-9192; Fax. (705)671-3031.

KOKA, Suman K; 102-1280 Lasalle Blvd, Sudbury ON P3A 1Y8; Saba(MA) (USA)'06; CCFP; (705)560-2227; Fax. (705)521-0729.

KOKAN, Peter A; 104-5512 Hastings St, Burnaby BC V5B 1R3; UBC'93; BSc; FRCSC; OrthSurg (Arthroplasty). Staff False Creek Surgical Centre, Burnaby Hospital; Langs: Croatian; (604)294-3265; Fax. (604)294-1473.

KOKE, Michael J; Grand River Hosp-Freeport HC, PO Box 9056 Stn C 3570 King St E, Kitchener ON N2G 1G3; McM'95; CCFP; CCFP(E.M.); Staff, Grand River Hospital - Freeport Site; Staff, Cambridge Memorial Hospital; (519)749-4300 x7366

KOKIS, Andre; CHUM-Hotel-Dieu, 3840 rue Saint-Urbain, Montreal QC H2W 1T8; Mon'95; FRCPC; IntMed (Echocardiography); Cardiol. Staff, Centre Hospitalier l'Université de Montréal (CHUM) - Hôtel-Dieu; assoc Prof, Universite de Montreal; Langs: English; Portuguese; (514)890-8315

KOKJE, Aron Eduard; Sussex Health Centre, 75 Leonard Dr, Sussex NB E4E 2P7; Netherlands (Netherlands)'85; Staff, Sussex Health Centre; (506)432-3100

KOKOSKI, Richard J; Psychotherapy & Counselling Ct, 102-2150 Bloor St W, Toronto ON M6S 1M8; Tor'00; PhD; CCFP; (416)516-6969; Fax. (416)516-8293.

KOKTA, Victor; Hôpital Ste-Justine, 3175 ch Cote-Sainte-Catherine, Montreal QC H3T 1C5; Sher'94; CSPQ; AnatPath. Staff, Hôpital Ste-Justine; Langs: English; Czech; (514)345-4649; victorkokta@yahoo.ca.

KOLABINSKI, Irene; Dr I Kolabinski Associates, 5 Spencer St, Picton ON K0K 2T0; Tor'77; Ac Staff, QHC Prince Edward County Memorial; Langs: Polish; (613)476-3298; Fax. (613)476-2770.

KOLADICH, Carol J; Chambers of Commerce Bldg, 201-345 Lakeshore Rd E, Oakville ON L6J 1J5; Tor'63; (905)339-0222; Fax. (905)339-0018.

KOLAKOWSKI, Anna A; Emerson Health Centre, PO Box 428, Emerson MB R0A 0L0; (Poland)'84; Staff, Emerson Health Centre; (204)373-2109; akolakowski@rha-central.mb.ca.

KOLAN, Christophe C P; CHUM-Hotel-Dieu, 3840 rue Saint-Urbain, Montreal QC H2W 1T8; Liege (Belgium)'01; Critical Care Medicine (P.Q.). Staff, Centre Hospitalier l'Université de Montréal (CHUM) - Hôtel-Dieu; (514)890-8000

KOLANO, Lori L; 120 Vidal St N, Sarnia ON N7T 5X5; Wes'86; CCFP; FCFP; Staff, Bluewater Health - Norman Site; Staff, Bluewater Health - Mitton Site; (519)339-1070; Fax. (519)339-1027.

KOLARI, Charis K; 1 King St, St Charles ON P0M 2W0; McM'01; CCFP; (705)867-0095; Fax. (705)867-0097.

KOLAWOLE, Olubukola F; St Joseph's Mountain H Serv, PO Box 585 Stn Lcd 100 West 5th St, Hamilton ON L8N 3K7; (Nigeria)'00; FRCPC; Psy. Staff, St Joseph's Healthcare Hamilton - West 5th Campus; (905)522-1155

KOLAWOLE, Rebecca O; Central Nfld Reg Hlth Centre, 50 Union St, Grnd-Falls-Windsor NL A2A 2E1; London (England)'02; Staff, Central Newfoundland Regional Health Centre; (709)292-2500

KOLB, Elena; 204-1950 Algonquin Ave, North Bay ON P1B 4Z2; Minsk State (Belarus)'84; (705)474-0060

KOLB, Martin R J; St Joseph's Healthcare, T2121-50 Charlton Ave E, Hamilton ON L8N 4A6; Wurzburg (Germany)'91; PhD; Staff, St Joseph's Healthcare - Charlton Campus; Teach Staff Med & Path, McMaster University; Langs: German; (905)522-1155 x5003; Fax. (905)521-6132; kolbm@mcmaster.ca.

KOLBASNIK, Alexandr; Centre for Family Medicine, 10B Victoria St S, Kitchener ON N2G 1C5; McM'01; CCFP; Staff Phys, Grand River Hospital - Kitchener/Waterloo Health Centre; Staff Phys, St Mary's General Hospital; Clinical Asst Prof, McMaster University; Clinical Asst Prof, University of Western Ontario; (519)783-0022; Fax. (519)783-0032.

KOLBASNIK, Jeffrey G; 210-400 Bronte St S, Milton ON L9T 0H7; Wes'95; FRCSC; GenSurg (Billing Disputes). Staff, Halton Healthcare Services Corporation - Milton District Hospital; (905)693-1338; Fax. (905)693-1351.

KOLBE, George A; Upper Canada Fam Hlth Team, 2-5 Home St, Brockville ON K6V 0A5; Pretoria (South Africa)'88; MB ChB; CCFP; FCFP; (613)423-1111

KOLBER, Michael R; Associate Med Clinic, PO Box 7590 Stn Main 10011 101 St, Peace River AB T8S 1T2; Alb'96; BSc; CCFP; FCFP; (780)624-2581; Fax. (780)624-4015.

KOLCHAK, Andriy; Waypoint Centre for Mental H C, 500 Church St, Penetanguishene ON L9M 1G3; Odessa (Ukraine)'94; FRCPC; Psy. Staff, Waypoint Centre for Mental Health Care; (705)549-3481

KOLDEWEY, Natalia; Carlington Comm Hlth Services, 900 Merivale Rd, Ottawa ON K1Z 5Z8; (Moldova)'90; CCFP; (613)722-2161; Fax. (613)722-8471.

KOLENDA, Jacek; 306-277 Lakeshore Rd E, Oakville ON L6J 6J3; Tor'96; FRCSC; Otol (Rhinology). Staff, Halton Healthcare Services Corporation - Oakville Site; Staff, St Joseph's Health Centre; (905)849-7560; Fax. (289)295-0113.

KOLES, Sarah L; Radiology Consultants Assoc, 120A-6707 Elbow Dr SW, Calgary AB T2V 0E3; Cal'00; MSc; ABR; FRCPC; DiagRad. (403)777-3003; sarah.koles@calgaryhealthregion.ca.

KOLESAR, Richard E; Hamilton HS-General Site, 237 Barton St E, Hamilton ON L8L 2X2; Tor'85; FRCPC; Anes. Coord, Hamilton Health Sciences Centre - Hamilton General Hospital; Clin Assoc Prof Anes, McMaster University; (905)527-0271

KOLESAR, Sharlene E; Aquarius Med Clinic, 179 Davie Dr, Vancouver BC V6Z 2Y1; UBC'07; CCFP; (604)669-7772

KOLESKY, Hendrey C; Melville Med Associates, PO Box 209, Melville SK S0A 2P0; Pretoria (South Africa)'95; MB ChB; CCFP; (306)728-4466

KOLIASKA, Kathryn M; Alberta Health Services, 101-14310 111 Ave NW, Edmonton AB T5M 3Z7; Alb'97; MPH; FRCPC; CommunMed;CCFP; koliaska@shaw.ca.

KOLISANG, Mohau P; 210-2155 10th Ave, Prince George BC V2M 5J6; Witwatersrand (South Africa)'90; MB BCh; FRCPC; Psy. (250)562-2661; Fax. (250)562-2664.

KOLIVAKIS, Theodore T; Allan Memorial Institute, 1025 av des Pins O, Montreal QC H3A 1A1; McG'96; FRCPC; Psy. Staff, Allan Memorial Institute; (514)934-1934

KOLIVAKIS, Thomas N; Allan Memorial Institute, 1025 av des Pins O, Montreal QC H3A 1A1; Athens (Greece)'57; Psy (P.Q.). Staff, McGill University Health Centre - Royal Victoria Hospital; (514)934-1934 x5515; Fax. (514)843-1644.

KOLK, Sarah J; Two Rivers FHT-Healthlink, 10-350 Conestoga Blvd, Cambridge ON N1R 7L7; Ott'02; CCFP; Staff Privil, Cambridge Memorial Hospital; (519)740-5010

KOLKIND, Kristie-Ann; Mill Creek Family Medicine, 101-1912 Enterprise Way, Kelowna BC V1Y 9S9; UBC'95; CCFP; (250)868-0700; Fax. (250)868-3003.

KOLL, Wayne A L; 1 Hospital Crt, Oshawa ON L1G 2B9; UBC'92; BSc; FRCPC; RadOncol (Brachy Therapy). Staff Durham Reg Cancer Centre, Lakeridge Health - Oshawa Site; Asst Prof, Queen's University; (905)576-8711 x4595; Fax. (905)721-6101.

KOLLA, Lee A; St Paul's Hosp, 1081 Burrard St, Vancouver BC V6Z 1Y6; Sask'07; OrthSurg. Staff, Providence Health Care - St Paul's Hospital; (604)682-2344 x66118

KOLLA, Nathan J; Addiction & Mental Hlth-Clarke, B26-250 College St, Toronto ON M5T 1R8; Sask'05; FRCPC; Psy. Staff, Centre for Addiction & Mental Health (CAMH) - College Street Site; (416)535-8501

KOLLEK, Daniel; Joseph Brant Mem Hosp, 1230 North Shore Blvd, Burlington ON L7S 1W7; Ott'86; CCFP; CCFP(E.M.); Staff, Joseph Brant Memorial Hospital; (905)336-4116

KOLLER, John P; University of Alberta Hosp, 1C1 04-8440 112 St NW, Edmonton AB T6G 2B7; Alb'90; FRCPC; Anes. Staff, University of Alberta Hospital; (780)407-7035

KOLLER, Katalin E; Abbie J Lane Mem Bldg, 3310-5955 Veterans Memorial La, Halifax NS B3H 2E1; Dal'03; FRCPC; IntMed (Palliative Medicine); GeriatricMed. (902)473-4995

KOLLER, Katalin E; Dr Everett Chalmers Reg Hosp, PO Box 9000 Stn A, Fredericton NB E3B 5N5; Semmelweis (Hungary)'73; FRCPC; AnatPath. Staff, Dr Everett Chalmers Regional Hospital; (506)452-5254; Fax. (506)443-2168.

KOLLER, Oscar L; Fredericton Med Clinic, 302-1015 Regent St, Fredericton NB E3B 6H5; Semmelweis (Hungary)'72; FRCPC; IntMed; Gastroent. (506)458-0216; Fax. (506)457-4758.

KOLLMANN, Tobias; CFRI A517-950 28th Ave W, Vancouver BC V5Z 4H4; Yeshiva(NY,USA) (USA)'98; PhD; Asst Prof, University of British Columbia; (604)875-2466

KOLLMANNSBERGER, Christian; BC Cancer Agency-Vancouver CC, 600 10th Ave W, Vancouver BC V5Z 4E6; Munich (Germany)'93; FRCPC; IntMed; MedOncol. Staff, BC Cancer Agency Vancouver Centre; Clin Assoc Prof Med, University of British Columbia; Langs: German; (604)877-6000 x2674

KOLOBOV, Anton; Thunder Bay Reg HSC-T-Bay, 980 Oliver Rd, Thunder Bay ON P7B 6V4; Sverdlovsk State (Other Foreign)'93; FRCPC; IntMed. Staff, Thunder Bay Regional Health Sciences Centre; (807)684-6030

KOLODENKO, Yuliya; Heritage Med Clinic, 105-2841 109 St NW, Edmonton AB T6J 6B7; Alb'07; CCFP; (780)436-3790; Fax. (780)434-8378.

KOLODINSKY, Steve D; Radiology Consultants Assoc, 120-6707 Elbow Dr SW, Calgary AB T2V 0E3; Alb'85; FRCPC; DiagRad. (403)777-3003; Fax. (403)777-3008.

KOLODZIEJ, Alexander W; Canadian Forces Services Ctre, 101 Colonel By Dr, Ottawa ON K1K 0T2; Wroclaw (Poland)'88; FRCPC; Psy (Forensic Psychiatry). Langs: Polish; (613)945-1060

KOLODZIEJCZYK, M Dean; Royal Jubilee Hosp, 1952 Bay St, Victoria BC V8R 1J8; UBC'01; CCFP; Staff, Royal Jubilee Hospital; (250)370-8000

KOLOSOWSKA-RYDLEWSKI, Anna; Univ Hlth Network-Princess M, 610 University Ave, Toronto ON M5G 2M9; Gdansk (Poland)'80; Staff, Princess Margaret Hospital - University Health Network; (416)946-2000

KOLOTYLUK, Timothy D; Misericordia Community Hosp, C-16940 87 Ave NW, Edmonton AB T5R 4H5; Alb'76; CCFP; FCFP; Staff, Covenant Health - Misericordia Community Hospital; Staff, Westlock Healthcare Centre; Clin Prof Family Med, University of Alberta; (780)735-2800; Fax. (780)735-2857.

KOLSKI, Hanna; Edmonton Clinic Health Academy, 4 588-11405 87 Ave NW, Edmonton AB T6G 1C9; Alb'95; FRCPC; Neur (Pediatrics). Staff Peds, University of Alberta Hospital; Staff, Edmonton Clinic Health Academy; (780)248-5630; Fax. (780)248-5627.

KOLTEK, Mark M; Manitoba Adolescent Trmt Ctr, 228 Maryland St, Winnipeg MB R3G 1L6; Man'93; FRCPC; Psy. mkoltek@matc.ca.

KOLTIN, Dror; The Credit Valley Hosp, 2200 Eglinton Ave W, Mississauga ON L5M 2N1; Tel Aviv (Israel)'98; Staff, The Credit Valley Hospital; (905)813-4120; Fax. (905)813-4128.

KOLTON, Michael; Anaesthesia Services, 807-61 Queen St E, Toronto ON M5C 2T2; Tor'74; FRCPC; Anes. Staff, St Michael's Hospital; (416)363-2858

KOLTUN, Ronald N; Whitehorse Med Services Ltd, 406 Lambert St, Whitehorse YT Y1A 1Z7; Sask'77; CCFP; CCFP(E.M.); FCFP; Staff, Whitehorse General Hospital; Staff, Whitehorse Medical Services Ltd; (867)393-6600; Fax. (867)393-6601.

KOLYN, Donna M; Cambridge Med Plaza, 2B-695 Coronation Blvd, Cambridge ON N1R 7J9; Qns'88; FRCSC; GenSurg. (519)740-1625; Fax. (519)740-0115; kolyn@rogers.com.

KOLYSHER, Paula L; Queen Elizabeth II HSC, 10F-1276 South Park St, Halifax NS B3H 2Y9; Sask'98; FRCPC; Anes. Staff, Queen Elizabeth II Health Sciences Centre - Victoria General Site; (902)473-2331

KOLYVAS, George; Saint John Reg Hosp, PO Box 2100 Stn Main, Saint John NB E2L 4L2; West Indies (Jamaica)'84; FRCSC; Neursurg. Staff, Saint John Regional Hospital; (506)648-6650; Fax. (506)648-6649; george.kolyvas@horizonnb.ca.

KOM MOGTO, Christelle A D; Dir Sante Publique de l'Outaou, 104 rue Lois, Gatineau QC J8Y 3R7; Cotonou (Benin)'99; Public Health & Preventive Med; CommunMed (P.Q.). (819)776-7660

KOMAR, Luba N V; The Hosp For Sick Children, 555 University Ave, Toronto ON M5G 1X8; Tor'83; FRCPC; Peds. Staff Div of EmergMed, The Hospital For Sick Children; Langs: Ukrainian; (416)813-5278; Fax. (416)813-5043; luba.komar@sickkids.ca.

KOMAR, Ronald R; 1A-163 Commissioners Rd W, London ON N6J 1X9; Wes'89; BSc; MSc; (519)657-2032; Fax. (519)657-3357.

KOMARANSKI, Norman; 40 Place Shellington, Brantford ON N3S 0C5; Tor'73; MD; FRCPC; EmergMed. (519)753-9581

KOMATSU, Teruya; Queen Elizabeth II HSC, 7S 012-1276 South Park St, Halifax NS B3H 2Y9; Osaka City (Japan)'99; Staff, Queen Elizabeth II Health Sciences Centre - Victoria General Site; (902)473-2281

KOMENDA, Ben W; Concordia Health Associates, 102-1155 Concordia Ave, Winnipeg MB R2K 2M9; Man'70; Staff, St Boniface General Hospital; Staff, Concordia General Hospital.

KOMENDA, Paul V J; Seven Oaks Gen Hosp, 2PD12-2300 McPhillips St, Winnipeg MB R2V 3M3; Man'01; FRCPC; IntMed; Nephrol. Staff, Seven Oaks General Hospital; (204)237-2613

KOMER, Lawrence D; Burlington Square, 408A-760 Brant St, Burlington ON L7R 4B8; Qns'72; FRCSC; ObstGyn (Andropause). Consultant, Joseph Brant Memorial Hospital; Founder/Dir, Peak Performance Institute; Asst Prof, McMaster University; (905)639-2571; Fax. (905)639-7647.

KOMER, William J; Regional Mental HC-St Thomas, PO Box 2004 Stn Main 467 Sunset Dr, St Thomas ON N5P 3V9; Wes'85; FRCPC; Psy (Forensic Psychiatry). Staff, Regional Mental Health Care-St Joseph's Health Care; Staff, Bluewater Health - Mitton Site; Physician, Ontario Review Board; Pt-Time Adjunct Ass't. Prof., Psy., University of Western Ontario; (519)631-8510

KOMOROWSKI, Laurie A; Happy Valley Family Hlth Team, PO Box 1120 Stn Main 268 Maiden Lane, St Marys ON N4X 1B7; Alb'00; CCFP; (519)284-3450; Fax. (519)284-4471; lkomorowski@stmmc.ca.

KOMOSKY, Judy A; Selkirk Mental Health Centre, PO Box 9600 Stn Main 825 Manitoba Ave, Selkirk MB R1A 2B5; Man'90; Staff, Selkirk Mental Health Centre; (204)482-3810

KON KAM KING, Christopher A; Boardwalk Prof Centre, 220 Water St, Charlottetown PE C1A 2M5; Dal'00; CCFP; (902)368-7602; Fax. (902)368-7605.

KONDAPANENI, Satyam; Lakeridge Hlth Corp-Oshawa, 1 Hospital Crt, Oshawa ON L1G 2B9; Poona (India)'70; Staff, Lakeridge Health - Oshawa Site; (905)576-8711 x3237

KONDEJEWSKI, Richard J; LL-240 Chapel St, Cobourg ON K9A 0E3; Ott'71; (905)372-1174; Fax. (905)372-7782.

KONDI, Joma; Eastwood Med Clinic, 7919 118 Ave NW, Edmonton AB T5B 0R5; Univ of Al Fateh (Libya)'95; ABIM; FRCPC; IntMed (Diabetes); Endocrin&Metab. Staff, Sturgeon Community Hospital; Teach Staff, University of Alberta; (780)756-3666; Fax. (780)756-2598.

KONDOR, Natalie M; Family Med Centre, PO Box 8888 Stn Main 220 Bagot St, Kingston ON K7L 5E9; UBC'04; CCFP.

KONDRA, Peter M; Hamilton Family Hlth Team, 3F-10 George St, Hamilton ON L8P 1C8; Man'81; BSc; MSc; FRCPC; Psy (Child & Adolescent Psychiatry). Court Staff, St Joseph's Healthcare - Charlton Campus; Staff, Hamilton Health Sciences Centre - McMaster Children's Hospital; Asst Clin Prof, McMaster University; Langs: Ukrainian; (905)667-4848 x143; Fax. (905)667-4873; peter.kondra@hamiltonfht.ca.

KONDRASHOV, Maxim V; Riverbend Med Clinic, 2735 Quance St, Regina SK S4V 3B7; Moscow (Russia (Federation))'85; CCFP; Langs: Russian; (306)347-2500; Fax. (306)347-2514; rbmedical@accesscomm.ca.

KONERU, Rama D; Lakeridge Health Corp-Oshawa, 1 Hospital Crt, Oshawa ON L1G 2B9; Gandhi (India)'98; MB BS; FRCPC; IntMed; MedOncol. Staff, Lakeridge Health - Oshawa Site; Staff, Durham Regional Cancer Centre; (905)576-8711 x3282; Fax. (905)721-4741.

KONFORTE-VASILJEVIC, Tilda; 451 Milltown Blvd, St Stephen NB E3L 1J9; Sarajevo (Bosnia-Herzegovina)'78; Langs: Serbian; Croatian.

KONG, Anna W S; Toronto East Gen Hosp Inc, 825 Coxwell Ave, Toronto ON M4C 3E7; Qns'94; FRCPC; Anes. Staff Anes, Toronto East General Hospital Inc; (416)469-6212; Fax. (416)469-6874.

KONG, Anne M C; Henderson Med Centre, 441 Henderson Hwy, Winnipeg MB R2K 2H5; Man'91; BSc; CCFP; FCFP; Acad Member Family Pract Obst, Health Sciences Centre; Lecturer Family Pract, University of Manitoba; (204)667-8650; Fax. (204)668-1928.

KONG, Audley L; Forest Hill Inst of Aesthetic, 1188B Eglinton Ave W, Toronto ON M6C 2E3; West Indies (Jamaica)'72; FRCPC; Anes. Staff, The Scarborough Hospital - Birchmount Campus; University of Toronto; (416)785-7864; Fax. (416)785-7207.

KONG, Iwa; The Juravinski Cancer Centre, 699 Concession St, Hamilton ON L8V 5C2; Alb'04; FRCPC; RadOncol. Staff, Hamilton Health Sciences Centre - Juravinski Cancer Centre; (905)387-9711

KONG, Jason M; 4104-2775 Laurel St, Vancouver BC V5Z 1M9; UBC'95; FRCPC; IntMed; Endocrin&Metab. (604)875-5920; Fax. (604)875-5925.

KONG, Kester; 205-4040 Finch Ave E, Scarborough ON M1S 4V5; Edinburgh (Scotland)'86; MB ChB; FRCPC; IntMed; Neur (Neuromuscular Diseases). Court Staff, The Scarborough Hospital - Birchmount Campus; Assoc Staff, Toronto Western Hospital - University Health Network; Langs: Cantonese; (416)754-1554; Fax. (416)754-0116.

KONG, Waitak; William Osler HC-Brampton, N 2 916-2100 Bovaird Dr E, Brampton ON L6R 3J7; Tor'92; ABIM; FRCPC; IntMed (Interventional Cardiology); Cardiol. Staff, William Osler Health System - Brampton Civic Hospital; Langs: Cantonese; (905)494-6221; Fax. (905)494-6717.

KONG, Wei Lin; CSSS Haut-Richelieu-Rouville, 920 boul du Seminaire N, St-Jean-sur-Richel QC J3A 1B7; Sher'04; FRCPC; IntMed; Endocrin&Metab. Staff, Hôpital du Haut-Richelieu; (450)359-5000

KONG, Y S Peter; York-Finch Med Centre, 302-2115 Finch Ave W, North York ON M3N 2V6; Seoul (Korea)'78; FRCSC; Urol (Surgical Oncology). Staff, Humber River Regional Hospital - Finch Avenue Site; (416)748-3237; Fax. (416)748-3277.

KONG, Yat Ming; Sunnybrook Hlth Sciences Ctre, 3M 200-2075 Bayview Ave, Toronto ON M4N 3M5; Tor'02; FRCPC; Anes. Staff Anes, Sunnybrook Health Sciences Centre; (416)480-4864; Fax. (416)480-6039.

KONG, Yuan; 307-164 Queen St E, Brampton ON L6V 1B4; Qns'07; Endocrin&Metab; IntMed.

KONG TING, Margaret C; Toronto East Gen Hosp Inc, 825 Coxwell Ave, Toronto ON M4C 3E7; Tor'77; Staff Emerg Dept, Toronto East General Hospital Inc; (416)461-8272

KONGKHAM, Paul N; Univ Hlth Network-Toronto Western Hosp, 4 450-399 Bathurst St, Toronto ON M5T 2S8; Tor'01; FRCSC; Neursurg. Staff, Toronto Western Hospital - University Health Network; (416)603-5428

KONIECZNA, Ewa M; MCI The Doctor's Office, PO Box 134 Stn Royal Bank 200 Bay St, Toronto ON M5J 2J3; (Poland)'75; Langs: Polish; (416)368-6787; Fax. (416)368-7632.

KONIECZNY, Stanislaw J; Humber River Reg Hosp-Church, 200 Church St, Toronto ON M9N 1N8; Bialystok (Poland)'77; FRCPC; Anes. Staff, Humber River Regional Hospital - Church Street Site; University of Toronto; (416)243-4154

KONIGSBERG, Esther; 18-1960 Appleby Line, Burlington ON L7L 0B7; McM'83; (905)319-2000

KONIOUCHINE, Vladimir; Clinique Med Belanger, 300-3871 rue Belanger, Montreal QC H1X 3M7; Laval'99; CCFP; Staff, CSSS du Coeur de l'Isle Hôpital Jean-Talon; (514)495-6767; Fax. (514)495-4569; vladimir@pharmaciegabriel.com.

KONKAL, P John; Phoenix Med Centre, 206-2155 10th Ave, Prince George BC V2M 5J6; Man'64; DrMedCh; FRCS; FRCSC; Ophth (Plastic Surgery). Ac Staff, University Hospital of Northern British Columbia; Asst Prof Northern Med Program, University of British Columbia; (250)562-9518; Fax. (250)562-8678; pjkonkal@shaw.ca.

KONKIN, D Jill; Edmonton Clinic Health Academy, 2 115-11405 87 Ave, Edmonton AB T6G 1C9; Cal'82; BA(Hons); CCFP; FCFP; Staff, Edmonton Clinic Health Academy; Assoc Prof Family Med/Assoc Dean Community Engagement Faculty of Med & Dentistry, University of Alberta; (780)492-0678; Fax. (780)492-1559.

KONKIN, David E; 208-250 Keary St, New Westminster BC V3L 5E7; UBC'01; FRCSC; GenSurg.

KONKIN, Thomas M; 2-32442 George Ferguson Way, Abbotsford BC V2T 4Y4; Alb'80; (604)853-6667; Fax. (604)853-6658; tt.konkin@shaw.ca.

KONN, George; Baywood Med Centre, 206-95 Bayly St W, Ajax ON L1S 7K8; Tor'80; FRCSC; GenSurg. (905)619-8778; Fax. (905)619-8998.

KONRAD, Gerald P; Family Med Centre, 500-400 Tache Ave, Winnipeg MB R2H 3E1; (Other Foreign)'84; CCFP.

KONSTANTATOS, Spiros; 101-855 Broadview Ave, Toronto ON M4K 3Z1; Wes'93; BSc; CCFP; CCFP(E.M.); Langs: Greek; (416)466-4828; Fax. (416)466-5394.

KONSTANTINOU, Chris; 11-398 Steeles Ave W, Thornhill ON L4J 6X3; Columbus(OH) (USA)'89; (905)881-0334; Fax. (905)881-1721.

KONSTANTYNOWICZ, Barbara R; Regina Med Centre, 103-2550 12th Ave, Regina SK S4P 3X1; Sask'81; CCFP; FCFP; Clin Prof, University of Saskatchewan; (306)566-4100

KONTIO, Ken; Children's Hosp Eastern Ont, 401 Smyth Rd, Ottawa ON K1H 8L1; McM'94; FRCSC; OrthSurg (Pediatrics). Staff, Children's Hospital of Eastern Ontario (CHEO); Langs: Finnish; (613)737-7600 x2426; Fax. (613)738-4840; kkontio@cheo.on.ca.

KONTOLEMOS, Mario; The Ottawa Hosp-Civic Campus, C120-1053 Carling Ave, Ottawa ON K1Y 4E9; McG'06; MDCM; CSPQ; FRCPC; DiagRad. Staff, The Ottawa Hospital - Civic Campus; (613)737-8899

KONTOR, Jurgen A; Polyclinic, 199 Grafton St, Charlottetown PE C1A 1L2; Tor'68; PlasSurg. (902)629-8810

KONTOZOGLOU, Theodosios; Nanaimo Reg Gen Hosp, 1200 Dufferin Cres, Nanaimo BC V9S 2B7; Athens (Greece)'75; FCAP; FRCPC; AnatPath. Staff, Nanaimo Regional General Hospital; (250)755-7691

KONTSIOTIS, Akatereny; 28-3806 Albert St, Regina SK S4S 3R2; Sask'90; CCFP; FCFP; Staff, Regina General Hospital; Staff, Pasqua Hospital; Langs: Greek; (306)584-1818; Fax. (306)584-5141.

KONWAY, Desmond C; Courtenay Med Associates, 201-1350 England Ave, Courtenay BC V9N 8X6; UBC'90; (250)334-4411; Fax. (250)338-1245.

KONYER, Alan T; B-40 Lindsay St S, Lindsay ON K9V 2L8; Tor'80; Assoc Staff, Peterborough Regional Health Centre - Hospital Drive; Staff, Ross Memorial Hospital; (705)324-5553; Fax. (705)324-7184.

KONYNENBELT, Susan; Associate Med Group, 4705 48 Ave, Red Deer AB T4N 3T1; Alb'89; Physician, Associate Medical Group; Med Examiner, City Of Red Deer; (403)755-7501; Fax. (403)347-2989; susan.konynenbelt@reddeer.ca.

KONZUK, Peter J; 216-350 Sparks St, Ottawa ON K1R 7S8; Ott'80; FRCSC; Ophth. (613)237-3166; Fax. (613)567-1160.

KOO, Anson; Fraser Health Authority, 4F-260 Sherbrooke St, New Westminster BC V3L 3M2; UBC'98; FRCPC; Psy. Staff, Royal Columbian Hospital; (604)520-4662

KOO, Betty K K; 211B-801 York Mills Rd, North York ON M3B 1X7; (Hong Kong)'75; MB BS; FRCPC; Neur (Electroencephalography). Ac Staff Neurol(Med & Peds)/Med Dir EEG & EMG, North York General Hospital; Langs: Chinese; Cantonese; Mandarin; (416)510-8810; Fax. (416)510-8010.

KOO, Catherine Y; 107-1428 Ouellette Ave, Windsor ON N8X 1K4; Tor'76; (519)256-2645; Fax. (519)256-2646.

KOO, David W K; G F Strong Rehabilitation Ctre, 4255 Laurel St, Vancouver BC V5Z 2G9; Cal'95; FRCPC; PhysMed&Rehab. Staff, G F Strong Rehabilitation Centre; (604)714-4112; Fax. (604)737-6251; david.koo@vch.ca.

KOO, Henry; 104B-10 Keith Ave, Collingwood ON L9Y 0W5; McM'98; BSc; FRCSC; OrthSurg (Sports Medicine). Ac Staff, Collingwood General & Marine Hospital; (705)446-1845; Fax. (705)446-1897.

KOO, Howan; 203-515 Main St, Vancouver BC V6A 2V1; (Taiwan)'60; Court Staff, Providence Health Care - Mount Saint Joseph Hospital; (604)685-3814

KOO, Jarley; St Michael's Hosp, 30 Bond St, Toronto ON M5B 1W8; Sheffield (England)'70; MB ChB; FACS; FRCS(Ed); MSc(Surg.); MBA; FRCSC; GenSurg (Endoscopy). Staff, St Michael's Hospital; Assoc Prof Surg, University of Toronto; (416)864-5955; Fax. (416)864-5239.

KOO, Jonathan J; Burrard Health Bldg, 505-1160 Burrard St, Vancouver BC V6Z 2E8; Cal'04; (604)683-0206

KOO, Karen; London HSC-Victoria Hosp, D2 521C-800 Commissioners Rd E, London ON N6A 5W9; McM'04; FRCPC; IntMed; Critical Care Medicine. Consultant, London Health Sciences Centre - Victoria Campus; (519)685-8500 x55150

KOOBAIR, Sandhya; 5565 Wyandotte St E, Windsor ON N8S 4T9; Witwatersrand (South Africa)'00; MB ChB; CCFP; (519)974-6147; Fax. (519)974-6920.

KOOCHESFAHANI, Kasra M; U of Toronto-Health Services, 111-214 College St, Toronto ON M5T 2Z9; Meshed Univ of Medical Sciences (Saint Kitts-Nevis)'96; FRCPC; Psy. Staff, Victoria General Hospital; (416)978-8070

KOOCHIN, Harvey L; E-2020 Falcon Rd, Kamloops BC V2C 4J3; UBC'90; (250)372-8003

KOODOO, Stanley R; Psychealth Centre, 771 Bannatyne Ave, Winnipeg MB R3E 3N4; Man'97; FRCPsy; BSc; BMedSci; PhC; FRCPC; Psy (Child & Adolescent Psychiatry). Chief Inpatient Child & Adolescent Psy, Psychealth Centre; Asst Prof Psy, University of Manitoba; (204)787-7191; Fax. (204)787-4975; skoodoo@exchange.hsc.mb.ca.

KOOIMAN, Edith D H; Midpark Family Med Centre, 100-290 Midpark Way SE, Calgary AB T2X 1P1; Stellenbosch (South Africa)'93; MB ChB; DRCOG; MRCGPract; CCFP; (403)254-8405; Fax. (403)254-6585.

KOOKA, Dara M; PO Box 192 Stn Main, Glace Bay NS B1A 5V2; Bombay (India)'63; DABR; FRCR; FRCPC; DiagRad. Consultant Radiol, Cape Breton Healthcare Complex; (902)849-5511; Fax. (902)849-0287.

KOOLE, Janice J; Rosedale Med Group, 280 Queenston Rd, Hamilton ON L8K 1H1; Tor'96; BScPharm; CCFP; FCFP; (905)547-0508; Fax. (905)547-6865.

KOONAR, Harvir S; Foothills Med Centre, C231-1403 29 St NW, Calgary AB T2N 2T9; Cal'91; CCFP; CCFP(E.M.); Staff EmergMed, Foothills Medical Centre; (403)944-8430

KOONER, Sukhdev S; 1558 Ouellette Ave, Windsor ON N8X 1K7; Guru Nanak Dev (India)'77; FRCPC; IntMed (Pulmonary Medicine). Staff, Windsor Regional Hospital - Tayfour Site; Langs: Punjabi; Hindi; (519)253-8507; Fax. (519)253-8336.

KOOP, V Gary; Lively Med Centre, 3-204 Sixth Ave, Lively ON P3Y 1M4; Wes'69; Hon Staff, Health Sciences North - Memorial Site; Langs: German; (705)692-4774; Fax. (705)692-0528.

KOOPMANN, Peter; Hop Brome-Missisquoi-Perkins, 950 rue Principale, Cowansville QC J2K 1K3; Geneva (Switzerland)'66; PhD(McG); Hem; IntMed (Oncology). ac Staff IntMed & HemOncol Service, Hôpital Brome-Missisquoi-Perkins; Langs: German; French; (450)266-4342; Fax. (450)263-2042.

KOOPMANS, Robert A; Victoria Gen Hosp, 1 Hospital Way, Victoria BC V8Z 6R5; Alb'90; FRCPC; DiagRad. Staff, Victoria General Hospital; (250)727-4208

KOOPMANS, Veronica D; 201-1 Hesperus Rd, Thornhill ON L4J 0G9; Nijmegen (Netherlands)'85; MB BS; CCFP; FCFP; (905)882-4949; Fax. (905)882-0560.

KOORJEE, Rajabali G; Village Med Centre, 9526 Erickson Dr, Burnaby BC V3J 1M9; Glasgow (Scotland)'66; Assoc Staff, Royal Columbian Hospital; (604)421-1821; Fax. (604)421-0524.

KOORTS, Sybil; Langley Mem Hosp, 22051 Fraser Hwy, Langley BC V3A 4H4; (Other Foreign)'97; CCFP; CCFP(E.M.); Staff Emerg, Langley Memorial Hospital; (604)534-4121

KOOY, Jacobus; Medical Arts Bldg, 5-626 Main St, Penticton BC V2A 5C8; Stellenbosch (South Africa)'87; MB ChB; CCFP; Staff, Penticton Regional Hospital; (250)492-0153; Fax. (250)492-3618.

KOPAC, Daniel S; 910 10th Ave W, Vancouver BC V5Z 1M9; Alb'06; FRCPC; GenSurg. (604)362-4259

KOPANIAK, Marguerite M; Four Villages Comm Health Ctr, 1700 Bloor St W, Toronto ON M6P 4C3; Tor'93; BSc; PhD; CCFP; Staff, Ross Memorial Hospital; Staff, St Joseph's Health Centre; Langs: Polish; French; (416)604-3361

KOPE, Teresa M; 301-5027 47A Ave, Delta BC V4K 1T9; UBC'77; FRCPC; Psy. Staff, Vancouver General Hospital - Centennial Pavillion; (604)946-1050

KOPECHANSKI, Lauren; Thames Valley Family Hlth Team, RR 5 22262 Mill Rd, Mount Brydges ON N0L 1W0; Wes'09; CCFP; (519)264-2800; laurenk@smhc.net.

KOPEK, Neil J; MUHC-Montreal Gen Hosp, 1650 av Cedar, Montreal QC H3G 1A4; Tor'02; FRCPC; RadOncol. Staff RadOncol, McGill University Health Centre - Montreal General Campus; (514)934-8040; Fax. (514)934-8425.

KOPEL, Tal; CHUM-Hop St-Luc, 1058 rue Saint-Denis, Montreal QC H2X 3J4; McG'03; FRCPC; IntMed; Nephrol. Staff, Centre Hospitalier l'Université De Montréal (CHUM) - Hôpital Saint-luc; (514)281-2085

KOPOLOVIC, Shirley; 303-2797 Bathurst St, North York ON M6B 4B9; Tor'79; BSc; CCFP; FCFP; Staff, Mount Sinai Hospital; (416)787-5646; Fax. (416)787-9049.

KOPONEN, Glynis M; North Bramalea Med Centre, 305-9780 Bramalea Rd, Brampton ON L6S 2P1; Tor'87; FRCPC; Neur (Electromyography). Staff, Norfolk General Hospital; (905)792-4362; Fax. (905)792-2449.

KOPP, Justin E J; Medicine Hat Reg Hosp, 666 5 St SW, Medicine Hat AB T1A 4H6; Alb'08; CCFP; CCFP(E.M.); Staff, Medicine Hat Regional Hospital; (403)529-8000

KOPP, Michael; 166 Main St, St Catharines ON L2N 4V5; Ott'88; CCFP; (905)935-6880

KOPPERT, George J; 410 Giles Blvd E, Windsor ON N9A 4C6; Wes'75; DABOS; FRCSC; OrthSurg. Staff Surg, Hôtel-Dieu Grace Hospital; Staff Surg, Windsor Regional Hospital - Metropolitan Site; (519)256-1823; Fax. (519)254-3849; rosemary@skypa.ca.

KOPPERT, Theresa M; Saint John Med Clinic, 299 Metcalf St, Saint John NB E2K 4P8; Wes'86; CCFP; (506)658-0994; Fax. (506)636-9002; dtees@nbnet.nb.ca.

KOPPLIN, Peter A; St Michael's Hosp, 30 Bond St, Toronto ON M5B 1W8; Tor'63; FRCPC; IntMed (Palliative Care). Consultant, Bridgepoint Health Centre; Ac Staff, St Michael's Hospital; Assoc Prof Med, University of Toronto; (416)864-5903; Fax. (416)864-5714; kopplinp@smh.ca.

KOPPULA, Sudha; Royal Alexandra Hosp, 10240 Kingsway NW, Edmonton AB T5H 3V9; Alb'02; CCFP; Staff, Royal Alexandra Hospital; (780)735-4201

KOPRIVA, David; Regina Qu'Appelle HR-Regina, 1440 14th Ave, Regina SK S4P 0W5; McG'92; FRCSC; GenSurg; VascSurg. Staff, Regina General Hospital; Clin Assoc Prof, University of Saskatchewan; Langs: Czech; (306)766-6900; Fax. (306)766-6920.

KOPROWICZ, Kinga T; Kirkfield Med Centre, 1699 Kirkfield Rd, Kirkfield ON K0M 2B0; Ott'94; CCFP; Langs: Polish; (705)438-3189; Fax. (705)438-5174.

KOPYLENKO, Eleonor; Mulock-Bayview Medical, 30-16700 Bayview Ave, Newmarket ON L3X 1W1; Tor'87; CCFP; FCFP; Staff, Southlake Regional Health Centre; Langs: French; Ukrainian; Russian; (905)830-0016; Fax. (905)830-0016.

KOPYTO, Allan A; Wentworth Limeridge Med Ctre, 300-849 Upper Wentworth St, Hamilton ON L9A 5H4; Tor'90; DOHS; MSc; CCFP; FCFP; Ac Staff, Hamilton Health Sciences Centre - McMaster University Medical Centre; Court Staff, St Joseph's Hospital - St Joseph's Health Care; (905)387-3667; Fax. (905)387-3545; allankopyto@aol.com.

KORADA, Srinivasa M; Simon Fraser Health Region, 600-22470 Dewdney Trunk Rd, Maple Ridge BC V2X 5Z6; Vijayawada (India)'96; FRCPC; Peds. (604)466-6082

KORAH, Nadine; University of Toronto, 602-500 University Ave, Toronto ON M5G 1V7; McG'08; Peds.

KORANTENG, Samuel; Northern Lights Health Region, 7 Hospital St, Fort McMurray AB T9H 1P2; (Ghana)'96; MB ChB; Staff, Northern Lights Regional Health Centre; (780)791-6161

KORANY, A Leyla; CLSC Boraux-Cartierville, 11822 av Du Bois-De-Boulogne, Montreal QC H3M 2X6; Mon'00; CCFP; (514)331-2572

KORB, Edwin J; 600-123 Edward St, Toronto ON M5G 1E2; Witwatersrand (South Africa)'79; FRCPC; DiagRad. Staff, Humber River Regional Hospital - Keele Street Site; (416)379-4481

KORBAN, Nadim; CHUM-Hop St-Luc, 1058 rue Saint-Denis, Montreal QC H2X 3J4; St. Joseph (Lebanon)'80; FRCSC; Otol. Otolaryngology, Centre Hospitalier l'Université De Montréal (CHUM) - Hôpital Saint-luc; Consultant, Centre Hospitalier l'Université de Montréal (CHUM) - Hôtel-Dieu; Clin Teacher, Universite de Montreal; Langs: English; Arabic; Spanish; (514)890-8000; Fax. (514)412-7328; nadimkorban@yahoo.ca.

KORBYL, Robert E; 300-4309 52 Ave, Red Deer AB T4N 6S4; Alb'96; FRCSC; OrthSurg. (403)309-2001

KORCAZ, Yves A; 100-235 boul René-Lévesque E, Montreal QC H2X 1N8; Grenoble (France)'74; ABOG; FACOG; FRCSC; ObstGyn. ac Staff, Centre Hospitalier l'Université de Montréal (CHUM) - Hôtel-Dieu; Ac Staff, Centre Hospitalier l'Université De Montréal (CHUM) - Hôpital Saint-luc; Lecturer ObstGyn, Universite de Montreal; Langs: Spanish; (514)866-2446; Fax. (514)866-4013.

KORCZAK, Daphne J; The Hosp for Sick Children, 555 University Ave, Toronto ON M5G 1X8; Qns'00; BSc; FRCPC; Peds (Child Psychiatry); Psy. Staff Psy, The Hospital For Sick Children; (416)813-7529

KORDA, Andrew; 1294 Weston Rd, York ON M6M 4R3; Tor'73; CCFP; Staff, West Park Healthcare Centre; Staff, Humber River Regional Hospital - Church Street Site; Langs: Hungarian; (416)243-0700

KORDA, Ryan N; 1294 Weston Rd, Toronto ON M6M 4R3; Tor'05; CCFP; (416)243-0700

KORDIC, Ljiljana; Delta Health Sciences Centre, 202-4515 Harvest Dr, Delta BC V4K 4L1; Sarajevo (Bosnia-Herzegovina)'81; MSc; CCFP; Staff, Delta Hospital; Physician, Delta Health Sciences Centre; Clin Instructor, University of British Columbia; Langs: Croatian; Serbian; (604)946-6411; Fax. (604)946-0372.

KORDICH, Miroslav; Polyclinique Masson, 200-3425 rue Masson, Montreal QC H1X 1R6; Guadalajara (Mexico)'71; FACS; GenSurg. Langs: Spanish; French; (514)376-9961; Fax. (514)376-8100.

KORDISH, Paul L; K W Urgent Care Clinic, 385 Fairway Rd S, Kitchener ON N2C 2N9; Wes'79; DBIM; Staff, St Mary's General Hospital; Pres, P L Kordish Consulting Ltd; (519)748-2327

KOREN, Gideon; The Hosp for Sick Children, 555 University Ave, Toronto ON M5G 1X8; Tel Aviv (Israel)'76; FRCPC; MedScient(Med) (Pediatrics). Staff, The Hospital For Sick Children; Prof Peds, University of Toronto; Langs: Hebrew; (416)813-5781; Fax. (416)813-7562; gkoren@sickkids.ca.

KOREN, Sharon; 210-4800 Leslie St, North York ON M2J 2K9; Dal'95; BSc; FRCPC; IntMed; Rheum. Court Staff, Sunnybrook Health Sciences Centre; (416)221-1061; Fax. (416)221-0534.

KORENBERG, Lela C; Medical & Dental Bldg, 907-1849 Yonge St, Toronto ON M4S 1Y2; McG'67; BSc; DPsy; FRCPC; Psy (Couples & Family Therapy). (416)440-0213

KORENBLUM, Marshall S; Silverman Bldg, 502-114 Maitland St, Toronto ON M4Y 1E1; Tor'75; DCP; FRCPC; Psy (Child & Adolescent Psychiatry). Chief Psychiatrist, The Hincks-Dellcrest Centre - Toronto; Consultant, Sunnybrook Health Sciences Centre; Chairman Education Committee, Canadian Academy Child Psychiatry; Dir Postgraduate Educ, University of Toronto; (416)972-1935 x3316; Fax. (416)924-9808.

KORIN-SKAMENE, Tamara; Westmount Med Bldg, 660-5025 rue Sherbrooke O, Montreal QC H4A 1S9; Frankfurt (Germany)'75; (514)932-1702; Fax. (514)932-8739.

KORITAR, Endre L; 530-999 Broadway W, Vancouver BC V5Z 1K5; McG'78; FRCPC; Psy (Psychoanalysis). Ac Staff, Vancouver General Hospital - Centennial Pavillion; Clinical Asst Prof, University of British Columbia; Langs: English; French; Hungarian; (604)733-3540; Fax. (604)737-2424.

KORITNIK, Angela R; 204-700 March Rd, Kanata ON K2K 2V9; Sask'82; FRCPC; Psy. (613)271-7056

KORKIS, Joseph A; 405-672 Brant St, Burlington ON L7R 2H3; Dublin (Ireland)'77; FRCSI; FRCSC; Otol (Facial & Cosmetic Surgery). Hd Otol, Joseph Brant Memorial Hospital; Langs: Arabic; (905)333-9255; Fax. (905)333-3414; drkorkis@lara.on.ca.

KORKMAZ, Paul; CSSS du Lac-des-Deux-Montagnes, 520 boul Arthur-Sauve, Saint-Eustache QC J7R 5B1; Mon'00; FRCPC; PhysMed&Rehab. Staff, Hôpital de Saint-Eustache; (450)473-6811

KORKOLA, Darrell; Barrie Family Medicine, 5-18 Cundles Rd E, Barrie ON L4M 2Z5; Wes'89; BSc; (705)737-1887; Fax. (705)735-6949.

KORKOLA, Michael L; Georgian Prof Centre, 300-125 Bell Farm Rd, Barrie ON L4M 6L2; Wes'96; BSc(Hon); FRCSC; OrthSurg. Ac Staff OrthSurg, Royal Victoria Regional Health Centre; (705)725-8295; Fax. (705)733-8350.

KORKOLA, Stephen J; Regina Qu'Appelle HR-Regina, 1440 14th Ave, Regina SK S4P 0W5; Wes'96; LMCC; FRCSC; CardSurg. Staff, Regina General Hospital; (306)766-6900; Fax. (306)766-6920.

KORKUCZANSKA, Svetlana; 414-837 Hastings St W, Vancouver BC V6C 3N6; Lodz (Poland)'81; FRCPC; Psy. Consultant, Vancouver General Hospital - Centennial Pavillion; Langs: Polish; Russian; (604)771-5687

KORLEY, Ebenezer K; Workers' Compensation Board, 200-1881 Scarth St, Regina SK S4P 4L1; London (England)'61; MB BS(Lond); FRCS(Eng & Ed); FWACS; Staff, Worker's Comp Board of SK; (306)787-4996; Fax. (306)787-7588; ekorley@ucbsnsk.com.

KORLEY, Robert; Alberta Hip & Knee Clinic, 335-401 9 Ave SW, Calgary AB T2P 3C5; McG'99; MDCM; OrthSurg (Trauma). Staff Surg, Foothills Medical Centre; Clin Lecturer Orthopedics, University of Calgary; (403)221-4363

KORLEY, Victoria J; St Michael's Hosp, 6050-30 Bond St, Toronto ON M5B 1W8; McG'93; BSc; FRCPC; IntMed (Electrophysiology); Cardiol. Dir Electrophysiol Fellowship Prog Div of Cardiol, St Michael's Hospital; Asst Prof Med, University of Toronto; (416)864-5152; Fax. (416)864-5283.

KORMAN, Mark J; Springdale Prof Bldg, 617-2250 Bovaird Dr, Brampton ON L6R 0W3; Tor'98; FRCSC; Otol. (905)792-6949; Fax. (905)792-6977.

KORMAN, S Bruce; McMaster Children's Hosp, PO Box 2000 Stn Lcd 1 4E1-1200 Main St W, Hamilton ON L8N 3Z5; Man'95; BSc; FRCSC; Otol (Pediatric Otolaryngology). Asst Prof, McMaster University; (905)521-2100; Fax. (905)521-9992; kormanb@mcmaster.ca.

KORMENDI, Ferenc; Toronto East Gen Hosp Inc, 825 Coxwell Ave, Toronto ON M4C 3E7; Debrecen (Hungary)'73; FRCPC; IntMed (Dementia); GeriatricMed. Staff, Toronto East General Hospital Inc; Asst Prof, Univ. of Massachusetts(USA); (416)461-8272

KORMOS, Arpad I; Aberdeen Hosp, 835 East River Rd, New Glasgow NS B2H 3S6; Semmelweis (Hungary)'86; Staff, Aberdeen Regional Hospital; (902)752-7600

KORN, Miriam; USTAT/Group Clinic, 1119 Pembroke St, Victoria BC V8T 1J3; Dal'97; BSc; FRCPC; Psy. Staff, Vancouver Island Health Authority; (250)213-4400; Fax. (250)213-4401.

KORN, Paul M A; Oakridge Centre South Tower, 207-650 41st Ave W, Vancouver BC V5Z 2M9; McM'82; DABPed; FRCPC; Peds. Staff, BC Children's Hospital; Staff, BC Women's Hospital & Health Centre; Staff, Vancouver General Hospital - Centennial Pavillion; Clin Instructor, University of British Columbia; (604)266-1874; Fax. (604)266-1583.

KORN, Sheryl F; Guildwood Village Shopping Ctr, 5-123 Guildwood Pky, Scarborough ON M1E 4V2; Tor'81; Ac Staff, Baycrest Centre for Geriatric Care; Ac Staff, Rouge Valley Health System - Centenary Health Centre Site; (416)269-5088; Fax. (416)261-3112.

KORNACKI, Joseph B; 4074 boul Lasalle, Verdun QC H4G 2A2; McG'79; FRCSC; OrthSurg (Joint Replacement). ac Staff, Centre Hospitalier de LaSalle; Langs: Polish; French; (514)362-8965; Fax. (514)362-8012.

KORNBLUTH, Murray; MUHC-Montreal Gen Hosp, 1650 av Cedar, Montreal QC H3G 1A4; Wes'91; FRCPC; IntMed; Cardiol. Staff, McGill University Health Centre - Montreal General Campus; (514)934-1934

KORNDER, Jan M; Surrey Med Arts Bldg, 203-13798 94A Ave, Surrey BC V3V 1N1; UBC'81; FACC; FRCPC; IntMed (Cardiology). Dir Cardiol Clin Trials/Member, Surrey Memorial Hospital; (604)584-2200; Fax. (604)584-4550; jmkornder@gmail.ca.

KORNECKI, Aleksander; Children's Hosp of Western Ont, 800 Commissioners Rd E, London ON N6C 2V5; Milano (Italy)'84; FRCPC; Peds. Staff Peds, Children's Hospital of Western Ontario; (519)685-8500

KORNECKI, Anat; St Joseph's Health Care, PO Box 5777 Stn B 268 Grosvenor St, London ON N6A 4V2; Tel Aviv (Israel)'95; FRCPC; DiagRad. Staff DiagRad & Nuclear Med, St Joseph's Hospital - St Joseph's Health Care; (519)646-6000

KORNELSEN, Jeffrey L; The Medical Group, 32243 Hurd St, Mission BC V2V 3J9; Sask'93; CCFP; Staff, Abbotsford Regional Hospital & Cancer Centre; Staff, Mission Memorial Hospital; (604)826-6231; Fax. (604)820-1174.

KORNGUT, Lawrence W; South Health Campus, 4448 Front St SE, Calgary AB T3M 1M4; Wes'02; FRCPC; Neur. Staff Holy Cross Ambulatory Care Centre, Rockyview General Hospital; (403)956-2462

KORNHAUSER, Danny S; Bayview-Finch Med Clinic, 301-3292 Bayview Ave, North York ON M2M 4J5; Tor'80; CCFP; FCFP; Ac Staff, North York General Hospital; Asst Prof Family & Commun Med, University of Toronto; (416)222-2200; Fax. (416)224-9880.

KOROL, Debra A; Regina Qu'Appelle HR-Pasqua, 4101 Dewdney Ave, Regina SK S4T 1A5; Man'87; FRCPC; GenPath. Staff, Pasqua Hospital; (306)766-2158

KOROSI, Judit; 201-5171 221A Street, Langley BC V2Y 1A0; Buenos Aires (Argentina)'75; ABIM; FRCPC; IntMed (Cardiology). Staff, Langley Memorial Hospital; Langs: Hungarian; Spanish; (604)514-1741

KOROSTIL, Michele C; Addiction & Mental Hlth-Queen, 1001 Queen St W, Toronto ON M6J 1H4; McM'00; FRCPC; Psy. Staff, Centre for Addiction & Mental Health (CAMH) - Queen Site; (416)535-8501

KOROWNYK, Christina S; Northeast Comm Health Centre, 14007 50 St NW, Edmonton AB T5A 5E4; Alb'03; CCFP; Staff, University of Alberta Hospital; (780)342-4038

KORPASSY, Andras; Centre Med Brunswick, 955 boul Saint-Jean, Pointe-Claire QC H9R 5K3; Szeged (Hungary)'64; Psy. (514)426-6677; Fax. (514)426-3323.

KORSHEED, Shvan; New Vision Family Health Team, 421 Greenbrook Dr, Kitchener ON N2M 4K1; (Other Foreign)'98; CCFP; (519)578-3510

KORTAN, Paul P; St Michael's Hosp, 16048-30 Bond St, Toronto ON M5B 1W8; McM'74; FRCPC; IntMed; Gastroent. Staff, St Michael's Hospital; (416)864-3094; Fax. (416)864-5619.

KORTAS, Claude; LHSC-Victoria Hosp, A2 342-800 Commissioners Rd E, London ON N6A 5W9; Cluj (Romania)'82; MEd; FRCPC; IntMed; Nephrol. Dir Adam Linton Dialysis Unit, London Health Sciences Centre - Victoria Campus; Prog Dir IntMed, University of Western Ontario; Langs: Romanian; Arabic; French; Greek; (519)685-8287; Fax. (519)685-8224; claude.kortas@lhsc.on.ca.

KORTBAOUI, Alain; CSSS de Laval, 1755 boul Rene-Laennec, Laval QC H7M 3L9; Laval'93; Staff, Hopital de la Cite de la santé; Université Laval; Universite de Montreal; (450)668-1010; alain.kort@sympatico.ca.

KORTBEEK, Frank B; Orthopaedic Consultants, 10972 124 St NW, Edmonton AB T5M 0H8; Alb'86; BMedSci; FRCSC; OrthSurg (Joint Arthroplasty). Site Chief, Royal Alexandra Hospital; Clin Assoc Prof, University of Alberta; Langs: Bilingual(English/French); (780)732-3711; Fax. (780)451-1437.

KORTBEEK, John B; Foothills Med Centre, 1403 29 St NW, Calgary AB T2N 2T9; Alb'84; FRCSC; GenSurg (Critical Care Medicine). Staff Surg, Foothills Medical Centre; Dept Head Surg, University of Calgary; Langs: Bilingual(English/French); (403)944-1697; Fax. (403)270-8409.

KORVEMAKER, Michelle L; Woodstock Gen Hosp, 310 Juliana Dr, Woodstock ON N4V 0A4; Ott'02; CCFP; Staff, Woodstock General Hospital; (519)421-4211

KORWAN, Claudia A; Rouge Valley-Ajax & Pickering, 580 Harwood Ave S, Ajax ON L1S 2J4; Tor'83; FRCPC; DiagRad (Ultrasound). Staff Radiol, Rouge Valley Health System - Ajax & Pickering Health Centre Site; Langs: German; (905)683-2320 x1468; Fax. (905)683-9906; akorwan@rogers.com.

KORZ, Linda T C; Hamilton HS-McMaster Site, PO Box 2000 Stn Lcd 1, Hamilton ON L8N 3Z5; McM'94; FRCPC; Anes. Staff, Hamilton Health Sciences Centre - McMaster Children's Hospital; (905)521-2100 x75166

KORZAN, Gregory J; Kelowna Gen Hosp, 2268 Pandosy St, Kelowna BC V1Y 1T2; Alb'75; DAB; Ac Staff, Kelowna General Hospital; (250)862-4495; Fax. (250)862-4361.

KORZAN, Jeffrey R; University of Alberta Hosp, 2A2 41-8440 112 St NW, Edmonton AB T6G 2B7; Alb'05; FRCPC; DiagRad. Staff, University of Alberta Hospital; (780)407-6810

KORZEKWA, Marilyn I; St Joseph's Healthcare, 50 Charlton Ave E, Hamilton ON L8N 4A6; Tor'82; FRCPC; Psy (Adult Psychiatry). Ac Staff, St Joseph's Healthcare - Charlton Campus; Consultant, St Joseph's Healthcare Hamilton - West 5th Campus; Asst Prof Psy, McMaster University; (905)521-6040; Fax. (905)521-6059; mkorzek@mcmaster.ca.

KORZENIEWSKI, Alexandra; 3-1032 17 Ave SW, Calgary AB T2T 0A5; Poznan (Poland)'82; (403)229-1771; Fax. (403)229-1812.

KORZENIEWSKI, Peter A; Foothills Med Centre, 1403 29 St NW, Calgary AB T2N 2T9; Lekarsky (Poland)'82; FRCPC; Anes. Staff, Foothills Medical Centre; (403)944-1430; Fax. (403)944-2425.

KORZENOWSKI, Donald W; Millwoods Family Clinic, 104-2551 Hewes Way NW, Edmonton AB T6L 6W6; Alb'78; Staff, Covenant Health - Grey Nuns Community Hospital; (780)462-2767; Fax. (780)463-7025.

KORZINSTONE, Clifford A; Oshawa Clinic, 117 King St E, Oshawa ON L1H 1B9; Sher'78; AB; FRCSC; Ophth. Staff, Lakeridge Health - Oshawa Site; Langs: Bilingual(English/French); (905)723-8551; Fax. (905)721-4916.

KOS, Antonio I; Timmins Family Health Team, 206 Fifth Ave, Timmins ON P4N 5L3; (Grenada)'94; CCFP; Langs: English; French; (705)264-6888; Fax. (705)264-6887.

KOSALKA, Tadeusz; Regency Medical Centre, 106-2737 Keele St, North York ON M6M 3E9; Cracow (Poland)'82; FRCSC; ObstGyn (Colposcopy). Staff, Humber River Regional Hospital - Church Street Site; Langs: Polish; (416)241-7988; Fax. (416)241-5528; tkosalka@rogers.com.

KOSAR, Katherine J; A1-3492 Weston Rd, North York ON M9M 2W1; Tor'90; CCFP; FCFP; Ac Staff, Humber River Regional Hospital - Finch Avenue Site; (416)744-8510; Fax. (416)744-7642.

KOSAR, Stephen E; Four Corners Med Bldg, 404-2009 Long Lake Rd, Sudbury ON P3E 6C3; Tor'81; FRCSC; Ophth (Medical Retina). Ac Staff, Health Sciences North-St Joseph's Health Centre; Four Corners Medical Bldg; Asst Prof Surg, Northern Ontario School of Medicine; Langs: Ukrainian; (705)523-4545; Fax. (705)523-4511.

KOSARIC, Alan; Ophthalmic Consultant Centers, 1880 Sismet Rd, Mississauga ON L4W 1W9; Wes'93; FRCSC; Ophth;CCFP; CCFP(E.M.); (905)212-9482 x400; Fax. (905)212-9821.

KOSATSKY, Thomas B; BC Centre for Disease Control, 655 12th Ave W, Vancouver BC V5Z 4R4; Man'75; CommunMed (P.Q.). Langs: Bilingual(French/English); (604)660-6630

KOSEFF, Howard D; 102-17770 56 Ave, Surrey BC V3S 1C7; Witwatersrand (South Africa)'86; MB ChB; (604)574-7883

KOSHAL, Arvind; University of Alberta Hosp, WMC 3H2 14-8440 112 St NW, Edmonton AB T6G 2B7; Ravishankar (India)'71; MB BS; MS(Surg.); FRCSC; GenSurg; Cardiovasc&ThorSurg. Sr Med Dir, Mazankowski Alberta Heart Institute; Clin Prof, University of Alberta; Langs: Hindi; (780)407-8058; Fax. (780)407-7657; akoshal@ualberta.ca.

KOSHI, Edvin; Halifax Spine & Pain Institute, 3-1574 Argyle St, Halifax NS B3J 2B3; Tirana (Albania)'89; FRCPC; PhysMed&Rehab (Pain Medicine). (902)422-0888; Fax. (902)422-0902.

KOSHY, Varghese C; 64 Ontario St, Trenton ON K8V 6H9; Kerala (India)'75; MB BS; BSc; MD(IntMed); FRCPC; IntMed. Ac Staff, QHC Trenton Memorial; Assoc Staff, QHC Belleville General; (613)392-2634; Fax. (613)392-0388.

KOSICK, Kevin B; North Island Medical, 1959 Cliffe Ave, Courtenay BC V9N 2L2; Wes'73; Vis Staff, Vancouver General Hospital - Centennial Pavillion; (250)338-5097

KOSICK, Thomas M; Northern Lights Health Region, 7 Hospital St, Fort McMurray AB T9H 1P2; UBC'07; Staff, Northern Lights Regional Health Centre; (780)791-6161; Fax. (780)791-6019.

KOSIUK, John P; MUHC-Royal Victoria Hosp, 687 av des Pins O, Montreal QC H3A 1A1; McG'83; FRCPC; DiagRad. Asst Prof Radiol, McGill University Health Centre - Royal Victoria Hospital; Teach Staff Radiol, McGill University; (514)934-1934

KOSKI, Sheryl L; Cross Cancer Institute, 11560 University Ave NW, Edmonton AB T6G 1Z2; Wes'94; MD; FRCP; MEd; FRCPC; IntMed (Gastrointestinal Cancer); MedOncol. Staff, Cross Cancer Institute; Assoc Prof Oncol, University of Alberta; (780)432-8221; sheryl.koski@albertahealthservices.ca.

KOSLOWSKI, Walter; 350 Main St E, Milton ON L9T 1P6; Wes'65; Staff, Halton Healthcare Services Corporation - Milton District Hospital; School Physician, E C Drury School For The Deaf; Langs: German; (905)636-0766; Fax. (905)636-0429; w.koslowski@look.ca.

KOSOWAN, Marisa R; Tuxedo Family Med Centre, 981 Corydon Ave, Winnipeg MB R3M 0X1; Man'08; CCFP; (204)988-6040

KOSOY, Martin H; 307 Sheppard Ave W, North York ON M2N 1N6; Tor'59; FRCPC; Peds (Pediatric Hematology). Sr Physician, The Hospital For Sick Children; Assoc Prof Peds, University of Toronto; (416)221-1177

KOSS, Erica; CHUM-Hotel-Dieu, 3840 rue Saint-Urbain, Montreal QC H2W 1T8; Mon'05; Staff, Centre Hospitalier l'Université de Montréal (CHUM) - Hôtel-Dieu; (514)890-8000

KOSS, Gary M; Medical Bldg, 120-6180 Blundell Rd, Richmond BC V7C 4W7; Cal'80; MSc; BSc; Staff, Richmond Hospital; Med Dir, Rosewood Manor Intermediate Care Home & Courtyard Gardens; (604)271-0654; Fax. (604)241-8615.

KOSS, Michael A; Guisachan Family Medicine, 105-2395 Gordon Dr, Kelowna BC V1W 3X7; UBC'84; CCFP; FCFP; Ac Staff, Kelowna General Hospital; (250)860-5888; Fax. (250)860-5880.

KOSSOWSKI, Alexandra; Dir de la Sante Publique Mtl, 1301 rue Sherbrooke E, Montreal QC H2L 1M3; Mon'01; FRCPC; CommunMed. (514)528-2400 x3898

KOST, Karen M; MUHC-Montreal Gen Hosp, A2 141-1650 av Cedar, Montreal QC H3G 1A4; McG'82; DAB; CSPQ; MDCM; FRCSC; Otol (Head & Neck Oncology). assoc Prof Otol, McGill University Health Centre - Montreal General Campus; Membre The Examination Board of Otolaryngology, College des Medecins du Quebec; Dir Lab & Assoc Prof, McGill University; Langs: English; French; (514)934-1934 x42273; Fax. (514)934-8422.

KOSTAMO, Timothy; 106-3825 Sunset St, Burnaby BC V5G 1T4; UBC'02; FRCSC; OrthSurg. (604)437-9600

KOSTASH, Mark A; Peter Lougheed Centre, 3500 26 Ave NE, Calgary AB T1Y 6J4; Alb'88; FRCPC; Anes. Staff, Peter Lougheed Centre; (403)943-5554

KOSTASHUK, Edmund C; BC Cancer Agency-Fraser Valley, 13750 96 Ave, Surrey BC V3V 1Z2; Qns'74; FRCPC; RadOncol. Staff, BC Cancer Agency Fraser Valley Centre; (604)930-2038

KOSTENUIK, Marcia A; 303-190 Cundles Rd E SS 103, Barrie ON L4M 4S5; Tor'00; CCFP; Staff, Royal Victoria Regional Health Centre; (705)728-3722

KOSTIC, Zlatko; 104-5009 48 St NW, Lloydminster AB T9V 0H7; Zagreb (Croatia)'89; FCP (SA); FRCPC; IntMed (Rheumatology). Staff, Lloydminster Hospital; Langs: Croatian; (780)875-7800

KOSTIUK, David P; Seaforth Med Bldg, 685-3550 ch de la Cote-des-Nei, Montreal QC H3H 1V4; McG'79; BSc; MSc; PhD; ABIM; FRCPC; IntMed (Clinical Cardiology); Cardiol. Staff, McGill University Health Centre - Montreal General Campus; adj Prof Med, McGill University; Langs: French; (514)934-6161; Fax. (514)934-5640.

KOSTOLOWSKI-KONDYSAR, M H; 303-1676 Martin Dr, Surrey BC V4A 6E7; Wroclaw (Poland)'74; MSc; MD; FRCPC; Psy. Langs: Polish; (604)560-5660

KOSTOPOULOS, Elen; 200-300 Main St N, Brampton ON L6V 4H6; Semmelweis (Hungary)'02; CCFP; (905)451-1806

KOSTOVIC, Biljana; William Osler HC-Etobicoke, 101 Humber College Blvd, Etobicoke ON M9V 1R8; Sarajevo (Bosnia-Herzegovina)'85; Staff, William Osler Health System - Etobicoke General Hospital; (416)494-2120

KOSTUK, William J; London HSC-University Hosp, PO Box 5339 Stn B 339 Windermere Rd, London ON N6A 5A5; Wes'65; FACC; FACP; FAHA; FRCPC; IntMed (Cardiology). Staff, London Health Sciences Centre - University Hospital; Prof, University of Western Ontario; (519)663-3263; Fax. (519)434-3278; bill.kostuk@lhsc.on.ca.

KOSTYK, Richard J; The Pas Health Complex, PO Box 240 Stn Main, The Pas MB R9A 1K4; Man'95; FRCPC; IntMed. Staff, St. Anthony General Hospital; (204)623-6431; Fax. (204)633-9263.

KOSTYNIUK, Ron W; Willowgrove Med Group, 2-527 Nelson Rd, Saskatoon SK S7S 1P4; Sask'76; Staff, Saskatoon City Hospital; Staff, St Paul's Hospital (Grey Nuns) of Saskatoon; Staff, Royal University Hospital; (306)653-1543; Fax. (306)653-0422.

KOSTYNUK, Carol D; 106-14727 87 Ave NW, Edmonton AB T5R 4E5; Alb'80; FRCPC; Psy (Eating Disorders). (780)488-1090

KOTA, Suzanne E; Humber River Reg Hosp-Church, 200 Church St, Toronto ON M9N 1N8; Tor'79; Staff, Humber River Regional Hospital - Church Street Site; (416)249-8111

KOTALIK, Jaroslav F; Lakehead University, 955 Oliver Rd, Thunder Bay ON P7B 5E1; Karlova (Czech Republic)'62; DMRT; MA(Med.Ethics); FRCPC; RadOncol (Biomedical Ethics). Court Staff, Thunder Bay Regional Health Sciences Centre Port-Arthur; Court Staff, St Joseph's Care Group - St Joseph's Hospital; Aj Prof Philosophy-Ctr for Hlth Care Ethics, Lakehead University / Library; Prof, Northern Ontario School of Medicine; (807)343-8126; Fax. (807)346-7935; jkotalik@lakeheadu.ca.

KOTALIK, Thomas; Guelph Family Health Team, 305-85 Norfolk St, Guelph ON N1H 4J4; Tor'97; CCFP; FCFP; Court Staff, Guelph General Hospital; Ac Staff, St Joseph's Hospital - St Joseph's Health Care; Med Dir, Village of Riverside Glen; (519)836-9440; Fax. (519)836-9530; tkotalik@gbhs.on.ca.

KOTARBA, Delani D; Ottawa Fertility Centre, 200-955 Green Valley Cres, Ottawa ON K2C 3V4; Tor'87; BSc; FRCSC; ObstGyn (Infertility). Assoc Staff, The Ottawa Hospital - Civic Campus; Chief Div of Reproductive Med/Assoc Prof, University of Ottawa; (613)686-3378 x622; Fax. (613)225-9736; dkotarba@conceive.ca.

KOTARBA, Jan A; The Ottawa Hosp-Civic Campus, 1053 Carling Ave, Ottawa ON K1Y 4E9; Ott'88; FRCPC; Peds (Neonatal & Perinatal Medicine). Staff, The Ottawa Hospital - Civic Campus; (613)761-4000; Fax. (613)761-5017; jkotarba@ottawahospital.on.ca.

KOTB, Rami; BC Cancer Agency-Vanc Isl Ctr, 2410 Lee Ave, Victoria BC V8R 6V5; Cairo (Egypt)'93; MB BCh; Staff, BC Cancer Agency Vancouver Island Centre; (250)519-5580

KOTCHETKOV, Rouslan I; Thunder Bay Reg HSC-T-Bay, 980 Oliver Rd, Thunder Bay ON P7B 6V4; Minsk State Med Inst (Belarus)'94; FRCPC; IntMed; Hem. Staff, Thunder Bay Regional Health Sciences Centre; (807)684-6000

KOTECHA, Suhas A; Headwaters Health Care Centre, 100 Rolling Hills Dr, Orangeville ON L9W 4X9; Tor'06; DiagRad. (519)941-2410

KOTECHA, Yatish J; Assiniboine Clinic, 633 Lodge Ave, Winnipeg MB R3J 0S9; Southampton (England)'80.

KOTHANDARAMAN, Maitreyi; HSC-Faculty of Med, 6D26-3280 Hospital Dr NW, Calgary AB T2N 4Z6; Ott'99; MSc; FRCPC; IntMed (Nutrition); Gastroent. Clinical Asst Prof, University of Calgary; (403)592-5020; Fax. (403)592-5090.

KOTHAPALLI, Anil; Saint John Reg Hosp, PO Box 2100 Stn Main, Saint John NB E2L 4L2; (India)'94; Staff, Saint John Regional Hospital; (506)648-6000; drkothapalli@yahoo.com.

KOTHARE, Dnyanada L; Fifth Avenue Medical, 3013 5th Ave, Regina SK S4T 0L6; Bombay (India)'82; MB BS; MD; DGO; Langs: Gujarati; Marathi; Arabic; Hindi; (306)757-2664; Fax. (306)757-1565.

KOTHARI, Kasiyal; PO Box 88568 Rpo Newton Town C, Surrey BC V3W 0X1; Wes'76; CCFP; Chair Credential Committee/Member, Surrey Memorial Hospital; (604)979-7741; Fax. (604)599-7029.

KOTIN, Svetlana N; Yorkton Mental Health Centre, 270 Bradbrooke Dr, Yorkton SK S3N 2K6; Vitebsk Medical Institute (Belarus)'89; FRCPC; Psy. Psychiatrist, Yorkton Mental Health & Addiction Centre; (306)786-0558; Fax. (306)786-0556; svetlana.kotin@shr.sk.ca.

KOTKAS, Lawrence J; 2402 20 Ave S, Lethbridge AB T1K 1G6; Alb'56; DPM(Lond & Leeds); MRCPsy(UK); FRSM(UK); Psy (Psychoanalysis). Langs: Finnish; French; Swedish; (403)328-6727; Fax. (403)327-0803.

KOTOWYCZ, Mark A; 500-491 Lawrence Ave W, North York ON M5M 1C7; McG'04; FRCPC; IntMed; Cardiol. (416)781-3500

KOTREC, Marian; Niagara H System-St Catharines, 142 Queenston St, St. Catharines ON L2R 7C6; Komenskeho (Slovakia)'98; Cardiol; IntMed. Staff, Niagara Health System - St Catharines General Site.

KOTSAKIS, Afrothite; The Hosp for Sick Children, 555 University Ave, Toronto ON M5G 1X8; McM'99; FRCPC; Peds (Critical Care Medicine). Staff, The Hospital For Sick Children; (416)813-6485; afrothite.kotsakis@sickkids.ca.

KOTTACHCHI, Dan; Guelph GI & Surgery Clinic, 105-21 Surrey St W, Guelph ON N1H 3R3; Ott'05; FRCPC; IntMed; Gastroent. Consultant, Groves Memorial Community Hospital; Staff, Guelph General Hospital; Staff, North Wellington Health Care - Palmerston & District Hospital; (519)836-8201; Fax. (519)836-1341.

KOTWALL, Zenobia A; Madrona Imaging Westhill Ctre, A-1804 Bowen Rd, Nanaimo BC V9S 5W4; Sask'82; FRCPC; DiagRad. Staff, Nanaimo Regional General Hospital; (250)753-4351; Fax. (250)753-0856.

KOTYLAK, Gregory S; 11664 223 St, Maple Ridge BC V2X 5X5; UBC'86; FRCSC; GenSurg. Consultant, Ridge Meadows Hospital & Health Care Centre; (604)466-9019; Fax. (604)467-0455.

KOTZE, Annegret; Village Mall Med Clinic, 6320 50 Ave, Red Deer AB T4N 4C6; (South Africa)'91; (403)314-5357

KOTZE, Charlene; Workers' Comp Board, 4980 Wills Rd, Nanaimo BC V9T 6C6; Pretoria (South Africa)'87; MB ChB; CCFP; (250)751-8033

KOTZE, Dirk A; 1001 110 Ave, Dawson Creek BC V1G 4X3; Stellenbosch (South Africa)'94; MB ChB; FCP (SA); Psy. (250)719-6525; Fax. (250)719-6540.

KOTZER, Eric J; Davisville Med & Dental Centre, 901-1849 Yonge St, Toronto ON M4S 1Y2; Tor'88; (416)921-9566; Fax. (416)921-7289.

KOU, Brenda S H M; Scarborough Prof Centre, 110-1371 Neilson Rd, Scarborough ON M1B 4Z8; Tor'93; FRCSC; Otol. (416)850-2416; Fax. (416)850-2415.

KOUBAESH, Yousery Y R; 94 Charing Cross St, Brantford ON N3R 2H6; Tanta (Egypt)'89; IntMed (Cardiology). (519)759-0010; Fax. (519)759-4310.

KOUCHAKAN, Mohsen; Dixon Med Centre, 209-531 Davis Dr, Newmarket ON L3Y 6P5; Tehran (Iran)'93; FRCPC; IntMed (Cardiology). Staff, Southlake Regional Health Centre; (905)895-4521

KOUDRA, Fahamia; Maitland Valley Family Hlth Team, 180 Cambria Rd N, Goderich ON N7A 4N8; Sher'08; CCFP; (519)524-6060

KOUDSI, Nasir M; 271 Bradbrooke Dr, Yorkton SK S3N 3L3; Istanbul (Turkey)'72; Chief Staff/Ac Staff, Yorkton Regional Health Centre; (306)782-9444

KOUDYS, Deborah; Thames Valley FHT-Whitehills M, 1225 Wonderland Rd N, London ON N6G 2V9; Wes'79; CCFP; FCFP; (519)472-0040; Fax. (519)472-7732.

KOUFOGIANIS, Vayia; Groupe Sante Physimed, 137-6363 rte Transcanadienne, Saint-Laurent QC H4T 1Z9; McG'95; FRCSC; ObstGyn. (514)747-8185

KOUIDER EL OUAHED, Ali; CSSS d'Antoine-Labelle-Mt Laur, 2561 ch de la Lievre S, Mont-Laurier QC J9L 3G3; Staff, CSSS d'Antoine-Labelle; (819)623-1234

KOUJOK, Khaldoun; Children's Hosp Eastern Ont, 401 Smyth Rd, Ottawa ON K1H 8L1; Damascus (Syria)'95; Staff, Children's Hospital of Eastern Ontario (CHEO); (613)737-7600 x3356

KOUL, Rashmi; Allan Blair Cancer Centre, 300-4101 Dewdney Ave, Regina SK S4T 7T1; Devi Ahilva Vishwavidyalaya (India)'94; FRCPC; RadOncol.

KOULACK, Joshua; Health Sciences Centre, GF548-820 Sherbrook St, Winnipeg MB R3A 1R9; Man'87; FRCS; MSc; FRCSC; GenSurg (Vasculities); VascSurg. Asst Prof, University of Manitoba; (204)787-2853; Fax. (204)787-3201.

KOUNCAR, Nathalie; Ctr Ortho Med Sportive de Lava, 255-300 boul de la Concorde E, Laval QC H7G 2E6; Mon'96; FRCSC; OrthSurg. Staff, CH Hôtel-Dieu d'Amos; Staff, Hopital de la Cite de la santé; (450)668-3840; Fax. (450)668-1157.

KOUNDE-TOGNIDE, Elisabeth; Hop de Sacre-Coeur de Mtl, 5400 boul Gouin O, Montreal QC H4J 1C5; Paris (France)'84; Staff, Hôpital du Sacre-Coeur de Montréal; (514)338-2050; Fax. (514)279-5647.

KOUNINE, Michael; Ontario Shores Ctr Mental HS, 7 2025-700 Gordon St, Whitby ON L1N 5S9; Donetsk (Ukraine)'78; DCPsy; MD; FRCPC; Psy (Emergency Psychiatry). Staff, Ontario Shores Centre for Mental Health Sciences; Langs: Russian; (905)430-4055 x6998; Fax. (905)430-4464; kouninem@ontarioshores.ca.

KOUROS, Evangelos P; 285 Riverside Dr, Welland ON L3C 5E6; Athens (Greece)'67; Ac Staff, Niagara Health System - Welland Hospital Site; Langs: Greek; (905)735-7667; Fax. (905)735-2997.

KOUROUKIS, Chrisostomos; The Juravinski Cancer Centre, 699 Concession St, Hamilton ON L8V 5C2; Tor'93; FRCPC; IntMed (Hematological Oncology); Hem. Staff Hematologist, Hamilton Health Sciences Centre - McMaster Children's Hospital; Head Service of Hematology, The Juravinski Cancer Centre; Assoc Prof, McMaster University; Langs: Greek; (905)575-7820; Fax. (905)575-6340; tom.kouroukis@jcc.hhsc.ca.

KOUSAIE, Kenneth N; 102-9123 Mary St, Chilliwack BC V2P 4H7; Ott'75; FRCSC; OrthSurg. (604)792-9104

KOUSONSAVATH, Ratana; West End Med Centre, 711 Sargent Ave, Winnipeg MB R3E 0B1; Moscow (Russia (Federation))'68; (204)775-5160

KOUTELAS, Nikolaos; 1366 Langois, Windsor ON N8X 4L7; (Dominica)'09; CCFP.

KOUTRAS, Nicholas P; Central Family Practice, C-3955 Tecumseh Rd E, Windsor ON N8W 1J5; Tor'91; (519)974-9778; Fax. (519)974-6479.

KOUTROULARAS, Ekaterine; CHUM-Hotel-Dieu, 3840 rue Saint-Urbain, Montreal QC H2W 1T8; Mon'95; Staff, Centre Hospitalier l'Université de Montréal (CHUM) - Hôtel-Dieu; Staff, Centre Hospitalier Pierre Boucher; Langs: Greek; English; (514)890-8159

KOUTSOGIANNIS, Dimitri; Niagara H System-St Catharines, PO Box 3018 Stn Main 142 Queenston St, St Catharines ON L2R 7C6; McG'03; FRCPC; AnatPath. Staff, Niagara Health System - St Catharines General Site; (905)378-4647 x46421

KOUTSOUKOS, Georgios; 104-1920 Yonge St, Toronto ON M4S 3E2; Tor'01; BSc; MSc; FRCPC; Psy. Langs: Greek; (416)481-8054; Fax. (416)481-8056.

KOUVELOS-FOSTER, Kallie L; Pine Valley Med Centre, 7700 Pine Valley Dr, Woodbridge ON L4L 2X4; Ott'87; (905)851-1234; Fax. (905)851-4548.

KOUYOUMDJIAN, Fiona; Hamilton Wentworth Detention C, 165 Barton St E, Hamilton ON L8L 2W6; Dal'05; FRCPC; Public Health & Preventive Med;CCFP.

KOUZ, Simon; CSSS du Nord de Lanaudière, 1000 boul Sainte-Anne, St-Charles-Brromee QC J6E 6J2; Aleppo (Syria),Paris (France)'82; FACC; FRCPC; Cardiol. Chef Div of Cardiol/Dir, Centre Hospitalier Régional de Lanaudière; Langs: Bilingual(French/English); (450)759-8222; Fax. (450)752-0651; simon.kouz@ssss.gouv.qc.ca.

KOVACINA, Nebojsa; St Mary's Hosp Centre, 3830 av Lacombe, Montreal QC H3T 1M5; McG'06; MDCM; CCFP; Staff, St Mary's Hospital Centre; (514)734-2677

KOVACS, Christopher S; Health Sciences Centre, 300 Prince Philip Dr, St. John's NL A1B 3V6; Qns'89; FACP; BA; LMCC; FACE; FRCPC; IntMed (Bone Metabolism); Endocrin&Metab. Att Physician Med & Endocrin, Health Sciences Centre; Consultant, St Clare's Mercy Hospital; Prof Endocrin & Metab, Memorial University Of Newfoundland; (709)777-6881; Fax. (709)777-8049; ckovacs@mun.ca.

KOVACS, Colin M; Maple Leaf Med Clinic, 301-14 College St, Toronto ON M5G 1K2; Man'83; FRCPC; EmergMed (AIDS/HIV). Physician, Maple Leaf Medical Clinic; University of Toronto; (416)465-3252 x2; Fax. (416)465-0792.

KOVACS, David P R; 304 Dundas St E, Belleville ON K8N 1E6; Qns'97; FRCSC; ObstGyn. (613)967-9900; Fax. (613)967-4882.

KOVACS, Eva; 406-2130 Lawrence Ave E, Scarborough ON M1R 3A6; Budapest (Hungary)'68; (416)298-0666; Fax. (416)298-7807.

KOVACS, George J; Queen Elizabeth II HSC-Halifax, 3021-1796 Summer St, Halifax NS B3H 3A7; Dal'89; FRCPC; EmergMed. Staff, Queen Elizabeth II Health Sciences Centre - Halifax Infirmary Site; (902)473-8769; Fax. (902)473-3617.

KOVACS, James F; 5230 South Service Rd, Burlington ON L7L 5K2; Wes'88; (905)331-7888; Fax. (905)331-0911.

KOVACS, Julie A J; Medical & Dental Bldg, 801-1849 Yonge St, Toronto ON M4S 1Y2; McG'87; BSc; FRCPC; IntMed; Rheum. Staff, St Michael's Hospital; University of Toronto; Langs: Hungarian; (416)482-4001; Fax. (416)482-4003; jajkovacs@look.ca.

KOVACS, Kalman T; St Michael's Hosp, 30 Bond St, Toronto ON M5B 1W8; Szeged (Hungary)'50; PhD; FRCPath; FCAP; FRCPC; AnatPath (Endocrinology Pathology - Pituitary)., St Michael's Hospital; Prof Path, University of Toronto; Langs: Hungarian; German; (416)864-5858; kovacsk@sm.ca.

KOVACS, Katalin; Queensway-Carleton Hosp, 3045 Baseline Rd, Nepean ON K2H 8P4; Dal'81; BSc; FRCPC; Psy (Crisis Intervention). Ac Staff, Queensway Carleton Hospital; (613)721-4708; Fax. (613)721-4773.

KOVACS, Katherine Ann; Hotel-Dieu Hosp, 166 Brock St, Kingston ON K7L 5G2; Qns'92; MSc(CommunHealth&Epidem); BSc; FRCPC; IntMed; Endocrin&Metab. Att Staff IntMed, Hotel-Dieu Hospital; Att Staff IntMed, Kingston General Hospital; Asst Prof, Queen's University; (613)544-3400 x2320; kovacsk@queensu.ca.

KOVACS, Lajos B; SMBD Jewish Gen Hosp, B605-3755 ch Cote-Ste-Catherin, Montreal QC H3T 1E2; McG'87; FRCP; FRCPC; Peds (Neonatology). Staff Neonatol, Sir Mortimer B Davis Jewish General; Staff, St Mary's Hospital Centre; Staff, McGill University Health Centre - Montreal Children's Hospital; Assoc Prof Peds, McGill University; Langs: French; (514)340-7598; Fax. (514)340-7566; lajos.kovacs@mcgill.ca.

KOVACS, Mark A; 400-1338 Broadway W, Vancouver BC V6H 1H2; Alb'89; FRCPC; Peds (Gastrointestinal Disorders). Staff, BC Children's Hospital; Clinical Asst Prof, University of British Columbia; (604)731-2102; info@kidscare.ca.

KOVACS, Susan V B; Medical & Dental Bldg, 801-1849 Yonge St, Toronto ON M4S 1Y2; McG'89; FRCPC; Peds (Pediatric Gastroenterology). Staff Consultant, North York General Hospital; Lecturer, University of Toronto; Langs: French; Hungarian; (416)482-4001; Fax. (416)482-4003.

KOVAL, Donald C; Picton Med Clinic, RR 2 4-389 Main St, Picton ON K0K 2T0; Qns'85; CCFP; FCFP; Ac Staff, QHC Prince Edward County Memorial; (613)476-3103; Fax. (613)476-1604.

KOVAL, Marilyn R; Sioux Lookout Zone Family, PO Box 4000, Sioux Lookout ON P8T 1K2; McM'93; CCFP; FCFP; Staff, Sioux Lookout Meno-Ya-Win Health Centre; University of Toronto; (807)737-5160; Fax. (807)737-4866.

KOVALEVA, Maria; William Osler HC-Etobicoke, 101 Humber College Blvd, Etobicoke ON M9V 1R8; (Tajikistan)'84; Staff, William Osler Health System - Etobicoke General Hospital; (416)494-2120

KOVARIK, Garrett G; SMBD Jewish Gen Hosp, 3755 ch Cote-Sainte-Catherine, Montreal QC H3T 1E2; Ott'99; CSPQ; FRCPC; Anes. Staff, Sir Mortimer B Davis Jewish General; (514)340-8222 x5701

KOVEN, Sheldon J; Simkin Centre, 1 Falcon Ridge Dr, Winnipeg MB R3Y 1V9; Man'79; PhD(Pharm); (204)586-9781

KOVESI, Thomas A; Children's Hosp Eastern Ont, 401 Smyth Rd, Ottawa ON K1H 8L1; Ott'85; FRCPC; Peds (Pediatric Respirology); Respir. Staff, The Ottawa Hospital - General Campus; Staff, Children's Hospital of Eastern Ontario (CHEO); Prof Peds & Respirol, University of Ottawa; Langs: Bilingual(French/English); (613)737-7600 x2868; Fax. (613)738-4886; kovesi@cheo.on.ca.

KOVITCH, Ingrid; Waskaganish Clinic, PO Box 390, Waskaganish QC J0M 1R0; McG'93; (819)895-8833 x4016; Fax. (819)895-8866.

KOVITHAVONGS, Carl S; Edmonton Mental Health Clinic, 5F-9942 108 St NW, Edmonton AB T5K 2J5; Alb'99; FRCPC; Psy. (780)342-7700

KOVITZ-LENSCH, Jessica M; Centre Hosp Honore-Mercier, 2750 boul Laframboise, Saint-Hyacinthe QC J2S 4Y8; Sher'06; Neur. Staff, Centre Hospitalier Honore-Mercier; (450)771-3333

KOVNATS, Sylvia F; St Boniface Gen Hosp, 409 Tache Ave, Winnipeg MB R2H 2A6; Man'74; FRCPC; Peds. Att Staff, St Boniface General Hospital; Att Staff, Health Sciences Centre; Asst Prof, University of Manitoba; (204)237-2278; Fax. (204)233-8825.

KOWAL, Caroline; Seven Oaks Gen Hosp, 2300 McPhillips St, Winnipeg MB R2V 3M3; Sask'01; CCFP; CCFP(E.M.); Staff, Seven Oaks General Hospital; (204)632-7133

KOWALCHUK, Glenn; 5-448 Welland Ave, St Catharines ON L2M 7V3; McM'91; (905)988-1323

KOWALCHUK, Ivan J; Country Club Plaza, 320-3025 Portage Ave, Winnipeg MB R3K 2E2; Man'68; FRCPC; Psy (General Adult Psychiatry). (204)832-8817; Fax. (204)888-9055.

KOWALCHUK, Shauna L; Cook Medical Bldg, 106-1175 Cook St, Victoria BC V8V 4A1; Man'90; FRCPC; Psy (Psychotherapy). (250)472-0060

KOWALCZYK, Amie J; Prairie North Specialist Clini, 107-4910 50th St, Lloydminster SK S9V 0Y5; Sask'06; FRCPC; Peds. (306)820-2599; Fax. (306)825-4774.

KOWALCZYK, Earl S; 3-5202 12 St, Lloydminster AB T9V 0W1; Sask'06; FRCSC; OrthSurg. (780)875-5200; Fax. (780)875-9258.

KOWALCZYK, Jill C; 206-7031 Westminster Hwy, Richmond BC V6X 1A3; Sask'04; FRCSC; ObstGyn. (604)821-0626

KOWALEWSKA-GROCHOWSKA, Kinga; University of Alberta Hosp, 2B3 09-8440 112 St NW, Edmonton AB T6G 2B7; Warsaw (Poland)'75; FRCPC; MedMicrobiol (Administration). Staff Med Microbiol, University of Alberta Hospital; Staff Med. Microbiol. & Parasitologist, Provincial Laboratory for Public Health for Northern Alberta; Assoc Prof Med Microbiol, University of Alberta; (780)407-7121; Fax. (780)407-3864; kkowalew@ualberta.ca.

KOWALEWSKI, Jerzy L; Vaughan Med Centre, H 26-9200 Weston Rd, Woodbridge ON L4H 2P8; Warsaw (Poland)'69; (905)417-2273; Fax. (905)417-7088.

KOWALSKI, Odile; Clinique Med L'Envolee, 5025 rue De Salaberry, Montreal QC H4J 1J1; Mon'91; Chef Neonatal Serv, Hôpital du Sacre-Coeur de Montréal; Universite de Montreal; Langs: English; (514)331-2323; Fax. (514)333-8534; obstetrique@cliniquelenvolee.com.

KOWALSKI, Stephen E; Health Sciences Centre, 820 Sherbrook St, Winnipeg MB R3A 1R9; Tor'78; FRCPC; Anes (Critical Care Medicine). Assoc Prof Anes, University of Manitoba; (204)787-2261; Fax. (204)787-4291.

KOWALSKY, Glenn D; Greenwood Fam Physicians, PO Box 5 709 1 St, Sundre AB T0M 1X0; Alb'83; Assoc Staff, Sundre Hospital & Care Centre; (403)638-2424; Fax. (403)638-3580.

KOWALUK, Bruce A; Kin Place Primary Health Care, PO Box 28 689 Main St, Oakbank MB R0E 1J0; Man'95; (204)444-2227

KOWAND, Linda M M; 7121 109 St NW, Edmonton AB T6G 1B9; Alb'76; AB; FRCPC; DiagRad (Mammography). (780)434-9147; Fax. (780)436-7650.

KOWBEL, Michael A M; Royal Inland Hosp, 311 Columbia St, Kamloops BC V2C 2T1; Sask'86; FRCPC; Anes (Pain Management). Staff, Royal Inland Hospital; Langs: Ukrainian; (250)374-5111

KOWE, Olajide O; Yorkton Reg Health Centre, 270 Bradbrooke Dr, Yorkton SK S3N 2K6; Staff, Yorkton Regional Health Centre; (306)786-0105; Fax. (306)786-0457.

KOYLE, Martin A; The Hosp for Sick Children, 555 University Ave, Toronto ON M5G 1X8; Man'76; Urol. Staff, The Hospital For Sick Children; (416)813-6581

KOZAK, Frederick K; Children's & Women's HC of BC, K2 184-4480 Oak St, Vancouver BC V6H 3V4; McM'85; MD; FRCSC; Otol (Pediatric Otolaryngology). Staff Ped Otol, BC Children's Hospital; Clin Assoc Prof Surg, University of British Columbia; (604)875-2113

KOZAK, Gregory N; Rockyview Gen Hosp, 6645-7007 14 St SW, Calgary AB T2V 1P9; Alb'91; FRCSC; Urol (Laparoscopy). Staff, Rockyview General Hospital; Staff, Foothills Medical Centre; (403)943-8987; Fax. (403)943-8990.

KOZAK, Joseph H; 305-3101 Bloor St W, Toronto ON M8X 2W2; Tor'73; BSc; CCFP; FCFP; Med Dir Occup Health Unit Ivan Nursing Home, West Park Healthcare Centre; Court Staff, Toronto Western Hospital - University Health Network; University of Toronto; Langs: Ukrainian; (416)231-9500; Fax. (416)231-4641; josephkozak@sympatico.ca.

KOZAK, Roman I; London X-Ray Associates, 104-450 Central Ave, London ON N6B 2E8; London (England)'78; MB BS; FRCPC; DiagRad (Interventional Radiology). Ac Staff, St Joseph's Hospital - St Joseph's Health Care; Ac Staff, Strathroy Middlesex General Hospital - Middlesex Hospital Alliance; Ac Staff, Tillsonburg District Memorial Hospital; Assoc Prof Radiol, University of Western Ontario; (519)672-5270

KOZAKAVICH, Ronald N; Herold Road Fam Physicians, 1-325 Herold Rd, Saskatoon SK S7V 1J7; Sask'71; LMCC; Ac Staff, St Paul's Hospital (Grey Nuns) of Saskatoon; Ac Staff, Saskatoon City Hospital; Ac Staff, Royal University Hospital; (306)374-2404

KOZAKIEWICZ, Richard; PO Box 1180, Onoway AB T0E 1V0; Wroclaw (Poland)'65.

KOZAN, James R; Bigelow Fowler Clinic West, 30 Jerry Potts Blvd W, Lethbridge AB T1K 5M5; Sask'87; BSc; MBA; CCFP; FCFP; (403)381-8444; Fax. (403)381-8166.

KOZANITIS, Chris D; CDK Family Medicine, 175 Princess St, Kingston ON K7L 1A9; Qns'06; CCFP; (613)766-0318

KOZAR, Walter J; The Ottawa Hosp-Gen Campus, 501 Smyth Rd, Ottawa ON K1H 8L6; Tor'91; CCFP; CCFP(E.M.); FCFP; Staff, The Ottawa Hospital - General Campus; (613)737-8899 x79002

KOZEL, Vitezslava V; Family Health Team, PO Box 1110 63 Fifth St, Englehart ON P0J 1H0; Karlova (Czech Republic)'79; Staff, Englehart & District Hospital Inc; Langs: Czech; Russian; Polish; (705)544-2321

KOZENKO, Mariya A; McMaster University, 3N 11F-1280 Main St W, Hamilton ON L8S 4K1; (Ukraine)'95; FRCPC; MedGenetics. (905)521-2100

KOZERAWSKI, G Margaret; 230-1560 Yonge St, Toronto ON M4T 2S9; Warsaw (Poland)'79; FRCPC; Psy. (416)944-9120

KOZERAWSKI, Waldemar J; 2240 Dixie Rd, Mississauga ON L4Y 1Z4; Warsaw (Poland)'79; (905)629-9414

KOZIAK, Steven J; 132 Parkdale Ave S, Hamilton ON L8K 3P3; McM'73; CCFP; FCFP; (905)547-8915; Fax. (905)547-3785.

KOZIAR, Mary L; Glazier Med Centre, 11 Gibb St, Oshawa ON L1H 2J9; Tor'74; CCFP; FCFP; (905)579-1212

KOZIARZ, Peter; 200 Meadowlark Shopping Ctr NW, Edmonton AB T5R 5W9; Ott'02; FRCPC; DiagRad. (780)489-8430

KOZIARZ, Piotr; 118-115 Maclean Pl, Welland ON L3B 5X9; Cal'93; MSc; BSc; FRCSC; GenSurg. Staff, Niagara Health System - Welland Hospital Site; Langs: English; French; Polish; (905)732-0121; Fax. (905)732-9783.

KOZIC, Jennifer R; 746 McLean St, Quesnel BC V2J 2P9; UBC'07; (604)682-2344 x66140

KOZIOL, Kathie A; 3-7865 Patterson Rd, Saanichton BC V8M 2C7; Alb'83; MSc; FRCPC; IntMed (Hepatology); Gastroent. Clinical Asst Prof, University of British Columbia; (250)652-7912; Fax. (250)652-7913; kkoziol@shaw.ca.

KOZLOVSKI, Christopher H; McLeod Medical Clinic, 229-100 Tabor Blvd, Prince George BC V2M 5T4; Monash (Australia)'92; MB BS; (250)562-5166

KOZLOWSKA, Marta D; PO Box 74018 Rpo Strathcona, Calgary AB T3H 3B6; Sydney (Australia)'07; CCFP; (403)404-0334

KOZLOWSKA, Urszula M; 425 Marlborough Way NE, Calgary AB T2A 7E7; (Poland)'74; CCFP; (403)272-6422; Fax. (403)272-4297.

KOZMA, David J; Queen Elizabeth Hosp, PO Box 6600 Stn Central, Charlottetown PE C1A 8T5; Mem'92; FRCPC; Anes. Staff, Queen Elizabeth Hospital; (902)894-2111

KOZMA, Stephanie A C; Med-Stop Heritage Plaza, B E-8330 Macleod Trail SE, Calgary AB T2H 2V2; Alb'72; BSc; CCFP; Assoc Prof Family Pract, University of Calgary; (403)258-3000; Fax. (403)258-0300; kozma@shaw.ca.

KOZMAN, Mervat N; May Fair Place, 303-6707 Elbow Dr SW, Calgary AB T2V 0E5; (Egypt)'90; MB BCh; MRCPsy(UK); FRCPC; Psy (Geriatric Psychiatry). Staff, Rockyview General Hospital; Langs: Arabic; (403)571-2480; Fax. (403)571-2499.

KOZMINSKI, Mary T; SCOHS-St Vincent Hospital, 60 Cambridge Ave N, Ottawa ON K1R 7A5; Tor'08; CCFP; Staff, Bruyère Continuing Care - Saint-Vincent Hospital; (613)233-4041

KOZODY, Raymond; Peter Lougheed Centre, 2230-3500 26 Ave NE, Calgary AB T1Y 6J4; Man'77; FRCPC; Anes. Staff, Peter Lougheed Centre; (403)943-5554

KOZORIZ, Kelsey D M; 101-777 Broadway W, Vancouver BC V5Z 4J7; UBC'08; CCFP; (604)734-8252

KOZOUSEK, Vladimir; Queen Elizabeth II HSC, 2035 2W-1276 South Park St, Halifax NS B3H 2Y9; Laval'80; MPH; FRCSC; Ophth. Staff Nova Scotia Eye Centre, Queen Elizabeth II Health Sciences Centre - Victoria General Site; Assoc Prof, Dalhousie University; (902)473-3473; Fax. (902)473-2839.

KOZROSKI, Clare J; PO Box 300, Gull Lake SK S0N 1A0; Wes'90; BSc; CCFP; (306)672-4034; Fax. (306)672-3464.

KOZYRA, Lesia M A; 2052 St. Joseph Blvd, Orleans ON K1C 1E6; Man'93; BSc; CCFP; CCFP(E.M.); Staff, The Ottawa Hospital - General Campus; Staff, Queensway Carleton Hospital; Staff, Carleton Place & District Memorial Hospital; (613)845-0084

KPOGO, Amos L; Pleasant Street Med Clinic, 6-250 Pleasant St, Miramichi NB E1V 1Y5; Geneva (Switzerland)'95; CCFP; Staff, Miramichi Regional Hospital; (506)836-0189

KRAAG, Gunnar R; The Ottawa Hosp-Riverside, 1967 Riverside Dr, Ottawa ON K1H 7W9; Qns'69; Rheum; IntMed. Staff Arthritis Centre, The Ottawa Hospital - Riverside Campus; Staff Div of Rheum, The Ottawa Hospital - Civic Campus; Staff, The Ottawa Hospital - General Campus; Prof Med, University of Ottawa; (613)738-8258; Fax. (613)738-8259; grkraag@toh.on.ca.

KRABBE, Marjorie E; 100-13009 Rosedale Ave PO Box 460, Summerland BC V0H 1Z0; California (USA)'94; CCFP; Langs: Bilingual(English/French); (250)404-4242

KRACKOVITCH, Stephanie; Centre Med Brunswick, 200-955 boul Saint-Jean, Pointe-Claire QC H9R 5K3; Cal'00; FRCSC; ObstGyn. Staff, Lakeshore General Hospital - Pointe Claire; (514)426-4966

KRAEKER, Christian B; Hamilton HS-Juravinski Site, A3 61-711 Concession St, Hamilton ON L8V 1C3; McM'06; FRCPC; IntMed. Staff, Hamilton Health Sciences Centre-Juravinski Site; Teach Staff, McMaster University; (905)389-4411

KRAEMER, Geoffrey T; St Thomas-Elgin Gen Hosp, PO Box 2007 Stn Main 189 Elm St, St Thomas ON N5R 5C4; Ott'03; BSc(Hon)Chemistry; CCFP; Staff, St Thomas Elgin General Hospital; (519)631-2020; gkraemermd@hotmail.com.

KRAEMER, James M; Caroline Family Hlth Team-CMG, 15-3305 Harvester Rd, Burlington ON L7N 3N2; McM'73; CCFP; FCFP; Staff, Joseph Brant Memorial Hospital; Clinical Asst Prof Family Med, McMaster University; Clinical Asst Prof Family Med, University of Toronto; (905)632-8007; Fax. (905)681-6341.

KRAEMER, William J; Medical & Dental Bldg, 604-586 Eglinton Ave E, Toronto ON M4P 1P2; Wes'89; FRCSC; OrthSurg (Spine). Ac Staff, Toronto East General Hospital Inc; Vis Staff, Sunnybrook Health Sciences Centre; Asst Prof, University of Toronto; (416)483-1444; Fax. (416)483-8856.

KRAFCHIK, Bernice R; 201-1466 Bathurst St, Toronto ON M5R 3S3; Cape Town (South Africa)'61; MB ChB; FRCPC; Derm (Pediatric Dermatology). Staff, St Joseph's Health Centre; Emeritus Prof Peds & Med, University of Toronto; (416)531-3331

KRAFT, Claudia S; Qikiqtani Gen Hosp, PO Box 1000, Iqaluit NU X0A 0H0; Qns'07; CCFP; Staff, Qikigtani General Hospital; (867)979-7343

KRAFT, John N; 210-5762 Highway 7, Markham ON L3P 1A8; Tor'06; FRCPC; Derm. (905)472-9950

KRAFT, Jouni P; Port Arthur Health Centre Inc, 194 Court St N, Thunder Bay ON P7A 4V7; Tor'76; Court Staff, Thunder Bay Regional Health Sciences Centre Port-Arthur; Langs: Finnish; (807)346-1000; Fax. (807)346-6206.

KRAFT, Scott W; Dept of Clinical Neurosciences, 3350 Hospital Dr NW, Calgary AB T2N 4Z5; Sask'97; FRCPC; Neur. (403)944-4364; Fax. (403)944-4063.

KRAFT, Stephen P; The Hosp For Sick Children, 555 University Ave, Toronto ON M5G 1X8; Tor'78; DABOphOphthSci; DOphthSci; FRCSC; Ophth (Strabismus). Staff Ophth, Toronto Western Hospital - University Health Network; Staff Ophth, The Hospital For Sick Children; Prof Med, University of Toronto; (416)813-6123; Fax. (416)813-5159; stephen.kraft@sickkids.ca.

KRAFTCHECK, Daniel J J; Family Med Centre, 102-155 James St S, Hamilton ON L8P 3A4; Qns'67; CCFP; FCFP; Sr Staff, St Joseph's Healthcare - Charlton Campus; Clin Assoc Prof, McMaster University; (905)528-8747; Fax. (905)528-9742.

KRAFTCHECK, Erin R; The U of Toronto-Mississauga, 3359 Mississauga Rd N, Mississauga ON L5L 1C6; McM'06; CCFP; Staff, St Joseph's Health Centre; (905)828-5255

KRAHN, Andrew D; Diamond Health Care Centre, 9173-2775 Laurel St, Vancouver BC V5Z 1M9; Man'88; FRCPC; IntMed (Arrhythmias); Cardiol. (604)875-5069

KRAHN, Corrie G; Richmond Health Science Ctre, 650-6091 Gilbert Rd, Richmond BC V7C 5L9; Man'87; BSc; FRCSC; Urol. (604)273-4320; Fax. (604)273-7599.

KRAHN, Curtis D N; Steinbach Family Med Centre, 10-333 Loewen Blvd, Steinbach MB R5G 0C3; Man'81; CCFP; FCFP; (204)326-3401; Fax. (204)326-3899.

KRAHN, James K H; Four Rivers Med Clinic, 647 Broadway, Winnipeg MB R3C 0X2; Man'82; CCFP; FCFP; Physician, Four Rivers Medical Clinic; Langs: German; (204)775-6226; Fax. (204)775-6446.

KRAHN, Marianne J; St Boniface Gen Hosp, 409 Tache Ave, Winnipeg MB R2H 2A6; Man'94; FRCPC; IntMed; MedOncol. Staff Oncol, St Boniface General Hospital; (204)237-2033; Fax. (204)237-6048; marianne.krahn@cancercare.mb.ca.

KRAHN, Murray D; Univ Hlth Network-The Toronto, EN14 207-200 Elizabeth St, Toronto ON M5G 2C4; Man'82; MSc(ClinEpidem); FRCPC; IntMed (Decision Analysis/Economic Evaluation). Staff Physician, Toronto General Hospital - UHN; Prof Med, University of Toronto; (416)978-6608; Fax. (416)595-5826; murray.krahn@theta.utoronto.ca.

KRAITBERG, Neil J; Queensway-Carleton Hosp, 3045 Baseline Rd, Nepean ON K2H 8P4; Man'90; FRCPC; Psy. Staff Psy, Queensway Carleton Hospital; (613)721-4700 x3991

KRAJBICH, Jana; South Calgary Med Clinic, 118-40 Sunpark Plaza SE, Calgary AB T2X 3X7; Tor'02; CCFP; Langs: Czech; Slovak; (403)254-4000; Fax. (403)254-1282.

KRAJDEN, Mel; BC Centre For Disease Control, 655 12th Ave W, Vancouver BC V5Z 4R4; McG'80; FRCPC; IntMed; MedMicrobiol; InfectDis. Prof Path & Lab Med, University of British Columbia; (604)707-2421; Fax. (604)707-2420; mel.krajden@bccdc.ca.

KRAJDEN, Selig; Springdale Prof Bldg, 508-2250 Bovaird Dr E, Brampton ON L6R 0W3; Wes'01; BSc; FRCSC; PlasSurg (Hand Surgery). Div Head Plastic Surg, William Osler Health System - Brampton Civic Hospital; Med Dir First Canadian Place, SpaMedica; Asst Prof, McMaster University; (905)453-1900; Fax. (905)453-0992; dr.krajden@doctor.com.

KRAJDEN, Sigmund; St Joseph's Health Centre, 30 The Queensway, Toronto ON M6R 1B5; McG'71; FRCPC; IntMed (Infectious Diseases); MedMicrobiol. Head Infectious Dis, St Joseph's Health Centre; Asst Prof Med & Med Microbiol, University of Toronto; (416)530-6268; Fax. (416)530-6590; krajds@stjoe.on.ca.

KRAJEWSKI, Adam; Humber River Reg Hosp-Finch, 2111 Finch Ave W, North York ON M3N 1N1; Warsaw (Poland)'79; PhD; ABIM; FRCPC; IntMed (Memory Disorders); GeriatricMed. Ac Staff, Humber River Regional Hospital - Finch Avenue Site; Ac Staff, Bridgepoint Health Centre; Langs: Polish; German; (416)747-3748; Fax. (416)747-3802.

KRAJEWSKI, Susan A; Renfrew Victoria Hosp, 499 Raglan St N, Renfrew ON K7V 1P6; Tor'05; FRCPC; GenSurg. Staff, Renfrew Victoria Hospital; (613)432-3135

KRAJINA, Vladimir P J; 203-3825 Sunset St, Burnaby BC V5G 1T4; Dal'75; (604)434-9515; Fax. (604)434-5984.

KRAJNY, Milos J; 470-5 Fairview Mall Dr, Toronto ON M2J 2Z1; Palacky (Czech Republic)'64; FRCPC; IntMed (Allergy & Immunology). Ac Staff, Rouge Valley Health System - Centenary Health Centre Site; Langs: Czech; Slovak; German; (416)499-2716; Fax. (416)499-1169.

KRAKE, Shelley M; Cardiac Wellness Institute, 2225 Macleod Trail SE, Calgary AB T2G 5B6; Cal'90; CCFP; FCFP; CCFP(E.M.); (403)571-6950

KRAKOFSKY, Sheldon L; 445 Hamilton Rd, London ON N5Z 1S2; Wes'76; Court Staff, St Joseph's Hospital - St Joseph's Health Care; Court Staff, London Health Sciences Centre - University Hospital; Court Staff, London Health Sciences Centre - Victoria Campus; (519)679-0131; Fax. (519)679-9514.

KRAKOWER, Sharlene B; 203-9123 Mary St, Chilliwack BC V2P 4H7; Wes'07; CCFP; Staff, Chilliwack General Hospital; (604)795-9161

KRAKOWSKY, Harry W; 710-2300 Yonge St, Toronto ON M4P 1E4; Tor'73; Ac Staff Family & CommunMed, Mount Sinai Hospital; (416)487-3427; Fax. (416)487-3428; hwkgb@aol.com.

KRALT, Douglas; Sturgeon Community Hosp, 201 Boudreau Rd, St. Albert AB T8N 6C4; Man'07; CCFP; CCFP(E.M.); Staff Emerg Med, Sturgeon Community Hospital; (780)418-8229; Fax. (780)418-7376.

KRAMARCHUK, Markijan W; Rehab & Wellness Centre, 7-77 Matheson Blvd E, Mississauga ON L4Z 2Y5; Tor'93; BSc; Dip SportMed; CCFP; Langs: Ukrainian; (905)712-3626; Fax. (905)712-4265.

KRAMER, Andreas H; Foothills Med Centre, 3134-1403 29 St NW, Calgary AB T2N 2T9; Man'97; Critical Care Medicine; IntMed. Staff, Foothills Medical Centre; Langs: German; (403)944-4749

KRAMER, Barry N; Peterborough Clinic, 302-26 Hospital Dr, Peterborough ON K9J 7C3; Wes'86; FRCSC; ObstGyn. Assoc Staff ObstGyn, Peterborough Regional Health Centre - Hospital Drive; (705)740-6882; Fax. (705)740-6891.

KRAMER, David; 320-301 Victoria St, Kamloops BC V2C 2A3; UBC'98; FRCSC; Otol. (250)374-1488

KRAMER, John; 41 CF Health Services Centre, CP 100 Succ Bureau-Chef, St-Jean-sur-Richel QC J0J 1R0; Mon'10; CCFP; (450)358-7099

KRAMER, Larry P; Brant Community HC-Brantford, 200 Terrace Hill St, Brantford ON N3R 1G9; Wes'73; Staff, The Brant Community Healthcare System - Brantford General Hospital Site; (519)752-7871

KRAMER, Matthias P A; St Boniface Gen Hosp, 409 Tache Ave, Winnipeg MB R2H 2A6; Man'94; FRCPC; IntMed. Staff, St Boniface General Hospital; (204)233-8563

KRAMER, Steven; Malvern Med Centre, 100-1333 Neilson Rd, Scarborough ON M1B 4Y9; Witwatersrand (South Africa)'81; MB BCh; BSc; Physician, Malvern Medical Centre; (416)291-7719; Fax. (416)287-3775.

KRAMER, Timothy A; 202-3330 Richter St, Kelowna BC V1W 4V5; Tor'82; DAB; FRCSC; Otol. Ac Staff, Kelowna General Hospital; Clin Instructor, University of British Columbia; (250)861-5578; Fax. (250)861-5979; takramer@telus.net.

KRAMPETZ, Ingrid K; Emo Community Health Service, PO Box 569, Emo ON P0W 1E0; Cal'95; PhD; (807)482-2323; Fax. (807)482-3089.

KRAMPL, Peter; Kootenay-Boundary Reg Hosp, 1200 Hospital Bench, Trail BC V1R 4M1; Tor'98; CCFP; CCFP(E.M.); Staff, Kootenay Boundary Regional Hospital; (250)368-3311

KRANE, Sam D; 309-2249 Carling Ave, Ottawa ON K2B 7E9; Ott'80; FRCPC; Psy. (613)236-3443

KRANEMANN, Christoph F; Lawrence Curlew Med Centre, 1260 Lawrence Ave E, North York ON M3A 1C4; Qns'90; FRCSC; Ophth (Refractive Surgery). Staff, St Michael's Hospital; Staff, The Scarborough Hospital - General Campus; Lecturer, University of Toronto; (416)289-4000; Fax. (416)289-2318; team@clearviewinstitute.com.

KRANENKA, Joan; 157A Minnesota Dr, Stephenville NL A2N 3Y3; Mem'91.

KRANJCEVIC, Joseph; Clinical Sciences Building, 8 120-152 University Campus NW, Edmonton AB T6G 2G3; Cal'97; CSPQ; FRCPC; Anes. (780)407-8861

KRANTZ, Roselynn A; Medical & Dental Bldg, 902-1849 Yonge St, Toronto ON M4S 1Y2; McM'91; (416)487-1060; Fax. (416)487-0137.

KRANZ, T Robert; Elaho Med Clinic, PO Box 10003 1337 Pemberton Ave, Squamish BC V8B 0R1; Poznan (Poland)'07.

KRASNIK, Catherine E; St Joseph's Healthcare, 50 Charlton Ave E, Hamilton ON L8N 4A6; McM'06; FRCPC; Psy. Staff, St Joseph's Healthcare - Charlton Campus; (905)572-1838

KRASNOPOLSKY, Marina; The Polyclinic, 5-4646 Dufferin St, North York ON M3H 5S4; New Jersey (USA)'02; Langs: Russian; (416)222-6160

KRASNY, Jiri L; Westmount Med Bldg, 637-5025 rue Sherbrooke O, Montreal QC H4A 1S9; Karlova (Czech Republic)'64; MSc(UBC); Rheum (P.Q.). assoc Médecin Rheum, McGill University Health Centre - Royal Victoria Hospital; Physician, Constance Lethbridge Rehabilitation Centre; adj Prof, McGill University; (514)488-7350; Fax. (514)488-8242.

KRASNY, Mark J; Hop Maisonneuve-Rosemont, 5415 boul de l'Assomption, Montreal QC H1T 2M4; McG'03; Derm. Staff, Hopital Maisonneuve-Rosemont; (450)466-5000

KRASOVEC, Barbara; Sexual Health Clinic, 101 17th St E, Owen Sound ON N4K 0A5; Tor'91; BSc; CCFP; (519)376-9420

KRASS, Melvin E; Niagara Med Group Fam Hlth Team, 65-4421 Queen St, Niagara Falls ON L2E 2L2; Man'70; PhD(Pharm); CCFP; FCFP; Ac Staff, Niagara Health System - Greater Niagara General Site; (905)356-2236; Fax. (905)356-2568; webmaster@niagaramedicalgroup.com.

KRASSIOUKOV, Andrei; Blusson-Spinal Cord Centre, 818 10th Ave W, Vancouver BC V5Z 1M9; Volgograd (Russia (Federation))'79; FRCPC; PhysMed&Rehab (Spinal Cord Injury). Staff, G F Strong Rehabilitation Centre; Assoc Prof Med, University of British Columbia; Langs: Russian; (604)875-4111 x69402

KRATKA, Lida; Carrefour Vanier Med Centre, 305-150 Montreal Rd, Vanier ON K1L 8H2; Ott'80; Physician Occupational Med Clinic, Royal Canadian Mounted Police; Langs: Czech; French; (613)744-4978; Fax. (613)744-2151.

KRATKY, Antonin; Highbury Med Clinic, 1345 Huron St, London ON N5V 2E3; Masaryk (Czech Republic)'60; Langs: Czech; (519)659-2331; Fax. (519)659-4617.

KRATKY, Vladimir; Hotel-Dieu Hosp, 262D-166 Brock St, Kingston ON K7L 5G2; Ott'82; FRCSC; Ophth (Oculo Plastic Surgery). Att Staff, Hotel-Dieu Hospital; Asst Prof Ophth, Queen's University; (613)544-3400

KRAUBNER, Davina; Vernon Jubilee Hosp, 2101 32 St, Vernon BC V1T 5L2; UBC'04; CCFP; CCFP(E.M.); Staff, Vernon Jubilee Hospital; (250)558-1200

KRAULIS, John E; Weeneebayko Gen Hosp, PO Box 34 19 Hospital Dr, Moose Factory ON P0L 1W0; Tor'73; FACS; DABS; FRCSC; GenSurg. Staff, Weeneebayko General Hospital; (705)658-4544

KRAUS, Daniel J; McGill U Mental Health Service, 3600 rue McTavish, Montreal QC H3A 1Y2; Rochester (USA)'72; FRCPC; Psy (Adult Psychiatry). Staff, Centre Hospitalier de Val d'Or; Langs: English; French; (514)938-6019; Fax. (514)398-5529.

KRAUS, Danielle; 240-315 boul Brunswick, Pointe-Claire QC H9R 5M7; McG'79; FRCSC; Ophth. Staff, Sir Mortimer B Davis Jewish General; Conférencier Med, McGill University; Langs: Bilingual(English/French); (514)694-2010; Fax. (514)694-0772; danielle.kraus@mcgill.ca.

KRAUS, Peter A; Hamilton HS-General Site, 403-237 Barton St E, Hamilton ON L8L 2X2; Johannesburg (South Africa)'81; FRCPC; IntMed (Critical Care Medicine). Chief Critical Care Med, Hamilton Health Sciences Centre - Hamilton General Hospital; (905)527-4322 x44051; Fax. (905)522-9782.

KRAUS, Peter J; Atrium Prof Bldg, SS 103 309-190 Cundles Rd E, Barrie ON L4M 4S5; Tor'71; FRCPC; Psy (Affective Disorders). (705)737-4641; peterj.kraus@sympatico.ca.

KRAUS, Steven J; Qikiqtani Gen Hosp, PO Box 1000, Iqaluit NU X0A 0H0; Qns'04; CCFP; (867)975-8600

KRAUS, Steven L; Cowichan Dist Hosp, 3045 Gibbins Rd, Duncan BC V9L 1E5; UBC'93; MSc; FRCPC; Anes. Staff, Cowichan District Hospital; (250)746-4141; Fax. (250)746-4247.

KRAUS DE CAMARGO, Olaf; McMaster University, HSC 3A-1280 Main St W, Hamilton ON L8S 4K1; Sao Paulo (Brazil)'89; FRCPC; Peds. Teach Staff, McMaster University; (905)521-2100

KRAUSE, Barbara E; PO Box 66 Stn Main, Edmonton AB T5J 2G9; Sask'77; FRCPC; RadOncol. Staff, Cross Cancer Institute; (780)436-6068

KRAUSE, Elizabeth; All Well Primary Care Centre, 1-2835 Mill Woods Rd NW, Edmonton AB T6K 4A9; Silesia (Poland)'68; Langs: Polish; (780)450-4550; Fax. (780)461-1985.

KRAUSE, Kevin L; Rockyview Gen Hosp, 7007 14 St SW, Calgary AB T2V 1P9; Cal'93; BSc; CCFP; CCFP(E.M.); Staff, Rockyview General Hospital; (403)943-3449; Fax. (403)943-3220.

KRAUSE, Richard A; St Thomas-Elgin Gen Hosp, PO Box 2007 Stn Main, St Thomas ON N5P 3W2; Wes'93; Staff, St Thomas Elgin General Hospital; (519)631-2020 x2063

KRAUSE, Vanessa S; Tom Baker Cancer Centre, 1331 29 St NW, Calgary AB T2N 4N2; Alb'00; BSc; FRCPC; IntMed; MedOncol. Staff Med, Tom Baker Cancer Centre; Clinical Asst Prof, University of Calgary; (403)521-3093; Fax. (403)283-1651.

KRAUSHAAR, Greg C; Radiology Associates Of Regina, 6-2727 Parliament Ave, Regina SK S4S 6X5; Sask'04; FRCPC; DiagRad. Staff, Radiology Associates of Regina; (306)352-7653; Fax. (306)522-4311.

KRAUSHAAR, Jacqueline; 2180 23rd Ave, Regina SK S4S 0A5; Sask'07; PhysMed&Rehab. (306)766-5402

KRAUSZ, R Michael; St Paul's Hospital, 620B-1081 Burrard St, Vancouver BC V6Z 1Y6; Hamburg (Germany)'84; FRCPC; Psy. Staff Ctr for Health Evaluation & Outcome Sciences, Providence Health Care - St Paul's Hospital; (604)806-9113

KRAUSZ, Samuel E; 505-1160 Burrard St, Vancouver BC V6Z 2E8; Wes'09; CCFP; (604)683-0206

KRAUT, Allen G; S108-750 Bannatyne Ave, Winnipeg MB R3E 0W2; Man'80; FRCPC; IntMed; OccupMed.

KRAVCHENKO, Olena; Airdrie Med Clinic, 10-620 1 Ave NW, Airdrie AB T4B 2R3; (Ukraine)'94; (403)948-6412; Fax. (403)948-6284.

KRAVCHENKO, Viktor; CSSS de la Haute-Gaspésie, 50 rue du Belvedere, Ste-Anne-des-Monts QC G4V 1X4; (Ukraine)'95; Staff, Centre Hospitalier des Monts; (418)763-2261

KRAVCIK, Stephen; The Ottawa Hosp-Gen Campus, LM 14-501 Smyth Rd, Ottawa ON K1H 8L6; McG'89; BSc; FRCPC; IntMed (HIV Infection). Staff Physician Div of General Med, The Ottawa Hospital - General Campus; Asst Prof, University of Ottawa; (613)737-8610; Fax. (613)737-8688; skravcik@ottawahospital.on.ca.

KRAVETZ, Arnold I; Medical Clinic Bldg, 112-89 Humber College Blvd, Etobicoke ON M9V 4B8; Tor'74; FRCSC; Ophth (Cataract). Staff, William Osler Health System - Etobicoke General Hospital; Staff, Trillium Health Centre - West Toronto; (416)746-1617; Fax. (416)746-1619.

KRAVIS, Marc M J; Halton HCS Corp-Oakville, 327 Reynolds St, Oakville ON L6J 3L7; Tor'88; FRCPC; DiagRad. Staff, Halton Healthcare Services Corporation - Oakville Site; (905)338-4601

KRAVITZ, Elliot; 401-1440 rue Sainte-Catherine, Montreal QC H3G 1R8; McG'76; ABIM; GeriatricMed; IntMed. adj Prof McGill Centre for Studies in Age & Aging, McGill University; (514)844-1000

KRAVITZ, Heidi; 200 Pleasant St, St. John's NL A1E 1L8; Mem'80; FRCSC; ObstGyn. (709)579-2464

KRAW, Nicholas M; Braithwaite & Assoc Eye Clinic, 250 Wincott Dr, Etobicoke ON M9R 2R5; Australia (Australia)'60; ABOph; Ophth. (416)241-1958; Fax. (416)241-4769.

KRAWCHUK, Margaret; Tsawwassen Fam Hlth Centre, 101-5461 12 Ave, Delta BC V4M 2B2; UBC'89; (604)943-3982; Fax. (604)943-8077.

KRAWCIW, Donald; 510-1230 Government St, Victoria BC V8W 3Y2; Alb'97; CCFP; (250)363-3566

KRAWCZUK, Daniel M; Medical Centre, 105-1122 Lasalle Blvd, Sudbury ON P3A 1Y4; Tor'87; CCFP; FCFP; (705)566-5151; Fax. (705)566-4981.

KRAWCZYK, Jan W; Whitney Med Centre, PO Box 280 1 Medical Centre St, Whitney ON K0J 2M0; Cracov (Poland)'80; CCFP; FCFP; (613)637-2170

KRAWCZYK, John G; St Martha's Reg Hosp, 3F-25 Bay St, Antigonish NS B2G 2G5; Warsaw (Poland)'85; Staff Child Youth Family Program, St Martha's Regional Hospital; (902)867-4500; Fax. (902)867-4761.

KRAWETZ, Michael; 1033 River St PO Box 228, Bala ON P0C 1A0; Wes'57; Court Staff, South Muskoka Memorial Hospital - Muskoka Algonquin Healthcare; Langs: Ukrainian; Polish; (705)762-3210; Fax. (705)762-1549.

KRAYACICH, Nicholas C; Lasalle Community Health Care, 2125 Front Rd, Windsor ON N9J 2C1; Tor'89; Staff, Windsor Regional Hospital - Metropolitan Site; Staff, Hôtel-Dieu Grace Hospital; (519)734-8790

KRCEK, Jerry P; Health Sciences Centre, GB103-820 Sherbrook St, Winnipeg MB R3A 1R9; Cal'86; PhD(Med Sci); FRCSC; Neursurg. Att Staff, Health Sciences Centre; Assoc Prof, University of Manitoba; (204)787-7267; Fax. (204)787-3851.

KREADEN, David A; Keele-Ingram Prof Centre, 203-2221 Keele St, North York ON M6M 3Z5; Tor'73; FRCPC; IntMed (Gastroenterology). Staff, Humber River Regional Hospital - Finch Avenue Site; (416)240-8616

KREBES, Andrew J; Rideau Med & Dental Centre, 1-1711 4 St SW, Calgary AB T2S 1V8; Alb'59; FRCSC; Ophth. (403)228-5235; Fax. (403)228-4481.

KREDENTSER, Jeremy V; Heartland Fertility & Gyne Cli, 701-1661 Portage Ave, Winnipeg MB R3J 3T7; Alb'77; ABOG(ReproEndocrin); FRCSC; ObstGyn (Reproductive Endocrinology & Infertility). Ac Staff, Health Sciences Centre; Ac Staff, The Salvation Army Grace Hospital; Assoc Prof ObstGyn, University of Manitoba; (204)779-8888; Fax. (204)779-8877.

KREDENTSER, Sarah E; Kildonan Med Centre, 2300 McPhillips St, Winnipeg MB R2V 3M3; Alb'80; CCFP; FCFP; Staff, Seven Oaks General Hospital; (204)632-3203; Fax. (204)694-5697.

KREDER, Hans J; Sunnybrook Hlth Sciences Ctre, MG 365-2075 Bayview Ave, Toronto ON M4N 3M5; Tor'85; MPH; FRCSC; OrthSurg (Arthroplasty). Staff, Sunnybrook Health Sciences Centre; Asst Prof, University of Toronto; Langs: German; (416)480-6816; Fax. (416)480-5886.

KREDER, Marion R; Rexdale Med Centre, 2-123 Rexdale Blvd, Etobicoke ON M9W 1P1; Tor'85; CCFP; FCFP; Ac Staff, William Osler Health System - Etobicoke General Hospital; (416)743-5853; Fax. (416)743-1358.

KREICHMAN, Daniel; 100-36 York Mills Rd, North York ON M2P 2E9; Tor'02; FRCSC; ObstGyn (Urogynecology). Staff, North York General Hospital; Lecturer, University of Toronto; (416)644-1404

KREIDSTEIN, Michael L; Cosmetic Plastic Surg Clinic, 211-300 York Mills Rd, Toronto ON M2L 2Y5; Tor'87; MSc; FRCS; FRCSC; PlasSurg (Cosmetic Surgery). Ac Staff Plastic Surg, The Scarborough Hospital - General Campus; (416)391-4452; Fax. (416)391-3031; drkreidstein@bellnet.ca.

KREIDSTEIN, Sharon H; Oakdale Med Bldg, 104-2065 Finch Ave W, North York ON M3N 2V7; Tor'90; FRCPC; IntMed; Rheum. Court Staff, Humber River Regional Hospital - Finch Avenue Site; Langs: Italian; (416)743-6372; Fax. (416)741-2276; skreidstein@yahoo.ca.

KREINDLER, David; Sunnybrook Hlth Sciences Ctre, FG 53-2075 Bayview Ave, Toronto ON M4N 3M5; Cincinnati(Ohio) (USA)'95; BSc; FRCPC; Psy (Child & Adolescent Psychiatry). Staff Physician & Interim Head Div of Youth Psy, Sunnybrook Health Sciences Centre; Asst Prof Psy, University of Toronto; (416)480-5225; Fax. (416)480-6818.

KREINDLER, Simon; 206 St Clair Ave W, Toronto ON M4V 1R2; McG'65; FRCPC; Psy (Child Psychiatry). (416)920-5546

KREISMAN, Stuart H; Burrard Health Bldg, 301-1160 Burrard St, Vancouver BC V6Z 2E8; McG'92; IntMed (Endocrinology & Metabolism). Staff Endocrin, Providence Health Care - St Paul's Hospital; Langs: English; French; (604)681-3501; Fax. (604)681-4508.

KRELINA, Michael; 301-117 Murray St, Ottawa ON K1N 5M5; Ott'78; DABPN; FRCPC; Neur; Psy. Staff, Royal Ottawa Mental Health Centre - Royal Ottawa Health Care Group; Asst Prof, University of Ottawa; (613)562-1972; Fax. (613)562-1973; michael.krelina@sympatico.ca.

KREMA, Muhammed H A A; Univ Hlth Network-Princess M, 18 606-610 University Ave, Toronto ON M5G 2M9; Cairo (Egypt)'89; Staff, Princess Margaret Hospital - University Health Network; (416)946-2000 x5524

KREMENCHUTZKY, C Marcelo M; London HSC-University Hosp, PO Box 5339 Stn B 339 Windermere Rd, London ON N6A 5A5; Buenos Aires (Argentina)'88; FRCPC; Neur. Staff/Assoc Prof Neurol, London Health Sciences Centre - University Hospital; Langs: Spanish; (519)663-3121; Fax. (519)663-3744; marc6363@hotmail.com.

KREMENIK, Terri L; Haig Clinic, 601 6 Ave S, Lethbridge AB T1J 0Z2; Cal'00; CCFP; (403)328-6641; Fax. (403)328-6118.

KREMER, Bernardo; SMBD Jewish Gen Hosp, 3755 ch Cote-Sainte-Catherine, Montreal QC H3T 1E2; (Other Foreign)'92; CCFP; Staff, Sir Mortimer B Davis Jewish General; (514)340-8222

KREMER, Richard B; MUHC-Royal Victoria Hosp, H4 61-687 av des Pins O, Montreal QC H3A 1A1; Paris (France)'77; FRCPC; MedBiochem (Endocrinology). principale Médecin, McGill University Health Centre - Royal Victoria Hospital; Membre Experimental Med, Boehringer-Engelheim Resch Cda; Consultant, MRC & DSL(Webster-TX); Prof Med, McGill University; Langs: English; French; (514)934-1934 x31632; richard.kremer@mcgill.ca.

KREMER, Sidney G J; Meadowvale Prof Centre, 220-6855 Meadowvale Town Ctre, Mississauga ON L5N 2Y1; Tor'93; BSc; MSc; FACP; FRCPC; IntMed; Cardiol. Staff Cardiol, The Credit Valley Hospital; (905)858-4883; Fax. (905)858-4839.

KREMER, Steven; Selkirk Mental Health Centre, PO Box 9600 Stn Main, Selkirk MB R1A 2B5; Man'94; FRCPC; Psy. Staff Psy, Selkirk Mental Health Centre; (204)482-3810

KREML, John A; Parkview Prof Centre, 203-2110 Main St, Winnipeg MB R2V 2C2; Man'78; (204)338-9349; Fax. (204)339-7260.

KREML, Marian J; Valley Med Imaging, 102-32475 Simon Ave, Abbotsford BC V2T 5E3; Man'82; FRCPC; DiagRad. (604)855-0112

KREML, Renee; Health Sciences Centre, 820 Sherbrook St, Winnipeg MB R3A 1R9; Man'05; FRCPC; DiagRad. Staff, Health Sciences Centre; (204)774-8511

KREPINSKY, Joan C; St Joseph's Healthcare, T3311-50 Charlton Ave E, Hamilton ON L8N 4A6; McM'96; FRCPC; IntMed; Nephrol. Staff, St Joseph's Healthcare - Charlton Campus; (905)522-1155 x34991; Fax. (905)540-6589.

KREPTUL, Dennis W; Sheldon Chumuik Centre, 8F-1213 4 St SW, Calgary AB T2R 0X7; Alb'70; CCFP; FCFP; (403)955-9300

KRESAN, Patricia J; Sudbury Med Centre, 402-65 Larch St, Sudbury ON P3E 1B8; McM'83; (705)670-8911

KRESS, Stephan G; Concordia Gen Hosp, 1095 Concordia Ave, Winnipeg MB R2K 3S8; Man'02; BSc; CCFP; CCFP(E.M.); Staff, Concordia General Hospital; Staff, Misericordia Health Centre; (204)667-1560

KRESTOW, Martin; Burnaby Hosp, 3935 Kincaid St, Burnaby BC V5G 2X6; Wes'97; Anes. Staff, Burnaby Hospital; (604)434-4211

KRESTOW, Michael; Burnaby Hosp, 3935 Kincaid St, Burnaby BC V5G 2X6; Heidelberg (Germany)'60; FRCPC; Anes. Staff, Burnaby Hospital; (604)412-6311

KRETE, Derek M; Peterborough Reg HC-Hospital, 1 Hospital Dr, Peterborough ON K9J 7C6; Medical University of the Americas (Other Foreign)'04; FRCPC; PhysMed&Rehab (Sports Medicine). Staff, Peterborough Regional Health Centre - Hospital Drive; (705)740-8351; dkrete@ptboclinic.com.

KRETSCHMANN, Richard J; Canadian Forces Base, PO Box 10500 Stn Forces 1 Field Ambulance, Edmonton AB T5J 4J5; UBC'07; CCFP; (780)973-4011

KRETZ, Patrice; Centre Med Fontainebleau, 102-10 boul des Chateaux, Blainville QC J7B 1Z5; McG'84; ac Staff Med, Centre Hospitalier Laurentien; (450)419-8811; Fax. (450)419-7758.

KRETZUL, Eugene M; Meadowlark Health Centre, 224 Meadowlark Shopping Ctr NW, Edmonton AB T5R 5W9; Alb'73; FRCPC; IntMed (Hypertension). Ac Staff, Royal Alexandra Hospital; Clin Prof, University of Alberta; (780)484-8474; Fax. (780)489-3836.

KREUTZER, Donovan R A; 204-2031 33 Ave SW, Calgary AB T2T 1Z5; Pretoria (South Africa)'97; MB ChB; (403)685-4520; Fax. (403)685-4525.

KREVIAZUK, Jessica L; Access River East, 975 Henderson Hwy, Winnipeg MB R2K 2M2; Man'04; FRCPC; Psy. Staff, St Boniface General Hospital.

KRIBS, Stewart W; London HSC-Victoria Hosp, PO Box 5010 Stn B 800 Commissioners Rd E, London ON N6A 5W9; Wes'89; FRCPC; DiagRad. Staff Radiol, London Health Sciences Centre - Victoria Campus; University of Western Ontario; (519)685-8300 x54965; Fax. (519)667-6771.

KRIEF, Olivier; CSSS de Laval, 1755 boul Rene-Laennec, Laval QC H7M 3L9; (France)'90; FRCPC; DiagRad. Staff, Hopital de la Cite de la santé; (450)668-1010

KRIEGEL PEREZ, Graciela Ruth R; Ontario Shores Ctr Mental HS, 700 Gordon St, Whitby ON L1N 5S9; Buenos Aires (Argentina)'85; FRCPC; Psy. (905)430-4055

KRIEGER, Charles; G F Strong Rehabilitation Ctr, 4255 Laurel St, Vancouver BC V5Z 2G9; Tor'78; MSc; PhD; FRCPC; Neur. Staff, G F Strong Rehabilitation Centre; (604)737-6320

KRIEGER, Henry; SGH Medical Mall, 318-3030 Lawrence Ave E, Scarborough ON M1P 2T7; Tor'70; FRCPC; IntMed (Medical Oncology); Hem. Staff, The Scarborough Hospital - General Campus; Staff, Sunnybrook Health Sciences Centre; University of Toronto; (416)289-2166; Fax. (416)289-2168.

KRIEGER, Howard M; 200-11 Ferris Lane, Barrie ON L4M 5N6; Tor'71; Assoc Staff, Royal Victoria Regional Health Centre; University of Toronto; (705)739-8667; Fax. (705)739-9341.

KRIEGER, Mark; 206-726 Bloor St W, Toronto ON M6G 4A1; Tor'76; Ac Staff, Toronto General Hospital - UHN; Ac Staff, West Park Healthcare Centre; Ac Staff, Humber River Regional Hospital - Church Street Site; Langs: Spanish; French; (416)516-5244; Fax. (416)516-3552.

KRIEGER, Michael P; PO Box 19, Malahat BC V0R 2L0; New York (USA)'68.

KRIEGLER, Johann C; Mediclinic, 101-3301 8th St E, Saskatoon SK S7H 5K5; Witwatersrand (South Africa)'83; MB ChB; (306)955-1530; Fax. (306)955-8811.

KRIEGLER, Stefan G; St Joseph's Gen Hosp, 2137 Comox Ave, Comox BC V9M 1P2; Stellenbosch (South Africa)'93; FRCPC; DiagRad. Staff, St Joseph's General Hospital; (250)890-3024

KRIEK, Gileam J; Riverheights Med Clinic, 2734 Montague St, Regina SK S4S 0J9; Pretoria (South Africa)'84; MB ChB; (306)584-3344

KRIEL, Adriaan P; Southridge Prof Centre, 5-1224 Strachan Rd SE, Medicine Hat AB T1B 4R2; Pretoria (South Africa)'89; MB ChB; CAFCI; CCFP; FCFP; Staff, Medicine Hat Regional Hospital; (403)580-3888; Fax. (403)504-1220; apkriel@krielcorp.com.

KRIEL, Johannes N; South Hill Med Centre, 5-2685 2nd Ave W, Prince Albert SK S6V 5E3; Pretoria (South Africa)'88; MB ChB; CCFP; FCFP; (306)922-9570; Fax. (306)922-2513.

KRIEL, Wessel J C; Mayfair Place, 236-6707 Elbow Dr SW, Calgary AB T2V 0E4; Pretoria (South Africa)'96; MB ChB; (403)259-3357

KRIEVINS, Matthew C; North York Gen Hosp, 1NE 126-4001 Leslie St, North York ON M2K 1E1; Qns'05; CCFP; CCFP(E.M.); Staff, North York General Hospital; (416)756-6165

KRIGSTEIN, Esther S; 55 Belmont St, Toronto ON M5R 1R1; Tor'73.

KRIIK, Vivian H; Care Point Med Centre, 528A Clarke Rd, Coquitlam BC V3J 3X5; UBC'82; (604)936-9874; Fax. (604)936-9741.

KRIKLER, Samuel H; Surrey Mem Hosp, 13750 96 Ave, Surrey BC V3V 1Z2; Rhodesia (Zimbabwe)'79; MB ChB; FRCPC; HemPath. Staff, Surrey Memorial Hospital; Asst Prof Path, University of British Columbia; (604)585-5666 x2580; Fax. (604)588-3322; sam.krikler@fraserhealth.ca.

KRIMLY, Ahmed M S; 4N 483-585 University Ave, Toronto ON M5G 2N2; King Abdul Aziz U (Saudi Arabia)'01; Cardiol; IntMed.

KRINGS, Timo; Univ Hlth Network-Toronto Western Hosp, 3MCL 429-399 Bathurst St, Toronto ON M5T 2S8; Rhenish-Westphalian (Germany)'98; FRCPC; DiagRad. Staff, Toronto Western Hospital - University Health Network; (416)603-5800 x5562

KRINKE, Valerie; MOMCare Docs, 10155 120 St NW, Edmonton AB T5K 2A2; Alb'89; CCFP; (780)482-7551

KRISDAPHONGS, Michoke; Conception Bay Med Clinic, 119-120 Conception Bay Hwy, Conception Bay S NL A1W 3A6; Shansi (China)'56; Fax. (709)834-3101; mkrisdaphongs@hotmail.com.

KRISHAN, Vivek T; Dr Vivek Tony Krishan, 110-13588 88 Ave, Surrey BC V3W 3K8; Sask'90; (604)594-4954; Fax. (604)572-3560.

KRISHANTHA, Mahadeva; Finch-Warden Med Walk-In Clin, 6A-3430 Finch Ave E, Scarborough ON M1W 2R5; (Latvia)'01; (416)496-1990

KRISHNA, Popuri M; Northeast Mental Hlth Centre, 680 Kirkwood Dr, Sudbury ON P3E 1X3; Kurnool (India)'80; Staff, North Bay Regional Health Centre - Kirkwood; (705)675-9192

KRISHNALINGAM, Chinniah; Mackenzie Richmond Hill Hosp, 10 Trench St, Richmond Hill ON L4C 4Z3; Ceylon (Sri Lanka)'75; FRCPC; Psy. Staff Mental Health Clinic, Mackenzie Richmond Hill Hospital; (905)832-1406 x2208; Fax. (905)737-5152; ckrishnalingam@yorkcentral.on.ca.

KRISHNAMOORTHY, Preetha; MUHC-Montreal Children's Hosp, E315-2300 rue Tupper, Montreal QC H3H 1P3; McG'96; FRCPC; Peds; Endocrin (P.Q.); Endocrin&Metab. Staff, McGill University Health Centre - Montreal Children's Hospital; Langs: English; French; (514)412-4400; preetha.krishnamoorthy@muhc.mcgill.ca.

KRISHNAMURTHY, Ashok B; St James Town Health Centre, 410 Sherbourne St, Toronto ON M4X 1K2; McG'03; CCFP; (416)864-3096

KRISHNAN, Mukta M; The Royal Victoria Hosp, 201 Georgian Dr, Barrie ON L4M 6M2; Nagpur (India)'89; FRCPC; IntMed. Staff IntMed, Royal Victoria Regional Health Centre; (705)739-5661; Fax. (705)739-5619.

KRISHNAN, Murali; Royal Court Med Centre, 205-1 Quarry Ridge Rd, Barrie ON L4M 7G1; Nagpur (India)'89; MB BS; FRCPC; IntMed (Nephrology). Ac Staff, Royal Victoria Regional Health Centre; Langs: Hindi; (705)728-1962; Fax. (705)728-9455.

KRISHNAN, Narayanan; Lindsay Prof Bldg, 12-65 Angeline St N, Lindsay ON K9V 5N7; Madras (India)'81; MB BS; FRCPC; IntMed (Cardiology). Staff, Ross Memorial Hospital; Langs: Tamil; (705)878-5337; Fax. (705)878-9798; krish@bellnet.ca.

KRISHNAN, Rajesh; Northumberland Hills Hosp, 1000 Depalma Dr, Cobourg ON K9A 5W6; Madras (India)'88; FRCPC; IntMed. Staff, Northumberland Hills Hospital; (905)372-6811; Fax. (905)373-6933.

KRISHNAN, Usha; Royal Court Medical Centre, 308-5 Quarry Ridge Rd, Barrie ON L4M 7G1; Madras (India)'81; FRCPC; IntMed. (705)797-1475

KRISHNAN, Venkataraman S G; Millbrook Mall, 304-2 Herald Ave, Corner Brook NL A2H 4B5; Madras (India)'79; MB BS; FRCPC; IntMed. Staff, Western Memorial Regional Hospital.

KRISHNAPRASAD, Degala V; Appletree Med Centre, 225 Preston St, Ottawa ON K1R 7R1; Andhra (India)'74; FRCPC; Psy. Staff, Waypoint Centre for Mental Health Care; (613)288-0279

KRISHNAR, Kannan; Bronte Health Clinic, 78 Jones St, Oakville ON L6L 6C5; Tor'95; CCFP; (905)827-9865; Fax. (905)827-3583.

KRISHNASWAMY, Ramaiyer; Fredericton Med Clinic, 403-1015 Regent St, Fredericton NB E3B 6H5; Mysore (India)'77; MB BS; FAAP(Peds); FAAP(Neonatology); FRCPC; Peds (Neonatology). Staff, Dr Everett Chalmers Regional Hospital; Hon. Teach. Staff, Dalhousie University; Langs: Hindi; Tamil; Malayalam; (506)458-0306; Fax. (506)458-0474.

KRISMAN, Avery A; 202-96 Harbord St, Toronto ON M5S 1G6; UBC'87; FRCPC; Psy. Staff Pt-Time, Toronto General Hospital - UHN; (416)966-9256

KRISTENSEN, John W; PO Box 298, Whaletown BC V0P 1Z0; Tor'73; CCFP.

KRISTJANSON, David N; Hamiota Dist Health Centre, 177 Birch Ave, Hamiota MB R0M 0T0; Man'90; CCFP; FCFP; Staff, Hamiota District Health Centre; Lecturer Family Med, University of Manitoba; (204)764-4218; Fax. (204)764-2325; dkristjanson@arha.ca.

KRISTJANSON, Mark R; Kildonan Med Centre, 2300 McPhillips St, Winnipeg MB R2V 3M3; Man'85; CCFP; (204)632-3203

KRISTOF, Arnold S; MUHC-Royal Victoria Hosp, L3 05-687 av des Pins O, Montreal QC H3A 1A1; McG'92; FRCPC; IntMed; Critical Care Medicine (P.Q.); Respir. Staff, McGill University Health Centre - Royal Victoria Hospital; (514)843-1664; Fax. (514)843-1686; arnold.kristof@muhc.mcgill.ca.

KRISTOF, Lorand; Wise Elephant Fam Health Team, 280 Main St S, Brampton ON L6V 1P6; (Romania)'01; (905)216-1065

KRISTOFFERSEN, Arthur N; 110 Crown St, Saint John NB E2L 2X7; Dal'76; Ac Staff, Saint John Regional Hospital; Ac Staff, St Joseph's Hospital; (506)634-6653; Fax. (506)634-1136.

KRITZINGER, Irma E; Bonnyville Health Centre, PO Bag 1008 Stn Main, Bonnyville AB T9N 2J7; (South Africa)'87; MB ChB; Staff, Bonnyville Healthcare Centre; (780)826-8271; Fax. (780)826-6530.

KRITZINGER, Johan F; 1025 103 Ave, Dawson Creek BC V1G 2G6; Stellenbosch (South Africa)'74; MB ChB; Langs: Afrikaans; (250)782-1186; Fax. (250)782-9447.

KRITZINGER, Johan J; Red Deer Reg Hosp Centre, PO Box 5030 Stn Postal Box Ctr 3942 50A Ave, Red Deer AB T4N 4E7; Pretoria (South Africa)'87; MB ChB; CCFP; CCFP(E.M.); Staff, Red Deer Regional Hospital Centre; (403)343-4444; Fax. (403)346-2205.

KRITZINGER, Philip M; York Vein & Laser Clinic, 647 Davis Dr, Newmarket ON L3Y 2R2; Cal'82; MD; BSc; CCFP; (905)853-3200; Fax. (905)853-7233; info@yorkvein.com.

KRIVY, Joel L; U of Toronto-Health Services, 214 College St, Toronto ON M5T 2Z9; Tor'82; Assoc Staff, Mackenzie Richmond Hill Hospital; (416)978-8034; Fax. (416)971-2089.

KRIZ, Robert P; Lakeridge Hlth Corp-Oshawa, 1 Hospital Crt, Oshawa ON L1G 2B9; Ott'05; FRCPC; Anes. Staff, Lakeridge Health - Oshawa Site; (905)576-8711

KRIZAJ-KAPLJIC, Davorka; 2290 Mississauga Rd, Mississauga ON L5H 2L1; Zagreb (Croatia)'82; Staff, The Credit Valley Hospital; (905)278-6737

KRIZAN, Igor; The Goodhouse Bldg, 312-93 West St, Corner Brook NL A2H 2Y6; Komensky (Slovakia)'68; Staff, Western Memorial Regional Hospital; Langs: Slovak; (709)634-8843

KRIZMANICH, William J; Hamilton HS-General Site, 237 Barton St E, Hamilton ON L8L 2X2; McM'90; CCFP; CCFP(E.M.); Staff, Hamilton Health Sciences Centre - Hamilton General Hospital; (905)527-4322 x6368

KROACH, Murray N; Medical Office, 208-840 Coxwell Ave, Toronto ON M4C 5T2; Tor'65; BSc(Med); FSOGC; FRCSC; ObstGyn (Infertility). Dir Life IVF Prog & IVF Canada Private Infertility Unit/Consultant ObstGyn, Toronto East General Hospital Inc; Asst Prof ObstGyn/Teach Staff, University of Toronto; (416)425-0112; Fax. (416)425-0229.

KROCHAK, Carla A M; Midtown Med Centre, 301-39 23rd St E, Saskatoon SK S7K 0H6; Sask'84; FRCPC; Peds. Ac Staff, Royal University Hospital; Asst Prof, University of Saskatchewan; (306)653-7741; Fax. (306)653-7743.

KROCZAK, Tadeusz J; Parkview Professional Centre, 102-2110 Main St, Winnipeg MB R2V 2C2; Cracow (Poland)'81; Langs: Polish; (204)633-7281; Fax. (204)694-0553.

KROEKER, Garth D; UBC Hospital, M334-2211 Wesbrook Mall, Vancouver BC V6T 2B5; Man'95; BSc(Med.); FRCPC; Psy. Staff, UBC Hospital - Koerner Pavillion; (604)822-7689; Fax. (604)822-7889.

KROEKER, Joel S; Keewatin Med Clinic, PO Box 847 904 Ottawa St, Keewatin ON P0X 1C0; Man'00; CCFP; (807)547-2818; Fax. (807)547-3285.

KROEKER, Karen I; Zeidler Ledcor Centre, 130 University Campus NW, Edmonton AB T6G 2X8; Cal'04; FRCPC; IntMed; Gastroent. (780)248-1433

KROEKER, L Robert; Medical Arts Bldg, 1405-233 Kennedy St, Winnipeg MB R3C 3J5; Man'80; FRCPC; IntMed (Cardiology). Ac Staff, Health Sciences Centre; Teach Staff Section of Cardiol, University of Manitoba; (204)947-2904; Fax. (204)943-3996; dr.bob@mts.net.

KROEKER, Leanne C M; Sunpark Prof Centre, 326-40 Sunpark Plaza SE, Calgary AB T2X 3X7; Cal'92; BSc; CCFP; Staff, Foothills Medical Centre; (403)278-1997; Fax. (403)278-2052.

KROEKER, Stanley G; Westland Fam Practice Clinic, 144-70 Mcleod Ave, Spruce Grove AB T7X 3C7; Alb'87; CCFP; FCFP; Med Staff, Covenant Health - Misericordia Community Hospital; (780)962-9393; Fax. (780)962-4295.

KROETSCH, Michael D; 204-2004 14 St NW, Calgary AB T2M 3N3; Alb'01; CCFP; (403)282-8200

KROEZE, Jan; 202-45425 Luckakuck Way, Chilliwack BC V2R 2T7; Pretoria (South Africa)'86; MB ChB; BMedSci; Langs: Afrikaans; (604)858-9461

KROFT, Cara D L; C200-123 Doncaster St, Winnipeg MB R3N 2B2; Man'87; FRCPC; Psy. (204)477-7442; Fax. (204)477-7450.

KROFT, Jamie; Sunnybrook Hlth Sciences Ctre, C703-2075 Bayview Ave, Toronto ON M4N 3M5; Tor'05; FRCSC; ObstGyn. Staff, Sunnybrook Health Sciences Centre; (416)480-6100

KROL-LASS, Justyna; Cumberland Health Authority, 34 Prince Arthur St, Amherst NS B4H 1V6; Silesian (Czech Republic)'86.

KROL-SZPAKOWSKI, Margaret; 255 Main St W, Hamilton ON L8P 1J5; Krakow (Poland)'84; Court Staff, St Joseph's Healthcare - Charlton Campus; (905)523-7944; Fax. (905)523-1597.

KROLL, Edward S; Lions Gate Hosp, 231 15th St E, North Vancouver BC V7L 2L7; Alb'78; Staff, Lions Gate Hospital; (604)988-3131

KROLL, Ian T; PO Box 20172 Rpo Bow Valley, Calgary AB T2P 4L2; Man'91; DABPN; FRCPC; Psy. Clin Lecturer, University of Calgary; Langs: German; (403)294-0948

KROLL, Michael M; Credit Valley Family Hlth Team, 105-2300 Eglinton Ave W, Mississauga ON L5M 2V8; Wes'81; CCFP; CCFP(E.M.); FCFP; Staff, The Credit Valley Hospital; Asst Prof, University of Toronto; (905)813-3850

KRONBERG, Jean E; Women's College Hosp, 76 Grenville St, Toronto ON M5S 1B2; Qns'80; FRCPC; Anes (Ambulatory Anesthesia). Assoc Prof, University of Toronto; (416)323-6269; Fax. (416)323-2666.

KRONBY, Michael H; Charlton Med Centre, 802-25 Charlton Ave E, Hamilton ON L8N 1Y2; McM'74; FRCPC; Neur. Staff, Hamilton Health Sciences Centre - McMaster University Medical Centre; Staff, Hamilton Health Sciences Centre - Hamilton General Hospital; Staff, Hamilton Health Sciences Centre-Juravinski Site; Staff, Hamilton Health Sciences Centre - McMaster Children's Hospital; Ac Staff, St Joseph's Healthcare - Charlton Campus; Asst Prof, McMaster University; (905)522-5401; Fax. (905)522-5550.

KRONENWALD, Alexander; 52 King St E, Dundas ON L9H 1B8; McM'78; Staff, Hamilton Health Sciences Centre - McMaster Children's Hospital; (905)627-1661; Fax. (905)627-1178.

KRONFLI, Risk; East Coast Forensic Psy Hosp, 88 Gloria Mccluskey Ave, Dartmouth NS B3B 2B8; Ain Shams (Egypt)'83; MB; FRCPC; Psy (Addiction Psychiatry). Chief Psy MIOUOffender Mental Hlth, The East Coast Forensic Psychiatry Hospital; Staff/Team Leader, Correction Mental Health Clinic; Asst Prof Psy, Dalhousie University; Langs: Arabic; French; (902)835-8993; Fax. (902)835-0981; risk.kronfli@cdha.nshealth.ca.

KRONGOLD, Israel J; Medical Arts Bldg, 202-233 Kennedy St, Winnipeg MB R3C 3J5; Ott'71; FRCPC; DiagRad. Ac Staff/Head Imaging Serv, Victoria General Hospital.

KRONGOLD, Penina H; Salvation Army Grace Hosp, 300 Booth Dr, Winnipeg MB R3J 3M7; McM'02; FRCPC; IntMed; Gastroent. Staff, The Salvation Army Grace Hospital; (204)837-0391

KRONICK, Jonathan B; The Hosp for Sick Children, 555 University Ave, Toronto ON M5G 1X8; McM'78; PhD; AB(Critical Care); FRCPC; Peds (Metabolic Genetics). Staff, The Hospital For Sick Children; (416)813-1500

KRONICK, Stanley H; Appletree Medical Group, 225 Preston St, Ottawa ON K1R 7R1; McG'70; FRCPC; IntMed. Staff IntMed & Respirol, Queensway Carleton Hospital; (613)288-2437; Fax. (613)288-2442.

KRONITZ, Naomi S; BC Women's Hosp & Health Ctre, 4500 Oak St, Vancouver BC V6H 3N1; McM'83; FRCPC; Anes. Staff, BC Women's Hospital & Health Centre; (604)875-2424; Fax. (604)875-2379.

KRONSTROM, Jean; Centre Med Christ-Roi, 102-40 rte du President-Kenned, Levis QC G6V 6C4; Laval'75; Staff, Hôtel-Dieu de Lévis; (418)833-4977; Fax. (418)833-9557.

KROP, Jozef; 6517A Mississauga Rd N, Mississauga ON L5N 1A6; Krakow (Poland)'68; Assoc Staff, St Joseph's Health Centre; Langs: Polish; Russian; (905)816-9657; Fax. (905)816-9661.

KROPELIN, Bruce W; Grey Nuns Community Hosp, 1100 Youville Drive West NW, Edmonton AB T6L 5X8; Man'93; BSc; FRCPC; Anes; Critical Care Medicine. Staff, Covenant Health - Grey Nuns Community Hospital; (780)735-7136

KROPYVNYTSKYY, Ivan; Canadian Sleep Institute, 300-295 Midpark Way SE, Calgary AB T2X 2A8; (Ukraine)'94; (403)254-6400; Fax. (403)254-6403.

KROTECKI, Lech; Centre Med Ormstown, GD 24 rue Gale, Ormstown QC J0S 1K0; Poznan (Poland)'73; CCFP; Staff, Barrie Memorial Hospital; Langs: Polish; French; (450)829-2331; Fax. (450)829-3636.

KROWITZ, Jason K; Powell River Gen Hosp, 5000 Joyce Ave, Powell River BC V8A 5R3; UBC'06; CCFP; Staff, Powell River General Hospital; (604)485-3211

KRSTICH, Desanka; 121 Howard Park Ave, Toronto ON M6R 1V7; Belgrade (Serbia)'66; FRCPC; Psy (Adult Psychiatry). Staff Sessional Psy, Centre for Addiction & Mental Health (CAMH) - Queen Site; Psy., The Review Board; (416)537-8256

KRUBA, Richard; Windsor Reg Hosp-Metropolitan, 1995 Lens Ave, Windsor ON N8W 1L9; Poznan (Poland)'05; Staff, Windsor Regional Hospital - Metropolitan Site; (519)254-5577

KRUCZYNSKI, Krystyna H; North York Gen Hosp, 4001 Leslie St, North York ON M2K 1E1; Tor'86; FRCPC; IntMed (Critical Care Medicine). Staff, North York General Hospital; (416)756-6000

KRUEGER-NAUG, Anne M; Queen Elizabeth II HSC-Halifax, 436-1276 South Park St, Halifax NS B3H 2Y9; Dal'06; FRCPC; IntMed. Staff, Queen Elizabeth II Health Sciences Centre - Victoria General Site; (902)473-7453

KRUGER, Alan M; William Osler HC-Etobicoke, 101 Humber College Blvd, Etobicoke ON M9V 1R8; Tor'69; Assoc Staff, William Osler Health System - Etobicoke General Hospital; Consultant, Xerox Canada; Consultant, Belgium Standard Canada; Consultant, Litton Systems Canada; (416)747-3500; alan.kruger@xerox.com.

KRUGER, Brian M; Radiology Consultants Assoc, 120-6707 Elbow Dr SW, Calgary AB T2V 0E3; Cal'97; FRCPC; DiagRad. (403)777-3005; Fax. (403)777-3008.

KRUGER, Frederick J; Aberdeen Med Centre, 1966 Harrison Way, Kamloops BC V1S 1M9; Pretoria (South Africa)'98; MB ChB; CCFP; Staff, Nicola Valley Health Centre; Staff, Royal Inland Hospital; Langs: Afrikaans; (250)314-5333

KRUGER, Garth; Mayfair Diagnostics, 1621 Albert St, Regina SK S4P 2S5; (South Africa)'79; MB ChB; (306)569-9729; Fax. (306)569-3337.

KRUGER, Gita; Westglen Med Centre, 108-30 Springborough Blvd SW, Calgary AB T3H 0N9; McM'97; CCFP; Staff, Rockyview General Hospital; (403)240-2221; Fax. (403)240-4670.

KRUGER, Gordon D; 101-527 Admiral St, Woodstock ON N4S 5B2; Wes'82; FRCSC; OrthSurg. (519)539-8581; Fax. (519)539-7817.

KRUGER, Jaco; Riley Park Primary Care Centre, 171-1402 8 Ave NW, Calgary AB T2N 1B9; (Other Foreign)'93; MB ChB; CCFP; (403)284-3272; Fax. (403)265-5503.

KRUGER, Kenneth; Wise Elephant Family Hlth Team, 247 Main St N, Brampton ON L6X 1N3; Ott'77; FRCPC; Psy (Anxiety Disorder). (905)459-4385; Fax. (905)459-6373; kkruger@ahealingplace.ca.

KRUGER, Marelise; Peter Lougheed Centre, 3500 26 Ave NE, Calgary AB T1Y 6J4; Pretoria (South Africa)'92; MB ChB; FRCA; FRCPC; Anes. Staff Anes, Peter Lougheed Centre; (403)943-5721

KRUGER, Petrus F; Royal Alexandra Hosp, 201-10240 Kingsway NW, Edmonton AB T5H 3V9; Stellenbosch (South Africa)'02; MB ChB; Staff, Royal Alexandra Hospital; Langs: Afrikaans; (780)735-4927; Fax. (780)735-4981.

KRUGER, Phil; Children's Hosp Eastern Ont, 401 Smyth Rd, Ottawa ON K1H 8L1; Orange Free State (South Africa)'00; FRCPC; Anes. Staff, Children's Hospital of Eastern Ontario (CHEO); (613)737-2431

KRUGER, Pieter Ernst; Morrison Centre, 202-9914 Morrison St, Fort McMurray AB T9H 4A4; (South Africa)'93; MB ChB; BMedSci; Langs: Afrikaans; Dutch; German; Zulu; (780)714-5763; Fax. (780)714-5765.

KRUGER, Schalk; 3F-65 Henry St, Miramichi NB E1V 2N4; Pretoria (South Africa)'90; Staff, Miramichi Regional Hospital; (506)623-3353; Fax. (506)623-3356.

KRUGER, Stephanus J; Clearview Med Clinic, 125-47 Clearview Market Way, Red Deer AB T4P 0M9; (South Africa)'06; MB ChB; Langs: Afrikaans; (403)356-0222; Fax. (403)356-0223.

KRUGER, Tamara L; Nortown Health Clinic, 875 Eglinton Ave W, Toronto ON M6C 3Z9; Tor'00; CCFP; (416)782-6111

KRUHLAK, Robert T; Grey Nuns Community Hosp, 1100 Youville Drive West NW, Edmonton AB T6L 5X8; Alb'85; Assoc Staff, Covenant Health - Grey Nuns Community Hospital; (780)735-7000; Fax. (780)438-4752.

KRUISSELBRINK, Rebecca J; McMaster University, 1-1280 Main St W, Hamilton ON L8S 4K1; McM'08; IntMed.

KRUK, Robert D; Dr Robert Kruk Med Corp, PO Box 728, Carman MB R0G 0J0; Man'98; BSc; CCFP; (204)745-2024

KRUL, L Edward; Main Floor, 1-353 Waverley St, Ottawa ON K2P 0W4; Palacky (Czech Republic)'65; DPsy; FRCPC; Psy (Andrology). Member Andrology Clinic, The Ottawa Hospital - Civic Campus; Cons. Roster Phys., W.C.B. & Cons., Zurich Insurance Co.; (613)235-8331

KRULEWITZ, Janet B; Flemingdon Health Centre, 10 Gateway Blvd, North York ON M3C 3A1; Tor'79; CCFP; FCFP; Court Staff Family Med, Sunnybrook Health Sciences Centre; Ac Staff, Toronto East General Hospital Inc; Asst Prof, University of Toronto; (416)429-3205; Fax. (416)422-3573; jkrulewitz@fhc-chc.com.

KRULL, Andreas; MUHC-Montreal Gen Hosp, 1650 av Cedar, Montreal QC H3G 1A4; Mon'95; FRCPC; EmergMed;CCFP; Staff, McGill University Health Centre - Montreal General Campus; (514)934-1934 x42501

KRUPA, Andrea M E; Kanata North Med Centre, 2-832 March Rd, Kanata ON K2W 0C9; Ott'02; MSc; BSc(Hon); CCFP; (613)599-5599

KRUPA, Norman K; The Spence Clinic, 500-1265 Arthur St E, Thunder Bay ON P7E 5H7; Tor'76; (807)626-1147; Fax. (807)626-1121.

KRUPSKI, Malgorzata H; Dr Charles S Curtis Mem Hosp, 178-200 West St, St. Anthony NL A0K 4S0; Poznan (Poland)'91; Staff, Charles S Curtis Memorial Hospital; (709)454-3333

KRUSE, Karen P; 1730 Kitchener St, Vancouver BC V5L 2W3; Cambridge (England)'79; (604)215-1334; pscott_argyle@yahoo.com.

KRUSHEL, Robert F; Stanton Terr Health Authority, PO Box 10 Stn Main, Yellowknife NT X1A 2N1; Alb'92; BSc; ObstGyn. Staff, Stanton Territorial Health Authority; (867)669-4111

KRUSZELNICKI, Dan; Kirkland & District Hosp, PO Box 300 Stn Main 145 Government Rd E, Kirkland Lake ON P2N 3P4; Qns'08; CCFP; Staff, Kirkland & District Hospital; (705)568-2245

KRUZYK, G Jurii K; 103-115 Bell Farm Rd, Barrie ON L4M 5G1; Tor'86; FRCSC; GenSurg. Staff, Royal Victoria Regional Health Centre; (705)722-9668; Fax. (705)726-1755.

KRYGIER, Darin S; 410-301 Columbia St E, New Westminster BC V3L 3W5; Alb'04; FRCPC; IntMed; Gastroent. (604)525-0155

KRYKORKA, Peter; Vancouver Gen Hosp, 3500-855 12th Ave W, Vancouver BC V5Z 1M9; Prague (Czech Republic)'71; CCFP; Staff, Vancouver General Hospital - Centennial Pavillion; Langs: Czech; (604)822-7121

KRYM, Valerie F; Sunnybrook Hlth Sciences Ctre, C Wing 7F-2075 Bayview Ave, Toronto ON M4N 3M5; McM'93; BScN; MPH; CCFP; CCFP(E.M.); FCFP; Staff, Sunnybrook Health Sciences Centre; (416)480-4037; Fax. (416)480-4074.

KRYSA, Clifford J; Heritage Village Medicentre, 2041 111 St NW, Edmonton AB T6J 4V9; Alb'80; (780)438-2306

KRYSHTALSKYJ, Nina; 1-2453 Bloor St W, Toronto ON M6S 1P7; Tor'86; CCFP; (416)760-0607; Fax. (416)760-7398.

KRYSKI, Albert; Calgary Heart Centre, 403-3280 Hospital Dr NW, Calgary AB T2N 4Z6; Cal'88; PhD; FRCPC; IntMed; Cardiol. Staff Cardiol, Foothills Medical Centre; Staff, Health Research Innovation Centre; (403)521-2227; Fax. (403)283-6360.

KRYSKOW, Pamela A; PO Box 5442 Stn B, Victoria BC V8R 6S4; UBC'06; CCFP.

KRYSL, Joseph; Campbell River & Dist Gen Hosp, 375 2nd Ave, Campbell River BC V9W 3V1; Tor'88; FRCPC; DiagRad (Interventional Radiology). Staff, Campbell River & District General Hospital; (250)287-7111

KRYSTOLOVICH, Leonard W; Unimedico Family Practice, 110-955 Major Mackenzie Dr, Maple ON L6A 4P9; Tor'68; Ac Staff/Med Dir Extendicare Nursing Home, Mackenzie Richmond Hill Hospital; (289)553-3300

KRYWULAK, Steven; 303-3330 Richter St, Kelowna BC V1W 4V5; Cal'95; FRCSC; OrthSurg (Shoulder & Joint Reconstruction). Clin Instructor, University of British Columbia; (250)763-6066; Fax. (250)862-5842; skrywulak@telus.net.

KRYWULAK-RIZZO, Natalia; 102-6955 boul Taschereau, Brossard QC J4Z 1A7; Man'79; (450)656-2310

KRYZANOWSKI, Julie A; Medical Officer of Health Offi, 101-310 Idylwyld Dr N, Saskatoon SK S7L 0Z2; Qns'06; FRCPC; Public Health & Preventive Med;CCFP; Staff Office of the MOH, Saskatoon Health Region Saskatoon Public Health; (306)655-3438

KRZECZUNOWICZ, Dominic E J; North Bay Regl Health Centre, 50 College Dr, North Bay ON P1B 0A4; Ott'07; FRCPC; DiagRad. Staff, North Bay Regional Health Centre - Regional Mental Health; (705)474-8600

KRZNARIC, Joseph; Medi-Kel Clinic, PO Box 2100 Rpo Banks Centre, Kelowna BC V1X 4K5; UBC'94; CCFP; (250)862-4996

KRZYWICKA, Maria H; Mission Med Clinic, 2303 4 St SW, Calgary AB T2S 2S7; Warsaw (Poland)'65; Langs: Polish; French; (403)229-1700; missionmedicalclinic@gmail.com.

KRZYZANIAK, Kelly M; Mountain Med Clinic, PO Box 1660, Neepawa MB R0J 1H0; Man'89; (204)476-3381; Fax. (204)476-2156.

KRZYZANOWSKA, Monika K; Univ Hlth Network-Princess M, 5-206-610 University Ave, Toronto ON M5G 2M9; Tor'95; MPH; FRCPC; IntMed (Gastrointestinal Oncology); MedOncol. Staff, Princess Margaret Hospital - University Health Network; Asst Prof, University of Toronto; Langs: Polish; (416)946-6542; Fax. (416)946-6546.

KSIAZEK, Danuta; Associated Med Specialists, 1555 Second Ave, Trail BC V1R 1M3; Szczecin (Poland)'84; FRCPC; IntMed (Cardiology). Staff, Kootenay Boundary Regional Hospital; Langs: Polish; (250)368-3301; Fax. (250)368-5053; imed@shawcable.com.

KSIENSKI, Asaph E; South Health Campus, 4448 Front St SE, Calgary AB T3M 1M4; Cal'09; CCFP; (403)956-3042

KSIENSKI, Doran S; BC Cancer Agency-Vanc Isl Ctr, 2410 Lee Ave, Victoria BC V8R 6V5; Alb'05; FRCPC; IntMed; MedOncol. Staff, BC Cancer Agency Vancouver Island Centre; (250)519-5572

KU, James L Y; Barrie Chronic Pain Clinic, 204-480 Huronia Rd, Barrie ON L4N 8Z1; Tor'91; (705)792-7890

KU, Nancy S N; Dorval Med Assoc Fam Hlth Team, 465 Morden Rd, Oakville ON L6K 3W6; Tor'86; Staff, Halton Healthcare Services Corporation - Oakville Site; (905)842-7154; Fax. (905)842-3604; nku@cogeco.ca.

KUA, Jimmy; 2168 Beaumont Rd, Ottawa ON K1H 5V3; Dublin (Ireland)'74; LRCPSI; FRCPC; Psy (Adult Psychiatry). (613)739-1059; Fax. (613)737-7053; jimmy.kua@sympatico.ca.

KUAN, Alano; Surrey Mem Hosp, 13750 96 Ave, Surrey BC V3V 1Z2; Alb'89; BSc; MSc; CCFP; CCFP(E.M.); FCFP; Staff Emerg, Surrey Memorial Hospital; Clin Instructor Emerg & Family Med, University of British Columbia; Langs: Chinese; (604)588-3369; Fax. (604)588-3377.

KUATE, Xaviere C; Medecine Familiale Montclair, 202-15 boul Montclair, Gatineau QC J8Y 2E2; Louvain (Belgium)'00; (819)777-2752

KUBACKI, Andrzej; Medical Arts Bldg, 115 Hazen St, Saint John NB E2L 3L3; Rokitnica (Poland)'63; PhD; FAB; FRCPC; Psy (Couple Therapy). (506)634-0874

KUBAZKY, Valerie T; Sheridan Med Associates, 1-1960 Dundas St W, Mississauga ON L5K 2R9; Ott'94; CCFP; (905)822-3993

KUBBA, Hayder S H; Dixie Road Med Associates, 2200 Dixie Rd, Mississauga ON L4Y 1Z4; Al-Mustansiriyah (Iraq)'84; LMCC; MB ChB; FRCS; CCFP; Ac Staff, Trillium Health Centre - Mississauga; Staff, Tamarack Health Centre; Langs: Arabic; (905)279-1700

KUBELIK, Dalibor; The Ottawa Hosp-Civic Campus, 1053 Carling Ave, Ottawa ON K1Y 4E9; McG'02; FRCSC; GenSurg (Critical Care Medicine); VascSurg. Staff, The Ottawa Hospital - Civic Campus; (613)722-7000

KUBIK, Stephanie J M; Crowfoot Village Fam Practice, 210-600 Crowfoot Cres NW, Calgary AB T3G 0B4; Cal'90; BSc; CCFP; Med Staff Member, Foothills Medical Centre; Clin Lecturer Family Med, University of Calgary; (403)239-9733; Fax. (403)241-8112.

KUBLIK, Harry E; Lions Gate Hosp, 231 15th St E, North Vancouver BC V7L 2L7; UBC'73; Anes. Staff, Lions Gate Hospital; (604)984-5709; Fax. (604)984-5729.

KUBOW, Janusz; Nova Scotia Rehab Centre, 1341 Summer St, Halifax NS B3H 4K4; Wroclaw (Poland)'79; Staff, Nova Scotia Rehabilitation Centre; (902)473-2702

KUC, Zenia N; Liberton Med Centre, 205-31 Liberton Dr, St. Albert AB T8N 3X6; Alb'76; CCFP; FCFP; Court Staff, Sturgeon Community Hospital; (780)458-5505; Fax. (780)460-1479.

KUCERAK, Martin; 8-2168 McCallum Rd, Abbotsford BC V2S 6R6; Tor'71; FRCPC; IntMed (Cardiology). (604)859-2212; Fax. (604)859-3508.

KUCEROVA, Lenka; 316 George St, Sarnia ON N7T 4P4; Karlova (Czech Republic)'81; Langs: Czech; (519)337-6200

KUCEY, Daryl S; 402-1881 Yonge St, Toronto ON M4S 3C4; Alb'86; MSc; MPH; FRCSC; GenSurg; VascSurg. Staff VascSurg, Sunnybrook Health Sciences Centre; Asst Prof, University of Toronto; (416)966-3886; Fax. (416)487-8746.

KUCHARCZYK, Walter; 1C 552-585 University Ave, Toronto ON M5G 2N2; Tor'79; FRCPC; DiagRad (Neuro Radiology)., Toronto General Hospital - UHN; Staff, The Hospital For Sick Children; Staff, Mount Sinai Hospital; Teach Staff, University of Toronto; (416)340-4656; Fax. (416)340-3900; w.kucharczyk@utoronto.ca.

KUCHARSKA, Agnes; Derry Heights Plaza, 201B-6941 Derry Rd, Milton ON L9T 7H5; McM'99; CCFP; Assoc Staff, Halton Healthcare Services Corporation - Milton District Hospital; Langs: Polish; Spanish; (905)876-3231; Fax. (905)876-3739.

KUCHARSKI, Edward A; Sherbourne Health Centre, 333 Sherbourne St, Toronto ON M5A 2S5; Ott'05; CCFP; (416)324-4103

KUCHEREPA, Nadia N A; Petawawa Centennial Family HC, 154 Civic Centre Rd, Petawawa ON K8H 3H5; Ott'09; CCFP; (613)687-8538; Fax. (613)687-6808.

KUCHINAD, Raul A; Gulf Canada Square, 335-401 9 Ave SW, Calgary AB T2P 3C5; Qns'05; FRCSC; OrthSurg. (403)221-4308; Fax. (403)221-4387.

KUCHTARUK, Andrew; 1935 Paris St, Sudbury ON P3E 3C6; Wes'82; CCFP; FCFP; Med Dir, Extendicare Falconbridge; Med Dir, Extendicare York Sudbury; Langs: Ukrainian; (705)523-4522; Fax. (705)523-4524.

KUCPARIC, Peter S; PO Box 460 Stn Main, Flin Flon MB R8A 1N3; Belgrade (Serbia)'69; LMCC; Staff, Flin Flon General Hospital Inc; (204)687-8271; Fax. (204)687-5624.

KUDEL, Robert M; 3000-700 9 Ave SW, Calgary AB T2P 3V4; Sask'69; FRCPC; DiagRad. (403)291-3315; Fax. (403)291-9308.

KUDEL, Timothy A; Wetaskiwin Hosp & Care Centre, 6910 47 St, Wetaskiwin AB T9A 3N3; Sask'76; FRCPC; DiagRad. Staff DiagRad, Wetaskiwin Hospital & Care Centre; (780)361-4149

KUDISH, Vitaly; SMBD Jewish Gen Hosp, 3755 ch Cote-Sainte-Catherine, Montreal QC H3T 1E2; Riga (Latvia)'79; CSPQ; Anes. Staff, Sir Mortimer B Davis Jewish General; (514)340-8222

KUDO, Patricia A; Workers' Comp Board, 6951 Westminster Hwy, Richmond BC V7C 1C6; Tor'97; MSc; CCFP; (604)273-2266

KYEI-ABOAGYE, Catherine F; MUHC-Royal Victoria Hosp, 687 av des Pins O, Montreal QC H3A 1A1; McG'62; Endocrin (P.Q.). Assoc Physician, McGill University Health Centre - Royal Victoria Hospital; adj Prof, McGill University; (514)843-1510; Fax. (514)843-2838.

KUDRYK, William H; University of Alberta Hosp, 1E4 32-8440 112 St NW, Edmonton AB T6G 2B7; Alb'68; FRCSC; Otol. Staff, University of Alberta Hospital; (780)407-6640; Fax. (780)407-1593; wkudryk@cha.ab.ca.

KUECHLER, Peter M; Surgical Associates, 405-1120 Yates St, Victoria BC V8V 3M9; Alb'73; FRCSC; GenSurg; VascSurg. Staff, Royal Jubilee Hospital; Staff, Victoria General Hospital; (250)592-4313

KUEGLE, Peter F X; Family Med Practice, 453 Selkirk Ave, Winnipeg MB R2W 2M4; Tor'87; CCFP; FCFP; Staff, Concordia General Hospital; (204)987-8440; Fax. (204)987-8445.

KUGANATHAN, Girudiha; Clinique Med des Trois Lacs, 585 av Saint-Charles, Vaudreuil-Dorion QC J7V 8P9; Sher'10; (450)455-3322

KUGELMASS, Michael I; Humber River Reg Hosp-Keele St, 2175 Keele St, North York ON M6M 3Z4; McG'68; DPsy; FRCPC; Psy. Staff, Humber River Regional Hospital - Keele Street Site; (416)658-2139

KUGELMASS, Robin; Children's Care Clinic, 100-14770 boul De Pierrefonds, Pierrefonds QC H9H 4Y6; Mon'86; FRCPC; Peds (Dermatology). Staff, McGill University Health Centre - Montreal Children's Hospital; Langs: Bilingual(French/English); (514)696-2442; Fax. (514)624-3099.

KUGLER, Pierre E A; 135 Union St E, Waterloo ON N2J 1C4; Tor'88; BSc(Psych); CCFP; FCFP; Court Staff, Grand River Hospital - Kitchener/Waterloo Health Centre; Court Staff, St Mary's General Hospital; (519)744-9693; Fax. (519)744-5258; kuglerpierre@yahoo.com.

KUGYELKA, Janet; Burnaby Hosp, 3935 Kincaid St, Burnaby BC V5G 2X6; Alb'87; CCFP; Staff, Burnaby Hospital; (604)434-4211

KUHL, David R; St Paul's Hosp, 1081 Burrard St, Vancouver BC V6Z 1Y6; McM'85; MHSc; Ac Staff, Providence Health Care - St Paul's Hospital; Asst Prof, University of British Columbia; (604)682-2344 x2099; Fax. (604)631-5764.

KUHLMANN, John C; 202-666 Burnhamthorpe Rd, Etobicoke ON M9C 2Z4; (Ireland)'73; Staff, Trillium Health Centre - West Toronto; (416)622-0933; Fax. (416)622-0409.

KUHLMANN, Peter A; 9833 Tecumseh Rd E, Windsor ON N8R 1A5; Melbourne (Australia)'66; Staff, Hôtel-Dieu Grace Hospital; Staff, Windsor Regional Hospital - Metropolitan Site; Staff, Windsor Regional Hospital - Tayfour Site; (519)735-6844; Fax. (519)735-5473.

KUHN, Craig J; Niagara Addiction Services, 260 Sugarloaf St, Port Colborne ON L3K 2N7; McM'81; ABAM; CSAM; CCFP; Staff, Niagara Health System - Port Colborne General Site; Asst Clin Prof Psy, McMaster University; (905)834-4501 x32542; Fax. (905)834-4493.

KUHN, Fernando H; Cannon Clinic, 4-2151 McCallum Rd, Abbotsford BC V2S 3N9; Stellenbosch (South Africa)'85; Member Family Pract & Obst, Abbotsford Regional Hospital & Cancer Centre; Langs: Afrikaans; German; Zulu; (604)853-3314; Fax. (604)853-2171.

KUHN, Magdalena; The Moncton Hosp, 135 Macbeath Ave, Moncton NB E1C 6Z8; Sask'78; FRCPC; MedMicrobiol. Staff, The Moncton Hospital; (506)857-5324; Fax. (506)857-5632.

KUHN, Susan M; Alberta Children's Hosp, 2888 Shaganappi Trail NW, Calgary AB T3B 6A8; Alb'88; MSc(ClinEpidemiol.); FRCPC; Peds (Tropical & Travel Medicine); InfectDis. Staff, Alberta Children's Hospital; Clinical Asst Prof Peds, University of Calgary; (403)955-7813; Fax. (403)955-3045.

KUHNERT, Peter E; Grand River Hosp-Freeport Site, PO Box 9056 3570 King St E, Kitchener ON N2A 2W1; Alb'90; CCFP; FCFP; Staff, Grand River Hospital - Freeport Site; (519)749-4300

KUJATH, Magdalena; Manitoba Clinic, 790 Sherbrook St, Winnipeg MB R3A 1M3; Man'06.

KUJAVSKY, Andrew S; The Westend Family Care Clinic, 80 Michael Cowpland Dr, Kanata ON K2M 1P6; Wes'00; CCFP; Staff, Westend Family Care Clinic Family Health Team; (613)596-3321; Fax. (613)599-3366.

KUJTAN, Peter W; Credit Valley Med Arts Centre, A508-2000 Credit Valley Rd, Mississauga ON L5M 4N4; Tor'87; PhD(Toxicology); Staff, The Credit Valley Hospital; Coroner, Ministry of the Solicitor-General; (905)828-2837; Fax. (905)820-1738.

KUK, Joda; Grand River Hosp-KW Hlth Ctre, PO Box 9056 Stn C 835 King St W, Kitchener ON N2G 1G3; McM'06; FRCPC; RadOncol. Staff RadOncol, Grand River Hospital - Kitchener/Waterloo Health Centre; (519)749-4380 x5489

KUKASWADIA, Sadiya S; Humber River Reg Hosp-Church, 200 Church St, Toronto ON M9N 1N8; Qns'05; FRCPC; IntMed; Hem. Staff, Humber River Regional Hospital - Church Street Site; (416)243-4505; Fax. (416)243-4580.

KUKHA-MOHAMAD, Shirwan; 201-626 Broadway Ave, Saskatoon SK S7N 1A9; Baghdad (Iraq)'79; FRCPC; Psy (Biological Psychiatry). Staff Contract Psy, Regional Psychiatric Centre - Prairies; Consultant Psy, Saskatoon Health Region Saskatoon Public Health; Assoc Prof Psy, University of Saskatchewan; (306)244-2421; Fax. (306)244-2436.

KUKHTA, Allison; CSSS de la Vallée de l'Or, 725 6e rue, Val-d'Or QC J9P 3Y1; McM'90; FRCPC; Peds; ClinImmunol&Allergy. Staff, Centre Hospitalier de Val d'Or; Langs: English; French; (819)825-5858 x2215

KUKKADI, Zaheer; Chatham Prof Bldg, 857 Grand Ave W, Chatham ON N7L 4T1; Mangalore (India)'89; MB BS; FRCS; FRCSC; OrthSurg.

KUKREJA, Kanwal; Homewood Health Centre, 150 Delhi St, Guelph ON N1E 6K9; Punjab (India)'90; FRCPC; Psy. Staff, Homewood Health Centre; (519)824-1010

KUKREJA, Tarvinder K; Toronto Sleep Institute, 208-390 Steeles Ave W, Thornhill ON L4J 6X2; Punjabi (India)'90; MB BS; CCFP; (905)709-9696; Fax. (905)709-9764.

KUKRETI, Asha; Medical Centre, 115-2100 Ellesmere Rd, Scarborough ON M1H 3B7; Delhi (India)'66; Court Staff, The Scarborough Hospital - Birchmount Campus; Court Staff, North York General Hospital; Langs: Hindi; Urdu; (416)439-8497

KUKRETI, Vinay; The Hosp for Sick Children, 555 University Ave, Toronto ON M5G 1X8; Gorakhpur (India)'02; Staff, The Hospital For Sick Children; (416)813-1500

KUKRETI, Vishal; Univ Hlth Network-Princess M, 5-227-610 University Ave, Toronto ON M5G 2M9; Cal'98; MD; MSc; FRCPC; IntMed (Hematological Oncology); Hem. Staff Hematologist, Princess Margaret Hospital - University Health Network; Langs: Hindi; Urdu; (416)946-4566; Fax. (416)946-2087.

KULAGA, Andrzej; Rockyview Gen Hosp, 7007 14 St SW, Calgary AB T2V 1P9; (Poland)'83; FRCPC; AnatPath. Staff Path, Rockyview General Hospital; (403)943-3411; Fax. (403)943-3333.

KULAK, Larry M; Associate Med Clinic, PO Box 1076 Stn Main, Whitecourt AB T7S 1P9; Alb'79; (780)778-2224; Fax. (780)778-2127; lmkulak@telusplanet.net.

KULANDAIVELU, Murugesan; Dr Charles S Curtis Mem Hosp, PO Box 1103 178-200 West St, St. Anthony NL A0K 4S0; Madurai (India)'80; MB BS; Staff, Charles S Curtis Memorial Hospital; (709)454-3333

KULAR, Kuldip S; North Bramalea Med Centre, 401-9780 Bramalea Rd, Brampton ON L6S 2P1; Amritsar (India)'73; MB BS; Ac Staff, William Osler Health System - Brampton Civic Hospital; (905)458-8898

KULASINGHAM, Shaneka; St Joseph's Healthcare, 50 Charlton Ave E, Hamilton ON L8N 4A6; Ott'95; Staff, St Joseph's Healthcare - Charlton Campus; (905)522-1155

KULBISKY, Gordon P; Medical Arts Bldg, 202-233 Kennedy St, Winnipeg MB R3C 3J5; Man'00; FRCPC; DiagRad.

KULCHYK, James S; Toronto East Gen Hosp Inc, 825 Coxwell Ave, Toronto ON M4C 3E7; Tor'88; FRCPC; Anes. Staff, Toronto East General Hospital Inc; (416)469-6212

KULD, Arvo; St Joseph's Health Centre, 30 The Queensway, Toronto ON M6R 1B5; Tor'76; AB; Ac Staff EmergMed, St Joseph's Health Centre; (416)530-6587

KULENKAMP, Anne C D; CSSS de la Cote-de-Gaspe, 215 boul de York O, Gaspe QC G4X 2W2; Laval'06; CCFP; Staff, Centre Hospitalier de Gaspe; Langs: German; English; (418)368-3301

KULESHA, Denis; 202-3271 Bloor St W, Etobicoke ON M8X 1E2; Tor'74; FRCPC; Psy. Staff Psy, Toronto Western Hospital - University Health Network; Asst Prof, University of Toronto; (416)233-4555; Fax. (416)239-3882.

KULIK, Dina M; The Hosp for Sick Children, 555 University Ave, Toronto ON M5G 1X8; McM'07; FRCPC; Peds; PedEmergMed. Staff, The Hospital For Sick Children; (416)813-1500

KULKARNI, Abhaya V; The Hosp for Sick Children, 555 University Ave, Toronto ON M5G 1X8; Tor'94; FRCSC; Neursurg. Staff, The Hospital For Sick Children; (416)813-6427; Fax. (416)813-4975; abhaya.kulkarni@sickkids.ca.

KULKARNI, Chetana A; The George Hull Centre, 600 The East Mall, Etobicoke ON M9B 4B1; McM'02; FRCPC; Psy. Staff, Hamilton Health Sciences Centre - McMaster Children's Hospital; (416)622-8833

KULKARNI, Girish S; Univ Hlth Network-Princess M, 610 University Ave, Toronto ON M5G 2M9; Tor'01; BSc; FRCSC; Urol (Bladder Cancer). Staff, Princess Margaret Hospital - University Health Network; (416)946-2246

KULKARNI, Jyothi; 550 King St E, Kitchener ON N2G 2L8; (Other Foreign)'95; CCFP; (519)224-0540

KULKARNI, Pradeep R; University of Alberta Hosp, 1C1 04-8440 112 St NW, Edmonton AB T6G 2B7; Bombay (India)'85; MB BS; FRCA; FRCPC; Anes (Pediatric Anesthesia). Staff Anes, University of Alberta Hospital; Asst Prof, University of Alberta; (780)407-7035; kulkarni@ualberta.ca.

KULKARNI, Ramesh; Medical & Dental Bldg, 307-1221 Algonquin Ave, North Bay ON P1B 4Y3; Mysore (India)'71; MB BS; BSc; FRCOG(UK); FRCSC; ObstGyn. Consultant ObstGyn, North Bay Regional Health Centre - Regional Mental Health; Staff, West Nipissing General Hospital; Preceptor ObstGyn, Laurentian University; Langs: Hindi; Kanarese; Marathi; (705)495-0844; Fax. (705)495-6698.

KULKARNI, Savita S; Humber River Reg Hosp-Finch, 2111 Finch Ave W, North York ON M3N 1N1; Poona (India)'69; MB BS; ABNPath; FRCPC; AnatPath. Associate Path, Humber River Regional Hospital - Finch Avenue Site; (416)744-2500 x2780; Fax. (416)747-3743.

KULKARNI, Sharmila N; Lifemark Health Institute, 154 Meadowlark Shopping Ctr NW, Edmonton AB T5R 5W9; Dal'96; FRCPC; PhysMed&Rehab. (780)429-4761

KULKARNI, Shobhana P; Dynacare Kasper Med Labs, 200-10150 102 St NW, Edmonton AB T5J 4C7; London (England)'86; MB BS; FRCPC; MedMicrobiol. (780)451-3702; Fax. (780)454-2845.

KULKARNI, Supriya R; Univ Hlth Network-Princess M, 3 963-610 University Ave, Toronto ON M5G 2M9; Pune (India)'91; Staff, Princess Margaret Hospital - University Health Network; (416)946-4501 x5840; Fax. (416)946-6564.

KULKARNI, Swati; 2220 Kildare Rd, Windsor ON N8W 2X3; (India)'92; FRCPC; IntMed; MedOncol. Staff, Windsor Regional Hospital - Windsor Regional Cancer Centre; Langs: Hindi; (519)253-5253; Fax. (519)253-4204.

KULLA, Steven B; Wellington Med Clinic, 84C-3200 Island Hwy N, Nanaimo BC V9T 1W1; UBC'08; CCFP; (250)740-2100

KULPAS, Leila; Business Bldg, 330-1200 Burrard St, Vancouver BC V6Z 2C7; New South Wales (Australia)'76; MB BS; FRCPC; Psy (Psychotherapy). (604)685-4518

KUM, Franklin N; Health Sciences Centre, 300 Prince Philip Dr, St. John's NL A1B 3V6; Dublin (Ireland)'72; LRCPS; DAB; FRCSC; ObstGyn. Staff Consultant, St Clare's Mercy Hospital; Ac Staff, Health Sciences Centre; Asst Prof ObstGyn, Memorial University Of Newfoundland; (709)777-8477

KUMALO, Thandanani G Q; Grand River Hosp-KW Hlth Ctre, PO Box 9056 Stn C 835 King St W, Kitchener ON N2G 1G3; Natal (South Africa)'75; MB ChB; GenPath (Oncology). Assoc Staff, Grand River Hospital - Kitchener/Waterloo Health Centre; Assoc Staff, St Mary's General Hospital; (519)749-4300; Fax. (519)749-4274.

KUMANAN, Mekalai; Two Rivers FHT-Healthlink, B10-350 Conestoga Blvd, Cambridge ON N1R 7L7; Dal'06; CCFP; (519)740-5010

KUMAR, Aalok; BC Cancer Agency-Vancouver CC, 600 10th Ave W, Vancouver BC V5Z 4E6; Tor'08; IntMed. Staff, BC Cancer Agency Vancouver Centre; (604)877-6000

KUMAR, Amit; Ellerslie Medicentre, 102-9404 Ellerslie Rd SW, Edmonton AB T6X 0K6; (Russia (Federation))'02; (780)466-8064; Fax. (780)466-8095.

KUMAR, Anand; Health Sciences Ctr Gen Hosp, JJ 399D-700 William Ave, Winnipeg MB R3E 0Z3; Tor'86; IntMed (Critical Care Medicine). Assoc Prof, Health Sciences Centre; (204)787-3112; Fax. (204)787-3069; akumar61@yahoo.com.

KUMAR, Anil; Cornwall Professional Bldg, 601-2125 11th Ave, Regina SK S4P 3X3; Punjab(India) (India)'80; FRCSC; Neursurg. Staff NeuroSurg, Regina General Hospital; (306)359-3489

KUMAR, Anu; Hys Med Centre, 202-11010 101 St NW, Edmonton AB T5H 4B9; Tor'95; FRCPC; DiagRad. (780)426-1121; Fax. (780)425-5979.

KUMAR, Aparna; Winnipeg Clinic, 425 St Mary Ave, Winnipeg MB R3C 0N2; Tor'86; Peds.

KUMAR, Ashesh; St Michael's Hosp, 30 Bond St, Toronto ON M5B 1W8; Ott'05; FRCSC; OrthSurg. Staff, St Michael's Hospital; (416)360-4000

KUMAR, Brinda C P; Bathurst Walk-In Clinic, 101-4430 Bathurst St, North York ON M3H 3S3; Mysore (India)'68; MB BS; (416)633-3629; Fax. (416)633-3624.

KUMAR, C L Prasanna; Rosedale Med Centre, 404-600 Sherbourne St, Toronto ON M4X 1W4; Bangalore (India)'61; MB BS; DABOG; FRCSC; ObstGyn. Court Staff ObstGyn, Toronto East General Hospital Inc; Langs: Telugu; Hindi; (416)921-2113

KUMAR, David; Southlake Reg Health Centre, 596 Davis Dr, Newmarket ON L3Y 2P9; Kurnool (India)'95; Staff, Southlake Regional Health Centre; (905)895-4521

KUMAR, Deepa; Credit Valley Surgical Assoc, 2207 Dunwin Dr, Mississauga ON L5L 1X1; Tor'97; FRCSC; GenSurg; General Surgical Oncology. Staff Gen Surgeon, The Credit Valley Hospital; (905)820-3633; Fax. (905)820-3352.

KUMAR, Deepali; Katz-Rexall Centre, 6 030-1A University Campus NW, Edmonton AB T6G 2E1; Ott'96; BMedSci; MMedSci; FRCP; FRCPC; IntMed (Transplantation); InfectDis. Staff, University of Alberta Hospital; (780)492-3885; Fax. (780)492-4805.

KUMAR, Ganraj; 2622 Eglinton Ave E, Scarborough ON M1K 2S3; McG'61; FACP; FRCPC; IntMed (Cardiology). Langs: Hindi; (416)755-7500; Fax. (416)755-7509.

KUMAR, Gautam; 1485 Bancroft Dr, Sudbury ON P3B 1R6; Ott'06; FRCPC; Peds. (705)523-7120; Fax. (705)523-8232.

KUMAR, Hullur V; Grand River Hosp-KW Hlth Ctre, PO Box 9056 Stn C 835 King St W, Kitchener ON N2G 1G3; Sri Venkateshwara (India)'81; MB; BSc; DPM(India); MRCPsy(UK); FRCPC; Psy. Staff, Grand River Hospital - Kitchener/Waterloo Health Centre; (519)749-4300

KUMAR, Krishna; Regina Qu'Appelle HR-Regina, 1440 14th Ave, Regina SK S4P 0W5; Agra (India)'53; MS; FRCS; FRCSC; Neursurg (Chronic Pain). Head Sect of NeurSurg, Regina General Hospital; Ac Staff, Pasqua Hospital; Clin Prof NeurSurg, University of Saskatchewan; Langs: Hindi; (306)781-6116; Fax. (306)781-6153; krishna.kumar@rqhealth.ca.

KUMAR, M M Sujana; London Med Dental Bldg, 412-450 Central Ave, London ON N6B 2E8; Bangalore (India)'70; MB BS; DPM; MRCPsy; FRCPC; Psy. (519)642-7958; Fax. (519)642-7580.

KUMAR, Manoj; Royal Alexandra Hosp, 5027-10240 Kingsway NW, Edmonton AB T5H 3V9; (India)'94; MB BS; MD; MScEpidemiol; Staff, Royal Alexandra Hospital; (780)735-4644; Fax. (780)735-4072; manojk@ualberta.ca.

KUMAR, Naresh; Whitby Cardiovascular Inst, 3020 Brock St N, Whitby ON L1R 3J7; Calcutta (India)'76; MB BS; MRCP(UK); FRCPC; IntMed (Cardiology). (905)668-0416; Fax. (905)668-8778.

KUMAR, Naresh; 202-83 Mill St, Georgetown ON L7G 5E9; Delhi (India)'79; CCFP; (905)873-2402

KUMAR, Patel R V; Regina Mental Health Clinic, 3F-2110 Hamilton St, Regina SK S4P 2E3; Osmania (India)'79; MB BS; (306)766-7800; Fax. (306)766-7811.

KUMAR, Pavan; CHUM-Hop Notre-Dame, 1560 rue Sherbrooke E, Montreal QC H2L 4M1; UBC'07; Anes. Staff, Centre Hospitalier l'Université de Montréal (CHUM) - Hôpital Notre-Dame; (514)890-8000

KUMAR, Puja R; Teaching Res & Wellness Centre, 3280 Hospital Dr NW, Calgary AB T2N 4Z6; Wes'06; FRCPC; IntMed; Gastroent. (403)592-5015; Fax. (403)592-5090.

KUMAR, Ragbir S; Diabetic Day Care Clinic, 700 Coronation Blvd, Cambridge ON N1R 3G2; New Delhi (India)'60; MB BS; FRCPC; IntMed (Diabetes). Staff Consultant, Cambridge Memorial Hospital; Langs: Hindi; (519)621-2330 x2345

KUMAR, Rajat; Cancercare Manitoba, ON2025-675 McDermot Ave, Winnipeg MB R3E 0V9; Delhi (India)'78; FRCPC; Hem.

KUMAR, Rajat; Royal Victoria Hosp, 201 Georgian Dr, Barrie ON L4M 6M2; Delhi (India)'03; Staff, Royal Victoria Regional Health Centre; (705)728-9090

KUMAR, Rajender; Northeast Mental Hlth Centre, 680 Kirkwood Ave, Sudbury ON P3E 1X3; Poona (India)'77; MPH; DPM; MRCPsy(Lond); FRCPC; Psy (Adult General Psychiatry). Staff, North Bay Regional Health Centre - Kirkwood; Staff, Health Sciences North-St Joseph's Health Centre; Lecturer Psy, University of Western Ontario; Lecturer, Northern Ontario School of Medicine; Langs: Hindi; Urdu; Punjabi; (705)675-5900; Fax. (705)671-3031; rkumar@hrsrh.on.ca.

KUMAR, Rakesh; Toronto East Gen Hosp Inc, 825 Coxwell Ave, Toronto ON M4C 3E7; (India)'83; CCFP; CCFP(E.M.); FCFP; Chief Emerg Med, Humber River Regional Hospital - Church Street Site; Staff Emerg Med, Toronto East General Hospital Inc; Staff Family Med, The Scarborough Hospital - General Campus; Staff, Providence Healthcare; (416)461-8272; kumar@on.aibn.com.

KUMAR, Ramneek; Grey Nuns Community Hosp & HC, 1100 Youville Drive West NW, Edmonton AB T6L 5X8; (India)'97; MB BS; Staff, Covenant Health - Grey Nuns Community Hospital; (780)966-5130

KUMAR, Rohini; Family Practice Health Centre, 77 Grenville St, Toronto ON M5S 1B3; Wes'10; CCFP; (416)323-6485

KUMAR, Rohit; Trillium Hlth Ctr-Mississauga, 100 Queensway W, Mississauga ON L5B 1B8; Dal'02; FRCPC; Anes. Staff, Trillium Health Centre - Mississauga; (905)848-7628

KUMAR, S Eshwar; Saint John Reg Hosp, PO Box 2100 Stn Main, Saint John NB E2L 4L2; Bangalore (India)'71; MB BS; FRCR; Staff, Saint John Regional Hospital; Co-CEO Dept of Health, New Brunswick Cancer Network; Asst Prof, Dalhousie University; (506)648-6884; Fax. (506)648-6880.

KUMAR, Sameer; The Credit Valley Hosp, 2200 Eglinton Ave W, Mississauga ON L5M 2N1; Tor'95; FRCPC; IntMed; Critical Care Medicine. Staff, The Credit Valley Hospital; (905)813-2200

KUMAR, Sameer; Sunnybrook Hlth Sciences Ctre, 2075 Bayview Ave, Toronto ON M4N 3M5; Qns'01; FRCPC; Psy. Staff, Sunnybrook Health Sciences Centre; (416)480-6100

KUMAR, Sandeep; 203-9425 94 Ave, Fort Saskatchewan AB T8L 1N6; (India)'98; MB BS; (780)998-7757

KUMAR, Saroj; 120-6345 120 St, Delta BC V4E 2A6; Kanpur (India)'75; MB BS; Langs: Hindi; Punjabi; (604)599-9401; Fax. (604)599-9389.

KUMAR, Shree; Queen Elizabeth II HSC, 5F-5788 University Ave, Halifax NS B3H 1V8; (India)'95; MB BS; Staff, Queen Elizabeth II Health Sciences Centre - Victoria General Site; (902)473-5160

KUMAR, S; Smith Clinic, 1-6601 48 Ave, Camrose AB T4V 3G8; (Pakistan)'88; MB BS; FRCSC; OrthSurg (Foot & Ankle Surgery). Staff, Covenant Health - St Mary's Hospital; (780)672-2420; Fax. (780)679-2630.

KUMAR, U Sujana; London Med Dental Bldg, 412-450 Central Ave, London ON N6B 2E8; Bangalore (India)'74; MB BS; CCFP; Langs: Tamil; Kanarese; (519)642-3364; Fax. (519)642-7580.

KUMAR, Vijay; Four Corners Med Bldg, 408-2009 Long Lake Rd, Sudbury ON P3E 6C3; Madras (India)'73; MB BS; DCH; DAB; FRCPC; Peds. Ac Staff, Health Sciences North-St Joseph's Health Centre; Asst Prof Peds, Northern Ontario School of Medicine-Laurentian University; Clinical Asst Prof Peds, University of Ottawa; (705)674-1499; Fax. (705)671-3649.

KUMAR, Vikaash N C; Cancer Centre of Southern Ont, 25 King St W, Kingston ON K7L 5P9; Wes'05; FRCPC; IntMed; MedOncol. Staff, Cancer Centre of Southeastern Ontario; (613)544-2631; Fax. (613)546-8209.

KUMAR, Vilas; Centennial CMH & Brain Injury, PO Box 1000 Stn Main, Ponoka AB T4J 1R8; Hyderabad (India)'88; MB BS; Staff, Centennial Centre for Mental Health & Brain Injury; (403)783-7646; Fax. (403)783-7790.

KUMARAN, Raghunath; 3-115 Maclean Pl, Welland ON L3B 5X9; Mysore (India)'70; MB BS; MRCPsy; FRCPC; Psy. Chief Psy, Niagara Health System - Welland Hospital Site; (905)735-8011

KUMARAN, Vazhkudai S; Royal Alexandra Hosp, 10240 Kingsway NW, Edmonton AB T5H 3V9; Madras (India)'90; Staff, Royal Alexandra Hospital; (780)735-4111

KUMARANAYAKE, Prasanna; 1385 Ontario St, Burlington ON L7S 1G2; McM'95; BSc; FRCPC; IntMed; Gastroent. Ac Staff, Joseph Brant Memorial Hospital; (905)633-7862; Fax. (905)633-8011.

KUMARASAMY, Jeyakumar; Musquodoboit Harbour Med Clini, 7907 Highway 7, Musquodoboit-Harbr NS B0J 2L0; Univ of Kelaniya (Sri Lanka)'97; MB BS; (902)889-2650

KUMARI, Amita; Family Med Clinic, 203-9425 94 Ave, Fort Saskatchewan AB T8L 1N6; (India)'00; (780)998-7757; Fax. (780)998-0636.

KUMBHARATHI, Ravi B; Burntwood Reg Health Authority, 867 Thompson Dr, Thompson MB R8N 1Z4; (India)'00; Staff, Northern Health Thompson Regional Office; (204)788-6375

KUMBHARE, Dinesh A; 240 James St S, Hamilton ON L8P 3B3; Dal'87; FRCPC; PhysMed&Rehab. (905)777-9389; Fax. (905)777-9399.

KUMKA, Gillian L; MUHC-Montreal Gen Hosp, B2 117 2-1650 av Cedar, Montreal QC H3G 1A4; Man'00; CCFP; CCFP(E.M.); Staff, McGill University Health Centre - Montreal General Campus; Lecturer, McGill University Health Centre - Royal Victoria Hospital; (514)934-1934 x42501

KUMLEBEN, Mark A; 9368 Southfort Dr, Fort Saskatchewan AB T8L 0C5; (South Africa)'81; MB ChB; (780)997-0177; Fax. (780)992-2065.

KUMPULA, Iris M; Primrose Med Clinic, 8436 182 St NW, Edmonton AB T5T 1Y7; Alb'73; BMedSci; FRCPC; Psy (Depression). (780)487-7532; Fax. (780)487-8862.

KUMPULA, Joseph V; Westgate Medicentre, 101-9540 163 St NW, Edmonton AB T5P 3M7; Alb'05; CCFP; (780)489-4976; Fax. (780)481-6761.

KUMRA, Rajiv; 5A-5230 Dundas St W, Etobicoke ON M9B 1A8; Tor'88.

KUN, Carmen; Medical Centre, 252-2100 Ellesmere Rd, Scarborough ON M1H 3B7; Timisoara (Romania)'80; Assoc Staff, The Scarborough Hospital - General Campus; Langs: Romanian; (416)438-8000; Fax. (416)289-2520.

KUNANITHY, Vitharani; Kingston Gen Hosp, 76 Stuart St, Kingston ON K7L 2V7; UBC'07; FRCPC; IntMed. Staff, Kingston General Hospital; (613)549-6666

KUNASHKO, Peter G; Brant Community HC-Brantford, 200 Terrace Hill St, Brantford ON N3R 1G9; Tor'85; FRCPC; DiagRad. Staff, The Brant Community Healthcare System - Brantford General Hospital Site; (519)752-7871

KUNCHERIA, Joy; Cambridge Mem Hosp, 700 Coronation Blvd, Cambridge ON N1R 3G2; Lille (France)'89; CCFP; FCFP; Staff, Cambridge Memorial Hospital; Langs: English; French; (519)621-2330

KUNDAPUR, Mirja; The Village of Erin Meadows, 2930 Erin Centre Blvd, Mississauga ON L5M 7M4; Mysore (India)'69; (905)569-7155

KUNDAPUR, Rekha; 207 2nd Ave N, Saskatoon SK S7K 3P2; Bangalore (India)'88; FRCPC; IntMed. (306)664-8833; Fax. (306)653-3166.

KUNDAPUR, Vijayananda; Saskatoon Cancer Centre, 20 Campus Dr, Saskatoon SK S7N 4H4; DMRT; FRCR; Staff RadOncol, Saskatoon Cancer Centre; Clin Assoc Prof, Royal University Hospital; (306)655-2712; Fax. (306)655-2639.

KUNDHAL, Kiran K; Trillium Hlth Ctr-Mississauga, 100 Queensway W, Mississauga ON L5B 1B8; Tor'01; FRCPC; IntMed; Nephrol. Staff, Trillium Health Centre - Mississauga; (905)848-7100

KUNDHAL, Prabhsharan S; 121-9401 Jane St, Vaughan ON L6A 4H7; Tor'04; FRCSC; GenSurg. (905)303-1080

KUNDI, Anjali; 5 Plymouth Rd, Welland ON L3B 3C4; Ott'06; CCFP.

KUNDI, Kusum; 5 Plymouth Rd, Welland ON L3B 3C4; Punjabi (India)'73; MB BS; CCFP; FCFP; Ac Staff, Niagara Health System - Welland Hospital Site; (905)735-1121; Fax. (905)735-5283.

KUNDI, Pran J; 5 Plymouth Rd, Welland ON L3B 3C4; Punjab (India)'70; CCFP; FCFP; Ac Staff, Niagara Health System - Welland Hospital Site; Court Staff, Niagara Health System - St Catharines General Site; Court Staff, Niagara Health System - Port Colborne General Site; (905)735-1121; Fax. (905)735-5283.

KUNDRA, Manu; Edmonton Clinic Health Academy, 11405 87 Ave NW, Edmonton AB T6G 1C9; (India)'95; Staff, Edmonton Clinic Health Academy; (780)248-5575

KUNDU, Sanjoy; The Vein Institute of Toronto, 217 Davenport Rd, Toronto ON M5R 1J3; Tor'94; FACPh; FRCPC; DiagRad (Venous Diseases). Staff, The Scarborough Hospital - General Campus; (416)929-0834; info@theveininstitute.com.

KUNG, Elizabeth Y L; Taunton Health Centre, SS 201 1290 Keith Ross Dr, Oshawa ON L1H 7K4; Monash (Australia)'98; CCFP; (905)721-6876

KUNG, F L Frank; Doctor's Office, 325 Bamburgh Cir, Scarborough ON M1W 3Y1; Tor'91; (416)492-8068; Fax. (416)497-7796.

KUNG, James H; Lion's Gate Hosp, 231 15th St E, North Vancouver BC V7L 2L7; UBC'01; FRCPC; EmergMed. Staff, Lions Gate Hospital; (604)988-3131

KUNG, Lina; 305-4625 Varsity Dr NW, Calgary AB T3A 0Z9; Cal'04; CCFP; (403)400-1363

KUNG, Rose C; Sunnybrook Hlth Sciences Ctre, B728-2075 Bayview Ave, Toronto ON M4N 3M5; Tor'86; MSc; FACOG; FRCSC; ObstGyn (Urological Gynecology). Staff, Sunnybrook Health Sciences Centre; Assoc Prof, University of Toronto; Langs: Cantonese; (416)480-5036; Fax. (416)480-5050; rose.kung@utoronto.ca.

KUNG, Tabitha N; The Joseph & Wolf Lebovic Bldg, 2 001-60 Murray St, Toronto ON M5T 3L9; Tor'05; Rheum; IntMed. Staff, Mount Sinai Hospital; (416)586-4800; Fax. (416)586-8228.

KUNG, Tania Y L; Affinity Med Clinic, 2186-3779 Sexsmith Rd, Richmond BC V6X 3Z9; UBC'06; CCFP; (778)297-7992

KUNGUROV, Maria; Carleton Place & Dist Hosp, 211 Lake Ave E, Carleton Place ON K7C 1J4; McG'01; CCFP; Staff, Carleton Place & District Memorial Hospital; (613)257-2200

KUNICA, Richard D; 9738 Fourth Line, Milton ON L9T 2X9; Tor'62; Court Staff, Halton Healthcare Services Corporation - Milton District Hospital; Court Staff, Halton Healthcare Services Corporation - Oakville Site; Physician, Maplehurst Correctional Inst. & Syl Apps Detention Centre; (905)878-9519; Fax. (905)878-3787; dick@kunica.com.

KUNICKI, Stephane; Clinique TDAH de Montreal, 300-5130 boul Saint-Laurent, Montreal QC H2T 1R8; Mon'95; BSc(Microbiol); FRCPC; Psy. Head Intensive Care Psy, Hopital Louis-H Lafontaine; (514)800-8324

KUNIMOTO, Brian T; Skin Care Centre, 835 10th Ave W, Vancouver BC V5Z 4E8; UBC'83; FRCPC; Derm. Consultant, Vancouver General Hospital - Centennial Pavillion; Clin Assoc Prof, University of British Columbia; (604)875-5151

KUNIMOTO, Dennis Y; University of Alberta Hosp, 2J2 03 WMC-8440 112 St NW, Edmonton AB T6G 2B7; Alb'80; FRCPC; IntMed (Infectious Diseases). Prof Med & InfectDis/Vice Dean Faculty Affairs (Acting), University of Alberta Hospital; (780)492-9727; Fax. (780)492-7303; dennis.kunimoto@ualberta.ca.

KUNJUKRISHNAN, Reghuvaran; Royal Ottawa Hlth Care Group, 1145 Carling Ave, Ottawa ON K1Z 7K4; Kerala (India)'67; FRANZCP; MRC(Psy); FRCPC; Psy (Education). Asst Dir Forensic Services & Psy, Royal Ottawa Mental Health Centre - Royal Ottawa Health Care Group; Assoc Prof, University of Ottawa; (613)722-6521

KUNKEL, Lucinda C; BC Children's Hosp, 4480 Oak St, Vancouver BC V6H 3V4; Wes'06; FRCPC; Psy. Staff, BC Children's Hospital; (604)875-2345

KUNNEMAN, Sara F; Heritage Plaza, 8330 MacLeod Trail SE, Calgary AB T2H 2V2; Omaha (USA)'07; BSc; (403)258-3000; Fax. (403)258-0300.

KUNTZ, Carolyn J; The Group Health Centre, 240 McNabb St, Sault Ste. Marie ON P6B 1Y5; Dal'06; CCFP; (705)759-1234; Fax. (705)759-5683.

KUNTZ, Christiane; 3844 Albion Rd, Gloucester ON K1T 1B1; Ott'81; CCFP; FCFP; Ac Staff Family Med, The Ottawa Hospital - General Campus; Ac Staff Family Med, The Ottawa Hospital - Riverside Campus; Asst Prof Family Med, University of Ottawa; Langs: German; Bilingual(French/English); (613)737-0340; Fax. (613)737-0395; docjock@rogers.com.

KUNTZ, M Eleanor; Medical Center, 203-974 Queen St E, Sault Ste Marie ON P6A 2C5; Wes'70; (705)759-1757

KUNTZ, Michael P; Medical Center, 203-974 Queen St E, Sault Ste. Marie ON P6A 2C5; Wes'70; Ac Staff, Sault Area Hospital - Sault Ste Marie; (705)759-1752

KUNYNETZ, Rodion A W; 104-125 Bell Farm Rd, Barrie ON L4M 6L2; Tor'77; DAB; BSc; FRCPC; Derm (Clinical Trials). Staff, Toronto Western Hospital - University Health Network; Staff, Georgian Bay General Hospital - Midland; Med Dir, Ultranova Skincare Clinical Trials; Asst Prof Med, University of Toronto; Langs: Ukrainian; (705)722-4044; Fax. (705)722-6578.

KUO, Brian Y; St Boniface Gen Hosp, L2035-409 Tache Ave, Winnipeg MB R2H 2A6; Man'94; FRCPC; Anes. Staff, St Boniface General Hospital; (204)233-8563

KUO, Carey P; Victoria Gen Hosp, 2340 Pembina Hwy, Winnipeg MB R3T 2E8; Man'96; Staff, Victoria General Hospital.

KUO, Eugene E C; Rouge Valley-Ajax & Pickering, 580 Harwood Ave S, Ajax ON L1S 2J4; Tor'93; CCFP; Staff, Rouge Valley Health System - Ajax & Pickering Health Centre Site; (905)683-2320

KUO, Kevin H; Univ Hlth Network-Toronto Gen, 8N 884-200 Elizabeth St, Toronto ON M5G 2C4; Wes'05; FRCPC; IntMed; Hem. Staff, Toronto General Hospital - UHN; (416)340-4800

KUO, Susan; 365-7031 Westminster Hwy, Richmond BC V6X 1A3; UBC'91; CCFP; FCFP; (604)270-6200

KUPER, Ayelet; Sunnybrook Hlth Sciences Ctre, HG62-2075 Bayview Ave, Toronto ON M4N 3M5; Tor'01; DPhil; FRCPC; IntMed. Staff/Asst Prof Med, Sunnybrook Health Sciences Centre; (416)480-5495

KUPERBERG, Karol; Centre Medical de la Plaza, 125-6700 ch de la Cote-des-Nei, Montreal QC H3S 2B2; Pomorski Coll. (Poland)'57; Langs: German; French; Polish; Russian; Czech; Serbian; Italian; Spanish; (514)342-2941; Fax. (514)342-3976.

KUPETS, Rachel S; Sunnybrook Hlth Sciences Ctre, T2 001-2075 Bayview Ave, Toronto ON M4N 3M5; Man'92; BSc; MSc; FRCSC; ObstGyn (Gynecologic Oncology). Staff, Sunnybrook Health Sciences Centre; (416)480-4378

KUPEYAN, Kristen A; Ouellette Health Centre, 1083 Ouellette Ave, Windsor ON N9A 4J8; St Matthew's University (Cayman Islands)'04; MHSA; MD; BSc; CCFP; Staff, Hôtel-Dieu Grace Hospital; (519)915-7125; Fax. (519)946-0557.

KUPFERT, Beverly; 103-3910 Bathurst St, North York ON M3H 5Z3; McM'78; FRCPC; Peds. Staff Pt-Time Peds, The Hospital For Sick Children; Court Staff, Sunnybrook Health Sciences Centre; Asst Prof, University of Toronto; Langs: English; French; (416)636-2203; Fax. (416)638-5286.

KUPROWSKI, Gary N; 600 Norfolk St, Windsor ON N9E 1H1; Tor'75; Staff, Hôtel-Dieu Grace Hospital; Staff, Windsor Regional Hospital - Metropolitan Site; Staff, Windsor Regional Hospital - Tayfour Site; (519)969-0580

KUPSH, Christine; Sudbury Reg Hosp-Laurentian, 41 Ramsey Lake Rd, Sudbury ON P3E 5J1; Qns'93; CCFP; CCFP(E.M.); FCFP; Staff, Health Sciences North-Laurentian Site; University of Ottawa; Langs: English; French; (705)675-4790

KUR, Jason K; 208-888 8th Ave W, Vancouver BC V5Z 3Y1; Alb'01; FRCPC; IntMed; Rheum. (604)875-0880

KURBAN, Henry M; Thunder Bay District Hlth Unit, 999 Balmoral St, Thunder Bay ON P7B 6E7; Wes'02; (807)625-8319

KURBIS, Carol A; Winnipeg Reg Health Authority, 2F-490 Hargrave St, Winnipeg MB R3A 0X7; Man'90; FRCPC; CommunMed;CCFP; (204)940-3610; Fax. (204)956-4494; ckurbis@wrha.mb.ca.

KURDYAK, Paul A; Addiction & Mental Hlth-Clarke, 250 College St, Toronto ON M5T 1R8; Tor'97; FRCPC; Psy. Staff, Centre for Addiction & Mental Health (CAMH) - College Street Site; (416)835-8501; Fax. (416)979-6815.

KURDYAK, Stephen A; 200-2475 Bayswater St, Vancouver BC V6K 4N3; Qns'88; CCFP; FCFP; (604)731-0091; Fax. (604)731-0081.

KURDYLA, Margaret T; CLSC des Mille-Iles, 4731 boul Levesque E, Laval QC H7C 1M9; McG'80; (450)661-5370; Fax. (450)661-6177.

KURESHI, Jamila; Royal Alexandra Hosp, 10240 Kingsway NW, Edmonton AB T5H 3V9; (Pakistan)'68; MB BS; Staff, Royal Alexandra Hospital; (780)735-4111

KURET, Verena; BC Women's Hosp & Health Ctre, 4500 Oak St, Vancouver BC V6H 3N1; UBC'05; ObstGyn. Staff, BC Women's Hospital & Health Centre; (604)875-2161

KURGANSKY, Vladimir; 16990 boul Hymus, Kirkland QC H9J 2W2; McG'77; CSPQ; FRCSC; Urol. Ac Staff, Lakeshore General Hospital - Pointe Claire; Langs: Czech; French; (514)695-8104; Fax. (514)426-5157.

KURIACHAN, Vikas P; Foothills Med Centre, C829-1403 29 St NW, Calgary AB T2N 2T9; Qns'01; FRCPC; IntMed; Cardiol. Fellow Cardiol, Foothills Medical Centre; (403)944-3282; Fax. (403)944-2906.

KURIAKOSE, Binny C; 204-595 Montreal Rd, Ottawa ON K1K 4L2; Ott'88; FRCPC; IntMed (Cardiology). Staff, Ottawa Cardiovascular Centre; (613)749-5421

KURIAKOSE, Renju; Saint John Reg Hosp, PO Box 2100 Stn Main, Saint John NB E2L 4L2; Kottayam (India)'98; MB BS; MD; Staff Neurology, Saint John Regional Hospital; Clinical Asst Prof, Memorial Univ of Newfoundland; Lecturer, Dalhousie University; (506)648-7556; Fax. (506)648-7924; renju.kuriakose@horizon.nb.ca.

KURIAN, Annie; Bluewater Health-Norman Site, 89 Norman St, Sarnia ON N7T 6S3; Lille (France)'92; FRCPC; AnatPath. Staff, Bluewater Health - Norman Site; (519)464-4400 x7201

KURIAN, Susan; 257-346 John St N, Arnprior ON K7S 2P6; Sydney (Australia)'97; CCFP; (613)623-2048; Fax. (613)623-6719.

KURIAN, Susannah; The Doctor's Office, 137-1829 Ranchlands Blvd NW, Calgary AB T3G 2A7; Lucknow (India)'58; LRCP(Lond); MRCS(Eng); (403)239-8888

KURIEN, Elizabeth C; Tom Baker Cancer Centre, 1331 29 St NW, Calgary AB T2N 4N2; McG'94; FRCPC; RadOncol (Lung Cancer). Staff RadOncol, Tom Baker Cancer Centre; Langs: Bilingual(French/English); (403)521-3095; Fax. (403)283-1651; elizabeth.kurien@albertahealthservices.ca.

KURITZKY, Robin A; Keary Med Centre, 102-245 Columbia St E, New Westminster BC V3L 3W4; McG'73; ABIM(IntMed&Cardiol); FRCPC; IntMed (Interventional Cardiology); Cardiol. Staff, Royal Columbian Hospital; Langs: Italian; French; (604)524-9571; Fax. (604)524-5322.

KURIYA, Bindee; 2F-60 Murray St, Toronto ON M5T 3L9; Tor'03; FRCPC; IntMed; Rheum. (416)586-4800

KURJI, Ayisha; Royal University Hosp, 103 Hospital Dr, Saskatoon SK S7N 0W8; Cal'04; FRCPC; Peds. Staff, Royal University Hospital; Asst Prof, University of Saskatchewan; (306)966-8552

KURJI, Karimmohamed H; Regional Municipality of York, 17250 Yonge St, Newmarket ON L3Y 6Z1; London (England)'78; MB BS; MSc; FRCPC; CommunMed (Family Medicine); Public Health & Preventive Med. Med Officer of Hlth, Regional Municipality of York; Aj Lecturer Prev Med & Biostats, University of Toronto; Aj Asst Prof, Queen's University; (905)830-4444 x4012

KURKJIAN, Paul S; Kelowna Medical Imaging, 101-3330 Richter St, Kelowna BC V1W 4V5; Tor'88; FRCPC; DiagRad. (250)762-4420; Fax. (250)860-3449.

KURREK, Matthias M; Scarborough Hosp-Birchmount, 3030 Birchmount Rd, Scarborough ON M1W 3W3; (Germany)'86; FRCPC; Anes. Staff, The Scarborough Hospital - Birchmount Campus; (416)399-7640

KURSELL, Paul H; Family Med Centre, 387 Cedar St, Simcoe ON N3Y 2J2; Wes'91; CCFP; (519)426-4821; Fax. (519)426-6649.

KURTZ, Ingrid L; 4004 Dewdney Ave, Regina SK S4T 1A2; Sask'84; FRCSC; GenSurg. (306)757-1606; Fax. (306)757-1607.

KURTZ, J Aube; Rouge Valley-Centenary HC, 6F-2867 Ellesmere Rd, Scarborough ON M1E 4B9; Qns'63; Staff, Rouge Valley Health System - Centenary Health Centre Site; (416)284-8131; Fax. (416)281-7320.

KURTZ, Martin J; Whites Road Med Clinic, 5A-750 Oklahoma Dr, Pickering ON L1W 3G9; Tor'73; Staff, The Scarborough Hospital - General Campus; Staff, Rouge Valley Health System - Centenary Health Centre Site; (905)831-8666; Fax. (905)831-8749.

KURTZ, Robert; William Osler HC-Brampton, 2100 Bovaird Dr E, Brampton ON L6R 3J7; Tor'96; FRCPC; DiagRad;CCFP; CCFP(E.M.); Staff, William Osler Health System - Brampton Civic Hospital; (905)494-2120; Fax. (905)494-6614.

KURTZ, Sonia; North York Family Health Team, 306-3292 Bayview Ave, North York ON M2M 4J5; Tor'80; MSc; Staff, North York General Hospital; University of Toronto; (416)225-8499; Fax. (416)225-1089.

KURTZ, Stuart F; Meadowlands Fam Health Centre, 888 Meadowlands Dr, Ottawa ON K2C 3R2; McG'88; CCFP; Physician, Meadowlands Family Health Centre; (613)228-2882; Fax. (613)228-2856.

KURTZER, Barry D; Drivercheck Inc, PO Box 1186 1 Manley St, Ayr ON N0B 1E0; Tor'75; MD; BSc; Med Dir/Chief Medical Review Officer, Drivercheck Inc; (519)632-9371; Fax. (519)632-9534; bkurtzer@drivercheck.ca.

KURUGANTY, Sailaja; Balmoral Med Arts Facility, 305-1366 Yonge St, Toronto ON M4T 3A7; Qns'96; BSc; CCFP; FCFP; (416)962-2964; Fax. (416)962-2526.

KURUKULA ARACHCHI, Sandhya; Grace Medical Clinic, B024-279 Wharncliffe Rd N, London ON N6H 2C2; Peradeniya (Sri Lanka)'91; MD; MB BS; CCFP; Langs: Sinhalese; (519)850-8774; Fax. (519)850-8775.

KURUNATHAN, Devayani; Medical Centre, 201A-1939 Kennedy Rd, Scarborough ON M1P 2L9; Ceylon (Sri Lanka)'83; MB BS; MRCS(Eng); LRCP(Lond); CCFP; (416)293-7700; Fax. (416)293-9684.

KURUP, Asha; Finch-Midland Med Centre, 218-4190 Finch Ave E, Scarborough ON M1S 4T7; (Singapore)'81; MB BS; MRCOG; FRCSC; ObstGyn. Ac Staff, The Scarborough Hospital - Birchmount Campus; (416)332-8128

KURUP, Lekha M G; Mackenzie Richmond Hill Hosp, 10 Trench St, Richmond Hill ON L4C 4Z3; Kerala (India)'92; FRCPC; Psy. Staff, Mackenzie Richmond Hill Hospital; (905)883-1212

KURUVILLA, John G; Univ Hlth Network-Princess M, 5 110-610 University Ave, Toronto ON M5G 2M9; Tor'98; FRCPC; IntMed; Hem. Staff, Princess Margaret Hospital - University Health Network; (416)946-2821; Fax. (416)946-4563; john.kuruvilla@uhn.on.ca.

KURUVILLA, Mridula S; London Reg Cancer Centre, 790 Commissioners Rd E, London ON N6A 4L6; Kerala (India)'99; MedOncol; IntMed. (519)685-8600

KURUVILLA, Philip G; The Oncology Group, 5F-2100 Bovaird Dr E, Brampton ON L6R 3J7; Tor'86; FRCPC; IntMed; MedOncol. Ac Staff, William Osler Health System - Brampton Civic Hospital; Staff, The Oncology Group; (905)494-6542; Fax. (905)494-6416.

KURWA, Habib A; Richmond Road Diag Trmt Ctre, 1820 Richmond Rd SW, Calgary AB T2T 5C7; (United Kingdom)'88; MB ChB; Staff/Dir Dermatology Surg, Foothills Medical Centre; Dir Dermatol Surg, Richmond Road Diagnostic & Treatment Centre; Assoc Prof Derm, University of Calgary; (403)955-8660

KURYTNIK, Ryan D; Wellington Med Clinic, 84C-3200 Island Hwy N, Nanaimo BC V9T 1W1; UBC'05; BSc; CCFP; Clin Assoc Prof, University of British Columbia; (250)740-2100

KURZ, Christine J; Northern Health Authority, 820-299 Victoria St, Prince George BC V2L 5B8; UBC'00; FRCSC; PlasSurg. Staff Plastic Surg, Women's College Hospital.

KURZENCWYG, David; Ctr Hosp de Lachine, 650 16e Av, Lachine QC H8S 3N5; McG'08; Staff, Centre Hospitalier de Lachine; (514)637-2351; david.kurzencwyg@mail.mcgill.ca.

KUS, Teresa K; Hop Du Sacre-Coeur de Mtl, 5400 boul Gouin O, Montreal QC H4J 1C5; McG'79; PhD; FACC; Cardiol (P.Q.); IntMed (P.Q.) (Cardiac Electrophysiology). Staff Cardiol, Hôpital du Sacre-Coeur de Montréal; Staff Cardiol, McGill University Health Centre - Montreal General Campus; Assoc Prof Pharmacol, Universite de Montreal; Langs: Polish; Bilingual(English/French); (514)338-2222 x2571; Fax. (514)338-2694; teresa.kus@umontreal.ca.

KUSCHKE, Johann M; Drumheller Assoc Physicians, PO Box 5600, Drumheller AB T0J 0Y0; Stellenbosch (South Africa)'85; (403)823-3345; Fax. (403)823-7823.

KUSENTHIRAN, Sri Kasthuri; Albany Med Clinic, 807 Broadview Ave, Toronto ON M4K 2P8; Saba (Netherlands Antilles)'07; (416)461-9471; Fax. (416)461-2710.

KUSHNER, Arthur M; 106-245 Dixon Rd, Etobicoke ON M9P 2M4; Wes'70; Chief Family Pract/Physician Co-Dir, Humber River Regional Hospital - Church Street Site; Court Staff, St Michael's Hospital; (416)247-2193; Fax. (416)247-0402.

KUSHNER KOW, Janet V; Mount St Joseph Hosp, 4E-3080 Prince Edward St, Vancouver BC V5T 3N4; Cal'95; FRCPC; IntMed; GeriatricMed. Staff, Providence Health Care - Mount Saint Joseph Hospital; Langs: Mandarin; (604)874-1411; jkow@canada.com.

KUSKA, Renee; Clinique Med Saint-Agapit, 105-125 rue Principale RR 1, Saint-Agapit QC G0S 1Z0; Laval'84; LMCC; Consultant Med, CSSS de la Mitis; Langs: English; (418)888-3951; Fax. (418)888-3952.

KUSKOWSKI, Agnes A; 201-3370 South Service Rd, Burlington ON L7N 3M6; McM'88; Ac Member, Hamilton Health Sciences Centre - McMaster University Medical Centre; (905)592-4261

KUSLER, Janet L; PO Box 539 Stn Main, Kamloops BC V2C 5L2; UBC'80; DABSM; BAP; ABPN; LMCC; FRCP; FRCPC; Psy (Adult Psychiatry). Assoc Staff, Royal Inland Hospital; (250)374-3222; Fax. (250)374-1256; jkusler@telus.net.

KUSMIREK, Dorothy J; Canmore Gen Hosp, 1100 Hospital Place, Canmore AB T1W 1N2; Jagiellonian (Poland)'06; CCFP; CCFP(E.M.); Staff, Canmore General Hospital; (403)678-5536; Fax. (403)678-5069.

KUSNIERCZYK, John; Northeastern On Reg Cancer Ctr, 41 Ramsey Lake Rd, Sudbury ON P3E 5J1; Tor'90; CCFP; CCFP(E.M.); Staff, Health Sciences North-Laurentian Site; Ac Staff EmergMed, Health Sciences North-St Joseph's Health Centre; (705)675-4700

KUSSIN, Dennis J; Univ Hlth Network-Toronto Western Hosp, 9E452-399 Bathurst St, Toronto ON M5T 2S8; Man'66; FRCPC; Psy. Staff, Toronto Western Hospital - University Health Network; (416)603-5983; Fax. (416)603-5490.

KUSTKA, Sonja S; 201-3910 Bathurst St, North York ON M3H 5Z3; Tor'84; (416)636-7018

KUSZEWSKI, Maciej J; Sunnyside Med Arts Centre, 507A-27 Roncesvalles Ave, Toronto ON M6R 3B2; (Poland)'74; Ac Staff, St Joseph's Health Centre; (416)531-1909; Fax. (416)531-7002.

KUTASH, Anola L; Senior's Clinic-Edmonton Clini, 11400 University Ave NW, Edmonton AB T6G 1Z1; Alb'89; CCFP; Staff, University of Alberta Hospital; (780)407-6947; Fax. (780)407-2006.

KUTCHER, R Walter W; Barrie GI Associates, 301-5 Quarry Ridge Rd, Barrie ON L4M 7G1; McM'84; BSc(Hon); MSc; ABIM; MD; FRCPC; IntMed (Gastroenterology). Staff, Stevenson Memorial Hospital; Staff, Royal Victoria Regional Health Centre; Langs: Ukrainian; (705)721-3344; Fax. (705)721-5522.

KUTCHER, Stanley P; IWK Health Centre, PO Box 9700 Rpo CSC 5850 University Ave, Halifax NS B3K 6R8; McM'79; DCPsy; FRCPC; Psy (Psycho Pharmacology). Staff, IWK Health Centre; Prof, Dalhousie University; (902)473-2464

KUTRYK, Michael J B; St Michael's Hosp, 30 Bond St, Toronto ON M5B 1W8; Man'90; FRCPC; IntMed. Dir Interventional Cardiol Research, St Michael's Hospital; Asst Prof Med, University of Toronto; (416)864-5733; Fax. (416)864-5989.

KUTSCHE, Reta A; Haugen Med Group, 23C-3300 Smith Dr, Armstrong BC V0E 1B1; UBC'05; CCFP; Staff, Vernon Jubilee Hospital; (250)546-8115; Fax. (250)546-2553.

KUTSKYY, Orest; PO Box 67215 Rpo Northland Vlg, Calgary AB T2L 2L2; (Ukraine)'00; CCFP; (403)556-3381

KUTSOGIANNIS, Demetrios J; Royal Alexandra Hosp, 616CSC-10240 Kingsway NW, Edmonton AB T5H 3V9; Qns'89; MHSc; FRCPC; IntMed (Critical Care Medicine). Staff, Royal Alexandra Hospital; Staff, University of Alberta Hospital; Assoc Prof Critical Care Med, University of Alberta; Langs: Greek; (780)735-4096; Fax. (780)735-4032; jim.kutsogiannis@ualberta.ca.

KUTSUKAKE, Paul M; Dixon Med Centre, 201-531 Davis Dr, Newmarket ON L3Y 6P5; Wes'80; Ac Staff, Southlake Regional Health Centre; (905)853-3353; Fax. (905)853-3353.

KUTT, Judith L; London HSC-University Hosp, PO Box 5339 Stn B 339 Windermere Rd, London ON N6A 5A5; Wes'68; FRCPC; Anes. Staff, London Health Sciences Centre - University Hospital; (519)685-8500 x34801; Fax. (519)663-2957.

KUTTY, P Karunakaran; Brampton Endoscopy Centre, 10886 Hurontario St N, Brampton ON L7A 3R9; Kerala (India)'68; MB BS; MRC(UK); AB; FACP; FRCPC; IntMed; Gastroent. Langs: Hindi; Malayalam; Tamil; (905)495-5200; dr.p.k.kutty@rogers.com.

KUTZNER, Morley R; Hys Med Centre, 611-11010 101 St NW, Edmonton AB T5H 4B9; Loma Linda(Calif.) (USA)'76; DAB; BSc; FRCSC; Ophth (Cataract & Glaucoma). Staff, Royal Alexandra Hospital; Clin Assoc Prof, University of Alberta; (780)429-3937

KUUSK, Urve; Seymour Med Clinic, 200-1530 7th Ave W, Vancouver BC V6J 1S3; UBC'76; FRCSC; GenSurg (Surgical Oncology). Staff, BC Cancer Agency Vancouver Centre; Staff, Providence Health Care - St Paul's Hospital; Clin Assoc Prof, University of British Columbia; (604)731-0522; Fax. (604)731-6938.

KUUTAN, Toivo; The Doctor's Office, 245 Eglinton Ave E, Toronto ON M4P 3B7; Tor'71; (416)488-1455; Fax. (416)488-8846.

KUWAHARA, Brian S; Alberta Children's Hosp, 2888 Shaganappi Trail NW, Calgary AB T3B 6A8; Alb'78; FRCPC; Anes (Pediatric Anesthesia). Head Div Pediatric Anes, Alberta Children's Hospital; Asst Prof, University of Calgary; (403)955-2286; Fax. (403)955-7606; kuwahara@ucalgary.ca.

KUWAHARA, Leonard S; 200-2494 Danforth Ave, Toronto ON M4C 1K9; Tor'80; Assoc Staff, Toronto East General Hospital Inc; (416)694-1171; Fax. (416)694-7885.

KUYUMJIAN, Jirair; 207-5855 boul Gouin O, Montreal QC H4J 1E5; Yerevan (Armenia (Republic))'75; Langs: Arabic; Armenian; Bilingual(French/English); Russian; Turkish; (514)335-0931; Fax. (514)335-3463; jirair@kuyumjian.com.

KUYUMJIAN, Raffi S; Agence Spatiale Canadienne, 6767 rte de l'Aeroport, Saint-Hubert QC J3Y 8Y9; Laval'97; CCFP; Langs: English; German; Armenian; (450)926-5785; Fax. (450)926-4707.

KUYUMJIAN, Rita; St Mary's Hosp Centre, 3830 av Lacombe, Montreal QC H3T 1M5; Yerevan (Russia (Federation))'75; FRCPC; Psy (Post Traumatic Stress Disorder). Dir Outpatient Psy Clinic, St Mary's Hospital Centre; Asst Prof Psy, McGill University; Langs: Armenian; Arabic; Turkish; (514)345-3511 x3850; Fax. (514)734-2609; rita.kuyumjian@ssss.gouv.qc.ca.

KUZAK, Nicholai D; Kelowna Gen Hosp, 2268 Pandosy St, Kelowna BC V1Y 1T2; Qns'01; FRCPC; EmergMed; Anes. Staff, Kelowna General Hospital; (250)862-4000

KUZENKO, Nina J L; PsycHealth Centre, PZ 202-771 Bannatyne Ave, Winnipeg MB R3E 3N4; Man'07; FRCPC; Psy.

KUZIK, Brian A; Royal Court Med Centre, 208-1 Quarry Ridge Rd, Barrie ON L4M 7G1; Qns'84; FRCPC; Peds (Respirology). (705)728-3766; Fax. (705)728-3757.

KUZMAR, Dusko N; 205-1223 St Clair Ave W, Toronto ON M6E 1B5; Tor'91; (416)652-7980

KUZMICZ, Jennifer E; Family Medicine Unit, 172-1621 Albert St, Regina SK S4P 2S5; Sask'99; BA; MCFP; CCFP; Staff, Regina General Hospital; Asst Prof Family Med, University of Saskatchewan; (306)766-0444; jennifer.kuzmicz@usask.ca.

KUZMIN, Yulia; The Medical Place, 799 Bloor St W, Toronto ON M6G 1L8; Tor'07; CCFP; (647)349-0053

KUZMINA, Alona; 21 Charles St, Newmarket ON L3Y 3V7; McM'09; CCFP; (905)235-4623

KUZMYK, Susan M; 136 John St W PO Box 809 Stn Main, Bradford ON L3Z 2B3; McM'88; CCFP; Staff, Southlake Regional Health Centre; (905)778-9901; Fax. (905)778-9902.

KUZNETSOV, Fiodar; Queen Elizabeth II HSC-Halifax, 1796 Summer St, Halifax NS B3H 3A7; (Belarus)'04; Staff, Queen Elizabeth II Health Sciences Centre - Halifax Infirmary Site; (902)473-3808

KUZYK, Cathryn J; 204-2004 14 St NW, Calgary AB T2M 3N3; Alb'79; BSc(Hon); CCFP; FCFP; Staff, Foothills Medical Centre; Asst Prof, University of Calgary; (403)282-1038; Fax. (403)282-1071.

KUZYK, Paul R T; Mount Sinai Hosp, 476-600 University Ave, Toronto ON M5G 1X5; Tor'02; FRCSC; OrthSurg. Staff, Mount Sinai Hospital; (416)586-4800; Fax. (416)586-8673.

KVAS, Richard G; Timmins Family Health Team, 208-38 Pine St N, Timmins ON P4N 6K6; Tor'91; BSc; CCFP; FCFP; Staff, Timmins & District Hospital; Staff, White Pines Health Network; (705)267-5111; Fax. (705)267-4212; rkvas@pht.ca.

KVERN, Brent L; Family Med Centre, 500-400 Tache Ave, Winnipeg MB R2H 3E1; Man'84; CCFP; FCFP; Staff, St Boniface General Hospital; (204)237-2863; Fax. (204)231-2648; bkvern@cc.umanitoba.ca.

KVINLAUG, Kylie E; 222-750 Spadina Cres E, Saskatoon SK S7K 3H3; Sask'04; VascSurg; GenSurg. (306)653-3366; Fax. (306)653-8832.

KWA, Poh Gin; Dr Charles A Janeway Child HC, 300 Prince Philip Dr, St. John's NL A1B 3V6; (Taiwan)'65; FRCPC; Peds (High Risk Infants). Staff, Janeway Children's Health & Rehabilitation Centre; Ac Staff, Health Sciences Centre; Asst Prof, Memorial University Of Newfoundland; Langs: Chinese; (709)777-8458; pgkwa@hotmail.com.

KWAK, John J; Surrey Med Arts Bldg, 213-13710 94A Ave, Surrey BC V3V 1N1; Cal'96; FRCSC; Otol (Head & Neck Surgery). Staff, Surrey Memorial Hospital; Langs: Korean; (604)582-9890; Fax. (604)582-9892.

KWAMIE, Yosef K; Lakeridge Hlth Corp-Oshawa, 1 Hospital Crt, Oshawa ON L1G 2B9; Accra (Ghana)'76; MB ChB; FRCPC; Psy. Staff, Lakeridge Health - Oshawa Site; (905)433-2206; Fax. (905)721-4742.

KWAN, Anthony L; Plaza 33, PO Box 23122 Rpo Plaza 33, Kelowna BC V1X 7K7; Tor'99; FRCPC; EmergMed. Staff, Kelowna General Hospital; (250)765-5500

KWAN, Bartholomew P; William Osler HC-Brampton, 2100 Bovaird Dr E, Brampton ON L6R 3J7; (Hong Kong)'80; FRCR; MB BS; DABR; FRCP; FRCPC; DiagRad (Interventional Radiology). Staff Radiol, William Osler Health System - Brampton Civic Hospital; Langs: Cantonese; (905)494-2120

KWAN, Charisse W; The Hosp for Sick Children, 555 University Ave, Toronto ON M5G 1X8; McM'06; FRCPC; Peds; PedEmergMed. Staff, The Hospital For Sick Children; (416)267-2642

KWAN, Christina Y; Polyclinic, 5-4646 Dufferin St, North York ON M3H 5S4; Cal'09; CCFP; (416)222-6160; Fax. (416)222-9604.

KWAN, Eddie; Lethbridge Centre Tower, 404-400 4 Ave S, Lethbridge AB T1J 4E1; Alb'85; FRCSC; Ophth. (403)320-2277; Fax. (403)320-2067.

KWAN, Francis S Y; 1533 Dundas St E, Whitby ON L1N 2K6; Man'68; Ac Staff, Lakeridge Health - Whitby Site; Ac Staff, Lakeridge Health - Oshawa Site; (905)668-6667; Fax. (905)668-6496.

KWAN, Helen H; Canadian Forces Services Ctre, 101 Colonel By Dr, Ottawa ON K1A 0K2; Sask'87; CCFP; (613)945-6545

KWAN, Herman C; 300-2099 152 St, Surrey BC V4A 4N7; UBC'01; FRCSC; Urol. Staff, Peace Arch Hospital; (604)536-1801

KWAN, Irene K W; First Markham Med Centre, 268-3255 Highway 7, Markham ON L3R 3P9; Tor'92; Court Staff Privil, The Scarborough Hospital - Birchmount Campus; (905)940-2882; Fax. (905)940-0262.

KWAN, Janice L; Mount Sinai Hosp, 427-600 University Ave, Toronto ON M5G 1X5; Tor'09; Staff, Mount Sinai Hospital; (416)586-5133

KWAN, Keith F; London HSC-University Hosp, PO Box 5339 Stn B 339 Windermere Rd, London ON N6A 5A5; Alb'88; FRCPC; GenPath. Staff Path, London Health Sciences Centre - University Hospital; (519)685-8500 x36358

KWAN, Kevin; Commercial Street Med Centre, 205-311 Commercial St, Milton ON L9T 3Z9; Wes'05; FRCPC; Urol. (905)875-3920; Fax. (905)875-4340.

KWAN, Lawrence W; Woodside Square, 508-1571 Sandhurst Cir, Scarborough ON M1V 1V2; (Hong Kong)'86; CCFP; FCFP; Langs: Chinese; Cantonese; (416)321-3322; lawrence@vex.net.

KWAN, Man Wai; Fairmont Med Bldg, 1113-750 Broadway W, Vancouver BC V5Z 1J1; McG'72; FRCPC; Psy. Assoc Staff, Vancouver General Hospital - Centennial Pavillion; Clinical Asst Prof, University of British Columbia; (604)879-0975; Fax. (604)879-0976.

KWAN, Manbun; Family Med Clinic, 1200 Lawrence Ave E, North York ON M3A 1C1; Tor'92; CCFP; FCFP; Assoc Member Family Med, North York General Hospital; (416)391-5155; Fax. (416)391-5286.

KWAN, Michael W H; Lakeridge Hlth Corp-Oshawa, 1 Hospital Crt, Oshawa ON L1G 2B9; Tor'84; FRCPC; IntMed; NuclearMed. Staff, Lakeridge Health - Oshawa Site; (905)433-4334; Fax. (905)433-4399.

KWAN, Peter O; University of Alberta Hosp, 8440 112 St NW, Edmonton AB T6G 2B7; Qns'06; Staff, University of Alberta Hospital; (780)407-8822

KWAN, Peter; 5153-2775 Laurel St, Vancouver BC V5Z 1M9; Wes'81; FRCPC; IntMed; Gastroent. (604)875-5862; Fax. (604)875-5447.

KWAN, Peter; Chinook Reg Hosp, 960 19 St S, Lethbridge AB T1J 1W5; Sask'94; BSc; CCFP; CCFP(E.M.); Staff, Foothills Medical Centre; Staff, Chinook Regional Hospital; (403)388-6300

KWAN, Raymond S H; 104-515 Main St, Vancouver BC V6A 2V1; UBC'84; (604)696-6138; Fax. (604)696-6128.

KWAN, Robert P K F; Scarborough North Med Arts, 200-4040 Finch Ave E, Scarborough ON M1S 4V5; NSW (Australia)'82; MB BS; Ac Staff, The Scarborough Hospital - Birchmount Campus; Langs: Cantonese; Chinese; (416)292-3498; Fax. (416)292-9978.

KWAN, Siu Ling; The Credit Valley Hosp, 2200 Eglinton Ave W, Mississauga ON L5M 2N1; Ott'79; FRCPC; Anes. Ac Staff, The Credit Valley Hospital; (905)813-4466; Fax. (905)608-9439.

KWAN, Stephen C K; Centennial CMH & Brain Injury, PO Box 1000 Stn Main, Ponoka AB T4J 1R8; Taipei (Taiwan)'74; Staff, Centennial Centre for Mental Health & Brain Injury; (403)783-7600; Fax. (403)783-7790.

KWAN, Stephen F; University of Lethbridge, PE100-4401 University Dr W, Lethbridge AB T1K 3M4; Alb'86; BSc; FRCSC; OrthSurg (Sports Medicine). Staff, Chinook Regional Hospital; (403)329-2059; Fax. (403)329-2106.

KWAN, Susan Y L; Dr Susan Kwan Inc, 501-4885 Kingsway, Burnaby BC V5H 4T2; (Hong Kong)'79; MB BS; MRCP(UK); FCCP; FRCPC; IntMed; Respir. Head Dept of Med/Ac Staff Respirol, Burnaby Hospital; Consultant, Vancouver Chest Clinic; Clinical Asst Prof Med, University of British Columbia; Langs: Cantonese; Mandarin; (604)432-9182; Fax. (604)432-9281.

KWAN, Tammi Y; The Moncton Hosp, 135 MacBeath Ave, Moncton NB E1C 6Z8; Cal'98; MSc; CCFP; Staff, The Moncton Hospital; (506)857-5111

KWAN, Terry; 402-101 Queensway W, Mississauga ON L5B 2P7; Alb'95; FRCPC; IntMed; Hem. Staff, Trillium Health Centre - Mississauga; (905)272-8159; Fax. (905)272-1043.

KWAN, Winkle B; BC Cancer Agency-Fraser Valley, 13750 96 Ave, Surrey BC V3V 1Z2; (Hong Kong)'86; FRCPC; RadOncol; IntMed. Staff RadOncol, BC Cancer Agency Fraser Valley Centre; (604)930-4032; wkwan@bccancer.bc.ca.

KWANTES, Lindsay N; 1-1230 Alward St, Prince George BC V2M 7B1; UBC'09; CCFP; (250)563-8151

KWAPISZ, Myron M; Queen Elizabeth II HSC, 1276 South Park St, Halifax NS B3H 2Y9; Justus Liebig (Germany)'96; Staff, Queen Elizabeth II Health Sciences Centre - Victoria General Site; (902)473-2331; Fax. (902)473-3820.

KWASNIK-KRAWCZYK, Anne M; 69 Abercrombie Rd, New Glasgow NS B2H 1K4; Warsaw (Poland)'85; CCFP; (902)752-7559; Fax. (902)752-1611.

KWEE, Jeffrey K; 1500 Foster St, White Rock BC V4B 3X8; UBC'04; FRCSC; OrthSurg. (604)531-1171

KWEE, Kai Liang; 1500 Foster St, White Rock BC V4B 3X8; (Singapore)'71; MB BS; FRCSC; OrthSurg. Ac Staff, Peace Arch Hospital; Vis Staff, Surrey Memorial Hospital; Langs: Dutch; Malay; (604)531-1171

KWEE, Roy T G; 2-141 King Rd, Richmond Hill ON L4E 3L7; Tor'84; Staff, Mackenzie Richmond Hill Hospital; (905)773-5566; Fax. (905)773-8464.

KWEE, Yee-Nga Yong; Surrey Med Arts Bldg, 206-13710 94A Ave, Surrey BC V3V 1N1; (Singapore)'71; MB BS; FRCPC; Peds (Pediatric Allergy). Staff Consultant, Peace Arch Hospital; Vis Consultant, Langley Memorial Hospital; Langs: Mandarin; Cantonese; (604)585-4477; Fax. (604)585-6265; ynkwee@gmail.com.

KWIATKOWSKA, Caroline; Clinique Medic Elle, 500-1980 rue Sherbrooke O, Montreal QC H3H 1E8; Wes'90; (514)788-7877

KWIATKOWSKI, Christopher J; Huntsville Prof Bldg, 203-348 Muskoka Rd 3 N, Huntsville ON P1H 1H8; Wes'84; CCFP; FamilyMed(EM). (705)789-2145

KWOK, Bruce C; Health Centre @ 80 Bond, 80 Bond St, Toronto ON M5B 1X2; McM'04; CCFP; (416)864-3011; Fax. (416)864-3099.

KWOK, Carson C C; Coborag Health Centre, 203-316 King St E, Cobourg ON K9A 5R8; Tor'87; (905)373-1280; Fax. (905)373-9335.

KWOK, Desmond C; Hamilton HS-General Site, 237 Barton St E, Hamilton ON L8L 2X2; Tor'76; FRCSC; OrthSurg. Staff, Hamilton Health Sciences Centre - Hamilton General Hospital; (905)527-0271; Fax. (905)381-4153.

KWOK, Edmund S H; The Ottawa Hosp-Civic Campus, 1053 Carling Ave, Ottawa ON K1Y 4E9; Qns'06; EmergMed. Staff, The Ottawa Hospital - Civic Campus; (613)798-5555

KWOK, Eva; 311-4040 Finch Ave E, Scarborough ON M1S 4V5; Tor'94; FRCPC; IntMed; Respir. Assoc Staff, The Scarborough Hospital - Birchmount Campus; Langs: Cantonese; Mandarin; (416)321-2879; Fax. (416)321-2855.

KWOK, Ezra; Aberdeen Health Centre, 2180-4151 Hazelbridge Way, Richmond BC V6X 4J7; McM'04; CCFP; Langs: Cantonese; (604)233-0068

KWOK, Harold K Y; Rosedale Med Centre, 712-600 Sherbourne St, Toronto ON M4X 1W4; Liverpool (England)'76; MB ChB; FRCS(Ed); FRCSC; Urol. Staff, Humber River Regional Hospital - Church Street Site; (416)922-2233

KWOK, Jason W; First Commercial Place, 339-4168 Finch Ave E, Scarborough ON M1S 5H6; (Hong Kong)'76; MB BS; FRCS(Edin); FRCS(Glas); CCFP; (416)291-0051; Fax. (416)291-0552; dr_jason_kwok@hotmail.com.

KWOK, Jimmy C W; 7007 14 St SW, Calgary AB T2V 1P9; Alb'89; BSc; FRCPC; IntMed (Acute Pain Management); GeriatricMed. Staff, Rockyview General Hospital; Langs: Cantonese; (403)943-3294; Fax. (403)212-1230; jimmy.kwok@calgaryhealthservices.ca.

KWOK, Juanita W; 201-600 Sherbourne St, Toronto ON M4X 1W4; (Taiwan)'73; (416)922-4173; Fax. (416)922-5652.

KWOK, Keith; Yee Hong Med Centre/Geriatric, 60 Scottfield Dr, Scarborough ON M1S 5T7; Tor'81; FRCPC; IntMed; Cardiol. Staff, North York General Hospital; Staff Cardiol, Yee Hong Medical Centre; Langs: Cantonese; Mandarin; (416)940-4818; kkwok@nygh.on.ca.

KWOK, Leung Sun; 455 2nd Ave N, Saskatoon SK S7K 2C2; National (Ireland)'86; MB ChB; (306)652-0300; Fax. (306)652-0682.

KWOK, M K Joseph; Keele-Ingram Prof Centre, 210-2221 Keele St, North York ON M6M 3Z5; Alb'75; FRCSC; OrthSurg. (416)242-7570; Fax. (416)242-3633.

KWOK, Matthew M K; The Richmond Hosp, 7000 Westminster Hwy, Richmond BC V6X 1A2; UBC'99; CCFP; CCFP(E.M.); FCFP; Staff, Richmond Hospital; (604)244-5585

KWOK, Raphael M B; 148B-2301 Brimley Rd, Scarborough ON M1S 5B8; (Hong Kong)'75; CCFP; FCFP; Assoc Staff, The Scarborough Hospital - General Campus; (416)291-9552

KWOK, Stephen T F; 175-8100 Ackroyd Rd, Richmond BC V6X 3K2; (Hong Kong)'88; MB BS; CCFP; FCFP; Ac Staff, Richmond Hospital; (604)273-1838; Fax. (604)273-8225.

KWOK, Trevor P H; Health Sciences Bldg, 210-15 Mountain Ave S, Stoney Creek ON L8G 2V6; Wes'87; CCFP; Ac Staff, St Joseph's Healthcare - Charlton Campus; (905)664-8599; Fax. (905)664-1140.

KWOK, Winnie W; Alan Cashmore Centre, 420-1669 Broadway E, Vancouver BC V5N 1V9; Man'98; BScMed; FRCPC; Psy (Child Psychiatry). (604)675-3996

KWOK-LIU, Josephine P Y; St Joseph's Healthcare, 50 Charlton Ave E, Hamilton ON L8N 4A6; Hongkong (Hong Kong)'73; FRCPC; DiagRad. Ac Staff, St Joseph's Healthcare - Charlton Campus; Asst Prof, McMaster University; (905)522-4941 x33110

KWON, Brian K; Blusson Spinal Cord Centre, 6196-818 10th Ave W, Vancouver BC V5Z 1M9; Qns'95; FRCSC; OrthSurg. (604)875-5857

KWON, Elena; Grey Nuns Community Hosp, 1100 Youville Drive West NW, Edmonton AB T6L 5X8; Alb'06; FRCPC; Anes. Staff, Covenant Health - Grey Nuns Community Hospital; (780)445-7264

KWON, Janice S; Leslie Diamond Health CC, 6F-2775 Laurel St, Vancouver BC V5Z 1M9; Qns'94; MPH; FRCSC; ObstGyn (Gynecologic Oncology). (604)875-4268

KWON, Sabrina; Palisades Med Clinic, 12808 137 Ave NW, Edmonton AB T5L 4Y8; Wes'05; (780)457-1100; Fax. (780)457-0033.

KWONG, Charles K F; 6-2 Antrim Cres, Scarborough ON M1P 2N3; Tor'90; Ac Staff, The Scarborough Hospital - Birchmount Campus; Ac Staff, Rouge Valley Health System - Centenary Health Centre Site; (416)321-8158

KWONG, Edward K B; Fairview Med Arts Centre, 201-2200 Fairview St, Burlington ON L7R 4H9; Ott'75; CCFP; Ac Staff, Joseph Brant Memorial Hospital; (905)632-9133; Fax. (905)632-2435.

KWONG, Eugene C K; 27-420 Highway 7 E, Richmond Hill ON L4B 3K2; (Hong Kong)'86; CCFP; (905)695-1133; eugene.kwong@carefirstfht.com.

KWONG, J Stephen; Kelowna Gen Hosp, 2268 Pandosy St, Kelowna BC V1Y 1T2; Sask'86; FRCPC; DiagRad (Thoracic Radiology); NuclearMed. Staff, Kelowna General Hospital; Ac Staff, Burnaby Hospital; Ac Staff, Richmond Hospital; (250)862-4454; Fax. (250)862-4456.

KWONG, Jeffrey C Y; Univ Hlth Network-Toronto Western Hosp, 2W404-399 Bathurst St, Toronto ON M5T 2S8; Tor'01; MSc; CCFP; CommunMed. Physician, Toronto Western Hospital - University Health Network; Scientist, Institute for Clinical Evaluative Sciences; Langs: Cantonese; (416)603-5888 x1; j.kwong@utoronto.ca.

KWONG, Jennifer M; William Osler HC-Brampton, 2100 Bovaird Dr E, Brampton ON L6R 3J7; Tor'03; CCFP; CCFP(E.M.); Staff Emerg, William Osler Health System - Brampton Civic Hospital; (905)494-2120; Fax. (905)451-2690.

KWONG, Juliet; 370-5740 Cambie St, Vancouver BC V5Z 3A6; UBC'99; BSc(Hon); CCFP; FCFP; (604)322-6658

KWONG, Patrick; Universite Concordia, ER 407-1455 boul de Maisonneuv, Montreal QC H3G 1M8; Alb'88; CCFP; (514)848-2424 x3565

KWONG, Sarah L; Heritage Med Research Centre, 362-107 University Campus NW, Edmonton AB T6G 2S2; Alb'02; FRCPC; IntMed; Endocrin&Metab. (780)407-3636

KWONG, Sher P B; Finch-Midland Med Centre, 209-4190 Finch Ave E, Scarborough ON M1S 4T7; Tor'86; Staff, The Scarborough Hospital - Birchmount Campus; (416)297-9225; Fax. (416)297-1075.

KWONG, T Y Paul; Westbram Family Physicians, 104-100 Pertosa Dr, Brampton ON L6X 0H9; Tor'77; Ac Staff, William Osler Health System - Brampton Civic Hospital; Langs: Chinese; Cantonese; (905)451-1244; Fax. (905)451-6955.

KYANZADEH, Fareiborz; Willowdale Med Clinic, 6023 Yonge St, North York ON M2M 3W2; Shiraz (Iran)'93; CCFP; (416)916-2733; Fax. (416)916-2315.

KYCIA, Katarzyna; Forest Hill Fam Health Centre, 2F-491 Eglinton Ave W, Toronto ON M5N 1A8; Alb'05; CCFP; (416)782-6111; Fax. (416)782-5515.

KYDD, Alison S; 206-1650 Terminal Ave N, Nanaimo BC V9S 0A3; Cal'07; FRCPC; IntMed; Rheum. (250)591-4293

KYDD, David W; The Moncton Hosp, 135 MacBeath Ave, Moncton NB E1C 6Z8; Dal'93; FRCPC; NeurPath (Neuro Radiology); DiagRad. Staff, The Moncton Hospital; (506)857-5111

KYDD, Richard W; Medical Arts Bldg, 202-42 Glen Allan Dr, Bridgewater NS B4V 3N2; Dal'80; BSc; Ac Staff, South Shore Regional Hospital; (902)543-6904; Fax. (902)527-1457.

KYEREMANTENG, Kwadwo S; The Ottawa Hosp-Gen Campus, 501 Smyth Rd, Ottawa ON K1H 8L6; Alb'05; FRCPC; IntMed (Palliative Medicine); Critical Care Medicine. Staff, The Ottawa Hospital - General Campus; (613)722-7000

KYEREMATENG, Doris; 10-414 Westmount Dr, Winnipeg MB R2J 1P2; (Other Foreign)'92; BSc; CCFP; (204)255-7430; Fax. (204)255-0643.

KYES, John H; 2234 Chancery Lane W, Oakville ON L6J 6A3; Wes'67; NuclearMed; DiagRad. Dir Dept of Radiol, Halton Healthcare Services Corporation - Oakville Site; (905)842-6449

KYI, Nyunt Nyunt; Northland Med Clinic, 101-4600 Crowchild Trail NW, Calgary AB T3A 2L6; (Burma)'01; MB BS; CCFP; (403)286-3700

KYLE, Beverley; 245-175 Av Stillview, Pointe-Claire QC H9R 4S3; McG'82; BSc; MDCM; CCFP; Langs: English; French; (514)694-6455; Fax. (514)697-4418.

KYLE, David W; Paterson Med Centre, RR 1 45 Wolsley St, Kenora ON P9N 3W7; Cork (Ireland)'10; MB BCh; BAO; CCFP; Staff, Lake of the Woods District Hospital; (807)468-3021

KYLE, Pamela J; 113-31 Sunpark Plaza SE, Calgary AB T2X 3W5; Ott'86; CCFP; FCFP; (403)254-2030; Fax. (403)254-2929; pkyle@shaw.ca.

KYLE, Robert J; Durham Region Health Dept, PO Box 730 Stn Main L2-605 Rossland Rd E, Whitby ON L1N 0B2; Tor'83; BSc; MHSc; FACPrevMed; FRCPC; CommunMed (Public Health & Preventive Medicine);CCFP; Staff, Markham Stouffville Hospital; Court Staff, Lakeridge Health - Whitby Site; Court Staff, Rouge Valley Health System - Ajax & Pickering Health Centre Site; (905)668-7711 x3110; Fax. (905)666-6229.

KYLE, Sharisse E L; Sports Med Centre, 376-2500 University Dr NW, Calgary AB T2N 1N4; Cal'82; CCFP; CCFP(E.M.); FCFP; (403)220-8518

KYNE, Julian A; 201-836 1 Ave NW, Airdrie AB T4B 0V2; Cal'85; CCFP; (403)948-6422; Fax. (403)948-4492.

KYNE, Peter T; Peace Arch Hosp, 15521 Russell Ave, White Rock BC V4B 2R4; Otago (New Zealand)'73; FRCPC; Psy. Consultant Psy, Peace Arch Hospital; Consultant Psy, Providence Health Care - St Paul's Hospital; (604)538-4240; Fax. (604)538-8500.

KYONE, Soe L; Dixie X-Ray Associates, 101-2115 Finch Ave W, North York ON M3N 2V6; Tor'96; FRCPC; DiagRad. Staff Radiol, St Michael's Hospital; (416)744-2655; Fax. (416)744-0581.

KYRIAKIDES, Christine P; 109A-11910 111 Ave NW, Edmonton AB T5G 0E5; Alb'91; BSc(Hons)(Physiol); PhD; FRCPC; Peds. Med Dir, Stollery Children's Hospital; Medical Site Leader, University of Alberta Hospital; Assoc Prof, University of Alberta; (780)455-5437; Fax. (780)452-3220; christine.kyriakides@albertahealthservices.ca.

KYRILLOS, Edmond; Caremedics Med Centre, 18-1910 St. Laurent Blvd, Ottawa ON K1G 1A4; Sher'07; CCFP; Langs: Spanish; Arabic; French; (613)523-5550; Fax. (613)523-5580.

KYRITSIS, Dimitrios; 22 Water St PO Box 40 Stn Main, Kirkland Lake ON P2N 3M6; McG'02; CCFP; Staff, Lady Minto Hospital Cochrane; (705)567-1414; Fax. (705)567-1422.

KYROLLOS, Adel G H; Centrepointe Family Health, 103-117 Centre Pointe Dr, Nepean ON K2G 5X3; Ain Shams (Egypt)'84; FRCPC; IntMed. (613)221-9765; Fax. (613)221-9805.

KYROLLOS, Maggy G H; Monfort Hosp, 713 Montreal Rd, Ottawa ON K1K 0T2; Cairo (Egypt)'84; MB ChB; BAO; FRCPC; GenPath. Staff, Montfort Hospital; Langs: Arabic; Bilingual(French/English); (613)746-4621

KYSELA, Alenia R; Yarmouth Reg Hosp, 60 Vancouver St, Yarmouth NS B5A 2P5; McM'97; CCFP; FCFP; Staff, Yarmouth Regional Hospital; (902)742-3542

KYSKAN, Robert; St Paul's Hosp, 1081 Burrard St, Vancouver BC V6Z 1Y6; McG'08; IntMed. Staff, Providence Health Care - St Paul's Hospital; (604)682-2344

L'ABBE, Daniel; 115-5345 boul de l'Asomption, Montreal QC H1T 4B3; Mon'93; Staff, Hopital de la Cite de la santé; (514)251-9331

L'ALLIER, Johanne; CHUS-Hop Fleurimont, 3001 12e av N, Sherbrooke QC J1H 5N4; Sher'83; FRCPC; Peds. Staff, Centre Hospitalier Universitaire de Sherbrooke-Hopital Fleurimont; (819)346-1110; Fax. (819)564-5398.

L'ANGLAIS, Marie-Eve; 867 av de Bougainville, Quebec QC G1S 3A5; Laval'10; CCFP.

L'ECUYER, Charles; Centre Med Cherbourg, 8150 boul Henri-Bourassa, Quebec QC G1G 4C9; Laval'78; (418)622-4392

L'ECUYER, Genevieve; CSSS du Lac-des-Deux-Montagnes, 520 boul Arthur-Sauve, Saint-Eustache QC J7R 5B1; Mon'10; CCFP; Staff, Hôpital de Saint-Eustache; (450)473-6811

L'ECUYER, Genevieve; Centre Med Laval, 1110 boul Vanier, Laval QC H7C 2R8; Mon'96; Staff, Hopital de la Cite de la santé; Langs: Bilingual(French/English); (450)661-2521; Fax. (450)661-7193.

L'ECUYER, Michel A; 171 Slater St, Ottawa ON K1A 5H7; Ott'86; CCFP; (613)789-3999

L'ECUYER, Serge; GMF de Mascouche, 100-880 Montee Masson, Mascouche QC J7K 2L7; Mon'78; Staff, Hopital de la Cite de la santé; (450)474-2493; Fax. (450)966-0156.

L'ECUYER, Vincent; Ctr Hosp Rouyn-Noranda, 4 9e rue, Rouyn-Noranda QC J9X 2B2; Sher'04; CCFP; Staff, Centre Hospitalier Rouyn-Noranda; Langs: Bilingual(French/English); (819)764-5131

L'ÉPICIER, Marilou; Clinique Med Trait-d'Union, 38 boul Marie-Victorin, Delson QC J5B 1A9; Mon'09; CCFP; (450)633-0123

L'ESPERANCE, Georges; Clinique Med 3000 Inc, 3000 rue Belanger, Montreal QC H1Y 1A9; Nancy (France)'78; FRCS; ATLS; MHA; MHSc; FRCSC; Neursurg. Prof adj clin Med, Universite de Montreal; Langs: Bilingual(French/English); (514)376-7313 x254; Fax. (514)376-2639; georges.lesperance@sympatico.ca.

L'ESPERANCE, Guy; Hotel-Dieu de Levis, 143 rue Wolfe, Levis QC G6V 3Z1; Laval'72; Gastroent (P.Q.). ac Staff, Hôtel-Dieu de Lévis; Langs: English; (418)835-7182; Fax. (418)835-7218.

L'ESPERANCE, Helene; Clinique Med Du Quartier, 1191 av Cartier, Quebec QC G1R 2S9; Laval'75; Langs: Bilingual(French/English); (418)522-1911; Fax. (418)522-1789.

L'ESPERANCE, Marion; CSSS De Sept-Iles, 45 rue du Pere-Divet, Sept-Iles QC G4R 3N7; Mon'04; FRCSC; GenSurg. Staff, Centre Hospitalier Regional de Sept-Iles; (418)962-9761

L'ESPERANCE, Monica; 303-2020 Richmond Rd, Victoria BC V8R 6R5; Qns'99; (250)380-2620; Fax. (250)380-2623.

L'ESPERANCE, Paul; CHUM-Hop Notre-Dame, 1560 rue Sherbrooke E, Montreal QC H2L 4M1; Mon'89; FRCPC; Psy. Staff, Centre Hospitalier l'Université de Montréal (CHUM) - Hôpital Notre-Dame; (514)890-8000; Fax. (514)412-7658; paul.lesperance@umontreal.ca.

L'ETOILE, Michel; Clin Perinatalitie Trois-Rivie, 100-4900 boul des Forges, Trois-Rivieres QC G8Y 1X1; Sher'77; CCFP; (819)373-2303

L'HEBREUX, Marie-Claude; Clinique Med Levis Metro, 150-5700 boul Etienne-Dallaire, Levis QC G6V 8R8; Laval'96; Staff, Hôtel-Dieu de Lévis; Langs: Bilingual(French/English); (418)833-4977

L'HEREAULT, Sylvie; CSSS de Papineau, 155 rue MacLaren E, Gatineau QC J8L 0C2; Laval'94; Staff, CH-CHSLD de Papineau - Pavillon du centre hospitalier; Staff, Hôpital de Papineau; (819)986-3341

L'HEUREUX, Bruno; GMF/CR Concorde, 300 boul de la Concorde E, Laval QC H7G 2E6; Laval'80; BSc; MSc; CSPQ; LMCC; hon Membre, Hopital de la Cite de la santé; (450)667-5310 x2464; Fax. (450)667-5248; lhebru20_siril@ssss.gouv.qc.ca.

L'HEUREUX, Caroline; CSSS de Montmagny-L'Islet, 350 boul Tache O RR 1, Montmagny QC G5V 3R8; Laval'95; Psy. Staff Psy, CSSS de Montmagny-L'Islet; (418)248-0630

L'HEUREUX, Christian; Centre Med St-Francois, 200-2125 boul Lemire, Drummondville QC J2B 8N8; Laval'85; (819)622-1414; Fax. (819)622-1418.

L'HEUREUX, Daniele; Clinique Medicale GMF-1851, 101-1851 rue Sherbrooke E, Montreal QC H2K 4L5; Mon'80; (514)524-7564; Fax. (514)527-5251.

L'HEUREUX, Francine; Centre Royal Comtois, 001-444 McGill St, Hawkesbury ON K6A 1R2; Mon'83; FRCPC; Psy. (613)632-0139; Fax. (613)632-4791.

L'HEUREUX, Jean; 203-1760 boul Jacques-Cartier, Longueuil QC J4N 1C2; Mon'58; MSc; DPH; FRSH; CCBOM; CommunMed (P.Q.); PH (P.Q.) (Aeronautical Medicine). (450)468-2946; Fax. (450)468-2540.

L'HEUREUX, Pierre R; Orleans Medical-Dental Centre, 100-2555 St. Joseph Blvd, Orleans ON K1C 1S6; Ott'74; CCFP; FCFP; (613)830-1298; Fax. (613)830-2170.

L'HEUREUX, Sophie; Ctr Hosp Affilie-Enfant-Jesus, 1401 18e rue, Quebec QC G1J 1Z4; Mon'93; FRCPC; Psy (Psychosis). Staff, Centre Hospitalier Affilié Universitaire de Québec - Hôpital De L'Enfant Jésus; Staff Inst Univ Sante Mentale, Institut Universitaire Sante; Langs: Bilingual(French/English); (418)649-5769; sophie.lheureux.cha@ssss.gouv.qc.ca.

L'ITALIEN, Helene; Centre Med Le Mesnil, 300-1300 boul Lebourgneuf, Quebec QC G2K 2N1; Laval'77; (418)624-1800

LA, Dong-Ky; 2100 rue Frontenac, Montreal QC H2K 2Z3; Saigon (Vietnam)'72; (514)527-9428; Fax. (514)527-8585.

LA, Thuy Phuong; CLSC Saint-Michel, 3355 rue Jarry E, Montreal QC H1Z 2E5; McG'05; CCFP; (514)374-8223

LA BARRE, Marc; Clinique Med Papineauville, GD 303 rue Papineau, Papineauville QC J0V 1R0; Mon'86.

LA BERGE, Shelley-Ann A; 3-1131 Lawson Ave, Kelowna BC V1Y 6T8; Ott'95; BSc; MSc; FRCSC; ObstGyn. Staff, Kelowna General Hospital; (250)763-0640; Fax. (250)763-0646.

LA BORDE, Heather Y; Bowmont Med Clinic, 6535 Bowness Rd NW, Calgary AB T3B 0E8; (Other Foreign)'05; CCFP; (403)247-9797

LA COCK, Mari C; North Battleford Med Clinic, 102-11427 Railway Ave, North Battleford SK S9A 3G8; MB ChB; Langs: Afrikaans; (306)445-4415

LA CROIX, Eileen L; Sunnybrook Hlth Sciences Ctre, 2075 Bayview Ave, Toronto ON M4N 3M5; Cal'95; FRCPC; Psy (General Adult Psychiatry). Staff Psy, Sunnybrook Health Sciences Centre; Consultant Psy, Sunnybrook Health Sciences Centre - Edmond Odette Cancer Centre; University of Toronto; (416)480-4693; Fax. (416)480-6878.

LA DELFA, Ignazio; St Michael's Hosp, 30 Bond St, Toronto ON M5B 1W8; Tor'82; ABIM; FACP; FRCPC; IntMed. Staff Div of Gen IntMed & Med Dir, St Michael's Hospital; Med Dir Palliative Care Unit, Bridgepoint Health Centre; Asst Prof Med, University of Toronto; Langs: Italian; (416)864-5361; Fax. (416)864-5714; ladelfai@smh.toronto.on.ca.

LA FONTAINE, Louise; CLSC Rivieres Et Marees, 22 rue Saint-Laurent, Riviere-du-Loup QC G5R 4W5; Sher'80; Staff, Centre Hospitalier Regional du Grand-Portage; (418)867-2642

LA FRANCE, Monique S; Inverness Consolid Mem Hosp, PO Box 610, Inverness NS B0E 1N0; Man'99; CCFP; Assoc Staff, Inverness Consolidated Memorial Hospital; Langs: English; French; (902)258-3589; Fax. (902)258-3631.

LA HAYE, Andre; Hop Charles Lemoyne, 3120 boul Taschereau, Greenfield Park QC J4V 2H1; Laval'83; FRCPC; Psy. Staff, Hopital Charles LeMoyne; (450)466-5020; Fax. (450)466-5015.

LA HAYE, Bruno; 3605 rue Foucher, Trois-Rivieres QC G8Y 1L1; Laval'79; FRCSC; OrthSurg. Staff, Centre Hospitalier Regional de Trois-Rivieres; (819)693-8389

LA HAYE, Stephen A; Hotel-Dieu Hosp, 166 Brock St, Kingston ON K7L 5G2; Tor'94; FRCPC; IntMed; Cardiol. Staff, Hotel-Dieu Hospital; (613)544-3400 x2155; Fax. (613)544-4749.

LA MERE, Elizabeth A; North York Gen Hosp, 4001 Leslie St, North York ON M2K 1E1; McM'84; FRCPC; DiagRad. Staff, North York General Hospital; (416)756-6289

LA RIVIERE, Christian G; Health Sciences Centre, 820 Sherbrook Ave, Winnipeg MB R3A 1R9; Man'02; FRCPC; EmergMed (Palliative Medicine). Staff, Health Sciences Centre; (204)774-6511

LA ROCHELLE, Pierre; Reseau Sante-Hop Notre-Dame, 1201 6e Av, La Pocatiere QC G0R 1Z0; Laval'90; Staff, CSSS de Kamouraska; (418)856-3540; Fax. (418)856-5916.

LA RUE, Leonard B; 481 1/2 William Ave., Winnipeg MB R3A 0J5; Man'77; BSc; (204)786-4444; Fax. (204)774-1157; hellarue@mts.net.

LA RUE, Suzanne; Inst U en Sante Mentale de QC, 2601 ch de la Canardiere, Quebec QC G1J 2G3; Laval'82; Staff, Institut Universitaire Sante; (418)663-5321; Fax. (418)661-6891.

LAATSCH, A Keith; Heritage Hill Prof Bldg, 330-8180 Macleod Trail SE, Calgary AB T2H 2B8; Alb'79; Staff, Rockyview General Hospital; (403)221-4350

LABA-KACZMAREC, Jessica A; The Roseland Family Med Ctre, 3840 Howard Ave, Windsor ON N9E 3N9; Poznan University (Poland)'07; (519)972-3944

LABADIE, Caroline; CHUM-Hop Notre-Dame, 1560 rue Sherbrooke E, Montreal QC H2L 4M1; Mon'04; Staff, Centre Hospitalier l'Université de Montréal (CHUM) - Hôpital Notre-Dame; (514)890-8000

LABAN, Premakanthie R; St Paul's Hosp, 1081 Burrard St, Vancouver BC V6Z 1Y6; Natal (South Africa)'86; MB ChB; Staff, Providence Health Care - St Paul's Hospital; (604)806-8320

LABARIAS-ROMEO, Jose; MUHC-Montreal Chest Institute, 3650 rue Saint-Urbain, Montreal QC H2X 2P4; Zaragoza (Spain)'71; ac Staff, McGill University Health Centre - Royal Victoria Hospital; Staff, McGill University Health Centre - Montreal Chest Institute; Coroner, Province of Quebec; (514)934-1934 x32574; jose_labarias-romeo@ssss.gouv.qc.ca.

LABART, Christian G; CSSS de la Haute-Gaspésie, 50 rue du Belvedere, Ste-Anne-des-Monts QC G4V 1X4; Mon'70; CSPQ; Anes. Staff, Centre Hospitalier des Monts; (418)763-2261

LABATEYA, Nabil; Centre Med Hochelaga, 9080 rue Hochelaga, Montreal QC H1L 2N9; Ein Shams (Egypt)'77; MB ChB; (514)353-8742; Fax. (514)353-2351.

LABBAF, Saeed; St Mary's Hosp, 4607 53 St, Camrose AB T4V 1Y5; (Germany)'88; Staff, Covenant Health - St Mary's Hospital; (780)679-6100

LABBE, Annie-Claude; Hop Maisonneuve-Rosemont, 5415 boul de l'Assomption, Montreal QC H1T 2M4; Sher'93; FRCPC; MedMicrobiol; InfectDis (P.Q.). Staff Microbiol, Hopital Maisonneuve-Rosemont; Prof, Universite de Montreal; (514)252-3400 x2693; Fax. (514)252-3898; ac.labbe@umontreal.ca.

LABBE, Caroline; Hotel-Dieu de Levis, 143 rue WOlfe, Levis QC G6V 3Z1; Laval'90; FRCSC; Otol (Pediatric Otolaryngology). Staff, Hôtel-Dieu de Lévis; Staff, Centre Hospitalier Paul-Gilbert; Langs: English; (418)835-7119; Fax. (418)835-7213.

LABBE, Gilles; Centre Med Christ-Roi, 102-40 Rte du Président-Kenned, Levis QC G6V 6C4; Laval'79; (418)833-4977; Fax. (418)833-9557.

LABBE, Janel; Ctr Hosp Trois-Riv-St-Joseph, 731 rue Sainte-Julie, Trois-Rivieres QC G9A 1Y1; Sher'98; CCFP; Staff, Centre Hospitalier Regional de Trois-Rivieres; (819)697-3333; Fax. (819)372-3592.

LABBE, Jean C; Medi-Ressources Inc, 506 rue Bonaventure, Trois-Rivieres QC G9A 2B4; Laval'81; MSc; Langs: English; (819)372-9580; Fax. (819)372-0074.

LABBE, Jean; Dir de la Sante Publique, 2400 av d'Estimauville, Quebec QC G1E 7G9; Laval'70; LMCC; FRCPC; Peds (Child Abuse). Médecin, Direction de la Sante Publique de Quebec; Prof Peds, Université Laval; Langs: Bilingual(French/English); (418)666-7000 x534; Fax. (418)666-2776; jean.labbe@ssss.gouv.qc.ca.

LABBE, Lionel J; Pavillon Vertefeuille, 305-311 McArthur Ave, Vanier ON K1L 8M3; Ott'71; Ac Staff, The Ottawa Hospital - General Campus; Lecturer Family Med, University of Ottawa; Langs: English; (613)745-9790; Fax. (613)745-2959.

LABBE, Mario; Clinique Med Familiale Clermon, 500-106 boul Notre-Dame, Clermont QC G4A 1G3; Laval'91; Langs: English; (418)439-3935; Fax. (418)439-4548; mario.labbe@ssss.gouv.qc.ca.

LABBE, Michel; CHUQ-st-Francois D'Assise, 10 rue de l'Espinay, Quebec QC G1L 3L5; Laval'76; IntMed. Chef méd int IntMed Services, Centre Hospitalier Universitaire De Québec - Pavillon De St-françois-d'assise; (418)525-4303

LABBE, Patrick; CSSS de Chicoutimi, 305 rue Saint-Vallier, Chicoutimi QC G7H 5H6; Laval'05; Critical Care Medicine; IntMed. Staff, Complexe hospitalier de la Sagamie; (418)541-1000

LABBE, Paule; CSSS Des Etchemins, RR 1 331 rue Du Sanatorium, Lac-Etchemin QC G0R 1S0; Laval'88; Staff, CSSS des Etchemins; (418)625-8001; Fax. (418)625-3020.

LABBE, Raymond; CHUQ-St-Francois D'Assise, 10 rue de l'Espinay, Quebec QC G1L 3L5; Laval'79; FRCSC; GenSurg (Thoracic Surgery); VascSurg. ac Staff, Centre Hospitalier Universitaire De Québec - Pavillon De St-françois-d'assise; ac Staff, Centre Hospitalier Affilié Universitaire de Québec - Hôpital du St-Sacrement; assoc Prof, Université Laval; Langs: English; (418)525-2279; Fax. (418)525-2264.

LABBE, Robert; Medicentre St-Remi, GD 901 rue Notre-Dame, Saint-Remi QC J0L 2L0; Mon'79; (450)454-3913; Fax. (450)454-3958.

LABBE, Sebastien; GMF Centre Med du Parc, 101-84 rue Court, Granby QC J2G 4Y5; Sher'99; Ophth. Staff, Centre Hospitalier de Granby; (450)375-2074; Fax. (450)375-8719.

LABBE, Sylvain; Clinique Med Notre-Dame Inc, 147 rue Notre-Dame E, Victoriaville QC G6P 3Z8; Sher'85; CCFP; assoc Prof, Universite de Sherbrooke; Langs: Bilingual(French/English); (819)758-3165; Fax. (819)758-0745.

LABBE, Sylvie; CLSC La Region-Sherbrookoise, 1200 rue King E, Sherbrooke QC J1G 1E4; Laval'97; (819)563-2572; Fax. (819)563-8502.

LABBE, Valerie; Hotel-Dieu de Levis, 143 rue Wolfe, Levis QC G6V 3Z1; Laval'98; FRCPC; Peds. Staff, Hôpital de Gatineau; (418)835-7121

LABELLE, Alain; Royal Ottawa Hlth Care Group, 1145 Carling Ave, Ottawa ON K1Z 7K4; Mon'83; FRCPC; Psy. Clin Dir Schizophrenia Prog & Psy, Royal Ottawa Mental Health Centre - Royal Ottawa Health Care Group; Assoc Prof, University of Ottawa; (613)722-6521 x6505; alabelle@rohcg.on.ca.

LABELLE, Andre; CHSLD Ermitage de la MRC, 61 rue de l'Ermitage, Victoriaville QC G6P 6X4; Laval'83; (819)751-8511 x2213

LABELLE, Celine; Inst de Readaptation de Mtl, 6300 av de Darlington, Montreal QC H3S 2J4; Mon'68; Staff, Institut de Réadaptation Gingras-Lindsay de Montréal; (514)340-2085

LABELLE, Eric R; Timmins & Dist Hosp, 1583-700 Ross Ave E, Timmins ON P4N 8P2; Ott'95; FRCSC; GenSurg. Staff, Anson General Hospital; Staff, Timmins & District Hospital; Langs: English; French; (705)360-6071; Fax. (705)360-6072; elabelle@tadh.com.

LABELLE, Genevieve; CSSS de la Haute-Yamaska, 205 boul Leclerc O, Granby QC J2G 1T7; Mon'97; FRCSC; ObstGyn. Staff Gyn, Centre Hospitalier de Granby; (450)372-5491

LABELLE, Hubert B; Hôpital Ste-Justine, 6830-3175 ch Cote-Sainte-Cathe, Montreal QC H3T 1C5; Mon'76; FRCSC; OrthSurg. Orthopedic Surgery, Hôpital Ste-Justine; (514)345-4876; Fax. (514)345-4755.

LABELLE, Jacquelin; Centre Med Jolibourg, 1271 boul Jolibourg, Laval QC H7Y 1Z8; Laval'65; (450)689-2424; Fax. (450)689-9548.

LABELLE, Jean-Francois; CSSS de Sept-Iles, 45 rue Du Pere-Divet, Sept-Iles QC G4R 3N7; Sher'94; Staff, Centre Hospitalier Regional de Sept-Iles; (418)962-9761

LABELLE, Jean-Philippe; Centre de Peri-Maternite, 575 rue Saint-Charles E, Longueuil QC J4H 1B8; Mon'10; CCFP; (450)332-9833

LABELLE, Marie-Esther; Clinique Med l'Envolee, 5025 rue de Salaberry, Montreal QC H4J 1J1; (Other Foreign)'06; (514)331-2323; Fax. (514)333-8534.

LABELLE, Martin J; 1000-1440 rue Sainte-Catherine, Montreal QC H3G 1R8; Mon'76; (514)878-1911; Fax. (514)878-4455.

LABELLE, Martine; CHUM-Hop Notre-Dame, 1560 rue Sherbrooke E, Montreal QC H2L 4M1; Mon'06; CCFP; CCFP(E.M.); Staff, Centre Hospitalier l'Université de Montréal (CHUM) - Hôpital Notre-Dame; (514)890-8000

LABELLE, Mathieu; CSSS du Lac-des-Deux-Montagnes, 520 boul Arthur-Sauve, Saint-Eustache QC J7R 5B1; Mon'00; Staff, Hôpital de Saint-Eustache; (450)473-6811

LABELLE, Maude; CHUM-Hotel-Dieu, 3840 rue Saint-Urbain, Montreal QC H2W 1T8; Mon'04; FRCPC; DiagRad. Staff, Centre Hospitalier l'Université de Montréal (CHUM) - Hôtel-Dieu; (514)890-8000

LABELLE, Paul D; St Paul's Hosp, 1702 20th St W, Saskatoon SK S7M 0Z9; Sask'91; CCFP; FCFP; Staff, St Paul's Hospital (Grey Nuns) of Saskatoon; (306)655-5113; Fax. (306)655-5963.

LABELLE, Pierre F; Bellevue Ophtalmologie, 4135 rue de Rouen, Montreal QC H1V 1G5; Mon'65; DABOph; FRCSC; Ophth. Ac Staff, Hopital Maisonneuve-Rosemont; Chief, Michel-Mathieu Eye Centre; (514)256-0007; plabelle.hmr@ssss.gouv.qc.ca.

LABELLE, Pierre; Centre Med de Chambly, 205-1101 boul Brassard, Chambly QC J3L 5R4; Mon'73; ac Staff, Hôpital du Haut-Richelieu; (450)658-6601; Fax. (450)658-7849.

LABELLE, Robert; Clinique Familiale la Providen, 16405 av Bourdages S, Saint-Hyacinthe QC J2T 4G9; Mon'88; Staff, Centre Hospitalier Honore-Mercier; Langs: English; (450)773-6734; Fax. (450)773-9909.

LABELLE, Sylvain; CLSC des Hautes Laurentides, 757 rue de la Madone, Mont-Laurier QC J9L 1T3; Mon'81; (819)623-6127 x6442; Fax. (819)623-1311.

LABELLE, Sylvie; Clinique Med de la Marine, 101-303 boul de la Marine, Varennes QC J3X 2G6; Sher'88; (450)652-9616; Fax. (450)652-4345.

LABERGE, Anne-Marie; Hôpital Ste-Justine, 3175 ch Cote-Sainte-Catherine, Montreal QC H3T 1C5; Mon'98; FRCPC; MedGenetics. Staff, Hôpital Ste-Justine; (514)345-4931 x4727; Fax. (514)345-4766.

LABERGE, Caroline; UMF Laurier, 2875 boul Laurier, Quebec QC G1V 2M2; Laval'03; CCFP; Staff Obst, Complexe hospitalier de la Sagamie; Langs: English; Spanish; (418)654-2701

LABERGE, Christiane; Centre De Sante de la Rive, 8809A boul LaSalle, LaSalle QC H8P 1Z4; Mon'76; (514)366-6004; Fax. (514)364-6297.

LABERGE, Claude; Min of Health & Social Service, RC 03-201 boul Cremazie E, Montreal QC H2M 1L2; Mon'83; Consultant Public Health, Ministry of Health & Social Services-Quebec; Langs: Bilingual(English/French); (514)873-9976; Fax. (514)873-9997; claude.laberge@msss.gouv.qc.ca.

LABERGE, Francis; Hôpital Laval, 2725 ch Sainte-Foy, Quebec QC G1V 4G5; Laval'77; FRCPC; IntMed; Respir. Head Pulmonary Med, Hôpital Laval; Consultant, CSSS de Quebec-Sud; Université Laval; (418)656-4747; Fax. (418)656-4762.

LABERGE, J Roger; Clinique Med Chateauguay, 120 boul Saint-Jean-Baptiste, Chateauguay QC J6K 3A9; Mon'63; ac Membre, Hôpital Anna-Laberge; hon Membre, Centre Hospitalier de LaSalle; Coroner, Province of Quebec; Langs: English; (450)691-8191; Fax. (450)691-8568; roger_laberge@ssss.gouv.qc.ca.

LABERGE, Janick; CSST Direction Reg de Quebec, CP 4900 Succ Terminus 4D59-425 rue du Pont, Quebec QC G1K 7S6; Laval'86; (418)266-4000 x4126; Fax. (418)266-4430.

LABERGE, Jean; Hotel-Dieu d'Arthabaska, 5 rue des Hospitalieres, Victoriaville QC G6P 6N2; Laval'70; DiagRad. Diagnostic-Radiology, Hotel-Dieu d'Arthabaska; (819)357-6043

LABERGE, Jean-Martin; MUHC-Montreal Children's Hosp, C 820-2300 rue Tupper, Montreal QC H3H 1P3; Laval'77; AB; FACS; FRCSC; GenSurg; PedGenSurg. Att Staff, McGill University Health Centre - Montreal Children's Hospital; Consultant, Hôpital Ste-Justine; Prof Surg, McGill University; Langs: Spanish; Bilingual(English/French); (514)412-4400 x24498; Fax. (514)412-4289; jean-martin.laberge@muhc.mcgill.ca.

LABERGE, Julie; CLSC Chateauguay, 95 av de la Verdure, Chateauguay QC J6K 0E8; Mon'99; CCFP; (450)699-3333

LABERGE, Lauren E; Parkdale Med Tower, 308-1081 Carling Ave, Ottawa ON K1Y 4G2; Ott'07; FRCPC; Derm. (613)722-8532

LABERGE, Louise; Clinique Med du Faubourg, 145-1160 boul Saint-Joseph, Gatineau QC J8Z 1T3; Mon'78; CCFP; FCFP; Consultant, Hull Hospital; (819)595-1991; Fax. (819)595-0486.

LABERGE, Marc Andre; CSSS Pierre Boucher, 1333 rue Jacques-Cartier E, Longueuil QC J4M 2A5; Mon'96; IntMed. Staff, Centre Hospitalier Pierre Boucher; (819)764-5131

LABERGE, Melanie; I R D P Q-Site Francois-Charon, D111 8-525 boul Wilfrid-Hamel, Quebec QC G1M 2S8; Laval'99; Staff, Hôpital Regional Rimouski; Staff, Centre Hospitalier Universitaire De Québec - Pavillon De St-françois-d'assise; (418)525-9141 x6312

LABERGE, Micheline; 407 rue Melancon, Saint-Jerome QC J7Z 4K3; Mon'76; (450)431-6977

LABERGE, Philippe-Yves; CHUQ-Ctr Hosp Univ Laval, 2705 boul Laurier, Quebec QC G1V 4G2; Laval'85; FRCSC; ObstGyn (Endoscopic Gynecology Surgery). Staff, Centre Hospitalier Universitaire de Quebec-CHUL; Dir, Centre Hospitalier Affilié Universitaire de Québec - Hôpital du St-Sacrement; (418)656-4141; Fax. (418)691-5717.

LABERGE, Pierre; Clinique de Med Familiale, 501-2120 rue Sherbrooke E, Montreal QC H2K 1C3; Laval'60; Psy (P.Q.). (514)521-7871

LABERGE, Pierre-R.; CSSS de Sept-Iles, 45 rue Du Pere-Divet, Sept-Iles QC G4R 3N7; Laval'75; Microbio & Infect Dis (P.Q.); MedMicrobiol. Staff, Centre Hospitalier Regional de Sept-Iles; Langs: Bilingual(French/English); (418)962-9761 x2567; pierre_laberge@ssss.gouv.qc.ca.

LABERGE, Renee; CLSC de Limoilou, 1405 ch de la Canardiere, Quebec QC G1J 0A7; Laval'94; Langs: Italian; English; (418)529-2572; Fax. (418)648-6736.

LABERGE, Robert C; Children's Hosp Eastern Ont, 401 Smyth Rd, Ottawa ON K1H 8L1; Wes'05; FRCPC; Peds. Staff Peds, Children's Hospital of Eastern Ontario (CHEO); (613)737-7600 x2108

LABERGE, Sophie; Hôpital Ste-Justine, 3175 ch Cote-Sainte-Catherine, Montreal QC H3T 1C5; Laval'85; FRCPC; Peds; Respir. Staff, Hôpital Ste-Justine; (514)345-4931 x5409; Fax. (514)345-4804.

LABERGE, Sophie; Ctr Hosp Anna-Laberge, 200 boul Brisebois, Chateauguay QC J6K 4W8; Mon'96; CCFP; Staff, Hôpital Anna-Laberge; (450)699-2425

LABERGE, Sophie; Ctr Hosp Affilie-St-Sacrement, 1050 ch Sainte-Foy, Quebec QC G1S 4L8; Sher'91; FRCPC; AnatPath. Staff, Centre Hospitalier Affilié Universitaire de Québec - Hôpital du St-Sacrement; (418)682-7511

LABERGE, Stephane; Centre Hosp Honore-Mercier, 2750 boul Laframboise, Saint-Hyacinthe QC J2S 4Y8; Mon'94; CSPQ; Anes (P.Q.). Staff, Centre Hospitalier Honore-Mercier; (450)771-3353

LABERGE-MALO, Marie E; Hôpital Ste-Justine, 3175 ch Cote-Sainte-Catherine, Montreal QC H3T 1C5; Mon'77; FRCPC; Peds; PhysMed&Rehab. Chief-Physical Med, Hôpital Ste-Justine; (514)345-4788 x5774

LABIB, Mohamed A M; The Ottawa Hosp-Civic Campus, C2 2246-1053 Carling Ave, Ottawa ON K1Y 4E9; McG'06; MDCM; Neursurg. Staff, The Ottawa Hospital - Civic Campus; (613)798-5555

LABIB, Noura A M E; St Joseph's Healthcare, 50 Charlton Ave E, Hamilton ON L8N 4A6; McG'08; (905)522-4941

LABIB, Yasser M A; Thunder Bay Reg HSC-T-Bay, 980 Oliver Rd, Thunder Bay ON P7B 6V4; Cairo (Egypt)'87; Staff, Thunder Bay Regional Health Sciences Centre; (807)684-6027

LABINAZ, Marino; Univ of Ottawa Heart Institute, H1264-40 Ruskin St, Ottawa ON K1Y 4W7; Qns'87; FRCPC; IntMed (Interventional Cardiology); Cardiol. Staff, University of Ottawa Heart Institute; Staff Cardiol, The Ottawa Hospital - Civic Campus; Prof Med, University of Ottawa; (613)761-5427; Fax. (613)761-4690.

LABINE, Robert; 200-30 rue de Martigny O, Saint-Jerome QC J7Y 2E9; Sher'80; Psy (P.Q.) (Psychoanalysis). Staff Psy, Centre Hospitalier Laurentien; Langs: Bilingual(French/English); (450)569-9922; Fax. (450)569-5399; dr.labine@net.ca.

LABISSONNIERE, Paul-Emile; Groupe Sante Physimed, 121-6363 rte Transcanadienne, Saint-Laurent QC H4T 1Z9; Mon'85; (514)747-8888; Fax. (514)747-4705.

LABIYARATNE, W W Chamindra P; Boyd Med Centre, 392 Portage Ave, Winnipeg MB R3C 0C7; (Other Foreign)'95; CCFP; (204)415-2740

LABONTE, Anne; CFB Borden, PO Box 1000, Borden ON L0M 1C0; Mon'81; FRCPC; Psy (Geriatric Psychiatry). Staff, Royal Victoria Regional Health Centre; (705)424-1200 x3523; Fax. (705)423-2088; labonte.am2@forces.gc.ca.

LABONTE, Chantal; CLSC Laurier-Station, RR 1 135 rue de la Station, Laurier-Station QC G0S 1N0; Laval'95; (418)728-3435; Fax. (418)728-2233.

LABONTE, Chantal; CLSC-CHSLD-Meilleur, 193 boul Lacombe, Repentigny QC J5Z 3C4; Mon'86; NuclearMed (P.Q.). (450)654-9012 x322; Fax. (450)654-0993.

LABONTE, Edith; Ctr Hosp Affilie-Enfant-Jesus, 1401 18e rue, Quebec QC G1J 1Z4; Laval'84; FRCPC; Psy. Staff, Centre Hospitalier Affilié Universitaire de Québec - Hôpital De L'Enfant Jésus; (418)649-5769; Fax. (418)649-5934.

LABONTE, Genevieve; Clin Med Familiale Plessisvill, 1971 rue Bilodeau, Plessisville QC G6L 3J1; Laval'07; CCFP; (819)362-6337; Fax. (819)362-9147.

LABONTE, Isabelle; Hôpital Laval, 2725 ch Sainte-Foy, Quebec QC G1V 4G5; Sher'90; FRCPC; IntMed (Cardiology). Staff, Hôpital Laval; adj Prof, Université Laval; Langs: Bilingual(French/English); (418)656-8711; Fax. (418)656-4587.

LABONTE, Pierre; Clinique Med Deux-Montagnes, 201 9e av, Deux-Montagnes QC J7R 3M1; Mon'77; Staff, Centre Hospitalier l'Université de Montréal (CHUM) - Hôtel-Dieu; (450)472-7520; Fax. (450)472-0886.

LABONTE, Roger A; Ctr Hosp Pierre-Janet, 20 rue Pharand, Gatineau QC J9A 1K7; Ott'98; FRCPC; Psy. Staff, Centre Hospitalier Pierre-Janet; (819)776-8001; Fax. (819)771-4727.

LABONTE, Roger E; Dr Roger Labonte Med Prof Corp, 2-1500 Paris St, Sudbury ON P3E 3B8; Ott'81; FACC; FRCPC; IntMed (Invasive Cardiology); Cardiol. Staff, Health Sciences North-Laurentian Site; Staff, West Nipissing General Hospital; Teacher Family Med Residency Prog, Northern Ontario School of Medicine; Langs: French; (705)522-7346; Fax. (705)523-6806; cardio@isys.ca.

LABONTE, Sebastien; CHUQ-Hotel-Dieu de Quebec, 11 Cote du Palais, Quebec QC G1R 2J6; Sher'95; CSPQ; FRCPC; AnatPath. Staff, Centre Hospitalier Universitaire de Québec (CHUQ) - Siege Social; (418)691-5233

LABOSSIERE, Emil J; 440 Comer St, Williams Lake BC V2G 1T7; UBC'89; Staff, Cariboo Memorial Hospital and Health Centre; (250)398-8499; Fax. (250)398-8692; emil_labossiere@telus.net.

LABOURDETTE, Annie; Hotel-Dieu de Levis, 143 rue Wolfe, Levis QC G6V 3Z1; Laval'98; DiagRad. Staff, Hôtel-Dieu de Lévis; (418)835-7121 x7901

LABOURDETTE, Claudine; CSSS de l'Hématite, GD 1 rue de l'Aquilon, Fermont QC G0G 1J0; Laval'78; Staff, CLSC de l'Hématite; (418)287-5461; Fax. (418)287-5465; clau_lab2@hotmail.com.

LABOW, Stanley S; Riverside Prof Centre, 402-1919 Riverside Dr, Ottawa ON K1H 1A2; Ott'61; FRCSC; PlasSurg (Plastic & Reconstructive Surgery). Staff, The Ottawa Hospital - Riverside Campus; University of Ottawa; (613)733-7817; Fax. (613)733-7817; stanley.labow@gmail.com.

LABRADOR FEBLES, Jose; Meadow Lake Assoc Clinic, PO Box 1510, Meadow Lake SK S9X 1Z1; Langs: Spanish; (306)236-5661

LABRANCHE, Rachelle S; Colborne Family Med Centre, 612 Colborne St, London ON N6B 2V2; Cal'98; CCFP; (519)673-1962; Fax. (519)673-3758.

LABRECHE, Jacques; CSSS Drummond-Hop Sainte-Croix, 570 rue Heriot, Drummondville QC J2B 1C1; Mon'92; FRCSC; GenSurg. Staff, Hôpital Sainte-croix; Langs: English; (819)478-6464; Fax. (819)472-3105.

LABRECQUE, Alain; CHUQ-Hotel-Dieu de Quebec, 11 Cote du Palais, Quebec QC G1R 2J6; Laval'84; CSPQ; FRCPC; Anes. Staff, Centre Hospitalier Universitaire de Québec (CHUQ) - Siege Social; (418)691-5323

LABRECQUE, Carole; CSSS de Beauce-Etchemin, 1515 17e rue, Saint-Georges QC G5Y 4T8; Laval'08; CCFP; Staff, Centre Hospitalier Beauce-Etchemin; (418)288-2031; Fax. (418)227-3825.

LABRECQUE, Catherine; Clin d'Endocrin Trois-Rivieres, 5050 boul des Forges, Trois-Rivieres QC G8Y 1X2; Mon'03; Endocrin&Metab; IntMed. (819)379-1442; Fax. (819)379-9708.

LABRECQUE, Denis; Clinique D'Urgence St-Denis, 101-8415 rue Saint-Denis, Montreal QC H2P 2H1; Laval'76; (514)388-5723; Fax. (514)388-3423.

LABRECQUE, Eric; Clinique Med De Montmagny, 100-83 av de la Fabrique, Montmagny QC G5V 2J3; Laval'94; (418)248-4933; Fax. (418)248-2778; eric.labrecque@gmf.gouv.qc.ca.

LABRECQUE, Gilles F; CSSS de Montmagny-l'Islet, RR 1 430 rue Jean-Leclerc, St-Jean-Port-Joli QC G0R 3G0; Laval'83; Staff, CSSS de Montmagny-l'Islet; Langs: Bilingual(English/French); (418)598-3355; gilleslabrecque@globetrotter.net.

LABRECQUE, Josee; CSSS des Iles, 430 ch Principal, Cap-aux-Meules QC G4T 1G7; Sher'96; Staff, Hôpital de l'Archipel; (418)986-2121

LABRECQUE, Judith; CHUQ-Ctr Hosp Univ Laval, 4221-2705 boul Laurier, Quebec QC G1V 4G2; Laval'89; FRCPC; Psy. Staff, Centre Hospitalier Universitaire de Quebec-CHUL; (418)654-2177; Fax. (418)654-2716.

LABRECQUE, Katherine; Carrefour Sante du Granit, 3569 rue Laval, Lac-Megantic QC G6B 1A5; Laval'09; Staff, Carrefour Sante Granit; (819)583-0330

LABRECQUE, Louise-Genevieve; CHUM-Hotel-Dieu, 3840 rue Saint-Urbain, Montreal QC H2W 1T8; Mon'82; ABIM; FRCPC; IntMed; InfectDis (P.Q.); MedMicrobiol. Staff, Centre Hospitalier l'Université de Montréal (CHUM) - Hôtel-Dieu; adj Prof, Universite de Montreal; (514)890-8000; Fax. (514)412-7290.

LABRECQUE, Manon; Hop Du Sacre-Coeur de Mtl, 5400 boul Gouin O, Montreal QC H4J 1C5; Mon'86; ABIM; FRCPC; IntMed; Respir. Staff, Hôpital du Sacre-Coeur de Montréal; (514)338-2162

LABRECQUE, Michel; CHUQ-St-Francois D'Assise, 10 rue de l'Espinay, Quebec QC G1L 3L5; Mon'77; CCFP; FCFP; Staff, Centre Hospitalier Universitaire De Québec - Pavillon De St-françois-d'assise; (418)525-4425; Fax. (418)525-4322.

LABRECQUE, Michele A; Hop Du Sacre-Coeur De Mtl, 532-5400 boul Gouin O, Montreal QC H4J 1C5; Mon'01; CCFP; CCFP(E.M.); Staff, Hôpital du Sacre-Coeur de Montréal; (514)338-2002; Fax. (514)338-3513.

LABRECQUE, Nancy; CHUQ-Ctr Hosp Univ Laval, 2705 boul Laurier, Quebec QC G1V 4G2; Laval'99; Staff, Centre Hospitalier Universitaire de Québec (CHUQ) - Siege Social; (418)525-4444; nancylabrecque73@hotmail.com.

LABRECQUE, Nathalie; Ctr Hosp Affilie-St-Sacrement, 1050 ch Sainte-Foy, Quebec QC G1S 4L8; Laval'85; FRCSC; Ophth. Staff, Centre Hospitalier Affilié Universitaire de Québec - Hôpital du St-Sacrement; Head Ophth, Université Laval; (418)682-7680; Fax. (418)682-7534.

LABRECQUE, Pascal; CHUQ-Hotel-Dieu De Quebec, 11 Cote Du Palais, Quebec QC G1R 2J6; Laval'80; FRCP; FRCPC; Anes. Chef, Centre Hospitalier Universitaire de Québec (CHUQ) - Siege Social; (418)691-5323; Fax. (418)691-5097; pascal.labrecque@chuq.qc.ca.

LABRECQUE, Paul A; Sheldon M Chumir Urgent Care, 1213 4 St SW, Calgary AB T2R 0X7; McM'95; BSc; MSc; CCFP; CCFP(E.M.); FCFP; (403)955-6011; Fax. (403)955-6023.

LABRECQUE, Paul; CSSS Haut-Richelieu-Rouville, 978 boul du Seminaire N, St-Jean-sur-Richel QC J3A 1E5; Sher'92; (450)358-2572

LABRECQUE, Raymonde; CHUM-Hop Notre-Dame, 1560 rue Sherbrooke E, Montreal QC H2L 4M1; Mon'73; FRCPC; Neur. Ac Staff, Institut Universitaire de Gériatrie de Montréal; ac Staff, Centre Hospitalier l'Université de Montréal (CHUM) - Hôpital Notre-Dame; adj Prof, Universite de Montreal; (514)890-8237

LABRECQUE, Susan; Univ de Sherbrooke, 2500 boul de l'Universite, Sherbrooke QC J1K 2R1; Sher'86; CCFP; (819)821-7593

LABRECQUE-SAUVE, Sebastien; Groupe Sante Physimed, 6363 rte Transcanadienne, Saint-Laurent QC H4T 1Z9; McG'08; CCFP; (514)747-8888

LABREQUE, Luc; Centre Med Acton, CP 1589 967 rue Boulay, Acton Vale QC J0H 1A0; Laval'71; ac Staff, Hôpital Sainte-croix; (450)546-4711; Fax. (450)546-4720; ll@actonmedical.com.

LABRIE, Christian; CSSS Pierre Boucher, 1333 boul Jacques-Cartier E, Longueuil QC J4M 2A5; Sher'89; Psy. Ac Member Psy, Centre Hospitalier Pierre Boucher; Langs: English; (450)468-8401; Fax. (450)468-8403; clabrie.md@sympatico.ca.

LABRIE, Christiane; CSSS du Val-Saint-Francois, 23 rue Ambroise-Dearden, Windsor QC J1S 1G8; Mon'96; Langs: English; (819)845-2751; Fax. (819)845-4269.

LABRIE, Claude; CHUQ-Ctr Hosp Univ Laval, 2705 boul Laurier, Quebec QC G1V 4G2; Laval'85; Staff, Centre Hospitalier Universitaire de Quebec-CHUL; Langs: Bilingual(French/English); (418)654-2296; Fax. (418)654-2761; claude.labrie@crchul.ulaval.ca.

LABRIE, Eric; CSSS de Trois-Rivières, 1991 boul du Carmel, Trois-Rivieres QC G8Z 3R9; Laval'96; Staff, CSSS de Trois-Rivières; (819)697-3333

LABRIE, Isabelle; CLSC Grande Riviere, 425 rue Leguerrier, Gatineau QC J9H 6N8; Laval'84; LMCC; Langs: English; (819)684-2251

LABRIE, Marie-Claude; Clinique Med Masson-Angers, 101-1100 Ch De Montreal O, Gatineau QC J8M 2A9; Laval'99; (819)281-1509; Fax. (819)281-1741.

LABRIE, Martin J; Foothills South Tower, 710-3031 Hospital Dr NW, Calgary AB T2N 2T8; Cal'81; CCFP; FCFP; Staff, Foothills Medical Centre; (403)944-2304; Fax. (403)270-9652.

LABRIE, Michel; Ctr Hosp Affilie-Enfant-Jesus, 1401 18e rue, Quebec QC G1J 1Z4; Laval'83; FRCPC; IntMed; Respir. Staff, Centre Hospitalier Affilié Universitaire de Québec - Hôpital De L'Enfant Jésus; (418)649-5743

LABRIE, Nicole; Maternity Care Clinic, 178 96 Ave NE, Calgary AB T3K 6G4; Qns'09; CCFP; Staff, Maternity Care Clinic; (403)735-4922

LABRIE, Robert; Clinique Med de Montmagny, 100-83 av de la Fabrique, Montmagny QC G5V 2J3; Laval'69; (418)248-4933; Fax. (418)248-2778; robert.labrie@gmf.gouv.qc.ca.

LABRIE, Vincent; Ctr Hosp Anna-Laberge, 200 boul Brisebois, Chateauguay QC J6K 4W8; Mon'06; CCFP; CCFP(E.M.); Staff, Hôpital Anna-Laberge; (450)699-2425

LABROSSE, Carl; CSSS Drummond-Hop Sainte-Croix, 570 rue Heriot, Drummondville QC J2B 1C1; Mon'05; FRCPC; Anes. Staff, Hôpital Sainte-croix; (819)478-6464

LABROSSE, Josee L; 1048 North River Rd, Ottawa ON K1K 3V4; McM'88; Langs: English; French; (613)842-8187; Fax. (613)842-8188.

LABROSSE, Julie M; CSSS du Sud de Lanaudière, 911 montee des Pionniers, Terrebonne QC J6V 2H2; Mon'03; FRCPC; DiagRad. Staff, Centre Hospitalier Pierre le Gardeur; (450)654-7525

LABROUSSE, Jean-Marie; CLSC des Faubourgs, 1250 rue Sanguinet, Montreal QC H2X 3E7; Mon'73; (514)527-2361

LABROUSSE, Yanouchka; UMF Charles Lemoyne, 201-299 boul Sir-Wilfrid-Lauri, Saint-Lambert QC J4R 2L1; Mon'01; Staff, Hopital Charles LeMoyne; (450)466-5630; Fax. (450)466-5631.

LABRUZZO, Peter; 729 Devonshire Ave, Woodstock ON N4S 5R3; Wes'92; Langs: Italian; (519)533-5485; Fax. (519)533-6444; drlabruzzo@execulink.com.

LABUDA, Anna; Halton HCS Corp-Oakville, 327 Reynolds St, Oakville ON L6J 3L7; Wes'05; FRCPC; PhysMed&Rehab. Staff, Halton Healthcare Services Corporation - Oakville Site; (905)845-2571; Fax. (905)338-4453.

LABUDA, Marcin; Lakeshore General Hosp, 160 av Stillview, Pointe-Claire QC H9R 2Y2; Mon'04; IntMed. Staff, Lakeshore General Hospital - Pointe Claire; (514)630-2225

LABUDA, Zuzanna; Ctr Hosp de LaSalle, 8585 Tsse Champlain, LaSalle QC H8P 1C1; Mon'10; CCFP; Staff, Centre Hospitalier de LaSalle; (514)362-8000

LABUSCHAGNE, Barend C J; Regina General Hosp, 1440 14th Ave, Regina SK S4P 0W5; Pretoria (South Africa)'93; Staff, Regina General Hospital.

LABUSCHAGNE, Pieter Willem; Vegreville Family Clinic, PO Box 219 136-4917 50 Ave, Vegreville AB T9C 1R2; (South Africa)'00; MB ChB; Staff, Covenant Health - St Joseph's General Hospital; (780)632-6414; Fax. (780)632-6404.

LACAILLE, Diane V; Arthritis Research Centre, 1F-5591 No. 3 Rd, Richmond BC V6X 2C7; McG'88; MHSc; FRCPC; IntMed; Rheum. Staff, Vancouver General Hospital - Centennial Pavillion; Asst Prof Rheum, University of British Columbia; Langs: Bilingual(English/French); (604)207-4025

LACAILLE, Jacques; Centre De Sante Carillon, 20 rue De Carillon, Sherbrooke QC J1J 2K8; Sher'77; (819)564-1331

LACAILLE, Luc; Clinique Ped La Courte Echelle, 101-86 boul Brien, Repentigny QC J6A 5K7; Mon'91; Peds. Staff, Centre Hospitalier Pierre le Gardeur; (450)657-1705; Fax. (450)657-1800.

LACAILLE, Marie-Claude; CSSS d'Antoine-Labelle-Mt Laur, RR 1 2561 ch de la Lievre S, Mont-Laurier QC J9L 3G3; Mon'99; Staff, CSSS d'Antoine-Labelle; (819)623-1234; Fax. (819)275-1520; lacaille71@hotmail.com.

LACAILLE-BELANGER, Pierre; CSSS du Sud de Lanaudière, 911 montee des Pionniers, Terrebonne QC J6V 2H2; Mon'93; FRCPC; DiagRad. Staff, Centre Hospitalier Pierre le Gardeur; (450)654-7525

LACAS, Alethea D; Dalhousie Fam Med Spryfield MC, 16 Dentith Rd, Halifax NS B3R 2H9; Dal'02; CCFP; (902)473-1234

LACASSE, Bernard; Institut Prive de Chirurgie, 180-801 Grande Allee O, Quebec QC G1S 1C1; Laval'85; OrthSurg (P.Q.). Staff, Centre Hospitalier Beauce-Etchemin; (418)681-3849

LACASSE, Diane; Clinique Haut Anjou, Suite 45 7500 boul Les Galeries d'Anjou, Anjou QC H1M 3M4; Mon'75; Universite de Montreal; Langs: Spanish; English; (514)493-1999

LACASSE, Jacqueline; Clinique Med Familiale Dolbeau, 1521 rue des Erables, Dolbeau-Mistassini QC G8L 1C4; Laval'75; Staff, Centre Maria-Chapdelaine - CH de Dolbeau-Mistassini; (418)276-0041; Fax. (418)276-7170.

LACASSE, Jacques E; CSSS de la Haute-Gaspésie, 50 rue du Belvedere, Ste-Anne-des-Monts QC G4V 1X4; Laval'75; ABR; DiagRad (Echography). Staff, Centre Hospitalier des Monts; Université Laval; Langs: Bilingual(English/French); (418)763-2261; Fax. (418)763-1250; jacques.lacasse@videotron.ca.

LACASSE, Lise; Clinique Med Jean Coutu, 1116A Mountain Rd, Moncton NB E1C 2T3; Laval'80; Langs: English; (506)857-1106; Fax. (506)855-7537.

LACASSE, Louis-Andre; Clinique Med St-Jerome, 102-450 boul Monseigneur-Duboi, Saint-Jerome QC J7Y 3L8; Mon'81; MBA; CCFP; Staff, Hôtel-Dieu de Saint-Jérôme; Pres, Juvencia Inc; Langs: English; French; (450)438-1518; Fax. (450)438-6119.

LACASSE, Marie-Andree; CSSS de Trois-Rivières, 1991 boul du Carmel, Trois-Rivieres QC G8Z 3R9; Sher'06; CSPQ; FRCPC; Anes. Staff, CSSS de Trois-Rivières; (819)697-3333

LACASSE, Marie-Eve; CSSS du Sud de Lanaudière, 911 montee des Pionniers, Terrebonne QC J6V 2H2; Mon'07; CCFP; Staff, Centre Hospitalier Pierre le Gardeur; (450)654-7525

LACASSE, Marie-Lynn; Englehart & District Hosp, PO Box 69 61 5th St, Englehart ON P0J 1H0; Ott'03; CCFP; Staff, Englehart & District Hospital Inc; (705)544-2301

LACASSE, Martin; Clinique Med de Buckingham, 200-620 av de Buckingham, Gatineau QC J8L 2H5; Ott'68; assoc Staff, CH-CHSLD de Papineau - Pavillon du centre hospitalier; (819)986-6006; Fax. (819)986-1616.

LACASSE, Melanie; Clinique Med de Buckingham, 200-620 av de Buckingham, Gatineau QC J8L 2H5; Ott'06; CCFP; (819)986-6006; Fax. (819)986-1616.

LACASSE, Yves; Hôpital Laval, 2725 ch Sainte-Foy, Quebec QC G1V 4G5; Laval'89; MSc; FRCPC; IntMed; Respir. Staff Pulmonologist, Hôpital Laval; assoc Prof Med, Université Laval; Langs: Bilingual(English/French); (418)656-8711 x4747; Fax. (418)656-4762; yves.lacasse@med.ulaval.ca.

LACAZE-MASMONTEIL, Thierry; Children's Hosp Eastern Ont, 3420-401 Smyth Rd, Ottawa ON K1H 8L1; (France)'91; Staff, Children's Hospital of Eastern Ontario (CHEO); (613)737-7600; Fax. (613)738-4847.

LACE DE ALMEIDA, Claudia; McMaster University, HSC 3A-1280 Main St W, Hamilton ON L8S 4K1; Rio De Janerio (Brazil)'96; Staff, Hamilton Health Sciences Centre - Chedoke Hospital; Teach Staff, McMaster University; (905)521-2100

LACELLE, Johanne; East End Health Centre, 2 Mount Cashel Rd, St. John's NL A1A 1X7; Mem'91; CCFP; FCFP; (709)753-1450; Fax. (709)722-3576.

LACELLE, Marie-Josee; CSSS du Lac-des-Deux-Montagnes, 520 boul Arthur-Sauve, Saint-Eustache QC J7R 5B1; Sher'03; FRCPC; IntMed. Staff, Hôpital de Saint-Eustache; (450)473-6811

LACERTE, Caroline; Clin Ped de Trois-Rivieres, 110-5725 Boul des Forges, Trois-Rivieres QC G8Y 5L5; Laval'95; FRCPC; Peds. Staff Ped, CSSS de Trois-Rivières; (819)375-0504

LACERTE, Jean-F.; Pavillon Rosemont, 5689 boul Rosemont, Montreal QC H1T 2H1; Laval'64; Psy (Pedology Psychiatry). Staff Psy, Hopital Maisonneuve-Rosemont; (514)252-3400 x2923; jflacerte@sympatico.ca.

LACERTE, Louise; CHUQ-St-Francois D'Assise, 10 rue de l'Espinay, Quebec QC G1L 3L5; Laval'85; CSPQ; FRCPC; Anes. Ac Staff, Centre Hospitalier Universitaire De Québec - Pavillon De St-françois-d'assise; (418)525-4340; Fax. (418)525-4434.

LACERTE, Marcel; 3E-575 rue Saint-Amable, Quebec QC G1R 2G4; Laval'57; MSc(McG); FRCPC; IntMed; Gastroent (P.Q.).

LACERTE, Martina M; Springfield Med Clinic, PO Box 10 559 Main St, Oakbank MB R0E 1J0; Man'00; CCFP.

LACERTE, Maxime; CSSS de Laval, 1755 boul Rene-Laennec, Laval QC H7M 3L9; Mon'03; FRCSC; ObstGyn. Staff, Hopital de la Cite de la santé; (450)668-1010; Fax. (450)975-5545.

LACERTE, Michel; 4520 Colonel Talbot Rd PO Box 10 Stn Lambeth, London ON N6P 1P9; McG'83; MSc(Rehab); FRCPC; PhysMed&Rehab. Assoc Prof, University of Western Ontario; Langs: Bilingual(French/English); (519)652-2141; Fax. (519)652-2138; mlacerte@uwo.ca.

LACEY, David E; St Clare's Mercy Hosp, 154 Lemarchant Rd, St. John's NL A1C 5B8; Mem'88; FRCPC; Anes. Staff, St Clare's Mercy Hospital; (709)777-5520

LACEY, Glen W; Lakeridge Hlth Corp-Oshawa, 1 Hospital Crt, Oshawa ON L1G 2B9; Man'88; FRCPC; DiagRad. Staff, Lakeridge Health - Oshawa Site; (905)686-6411 x4305

LACEY, James D; Kanata Plastic & Cosmetic Surg, 895 March Rd, Kanata ON K2K 1X7; McG'94; FRCSC; PlasSurg (Hand Surgery). Assoc Prof, McMaster University; Langs: French; (613)591-1099

LACEY, Kendrick R; Health Services Centre, PO Box 340, Stanley NB E6B 2K5; Qns'85; CCFP; Staff Family Pract, Dr Everett Chalmers Regional Hospital; Med Dir, Nashwaak Villa Nursing Home; Lecturer, Dalhousie University; (506)367-7730; Fax. (506)367-7738.

LACH, Boleslaw; Hamilton HS-General Site, 237 Barton St E, Hamilton ON L8L 2X2; Lodz (Poland)'66; PhD; FRCPC; AnatPath; NeurPath. Pathologist, Hamilton Health Sciences Centre - Hamilton General Hospital; Prof Lab Med & Path, McMaster University; Langs: Polish; (905)527-0271 x46168

LACH, Lori-Ann D; University Health Service, 104-65 Chancellors Cir, Winnipeg MB R3T 2N2; Man'97; CCFP; Langs: English; French; Fax. (204)474-7573.

LACHAINE, Colette; Ctr Hosp Laurentien, 234 rue Saint-Vincent, Ste-Agathe-Des-Mts QC J8C 2B8; McG'86; Staff, Centre Hospitalier Laurentien; (819)324-4000; Fax. (819)324-4010.

LACHAINE, Lynda; CLSC des Hautes-Laurentides, 515 boul Albiny-Paquette, Mont-Laurier QC J9L 1K8; Mon'90; Langs: English; (819)623-1228; Fax. (819)623-1311.

LACHAINE, Marie-Pierre; CSSS de Papineau, 155 rue MacLaren E, Gatineau QC J8L 0C2; Sher'99; CCFP; Staff, Hôpital de Papineau; Langs: English; (819)986-3341; Fax. (819)986-4000.

LACHANCE, Alain; Clinique d'Ophthalmologie & La, 11505 1re av, Saint-Georges QC G5Y 2C7; Laval'73; FRCS; FRCSC; Ophth (Contact Lenses). ac Staff, Centre Hospitalier Beauce-Etchemin; Langs: Bilingual(French/English); (418)228-3533; Fax. (418)228-9758; support@colbi.ca.

LACHANCE, Andre; Ctr Hosp Affilie-St-Sacrement, 1050 ch Sainte-Foy, Quebec QC G1S 4L8; Laval'78; MCFP(E.M.); EmergMed (P.Q.) (Emergency Family Medicine). Chef méd urgence Emerg Serv, Centre Hospitalier Affilié Universitaire de Québec - Hôpital du St-Sacrement; Université Laval; (418)682-7515; Fax. (418)682-7970.

LACHANCE, Benoit; CLSC Haute-Ville-des-Rivieres, 2400 av d'Estimauville, Quebec QC G1E 7G9; Laval'75; Staff, Centre Hospitalier Affilié Universitaire de Québec - Hôpital De L'Enfant Jésus; (418)623-1010 x251; Fax. (418)623-7513; benoit.lachance@ssss.gouv.qc.ca.

LACHANCE, Carl-Hugo; CHUQ-St-Francois d'Assise, 10 rue de l'Espinay, Quebec QC G1L 3L5; Sher'00; FRCPC; IntMed. Staff, Centre Hospitalier Universitaire De Québec - Pavillon De St-françois-d'assise; (418)525-4444

LACHANCE, Carole; Centre Med Le Mesnil, 300-1300 boul Lebourgneuf, Quebec QC G2K 2N1; Laval'85; (418)624-1800

LACHANCE, Christian; Hôpital Ste-Justine, 3175 ch Cote-Sainte-Catherine, Montreal QC H3T 1C5; Mon'88; FRCPC; Peds (Neonatology). Staff Neonatol, Hôpital Ste-Justine; (514)345-4685; Fax. (514)345-7725.

LACHANCE, Claude; Hop Jean-Talon, 1385 rue Jean-Talon E, Montreal QC H2E 1S6; Laval'85; Staff, CSSS du Coeur de l'Isle Hôpital Jean-Talon; (514)495-6767

LACHANCE, Danielle; Centre Med Pour Enfants, 1791 av Dollard, LaSalle QC H8N 1T9; Laval'85; Staff, McGill University Health Centre - Montreal Children's Hospital; adj Prof, McGill University; Langs: Bilingual(French/English); (514)368-0441; Fax. (514)368-0445.

LACHANCE, Eric; CLSC La Region-Sherbrookoise, 1200 rue King E, Sherbrooke QC J1G 1E4; Mon'93; CCFP; (819)563-2572; Fax. (819)563-8502; elachance.dr@gmf.gouv.qc.ca.

LACHANCE, Guy; Centre Oculaire de Quebec, 050-2480 ch Sainte-Foy, Quebec QC G1V 1T6; Laval'68; FRCSC; Ophth. Ac Staff, Centre Hospitalier Universitaire de Québec (CHUQ) - Siege Social; Consultant, Rehabilitation Centre of Quebec; (418)780-6345

LACHANCE, Isabelle; Polyclinique St-Eustache, 75 rue Grignon, Saint-Eustache QC J7P 4J2; Laval'98; Staff, Hôpital de Saint-Eustache; (450)473-6882; isabellelachance@hotmail.com.

LACHANCE, Jacques R; CSSS de Montmagny-l'Islet, 430 rue Jean-Leclerc RR 1, St-Jean-Port-Joli QC G0R 3G0; Sher'72; Gen Practice, CSSS de Montmagny-l'Islet; Langs: English; (418)598-3355; Fax. (418)598-9794.

LACHANCE, Jean-Guy; CHUQ-Hotel-Dieu De Quebec, 11 Cote Du Palais, Quebec QC G1R 2J6; Laval'67; Nephrol (P.Q.). Staff, Centre Hospitalier Universitaire de Québec (CHUQ) - Siege Social; (418)691-5464; Fax. (418)691-5757.

LACHANCE, Jean-Rene; Hop Maisonneuve-Rosemont, 5415 boul de l'Assomption, Montreal QC H1T 2M4; Laval'76; Gastroent (P.Q.). Staff, Hopital Maisonneuve-Rosemont; Langs: English; (514)252-3400; Fax. (514)252-3486.

LACHANCE, Lucie; UMF de Laval, 2690 ch des Quarter-Bourgeois, Quebec QC G1V 0B7; Laval'76; Staff UMF, Hôpital Laval; Staff, CSSS Haute-Ville; Clin Prof, Université Laval; Langs: English; (418)656-8711; lucie.lachance@irdpq.qc.ca.

LACHANCE, Maggie; Clinique familiale de Thetford, RR 2 1001-926 rue Labbe, Thetford Mines QC G6G 2A8; Laval'05; (418)338-3521

LACHANCE, Marc; Centre Med Drummond, 60 rue Loring, Drummondville QC J2C 7Y9; Laval'73; Langs: Bilingual(French/English); (819)477-2500; Fax. (819)477-6249.

LACHANCE, Marianne; CSSS de Beauce-Etchemin, 1515 17e rue, Saint-Georges QC G5Y 4T8; Laval'04; FRCSC; Otol (Head & Neck Surgery). Staff, Centre Hospitalier Beauce-Etchemin; (418)228-2031; Fax. (418)227-3825.

LACHANCE, Marie-Josee; Clin Med Riviere du Moulin, 1388 boul du Saguenay E, Chicoutimi QC G7H 1G8; Laval'10; (418)549-3564

LACHANCE, Marie-Noelle; CSSS Pierre Boucher, 1333 boul Jacques-Cartier E, Longueuil QC J4M 2A5; Mon'05; Staff, Centre Hospitalier Pierre Boucher; (450)468-8111

LACHANCE, Martin; Clinique Metro-Medic, 1538 rue Sherbrooke O, Montreal QC H3G 1L5; McG'04; CCFP; (514)932-2122

LACHANCE, Nadia; Clin Ortho Du Haut-Richelieu, 320-900 boul du Seminaire N, St-Jean-sur-Richel QC J3A 1C3; Laval'99; FRCSC; OrthSurg. Staff, Centre Hospitalier Régional du Suroît; (450)348-6966

LACHANCE, Nadine; Centre Med Fusion, 200-2035 av Sainte-Anne, Saint-Hyacinthe QC J2S 5H3; Sher'90; Staff, Centre Hospitalier Honore-Mercier; Langs: Bilingual(French/English); (450)773-6023

LACHANCE, Nathalie; CSSS Maria-Chapdelaine, 2000 boul du Sacre-Coeur, Dolbeau-Mistassini QC G8L 2R5; Mon'92; IntMed (P.Q.). Staff, Centre Maria-Chapdelaine - CH de Dolbeau-Mistassini; (418)276-1234

LACHANCE, Nicole; RAMD Drummond, 2125 boul Lemire, Drummondville QC J2B 8N8; Sher'83; Associate, Hôpital Sainte-croix; (819)475-5151

LACHANCE, Paul; CLSC de Limoilou, 1405 ch de la Canardiere, Quebec QC G1J 0A7; Laval'72; LMCC; (418)529-2573; Fax. (418)648-6736.

LACHANCE, Paul-Andre; CSSS de Laval, 413-1755 boul Rene-Laennec, Laval QC H7M 3L9; McG'83; EmergMed. Staff, Hopital de la Cite de la santé; (450)668-1010 x24106

LACHANCE, Philippe; CSSS de Montmagny-L'Islet, 350 boul Tache O RR 1, Montmagny QC G5V 3R8; Laval'05; Anes. Staff, CSSS de Montmagny-L'Islet; (418)248-0630

LACHANCE, Pierre; Clinique Med St-Louis, 220-3165 ch Saint-Louis, Quebec QC G1W 4R4; Laval'81; Staff, Centre Hospitalier Universitaire de Québec (CHUQ) - Siege Social; (418)653-1970

LACHANCE, Pierre; Hotel-Dieu de Levis, 143 rue Wolfe, Levis QC G6V 3Z1; Laval'89; FRCPC; MedBiochem (Lipidology). Staff, Hôtel-Dieu de Lévis; (418)835-7121 x3210; Fax. (418)835-7139; pierre.lachance@ssss.gouv.qc.ca.

LACHANCE, Raymond; CHUM-Hotel-Dieu, 3840 rue Saint-Urbain, Montreal QC H2W 1T8; Mon'71; ac Staff, Centre Hospitalier l'Université de Montréal (CHUM) - Hôtel-Dieu; (514)890-8149

LACHANCE, Richard; CSSS du Nord de Lanaudière, 1000 boul Sainte-Anne, St-Charles-Brromee QC J6E 6J2; Mon'84; Respir (P. Q.); IntMed. Staff, Centre Hospitalier Régional de Lanaudière; (450)759-8222; Fax. (450)759-5308.

LACHANCE, Sabrina; GMF de l'Assomption, CP 3406 814 boul l'Ange-Gardien N, L'Assomption QC J5W 4M9; Mon'07; (450)589-5778; Fax. (450)589-5779.

LACHANCE, Sophie; CHUQ-Ctr Hosp Univ Laval, 2705 boul Laurier, Quebec QC G1V 4G2; Laval'07; Otol. Staff, Centre Hospitalier Universitaire de Quebec-CHUL; (418)525-4444 x47221

LACHANCE, Suzelle; Inst U en Sante Mentale de QC, 2601 ch de la Canardiere, Quebec QC G1J 2G3; Laval'76; Staff, Institut Universitaire Sante; (418)663-5000

LACHANCE, Sylvain; Centre Med de l'Hetriere, 201-3520 rue de l'Hetriere, St-Augustin-D-Desm QC G3A 0B4; Mon'95; (418)651-3933

LACHANCE, Sylvie; Hop Maisonneuve-Rosemont, 5415 boul de l'Assomption, Montreal QC H1T 2M4; Sher'87; FRCPC; IntMed; Hem. Staff, McGill University Health Centre - Montreal General Campus; (514)252-3400 x3743

LACHANCE, Yves; Ctr Hosp de Verdun, 4000 boul Lasalle, Verdun QC H4G 2A3; Laval'80; FRCPC; IntMed; Respir. Staff, Centre Hospitalier de Verdun; (514)362-1000

LACHANCE-FORTIN, Geraldine; CSSS de la Cote-de-Gaspe, 215 boul de York O, Gaspe QC G4X 2W2; Laval'08; CCFP; Staff, Centre Hospitalier de Gaspe; (418)368-6663

LACHAPELLE, Anne; CSSS de Port-Cartier, 3 rue de Shelter Bay, Port-Cartier QC G5B 2W9; Mon'02; Staff, CLSC-CSSS de Port-Cartier; (418)766-2572

LACHAPELLE, Jacques; 205-6070 rue Sherbrooke E, Montreal QC H1N 1C1; Mon'71; Electroenceph (P.Q.); Neur. Ac Staff, Hopital Maisonneuve-Rosemont; (514)251-4790

LACHAPELLE, Jean; Hop Maisonneuve-Rosemont, 5415 boul de l'Assomption, Montreal QC H1T 2M4; Mon'87; FRCPC; Peds (Neonatology). Staff, Hopital Maisonneuve-Rosemont; Langs: Bilingual(French/English); (514)252-3400

LACHAPELLE, Kevin J; MUHC-Royal Victoria Hosp, 8 30-687 av des Pins O, Montreal QC H3A 1A1; McG'88; FRCSC; GenSurg; Cardiovasc&ThorSurg (P.Q.); CardiothorSurg. Staff, McGill University Health Centre - Royal Victoria Hospital; (514)843-1519

LACHAPELLE, Kevin R; 2-1 Frankford Cres, Trenton ON K8V 6H8; Qns'94; FRCSC; Ophth. Staff, QHC Trenton Memorial; (613)965-5777; Fax. (613)965-5756.

LACHAPELLE, Lucie; CSSS Rimouski-Neigette, 165 rue des Gouverneurs, Rimouski QC G5L 7R2; Mon'81; (418)724-3000

LACHAPELLE, Marie-France; 202-5858 ch de la Cote-des-Nei, Montreal QC H3S 1Y9; McG'88; FRCSC; ObstGyn (Maternal Fetal Medicine). Staff, Sir Mortimer B Davis Jewish General; (514)739-1309

LACHAPELLE, Michel; CHSLD Manoir Trinite, 1275 boul Jacques-Cartier E, Longueuil QC J4M 2Y8; Mon'81; (450)674-4948; Fax. (450)674-8571; m_lachap@hotmail.com.

LACHARITE, Karine; CSSS de Portneuf, 700 rue Saint-Cyrille, Saint-Raymond QC G3L 1W1; Laval'08; Staff, Centre Hospitalier Portneuf; (418)337-4611

LACHARITE, Sophie; Hop du Sacre-Coeur de Mtl, 5400 boul Gouin O, Montreal QC H4J 1C5; Sher'83; FRCSC; GenSurg (Intensive Care). Staff, Hôpital du Sacre-Coeur de Montréal; (514)338-2050; Fax. (514)333-3379.

LACHMAN, Matthew; Forbes Park Med Centre, 26 Forbes St, Cambridge ON N3C 2E2; (Other Foreign)'00; (519)658-4615; Fax. (519)658-4630.

LACHMANN, Mark H; Rouge Valley HS-Ajax/Pickering, 580 Harwood Ave S, Ajax ON L1S 2J4; UBC'96; MHSc(Bioethics); CCFP; FCFP; Psy. Staff, Rouge Valley Health System - Ajax & Pickering Health Centre Site; (905)683-2320

LACHOWSKI, Richard J; Medical Arts Bldg, 408-1 Young St, Hamilton ON L8N 1T8; Tor'78; FRCSC; OrthSurg (Trauma/Joint Replacement). Clin Assoc Prof Surg, McMaster University; (905)528-1305; Fax. (905)528-0222.

LACKIE, Elyse G; North York Med Arts Bldg, 315-1333 Sheppard Ave E, North York ON M2J 1V1; Wes'93; FRCSC; ObstGyn. Ac Staff, North York General Hospital; University of Toronto; (416)494-0007; Fax. (416)494-8758.

LACKMAN, Felice D; 3-106 Cornell Park Ave, Markham ON L6B 1B6; McG'96; FRCSC; ObstGyn (Gynecologic Oncology). Med Staff, Markham Stouffville Hospital; (905)471-1945; Fax. (905)471-6315.

LACKNER, Colin R; Grey Bruce HS-Owen Sound, PO Box 1800 Stn Main 1800 8th St E, Owen Sound ON N4K 6M9; Wes'96; BSc; CCFP; CCFP(E.M.); Staff, Grey Bruce Health Services - Owen Sound; (519)376-2121

LACKO, Cyril J; Medical Clinic Bldg, 217-89 Humber College Blvd, Etobicoke ON M9V 4B8; Tor'81; Staff, William Osler Health System - Etobicoke General Hospital; (416)746-0304; Fax. (416)746-0309.

LACNY, Andrew M; Mediclinic, 101-3301 8th St E, Saskatoon SK S7H 5K5; Sask'80; Ac Staff, St Paul's Hospital (Grey Nuns) of Saskatoon; Ac Staff, Royal University Hospital; Ac Staff, Saskatoon City Hospital; Clinical Asst Prof Family Med, University of Saskatchewan; (306)955-1530; Fax. (306)955-8811; andrew.lacny@cic.gc.ca.

LACOMBE, Annie; Centre Med des Generations, 200-465 rue Bibeau, Saint-Eustache QC J7R 0C8; Mon'09; Staff, Hopital Maisonneuve-Rosemont; (450)472-1955

LACOMBE, Christina; Field Ambulance Det Yellowknif, PO Box 6666 Stn Main, Yellowknife NT X1A 2R3; Laval'07; CCFP; (867)873-0700

LACOMBE, Danyele; Clinique Med Champlain, 103-195 rue de l'Atmosphere, Gatineau QC J9A 0A3; Ott'06; (819)777-7270

LACOMBE, Francois; GMF Concorde, 300 boul de la Concorde E, Laval QC H7G 2E6; Mon'82; Staff, Hopital de la Cite de la santé; (450)667-5310; Fax. (450)667-5248; flacombe@lajacombe.com.

LACOMBE, Guy; Inst U Geriatrie Sherbrooke, 375 rue Argyll, Sherbrooke QC J1J 3H5; Sher'80; FRCPC; IntMed (Dementia); GeriatricMed (P.Q.). Staff, Institut Universitaire de Geriatrie de Sherbrooke-Pavillon Argyll; Langs: Bilingual(English/French); (819)821-1170 x46254; Fax. (819)829-7145; guy.lacombe@usherbrooke.ca.

LACOMBE, Jean-Guy; Clinique Du Havre, 79A rue Jacques-Cartier, Gaspe QC G4X 1M5; Mon'73; (418)368-5609; Fax. (418)368-6498.

LACOMBE, Jose; CSSS de Saint-Jerome, 290 rue de Montigny, Saint-Jerome QC J7Z 5T3; Mon'91; CCFP; Staff, Hôtel-Dieu de Saint-Jérôme; (450)431-8200

LACOMBE, Louis; CHUQ-Hotel-Dieu De Quebec, 11 Cote-du-Palais, Quebec QC G1R 2J6; Sher'88; FRCSC; Urol (Oncology). Staff, Centre Hospitalier Universitaire de Québec (CHUQ) - Siege Social; Langs: Bilingual(French/English); (418)525-4444; Fax. (418)691-5331; louis.lacombe@crhdq.ulaval.ca.

LACOMBE, Louise; 2404 av Saint-Marc, Shawinigan QC G9N 2J7; Laval'77; (819)539-4524; Fax. (819)539-9819.

LACOMBE, Marc-Andre; CSSS du Haut-Saint-Maurice, 885 boul Ducharme, La Tuque QC G9X 3C1; Sher'04; Staff, Centre Hospitalier Saint-Joseph de la Turque; (819)523-4581

LACOMBE, Marie-Claude; Dir Sante Publique Laurentides, 210-1000 rue Labelle, Saint-Jerome QC J7Z 5N6; Mon'95; Staff, Direction de la Sante Publique Laurentides; (450)432-8735; Fax. (450)569-6305; marie-claude.lacombe@ssss.gouv.qc.ca.

LACOMBE, Paméla; Clinique de Med Familiale, 6e-2120 rue Sherbrooke E, Montreal QC H2K 1C3; Mon'06; (514)527-1958; Fax. (514)527-1649.

LACOMBE, Real; Dir de la Sante Publique, 1 9e rue, Rouyn-Noranda QC J9X 2A9; Mon'72; Ac Staff Sante Commun, Centre Hospitalier Affilié Universitaire de Québec - Hôpital du St-Sacrement; (819)764-3264; Fax. (819)797-1947.

LACOSTE, Daniel; CSSS de la Haute-Gaspésie, 50 rue du Belvedere, Ste-Anne-des-Monts QC G4V 1X4; Mon'94; CCFP; Staff, Centre Hospitalier des Monts; (418)763-2261

LACOSTE, Lucie; Ctr Hosp Anna-Laberge, 200 boul Brisebois, Chateauguay QC J6K 4W8; Mon'99; CCFP; Staff, Hôpital Anna-Laberge; (450)649-2436; Fax. (450)649-2525.

LACOSTE, Pierre; Clinique Med Ste-Adele, 1150 rue Du Bourg-Joli, Sainte-Adele QC J8B 1W8; Mon'75; FRCPC; PhysMed&Rehab (Consultation). (450)229-6633; Fax. (450)229-5765.

LACOSTE, Sophie; CSSS de la Haute-Yamaska, 205 boul Leclerc O, Granby QC J2G 1T7; Mon'90; Staff, Centre Hospitalier de Granby; (450)375-8000

LACOURCIERE, Yves; Institut Prive de Chirurgie, 801 Grande Allee O, Quebec QC G1S 1C1; Laval'65; IntMed; NuclearMed (P.Q.). Staff, Centre Hospitalier Universitaire de Quebec-CHUL; Langs: English; (418)687-7328; yves.lacourciere@crchul.ulaval.ca.

LACOURSIERE, Jean-Pierre; Clinique D'Orthopedie de Levis, 6620 rue Saint-Georges, Levis QC G6V 4H1; Laval'64; FRCSC; OrthSurg. Staff, Hôtel-Dieu de Lévis; (418)837-8251; Fax. (418)837-2033.

LACOURSIERE, Joan E; Queen University, 146 Stuart St, Kingston ON K7L 2V8; Tor'91; CCFP; FCFP; (613)533-2506; Fax. (613)533-6740.

LACOURSIERE, Josiane; Clinique Medicale 1851, 101-1851 rue Sherbrooke E, Montreal QC H2K 4L5; Sher'04; Staff, Centre Hospitalier Trois-Pistoles; (514)524-7564

LACOURSIERE, Luc; Hotel-Dieu de Levis, 143 rue Wolfe, Levis QC G6V 3Z1; Laval'92; FRCPC; DiagRad. Staff, Hôtel-Dieu de Lévis; (418)835-7101

LACOURSIERE, Sylvie; Direction de la Sante Publique, 550 rue Bonaventure, Trois-Rivieres QC G9A 2B5; Laval'84; Langs: English; (819)693-3636; Fax. (819)373-1627.

LACOUTURE QUINTERO, Astrid P; Polyclinique Coeur de l'Ile, 201-529 rue Jarry E, Montreal QC H2P 1V4; Bogota (Colombia)'02; CCFP; (514)277-4111

LACROIX, Andre; CHUM-Hotel-Dieu, 3840 rue Saint-Urbain, Montreal QC H2W 1T8; Mon'72; Endocrin (P.Q.) (Cushing's Syndrome). adj Chef endo, Centre Hospitalier l'Université de Montréal (CHUM) - Hôtel-Dieu; Prof Med, Universite de Montreal; (514)890-8100 x14930; Fax. (514)412-7128; andre.lacroix@umontreal.ca.

LACROIX, Anne; 100-750 13e Av N, Sherbrooke QC J1E 3L7; Sher'81; CSPQ; FRCPC; Anes. Staff, Centre Hospitalier Universitaire de Sherbrooke-Hopital Fleurimont; adj Prof, Universite de Sherbrooke; (819)822-0442

LACROIX, Annie; CSSS Haut-Richelieu-Rouville, 920 boul du Seminaire N, St-Jean-sur-Richel QC J3A 1B7; Sher'06; MedOncol; Hem; IntMed. Staff, Hôpital du Haut-Richelieu; (450)359-5000 x5205; Fax. (450)359-5251.

LACROIX, Chantal; Dir de la Sante des femmes, 5180 boul Gouin O, Montreal QC H4J 1C3; Mon'87; (514)333-8105; Fax. (514)333-8150; clacroix@santepub-mtl.qc.ca.

LACROIX, Christine; Dir de la Sante Publique, 1255 rue Beauregard, Longueuil QC J4K 2M3; Mon'94; FRCPC; CommunMed. (450)928-6777

LACROIX, Daniel; Moose Creek Med Centre, PO BOX 70 66 Sabourin St, Moose Creek ON K0C 1W0; Ott'84; Court Staff, Glengarry Memorial Hospital; Langs: English; French; (613)538-2710; Fax. (613)538-2258.

LACROIX, Ghyslain; CSSS Drummond-Hop Sainte-Croix, 570 rue Heriot, Drummondville QC J2B 1C1; Laval'69; Ac Staff, Hôpital Sainte-croix; (819)478-6464

LACROIX, Gilles; Ctr Hosp Affilie-Enfant-Jesus, 1401 18e rue, Quebec QC G1J 1Z4; Laval'91; CSPQ; FRCPC; Anes (Intensive Care). Staff, Centre Hospitalier Affilié Universitaire de Québec - Hôpital De L'Enfant Jésus; (418)649-0252; Fax. (418)649-5918; glac@videotron.ca.

LACROIX, J L Denis; 1425 Front St PO Box 20, Hearst ON P0L 1N0; Ott'83; Staff, Hôpital Notre Dame Hospital - Hearst; Langs: English; (705)372-1043; Fax. (705)362-4551.

LACROIX, Jacques; Hôpital Ste-Justine, 3175 ch Cote-Sainte-Catherine, Montreal QC H3T 1C5; Mon'74; FAAP; FRCPC; Peds (Critical Care Medicine). Staff Ped Intensive Care, Hôpital Ste-Justine; Prof Peds, Universite de Montreal; Langs: English; (514)345-4931 x5556; Fax. (514)345-7731; jacques_lacroix@ssss.gouv.qc.ca.

LACROIX, Julie D M; The Ottawa Hosp-Civic Campus, 1053 Carling Ave, Ottawa ON K1Y 4E9; Ott'03; CCFP; Staff, The Ottawa Hospital - Civic Campus; (613)761-4774

LACROIX, Lianne; Glenmore Clinic, 1605 Gordon Dr, Kelowna BC V1Y 3G8; Ott'72; Assoc Staff, Kelowna General Hospital; Langs: English; (250)861-3120; Fax. (250)861-3603; lianne.lacroix@shaw.ca.

LACROIX, Linda A M; 302-595 Montreal Rd, Ottawa ON K1K 4L2; McG'83; FRCPC; IntMed; Hem. Staff, The Ottawa Hospital - Civic Campus; Staff, Montfort Hospital; Assoc Prof Med, University of Ottawa; Langs: Italian; Spanish; French; (613)725-9374; drllacroix@bellnet.ca.

LACROIX, Luc-Phillippe J; CSSSG-Hop de Gatineau, CP 2000 succ Bureau-chef 909 boul de la Verendrye O, Gatineau QC J8P 7H2; Ott'89; CCFP; FCFP; Staff, Hôpital de Gatineau; Langs: French; (819)966-6333

LACROIX, Marc; Clinique Med Lacroix, 300-795 boul du Lac, Quebec QC G2M 0E4; Laval'98; CCFP; Langs: Bilingual(French/English); (418)841-1911; marclacroixmd@hotmail.com.

LACROIX, Melanie; Hotel-Dieu de Levis, 143 rue Wolfe, Levis QC G6V 3Z1; Laval'97; CSPQ; FRCPC; Anes. Staff, Hôtel-Dieu de Lévis; (418)835-7121 x3218; Fax. (418)835-3969.

LACROIX, Mylene H; Clinique Med Pierre-Bertrand, 212-303 boul Pierre-Bertrand, Quebec QC G1M 3L7; Cayetano Heredia (Peru)'94; CCFP; Langs: French; Spanish; (418)683-2724; Fax. (418)683-8861.

LACROIX, Patrick; Hotel-Dieu De Sorel, 400 av de l'Hotel-Dieu, Sorel-Tracy QC J3P 1N5; Mon'04; CCFP; Staff, Hôtel-Dieu de Sorel; (450)746-6000

LACROIX, Remi; Ctr Hosp Affilie-Enfant-Jesus, 1401 18e rue, Quebec QC G1J 1Z4; Mon'05; FRCPC; PhysMed&Rehab (Sports Medicine). Staff, Centre Hospitalier Affilié Universitaire de Québec - Hôpital De L'Enfant Jésus; Langs: Bilingual(French/English); (418)649-0252

LACROIX, Sebastien; Hôtel-Dieu de Saint-Jérôme, 290 rue de Montigny, Saint-Jerome QC J7Z 5T3; Mon'07; CCFP; CCFP(E.M.); Staff, Hôtel-Dieu de Saint-Jérôme; (450)431-8266; Fax. (450)431-8244.

LACROIX, Thomas B; St Clair Corporate Centre, 110-265 Front St N, Sarnia ON N7T 7X1; McG'93; FRCPC; Peds (Neonatology). Ac Staff, Bluewater Health - Mitton Site; Asst Prof Peds, University of Western Ontario; Langs: English; French; (519)344-4868; Fax. (519)344-4848.

LACROIX, Vincent J; MUHC-Montreal Gen Hosp, 1650 av Cedar, Montreal QC H3G 1A4; McG'90; CCFP; Staff Emerg, McGill University Health Centre - Montreal General Campus; Dir, Primary Care Sports Med. Fellowship Program; McGill University; (514)934-8041; Fax. (514)934-8394.

LACROIX, Yolene; MUHC-Montreal Children's Hosp, 2300 rue Tupper, Montreal QC H3H 1P3; Laval'01; FRCSC; Otol. Staff, McGill University Health Centre - Montreal Children's Hospital; (514)412-4303

LACROIX, Yvon; Hôpital Ste-Justine, 3175 ch de la Cote-Sainte-Cath, Montreal QC H3T 1C5; Laval'70; Psy (P.Q.). Staff, Hôpital Ste-Justine; (514)345-4931

LACSON, Atilano G; University of Alberta Hosp, 5B4 18-8440 112 St NW, Edmonton AB T6G 2B7; Manila (Philippines)'72; AB(AP&CP); AB(N); FRCPC; NeurPath (Pediatric Pathology). Staff Path, University of Alberta Hospital; Langs: Tagalog; (780)407-2716; Fax. (780)407-3009.

LACUESTA, Gina A; Park Lane Mall, 503-5657 Spring Garden Rd, Halifax NS B3J 3R4; Mem'97; BMedSci; FRCPC; IntMed; ClinImmunol&Allergy. Staff Capital Health District, Queen Elizabeth II Health Sciences Centre - Victoria General Site; Asst Prof IntMed, Dalhousie University; (902)425-3927; lacuesta@dal.ca.

LACUNA, Julie B D; 350-507 Broadway W, Vancouver BC V5Z 1E6; McG'04; CCFP; Langs: Vietnamese; French; (604)568-7229

LACY, Richard A; Active Care Med Group, A-1108 Klondike Rd, Kanata ON K2K 0G1; Wes'72; (613)254-9777; Fax. (613)254-9778.

LAD, Mohanlal; 433B King St E, Hamilton ON L8N 1C5; Aberdeen (Scotland)'63; MB ChB; Ac Staff, St Joseph's Healthcare - Charlton Campus; Court Staff, Hamilton Health Sciences Centre - McMaster University Medical Centre; Langs: Gujarati; Hindi; (905)526-9904; Fax. (905)526-9904.

LAD, Rameeta J; 428-2289 Fairview St, Burlington ON L7R 2E3; Tor'94; MSc(Epid); FRCPC; IntMed; Gastroent. Staff, Joseph Brant Memorial Hospital; (905)681-1103; Fax. (905)681-0052.

LAD, Shilpa V; The Ottawa Hosp-Civic Campus, C159-1053 Carling Ave, Ottawa ON K1Y 4E9; Bombay (India)'99; Staff, The Ottawa Hospital - Civic Campus; (613)761-4623

LAD, Tara L; 428-2289 Fairview St, Burlington ON L7R 2E3; McM'99; FRCPC; Neur. (905)681-1103; Fax. (905)681-0052.

LADAK, Rahim A; 302-222 King St E, Bowmanville ON L1C 1P6; Wes'04; CCFP; (905)697-8847

LADAK, Shenif; Lakeridge Health Corp-Oshawa, 1 Hospital Crt, Oshawa ON L1G 2B9; McM'98; Staff, Lakeridge Health - Oshawa Site; (905)576-8711

LADAK, Yasmin; Stouffville Med Centre, 34 Civic Ave, Stouffville ON L4A 1H2; McM'04; CCFP; (905)640-3100

LADDADA, Kherdine; CSSS de la Matapedia, 135 av Gaetan-Archambault, Amqui QC G5J 2K5; (Algeria)'91; Staff, CSSS de la Matapedia; (418)629-2211

LADHA, Al-Karim; Fairview Med Arts Centre, 204-2200 Fairview St, Burlington ON L7R 4H9; McM'96; FRCPC; IntMed. Staff, Joseph Brant Memorial Hospital; (905)637-8672; Fax. (905)639-3076.

LADHA, Nizar B; Waterford Hosp, 306 Waterford Bridge Rd, St. John's NL A1E 4J8; RCS (Ireland)'72; LRCP; LRCS; DABPN; FRCPC; Psy. Staff Psy, Waterford Hospital; Assoc Prof Psy, Memorial University Of Newfoundland; (709)777-3029

LADHA, Tehseen S; Hys Med Centre, 505-11010 101 St NW, Edmonton AB T5H 4B9; Alb'06; FRCPC; Peds. (780)414-6812

LADHAM, Shaun A; Saskatoon City Hosp, 701 Queen St, Saskatoon SK S7K 0M7; Dal'92; Staff, Saskatoon City Hospital; (306)964-1677; shaun.ladham@saskatoonhealthregion.ca.

LADHANI, Azim; Metrotown Med Centre, 201-6411 Nelson Ave, Burnaby BC V5H 4H3; Edinburgh (Scotland)'78; MB ChB; DRCOG; CCFP; Staff, Burnaby Hospital; (604)451-4100; Fax. (604)451-4101.

LADHANI, Moyez; McMaster University, HSC 3N11-1280 Main St W, Hamilton ON L8S 4K1; Tor'89; FRCPC; Peds. Staff, St Joseph's Healthcare - Charlton Campus; Staff, Hamilton Health Sciences Centre - McMaster Children's Hospital; Dep Chief/Dir Pediatric Postgrad Medicine/Assoc Prof, McMaster University; (905)521-2100 x75639; Fax. (905)521-4981.

LADHANI, Noor N N; Sunnybrook Hlth Sciences Ctre, M4 172-2075 Bayview Ave, Toronto ON M4N 3M5; Wes'04; FRCSC; ObstGyn (Maternal Fetal Medicine). Staff, Sunnybrook Health Sciences Centre; (416)480-4920

LADKI, Alena; 104-145 15th St W, North Vancouver BC V7M 1R9; Prague (Czech Republic)'79; FRCPC; Peds (Neonatology). Staff, Lions Gate Hospital; Langs: Czech; Arabic; (604)924-3133

LADORA, Marie-Josee; 200-4 Beechwood Ave, Vanier ON K1L 8L9; Laval'80; Langs: Bilingual(French/English); (613)741-7580; Fax. (613)741-0176.

LADOUCEUR, Denis; C-122 rue Saint-Laurent, Saint-Eustache QC J7P 5G1; Sher'81; FRCSC; Neursurg. Staff, Hôpital du Sacre-Coeur de Montréal; (450)623-3850

LADOUCEUR, Diane; Clin de Gynecologie et Obst, 350-1215 ch du Tremblay, Longueuil QC J4N 1R4; Mon'79; ObstGyn. Staff, Centre Hospitalier Pierre Boucher; Langs: Bilingual(French/English); (450)468-6866; Fax. (450)468-6836; clinique.ladouceur@bellnet.ca.

LADOUCEUR, Robert; Polyclinique Med de Terrebonne, 201-901 boul des Seigneurs, Terrebonne QC J6W 1T8; Mon'80; (450)471-1117; Fax. (450)471-8043.

LADOUCEUR, Roger; College des Med du Quebec, 2170 boul Rene-Levesque O, Montreal QC H3H 2T8; Mon'76; CCFP; FCFP; Staff, Centre Hospitalier de Verdun; (514)933-4441 x5296; Fax. (514)933-4668.

LADOUCEUR, Sylvain; Centre Hosp Honore-Mercier, 2750 boul Laframboise, Saint-Hyacinthe QC J2S 4Y8; Sher'92; Dip SportMed; Staff, Centre Hospitalier Honore-Mercier; (450)778-3238; Fax. (450)778-3308.

LAEVSKI, Aleksandar L; Campbellton Reg Hosp, PO Box 880 Stn Main 189 Lily Lake Rd, Campbellton NB E3N 3H3; Skopje (Macedonia)'93; FRCPC; Psy. Staff, Hôpital Régional Campbellton; (506)753-5717

LAEVSKI, Hristo L; PO Box 1002 Stn Main, Campbellton NB E3N 3H4; St Cyril (Macedonia)'93; BSc; DPMRA; FRCP; FRCPC; Anes (Pain Management). Staff Anesthetist, Hôpital Régional Campbellton; (506)759-7292; Fax. (506)789-0574.

LAEVSKI, Lefter M; 114 Roseberry St PO Box 1002, Campbellton NB E3N 3H4; Skopje (Macedonia)'66; Staff Pt-Time, Centre Hospitalier Restigouche; Staff, Hôpital Régional Campbellton; (506)759-7292; Fax. (506)789-0574.

LAFAILLE, Philippe; Hop Maisonneuve-Rosemont, 5415 boul de l'Assomption, Montreal QC H1T 2M4; Mon'04; FRCPC; Derm (Moles Surgery). Staff, Hopital Maisonneuve-Rosemont; (514)252-3400

LAFARGE, Muriel; Direction de Sante Publique, 245 rue du Cure-Majeau, Joliette QC J6E 8S8; Mon'84; Staff, Centre Hospitalier Régional de Lanaudière; (450)759-1157; Fax. (450)759-0281.

LAFAY-COUSIN, Lucie E; Alberta Children's Hosp, 2888 Shaganappi Trail NW, Calgary AB T3B 6A8; Lille (France)'98; Staff, Alberta Children's Hospital; Asst Prof Ped Oncol, University of Calgary; Langs: Bilingual(English/French); (403)955-7203

LAFERRIERE, Albert Real; 34 rue De Juan-Les-Pins, Gatineau QC J8T 6H2; Laval'51; DiagRad; RadOncol. (819)568-0638; Fax. (819)568-1443.

LAFERRIERE, Celine; Hôpital Ste-Justine, 3175 ch Cote-Sainte-Catherine, Montreal QC H3T 1C5; Laval'73; FRCPC; Peds; InfectDis; MedMicrobiol (P.Q.). MicroBiology, Hôpital Ste-Justine; Langs: Bilingual(English/French); (514)345-4931 x4643; celine_laferriere@ssss.gouv.qc.ca.

LAFERRIERE, Edith; Centre Med St Basile, 101-275 boul Sir-Wilfrid-Lauri, St-Basile-Le-Grand QC J3N 1V6; Laval'76; (450)653-7323; Fax. (450)653-3021.

LAFERRIERE, Gilles; Clin d'Urgence Pincourt, 430 boul Don-Quichotte, N-D-D-L'Ile-Perrot QC J7V 0J9; McG'76; (514)453-0884

LAFERRIERE, Jacques; Clinique Medicale, 100-2200 ch de Chambly, Longueuil QC J4J 3Z3; Mon'65; Otol. (450)674-3042

LAFERRIERE, Luc; Clinique Med St-Etienne, 2-965 rte Lagueux, St-Etienne-de Lauz QC G6J 1T5; Laval'79; (418)831-9538; Fax. (418)831-8552.

LAFERRIERE, Nicole B; NWORCC, 980 Oliver Rd, Thunder Bay ON P7B 6V4; McM'99; FRCPC; IntMed; Hem. (807)684-7200

LAFERRIERE, Sophie; Clinique Med L'Envolee, 5025 rue De Salaberry, Montreal QC H4J 1J1; Mon'98; (514)331-2323; Fax. (514)333-8534.

LAFERTE, Noemie; Unite de Med Familiale, 80 118e rue, Shawinigan-Sud QC G9P 3E4; Sher'07; CCFP; Langs: Bilingual(French/English); (819)536-7500 x7511; Fax. (819)537-3489.

LAFFERTY, Kathleen B; Broadway Family Health Centre, 3 Herald Ave, Corner Brook NL A2H 4B8; Ott'98; BSc(Hons.); CCFP; FCFP.

LAFFEY, John G; St Michael's Hosp, 30 Bond St, Toronto ON M5B 1W8; Dublin (Ireland)'92; Staff, St Michael's Hospital; (416)360-4000

LAFKOVICI, Vladimir; Digby Prof Centre, PO Box 228, Digby NS B0V 1A0; Bucharest (Romania)'72; CCFP; Langs: Romanian; (902)245-6611; Fax. (902)245-6309.

LAFLAMME, Ann; CLSC Ste-Foy-Sillery, 3108 ch Sainte-Foy, Quebec QC G1X 1P8; Laval'82; Staff, Centre Hospitalier Universitaire de Quebec-CHUL; Physician, RAMQ; (418)651-2572; Fax. (418)651-3133.

LAFLAMME, Benoit; CSSS Pierre Boucher, 1333 boul Jacques-Cartier E, Longueuil QC J4M 2A5; Mon'88; Staff, Centre Hospitalier Pierre Boucher; (450)468-8111

LAFLAMME, Caroline; CSSS d'Antoine-Labelle, RR 4 1525 rue l'Annonciation N, Riviere-Rouge QC J0T 1T0; Laval'09; CCFP; Staff, Centre de L'Annonciation; (819)275-2118

LAFLAMME, Chantal; 100-900 Boul Moody, Terrebonne QC J6W 3K8; Mon'83; (450)471-1212; Fax. (450)471-5795.

LAFLAMME, Claude; Sunnybrook Hlth Sciences Ctre, M3 200-2075 Bayview Ave, Toronto ON M4N 3M5; Sher'86; CSPQ; FRCPC; Anes (Cardiac Anesthesia). Med Dir Cardiovascular Anes, Sunnybrook Health Sciences Centre; Langs: Bilingual(English/French); (416)480-6100 x4864; Fax. (416)480-6039; claude.laflamme@sunnybrook.ca.

LAFLAMME, David; Hotel-Dieu de Levis, 143 rue Wolfe, Levis QC G6V 3Z1; Laval'92; Staff, Hôtel-Dieu de Lévis; (418)835-7122

LAFLAMME, David; CHUS-Hop Fleurimont, 3001 12E av N, Sherbrooke QC J1H 5N4; Sher'06; Cardiol; IntMed. Staff, Centre Hospitalier Universitaire de Sherbrooke-Hopital Fleurimont; (819)346-1110

LAFLAMME, Denis; Clinique Med Saint-Nicephore, 4534 Boul Saint-Joseph, Saint-Nicephore QC J2A 1B5; Mon'82; CCFP; (819)472-3350; Fax. (819)472-0315.

LAFLAMME, Denis; Clinique d'Orthopedie de Levis, 6620 rue Saint-Georges, Levis QC G6V 4H1; Laval'61; OrthSurg (P.Q.). Staff, Hôtel-Dieu de Lévis; (418)837-8251; Fax. (418)837-2033.

LAFLAMME, George-Yves; Hop du Sacre-Coeur de Mtl, 5400 boul Gouin O, Montreal QC H4J 1C5; Sher'93; FRCSC; OrthSurg. assoc Prof, Universite de Montreal; (514)338-2222 x2060; gylaflamme@videotron.ca.

LAFLAMME, Georges; 480-1575 boul Henri-Bourassa O, Montreal QC H3M 3A9; Laval'68; MSc; DABOS; CSPQ; FRCS; FRCSC; OrthSurg (Trauma Adult Reconstructive Surgery). Staff OrthSurg, Hôpital du Sacre-Coeur de Montréal; Prof, Universite de Montreal; Langs: English; (514)332-6025; Fax. (514)332-4243.

LAFLAMME, Jean-Claude; 100-900 Boul Moody, Terrebonne QC J6W 3K8; Mon'83; (450)471-1212; Fax. (450)471-5795.

LAFLAMME, Julie; CHUQ-Ctr Hosp Univ Laval, 2705 boul Laurier, Quebec QC G1V 4G2; Sher'01; FRCPC; Peds (Palliative Medicine). Staff, Centre Hospitalier Universitaire de Quebec-CHUL; (418)654-2282

LAFLAMME, Louis; 420-900 boul Du Seminaire N, St-Jean-Sur-Richel QC J3A 1C3; Mon'69; DiagRad. Staff, Hôpital du Haut-Richelieu; Dir, Clinique Radiologie du Haut-Richelieu; Langs: English; French; (450)348-1111; Fax. (450)348-8585.

LAFLAMME, Louis; Hop Maisonneuve-Rosemont, 5415 boul de l'Assomption, Montreal QC H1T 2M4; Laval'83; AB; FRCPC; NuclearMed. Staff, Hopital Maisonneuve-Rosemont; adj Prof, Universite de Montreal; (514)252-3424

LAFLAMME, Marie; Clinique du Village, 382 rue Principale, St-Donat-De-Mtcalm QC J0T 2C0; Laval'87; (819)419-0123; Fax. (819)419-0126; marie.laflamme.gmf14@ssss.gouv.qc.ca.

LAFLAMME, Marie-Pierre; Clinique Medicale 3000, 3000 rue Belanger, Montreal QC H1Y 1A9; Mon'91; Langs: English; Italian; (514)376-7702; Fax. (514)376-2639.

LAFLAMME, Melissa; CHUQ-Ctr Hosp Univ Laval, 1211-2705 boul Laurier, Quebec QC G1V 4G2; Laval'06; FRCSC; OrthSurg. Staff, Centre Hospitalier Universitaire de Quebec-CHUL; Langs: Bilingual(French/English); (418)525-4444

LAFLAMME, Michel-Yves; Ctr Hosp de Lachine, 650 16e Av, Lachine QC H8S 3N5; Mon'65; Ophth. Staff, Centre Hospitalier de LaSalle; Consultant, Hôpital Ste-Justine; (514)637-2351

LAFLAMME, Nadia; CSSS de Trois-Rivieres, 155 rue Toupin, Trois-Rivieres QC G8T 3Z8; Laval'92; Staff Med, Centre de santé Cloutier-du-Rivage; Langs: Bilingual(French/English); (819)370-2100; Fax. (819)370-2362.

LAFLAMME, Nathalie; Clin Med du Vieux St-Eustache, 136 rue Saint-Louis, Saint-Eustache QC J7R 1Y2; Mon'03; CCFP; Langs: Bilingual(French/English); (514)370-2112

LAFLAMME, Patrice; Clinique Med Notre-Dame, 138 rue Notre-Dame S, Sainte-Marie QC G6E 4A4; Mon'90; MSc; LMCC; CommunMed (P.Q.). Langs: Bilingual(French/English); (418)387-5280; patrice_laflamme@ssss.gouv.qc.ca.

LAFLAMME, Paule; 582 rue Principale CP 29, St-Sebast-De-Front QC G0Y 1M0; Laval'85; Physician, Maison Paternelle-Foyer; (819)652-2402

LAFLAMME, Paule; Clin du Carrefour, 1005 rte Lagueux, St-Etienne-De-Lauz QC G6J 1J8; Laval'91; Staff, Hôtel-Dieu de Lévis; (418)836-2002

LAFLAMME, Pierre J; Hop Du Sacre-Coeur De Mtl, 5400 boul Gouin O, Montreal QC H4J 1C5; Mon'81; FRCPC; MedMicrobiol; Microbio & Infect Dis (P.Q.). Staff, Hôpital du Sacre-Coeur de Montréal; (514)338-2222 x2157; Fax. (514)338-2909.

LAFLAMME, Pierre; Hôpital Laval, 2725 ch Sainte-Foy, Quebec QC G1V 4G5; Laval'83; CSPQ; Anes. Staff, Hôpital Laval; (418)656-8711

LAFLAMME, Pierre; Clinique De Gastro-Enterologie, 90 rue Bernard, St-Charles-Brromee QC J6E 2C3; Mon'81; Gastroent (P. Q.); IntMed (P.Q.). Staff Gastroent, Centre Hospitalier Régional de Lanaudière; (450)752-6667; Fax. (450)752-5507.

LAFLAMME, Pierre; Polyclinique Med Concorde, 300 boul de la Concorde E, Laval QC H7G 2E6; Mon'68; DABOph; Ophth. Prof adj clin/Staff, Centre Hospitalier l'Université de Montréal (CHUM) - Hôpital Notre-Dame; adj Prof, Universite de Montreal; (450)667-5310

LAFLAMME, Sebastien; Centre Hosp de Charlevoix, 74 rue Ambroise-Fafard, Baie-Saint-Paul QC G3Z 2J6; Laval'07; CCFP; Staff, CSSS de Charlevoix; (418)435-5150 x2106

LAFLAMME, Sophie; CHUS-Hop Fleurimont, 3001 12e Av N, Sherbrooke QC J1H 5N4; Laval'94; FRCPC; Peds; Critical Care Medicine (P.Q.). Staff, Centre Hospitalier Universitaire de Sherbrooke-Hopital Fleurimont; Sec Faculty/vice Doyen Student Services, Universite de Sherbrooke; (819)346-1110; Fax. (819)820-6420.

LAFLAMME-FILLION, Annie; Hôpital régional Chaleur, 1750 Sunset Dr, Bathurst NB E2A 4L7; Sher'09; CCFP; Staff, Hopital Regional Chaleur; (506)544-3000

LAFLECHE, Claire M; 306-595 Montreal Rd, Ottawa ON K1K 4L2; McM'79; CCFP; FCFP; Vis Staff Privil, Montfort Hospital; (613)744-3236; Fax. (613)744-5624.

LAFLECHE, Francois E J; McArthur Med Centre, 390 McArthur Ave, Vanier ON K1L 6N6; Ott'80; CCFP; FCFP; (613)741-1134; Fax. (613)741-4276.

LAFLECHE, J J Rene; NORD-ASKI Family Health Team, PO Box 727 1403 Edward St, Hearst ON P0L 1N0; Ott'82; CCFP; FCFP; Ac Staff, Hôpital Notre Dame Hospital - Hearst; Langs: English; French; (705)362-7363; Fax. (705)372-6177.

LAFLECHE, Jean-Pierre; 202-595 Montreal Rd, Ottawa ON K1K 4L2; Ott'75; FACS; FRCSC; OrthSurg. Ac Staff Orthop Surg, Montfort Hospital; (613)746-6745; Fax. (613)746-6008.

LAFLECHE, Robert A; Clinique Med Memphre, 200-323 rue Sherbrooke, Magog QC J1X 2R9; Ott'76; (819)847-1313; lafleche.robert@sympatico.ca.

LAFLEUR, Alexandra; CHUQ-Ctr Hosp Univ Laval, D1207-2705 boul Laurier, Quebec QC G1V 4G2; Laval'07; IntMed. Staff, Centre Hospitalier Universitaire de Quebec-CHUL; (418)525-4444

LAFLEUR, Daniel; CSSS Drummond-Hop Sainte-Croix, 570 rue Heriot, Drummondville QC J2B 1C1; Sher'97; CCFP; Staff, Hôpital Sainte-croix; (819)478-6464

LAFLEUR, Daniel L; Children's & Women's HC of BC, 4500 Oak St, Vancouver BC V6H 3N1; McG'03; FRCPC; Psy. Staff, BC Women's Hospital & Health Centre; (604)875-2345; dlafleur@cw.bc.ca.

LAFLEUR, Edith P; Woodlawn Med Clinic, 92 Main St, Dartmouth NS B2X 1R5; Ott'99; CCFP; FCFP; (902)434-1500

LAFLEUR, J Richard; 202-189 boul Hymus, Pointe-Claire QC H9R 1E9; Ott'64; FRCSC; Otol. Staff, Lakeshore General Hospital - Pointe Claire; (514)695-5993; Fax. (514)695-3807.

LAFLEUR, Jacques O J; Delta Hosp, 5800 Mountain View Blvd, Delta BC V4K 3V6; Ott'76; CCFP; CCFP(E.M.); FCFP; Staff Emerg, Delta Hospital; (604)946-1121

LAFLEUR, Jean; 150-930 ch Sainte-Foy, Quebec QC G1S 2L4; Laval'69; Electroenceph (P.Q.); Neur. Ac Staff, Centre Hospitalier Universitaire De Québec - Pavillon De St-françois-d'assise; Teach Staff Neurol, Université Laval; (418)687-1311

LAFLEUR, Jean-Marc; GMF Concorde, 300 boul de la Concorde E, Laval QC H7G 2E6; Mon'67; Staff, Centre Hospitalier Fleury; (450)667-5310; Fax. (450)667-5248.

LAFLEUR, Julie; Clinique Pierre-Boucher, 1615 boul Jacques-Cartier E, Longueuil QC J4M 2X1; Sher'97; Staff, Hôpital Brome-Missisquoi-Perkins; (450)468-2488

LAFLEUR, Marie-Eve; CSSS du Lac-des-Deux-Montagnes, 520 boul Arthur-Sauve, Saint-Eustache QC J7R 5B1; Mon'08; CCFP; Staff, Hôpital de Saint-Eustache; (450)473-6811; Fax. (450)473-6966.

LAFLEUR, Martine; CHUM-Hop Notre-Dame, 1560 rue Sherbrooke E, Montreal QC H2L 4M1; Mon'94; BSc(Nutrition); MSc(Nutrition); FRCPC; IntMed; GeriatricMed. Staff, Centre Hospitalier l'Université de Montréal (CHUM) - Hôpital Notre-Dame; Langs: English; Italian; (514)890-8000 x26769

LAFLEUR, Paul-Andre; Clinique Med Chamberland, 641 av Beaumont, Montreal QC H3N 1V7; Mon'83; FRCPC; Psy. adj Prof, Universite de Montreal; (514)385-1977

LAFLEUR, Pierre; CLSC Jacques-Cartier, 11150 boul Valcartier, Quebec QC G2A 2M5; Laval'84; (418)843-3001

LAFOND, Chantal; Centre de Sante Rene-Ricard, CP 1300 32 3e av, Chapais QC G0W 1H0; Sher'90; LMCC; (418)745-2591

LAFOND, Chantal; Hop Du Sacre-Coeur De Mtl, 5400 boul Gouin O, Montreal QC H4J 1C5; Mon'87; FRCPC; IntMed (Asthma); Respir. Staff, Hôpital du Sacre-Coeur de Montréal; (514)338-2162

LAFOND, Daniel; Ctr Hosp De Verdun, 4000 boul Lasalle, Verdun QC H4G 2A3; Mon'84; Staff, Centre Hospitalier de Verdun; (514)765-8121

LAFOND, Elaine; Hop Brome-Missisquoi-Perkins, 950 rue Principale, Cowansville QC J2K 1K3; Mon'01; Staff, Hôpital Brome-Missisquoi-Perkins; (450)266-4342

LAFOND, Gilles-Philippe; Clinique D'Ophtalmologie, 200-2875 boul Laurier, Quebec QC G1V 2M2; Laval'78; AB; FRCSC; Ophth (Refractive Surgery). Staff, Centre Hospitalier Affilié Universitaire de Québec - Hôpital du St-Sacrement; Langs: English; German; Italian; Spanish; (418)658-2010; Fax. (418)658-8310.

LAFOND, Guillaume; CSSS Haut-Richelieu-Rouville, 920 boul du Seminaire N, St-Jean-sur-Richel QC J3A 1B7; Mon'03; FRCPC; IntMed; Gastroent. Staff, Hôpital du Haut-Richelieu; (450)359-5000

LAFOND, Jean-Robert; CSSS de Rimouski-Neigette, CP 3150 Succ A 150 av Rouleau, Rimouski QC G5L 5T1; Laval'78; CSPQ; Anes. Staff, Hôpital Regional Rimouski; (418)724-8282; Fax. (418)723-7668.

LAFOND, Johanne; Clinique Med Pierre-Boucher, 1615 boul Jacques-Cartier E, Longueuil QC J4M 2X1; Mon'84; Langs: Bilingual(French/English); (450)468-6223; Fax. (450)468-5041.

LAFOND, Lucie; Clin Med Pediatrique Lafond, 111-10 rue Notre-Dame, Repentigny QC J6A 2N9; Mon'85; Peds (Neonatology). Pediatrics, Centre Hospitalier Pierre le Gardeur; (450)657-2544

LAFOND, Michel; Clinique Med de la Rive, 169 av Prince Albert, Otterburn Park QC J3H 1L4; Mon'92; (450)446-7333; Fax. (450)446-3420.

LAFOND, Michel; Clinique Med Shawinigan-Sud, 200-2355 5e av, Shawinigan-Sud QC G9P 1P4; Sher'86; CCFP; FCFP; (819)537-6205; Fax. (819)537-5596; michel.lafond@gmf.gouv.qc.ca.

LAFOND, Sylvain; Clinique Med Antoine-Labelle, 555 boul Saint-Antoine, Saint-Jerome QC J7Z 3B8; Mon'96; (450)438-1252; Fax. (450)438-6441.

LAFONTAINE, Alika; Queen Elizabeth II Hosp, 10409 98 St, Grande Prairie AB T8V 2E8; Sask'06; FRCPC; Anes. Staff, Queen Elizabeth II Hospital; (780)538-7100

LAFONTAINE, Anne-Louise; MUHC-Montreal Gen Hosp, L7 312-1650 av Cedar, Montreal QC H3G 1A4; McM'93; FRCPC; Neur (Movement Disorders). Staff, McGill University Health Centre - Montreal General Campus; (514)934-8026; Fax. (514)934-8265.

LAFONTAINE, Danielle; Clinique Med Boisbriand, 877 boul de la Grande-Allee, Boisbriand QC J7G 1W6; Laval'83; (450)437-4600; Fax. (450)437-7038.

LAFONTAINE, Edwin R; CHUM-Hotel-Dieu, 3840 rue Saint-Urbain, Montreal QC H2W 1T8; Sher'74; FRCSC; GenSurg; Cardiovasc&ThorSurg. ac Staff, Centre Hospitalier l'Université de Montréal (CHUM) - Hôtel-Dieu; (514)890-8000

LAFONTAINE, Gilles; CRSSS Baie-James-Sante Lebel, GD 950 boul Quevillon N, Lebel-s-Quevillon QC J0Y 1X0; Sher'84; CCFP; Fam Med, Centre de santé Lebel; (819)755-4881; Fax. (819)755-3779.

LAFONTAINE, J A Guy; CSSS de Trois-Rivieres, 155 rue Toupin, Trois-Rivieres QC G8T 3Z8; Laval'63; FRCPC; DiagRad. Staff, Centre de santé Cloutier-du-Rivage; (819)370-2285; Fax. (819)370-2182.

LAFONTAINE, Laurie; CSSS Pierre Boucher, 1333 boul Jacques-Cartier E, Longueuil QC J4M 2A5; McG'08; CCFP; CCFP(E.M.); Staff, Centre Hospitalier Pierre Boucher; (450)468-8111

LAFONTAINE, Lucie; Hop Charles LeMoyne, 3120 boul Taschereau, Greenfield Park QC J4V 2H1; Mon'97; DiagRad. Staff, Hopital Charles LeMoyne; (450)466-5000

LAFONTAINE, Marc; Medisys, 500 rue Sherbrooke O, Montreal QC H3A 3C6; Laval'81; FRCPC; DiagRad. Staff, Lakeshore General Hospital - Pointe Claire; (514)499-2782

LAFONTAINE, Nancy; Polyclinique du Cap, 110-700 boul Thibeau, Trois-Rivieres QC G8T 7A1; Sher'90; FRCPC; Derm. Staff/Médecin, CSSS de Trois-Rivières; (819)373-4551; Fax. (819)373-6516.

LAFONTAINE, Robert E; D-640 Ross Ave E, Timmins ON P4N 0A2; Mon'97; FRCSC; OrthSurg. Staff OrthSurg, Timmins & District Hospital; Langs: Bilingual(French/English); (705)267-2131

LAFONTAINE, Sylvain-Louis; Medisys, 5e-500 rue Sherbrooke O, Montreal QC H3A 3C6; Mon'82; FRCPC; Psy. Staff, Hopital Louis-H Lafontaine; (514)499-2777; Fax. (514)499-8004.

LAFONTAINE-GODBOUT, Matthieu; Inst U Geriatrie Sherbrooke, 1036 rue Belvedere S, Sherbrooke QC J1H 4C4; Sher'09; CCFP; Staff, CSSS Institut universitaire de gériatrie de Sherbrooke.

LAFORCE, Paul C; 26 CF Health Services Centre, PO Box 5000 Greenwood Rpo, Greenwood NS B0P 1N0; Dal'93.

LAFORCE, Robert; Ctr Hosp Affilie-Enfant-Jesus, 1401 18e rue, Quebec QC G1J 1Z4; Laval'06; FRCPC; Neur. Staff, Centre Hospitalier Affilié Universitaire de Québec - Hôpital De L'Enfant Jésus; (418)649-0252

LAFOREST, Carole; Clinique de Mistissini, GD 395 boul Mistissini, Mistissini QC G0W 1C0; Sher'91; Staff, CSSS de la Basse Côté-Nord; (418)923-3376

LAFOREST, Jacques J; Angus Family Med Centre, PO Box 2042 1-38 Margaret St, Angus ON L0M 1B0; Laval'67; Ac Staff, Stevenson Memorial Hospital; Preceptor Undergrad Student, University of Toronto; Langs: English; French; (705)424-5700; Fax. (705)424-1868.

LAFOREST-RENALD, Alexandra; Hop Du Sacre-Coeur De Mtl, 5400 boul Gouin O, Montreal QC H4J 1C5; Laval'98; FRCPC; IntMed; Nephrol. Staff, Hôpital du Sacre-Coeur de Montréal; (514)338-2050

LAFORGE, Jacques M; Hôpital Laval, 2725 ch Sainte-Foy, Quebec QC G1V 4G5; Laval'71; Respir (Apnea). Staff Home Care Prog, Hôpital Laval; Clin Adj, Université Laval; Langs: Bilingual(French/English); (418)656-4747

LAFORGE, Marlene; CRSSS Baie-James-Chibougamau, 51 3e rue, Chibougamau QC G8P 1N1; Laval'03; CCFP; Staff, CRSSS de la Baie-James; (418)748-2676

LAFORME, Lucie; CSSS de l'Energie-Ste-Therese, 1705 av Georges, Shawinigan QC G9N 2N1; Laval'85; Staff, CH du Centre-de-la-Mauricie (Ste-Thérèse de Shawinigan); (819)536-7575 x4276; Fax. (819)539-0078; lucie_laforme@ssss.gouv.qc.ca.

LAFORTE, Anne R; Bluewater Health-Norman Site, 89 Norman St, Sarnia ON N7T 6S3; West Indies (Jamaica)'80; MB BS; CABAP; DABFE; FRCPC; Psy (Child & Adolescent Psychiatry). Staff, Bluewater Health - Norman Site; Consultant Psy, Chatham Kent Integrated Children's Services; (519)464-4500; Fax. (519)464-4516.

LAFORTE, Mario; 644 rue Jacques-Cartier E, Chicoutimi QC G7H 2A4; Laval'73; FCCP; FRCPC; Respir (Pneumology). Ac Staff, Complexe hospitalier de la Sagamie; adj Prof, Universite de Sherbrooke; Langs: Bilingual(French/English); (418)549-1512; Fax. (418)549-6965.

LAFORTUNE, Chantal; Clin de Gyn et de Maternite, 1811 av Dollard, Lasalle QC H8N 1T9; Mon'95; FRCSC; ObstGyn. Langs: Bilingual(French/English); (514)364-3700; chantal.lafortune@hotmail.com.

LAFORTUNE, Claude; CLSC Naskapi, CP 5154, Kawawachikamach QC G0G 2Z0; Mon'91; Staff, CSSS de la Minganie; (418)585-2897

LAFORTUNE, Donald; GMF de l'Assomption, CP 3406 814 boul l'Ange-Gardien N, L'Assomption QC J5W 4M9; Mon'77; (450)589-5778

LAFORTUNE, Jacques; Ctr Hosp De Verdun, 4000 boul Lasalle, Verdun QC H4G 2A3; Mon'95; CCFP; Staff Emerg Services & Cardiol, Centre Hospitalier de Verdun; (514)362-1000

LAFORTUNE, Pascale; CSSS de Sept-Iles, 45 rue Du Pere-Divet, Sept-Iles QC G4R 3N7; Mon'92; FRCPC; IntMed. Staff, Centre Hospitalier Regional de Sept-Iles; (418)962-9761

LAFORTUNE, Valerie; Clinique Medicale, CP 1000 Succ Forces, Shannon QC G0A 4N0; Ott'06; CCFP; (418)844-5000

LAFORTUNE-PAYETTE, Annie; CSSS de Chicoutimi, 305 rue Saint-Vallier, Chicoutimi QC G7H 5H6; Mon'07; GenSurg. Staff, Complexe hospitalier de la Sagamie; (418)541-1000

LAFORTY, Jack M; 4319 Cove Rd PO Box 58, Portland ON K0G 1V0; Tor'91; Staff, Brockville Mental Health Centre - Royal Ottawa Health Care Group; (613)272-3302; jlaforty@crchc.on.ca.

LAFOURNAISE, Carrie L; Pritchard Farm Health Centre, 5-3014 Henderson Hwy, East St Paul MB R2E 0H9; Man'07; CCFP.

LAFRAMBOISE, Karen F; Royal University Hosp, 103 Hospital Dr, Saskatoon SK S7N 0W8; Ott'89; FRCPC; Respir; Critical Care Medicine; IntMed. Staff, Royal University Hospital; Assoc Prof, University of Saskatchewan; Langs: French; (306)966-8274; Fax. (306)966-8694; karen.laframboise@usask.ca.

LAFRAMBOISE, Patrice; Clinique Medicale du Granit, 110-3700 rue Laval, Lac-Megantic QC G6B 1A4; Sher'90; CCFP; FCFP; Chef IntMed, Carrefour Sante Granit; (819)583-0075; Fax. (819)583-0056.

LAFRAMBOISE, Rachel; CHUQ-Ctr Hosp Univ Laval, H1336-2705 boul Laurier, Quebec QC G1V 4G2; Sher'74; MedGenetics (P.Q.). Staff, Centre Hospitalier Universitaire de Quebec-CHUL; Langs: English; (418)656-4141 x47130

LAFRAMBOISE, Stephane; Univ Hlth Network-Princess M, M 700-610 University Ave, Toronto ON M5G 2M9; Tor'90; BSc; MSc; FRCSC; ObstGyn (Chemotherapy). Staff Gyn Oncol, Princess Margaret Hospital - University Health Network; Asst Prof, University of Toronto; Langs: English; French; (416)946-2254; Fax. (416)946-2288.

LAFRANCE, Dominique; CHUM-Hop Notre-Dame, 1560 rue Sherbrooke E, Montreal QC H2L 4M1; Mon'02; FRCPC; IntMed; Critical Care Medicine (P.Q.). Staff, Centre Hospitalier l'Université de Montréal (CHUM) - Hôpital Notre-Dame.

LAFRANCE, Elise; 894 boul Maloney E, Gatineau QC J8P 1H5; Laval'85; FRCPC; Peds. (819)643-3566

LAFRANCE, Gilles; Clinique Medicale Du Jardin, 200-15094 boul Henri-Bourassa, Quebec QC G1G 3Z4; Laval'80; Ac Staff, Centre Hospitalier Universitaire De Québec - Pavillon De St-françois-d'assise; (418)628-9074; Fax. (418)628-0267.

LAFRANCE, Jean-Philippe; Hop Maisonneuve-Rosemont, 5415 boul de l'Assomption, Montreal QC H1T 2M4; Mon'01; FRCPC; IntMed; Nephrol. Staff, Hopital Maisonneuve-Rosemont; (514)252-3400

LAFRANCE, Julie; Hop Maisonneuve-Rosemont, 5415 boul de l'Assomption, Montreal QC H1T 2M4; Mon'04; DiagRad. Staff, Hopital Maisonneuve-Rosemont; (514)252-3400

LAFRANCE, Justine; Clinique Med de l'Assomption, 201-814 boul l'Ange-Gardien N, L'Assomption QC J5W 4M9; Laval'09; (450)589-5778

LAFRANCE, Rena S; Misericordia Community Hosp, 2F-16940 87 Ave NW, Edmonton AB T5R 4H5; Man'00; FRCPC; Psy. Staff, Covenant Health - Misericordia Community Hospital; (780)735-2731; Fax. (780)735-2794.

LAFRANCE, Serge; CSST, CP 1200 Succ Terminus 280-524 rue Bourdages, Quebec QC G1K 7E2; Laval'79; LMCC; Médecin, Commission de la Sante Securite du Travail; (418)266-4670

LAFRANCHISE, Karine; CSSS de Quebec-Sud, 900 boul Wilfrid-Hamel, Quebec QC G1M 2R9; Laval'07; Staff, CSSS de Quebec-Sud; (418)682-1762

LAFRANCHISE, Luc; Clinique Sante de Thetford, 926 rue Labbe, Thetford Mines QC G6G 2A8; Laval'99; (418)338-4619

LAFRENAYE, Sylvie; CHUS-Hop Fleurimont, 3001 12e Av N, Sherbrooke QC J1H 5N4; Sher'84; FRCPC; Peds. Staff, Centre Hospitalier Universitaire de Sherbrooke-Hopital Fleurimont; (819)346-1110; Fax. (819)564-5398; sylvie.lafrenaye@usherbrooke.ca.

LAFRENIERE, Anne-Marie; Ctr Hosp du Centre la Mauricie, 50 119e rue, Shawinigan-Sud QC G9P 5K1; Mon'02; FRCPC; IntMed. Staff, Centre Hospitalier du Centre la Mauricie; (819)536-7500

LAFRENIERE, Bernard; Centre d'Urgence St-Laurent, 200-1605 boul Marcel-Laurin, Saint-Laurent QC H4R 0B7; Mon'66; Staff, Hôpital du Sacre-Coeur de Montréal; (514)747-2555

LAFRENIERE, Celine; CLSC des Seigneuries, RR 102 555 rue Principale, Saint-Amable QC J0L 1N0; Mon'78; Med Dir-Pub Hlth, Hopital Charles LeMoyne; (450)468-5250; Fax. (450)468-5251.

LAFRENIERE, Lynn M; Halton HCS Corp-Oakville, 327 Reynolds St, Oakville ON L6J 3L7; Leeds (England)'88; FRCPC; Anes. Staff Anes, Halton Healthcare Services Corporation - Oakville Site; (905)845-2571

LAFRENIERE, Marie; 2400-504 rue Notre-Dame, Repentigny QC J6A 2T8; Mon'86; Staff, Centre Hospitalier Pierre le Gardeur; (450)582-3992; Fax. (450)582-7412.

LAFRENIERE, Marie-France; CSSS de Saint-Jerome, 290 rue de Montigny, Saint-Jerome QC J7Z 5T3; Mon'94; Psy (P.Q.). Staff, Hôtel-Dieu de Saint-Jérôme; Langs: Bilingual(French/English); (450)431-8200

LAFRENIERE, Michel; La Cite Medicale, 295-2600 boul Laurier, Quebec QC G1V 4T3; Laval'83; Staff, Centre Hospitalier Universitaire de Québec (CHUQ) - Siege Social; assoc Staff, Centre Hospitalier Affilié Universitaire de Québec - Hôpital De L'Enfant Jésus; (418)781-0480; Fax. (418)780-1843; michel.lafreniere@sympatico.ca.

LAFRENIERE, Rene; Foothill Med Centre, 1403 29 St NW, Calgary AB T2N 2T9; McG'77; FACS; FRCSC; GenSurg (Surgical Oncology). Staff Surg Calgary Health Region, Foothills Medical Centre; Staff, Tom Baker Cancer Centre; Teach Staff, University of Calgary; Langs: English; French; (403)944-2835; Fax. (403)270-0671; rene.lafreniere@albertahealthservices.ca.

LAFRENIERE, Renee; Clin Med Saint-Chrysostome, GD 23 rang Sainte-Anne, Saint-Chrysostome QC J0S 1R0; Mon'75; (450)826-3154

LAFRENIERE, Robert W; Foothills Med Centre, C231-1403 29 St NW, Calgary AB T2N 2T9; UBC'03; Staff EmergMed, Foothills Medical Centre; (403)944-8430

LAFRENIERE, Ronald T J; Victoria Gen Hosp, 1 Hospital Way, Victoria BC V8Z 6R5; Ott'74; BSc; MSc; FRCPC; PhysMed&Rehab. Staff, Victoria General Hospital; Langs: English; French; (250)727-4221; Fax. (250)727-4225.

LAFTAH, Abdulrahem L A; 535 Granville St, Summerside PE C1N 6N4; Baghdad (Iraq)'69; PhmB; CCFP; Staff, Community Hospital Inc; Langs: Russian; Arabic.

LAGACÉ, Anne-Renée; Clinique Med Nepisiguit, 950 Picot Ave, Bathurst NB E2A 4Z9; Mon'07; CCFP; (506)544-3000

LAGACE, Annie; Hop Du Sacre-Coeur De Mtl, 5400 boul Gouin O, Montreal QC H4J 1C5; Sher'96; CSPQ; FRCPC; Anes. Staff, Hôpital du Sacre-Coeur de Montréal; (514)338-2222

LAGACE, Catherine; Clin Dermatologique de Lachena, 345-950 montee des Pionniers, Terrebonne QC J6V 1S8; Mon'01; Derm. Langs: Bilingual(French/English); (450)470-1221; Fax. (450)470-1586.

LAGACE, Dannie; CSSS de la Mitis, 800 av du Sanatorium, Mont-Joli QC G5H 3L6; Sher'93; CCFP; Staff, CSSS de la Mitis; (418)775-7261 x3100; Fax. (418)775-6487; dannie.lagace@cgocable.ca.

LAGACE, Gilles; 200-3030 boul Le carrefour, Laval QC H7T 2P5; McG'73; (450)686-8899; Fax. (450)686-7466.

LAGACE, Jean; CSSS de l'Energie, 1265 rue Trudel, Shawinigan QC G9N 8T3; Sher'72; (819)539-8371 x8290

LAGACE, Louis-Marie; Clinique Med 201, 104 rue Sainte-Agathe, Ste-Agathe-Des-Mts QC J8C 2K3; Laval'77; Chef, Centre Hospitalier Laurentien; Langs: English; (819)326-2020; Fax. (819)326-8801.

LAGACE, Marc; Campbellton Med Clinic, PO Box 246 Snt Main, Campbellton NB E3N 3G4; Laval'91; DDS; FRCSC; GenSurg (Oncology). Staff Surgeon, Hôpital Régional Campbellton; Langs: English; (506)753-2292; Fax. (506)789-7641.

LAGACE, Real; CSSS de Rimouski-Neigette, CP 3150 succ A 150 av Rouleau, Rimouski QC G5L 5T1; Laval'66; CSPQ; FRCPC; AnatPath (Soft Tissue Disorders). Staff, Hôpital Regional Rimouski; Prof Path, Université Laval; Langs: German; English; (418)724-3000 x8535; real.lagace@hotmail.com.

LAGACE-WIENS, Philippe R; St Boniface Gen Hosp, L4025-409 Tache Ave, Winnipeg MB R2H 2A6; Man'03; FRCPC; MedMicrobiol. Asst Prof, Health Sciences Centre; Staff, St Boniface General Hospital; (204)233-8563

LAGANIERE, Louise; Clinique Med Chemin Chambly, 101-3090 ch de Chambly, Longueuil QC J4L 4N5; Sher'77; Langs: English; (450)670-5700; Fax. (450)670-8830.

LAGANIERE, Marie-Josee; 50 ch du Golf E, St-Charles-Brromee QC J6E 2B4; Mon'08; CCFP; (450)759-3060; Fax. (450)759-7799.

LAGANIERE, Michel; Hotel-Dieu d'Arthabaska, 5 rue des Hospitalieres, Victoriaville QC G6P 6N2; Laval'72; GenSurg (P.Q.). Staff Surg, Hotel-Dieu d'Arthabaska; Asst Prof Surg, Universite de Sherbrooke; (819)357-2030 x2108

LAGANIERE, Yves; CSSS Haut-Richelieu-Rouville, 920 boul Du Seminaire N, St-Jean-Sur-Richel QC J3A 1B7; Mon'83; Staff, Hôpital du Haut-Richelieu; (450)359-5000

LAGARE, Bahubali D; 112-377 Burnhamthorpe Rd E, Mississauga ON L5A 3Y1; Karnataka (India)'97; CCFP; Langs: Marathi; Hindi; Urdu; Kanarese; (905)896-3777; Fax. (905)896-7847.

LAGE, Karen L; Springfield Heights Med Centre, 4-963 Henderson Hwy, Winnipeg MB R2K 2M3; Man'93; CCFP; (204)663-4404; Fax. (204)663-3671.

LAGEIX, Philippe; Douglas Mental Hlth Univ Inst, 6875 boul Lasalle, Verdun QC H4H 1R3; Paris (France)'84; Staff, Douglas Mental Health University Institute; adj Prof, Universite de Montreal; adj Prof, McGill University; Langs: Bilingual(English/French); Creole; Spanish; (514)761-6131 x4604; Fax. (514)769-1745; lagphi@douglas.mcgill.ca.

LAGODICH, Marina; Hôp Santa Cabrini Ospedale, 5655 av Saint-Zotique E, Montreal QC H1T 1P7; McG'10; MDCM; Staff, Hôpital Santa Cabrini Ospedale; (514)252-6000

LAGOWSKI, Michael C; Norwood Family Med Centre, 43A Marion St, Winnipeg MB R2H 0S8; (Poland)'64.

LAGRENADE-VERDANT, Colin; Hop Du Sacre-Coeur De Mtl, 5400 boul Gouin O, Montreal QC H4J 1C5; Mon'97; FRCPC; IntMed; Critical Care Medicine (P.Q.). Staff, Hôpital du Sacre-Coeur de Montréal; (514)338-2222 x2050

LAGROTTERIA, Danny D; 2C Renal Clinic, 155 Ontario St, St Catharines ON L2R 5K3; Cal'02; FRCPC; IntMed; Nephrol. (905)682-6411

LAGROTTERIA, David M; Niagara H System-St Catherine, PO Box 3018 Stn Main 142 Queenston St, St. Catharines ON L2R 7C6; Tor'07; FRCPC; Anes. Staff, Niagara Health System - St Catharines General Site; (905)684-7271

LAGROTTERIA, Leda C; Westmount Comm Health Ctr, 800-723 Rymal Rd W, Hamilton ON L9B 2W2; McM'86; CCFP; FCFP; Staff, St Joseph's Healthcare - Charlton Campus; Asst Prof Family Med, McMaster University; Langs: Italian; French; (905)574-1115; Fax. (905)574-2283.

LAGROTTERIA, Lino P; Westmount Community Health Ctr, 800-723 Rymal Rd W, Hamilton ON L9B 2W2; McM'86; BSc(Hon.); MSc; CCFP; FCFP; Langs: Italian; French; (905)574-1115; Fax. (905)574-2283.

LAGUE, Guylaine; GMF Centre de santé, 3745 rue Georges-Couture, Drummondville QC J2B 7P4; Sher'05; CCFP; (819)477-2231; Fax. (819)477-1122.

LAGUE, Johanne; Inst Nat'l Sante Publique, 190 boul Cremazie E, Montreal QC H2P 1E2; Sher'80; MRCP; CSPQ; MPH; FRCPC; CommunMed (Health Promotion). Med Consultant Preventive Med, Hopital Charles LeMoyne; Coord Scientific, Unite Habitudes de Vie, Inst. Nat'l. de Sante Publique du Quebec; Clinical Asst Prof Social & Preventive Med, Universite de Montreal; assoc Prof Med, Universite de Sherbrooke; (514)864-1600 x3536; Fax. (514)864-1616; johanne.lague@inspq.qc.ca.

LAGUE, Nadine; Ctr Hosp Laurentien, 234 rue Saint-Vincent, Ste-Agathe-des-Mts QC J8C 2B8; Mon'97; ObstGyn. Staff, Centre Hospitalier Laurentien; (819)324-4000

LAGUE, Normand; Centre medical de Cowansville, 101-370 rue de la Riviere, Cowansville QC J2K 1N3; Mon'70; Langs: English; (450)263-0774

LAGUEUX, Viviane; Polyclinique Med de La Lievre, 536 rue de la Madone, Mont-Laurier QC J9L 1S7; Mon'78; (819)440-2345; Fax. (819)440-2330.

LAHAIE, Pascale; CSSS de Trois-Rivieres, 155 rue Toupin, Trois-Rivieres QC G8T 3Z8; Mon'83; Staff, Centre de santé Cloutier-du-Rivage; (819)370-2200 x3239

LAHAIE, Raymond; CHUM-Hop St-Luc, 1058 rue Saint-Denis, Montreal QC H2X 3J4; Sher'74; Gastroent; IntMed. Gastroent, Centre Hospitalier l'Université De Montréal (CHUM) - Hôpital Saint-luc; assoc Prof Med, Universite de Montreal; (514)890-8000 x36383; Fax. (514)412-7372; lahaier@sympatico.ca.

LAHAM, Robert S; Appletree Medical Centre, 4700 Keele St, North York ON M3J 1P3; Tor'86; BSc; Staff EmergMed, Humber River Regional Hospital - Keele Street Site; (416)736-5525; Fax. (416)736-5523.

LAHAYE, Pierre-Andre; Clinique Med Douville, 5460 boul Laurier O, Saint-Hyacinthe QC J2S 3V7; Laval'79; (450)773-8777; Fax. (450)771-7530.

LAHENS, Pierre; Clinique Med Viau, 4750 rue Jarry E, Saint-Leonard QC H1R 1X8; (Haiti)'69; Staff, Hôpital Riviere des Prairies; (514)326-7203

LAHENS, Roger; Clinique Med Chemin Chambly, 101-3090 ch de Chambly, Longueuil QC J4L 4N5; (Haiti)'71; (450)670-5700; Fax. (450)670-8830.

LAHEY, Sandra K; Lahey Med Centre, 2204-120 5 Ave W, Cochrane AB T4C 0A4; Witwatersrand (South Africa)'97; MB ChB; (403)981-6000; Fax. (403)981-6001.

LAHIFFE, Brian F; 615-1641 Lonsdale Ave, North Vancouver BC V7M 2J5; Qns'00; CCFP; CCFP(E.M.).

LAHLOU, Hala; Ctr Hosp de Verdun, 4000 boul Lasalle, Verdun QC H4G 2A3; McG'03; BSc; CCFP; Staff, Centre Hospitalier de Verdun; (514)362-1000

LAHNSTEINER, Eric P; Mississauga Med Centre, 410-1420 Burnhamthorpe Rd E, Mississauga ON L4X 2Z9; Tor'80; CCFP; (905)624-1597; Fax. (905)624-6853.

LAHOUD, Nadine J; Ctr Hosp de Lasalle, 8585 Tsse Champlain, Lasalle QC H8P 1C1; Beirut (Lebanon)'90; FRCPC; IntMed. Staff, Centre Hospitalier de LaSalle; Langs: Arabic; French; (514)362-8000; Fax. (514)731-2708.

LAHOUD, Salim; CHUM-Hop Notre-Dame, 1560 rue Sherbrooke E, Montreal QC H2L 4M1; St. Joseph (Lebanon)'82; FRCSC; Ophth (Ophthalmology Pathology). Chef opthal, Centre Hospitalier l'Université de Montréal (CHUM) - Hôpital Notre-Dame; Langs: Arabic; English; (514)890-8000 x27103; salimlahoud@videotron.ca.

LAI, Albert I; 201-390 Steeles Ave W, Thornhill ON L4J 6X2; Wes'92; Langs: Cantonese; Mandarin; (905)707-8682; Fax. (905)707-8415.

LAI, Alice M; 347 Spadina Ave, Toronto ON M5T 2G3; Tor'77; Court Staff Family Pract, Mount Sinai Hospital; Court Staff, The Scarborough Hospital - Birchmount Campus; Court Staff, The Scarborough Hospital - General Campus; (416)977-1560

LAI, Alvin Y W; Baywood Med Centre, 205-95 Bayly St W, Ajax ON L1S 7K8; Tor'00; CCFP; (905)683-2900; Fax. (905)683-2904.

LAI, Andrea S L P; Vital Health Med & Aesthetic, 1855 4th Ave W, Vancouver BC V6J 1M5; Man'05; CCFP; (604)558-4825

LAI, Chi Kien; The Ottawa Hosp-Gen Campus, 4114-501 Smyth Rd, Ottawa ON K1H 8L6; McG'99; FRCPC; AnatPath. Staff, The Ottawa Hospital - General Campus; (613)737-8899

LAI, Christopher C; Curans Health Centre, 384 Fort William Rd, Thunder Bay ON P7B 2Z3; Tor'77; FRCPC; IntMed; Cardiol. Consultant Cardiol, Thunder Bay Regional Health Sciences Centre; Med Dir for Translational Research, Thunder Bay Regional Health; Pres, Curans Health Centre Corp; Assoc Prof, Northern Ontario School of Medicine; Clin Assoc Prof, McMaster University; Aj Prof, Lakehead University / Library; Langs: English; Cantonese; (807)345-3355; Fax. (807)345-0099; chrislai@tbaytel.net.

LAI, Crystal Y C; Markham Stouffville Hosp, PO Box 1800 Stn Main 381 Church St, Markham ON L3P 7P3; Wes'10; CCFP; Staff, Markham Stouffville Hospital; (905)472-7373

LAI, David K F; 1757 Robson St, Vancouver BC V6G 1C9; Cal'93; CCFP; Langs: Cantonese; (604)689-1828; Fax. (604)689-1849.

LAI, Eliza P Y; Ashgrove Med Centre, 210-6633 Highway 7, Markham ON L3P 7P2; (Hong Kong)'89; CCFP; FCFP; Ac Staff, Markham Stouffville Hospital; Langs: Chinese; (905)294-3170; Fax. (905)294-3379.

LAI, Emily J; Univ Hlth Network-Toronto Gen, 3 805-200 Elizabeth St, Toronto ON M5G 2C4; Tor'06; Cardiol; IntMed. Staff, Toronto General Hospital - UHN; (416)978-2645

LAI, Emily J; Royal Columbian Hosp, 330 Columbia St E, New Westminster BC V3L 3W7; UBC'05; FRCPC; IntMed. Staff, Royal Columbian Hospital; (604)520-4253

LAI, Enoch K Y; North York Gen Hosp, 4001 Leslie St, North York ON M2K 1E1; Alb'94; LMCC; FRCPC; DiagRad. Staff Medical Imaging, North York General Hospital; Langs: Chinese; (416)756-6186; Fax. (416)756-6370; enoch.lai@nygh.on.ca.

LAI, Godwin; St Joseph's Health Centre, 30 The Queensway, Toronto ON M6R 1B5; Tor'96; CCFP; Staff, St Joseph's Health Centre; (416)530-6004

LAI, Grace H K; 302-8055 Anderson Rd, Richmond BC V6Y 1S2; UBC'87; (604)273-9392

LAI, Henry H C; Oak Ridges Urgent Care Centre, 13291 Yonge St, Richmond Hill ON L4E 4L6; Tor'04; CCFP; CCFP(E.M.); (905)773-7759

LAI, Ho-Yin; Malton Med Arts Bldg, 107-3530 Derry Rd E, Mississauga ON L4T 4E3; Qns'92; CCFP; FCFP; (905)677-6532; Fax. (905)677-6533.

LAI, Jacob K T; Univ Hlth Network-Toronto Western Hosp, 399 Bathurst St, Toronto ON M5T 2S8; Tor'79; FRCPC; Anes. Staff, Toronto Western Hospital - University Health Network; (416)603-5118; Fax. (416)603-6494.

LAI, James K; 620-943 Broadway W, Vancouver BC V5Z 1K3; UBC'83; CAFCI; CCFP; FCFP; Ac Staff, Providence Health Care - Mount Saint Joseph Hospital; Ac Staff, BC Women's Hospital & Health Centre; Clin Assoc Prof Family Pract, University of British Columbia; Langs: Cantonese; (604)738-8030; Fax. (604)738-8021.

LAI, Jatina; Lions Gate Hosp, 231 15th St E, North Vancouver BC V7L 2L7; UBC'06; CCFP; CCFP(E.M.); Staff, Lions Gate Hospital; Langs: Cantonese; (604)984-5799

LAI, Joe H; Oak Ridges Med Centre, 13291 Yonge St, Richmond Hill ON L4E 4L6; Tor'07; FRCPC; IntMed. Staff, North York General Hospital; (905)773-7759

LAI, John T W; 200-5503 206 St, Langley BC V3A 2C6; UBC'96; MD; BSc; FRCPC; DiagRad. Staff, Langley Memorial Hospital; (604)534-4114; Fax. (604)534-7877; johnlai88@hotmail.com.

LAI, Kai-Fai; 202-8035 120 St, Delta BC V4C 6P8; (Taiwan)'62; FRCSC; GenSurg (Vascular Surgery). Chief GenSurg, Surrey Memorial Hospital; Clin Instructor, University of British Columbia; Langs: Chinese; (604)596-3243; Fax. (604)589-1538.

LAI, Ken K K; 5017 47A Ave, Delta BC V4K 1T9; Monash (Australia)'69; MB BS; (604)946-1168; Fax. (604)946-4251.

LAI, Kenneth K K; C-17215 Leslie St, Newmarket ON L3Y 8E4; Tor'87; DIMOH; Staff, Southlake Regional Health Centre; Med Dir, York Medical; Med Dir, Bradford Valley LTC; Med Dir, Elginwood LTC; Med Dir, Sherwood Court LTC; Langs: Cantonese; (905)853-0404; Fax. (905)853-3702; klai@yorkmed.ca.

LAI, Kevin C Y; 5-4646 Dufferin St, North York ON M3H 5S4; Tor'05; CCFP; (416)222-6160; Fax. (416)222-9604.

LAI, Kevin; 16-1529 Dufferin Cres, Nanaimo BC V9S 5H6; Witwatersrand (South Africa)'79; MB BCh; FRCPC; IntMed (Critical Care Medicine). Staff, Nanaimo Regional General Hospital; (250)753-3646; Fax. (250)753-3548.

LAI, Lillian S; Children's Hosp Eastern Ont, 401 Smyth Rd, Ottawa ON K1H 8L1; Qns'97; FRCPC; Peds; Cardiol. Staff, Children's Hospital of Eastern Ontario (CHEO); (613)737-7600 x2889

LAI, Mark K K; Baywood Med Centre, 205-95 Bayly St W, Ajax ON L1S 7K8; (Taiwan)'68; Staff, Rouge Valley Health System - Ajax & Pickering Health Centre Site; Langs: Chinese; (905)683-2900; Fax. (905)683-2904.

LAI, Michael W K; 347 Spadina Ave, Toronto ON M5T 2G3; Tor'76; Assoc Staff, Toronto Western Hospital - University Health Network; Assoc Staff, The Scarborough Hospital - Birchmount Campus; Assoc Staff, Mount Sinai Hospital; (416)977-1560

LAI, Ming; North Rd Plaza II, 370-9940 Lougheed Hwy, Burnaby BC V3J 1N3; Cape Town (South Africa)'67; Staff, Royal Columbian Hospital; (604)421-5544

LAI, Patrick C W; Brentwood Family Med Centre, 810-3630 Brentwood Rd NW, Calgary AB T2L 1K8; Cal'81; (403)289-1901; Fax. (403)289-6575.

LAI, Paul F S; 106-3530 Derry Rd E, Mississauga ON L4T 4E3; Tor'94; CCFP; FCFP; (905)671-1052

LAI, Philip; 306-277 Lakeshore Rd E, Oakville ON L6J 6J3; Ott'05; FRCSC; Otol. (905)849-7560

LAI, Raymond K C; Cross Cancer Institute, 11560 University Ave NW, Edmonton AB T6G 1Z2; Alb'92; FRCPC; GenPath. Staff Lab Med & Path, Cross Cancer Institute; (780)432-8338; Fax. (780)432-8214.

LAI, Raymond P C; Cornwall Prof Bldg, 515-2125 11th Ave, Regina SK S4P 3X3; Dublin (Ireland)'78; MB ChB; LRCPSI; MCFPCanada; Ac Staff, Regina General Hospital; Ac Staff, Pasqua Hospital; Ac Staff, Wascana Rehabilitation Centre; Langs: Chinese; (306)525-2888; Fax. (306)525-8255; irene_raymond_lai@hotmail.com.

LAI, Roxanne; PO Box 20522 Rpo Howe Street, Vancouver BC V6Z 2N8; Qns'07; CCFP.

LAI, Samuel; 11F-151 Yonge St, Toronto ON M5C 2W7; Tor'01; BSc; CCFP; Staff, The Medical Clinic for Person-Centred Psychotherapy; (647)498-8583; Fax. (647)494-7788.

LAI, Sio Mei; CSSSG-Hop de Hull, 116 boul Lionel-Emond, Gatineau QC J8Y 1W7; Mon'09; CCFP; Staff, Hull Hospital; (819)966-6300

LAI, Stephen I H; 10 Royal Orchard Blvd, Thornhill ON L3T 3C3; Wes'94; CCFP; FCFP; (905)771-7600

LAI, The Hung; Centre Med de Chambly, 205-1101 boul Brassard, Chambly QC J3L 5R4; Saigon (Vietnam)'78; (450)658-6601

LAI, Wayne W; 202-436 Cedar Ave, Kelowna BC V1Y 4X3; Ross (Dominica)'02; (250)850-8400

LAI, Wendy A; Humber River Reg Hosp-Church, 200 Church St, Toronto ON M9N 1N8; Wes'03; CCFP; CCFP(E.M.); Staff, Humber River Regional Hospital - Church Street Site; (416)243-4251

LAI, Yew H; Tuxedo Centre Med Clinic, 2201 Centre St SW, Calgary AB T2E 2T4; Alb'02; (403)984-3877; Fax. (403)453-8588.

LAI FATT, Peter H; Oshawa Clinic, 117 King St E, Oshawa ON L1H 1B9; (Jamaica)'80; FRCPC; Peds (Neonatology). Staff, Lakeridge Health - Oshawa Site; Med Dir, Oshawa Clinic; (905)723-8551; Fax. (905)721-4329.

LAIB-BARAMA, Dalila; Lakeshore Gen Hosp, 160 av Stillview, Pointe-Claire QC H9R 2Y2; Alger (Algeria)'80; Endocrin&Metab (P.Q.). Staff, Lakeshore General Hospital - Pointe Claire; (514)630-2225 x1821; Fax. (514)630-4704.

LAIDLAW, Carla S; Westgrove Clinic, 210-505 Queen St, Spruce Grove AB T7X 2V2; Alb'04; CCFP; (780)962-9888

LAIDLAW, Susan M; Med Emerg Inc, 9-6400 Millcreek Dr, Mississauga ON L5N 3E7; Tor'79; BSc; CCFP; CCFP(E.M.); FCFP; (905)858-1368

LAIDLOW, Duncan M; 190-2300 Carrington Rd, West Kelowna BC V4T 2N6; Qns'78; FRCPC; PhysMed&Rehab (Electromyography). (250)768-2122; Fax. (250)768-1959; duncan.laidlow@interiorhealth.ca.

LAIFER, Elizabeth; Manchenda Medical, 106-7550 King George Blvd, Surrey BC V3W 2T2; (Russia (Federation))'69; (604)598-9880

LAIL, Harajit S; Blueridge Med Clinic, 102-30461 Blueridge Dr, Abbotsford BC V2T 0B1; Alb'85; CCFP; FCFP; Staff, Surrey Memorial Hospital; Staff, Abbotsford Regional Hospital & Cancer Centre; (604)870-8707; Fax. (604)870-8708.

LAIL, Vanindar J; 100-5791 No. 3 Rd, Richmond BC V6X 2C9; UBC'83; ABR; FRCPC; DiagRad. Staff Radiol, Richmond Hospital; Staff, Burnaby Hospital; Physician, Brooke Radiology Associates; (604)278-9152; Fax. (604)278-9291.

LAILEY, Jennifer A; Lakehead University, 955 Oliver Rd, Thunder Bay ON P7B 5E1; Qns'96; BSc; CCFP; FCFP; Staff, Thunder Bay Regional Health Sciences Centre; (807)343-8361; Fax. (807)346-7740.

LAINE, Roy E; Geraldton Med Group, PO Box 1240 510 Hogarth Ave W, Geraldton ON P0T 1M0; Qns'68; Staff, Geraldton District Hospital; (807)854-0363; Fax. (807)854-0227.

LAINE-GOSSIN, Joanne; 501-1110 Sheppard Ave E, North York ON M2K 2W2; Tor'78; CCFP; FCFP; Staff, North York General Hospital; Staff, North York General Hospital - Branson Division; Lecturer, University of Toronto; (416)223-0555; Fax. (416)223-0540.

LAINESSE, Andre; CSSS de Trois-Rivieres, 155 rue Toupin, Trois-Rivieres QC G8T 3Z8; Laval'66; Cardiol (P.Q.). Staff, Centre de santé Cloutier-du-Rivage; Langs: English; (819)370-2245; Fax. (819)370-2180.

LAINESSE, Michel; Hotel-Dieu de Levis, 143 rue Wolfe, Levis QC G6V 3Z1; Laval'69; FRCPC; DiagRad. Staff, Hôtel-Dieu de Lévis; (418)535-7121

LAING, Bryce J; UBC-Dept of Surgery, 11265-2775 Laurel St, Vancouver BC V5Z 1M9; Sask'02; FRCSC; CardSurg; ThorSurg. (604)875-4111

LAING, James A; 918 Esquimalt Rd, Victoria BC V9A 3M6; Wes'69; (250)382-4296; Fax. (250)382-0023.

LAING, Kara E T; Dr H Bliss Murphy Cancer Ctr, 300 Prince Philip Dr, St. John's NL A1B 3V6; Mem'93; FRCPC; IntMed; MedOncol. Staff, Dr H Bliss Murphy Cancer Centre; Assoc Prof, Memorial University Of Newfoundland; (709)777-8095; Fax. (709)753-0927.

LAIRD, John L; Guelph Family Health Team, 207-55 Wyndham St N, Guelph ON N1H 7T8; Tor'92; BSc; Court Staff, Guelph General Hospital; (519)836-1455; Fax. (519)836-1321.

LAIRD, Philip R; 24 CF Health Services Centre, PO Box 1000 Stn Forces 50 Yukon St, Astra ON K0K 3W0; Cal'08; CCFP; (613)392-2811

LAISHRAM, Haladhra P S; Markham Endoscopy Diag Inc, 130-100 Renfrew Dr, Markham ON L3R 9R6; Punjab (India)'76; FRCS(Ed); FRCSC; GenSurg. (905)948-9119

LAITY, Alan H; London Medical-Dental Bldg, 202-450 Central Ave, London ON N6B 2E8; Wes'93; CCFP; (519)433-4150; Fax. (519)433-4231.

LAJEUNESSE, Charles; Hotel-Dieu de Levis, 143 rue Wolfe, Levis QC G6V 3Z1; Paris (France)'82; CSPQ; FRCPC; Psy. Psychiatre, Hôtel-Dieu de Lévis; assoc Prof Psy, Université Laval; (418)835-7155; Fax. (418)835-7199.

LAJEUNESSE, Judith; CSSS Manicouagan, 635 boul Jolliet, Baie-Comeau QC G5C 1P1; Sher'06; CCFP; Staff, Centre Hospitalier Régional Baie-Comeau; (418)589-3701

LAJEUNESSE, Julie; Clinique de Med Familiale, 6e-2120 rue Sherbrooke E, Montreal QC H2K 1C3; Sher'90; MSc; CCFP; FCFP; Staff, Centre Hospitalier l'Université De Montréal (CHUM) - Hôpital Saint-luc; Prof clin agrégé, Universite de Montreal; (514)527-1958; Fax. (514)527-1649.

LAJEUNESSE, Simon; CSSS des Iles, 430 ch Principal, Cap-aux-Meules QC G4T 1R9; Laval'97; FRCSC; ObstGyn. Staff, Hôpital de l'Archipel; (418)986-2121; Fax. (418)986-7001.

LAJEUNESSE, Yvette; Inst U Geriatrie De Montreal, 4565 ch Queen-Mary, Montreal QC H3W 1W5; Mon'76; Staff, Institut Universitaire de Gériatrie de Montréal; (514)340-1424; Fax. (514)340-2832.

LAJEUNESSE VIENS, Guylaine; Centre Bois De Boulogne, 2e-1575 boul Henri-Bourassa O, Montreal QC H3M 3A9; Mon'10; CCFP; (514)338-2383

LAJILI, Fathi Abdalla; La Crete Med Clinic, PO Box 2489, La Crete AB T0H 2H0; (Libya)'95; (780)926-2286; Fax. (780)926-3550.

LAJOIE, Carole; Clinique Med Frontenac, 24 rue Frontenac, Riviere-du-Loup QC G5R 1S5; Laval'01; (418)862-0333; Fax. (418)868-0505.

LAJOIE, Caroline; Ctr Hosp Affilie-St-Sacrement, 1050 ch Sainte-Foy, Quebec QC G1S 4L8; Laval'95; FRCSC; Ophth (Cataract & Glaucoma). Staff, Centre Hospitalier Affilié Universitaire de Québec - Hôpital du St-Sacrement; (418)682-7511; Fax. (418)682-7534.

LAJOIE, Christine; CSSS Cap-Rouge-St-Augustin, 115-1100 boul de la Chaudiere, Quebec QC G1Y 0A1; Laval'87; LMCC; Langs: Bilingual(French/English); (418)651-2572 x8219; Fax. (418)872-9245; christine.lajoie@ssss.gouv.qc.ca.

LAJOIE, Claude; Source Unique Clinic, 219 Main St E, Hawkesbury ON K6A 1A1; Mon'82; (613)632-4185

LAJOIE, Danielle; 214-848 rue Commerciale, St-J-Chrysostome QC G6Z 2T6; Sher'80 Sherbrooke; DOHS; ac Membre, CSSS de Montmagny-L'Islet; assoc Membre, CSSS Alphonse-Desjardins; Langs: French; (418)839-2070 x2287; Fax. (418)839-9161; daniellelajoie@ssss.gouv.qc.ca.

LAJOIE, Elisabeth; Direction de la Sante Publique, 1255 rue Beauregard, Longueuil QC J4K 2M3; Sher'97; FRCPC; CommunMed. Med Consultant Public Health, Agence de santé et des services sociaux de la Montérégie; Langs: Bilingual(French/English); (450)928-6777 x4077; Fax. (450)928-3783.

LAJOIE, Francois; 3001 12e Av N, Sherbrooke QC J1H 5N4; Sher'74; CSPQ; FRCSC; ObstGyn (Urological Gynecology). ac Staff, Centre Hospitalier Universitaire de Sherbrooke-Hopital Fleurimont; Prof, Universite de Sherbrooke; Langs: Bilingual(French/English); (819)820-6868 x12495; Fax. (819)820-6434; francois.lajoie@usherbrooke.ca.

LAJOIE, Genevieve C; Ctr Hosp Affilie-Enfant-Jesus, 1401 18e rue, Quebec QC G1J 1Z4; Laval'03; FRCPC; Psy. Staff, Centre Hospitalier Affilié Universitaire de Québec - Hôpital De L'Enfant Jésus; (418)649-0252

LAJOIE, Ginette; William Osler HC-Brampton Civi, 2100 Bovaird Dr E, Brampton ON L6R 3J7; Mon'88; FRCPC; AnatPath (Renal Pathology). Assoc Staff Path, Mount Sinai Hospital; Staff Path, William Osler Health System - Brampton Civic Hospital; Asst Prof, University of Toronto; Langs: Italian; French; (905)494-2120 x58706

LAJOIE, Jean-Francois; CHUS-Hop Fleurimont, 3001 12e Av N, Sherbrooke QC J1H 5N4; Sher'81; FRCPC; IntMed. Staff, Centre Hospitalier Universitaire de Sherbrooke-Hopital Fleurimont; assoc Prof, Universite de Sherbrooke; (819)346-1110; Fax. (819)820-6406; jean-francois.lajoie@usherbrooke.ca.

LAJOIE, Jennifer M; 201-1801 Bowen Rd, Nanaimo BC V9S 1H1; UBC'00; MSc; FRCSC; ObstGyn. (250)755-2012; Fax. (250)755-2032.

LAJOIE, Julie J M; St Joseph's Healthcare, 50 Charlton Ave E, Hamilton ON L8N 4A6; Tor'02; FRCPC; Anes. Staff, St Joseph's Healthcare - Charlton Campus; (905)522-1155

LAJOIE, Louise; Direction de la Sante Publique, 1255 rue Beauregard, Longueuil QC J4K 2M3; Mon'91; MSc; Langs: German; English; (450)928-6777 x4051; Fax. (450)928-3760.

LAJOIE, Luce; CLSC LaSalle, 8550 boul Newman, LaSalle QC H8N 1Y5; Sher'85; (514)364-2572; Fax. (514)364-6365.

LAJOIE, Lucie; 20260 Country Rd 43 PO Box 1630, Alexandria ON K0C 1A0; McM'99; CCFP; (613)525-0161; lajoielucie@hotmail.com.

LAJOIE, Marc; CLSC Jardin Du Quebec, 509 rue Saint-Jacques RR 1, Napierville QC J0J 1L0; Mon'88; (450)245-3336; Fax. (450)245-0278.

LAJOIE, Mireille; CSSS de Laval, 280 boul Roi-du-Nord, Laval QC H7L 4L2; Sher'70; FRCPC; Peds; CommunMed (P.Q.). (450)622-4478

LAJOIE, Pierre; Inst Nat'l De Sante Publique, 945 av Wolfe, Quebec QC G1V 5B3; Laval'69; FRCPC; CommunMed; Public Health & Preventive Med. ac Staff, Centre Hospitalier Universitaire de Quebec-CHUL; Consultant, Centre Hospitalier Affilié Universitaire de Québec - Hôpital De L'Enfant Jésus; (418)650-5115; pierre.lajoie@inspq.qc.ca.

LAJOIE, Yves; CHUS-Hop Fleurimont, 3001 12e Av N, Sherbrooke QC J1H 5N4; Sher'82; FRCPC; Psy (Pediatric Psychiatry). Staff, Centre Hospitalier Universitaire de Sherbrooke-Hopital Fleurimont; adj Prof, Universite de Sherbrooke; Langs: English; (819)346-1110 x14000

LAJZEROWICZ, Michelle; Centre De Med Fam De Wakefield, CP 400 777 Riverside Dr, Wakefield QC J0X 3G0; McG'94; CCFP; Langs: French; (819)459-2363; Fax. (819)459-2997.

LAKDAWALLA, Fakhrudin; 400-1100 Sheppard Ave E, North York ON M2K 2W1; RCS (Ireland)'63; DPM; Ac Staff, Centre for Addiction & Mental Health (CAMH) - Queen Site; (416)221-6030

LAKDAWALLA, Nadira F; 405-1100 Sheppard Ave E, North York ON M2K 2W1; Bombay (India)'66; MB BS; FRCPC; Peds. Ac Staff, North York General Hospital; (416)221-6588

LAKE, David M; Cowichan Dist Hosp, 3045 Gibbins Rd, Duncan BC V9L 1E5; UBC'80; OrthSurg. Staff, Cowichan District Hospital; (250)709-3000

LAKE, H Russell; Vale of Avoca Med Clinic, PO Box 10, Avondale NL A0A 1B0; Mem'87; BMedSci; LMCC; PhC; BSc; Member Interchangeable Drug Committee, Health Canada; (709)229-3531; Fax. (709)229-1104.

LAKE, Karen F; Cabot Square Med Clinic, 55 Stavanger Dr, St. John's NL A1A 5E8; Mem'01; CCFP; (709)576-7075

LAKE, Peter R; Queen Charlotte Med Clinic, PO Box 430 3209 Oceanview Dr, Queen Charlotte BC V0T 1S0; Cal'89; BASc; MD; CCFP; FCFP; Clinical Asst Prof Family Pract, University of British Columbia; (250)559-4447; Fax. (250)559-8037.

LAKE, Rae G; Wellpoint Family Practice, 900-1240 Bay St, Toronto ON M5R 2A7; Tor'72; CCFP; FCFP; Court Staff, Women's College Hospital; Asst Prof Family & CommunMed, University of Toronto; (416)969-3240; Fax. (416)971-7718.

LAKE-RICHARDS, Ruby B V; Douglas Mental Hlth Univ Inst, 6875 boul Lasalle, Verdun QC H4H 1R3; West Indies (Jamaica)'56; MB BS; FRCPC; Psy (Child & Adolescent Psychiatry). Ac Staff, Douglas Mental Health University Institute; Lecturer Psy, McGill University; (514)761-6131; Fax. (514)888-4063.

LAKEY, William H; Occupational Health Programs, 707-808 Nelson St, Vancouver BC V6Z 2H2; Alb'85; Med Dir Occupational Health Programs, BC Health Services; (604)660-2587; Fax. (604)775-0697.

LAKHA, Anis H; Plaza 15 Family Practice, 100-145 15th St W, North Vancouver BC V7M 1R9; Sheffield (England)'85; MB ChB; Ac Staff Privil, Lions Gate Hospital; Langs: Gujarati; (604)983-9832

LAKHANI, Aly; Univ Hlth Network-Toronto Gen, 14EN 208A-200 Elizabeth St, Toronto ON M5G 2C4; Aga Khan (Pakistan)'02; FRCPC; IntMed (Pain Pharmacotherapy). Staff, Toronto General Hospital - UHN; (416)340-4800

LAKHANI, Amin; University Hosp of Northern BC, 1475 Edmonton St, Prince George BC V2M 1S2; Karachi (Pakistan)'90; MB BS; Staff, University Hospital of Northern British Columbia; (250)981-9219

LAKHANI, Shahnavaz; Toronto Poly Clinic, 298 John St, Thornhill ON L3T 6M8; Sind (Pakistan)'74; MB BS; Staff, The Scarborough Hospital - Birchmount Campus; (905)482-8648

LAKHANI, Zaheerali; Circle Square Prof Centre, 202-11808 St Albert Trail NW, Edmonton AB T5L 4G4; Leeds (England)'75; MB ChB(Hons); MRCP; FACP; FACC; FRCPC; IntMed; Cardiol. (780)454-6601; Fax. (780)454-6651.

LAKHANI, Zubair; 368 College St N, Durham ON N0G 1R0; Wes'02; CCFP; (519)369-2510; Fax. (519)369-3831.

LAKHANPAL, Neeraj; Halton HCS Corp-Milton, 7030 Derry Rd, Milton ON L9T 7H6; Dal'98; CCFP; FCFP; Staff, Halton Healthcare Services Corporation - Milton District Hospital; (905)878-2383

LAKHEERAM, Indrani; MUHC-Montreal Children's Hosp, 2300 rue Tupper, Montreal QC H3H 1P3; McG'95; CSPQ; FRCPC; Anes. Staff Anes, McGill University Health Centre - Montreal Children's Hospital; (514)412-4463

LAKHER, Vladimir; Able-Care Med Clinic, 56-2991 Lougheed Hwy, Coquitlam BC V3B 6J6; McG'97; Langs: Russian; (604)945-7819; Fax. (604)945-2884.

LAKHOO, Parbhoobhai; 301-2155 10th Ave, Prince George BC V2M 5J6; Witwatersrand (South Africa)'82; MB ChB; (250)562-6569

LAKHOO, Sheila; St James Town Health Centre, 410 Sherbourne St, Toronto ON M4X 1K2; Alb'04; CCFP; (416)864-3096

LAKINS, Jill E; Lloydminster Clinic, 5120 46 St, Lloydminster AB T9V 2P7; Leeds (England)'59; DObst; DRCOG; DA; (780)875-2221; Fax. (780)875-0605.

LAKIS, Nicolaos; Hys Med Centre, 202-11010 101 St NW, Edmonton AB T5H 4B9; (South Africa)'79; MB ChB; (780)426-1121

LAKOSHA, Hesham M M A; Halifax Prof Centre, 520-5991 Spring Garden Rd, Halifax NS B3H 1Y6; Tanta (Egypt)'86; MB ChB; FRCSEd; FRCSC; Ophth (Ocular Oncology). Staff, Queen Elizabeth II Health Sciences Centre - Victoria General Site; Langs: Arabic; (902)423-4423

LAKRA, Arun; 101-49 Richard Way SW, Calgary AB T3E 7M8; Tor'90; DAB; FRCSC; Ophth (Refractive Surgery). (403)264-0141; Fax. (403)265-9279.

LAKRA, Prem P; 207 Pump Hill View SW, Calgary AB T2V 4R7; Durham (England)'57; Langs: Hindi; (403)253-9084

LAKRA, Roopa K S; 630 9 Ave SE, Calgary AB T2G 4V9; Cal'94; CCFP; (403)920-0011; Fax. (403)920-0014.

LAKROUF, El-Hadi; CSSS de Haut Saint-Maurice, 885 boul Ducharme, La Tuque QC G9X 3C1; (Algeria)'83; Staff, Centre Hospitalier Saint-Joseph de la Turque; (819)523-4581

LAKSHMI, Santhosh; Prince County Hosp, PO Box 3000 Stn Main, Summerside PE C1N 2A9; Staff, Prince County Hospital.

LAKSMAN, Zachary W; Univ of Toronto, 602-500 University Ave, Toronto ON M5G 1V7; Tor'06; FRCPC; IntMed; Cardiol.

LAKUSTA, Cherelyn M; Adolescent Day Treatment Prog, 200-2204 2 St SW, Calgary AB T2S 3C2; Cal'99; FRCPC; Psy (Adolescent Psychiatry). (403)802-2265; Fax. (403)244-7964.

LAL, Anita; Ontario Forensic Pathology Ser, 26 Grenville St, Toronto ON M7A 2G9; (Dominica)'04; DABPath.

LAL, Justiene; 1-160 The Westway, Etobicoke ON M9P 2C1; Dublin (Ireland)'07; CCFP; (647)547-8181

LAL, Kartar; Queen Elizabeth II Hosp, 10409 98 St, Grande Prairie AB T8V 2E8; (Pakistan)'86; MCPSPsy; MB BS; Staff, Queen Elizabeth II Hospital; Langs: Sindhi; Urdu; Punjabi; Hindi; (780)538-7100; Fax. (780)538-7600.

LAL, Moti; Clareview Med Office, 3504 137 Ave NW, Edmonton AB T5Y 1Y7; (India)'89; CCFP; (780)456-8552; Fax. (780)456-8505.

LAL, Rekha B; Maitland Valley Family Hlth Team, 180 Cambria Rd N, Goderich ON N7A 4N8; Delhi (India)'72; Staff, Alexandra Marine & General Hospital; (519)524-6060; Fax. (519)524-5225.

LAL, Shirin B; 5230 Mitch Owens Rd RR 1, Manotick ON K4M 1B2; Ott'02; CCFP; (613)692-2571

LAL, Smita J; Fleetwood Med Clinic, 108-8927 152 St, Surrey BC V3R 4E5; Bombay (India)'84; MB BS; Staff, Surrey Memorial Hospital; (604)589-8900

LAL, Sunita T; 304-1580 Merivale Rd, Ottawa ON K2G 4B5; Qns'96; FRCSC; ObstGyn. (613)686-7580

LAL, Sushma; West Hill Med Clinic, 1A-2995 2nd Ave W, Prince Albert SK S6V 5V5; (Other Foreign)'96; (306)765-8500; Fax. (306)765-8501.

LALA, Shantilal M; Radiology Associates of Regina, 6-2727 Parliament Ave, Regina SK S4S 6X5; Mysore (India)'78; FFR(S.A.); FRCPC; DiagRad. Staff, Radiology Associates of Regina; (306)352-7653; Fax. (306)522-4311; lalashanti@hotmail.com.

LALANCETTE, Christian; CSSS de Chicoutimi, 305 rue Saint-Vallier, Chicoutimi QC G7H 5H6; Laval'84; Staff, Complexe hospitalier de la Sagamie; (418)541-1000

LALANCETTE, Julie; CSSS du Lac-des-Deux-Montagnes, 520 boul Arthur-Sauve, Saint-Eustache QC J7R 5B1; Mon'87; Staff, Hôpital de Saint-Eustache; (450)472-1955; jlalancette@cm25.ca.

LALANCETTE, Linda; CSSS du Lac-des-Deux-Montagnes, 520 boul Arthur-Sauve, Saint-Eustache QC J7R 5B1; Mon'95; FRCPC; MedMicrobiol; Microbio & Infect Dis (P.Q.). Staff, Hôpital de Saint-Eustache; (450)473-6811 x2075; Fax. (450)473-4381; linda.lalancette@ssss.gouv.qc.ca.

LALANCETTE, Marc; CHUQ-Hotel-Dieu De Quebec, 11 Cote Du Palais, Quebec QC G1R 2J6; Ott'89; FRCPC; IntMed; MedOncol; Hem. Staff, Centre Hospitalier Universitaire de Québec (CHUQ) - Siege Social; (418)691-5280; Fax. (418)691-5383.

LALANCETTE, Mathieu; CSSS Drummond-Hop Sainte-Croix, 570 rue Heriot, Drummondville QC J2B 1C1; Sher'01; FRCSC; GenSurg. Staff, Hôpital Sainte-croix; (819)478-6464

LALANDA, Carmen; Clin Externe De Psychiatrie, 203-100 rue Grenier, Charlemagne QC J5Z 4C6; Paris (France)'82; Staff, Centre Hospitalier Pierre le Gardeur; Langs: Spanish; (450)585-9010; Fax. (450)585-2709.

LALANDE, Bruno; CSSS de Sept-Iles, 45 rue du Pere-Divet, Sept-Iles QC G4R 3N7; Mon'94; Staff, Centre Hospitalier Regional de Sept-Iles; (418)962-9761

LALANDE, Johanne; Maternity & Gynecology Centre, 1811 av Dollard, Lasalle QC H8N 1T9; Laval'96; FRCSC; ObstGyn. Staff, Centre Hospitalier de LaSalle; (514)364-3700

LALANDE, Johanne; Clin Med Plateau Mont-Royal, 103-1374 av du Mont-Royal E, Montreal QC H2J 1Y7; Mon'81; (514)527-3997

LALANDE, Phillip D N; Grey Bruce HS-Owen Sound, PO Box 1800 Stn Main 1800 8th St E, Owen Sound ON N4K 6M9; Dal'84; BSc; FRCPC; Anes. Staff Anes, Grey Bruce Health Services - Owen Sound; (519)376-2121

LALANDE, Raymond; Univ de Montreal, CP 6128 Succ Centre Ville, Montreal QC H3C 3J7; Mon'83; CCFP; FCFP; Staff, Hopital de la Cite de la santé; Vice-Rector Academic Affairs, Universite de Montreal; (514)343-6111 x3606; Fax. (514)343-5750; raymond.lalande@umontreal.ca.

LALANI, Akbar V; Keary Med Centre, 103-245 Columbia St E, New Westminster BC V3L 3W4; London (England)'71; MB BS; MSc(Exp.Med.); ABIM; FRCPC; IntMed (Interventional Cardiology); Cardiol. Staff Cardiol, Royal Columbian Hospital; Clinical Asst Prof Med, University of British Columbia; Langs: Hindi; (604)522-1644; Fax. (604)522-7848.

LALANI, Aleem; Orthopaedic Consultants, 10972 124 St NW, Edmonton AB T5M 0H8; Cal'95; FRCSC; OrthSurg (Upper Extremity Surgery). Clinical Asst Prof, Sturgeon Community Hospital; Clin. Lect., Div. of OrthSurg., University of Alberta; (780)454-0311; Fax. (780)454-0920; laurap@edmontonortho.com.

LALANI, Amin; Radiology Consultants Assoc, 120-6707 Elbow Dr SW, Calgary AB T2V 0E3; Alb'95; FRCPC; DiagRad. (403)777-3003; Fax. (403)777-3008.

LALANI, Amina P; The Hosp For Sick Children, 555 University Ave, Toronto ON M5G 1X8; UBC'96; FRCPC; Peds (Pediatric Emergency Medicine). Staff Physician, The Hospital For Sick Children; (416)813-7832; Fax. (416)813-5043; amina.lalani@sickkids.ca.

LALANI, Fereshte N; 303-343 Wilson Ave, North York ON M3H 1T1; Tor'09; CCFP; Staff Family Practice Obst, Mount Sinai Hospital; (416)785-8412; wilsonmedicalgroup@gmail.com.

LALANI, Nadim J; St Paul's Hosp, 1702 20th St W, Saskatoon SK S7M 0Z9; Cal'04; FRCPC; EmergMed. Staff, St Paul's Hospital (Grey Nuns) of Saskatoon; (306)655-5113; Fax. (306)655-5963.

LALANI, Naznin; Scarborough Med Centre, 2680 Lawrence Ave E, Scarborough ON M1P 4Y4; Newcastle-upon-Tyne (England)'80; MB BS; MHSc; CCFP; FCFP; Staff, The Scarborough Hospital - General Campus; Asst Prof Family & Commun Med/Preceptor, University of Toronto; Langs: Gujarati; (416)755-2242; Fax. (416)755-8412.

LALANI, Salim; 3809 Sunset St, Burnaby BC V5G 1T4; Cal'04; ObstGyn. (604)565-9447

LALANI, Sartajali G; King Street Med Arts Centre, 206-71 King St W, Mississauga ON L5B 4A2; Makerere (Uganda)'68; MB ChB; FRCPC; Psy (General Adult Psychiatry). Consultant Psy, Trillium Health Centre - Mississauga; (905)848-8702

LALIBERTE, Alain L; CSSS de la Baie-des-Chaleurs, RR 2 419 boul Perron, Maria QC G0C 1Y0; Mon'84; FRCPC; IntMed. Staff, CSSS de la Baie-des-Chaleurs; (418)759-3443

LALIBERTE, Anne; Clinique Med St-Anselme, 1-706 Rte Begin, Saint-Anselme QC G0R 2N0; Laval'90; Staff, Hôtel-Dieu de Lévis; Physician, CLSC Bellechasse; Confér Clin, Université Laval; Langs: Bilingual(French/English); (418)885-9625; Fax. (418)885-9826; annelaliberte@globetrotter.net.

LALIBERTE, Ariane; Clinique Med Desy, 5636 boul Henri-Bourassa E, Montreal-Nord QC H1G 2T2; Mon'06; (514)326-9060

LALIBERTE, Audrey; CSSS Becancour-Nicolet-Yamaska, 216 rue Principale, Fortierville QC G0S 1J0; Mon'09; (819)287-4442; Fax. (819)287-4017.

LALIBERTE, Benoit; Hop Maisonneuve-Rosemont, 5415 boul de l'Assomption, Montreal QC H1T 2M4; Mon'99; FRCPC; RadOncol. Staff, Hopital Maisonneuve-Rosemont; (514)252-3425

LALIBERTE, Bernard; Ctr Hosp Affilie-Enfant-Jesus, 1401 18e rue, Quebec QC G1J 1Z4; Laval'96; FRCSC; OrthSurg. Staff, Centre Hospitalier Affilié Universitaire de Québec - Hôpital De L'Enfant Jésus; Langs: English; (418)649-0252; Fax. (418)649-5567.

LALIBERTE, Carmen; Clinique Med St-Louis, 504 rue Saint-Louis, Joliette QC J6E 2Z2; Sher'82; (450)759-0581; Fax. (450)759-0584.

LALIBERTE, Christian; CSSS de la Baie-des-Chaleurs, RR 2 419 boul Perron, Maria QC G0C 1Y0; Mon'89; Staff, CSSS de la Baie-des-Chaleurs; (418)759-3443

LALIBERTE, Daniel; Clinique Les Jardins Dorval, 204-352 av Dorval, Dorval QC H9S 3H8; Laval'94; LMCC; CCFP; Staff Emerg, CSSS de Dorval-Lachine-Lasalle; Langs: English; (514)631-6086; Fax. (514)631-6691; danl12md@hotmail.com.

LALIBERTE, Denis; Direction de Sante Publique, 2400 av d'Estimauville, Quebec QC G1E 7G9; Laval'77; MPH; FRCPC; CommunMed (Public Health). Ac Staff, Centre Hospitalier Universitaire de Quebec-CHUL; Prog Dir Occupational Health, Université Laval; Langs: Bilingual(French/English); (418)666-7000 x355; Fax. (418)666-2776; denis.laliberte@ssss.gouv.qc.ca.

LALIBERTE, Diane; Clin Medico-Dentaire Pasteur, 770 1re av, Quebec QC G1L 3K2; Laval'82; (418)529-0042; Fax. (418)529-4924.

LALIBERTE, Isabelle; CHUQ-Ctr Hosp Univ Laval, 2705 boul Laurier, Quebec QC G1V 4G2; Laval'00; FRCSC; Ophth (Pediatrics). Staff, Centre Hospitalier Universitaire de Quebec-CHUL; Langs: Bilingual(French/English); (418)654-2119; Fax. (418)654-2188.

LALIBERTE, Jean; Hotel-Dieu de Levis, 143 rue Wolfe, Levis QC G6V 3Z1; Laval'83; FRCSC; GenSurg (Cardio & Thoracic Surgery). gén Chirurgien, Hôtel-Dieu de Lévis; (418)835-7121

LALIBERTE, Josette; CSSS Becancour-Nicolet-Yamaska, 216 rue Principale GD, Fortierville QC G0S 1J0; Laval'95; Staff, Carrefour Sante Granit; (819)287-4442; Fax. (819)287-4017.

LALIBERTE, Laura; CSST Chaudieres-Appalaches, 835 rue de la Concorde, SAint-Romuald QC G6W 7P7; Laval'83; DiagRad (P.Q.); Neursurg. (418)839-2500

LALIBERTE, Lyne; CSSS de Saint-Jerome, 290 rue de Montigny, Saint-Jerome QC J7Z 5T3; Mon'90; FRCPC; IntMed; Gastroent (P.Q.). Staff, Hôtel-Dieu de Saint-Jérôme; (450)431-8200

LALIBERTE, Marc-Andre; Institut de Cardiologie de Mtl, 5000 rue Belanger, Montreal QC H1T 1C8; Laval'83; FRCPC; Psy (Consultation-Liaison). Staff, Institut de Cardiologie de Montréal; Langs: English; (514)593-2571

LALIBERTE, Marie; CHUQ-Hotel-Dieu De Quebec, 11 Cote du Palais, Quebec QC G1R 2J6; Laval'05; CCFP; CCFP(E.M.); Staff, Centre Hospitalier Universitaire de Québec (CHUQ) - Siege Social; (418)691-5042

LALIBERTE, Martin; MUHC-Royal Victoria Hosp, 687 av des Pins O, Montreal QC H3A 1A1; Laval'85; FRCPC; EmergMed. Staff, McGill University Health Centre - Royal Victoria Hospital; (514)934-1934 x34277

LALIBERTE, Matthieu; CLSC du Richelieu, 300 ch de Marieville, Richelieu QC J3L 3V8; McG'05; CCFP; (450)658-7561

LALIBERTE, Pierre; CHUQ-St-Francois D'Assise, 10 rue de l'Espinay, Quebec QC G1L 3L5; Laval'89; CSPQ; FRCPC; Anes. Staff, Centre Hospitalier Universitaire De Québec - Pavillon De St-françois-d'assise; (418)525-4340; Fax. (418)525-4434.

LALIBERTE, Pierre; Inst U en Sante Mentale de QC, 2601 ch de la Canardiere, Quebec QC G1J 2G3; Laval'84; Staff, Institut Universitaire Sante; (418)663-5142; pierre.laliberte@institutsmq.qc.ca.

LALIBERTE, Richard; Hotel-Dieu de Levis, 143 rue Wolfe, Levis QC G6V 3Z1; Laval'78; FRCPC; Psy. Staff, Hôtel-Dieu de Lévis; (418)835-7155

LALIBERTE, Serge A; Lorraine Wing Tower C, 139-201 Deacon St, Pembroke ON K8A 2J6; Ott'75; Staff, Pembroke Regional Hospital Inc; (613)732-3645; Fax. (613)732-3498.

LALIC, Vesna; Sturgeon Community Hosp, 201 Boudreau Rd, St. Albert AB T8N 6C4; (Bosnia-Herzegovina)'78; Staff, Sturgeon Community Hospital; (780)418-8200

LALIK, Christopher A; Dr Christopher Lalik Fam Clini, 202-5 Quarry Ridge Rd, Barrie ON L4M 7G1; Lodz (Poland)'97; CCFP; (705)792-4800

LALIK, Jolanta M; B-101 King St, St Stephen NB E3L 2C6; Jagiellonski (Poland)'85; Staff, Charlotte County Hospital; Langs: Polish; (506)466-9254

LALINEC, Martine; Douglas Hosp, 6875 boul Lasalle, Verdun QC H4H 1R3; Paris (France)'59; FRCPC; Psy (Administration). Chief Med, Douglas Mental Health University Institute; Assoc Prof Psy, McGill University; (514)761-6131 x2749; Fax. (514)888-4063.

LALINEC-MICHAUD, Martin; CLSC Haute-Ville, 55 ch Sainte-Foy, Quebec QC G1R 1S9; McG'84; Staff, Centre Hospitalier Affilié Universitaire de Québec - Hôpital du St-Sacrement; Staff, CLSC Haute-Ville des Rivieres; Asst Teacher, Université Laval; Langs: English; French; (418)641-2572; Fax. (418)522-5437.

LALJI, Ronil S; Workers' Comp Board, 6951 Westminster Hwy, Richmond BC V7C 1C6; Alb'93; FRCPC; CommunMed; Public Health & Preventive Med. (604)276-3100

LALJI, Sayrin S; BC Women's Hosp & Health Ctre, 1U3-4500 Oak St, Vancouver BC V6H 3N1; UBC'96; FRCSC; ObstGyn (Perinatology). Staff Maternal Fetal Med, BC Women's Hospital & Health Centre; Clinical Asst Prof, University of British Columbia; (604)875-3174

LALL, Frank R; Shoal Lake Med Associates, PO Box 490, Shoal Lake MB R0J 1Z0; Dublin (Ireland)'66.

LALL, Rohan N; Foothills Med Centre, 1403 29 St NW, Calgary AB T2N 2T9; Tor'98; ABS; BSc(Hon); FACS; MSc; FRCSC; GenSurg (Trauma). Staff, Foothills Medical Centre; (403)944-3417; Fax. (403)944-8799.

LALL, Rosemarie N; Platinum Med Clinic, 3170 Eglinton Ave E, Scarborough ON M1J 2H3; Qns'92; CCFP; FCFP; Staff, The Scarborough Hospital - General Campus; Staff, Rouge Valley Health System - Centenary Health Centre Site; Langs: French; (416)265-2255; Fax. (416)265-6737.

LALL, Vipin; Lasalle Community Health Care, 2125 Front Rd, Windsor ON N9J 2C1; Wes'89; CCFP; (519)734-1234; Fax. (519)734-8674.

LALLA, Angela; B12-350 Conestoga Blvd, Cambridge ON N1R 7L7; Ott'09; CCFP; (519)629-4615

LALLA, Daniel E; Clinique Med Cowansville, 1001-101 rue Albert, Cowansville QC J2K 2W4; McG'92; CCFP; FCFP; Staff, Hôpital Brome-Missisquoi-Perkins; Lecturer, McGill University; (450)266-4060; Fax. (450)266-5335; daniel_lalla@hotmail.com.

LALLA, Fiore R; Lakeshore Gen Hosp, 160 av Stillview, Pointe-Claire QC H9R 2Y2; McG'91; BSc(Hon.); FRCPC; Psy. Staff, Lakeshore General Hospital - Pointe Claire; Langs: Italian; French; (514)630-2225 x4036; frlalla@videotron.ca.

LALLA, Leonora; St Mary's Hosp Centre, 3830 av Lacombe, Montreal QC H3T 1M5; McG'96; CCFP; Staff Family Med, St Mary's Hospital Centre; Langs: English; French; (514)734-2677

LALLI, Eleonora C; 3051 Homestead Dr PO Box 40, Mount Hope ON L0R 1W0; McM'84; Vis Physician, Hamilton Health Sciences Centre - McMaster Children's Hospital; Vis Physician, St Joseph's Healthcare - Charlton Campus; (905)679-4241; Fax. (905)679-6100.

LALLIER, Michel; Hôpital Ste-Justine, 3175 ch Cote-Sainte-Catherine, Montreal QC H3T 1C5; Mon'91; BSc; FRCSC; GenSurg (Transplantation); PedGenSurg. Staff, Hôpital Ste-Justine; adj Prof, Universite de Montreal; Langs: English; Spanish; (514)345-4915; Fax. (514)345-4964.

LALLO, Alexandre; CHUM-Hop Notre-Dame, 1560 rue Sherbrooke E, Montreal QC H2L 4M1; Sher'00; CSPQ; FRCPC; Anes. Staff, Centre Hospitalier l'Université de Montréal (CHUM) - Hôpital Notre-Dame; (514)890-8000 x26876

LALONDE, Alain-Paul; Centre Medical Familiale, 552 av Saint-Alphonse SS 1, St-Bruno-LSJ QC G0W 2L0; Laval'87; CCFP; FCFP; Staff Pt-Time, CRSSS de la Baie-James; (418)343-2444; Fax. (418)343-2448.

LALONDE, Andre; Clinique Med Duvernay, 3333 boul de la Concorde E, Laval QC H7E 2C3; Mon'78; (450)661-2444; Fax. (450)661-2411.

LALONDE, Andrea E S; CSSS-Hop de Hull, 116 boul Lionel-Emond, Gatineau QC J8Y 1W7; McG'05; IntMed. Staff, Hull Hospital; (819)966-6200

LALONDE, Bernard G; Sports & Spinal Injury Clinic, 602-1335 Carling Ave, Ottawa ON K1Z 8N8; Ott'70; Staff/Med Dir, Carleton Sports Med Clinic; Staff, Ray Friel Sports Medicine Facility; Langs: Bilingual(English/French); (613)729-8098; bglake@sympatico.ca.

LALONDE, Carlos D; Homewood Health Centre, 150 Delhi St, Guelph ON N1E 6K9; McM'05; FRCPC; Psy. Staff, Homewood Health Centre; (519)824-1010

LALONDE, Carole; Clinique Med Havre Sante, 521 boul Du Havre, Salaber-de-Valleyf QC J6S 4Z5; Sher'85; FRCSC; ObstGyn. Langs: English; (450)370-1300; Fax. (450)370-1314.

LALONDE, Catherine; Hôpital Laval, 2725 ch Sainte-Foy, Quebec QC G1V 4G5; Laval'06; DiagRad. Staff, Hôpital Laval; (418)656-8711

LALONDE, Catherine; Hop Santa Cabrini Ospedale, 5655 rue Saint-Zotique E, Montreal QC H1T 1P7; Mon'95; Staff, Hôpital Santa Cabrini Ospedale; (514)252-6000

LALONDE, Christine; CSSS de Quebec Nord, 3666 ch Royal, Quebec QC G1E 1X5; Mon'91; (418)663-2572; Fax. (418)663-2939; christine.lalonde@ssss.gouv.qc.ca.

LALONDE, Daniel; CSSSG-Hop de Gatineau, CP 2000 Succ Bureau-Chef 909 boul de la Verendrye O, Gatineau QC J8P 7H2; Mon'87; AB; NuclearMed. Staff, Hôpital de Gatineau; Staff, Queensway Carleton Hospital; (819)561-8166; Fax. (819)561-8119.

LALONDE, Donald H; C204-600 Main St, Saint John NB E2K 1J5; Qns'79; ABPlasSurg; ABHandSurg; MSc(Exp.Surg); FRCSC; PlasSurg (Hand Surgery). Staff, Saint John Regional Hospital; Prof, Dalhousie University; Langs: English; French; Spanish; (506)648-7950; Fax. (506)652-8042.

LALONDE, Eric; Hop Du Sacre-Coeur De Mtl, 5400 boul Gouin O, Montreal QC H4J 1C5; Sher'99; CCFP; CCFP(E.M.); Staff, Hôpital du Sacre-Coeur de Montréal; (514)352-1252

LALONDE, Gilles; Centre Oculairede Quebec, 050-2480 ch Sainte-Foy, Quebec QC G1V 1T6; Laval'75; DABOph; Ophth (Medical Retina). ac Staff, Centre Hospitalier Universitaire de Québec (CHUQ) - Siege Social; Langs: Bilingual(French/English); (418)780-6345; Fax. (418)780-3345.

LALONDE, Gilles; Medi-Centre Chomedey, 610 boul Cure-Labelle, Laval QC H7V 2T7; Mon'83; Staff, Hopital de la Cite de la santé; (450)687-6452; Fax. (450)687-3243.

LALONDE, Guy; Hop Du Sacre-Coeur De Mtl, 5400 boul Gouin O, Montreal QC H4J 1C5; Mon'77; FRCPC; IntMed; Cardiol. Ac Staff, Hôpital du Sacre-Coeur de Montréal; assoc Prof Med, Universite de Montreal; (514)338-2200; Fax. (514)338-3226; glalonde@ssss.gouv.qc.ca.

LALONDE, Jacques; Clinique Med Urgence Rive-Sud, 3200 boul Taschereau, Greenfield Park QC J4V 2H3; Mon'68; Staff, Centre Hospitalier de Verdun; Staff, Centre Hospitalier de LaSalle; adj Prof, Universite de Montreal; (450)672-5577

LALONDE, Jean; CSSS du Lac-Témiscamingue, 22 rue Notre-Dame N, Ville-Marie QC J9V 1W8; Mon'68; Staff, CSSS du Témiscamingue; Langs: English; (819)629-2420 x4243; Fax. (819)629-3069; jean_lalonde@ssss.gouv.qc.ca.

LALONDE, Jean-Serge; 170-455 Montee Paiement, Gatineau QC J8P 0B1; Ott'76; Ac Staff, Hull Hospital; (819)665-9000; Fax. (819)665-9008.

LALONDE, Jocelyne; Clinique Familiale Montclair, 207-15 boul Montclair, Gatineau QC J8Y 2E2; Laval'86; Langs: English; (819)772-2003; Fax. (819)772-4880.

LALONDE, Karl-Andre R; The Ottawa Hosp-Gen Campus, 501 Smyth Rd, Ottawa ON K1H 8L6; Ott'99; FRCSC; OrthSurg. Staff, The Ottawa Hospital - General Campus; (613)737-8899 x79147

LALONDE, Laurent; Inst de l'Oeil de Laurentides, 4800 rue Ambroise-Lafortune, Boisbriand QC J7H 1S6; Mon'87; DAB; FRCSC; Ophth. Staff, Hôtel-Dieu de Saint-Jérôme; (450)419-6345; Fax. (450)434-9389.

LALONDE, Lisa M; Carleton Univ Health Services, 1125 Colonel By Dr, Ottawa ON K1S 5B6; Ott'89; (613)520-6674

LALONDE, Lise; Clinique Med Rock Forest, 1-4870 boul Bourque, Sherbrooke QC J1N 3S5; Mon'76; CCFP; Langs: English; (819)820-2673; Fax. (819)820-2112.

LALONDE, Louise; 111-1919 Southland Dr SW, Calgary AB T2W 0K1; Cal'90; CCFP; (403)258-2133

LALONDE, Lucie; CHUM-Hotel-Dieu, 3e-3840 rue Saint-Urbain, Montreal QC H2W 1T8; Mon'85; FRCPC; DiagRad. Staff, Centre Hospitalier l'Université de Montréal (CHUM) - Hôtel-Dieu; (514)890-8059

LALONDE, Lucille D; University of Alberta Hosp, 2C2-8440 112 St NW, Edmonton AB T6G 2B7; Sask'75; Cardiol. Staff, University of Alberta Hospital; (780)407-7929; Fax. (780)407-6918.

LALONDE, Maryse H; 10134 111 Ave NW, Edmonton AB T5G 0B3; Alb'92; CCFP; (780)474-3712

LALONDE, Megan M; Royal Alexandra Hosp, 10240 Kingsway NW, Edmonton AB T5H 3V9; Alb'01; FRCPC; Anes. Staff, Royal Alexandra Hospital; (780)735-4010

LALONDE, Michel; CSSSG-Hop De Gatineau, CP 2000 succ Bureau-chef, Gatineau QC J8P 7H2; Sher'90; FRCSC; Otol. Staff, Hôpital de Gatineau; (819)561-8100

LALONDE, Pierre; Hop Louis-H Lafontaine, 7401 rue Hochelaga, Montreal QC H1N 3M5; Mon'68; FRCPC; Psy (Schizophrenia). Ac Staff, Hopital Louis-H Lafontaine; Prof, Universite de Montreal; Langs: French; (514)251-4000 x3880; Fax. (514)899-0862; lalonde.md@videotron.ca.

LALONDE, Richard A; 4484 rue Sherbrooke O, Westmount QC H3Z 1E6; McG'79; Peds (P.Q.). Pediatrics, McGill University Health Centre - Royal Victoria Hospital; Staff, McGill University Health Centre - Montreal Children's Hospital; (514)933-4490; Fax. (514)933-6934.

LALONDE, Richard G J; MUHC-Royal Victoria Hosp, 687 av des Pins O, Montreal QC H3A 1A1; Ott'71; FRCPC; IntMed (Chronic Viral Ilnesses); InfectDis. principale Médecin, McGill University Health Centre - Royal Victoria Hospital; assoc Prof Med, McGill University; Langs: English; French; (514)843-2090

LALONDE, Serge R; Medicentre Pincourt, 88 5e Av, Pincourt QC J7V 5K7; Mon'78; (514)425-1000; Fax. (514)425-1288.

LALONDE, Stephanie; CSSS de Papineau, 155 rue Maclaren E, Gatineau QC J8L 0C2; Ott'06; CCFP; CCFP(E.M.); Staff, Hôpital de Papineau; (819)986-4115

LALONDE, Suzanne; Hop Du Sacre-Coeur De Mtl, 5400 boul Gouin O, Montreal QC H4J 1C5; Mon'88; LMCC; Staff, Hôpital du Sacre-Coeur de Montréal; Langs: Bilingual(French/English); (514)338-2383; Fax. (514)338-3155.

LALONDE-KONTIO, Ginette; Groupe Sante Sentinelle, 232 boul Saint-Joseph, Gatineau QC J8Y 3X4; McM'00; CCFP; (819)778-1330; Fax. (819)778-3455.

LALOR, Eoin A G; 301-5 Quarry Ridge Rd, Barrie ON L4M 7G1; Auckland (New Zealand)'83; FRCPC; IntMed; Gastroent. Staff, Royal Victoria Regional Health Centre; (705)721-3344

LALUCK, Bohdan; Univ Hlth Network-Toronto Western Hosp, 8E 419-399 Bathurst St, Toronto ON M5T 2S8; Qns'97; FRCPC; IntMed. Staff, Toronto Western Hospital - University Health Network; Instructor, University of Toronto; Langs: Ukrainian; (416)603-5853; Fax. (416)603-6495.

LALUMIERE, Eric; CSSS de Laval, 1755 boul Rene-Laennec, Laval QC H7M 3L9; Mon'90; Electroenceph (P.Q.); Neur. Staff, Hopital de la Cite de la santé; (450)668-1010; Fax. (450)975-5545.

LALUMIERE, Robert; CSST Saint-Jerome, 85 rue de Martigny O, Saint-Jerome QC J7Y 3R8; Mon'66; (450)431-4000 x5322

LAM, Alan J; Squamish Med Clinic, PO Box 389 Stn Main, Squamish BC V8B 0A3; McG'69; Staff, Squamish General Hospital / Hilltop House; Langs: Cantonese; (604)892-3535; Fax. (604)892-3545.

LAM, Allen K L; 525 Colborne St, Brantford ON N3S 3P3; Ott'99; FRCSC; Otol. (519)756-6770

LAM, Andrew J Y W; MCI The Doctor's Office, PO Box 134 Stn Royal Bank LR8-200 Bay St, Toronto ON M5J 2J3; Tor'86; CCFP; Court Staff, St Michael's Hospital; Court Staff, Toronto General Hospital - UHN; Assoc Staff, Mount Sinai Hospital; Court Staff, Women's College Hospital; Lecturer Med(DFCM), University of Toronto; (416)368-6787; Fax. (416)368-7632.

LAM, Andrew W K; Rosedale Med Centre, 801-600 Sherbourne St, Toronto ON M4X 1W4; New South Wales (Australia)'83; CCFP; Staff, St Joseph's Health Centre; Lecturer Med, University of Toronto; (416)975-1485; Fax. (416)975-8244.

LAM, Andy S C; West Lincoln Mem Hosp, 169 Main St E, Grimsby ON L3M 1P3; Tor'84; ABIM(IntMed,Pulmonary); FACP; FRCPC; IntMed; Respir. Staff, West Lincoln Memorial Hospital; Langs: Chinese; (905)945-8609; Fax. (905)945-2019; alam1@cogeco.ca.

LAM, Angela W W; Heritage Med Centre, 2 Wootten Way N, Markham ON L3P 5T7; Alb'86; Ac Staff, The Scarborough Hospital - General Campus; Langs: Chinese; (905)294-4990

LAM, Anthony K S; Olive Med Clinic, 101-117 17 Ave NE, Calgary AB T2E 1L7; McG'62; BSc; MS; MDCM; CCFP; Langs: Mandarin; Cantonese; (403)276-8866; Fax. (403)230-2000.

LAM, Augustine S K; Parker Place Med Clinic, 1550-4380 No. 3 Rd, Richmond BC V6X 3V7; Melbourne (Australia)'69; (604)303-0799

LAM, Benjamin; Sunnybrook Hlth Sciences Ctre, 2075 Bayview Ave, Toronto ON M4N 3M5; Tor'03; Neur. Staff, Sunnybrook Health Sciences Centre; (416)480-4551

LAM, Buu-Khanh; Univ of Ottawa Heart Institute, H340A-40 Ruskin St, Ottawa ON K1Y 4W7; McG'94; FRCSC; CardSurg. Staff, University of Ottawa Heart Institute; (613)761-5001; Fax. (613)761-5217.

LAM, C Allan; I S T O P, LF-5655 Cambie St, Vancouver BC V5Z 3A4; Tor'79; Langs: Cantonese; (604)264-7867

LAM, Calvin; Foothills Med Centre, 1403 29 St NW, Calgary AB T2N 2T9; Ott'83; FRCPC; IntMed; Critical Care Medicine. Staff, Peter Lougheed Centre; Staff, Foothills Medical Centre; Staff, Calgary Regional Health Authority; (403)944-8094; calvin.lam@calgaryhealthregion.ca.

LAM, Charles C K; 110 Isabel St, Winnipeg MB R3A 1G4; Nashville(TN) (USA)'64; (204)786-4653; Fax. (204)772-3262.

LAM, Charles N H; Caledonian Med Clinic, 340 Campbell St, Nanaimo BC V9R 3G7; McM'89; Assoc Staff Privil, Nanaimo Regional General Hospital; Langs: Cantonese; Mandarin; (250)753-3202; Fax. (250)753-1039.

LAM, Christopher; 105-2020 Richmond Rd, Victoria BC V8R 6R5; UBC'72; BSc; CAFCI; CCFP; Clinical Asst Prof, University of British Columbia; Clinical Asst Prof, University of Victoria; Langs: Chinese; Cantonese; (250)472-3338; Fax. (250)472-3290.

LAM, Clement; Humber Valley Med Centre, 6-2630 Kipling Ave, Etobicoke ON M9V 4B9; Tor'76; Assoc Staff, William Osler Health System - Etobicoke General Hospital; Assoc Staff, Humber River Regional Hospital - Church Street Site; (416)743-7424; Fax. (416)743-9923.

LAM, David B W; Halton Geriatric Mental Health, 5230 South Service Rd, Burlington ON L7L 5K2; Mem'96; FRCPC; Psy. (905)681-8233

LAM, David D W; 301-240 Alton Towers Cir, Scarborough ON M1V 3Z3; (Hong Kong)'82; MRCP(UK); DCH(Glas); CCFP; FCFP; Ac Staff Family Pract, The Scarborough Hospital - General Campus; (416)321-6001

LAM, David L; Strathroy Middlesex Gen Hosp, 395 Carrie St, Strathroy ON N7G 3C9; Ott'06; Staff, Strathroy Middlesex General Hospital - Middlesex Hospital Alliance; (519)245-5295

LAM, David S C; Winnipeg Clinic, 2855 Pembina Hwy, Winnipeg MB R3T 2H5; Man'94; (204)949-1447

LAM, Desmond K; Toronto East Gen Hosp Inc, 825 Coxwell Ave, Toronto ON M4C 3E7; Tor'94; FRCPC; Anes. Staff, Toronto East General Hospital Inc; (416)469-6212

LAM, Doan Trang; CSSS de Vaudreuil-Soulanges, 408 av Saint-Charles, Vaudreuil-Dorion QC J7V 7M9; Sher'91; CCFP; FCFP; (450)455-6177

LAM, Emilie Y; Markham Walk In Clinic, 3606 Highway 7, Markham ON L3R 8W3; Tor'10; CCFP; (905)474-5764

LAM, Eric C S; Pacific Gastroenterology Assoc, 770-1190 Hornby St, Vancouver BC V6Z 2K5; Mem'97; FRCPC; IntMed; Gastroent. (604)688-6332 x224

LAM, Gail; Rockyview Gen Hosp, 7007 14 St SW, Calgary AB T2V 1P9; Qns'94; FRCSC; ObstGyn. Staff ObstGyn, Rockyview General Hospital; (403)943-3870; Fax. (403)212-1231.

LAM, Herman P Y; Health Sciences Centre, GF621F-820 Sherbrook St, Winnipeg MB R3A 1R9; Man'99; FRCPC; IntMed; Nephrol. Staff, Health Sciences Centre; (204)774-6511

LAM, Irina C Y; Danforth Med Centre, 1473 Danforth Ave, Toronto ON M4J 1N5; Tor'84; Staff, Toronto East General Hospital Inc; Staff, The Scarborough Hospital - Birchmount Campus; (416)461-0785

LAM, James H C; 60 Colborne St W, Orillia ON L3V 2Y4; Wes'73; BSc; Ac Staff, Orillia Soldiers' Memorial Hospital; Langs: Chinese; Cantonese; (705)325-7272; Fax. (705)325-9271.

LAM, James S M; 103-22720 119 Ave, Maple Ridge BC V2X 2Z8; UBC'88; CCFP; CCFP(E.M.); FCFP; (604)467-2133; Fax. (604)466-8933.

LAM, Jasmine C; Oakridge Centre-South Tower, 222-650 41st Ave W, Vancouver BC V5Z 2M9; UBC'07; CCFP; Langs: Cantonese; (604)261-2633

LAM, Jennifer K; North York Gen Hosp, 4001 Leslie St, North York ON M2K 1E1; Nottingham (United Kingdom)'10; CCFP; Staff, North York General Hospital; (416)714-4049

LAM, Jennifer K; Ryerson Med Centre, 350 Victoria St, Toronto ON M5B 2K3; Tor'09; CCFP; (416)979-5070; Fax. (416)979-5073.

LAM, Joseph K P; Main & Marine Med Clinic, 235 Marine Dr SE, Vancouver BC V5X 2S4; (Hong Kong)'79; MB BS; CCFP; Langs: Mandarin; Cantonese; (604)322-3011; Fax. (604)322-2827.

LAM, Joseph M; Pediatric Allergy Derm Clinic, 1803-805 Broadway W, Vancouver BC V5Z 1K1; McG'01; BSc; FRCPC; Peds (Pediatric Dermatology). Clinical Asst Prof Peds/Assoc Member Derm, University of British Columbia; (604)876-4433; joseph.lam@ubc.ca.

LAM, K S Kenneth; Foothills Med Centre, AC 142-1403 29 St NW, Calgary AB T2N 2T9; (Hong Kong)'85; FRCS(Glas); FRCPC; PhysMed&Rehab. Staff Div of PhysMed & Rehab, Foothills Medical Centre; Langs: Cantonese; (403)944-4226; Fax. (403)283-2526.

LAM, Kenneth H M; Royal Alexandra Hosp, 541-10240 Kingsway NW, Edmonton AB T5H 3V9; Cal'98; FRCPC; CCFP; EmergMed. Staff Community Services Centre, Royal Alexandra Hospital; (780)735-4442; Fax. (780)735-4916.

LAM, Kenneth W K; 797 Broadview Ave, Toronto ON M4K 2P8; Tor'87; (416)463-3228; Fax. (416)463-7868.

LAM, Leo T Y; 202-100 Colborne St W, Orillia ON L3V 2Y9; Alb'84; FRCPC; IntMed (Dialysis); Nephrol. Media Dir Dialysis, Stevenson Memorial Hospital; Med Dir Dialysis, Collingwood General & Marine Hospital; Staff Med Dir Dialysis, Orillia Soldiers' Memorial Hospital; Med Dir, Huntsville District Memorial Hospital - Muskoka Algonquin Healthcare; Clinical Asst Prof, McMaster University; (705)329-0644; Fax. (705)329-4987.

LAM, Man-Hoa; MUHC-Royal Victoria Hosp, 687 av des Pins O, Montreal QC H3A 1A1; Mon'99; CCFP; Staff, McGill University Health Centre - Royal Victoria Hospital; (514)843-1610

LAM, Mayda; Hazelwood Med Clinic, 102-16088 84 Ave, Surrey BC V4N 0V9; UBC'86; Staff, Surrey Memorial Hospital; (604)507-2527

LAM, Michael Chi-Kwok; 2-9640 Bayview Ave, Richmond Hill ON L4C 9P7; (Hong Kong)'74; FRCS(Glas); FRACS; CCFP; FCFP; Court Staff, Mackenzie Richmond Hill Hospital; (905)737-0509; Fax. (905)737-4889.

LAM, Michael Y C; 9-1170 Burnhamthorpe Rd W, Mississauga ON L5C 4E6; (Hong Kong)'78; MB BS; MRCP(UK); FRACGP(Australia); CCFP; FCFP; Langs: Mandarin; Cantonese; (905)281-9337; Fax. (905)281-9849.

LAM, Ngan; London HSC-South St, PO Box 5375 Stn B 800 Commissioners Rd E, London ON N6A 4G5; Tor'07; FRCPC; IntMed; Nephrol. Staff, London Health Sciences Centre - South Street; (519)685-8500 x56044

LAM, Ngoc Nga; CHUM-Hop St-Luc, 1058 rue Saint-Denis, Montreal QC H2X 3J4; Sher'94; Staff, Centre Hospitalier l'Université De Montréal (CHUM) - Hôpital Saint-luc; Langs: Vietnamese; (514)890-8000

LAM, Ni T; University of Alberta Hosp, 1G1 50-8440 112 St NW, Edmonton AB T6G 2B7; Alb'06; FRCPC; EmergMed. Staff, University of Alberta Hospital; (780)407-8432

LAM, Paul H S; Baker Clinic, 290-10405 Jasper Ave NW, Edmonton AB T5J 3N4; Ott'93; FRCPC; IntMed. (780)944-9587; Fax. (780)944-1165; phl1@telusplanet.net.

LAM, Pei-Yoong; Children's & Women's HC of BC, 4500 Oak St, Vancouver BC V6H 3N1; Melbourne (Australia)'94; Staff, BC Women's Hospital & Health Centre; (604)875-2200; plam@cw.bc.ca.

LAM, Peter C Y; Peter Lougheed Centre, 25-3500 26 Ave NE, Calgary AB T1Y 6J4; UBC'78; FRCPC; Psy. Ac Staff, Peter Lougheed Centre; Asst Prof, University of Calgary; (403)943-4555

LAM, Peter J; Trillium Hlth Ctr-West Toronto, 2F-150 Sherway Dr, Etobicoke ON M9C 1A5; Tor'92; ABIM; FRCPC; IntMed. Staff, Trillium Health Centre - Mississauga; Staff Consultant, Trillium Health Centre - West Toronto; (416)521-4196

LAM, Quoc Hung; CH Manoir de l'Age d'Or, 3430 rue Jeanne-Mance, Montreal QC H2X 2J9; Saigon (Vietnam)'78; Staff, Centre Hospitalier Rouyn-Noranda; (514)842-1147

LAM, Quoc Tru; Polyclinique Rosemont, 3377 boul Rosemont, Montreal QC H1X 1H4; Sher'97; (514)798-8688

LAM, Quyen Kim; Alberta Children's Hosp, 2888 Shaganappi Trail NW, Calgary AB T3B 6A8; Cal'98; FRCPC; Peds. Staff, Alberta Children's Hospital; (403)955-2953

LAM, Raymond W; UBC-Dept of Psychiatry, 7-2255 Wesbrook Mall, Vancouver BC V6T 2A1; UBC'81; FRCPC; Psy (Mood Disorders). Dir Mood Disorders Clinic, UBC Hospital - Koerner Pavillion; Prof, University of British Columbia; (604)822-7325; Fax. (604)822-7922.

LAM, Richard P; Dragon City Plaza, 219-328 Centre St SE, Calgary AB T2G 4X6; Cal'85; BSc; MSc; CCFP; FCFP; Langs: Chinese; (403)266-3331; Fax. (403)266-3346.

LAM, Richard P; 2F-607 Gerrard St E, Toronto ON M4M 1Y2; Man'71; Court Staff, St Michael's Hospital; Med Dir, Fairview Nursing Home; (416)461-7547

LAM, Robert E; Univ Hlth Network-Toronto Western Hosp, 2W 404-399 Bathurst St, Toronto ON M5T 2S8; Wes'91; MSc; DAB; CCFP; FCFP; Ac Staff, Toronto Western Hospital - University Health Network; Staff, Toronto Rehabilitation Institute - University Centre; Asst Prof, University of Toronto; (416)603-5888 x2; Fax. (416)603-5448.

LAM, Roger H C; Toronto Poly Clinic, 298 John St, Thornhill ON L3T 6M8; Tor'91; Med Dir, Rejuvena Skin & Laser Centre; (905)482-8648

LAM, Russell A; Alberta Children's Hosp, 2888 Shaganappi Trail NW, Calgary AB T3B 6A8; Cal'08; Peds. Staff, Alberta Children's Hospital; (403)955-7070

LAM, Selay; London HSC-Victoria Hosp, PO Box 5010 Stn B A2 401-800 Commissioners Rd E, London ON N6A 5W9; Ott'08; FRCPC; IntMed. Staff, London Health Sciences Centre - Victoria Campus; (519)685-8500

LAM, Sheung L L; Niagara H System-St Catharines, PO Box 3018 Stn Main 142 Queenston St, St Catharines ON L2R 7C6; McM'83; BSc; MSc; FRCPC; Anes. Ac Staff Anes, Niagara Health System - St Catharines General Site; Ac Staff Anes, Niagara Health System - Ontario Street Site; Langs: Chinese; Cantonese; (905)684-7271 x45561; lsl_lam@hotmail.com.

LAM, Sheung-Ying S; LL-1107 37 St SW, Calgary AB T3C 1S5; Cal'89; CCFP; FCFP; Med Dir, Extendicare Calgary; Clinical Asst Prof, University of Calgary; (403)246-7788; Fax. (403)242-8850.

LAM, Simon R; 200-555 Sixth St, New Westminster BC V3L 5H1; London (England)'84; MRCP; FRCS; FRCSC; Ophth (Vitreo Retinal Surgery). Ac Staff, Surrey Memorial Hospital; Clinical Asst Prof, University of British Columbia; Langs: Chinese; Cantonese; (604)521-4144; Fax. (604)521-4129.

LAM, Stephen C T; 675 10th Ave W, Vancouver BC V5Z 1L3; Tor'74; FRCPC; IntMed (Lung Cancer); Respir. Staff/Chair Lung Tumor Group, BC Cancer Agency Vancouver Centre; Prof Med, University of British Columbia; Langs: Chinese; (604)675-8094; slam2@bccancer.bc.ca.

LAM, Sui-Sang; Keary Med Centre, 203-245 Columbia St E, New Westminster BC V3L 3W4; (Hong Kong)'81; MB BS; FRCPC; IntMed (Hypertension); Nephrol. (604)525-9666; Fax. (604)525-2173.

LAM, Tai-Thuong; Hop Louis-H Lafontaine, 7401 rue Hochelaga, Montreal QC H1N 3M5; Saigon (Vietnam)'69; Ac Staff, Hopital Louis-H Lafontaine; (514)251-4000; Fax. (514)251-8474.

LAM, Terena P T; 299 Main St, Callander ON P0H 1H0; Wes'98; (705)752-1004

LAM, Thu Loan; Clinique Med Jardins Dorval, 204-352 rue Dorval, Dorval QC H9S 3H8; McG'85; CCFP; Staff, McGill University Health Centre - Montreal General Campus; (514)631-6086; Fax. (514)631-6691.

LAM, Thuc Bao; CSSS du Suroît, 150 rue Saint-Thomas, Salaber-de-Valleyf QC J6T 6C1; Mon'94; IntMed (P.Q.) (Pharmacology). Staff, Centre Hospitalier Régional du Suroît; (450)371-9920

LAM, Tong V; University of Alberta Hosp, 8440 112 St NW, Edmonton AB T6G 2B7; Alb'08; Staff, University of Alberta Hospital; (780)407-8822

LAM, Tukien M; Mackenzie Richmond Hill Hosp, 10 Trench St, Richmond Hill ON L4C 4Z3; Chicago(IL,USA) (USA)'93; FRCPC; IntMed. Staff Internist, Rouge Valley Health System - Ajax & Pickering Health Centre Site; Staff Internist, Mackenzie Richmond Hill Hospital; Langs: Cantonese; (905)883-1212

LAM, Vincent H C; Toronto East Gen Hosp Inc, 825 Coxwell Ave, Toronto ON M4C 3E7; Tor'99; CCFP; Staff Emerg, Toronto East General Hospital Inc; (416)461-8272

LAM, Vincent Y Y; 74 Finch Ave E, North York ON M2N 4R3; Tor'88; Ac Staff, Rouge Valley Health System - Centenary Health Centre Site; Court Staff, The Scarborough Hospital - General Campus; Langs: Cantonese; Mandarin; (416)222-6822; Fax. (416)222-8021.

LAM, Vo-Hoa; Grace Dart Extended Care Ctr, 5155 rue Sainte-Catherine E, Montreal QC H1V 2A5; Sher'00; CCFP; Fam Med, Grace Dart Extended Care Centre; (514)255-2833; vlam@ssss.gouv.qc.ca.

LAM, Wai-Arm; 207-236 Georgia St E, Vancouver BC V6A 1Z7; Tor'82; Assoc Staff, Providence Health Care - Mount Saint Joseph Hospital; Villa Cathay Care Home; Langs: Cantonese; Mandarin; Teochew; (604)688-6415; Fax. (604)688-5037.

LAM, Wai-Ching; Univ Hlth Network-Toronto Western Hosp, 6 432EW-399 Bathurst St, Toronto ON M5T 2S8; Man'82; FRCSC; Ophth (Vitreo Retina). Staff, Toronto Western Hospital - University Health Network; Staff, The Hospital For Sick Children; Assoc Prof, University of Toronto; Langs: Chinese; (416)603-5376; Fax. (416)603-5059; waiching.lam@utoronto.ca.

LAM, Wendy Y H; Kingsway Plaza Phase III, 705-4980 Kingsway, Burnaby BC V5H 4K7; UBC'91; BScPharm; FRCPC; IntMed; Hem. (604)434-5001; Fax. (604)434-5053.

LAM, Wilson L T; Manitoba X-Ray Clinic, 3263 Portage Ave, Winnipeg MB R3K 0W6; Man'83; PhmB; FRCPC; DiagRad. Att Staff Radiol, The Salvation Army Grace Hospital; Att Staff Radiol, St Boniface General Hospital; Lecturer Radiol, University of Manitoba; (204)832-0273

LAM, Yuen-Ming; South Huron Med Centre, SS 2 23 Huron St W, Exeter ON N0M 1S2; Wes'79; BSc; Hospitalist, South Huron Hospital Association; Langs: Cantonese; (519)235-3343; Fax. (519)235-3845.

LAM ANTONIADES, Margarita; St James Town Health Centre, G/F-410 Sherbourne St, Toronto ON M4X 1K2; Tor'01; MHSc; BSc; CCFP; Langs: Greek; (416)864-3096; Fax. (416)864-6035; margarita.antoniades@utoronto.ca.

LAM POYUEN, Hian Kow; Clinique MEd Alexandre, A-8100 boul Taschereau, Longueuil QC J4X 1C2; Grenoble (France)'76; (450)465-5589; Fax. (450)465-0092.

LAM-YUK-TSEUNG, Jules C C; Institut de Cardiologie de Mtl, 5000 rue Belanger, Montreal QC H1T 1C8; McG'79; FRCPC; IntMed (Coronary Care); Cardiol. Staff Cardiol, Institut de Cardiologie de Montréal; assoc Prof Med, Universite de Montreal; (514)376-3330; Fax. (514)593-7461.

LAM-YUK-TSEUNG, Y Sophie; CSD & DSS du Rocher-Perce, GD 633 av Daigneault, Chandler QC G0C 1K0; Mon'85; LMCC; CCFP; Staff, Centre Hospitalier de Chandler; Langs: English; (418)689-2572; Fax. (418)689-2840.

LAMANQUE, Pascal; CSSS Pierre Boucher, 1333 boul Jacques-Cartier E, Longueuil QC J4M 2A5; Mon'02; Staff, Centre Hospitalier Pierre Boucher; (450)468-8111

LAMARCHE, Jean; GMF du Carrefour Beauport, 210-3333 rue du Carrefour, Quebec QC G1C 5R9; Laval'80; LMCC; (418)663-6345; Fax. (418)663-8621; jeanlamarche@ssss.gouv.qc.ca.

LAMARCHE, Maurice; Clinique médicale de Shawville, CP 700 269 rue Main, Shawville QC J0X 2Y0; Ott'73; ac Staff, Pontiac Hospital Centre; Langs: English; (819)647-2924; Fax. (819)647-2845.

LAMARCHE, Robert A; Casselman Med Centre, PO Box 380 2-629 rue Principale, Casselman ON K0A 1M0; Ott'77; Langs: Bilingual(English/French); (613)764-5440; Fax. (613)764-9974.

LAMARCHE, Yoan; Institut de Cardiologie de Mtl, 5000 rue Belanger, Montreal QC H1T 1C8; Mon'01; FRCSC; CardSurg; Critical Care Medicine (P.Q.). Staff, Institut de Cardiologie de Montréal; (514)376-3330

LAMARGESE, Isabella; CSSS du Sud de Lanaudière, 911 montee des Pionniers, Terrebonne QC J6V 2H2; Mon'96; FRCPC; NuclearMed; IntMed (P.Q.). Staff, Centre Hospitalier Pierre le Gardeur; Langs: English; Italian; (450)654-7525 x31263

LAMARRE, Alexandre; Hop du Sacre-Coeur de Mtl, 5400 boul Gouin O, Montreal QC H4J 1C5; Sher'00; FRCPC; DiagRad. Staff, Hôpital du Sacre-Coeur de Montréal; (514)338-2222 x2853

LAMARRE, Andre; CHUQ-Ctr Hosp Univ Laval, 2100-2705 boul Laurier, Quebec QC G1V 4G2; Laval'94; FRCPC; DiagRad. Staff, Centre Hospitalier Universitaire de Quebec-CHUL; Chef Radiology(Interim), Université Laval; (418)654-2258

LAMARRE, Angele; CLSC Saint-Hubert, 6800 boul Cousineau, Saint-Hubert QC J3Y 8Z4; Mon'86; CCFP; FCFP; (450)443-7400; Fax. (450)676-3488.

LAMARRE, Caroline; Clinique Med de Mont-Joli, 1385 boul Benoit-Gaboury, Mont-Joli QC G5H 4B1; Laval'01; Staff, Centre Hospitalier de Chandler; (418)775-5353

LAMARRE, Celine; Inst De Readaptation De Mtl, 6300 av De Darlington, Montreal QC H3S 2J4; Laval'67; PhysMed&Rehab. Staff Physiatrist, Hôpital Ste-Justine; Staff Physiatrist, Institut de Réadaptation Gingras-Lindsay de Montréal; (514)340-2146

LAMARRE, Claude; GMF de Lorraine, 99 boul De Gaulle, Lorraine QC J6Z 3Z9; Sher'87; Staff, Hopital de la Cite de la santé; Staff, Clinique Santé Voyage Vacsan; (450)621-1444; Fax. (450)621-7183; claude@vascan.com.

LAMARRE, Claudine; Ctr Hosp Anna Laberge, 200 boul Brisebois, Chateauguay QC J6K 4W8; McG'97; GenSurg. Staff, Hôpital Anna-Laberge; (450)699-2425

LAMARRE, Edmond; CSSS de Laval, 1755 boul Rene-Laennec, Laval QC H7M 3L9; McG'85; Staff, Hopital de la Cite de la santé; (450)668-1010

LAMARRE, Elisabeth; Hop du Sacre-Coeur de Mtl, 5400 boul Gouin O, Montreal QC H4J 1C5; Sher'02; FRCPC; DiagRad. Staff, Hôpital du Sacre-Coeur de Montréal; (514)338-2222

LAMARRE, Hans; Pavillon Rosemont, 5689 boul Rosemont, Montreal QC H1T 2H1; (Haiti)'88; Psy. (514)252-3400 x4766; Fax. (514)252-3810.

LAMARRE, Jean; CSSS Chicoutimi-CLSC, 411 rue de l'Hotel-Dieu, Chicoutimi QC G7H 7Z5; Laval'72; ac Staff, Complexe hospitalier de la Sagamie; (418)690-3924 x3864; Fax. (418)690-3241.

LAMARRE, Leo-Yves; 650 av Hartland, Outremont QC H2V 2X3; Mon'60; PhD; Staff, Hôpital du Sacre-Coeur de Montréal; Prof Physiol, Universite de Montreal.

LAMARRE, Louis P; Hop Charles Lemoyne, 3120 boul Taschereau, Greenfield Park QC J4V 2H1; Mon'80; ABPath; CSPQ; FRCPC; AnatPath. Staff, Hopital Charles LeMoyne; Clin Assoc Prof, Universite de Montreal; (450)466-5000 x2343; louis.lamarre@rrsss16.gouv.qc.ca.

LAMARRE, Marc; CSSS de Rimouski-Neigette, CP 3150 Succ A 150 av Rouleau, Rimouski QC G5L 5T1; Laval'84; FRCPC; Psy. Staff, Hôpital Regional Rimouski; (418)724-8315; Fax. (418)724-8652.

LAMARRE, Marie-Lise; Hop Charles LeMoyne, 3120 boul Taschereau, Greenfield Park QC J4V 2H1; Mon'07; FRCPC; EmergMed. Staff, Hopital Charles LeMoyne.

LAMARRE, Martin; Place de la Cite-Medicale, 295-2600 boul Laurier, Quebec QC G1V 4T3; McG'96; Staff, Centre Hospitalier de Gaspe; (418)781-0480; Fax. (418)659-7072; martin.lamarre.chgaspe@ssss.gouv.qc.ca.

LAMARRE, Michelle A; Rainbow Centre, 109-40 Elm St, Sudbury ON P3C 1S8; Laval'81; CCFP; FCFP; Langs: Spanish; French; (705)522-9200

LAMARRE, Monique; Ctr Hosp du Centre la Mauricie, 50 119e rue, Shawinigan-Sud QC G9P 5K1; Mon'83; FRCPC; Psy. Staff, Centre Hospitalier du Centre la Mauricie; Universite de Montreal; (819)536-7500

LAMARRE, Pascal; Centre Med Brunswick, 203-955 rue Saint-Jean, Pointe-Claire QC H9R 5K3; McG'04; FRCSC; GenSurg; Critical Care Medicine (P.Q.). Staff, Lakeshore General Hospital - Pointe Claire; (514)459-0248; Fax. (514)426-9059.

LAMARRE, Paul; CSSS de Saint-Jerome, 290 rue de Montigny, Saint-Jerome QC J7Z 5T3; Laval'69; DiagRad. Staff Radiol, Hôtel-Dieu de Saint-Jérôme; (450)431-8300

LAMARRE, Suzanne; St Mary's Hosp Centre, 3830 av Lacombe, Montreal QC H3T 1M5; Laval'65; FAPA; FRCPC; Psy. Hd Psy, St Mary's Hospital Centre; adj Prof, McGill University; (514)345-3511 x3358; Fax. (514)734-2609; suzanne.lamarre@ssss.gouv.qc.ca.

LAMARRE, Valerie; Hôpital Ste-Justine, 3175 ch Cote-Sainte-Catherine, Montreal QC H3T 1C5; McG'91; FRCPC; Peds; InfectDis. Staff, Hôpital Ste-Justine; (514)345-4931 x5566; Fax. (514)345-4908; valerie_lamarre@ssss.gouv.qc.ca.

LAMARRE-CLICHE, Maxime; CHUM-Hotel-Dieu, 3840 rue Saint-Urbain, Montreal QC H2W 1T8; Mon'95; MSc; FRCPC; IntMed (Cardiology). Spécialiste IntMed, Centre Hospitalier l'Université de Montréal (CHUM) - Hôtel-Dieu; Clin Assoc Prof, Universite de Montreal.

LAMB, David J; Medical Arts Bldg, 4-165 Plymouth Rd, Welland ON L3B 3E1; Mem'84; Ac Staff, Niagara Health System - Welland Hospital Site; (905)732-3087; Fax. (905)732-9011.

LAMB, Fanny; Ctr Hosp de LaSalle, 8585 tsse Champlain, LaSalle QC H8P 1C1; Sher'05; FRCSC; ObstGyn. Staff, Centre Hospitalier de LaSalle; (514)362-8000

LAMB, Blair; 5230 South Service Rd, Burlington ON L7L 5K2; Wes'88; CCFP; FCFP; Pres, The Pain Reliever Corporation; Pres, The IASIS Corporation; Pres, The Lamb Pain Clinic; (905)331-7888; Fax. (905)331-0911.

LAMB, Howard F; Tillsonburg Med Centre, 200 Broadway St, Tillsonburg ON N4G 5A7; Dal'81; Staff, Tillsonburg District Memorial Hospital; (519)842-4231; Fax. (519)842-7579.

LAMB, Jonathan D; Saskatoon City Hosp, 701 Queen St, Saskatoon SK S7K 0M7; Sask'75; DABA; FRCPC; Anes. Staff, Saskatoon City Hospital; (306)655-8371; Fax. (306)655-8817.

LAMB, Julie A; Autumnwood Med Centre, 10-414 Westmount Dr, Winnipeg MB R2J 1P3; Man'91; CCFP; (204)255-7430; Fax. (204)255-0643.

LAMB, Kendra M; Maternity Care Clinic, 201-178 96 Ave NE, Calgary AB T3K 6G4; Cal'03; FRCSC; ObstGyn. Staff, Foothills Medical Centre; Staff, Maternity Care Clinic; (403)806-2496; Fax. (403)806-2497.

LAMB, M Nicholas; Phoenix Medical XRay Clinic, 101-2155 10th Ave, Prince George BC V2M 5J6; Ott'91; FRCPC; DiagRad., University Hospital of Northern British Columbia; (250)563-0635

LAMB, Sandra I; University Hosp of Northern BC, 1475 Edmonton St, Prince George BC V2M 1S2; Ott'91; Staff, University Hospital of Northern British Columbia; (250)565-2000

LAMB, Sheilah B; Harvard Square Mall, 202-801 Mohawk Rd W, Hamilton ON L9C 6C2; McM'80; CCFP; FCFP; Ac Staff, Hamilton Health Sciences Centre - McMaster University Medical Centre; (905)383-8431; Fax. (905)387-3965.

LAMB, Tasha H; BC Women's Hosp & Health Ctre, 4500 Oak St, Vancouver BC V6H 3N1; UBC'02; CCFP; Staff, BC Women's Hospital & Health Centre; (604)875-2029; Fax. (604)875-3197.

LAMBA, Geetinder K; St James Street Med Clinic, 1600 Portage Ave, Winnipeg MB R3J 0C6; Man'91.

LAMBA, Kiraninder S; Health Sciences Centre, GC419-820 Sherbrook St, Winnipeg MB R3A 1R9; Man'98; FRCPC; IntMed. Staff IntMed, Health Sciences Centre; (204)774-6511

LAMBA, Manisha; The Ottawa Hosp-Gen Campus, 501 Smyth Rd, Ottawa ON K1H 8L6; Delhi (India)'78; DAB(AnatPath); DAB(Hem); FRCPC; GenPath (Hematology Pathology). Staff, The Ottawa Hospital - General Campus; Consultant, MDS Laboratories; Asst Prof, University of Ottawa; Langs: Hindi; (613)737-8288

LAMBA, Rakesh K; Regional Treatment Centre, PO Box 3000 Stn Del Ctr 33344 King Rd, Abbotsford BC V2S 4P4; Gujarat (India)'86; MB BS; FRCPC; Psy (Forensic Psychiatry). Staff, Regional Treatment Centre & Pacific Institution; Clinical Asst Prof Psy, University of British Columbia; Langs: Gujarati; Hindi; Punjabi; (604)851-7675; rakeshl@telus.net.

LAMBA, Wiplove R; 3227-100 Stokes St, Toronto ON M6J 1H4; Ott'06; Psy. Staff, Centre for Addiction & Mental Health (CAMH) - Queen Site; (416)535-8501

LAMBERT, A Wayne; Health Sciences North-Laurenti, 41 Ramsey Lake Rd, Sudbury ON P3E 5J1; Qns'72; FRCPC; Anes. Staff, Health Sciences North-Laurentian Site; Consultant, Health Sciences North-St Joseph's Health Centre; Section Leader Anaes, Northern Ontario School of Medicine; (705)522-2200

LAMBERT, Andre-Stephane; Univ of Ottawa Heart Institute, H 2410-40 Ruskin St, Ottawa ON K1Y 4W7; McG'90; FRCPC; Anes;CCFP; Staff, University of Ottawa Heart Institute; (613)761-4379; Fax. (613)761-4925.

LAMBERT, Bernard; CHUM-Hotel-Dieu, 3840 rue Saint-Urbain, Montreal QC H2W 1T8; Mon'55; FACOG; ObstGyn (Colposcopy). Staff, Centre Hospitalier l'Université de Montréal (CHUM) - Hôtel-Dieu; assoc Prof, Universite de Montreal; (514)890-8000 x12685; Fax. (514)412-7093.

LAMBERT, Carole; CHUM-Hop Notre-Dame, 1560 rue Sherbrooke E, Montreal QC H2L 4M1; Sher'96; MScEd; FRCPC; RadOncol (Neuro Oncology). Staff, Centre Hospitalier l'Université de Montréal (CHUM) - Hôpital Notre-Dame; (514)890-8254; Fax. (514)412-7537; carole.lambert.chum@ssss.gouv.qc.ca.

LAMBERT, Christine; MUHC-Montreal Gen Hosp, 1650 av Cedar, Montreal QC H3G 1A4; Laval'90; FRCPC; RadOncol. Staff, McGill University Health Centre - Montreal General Campus; (514)934-8040

LAMBERT, David A; Health Sciences Centre, GH611-820 Sherbrook St, Winnipeg MB R3A 1R9; Man'00; FRCPC; Anes. Staff Anes, Health Sciences Centre; (204)774-6511

LAMBERT, David C; Concorde Physio Sport, 262-7005 boul Taschereau, Brossard QC J4Z 1A7; Durham (England)'65; OrthSurg (P.Q.). Langs: French; Spanish; (450)445-1556

LAMBERT, Diane; Centre Med St-Jean, 202-1018 rue de la Prairie O, St-J-Chrysostome QC G6Z 0A7; Laval'85; Teach Staff Clin de Med du Sport, Université Laval; Langs: Bilingual(French/English); (418)839-4433; Fax. (418)839-3574.

LAMBERT, Diane; Direction de la Santé publique, 210-1000 rue Labelle, Saint-Jerome QC J7Z 5N6; Mon'80; Staff, Hôtel-Dieu de Saint-Jérôme; (450)436-8622; Fax. (450)569-6305.

LAMBERT, France; CSSS de Trois-Rivières, 1991 boul du Carmel, Trois-Rivieres QC G8Z 3R9; Sher'72; DrMedCh; Nephrol (P.Q.) (Clinical Nephrology). Staff, CSSS de Trois-Rivières; Langs: English; (819)697-3333; Fax. (819)693-1845.

LAMBERT, Gilles; Dir de la Sante Publique-Mtl, 1301 rue Sherbrooke E, Montreal QC H2L 1M3; Laval'76; (514)528-2400

LAMBERT, Jacinthe; CHUQ-St-Francois d'Assise, 10 rue de l'Espinay, Quebec QC G1L 3L5; Laval'97; Staff, Centre Hospitalier Universitaire De Québec - Pavillon De St-françois-d'assise; (418)525-4444

LAMBERT, Jacques; Clinique Familiale St-Lambert, 201-209 rue Woodstock, Saint-Lambert QC J4P 1W7; Sher'79; Dep Head, Centre Hospitalier Pierre Boucher; (450)466-3865; Fax. (450)466-4072.

LAMBERT, Jean-Marie; CLSC Le Minordet, CP 4000 961 de la Clinique, Senneterre QC J0Y 2M0; Mon'75; (819)737-2243; Fax. (819)737-3122.

LAMBERT, Kerri L; 218-2025 Corydon Ave, Winnipeg MB R3P 0N5; Man'00; FRCPC; Psy.

LAMBERT, Linda A; 201-6628 Crowchild Trail SW, Calgary AB T3E 5R8; Cal'78; CCFP; FCFP; Ac Staff Privil, Rockyview General Hospital; (403)240-9350; Fax. (403)240-9783.

LAMBERT, Louise; Direction de la Sante Publique, 1255 rue Beauregard, Longueuil QC J4K 2M3; Mon'77; MSc; Med Consultant, Agence de santé et des services sociaux de la Montérégie; (450)676-6772; Fax. (450)928-3023.

LAMBERT, Louise; CHUM-Hôp Notre-Dame, 1560 rue Sherbrooke E, Montreal QC H2L 4M1; Mon'03; FRCPC; RadOncol. Staff, Centre Hospitalier l'Université de Montréal (CHUM) - Hôpital Notre-Dame; (514)890-8254

LAMBERT, Louise; Regie des Rentes Du Quebec, CP 5200 Succ Terminus, Quebec QC G1K 7S9; Laval'84; (418)657-8709 x3239; Fax. (418)646-7609.

LAMBERT, Luc; Clinique Med Maskinonge, 147 A boul Est, Maskinonge QC J0K 1N0; Laval'78; Staff, CSSS de Maskinongé; (819)227-2228; Fax. (819)227-3737.

LAMBERT, Lynn A C; Health Science Centre, 1413-3330 Hospital Dr NW, Calgary AB T2N 4N1; (United Kingdom)'85; MB ChB; Staff, Foothills Medical Centre; (403)592-5010

LAMBERT, Marie; Hôpital Ste-Justine, 3175 ch Cote-Sainte-Catherine, Montreal QC H3T 1C5; Mon'77; FRCPC; Peds; MedGenetics. Staff, Hôpital Ste-Justine; (514)345-4736; Fax. (514)345-4766.

LAMBERT, Marie-France; CSSS de Rivière-de-Loup, 75 rue Saint-Henri, Riviere-Du-Loup QC G5R 2A4; Tor'89; FRCSC; ObstGyn. Staff, Centre Hospitalier Regional du Grand-Portage; (418)868-1000

LAMBERT, Michel; Clinique Med Plateau Marquette, 200-731 rue Galt O, Sherbrooke QC J1H 1Z1; Laval'84; Ac Member, Centre Hospitalier Universitaire de Sherbrooke-Hôpital Hôtel-Dieu; Langs: English; (819)564-8662; Fax. (819)564-1294.

LAMBERT, Nicole; CLSC Villeray, 1425 rue Jarry E, Montreal QC H2E 1A7; Mon'95; (514)376-4141 x320

LAMBERT, Nicole; CSSS de la Vieille-Capitale, 5100-2400 av d'Estimauville, Quebec QC G1E 7G9; Mon'83; MSc(Commun.); OccupMed (P.Q.). Staff CommunHealth & Public Health, Centre Hospitalier Universitaire de Quebec-CHUL; (418)623-1010 x281; Fax. (418)623-7513.

LAMBERT, Raymond; Hôpital Ste-Justine, 3175 ch Cote-Sainte-Catherine, Montreal QC H3T 1C5; Sher'82; ABNM; FRCPC; NuclearMed. Chef méd nucl, Hôpital Ste-Justine; Universite de Montreal; (514)345-4931 x6879; Fax. (514)345-2120.

LAMBERT, Richard; CHUM-Hop Notre-Dame, 1560 rue Sherbrooke E, Montreal QC H2L 4M1; Mon'80; FRCPC; PhysMed&Rehab. ac Staff, Centre Hospitalier l'Université de Montréal (CHUM) - Hôpital Notre-Dame; Physician, Centre de Physiatrie Val-des-Arbres Inc.; Langs: Bilingual(French/English); (514)890-8201; Fax. (514)412-7610.

LAMBERT, Robert G W; University of Alberta Hosp, 2A2 41 WCM-8440 112 St NW, Edmonton AB T6G 2B7; Queen's (United Kingdom)'80; FRCR(Lond); MB ChB; FRCPC; DiagRad (Diagnostic Radiology). Ac Staff Radiol, University of Alberta Hospital; Dept Chair Radiol & DiagImaging/Assoc Prof, University of Alberta; (780)407-6907; Fax. (780)407-3853; rlambert@ualberta.ca.

LAMBERT, Roch; Centre Med de St-Lambert, RR 3 1329 rue des Erables, St-Lambert-de-Lauz QC G0S 2W0; Laval'73; Langs: English; (418)889-9745; Fax. (418)889-0807.

LAMBERT, Todd B; 160-600 Main St, Saint John NB E2K 1J5; Mem'97; FRCPC; Peds. Staff, Saint John Regional Hospital; Acting Asst Dean Graduate Med Educ New Brunswick, Dalhousie University; (506)648-6936

LAMBERT, Waide T; Sudbury Reg Hosp-Laurentian, 41 Ramsey Lake Rd, Sudbury ON P3E 5J1; Qns'85; FRCPC; Anes. Court Staff, Health Sciences North-Laurentian Site; Court Staff, North Bay Regional Health Centre - Kirkwood; (705)671-5492

LAMBERT, Wendy C L; The Ottawa Hosp-Gen Campus, 501 Smyth Rd, Ottawa ON K1H 8L6; Ott'94; CCFP; Staff, The Ottawa Hospital - General Campus; Staff, Children's Hospital of Eastern Ontario (CHEO); (613)737-7700 x70166

LAMBERT, Yves; Ctr Jeunesse de la Monteregie, 1251 rue Beauregard, Longueuil QC J4K 2M3; Mon'80; CCFP; FCFP; Clin Prof Family Med, Universite de Montreal; Langs: Bilingual(French/English); (450)646-6631; Fax. (450)928-3857; yves.lambert@rrsss16.gouv.qc.ca.

LAMBERT-PERRAULT, Anne-Marie; Hotel-Dieu de Levis, 143 rue Wolfe, Levis QC G6V 3Z1; Laval'06; CCFP; Staff, Hôtel-Dieu de Lévis; (418)835-7121

LAMBETH, Michelle A; Canadian Forces Hlth Serv Ctr, PO Box 99000 Stn Forces, Halifax NS B3K 5X5; UBC'97; CCFP; Staff CF Health Services Centre(A), Canadian Forces Health Services Centre (Atlantic); (902)427-8700

LAMBOS, Peggy; Victoria Square Med Clinic, PO Box 5700 Stn Main 217-2345 10th Ave W, Prince Albert SK S6V 7V6; Man'95; FRCPC; Peds. (306)953-5664; Fax. (306)922-9394.

LAMBOTHARAN, Aruna; Legacy Med Centre, 7-5637 Finch Ave E, Scarborough ON M1B 5K9; Jaffna (Sri Lanka)'91; MB BS; CCFP; (416)299-8100

LAMBOTHARAN, Ramanathan; Legacy Med Centre, 7-5637 Finch Ave E, Scarborough ON M1B 5K9; Jaffna (Sri Lanka)'91; MB BS; CCFP; (416)299-8100; Fax. (416)299-4620.

LAMBRECHTS, Hugo; Fort Alexander Health Centre, PO Box 70, Pine Falls MB R0E 1M0; (South Africa)'89; MB ChB; Langs: Afrikaans; (204)367-2208 x224; Fax. (204)367-4587.

LAMBRINOS, Dimitrios J; 107-915 rue Jean-Talon O, Montreal QC H3N 1S7; McG'79; (514)277-8088; Fax. (514)777-1901.

LAMBROPOULOS, Cristos; 207-640 Prospect St, Fredericton NB E3B 9M7; Dal'01; CCFP; (506)458-0483

LAMBROS, George A; The Sports Injury Clinic, 2225 Macleod Trail SE, Calgary AB T2G 5B6; Qns'89; Dip SportMed; CCFP; FCFP; (403)237-5633; Fax. (403)237-5142.

LAMENSA, John W E; Harmony Med Centre, 101-152 Cleopatra Dr, Nepean ON K2G 5X2; Tor'96; FRCSC; ObstGyn. Staff, The Ottawa Hospital - Civic Campus; (613)728-6533; Fax. (613)728-4745.

LAMENT, Richard; St Paul's Hosp, 1081 Burrard St, Vancouver BC V6Z 1Y6; London (England)'66; FRCPC; Psy. Staff, Providence Health Care - St Paul's Hospital; (604)682-2344

LAMENZA, Cecilia; Markham College Med Clinic, 306-474 College St, Toronto ON M6G 1A4; National (Colombia)'58; FRCPC; Peds (Clinical Immunology & Allergy). Langs: Italian; Spanish; French; (416)922-0818; Fax. (416)922-5188.

LAMER, Danielle; Clinique Santé-Voyage de Mtl, 2E-6865 rue Sherbrooke E, Montreal QC H1N 1C7; Mon'84; Staff, Hopital Maisonneuve-Rosemont; Langs: Bilingual(French/English); (514)252-0943

LAMER, Mark; CSSS Des Etchemins, RR 1 331 rue Du Sanatorium, Lac-Etchemin QC G0R 1S0; Laval'97; Staff, CSSS des Etchemins; (418)675-8001; Fax. (418)625-3020.

LAMIRANDE, Maxime; CSSS de Trois-Rivières, 1991 boul du Carmel, Trois-Rivieres QC G8Z 3R9; Mon'05; CCFP; Staff, CSSS de Trois-Rivières; (819)697-3333

LAMIRANDE, Yves; Clinique Med Familiale, 101-940 boul des Recollets, Trois-Rivieres QC G8Z 3W9; Mon'82; Staff, CSSS de Trois-Rivières; (819)373-0303; Fax. (819)373-8431.

LAMMERSE, Christine; Surrey Mem Hosp, 13750 96 Ave, Surrey BC V3V 1Z2; Wes'83; CCFP; Staff Youth Clinic, Surrey Memorial Hospital; (604)585-5999

LAMON, Richard D; 28 Rosedale Rd, Toronto ON M4W 2P3; Wes'68; DPsy; FRCPC; Psy. Staff, St Michael's Hospital; (416)928-0307; Fax. (416)928-1699; rlamon@on.aibn.com.

LAMOND, Shawna M; Alexandra Comm Health Centre, 101-1318 Centre St NE, Calgary AB T2E 2R7; Cal'06; CCFP; (403)266-2622

LAMONDE-BOULET, Guillaume; Hotel-Dieu D'Arthbaska, 5 rue des Hospitalieres, Victoriaville QC G6P 6N2; Sher'02; Staff, Hotel-Dieu d'Arthabaska; (819)357-2030

LAMONT, A Margaret; 103-2025 Broadway W, Vancouver BC V6J 1Z6; Glasgow (Scotland)'84; MB ChB; CCFP; (604)730-9769

LAMONT, D David; Medical & Dental Bldg, 202-1221 Algonquin Ave, North Bay ON P1B 4Y3; Wes'85; FRCSC; GenSurg. Staff, North Bay Regional Health Centre - Regional Mental Health; (705)495-8854; Fax. (705)495-0874.

LAMONT, Barry J B; Windsor Med Clinic, 1608 Tecumseh Rd W, Windsor ON N9B 1T8; Belfast (Ireland)'77; MB ChB; BAO; Affil Staff, Windsor Regional Hospital - Tayfour Site; (519)258-4400

LAMONT, Jennifer; Arbour Family Medicine, 201-770 Broadview Ave, Ottawa ON K2A 3A3; Dal'07; CCFP; Staff, Arnprior & District Memorial Hospital; (613)739-3700

LAMONT, John A; Hamilton HS-Henderson Site, 711 Concession St, Hamilton ON L8V 1C3; Wes'66; FACOG; FSOGC; MSc; FRCSC; ObstGyn (Sexual Medicine). Ac Staff, Hamilton Health Sciences Centre-Juravinski Site; Emeritus Prof ObstGyn, McMaster University; (905)574-8606; Fax. (905)575-2587; lamontj@hhsc.ca.

LAMONT, R Neil; Grey Bruce HS-Owen Sound, PO Box 1800 Stn Main 7207-1800 8th St E, Owen Sound ON N4K 6M9; McM'87; BSc; FRCSC; GenSurg. Staff, Grey Bruce Health Services - Owen Sound; Asst Prof Surg, McMaster University; (519)372-3388; Fax. (519)372-0405.

LAMONT, Robert W; Scarborough Hosp-General Div, 3050 Lawrence Ave E, Scarborough ON M1P 2V5; Tor'63; DA; FRCPC; Anes (Chronic Pain). Ac Staff, The Scarborough Hospital - General Campus; Court Staff, Rouge Valley Health System - Centenary Health Centre Site; Court Staff, William Osler Health System - Brampton Civic Hospital; Langs: English; French; (416)438-2911; Fax. (416)445-8438.

LAMONT, Samantha J; Brightstar Clinic, 472 Woodlawn Rd E, Guelph ON N1E 1B9; McM'06; CCFP; Staff, Guelph General Hospital; (519)821-9449

LAMONTAGNE, Alain; CSSS de Saint-Jerome, 290 rue de Montigny, Saint-Jerome QC J7Z 5T3; Mon'06; CSPQ; FRCPC; Anes. Staff, Hôtel-Dieu de Saint-Jérôme; (450)432-2777

LAMONTAGNE, Annie; Les Gynecologues Ass Laval, 1299 boul de la Concorde O, Laval QC H7N 5T4; Mon'03; FRCSC; ObstGyn. Staff, Hôpital Anna-Laberge; (450)668-3250

LAMONTAGNE, Christine; Children's Hosp Eastern Ont, 401 Smyth Rd, Ottawa ON K1H 8L1; McG'94; FRCPC; Anes. Staff, Children's Hospital of Eastern Ontario (CHEO); (613)737-2431

LAMONTAGNE, Claude; Clinique Dr Claude Lamontagne, 1955 rue Bonin, Quebec QC G1S 4J1; Laval'64; CCFP; FCFP; (418)956-2770

LAMONTAGNE, Daniel; CSSS de Quebec-Nord, 791 rue de Sherwood, Quebec QC G2N 1X7; Sher'89; Langs: English; (418)849-2572; Fax. (418)841-5110.

LAMONTAGNE, Dominique; Clinique De Med Fam Mailloux, 130-1900 av Mailloux, Quebec QC G1J 5B9; Laval'71; Staff, Centre Hospitalier Universitaire de Québec (CHUQ) - Siege Social; Staff, Centre d'hebergement Saint-Augustin; Staff, Centre Hospitalier Affilié Universitaire de Québec - Hôpital De L'Enfant Jésus; (418)667-7014; Fax. (418)667-5808.

LAMONTAGNE, Francois; CHUS-Hop Fleurimont, 3001 12e av N, Sherbrooke QC J1H 5N4; Mon'00; FRCPC; IntMed; Critical Care Medicine (P.Q.). Staff, Centre Hospitalier Universitaire de Sherbrooke-Hopital Fleurimont; (819)346-1110 x74977

LAMONTAGNE, G Albert; CHUS-Hop Fleurimont, 3001 12e Av N, Sherbrooke QC J1H 5N4; Laval'60; Electroenceph (P.Q.); Neur (Electromyography). Staff, Centre Hospitalier Universitaire de Sherbrooke-Hopital Fleurimont; Neurology, Centre Hospitalier Universitaire de Sherbrooke-Hôpital Hôtel-Dieu; assoc Prof, Universite de Sherbrooke; Langs: English; (819)812-3331; Fax. (819)812-3337; albert.lamontagne@usherbrooke.ca.

LAMONTAGNE, Hugo; CSSS du Sud de Lanaudière, 911 montee des Pionniers, Terrebonne QC J6V 2H2; Mon'03; Staff, Centre Hospitalier Pierre le Gardeur; (450)654-7525

LAMONTAGNE, Janie M F; Hotel-Dieu d'Arthabaska, 5 rue des Hospitalieres, Victoriaville QC G6P 6N2; Sher'04; FRCSC; OrthSurg. Staff, Hotel-Dieu d'Arthabaska; (819)357-2030

LAMONTAGNE, Jean; Ctr Hosp Affilie-Enfant-Jesus, 1401 18e rue, Quebec QC G1J 1Z4; Laval'93; FRCSC; OrthSurg (Trauma). Orthopedic Surgery, Centre Hospitalier Affilié Universitaire de Québec - Hôpital De L'Enfant Jésus; (418)649-0252; Fax. (418)649-5567.

LAMONTAGNE, Lysanne; CLSC Gatineau, 777 boul de la Gappe, Gatineau QC J8T 8R2; Laval'04; CCFP; (819)561-2550

LAMONTAGNE, Martin; CHUM-Hop Notre-Dame, 1560 rue Sherbrooke E, Montreal QC H2L 4M1; Laval'95; FRCPC; PhysMed&Rehab (Sports Medicine). Staff, Centre Hospitalier l'Université de Montréal (CHUM) - Hôpital Notre-Dame; Staff, Institut de Réadaptation Gingras-Lindsay de Montréal; Langs: Bilingual(French/English); (514)890-8201

LAMONTAGNE, Philippe; Clinique du Plateau Marquette, 200-731 rue Galt O, Sherbrooke QC J1H 1Z1; Sher'85; (819)564-8542

LAMONTAGNE, Renee; Ctr Hosp Rouyn-Noranda, 4 9e rue, Rouyn-Noranda QC J9X 2B2; Sher'85; FRCPC; Psy. Staff, Centre Hospitalier Rouyn-Noranda; (819)764-5131; Fax. (819)762-8887; nguyendn@cablevision.qc.ca.

LAMONTAGNE, Roland; Polyclinique Boreale, 668 rue De Parfondeval, Baie-Comeau QC G5C 3R3; Mon'85; (418)589-2222; Fax. (418)589-8302.

LAMONTAGNE, Serge; Clinique Med Soleil, 64 1re Av O, Amos QC J9T 1T8; Sher'77; LMCC; CCFP; FCFP; Admin, CH Hôtel-Dieu d'Amos; (819)732-8341; Fax. (819)732-1642; slamontagne@hotmail.com.

LAMONTAGNE, Suzanne; CLSC Du Val St-Francois, 23 rue Ambroise-Dearden, Windsor QC J1S 1G8; Sher'88; Staff, Carrefour de Sante et Services Sociaux-Pavillon St-Louis; (819)845-2751

LAMONTAGNE, Yvan; SMBD Jewish Gen Hosp, 3755 ch Cote-Sainte-Catherine, Montreal QC H3T 1E2; Laval'79; GenSurg. Staff, Sir Mortimer B Davis Jewish General; (514)340-8222 x5598; Fax. (514)340-7561.

LAMONTAGNE, Yves; College des Med Du Quebec, 904-333 Sherbrooke est, Montreal QC H2X 4E3; Mon'68; FRCPC; Psy (Administration). Pres, Gestion Y L Inc; Prés, College des Medecins du Quebec; Langs: English; French; (514)543-8370; Fax. (514)543-8370; lamontagne.yves@videotron.ca.

LAMOTHE, Bruno; Clin Medicale du Manoir, 1441 av du Manoir, Alma QC G8B 4X3; Laval'02; Langs: Bilingual(French/English); (418)662-3944; Fax. (418)662-2607.

LAMOTHE, Francis; Mango Tree Fam Health Team, 550 King St E, Kitchener ON N2G 2L8; (Haiti)'76; (519)224-0540

LAMOTHE, Francois; CSSS du Lac-des-Deux-Montagnes, 520 boul Arthur-Sauve, Saint-Eustache QC J7R 5B1; Mon'71; FRCPC; MedMicrobiol; InfectDis (P.Q.). Staff, Hôpital de Saint-Eustache; (450)473-6811; Fax. (450)473-6966; francois.lamothe.chum@ssss.gouv.qc.ca.

LAMOTHE, J P Andre; The Ottawa Hosp-Gen Campus, 501 Smyth Rd, Ottawa ON K1H 8L6; Sher'77; FRCSC; Otol (Head & Neck Surgery). Head Dept of ENT, The Ottawa Hospital - General Campus; Ass't. Prof. & Prog. Dir., University of Ottawa; (613)737-8372

LAMOTHE, Marc; 101-39 rue Laurier E, Victoriaville QC G6P 6P6; Sher'80; IntMed. Langs: Spanish; English; (819)357-3930; Fax. (819)357-4310.

LAMOTHE, Marcel; Place Bonaventure, 6505-800 rue de la Gauchetiere, Montreal QC H5A 1L8; Mon'58; Ac Member, Hopital Ste-Anne; Langs: Bilingual(French/English); (514)496-6127; Fax. (514)496-2893.

LAMOTHE, Sylvie; 200-2235 rue Galt O, Sherbrooke QC J1K 1K6; Sher'89; CCFP; CCFP(E.M.); Staff, Centre Hospitalier Universitaire de Sherbrooke-Hopital Fleurimont; Prof, Universite de Sherbrooke; (819)821-0088

LAMOTHE-GUAY, Monique C; CHUM-Hop Notre-Dame, 1560 rue Sherbrooke E, Montreal QC H2L 4M1; Mon'68; Staff Surg, Centre Hospitalier l'Université de Montréal (CHUM) - Hôpital Notre-Dame; (514)890-8282; Fax. (514)412-7680.

LAMOUR, Dominique; Restigouche Hosp Centre, PO Box 10 63 Galland Dr, Campbellton NB E3N 3G2; Tours (France)'82; Psychiatrist, Centre Hospitalier Restigouche; (506)789-7000; Fax. (506)789-6726.

LAMOUREUX, Alain; 300 rue Paradis, Sorel-Tracy QC J3P 3G6; Sher'77; FRCSC; Ophth. (450)746-4464

LAMOUREUX, Alain G; Burlington Prof Centre, 101-3155 Harvester Rd, Burlington ON L7N 3V2; Alb'80; Ac Staff, Joseph Brant Memorial Hospital; Assoc Staff, Hamilton Health Sciences Centre - McMaster Children's Hospital; Court Staff, St Joseph's Healthcare - Charlton Campus; (905)639-1142

LAMOUREUX, Christian; Clinique Med Notre-Dame Inc, 147 rue Notre-Dame E, Victoriaville QC G6P 3Z8; Sher'87; Staff, Hotel-Dieu d'Arthabaska; Langs: English; (819)758-3165; Fax. (819)758-0745.

LAMOUREUX, Claude; Clinique Med St-Redempteur, 266 rue Thibault, Matane QC G4W 2V9; Sher'89; Staff, Centre Hospitalier de Matane; (418)562-6133; Fax. (418)562-6947.

LAMOUREUX, Daniel; CSSS de Laval, 1755 boul Rene-Laennec, Laval QC H7M 3L9; Mon'83; Psy (P.Q.). Staff, Hopital de la Cite de la santé; (450)668-1010; Fax. (450)975-5545.

LAMOUREUX, Diane; CSSS Pierre Boucher, 1333 boul Jacques-Cartier E, Longueuil QC J4M 2A5; Sher'85; CSPQ; FRCPC; AnatPath. Staff, Centre Hospitalier Pierre Boucher; Langs: English; Spanish; (450)468-8111 x82938; diane.lamoureux@rrsss16.gouv.qc.ca.

LAMOUREUX, Francois; Hop Santa Cabrini Ospedale, 5655 rue Saint-Zotique E, Montreal QC H1T 1P7; Sher'72; MSc; ABNM; LMCC; NuclearMed. Chef méd nucl, Hôpital Santa Cabrini Ospedale; Clin Assoc Prof Radiol, Universite de Montreal; (514)252-6112; Fax. (514)252-6588; lamoureux@sympatico.ca.

LAMOUREUX, Gilles; 204-100 rue King E, Sherbrooke QC J1G 1A4; Laval'63; FRCSC; OrthSurg. Orthopedic Surgery, Centre Hospitalier Universitaire de Sherbrooke-Hôpital Hôtel-Dieu; Prof, Universite de Sherbrooke; (819)566-5959; Fax. (819)566-1262.

LAMOUREUX, Guy A; Bonnyville Med Clinic, PO Box 1007 Stn Main 4610 50 St, Bonnyville AB T9N 2J7; Cal'79; CCFP; FCFP; Clin Instructor Rural Family Pract Prog, University of Alberta; (780)826-3346; Fax. (780)826-6362.

LAMOUREUX, Guy; CHUS-Hop Fleurimont, 3001 12e Av N, Sherbrooke QC J1H 5N4; Sher'76; FRCPC; NuclearMed. Assoc Prof Nuclear Med, Centre Hospitalier Universitaire de Sherbrooke-Hopital Fleurimont; Consultant, Centre Hospitalier Universitaire de Sherbrooke-Hôpital Hôtel-Dieu; assoc Prof, Universite de Sherbrooke; (819)346-1110 x14624; Fax. (819)820-6462.

LAMOUREUX, Michel; Clin De Med Family D'Embrun, PO Box 1259 869 rue Notre Dame, Embrun ON K0A 1W0; Ott'74; Ac Staff, Montfort Hospital; Langs: Spanish; (613)443-3311; Fax. (613)443-0142.

LAMOUREUX, Louis; Ctr Hosp de Verdun, 4000 boul Lasalle, Verdun QC H4G 2A3; Mon'93; Gastroent (P.Q.). Staff, Centre Hospitalier de Verdun; (514)362-1000

LAMOUREUX, Louise; Clinique Med Le Champetre, RR 2 3220 ch de la Visitation, St-Ambroise-d-Kild QC J0K 1C0; Sher'87; FRCPC; Neur (Adult Neurology); Electroenceph (P.Q.). (450)760-9696

LAMOUREUX, Manon; Pavillon Rosemont, 5689 boul Rosemont, Montreal QC H1T 2H1; Mon'88; CCFP; Staff, Hopital Maisonneuve-Rosemont; (514)252-3400

LAMOUREUX, Marie-Catherine; Dr Georges-L Dumont Reg Hosp, 330 av Universite, Moncton NB E1C 2Z3; Mon'04; FRCSC; ObstGyn. Staff, Dr Georges-L-Dumont University Hospital Centre; (506)862-4000

LAMOUREUX, Michelle; Clin Sante Beaute de la Montag, 400-1538 rue Sherbrooke O, Montreal QC H3G 1L5; Mon'79; (514)286-5555; Fax. (514)286-0707.

LAMOUREUX, Patrice; CSSS de Laval, 1755 boul Rene-Laennec, Laval QC H7M 3L9; Mon'88; FRCSC; GenSurg (Hepatobiliary Surgery). Staff, Hopital de la Cite de la santé; Asst Prof Surg, Universite de Montreal; (450)668-1010

LAMOUREUX, Pierre; Institut de Cardiologie de Mtl, 5000 rue Belanger, Montreal QC H1T 1C8; Laval'72; FRCPC; Psy. Staff, Institut de Cardiologie de Montréal; (514)593-2571

LAMOUREUX, Pierre; Centre Med St Basile, 101-275 boul Sir-Wilfrid-Lauri, St-Basile-Le-Grand QC J3N 1V6; Mon'72; Staff, Hôpital Laval; (450)653-7323; Fax. (450)653-3021.

LAMOUREUX, Robin A J; 1 Field Ambulance Edmonton, PO Box 10500 Stn Forces, Edmonton AB T5J 4J5; Alb'02; CCFP; (780)973-4011

LAMOUREUX-ROBERT, Marie-Josee; Direction de la Sante Publique, 1255 rue Beauregard, Longueuil QC J4K 2M3; Sher'07; CCFP; Staff, Hôtel-Dieu de Sorel; (450)928-6777 x3136

LAMPA, Martin J; UBC-Dept of Anes, 2449-910 10th Ave W, Vancouver BC V5Z 1M9; UBC'93; FRCPC; Anes. Staff, Vancouver General Hospital - Centennial Pavillion; (604)875-4304; Fax. (604)875-5209.

LAMPARD, J Robert; 12-26540 Hwy 11, Red Deer County AB T4E 1A3; Alb'64; BSc; MSc(Surg); MBA; (403)340-5736; Fax. (403)340-7521; robert.lampard@gov.ab.ca.

LAMPARD, Robert B; Univ Hlth Network-Toronto Gen, 200 Elizabeth St, Toronto ON M5G 2C4; Cal'94; FRCPC; EmergMed. Staff, Toronto General Hospital - UHN; (416)340-4800

LAMPE, K Mary; PO Box 1192, Grand Bend ON N0M 1T0; Wes'78; FRCPC; Anes (Neuro Anesthesia). Staff, London Health Sciences Centre - University Hospital; Consultant, St Joseph's Hospital - St Joseph's Health Care; Assoc Prof, University of Western Ontario; (519)238-8924; mary.lampe@lhsc.on.ca.

LAMPEN, Ockert; 11664 223 St, Maple Ridge BC V2X 5X5; Stellenbosch (South Africa)'95; MB ChB; FRCOG; FRCSC; ObstGyn. Specialist ObstGyn, Ridge Meadows Hospital & Health Care Centre; (604)463-5450; Fax. (604)467-0455.

LAMPRECHT, Albertus J; Peace Arch Hosp, 15521 Russell Ave, White Rock BC V4B 2R4; Stellenbosch (South Africa)'89; MB ChB; CCFP; CCFP(E.M.); Staff, Peace Arch Hospital; (604)541-7133

LAMPRECHT, Gideon P; Omineca Clinic, RR 2 3348 Hospital Rd, Vanderhoof BC V0J 3A2; Orange Free State (South Africa)'75; MB ChB; Chief Staff, St John Hospital; Langs: Afrikaans; (250)567-2201; Fax. (250)567-2105.

LAMPRON, Carmen; Centre Hosp Honore-Mercier, 2750 boul Laframboise, Saint-Hyacinthe QC J2S 4Y8; Mon'92; FRCSC; PlasSurg. Staff, Centre Hospitalier Honore-Mercier; (450)778-2572

LAMPRON, Jacinthe; The Ottawa Hosp-Civic Campus, 1053 Carling Ave, Ottawa ON K1Y 4E9; Laval'01; FRCSC; GenSurg (Critical Care Medicine). Staff, The Ottawa Hospital - Civic Campus; (613)722-7000

LAMPRON, Noel; Hôpital Laval, 2725 ch Sainte-Foy, Quebec QC G1V 4G5; Laval'75; Respir; IntMed. Dir ICU, Hôpital Laval; (418)656-4747; Fax. (418)656-4762.

LAMPRON, Sebastien; CSSS de Trois-Rivieres, 155 rue Toupin, Trois-Rivieres QC G8T 3Z8; Mon'08; Staff, Centre de santé Cloutier-du-Rivage; (819)370-2100

LAMPRON-GOULET, Eric; ASSS de l'Abitibi-Temiscamingu, 1 9e rue, Rouyn-Noranda QC J9X 2A9; Sher'07; CommunMed (P.Q.); Public Health & Preventive Med. (819)764-3264

LAMPTEY, Na-Koshie; Sudbury & District Health Uni, 1300 Paris St, Sudbury ON P3E 3A3; Tor'05; MPH; FRCPC; CommunMed;CCFP; Assoc Med Officer of Hlth, Sudbury & District Health Unit Corporate Office; Prog Dir Public Health & Preventive Med, Northern Ontario School of Medicine; (705)522-9200 x291; Fax. (705)677-9606.

LAMSCHTEIN, Claudia; Saint John Reg Hosp, PO Box 2100, Saint John NB E2L 4L2; University of the Republic (Uruguay)'88; Staff, Saint John Regional Hospital; (506)648-6000

LAMSWOOD, F Scott S; Bay St George Med Centre, 129 Montana Dr, Stephenville NL A2N 2T4; Mem'94; Staff, Sir Thomas Roddick Hospital; (709)643-6635; Fax. (709)643-6575.

LAMY, Andre; Hamilton HS-General Site, C1 112-237 Barton St E, Hamilton ON L8L 2X2; Laval'85; MHSc(ClinEpidem); FRCSC; GenSurg (Clinical Epidemiology); Cardiovasc&ThorSurg (P.Q.); CardiothorSurg. Staff, Hamilton Health Sciences Centre - Hamilton General Hospital; Assoc Prof, McMaster University; Langs: French; (905)522-0175; Fax. (905)522-2029.

LAMY, Marie-Eve; Unite de Medecine Familiale, 80 118e rue, Shawinigan-Sud QC G9P 3E4; Sher'08; CCFP; Langs: Bilingual(French/English); (819)536-7511; Fax. (819)537-3489.

LAMY, Mario; Clinique Med Valmont, 101-783 rue Notre-Dame, Repentigny QC J5Y 1B4; Mon'82; Ac Staff, Centre Hospitalier Pierre le Gardeur; (450)582-1260; Fax. (450)582-0677.

LAMY, Martin; CSSS de Trois-Rivières, 1991 boul du Carmel, Trois-Rivieres QC G8Z 3R9; Sher'93; FRCSC; GenSurg. Staff, CSSS de Trois-Rivières; (819)697-3333; Fax. (819)375-3010.

LAMY-MONNOT, Lianne; Medi Centre Chomedey, 610 boul Cure-Labelle, Laval QC H7V 2T7; Sher'83; LMCC; CCFP; Langs: Bilingual(French/English); (450)687-6452; Fax. (450)687-3243.

LAMYKINA, Olga; Courtenay Med Clinic, 788 Grant Ave, Courtenay BC V9N 2T3; Novosibirsk (Russia (Federation))'95; CCFP; (250)334-2445

LAN, Frederick P; Mackenzie Richmond Hill Hosp, 10 Trench St, Richmond Hill ON L4C 4Z3; Tor'98; FRCPC; DiagRad. Staff, Mackenzie Richmond Hill Hospital; (905)883-1212

LAN, John S F; Alexander Prof Bldg, 209-849 Alexander Crt, Peterborough ON K9J 7H8; Dublin (Ireland)'72; LRCPSI; FRCPC; Neur (Electromyography). (705)743-9626; Fax. (705)743-8664.

LAN, Robert H M; Medical Bldg, 144-600 Tecumseh Rd E, Windsor ON N8X 4X9; National (Ireland)'64; MB ChB; BAO; DLO(Lond); FRCS(E); FRCSC; Otol. Ac Staff, Hôtel-Dieu Grace Hospital; Ac Staff, Windsor Regional Hospital - Metropolitan Site; (519)258-6665

LAN, Steven C; Campbell River & Dist Gen Hosp, 375 2nd Ave, Campbell River BC V9W 3V1; Tor'01; CCFP; CCFP(E.M.); Staff, Campbell River & District General Hospital; (250)850-2671

LAN-HING-MING, Rose-Marie; Amherstburg Med Associates, 71 Sandwich St S, Amherstburg ON N9V 1Z5; Qns'88; (519)736-5444; Fax. (519)736-7687.

LANCIAULT, Diane; CSSS D'Argenteuil, 145 av de la Providence, Lachute QC J8H 4C7; Mon'87; Staff, Centre Hospitalier d'Argenteuil; Langs: English; (450)562-3761; Fax. (450)562-2111.

LANCTOT, Claude; Clinique Med Belanger, 405-3871 rue Belanger, Montreal QC H1X 3M7; Mon'69; Derm. Staff Derm, Hopital Maisonneuve-Rosemont; Clin Prof, Universite de Montreal; Langs: Bilingual(French/English); (514)722-2042; Fax. (514)722-5693; claude@pharmaciegabriel.com.

LANCTOT, Francine; Clinique Med L'Avenir, 200-1150 boul de l'Avenir, Laval QC H7N 6L2; Mon'83; Staff, Hopital Maisonneuve-Rosemont; (450)680-1150

LANCTOT, Guy; Clinique Med Havre Sante, 521 boul Du Havre, Salaber-de-Valleyf QC J6S 4Z5; Mon'83; Peds. Staff, Centre Hospitalier Régional du Suroît; Langs: Bilingual(French/English); (450)371-6444

LANCTOT, Guy R; Ctr Hosp Affilie-Enfant-Jesus, 1401 18e rue, Quebec QC G1J 1Z4; Laval'84; FRCPC; Psy. Staff, Centre Hospitalier Affilié Universitaire de Québec - Hôpital De L'Enfant Jésus; (418)649-5769; Fax. (418)649-5934.

LANCTOT, Jean-Francois; Hop Charles LeMoyne, 3120 boul Taschereau, Greenfield Park QC J4V 2H1; Mon'01; CCFP; CCFP(E.M.); Staff, Hopital Charles LeMoyne; (450)466-5000; Fax. (450)466-8887.

LANCTOT, Jean-Francois; Les Gynecologues Ass Laval, 1299 boul de la COncorde O, Laval QC H7N 5T4; Mon'89; ObstGyn. Staff, Hopital de la Cite de la santé; (450)668-3250

LANCTOT, Jean-Luc; Hop Brome-Missisquoi-Perkins, 950 rue Principale, Cowansville QC J2K 1K3; Mon'01; CCFP; Staff, Hôpital Brome-Missisquoi-Perkins; (450)266-5500

LANCTOT, Robert; Clinique D'Urgence St-Denis, 101-8415 rue Saint-Denis, Montreal QC H2P 2H1; Mon'73; (514)388-5723; Fax. (514)388-3423.

LANCTOT, Rosaire; Medicentre St-Remi, CP 426 901 rue Notre-Dame, Saint-Remi QC J0L 2L0; Mon'79; Physician-in-Charge, Centre d'Accueil La Prairie; Langs: Bilingual(French/English); (450)454-3913; Fax. (450)454-3958.

LANDA, Jean-Claude; 123-151 Main St E, Hawkesbury ON K6A 1A1; Pécs (Hungary)'91; LMCC; CCFP; Staff, Hawkesbury & District General Hospital; Langs: English; Hungarian; (613)632-0151; Fax. (613)632-1073.

LANDAU, Petr; Fredericton Med Clinic, 201-1015 Regent St, Fredericton NB E3B 6H5; Dal'77; ObstGyn. Staff, Dr Everett Chalmers Regional Hospital; Teach Staff Med, Dalhousie University; (506)457-2113; Fax. (506)459-7073.

LANDECKER, Elizabeth A M; Moog & Friends Hospice House, 1701 Government St, Penticton BC V2A 8J7; Sydney (Australia)'66; (250)492-9071

LANDECKER, Leslie S; Dixon Med Centre, 308-531 Davis Dr, Newmarket ON L3Y 6P5; Cape Town (South Africa)'71; MB ChB; DAB; FRCSC; Ophth (Cataract Surgery). Ac Staff, Southlake Regional Health Centre; Court Staff, Mackenzie Richmond Hill Hospital; Court Staff, Markham Stouffville Hospital; (905)898-7414; Fax. (905)898-7792.

LANDELLS, Colin D; Rebalance MD, 104-3551 Blanshard St, Victoria BC V8Z 0B9; Mem'79; BMedSci; FRCSC; OrthSurg (Sports Medicine). Ac Staff, Royal Jubilee Hospital; (250)940-4444

LANDELLS, Ian D R; 103-120 Stavanger Dr, St. John's NL A1A 5E8; Mem'88; BMedSci; FRCPC; Derm (Cosmetic Dermatology). Clinical Asst Prof Med, Memorial University Of Newfoundland; (709)726-7546; Fax. (709)726-7575; landells@landellsclinic.com.

LANDER, Debra A; Psychealth Centre, PZ202-771 Bannatyne Ave, Winnipeg MB R3E 3N4; Man'87; BSc; FRCPC; Psy (Consultant Liaison Psychiatry). Staff, Health Sciences Centre; Asst Prof, University of Manitoba; (204)787-7253; Fax. (204)787-7480.

LANDER, S Mark; Psychealth Centre, PZ202-771 Bannatyne Ave, Winnipeg MB R3E 3N4; Man'79; BSc; FRCPC; Psy (Mood Disorders). Staff Psy, Health Sciences Centre; Assoc Prof, University of Manitoba; (204)787-7253; Fax. (204)787-7480.

LANDERO, Jennifer L; Foothills Med Centre, 1403 29 St NW, Calgary AB T2N 2T9; UBC'08; Staff, Foothills Medical Centre; (403)944-1110

LANDES, Megan; Univ Hlth Network-Toronto Gen, 200 Elizabeth St, Toronto ON M5G 2C4; McG'04; CCFP; CCFP(E.M.); Staff, Toronto General Hospital - UHN; (416)340-3856

LANDINE, James K; Kingston Gen Hosp, 76 Stuart St, Kingston ON K7L 2V7; Dal'96; FRCPC; EmergMed. Staff EmergMed, Kingston General Hospital; (613)548-2368 x3530

LANDIS, Mark S; London HSC-Victoria Hosp, PO Box 5010 Stn B 800 Commissioners Rd E, London ON N6A 5W9; Tor'06; FRCPC; DiagRad. Staff, London Health Sciences Centre - Victoria Campus; (519)685-8500

LANDIS, Stephan J; Guelph Gen Hosp, 115 Delhi St, Guelph ON N1E 4J4; Ott'74; ABIM; FRCPC; IntMed (Infectious Diseases). Physician Wound Care, Women's College Hospital; Staff, Guelph General Hospital; Langs: French; Polish; (519)837-6440

LANDOLT, Sandra J; Thornhill Dermatology Centre, 302-1137 Centre St, Thornhill ON L4J 3M6; Tor'86; FRCPC; IntMed (Internal Medicine-Pertains to Skin); Derm. Assoc Consultant, Trillium Health Centre - Mississauga; Instructor, University of Toronto; (905)695-2020; Fax. (905)695-3800.

LANDOLT-MARTICORENA, C Maria; Univ Hlth Network-Toronto Western Hosp, 399 Bathurst St, Toronto ON M5T 2S8; Tor'99; FRCPC; IntMed; Rheum. Staff, Toronto Western Hospital - University Health Network; (416)603-5800 x5894; Fax. (416)603-4348.

LANDONI, Thomas A; Arthur Family Health Centre, 110 Charles St E, Arthur ON N0G 1A0; Tor'77; Ac Staff, Groves Memorial Community Hospital; (519)848-3798; Fax. (519)848-6373.

LANDREVILLE, Marie-Helene; CSSSG-Hop De Gatineau, CP 2000 Succ Bureau-Chef, Gatineau QC J8P 7H2; Sher'90; Peds. Staff, Hôpital de Gatineau; (819)561-8100; Fax. (819)561-8103.

LANDRIAULT, Eric; Orleans Medical-Dental Centre, 402-2555 St. Joseph Blvd, Orleans ON K1C 1S6; Ott'99; CCFP; (613)830-1693; Fax. (613)841-6550.

LANDRY, Aline; CSSS des Iles, 430 ch Principal, Cap-aux-Meules QC G4T 1R9; Laval'97; CCFP; Staff, Hôpital de l'Archipel; (418)986-2121

LANDRY, Audrey; Clinique Med de la Marine, 101-303 boul de la Marine, Varennes QC J3X 2G6; Mon'88; Staff Family Med, Centre Hospitalier Pierre Boucher; (450)652-9616; Fax. (450)652-4345.

LANDRY, Caroline; CSSS Des Etchemins, 331 rue du Sanatorium, Lac-Etchemin QC G0R 1S0; Laval'04; Staff, CSSS des Etchemins; (418)625-8001

LANDRY, Chantal; Clinique Med Amos, 641 4e rue O, Amos QC J9T 2S1; Laval'92; (819)732-0717; Fax. (819)732-4646.

LANDRY, Charles; Mediclub du Sanctuaire, 6100 av du Boise, Montreal QC H3S 2W1; Mon'99; Staff, Centre Hospitalier l'Université De Montréal (CHUM) - Hôpital Saint-luc; (514)739-5646

LANDRY, Claude; Clinique Maisonneuve-Rosemont, 60-5345 boul de l'Assomption, Montreal QC H1T 4B3; Sher'89; CCFP; Staff, CSSS de Maskinongé; (514)257-7000

LANDRY, Cynthia; Ctr Hosp Anna-Laberge, 200 boul Brisebois, Chateauguay QC J6K 4W8; Sher'10; Staff, Hôpital Anna-Laberge; (450)699-2425

LANDRY, Daniel A; Moncton Med Centre, 205-1789 Mountain Rd, Moncton NB E1G 5C4; Dal'85; CCFP; FCFP; Member Bd of Directors, New Brunswick Lung Association; Langs: English; French; (506)387-4403; Fax. (506)387-4457.

LANDRY, Daniel; Clinique Medicale 910, 910 boul Saint-Joseph E, Montreal QC H2J 1K6; Mon'82; FRCSC; ObstGyn (Endoscopy). Clin Prof, Centre Hospitalier l'Université de Montréal (CHUM) - Hôpital Notre-Dame; Staff, Centre Hospitalier l'Université De Montréal (CHUM) - Hôpital Saint-luc; Langs: English; (514)590-0910; Fax. (514)590-0448.

LANDRY, Daniel; 210-3333 rue du Carrefour, Quebec QC G1C 5R9; Mon'92; (418)663-6345

LANDRY, Daniel; CFB Gagetown, PO Box 17000 Stn Forces, Oromocto NB E2V 4J5; Ott'10; CCFP.

LANDRY, Danielle; Inst Nat Sante Pub Qebec, 945 av Wolfe, Quebec QC G1V 5B3; McG'90; (418)650-5115 x5511

LANDRY, David; CSSS de la Baie-des-Chaleurs, RR 2 419 boul Perron, Maria QC G0C 1Y0; Mon'08; Staff, CSSS de la Baie-des-Chaleurs; (418)759-3443

LANDRY, David J; Hamilton HS-General Site, 237 Barton St E, Hamilton ON L8L 2X2; McM'02; FRCPC; DiagRad. Staff Radiol, Hamilton Health Sciences Centre - Hamilton General Hospital; (905)527-4322 x46521

LANDRY, Diane; CLSC Amos, 632 1ere rue O, Amos QC J9T 2N2; Laval'88; Staff Psy, CH Hôtel-Dieu d'Amos; (819)732-3271

LANDRY, Elaine; 205-387 Main St, Shediac NB E4P 2B5; Mon'82; Staff, Dr Georges-L-Dumont University Hospital Centre; (506)532-1479; Fax. (506)532-1569.

LANDRY, Esther; Clinique Med Centre-Ville, 5-167 rue de la Reine, Gaspe QC G4X 2W6; Mon'86; Staff, Centre Hospitalier de Gaspe; (418)368-1811; Fax. (418)368-2616.

LANDRY, France; SAAQ, S2 1-333 boul Jean-Lesage, Quebec QC G1K 8Z2; Laval'81; (418)528-3888; france.landry@saaq.gouv.qc.ca.

LANDRY, Gabrielle; Clinique A rue McGill Inc, 900-407 rue McGill, Montreal QC H2Y 2G3; Mon'10; (514)787-0055

LANDRY, Gerard; 630 Boul Du Seminaire N, St-Jean-Sur-Richel QC J3B 7X6; Mon'81; ObstGyn (P.Q.). (450)348-1171; Fax. (450)348-1172.

LANDRY, Helene; CSSS de la Baie-des-Chaleurs, RR 2 419 boul Perron, Maria QC G0C 1Y0; Mon'03; Staff, CSSS de la Baie-des-Chaleurs; (418)759-3443

LANDRY, Hubert; Ctr Hosp Anna-Laberge, 200 boul Brisebois, Chateauguay QC J6K 4W8; Laval'06; CSPQ; FRCSC; Ophth. Staff, Hôpital Anna-Laberge; (450)699-2425

LANDRY, Isabelle; CLSC Rimouski-Neigette-UMF, 165 rue des Gouverneurs, Rimouski QC G5L 7R2; Laval'06; CCFP; (418)727-5493

LANDRY, Ivan; Polyclinique Concorde, 222-300 boul de la Concorde E, Laval QC H7G 2E6; Mon'68; FRCSC; Otol. Otolaryngology, Centre Hospitalier Pierre le Gardeur; Langs: Bilingual(French/English); (450)667-5310 x2424; Fax. (450)669-5409.

LANDRY, J Sylvain; Ctr Hosp Trois-Riv-St-Joseph, 731 rue Sainte-Julie, Trois-Rivieres QC G9A 1Y1; Laval'86; Staff, Centre Hospitalier Regional de Trois-Rivieres; (819)697-3333 x59849

LANDRY, Jacques; 101-185 av Acadie, Dieppe NB E1A 1G6; Sher'92; CCFP; Ac Member, Dr Georges-L-Dumont University Hospital Centre; (506)855-8805; Fax. (506)388-9109.

LANDRY, Jean-Francois; CSSS de Rivière-de-Loup, 75 rue Saint-Henri, Riviere-Du-Loup QC G5R 2A4; Laval'94; FRCPC; IntMed. Staff, Centre Hospitalier Regional du Grand-Portage; (418)868-1000; Fax. (418)868-1059.

LANDRY, Jennifer M; Westbrook Prof Bldg, 215-1610 37 St SW, Calgary AB T3C 3P1; UBC'97; FRCPC; IntMed., University of Calgary; (403)685-9499; Fax. (403)685-9422.

LANDRY, Jennifer S; MUHC-Montreal Chest Institute, K1 18-3650 rue Saint-Urbain, Montreal QC H2X 2P4; McG'97; ABIM; FRCP; FRCPC; IntMed; Critical Care Medicine (P.Q.); Respir (Cystic Fibrosis). Staff, McGill University Health Centre - Montreal Chest Institute; Langs: French; (514)934-1934 x32152; jennifer.landry@mcgill.ca.

LANDRY, Johanne; Ctr Hosp Affilie-St-Sacrement, 1050 ch Sainte-Foy, Quebec QC G1S 4L8; Sher'96; Staff, Centre Hospitalier Affilié Universitaire de Québec - Hôpital du St-Sacrement; (418)682-7511

LANDRY, Josee; UMF Laurier, 2875 boul Laurier, Quebec QC G1V 2M2; Mon'96; (418)654-2701

LANDRY, Kerri L; Alberta Children's Hosp, 2888 Shaganappi Trail NW, Calgary AB T3B 6A8; McG'02; FRCPC; Peds; PedEmergMed. Staff, Alberta Children's Hospital; (403)955-7211

LANDRY, Linda; 102-2387 rue Commerciale S GD, Notre-Dame-du-Lac QC G0L 1X0; Laval'78; ac Staff, Centre Hospitalier Notre-Dame-du-Lac; (418)899-6703; Fax. (418)899-6337.

LANDRY, Lynda; Siege Social & CLSC, 757 rue de la Madone, Mont-Laurier QC J9L 1T3; Mon'96; Médecin, CSSS d'Antoine-Labelle; Clin Prof, Universite de Montreal; Langs: Bilingual(French/English); (819)623-1228

LANDRY, Lyse; CSSS Les Eskers de l'Abitibi, 622 4e rue O, Amos QC J9T 2S2; Laval'77; Dir Prof Services, CH Hôtel-Dieu d'Amos; (819)732-3341; Fax. (819)732-7054; lyse_landry@ssss.gouv.qc.ca.

LANDRY, Marc-Antoine; Foothills Med Centre, 780-1403 29 St NW, Calgary AB T2N 2T9; Sher'02; Peds (Neonatal & Perinatal Medicine). Staff, Rockyview General Hospital; (403)944-4638

LANDRY, Marlene; CSSS de Chicoutimi, 305 rue Saint-Vallier, Chicoutimi QC G7H 5H6; Mon'96; Staff, Complexe hospitalier de la Sagamie; (418)541-1010

LANDRY, Martine; I R D P Q-Site Francois-Charon, 525 boul Wilfrid-Hamel, Quebec QC G1M 2S8; Laval'85; Evaluateur Med, Societe Assurance Automobile du Quebec; Physician, Centre Francois-Charon; (418)529-9141; Fax. (418)649-3703.

LANDRY, Martine; Clin Pediatrique Rive-Sud, 405-5811 boul Taschereau, Brossard QC J4Z 1A5; Mon'82; Peds (P.Q.). assoc Staff, Hopital Charles LeMoyne; Langs: English; (450)443-6585; Fax. (450)443-9002.

LANDRY, Michel E; 469 rang Saint-Georges CP 286, L'Ange-Gardien QC J0E 1E0; Sher'73; (450)293-7324

LANDRY, Michel; 105-185 av Acadie, Dieppe NB E1A 1G6; Sher'85; CCFP; FCFP; Physician, Unite de Medicine Familiale; (506)862-4182; Fax. (506)862-4179; pierrette.morton@vitalitenb.ca.

LANDRY, Michel; CSSS de Saint-Jerome, 290 rue de Montigny, Saint-Jerome QC J7Z 5T3; Mon'82; CSPQ; FRCPC; Anes. Staff, Hôtel-Dieu de Saint-Jérôme; (450)431-8200

LANDRY, Michel P; Unite Med Familiale Maizerets, 2480 ch de la Canardiere, Quebec QC G1J 2G1; Sher'85; (418)661-1413

LANDRY, Monique; MSSS, 2F-201 boul Cremazie E, Montreal QC H2M 1L2; Mon'80; Langs: Bilingual(English/French); (514)873-1296; Fax. (514)864-2778; monique.landry@msss.gouv.qc.ca.

LANDRY, Nicole; Hop Maisonneuve-Rosemont, 5415 boul de l'Assomption, Montreal QC H1T 2M4; Mon'77; CSPQ; FRCPC; Anes. Staff, Hopital Maisonneuve-Rosemont; (514)252-3808

LANDRY, Patrice; Dr Georges-L Dumont Reg Hosp, 330 av Universite, Moncton NB E1C 2Z3; Sher'06; CCFP; Staff, Dr Georges-L-Dumont University Hospital Centre; (506)862-4000

LANDRY, Patricia; Clin Familiale De Coaticook, 206-18 rue du Manege, Coaticook QC J1A 3B3; Sher'93; CCFP; Staff, Centre Hospitalier de Coaticook; (819)849-4808; Fax. (819)849-7400.

LANDRY, Philip; Centre Med de la Vallee, 1-22 rue du Pont, Amqui QC G5J 3T5; Mon'94; (418)629-6611

LANDRY, Pierre; Hop Louis-H Lafontaine, 7401 rue Hochelaga, Montreal QC H1N 3M5; Mon'88; PhD; FRCPC; Psy (Pharmacotherapy). Staff, Hopital Louis-H Lafontaine; Asst Prof Research, Universite de Montreal; (514)251-4000 x3070; Fax. (514)251-7527; plandry@ssss.gouv.qc.ca.

LANDRY, Pierre; CSSS du Nord de Lanaudière, 1000 boul Sainte-Anne, St-Charles-Brromee QC J6E 6J2; Sher'93; Nephrol; IntMed. Staff, Centre Hospitalier Régional de Lanaudière; (450)759-8222

LANDRY, Rachelle; 204-565 Elmwood Dr, Moncton NB E1A 2X4; Laval'00; CCFP; Staff, Dr Georges-L-Dumont University Hospital Centre; (506)388-8851; Fax. (506)388-8805.

LANDRY, Rene; CSSS des Sources, 475 3e Av, Asbestos QC J1T 1X6; Sher'98; CCFP; Staff, CSSS des Sources d'Asbestos; (819)879-7151; Fax. (819)879-7433.

LANDRY, Sarah; CSSS de Rimouski-Neigette, CP 3150 Succ A 150 av Rouleau, Rimouski QC G5L 5T1; Laval'93; FRCPC; Psy (Schizophrenia). Staff, Hôpital Regional Rimouski; Université Laval; Langs: Bilingual(French/English); (418)724-8315; Fax. (418)724-8652.

LANDRY, Serge M; The Moncton Hosp, 135 MacBeath Ave, Moncton NB E1C 6Z8; Sher'93; CCFP; Staff, The Moncton Hospital; (506)857-5520

LANDRY, Serge; Clinique Medicale Landry, 317 rue Fournier, Matane QC G4W 4G1; Laval'86; (418)562-1228

LANDRY, Simon-Pierre; Ctr Hosp Laurentien, 234 rue Saint-Vincent, Ste-Agathe-des-Mts QC J8C 2B8; Sher'09; CCFP; CCFP(E.M.); Staff, Centre Hospitalier Laurentien; (819)324-4000

LANDRY, Sonia; Clinique Fam de Coaticook, 206-18 rue du Manege, Coaticook QC J1A 3B3; Mon'05; (819)849-4808

LANDRY, Steeve; Campbellton Reg Hosp, PO Box 880 Stn Main 189 Lily Lake Rd, Campbellton NB E3N 3H3; Sher'00; CCFP; Staff, Hôpital Régional Campbellton; (506)789-5000

LANDRY, Stephanie; Hotel-Dieu de Levis, 143 rue Wolfe, Levis QC G6V 3Z1; Laval'99; FRCPC; IntMed. Staff, Hôtel-Dieu de Lévis; Langs: Bilingual(French/English); (418)835-7121

LANDRY, Suzanne; Clinique Med Le Champetre, RR 2 3220 A ch de la Visitation, St-Ambroise-d-Kild QC J0K 1C0; McG'95; Staff, Centre Hospitalier Régional de Lanaudière; (450)760-3706

LANDRY, V L Joseph; Montfort Hosp, 713 Montreal Rd, Ottawa ON K1K 0T2; Ott'00; FRCPC; Anes. Staff, Montfort Hospital; (613)746-4621; drvlandry@rogers.com.

LANDRY, Yves; Clinique Med Joliette, 3841 rue Ontario E, Montreal QC H1W 1S5; Mon'68; (514)524-3731

LANDRY-FRECHETTE, Guylaine; 890 10e Rang RR 2, Saint-Wenceslas QC G0Z 1J0; Laval'78; MPH; MSc; Clin Staff Public Health, Hôpital Sainte-croix; (819)224-7577; Fax. (819)224-4277; clinique.landry.frechette@lino.com.

LANDS, Larry C; MUHC-Montreal Children's Hosp, D 380-2300 rue Tupper, Montreal QC H3H 1P3; McG'81; PhD; Respir (P.Q.); Peds (Pediatric Pulmonology). Asst Dir Div of RespMed, McGill University Health Centre - Montreal Children's Hospital; Assoc Prof Peds, McGill University; (514)412-4400; Fax. (514)412-4364; larry.lands@muhc.mcgill.ca.

LANDSBERG, David N; St Paul's Hosp, 542-1081 Burrard St, Vancouver BC V6Z 1Y6; Tor'77; FRCPC; IntMed (Transplantation); Nephrol. Ac Staff, Providence Health Care - St Paul's Hospital; Consultant, Vancouver General Hospital - Centennial Pavillion; (604)806-8970; dlandsberg@providencehealth.bc.ca.

LANDSBERG, Hester C; Community Medi Centre, 2707 50 Ave, Lloydminster SK S9V 2A8; Stellenbosch (South Africa)'04; MB ChB; DA(SA); Staff GP Anes, Lloydminster Hospital; (306)825-4427; Fax. (306)825-2028.

LANDSBERGEN, Eugene P; Greenwood Fam Physicians, PO Box 5 709 1 St NE, Sundre AB T0M 1X0; (Netherlands)'85; Langs: Dutch; German; French; (403)638-2424; Fax. (403)638-3580.

LANDSIEDEL, Trevor M; PO Box 543 Stn A, Abbotsford BC V2T 6Z8; UBC'82; Staff EmergMed, Abbotsford Regional Hospital & Cancer Centre; (604)864-3909; Fax. (604)864-3970.

LANDY, Cynthia J; Circle Med at Copperfield, 123-15566 McIvor Blvd SE, Calgary AB T2Z 4Y2; Cal'01; CCFP; (403)726-0524; Fax. (403)726-0579.

LANDY, Gerald J; Care Point Med Centre, 528A Clarke Rd, Coquitlam BC V3J 3X5; Dublin (Ireland)'70; (604)936-9874; Fax. (604)936-9741.

LANDY, Joshua S; Div of Critical Care Med, 11C 1170-585 University Ave, Toronto ON M5G 2N2; Wes'06; FRCPC; IntMed; Critical Care Medicine. (416)340-4485

LANDY, Patrick M P M; Northfield Family Health Ctre, 99 Northfield Dr E, Waterloo ON N2K 3P9; Dublin (Ireland)'79; MRCGPract; DCH; DObst; CCFP; Staff, St Mary's General Hospital; Staff, Grand River Hospital - Kitchener/Waterloo Health Centre; (519)746-3378; Fax. (519)746-3380.

LANDY, Philip J; Homewood Health Centre, 150 Delhi St, Guelph ON N1E 6K9; Tor'84; ASAM; CCFP; FCFP; Ac Staff, Homewood Health Centre; (519)824-1010 x2120; Fax. (519)767-3536.

LANE, Alan T; The Ottawa Hosp-Gen Campus, 501 Smyth Rd, Ottawa ON K1H 8L6; Dublin (Ireland)'93; FRCPC; Anes. Staff, The Ottawa Hospital - General Campus; (613)737-8187

LANE, Anthony P; Medical Arts Centre, 103-650 Terminal Ave, Nanaimo BC V9R 5E2; National (Ireland)'69; MB ChB; BAO; CCFP; FCFP; Ac Staff, Nanaimo Regional General Hospital; Asst Prof Med & Family Practice, University of British Columbia; (250)753-3431; Fax. (250)754-6897.

LANE, Carolyn A; Maternal Child Clinic, 130-1402 8 Ave NW, Calgary AB T2N 1B8; Tor'80; CCFP; FCFP; Ac Staff, Foothills Medical Centre; Clinical Asst Prof, University of Calgary; (403)509-3080; Fax. (403)509-3082.

LANE, Christopher J; 335-1900 Richmond Rd, Victoria BC V8R 4R2; Tor'04; Cardiol; IntMed. (250)951-1551

LANE, David P P; 39 Commerce Rd, Lindsay ON K9V 5Y3; Sask'95; FRCSC; Ophth. (705)320-8080; Fax. (705)320-8082.

LANE, Debra; Canadian Blood Services, 777 William Ave, Winnipeg MB R3E 3R4; Cal'80; FRCP; FRCPC; HemPath. Med Dir, Canadian Blood Services; Assoc Prof Path, University of Manitoba; (204)789-1075; Fax. (204)783-6780; debra.lane@blood.ca.

LANE, Eric S; Dr CW Wiebe Med Centre, 385 Main St, Winkler MB R6W 1J2; Cape Town (South Africa)'85; LMCC; CCFP; FCFP; Staff, Boundary Trails Health Centre; (204)325-4312; Fax. (204)325-4594.

LANE, James E; 510 Ascot St, Coquitlam BC V3J 6H5; UBC'73; (604)942-7292; Fax. (604)942-9698.

LANE, James G A; Stayner Med Centre, PO Box 220 7477 Hwy 26, Stayner ON L0M 1S0; Wes'85; CCFP; Ac Staff, Collingwood General & Marine Hospital; Asst Prof, McMaster University; University of Toronto; (705)428-3246; Fax. (705)428-5652.

LANE, Jeremy J; Joseph Brant Mem Hosp, 1230 North Shore Blvd E, Burlington ON L7S 1W7; Qns'99; BSc(Hons); FRCPC; Anes. Staff, Joseph Brant Memorial Hospital; (905)632-3730

LANE, Joanne E L; Southern Med Clinic, 390 Topsail Rd, St. John's NL A1E 2B8; Mem'01; CCFP; (709)364-9556

LANE, John; Superior Family Health Team, 48-44 Great Northern Rd, Sault Ste. Marie ON P6B 4Y5; Alb'88; Staff, Sault Area Hospital - Sault Ste Marie; (705)253-6599

LANE, Judith I; Churchill Med Clinic, 6750 Winston Churchill Blvd, Mississauga ON L5N 4C4; Tor'85; CCFP; (905)824-3700; Fax. (905)824-9956.

LANE, Keith M; St Joseph Family Med Clinic, 402-2555 St Joseph Blvd, Orleans ON K1C 1S6; Dal'99; BSc; (613)830-1298; Fax. (613)830-6500.

LANE, Lynsay R; Petawawa Fam Health Centre, 154 Civic Centre Rd, Petawawa ON K8H 3H5; Ott'10; CCFP; Staff Family Med Teaching Unit, Pembroke Regional Hospital Inc; (613)687-7641

LANE, Margo A; Children's Hosp, CH102-840 Sherbrook St, Winnipeg MB R3A 1S1; Sask'88; FRCPC; Peds. Staff, Health Sciences Centre.

LANE, Martin P; St Anthony's Med Centre, 206-582 Goldstream Ave, Victoria BC V9B 2W7; UBC'86; Staff, Vancouver Island Health Authority; (250)474-3311; Fax. (250)474-2783.

LANE, Michael D; Radiology Associates, 1122 Scenic Dr, Lethbridge AB T1K 7E5; UBC'07; DiagRad. (403)328-1122

LANE, Robert A; Bowmanville Prof Bldg, 3101-222 King St E, Bowmanville ON L1C 1P6; McM'76; BSc; FACS; FRCSC; GenSurg. Medical Staff, Lakeridge Health - Bowmanville Site; (905)697-6446; Fax. (905)623-1835.

LANE-SMITH, D Mark; 152-150 Rolling Hills Dr, Orangeville ON L9W 4X8; McM'90; FRCSC; GenSurg. Ac Staff, Headwaters Health Care Centre - Orangeville Site; (519)941-0700; Fax. (519)938-5640.

LANEUVILLE, Louis; CLSC La Vallee des Patriotes, 300 boul Serge-Pepin, Beloeil QC J3G 0B8; Sher'88; (450)536-2572

LANEUVILLE, Pierre J; MUHC-Royal Victoria Hosp, C6 90-687 av des Pins O, Montreal QC H3A 1A1; Ott'82; Hem; IntMed (Malignant Hematology). Dir Div of Hem, McGill University Health Centre - Montreal General Campus; Dir Div of Hem, McGill University Health Centre - Royal Victoria Hospital; (514)934-1934 x31558; Fax. (514)843-1418; laneuvillep@muhchem.mcgill.ca.

LANFEAR, Paul C; Medical Arts Centre, 30-650 Terminal Ave, Nanaimo BC V9R 5E2; Sheffield (England)'75; MB ChB; CCFP; (250)753-3431

LANFRANCHI, Paola A; Hop du Sacre-Coeur de Mtl, 5400 boul Gouin O, Montreal QC H4J 1C5; Di Pavia (Italy)'89; Staff, Hôpital du Sacre-Coeur de Montréal; (514)338-2222 x7710

LANG, Anik; Clinique de Med Interne, 20 rue Carrier, Edmundston NB E3V 3Y1; Sher'06; FRCPC; IntMed. Staff, Hôpital regional d'Edmundston; (506)739-9511

LANG, Anthony E T; Univ Hlth Network-Toronto Western Hosp, 7MCL-399 Bathurst St, Toronto ON M5T 2S8; Tor'75; FRCPC; IntMed (Movement Disorders); Neur. Dir Movement Disorders Centre/Ac Staff, Toronto Western Hospital - University Health Network; Prof Joch Clarke Chair for Parkinson's Dis Res, University of Toronto; (416)603-6422; lang@uhnres.utoronto.ca.

LANG, Bianca A; IWK Health Centre, PO Box 9700 Rpo CSC, Halifax NS B3K 6R8; Dal'83; FAAP; FRCPC; Peds; Rheum. Ac Staff, IWK Health Centre; Assoc Prof, Dalhousie University; (902)470-8827; Fax. (902)470-7217; bianca.lang@iwk.nshealth.ca.

LANG, Brian A; Medical Centre, C03-3000 Lawrence Ave E, Scarborough ON M1P 2V1; McG'88; CCFP; Staff Family Pract, The Scarborough Hospital - General Campus; Langs: English; French; (416)431-2033; Fax. (416)431-4857.

LANG, Bridget Y C; 308-237 Keefer St, Vancouver BC V6A 1X6; Monash (Australia)'77; Court Staff, BC Women's Hospital & Health Centre; Court Staff, Providence Health Care - Mount Saint Joseph Hospital; Langs: Cantonese; (604)669-3994; Fax. (604)669-5511.

LANG, Clement; Lang Med Clinic, 132 Horace St, Winnipeg MB R2H 0W1; Man'87; BSc; MSc(Path.); PhD(Physiol); (204)237-3850; Fax. (204)237-9988.

LANG, Eddy S; 1633-1632 14 Ave NW, Calgary AB T2N 1M7; McG'90; CCFP; CCFP(E.M.); EmergMed (P.Q.). (403)944-8430

LANG, Francis K L; Lincoln Plaza, 110 Weber St N, Waterloo ON N2J 3G8; Man'82; (519)746-4344; Fax. (519)746-3334.

LANG, H Benno; Tantallon Family Practice, 202-5110 St Margarets Bay Rd, Upper Tantallon NS B3Z 1E2; Dal'93; CCFP; Langs: German; (902)826-2744

LANG, Isabelle; CLSC Point de Service, GD 211 rue du Couvent, Saint-Epiphane QC G0L 2X0; Laval'99; (418)868-2572

LANG, J Michael; Halton HCS Corp-Oakville, 327 Reynolds St, Oakville ON L6J 3L7; Wes'99; FRCPC; PhysMed&Rehab. Staff, Halton Healthcare Services Corporation - Oakville Site; (905)845-2571

LANG, Jefferey D; Burlington Prof Centre, 302-3155 Harvester Rd, Burlington ON L7N 3V2; Wes'90; FRCPC; IntMed (Critical Care Medicine). Ac Staff Med, Joseph Brant Memorial Hospital; (905)634-0800; Fax. (905)634-0825.

LANG, Maria T; Tantallon Family Practice, 202-5110 St Margarets Bay Rd, Upper Tantallon NS B3Z 1E2; Dal'86; BSc; (902)826-2744; Fax. (902)826-2887.

LANG, Mia E; Royal Alexandra Hosp, 2F-10240 Kingsway NW, Edmonton AB T5H 3V9; Alb'99; PhD; MSc; FRCPC; Peds. Staff, Royal Alexandra Hospital; Asst Prof, University of Alberta; (780)735-4605

LANG, Michael L; Regina Qu'Appelle HR-Regina, 1440 14th Ave, Regina SK S4P 0W5; Cape Town (South Africa)'75; MB ChB; MMed(Anes); DABA; DABPainMed; FRCPC; Anes (Pain Management). Staff Anes, Regina General Hospital; Asst Prof, University of Saskatchewan; Langs: Afrikaans; (306)545-6532; Fax. (306)766-4443.

LANG, Michael P; Nanaimo Reg Gen Hosp, 1200 Dufferin St, Nanaimo BC V9S 2B7; New York (USA)'04; IntMed. Staff, Nanaimo Regional General Hospital; (250)755-7691

LANG, Peter J; 22 Water St S, Kitchener ON N2G 4K4; Tor'75; FRCPC; Psy (Child & Adolescent Psychiatry). Staff, St Mary's General Hospital; (519)570-4572

LANG, Robert M; 1428 20 Ave NW, Calgary AB T2M 1G5; Cal'74; Ophth. Ac Staff, Foothills Medical Centre; (403)284-1136; Fax. (403)282-2031.

LANG, Roger L; Clin Med Du Haut-Madawaska, H-809 rue Principale, Clair NB E7A 2H7; Laval'81; (506)992-0040; Fax. (506)992-0044.

LANG, Sandra R; Canadian Med Protective Assoc, 875 Carling Ave, Ottawa ON K1S 5P1; Tor'81; Assoc Staff, Northumberland Hills Hospital; Court Staff Surgical Ass't, Lakeridge Health - Oshawa Site.

LANG, William J; Vancouver Gen Hosp, 855 12th Ave W, Vancouver BC V5Z 1M9; Tor'68; FRCPC; EmergMed. Staff Emerg, Vancouver General Hospital - Centennial Pavillion; Assoc Prof Surg, University of British Columbia; (604)875-5242; Fax. (604)875-4872.

LANG BAYONA, Francisco; Davidson Family Practise, PO Box 1058, Davidson SK S0G 1A0; (306)567-5550

LANG HANG YEE, Sam; Norburn Med Clinic, 200-4012 Hastings St, Burnaby BC V5C 2H9; Dublin (Ireland)'85; MB ChB; CCFP; FCFP; Staff, Burnaby Hospital; Langs: Mandarin; French; (604)299-2677; Fax. (604)298-6656.

LANG-HODGE, Brian J; South Okanagan Gen Hosp, RR 3 7169 362nd Ave, Oliver BC V0H 1T0; Alb'86; FRCPC; EmergMed. Staff, South Okanagan General Hospital; (250)498-5010; lang-hodgeb@shaw.ca.

LANGAN, John T; 404-225 Vaughan St, Winnipeg MB R3C 1T7; Galway (Ireland)'67; MB ChB; DCH; DRCOG; DOphth; (204)943-7969

LANGBURT, Wayne; 313-7368 Yonge St, Thornhill ON L4J 8H9; McG'91; FRCPC; Peds (Child Neurology); Neur. Assoc Staff, The Hospital For Sick Children; Staff Ped, North York General Hospital; (905)707-8343; Fax. (905)707-8344.

LANGE, Alden W; Orchard Med Centre, 104-1990 Cooper Rd, Kelowna BC V1Y 8K5; UBC'96; BSc; CCFP; CCFP(E.M.); Associate Privileges, Kelowna General Hospital; Staff, Orchard Medical Center; (250)861-3235; Fax. (250)861-3448.

LANGE, Elizabeth J; South Health Campus, 4448 Front St SE, Calgary AB T3M 1M4; Otago (New Zealand)'75; MB ChB; FRCSC; Otol (AIDS/HIV). Ac Staff, Foothills Medical Centre; Ac Staff, Alberta Children's Hospital; Clinical Asst Prof, University of Calgary; (403)956-3462; Fax. (403)956-3494; blange@arczone.com.

LANGE, Ian R; Foothills Med Centre, 4F-1403 29 St NW, Calgary AB T2N 2T9; Otago (New Zealand)'72; MRC; FSOGC; FRCSC; ObstGyn. Staff, Foothills Medical Centre; Prof, University of Calgary; (403)944-1636; Fax. (403)270-4249.

LANGE, Jennifer; New Waterford Consolidated Hos, 716 King St, New Waterford NS B1H 3Z5; Sask'05; BSc; CCFP; Staff, New Waterford Consolidated Hospital; (902)592-3400

LANGE, Lisa M M; 200-1330 8th Ave W, Vancouver BC V6H 4A6; UBC'09; CCFP; (604)734-7125

LANGE-MECHLEN, Ilse; Trillium Hlth Ctr-Mississauga, 100 Queensway W, Mississauga ON L5B 1B8; Tor'72; FRCPC; IntMed. Staff, Trillium Health Centre - Mississauga; (905)848-7100

LANGELIER, Diane; CHUS-Hop Hotel-Dieu, 580 rue Bowen S, Sherbrooke QC J1G 2E8; Sher'88; LMCC; Gastroent (P.Q.); IntMed (Nutrition). Staff, Centre Hospitalier Universitaire de Sherbrooke-Hôpital Hôtel-Dieu; assoc Prof, Universite de Sherbrooke; Langs: English; (819)346-1110; Fax. (819)822-6797.

LANGELIER, Marlene; Centre Med Chambly-Latour, B-5580 ch de Chambly, Saint-Hubert QC J3Y 3P5; Mon'84; (450)926-2236

LANGELIER, Michel; Ctr Hosp Affilie-Enfant-Jesus, 1401 18e rue, Quebec QC G1J 1Z4; Laval'69; FRCPC; IntMed. Staff, Centre Hospitalier Affilié Universitaire de Québec - Hôpital De L'Enfant Jésus; (418)649-0252 x3575; Fax. (418)649-5913.

LANGER, Anatoly I; St Michael's Hosp, 30 Bond St, Toronto ON M5B 1W8; Man'82; MSc; FACC; FRCPC; IntMed; Cardiol. Chair Canadian Heart Res Centre, St Michael's Hospital; Prof Med, University Of Toronto; (416)864-5951; langera@smh.toronto.on.ca.

LANGER, Frederick; 1301-123 Edward St, Toronto ON M5G 1E2; Tor'64; FRCSC; OrthSurg. Assoc Prof Surg, University of Toronto; (416)598-0474; Fax. (416)598-8928.

LANGER, Galina; 398 Steeles Ave W, Thornhill ON L4J 6X3; Man'83; FACC(Cardiol); FRCPC; IntMed; Cardiol. Langs: Russian; Ukrainian; (905)881-0334; Fax. (905)881-1721.

LANGER, Howard M; 30 Berwick Ave, Toronto ON M5P 1H1; Tor'66; DABIM; FAAA; FRCPC; Peds. Staff, The Hospital For Sick Children; Staff, Trillium Health Centre - Mississauga; Staff, The Credit Valley Hospital; Assoc Prof, University of Toronto; (416)483-3866; Fax. (905)279-1064.

LANGER, Jacob C; The Hosp for Sick Children, 1526-555 University Ave, Toronto ON M5G 1X8; Tor'80; FRCSC; GenSurg; PedGenSurg. Staff GenSurg, The Hospital For Sick Children; Prof Surg, University of Toronto; (416)813-7340; Fax. (416)813-7477; jacob.langer@sickkids.ca.

LANGER, Joseph; 82 Chatham St, Belleville ON K8N 3S6; Wes'56; BSc; OrthSurg. Langs: Spanish; (613)962-0250; Fax. (613)966-0250; joelanger@hotmail.com.

LANGER, Lorne J; Dr Langer & Associates, 180 Sandalwood Pky E, Brampton ON L6Z 1Y4; Tor'79; Staff, William Osler Health System - Brampton Civic Hospital; (905)846-9255; Fax. (905)846-2525; mdclinic@rogers.com.

LANGER, Pearl S; Colborne Family Med Centre, 612 Colborne St, London ON N6B 2V2; Cal'87; CCFP; FCFP; (519)673-1962; Fax. (519)673-3758.

LANGEVIN, Anny; Clin De Gynecologie du Lac St-, 24 rue Melancon E, Alma QC G8B 6W3; Mon'91; FRCSC; ObstGyn. Staff, CSSS de Lac-Saint Jean-Est; Langs: Bilingual(French/English); (418)662-6553; Fax. (418)662-3731.

LANGEVIN, Benoit; CSSS Maria-Chapdelaine, 2000 boul du Sacre-Coeur, Dolbeau-Mistassini QC G8L 2R5; Laval'65; FRCPC; DiagRad. Staff, Centre Maria-Chapdelaine - CH de Dolbeau-Mistassini; (418)276-1234 x4245

LANGEVIN, Catherine; Centre Prof Gerard-Blain, 175 rue Doody, Chambly QC J3L 1K7; Mon'87; FRCPC; Psy. (450)658-9650

LANGEVIN, Dominique; CLSC Verdun/Cote-St-Paul, 400 rue de l'Eglise, Verdun QC H4G 2M4; Mon'87; (514)766-0546

LANGEVIN, Gilles; Clinique Med De Courville, 1049 av Larue, Quebec QC G1C 1J5; Laval'81; LMCC; Staff Emerg, Centre Hospitalier Universitaire de Quebec-CHUL; Staff, Centre Hospitalier Affilié Universitaire de Québec - Hôpital De L'Enfant Jésus; (418)661-0097; Fax. (418)661-0307; glangevin@dr.com.

LANGEVIN, Jacques; Ctr Hosp Affilie-Enfant-Jesus, 1401 18e rue, Quebec QC G1J 1Z4; Laval'92; CSPQ; Critical Care Medicine (P.Q.); Anes. Staff, Centre Hospitalier Affilié Universitaire de Québec - Hôpital De L'Enfant Jésus; (418)649-5807; Fax. (418)649-5918.

LANGEVIN, Jean; 200-300 Columbia St, Kamloops BC V2C 6L1; Mon'94; FRCSC; OrthSurg. (250)374-1448

LANGEVIN, Julie; Base Militaire Valcartier, CP 1000 Bdp Succ Forces 5e Ambulance de Campagne, Courcelette QC G0A 4Z0; Laval'07; CCFP; (418)844-5000

LANGEVIN, Melissa K; Children's Hosp Eastern Ont, 401 Smyth Rd, Ottawa ON K1H 8L1; Ott'07; FRCPC; Peds. Staff EmergMed, Children's Hospital of Eastern Ontario (CHEO); (613)737-7600

LANGEVIN, Pierre L; CHUQ-Ctr Hosp Univ Laval, 1235-2705 boul Laurier, Quebec QC G1V 4G2; Laval'65; FRCPC; Peds; Neur (P.Q.); Electroenceph (P.Q.). Staff, Centre Hospitalier Universitaire de Quebec-CHUL; Staff, Hotel-Dieu du Sacre-Coeur de Jesus de Quebec; Langs: Bilingual(French/English); (418)654-2708

LANGEVIN, Serge; CHUS-Hop Fleurimont, 3001 12e av, Sherbrooke QC J1H 5N4; Sher'83; FRCPC; IntMed; Gastroent. Staff, Centre Hospitalier Universitaire de Sherbrooke-Hopital Fleurimont; vice Doyen Postgraduate Med Studies, Universite de Sherbrooke; Langs: English; (819)564-5206; Fax. (819)564-5293.

LANGEVIN, Stephan; Ctr Hosp Affilie-Enfant-Jesus, 1401 18e rue, Quebec QC G1J 1Z4; Mon'93; FRCPC; Anes (Intensive Care); Critical Care Medicine (P.Q.). Staff, Centre Hospitalier Affilié Universitaire de Québec - Hôpital De L'Enfant Jésus; (418)649-0252; Fax. (418)649-5918.

LANGFORD, E Robert; PH8-398 Eglinton Ave E, Toronto ON M4P 3H8; Qns'58; DPH; CM; Court Staff, Mount Sinai Hospital; Assoc Prof Community Health, University of Toronto; (416)483-8337; Fax. (416)483-7100; robert.langford@utoronto.ca.

LANGFORD, Grace M; GM Langford Med Prof Corp, C-59 Lorne Ave E, Stratford ON N5A 6S4; Wes'89; CCFP; FCFP; Ac Staff, Stratford General Hospital - Huron Perth Healthcare Alliance; (519)271-3200; Fax. (519)271-3124.

LANGFORD, Mark E; Royal Inland Hosp, 311 Columbia St, Kamloops BC V2C 2T1; UBC'92; CCFP; CCFP(E.M.); Staff, Royal Inland Hospital; (250)374-5111

LANGFORD, Steve; 27 Third St, Collingwood ON L9Y 1K4; McM'87; CCFP; Staff, Collingwood General & Marine Hospital; (705)445-4111; Fax. (705)445-8250; cmc@cois.on.ca.

LANGHAN, Trevor S; Foothills Med Centre, C231-1403 29 St NW, Calgary AB T2N 2T9; Man'03; FRCPC; EmergMed. Staff, Foothills Medical Centre; (403)944-1635

LANGHANS, J Marcus; Valley Care Med Clinic, E-310 8th St, Courtenay BC V9N 1N3; Friedrich Alexander (Germany)'96; CCFP; (250)331-0500

LANGHORNE, Noel B; 102-955 Major Mackenzie Dr, Vaughn ON L6A 4P9; Qns'94; FRCPC; DiagRad (Interventional Radiology). Staff, Mackenzie Richmond Hill Hospital; (289)553-6336; Fax. (289)553-6339.

LANGILL, Marc V; 100-190 Main St, Ottawa ON K1S 1C2; Ott'87; CCFP; Langs: English; French; (613)235-2685; Fax. (613)235-2688.

LANGILLE, Donald B; Community Hlth & Epidemiology, 5790 University Ave, Halifax NS B3H 1V7; Dal'74; (902)494-1312; Fax. (902)494-1597.

LANGILLE, Heather I; Civil Aviation Medicine, 617-330 Sparks St, Ottawa ON K1A 0N8; Dal'93; CCFP; CCFP(E.M.); Langs: English; French; (613)990-1305; Fax. (613)990-6623.

LANGILLE, Kenneth R; 121 Orchard St PO Box 578, Berwick NS B0P 1E0; Dal'75.

LANGILLE, Morgan A; University of Alberta Hosp, 8440 112 St NW, Edmonton AB T6G 2B7; Dal'08; Staff, University of Alberta Hospital; (780)407-8822

LANGIS, Denis; Hotel-Dieu de Levis, 143 rue Wolfe, Levis QC G6V 3Z1; Laval'84; FRCSC; Otol. Staff, Hôtel-Dieu de Lévis; (418)835-7121

LANGIS, Denis; CSSS de Laval, 280 boul Du Roi-Du-Nord, Laval QC H7L 4L2; Mon'80; Langs: English; (450)622-5110; Fax. (450)622-4150.

LANGIS, Lise; Centre De Sante Bouctouche, 201-101 Evangeline St, Bouctouche NB E4S 5L4; Laval'95; CCFP; Langs: Bilingual(French/English); (506)743-8941; Fax. (506)743-8405.

LANGIS, Louis; CHUQ-Hotel-Dieu De Quebec, 11 Cote Du Palais, Quebec QC G1R 2J6; Laval'66; DiagRad. Staff, Centre Hospitalier Universitaire de Québec (CHUQ) - Siege Social; (418)691-5453

LANGIS, Paul-Andre; CHUQ-St-Francois D'Assise, 10 rue de l'Espinay, Quebec QC G1L 3L5; Sher'77; FRCPC; DiagRad. ac Staff, Centre Hospitalier Universitaire De Québec - Pavillon De St-françois-d'assise; (418)525-4462; paul.langis@rad.ulaval.ca.

LANGLAIS, Albert; Clinique Medicale de l'Est, 203-100 rue King E, Sherbrooke QC J1G 1A4; Sher'73; Med Consultant, Centre Jean-Patrice Chiasson; Langs: Bilingual(French/English); (819)563-7225; Fax. (819)563-7271.

LANGLAIS, Caroline; CSSS de Memphremagog, 50 rue Saint-Patrice E, Magog QC J1X 3X3; Sher'04; Staff, Centre Hospitalier et CLSC de Memphremagog; (819)843-2572

LANGLAIS, Caroline; CHUS-Hop Fleurimont, 3001 12e av N, Sherbrooke QC J1H 5N4; McG'01; FRCPC; Peds. Staff, Centre Hospitalier Universitaire de Sherbrooke-Hopital Fleurimont; (819)345-1110

LANGLAIS, Francois; Ctr Hosp de Lasalle, 8585 Tsse Champlain, Lasalle QC H8P 1C1; Mon'92; FRCPC; IntMed. Staff, Centre Hospitalier de LaSalle; (514)362-8000; Fax. (514)367-8635.

LANGLAIS, Marc; CHUQ-St-Francois d'Assise, 10 rue de l'Espinay, Quebec QC G1L 3L5; Laval'93; BSc; LMCC; CCFP; Staff, Centre Hospitalier Universitaire De Québec - Pavillon De St-françois-d'assise; (418)525-4388

LANGLAIS, Mario; CHUQ-Ctr Hosp Univ Laval, 219-2705 boul Laurier, Quebec QC G1V 4G2; Laval'80; Cardiol; IntMed. ac Staff, Centre Hospitalier Universitaire de Quebec-CHUL; (418)654-2110; Fax. (418)654-2268.

LANGLAIS, Nathalie; CSSS du Nord de Lanaudière, 1000 boul Sainte-Anne, St-Charles-Brromee QC J6E 6J2; Mon'88; FRCPC; IntMed; Rheum. Staff Rheumatology, Centre Hospitalier Régional de Lanaudière; (450)759-8222; Fax. (450)759-5308.

LANGLAIS, Rebecca; CSSS de Laval, 1755 boul Rene-Laennec, Laval QC H7M 3L9; Laval'99; Respir; IntMed. Staff, Hopital de la Cite de la santé; (450)668-1010

LANGLEBEN, Adrian; St Mary's Hosp Centre, 3830 av Lacombe, Montreal QC H3T 1M5; McG'76; FRCPC; IntMed (Bone Marrow Transplant); MedOncol (P.Q.); Hem (P.Q.). Staff, St Mary's Hospital Centre; Asst Prof MedOncol, McGill University; (514)734-2679; Fax. (514)734-2795.

LANGLEBEN, David; SMBD Jewish Gen Hosp, 3755 ch Cote-Sainte-Catherine, Montreal QC H3T 1E2; McG'77; FRCPC; IntMed (Pulmonary Hypertention); Cardiol. Chief Cardiol, Sir Mortimer B Davis Jewish General; Prof Med, McGill University; Langs: French; (514)340-7531; Fax. (514)340-7534; david.langleben@mcgill.ca.

LANGLEY, Christine E; Bedford Waterfront Hlth Clinic, 207-967 Bedford Hwy, Bedford NS B4A 1A9; Dal'90; (902)835-6444; Fax. (902)832-1193.

LANGLEY, Hugh G; 370 Select Dr, Kingston ON K7M 8T4; Qns'85; CCFP; Staff, Hotel-Dieu Hospital; Staff, Kingston General Hospital; Family Medicine, Ongwanada Resource Centre; Med Consultant Long Term Care & Health Services, Ministry Of Health; Lecturer Med, Queen's University; hlangley@kflapublichealth.ca.

LANGLEY, Jean E; Telus Plaza South, 2700-10020 100 St NW, Edmonton AB T5J 0N3; Qns'80; CCFP; FCFP; (780)423-4764

LANGLEY, Joanne M; IWK Health Centre, PO Box 9700 Rpo CSC, Halifax NS B3K 6R8; Dal'84; MSc(Epidem.); FRCPC; Peds; InfectDis. Ac Staff, IWK Health Centre; Prof Peds & Commun Health & Epidemiol, Dalhousie University; (902)470-8141; Fax. (902)470-7232.

LANGLEY, John H; St Michael's Hosp, 17006-30 Bond St, Toronto ON M5B 1W8; McM'92; FRCPC; Psy. Staff, St Michael's Hospital; Lecturer Psy, University of Toronto; (416)864-3084; Fax. (416)864-5480; john.langley@utoronto.ca.

LANGLEY, Richard G B; 5743 University Ave, Halifax NS B3H 0A2; Dal'90; FRCPC; Derm (Psoriasis). (902)425-8038

LANGLEY, Stephanie A; 3-131 King St, North Sydney NS B2A 3S1; Dal'95; CCFP; Hd Fam Practice, Northside General Hospital; MD-MLA Contact, Medical Society of Nova Scotia; Clin Preceptor Family Med, Dalhousie University; (902)794-5900; Fax. (902)794-5930; slangley@ns.sympatico.ca.

LANGLEY, Suzanne M; 6412 Bay St, West Vancouver BC V7W 2H1; Tor'73; (604)921-7120

LANGLOIS, Alexis; CSSS de Papineau, 155 rue MacLaren E, Gatineau QC J8L 0C2; Laval'04; CCFP; Staff, CH-CHSLD de Papineau - Pavillon du centre hospitalier; Staff, Hôpital de Papineau; (819)986-3341

LANGLOIS, Andre; Centre Radiol de Sherbrooke, 250 rue King E, Sherbrooke QC J1G 1A9; Sher'81; DiagRad. (819)563-1443

LANGLOIS, Claude; CLSC-CHSLD de L'Erable, 1331 rue Saint-Calixte, Plessisville QC G6L 1P4; Laval'73; Staff, CLSC de l'Erable; Staff, Hopital St-Julien; (819)362-6301

LANGLOIS, Daniel; Clinique Med Brien, 223 boul Brien, Repentigny QC J6A 6M4; Mon'81; FRCSC; ObstGyn. (450)585-9810; Fax. (450)585-8538.

LANGLOIS, David A; Victoria Park Clinic, 95 Darling St, Brantford ON N3T 2K7; Wes'98; MSc; BSc; FSOGC; BA; FRCOG; FRCSC; ObstGyn (Minimal Invasive Surgery). Staff Consultant, London Health Sciences Centre - Victoria Campus; (519)720-0712; davidallanlanglois@hotmail.com.

LANGLOIS, Denis; CHUQ-St-Francois D'Assise, 10 rue de l'Espinay, Quebec QC G1L 3L5; Laval'81; CSPQ; Anes. Ac Staff, Centre Hospitalier Universitaire De Québec - Pavillon De St-françois-d'assise; (418)525-4340; Fax. (418)525-4434.

LANGLOIS, E Anne; Mount Sinai Hosp, 1001B-600 University Ave, Toronto ON M5G 1X5; McG'79; BSc; CCFP; Staff Palliative Med, Mount Sinai Hospital; Asst Prof, University of Toronto; Langs: French; (416)586-4800 x6771; Fax. (416)586-4804; alanglois@mtsinai.on.ca.

LANGLOIS, Fabienne; Hop Charles Lemoyne, 3120 boul Taschereau, Greenfield Park QC J4V 2H1; Sher'05; Endocrin&Metab; IntMed. Staff, Hopital Charles LeMoyne; (450)466-5000

LANGLOIS, Francois; Clinique Med de Buckingham, 200-620 av De Buckingham, Gatineau QC J8L 2H5; McG'78; Langs: Bilingual(French/English); (819)986-6006; Fax. (819)986-1616; francois.langlois@sympatico.ca.

LANGLOIS, Gaetan; CHUS-Hop Fleurimont, 3001 12e av N, Sherbrooke QC J1H 5N4; Mon'71; FRCSC; OrthSurg. Staff, Centre Hospitalier Universitaire de Sherbrooke-Hopital Fleurimont; Chef Surg, Universite de Sherbrooke; (819)346-1110 x14460; Fax. (819)564-5387.

LANGLOIS, Guillaume; Coop de Solidarite Ste-Gertrud, 6445 rue des Pins, Becancour QC G9H 3K9; Mon'04; CCFP; Staff, Hôpital de Christ-Roi; (819)297-2911

LANGLOIS, Isabelle; CSSS de Laval, 1755 boul Rene-Laennec, Laval QC H7M 3L9; Mon'86; Staff, Hopital de la Cite de la santé; (450)975-5444

LANGLOIS, J L Jean; CHUS-Hop Fleurimont, 3001 12e av N, Sherbrooke QC J1H 5N4; Laval'81; CSPQ; FRCPC; EmergMed. Staff, Centre Hospitalier Universitaire de Sherbrooke-Hopital Fleurimont; (819)346-1110

LANGLOIS, Janick; Clinique Med de L'Or, 228 2e rue E, La Sarre QC J9Z 2G9; Laval'92; CCFP; (819)339-5617; Fax. (819)339-2729.

LANGLOIS, Jean; CSSS Becancour-Nicolet-Yamaska, 216 rue Principale, Fortierville QC G0S 1J0; Laval'96; Staff, Carrefour Sante Granit; (819)287-4442; Fax. (819)287-4017.

LANGLOIS, Julie; Clinique Med Belvedere, 202-2235 rue Galt O, Sherbrooke QC J1K 1K6; Sher'06; CCFP; CCFP(E.M.); (819)566-8616

LANGLOIS, Julie; Clinique Med Nepisiguit, 950 av Picot, Bathurst NB E2A 4Z9; Sher'98; CCFP; Langs: English; (506)546-6696; Fax. (506)545-7723.

LANGLOIS, Line; 8 rue Speid, Sherbrooke QC J1M 1R6; Laval'79; CCFP; Teach Staff, Universite de Sherbrooke; Langs: English; (819)780-2222; Fax. (819)566-8059.

LANGLOIS, Louis-Charles; Ctr Medico Prof De Brossard, 101-2424 boul Lapiniere, Brossard QC J4Z 2K9; Mon'74; (450)678-9033; Fax. (450)678-8274; lclanglois@videotron.ca.

LANGLOIS, Lyne; CLSC des Maskoutins, 1015 rue Gauthier, Saint-Hyacinthe QC J2S 8T2; Sher'88; (450)778-2572 x6154; Fax. (450)778-1899.

LANGLOIS, Marie-Eve; Starpoint Health Corp, 202-3716 61 Ave SE, Calgary AB T2C 1Z4; Mon'01; LMCC; CCFP; Langs: Bilingual(French/English); (403)236-8400; Fax. (403)236-8806; marilanca@yahoo.ca.

LANGLOIS, Marie-France; CHUS-Hop Fleurimont, 3001 12e Av N, Sherbrooke QC J1H 5N4; Sher'90; FRCPC; IntMed (Thyroid Diseases); Endocrin (P.Q.); Endocrin&Metab. Staff Endocrin, Centre Hospitalier Universitaire de Sherbrooke-Hopital Fleurimont; adj Prof, Universite de Sherbrooke; Langs: Bilingual(English/French); (819)564-5223; marie-france.langlois@usherbrooke.ca.

LANGLOIS, Marie-Josee; CSSS de Saint-Jerome, 290 rue de Montigny, Saint-Jerome QC J7Z 5T3; Mon'05; FRCPC; Neur. Staff, Hôtel-Dieu de Saint-Jérôme; (450)432-2777

LANGLOIS, Martine; CHSLD de la MRC De Champlain, 831 av Notre-Dame, Saint-Lambert QC J4R 1S1; Mon'83; Staff, CHSLD de la MRC de Champlain-Centre Saint-Lambert; Universite de Montreal; (450)672-3328 x2009; Fax. (450)672-1707; martine.langlois@rrsss16.gouv.qc.ca.

LANGLOIS, Melanie; Ctr Hosp Affilie-Enfant-Jesus, 1401 18e rue, Quebec QC G1J 1Z4; Laval'98; FRCPC; Neur (Parkinson's Disease). Neurology, Centre Hospitalier Affilié Universitaire de Québec - Hôpital De L'Enfant Jésus; Langs: Bilingual(French/English); (418)649-0252; Fax. (418)649-5915.

LANGLOIS, Michel; 19 rue Vachon GD, St-Jacques-D-Leeds QC G0N 1J0; Laval'70; Staff, Hopital du CSS de la Region de Thetford; Langs: English; (418)424-3663

LANGLOIS, Michel; Clinique Med Fabreville, 380 boul Cure-Labelle, Laval QC H7P 5L3; Laval'67; FRCPC; Peds (P.Q.). Staff, Hôpital Ste-Justine; (450)628-5800; Fax. (450)628-0217.

LANGLOIS, Nadine; Clinique Med St-Louis, 220-3165 ch Saint-Louis, Quebec QC G1W 4R4; Laval'97; (418)653-1970

LANGLOIS, Nathalie; CHUS-Hop Fleurimont, 3001 12e av N, Sherbrooke QC J1H 5N4; Sher'95; FRCPC; IntMed; Nephrol. Staff, Centre Hospitalier Universitaire de Sherbrooke-Hopital Fleurimont; Langs: Bilingual(French/English); (819)346-1110 x12389; Fax. (819)564-5369.

LANGLOIS, Patrice; Kilborn Med Clinic, 315-1385 Bank St, Ottawa ON K1H 8N4; Laval'94; CSPQ; FRCPC; Anes (Chronic Pain). Langs: Bilingual(French/English); (613)860-6777; Fax. (613)860-1777; drpatricelanglois@hotmail.com.

LANGLOIS, Richard; CSSS-Baie-des-Chaleurs, GD 48 boul Inter-Provincial, Pointe-a-la-Croix QC G0C 1L0; Laval'89; FRCPC; CommunMed (Mental Illness). Staff, Centre de santé Cloutier-du-Rivage; (418)788-5454

LANGLOIS, Robert P; Hop Louis-H Lafontaine, 7401 rue Hochelaga, Montreal QC H1N 3M5; Mon'73; FRCPC; Nephrol; IntMed. Staff, Hopital Louis-H Lafontaine; (514)251-4000 x2945

LANGLOIS, Serge; 11 Cote Du Palais, Quebec QC G1R 2J6; Laval'72; FRCPC; IntMed; Nephrol (P.Q.). ac Staff, Centre Hospitalier Universitaire de Québec (CHUQ) - Siege Social; Prof, Université Laval; Langs: English; (418)691-5464; Fax. (418)691-5757; serge.langlois@med.ulaval.ca.

LANGLOIS, Stephanie F; Renfrew Med Group, 510 Raglan St N, Renfrew ON K7V 1P5; Ott'87; Med Dir, Renfrew Victoria Hospital; Langs: Bilingual(French/English); (613)432-4815; Fax. (613)433-9154.

LANGLOIS, Sylvie; Children's & Women's Hlth Ctre, C234-4500 Oak St, Vancouver BC V6H 3N1; Sher'81; CCMG(Genetics); FRCPC; Peds (Medical Genetics). Staff, BC Children's Hospital; Prof, University of British Columbia; Langs: Bilingual(French/English); (604)875-2157; Fax. (604)875-2376; slanglois@cw.bc.ca.

LANGLOIS, Valerie; The Hosp For Sick Children, 555 University Ave, Toronto ON M5G 1X8; Sher'94; FRCPC; Peds; Nephrol. Staff, The Hospital For Sick Children; (416)813-7654 x1424; valerie.langlois@sickkids.ca.

LANGLOIS, Veronique; Med Privee Notre-Dame, 597 av Notre-Dame, Longueuil QC J4P 2K8; Mon'00; (450)766-0766

LANGLOIS, W John; Credit Valley Med Bldg, 505-2300 Eglinton Ave W, Mississauga ON L5M 2V8; Tor'88; FRCPC; IntMed; Endocrin&Metab. Ac Staff, The Credit Valley Hospital; (905)569-3007

LANGLOIS, Yves P; Ctr Medi Soleil St-Jean-Sur-Ri, 120-383 boul du Seminaire N, St-Jean-sur-Richel QC J3B 8C5; Mon'82; Staff, Hôpital du Haut-Richelieu; (450)347-7557; Fax. (450)347-3099.

LANGLOIS, Yves; SMBD Jewish Gen Hosp, A520-3755 Cote-Ste-Catherine, Montreal QC H3T 1E2; Mon'75; FRCSC; GenSurg (Adult Cardiac Surgery); Cardiovasc&ThorSurg. Ac Staff, Sir Mortimer B Davis Jewish General; Assoc Prof Surg, McGill University; Langs: English; (514)340-8222 x5598; Fax. (514)340-7561; ylanglois@surg.jgh.mcgill.ca.

LANGMANN, Caillin; Hamilton HS-General Site, 237 Barton St E, Hamilton ON L8L 2X2; Qns'08; Staff, Hamilton Health Sciences Centre - Hamilton General Hospital; (905)522-9017

LANGNER, Sabine M; 5017 47A Ave, Delta BC V4K 1T9; Man'93; CCFP; FCFP; (604)946-1168

LANGRIDGE, James K; Pam Am Sports Med Centre, 75 Poseidon Bay, Winnipeg MB R3M 3E4; Man'91; CCFP; FCFP; (204)925-2699; Fax. (204)452-5362.

LANGRIDGE, Jonathon M D; 202-535 Belmont Ave W, Kitchener ON N2M 5E9; Wes'99; FRCPC; IntMed (Intensive Care); Respir. Staff, St Mary's General Hospital; (519)894-9825; Fax. (519)896-0997.

LANGTON, E Michelle; North Woodlands Med Clinic, 204-40 Shellington Place, Brantford ON N3S 0C5; Tor'84; BFA; CAFCI; CCFP; FCFP; Clinical Asst Prof Family Med, McMaster University; (519)759-6116

LANGTON, Stephen R; Allin Clinic, 10155 120 St NW, Edmonton AB T5K 2A2; Alb'69; FRCSC; ObstGyn. Staff, Royal Alexandra Hospital; Full Clin Prof, University of Alberta; (780)482-7551; Fax. (780)488-2056.

LANGUEDOC, Francine; 103-10302 rue Chambord, Montreal QC H2C 2R5; Mon'81; (514)383-6646; Fax. (514)383-7686.

LANIEL, Chantal; Hop Santa Cabrini Ospedale, 5655 rue Saint-Zotique E, Montreal QC H1T 1P7; Sher'98; CSPQ; FRCPC; Anes. Staff, Hôpital Santa Cabrini Ospedale; (514)252-6000

LANIEL, Christian; Sudbury Reg Hosp-Laurentian Si, 41 Ramsey Lake Rd, Sudbury ON P3E 5J1; Ott'09; CCFP; Staff, Health Sciences North-Laurentian Site; (705)523-7100

LANIEL, Sylvain; Inst Albert Prevost, 6555 boul Gouin O, Montreal QC H4K 1B3; Sher'96; FRCPC; Psy. (514)338-2222

LANIGAN, Dennis T; 601 The Tower at Midtown, 201 1st Ave S, Saskatoon SK S7K 1J5; Sask'77; DMD; Ac Staff PlasSurg & Dentistry, Saskatoon Health Region Saskatoon Public Health; Clin Prof, University of Saskatchewan; (306)652-9454; Fax. (306)665-8778.

LANIUS, Ruth A; London HSC-University Hosp, PO Box 5339 Stn B 339 Windermere Rd, London ON N6A 5A5; UBC'96; FRCPC; Psy. Staff, London Health Sciences Centre - University Hospital; (519)663-3306

LANKTREE, Bruce B; 3-715 Coronation Blvd, Cambridge ON N1R 7R1; Wes'70; (519)740-1700; Fax. (519)740-8487.

LANNES, Marcelo; MUHC-Montreal Neurology Inst, 548-3801 rue University, Montreal QC H3A 2B4; (Brazil)'86; CSPQ; FRCPC; Anes; Critical Care Medicine (P.Q.). Anes & Critical Care, McGill University Health Centre - Montreal Neurological Hospital; Langs: Spanish; Portuguese; French; Italian; (514)398-1917; Fax. (514)398-1352; marcelo.lannes@muhc.mcgill.ca.

LANNEVILLE, Pascale; Ctr Hosp du Centre la Mauricie, 50 119e rue, Shawinigan-Sud QC G9P 5K1; Laval'94; CSPQ; AnatPath. Staff, Centre Hospitalier du Centre la Mauricie; (819)536-7575 x7663; p.lanneville@tr.cgocable.ca.

LANNIGAN, Robert; London HSC-Victoria Hosp, PO Box 5010 Stn B 800 Commissioners Rd E, London ON N6A 5W9; McG'74; FRCPC; IntMed; MedMicrobiol. Chief Dept of Microbiol & Infect Control, London Health Sciences Centre - Victoria Campus; Prof, University of Western Ontario; (519)685-8213; robert.lannigan@lhsc.on.ca.

LANNON, Karen P; 855 Ross Ave, Penticton BC V2A 3A5; Cal'84; FRCPC; Peds. Consultant Staff Peds, Princeton General Hospital; Assoc Staff Peds, Penticton Regional Hospital; (250)492-4247; drlannon@telus.net.

LANOIE, Genevieve; CSSSG-Hop de Hull, 116 boul Lionel-Emond, Gatineau QC J8Y 1W7; Mon'92; FRCPC; IntMed; Endocrin (P.Q.); Endocrin&Metab. Staff, Hull Hospital; (819)595-6103; Fax. (819)966-6221; genevieve_lanoie@ssss.gouv.qc.ca.

LANOIE, Leo O; Prince Albert Commun Clinic, 110 8th St E, Prince Albert SK S6V 0V7; Sask'73; MPH; ASAM; CASM; CCFP; FCFP; Staff Family Med & Addiction, Prince Albert Parkland Health Region; Med Dir, Prince Albert Co-Op Health Centre; (306)763-6464; Fax. (306)763-2101; llanoie@paphr.sk.ca.

LANOIE, Marie-Claude; CSSS de Saint-Jerome, 290 rue de Montigny, Saint-Jerome QC J7Z 5T3; Mon'93; FRCSC; Otol. Staff, Hôtel-Dieu de Saint-Jérôme; (450)431-8200

LANOIE, Nathalie; CSSSG-Hop de Hull, 116 boul Lionel-Emond, Gatineau QC J8Y 1W7; Sher'95; FRCPC; PhysMed&Rehab. Staff, Hull Hospital; (819)595-6000

LANOIX, Pierre J; Clarence-Rockland Fam Hlth Team, 2741 rue Chamberland, Rockland ON K4K 0B4; Ott'85; ATLS; ACLS; CCFP; FCFP; Staff, Montfort Hospital; Langs: English; French.

LANOUE, Danielle; Clinique Santé-Voyage de Mtl, 2E-6865 rue Sherbrooke E, Montreal QC H1N 1C7; Mon'79; Staff, Hopital Maisonneuve-Rosemont; Physician, Clinique Sante Voyage de Montreal; Langs: Bilingual(French/English); (514)252-0943; Fax. (514)252-1370.

LANOUE, Linda; CLSC Du Richelieu, 300 ch de Marieville, Richelieu QC J3L 3V8; Laval'80; LMCC; (450)658-7561; Fax. (450)658-4390.

LANOUE, Martin; Centre Med St-Leonard, 360 rue Beliveau, St-Leonard-d'Aston QC J0C 1M0; Mon'08; CCFP; Staff, Hôpital Sainte-croix; Langs: Bilingual(French/English); (819)399-4020; Fax. (819)399-2343; martin_lanoue@gmf.gouv.qc.ca.

LANOUETTE, Pierre; Clinique Med Du Centre, 15-2020 boul Rene-Gaultier, Varennes QC J3X 1N9; Sher'94; MSc(Biochem); BSc(BioChem); Staff Family Med, CA Jeanne-Crevier Boucherville; Clin Researcher, Innovaderm Rechercher Inc; Langs: English; (450)652-2222; Fax. (450)652-3970; lapie66@sympatico.ca.

LANPHEAR, Nancy E; Sunny Hill Health Ctre for Chi, 3644 Slocan St, Vancouver BC V5M 3E8; Missouri (USA)'87; Staff, Sunny Hill Health Centre for Children; (604)453-8383

LANSANG, Edward P; Univ Hlth Network-Toronto Western Hosp, 399 Bathurst St, Toronto ON M5T 2S8; (Philippines)'98; OrthSurg. Staff, Toronto Western Hospital - University Health Network; (416)603-2581

LANSANG, Perla; Sunnybrook Hlth Sciences Ctre, 2075 Bayview Ave, Toronto ON M4N 3M5; (Philippines)'98; FRCPC; Derm (Pediatric Dermatology). Staff, Sunnybrook Health Sciences Centre; Staff, Women's College Hospital; Staff, The Hospital For Sick Children; (416)480-6100 x4995; Fax. (416)480-6897.

LANSING, Barbara E; 2604 Kensington Rd NW PO Box 63040 RPO Stadium, Calgary AB T2N 4S5; Cal'83; BSc; CCFP; FCFP; (403)270-8988

LANSING, Davina R J; Hinton Med Clinic, 102 Allen Cove, Hinton AB T7V 2A6; Tor'10; CCFP; (780)865-3338; Fax. (780)865-4541.

LANTAGNE, Christiane; Curateur Public, 600 boul Rene-Levesque O, Montreal QC H3B 4W9; Sher'82; (514)873-9153

LANTAGNE, Louise; Clinique Med Saint-Prosper, 2475 28e rue, St-Prosper-D-Dorch QC G0M 1Y0; Laval'85; (418)594-8218; Fax. (418)594-8294.

LANTAGNE, Marie-Josee; Clinique Mediacle St-Prosper, 2475 28e rue, St-Prosper-d-Dorch QC G0M 1Y0; Mon'97; Staff, Centre Hospitalier Beauce-Etchemin; (418)594-8218

LANTEIGNE, Jean-Pierre; Centre Medical Vanier, 3-325 Vanier Blvd, Bathurst NB E2A 3N1; Laval'71; Ac Member, Centre Hospitalier Regional Chaleur-Bathurst; Ac Member, Réseau De Santé Vitalité; Langs: English; (506)548-8861; Fax. (506)549-4242; jean-pierrel@rrsb.nb.ca.

LANTEIGNE, Solange; Polyclinique Isabell-sur-Mer, 8224 rue St-Paul, Bas-Caraquet NB E1W 6E2; Mon'07; CCFP; Staff, Hôpital de l'Enfant-Jésus RHSJ; (506)727-7549; Fax. (506)727-7320.

LANTHIER, Annie; Centre Med Christ-Roi, 102-40 rte du Président-Kenned, Levis QC G6V 6C4; Laval'09; CCFP; (418)833-4977

LANTHIER, Luc; CHUS-Hop Hotel-Dieu, 580 rue Bowen S, Sherbrooke QC J1G 2E8; Sher'94; FRCPC; IntMed. Staff, Centre Hospitalier Universitaire de Sherbrooke-Hôpital Hôtel-Dieu; (819)346-1110 x28303

LANTHIER, Nathalie; Centre Med Saint-Charles, 101-1740 ch Saint-Charles, Terrebonne QC J6W 3R3; Mon'89; Staff, Centre Hospitalier Pierre le Gardeur; (450)492-2277; Fax. (450)492-1030.

LANTHIER, Sylvain; CHUM-Hop Notre-Dame, 1560 rue Sherbrooke E, Montreal QC H2L 4M1; Mon'93; Neur (P.Q.) (Cerebrovascular Disease). Staff, Centre Hospitalier l'Université de Montréal (CHUM) - Hôpital Notre-Dame; (514)890-8000 x26260; Fax. (514)412-7556.

LANTHIER-VEILLEUX, Marie-Soleil; CSSS de Rimouski-Neigette, 150 av Rouleau, Rimouski QC G5L 5T1; Laval'06; Staff, Hôpital Regional Rimouski; (418)724-3000; Fax. (418)724-8632.

LANTING, Brent A; London HSC-University Hosp, PO Box 5339 Stn B 339 Windermere Rd, London ON N6A 5A5; Wes'06; FRCSC; OrthSurg. Staff, London Health Sciences Centre - University Hospital; (519)685-8500

LANTOS, Gabor; 12F-95 St Clair Ave W, Toronto ON M4V 1N6; Tor'87; BEng; MBA; Staff, St Joseph's Health Centre; Med Dir Occup Health, Medisys Group; Med Consultant, The Equitable Life Ins Co. Cda; Consultant Occup Health, York University; Consultant Occup Health/Site Supvr, University of Toronto; Langs: Hungarian; Spanish; Portuguese; French; (416)410-5018; Fax. (416)229-2669.

LANTOS, Veronica M; 311-1390 Prince of Wales Dr, Ottawa ON K2C 3N6; Semmelweis (Hungary)'69; FRCPC; Psy. Consultant, The Ottawa Hospital - General Campus; (613)233-2298

LANTZ, Andrea G; St Michael's Hosp, 30 Bond St, Toronto ON M5B 1W8; Dal'07; FRCSC; Urol. Staff, St Michael's Hospital; (416)864-6060

LANTZ, Christopher J; Queen Elizabeth Hosp, PO Box 6600 Stn Central, Charlottetown PE C1A 8T5; Dal'90; Staff, Queen Elizabeth Hospital; (902)894-2200

LANTZ, J Brodie; Polyclinic Prof Centre Inc, 199 Grafton St, Charlottetown PE C1A 1L2; Dal'65; (902)629-8806; Fax. (902)626-3489.

LANUKE, Kathryn M; 2002D Comox Ave, Comox BC V9M 3M6; Alb'05; FRCSC; GenSurg. (250)339-7115

LAO, Victor K C; 28 Langstaff Rd E, Thornhill ON L3T 3P8; Tor'88; (905)709-9955

LAOSEBIKAN, Adeyemi O; Melfort Hosp, PO Box 1480 510 Broadway Ave, Melfort SK S0E 1A0; Ilorin (Nigeria)'92; MB BS; FRCS(Ed); FRCSC; GenSurg. Staff, Melfort Hospital; (306)752-8775; Fax. (306)752-8777.

LAPAIGE, Veronique; Hop Louis-H Lafontaine, 7401 rue Hochelaga, Montreal QC H1N 3M5; (Belgium)'93; Staff, Hopital Louis-H Lafontaine; (514)251-4015 x3280

LAPALME, Sophie; CSSS de Trois-Rivières, 1991 boul du Carmel, Trois-Rivieres QC G8Z 3R9; Laval'99; FRCPC; Neur. Staff, CSSS de Trois-Rivières; Langs: Bilingual(French/English); (819)697-3333

LAPENA, Hilario S; Taunton Health Centre, SS 201 1290 Keith Ross Dr, Oshawa ON L1H 7K4; University of the East (Philippines)'87; CCFP; Langs: Tagalog; (905)721-4165

LAPENA, U Elsa O; Taunton Health Centre, 1290 Keith Ross Dr, Oshawa ON L1H 7K4; University of the East (Philippines)'84; CCFP; Langs: Tagalog; (905)721-4164; Fax. (905)721-6687.

LAPENSEE, Louise; Clinique de Fertilite OVO, 100-8000 boul Decarie, Montreal QC H4P 2S4; Laval'89; FRCSC; ObstGyn (Infertility).

LAPERRIERE, Daniel; CHUQ-Ctr Hosp Univ Laval, 2705 boul Laurier, Quebec QC G1V 4G2; Mon'97; Staff, Centre Hospitalier Universitaire de Quebec-CHUL; (418)656-4141

LAPERRIERE, Gilles; CSSS de Trois-Rivières, 1991 boul du Carmel, Trois-Rivieres QC G8Z 3R9; Laval'79; CSPQ; FRCPC; Anes. Staff, CSSS de Trois-Rivières; (819)697-3333

LAPERRIERE, Helene; CSSS Jeanne-Mance, 100-15 av du Mont-Royal O, Montreal QC H2T 2R9; Mon'77; CCFP; FCFP; Conférencier Family Med, McGill University; (514)286-9657

LAPERRIERE, J Normand; Univ Hlth Network-Princess M, 610 University Ave, Toronto ON M5G 2M9; Tor'78; AB; FRCPC; RadOncol (Brain Tumors). Staff Radiol, Princess Margaret Hospital - University Health Network; Staff, The Hospital For Sick Children; Assoc Prof, University of Toronto; (416)946-2127; Fax. (416)946-2227; norm.laperriere@rmp.uhn.on.ca.

LAPERRIERE, Jean; CHUM-Hotel-Dieu, 3840 rue Saint-Urbain, Montreal QC H2W 1T8; Mon'70; DiagRad. Staff, Centre Hospitalier l'Université de Montréal (CHUM) - Hôtel-Dieu; adj Prof, Universite de Montreal; (514)890-8150

LAPERRIERE, Luc; Clinique Med de Mirabel, CP 1059 Succ St-Janvier 13714 boul du Curé-Labelle, Mirabel QC J7J 1A1; Mon'88; Langs: English; (450)435-7666

LAPERRIERE, Rene; 2-4074 boul Lasalle, Verdun QC H4G 2A2; Laval'68; Psy. (514)765-8177; Fax. (514)658-1181.

LAPERRIERE-NGUYEN, Eric V; Ctr Hosp de Verdun, 4000 boul Lasalle, Verdun QC H4G 2A3; McG'94; Staff, Centre Hospitalier de Verdun; Consultant, CMDP & CMA Administration; Langs: English; Spanish; (514)362-1000

LAPETSKY, Angela M; Lakeside Med Clinic, 3919 8th St E, Saskatoon SK S7H 5M7; Sask'03; BSc(Biol); CCFP; Teach Staff College of Med, University of Saskatchewan; (306)374-6884; Fax. (306)374-2552.

LAPEYRAQUE, Anne-Laure; Hôpital Ste-Justine, 3175 ch Cote-Sainte-Catherine, Montreal QC H3T 1C5; Paris (France)'96; Clinical Asst Prof, Hôpital Ste-Justine; (514)345-4931; alapeyraque@sympatico.ca.

LAPIE, Frederique; Centre Med de Chambly, 205-1101 boul Brassard, Chambly QC J3L 5R4; Sher'89; Staff General Med, Hôpital du Haut-Richelieu; (450)658-6601; Fax. (450)658-7849.

LAPIE, Veronique; CHUS-Hop Fleurimont, 3001 12e av N, Sherbrooke QC J1H 5N4; Mon'90; FRCSC; GenSurg; VascSurg. Consultant Vascular Surg, Centre Hospitalier de Granby; Chef chir gén, Centre Hospitalier Universitaire de Sherbrooke-Hopital Fleurimont; adj Prof Med, Universite de Sherbrooke; Langs: English; (819)346-1110 x14356; Fax. (819)820-6871; veronique.lapie@usherbrooke.ca.

LAPIERRE, Andre J; Hop Maisonneuve-Rosemont, 5415 boul de l'Assomption, Montreal QC H1T 2M4; Mon'69; Cardiol. Staff, Hopital Maisonneuve-Rosemont; Langs: English; (514)252-3812; Fax. (514)252-3835.

LAPIERRE, Benoit; CLSC Notre-Dame-De-Grace, 110-2525 boul Cavendish, Montreal QC H4B 2Y4; Sher'86; CCFP; FCFP; (514)485-1670; Fax. (514)485-6406.

LAPIERRE, Bernard; Clinique Med Adoncour, 505 rue Adoncour, Longueuil QC J4G 2M6; Mon'71; LMCC; Staff GenMed & Perinatal, Centre Hospitalier Pierre Boucher; Langs: English; (450)646-4445; Fax. (450)646-5526.

LAPIERRE, Chantale; Hôpital Ste-Justine, 3175 ch Cote-Sainte-Catherine, Montreal QC H3T 1C5; Sher'93; FRCPC; DiagRad (Pediatric Radiology). Staff, Hôpital Ste-Justine; (514)345-4637; Fax. (514)345-4816; lapierrechantale@hotmail.com.

LAPIERRE, Claude; 13e-935 rue de la Gauchetiere, Montreal QC H3B 2M9; Mon'65; Langs: Bilingual(French/English); (514)696-5802; Fax. (514)696-2952; domicileclaude.lap@videotron.ca.

LAPIERRE, Claudie; CLSC Simonne-Monet-Chartrand, 1303 boul Jacques-Cartier E, Longueuil QC J4M 2Y8; Laval'92; (450)463-2850 x2240; Fax. (450)463-1879.

LAPIERRE, Harry; Univ of Ottawa Heart Institute, H 3413-40 Ruskin St, Ottawa ON K1Y 4W7; Mon'94; FRCSC; CardSurg. Staff, University of Ottawa Heart Institute; (613)761-4125; Fax. (613)761-4712.

LAPIERRE, Jean-Guy; Hôpital Ste-Justine, 3175 ch Cote-Sainte-Catherine, Montreal QC H3T 1C5; Mon'69; FRCPC; Peds; Respir (P.Q.). Staff, Hôpital Ste-Justine; Langs: Bilingual(French/English); (514)345-4931 x5409; Fax. (514)345-4804; guylapierre@videotron.ca.

LAPIERRE, Julie; Inst U Geriatrie Sherbrooke, 375 rue Argyll, Sherbrooke QC J1J 3H5; Mon'94; FRCPC; IntMed; GeriatricMed. Staff, Institut Universitaire de Geriatrie de Sherbrooke-Pavillon Argyll; (819)821-1150; Fax. (819)829-7145; jlapierre.iugs@ssss.gouv.qc.ca.

LAPIERRE, Louis; Centre Eva Sante, 1001 rue Saint-Denis, Montreal QC H2X 3H9; Mon'56; FRCPC; IntMed. Consultant Hlth Assessment Ctre de la Fondation, Centre Hospitalier l'Université de Montréal (CHUM) - Hôpital Notre-Dame; Langs: English; (514)890-8323; Fax. (514)412-7362.

LAPIERRE, Luc; Clinique Nouveau Depart, 1110 av Beaumont, Mont-Royal QC H3P 3E5; Mon'05; CCFP; (514)521-9023

LAPIERRE, Melanie; Clinique Med de l'Ouest, 2200 boul Dionne, Saint-Georges QC G5Y 3X3; Sher'08; (418)228-2024

LAPIERRE, Michel; GMF Jacques-Cartier, 200-1815 rue King O, Sherbrooke QC J1J 2E3; Sher'78; (819)565-7557

LAPIERRE, Nathalie; Clinique De Med Fam Montcalm, 309 rue Montcalm, Chicoutimi QC G7J 2V1; Laval'97; (418)545-4211; Fax. (418)545-2920.

LAPIERRE, Odile; Inst Albert Prevost, 6555 boul Gouin O, Montreal QC H4K 1B3; Mon'90; FRCPC; Psy. Staff, Hôpital du Sacre-Coeur de Montréal; (514)338-4356; Fax. (514)338-4357.

LAPIERRE, Patricia; CHSLD Chanoine-Audet, 2155 ch du Salt, Saint-Romuald QC G6W 2K7; Laval'96; Staff, Centre Hospitalier Paul-Gilbert; Langs: English; (418)834-5322

LAPIERRE, Patrick; CHUS-Hop Hotel-Dieu, 580 rue Bowen S, Sherbrooke QC J1G 2E8; Sher'99; FRCPC; Psy. Staff Psy, Centre Hospitalier Universitaire de Sherbrooke-Hôpital Hôtel-Dieu; (819)346-1110 x26546; Fax. (819)829-6259.

LAPIERRE, Paul D; Lasik MD, 330 Torbay Rd, St. John's NL A1A 4E1; Mon'90; DAB; FRCSC; Ophth (General Ophthalmic Surgery).

LAPIERRE, Sylvain; CSSS de Trois-Rivières, 1991 boul du Carmel, Trois-Rivieres QC G8Z 3R9; Laval'95; FRCSC; Urol. Staff, CSSS de Trois-Rivières; (819)697-3333

LAPIERRE, Yves L; MUHC-Montreal Neurology Inst, 267-3801 rue University, Montreal QC H3A 2B4; Mon'66; CSPQ; Neur (Multiple Sclerosis). Staff, McGill University Health Centre - Montreal Neurological Hospital; assoc Prof, McGill University; Langs: English; French; (514)398-1931; Fax. (514)398-7454.

LAPIERRE, Yves; CSSS de Beauce-Etchemin, 1515 17e rue, Saint-Georges QC G5Y 4T8; Mon'04; FRCPC; Psy. Staff, Centre Hospitalier Beauce-Etchemin; Langs: Bilingual(French/English); (418)228-2068; Fax. (418)227-1081.

LAPIN, Henry D; Ctr Hosp de Lasalle, 8585 Tsse Champlain, Lasalle QC H8P 1C1; McG'93; FRCPC; IntMed. Staff, Centre Hospitalier de LaSalle; (514)362-8000

LAPIN, Jonathan L; 53 Farnham Ave, Toronto ON M4V 1H6; McG'88; FRCPC; DiagRad. Langs: Bilingual(English/French); (416)691-5071

LAPINSKY, Anne S; Queenston Med & Dental Centre, 202-631 Queenston Rd, Hamilton ON L8K 6R5; Qns'69; Staff, St Joseph's Healthcare - Charlton Campus; (905)560-4600; Fax. (905)560-2644.

LAPINSKY, J Gerald; Queenston Med & Dental Centre, 202-631 Queenston Rd, Hamilton ON L8K 6R5; Qns'68; Ac Staff, St Joseph's Healthcare - Charlton Campus; (905)560-4600; Fax. (905)560-2644.

LAPINSKY, Nicola-Ann; Vancouver Breast Centre, 505-750 Broadway W, Vancouver BC V5Z 1H4; Witwatersrand (South Africa)'85; FRCPC; DiagRad. (604)879-4177; Fax. (604)879-4147.

LAPINSKY, Stephen E; Mount Sinai Hosp, 18-214-600 University Ave, Toronto ON M5G 1X5; Witwatersrand (South Africa)'81; MSc; MB BS; FRCPC; IntMed (Critical Care Medicine). Ac Staff, Mount Sinai Hospital; Assoc Prof, University of Toronto; (416)586-4800 x3211; Fax. (416)586-8480; stephen.lapinsky@utoronto.ca.

LAPLANTE, Alain; CSSS de Rimouski-Neigette, CP 3150 Succ A 150 av Rouleau, Rimouski QC G5L 5T1; Laval'02; FRCSC; Ophth. Staff, Hôpital Regional Rimouski; (418)724-3000

LAPLANTE, Bernard; CSSS de Sept-Iles, 45 rue du Pere-Divet, Sept-Iles QC G4R 3N7; Mon'79; Staff, Centre Hospitalier Regional de Sept-Iles; Langs: English; (418)968-8274; Fax. (418)962-8121; bjlaplante@hotmail.com.

LAPLANTE, Bruno T; Expertise Psycho-Med de Quebec, 989 av Casot, Quebec QC G1S 2Y2; Laval'74; FRCPC; Psy. (418)524-6484

LAPLANTE, Claude; CHUS-Hop Fleurimont, 3001 12e av N, Sherbrooke QC J1H 5N4; Sher'97; FRCPC; AnatPath. Staff, Centre Hospitalier Universitaire de Sherbrooke-Hopital Fleurimont; (819)346-1110 x15331

LAPLANTE, Francine; CSSS Drummond-Hop Sainte-Croix, 570 rue Heriot, Drummondville QC J2B 1C1; Sher'93; CSPQ; Anes. Staff, Hôpital Sainte-croix; (819)478-6464; Fax. (819)478-6465.

LAPLANTE, Francois; Clinique Med Du Quartier Latin, 905 boul Rene-Levesque E, Montreal QC H2L 5B1; Mon'81; LMCC; (514)285-5500; Fax. (514)285-2226.

LAPLANTE, Gerald; Centre medical Le Mesnil, 300-1300 boul Lebourgneuf, Quebec QC G2K 2N1; Sher'87; (418)624-1800

LAPLANTE, Jacques; Hop Du Sacre-Coeur De Mtl, 5400 boul Gouin O, Montreal QC H4J 1C5; Mon'83; FRCPC; IntMed; MedOncol (P.Q.); Hem (P.Q.). Dir Prof Services/Staff, Hôpital du Sacre-Coeur de Montréal; (514)338-2050

LAPLANTE, Joanne; Clinique Med Du Coteau, 100-440 boul Saint-Luc, St-Jean-sur-Richel QC J2W 0E2; Mon'96; (450)359-6819

LAPLANTE, Lise; Tour A-800 Boul Chomedey, Laval QC H7V 3Y4; Mon'83; MSc(CommunHealth); Med Consultant Environmental & Industrial Med, Hopital de la Cite de la santé; Physician Dir de Sante Publique, Agence de Sante et des Service Sociaux de Laval; Clin Prof Social & Preventive Med, Universite de Montreal; (450)978-2101; Fax. (450)978-2100; lise_laplante@ssss.gouv.qc.ca.

LAPLANTE, Lucie; CHUM-Hop Notre-Dame, 1560 rue Sherbrooke E, Montreal QC H2L 4M1; Laval'78; Membre Palliative Care Serv, Centre Hospitalier l'Université de Montréal (CHUM) - Hôpital Notre-Dame; Clin Prof, Universite de Montreal; Langs: English; (514)890-8000 x24444; lucie.laplante.chum@ssss.gouv.qc.ca.

LAPLANTE, Odette; ASSS Chaudière-Appalaches, 12e-373 rte Cameron, Sainte-Marie QC G6E 3E2; Ott'75; FRCPC; CommunMed. Ac Member DSC, Hôtel-Dieu de Lévis; (418)266-6770; Fax. (418)266-6779; odette.laplante@msss.gouv.qc.ca.

LAPLANTE, Patrice; Clinique médicale de Fleurimon, 210-2140 rue King E, Sherbrooke QC J1G 5G6; Sher'86; CCFP; Staff, Centre Hospitalier Universitaire de Sherbrooke-Hopital Fleurimont; (819)563-4462; Fax. (819)563-4464.

LAPLANTE, Patrick; CSSS de la Haute-Yamaska, 205 boul Leclerc O, Granby QC J2G 1T7; Laval'97; Staff Med, Centre Hospitalier de Granby; Clinical Asst Prof, Universite de Sherbrooke; (450)372-5491 x2122

LAPLANTE, Pierre; Clinique Med Saint-Sauveur, 70 rue Principale, Saint-Sauveur QC J0R 1R6; Mon'63; Derm. (450)227-8436

LAPLANTE, Pierre; Hop Maisonneuve-Rosemont, 5415 boul de l'Assomption, Montreal QC H1T 2M4; Mon'78; Neur. Staff, Hopital Maisonneuve-Rosemont; adj Prof Med, Universite de Montreal; (514)252-3528; Fax. (514)252-3529.

LAPLANTE, Raymonde; CLSC Ste-Therese de Blainville, 125 rue Duquet, Sainte-Therese QC J7E 0A5; Mon'83; (450)430-4553; Fax. (450)430-3859.

LAPLANTE, Renaud; Dr Georges-L Dumont Reg Hosp, 330 Av Universite, Moncton NB E1C 2Z3; Laval'96; FRCPC; Anes. Staff Anes, Dr Georges-L-Dumont University Hospital Centre; (506)862-4000; Fax. (506)862-4256.

LAPLANTE, Richard; CSSS Drummond-Hop Sainte-Croix, 570 rue Heriot, Drummondville QC J2B 1C1; Laval'89; FRCSC; GenSurg (Surgical Oncology). Staff, Hôpital Sainte-croix; Langs: English; (819)478-6464; Fax. (819)850-0822.

LAPLANTE, Severine; St Mary's Hosp Centre, 3830 av Lacombe, Montreal QC H3T 1M5; McG'01; CCFP; Staff, St Mary's Hospital Centre; (514)734-2677; Fax. (514)734-2602.

LAPLANTE, Sophie; Radiologie Laennec Inc, 104-1100 av Beaumont, Mont-Royal QC H3P 3H5; Mon'87; FRCPC; DiagRad (Abdominal Radiology). Directrice Med Board, Imagix Imaging Medicale; Langs: English; (514)738-6866; slaplante@imagixmedical.com.

LAPLANTE PAQUIN, Tristan; CSSS du Lac-des-Deux-Montagnes, 520 boul Arthur-Sauve, Saint-Eustache QC J7R 5B1; Mon'10; Staff, Hôpital de Saint-Eustache; (450)473-6811

LAPNER, Manfred; Riverside Prof Centre, 205-1919 Riverside Dr, Ottawa ON K1H 1A2; Qns'69; FRCPC; Peds (Community Pediatrics). Emeritus Staff, Children's Hospital of Eastern Ontario (CHEO); Sec Head Medical Devices Bureau, Health Canada; Asst Prof, University of Ottawa; Langs: German; French; (613)737-3121; Fax. (613)737-6048.

LAPNER, Michael A C; St Joseph's Health Care, PO Box 5777 Stn B 268 Grosvenor St, London ON N6A 4V2; McM'06; OrthSurg. Staff, St Joseph's Hospital - St Joseph's Health Care; Langs: Bilingual(English/French); (519)646-6100

LAPNER, Peter L C; The Ottawa Hosp-Gen Campus, Box 502 CCW 1648-501 Smyth Rd, Ottawa ON K1H 8L6; Tor'96; FRCSC; OrthSurg (Shoulder). Staff, The Ottawa Hospital - General Campus; Langs: French; (613)737-8377; Fax. (613)737-8837.

LAPOINTE, Andre; Ctr Hosp Laurentien, 234 rue Saint-Vincent, Ste-Agathe-Des-Mts QC J8C 2B8; Mon'81; DSc; Staff Commun Med, Centre Hospitalier Laurentien; Staff, Hôtel-Dieu de Saint-Jérôme; Coroner, Occupational Health & Safety; (819)326-3111

LAPOINTE, Andre; Clin d'Ophtalmologie Saguenay, 150 boul Barrette, Chicoutimi QC G7H 7W8; Laval'88; FRCSC; Ophth. (418)545-2571; Fax. (418)545-0774.

LAPOINTE, Anie; Hôpital Ste-Justine, 3175 ch Cote-Sainte-Catherine, Montreal QC H3T 1C5; Laval'05; FRCPC; Peds (Neonatal & Perinatal Medicine). Staff, Hôpital Ste-Justine; (514)345-4931

LAPOINTE, Annie; Hôpital Ste-Justine, 3175 ch Cote-Sainte-Catherine, Montreal QC H3T 1C5; Laval'96; FRCSC; Otol (Head & Neck Surgery). Staff, Hôpital Ste-Justine; (514)345-4788

LAPOINTE, Annie-Pier; Centre Medical Des Generations, 200-465 rue Bibeau, Saint-Eustache QC J7R 0C8; Laval'10; (450)472-1955

LAPOINTE, Bernard; SMBD Jewish Gen Hosp, 3755 ch Cote-Sainte-Catherine, Montreal QC H3T 1E2; Sher'80; Staff, Sir Mortimer B Davis Jewish General; (514)340-8222; blapoint@onc.jgh.mcgill.ca.

LAPOINTE, Carole; CSSS de Laval, 1755 boul Rene-Laennec, Laval QC H7M 3L9; Mon'92; FRCPC; IntMed; MedOncol; Hem. Staff, Hopital de la Cite de la santé; (450)668-1010; Fax. (450)975-5044.

LAPOINTE, Carole S M; 444 Algoma St N, Thunder Bay ON P7A 5B9; Mon'75; FRCPC; Psy (Consultation). Langs: Bilingual(French/English); (807)766-8239; Fax. (807)766-9401.

LAPOINTE, Caroline; Rockland MD, 110-100 ch Rockland, Mont-Royal QC H3P 2V9; Laval'04; Staff, Centre Hospitalier Notre-Dame-du-Lac; (514)667-3383

LAPOINTE, Claude; Clinique Med Havre Sante, 521 boul Du Havre, Salaber-de-Valleyf QC J6S 4Z5; Laval'78; Staff, Centre Hospitalier Régional du Suroît; Physician, Royal Canadian Mounted Police; (450)371-6444; Fax. (450)371-5315.

LAPOINTE, Claude; Centre Hosp Honore-Mercier, 2750 boul Laframboise, Saint-Hyacinthe QC J2S 4Y8; Laval'80; Consultant, Centre Hospitalier Honore-Mercier; (450)771-3333

LAPOINTE, Claude; Clinique Med Fam des Recollets, 101-940 boul des Recollets, Trois-Rivieres QC G8Z 3W9; Laval'78; Staff, Centre de santé Cloutier-du-Rivage; (819)373-0303

LAPOINTE, Daniel; CHUQ-Ctr Hosp Univ Laval, 2705 boul Laurier, Quebec QC G1V 4G2; Laval'99; CSPQ; FRCPC; Anes. Staff, Centre Hospitalier Universitaire de Quebec-CHUL; (418)525-4444

LAPOINTE, Elise S; Inst de Readaptation de Mtl, 6300 av de Darlington, Montreal QC H3S 2J4; McG'06; MDCM; CCFP; Staff, Institut de Réadaptation Gingras-Lindsay de Montréal; (514)340-2085

LAPOINTE, Genevieve; Ctr Hosp Affilie-Enfant-Jesus, 1401 18e rue, Quebec QC G1J 1Z4; Laval'02; FRCSC; Neursurg. Staff, Centre Hospitalier Affilié Universitaire de Québec - Hôpital De L'Enfant Jésus; (418)649-5882

LAPOINTE, Gerald; Clinique Med Varennes, 201-2082 rte Marie-Victorin, Varennes QC J3X 2C7; Mon'71; Langs: Bilingual(French/English); (450)652-2959; Fax. (450)652-3792; dr_lapointe@yahoo.ca.

LAPOINTE, Helene; Clinique Medicale d'Alma, 935 av du Pont S, Alma QC G8B 2V5; Laval'09; CCFP; (418)668-6121

LAPOINTE, Isabelle; CHUQ-Hotel-Dieu de Quebec, 11 Cote du Palais, Quebec QC G1R 2J6; Laval'04; FRCPC; IntMed; Nephrol. Staff, Centre Hospitalier Universitaire de Québec (CHUQ) - Siege Social; (418)525-4444; Fax. (418)691-5757.

LAPOINTE, Jacques; CHUM-Montreal Gen Hosp, 1650 av Cedar, Montreal QC H3G 1A4; Laval'92; CCFP; Staff, McGill University Health Centre - Montreal General Campus; (514)934-1934

LAPOINTE, Jacques; Hop Maisonneuve-Rosemont, 5415 boul de l'Assomption, Montreal QC H1T 2M4; Mon'81; Cardiol (P.Q.); IntMed. Staff, Hopital Maisonneuve-Rosemont; Universite de Montreal; (514)252-3812; Fax. (514)252-3835.

LAPOINTE, Jean; Hotel-Dieu de Levis, 143 rue Wolfe, Levis QC G6V 3Z1; Laval'87; CCFP; CCFP(E.M.); EmergMed (P.Q.). Staff, Hôtel-Dieu de Lévis; Staff, Centre Hospitalier Affilié Universitaire de Québec - Hôpital De L'Enfant Jésus; Member, Aeromedicale de Quebec; adj Prof, Université Laval; (418)835-7122

LAPOINTE, Jessica; Clinique Med Grande Ourse, 534 3e rue, Chibougamau QC G8P 1N9; Sher'09; CCFP; (418)748-3469

LAPOINTE, Joris; Centre Med Jonquiere, CP 1500 Succ Pdf Jonquiere 1955 boul Mellon, Jonquiere QC G7S 4L2; Sher'84; LMCC; CASM(DipSportMed); Staff, Centre Hospitalier Jonquiere; (418)699-2111

LAPOINTE, Louis; CSSS de Rivière-de-Loup, 75 rue Saint-Henri, Riviere-Du-Loup QC G5R 2A4; Mon'82; GenSurg. Ac Staff, Centre Hospitalier Regional du Grand-Portage; (418)868-1000; Fax. (418)868-3336.

LAPOINTE, Luc; Ctr Hosp de Verdun, 4000 boul Lasalle, Verdun QC H4G 2A3; Mon'84; CCFP; Staff, Centre Hospitalier de Verdun; (514)765-7325; Fax. (514)765-7306.

LAPOINTE, Lucie; Clin Med Plateau Mont-Royal, 103-1374 av Mont-Royal E, Montreal QC H2J 1Y7; Mon'93; Staff, Hôpital de Saint-Eustache; (514)527-3997

LAPOINTE, Marc; CLSC-CHSLD de Gatineau, 80 av Gatineau, Gatineau QC J8T 4J3; Ott'85; (819)561-2001

LAPOINTE, Marc-Henry; CSSS du Lac-Temiscamingue, 22 rue Notre-Dame N, Ville-Marie QC J9V 1W8; Laval'76; FRCPC; Psy. Staff, CSSS du Témiscamingue; Langs: English; (819)629-2420; Fax. (819)629-3257.

LAPOINTE, Marie; CSSS de Chicoutimi, 305 rue Saint-Vallier, Chicoutimi QC G7H 5H6; Laval'79; Staff Unite de Med de Famille, Complexe hospitalier de la Sagamie; Prof Full-Time Geog, Universite de Sherbrooke; (418)541-1079; Fax. (418)541-1129.

LAPOINTE, Marie; Clinique Med Blainville, 519 boul du Curé-Labelle, Blainville QC J7C 2H6; Mon'74; Staff, Hôtel-Dieu de Saint-Jérôme; (450)430-2431; Fax. (450)430-1274.

LAPOINTE, Marie-Louise; 507-595 Montreal Rd, Ottawa ON K1K 4L2; McG'78; FRCSC; Ophth. Staff, The Ottawa Hospital - Riverside Campus; Staff, The Ottawa Hospital - General Campus; Asst Prof Ophth, University of Ottawa; (613)741-2020; Fax. (613)741-5997.

LAPOINTE, Marie-Noel; Ctr Hosp Affilie-Enfant-Jesus, 1401 18e rue, Quebec QC G1J 1Z4; Laval'04; FRCPC; DiagRad. Staff, Centre Hospitalier Affilié Universitaire de Québec - Hôpital De L'Enfant Jésus; (418)649-5782

LAPOINTE, Mario; Centre Hosp Honore-Mercier, 2750 boul Laframboise, Saint-Hyacinthe QC J2S 4Y8; Mon'87; MSc; Staff, Centre Hospitalier Honore-Mercier; (450)771-3335; Fax. (450)467-0946.

LAPOINTE, Mario; 1217 Boul Sainte-Genevieve, Chicoutimi QC G7G 2G8; Laval'78; Ac Staff, Complexe hospitalier de la Sagamie; (418)693-0036; Fax. (418)693-0036.

LAPOINTE, Martin; Clinique Med St-Sauveur, 70 rue Principale RR 6, Saint-Sauveur QC J0R 1R6; Mon'90; Staff, Hôpital du Sacre-Coeur de Montréal; (450)227-8436; Fax. (450)227-7222.

LAPOINTE, Michel A; 4225 boul Dorchester O, Westmount QC H3Z 1V5; Mon'83; CCFP; Physician, Citizenship & Immigration Canada; Langs: Italian; English; (514)939-8303

LAPOINTE, Michel; CSSS de Trois-Rivières, 1991 boul du Carmel, Trois-Rivieres QC G8Z 3R9; Laval'81; Respir; IntMed. Staff, CSSS de Trois-Rivières; (819)697-3333; Fax. (819)371-1360.

LAPOINTE, Nicole; CSSS de la Vallée de l'Or, 725 6e rue, Val-d'Or QC J9P 3Y1; Laval'67; DPsy; Psy (Pedology Psychiatry). Consultant PedoPsy, Hôpital de l'Archipel; Consultant PedoPsy, Centre Hospitalier Rouyn-Noranda; Consultant PedoPsy, Centre Hospitalier de Val d'Or; (819)825-5858

LAPOINTE, Normand; Hôpital Ste-Justine, 3175 ch Cote-Sainte-Catherine, Montreal QC H3T 1C5; Mon'63; MSc; FRCPC; Peds (Clinical Immunology & Allergy). Staff, Hôpital Ste-Justine; Langs: English; (514)345-4713; Fax. (514)345-4897.

LAPOINTE, Pierre; Coop Sante Val-Morin, GD 6162 rue Morin, Val-Morin QC J0T 2R0; Paris (France)'81; Staff, Centre Hospitalier Laurentien; (819)320-0488

LAPOINTE, Pierre; 143 rue Wolfe, Levis QC G6V 3Z1; Laval'98; CRCP; CSPQ; FRCSC; OrthSurg (Upper Extremity Surgery). Staff, Hôtel-Dieu de Lévis; Langs: French; English; (418)835-7121; pslapointe@hotmail.com.

LAPOINTE, Pierre; Clinique Med De Matane, 101-548 av Du Phare E, Matane QC G4W 1A7; Laval'74; Staff, Centre Hospitalier de Matane; (418)562-4530; Fax. (418)562-4532.

LAPOINTE, Real; CHUM-Hop St-Luc, 9304 B-1058 rue Saint-Denis, Montreal QC H2X 3J4; Laval'76; FRCSC; GenSurg (Hepatobiliary & Pancreatic Surgery). Chef chir gén, Centre Hospitalier l'Université De Montréal (CHUM) - Hôpital Saint-luc; Chef Div of Surg, Universite de Montreal; Langs: Bilingual(French/English); (514)890-8000 x36146; Fax. (514)412-7380; real.lapointe.chum@ssss.gouv.qc.ca.

LAPOINTE, Richard H; 200 boul Henri-Bourassa E, Montreal QC H3L 1B8; Mon'83; PlasSurg (Esthetic Plastic Surgery). Langs: Bilingual(French/English); (514)744-3377

LAPOINTE, Richard; Clinique Med d'Asbestos, 605 boul Simoneau, Asbestos QC J1T 4G7; Mon'76; (819)879-7447

LAPOINTE, Richard; Clinique Med du Cuivre, 12 rue Gamble E, Rouyn-Noranda QC J9X 3B7; Sher'83; Langs: Bilingual(French/English); (819)764-9441; Fax. (819)764-5792.

LAPOINTE, Romuald; Clin Med du Faubourg, 2655 boul du Royaume, Jonquiere QC G7S 4S9; Laval'75; Staff, Complexe hospitalier de la Sagamie; (418)699-0005; Fax. (418)699-1220.

LAPOINTE, Stephanie; UMF de Repentigny, 135 boul Claude-David, Repentigny QC J6A 1N6; Mon'08; CCFP; (450)654-2911

LAPOINTE, Steven P; Polyclinique Med Concorde, 300 boul de la Concorde E, Laval QC H7G 2E6; Mon'92; FRCSC; Urol. Staff, Hôpital Ste-Justine; (450)667-5310

LAPOINTE, Steven; College des Med du Quebec, 2170 boul Rene-Levesque O, Montreal QC H3H 2T8; Mon'78; FRCSC; Urol. Asst Prof Urol, Universite de Montreal; (514)933-4441

LAPOINTE, Veronique; CSSS de Manicouagan, 635 boul Jolliet, Baie-Comeau QC G5C 1P1; Sher'07; IntMed. Staff, Centre Hospitalier Régional Baie-Comeau.

LAPOINTE, Veronique; 500 boul de l'Hopital, Gatineau QC J8V 2P5; Laval'08; CCFP; (819)966-6171

LAPOINTE, Veronique; CSSS de Saint-Jerome, 290 rue de Montigny, Saint-Jerome QC J7Z 5T3; Sher'07; FRCPC; MedMicrobiol. Staff, Hôtel-Dieu de Saint-Jérôme; (450)432-2777

LAPOINTE, Yves J; 929 3e Av, Val-d'Or QC J9P 1T4; Laval'81; (819)825-3975; Fax. (819)874-9191.

LAPOINTE, Yves; CHUM-Hop Notre-Dame, 1560 rue Sherbrooke E, Montreal QC H2L 4M1; Mon'68; HemPath (Transfusion Medicine). ac Staff, Centre Hospitalier l'Université de Montréal (CHUM) - Hôpital Notre-Dame; (514)890-8000 x28228; Fax. (514)412-7530.

LAPOINTE-MILOT, Korine; The Ottawa Hosp-Gen Campus, 501 Smyth Rd, Ottawa ON K1H 8L6; Sher'05; ObstGyn. Staff, The Ottawa Hospital - General Campus; (613)737-8560

LAPOINTE-SHAW, Lauren; Univ Hlth Network-Toronto Gen, 14 217-200 Elizabeth St, Toronto ON M5G 2C4; McG'09; Staff, Toronto General Hospital - UHN; (416)340-3155

LAPORTA, Donald P; SMBD Jewish Gen Hosp, 3755 ch Cote-Sainte-Catherine, Montreal QC H3T 1E2; McG'77; ABIM; FRCPC; IntMed; Critical Care Medicine (P.Q.); Respir. Staff IntMed, Sir Mortimer B Davis Jewish General; adj Prof, McGill University; (514)340-7500; Fax. (514)340-8133; dlaporta@icu.jgh.mcgill.ca.

LAPORTA, Marc; Allan Memorial Institute, 1025 av des Pins O, Montreal QC H3A 1A1; McG'82; FRCPC; Psy (Mood Disorders). Staff, McGill University Health Centre - Royal Victoria Hospital; adj Prof, McGill University; Langs: French; Italian; (514)934-1934 x34393; Fax. (514)843-2958.

LAPORTE, Bertrand; PO Box 870, Campbellton NB E3N 3H3; Mon'81; Staff, Hôpital Régional Campbellton; (506)789-0991; Fax. (506)789-7641; blaporte@nbnet.nb.ca.

LAPORTE, Diane; CLSC Lamater, 1317 boul des Seigneurs, Terrebonne QC J6W 5B1; Sher'88; (450)471-2881 x4056

LAPORTE, Guy; CSSS De Sept-Iles, 45 rue du Pere-Divet, Sept-Iles QC G4R 3N7; Laval'05; Staff, Centre Hospitalier Regional de Sept-Iles; (418)962-9761

LAPORTE, Helene; Clinique Med Lanaudiere, 222 rue Bernard, St-Charles-Brromee QC J6E 2C5; Mon'82; assoc Staff, Centre Hospitalier Régional de Lanaudière; (450)755-1033; Fax. (450)753-5558.

LAPORTE, Jean-Luc B; Laboratoire De Med Legale, 12e-1701 rue Parthenais, Montreal QC H2K 3S7; Paris (France)'95; Staff, Centre Hospitalier l'Université de Montréal (CHUM) - Hôpital Notre-Dame; (514)873-3300; jeanluc_laporte@hotmail.com.

LAPORTE, Julie; CSSS Drummond-Hop Sainte-Croix, 570 rue Heriot, Drummondville QC J2B 1C1; Laval'95; DiagRad. Staff, Hôpital Sainte-croix; (819)478-6464

LAPORTE, Nathalie; Ctr Hosp de LaSalle, 8585 Tsse Champlain, LaSalle QC H8P 1C1; Sher'07; ObstGyn. Staff, Centre Hospitalier de LaSalle; (514)362-8000

LAPORTE, Noel P; Regional Mental HC-London, PO Box 5532 Stn B K161-850 Highbury Ave, London ON N6A 4H1; Sask'01; FRCPC; Psy. Staff, Regional Mental Health Care-St Joseph's Health Care; (519)455-5110 x47604

LAPORTE, Pierre; Clin Med Racicot, 520 rue d'Avaugour, Boucherville QC J4B 0G6; Mon'04; Staff, Centre Hospitalier l'Université de Montréal (CHUM) - Hôtel-Dieu; Langs: English; (450)449-7525

LAPORTE, Sophie; CLSC Montreal-Nord, 11441 boul Lacordaire, Montreal-Nord QC H1G 4J9; Mon'92; (514)327-0400; Fax. (514)340-1387.

LAPORTE, Sophie; CSSS de Saint-Jerome, 290 rue de Montigny, Saint-Jerome QC J7Z 5T3; Mon'91; Staff, Hôtel-Dieu de Saint-Jérôme; (450)431-8200

LAPORTE-PROULX, Joanie; Clinique Med de Lavaltrie, 1400 rue Notre-Dame, Lavaltrie QC J5T 1M6; Mon'10; (450)586-1033

LAPOSTOLLE, Annie-Claude; CSSS Haut-Richelieu-Rouville, 920 boul du Seminaire N, St-Jean-sur-Richel QC J3A 1B7; Mon'01; FRCSC; GenSurg. Staff, Hôpital du Haut-Richelieu; (450)359-5000

LAPP, Jonathan F; Halton Healthcare, 327 Reynolds St, Oakville ON L6J 3L7; Qns'81; MCFP(EM); CCFP; CCFP(E.M.); FCFP; Member, Trafalgar Ethics Board; (905)845-2571; jfl@cogeco.ca.

LAPP, Ralph A; Victoria Prof Bldg, 200-1120 Yates St, Victoria BC V8V 3M9; Alb'71; MD; LMCC; BSc; FRCSC; OrthSurg (Arthroplasty). Vis Staff Cons OrthSurg, Victoria General Hospital; Vis Staff Cons OrthSurg, Saanich Peninsula Hospital; Vis Staff Cons OrthSurg, Royal Jubilee Hospital; (250)384-4121; Fax. (250)385-9600.

LAPP, Timothy J; Huntsville Prof Bldg, 206-348 Muskoka Rd 3 N, Huntsville ON P1H 1H8; McM'89; BPHE; MSc; BA; FRCPC; PhysMed&Rehab (Electrodiagnosis). Staff, South Muskoka Memorial Hospital - Muskoka Algonquin Healthcare; Staff, West Parry Sound Health Centre; Evaluator Non-Economic Loss-WCB & Designated Assessment Centre, Med-Rehab Insurance Industry; Asst Prof Med/Member Med, Northern Ontario School of Medicine-Lakehead University; Asst Prof, Laurentian University; (705)787-0333; Fax. (705)787-1808.

LAPPA, Scot V; Northeast Comm Health Ctre, 14007 50 St NW, Edmonton AB T5A 5E4; Sask'90; FRCPC; Peds (Adolescent Medicine). (780)342-4033; Fax. (780)472-5196.

LAPPA-WALKER, Tracy A; Stonegate Comm Health Centre, 150 Berry Rd, Etobicoke ON M8Y 1W3; McM'93; BSc; CCFP; (416)231-7070; Fax. (416)231-6903.

LAPPANO, Sergio; Mitchell Family Doctors, PO Box 790 7 Francis St, Mitchell ON N0K 1N0; Wes'85; BSc; MSc; CCFP; FCFP; (519)348-8402; Fax. (519)348-8400.

LAPPI, Vernon G; Workers' Comp Board, 9912 107 St NW, Edmonton AB T5K 1G5; Sask'78; MSc; FCBOM; FRCPC; OccupMed. Dir Medical Services, Workers' Comp Board; (780)498-3999; Fax. (780)498-7807; vernon.lappi@wcb.ab.ca.

LAPPIN, Susan F; Lockview Med Clinic, 207-159 Cobequid Rd, Lower Sackville NS B4C 2N1; Dal'87; Staff, IWK Health Centre; Lecturer, Dalhousie University; (902)865-7549; Fax. (902)865-7617.

LAPRISE, Benoit; CSSS de Lac-Saint Jean-Est, CP 1300 succ Bureau-Chef 300 boul Champlain S, Alma QC G8B 5W3; Laval'76; FRCSC; OrthSurg (P.Q.) (Trauma). Staff, CSSS de Lac-Saint Jean-Est; (418)669-2000; Fax. (418)344-1299; benoitlaprise@me.com.

LAPRISE, Christine; CSSS de Montmagny-L'Islet, 350 boul Tache O RR 1, Montmagny QC G5V 3R8; Laval'91; FRCSC; GenSurg. Staff, CSSS de Montmagny-L'Islet; (418)884-3240

LAPRISE, Genevieve; CSSS Drummond-Hop Sainte-Croix, 570 rue Heriot, Drummondville QC J2B 1C1; Laval'99; FRCPC; Psy. Staff, Hôpital Sainte-croix; Langs: Bilingual(French/English); (819)478-6464

LAPRISE-DEMERS, Audrey; CSSS de Chicoutimi, 305 rue Saint-Vallier, Chicoutimi QC G7H 5H6; Mon'07; FRCPC; Anes. Staff, Complexe hospitalier de la Sagamie; (418)541-1000

LAPSLEY, Peter K; Caledonia Med Centre, 14 Caithness St E, Caledonia ON N3W 1L4; McM'72; Staff, Hamilton Health Sciences Centre-Juravinski Site; Staff, Hamilton Health Sciences Centre - McMaster University Medical Centre; (905)765-4061; Fax. (905)765-0584.

LAPUSTE, Mihaela F; Vancouver Family Health Centre, 100-2732 Hastings St E, Vancouver BC V5K 1Z9; Cluj-Napoca (Romania)'97; CCFP; Langs: Romanian; (604)253-3166

LAQUERRE, Chantal; CSSS Gatineau-Hull Hosp, 6eN-116 boul Lionel-Emond, Gatineau QC J8Y 1W7; Laval'82; CCFP; FCFP; Staff, Hull Hospital; Langs: Bilingual(French/English); (819)777-2111

LARA CORRALES, Irene; The Hosp for Sick Children, 555 University Ave, Toronto ON M5G 1X8; (Costa Rica)'99; Staff, The Hospital For Sick Children; Asst Prof Peds, University of Toronto; (416)813-7654 x4864; Fax. (416)813-7909.

LARABEE, Sonia; CSSS du Nord de Lanaudière, 1000 boul Sainte-Anne, St-Charles-Brromee QC J6E 6J2; Sher'95; CSPQ; Anes. Staff Anes, Centre Hospitalier Régional de Lanaudière; (450)759-8222 x2960

LARABIE, Lynn M; 411-797 Princess St, Kingston ON K7L 1G1; McM'83; (613)544-8391

LARAMÉE, Benoit; 220-504 rue Notre-Dame, Repentigny QC J6A 2T8; Mon'81; FRCPC; IntMed; ClinImmunol&Allergy. Staff, Centre Hospitalier l'Université de Montréal (CHUM) - Hôpital Notre-Dame; (450)582-2066; Fax. (450)582-6589.

LARAMEE, Delphine; CMF Gatineau, 201-908 boul Maloney E, Gatineau QC J8P 1H5; Mon'04; CCFP; (819)663-7711; Fax. (819)663-9326.

LARAMEE, Jani; Vancouver Native Hlth Society, 449 Hasting St E, Vancouver BC V6A 1P5; McG'08; CCFP; (604)255-9766

LARAMEE, Louise A; Univ of Ottawa Heart Institute, 40 Ruskin St, Ottawa ON K1Y 4W7; Mon'81; FRCPC; IntMed (Interventional Cardiology); Cardiol. Staff, University of Ottawa Heart Institute; Asst Prof Med, The Ottawa Hospital - Civic Campus; Asst Dean Student Affairs, University of Ottawa; (613)593-7532

LARAMEE, Michel; 4-426 boul Saint-Joseph E, Montreal QC H2J 1J5; Mon'92; Psy (P.Q.). (514)656-3340; Fax. (514)656-3341.

LARAMEE, Pierre; CHUM-Hotel-dieu, 3840 rue Saint-Urbain, Montreal QC H2W 1T8; Mon'77; FRCPC; IntMed; Cardiol. Staff, Centre Hospitalier l'Université de Montréal (CHUM) - Hôtel-Dieu; (514)890-8000 x14444

LARANJEIRO, Joao M V; Markham College Med Clinic, 104-474 College St, Toronto ON M6G 1A4; Tor'81; FRCPC; IntMed. (416)961-1326

LARAYA, Jose F G; Ctr Hospitalier de Lasalle, 8585 Tsse Champlain, LaSalle QC H8P 1C1; Qns'07; Anes. Staff, Centre Hospitalier de LaSalle; (514)362-8000

LARAYA, Nadine; 1-523 The Queensway, Etobicoke ON M8Y 1J7; Qns'06; CCFP; Staff Family Med, St Joseph's Health Centre; (416)760-8367

LARBRISSEAU, Albert; Hôpital Ste-Justine, 3175 ch Cote-Sainte-Catherine, Montreal QC H3T 1C5; Mon'67; FRCPC; Peds (P.Q.) (Pediatric Neurology); Neur. ac Staff Ped Neurol, Hôpital Ste-Justine; Prof Peds, Universite de Montreal; Langs: French; Spanish; (514)345-4894; Fax. (514)345-4787; albert_larbrisseau@ssss.gouv.qc.ca.

LARCHE, Margaret J; Charlton Med Centre, 702-25 Charlton Ave E, Hamilton ON L8N 1Y2; Bristol (England)'93; BSc; MB ChB; PhD; Assoc Prof, McMaster University; (905)528-0489; Fax. (905)528-0450.

LARDER, Andrew P; Kelowna Health Centre, 1340 Ellis St, Kelowna BC V1Y 9N1; Cambridge (England)'87; FRCPC; CommunMed; Public Health & Preventive Med. (250)868-7729

LARDNER, David R R; Alberta Children's Hosp, 2888 Shaganappi Trail NW, Calgary AB T3B 6A8; Auckland (New Zealand)'92; MB ChB; Staff Div of Ped Anes, Alberta Children's Hospital; (403)955-7810

LAREAU, Christian; Pontiac Health Centre, 200 rue Argue, Shawville QC J0X 2Y0; Sher'82; FRCPC; DiagRad. Staff, Pontiac Hospital Centre; Langs: Bilingual(French/English); (819)647-2211; Fax. (819)647-6814.

LAREAU, Ross; Clinique Dr Lareau et Dr Larou, 104-2025 boul Hébert, Salaber-de-Valleyf QC J6S 5Y5; Mon'81; (450)373-3365; Fax. (450)373-3282.

LAREDO, E Sheila; Women's College Hosp, 76 Grenville St, Toronto ON M5S 1B2; Tor'91; FRCPC; IntMed; Endocrin&Metab. Staff, Women's College Hospital; Langs: Spanish; French; (416)323-6013

LARENTE, Amelie; Clin de Gynecology et d'Obst, 630 boul du Seminaire N, St-Jean-sur-Richel QC J3B 7X6; Mon'06; ObstGyn. (450)348-1171

LARENTE, Nadine; MUHC-Montreal Gen Hosp, D17 173-1650 av Cedar, Montreal QC H3G 1A4; Sher'90; FRCPC; IntMed (External Clinic); GeriatricMed. Staff, McGill University Health Centre - Montreal General Campus; Staff, CSSS Institut universitaire de gériatrie de Sherbrooke; Staff, Centre Hospitalier Universitaire de Sherbrooke-Hôpital Hôtel-Dieu; adj Prof, Universite de Sherbrooke; (514)934-8015; Fax. (514)934-8286; nadine.larente@muhc.mcgill.ca.

LARGE, Barbara J; Kenderdine Med Clinic, 110-1804 McOrmond Dr, Saskatoon SK S7S 0A6; Sask'81; (306)934-6606; Fax. (306)955-3180.

LARGE, Gregory W; Western Med Clinic, 144 6th St, Brandon MB R7A 3N2; Man'81; (204)727-6451; Fax. (204)727-4150.

LARGOZA, Josef P; Northern Lights Health Region, 7 Hospital St, Fort McMurray AB T9H 1P2; Santo Tomas (Philippines)'73; Northern Lights Regional Health Centre; (780)791-6161; largoza@shaw.ca.

LARI, Harris; Fraser Health Authority, 4F-260 Sherbrooke St, New Westminster BC V3L 3M2; Karachi (Pakistan)'95; MB BS; FRCPC; Psy. (604)520-4662

LARIGAKIS, Steven; Morgan Creek Site Clinic, 106-15252 32 Ave, Surrey BC V3S 0R7; UBC'86; CCFP; CCFP(E.M.); Staff, Peace Arch Hospital; Langs: Greek; (604)542-4885; Fax. (604)542-4225.

LARIN, Pierre; 103-130 rue Saint-Nicolas, Sorel-Tracy QC J3P 6X9; Mon'74; Cardiol. Ac Staff Cardiol, Hôtel-Dieu de Sorel; Langs: Bilingual(French/English); (450)730-0020

LARIOS, Oscar; South Health Campus, 210030-4448 Front St SE, Calgary AB T3M 1M4; Sask'03; BSc(Hons); FRCPC; IntMed; MedMicrobiol (Infection Control); InfectDis. Staff, Foothills Medical Centre; Staff, South Health Campus; Langs: Spanish; (403)956-2888; Fax. (403)956-2966.

LARIVEE, Pierre; CHUS-Hop Fleurimont, 3001 12e Av N, Sherbrooke QC J1H 5N4; Sher'85; FRCPC; IntMed (Pneumology); Respir. Staff, Centre Hospitalier Universitaire de Sherbrooke-Hopital Fleurimont; Staff, Centre Hospitalier Universitaire de Sherbrooke-Hôpital Hôtel-Dieu; Asst Prof Med Service, Universite de Sherbrooke; (819)346-1110 x14463; Fax. (819)820-6422.

LARIVEE, Yanick; CSSS de la Haute-Yamaska, 205 boul Leclerc O, Granby QC J2G 1T7; Mon'96; FACO; MRCS; FRCS; FRCSC; Otol (Hearing Loss). Prés CMDP, Centre Hospitalier de Granby; Clin Prof, Universite de Sherbrooke; Langs: English; French; (450)375-8000; Fax. (450)770-8567.

LARIVIERE, France; CLSC-CHSLD des Maskoutains, 1015 rue Gauthier, Saint-Hyacinthe QC J2S 8T2; Sher'91; (450)778-2572

LARIVIERE, Francois; CHUM-Hotel-Dieu, 3840 rue Saint-Urbain, Montreal QC H2W 1T8; Mon'79; FRCPC; MedBiochem. Staff, Centre Hospitalier l'Université de Montréal (CHUM) - Hôtel-Dieu; Clin Assoc Prof, Universite de Montreal; Langs: English; Italian; (514)890-8000 x15392; francois.lariviere.chum@ssss.gouv.qc.ca.

LARIVIERE, J Louis R; 206-260 Dalhousie St, Ottawa ON K1N 7E4; Ott'76; Langs: Bilingual(French/English); (613)241-2278; Fax. (613)241-3206.

LARIVIERE, Katherine E; The Ottawa Hosp Academic FHT, 210 Melrose Ave, Ottawa ON K1Y 4K7; Ott'06; CCFP; Langs: Bilingual(English/French); (613)761-4334; Fax. (613)761-4200.

LARIVIERE, Luc; CSSS Pierre Boucher, 1333 boul Jacques-Cartier E, Longueuil QC J4M 2A5; Mon'89; CSPQ; GenPath (P.Q.) (Anatomical Pathology). Staff, Centre Hospitalier Pierre Boucher; (450)468-8111 x2274; Fax. (450)468-8201.

LARIVIERE, Michele; 208-260 Dalhousie St, Ottawa ON K1N 7E4; Mon'82; Langs: Bilingual(French/English); (613)241-0888; Fax. (613)241-6201.

LARKAI, Edwin N L; 202-203 Stonebridge Blvd, Saskatoon SK S7T 0G3; Cambridge (England)'76; MB ChB; MRCP; FRCPC; IntMed; Gastroent. Ac Staff, Royal University Hospital; Ac Staff, Saskatoon City Hospital; (306)244-2977; Fax. (306)665-0717.

LARKE, David P; Cambridge Mem Hosp, 700 Coronation Blvd, Cambridge ON N1R 3G2; Wes'91; CCFP; CCFP(E.M.); Staff, Cambridge Memorial Hospital; (519)621-2330

LARKIN, Anne-Marie; Clinique Os'ceans, 34 Place la Salle, Baie-Comeau QC G4Z 1K3; Laval'01; CCFP; CCFP(E.M.); Langs: Bilingual(French/English); (418)296-8881; Fax. (418)296-8870; anne-marie.larkin.1@ulaval.ca.

LARKIN, Emilie; Ctr de Med Familiale de Granby, 48 rue Denison E, Granby QC J2G 4C6; Sher'10; Staff, Centre de médecine familiale de Granby; (450)372-3996

LARKIN, Tara L; Eastside Health Centre, 688A East River Rd, New Glasgow NS B2H 3S1; Dal'05; CCFP; Staff, Aberdeen Regional Hospital; (902)752-3632

LARKIN-CHAGNON, Anne; Clinique Med de Waterloo, GD 100-4900 Foster, Waterloo QC J0E 2N0; Sher'78; Assoc Member, Hôpital Brome-Missisquoi-Perkins; Langs: Spanish; English; (450)539-1102; Fax. (450)539-2551.

LARMER, James; Brighton Family Health Team, PO Box 1510 170 Main St, Brighton ON K0K 1H0; McM'09; CCFP; (613)475-1555; Fax. (613)475-5556.

LAROCHE, Andre M; The Ottawa Hosp-Gen Campus, 501 Smyth Rd, Ottawa ON K1H 8L6; Sher'07; FRCSC; ObstGyn. Staff, The Ottawa Hospital - General Campus; (613)737-8899 x73254

LAROCHE, Annie; Centre Med Saint-Denis, RR 2 202-620 ch des Patriotes, St-Denis-sur-Rich QC J0H 1K0; Laval'00; CCFP; (450)787-3233

LAROCHE, Bruno; CHUQ-St-Francois D'Assise, 10 rue de l'Espinay, Quebec QC G1L 3L5; Laval'72; Urol (Endoscopy Urology). Ac Staff, Centre Hospitalier Universitaire De Québec - Pavillon De St-françois-d'assise; Langs: French; (418)525-4444; Fax. (418)266-2879.

LAROCHE, Caroline; Horizon Feminin, 206-200 rue Durand, Saint-Jerome QC J7Z 7E2; McG'04; FRCSC; ObstGyn. Staff, Hôtel-Dieu de Saint-Jérôme; (450)432-2777

LAROCHE, Catherine; North Shore Health Region, 132 Esplanade W, North Vancouver BC V7M 1A2; UBC'57; FRCPC; Psy (P.Q.). (604)983-6719; Fax. (604)983-6839.

LAROCHE, Chantal; Clinique Med Pelletier, 300-8330 boul Taschereau, Brossard QC J4X 1C2; Sher'90; (450)465-5379; Fax. (450)465-5615.

LAROCHE, Claude; Clinique Med Cadillac, 3435 rue Bossuet, Montreal QC H1M 2M1; Mon'76; (514)253-1211; Fax. (514)253-5091.

LAROCHE, Esther; Polyclinique Med Terrebonne, 201-901 boul des Seigneurs, Terrebonne QC J6W 1T8; Mon'99; Staff, Centre Hospitalier Pierre le Gardeur; Langs: English; (450)471-1117

LAROCHE, Francois; Centre Med St-Redempteur, 210-600 116 Rte, Saint-Nicolas QC G7A 4X8; Laval'85; CCFP; FCFP; (418)831-4455; francois.laroche@gmf.gouv.qc.ca.

LAROCHE, Francois; Centre Med Berger, 208-1000 ch Sainte-Foy, Quebec QC G1S 2L6; Laval'60; FRCPC; DiagRad. Diag Radiol, Hotel-Dieu du Sacre-Coeur de Jesus de Quebec; Staff Radiol, Centre Hospitalier Affilié Universitaire de Québec - Hôpital du St-Sacrement; Diagnostic-Radiology, CSSS de Quebec-Sud; (418)681-6121; Fax. (418)681-0125.

LAROCHE, G Robert; IWK Health Centre, PO Box 9700 Rpo CSC 5850-5980 University Ave, Halifax NS B3K 6R8; Laval'75; FRCSC; Ophth (Ophthalmology Pediatrics & Adult Strabismus). Staff Ped Ophth, IWK Health Centre; Assoc Prof Ophth/Dir Residency Training, Dalhousie University; (902)470-8008

LAROCHE, Jean-Pierre; Clinique Med 201, 104 rue Sainte-Agathe, Ste-Agathe-Des-Mts QC J8C 2K3; Mon'79; Staff, Centre Hospitalier Laurentien; (819)326-1555; Fax. (819)326-8801.

LAROCHE, Julie C; Polyclinique Med des Ponts, 120-1100 boul de la Rive-Sud, Saint-Romuald QC G6W 5M6; Laval'84; Staff, CSSS du Grand Littoral; (418)834-1177; Fax. (418)834-9275.

LAROCHE, Julie; CSSS de la Baie-des-Chaleurs, RR 2 419 boul Perron, Maria QC G0C 1Y0; Mon'94; Psy. Staff, CSSS de la Baie-des-Chaleurs; (418)759-3443

LAROCHE, Liny; UMF Laval, 2690 ch des Quatre-Bourgeois, Quebec QC G1V 0B7; Mon'04; CCFP; (418)656-4795

LAROCHE, Marc C; Hop Santa Cabrini Ospedale, 5655 rue Saint-Zotique E, Montreal QC H1T 1P7; McG'93; FRCPC; IntMed; MedMicrobiol; InfectDis. Staff, Hôpital Santa Cabrini Ospedale; (514)252-6000 x7203; Fax. (514)252-6592.

LAROCHE, Mathieu; Hop du Sacre-Coeur de Mtl, 5400 boul Gouin O, Montreal QC H4J 1C5; Sher'04; FRCSC; Neursurg. Staff, Hôpital du Sacre-Coeur de Montréal; (514)338-2222

LAROCHE, Maxime; Hotel-Dieu de Roberval, 450 rue Brassard, Roberval QC G8H 1B9; Mon'07; Ophth. Staff, Hotel-Dieu de Roberval; (418)275-0110

LAROCHE, P A Paul; Brooklin Med Centre, 1A-5959 Anderson St, Whitby ON L1M 2E9; Tor'90; CCFP; (905)655-3321; Fax. (905)655-4848.

LAROCHE, Robert; 1901 rue Claude, Longueuil QC J4G 1Y5; Sher'76; Langs: English; (450)651-2210; Fax. (450)670-7731; rlaroche@msn.com.

LAROCHE, Steve; CSSS du Sud de Lanaudière, 911 montee des Pionniers, Terrebonne QC J6V 2H2; Sher'95; Psy. Staff, Centre Hospitalier Pierre le Gardeur; (450)654-7525; Fax. (450)470-2640.

LAROCHE, Vincent; Hôpital Laval, 2725 ch Sainte-Foy, Quebec QC G1V 4G5; Laval'98; FRCPC; IntMed (Medical Oncology); Hem. Hematologist, Hôpital Laval; Staff, Centre Hospitalier Affilié Universitaire de Québec - Hôpital De L'Enfant Jésus; Langs: English; (418)656-8711 x5588; vincent.laroche@ssss.gouv.qc.ca.

LAROCHE SAVARD, Amelie; Ctr Hosp Affilie-St-Sacrement, 1050 ch Sainte-Foy, Quebec QC G1S 4L8; Laval'05; FRCPC; Psy. Staff, Centre Hospitalier Affilié Universitaire de Québec - Hôpital du St-Sacrement; (418)682-7898

LAROCHELLE, Andre; CSSS de Jonquiere, CP 1200 Succ Pdf Jonquiere 2230 rue de l'Hopital, Jonquiere QC G7X 7X2; Laval'70; CSPQ; ObstGyn. Staff, Centre Hospitalier Jonquiere; Langs: Spanish; English; (418)695-7700 x2973

LAROCHELLE, Annick; 200-1760 boul Jacques-Cartier, Longueuil QC J4N 1C2; Mon'99; FRCSC; ObstGyn (Urogynecology). Staff, Hôpital Ste-Justine; Langs: Bilingual(French/English); (450)468-2151

LAROCHELLE, Bernard; CHUQ-Ctr Hosp Univ Laval, 2705 boul Laurier, Quebec QC G1V 4G2; Laval'02; FRCPC; IntMed. Staff, Centre Hospitalier Universitaire de Quebec-CHUL; (418)654-2160

LAROCHELLE, Catherine A; Toronto Sunnybrook Reg Cancer, T2 128-2075 Bayview Ave, Toronto ON M4N 3M5; Tor'79; Staff, Sunnybrook Health Sciences Centre; (416)480-6165; Fax. (416)480-6002.

LAROCHELLE, Catherine; CHUM-Hop Notre-Dame, 1560 rue Sherbrooke E, Montreal QC H2L 4M1; Laval'04; FRCPC; Neur. Staff, Centre Hospitalier l'Université de Montréal (CHUM) - Hôpital Notre-Dame; (514)930-9276

LAROCHELLE, Daniel; Polyclinique de l'Oreille, 252-1111 rue Saint-Charles O, Longueuil QC J4K 5G4; Laval'68; FAAO; Otol (Head & Neck). Langs: Bilingual(French/English); (450)651-9000; Fax. (450)679-1651.

LAROCHELLE, Denis; Hotel-Dieu de Levis, 143 rue Wolfe, Levis QC G6V 3Z1; Mon'96; CSPQ; FRCPC; Anes (Intensive Care). Staff, Hôtel-Dieu de Lévis; Langs: English; (418)835-7121; Fax. (418)835-3969.

LAROCHELLE, Gerard; GMF du Chatel, 200-9465 boul de l'Ormiere, Quebec QC G2B 3K7; Laval'73; (418)843-5141; Fax. (418)843-5343.

LAROCHELLE, Guillaume; CSSS de Chicoutimi, 305 rue Saint-Vallier, Chicoutimi QC G7H 5H6; Sher'04; FRCSC; GenSurg. Staff, Complexe hospitalier de la Sagamie; (418)541-1000

LAROCHELLE, Isabel; Polyclinique Ancienne-Lorette, 204-6385 boul Wilfrid-Hamel, L'Ancienne-Lorette QC G2E 5W2; Laval'95; ac Staff Med, Centre Hospitalier Universitaire De Québec - Pavillon De St-françois-d'assise; Langs: Bilingual(French/English); (418)872-2012

LAROCHELLE, Josee; CLSC Naskapi, CP 5154, Kawawachikamach QC G0G 2Z0; Laval'90; Staff, CSSS de la Minganie; (418)585-2110; Fax. (418)585-3795.

LAROCHELLE, Julie; UMF Grand Littoral, 100-1205 boul de la Rive-Sud, Saint-Romuald QC G6W 0J4; Sher'02; Physician, Hôtel-Dieu de Lévis; Langs: English; (418)380-8597; Fax. (418)380-8596.

LAROCHELLE, Julie; CLSC Kateri, 90 boul Marie-Victorin, Candiac QC J5R 1C1; Mon'91; (450)659-7661; Fax. (450)444-6276.

LAROCHELLE, Leandre; Clinique Med Lauzon, 213 rue Saint-Joseph, Levis QC G6V 1C8; Laval'71; Staff, Hôtel-Dieu de Lévis; (418)833-5040; Fax. (418)833-6954.

LAROCHELLE, Olivier; CHUQ-Hotel-Dieu de Quebec, 11 Cote du Palais, Quebec QC G1R 2J6; Mon'01; FRCPC; DiagRad. Staff, Centre Hospitalier Universitaire de Québec (CHUQ) - Siege Social; (418)691-5151

LAROCHELLE, Pascale; Hotel-Dieu D'arthabaska, 5 rue des Hospitalieres, Victoriaville QC G6P 6N2; Laval'94; FRCSC; OrthSurg. Staff OrthSurg, Hotel-Dieu d'Arthabaska; Langs: Bilingual(French/English); (819)357-2030; pascalelarochelle@videotron.ca.

LAROCHELLE, Pierre; Inst de Recherche Clin de Mtl, 110 av des Pins O, Montreal QC H2W 1R7; Laval'68; PhD; FACP; FRCPC; IntMed (Hypertension). Dir clinical Research, Institut de Recherche Clin de Montreal; Prof Pharmacology, Universite de Montreal; (514)987-5550; larochp@ircm.qc.ca.

LAROCHELLE, Real; Polyclinique Ancienne-Lorette, 204-6385 boul Wilfrid-Hamel, L'Ancienne-Lorette QC G2E 5W2; Laval'66; (418)872-2012; Fax. (418)872-2349.

LAROCHELLE, Roger E J; Spanish Med Clinic, PO Box 279 16 Trunk Rd, Spanish ON P0P 2A0; Laval'91; Court Staff, Espanola Regional Hospital and Health Centre; Court Staff, St Joseph's General Hospital Elliot Lake; Langs: Spanish; French; (705)844-2263; Fax. (705)844-2028; rlarochelle@bellnet.ca.

LAROCHELLE-BELAND, Marie; ASSS de la Capitale-Nationale, 2400 av d'Estimauville, Quebec QC G1E 7G9; Laval'74; FRCPC; RadOncol (Breast Cancer). Staff, Agence de la santé et des services sociaux de la Capitale-Nationale; Langs: Bilingual(English/French); (418)666-7000 x400

LAROCHELLE-GIRARD, Marie-Noelle; CHUS-Hop Fleurimont, 3001 12e av N, Sherbrooke QC J1H 5N4; Laval'06; Anes. Staff, Centre Hospitalier Universitaire de Sherbrooke-Hopital Fleurimont; (819)346-1110 x14403

LAROCQUE, Alexandre; CHUM-Hotel-Dieu de Montreal, 3840 rue Saint-Urbain, Montreal QC H2W 1T8; Mon'03; FRCPC; EmergMed. Staff, Centre Hospitalier l'Université de Montréal (CHUM) - Hôtel-Dieu; (514)890-8000

LAROCQUE, Amelie; Ctr Hosp De Verdun, 4000 boul Lasalle, Verdun QC H4G 2A3; Mon'05; CCFP; Staff, Centre Hospitalier de Verdun; (514)765-7325

LAROCQUE, Annie; IMSL, 103-1875 rue Maurice-Gauvin, Laval QC H7S 2M5; Sher'93; FRCPC; Derm. Langs: Bilingual(French/English); (450)902-4675; Fax. (450)902-9978.

LAROCQUE, Brian J; St Joseph's Health Care, PO Box 5777 Stn B 268 Grosvenor St, London ON N6A 4V2; Wes'86; FRCPC; IntMed. Staff, St Joseph's Hospital - St Joseph's Health Care; Assoc Prof Med, University of Western Ontario; (519)646-6117; Fax. (519)646-6064; larocque@uwo.ca.

LAROCQUE, Celine; Ctr Hosp du Centre la Mauricie, 50 119e rue, Shawinigan-Sud QC G9P 5K1; Sher'88; CSPQ; FRCPC; AnatPath. Staff, Centre Hospitalier du Centre la Mauricie; (819)536-7500 x2506; Fax. (819)536-6172; celine_larocque_energie@ssss.gouv.qc.ca.

LAROCQUE, David J; Castlegar Med Clinic, 1101 3rd St, Castlegar BC V1N 2A1; McG'91; BSc; CCFP; CCFP(E.M.); FCFP; (250)365-7717; Fax. (250)365-0347.

LAROCQUE, Isabelle; CLSC Des Faubourgs, 2260 rue Parthenais, Montreal QC H2K 3T5; Sher'96; Langs: Spanish; English; (514)527-2361 x2356; Fax. (514)527-6016; isabelle_larocque@ssss.gouv.qc.ca.

LAROCQUE, Isabelle; GMF de l'Assomption, CP 3406 814 boul l'Ange-Gardien N, L'Assomption QC J5W 4M9; Mon'04; Médecin, Centre Hospitalier Pierre le Gardeur; Langs: Bilingual(French/English); (450)589-5778

LAROCQUE, Jean-Francois; CSSS De Saint-Jerome, 290 rue de Montigny, Saint-Jerome QC J7Z 5T3; Mon'01; FRCPC; NuclearMed. Staff, Hôtel-Dieu de Saint-Jérôme; (450)431-8284 x2297

LAROCQUE, Marc; Hotel-Dieu De Roberval, 450 rue Brassard, Roberval QC G8H 1B9; Sher'89; Instructor ATLS, Centre Hospitalier Universitaire de Sherbrooke-Hopital Fleurimont; Staff, Hotel-Dieu de Roberval; (418)275-0110

LAROCQUE, Martin; CSSS Haut-Richelieu-Rouville, 920 boul du Seminaire N, St-Jean-sur-Richel QC J3A 1B7; McG'01; FRCPC; IntMed; Gastroent. Staff, Hôpital du Haut-Richelieu; (450)359-5000

LAROCQUE, Martine; CSSS du Rocher-Perce, CP 3300 451 rue Mgr Ross E, Chandler QC G0C 1K0; Mon'97; FRCSC; OrthSurg. Staff, Centre Hospitalier de Chandler; (418)689-2261

LAROCQUE, Maurice; 401-1303 av Greene, Westmount QC H3Z 2A7; Mon'69; (514)931-5252; Fax. (514)931-4655.

LAROCQUE, Monique; Clinique Med Nesipiguit, 950 Picot Ave, Bathurst NB E2A 4Z9; Laval'04; CCFP; (506)546-6696; Fax. (506)545-7723.

LAROCQUE, Rene; GMF de Grand-Mere, 200-1050 8e rue, Grand-Mere QC G9T 4L4; Laval'72; Langs: Bilingual(French/English); (819)538-6669; Fax. (819)538-6970.

LAROCQUE, Robert; 173 rue Saint-Vincent, Ste-Agathe-des-Mts QC J8C 2B5; Mon'72; Langs: English; (819)326-2441

LAROCQUE LAPLANTE, Sylvie; CSSS du Rocher-Perce, CP 3300 451 rue Mgr Ross, Chandler QC G0C 1K0; Sher'05; Staff, Centre Hospitalier de Chandler; (418)689-2261

LAROSE, Andre; CSSS de Rimouski-Neigette, CP 3150 Succ A 150 av Rouleau, Rimouski QC G5L 5T1; Mon'75; FRCPC; Gastroent. Staff, Hôpital Regional Rimouski; (418)723-7851

LAROSE, Andre; CSSS Drummond-Hop Sainte-Croix, 570 rue Heriot, Drummondville QC J2B 1C1; Sher'79; IntMed. ac Staff, Hôpital Sainte-croix; (819)478-6464

LAROSE, Annie; Hop Jean-Talon, 1385 rue Jean-Talon E, Montreal QC H2E 1S6; Sher'94; CSPQ; AnatPath. Staff, CSSS du Coeur de l'Isle Hôpital Jean-Talon; (514)495-6767

LAROSE, Dominic; Institut de Cardiologie de Mtl, 5000 rue Belanger, Montreal QC H1T 1C8; Mon'80; FACEP; MCFP(EM)(E.M.); Staff, Institut de Cardiologie de Montréal; Physician, Centre Hospitalier de Granby; Asst Prof FamMed, Universite de Sherbrooke; Langs: English; (514)376-3330; domlarose@videotron.ca.

LAROSE, Dwaine L; 192-17010 90 Ave NW, Edmonton AB T5T 1L6; Alb'01; FRCSC; ObstGyn. (780)483-2901

LAROSE, Eric; Hôpital Laval, 2725 ch Sainte-Foy, Quebec QC G1V 4G5; Mon'97; FRCPC; IntMed; Cardiol. Staff, Hôpital Laval; adj Prof, Université Laval; Langs: English; (418)656-8711 x4657

LAROSE, Gontran; 200-85 rue Saint-Pierre, Saint-Constant QC J5A 1G8; Mon'77; Langs: English; (450)632-1630; Fax. (450)632-5242.

LAROSE, Guylaine; Hôpital Ste-Justine, 3175 ch de la Cote-Sainte-Cath, Montreal QC H3T 1C5; Mon'99; FRCPC; Peds; PedEmergMed (P.Q.). Staff, Hôpital Ste-Justine; (514)345-4931

LAROSE, Marie; Clinique Med des Sommets, 1070 rue Principale, Ste-Agathe-des-Mts QC J8C 1L6; Mon'99; (819)321-1212; Fax. (819)321-3232.

LAROSE, Michel; Dir Regionale de Montreal, 17401-500 Boul Rene-Levesque O, Montreal QC H2Z 1W7; Mon'65; Consultant, Centre Hospitalier l'Université de Montréal (CHUM) - Hôpital Notre-Dame; Physician, Tribunal de l'Aviation Civile du Canada; Langs: Bilingual(French/English); (514)873-8349; Fax. (514)873-0232.

LAROSE, Michel; Inst U en Sante Mentale de QC, 2601 ch de la Canardiere, Quebec QC G1J 2G3; Laval'82; Psy. Staff, Institut Universitaire Sante; (418)663-5321

LAROSE, Michele; MUHC-Montreal's Children's Hos, D573-2300 rue Tupper, Montreal QC H3H 1P3; Laval'82; FRCPC; Psy. Staff, McGill University Health Centre - Montreal Children's Hospital; (514)412-4400 x22973

LAROSE, Milie-Ève; CSSS Kamouraska-Hop-Notre Dame, CP 460 1201 6e av, La Pocatiere QC G0R 1Z0; Mon'09; Staff, CSSS de Kamouraska; (418)856-7000

LAROSE, Pierre; 3120 boul Taschereau, Greenfield Park QC J4V 2H1; Mon'88 UNIVERSITE DE MONTREAL; FRCSC; GenSurg; VascSurg. Chef Dept of Surg, Hopital Charles LeMoyne; Langs: English; (450)466-5000 x2965; Fax. (450)466-5081; larose.vasc@sympatico.ca.

LAROSE, Pierre-Philippe; Ctr Hosp Anna-Laberge, 200 boul Brisebois, Chateauguay QC J6K 4W8; Mon'85; Otol. Staff, Hôpital Anna-Laberge; (450)699-2425

LAROSE, Robert; Clinique Med De Matane, 101-548 av Du Phare E, Matane QC G4W 1A7; Laval'74; ac Staff, Centre Hospitalier de Matane; (418)562-4530; Fax. (418)562-4532.

LAROSE, Sebastien; CHUQ-Ctr Hosp Univ Laval, 2705 boul Laurier, Quebec QC G1V 4G2; Laval'01; CCFP; CCFP(E.M.); Staff, Centre Hospitalier Universitaire de Quebec-CHUL; (418)656-4141

LAROUCHE, Alain; 3492 Av Royale RR 4, St-Ferreol-L-Neig QC G0A 3R0; Laval'75; Physician, Groupe Conseil Sante Concerto; Langs: English; (418)826-1084; larouche_alain_md@hotmail.com.

LAROUCHE, Alain L; Polyclinique St-Jerome, 204-200 rue Durand, Saint-Jerome QC J7Z 7E2; Mon'69; FRCSC; GenSurg. Staff, Hôtel-Dieu de Saint-Jérôme; (450)438-5922

LAROUCHE, Andre; Polyclinique De Trois-Rivieres, 375-1900 boul des Recollets, Trois-Rivieres QC G8Z 4K4; Laval'72; ABOtol; FRCSC; Otol (Vertigo). Associé Surg, Centre de santé Cloutier-du-Rivage; Associé Surg, Centre Hospitalier Regional de Trois-Rivieres; Associé Surg, CSSS de Trois-Rivières; (819)371-2085; Fax. (819)371-2390.

LAROUCHE, Darie; Clinique Med Legendre, 201-1650 av Jules-Verne, Quebec QC G2G 2R1; Laval'82; (418)872-5600; Fax. (418)872-8408.

LAROUCHE, Gilles; CSSS Cleophas-Claveau, CP 38 succ La Baie 1000 rue du Docteur-Desgagne, La Baie QC G7B 3P9; Laval'85; NBME; LMCC; Staff, CHSLD-CLSC Cleophas-Claveau; Langs: English; German; (418)544-3381

LAROUCHE, Isabelle; 204A-860 Mountain Rd, Moncton NB E1C 2N7; Mon'05; BScMicrobiol; MSc; CCFP; Staff Family Med, The Moncton Hospital; Langs: Bilingual(French/English); (506)855-5345

LAROUCHE, Jacynthe; Polyclinique De Trois-Rivieres, 100-1900 boul des Recollets, Trois-Rivieres QC G8Z 4K4; Mon'89; FRCPC; IntMed; Gastroent. Staff, CSSS de Trois-Rivières; Langs: Bilingual(French/English); (819)373-1538; Fax. (819)373-2138.

LAROUCHE, Jean-Francois; Ctr Hosp Affilie-Enfant-Jesus, 1401 18e rue, Quebec QC G1J 1Z4; Laval'00; FRCPC; IntMed; MedOncol; Hem. Staff, Centre Hospitalier Affilié Universitaire de Québec - Hôpital De L'Enfant Jésus; (418)649-5727

LAROUCHE, Leon; 991 3e rue, La Baie QC G7B 2C3; Laval'71; Consultant Environment Health, Regie Reg de la Sante et des Services Sociaux(RRSSS); Langs: French; (418)544-5181; Fax. (418)544-8926; leonlaro@royaume.com.

LAROUCHE, Leon-Maurice; Clinique Bois de Boulogne, 505-1575 boul Henri-Bourassa O, Montreal QC H3M 3A9; Laval'66; CSPQ; Psy (Affective Disorders). Staff, Hôpital du Sacre-Coeur de Montréal; Clinical Asst Prof, Universite de Montreal; (514)338-4300; Fax. (514)338-4493.

LAROUCHE, Lucie; Clinique Sante Femme, 31 rue Drummond, Granby QC J2G 2S3; Laval'87; FRCSC; ObstGyn (Colposcopy). Staff ObstGyn, Centre Hospitalier de Granby; Langs: Bilingual(French/English); (450)372-4008; Fax. (450)372-0068.

LAROUCHE, Michel; Clinique Maisonneuve-Rosemont, 60-5345 boul de l'Assomption, Montreal QC H1T 4B3; Laval'78; (514)257-7000; Fax. (514)257-7003.

LAROUCHE, Nathalie; GMF de Lorraine, 99 boul de Gaulle, Lorraine QC J6Z 3Z9; Sher'92; (450)621-1444; Fax. (450)621-7193.

LAROUCHE, Nicole; CHUM-Hotel-Dieu, 3840 rue Saint-Urbain, Montreal QC H2W 1T8; Mon'77; Staff, Centre Hospitalier l'Université de Montréal (CHUM) - Hôtel-Dieu; Langs: Bilingual(French/English); (514)890-8066; Fax. (514)412-7117.

LAROUCHE, Pierre; Clinique Dr Lareau et Dr Larou, 104-2055 boul Hébert, Salaber-de-Valleyf QC J6S 5Y5; Mon'82; Staff, Centre Hospitalier Régional du Suroît; Langs: English; Italian; (450)373-0100; Fax. (450)373-3282; cliniquelarouche@hotmail.com.

LAROUCHE, Renee; Clinique Med Fam Saint-Bruno, SS 1 552 av Saint-Alphonse, St-Bruno-du-L-St-J QC G0W 2L0; Laval'80; (418)343-2444; Fax. (418)343-2448.

LAROUCHE, Richard; Anapharm, 800-5160 Boul Decarie, Montreal QC H3X 2H9; Laval'84; PhmB; Dir Medical Affairs, Anapharm Inc; Langs: French; (514)485-7500 x7577; rlarouche@anapharm.com.

LAROUCHE, Valerie; CHUQ-Ctr Hosp Univ Laval, 2705 boul Laurier, Quebec QC G1V 4G2; Laval'00; FRCPC; Peds (Neuro Oncology); Hem. Staff, Centre Hospitalier Universitaire de Quebec-CHUL; Langs: Bilingual(French/English); (418)656-4141 x47191; valerie.larouche@mail.chuq.qc.ca.

LAROUCHE-MARCHESSEAULT, Line; Clinique Med Fusion, 200-2035 av Sainte-Anne, Saint-Hyacinthe QC J2S 5H3; Laval'77; (450)773-9554

LAROUSSI, Leila; CSSS Haut-Richelieu-Rouville, 920 boul du Seminaire N, St-Jean-sur-Richel QC J3A 1B7; Mon'07; IntMed. Staff, Hôpital du Haut-Richelieu; (450)359-5000

LAROYE, Guy Jean; Mills Memorial Hosp, 4720 Haugland Ave, Terrace BC V8G 2W7; Ghent (Belgium)'61; FRCPC; GenPath (Anatomical Pathology). Staff, Mills Memorial Hospital; Langs: Dutch; German; French; (250)635-2211 x4427; Fax. (250)638-4037; guy.laroye@northernhealth.ca.

LARRATT, Loree M; 13 106B-152 University Campus, Edmonton AB T6G 2G3; Alb'80; FRCPC; IntMed; Hem. Staff, University of Alberta Hospital; Staff, Cross Cancer Institute; Staff, Canadian Blood Services; Prof, University of Alberta; (780)407-7021; Fax. (780)407-2680; loree.larratt@ualberta.ca.

LARRAZABAL, Ramiro A; Hamilton HS-General Site, 237 Barton St E, Hamilton ON L8L 2X2; Colombia (Colombia)'91; Staff, Hamilton Health Sciences Centre - Hamilton General Hospital; Langs: Spanish; (905)527-4322

LARRIGAN, John R C; Foothills Med Centre, 1403 29 St NW, Calgary AB T2N 2T9; Man'96; FRCPC; DiagRad. Staff Diag Imaging, Foothills Medical Centre; (403)944-1344

LARRIVEE, Claude; Clinique Med de l'Or, 228 2e rue E, La Sarre QC J9Z 2G9; Sher'97; (819)333-0445

LARRIVEE, Luc; CSSS de Memphremagog, 50 rue Saint-Patrice E, Magog QC J1X 3X3; Laval'92; Staff, Centre Hospitalier et CLSC de Memphremagog; (819)843-3381

LARRIVEE, Marie-Pier; Hôpital Ste-Justine, 3175 ch Cote-Sainte-Catherine, Montreal QC H3T 1C5; Laval'00; FRCPC; Psy. Staff, Hôpital Ste-Justine; (514)345-4931

LARRIVEE, Mathieu; Centre Med Saint-Francois, 2125 boul Lemire, Drummondville QC J2B 8N8; Sher'08; CCFP; (819)477-6793

LARSEN, Bjorn R; Salveo Family Med Clinic, B8-6455 Macleod Trail SW, Calgary AB T2H 0K8; Cal'07; CCFP; (403)444-0428; Fax. (403)537-0029.

LARSEN, Carmen H; PO Box 21189 Rpo Terwillegar, Edmonton AB T6R 2V4; Dal'06; CCFP.

LARSEN, Charles J; 301-11001 13 St, Dawson Creek BC V1G 4Z8; Cape Town (South Africa)'74; MB ChB; Staff, Dawson Creek & District Hospital; (250)782-8501

LARSEN, Darren A; Thornhill Village Fam Health, 18 Centre St, Thornhill ON L4J 1E9; Cal'89; CCFP; Staff/Pres Med Assoc, Mackenzie Richmond Hill Hospital; (905)889-3634; Fax. (905)889-3986; info@tmcdocs.info.

LARSEN, David P F; Bonavista Peninsula Health Ctr, Postal Service 1, Bonavista NL A0C 1B0; (England)'90; MB BS; Med Advisor, Bonavista Peninsula Health Centre; (709)468-1967

LARSEN, Erik T; Rockyview Gen Hosp, 4N04-7007 14 St SW, Calgary AB T2V 1P9; Alb'88; BSc; GenPath; AnatPath (Laboratory Medicine). Staff, Foothills Medical Centre; Staff Calgary Lab Serv, Rockyview General Hospital; Staff, Calgary Health Region; Teach Staff, University of Calgary; (403)943-3712; Fax. (403)943-3333; erik.larsen@cls.ab.ca.

LARSEN, Grant A; 975 Kye Bay Rd, Comox BC V9M 3T9; Sask'97; FRCPC; DiagRad. Staff Radiol, St Joseph's General Hospital; (250)218-4708

LARSEN, Joanne H; Hollyburn Med Bldg, 201-520 17th St, West Vancouver BC V7V 3S8; UBC'89; (604)913-8183

LARSEN, Sean S; Gaetz Family Practice, 104-45744 Gaetz St, Chilliwack BC V2R 3P1; Alb'00; CCFP; (604)824-1588

LARSEN-PASSE, Marie-Andree; Polyclinique Metro Longueuil, 100-1144 rue Saint-Laurent O, Longueuil QC J4K 1E2; (Haiti)'68; (450)651-5700; Fax. (450)679-4333.

LARSEN SOLES, Trina M; Golden Med Clinic, PO Box 1170, Golden BC V0A 1H0; UBC'86; (250)344-6863

LARSON, Alfhild J; IWK Health Centre, PO Box 9700 Rpo CSC, Halifax NS B3K 6R8; San Diego(CA) (USA)'79; FRCPC; Peds. Staff, IWK Health Centre; (902)470-8529; Fax. (902)470-6913.

LARSON, Berwyn L; McEown Med Clinic, 102-2315 McEown Ave, Saskatoon SK S7J 2H1; Sask'78; CCFP; (306)374-2438; Fax. (306)374-8262.

LARSON, Bonnie; Sheldon Chumir Centre, 7F-1213 4 St SW, Calgary AB T2R 0X7; McM'06; CCFP; Clin Lecturer, University of Calgary; (403)955-6600; Fax. (403)955-6601.

LARSON, Jacelyn M; Royal University Hosp, 103 Hospital Dr, Saskatoon SK S7N 0W8; Sask'98; FRCPC; Anes. Staff Anes, Royal University Hospital; (306)655-1183; Fax. (306)655-1279; j_kolman@hotmail.com.

LARSSON, Stephan N; BC Cancer Agency-Vanc Isl Ctr, 2410 Lee Ave, Victoria BC V8R 6V5; Birmingham (England)'78; MRCP; FRCR; LMCC; FRCP; FRCPC; RadOncol. Staff Rad Oncologist, BC Cancer Agency Vancouver Island Centre; Ac Staff, Vancouver Island Health Authority; Asst Prof Surg, University of British Columbia; Asst Prof Med, University of Victoria; (250)519-5576; Fax. (250)519-2018; slarsson@bccancer.bc.ca.

LARTON, Heather A; Univ of Waterloo Hlth Services, 200 University Ave W, Waterloo ON N2L 3G1; McM'96; Langs: Bilingual(English/French); (519)888-4096

LARUE, Bernard; CHUS-Hop Fleurimont, 3001 12e av N, Sherbrooke QC J1H 5N4; Sher'01; FRCSC; OrthSurg. Staff, Centre Hospitalier Universitaire de Sherbrooke-Hopital Fleurimont; (819)346-1110

LARUE, Bertrand; Clinique Med Pierre-Boucher, 110-1615 boul Jacques-Cartier, Longueuil QC J4M 2X1; Mon'81; (450)468-6177; Fax. (450)468-5041.

LARUE, Frank J; 381 boul Maloney E, Gatineau QC J8P 1E3; Laval'68; DrMedCh; Langs: Bilingual(English/French); (819)669-7393

LARUE, Jordan M; Sylvan Family Health Centre, 101-190 Pelican Pl, Sylvan Lake AB T4S 1K2; Alb'09; CCFP; (403)887-2224; Fax. (403)887-2261.

LARUE, Louis; Hotel-Dieu de Levis, 143 rue Wolfe, Levis QC G6V 3Z1; Laval'92; Staff, Hôtel-Dieu de Lévis; (418)835-7121

LARUE, Marie; CSSS de la Baie-des-Chaleurs, RR 2 419 boul Perron, Maria QC G0C 1Y0; Laval'94; FRCS; DGS; FRCSC; GenSurg (Gastroenterology). Staff Surg, CSSS de la Baie-des-Chaleurs; Langs: French; English; (418)759-3443; Fax. (418)759-5537.

LARUE, Nathalie; 950 Principale, Cowansville QC J2K 1K3; Laval'94; FRCSC; GenSurg. Staff General Surg, Hôpital Brome-Missisquoi-Perkins; Langs: English; French; (450)266-4342

LARUE, Nicole; Clinique de l'Alternative, 2034 rue Saint-Hubert, Montreal QC H2L 3Z5; Laval'76; (514)281-9848

LARUE, Sandrine; Clinique Neuro Rive-Sud, 250-4896 boul Taschereau, Greenfield Park QC J4V 2J2; Mon'01; FRCPC; Neur (Neuromuscular Diseases). Staff Neurol, Hopital Charles LeMoyne; Staff Neurol, Centre Hospitalier l'Université de Montréal (CHUM) - Hôpital Notre-Dame; Langs: Bilingual(French/English); (450)672-1931; larue@neurorivesud.ca.

LARYEA, Horace D; Hopital General du Lakeshore, 160 av Stillview, Pointe-Claire QC H9R 2Y2; McG'73; CSPQ; FRCPC; IntMed; MedOncol (P.Q.) (Sickle Cell). Staff IntMed, Lakeshore General Hospital - Pointe Claire; assoc Staff, McGill University Health Centre - Royal Victoria Hospital; Member/Member Advisory Board, Canadian Blood Committee; Member, International Bulletin of Sickle-Cells; Aj Prof, McGill University; Langs: Ghanaian; (514)630-2225; henaa@total.net.

LARYEA, Marie A; Queen Elizabeth II HSC, 6 291B-1278 South Park St, Halifax NS B3H 2Y9; McG'99; FRCPC; IntMed; Gastroent. Staff, Queen Elizabeth II Health Sciences Centre - Victoria General Site; (902)473-1150

LASALETA, Moises S; Pacific Place Mall, 958-999 36 St NE, Calgary AB T2A 7X6; Manila (Philippines)'83; Langs: Tagalog; (403)387-3300

LASALLE, Leo; Clinique Med De Verdun, 42-55 av de l'Eglise, Verdun QC H4G 3E7; Sher'70; Langs: English; (514)766-9405

LASALLE, Luc; Polyclinique Med Pierre LeGard, 300-1000 montee des Pionniers, Terrebonne QC J6V 1S8; Mon'84; Staff, Centre Hospitalier Pierre le Gardeur; (450)657-5799

LASALLE-FOLOT, Marie-Helene; CSSSG-Hop de Gatineau, CP 2000 Succ Bureau-Chef 909 boul de la Verendrye O, Gatineau QC J8P 7H2; Mon'00; Staff, Hôpital de Gatineau; (819)561-8222

LASCHUK, Bohdan S; Windsor Health Unit, 350-1720 Howard Ave, Windsor ON N8X 5A6; Wes'81; FRCSC; GenSurg (Surgical Oncology). Staff, Windsor Regional Hospital - Metropolitan Site; (519)255-9792; Fax. (519)255-9908.

LASCHUK, Maria J; Windsor Health Unit, 350-1720 Howard Ave, Windsor ON N8X 5A6; Wes'81; FRCPC; Anes. Staff, Hôtel-Dieu Grace Hospital; Staff, Windsor Regional Hospital - Metropolitan Site; Langs: German; (519)255-9792; Fax. (519)255-9908; laschuk@mnsi.net.

LASEINDE, Olufunto O; Medical Bldg, 409-250 Harding Blvd W, Richmond Hill ON L4C 9M7; Ibadan (Nigeria)'82; MB BS; MRCOG; FRCSC; ObstGyn. (905)508-3570; Fax. (905)508-3784.

LASH, Vynka C; MUHC-Royal Victoria Hosp, S5 05-687 av des Pins O, Montreal QC H3A 1A1; Cal'99; CSPQ; FRCPC; Anes. Staff, McGill University Health Centre - Royal Victoria Hospital; (514)934-1934 x34880

LASHEVSKY, Ilan; Sunnybrook Hlth Sciences Ctre, D374A-2075 Bayview Ave, Toronto ON M4N 3M5; Tel Aviv (Israel)'89; Staff Cardiol, Sunnybrook Health Sciences Centre; Langs: Italian; Hebrew; (416)480-6100 x7383; Fax. (416)480-6913.

LASICH, Jonathan F; Brockville Gen Hosp, 75 Charles St, Brockville ON K6V 1S8; McG'85; Staff, Brockville General Hospital - Charles Street; Langs: Bilingual(English/French); (613)345-5649 x1256

LASKEY, Jennifer D; Centennial Med Centre, 299 Lake Ave E, Carleton Place ON K7C 1J3; Tor'92; CCFP; FCFP; (613)257-2311; Fax. (613)257-4435.

LASKI, Jennifer B; Onaping Falls Med Centre, PO Box 160 24 Nickel St, Levack ON P0M 2C0; Dublin (Ireland)'87; ATLS; ACLS; CCFP; Staff, Health Sciences North-St Joseph's Health Centre; Staff, Health Sciences North-Laurentian Site; Staff, Health Sciences North - Memorial Site; (705)966-3426; Fax. (705)966-0252.

LASKIN, Carl A; 1800-655 Bay St, Toronto ON M5G 2K4; McM'75; FACRheum; FRCPC; Rheum (Infertility); IntMed. Consultant, Toronto General Hospital - UHN; Consultant, Mount Sinai Hospital; Consultant, Women's College Hospital; Assoc Prof Med, University of Toronto; (416)593-9220; Fax. (416)599-8624.

LASKIN, Janessa J; BC Cancer Agency-Vancouver CC, 600 10th Ave W, Vancouver BC V5Z 4E6; UBC'97; FRCPC; IntMed; MedOncol. Staff, BC Cancer Agency Vancouver Centre; (604)877-6000

LASKIN, Matthew D; Lifequest, 1800-655 Bay St, Toronto ON M5G 2K4; Qns'06; FRCSC; ObstGyn.

LASKINE, Mikhael; CHUM-Hotel-Dieu, 4414-3840 rue Saint-Urbain, Montreal QC H2W 1T8; Geneva (Switzerland)'99; Critical Care Medicine (P.Q.). Staff, Centre Hospitalier l'Université de Montréal (CHUM) - Hôtel-Dieu; (514)890-8000

LASKO, Benjamin H; Kipling Heights Med Centre, 117B-2291 Kipling Ave, Etobicoke ON M9W 4L6; Tor'71; Langs: Italian; Yiddish; (416)740-2895; Fax. (416)740-4517.

LASKOWSKA, Barbara E; Active Care Carlingwood, 35B-2121 Carling Ave, Ottawa ON K2A 1H2; Pomeranian (Poland)'80; Langs: Polish; (613)761-6777; Fax. (613)761-7744.

LASKOWSKI, Alexandra; Aberdeen Hosp, 835 East River Rd, New Glasgow NS B2H 3S6; Wroclaw (Poland)'81; Staff, Aberdeen Regional Hospital; (902)752-7600; Fax. (902)755-4549.

LASKOWSKI, Alfred E; 950 Oak Cres PO Box 129, Telkwa BC V0J 2X0; Cal'95; BSc; CCFP; Wrinch Memorial Hospital; (250)842-5234; Fax. (250)842-5065.

LASKOWSKI, Derek; The Nova Scotia Hosp, PO Box 1004 Stn Main, Dartmouth NS B2Y 3Z9; Wroclaw (Poland)'82; CCFP; Staff, The Nova Scotia Hospital; (902)464-3111

LASKOWSKI, Kevin B; Royal University Hosp, 103 Hospital Dr, Saskatoon SK S7N 0W8; Alb'05; FRCPC; Anes. Staff, Royal University Hospital; (306)655-1183; Fax. (306)655-1279.

LASKOWSKI, Wojciech; Active Care, 35B-2121 Carling Ave, Ottawa ON K2A 1H2; Pomeranian (Poland)'80; Physician, CLSC Quyon; Langs: Polish; French; (613)761-6777; Fax. (613)761-7744.

LASNER, Brian R W; True Balance, 203-52 Sioux Rd, Sherwood Park AB T8A 4X1; (Netherlands Antilles)'00; (780)464-4506

LASNIER, Frederic; Ctr de Sante Basse Cote Nord, CP 130 1070 boul Dr Camilee-Marcoux, Lourdes-d-Bl-Sabl QC G0G 1W0; Laval'07; CCFP; Staff, CSSS de la Basse Côté-Nord; (418)461-2144

LASNIER, Luc; 35 rue Principale, Granby QC J2G 2T7; McG'79; (450)372-4211; Fax. (450)372-5374.

LASORE, Dapo; Lethbridge Med Clinic, 300 3 St S, Lethbridge AB T1J 1Y9; (Nigeria)'85; MB BS; LMCC; (403)394-2002; Fax. (403)394-2066.

LASRY, David A; MUHC-Montreal Gen Hosp, 1650 av Cedar, Montreal QC H3G 1A4; Sher'96; CCFP; CCFP(E.M.); FCFP; Staff, McGill University Health Centre - Montreal General Campus; Langs: French; (514)934-1934

LASS, Rowena; Paterson Med Centre, RR 1 45 Wolsley St, Kenora ON P9N 3W7; Bristol (England)'73; MB ChB; Court Staff Privil, Lake of the Woods District Hospital; Coroner, City Of Kenora; Physician, North West Health Unit; Langs: Bilingual(English/French); (807)468-3021; rlass@kenora.ca.

LASSEY, Steve; Pictou Med Clinic, PO Box 520, Pictou NS B0K 1H0; Cambridge (England)'76; MB ChB; LMCC; Langs: German; Italian; (902)485-4302; Fax. (902)485-4049.

LASSILA, Laura L; Alexandra Comm Health Centre, 101-1318 Centre St NE, Calgary AB T2E 2R7; Ott'99; CCFP; (403)266-2622

LASSONDE, Anick; Ctr Hosp Affilie-Enfant-Jesus, 1401 18e rue, Quebec QC G1J 1Z4; Mon'97; LMCC; Staff, Centre Hospitalier Affilié Universitaire de Québec - Hôpital De L'Enfant Jésus; (418)649-0252

LASSONDE, Pierre; 12450 rue Notre-Dame E, Pte-aux-Trembles QC H1B 2Z1; Sher'73; (514)645-1500; Fax. (514)645-9007.

LASSONDE, Sophie; Clinique Externe des Moulins, 101-1355 Grande Allee, Terrebonne QC J6W 4K6; Mon'95; FRCPC; Psy. Staff, Centre Hospitalier Pierre le Gardeur; (450)964-6418

LASUTA, Sarah A M; 5531 Inlet Ave PO Box 638, Sechelt BC V0N 3A0; UBC'05; CCFP; (604)885-2257

LASWICK, Alison J; The Ctre for Child Development, 9460 140 St, Surrey BC V3V 5Z4; McM'85; ABPeds; FRCPC; Peds (Developmental Pediatrics). (604)584-1361

LASZLO, Theodore A; Old Quebec Street Mall, 201-55 Wyndham St N, Guelph ON N1H 7T8; Ott'60; Peds. (519)822-7581

LATA, Andrew C; Albany Med Clinic, 807 Broadview Ave, Toronto ON M4K 2P8; Wes'80; FRCPC; DiagRad. Staff Radiol, St Michael's Hospital; (416)461-9471

LATAKGOMO, Lehlohonolo; Watrous Med Clinic, PO Box 1059, Watrous SK S0K 4T0; (306)946-2075; Fax. (306)946-2072.

LATCHFORD, Kevin J; Anaesthesia Associates, 439 Park St, Kitchener ON N2G 1N4; Qns'05; Anes. (519)744-7361

LATCHMAN, Andrew R; Hamilton HS-McMaster Site, PO Box 2000 Stn Lcd 1 2G-1200 Main St W, Hamilton ON L8N 3Z5; McM'01; FRCPC; Peds. Clinical Asst Prof, Hamilton Health Sciences Centre - McMaster Children's Hospital; Teach Staff, McMaster University; (905)521-2100 x75774

LATEGAN, Belinda; St Boniface Gen Hosp, 409 Tache Ave, Winnipeg MB R2H 2A6; Pretoria (South Africa)'00; FRCPC; AnatPath. Staff, St Boniface General Hospital; (204)233-8563

LATEGAN, Jan H J; Associate Specialist Clinic, 203-10030 106 St, Westlock AB T7P 2K4; (South Africa)'86; MB ChB; MMed(Orth); Consultant Orth, Westlock Healthcare Centre; Langs: Afrikaans; (780)349-3341; Fax. (780)349-6686.

LATEGAN, Johannes C; Peter Lougheed Centre, 3500 26 Ave NE, Calgary AB T1Y 6J4; Stellenbosch (South Africa)'88; MMed; Staff IntMed, Peter Lougheed Centre; (403)943-5423

LATELLA, Jennifer; Thunder Bay Reg HSC T-Bay, 980 Oliver Rd, Thunder Bay ON P7B 6V4; Sher'99; FRCPC; IntMed. Staff, Thunder Bay Regional Health Sciences Centre; Langs: Italian; French; (807)684-6030

LATENDRESSE, Helene; Hotel-Dieu D'Arthabaska, 5 rue des Hospitalieres, Victoriaville QC G6P 6N2; Mon'88; CSPQ; AnatPath (P.Q.). Staff, Hotel-Dieu d'Arthabaska; (819)357-1151; Fax. (819)357-6022.

LATENDRESSE, Myriam; Kootenay-Boundary Reg Hosp, 1200 Hospital Bench, Trail BC V1R 4M1; Sher'98; CCFP; CCFP(E.M.); Staff, Kootenay Boundary Regional Hospital; (250)368-3311

LATERREUR, Marie-Eve; Ctr Hosp Affilie-Enfant-Jesus, 1401 18e rue, Quebec QC G1J 1Z4; Laval'02; FRCPC; IntMed. Staff, Centre Hospitalier Affilié Universitaire de Québec - Hôpital De L'Enfant Jésus; (418)649-0252

LATHAM, Timothy B; Keary Med Centre, 105-245 Columbia St E, New Westminster BC V3L 3W4; Wes'92; FRCSC; CardSurg (Adult Cardiac Surgery). Ac Staff, Royal Columbian Hospital; Clin Instructor, University of British Columbia; (604)522-6800; Fax. (604)540-8126; tbl@telus.net.

LATHAM, Warren C W; 206-385 Silverstar Blvd, Scarborough ON M1V 0E3; UBC'01; FRCSC; OrthSurg. Staff Orth Surg, Toronto Western Hospital - University Health Network; Langs: Bilingual(English/French); (416)412-3535; Fax. (416)412-3536.

LATHIA, Anita; 3A-2650 Lawrence Ave E, Scarborough ON M1P 2S1; McM'06; CCFP; (416)289-0593

LATHWELL, Margaret J S; Regent Park Comm Health Centre, 465 Dundas St E, Toronto ON M5A 2B2; Pennsylvania (USA)'83; (416)364-2261; Fax. (416)364-0822.

LATIF, Shazia; Milton Med Centre, 200-1225 Maple Ave, Milton ON L9T 0A5; Punjab (Pakistan)'96; CCFP; Langs: Punjabi; Urdu; (905)693-6400

LATIF, Zahid; Alberta Hosp Edmonton, PO Box 307 Stn Main, Edmonton AB T5J 2J7; (Pakistan)'93; Staff, Alberta Hospital Edmonton; (780)342-5438; Fax. (780)342-5233.

LATIMER, Bradley R; Appletree Med Centre, 225 Preston St, Ottawa ON K1R 7R1; Wes'85; (613)288-2437

LATIMER, Paul R; Okanagan Clinical Trials, 204-1353 Ellis St, Kelowna BC V1Y 1Z9; Qns'72; PhD; FRCPC; Psy (Clinical Trials). CEO, Okanagan Clinical Trials; (250)862-8141; Fax. (250)862-8130; dr@oktrials.ca.

LATMAN, Irit-Irina; 802-19369 Sheriff King St SW, Calgary AB T2X 0T9; (Other Foreign)'84; CCFP; (403)873-7300; Fax. (403)873-8880.

LATORTUE, Nicole; Ctr Hosp de Lasalle, 8585 Tsse Champlain, Lasalle QC H8P 1C1; (Haiti)'63; CSPQ; Anes. Staff, Centre Hospitalier de LaSalle; (514)362-8000 x1871

LATOSINSKY, Steven; London Reg Cancer Centre, A3 931C-790 Commissioners Rd E, London ON N6A 4L6; Tor'90; BSc; MSc; FRCSC; GenSurg (Breasts). Staff, London Health Sciences Centre - Children's Hospital; Assoc Prof, University of Western Ontario; (519)685-8740; Fax. (519)685-8744; steven.latosinsky@lhsc.on.ca.

LATOUCHE, Marie-Josee; Unite Med Familiale Maizerets, 2480 ch de la Canardiere, Quebec QC G1J 2G1; Laval'90; CCFP; (418)661-1413; Fax. (418)661-7504.

LATOUR, Anne H; Cape Breton Hlthcare Complex, 1482 George St, Sydney NS B1P 1P3; McG'68; DiagRad. Staff, Cape Breton Healthcare Complex; (902)567-8000

LATOUR, John A; Riverview Surgical Centre, 3127 Bowwood Dr NW, Calgary AB T3B 2E7; Cal'82; FRCPC; Anes. Staff, Rockyview General Hospital; (403)288-9400

LATOUR, M P Judith; CHUM-Hop St-Luc, 1058 rue Saint-Denis, Montreal QC H2X 3J4; Sher'75; FRCPC; IntMed; GeriatricMed. Staff Geriatric, Institut Universitaire de Gériatrie de Montréal; Geriatric Med/Int Med, Centre Hospitalier l'Université De Montréal (CHUM) - Hôpital Saint-luc; (514)890-8000 x34980; Fax. (514)412-7376.

LATOUR, Marc-Andre; Clin Orth Roy & Montminy, 150-1165 boul Lebourgneuf, Quebec QC G2K 2C9; Laval'83; FRCSC; OrthSurg (Spine Surgery). Langs: Bilingual(French/English); (418)627-3330

LATOUR, Mathieu; CHUM-Hop Saint-Luc, 1058 rue Saint-Denis, Montreal QC H2X 3J4; Mon'01; CSPQ; FRCPC; AnatPath. Staff, Centre Hospitalier l'Université De Montréal (CHUM) - Hôpital Saint-luc; (514)890-8000 x36217

LATOUR, Sonia; Clinique Med Acces-Sante, 8 rue Du Terminus E, Rouyn-Noranda QC J9X 3B4; Mon'96; Staff, Centre Hospitalier Rouyn-Noranda; (819)762-2130; Fax. (819)762-5130.

LATOWSKY, Mark L; 207-3447 Kennedy Rd, Scarborough ON M1V 3S1; Tor'85; University of Toronto; (416)332-2757; Fax. (416)332-3747.

LATRAVERSE, Frederique; Ctr Hosp Anna-Laberge, 200 boul Brisebois, Chateauguay QC J6K 4W8; Mon'89; ObstGyn. Staff ObstGyn, Hôpital Anna-Laberge; (450)699-2425

LATRAVERSE, Veronique; CSSS Pierre Boucher, 1333 boul Jacques-Cartier E, Longueuil QC J4M 2A5; Mon'07; Peds. Staff, Centre Hospitalier Pierre Boucher; (450)468-8111

LATREILLE, Isabelle; Groupe Sante Physimed, 121-6363 rte Transcanadienne, Saint-Laurent QC H4T 1Z9; Mon'01; CCFP; (514)747-8888

LATREILLE, Jean; Hop Charles Lemoyne, 3120 boul Taschereau, Greenfield Park QC J4V 2H1; McG'73; FRCPC; IntMed (Breast Cancer); MedOncol (P.Q.); Hem (P.Q.). Dir CICM, Hopital Charles LeMoyne; Langs: Bilingual(English/French); (450)466-5009 x2318; Fax. (450)466-5066; jean.latreille@cicm.hclm.qc.ca.

LATREILLE, Jean-Marie; Comm Lesions Prof, 116-157 rue Victoria, Salaber-de-Valleyf QC J6T 1A5; Mon'66; FRCPC; PhysMed&Rehab. Staff, Centre Hospitalier Régional du Suroît; (450)370-6862

LATTA, Eleanor K; St Michael's Hosp, 2 085-30 Bond St, Toronto ON M5B 1W8; Tor'96; FRCPC; AnatPath. Staff Lab Med & Pathobiol, St Michael's Hospital; (416)360-4000 x5858; lattae@smh.toronto.on.ca.

LATTER, David A; St Michael's Hosp, 30 Bond St, Toronto ON M5B 1W8; McG'82; FRCSC; GenSurg (Cardiac Surgery); Cardiovasc&ThorSurg. Chief Cardiovascular & Thoracic Surg, St Michael's Hospital; Assoc Prof Surg, University of Toronto; Langs: English; French; (416)864-5366; Fax. (416)864-6067; latterd@smh.toronto.on.ca.

LATTER, John E; Alberta Children's Hosp, C4 650-2888 Shaganappi Trail N, Calgary AB T3B 6A8; Qns'71; MPA; FRCPC; PhysMed&Rehab (Pediatric Rehabilitation). Staff, Alberta Children's Hospital; Prof/Head Div of PhysMed & Rehab, University of Calgary; (403)955-7251; Fax. (403)955-3045; jlatter@ucalgary.ca.

LATTERMANN, Ralph B; MUHC-Royal Victoria Hosp, 687 av des Pins O, Montreal QC H3A 1A1; Ulm (Germany)'97; Staff, McGill University Health Centre - Royal Victoria Hospital; (514)934-1934 x34880

LATTOUF, Jean-Baptiste; CHUM-Hop St-Luc, 1058 rue Saint-Denis, Montreal QC H2X 3J4; Mon'99; FRCSC; Urol (Oncology). Staff/Prof adj clin, Centre Hospitalier l'Université De Montréal (CHUM) - Hôpital Saint-luc; Langs: English; Arabic; (514)890-8000 x27466; Fax. (514)412-7620; jean-baptiste.lattouf@umontreal.ca.

LATULIPPE, Dany; 880 av Painchaud, Quebec QC G1S 0A3; Laval'91; CCFP; Staff, Centre Hospitalier Universitaire de Quebec-CHUL; (418)688-1221

LATULIPPE, Denise; 110-4850 boul Henri-Bourassa, Quebec QC G1H 3A7; Laval'78; (418)628-3517; Fax. (418)628-0000.

LATULIPPE, Eva; CHUQ-Hotel-Dieu De Quebec, 11 Cote Du Palais, Quebec QC G1R 2J6; Laval'94; CSPQ; FRCPC; AnatPath. Staff, Centre Hospitalier Universitaire de Québec (CHUQ) - Siege Social; (418)691-5233; Fax. (418)691-5226; eva.latulippe@chuq.qc.ca.

LATULIPPE, Isabelle; CSSS de la Haute-Yamaska, 205 boul Leclerc O, Granby QC J2G 1T7; Sher'00; CCFP; CCFP(E.M.); Staff, Centre Hospitalier de Granby; (450)375-8000

LATULIPPE, Jean-Francois; Hop Maisonneuve-Rosemont, 5415 boul de l'Assomption, Montreal QC H1T 2M4; Laval'91; FRCSC; GenSurg. Staff, Hopital Maisonneuve-Rosemont; (514)252-3400

LATULIPPE, Louis G; CSSS de Memphremagog, 50 rue Saint-Patrice E, Magog QC J1X 3X3; Laval'76; MSc; Staff, Centre Hospitalier et CLSC de Memphremagog; Langs: Bilingual(French/English); (819)843-3381

LATULIPPE, Maude; CSSS de Saint-Jerome, 290 rue de Montigny, Saint-Jerome QC J7Z 5T3; Mon'07; CCFP; CCFP(E.M.); Staff, Hôtel-Dieu de Saint-Jérôme; (450)431-8200

LATULIPPE, Richard; CSSS d'Antoine-Labelle-Mt Laur, RR 1 2561 ch de la Lièvre S, Mont-Laurier QC J9L 3G3; Mon'78; Staff, CSSS d'Antoine-Labelle; (819)623-1234; latulipper@hotmail.com.

LATULIPPE, Sebastien M; CSSS de Trois-Rivières, 1991 boul du Carmel, Trois-Rivieres QC G8Z 3R9; Sher'06; FRCPC; Anes. Staff, CSSS de Trois-Rivières; (819)697-3333

LATUS, Andrew M; Dr Charles A Janeway Child HC, 300 Prince Philip Dr, St. John's NL A1B 3V6; Mem'07; FRCPC; Psy. Staff, Janeway Children's Health & Rehabilitation Centre; (709)777-6300

LATUSKIE, Russell H K; 185 Inkerman St E, Listowel ON N4W 2N1; Leicester (England)'82; DObst(Auckland); CCFP; Listowel Memorial Hospital - Listowel Wingham Hospitals Alliance; (519)291-4200; Fax. (519)291-5947.

LAU, Agatha; 004B-6633 Highway 7, Markham ON L3P 7P2; Tor'03; FRCPC; IntMed; Gastroent. Staff IntMed & Gastroent, Markham Stouffville Hospital; Langs: Cantonese; (905)294-8008

LAU, Albert; St Joseph's Health Centre, 30 The Queensway, Toronto ON M6R 1B5; Tor'00; CCFP; CCFP(E.M.); Staff, St Joseph's Health Centre; (416)530-6000

LAU, Alvin W W; Rapids Family Health Team, 1-1150 Pontiac Dr, Sarnia ON N7S 3A7; Tor'03; (519)339-8949; Fax. (519)339-9022; alau@rapidsfhteam.ca.

LAU, Amanda W M; Oakridge Centre, 222-650 41 St W, Vancouver BC V5Z 2M9; UBC'08; CCFP; Langs: Cantonese; (604)261-2633

LAU, Ambrose K; Univ Hlth Network-Toronto Western Hosp, EW 7F-399 Bathurst St, Toronto ON M5T 2S8; Wes'05; FRCPC; IntMed; Respir. Staff, Toronto Western Hospital - University Health Network; Teach Staff, University of Toronto; (416)603-5499; Fax. (416)603-3456.

LAU, Andrew H C; 8860 Moore Rd, Richmond BC V6Y 2J1; Man'91; CCFP; (604)232-9581

LAU, Anita S; Children's Hosp Eastern Ont, 401 Smyth Rd, Ottawa ON K1H 8L1; Qns'03; FRCPC; Peds; PedEmergMed. Staff, Children's Hospital of Eastern Ontario (CHEO); (613)737-7600

LAU, Arthur; Charlton Med Centre, 708-25 Charlton Ave E, Hamilton ON L8N 1Y2; McM'08; IntMed. Staff, Charlton Medical Centre; (905)521-9034; Fax. (905)521-1863.

LAU, B Chung; 202-943 Broadway W, Vancouver BC V5Z 4E1; Ott'06; FRCSC; Otol (Head & Neck Surgery). (604)879-3223

LAU, Benson P S; 6B-3430 Finch Ave E, Scarborough ON M1W 2R5; Tor'85; Langs: Chinese; (416)497-2096

LAU, Bertrand P; Burnaby Hosp, 3935 Kincaid St, Burnaby BC V5G 2X6; UBC'01; FRCPC; Anes. Staff, Burnaby Hospital.

LAU, Bienca; Royal Univerity Hosp, 103 Hospital Dr, Saskatoon SK S7N 0W8; UBC'99; FRCPC; Psy. Staff, Royal University Hospital; Consultant Psy, University of Saskatchewan; (306)966-8232; Fax. (306)966-8761.

LAU, Brenda W; Pain Management Clinic, 9750 140 St, Surrey BC V3T 0G9; Cal'98; BSc; FRCPC; Anes. Staff, Surrey Memorial Hospital; Staff, Providence Health Care - St Paul's Hospital; Staff, Dr Brenda Lau Medical Inc; Langs: Cantonese; (604)582-4587

LAU, Ching; Sunnybrook Hlth Sciences Ctre, E254-2075 Bayview Ave, Toronto ON M4N 3M5; Tor'84; FRCPC; IntMed; Cardiol. Staff, Sunnybrook Health Sciences Centre; Langs: Cantonese; Mandarin; (416)480-6100

LAU, Chuen-Ping; Royal Oak Med Centre, 201-6440 Royal Oak Ave, Burnaby BC V5H 3P2; (Hong Kong)'69; DABIM; FRCPC; IntMed. Staff Consultant, Burnaby Hospital; Langs: Chinese; (604)433-7372; Fax. (604)433-7003; cp.lau@fraserhealth.ca.

LAU, Yan; Manitoba Clinic, 790 Sherbrook St, Winnipeg MB R3A 1M3; McM'94; FRCPC; IntMed; Gastroent. Langs: Cantonese; (204)774-6541 x434; Fax. (204)775-6373; lauyan@hotmail.com.

LAU, David C W; Julia McFarlane Diab Research, 2998-3330 Hospital Dr NW, Calgary AB T2N 4N1; Tor'75; PhD; ABIM; FRCPC; IntMed (Diabetes). Att Staff Calgary Health Region, Foothills Medical Centre; Prof Med Biochem & Molec Biol, University of Calgary; (403)220-2261; Fax. (403)210-8113; dcwlau@ucalgary.ca.

LAU, David Y M; Parkway Mall, 204-85 Ellesmere Rd, Scarborough ON M1R 4B8; Liverpool (England)'80; MB ChB; DRCOG; DCH(Ire); Ac Staff, Rouge Valley Health System - Centenary Health Centre Site; Court Staff, The Scarborough Hospital - General Campus; Court Staff, The Scarborough Hospital - Birchmount Campus; Langs: Cantonese; (416)446-1661; Fax. (416)446-1872.

LAU, Eddy C H; Village Park Paediatrics, 405-27 Roncesvalles Ave, Toronto ON M6R 3B2; Qns'96; BSc; FRCPC; Peds. Ac Staff/Chief Peds, St Joseph's Health Centre; Assoc Staff, The Hospital For Sick Children; Langs: Cantonese; (416)516-4111; Fax. (416)516-1104; eddy.lau@utoronto.ca.

LAU, Edgar S T; 365-7031 Westminster Hwy, Richmond BC V6X 1A3; UBC'87; FRCPC; IntMed; Respir. (604)270-3760

LAU, Edward T; 7347A 120 St, Delta BC V4C 6P5; (Hong Kong)'70; Staff, Surrey Memorial Hospital.

LAU, Eunice; King Street Med Arts Centre, 403-71 King St W, Mississauga ON L5B 4A2; McM'85; CCFP; Langs: Chinese; (905)949-4017

LAU, Francis T Y; 230-3476 Glen Erin Dr, Mississauga ON L5L 3R4; Tor'82; CCFP; Langs: Chinese; (905)820-3822; Fax. (905)820-7623.

LAU, Gary K L; A6-3300 Mcnicoll Ave, Scarborough ON M1V 5J6; (Hong Kong)'76; FRCS(Glas & Ed); Court Staff, The Scarborough Hospital - Birchmount Campus; Langs: Cantonese; (416)609-8999; Fax. (416)609-8994.

LAU, H K Henry; Times Medical Clinic, 96-550 Highway 7 E, Richmond Hill ON L4B 3Z4; Tor'90; (905)707-8181

LAU, Harold Y H; Tom Baker Cancer Centre, 1331 29 St NW, Calgary AB T2N 4N2; UBC'86; FRCPC; RadOncol. Staff Rad Oncol, Tom Baker Cancer Centre; Langs: Chinese; (403)521-3012; Fax. (403)283-1651.

LAU, Helena L W; Oakville Med Centre, 300-690 Dorval Dr, Oakville ON L6K 3W7; Tor'93; FRCPC; IntMed; Gastroent. Ac Staff, Halton Healthcare Services Corporation - Oakville Site; (905)338-5428; Fax. (905)845-3996.

LAU, Herman H M; Burrard Health Bldg, 502-1160 Burrard St, Vancouver BC V6Z 2E8; Man'92; FRCPC; PhysMed&Rehab. Staff, Providence Health Care - Holy Family Hospital; Staff, Providence Health Care - St Paul's Hospital; Clin Instructor PhysMed&Rehab, University of British Columbia; Langs: Cantonese; (604)668-2580; Fax. (604)688-2507.

LAU, Ho-Yin; Meadowbrook Lanes Med Centre, 109-4591 Highway 7, Unionville ON L3R 1M6; (Hong Kong)'80; MB BS; MRCP(UK); DCH(Glas); FAAP; FRCPC; Peds. Staff Peds, Markham Stouffville Hospital; (905)940-0112

LAU, Ian T; North Simcoe Fam Health Networ, 240 Old Penetanguishene Rd, Midland ON L4R 4P4; (Other Foreign)'10; CCFP.

LAU, Jacqueline C O; The Ottawa Hosp-Civic Campus, C120-1053 Carling Ave, Ottawa ON K1Y 4E9; Qns'06; DiagRad. Staff, The Ottawa Hospital - Civic Campus; (613)761-4054

LAU, Johnny T; Univ Hlth Network-Toronto Western Hosp, 1E 438-399 Bathurst St, Toronto ON M5T 2S8; Tor'94; FRCSC; OrthSurg. Staff, Toronto Western Hospital - University Health Network; (416)603-6292; Fax. (416)603-6293.

LAU, Juliet Y; 5633 177B St, Surrey BC V3S 4H9; (Hong Kong)'73; CCFP; FCFP; Ac Staff, Surrey Memorial Hospital; (604)576-2828; Fax. (604)576-6911.

LAU, Keith K H; McMaster Unversity, 3A-1280 Main St W, Hamilton ON L8S 4K1; (Hong Kong)'87; Nephrol. Staff, Hamilton Health Sciences Centre - McMaster Children's Hospital; (905)521-2100

LAU, Lawrence C Y; Rouge Valley-Centenary Hc, 2867 Ellesmere Rd, Scarborough ON M1E 4B9; Tor'81; FRCPC; Anes. Staff, Rouge Valley Health System - Centenary Health Centre Site; Court Staff, The Scarborough Hospital - General Campus; (416)284-7454; Fax. (416)281-7453.

LAU, Man Pang; 102-4631 Steeles Ave E, Scarborough ON M1V 4S5; (Hong Kong)'60; MB BS(Hongkong); MRCPsy; MD; FRCPC; Psy. Court Staff Psy, The Scarborough Hospital - Birchmount Campus; Langs: Chinese; (416)979-7455; Fax. (416)293-5410.

LAU, Michael C K; 381 Church St PO Box 1800 Stn Main, Markham ON L3P 7P3; Liverpool (England)'82; MB ChB(Path.); FRCPC; GenPath; AnatPath. Assoc Staff Path, Markham Stouffville Hospital; Langs: Cantonese; Mandarin; (905)472-7044

LAU, Micheline C; 22 Hoseyhill Cres, Scarborough ON M1S 2X4; Tubingen (Germany)'68; Langs: Mandarin; German; Cantonese; Italian; Bilingual(French/English).

LAU, Ming-Jarm; 705-5799 Yonge St, North York ON M2M 3V3; Mem'82; Ac Staff/Member CME Committee, North York General Hospital; Ac Staff/Med Examiner Civil Aviation, Bayview Extendicare Nursing Home; (416)221-8612; Fax. (416)221-8784.

LAU, Paul P L; York Medical, 17215 Leslie St, Newmarket ON L3Y 8E4; Qns'94; BSc; CCFP; FCFP; (905)853-0404; Fax. (905)853-3702; paulpllau@hotmail.com.

LAU, Peter C K; Medical Arts Bldg, 537-750 Spadina Cres E, Saskatoon SK S7K 3H3; Sidney (Australia)'86; MB BS; FRCS(Edin); FRCSC; Urol. (306)653-3255; Fax. (306)653-4386.

LAU, Peter P T; 3 G/F-260 Spadina Ave, Toronto ON M5T 2E4; Tor'94; CCFP; FCFP; Langs: Cantonese; Mandarin; (416)979-9988; Fax. (416)979-8774.

LAU, Rick L; Kingston Gen Hosp, 76 Stuart St, Kingston ON K7L 2V7; Dal'05; FRCSC; OrthSurg. Staff, Kingston General Hospital; (613)533-6302; Fax. (613)544-9174.

LAU, Robert C; Medical Clinic Bldg, 303-89 Humber College Blvd, Etobicoke ON M9V 4B8; West Indies (Jamaica)'84; FRCPC; Peds (Pediatric Hematology Oncology); Hem. Staff Physician Peds, The Hospital For Sick Children; Court Staff Peds, William Osler Health System - Etobicoke General Hospital; Asst Prof Peds, University of Toronto; (416)743-6063; Fax. (416)743-0101.

LAU, Susie K S; SMBD Jewish Gen Hosp, 3755 ch Cote-Sainte-Catherine, Montreal QC H3T 1E2; McM'95; MSc; FRCSC; ObstGyn (Surgical Oncology); GynOnco (P.Q.). Staff, Sir Mortimer B Davis Jewish General; adj Prof, McGill University; Langs: Chinese; (514)340-8222 x3114

LAU, Tain Ming; Associated Anaes Services, M2A-601 Broadway W, Vancouver BC V5Z 4C2; (Taiwan)'62; Anes. Ac Staff, Vancouver General Hospital - Centennial Pavillion; Clinical Asst Prof Anes, University of British Columbia; Langs: Cantonese; (604)874-1626

LAU, Tak Sang; Dufferin Med Clinic, 2045 Dufferin St, Toronto ON M6E 3R4; (Hong Kong)'61; FRCS(Glas); FACS; FRCSC; GenSurg. Ac Staff Surg, St Michael's Hospital; Lecturer, University of Toronto; (416)656-6500

LAU, Timothy E; Royal Ottawa Hlth Care Group, 1145 Carling Ave, Ottawa ON K1Z 7K4; Ott'97; FRCPC; Psy. Staff Psy, Royal Ottawa Mental Health Centre - Royal Ottawa Health Care Group; (613)722-6521

LAU, Wayne C; Summerville Family Health Team, 1221 Bloor St, Mississauga ON L4Y 2N8; Tor'97; CCFP; FCFP; (905)625-1241; Fax. (905)625-9514.

LAU, Wendy W; The Hosp for Sick Children, 555 University Ave, Toronto ON M5G 1X8; (Hong Kong)'80; FRCPC; HemPath. Dir Transfusion Med Dept of Paediatric Lab Med, The Hospital For Sick Children; Assoc Med Dir, Canadian Blood Services; Asst Prof Lab Med & Pathol, University of Toronto; (416)813-5440

LAU, William W L; 100-4415 boul Notre-Dame, Laval QC H7W 1T7; Tor'73; Langs: Cantonese; French; Mandarin; (450)687-2221; Fax. (450)687-0117.

LAU, William W L; Royal Columbian Hosp, 330 Columbia St E, New Westminster BC V3L 3W7; UBC'96; FRCPC; GenPath. Staff, Royal Columbian Hospital; (604)520-4940

LAU, Yiu-Keung; Cancer Care Manitoba, 675 McDermot Ave, Winnipeg MB R3E 0V9; Houston(TX) (USA)'98.

LAUBENSTEIN, Susan; Guildford Med Dental Centre, 37-15300 105 Ave, Surrey BC V3R 6A7; UBC'77; BSc; (778)395-6400

LAUBSCHER, Tessa A; Mediclinic, 101-3333 8th St E, Saskatoon SK S7H 4K1; Cape Town (South Africa)'87; MB ChB; CCFP; FCFP; Physician, Saskatoon Health Region Saskatoon Public Health; Asst Prof, University of Saskatchewan; (306)955-1530; Fax. (306)955-8811.

LAUDANSKI, Gerald J; Beaverton Thorah Med Centre, 468 Main St E, Beaverton ON L0K 1A0; McM'84; Physician, Don Valley Med Centre; (705)426-7332; dr.laundanski@hotmail.com.

LAUDER, Gillian R; Children's & Wome's HC of BC, 4480 Oak St, Vancouver BC V6H 3V4; (Wales)'85; MB BCh; FRCPC; Anes. Staff, BC Children's Hospital; (604)875-2711

LAUF, George R; Hys Med Centre, 202-11010 101 St NW, Edmonton AB T5H 4B9; Alb'80; FRCPC; DiagRad. (780)426-1121; Fax. (780)425-5979.

LAUF, Ulrich S; 7020 4 St NW, Calgary AB T2K 1C4; Alb'92; CCFP; Staff, Foothills Medical Centre; Langs: French; German; (403)730-7663

LAUF, Walter W; CPHC Brockville Commu Fam Hlth, 204-309 Park St, Brockville ON K6V 6E5; Tor'78; Staff Privil, Brockville General Hospital - Charles Street; Staff Privil, Providence Continuing Care Centre (PCCC) - St Vincent de Paul Hospital; (613)498-2761; Fax. (613)345-7787.

LAUFER, Brian; Hop Maisonneuve-Rosemont, 5415 boul de l'Assomption, Montreal QC H1T 2M4; Mon'80; FRCPC; IntMed; Critical Care Medicine (P.Q.). Staff, Hopital Maisonneuve-Rosemont; Langs: French; Spanish; (514)252-3822; brian.laufer@sympatico.ca.

LAUFER, Jerome R; SMBD Jewish Gen Hosp, 3755 ch Cote-Sainte-Catherine, Montreal QC H3T 1E2; Angers (France)'84; FRCPC; NuclearMed. Staff, Sir Mortimer B Davis Jewish General; Langs: Bilingual(French/English); (514)340-8222; Fax. (514)340-8720.

LAUGHLAND, Lori A; Sardis Family Practice, 202-45425 Luckakuck Way, Chilliwack BC V2R 2T7; McM'95; BSc; MSc; CCFP; (604)858-9461; Fax. (604)858-9921.

LAUGHLIN, Robert; High Prairie Med Clinic, PO Box 449 4620 53 Ave, High Prairie AB T0G 1E0; Glasgow (Scotland)'68; MB ChB; Teacher, University of Alberta; (780)523-4501; Fax. (780)523-4800; hpmed@telusplanet.net.

LAUGHLIN, Sharyn A; Medical Towers, 650-1600 Carling Ave, Ottawa ON K1Z 1G3; Ott'76; DABD; FRCPC; Derm (Photobiol & Laser Med). (613)722-4436; Fax. (613)722-2877; info@laserderm.ca.

LAUGHLIN, Suzanne; The Hosp for Sick Children, 2136 EW-555 University Ave, Toronto ON M5G 1X8; Wes'91; FRCPC; DiagRad (Neuro Radiology). Staff, The Hospital For Sick Children; Asst Prof Medical Imaging, University of Toronto; (416)813-6033; suzanne.laughlin@sickkids.ca.

LAUGHLIN, Thomas A; Moncton Med Clinic, 301-860 Mountain Rd, Moncton NB E1C 2N7; Dal'78; CCFP; FCFP; (506)853-5150; laughlint@nbnet.nb.ca.

LAUGHREA, John B; Ctr Hosp Affilie-Enfant-Jesus, 1401 18e rue, Quebec QC G1J 1Z4; Laval'82; NBME; FRCPC; IntMed (Infectious Diseases); Respir. Staff, Centre Hospitalier Affilié Universitaire de Québec - Hôpital De L'Enfant Jésus; Staff, Centre Hospitalier Affilié Universitaire de Québec - Hôpital du St-Sacrement; Université Laval; Langs: Bilingual(French/English); (418)649-0252 x5743; Fax. (418)649-5928; laughrea@videotron.ca.

LAUGHREA, Patricia A; Ctr Hosp Affilie-St-Sacrement, D1 45-1050 ch Sainte-Foy, Quebec QC G1S 4L8; Laval'78; AB; FACS; FRCSC; Ophth (Cornea & Anterior Segment). Staff, Centre Hospitalier Affilié Universitaire de Québec - Hôpital du St-Sacrement; Prof, Université Laval; Langs: English; (418)682-7511; Fax. (418)682-7534.

LAUGHTON, Angela F; Bruyere Family Med Centre, 75 Bruyere St, Ottawa ON K1N 5C8; McM'07; CCFP; (613)241-3344

LAUKKANEN, Ethan; Queen Elizabeth Hosp, PO Box 6600 Stn Central, Charlottetown PE C1A 8T5; McM'80; FRCPC; RadOncol. Ac Staff, Queen Elizabeth Hospital; Dir, PenCentric Health System Inc; (902)894-2951; Fax. (902)894-2187; ethan.laukkanen@pencentric.net.

LAUNAY, Marc P; 4840 Circle Rd, Montreal QC H3W 1Z4; Mon'61; MSc(InvestMed.); Endocrin (P.Q.); IntMed (P.Q.) (Medico Legal Consultant). Langs: English; French; (514)481-2247; Fax. (514)481-5761.

LAUNCELOTT, Gordon O; Queen Elizabeth II HSC, 1276 South Park St, Halifax NS B3H 2Y9; Ott'78; FRCPC; Anes. Staff, Queen Elizabeth II Health Sciences Centre - Victoria General Site; (902)473-2331; Fax. (902)423-9454.

LAUPACIS, Andreas; 30 Bond St, Toronto ON M5B 1W8; Qns'79; FRCPC; IntMed (Palliative Care). Dir Li Ka Shing Knowledge Institute, St Michael's Hospital; (416)864-5780; Fax. (416)864-5117; laupacisa@smh.ca.

LAUPLAND, Brenda R; Royal Inland Hosp, 311 Columbia St, Kamloops BC V2C 2T1; Tor'96; CCFP; FCFP; Staff, Royal Inland Hospital; (250)374-5111

LAUPLAND, Kevin B; Peter Lougheed Centre, 3500 26 Ave NE, Calgary AB T1Y 6J4; Tor'96; FRCPC; IntMed; Critical Care Medicine; InfectDis. Staff, Foothills Medical Centre; Staff, Peter Lougheed Centre; (403)943-5785; Fax. (403)291-1491.

LAURANS, Muriel; Hop Jean-Talon, 1385 rue Jean-Talon E, Montreal QC H2E 1S6; Mon'98; CCFP; Staff, CSSS du Coeur de l'Isle Hôpital Jean-Talon; (514)495-6733

LAUREIJS, Pauweliena P M; Stanton Terr Health Authority, PO Box 10 Stn Main 550 Byrne Rd, Yellowknife NT X1A 2N1; Dal'96; FRCPC; Psy. Staff, Stanton Territorial Health Authority; (867)445-8753

LAURENCE, Craig; Whitecourt Med Clinic, PO Box 1076 Stn Main 5035 51 Ave, Whitecourt AB T7S 1P9; (South Africa)'05; MB ChB; (780)778-2224; Fax. (780)778-2127.

LAURENCE, Jennifer; 2720 Mill Bay Rd PO Box 76, Mill Bay BC V0R 2P0; McM'06; CCFP; CCFP(E.M.); (250)732-6176

LAURENCE, Kelly H; Peterborough Reg HC-Hospital, 1 Hospital Dr, Peterborough ON K9J 7C6; Dal'93; FRCPC; AnatPath. Staff, Peterborough Regional Health Centre - Hospital Drive; (705)876-5014 x3082; Fax. (705)876-5008.

LAURENCE, Michel; CSSS Pierre Boucher, 1333 boul Jacques-Cartier E, Longueuil QC J4M 2A5; Mon'74; Staff, Centre Hospitalier Pierre Boucher; (450)468-8239

LAURENCIC, Djurdjica; Trillium Hlth Ctr-Mississauga, 100 Queensway W, Mississauga ON L5B 1B8; Belgrade (Serbia)'99; FRCPC; Psy. Staff, Trillium Health Centre - Mississauga; (905)848-7585

LAURENDEAU, Catherine; Clinique Medicale Angus, 101-4101 rue Molson, Montreal QC H1Y 3L1; Mon'98; Staff, Hôpital Ste-Justine; (514)807-2333

LAURENDEAU, Denis; Pavillon Albert Prevost, 6555 boul Gouin O, Montreal QC H4K 1B3; Mon'67; FRCPC; Psy (Pedology Psychiatry). Staff, Hôpital du Sacre-Coeur de Montréal; Asst Prof Psy, Universite de Montreal; (514)338-4356; Fax. (514)338-4357.

LAURENDEAU, Francois; CLSC Les Eskers de l'Abitibi, 612 5e av O, Amos QC J9T 4L3; Mon'77; Langs: Bilingual(French/English); (819)732-6696 x3234; Fax. (819)732-0038; francois.l@cableamos.com.

LAURENDEAU, Louis; Ctr Medico Prof de Brossard, 2424 boul Lapiniere, Brossard QC J4Z 2K9; Mon'69; (450)678-9033

LAURENDEAU, Lyne; CSSS Champlain-CLSC St Hubert, 6800 boul Cousineau, Saint-Hubert QC J3Y 8Z4; Mon'87; CCFP; FCFP; Universite de Montreal; Langs: English; (450)443-7400; Fax. (450)676-3488; lyne.laurendeau@rrsss16.gouv.qc.ca.

LAURENDEAU, Steve; CSSS de Chicoutimi, 305 rue Saint-Vallier, Chicoutimi QC G7H 5H6; Laval'02; CardSurg. Staff, Complexe hospitalier de la Sagamie; (418)541-1000

LAURENS, Jean-Pierre; CHUM-Hop Notre-Dame, 1560 rue Sherbrooke E, Montreal QC H2L 4M1; Sher'92; Staff, Centre Hospitalier l'Université de Montréal (CHUM) - Hôpital Notre-Dame; (514)890-8000

LAURENT, Guy; Polyclinique Med Concorde, 300 boul de la Concorde E, Laval QC H7G 2E6; Mon'62; Urol. ac Staff, Hôpital de Saint-Eustache; Langs: Bilingual(French/English); (450)667-5310; Fax. (450)667-2163; urolaval@videotron.ca.

LAURIE, Alexa M M; Dr Walter Templeman Hlth Ctr, PO Box 580, Bell Island NL A0A 4H0; London (England)'73; MRCS; LRCP; DCH; CCFP; Staff, Dr Walter Templeman Health Centre; Clin Preceptor, Memorial University Of Newfoundland; (709)488-2774; Fax. (709)488-2600.

LAURIE, Scott A; Ottawa Reg Cancer Centre, 501 Smyth Rd, Ottawa ON K1H 8L6; Ott'94; FRCPC; IntMed (Thoracic Oncology); MedOncol. Staff Ottawa Reg Cancer Centre, The Ottawa Hospital - General Campus; (613)737-7700 x70175; Fax. (613)247-3511.

LAURIER, Danielle; Direction Sante et Securite, 7E-75 boul Rene-Levesque O, Montreal QC H2Z 1A4; Mon'80; (514)289-2265; Fax. (514)289-4507; laurier.danielle@hydro.qc.ca.

LAURIER, Louis; Polyclinique St-Jerome, 302-200 rue Durand, Saint-Jerome QC J7Z 7E2; Mon'80; FRCPC; IntMed; Gastroent. Staff, Hôtel-Dieu de Saint-Jérôme; (450)438-0404; Fax. (450)431-8244.

LAURIER, Michel; Hop Du Sacre-Coeur De Mtl, 5400 boul Gouin O, Montreal QC H4J 1C5; Mon'73; FRCPC; IntMed. Ac Staff, Hôpital du Sacre-Coeur de Montréal; Clin Teacher, Universite de Montreal; (514)338-2222

LAURIN, Daniel; Centre Med Laval, 1110 boul Vanier, Laval QC H7C 2R8; Mon'86; Staff, Hopital de la Cite de la santé; Langs: English; (450)661-2521; Fax. (450)661-7193.

LAURIN, Gilles; Hop Charles Lemoyne, 3120 boul Taschereau, Greenfield Park QC J4V 2H1; Mon'54; GenSurg (P.Q.). Staff Surg, Hopital Charles LeMoyne; (450)466-5000

LAURIN, Gilles; Clin Med Privee des Mille-Iles, 200-230 ch de la Grande-Cote, Boisbriand QC J7G 1B5; Mon'77; Langs: English; (450)437-1111

LAURIN, Luc; Polyclinique Med de La Lievre, 536 rue de la Madone, Mont-Laurier QC J9L 1S7; Mon'79; Staff, CSSS d'Antoine-Labelle; (819)440-2345

LAURIN, Michel A; Centre Hosp Honore-Mercier, 2750 boul Laframboise, Saint-Hyacinthe QC J2S 4Y8; Sher'80; CSPQ; FRCPC; GenPath; AnatPath. Staff, Centre Hospitalier Honore-Mercier; Langs: Spanish; French; (450)771-3333

LAURIN, Norman R; CSSS de Trois-Rivières, 1991 boul du Carmel, Trois-Rivieres QC G8Z 3R9; Sher'84; NuclearMed. Staff, CSSS de Trois-Rivières; Staff, Centre Hospitalier Regional de Trois-Rivieres; Clinical Asst Prof, Universite de Sherbrooke; Langs: English; (819)697-3333 x69854

LAURIN, Pierre-Michel; GMF du Grand Saint-Jerome, 2100 boul du Cure-Labelle, Saint-Jerome QC J7Y 1S8; Mon'78; Staff, Hôtel-Dieu de Saint-Jérôme; Langs: Spanish; English; (450)565-6493; Fax. (450)565-1099.

LAURIN, Suzanne; Hop Du Sacre-Coeur De Mtl, 5400 boul Gouin O, Montreal QC H4J 1C5; Mon'84; CCFP; FCFP; Staff, Hôpital du Sacre-Coeur de Montréal; (514)338-2383; Fax. (514)338-3155.

LAURION, Marcel; CSSS de Laval, 1755 boul Rene-Laennec, Laval QC H7M 3L9; Mon'74; FRCSC; GenSurg (Surgical Oncology). Staff GenSurg, Hopital de la Cite de la santé; Confér Clin Surg, Universite de Montreal; Langs: Bilingual(French/English); (450)668-1010; Fax. (450)629-4704; famillelaurion@videotron.ca.

LAURION, Monique; CSSS de Quebec Nord, 3666 ch Royal, Quebec QC G1E 1X5; Laval'84; Langs: Bilingual(French/English); (418)663-3099; Fax. (418)663-2939; monique.laurion@ssss.gouv.qc.ca.

LAURISTON, Christian; Clinique Med Perrier, 10-10794 rue Lajeunesse, Montreal QC H3L 2E8; (Mexico)'80; Staff, Hôpital Santa Cabrini Ospedale; ac Staff, CSSS Saint-Leonard et Saint-Michel; Langs: Spanish; English; (514)383-0559; Fax. (514)383-3430.

LAURORE, Yardley; Clinique Privee du Dr Savaria, 75 boul des Chateaux, Blainville QC J7B 2A4; Sher'05; CCFP; (450)434-2009

LAURSEN, Brian W; Northgate Med Centre, 2711 Avonhurst Dr, Regina SK S4R 3J3; Glasgow (Scotland)'72; MB ChB; VP Medical Serv, Regina General Hospital; Clin Teacher Family Med, University of Saskatchewan; (306)543-4566; Fax. (306)543-4441.

LAUSMAN, Andrea Y; St Michael's Hosp, 15 018B-30 Bond St, Toronto ON M5B 1W8; Wes'00; FRCSC; ObstGyn (Maternal Fetal Medicine). Staff, St Michael's Hospital; Asst Prof, University of Toronto; (416)864-6060 x2395

LAUSSEN, Peter C; The Hosp for Sick Children, 555 University Ave, Toronto ON M5G 1X8; Melbourne (Australia)'80; Staff, The Hospital For Sick Children; (416)813-1500

LAUTATZIS, Miltiade; Legacy X-Ray Clinic, 14-160 Meadowood Dr, Winnipeg MB R2M 5L6; Modena (Italy)'62; DMRD(Lond); DiagRad. Staff, St Boniface General Hospital.

LAUTNER, David; Foothills Med Centre, 1403 29 St NW, Calgary AB T2N 2T9; Sask'90; FRCPC; IntMed; DiagRad. Staff Diag Imaging, Foothills Medical Centre; (403)944-4530; Fax. (403)944-1687.

LAUWERS, Albert E; Office of the Coroner, 26 Grenville St, Toronto ON M7A 2G9; Tor'82; CCFP; FCFP; Dist Coroner, District Area 12; (416)326-4805; Fax. (416)314-4030; albert@hhfht.com.

LAUZE, Michelle; Regie des Rentes du Quebec, CP 5200 Succ Terminus 348-2600 boul Laurier, Quebec QC G1K 7S9; Laval'83; (418)657-8709 x3552

LAUZIER, Francois; Ctr Hosp Affilie-Enfant-Jesus, 1401 18e rue, Quebec QC G1J 1Z4; Sher'99; FRCPC; IntMed (Intensive Care); Critical Care Medicine (P.Q.). Staff, Centre Hospitalier Affilié Universitaire de Québec - Hôpital De L'Enfant Jésus; (418)649-0252 x3575; Fax. (418)649-5913.

LAUZIER, Nathalie; CLSC des Faubourgs, 1250 rue Sanguinet, Montreal QC H2X 3E7; Laval'98; LMCC; Langs: Bilingual(French/English); (514)527-2361 x3771

LAUZIER, Sylvie; Hop du Sacre-Coeur de Mtl, 5400 boul Gouin O, Montreal QC H4J 1C5; Mon'79; FRCPC; Neur (Cerebrovascular Disease). Staff, Hôpital du Sacre-Coeur de Montréal; (514)338-2050

LAUZIERE, Maurice; Clinique Dr Maurice Lauziere, 497 114e rue, Shawinigan-Sud QC G9P 2X6; Laval'74; Staff, Centre Hospitalier du Centre la Mauricie; (819)537-0749

LAUZON, Andre; Laboratoire De Med Legale, 12e-1701 rue Parthenais, Montreal QC H2K 3S7; Mon'70; CSPQ; GenPath (P.Q.) (Anatomical Pathology). Médecin traitant, Laboratoire De Med Legale; adj Prof, Universite de Montreal; (514)873-3300

LAUZON, Claude; CSSS de la Region de Thetford, 1717 rue Notre-Dame E, Thetford Mines QC G6G 2V4; Laval'83; ABIM; FRCPC; IntMed. Consultant Intensive Care, Hopital du CSS de la Region de Thetford; (418)338-7777

LAUZON, Dominique; CSSS Haut-Richelieu-Rouville, 920 boul Du Seminaire N, St-Jean-Sur-Richel QC J3A 1B7; Sher'79; FRCPC; MedMicrobiol; InfectDis (P.Q.). Staff, Hôpital du Haut-Richelieu; (450)359-5000 x5241; dominique.lauzon@rrsss16.gouv.qc.ca.

LAUZON, France; Centre Med Saint-Charles, 1740 ch Saint-Charles, Terrebonne QC J6W 3R3; Laval'89; Staff, Centre Hospitalier Pierre le Gardeur; Langs: Bilingual(French/English); (450)492-2277

LAUZON, Francine; Clinique Med Dagenais, 2065 boul des Laurentides, Laval QC H7M 4M2; Mon'87; (450)975-1557; Fax. (450)975-1557.

LAUZON, Genevieve; 202-520 17th St, West Vancouver BC V7V 3S8; Ott'91; Langs: Bilingual(English/French); (604)913-8183

LAUZON, Ghyslain; CSSS de la Vallée de l'Or, 725 6e rue, Val-d'Or QC J9P 3Y1; Sher'90; FRCPC; IntMed; Respir. Staff, Centre Hospitalier de Val d'Or; (819)825-6711 x2320; Fax. (819)825-7948.

LAUZON, Gilles; 522-2600 av Pierre-Dupuy, Montreal QC H3C 3R6; Mon'59 UniversitÃ© de MontrÃ©al; BA; FRCSC; GenSurg; PlasSurg. Staff, Centre Metropolitan de Chirurgie Plastique; Langs: Bilingual(English/French); Chavacano; (514)933-8441; gillauzon@gmail.com.

LAUZON, Guylaine; CSSS de la Matapedia, 135 av Gaetan-Archambault, Amqui QC G5J 2K5; Laval'91; LMCC; Staff, CSSS de la Matapedia; (418)629-2211

LAUZON, Jean G; 100-1647 140 St, Surrey BC V4A 4H1; Ott'87; FRCSC; GenSurg. Staff, Peace Arch Hospital; Staff, Cambie Surgery Centre; Langs: English; French; (604)538-8015; Fax. (604)538-8037.

LAUZON, Julie L; Alberta Children's Hosp, 2888 Shaganappi Trail NW, Calgary AB T3B 6A8; Ott'01; FRCPC; MedGenetics. Staff Med Genetics, Alberta Children's Hospital; Langs: Bilingual(French/English); (403)955-7373; Fax. (403)955-2701; julie.lauzon@albertahealthservices.ca.

LAUZON, Lucie; GMF de Lorraine, 99 boul de Gaulle, Lorraine QC J6Z 3Z9; Mon'81; (450)621-1444; Fax. (450)621-7193.

LAUZON, Marguerite; Clinique Domus Medica, 5601 rue Belanger, Montreal QC H1T 1G3; Mon'77; (514)256-5011

LAUZON, Matthew A; 5-30 University Terrace, 8303 112 St NW, Edmonton AB T6G 1K4; Cal'07; FRCPC; IntMed; OccupMed.

LAUZON, Michel; Centre Serv Sante F C, 6560 rue Hochelaga, Montreal QC H1N 1X9; Mon'70; Staff, Centre Hospitalier d'Argenteuil; (514)252-2777 x4920

LAUZON, Pierre P E; CLSC de Dorval-Lachine, 1900 rue Notre-Dame, Lachine QC H8S 2G2; Mon'75; Ac Staff, CSSS de Dorval-Lachine-Lasalle; (514)639-0063

LAUZON, Pierre; CHUM-Hop St-Luc, 1058 rue Saint-Denis, Montreal QC H2X 3J4; Mon'71; Staff, Centre Hospitalier l'Université De Montréal (CHUM) - Hôpital Saint-luc; (514)890-8316; Fax. (514)412-7295.

LAUZON, Robert; Ctr Hosp Affilie-Enfant-Jesus, 1401 18e rue, Quebec QC G1J 1Z4; Laval'82; EmergMed (P.Q.). Ac Staff, Centre Hospitalier Affilié Universitaire de Québec - Hôpital De L'Enfant Jésus; (418)649-5632; Fax. (418)649-5975.

LAUZON-LAURIN, Anais; CSSS du Nord de Lanaudière, 1000 boul Sainte-Anne, St-Charles-Brromee QC J6E 6J2; Laval'07; CSPQ; MedMicrobiol. Staff, Centre Hospitalier Régional de Lanaudière; (450)759-8222

LAVALLEE, Barry D A; St Jame Street Med Clinic, 1600 Portage Ave, Winnipeg MB R3J 0C6; Man'88; CCFP; FCFP; (204)925-3700

LAVALLEE, Carol L; North Bay Reg Health Centre, 680 Kirkwood Dr, Sudbury ON P3E 1X3; RCS (Ireland)'82; MB ChB; BSc(Hons); BA(Hons Philosophy); MRCPsy; FRCPC; Psy. Staff, North Bay Regional Health Centre - Regional Mental Health; Staff, North Bay Regional Health Centre - Kirkwood; Langs: English; French; (705)675-9193; clavallee@nemhe.on.ca.

LAVALLEE, Catherine; Hop Charles Lemoyne, 3120 boul Taschereau, Greenfield Park QC J4V 2H1; McG'07; MDCM; CSPQ; FRCPC; Anes. Staff, Hopital Charles LeMoyne; (450)466-5000

LAVALLEE, Chad M; St Mary's Gen Hosp, 911 Queens Blvd, Kitchener ON N2M 1B2; Wes'96; FRCPC; DiagRad. Staff, St Mary's General Hospital; (519)749-6455; Fax. (519)749-6513; dr_chad_l@hotmail.com.

LAVALLEE, Christian; Hop Maisonneuve-Rosemont, 5415 boul de l'Assomption, Montreal QC H1T 2M4; Mon'05; CSPQ; FRCPC; MedMicrobiol; InfectDis (P.Q.). Staff, Hopital Maisonneuve-Rosemont; (514)252-3400 x4524

LAVALLEE, Claude H; Clinique Med Ste-Therese, 101-233 rue Turgeon, Sainte-Therese QC J7E 3J8; Mon'91; CCFP; Staff, Hôpital de Saint-Eustache; (450)430-4301; Fax. (450)430-7258.

LAVALLEE, Emilie; Reseau de sante des Basques, 550 rue Notre-Dame E, Trois-Pistoles QC G0L 4K0; Laval'09; (418)851-3700

LAVALLEE, Gilles; Hop Du Sacre-Coeur De Mtl, 5400 boul Gouin O, Montreal QC H4J 1C5; Mon'71; ABR; FRCPC; DiagRad. Staff, Hôpital du Sacre-Coeur de Montréal; (514)338-2222 x2131

LAVALLEE, Jean; Clinique Reseau Val-Belair, 1147 boul Pie XI N, Quebec QC G3K 2P8; Laval'68; (418)843-2473

LAVALLEE, Jean-Pierre; Hop Brome-Missisquoi-Perkins, 950 rue Principale, Cowansville QC J2K 1K3; Sher'70; FCCP; Cardiol (P.Q.). Dir Div of Cardiol, Hôpital Brome-Missisquoi-Perkins; Langs: English; (450)266-4342 x5195; Fax. (450)266-5049.

LAVALLEE, Lucie; Coop Sante-L'Islet, 82 10e rue, L'Isletville QC G0R 2C0; Laval'94; (418)247-5065

LAVALLEE, Lucie; Centre Med Donnacona, 420 rte 138, Donnacona QC G3M 1C2; Laval'96; (418)285-1122

LAVALLEE, Melvyn R; 216A Fourth Ave, Strathmore AB T1P 1B9; Sask'70; MD; Med Examiner Civil Aviation, Transport Canada; (403)361-2422

LAVALLÉE, Philippe; CSSS de Trois-Rivières, 1991 boul du Carmel, Trois-Rivieres QC G8Z 3R9; Mon'09; Staff, CSSS de Trois-Rivières; (819)697-3333

LAVALLEE, Pierre; Clinique Med 6930 Papineau Inc, 6930 av Papineau, Montreal QC H2G 2X7; Mon'66; Staff, CSSS du Coeur de l'Isle Hôpital Jean-Talon; (514)722-0000; Fax. (514)722-2431.

LAVALLEE, Pierre; Ctr Hosp Affilie-Enfant-Jesus, 1401 18e rue, Quebec QC G1J 1Z4; Laval'80; FRCSC; OrthSurg. Assoc Staff, CSSS de Quebec-Sud; Ac Staff, Centre Hospitalier Affilié Universitaire de Québec - Hôpital De L'Enfant Jésus; (418)649-0252; Fax. (418)649-5567.

LAVALLEE, Sophie; 207-468 boul Sir-Wilfrid-Lauri, Mont-Saint-Hilaire QC J3H 6K3; Mon'96; LMCC; Langs: English; (450)281-2121

LAVALLEE, Vincent P; Hop Maisonneuve-Rosemont, 5415 boul de l'Assomption, Montreal QC H1T 2M4; Mon'07; Hem; IntMed. Staff, Hopital Maisonneuve-Rosemont; (514)252-3400

LAVALLEE, Yvon-Jacques; CSSS de Chicoutimi, CP 264 305 rue Saint-Vallier, Chicoutimi QC G7H 5H6; Mon'70 Université de Montréal; FRCPC; Psy. Staff, Complexe hospitalier de la Sagamie; Langs: English; (418)549-5477; Fax. (418)549-7604.

LAVALLEY, J William; Medical Wellness Centre, PO Box 2020 227 Central St, Chester NS B0J 1J0; Baylor College of Medicine-Houston (TX) (USA)'86; Chairman Integrated & Complementary Med Section, Doctors Nova Scotia; Member, Society for Integrative Oncology; Member, Canadian Medical Association; (902)275-4555; Fax. (902)273-3303; MedicalWellness@eastlink.ca.

LAVANCHY, Marcel C; 107-3500 Carrington Rd, Westbank BC V4T 3C1; (Chile)'95; CCFP; Staff, Travel Medicine Clinic; Langs: Spanish; (250)452-6742

LAVELLE, Nancy L; Workers' Compensation Board, 200-1881 Scarth St, Regina SK S4P 4L1; Alb'84; (306)787-4458; nlavelle@wcbsask.com.

LAVELLE, Peter R; Medical Arts Bldg, 353 St Paul Ave, Brantford ON N3R 4N3; Dublin (Ireland)'71; Assoc Staff, The Brant Community Healthcare System - Brantford General Hospital Site; (519)756-8601; Fax. (519)756-8601.

LAVENDER, S Jo Anne; Foothills Family Practice, 102-30 Crystalridge Dr, Okotoks AB T1S 2C3; Alb'71; (403)938-5455

LAVENS, M Timothy; Beiseker Med Clinic, PO Box 100 319 6th Ave, Beiseker AB T0M 0G0; Alb'71; CCFP; CCFP(E.M.); Staff ER, Rockyview General Hospital; (403)947-3440; Fax. (403)947-3440.

LAVENS, Nathan T; 100-1410 Mayor Magrath Dr S, Lethbridge AB T1K 2R3; Cal'03; FRCSC; Urol. Staff UroOncology, Jack Ady Cancer Centre; (403)524-1411; Fax. (403)524-1403.

LAVERDIERE, Annie; CSSS de Trois-Rivières, 1991 boul du Carmel, Trois-Rivieres QC G8Z 3R9; Laval'01; CCFP; CCFP(E.M.); Staff Emerg, CSSS de Trois-Rivières; Langs: English; (819)697-3333

LAVERDIERE, Caroline; Hôpital Ste-Justine, 3175 ch Cote-Sainte-Catherine, Montreal QC H3T 1C5; Mon'96; FRCPC; Peds; Hem. Staff, Hôpital Ste-Justine; (514)345-4931 x4639; josee.robert.hsj@ssss.gouv.qc.ca.

LAVERDIERE, David; CSSS de Chicoutimi, 305 rue Saint-Vallier, Chicoutimi QC G7H 5H6; Mon'98; FRCPC; IntMed. Staff, Complexe hospitalier de la Sagamie; (418)541-1013

LAVERDIERE, Francois M; 104-201 rue Dupont, Pont-Rouge QC G3H 1N7; Laval'82; (418)873-4197; Fax. (418)873-5117.

LAVERDIERE, Ginette M B; Lincoln Med Centre, 4413 Ontario St, Beamsville ON L0R 1B5; McM'99; BScN; CCFP; Staff, West Lincoln Memorial Hospital; (905)563-1212; Fax. (905)563-4404; glaverd@hotmail.com.

LAVERDIERE, Ines; CLSC-CHSLD de la Petite Nation, 14 rue St-Andre, St-Andre-Avellin QC J0V 1W0; Laval'02; (819)983-7341; Fax. (819)983-1315.

LAVERDIERE, Marianne; CSSS de l'Energie-Ste-Therese, 1705 av Georges, Shawinigan QC G9N 2N1; Laval'07; FRCPC; Psy. Staff, CH du Centre-de-la-Mauricie (Ste-Thérèse de Shawinigan); (819)536-7500; marianne_laverdiere@ssss.gouv.qc.ca.

LAVERDIERE, Maryse; Clinique Med Saint-Louis, 220-3165 ch Saint-Louis, Quebec QC G1W 4R4; Laval'82; LMCC; Physician, Clinique Medicale Domaine des Soeurs; (418)653-1970

LAVERDIERE, Melanie; Hotel-Dieu de Levis, 143 rue Wolfe, Levis QC G6V 3Z1; Laval'04; FRCPC; Anes. Staff, Hôtel-Dieu de Lévis; (418)835-7121 x3217

LAVERDIERE, Michel; Hop Maisonneuve-Rosemont, 5415 boul de l'Assomption, Montreal QC H1T 2M4; Mon'71; InfectDis (P.Q.); MedMicrobiol (P.Q.). Staff, Hopital Maisonneuve-Rosemont; Langs: English; (514)252-3817; Fax. (514)252-3898.

LAVERDIERE, Michel-Andre; Hop Maisonneuve-Rosemont, 5415 boul de l'Assomption, Montreal QC H1T 2M4; Mon'81; Cardiol (P.Q.); IntMed (Echocardiography). Staff, Hopital Maisonneuve-Rosemont; Langs: English; (514)252-3812

LAVERDIERE, Patrick; CSSS de la Cote-De-Gaspe, 215 boul de York O, Gaspe QC G4X 2W2; Laval'07; FRCPC; IntMed. Staff, Centre Hospitalier de Gaspe; (418)368-3301

LAVERDURE, Julie; Clin Externe Psychiatrie, 7345 rue Garnier, Montreal QC H2E 2A1; Sher'01; Psy. (514)729-3425

LAVERGNE, Genevieve; 101-3195 boul de la Piniere, Terrebonne QC J6X 4P7; Laval'98; CCFP; Staff, Hopital de la Cite de la santé; (450)824-1515

LAVERGNE, Louis J; CSSS Pierre de Saurel, 30 rue Ferland, Sorel-Tracy QC J3P 3C7; Sher'94; (450)746-4545

LAVERGNE, Martine; CSSS du Nord de Lanaudière, 1000 boul Sainte-Anne, St-Charles-Brromee QC J6E 6J2; Mon'87; CSPQ; FRCPC; MedMicrobiol; Microbio & Infect Dis (P.Q.). Staff Microbiol & InfectDis, Centre Hospitalier Régional de Lanaudière; (450)759-8222 x2673

LAVERGNE, Valery; Hop du Sacre-Coeur de Mtl, 5400 boul Gouin O, Montreal QC H4J 1C5; Mon'01; FRCPC; MedMicrobiol; Microbio & Infect Dis (P.Q.). Staff, Hôpital du Sacre-Coeur de Montréal; (514)338-2222

LAVERTU, Caroline; Clinique Med St-Louis, 220-3165 ch Saint-Louis, Quebec QC G1W 4R4; Laval'98; (418)653-1970

LAVERTU, Denis J R; 625-2590 boul Laurier, Quebec QC G1V 4M6; Laval'67; FRCSC; PlasSurg. (418)623-2300

LAVERTU, Real; Clinique Med Saint-Marc, 1295 boul Saint-Sacrement, Shawinigan QC G9N 3M8; Mon'78; Staff, CH du Centre-de-la-Mauricie (Ste-Thérèse de Shawinigan); (819)539-2999; Fax. (819)539-0078; real_lavertu@ssss.gouv.qc.ca.

LAVERTU, Sophie; CHUM-Hop Notre-Dame, 1560 rue Sherbrooke E, Montreal QC H2L 4M1; Laval'94; FRCPC; RadOncol. Staff RadOncol, Centre Hospitalier l'Université de Montréal (CHUM) - Hôpital Notre-Dame; Clin Teacher, Universite de Montreal; (514)890-8254; Fax. (514)412-7537; sophielavertu@hotmail.com.

LAVERTY, H K Kay; 2704 48 St NW, Edmonton AB T6L 6B8; (India)'85; MB BS; CCFP; (587)520-8788

LAVERTY, Lee-Anne; Riverside Med Clinic, 305-1101 Dewdney Ave, Trail BC V1R 4T1; Qns'95; FRCSC; OrthSurg (Hand & Upper Extremity Surgery). Langs: French; (250)364-1599; Fax. (250)368-8886; lalaverty@hotmail.com.

LAVI, Ronit; London HSC-University Hosp, PO Box 5339 Stn B C3 104-399 Windermere Rd, London ON N6A 5A5; (Israel)'99; Staff, London Health Sciences Centre - University Hospital; (519)663-3270

LAVI, Sasson; 207-398 Steeles Ave W, Thornhill ON L4J 6X3; Hebrew (Israel)'78; ABAI; FRCPC; Peds (Allergy & Immunology). Staff, The Hospital For Sick Children; Asst Prof, University of Toronto; Langs: Hebrew; Arabic; (905)709-4604; Fax. (905)709-4610.

LAVI, Shahar; London HSC-University Hosp, PO Box 5339 Stn B 339 Windermere Rd, London ON N6A 5A5; (Israel)'97; Staff, London Health Sciences Centre - University Hospital; (519)663-3611

LAVIGNE, Alexandre; CSSS de Montmagny-L'Islet, RR 1 350 boul Tache O, Montmagny QC G5V 3R8; Laval'00; FRCSC; GenSurg (Laparoscopy). Staff, CSSS de Montmagny-L'Islet; (418)248-0630; Fax. (418)248-0947; saxalex@hotmail.com.

LAVIGNE, Annie; Hop Charles Lemoyne, 3120 boul Taschereau, Greenfield Park QC J4V 2H1; Sher'90; FRCPC; IntMed; Critical Care Medicine (P.Q.). Staff, Hopital Charles LeMoyne; (450)466-5000 x2880

LAVIGNE, Caroline; Polyclinique St-Eustache, 75 rue Grignon, Saint-Eustache QC J7P 4J2; McG'07; MDCM; CCFP; Staff, Hôpital de Saint-Eustache; Staff Planning, CLSC Jean-Olivier-Chenier; Langs: Bilingual(French/English); (450)473-6777; Fax. (450)473-1916; caroline_lavigne@ssss.gouv.qc.ca.

LAVIGNE, Dominique; Hôpital Laval, 2725 ch Sainte-Foy, Quebec QC G1V 4G5; Mon'02; FRCPC; Anes. Staff, Hôpital Laval; (418)656-8711

LAVIGNE, Francois G; Institut ORL De Montreal, 201-1361 av Beaumont, Mont-Royal QC H3P 2W3; Sher'81; FRCSC; Otol (Rhinology). ac Staff, Centre Hospitalier l'Université de Montréal (CHUM) - Hôpital Notre-Dame; (514)343-5244; Fax. (514)738-4668; orl@medilyfe.com.

LAVIGNE, Gisele; CLSC-CHSLD PAT Montreal Est, 13926 rue Notre-Dame E, Pte-aux-Trembles QC H1A 1T5; Mon'78; (514)642-4050; Fax. (514)498-7505.

LAVIGNE, Jean-Pierre; Clin Med Du Vieux-Terrebonne, 883 rue Saint-Pierre, Terrebonne QC J6W 1E6; Mon'94; BSc(BioChem.); MSc(MolecularBiol.); CCFP; Staff, Centre Hospitalier Pierre le Gardeur; (450)964-9111; Fax. (450)964-1450.

LAVIGNE, Jocelyn; Centre Hosp Honore-Mercier, 2750 boul Laframboise, Saint-Hyacinthe QC J2S 4Y8; Mon'86; FRCPC; Peds. Staff, Centre Hospitalier Honore-Mercier; (450)771-3333; Fax. (450)771-3557.

LAVIGNE, Louise; Hôpital Ste-Justine, 3175 ch Cote-Sainte-Catherine, Montreal QC H3T 1C5; Laval'67; DPsy(McG.); Psy. Staff, Hôpital Ste-Justine; (514)345-4695

LAVIGNE, Marie-Aimee; Ctr Hosp Rouyn-Noranda, 4 9e rue, Rouyn-Noranda QC J9X 2B2; Laval'05; Staff, Centre Hospitalier Rouyn-Noranda; Langs: Bilingual(French/English); (819)764-5131

LAVIGNE, Marie-Claude; Centre Med Laval, 1110 boul Vanier, Laval QC H7C 2R8; Mon'98; (450)661-2521; Fax. (450)661-7193.

LAVIGNE, Martin; Hop Maisonneuve-Rosemont, 5415 boul de l'Assomption, Montreal QC H1T 2M4; Sher'95; FRCSC; OrthSurg (Hip & Knee Reconstruction). Staff, Hopital Maisonneuve-Rosemont; Clin Associé Prof of Orthopaedics, Universite de Montreal; Langs: English; (514)254-6161; Fax. (514)254-1596; secortho@yahoo.fr.

LAVIGNE, Melanie; CSSS du Lac-Des-Deux-Montagnes, 520 boul Arthur-Sauve, Saint-Eustache QC J7R 5B1; McG'06; MDCM; Staff, Hôpital de Saint-Eustache; (450)473-6811

LAVIGNE, Patrick; Clinique Maisonneuve-Rosemont, 320-5345 boul de l'Assomption, Montreal QC H1T 4B3; Mon'99; PhD; FRCS; DSc; FRCSC; OrthSurg (Arthroscopy & Knee Ligament Reconstruction). Prof adj clin, Universite de Montreal; Langs: English; French; (514)254-6161; Fax. (514)254-1596.

LAVIGNE, Paul A; Pembroke Regional Hosp, 705 MacKay St, Pembroke ON K8A 1G8; Qns'08; CCFP; Staff, Pembroke Regional Hospital Inc; (613)732-2811

LAVIGNE, Philippe; CSSS de la Region de Thetford, 1717 rue Notre-Dame E, Thetford Mines QC G6G 2V4; Laval'06; CCFP; Staff, Hopital du CSS de la Region de Thetford; (418)338-7777

LAVIGNE, Ronald F; 494 Raglan St S, Renfrew ON K7V 1R8; Ott'68; CCFP; Langs: Bilingual(English/French); (613)432-5828; Fax. (613)432-9147.

LAVIGUEUR, Catherine; Centre Hosp Honore-Mercier, 2750 boul Laframboise, Saint-Hyacinthe QC J2S 4Y8; Mon'04; FRCPC; Psy. Staff, Centre Hospitalier Honore-Mercier; (450)771-3333

LAVIGUEUR, Denis; 4290 rue Beaubien E, Montreal QC H1T 1S6; Mon'81; Ac Staff, CSSS Saint-Leonard et Saint-Michel; (514)374-6711; Fax. (514)374-2051.

LAVIGUEUR, Denis; Polyclinique St-Eustache, 75 rue Grignon, Saint-Eustache QC J7P 4J2; Mon'89; ABAM; Staff, Centre Hospitalier Régional de Lanaudière; Staff Medecin, Centre de Desintoxication "Le Tremplin"(Joliette); Langs: English; (450)473-6882; Fax. (450)473-1916.

LAVIGUEUR, Michel; Clinique Med Chaumont, 8641 Av Chaumont, Anjou QC H1K 1N4; Mon'79; Ac Staff, CSSS Saint-Leonard et Saint-Michel; (514)352-3434; Fax. (514)351-6866.

LAVIGUEUR, Rene; Clinique Med Sainte-Anne, 11B boul Sainte-Anne E, Ste-Anne-des-Monts QC G4V 1M4; Sher'78; Dir-svcs prof, Centre Hospitalier des Monts; (418)763-2112

LAVINE, Elana S; Medical & Dental Bldg, 404-586 Eglinton Ave E, Toronto ON M4P 1P2; Tor'02; FRCPC; Peds; ClinImmunol&Allergy. (416)489-3273

LAVIOLETTE, Eric L; Hawkesbury Dist Gen Hosp, 1111 Ghislain St, Hawkesbury ON K6A 3G5; Sher'94; CCFP; CCFP(E.M.); Staff, Hawkesbury & District General Hospital; Langs: Bilingual(French/English); (613)632-1111

LAVIOLETTE, Genevieve; Clinique Med du Plateau, 300-195 rue de l'Atmosphere, Gatineau QC J9A 0A3; Laval'06; CCFP; (819)776-0001

LAVIOLETTE, Michel; Hôpital Laval, 2725 ch Sainte-Foy, Quebec QC G1V 4G5; Laval'73; Respir. Staff, Hôpital Laval; Université Laval; (418)656-4747; Fax. (418)656-4762; michel.laviolette@med.ulaval.ca.

LAVIS, John N; McMaster University, CRL 209-1280 Main St W, Hamilton ON L8S 4K1; Qns'89; PhD; MSc; Prof Epidemiol & Biostatistic/Chair Canada Research Knowledge Transfer & Exchange/Dir McMaster Health Forum, McMaster University; (905)525-9140 x22521; lavisj@mcmaster.ca.

LAVITT, Gail B; 2429-85 Garry St, Winnipeg MB R3C 4J5; Man'84; BSc; FRCPC; Psy. (204)942-5585

LAVOIE, Alain; Clinique Med Mont Ste-Anne, RR 1 100-10974 boul Ste-Anne, Beaupre QC G0A 1E0; Laval'77; (418)827-4022; Fax. (418)827-4964.

LAVOIE, Andre; Hôtel-Dieu de Lévis, 143 rue Wolfe, Levis QC G6V 3Z1; Laval'67; MedOncol (P.Q.); Hem (P.Q.). ac Staff, Hôtel-Dieu de Lévis; Clin Teach Staff Med, Université Laval; (418)835-7121 x1755

LAVOIE, Andre; Clinique Med Marieville, 301-2211 rue Du Pont, Marieville QC J3M 1K8; Mon'71; (450)460-4401; Fax. (450)460-7116.

LAVOIE, Andrea J; Regina Cardiology Associates, 701-2125 11th Ave, Regina SK S4P 3X3; Sask'99; BSc; FRCPC; IntMed (Interventional Cardiology); Cardiol. Dir Coronary Unit/Cardiac Rehab, Mosaic Heart Centre; (306)781-7944

LAVOIE, Anne; CHUM-Hop St-Luc, 1058 rue Saint-Denis, Montreal QC H2X 3J4; Mon'06; CSPQ; FRCPC; Anes. Staff, Centre Hospitalier l'Université De Montréal (CHUM) - Hôpital Saint-luc; (514)890-8000

LAVOIE, Annick; CHUM-Hotel-Dieu, 3840 rue Saint-Urbain, Montreal QC H2W 1T8; Mon'88; FRCPC; IntMed; Critical Care Medicine (P.Q.); Respir. Staff, Centre Hospitalier l'Université de Montréal (CHUM) - Hôtel-Dieu; (514)890-8000

LAVOIE, Annie; Ctr Hosp de Matane, 333 rue Thibault, Matane QC G4W 2W5; Sher'94; Staff, Centre Hospitalier de Matane; (418)562-3135

LAVOIE, Aubert; CHUQ-Ctr Hosp Univ Laval, 2705 boul Laurier, Quebec QC G1V 4G2; Laval'80; FRCPC; IntMed; ClinImmunol&Allergy. Ac Staff, Centre Hospitalier Universitaire de Quebec-CHUL; (418)654-2240; Fax. (418)654-2770.

LAVOIE, Bernadette; CSSS de Témiscouta, 103 7e rue E, Degelis QC G5T 1Y6; Laval'84; (418)853-2572; Fax. (418)853-3852.

LAVOIE, Bertrand; Clinique Med Soleil, 64 1re Av O, Amos QC J9T 1T8; Laval'77; Staff, CH Hôtel-Dieu d'Amos; Langs: English; (819)732-8341; Fax. (819)732-1642.

LAVOIE, Caroline; CHUQ-Hotel-Dieu De Quebec, 11 Cote du Palais, Quebec QC G1R 2J6; Laval'03; FRCPC; RadOncol. Staff, Centre Hospitalier Universitaire de Québec (CHUQ) - Siege Social; (418)691-5264; Fax. (418)691-5268; caroline.lavoie@mail.chuq.qc.ca.

LAVOIE, Catherine; CSSS de Laval, 1755 boul Rene-Laennec, Laval QC H7M 3L9; Mon'98; MedOncol (P.Q.); Hem (P.Q.). Staff, Hopital de la Cite de la santé; (450)668-1010

LAVOIE, Catherine; CLSC du Grand Chicoutimi, 411 rue de l'Hotel-Dieu, Chicoutimi QC G7H 7Z5; Mon'89; (418)543-2221

LAVOIE, Cecile R; Bonnyville Med Clinic, PO Box 1007 Stn Main 4610 50 St, Bonnyville AB T9N 2J7; Alb'83; BSc; Staff, Bonnyville Healthcare Centre; Langs: English; French; (780)826-3346; Fax. (780)826-6362.

LAVOIE, Christiane-Elise; IVAC, 1199 rue de Bleury, Montreal QC H3B 3J1; Laval'82; (514)906-3019; Fax. (514)906-3029.

LAVOIE, Claire; CHUM-Hotel-Dieu, 3840 rue Saint-Urbain, Montreal QC H2W 1T8; Mon'75; CSPQ; FRCPC; Anes. Staff Anes, Centre Hospitalier l'Université de Montréal (CHUM) - Hôtel-Dieu; Staff Teacher, Universite de Montreal; (514)890-8158; Fax. (514)412-7222.

LAVOIE, Claude A; Ctr Hosp Affilie-St-Sacrement, 1050 ch Sainte-Foy, Quebec QC G1S 4L8; Laval'66; Psy (P.Q.) (Adult Clinics). Staff, Centre Hospitalier Affilié Universitaire de Québec - Hôpital du St-Sacrement; Langs: Bilingual(French/English); (418)682-7898; Fax. (418)682-7959.

LAVOIE, Curtis F; Montfort Hosp, 713 Montreal Rd, Ottawa ON K1K 0T2; Cal'93; CCFP; CCFP(E.M.); FCFP; Staff, Montfort Hospital; (613)746-4621; Fax. (613)748-4949.

LAVOIE, Daniel C G; 15169 rue Maurice, Mirabel QC J7N 1Y8; Mon'77; (450)475-8759; Fax. (450)475-8265.

LAVOIE, Daniel; CSSS Haut-Richelieu-Rouville, 920 boul Du Seminaire N, St-Jean-Sur-Richel QC J3A 1B7; Laval'96; Staff, Hôpital du Haut-Richelieu; (450)359-5000; Fax. (450)359-5251.

LAVOIE, Danielle; Ctr Obstetrique et Gynecologie, 4250 1Re av, Quebec QC G1H 2S5; Laval'75.

LAVOIE, Danielle; CSSS de Sept-Iles, 45 rue du Pere-Divet, Sept-Iles QC G4R 3N7; St George's (Grenada)'01; Staff, Centre Hospitalier Regional de Sept-Iles; (418)962-9761

LAVOIE, Denis J; 201-3301 24 Ave, Vernon BC V1T 9S8; McG'83; DABU; FACS; FRCSC; Urol (Prostate Cancer). Staff, Queen Victoria Hospital; Ac Staff, Vernon Jubilee Hospital; Consultant, Shuswap Lake General Hospital; Consultant, Kelowna General Hospital; Langs: Bilingual(French/English); (250)542-8715; Fax. (250)542-2798.

LAVOIE, Eric; CHUS-Hop Fleurimont, 3001 12e Av N, Sherbrooke QC J1H 5N4; Sher'89; FRCPC; Peds (Adolescent Medicine). Staff Peds, Centre Hospitalier Universitaire de Sherbrooke-Hopital Fleurimont; adj Prof Med, Universite de Sherbrooke; Langs: Bilingual(French/English); (819)346-1110 x14464; Fax. (819)564-5398; eric.lavoie@usherbrooke.ca.

LAVOIE, Eric; CSSS des Basques, 550 rue Notre-Dame E RR 1, Trois-Pistoles QC G0L 4K0; Laval'99; CCFP; Staff, Centre Hospitalier Trois-Pistoles; (418)851-3301; Fax. (418)851-2944; eric.lavoie.rsssbasques@gmf.gouv.qc.ca.

LAVOIE, Fabien; 305-2954 boul Laurier, Quebec QC G1V 4T2; Laval'99; ABPh; (418)653-2226; info@cliniqueparetre.com.

LAVOIE, Frederic; Ctr Hosp du Centre la Mauricie, 50 119e rue, Shawinigan-Sud QC G9P 5K1; Laval'92; GenSurg. Staff, Centre Hospitalier du Centre la Mauricie; (819)536-7500; Fax. (819)536-7611.

LAVOIE, Frederic; CHUM-Hop Notre-Dame, 1560 rue Sherbrooke E, Montreal QC H2L 4M1; Laval'01; MSc; FRCSC; OrthSurg (General Surgery). ac Staff, Centre Hospitalier l'Université de Montréal (CHUM) - Hôpital Notre-Dame; (514)890-8000 x25900

LAVOIE, Gaetan; CLSC Longueuil-Ouest, 201 boul Cure-Poirier O, Longueuil QC J4J 2G4; Mon'77; (450)651-9830

LAVOIE, Gaetan Y; Cooperative Solidarite, GD 200 boul Perron, Sainte-Felicite QC G0J 2K0; Laval'88; MScSanteCom; MScMicrobiol; CCFP; FCFP; Staff, Centre Hospitalier de Matane; (418)733-1337

LAVOIE, Gilles; 216 av de la Cathedrale, Rimouski QC G5L 5J2; Laval'75; FRCPC; Derm. (418)723-0181; gilles.lavoie3@cgocable.ca.

LAVOIE, Ginette; 485-2 Place Laval, Laval QC H7N 5N6; Mon'86; FRCPC; Psy (Pedology Psychiatry) (General Psychiatry). Staff, Hôpital du Sacre-Coeur de Montréal; (450)669-5600; Fax. (450)669-0997; dreginettelavoie@hotmail.com.

LAVOIE, Guy J; Guy J Lavoie Prof Corp, 172 Meadowlark Shopping Ctr NW, Edmonton AB T5R 5W9; Alb'82; FRCSC; OrthSurg (Joint Reconstruction). Staff, University of Alberta Hospital; Staff, Cross Cancer Institute; Staff, Covenant Health - Misericordia Community Hospital; Langs: Bilingual(English/French); (780)481-4194; Fax. (780)444-6936.

LAVOIE, Guylaine; 204-2075 Boul Mellon, Jonquiere QC G7S 5Z8; Laval'81; Staff, Complexe hospitalier de la Sagamie; (418)548-8281

LAVOIE, Helene B; Clinique Procrea, 301-1361 Av Beaumont, Mont-Royal QC H3P 2W3; Mon'90; FRCPC; IntMed; Endocrin (P. Q.); Endocrin&Metab. Endocrin, Centre Hospitalier l'Université De Montréal (CHUM) - Hôpital Saint-luc; Consultant, Endocrin. Reproduction, Procrea Cliniques; Clinical Asst Prof Med, Universite de Montreal; (514)345-8535; Fax. (514)345-8978.

LAVOIE, Janie; CSSS de Chicoutimi, 305 rue Saint-Vallier, Chicoutimi QC G7H 5H6; Sher'03; FRCSC; Otol. Staff, Complexe hospitalier de la Sagamie; (418)541-1000

LAVOIE, Jean-Denis; Clinique Med St-Damase, 192 rue Principale, St-Damase QC J0H 1J0; Mon'86; Staff, Centre Hospitalier Honore-Mercier; (450)797-3385; Fax. (450)797-1062.

LAVOIE, Jean-Jacques; 565 rue Tache GD, Saint-Pascal QC G0L 3Y0; Laval'77; (418)492-2148; Fax. (418)492-6053.

LAVOIE, Jean-Pierre; Centre Cardio Rive-Sud, 200-1615 boul Jacques-Cartier, Longueuil QC J4M 2X1; Mon'97; Cardiol (P.Q.); IntMed (P.Q.) (Echography). Cardiology, Centre Hospitalier St-Jean; Cardiology/Int'l Med, Hôpital du Haut-Richelieu; Staff Cardiol, Centre Hospitalier Pierre Boucher; (450)674-2345; Fax. (450)674-1622.

LAVOIE, Jerome; CLSC Saint-Hubert, 6800 boul Cousineau, Saint-Hubert QC J3Y 8Z4; Sher'99; (450)443-7400; Fax. (450)676-3488.

LAVOIE, Joel; Ctr de Readaptation l'Interval, 3450 rue Sainte-Marguerite, Trois-Rivieres QC G8Z 1X3; Mon'10; CCFP; (819)375-4624

LAVOIE, Johanne; Clinique Med Mercier, 101-464 boul Saint-Jean-Baptis, Mercier QC J6R 2B1; Sher'78; (450)699-0539; Fax. (450)699-8438.

LAVOIE, Josee; MUHC-Montreal Children's Hosp, 2300 rue Tupper, Montreal QC H3H 1P3; Sher'87; CSPQ; FRCPC; Anes (Pediatric Cardiac Anesthesia). Staff, McGill University Health Centre - Montreal Children's Hospital; Assoc Member Anes, McGill University; Langs: Bilingual(English/French); (514)412-4400 x22463; Fax. (514)412-4341; josee.lavoie@muhc.mcgill.ca.

LAVOIE, Julie; Carrefour Med Vallee Richelieu, 665 boul Sir-Wilfrid-Laurier, Beloeil QC J3G 4J1; Mon'99; Staff, Centre Hospitalier Pierre Boucher; (450)467-0088; Fax. (450)467-4936.

LAVOIE, Line; CSSS de la Vallée de l'Or, 725 6e rue, Val-d'Or QC J9P 3Y1; Sher'91; FRCPC; IntMed; Gastroent. Staff Gastroent, Centre Hospitalier de Val d'Or; (819)825-6711

LAVOIE, Lionel A; Associate Med Clinic, PO Box 1690 805 Main St, Melfort SK S0E 1A0; Ott'64; BA; CCFP; FCFP; Chief Med Officer of Hlth, Bourgault Industries; Staff, Associate Medical Clinic; Clin Prof Family Med, University of Saskatchewan; Langs: English; French; (306)752-4866; Fax. (306)752-4609; lionelmarylavoie@hotmail.com.

LAVOIE, Lise; CSSS de Chicoutimi, 305 rue Saint-Vallier, Chicoutimi QC G7H 5H6; Laval'94; FRCPC; Psy. Staff, Complexe hospitalier de la Sagamie; (418)541-1234 x5151

LAVOIE, Lucie; CSSS de Trois-Rivières, 1991 boul du Carmel, Trois-Rivieres QC G8Z 3R9; Laval'98; GeriatricMed; IntMed. Staff, CSSS de Trois-Rivières; (819)697-3333

LAVOIE, Marc-Andre; Institut de Cardiologie de Mtl, 5000 rue Belanger, Montreal QC H1T 1C8; Mon'78; IntMed (Lipidology). Staff, Institut de Cardiologie de Montréal; adj Prof, Universite de Montreal; (514)593-2552; Fax. (514)593-2567.

LAVOIE, Marcel; CLSC-CHSLD PAT Montreal Est, 13926 rue Notre-Dame E, Pte-aux-Trembles QC H1A 1T5; Laval'69; (514)642-2121 x321; Fax. (514)642-1684; marcel.lavoie@ssss.gouv.qc.ca.

LAVOIE, Marianne; CHUQ-Hotel-Dieu De Quebec, 11 Cote du Palais, Quebec QC G1R 2J6; Laval'02; FRCPC; IntMed; MedOncol; Hem. Staff, Centre Hospitalier Universitaire de Québec (CHUQ) - Siege Social; (418)525-4444

LAVOIE, Marie-Andree; 33e CF Health Services, PO Box 17000 Stn Forces, Kingston ON K7K 7B4; Sher'10; CCFP; (613)541-5010

LAVOIE, Marie-Eve; Ctr Hosp du Centre la Mauricie, 50 119e rue, Shawinigan-Sud QC G9P 5K1; Mon'08; CCFP; Staff, Centre Hospitalier du Centre la Mauricie; (819)536-7500

LAVOIE, Marie-Josee; CSSS de Beauce-Etchemin, 1515 17e rue, Saint-Georges QC G5Y 4T8; Laval'93; CSPQ; FRCPC; Anes. Staff, Centre Hospitalier Beauce-Etchemin; (418)228-2031 x5000

LAVOIE, Martin; Alberta Health & Wellness, PO Box 1360 Stn Main 24F-10025 Jasper Ave NW, Edmonton AB T5J 2N3; Mon'91; RC; FRCPC; CommunMed (Public Health). Langs: Bilingual(French/English); (780)427-5263; Fax. (780)427-7683.

LAVOIE, Maryse; 52 av Bateman, Edmundston NB E3V 4A4; Sher'07; CCFP; (506)735-8442

LAVOIE, Maurice; 100-400 boul Jean-Lesage, Quebec QC G1K 8W1; Laval'74; Assoc Staff, Centre Hospitalier Affilié Universitaire de Québec - Hôpital du St-Sacrement; (418)529-9323; Fax. (418)529-9722.

LAVOIE, Michel; Pavillon Rosemont, 5689 boul Rosemont, Montreal QC H1T 2H1; Mon'82; FRCPC; Psy. Staff, Centre Hospitalier Pierre Boucher; (514)252-3914; Fax. (514)252-3810.

LAVOIE, Michel; Centre de Sante Publique, 2400 av d'Estimauville, Quebec QC G1E 7G9; Laval'78; CommunMed (Security/Prevention Traumatization). Staff, Centre Hospitalier Affilié Universitaire de Québec - Hôpital De L'Enfant Jésus; (418)666-7000 x421

LAVOIE, Michel V M; 11202 76 Ave NW, Edmonton AB T6G 0K1; Alb'78; FRCSC; OrthSurg (Spine). (780)483-8311

LAVOIE, Michele; CHUQ-Hotel-Dieu de Quebec, 11 Cote-du-Palais, Quebec QC G1R 2J6; Mon'90; CCFP; Staff, Centre Hospitalier Universitaire de Québec (CHUQ) - Siege Social; Prof Family Med Unit, Université Laval; (418)525-4444

LAVOIE, Mireille; CSSS de la Minganie, CP 190 1035 Prom des Anciens, Havre-Saint-Pierre QC G0G 1P0; Sher'87; Staff, CSSS de la Minganie; (418)538-2212

LAVOIE, Mona; Hotel-Dieu de Levis, 143 rue Wolfe, Levis QC G6V 3Z1; Laval'87; FRCPC; AnatPath. Staff, Hôtel-Dieu de Lévis; Langs: English; French; (418)835-7121 x3282

LAVOIE, Myriam; CSSS de Chicoutimi, 305 rue Saint-Vallier, Chicoutimi QC G7H 5H6; Mon'04; FRCPC; MedMicrobiol; Microbio & Infect Dis (P.Q.). Staff, Complexe hospitalier de la Sagamie; (418)541-1000

LAVOIE, Nicole; Hop Sacre-Coeur de Mtl, 5400 boul Gouin O, Montreal QC H4J 1C5; Mon'79; CSPQ; FRCPC; Anes. Staff Anes, Hôpital du Sacre-Coeur de Montréal; (514)338-2222 x2140

LAVOIE, Normand; Clinique Serv Sante Rosemere, 400 ch de la Grande-Cote, Rosemere QC J7A 1K7; Mon'79; Langs: English; (450)621-1292; Fax. (450)621-1296.

LAVOIE, Pascal; Children's & Women's HC of BC, 1R47-4480 Oak St, Vancouver BC V6H 3V4; McG'01; FRCPC; Peds (Neonatal & Perinatal Medicine). Staff, BC Children's Hospital; Langs: Bilingual(French/English); (604)875-2345 x7318

LAVOIE, Pascale; Ctr Hosp Affilie-Enfant-Jesus, 1401 18e rue, Quebec QC G1J 1Z4; Sher'00; FRCSC; Neursurg. Staff, Centre Hospitalier Affilié Universitaire de Québec - Hôpital De L'Enfant Jésus; (418)649-0252

LAVOIE, Pauline; Clinique Orthopedique Duval, 1487 boul des Laurentides, Vimont QC H7M 2Y3; Laval'83; Gen Dir/Physician, Clinique Orthopedique Duval; Langs: English; (450)663-3901; Fax. (450)663-0776.

LAVOIE, Perrine; CSSS de Beauce-Etchemin, 1515 17e rue, Saint-Georges QC G5Y 4T8; Laval'03; FRCSC; GenSurg. Staff, Centre Hospitalier Beauce-Etchemin; (418)228-2031

LAVOIE, Raynald; Clinique St-Georges, 3-1000 rue Chabanel, Chicoutimi QC G7H 2R3; Laval'58; ABOtol(USA); FRCSC; Otol (Otolaryngology & Plasty). Member, Canadian Institue of Facial Plastic Surgery; Langs: Bilingual(French/English); (418)549-0292; Fax. (418)549-4180; ray.lavoie@videotron.ca.

LAVOIE, Regis; Clinique Med Delisle, 94 rue Joseph-W.-Fleury, Alma QC G8E 2K2; Laval'78; Staff, CSSS de Lac-Saint Jean-Est; (418)347-4696; Fax. (418)347-4697.

LAVOIE, Remi; Hotel-Dieu de Levis, 143 rue Wolfe, Levis QC G6V 3Z1; Sher'98; FRCPC; IntMed; Gastroent. Staff, Hôtel-Dieu de Lévis; Langs: English; (418)835-7121; Fax. (418)835-7218.

LAVOIE, Robert; Hôpital Laval, 2725 ch Sainte-Foy, Quebec QC G1V 4G5; Laval'80; MedBiochem. Staff, Hôpital Laval; (418)656-4860; Fax. (418)656-4659.

LAVOIE, Roberto; 502-222 McIntyre St W, North Bay ON P1B 2Y8; Laval'02; FRCPC; IntMed (Cardiology). Ac Staff, North Bay Regional Health Centre - Regional Mental Health; Langs: Bilingual(French/English); (705)494-7670; Fax. (705)494-4861.

LAVOIE, Sebastien; Clinique Med Blainville, 519 boul du Cure-Labelle, Blainville QC J7C 2H6; Sher'03; CCFP; (450)430-2222

LAVOIE, Stephane; Clinique Med l'Actuel, 1130-1001 Boul De Maisonneuve, Montreal QC H2L 4P9; Mon'90; (514)524-1001; Fax. (514)524-3831.

LAVOIE, Susan D; The Ottawa Hosp-Riverside, 5F-1967 Riverside Dr, Ottawa ON K1H 7W9; McG'77; FRCPC; IntMed (Nephrology). Staff Nephrol, The Ottawa Hospital - Riverside Campus; Assoc Prof Med, University of Ottawa; Langs: English; French; (613)738-8400 x82528; Fax. (613)738-8337; sdlavoie@ottawahospital.on.ca.

LAVOIE, Suzanne; Clinique Med Millenia Sante, 295-2600 boul Laurier, Quebec QC G1V 4T3; Laval'84; FRCPC; PhysMed&Rehab (Medico Legal Issues). Staff, Jeffery Hale Hospital-Saint Brigid's; Langs: Bilingual(French/English).

LAVOIE, Sylvain; Ctr Hosp Affilie-Enfant-Jesus, 1401 18e rue, Quebec QC G1J 1Z4; Laval'72; LMCC; FACG; FRCPC; Gastroent. Consultant, Institut Universitaire Sante; Staff, Centre Hospitalier Affilié Universitaire de Québec - Hôpital De L'Enfant Jésus; Université Laval; Langs: English; (418)649-5732; Fax. (418)649-5570.

LAVOIE, Sylvain; CSSS de Trois-Rivières, 1991 boul du Carmel, Trois-Rivieres QC G8Z 3R9; Sher'97; FRCPC; DiagRad. Staff, CSSS de Trois-Rivières; (819)697-3333

LAVOIE, Valerie; Clinique Med Racicot, 520 rue d'Avaugour, Boucherville QC J4B 0G6; Mon'03; (450)449-7525

LAVOIE, Vincent; Hop Jean-Talon, 1385 rue Jean-Talon E, Montreal QC H2E 1S6; Laval'64; Cardiol (P.Q.). Staff, CSSS du Coeur de l'Isle Hôpital Jean-Talon; Langs: Spanish; English; (514)495-6767; Fax. (514)495-6785.

LAVOIE, Yannick; CLSC Du Marigot, 1351 boul des Laurentides, Vimont QC H7M 2Y2; Sher'93; CCFP; (450)668-1803; Fax. (450)668-1507; yannick.lavoie@videotron.ca.

LAVOIE, Yvan; Clinique Med Notre-Dame, 138 rue Notre-Dame S, Sainte-Marie QC G6E 4A4; Laval'79; (418)387-5280; Fax. (418)387-5283; yvan_lavoie@ssss.gouv.qc.ca.

LAVOIE COUTU, Christine; CSSS les Eskers de l'Abitibi, 622 4e rue O, Amos QC J9T 2S2; Sher'08; Staff, CH Hôtel-Dieu d'Amos; (819)732-3341

LAVOIE-DUFOUR, Line; 200-441 ch Madawaska, Grand Falls NB E3Y 1A3; Laval'88; Staff, Hôpital Général de Grand-Falls; Physician Family Med, Clinique Medicale Grand-Sault; Langs: English.

LAVOIE-FERLAND, Helene; Centre Med Racine, 201-900 boul Raymond, Quebec QC G1B 3G3; Laval'78; (418)667-8066; Fax. (418)667-8131.

LAVOIE-LEVESQUE, Josiane; CSSS de Trois-Rivieres, 155 rue Toupin, Trois-Rivieres QC G8T 3Z8; Sher'07; Staff, Centre de santé Cloutier-du-Rivage; (819)370-2100

LAVOIE-ST-GELAIS, Genevieve; Hop du Sacre-Coeur de Mtl, 5400 boul Gouin O, Montreal QC H4J 1C5; McG'05; CSPQ; ObstGyn. Staff, Hôpital du Sacre-Coeur de Montréal; (514)338-2222

LAVOIE-L'ALLIER, Philippe; Institut de Cardiologie de Mtl, 5000 rue Belanger, Montreal QC H1T 1C8; Sher'92; FRCPC; IntMed (Angioplasty); Cardiol. Staff, Institut de Cardiologie de Montréal; adj Prof, Universite de Montreal; (514)376-3330; Fax. (514)593-2567; philippe.lallier@sympatico.ca.

LAVORATO, Amy; One Care Family Clinic, 1755 Brimley Rd, Scarborough ON M1P 0A3; St George's U (Grenada)'06; Physician, One Care Medical Clinic; (416)290-0361

LAW, Angeline; The Ottawa Hosp-Gen Campus, W1683-501 Smyth Rd, Ottawa ON K1H 8L6; McG'00; FRCPC; IntMed; Cardiol. Staff, The Ottawa Hospital - General Campus; Langs: Bilingual(French/English); (613)737-8859; Fax. (613)739-6727.

LAW, Anthony C H; Royal Columbian Hosp, 330 Columbia St E, New Westminster BC V3L 3W7; Alb'69; FRCPA; FRCPC; AnatPath. Staff, Ridge Meadows Hospital & Health Care Centre; Staff Path, Royal Columbian Hospital; Staff, Eagle Ridge Hospital & Health Care Centre; (604)520-4310

LAW, Barbara J; Public Health Agency of Canada, 292A-130 Colonnade Rd, Nepean ON K2E 1B6; Cal'75; FRCPC; Peds; InfectDis. Staff Consultant, St Boniface General Hospital; Ac Staff, Health Sciences Centre; Prof, University of Manitoba, Peds. & Med. Microbiol. & Section Hd.; Prof Peds & Med Microbiol/Sec Head, University of Manitoba; blaw@ms.umanitoba.ca.

LAW, Bonnie; Oakridge Centre South Tower, 203-650 41st Ave W, Vancouver BC V5Z 2M9; UBC'95; CCFP; Langs: Cantonese; (604)263-6232; Fax. (604)263-9297.

LAW, Calvin H L; Toronto Sunnybrook Reg Cancer, T2 001-2075 Bayview Ave, Toronto ON M4N 3M5; Tor'94; MPH; FRCSC; GenSurg; General Surgical Oncology. Staff Surg Oncol, Sunnybrook Health Sciences Centre - Edmond Odette Cancer Centre; Assoc Staff, Sunnybrook Health Sciences Centre; Aj Scientist, Institute for Clinical Evaluative Sciences; Asst Prof, University of Toronto; Langs: Cantonese; (416)480-4329; Fax. (416)480-6002.

LAW, Charles C S; Oakridge Centre South Tower, 360-650 41st Ave W, Vancouver BC V5Z 2M9; (Taiwan)'70; Langs: Cantonese; Fookien; Hakka; Hokkin; Indonesian; Malay; Taiwanese; (604)261-6000

LAW, David T S; Hillside Med Centre, 2867 Lawrence Ave E, Scarborough ON M1P 2T2; Tor'94; BSc; PhD; CCFP; Staff, Rouge Valley Health System - Centenary Health Centre Site; Staff, The Scarborough Hospital - General Campus; Staff, The Scarborough Hospital - Birchmount Campus; Asst Prof Family & Commun Med, University of Toronto; (416)261-7223; Fax. (416)261-6374.

LAW, Francis C H; 408-1338 Broadway W, Vancouver BC V6H 1H2; UBC'86; DABOph; FAAO; FRCSC; Ophth. Assoc Staff, Vancouver General Hospital - Centennial Pavillion; Clin Instructor, University of British Columbia; Langs: Cantonese; Mandarin; (604)732-0328; Fax. (604)732-0809.

LAW, Genevieve; 2680 Richmond Rd, Victoria BC V8R 4S9; Alb'06; Rheum; IntMed. (250)598-2277

LAW, Graham R; Sunridge Family Med Teaching C, 2685 36 St NE, Calgary AB T1Y 5S3; Cal'75; CCFP; CCFP(E.M.); FCFP; Staff, Sunridge Family Medicine Teaching Centre; Clinical Asst Prof, University of Calgary; (403)943-5000; Fax. (403)476-8784.

LAW, Hugo K C; 106-350 Highway 7 E, Richmond Hill ON L4B 3N2; Wes'74; Court Staff, Toronto Western Hospital - University Health Network; Court Staff, The Scarborough Hospital - Birchmount Campus; Court Staff, The Scarborough Hospital - General Campus; Langs: Chinese; (416)291-9007

LAW, Jaimie R; Pritchard Farm Health Centre, 5-3014 Henderson Hwy, East St Paul MB R2E 0H9; Man'09; CCFP.

LAW, Joanna K Y; 250-5780 Cambie St, Vancouver BC V5Z 3A7; UBC'03; FRCPC; IntMed; Gastroent. (604)324-4849

LAW, John A; Queen Elizabeth II HSC-Halifax, 1796 Summer St, Halifax NS B3H 3A7; Dal'83; FRCPC; Anes (Neuro Anesthesia). Staff, Queen Elizabeth II Health Sciences Centre - Halifax Infirmary Site; Prof Anes, Dalhousie University; (902)473-4326; Fax. (902)473-3820; jlaw@dal.ca.

LAW, John O; Courtenay Med Clinic, 788 Grant Ave, Courtenay BC V9N 2T3; UBC'90; Staff, St Joseph's General Hospital; Examiner Commercial Scuba, Work Safe BC; Med Examiner Aviation & Marine, Ministry Of Transportation; (250)334-2445; Fax. (250)334-2642; jlaw@shawbiz.ca.

LAW, Joyce S; Labrador Grenfell Health, PO Bix 7000 Stn C 227 Hamilton River Rd, Happy-Valley-Goose NL A0P 1C0; UBC'06; CCFP; Staff, Labrador Health Centre; (709)897-2000

LAW, Lorraine T; Scarborough Hosp-Gen Site, 3050 Lawrence Ave E, Scarborough ON M1P 2V5; McG'03; FRCSC; GenSurg; Critical Care Medicine., The Scarborough Hospital - General Campus; (416)438-2911

LAW, Marcus; South East Toronto FHT, 1871 Danforth Ave, Toronto ON M4C 1J3; Tor'00; CCFP; (416)699-7775; Fax. (416)699-7776.

LAW, Michael K; 223 Gladys Allison Place, North York ON M2N 4T5; Tor'73; Court Staff, North York General Hospital; (416)221-0136; Fax. (416)221-0509.

LAW, Michael W; Royal Columbian Hosp, 330 Columbia St E, New Westminster BC V3L 3W7; UBC'98; FRCPC; Anes. Staff, Royal Columbian Hospital; (604)520-4603

LAW, Peter; Mackenzie Richmond Hill Hosp, 10 Trench St, Richmond Hill ON L4C 4Z3; Ott'95; FRCPC; DiagRad. Staff, Mackenzie Richmond Hill Hospital; (905)883-1212

LAW, Sally S C; 3809 Main St, Vancouver BC V5V 3P1; Tor'91; BSc; CCFP; Court Staff Privil, Providence Health Care - Mount Saint Joseph Hospital; Court Staff Privil, Providence Health Care - St Paul's Hospital; Langs: Mandarin; Cantonese; (604)872-4025; Fax. (604)872-2252.

LAW, Samuel F; St Michael's Hosp, 17F-30 Bond St, Toronto ON M5B 1W8; McG'94; FRCPC; Psy. Staff, St Michael's Hospital; Langs: Cantonese; Mandarin; (416)864-6060 x2415; Fax. (416)864-3091.

LAW, Teresa H L; Clinique Med Carron, 995 boul Saint-Laurent, Montreal QC H2Z 1J4; McG'79; MSc; ABD; CSPQ; Derm (P.Q.). Langs: Chinese; (514)861-9154; Fax. (514)861-8447.

LAW, Tommy; CLSC De Hull, 85 rue Saint-Redempteur, Gatineau QC J8X 4E6; Laval'94; CCFP; (819)966-6510 x4306; Fax. (819)966-6513.

LAW, Warren C; Grand River Hosp-KW Hlth Ctre, PO Box 9056 Stn C 835 King St W, Kitchener ON N2G 1G3; Tor'73; AB; PlasSurg. Ac Staff, Grand River Hospital - Kitchener/Waterloo Health Centre; Ac Staff, St Mary's General Hospital; (519)742-3611

LAWAL, Waheed O; Cape Breton Hlthcare Complex, 1482 George St, Sydney NS B1P 1P3; Ilorin (Nigeria)'98; MB BS; Staff, Cape Breton Healthcare Complex; (902)794-8551; Fax. (902)794-2149.

LAWALE, Dag L; Living Spring Med Centre, 379 Parkview Rd, Yorkton SK S3N 2L4; Ibadan (Nigeria)'90; MRCGPract; MRCOG(UK); BSc; MB BS; CCFP; (306)890-0405; Fax. (306)890-0408; dlawale@livingspringsmedical.com.

LAWAND, Christopher; Pier Med Clinic, 788 Victoria Rd, Sydney NS B1N 1J7; Dal'05; CCFP; CCFP(E.M.); (902)567-6161

LAWANDI, Philip; 383-1255 Boul Laird, Mont-Royal QC H3P 2T1; Cairo (Egypt)'65; FRCPC; Peds. Assoc Staff, McGill University Health Centre - Montreal Children's Hospital; Assoc Staff, St Mary's Hospital Centre; McGill University; (514)733-0681; Fax. (514)341-2872.

LAWE, Andrew D; Riverside Med Clinic, 306-1101 Dewdney Ave, Trail BC V1R 4T1; UBC'00; FRCSC; GenSurg. Staff, Penticton Regional Hospital; (250)493-0134; andrea.louwe@kscu.com.

LAWEE, David; Yonge-Eglinton Med Centre, 209-2401 Yonge St, Toronto ON M4P 3H1; Paris (France)'55; BSc; CCFP; FCFP; Consultant Family Med, Toronto Western Hospital - University Health Network; Emeritus Prof Family & Commun Med, University of Toronto; Langs: Italian; French; (416)322-9933

LAWEN, Joseph G; Urology Consultants, 602-5991 Spring Garden Rd, Halifax NS B3H 1Y6; Dal'78; DAB; FRCSC; Urol (Kidney Transplantation). Staff, Queen Elizabeth II Health Sciences Centre - Victoria General Site; Assoc Prof Urol, Dalhousie University.

LAWENDY, Abdel-Rahman; London HSC-Victoria Hosp, E4 126-800 Commissioner Rd E, London ON N6A 5W9; Wes'03; OrthSurg. Staff, London Health Sciences Centre - Victoria Campus; (519)685-8218

LAWLER, Michelle C; West Carleton Family Hlth Team, PO Box 218 119 Langstaff Dr, Carp ON K0A 1L0; Ott'94; CCFP; FCFP; Ac Staff, Queensway Carleton Hospital; (613)839-3271; Fax. (613)839-3273.

LAWLESS, Bernard W; St Michael's Hosp, 3 073 QW-30 Bond St, Toronto ON M5B 1W8; Wes'95; FRCSC; GenSurg. Staff, St Michael's Hospital; (416)864-5481; Fax. (416)864-3083.

LAWLESS, Jill; Dartmouth Gen Hosp, 325 Pleasant St, Dartmouth NS B2Y 4G8; Dal'04; CCFP; CCFP(E.M.); Staff, Dartmouth General Hospital; (902)465-8338

LAWLESS, John; Centre Medical de l'Hetriere, 201-3520 rue de l'Hetriere, St-Augustin-D-Desm QC G3A 0B4; Laval'85; Langs: English; (418)651-3933; Fax. (418)651-0256.

LAWLESS, Kevin; Villa Caritas, 16515 88 Ave NW, Edmonton AB T5R 0A4; Alb'89; FRCPC; Psy (Geriatric Psychiatry). Staff, Alberta Hospital Edmonton; Asst Prof, University of Alberta; (780)342-6552; Fax. (780)342-6579; kevin.lawless@convenanthealth.ca.

LAWLEY, Thomas; Syncrude Canada Ltd, Mail Drop 1050 PO Box 4009 Stn Main, Fort McMurray AB T9H 3L1; Dal'91; MSc(PublicHealthScience; FRCPC; OccupMed (Disability Management & Rehabilitation)., Syncrude Canada Ltd; (780)790-4278; Fax. (780)790-4334; lawley.tom@syncrude.com.

LAWLIS, Catherine M; Grist Mill Family Physicians, 3-45 Grist Mill Rd, Holland Landing ON L9N 1M7; McM'95; BScN; CCFP; FCFP; Ac Staff, Southlake Regional Health Centre; (905)853-8966; Fax. (905)853-2953; c.lawlis@sympatico.ca.

LAWLOR, Cindy J; Kingston Reg Cancer Centre, 25 King St W, Kingston ON K7L 5P9; Dal'92; (613)544-2630

LAWLOR, Colleen E; Hollyburn Med Bldg, 202A-520 17th St, West Vancouver BC V7V 3S8; San Antonio (USA)'01; CCFP; Langs: Bilingual(English/French); (604)913-8183

LAWLOR, D Kirk; 205-616 K.L.O. Rd, Kelowna BC V1Y 4X4; Wes'96; BSc; FRCSC; GenSurg; VascSurg. (250)762-7731

LAWLOR, Krista A; MUHC-Montreal Gen Hosp, E10 220 1-1650 av Cedar, Montreal QC H3G 1A4; McG'93; CCFP; Staff, McGill University Health Centre - Montreal General Campus; Dir Residency Prog, McGill University; (514)934-1934 x43993

LAWLOR, Peter G; SCOHS-Elisabeth Bruyere Hosp, 43 Bruyere St, Ottawa ON K1N 5C8; Dublin (Ireland)'83; CCFP; Staff, SCO Health Service - Élisabeth Bruyère Hospital.

LAWRENCE, D'Arcy D; Royal Jubilee Hosp, 1952 Bay St, Victoria BC V8R 1J8; Tor'65; FRCPC; DiagRad. Staff Imaging Services/Chief Med Imaging, Royal Jubilee Hospital; (250)370-8238

LAWRENCE, Elizabeth L; Maple Family Hlth Team-Clergy, 71 Clergy St, Kingston ON K7L 3J3; Wes'09; CCFP; (613)542-7858

LAWRENCE, Janet A; The Credit Valley Hosp, 2200 Eglinton Ave W, Mississauga ON L5M 2N1; Wes'87; FRCPC; DiagRad. Staff, The Credit Valley Hospital; (905)813-4045; Fax. (905)813-3042.

LAWRENCE, Julie B H; 525 Broadway Ave W PO Box 20011 Rpo Fairview, Vancouver BC V5Z 0C1; Cal'08; CCFP; (604)220-5341

LAWRENCE, Kathrine J; Academic Family Medicine, 172-1621 Albert St, Regina SK S4P 2S5; Sask'94; CCFP; FCFP; Staff Family Medicine Unit, Regina General Hospital; (306)766-0444; Fax. (306)766-0471.

LAWRENCE, Kim C; Bow River Prof Centre, 218-4411 16 Ave NW, Calgary AB T3B 0M3; Alb'80; (403)234-8008

LAWRENCE, Michael R; Fairmont Med Bldg, 1404-750 Broadway W, Vancouver BC V5Z 1J4; London (England)'65; CCFP; Staff, Vancouver General Hospital - Centennial Pavillion; Staff, BC Children's Hospital; (604)873-4851; Fax. (604)879-4266.

LAWRENCE, Patrick H; St Boniface Gen Hosp, 409 Tache Ave, Winnipeg MB R2H 2A6; Man'90; FRCPC; DiagRad (Pediatric Radiology). Staff Ultrasound Dept, St Boniface General Hospital; (204)233-8563; Fax. (204)231-0640.

LAWRENCE, Sarah E; Children's Hosp Eastern Ont, 401 Smyth Rd, Ottawa ON K1H 8L1; Dal'87; FRCPC; Peds; Endocrin&Metab. Prof, Children's Hospital of Eastern Ontario (CHEO); Court Staff Privil, The Ottawa Hospital - General Campus; Court Staff Privil, The Ottawa Hospital - Civic Campus; Assoc Prof, University of Ottawa; Langs: Bilingual(English/French); (613)737-7600 x2434; Fax. (613)738-4236; slawrence@cheo.on.ca.

LAWRENCE, Sarah L; Children's Hosp Eastern Ont, 401 Smyth Rd, Ottawa ON K1H 8L1; Dal'99; FRCPC; Peds (Neonatal & Perinatal Medicine). Staff, Children's Hospital of Eastern Ontario (CHEO); Langs: Bilingual(English/French); (613)737-7600 x2415; Fax. (613)738-4847.

LAWRENCE, Stephen S; Professional Arts Bldg, 1F-570 King St, Welland ON L3B 3L2; Tor'86; BSc; Staff, Niagara Health System - Welland Hospital Site; (519)735-3900; Fax. (519)735-2588.

LAWRENCE-PATEL, Giselle M T; 1-4175 Confederation Pky, Mississauga ON L5B 0H1; Bangalore (India)'00; CCFP; (905)848-4880

LAWRIE, Michael E; 5-350 Hespeler Rd, Cambridge ON N1R 7N7; Tor'75; BSc; CCFP; FCFP; Chief of Staff, Cambridge Memorial Hospital; (519)621-4071; Fax. (519)621-6206.

LAWRIE, Selena; Aberdeen Med Clinic, 1966 Harrison Way, Kamloops BC V1S 1M9; UBC'94; BSc; CCFP; (250)314-5314

LAWRIE, Susan L; Surrey Med Arts Bldg, 304-13798 94A Ave, Surrey BC V3V 1N1; Alb'82; (604)681-5261 x121

LAWRIE, W Mark; Sage Med Clinic, 101-2210 Main St, Penticton BC V2A 5H8; UBC'83; Ac Staff, Penticton Regional Hospital; (250)492-0990; Fax. (250)492-0992.

LAWRIMORE, Tara M; Gulf Canada Square, 300-401 9 Ave SW, Calgary AB T2P 3C5; Tor'00; FRCPC; DiagRad. (403)284-0230

LAWS, Anthony R E; 357 Main St E, Hamilton ON L8N 1J4; McM'82; Med Officer DND, Government of Canada; (905)522-0999

LAWS, Margaret-Anne; Perth-Smiths Falls Dist Hosp, 33 Drummond St W, Perth ON K7H 2K1; McM'91; FRCPC; DiagRad. Chair Diagnostic Imaging, Perth & Smiths Falls District Hospital - Perth Site (Great War Memorial Site); (613)267-1500 x4320

LAWSON, Andrea L; West Lincoln Mem Hosp, 169 Main St E, Grimsby ON L3M 1P3; McM'99; CCFP; Staff, West Lincoln Memorial Hospital; (905)945-2253

LAWSON, Dennis M; Royal University Hosp, 103 Hospital Dr, Saskatoon SK S7N 0W8; Sask'00; BScBiology; FRCPC; Psy. Staff Psy, Royal University Hospital; (306)655-1000

LAWSON, Edward J; Surrey Med Arts Bldg, 210-13710 94A Ave, Surrey BC V3V 1N1; Wes'94; FRCPC; IntMed; Respir (Critical Care Medicine). Staff Physician, Surrey Memorial Hospital; (604)582-2100

LAWSON, Fiona M E; Clinical Sciences Bldg, 108-11350 83 Ave NW, Edmonton AB T6G 2P4; Glasgow (Scotland)'91; MB ChB; BSc; FRCPC; IntMed; GeriatricMed. Staff, University of Alberta Hospital; (780)492-3917

LAWSON, Glasine O; Stevenson Mem Hosp, PO Box 4000 Stn Main 200 Fletcher Cres, Alliston ON L9R 1W7; Washington (USA)'92; MD; Staff, Stevenson Memorial Hospital; (705)435-6281; Fax. (705)434-5138.

LAWSON, Jennifer J; Dilico Anishinabek Family Care, 198 Anemki Dr, Thunder Bay ON P7J 1L6; Ott'06; CCFP; CCFP(E.M.); (807)623-8511

LAWSON, Laurie E M; Lions Gate Maternity Clinic, 302-231 15th St E, North Vancouver BC V7L 2L7; UBC'95; CCFP; Staff, Lions Gate Hospital; (604)985-6408

LAWSON, Margaret L; Children's Hosp Eastern Ont, 2291A-401 Smyth Rd, Ottawa ON K1H 8L1; McM'89; MSc; FRCPC; Peds (Pediatric Endocrinology); Endocrin&Metab. Chief Div of Endocrin & Metab, Children's Hospital of Eastern Ontario (CHEO); Assoc Prof Peds, University of Ottawa; (613)737-2411; Fax. (613)738-4236; lawson@cheo.on.ca.

LAWSON, Thomas; St Mary's Hosp Centre, 3830 av Lacombe, Montreal QC H3T 1M5; McG'77; Staff, St Mary's Hospital Centre; (514)345-3511

LAWTON, Louis J; Children's Hosp Eastern Ont, 3369-401 Smyth Rd, Ottawa ON K1H 8L1; Mem'76; BMedSci; MD; FRCSC; OrthSurg (Pediatric Orthopedics). Staff, Children's Hospital of Eastern Ontario (CHEO); Staff, Ottawa Children's Treatment Centre; Asst Prof Surg, University of Ottawa; Langs: Bilingual(English/French); (613)737-7600 x2676; Fax. (613)738-4840; lawton@cheo.on.ca.

LAX, Matthew J; Mount Sinai Hosp, 569-600 University Ave, Toronto ON M5G 1X5; Tor'94; FRCPC; DiagRad. Staff, Mount Sinai Hospital; (416)586-4800 x5104; Fax. (416)586-8695.

LAX, Steven A; Pine Plaza Med Centre, 201-119 Pine St S, Timmins ON P4N 2K3; Tor'82; CCFP; FCFP; Staff, Timmins & District Hospital; (705)264-8840; Fax. (705)267-4181.

LAX, Stuart A; Forensic Psychiatric Hosp, 70 Colony Farm Rd, New Westminster BC V3C 5X9; Tor'05; FRCPC; Psy. Staff, Forensic Psychiatric Hospital; (604)524-7700; slax@forensic.bc.ca.

LAXDAL, Grant M; Campbell River & Dist Gen Hsp, 375 2nd Ave, Campbell River BC V9W 3V1; Sask'02; CCFP; CCFP(E.M.); Staff, Campbell River & District General Hospital; (250)287-7111

LAXDAL, Muriel L; PO Box 218, Biggar SK S0K 0M0; Pretoria (South Africa)'90; MB ChB; Langs: Afrikaans; (306)948-3331; Fax. (306)948-5060; muriell@sasktel.net.

LAXER, Ronald M; The Hosp For Sick Children, 8253A-555 University Ave, Toronto ON M5G 1X8; McG'77; FRCPC; Peds; Rheum. Staff Rheumatologist, The Hospital For Sick Children; Staff, Holland Bloorview Kids Rehabilitation Hospital; Prof Peds & Med, University of Toronto; (416)813-7711; Fax. (416)813-4989.

LAY, Christine L; Women's College Hosp, W571-76 Grenville St, Toronto ON M5S 1B2; Tor'92; FRCPC; Neur. Staff, Women's College Hospital; (416)323-6400

LAYCOCK, Tyler M; Concordia Gen Hosp, 1095 Concordia Ave, Winnipeg MB R2K 3S8; McM'08; CCFP; CCFP(E.M.); Staff, Concordia General Hospital; (204)667-1560

LAYHER, Corrie R; 3-177 Fourth St, Duncan BC V9L 5J8; UBC'99; BSc; CCFP; FCFP; (250)746-6557

LAYNE, Elizabeth C; 203-345 Lakeshore Rd E, Oakville ON L6J 1J5; McM'00; FRCPC; Psy. Staff, Trillium Health Centre - Mississauga; (905)844-7770

LAYTON, Zeinab A; William Osler HC-Brampton, 2100 Bovaird Dr E, Brampton ON L6R 3J7; Wes'99; FRCPC; DiagRad. Staff, William Osler Health System - Brampton Civic Hospital; (905)494-2120

LAZA, Diana C; William Osler HC-Etobicoke, 101 Humber College Blvd, Etobicoke ON M9V 1R8; Timisoara (Romania)'85; CCFP; Staff, Mackenzie Richmond Hill Hospital; William Osler Health System - Etobicoke General Hospital; Langs: Romanian; Hungarian; (416)747-3400; diana.laza@rogers.com.

LAZAR, Edward R; Grey Nuns Community Hosp, 1100 Youville Drive West NW, Edmonton AB T6L 5X8; Dal'94; FRCPC; Anes. Staff Anes, Covenant Health - Grey Nuns Community Hospital; (780)735-7020; Fax. (403)735-7279.

LAZAR, Gary A; Medical Bldg, 1503-805 Broadway W, Vancouver BC V5Z 1K1; Man'84; FRCPC; Psy. Staff, BC Children's Hospital; (604)879-1503; Fax. (604)879-1594; glazar@cw.bc.ca.

LAZAR, Matthew H; Sterling Lyon Pediatrics, 401-1020 Lorimer Blvd, Winnipeg MB R3P 1C7; Man'86; FRCPC; Peds (Consultant & Primary Care). Ac Staff Children's Hosp, Health Sciences Centre; Staff Peds, St Boniface General Hospital; Staff, Victoria General Hospital; Teach Staff Peds & Child Health, University of Manitoba; (204)942-0949; Fax. (204)943-2666.

LAZAR, Neil M; 11C 1174-585 University Ave, Toronto ON M5G 2N2; Man'77; FRCPC; IntMed (Critical Care Medicine); Respir. Dir MSICU Site, Toronto General Hospital - UHN; Assoc Prof Med, University of Toronto; (416)340-3438; Fax. (416)340-3359; neil.lazar@uhn.on.ca.

LAZAR, Susan F; BC Women's Hosp & Health Ctre, C433-4500 Oak St, Vancouver BC V6H 3N1; Man'96; FRCPC; Psy. Staff, BC Women's Hospital & Health Centre; (604)875-2161

LAZARE, Darren M; Crossroads Med Clinic, 330-507 Broadway W, Vancouver BC V5Z 1E6; Ross (Dominica)'02; FRCSC; ObstGyn (Urogynecology). (604)708-0788

LAZARE, Nancy M; Stittsville Dist Med Centre, 1-1339 Stittsville Main St, Stittsville ON K2S 1C6; McG'81; (613)836-5083; Fax. (613)836-2451; nlazare@gmail.com.

LAZARE, Samuel J; City Centre Family Physicians, 500-71 King St W, Mississauga ON L5B 4A2; McG'80; Ac Staff, Trillium Health Centre - Mississauga; (905)270-0415; Fax. (905)848-1500.

LAZARENKO, Gerald C; Rockyview Gen Hosp, 7007 14 St SW, Calgary AB T2V 1P9; Cal'85; FRCPC; EmergMed. Staff, Rockyview General Hospital; (403)943-3450

LAZARESCU, Adriana; Zeidler Ledcor Centre, 22 30A-130 University Campus N, Edmonton AB T6G 2X8; Tor'02; FRCPC; IntMed; Gastroent. (780)248-1498; Fax. (780)248-1499.

LAZARIC, Daniel M; PO Box 99, Port Williams NS B0P 1T0; Dal'94; BSc; FRCPC; Anes (Acute Pain Management). (902)679-9255

LAZARIDIS, Sofia; Workplace Hlth & Public Safety, Pl 3712A-171 Slater St, Ottawa ON K1A 0L3; McG'94; CCFP; Langs: English; French; (613)946-6583; Fax. (613)990-9397; sofia_lazaridis@hc-sc.gc.ca.

LAZARO-LOPEZ, Francisco J; Clinique Med Nova, 3755 boul Saint-Laurent, Montreal QC H2W 1X8; Zaragoza (Spain)'72; FAAP; FRCPC; Peds. ac Staff, Centre Hospitalier l'Université de Montréal (CHUM) - Hôpital Notre-Dame; adj Prof, Universite de Montreal; (514)987-0080

LAZAROU, Jason; The Joseph & Wolf Lebovic Bldg, L2 411-60 Murray St, Toronto ON M5T 3L9; Tor'01; FRCPC; Neur. Staff, Mount Sinai Hospital; (416)586-4800

LAZAROU, Lazaros P; Ellesmere X-Ray Associates, 2880 Ellesmere Rd, Scarborough ON M1E 4B8; Salonica (Greece)'52; FRCPC; DiagRad. (416)284-1697; Fax. (416)284-1780.

LAZARUS, Arie; Pembina Med Clinic, 2251 Pembina Hwy, Winnipeg MB R3T 2H1; Witwatersrand (South Africa)'96; MB ChB.

LAZARUS, Michael; Dr B Russillo & M Rappaport Cl, 206-5450 Ch de la Cote-des-Nei, Montreal QC H3T 1Y6; Ott'77; assoc Staff, St Mary's Hospital Centre; (514)731-3249; Fax. (514)731-0395.

LAZENBY, Anne L; 362-21 St Clair Ave E, Toronto ON M4T 1L9; Tor'67; FRCPC; Psy (Child & Adolescent Psychiatry). (416)923-2131; Fax. (416)923-2131.

LAZEO, Sharon R; Klondyke Med Clinic, 1-3089 3rd Ave, Whitehorse YT Y1A 5B3; McM'91; Med Staff, Whitehorse General Hospital; Staff, Klondyke Medical Clinic; (867)688-4046

LAZIER, Kate; Toronto East Gen Hosp Inc, B 112-825 Coxwell Ave, Toronto ON M4C 3E7; Dal'03; CCFP; CCFP(E.M.); Staff Emerg Med, Toronto East General Hospital Inc; (416)469-6580 x6545

LAZIER, Lorraine L; Hants Community Hosp, 89 Payzant Dr, Windsor NS B0N 2T0; McM'91; FRCPC; Psy (Child & Adolescent Psychiatry). Staff, Hants Community Hospital; Staff, IWK Health Centre; Asst Prof Psy, Dalhousie University; (902)792-2198; Fax. (902)798-0709.

LAZINSKI, Dorothy; Univ Hlth Network-Princess M, 3F-610 University Ave, Toronto ON M5G 2M9; Tor'90; FRCPC; DiagRad (Neuro Radiology)., Princess Margaret Hospital - University Health Network; Staff, Toronto Western Hospital - University Health Network; (416)946-4501

LAZO LANGNER, Alejandro; London HSC-Victoria Hosp, PO Box 5010 Stn B A2 401-800 Commissioners Rd E, London ON N6A 5W9; (Mexico)'93; Staff, London Health Sciences Centre - Victoria Campus; (519)685-8500; Fax. (519)685-8477.

LAZONGAS, Chris; Scarborough Hosp-General Div, 3050 Lawrence Ave E, Scarborough ON M1P 2V5; Tor'06; FRCPC; IntMed; Critical Care Medicine. Staff Intensivist, The Scarborough Hospital - General Campus; (416)438-2911

LAZOVSKIS, Juris; Riverside Prof Centre, 31 Riverside Dr, Sydney NS B1S 3N1; Riga (Latvia)'85; Staff, Cape Breton Healthcare Complex; Langs: Latvian; German; French; (902)539-7875; Fax. (902)539-8033.

LAZOWSKI, Waldemar; PO Box 640, Souris PE C0A 2B0; Lublinie (Poland)'67; MB ChB; CCFP; Langs: Polish; Russian; (902)687-7096

LAZURE, Rene; Clinique Med L'Azur, 2689 rue Laval, Nantes QC G6B 1A2; Mon'87; Staff, Carrefour Sante Granit; (819)583-6565; Fax. (819)583-0645.

LAZZAM, Charles; 206-101 Queensway W, Mississauga ON L5B 2P7; Mon'81; FRCPC; IntMed (Interventional Cardiology); Cardiol. Staff Cardiol, Trillium Health Centre - Mississauga; Asst Prof, University of Toronto; Langs: English; French; (905)615-0012; Fax. (905)615-8537; charles.lazzam@sympatico.ca.

LAZZARA, Frank T; Centre Med Nazareth, 101-1771 av Dollard, LaSalle QC H8N 1T9; Padua (Italy)'80; Langs: French; Italian; (514)368-5500; Fax. (514)368-0056.

LE, Anh-Tai; Hop du Sacre-Coeur de Mtl, 5400 boul Gouin O, Montreal QC H4J 1C5; Sher'88; CSPQ; FRCPC; Anes. Staff, Hôpital du Sacre-Coeur de Montréal; (514)338-2222 x2680

LE, Anh-Thu; UMF Legardeur, 135 rue Claude-David, Repentigny QC J6A 1N6; Mon'09; (450)654-2911; Fax. (450)654-0359.

LE, Binh Quoc Huy; SMBD Jewish Gen Hosp, 3755 ch Cote-Sainte-Catherine, Montreal QC H3T 1E2; McG'03; FRCPC; DiagRad. Staff, Sir Mortimer B Davis Jewish General; (514)340-8222; Fax. (514)340-7907.

LE, Binh-Dang; CLSC-CHSLD du Marigot, 250 boul Cartier O, Laval QC H7N 5S5; Saigon (Vietnam)'74; Staff, CSSS de Dorval-Lachine-Lasalle; Médecin, CLSC-CHSLD du Marigot; Physician, CLSC-CHSLD du Ruisseau Papineau; Langs: English; Vietnamese; (450)668-6750

LE, Brian B; Scarborough Hosp-Birchmount, 3030 Birchmount Rd, Scarborough ON M1W 3W3; McM'03; FRCPC; IntMed (Respirology). Staff, The Scarborough Hospital - Birchmount Campus; Langs: Vietnamese; (416)495-2465; Fax. (416)495-2420.

LE, Brian V; Regina Gen Hosp, 1440 14th Ave, Regina SK S4P 0W5; Dal'00; FRCPC; DiagRad. Staff, Regina General Hospital; (306)766-4444

LE, Chu Quang; 203-474 College St, Toronto ON M6G 1A4; Tor'84; PhD; Langs: Vietnamese; French; (416)532-2958; Fax. (416)532-1812.

LE, David; 6A-3585 Keele St, North York ON M3J 3H5; (Vietnam)'78; (416)635-7131

LE, De Quang; 203-987 King St E, Hamilton ON L8M 1C6; Tor'91; CCFP; (905)544-9922; Fax. (905)544-5825.

LE, Doan Thuy; Alberta Children's Hosp, 2888 Shaganappi Trail NW, Calgary AB T3B 6A8; Cal'96; FRCPC; Peds (Pediatric Hematology); Hem. Staff, Alberta Children's Hospital; (403)955-3035

LE, Duc M; Saskaton Cancer Centre, 20 Campus Dr, Saskatoon SK S7N 4H4; Tor'05; MSc; BSc; FRCPC; RadOncol. (306)655-2740; Fax. (306)655-2639.

LE, Grace; Olive Med Clinic, 101-117 17 Ave NE, Calgary AB T2E 1L7; Alb'00; CCFP; Langs: Vietnamese; (403)276-8866; Fax. (403)230-2000; gle@calgaryhealthregion.ca.

LE, Han; Clinique Domus Medica, 214-5601 rue Belanger, Montreal QC H1T 1G3; Laval'95; Staff, CHSLD Lucille-Teasdale; (514)256-5011; Fax. (514)254-1114.

LE, Hoang Yen; 1218 King St W, Toronto ON M6K 1G4; Wes'92; FRCPC; Peds. Staff Pt-Time, Toronto General Hospital - UHN; Clin Asst, The Hospital For Sick Children; Langs: Vietnamese; (416)538-8833; Fax. (416)538-7685.

LE, Huu Phuong; CHSLD Lucille-Teasdale, 3095 rue Sherbrooke E, Montreal QC H1W 1B2; Saigon (Vietnam)'73; Staff, CHSLD Lucille-Teasdale; (514)523-1173

LE, Ian L D; Life Mark Health Centre, 2225 Macleod Trail SE, Calgary AB T2G 5B6; Alb'00; FRCSC; OrthSurg (Foot & Ankle Surgery). (403)291-0045

LE, Khoa-Anh; Markham Stouffville Hosp, 381 Church St, Markham ON L3P 7P3; Qns'95; FRCPC; IntMed. Staff, The Scarborough Hospital - Birchmount Campus; Langs: Vietnamese; French; (905)472-7000

LE, Luan B; St Martins Med Clinic, 1-73 Main St, St Martins NB E5R 1B4; Saba (Netherlands Antilles)'07; CCFP; (506)833-2012

LE, Lyly H; BC Cancer Agency-Fraser Valley, 13750 96 Ave, Surrey BC V3V 1Z2; McG'97; FRCP; ABIM; ABMO; FRCPC; IntMed (Gastroenterology & Genitourinary); MedOncol. Staff Med Oncologist, Surrey Memorial Hospital; Staff Med Oncologist, BC Cancer Agency Fraser Valley Centre; Clin Asst Prof, University Of British Columbia; Langs: Vietnamese; Bilingual(French/English); (604)930-4028; Fax. (604)587-4312; lle@bccancer.bc.ca.

LE, Melissa; MUHC-Royal Victoria Hosp, S7 64A-687 av des Pins O, Montreal QC H3A 1A1; Mon'08; CCFP; Staff, McGill University Health Centre - Royal Victoria Hospital; (514)934-1934

LE, Minh Tien; Clinique Med Jarry-Lajeunesse, 201-529 rue Jarry E, Montreal QC H2P 1V4; Saigon (Vietnam)'64; (514)277-4111; Fax. (514)277-0387; info@polycdi.com.

LE, Minh Van; 1450 Queen St W, Toronto ON M6K 1M2; Saigon (Vietnam)'74; (416)532-8277; Fax. (416)532-9104.

LE, Ngoc Duy; CSSS du Suroît, 150 rue Saint-Thomas, Salaber-de-Valleyf QC J6T 6C1; Sher'93; Staff, Centre Hospitalier Régional du Suroît; (450)371-9925; Fax. (450)371-7454.

LE, Ngoc Quan; CLSC Ahuntsic, 1165 boul Henri-Bourassa E, Montreal QC H2C 3K2; Sher'93; Staff, Centre Hospitalier l'Université de Montréal (CHUM) - Hôpital Notre-Dame; (514)381-4221 x346

LE, Nhan Trung; CSSS de Laval, 280 boul du Roi-du-Nord, Laval QC H7L 4L2; Sher'88; (450)622-5110

LE, Pham D T; SMBD Jewish Gen Hosp, 3755 ch Cote-Sainte-Catherine, Montreal QC H3T 1E2; McG'00; CCFP; CCFP(E.M.); Staff, Sir Mortimer B Davis Jewish General; (514)340-8222

LE, Philippe; SMBD Jewish Gen Hosp, 3755 ch Cote-Sainte-Catherine, Montreal QC H3T 1E2; McG'08; IntMed. Staff, Sir Mortimer B Davis Jewish General; (514)340-8222

LE, Phu-Tao; CLSC Saint-Michel, 3355 rue Jarry E, Montreal QC H1Z 2E5; Mon'86; (514)374-8223

LE, Phuoc Hoang; Clin Med Metro Beaubien, 300 rue Beaubien E, Montreal QC H2S 1R8; Mon'79; (514)276-2020; Fax. (514)273-1586.

LE, Phuoc-Hai; Saint Thomas Comm Health Ctre, 9040 84 Ave NW, Edmonton AB T6C 1E4; Mon'97; CCFP; Langs: Vietnamese; English; (780)434-2778; Fax. (780)466-8702.

LE, Quang Tien; Clinique Med Physimed, 6363 Rte Transcanadienne, Saint-Laurent QC H4T 1Z9; Hue (Vietnam)'73; Médecin, CLSC Ahuntsic; Langs: English; (514)747-8888

LE, Quynh M T; Peel Med Arts Bldg, 219-2120 North Park Dr, Brampton ON L6S 0C9; Tor'95; MD; FACOG; DABOG; FRCSC; ObstGyn. Staff ObstGyn, William Osler Health System - Brampton Civic Hospital; Langs: French; Vietnamese; (905)452-1951; Fax. (905)452-0478.

LE, Thanh Long; 958-999 36 St NE, Calgary AB T2A 7X6; Saigon (Vietnam)'75; Langs: Vietnamese; (403)273-3122; Fax. (403)273-3866.

LE, Thanh-Minh; 2547 rue des Ormeaux, Montreal QC H1L 4X4; Sher'87; (514)355-5755

LE, Thanh-Y.; CLSC des Seigneuries, RR 102 555 rue Principale, Saint-Amable QC J0L 1N0; Saigon (Vietnam)'69; (450)468-5250

LE, Thi Qui; Clinique Medicale 3600, 3600 rue Ontario E, Montreal QC H1W 1R7; Saigon (Vietnam)'82; Langs: Vietnamese; English; (514)523-8775; Fax. (514)526-9212.

LE, Thi Som Mai; CHUM-Hotel-Dieu, 3840 rue Saint-Urbain, Montreal QC H2W 1T8; Mon'06; FRCPC; DiagRad. Staff, Centre Hospitalier l'Université de Montréal (CHUM) - Hôtel-Dieu; (514)890-8150

LE, Thi Xuan Mai; Clinique Familiale Pas-A-Pas, 3650 boul Henri-Bourassa E, Montreal-Nord QC H1H 1J6; Mon'03; Chef méd interne, Hôpital du Sacre-Coeur de Montréal; Langs: English; Vietnamese; (514)328-9797; Fax. (514)328-2672.

LE, Thien Nhan; CLSC Saint-Henri, 3833 rue Notre-Dame O, Montreal QC H4C 1P8; Saigon (Vietnam)'74; Langs: Vietnamese; English; (514)933-7541; Fax. (514)933-2411; n.le@videotron.ca.

LE, Tien Dung; The Ottawa Hosp-Gen Campus, 8130-501 Smyth Rd, Ottawa ON K1H 8L6; Tor'89; FRCSC; ObstGyn; GynOnco. Staff, The Ottawa Hospital - General Campus; Langs: Vietnamese; (613)737-8560; Fax. (613)737-8828.

LE, Tung Trong; 346 Bronson Ave, Ottawa ON K1R 6J3; Ott'92; CCFP; (613)233-9505; Fax. (613)233-1872.

LE, Tuyet-Diem; Hop Maisonneuve-Rosemont, 5415 boul de l'Assomption, Montreal QC H1T 2M4; Hue (Vietnam)'75; FRCPC; Peds. Staff, Hopital Maisonneuve-Rosemont; Langs: Bilingual(French/English); (514)374-7940; Fax. (514)374-8101.

LE, Van Hoai V; Hop du Sacre-Coeur de Mtl, 5400 boul Gouin O, Montreal QC H4J 1C5; Mon'04; FRCPC; IntMed; Cardiol. Staff, Hôpital du Sacre-Coeur de Montréal; (514)338-2222

LE, Vanessa H; Clinique Med Diamant, 204-5512 ch de la Cote-des-Nei, Montreal QC H3T 1Y9; McM'04; CCFP; (514)737-3782

LE, Vy-Van; CHUM-Hotel-Dieu, 3840 rue Saint-Urbain, Montreal QC H2W 1T8; Sher'01; FRCPC; IntMed; Cardiol. Staff, Centre Hospitalier l'Université de Montréal (CHUM) - Hôtel-Dieu; (514)890-8000

LE BEL, Lucie; CHUQ-St-Francois D'Assise, 10 rue de l'Espinay, Quebec QC G1L 3L5; Laval'95; CSPQ; FRCPC; Anes. Staff, Centre Hospitalier Universitaire De Québec - Pavillon De St-françois-d'assise; (418)525-4303; Fax. (418)525-4434.

LE BEL, Roger E; 202-189 boul Hymus, Pointe-Claire QC H9R 1E9; Ott'71; DAB; BA; FRCSC; Otol. ac Staff Surg, Lakeshore General Hospital - Pointe Claire; Consultant Surg, Centre Hospitalier d'Argenteuil; Langs: French; (514)695-5993; Fax. (514)695-3807; r.l.lebel@hotmail.ca.

LE BEL, Stephane; Ctr Hosp du Centre la Mauricie, 50 119e rue, Shawinigan-Sud QC G9P 5K1; Mon'96; FRCSC; Ophth. Staff, Centre Hospitalier du Centre la Mauricie; (819)536-7640

LE BIRE, Francois; 115-5345 Boul de l'Assomption, Montreal QC H1T 4B3; Mon'72; (514)251-9331; Fax. (514)251-0511.

LE BLANC, Elsa; CSSS Pierre Boucher, 1333 boul Jacques-Cartier E, Longueuil QC J4M 2A5; Mon'97; Staff, Centre Hospitalier Pierre Boucher; (450)468-8111

LE BLANC, Richard; CHUS-Hop Fleurimont, 3001 12e Av N, Sherbrooke QC J1H 5N4; Mon'95; FRCPC; IntMed (Dermatology); Hem. Hématologue, Centre Hospitalier Universitaire de Sherbrooke-Hopital Fleurimont; Fax. (819)564-5369.

LE BOUTHILLIER, Annie-Josee; 102-4275 Innes Rd, Orleans ON K1C 1T1; Laval'00; CCFP; Langs: Bilingual(French/English); (613)837-3853; Fax. (613)837-6212.

LE BOUTHILLIER, Guy; CSSS du Nord de Lanaudière, 1000 boul Sainte-Anne, St-Charles-Brromee QC J6E 6J2; Mon'90; OrthSurg. Staff, Centre Hospitalier Régional de Lanaudière; (450)759-8222; Fax. (450)759-8289.

LE BOUTHILLIER, Pierre; Ctr Hosp Affilie-St-Sacrement, 1050 ch Sainte-Foy, Quebec QC G1S 4L8; Laval'83; FRCPC; IntMed; Cardiol. ac Staff, Centre Hospitalier Affilié Universitaire de Québec - Hôpital du St-Sacrement; (418)682-7985

LE BRETON, Michel A; 210-211 rue Champlain, Dieppe NB E1A 1N9; Ott'03; FRCSC; OrthSurg. Langs: Bilingual(English/French); (506)855-4481; Fax. (506)855-4372.

LE BRUN, David P; Queen's Univ-Richardson Lab, 99 University Ave, Kingston ON K7L 3N5; Qns'84; FRCPC; AnatPath (Hematology Pathology). Asst Prof, Queen's University; (613)533-3209

LE CLAIR, J Kenneth; Providence Care Mental Health, PO Box 603 Stn Main 752 King St W, Kingston ON K7L 4X3; Ott'77; BSc; FRCPC; Psy (Geriatric Psychiatry). Clin Dir Reg Geriatric Psy Prog, Providence Care - Mental Health Services; Clin Prof, University of Western Ontario; Prof, Queen's University; (613)548-5567 x5928; Fax. (613)540-6128; albertm@providencecare.ca.

LE CLERCQ, Sharon; South Health Campus, 4448 Front St SE, Calgary AB T3M 1M4; Alb'75; FRCPC; IntMed; Rheum. Ac Staff, Rockyview General Hospital; Clin Assoc Prof, University of Calgary; (403)956-2493; Fax. (403)956-2994.

LE CORFF, Joelle; CLSC Ruisseau Papineau, 1665 rue Du Couvent, Laval QC H7W 3A8; Mon'83; Physician, Maison Notre Dame de Laval; (450)687-5690

LE CORRE, Isabelle; Hop Charles Lemoyne, 3120 boul Taschereau, Greenfield Park QC J4V 2H1; Mon'85; FRCPC; MedMicrobiol; Microbio & Infect Dis (P.Q.). Ac Staff, Hopital Charles LeMoyne; (450)466-5000; isabelle.lecorre@rrsss16.gouv.qc.ca.

LE DEIST, Francoise; Hôpital Ste-Justine, 3175 ch de la Cote-Sainte-Cath, Montreal QC H3T 1C5; Paris (France)'82; Staff, Hôpital Ste-Justine; (514)345-4931 x3534

LE DU, Sylvain; Polyclinique Med de la Lievre, 536 rue de la Madone, Mont-Laurier QC J9L 1S7; Laval'05; (819)440-2345

LE DUC, Tam; Centre Medical 425, 425 Boul Cure-Poirier O, Longueuil QC J4J 2H3; Mon'83; Respir (P.Q.). Staff, Centre Hospitalier Pierre Boucher; Langs: Vietnamese; (450)679-6666; Fax. (450)679-6446.

LE FEUVRE, Catherine A; 206-101 Queensway W, Mississauga ON L5B 2P7; McM'88; BSc(Hons); ABIM; FRCPC; IntMed (Cardiac Electrophysiology); Cardiol., Trillium Health Centre - Mississauga; Asst Prof Med, McMaster University; Langs: English; French; (905)615-1441; Fax. (905)615-8537.

LE FRANCOIS, Michel; Polyclinique St-Martin, 300-1435 boul Saint-Martin O, Laval QC H7S 2C6; Mon'69; FRCSC; Ophth. (450)668-1211

LE GAL, Gregoire; The Ottawa Hosp-Gen Campus, 501 Smyth Rd, Ottawa ON K1H 8L6; (France)'03; Staff, The Ottawa Hospital - General Campus; (613)798-5555

LE GOFF, Gilbert; CSSSG-Hop de Gatineau, CP 2000 Succ Bureau-Chef, Gatineau QC J8P 7H2; Sher'80; FRCSC; ObstGyn. Staff, Hôpital de Gatineau; (819)561-8100

LE GOUEFF, Real J; CLSC St-Michel des Saints, 171 rue Archambault RR 1, St-Mich-D-Sts QC J0K 3B0; Mon'85; (450)833-6334; Fax. (450)833-6009.

LE GRESLEY, Jovain; CSSS De La Haute-Yamaska, 205 boul Leclerc O, Granby QC J2G 1T7; Sher'06; Staff, Centre Hospitalier de Granby; (450)375-8000

LE GUERRIER, Paul; Dir de la Sante Publique-Mtl, 1301 rue Sherbrooke E, Montreal QC H2L 1M3; McG'84; LMCC; MPH; CCFP; Med Consultant, Direction de la Sante Publique de Montreal; Prof, Universite de Montreal; Langs: English; (514)528-2400 x3801; Fax. (514)528-2452; pleguerr@santepub-mtl.qc.ca.

LE GUILLAN, Marie-Pierre; Hop Charles Lemoyne, 3120 boul Taschereau, Greenfield Park QC J4V 2H1; Sher'95; FRCSC; GenSurg; VascSurg. Staff, Hopital Charles LeMoyne; (450)466-5000

LE GUILLAN, Soazig; 100-100 ch Rockland, Mont-Royal QC H3P 2V9; Mon'02; GenSurg. (514)331-4322

LE JOUR, Caroline; Foothills Med Centre, 1403 29 St NW, Calgary AB T2N 2T9; McG'07; MDCM; FRCSC; ObstGyn. Staff, Foothills Medical Centre; (403)944-1437

LE LIEVRE, Christine M; The Juravinski Cancer Centre, 699 Concession St, Hamilton ON L8V 5C2; Wes'88; CCFP; Ac Staff, Joseph Brant Memorial Hospital; (905)336-4103

LE LORIER, Jacques; CHUM-Hotel-Dieu, 3840 rue Saint-Urbain, Montreal QC H2W 1T8; (Mexico)'66; PhD(Pharm); ABIM; IntMed. Staff, Centre Hospitalier l'Université de Montréal (CHUM) - Hôtel-Dieu; Head Med, Universite de Montreal; (514)890-8000 x12918; Fax. (514)412-7174; jacques.le.lorier@umontreal.ca.

LE MAY, Claude; CSSS De Quebec-Sud, 300 boul Wilfrid-Hamel, Vanier QC G1M 2R9; Laval'72; Urol (Prostate Laser Therapy). Staff, CSSS de Quebec-Sud; Consultant, Institut Prive d'Urologie de Quebec; (418)682-1711

LE MAY, J Michel R; Univ of Ottawa Heart Institute, H150-40 Ruskin St, Ottawa ON K1Y 4W7; Ott'78; FRCPC; IntMed (Interventional Cardiology); Cardiol. Staff, University of Ottawa Heart Institute; (613)761-4223

LE MAY, Jacques P; Hop du Sacre-Coeur de Mtl, 5400 boul Gouin O, Montreal QC H4J 1C5; Mon'66; FRCPC; HemPath; MedOncol (P.Q.); Hem (P.Q.). Ac Staff, Hôpital du Sacre-Coeur de Montréal; adj Prof, Universite de Montreal; (514)338-2150

LE MELLEDO, Jean-Michel; University of Alberta Hosp, 1E7 14-8440 112 St NW, Edmonton AB T6G 2B7; (France)'92; Staff, University of Alberta Hospital; Langs: English; French; (780)407-6578; Fax. (780)407-6672.

LE MEVEL-MOREIRA, Francoise; Clinique MRC des Moulins, 101-1355 Grande Allee, Terrebonne QC J6W 4K6; Paris (France)'82; Psy (P.Q.). Staff, Centre Hospitalier Pierre le Gardeur; Langs: English; Spanish; (450)964-6418; Fax. (450)964-9260.

LE MOINE, Lindsay; Clinique Med Racine, 201-900 boul Raymond, Quebec QC G1B 3G3; Laval'72; ac Staff, Centre Hospitalier Affilié Universitaire de Québec - Hôpital De L'Enfant Jésus; (418)667-8066; Fax. (418)667-8131.

LE-NGOC, A Anne; MUHC-Montreal Gen Hosp, 1650 av Cedar, Montreal QC H3G 1A4; McG'07; MDCM; IntMed. Staff, McGill University Health Centre - Montreal General Campus; (514)934-1934

LE NOBEL, John C; Northmount Med Centre, 601-145 13th St E, North Vancouver BC V7L 2L4; Tor'75; FRCPC; PhysMed&Rehab. Staff, Lions Gate Hospital; Court Staff, G F Strong Rehabilitation Centre; (604)985-3018; Fax. (604)985-6899.

LE QUOC, Thuy Linh; Centre de Peri-Maternite, 575 rue Saint-Charles E, Longueuil QC J4H 1B8; Sher'02; CCFP; (450)332-9833

LE REGENT, Linda; CSSS les Eskers de l'Abitibi, 622 4e rue O, Amos QC J9T 2S2; Laval'05; FRCSC; GenSurg. Staff, CH Hôtel-Dieu d'Amos; (819)732-3341

LE RICHE, Nicole G H; St Joseph's Health Care, PO Box 5777 Stn B 268 Grosvenor St, London ON N6A 4V2; Qns'77; FRCPC; IntMed (Adult Rheumatology); Rheum. Staff, St Joseph's Hospital - St Joseph's Health Care; Assoc Prof Med, Schulich School of Medicine & Dentistry; (519)646-6119; Fax. (519)646-6216; nicole.leriche@sjhc.london.on.ca.

LE ROUX, Andries; Sain John Reg Hosp, PO Box 2100 Stn Main, Saint John NB E2L 4L2; 80Stellenbosch (South Africa)'92; MB ChB; Staff, Saint John Regional Hospital; (506)648-6650

LE ROUX, Bartholomeus J M; Professional Bldg, 304-5400 Portage Rd, Niagara Falls ON L2G 5X7; Pretoria (South Africa)'97; FRCSC; OrthSurg. (905)353-8833

LE ROUX, Carinca; Dr CW Wiebe Med Centre, 385 Main St, Winkler MB R6W 1J2; Stellenbosch (South Africa)'98; MB ChB; CCFP; (204)325-4312

LE ROUX, Carl J; Erindale Health Centre, 2-50 Kenderdine Rd, Saskatoon SK S7N 3A1; Stellenbosch (South Africa)'90; MB ChB; Langs: Afrikaans; (306)934-6601; Fax. (306)934-6615.

LE ROUX, Cindy-Anne; Eastport Shopping Centre, 3-200 52 St NE, Calgary AB T2A 4K8; Cape Town (South Africa)'81; MB ChB; (403)569-7464; Fax. (403)248-6896.

LE ROUX, Eric W; Regina Qu'Appelle HR-Regina, 1440 14th Ave, Regina SK S4P 0W5; Orange Free State (South Africa)'85; MB ChB; LMCC; Staff, Regina General Hospital; (306)766-4444

LE ROUX, Jacobus F; 3310 32nd Ave, Vernon BC V1T 2M6; Stellenbosch (South Africa)'83; MB ChB; (250)545-5321

LE ROUX, Jacobus J; Holley Clinic, 348 Front St, Quesnel BC V2J 2K3; Pretoria (South Africa)'89; MB ChB; CCFP; Langs: Afrikaans; (250)992-2158; Fax. (250)992-9391.

LE ROUX, Johannes L; 504-3 Stonegate Dr NEW, Airdrie AB T4B 0N2; (South Africa)'98; BSc; MB ChB; CCFP; Langs: Afrikaans; (403)945-8216; Fax. (403)945-8276.

LE ROUX, Johannes M; The Malone Med Clinic, 4955 41 Ave, Drayton Valley AB T7A 1V4; Stellenbosch (South Africa)'81; (780)542-3366

LE ROUX, Jolene; 3-4402 37 St, Stony Plain AB T7Z 2A9; (South Africa)'08; MB ChB; (780)963-7800

LE ROUX, Kriegler; Family Practice Associates, PO Box 2010 223 16th Ave, Creston BC V0B 1G0; Pretoria (South Africa)'85; MB ChB; CCFP; (250)428-9371; Fax. (250)428-9350.

LE ROUX, Marion A; Victoria East Med Clinic, 2068 Prince of Wales Dr, Regina SK S4V 3A6; Pretoria (South Africa)'89; LMCC; MB ChB; (306)789-4677; Fax. (306)789-3422.

LE ROUX, Marius N; PO Box 306, Fort Vermilion AB T0H 1N0; (780)927-3213

LE ROUX, Noelene; Prince Albert Med Clinic, 681 15th St W, Prince Albert SK S6V 7H9; Pretoria (South Africa)'96; MB ChB; Langs: Afrikaans; (306)764-1505 x216; Fax. (306)764-7775.

LE ROUX, Pieter C; PO Box 1828, Swan River MB R0L 1Z0.

LE ROUX, Theodorus; Regina Qu'Appelle HR-Regina, 1440 14th Ave, Regina SK S4P 0W5; Pretoria (South Africa)'89; MB ChB; FRCPC; Anes. Staff, Regina General Hospital; (306)766-2295

LE ROY, Marie-Claire; 388 rue Saint-Vallier O, Quebec QC G1K 1K6; Caen (France)'76; (418)522-1555; Fax. (418)683-1935.

LE SAGE, Natalie; Ctr Hosp Affilie-Enfant-Jesus, 1401 18e rue, Quebec QC G1J 1Z4; Laval'87; MSc; EmergMed (P.Q.). Ac Staff Emerg, Centre Hospitalier Affilié Universitaire de Québec - Hôpital De L'Enfant Jésus; Teach Staff, Université Laval; Langs: English; (418)649-5632; Fax. (418)649-5975.

LE SAUX, Nicole M A; Children's Hosp Eastern Ont, 401 Smyth Rd, Ottawa ON K1H 8L1; Ott'81; BSc; FRCPC; IntMed; AnatPath; InfectDis. Staff InfectDis, Children's Hospital of Eastern Ontario (CHEO); Assoc Prof, University of Ottawa; Langs: English; French; (613)737-7600 x2651; Fax. (613)738-4832; lesaux@cheo.on.ca.

LE SIEGE, Michele; Place Val des Arbres, 175-1600A boul Saint-Martin E, Laval QC H7G 4R8; Mon'78; FRCPC; Peds. Staff, Hopital de la Cite de la santé; (450)669-6666; Fax. (450)669-5412.

LE TEMPLIER, Genevieve; CHUS-Hop Fleurimont, 3001 12e av N, Sherbrooke QC J1H 5N4; Mon'01; FRCPC; IntMed. Staff, Centre Hospitalier Universitaire de Sherbrooke-Hopital Fleurimont; (819)346-1110 x28303

LE THI, Minh-Tri; Clinique d'Urgence Forcemedic, 200-1021 rue Jean-Talon E, Montreal QC H2R 1V6; Saigon (Vietnam)'72; (514)787-1818

LE TIEN HO THI, Kim H; Ctr Hosp Affilie-Enfant-Jesus, 1401 18e rue, Quebec QC G1J 1Z4; Pierre & Marie Curie (France)'79; Staff, Centre Hospitalier Affilié Universitaire de Québec - Hôpital De L'Enfant Jésus; (418)649-5604

LE TRUONG, Hong Hanh; CSSSG-Hop de Gatineau, CP 2000 Succ Bureau-Chef 909 boul de la Verendrye O, Gatineau QC J8P 7H2; Sher'95; FRCPC; Anes. Staff, Hôpital de Gatineau; (819)561-8299; Fax. (819)246-0314.

LE VAN, Mai Anh; MUHC-Montreal Gen Hosp, B2 117-1650 av Cedar, Montreal QC H3G 1A4; McG'99; CCFP; CCFP(E.M.); Staff, McGill University Health Centre - Montreal General Campus; McGill University; Langs: Spanish; English; (514)934-1934 x42501

LE VAN LONG, Maurice; Hop Louis-H Lafontaine, 7401 rue Hochelaga, Montreal QC H1N 3M5; Paris (France)'83; IntMed (P.Q.) (Digestive Endoscopy). Staff, Hopital Louis-H Lafontaine; (514)251-4000 x2260; Fax. (514)251-4054.

LEA, David E; BC Women's Hosp & Health Ctre, 1Q72-4500 Oak St, Vancouver BC V6H 3N1; Ott'79; FRCPC; Anes. Staff Anes, BC Women's Hospital & Health Centre; (604)875-2158

LEA, Denise A; Prov Addictions Treatment Faci, PO Box 2000 Stn Central, Charlottetown PE C1A 7N8; Sask'90; CCFP; (902)569-0508; Fax. (902)368-6229.

LEA, Jane; St Paul's Hosp, 1081 Burrard St, Vancouver BC V6Z 1Y6; Tor'05; FRCSC; Otol. Staff, Providence Health Care - St Paul's Hospital; (604)806-8540

LEA, Janice F C; York Medical, 123-14800 Yonge St, Aurora ON L4G 1N3; Tor'94; CCFP; (905)713-0404; Fax. (905)713-6341.

LEA, John N; Lions Gate Hosp, 231 15th St E, North Vancouver BC V7L 2L7; UBC'79; Staff, Lions Gate Hospital; (604)985-4545

LEA, Norman; Saddle Mountain Med Clinic, PO Box 159, Nakusp BC V0G 1R0; Cal'86; CCFP; FCFP; Chief of Staff, Arrow Lakes Hospital; (250)265-3694; Fax. (250)265-3050.

LEA-MAKENNY, Susan J; 217-1111 Olympic Way SE, Calgary AB T2G 0E6; Cal'85; CCFP; FCFP; Clin Assoc Prof Family Med, University of Calgary; (403)538-8881; slea@foothills-health.com.

LEACH, Alan J; Bank Med Centre, 1935 Bank St, Ottawa ON K1V 8A3; Wes'71; FRCPC; Cardiol. (613)521-2391 x140; Fax. (613)521-5443; alan@terapia.ca.

LEACH, James D; Dr Everett Chalmers Hosp, PO Box 9000 Stn A, Fredericton NB E3B 5N5; Dal'01; Anes. Staff, Dr Everett Chalmers Regional Hospital; (506)452-5400

LEACH, Leslie A; Avenue Med Centre, 1-221 Brant Ave, Brantford ON N3T 3J2; McM'82; CCFP; FCFP; Staff, The Brant Community Healthcare System - Brantford General Hospital Site; Staff, The Brant Community Healthcare System - Willett Hospital Site; (519)753-8666; Fax. (519)753-6880.

LEACOCK, Susan L; Anaesthetic Services, 213-2186 Oak Bay Ave, Victoria BC V8R 1G3; Alb'76; FRCPC; Anes. Staff, Victoria General Hospital; (250)595-7211

LEACY, James W B; Pittsburgh Institution, GD Highway 15, Joyceville ON K0H 1Y0; Qns'60; Med Advisor Bd/Board Member, Hotel-Dieu Hospital; (613)536-2148

LEADER, Arthur; Ottawa Fertility Centre, 200-955 Green Valley Cres, Ottawa ON K2C 3V4; McM'72; BAHon; FRCSC; ObstGyn (Reproductive Endocrinology & Infertility). Ac Staff, The Ottawa Hospital - Civic Campus; Prof Obst, University of Ottawa; Langs: Bilingual(French/English); (613)686-3378 x624; Fax. (613)225-9736; aleader@conceive.ca.

LEADER, Rolland M; Baywood Med Centre, 305-95 Bayly St W, Ajax ON L1S 7K8; Tor'76; FRCPC; IntMed (Cardiology). Consultant, Rouge Valley Health System - Ajax & Pickering Health Centre Site; (905)686-3211; Fax. (905)686-8564; leadermd@rogers.com.

LEADER, Susan M A; Oak Ridges Med Centre, 100-13291 Yonge St, Richmond Hill ON L4E 4L6; Tor'89; CCFP; FCFP; Court Staff, Trillium Health Centre - Mississauga; (905)773-7759; Fax. (905)773-1325.

LEADMAN, Martha L; Leamington Dist Mem Hosp, 194 Talbot St W, Leamington ON N8H 1N9; Ott'79; AB; FRCPC; DiagRad. Chief DiagRad, Leamington District Memorial Hospital; Staff, Windsor Regional Hospital - Tayfour Site; (519)322-2501 x417

LEAF, Suzanne C; Musculoskeletal Centre, 189 Elm St, St Thomas ON N5R 5C4; Minnesota(MN) (USA)'97; DABIM; FRCPC; IntMed; Rheum. Staff, St Thomas Elgin General Hospital; (519)637-7171

LEAHEY, Shelagh M; Ocean View Family Practice, 306C-60 Vancouver St, Yarmouth NS B5A 2P5; Dal'75; Staff, Yarmouth Regional Hospital; Board Member, CPSNS & Cardiac Advisory Committee; (902)742-4365; Fax. (902)742-9234.

LEAHY, James R; Payzant Med Clinic, PO Box 2498 59 Payzant Dr, Windsor NS B0N 2T0; Dal'79; (902)798-5791; Fax. (902)798-4668.

LEAHY, Marilyn T; The Group Health Centre, 240 McNabb St, Sault Ste. Marie ON P6B 1Y5; Wes'86; CCFP; (705)759-1234; Fax. (705)759-7469.

LEAHY, Martin F; Queensway Carleton Hosp, 3045 Baseline Rd, Nepean ON K2H 8P4; Dublin (Ireland)'03; CCFP; CCFP(E.M.); Staff Family Med, Queensway Carleton Hospital; (613)721-2000

LEAHY, Natalie C; Taunton Health Centre, SS 201 1290 Keith Ross Dr, Oshawa ON L1H 7K4; McM'04; BSc; CCFP; (905)721-4160; Fax. (905)721-6689.

LEAHY, Patrick J; Kemptville Med Centre, PO Box 1859 2670 Highway 43, Kemptville ON K0G 1J0; Wes'92; CCFP; FCFP; Staff, Kemptville District Hospital; Langs: French; (613)258-4600; Fax. (613)258-2799.

LEAKER, Michael T; Alberta Children's Hosp, C4 417-2888 Shaganappi Trail N, Calgary AB T3B 6A8; Alb'85; FRCPC; Peds (Oncology); Hem. Staff, Alberta Children's Hospital; (403)955-3035; Fax. (403)955-3055.

LEAKOS, Richard J; Lakeside Med Clinic, 3919 8th St E, Saskatoon SK S7H 5M7; Sask'95; CCFP; (306)374-6884; Fax. (306)374-2552.

LEAL, Gregory R J; Hilden Square, 2-393 Sidney St, Belleville ON K8P 3Z9; Ott'95; FRCSC; Urol (Incontinence). Staff, QHC Belleville General; Staff/Chief Urol, QHC Trenton Memorial; Staff, Kingston General Hospital; Queen's University; (613)967-5916; Fax. (613)967-4274; gregleal@hotmail.com.

LEAM, Howe; Haig Clinic, 601 6 Ave S, Lethbridge AB T1J 0Z2; Alb'88; CCFP; FCFP; Langs: Chinese; Cantonese; Mandarin; (403)328-6641; Fax. (403)328-6118.

LEANOFF, Dimitri; Golfdale Med Centre, 3750 Lawrence Ave E, Scarborough ON M1G 1R1; Sofia (Bulgaria)'70; (416)438-1664

LEAR, N Adrian; Dr H Bliss Murphy Cancer Ctr, 300 Prince Philip Dr, St. John's NL A1B 3V6; Mem'75; Clin Associate RadOncol, Dr H Bliss Murphy Cancer Centre; (709)777-7805; Fax. (709)777-8756.

LEAR, Naomi D; Bathurst Walkin & Family Pract, 101-4430 Bathurst St, North York ON M3H 3S3; McG'07; MDCM; CCFP; (416)633-3629; Fax. (416)633-3624.

LEARY, Courtney C; Thompson Gen Hosp, 871 Thompson Dr, Thompson MB R8N 0C8; Man'08; Staff, Thompson General Hospital; (204)677-2381

LEARY, Tara J; Sudbury Reg Hosp, 41 Ramsey Lake Rd, Sudbury ON P3E 5J1; Qns'99; CCFP; Staff Hospitalist, Health Sciences North-Laurentian Site; Clin Lecturer, Northern Ontario School of Medicine; (705)526-7147

LEASA, David J; London HSC-University Hosp, PO Box 5339 Stn B B2 194E-339 Windermere Rd, London ON N6A 5A5; Wes'79; BSc; ABIM(CriticalCare); FRCPC; IntMed (Critical Care Medicine); Respir. Staff, London Health Sciences Centre - University Hospital; Prof Med, University of Western Ontario; (519)663-3921; Fax. (519)663-8813; david.leasa@lhsc.on.ca.

LEASK, Barbara E; Sunlife Financial, 227 King St S, Waterloo ON N2J 1R3; Wes'70; Med Dir, Sunlife Financial; (519)888-2947

LEATHER, Richard A; Fort Royal Med Centre, 335-1900 Richmond Ave, Victoria BC V8R 4R2; Qns'84; BSc; FRCPC; IntMed (Cardiac Electrophysiology); Cardiol. Assoc Prof Med, University of British Columbia; (250)595-1551; Fax. (250)595-1000.

LEATHERBARROW, Zoe A; 4500 Oak St, Vancouver BC V6H 3N1; UBC'97; PhC; FRCPC; Peds (Pediatric Emergency Medicine). Staff, BC Women's Hospital & Health Centre; (604)875-2045

LEATHERDALE, Charles L; 61 Victoria St PO Box 220, Port Burwell ON N0J 1T0; Wes'60; (519)874-4242; Fax. (519)874-4518.

LEAVITT, Blair R; UBC Hospital, S179-2211 Wesbrook Mall, Vancouver BC V6T 2B5; McG'92; FRCPC; Neur (Neuro Genetics). Staff HD Medical Clinic/Staff Neurogenetics Clinc/Staff Medical Genetics & Neurology, UBC Hospital - Koerner Pavillion; Prof, Centre for Molecular Medecine & Therapeutics Medical Genetics; (604)822-7738; slanglois@cw.bc.ca.

LEBEAU, Annie; Cite de la Sante de Laval, 1755 boul Rene-Laennec, Laval QC H7M 3L9; Mon'96; FRCPC; AnatPath; GenPath (P.Q.). Staff, Hopital de la Cite de la santé; (450)668-1010 x23140; lebeauannie@hotmail.com.

LEBEAU, Johanne; Clinique Med Saint-Hippolyte, CP 29 780 ch des Hauteurs, Saint-Hippolyte QC J8A 3P4; Sher'83; Médecin Family Med, CLSC Arthur Buies; (450)224-8271; Fax. (450)224-1985; johanne.lebeau@ssss.gouv.qc.ca.

LEBEAU, Marc; St Michael's Hosp, 30 Bond St, Toronto ON M5B 1W8; Ott'85; CCFP; FCFP; Staff, St Michael's Hospital; Langs: French; (416)867-7428; Fax. (416)867-7498.

LEBEAU, Marie-Claude; CSSS de la Cote-De-Gaspe, 215 boul de York O, Gaspe QC G4X 2W2; Sher'85; FRCPC; Peds (Developmental). Staff, Centre Hospitalier de Gaspe; Langs: English; (418)368-3301 x3308

LEBEAU, Real; Hop Du Sacre-Coeur De Mtl, 5400 boul Gouin O, Montreal QC H4J 1C5; Mon'73; Cardiol (P.Q.) (Ultrasound). Staff, Hôpital du Sacre-Coeur de Montréal; Langs: Bilingual(French/English); (514)338-2200

LEBEAU, Thierry; Hop Maisonneuve-Rosemont, 5415 boul de l'Assomption, Montreal QC H1T 2M4; Laval'03; FRCSC; Urol. Staff, Hopital Maisonneuve-Rosemont; (514)252-3400

LEBEDIN, Walter W; Seven Oaks Gen Hosp, 2300 McPhillips St, Winnipeg MB R2V 3M3; Man'70; FRCPC; Psy. Head Dept of Psy, Seven Oaks General Hospital; (204)632-3523; Fax. (204)697-3043.

LEBEL, Alain; Inst Albert Prevost, 6555 boul Gouin O, Montreal QC H4K 1B3; Mon'85; FRCPC; Psy (Child Psychiatry). Clin Staff Pavillon Albert-Prevost, Hôpital du Sacre-Coeur de Montréal; Langs: Bilingual(French/English); (514)338-4356; Fax. (514)338-4357.

LEBEL, Annie; CSSS de Sept-Iles, 45 rue Du Pere-Divet, Sept-Iles QC G4R 3N7; Sher'94; Staff, Centre Hospitalier Regional de Sept-Iles; (418)962-9761

LEBEL, Catherine; CSSS de Rimouski-Neigette, CP 3150 Succ A 150 av Rouleau, Rimouski QC G5L 5T1; Laval'07; Psy. Staff, Hôpital Regional Rimouski.

LEBEL, Daniel; Falls Med Clinic, 107 Kelly Rd, Smooth Rock Falls ON P0L 2B0; Laval'89; Chief Medical Staff, Smooth Rock Falls Hospital; Langs: Bilingual(French/English); (705)338-2788; Fax. (705)338-2933.

LEBEL, Jean-Philippe; Polyclinique Med Pierre LeGard, 300-1000 montee des Pionniers, Terrebonne QC J6V 1S8; Mon'00; CCFP; Staff, Centre Hospitalier Pierre le Gardeur; (450)657-5799; Fax. (450)657-1809.

LEBEL, Jocelyn J; Clin Med Riviere des Mille-Ile, 200A-230 ch de la Grande-Cote, Boisbriand QC J7G 1B5; Laval'74; (450)437-1111

LEBEL, Laurie; Delta Health Sciences Centre, 202-4515 Harvest Dr, Delta BC V4K 4L1; UBC'04; CCFP; Physician, Delta Health Sciences Centre; (604)946-6411

LEBEL, Lisa; CSSS du Nord de Lanaudière, 1000 boul Sainte-Anne, St-Charles-Brromee QC J6E 6J2; Sher'84; NuclearMed (P.Q.). Staff Nuclear Med, Centre Hospitalier Régional de Lanaudière; (450)759-8222; Fax. (450)759-9075.

LEBEL, Marc; Hôpital Ste-Justine, 3175 ch Cote-Sainte-Catherine, Montreal QC H3T 1C5; Mon'81; NBME; ABPeds; InfectDis (P.Q.); Peds. Att Staff, Hôpital Ste-Justine; assoc Prof, Universite de Montreal; (514)349-4931 x5566; Fax. (514)345-4908; marc_lebel@ssss.gouv.qc.ca.

LEBEL, Marie-Claude; CSSS de Manicouagan, 635 boul Jolliet, Baie-Comeau QC G5C 1P1; Mon'93; FRCSC; ObstGyn. Staff, Centre Hospitalier Régional Baie-Comeau; (418)589-3701; Fax. (418)589-3659.

LEBEL, Marie-Eve; Univ of Western Ontario, 3M-1151 Richmond Rd, London ON N6A 3K7; Laval'99; FRCSC; OrthSurg. (519)661-4003

LEBEL, Mario; 565 rue Tache GD, Saint-Pascal QC G0L 3Y0; Mon'84; Staff, CSSS de Kamouraska; (418)492-6234; Fax. (418)492-6053.

LEBEL, Martine; 9923 Jubilee Rd PO Box 218, Summerland BC V0H 1Z0; Sher'79; (250)494-0521

LEBEL, Maude; CHUQ-Ctr Hosp Univ Laval, 2705 boul Laurier, Quebec QC G1V 4G2; McG'98; Staff, Centre Hospitalier Universitaire de Quebec-CHUL; (418)654-2114

LEBEL, Michel H; 307-176 av Rouleau, Rimouski QC G5L 8W1; Laval'05; CSPQ; FRCSC; Urol. Staff, Hôpital Regional Rimouski; Langs: Bilingual(French/English); (418)724-6262; Fax. (418)722-6265.

LEBEL, Michel L; 237-1055 12e Av N, Sherbrooke QC J1E 2X4; Sher'72; AB; FRCPC; Electroenceph (P.Q.) (Neuro Physiology); Neur. assoc Prof, Universite de Sherbrooke; (819)565-1224; Fax. (819)565-1423.

LEBEL, Monique; 8747 rue Hochelaga, Montreal QC H1L 2M8; Mon'79; FRCPC; Derm. (514)354-4830

LEBEL, Paule T; Universite de Montreal, CP 6128 succ Centre ville, Montreal QC H3C 3J7; Mon'77; FRCPC; CommunMed. assoc Staff, Hôpital Ste-Justine; Prof, Universite de Montreal; (514)343-6111 x0556; plebel@sympatico.ca.

LEBEL, Pierre; A5 156-1650 av Cedar, Montreal QC H3G 1A4; Mon'82; FRCPC; MedMicrobiol; Microbio & Infect Dis (P.Q.). Staff, McGill University Health Centre - Montreal General Campus; Langs: English; French; (514)934-1934 x42812; Fax. (514)934-8423; pierre.lebel@muhc.mcgill.ca.

LEBEL, Rejean; CSSS des Aurores Boreales, CP 6000 Succ Bureau-Chef 679 2e rue E, La Sarre QC J9Z 2X7; Mon'89; CCFP; Chef méd fam, Centre Hospitalier La Sarre; Staff, Centre Hospitalier St-Jean; (819)333-2311; Fax. (819)333-4227.

LEBEL, Roseline; GMF Concorde, 300 boul de la Concorde E, Laval QC H7G 2E6; Mon'75; (450)667-5310; Fax. (450)667-5248.

LEBEL, Stefane; Hôpital Laval, 2725 ch Sainte-Foy, Quebec QC G1V 4G5; Mon'89; FRCSC; GenSurg. Staff, Hôpital Laval; (418)656-4810; Fax. (418)656-4825.

LEBEL, Suzanne; CLSC des Hautes Laurentides, 757 rue de la Madone, Mont-Laurier QC J9L 1T3; Mon'77; Gen Practice, CSSS d'Antoine-Labelle; (819)623-1228

LEBEL, Tania C; Owen Sound Fam Health Team, 1415 1st Ave W, Owen Sound ON N4K 4K8; McG'03; CCFP; (519)470-3030

LEBELLE DEJARIO, Nadine; PO Box 1017 Stn Main, Campbellton NB E3N 3H4; Sher'94; Med Dir Emerg Med/Staff, Hôpital Régional Campbellton; (506)759-7113; Fax. (506)759-7118.

LEBER, Brian F; Hamilton HS-Juravinski Site, B3 147-711 Concession St, Hamilton ON L8V 1C3; McG'81; FRCPC; IntMed; Hem. Att Physician, Hamilton Health Sciences Centre-Juravinski Site; Prof Health Sciences, McMaster University; (905)521-2100 x76384; leberb@mcmaster.ca.

LEBER, Wolfgang A; Sunnybrook Hlth Sciences Ctre, A253-2075 Bayview Ave, Toronto ON M4N 3M5; (Germany)'98; Staff, Sunnybrook Health Sciences Centre; (416)480-5687

LEBERT, Phyllis A; Hamilton HS-General Site, 237 Barton St E, Hamilton ON L8L 2X2; Wes'84; BSc; MSc; FRCPC; IntMed; ClinImmunol&Allergy. Staff, Hamilton Health Sciences Centre - Hamilton General Hospital; (905)527-4322

LEBEUF, Christine; Foothills Prof Bldg, 245-1620 29 St NW, Calgary AB T2N 4L7; Mon'85; CCFP; FCFP; Staff, Foothills Medical Centre; Teach Staff Family Med, University of Calgary; (403)289-0069; Fax. (403)289-0533.

LEBEUF, Stephen J; Alder Med Centre, 277 Evergreen Rd, Campbell River BC V9W 5Y4; Sask'96; BSc; CCFP; (250)287-7441; Fax. (250)287-4384.

LEBL, Martin G; Morgan Creek Site Clinic, 106-15252 32 Ave, Surrey BC V3S 0R7; Prague (Czech Republic)'98; CCFP; (604)542-4885

LEBLANC, Benoit; Clin Chirurgie Esthetique Carp, 5270 rue de Bellechasse, Montreal QC H1T 2A9; Mon'02; BEng; MEng; FRCSC; PlasSurg (Anesthesia). Staff Plastic Surg, Hopital Maisonneuve-Rosemont; Prof Plastic Surg, Universite de Montreal; Langs: Bilingual(French/English); (514)257-1860; Fax. (514)257-1326; cliniquecarpediem@gmail.com.

LEBLANC, Bruno; Polyclinique St-Jerome, 304-200 rue Durand, Saint-Jerome QC J7Z 7E2; Sher'90; Urol. (450)436-7173

LEBLANC, Carole; 516-100 Arden St, Moncton NB E1C 4B7; Mon'00; FRCSC; ObstGyn. Staff, The Moncton Hospital; Langs: English; (506)857-4242; Fax. (506)854-2556; carleb@nb.aibn.com.

LEBLANC, Claire; MUHC-Montreal Children's Hosp, C504-2300 rue Tupper, Montreal QC H3H 1P3; Dal'83; FRCPC; Peds (Sports Medicine); Rheum. Staff, McGill University Health Centre - Montreal Children's Hospital; Langs: English; French; (514)412-4400 x23171

LEBLANC, Claude J; Polyclinique de la Sante, 105-1688 boul des Laurentides, Vimont QC H7M 2P4; Mon'77; (450)663-9950; Fax. (450)663-9956.

LEBLANC, Constance; Queen Elizabeth II HSC-Halifax, 3021-1796 Summer St, Halifax NS B3H 3A7; Laval'87; CCFP; CCFP(E.M.); FCFP; Staff, Queen Elizabeth II Health Sciences Centre - Halifax Infirmary Site; Assoc Prof, Dalhousie University; Langs: English; French; (902)473-3562; Fax. (902)473-3617.

LEBLANC, Daniel; Clinique Med Havre Sante, 521 boul Du Havre, Salaber-de-Valleyf QC J6S 4Z5; McG'78; Staff, Centre Hospitalier Régional du Suroît; (450)371-6444; Fax. (450)371-5315.

LEBLANC, Danielle; Clinique de Med Familiale, 6e-2120 rue Sherbrooke E, Montreal QC H2K 1C3; Laval'82; Clin Prof Family Med, Centre Hospitalier l'Université de Montréal (CHUM) - Hôpital Notre-Dame; Langs: English; (514)527-1958; Fax. (514)527-1649.

LEBLANC, Diane; Inst U en Sante Mentale de QC, 2601 ch de la Canardiere, Quebec QC G1J 2G3; Mon'88; FRCPC; Psy. Staff, Institut Universitaire Sante; (418)663-5321

LEBLANC, Emilie; Hop Brome-Missisquoi-Perkins, 950 rue Principale, Cowansville QC J2K 1K3; Sher'10; Staff, Hôpital Brome-Missisquoi-Perkins; (450)266-4342

LEBLANC, Francis E; Elbow Drive Med Centre, 5116 Elbow Dr SW, Calgary AB T2V 1H1; Ott'59; PhD; FACS; Neursurg. (403)255-6647; Fax. (403)255-6547.

LEBLANC, Francois; Ctr Hosp Affilie-Enfant-Jesus, 1401 18e rue, Quebec QC G1J 1Z4; Laval'92; FRCPC; IntMed; Critical Care Medicine (P.Q.). Staff, Centre Hospitalier Affilié Universitaire de Québec - Hôpital De L'Enfant Jésus; (418)649-0252 x3575; Fax. (418)649-5913.

LEBLANC, Francois; GMF Centre Med du Parc, 101-84 rue Court, Granby QC J2G 4Y5; Sher'83; Staff, Centre Hospitalier de Granby; Langs: English; (450)375-1161; Fax. (450)375-7740.

LEBLANC, Genevieve; 105A-667 rue Champlain, Dieppe NB E1A 1P6; Sher'95; AB; FRCPC; Peds. Pediatrics, Dr Georges-L-Dumont University Hospital Centre; (506)869-2150; Fax. (506)869-2147.

LEBLANC, Gerard A; Ctr Hosp Affilie-St-Sacrement, 1050 ch Sainte-Foy, Quebec QC G1S 4L8; Laval'84; FRCPC; Psy. Staff, Centre Hospitalier Affilié Universitaire de Québec - Hôpital du St-Sacrement; Clin Assoc Prof, Université Laval; (418)682-7898; Fax. (418)682-7959; gerardleblanc@sympatico.ca.

LEBLANC, Germain; CSSS-Hop de Hull, 116 boul Lionel-Emond, Gatineau QC J8Y 1W7; Sher'00; Staff, Hull Hospital; (819)595-6000

LEBLANC, Guy D; 201-51 Highfield St, Moncton NB E1C 5N2; Laval'76; Ophth (P.Q.). (506)857-4084; Fax. (506)862-1897.

LEBLANC, Guy; Hop Maisonneuve-Rosemont, 5415 boul de l'Assomption, Montreal QC H1T 2M4; Mon'97; General Surgical Oncology (P.Q.); GenSurg. Staff, Hopital Maisonneuve-Rosemont; (514)252-3822

LEBLANC, Guy; Professional Arts Bldg, 410-100 Arden St, Moncton NB E1C 4B7; Mon'92; FRCSC; Urol. Staff, The Moncton Hospital; Langs: English; (506)387-7871; Fax. (506)387-7872; guycarol2002@yahoo.ca.

LEBLANC, Guy; 2F-460 Main St E, Hamilton ON L8N 1K4; Dal'06; CCFP; (905)528-0163; Fax. (905)528-9196.

LEBLANC, Guy; Hop Louis-H Lafontaine, 7401 rue Hochelaga, Montreal QC H1N 3M5; Mon'56; Psy (P.Q.). Ac Staff Psy, Hopital Louis-H Lafontaine; (514)251-4000 x2624; Fax. (514)251-2744; guyleblanc@hotmail.com.

LEBLANC, Helene; Inst Philippe Pinel De Mtl, 10905 boul Henri-Bourassa E, Montreal QC H1C 1H1; Mon'78; FRCPC; Psy. Staff, Institut Philippe-Pinel de Montreal; (514)648-8461

LEBLANC, Isabelle; St Mary's Hosp Centre, 3830 av Lacombe, Montreal QC H3T 1M5; Ott'04; CCFP; Staff, St Mary's Hospital Centre; (514)734-2628

LEBLANC, Jacques G; Children's & Women's HC of BC, AB307-4480 Oak St, Vancouver BC V6H 3V4; Laval'75; LMCC; FRCSC; Cardiovasc&ThorSurg (Adult Congenital Heart Disease). Staff, BC Children's Hospital; Langs: Bilingual(English/French); (604)875-3165

LEBLANC, Jacques-F.; Centre Medical de l'Hetriere, 201-3520 rue de l'Hetriere, St-Augustin-D-Desm QC G3A 0B4; Laval'77; Staff, Centre Hospitalier Affilié Universitaire de Québec - Hôpital De L'Enfant Jésus; Staff, Hôpital général de Québec - CHSLD; (418)651-3933; Fax. (418)651-0256.

LEBLANC, Jean; Centre Bois de Boulogne, 505-1575 boul Henri-Bourassa O, Montreal QC H3M 3A9; Laval'60; FRCPC; Psy (Mood Disorders). Ac Staff, Hôpital du Sacre-Coeur de Montréal; assoc Prof, Universite de Montreal; Langs: Bilingual(French/English); (514)338-4300; Fax. (514)338-4493.

LEBLANC, Jean; 25 boul St-Pierre CP 5534, Caraquet NB E1W 1B7; Sher'91; CCFP; (506)727-2299; Fax. (506)727-4570.

LEBLANC, Jean-Bernard; 200B-140 rue Champlain, Dieppe NB E1A 1N8; Sher'77; (506)853-3911; Fax. (506)853-8866.

LEBLANC, Jean-Paul M; 395 boul Jessop, Rimouski QC G5L 1M9; Laval'71; FRCSC; Ophth. Langs: Bilingual(French/English); (418)723-0488; Fax. (418)723-6583.

LEBLANC, Jean-Paul R; Hotel-Dieu de Levis, 143 rue Wolfe, Levis QC G6V 3Z1; Laval'71; CSPQ; FRCPC; Anes. Staff, Hôtel-Dieu de Lévis; (418)835-7121 x3218

LEBLANC, Jean-Pierre; CSSS de Chicoutimi, 305 rue Saint-Vallier, Chicoutimi QC G7H 5H6; Sher'83; FRCPC; IntMed; Respir. Staff, Complexe hospitalier de la Sagamie; (418)549-2195

LEBLANC, Joanne; Edmundston Reg Hosp, 275 Hebert Blvd, Edmundston NB E3V 4E4; Sher'05; CCFP; Staff, Hôpital regional d'Edmundston; (506)739-2200

LEBLANC, John C; IWK Health Centre, PO Box 9700 Rpo CSC 5850-5980 University Ave, Halifax NS B3K 6R8; McM'81; AB; MSc; FRCPC; Peds (Epidemiology). Ac Staff, IWK Health Centre; Assoc Prof Peds & Psy, Dalhousie University; (902)470-8930; Fax. (902)470-6913.

LEBLANC, John L; Hôpital régional Chaleur, 1750 Sunset Dr, Bathurst NB E2A 4L7; Laval'89; FRCPC; NuclearMed (Diagnostic Radiology). (506)544-3000; Fax. (506)545-1427.

LEBLANC, Josee; CHUQ-Ctr Hosp Univ Laval, 2705 boul Laurier, Quebec QC G1V 4G2; Laval'97; Staff Emerg, Centre Hospitalier Universitaire de Quebec-CHUL; (418)656-4141 x70553

LEBLANC, Karine; 1116 Mountain Rd, Moncton NB E1C 2T3; Sher'09; CCFP; (506)853-3911; Fax. (506)853-8866.

LEBLANC, Karine; 205-565 Elmwood Dr, Moncton NB E1A 2X4; Sher'01; CCFP; Staff, Dr Georges-L-Dumont University Hospital Centre; (506)859-6803; Fax. (506)859-6818.

LEBLANC, Linda M; Dr Leon Richard Oncology Ctre, 37 Providence St, Moncton NB E1C 8X3; McM'95; FRCPC; RadOncol. Langs: French; (506)862-4030; Fax. (506)862-4222.

LEBLANC, Louis-Paul; 19 rue Bellevue CP 189, Matapedia QC G0J 1V0; Laval'65; Ac Staff, Hôpital Régional Campbellton; (418)865-2175; Fax. (418)865-2711.

LEBLANC, Louise; CLSC-CHSLD Du Haut St-Francois, RR 3 460 2E Avenue, Weedon QC J0B 3J0; Laval'75; (819)877-3434; Fax. (819)877-5272.

LEBLANC, Louiselle; Surrey Mem Hosp, 13750 96 Ave, Surrey BC V3V 1Z2; Sher'01; FRCPC; IntMed; MedMicrobiol; InfectDis. Staff, Surrey Memorial Hospital; (778)840-7474

LEBLANC, Marc; CSSS de Laval, 1755 boul Rene-Laennec, Laval QC H7M 3L9; Mon'83; FRCPC; DiagRad. Staff, Tomo Concorde & Polyclinique Concorde; (450)975-5406

LEBLANC, Marie-Andree; Clinique Med Privee, 75 boul des Chateaux, Blainville QC J7B 2A4; Sher'06; CCFP; Staff, Centre Hospitalier Pierre le Gardeur; (450)434-2009

LEBLANC, Marie-Claude; Hop Maisonneuve-Rosemont, 5415 boul de l'Assomption, Montreal QC H1T 2M4; Mon'88; CCFP; FCFP; Teach Staff-Fam Med, Hopital Maisonneuve-Rosemont; Universite de Montreal; (514)252-3814; Fax. (514)252-3854.

LEBLANC, Marie-Helene; CSSS de Rivière-du-Loup, 75 rue Saint-Henri, Riviere-du-Loup QC G5R 2A4; Laval'08; CCFP; Staff, Centre Hospitalier Regional du Grand-Portage; (418)868-1000; Fax. (418)868-1032.

LEBLANC, Marie-Helene; Hôpital Laval, 2725 ch Sainte-Foy, Quebec QC G1V 4G5; Laval'76; FRCPC; Cardiol. Ac Staff, Hôpital Laval; (418)656-8711

LEBLANC, Marie-Josee; UMF de Chicoutimi, 305 rue Saint-Vallier, Chicoutimi QC G7H 5H6; Sher'01; CCFP; Staff, Complexe hospitalier de la Sagamie; (418)541-1079; Fax. (418)541-1129.

LEBLANC, Martin; CSSS du Sud de Lanaudière, 911 montee des Pionniers, Terrebonne QC J6V 2H2; Laval'98; CCFP; Staff, Centre Hospitalier Pierre le Gardeur; (450)654-7525

LEBLANC, Martin; Ctr Hosp Affilie-Enfant-Jesus, 1401 18e rue, Quebec QC G1J 1Z4; Laval'96; CCFP; CCFP(E.M.); Staff, Centre Hospitalier Affilié Universitaire de Québec - Hôpital De L'Enfant Jésus; (418)649-0252

LEBLANC, Martin R; Queen Elizabeth II HSC-Halifax, 4437-1796 Summer St, Halifax NS B3H 3A7; Dal'05; FRCSC; PlasSurg. Staff, Queen Elizabeth II Health Sciences Centre - Halifax Infirmary Site; (902)473-6487

LEBLANC, Martine; Hop Maisonneuve-Rosemont, 5415 boul de l'Assomption, Montreal QC H1T 2M4; Mon'89; FACP; FRCPC; IntMed (Dialysis); Nephrol. Staff, Hopital Maisonneuve-Rosemont; assoc Prof, Universite de Montreal; (514)252-3489; Fax. (514)255-3026; martine.leblanc@sympatico.ca.

LEBLANC, Melanie; CSSS de Laval, 1755 boul Rene-Laennec, Laval QC H7M 3L9; Mon'05; CCFP; Staff, Hopital de la Cite de la santé; (450)975-5445

LEBLANC, Michel; 101-233 rue Turgeon, Sainte-Therese QC J7E 3J8; Mon'81; (450)430-1030

LEBLANC, Michel; CSSS de Trois-Rivières, 1991 boul du Carmel, Trois-Rivieres QC G8Z 3R9; Mon'87; FRCPC; NuclearMed. Staff, CSSS de Trois-Rivières; (819)697-3333 x69854

LEBLANC, Michel; Clinique Familiale St-Lambert, 209 rue Woodstock, Saint-Lambert QC J4P 1W7; Sher'79; (450)466-8583; Fax. (450)466-4072.

LEBLANC, Michel; Clinique Med Lanaudiere, 222 rue Bernard, St-Charles-Brromee QC J6E 2C5; Mon'85; ac Staff, Centre Hospitalier Régional de Lanaudière; (450)755-1033

LEBLANC, Michelle M; Health Services Centre, 33 Main St, Rexton NB E4W 0E5; Sher'97; CCFP; Mgr, The Moncton Hospital; (506)523-7943; Fax. (506)523-7949; denise.leblanc@ncc-ccn.ca.

LEBLANC, Michelle; Direction de la Sante Publique, 1-205 boul de York O, Gaspe QC G4X 2W5; Sher'90; Staff, Installation CLSC Gaspe; Langs: Bilingual(French/English); (418)368-2443; Fax. (418)368-1317.

LEBLANC, Milaine; CSSS du Lac-des-Deux-Montagnes, 520 boul Arthur-Sauve, Saint-Eustache QC J7R 5B1; Sher'08; CCFP; Staff, Hôpital de Saint-Eustache; (450)473-6811

LEBLANC, Nadine; CSSS de la Haute Yamaska, 294 rue Deragon, Granby QC J2G 5J5; Mon'98; (450)375-1442

LEBLANC, Nicole; CSSS de Trois-Rivieres, 155 rue Toupin, Trois-Rivieres QC G8T 3Z8; Sher'86; CCFP; Staff, Centre de santé Cloutier-du-Rivage; (819)370-2108; Fax. (819)370-2010.

LEBLANC, Nicole; 105A-667 rue Champlain, Dieppe NB E1A 1P6; Sher'93; FRCPC; Peds. Staff, Dr Georges-L-Dumont University Hospital Centre; (506)869-2150; nicoleleb@rrsb.nb.ca.

LEBLANC, P Nicole; Montfort Hosp, 713 Montreal Rd, Ottawa ON K1K 0T2; Ott'10; CCFP; (613)746-4621

LEBLANC, Paul E; Westbrook Prof Bldg, 215-1610 37 St SW, Calgary AB T3C 3P1; Cal'90; MSc; FRCPC; IntMed. Ac Staff, Peter Lougheed Centre; Clin Lecturer, University of Calgary; (403)284-0777; Fax. (403)284-0711.

LEBLANC, Paulette M; Clinique Med Jean Coutu, 1116B Mountain Rd, Moncton NB E1C 2T3; Mem'81; ACLS; ATLS; Staff, Dr Georges-L-Dumont University Hospital Centre; Langs: French; (506)853-8812; lebpau@health.nb.ca.

LEBLANC, Pierre; Hôpital Laval, 2725 ch Sainte-Foy, Quebec QC G1V 4G5; Laval'78; FRCP; FRCPC; Respir (Administration). Consultant, Centre Hospitalier Universitaire De Québec - Pavillon De St-françois-d'assise; Staff, Hôpital Laval; Consultant, CSSS de Quebec-Sud; Chef Dept of Med, Institut Universitaire De Cardiologie et de Pneumologie de Quebec; Chef Med, Université Laval; (418)656-4790; Fax. (418)656-4762; pierre.leblanc@med.ulaval.ca.

LEBLANC, Pierre-P.; CHUM-Hotel-Dieu, 6 106-3840 rue Saint-Urbain, Montreal QC H2W 1T8; Mon'63; Respir (P.Q.). Staff, Centre Hospitalier l'Université de Montréal (CHUM) - Hôtel-Dieu; (514)890-8000 x12761

LEBLANC, Remi; Dr Georges-L Dumont Reg Hosp, 330 av Universite, Moncton NB E1C 2Z3; Mon'07; FRCSC; IntMed. Staff, Dr Georges-L-Dumont University Hospital Centre; (506)862-4000

LEBLANC, Renee M; Hop du Saint-Sacrement, 1050 ch Sainte-Foy, Quebec QC G1S 4L8; Mon'93; Staff, Centre Hospitalier Affilié Universitaire de Québec - Hôpital du St-Sacrement; (514)281-1722; Fax. (514)281-6697.

LEBLANC, Richard; Hop Maisonneuve-Rosemont, 5415 boul de l'Assomption, Montreal QC H1T 2M4; Laval'95; FRCPC; IntMed; MedOncol; Hem (P.Q.). Staff, Hopital Maisonneuve-Rosemont; assoc Prof, Université Laval; Langs: English; (514)252-3404

LEBLANC, Richard; MUHC-Montreal Neurology Inst, 3801 rue University, Montreal QC H3A 2B4; Ott'76; FRCSC; Neursurg. Ac Staff, McGill University Health Centre - Montreal Neurological Hospital; Prof Neurosurg, McGill University; (514)398-1939; Fax. (514)398-8540.

LEBLANC, Robert E M; Grey Bruce HS-Southampton, RR 1 340 High St, Southampton ON N0H 2L0; Mem'89; Staff, Grey Bruce Health Services - Southampton Site; (519)797-3230

LEBLANC, Robin B; Dartmouth ENT Associates, 100-35 Baker Dr, Dartmouth NS B2W 0H3; Dal'97; FRCSC; Otol. (902)435-8585; Fax. (902)435-8695.

LEBLANC, Roger P; 023-3545 Ch de la Cote-des-Nei, Montreal QC H3H 1V1; McG'78; BSc; MDCM; FRCPC; IntMed (Infectious Diseases). Att Physician IntMed & InfectDis, McGill University Health Centre - Montreal Chest Institute; adj Prof, McGill University; Langs: English; French; (514)935-1197; Fax. (514)935-1310.

LEBLANC, Serge R; Richmond Street Clinic, 200-862 Richmond St W, Toronto ON M6J 1C9; Ott'07; FRCPC; Psy. (416)535-8501

LEBLANC, Sophie; Dr Georges-L Dumont Reg Hosp, 330 av Universite, Moncton NB E1C 2Z3; Sher'02; FRCPC; Anes. Staff, Dr Georges-L-Dumont University Hospital Centre; (506)862-4000

LEBLANC, Steve; Polyclinique des Prairies, 980 Boul Thibeau, Trois-Rivieres QC G8T 7B2; Sher'87; Staff, CSSS de Trois-Rivières; (819)378-3433; Fax. (819)378-9581.

LEBLANC, Sylvie J; 203-860 Mountain Rd, Moncton NB E1C 2N7; Sher'02; CCFP; Langs: Bilingual(French/English); (506)853-5135

LEBLANC, Valerie; CSSS du Nord de Lanaudière, 1000 boul Sainte-Anne, St-Charles-Brromee QC J6E 6J2; Sher'10; CCFP; Staff, Centre Hospitalier Régional de Lanaudière; (450)759-8222

LEBLANC, Valerie; CHUS-Hop Hotel-Dieu, 580 rue Bowen S, Sherbrooke QC J1G 2E8; Sher'01; FRCSC; GenSurg. Staff, Centre Hospitalier Universitaire de Sherbrooke-Hôpital Hôtel-Dieu; (819)346-1110

LEBLANC, Veronique; 204-123 Champlain St, Dieppe NB E1A 1N5; Mon'98; LMCC; CCFP; (506)862-1887; Fax. (506)862-1898.

LEBLANC-BOUCHER, Nicole; CLSC Arthur-Buies, 1000 rue Labelle, Saint-Jerome QC J7Z 5N6; Mon'87; Staff, Hôpital de Saint-Eustache; (450)432-2777; Fax. (450)431-6538.

LEBLANC-HIDEBRAND, Julie; 209-199 Chesley Dr, Saint John NB E2K 4S9; Laval'09; (506)643-8343

LEBLANC-SIMARD, Virginie; Hotel-Dieu de Levis, 143 rue Wolfe, Levis QC G6V 3Z1; Laval'00; FRCSC; Ophth. Staff, Hôtel-Dieu de Lévis; (418)835-7121

LEBLOND, Antoine; CHUM-Hotel-Dieu, 3840 rue Saint-Urbain, Montreal QC H2W 1T8; Laval'02; FRCPC; NuclearMed. Staff, Centre Hospitalier l'Université de Montréal (CHUM) - Hôtel-Dieu; (514)890-8380

LEBLOND, Caroline; Ctr de Services de Riviere-Rou, 1525 rue l'Annonciation N, Riviere-Rouge QC J0T 1T0; Mon'09; Staff, Centre de L'Annonciation; (819)275-2118

LEBLOND, Christian; CSSS de la Baie-des-Chaleurs, RR 2 419 boul Perron, Maria QC G0C 1Y0; Sher'98; FRCSC; OrthSurg. Staff, CSSS de la Baie-des-Chaleurs; (418)759-3443

LEBLOND, Daniel; St Michael's Health Centre, 1400 9 Ave S, Lethbridge AB T1J 4V5; Ott'83; FRCP; FRCPC; PhysMed&Rehab (Electromyography). Staff/Med Dir Rehabilitation, Covenant Health - St Michael's Health Centre; Staff, Chinook Regional Hospital; Langs: Bilingual(English/French); (403)382-6466; Fax. (403)382-6451.

LEBLOND, Denis; Clinique Med De Bernieres, 479A ch Saint-Joseph, Saint-Nicolas QC G7A 1N3; Laval'76; (418)831-9228; Fax. (418)831-0249.

LEBLOND, Helene; Hop Maisonneuve-Rosemont, 5415 boul de l'Assomption, Montreal QC H1T 2M4; Laval'74; FRCPC; Peds (Asthma). Staff, Hopital Maisonneuve-Rosemont; Langs: Bilingual(French/English); (514)374-7940; Fax. (514)374-8101.

LEBLOND, Marie-Josee; Ctr D'Accueil Le Vaisseau D'Or, 55 rue Saint-Andre, Beauharnois QC J6N 3G7; Mon'88; (450)429-6403; Fax. (450)429-6602.

LEBLOND, Martin; Ctr Hosp Affilie-St-Sacrement, 1050 ch Sainte-Foy, Quebec QC G1S 4L8; Laval'92; FRCPC; IntMed. Staff, Centre Hospitalier Affilié Universitaire de Québec - Hôpital du St-Sacrement; (418)682-7511; Fax. (418)682-7977.

LEBLOND, Martin; Hop Charles Lemoyne, 3120 boul Taschereau, Greenfield Park QC J4V 2H1; Sher'99; FRCPC; Psy. Staff, Hopital Charles LeMoyne; Langs: English; (450)466-5000

LEBLOND, Pierre F; Ctr Hosp Affilie-Enfant-Jesus, 1401 18e rue, Quebec QC G1J 1Z4; Laval'65; Hem (P.Q.) (Clinical Hematology). Staff, Centre Hospitalier Affilié Universitaire de Québec - Hôpital De L'Enfant Jésus; Consultant, Centre Hospitalier Regional de Sept-Iles; Prof Med, Université Laval; Langs: English; (418)649-5726; Fax. (418)649-5720; pierre.leblond@med.ulaval.ca.

LEBLOND, Richard; CSSS Haute Gaspésie, 50 rue du Belvedere, Ste-Anne-des-Monts QC G4V 1X4; Laval'91; IntMed (P.Q.). Staff, Centre Hospitalier des Monts; (418)763-2261

LEBLOND, Richard; CSSS de Chicoutimi, 305 rue Saint-Vallier, Chicoutimi QC G7H 5H6; Laval'75; MBA; DR; FRCPC; NuclearMed. Médecin, Hotel-Dieu de Roberval; Staff, Complexe hospitalier de la Sagamie; (418)541-1034; Fax. (418)541-1101; richard@leblond.com.

LEBOEUF, Andreanne; Centre Med Donnacona, 420 138 Rte, Donnacona QC G3M 1C2; Laval'02; Staff, Centre Hospitalier Portneuf; (418)285-1122

LEBOEUF, Gilles; Clinique Med Adoncour, 200-505 rue Adoncour, Longueuil QC J4G 2M6; Mon'80; (450)646-4445; Fax. (450)646-5526.

LEBOEUF, Jean-Louis; COOP Sante Gatineau, 200 boul Greber, Gatineau QC J8T 6K2; Laval'64; Langs: English; (819)568-0444; Fax. (819)568-1356.

LEBOEUF, Line; Hop Maisonneuve-Rosemont, 5415 boul de l'Assomption, Montreal QC H1T 2M4; Mon'96; FRCSC; Urol. Staff, Hopital Maisonneuve-Rosemont; (514)255-9006

LEBOEUF, Mathieu; CHUQ-Ctr Hosp Univ Laval, 2705 boul Laurier, Quebec QC G1V 4G2; Laval'98; FRCSC; ObstGyn (Reproductive Medicine). Staff, Centre Hospitalier Universitaire de Quebec-CHUL; (418)654-2738; Fax. (418)525-4281.

LEBOEUF, Rebecca; CHUM-Hop Notre-Dame, Z9902-1560 rue Sherbrooke E, Montreal QC H2L 4M1; McG'00; FRCPC; IntMed; Endocrin&Metab. Staff, Centre Hospitalier l'Université de Montréal (CHUM) - Hôpital Notre-Dame; Langs: English; (514)890-8000 x26818

LEBOLDUS, Gordon M; 108-396 Queens Ave, London ON N6B 1X7; Wes'60; FRCSC; Otol. Staff, London Health Sciences Centre - University Hospital; Staff, St Joseph's Hospital - St Joseph's Health Care; Staff, London Health Sciences Centre - Victoria Campus; Emeritus Prof, University of Western Ontario; (519)434-9151; Fax. (519)434-9152.

LEBON, Jean-Sebastien; Montreal Heart Institute, 5000 rue Belanger, Montreal QC H1T 1C8; Mon'01; CSPQ; FRCPC; Anes. Staff, Institut de Cardiologie de Montréal; (514)376-3330 x3732

LEBOUCHE, Bertrand P; MUHC-Montreal Chest Institute, R803-3650 rue Saint-Urbain, Montreal QC H2X 2P4; Staff, McGill University Health Centre - Montreal Chest Institute; (514)843-2090

LEBOUTHILLIER, Anne; 103-1850 Vanier Blvd, Bathurst NB E2A 7B7; Mon'98; FRCSC; ObstGyn. Chief Surg, Hopital Regional Chaleur; Langs: Bilingual(French/English); (506)548-4485; Fax. (506)548-4495.

LEBOVICH, Irith; Hop Charles Lemoyne, 3120 boul Taschereau, Greenfield Park QC J4V 2H1; McM'02; FRCPC; IntMed; Nephrol. Staff, Hopital Charles LeMoyne; (450)466-5000

LEBRETON, Nathalie J; 202-185 av Acadie, Dieppe NB E1A 1G6; Sher'97; CCFP; Staff, Dr Georges-L-Dumont University Hospital Centre; Langs: English; Spanish; (506)862-1260; Fax. (506)862-1265.

LEBREUX, Elie; CSSS de Rimouski-Neigette, CP 3150 Succ A 150 av Rouleau, Rimouski QC G5L 5T1; Sher'77; ABIM; FACCP; FRCPC; IntMed; Respir. Chef thérap resp, Hôpital Regional Rimouski; (418)724-8122; Fax. (418)724-6889; elebreux@globetrotter.net.

LEBRUN, Andre; Hema-Quebec, 4045 boul de la Cote-Vertu, Saint-Laurent QC H4R 2W7; Mon'64; MedOncol (P.Q.); Hem (P.Q.) (Transfusion Medicine). Consultant Med, Hôpital du Sacre-Coeur de Montréal; VP Med Affaires Hematol, Hema-Quebec; adj Prof, Universite de Montreal; Langs: Bilingual(French/English); (514)832-5000 x250; Fax. (514)904-4896; andre.lebrun@hema-quebec.qc.ca.

LEBRUN, Benoit; CSSS de Trois-Rivières, 1991 boul du Carmel, Trois-Rivieres QC G8Z 3R9; Laval'00; FRCPC; RadOncol. Staff, CSSS de Trois-Rivières; (819)371-5002

LEBRUN, Constance M; Glen Sather Sports Med Clinic, L 2-11400 University Ave NW, Edmonton AB T6G 1Z1; McG'81; BSc; Dip SportMed; CCFP; Dir, Glen Sather Sports Medical Clinic; (780)407-5160

LEBRUN, G Paul; Queen Elizabeth II HSC, 1276 South Park St, Halifax NS B3H 2Y9; Dal'69; FRCPC; DiagRad. Head Dept of Radiol, Queen Elizabeth II Health Sciences Centre - Victoria General Site; Prof, Dalhousie University; (902)473-5452; Fax. (902)473-2018; plebrun@dal.ca.

LEBRUN, John B; 403-1200 Lonsdale Ave, North Vancouver BC V7M 3H6; Man'90; Staff Outreach Prog & Sunshine Coast, Providence Health Care - St Paul's Hospital; Med Staff, Lions Gate Hospital; Clin Teacher Family Pract, University of British Columbia; (604)987-5250

LEBRUN, Josee; Ctr Hosp Affilie-St-Sacrement, 1050 ch Sainte-Foy, Quebec QC G1S 4L8; Laval'89; CSPQ; FRCPC; NuclearMed. Staff, Centre Hospitalier Affilié Universitaire de Québec - Hôpital du St-Sacrement; (418)682-7511; Fax. (418)682-7956.

LEBRUN, Louise-Helene; CHUM-Hop Notre-Dame, RG 1165-1560 rue Sherbrooke E, Montreal QC H2L 4M1; Mon'71; FRCPC; Neur; Electroenceph (P.Q.). Staff, Centre Hospitalier l'Université de Montréal (CHUM) - Hôpital Notre-Dame; adj Prof, Universite de Montreal; (514)890-8000 x26268; Fax. (514)412-7556.

LEBRUN, Manon; Clinique Med Lemoyne, 202-2499 rue Saint-Georges, Lemoyne QC J4R 2T4; Mon'86; MSc(Microbiol.); FRCSC; ObstGyn. Staff, Hopital Charles LeMoyne; (450)923-3060; Fax. (450)923-3072.

LEBRUN, Natalie; Centre médicale Centrale, 4-135 rue Saint-Antoine N, Granby QC J2G 5G7; Mon'90; Staff, Centre Hospitalier de Granby; (450)372-5401; Fax. (450)372-4174.

LEBRUN, Paul J; Ottawa Trainyards Health & WC, B22-550 Terminal Ave, Ottawa ON K1G 0Z3; Qns'93; (613)731-4770

LEBRUN, Philippe; CSSS de l'Energie-Ste-Therese, 1705 av Georges, Shawinigan QC G9N 2N1; Mon'10; CCFP; Staff, CH du Centre-de-la-Mauricie (Ste-Thérèse de Shawinigan); (819)536-7500; philippe_lebrun@ssss.gouv.qc.ca.

LECAULT, Melanie; CSSSG-Hop De Gatineau, 909 boul de la Verendrye, Gatineau QC J8P 7H2; McG'06; MDCM; Staff, Hôpital de Gatineau; (819)966-6100

LECAVALIER, Danielle; CLSC Riviere-des-Prairies, 8655 boul Perras, Montreal QC H1E 4M7; Mon'81; (514)494-4924

LECCIA, Jean-Dominique; Ctr Hosp Anna-Laberge, 200 boul Brisebois, Chateauguay QC J6K 4W8; Marseille (France)'75; Staff, Hôpital Anna-Laberge; (450)699-2425; Fax. (450)699-2525.

LECHELT, David P; St Mary's Hosp, 4607 53 St, Camrose AB T4V 1Y5; Alb'99; BSc(Hons); CCFP; FCFP; CCFP(E.M.); Staff, Covenant Health - St Mary's Hospital; (780)679-6111

LECHELT, Katherine; Glenrose Rehab Hosp, 1259-10230 111 Ave NW, Edmonton AB T5G 0B7; Alb'83; FRCPC; IntMed; GeriatricMed. Staff, Glenrose Rehabilitation Hospital; Ac Staff, Caritas Health Group-Edmonton; Assoc Prof, University of Alberta; (780)735-8828; Fax. (780)735-8846; kathy.lechelt@albertahealthservices.ca.

LECHTER, Mortimer; Westmount Square Med Centre, 550-1 Car Westmount, Westmount QC H3Z 2P9; Qns'62; FAAN; Neur (P.Q.) (Adult Neurology). Consultant, McGill University Health Centre - Royal Victoria Hospital; Associate Neurol, Sir Mortimer B Davis Jewish General; Consultant Neurol, St Mary's Hospital Centre; adj Prof, McGill University; Langs: English; French; (514)934-2334; Fax. (514)931-2929; mortlechter@yahoo.com.

LECKEY, J Robert; Stan Cassidy Centre For Rehab, Stan Cassidy Centre 800 Priestman St, Fredericton NB E3B 0C7; Dal'88; BSc; FRCPC; PhysMed&Rehab (Bone Joint Injuries). Med Dir, Stan Cassidy Centre for Rehabilitation; Dalhousie University; Langs: English; (506)452-5225

LECKEY, Naida L; 8-225 Cobequid Rd, Lower Sackville NS B4C 3J7; Dal'87; (902)864-9400

LECKEY, Richard N; Bedford Waterfront Hlth Clinic, 207-967 Bedford Hwy, Bedford NS B4A 1A9; Dal'94; BSc; FRCPC; Neur (Electrodiagnostic). Staff, South Shore Regional Hospital; Staff, Aberdeen Regional Hospital; Staff, Cobequid Multiservice Centre; Staff, Multiple Sclerosis Clinic; (902)835-6444

LECKIE, Michael; Near North Med Clinic, 201-66 Josephine St, North Bay ON P1B 0A7; McG'82; Staff, North Bay Regional Health Centre - Regional Mental Health; (705)495-2685; Fax. (705)495-4128.

LECKIE, Peter A; 3-271 Ingram St, Duncan BC V9L 1P3; McG'76; FRCSC; GenSurg. (250)746-7181; Fax. (250)746-4202.

LECLAIR, Jason M; 500-267 O'Connor St, Ottawa ON K2P 1V3; Ott'08; CCFP; (613)760-3727; Fax. (613)232-4818.

LECLAIR, Jean; I R D P Q-Site Francois-Charon, F 137-525 boul Wilfrid-Hamel, Quebec QC G1M 2S8; Laval'77; Physician, CHSLD St-Antoine; Physician, I R D P Q; Langs: Bilingual(French/English); (418)529-9141 x6618; Fax. (418)649-3738; jean.leclair@irdpq.qc.ca.

LECLAIR, Marc-Andre; CHUS-Hop Hotel-Dieu, 580 rue Bowen S, Sherbrooke QC J1G 2E8; Mon'03; FRCPC; IntMed. Staff, Centre Hospitalier Universitaire de Sherbrooke-Hôpital Hôtel-Dieu; (819)346-1110 x28303

LECLAIR, Marcel; 8641 Av Chaumont, Anjou QC H1K 1N4; Mon'77; CCFP; Staff, CSSS Saint-Leonard et Saint-Michel; (514)352-8013; Fax. (514)351-6866.

LECLAIR, Marie Ann; Hudson Medicentre, RR 1 200-465 rue Main, Hudson QC J0P 1H0; Ott'78; (450)458-5393; Fax. (450)458-8041.

LECLAIR, Normand; Clinique Med Fam des Recollets, 101-940 boul des Recollets, Trois-Rivieres QC G8Z 3W9; Laval'76; (819)373-0303; Fax. (819)373-8431.

LECLAIR, Patrick W; 2F-750 Taylor Creek Dr, Orleans ON K1C 1T1; Mon'05; MScPharm; BScBiology; CCFP; Staff, Montfort Hospital; Langs: Bilingual(French/English); (613)830-8388; patrick.leclair@hotmail.com.

LECLAIR, Sabrina; UMF Nord de Lanaudiere, 50 ch du Golf E, St-Charles-Brromee QC J6E 2B4; Sher'00; Ac Staff Geriatrie, Centre Hospitalier Régional de Lanaudière; (450)759-3060

LECLAIR, Suzanne E; CHUM-Hop St-Luc, 1058 rue Saint-Denis, Montreal QC H2X 3J4; Sher'77; FRCPC; Psy. Staff, Centre Hospitalier l'Université De Montréal (CHUM) - Hôpital Saint-luc; (514)890-8000

LECLAIRE, Luc; Ctr Multiphysio de Blainville, 101-920 boul du Cure-Labelle, Blainville QC J7C 2L2; Mon'78; (450)434-1334; Fax. (450)434-0337.

LECLAIRE, Richard; Inst De Physiatrie Du Quebec, 2049 rue Sherbrooke E, Montreal QC H2K 1C1; Mon'66; FRCPC; PhysMed&Rehab. (514)527-4155

LECLERC, Alexandre; CHUQ-Ctr Hosp Univ Laval, 2705 boul Laurier, Quebec QC G1V 4G2; Laval'05; OrthSurg. Staff, Centre Hospitalier Universitaire de Quebec-CHUL; (418)525-4444

LECLERC, Andre; CSSS de Montmagny-L'Islet, 350 boul Tache O RR 1, Montmagny QC G5V 3R8; Sher'06; CCFP; CCFP(E.M.); Staff, CSSS de Montmagny-L'Islet; (418)248-0630

LECLERC, Andre; Clinique Med Neufchatel, 101-2425 boul Bastien, Quebec QC G2B 1B3; Laval'66; (418)843-3771; Fax. (418)843-3865.

LECLERC, Anne; Halles Fleur de Lys, 298-245 rue Soumande, Quebec QC G1M 3H6; Laval'92; Langs: English; (418)780-0122; Fax. (418)780-4778; info@medicina.ca.

LECLERC, Celine; CLSC Haute-Ville, 55 ch Sainte-Foy, Quebec QC G1R 1S9; Laval'81; CCFP; FCFP; Teach Staff Family Med, Université Laval; Langs: English; (418)641-2572; Fax. (418)522-5437.

LECLERC, Claude; 250 boul La Salle, Baie-Comeau QC G4Z 1S8; Laval'63; hon Membre CMDP, Centre Hospitalier Régional Baie-Comeau; Langs: English; (418)296-9681; Fax. (418)296-5551.

LECLERC, Claude; Clinique Med St-Alexandre, 200-2310 rue Saint-Louis, Gatineau QC J8T 5L7; Mon'82; Staff, Hôpital de Gatineau; (819)243-4500; Fax. (819)243-1369; cleclerc@medecinefamiliale.com.

LECLERC, Claude E; 210-900 Boul Du Seminaire N, St-Jean-Sur-Richel QC J3A 1C3; Mon'71; Staff, Hôpital du Haut-Richelieu; Langs: English; (450)348-1118; Fax. (450)348-9998.

LECLERC, Clement; Clin Med Bat 150 Garrison St-J, CP 100 Succ Bureau Chef, Richelain QC J0J 1R0; Mon'69; Ac Staff, Hopital Charles LeMoyne.

LECLERC, Denise; CSSS d'Antoine-Labelle, 1525 rue de l'Annonciation N, Riviere-Rouge QC J0T 1T0; Laval'72; LMCC; (819)275-2118 x3418; Fax. (819)686-9301; gmfrouge@hotmail.ca.

LECLERC, Etienne; Hop Brome-Missisquoi-Perkins, 950 rue Principale, Cowansville QC J2K 1K3; Sher'06; OrthSurg. Staff, Hôpital Brome-Missisquoi-Perkins; (450)266-4342

LECLERC, Georges-Edouard; 320-900 Boul Du Seminaire N, St-Jean-Sur-Richel QC J3A 1C3; Mon'65; FRCSC; OrthSurg. Staff, Hôpital du Haut-Richelieu; Consultant, CFB St-Jean; (450)348-6966; Fax. (450)348-0664.

LECLERC, Georgette; 644 rue Jacques-Cartier E, Chicoutimi QC G7H 2A4; Laval'75; FRCPC; Derm. Ac Staff, Complexe hospitalier de la Sagamie; (418)545-1542; Fax. (418)549-6965.

LECLERC, Gilles; Clinique Med Centrale, 2050 rue Regent, Saint-Hubert QC J4T 3R5; Mon'79; (450)678-9194; Fax. (450)678-0915.

LECLERC, Guy; CHUM-Hotel-Dieu, 3840 rue Saint-Urbain, Montreal QC H2W 1T8; Mon'83; FRCPC; IntMed; Cardiol (P.Q.). Staff, Centre Hospitalier l'Université de Montréal (CHUM) - Hôtel-Dieu; (514)890-8000 x15446

LECLERC, Jacinthe; Clinique Med Legendre, 201-1650 av Jules-Verne, Quebec QC G2G 2R1; Laval'88; (418)872-5600; Fax. (418)872-8408.

LECLERC, Jacques; 213 rte du Long-Sault, St-Andr-Argenteuil QC J0V 1X0; Mon'79; (450)537-8557

LECLERC, Jacques-Ernest; CHUQ-Ctr Hosp Univ Laval, 2705 boul Laurier, Quebec QC G1V 4G2; Laval'79; ABOtol; FACS; FRCSC; Otol. Staff, Centre Hospitalier Universitaire de Quebec-CHUL; Staff, Jeffery Hale Hospital-Saint Brigid's; (418)654-2118; Fax. (418)654-2214.

LECLERC, Jean; Centre Med Hochelaga, 9080 rue Hochelaga, Montreal QC H1L 2N9; Mon'72; Med Consultant, Sun Life Financial; Langs: Bilingual(French/English); (514)353-8742; Fax. (514)353-2351; jujleclerc@videotron.ca.

LECLERC, Jean-Louis; Hotel-Dieu De Sorel, 400 av de l'Hotel-Dieu, Sorel-Tracy QC J3P 1N5; Laval'66; GenPath (P.Q.). Staff Med Labs, Hôtel-Dieu de Sorel; (450)746-6000 x7573

LECLERC, Jean-Marie; Hôpital Ste-Justine, 3175 ch Cote-Sainte-Catherine, Montreal QC H3T 1C5; Mon'77; FRCPC; HemPath; Hem (P.Q.); MedOncol (P.Q.). Staff, Hôpital Ste-Justine; (514)345-4969

LECLERC, Jonathan; CSSS du Lac-des-Deux-Montagnes, 520 boul Arthur-Sauve, Saint-Eustache QC J7R 5B1; McG'09; CCFP; Staff, Hôpital de Saint-Eustache; (450)473-6811

LECLERC, Julie; Clinique Med la Perade, 81 rue Ricard, Ste-Anne-de-la-Per QC G0X 2J0; Laval'01; CCFP; (418)325-2777

LECLERC, Louise; Reseau Sante Richelieu-Yamaska, 1800 rue Dessaulles, Saint-Hyacinthe QC J2S 2T2; Mon'82; Staff, Centre d hebergement de l Hôtel-Dieu de Saint-Hyacinthe; (450)771-3333

LECLERC, Lucie; Clinique Med de Mistassini, 148 boul Saint-Michel, Dolbeau-Mistassini QC G8L 5J8; Laval'86; LMCC; (418)276-3161; Fax. (418)276-4581.

LECLERC, Marc-Yves; CSSS de Chicoutimi, 305 rue Saint-Vallier, Chicoutimi QC G7H 5H6; Nantes (France)'71; Staff, Complexe hospitalier de la Sagamie; (418)541-1000 x5151; Fax. (418)549-5706.

LECLERC, Marie-Josee; 5100-2400 av D'Estimauville, Quebec QC G1E 7G9; Laval'89; Assoc Member Obstetric Priv, Jeffery Hale Hospital-Saint Brigid's; Staff, Hôpital Laval; Teach Staff Auxillaire, Université Laval; (418)623-1010; Fax. (418)623-7513.

LECLERC, Martin; Centre Sante Rene-Richard, 32 3e Av E CP 1300, Chapais QC G0W 1H0; Laval'87; (418)745-2591

LECLERC, Michel; CSSS de Rivière-de-Loup, 75 rue Saint-Henri, Riviere-du-Loup QC G5R 2A4; Laval'69; CSPQ; Anes (P.Q.) (Pain Management). Staff, Centre Hospitalier Regional du Grand-Portage; Langs: English; (418)868-1000

LECLERC, Michele; 2570 av Vanier, Saint-Hyacinthe QC J2S 6L7; Sher'75; FRCSC; Ophth (Glaucoma). Chief Ophth, Centre Hospitalier Honore-Mercier; Langs: English; (450)774-6224; mich@maskatel.net.

LECLERC, Olga; Hopital Reg D'Edmundston, 275 Hebert Blvd, Edmundston NB E3V 4E4; Sher'06; FRCPC; DiagRad. Staff, Hôpital regional d'Edmundston; (506)739-2200

LECLERC, Pierre J A; CSSS de la Cote-de-Gaspe, 215 boul de York O, Gaspe QC G4X 2W2; Laval'77; FRCSC; GenSurg (Bariatric Surgery). Staff, Centre Hospitalier de Gaspe; Langs: Bilingual(French/English); (514)677-3092

LECLERC, Pierre; Ctr Hosp Affilie-St-Sacrement, 1050 ch Sainte-Foy, Quebec QC G1S 4L8; Laval'78; FRCPC; MedBiochem. Ac Staff MedBiochem, Centre Hospitalier Affilié Universitaire de Québec - Hôpital du St-Sacrement; Chef Molecular Biology Med Biochem & Pathology, Université Laval; (418)682-7659; Fax. (418)682-7712.

LECLERC, Rachel; CSSS des Aurores Boreales, 679 2e rue E, La Sarre QC J9Z 2X7; Mon'08; CCFP; Staff, Centre Hospitalier La Sarre; (819)333-2311

LECLERC, Renee; Ctr Hosp Affilie-Enfant-Jesus, 1401 18e rue, Quebec QC G1J 1Z4; Laval'02; FRCPC; IntMed. Staff, Centre Hospitalier Affilié Universitaire de Québec - Hôpital De L'Enfant Jésus; (418)649-0252

LECLERC, Roland; Ctr Hosp Rouyn-Noranda, 4 9e rue, Rouyn-Noranda QC J9X 2B2; Laval'61; FRCPC; Peds. Staff, Centre Hospitalier Rouyn-Noranda; (819)764-5131; Fax. (819)764-2901.

LECLERC, Roselyn; CSSS de Becancour-Nicolet-Yama, 675 rue Saint-Jean-Baptiste, Nicolet QC J3T 1S4; Laval'07; CCFP; Staff Emerg, Hôpital de Christ-Roi; Langs: Bilingual(French/English); (819)293-2071; Fax. (819)293-6160.

LECLERC, Suzanne G; CHUQ-Ctr Hosp Univ Laval, 2211-2705 boul Laurier, Quebec QC G1V 4G2; Laval'86; FRCSC; GenSurg (Pediatric Surgery); PedGenSurg. Staff, Centre Hospitalier Universitaire de Quebec-CHUL; (418)654-2259; Fax. (418)654-2247.

LECLERC, Suzanne; Clin Medico-Sportive du CNMM, CP 1000 Succ M 4545 av Pierre de Coubertin, Montreal QC H1V 0B2; Laval'85; PhD; Staff, Centre Hospitalier l'Université de Montréal (CHUM) - Hôpital Notre-Dame; Langs: English; (514)255-1000 x301; Fax. (514)527-1649.

LECLERC, Sylvie; CHUQ-St-Francois D'Assise, 10 rue de l'Espinay, Quebec QC G1L 3L5; Laval'80; Staff Med/Prof, Centre Hospitalier Universitaire De Québec - Pavillon De St-françois-d'assise; adj Prof Family Med/prog Dir Family Med, Université Laval; Langs: Bilingual(French/English); (418)525-4351; Fax. (418)525-4322; sylvie.leclerc@videotron.ca.

LECLERC, Sylvie; Hop Maisonneuve-Rosemont, 5415 boul de l'Assomption, Montreal QC H1T 2M4; Mon'81; LMCC; Staff, Hopital Maisonneuve-Rosemont; (514)252-3400

LECLERC, Valerie; CHUQ-Ctr Hosp Univ Laval, 2705 boul Laurier, Quebec QC G1V 4G2; Laval'06; Rheum; IntMed. Staff, Centre Hospitalier Universitaire de Quebec-CHUL; (418)525-4444

LECLERC, Yves E; Hop Maisonneuve-Rosemont, 5415 boul de l'Assomption, Montreal QC H1T 2M4; Laval'79; ABS; FACS; FRCSC; GenSurg; General Surgical Oncology (P.Q.). Staff GenSurg, Hopital Maisonneuve-Rosemont; Clin Lecturer GenSurg, Universite de Montreal; (514)252-3400

LECLERC, Yves; St Mary's Reg Cardiac CC, 911 Queens Blvd, Kitchener ON N2M 1B2; Laval'73; AB; FACS; FRCS; FRCSC; Cardiovasc&ThorSurg (Adult Cardiac Surgery). Chief Cardiac Surg St Mary's Reg Cardiac Care Ctr, St Mary's General Hospital; Staff, Grand River Hospital - Kitchener/Waterloo Health Centre; Staff, Grey Bruce Health Services - Owen Sound; Langs: Bilingual(English/French); (519)749-6937; Fax. (519)749-6492; yleclerc@smgh.ca.

LECLERC, Yves; CHUS-Hop Fleurimont, 3001 12e Av N, Sherbrooke QC J1H 5N4; Sher'85; FRCPC; NuclearMed. Staff, Centre Hospitalier Universitaire de Sherbrooke-Hopital Fleurimont; (819)346-1110 x15598; yves.leclerc@usherbrooke.ca.

LECLERC-SOUBRIER, Annie; CLSC la Source Nord, 791 rue Sherwood, Quebec QC G2N 1X7; Laval'99; CCFP; Staff, Centre Hospitalier Regional de Trois-Rivieres; (418)628-2572; Fax. (418)841-5110.

LECLERCQ, Corinne; Clinique Gynecologique, 102-39 rue Laurier E, Victoriaville QC G6P 6P6; Sher'94; FRCSC; ObstGyn (Maternal Fetal Medicine). Staff, Hotel-Dieu d'Arthabaska; (819)357-4073

LECO, Pamela A; BC Cancer Ctre-Southern Interi, 399 Royal Ave, Kelowna BC V1Y 5L3; Cal'96; BSc(Hons); MSc; FRCP; FRCPC; RadOncol (Oncology). Staff, Royal Inland Hospital; BC Cancer Agency Sindi Ahluwalia Hawkins Centre for the Southern Interior; Staff, Kelowna General Hospital; Teach Staff Surg, University of British Columbia; (250)979-6645; Fax. (250)712-3911.

LECOEUR, Daniel; CSSS de Trois-Rivières, 1991 boul Du Carmel, Trois-Rivieres QC G8Z 3R9; Reims (France)'78; Staff, CSSS de Trois-Rivières; Langs: Bilingual(French/English); (819)697-3333 x69849; daniel_lecoeur@ssss.gouv.qc.ca.

LECOMPTE, Brigitte; CSSS d'Antoine-Labelle-Mt Laur, RR 1 2561 ch de la Lièvre S, Mont-Laurier QC J9L 3G3; Mon'78; Staff, CSSS d'Antoine-Labelle; (819)623-1234

LECOMPTE, Martin; CSSSG-Hop de Gatineau, CP 2000 Succ Bureau-Chef 909 boul de la Verendrye O, Gatineau QC J8P 7H2; Laval'90; FRCPC; DiagRad. Staff, Hôpital de Gatineau; Langs: Spanish; English; (819)561-8100

LECOMPTE, Michele; 123-70 rue O'Keefe, Salaber-de-Valleyf QC J6S 5C6; Mon'81; Staff, Centre Hospitalier Régional du Suroît; (450)371-5412

LECOMTE, Caroline; Clinique médicale de Fleurimon, 210-2140 rue King E, Sherbrooke QC J1G 5G6; Sher'92; CCFP; CCFP(E.M.); Médecin, Centre Hospitalier Universitaire de Sherbrooke-Hôpital Hôtel-Dieu; Langs: Bilingual(French/English); (819)563-4462

LECOMTE, Veronique; CSSS de Jonquiere, 2230 rue de l'Hopital, Jonquiere QC G7X 4H6; Mon'08; CCFP; Staff, Centre Hospitalier Jonquiere; (418)695-7700

LECOQ, Henri; 5704 rue Laurendeau, Montreal QC H4E 3W4; Mon'59; (514)766-5114

LECOURS, Brigitte; Hop Charles LeMoyne, 3120 boul Taschereau, Greenfield Park QC J4V 2H1; Mon'99; CSPQ; FRCPC; Anes. Staff, Hopital Charles LeMoyne; (450)466-5000

LECOURS, Catherine; Clin de Chir Plastique-Estheti, 300-34 cote de la Fabrique, Quebec QC G1R 3V7; Sher'05; PlasSurg. Staff Plastic Surg, Centre Hospitalier Universitaire de Sherbrooke-Hôpital Hôtel-Dieu; Staff Plastic Surg, Centre Hospitalier Affilié Universitaire de Québec - Hôpital De L'Enfant Jésus; Langs: Bilingual(French/English); (418)692-3843; Fax. (418)692-5872; info@chirurgieesthetiquequebec.com.

LECOURS, Isabelle; CLSC Ahuntsic, 1165 boul Henri-Bourassa E, Montreal QC H2C 3K2; Mon'08; CCFP; (514)381-4221

LECOURS, Junie; CHUS-Hop Fleurimont, 3001 12e av N, Sherbrooke QC J1H 5N4; Mon'04; FRCPC; DiagRad. Staff, Centre Hospitalier Universitaire de Sherbrooke-Hopital Fleurimont; (819)346-1110; Fax. (819)820-6423.

LECOURS, Mireille; 5 Brighton Rd, Charlottetown PE C1A 8T6; Sher'92; CCFP; Staff Paliative Care, Queen Elizabeth Hospital; (902)368-4781

LECOURS, Mylene; Ctr Hosp Affilie-Enfant-Jesus, 1401 18e Rue, Quebec QC G1J 1Z4; Mon'07; CSPQ; Anes. Staff, Centre Hospitalier Affilié Universitaire de Québec - Hôpital De L'Enfant Jésus; (418)649-5807

LECOURS, Rene; CHUM-Hop St-Luc, 11301-1058 rue Saint-Denis, Montreal QC H2X 3J4; Mon'75; ABIM; LMCC; IntMed (Vascular Medicine). Staff Internist, Centre Hospitalier l'Université De Montréal (CHUM) - Hôpital Saint-luc; Langs: English; (514)890-8000 x34599; Fax. (514)412-7417.

LECOURS, Richard; Hotel-Dieu de Levis, 143 rue Wolfe, Levis QC G6V 3Z1; Laval'79; FRCPC; Respir. Ac Staff, Hôtel-Dieu de Lévis; (418)835-7121

LECOURS, Serge; Clin Toxicologie De Montreal, 27-55 av de l'Eglise, Verdun QC H4G 3E7; Mon'77; MPH; CommunMed (P.Q.) (Public Health). Ac Staff, Centre Hospitalier de Verdun; Dir, Clinique de Toxicologie de Montreal; (514)362-8530; Fax. (514)362-7343; lecours@clintox1.com.

LECOURS, Simon; Clinique Med Interne Laurier, 101-39 rue Laurier E, Victoriaville QC G6P 6P6; Sher'77; IntMed. Ac Staff, Hotel-Dieu d'Arthabaska; (819)357-3933; Fax. (819)357-4310.

LECUYER, Nadine S; Family Matters Med Centre, X-730 St Anne's Rd, Winnipeg MB R2N 0A2; Man'00; CCFP; Langs: French; (204)253-5320

LEDDIN, Desmond J; Queen Elizabeth II HSC, 912-1276 South Park St, Halifax NS B3H 2Y9; Dublin (Ireland)'78; MRCP; MSc; FRCPC; IntMed; Gastroent. Staff, Queen Elizabeth II Health Sciences Centre - Victoria General Site; Prof, Dalhousie University; (902)473-4585; Fax. (902)473-4406.

LEDDING, Edward C; St Paul's Hosp, 1702 20th St W, Saskatoon SK S7M 0Z9; Sask'81; Staff Emerg, St Paul's Hospital (Grey Nuns) of Saskatoon; (306)655-5113; Fax. (306)655-5963.

LEDDING, James D; Rosetown Med Group, PO Box 340, Rosetown SK S0L 2V0; Sask'70; Fam Med, Rosetown & District Health Centre; Med Examiner, Saskatchewan Min. of Transport; (306)882-2631; Fax. (306)882-4488.

LEDDING, Kristopher M W; Cornwall Prof Bldg, 506-2125 11th Ave, Regina SK S4P 3X3; Sask'96; FRCSC; PlasSurg. (306)780-3650; Fax. (306)780-3718.

LEDDING, M David; Rosetown Med Group, PO Box 995, Rosetown SK S0L 2V0; Sask'67; Ac Staff, Rosetown & District Health Centre; Sr Mgr Medical, Heartland Health Region Corporate Office; Assessor, Practice Enhancement Program; Preceptor Family Med, University of Saskatchewan; (306)882-2631; Fax. (306)882-4488.

LEDDY, Danielle S; St Mary's Gen Hosp, 911 Queens Blvd, Kitchener ON N2M 1B2; Ott'85; FRCPC; IntMed (Interventional Cardiology); Cardiol. Staff, St Mary's General Hospital; Langs: English; French; (519)749-6924; Fax. (519)749-6982.

LEDDY, Maire; Highlands Health Network, 140 Rolling Hills Dr, Orangeville ON L9W 4X8; Dublin (Ireland)'73; (519)941-7575; Fax. (519)941-7060.

LEDERER, David; Eye Health MD, 440-8000 boul Decaire, Montreal QC H4P 2S4; Tufts(MA) (USA)'02; FRCSC; Ophth (Retina). (514)340-3937; Fax. (514)340-2729.

LEDESMA-CADHIT, Christina J; Abha Family Med Clinic, 2163 Danforth Ave, East York ON M4C 1K2; Manila (Philippines)'89; CCFP; Langs: Tagalog; (416)691-3030; Fax. (416)691-3031; mccadhit@hotmail.com.

LEDEZ, Kenneth M; Health Sciences Centre, 300 Prince Philip Dr, St. John's NL A1B 3V6; Dundee (Scotland)'80; MB ChB; FRCPC; Anes. Staff Anes, Health Sciences Centre; Chair Dept of Anes, Memorial University Of Newfoundland; (709)777-6540; Fax. (709)777-6506.

LEDEZMA, Jose; Dr Jose Ledezma Prof Corp Inc, 106 Doncaster Dr, Quispamsis NB E2E 1R2; U.N.A.M. (Mexico)'80; ABIME; Member, American Academy of Pain Management; Member, International Association for the Study of Pain; Langs: Spanish; French; (506)738-4354; Fax. (506)847-2880; maverick2013@bellaliant.net.

LEDGER, Gabrielle H; 201-60 Liberty St S, Bowmanville ON L1C 2N5; McM'03; FRCPC; Psy. Staff, Ontario Shores Centre for Mental Health Sciences; (905)419-5900

LEDGER, J Douglas; Victoria Health Centre, 2F-521 Victoria Park Ave, Scarborough ON M4C 5H1; Tor'73; CCFP; FCFP; Staff, Providence Healthcare; Lecturer Family & CommunMed, University of Toronto; (416)694-1400; Fax. (416)694-1985.

LEDINGHAM, Donna L; Regina Qu'Appelle HR-Regina, 1440 14th Ave, Regina SK S4P 0W5; Sask'07; HemPath. Staff, Regina General Hospital; (306)766-4444

LEDOUX, Elisabeth; CSSS du Nord de Lanaudière, 1000 boul Sainte-Anne, St-Charles-Brromee QC J6E 6J2; Sher'96; FRCPC; DiagRad. Staff, Centre Hospitalier Régional de Lanaudière; (450)755-1609 x2844; Fax. (450)759-8222.

LEDOUX, Isabelle; CSSS du Lac-des-Deux-Montagnes, 520 boul Arthur-Sauve, Saint-Eustache QC J7R 5B1; Mon'06; CCFP; Staff, Hôpital de Saint-Eustache; (450)473-6811; Fax. (450)473-6966.

LEDOUX, Stephane; CSSS de Laval, 1755 boul Rene-Laennec, Laval QC H7M 3L9; Mon'85; Neur. Staff, Hopital de la Cite de la santé; (450)668-1010; Fax. (450)975-5550.

LEDRAY, Lynda L; City Centre Fam Physicians, 100-514 Queen St, Saskatoon SK S7K 0M5; Sask'88; CCFP; FCFP; (306)244-3016; Fax. (306)244-4737.

LEDREW, Kellie K; Waterford Hosp, 306 Waterford Bridge Rd, St. John's NL A1E 4J8; Mem'94; FRCPC; Psy (Early Psychosis). Co-Dir Early Psychosis Prog & Gen Adult Inpatient & Outpatient/Staff Psy & Educ Coord, Waterford Hospital; Assoc Prof Psy, Memorial University Of Newfoundland; (709)777-3534; Fax. (709)777-3553; kellie.ledrew@eastlink.ca.

LEDREW, Ruth L J; Paradise Med Clinic, 7 Elizabeth Dr, Paradise NL A1L 1E5; Mem'85.

LEDSOME, John R; Delta Hosp, 5800 Mountain View Blvd, Delta BC V4K 3V6; Edinburgh (Scotland)'55; MB ChB; DSc; Dir Pulmonary Lab, Delta Hospital; Emeritus Prof Physiol, University of British Columbia; (604)946-1121; Fax. (604)921-9641.

LEDUC, Bernard; Montfort Hosp, 713 Montreal Rd, Ottawa ON K1K 0T2; Mon'81; CCFP; Ac Member, Montfort Hospital; (613)746-4621

LEDUC, Bernard E; CHUM-Hotel-Dieu, 3840 rue Saint-Urbain, Montreal QC H2W 1T8; Mon'69; CSPQ; FRCPC; PhysMed&Rehab. ac Staff, Centre Hospitalier l'Université de Montréal (CHUM) - Hôtel-Dieu; Ac Staff, Institut de Réadaptation Gingras-Lindsay de Montréal; Langs: Bilingual(French/English); (514)890-8101

LEDUC, Christian; Clinique Med des Trois Lacs, 160-585 av Saint-Charles, Vaudreuil-Dorion QC J7V 8P9; Mon'94; Staff, Centre Hospitalier Régional du Suroît; (450)455-3322; Fax. (450)455-0756.

LEDUC, Christian; Centre Med Berger, 116-1000 ch Sainte-Foy, Quebec QC G1S 2L6; Laval'86; (418)688-1385

LEDUC, Claude; Clinique Med Sainte-Dorothee, 102-1 boul Samson, Laval QC H7X 3S5; Mon'83; CCFP; Staff, Hopital de la Cite de la santé; Langs: English; (450)689-6334; Fax. (450)689-6339.

LEDUC, David A; Queensway Med Centre, 300-5307 Canotek Rd, Gloucester ON K1J 9M2; Ott'83; (613)746-6223; Fax. (613)746-6018.

LEDUC, Dean C; Orleans Medical-Dental Centre, 100-2555 St. Joseph Blvd, Orleans ON K1C 1S6; Ott'91; CCFP; Langs: English; French; (613)830-1298; Fax. (613)830-2170.

LEDUC, Denis G; Melville Pediatric Centre, 4500 rue Sherbrooke O, Westmount QC H3Z 1E6; Alb'71; FAAP; FRCPC; Peds (Family Medicine). Staff, McGill University Health Centre - Montreal Children's Hospital; Staff, McGill University Health Centre - Royal Victoria Hospital; assoc Prof Peds, McGill University; Langs: Bilingual(English/French); (514)932-4975; Fax. (514)932-9984; denis.leduc@mcgill.ca.

LEDUC, Eugene R J; Lansdowne Professional II, 215-3066 Shelbourne St, Victoria BC V8R 6T9; UBC'85; CCFP; FCFP; Clin Instructor Med, University of British Columbia; (250)388-4211; Fax. (250)383-4119.

LEDUC, Francois A; CSSS Pierre Boucher, 1333 boul Jacques-Cartier E, Longueuil QC J4M 2A5; Ott'92; BSc(Biology); MSc(MolecularBiol); Cardiol; IntMed. Staff, Centre Hospitalier Pierre Boucher; (450)468-8111

LEDUC, Genevieve; CSSS de Saint-Jerome, 290 rue de Montigny, Saint-Jerome QC J7Z 5T3; Mon'01; CCFP; CCFP(E.M.); Staff, Hôtel-Dieu de Saint-Jérôme; (450)431-8200

LEDUC, Genevieve; Centre Med Hochelaga, 9080 rue Hochelaga, Montreal QC H1L 2N9; Laval'09; (514)353-8742

LEDUC, Ghyslain; CHUS-Hop Fleurimont, 3001 12e Av N, Sherbrooke QC J1H 5N4; Sher'97; CCFP; CCFP(E.M.); Staff, Centre Hospitalier Universitaire de Sherbrooke-Hopital Fleurimont; (819)346-1110

LEDUC, Jean-Sebastien; Carrefour Med Vallee Richelieu, 665 boul Sir-Wilfrid-Laurier, Beloeil QC J3G 4J1; Mon'95; (450)467-0088

LEDUC, Julie; CHAQ-Hop du St-Sacrement, 1050 ch Sainte-Foy, Quebec QC G1S 4L8; Mon'01; CCFP; CCFP(E.M.); Staff, Centre Hospitalier Affilié Universitaire de Québec - Hôpital du St-Sacrement; (418)682-7684

LEDUC, Line; Hôpital Ste-Justine, 3175 ch Cote-Sainte-Catherine, Montreal QC H3T 1C5; Mon'83; DABOG; FRCSC; ObstGyn (Maternal Fetal Medicine). ac Staff, Hôpital Ste-Justine; dép Chef ObstGyn, Universite de Montreal; Langs: English; (514)345-4706; Fax. (514)345-4648; l.leduc@umontreal.ca.

LEDUC, Louis-Joseph; Hop Maisonneuve-Rosemont, 5415 boul de l'Assomption, Montreal QC H1T 2M4; Mon'82; MSc; FRCPC; AnatPath (Cytology)., Hopital Maisonneuve-Rosemont; Coroner, Province of Quebec; (514)252-3400 x7270; Fax. (514)252-3538.

LEDUC, Manon; CSSS Vaudreuil-Soulanges, 4-401 boul Harwood, Vaudreuil-Dorion QC J7V 7W1; Sher'98; Staff, CSSS de Vaudreuil-Soulanges; (450)424-1812 x221

LEDUC, Marie-Claude; UMF Charles Lemoyne, 201-299 boul Sir-Wilfrid-Lauri, Saint-Lambert QC J4R 2L1; Laval'92; (450)466-5630; Fax. (450)466-5631.

LEDUC, Martin; CSSS de Beauce-Etchemin, 1515 17e rue, Saint-Georges QC G5Y 4T8; Laval'93; Psy. Staff Psy, Centre Hospitalier Beauce-Etchemin; (418)228-2068; Fax. (418)227-1081; tintinmylou@videotron.ca.

LEDUC, Michel; Clinique Med des Trois Lacs, 160-585 av Saint-Charles, Vaudreuil-Dorion QC J7V 8P9; Mon'65; Staff, Centre Hospitalier de LaSalle; (450)455-3322; Fax. (450)455-0756.

LEDUC, Michel; CLSC-CHSLD D'Autray, 30 rue Saint-Gabriel CP 870, St-Gabriel-D-Brand QC J0K 2N0; Mon'77; (450)835-4705; Fax. (450)835-7217.

LEDUC, Pierre; Medi-Centre Chomedey, 610 boul Cure-Labelle, Laval QC H7V 2T7; Mon'65; Staff, Hôpital du Sacre-Coeur de Montréal; (450)687-6452; Fax. (450)687-3243.

LEDUC, Raymond; CHUM-Hotel-Dieu, 3840 rue Saint-Urbain, Montreal QC H2W 1T8; Mon'80; FRCPC; IntMed; Gastroent. Staff, Centre Hospitalier l'Université de Montréal (CHUM) - Hôtel-Dieu; (514)890-8000 x14980; Fax. (514)412-7206.

LEDUC, Sophie M; Hop Du Sacre-Coeur De Mtl, 5400 boul Gouin O, Montreal QC H4J 1C5; Mon'95; FRCSC; Ophth. Staff, Hôpital du Sacre-Coeur de Montréal; (514)338-2222 x2679; Fax. (514)338-2614.

LEDUC, Stephane; Hop du Sacre-Coeur de Mtl, 5400 boul Gouin O, Montreal QC H4J 1C5; Mon'00; OrthSurg. Staff, Hôpital du Sacre-Coeur de Montréal; (514)338-2050

LEDUC, Sylvain; CSSS de Rimouski-Neigette, CP 3150 Succ A 150 av Rouleau, Rimouski QC G5L 5T1; Laval'91; FRCPC; CommunMed. Staff, Hôpital Regional Rimouski; (418)724-8177

LEDUC, Yolande; 183 rue Sainte-Catherine, Longueuil QC J4H 2B4; Mon'74; Ac Member Perinatal, Centre Hospitalier Pierre Boucher; (450)677-5247; Fax. (450)677-5248.

LEDUC, Yvan; Unite Med Familiale Maizerets, 2480 ch de la Canardiere, Quebec QC G1J 2G1; Laval'90; CCFP; FCFP; (418)661-1413; Fax. (418)661-7504.

LEDUC, Yves; CSSS De La Haute-Yamaska, 205 boul Leclerc O, Granby QC J2G 1T7; Sher'06; Staff, Centre Hospitalier de Granby; (450)375-8000

LEDUC-ARBOUR, Nathael; Clinique Med des Sommets, 1070 rue Principale, Ste-Agathe-des-Mts QC J8C 1L6; Mon'04; (819)321-1212; Fax. (819)321-3232.

LEE, Adrian T; Surrey Med Arts Bldg, 308-13710 94A Ave, Surrey BC V3V 1N1; UBC'95; FRCSC; PlasSurg. Chair Plastic Surg, Surrey Memorial Hospital; Ac Staff, Royal Columbian Hospital; Ac Staff, Peace Arch Hospital; (604)589-1151; Fax. (604)589-6841.

LEE, Adrienne; Foothills Med Centre, 1403 29 St NW, Calgary AB T2N 2T9; UBC'07; FRCPC; IntMed; Hem. Staff, Foothills Medical Centre; (403)944-1564

LEE, Agnes S; 2921 66 St NW, Edmonton AB T6K 4C1; Alb'86; FRCSC; ObstGyn. Staff, Covenant Health - Grey Nuns Community Hospital; Langs: Cantonese; (780)450-9668; Fax. (780)465-7239.

LEE, Agnes Y Y; Gordon & Leslie Diamond HCC, 10F-2775 Laurel St, Vancouver BC V5Z 1M9; UBC'89; MSc; FRCPC; IntMed (Thrombosis); Hem. Staff, Vancouver General Hospital - Centennial Pavillion; Dir Thrombosis, University of British Columbia; Langs: Cantonese; (604)875-4863; Fax. (604)875-4763.

LEE, Aimee W; PO Box 15045 Rpo Aspenwoods, Calgary AB T3H 0N8; Alb'05; CCFP.

LEE, Alan Y; Foothills Med Centre, 1403 29 St NW, Calgary AB T2N 2T9; Tor'96; MD; LMCC; FRCPC; Anes. Staff Anes, Foothills Medical Centre; (403)944-1430; Fax. (403)944-2425; alan.lee@calgaryhealthregion.ca.

LEE, Alexander L; York Thoracic Surgery Assoc, 56 Prospect St, Newmarket ON L3Y 3S9; Wes'99; BSc; MSc; FRCSC; CardSurg; ThorSurg. Staff Div of Thoracic Surg, Southlake Regional Health Centre; (905)853-5864

LEE, Allan; William Osler HC-Etobicoke, 101 Humber College Blvd, Etobicoke ON M9V 1R8; Tor'01; Staff, William Osler Health System - Etobicoke General Hospital; (416)747-3400

LEE, Allan K L; Halton HCS Corp-Oakville, 327 Reynolds St, Oakville ON L6J 3L7; Tor'05; CCFP; Staff, Halton Healthcare Services Corporation - Oakville Site; (905)845-2571

LEE, Ambrose W M; 306-250 Harding Blvd W, Richmond Hill ON L4C 9M7; Qns'94; FRCSC; Otol;CCFP; CCFP(E.M.); FCFP; (905)508-6516; Fax. (905)508-6515.

LEE, Andrea; 118-1060 Speers Rd, Oakville ON L6L 2X4; Wes'06; FRCPC; IntMed; Hem. (905)815-8914; Fax. (905)815-8920.

LEE, Andrew G; Foothills Med Centre, 1403 29 St NW, Calgary AB T2N 2T9; Cal'94; FRCPC; DiagRad. Staff, Foothills Medical Centre; (403)944-4530

LEE, Andrew S Y; Royal City Med Bldg, 304-250 Keary St, New Westminster BC V3L 5E7; Wes'90; FRCSC; Neursurg. (604)526-8979; Fax. (604)526-7317.

LEE, Andrew W Y; Royal Victoria Hosp, 201 Georgian Dr, Barrie ON L4M 6M2; Tor'06; FRCPC; Anes. Staff, Royal Victoria Regional Health Centre; (705)728-9802

LEE, Angela Y M; Cross Roads Clinics, 350-507 Broadway W, Vancouver BC V5Z 1E6; UBC'91; (604)568-7229

LEE, Anita K; Mid-Main Comm Health Centre, 3998 Main St, Vancouver BC V5V 3P2; UBC'96; CCFP; (604)873-3666; Fax. (604)875-8790.

LEE, Ann E; Richmond Road Fam Med Ctre, 290-5255 Richmond Rd SW, Calgary AB T3E 7C4; (Ireland)'04; CCFP; (403)249-3165

LEE, Ann S O; Misericordia Community Hosp, 16940 87 Ave NW, Edmonton AB T5R 4H5; UBC'06; CCFP; Staff, Covenant Health - Misericordia Community Hospital; (780)735-2800; Fax. (780)735-2857.

LEE, Annesse Y; Southlake Med Centre, 104-581 David Dr, Newmarket ON L3Y 2P6; McM'06; FRCSC; Otol (Head & Neck Surgery). (905)898-5558

LEE, B Craig; The Ottawa Hosp-Gen Campus, G 12-501 Smyth Rd, Ottawa ON K1H 8L6; Man'73; FRCPC; IntMed; InfectDis. Staff Med, The Ottawa Hospital - General Campus; Teach Staff Biochem, University of Ottawa; (613)737-8051; Fax. (613)737-8009; clee@ottawahospital.on.ca.

LEE, Barbara A; 1-48 Water St S PO Box 1259 Stn Main, St Marys ON N4X 1B8; Tor'84; CAFCI; (519)284-1006

LEE, Benita S M; Surrey Mem Hosp, 13750 96 Ave, Surrey BC V3V 1Z2; Man'96; FRCPC; GenPath. Staff, Surrey Memorial Hospital; (604)588-3384

LEE, Betty; William Osler HC-Brampton, 2100 Bovaird Dr E, Brampton ON L6R 3J7; Cal'86; FRCPC; DiagRad. Staff, William Osler Health System - Brampton Civic Hospital; (905)494-2120 x58560

LEE, Betty H; London Reg Cancer Centre, 790 Commissioners Rd E, London ON N6A 4L6; Wes'06; CCFP; (519)685-8650

LEE, Bobby S; St Paul's Hosp, 1081 Burrard St, Vancouver BC V6Z 1Y6; Qns'97; FRCPC; Anes. Staff Anes, Providence Health Care - St Paul's Hospital; (604)682-2344

LEE, Bonita E; Edmonton Clinic Health Academy, 3 593-11405 87 Ave NW, Edmonton AB T6G 1C9; Alb'92; FRCPC; Peds; InfectDis. Staff, University of Alberta Hospital; (780)248-5540; Fax. (780)248-5625.

LEE, Bonnie P Y; Windsor Reg Hosp-Metropolitan, 1995 Lens Ave, Windsor ON N8W 1L9; Qns'93; CCFP; CCFP(E.M.); FCFP; Staff, Windsor Regional Hospital - Metropolitan Site; Langs: Cantonese; (519)254-1661

LEE, Boyd S; ENT Consultants, 219-1 Paton St, St. John's NL A1B 4S8; Dal'98; FRCSC; Otol. (709)579-1003

LEE, Brenda C; Rockyview Gen Hosp, 7007 14 St SW, Calgary AB T2V 1P9; UBC'83; FRCPC; Anes. Ac Staff, Rockyview General Hospital; (403)943-3410; Fax. (403)255-7858.

LEE, Brent R; Royal Jubilee Hosp, 1952 Bay St, Victoria BC V8R 1J8; UBC'95; FRCPC; DiagRad. Staff, Royal Jubilee Hospital; (250)370-8272

LEE, Brian P; Tower Prof Centre, 5520 50 Ave, Wetaskiwin AB T9A 0T3; (South Africa)'79; MB ChB; DA; Staff, Drayton Valley Hospital & Care Centre; Langs: Afrikaans; (780)352-9700

LEE, Bryan C W; Brant Community HC-Brantford, 200 Terrace Hill St, Brantford ON N3R 1G9; Wes'06; MedOncol; IntMed. Staff, The Brant Community Healthcare System - Brantford General Hospital Site; (519)751-5585; Fax. (519)751-5588.

LEE, C T Andy; Pape Village Med Centre, 1032A Pape Ave, Toronto ON M4K 3W2; Tor'88; Court Staff, Toronto Western Hospital - University Health Network; (416)467-5787

LEE, Calvin; Simon Fraser University, 300-515 Hastings St W, Vancouver BC V6B 5K3; Wes'96; (604)291-5200

LEE, Candace Y W; Cardiology Clinic, 4987 boul des Sources, Pierrefonds QC H8Y 3E3; Qns'96; FRCPC; IntMed; Cardiol. (514)685-3511

LEE, Carl H; 307A Bridge St W, Napanee ON K7R 3V3; McM'99; CCFP; CCFP(E.M.); Ac Staff, Lennox & Addington County General Hospital; (613)354-5361; Fax. (613)354-3283.

LEE, Carol; 11022 101 St NW, Edmonton AB T5H 2T1; Alb'82; CCFP; Staff, Royal Alexandra Hospital; (780)424-5417; Fax. (780)425-8297.

LEE, Carol K; Vancouver Gen Hosp, 855 12th Ave W, Vancouver BC V5Z 1M9; UBC'02; FRCPC; AnatPath. Staff, Vancouver General Hospital - Centennial Pavillion; Langs: Cantonese; (604)875-4024

LEE, Catherine M; PO Box 3591 Stn Main, Vancouver BC V6B 3Y6; Qns'06; CCFP; (604)261-8177

LEE, Chen; 100-4055 rue Sainte-Catherine, Montreal QC H3Z 3J8; Tor'86; MSc; FRCSC; PlasSurg (Aesthetic Surgery). Staff, McGill University Health Centre - Montreal General Campus; Plastic Surgery, McGill University Health Centre - Royal Victoria Hospital; Staff, McGill University Health Centre - Montreal Children's Hospital; Chair Div of Plastic Surg, McGill University; (514)932-7667

LEE, Cheng-Han; Vancouver Gen Hosp, 855 12th Ave W, Vancouver BC V5Z 1M9; UBC'04; FRCPC; AnatPath. Staff, Vancouver General Hospital - Centennial Pavillion; Langs: Cantonese; Taiwanese; (604)875-4111

LEE, Ching Sang; Lansdowne Professional Ctr II, 315-3066 Shelbourne St, Victoria BC V8R 6T9; UBC'99; FRCPC; IntMed; ClinImmunol&Allergy. (250)370-0318

LEE, Chiu-Ying; 302-4190 Finch Ave E, Scarborough ON M1S 4T7; Tor'85; (647)765-9226

LEE, Christie M; Mount Sinai Hosp, 18 210-600 University Ave, Toronto ON M5G 1X5; Tor'04; FRCPC; IntMed; Critical Care Medicine; Respir. Staff, Mount Sinai Hospital; (416)586-4800

LEE, Christina D; The Credit Valley Hospital, 2200 Eglinton Ave W, Mississauga ON L5M 2N1; McM'05; FRCPC; IntMed; Hem. Staff, The Credit Valley Hospital; (905)813-1100 x3905

LEE, Christina L Y; Carefirst Family Health Team, 27-420 Highway 7 E, Richmond Hill ON L4B 3K2; Tor'07; (905)695-1133; christina.lee@carefirstfht.com.

LEE, Christine H C; St Joseph's Healthcare, 50 Charlton Ave E, Hamilton ON L8N 4A6; Tor'94; BSc; FRCPC; IntMed; InfectDis; MedMicrobiol. Staff, St Joseph's Healthcare - Charlton Campus; Langs: Korean; (905)521-6143; clee@mcmaster.ca.

LEE, Christopher T; 4904 48 St, Leduc AB T9E 6X4; Alb'07; CCFP; (780)986-2712

LEE, Christopher W K; BC Cancer Agency-Fraser Valley, 13750 96 Ave, Surrey BC V3V 1Z2; Dal'91; FRCPC; IntMed; MedOncol. Staff, Surrey Memorial Hospital; Medical Staff Oncologist, BC Cancer Agency Fraser Valley Centre; (604)930-4017; Fax. (604)587-4312; clee@bccancer.bc.ca.

LEE, Cinda B S; North Scarborough Prof Bldg, 408-3420 Finch Ave E, Scarborough ON M1W 2R6; UBC'75; BSc; FAAP; FRCP; FRCPC; Peds (Consultant Pediatrics). Ac Staff, The Hospital For Sick Children; Staff Privil Nursery, North York General Hospital; Clin Teacher, University of Toronto; (416)491-3331

LEE, Cindy H Y; 507-586 Eglinton Ave E, Toronto ON M4P 1P2; Tor'04; FRCPC; IntMed; Respir. (416)488-6980

LEE, Cindy W; Midtown Med Clinic, 130-8780 Blundell Rd, Richmond BC V6Y 3Y8; Albany (USA)'10; CCFP; (604)277-9006

LEE, Clifton R; 3575 20 Ave NE, Calgary AB T1Y 6R3; Sask'95; CCFP; (403)248-7955

LEE, Clive C M; Oakdale Med Bldg, 408-2065 Finch Ave W, North York ON M3N 2V7; London (England)'88; FRCSC; ObstGyn (Infertility). Ac Staff, Humber River Regional Hospital - Church Street Site; Court Staff, Women's College Hospital; (416)742-6848; Fax. (416)744-9800.

LEE, Colin Q T; 15 Sperling Dr, Barrie ON L4M 6K9; Tor'98; BSc; FRCPC; CommunMed;CCFP; CCFP(E.M.); Staff Emerg, Toronto East General Hospital Inc.

LEE, Colleen M Y M; Tsawwassen Med Clinic, 201-1077 56 St, Delta BC V4L 2A2; Dal'90; (604)943-1131; Fax. (604)943-2617.

LEE, Connie N; Univ Hlth Network-Toronto Gen, 200 Elizabeth St, Toronto ON M5G 2C4; Tor'85; CCFP; CCFP(E.M.); Staff Physician Emerg, Toronto General Hospital - UHN; (416)340-3856; Fax. (416)340-4312.

LEE, D Dae-Won; 1102-160 14th St E, North Vancouver BC V7L 2N3; Tor'83; FRCPC; IntMed; Endocrin&Metab. Langs: Korean; (604)980-0018; Fax. (604)987-3699.

LEE, Daniel K; Georgian Bay Gen Hosp, PO Box 760 Stn Main 1112 St Andrews Dr, Midland ON L4R 4P4; Ott'07; CCFP; CCFP(E.M.); Staff, Georgian Bay General Hospital - Midland; (705)526-1330

LEE, David C; 305-2051 McCallum Rd, Abbotsford BC V2S 3N5; Connecticut (USA)'03; FRCSC; OrthSurg. (604)852-8875

LEE, David; CSSS de Manicouagan, 635 boul Jolliet, Baie-Comeau QC G5C 1P1; Laval'08; CCFP; Staff, Centre Hospitalier Régional Baie-Comeau; (418)589-3701

LEE, David H; Queen's Univ-Etherington Hall, 2025-94 Stuart St, Kingston ON K7L 3N6; Wes'90; FRCPC; IntMed; Hem. Assoc Prof, Queen's University; (613)533-6803; dlee@queensu.ca.

LEE, David S; Lonsdale Med Dental Bldg, 108-1940 Lonsdale Ave, North Vancouver BC V7M 2K2; Alb'89; (604)987-3357

LEE, David S C; London HSC-Victoria Campus, PO Box 5010 Stn B D4 212-800 Commissioners Rd E, London ON N6A 5W9; London (England)'76; BA(Oxon); MB BS; MRC; DCH; FRCPC; Peds (Clinical Neonatology). Staff, London Health Sciences Centre - Victoria Campus; Asst Prof Peds, University of Western Ontario; Langs: Chinese; Cantonese; Mandarin; (519)685-8500; dsclee@uwo.ca.

LEE, Deborah; North Burlington Med Centre, 18-1960 Appleby Line, Burlington ON L7L 0B7; Ott'04; CCFP; (905)319-2000

LEE, Della D; Wawanesa Health Centre, PO Box 309 506 George St, Wawanesa MB R0K 2G0; Man'89; CCFP; FCFP; Staff, Brandon Regional Health Centre; (204)726-2119; Fax. (204)728-8298.

LEE, Dennis; 578 St Clair Ave W, Toronto ON M6C 1A6; Tor'78; (416)654-4552; Fax. (416)656-2897.

LEE, Dennis Y L; Surrey Mem Hosp, 13750 96 Ave, Surrey BC V3V 1Z2; UBC'06; FRCPC; DiagRad. Staff Radiol, Surrey Memorial Hospital; (604)585-5666

LEE, Diana W K; PO Box 62045 Rpo Hawkwood, Calgary AB T3G 5S7; Alb'08; CCFP.

LEE, Donald D; Vancouver Gen Hosp, 855 12th Ave W, Vancouver BC V5Z 1M9; UBC'87; Staff, Vancouver General Hospital - Centennial Pavillion; Langs: Cantonese; (604)822-7121

LEE, Donald H; London HSC-University Hosp, PO Box 5339 Stn B 339 Windermere Rd, London ON N6A 5A5; Witwatersrand (South Africa)'78; FRCPC; DiagRad (Neuro Radiology). Staff, London Health Sciences Centre - University Hospital; Prof, University of Western Ontario; (519)663-3203; Fax. (519)663-8803; dlee@uwo.ca.

LEE, Donna S H; Vancouver Gen Hosp, 855 12th Ave W, Vancouver BC V5Z 1M9; UBC'06; FRCPC; EmergMed. Staff, Vancouver General Hospital - Centennial Pavillion; (604)875-4111

LEE, Doris S; 3-3269A Bloor St W, Etobicoke ON M8X 1E2; Tor'88; BSc; Staff, St Joseph's Health Centre; Langs: Chinese; (416)236-4952; Fax. (416)236-0558.

LEE, Douglas J; 7204 Main St, Vancouver BC V5X 3J4; UBC'90; (604)325-3331

LEE, Douglas S Y; 482 4NU-200 Elizabeth St, Toronto ON M5G 2C4; Tor'94; FRCPC; IntMed; Cardiol. Staff Cardiologist, Toronto General Hospital - UHN; Langs: Korean; (416)340-3861

LEE, Edward; Chinook Reg Hosp, 960 19 St S, Lethbridge AB T1J 1W5; McG'04; FRCPC; DiagRad; NuclearMed. Staff, Chinook Regional Hospital; (403)388-6135

LEE, Edward S C; 204-174 Harwood Ave S, Ajax ON L1S 2H6; Man'69; BSc; CCFP; FCFP; Court Staff, Rouge Valley Health System - Ajax & Pickering Health Centre Site; Assoc Staff, The Salvation Army Toronto Grace Health Centre; Langs: Cantonese; (905)683-3572; Fax. (905)683-3578.

LEE, Edward T; Parkdale Comm Health Centre, 1299 Queen St W, Toronto ON M6K 1L2; McG'88; BSc; Staff, St Joseph's Health Centre; Staff, Parkdale Community Health Centre; (416)537-2455; Fax. (416)537-3526; edward.lee@pchc.on.ca.

LEE, Edward Y; 106-1 Quarry Ridge Rd, Barrie ON L4M 7G1; (Ireland)'05; CCFP; (705)725-9922; Fax. (705)725-8622.

LEE, Ellen F F; Maple Family Health Team, 7-730 Front Rd, Kingston ON K7M 6P7; Qns'09; CCFP.

LEE, Elliott K; Royal Ottawa Hlth Care Group, 3125-1145 Carling Ave, Ottawa ON K1Z 7K4; Alb'99; DABPNAddictionPsy; DABPNSleepMed; FRCPC; Psy (Sleep Medicine). Staff, Royal Ottawa Mental Health Centre - Royal Ottawa Health Care Group; (613)722-6521 x6226; e.lee@rohcg.on.ca.

LEE, Elmer C C; Trillium Hlth Ctr-Mississauga, 100 Queensway W, Mississauga ON L5B 1B8; Tor'96; FRCPC; IntMed; Endocrin&Metab. Staff, Trillium Health Centre - Mississauga; (905)848-7100

LEE, Emil J Y; 200-5503 206 St, Langley BC V3A 2C6; UBC'94; FRCPC; DiagRad. Staff, Abbotsford Regional Hospital & Cancer Centre; Staff, Langley Memorial Hospital; Staff, Mission Memorial Hospital; (604)534-4114

LEE, Eunice; 120-1315 Finch Ave W, North York ON M3J 2G6; Tor'85; (416)661-7000

LEE, F Joseph; The Centre for Family Medicine, 10B Victoria St S, Kitchener ON N2G 1C5; Wes'86; CCFP; FCFP; Staff, St Mary's General Hospital; Staff, Grand River Hospital - Kitchener/Waterloo Health Centre; (519)783-0021; Fax. (519)783-0031.

LEE, Francis F W; Heartland Fertility & Gyn Clin, 701-1661 Portage Ave, Winnipeg MB R3J 3T7; Man'77; BSc; MSc; FACOG; FRCSC; ObstGyn (Reproductive Endocrinology & Infertility). Staff, Grace General Hospital; Staff, Seven Oaks General Hospital; Staff, Health Sciences Centre; Staff, St Boniface General Hospital; Langs: Chinese; (204)779-8888; Fax. (204)779-8877.

LEE, Francis K; 208-1110 Sheppard Ave E, North York ON M2K 2W2; Alb'91; FRCPC; Psy (Addiction Medicine). (416)222-7040

LEE, Frank R; Broadway Med Clinic, 220-41 Broadway St W, Yorkton SK S3N 0L6; Glasgow (Scotland)'71; MB ChB; FFARCSI; LMCC; Reg Educational Coord Sunrise Region/Medical Staff, Yorkton Regional Health Centre; (306)782-4840; Fax. (306)782-4220.

LEE, Frank S; The Ottawa Hosp-Riverside, 1967 Riverside Dr, Ottawa ON K1H 7W9; Qns'95; FRCPC; DiagRad. Staff Radiol, The Ottawa Hospital - Riverside Campus; (613)738-8400 x2321; Fax. (613)738-8540.

LEE, Gary L; MUHC-Montreal Gen Hosp, 1650 av Cedar, Montreal QC H3G 1A4; Alb'90; CSPQ; BMedSci; DABEM; FRCPC; EmergMed;CCFP; CCFP(E.M.); Médecin EmergMed, McGill University Health Centre - Montreal General Campus; Médecin EmergMed, McGill University Health Centre - Montreal Children's Hospital; Médecin, Donald Berman Maimonides Geriatric Centre; Conférencier Family Med, McGill University; Langs: French; Cantonese; Toishan; (514)934-1934 x42501; gary.lee@mcgill.ca.

LEE, George T W; Dalhousie Univ Hlth Services, PO Box 15000 Lcd 2 6230 Coburg Rd, Halifax NS B3H 4R2; Dal'90; (902)494-2171

LEE, Gilbert; Chancellor Medical, 820 9th St, Brandon MB R7A 4B8; Man'86; FRCPC; Psy (Adult Psychiatry). (204)571-6876; Fax. (204)728-1987.

LEE, Hank C; Regency Med Centre, 108-2737 Keele St, North York ON M3M 2E9; Tor'94; FRCPC; IntMed; Endocrin&Metab. Staff, Humber River Regional Hospital - Church Street Site; (416)240-0206; Fax. (416)240-9720.

LEE, Harvey B; Medical Arts Bldg, 711-233 Kennedy St, Winnipeg MB R3C 3J5; Man'72; FRCPC; IntMed (Diabetology). Staff, St Boniface General Hospital; Staff, Concordia General Hospital; (204)953-1270; Fax. (204)953-1273.

LEE, Hayvin; Woodbine Med Centre, 233-8787 Woodbine Ave, Markham ON L3R 9S2; Tor'94; CCFP; FCFP; Court Staff Privil, The Scarborough Hospital - Birchmount Campus; Langs: Cantonese; (905)415-0800; Fax. (905)415-0801.

LEE, Helen H K; Southlake Reg Health Centre, 596 Davis Dr, Newmarket ON L3Y 2P9; Tor'97; CCFP; Staff, Southlake Regional Health Centre.

LEE, Henderson; Toronto East Gen Hosp Inc, 825 Coxwell Ave, Toronto ON M4C 3E7; Wes'90; FRCPC; Anes. Ac Staff Anes, Toronto East General Hospital Inc; Asst Prof, University of Toronto; (416)462-6212; Fax. (416)469-6874.

LEE, Herman; 1612-4500 Kingsway Ave, Burnaby BC V5H 2V9; Alb'85; CCFP; FCFP; Langs: Cantonese; Mandarin; (604)436-1231

LEE, Hoi Kwan; Brockville Gen Hosp, 75 Charles St, Brockville ON K6V 1S8; Qns'02; Staff, Brockville General Hospital - Charles Street; (613)345-5649

LEE, Howard C; Port Hardy Med Clinic, 7090 Thunderbird Way, Port Hardy BC V0N 2P0; Witwatersrand (South Africa)'03; MB BCh; Langs: Mandarin; (250)949-7117; Fax. (250)949-7110; phmedicalclinic@hotmail.com.

LEE, Ik Ju; CLSC de Montreal-Nord, 11441 boul Lacordaire, Montreal-Nord QC H1G 4J9; Mon'08; (514)327-0400

LEE, Jacqueline A; Stollery Children's Hosp, 1D1-8440 112 St NW, Edmonton AB T6G 2B7; Alb'99; BSc; FRCPC; Peds. Staff/Asst Prof Peds, University of Alberta Hospital; Staff, Stollery Children's Hospital; (780)407-6370; Fax. (780)407-6414.

LEE, Jacques S; Sunnybrook Hlth Sciences Ctre, 2075 Bayview Ave, Toronto ON M4N 3M5; Alb'88; EmergMed. Staff, Sunnybrook Health Sciences Centre; (416)480-4037

LEE, James L; Urology Clinic, 202-180 Vine St S, St Catharines ON L2R 7P3; Tor'71; DAB; FRCSC; Urol. Ac Staff, Hôtel Dieu Shaver Health & Rehabilitation Centre; Ac Staff, Niagara Health System - Ontario Street Site; Ac Staff, Niagara Health System - St Catharines General Site; (905)688-2761; Fax. (905)688-6638.

LEE, Jason K; 920-123 Edward St, Toronto ON M5G 1E2; Tor'05; FRCPC; IntMed; ClinImmunol&Allergy. (647)352-2554

LEE, Jason K C; Nanaimo Reg Gen Hosp, 1200 Dufferin Cres, Nanaimo BC V9S 2B7; Alb'06; FRCPC; Anes. Staff, Nanaimo Regional General Hospital; (250)754-2141

LEE, Jason Y; 9 103-61 Queen St E, Toronto ON M5C 2T2; Tor'04; FRCSC; Urol.

LEE, Jay C H; Rockyview Gen Hosp, 6610-7007 14 St SW, Calgary AB T2V 1P9; Cal'94; FRCSC; Urol (Andrology). Staff Urologist, Rockyview General Hospital; (403)943-8985; Fax. (403)943-8984.

LEE, Jeffrey W; Radiology Consultants Assoc, 120-6707 Elbow Dr SW, Calgary AB T2V 0E3; Alb'02; FRCPC; DiagRad. (403)777-3007

LEE, Jennifer L; Co-Op Commun Health Centre, 547 Michigan St, Victoria BC V8V 1S5; UBC'96; CCFP; FCFP; (250)388-6811; Fax. (250)380-0245.

LEE, Jenny; Wrinch Mem Hosp, PO Bag 999, Hazelton BC V0J 1Y0; Sask'92; CCFP; Wrinch Memorial Hospital; Clin Instructor Med, University of British Columbia; (250)842-5234; Fax. (250)842-5865.

LEE, Jerome B; Burnaby Mental Health Services, 3935 Kincaid St, Burnaby BC V5G 2X8; UBC'05; FRCPC; Psy. Staff, Providence Health Care - St Paul's Hospital; (604)453-1960

LEE, John J Y; St Boniface Gen Hosp, Y3521-409 Tache Ave, Winnipeg MB R2H 2A6; Tor'88; FRCSC; GenSurg; CardSurg. Staff, St Boniface General Hospital; (204)237-2572; Fax. (204)233-4853; jlee@sbgh.mb.ca.

LEE, John; St Michael's Hosp, 8F-30 Bond St, Toronto ON M5B 1W8; Wes'03; FRCSC; Otol (Rhinology). Staff, St Michael's Hospital; (416)864-5206; Fax. (416)864-5469.

LEE, John O; Ottawa West Travel Med Clinic, 2F-760 Eagleson Rd, Kanata ON K2M 0A7; Alb'90; BSc(Hon); CCFP; FCFP; Ac Staff, Queensway Carleton Hospital; Langs: Korean; French; (613)592-9081; Fax. (613)592-6554.

LEE, John P L; Baywood Clinic, 5-75 Bayly St W, Ajax ON L1S 7K7; Wes'76; CCFP; FCFP; Ac Staff, Rouge Valley Health System - Ajax & Pickering Health Centre Site; (905)428-6495

LEE, John S; North Whitby Med Centre, 3975 Garden St, Whitby ON L1R 3A4; Tor'91; CCFP; Staff, Lakeridge Health - Oshawa Site; (905)430-2400; Fax. (905)430-1599.

LEE, John Y C; 102-1300 Don Mills Road, North York ON M3B 2W6; Tor'75; FAAP; FRCPC; Peds. Asst Prof, University of Toronto; (416)445-4611; Fax. (416)445-5025; john.lee@utoronto.ca.

LEE, John Y H; Quinte HC Corp-Trenton Mem, PO Box 1600 Stn Main 242 King St, Trenton ON K8V 5S6; McG'65; AB; FRCSC; Otol. Consultant, QHC Trenton Memorial; (613)392-2540

LEE, Jonathan P; MacLeod Trail Plastic Surgery, 7425 MacLeod Trail SW, Calgary AB T2H 0L8; Alb'03; FRCPC; PlasSurg. (403)286-4263; Fax. (403)242-5090.

LEE, Joseph S K; Bathurst Med Centre, 303-4256 Bathurst St, North York ON M3H 5Y8; Tor'74; ObstGyn. (416)630-7015; Fax. (416)730-9144.

LEE, Joseph Y; NewLife Fertility Centre, 4250 Sherwoodtowne Blvd, Mississauga ON L4Z 2G6; Qns'92; BSc(BioChem.); ObstGyn. Langs: English; French; (905)896-7100

LEE, Joyce W Y; Seniors Health Centre, 2 Buchan Crt, North York ON M2J 5A3; Tor'01; CCFP; Staff, North York General Hospital; Langs: Cantonese; (416)756-6050 x8093

LEE, Judy K M; Kerrisdale Prof Centre, 235-2025 42nd Ave W, Vancouver BC V6M 2B5; UBC'76; Langs: Cantonese; (604)873-4491

LEE, Judy S M; 204-73 7 St SE, Medicine Hat AB T1A 1J2; National (Taiwan)'71; Court Staff, Medicine Hat Regional Hospital; (403)527-3121; Fax. (403)527-9694.

LEE, Julia; 10886 Hurontario St, Brampton ON L7A 3R9; Tor'02; CCFP; (905)846-9911

LEE, Julian S; 311-233 Nelson's Cres, New Westminster BC V3L 0E3; Wes'06; FRCPC; Neur. (604)527-0008

LEE, Julie; 202-250 Keary St, New Westminster BC V3L 5E7; UBC'00; BSc; FRCPC; IntMed; Endocrin&Metab. Postgrad Education Dir Endocrin & Medical Dir, Royal Columbian Hospital; Clinical Asst Prof, University of British Columbia; (604)520-1135; Fax. (604)520-1132; endo.mds@gmail.com.

LEE, Julietta C T; Scarborough Prof Centre, 319-1371 Neilson Rd, Scarborough ON M1B 4Z8; (Hong Kong)'87; MB BS; MRCP(UK); FACR; FRCPC; IntMed; Rheum. Court Staff, The Scarborough Hospital - Birchmount Campus; Langs: Cantonese; (416)284-7227; Fax. (416)284-7102.

LEE, Jung Hwa; Market Mall, 3625 Shaganappi Trail NW, Calgary AB T3A 0E2; McG'06; MDCM; CCFP.

LEE, Justin T; 201-10168 Yonge St, Richmond Hill ON L4C 1T6; Tor'81; FRCSC; GenSurg (Endoscopy). Ac Staff, Mackenzie Richmond Hill Hospital; Langs: Mandarin; (905)770-1266; Fax. (905)770-1270.

LEE, Justin W; Odette Cancer Centre, 2075 Bayview Ave, Toronto ON M4N 3M5; McM'02; FRCPC; RadOncol. (416)480-5000

LEE, K Dick; Surrey Mem Hosp, 13750 96 Ave, Surrey BC V3V 1Z2; Wes'81; DAB; FRCPC; Anes. Staff, Surrey Memorial Hospital; University of British Columbia; (604)588-3367; Fax. (604)585-5644.

LEE, Tom; 6683 Victoria Dr, Vancouver BC V5P 3Y2; Newcastle (England)'86; Staff, Richmond Hospital; Langs: Mandarin; Cantonese; (604)301-1666

LEE, Kan Chee; West End Prof Bldg, 210-9509 156 St NW, Edmonton AB T5P 4J5; Tor'77; FRCPC; Peds. (780)483-6884; Fax. (780)486-5725.

LEE, Kar Cheong; Mackenzie Richmond Hill Hosp, 10 Trench St, Richmond Hill ON L4C 4Z3; Wes'05; FRCPC; IntMed. Staff, Mackenzie Richmond Hill Hospital; (905)883-1212; Fax. (905)883-2455.

LEE, Karr-Hong; University of Alberta Hosp, 8440 112 St NW, Edmonton AB T6G 2B7; Alb'07; EmergMed. Staff, University of Alberta Hospital; (780)407-8822

LEE, Kathy K; 205-9656 King George Blvd, Surrey BC V3T 2V5; UBC'05; FRCSC; GenSurg. (604)582-3004

LEE, Kelvin H Y; Hys Med Centre, 202-11010 101 St NW, Edmonton AB T5H 4B9; Qns'96; FRCPC; DiagRad (Abdominal Imaging). Active Staff-Non-Admitting, University of Alberta Hospital; Ac Staff, Royal Alexandra Hospital; Ac Staff, Covenant Health - Grey Nuns Community Hospital; (780)426-1121; Fax. (780)425-5979.

LEE, Kenneth W; WOTCH Comm Mental Health Serv, 534 Queens Ave, London ON N6B 1Y6; Wes'86; Staff Family Med, St Joseph's Hospital - St Joseph's Health Care; Staff, Parkwood Hospital - St Joseph's Health Care; Staff, London Health Sciences Centre - University Hospital; (519)668-0624; Fax. (519)668-2227.

LEE, Kenny; Laurel Med Centre Ltd, 215-888 8th Ave W, Vancouver BC V5Z 3Y1; UBC'84; LMCC; Staff, Vancouver General Hospital - Centennial Pavillion; Langs: Mandarin; Spanish; (604)872-0345; Fax. (604)639-2689.

LEE, Kevin A; 105-3950 14th Ave, Markham ON L3R 0A9; Tor'89; FAAP; FRCPC; Peds (Neurology). Staff, Markham Stouffville Hospital; Langs: Cantonese; (905)305-1700; Fax. (905)305-1706.

LEE, Kevin K; 252 Ester St, Sudbury ON P3E 5C3; Tor'91; FRCSC; Ophth. (705)522-3393; Fax. (705)522-3369.

LEE, Khong-Yam; Bramalea Med Centre, 304-18 Kensington Rd, Brampton ON L6T 4S5; National (Taiwan)'74; Staff, William Osler Health System - Brampton Civic Hospital; (905)791-3373; Fax. (905)791-3373.

LEE, King Siu; Humber River Reg Hosp-Finch, 2111 Finch Ave W, North York ON M3N 1N1; (Taiwan)'72; FRCPC; AnatPath. Staff, Humber River Regional Hospital - Finch Avenue Site; (416)744-2500; klee@hrrh.on.ca.

LEE, Kingsley R; 4092 Shelbourne St, Victoria BC V8N 4P6; Man'92; ABIM; FRCPC; IntMed; ClinImmunol&Allergy. (250)595-8111

LEE, Kit Shan; South East Toronto Fam Health, 1871 Danforth Ave, Toronto ON M4C 1J3; UBC'07; CCFP; (416)699-7775; Fax. (416)699-7776.

LEE, Kut Yau; 406-302 Spadina Ave, Toronto ON M5T 2E7; Kyushu (Japan)'61; FRCPC; IntMed (Rheumatology). Staff, St Michael's Hospital; (416)260-2002

LEE, Kwok Ching; North York Gen Hosp, 4001 Leslie St, North York ON M2K 1E1; McM'79; FRCPC; Anes (Intensive Care). Chief Anes, North York General Hospital; Langs: Chinese; French; (416)756-6265; kwokching.lee@nygh.on.ca.

LEE, Kyong-Jin; The Hosp For Sick Children, 555 University Ave, Toronto ON M5G 1X8; Tor'89; FRCPC; Peds; PedCardiol. Staff Cardiologist Div of Cardiology-The Labatt Family Heart Ctr, The Hospital For Sick Children; Assoc Prof Med, University of Toronto; (416)813-7326; Fax. (416)813-5857.

LEE, Kyong-Soon; The Hosp for Sick Children, 555 University Ave, Toronto ON M5G 1X8; Tor'86; MSc(ClinEpidemiol); FRCPC; Peds (Neonatology). Staff Div of Neonatol, The Hospital For Sick Children; Assoc Prof Peds, University of Toronto; (416)813-7488; Fax. (416)813-5245.

LEE, Lap Cheung; 311-1100 Sheppard Ave E, North York ON M2K 2W1; Tor'75; Court Staff, The Scarborough Hospital - General Campus; Ac Staff, Toronto East General Hospital Inc; Court Staff, North York General Hospital; Langs: Cantonese; Hakka; Mandarin; (416)222-2800

LEE, Lawrence C F; Burnaby Hosp, 3935 Kincaid St, Burnaby BC V5G 2X6; Tor'86; CCFP; CCFP(E.M.); Staff, Burnaby Hospital; (604)434-4211

LEE, Lawrence C H; 1090 Youville Drive West NW, Edmonton AB T6L 0A3; Alb'07; (780)735-7834; Fax. (780)735-7640.

LEE, Lawrence L M; 2F-607 Gerrard St E, Toronto ON M4M 1Y2; Man'71; Court Staff, St Michael's Hospital; (416)461-7547; Fax. (416)461-7548.

LEE, Liesly; Sunnybrook Hlth Sciences Ctre, A411-2075 Bayview Ave, Toronto ON M4N 3M5; Tor'93; BSc; MSc; FRCPC; Neur (Multiple Sclerosis). Staff, Sunnybrook Health Sciences Centre; Asst Prof Med, University of Toronto; Langs: Chinese; Cantonese; (416)480-4114; Fax. (416)480-4199.

LEE, Linda L W; Centre for Family Medicine, 10B Victoria St S, Kitchener ON N2G 1C5; Wes'86; CCFP; FCFP; Staff Fam Pract, Grand River Hospital - Kitchener/Waterloo Health Centre; Staff, St Mary's General Hospital; (519)783-0023; Fax. (519)783-0033.

LEE, Linda M; 201-112 Queenston St, St. Catharines ON L2R 2Z4; Alb'04; FRCPC; IntMed; MedOncol. Staff, Toronto East General Hospital Inc; (905)685-8082

LEE, Livia K Y; 301-16 O'Brien St, Orillia ON L3V 5S2; Wes'05; FRCSC; Urol.

LEE, Loretta E; 9 Haineault St, Fort McMurray AB T9H 1R8; Mem'86; CCFP; (780)799-4477; Fax. (780)799-4544.

LEE, Lorraine P H; South Riverdale Comm Hlth Ctr, 955 Queen St E, Toronto ON M4M 3P3; Qns'09; CCFP; (416)461-2493; Fax. (416)461-8245.

LEE, M Anne F; The Group Health Centre, 240 McNabb St, Sault Ste. Marie ON P6B 1Y5; Qns'90; CCFP; FCFP; Staff, Sault Area Hospital - Sault Ste Marie; (705)759-1234; Fax. (705)759-7487; lee_a@ghc.on.ca.

LEE, Mabel M F; Pavillon Vertefeuille, 103-311 McArthur Ave, Vanier ON K1L 8M3; Alb'93; CCFP; (613)749-1678

LEE, Mao-Cheng; Dynalife Diagnostic Lab Servic, 200-10150 102 St NW, Edmonton AB T5J 5E2; McG'02; BSc; MSc; MDCM; FRCPC; IntMed (Infectious Diseases); MedMicrobiol. Staff, University of Alberta Hospital; Langs: Spanish; French; Mandarin; Taiwanese; (780)451-3702 x8365; Fax. (780)454-2845; mao-cheng.lee@albertahealthservices.ca.

LEE, Marc F; CSSS de la Vallée de l'Or, 725 6e rue, Val-d'Or QC J9P 3Y1; Sher'94; CCFP; Staff, Centre Hospitalier de Val d'Or; (819)825-6711

LEE, Marette H; Div of Gynecologic Oncology, 6F-2775 Laurel St, Vancouver BC V5Z 1M9; Alb'04; FRCSC; ObstGyn. (604)875-4268

LEE, Marilyn; Riverside Med Clinic, 121-4411 16 Ave NW, Calgary AB T3B 0M3; Cape Town (South Africa)'78; (403)286-7211; Fax. (403)247-6838.

LEE, Mark H; 102-22 Richmond St, Richmond Hill ON L4C 3Y1; Tor'87; FRCSC; GenSurg; ThorSurg. Staff Surg, Mackenzie Richmond Hill Hospital; Langs: Korean; (905)780-6626; Fax. (905)780-6623.

LEE, Mark J; Valley Med Imaging, 404A-2151 McCallum Rd, Abbotsford BC V2S 3N8; UBC'05; FRCPC; DiagRad. (604)859-4810

LEE, Mark J; 201-20 Hobson St, Cambridge ON N1S 2M6; Ott'02; FRCPC; IntMed; Gastroent. (519)624-8589

LEE, Mark K; Trillium Hlth Ctr-Mississauga, 100 Queensway W, Mississauga ON L5B 1B8; McG'96; CCFP; CCFP(E.M.); FCFP; Ac Staff, Trillium Health Centre - Mississauga; (905)848-7600

LEE, Mark W; Royal Alexandra Hosp, 10240 Kingsway NW, Edmonton AB T5H 3V9; Cal'89; FRCPC; AnatPath. Staff, Royal Alexandra Hospital; (780)735-6933; Fax. (780)735-4715.

LEE, Martin M S; Pickering Med Centre, 108-1885 Glenanna Rd, Pickering ON L1V 6R6; Tor'89; FACP; FRCPC; IntMed; Rheum. (905)839-6309

LEE, Mary C Y; Doctors Hosp Phase 1, 220-340 College St, Toronto ON M5T 3A9; Tor'91; FRCPC; IntMed; Rheum. Langs: Mandarin; Portuguese; (416)323-9440; Fax. (416)323-9545.

LEE, Mary; Com El Med Bldg, 309-2620 Commercial Dr, Vancouver BC V5N 4C4; Karachi (Pakistan)'63; MB BS; MRCOG; FRCSC; ObstGyn. Consultant, Vancouver General Hospital - Centennial Pavillion; Langs: Chinese; (604)873-1541; Fax. (604)873-1199.

LEE, Mervin M F; 315-5000 Kingsway, Burnaby BC V5H 2E4; UBC'96; FRCPC; IntMed. (604)432-9222

LEE, Michael C; 306-1160 Burrard St, Vancouver BC V6Z 2E8; Wes'06; CCFP; (604)685-7747

LEE, Michael C F; 230 Ridge Rd N PO Box 730, Ridgeway ON L0S 1N0; Tor'82; Staff, Niagara Health System - Douglas Memorial Hospital Site; Langs: Cantonese; Chinese; (905)894-4043; Fax. (905)894-1094; mlee10q@yahoo.ca.

LEE, Michael D; 102-15122 72 Ave, Surrey BC V3S 2G2; UBC'91; Staff, Surrey Memorial Hospital; (604)572-9110; Fax. (604)572-6770.

LEE, Michael R; Palliser Health Authority, 666 5 St SW, Medicine Hat AB T1A 4H6; Alb'72; FACEP; MCFP(EM); Staff, Medicine Hat Regional Hospital; (403)529-8000

LEE, Michael R; South Calgary Med Clinic, 118-40 Sunpark Plaza SE, Calgary AB T2X 3X7; Alb'95; BMedSci; CCFP; FCFP; (403)254-4000; Fax. (403)254-1282; mikerana@telus.net.

LEE, Michael S W; 403-265 Yorkland Blvd, North York ON M2J 5C7; (Hong Kong)'68; MB BS; FRCPC; Psy (Adult General Psychiatry). (416)229-2399

LEE, Min Sun; Queen Elizabeth II HSC-Halifax, 4F-1796 Summer St, Halifax NS B3H 3A7; Dal'99; FRCSC; GenSurg; VascSurg. Staff, Queen Elizabeth II Health Sciences Centre - Halifax Infirmary Site; (902)473-8512; Fax. (902)473-8513.

LEE, Mona; Mount Seymour Clinic, 2F-333 Seymour Blvd, North Vancouver BC V7J 2J4; Man'88; CCFP; FCFP; Physician Student Health Services, Capilano University; Langs: Cantonese; (604)904-7712; Fax. (604)904-7714.

LEE, Moo-Hyung; York Prof Bldg, 208-679 Davis Dr, Newmarket ON L3Y 5G8; McG'89; FRCSC; OrthSurg (Arthroplasty). Staff, Southlake Regional Health Centre; (905)853-0731; Fax. (905)853-0226.

LEE, Nancy B; St Joseph's Mountain H Serv, PO Box 585 Stn Lcd 1 100 West 5th St, Hamilton ON L8N 3K7; Sask'76; CCFP; Staff, St Joseph's Healthcare Hamilton - West 5th Campus; (905)522-1155

LEE, Norman J; Memorial U-Student Hlth Serv, PO Box 4200 Stn C, St. John's NL A1C 5S7; Mem'98; CCFP; (709)737-3507; Fax. (709)737-2087.

LEE, Norman K K; Lakeridge Hlth Corp-Oshawa, 1 Hospital Crt, Oshawa ON L1G 2B9; (Hong Kong)'81; MB BS; FRCPC; NuclearMed. Staff NuclearMed, Lakeridge Health - Oshawa Site; Asst Prof, University of Connecticut; (905)576-8711 x3571; Fax. (905)721-4762.

LEE, Oscar I; 207-800 Bathurst St, Toronto ON M5R 3M8; (Jamaica)'67; MB BS; Ac Staff, St Joseph's Health Centre; (416)536-0207; Fax. (416)532-6649.

LEE, Patricia A; Nottingham Medical, 310-664 Wye Rd, Sherwood Park AB T8A 6G3; Alb'01; CCFP; (780)416-3220; Fax. (780)416-3224.

LEE, Patricia E; Sunnybrook Hlth Sciences Ctre, B732-2075 Bayview Ave, Toronto ON M4N 3M5; McG'87; FRCSC; ObstGyn (Urogynecology). Staff, Sunnybrook Health Sciences Centre; Asst Prof, University of Toronto; (416)480-6740; Fax. (416)480-6741.

LEE, Patricia H; Ridgeview Med Centre, 212-1240 Railway Ave, Canmore AB T1W 1P4; Wes'07; CCFP; (403)609-8333; Fax. (403)609-3666.

LEE, Patricia P S; Westway Women & Children's HC, 2G-1723 Kipling Ave, Etobicoke ON M9R 2Y8; Wes'05; MSc; CCFP; Langs: Cantonese; (416)279-0840

LEE, Patricia; Fairmont Med Bldg, 1311-750 West Broadway, Vancouver BC V5Z 1J3; UBC'99; FRCSC; Otol. Clinical Asst Prof/Dir Undergrad Educ for Div of Otol, University of British Columbia; Langs: Cantonese; (604)875-4126; Fax. (604)875-5533.

LEE, Patrick F T; Sheldon Chumir Centre, 1213 4 St SW, Calgary AB T2R 0X7; Man'84; CCFP; FCFP; (403)955-9300; Fax. (403)476-8766; patrickftlee@gmail.com.

LEE, Patrick; Com El Med Bldg, 309-2620 Commercial Dr, Vancouver BC V5N 4C4; Punjab (India)'62; FRCSC; ObstGyn. Consultant, Vancouver General Hospital - Centennial Pavillion; (604)873-1541; Fax. (604)873-1199.

LEE, Peter C K; Woodlawn Med Clinic, 92 Main St, Dartmouth NS B2X 1R5; Dal'99; CCFP; Langs: Chinese; Cantonese; (902)434-1500; Fax. (902)434-4368.

LEE, Peter K O; Kanata Prof Centre, 212-99 Kakulu Rd, Kanata ON K2L 3C8; Qns'86; FRCPC; Peds; ClinImmunol&Allergy. (613)599-4452; Fax. (613)599-6413.

LEE, Peter; The Joseph & Wolf Lebovic Bldg, Box 9 2 004-60 Murray St, Toronto ON M5T 3L9; Otago (New Zealand)'66; MB ChB; MD; FRCPC; IntMed (Adult Rheumatology); Rheum. Assoc Staff, University Health Network; Assoc Staff, Mount Sinai Hospital; Langs: Cantonese; (416)586-4800 x8247; Fax. (416)586-8766.

LEE, Peter; 503-1200 Burrard St, Vancouver BC V6Z 2C7; UBC'04; FRCSC; Ophth. (604)609-2022

LEE, Peter T C; 69 Abercrombie Rd, New Glasgow NS B2H 1K4; Dal'80; Ac Staff, Aberdeen Regional Hospital; Prov Med Examiner/Pres, Pictou Co. Med. Soc.; (902)752-5612

LEE, Philip E; St Paul's Hosp, 9B-1081 Burrard St, Vancouver BC V6Z 1Y6; UBC'97; FRCPC; IntMed; GeriatricMed. Staff, Providence Health Care - St Paul's Hospital; (604)806-8029

LEE, Pi Kay; Somerset West Commun Hlth Ctre, 55 Eccles St, Ottawa ON K1R 6S3; Dal'84; BSc; MSc; CCFP; FCFP; Asst Prof Family Med, University of Ottawa; (613)238-1220; Fax. (613)235-2982.

LEE, Pui-Kee; Gordon & Leslie Diamond HCC, F9-2775 Laurel St, Vancouver BC V5Z 1M9; (Hong Kong)'74; FRCPC; IntMed; Cardiol. Staff Cardiol, Vancouver General Hospital - Centennial Pavillion; Asst Prof, University of British Columbia; Langs: Mandarin; Cantonese; (604)875-5485; Fax. (604)875-5632.

LEE, Rachel N; 5570 Joyce St, Vancouver BC V5R 4H6; UBC'76; Langs: Cantonese; Mandarin; (604)430-2311; Fax. (604)430-2350.

LEE, Ralph F; The Ottawa Hosp-Civic Campus, 1053 Carling Ave, Ottawa ON K1Y 4E9; Ott'02; FRCPC; IntMed; Gastroent. Staff, The Ottawa Hospital - Civic Campus.

LEE, Randall T; Professional Place, 201-2901 Lawrence Ave E, Scarborough ON M1P 2T4; Tor'88; BSc; MEd; CCFP; FCFP; Ac Staff Family Med, The Scarborough Hospital - General Campus; Court Staff Family Med, Women's College Hospital; Asst Prof Family Med, University of Toronto; (416)266-4543; Fax. (416)267-4050.

LEE, Randolph; Discovery Medical Centre, 1477 Island Hwy, Campbell River BC V9W 8E5; Tor'63; MSc; FRCPC; IntMed (Endocrinology). Ac Medical Staff, Campbell River & District General Hospital; (250)850-4505; drlee3@telus.net.

LEE, Raymond; Southlake Reg Health Centre, 596 Davis Dr, Newmarket ON L3Y 2P9; Saba (Netherlands Antilles)'02; CCFP; CCFP(E.M.); Staff EmergMed, Southlake Regional Health Centre; (905)895-4521; Fax. (905)830-5972.

LEE, Raymond S Y; Meadowlark Prof Bldg, 205-8702 Meadowlark Rd NW, Edmonton AB T5R 5W5; Alb'74; (780)489-5885; Fax. (780)483-1809.

LEE, Richard D; Hamilton HS-General Site, 237 Barton St E, Hamilton ON L8L 2X2; Tor'85; MHSc; FRCPC; DiagRad. Ac Staff, Hamilton Health Sciences Centre - Hamilton General Hospital; Assoc Prof, McMaster University; (905)521-2100 x46521; Fax. (905)527-5761.

LEE, Richard J; Children's & Women's HC of BC, 1L7-4480 Oak St, Vancouver BC V6H 3V4; London (England)'69; LRCP; MRCS; DRCOG; FRCPC; Anes (Cardiovascular Anesthesia). Staff Anes, BC Children's Hospital; (604)875-2711

LEE, Richard; Mount St Joseph Hosp, 3080 Prince Edward St, Vancouver BC V5T 3N4; (Singapore)'78; MB BS; FRCR; DMRD(Lond); DABR; FRCPC; DiagRad. Staff Diag Imaging Services, Providence Health Care - Mount Saint Joseph Hospital; Langs: Hokkin; Malay; (604)874-1141; Fax. (604)872-0388.

LEE, Rina; 203-140 Champlain St, Dieppe NB E1A 1N8; Sher'90; FACC; FRCPC; IntMed; Cardiol. Staff Cardiologist, Dr Georges-L-Dumont University Hospital Centre; (506)862-0110; Fax. (506)855-2324.

LEE, Robert K W; Waterloo Sports Med Centre, 10-65 University Ave E, Waterloo ON N2J 2V9; Tor'87; (519)746-2220; Fax. (519)746-2295; rlee@wsm.ca.

LEE, Robin; Heart Lake Med Centre, 204-10425 Kennedy Rd, Brampton ON L6Z 0A4; Wes'91; (905)846-3777; Fax. (905)846-4498.

LEE, Ronita S M; The Scarborough Hosp-General, 3050 Lawrence Ave E, Scarborough ON M1P 2V5; Tor'07; FRCPC; IntMed; MedOncol. (416)438-2911

LEE, Rose; True North Imaging, 120-7330 Yonge St, Thornhill ON L4J 7Y7; Tor'94; FRCPC; DiagRad. (905)707-1777; Fax. (905)707-0616; rose.lee@utoronto.ca.

LEE, Sabrina K; North York Med Arts Bldg, 315-1333 Sheppard Ave E, North York ON M2J 1V1; Tor'01; FRCSC; ObstGyn (Minimal Invasive Surgery). Staff, North York General Hospital; (416)494-2400

LEE, Sai-Kui; 301-713 Davis Dr, Newmarket ON L3Y 2R3; (Hong Kong)'65; FRCPC; Peds. Ac Staff, Southlake Regional Health Centre; (905)898-2422; Fax. (905)898-6839.

LEE, Sai-Ping; 1483 Gerrard St E, Toronto ON M4L 2A4; (Hong Kong)'68; MB BS; FRCPC; DiagRad. (416)461-1516; Fax. (416)461-8812.

LEE, Sammy S H; Continental Shopping Centre, 1193-3779 Sexsmith Rd, Richmond BC V6X 3Z9; Man'88; BSc(Hons); Langs: Chinese; Malay; (604)821-1193; Fax. (604)231-8971.

LEE, Samuel S; 3330 Hospital Dr NW, Calgary AB T2N 4N1; Mem'78; ABIM; FRCPC; IntMed (Hepatology). Ac Staff, Foothills Medical Centre; Prof, University of Calgary; (403)220-8457; Fax. (403)270-0995.

LEE, Sandra L; Foothills Med Centre, 1403 29 St NW, Calgary AB T2N 2T9; Alb'06; AnatPath. Staff, Foothills Medical Centre; (403)944-3395

LEE, Sandra S L; Medical Corporation, 5 St Anne's Rd, Winnipeg MB R2M 2X9; Man'84; CCFP; FCFP; (204)231-3355; Fax. (204)233-6801.

LEE, Sandra W; 515-757 Hastings St W, Vancouver BC V6C 1A1; UBC'97; CCFP; Staff, Delta Health Sciences Centre; Langs: Cantonese; (604)666-6179

LEE, Sharon J; PO Box 1102 Stn Main, Nelson BC V1L 6H3; UBC'83; Ac Staff, Mills Memorial Hospital.

LEE, Shelter S; Chilliwack Gen Hosp, 45600 Menholm Rd, Chilliwack BC V2P 1P7; UBC'05; CCFP; CCFP(E.M.); Staff, Chilliwack General Hospital; (604)795-4141

LEE, Shirley; Mount Sinai Hosp, 206-600 University Ave, Toronto ON M5G 1X5; Wes'92; CCFP; CCFP(E.M.); FCFP; Staff Emerg Med, Mount Sinai Hospital; (416)586-4800 x5058; Fax. (416)586-4719.

LEE, Shoo Kim; Mount Sinai Hosp, 782-600 University Ave, Toronto ON M5G 1X5; (Singapore)'80; MB BS; DAB; LMCC; PhD; FRCPC; Peds (Neonatology). Staff, Mount Sinai Hospital; (416)586-8379

LEE, Shui Hing; Central Square Med Centre, 255-4231 Hazelbridge Way, Richmond BC V6X 3L7; New South Wales (Australia)'72; MB BS; DAB; FAAO; FRCSC; Ophth (Cataract). CEO/Med Dir, Sunray Surgical Centre; Clin Teacher Med, University of British Columbia; Langs: Cantonese; Mandarin; (604)273-6767; Fax. (604)273-6730.

LEE, Shung; Victoria Prof Bldg, 405-1120 Yates St, Victoria BC V8V 3M9; Alb'95; BSc; FRCSC; GenSurg; VascSurg. Staff VascSurg, Royal Jubilee Hospital; Staff VascSurg, Victoria General Hospital; Clin Instructor, University of British Columbia; (250)220-8931; Fax. (250)220-8925.

LEE, Simon K W; 2-160 East Beaver Creek Rd, Richmond Hill ON L4B 3L4; McG'86; FRCPC; Derm. Clin Associate Derm, Toronto Western Hospital - University Health Network; (905)886-7546

LEE, Sonya M; Sheldon M Chumir Health Centre, 8F-1213 4 St SW, Calgary AB T2R 0X7; Tor'96; CCFP; FCFP; (403)955-9300

LEE, Stella; 110-200 St Clair Ave W, Toronto ON M4V 1R1; McM'06; CCFP; Staff, St Joseph's Health Centre; (416)928-9343; Fax. (416)928-9368.

LEE, Stephen G; Family Med Clinic, 17-141 Torbay Rd, St. John's NL A1A 2H1; Mem'89; CCFP; FCFP; (709)579-4400

LEE, Stephen L; St Joseph's Health Centre, 30 The Queensway, Toronto ON M6R 1B5; Wes'00; FRCPC; Anes. Staff, St Joseph's Health Centre; (416)530-6000 x4090

LEE, Stephen; 2F-4410 17 St NW, Edmonton AB T6T 0C1; RCS (Ireland)'88; BSc(Eng.); MSc(Eng.); Med Dir, RediCare Clinic; Med Consultant, The Great-West Life Assurance; Med Consultant, Sun Life Financial; Med Consultant Appeals Commission & Board, Workers' Comp Board of AB; Board Member, Edmonton Public Schools; (780)468-1884; Fax. (780)468-1868; stephen.lee@gwl.com.

LEE, S-K; PO Box 35005 Rpo Midtown, Edmonton AB T5J 0B7; Alb'97; FRCPC; IntMed.

LEE, Susan M; Woodstock Gen Hosp, 310 Juliana Dr, Woodstock ON N4V 0A4; Tor'07; FRCPC; Anes. Staff, Woodstock General Hospital; (519)421-4211

LEE, Susan; Saunte Medical Clinic, 101-15850 26 Ave, Surrey BC V3S 2N6; UBC'04; MEd; BSc(Hon); CCFP; Med Dir, Peninsula Medical Clinic; (604)542-7788

LEE, Susan; Saint John Reg Hosp, PO Box 2100 Stn Main, Saint John NB E2L 4L2; Qns'87; FRCPC; Anes. Staff, Saint John Regional Hospital; (506)648-6861; Fax. (506)648-6860.

LEE, Suzie; Children's Hosp Eastern Ont, 401 Smyth Rd, Ottawa ON K1H 8L1; Alb'95; FRCPC; Peds; Cardiol. Staff, Children's Hospital of Eastern Ontario (CHEO); (613)737-7600

LEE, Sze Lap; Misericordia Community Hosp, 304-16940 87 Ave NW, Edmonton AB T5R 4H5; Alb'92; FRCPC; Peds (Neonatal & Perinatal Medicine). Staff, Covenant Health - Misericordia Community Hospital; (780)735-2744; Fax. (780)735-2936.

LEE, T Joseph; Markham Stouffville Hosp, PO Box 1800 Stn Main 381 Church St, Markham ON L3P 7P3; Tor'04; FRCPC; AnatPath. Staff, Markham Stouffville Hospital; (905)472-7000

LEE, Tara S; Associate Fam Physicians Clini, 262 2nd Ave NE, Swift Current SK S9H 2C8; Sask'06; CCFP; Rural Coord Family Med Residency Program, University of Saskatchewan; (306)773-1555; Fax. (306)773-6817.

LEE, Thomas F; Vancouver Gen Hosp, 855 12th Ave W, Vancouver BC V5Z 1M9; Man'78; FRCPC; EmergMed. Ac Staff, Vancouver General Hospital - Centennial Pavillion; Clinical Asst Prof, University of British Columbia; (604)875-4700; Fax. (604)875-4872.

LEE, Thomas K M; Retina Center of Ottawa, 500-1565 Carling Ave, Ottawa ON K1Z 8R1; Alb'03; FRCSC; Ophth. (613)226-7061; Fax. (613)226-9478.

LEE, Tih-Shih W; UBC Hospital, 2211 Wesbrook Mall, Vancouver BC V6T 2B5; Yale(CT) (USA)'87; FRCPC; Psy. Staff, UBC Hospital - Koerner Pavillion; (604)822-7121

LEE, Todd C; MUHC-Royal Victoria Hosp, A 423A-687 av des Pins O, Montreal QC H3A 1A1; Tor'05; FRCPC; IntMed; InfectDis. Staff, McGill University Health Centre - Royal Victoria Hospital; (514)934-1934

LEE, Tony C L; Queen Elizabeth II HSC-Halifax, 6896-1796 Summer St, Halifax NS B3H 3A7; Tor'04; FRCPC; IntMed; Cardiol. Staff, Queen Elizabeth II Health Sciences Centre - Halifax Infirmary Site; (902)473-2292; Fax. (902)473-7277.

LEE, Tracy Y; The Richmond Hosp, 7000 Westminster Hwy, Richmond BC V6X 1A2; UBC'05; CCFP; Staff, Richmond Hospital; (604)244-5170

LEE, Trevor J; Assiniboine Clinic, 633 Lodge Ave, Winnipeg MB R3J 0S9; Man'96; FRCSC; GenSurg.

LEE, Trevor W R; St Boniface Gen Hosp, 409 Tache Ave, Winnipeg MB R2H 2A6; Man'96; FRCPC; Anes. Head Dept of Anes, St Boniface General Hospital; (204)237-2580; Fax. (204)231-0425.

LEE, Tzu-Kuang; 205-9148 23 Ave NW, Edmonton AB T6N 1H9; (Singapore)'71; MSc; MB BS; FRCP(UK); FACP; FRCPC; IntMed. Ac Staff, Covenant Health - Grey Nuns Community Hospital; Clin Prof Med/Assoc Dean Clinical Faculty, University of Alberta; Langs: Cantonese; Mandarin; (780)462-3010; Fax. (780)440-2911.

LEE, Ursula J Y M; BC Cancer Agency-Fraser Valley, 13750 96 Ave, Surrey BC V3V 1Z2; UBC'89; FRCPC; IntMed; MedOncol. Staff Oncol, BC Cancer Agency Fraser Valley Centre; Asst Prof Med, University of British Columbia; (604)930-4028

LEE, Vansen M; 408-800 Bathurst St, Toronto ON M5R 3M8; Tor'79; Langs: Chinese; (416)733-8800

LEE, Victor Chee Choon; 207-4190 Finch Ave E, Scarborough ON M1S 4T7; (Taiwan)'81; BSc; DABFP; FAAFP; Langs: Mandarin; Cantonese; Hakka; (416)298-3883; Fax. (416)298-9849; victorlee@sympatico.ca.

LEE, Victor K G; The Medical Centre, PO Box 4200 Stn Main 707 Charlotte St, Peterborough ON K9J 7B3; Tor'75; FRCPC; IntMed; Gastroent. Staff, Peterborough Regional Health Centre - Hospital Drive; Langs: Cantonese; (705)876-4539

LEE, Victoria E H; Pine Clinic, 1985 4th Ave W, Vancouver BC V6J 1M7; Wes'04; FRCPC; CommunMed;CCFP; Med Officer of Hlth, Office of the Medical Health Officer; Langs: Korean; (604)736-2391

LEE, Victoria; 1001-123 Edward St, Toronto ON M5G 1E2; McM'82; BSc; FRCPC; Psy (Geriatric Psychiatry). Ac Staff Psy, Toronto East General Hospital Inc; (416)485-5768; Fax. (416)485-0812; victorialeemd@rogers.com.

LEE, Virginia; 103-3325 Kingsway, Vancouver BC V5R 5K6; (Hong Kong)'87; MB BS; (604)431-5008

LEE, Vivian K; Manitoba Clinic, 790 Sherbrook St, Winnipeg MB R3A 1M3; Man'92; FRCSC; ObstGyn. Lecturer ObstGyn, University of Manitoba; leev@cc.umanitoba.ca.

LEE, Vivian T P; 303-1100 Sheppard Ave E, North York ON M2K 2W1; Wes'87; FRCPC; IntMed; Critical Care Medicine; InfectDis. Ac Staff, North York General Hospital; (416)223-9284; Fax. (416)223-3320.

LEE, W Leslie; Grand River Comm Hlth Centre, 347 Colborne St, Brantford ON N3S 3N2; West Indies (Jamaica)'64; MB BS; (519)754-0777

LEE, W J Kenny; Fowler Kennedy Sports Med Clin, 1151 Richmond St, London ON N6A 3K7; UBC'07; FRCSC; OrthSurg.

LEE, Warren L; St Michael's Hospital, 4071 QW-30 Bond St, Toronto ON M5B 1W8; Tor'97; FRCPC; IntMed (Critical Care Medicine); Respir. Staff Physician Phy, St Michael's Hospital; Langs: Bilingual(French/English); (416)864-6060 x3970; warren.lee@utoronto.ca.

LEE, William R; Dartmouth Med Centre, 201-46 Portland St, Dartmouth NS B2Y 1H4; McG'76; CCFP; CCFP(E.M.); FCFP; (902)465-4542; Fax. (902)465-4537.

LEE, William W; Lakeshore Village Walk in Clin, 2885 Lake Shore Blvd W, Etobicoke ON M8V 1J1; Tor'78; Ac Staff FamPract, St Joseph's Health Centre; Court Staff, Trillium Health Centre - West Toronto; (416)259-5100

LEE, William; 506-1750 10th Ave E, Vancouver BC V5N 5K4; Alb'87; Assoc Staff Privil, Vancouver General Hospital - Centennial Pavillion; (604)325-9221

LEE, Wilson; 203-4603 Kingsway, Burnaby BC V5H 4M4; Wes'98; FRCPC; IntMed; Cardiol. (604)438-1382

LEE, Winifred; Woodlawn Med Consultants, 92 Main St, Dartmouth NS B2X 1R5; UBC'99; FRCSC; ObstGyn. Staff ObstGyn, IWK Health Centre; Lecturer, Dalhousie University; Langs: Chinese; Cantonese; Mandarin; (902)434-1500; Fax. (902)434-7360.

LEE, Winnie W S; Bay College Med Centre, C216-777 Bay St, Toronto ON M5G 2C8; Tor'94; Physician, Vermont Square Medical Clinic; Langs: Cantonese; Mandarin; (416)977-8878; Fax. (416)977-0118.

LEE, Winnie; Cambridge Mem Hosp, 700 Coronation Blvd, Cambridge ON N1R 3G2; Tor'02; FRCPC; DiagRad. Staff, Cambridge Memorial Hospital; (519)621-2330

LEE, Winston; Dr Winston Lee Prof Clinic, 299 Metcalf St, Saint John NB E2K 4P8; Dal'84; Staff Family Med, Saint John Regional Hospital; Staff, St Joseph's Hospital; Physician, Thumball Nursing Home; Lecturer Faculty Advisor, Dalhousie University; (506)634-3099; Fax. (506)634-2114.

LEE, Young M; 15-9555 Yonge St, Richmond Hill ON L4C 9M5; Tor'80; (905)884-6450

LEE, Yuna; St Michael's Hosp, 4CCW 4 149-30 Bond St, Toronto ON M5B 1W8; McG'95; FRCPC; IntMed (Osteoporosis). Staff, St Michael's Hospital; Langs: Korean; English; (416)864-6060 x3109

LEE-CHEN, Beverley; Richmond Central Med Clinic, 150-7997 Westminster Hwy, Richmond BC V6X 4J4; Man'05; CCFP; (778)297-4700

LEE CHEONG, Noel L; 8-2155 Lawrence Ave E, Scarborough ON M1R 5G9; Glasgow (Scotland)'81; MB BS; Staff, The Scarborough Hospital - General Campus; (416)751-0052; cdnmdlee@yahoo.ca.

LEE CHOI, Kenneth; 302-4190 Finch Ave E, Scarborough ON M1S 4T7; Tor'78; FRCPC; IntMed; Derm. Staff, Toronto General Hospital - UHN; Staff, The Scarborough Hospital - Birchmount Campus; (416)321-5667; Fax. (416)321-9191.

LEE KIM KOON, Andrew C; Parkgate Med Centre, 220-3650 Mt Seymour Pky, North Vancouver BC V7H 2Y5; London (England)'74; MB BS; LRCP; MRCS; (604)929-7321; Fax. (604)929-7329.

LEE-KWEN, Johnson; Brandon Reg Health Centre, 150 McTavish Ave E, Brandon MB R7A 2B3; Dublin (Ireland)'66; MB ChB; BAO; FACOG; FRCSC; ObstGyn. Ac Staff, Brandon Regional Health Centre; jleekwen@mts.net.

LEE MEI SI, Sylvana; Clin Medicale Adoncour, 200-505 rue Adoncour, Longueuil QC J4G 2M6; Mon'00; Staff, Centre Hospitalier Pierre le Gardeur; (450)646-4445; Fax. (450)646-5526.

LEE-NG, M Madeleine; 208-2863 Ellesmere Rd, Scarborough ON M1E 5E9; RCS (Ireland)'67; Staff, Rouge Valley Health System - Centenary Health Centre Site; Staff, The Scarborough Hospital - Birchmount Campus; Langs: Mandarin; Cantonese; French; (416)281-8618; Fax. (416)724-0369.

LEE NG, Vicky; The Hosp for Sick Children, 8F 8262-555 University Ave, Toronto ON M5G 1X8; Tor'93; FRCPC; Peds; Gastroent. Staff, The Hospital For Sick Children; (416)813-7733; Fax. (416)813-4972; vicky.ng@sickkids.ca.

LEE PONG, Noella M I; Baker Clinic, 100-10405 Jasper Ave NW, Edmonton AB T5J 3N4; Alb'87; CCFP; (780)944-9584; Fax. (780)944-9534.

LEE-POY, Michael F; Centre for Family Medicine, 10B Victoria St S, Kitchener ON N2G 1C5; Wes'03; CCFP; Clinical Asst Prof, McMaster University; Aj Prof, University of Western Ontario; (519)783-0022

LEE SANG, Ivan A; North Whitby Med Centre, 3975 Garden St, Whitby ON L1R 3A4; London (England)'63; (905)430-2400

LEE SANG, Katherine A; North Whitby Med Centre, 3975 Garden St, Whitby ON L1R 3A4; Wes'83; (905)430-2400; Fax. (905)430-1599.

LEE-SING, Richard A; 205-294 Main St, Toronto ON M4C 4X5; McG'68; (416)690-5354; Fax. (416)690-5362.

LEE SON, Archie; East Van Med Bldg, 506-1750 10th Ave E, Vancouver BC V5N 5K4; Cape Town (South Africa)'75; Ac Staff, Vancouver General Hospital - Centennial Pavillion; Langs: Afrikaans; (604)874-2211; Fax. (604)874-2677.

LEE-SON, Kathy K Y; Children's & Women's HC of BC, K4 158-4480 Oak St, Vancouver BC V6H 3V4; UBC'06; FRCPC; Peds; Nephrol. Staff, BC Children's Hospital; Langs: Cantonese; (604)875-2345 x5222

LEE-SON, Llewellyn; 300-7031 Westminster Hwy, Richmond BC V6X 1A3; Cape Town (South Africa)'69; MB ChB; FRCPC; IntMed. Consultant, Richmond Hospital; (604)273-1281; Fax. (604)273-6722.

LEE-WING, Matthew; Medical Arts Bldg, 1010-233 Kennedy St, Winnipeg MB R3C 3J5; Man'88; FRCOphth; ABOph; FACS; FRCSC; Ophth (Orbital, Lacrimal & Eyelid Surgery). Asst Prof, University of Manitoba; (204)946-0649; Fax. (204)957-0294; leewingm@ms.umanitoba.ca.

LEECE, Pamela N; Dana Lana School of Public Hlt, 10F-155 College St, Toronto ON M5T 3M7; Ott'09; CCFP; (416)978-0952

LEECH, Judith A; The Ottawa Hosp-Civic Campus, 1053 Carling Ave, Ottawa ON K1Y 4E9; Qns'75; ABSM; FRCPC; IntMed (Sleep Medicine); Respir. Staff Consultant, The Ottawa Hospital - General Campus; Att Staff Respiratory Div, The Ottawa Hospital - Civic Campus; Staff Consultant, Renfrew Victoria Hospital; Med Staff, Health Canada; Assoc Prof, University of Ottawa; (613)761-4636; Fax. (613)761-5333; jleech@ottawahospital.on.ca.

LEECH-PORTER, J Colin G; 7-3596 27th Ave W, Vancouver BC V6S 1P8; Wes'67; FRCPC; Psy (Traumatic Brain Injuries). Pres/CEO, Immunis Corporation; (604)737-0600; Fax. (604)737-1671; colinlp@shaw.ca.

LEEDER, David G; 580 Ofield Rd North, Dundas ON L9H 5E2; Tor'99.

LEEKAM, Roger N; West End Diagnostic Imaging, 2425 Bloor St W, Toronto ON M6S 4W4; RCS (Ireland)'75; FRCPC; DiagRad. Ac Staff, St Joseph's Health Centre; Court Staff, Peterborough Regional Health Centre - Rogers St Site; Asst Prof, University of Toronto; (416)763-4331

LEENEN, Frans H H; Univ of Ottawa Heart Institute, H3238-40 Ruskin St, Ottawa ON K1Y 4W7; Utrecht (Netherlands)'73; PhD; FRCPC; MedScient(Med) (Cardiology). Dir Hypertension Unit, University of Ottawa Heart Institute; Prof, University of Ottawa; (613)761-4521; Fax. (613)761-5105; fleenen@ottawaheart.ca.

LEEPER, William R; London HSC-Victoria Hosp, PO Box 5010 Stn B 800 Commissioners Rd E, London ON N6A 5W9; Wes'07; FRCSC; GenSurg. Staff, London Health Sciences Centre - Victoria Campus; (519)685-8500

LEES, Gordon; University of Alberta Hosp, 2C3.62-8440 112 St NW, Edmonton AB T6G 2B7; Alb'74; FRCSC; GenSurg (Inflammatory Bowel Disease); PedGenSurg. Staff, Stollery Children's Hospital; Staff, University of Alberta Hospital; Staff, Children's Health Centre of Northern Alberta; Clin Assoc Prof Surg, University of Alberta; (780)407-1843; Fax. (780)407-8500; glees@ualberta.ca.

LEES, Mark; West Winds Primary Health Ctr, 3311 Fairlight Dr, Saskatoon SK S7M 3Y5; Sask'02; CCFP; Asst Prof Academic Fam Med, West Winds Health Centre; (306)655-4244

LEES, Martin G J; Chatham-Kent Hlth Alliance, PO Box 2030 Stn Main 80 Grand Ave W, Chatham ON N7M 5L9; Ott'86; Staff, Chatham-Kent Health Alliance; Associate Faculty & Administration Prog, Central Michigan University; (519)354-6400

LEES, Nicholas M; 360 Springbank Dr PO Box 26021 Rpo Southcrest, London ON N6J 4Y9; Wes'10; CCFP; (519)319-2566

LEES, Sharon A; Northmount Med Centre, 502-145 13th St E, North Vancouver BC V7L 2L4; UBC'81; (604)988-4744; Fax. (604)988-4725.

LEET, Carol A; North Bramalea Med Centre, 301-9780 Bramalea Rd, Brampton ON L6S 2P1; Qns'83; FRCPC; Peds. Ac Staff, William Osler Health System - Brampton Civic Hospital; (905)458-0910; Fax. (905)458-9807.

LEETE, Stanley F; Georgia Quay Surgical Assoc, 103-901 Island Hwy, Campbell River BC V9W 2C2; London (England)'61; MRCS; LRCP; FRCSC; OrthSurg (Spine Surgery). Staff, Campbell River & District General Hospital; Assoc Staff, Port McNeill & District Hospital; Assoc Staff, Port Hardy Hospital; (250)286-0767; fleet@connected.bc.ca.

LEEUWNER, Isabel; 1-11116 100 Ave, Fort St. John BC V1J 1Z8; Stellenbosch (South Africa)'02; MB ChB; (250)787-0010; Fax. (250)787-0018.

LEFAIVRE, Dominique; Hôpital Laval, 2725 ch Sainte-Foy, Quebec QC G1V 4G5; Mon'00; Staff, Hôpital Laval; (418)656-8711

LEFAIVRE, Kelly A; Orthopedic Trauma Office, 3F-2775 Laurel St, Vancouver BC V5Z 1M9; UBC'02; FRCSC; OrthSurg.

LEFAIVRE, Robert; 101-171 6e rue, La Baie QC G7B 0A3; Laval'71; (418)544-3331; Fax. (418)544-7571.

LEFCOE, Daniel H; London HSC-Victoria Campus, PO Box 5010 Stn B AD649-800 Commissioners Rd E, London ON N6A 5W9; Dublin (Ireland)'79; MB ChB; FRCPC; Psy. Staff, London Health Sciences Centre - South Street; Assoc Prof, University of Western Ontario; (519)667-6868; Fax. (519)667-6836.

LEFEBRE, Harry J; Lefebre & Burke Weight Loss &, 100-10655 Southport Rd SW, Calgary AB T2W 4Y1; Alb'73; BMedSci; (403)278-3411; Fax. (403)278-3414; lefebreclinic@telus.net.

LEFEBVRE, Andreanne; CSSS de la Cote-de-Gaspe, 215 boul York O, Gaspe QC G4X 2W2; Mon'08; CCFP; Staff, Centre Hospitalier de Gaspe; (418)368-3301

LEFEBVRE, Anika; CHUM-Hop Notre-Dame, 1560 rue Sherbrooke E, Montreal QC H2L 4M1; Mon'95; CCFP; CCFP(E.M.); Staff, Centre Hospitalier l'Université de Montréal (CHUM) - Hôpital Notre-Dame; (514)890-8000 x26767

LEFEBVRE, Arlette M L; The Hosp For Sick Children, 1157-555 University Ave, Toronto ON M5G 1X8; Tor'70; MRCP; FRCPsy; DCH; FRCPC; Psy (Child Psychiatry). Staff, Holland Bloorview Kids Rehabilitation Hospital; Staff Psy, The Hospital For Sick Children; Assoc Prof, University of Toronto; Langs: Bilingual(French/English); (416)813-7526; Fax. (416)813-5326; arlette.lefebvre@sickkids.ca.

LEFEBVRE, Bernard; Hotel-Dieu de Levis, 143 rue Wolfe, Levis QC G6V 3Z1; Mon'76; FRCPC; NuclearMed. Staff, Hôtel-Dieu de Lévis; (418)835-7121; Fax. (819)820-6420; bernard_lefebvre@ssss.gouv.qc.ca.

LEFEBVRE, Chantal; Centre Med & Prof de Dorval, 667 Ch Bord-Du-Lac Lakeshore, Dorval QC H9S 2B7; Sher'86; (514)633-1510

LEFEBVRE, Charlotte; PO Box 72091 Rpo Glenmore Land, Calgary AB T2V 5H9; Mon'02; CCFP.

LEFEBVRE, Christian; 79 rue Leblanc O, Longueuil QC J4J 1K1; Mon'88; FRCPC; Derm. (450)463-3881; Fax. (450)463-0908.

LEFEBVRE, Claudette; Clinique Med de Repentigny, 205-579A rue Notre-Dame, Repentigny QC J6A 7L4; Mon'84; (450)654-0089

LEFEBVRE, Daniel L; CSSS de Sept-Iles, 45 rue Du Pere-Divet, Sept-Iles QC G4R 3N7; Mon'86; BSc; FRCPC; Anes. Staff, Centre Hospitalier Regional de Sept-Iles; (418)962-9761

LEFEBVRE, Denis; 335-900 Boul Du Seminaire N, St-Jean-Sur-Richel QC J3A 1C3; Mon'78; Peds. (450)349-2701; Fax. (450)349-3012.

LEFEBVRE, Denis; Ctr Hosp Affilie-Enfant-Jesus, 1401 18e rue, Quebec QC G1J 1Z4; Laval'86; Staff, Centre Hospitalier Affilié Universitaire de Québec - Hôpital De L'Enfant Jésus; (418)649-0252

LEFEBVRE, Dennis C; Royal Alexandra Hosp, 541CSC-10240 Kingsway NW, Edmonton AB T5H 3V9; UBC'07; EmergMed. Staff, Royal Alexandra Hospital; (780)735-4442

LEFEBVRE, Diane; CSSS du Lac-Temiscamingue, 22 rue Notre-Dame N, Ville-Marie QC J9V 1W8; Mon'97; Staff, CSSS du Témiscamingue; (819)629-2420

LEFEBVRE, Francine; Hôpital Ste-Justine, 3175 ch Cote-Sainte-Catherine, Montreal QC H3T 1C5; Mon'73; FAAP; FRCPC; Peds (Neonatology). Ac Staff Peds, Hôpital Ste-Justine; Asst Prof Peds, Universite de Montreal; (514)345-4788; Fax. (514)345-7725; francine.lefebvre.2@umontreal.ca.

LEFEBVRE, Francine; Clinique Med Legendre, 201-1650 av Jules-Verne, Quebec QC G2G 2R5; Laval'97; Staff, Hôtel-Dieu de Lévis; Langs: English; (418)872-5600

LEFEBVRE, Francois; CSSS de Chicoutimi, 305 rue Saint-Vallier, Chicoutimi QC G7H 5H6; Laval'94; OrthSurg (Musculoskeletal). Staff, Complexe hospitalier de la Sagamie; (418)541-1000

LEFEBVRE, Genevieve; 584 Riverbend Square NW PO Box 21152 Rpo Terwillegar, Edmonton AB T6R 2V4; Mon'79; Psy. Staff, University of Alberta Hospital; Staff, University of Alberta.

LEFEBVRE, Guy R B; La Loche Health Centre, PO Box 1, La Loche SK S0M 1G0; (306)822-3201; Fax. (306)822-2112.

LEFEBVRE, Guylaine G; St Michael's Hosp, 30 Bond St, Toronto ON M5B 1W8; Ott'85; FACOG; FRCSC; ObstGyn (Gynecological Surgery). Chief ObstGyn, St Michael's Hospital; Assoc Prof ObstGyn, University of Toronto; Langs: Bilingual(French/English); (416)864-5384; Fax. (416)864-6073; lefebvreg@smh.ca.

LEFEBVRE, Helene; Clinique Med Du Quartier Latin, 905 boul Rene-Levesque E, Montreal QC H2L 5B1; Mon'79; CCFP; Physician, Clinique Morgentaler; (514)285-5500; Fax. (514)285-2226; lefebvrelapointe@videotron.ca.

LEFEBVRE, Jean; Clinique Drs Lefevbre et Tousi, 513 5e Av, Grand-Mere QC G9T 2M5; Laval'78; Staff, Centre Lafleche Grand-Mere; Physician, Domaine Forestier Stone-Consolidated Inc; (819)533-5721; Fax. (819)533-5337.

LEFEBVRE, Jean-Claude; Ctr Hosp Affilie-Enfant-Jesus, 1401 18e rue, Quebec QC G1J 1Z4; Laval'04; FRCPC; IntMed; Critical Care Medicine (P.Q.). Staff, Centre Hospitalier Affilié Universitaire de Québec - Hôpital De L'Enfant Jésus; (418)649-0252

LEFEBVRE, Jean-Francois; CSSS de la Cote-De-Gaspe, 215 boul De York O, Gaspe QC G4X 2W2; Mon'02; CCFP; Staff, Centre Hospitalier de Gaspe; (418)368-6663; Fax. (418)368-5358.

LEFEBVRE, Jeanne M J; Scarborough Hosp-General Div, 3050 Lawrence Ave E, Scarborough ON M1P 2V5; Wes'86; FRCPC; IntMed. Staff, The Scarborough Hospital - General Campus; (416)438-2911

LEFEBVRE, Jocelyn; Clinique Med Lariviere, 423 av Lariviere, Rouyn-Noranda QC J9X 4H9; Sher'84; Staff, Centre Hospitalier Rouyn-Noranda; Universite de Sherbrooke; Langs: English; (819)762-4004

LEFEBVRE, Jonathan; UMF-CLSC du Marigot, 1351 boul des Laurentides, Laval QC H7M 2Y2; Mon'09; CCFP; (450)668-1804; Fax. (450)668-1507.

LEFEBVRE, Josee; Polyclinique Ile-Des-Soeurs, 2010 boul Rene Levesque, Verdun QC H3E 1Z7; Mon'84; FRCSC; ObstGyn. Staff Gyn, CSSS de Dorval-Lachine-Lasalle; Staff Gyn, St Mary's Hospital Centre; Langs: Bilingual(French/English); (514)767-2683; Fax. (514)767-7351; lefebvrejosee@gmail.com.

LEFEBVRE, Julie; CSSS Pierre Boucher, 1333 boul Jacques-Cartier E, Longueuil QC J4M 2A5; Sher'98; FRCPC; Psy (General Adult Psychiatry). Staff, Centre Hospitalier Pierre Boucher; (450)468-8401 x2426; Fax. (450)468-8403.

LEFEBVRE, Kevin L; 589 West Gore St, Stratford ON N5A 1L4; Ott'98; BSc; FRCSC; GenSurg (Endoscopy). Staff, Stratford General Hospital - Huron Perth Healthcare Alliance; (519)273-4100 x5; Fax. (519)273-3208; klefebvremd@hotmail.com.

LEFEBVRE, Leon A J; Associate Med Clinic, 25 St Michael St, St. Albert AB T8N 1C7; Alb'81; Head Family Pract & RehabMed, Sturgeon Community Hospital; (780)458-1234; Fax. (780)460-7941.

LEFEBVRE, Lisa G; Addiction & Mental Hlth-ARF, 33 Russell St, Toronto ON M5S 2S1; McG'03; CCFP; Staff, Centre for Addiction & Mental Health (CAMH) - Russell Street Site; Staff, St Joseph's Health Centre; Lecturer, University of Toronto; (416)535-8501 x6019

LEFEBVRE, Manon; Centre Med Laval, 1110 boul Vanier, Laval QC H7C 2R8; Mon'87; (450)661-2521; Fax. (450)661-7193.

LEFEBVRE, Marc; CSSS du Nord de Lanaudière, 1000 boul Sainte-Anne, St-Charles-Brromee QC J6E 6J2; Sher'94; FRCPC; Psy. Staff, Centre Hospitalier Régional de Lanaudière; Langs: English; (450)834-5407; Fax. (450)834-5400.

LEFEBVRE, Marie-Claude; 5689 boul Rosemont, Montreal QC H1T 2H1; Mon'94; CCFP; Staff, Hopital Maisonneuve-Rosemont; Staff Teacher, Universite de Montreal; Langs: English; (514)252-3400 x4513; Fax. (514)252-3854.

LEFEBVRE, Marie-Eve; Clinique Med Les Gres, RR 1 104-190 rue Saint-Honore, St-Etienne-de-Gres QC G0X 2P0; Sher'05; (819)535-6512

LEFEBVRE, Marie-Pierre; CSSS du Nord de Lanaudière, 1000 boul Sainte-Anne, St-Charles-Brromee QC J6E 6J2; Mon'97; Staff, Centre Hospitalier Régional de Lanaudière; (450)759-8222; marie-pierre.lefebvre@ssss.gouv.qc.ca.

LEFEBVRE, Marieve; CSSS de Saint-Jerome, 290 rue de Montigny, Saint-Jerome QC J7Z 5T3; Mon'08; CCFP; Staff, Hôtel-Dieu de Saint-Jérôme; (450)432-2777

LEFEBVRE, Martin; CSSS de Rivière-de-Loup, 75 rue Saint-Henri, Riviere-Du-Loup QC G5R 2A4; Laval'88; IntMed. Staff, Centre Hospitalier Regional du Grand-Portage; (418)862-1000; Fax. (418)868-1059.

LEFEBVRE, Martin; Clinique Familiale, 13555 boul Lacroix, Saint-Georges QC G5Y 1P1; Laval'76; (418)288-8001

LEFEBVRE, Martine; CSST Direction Reg de Quebec, CP 4900 Succ Terminus 425 rue du Pont, Quebec QC G1K 7S6; Laval'89; (418)266-4000

LEFEBVRE, Maude; Hydro Place Bldg, 700 University Ave, Toronto ON M5G 1Z5; Mon'07; MedGenetics.

LEFEBVRE, Patrick; Hop Charles LeMoyne, 3120 boul Taschereau, Greenfield Park QC J4V 2H1; Mon'97; Staff, Hopital Charles LeMoyne; (450)466-5000

LEFEBVRE, Pierre D; Hop Maisonneuve-Rosemont, 5415 boul de l'Assomption, Montreal QC H1T 2M4; Laval'82; ABR; RadOncol. Staff, Hopital Maisonneuve-Rosemont; Universite de Montreal; (514)252-3425; Fax. (514)252-3556.

LEFEBVRE, Richard T; Clinique Med de Lambton, 230A rue Du College, Lambton QC G0M 1H0; Laval'75; (418)486-7480

LEFEBVRE, Sebastien; CSSS de Saint-Jerome, 290 rue de Montigny, Saint-Jerome QC J7Z 5T3; Laval'04; FRCPC; AnatPath. Staff, Hôtel-Dieu de Saint-Jérôme; (450)432-2777

LEFEBVRE, Sebastien; CSSS de Chicoutimi, 305 rue Saint-Vallier, Chicoutimi QC G7H 5H6; Sher'07; CCFP; CCFP(E.M.); Staff, Complexe hospitalier de la Sagamie; (418)541-1088; Fax. (418)541-1129.

LEFEBVRE, Sonia; CSSSG-Hop de Gatineau, CP 2000 succ Bureau-Chef 909 boul la Verendrye O, Gatineau QC J8P 7H2; Mon'94; FRCPC; IntMed; Gastroent. Staff, Hôpital de Gatineau; (819)561-8100

LEFEBVRE, Stephane; GMF Centre Med du Parc, 101-84 rue Court, Granby QC J2G 4Y5; Laval'90; Staff, Centre Hospitalier de Granby; (450)375-1161; Fax. (450)375-7740.

LEFEBVRE, Veronique; CHUQ-Hotel-Dieu de Quebec, 11 Cote du Palais, Quebec QC G1R 2J6; Laval'04; FRCPC; AnatPath. Staff, Centre Hospitalier Universitaire de Québec (CHUQ) - Siege Social; (418)691-5233

LEFEBVRE, Yves A; Clarence-Rockland Fam Hlth Team, 2741 rue Chamberland, Rockland ON K4K 0B4; Ott'94; CCFP; CCFP(E.M.); FCFP; Staff, Montfort Hospital; (613)446-7677; Fax. (613)446-5737.

LEFEL, Oleg; Yarmouth Reg Hosp, 304C-60 Vancouver St, Yarmouth NS B5A 2P5; Riga (Latvia)'87; GenSurg. Staff, Yarmouth Regional Hospital; (902)881-3202

LEFEUVRE, Philip A; Carboner Gen Hosp, 86 Highroad South, Carbonear NL A1Y 1A4; Dal'72; Staff, Carbonear General Hospital.

LEFEVRE, Alain; Dir de la Sante Publique-Mtl, 1301 rue Sherbrooke E, Montreal QC H2L 1M3; Bordeaux (France)'77; (514)528-2400

LEFEVRE, Gerald R; Physician Anes Services, 303-400 Tache Ave, Winnipeg MB R2H 3C3; Sask'77; FRCPC; EmergMed; Anes. Staff, Health Sciences Centre; Staff, St Boniface General Hospital; (204)233-3413; Fax. (204)233-9763.

LEFEVRE, Kim M; 303-3320 Richter St, Kelowna BC V1W 4V5; Sask'85; FRCSC; Neursurg (Spine Surgery). (250)763-2782; Fax. (250)763-2912; kimlefevre@shaw.ca.

LEFKO-SINGH, Karen J; CASA Center, 10645 63 Ave NW, Edmonton AB T6H 1P7; Alb'93; FRCPC; Psy. Staff, Glenrose Rehabilitation Hospital; (780)438-0011

LEFKOWITZ, A Charles J; K403-650 Sammon Ave, East York ON M4C 5M5; Tor'79; FRCPC; IntMed; Cardiol. Ac Staff Cardiol, Toronto East General Hospital Inc; Att Staff, St Michael's Hospital; Asst Prof, University of Toronto; (416)778-0000; Fax. (416)778-5852.

LEFKOWITZ, Jack M; North Med Centre, 303-7131 Bathurst St, Thornhill ON L4J 7Z1; Tor'83; CCFP; Ac Staff, North York General Hospital - Branson Division; Physician, Sports Clinic; (905)731-5554; Fax. (905)709-7722.

LEFORT, Louise A; Canadian Med Protective Assoc, 875 Carling Ave, Ottawa ON K1S 5P1; Mon'75; BSc(Hon); FCFP; CGPP; CCFP; CCFP(E.M.); FCFP; Staff, Canadian Medical Protective Association; Vol. Pt-Time Staff, University of Ottawa; Langs: Bilingual(French/English); (613)725-2000; louise.lefort@ontariomd.ca.

LEFORT, Pierre; CSSS de la Vallée de l'Or, 725 6e rue, Val-d'Or QC J9P 3Y1; Mon'68; Gastroent (P.Q.). Staff, Centre Hospitalier de Val d'Or; (819)825-6711; Fax. (819)825-5624.

LEFRANCOIS, Daniel P; CSSS Pierre Boucher, 1333 boul Jacques-Cartier E, Longueuil QC J4M 2A5; Mon'80; EmergMed (P.Q.). Emergency Medicine, Centre Hospitalier Pierre Boucher; Med Dir EMS, Ministry of Health & Social Services-Quebec; Langs: Bilingual(English/French); Bilingual(French/English); (450)468-8111; daniel.lefrancois@msss.gouv.qc.ca.

LEFRANCOIS, Katleen; Centre Med De Beauport, 737 av Royale, Quebec QC G1E 1Z1; Laval'85; LMCC; Langs: Bilingual(French/English); (418)667-7114; Fax. (418)667-5843.

LEFRANCOIS, Nil; Centre Med Du Beauport, 737 av Royale, Quebec QC G1E 1Z1; Laval'71; (418)667-7114; Fax. (418)667-5843.

LEFRANCOIS, Tina I; Queen Elizabeth II HSC-Halifax, 4520-1796 Summer St, Halifax NS B3H 3A7; Wes'07; FRCSC; OrthSurg. Staff, Queen Elizabeth II Health Sciences Centre - Halifax Infirmary Site; (902)473-6156; Fax. (902)473-3563.

LEFSON, Michael A; Ctr Hosp Reg Chisasibi CP 250, Chisasibi QC J0M 1E0; McG'89; CCFP; FCFP; Staff, Cree Board of Health & Social Services James Bay; (819)855-9001 x4002; Fax. (819)855-2867; mikelefson@hotmail.com.

LEGA, Iliana C; Women's College Hosp, 4F-76 Grenville St, Toronto ON M5S 1B6; Wes'04; FRCPC; IntMed; Endocrin&Metab. (416)323-6013

LEGARE, Alain; CSSS du Sud de Lanaudière, 911 montee des Pionniers, Terrebonne QC J6V 2H2; Sher'89; GenSurg. Staff, Centre Hospitalier Pierre le Gardeur; (450)654-7525; Fax. (450)585-5939.

LEGARE, Carole; Health Canada-Tunney's Pasture, AL 0701A-200 Tunney's Pasture, Ottawa ON K1A 0K9; Ott'86; BSc(Hon); MCFP; LMCC; CCFP; Langs: French; (613)946-6506; Fax. (613)954-2354; carole.legare@hc-sc.gc.ca.

LEGARE, Denis; Clinique Med Saint-Louis, 220-3165 ch Saint-Louis, Quebec QC G1W 4R4; Laval'83; FRCSC; ObstGyn. Staff, Centre Hospitalier Affilié Universitaire de Québec - Hôpital du St-Sacrement; (418)653-1970; Fax. (418)653-9956.

LEGARE, France; CHUQ-St-Francois D'Assise, 10 rue de l'Espinay, Quebec QC G1L 3L5; Laval'88; PhD; CCFP; FCFP; Ac Member, Centre Hospitalier Universitaire De Québec - Pavillon De St-françois-d'assise; Clin Prof, Université Laval; (418)525-4351; Fax. (418)525-4322; france.legare@mfa.ulaval.ca.

LEGARE, Genevieve; CSSS Haut-Richelieu-Rouville, 920 boul du Seminaire N, St-Jean-sur-Richel QC J3A 1B7; Mon'92; FRCSC; GenSurg. Staff, Hôpital du Haut-Richelieu; (450)359-5000 x5234; Fax. (450)359-5251.

LEGARE, Jean-Francois; Maritime Heart Center, 2269-1796 Summer St, Halifax NS B3H 3A7; McG'95; FRCSC; CardSurg. Assoc Prof Surg, Dalhousie University; Langs: English; (902)473-7597; Fax. (902)473-4448; jean.legare@cdha.nshealth.ca.

LEGARE, Jean-Jacques; Polyclinique St-Eustache, 75 rue Grignon, St-Eustache QC J7P 4J2; Mon'76; Staff Obst, Hôpital de Saint-Eustache; (450)472-0116; Fax. (450)473-1916.

LEGARE, Louise; Clin Med de la Cite, 150-175 rue de la Visitation, St-Charles-Brromee QC J6E 4N4; Mon'84; Staff, Centre Hospitalier Régional de Lanaudière; Gen Med, CHSLD Le Chateau; (450)759-1444; Fax. (450)759-2036.

LEGARE, Louise; Clinique Med Saint-Marc, 1295 boul Saint-Sacrement, Shawinigan QC G9N 3M8; Laval'78; (819)539-2999; Fax. (819)539-0078.

LEGARE, Lyne; Niagara H System-G Niagara, PO Box 1018 Stn Main 5546 Portage St, Niagara Falls ON L2E 6X2; Mon'00; FRCPC; DiagRad. Staff, Niagara Health System - Greater Niagara General Site; Langs: English; (905)358-4937; Fax. (905)358-4908; lyne.legare@hotmail.com.

LEGARE, Marie-Christine; CHUS-Hop Fleurimont, 3001 12e av N, Sherbrooke QC J1H 5N4; Sher'04; FRCPC; Psy. Staff, Centre Hospitalier Universitaire de Sherbrooke-Hopital Fleurimont; (819)346-1110 x13185

LEGARE, Marie-Eve; Ctr Hosp Affilie-St-Sacrement, 1050 ch Sainte-Foy, Quebec QC G1S 4L8; Laval'04; CSPQ; FRCSC; Ophth. Staff, Centre Hospitalier Affilié Universitaire de Québec - Hôpital du St-Sacrement; (418)682-7680

LEGARE, Martin; Hop Maisonneuve-Rosemont, 5415 boul de l'Assomption, Montreal QC H1T 2M4; Laval'82; FRCPC; IntMed; Critical Care Medicine (P.Q.); Respir. Staff Pneumology & Intensive Care, Hopital Maisonneuve-Rosemont; Universite de Montreal; (514)252-3822; Fax. (514)252-3434; martinlegare@videotron.ca.

LEGASPI, Ofelia; Langley Mental Health Centre, 305-20300 Fraser Hwy, Langley BC V3A 4E6; Manila (Philippines)'62; Langs: Tagalog; (604)514-7940

LEGASSIE, Jenny M; St Joseph's Healthcare, 50 Charlton Ave E, Hamilton ON L8N 4A6; Dal'04; FRCPC; IntMed (Palliative Medicine). Staff, St Joseph's Healthcare - Charlton Campus; (905)522-1155

LEGAULT, Catherine; UMF Legardeur, 135 boul Claude-David, Repentigny QC J6A 1N6; Mon'09; Staff, Centre Hospitalier Pierre le Gardeur; (450)654-2911

LEGAULT, Christian; CSSS Pierre Boucher, 1333 boul Jacques-Cartier E, Longueuil QC J4M 2A5; Sher'98; Cardiol; IntMed. Staff, Centre Hospitalier Pierre Boucher; (450)468-8111

LEGAULT, Claude; COOP Sante TemiscaVie, 19 rue Dollard, Ville-Marie QC J9V 1L1; Laval'92; Staff, CSSS du Témiscamingue; (819)622-2773; Fax. (819)622-0441; claude_legault@ssss.gouv.qc.ca.

LEGAULT, Danielle; Clinique Med l'Actuel, 1130-1001 boul De Maisonneuve, Montreal QC H2L 4P9; Mon'94; CCFP; Langs: English; (514)524-1001; Fax. (514)524-3831.

LEGAULT, Dominic; CSSS du Lac des deux Montagnes, 520 boul Arthur-Sauve, Saint-Eustache QC J7R 5B1; Sher'08; CCFP; Staff, Hôpital de Saint-Eustache; (450)473-6811

LEGAULT, Jean-Pierre J G; Centre Med de Maniwaki, 163 rue des Oblats, Maniwaki QC J9E 1G4; Ott'82; Physician, Royal Canadian Mounted Police; (819)449-5583

LEGAULT, Jean-Pierre; 310 rte de Sainte-Beatrix RR 2, St-Alphonse-Rodrig QC J0K 1W0; Mon'80; Assoc Staff, Centre Hospitalier Régional de Lanaudière; (450)883-0711; Fax. (450)883-0712.

LEGAULT, Kimberly J; 187 Hughson St S, Hamilton ON L8N 2B6; Wes'07; FRCPC; IntMed; Rheum. (905)528-1123

LEGAULT, Laurent; MUHC-Montreal Children's Hosp, C 244-2300 rue Tupper, Montreal QC H3H 1P3; Mon'84; FRCPC; Peds (Diabetology); Endocrin&Metab. Staff, McGill University Health Centre - Montreal Children's Hospital; Universite de Montreal; Asst Prof Peds, McGill University; (514)412-4400 x22864; Fax. (514)412-4405.

LEGAULT, Louis; Carrefour Med Vallee Richelieu, 665 boul Sir-Wilfrid-Laurier, Beloeil QC J3G 4J1; Mon'75; (450)467-0088; Fax. (450)467-4938.

LEGAULT, Louis; 4110 av d'Oxford, Montreal QC H4A 2Y4; Mon'78; LMCC; Psy (Adult Psychiatry). Langs: Bilingual(French/English); (514)827-4122; louislegault@hotmail.com.

LEGAULT, Louis; CHUM-Hop St-Luc, 1058 rue Saint-Denis, Montreal QC H2X 3J4; Mon'83; FRCPC; IntMed; Nephrol. Nephrol, Centre Hospitalier l'Université De Montréal (CHUM) - Hôpital Saint-luc; adj Prof Med, Universite de Montreal; (514)890-8000 x32588

LEGAULT, Luc; 210 rue Beaudry N CP 422 Succ Bureau-Chef, Joliette QC J6E 3Z9; Mon'75; FRCPC; Peds. (450)759-3030; Fax. (450)759-3038.

LEGAULT, Lucie; Inst Philippe Pinel De Mtl, 10905 boul Henri-Bourassa E, Montreal QC H1C 1H1; Mon'84; Psy. Staff, Institut Philippe-Pinel de Montreal; (514)648-8461; Fax. (514)881-3704.

LEGAULT, M Suzanne E; Trillium Hlth Ctr-Mississauga, 100 Queensway W, Mississauga ON L5B 1B8; Qns'82; BSc(Hon); MSc; FRCPC; Psy. Ac Staff Psy, Trillium Health Centre - West Toronto; Staff, Trillium Health Centre - Mississauga; (905)848-7585

LEGAULT, Marie-Jose; Dir de la Sante Publique-Mtl, 1301 rue Sherbrooke E, Montreal QC H2L 1M3; Mon'83; CCFP; FCFP; (514)528-2400 x3356; Fax. (514)528-2426.

LEGAULT, Mathieu; Hotel-Dieu de Saint-Jerome, 290 rue de Montigny, Saint-Jerome QC J7Z 5T3; Mon'07; CCFP; Staff, Hôtel-Dieu de Saint-Jérôme; (450)431-8266; Fax. (450)431-8244.

LEGAULT, Maurice; Clinique Med Esthe-Novo, 208-620 boul Saint-Jean, Pointe-Claire QC H9R 3K2; Mon'63; (450)694-0160

LEGAULT, Michel; CSSS du Nord de Lanaudière, 1000 boul Sainte-Anne, St-Charles-Brromee QC J6E 6J2; Sher'87; FACS; CSPQ; FRCSC; GenSurg (Vascular Surgery). Staff Vasc & ThorSurg Serv, Centre Hospitalier Régional de Lanaudière; Langs: Bilingual(French/English); (450)759-8222; Fax. (450)759-5308.

LEGAULT, Paul J W; Appletree Med Centre, 3001 Carling Ave, Ottawa ON K2B 7Y6; Ott'85; BSc; FSOGC; FACOG; FRCSC; ObstGyn. Ac Staff, Queensway Carleton Hospital; Consultant, The Ottawa Hospital - Civic Campus; (613)596-2323; Fax. (613)596-6569.

LEGAULT, Pierre; Clinique Med Sainte-Dorothee, 102-1 boul Samson, Laval QC H7X 3S5; Mon'81; Langs: English; (450)689-6334; Fax. (450)689-6339.

LEGAULT, Pierre-Marc B; 716-1849 Yonge St, Toronto ON M4S 1Y2; Ott'03; BSc; MB; CCFP; Langs: Bilingual(French/English); (416)487-3668; Fax. (416)487-8886; pierremarcmd@hotmail.com.

LEGAULT, Serge; CSSS de Laval, 1755 boul Rene-Laennec, Laval QC H7M 3L9; Mon'86; FRCSC; GenSurg. Staff, Hopital de la Cite de la santé; (450)668-1010; Fax. (450)975-5545.

LEGAULT, Sylvie; CHUM-Hotel-Dieu, 3840 rue Saint-Urbain, Montreal QC H2W 1T8; Mon'99; FRCPC; IntMed; Cardiol. Staff, Centre Hospitalier l'Université de Montréal (CHUM) - Hôtel-Dieu; Langs: English; (514)890-8000

LEGAULT, Teisha; Nation River Health Clinic, PO Box 519 494 Fred St, Winchester ON K0C 2K0; Ott'03; BSc; CCFP; Staff Family Emerg Med, Winchester District Memorial Hospital; Langs: French; (613)774-0915; Fax. (613)774-0916.

LEGAULT, Veronique; Family & Primary Care Physicia, 201-1789 Mountain Rd, Moncton NB E1G 1A7; Sher'00; CCFP; Staff, The Moncton Hospital; Langs: Bilingual(French/English); (506)870-2811; Fax. (506)870-2808.

LEGAY, Douglas A; Queens Square, 1802-45 Alderney Dr, Dartmouth NS B2Y 2N6; Dal'84; BSc; Dip SportMed; FRCSC; OrthSurg (Arthroscopic Surgery). Consultant, Stadacona Hospital; Consultant, Halifax Moosehead Hockey Team Major Junior; Asst Prof Div of OrthSurg, Dalhousie University; (902)466-2555; Fax. (902)469-4753; dlegay@eastlink.ca.

LEGENDRE, Andree; Hop Louis-H Lafontaine, 7401 rue Hochelaga, Montreal QC H1N 3M5; Mon'92; FRCPC; Psy. Staff, Hopital Louis-H Lafontaine; (514)251-4000 x3060; Fax. (514)251-1604.

LEGENDRE, Eric; Hotel-Dieu de Levis, 143 rue Wolfe, Levis QC G6V 3Z1; Laval'02; CCFP; CCFP(E.M.); Staff, Hôtel-Dieu de Lévis; (418)835-7121 x6178

LEGENDRE, Luc; CHUQ-St-Francois D'Assise, 10 rue de l'Espinay, Quebec QC G1L 3L5; Laval'80; Anes. Ac Staff, Centre Hospitalier Universitaire De Québec - Pavillon De St-françois-d'assise; (418)525-4340; Fax. (418)525-4434.

LEGENDRE, Robert; CLSC Beauce-Sartigan, 763 14e Av RR 1, La Guadeloupe QC G0M 1G0; Laval'83; (418)459-3441; Fax. (418)459-3142.

LEGER, Alain; Centre Med Normandie, 479 rue Notre-Dame, Saint-Tite QC G0X 3H0; Mon'73; Langs: English; (418)365-3666; Fax. (418)365-3664.

LEGER, Annie; Ctr Hosp Rouyn-Noranda, 4 9e rue, Rouyn-Noranda QC J9X 2B2; Sher'89; Staff, Centre Hospitalier Rouyn-Noranda; (819)764-5131; Fax. (819)764-2900; annie_leger@ssss.gouv.qc.ca.

LEGER, Caroline; Le Mediclub, 6100 av Du Boise, Montreal QC H3S 2W1; Sher'92; FRCPC; Psy. Staff, Centre Hospitalier l'Université De Montréal (CHUM) - Hôpital Saint-luc; (514)739-5646

LEGER, Caroline; Hop Maisonneuve-Rosemont, 5415 boul de l'Assomption, Montreal QC H1T 2M4; Mon'08; Staff, Hopital Maisonneuve-Rosemont; (514)252-3400; Fax. (514)252-3506.

LEGER, Chantal S; Burrard Med Bldg, 440-1144 Burrard St, Vancouver BC V6Z 2A5; Ott'96; FRCPC; IntMed; Hem. Langs: Bilingual(English/French); (604)684-5794; Fax. (604)684-5705.

LEGER, Christian; CLSC de Bedford, GD 34 rue Saint-Joseph, Bedford QC J0J 1A0; Mon'90; Staff, Hôpital Brome-Missisquoi-Perkins; (450)248-4321

LEGER, Claude; Clinique Radiol de Valleyfield, 521 boul Du Havre, Salaber-de-Valleyf QC J6S 4Z5; Mon'69; FRCPC; DiagRad (Angioradiology). Radiologiste, Centre Hospitalier Régional du Suroît; ac Membre, Barrie Memorial Hospital; Staff, Clinique Radiologique de Valleyfield; Langs: Bilingual(English/French); (450)371-6444; Fax. (450)371-5062; crv@cgocable.ca.

LEGER, Claude; CSSS de la Haute-Cote-Nord, RR 1 4 rue de l'Hopital, Les Escoumins QC G0T 1K0; Mon'85; (418)233-2931

LEGER, Daniel; CSSS Institut Universitaire, 500-500 rue Murray, Sherbrooke QC J1G 2K6; Mon'78; (819)780-2220 x47048

LEGER, Daniel; Thames Valley FHT-Strathroy Me, 74 Front St E, Strathroy ON N7G 1Y7; Ott'06; CCFP.

LEGER, Francine; CSSS Haut-Richelieu-Rouville, 920 boul du Seminaire N, St-Jean-sur-Richel QC J3A 1B7; Sher'87; Ac Staff Gen Med, Hôpital du Haut-Richelieu; Langs: English; (450)359-5000

LEGER, Francine; Clinique Med Du Quartier Latin, 905 boul Rene-Levesque E, Montreal QC H2L 5B1; Mon'81; FCFP; Clin Prof Family Med, Universite de Montreal; Langs: Bilingual(French/English); (514)285-5500; Fax. (514)285-2226.

LEGER, Gabriel R; 185 Av Universite, Moncton NB E1C 5K4; Lille (France)'66; FRCPC; Peds. Staff, Dr Georges-L-Dumont University Hospital Centre; Staff, The Moncton Hospital; (506)857-2027; Fax. (506)860-6448.

LEGER, Roland; 208-260 Dalhousie St, Ottawa ON K1N 7E4; Mon'82; (613)241-0888

LEGER, John; Sussex Health Centre, 75 Leonard Dr, Sussex NB E4E 2P7; Dal'73; FRCPC; DiagRad. Staff, Sussex Health Centre; (506)432-3225

LEGER, Julie; Clinique Med Vents et Marees, 201-391 av Brochu, Sept-Iles QC G4R 4S7; Sher'05; CCFP; Staff, Centre Hospitalier Regional de Sept-Iles; Langs: Bilingual(French/English); (418)962-9761; julieleger@hotmail.com.

LEGER, Paul S; Dixon Med Centre, 201-581 Davis Dr, Newmarket ON L3Y 2P6; Tor'87; CCFP; FCFP; (905)853-3103; Fax. (905)853-3196.

LEGER, Richard; Lasik MD Inc, 900-734 7 Ave SW, Calgary AB T2P 3P8; Sher'92; FRCSC; Ophth (Refractive Surgery). Langs: Bilingual(English/French); (403)539-2020

LEGER, Roger J; 115 Pacific Ave, Moncton NB E1E 2G2; Ott'69; Ac Staff, The Moncton Hospital; (506)857-9277; Fax. (506)854-7961.

LEGER, Yves A; Public Health Services, PO Box 5001 Stn Lcd 1 81 Albert St, Moncton NB E1C 8R3; Sher'02; FRCPC; CommunMed. Staff, Vitalité Health Network Public Health Office Moncton; Langs: Bilingual(French/English); (506)869-6287; Fax. (506)869-6122.

LEGER, Yves; CSSS des Sources, 475 3e av, Asbestos QC J1T 1X6; Sher'02; CCFP; Staff, CSSS des Sources d'Asbestos; (819)879-7151

LEGER-BERNIER, Monique; CSSS de la Mitis, 800 av du Sanatorium, Mont-Joli QC G5H 3L6; Sher'88; CCFP; FCFP; Staff, CSSS de la Mitis; (418)775-7261 x3100; Fax. (418)775-6487.

LEGER-NOLET, Celine N; Temiskaming Hospital 421 Shepherdson Rd, New Liskeard ON P0J 1P0; Ott'96; FRCPC; IntMed (Echocardiography). Assoc Staff, Englehart & District Hospital Inc; Ac Staff, Temiskaming Hospital; Langs: French; (705)647-1088 x2434; Fax. (705)647-1065.

LEGERE, Janice M; 200 Terrace Hill St, Brantford ON N3R 1G9; McM'95; Hospitalist, The Brant Community Healthcare System - Brantford General Hospital Site; Med Dir, John Noble Home for Aged; Langs: French; (519)751-5544 x2268; legja@bchsys.org.

LEGERE, Paul W; Yarmouth Reg Health Centre, 60 Vancouver St, Yarmouth NS B5A 2P5; Dal'89; Ac Staff EmergMed, Yarmouth Regional Hospital; (902)742-3541

LEGG, Karen K; UBC Hospital, M334-2211 Wesbrook Mall, Vancouver BC V6T 2B5; McG'91; Dip SportMed; Vis Staff Privil, Vancouver General Hospital - Centennial Pavillion; Vis Staff Privil, UBC Hospital - Koerner Pavillion; (604)822-7011

LEGGATT, Suzanne; 304-4420 Chatterton Way, Victoria BC V8X 5J2; UBC'95; BSc; MSc; CCFP; FCFP; Staff, Victoria General Hospital; (250)727-9664; Fax. (250)727-9445; suzilegg@telus.net.

LEGGATT, W Ker; Queen Square Doctors FHT, 201-366 Main St N, Brampton ON L6V 1P8; Tor'75; CCFP; FCFP; Ac Staff/Corp Chief FamilyMed, William Osler Health System - Brampton Civic Hospital; Lecturer Family & Commun Med, University of Toronto; Clinical Asst Prof Family Med, McMaster University; (905)455-1331; Fax. (905)455-5498.

LEGGE, A Murray; Orillia Soldiers' Mem Hosp, 170 Colborne St W, Orillia ON L3V 2Z3; Tor'75; FRCPC; DiagRad. Staff, Orillia Soldiers' Memorial Hospital; (705)325-2201

LEGGE, Rebecca J; PO Box 50030 Rpo South Slope, Burnaby BC V5J 5G3; UBC'04; CCFP.

LEGGETT, Alison A; Rockyview Gen Hosp, 7007 14 St SW, Calgary AB T2V 1P9; Tor'94; CCFP; Staff, Rockyview General Hospital; (403)619-2373

LEGGETT, Peter J; 10-1423 Upper Ottawa St, Hamilton ON L8W 3J6; McM'84; CCFP; FCFP; Med Dir, Grace Villa Nursing Home; (905)575-0228; Fax. (905)575-3384.

LEGIEHN, Gerald M; Vancouver Gen Hosp, 855 12th Ave W, Vancouver BC V5Z 1M9; Man'90; DABR; LMCC; FRCPC; DiagRad (Interventional Radiology). Staff Radiol, Vancouver General Hospital - Centennial Pavillion; Asst Prof, University of British Columbia; (604)875-4111 x63711; Fax. (604)875-4723; gerald@telus.net.

LEGLER, Christine M; MUHC-Montreal Gen Hosp, A7 130-1650 av Cedar, Montreal QC H3G 1A4; McG'89; FRCPC; IntMed; MedOncol. Staff, McGill University Health Centre - Montreal General Campus; Langs: French; (514)934-8007; Fax. (514)934-8379; christine.legler@muhc.mcgill.ca.

LEGNINI, Veronica M G; Greenwood Med Centre, 10-496 Discovery Ave, Kingston ON K7K 7E9; Tor'08; CCFP; (613)507-7003

LEGRAND, Jacques; 100-400 boul Jean-Lesage, Quebec QC G1K 8W1; Laval'72; Staff, Centre Hospitalier Affilié Universitaire de Québec - Hôpital du St-Sacrement; (418)529-9323

LEGRAND, Jean-Claude; Hop Charles Lemoyne, 3120 boul Taschereau, Greenfield Park QC J4V 2H1; Mon'81; Anes. Staff, Hopital Charles LeMoyne; (450)466-5000; Fax. (450)466-5007.

LEGRAND WESTFALL, Lorraine; Canadian Med Protective Assn, PO Box 8225 Stn T Csc, Ottawa ON K1G 3H7; Mon'81; FRCSC; GenSurg (Breast Oncology). Physician Risk Manager, Canadian Medical Protective Association; Langs: English; French; Fax. (613)725-1300.

LEGRESLEY, Conrad; 206-387 Main St, Shediac NB E4P 2B5; Sher'77; Staff, Dr Georges-L-Dumont University Hospital Centre; (506)533-3008

LEGRESLEY, Lisa B; 302-9200 Mary St, Chilliwack BC V2P 4H6; McM'90; (604)793-8444; Fax. (604)793-8434.

LEGRIS, Celine; 200-900 boul Du Seminaire N, St-Jean-sur-Richel QC J3A 1C3; Laval'88; FRCSC; Ophth. Langs: Bilingual(French/English); (450)348-6155

LEGRIS, Genevieve; CHUQ-Ctr Hosp Univ Laval, 2705 boul Laurier, Quebec QC G1V 4G2; Laval'98; FRCPC; Psy. Staff, Centre Hospitalier Universitaire de Quebec-CHUL; (418)654-2121

LEGROS, Guy; Hop Marie Clarac, 3530 boul Gouin E, Montreal-Nord QC H1H 1B7; Mon'63; GenSurg. Staff, Institut de Cardiologie de Montréal; assoc Dir serv, College des Medecins du Quebec; (514)321-8800 x324

LEGROS, Marie-Florence; Clinique Med Vita-Nor, 6892 boul Gouin E, Montreal-Nord QC H1G 6M2; Port-au-Prince (Haiti)'80; CCFP; Médecin, CSSS Saint-Leonard et Saint-Michel; Médecin, CLSC St-Leonard; Langs: English; Creole; (514)325-7241; Fax. (514)798-0698.

LEGROW, Jennifer L; Family First Medical, 207-496 Topsail Rd, St. John's NL A1E 2C2; Mem'07; CCFP; Clin Asst, Health Sciences Centre.

LEHAN, Anne E; 2-210 Lorraine Ave, Kitchener ON N2B 3T4; McM'86; CCFP; FCFP; (519)570-1223; Fax. (519)570-9367.

LEHMAN, Anna M; BC Women's Hosp & Health Ctre, C234-4500 Oak St, Vancouver BC V6H 3N1; UBC'05; FRCPC; MedGenetics. Staff Adult Metabolic Diseases Clinic, Vancouver General Hospital - Centennial Pavillion; Staff Provincial Medical Genetics Program, BC Women's Hospital & Health Centre; (604)875-2157

LEHMAN, Robert M; Gibsons Med Clinic, 211-1100 Sunshine Coast Hwy, Gibsons BC V0N 1V7; UBC'76; MClSc; CCFP; FCFP; Staff, St Mary's Hospital; Clin Associate Family Med, University of British Columbia; (604)886-2870; Fax. (604)886-9716.

LEHMANN, Carmen; Westglen Med Centre, 108-30 Springborough Blvd SW, Calgary AB T3H 0N9; Cal'89; BScPharm; CCFP; FCFP; Clin Associate, Rockyview General Hospital; Clin Associate, Peter Lougheed Centre; (403)240-2221; Fax. (403)240-4670.

LEHMANN, Christian; Queen Elizabeth II HSC, 1276 South Park St, Halifax NS B3H 2Y9; Berlin (Germany)'91; FRCPC; Anes. Staff Anes, Queen Elizabeth II Health Sciences Centre - Victoria General Site; (902)473-2331

LEHMANN, Francois; Ctr Hosp de Verdun, 4000 boul Lasalle, Verdun QC H4G 2A3; McG'68; CCFP; FCFP; Staff, Centre Hospitalier de Verdun; Dir Family Med, Universite de Montreal; Langs: English; (514)362-1000; Fax. (514)765-7306; francois.lehmann@umontreal.ca.

LEHMANN, Heather C; Dr C W Wiebe Med Centre, 385 Main St, Winkler MB R6W 1J2; Man'06; CCFP; (204)325-4312

LEHMANN, Ordan J; Royal Alexandra Hosp, 2318-10240 Kingsway NW, Edmonton AB T5H 3V9; (United Kingdom)'89; MB BS; PhD; Staff Ophth, Royal Alexandra Hospital; Staff, University of Alberta Hospital; Assoc Prof Ophth & Med Genetics, University of Alberta; (780)735-4720; Fax. (780)735-4969.

LEHNERT, Dominic C; St Joseph's Health Centre, 30 The Queensway, Toronto ON M6R 1B5; Tor'96; FRCPC; IntMed. Staff, St Joseph's Health Centre; (416)530-6573

LEHNERT, Thomas B; 11-679 King George Hwy, Miramichi NB E1V 1N9; Essen (Germany)'84; CCFP; FCFP; Staff, Miramichi Regional Hospital; (506)627-7511

LEHOUILLIER, Philippe; CHUS-Hop Fleurimont, 3001 12e av N, Sherbrooke QC J1H 5N4; Laval'00; FRCPC; MedBiochem. Staff, Centre Hospitalier Universitaire de Sherbrooke-Hopital Fleurimont; (418)723-7851

LEHOUX, Martine; 101-2880 ch des Quatre-Bourgeo, Quebec QC G1V 4X7; Laval'76; Langs: Bilingual(English/French); (418)650-3109; Fax. (418)650-6091; ma.lehoux@sympatico.ca.

LEHOUX, Suzie; Regie l'Assurance Maladie QC, Q044-1125 Grande Allee O, Quebec QC G1S 1E7; Laval'76; Médecin, Regie de l'Assurance Maladie du Quebec; (418)682-5144 x4758; Fax. (418)643-3858.

LEHOUX, Virginie; CLSC Rimouski-Neigette-UMF, 165 rue des Gouverneurs, Rimouski QC G5L 7R2; Laval'04; CCFP; (418)727-5493

LEHUQUET, John B; Abbotsford Reg Hosp & Cancer C, 32900 Marshall Rd, Abbotsford BC V2S 0C2; UBC'78; FCAP; FRCPC; GenPath;CCFP; Staff, Abbotsford Regional Hospital & Cancer Centre; (604)851-4700 x646539

LEHUQUET, Leslie A; Surrey Mem Hosp, 13750 96 Ave, Surrey BC V3V 1Z2; Dal'80; BSc; FRCPC; GenPath;CCFP; Staff, Surrey Memorial Hospital; (604)585-5609

LEHUU, Phung; 1260 rue Sainte-Helene, Longueuil QC J4K 3S6; Montpellier (France)'70; Peds (P.Q.). (450)670-7700; Fax. (450)928-0085.

LEI, Calvin Z H; 108-790 Bay St, Toronto ON M5G 1N8; McG'89; (416)929-1900; Fax. (416)929-7316.

LEI, K K Lourenco; Saunte Medical Clinic, 101-15850 26 Ave, Surrey BC V3S 2N6; (Ireland)'91; MB BCh; BAO; (604)542-7788

LEI, T C Benny; 11-1099 Kingsbury Ave, Winnipeg MB R2P 2P9; Alb'84; Langs: Chinese; Cantonese; (204)697-9214; Fax. (204)697-9213.

LEIA, Allan P; Campbell River & Dist Gen Hosp, 375 2nd Ave, Campbell River BC V9W 3V1; Sask'92; FRCPC; GenPath. Staff, Campbell River & District General Hospital; (250)850-2968

LEIA-STEPHEN, Maureen; 114-436 Lorne St, Kamloops BC V2C 1W3; Sask'81; FRCSC; GenSurg (Phlebology). Staff, Royal Inland Hospital; (250)372-9995; Fax. (250)372-7801.

LEIBEL, Sandra L; Mount Sinai Hosp, 600 University Ave, Toronto ON M5G 1X5; Jagiellonian U (Poland)'06; Staff, Mount Sinai Hospital; (416)596-4200

LEIBEL, Sharon M; Hillsdale Med Clinic, 1380G 23rd Ave, Regina SK S4S 3S5; Sask'83; Ac Staff, Regina General Hospital; Ac Staff, Pasqua Hospital; Member Child Abuse Team, Regina Health District; Clin Asst Teacher, University of Saskatchewan; (306)584-1533; Fax. (306)584-1767.

LEIBEL, Sydney A; Kindercare Paediatrics, 200-491 Eglinton Ave, Toronto ON M5N 1A8; (Australia)'05.

LEIBFRIED, Bryan L; Garden City Family Health Team, 22 Ontario St, St Catharines ON L2R 7M3; Man'90; CCFP; (905)984-5210; Fax. (905)984-5491.

LEIBOVICI, Dalila; 215 rue Dante, Montreal QC H2S 1K2; Bologna (Italy)'75; Staff, Douglas Mental Health University Institute; (514)273-4808

LEIBOVICI, Theodore; 215 rue Dante, Montreal QC H2S 1K2; Bologna (Italy)'75; (514)273-4808

LEIBOVITZ, Neil V; CPM Brampton, 4-2 Kennedy Rd S, Brampton ON L6W 3E1; Tor'86; CCFP; FCFP; Ac Staff, Rouge Valley Health System - Centenary Health Centre Site; (905)458-7377

LEIBOW, Deborah F; 41 Ava Rd, Toronto ON M5P 1Y7; Tor'78; FRCPC; Psy. (416)487-2743

LEIBOW, Stephen R; Park Towers, 125-400 Walmer Rd, Toronto ON M5P 2X7; Tor'78; FRCPC; Psy. (416)967-1871; Fax. (416)488-6087.

LEICHT, Krista K; Alberta Mental Health Board, PO Box 307 Stn Main, Edmonton AB T5J 2J7; Alb'97; Psy (Developmental Delay). Staff, Alberta Hospital Edmonton; Staff, Alberta Mental Health Board; (780)342-5449; leicht@telusplanet.net.

LEICHT, Richard T; Winnipeg Clinic, 425 St Mary Ave, Winnipeg MB R3C 0N2; Tor'83; FRCSC; Ophth (Retina Vitreous Surgery). Asst Prof, University of Manitoba; (204)957-3343; Fax. (204)942-0677.

LEIFER, Randy J; 20 Doctors Lane PO Box 370 Stn Main, King City ON L7B 1A6; Tor'87; Assoc Staff, Mackenzie Richmond Hill Hospital; (905)833-5381; Fax. (905)833-5649; kcma@bigfoot.com.

LEIFSO, Kirk R; Children's Hosp Eastern Ont, 401 Smyth Rd, Ottawa ON K1H 8L1; Cal'08; Peds. Staff, Children's Hospital of Eastern Ontario (CHEO); (416)737-7600

LEIFSO, Lowell R; 100-5500 152 St, Surrey BC V3S 5J9; Tor'83; ASAM; Med Advisor Disablity Award, Workers' Comp Board of BC; (604)232-7022

LEIGH, Clara P; 5-30 Thirteenth St E, Cornwall ON K6H 6V9; McG'09; CCFP; Staff, SCO Health Service - Élisabeth Bruyère Hospital; (613)933-2493

LEIGH, John D; 197 St Clair St, Chatham ON N7L 3J4; Wes'79; Staff, Chatham-Kent Health Alliance; (519)351-6570; Fax. (519)351-2867.

LEIGH, Richard; Health Research Innovation Ctr, 4C62-3280 Hospital Dr NW, Calgary AB T2N 4Z6; Cape Town (South Africa)'87; MB BS; MSc; PhD; FRCPC; IntMed (Respirology). Med Dir, Calgary COPD & Asthma Program; Assoc Prof, University of Calgary; (403)220-8981; Fax. (403)210-7944.

LEIGHL, Natasha B; Univ Hlth Network-Princess M, 5 105-610 University Ave, Toronto ON M5G 2M9; Tor'94; FRCPC; IntMed (Lung Cancer); MedOncol. Staff, Princess Margaret Hospital - University Health Network; Assoc Prof Med, University of Toronto; Langs: Hindi; Punjabi; Spanish; (416)946-4645; Fax. (416)946-6546.

LEIGHTON, Alasdair I M; Phoenix Med Centre, 101-2155 10th Ave, Prince George BC V2M 5J6; UBC'79; FRCPC; DiagRad. (250)563-0635

LEIGHTON, Christopher C; University of Windsor, 401 Sunset Ave, Windsor ON N9B 3P4; Tor'92; FRCPC; RadOncol (Brain Tumors). (519)253-3000

LEIGHTON, Margaret M; 307-5880 Spring Garden Rd, Halifax NS B3H 1Y1; Dal'77; CCFP; FCFP; Court Staff Halifax Infirmary, Queen Elizabeth II Health Sciences Centre - Victoria General Site; Court Staff, IWK Health Centre; (902)425-4990; Fax. (902)422-5243.

LEIGHTON, Ross K; Queen Elizabeth II HSC-Halifax, 4873-1796 Summer St, Halifax NS B3H 3A7; Dal'79; FRCSC; OrthSurg (Arthroplasty). Staff, Queen Elizabeth II Health Sciences Centre - Halifax Infirmary Site; Staff Div of OrthSurg, Queen Elizabeth II Health Sciences Centre - Victoria General Site; Prof Surg, Dalhousie University; (902)473-4035; Fax. (902)473-4490.

LEIGHTON-LANE, Dayna R; Grey Nuns Community Hosp, 1100 Youville Drive West NW, Edmonton AB T6L 5X8; Alb'03; FRCPC; Anes. Staff, Covenant Health - Grey Nuns Community Hospital; (780)735-7020; Fax. (780)735-7279.

LEIPER, Thomas R; Edmonton Mental Health Clinic, 3F-9942 108 St NW, Edmonton AB T5K 2J5; Alb'93; Psy. Staff, Alberta Hospital Edmonton; (780)342-7788; Fax. (780)425-9317.

LEIPOLDT, Carl C P; Victoria Gen Hosp, 1 Hospital Way, Victoria BC V8Z 6R5; Pretoria (South Africa)'93; MB ChB; FRCPC; Anes. Staff, Victoria General Hospital; (250)727-4212

LEIPSIC, Jonathon A; St Paul's Hosp, 1081 Burrard St, Vancouver BC V6Z 1Y6; Man'99; FRCPC; DiagRad. Staff, Providence Health Care - St Paul's Hospital; (604)806-8006

LEIS, Jerome A; Univ Hlth Network-Toronto Gen, 13EN 213-200 Elizabeth St, Toronto ON M5G 2C4; Ott'08; FRCPC; IntMed. Staff, Toronto General Hospital - UHN; (416)340-3505

LEIS, Karen S; Royal University Hosp, 103 Hospital Dr, Saskatoon SK S7N 0W8; Sask'05; FRCPC; Peds. Staff, Royal University Hospital; (306)966-8112

LEISHMAN, David J; Royal Jubilee Hosp, 1952 Bay St, Victoria BC V8R 1J8; McM'85; FRCPC; Psy (Geriatric Psychiatry). Staff/Vice Chief Geriatric Psy, Royal Jubilee Hospital; Staff Psy, Vancouver Island Health Authority; (250)370-8354; dleishman@shaw.ca.

LEISHMAN, Donald M; Port Arthur Health Centre Inc, 194 Court St N, Thunder Bay ON P7A 4V7; Man'74; (807)346-1000; Fax. (807)346-6206.

LEISHMAN, Fraser T; Claresholm Med Centre, PO Box 2050, Claresholm AB T0L 0T0; Alb'08; CCFP; (403)625-4484; Fax. (403)625-3969.

LEISHMAN, Robert G; 108-1410 Mayor Magrath Dr S, Lethbridge AB T1K 2R3; Alb'77; FRCSC; Ophth. (403)320-0700; Fax. (403)320-0091.

LEISHMAN, William R; Family Med Centre, PO Box 460, Picture Butte AB T0K 1V0; Alb'81; CCFP; (403)732-4542; Fax. (403)732-5298.

LEITAO, Darren J; Health Sciences Centre, GB421-820 Sherbrook St, Winnipeg MB R3A 1R9; Sask'97; FRCSC; Otol (Pediatric Otolaryngology). Staff Otolaryngology, Health Sciences Centre; (204)787-3349; Fax. (204)787-1727.

LEITCH, Heather A; Burrard Med Bldg, 440-1144 Burrard St, Vancouver BC V6Z 2A5; UBC'95; FRCPC; IntMed (Hematological Oncology); Hem. Staff Hem, Providence Health Care - St Paul's Hospital; Clin Assoc Prof, University of British Columbia; (604)684-5794; Fax. (604)684-5705.

LEITCH, K Kellie; The Hosp for Sick Children, 555 University Ave, Toronto ON M5G 1X8; Tor'94; MBA; FRCSC; OrthSurg (Pediatric Orthopedics). Staff, The Hospital For Sick Children; Member Parliament Simcoe-Grey, City of Simcoe-Grey; Asst Prof Surg, University of Toronto; (416)813-7654; kellie.leitch@utoronto.ca.

LEITE VIEIRA COSTA, Ricardo; CSSS de Trois-Rivières, 1991 boul du Carmel, Trois-Rivieres QC G8Z 3R9; (Brazil)'93; Staff, CSSS de Trois-Rivières; (819)697-3333

LEITENBERG, Samuel; 545 Eglinton Ave E, Toronto ON M4P 1N7; Tor'74; CCFP; Staff, Sunnybrook Health Sciences Centre; Staff, Humber River Regional Hospital - Keele Street Site; Physician, FMC Canada Ltd.; Teach Staff Family Pract/Lecturer, University of Toronto; (416)482-9533; Fax. (416)482-9535.

LEITER, Lawrence A; 6121Q-61 Queen St E, Toronto ON M5C 2T2; McG'76; FACP; FRCP; FRCPC; IntMed (Academic & Research Practice); Endocrin&Metab. Staff Div of Endocrinology & Metab, St Michael's Hospital; Prof Med & Nutritional Sciences, University of Toronto; (416)867-7441; Fax. (416)867-3696.

LEITH, Diane B; 401-960 Lawrence Ave W, North York ON M6A 3B5; McG'80; Ac Staff, Humber River Regional Hospital - Keele Street Site; Court Staff, Women's College Hospital; (416)256-1150

LEITH, Eric S; 302-331 Sheddon Ave, Oakville ON L6J 1X8; RCS (Ireland)'77; FACP; FAAAI; FRCPC; ClinImmunol&Allergy; IntMed. Ac Staff Med, Women's College Hospital; Ac Staff, Halton Healthcare Services Corporation - Oakville Site; Lecturer, University of Toronto; (905)842-6555

LEITH, Jordan M; Joint Preservation Centre, 2C-2211 Wesbrook Mall, Vancouver BC V6T 2B5; UBC'94; FRCSC; OrthSurg (Arthroscopic Surgery). Staff, UBC Hospital - Koerner Pavillion; Clin Instructor, University of British Columbia; (604)822-5601; Fax. (604)822-1999.

LEITH, Mark G; Medical & Dental Bldg, 510-586 Eglinton Ave E, Toronto ON M4P 1P2; Wes'77; FRCPC; Psy. Staff Teacher, Sunnybrook Health Sciences Centre; Active Teach. Staff, University of Toronto; (416)486-6818

LEITNER, Douglas M; Sage Med Clinic, 101-2210 Main St, Penticton BC V2A 5H8; Sask'91; BSc; Staff Privil, Penticton Regional Hospital; Langs: Bilingual(English/French); (250)492-0990; Fax. (250)492-0992.

LEITNER, Fredric S; Promenade Village Hlth Centre, 3-7700 Bathurst St, Thornhill ON L4J 7Y3; Wes'76; CCFP; Asst Prof, University of Toronto; (905)660-9760

LEIVA, Rene A; SCOHS-Elisabeth Bruyere Hosp, 43 Bruyere St, Ottawa ON K1N 5C8; McG'00; CCFP; Staff, SCO Health Service - Élisabeth Bruyère Hospital; (613)562-4262

LEIVO, Raymond D; Saddle Lake Health Centre, PO Box 160, Saddle Lake AB T0A 3T0; Tor'79; (780)726-3930; Fax. (780)726-3976.

LEJAY, P Sue; 310-6411 Buswell St, Richmond BC V6Y 2G4; UBC'88; (604)278-6838

LEJEUNE, Dominique; Commission des Lesons Prof, 700-900 Pl D'Youville, Quebec QC G1R 3P7; Laval'81; (418)643-5491; Fax. (418)644-8237.

LEJTENYI, M Christine; MUHC-Montreal Children's Hosp, C 510-2300 rue Tupper, Montreal QC H3H 1P3; McG'64; MSc; FRCPC; Peds; ClinImmunol&Allergy (P.Q.). Clin Div of Allergy & Immunization/prog Dir Ped Allergy & Immunology, McGill University Health Centre - Montreal Children's Hospital; Vis Staff, Centre Hospitalier de Val d'Or; adj Prof, McGill University; Langs: English; French; (514)412-4470; Fax. (514)412-4390; christine.lejtenyi@muhc.mcgill.ca.

LEKAS, Poli; Humber River Reg Hosp-Keele St, 2175 Keele St, North York ON M6M 3Z4; Tor'04; FRCPC; IntMed; Nephrol. Staff, Humber River Regional Hospital - Keele Street Site; (416)658-2241

LEKNICKAS, Liuda R; Kipling Med Centre, 6-1570 Kipling Ave, Etobicoke ON M9R 2Y1; Tor'64; Ac Staff, William Osler Health System - Etobicoke General Hospital; (416)247-8400; Fax. (416)247-8400.

LEKOTA, Phuma J; Municipal Med Clinic, PO Box 70, Wakaw SK S0K 4P0; (306)233-4443; Fax. (306)233-4433.

LELACHEUR, Ruth C; PO Box 818, Middleton NS B0S 1P0; Dal'69.

LELIEVRE, Andre; Hop Du Sacre-Coeur De Mtl, 5400 boul Gouin O, Montreal QC H4J 1C5; Laval'78; Psy. Staff, Hôpital du Sacre-Coeur de Montréal; (514)338-2070; Fax. (514)338-3187.

LELIEVRE, Rejean; CSSS de Chicoutimi, 305 rue Saint-Vallier, Chicoutimi QC G7H 5H6; Laval'00; FRCPC; Anes. Staff, Complexe hospitalier de la Sagamie; (418)541-1000

LELLOUCHE, Francois; Hôpital Laval, 2725 ch Sainte-Foy, Quebec QC G1V 4G5; Paris (France)'99; Critical Care Medicine (P.Q.). Staff, Hôpital Laval; (418)656-8711

LELOKA, Clare M; Four Rivers Med Clinic, 647 Broadway, Winnipeg MB R3C 0X2; Witwatersrand (South Africa)'87; Staff, Seven Regions Health Centre.

LEM, Marcus E; 102-34194 Marshall Rd, Abbotsford BC V2S 5E4; McM'96; FRCPC; CommunMed. (604)556-5070

LEM, Melissa M P; U of Toronto-Health Services, 214 College St, Toronto ON M5T 2Z9; Ott'05; CCFP; (416)978-8030

LEM, Selina L; 3-2630 Kipling Ave, Etobicoke ON M9V 4B9; Qns'99; FRCPC; DiagRad. (416)748-8434

LEMAIRE, Celine; Hop Maisonneuve-Rosemont, 5415 boul de l'Assomption, Montreal QC H1T 2M4; Mon'86; RadOncol (P.Q.). Ac Staff, Hopital Maisonneuve-Rosemont; Langs: English; (514)252-3425; Fax. (514)252-3556.

LEMAIRE, Daniel; GMF Centre de santé, 3745 rue Georges-Couture, Drummondville QC J2B 7P4; Mon'74; ac Staff, Hôpital Sainte-croix; (819)477-2231; Fax. (819)477-1122.

LEMAIRE, David; 420 Champlain St, Dieppe NB E1A 1P3; Sher'95; FRCSC; Otol. Staff Otol, The Moncton Hospital; Otolaryngology, Dr Georges-L-Dumont University Hospital Centre; Langs: Bilingual(French/English); (506)204-4448; Fax. (506)389-4321.

LEMAIRE, Frédéric B; Hop Charles Lemoyne, 3120 boul Taschereau, Greenfield Park QC J4V 2H1; Mon'09; CCFP; CCFP(E.M.); Staff, Hopital Charles LeMoyne; (450)466-5000

LEMAIRE, Jane B; Health Sciences Centre, 3330 Hospital Dr NW, Calgary AB T2N 4N1; Ott'86; FRCPC; IntMed. Staff Med, Foothills Medical Centre; Clin Prof, University of Calgary; Langs: English; French; (403)220-4506; Fax. (403)283-6151.

LEMAIRE, Jean-Rene; Ctr Hosp Affilie-Enfant-Jesus, 1401 18e rue, Quebec QC G1J 1Z4; Laval'66; IntMed (P.Q.). Ac Staff, Centre Hospitalier Affilié Universitaire de Québec - Hôpital De L'Enfant Jésus; (418)649-0252 x3575

LEMAIRE, Julie; GMF Centre de santé, 3745 rue Georges-Couture, Drummondville QC J2B 7P4; Sher'06; CCFP; (819)477-2231

LEMAITRE, Jean-Luc; Ctr Hosp de Matane, 333 rue Thibault, Matane QC G4W 2W5; Staff, Centre Hospitalier de Matane; (418)562-3135

LEMAITRE, John P; 110-245 Columbia St E, New Westminster BC V3L 3W4; Edinburgh (Scotland)'07; MB ChB; (604)522-5727

LEMAITRE-AUGER, Michele; Clinique Med des Laurentides, 1950 boul du Cure-Labelle, Saint-Jerome QC J7Y 1S1; Mon'76; (450)432-1442; Fax. (450)432-6814.

LEMARQUAND, Janique; Clinique Med En Route, F5-895 rue de la Gauchetiere O, Montreal QC H3B 4G1; Sher'88; CCFP; Staff, CSSS de Dorval-Lachine-Lasalle; (514)954-1444; Fax. (514)954-1619.

LEMAY, Andre; CHUQ-St-Francois D'Assise, 10 rue de l'Espinay, Quebec QC G1L 3L5; Laval'68; PhD; MedBiochem (P.Q.); Endocrin (P.Q.) (Infertility). Dir Endocrinology & Reproduction Unit, Centre Hospitalier Universitaire De Québec - Pavillon De St-françois-d'assise; Prof ObstGyn, Université Laval; Langs: English; (418)525-4307; andre.lemay@ogy.ulaval.ca.

LEMAY, Andree; Inst U en Sante Mentale de QC, 2601 ch de la Canardiere, Quebec QC G1J 2G3; Laval'82; FRCPC; Psy. Ac Staff Psy, Institut Universitaire Sante; Université Laval; (418)663-5020; Fax. (418)661-6891.

LEMAY, Catherine; Polyclinique De Trois-Rivieres, 305-1900 boul des Recollets, Trois-Rivieres QC G8Z 4K4; Mon'89; Cardiol (P.Q.); IntMed. Staff, CSSS de Trois-Rivières; (819)375-4313

LEMAY, Catherine; Clinique du Plateau Marquette, 200-731 rue Galt O, Sherbrooke QC J1H 1Z1; Sher'08; (819)564-8662

LEMAY, Chantal; Clinique Med Grande Ourse, 534 3e rue, Chibougamau QC G8P 1N9; Sher'00; CCFP; (418)748-3469; Fax. (418)748-6983.

LEMAY, Christine; Hop Ste-Anne-De-Beaupre, 11000 rue des Montagnards, Beaupre QC G0A 1E0; Laval'98; CCFP; Staff, Hôpital Sainte Anne de Beaupré; (418)827-3738; Fax. (418)827-7365.

LEMAY, Diane; Centre De Med Fam De Wakefield, CP 400, Wakefield QC J0X 3G0; Mon'92; Staff, Centre Hospitalier Gatineau Mémorial; (819)459-2363; Fax. (819)459-2997.

LEMAY, Erik; Vernon Jubilee Hosp, 2101 32 St, Vernon BC V1T 5L2; Mon'96; FRCPC; Anes. Staff, Vernon Jubilee Hospital; (250)545-2211; Fax. (250)545-5602.

LEMAY, Frederic; CHUS-Hop Hotel-Dieu, 580 rue Bowen S, Sherbrooke QC J1G 2E8; Sher'03; FRCPC; IntMed; Gastroent (Oncology). Staff/adj Prof, Centre Hospitalier Universitaire de Sherbrooke-Hôpital Hôtel-Dieu; Langs: Bilingual(French/English); (819)346-1110; Fax. (819)822-6797.

LEMAY, Gabriel; CSSS de Manicouagan, 635 boul Jolliet, Baie-Comeau QC G5C 1P1; Sher'04; Anes. Staff, Centre Hospitalier Régional Baie-Comeau; (418)589-3701

LEMAY, Genevieve; The Ottawa Hosp-Civic Campus, 1053 Carling Ave, Ottawa ON K1Y 4E9; Ott'08; FRCPC; IntMed. Staff, The Ottawa Hospital - Civic Campus; (613)761-4795

LEMAY, Gerard; Hop Charles-Lemoyne, 3120 boul Taschereau, Greenfield Park QC J4V 2H1; Mon'75; Staff, Hopital Charles LeMoyne; (450)466-5000

LEMAY, Gilbert; Centre Sante Chibougamau, 215 3e rue, Chibougamau QC G8P 1N3; Laval'74; Staff, CRSSS de la Baie-James; (418)748-4486 x306; Fax. (418)748-2961; gilbert_lemay@ssss.gouv.qc.ca.

LEMAY, Guillaume; Centre Med McMasterville, 785 rue Tetreault, Beloeil QC J3G 1A7; Mon'07; CCFP; Langs: Bilingual(French/English); (450)464-1156

LEMAY, Guy; 32 rue Lionel-Groulx, Gatineau QC J8T 1T6; Laval'63; Assoc CEO, Canadian Medical Protective Association.

LEMAY, Isabelle; Centre Hosp Trois-Pistoles, RR 1 550 rue Notre-Dame E, Trois-Pistoles QC G0L 4K0; Mon'07; CCFP; Staff, Centre Hospitalier Trois-Pistoles; (418)851-1111; Fax. (418)851-4546.

LEMAY, Jean-Francois; Ctr Hosp du Centre la Mauricie, 50 119e rue, Shawinigan-Sud QC G9P 5K1; Mon'08; CCFP; Staff, Centre Hospitalier du Centre la Mauricie; (819)536-7500

LEMAY, Jean-Francois; Alberta Children's Hosp, C4 627-2888 Shaganappi Trail N, Calgary AB T3B 6A8; Laval'84; FRCPC; Peds (Asthma). Ac Staff, Alberta Children's Hospital; (403)955-2911; Fax. (403)955-7649.

LEMAY, Julie; CHUQ-Hotel-Dieu de Quebec, 11 Cote du Palais, Quebec QC G1R 2J6; Laval'05; Respir; IntMed. Staff, Centre Hospitalier Universitaire de Québec (CHUQ) - Siege Social; (418)525-4444

LEMAY, Julie; Ctr Hosp de Charlevoix, 74 boul Ambroise-Fafard, Baie-Saint-Paul QC G3Z 2J6; Laval'07; CCFP; Staff, CSSS de Charlevoix; (418)435-5150

LEMAY, Keith D; Queen Elizabeth II Hosp, 10409 98 St, Grande Prairie AB T8V 2E8; Alb'91; BMedSci; FRCPC; DiagRad. Staff, Queen Elizabeth II Hospital; (780)538-7676

LEMAY, Line; 200-1055 boul des Forges, Trois-Rivieres QC G8Z 4J9; Laval'85; (819)372-3400 x3407; Fax. (819)372-3288.

LEMAY, Louise; CSSS du Lac-des-Deux-Montagnes, 520 boul Arthur-Sauve, Saint-Eustache QC J7R 5B1; Mon'09; Staff, Hôpital de Saint-Eustache; (450)473-6811

LEMAY, Marianne; Clinique Fam d'Arthabaska, 2-39 rue Laurier E, Victoriaville QC G6P 6P6; Mon'06; Médecin, Hotel-Dieu d'Arthabaska; Staff, CSSS des Sources d'Asbestos; Langs: English; (819)357-7926; Fax. (819)357-7926; auloscience@hotmail.com.

LEMAY, Marie-Claire; UMF Laval, 2690 ch des Quatre-Bourgeois, Quebec QC G1V 0B7; Laval'07; CCFP; (418)656-4795; Fax. (418)656-4503.

LEMAY, Marjorie; Clinique Med Notre-Dame Inc, 147 rue Notre-Dame E, Victoriaville QC G6P 3Z8; Sher'05; (819)758-3165

LEMAY, Martin; CHUQ-Ctr Hosp Univ Laval, 2705 boul Laurier, Quebec QC G1V 4G2; Laval'71; AnatPath. Ac Staff, Centre Hospitalier Universitaire de Quebec-CHUL; (418)654-2101; Fax. (418)654-2199.

LEMAY, Michel; Hop Brome-Missisquoi-Perkins, 950 rue Principale, Cowansville QC J2K 1K3; Mon'70; FRCSC; ObstGyn. Staff, Hôpital Brome-Missisquoi-Perkins; assoc Prof, Universite de Montreal; Langs: English; (450)266-4342

LEMAY, Michel; Hôpital Ste-Justine, 3175 ch Cote-Sainte-Catherine, Montreal QC H3T 1C5; Rennes (France)'60; Psy (P.Q.). Assoc Staff, Hôpital Ste-Justine; Prof Med, Universite de Montreal; (514)345-4931 x5695

LEMAY, Michele; Ctr Hosp Anna-Laberge, 200 boul Brisebois, Chateauguay QC J6K 4W8; Laval'79; CCFP; Staff, Hôpital Anna-Laberge; (450)699-2425

LEMAY, Mireille D; Alberta Children's Hosp, 2888 Shaganappi Trail NW, Calgary AB T3B 6A8; Ott'80; FRCPC; Peds; InfectDis. Staff, Alberta Children's Hospital; (403)955-7211

LEMAY, Nadia; Polyclinique Pierre Le Gardeur, 300-1000 montee des Pionniers, Terrebonne QC J6V 1S8; Sher'99; ObstGyn. Staff, Centre Hospitalier Pierre le Gardeur; Langs: Bilingual(French/English); (450)657-1313; Fax. (450)657-1809.

LEMAY, Nathalie; Clin Pediatrique des Mille-aZl, 230-233 rue Turgeon, Sainte-Therese QC J7E 3J8; Laval'93; Peds. Staff, Hôpital de Saint-Eustache; (450)430-8009

LEMAY, Odette; Centre de Med Fam St-Laurent, 200-1605 boul Marcel-Laurin, Saint-Laurent QC H4R 0B7; Laval'78; Staff, Hôpital du Sacre-Coeur de Montréal; (514)331-9222

LEMAY, Robert; CHUM-Hop Notre-Dame, 1560 rue Sherbrooke E, Montreal QC H2L 4M1; Mon'65; Electroenceph (P.Q.); Neur (Dystonia). Chef EMG Lab & Neuro-Musculaire Clin/ac Membre, Centre Hospitalier l'Université de Montréal (CHUM) - Hôpital Notre-Dame; Asst Prof Neurol, Universite de Montreal; (514)890-8237; Fax. (514)412-7554; neurolem@hotmail.com.

LEMAY, Serge; MUHC-Royal Victoria Hosp, R2 38-687 av des Pins O, Montreal QC H3A 1A1; Mon'89; Nephrol (P.Q.); IntMed. Staff, McGill University Health Centre - Royal Victoria Hospital; (514)843-1586; Fax. (514)843-2815.

LEMAY, Yvan; Univ De Sherbrooke, 201-2500 boul de l'Universite, Sherbrooke QC J1K 2R1; Sher'77; Staff, Centre Hospitalier Universitaire de Sherbrooke-Hopital Fleurimont; (819)821-7667; Fax. (819)821-7577.

LEMAY-GERVAIS, Francois; Hop Brome-Missisquoi-Perkins, 950 rue Principale, Cowansville QC J2K 1K3; Mon'01; CCFP; Staff, Hôpital Brome-Missisquoi-Perkins; (450)266-4342

LEMAY-ROY, Claudia; CSSS de Rivière-de-Loup, 75 rue Saint-Henri, Riviere-du-Loup QC G5R 2A4; Laval'10; Staff, Centre Hospitalier Regional du Grand-Portage; (418)868-1010

LEMBKE, Edward C; Radiology Associates of Regina, 6-2727 Parliament Ave, Regina SK S4S 6X5; Man'77; FRCPC; DiagRad. Staff, Pasqua Hospital; Staff, Radiology Associates of Regina; Assoc Prof/Clin Teacher, University of Saskatchewan; (306)352-7653; Fax. (306)522-4311.

LEMBOYE, Adeola; Mental Health Centre, 65 Brunswick St, Fredericton NB E3B 1G5; (Nigeria)'00; (506)444-3720; Fax. (506)444-3271; dr.adeola.lemboye@gnb.ca.

LEMCKERT, Ronald; Dundas Derm Otolaryngology, 102-17 King St E, Dundas ON L9H 1B7; Mem'92; BMedSci; FRCSC; Otol (Facial Cosmetic). Court Staff, St Joseph's Healthcare - Charlton Campus; Court Staff, Joseph Brant Memorial Hospital; Staff, Hamilton Health Sciences Centre - Chedoke Hospital; Clin Assoc Prof Surg(ENT), McMaster University; (905)628-3377; Fax. (905)628-8833; rlemckert@dundasderm.ca.

LEMELIN, François; Hotel-Dieu de Levis, 143 rue Wolfe, Levis QC G6V 3Z1; Laval'93; FRCSC; Urol. Staff, Hôtel-Dieu de Lévis; Langs: English; (418)835-7121; flemelin@sympatico.ca.

LEMELIN, Jacques; Family Med Centre, 210 Melrose Ave, Ottawa ON K1Y 4K7; McG'74; CCFP; FCFP; Staff, SCO Health Service - Élisabeth Bruyère Hospital; Head Family Med, University of Ottawa; (613)761-4334; Fax. (613)761-4200.

LEMELIN, Jean-Luc; GMF des Seigneuries, 2220 boul Rene-Gaultier, Varennes QC J3X 1E3; Mon'91; (450)652-2917; Fax. (450)652-6418.

LEMELIN, Michel J R; Ctr Hosp Affilie-St-Sacrement, 1515 17e rue, Saint-Georges QC G5Y 4T8; Laval'71; Otol. Staff, Centre Hospitalier Beauce-Etchemin; (418)228-2031

LEMELIN, Myra M; Monfort Hosp, 713 Montreal Rd, Ottawa ON K1K 0T2; Sher'00; CCFP; CCFP(E.M.); Staff, Montfort Hospital; Langs: Bilingual(French/English); (613)746-4621 x4212

LEMELIN, Pierre-Paul; CSSS de la Mitis, 800 av du Sanatorium, Mont-Joli QC G5H 3L6; Sher'88; Staff, CSSS de la Mitis; (418)775-7261; Fax. (418)775-1989.

LEMELIN, Richard; Centre Med De Beauport, 737 av Royale, Quebec QC G1E 1Z1; Laval'85; (418)667-7114; Fax. (418)667-5843.

LEMELIN, Tania; Wakefield Family Med Centre, RR 2 777 ch Riverside, Wakefield QC J0X 3G0; McG'02; CCFP; Langs: Bilingual(French/English); (819)459-2363; Fax. (819)459-2997.

LEMELIN, Valery; CHUQ-Ctr Hosp Univ Laval, RC575-2705 boul Laurier, Quebec QC G1V 4G2; Laval'99; EUS; FRCP; LMCC; Gastroent; IntMed (Digestive Endoscopy). Staff, Centre Hospitalier Universitaire de Quebec-CHUL; Langs: Bilingual(English/French); (418)654-2168; Fax. (418)654-2164; valery.lemelin@mail.chuq.qc.ca.

LEMERY, Robert; Univ of Ottawa Heart Institute, H123-40 Ruskin St, Ottawa ON K1Y 4W7; Sher'79; FACC; FACP; FRCPC; IntMed (Electrophysiology); Cardiol. Staff, University of Ottawa Heart Institute; Langs: English; (613)761-4978; Fax. (613)761-4407; rlemery@ottawaheart.ca.

LEMIERE, Catherine; Hop Du Sacre-Coeur De Mtl, 5400 boul Gouin O, Montreal QC H4J 1C5; Marseille (France)'89; MSc; Staff Pneumol, Hôpital du Sacre-Coeur de Montréal; Asst Researcher, Universite de Montreal; (514)338-2162

LEMIEUX, Alain-P; Hotel-Dieu Du Sacre-Coeur, 1 av Du Sacre-Coeur, Quebec QC G1N 2W1; Laval'76; Geriatric Med, Hotel-Dieu du Sacre-Coeur de Jesus de Quebec; (418)691-0743; Fax. (418)691-0744; a-p.lemieux@ssss.gouv.qc.ca.

LEMIEUX, Andree; CSSS de Trois-Rivières, 1991 boul du Carmel, Trois-Rivieres QC G8Z 3R9; Laval'84; Anes. Staff, CSSS de Trois-Rivières; (819)697-3333

LEMIEUX, Anne-Marie; Spence Family Med Centre, 400 Spence Ave, Hawkesbury ON K6A 2Y3; Mon'95; Staff, Hawkesbury & District General Hospital; (613)632-0997; Fax. (613)632-9297.

LEMIEUX, Annie; CHUQ-Ctr Hosp Univ Laval, 2705 boul Laurier, Quebec QC G1V 4G2; Sher'04; FRCPC; IntMed; Cardiol. Staff, Centre Hospitalier Universitaire de Quebec-CHUL; (418)525-4444

LEMIEUX, Ariane; Hotel-Dieu de Levis, 143 rue Wolfe, Levis QC G6V 3Z1; Laval'04; FRCPC; IntMed; Cardiol. Staff, Hôtel-Dieu de Lévis; (418)835-7121

LEMIEUX, Barbara; Regie des Rentes du Quebec, CP 5200 succ Terminus 348-2600 boul Laurier, Quebec QC G1K 7S9; Laval'85; LMCC; (418)657-8709 x3252

LEMIEUX, Bernard; CHUM-Hop Notre-Dame, 1560 rue Sherbrooke E, Montreal QC H2L 4M1; Mon'96; FRCPC; IntMed; MedOncol; Hem. Staff, Centre Hospitalier l'Université de Montréal (CHUM) - Hôpital Notre-Dame; (514)890-8000

LEMIEUX, Bruno; Inst de Readaptation de Mtl, 6300 av de Darlington, Montreal QC H3S 2J4; Mon'68; Staff, Institut de Réadaptation Gingras-Lindsay de Montréal; Langs: Bilingual(French/English); (514)340-2085; bruno.lemieux.chum@ssss.gouv.gc.ca.

LEMIEUX, Camille M; Univ Hlth Network-Toronto Western Hosp, 2F-399 Bathurst St, Toronto ON M5T 2S8; Qns'94; CCFP; Staff, Toronto Western Hospital - University Health Network; (416)603-5888

LEMIEUX, Claire; CSSS de Montmagny-L'Islet, 350 boul Tache O RR 1, Montmagny QC G5V 3R8; Laval'76; Staff, CSSS de Montmagny-L'Islet; (418)248-0630 x5108; claire_lemieux@ssss.gouv.qc.ca.

LEMIEUX, Claude; CHUM-Hop Notre-Dame, 1560 rue Sherbrooke E, Montreal QC H2L 4M1; Mon'77; FRCPC; MedMicrobiol; InfectDis (P.Q.). Staff, Centre Hospitalier l'Université de Montréal (CHUM) - Hôpital Notre-Dame; (514)890-8000 x25103

LEMIEUX, Daniele; CLSC Riviere des Prairies, 8655 boul Perras, Montreal QC H1E 4M7; Mon'81; Chief Med, CSSS de la Pointe de Île; Langs: English; (514)494-4924; Fax. (514)494-4235.

LEMIEUX, Francine; CSSS Pierre Boucher, 1333 boul Jacques-Cartier E, Longueuil QC J4M 2A5; Mon'85; Anes (P.Q.). Staff, Centre Hospitalier Pierre Boucher; (450)468-8111

LEMIEUX, Francois; Clinique Medicale Sainte-Julie, 286 rue de Normandie, Sainte-Julie QC J3E 1A7; Laval'69; (450)649-1593

LEMIEUX, Francois; CSSS du Suroît, 150 rue Saint-Thomas, Salaber-de-Valleyf QC J6T 6C1; Mon'95; FRCSC; GenSurg. Staff, Centre Hospitalier Régional du Suroît; (450)371-9920

LEMIEUX, Gaetan; Clinique Med De Bernieres, 479A ch Saint-Joseph, Saint-Nicolas QC G7A 1N3; Laval'74; (418)831-9228; Fax. (418)831-0249.

LEMIEUX, Ghislain; 74A rue Principale CP 130, Lac-Des-Aigles QC G0K 1V0; Mon'75; (418)779-2324; Fax. (418)779-2305.

LEMIEUX, Isabelle; Clinique Med Kingsey Falls, RR 1 19 rue Comeau, Kingsey Falls QC J0A 1B0; Sher'04; (819)363-3030

LEMIEUX, Jacinthe C; Clinique Med Les Gres, 104-190 rue St Honore, St-Etienne-Ds-Gres QC G0X 2P0; Sher'84; Staff, Centre Hospitalier Regional de Trois-Rivieres; Langs: English; (819)535-6512; Fax. (819)535-1627.

LEMIEUX, Jacques; CSSSG-Hop de Gatineau, CP 2000 Succ Bureau-Chef 909 boul la Verendrye O, Gatineau QC J8P 7H2; Sher'80; FRCPC; DiagRad (General Radiology & Ultrasound). Staff Radiol, Hôpital de Gatineau; Langs: English; (819)561-8297; Fax. (819)561-8109.

LEMIEUX, Jean; Inst U en Sante Mentale de QC, 2601 ch de la Canardiere, Quebec QC G1J 2G3; Mon'79; Staff, Institut Universitaire Sante; (418)663-5321

LEMIEUX, Jerome; Hôpital Laval, 2725 ch Sainte-Foy, Quebec QC G1V 4G5; Laval'99; FRCSC; Anes. Staff, Hôpital Laval; (418)656-8711

LEMIEUX, Julie; Ctr Hosp Affilie-St-Sacrement, 1050 ch Sainte-Foy, Quebec QC G1S 4L8; Laval'97; FRCPC; IntMed (Breast Cancer); MedOncol; Hem. Staff, Centre Hospitalier Affilié Universitaire de Québec - Hôpital du St-Sacrement; Langs: English; (418)682-7511; Fax. (418)682-7912.

LEMIEUX, Kathleen; UMF du Grand Littoral, 100-1205 boul de la Rive-Sud, Saint-Romuald QC G6W 0J4; Laval'06; CCFP; (418)380-8597; Fax. (418)380-8596.

LEMIEUX, Lisa B; Alberta Children's Hosp, 2888 Shaganappi Trail NW, Calgary AB T3B 6A8; Alb'05; FRCPC; Peds. Staff, Alberta Children's Hospital; (403)955-7211

LEMIEUX, Lucie; Institut National Sante Publiq, 190 boul Cremazie E, Montreal QC H2P 1E2; Ott'76; (514)864-1600 x3747

LEMIEUX, Marc-Andre; CLSC des Patriotes, 300 boul Serge-Pepin, Beloeil QC J3G 0B8; Sher'91; (450)536-2572; Fax. (450)536-6367.

LEMIEUX, Marguerite; Hotel-Dieu D'Arthabaska, 5 rue des Hospitalieres, Victoriaville QC G6P 6N2; Mon'85; Urol (P.Q.) (Oncology). Staff, Hotel-Dieu d'Arthabaska; Staff, Hôpital de Christ-Roi; (819)357-2030; Fax. (819)357-6027.

LEMIEUX, Marie-Claude; Clinique Maisonneuve-Rosemont, 340-5345 boul de l'Assomption, Montreal QC H1T 4B3; McG'85; FRCSC; ObstGyn (Urogynecology). Consultant, Sir Mortimer B Davis Jewish General; Staff, Hopital Maisonneuve-Rosemont; adj Prof, Universite de Montreal; Langs: French; (514)257-0961

LEMIEUX, Marie-Eve; CSSS de Trois-Rivières, 1991 boul du Carmel, Trois-Rivieres QC G8Z 3R9; Laval'08; Staff, CSSS de Trois-Rivières; (819)697-3333

LEMIEUX, Marie-France; CLSC Du Richelieu, 300 ch de Marieville, Richelieu QC J3L 3V8; Sher'76; Physician, Centre de Detention-Sorel; (450)658-7561; Fax. (450)658-4390.

LEMIEUX, Marie-Josee; CSSS Pierre Boucher, 1333 boul Jacques-Cartier E, Longueuil QC J4M 2A5; Laval'84; FRCPC; DiagRad. Staff, Centre Hospitalier Pierre Boucher; (450)468-8111

LEMIEUX, Marie-Pier; UMF Horizon, 3 9e rue, Rouyn-Noranda QC J9X 2A9; Sher'10; CCFP; (819)797-4535

LEMIEUX, Martin; CSSS de Chicoutimi, 263-305 rue Saint-Vallier, Chicoutimi QC G7H 5H6; Sher'04; CCFP; Staff, Complexe hospitalier de la Sagamie; (418)541-1079

LEMIEUX, Maryse C; CSSS de la Region de Thetford, 1717 rue Notre-Dame E, Thetford Mines QC G6G 2V4; Sher'86; Staff, Hopital du CSS de la Region de Thetford; (418)338-7777

LEMIEUX, Maryse D; CSSS de la Mitis, 800 av du Sanatorium, Mont-Joli QC G5H 3L6; Sher'83; Staff, CSSS de la Mitis; (418)775-2251 x3100; Fax. (418)775-6487.

LEMIEUX, Maude; CHUQ-Ctr Hosp Univ Laval, 2705 boul Laurier, Quebec QC G1V 4G2; Laval'04; FRCPC; Psy. Staff, Centre Hospitalier Universitaire de Quebec-CHUL; (418)525-4444

LEMIEUX, Michel D; Sante et Services Sociaux, 1075 ch Sainte-Foy, Quebec QC G1S 2M1; Laval'62; FACS; Cardiovasc&ThorSurg (P.Q.); GenSurg. (418)226-6952

LEMIEUX, Nathalie; Hop Maisonneuve-Rosemont, 5415 boul de l'Assomption, Montreal QC H1T 2M4; Mon'98; CCFP; Staff, Hopital Maisonneuve-Rosemont; (514)252-3400; Fax. (514)252-3482.

LEMIEUX, Patrice; CSSS du Nord de Lanaudière, 1000 boul Sainte-Anne, St-Charles-Brromee QC J6E 6J2; Mon'04; FRCSC; GenSurg. Staff, Centre Hospitalier Régional de Lanaudière; (450)759-8222

LEMIEUX, Pierre; Clinique De Medecine Generale, 2000-926 rue Labbe, Thetford Mines QC G6G 2A8; Laval'79; Staff, Hopital du CSS de la Region de Thetford; (418)338-4581; Fax. (418)338-4584.

LEMIEUX, Raymond G; 275-45 rue Saint-Patrice E, Magog QC J1X 1T5; Sher'71; Psy., McGill University; Langs: English; (819)843-2804

LEMIEUX, Raymond J; Hop du Sacre-Coeur de Mtl, 5400 boul Gouin O, Montreal QC H4J 1C5; Ott'71; FRCPC; Cardiol; NuclearMed. Staff Nuclear Med, Hôpital du Sacre-Coeur de Montréal; Clin Assoc Prof, Universite de Montreal; (514)338-2244; Fax. (514)338-3686.

LEMIEUX, Raymond; Centre Medical de Huntington, RR 3 72A rue Chateauguay, Huntingdon QC J0S 1H0; Mon'75; assoc Staff, Huntingdon County Hospital Centre; assoc Staff, Barrie Memorial Hospital; (450)264-6101

LEMIEUX, Real; CSST Laval, 200-1700 boul Laval, Laval QC H7S 2G6; Mon'60; FRCSC; OrthSurg (Sports Medicine). Staff OrthSurg, Hôpital de Saint-Eustache; Staff, Hopital de la Cite de la santé; Langs: English; (450)967-3200 x3283

LEMIEUX, Rejean; Clinique Med de Pintendre, 5-792 rte du President-Kennedy, Pintendre QC G6C 1C8; Laval'93; ObstGyn. Staff, Hôtel-Dieu de Lévis; (418)837-6943; Fax. (418)837-0487.

LEMIEUX, Remy; Place Barrette, 270 rue Malraux, Chicoutimi QC G7H 6R9; Laval'83; FRCSC; OrthSurg. Orthopedic Surg, Hotel-Dieu de Roberval; (418)690-1014

LEMIEUX, Sebastien; CSSS du Lac-des-Deux-Montagnes, 520 boul Arthur-Sauve, Saint-Eustache QC J7R 5B1; Laval'03; FRCPC; Anes. Staff, Hôpital de Saint-Eustache; (450)473-6811

LEMIEUX, Sylvie; C M F Chicoutimi-Nord, 2185 boul de Tadoussac, Chicoutimi QC G7G 4X2; Mon'88; Ac Staff, Complexe hospitalier de la Sagamie; (418)698-2414; Fax. (418)698-2413.

LEMIEUX, Sylvie; ASSS Chaudière-Appalaches, 363 route Cameron, Sainte-Marie QC G6E 3E2; Laval'80; Staff, Agence de la santé et des services sociaux de Chaudière-Appalaches; Langs: French; Bilingual(French/English); (418)389-1520; sylvie_lemieux@ssss.gouv.qc.ca.

LEMIEUX-BLANCHARD, Emilie; CHUM-Hop Notre-Dame, 1560 rue Sherbrooke E, Montreal QC H2L 4M1; Mon'04; FRCPC; IntMed; MedOncol; Hem. Staff, Centre Hospitalier l'Université de Montréal (CHUM) - Hôpital Notre-Dame; (514)890-8000 x25831

LEMIEUX POTVIN, Frédérique; CSSS de Sept-Iles, 45 rue du Pere-Divet, Sept-Iles QC G4R 3N7; Mon'09; CCFP; CCFP(E.M.); Staff, Centre Hospitalier Regional de Sept-Iles; (418)962-9761

LEMIEUX-ROY, Marie-Josee; CSSS de Beauce-Etchemin, 1515 17e rue, Saint-Georges QC G5Y 4T8; Laval'99; Peds. Staff, Centre Hospitalier Beauce-Etchemin; (418)228-2031; Fax. (418)227-1270.

LEMIRE, Anouc; Polyclinique de l'Oreille, 310-6020 rue Jean-Talon E, Saint-Leonard QC H1S 3B1; Mon'90; FRCSC; Otol. ac Membre Otol, Hôpital de Saint-Eustache; (514)721-6299; Fax. (514)721-6299.

LEMIRE, Caroline; Centre Med des Laurentides, 102-1100 rue Saint-Isidore, St-Lin-Laurentides QC J5M 2V6; Mon'07; CCFP.

LEMIRE, Chantal; CHUS-Hop Fleurimont, 3001 12e av N, Sherbrooke QC J1H 5N4; Mon'92; FRCPC; Peds; ClinImmunol&Allergy (P.Q.). Staff, Centre Hospitalier Universitaire de Sherbrooke-Hopital Fleurimont; Langs: English; (819)346-1110; Fax. (819)564-5215.

LEMIRE, Edmond G; Royal University Hosp, 515-103 Hospital Dr, Saskatoon SK S7N 0W8; Laval'92; PhD; BSc(Hon); LMCC; CCMG; FRC; FRCPC; MedGenetics. Head Div of Med Genetics, Royal University Hospital; Staff, Regina General Hospital; Staff, Saskatoon Health Region Saskatoon Public Health; Assoc Prof Peds, University of Saskatchewan; Langs: Bilingual(English/French); (306)655-1692; Fax. (306)655-1736; edmond.lemire@saskatoonhealthregion.ca.

LEMIRE, Eliane; Centre Med St-Bruno, 1435 rue Roberval, Saint-Bruno QC J3V 3P7; Mon'91; (450)653-3631; Fax. (450)653-5518.

LEMIRE, Francine L; College of Fam Phys of Canada, 2630 Skymark Ave, Mississauga ON L4W 5A4; McG'76; CCFP; FCFP; Physician, College Of Family Physicians Of Canada-Ontario; (905)629-0900; Fax. (905)629-0893.

LEMIRE, Francois; CHUM-Hotel-Dieu, 3840 rue Saint-Urbain, Montreal QC H2W 1T8; Laval'69; FRCPC; Cardiol. ac Staff Cardiol Serv, Centre Hospitalier l'Université de Montréal (CHUM) - Hôtel-Dieu; adj Prof Med, Universite de Montreal; Langs: English; (514)890-8000 x14765

LEMIRE, Isabelle; Serv Psy Enfants Pour et Adole, 204-465 rue Notre-dame, Repentigny QC J6A 2T3; Mon'86; FRCPC; Psy (Pediatric Psychiatry). Staff PedPsy, Centre Hospitalier Régional de Lanaudière; Langs: English; (450)581-5100; Fax. (450)581-2302.

LEMIRE, Luc; Ctr Hosp Affilie-Enfant-Jesus, 1401 18e rue, Quebec QC G1J 1Z4; Laval'77; FRCSC; GenSurg (P.Q.); OrthSurg. Staff, Centre Hospitalier Affilié Universitaire de Québec - Hôpital De L'Enfant Jésus; (418)649-0252

LEMIRE, Magali; CSSS du Nord de Lanaudière, 1000 boul Sainte-Anne, St-Charles-Brromee QC J6E 6J2; Mon'03; FRCPC; Psy. Staff, Centre Hospitalier Régional de Lanaudière; (450)759-8222

LEMIRE, Marie L C; Cornwall Comm Hosp-Mcconnell, PO Box 100 Stn Main 840 McConnell Ave, Cornwall ON K6H 5S5; McG'06; MDCM; CCFP; Staff, Cornwall Community Hospital; Langs: Bilingual(English/French); (613)938-4240

LEMIRE, Martine; CHUS-Hop Fleurimont, 3001 12e av N, Sherbrooke QC J1H 5N4; Laval'94; FRCPC; IntMed; ClinImmunol&Allergy. Staff Service d'Immunologie, Centre Hospitalier Universitaire de Sherbrooke-Hopital Fleurimont; Langs: Bilingual(French/English); (819)821-8000 x14892; martine_lemire@hotmail.com.

LEMIRE, Myriam; Hop Charles Lemoyne, 3120 boul Taschereau, Greenfield Park QC J4V 2H1; Mon'93; FRCPC; Psy. Staff, Hopital Charles LeMoyne; Langs: Bilingual(French/English); (450)466-5453

LEMIRE, Pierre-Luc; CSSS de Trois-Rivières, 1991 boul du Carmel, Trois-Rivieres QC G8Z 3R9; Laval'08; CCFP; Staff, CSSS de Trois-Rivières; (819)697-1333

LEMISKI, William M; 101-3607 31 St, Vernon BC V1T 5J4; UBC'88; (250)545-1329; Fax. (250)549-1247.

LEMKE, Krista K; Toronto East Gen Hosp Inc, 825 Coxwell Ave, Toronto ON M4C 3E7; Cal'94; FRCPC; Psy. Staff, Toronto East General Hospital Inc; (416)469-6580 x3298; Fax. (416)469-6179; klemk@tegh.on.ca.

LEMKE, Marvin G; Royal Oak Med Centre, 205-6440 Royal Oak Ave, Burnaby BC V5H 3P2; Alb'90; Staff, Burnaby Hospital; (604)433-1268; Fax. (604)433-0366.

LEMKE, Robert P; University of Alberta Hosp, 3A3-8440 112 St NW, Edmonton AB T6G 2B7; Alb'89; BSc; FRCPC; Peds (Neonatal & Perinatal Medicine). Staff, University of Alberta Hospital; Clinical Asst Prof Peds, University of Alberta; (780)407-1305; Fax. (780)407-3030; rlemke@cha.ab.ca.

LEMLIN, Pierre; CSSS du Nord de Lanaudière, 1000 boul Sainte-Anne, St-Charles-Brromee QC J6E 6J2; Mon'66; CSPQ; Otol. Staff, Centre Hospitalier Régional de Lanaudière; Langs: English; (450)759-8222 x2525; lemlin@sympatico.ca.

LEMMEX, Byron W G; 309-1580 Merivale Rd, Nepean ON K2G 4B5; McM'83; (613)226-4030; Fax. (613)225-3891.

LEMOINE, Bernard; Centre Hosp Honore-Mercier, 2750 boul Laframboise, Saint-Hyacinthe QC J2S 4Y8; Mon'81; Respir (P.Q.); IntMed. Staff, Centre Hospitalier Honore-Mercier; (450)771-3251

LEMOINE, Gabriel J G; Seine Med Centre, 110-142 Centrale Ave, Ste Anne MB R5H 1C3; Ott'66; Staff, Ste Anne Hospital; Med Examiner, Pediatric Health Standard; (204)422-8811; Fax. (204)422-5876; glemoine@sehealth.mb.ca.

LEMOINE, Marie-Helene; Centre Hosp Honore-Mercier, 2750 boul Laframboise, Saint-Hyacinthe QC J2S 4Y8; Sher'00; Peds. Staff, Centre Hospitalier Honore-Mercier; Langs: English; Spanish; (450)771-3335

LEMON, Peter W; Salvation Army Grace Gen Hosp, 300 Booth Dr, Winnipeg MB R3J 3M7; Man'77; DAB; FRCPC; Anes. Staff, The Salvation Army Grace Hospital; (204)837-8311; Fax. (204)831-0029.

LEMON-MULE, Heather F; Taunton Health Centre, SS 201 1290 Keith Ross Dr, Oshawa ON L1H 7K4; Mem'02; ClinImmunol&Allergy; Peds (Asthma). (905)721-4980; Fax. (905)721-6633.

LEMONDE, Jean; Le Centre Medicale, 427-4 rue Taschereau, Gatineau QC J8Y 2V5; Sher'70; Peds. Ac Staff, Hull Hospital; Langs: English; (819)771-8367; Fax. (819)771-9930; jean_lemonde@ssss.gouv.qc.ca.

LEMONNIER, Marie-Chantal; Clinique Sante Femme, 31 rue Drummond, Granby QC J2G 2S3; Sher'81; FRCSC; ObstGyn. (450)372-4008

LEMOS, Vivienne M; Univ Hlth Network-Toronto Western Hosp, 2F-399 Bathurst St, Toronto ON M5T 2S8; McG'10; MDCM; CCFP; Staff, Toronto Western Hospital - University Health Network; (416)603-5800

LEMOYNE, Jean; CRSSS de la Baie-James, 312 3e rue, Chibougamau QC G8P 1N5; Laval'82; Staff, CRSSS de la Baie-James; (418)748-3575

LEMOYNE, Michel M; CHUM-Hop St-Luc, 1058 rue Saint-Denis, Montreal QC H2X 3J4; Sher'78; FRCPC; Gastroent (Nutrition). Staff, Centre Hospitalier l'Université De Montréal (CHUM) - Hôpital Saint-luc; adj Prof, Universite de Montreal; Langs: Bilingual(French/English); (514)890-8356; Fax. (514)412-7372; michel.lemoyne@sympatico.ca.

LEMYRE, Brigitte; Children's Hosp Eastern Ont, 401 Smyth Rd, Ottawa ON K1H 8L1; Sher'93; FRCPC; Peds (Neonatal & Perinatal Medicine). Staff, The Ottawa Hospital - General Campus; Staff, Children's Hospital of Eastern Ontario (CHEO); (613)737-8561; Fax. (613)737-8889.

LEMYRE, Emmanuelle; 7-3175 ch de la Côte-Sainte-Ca, Montreal QC H3T 1C5; McG'92; FRCPC; Peds; MedGenetics. Staff, Hôpital Ste-Justine; (514)345-4727; Fax. (514)345-4766.

LEMYRE, Karine; Pontiac Health Centre, 200 rue Argue, Shawville QC J0X 2Y0; Laval'10; CCFP; Staff, Pontiac Hospital Centre; (819)647-2211

LEMYRE, Madeleine; CHUQ-Ctr Hosp Univ Hop Laval, S 762-2705 boul Laurier, Quebec QC G1V 4G2; Laval'02; FRCSC; ObstGyn (Endoscopy). Staff, Centre Hospitalier Universitaire de Quebec-CHUL; (418)654-2738; Fax. (418)525-4281; madeleine.lemyre@fmed.ulaval.ca.

LEMYRE, Reine; CLSC La Pommeraie, 397 rue de la Riviere, Cowansville QC J2K 1N4; Sher'78; CCFP; (450)266-2522; Fax. (450)263-4985; reine.lemyre@rrsss16.gouv.qc.ca.

LENA, Anthony I; Bluewater Health-Norman Site, 89 Norman St, Sarnia ON N7T 6S3; Ceylon (Sri Lanka)'75; MRCS(Ed); MB BS; FFARCS(Ire); LRCPS(Ed & Glas); FRCPC; Anes. Staff, Bluewater Health - Norman Site; (519)464-4500 x5407

LENA, Boneventure; U of Ottawa Health Services, 302-1 Nicholas St, Ottawa ON K1N 7B7; (Sri Lanka)'68; DABPN; MRCPsy; FRANZCP; FRCPC; Psy (Youth Psychiatry). Clinical Asst Prof Psy, University of Ottawa; (613)564-3950 x296; Fax. (613)564-6627.

LENA, Sujatha M; 5-2430 Bank St, Ottawa ON K1V 0T7; (Sri Lanka)'67; MB BS; DCH(Lond); MRC(UK); FAAP; Peds (Adolescent Medicine). Ac Staff Peds, Children's Hospital of Eastern Ontario (CHEO); Co-Dir Eating Disorders Clinic, Smyth Medical Centre; Asst Clin Prof, University of Ottawa; Langs: Sinhalese; (613)737-7119

LENA, Tanya S; Addiction & Mental Hlth-Queen, 1001 Queen St W, Toronto ON M6J 1H4; Ott'05; FRCPC; Neur. Staff, Centre for Addiction & Mental Health (CAMH) - Queen Site; (416)535-8501; Fax. (416)583-1296.

LENAUSKAS, Daiva A; Adelaide Health Clinic, PO Box 228 Stn 1st Can Place 1 First Canadian Plave, Toronto ON M5X 1C8; (Other Foreign)'09; CCFP; (416)367-5200

LENCSES, Kathy A; Health Services, 599 Brealey Dr, Peterborough ON K9J 7B1; Cal'05; CCFP; (705)749-5504

LENCZNER, Eric M; MUHC-Montreal Gen Hosp, B5 1585-1650 av Cedar, Montreal QC H3G 1A4; Tor'69; FRCSC; OrthSurg. Ac Staff, McGill University Health Centre - Montreal General Campus; adj Prof, McGill University; Langs: English; French; (514)934-1934 x42264; Fax. (514)934-8283; eric.lenczner@muhc.mcgill.ca.

LENDRUM, David A; Foothills Med Centre, C231-1403 29 St NW, Calgary AB T2N 2T9; Cal'03; FRCPC; EmergMed. Staff, Foothills Medical Centre; (403)944-1635; Fax. (403)944-2419.

LENECK, Charles M; 511-4430 Bathurst St, North York ON M3H 3S3; Tor'65; FRCPC; Derm. Ac Staff, Sunnybrook Health Sciences Centre; University of Toronto; (416)636-9971

LENEMAN, Michal; William Osler HC-Etobicoke, 101 Humber College Blvd, Etobicoke ON M9V 1R8; Ott'00; CCFP; Staff, William Osler Health System - Etobicoke General Hospital; (416)747-3400

LENFERNA DE LA MOTTE, Alain; Weyburn Health Centre, 36 4th St, Weyburn SK S4H 0X7; Witwatersrand (South Africa)'84; MB ChB; LMCC; Staff, Weyburn General Hospital; (306)842-5444 x302; Fax. (306)842-5449; a.lenferna@weyburnhealthcentre.com.

LENGA, Ilan; Oshawa Clinic, 117 King St E, Oshawa ON L1H 1B9; Tor'98; FRCPC; IntMed (Dialysis); Nephrol. Staff Nephrol, Lakeridge Health - Oshawa Site; Lecturer, University of Toronto; (905)721-4339; Fax. (905)723-1495.

LENIS, Serge G; Fed des Med Specialistes du QC, CP 216 Succ Pl-Desjardins 3000-2 Complexe Desjardins, Montreal QC H5B 1G8; McG'77; FRCPC; Anes (Intensive Care). Chief Dept of Anes, St Mary's Hospital Centre; Assoc Prof Anes, McGill University; (514)350-5002; serge.lenis@mcgill.ca.

LENKOV, Pamela L; U Of Toronto-Health Services, 214 College St, Toronto ON M5T 2Z9; McG'86; CCFP; Staff GP Oncol, Sunnybrook Health Sciences Centre; (416)978-8030; Fax. (416)971-2089.

LENNOX, Arthur S; 202-26 North St, Bridgewater NS B4V 2V6; Dundee (Scotland)'86; MB ChB; (902)543-9624

LENNOX, Carla; East Wellington Family Hlth Team, SS 1 6 Thompson Cres, Erin ON N0B 1T0; Qns'77; Court Staff, William Osler Health System - Brampton Civic Hospital; (519)833-9396

LENNOX, Catherine L; Lakeridge HC-Bowmanville Site, 47 Liberty St S, Bowmanville ON L1C 2N4; Wes'96; CCFP; Staff, Lakeridge Health - Bowmanville Site; (905)623-3331

LENNOX, Harriet A; Sioux Lookout Zone Fam Phys, PO Box 4000 Stn Main, Sioux Lookout ON P8T 1K2; Tor'80; CCFP; FCFP; Ac Staff Privil, Sioux Lookout Meno-Ya-Win Health Centre; Asst Prof, Northern Ontario School of Medicine-Lakehead University; Clinical Asst Prof Family Med, McMaster University; (807)737-5165; Fax. (807)737-3384; hlennox@slmhc.on.ca.

LENNOX, Joanne S; 26 Hiscott St, St Catharines ON L2R 1C6; Tor'66; (905)688-4640

LENNOX, Pamela H; Dept Of Anaes, 2449-910 10th Ave W, Vancouver BC V5Z 1M9; Ireland (Ireland)'93; FRCPC; Anes. (604)875-4304

LENNOX, Peter A; Vancouver Plastic Surg Centre, 1000-777 Broadway W, Vancouver BC V5Z 4J7; UBC'91; FRCSC; PlasSurg (Aesthetic Surgery). (604)876-1300

LENNY, David B; Centennial Med Centre, 299 Lake Ave E, Carleton Place ON K7C 1J3; Tor'76; Staff, Carleton Place & District Memorial Hospital; (613)257-2311; Fax. (613)257-4435.

LENSER, Rose E; Doctor's Med Clinic, 215-3066 Shelbourne St, Victoria BC V8R 6T9; UBC'99; CCFP; (250)388-4211; Fax. (250)383-4119.

LENT, Barbara P; Victoria Family Med Centre, 60 Chesley Ave, London ON N5Z 2C1; Wes'78; CCFP; FCFP; (519)433-8424

LENTINI, Anthony C; 218-223 Colonnade Rd, Nepean ON K2E 7K3; McM'96; BPE; MSc; FRCPC; PhysMed&Rehab. Staff Physical Med & Rehab, The Ottawa Hospital Rehabilitation Centre; (613)792-1525; Fax. (613)792-3648.

LENTINI, Vittorio; Veterans Affiars Canada, 205-55 Town Centre Crt, Scarborough ON M1P 4X4; Dal'88; BSc; MHSc; DTMH; Langs: Italian; French; (416)954-0912

LENTZ, John S; Mackenzie Richmond Hill Hosp, 10 Trench St, Richmond Hill ON L4C 4Z3; Tor'82; FRCPC; AnatPath (Hematology Pathology). Staff, Mackenzie Richmond Hill Hospital; (905)883-1212; jlentz@yorkcentral.on.ca.

LENZ, David G; Associate Med Clinic, 123 10th Ave S, Cranbrook BC V1C 2N1; Wes'78; Staff, East Kootenay Regional Hospital; (250)426-4231; Fax. (250)426-4357.

LENZ, Radomila; Smyth Med Centre, 326-1929 Russell Rd, Ottawa ON K1G 4G3; Wes'90; FRCPC; Psy (Women's Mental Health). Langs: Czech; (613)789-1299; Fax. (613)789-7237.

LEON, Chloe M; CAMH Bell Gateway Bldg, 4207-100 Stokes St, Toronto ON M6J 1H4; McM'07; FRCPC; Psy. (416)535-8501

LEON, Magda M; 305-233 Nelson's Cres, New Westminster BC V3L 0E4; (Venezuela)'79; CCFP; (604)533-1804

LEON, Malcolm; Cedar Hills Med Clinic, 12860 96 Ave, Surrey BC V3V 6A8; Witwatersrand (South Africa)'98; MSc; MB ChB; CCFP; (604)584-3531

LEON, Paola; 201-96 Harbord St, Toronto ON M5S 1G6; McG'85; FRCPC; Psy. (416)962-9101

LEON, Roberto; 3-1131 Lawson Ave, Kelowna BC V1Y 6T8; Paraguay (Paraguay)'80; FCOG(SA)(SA); FRCOG(UK); FACOG; FRC; FRCSC; ObstGyn (Quality Improvement). Staff, Kelowna General Hospital; Clin Assoc Prof, University of British Columbia; Langs: Spanish; (250)763-0640; Fax. (250)763-0646.

LEON, Sebastian B; CFB Trenton, PO Box 1000 Stn Forces 190-95 RCAF Rd, Astra ON K0K 3W0; Alb'94; (613)955-8714; Fax. (613)955-8656.

LEON ARDILA, Hernando; University of Alberta Hosp, 8440 112 St NW, Edmonton AB T6G 2B7; (Colombia)'98; Staff, University of Alberta Hospital; (780)407-8822

LEON REY-SANCHEZ, Raul A; Central Nfld Reg Health Ctr, 50 Union St, Grnd-Falls-Windsor NL A2A 2E1; Peruana Cayetano Heredia (Peru)'93; Staff, Central Newfoundland Regional Health Centre; (709)292-2500

LEONARD, Allison M; 403-1 Centrepointe Dr, Nepean ON K2G 6E2; Mem'09; CCFP.

LEONARD, Blair J N; M14-414 Victoria Ave N, Hamilton ON L8L 5G8; Tor'05; FRCPC; IntMed; Hem. (905)527-7663

LEONARD, Brian C; The Ottawa Hosp-Gen Campus, 501 Smyth Rd, Ottawa ON K1H 8L6; Ott'70; FRCSC; Ophth (Retina). Staff, Children's Hospital of Eastern Ontario (CHEO); Staff, The Ottawa Hospital - General Campus; Staff, University of Ottawa Eye Institute; Prof Ophth, University of Ottawa; (613)737-8574; Fax. (613)739-6645; brian@fishermansmarket.com.

LEONARD, Celine; Clinique Med De Saint-Jovite, CP 19069 CSP Place Ouimet 992 rue Saint-Jovite, Mont-Tremblant QC J8E 3C1; Mon'85; (819)425-2728; Fax. (819)425-8012.

LEONARD, Deanne M; Anderson Avenue Fam Practice, B-25 Anderson Ave, St. John's NL A1B 3E4; Mem'09; CCFP.

LEONARD, Gregory J; 2670 Highway 43 PO Box 1673, Kemptville ON K0G 1J0; Ott'79; CCFP; Ac Staff, Kemptville District Hospital; (613)258-4947; Fax. (613)258-2799.

LEONARD, Heather E; Edmonton Clinic Health Aacdemy, 3 575-11405 87 Ave NW, Edmonton AB T6G 1C9; Mem'06; FRCPC; Peds (Hospitalist). (780)248-5510

LEONARD, Jennifer R; Health Sciences Centre, 300 Prince Philip Dr, St. John's NL A1B 3V6; Mem'01; FRCPC; IntMed; Gastroent. Staff, Health Sciences Centre; (709)777-6300

LEONARD, Julie; CSSS du Suroît, 150 rue Saint-Thomas, Salaber-de-Valleyf QC J6T 6C1; Mon'05; CCFP; Staff, Centre Hospitalier Régional du Suroît; (450)371-9920

LEONARD, Marie; Clinique Familiale St-Lambert, 209 rue Woodstock, Saint-Lambert QC J4P 1W7; McG'85; Staff, Centre Hospitalier Pierre Boucher; (450)466-8583; Fax. (450)466-4072.

LEONARD, Michael P G; Children's Hosp Eastern Ont, 401 Smyth Rd, Ottawa ON K1H 8L1; Qns'83; FAAP; Urol; FRCS; FRCSC; Urol (Pediatric Urology). Staff, Children's Hospital of Eastern Ontario (CHEO); Prof Surg, University of Ottawa; (613)737-7600 x1353; Fax. (613)738-4271; mleonard@cheo.on.ca.

LEONARD, Norma J; Medical Sciences Building, 8 53-131 University Campus NW, Edmonton AB T6G 2H7; Cal'89; FRCPC; MedGenetics. Staff Med Genetics, University of Alberta Hospital; (780)407-7333; Fax. (780)407-6845; norma.leonard@ualberta.ca.

LEONARD, Rebecca L; PO Box 1690 Stn Main, Cochrane AB T4C 1B6; Cal'06; CCFP; (403)702-2196

LEONARD, Russell K; 204-1676 Martin Dr, Surrey BC V4A 6E7; UBC'84; FRCPC; IntMed. (604)536-2188; Fax. (604)538-6317.

LEONARD, Sophie; Hop Charles Lemoyne, 3120 boul Taschereau, Greenfield Park QC J4V 2H1; Sher'92; FRCPC; IntMed; Cardiol. Staff, Hopital Charles LeMoyne; (450)466-5000

LEONE, Ercole F; Burrard Med Bldg, 400-1144 Burrard St, Vancouver BC V6Z 2A5; UBC'90; FRCSC; Urol. Langs: Italian; (604)688-5116; Fax. (604)688-5608; ercoleleone@shaw.ca.

LEONE, James M; B4D-350 Conestoga Blvd, Cambridge ON N1R 7L7; McM'99; FRCSC; OrthSurg (Hips Surgery). Staff, Cambridge Memorial Hospital; (519)624-5999; Fax. (519)624-1917.

LEONE, Karen L; Cambridge Mem Hosp, 700 Coronation Blvd, Cambridge ON N1R 3G2; Tor'04; FRCPC; Anes. Staff, Cambridge Memorial Hospital; (519)621-2330

LEONE, Rosa; Keele Med Place, 305-2830 Keele St, North York ON M3M 3E5; Palermo (Italy)'83; Court Staff, Humber River Regional Hospital - Finch Avenue Site; Langs: Italian; (416)243-2939; Fax. (416)243-0733.

LEONE, Sylvie; Credit Valley Med Arts Centre, 502-2000 Credit Valley Rd, Mississauga ON L5M 4N4; McG'84; FACOG; FRCSC; ObstGyn. Staff, The Credit Valley Hospital; Langs: Hebrew; Spanish; French; (905)820-8748; Fax. (905)820-0255; s_leonet@yahoo.ca.

LEONG, Aaron; Montreal Chinese Hosp, 189 av Viger E, Montreal QC H2X 3Y9; McG'07; MDCM; Endocrin&Metab; IntMed. Staff, Hôpital Chinois de Montréal; (514)871-0961; Fax. (514)871-0966.

LEONG, Baldwin J; 304-980 Queenston Rd, Stoney Creek ON L8G 1B9; Wes'84; CCFP; FCFP; Ac Staff, St Joseph's Healthcare - Charlton Campus; (905)662-5775; Fax. (905)662-1122.

LEONG, Carson; BC Cancer Agency-Fraser Valley, 13750 96 Ave, Surrey BC V3V 1Z2; UBC'89; FRCPC; RadOncol. Staff, BC Cancer Agency Fraser Valley Centre; Clinical Asst Prof Div of RadOncol, University of British Columbia; (604)930-4033; Fax. (604)675-7207.

LEONG, Eric W H; Humber River Reg Hosp-Church, 200 Church St, Toronto ON M9N 1N8; Tor'93; DABIM(IntMed&Gastroent); FRCPC; IntMed (Hepatology); Gastroent. Ac Staff, Humber River Regional Hospital - Church Street Site; Langs: Cantonese; French; (416)249-8111

LEONG, James P; Rockyview Gen Hosp, 6618-7007 14 St SW, Calgary AB T2V 1P9; Alb'74; FRCSC; Urol. Court Staff, Foothills Medical Centre; Ac Staff, Rockyview General Hospital; Lecturer, University of Calgary; (403)943-8966

LEONG, John C S; 110-100 Humber College Blvd, Etobicoke ON M9V 5G4; Tor'76; BSc(Hons.); Ac Staff, William Osler Health System - Etobicoke General Hospital; (416)745-5459

LEONG, Judith M; Venture House, 220 13 Ave E, Vancouver BC V5T 2K4; Alb'85; FRCPC; Psy (Community Mental Health). Staff, Venture -VCMHS; (604)879-8222

LEONG, L Anthony; 205-648 Herald St, Victoria BC V8W 1S7; UBC'73; Dip SportMed(CASM); CCFP; Staff, Vancouver Island Health Authority; Staff, Aberdeen Hospital; Med Examiner Civil Aviation Marine & Pacific Pilotage, Transport Canada; (250)384-3241

LEONG, Philip W T; 207-236 Georgia St E, Vancouver BC V6A 1Z7; UBC'73; Langs: Chinese; (604)681-4709

LEONG, Renata M W; St Michael's Hosp, 30 Bond St, Toronto ON M5B 1W8; McG'97; CAFCI; MHSc; CCFP; FCFP; Staff Family Pract Unit, St Michael's Hospital; Asst Prof, University of Toronto; Langs: Cantonese; Mandarin; (416)867-7428; Fax. (416)867-7498.

LEONG, Roger; Quinte HC Corp-Belleville Gen, 265 Dundas St E, Belleville ON K8N 5A9; Qns'02; FRCPC; IntMed. Staff, QHC Belleville General; (613)969-7400

LEONG, Wey-Liang; Univ Hlth Network-Princess M, 3 130-610 University Ave, Toronto ON M5G 2M9; Dal'94; FRCSC; GenSurg (Breasts). Staff, Mount Sinai Hospital; Staff, Toronto General Hospital - UHN; Staff GenSurg, Princess Margaret Hospital - University Health Network; (416)946-2992; Fax. (416)946-4429; wey.leong@uhn.on.ca.

LEONG, Yuen-Moi; Burnaby Med Centre, M37-4277 Kingsway, Burnaby BC V5H 3Z2; Taipe (Taiwan)'72; (604)438-9991

LEONG, Yvonne W; Mount Sinai Hosp, 600 University Ave, Toronto ON M5G 1X5; Wes'07; FRCSC; ObstGyn. Staff, Mount Sinai Hospital; (416)596-4200

LEONG-POI, Brian C; The Doctor's Office, 5230 Dundas St W, Etobicoke ON M9B 1A8; Tor'90; (416)234-8668; Fax. (416)234-8720.

LEONG-POI, Howard M; St Michael's Hosp, 6 044QW-30 Bond St, Toronto ON M5B 1W8; Tor'92; FRCPC; IntMed; Cardiol. Head Div of Cardiol/Dir Echocardiography & Vascular Ultrasound, St Michael's Hospital; Assoc Prof Med, University of Toronto; (416)864-5642; Fax. (416)864-5989.

LEONG-SIT, Fook Lin; EYE Q Premium Laser, 10565 124 St NW, Edmonton AB T5N 1R8; Edinburgh (Scotland)'65; MB ChB; DOphth; FRCSC; Ophth (Anterior Segment Surgery). Ac Staff, Capital Health Region 10 Hospitals; Clin Prof, University of Alberta; Langs: Cantonese; Hakka; French; (780)432-1261; Fax. (780)433-2247.

LEONG-SIT, Joseph P T; EYE Q Premium Laser, 10565 124 St NW, Edmonton AB T5N 1R8; Alb'90; FRCSC; Ophth (Cornea/External Disease). Staff, Royal Alexandra Hospital; (780)429-2015; Fax. (780)429-2010.

LEONG-SIT, Kee Sheen; 202-3811 Chatham St, Richmond BC V7E 2Z4; Glasgow (Scotland)'71; (604)275-6652; Fax. (604)271-1612.

LEONG-SIT, Peter; London HSC-University Hosp, PO Box 5339 Stn B 339 Windermere Rd, London ON N6A 5A5; UBC'01; FRCPC; IntMed; Cardiol. Staff, London Health Sciences Centre - University Hospital; (519)685-8500 x19943

LEONG-SIT, Philip P; Allin Clinic, 10155 120 St NW, Edmonton AB T5K 2A2; Alb'00; CCFP; (780)482-7551

LEONHARDT, Charlene M; 408-658 Danforth Ave, Toronto ON M4J 5B9; Wes'84; FRCPC; DiagRad. Staff, Joseph Brant Memorial Hospital; (905)330-1853; Fax. (905)335-1165.

LEONI, Franco E; Smith Clinic, 1-6601 48 Ave, Camrose AB T4V 3G8; Genoa (Italy)'73; FRCSC; GenSurg. (780)672-2425; Fax. (780)679-2640.

LEONOR, Rosario S; Royal Oak Med Centre, 204-6440 Royal Oak Ave, Burnaby BC V5H 3P2; UBC'05; CCFP; (604)482-6163

LEONTIADIS, Grigorios I; McMaster University HSC, 4W8B-1200 Main St W, Hamilton ON L8N 3Z5; Thessaloniki (Greece)'92; Teach Staff, McMaster University; (905)521-2100

LEOUFFRE, Pierre J; Hop Louis-H Lafontaine, 7401 rue Hochelaga, Montreal QC H1N 3M5; Nice (France)'85; Psy (P.Q.). Staff, Hopital Louis-H Lafontaine; Universite de Montreal; Langs: Bilingual(French/English); (514)251-4000 x2584

LEPADATU, Silvia I; Bank Street Prof Centre, 208-1355 Bank St, Ottawa ON K1H 8K7; Bucharest (Romania)'98; Psy. (613)737-8069

LEPAGE, Anik; The Moncton Hosp, 135 MacBeath Ave, Moncton NB E1C 6Z8; Laval'99; FRCPC; Derm. Staff, The Moncton Hospital; Langs: Bilingual(English/French); (506)857-5066; Fax. (506)867-6556.

LEPAGE, Caroline; Ctr Hosp Affilie-Enfant-Jesus, 1401 18e rue, Quebec QC G1J 1Z4; Sher'98; Staff, Centre Hospitalier Affilié Universitaire de Québec - Hôpital De L'Enfant Jésus; (418)649-0252

LEPAGE, Caroline; CHUM-Hop St-Luc, 1058 rue Saint-Denis, Montreal QC H2X 3J4; Mon'95; FRCPC; Anes. Staff, Centre Hospitalier l'Université De Montréal (CHUM) - Hôpital Saint-luc; (514)890-8000 x36581; Fax. (514)412-7310; carolipe@yahoo.com.

LEPAGE, Christiane; CHUM-Hop Notre-Dame, 1560 rue Sherbrooke E, Montreal QC H2L 4M1; Laval'78; Staff, Centre Hospitalier l'Université de Montréal (CHUM) - Hôpital Notre-Dame; Langs: Bilingual(French/English); (514)890-8000; Fax. (514)412-7139.

LEPAGE, Denis J B; 1635 rue Galt O, Sherbrooke QC J1H 2B3; Sher'70; CSPQ; FRCPC; Psy (Medico Legal Psychiatry). Langs: Bilingual(English/French); (819)566-2524; Fax. (819)566-6409.

LEPAGE, Dominique; CSSS Kamouraska-Hop Notre-Dame, 1201 6e Av CP 460, La Pocatiere QC G0R 1Z0; Laval'01; Staff, CSSS de Kamouraska; (418)856-7000; Fax. (418)856-4737.

LEPAGE, France; Clinique Med Nepisiguit, 950 Picot Ave, Bathurst NB E2A 4Z9; Mon'99; FRCPC; Derm;CCFP; Dermatol, Hopital Regional Chaleur; Staff Dermatol, Hôpital de l'Enfant-Jésus RHSJ; Langs: Bilingual(French/English); (506)546-6699; Fax. (506)548-4124; cmni@nbnet.nb.ca.

LEPAGE, Ghislain; Clinique Med De Montmagny, 100-83 av de la Fabrique, Montmagny QC G5V 2J3; Laval'74; assoc Staff, CSSS de Montmagny-L'Islet; (418)248-4933; Fax. (418)248-2778; ghislain.lepage@gmf.gouv.qc.ca.

LEPAGE, Jean-Marc; 301 rue Dufort, La Prairie QC J5R 2X6; Mon'65; Staff, Hopital Charles LeMoyne; Langs: English; (450)659-9193

LEPAGE, Marie-Aline; Ctr Hosp Fleury, 2180 rue Fleury E, Montreal QC H2B 1K3; Laval'74; LMCC; Anes (P.Q.). Staff, Centre Hospitalier Fleury; Langs: English; Spanish; (514)383-5074

LEPAGE, Marie-Christine; CSSS d'Argenteuil, 145 av de la Providence, Lachute QC J8H 4C7; Mon'97; Staff, Centre Hospitalier d'Argenteuil; Langs: Bilingual(French/English); (450)562-3761; Fax. (450)562-2111.

LEPAGE, Martin; CSSSG-Hop de Hull, 116 boul Lionel-Emond, Gatineau QC J8Y 1W7; Mon'93; LMCC; FRCPC; DiagRad (Angiography). Staff, Hull Hospital; Staff Radiol, Hopital Maisonneuve-Rosemont; (819)595-6000; Fax. (819)595-6076; martin_lepage@ssss.gouv.qc.ca.

LEPAGE, Patrice; Clinique Med St-Lazare, 1771B ch Ste-Angelique, Saint-Lazare QC J7T 2N7; Mon'95; Staff, Centre Hospitalier Régional du Suroît; Langs: Bilingual(French/English); (450)455-3322; Fax. (450)455-0756.

LEPAGE, Patricia A; Lakehead Psychiatric Hosp, PO Box 2930 Stn P 580 Algoma St N, Thunder Bay ON P7B 5G4; McM'86; FRCPC; Psy. Staff, Lakehead Psychiatric Hospital - St. Joseph's Care Group; (807)343-4300

LEPAGE, Philippe A; 3591 31 St, Vernon BC V1T 5J4; McG'91; CCFP; (778)475-7511; Fax. (250)542-0160.

LEPAGE, Robert; CLSC La Source, 190 76e rue E, Quebec QC G1H 7K4; Laval'80; (418)628-2572; Fax. (418)628-8668.

LEPAGE, Robert; Inst de l'Oeil de Laurentides, 4800 rue Ambroise-Lafortune, Boisbriand QC J7H 1S6; Mon'92; Ophth (Retinal Disease). Staff, Hôtel-Dieu de Saint-Jérôme; (450)419-6345; Fax. (450)434-9389.

LEPAGE, Robert S; Sudbury Reg Hosp-Laurentian, 41 Ramsey Lake Rd, Sudbury ON P3E 5J1; McM'87; CCFP; CCFP(E.M.); FCFP; Staff, Health Sciences North-Laurentian Site; Langs: English; French; (705)675-4700; robleah@neilnet.com.

LEPAGE, Serge; CHUS-Hop Fleurimont, 3001 12e Av N, Sherbrooke QC J1H 5N4; Sher'85; FRCPC; IntMed; Cardiol. Staff Cardiol Serv, Centre Hospitalier Universitaire de Sherbrooke-Hopital Fleurimont; Langs: English; (819)346-1110 x14947; Fax. (819)820-6897; mcloutier.chus@ssss.gouv.qc.ca.

LEPAGE, Sylvie; Clinique Medicale, 157 rue Water, Campbellton NB E3N 3L4; Sher'00; CCFP; Langs: Bilingual(French/English); (506)753-0130; Fax. (506)753-0139.

LEPAGE, Veronik; The Ravines Med Centre, 535 Larry Uteck Blvd, Halifax NS B3M 0E3; Sher'10; CCFP; (902)407-4382

LEPANTO, Luigi; CHUM-Hop St-Luc, 1058 rue Saint-Denis, Montreal QC H2X 3J4; Mon'84; FRCPC; NuclearMed; DiagRad. Staff, Centre Hospitalier l'Université De Montréal (CHUM) - Hôpital Saint-luc; (514)890-8000

LEPARD, Linda; 211-2223 Broadway W, Vancouver BC V6K 2E4; Birmingham (England)'71; Vis Staff, Vancouver General Hospital - Centennial Pavillion; (604)266-1191

LEPARD, Timothy; West Fraser Mills, 501-858 Beatty St, Vancouver BC V6B 1C1; London (England)'69; MRCS; LRCP; Physician, West Fraser Pulp Sales; (604)895-2747

LEPIC, Kylie L; Hamilton HS-Henderson Site, 144-711 Concession St, Hamilton ON L8V 1C3; McM'06; FRCPC; IntMed; Hem. Staff, Hamilton Health Sciences Centre-Juravinski Site; (905)521-2100

LEPINE, Jean; CSSS de Rimouski-Neigette, CP 3150 Succ A 150 av Rouleau, Rimouski QC G5L 5T1; Sher'72; FRCPC; IntMed; MedOncol; Hem. Staff HemOncol, Hôpital Regional Rimouski; (418)724-8465; Fax. (418)724-8659; jean.lepine@ssss.gouv.qc.ca.

LEPINE, Jean-Marc; CHUQ-Hotel-Dieu de Quebec, 11 Cote du Palais, Quebec QC G1R 2J6; Laval'70; CSPQ; LMCC; FRCSC; OrthSurg (Spine Surgery). Staff, Centre Hospitalier Universitaire de Québec (CHUQ) - Siege Social; Staff Medical Expert, Bureau D'Expertise Lepine Bass; Clin Prof, Université Laval; Langs: English; (418)658-5320; Fax. (418)652-8313; jeanlepine@videotron.ca.

LEPINE, Martin; Clinique Med Grande Ours, 534 3e rue, Chibougamau QC G8P 1N9; Mon'96; CCFP; Fam Med, CRSSS de la Baie-James; Langs: Bilingual(French/English); (418)748-3469; Fax. (418)748-6983.

LEPINE, Suzanne; Hôpital Ste-Justine, 3175 ch Cote-Sainte-Catherine, Montreal QC H3T 1C5; Sher'72; CRCP; FRCPC; Psy (Child & Adolescent Psychiatry). Ac Staff, Hôpital Ste-Justine; Clin Asst, Universite de Montreal; Langs: Bilingual(English/French); (514)345-4931 x5737; Fax. (514)345-2187; suzanne_lepine@ssss.gouv.qc.ca.

LEPINE, Sylviane; CSSS du Sud de Lanaudière, 911 montee des Pionniers, Terrebonne QC J6V 2H2; Sher'04; ObstGyn. Staff, Centre Hospitalier Pierre le Gardeur; (450)654-7525; Fax. (450)470-2640.

LEPINE-MARTIN, Mariette; CHUS-Hop Fleurimont, 3001 12e Av N, Sherbrooke QC J1H 5N4; Sher'73; FRCPC; IntMed; MedOncol (P.Q.); Hem. Staff HemOncol, Centre Hospitalier Universitaire de Sherbrooke-Hopital Fleurimont; assoc Prof, Universite de Sherbrooke; Langs: English; (819)346-1110 x14816

LEPPARD, Jennifer L A; The Ottawa Hosp-Civic Campus, 1053 Carling Ave, Ottawa ON K1Y 4E9; Ott'07; CCFP; CCFP(E.M.); Staff, The Ottawa Hospital - Civic Campus; (613)737-8899

LEQUIER, Laurance; University of Alberta Hosp, 3A3.02 WMC-8440 112 St NW, Edmonton AB T6G 2B7; Alb'92; ABPeds; FRCP; FRCPC; Peds (Pediatric Critical Care). Staff, Stollery Children's Hospital; Staff, University of Alberta Hospital; Teach Staff Peds, University of Alberta; (780)407-1673; Fax. (780)407-3214; laurance.lequier@albertahealthservices.ca.

LEQUOC, Stephane; Ctr Hosp Fleury, 2180 rue Fleury E, Montreal QC H2B 1K3; Mon'94; CCFP; CCFP(E.M.); Staff, Centre Hospitalier Fleury; (514)384-2000

LERAT, Jean-Paul; CLSC Saint-Tite, 750 rue du Couvent, Saint-Tite QC G0X 3H0; Bordeaux (France)'88; (418)365-7556 x5581

LERICHE, Tammy G; Brockville Gen Hosp, 1F-75 Charles St, Brockville ON K6V 1S8; Ott'07; ObstGyn. Staff, Brockville General Hospital - Charles Street; (613)498-0740

LERM, Leon B; Ross Mem Hosp, 10 Angeline St N, Lindsay ON K9V 4M8; Pretoria (South Africa)'98; MB ChB; CCFP; Staff, Ross Memorial Hospital; Langs: Afrikaans; (705)324-6111

LERMER, Bram; Ultima Med Services, 300-4440 Stark St, Richmond BC V7B 1A1; McG'79; CCFP; FCFP; Asst Prof Family Pract, University of British Columbia; Langs: French; Yiddish; (604)270-1370; Fax. (604)270-3306.

LERNER, Edward C; Tsawwassen Med Clinic, 201-1077 56 St, Delta BC V4L 2A2; UBC'80; (604)943-1131; Fax. (604)943-2617.

LERNER, Lawrence; Malvern Med Arts Bldg, 100-1333 Neilson Rd, Scarborough ON M1B 4Y9; Tor'73; CCFP; FCFP; Staff, Rouge Valley Health System - Centenary Health Centre Site; (416)291-7719; Fax. (416)287-3775.

LERNER, Moe; Four Rivers Med Clinic, 878 Main St, Winnipeg MB R2W 3P1; Man'77; DABEM; CCFP; CCFP(E.M.); FCFP; Staff Emerg, Selkirk & District General Hospital; Staff Emerg, Stonewall & District Health Centre; Med Dir, Four Rivers Medical Clinic; Med Staff, CBC Information Radio; Assoc Prof, University of Manitoba; (204)586-5592; Fax. (204)586-5713.

LERNER, Neal Z; Seven Oaks Gen Hosp, 2300 McPhillips St, Winnipeg MB R2V 3M3; Man'81; FRCPC; IntMed. Ac Staff Med, Misericordia Health Centre; Ac Staff Med, Seven Oaks General Hospital; Ac Staff, St Boniface General Hospital; University of Manitoba; (204)632-7133

LEROUX, Andre-Marie; Montfort Hosp, 713 Montreal Rd, Ottawa ON K1K 0T2; Sher'77; FACOG; DAB; FRCSC; ObstGyn (Endocrinology). Staff, Centre Hospitalier l'Université de Montréal (CHUM) - Hôpital Notre-Dame; Staff, Montfort Hospital; Med. Evaluateur, Sante Canada; Langs: English; (613)746-4621

LEROUX, Claudie; Clin de Med Familiale Saguenay, 220-874 boul de l'Universite E, Chicoutimi QC G7H 6B9; Laval'09; CCFP; (418)545-1217

LEROUX, Elise; Clinique Med Lanaudiere, 222 rue Bernard, St-Charles-Brromee QC J6E 2C5; Mon'90; (450)755-1033; Fax. (450)753-5558.

LEROUX, Elizabeth; CHUM-Hop Notre-Dame, 1560 rue Sherbrooke E, Montreal QC H2L 4M1; Mon'01; FRCPC; Neur. Staff, Centre Hospitalier l'Université de Montréal (CHUM) - Hôpital Notre-Dame; (514)890-8000

LEROUX, Eric; Clinique Med 201, 104 rue Sainte-Agathe, Ste-Agathe-Des-Mts QC J8C 2K3; Mon'88; Staff Emerg, Hôpital du Sacre-Coeur de Montréal; Universite de Montreal; (819)326-2020; Fax. (819)326-8801.

LEROUX, Genevieve; Clarence-Rockland Fam Hlth Team, 2741 rue Chamberland, Rockland ON K4K 0B4; Ott'00; Dip SportMed; CCFP; Langs: English; (613)446-7677; Fax. (613)446-5737.

LEROUX, Helene; Clinique Fam d'Arthabaska, 2-39 rue Laurier E, Victoriaville QC G6P 6P6; Sher'80; assoc Staff, Hotel-Dieu d'Arthabaska; Clin Prof, Universite de Sherbrooke; (819)357-9322; Fax. (819)357-7926.

LEROUX, J Robert; Hop Louis-H Lafontaine, 7401 rue Hochelaga, Montreal QC H1N 3M5; Mon'69; FRCPC; Psy (Consultation-Liaison). Staff, Hopital Louis-H Lafontaine; (514)251-4000 x3036

LEROUX, Jacques-Rene; Hôpital Riviere des Prairies, 7070 boul Perras, Montreal QC H1E 1A4; Mon'77; FRCPC; Peds. Staff Peds, Hôtel-Dieu de Saint-Jérôme; Staff, Hôpital Riviere des Prairies; (514)323-7260; Fax. (514)328-3534.

LEROUX, Jean-Francois; Inst ORL et Chir de Monteregi, 230 rue Champlain, St-Jean-sur-Richel QC J3B 6V8; Sher'89; Otol. Langs: Bilingual(French/English); (450)741-0905

LEROUX, Karine; CMF Chicoutimi-Nord, 2185 boul de Tadoussac, Chicoutimi QC G7G 4X2; Sher'96; LMCC; (418)698-2414; Fax. (418)698-2413.

LEROUX, Manon; 125-667 Champlain St, Dieppe NB E1A 1P6; Sher'87; Staff, Dr Georges-L-Dumont University Hospital Centre; Langs: Bilingual(French/English); (506)855-6266; Fax. (506)855-6603.

LEROUX, Maude A; CSSS du Suroît, 150 rue Saint-Thomas, Salaber-de-Valleyf QC J6T 6C1; Mon'05; Staff, Centre Hospitalier Régional du Suroît; (450)371-9920

LEROUX, Michel; 320-900 Boul Du Seminaire N, St-Jean-Sur-Richel QC J3A 1C3; Laval'95; FRCSC; OrthSurg (Arthroplasty). Staff OrthSurg, Hôpital du Haut-Richelieu; (450)348-6966

LEROUX, Nathalie; Hôpital Ste-Justine, 3175 ch Cote-Sainte-Catherine, Montreal QC H3T 1C5; Mon'94; FRCSC; ObstGyn (Urogynecology). Staff ObstGyn, Hôpital Ste-Justine; Langs: Bilingual(French/English); (514)345-4931; Fax. (514)344-1991.

LEROUX, Patrick; CSSS de Saint-Jerome, 290 rue Montigny, Saint-Jerome QC J7Z 5T3; Mon'06; DiagRad. Staff, Hôtel-Dieu de Saint-Jérôme; (450)431-8200

LEROUX, Pierre H; Centre Med Montreal-Est, 201-11370 rue Notre-Dame E, Montreal-Est QC H1B 2W6; Mon'73; (514)645-7426

LEROUX, Robert; Polyclinique Med Fabreville, 380 boul Cure-Labelle, Laval QC H7P 5L3; Mon'78; (450)628-5800; Fax. (450)628-0217.

LEROUX-LEVESQUE, Raphaelle; Centre Hosp Honore-Mercier, 2750 boul Laframboise, Saint-Hyacinthe QC J2S 4Y8; Sher'04; CCFP; CCFP(E.M.); Staff, Centre Hospitalier Honore-Mercier; Langs: Bilingual(French/English); (450)771-3333

LEROYER, Valerie; CSSS de Maskinonge, GD 10 rue Jonathan, St-Alexis-D-Monts QC J0K 1V0; Mon'93; MSc; Langs: Bilingual(French/English); (819)265-2572; Fax. (819)265-4240; mosaikmd@yahoo.ca.

LES, Jacob E; Alberta Children's Hosp, 2888 Shaganappi Trail NW, Calgary AB T3B 6A8; Cal'98; FRCPC; Peds (Emergency Medicine). Staff EmergMed, Alberta Children's Hospital; (403)955-7211; Fax. (403)955-7398.

LESACK, David W; Kelowna Gen Hosp, 2268 Pandosy St, Kelowna BC V1Y 1T2; UBC'91; FRCPC; GenPath. Staff, Kelowna General Hospital; (250)862-4433

LESAGE, Alain; Centre Med De Mont-Laurier, 304 rue de la Madone, Mont-Laurier QC J9L 1R7; Mon'77; Assoc Staff, CSSS d'Antoine-Labelle; Langs: Bilingual(French/English); (819)623-1520; Fax. (819)623-9637; centre.medical.ml@tlb.sympatico.ca.

LESAGE, Alain D; Hop Louis-H Lafontaine, 218-7401 rue Hochelaga, Montreal QC H1N 3M5; Sher'78; MPhil(London,UK); FRCPC; Psy. Staff, Hopital Louis-H Lafontaine; Prof, Universite de Montreal; Langs: Italian; English; (514)251-4015 x2365; Fax. (514)251-5404; alesage@ssss.gouv.qc.ca.

LESAGE, David; Correctional Service of Canada, 400 rue Fordyce, Cowansville QC J2K 3G6; Mon'00; Staff, Hopital Maisonneuve-Rosemont; (450)263-3073

LESAGE, Jacques; Hop Charles Lemoyne, 3120 boul Taschereau, Greenfield Park QC J4V 2H1; Laval'69; FRCPC; DiagRad. Staff, Hopital Charles LeMoyne; (450)466-5000

LESAGE, Jacques; 103-7811 boul Louis-H. Lafonta, Anjou QC H1K 4E4; Mon'76; FRCPC; Psy (Disability Assessment). Langs: Bilingual(French/English); (514)984-9269

LESAGE, Marie-Eve; CSSS de Portneuf, 700 rue Saint-Cyrille, Saint-Raymond QC G3L 1W1; Laval'10; Staff, Centre Hospitalier Portneuf; (418)337-4611

LESAGE, Michel; Comm Lesions Prof, 530 rue Notre-Dame, Joliette QC J6E 3H7; Laval'62; Public Health & Preventive Med; CommunMed (P.Q.). Langs: Bilingual(French/English); (450)757-7972; michellesage@clp.gouv.qc.ca.

LESAGE, Sandra; Hôpital Ste-Justine, 3175 ch Cote-Sainte-Catherine, Montreal QC H3T 1C5; Mon'03; FRCPC; Anes. Staff, Hôpital Ste-Justine; (514)345-4733

LESCELLEUR, Odette; Hôpital Laval, 2725 ch Sainte-Foy, Quebec QC G1V 4G5; Laval'90; FRCSC; GenSurg. Staff, Hôpital Laval; (418)656-4810

LESCHEID, Jonathan M; Surrey Mem Hosp, 13750 96 Ave, Surrey BC V3V 1Z2; Qns'03; FRCSC; OrthSurg. Staff, Surrey Memorial Hospital; (604)539-4320

LESER, Michael; Main Square Med Centre, 2575 Danforth Ave, Toronto ON M4C 1L5; RCS (Ireland)'59; LRCPSI; LM; (416)694-0500; Fax. (416)694-9767.

LESIEGE, Daniel; Centre Hosp le Gardeur, 911 montee des Pionniers, Terrebonne QC J6V 2H2; Mon'89; MSc; BSc; FRCPC; MedBiochem (Lipid Disorders/Obesity). Chef Biologie Médicale, Centre Hospitalier Pierre le Gardeur; Consultant, Hotel-Dieu de Roberval; Consultant, Centre Hospitalier Jonquiere; Langs: English; (450)654-7525 x32279; daniel.lesiege@cssssl.ca.

LESIEUR, Denis; Centre de sante Sutton, 33 rue Principale S, Sutton QC J0E 2K0; Sher'79; ac Staff, CSSS la Pommeraie; Clin Prof, Universite de Sherbrooke; Langs: English; (450)538-3983; Fax. (450)538-8396.

LESIEUR, Martin; Ctr Hosp Affilie-Enfant-Jesus, 1401 18e rue, Quebec QC G1J 1Z4; Laval'07; OrthSurg. (418)649-0252

LESIEUR, Rene; Centre Med Ste-Foy Inc, 802 av Du Chanoine-Scott, Quebec QC G1V 3N4; Laval'77; assoc Staff, Hôpital Laval; assoc Staff, Centre Hospitalier Affilié Universitaire de Québec - Hôpital du St-Sacrement; Université Laval; (418)653-4931; Fax. (418)653-4797.

LESIUK, Howard J; The Ottawa Hosp-Civic Campus, C 2218-1053 Carling Ave, Ottawa ON K1Y 4E9; Man'82; FRCSC; Neursurg. Att Staff, The Ottawa Hospital - Civic Campus; Clin Assoc Staff, The Ottawa Hospital - General Campus; Assoc Prof Surg, University of Ottawa; (613)761-5383 x2; Fax. (613)761-4332.

LESIUK, Lawrence S; Hamilton HS-General Site, 237 Barton St E, Hamilton ON L8L 2X2; Alb'84; FRCPC; Anes. Ac Staff Anes, Hamilton Health Sciences Centre - Hamilton General Hospital; (905)527-0271

LESIUK, Thomas P; Western Med Assessments, 17204 106A Ave NW, Edmonton AB T5S 1E6; Man'87; BSc(Hons); MSc; FRCPC; PhysMed&Rehab. (780)453-1727

LESK, Mark R; Hop Maisonneuve-Rosemont, 5415 boul de l'Assomption, Montreal QC H1T 2M4; McG'89; BSc(Hon.); MSc; FRCSC; Ophth (Cataract). Att Staff Surg, Hopital Maisonneuve-Rosemont; assoc Prof Ophth, Universite de Montreal; Langs: Bilingual(English/French); (514)252-3878; Fax. (514)252-3905.

LESLEY, Peter A; Hampton Med Centre, 216-1419 Carling Ave, Ottawa ON K1Z 7L6; Ott'87; Med Dir, Canadian Blood Services; (613)728-8880; peter.lesley@blood.ca.

LESLIE, Allan S; 918 Esquimalt Rd, Victoria BC V9A 3M6; UBC'85; (250)382-4296; Fax. (250)382-0023.

LESLIE, Jasmine J T; Alder Med Centre, 277 Evergreen Rd, Campbell River BC V9W 5Y4; UBC'09; CCFP; (250)287-7441

LESLIE, Karen M; The Hosp For Sick Children, 555 University Ave, Toronto ON M5G 1X8; McM'86; FRCPC; Peds (Adolescent Medicine). Staff Peds, The Hospital For Sick Children; Court Staff, St Michael's Hospital; Assoc Prof Peds, University of Toronto; (416)813-6083; Fax. (416)813-5392.

LESLIE, Kenneth A; London HSC-Victoria Hosp, PO Box 5010 Stn B 800 Commissioners Rd E, London ON N6A 5W9; Wes'88; FRCSC; GenSurg. Staff, London Health Sciences Centre - Victoria Campus; (519)667-6778; Fax. (519)667-6764.

LESLIE, Michele I; Masset Med Clinic, PO Box 619, Masset BC V0T 1M0; McM'99; CCFP; (250)626-4702

LESLIE, Neil G; Selkirk Med Group, PO Box 590, Revelstoke BC V0E 2S0; Alb'80; CCFP; FCFP; Staff, Queen Victoria Hospital; Clin Instructor, University of British Columbia.

LESLIE, William D; St Boniface Gen Hosp, C5121-409 Tache Ave, Winnipeg MB R2H 2A6; Man'81; FRCPC; IntMed; NuclearMed. Ac Staff, St Boniface General Hospital; (204)233-8563; Fax. (204)231-0640.

LESOLA, Dasual S; Arcola Family Health Clinic, PO Box 479, Arcola SK S0C 0G0; (306)455-2287

LESOWAY, Robert N; Bridgeland Med Bldg, 306-803 1 Ave NE, Calgary AB T2E 7C5; Alb'76; BSc; FRCPC; IntMed (Angiography); Cardiol. Ac Staff, Rockyview General Hospital; Ac Staff, Foothills Medical Centre; Clin Associate Prof, University of Calgary; (403)571-8600; Fax. (403)571-8659.

LESPERANCE, Bernard; Hop Du Sacre-Coeur De Mtl, 5400 boul Gouin O, Montreal QC H4J 1C5; Mon'82; FRCPC; IntMed; MedOncol; Hem. Staff, Hôpital du Sacre-Coeur de Montréal; (514)338-2150; Fax. (514)338-2631.

LESPERANCE, Francois; CHUM-Hopital Notre-Dame, 1560 rue Sherbrooke E, Montreal QC H2L 4M1; Mon'85; FRCPC; Psy. Staff, Centre Hospitalier l'Université de Montréal (CHUM) - Hôpital Notre-Dame; Staff Teacher Psy, Universite de Montreal; (514)890-8000 x14799; Fax. (514)473-8017; francois.lesperance@umontreal.ca.

LESPERANCE, Jacques; Institut de Cardiologie de Mtl, 5000 rue Belanger, Montreal QC H1T 1C8; Mon'56; DiagRad (Cardiac Radiology). Staff, Institut de Cardiologie de Montréal; (514)376-3330 x3295; Fax. (514)593-2580; jacqueslesper@icm-mhi.org.

LESPERANCE, Jean; CSSS de la Region de Thetford, 1717 rue Notre-Dame E, Thetford Mines QC G6G 2V4; Sher'80; FRCPC; Psy. Staff, Hopital du CSS de la Region de Thetford; (418)338-7707; Fax. (418)338-7705.

LESPERANCE, M Jose O; Castlegar Med Clinic, 1840 8th Ave, Castlegar BC V1N 2Y2; McM'87; CCFP; FCFP; (250)365-7255; Fax. (250)365-0285; kmc@shawcable.com.

LESPERANCE, Sylvie; Polyclinique 640, 104-2000 rue Cours Le Corbusie, Boisbriand QC J7G 3E8; Mon'84; CCFP; Staff, Hôpital du Sacre-Coeur de Montréal; Universite de Montreal; (450)434-3434; Fax. (450)434-6494.

LESSARD, Andre; CHUS-Hop Hotel-Dieu, 580 rue Bowen S, Sherbrooke QC J1G 2E8; Mon'79; IntMed (P.Q.). Staff, Centre Hospitalier Universitaire de Sherbrooke-Hôpital Hôtel-Dieu; (819)346-1110; alesr@videotron.ca.

LESSARD, Andréa; CSSS de Chicoutimi, 305 rue Saint-Vallier, Chicoutimi QC G7H 5H6; Laval'09; CCFP; Staff, Complexe hospitalier de la Sagamie; (418)541-1079; Fax. (418)541-1129.

LESSARD, Anne-Marie; Ctr Hosp Anna-Laberge, 200 boul Brisebois, Chateauguay QC J6K 4W8; Mon'94; FRCPC; DiagRad. Staff Emerg, Hôpital Anna-Laberge; (450)699-2425; Fax. (450)692-3535; amlessard@videotron.ca.

LESSARD, Annie; Centre Hosp Honore-Mercier, 2750 boul Laframboise, Saint-Hyacinthe QC J2S 4Y8; Mon'99; FRCSC; Urol. Staff, Centre Hospitalier Honore-Mercier; (450)771-3333

LESSARD, Ariane; Clinique Med Notre-Dame, 147 rue Notre-Dame E, Victoriaville QC G6P 3Z8; Laval'09; CCFP; (819)758-3165; Fax. (819)758-0745.

LESSARD, Audrey; CSSS du Suroit, 150 rue Saint-Thomas, Salaber-de-Valleyf QC J6T 6C1; Mon'09; CCFP; Staff, Centre Hospitalier Régional du Suroît; (450)371-9920

LESSARD, Bernard; Clinique Med Du Quartier Latin, 905 boul Rene-Levesque E, Montreal QC H2L 5B1; Mon'91; CCFP; FCFP; Langs: Spanish; English; (514)285-5500; Fax. (514)285-2226.

LESSARD, Caryne; CSSS-Hopital De Hull, 116 boul Lionel-Emond, Gatineau QC J8Y 1W7; Laval'98; FRCSC; GenSurg. Staff, Hull Hospital; (819)966-6200

LESSARD, Charles; CSSS Maria-Chapdelaine, 2000 boul du Sacré-Coeur, Dolbeau-Mistassini QC G8L 2R5; Sher'04; Staff, Centre Maria-Chapdelaine - CH de Dolbeau-Mistassini; (418)276-1234

LESSARD, Christian; Clinique Med Notre-Dame, 138 rue Notre-Dame S, Sainte-Marie QC G6E 4A4; Mon'81; (418)387-5200; Fax. (418)387-5283; christian_lessard@ssss.gouv.qc.ca.

LESSARD, Clode; Clinique Enumatologie Centre, 1119 rue Sainte-Marguerite, Trois-Rivieres QC G8Z 1Y2; Sher'02; FRCPC; IntMed; Rheum. (819)370-8106

LESSARD, Daniel; Clinique Med Notre-Dame Inc, 147 rue Notre-Dame E, Victoriaville QC G6P 3Z8; Laval'73; (819)758-3165; Fax. (819)758-0745.

LESSARD, Francois Y; CHUM-Hop St-Luc, 1058 rue Saint-Denis, Montreal QC H2X 3J4; Laval'74; FRCPC; MedBiochem (Lipid Disorders). Chef biochimie, Centre Hospitalier l'Université De Montréal (CHUM) - Hôpital Saint-luc; Teach Staff, Universite de Montreal; (514)890-8000 x35998; Fax. (514)412-7420.

LESSARD, Gerard; 6420 rue des Pins, Becancour QC G9H 3K7; Laval'68; (819)297-2542; Fax. (819)297-2942.

LESSARD, Janice E; Scarborough Prof Centre, 305-1371 Neilson Rd, Scarborough ON M1B 4Z8; Mem'82; BSc; BMedSci; FRCPC; IntMed (Memory Disorders); GeriatricMed. Staff, Rouge Valley Health System - Centenary Health Centre Site; University of Toronto; (416)724-8531

LESSARD, Jean; Clinique Med de la Rive, 169 rue du Prince-Albert, Otterburn Park QC J3H 1L4; Sher'89; Staff, Hopital Charles LeMoyne; (450)446-7333

LESSARD, Julie; CSSS de Rimouski-Neigette, CP 3150 Succ A 150 av Rouleau, Rimouski QC G5L 5T1; Laval'04; Staff, Hôpital Regional Rimouski; (418)723-7851

LESSARD, Julie; CHUQ-Ctr Hosp Univ Laval, 2705 boul Laurier, Quebec QC G1V 4G2; Laval'90; FRCPC; Peds (Developmental Pediatrics). Staff, Centre Hospitalier Universitaire de Quebec-CHUL; Langs: Bilingual(French/English); (418)654-2282; Fax. (418)654-2137; julie.lessard@mail.chuq.qc.ca.

LESSARD, Louise; CSSS Jeanne-Mance, 100-15 av du Mont-Royal O, Montreal QC H2T 2R9; Sher'70; (514)286-9657

LESSARD, Lucie; Clinique Med Val-Belair, 202-1147 boul Pie-XI N, Quebec QC G3K 2P8; Laval'88; Langs: English; (418)843-2473; Fax. (418)843-0224.

LESSARD, Lyne; Plexi-Mediclub, 201-6100 av du Boise, Montreal QC H3S 2W1; Mon'87; Staff, Centre Hospitalier de LaSalle; Langs: Bilingual(French/English); (514)739-5646

LESSARD, M Lucie; MUHC-Montreal Gen Hosp, D6 269-1650 Cedar Ave, Montreal QC H3G 1A4; Laval'80; BSc; FACS; CSPQ; FRCSC; Otol (P.Q.) (Cranio Maxillofacial Surgery); PlasSurg (P.Q.). Chief Plastic Surg, Shriners Hospitals For Children - Canada; Chief Div of Plastic Surg, McGill University Health Centre - Montreal General Campus; Che oto-rhino-lary, McGill University Health Centre - Royal Victoria Hospital; Chef, McGill University Health Centre - Montreal Children's Hospital; assoc Prof, McGill University; Langs: French; (514)934-1934 x44341; Fax. (514)934-8203.

LESSARD, Marie-Claude; CSSS Becancour-Nicolet-Yamaska, 216 rue Principale GD, Fortierville QC G0S 1J0; Laval'95; Staff, CLSC Les Bles d'Or; (819)287-4442; Fax. (819)287-4017.

LESSARD, Marie-Claude; CSSS De Saint-Jerome, 290 rue de Montigny, Saint-Jerome QC J7Z 5T3; Sher'01; MedOncol; Hem; IntMed. Staff, Hôtel-Dieu de Saint-Jérôme; (450)431-8200 x8366

LESSARD, Marie-Eve; Centre de Sante Integrale, RR 5 160 rue Pope, Cookshire QC J0B 1M0; Mon'07; CCFP; (819)875-5535

LESSARD, Marquis; 891 rue Perron RR 2, Maria QC G0C 1Y0; Laval'71; Ac Staff, CSSS de la Baie-des-Chaleurs; (418)259-3944

LESSARD, Marthe; CHUM-Hop St-Luc, 1058 rue Saint-Denis, Montreal QC H2X 3K4; Laval'79; Staff, Centre Hospitalier l'Université De Montréal (CHUM) - Hôpital Saint-luc; (514)890-8444

LESSARD, Martin; Ctr Hosp Affilie-Enfant-Jesus, 1401 18e rue, Quebec QC G1J 1Z4; Laval'85; FRCPC; Anes (Intensive Care); Critical Care Medicine (P.Q.). Staff, Centre Hospitalier Affilié Universitaire de Québec - Hôpital De L'Enfant Jésus; Head Dept of Anes, Université Laval; (418)649-5803; Fax. (418)649-5936.

LESSARD, Melanie; CSSS de Drummond, 350 rue Saint-Jean, Drummondville QC J2B 5L4; Mon'05; FRCPC; Psy. (819)474-2572

LESSARD, Michel; CSSS de Chicoutimi, 305 rue Saint-Vallier, Chicoutimi QC G7H 5H6; Sher'82; AnatPath. Staff, Complexe hospitalier de la Sagamie; Langs: English; French; (418)541-1000 x2591

LESSARD, Monique; Hop Maisonneuve-Rosemont, 5415 boul de l'Assomption, Montreal QC H1T 2M4; Laval'79; FRCPC; RadOncol. Staff, Hopital Maisonneuve-Rosemont; Langs: English; (514)252-3425; Fax. (514)252-3556.

LESSARD, Myriam; Hop du Sacre-Coeur de Mtl, 5400 boul Gouin O, Montreal QC H4J 1C5; Mon'05; FRCPC; IntMed; Nephrol. Staff, Hôpital du Sacre-Coeur de Montréal; Langs: Bilingual(French/English); (514)338-2222 x2883; Fax. (514)338-2182; myriamlessard@yahoo.fr.

LESSARD, Nathalie J; CHUQ-Hotel-Dieu de Quebec, 11 Cote du Palais, Quebec QC G1R 2J6; Sher'02; FRCPC; RadOncol. Staff, Centre Hospitalier Universitaire de Québec (CHUQ) - Siege Social; (418)691-5264; Fax. (418)691-5268.

LESSARD, Nathalie R; Hotel-Dieu D'Arthabaska, 5 rue des Hospitalieres, Victoriaville QC G6P 6N2; Sher'02; Staff, Hotel-Dieu d'Arthabaska; (819)357-2030

LESSARD, Nicole; Hop Maisonneuve-Rosemont, 5415 boul de l'Assomption, Montreal QC H1T 2M4; Laval'79; FRCPC; Anes. Staff, Hopital Maisonneuve-Rosemont; (514)252-3808; Fax. (514)252-3542; nc.lessard@sympatico.ca.

LESSARD, Nicole; CLSC des Mille-Iles, 4731 boul Levesque E, Laval QC H7C 1M9; Mon'84; (450)661-5370; Fax. (450)661-9147.

LESSARD, Pascal; Centre Med Le Mesnil, 300-1300 boul Lebourgneuf, Quebec QC G2K 2N1; Laval'98; Langs: English; French; (418)624-1800; Fax. (418)624-1820.

LESSARD, Philippe; Dir de la Sante Publique, 363 Rte Cameron, Sainte-Marie QC G6E 3E2; Laval'76; MSc; Ac Staff DSC, Centre d'hébergement de Beauceville; Ac Staff Public Health, Centre Hospitalier Beauce-Etchemin; (418)386-3546

LESSARD, Pierre; Clinique D'Orthopedie de Levis, 6620 rue Saint-Georges, Levis QC G6V 4H1; Laval'81; CSPQ; FRCSC; OrthSurg (Reconstructive Surgery). Ac Staff, Centre Hospitalier Paul-Gilbert; Ac Staff, Hôtel-Dieu de Lévis; Langs: English; (418)837-8251; Fax. (418)837-2033.

LESSARD, Richard; Dir de la Sante Publique-Mtl, 1301 rue Sherbrooke E, Montreal QC H2L 1M3; Sher'71; FRCPC; CommunMed (Public Health). Dir, Public Health de Montreal; (514)528-2400 x3543; Fax. (514)528-2453.

LESSARD, Rupert; CSSS de Chicoutimi, 305 rue Saint-Vallier, Chicoutimi QC G7H 5H6; Laval'76; FRCPC; Psy. Staff, Complexe hospitalier de la Sagamie; (418)549-5474; Fax. (418)549-8143.

LESSARD, Serge; Montford Hosp, 713 Montreal Rd, Ottawa ON K1K 0T2; McM'96; FRCPC; Psy (Anxiety & Mood Disorders). Staff, Montfort Hospital; (613)746-4621 x2234; Fax. (613)748-4934.

LESSARD, Sophie; Clinique du Plateau Marquette, 200-731 rue Galt O, Sherbrooke QC J1H 1Z1; Sher'02; FRCPC; Peds. Staff, GMF Centre de sante; (819)564-8662

LESSARD, Stephanie; Clinique Externe Sante Mentale, 26 rue Sainte-Pierre, Saint-Constant QC J5A 1B8; Mon'07; FRCPC; Psy. (450)635-8807

LESSARD, Steve; CSSS de l'Arhipel, 430 ch Principal, Cap-aux-Meules QC G4T 1R9; Laval'09; Staff, Hôpital de l'Archipel; (418)986-2121

LESSARD, Sylvain; Ctr de Sante Paul-Gilbert, 9330 du Centre-Hospitalier, Charny QC G6X 1L6; Laval'03; CCFP; Staff Emerg Med, Centre Hospitalier Paul-Gilbert; (418)380-8993 x2064

LESSARD, Sylvain; CSSS de Trois-Rivières, 1991 boul du Carmel, Trois-Rivieres QC G8Z 3R9; Mon'84; FRCPC; Anes. Staff, CSSS de Trois-Rivières; (819)697-3333

LESSER, Sharolyn R; Courtice Health Centre, 1450 Highway 2, Courtice ON L1E 3C3; Qns'89; CCFP; FCFP; Staff, Lakeridge Health - Oshawa Site; (905)723-8551 x4317; Fax. (905)721-6179.

LESTER, Beverley H; Abbotsford Reg Hosp & Cancer C, 32900 Marshall Rd, Abbotsford BC V2S 0C2; Witwatersrand (South Africa)'92; FRCPC; RadOncol. Staff, Abbotsford Regional Hospital & Cancer Centre; (604)851-4710

LESTER, Frances T; Hamilton HS-McMaster Site, 4V2-1200 Main St W, Hamilton ON L8N 3Z5; Qns'66; MPhil; FRCPC; IntMed. Staff, Hamilton Health Sciences Centre - McMaster University Medical Centre; Staff, General Internal Medicine Rapid Assesstment Clinic; (905)521-2100

LESTER, Michael D; 1204 King St W, Toronto ON M6K 1G4; Tor'85; (416)923-2330

LESTER, Michael L; King Street Med Arts Centre, 204-71 King St W, Mississauga ON L5B 4A2; Tor'64; FRCPC; Peds. Consultant, The Hospital For Sick Children; Consultant, Trillium Health Centre - Mississauga; Asst Prof Peds, University of Toronto; (905)279-0212; Fax. (905)279-1447.

LESTER, Richard; Div of STI/HIV Control, 655 12th Ave W, Vancouver BC V5Z 4R4; Alb'99; FRCPC; IntMed; InfectDis. Staff Division of Infectious Diseases, Vancouver General Hospital - Centennial Pavillion; (604)707-5600

LESUR, Olivier J; CHUS-Hop Fleurimont, 3001 12e Av N, Sherbrooke QC J1H 5N4; (France)'88; PhD; Critical Care Medicine (P.Q.); Respir. Asst Prof Respiratory Med, Centre Hospitalier Universitaire de Sherbrooke-Hopital Fleurimont; Prof, Universite de Sherbrooke; (819)346-1110; Fax. (819)820-6420.

LESWICK, David A; Royal University Hosp, 103 Hospital Dr, Saskatoon SK S7N 0W8; Man'00; FRCPC; DiagRad. Staff, Royal University Hospital; (306)655-2371

LESZCZ, Molyn; Mount Sinai Hosp, 925-600 University Ave, Toronto ON M5G 1X5; Man'76; FRCPC; Psy. Chief Psy, Mount Sinai Hospital; University of Toronto; (416)586-4800 x4555; Fax. (416)586-8654; mleszcz@mtsinai.on.ca.

LETAL, Michael D; Alberta Children's Hosp, 2888 Shaganappi Trail NW, Calgary AB T3B 6A8; Alb'00; FRCPC; Anes. Staff, Alberta Children's Hospital; (403)955-7810; Fax. (403)955-7606.

LETARTE, Helene; CSSS Vieille Capitale, 2400 av d'Estimauville, Quebec QC G1E 7G9; Laval'84; (418)623-1010

LETARTE, Pierre; Chatham-Kent Health Alliance, PO Box 2030 Stn Main 80 Grand Ave W, Chatham ON N7M 5L9; Laval'69; FRCPC; IntMed. Staff, Chatham-Kent Health Alliance - Sydenham Hospital Campus; (519)352-6400

LETARTRE, Laurence; Ctr Hosp Affilie-St-Sacrement, 1050 ch Sainte-Foy, Quebec QC G1S 4L8; Laval'05; FRCPC; Ophth. Staff, Centre Hospitalier Affilié Universitaire de Québec - Hôpital du St-Sacrement; (418)682-7511; laurence.letartre@orlo.ulaval.ca.

LETCHER, Kevin V; Hamilton HS-Henderson Site, 711 Concession St, Hamilton ON L8V 1C3; McM'98; FRCPC; PhysMed&Rehab. Staff, Hamilton Health Sciences Centre-Juravinski Site; (905)385-9894

LETELLIER, Francois; CSSS Pierre Boucher, 1333 boul Jacques-Cartier E, Longueuil QC J4M 2A5; Mon'68; GenSurg (P.Q.) (Laparoscopic Surgery). Staff, Centre Hospitalier Pierre Boucher; Langs: English; Spanish; (450)468-8111; Fax. (450)468-0408; fran.letellier@gmail.com.

LETELLIER, Manon; Clin De Pediatrie De St-Jean, 335-900 boul Du Seminaire N, St-Jean-Sur-Richel QC J3A 1C3; Sher'92; Peds (P.Q.). (450)349-2701

LETELLIER, Monique; Dir de la Sante Publique-Mtl, 1301 rue Sherbrooke E, Montreal QC H2L 1M3; Mon'70; MEd; BPs; Consultant Preventive Med, McGill University Health Centre - Montreal General Campus; (514)528-2400 x3670; Fax. (514)528-2452; mletelli@santepub-mtl.qc.ca.

LETENDRE, Elaine; CHUM-Hop Notre-Dame, 1560 rue Sherbrooke E, Montreal QC H2L 4M1; Mon'90; PhD(McG); FRCPC; MedBiochem (Lipidology). Staff Metabolism Clinic/Chef Metanolic Med Service, Centre Hospitalier l'Université de Montréal (CHUM) - Hôpital Notre-Dame; Clin Prof Med, Universite de Montreal; Langs: Spanish; English; (514)890-8000 x27497; Fax. (514)412-7553; elaine.letendre.chum@ssss.gouv.qc.ca.

LETENDRE, Francois; Hop Maisonneuve-Rosemont, 5415 boul de l'Assomption, Montreal QC H1T 2M4; Mon'78; FRCPC; IntMed; MedOncol; Hem. Staff, Hopital Maisonneuve-Rosemont; Langs: English; (514)252-3404 x3404; Fax. (514)254-5094.

LETENDRE, Julien; 220-5345 boul de l'Assomption, Montreal QC H1T 4B3; Mon'07; FRCSC; Urol. (514)255-9006

LETENDRE, Marie; CLSC de Chateauguay, 95 av de la Verdure, Chateauguay QC J6K 5G4; Laval'95; (450)699-3333

LETENDRE, Michel; Centre Bois De Boulogne, 475-1575 boul Henri-Bourassa O, Montreal QC H3M 3A9; Laval'68; Endocrin (P.Q.); IntMed. Staff, Hôpital du Sacre-Coeur de Montréal; Universite de Montreal; (514)336-3411

LETENDRE, Micheline; CSSS Les Eskers de l'Abitibi, 622 4e rue O, Amos QC J9T 2S2; Laval'91; CCFP; FCFP; Staff, CH Hôtel-Dieu d'Amos; (819)732-3341

LETHOLE, Gabriel M; Biggar & Dist Health Centre, PO Box 70, Biggar SK S0K 0M0.

LETKEMAN, Jacob A; Meadow Lake Associate Clinic, PO Box 1510, Meadow Lake SK S9X 1Z1; Sask'66; Assoc Staff, Meadow Lake Hospital; (306)236-5661; Fax. (306)236-4355.

LETKEMAN, Richard L; Four Rivers Med Clinic, 878 Main St, Winnipeg MB R2W 3P1; Man'02; CCFP.

LETKEMANN, K Lisa; Sioux Lookout Zone Fam Phys, PO Box 4000, Sioux Lookout ON P8T 1K2; Man'02; CCFP; (807)737-5161

LETLEY, Kevyn; Smith Clinic, 1-6601 48 Ave, Camrose AB T4V 3G8; (South Africa)'03; MB ChB; (780)672-2425

LETO, Daniela L; Hamilton HS-Henderson Site, A3 70-711 Concession St, Hamilton ON L8V 1C3; McM'05; InfectDis; MedMicrobiol; IntMed. Staff, Hamilton Health Sciences Centre-Juravinski Site; (905)521-2100

LETOURNEAU, Anne; Clinique Med St-Laurent, 202-500 rte Marie-Victorin, Sorel-Tracy QC J3R 1K7; Mon'06; (450)724-9818

LETOURNEAU, Annie; Clinique Med Cap-St-Ignace, 40 ch des Pionniers E RR 1, Cap-Saint-Ignace QC G0R 1H0; Mon'96; (418)246-5347; Fax. (418)246-3325; annie.letourneau@gmf.gouv.qc.ca.

LETOURNEAU, Dany-Roch; CHUQ-Ctr Hosp Univ Laval, 2705 boul Laurier, Quebec QC G1V 4G2; Laval'97; FRCPC; Anes. Staff, Centre Hospitalier Universitaire de Quebec-CHUL; (418)525-4444; Fax. (418)654-2774; drletour@hotmail.com.

LETOURNEAU, Francois; Centre Med St-Redempteur, 210-600 116 Rte, Saint-Nicolas QC G7A 4X8; Sher'86; CCFP; (418)831-4455; francois.letourneau@gmf.gouv.qc.ca.

LETOURNEAU, Genevieve; Hop Louis-H Lafontaine, 7401 rue Hochelaga, Montreal QC H1N 3M5; Mon'06; Psy. Staff, Hopital Louis-H Lafontaine; (514)251-4000

LETOURNEAU, Gerald; CSSS de Rouyn-Noranda, 1 9e rue, Rouyn-Noranda QC J9X 2A9; Laval'72; FRCPC; CommunMed (P.Q.); Public Health & Preventive Med. Staff, CSSS de Rouyn-Noranda; (819)764-3264 x49339; Fax. (819)797-1947; gerald_letourneau@ssss.gouv.qc.ca.

LETOURNEAU, Isabelle; CSSS du Nord de Lanaudière, 1000 boul Sainte-Anne, St-Charles-Brromee QC J6E 6J2; Sher'97; FRCPC; IntMed (Transplantation); Nephrol. Staff Nephrol, Centre Hospitalier Pierre le Gardeur; Staff Nephrol, Centre Hospitalier Régional de Lanaudière; Langs: Bilingual(French/English); (450)759-8222 x2136; Fax. (450)759-1389.

LETOURNEAU, Jean-Marie; Clinique Medi-Plus, 4100 3e av O, Quebec QC G1H 6E1; Laval'71; (418)622-6969; Fax. (418)622-2037.

LETOURNEAU, Joel; CRSSS Baie-James-Chibougamau, 51 3e rue, Chibougamau QC G8P 1N1; Mon'94; Staff, CRSSS de la Baie-James; (418)748-2676; Fax. (418)748-7123.

LETOURNEAU, Justin; MUHC-Royal Victoria Hosp, 687 av des Pins O, Montreal QC H3A 1A1; McG'08; Staff, McGill University Health Centre - Royal Victoria Hospital; (514)934-1934

LETOURNEAU, Karine; Hotel-Dieu de-Levis, 143 rue Wolfe, Levis QC G6V 3Z1; Laval'04; FRCPC; Neur. Staff, Hôtel-Dieu de Lévis; (418)835-7121; Fax. (418)835-7212.

LETOURNEAU, Louis; CSSS de la Cote-de-Gaspe, 215 boul de York O, Gaspe QC G4X 2W2; Laval'86; DiagRad. Staff, Centre Hospitalier de Gaspe; (418)368-3301; Fax. (418)368-1824.

LETOURNEAU, Malorie; CSSS de Montmagny-L'Islet, 350 boul Tache O RR 1, Montmagny QC G5V 3R8; Laval'05; CSPQ; FRCPC; Anes. Staff, CSSS de Montmagny-L'Islet; (418)248-0630; Fax. (418)248-6838.

LETOURNEAU, Marc; 5 Av Saint-Georges, St-Charles-De-Bell QC G0R 2T0; Laval'70; (418)887-3415; Fax. (418)887-3429.

LETOURNEAU, Richard; CHUM-Hop St-Luc, 1058 rue Saint-Denis, Montreal QC H2X 3J4; Mon'89; FRCSC; GenSurg (Hepatobiliary Surgical Oncology). Staff, Centre Hospitalier l'Université De Montréal (CHUM) - Hôpital Saint-luc; Langs: English; (514)890-8000

LETOURNEAU, Sandra; CSSS de Beauce-Etchemin, 1515 17e rue, Saint-Georges QC G5Y 4T8; Mon'00; Staff, Centre Hospitalier Beauce-Etchemin; (418)228-2031 x7800

LETOURNEAU, Serge; Ctr Hosp St-Joseph La Malbaie, CP 340 Succ Bureau-Chef 303 rue St-Etienne, La Malbaie QC G5A 1T8; Laval'68; GenSurg. Staff, Hôpital de la Malbaie; (418)665-1700

LETOURNEAU, Steeve; Polyclinique De Trois-Rivieres, 250-1900 boul des Recollets, Trois-Rivieres QC G8Z 4K4; Laval'89; AB; FRCSC; Ophth. Staff, CSSS de Trois-Rivières; Clin Prof Ophth, Universite de Sherbrooke; (819)371-3333

LETOURNEAU, Yves; CSSS de Rimouski-Neigette, CP 3150 Succ A 150 av Rouleau, Rimouski QC G5L 5T1; Laval'73; MedOncol (P. Q.); Hem. Staff, Hôpital Regional Rimouski; (418)724-8465; Fax. (418)724-8659.

LETOURNEAU-GUILLON, Laurent; CHUM-Hop Notre-Dame, 1560 rue Sherbrooke E, Montreal QC H2L 4M1; Mon'05; FRCPC; DiagRad (Neuro Radiology). Staff, Centre Hospitalier l'Université de Montréal (CHUM) - Hôpital Notre-Dame; (514)890-8250

LETOVANEC, Sylvie; Centre Med Iberville, 101-235 2e Av, St-Jean-Sur-Richel QC J2X 2B2; Mon'83; Staff, Hôpital du Haut-Richelieu; Langs: Bilingual(French/English); (450)347-5548; Fax. (450)347-4091.

LETOVSKY, Eric E; The Credit Valley Hosp, 2200 Eglinton Ave W, Mississauga ON L5M 2N1; McG'78; MCFP(EM); FRCPC; EmergMed (Emergency Family Medicine). Chief EmergMed, The Credit Valley Hospital; Prof, University of Toronto; (905)813-4530; Fax. (905)813-4548.

LETT, Christine D; Queen City Obst & Gyn, 3271 Quance St E, Regina SK S4V 3B7; Sask'03; FRCSC; ObstGyn. Staff, Regina General Hospital; Physician, Queen City Obstetrics & Gynecology; (306)585-9565; Fax. (306)585-9209.

LETT, Darren A; 7A-389 Main St, Picton ON K0K 2T0; Qns'02; CCFP; CCFP(E.M.); (613)476-5744

LETT, Ronald R; 105-1985 Broadway W, Vancouver BC V6J 4Y3; Alb'76; FRCSC; GenSurg. Staff, University Hospital of Northern British Columbia; Langs: Bilingual(English/French); (604)739-4708

LETT, Ryan C; Regina Qu'Appelle HR-Regina, 1440 14th Ave, Regina SK S4P 0W5; Sask'04; FRCPC; Anes. Staff, Regina General Hospital; (306)766-4444

LETTE, Jean L; Hop Maisonneuve-Rosemont, 5415 boul de l'Assomption, Montreal QC H1T 2M4; McG'77; ABIM; ABNM; FACC; FCCP; FRCPC; NuclearMed. Staff, Hopital Maisonneuve-Rosemont; Staff, Institut de Cardiologie de Montréal; Prof Med, Universite de Montreal; Langs: Spanish; German; Japanese; (514)252-3400 x3219; Fax. (514)289-1813; jlette@lette.com.

LETTNER, Deborah M; Taunton Health Centre, SS 201 1290 Keith Ross Dr, Oshawa ON L1H 7K4; Tor'84; CCFP; (905)723-8551

LETWIN, Ken; 206-125 Bell Farm Rd, Barrie ON L4M 6L2; Tor'95; PhD; Ophth. Staff, Orillia Soldiers' Memorial Hospital; Staff, Royal Victoria Regional Health Centre; (705)725-5443; Fax. (705)725-5442.

LETWIN, Nadine M; Lakeside Med Clinic, 202-15379 Castle Downs Rd NW, Edmonton AB T5X 3Y7; Alb'00; CCFP; (780)472-7575

LEU, Eric D H; South Markham Med Centre, 6-2002 Middlefield Rd, Markham ON L3S 1Y5; Tor'89; (905)201-8222; Fax. (905)201-8238.

LEUCHT, Stephan T; The Hosp for Sick Children, 555 University Ave, Toronto ON M5G 1X8; Berlin (Germany)'00; Staff, The Hospital For Sick Children; (416)813-1500

LEUNG, Albert S H; York-Med Medical Arts Centre, 407-250 Harding Blvd W, Richmond Hill ON L4C 9M7; (Hong Kong)'63; MB BS; DPM; MRCPsy; FRCPC; Psy (Affective Disorders). Hon Consultant, Mackenzie Richmond Hill Hospital; Langs: Cantonese; Mandarin; (905)884-5999; Fax. (905)884-3301.

LEUNG, Alexander A; HSC-Faculty of Medicine, 1404-3330 Hospital Dr NW, Calgary AB T2N 4N1; Alb'06; FRCPC; IntMed.

LEUNG, Alexander K C; 200-233 16 Ave NW, Calgary AB T2M 0H5; (Hong Kong)'73; FRCP(UK&Ire); FRCPCH; FRSH; FRAM; FRCPC; Peds. Consultant Peds, Alberta Children's Hospital; Med Dir, Asian Medical Centre; Clin Prof, University of Calgary; Langs: Chinese; (403)230-3300; Fax. (403)230-3322; aleung@ucalgary.ca.

LEUNG, Alfred K; The Tannery Centre, 311-465 Davis Dr, Newmarket ON L3Y 7T9; Mem'76; Ac Staff, Southlake Regional Health Centre.

LEUNG, Alice C; CASA Downtown, 406-10011 109 St NW, Edmonton AB T5J 3S8; Alb'95; PhC; FRCPC; Psy (Child & Adolescent Psychiatry). Clinical Asst Prof, University of Alberta Hospital; Consultant, CASA Downtown; Consultant, CASA House; Consultant, Morinville Mental Health Clinic; (780)415-6684; Fax. (780)415-6050.

LEUNG, Allan H H; 2526A Jane St, North York ON M3L 1S1; Tor'76; Ac Staff Family Med, Humber River Regional Hospital - Church Street Site; Ac Staff, Humber River Regional Hospital - Finch Avenue Site; (416)746-4014; Fax. (416)749-5305.

LEUNG, Andrew E; London HSC-Victoria Hosp, PO Box 5010 Stn B C1 649-800 Commissioners Rd E, London ON N6A 5W9; Wes'98; FRCPC; DiagRad. Staff, London Health Sciences Centre - Victoria Campus; (519)685-8500 x56190

LEUNG, Andy W C; First Markham Med Centre, 268-3255 Highway 7, Markham ON L3R 3P9; Tor'92; (905)940-2882; Fax. (905)940-0262.

LEUNG, Benjamin Y; 214-3030 Lincoln Ave, Coquitlam BC V3B 6B4; UBC'05; FRCPC; IntMed; Cardiol. (604)474-2505

LEUNG, Bess; 306-9808 King George Blvd, Surrey BC V3T 2V6; UBC'83; Assoc Staff, Surrey Memorial Hospital; (604)588-0678

LEUNG, Bill P Y; Pelham Group Health Centre, 102-245 Pelham Rd, St Catharines ON L2S 1X8; Tor'79; BSc; Langs: Cantonese; (905)704-1331; Fax. (905)704-1137.

LEUNG, Ceta M Y; 4023 Sheppard Ave E, Scarborough ON M1S 1S7; Tor'90; (416)609-9072; Fax. (416)609-3193.

LEUNG, Cheryl S Y; South Riverdale Comm Hlth Ctr, 955 Queen St E, Toronto ON M4M 3P3; Wes'07; CCFP; (416)461-2493; Fax. (416)461-8245.

LEUNG, Chi Tak; Rosedale Med Centre, 303-600 Sherbourne St, Toronto ON M4X 1W4; National (Taiwan)'70; (416)922-0840; Fax. (416)922-2818.

LEUNG, Cho Yau; Douglas Med Centre, 238 Bertie St, Fort Erie ON L2A 1Z3; Manchester (England)'76; (905)871-2233

LEUNG, Christina C W; Univ Hlth Network-Toronto Western Hosp, 432-399 Bathurst St, Toronto ON M5T 2S8; McM'06; FRCSC; Ophth. Staff, Toronto Western Hospital - University Health Network; (416)603-5376

LEUNG, Christopher P; 320 Adelaide St S, London ON N5Z 3L2; Wes'75; (519)672-1530

LEUNG, Chung-Shan; North York Gen Hosp, 4SE 108-4001 Leslie St, North York ON M2K 1E1; (Hong Kong)'84; MB BS; FRCPC; AnatPath. Staff Path, North York General Hospital; Lecturer Path, University of Toronto; Langs: Cantonese; (416)756-6252

LEUNG, Constant H; Collingwood Med Clinic, 350-3150 54th Ave E, Vancouver BC V5S 1Z1; UBC'01; BSc(Hon); CCFP; (604)435-3388; Fax. (604)433-2323.

LEUNG, Cosmas W M; St Paul's Hosp, 1081 Burrard St, Vancouver BC V6Z 1Y6; Sydney (Australia)'68; AB; FRCPC; EmergMed (Administration). Physician Emerg, Providence Health Care - St Paul's Hospital; Clinical Asst Prof Emerg Med, University of British Columbia; Langs: Cantonese; (604)806-8480; Fax. (604)806-8488; cosmas_leung@providencehealth.bc.ca.

LEUNG, D Man-Sun; West End Prof Bldg, 211-9509 156 St NW, Edmonton AB T5P 4J5; Alb'75; FAAFP; CCFP; FCFP; Ac Staff, Covenant Health - Misericordia Community Hospital; Clin Lecturer Family Med, University of Alberta; (780)483-3253; Fax. (780)483-3212.

LEUNG, Daniel L; The Doctor's Office, 13-205 Marycroft Ave, Woodbridge ON L4L 5X8; Tor'75; (905)856-2100; Fax. (905)856-2101.

LEUNG, Daniel P; 1-17 Frank St, Strathroy ON N7G 2R2; Wes'77; BSc(Hon); Med Staff, Strathroy Middlesex General Hospital - Middlesex Hospital Alliance; Langs: Chinese; (519)245-3370; Fax. (519)245-5533; Dan.Leung@mha.tvh.ca.

LEUNG, Debbie W S; Ontario Shores Ctr Mental HS, 700 Gordon St, Whitby ON L1N 5S9; Ott'04; FRCPC; Psy. Staff, Ontario Shores Centre for Mental Health Sciences; (905)430-4055

LEUNG, Deborah K B; Sunnybrook Hlth Sciences Ctre, 2075 Bayview Ave, Toronto ON M4N 3M5; McM'08; CCFP; CCFP(E.M.); Staff, Sunnybrook Health Sciences Centre; (416)480-4037

LEUNG, Desmond D; North York Gen Hosp, 375-4001 Leslie St, North York ON M2K 1E1; Qns'08; CCFP; Staff, North York General Hospital; (416)756-6000

LEUNG, Edmond Y H; CML Health Care Imaging Inc, LL-4800 Leslie St, North York ON M2J 2K9; Tor'78; FRCPC; DiagRad. (416)493-1011

LEUNG, Edward C W; Health Sciences Centre, AE208-820 Sherbrook St, Winnipeg MB R3A 1R9; Tor'02; FRCPC; Peds; Neur. Staff, Health Sciences Centre; (204)774-6511

LEUNG, Elaine W Y; Children's Hosp Eastern Ont, 401 Smyth Rd, Ottawa ON K1H 8L1; Ott'96; FRCPC; Peds; HemPath. Staff, Children's Hospital of Eastern Ontario (CHEO); Fax. (613)738-4837.

LEUNG, Ellen P; 9-1170 Burnhamthorpe Rd W, Mississauga ON L5C 4E6; (Hong Kong)'79; MB BS; MRC(UK); DCH(Lond); CCFP; FCFP; Langs: Cantonese; Mandarin; (905)281-9337; Fax. (905)281-9849; ellenleung79@gmail.com.

LEUNG, Eric; Albert Park Family Med Centre, 3992 Albert St, Regina SK S4S 3R1; Sask'92; BScPharm; CCFP; FCFP; (306)584-3833; Fax. (306)585-3833.

LEUNG, Ernest Yuen-Lun; Chalmers Gate Med Bldg, 301-328 Highway 7 E, Richmond Hill ON L4B 3P7; (Hong Kong)'88; DCH(Ire); FRACGP(Australia); CCFP; FCFP; Langs: Cantonese; (905)882-0923; Fax. (905)882-7775.

LEUNG, Eugene Y C; The Ottawa Hosp-Civic Campus, 1053 Carling Ave, Ottawa ON K1Y 4E9; Ott'00; FRCPC; NuclearMed. Staff, The Ottawa Hospital - Civic Campus; (613)761-4280

LEUNG, F Edmund; St Michael's Health Centre, 80 Bond St, Toronto ON M5B 1X2; Tor'04; CCFP; Staff Family Med, St Michael's Hospital; (416)864-3011; Fax. (416)864-3099.

LEUNG, Fay; Richmond Health Sciences Ctre, 310-6091 Gilbert Rd, Richmond BC V7C 5L9; UBC'04; FRCSC; OrthSurg. Staff, UBC Hospital - Koerner Pavillion; (604)273-6148

LEUNG, Felix K Y; SGH Medical Mall, 502-3030 Lawrence Ave E, Scarborough ON M1P 2T7; Sask'98; FRCPC; IntMed; Rheum. Staff, Toronto Western Hospital - University Health Network; (416)439-4827; Fax. (416)439-7807.

LEUNG, Frances Y K; 202-855 Broadview Ave, Toronto ON M4K 3Z1; Alb'77; DABIM; MSc; FRCPC; Rheum (Fibromyalgia); IntMed. Ac Staff, Sunnybrook Health Sciences Centre; Court Staff, Sault Area Hospital - Sault Ste Marie; Lecturer Med, University of Toronto; Langs: Taishanese; Cantonese; Mandarin; (416)462-1220; Fax. (416)462-1220.

LEUNG, Frederick C C; 204-174 Harwood Ave S, Ajax ON L1S 2H6; Tor'91; CCFP; Langs: Cantonese; (905)683-3572; Fax. (905)683-3578.

LEUNG, Fung; Winterton Clinic, PO Box 100 99 Main St, Winterton NL A0B 3M0; (Taiwan)'64; MD; (709)583-2832

LEUNG, Gregory H Y; 10 Clark St W, Leamington ON N8H 1E4; Wes'77; Ac Staff, Leamington District Memorial Hospital; (519)326-6621

LEUNG, Helen K; 206-236 Georgia St E, Vancouver BC V6A 1Z7; UBC'77; Staff, Providence Health Care - Mount Saint Joseph Hospital; Staff, BC Women's Hospital & Health Centre; (604)681-5831; Fax. (604)683-6996.

LEUNG, Henry H K; 411 Broadway W, Vancouver BC V5Y 1R4; UBC'74; Assoc Staff, Providence Health Care - St Paul's Hospital; Langs: Cantonese; (604)875-1216; Fax. (604)875-1201.

LEUNG, Henry H Y; Alberta Health Services, 4733 49 St, Red Deer AB T4N 1T6; Alb'86; FRCPC; Psy. (403)340-7046; Fax. (403)340-5217; leungh@sah.on.ca.

LEUNG, James C K; 3636 Victoria Park Ave, North York ON M2H 3B2; (Hong Kong)'85; MRCGPract; DDerm; CCFP; FCFP; Court Staff, North York General Hospital; Court Staff, The Scarborough Hospital - Birchmount Campus; Langs: Cantonese; (416)493-1314; Fax. (416)502-3984.

LEUNG, James K H; 105-4235 Sheppard Ave E, Scarborough ON M1S 1T7; Tor'84; (416)298-2088; Fax. (416)298-2188.

LEUNG, Janice M; St Paul's Hosp, 1081 Burrard St, Vancouver BC V6Z 1Y6; Baltimore (USA)'06; Respir; IntMed. Staff, Providence Health Care - St Paul's Hospital; (604)682-2344

LEUNG, Jason K; 118-10151 No. 3 Rd, Richmond BC V7A 4R6; Alb'01; BSc; CCFP; Clin Instructor, University of British Columbia; Langs: Cantonese; (604)273-9920; Fax. (604)273-9924.

LEUNG, Jean-Pierre; Midpark Family Med Centre, 150-290 Midpark Way SE, Calgary AB T2X 1P1; Cal'98; BSc; CCFP; Clin Lecturer, University of Calgary; Langs: Cantonese; Chinese; Bilingual(French/English); (403)201-2726; Fax. (403)201-2710.

LEUNG, Jessica E; Saugeen Shores Med Bldg, RR 1 36 Grey St N, Southampton ON N0H 2L0; UBC'05; CCFP; (519)797-9940; Fax. (519)797-1225.

LEUNG, Kam Kong; North Scarborough Prof Bldg, 406-3420 Finch Ave E, Scarborough ON M1W 2R6; (Australia)'83; (416)494-2847; Fax. (416)494-2847.

LEUNG, Karen M C; 409-2333 Dundas St W, Toronto ON M6R 3A6; Wes'79; Langs: Cantonese; (416)533-5554; Fax. (416)537-9810.

LEUNG, Kelvin W; Thornlea Med Centre, 4A-62 Overlea Blvd, Toronto ON M4H 1C4; Tor'92; (416)425-8800

LEUNG, Kenneth K Y; Foothills Med Centre, 1403 29 St NW, Calgary AB T2N 2T9; Cal'03; CCFP; Staff, Foothills Medical Centre; (403)212-8223

LEUNG, Kent K K; T33A-1661 Denison St, Markham ON L3R 6E4; Alb'93; MD; BScPharm; Langs: Chinese; Cantonese; Mandarin; (905)470-6778; Fax. (905)470-6779.

LEUNG, Kevin K; 105-372 Hollandview Trail, Aurora ON L4G 0A5; Tor'98; CCFP; Staff, Southlake Regional Health Centre; Staff, Markham Stouffville Hospital; (905)726-8332

LEUNG, Kevin M K; 339-4168 Finch Ave E, Scarborough ON M1S 5H6; (Hong Kong)'76; MB BS; DPH(UK); LMCC; Court Staff, The Scarborough Hospital - Birchmount Campus; Court Staff, North York General Hospital; Langs: Chinese; (416)291-0051; Fax. (416)291-0552.

LEUNG, Kevin S N; Doctors Bldg, 40-955 Queen St E, Sault Ste. Marie ON P6A 2C3; (Hong Kong)'63; FRCPC; Peds. (705)949-7400

LEUNG, Man K; East Van Med Bldg, 403-1750 10th Ave E, Vancouver BC V5N 5K4; Sask'89; Langs: Chinese; German; Japanese; (604)873-2223; Fax. (604)874-0034.

LEUNG, Mark D; Collingwood Gen & Marine Hosp, 459 Hume St, Collingwood ON L9Y 1W9; Tor'00; FRCPC; DiagRad. Staff, Collingwood General & Marine Hospital; (705)444-8626

LEUNG, Mark; Rosedale Med Centre, 303-600 Sherbourne St, Toronto ON M4X 1W4; Wes'06; CCFP; (416)922-0840; Fax. (416)922-2818.

LEUNG, Max; Oshawa Clinic, 117 King St E, Oshawa ON L1H 1B9; Aberdeen (Scotland)'72; CCFP; CCFP(E.M.); FCFP; Ac Staff, Lakeridge Health - Oshawa Site; Langs: English; French; (905)723-8551; Fax. (905)721-3562.

LEUNG, Michael; 188 Giles Blvd E, Windsor ON N9A 4B9; Tor'77; CCFP; FCFP; Court Staff, Hôtel-Dieu Grace Hospital; Court Staff, Windsor Regional Hospital - Metropolitan Site; Staff Designated Med. Practitioner, Citizenship & Immigration Canada; (519)258-9314; michael.leung@cic.gc.ca.

LEUNG, Michael N F; 5731 Victoria Dr, Vancouver BC V5P 3W5; UBC'84; Assoc Staff, Providence Health Care - Mount Saint Joseph Hospital; Langs: Cantonese; (604)879-8919

LEUNG, Miriam M L; Market Mall Prof Bldg, 313-4935 40 Ave NW, Calgary AB T3A 2N1; (Hong Kong)'74; FCAP; FRCPC; CCFP; FCFP; AnatPath. (403)235-2450; Fax. (403)235-2453.

LEUNG, Nathalie M C; Hillcrest Mall, 212A-9350 Yonge St, Richmond Hill ON L4C 5G2; Ott'96; FRCPC; IntMed; Endocrin&Metab. Staff, Mackenzie Richmond Hill Hospital; Langs: English; French; (905)770-8034; Fax. (905)770-5637.

LEUNG, N L Eillen; 4-3039 Kingsway, Vancouver BC V5R 5J6; Tor'81; Langs: Cantonese; Mandarin; (604)435-4441

LEUNG, Nin-Ming; 123-8787 Woodbine Ave, Markham ON L3R 9S2; (Hong Kong)'76; MB BS; MRCP(UK); LMCC; CCFP; FCFP; Langs: Cantonese; (905)513-8795; Fax. (905)513-9497.

LEUNG, Patrick P; Wilson Centre Family Practice, 1-2185 Wilson Ave, Port Coquitlam BC V3C 6C1; Cal'90; MSc; BSc(Hons.); CCFP; Ac Staff, Royal Columbian Hospital; Staff, Fraser Health Authority Fraser North Service New Port Public Health; Staff, Community Maternity Centre; Staff Clin Faculty, University Of British Columbia; Langs: Mandarin; Cantonese; (604)942-7227; Fax. (604)942-7058.

LEUNG, Paul M K; Aberdeen Centre, 2180-4151 Hazelbridge Way, Richmond BC V6X 4J7; (Hong Kong)'66; Ac Staff, Vancouver General Hospital - Centennial Pavillion; (604)233-0068; Fax. (604)233-0078.

LEUNG, Paul M K; Strathcona Medical Dental Bldg, 200-8225 105 St NW, Edmonton AB T6E 4H2; Alb'80; FRCSC; OrthSurg (Knee Surgery). Staff, Royal Alexandra Hospital; Staff, Covenant Health - Grey Nuns Community Hospital; (780)439-5858; Fax. (780)433-1344.

LEUNG, Peter C S; Sheppard Med Bldg, 312-701 Sheppard Ave E, North York ON M2K 2Z3; Tor'77; FRCSC; ObstGyn (Infertility). Staff Life Programme, Toronto East General Hospital Inc; (416)733-2037; Fax. (416)445-0429.

LEUNG, Peter M P; PO Box 33101 RPO Glenwood, Edmonton AB T5P 4V8; Alb'84; (780)996-8836

LEUNG, Peter T; St Michael's Hosp, 30 Bond St, Toronto ON M5B 1W8; Tor'79; FRCPC; Anes. Staff Anes & Pain Management Serv, St Michael's Hospital; Asst Prof, University of Toronto; (416)864-5071; Fax. (416)864-6014.

LEUNG, Randy M H; Georgian Prof Centre, 203-125 Bell Farm Rd, Barrie ON L4M 6L2; Tor'05; FRCSC; Otol (Rhinology). (705)728-8066; Fax. (705)725-7330.

LEUNG, Raymond C M; Hys Med Centre, 350-11010 101 St NW, Edmonton AB T5H 4B9; McG'97; FRCPC; IntMed (Coronary Intervention); Cardiol. (780)428-3246; Fax. (780)425-0487.

LEUNG, Richard S T; St Michael's Hosp, 6 045-30 Bond St, Toronto ON M5B 1W8; UBC'93; PhD; FRCPC; IntMed (Sleep Medicine); Respir. Staff Physician, St Michael's Hospital; Asst Prof, University of Toronto; Langs: Cantonese; (416)864-6026; Fax. (416)864-5649.

LEUNG, Rico P N; St Michael's Hosp, 30 Bond St, Toronto ON M5B 1W8; Tor'07; FRCPC; Anes. Staff, St Michael's Hospital; (416)864-5071; leungr@smh.toronto.on.ca.

LEUNG, Robert O; Orleans Family Health Clinic, 101-210 Centrum Blvd, Orleans ON K1E 3V7; Ott'77; (613)837-5454; Fax. (613)837-3781.

LEUNG, Robert S L; 303-3415 Dixie Rd, Mississauga ON L4Y 2B1; McG'70; Ac Staff, Trillium Health Centre - Mississauga; Langs: Cantonese; Mandarin; Toishan; (905)625-1681; Fax. (905)625-0761.

LEUNG, See-Lap; 12-720 Bristol Rd W, Mississauga ON L5R 4A3; Tor'87; PhD; Court Staff, Trillium Health Centre - Mississauga; Langs: Chinese; (905)501-7132; Fax. (905)501-7138.

LEUNG, Sher-Ping; 1165 Dufferin Cres, Nanaimo BC V9S 2B5; Cal'03; FRCSC; GenSurg. Langs: Mandarin; (250)754-3315

LEUNG, Sophia S Y; Credit Valley Med Arts Centre, 213-2000 Credit Valley Rd, Mississauga ON L5M 4N4; Tor'78; Court Staff, Trillium Health Centre - Mississauga; Langs: Cantonese; Mandarin; (905)569-0103; Fax. (905)569-0104.

LEUNG, Stephen T Y; 8-2111 Centre St NW, Calgary AB T2E 2T2; Cal'76; CCFP; Staff, Peter Lougheed Centre; Physician, SAIT Health Services; Langs: Chinese; (403)277-3333; Fax. (403)277-5540.

LEUNG, Tack Ki; Institut de Cardiologie de Mtl, 5000 rue Belanger, Montreal QC H1T 1C8; Lyon (France)'68; GenPath (P.Q.). Pathologist, Institut de Cardiologie de Montréal; Consultant, Hôpital Ste-Justine; tack.leung@icm-mhi.org.

LEUNG, Tamara J; Crestwood Med & Dental Bldg, 208-6051 Gilbert Rd, Richmond BC V7C 3V3; UBC'86; Ac Staff, Richmond Hospital; (604)278-0090

LEUNG, Tanya M; Royal Alexandra Hosp, 10240 Kingsway NW, Edmonton AB T5H 3V9; Alb'00; FRCPC; Anes. Staff, Royal Alexandra Hospital; (780)735-4010

LEUNG, Terence L N; 1287 Gerrard St E, Toronto ON M4L 1Y5; Tor'85; Staff, Toronto East General Hospital Inc; Staff, The Scarborough Hospital - Birchmount Campus; Langs: Cantonese; Mandarin; (416)463-4220; Fax. (416)463-4220.

LEUNG, Tin-Chung; 203-725 Coronation Blvd, Cambridge ON N1R 7S9; Tor'80; Ac Staff, Cambridge Memorial Hospital; (519)624-2262

LEUNG, Vicki W K; King Edward Pediatrics Clinic, 926 King Edward Ave W, Vancouver BC V5Z 2E2; UBC'05; FRCPC; Peds. Langs: Cantonese; Mandarin; (604)600-7282

LEUNG, Victor; St Paul's Hosp, 1081 Burrard St, Vancouver BC V6Z 1Y6; UBC'05; FRCPC; IntMed; MedMicrobiol; InfectDis. Staff, Providence Health Care - St Paul's Hospital; Langs: Cantonese; (604)682-2344

LEUNG, Wai Ming; Leamington Dist Mem Hosp, 3F-194 Talbot St W, Leamington ON N8H 1N9; Tor'81; FRCPC; IntMed. Staff, Leamington District Memorial Hospital; (519)326-3330; Fax. (519)326-0104.

LEUNG, Wesley D C Y; Univ Hlth Network-Toronto Gen, 200 Elizabeth St, Toronto ON M5G 2C4; Tor'06; FRCPC; IntMed; Gastroent. Staff, Toronto General Hospital - UHN; (416)340-4800

LEUNG, Wilson L; Rosedale Med Centre, 709-600 Sherbourne St, Toronto ON M4X 1W4; Tor'79; Ac Staff, Toronto East General Hospital Inc; Langs: Chinese; (416)961-7499; Fax. (416)961-2050.

LEUNG, Wilson W S; 305-5400 Portage Rd, Niagara Falls ON L2G 5X7; Tor'86; BSc; CCFP; Ac Staff FamMed, Niagara Health System - Greater Niagara General Site; Clinical Asst Prof, McMaster University; Langs: Chinese; (905)356-4044; Fax. (905)356-4042.

LEUNG, Wilson W S; Medical Arts Bldg, 353 St Paul Ave, Brantford ON N3R 4N3; UBC'78; BSc; FACS; FRCSC; Urol. Staff, The Brant Community Healthcare System - Brantford General Hospital Site; Staff, The Brant Community Healthcare System - Willett Hospital Site; (519)753-9221; Fax. (519)756-8839; w. leung2008@rogers.com.

LEUNG, Wing Yee V; 3550 18th Ave W, Vancouver BC V6S 1B1; NY (USA)'68; LMCC; Clin Instructor Surg, University of British Columbia; Langs: Chinese; (604)737-1835; Fax. (604)737-1835; wyvleung@dr.com; Semi-Retired.

LEUNG, Winnie M W; College Plaza 3, 225-8215 112 St NW, Edmonton AB T6G 2C8; Qns'04; BSc; FRCPC; IntMed; Respir. Staff, University of Alberta Hospital; (780)407-1732; Fax. (780)407-3027.

LEUNG, Winnie W C; Finch-Midland Med Centre, 402-4190 Finch Ave E, Scarborough ON M1S 4T7; Qns'93; FRCSC; GenSurg (Colon & Rectal Surgery). Ac Staff, The Scarborough Hospital - Birchmount Campus; Langs: Cantonese; (416)291-1900; Fax. (416)291-9469.

LEUNG, Wynne I; Chrysalis Obst & Gyn Clinic, 21-10 Richard Way SW, Calgary AB T3E 7M9; Alb'02; FRCSC; ObstGyn. Staff, Foothills Medical Centre; (403)242-0770; Fax. (403)242-0711.

LEUNG, Yvette P Y; 3330 Hospital Dr NW, Calgary AB T2N 4N1; Cal'99; FRCPC; IntMed; Gastroent. Staff, Foothills Medical Centre; (403)210-9325

LEUNG SHING, Louis P; Charleswood Med Clinic, 3360 Roblin Blvd, Winnipeg MB R3R 0C5; RCS (Ireland)'80; Med Staff, The Salvation Army Grace Hospital; (204)889-7200; Fax. (204)896-5081.

LEVAC, Caroline; Centre Med des Laurentides, 102-1100 rue Saint-Isidore, St-Lin-Laurentides QC J5M 2V6; Mon'04; Langs: Bilingual(French/English); (450)439-3870

LEVAC, Eric; Direction de la Sante Publique, 1255 rue Beauregard, Longueuil QC J4K 2M3; Sher'89; (450)928-6777; Fax. (450)928-3023; e.levac@rrsss16.gouv.qc.ca.

LEVAC, Francine; Direction de la Santé publique, 210-1000 rue Labelle, Saint-Jerome QC J7Z 5N6; Laval'82; (450)436-8622; Fax. (450)436-1761.

LEVAC, Francois; Societe Med Montarvillois, 1435 rue Roberval, Saint-Bruno QC J3V 3P7; Sher'87; Physician, CHSLD Montarville; Langs: English; (450)653-3631; Fax. (450)653-5518.

LEVAC, Marie-France; 213-820 McConnell Ave, Cornwall ON K6H 4M4; Ott'98; BSc; FRCPC; IntMed; Endocrin&Metab. Assoc Staff IntMed, Cornwall Community Hospital; Langs: English; (613)933-0529

LEVAC, Sylvain; CSSS de la Baie-des-Chaleurs, RR 2 419 boul Perron, Maria QC G0C 1Y0; Laval'00; CCFP; CCFP(E.M.); Staff, CSSS de la Baie-des-Chaleurs; (418)759-3164

LEVALLOIS, Patrick J; Inst Nat'l De Sante Publique, 945 av Wolfe, Quebec QC G1V 5B3; Caen (France)'80; FRCPC; CommunMed (Environmental Health); Public Health & Preventive Med. Staff, Centre Hospitalier Universitaire de Quebec-CHUL; Assoc Prof Social & Preventive Med, Université Laval; (418)650-5115 x5216; Fax. (418)654-3144; patrick.levallois@msp.ulaval.ca.

LEVALLOIS-GIGNAC, Jasmin; CSSS du Nord de Lanaudière, 1000 boul Sainte-Anne, St-Charles-Brromee QC J6E 6J2; Mon'07; Nephrol; IntMed. Staff, Centre Hospitalier Régional de Lanaudière; (450)759-8222

LEVAN, Cathy-Mai; Centre Sante de Rigaud, 1 rue Hotel-de-Ville, Rigaud QC J0P 1P0; Mon'06; CCFP; (450)451-5336

LEVAN, Chau; Clinique Med De Castelnau, 785 rue De Castelnau E, Montreal QC H2R 3A3; Saigon (Vietnam)'68; LMCC; Médecin, Clinique Medicale Anjou; Langs: English; Vietnamese; (514)277-4143; Fax. (514)277-4144.

LEVASSEUR, Andre; Hop Maisonneuve-Rosemont, 5415 boul de l'Assomption, Montreal QC H1T 2M4; Laval'68; ABNM; NuclearMed (P.Q.). Staff, Hopital Maisonneuve-Rosemont; (514)252-3400 x3661

LEVASSEUR, Eric; Clin Med Fam D'Edmundston, 50 Av Bateman, Edmundston NB E3V 4A4; Laval'89; CCFP; (506)739-5929; Fax. (506)739-1008; ericlevasseur@msn.com.

LEVASSEUR, Isabelle; Clinique Med Du Vieux-Limoilou, 755 3e Av, Quebec QC G1L 2W7; Laval'76; (418)266-0500; Fax. (418)266-0501.

LEVASSEUR, Jacques; Clinique Med St-Henri, 223 rue Commerciale RR 1, St-Henri-De-Levis QC G0R 3E0; Laval'72; Staff, Hôtel-Dieu de Lévis; (418)882-2268; Fax. (418)882-3561.

LEVASSEUR, Jean; CSSS du Nord de Lanaudière, 1000 boul Sainte-Anne, St-Charles-Brromee QC J6E 6J2; Mon'86; Staff Emerg Med, Centre Hospitalier Régional de Lanaudière; (450)759-2222

LEVASSEUR, Judith L; Oakville Health Centre, 208-1060 Speers Rd, Oakville ON L6L 2X4; Tor'87; PhD; MPs; Staff, Halton Healthcare Services Corporation - Oakville Site; Langs: English; French; (905)842-3735; Fax. (905)842-8001.

LEVASSEUR, Liisa K; City of Lakes Fam Health Team, 25 Black Lake Rd, Lively ON P3Y 1J3; Tor'08; CCFP; Langs: Bilingual(English/French); (705)692-1018

LEVASSEUR, Louis; Ass Entraide Sante Mentale, GD 198 boul Perron O, New Richmond QC G0C 2B0; Mon'93; (418)392-4888

LEVASSEUR, Louis-Bernard; CSSS de Coaticook, 138 rue Jeanne-Mance, Coaticook QC J1A 1W3; Sher'10; Staff, Centre Hospitalier de Coaticook; (819)849-4876

LEVASSEUR, Marie-Eve; Hotel-Dieu de Levis, 143 rue Wolfe, Levis QC G6V 3Z1; Laval'01; FRCPC; PhysMed&Rehab. Staff, Hôtel-Dieu de Lévis; (418)835-7121

LEVECK, David E; St Mary's Gen Hosp, 911 Queens Blvd, Kitchener ON N2M 1B2; Qns'04; CCFP; Staff ER, St Mary's General Hospital; Staff, Grand River Hospital - Kitchener/Waterloo Health Centre; (519)744-3311

LEVEILLE, Alain; 10300 ch Ste-Marguerite CP 4099 succ A, Trois-Rivieres QC G9B 7Y6; Laval'76; Staff, Centre de santé Cloutier-du-Rivage; (819)377-5015; joan.t@videotron.ca.

LEVEILLE, Andre; Clinique Medicale Levis, 300-4975 boul de la Rive-Sud, Levis QC G6V 4Z5; Laval'79; FRCSC; PlasSurg. (418)837-4212; clinique@ccpmtl.com.

LEVEILLE, Claude; Clinique de Chir Esthetique, 300-4975 boul de la Rive-Sud, Levis QC G6V 4Z5; Laval'76; PlasSurg (P.Q.). (418)837-1015

LEVEILLE, Daniel; Polyclinique Med de Terrebonne, 201-901 boul des Seigneurs, Terrebonne QC J6W 1T8; Laval'97; Staff, Centre Hospitalier Pierre le Gardeur; (450)471-1117; Fax. (450)471-8043.

LEVEILLE, Francois; CSSS Drummond-Hop Sainte-Croix, 570 rue Heriot, Drummondville QC J2B 1C1; Mon'99; AnatPath. Pathologist, Hôpital Sainte-croix.

LEVEILLE, Germaine; CSSS de Montmagny-L'Islet, 350 boul Tache O RR 1, Montmagny QC G5V 3R8; Mon'80; GenSurg (P.Q.). Staff, CSSS de Montmagny-L'Islet; (418)248-0630; Fax. (418)248-0820.

LEVEILLE, J E Guy; CHUM-Hop Notre-Dame, 1560 rue Sherbrooke E, Montreal QC H2L 4M1; Laval'82; FRCPC; Psy. Staff, Centre Hospitalier l'Université de Montréal (CHUM) - Hôpital Notre-Dame; (514)890-8000 x26333; Fax. (514)412-7662.

LEVEILLE, Jean; Hotel-Dieu de Sorel, 400 av de L'Hotel-Dieu, Sorel-Tracy QC J3P 1N5; Mon'65; ABNM; FRCPC; Peds (Neurology); NuclearMed. Staff, Hôtel-Dieu de Sorel; Consultant, Hôpital Ste-Justine; Pres, Med. Specialist Assoc. for Nuclear Med. & Pres., Association Med. de Langue Francaise du Canada; Prof Nuclear Med & Radiol, Universite de Montreal; (450)746-6000 x7134

LEVEILLE, Josianne; Ctr Hosp du Centre la Mauricie, 50 119e rue, Shawinigan-Sud QC G9P 5K1; Laval'01; FRCPC; Anes. Staff, Centre Hospitalier du Centre la Mauricie; (819)536-7500 x3141

LEVEILLE, Kimberley L; 7-3353 The Credit Woodlands, Mississauga ON L5C 2K1; McM'82; CCFP; FCFP; Ac Staff, The Credit Valley Hospital; Lecturer, University of Toronto; (905)615-0990; Fax. (905)615-0995.

LEVEILLE, Marie-Eve; Ctr Hosp du Centre la Mauricie, 50 119e rue, Shawinigan-Sud QC G9P 5K1; Laval'02; Staff, Centre Hospitalier du Centre la Mauricie; (819)536-7575

LEVEILLE, Michel P; CHUM-Hop Notre-Dame, 1560 rue Sherbrooke E, Montreal QC H2L 4M1; Mon'72; Nephrol (P.Q.); IntMed (Clinical Nephrology). Staff, Centre Hospitalier l'Université de Montréal (CHUM) - Hôpital Notre-Dame; adj Prof, Universite de Montreal; Langs: English; Spanish; (514)890-8000 x26616

LEVEILLE, Pierre; Ctr Hosp du Centre la Mauricie, 50 119e rue, Shawinigan-Sud QC G9P 5K1; Laval'76; DiagRad. Staff, Centre Hospitalier du Centre la Mauricie; (819)536-7523; Fax. (819)536-7557.

LEVEILLE, Rheal J; 7-3353 The Credit Woodlands, Mississauga ON L5C 2K1; Tor'84; Court Staff, The Credit Valley Hospital; (905)615-0990; Fax. (905)615-0995.

LEVEILLEE, Felix; Hotel-Dieu D'arthabaska, 5 rue des Hospitalieres, Victoriaville QC G6P 6N2; Sher'03; FRCPC; NuclearMed. Staff, Hotel-Dieu d'Arthabaska; (819)357-2030

LEVEJAC, Chantal; CLSC Du Plateau Mont-Royal, 4625 av de Lorimier, Montreal QC H2H 2B4; Mon'85; (514)521-7663

LEVENBERG, Melissa; CLSC-CHSLD PAT Montreal Est, 13926 rue Notre-Dame E, Pte-aux-Trembles QC H1A 1T5; Mon'02; CCFP; (514)642-4050 x515; Fax. (514)642-5438.

LEVENDALL, Tamzyn D T; Family Physicians Group, PO Box 2170, Melfort SK S0E 1A0; (306)752-5757; Fax. (306)752-7252.

LEVENE, Richard G; St Michael's Hosp, 30 Bond St, Toronto ON M5B 1W8; McG'86; FRCPC; Anes (Critical Care Medicine); IntMed. Staff, St Michael's Hospital; Asst Prof Anes/Lecturer, University of Toronto; (416)926-5071; Fax. (416)864-6014.

LEVENSTADT, Jeremy S; Orleans Urgent Care, 1220 Place d'Orleans Dr, Orleans ON K1C 7K3; Tor'10; CCFP; (613)841-5389

LEVENTAL, Mark; SMBD Jewish Gen Hosp, 3755 ch Cote-Sainte-Catherine, Montreal QC H3T 1E2; McG'88; FRCPC; CCFP; DiagRad. Att Staff Radiol, Sir Mortimer B Davis Jewish General; Asst Prof Radiol, McGill University; (514)349-8222 x5348; Fax. (514)340-7907; mark.levental@mcgill.ca.

LEVENTHAL, Joseph I; Sports Med & Rehabilitation, 1539 Bloor St W, Toronto ON M6P 1A5; Tor'50; CCFP; FCFP; Langs: French; (416)539-0302; Fax. (416)539-0395.

LEVENTIS, Anastasios; Oak Ridges Med Centre, 100-13291 Yonge St, Richmond Hill ON L4E 4L6; Tor'00; CCFP; Staff, The Scarborough Hospital - General Campus; (905)773-7759 x2228

LEVER, Christopher G; Sunnyhill Pediatric Clinic, 200-1632 14 Ave NW, Calgary AB T2N 1M7; Cal'92; FRCPC; Peds. Staff, Alberta Children's Hospital; Staff, Foothills Medical Centre; (403)284-0001

LEVER, James P; 204A-849 Alexander Court, Peterborough ON K9J 7H8; Ott'95; FRCSC; OrthSurg. (705)743-3332; Fax. (705)743-5893.

LEVER, Paule; Clinique Saint-Sauveur, 70 rue Principale, Saint-Sauveur QC J0R 1R6; Laval'84; (450)227-8436

LEVERE, Kevin C; Alberta Children's Hosp, 2888 Shaganappi Trail NW, Calgary AB T3B 6A8; Qns'98; FRCPC; Peds. Staff, Alberta Children's Hospital; (403)955-7211; Fax. (403)955-7865.

LEVERETTE, John S; Kingston Gen Hosp, 76 Stuart St, Kingston ON K7L 2V7; Qns'69; FRCPC; Psy. Dep Chief Psy/Att Staff, Kingston General Hospital; Dep Head Chair/Chair, Queen's University; (613)549-6666

LEVERIDGE, Michael J; Kingston Gen Hosp, 76 Stuart St, Kingston ON K7L 2V7; Tor'03; FRCSC; Urol. Staff, Kingston General Hospital; (613)548-2502; Fax. (613)545-1970.

LEVERMAN, Jennifer; Cobequid Commun Health Centre, 40 Freer Lane, Lower Sackville NS B4C 0A2; Dal'02; CCFP; CCFP(E.M.); Staff, Cobequid Community Health Centre; (902)869-6101

LEVERT, Valerie; Hop du Sacre-Coeur de Mtl, 5400 boul Gouin O, Montreal QC H4J 1C5; Laval'99; CSPQ; NuclearMed. Staff, Hôpital du Sacre-Coeur de Montréal; (514)338-2222

LEVESQUE, Alain; Hop Riviere-des-Prairies, 7070 boul Perras, Montreal QC H1E 1A4; Laval'72; FRCPC; Psy. Staff, Hôpital Riviere des Prairies; (514)251-1551; Fax. (514)251-1651.

LEVESQUE, Andre; Clinique Med Lauzon, 213 rue Saint-Joseph, Levis QC G6V 1C8; Laval'65; Staff, Hôtel-Dieu de Lévis; (418)833-5040; Fax. (418)833-6954.

LEVESQUE, Andree; Dr Georges-L Dumont Reg Hosp, 330 av Universite, Moncton NB E1C 2Z3; Sher'01; FRCPC; Psy. Staff, Dr Georges-L-Dumont University Hospital Centre; (506)862-4587; Fax. (506)862-4325.

LEVESQUE, Anne; GMF des Seigneuries, 2220 boul Rene-Gaultier, Varennes QC J3X 1E3; Mon'88; (450)652-2917; Fax. (450)652-9902.

LEVESQUE, Anny; Clinique Med Pierre-Bertrand, 212-303 boul Pierre-Bertrand, Quebec QC G1M 3L7; Sher'96; Staff Emerg, Hôpital Sainte Anne de Beaupré; (418)683-2724

LEVESQUE, Benoit; Inst Nat'l De Sante Publique, 945 av Wolfe, Quebec QC G1V 5B3; Laval'83; FRCPC; CommunMed; Public Health & Preventive Med. Staff, Centre Hospitalier Universitaire de Quebec-CHUL; (418)650-5115 x5214; benoit.levesque@inspq.qc.ca.

LEVESQUE, Chantale; 101-4101 rue Molson, Montreal QC H1Y 3L1; Mon'91; CCFP; FCFP; Staff, CSSS du Coeur de l'Isle Hôpital Jean-Talon; Langs: English; French; (514)807-2333

LEVESQUE, Charles; Clinique De Med Familiale, 1971 rue Bilodeau, Plessisville QC G6L 3J1; Laval'75; Prés Council of Phys & Dentists, CLSC de l'Erable; (819)362-6337; Fax. (819)362-9147.

LEVESQUE, Christian; TB 200-800 boul Chomedey, Laval QC H7V 3Y4; Laval'83; DrMedChOccupHealth; CSPQ; OccupMed (P. Q.) (Public Health). ac Staff Public Health, Hopital de la Cite de la santé; Consultant Med, Hydro-Quebec; Langs: English; Spanish; (450)687-5691

LEVESQUE, Christian; Ctr Hosp Anna-Laberge, 200 boul Brisebois, Chateauguay QC J6K 4W8; Laval'92; GenSurg. Staff, Hôpital Anna-Laberge; (450)699-2425; Fax. (450)699-2525.

LEVESQUE, Christopher B; Cameron Street Clinic, PO Box 792 Stn Main 107 Cameron St, Moncton NB E1C 8N6; Mem'82; BL; LLM; BSc; BMedSci; Staff, The Moncton Hospital; (506)384-1894; cbl@nbnet.nb.ca.

LEVESQUE, Clairmont; Clinique Med Du Carrefour, 8585 boul Lacroix, Saint-Georges QC G5Y 5L6; Laval'88; (418)227-1271; Fax. (418)227-2781.

LEVESQUE, Claude; CSSSG-Hop de Hull, 116 boul Lionel-Emond, Gatineau QC J8Y 1W7; Laval'88; FRCPC; IntMed; Cardiol. Staff, Hull Hospital; (819)595-6054

LEVESQUE, Daniel; Clinique Med D'Amos, 106-641 4e rue O, Amos QC J9T 2S1; Sher'91; FRCSC; Otol. Staff, CH Hôtel-Dieu d'Amos; (819)732-3341; Fax. (819)732-4773.

LEVESQUE, Denise; CSSS de Rimouski-Neigette, CP 3150 Succ A 150 av Rouleau, Rimouski QC G5L 5T1; Sher'76; Staff, Hôpital Regional Rimouski; (418)724-8315; Fax. (418)724-8652.

LEVESQUE, Dominique; MUHC-Montreal Children's Hosp, D562-2300 rue Tupper, Montreal QC H3H 1P3; Laval'94; FRCPC; Peds (Motility Disease); Gastroent. Staff Ped Gastroent, McGill University Health Centre - Montreal Children's Hospital; Langs: Bilingual(French/English); (514)412-4474; Fax. (514)412-4392.

LEVESQUE, Eric; CHUQ-Hotel-Dieu de Quebec, 11 Cote du Palais, Quebec QC G1R 2J6; Laval'01; FRCPC; IntMed; MedOncol; Hem. Staff, Centre Hospitalier Universitaire de Québec (CHUQ) - Siege Social; (418)525-4444 x15280

LEVESQUE, France; Clinique Med Pierre-Bertrand, 212-303 boul Pierre-Bertrand, Quebec QC G1M 3L7; Mon'96; (418)683-2724; Fax. (418)683-8861.

LEVESQUE, Francine; CSSS de la Haute-Gaspésie, 50 rue du Belvedere, Ste-Anne-des-Monts QC G4V 1X4; Sher'80; ObstGyn (P.Q.). Staff, Centre Hospitalier des Monts; (418)763-2261 x2120; Fax. (418)763-9477.

LEVESQUE, Gaetan; 565 rue Tache RR 1, Saint-Pascal QC G0L 3Y0; Laval'74; Dir-Serv Prof/Occup Ther, CSSS de Kamouraska; (418)492-6234; Fax. (418)492-6053.

LEVESQUE, Genevieve; Unite De Med Familiale, 165 rue des Gouverneurs, Rimouski QC G5L 7R2; Laval'90; CCFP; FCFP; (418)723-1222; Fax. (418)723-7668.

LEVESQUE, Georges; Institut de Cardiologie de Mtl, 5000 rue Belanger, Montreal QC H1T 1C8; Sher'74; FRCPC; EmergMed. Staff, Institut de Cardiologie de Montréal; (514)376-3330 x3000

LEVESQUE, Georges; CSSS de Rimouski-Neigette, CP 3150 Succ A 150 av Rouleau, Rimouski QC G5L 5T1; Laval'73; MedOncol; Hem (P.Q.). Staff, Hôpital Regional Rimouski; (418)724-8465

LEVESQUE, Ghislain; 565 rue Tache GD, Saint-Pascal QC G0L 3Y0; Laval'69; (418)492-2148

LEVESQUE, Ghislain; CSSS de Laval, 280 boul Du Roi-Du-Nord, Laval QC H7L 4L2; Mon'83; (450)622-5110; Fax. (450)622-4150.

LEVESQUE, Gilles; Medicentre Kirkland, 2971 Boul Saint-Charles, Kirkland QC H9H 3B5; Sher'80; (514)693-5505; Fax. (514)697-3929.

LEVESQUE, Isabelle; CSSS Haut-Richelieu-Rouville, 920 boul du Seminaire N, St-Jean-sur-Richel QC J3A 1B7; Sher'04; Staff, Hôpital du Haut-Richelieu; (450)359-5000

LEVESQUE, Isabelle; Ctr Obstetrique et Gynecologie, 4250 1re av, Quebec QC G1H 2S5; Mon'05; FRCSC; ObstGyn. Staff, Centre Hospitalier Universitaire De Québec - Pavillon De St-françois-d'assise; (418)654-0555

LEVESQUE, Jacques; Clinique Radiologique Capitale, 4225 4e av O, Quebec QC G1H 6P3; Laval'75; FRCPC; DiagRad (Mammography). Langs: Bilingual(French/English); (418)628-8291; Fax. (418)628-2976.

LEVESQUE, Jacques P; Direction de la Sante Publique, 1-205 boul de York O, Gaspe QC G4X 2W5; Mon'66; MSc; (418)368-4623

LEVESQUE, Jean; Clin Med Sherbrooke-Dickson, 5696 rue Sherbrooke E, Montreal QC H1N 1A1; Mon'84; (514)254-0909

LEVESQUE, Jean-Charles; Ctr Hosp Fleury, 2180 rue Fleury E, Montreal QC H2B 1K3; Sher'83; Anes. Staff, Centre Hospitalier Fleury; Langs: English; (514)384-4200

LEVESQUE, Jean-Daniel; Ctr Hosp du Centre la Mauricie, 50 119e rue, Shawinigan-Sud QC G9P 5K1; Sher'05; FRCPC; DiagRad. Staff, Centre Hospitalier du Centre la Mauricie; (819)536-7500

LEVESQUE, Jean-Frederic; Inst Nat'l Sante Publique du Q, 190 boul Cremazie E, Montreal QC H2P 1E2; Mon'97; FRCPC; CommunMed (Epidemiology); Public Health & Preventive Med. Ac Member, Hopital Maisonneuve-Rosemont; (514)864-1600; jflevesq@santepub-mtl.qc.ca.

LEVESQUE, Jean-Louis; 116 boul Gerard-D.-Levesque O GD, Paspebiac QC G0C 2K0; Laval'75; Staff Family Med, CLSC de Paspebiac; (418)752-6331; Fax. (418)752-6981.

LEVESQUE, Jean-Luc; CSSS Haut-Richelieu-Rouville, 920 boul du Seminaire N, St-Jean-sur-Richel QC J3A 1B7; Mon'04; FRCSC; GenSurg (Gastroenterology). Staff, Hôpital du Haut-Richelieu; (450)359-5000

LEVESQUE, Jean-Marc; Ctr Hosp Anna-Laberge, 200 boul Brisebois, Chateauguay QC J6K 4W8; Mon'88; OrthSurg (P.Q.) (Sports Medicine). Staff, Hôpital Anna-Laberge; Langs: English; (450)699-2425; Fax. (450)699-2525.

LEVESQUE, Jennifer; CSSS Pierre Boucher, 1333 boul Jacques-Cartier E, Longueuil QC J4M 2A5; Laval'10; Staff 1, Centre Hospitalier Pierre Boucher; (450)468-8111

LEVESQUE, Jerome; Credit Valley Prof Bldg, 406-2300 Eglinton Ave W, Mississauga ON L5M 2V8; McM'89; FRCSC; OrthSurg. Staff, The Credit Valley Hospital; (905)569-7952; Fax. (905)828-5136.

LEVESQUE, Josette; Hop Santa Cabrini Ospedale, 5655 rue Saint-Zotique E, Montreal QC H1T 1P7; Sher'81; Anes (P.Q.). Staff, Hôpital Santa Cabrini Ospedale; (514)252-6000

LEVESQUE, Josée; Jacquet River Health Centre, 41 Mack St, Belledune NB E8G 2R3; Sher'96; CCFP; FCFP; Staff, Jacquet River Health Centre; (506)237-3222

LEVESQUE, Julie; CLSC Laurier-Station, 135 rue de la Station, Laurier-Station QC G0S 1N0; Laval'94; (418)728-3435

LEVESQUE, Julie; St Boniface Gen Hosp, D 1048-409 Tache Ave, Winnipeg MB R2H 2A6; Laval'98; CCFP; FCFP; Staff, St Boniface General Hospital; Langs: English; (204)235-3910; Fax. (204)237-9057; jlevesque@centredesante.mb.ca.

LEVESQUE, Lise; Clinique Med Soleil, 64 1re Av O, Amos QC J9T 1T8; Mon'00; (819)732-8341; Fax. (819)732-1642.

LEVESQUE, Marianne; Hop du Sacre-Coeur de Mtl, 5400 boul Gouin O, Montreal QC H4J 1C5; Mon'07; FRCPC; IntMed; Respir. Staff, Hôpital du Sacre-Coeur de Montréal; (514)338-2222

LEVESQUE, Marie-Helene; CSSS de Rimouski-Neigette, CP 3150 Succ A 150 av Rouleau, Rimouski QC G5L 5T1; Mon'93; FRCPC; Derm (External Clinic). Staff, Hôpital Regional Rimouski; (418)723-7851 x8056

LEVESQUE, Marise; Clinique De Med Fam Montcalm, 309 rue Montcalm, Chicoutimi QC G7J 2V1; Sher'10; CCFP; (418)545-4211

LEVESQUE, Martine; Centre Med Fam de Baie-Comeau, 189 av Damase-Potvin, Baie-Comeau QC G4Z 2Y9; Laval'91; Staff Family Med, Centre Hospitalier Régional Baie-Comeau; (418)296-9119; Fax. (418)296-9446.

LEVESQUE, Martine; Ctr Hosp Fleury, 2180 rue Fleury E, Montreal QC H2B 1K3; Mon'89; FRCSC; OrthSurg. Staff, Centre Hospitalier Fleury; (514)384-2000

LEVESQUE, Michael A; 201-112 Queenston St, St Catharines ON L2R 2Z4; Tor'03; FRCPC; IntMed; MedOncol. (905)685-8082; Fax. (905)988-5776.

LEVESQUE, Michel; Clinique Med Gen D'Alma, 22 rue Melancon E, Alma QC G8B 6W3; Laval'73; ac Staff, CSSS de Lac-Saint Jean-Est; (418)668-2377; michel.levesque@ssss.gouv.qc.ca.

LEVESQUE, Nancy; CSSS Becancour-Nicolet-Yamaska, 216 rue Principale GD, Fortierville QC G0S 1J0; Laval'95; Langs: English; (819)287-4442; Fax. (819)287-4017.

LEVESQUE, Normand; Clinique Med Du Boise Langevin, 130-288 rue Pierre-Saindon, Rimouski QC G5L 9A8; Sher'89; (418)724-4672; Fax. (418)724-4753.

LEVESQUE, Paul; Hop Maisonneuve-Rosemont, 5415 boul de l'Assomption, Montreal QC H1T 2M4; Mon'86; Staff, Hopital Maisonneuve-Rosemont; (514)252-3523; Fax. (514)252-3566.

LEVESQUE, Philippe; Hôpital Laval, 2725 ch Sainte-Foy, Quebec QC G1V 4G5; Laval'08; CCFP; Staff, Hôpital Laval; (418)656-8711

LEVESQUE, Pierre; CHUQ-Hotel-Dieu De Quebec, 11 Cote Du Palais, Quebec QC G1R 2J6; Laval'75; Cardiol (P.Q.). Staff, Centre Hospitalier Universitaire de Québec (CHUQ) - Siege Social; (418)691-5151

LEVESQUE, Rejean-Yves; CSSS de Jonquiere, CP 1200 Succ Pdf Jonquiere 2230 rue de l'Hopital, Jonquiere QC G7X 7X2; Sher'72; LMCC; DiagRad (Radiology). Staff, Centre Hospitalier Jonquiere; Langs: English; (418)695-7700

LEVESQUE, Renee; CHUM-Hop St-Luc, 1058 rue Saint-Denis, Montreal QC H2X 3J4; Mon'96; FRCPC; IntMed; Nephrol. Staff, Centre Hospitalier l'Université De Montréal (CHUM) - Hôpital Saint-luc; Langs: English; (514)890-8000 x32588; Fax. (514)412-7831; renee.1.levesque.chum@ssss.gouv.qc.ca.

LEVESQUE, Robin; 183 Boul Sainte-Anne, Ste-Anne-Plai QC J0N 1H0; Sher'77; Staff Obst, Hôtel-Dieu de Saint-Jérôme; (450)478-4243

LEVESQUE, Roger; Quinte Health CC-Belleville Si, 607-265 Dundas St E, Belleville ON K8N 5A9; Ott'89; FRCPC; IntMed (Hematology); MedOncol. Staff, QHC Belleville General; Asst Prof Oncol, Queen's University; (613)969-7400

LEVESQUE, Samuel; CSSS de Rimouski-Neigette, CP 3150 Succ A 150 av Rouleau, Rimouski QC G5L 5T1; McG'06; MDCM; FRCPC; DiagRad. Staff, Hôpital Regional Rimouski; (418)724-3000

LEVESQUE, Sebastien; CHUS-Hop Fleurimont, 3001 12e av N, Sherbrooke QC J1H 5N4; Laval'05; FRCPC; MedGenetics. Staff, Centre Hospitalier Universitaire de Sherbrooke-Hopital Fleurimont; (819)346-1110 x16640; Fax. (819)564-5217.

LEVESQUE, Simon; Ctr Hosp Affilie-Enfant Jesus, 1401 18e rue, Quebec QC G1J 1Z4; Laval'98; FRCPC; Anes. Staff, Centre Hospitalier Affilié Universitaire de Québec - Hôpital De L'Enfant Jésus; (418)649-0252; Fax. (418)649-5918.

LEVESQUE, Sonia; Centre Hosp Honore-Mercier, 2750 boul Laframboise, Saint-Hyacinthe QC J2S 4Y8; Mon'92; FRCSC; GenSurg. Staff, Centre Hospitalier Honore-Mercier; Langs: English; (450)771-3333

LEVESQUE, Stephane; CSSS du Lac-des-Deux-Montagnes, 520 boul Arthur-Sauve, Saint-Eustache QC J7R 5B1; Mon'91; CCFP; Staff, Hôpital de Saint-Eustache; (450)473-6811

LEVESQUE, Stephanie; CSSS de Rimouski-Neigette, CP 3150 Succ A 150 av Rouleau, Rimouski QC G5L 5T1; Laval'00; FRCSC; ObstGyn. Staff, Hôpital Regional Rimouski; (418)724-8147; Fax. (418)724-8632; stleve@hotmail.com.

LEVESQUE, Suzie L; CHUQ-Ctr Hosp Univ Laval, 2705 boul Laurier, Quebec QC G1V 4G2; Laval'84; FRCPC; Psy. Ac Staff, Centre Hospitalier Universitaire de Quebec-CHUL; (418)654-2121; Fax. (418)691-5717.

LEVESQUE, Sylvie; Club Tiny Tots, 3170-6900 boul Decarie, Montreal QC H3X 2T8; Sher'91; FRCPC; Psy (Medico Legal Psychiatry). Staff, Hopital Ste-Anne; Langs: Bilingual(French/English); (514)283-1726

LEVESQUE, Yvan; CSST Chaudieres-Appalaches, 835 rue de la Concorde, Saint-Romuald QC G6W 7P7; Laval'84; Staff, Centre Hospitalier Regional du Grand-Portage; (418)839-2500 x2343

LEVESQUE, Yves A; 924 rue Richelieu, Beloeil QC J3G 4P9; Mon'77; Langs: English; (450)467-8788; Fax. (450)467-0030.

LEVESQUE, Yves; Hotel-Dieu D'arthabaska, 5 rue des Hospitalieres, Victoriaville QC G6P 6N2; Laval'03; FRCSC; GenSurg. Staff, Hotel-Dieu d'Arthabaska; (819)357-2030

LEVESQUE-CHOUINARD, Annabelle; Clinique Med Champlain, 103-195 rue de l'Atmosphere, Gatineau QC J9A 0A3; Laval'07; CCFP; Staff, Hôpital de Gatineau; Langs: Bilingual(French/English); (819)777-7270

LEVESQUE-HALIMI, Carole; Ctr Hosp Anna-Laberge, 200 boul Brisebois, Chateauguay QC J6K 4W8; Laval'89; Staff, Hôpital Anna-Laberge; (450)699-2425

LEVESQUE ROULEAU, Maude; CSSS de Saint-Jerome, 290 rue de Montigny, Saint-Jerome QC J7Z 5T3; Mon'00; FRCPC; IntMed; Nephrol. Staff, Hôtel-Dieu de Saint-Jérôme; Langs: English; (450)431-8420

LEVI, Aline; 26 rue Silverbirch, Dollard-D-Ormeaux QC H9A 2L3; McG'84; Chef Gen Med, Jewish Rehabilitation Hospital; Langs: English; French; (514)683-2928; Fax. (514)684-0611.

LEVI, Clifford S; Health Sciences Centre, GF307-820 Sherbrook St, Winnipeg MB R3A 1R9; Man'75; FRCPC; DiagRad (Diagnostic Ultrasound). Med Staff, Health Sciences Centre; Med Cons/Radiol, Beausejour District Hospital; Prof Radiol, University of Manitoba; (204)787-3103; clevi@exchange.hsc.mb.ca.

LEVI, Dahlia; Clinique Med Ahuntsic, 241 rue Fleury O, Montreal QC H3L 1V2; McG'08; (514)381-8418; Fax. (514)381-1741.

LEVI, Yves; Clinique Med Ahuntsic, 118-241 rue Fleury O, Montreal QC H3L 1V2; McG'81; (514)381-8418

LEVICHEK, Zinaida; North York Gen Hosp-Branson, 5F-555 Finch Ave W, North York ON M2R 1N5; Chernovzy (Russia (Federation))'84; FRCPC; Peds. Staff, North York General Hospital - Branson Division; (416)632-8703

LEVICK, Carrie A; Humboldt Med Clinic, PO Box 220, Humboldt SK S0K 2A0; Sask'97; CCFP; (306)682-2618; Fax. (306)682-4499; humboldtclinic@sasktel.net.

LEVIN, Adeera; St Paul's Hosp, 6010A-1081 Burrard St, Vancouver BC V6Z 1Y6; McM'84; FRCPC; IntMed; Nephrol. Staff Nephrol, Providence Health Care - St Paul's Hospital; Dir, BC Provincial Renal Agency; Staff, Burrard Health Centre; Prof Med, University of British Columbia; Langs: Bilingual(English/French); (604)682-2344

LEVIN, Alexander L; 1702-805 Broadway W, Vancouver BC V5Z 1K1; Russia (Russia (Federation))'81; MD; FRCPC; Psy (Inpatient Psychiatry). Physician, Forensic Psychiatric Hospital; Asst Staff Departmental, University of British Columbia; Langs: Russian; (604)568-6688; alevin@forensic.bc.ca.

LEVIN, Brenda L; 602-400 Tache Ave, Winnipeg MB R2H 3C3; Man'84; FRCSC; Otol.

LEVIN, Daniel P; Health Sciences Centre, 820 Sherbrook St, Winnipeg MB R3A 1R9; Man'83; FRCPC; NuclearMed. Head Section of Nuclear Med, The Salvation Army Grace Hospital; Staff, Health Sciences Centre; Asst Prof, University of Manitoba; Langs: French; (204)787-3375; Fax. (204)787-3090; dlevin@exchange.hsc.mb.ca.

VANNA V DE AMORIN LEVIN, Gio; Psych Health Centre, PX362-771 Bannatyne Ave, Winnipeg MB R3E 3N4; Goias (Other Foreign)'92; FRCPC; Psy.

LEVIN, Heather A; Manitoba Clinic, 790 Sherbrook St, Winnipeg MB R3A 1M3; Man'77; FRCSC; Otol. (204)774-6541; Fax. (204)783-6558.

LEVIN, Ilona; Chinook Paediatric Clinic, 951 19 St S, Lethbridge AB T1J 3H5; (Russia (Federation))'91; Consultant Pediatrician, Chinook Regional Hospital; Langs: Russian; Hebrew; (403)320-7825; Fax. (403)320-8613.

LEVIN, Iwan; Brandon Reg Health Centre, 150 McTavish Ave E, Brandon MB R7A 2B3; (South Africa)'97; MB ChB; Staff, Brandon Regional Health Centre; (204)578-4000

LEVIN, Leo; 207-5293 Highway 7, Markham ON L3P 7M7; Man'80; FRCPC; Peds. Chief Peds, Markham Stouffville Hospital; Staff PartTime, The Hospital For Sick Children; (905)471-7787; Fax. (905)472-5148.

LEVIN, Leonard A; Hop Maisonnuve-Rosemont, 5415 boul de l'Assomption, Montreal QC H1T 2M4; Harvard,Boston(MA) (USA)'89; Ophth (P.Q.). Staff, Hopital Maisonneuve-Rosemont; Chef Ophthalmology, McGill University.

LEVIN, Leslie; Univ Hlth Network-Princess M, 5F-610 University Ave, Toronto ON M5G 2M9; Birmingham (England)'70; MB ChB; MRC; FRCPC; IntMed (Medical Oncology). Staff, Princess Margaret Hospital - University Health Network; Prov Coord Cancer Diseases, Ministry of Health; Prof/Chair, University of Western Ontario; (416)946-2000; Fax. (416)946-6556.

LEVIN, Martin R; Dr Levin's Teen Clinic, 314-250 Harding Blvd W, Richmond Hill ON L4C 9M7; Man'82; FRCPC; Peds (Acne Treatment). (905)508-5545; Fax. (905)508-9953.

LEVIN, Morris F; St Thomas-Elgin Gen Hosp PO Box 2007 Stn Main, St Thomas ON N5P 3W2; Witwatersrand (South Africa)'81; FRCPC; DiagRad. Staff, St Thomas Elgin General Hospital; (519)631-2020 x2009; Fax. (519)631-8842; mlevin@stegh.on.ca.

LEVIN, Moses; Jewish Rehab Hosp, 3205 Place Alton-Goldbloom, Laval QC H7V 1R2; McG'74; CCFP; Staff, Jewish Rehabilitation Hospital; (450)688-9550

LEVIN, Richard; MUHC-Royal Victoria Hosp, 687 av des Pins O, Montreal QC H3A 1A1; New York(NY) (USA)'74; ABIM; ABCD; BSc(Hon); DABIM; FACP; FACC; Staff, McGill University Health Centre - Royal Victoria Hospital; Emeritus Prof, New York State University; Doyen/Prof Vice-Principal Health Affairs, McGill University; Langs: Spanish; Bilingual(English/French); (514)398-3524; Fax. (514)937-6463; richard.levin@mcgill.ca.

LEVIN, Simon; Children's Hosp, PO Box 5010 Stn B B1 176-800 Commissioners Rd E, London ON N6A 5W9; Birmingham (England)'73; MB ChB; FRCP(E); FRCPC; Peds (Birth Asphyxia). Consultant Paediatric Neurol, London Health Sciences Centre - Victoria Campus; Assoc Prof, University of Western Ontario; (519)685-8332; Fax. (519)685-8350.

LEVIN, Wilfred; Univ Hlth Network-Princess M, 610 University Ave, Toronto ON M5G 2M9; Cape Town (South Africa)'66; MB ChB; MMed(Radiol.); FFR(T); FRCPC; RadOncol (Breasts)., Princess Margaret Hospital - University Health Network; Asst Prof RadOncol, University of Toronto; Langs: Afrikaans; (416)946-4501 x2127; Fax. (416)946-4442; wilfred.levin@mp.uhn.on.ca.

LEVINE, Daniel S; Centre Med Ste-Anne, 500 Old St. Patrick St, Ottawa ON K1N 9G4; McG'83; CCFP; FCFP; Staff, The Ottawa Hospital Rehabilitation Centre; Langs: English; French; (613)789-1552; Fax. (613)789-0659.

LEVINE, David Z; 403-265 Yorkland Blvd, North York ON M2J 5C7; McG'63; FRCPC; Nephrol (P.Q.); MedScient(Med). Court Staff, St Michael's Hospital; (416)229-2399; Fax. (416)229-9771.

LEVINE, Gerald M; Atrium Prof Bldg, 203-190 Cundles Rd E, Barrie ON L4M 4S5; Tor'82; CCFP; Ac Staff, Royal Victoria Regional Health Centre; (705)728-4242; Fax. (705)728-5703.

LEVINE, Mark F; The Hosp for Sick Children, 555 University Ave, Toronto ON M5G 1X8; Witwatersrand (South Africa)'82; FRCPC; Anes (Pediatric Anesthesia). Staff Aens, The Hospital For Sick Children; Asst Prof, University of Toronto; (416)813-7445; mark.levine@sickkids.on.ca.

LEVINE, Mark N; The Juravinski Cancer Centre, 699 Concession St, Hamilton ON L8V 5C2; McG'76; FRCPC; Hem; MedOncol. Mgr, Hamilton Health Sciences Centre-Juravinski Site; McMaster University; (905)387-9711 x64604; Fax. (905)575-6326.

LEVINE, Noah C; Dr Langer & Associates, 180 Sandalwood Pky E, Brampton ON L6Z 1Y4; Tor'96; CCFP; FCFP; (905)846-9255; Fax. (905)846-2525.

LEVINE, Norman B; 77 Maclaren St, Ottawa ON K2P 0K5; McG'72; FRCPC; Psy. (613)235-4692

LEVINE, Richard H; 202-149 Second Ave, Ottawa ON K1S 2H6; Tor'80; FRCPC; Psy. (613)594-4935

LEVINE, Richard J; Lakeridge Hlth Corp-Oshawa, 1 Hospital Crt, Oshawa ON L1G 2B9; Wes'97; BSc; FRCPC; DiagRad (Abdominal Imaging). Staff, Lakeridge Health - Oshawa Site; Partner, Durham Radiology Associates; (905)576-8711; Fax. (905)721-4770.

LEVINE, Ronald H; 650-56 Aberfoyle Cres, Etobicoke ON M8X 2W4; McG'79; FRCSC; PlasSurg. Head Plastic Surg, St Joseph's Health Centre; University of Toronto; (416)236-2581; Fax. (416)236-2695; ronald.levine@utoronto.ca.

LEVINE, Sharon S; Royal Ottawa Hlth Care Group, 1145 Carling Ave, Ottawa ON K1Z 7K4; McG'76; MPH; FRCPC; Psy (Geriatric Psychiatry). Staff Geriatric Psy, Royal Ottawa Mental Health Centre - Royal Ottawa Health Care Group; Langs: English; French; (613)722-6521; Fax. (613)798-2999.

LEVINE, Zachary A; MUHC-Montreal Gen Hosp, B2 117-1650 av Cedar, Montreal QC H3G 1A4; Qns'00; CCFP; CCFP(E.M.); Staff, McGill University Health Centre - Montreal General Campus; (514)934-1934 x42501

LEVINS, James P; Salmon Arm Med Clinic, PO Box 730 Stn Main, Salmon Arm BC V1E 4N8; UBC'95; CCFP; FCFP; (250)832-2321; Fax. (250)832-6095.

LEVINSKY, Elyse S; Hydro Place Bldg, 3155-700 University Ave, Toronto ON M5G 1Z5; Tor'95; MHSc; FRCSC; ObstGyn. Physician, Mount Sinai Hospital; Physician, St Michael's Hospital; (416)586-3108

LEVINSKYY, Mykhaylo V; Grey Nuns Community Hosp, 23A-1100 Youville Drive West N, Edmonton AB T6L 5X8; (Ukraine)'81; PhD; Staff Consultant Child & Adolescent Psy, Covenant Health - Grey Nuns Community Hospital; Clin Assoc Prof Psy, University of Alberta; Langs: Ukrainian; Russian; Polish; (780)735-7346

LEVINSON, Andrea J; Addiction & Mental Hlth-Queen, 1001 Queen St W, Toronto ON M6J 1H4; McM'99; FRCPC; Psy. Staff, Centre for Addiction & Mental Health (CAMH) - Queen Site; (416)535-8501 x33640

LEVINSON, Anthony J; McMaster University, MDCL 3117-1280 Main St W, Hamilton ON L8S 4K1; McM'97; FRCPC; Psy. Staff, Hamilton Health Sciences Centre - McMaster Children's Hospital; (905)525-9140

LEVINSON, Ari D; 206-840 Coxwell Ave, Toronto ON M4C 5T2; Cape Town (South Africa)'87; MB ChB; BSc(Med); DABIM; FRCPC; IntMed; Cardiol. Staff Cardiol, Toronto East General Hospital Inc; (416)691-3111; Fax. (416)691-9957; arilevinson@sympatico.ca.

LEVINSON, Edward D; 48-4324 rue Sherbrooke O, Westmount QC H3Z 1E1; McG'53; FRCPC; Psy. Staff, Sir Mortimer B Davis Jewish General; adj Prof, McGill University; (514)933-3376

LEVINSON, Steven D; Port Hope Med Centre, 202-249 Ontario St, Port Hope ON L1A 3Y9; Tor'71; (905)885-8371

LEVINSON, Wendy; St Michael's Hosp, RFE 3 805-190 Elizabeth St, Toronto ON M5G 2C4; McM'76; FRCPC; IntMed. Chair Medicine, University of Toronto; (416)946-8071

LEVIS, Carolyn M; St Joseph's Healthcare, 820-50 Charlton Ave E, Hamilton ON L8N 4A6; Wes'91; MSc; FRCSC; PlasSurg (Hand Microsurgery). Staff, St Joseph's Healthcare - Charlton Campus; Staff, Hamilton Health Sciences Centre - McMaster University Medical Centre; Assoc Prof Surg, McMaster University; (905)308-9419; Fax. (905)525-6424; levisc@mcmaster.ca.

LEVIS, Michael D; The Hosp for Sick Children, 555 University Ave, Toronto ON M5G 1X8; UBC'83; DAB; MHSc; FRCPC; Anes (Critical Care Medicine). Staff, The Hospital For Sick Children; (416)813-7445

LEVIS, Nicole D; Kensington Med Clinic, 6548 Hastings St, Burnaby BC V5B 1S2; UBC'00; CCFP.

LEVITAN, Deborah E; Women's College Hosp, 76 Grenville St, Toronto ON M5S 1B2; McG'80; CCFP; FCFP; Court Staff, Mackenzie Richmond Hill Hospital; Ac Staff Family Med, Women's College Hospital; Asst Prof Family Med, University of Toronto; (416)323-6060; Fax. (416)323-6402.

LEVITAN, Maurice D; 403-4430 Bathurst St, North York ON M3H 3S3; McG'81; FRCPC; Neur. Med Staff, North York General Hospital; Assoc Staff/Clin Instructor Neurol, Toronto Western Hospital - University Health Network; (416)633-2725; Fax. (416)633-4465.

LEVITAN, Riva E; Carling-Broadview Med Bldg, 205-770 Broadview Ave, Ottawa ON K2A 3Z3; Tor'93; CCFP; FCFP; (613)729-1324; Fax. (613)729-5870.

LEVITAN, Robert D; 4289-100 Stokes St, Toronto ON M6J 1H4; McG'86; FRCPC; Psy. Staff, Centre for Addiction & Mental Health (CAMH) - College Street Site; Prof, University of Toronto; (416)535-8501 x34020; Fax. (416)979-6864.

LEVITIN, Bryna S; Scarborough Hosp-General Div, 3050 Lawrence Ave E, Scarborough ON M1P 2V5; McG'74; FRCPC; DiagRad (Ultrasound). Staff Radiol, The Scarborough Hospital - General Campus; (416)431-8107

LEVITSKY, Neil S; 301-343 Wilson Ave, North York ON M3H 1T1; Wes'86; FRCPC; Psy (Cognitive Behaviour Therapy). Staff, North York General Hospital; (416)515-7741; Fax. (416)515-0241; drlevitsky@rogers.com.

LEVITT, Anthony J; Sunnybrook Hlth Sciences Ctre, 2075 Bayview Ave, Toronto ON M4N 3M5; Perth (Australia)'83; FRCPC; Psy. Staff, Sunnybrook Health Sciences Centre; (416)480-4089

LEVITT, Cheryl A; McMaster University, 201A-175 Longwood Rd S, Hamilton ON L8P 0A1; Witwatersrand (South Africa)'75; MB BCh; CCFP; FCFP; Staff, Hamilton Health Sciences Centre - McMaster Children's Hospital; Prof Family Med, McMaster University; (905)525-9140 x28500; Fax. (905)527-4440.

LEVITT, David S; Humber River Reg Hosp-Finch, 2111 Finch Ave W, North York ON M3N 1N1; Tor'87; Staff, Humber River Regional Hospital - Finch Avenue Site; (416)744-2500

LEVITT, Nirvair K; Sprectrum Health Med Clinic, 702-1080 Howe St, Vancouver BC V6Z 2T1; Lusaka (Zambia)'78; BSc; MB ChB; CCFP; FCFP; Clinical Asst Prof Family & CommunMed, University of British Columbia; Langs: Punjabi; (604)681-1080

LEVITT, Ralph; 908-38 William Carson Cres, North York ON M2P 2H2; Tor'66; Ac Staff Family & Commun Med, North York General Hospital; (416)733-9877; ralphlevitt@rogers.com.

LEVITZ, Suzanne F; Mount Sinai Hosp Centre, 5690 boul Cavendish, Cote Saint-Luc QC H4W 1S7; McG'86; CCFP; Staff, Mount Sinai Hospital Center; adj Prof, St Mary's Hospital Centre; adj Prof, McGill University; (514)369-2222; Fax. (514)369-6187.

LEVREAULT, Jean-Guy; CSSS de Saint-Jerome, 290 rue de Montigny, Saint-Jerome QC J7Z 5T3; Mon'93; Microbio & Infect Dis (P.Q.); MedMicrobiol (P.Q.). Staff, Hôtel-Dieu de Saint-Jérôme; (450)431-8200

LEVREAULT, Marie-Pier D; CSSS Haut-Richelieu-Rouville, 920 boul du Seminaire N, St-Jean-sur-Richel QC J3A 1B7; McG'09; CCFP; Staff, Hôpital du Haut-Richelieu; (450)359-5000

LEVROS, Louis-Charles; Clinique Med Perrier, 10-10794 rue Lajeunesse, Montreal QC H3L 2E8; (Haiti)'72; Médecin, CSSS Saint-Leonard et Saint-Michel; Langs: Creole; English; (514)383-0559; Fax. (514)383-3430.

LEVSTIK, Mark A; London HSC-University Hosp, PO Box 5339 C4 211C-339 Windermere Rd, London ON N6A 5A5; (Ireland)'90; FRCPC; IntMed (Hepatology). Staff, St Joseph's Hospital - St Joseph's Health Care; Staff, London Health Sciences Centre - University Hospital; Assoc Prof, University of Western Ontario; Langs: German; (519)663-3165; Fax. (519)663-3858.

LEVY, Arielle R; Hôpital Ste-Justine, 3175 ch Cote-Sainte-Catherine, Montreal QC H3T 1C5; Mon'92; FAAP; LMCC; FRCPC; Peds (Emergency Medicine). Staff, Hôpital Ste-Justine; (514)345-4931 x4919

LEVY, David; Clinique MD Sante, 200-8127 boul Saint-Laurent, Montreal QC H2P 2M1; McG'02; BSc; Dir méd, Clinique MD Sante; Langs: Hebrew; English; (514)687-4372; Fax. (514)687-4376; info@cliniquemdsante.com.

LEVY, David R; Dr Daniel Levy Mem Sports MC, 810 King St E, Hamilton ON L8M 1A9; McM'75; DOHS(McM); Dip SportMed; CCFP; FCFP; Dir Primary Care Sport Med Clinic, Hamilton Health Sciences Centre-Juravinski Site; Dir Primary Care Sport Med Clinic, Hamilton Health Sciences Centre - McMaster Children's Hospital; Court Staff, Joseph Brant Memorial Hospital; Chair Advisory Committee Athletic Therapy, Sheridan College; Clin Assoc Prof Family Med & Internal Med, McMaster University; (905)549-9242; Fax. (905)548-0003.

LEVY, Deborah M; The Hosp For Sick Children, 555 University Ave, Toronto ON M5G 1X8; Tor'95; FRCPC; Peds. Staff, The Hospital For Sick Children; Vis Staff, Health Sciences North-Laurentian Site; (416)813-7654 x28108; deborah.levy@sickkids.ca.

LEVY, Donald M; Hotel Dieu Grace Hosp, 1030 Ouellette Ave, Windsor ON N9A 1E1; Dal'98; CCFP; CCFP(E.M.); FCFP; Staff, Hôtel-Dieu Grace Hospital; (519)973-4401

LEVY, Emmanuelle; Douglas Mental Hlth Univ Inst, 6875 boul Lasalle, Verdun QC H4H 1R3; Sher'97; FRCPC; Psy. Staff, Douglas Mental Health University Institute; (514)761-6131

LEVY, Gary A; Multi Organ Transplant Program, NCSB11 123-585 University Ave, Toronto ON M5G 2N2; Tor'73; FRCPC; IntMed (Hepatology); Gastroent. Sr Scientist, Toronto General Hospital - UHN; Dir, Multi Organ Transplant Program; Prof Med, University of Toronto; Fax. (416)340-3378.

LEVY, Harold L; 610-101 Queensway W, Mississauga ON L5B 2P7; Ott'72; MBA; CHE; FRCPC; IntMed (Respirology)., Trillium Health Centre - Mississauga; University of Toronto; (905)276-2052; Fax. (905)276-0216; drchest@aol.com.

LEVY, Isra G; Ottawa Public Health, 100 Constellation Cres, Nepean ON K2G 6J8; Witwatersrand (South Africa)'86; BSc(Hons); MSc; FRCPC; CommunMed. Aj Prof, University of Ottawa; (613)580-6744 x23681

LEVY, J Mark; Vancouver Gen Hosp, 855 12th Ave W, Vancouver BC V5Z 1M9; UBC'80; FRCPC; Psy. Staff Psy, Vancouver General Hospital - Centennial Pavillion; Staff, Vancouver Regional Forensic Clinic; (604)875-4009; Fax. (604)875-4226; mlevy@forensic.bc.ca.

LEVY, Lance D; 174 Duplex Ave, Toronto ON M5P 2A9; Glasgow (Scotland)'78; MB ChB; MSc; FRCPC; Peds (Bariatric Medicine). (416)489-0180; drlancelevy@rogers.com.

LEVY, Lyall A; 8675 Granville St, Vancouver BC V6P 5A3; UBC'61; Staff, Vancouver General Hospital - Centennial Pavillion; Staff, BC Children's Hospital; Staff, BC Women's Hospital & Health Centre; (604)263-2646; Fax. (604)263-2649.

LEVY, Mark E; 325 Dundurn St S, Hamilton ON L8P 4L5; Tor'71; (905)526-1255

LEVY, Maurice; Bathurst Med Centre, 205-7117 Bathurst St, Thornhill ON L4J 2J6; Tel-Aviv (Israel)'81; FRCPC; Peds. (905)886-9033; Fax. (905)886-5001.

LEVY, Michelle H; Thames Valley FHT-Byron Fam Me, 1228 Commissioners Rd W, London ON N6K 1C7; McM'98; CCFP; FCFP; (519)472-9670

LEVY, Michelle; Sheppard Med Bldg, 304-701 Sheppard Ave E, North York ON M2K 2Z3; Tor'99; FRCPC; Derm. (416)590-9918

LEVY, Michelle R; Sherman Health & Wellness Ctr, 3F-9600 Bathurst St, Maple ON L6A 3Z8; Tor'07; CCFP; (289)269-1522

LEVY, Mortimer; MUHC-Royal Victoria Hosp, 687 av des Pins O, Montreal QC H3A 1A1; McG'61; FRCPC; IntMed; Nephrol (P.Q.). Sr Physician Nephrol, McGill University Health Centre - Royal Victoria Hospital; Prof, McGill University; (514)934-1934 x35203; Fax. (514)843-2815; mortimer.levy@mcgill.ca.

LEVY, Richard M; Levy Med Clinic, 1390 Main St E, Hamilton ON L8K 1C1; Tor'74; CCFP; FCFP; (905)549-1244; Fax. (905)549-4089.

LEVY, Robert D; Respiratory Division, 7F-2775 Laurel St, Vancouver BC V5Z 1M9; McG'79; FRCPC; IntMed (Pulmonary Medicine); Respir. Staff RespMed, Providence Health Care - St Paul's Hospital; Staff, Vancouver General Hospital - Centennial Pavillion; (604)875-4122; rlevy@providencehealth.bc.ca.

LEVY, Ron; Kingston Gen Hosp, 304-76 Stuart St, Kingston ON K7L 2V7; Qns'05; FRCSC; Neursurg. Staff, Kingston General Hospital.

LEVY, Sharon L; Don Valley Med Associates Inc, 144-1333 Sheppard Ave E, North York ON M2J 1V1; Tor'81; CCFP; FCFP; Court Staff, North York General Hospital; (416)491-5900; Fax. (416)491-1149.

LEVY, Shauna B; Victoria Gen Hosp, 2340 Pembina Hwy, Winnipeg MB R3T 2E8; Man'89; FRCPC; Anes. Staff, Victoria General Hospital; (204)269-3570

LEVY, Sheldon L; 1050-180 Dundas St W, Toronto ON M5G 1Z8; Wes'91; (416)599-5991 x19; Fax. (416)599-6169; sllevy@riverfront.com.

LEVY, Shirley; Uptown Health Centre, 243 Eglinton Ave W, Toronto ON M4R 1B1; McG'03; CCFP; (416)489-2106; Fax. (416)489-2981.

LEVY, Todd; 202-80 Finch Ave W, North York ON M2N 2H4; Tor'85; Court Staff, North York General Hospital; Med Consultant Rehab Solutions, Toronto Western Hospital - University Health Network; (416)222-6154; Fax. (416)224-8684.

LEVYTSKY, Adrian A; Guelph Gen Hosp, 115 Delhi St, Guelph ON N1E 4J4; Qns'95; CCFP; CCFP(E.M.); FCFP; Staff, Guelph General Hospital; (519)822-5350

LEW, Jason W L; 130-8191 Westminster Hwy, Richmond BC V6X 1A7; UBC'10; CCFP; (604)716-1527

LEW, Viviane A; CSSS de la Haute-Gaspésie, 50 rue du Belvedere, Ste-Anne-des-Monts QC G4V 1X4; Mon'86; FRCPC; Psy. Staff, Centre Hospitalier des Monts; (418)763-2261

LEWALL, Mark D; Palliser Health Authority, 666 5 St SW, Medicine Hat AB T1A 4H6; Cal'96; FRCPC; DiagRad. (403)529-8850; Fax. (403)529-8078.

LEWANCZUK, Richard Z; Heritage Med Research Centre, 362-107 University Campus NW, Edmonton AB T6G 2S2; Alb'83; PhD(MedSci); FRCPC; IntMed (Hypertension); Endocrin&Metab. Prof, University of Alberta; (780)407-3636; Fax. (780)407-6702; rlewancz@ualberta.ca.

LEWANDOWSKI, Bernard J; The Ottawa Hosp-Civic Campus, 1053 Carling Ave, Ottawa ON K1Y 4E9; McG'71; FRCPC; DiagRad. Staff/Head Ultrasound, The Ottawa Hospital - Civic Campus; (613)798-5555 x13255

LEWANS, Raymond L; Saanich Plaza Med Clinic, 3544 Blanshard St, Victoria BC V8X 1W3; Sask'73; (250)475-1101

LEWELL, Michael P; London HSC-Victoria Hosp, 800 Commissioners Rd E, London ON N6A 5W9; Wes'95; FRCPC; EmergMed. Staff, London Health Sciences Centre - Victoria Campus; (519)685-8500 x76538

LEWI, Renee; Norfinch Med Centre, 301-2100 Finch Ave W, North York ON M3N 2Z9; Tor'77; CCFP; FCFP; Staff, Humber River Regional Hospital - Finch Avenue Site; (416)739-8700

LEWICKE, Shannon M; 1050 91 St SW, Edmonton AB T6X 0P2; Cal'09; CCFP; (780)463-7050; Fax. (780)463-7551.

LEWICKI, Mark; North Oshawa Med Centre, 101-1400 Ritson Rd N, Oshawa ON L1G 7W4; Tor'90; Staff, Lakeridge Health - Oshawa Site; (905)433-5027; Fax. (905)721-1368.

LEWIN, Gabriela A; Kemptville Health Centre, RR 5 2671 Concession Rd, Kemptville ON K0G 1J0; Buenos Aires (Argentina)'95; CCFP; (613)258-0100

LEWIN, Laura L; 207-770 Broadview Ave, Ottawa ON K2A 3Z3; Ott'87; CCFP; (613)224-1248

LEWIN, Michael C; 344 Hume St, Collingwood ON L9Y 1W3; Tor'94; CCFP; Langs: Spanish; (705)445-9044

LEWIN, R Simon; Haugen Med Group, 23C-3300 Smith Dr, Armstrong BC V0E 1B1; Liverpool (England)'73; MB ChB; (250)546-8115

LEWIN, Sheila; 1388 Eglinton Ave W, Toronto ON M6C 2E4; Cape Town (South Africa)'65; MB ChB; Langs: Afrikaans; Yiddish; (416)789-0537; Fax. (416)780-0861.

LEWINGTON, Danielle C; The Ravines Med Centre, 2-535 Larry Uteck Blvd, Halifax NS B3M 0E3; Ott'87; Langs: English; French; (902)407-4380; Fax. (902)407-4381.

LEWINGTON, Richard B; The Ravines Med Centre, 2-535 Larry Uteck Blvd, Halifax NS B3M 0E3; UBC'87; (902)407-4382; Fax. (902)407-4381.

LEWINSHTEIN, Daniel J; CSSS de Saint-Jerome, 290 rue de Montigny, Saint-Jerome QC J7Z 5T3; McG'04; Urol. Staff, Hôtel-Dieu de Saint-Jérôme; (450)431-8777

LEWIS, Andrea P; 1-2379 Bevan Ave, Sidney BC V8L 4M9; UBC'94; (250)656-4143; Fax. (250)656-9285.

LEWIS, Anna M; CLSC Lamater, 1317 boul des Seigneurs, Terrebonne QC J6W 5B1; McG'00; CCFP; (450)471-2881 x4056

LEWIS, Anthony B; Portage Med Clinic, 3-140 9th St SE, Portage la Prairie MB R1N 3V5; Man'08; CCFP.

LEWIS, Brendan D; Western Mem Reg Hosp, PO Box 2005 Stn Main 1 Brookfield Ave, Corner Brook NL A2H 6J7; Mem'83; BMedSci; Dip SportMed; AB; FAAOS; FRCSC; OrthSurg (Arthroplasty). Ortho Surg, Western Memorial Regional Hospital; Asst Prof Surg, Memorial University Of Newfoundland; (709)637-5000

LEWIS, Cledwyn E; Prairie Med Clinic, 10309 98 St, Grande Prairie AB T8V 2E7; Cardiff (Wales)'67; MB ChB; LRCP; MRCS; Staff, Queen Elizabeth II Hospital; Physician Plant, Weyerheuser; Med Dir, Northern Alberta EMS Zone; (780)539-4010

LEWIS, David A R; Malton Med Centre, 22-7330 Goreway Dr, Mississauga ON L4T 4J2; Newcastle (England)'70; DCH; DObstRCOG; MRC; Ac Staff Emerg, William Osler Health System - Etobicoke General Hospital; Staff Designated Med Practitioner, Citizenship & Immigration Canada; (905)677-4200; Fax. (905)677-0541; david.lewis@cic.gc.ca.

LEWIS, David C; 990 3rd Ave W, Owen Sound ON N4K 4P6; Aberdeen (Scotland)'68; MB ChB; DABOph; FACS; FRCSC; Ophth (Cataract). (519)376-9144; Fax. (519)376-8249; drlewis@bellnet.ca.

LEWIS, David; Saint John Reg Hosp, PO Box 2100 Stn Main, Saint John NB E2L 4L2; London (England)'91; Staff, Saint John Regional Hospital; (506)648-6000

LEWIS, Douglas C; Canada Life Assurance Co, S8-330 University Ave, Toronto ON M5G 1R8; Tor'75; Med Dir, Canada Life Assurance Company; (416)552-5893; Fax. (416)552-5893.

LEWIS, Gary F; Univ Hlth Network-Toronto Gen, EN12-218-200 Elizabeth St, Toronto ON M5G 2C4; Witwatersrand (South Africa)'82; ABIM; FRCPC; IntMed (Diabetes Mellitus). Head Div of Endocrin & Metabolism, Mount Sinai Hospital; Prof, University of Toronto; (416)340-4270; Fax. (416)340-3314; gary.lewis@uhn.ca.

LEWIS, Geraint W; The Ottawa Hosp-Civic Campus, 1053 Carling Ave, Ottawa ON K1Y 4E9; Cardiff (Wales)'76; FRCPC; Anes. Staff Anes, The Ottawa Hospital - Civic Campus; Asst Prof Anes, University of Ottawa; (613)761-4169

LEWIS, Gregory M; Gateway Med Clinic, 308-2051 McCallum Rd, Abbotsford BC V2S 3N5; Cape Town (South Africa)'81; MB ChB; FRCSC; GenSurg; VascSurg. (604)852-0238; drlewis@shawbiz.ca.

LEWIS, Jacqueline E; Sheldon Chumuik Centre, 8F-1213 4 St SW, Calgary AB T2R 0X7; McM'74; MSc(Epid.); CCFP; FCFP; Assoc Prof Family Med, University of Calgary; (403)955-9300; Fax. (403)476-8766.

LEWIS, James F; St Joseph's Health Care, PO Box 5777 Stn B A3 003-268 Grosvenor St, London ON N6A 4V2; Wes'82; FRCPC; IntMed (Lung Injury); Respir. Staff, St Joseph's Hospital - St Joseph's Health Care; Prof Med & Physiology, University of Western Ontario; (519)646-6288; Fax. (519)646-6404; cathy.ede@sjhc.london.on.ca.

LEWIS, James R; Royal Alexandra Hosp, 1111-10240 Kingsway NW, Edmonton AB T5H 3V9; Alb'83; BSc(Hon); AB; FRCSC; Ophth (Adult & Pediatric Neuro Ophthalmology). Ac Staff Ophth, Royal Alexandra Hospital; Ac Staff, University of Alberta Hospital; Clin Assoc Prof, University of Alberta; (780)735-5754

LEWIS, Jennifer E; St Joseph's Healthcare, 50 Charlton Ave E, Hamilton ON L8N 4A6; Tor'07; FRCPC; Psy. Staff Emerg Psy, St Joseph's Healthcare - Charlton Campus; (905)522-1155

LEWIS, Jennifer J; Klinic Commun Health Centre, 870 Portage Ave, Winnipeg MB R3G 0P1; Man'04; CCFP.

LEWIS, Jillian M; The Hosp for Sick Children, 555 University Ave, Toronto ON M5G 1X8; West Indies (Jamaica)'97; Staff, The Hospital For Sick Children; (416)813-6925

LEWIS, Jlee; Peterborough Reg Hc-Hospital, 1 Hospital Dr, Peterborough ON K9J 7C6; Man'86; FRCPC; Anes. Ac Staff, Peterborough Regional Health Centre - Hospital Drive; Ac Staff, Peterborough Regional Health Centre - Rogers St Site; (705)876-5038

LEWIS, John R; St Mary's Hosp Centre, 3830 av Lacombe, Montreal QC H3T 1M5; Mem'93; CCFP; CCFP(E.M.); FCFP; Staff, St Mary's Hospital Centre; Staff, Hawkesbury & District General Hospital; Staff, Sioux Lookout Meno-Ya-Win Health Centre; McGill University; Langs: French; Spanish; (514)345-3511 x2690

LEWIS, Laura C; Huntsville Prof Bldg, 104-348 Muskoka Rd 3 N, Huntsville ON P1H 1H8; Wes'92; CCFP; Staff, Huntsville District Memorial Hospital - Muskoka Algonquin Healthcare; (705)789-2355; Fax. (705)789-1051.

LEWIS, Lorraine N; Cole Harbour Family Med Centre, 203A-240 Baker Dr, Dartmouth NS B2W 6L4; Dal'86; CCFP; (902)435-6312

LEWIS, Marion E S; BC Women's Hosp & Hlth Ctr, C234-4500 Oak St, Vancouver BC V6H 3N1; Wes'86; Staff, BC Women's Hospital & Health Centre; (604)875-2157

LEWIS, Mark P; Royal Victoria Hosp, 201 Georgian Dr, Barrie ON L4M 6M2; Tor'04; FRCPC; Anes. Staff, Royal Victoria Regional Health Centre.

LEWIS, Maxine A; St Joseph's Mountain H Serv, PO Box 585 Stn Lcd 1 100 West 5th St, Hamilton ON L8N 3K7; Cardiff (Wales)'89; Staff, St Joseph's Healthcare Hamilton - West 5th Campus; (905)522-1155; Fax. (905)540-6533; mlewis@mcmaster.ca.

LEWIS, Melanie A; 1D1 WCM-132 University Campus, Edmonton AB T6G 2R7; Cal'97; MMed; FRCPC; Peds. Staff Peds, University of Alberta Hospital; Assoc Dean Learner Advocacy & Wellness, University of Alberta; (780)407-6370; mlewis@cha.ab.ca.

LEWIS, Michael E; 110-200 St Clair Ave W, Toronto ON M4V 1R1; Tor'00; CCFP; (416)928-9343; Fax. (416)928-9368.

LEWIS, Paul J; Chinook Reg Hosp, 960 19 St S, Lethbridge AB T1J 1W5; McM'96; BScN; BMus; CCFP; CCFP(E.M.); Dir Resident Education/Staff, Chinook Regional Hospital; (403)388-6301; Fax. (403)388-6183.

LEWIS, Ralph B; Sunnybrook Hlth Sciences Ctre, FG 62-2075 Bayview Ave, Toronto ON M4N 3M5; Witwatersrand (South Africa)'90; MD; MSc; FRCPC; Psy (Child & Adolescent Psychiatry). Staff Psy, Sunnybrook Health Sciences Centre; Asst Prof, University of Toronto; (416)480-4098; Fax. (416)480-6818.

LEWIS, Renata Y; Town Plaza Med Clinic, RR 4 40-4314 Main St, Whistler BC V0N 1B4; UBC'99; (604)905-7089

LEWIS, Richard H; 206-135 15th St E, North Vancouver BC V7L 2P7; Wes'85; FRCSC; GenSurg. Staff GenSurg, Lions Gate Hospital; (604)980-5141

LEWIS, Robert J; Christina Lake Med Clinic, PO Box 570, Christina Lake BC V0H 1E0; UBC'07; CCFP; (250)447-6262

LEWIS, Ronald T; A280-1053 Carling Ave, Ottawa ON K1Y 4E9; (Jamaica)'66; MSc(McGill); FRCSC; GenSurg; VascSurg. Staff, The Ottawa Hospital - Civic Campus; Assoc Prof Surg, University of Ottawa; Langs: English; French; (613)761-4766; Fax. (613)761-5362; rlewis@ottawahospital.on.ca.

LEWIS, Rosamund F; Ottawa Public Health, 7F-100 Constellation Cres, Ottawa ON K2G 6J8; McG'88; FRCPC; CommunMed;CCFP; (613)580-2424 x23681

LEWIS, Ruby S; Family Care Med Clinic, 106-1265 Morningside Ave, Scarborough ON M1B 3V9; Jaffna (Sri Lanka)'97; MB BS; CCFP; (416)282-8000; rubysl18@hotmail.com.

LEWIS, Sheila M; Stephenville Comm Med Clinic, 1 Washington Dr, Stephenville NL A2N 2V5; Mem'09; CCFP; (709)643-5656

LEWIS, Sheldon D; Jackson Park Health Centre, 230-2475 McDougall St, Windsor ON N8X 3N9; Ott'88; FRCPC; IntMed; Cardiol. (519)258-2230; Fax. (519)258-5883; slewis@kelcom.net.

LEWIS, Stephen J; Univ Hlth Network-Toronto Western Hosp, 1 E442-399 Bathurst St, Toronto ON M5T 2S8; McG'90; MSc; FRCSC; OrthSurg (Spine). Staff, The Hospital For Sick Children; Staff, Toronto Western Hospital - University Health Network; (416)603-5851; Fax. (416)603-3437.

LEWIS, Timothy E; 205-1221 Algonquin Ave, North Bay ON P1B 4Y3; Sask'04; FRCSC; OrthSurg. Staff, North Bay Regional Health Centre - Regional Mental Health; (705)497-0110

LEWIS, Valerie K; Maternity Care Clinic, 109-178 96 Ave NE, Calgary AB T3K 6G4; Cal'91; BSc; CCFP; FCFP; Physician, Maternity Care Clinic; (403)735-4922; Fax. (403)735-4901.

LEWIS, Valerie S; Baywood Med Centre, 202-95 Bayly St W, Ajax ON L1S 7K8; Tor'87; BSc(Hon); FRCPC; Peds (Consultant Pediatrics). Staff, Rouge Valley Health System - Ajax & Pickering Health Centre Site; (905)683-7593; Fax. (905)683-7669.

LEWIS, Valerie; 100-65 Prestwick Close, Halifax NS B3S 0C1; Dal'85; BSc; CCFP; Med Advisor, Shannex Health Care; Lecturer Family Med, Dalhousie University; (902)429-2722; docval@hfx.eastlink.ca.

LEWIS, Victor A; Alberta Children's Hosp, 2888 Shaganappi Trail NW, Calgary AB T3B 6A8; Lahore (Pakistan)'88; MB BS; AB; Staff, Alberta Children's Hospital; (403)955-7272

LEWIS, William F; Regina Internal Med Specialist, 1821 Rose St, Regina SK S4P 1Z7; Wes'77; FRCPC; IntMed; Gastroent. (306)522-5659; Fax. (306)359-1068.

LEWIS-WATTS, Robert J; Atrium Prof Bldg, SS 103 305-190 Cundles Rd E, Barrie ON L4M 4S5; Wes'78; CCFP; Staff, Royal Victoria Regional Health Centre; (705)737-1160; Fax. (705)726-8414.

LEWITTES, Leora R; Mount Sinai Hosp, 1266A-600 University Ave, Toronto ON M5G 1X5; Tor'88; BSc; MHSc; CCFP; FCFP; Staff Courtesy Privil, Mount Sinai Hospital; Langs: Hebrew; (416)586-4800 x5264; Fax. (416)586-8847.

LEWITZKA, Ute; IWK Health Centre, PO Box 9700 Rpo CSC 5850 University Ave, Halifax NS B3K 6R8; (Germany)'04; Staff, IWK Health Centre; (902)470-8377

LEWKE, Bernard O; 2423 Apollo Rd, Westbank BC V4T 1P6; Cal'81; CCFP; (250)768-9515

LEWKE-BOGLE, Elisabeth; Milk River Med Clinic, PO Box 177, Milk River AB T0K 1M0; Alb'71; CCFP; FCFP; Staff/Chief of Staff, Milk River Health Centre; Langs: German; (403)647-3599; Fax. (403)647-3534; mrclinic@mrcable.ca.

LEWKONIA, Peter D; Crowfoot West Business Centre, 340-600 Crowfoot Cres NW, Calgary AB T3G 0B4; Cal'05; FRCSC; OrthSurg. (403)452-0999; Fax. (403)452-0995.

LEWKONIA, Raymond M; Richmond Road Diag & Trmt Ctr, 1820 Richmond Rd SW, Calgary AB T2T 5C7; Liverpool (England)'66; DCH; FRCP; DABIM; FACP; FRCPC; IntMed (Medical Genetics); Rheum. Prof Dept of IntMed, University of Calgary; (403)955-8733; Fax. (403)955-8029.

LEWTAS, Jody L; Markham Stouffville Health Ctr, 306-377 Church St, Markham ON L6B 1A1; Columbia(NY) (USA)'87; FRCPC; IntMed; Rheum. Staff, Markham Stouffville Hospital; Assoc Staff, Sunnybrook Health Sciences Centre; Assoc Staff, Women's College Hospital; (905)201-0800; Fax. (905)201-0018.

LEXIER, Reuven R; B100-340 College St, Toronto ON M5T 3A9; UBC'79; FRCSC; OrthSurg. Staff, Toronto Western Hospital - University Health Network; (416)972-0206; Fax. (416)972-6229.

LEY, David A; Sault Area Hosp, 750 Great Northern Rd, Sault Ste. Marie ON P6B 0A8; Bristol (England)'71; FRCPC; Anes. Staff, Sault Area Hospital - Sault Ste Marie; (705)759-3434

LEY, Sebastian; Mount Sinai Hosp, 562-600 University Ave, Toronto ON M5G 1X5; Mainz (Germany)'01; Staff, Mount Sinai Hospital; (416)340-4800

LEYEN, Heather A; Southgate Mall, 50-45905 Yale Rd, Chilliwack BC V2P 2M6; Cal'91; (604)792-2266; Fax. (604)792-2264; heatheranneleyen@gmail.com.

LEYENAAR, Laurina K; Saint John Reg Hosp, PO Box 2100 Stn Main, Saint John NB E2L 4L2; Mem'05; BSc; ObstGyn. Staff, Saint John Regional Hospital; (506)648-6741; Fax. (506)648-6878.

LEYLAND, Nicholas A; Hamilton HS-McMaster Site, PO Box 2000 stn Lcd 1 2F 39-1200 Main St W, Hamilton ON L8N 3Z5; Tor'83; BASc; FSOGC; FRCSC; ObstGyn (Gynecological Surgery). Chief, Hamilton Health Sciences Centre - McMaster University Medical Centre; Staff, Toronto General Hospital - UHN; Staff, Mount Sinai Hospital; Prof ObstGyn, McMaster University; (905)521-2100; Fax. (905)577-0471; drleyland@rogers.com.

LEYLAND, Steven; Links Clinic Office, 104-11910 111 Ave NW, Edmonton AB T5G 3G6; Sask'94; CCFP; (780)454-0351; Fax. (780)452-6767.

LEYLEK, Ahmet S; Cancercare Manitoba, 675 McDermot Ave, Winnipeg MB R3E 0V9; Istanbul (Turkey)'80; AB; Staff, Health Sciences Centre; Staff, St Boniface General Hospital; University of Manitoba; (204)787-2117; Fax. (204)786-0194.

LEZACK, Jack D; Manitoba Clinic, 790 Sherbrook St, Winnipeg MB R3A 1M3; Man'71; FRCPC; IntMed (Medical Oncology); Hem. Ac Staff, Seven Oaks General Hospital; (204)788-5736

LEZACK, Lisa J; U of Ottawa Health Services, 300-100 Marie Curie Pvt, Ottawa ON K1N 1A2; Man'02; CCFP; (613)564-3950

LEZNOFF, Arthur; 57 Patina Dr, Toronto ON M2H 1R3; McG'55; BSc; MSc; MDCM; FRCPC; IntMed (Environmental Health); ClinImmunol&Allergy. Hon Consultant Med, St Michael's Hospital; Langs: English; French; (416)497-2816; Fax. (416)497-3129.

LEZON-GIACOMELLI, Dianne; The Credit Valley Hospital, 2200 Eglinton Ave W, Mississauga ON L5M 2N1; Tor'85; FRCPC; Psy (Geriatric Psychiatry). Court Staff, Hamilton Health Sciences Centre; Court Staff, St Joseph's Healthcare - Charlton Campus; Ac Staff, The Credit Valley Hospital; (905)813-2398; Fax. (905)813-4284.

LHO, Hyoung-Zin; North York Gen Hosp, 4001 Leslie St, North York ON M2K 1E1; Tor'01; CCFP; CCFP(E.M.); Staff, North York General Hospital; (416)756-6000

LHOTSKY, Miroslava; Anne Johnston Health Station, 1F-2398 Yonge St, Toronto ON M4P 2H4; Ott'71; CCFP; Court Staff Privil Family Prac, Sunnybrook Health Sciences Centre; Langs: Czech; (416)486-8666; Fax. (416)486-8660; lhotsky@sympatico.ca.

LI, Alan T W; Regent Park Comm Health Centre, 465 Dundas St E, Toronto ON M5A 2B2; Tor'85; Staff, St Michael's Hospital; Langs: Cantonese; Mandarin; (416)364-2261; Fax. (416)364-0822; alanl@regentparkchc.org.

LI, Andrew W; 201-178 96 Ave NE, Calgary AB T3K 6G4; Wes'01; FRCSC; ObstGyn. (403)219-4243

LI, Ann L; 380-5 Fairview Mall Dr, North York ON M2J 2Z1; Tor'87; CCFP; FCFP; Staff, North York General Hospital; University of Toronto; (416)222-0833; Fax. (416)222-6895.

LI, Anson H Y; Specialized Geriatric Clinic, 232 Ross Dr, New Westminster BC V3L 0B2; UBC'06; FRCPC; IntMed. (604)528-5031

LI, Audrey M W; Lakeridge Health Corp-Oshawa, 1 Hospital Crt, Oshawa ON L1G 2B9; McM'03; FRCPC; RadOncol. Staff, Lakeridge Health - Oshawa Site; (905)576-8711 x4595

LI, Bernard Y T; Professional Place, 201-2901 Lawrence Ave E, Scarborough ON M1P 2T4; Tor'79; CCFP; Staff, The Scarborough Hospital - General Campus; (416)266-4543; Fax. (416)267-4050.

LI, Bessie P T; 22-7010 Warden Ave, Markham ON L3R 5Y3; Tor'98; BSc; CCFP; Langs: Cantonese; Mandarin; (905)944-0270

LI, Bing; 9534 87 St NW, Edmonton AB T6C 3J1; (China)'83; MSc; CCFP; Staff, Covenant Health - Grey Nuns Community Hospital; Langs: Chinese; (780)440-8274; Fax. (780)469-6495.

LI, Charles H; Gordon & Leslie Diamond HCC, 10241-2775 Laurel St, Vancouver BC V5Z 1M9; Alb'91; BMedSci; FRCPC; IntMed (Clinical Hematology); Hem. Staff, Vancouver General Hospital - Centennial Pavillion; Staff, Gordon & Leslie Diamond Health Care Centre; Clinical Asst Prof Med, University of British Columbia; Langs: Chinese; Cantonese; Mandarin; (604)875-4952

LI, Cheuk-Hon; Silverthorn Med Centre, 1707 St Clair Ave W, Toronto ON M6N 1J2; (Taiwan)'70; Staff, St Joseph's Health Centre; Langs: Chinese; (416)656-1944; Fax. (416)653-0515.

LI, Chien-Chuang; Taunton Health Centre, SS 201 1290 Keith Ross Dr, Oshawa ON L1H 7K4; Wes'95; CCFP; FCFP; (905)723-8551 x5401

LI, Christopher K; St Michael's Hosp, 6 045-30 Bond St, Toronto ON M5B 1W8; Cal'98; ABIM; DABSM; FRCPC; IntMed (Sleep Medicine); Respir. Staff Respirol, St Michael's Hospital; Langs: Cantonese; (416)864-6026; Fax. (416)864-5649; lic@smh.ca.

LI, Christopher W H; Scarborough Hosp-Birchmount, 3030 Birchmount Rd, Scarborough ON M1W 3W3; Tor'93; BSc; FRCPC; IntMed; Cardiol. Staff Cardiol, The Scarborough Hospital - Birchmount Campus; Staff Interventional Cardiol, Rouge Valley Health System - Centenary Health Centre Site; Langs: Cantonese; (416)495-2400

LI, Chumei; McMaster University HSC, 3N18-1200 Main St W, Hamilton ON L8N 3Z5; (China)'83; PhD; FRCPC; MedGenetics (Cancer Genetics Research). Staff, Toronto Western Hospital - University Health Network; Staff, Princess Margaret Hospital - University Health Network; Assoc Staff, The Hospital For Sick Children; Staff, Toronto General Hospital - UHN; Langs: Chinese; (905)521-2100 x73246

LI, Daniel M; Alberta Hosp Edmonton, PO Box 307 Stn Main 17480 Fort Rd, Edmonton AB T5J 2J7; Alb'96; FRCPC; Psy. Staff, Alberta Hospital Edmonton; (780)472-5473; Fax. (780)472-5411.

LI, David K B; UBC Hospital, 2211 Wesbrook Mall, Vancouver BC V6T 2B5; UBC'75; ABR; FRCPC; DiagRad. Staff Radiologist, Vancouver General Hospital - Centennial Pavillion; Staff Radiol, UBC Hospital - Koerner Pavillion; Staff Radiologist, Vancouver Coastal Health; Prof, University of British Columbia; (604)822-7071; Fax. (604)822-1779; david.li@ubc.ca.

LI, David W; The Richmond Hosp, 7000 Westminster Hwy, Richmond BC V6X 1A2; Alb'04; CCFP; Staff, Richmond Hospital; (604)278-9711

LI, Dominic W; 701-123 Edward St, Toronto ON M5G 1E2; Tor'88; (416)977-2833; Fax. (416)977-1335.

LI, Donna R; Westney Heights Med Centre, 2-15 Westney Rd N, Ajax ON L1T 1P4; (Guyana)'00; CCFP; (905)428-8055

LI, Dorothy Y Y; Univ Hlth Network-Toronto Western Hosp, 326-399 Bathurst St, Toronto ON M5T 2S8; Tor'08; IntMed. Staff, Toronto Western Hospital - University Health Network; (647)802-9403

LI, Francis; Pape Med Centre, 751 Pape Ave, Toronto ON M4K 3T1; Tor'89; BSc; (416)778-1810

LI, Gene S J; Bramalea Med Centre, 509-18 Kensington Rd, Brampton ON L6T 4S5; Tor'83; CCFP; FCFP; Ac Staff, William Osler Health System - Brampton Civic Hospital; Langs: Mandarin; (905)799-9875; Fax. (289)298-5339; geneli2000@hotmail.com.

LI, Gisele; Hopl Maisonneuve-Rosemont, 5415 boul de l'Assomption, Montreal QC H1T 2M4; McG'00; CSPQ; FRCSC; Ophth (Glaucoma). Staff, Hopital Maisonneuve-Rosemont; Langs: Bilingual(French/English); (514)252-3400; gisele.li@umontreal.ca.

LI, Heung-Wing; Birchwood Clinics, 204-2950 Birchmount Rd, Scarborough ON M1W 3G5; Tor'79; Langs: Chinese; (416)499-4499

LI, Hui; 110-101 Queensway W, Mississauga ON L5B 2P7; Shandong (China)'85; FRCSC; Neursurg. Staff, Trillium Health Centre - Mississauga; (905)272-9777; Fax. (905)272-9100.

LI, Hui-Wah; Cambie Plaza Med Clinic, 180-11700 Cambie Rd, Richmond BC V6X 1L5; UBC'09; CCFP; (604)270-9833

LI, Isabel; Royal Victoria Hosp, 201 Georgia Dr, Barrie ON L4M 6M2; Peking (China)'97; FRCPC; IntMed; MedOncol. Staff, Royal Victoria Regional Health Centre; (705)739-5661; Fax. (705)739-5619.

LI, Janice C Y; Markham Stouffville Hosp, PO Box 1800 Stn Main 381 Church St, Markham ON L3P 7P3; Tor'84; CCFP; FCFP; Ac Staff Family Pract, Markham Stouffville Hospital; (905)472-7000

LI, Jason; 7-5550 Lawrence Ave E, Scarborough ON M1C 3B2; Tor'90; CCFP; FCFP; Langs: Cantonese; Mandarin; (416)283-3700; Fax. (416)283-1453.

LI, Jian; Royal Columbian Hosp, 330 Columbia St E, New Westminster BC V3L 3W7; McG'06; MDCM; DiagRad. Staff, Royal Columbian Hospital; (604)941-7611 x766

LI, Jing; Toronto East Gen Hosp Inc, 825 Coxwell Ave, Toronto ON M4C 3E7; McM'00; FRCPC; IntMed; MedOncol. Staff, Toronto East General Hospital Inc; (416)469-3325; Fax. (416)469-6420.

LI, Jiwei; 6405 Knight St, Vancouver BC V5P 2V9; UBC'01; CCFP; (604)321-6151

LI, John H S; 207-1789 Mountain Rd, Moncton NB E1G 1A7; Dal'85; Ac Staff, The Moncton Hospital; Langs: Cantonese; Chinese; (506)859-8696; Fax. (506)383-8224.

LI, Judy W S; Hewes Way Med Clinic, 206-2603 Hewes Way NW, Edmonton AB T6L 6W6; Alb'88; BSc; CCFP; Langs: Chinese; (780)462-4210

LI, Kan Wen; Mackenzie Richmond Hill Hosp, 10 Trench St, Richmond Hill ON L4C 4Z3; Tor'94; BSc; Staff Emerg, Mackenzie Richmond Hill Hospital; Teach Staff Family & Commun Med, University of Toronto; Langs: Hakka; Chinese; (905)883-2041; Fax. (905)883-2138; kli@yorkcentral.on.ca.

LI, Kong Ching; 240 Mackay St, Pembroke ON K8A 1C5; Tor'74; FRCPC; IntMed. Staff/Chief IntMed, Pembroke Regional Hospital Inc; Langs: Chinese; (613)735-3109; Fax. (613)735-7132.

LI, Madeline T; Univ Hlth Network-Princess M, 610 University Ave, Toronto ON M5G 2M9; Tor'99; FRCPC; Psy. Staff, Princess Margaret Hospital - University Health Network; (416)946-2000

LI, Maria S; Hop Maisonneuve-Rosemont, 5415 boul de l'Assomption, Montreal QC H1T 2M4; McG'90; Neursurg. Staff, Hopital Maisonneuve-Rosemont; (514)252-3400

LI, Marilyn M; 301-272 Charlotte St, Peterborough ON K9J 2V4; Ott'04; FRCPC; IntMed; Gastroent.

LI, Mok-Dock; Worley Village Med Centre, 103-190 Wortley Rd, London ON N6C 4Y7; Taiwan National Univ (Taiwan)'58; FACC; ABPeds; FRCPC; Peds (Pediatric Cardiology). Physician, Wortley Village Medical Centre; Emeritus Prof Ped, University of Western Ontario; Langs: Chinese; (519)642-1101; Fax. (519)681-1158; mdli@sympatico.ca.

LI, Nan; CLSC de Saint-Michel, 3355 rue Jarry E, Montreal QC H1Z 2E5; Sher'09; (514)722-3000

LI, Olga; 1-2060 Ellesmere Rd, Scarborough ON M1H 2Y6; Wes'09; CCFP; (416)439-2273

LI, Patricia T; MUHC-Montreal Children's Hosp, 2300 rue Tupper, Montreal QC H3H 1P3; McM'04; FRCPC; Peds. Staff, McGill University Health Centre - Montreal Children's Hospital; (514)412-4400

LI, Pin; Health Sciences Centre, 3330 Hospital Dr NW, Calgary AB T2N 4N1; Shanghai (China)'95; FRCPC; IntMed. Clinical Asst Prof, Alberta Health Services; Clinical Asst Prof, University of Calgary; (403)210-6564; Fax. (403)283-6151.

LI, Qin; Univ Hlth Network-Toronto Western Hosp, 470-399 Bathurst St, Toronto ON M5T 2S8; McM'06; FRCPC; IntMed; Cardiol. Staff, Toronto Western Hospital - University Health Network; (416)603-5815

LI, Qinglu; Atrium Prof Bldg, SS 103 305-190 Cundles Rd E, Barrie ON L4M 4S5; Dal'99; CCFP; Langs: Chinese; (705)726-2060; Fax. (705)726-4826; chingluli@hotmail.com.

LI, Qiuyan; Kelowna Gen Hosp, 2268 Pandosy St, Kelowna BC V1Y 1T2; Harbin (China)'77; MSc; FRCPC; AnatPath. Staff, Kelowna General Hospital; Langs: Chinese; (250)362-4300 x7341

LI, Qiyu A; Humber River Reg Hosp-Finch, 2111 Finch Ave W, North York ON M3N 1N1; Harbin (China)'94; FRCPC; Anes. Staff, Humber River Regional Hospital - Finch Avenue Site; (416)744-2500

LI, Siu Hung C; 214-99 Sinclair Ave, Georgetown ON L7G 5G1; Tor'79; BSc; Court Staff, The Credit Valley Hospital; Langs: Cantonese; (905)873-0125; Fax. (905)873-3399.

LI, Stephanie K; 11202 76 Ave NW, Edmonton AB T6G 0K1; Tor'95; FRCPC; IntMed; Endocrin&Metab. (780)439-4945; Fax. (780)439-0396.

LI, Thomas C H; Niagara H System-G Niagara, PO Box 1018 Stn Main 5546 Portage Rd, Niagara Falls ON L2E 6X2; Wes'90; FRCPC; DiagRad. Staff, Niagara Health System - Greater Niagara General Site; (905)358-0171 x3422; Fax. (905)358-4908; tli9@cogeco.ca.

LI, Wei; Brentwood Shopping Centre, 38-4567 Lougheed Hwy, Burnaby BC V5C 3Z6; (China)'82; CCFP; Staff, Burnaby Hospital; Langs: Mandarin; (604)294-8540

LI, Xiao Y; Stadium Med Centre, 21-1941 Uxbridge Dr NW, Calgary AB T2N 2V2; McG'08; CCFP; (403)248-8807; Fax. (403)248-8897.

LI, Xiao Qing; All About Health, E-1070 Major Mackenzie Dr E, Richmond Hill ON L4S 1P3; (Other Foreign)'93; CCFP; (905)884-0666

LI, Xiaobin; Minto Health Service, PO Box 1600 233 8th St, Cochrane ON P0L 1C0; North Carolina (USA)'07; CCFP; (705)272-4276

LI, Xin-Min; Univ of Manitoba, S203-750 Bannatyne Ave, Winnipeg MB R3E 0W2; Jilin (China)'82; MD; PhD; FRCPC; Psy. Dir Int'l Med Graduate Education, University of Manitoba; Langs: Mandarin; (204)789-3616; Fax. (204)789-3911; xinmin.li@umanitoba.ca.

LI, Yang; University of Alberta Hosp, 8440 112 St NW, Edmonton AB T6G 2B7; Alb'08; Staff, University of Alberta Hospital; (780)407-8822

LI, Yunru; Markham Stouffville Hosp, PO Box 1800 Stn Main 381 Church St, Markham ON L3P 7P3; (China)'98; FRCPC; AnatPath. Staff, Markham Stouffville Hospital; (905)472-7000

LI, Zhi; 9534 87 St NW, Edmonton AB T6C 3J1; (China)'83; CCFP; Att Physician, Covenant Health - Misericordia Community Hospital; Clin Lecturer Med & Dentistry, University of Alberta; Langs: Chinese; (780)440-8274; Fax. (780)469-6495; drzhili2000@yahoo.com.

LI CHANG, Hector H; Univ of Toronto, 602-500 University Ave, Toronto ON M5G 1V7; Wes'07; FRCPC; AnatPath. (416)978-6976

LI PI SHAN, Rodney; Foothills Med Centre, AC142-1403 29 St NW, Calgary AB T2N 2T9; Sask'98; FRCPC; PhysMed&Rehab. Staff, Foothills Medical Centre; (403)944-1260; Fax. (403)270-7878; rodney.lipishan@albertahealthservices.ca.

LI PI SHAN, William; MUHC-Royal Victoria Hosp, S5 05-687 av des Pins O, Montreal QC H3A 1A1; Sask'98; FRCPC; Anes. Staff, McGill University Health Centre - Royal Victoria Hospital; (514)934-1934 x34883; Fax. (514)843-1753.

LI WAN PO, Ah-King; 4239 Petrolia Line PO Box 1179, Petrolia ON N0N 1R0; National U. (Ireland)'66; MB ChB; BAO; Assoc Staff, Bluewater Health - Charlotte Eleanor Englehart Hospital; (519)882-0190; Fax. (519)882-3776.

LI WAN PO, James Y L; 467 Notre Dame St PO Box 219, Belle River ON N0R 1A0; Galway (Ireland)'58; (519)728-3355; Fax. (519)728-4946.

LIABOTIS, Stephanie A; 701-440 Central Ave, London ON N6B 2E5; Dal'98; CCFP; FCFP; Clin Associate Cardiac Rehab Prog, London Health Sciences Centre - University Hospital; (519)601-7577

LIACONIS, Haralambos; 202-217 Terrace Hill St, Brantford ON N3R 1G8; McM'00; BEng; MBA; FRCSC; GenSurg. Staff, The Brant Community Healthcare System - Brantford General Hospital Site; Langs: Greek; (519)753-2200; Fax. (519)753-2202; surgeon@drliaconis.ca.

LIAGHATI NASSERI, Navid; The Credit Valley Hosp, 2200 Eglinton Ave W, Mississauga ON L5M 2N1; Azerbaijan (Iran)'92; FRCPC; AnatPath. Staff, The Credit Valley Hospital; (905)813-1100 x5447

LIAGHATI-NASSERI, Negin; Pinnacle Health Science Ctr, 2-9651 Yonge St, Richmond Hill ON L4C 1V7; Tor'03; CCFP; Langs: Persian; (905)780-8823

LIAGHATI-NASSERI, Omid; Brookfield Bonnews HC Centre, PO Box 209 57 Main St, Brookfield NL A0G 1J0; Shahid Beheshti U (Iran)'96; Staff, Brookfield Bonnews Health Care Centre; (709)536-2405

LIAN, Calvin T; Univ Hlth Network-Toronto Gen, 200 Elizabeth St, Toronto ON M5G 2C4; Tor'96; CCFP; CCFP(E.M.); FCFP; Staff, Toronto Western Hospital - University Health Network; Toronto General Hospital - UHN; Asst Prof Family & Commun Med, University of Toronto; Langs: Mandarin; Spanish; (416)340-3947

LIAN, Jidong; The Credit Valley Hosp, 2200 Eglinton Ave W, Mississauga ON L5M 2N1; China (China)'84; FRCPC; RadOncol. Staff, The Credit Valley Hospital; (905)813-1100; Fax. (905)813-3962.

LIANDIER, Frederic; Ctr Hosp Rouyn-Noranda, 4 9e rue, Rouyn-Noranda QC J9X 2B2; Sher'95; FRCSC; Urol. Staff, Centre Hospitalier Rouyn-Noranda; (819)764-5131

LIANG, Charles; 10014 Yonge St, Richmond Hill ON L4C 1T8; Tor'87; (905)884-8733; Fax. (905)884-9187.

LIANG, Dana Y; 506-1110 Sheppard Ave E, North York ON M2K 2W2; Qns'86; ABIM; FRCPC; IntMed (Gastroenterology). Ac Staff Med, North York General Hospital; (416)229-2201; Fax. (416)229-2261.

LIANG, Edmund K K; 403-9555 Yonge St, Richmond Hill ON L4C 9M5; Wes'84; FRCSC; Ophth. Staff, Mackenzie Richmond Hill Hospital; (905)737-4853

LIANG, Howard S H; Oakridge Plaza, 120-5780 Cambie St, Vancouver BC V5Z 3A7; g Kong (Hong Kong)'79; MB BS; MRCP(UK); DCH(Lond Glas); FRCPC; Peds. Staff, BC Children's Hospital; Staff, Providence Health Care - Mount Saint Joseph Hospital; Clinical Asst Prof, University of British Columbia; Langs: Mandarin; Cantonese; (604)323-2982; Fax. (604)323-2923.

LIANG, Hsien-Cheng; 212-2425 Tecumseh Rd E, Windsor ON N8W 1E6; Tor'76; CCFP; Head Family Pract, Windsor Regional Hospital - Metropolitan Site; (519)974-9700; Fax. (519)974-3554.

LIANG, Kenneth K C; All Med Health, 1-16880 Yonge St, Newmarket ON L3Y 0A3; Wes'86; (905)895-9777; Fax. (905)895-9720.

LIANG, Lily S; Rouge Valley-Ajax & Pickering, 580 Harwood Ave S, Ajax ON L1S 2J4; Wes'02; FRCPC; Anes. Staff, Rouge Valley Health System - Ajax & Pickering Health Centre Site; (905)683-2320

LIANG, Lorna L K; North Scarborough Prof Bldg, 309-3420 Finch Ave E, Scarborough ON M1W 2R6; (Hong Kong)'71; Staff, The Scarborough Hospital - General Campus; (416)499-1157; Fax. (416)499-4604.

LIANG, Patrick; CHUS-Hop Hotel-Dieu, 580 rue Bowen S, Sherbrooke QC J1G 2E8; Sher'91; FRCPC; IntMed (Vasculities); Rheum. Staff, Centre Hospitalier Universitaire de Sherbrooke-Hôpital Hôtel-Dieu; Langs: Bilingual(French/English); (819)564-5261; Fax. (819)564-5265; patrick.liang@usherbrooke.ca.

LIANG, Raymond A; Broadway Med Centre, 438-943 Broadway W, Vancouver BC V5Z 4E1; Manila (Philippines)'82; FRCPC; Psy (Personal Injury Management Assessment). Clin Assoc Prof, University of British Columbia; Langs: Mandarin; Cantonese; Taishanese; (604)731-7731; Fax. (604)733-8896; drraymondliang@yahoo.com.

LIANG, Stephen; 6173 Ravine Way, Orleans ON K1C 7E8; Ott'73; (613)824-8966

LIANG, William; 2-1447 Uper Ottawa St, Hamilton ON L8W 3J6; Tor'79; Staff Emerg & Family Pract, Hamilton Health Sciences Centre - Hamilton General Hospital; Staff Emerg, West Haldimand General Hospital; Staff, Halton Healthcare Services Corporation - Milton District Hospital; Clinical Asst Prof, McMaster University; Langs: Cantonese; Italian; Mandarin; (905)522-2171; Fax. (905)523-1250.

LIAO, H Robert; Scarborough North Med Arts, 310B-4040 Finch Ave E, Scarborough ON M1S 4V5; Kaohsiung (Taiwan)'76; FRCSC; Ophth. Staff, The Scarborough Hospital - Birchmount Campus; Langs: Mandarin; Cantonese; Taiwanese; (416)299-1484; Fax. (416)299-3583.

LIAO, Janice Y; Dermatology & Hair Transplant, 11516 Jasper Ave NW, Edmonton AB T5K 0M8; Kuala Lumpur (Malaysia)'70; FRCPC; Derm. Assoc Staff, University of Alberta Hospital; Assoc. Clin. Prof., Derm., University of Alberta; Langs: Chinese; (780)488-8798; Fax. (780)482-1317; jyliao@telusplanet.net.

LIAO, Joy; Mount St Joseph Hosp, 3080 Prince Edward St, Surrey BC V3T 3N4; McM'05; FRCPC; IntMed; GeriatricMed. Staff, Providence Health Care - Mount Saint Joseph Hospital; (604)877-1141

LIAO, Liang Ying; South Muskoka Med Centre, 230 Manitoba St, Bracebridge ON P1L 2E1; Tor'89; (705)646-7634; Fax. (705)646-0476; liang.liao@sympatico.ca.

LIAO, Patrick M; King Street Med Arts Centre, 302-71 King St W, Mississauga ON L5B 4A2; Cebu (Philippines)'77; FRCSC; ObstGyn. Ac Staff, Trillium Health Centre - Mississauga; (905)566-0905; Fax. (905)270-2826.

LIAO, Sunu M; Professional Place, 306-2901 Lawrence Ave E, Scarborough ON M1P 2T3; Madras (India)'82; FRCPC; PhysMed&Rehab. (416)266-6155; Fax. (416)266-2827.

LIASCHKO, Alexander A; Sunningdale Hlth & Wellness Ct, 1695 Wonderland Rd N, London ON N6G 4W3; (Russia (Federation))'84.

LIASHKO, Vitaly A; The Moncton Hosp, 135 MacBeath Ave, Moncton NB E1C 6Z8; Lennigrad (Russia (Federation))'88; FRCPC; Psy (Child & Adolescent Psychiatry). Staff, The Moncton Hospital; Asst Prof Psy, Dalhousie University; Langs: Ukrainian; Russian; (506)857-5780; Fax. (506)857-5751; dr.vitaly.liashko@horizonnb.ca.

LIBBUS, Yvonne E; Cape Breton Hlthcare Complex, 1482 George St, Sydney NS B1P 1P3; Dal'93; BSc; FRCPC; Psy. Staff, Cape Breton Healthcare Complex; (902)567-8092; Fax. (902)567-7905.

LIBBY, T Phillip; Brooklin Med Centre, 1A-5959 Anderson St, Brooklin ON L1M 2E9; Tor'93; BSc(Hons); CCFP; Med Dir, Community Nursing Home-Port Perry; Med Dir, Fairview Lodge; (905)655-3321; Fax. (905)655-4848.

LIBEN, Stephen B; MUHC-Montreal Children's Hosp, F122-2300 rue Tupper, Montreal QC H3H 1P3; McG'87; FAAP; FRCPC; Peds (Palliative Care); Critical Care Medicine (P.Q.). Dir Ped Palliative Care Services, McGill University Health Centre - Montreal Children's Hospital; adj Prof, McGill University; (514)412-4400

LIBERATORE, Anne M; Burlington Prof Centre, 402-3155 Harvester Rd, Burlington ON L7N 3V2; McM'83; Langs: Italian; (905)632-3000; Fax. (905)632-7960.

LIBERGE, Johanne; CHUM-Hop St-Luc, 1058 rue Saint-Denis, Montreal QC H2X 3J4; Mon'00; FRCPC; IntMed; Nephrol. Staff, Centre Hospitalier l'Université De Montréal (CHUM) - Hôpital Saint-luc; (514)890-8000 x32588

LIBERMAN, A Moishe; CHUM-Hop Notre-Dame, 1560 rue Sherbrooke E, Montreal QC H2L 4M1; McG'00; FRCSC; GenSurg; ThorSurg. Staff, Centre Hospitalier l'Université de Montréal (CHUM) - Hôpital Notre-Dame; Langs: Bilingual(French/English); (514)890-8000 x26252

LIBERMAN, Alexander S; MUHC-Montreal Gen Hosp, D16 173-1650 av Cedar, Montreal QC H3G 1A4; McG'00; CSPQ; FRCSC; GenSurg (Colon & Rectal Surgery). Staff, McGill University Health Centre - Montreal General Campus; Staff, St Mary's Hospital Centre; (514)934-8486

LIBERMAN, Dan; Sunnybrook Hlth Sciences Ctre, H479-2075 Bayview Ave, Toronto ON M4N 3M5; McG'08; IntMed. Staff Geriatric Med, Sunnybrook Health Sciences Centre; (416)480-6766

LIBICH, William G; Winnipeg Reg Health Authority, 2F-490 Hargrave St, Winnipeg MB R3A 0X7; Man'00; CommunMed. (204)940-3610

LIBIN, Michael A; Foothills Med Centre, G28-1403 29 St NW, Calgary AB T2N 2T9; Tor'96; CCFP; Staff, Foothills Medical Centre; Physician, Sheldon M Chumir Urgent Care Physician Group; (403)944-2800; michael.libin@albertahealthservices.ca.

LIBMAN, Esther R; Shops on Steeles Med Centre, 206-2900 Steeles Ave E, Thornhill ON L3T 4X1; Tor'80; CCFP; FCFP; Ac Staff, North York General Hospital; (905)881-6667; Fax. (905)731-1298.

LIBMAN, Jamie; Le Plein Ciel, 475 boul de la Cote-Vertu, Saint-Laurent QC H4L 1X7; McG'00; FRCSC; Urol. (514)337-3171

LIBMAN, Michael D; MUHC-Montreal Gen Hosp, A5 156-1650 av Cedar, Montreal QC H3G 1A4; McG'85; CSPQ; ABIM; BA; FRCP; FRCPC; IntMed (Infection Control); InfectDis; MedMicrobiol. Dir InfectDis, McGill University Health Centre - Montreal General Campus; Chef Centre for Tropical Diseases, McGill University; Langs: French; (514)934-1934 x42811; michael.libman@mcgill.ca.

LIBMAN, Robert N; Medical Centre, 2550A Finch Ave W, Toronto ON M9M 2G3; Ott'72; CCFP; FCFP; Ac Staff, Humber River Regional Hospital - Finch Avenue Site; (416)749-5291; Fax. (416)749-6598.

LIBOIRON, Gilles; Clinique Drs Gilles et Pierre, 378 Boul Cartier O, Laval QC H7N 2K2; Mon'63; CCFP; FCFP; Staff, Centre Hospitalier Fleury; (450)669-2944

LIBOIRON, Pierre; Clinique Drs Gilles et Pierre, 378 Boul Cartier O, Laval QC H7N 2K2; Mon'84; CCFP; Staff, Centre Hospitalier Fleury; (450)669-2944

LIBRACH, Clifford L; Fertility Centre, 1100-790 Bay St, Toronto ON M5G 1N8; Tor'83; FACOG(Obs/Gyn & Repro End; FRCSC; ObstGyn (Reproductive Endocrinology & Infertility). Ac Staff, Women's College Hospital; Asst Prof, University of Toronto; (416)323-7727; Fax. (416)323-7334.

LIBRACH, Kevin S; Guelph Family Health Team, 83 Dawson Rd, Guelph ON N1H 1B1; Cal'91; BMath; FCFP; CCFP; FCFP; Court Staff, Guelph General Hospital; (519)837-2242; Fax. (519)763-4315.

LIBRACH, S Lawrence; Joint Centre for Bioethics, 754-155 College St, Toronto ON M5T 1P8; Tor'70; CCFP; FCFP; Dir Temmy Latner Ctr for Palliative, Mount Sinai Hospital; Prof Family & Commun Med & W Gifford-Jones/Prof Pain Control & Palliative Care, University of Toronto; (416)978-1906; Fax. (416)978-1911.

LIBRACH, Samuel; Kensington Health Centre, 320-340 College St, Toronto ON M5T 3A9; Tor'52; FACOG; FSOGC; FRCSC; ObstGyn (Gynecological Surgery). Langs: Italian; (416)923-7311; Fax. (416)923-1287; slibrach@rogers.com.

LIBSEKAL, Kebreab; 214 Med Place, 12F-9909 102 St, Grande Prairie AB T8V 2V4; Ethiopia (Ethiopia)'72; FAAP; FRCPC; Peds. Ac Staff, Queen Elizabeth II Hospital; (780)538-2921; Fax. (780)539-3909.

LICHON, Marek; Mission Med Clinic, 2303 4 St SW, Calgary AB T2S 2S7; Wroclaw (Poland)'84; (403)229-1700

LICHT, Christoph P B; The Hosp for Sick Children, 555 University Ave, Toronto ON M5G 1X8; Albert-Ludwigs Univ at Freiburg (Germany)'92; Nephrol; Peds. Staff, The Hospital For Sick Children; Asst Prof, University of Toronto; Langs: German; (416)813-7654 x2058; Fax. (416)813-6271; christoph.licht@sickkids.ca.

LICHTBLAU, Ethan; 100-5252 boul de Maisonneuve O, Montreal QC H4A 3S5; McG'89; FRCSC; OrthSurg (Joint Replacement). (514)939-1416

LICHTENSTEIN, Samuel V; St Paul's Hosp, 1081 Burrard St, Vancouver BC V6Z 1Y6; Baltimore(MD) (USA)'77; FACS; FRCSC; GenSurg; Cardiovasc&ThorSurg. Dir Cardiol & ThorSurg, Providence Health Care - St Paul's Hospital; Head Cardiovascular Surg, University of British Columbia; (604)806-8501; Fax. (604)806-8375.

LICHTENSTEIN, Tersia; 102-1100 Lawrence Ave, Kelowna BC V1Y 6M4; Pretoria (South Africa)'86; MB ChB; Langs: Afrikaans; (250)763-1183

LICHTENWALD, Duane J; Midtown Med Centre, 211-39 23rd St E, Saskatoon SK S7K 0H6; Sask'84; FRCPC; Derm. Clinical Asst Prof, University of Saskatchewan; (306)653-3348; Fax. (306)653-5774.

LICHTER, Myrna; Medical & Dental Bldg, 218-1849 Yonge St, Toronto ON M4S 1Y2; Man'77; BSc(Med); FACS; FRCSC; Ophth. Att Staff, St Michael's Hospital; Lecturer, University of Toronto; (416)481-4433; Fax. (416)481-7011.

LICHTMAN, Sharla F; Genesis Prof Group Inc, 420-1600 Steeles Ave W, Concord ON L4K 4M2; Cal'86; CCFP; FCFP; Ac Staff, North York General Hospital; (905)760-1415; Fax. (905)760-2735.

LICKLEY, H Lavina A; Women's College Hosp, 7F-76 Grenville St, Toronto ON M5S 1B2; Tor'62; PhD; DAB; FACS; LRCPS; FRCSC; GenSurg (Breast Disease). Staff, Princess Margaret Hospital - University Health Network; Staff, Women's College Hospital; Prof Surg & Physiol, University of Toronto; (416)323-6225; Fax. (416)323-7730; lavina.lickley@utoronto.ca.

LICKRISH, Gordon M; 601-123 Edward St, Toronto ON M5G 1E2; Glasgow (Scotland)'64; MB ChB; FRCSC; ObstGyn (Gynecologic Oncology). Prof Emeritus, University of Toronto; (416)813-4178; Fax. (416)813-4179; gordon.lickrish@medisys.ca.

LICORISH, Paulette M; 15-9555 Yonge St, Richmond Hill ON L4C 9M5; McM'99; FRCPC; Neur. Staff Neurol, Mackenzie Richmond Hill Hospital; (647)385-3363

LICSKAI, Christopher J; St Joseph's Health Care, PO Box 5777 Stn B 268 Grosvenor St, London ON N6A 4V2; Tor'89; FRCPC; IntMed; Respir. Staff, St Joseph's Hospital - St Joseph's Health Care; Staff, London Health Sciences Centre - South Street; (519)646-6405; Fax. (519)646-6064.

LIDDLE, Jane E; 107-900 Greenbank Rd, Nepean ON K2J 1S8; Tor'90; FRCPC; Peds. (613)825-4655; Fax. (613)825-2816.

LIDDY, Clare E; The Ottawa Hosp-Riverside, 1967 Riverside Dr, Ottawa ON K1H 7W9; McM'93; CCFP; FCFP; Staff, The Ottawa Hospital - Riverside Campus; Langs: English; French; (613)738-8219; Fax. (613)738-8217.

LIDKEA, Marlene R; Liberton Med Centre, 212-31 Liberton Dr, St. Albert AB T8N 3X6; Alb'79; CCFP; FCFP; Clin Assoc Prof, Sturgeon Community Hospital; Teach Staff, University of Alberta; (780)459-7760; Fax. (780)460-1799.

LIDMAN, Per G L; College Plaza, 903-8215 112 St NW, Edmonton AB T6G 2C8; Alb'93; FRCPC; Peds; ClinImmunol&Allergy. Staff, University of Alberta Hospital; (780)413-6689

LIE, Kay I; 605-700 Bay St, Toronto ON M5G 1Z6; Heidelberg (Germany)'70; FRCSC; ObstGyn (Endometriosis). Ac Staff, Sunnybrook Health Sciences Centre; Ac Staff, Women's College Hospital; Assoc Prof, University of Toronto; Langs: Dutch; German; Indonesian; (416)595-1311; Fax. (416)979-0238.

LIE, Lie Ming; North York Gen Hosp, 4001 Leslie St, North York ON M2K 1E1; Munich (Germany)'74; FRCPC; Anes. Ac Staff, North York General Hospital; Langs: Chinese; German; (416)756-6262

LIEBERMAN, Diane K; Salvation Army Grace Gen Hosp, 300 Booth Dr, Winnipeg MB R3J 3M7; Man'91; FRCPC; Anes. Staff Anes, The Salvation Army Grace Hospital; (204)837-8311; Fax. (204)831-0029.

LIEBERMAN, Esther J; 1-2810 Major Mackenzie Dr, Maple ON L6A 3L2; Tor'10; CCFP; (905)832-3838

LIEBERMAN, Lani D; Rouge Valley-Centenary HC, 2867 Ellesmere Rd, Scarborough ON M1E 4B9; Tor'99; FRCPC; Peds. Staff, Rouge Valley Health System - Centenary Health Centre Site; (416)281-8481

LIEBERMAN, Murray; Meadowlark Health Centre, 162 Meadowlark Shopping Ctr NW, Edmonton AB T5R 5W9; Alb'68; FRCSC; ObstGyn (Menopause). Ac Staff, Covenant Health - Misericordia Community Hospital; Clin Prof, University of Alberta; (780)428-9516; Fax. (780)428-0629; mlieberman@incenter.net.

LIEBICH, Anne-Marie; Clin Med Maisonneuve-Rosemont, RC60-5345 boul de l'Assomption, Montreal QC H1T 4B3; Tucuman (Argentina)'69; Langs: Spanish; English; (514)257-7000; Fax. (514)257-7003.

LIEBMAN, Mira F; Mount Sinai Hosp, 6 500-600 University Ave, Toronto ON M5G 1X5; McG'05; FRCPC; Peds; PedHemaOncol. Staff, Mount Sinai Hospital; (416)596-4200

LIEBMAN, S; Windsor Health Unit, 350-1720 Howard Ave, Windsor ON N8X 5A6; McM'89; FRCSC; GenSurg. Staff, Windsor Regional Hospital - Metropolitan Site; Aj Prof, University of Western Ontario; (519)255-9584; Fax. (519)255-9908.

LIEBSCHER, Josephine S; 108-284 Helmcken Rd, Victoria BC V9B 1T2; Sask'07; CCFP; (250)480-7333

LIEBSCHER, Ryan S; Royal Jubilee Hosp, 1952 Bay St, Victoria BC V8R 1J8; Sask'07; CCFP; Staff, Royal Jubilee Hospital; (250)981-4505

LIEDEMAN, Mandy; York Med Health Centre, 3-17215 Leslie St, Newmarket ON L3Y 8E4; Tor'92; BSc; (905)853-0404; Fax. (905)853-3702; dr.liedeman@yahoo.com.

LIEFF, Susan J; Baycrest Ctre/Geriatric Care, 3560 Bathurst St, Toronto ON M6A 2E1; Tor'81; FRCPC; Psy. Staff Psy, Baycrest Centre for Geriatric Care; Asst Prof Psy, University of Toronto; (416)785-2500 x2452; Fax. (416)785-2450; s.lieff@utoronto.ca.

LIEKE, Anau; CSSS de la Haute-Cote-Nord, CP 1000 4 rue de l'Hopital, Les Escoumins QC G0T 1K0; (Other Foreign)'85; Staff, Centre de santé des Côté-Nord; (418)233-2931

LIELMANIS, Andris; Bramalea Med Centre, 201-18 Kensington Rd, Brampton ON L6T 4S5; Cardiff (Wales)'67; CCFP; (905)792-2236; Fax. (905)792-1349.

LIEM, Joel J; Windsor Allergy Asthma Assoc, 1407 Ottawa St, Windsor ON N8X 2G1; Ott'00; FRCPC; Peds; ClinImmunol&Allergy. (519)258-4356; Fax. (519)258-9918.

LIEM, Nathania R; Windsor Reg Hosp-Western Camp, 1453 Prince Rd, Windsor ON N9C 3Z4; Ott'98; MSc; FRCPC; PhysMed&Rehab. Staff, Windsor Regional Hospital - Tayfour Site; Staff, Hôtel-Dieu Grace Hospital; Langs: French; (519)257-5184; Fax. (519)257-5137.

LIEM, Daniel T H; Windsor Allergy & Asthma Assoc, 1407 Ottawa St, Windsor ON N8X 2G1; Wilhelms (Germany)'63; PhD; FRCPC; IntMed. Ac Staff, Hôtel-Dieu Grace Hospital; Assoc Staff, Windsor Regional Hospital - Metropolitan Site; Langs: Indonesian; Dutch; German; (519)258-4356; Fax. (519)258-9918.

LIEN, Dale C; University of Alberta Hosp, 2E4 33-8440 112 St NW, Edmonton AB T6G 2B7; Alb'78; BSc; FRCPC; IntMed; Respir. Staff Pulmonary Div, University of Alberta Hospital; Prof Med, University of Alberta; (780)407-7359; Fax. (780)407-6384; dale.lien@ualberta.ca.

LIEPERT, David J; Rockyview Gen Hosp, 7007 14 St SW, Calgary AB T2V 1P9; Sask'85; FRCPC; Anes. Staff Anes, Rockyview General Hospital; (403)943-8720

LIESEGANG, Nadine; MUHC-Montreal Gen Hosp, 1650 av Cedar, Montreal QC H3G 1A4; McG'90; FRCPC; EmergMed. Staff, McGill University Health Centre - Montreal General Campus; (514)934-8090; Fax. (514)934-8093.

LIEU, Hung-Ba; CSSSG-Hop de Hull, 116 boul Lionel-Emond, Gatineau QC J8Y 1W7; Sher'79; FRCSC; Neursurg. Staff, Hull Hospital; Langs: Bilingual(French/English); (819)595-6000; Fax. (819)595-6039.

LIEW, Allan S L; The Ottawa Hosp-Civic Campus, ORCC J135-1053 Carling Ave, Ottawa ON K1Y 4E9; Tor'93; FRCSC; OrthSurg. Staff Trauma & Sports, The Ottawa Hospital - Civic Campus; (613)761-4534; Fax. (613)761-4637; aliew@ottawahospital.on.ca.

LIEW, Chiam L; Slot 3009, PO Box 5053 Stn Forces, Belleville ON K8N 5W6; McM'98; BSc(Hon); MSc(Biol.); CCFP; Langs: Cantonese; Malay; (613)842-8122

LIEW, Elena; Univ Hlth Network-Princess M, 5 216-610 University Ave, Toronto ON M5G 2M9; Alb'06; FRCPC; IntMed; Hem. Staff, Princess Margaret Hospital - University Health Network; (416)946-4501 x3433

LIEW, Javier; 830-3630 Brentwood Rd NW, Calgary AB T2L 1K8; Alb'98; FRCPC; DiagRad. (403)338-4000

LIEW, Kenneth Y K; 306-8077 Islington Ave, Woodbridge ON L4L 7X7; Tor'04; FRCPC; Peds; ClinImmunol&Allergy. (905)856-8714

LIEW, Kim L; Oakridge Centre South Tower, 360-650 41st Ave W, Vancouver BC V5Z 2M9; Alb'76; Langs: Mandarin; Cantonese; (604)261-6000; Fax. (604)261-6667.

LIEW, Trina X; One-Stop Med Centre, 1A-3585 Lawrence Ave E, Scarborough ON M1G 1P4; Cal'00; BSc; CCFP; Langs: French; (416)431-0736; Fax. (416)431-0648.

LIGATE, Lora V; Parkland Med Clinic, 6-5030 47 Ave, Red Deer AB T4N 3P7; UBC'78; Staff, Red Deer Regional Hospital Centre; (403)346-4206; Fax. (403)346-4207.

LIGATE, Loys J; 43 Mistry River Dr SS 6, Conestogo ON N0B 1N0; UBC'76; BSc; MSc; FRCPC; Psy (Women's Issues). Affil Staff Psy-In-Charge of Aftercare Prog, Cambridge Memorial Hospital; Staff Psy., Grand Valley Inst. for Women; (519)206-0100

LIGGETT, Brian A; PO Box 62014 Rpo Hawkwood, Calgary AB T3G 5S7; Cal'75; CCFP; FCFP.

LIGHT, Robert B; St Boniface Gen Hosp, C5124-409 Tache Ave, Winnipeg MB R2H 2A6; Cal'75; FRCPC; IntMed. Ac Staff, St Boniface General Hospital; (204)233-8563; Fax. (204)231-0640.

LIGHT, Thurairajan; Forbes Park Med Centre, 26 Forbes St, Cambridge ON N3C 2E2; (Malaysia)'93; CCFP; Langs: Malay; Tamil; (519)658-4615; Fax. (519)658-4630.

LIGHTBODY, Peter; East Calgary Health Centre, 4715 8 Ave SE, Calgary AB T2A 3N4; Qns'93; CCFP; CCFP(E.M.); (403)955-1000

LIGHTER, Mark D; Brant Community HC-Brantford, 200 Terrace Hill St, Brantford ON N3R 1G9; McM'84; FRCPC; DiagRad. Staff, St Joseph's Healthcare - Charlton Campus; (519)752-7871

LIGHTFOOT, Christopher B; Queen Elizabeth II HSC, 1276 South Park St, Halifax NS B3H 2Y9; Dal'05; DiagRad. Staff, Queen Elizabeth II Health Sciences Centre - Victoria General Site; (902)473-2700

LIGHTFOOT, Peter D; Professional Arts Bldg, 616-100 Arden St, Moncton NB E1C 4B7; Dal'70; FRCPC; IntMed (Gastroenterology). Sr Active Staff, The Moncton Hospital; Lecturer, Dalhousie University; (506)854-0931

LIGHTHEART, Margaret R; 2-1216 Upper Wentworth St, Hamilton ON L9A 4W2; Ott'84; FRCSC; ObstGyn. Ac Staff, Hamilton Health Sciences Centre-Juravinski Site; Clin Assoc Prof, McMaster University; Langs: English; French; (905)389-5657; Fax. (905)389-3113.

LIGHTLE, Angela N; Downey Family Med Centre, 2-115 Downey Rd, Guelph ON N1C 1A2; McM'02; CCFP; (519)827-9779; Fax. (519)827-0162.

LIGIER, Bruno; Foothills Med Centre, 1403 29 St NW, Calgary AB T2N 2T9; McG'84; FRCPC; Anes (Critical Care Medicine). Staff Anes, Foothills Medical Centre; (403)944-1430; Fax. (403)944-2425.

LIGIER, Sophie; Hop Maisonneuve-Rosemont, 5415 boul de l'Assomption, Montreal QC H1T 2M4; McG'92; FRCPC; IntMed; Rheum. Staff, Hopital Maisonneuve-Rosemont; Langs: English; French; (514)252-3400 x4925; Fax. (514)252-3889.

LIGON, Inocencio R; 303-3034 Palstan Rd, Mississauga ON L4Y 2Z6; Quezon City (Philippines)'61; Court Staff, Trillium Health Centre - Mississauga; (905)270-5708

LIGORI, Tania; St Joseph's Healthcare, 50 Charlton Ave E, Hamilton ON L8N 4A6; Tor'03; FRCPC; Anes; Critical Care Medicine. Staff, St Joseph's Healthcare - Charlton Campus; (905)522-1155

LIKAR, Ivan; Kingsway Med Bldg, 15-2917 Bloor St W, Etobicoke ON M8X 1B4; London (England)'62; MB BS; LRCP; MRCS; FACP; FRCPC; IntMed (Cardiology). (647)352-6646

LIKAVCANOVA, Elena; L'Omniclinique de l'Outaouais, 202-28 boul du Mont-Bleu, Gatineau QC J8Z 1J1; Mon'97; MSc(Microbiolmmunol.); BSc(Biol.); CCFP; Physician, CHLSD Foyer du Bonheur; (819)669-7393; Fax. (819)669-0077.

LIKWORNIK, Gunilla; St Clair Med Clinic, 2F-50 St Clair Ave E, Toronto ON M4T 1M9; Tor'77; MHSc(CommunMed); Court Staff, Women's College Hospital; (416)921-1066; Fax. (416)921-8459.

LIKWORNIK, Victor; Nanaimo Sleep Clinic, 130-2124 Bowen Rd, Nanaimo BC V9S 1H7; Tor'73; DPsy; AB; DABPN; FRCPC; Psy (Psychotherapy). (250)758-0060

LILANI, Rizwana; Peace Med Centre, 20-9699 Jane St, Maple ON L6A 0A5; Ziauddin Medical University (Other Foreign)'03; AAFPhys; CCFP; Langs: Farsi; Urdu; Punjabi; Gujarati; (905)303-1700; Fax. (905)303-1727.

LILES, W Conrad; Univ Hlth Network-Toronto Gen, FE3 805-200 Elizabeth St, Toronto ON M5G 2C4; Washington(WA) (USA)'87; ABIM; PhD; FRCPC; IntMed; InfectDis. Dir Div of InfectDis/Staff, Toronto General Hospital - UHN; Sr Scientist Global Health, McLaughlin-Rotman Centre; Dir Div of InfectDis, University of Toronto; (416)340-4800 x3624; conrad.liles@uhn.on.ca.

LILIC, Nenad; Royal Alexandra Hosp, 10240 Kingsway NW, Edmonton AB T5H 3V9; (Serbia)'92; Staff, Royal Alexandra Hospital; (780)735-4737; Fax. (780)735-4715.

LILKER, Emmanuel S; 1-213 St Clair Ave W, Toronto ON M4V 1R3; Tor'62; FRCPC; IntMed (Respirology). Ac Staff, St Joseph's Health Centre; Asst Prof, University of Toronto; (416)920-3737; Fax. (416)920-7848.

LILKER, Suzanne J; St Joseph's Health Centre, 30 The Queensway, Toronto ON M6R 1B5; Tor'92; FRCPC; Anes. Staff, St Joseph's Health Centre; Langs: Spanish; (416)530-6000

LILLA, Mogamad N; Chilliwack Gen Hosp, 45600 Menholm Rd, Chilliwack BC V2P 1P7; Cape Town (South Africa)'01; MB BS; FRCPC; Psy. Staff, Chilliwack General Hospital; Langs: Afrikaans; (604)795-4141

LILLEY, John T; Royal Alexandra Hosp, 10240 Kingsway NW, Edmonton AB T5H 3V9; Alb'80; DAB; FRCPC; Anes (Pediatric Anesthesia). Staff Anes, Royal Alexandra Hospital; (780)735-4010; Fax. (780)735-4386; jtlilley@shaw.ca.

LILLEY, Kenneth; 3C-1218 Langley St, Victoria BC V8W 1W2; Liverpool (England)'58; MB ChB; FRCPC; Psy (General Adult Psychiatry). Ac Staff, Royal Jubilee Hospital; (250)383-4704; Fax. (250)383-4704.

LILLEY, Mary M; 2F-333 Eglinton Ave E, Toronto ON M4P 1L7; Alb'77; FRCPC; Psy (Child Psychiatry). (416)323-1852

LILLICRAP, David P; Queen's University, 115 Barrack St, Kingston ON K7L 3N6; London (England)'75; FRCPC; Hem; IntMed. (613)548-1304; lillicrap@cliff.path.queensu.ca.

LILLIE, Eric; 72D rue Sainte-Anne, Ste-Anne-de-Bellev QC H9X 1L8; McG'85; AB; Ac Staff Family Pract & EmergMed, Lakeshore General Hospital - Pointe Claire; Consultant Clinical Research, Phoenix International; (514)457-9355; Fax. (514)457-3061.

LILLQUIST, Yolanda P; Children's & Women's Hc Of Bc, K3 205-4480 Oak St, Vancouver BC V6H 3V4; New York (USA)'77; FRCPC; Peds (Cystic Fibrosis). Clinical Asst Prof, BC Children's Hospital; (604)875-2628

LILLY, Erica J; Clarence-Rockland Fam Hlth Team, 2741 Chamberland St, Rockland ON K4K 0B4; Ott'09; CCFP; (613)446-7677

LILLY, Leslie B; 11NCSB1241-585 University Ave, Toronto ON M5G 2N2; McM'86; BSc; MSc; FRCPC; IntMed (Hepatology); Gastroent. Staff Physician, Toronto General Hospital - UHN; Consultant, The Hospital For Sick Children; Asst Prof, University of Toronto; (416)340-4629; Fax. (416)340-3511; les.lilly@uhn.on.ca.

LILLY, Roy A; The Health Plex, 114 Empire Ave, St. John's NL A1C 3G2; Mem'93; BMedSci; CCFP; FCFP; (709)738-1919; Fax. (709)722-6029.

LILY, Muriel; Dr Langer & Associates, 180 Sandalwood Pky E, Brampton ON L6Z 1Y4; Mem'09; CCFP; (905)846-9255

LIM, Allen W K; Meadowlark Place Prof Centre, 408-8708 155 St NW, Edmonton AB T5R 1W2; Alb'04; Gastroent; IntMed. Staff, Foothills Medical Centre; (780)930-1915

LIM, Andrew S; Sunnybrook Hlth Sciences Ctre, M1 600-2075 Bayview Ave, Toronto ON M4N 3M5; Tor'03; FRCPC; Neur. Staff, Sunnybrook Health Sciences Centre; (416)480-6100

LIM, Audrey Y; McMaster University, 3A-1280 Main St W, Hamilton ON L8S 4K1; McM'94; MSc; FRCPC; Peds; Critical Care Medicine. Staff, Hamilton Health Sciences Centre - McMaster Children's Hospital; (905)521-2100

LIM, Beatriz T; Peter Lougheed Centre, 3500 26 Ave NE, Calgary AB T1Y 6J4; Mem'95; FRCPC; Anes. Staff Anes, Peter Lougheed Centre; (403)291-8555; btzlim@hotmail.com.

LIM, Bee K; Nokomis Health Care Centre, PO Box 98, Nokomis SK S0G 3R0; Glasgow (Scotland)'86; MB ChB; (306)528-2114; Fax. (306)528-4655.

LIM, Benito C; Lakeshore Med & Prof Bldg, 307-3170 Lake Shore Blvd W, Etobicoke ON M8V 3X8; Manila (Philippines)'62; Staff, St Joseph's Health Centre; (416)259-5238

LIM, Bill Y B; 302B-280 Spadina Ave, Toronto ON M5T 3A5; Tor'79; Staff, The Scarborough Hospital - Birchmount Campus; Physician, A C Nielson; (416)977-9888

LIM, Bin-Keng; Burrard Health Bldg, 306-1160 Burrard St, Vancouver BC V6Z 2E8; McG'78; CCFP; CCFP(E.M.); FCFP; Ac Staff, Providence Health Care - St Paul's Hospital; (604)685-7747; Fax. (604)844-2283.

LIM, Chern W; Rouge Valley-Centenary HC, 2867 Ellesmere Rd, Scarborough ON M1E 4B9; Mem'05; FRCPC; Neur. Staff, Rouge Valley Health System - Centenary Health Centre Site; (416)284-8131

LIM, Chong Won; University Hosp of Northern BC, 1475 Edmonton St, Prince George BC V2M 1S2; Seoul (Korea)'57; FRCPC; DiagRad. Staff Radiol, University Hospital of Northern British Columbia; (250)563-2000

LIM, Chong-Ha; Radiology Associates of Regina, 6-2727 Parliament Ave, Regina SK S4S 6X5; Mem'82; FRCPC; DiagRad. Staff, Radiology Associates of Regina; (306)352-7653; Fax. (306)522-4311.

LIM, David C; Rosedale Med Centre, 505-600 Sherbourne St, Toronto ON M4X 1W4; (Philippines)'79; Ac Staff Family Pract, Toronto East General Hospital Inc; Langs: Mandarin; Fookien; Tagalog; (416)469-8255; Fax. (416)469-2248.

LIM, Dawn Y; Univ Hlth Network-Toronto Gen, Gs 480-200 Elizabeth St, Toronto ON M5G 2C4; Tor'05; FRCPC; EmergMed. Staff, Toronto General Hospital - UHN; (416)340-3947

LIM, Diane; Bridlewood Prof Centre, 203-3443 Finch Ave E, Scarborough ON M1W 2S1; Man'89; BSc; Ac Staff, Rouge Valley Health System - Centenary Health Centre Site; Ac Staff, The Scarborough Hospital - General Campus; (416)493-4424; Fax. (416)490-8180.

LIM, Elizabeth S; 350-507 Broadway W, Vancouver BC V5Z 1E6; UBC'03; CCFP; (604)568-7229

LIM, Frank F S; 4-22932 Lougheed Hwy, Maple Ridge BC V2X 2W3; UBC'74; BSc(Hons); Langs: Malay; Mandarin; (604)466-5767

LIM, Gerald W K; Tom Baker Cancer Centre, 1331 29 St NW, Calgary AB T2N 4N2; Alb'02; FRCPC; RadOncol. Staff, Tom Baker Cancer Centre; (403)521-3012; Fax. (403)283-1651.

LIM, Gloria; Crestwood Medical Dental, 205-6051 Gilbert Rd, Richmond BC V7C 3V3; Qns'07; FRCPC; IntMed; Hem. (604)278-9116

LIM, Henry; Wentworth Limeridge Med Ctre, 204-849 Upper Wentworth St, Hamilton ON L9A 5H4; Tor'96; CCFP; (905)383-3115; Fax. (905)383-6581.

LIM, Hilda H; 4631 Steeles Ave E, Scarborough ON M1V 4S5; Tor'08; CCFP; (416)293-6600; Fax. (416)293-5410.

LIM, Howard J; BC Cancer Agency-Vancouver CC, 600 10th Ave W, Vancouver BC V5Z 4E6; UBC'02; FRCPC; IntMed; MedOncol. Staff, BC Cancer Agency Vancouver Centre; (604)877-6000 x5459

LIM, Jan T W; BC Cancer Agency-Vanc Isl Ctr, 2410 Lee Ave, Victoria BC V8R 6V5; Manchester (England)'84; FRCPC; RadOncol (Oncology). Staff, BC Cancer Agency Vancouver Island Centre; Clinical Asst Prof Surg, University of British Columbia; (250)519-5575; Fax. (250)519-2018; jlim@bccancer.bc.ca.

LIM, Jean-Paul; Park Avenue Med Centre, 500-4634 Park Ave, Terrace BC V8G 1V7; UBC'06; FRCPC; IntMed. (250)615-5088

LIM, Julie; CSSS du Sud de Lanaudière, 911 montee des Pionniers, Terrebonne QC J6V 2H2; Sher'04; CCFP; Staff, Centre Hospitalier Pierre le Gardeur; (450)654-7525

LIM, Ka-Chee; 210 Second Ave, Timmins ON P4N 1G2; RCS (Ireland)'73; LRCPSI; Staff GP, Timmins & District Hospital; (705)264-6118; Fax. (705)267-5544.

LIM, Kenneth I; BC Women's Hosp & Health Ctre, 1T60-4500 Oak St, Vancouver BC V6H 3N1; UBC'89; FRCSC; ObstGyn (Fetal & Maternal Medicine). Staff, BC Women's Hospital & Health Centre; Clinical Asst Prof, University of British Columbia; (604)875-3174; klim@cw.bc.ca.

LIM, Khian-Kok; 20-3360 rue Notre-Dame, Lachine QC H8T 3E2; (Taiwan)'65; Ophth (P.Q.). Staff Ophth, Hôpital Chinois de Montréal; Langs: French; Chinese; (514)637-3003

LIM, Ki Dong; Brampton Cardiopulmonary Clini, 31 Centre St S, Brampton ON L6W 2X7; McM'04; FRCPC; IntMed. (905)455-3010; Fax. (905)455-3011.

LIM, Larry F T; Pitt Meadows Prof Centre, 101-12195 Harris Rd, Pitt Meadows BC V3Y 2E9; UBC'88; Langs: Mandarin; (604)465-9977

LIM, Lawrence; Misericordia Community Hosp, 16940 87 Ave NW, Edmonton AB T5R 4H5; Alb'93; FRCPC; IntMed. Staff, Covenant Health - Misericordia Community Hospital; (780)735-2000; Fax. (780)735-2511.

LIM, Leonard; Red Deer Reg Hosp Centre, PO Box 5030 Stn Postal Box Ctr, Red Deer AB T4N 6R2; Alb'07; FRCPC; IntMed. Staff, Red Deer Regional Hospital Centre; (403)343-4422

LIM, Maileen M; Meadows Med Clinic, 2362 24 St NW, Edmonton AB T6T 0G9; (Other Foreign)'97; CCFP; (780)465-7335

LIM, May-Ling J; 104-515 Main St, Vancouver BC V6A 2V1; UBC'89; Langs: Cantonese; (604)696-6138; Fax. (604)696-6128.

LIM, Meng Chee; Hotel-Dieu Grace Hosp, 1030 Ouellette Ave, Windsor ON N9A 1E1; Mem'98; FRCPC; DiagRad;CCFP; CCFP(E.M.); Staff, Hôtel-Dieu Grace Hospital; (519)973-4411 x3477

LIM, Meng Eng; 205-135 15th St E, North Vancouver BC V7L 2P7; (Singapore)'68; MB BS; FRCPC; Psy. Clin Dir Adolesc Program & Psy Outpatient Serv, Lions Gate Hospital; Langs: Cantonese; Fookien; Malay; Mandarin; (604)988-8383; Fax. (604)988-2185; melim@direct.ca.

LIM, Michael D; Cambridge Mem Hosp, 700 Coronation Blvd, Cambridge ON N1R 3G2; Wes'08; CCFP; Staff, Cambridge Memorial Hospital; (519)621-2330

LIM, Nathan E; Eagle Ridge Hosp & Hlth CC, 475 Guildford Way, Port Moody BC V3H 3W9; UBC'08; CCFP; CCFP(E.M.); Staff Emerg, Eagle Ridge Hospital & Health Care Centre; (604)469-3191

LIM, Peter; BC Cancer Agency-Vancouver CC, 600 10th Ave W, Vancouver BC V5Z 4E6; UBC'89; FRCPC; RadOncol. Staff, BC Cancer Agency Vancouver Centre; (604)877-6000; Fax. (604)708-2000.

LIM, Peter S H; Lions Gate Hosp, 231 15th St E, North Vancouver BC V7L 2L7; Alb'94; FRCPC; Psy. Staff Psy, Lions Gate Hospital; Staff Psy, Coast Health Services; Langs: Korean; (604)453-1913

LIM, Princeton H; Metro Health Clinic, 4879 Kingsway, Burnaby BC V5H 4T6; UBC'84; BSc(Hons); PhD; Ac Staff, Burnaby Hospital; Staff Designated Med. Practitioner, Canadian Immigration; Langs: Mandarin; (604)433-8888; Fax. (604)433-8618; princeton_lim@telus.net.

LIM, Raymond T; The Credit Valley Hosp, 2200 Eglinton Ave W, Mississauga ON L5M 2N1; Wes'05; CCFP; CCFP(E.M.); Staff, The Credit Valley Hospital; (905)813-4530

LIM, Rodrick K; Children's Hosp of Western Ont, 800 Commissioners Rd E, London ON N6C 2V5; Qns'95; FRCPC; Peds. Staff, Children's Hospital of Western Ontario; (519)685-8500 x8131

LIM, Ronald T H; Westglen Med Clinic, 108-30 Springborough Blvd SW, Calgary AB T3H 0N9; UBC'84; CCFP; Ac Staff, Rockyview General Hospital; (403)240-2221

LIM, Rosemary Dy; 8630 120 St, Surrey BC V3W 3N6; (Philippines)'75; (604)591-2322; Fax. (604)591-9053.

LIM, Sen-Mei; Meadowlands Fam Health Centre, 888 Meadowlands Dr, Ottawa ON K2C 3R2; Qns'95; CCFP; Physician, Meadowlands Family Health Centre; (613)228-2882; Fax. (613)228-2856.

LIM, Teddy A; Rouge Valley-Centenary HC, 2867 Ellesmere Rd, Scarborough ON M1E 4B9; Man'97; FRCPC; Anes. Staff, Rouge Valley Health System - Centenary Health Centre Site; (416)284-8131 x4054

LIM, Thomas W P; South Health Campus, 4448 Front St SE, Calgary AB T3M 1M4; Alb'04; FRCPC; IntMed; Respir. (403)956-2800; Fax. (403)956-2848.

LIM, Wendy P W; St Joseph's Healthcare, L 208-50 Charlton Ave E, Hamilton ON L8N 4A6; Tor'98; FRCPC; IntMed; Hem. Staff, St Joseph's Healthcare - Charlton Campus; (905)521-6024; Fax. (905)540-6568.

LIM, Wi-Guan; Collingwood Medical, 350-3150 54th Ave E, Vancouver BC V5S 1Z1; UBC'87; Ac Staff, Burnaby Hospital; (604)435-3388; Fax. (604)433-2323.

LIM, Wing F; Synergy Med Plus, 229-501 Bethel Dr, Sherwood Park AB T8H 0N2; Alb'91; BMedSci; CCFP; FCFP; Langs: Chinese; Cantonese; Mandarin; Fukinese; (780)416-8747; Fax. (780)449-5461.

LIM, Y C Ben; Royal University Hosp, 103 Hospital Dr, Saskatoon SK S7N 0W8; Sask'97; FRCPC; Anes. Staff, Royal University Hospital; (306)655-1183; Fax. (306)655-1279.

LIM, Yen L; 4349 Hastings St, Burnaby BC V5C 2J8; UBC'03; CCFP; (604)299-4388

LIMA, Rosanna V; Dr Roanna V Lima Inc, 1017-750 Broadway W, Vancouver BC V5Z 1H9; Sao Paulo (Brazil)'79; CCFP; Preceptor, University of British Columbia; Langs: Portuguese; Italian; Spanish; (604)708-4333; Fax. (604)708-4680.

LIMA FILHO, Jose H C; Centre for Family Medicine, 3017-10B Victoria St S, Kitchener ON N2G 1C5; Ceara (Brazil)'89; FRCPC; ClinImmunol&Allergy; Derm. (519)885-5426

LIMAYE, Navika P; St Joseph's Health Centre, 30 The Queensway, Toronto ON M6R 1B5; Dal'04; CCFP; Staff, St Joseph's Health Centre; (416)530-6860; Fax. (416)530-6160.

LIMBOMBE, Basunga; Tilbury District Family Hlth Team, PO Box 760 22 Mill St W, Tilbury ON N0P 2L0; (519)682-2307

LIMOGES, Michel; Clinique Medicale 3000, 3000 rue Belanger, Montreal QC H1Y 1A9; Mon'80; Langs: English; (514)376-7702; Fax. (514)376-2639.

LIMOGES, Patrick; Hop Du Sacre-Coeur De Mtl, 5400 boul Gouin O, Montreal QC H4J 1C5; Mon'95; FRCPC; Anes. Staff, Hôpital du Sacre-Coeur de Montréal; (514)338-2222

LIN, Alan N; Market Mall Prof Bldg, 329-4935 40 Ave NW, Calgary AB T3A 2N1; Cal'91; BSc; FRCSC; PlasSurg. Ac Staff, Peter Lougheed Centre; (403)288-6666; Fax. (403)288-6624.

LIN, Andrew N; Edmonton Clinic, 3C-11400 University Ave NW, Edmonton AB T6G 1Z1; UBC'78; FRCPC; Derm. Ac Staff, University of Alberta Hospital; Assoc Prof Div of Derm, University of Alberta; (780)407-1257; Fax. (780)407-3003.

LIN, Betty P; 4419 Hastings St, Burnaby BC V5C 2K1; UBC'96; CCFP; FCFP; (604)299-3457; Fax. (604)299-3492.

LIN, Cassie W; Columbia Med Bldg, 410-301 Columbia St E, New Westminster BC V3L 3W5; Wes'97; BSc; FRCPC; IntMed; Gastroent. Langs: Mandarin; (604)525-0155; Fax. (604)525-1699.

LIN, Daniel C; St Paul's Hosp, 1081 Burrard St, Vancouver BC V6Z 1Y6; UBC'03; BSc; FRCPC; Psy. Staff, Providence Health Care - St Paul's Hospital; (604)806-8004

LIN, Daren; Hamilton HS-General Site, 260-237 Barton St E, Hamilton ON L8L 2X2; Wes'07; CCFP; CCFP(E.M.); Staff, Hamilton Health Sciences Centre - Hamilton General Hospital; (905)521-2100 x46368

LIN, David T; Pacific Laser Eye Centre, 5F-1401 Broadway W, Vancouver BC V6H 1H6; McG'83; MDCM; FRCSC; Ophth (Refractive Surgery). Court Staff, Vancouver General Hospital - Centennial Pavillion; Court Staff, BC Children's Hospital; Clin Assoc Prof, University of British Columbia; Langs: Fookien; French; (604)736-2625; Fax. (604)736-2699.

LIN, Denny; Old Quebec Street Mall, T28-55 Wyndham St N, Guelph ON N1H 7T8; McM'00; FRCSC; Otol. (519)766-0917

LIN, Edward D H; Dr Edward Lin Med Prof Corp, 702-2075 Kennedy Rd, Scarborough ON M1T 3V3; Tor'86; FRCPC; IntMed; Gastroent. Ac Staff, Rouge Valley Health System - Centenary Health Centre Site; (416)292-6509; Fax. (416)292-0797.

LIN, Frank Y; Medical Arts Bldg, 305-581 Davis Dr, Newmarket ON L3Y 2P6; Ott'96; FRCPC; IntMed; Gastroent. Staff, Southlake Regional Health Centre; (905)895-4521; Fax. (905)836-6920.

LIN, Hong; 103-7110 120 St, Surrey BC V3W 3M8; (China)'99; CCFP; (604)591-8008

LIN, I C John; 370-5740 Cambie St, Vancouver BC V5Z 3A6; Man'89; Langs: Mandarin; (604)322-6658; Fax. (604)321-8771.

LIN, Jackson M K; Atrium Prof Bldg, SS 103 303-190 Cundles Rd E, Barrie ON L4M 4S5; Tor'89; CCFP; Staff, Royal Victoria Regional Health Centre; (705)728-3722

LIN, Jenny C; Hôpital Ste-Justine, 3175 ch Cote-Sainte-Catherine, Montreal QC H3T 1C5; McG'00; FRCSC; PlasSurg. Staff, Hôpital Ste-Justine; (514)345-4771

LIN, Judy; North York Gen Hosp, 4001 Leslie St, North York ON M2K 1E1; Tor'07; FRCPC; Psy. Staff, North York General Hospital; (416)756-6655

LIN, Karen W; 3477 Kingston Rd, Scarborough ON M1M 1R4; McG'94; Court Staff, North York General Hospital; Court Staff Privil, The Scarborough Hospital - General Campus; Langs: French; Mandarin; (416)261-0588; Fax. (416)261-8520.

LIN, Ken C.; St Michael's Hosp, 30 Bond St, Toronto ON M5B 1W8; Tor'96; DABA; NBEchoTestamur; BSc; LRCPS; FRCPC; Anes (Cardiovascular Anesthesia). Staff Anes, St Michael's Hospital; (416)360-4000; Fax. (416)864-6014; link@smh.toronto.on.ca.

LIN, Leslie P S; Misericordia Community Hosp, 16940 87 Ave NW, Edmonton AB T5R 4H5; Birmingham (England)'75; MB ChB; FRCA(Eng); FRCPC; Anes (Chronic Pain Management). Staff Anes, Covenant Health - Misericordia Community Hospital; (780)735-2863; Fax. (780)735-2967.

LIN, Liping; St Michael's Hosp, 3F-30 Bond St, Toronto ON M5B 1W8; Tor'94; BSc; FRCPC; Neur (Neuromuscular Diseases). Staff Neurophysiology Lab, St Michael's Hospital; Physician, First Canadian Medical Centre; (416)864-5193; Fax. (416)864-6095.

LIN, Mary M L; Hotel-Dieu Grace Hosp, 1030 Ouellette Ave, Windsor ON N9A 1E1; Wes'89; FRCPC; Anes. Staff, Hôtel-Dieu Grace Hospital; (519)973-4421; Fax. (519)255-2130.

LIN, Michael C; 280-10405 Jasper Ave NW, Edmonton AB T5J 3N4; Alb'02; FRCPC; Peds; ClinImmunol&Allergy. (780)944-9588; Fax. (780)944-9586.

LIN, Peter J; 202-3609 Sheppard Ave E, Scarborough ON M1T 3K8; Tor'88; CCFP; Dir Primary Care Initiatives, Canadian Heart Research Centre; Past Med Dir, Health & Wellness Centre at Scarborough; Langs: Chinese; (416)321-2643; linp@smh.toronto.on.ca.

LIN, Roberto; CLSC Metro, 1801 boul de Maisonneuve O, Montreal QC H3H 1J9; Laval'07; CCFP; (514)934-0354

LIN, Susy; Medcan Health Mgmt Inc, 1500-150 York St, Toronto ON M5H 3S5; Tor'95; BSc; Staff, Medcan Health Management Inc; (416)350-5906; Fax. (416)350-5927.

LIN, Vincent Y; Sunnybrook Hlth Sciences Ctre, M1 102-2075 Bayview Ave, Toronto ON M4N 3M5; Qns'00; FRCSC; Otol. Staff, Sunnybrook Health Sciences Centre; (416)480-4141; Fax. (416)480-5761.

LIN, Jameson; Malton Med Arts Bldg, 107-3530 Derry Rd E, Mississauga ON L4T 4E3; Tor'89; Staff, William Osler Health System - Etobicoke General Hospital; (905)677-6532; Fax. (905)677-6533.

LIN, Yulia; Sunnybrook Hlth Sciences Ctre, B 204-2075 Bayview Ave, Toronto ON M4N 3M5; Tor'99; FRCPC; IntMed (Transfusion Medicine); Hem. Staff, Sunnybrook Health Sciences Centre; (416)480-4042

LINASSI, A Gary; Saskatoon City Hosp, 701 Queen St, Saskatoon SK S7K 0M7; Cork (Ireland)'96; MB ChB; BAO; BSc(Hons); LMCC; FRCPC; PhysMed&Rehab (Spinal Cord Injury). Staff, Saskatoon City Hospital; Assoc Prof/Asst Dean Undergraduate Med Education, University of Saskatchewan; (306)655-8736

LINCOLN, Lawrence; 5107 Boul De Maisonneuve O, Montreal QC H4A 1Z1; McG'79; FRCSC; OrthSurg. (514)369-0010; lincolnl@videotron.ca.

LINCOLN, Maximillian C; Aberdeen Reg Hosp, 835 East River Rd, New Glasgow NS B2H 3S6; Qns'02; OrthSurg. Staff, Aberdeen Regional Hospital; (902)752-8311

LINCOURT, Isabelle; CSSS Drummond-Hop Sainte-Croix, 570 rue Heriot, Drummondville QC J2B 1C1; Mon'01; CSPQ; FRCSC; ObstGyn. Staff, Hôpital Sainte-croix; (819)478-6464

LIND, Daren B; PO Box 45016 Rpo Brentwood, Calgary AB T2L 1Y4; Alb'97; CCFP; CCFP(E.M.); FCFP.

LINDA, Dorota; Mount Sinai Hosp, 600 University Ave, Toronto ON M5G 1X5; Man'06; FRCPC; DiagRad. Staff, Mount Sinai Hospital; (416)586-4800

LINDBERG, Alexandra L; Harrow H C Inc-A Family Hlth Team, PO Box 430 1480 Erie St, Harrow ON N0R 1G0; UBC'87; CCFP; (519)738-2000; Fax. (519)738-9944.

LINDEN, Paul N; Kelowna Gen Hosp, 2268 Pandosy St, Kelowna BC V1Y 1T2; UBC'87; CCFP; CCFP(E.M.); FCFP; Staff, Kelowna General Hospital; (250)862-4300

LINDEN, Ron; North York Gen Hosp-Branson, 2F-555 Finch Ave W, Toronto ON M2R 1N5; Tor'80; DrMedCh; BSc; CCFP; Att Staff, Toronto General Hospital - UHN; Court Staff, North York General Hospital - Branson Division; Lecturer, University of Toronto; (416)223-6600; Fax. (416)223-6764; drlinden@ontariowoundcare.com.

LINDENER, Margo; Springview Family Practice, 106-5675 Spring Garden Rd, Halifax NS B3J 1H1; Dal'85; (902)429-9146

LINDENSCHMIDT, Richard B; Selkirk Med Centre, 353 Eveline St, Selkirk MB R1A 1N1; Man'09; CCFP.

LINDENSCHMIDT, Richard R; Selkirk Med Centre, 353 Eveline St, Selkirk MB R1A 1N1; Man'80; CCFP; FCFP; Ac Staff, Selkirk & District General Hospital; (204)785-2550; Fax. (204)785-1087.

LINDENSMITH, Jorin M; Dartmouth Gen Hosp, 325 Pleasant St, Dartmouth NS B2Y 4G8; Dal'00; BSc; FRCPC; IntMed (Allergy & Immunology). Staff IntMed, Dartmouth General Hospital; Langs: French; (902)460-4152; Fax. (902)460-4154.

LINDER, Mark R; King West Village Med Centre, 2F-626 King St W, Toronto ON M5V 1M7; UBC'04; CCFP; (416)703-1313

LINDERS, Patricia M; Medical & Dental Bldg, 602-586 Eglinton Ave E, Toronto ON M4P 1P2; Dublin (Ireland)'80; FRCPC; Peds (Emergency Medicine). Staff, The Hospital For Sick Children; Staff, Mount Sinai Hospital; Staff, Women's College Hospital; University of Toronto; (416)489-3263; Fax. (416)489-7808.

LINDHOLM, James N T K; 1-160 The Westway, Etobicoke ON M9P 2C1; Dublin (Ireland)'06; CCFP; (647)547-8181

LINDLEY, Janette I; St Paul's Hosp, 1081 Burrard St, Vancouver BC V6Z 1Y6; Mem'81; ABOph; FRCSC; Ophth (Neuro Ophthalmology). Consultant, Vancouver General Hospital - Centennial Pavillion; Ac Staff, Providence Health Care - St Paul's Hospital; Consultant, UBC Hospital - Koerner Pavillion; Staff, Burrard Health Centre; Clin Prof, University of British Columbia; Langs: Bilingual(English/French); (604)806-8168; Fax. (604)806-8058.

LINDLEY, Rebecca J; Pemberton Med Clinic, PO Box 69, Pemberton BC V0N 2L0; McM'97; CCFP; Langs: French; (604)894-6454; Fax. (604)894-6721.

LINDLEY, Susan K; MUHC-Montreal Gen Hosp, L4 309-1650 av Cedar, Montreal QC H3G 1A4; McG'80; BSc; MSc; FRCSC; Ophth (Cataract Surgery). Staff, St Mary's Hospital Centre; Sr Staff Ophth, McGill University Health Centre - Montreal General Campus; assoc Prof, McGill University; Langs: French; (514)934-1934 x44060; Fax. (514)934-8223.

LINDNER, Kirsten K V; 110-231 Oak Park Blvd, Oakville ON L6H 7S8; McM'01; CCFP; Staff, Halton Healthcare Services Corporation - Oakville Site; (905)901-5111

LINDOR, Marie-Helene; Clinique Med Perrier, 101-10794 rue Lajeunesse, Montreal QC H3L 2E8; Port-au-Prince (Haiti)'74; (514)383-0559; Fax. (514)383-0555.

LINDQUIST, Larry V; Medical Arts Bldg, 202-233 Kennedy St, Winnipeg MB R3C 3J5; Man'79; DiagRad. (204)942-6453; Fax. (204)944-8101.

LINDSAY, A Morgan; Kootenay Lake Hosp, 3 View St, Nelson BC V1L 2V1; UBC'07; CCFP; Staff, Kootenay Lake General Hospital; (250)352-3111

LINDSAY, Ardis B; Central Park Med Centre, 108-309 Park St, Brockville ON K6V 6E5; McG'72; FRCSC; Ophth. Ac Staff, Brockville General Hospital - Charles Street; (613)342-9756; Fax. (613)342-1119.

LINDSAY, Brian G; Peterborough Reg HC-Hospital, 1 Hospital Dr, Peterborough ON K9J 7C6; Qns'99; CCFP; Staff, Peterborough Regional Health Centre - Hospital Drive; (705)743-2121

LINDSAY, Christopher S; York Prof Bldg, 204-679 Davis Dr, Newmarket ON L3Y 5G8; Wes'94; BSc(Chem.); FRCSC; OrthSurg (Lower Extremity Reconstruction). Staff, Southlake Regional Health Centre; (905)830-9797; Fax. (905)830-5107.

LINDSAY, D Ian; Downtown Med Place, 302-49 High St, Barrie ON L4N 5J4; Tor'74; Assoc Staff, Royal Victoria Regional Health Centre; (705)722-3443

LINDSAY, Daniel J; Serlkirk & Dist Gen Hosp, PO Box 5000 Stn Main 100 Easton Dr, Selkirk MB R1A 2M2; Man'80; FRCPC; DiagRad. Ac Staff, Selkirk & District General Hospital; Ac Staff/Hd DiagRad, Beausejour District Hospital; Asst Prof, University of Manitoba; Langs: French; (204)482-5800

LINDSAY, David R; St Joseph's Health Centre, 415-30 The Queensway, Toronto ON M6R 1B5; Tor'93; FRCSC; GenSurg. Staff Surg, St Joseph's Health Centre; Lecturer, University of Toronto; (416)530-6180; Fax. (416)530-6181.

LINDSAY, Deborah A; Pediatric Adolescent Clinic, 102-200 Goulet St, Winnipeg MB R2H 0R8; Man'80; FRCPC; Peds (Child Abuse). Staff Children's Hosp, Health Sciences Centre; Assoc Dir Child Protection Centre/Assoc Prof, University of Manitoba; dlindsay@hsc.mb.ca.

LINDSAY, Gary M; HCFHSC CFB Shilo, PO Box 5000, Shilo MB R0K 2A0; Man'75; CCFP; FCFP; Lecturer, University of Manitoba; (204)765-3000 x3153; glindsay@mts.net.

LINDSAY, George E; West Lincoln Mem Hosp, 169 Main St E, Grimsby ON L3M 1P3; Tor'56; FRCPC; DiagRad. Staff, West Lincoln Memorial Hospital; (905)945-2253; Fax. (905)945-5148.

LINDSAY, J E Gordon; Ross Mem Hosp, 10 Angeline St N, Lindsay ON K9V 4M8; Sask'61; Head Dept of Anes, Ross Memorial Hospital; (705)324-6111 x4228

LINDSAY, John S; 836 2nd Ave E, Owen Sound ON N4K 2H3; Tor'72.

LINDSAY, Krystaleah; St Paul's Hosp, 1081 Burrard St, Vancouver BC V6Z 1Y6; Wes'91; AB; Staff, Providence Health Care - St Paul's Hospital; (604)682-2344

LINDSAY, Leigh J; The Richmond Hosp, 7000 Westminster Hwy, Richmond BC V6X 1A2; Sask'88; FRCPC; GenPath. Staff Path, Richmond Hospital; (604)244-5296

LINDSAY, Mary E; BC Cancer Agency-Vanc Isl Ctr, 2410 Lee Ave, Victoria BC V8R 6V5; Qns'78; Staff, BC Cancer Agency Vancouver Island Centre; (250)519-5575

LINDSAY, Peter A; 315-800 Commissioners Rd E, London ON N6C 6B5; Tor'74; FRCPC; Anes.

LINDSAY, Peter K; 101-10104 97 Ave, Grande Prairie AB T8V 7X6; Man'69; CCFP; FCFP; (780)532-0300

LINDSAY, R Alexander; Oshawa Clinic, 117 King St E, Oshawa ON L1H 1B9; Tor'81; Staff, Lakeridge Health - Oshawa Site; (905)721-3545; Fax. (905)721-6644.

LINDSAY, Robert L; 101-7 Glenbrook Pl SW, Calgary AB T3E 6W4; Aberdeen (Scotland)'71; FRCSC; PlasSurg. Ac Staff, Foothills Medical Centre; Ac Staff, Alberta Children's Hospital; Asst Prof Surg, University of Calgary; (403)571-3155; Fax. (403)571-3138.

LINDSAY, Robert M; London HSC-South Street Hosp, PO Box 5375 Stn B 418W-375 South St, London ON N6A 4G5; Glasgow (Scotland)'65; MB ChB; MD; FRCP(Ed); FACP; FRCPC; IntMed (Nephrology). Staff, London Health Sciences Centre - South Street; Prof, University of Western Ontario; (519)685-8349; Fax. (519)685-8395.

LINDSAY, Shanna L; St Joseph's Health Centre, SWE414-30 The Queensway, Toronto ON M6R 1B5; Mem'94; FRCPC; Neur (Pediatric Neurology). Staff, St Joseph's Health Centre; Staff, Toronto East General Hospital Inc; (416)530-6180; Fax. (416)530-6181.

LINDSAY, Shelagh S; Cochrane Primary Care Centre, 103-100 Grande Blvd NW, Cochrane AB T4C 0S4; Cal'76; BSc(Hons); (403)932-2089; Fax. (403)932-1820.

LINDSAY, Thomas F; Univ Hlth Network-Toronto Gen, EW 6 228-200 ELizabeth St, Toronto ON M5G 2C4; McG'83; MSc; FRCSC; GenSurg; VascSurg. Sr Scientist, Toronto General Hospital - UHN; Assoc Prof, University of Toronto; (416)340-4620; Fax. (416)340-5029; thomas.lindsay@uhn.on.ca.

LINDSKOOG, Ross T; 1931 105 St NW, Edmonton AB T6J 5V9; Alb'79; (780)438-3241

LINDZON, Aaron J; Davisville Med & Dental Centre, 204-1849 Yonge St, Toronto ON M4S 1Y2; Qns'96; FRCPC; Peds. (416)488-8876; Fax. (416)488-7777.

LINDZON, Ronald D; Markham Mews Med Clinic, 7-4997 Highway 7, Unionville ON L3R 1N1; Tor'79; DABEM; EmergMed (Family Medicine). (905)475-3995; Fax. (905)475-3581.

LINEHAN, Patrick T; Westview Health Centre, 4405 South Park Dr, Stony Plain AB T7Z 2M7; McG'87; CCFP; CCFP(E.M.); Staff, Covenant Health - Grey Nuns Community Hospital; (780)968-3600

LINEKIN, Michelle J; Laurel Med Centre Ltd, 304-888 8th Ave W, Vancouver BC V5Z 3Y1; UBC'98; BSc; MSc; CCFP; Staff Family Pract Maternity, BC Women's Hospital & Health Centre; Clinical Asst Prof, University of British Columbia; (604)874-0261; Fax. (604)874-3099.

LINES, Alfred J; Brochet Nursing Station, GD, Brochet MB R0B 0B0; London (England)'61; MB BS; MRCS; LRCP; FRCS(Ed); Staff, Brochet Nursing Station; (204)323-2120

LINES, Jolyon B; Dr C W Wiebe Med Centre, 385 Main St, Winkler MB R6W 1J2; Man'06; CCFP; CCFP(E.M.); (204)325-4312

LINES, Matthew A; The Hosp for Sick Children, 555 University Ave, Toronto ON M5G 1X8; Cal'07; MedGenetics.

LINETT, Lauren J; Lakeridge Hlth Corp-Oshawa, 2D-1 Hospital Crt, Oshawa ON L1G 2B9; Ott'05; CCFP; Staff, Lakeridge Health - Oshawa Site; (905)576-8711

LING, Alison K W; Cambridge Mem Hosp, 700 Coronation Blvd, Cambridge ON N1R 3G2; Tor'05; FRCPC; Anes. Staff, Cambridge Memorial Hospital; (519)621-2330

LING, Audrey L H; Carleton Univ Health Services, 2600-1125 Colonel By Dr, Ottawa ON K1S 5B6; Dal'98; CCFP; CCFP(E.M.); (613)520-6674; Fax. (613)520-3851.

LING, Bernice C; Hys Medical Centre, MF-11010 101 St NW, Edmonton AB T5H 4B9; UBC'00; FRCPC; DiagRad; NuclearMed. Staff Diagnostic Radiol, University of Alberta Hospital; (780)426-1121

LING, Brian M Y; Ajax Family Care Centre, 30 Kingston Rd W, Ajax ON L1T 4K8; Tor'91; (905)426-2501; Fax. (905)426-4852.

LING, Chee K; Richmond Health Science Ctr, 315-6051 Gilbert Rd, Richmond BC V7C 3V3; Tor'66; BSc; Ac Staff, Richmond Hospital; Clin Instructor Med, University of British Columbia; (604)273-3218

LING, Constance M; Harmony Med Centre, 110-152 Cleopatra Dr, Nepean ON K2G 5X2; Tor'93; FRCSC; ObstGyn (Advanced Gyn Surg). Asst Prof, The Ottawa Hospital - Civic Campus; University of Ottawa; (613)725-1870 x2; Fax. (613)725-1647.

LING, Elaine B; 33 Church St S, Ajax ON L1S 6A6; Tor'74; Langs: Cantonese; (905)083-0200; Fax. (905)083-0636.

LING, Elisabeth; CHUM-Hop Notre-Dame, 1560 rue Sherbrooke E, Montreal QC H2L 4M1; Laval'96; FRCPC; PhysMed&Rehab. Staff Physiatrie, Centre Hospitalier l'Université de Montréal (CHUM) - Hôpital Notre-Dame; (514)890-8201; Fax. (514)412-7610.

LING, Elizabeth; Hamilton HS-General Site, 237 Barton St E, Hamilton ON L8L 2X2; McM'90; BSc; MSc; FRCPC; Anes. Ac Staff Anes, Hamilton Health Sciences Centre - Hamilton General Hospital; Clin Assoc Prof Anes, McMaster University; (905)527-0271 x46698; Fax. (905)577-8023; linge@mcmaster.ca.

LING, Eng T; Guelph Gen Hosp, 115 Delhi St, Guelph ON N1E 4J4; (Singapore)'66; MB BS; GenPath. Ac Staff, Guelph General Hospital; Consultant, Groves Memorial Community Hospital; Consultant, Homewood Health Centre; (519)837-6403

LING, Francis T K; Jackson Park Health Centre, 210-2475 McDougall St, Windsor ON N8X 3N9; Tor'00; FRCSC; Otol.

LING, Franklin C K; Grand River Hosp-KW Hlth Ctre, PO Box 9056 Stn C 835 King St W, Kitchener ON N2G 1G3; (Hong Kong)'85; MB BS; FRCPC; AnatPath; GenPath. Associate Path, Grand River Hospital - Kitchener/Waterloo Health Centre; (519)749-4300 x2261; Fax. (519)749-4221.

LING, Herbert S C; 303-210 Dundas St E, Belleville ON K8N 5G8; McG'82; FRCSC; OrthSurg (Arthroplasty). Consultant, QHC Belleville General; Court Consultant, QHC Trenton Memorial; Court Consultant, Northumberland Hills Hospital; (613)968-4808; Fax. (613)968-7834.

LING, Hilton; St Paul's Hosp, 488-1081 Burrard St, Vancouver BC V6Z 1Y6; Witwatersrand (South Africa)'68; FRCS(Ed); FRCSC; Cardiovasc&ThorSurg. Ac Staff, Providence Health Care - St Paul's Hospital; Langs: Afrikaans; (604)806-9305

LING, Hubert H F; Scarborough Hosp-General Div, 3050 Lawrence Ave E, Scarborough ON M1P 2V5; Man'87; FRCPC; Anes. Staff, The Scarborough Hospital - General Campus; (416)438-2911

LING, Michael C; 404-4040 Finch Ave E, Scarborough ON M1S 4V5; Wes'00; FRCPC; IntMed (Adult Cardiology); Cardiol. Langs: Cantonese; (416)297-7277; michael_ling@rogers.com.

LING, Patrick M C; St Paul's Hosp, 1702 20th St W, Saskatoon SK S7M 0Z9; Qns'94; CCFP; CCFP(E.M.); FCFP; Staff Emerg, St Paul's Hospital (Grey Nuns) of Saskatoon; (306)655-5113; Fax. (306)655-5963.

LING, Rosalind L L; 308-260 Spadina Ave, Toronto ON M5T 2E4; Melbourne (Australia)'71; MB BS; Court Staff, Toronto Western Hospital - University Health Network; (416)591-8940

LING, Simon C; The Hosp for Sick Children, 555 University Ave, Toronto ON M5G 1X8; Edinburgh (Scotland)'88; MB ChB; MRCP(UK); Staff Peds, The Hospital For Sick Children; (416)813-8757; Fax. (416)813-6531; simon.ling@sickkids.ca.

LING, T Donald; Provincial Addiction Facility, PO Box 2000 Stn Central, Charlottetown PE C1A 7N8; Dal'73; BSc; (902)368-4120; Fax. (902)368-6229.

LINGAS, Rania I; St Joseph's Health Centre, 30 The Queensway, Toronto ON M6R 1B5; Tor'04; FRCPC; IntMed; MedOncol. Staff, St Joseph's Health Centre; Langs: Greek; (416)530-6235; Fax. (416)530-6656.

LINGERTAT, John R; Haliburton High Hlth Serv-Mide, PO Box 30 6 McPherson St, Minden ON K0M 2K0; Tor'93; BScPharm; CCFP; Staff, Haliburton Highlands Health Services - Miden Site; (705)286-2288; john@hhfht.com.

LINGLEY, Michael D; Round Trip Travel Hlth Clinic, 2-96 Cornell Park Ave, Markham ON L6B 1B6; Ott'90; FRCPC; IntMed; InfectDis (Travel Medicine). Dir Infection Control Program, Southlake Regional Health Centre; (905)910-1194; Fax. (905)910-1195.

LINGURAR, Maxine A; The Group Health Centre, 240 McNabb St, Sault Ste. Marie ON P6B 1Y5; Qns'89; FRCSC; ObstGyn. (705)759-5605

LINGYS, Aukse T; Urgent Care Clinic, 1550 Dundas St E, Mississauga ON L4X 1L4; Tor'67; Ac Staff, Trillium Health Centre - Mississauga; Court Staff, William Osler Health System - Etobicoke General Hospital; Langs: Lithuanian; German; (416)621-2220

LINK, Catherine A; Cardiology Services Group, 303-274 Dundas St E, Belleville ON K8N 1E6; Wes'93; FRCPC; IntMed. (613)966-4377; Fax. (613)966-4730.

LINK, Margot; Kootenay Lake Med Clinic, 1140 Lakeside Dr, Nelson BC V1L 5Z3; Alb'79; (250)352-4666

LINKENHEIL, Edith; Markham Stouffville Health Ctr, 208-377 Church St, Markham ON L6B 1A1; Tor'80; FRCSC; ObstGyn. Ac Staff, Markham Stouffville Hospital; (905)294-8505; Fax. (905)294-8523.

LINKLATER, David M; First Edmonton Place, 350-10665 Jasper Ave NW, Edmonton AB T5J 3S9; Alb'83; CCFP; FCFP; Pres, Physician Management Inc; (780)421-7711; Fax. (780)421-9744.

LINKS, Paul S; London HSC-Victoria Hosp, B8 132-800 Commissioners Rd E, London ON N6A 4G5; Alb'73; FRCPC; Psy. Staff, London Health Sciences Centre - Victoria Campus; Dept Chair Psychiatry, University of Western Ontario; (519)685-8500 x76667

LINN III, George F; 200-11 Princess St, Kingston ON K7L 1A1; Qns'87; FRCPC; Psy (Consultant Liaison Psychiatry). Consultant Psy, Pembroke Regional Hospital Inc; Consultant Psy, St Francis Memorial Hospital; Staff Psy, Kingston Regional Cancer Centre; Teacher Oncol, Queen's University; (613)548-4848; Fax. (613)548-0856.

LINNEY, Louise M; 200-110 Bearbrook Rd, Gloucester ON K1B 5R2; McM'86; CCFP; CCFP(E.M.); FCFP; (613)824-6318; Fax. (613)824-0521.

LINT, Donald W; Brandon Reg Health Centre, 150 McTavish Ave E, Brandon MB R7A 2B3; Man'93; BSc; MSc; FRCPC; Psy. Staff, Brandon Regional Health Centre; (204)726-2901; Fax. (204)725-0911.

LINTERN, David; St Anthony's Med Centre, 203-582 Goldstream Ave, Victoria BC V9B 2W7; RCS (Ireland)'68; Staff, Victoria General Hospital; Staff, Royal Jubilee Hospital; (250)478-1423; Fax. (250)478-7912.

LINTON, Carol A V; Liberton Med Clinic, 112-31 Liberton Dr, St. Albert AB T8N 3X6; Alb'86; FRCSC; ObstGyn (High Risk Obstetrics). Staff, Sturgeon Community Hospital; (780)459-0500; Fax. (780)460-8828.

LINTON, Gregory J; Park Avenue Med Centre, 4F-4634 Park Ave, Terrace BC V8G 1V7; Cal'92; CCFP; (250)615-5090; Fax. (250)615-5049.

LINTOTT, Dale N; Medicine Hat College, 299 College Dr SE, Medicine Hat AB T1A 3Y6; Alb'73; Ac Staff, Medicine Hat Regional Hospital; Teach Staff, Medicine Hat College; (403)502-8437

LINZON, Charlene D; Forest Hill Dermatology, G 5-250 St Clair Ave W, Toronto ON M4V 1R6; Tor'81; FRCPC; Derm (Cosmetic Dermatology). Staff Teacher Diseases of Hair Clinic, Women's College Hospital; (416)840-3339; Fax. (416)840-0019.

LINZON, Ernest K; Malvern Med Arts Bldg, 100-1333 Neilson Rd, Scarborough ON M1B 4Y9; Tor'77; CCFP; FCFP; Assoc Staff, Rouge Valley Health System - Centenary Health Centre Site; Court Staff, The Scarborough Hospital - General Campus; Court Staff, North York General Hospital; (416)291-7719; Fax. (416)287-3775.

LIOLLI, Americo; Windsor Reg Hosp-Metropolitan, 1995 Lens Ave, Windsor ON N8W 1L9; Tor'94; BSc; FRCPC; Anes. Ac Staff Anes, Windsor Regional Hospital - Metropolitan Site; (519)254-1661 x52201

LIONEL, Jesuraj; Regina Qu'Appelle HR-Regina, NICU-1440 14th Ave, Regina SK S4P 0W5; Staff, Regina General Hospital; (306)766-6161; Fax. (306)766-4557.

LIPA, Joan; Univ Hlth Network-Toronto Gen, M1 514-200 Elizabeth St, Toronto ON M5G 2C4; Wes'92; MSc; FRCSC; PlasSurg (Breast Reconstruction). Staff, Toronto General Hospital - UHN; Staff Breast Surgical Team, Sunnybrook Health Sciences Centre - Edmond Odette Cancer Centre; (416)340-3111

LIPAN, Carla B; Brockville Gen Hosp, 75 Charles St, Brockville ON K6V 1S8; Bucharest (Romania)'97; FRCPC; Anes. Staff, Brockville General Hospital - Charles Street; (613)345-5645

LIPCSEI, Julie A; Toronto Ctr-Cognitive Therapy, 850-36 Toronto St, Toronto ON M5C 2C5; Tor'89; CCFP; FCFP; (416)777-6699

LIPES, Jed; SMBD Jewish Gen Hosp, 3755 ch Cote-Sainte-Catherine, Montreal QC H3T 1E2; McG'05; FRCPC; IntMed; Critical Care Medicine. Staff, Sir Mortimer B Davis Jewish General; (514)340-8222 x4974

LIPES, Peter M; 305-5858 Ch de la Cote-des-Nei, Montreal QC H3S 1Z1; McG'69; Clin Associate, McGill University; (514)735-1604; Fax. (514)735-1605.

LIPINSKI, Grazyna B; Parkview Prof Centre, 207-2110 Main St, Winnipeg MB R2V 2C2; Cracow (Poland)'76; (204)982-4650; Fax. (204)982-4651.

LIPINSKI, J Kenneth; 519-4916 130 Ave SE, Calgary AB T2Z 0G4; Alb'74; FRCPC; DiagRad. (403)726-9729; Fax. (403)726-8883.

LIPKOWITZ, Lana G; 202-179 Davie St, Vancouver BC V6Z 2Y1; Man'84; Assoc Staff, Providence Health Care - St Paul's Hospital; (604)669-7772

LIPMAN, Ellen L; McMaster University, 213-1280 Main St W, Hamilton ON L8S 4K1; McM'85; MSc; FRCPC; Psy (Child Psychiatry). Ac Staff, Hamilton Health Sciences Centre - McMaster University Medical Centre; Court Staff, St Joseph's Healthcare - Charlton Campus; Prof, McMaster University; (905)521-2100 x77359; Fax. (905)574-6665; lipmane@mcmaster.ca.

LIPMAN, Mark L; SMBD Jewish Gen Hosp, 3755 Ch Cote-Sainte-Catherine, Montreal QC H3T 1E2; McG'86; FRCPC; IntMed; Nephrol. Staff, Sir Mortimer B Davis Jewish General; Staff, McGill University Health Centre - Royal Victoria Hospital; adj Prof, McGill University; (514)340-8229; Fax. (514)340-8147.

LIPNOWSKI, Martin; SMBD Jewish Gen Hosp, 3755 ch Cote-Sainte-Catherine, Montreal QC H3T 1E2; McG'77; FRCPC; IntMed (Endocrinology). Clin Asst Endocrin & Health Service, Sir Mortimer B Davis Jewish General; (514)340-8222 x5115; Fax. (514)340-7512.

LIPNOWSKI, Stan; Manitoba Clinic, 790 Sherbrook St, Winnipeg MB R3A 1M3; McM'87; FAAP; FRCPC; Peds. Staff, Health Sciences Centre; Staff, St Boniface General Hospital; Physician, Ste Amant Centre; Asst Prof, University of Manitoba; Langs: English; French; (204)788-5521; slipnow@mts.net.

LIPOWSKA, Magdalena M; Lions Gate Hosp, 231 15th St E, North Vancouver BC V7L 2L7; Wes'05; FRCPC; Anes. Staff, Lions Gate Hospital; Langs: Polish; (604)984-5785

LIPP, Michele M; 103-1221 Lonsdale Ave, North Vancouver BC V7M 2H5; Cal'96; FRCSC; ObstGyn. (604)980-2800

LIPP, Olivier R; Hop Louis-H Lafontaine, 7401 rue Hochelaga, Montreal QC H1N 3M5; Sher'85; MPH; Psy (Medical Genetics). Staff Psy, Hopital Louis-H Lafontaine; Physician, Centre de Recherche Fernand-Seguin; adj Prof, Universite de Montreal; (514)251-4000; olipp@total.net.

LIPPA, Jodie L; Gaetz Family Practice, 104-45744 Gaetz St, Chilliwack BC V2R 3P1; UBC'92; CCFP; FCFP; (604)824-1588; Fax. (604)824-8743.

LIPPE, Julie; 230-1055 12e Av N, Sherbrooke QC J1E 2X4; Sher'75; FRCPC; Peds. (819)563-6232; Fax. (819)563-0159.

LIPPOLT, Gordon B; Associated Med Clinic, PO Box 510, Lac La Biche AB T0A 2C0; Alb'72; (780)623-4421; Fax. (780)623-1920.

LIPSCHITZ, Jeremy; Health Sciences Centre, GF442-820 Sherbrook St, Winnipeg MB R3A 1R9; Witwatersrand (South Africa)'79; MB ChB; FRCSC; GenSurg (Endoscopy). Chief Gastrointestinal Surgical Serv, Health Sciences Centre; Head Section of General Surg/Assoc Prof, University of Manitoba; (204)787-3125; Fax. (204)787-4063; jlipschitz@hsc.mb.ca.

LIPSCOMBE, Jennifer B; 132-101 Queensway W, Mississauga ON L5B 2P7; McG'96; BSc; FRCPC; IntMed; Nephrol. Staff, The Credit Valley Hospital; Staff, Trillium Health Centre - Mississauga; Langs: English; French; (905)272-1104; Fax. (905)272-1105.

LIPSCOMBE, Lorraine L; 741-790 Bay St, Toronto ON M5G 1N8; McG'98; FRCPC; IntMed; Endocrin&Metab. Langs: French; (416)323-6400

LIPSETT, William G C; Twin City Med Clinic, 1102 103rd St, North Battleford SK S9A 1K6; Belfast (Ireland)'67; MB ChB; BAO; MRC; DRCOG; (306)445-1066; Fax. (306)445-1266.

LIPSEY, Philip; Parksville Med Clinic, PO Box 250 Stn Main 154 Memorial Ave, Parksville BC V9P 2G4; McM'77; BSc; MSc; CCFP; FCFP; Staff, Nanaimo Regional General Hospital; Staff, Trillium Lodge Extended Care Hospital; (250)248-5757; Fax. (250)248-2128.

LIPSIT, Sharon E; 407-672 Brant St, Burlington ON L7R 2H3; Tor'81; BSc; FRCPC; IntMed (Clinical Immunology & Allergy). Ac Staff, Joseph Brant Memorial Hospital; (905)632-9288; Fax. (905)632-8810.

LIPSITZ, Jeffrey J; Sleep Disorders Centre, 2888 Bathurst St, Toronto ON M6B 4H6; Tor'83; PhC; Physician, Specialty Med Clinics Inc; Med Dir, Sleep Disorders Centre of Metropolitan Toronto; (416)785-1128 x301; Fax. (416)782-2740; sleepservices@gmail.com.

LIPSON, Adrienne; Royal Columbian Hosp, 330 Columbia St E, New Westminster BC V3L 3W7; Qns'00; FRCPC; Anes. Staff, Royal Columbian Hospital; (604)520-4602

LIPSON, Alisa B; Oakridge Centre South Tower, 207-650 41st Ave W, Vancouver BC V5Z 2M9; UBC'80; FRCPC; Peds. Langs: Hebrew; (604)266-1874; Fax. (604)266-1583; oakpeds@gmail.com.

LIPSON, David; Providence Healthcare, 3276 St Clair Ave E, Scarborough ON M1L 1W1; Wes'05; Staff, Providence Healthcare; (416)285-3666

LIPSON, Frank; 306-2021 Cliff Rd, Mississauga ON L5A 3N7; Tor'64; FRCPC; IntMed; PhysMed&Rehab. Staff, Trillium Health Centre - Mississauga; (905)897-7777; Fax. (905)897-5913.

LIPSON, Jennifer E; Parkdale Med Tower, 308-1081 Carling Ave, Ottawa ON K1Y 4G2; Ott'06; FRCPC; Derm. (613)722-8532

LIPSON, Martin H; 203-1223 St Clair Ave W, Toronto ON M6E 1B5; Tor'62; Staff, Mount Sinai Hospital; (416)652-3133; Fax. (416)652-7828.

LIPSZYC, Eli; 254 Franklin Ave, Thornhill ON L4J 7L6; Santiago (Chile)'79; (905)731-8247

LIPTAY, Christine M; Branksome Hall Centre, 10 Elm Ave, Toronto ON M4W 1N4; McM'92; MSc; CCFP; FCFP; (416)920-6265 x229; Fax. (416)927-0960.

LIPTON, Jeffrey H; Univ Hlth Network-Princess M, 610 University Ave, Toronto ON M5G 2M9; Cal'84; BSc; PhD(Biochem); ABIM; FRCPC; IntMed (Leukemia); MedOncol (P.Q.). Staff Allogeneic BMT Service & Leukemia Services, Princess Margaret Hospital - University Health Network; Prof Med, University of Toronto; Langs: Hebrew; (416)946-2266

LIPTON, Myles; 554 Spadina Cres, Toronto ON M5S 2J9; Tor'80.

LIQUORNIK, Karen N; Southlake Reg Health Centre, 596 Davis Dr, Newmarket ON L3Y 2P9; McG'91; FRCPC; Peds. Staff, Southlake Regional Health Centre; (905)895-4521

LIQUORNIK, Morrie S; Bayview Business Centre, 216-16700 Bayview Ave, Newmarket ON L3X 1W1; McG'89; BSc; FRCSC; Urol (Oncology). Staff Urol, Southlake Regional Health Centre; (905)836-4696; Fax. (905)836-9038.

LIRENMAN, Michael A; Langley Mem Hosp, 22051 Fraser Hwy, Langley BC V3A 4H4; UBC'90; CCFP; CCFP(E.M.); Staff, Langley Memorial Hospital; (604)534-4121

LIRETTE, Andree; Dr L Richard Ctre D'Oncologie, 37 Providence St, Moncton NB E1C 8X3; Laval'92; FRCPC; RadOncol. Staff, Dr Georges-L-Dumont University Hospital Centre; Langs: Bilingual(French/English); (506)862-3768; Fax. (506)862-4222.

LIRETTE, Richard; Place de la Cite, 295-2600 boul Laurier, Quebec QC G1V 4T3; Laval'80; FRCSC; OrthSurg. Staff, Centre Hospitalier Paul-Gilbert; (418)658-7888; Fax. (418)659-7070.

LISANU, Mesfin G; Polyclinique Coeur de l'Ile, 529 rue Jarry E, Montreal QC H2P 1V4; Rome (Italy)'80; Staff Emerg Med, McGill University Health Centre - Montreal General Campus; (514)277-4111

LISBONA, Andre; SMBD Jewish Gen Hosp, 3755 ch Cote-Sainte-Catherine, Montreal QC H3T 1E2; Mon'64; FRCPC; DiagRad (Breasts). Chief Dept of Radiol, Sir Mortimer B Davis Jewish General; assoc Prof, McGill University; (514)340-8222; Fax. (514)738-1165.

LISBONA, Robert; MUHC-Royal Victoria Hosp, 687 av des Pins O, Montreal QC H3A 1A1; McG'70; FRCPC; DiagRad; NuclearMed. Diagnostic-Radiology, McGill University Health Centre - Royal Victoria Hospital; Chef Diagnostic Rad, McGill University; (514)934-1934 x34102

LISERANI, P Donna M; 230-151 Walden Gate SE, Calgary AB T2X 0R2; Mem'90; (403)264-6372; Fax. (403)264-6399.

LISI, Michael P; Collingwood Health Centre, 203-186 Erie St, Collingwood ON L9Y 4T3; McM'03; FACS; FRCSC; GenSurg. Staff General Surgeon, Collingwood General & Marine Hospital; Staff, Collingwood Health Centre; Clinical Asst Prof Dept of Surgery, McMaster University; Clinical Asst Prof, University of Toronto; (705)444-0089; dr_michael_lisi@hotmail.com.

LISIAK, Elena; Midtown Mental Health Team, 3F-2450 Ontario St, Vancouver BC V5T 4T7; '75; FRCPsy; FRCPC; Psy. Ac Staff, Vancouver General Hospital - Centennial Pavillion; Asst Prof, University of British Columbia; Langs: Polish; Slovak; (604)822-8441

LISING, Jean B C; 155 Bright St, Sarnia ON N7T 4E8; RCS (Ireland)'74; LRCP; Ac Staff, Bluewater Health - Mitton Site; Ac Staff, Bluewater Health - Norman Site; (519)336-7102

LISINSKI, Julian T; Hillside Med Centre, PO Box 700 Stn Main 541 3 Ave, Ladysmith BC V9G 1A5; London (England)'76; MB BS; DA; CCFP; FCFP; Ac Staff Member, Ladysmith Community Health Centre; (250)245-2235; Fax. (250)245-3094.

LISKE, Sabine I; Oakville Med Centre, 204-331 Sheddon Ave, Oakville ON L6J 1X8; Tor'91; BSc; MSc; FRCSC; ObstGyn. Staff, Halton Healthcare Services Corporation - Oakville Site; (905)337-1995; Fax. (905)337-1994.

LISKOWICH, Sarah; Academic Family Medicine, 172-1621 Albert St, Regina SK S4P 2S5; Sask'10; BSc; CCFP; (306)766-0444; Fax. (306)766-0471; spl106@mail.usask.ca.

LISNEVSKAIA, Larissa A; Oshawa Clinic, 117 King St E, Oshawa ON L1H 1B9; Kuban (Russia (Federation))'90; FRCPC; IntMed. Staff, Kingston General Hospital; (905)721-4986; Fax. (905)721-6602.

LISOWSKI, David F J; 205-274 Dundas St E, Belleville ON K8N 1E6; Ott'72; BSc(Hon); Att Staff, QHC Belleville General; (613)962-5844; Fax. (613)962-7406.

LISS, Gary M; 401-960 Lawrence Ave W, North York ON M6A 3B5; Tor'76; AB; FRCPC; CommunMed; OccupMed. Court Staff, Sunnybrook Health Sciences Centre; Staff Family Pract, Humber River Regional Hospital - Keele Street Site; Med Consultant, Ministry of Labour; Asst Prof Preventive Med, University of Toronto; (416)256-1150; Fax. (416)256-0742.

LIST, Stephen J; Hamilton Schizophrenia Program, 102-350 King St E, Hamilton ON L8N 3Y3; McM'85; MSc; PhD; FRCPC; Psy (Schizophrenia). Staff, St Joseph's Healthcare Hamilton - West 5th Campus; Medical Officer, Health Protection Branch, Health Canada; Asst Prof Psy, McMaster University; (905)525-2832; Fax. (905)546-0055.

LISTA, Francesco R; The Plastic Surgery Clinic, 1421 Hurontario St, Mississauga ON L5G 3H5; Tor'81; FRCSC; PlasSurg. Staff, Trillium Health Centre - Mississauga; (905)278-7077; drlista@theplasticsurgeryclinic.com.

LISTER, David R A; 7871 Westminster Hwy PO Box 97126 Stn Main, Richmond BC V6X 8H3; UBC'86; FRCPC; Anes. Staff, Richmond Hospital; (604)278-9711 x4200

LISTER, Norman A; 89 Prince William St, St Stephen NB E3L 1S8; Dal'78; CCFP; FCFP; Staff Chief Family Med, Charlotte County Hospital; (506)466-2457; Fax. (506)466-6094.

LISTER, William S; Peace Arch Hosp, 15521 Russell Ave, White Rock BC V4B 2R4; Tor'95; FRCPC; DiagRad. Staff Med Imaging, Peace Arch Hospital; (604)531-5512; Fax. (604)535-4559.

LISTGARTEN, Charles; The Doctor's Office, 13-205 Marycroft Ave, Woodbridge ON L4L 5X8; Tor'64; FRCPC; IntMed (Clinical Immunology & Allergy). Court Staff, Humber River Regional Hospital - Church Street Site; Langs: Yiddish; Italian; German; French; (905)856-2100

LISTOE, Gregory B; 532 Lake St, St. Catharines ON L2N 4H4; Wes'89; CCFP; (905)646-0015

LISTON, Fiona A; 190 Ingram St, Duncan BC V9L 1P1; Dal'07; ObstGyn. (250)748-2422

LISTON, James P; Millbrook Med Centre, RR 2 1 Lisa Court, Millbrook ON L0A 1G0; Tor'77; CCFP; FCFP; (705)932-2772; Fax. (705)932-4089.

LISTON, Robert M; BC Women's Hosp & Health Ctre, 2H30-4500 Oak St, Vancouver BC V6H 3N1; Dundee (Scotland)'71; MB ChB; MRC; FACOG; FRCOG; FRCSC; ObstGyn (Maternal Fetal Medicine). Chief Obst, BC Women's Hospital & Health Centre; Assoc Prof/Dept Head ObstGyn/Exec Associate Deans Clinical Affairs, University of British Columbia; (604)875-3265; Fax. (604)875-2987; rliston@cw.bc.ca.

LISZAUER, Allan D; 88 Wentworth St S, Hamilton ON L8N 2Y9; McG'85; FRCSC; Ophth. Ac Staff, St Joseph's Healthcare - Charlton Campus; Court Staff, Hamilton Health Sciences Centre - McMaster University Medical Centre; (905)522-3563; Fax. (905)522-3564.

LISZKOWSKI, Mark; Institut de Cardiologie de Mtl, 5000 rue Belanger, Montreal QC H1T 1C8; McG'01; FRCPC; IntMed; Critical Care Medicine; Cardiol. Staff, Institut de Cardiologie de Montréal; (514)376-3330

LISZTWAN, Magdalena; Chinook Reg Hosp, 960 19 St S, Lethbridge AB T1J 1W5; Alb'03; CCFP; CCFP(E.M.); Staff, Chinook Regional Hospital; (403)388-6301; Fax. (403)388-6183.

LITALIEN, Albert; CSSS de Kamouraska, RR 1 575 av Martin, Saint-Pascal QC G0L 3Y0; Laval'66; FRCPC; Anes. Staff, CSSS de Kamouraska; (418)856-7000

LITALIEN, Catherine; Hôpital Ste-Justine, 3175 ch Cote-Sainte-Catherine, Montreal QC H3T 1C5; McG'93; FRCPC; Peds (Intensive Care); Critical Care Medicine. Staff, Hôpital Ste-Justine; (514)345-4788; Fax. (514)345-7731.

LITCH, Stanley W; Homewood Health Centre, 150 Delhi St, Guelph ON N1E 6K9; Tor'64; Psy. Staff, Homewood Health Centre; (519)824-1010 x2282

LITCHFIELD, Robert B; Fowler Kennedy Sport Clinic-UW, 3M Centre-1151 Richmond St, London ON N6A 3K7; Wes'86; FRCSC; OrthSurg (Arthroscopic Knee & Shoulder Surgery). Staff, London Health Sciences Centre - University Hospital; Assoc Prof Med, University of Western Ontario; (519)661-4156; Fax. (519)850-2497.

LITMAN, Melvin; Islington Med Clinic, 800-1243 Islington Ave, Etobicoke ON M8X 1Y9; Tor'80; (416)767-2525

LITNER, Geoffrey M; 200-236 Avenue Rd, Toronto ON M5R 2J4; Tor'98; CCFP; (416)922-2000; Fax. (416)922-2005.

LITNER, Michelle S; Medical Office, 8000 Bathurst St, Thornhill ON L4J 0B8; Ott'01; CCFP; (905)709-9709; Fax. (905)709-9701.

LITSAS, Steven; Woodbridge Med Centre, A13-9600 Islington Ave, Woodbridge ON L4H 2T1; Tor'97; CCFP; Langs: Macedonian; (905)893-8085; Fax. (905)893-8218.

LITTELJOHN, Cynthia; 471 Burlington Ave, Burlington ON L7S 1R6; McG'71; Langs: Chinese; (905)632-9700; Fax. (905)637-2516.

LITTLE, Albert W; Richmond Med Centre, 307 Bridge St W, Napanee ON K7R 2G3; Wes'72; Ac Staff, Lennox & Addington County General Hospital; (613)354-7486; Fax. (613)354-6992.

LITTLE, Cameron D; College of Phys & Surg of NS, 5005-7071 Bayers Rd, Halifax NS B3L 2C2; Alb'71; FACP; FRCPC; IntMed; MedOncol. Registrar, College of Physicians & Surgeons of Nova Scotia; (902)422-5823; Fax. (902)422-5035; clittle@cpsns.ns.ca.

LITTLE, D'Arcy L; Orillia Soldier's Mem Hosp, 170 Colborne St W, Orillia ON L3V 2Z3; Tor'95; FRCP; FRCPC; DiagRad;CCFP; Staff, Orillia Soldiers' Memorial Hospital; (705)327-9127; Fax. (705)330-3224; darcy.little@sympatico.ca.

LITTLE, Janet G; Commercial Street Med Centre, 205-311 Commercial St, Milton ON L9T 3Z9; Wes'91; CCFP; (905)878-2700; Fax. (905)878-4050.

LITTLE, John M; MUHC-Montreal Children's Hosp, D175-2300 rue Tupper, Montreal QC H3H 1P3; McG'61; DABOph; FACS; FAAO; FRCSC; Ophth (Pediatric Ophthalmology). Sr Staff Ophth & Ped Ophth, McGill University Health Centre - Montreal General Campus; Consultant, McGill University Health Centre - Royal Victoria Hospital; assoc Prof, McGill University; Langs: French; (514)412-4486; Fax. (514)412-4443.

LITTLE, Kyrie; Old Quebec Street Mall, 208-55 Wyndham St N, Guelph ON N1H 7T8; McM'90; CCFP; FCFP; Staff, Guelph General Hospital; (519)837-2283; Fax. (519)767-2262.

LITTLE, Michelle J; Ridge Meadows Hosp & Hlth CC, 11666 Laity St, Maple Ridge BC V2X 5A3; Queensland (Australia)'00; MB; BSc; Staff, Ridge Meadows Hospital & Health Care Centre; (604)463-4111

LITTLE, Richard H; Victoria Emergency Phys Assoc, 325-1627 Fort St, Victoria BC V8R 1H8; UBC'94; CCFP; CCFP(E.M.); FCFP; Staff Emerg Med, Victoria General Hospital; (250)479-6442

LITTLE, Sian C C; Hincks-Dellcrest Centre, 402-114 Maitland St, Toronto ON M4Y 1E1; McM'80; MPH(Harvard); FRCPC; Psy (Child Psychiatry). (416)631-2686; Fax. (416)924-9915.

LITTLEFORD, Judith A; Health Sciences Ctr Gen Hosp, 2F-671 William Ave, Winnipeg MB R3E 0Z2; Cal'87; FRCPC; Anes (Palliative Medicine).

LITTLEJOHN, Peter W; 469 Smith St, New Waterford NS B1H 3R5; Liverpool (England)'72; (902)862-3882; Fax. (902)862-2137.

LITTMAN, Charles D; Health Sciences Centre, MS4-820 Sherbrook St, Winnipeg MB R3A 1R9; Glasgow (Scotland)'73; MB ChB; FRCPC; AnatPath (Forensic Pathology). Staff Section Hd, Health Sciences Centre; Med Examiner, Province of Manitoba; Assoc Prof, University of Manitoba; (204)783-4715; Fax. (204)787-4942; clittman@hsc.mb.ca.

LITVAK, Eric; Dir de la Sante Publique-Mtl, 1301 rue Sherbooke E, Montreal QC H2L 1M3; Laval'00; FRCPC; CommunMed. (514)528-2400

LITWIN, Craig M E S; Royal Columbian Hosp, B130-330 Columbia St E, New Westminster BC V3L 3W7; Tor'96; FRCPC; GenPath (Forensic Pathology). Staff, Royal Columbian Hospital; (604)520-4818; Fax. (604)520-4409.

LITWIN, Crystal D; Wynward Commun Health Centre, PO Box 1539, Wynyard SK S0A 4T0; Sask'93; CCFP; Med Staff, Wynyard Hospital; (306)554-3363; Fax. (306)554-2994; crystal.litwin@saskatoonhealthregion.ca.

LITWIN, Shlomo; Dr S Litwin Med Clinic, 406-1081 Carling Ave, Ottawa ON K1Y 4G2; Wes'78; CCFP; FCFP; (613)725-2993; Fax. (613)725-1138.

LITWINSON, Laurie; Misericordia Community Hosp, 16940 87 Ave NW, Edmonton AB T5R 4H5; Alb'96; FRCPC; Psy. Staff, Covenant Health - Misericordia Community Hospital; (780)735-2594; Fax. (780)735-2595.

LITZ, D Sharon; IWK Health Centre, PO Box 9700 Rpo CSC, Halifax NS B3K 6R8; Dal'81; FRCPC; Anes (Intensive Care). Chief Ped Anes/Staff Intensivist Anes & ICU, IWK Health Centre; Asst Prof, Dalhousie University; (902)470-8251

LITZ, Henry A R; 120 Main St, Plaster Rock NB E7G 2E5; Dal'74; (506)356-6648

LIU, Allen T L; Grey Nuns Community Hosp, 1100 Youville Drive West NW, Edmonton AB T6L 5X8; Alb'88; FRCPC; IntMed; Critical Care Medicine; Respir. Staff, Covenant Health - Grey Nuns Community Hospital; Asst Prof, University of Alberta; Langs: Chinese; (780)735-7000; Fax. (780)735-7668.

LIU, Barbara A; Sunnybrook Hlth Sciences Ctre, HG69-2075 Bayview Ave, Toronto ON M4N 3M5; Tor'87; FRCPC; IntMed (Clinical Pharmacology); GeriatricMed. Consultant Med Staff, Baycrest Centre for Geriatric Care; Staff, Sunnybrook Health Sciences Centre; Assoc Prof Med, University of Toronto; (416)480-4076; Fax. (416)480-4778.

LIU, Bin; Nepean Clinical Associates, 1437 Woodroffe Ave, Nepean ON K2G 1W1; Nanjing (China)'82; MB; FRCPC; IntMed; Rheum. Langs: Chinese; (613)225-5532; Fax. (613)225-0540; bin_liu12345@yahoo.com.

LIU, Chin Kee; Evergold Centre, J-3833 Midland Ave, Scarborough ON M1V 5L6; Tor'79; (416)299-0820

LIU, Chongen; 20-1615 Dundas St E, Whitby ON L1N 2L1; (China)'99; CCFP; (905)436-2273; Fax. (905)436-2263.

LIU, Dong Feng; Woodstock Gen Hosp, 310 Juliana Dr, Woodstock ON N4V 0A4; Henan (China)'83; Chief Lab Med, Woodstock General Hospital.

LIU, Dora M; Endocrine and Diabetes Centre, 4F-1967 Riverside Dr, Ottawa ON K1H 7W9; Ott'00; FRCPC; IntMed; Endocrin&Metab. (613)738-8333

LIU, Edmond K H; 111-233 16 Ave NW, Calgary AB T2M 0H5; (Ireland)'92; MB ChB; DCH; DObst; Staff, Calgary Health Region; Clin Lecturer Family Med, University of Calgary; (403)230-8883; Fax. (403)230-2800; edmondliu@telusplanet.net.

LIU, Eugene S; 53 Prospect St, Newmarket ON L3Y 3T1; Tor'96; FRCSC; Ophth. Staff, Southlake Regional Health Centre; Staff, Mount Sinai Hospital; Clin Instructor, University of Toronto; (905)895-8738; Fax. (905)895-8227.

LIU, Fay F V; Medical Dental Centre, 10057 Yonge St, Richmond Hill ON L4C 1T7; Man'81; Staff Community Privil, Mackenzie Richmond Hill Hospital; Court Staff Privil, The Scarborough Hospital - Birchmount Campus; (905)737-9099; Fax. (905)737-9022.

LIU, Fei-Fei; Univ Hlth Network-Princess M, 610 University Ave, Toronto ON M5G 2M9; Tor'80; FRCPC; IntMed; RadOncol. Head/Sr Scientist Div AMP/OCI, Princess Margaret Hospital - University Health Network; Dept Chair Radiation Oncology, University of Toronto; (416)946-2123; fei-fei.liu@rmp.uhn.on.ca.

LIU, Geoffrey; Univ Hlth Network-Princess M, 7 124-610 University Ave, Toronto ON M5G 2M9; Tor'93; FRCPC; IntMed. Scientist, Princess Margaret Hospital - University Health Network; geoffliu@uhnres.utoronto.ca.

LIU, Grace; Sunnybrook Hlth Sciences Ctre, 6F B627-2075 Bayview Ave, Toronto ON M4N 3M5; Tor'95; FRCSC; ObstGyn. Staff, Sunnybrook Health Sciences Centre; (416)480-6100; Fax. (416)480-4317.

LIU, H K Kenneth; 302-280 Spadina Ave, Toronto ON M5T 3A5; Tor'78; (416)977-9888

LIU, Hongwei; Tom Baker Cancer Centre, CC110-1331 29 St NW, Calgary AB T2N 4N2; (China)'87; RadOncol. Staff, Tom Baker Cancer Centre; (403)521-3997

LIU, Hwayue; York Med Centre, 2-10660 Yonge St, Richmond Hill ON L4C 3C9; Magadh (India)'85; DAB; CCFP; Langs: Chinese; Hindi; (905)770-9096; Fax. (905)770-4703.

LIU, Jenny Y; 250-2184 Broadway W, Vancouver BC V6K 2E1; UBC'01; CCFP; Langs: Cantonese; (604)733-5181

LIU, Jimin; Halton HCS Corp-Oakville, 327 Reynolds St, Oakville ON L6J 3L7; Zhejiang (China)'83; FRCPC; AnatPath. Staff Path, Halton Healthcare Services Corporation - Oakville Site; Staff, Halton Healthcare Services Corporation - Georgetown Hospital; Staff, Halton Healthcare Services Corporation - Milton District Hospital; (905)338-4675 x3140

LIU, Joanne; Hôpital Ste-Justine, 3175 ch Cote-Sainte-Catherine, Montreal QC H3T 1C5; McG'91; FRCPC; Peds. Staff, Hôpital Ste-Justine; (514)345-4931

LIU, Julia J; Zeidler Ledcor Centre, 1 10-130 University Campus NW, Edmonton AB T6G 2X8; Tor'95; FRCPC; IntMed; Gastroent. Staff, University of Alberta Hospital; (780)492-7062; Fax. (780)492-7115.

LIU, Junliang; Cancercare Manitoba, 675 McDermot Ave, Winnipeg MB R3E 0V9; (China)'84; FRCPC; RadOncol.

LIU, Kimberly E; Ctr for Fertility & Reproducti, 700-250 Dundas St W, Toronto ON M5T 2Z5; Wes'01; FRCSC; ObstGyn.

LIU, L Felix; York-Med Medical Arts Centre, 302-250 Harding Blvd W, Richmond Hill ON L4C 9M7; Tor'78; FRCPC; IntMed; Respir. Ac Staff, Mackenzie Richmond Hill Hospital; (905)883-5580; Fax. (905)883-7824.

LIU, Li; Baywood Med Centre, 207-95 Bayly St W, Ajax ON L1S 7K8; Man'04; CCFP; Staff, North York General Hospital; (289)660-2888

LIU, Louis W C; Univ Hlth Network-Toronto Western Hosp, 8 M P 329-399 Bathurst St, Toronto ON M5T 2S8; McM'98; PhD; FRCPC; IntMed; Gastroent. Staff, Toronto Western Hospital - University Health Network; Langs: Chinese; (416)603-5276

LIU, Mitchell C C; BC Cancer Agency, 600 10th Ave W, Vancouver BC V5Z 4E6; McG'91; FRCPC; RadOncol. Staff, BC Cancer Agency Vancouver Centre; Langs: Cantonese; (604)877-6000 x2668

LIU, Pamela Y; Lakefront Clinics, 14-550 Queen's Quay W, Toronto ON M5V 3M8; UBC'07; CCFP; (647)347-0576

LIU, Peter C F; KMH-MRI & Health Care, 101-50 Minthorn Blvd, Thornhill ON L3T 7X8; Man'78; FRCPC; DiagRad. (905)731-7856; Fax. (905)855-1863.

LIU, Peter P; Univ of Ottawa Heart Institute, 40 Ruskin St, Ottawa ON K1Y 4W7; Tor'78; FACC; FRCPC; Cardiol (Cardiovascular Research). Langs: Mandarin; (613)761-5000; Fax. (613)761-5323.

LIU, Regina C Y; Scarborough Hosp-Birchmount, 3030 Birchmount Rd, Scarborough ON M1W 3W3; Cal'01; FRCPC; Psy. Staff, The Scarborough Hospital - Birchmount Campus; (416)495-2701 x5376

LIU, Richard; Meridian Plaza, 10130 111 St NW, Edmonton AB T5K 1K6; Alb'94; BSc; FRCSC; Otol (Neuro Otology). Staff, University of Alberta Hospital; Staff, Royal Alexandra Hospital; University of Alberta; Langs: Mandarin; Chinese; French.

LIU, Sandra A; Clin Fam Basses-Laurentides, 2100 boul du Cure-Labelle, Saint-Jerome QC J7Y 1S8; McG'89; CCFP; (450)565-4320; Fax. (450)565-1099.

LIU, Selina L; St Joseph's Health Care, PO Box 5777 Stn B 268 Grosvenor St, London ON N6A 4V2; Qns'06; FRCPC; IntMed; Endocrin&Metab. Staff, St Joseph's Hospital - St Joseph's Health Care.

LIU, Shi-Kai; Addiction & Mental Hlth-Queen, 1001 Queen St W, Toronto ON M6J 1H4; (Taiwan)'88; Staff, Centre for Addiction & Mental Health (CAMH) - Queen Site.

LIU, Stanley K; Odette Cancer Centre, T2 142-2075 Bayview Ave, Toronto ON M4N 3M5; Tor'04; FRCPC; RadOncol. Staff, Sunnybrook Health Sciences Centre; (416)480-4998

LIU, Suzy; Medical Dental Centre, 10057 Yonge St, Richmond Hill ON L4C 1T7; Man'85; (905)737-9099; Fax. (905)737-9022.

LIU, Tanya; 115-8600 Cambie Rd, Richmond BC V6X 4J9; Shanghai (China)'69; (604)270-6966

LIU, Theresa T; Grand River Hosp-Kw Hlth Ctre, PO Box 9056 Stn C 835 King St W, Kitchener ON N2G 1G3; Qns'05; FRCPC; IntMed; InfectDis. Staff, Grand River Hospital - Kitchener/Waterloo Health Centre; (519)749-4348

LIU, Tom T T; Grand River Hosp-KW Hlth Ctre, PO Box 9056 Stn C C706-835 King St W, Kitchener ON N2G 1G3; Sydney (Australia)'67; BSc(Path); FRACP; MB BS; FRCPC; IntMed (Nephrology). Ac Staff, Grand River Hospital - Kitchener/Waterloo Health Centre; Court Staff, St Mary's General Hospital; (519)743-6396; Fax. (519)746-0693; tomliu@sympatico.ca.

LIU, Vivian W; Wellpoint Family Practice, 9F-1240 Bay St, Toronto ON M5R 2A7; Tor'92; BSc; MSc; CCFP; FCFP; Langs: Mandarin; (416)969-3250; Fax. (416)971-7718.

LIU, Weldon; William Osler HC-Etobicoke, 101 Humber College Blvd, Etobicoke ON M9V 1R8; Tor'95; ABR; FRCPC; DiagRad. Staff, William Osler Health System - Etobicoke General Hospital; Langs: Cantonese; (416)747-3400 x33320; weldon.liu@utoronto.ca.

LIU, Yan; 16B-3221 Derry Rd W, Mississauga ON L5N 7L7; McM'99; FRCPC; IntMed (Arthritis); Rheum. Staff, Toronto Western Hospital - University Health Network; (289)897-3075; Fax. (905)824-7440.

LIU, Yi; Village Square Med Centre, 2942 Finch Ave E, Scarborough ON M1W 2T4; Fujian (China)'90; CCFP; (416)756-2725

LIU, Yuen Chi; Scarborough Hosp-General Div, 3050 Lawrence Ave E, Scarborough ON M1P 2V5; Tor'76; AB(Spec.Comp. ,NuclearM; FRCPC; DiagRad (Nuclear Medicine). Staff, The Scarborough Hospital - General Campus; (416)431-8100

LIU CHEN KIOW, Gilbert T S; CSSS Haut-Richelieu-Rouville, 920 boul Du Seminaire N, St-Jean-Sur-Richel QC J3A 1B7; Lyon (France)'90; FRCPC; Anes. Staff, Hôpital du Haut-Richelieu; (450)359-5212; Fax. (450)359-5251.

LIU CHEN KIOW, Khim Sew H; CSSS d'Argenteuil, 145 av de la Providence, Lachute QC J8H 4C7; Lyon (France)'88; FRCPC; IntMed. Staff, Centre Hospitalier d'Argenteuil; (450)562-3761; Fax. (450)566-3325.

LIU CHEN KIOW, Lee Ha; CHUM-Hotel-Dieu, 3840 rue Saint-Urbain, Montreal QC H2W 1T8; Lyon (France)'94; CCFP; Staff, Centre Hospitalier l'Université de Montréal (CHUM) - Hôtel-Dieu; Langs: English; French; (514)890-8759

LIU-SHUM, Alice T; 835-9700 Jasper Ave NW, Edmonton AB T5J 4C3; Alb'96; FRCPC; OccupMed. (780)495-6695; Fax. (780)495-2743; alice.liu-shum@hc.sc.gc.ca.

LIU-P'NG, Tina T S; 3-2083 Lake Shore Blvd W, Etobicoke ON M8V 4G2; Alb'87; CCFP; Court Staff, Trillium Health Centre - West Toronto; (416)255-1161; Fax. (416)255-1166.

LIU-TERTIL, Limin; Foothills Med Centre, 1403 29 St NW, Calgary AB T2N 2T9; (China)'85; Staff, Foothills Medical Centre; (403)944-1137

LIUTKUS, Joanne F; Cambridge Place Business Bldg, 601-73 Water St N, Cambridge ON N1R 7L6; McM'90; FRCPC; IntMed (Medical Complication Pregnancy). (519)624-8977

LIVERMORE, Craig A; Waypoint Centre for Mental H C, 500 Church St, Penetanguishene ON L9M 1G3; Tor'04; FRCPC; Psy. Staff, Waypoint Centre for Mental Health Care; (705)549-3181

LIVERNOCHE, Marie; CSSS Becancour-Nicolet-Yamaska, 675 rue Saint-Jean-Baptiste, Nicolet QC J3T 1S4; Laval'09; Staff, Hôpital de Christ-Roi; (819)293-2071

LIVESLEY, W John; UBC-Dept of Psychiatry, 7-2255 Wesbrook Mall, Vancouver BC V6T 2A1; Liverpool (England)'74; MB ChB; MRCPsy; FRCPC; Psy. Staff, UBC Hospital - Koerner Pavillion; Staff, Vancouver General Hospital - Centennial Pavillion; University of British Columbia; (604)822-7879; Fax. (604)822-7756; livesley@interchange.ubc.ca.

LIVINGSTON, Christopher; 203-2689 Pandosy St, Kelowna BC V1Y 9V9; Edinburgh (Scotland)'83; MB ChB; DCH; DA; (250)762-9058; Fax. (250)762-8939.

LIVINGSTON, Patricia L; Queen Elizabeth II HSC, 1276 South Park St, Halifax NS B3H 2Y9; Denver(CO) (USA)'85; FRCPC; Anes. Staff, Queen Elizabeth II Health Sciences Centre - Victoria General Site; (902)473-4130

LIVINGSTONE, Arthur G; Radiology Associates, 1122 Scenic Dr S, Lethbridge AB T1K 7E5; Cal'79; FRCPC; DiagRad. Ac Staff Radiol, Chinook Regional Hospital; (403)328-1122; Fax. (403)328-1218; arthur.livingstone@interiorhealth.ca.

LIVINGSTONE, Christopher J; Bayview Mall Medical Offices, 470 Dundas St E, Belleville ON K8N 1G1; Man'07; CCFP; (613)966-4045

LIVINGSTONE, Donald J; Sunnybrook Hlth Sciences Ctre, 2075 Bayview Ave, Toronto ON M4N 3M5; Qns'79; FRCPC; IntMed. Ac Staff, Sunnybrook Health Sciences Centre; Assoc Prof Med, University of Toronto; (416)480-4121; donald.livingstone@sw.ca.

LIVINGSTONE, James B; 200-26 North St, Bridgewater NS B4V 2V6; Dal'79; (902)543-7496; Fax. (902)530-3610.

LIVINGSTONE, Ronald A; 601-123 Edward St, Toronto ON M5G 1E2; Belfast (Ireland)'63; MB ChB; BSc(Physiol); FRCOG; FRCS(Ed); FRCSC; ObstGyn (Maternal Fetal Medicine). Assoc Chief Dept of ObstGyn, Mount Sinai Hospital; Emeritus Prof, University of Toronto; (416)813-2288; Fax. (416)813-4179; livingstone@mtsinai.on.ca.

LIVINGSTONE, Roy R; Medical Clinic, 1500 Cedar Ave, Trail BC V1R 4C6; Cape Town (South Africa)'77; MB ChB; FRCSC; Urol. (250)364-2777; Fax. (250)364-2757.

LIVINGSTONE, Verity H; Broadway Med Centre, 340-943 Broadway W, Vancouver BC V5Z 4E1; London (England)'74; MB BS; CCFP; FCFP; Med Dir, Vancouver Breasfeeding Centre; Assoc Prof, University of British Columbia; (604)738-1912; Fax. (604)738-1231.

LIVINGSTONE, William D; Lifemark Health Centre, 2121 29 St NE, Calgary AB T1Y 7H8; Ott'75; BSc(Hons.); CCFP; FCFP; (403)297-9500; Fax. (403)219-5345.

LIVSHIN, Oleg; North Med Centre, 304-7131 Bathurst St, Thornhill ON L4J 7Z1; Moscow (Russia (Federation))'64; PhD; VP Family Pract, North York General Hospital - Branson Division; (905)882-1400; Fax. (905)882-1406.

LIWANPO, Paul T F; 35 Wolf St, Tillsonburg ON N4G 1S5; U of St Andrews (Scotland)'72; MB ChB; ABIM; FRCPC; IntMed (Cardiology). Consultant IntMed, Tillsonburg District Memorial Hospital; Aj Prof Schulich School of Med, University of Western Ontario; (519)842-6056; Fax. (519)842-8255.

LIWSKI, Robert S; Mackenzie Bldg, 206E-5788 University Ave, Halifax NS B3H 1V8; Dal'03; FRCPC; HemPath.

LIYANAARACHCHI, Ravini; Capilano Med Centre, 5818 Terrace Rd NW, Edmonton AB T6A 3Y8; (Other Foreign)'04; CCFP; (780)761-3330

LIZE, Jean-Francois; CHUM-Hop Notre-Dame, 1560 rue Sherbrooke E, Montreal QC H2L 4M1; Mon'98; BSc(BioChem); FRCPC; IntMed (Intensive Care); Critical Care Medicine (P.Q.); Respir. Staff, Centre Hospitalier l'Université de Montréal (CHUM) - Hôpital Notre-Dame; (514)890-8000

LIZON, Marina J; Regency Centre, 502-333 25th St E, Saskatoon SK S7K 0L4; Nuevo Leon (Mexico)'82; FRCPC; Psy (Psychotherapy). Langs: Spanish; (306)665-8989; Fax. (306)244-3501.

LIZONDO, Enrique E; St Mary's Hosp Centre, 3830 av Lacombe, Montreal QC H3T 1M5; Tucuman (Argentina)'73; FRCPC; Psy. Staff, St Mary's Hospital Centre; assoc Prof, McGill University; (514)345-3511 x3826; Fax. (514)734-2663.

LIZOTTE, Jessica; CSSS de la Region de Thetford, 1717 rue Notre-Dame E, Thetford Mines QC G6G 2V4; Laval'08; CCFP; CCFP(E.M.); Staff, Hopital du CSS de la Region de Thetford; (418)338-7715; Fax. (418)335-7616.

LIZOTTE, Marie-Eve; CSSS Maria-Chapdelaine, 2000 boul du Sacre-Coeur, Dolbeau-Mistassini QC G8L 2R5; Mon'06; IntMed. Staff, Centre Maria-Chapdelaine - CH de Dolbeau-Mistassini; (418)276-1234; Fax. (418)276-4355.

LIZOTTE, Michel; Clin D'Expertises Med Du QC, 440-979 av de Bourgogne, Quebec QC G1W 2L4; Laval'72; Langs: Bilingual(French/English); (418)654-3268; Fax. (418)654-3271.

LIZOTTE, Pierre; Clinique De Med/Psychotherapie, 5839 rue Madore, Montreal QC H1M 1H3; Mon'68; Langs: English; (514)252-0898; Fax. (514)252-1405.

LLANO-FERRO, Miguel A; Wellness Centre, 6F-60 Murray St, Toronto ON M5G 1X5; Bogota (Colombia)'82; Staff Clin Urologist, Mount Sinai Hospital; Langs: Spanish; (416)586-6367; Fax. (416)586-4776; mllano@mtsinai.on.ca.

LLANOS, Romeo B; Thompson Gen Hosp, 871 Thompson Dr, Thompson MB R8N 0C8; Far Eastern (Philippines)'76; Staff, Thompson General Hospital; (204)677-1777

LLEWELLYN, M Evan; Albany Med Clinic, 807 Broadview Ave, Toronto ON M4K 2P8; Wes'02; CCFP; (416)461-9471

LLEWELLYN, Patrick A; North Shore Med Imaging, 139 16th St W, North Vancouver BC V7M 1T3; UBC'86; FRCPC; DiagRad. Staff, Lions Gate Hospital; (604)987-9729

LLEWELYN-WILLIAMS, Warwick; Golden Mile Centre, 27-3806 Albert St, Regina SK S4S 3R2; Cape Town (South Africa)'87; MB ChB; (306)789-3200; Fax. (306)789-3154.

LLOYD, David A; Manitoba Clinic, 790 Sherbrook St, Winnipeg MB R3A 1M3; Witwatersrand (South Africa)'67; MB ChB; FRCPC; IntMed; Gastroent.

LLOYD, Geoffrey J; Canadian Trauma Consultants, 1125-65 Queen St W, Toronto ON M5H 2M5; Sheffield (England)'57; MB ChB; FRCS(Eng); FRCSC; OrthSurg. Hon Staff, Toronto General Hospital - UHN; Assoc Prof Surg, University of Toronto; (416)863-1581; Fax. (416)863-1905; gjlblt@sympatico.ca.

LLOYD, John C; Sunnybrook Hlth Sciences Ctre, M1 302C-2075 Bayview Ave, Toronto ON M4N 3M5; Wes'89; FRCSC; Ophth (Cataract Surgery). Staff Ophthalmologist, Sunnybrook Health Sciences Centre; (416)480-4424; Fax. (416)480-4481; john.lloyd@sunnybrook.ca.

LLOYD, R Grayson; Valley Reg Hosp, 150 Exhibition St, Kentville NS B4N 5E3; UBC'04; FRCPC; Anes. Staff, Valley Regional Hospital; (902)678-7381

LLOYD, Robert J; McMaster University, HSC 3Y-1280 Main St W, Hamilton ON L8S 4K1; Tor'91; FRCPC; Peds (Pediatric Critical Care). Ac Staff Ped Intensivist, Hamilton Health Sciences Centre - McMaster Children's Hospital; Assoc Prof Peds & Critical Care, McMaster University; (905)521-2100 x76610; Fax. (905)524-5707; rlloyd@mcmaster.ca.

LLOYD, Robert L; Boundary Trails Health Centre, PO Box 2000 Stn Main, Winkler MB R6W 1H8; Man'74; DiagRad. Staff, Boundary Trails Health Centre; (204)331-8800

LLOYD, Ronald M; CFB Petawawa Bldg N-109, PO Box 9999 Stn Main, Petawawa ON K8H 2X3; Liverpool (England)'63; MD; DRCOG; MRC; (613)687-5511 x6356

LLOYD, Stephen R; McMaster University Med Centre, 1200 Main St W, Hamilton ON L8N 3Z5; McM'81; FACEP; MCFP(E.M.); Staff, Hamilton Health Sciences Centre - McMaster Children's Hospital; Staff, Hamilton Health Sciences Centre - McMaster University Medical Centre; Chief Div of Emerg Med, McMaster University; (905)521-2100 x76207; Fax. (905)528-5337.

LLOYD-JONES, Philip M; Summit View Med Centre, 100B-3300 Boundary Rd, Burnaby BC V5M 4A4; London (England)'66; MB BS; MRCS; MRC; FRCP; Peds (Asthma). Att Staff, BC Children's Hospital; Att Staff, Providence Health Care - Mount Saint Joseph Hospital; Att Staff, BC Women's Hospital & Health Centre; Asst Prof, University of British Columbia; (604)437-7001

LLOYD-SMITH, D Robertson; Allan McGavin Sports Med Ctr, 3055 Wesbrook Mall, Vancouver BC V6T 1Z3; McG'77; Ac Staff, UBC Hospital - Koerner Pavillion; Clin Prof, University of British Columbia; Langs: Bilingual(English/French); (604)822-3614; Fax. (604)822-9058; rob.lloyd-smith@ubc.ca.

LO, Ada Y T; Toronto North Med Arts Centre, 121-7155 Woodbine Ave, Markham ON L3R 1A3; Tor'93; CCFP; FCFP; Langs: Cantonese; (416)628-7702; Fax. (416)628-7708.

LO, Adrian W; Beczy Med Clinic, 3-20 Bur Oak Ave, Markham ON L6C 0A2; Tor'94; CCFP; FCFP; Langs: Cantonese; (905)887-3399; Fax. (905)887-0462.

LO, Alexander J; Toronto Rehab Inst-Univ Ctr, 550 University Ave, Toronto ON M5G 2A2; Qns'06; FRCPC; PhysMed&Rehab. Staff, Toronto Rehabilitation Institute - University Centre; (416)597-3422

LO, Anne; Finch-Midland Med Centre, 207-4190 Finch Ave E, Scarborough ON M1S 4T7; Tor'94; CCFP; FCFP; Langs: Cantonese; (416)497-9868

LO, Benjamin W Y; St Michael's Hosp, 30 Bond St, Toronto ON M5B 1W8; Ott'03; FRCSC; Neursurg; Critical Care Medicine. Staff, St Michael's Hospital; (416)360-4000

LO, Charles D; Queen Elizabeth II HSC-Halifax, 1796 Summer St, Halifax NS B3H 3A7; Dal'75; DABR; NBME; FRCPC; DiagRad (Cardiac Radiology). Staff Radiol, Queen Elizabeth II Health Sciences Centre - Halifax Infirmary Site; Prof, Dalhousie University; (902)473-2663; Fax. (902)473-2018; clo@dal.ca.

LO, Charles Y; St Paul's Hosp, 1081 Burrard St, Vancouver BC V6Z 1Y6; Tor'05; FRCPC; Anes. Staff, Providence Health Care - St Paul's Hospital; (604)806-8337

LO, Christina K Y; 302-4040 Finch Ave E, Scarborough ON M1S 4V5; Tor'93; CCFP; Court Staff, The Scarborough Hospital - Birchmount Campus; Court Staff, Rouge Valley Health System - Centenary Health Centre Site; Langs: Cantonese; (416)848-7788; christopher_li@rogers.com.

LO, Cynthia C Y; 6683 Victoria Dr, Vancouver BC V5P 3Y2; (Hong Kong)'88; MB BS; (604)301-1666

LO, Cynthia Y W; 250-2184 Broadway W, Vancouver BC V6K 2E1; McM'05; CCFP; Langs: Cantonese; (604)733-5181

LO, Dennis L; Langley Mem Hosp, 22051 Fraser Hwy, Langley BC V3A 4H4; Qns'87; FRCPC; Anes. Staff, Langley Memorial Hospital; (604)514-6009

LO, Dorothy S; St Joseph's Health Centre, 30 The Queensway, Toronto ON M6R 1B5; Tor'02; FRCPC; IntMed; MedOncol. Staff, St Joseph's Health Centre; (416)530-6000

LO, Eddie S; Rathburn Med Clinic, 4-592 Rathburn Rd W, Mississauga ON L5B 3A4; McG'69; Ac Staff, The Credit Valley Hospital; Staff, Trillium Health Centre - Mississauga; (905)896-0880; Fax. (905)896-0878.

LO, Edmond K W; Scarborough North Med Arts, 409-4040 Finch Ave E, Scarborough ON M1S 4V5; McG'63; MDCM; Langs: Chinese; Mandarin; Cantonese; (416)297-9592; Fax. (416)297-7552; dredmond.lo@gmail.com.

LO, Evelyn; St Boniface Gen Hosp, C5002-409 Tache Ave, Winnipeg MB R2H 2A6; Tor'97; InfectDis; IntMed. Staff, St Boniface General Hospital; elo@sbgh.mb.ca.

LO, Frank L; Public Gardens Med Group, 200-5675 Spring Garden Rd, Halifax NS B3J 1H1; Dal'77; Court Staff, Queen Elizabeth II Health Sciences Centre - Victoria General Site; Court Staff, IWK Health Centre; (902)429-7910

LO, Freda H F; LA Medical Clinic, 30-5201 50 St, Leduc AB T9E 6T4; Alb'04; CCFP; Staff, Covenant Health - Grey Nuns Community Hospital; Staff/Physician ER, Leduc Community Hospital; (780)986-9600; Fax. (780)986-9732.

LO, George Y K; Standard Life Centre, 100-10405 Jasper Ave NW, Edmonton AB T5J 3N4; Man'78; CCFP; (780)944-9583; Fax. (780)944-9534.

LO, Gregory K; Lakeridge Hlth Corp-Oshawa, 2C169-1 Hospital Crt, Oshawa ON L1G 2B9; McM'01; FRCPC; IntMed; MedOncol. Staff, Lakeridge Health - Oshawa Site; (905)576-8711 x4815

LO, Hanson K C; Byron Street Med Centre, 320 Byron St S, Whitby ON L1N 4P8; (Ireland)'90; MB BS; BAO; Langs: Cantonese; (905)668-5835; Fax. (905)668-8942.

LO, Henry; South Health Campus, 4448 Front St SE, Calgary AB T3M 1M4; Cal'09; CCFP; Staff, Peter Lougheed Centre; (403)956-3038

LO, Hung-Tat; Scarborough North Med Arts, 409-4040 Finch Ave E, Scarborough ON M1S 4V5; (Hong Kong)'71; MB BS; MRCPsy; FRCPC; Psy. Asst Prof, University of Toronto; Langs: Cantonese; Mandarin; (416)297-4807; Fax. (416)297-9592.

LO, Ian K Y; Health Research Innovation Ctr, 3280 Hospital Dr NW, Calgary AB T2N 4Z6; Wes'94; FRCSC; OrthSurg. Staff, Health Research Innovation Centre; (403)220-2745; Fax. (403)210-8197.

LO, James W; Stevenson Mem Hosp, PO Box 4000 Stn Main 200 Fletcher Cres, Alliston ON L9R 1W7; Qns'06; CCFP; Staff, Stevenson Memorial Hospital; (705)435-6281

LO, Jason H T; Village Square Med Centre, A202-3000 Highway 7, Markham ON L3R 6E1; Tor'98; CCFP; Staff, Markham Stouffville Hospital; Langs: Cantonese; (905)480-1050; Fax. (905)480-0898; jasonlo13@hotmail.com.

LO, Jeremy C K; 71B Willow St, Ottawa ON K1R 6V9; Tor'90; CCFP; Langs: Chinese; (613)238-6818; Fax. (613)238-1638.

LO, Julian K; Sunnybrook Hlth Sciences Ctre, 2075 Bayview Ave, Toronto ON M4N 3M5; Qns'93; FAAPMR; FRCPC; PhysMed&Rehab (Neuromuscular Diseases). Staff, Sunnybrook Health Sciences Centre; Teach Staff, University of Toronto; (416)480-4685

LO, Karen K W; 355 MCGarrell Dr, London ON N6G 0B1; Wes'95; CCFP; FCFP; Med Dir, McGarrell Place.

LO, Katherine A; Sunnybrook Hlth Sciences Ctre, M4176-2075 Bayview Ave, Toronto ON M4N 3M5; Alb'06; FRCSC; ObstGyn. Staff, Sunnybrook Health Sciences Centre; (416)480-5163

LO, Kirk C L; Murray Koffler Urology Wellnes, 6F-60 Murray St, Toronto ON M5T 3L9; McG'96; FRCSC; Urol. Langs: Chinese; (416)586-4613; Fax. (416)586-8354.

LO, Lawrence S; Mount St Joseph Hosp, 3080 Prince Edward St, Vancouver BC V5T 3N4; Tor'07; FRCPC; IntMed; GeriatricMed. Staff, Providence Health Care - Mount Saint Joseph Hospital; (604)874-1141

LO, Louis Y C; 9 Brandy Crt, North York ON M3B 3L3; Man'61; DAB; FRCPC; Peds (Consultant Pediatrics). Ac Staff, The Scarborough Hospital - General Campus; (416)297-8822; Fax. (416)297-8822.

LO, Lydia C L; Cornerstone Family Med Centre, 106-100 Strowger Blvd, Brockville ON K6V 5J9; Wes'91; CCFP; FCFP; Langs: Cantonese; (613)498-0444; Fax. (613)498-4850.

LO, Marco C; Ryerson Med Centre, W181-350 Victoria St, Toronto ON M5B 2K3; (Other Foreign)'10; CCFP; (416)979-5070

LO, Michael; Tecumseh Life Centre, 102A-11811 Tecumseh Rd E, Windsor ON N8N 4M7; Tor'76; (519)735-7755

LO, Nicholas T K L; St Michael's Hosp, 30 Bond St, Toronto ON M5B 1W8; Tor'04; FRCPC; Anes. Staff, St Michael's Hospital; (416)864-5071

LO, Patrick C C; Trillium Hlth Ctr-West Toronto, 150 Sherway Dr, Etobicoke ON M9C 1A5; Tor'90; FRCPC; DiagRad. Staff, Trillium Health Centre - West Toronto; (416)521-4047

LO, Raymond C T; Medical Arts Bldg, 406-1 Young St, Hamilton ON L8N 1T8; Tor'77; ABIM; FRCPC; IntMed; Neur. Consultant Neurol, Hamilton Health Sciences Centre - McMaster University Medical Centre; Clinical Asst Prof Med, McMaster University; (905)521-2737; Fax. (905)521-2739.

LO, Reginald W W; East Van Med Bldg, 202-1750 10th Ave W, Vancouver BC V5N 5K4; UBC'76; Assoc Staff, BC Women's Hospital & Health Centre; Assoc Staff, Vancouver General Hospital - Centennial Pavillion; Assoc Staff, Providence Health Care - Mount Saint Joseph Hospital; Assoc Staff, BC Children's Hospital; Langs: Cantonese; (604)251-1833

LO, Ronnie Y K; North Ajax Med Centre, 475 Westney Rd N, Ajax ON L1T 3H4; Tor'90; Ac Staff, Rouge Valley Health System - Ajax & Pickering Health Centre Site; (905)427-7767; Fax. (905)427-4339.

LO, Shirley M H; Niagara Health Centre, 302-180 Vine St S, St Catharines ON L2R 7P3; Wes'92; FRCSC; Otol. Staff, Niagara Health System - St Catharines General Site; Staff, Niagara Health System - Ontario Street Site; (905)684-9237; Fax. (905)684-4178.

LO, Stephen C W; Erindale Med Centre, 1101 McBride Ave, Mississauga ON L5C 1M6; Wes'91; Court Staff, Trillium Health Centre - Mississauga; Langs: Cantonese; (905)270-4020

LO, Tak-Shing; 105-1711 McCowan Rd, Scarborough ON M1S 2Y3; Tor'82; Ac Staff, Rouge Valley Health System - Centenary Health Centre Site; Langs: Chinese; (416)299-6601; Fax. (416)299-6601.

LO, Tony H; Geriatric Mental Health, 6F-1213 4 St SW, Calgary AB T2R 0X7; Alb'01; FRCPC; Psy. Langs: Cantonese; (403)955-6155

LO, Vivian K W; 103-174 Harwood Ave S, Ajax ON L1S 2H6; Wes'88; Staff, Rouge Valley Health System - Ajax & Pickering Health Centre Site; (905)683-0690

LO, W Alex; RCMP Med Clinic, 410-73 Leikin Dt, Ottawa ON K1A 0R2; McM'81; Physician, Royal Canadian Mounted Police; (613)843-6544

LOACH, David W; Univ Hlth Network-Princess M, 610 University Ave, Toronto ON M5G 2M9; Tor'90; Clin Associate, Princess Margaret Hospital - University Health Network; (416)946-2000; Fax. (416)946-4456.

LOADER, Kenneth R; The Brandon Clinic, 620 Dennis St, Brandon MB R7A 5E7; Man'77; PhD(Anat); Staff, Brandon Regional Health Centre; (204)728-4440; Fax. (204)726-1765.

LOANE, Thomas D; Halifax Prof Centre, 585-5991 Spring Garden Rd, Halifax NS B3H 1Y6; Dal'76; FRCPC; PhysMed&Rehab (Rehabilitation Medicine). Court Staff, Queen Elizabeth II Health Sciences Centre - Victoria General Site; (902)422-5808; Fax. (902)425-6388.

LOARING, Jaimie M; 1550-2109 Ottawa St, Windsor ON N8Y 1R8; Tor'86; CCFP; Staff, Windsor Regional Hospital - Metropolitan Site; (519)944-0683; Fax. (519)944-3005.

LOBACK, Dwight R; 117 Slimmon Rd, Saskatoon SK S7V 0B8; Sask'74; FRCSC; OrthSurg. Staff, St Paul's Hospital (Grey Nuns) of Saskatoon; Staff, Saskatoon City Hospital; Clinical Asst Prof, University of Saskatchewan; (306)244-1247; Fax. (306)934-3330.

LOBACK, Trevor J; Orthopedic Associates, 117 Slimmon Rd, Saskatoon SK S7V 0B8; Sask'06; FRCSC; OrthSurg. (306)244-1247; Fax. (306)934-3330.

LOBATO DE FARIA, Ricardo J L; Seven Oaks Gen Hosp, 2300 McPhillips St, Winnipeg MB R2V 3M3; Witwatersrand (South Africa)'87; MB ChB; Chief/Med Officer of Hlth, Seven Oaks General Hospital; (204)632-7133; Fax. (204)694-8276.

LOBAY, Gerald L W; Garneau Prof Centre, 201-11044 82 Ave NW, Edmonton AB T6G 0T2; Alb'68; FRCSC; PlasSurg (Hand Surgery). Ac Staff, University of Alberta Hospital; Ac Staff, Covenant Health - Misericordia Community Hospital; Clin Prof, University of Alberta; (780)433-4225; Fax. (780)439-6732.

LOBAY, Lori A; Valley Med Clinic, PO Box 2932 Stn Main 231 2 Ave, Strathmore AB T1P 1L5; Alb'82; Staff, Strathmore District Health Services; (403)934-4444; Fax. (403)934-5218.

LOBB, Trevor R; London HSC-Victoria Hosp, PO Box 5010 Stn B 800 Commissioners Rd E, London ON N6A 5W9; Wes'69; FRCPC; Anes (Cardiovascular Anesthesia). Staff Anes, London Health Sciences Centre - Victoria Campus; Clin Assoc Prof, University of Western Ontario; (519)685-8525; Fax. (519)685-8275.

LOBLAW, Douglas A B; Toronto Sunnybrook Reg Cancer, 2075 Bayview Ave, Toronto ON M4N 3M5; Qns'95; FRCPC; RadOncol. (416)480-4806; Fax. (416)480-6002.

LOBLEY, Jarrett; MINE Addictions Clinic, 25 Sherbrooke St, Winnipeg MB R3C 2B1; (Other Foreign)'08.

LOBO, A L Charlotte; Montfort Hosp, 713 Montreal Rd, Ottawa ON K1K 0T2; Ott'98; FRCPC; DiagRad. Staff, Montfort Hospital; (613)746-4621

LOBO, Andrea N; Queen-Spadina Med Centre, 455 Queen St W, Toronto ON M5V 2A9; Ott'99; CCFP; (416)869-3627; Fax. (416)703-3962.

LOBO, Joel J A; Ajax Med Arts Bldg, 200-601 Harwood Ave S, Ajax ON L1S 2J5; Tor'97; FRCSC; OrthSurg (Arthroscopic Knee & Shoulder Surgery). Orthopaedic Surg, Rouge Valley Health System - Ajax & Pickering Health Centre Site; (905)426-5460; Fax. (905)426-6667.

LOBO, Kevin A; Halton HCS Corp-Oakville, 327 Reynolds St, Oakville ON L6J 3L7; UBC'90; FACR; FRCPC; DiagRad. Ac Staff Radiol, Halton Healthcare Services Corporation - Oakville Site; Ac Staff, Halton Healthcare Services Corporation - Milton District Hospital; (905)338-4601

LOBO, Louella S; Brameast Family Health Org, 38-2130 North Park Dr, Brampton ON L6S 0C9; Tor'93; BSc; CCFP; FCFP; Staff, William Osler Health System - Brampton Civic Hospital; (905)792-2211; Fax. (905)792-2901.

LOBOS, Anna-Theresa; Children's Hosp Eastern Ont, 401 Smyth Rd, Ottawa ON K1H 8L1; McM'01; FRCPC; Peds (Critical Care Medicine). Staff Peds, Children's Hospital of Eastern Ontario (CHEO); (613)737-7600

LOBSINGER, Meghan P; Royal Jubilee Hosp, 1952 Bay St, Victoria BC V8R 1J8; Ott'10; CCFP; Staff, Royal Jubilee Hospital; (250)370-8699

LOBSINGER, Thomas R; 31 Frederick St, Orillia ON L3V 5W5; Tor'85; CCFP; (705)327-5225; Fax. (705)327-5226.

LOCAS, Francois; Clinique Med Angus, 4101 rue Molson, Montreal QC H1Y 3L1; Mon'92; Chief Emerg Services, Centre Hospitalier Fleury; (514)807-2333

LOCH, Simone R M; Ridge Meadows Maternity Clinic, 20580 Lougheed Hwy, Maple Ridge BC V2X 2P8; UBC'09; CCFP; (604)460-4444

LOCHNAN, Heather A; The Ottawa Hosp-Riverside Camp, 1967 Riverside Dr, Ottawa ON K1H 7W9; Tor'85; BSc; FRCPC; IntMed; Endocrin&Metab. Att Staff, The Ottawa Hospital - Riverside Campus; Assoc Prof Med, University of Ottawa; (613)738-8400 x81950; Fax. (613)738-8396.

LOCHRIN, Catherine A; The Ottawa Hosp-Gen Campus, 501 Smyth Rd, Ottawa ON K1H 8L6; Dublin (Ireland)'81; MB BCh; BAO; FRCPC; RadOncol (Breasts). Staff Ottawa Reg Cancer Centre, The Ottawa Hospital - General Campus; Assoc Prof Radiol, University of Ottawa; (613)737-7700 x6804; Fax. (613)247-3511.

LOCHT, Randall C; 110-9181 Main St, Chilliwack BC V2P 4M9; Man'74; FRCSC; OrthSurg. (604)792-7379

LOCK, E; Cumberland Med Hlth Services, 33 Havelock St, Amherst NS B4H 4W1; Dal'99; FRCPC; Psy. Langs: French; Sign Language; (902)667-3879

LOCK, Malcolm S; Brant County Health Unit, 194 Terrace Hill St, Brantford ON N3R 1G7; RCS (Ireland)'73; LRCPSI; MPH; (519)753-4937; Fax. (519)753-2140.

LOCK, Michael I; London Reg Cancer Centre, 790 Commissioners Rd E, London ON N6A 4L6; McM'94; BSc(Hon.); FRCPC; RadOncol;CCFP; Assoc Prof, London Regional Cancer Centre; University of Western Ontario; (519)685-8650; Fax. (519)685-8627.

LOCK, Walter A; 280 Main St PO Box 880, Lucan ON N0M 2J0; Tor'71; BSc; Med Dir, Chateau Gardens Nursing Home; (519)227-4015; Fax. (519)227-4215.

LOCK O'BRIEN, Jodi; William Osler HC-Etobicoke, 101 Humber College Blvd, Etobicoke ON M9V 1R8; Tor'01; CCFP; Staff, William Osler Health System - Etobicoke General Hospital; (416)494-2120

LOCKE, Carolynne; Brant Community HC-Brantford, 200 Terrace Hill St, Brantford ON N3R 1G9; Tor'78; Staff, The Brant Community Healthcare System - Brantford General Hospital Site; (519)752-7871

LOCKE, Jake J; Bc Women's Hosp & Health Ctre, P4 120-4500 Oak St, Vancouver BC V6H 3N1; UBC'80; FRCPC; Psy. Staff, BC Women's Hospital & Health Centre; (604)875-2007

LOCKE, Kenneth A; Mount Sinai Hosp, 457-600 University Ave, Toronto ON M5G 1X5; Tor'94; FRCPC; IntMed. Staff, Mount Sinai Hospital; (416)586-4800

LOCKE, Trevor A; Physicians Incorporated, 204-316 Willow St, Truro NS B2N 5A4; Dal'89; BSc; Ac Staff, Colchester East Hants Health Centre.

LOCKHART, Alexander S; 800-15355 24 Ave PO Box 203 Stn Main, Surrey BC V3T 4W8; UBC'71; Fax. (604)535-0249.

LOCKHART, Bruce F; Bath Med Clinic, 82 Hospital St, Bath NB E7J 1B9; Dal'79; Staff, Upper River Valley Hospital - Waterville; (506)278-5200; Fax. (506)278-3290.

LOCKHART, Colin E; Bath Med Clinic, 82 Hospital St, Bath NB E7J 1B9; Dal'81; (506)278-5200; Fax. (506)278-3290.

LOCKHART, Michelle A; Thames Valley FHT-Whitehills M, 1225 Wonderland Rd N, London ON N6G 2V9; Wes'88; CCFP; FCFP; Staff, St Joseph's Hospital - St Joseph's Health Care; (519)472-0040; Fax. (519)472-7732.

LOCKHART, Pamela J; 800-15355 24 Ave PO Box 512 Stn Main, Surrey BC V3T 5B7; UBC'72; Fax. (604)535-0249.

LOCKHART, Robert J M; 10301 Melrose Dr RR 3, Komoka ON N0L 1R0; Tor'84; FRCPC; Psy. (519)474-1498

LOCKHAT, Hassan S; 4825 50 St PO Box 939, Stettler AB T0C 2L0; (Ireland)'82; MB ChB; BAO; LRCP; LRCS; Ac Staff, Stettler Hospital and Care Centre; (403)742-4011; Fax. (403)742-4013; hlockhat@dthr.ab.ca.

LOCKINGTON, Kathryn; Maple Key Clinic Fam Hlth Team, D2-1036 Princess St, Kingston ON K7L 1H2; Qns'86; CCFP; FCFP; Staff Family Med, Kingston General Hospital; Staff, Hotel-Dieu Hospital; Staff Family Med, Queen's University; (613)546-9721; Fax. (613)546-2799.

LOCKMAN, Denis; 204-2339 Ogilvie Rd, Ottawa ON K1J 8M6; Ott'88; CSPQ; CCFP; CCFP(E.M.); FCFP; EmergMed (P.Q.). Ac Member Emerg, Montfort Hospital; Teach Staff Family Med, University of Ottawa; Langs: Bilingual(French/English); (613)842-9740; Fax. (613)842-4428.

LOCKMAN, Julie M I; 869 rue Notre Dame PO Box 1259, Embrun ON K0A 1W0; Sher'94; (613)443-3311; Fax. (613)443-0142.

LOCKMAN, Leonard E; St Vital Family Medical, 1087 St Mary's Rd, Winnipeg MB R2M 3T2; Natal (South Africa)'86; MB ChB; MCFP(SA); CCFP; FCFP; (204)255-2835; Fax. (204)255-3840; dr.lockman@stvitalfamilymedical.com.

LOCKNER, Charlene A; Oshawa Clinic, 117 King St E, Oshawa ON L1H 1B9; UBC'82; CCFP; FCFP; Staff, Lakeridge Health - Oshawa Site; (905)723-8551 x5222; Fax. (905)721-6646.

LOCKWOOD, Anthony P F; First Glance Aesthetic Clinic, 1851 Grant Ave, Winnipeg MB R3N 1Z2; Mem'79; FRCSC; PlasSurg (Cosmetic & Laser Surgery). Staff, Seven Oaks General Hospital; University of Manitoba; (204)885-1419; Fax. (204)885-1552; info@thefirstglance.ca.

LOCKWOOD, Evan E; Hys Med Centre, 350-11010 101 St NW, Edmonton AB T5H 4B9; Sask'99; FRCPC; IntMed (Telehealth); Cardiol. Staff, University of Alberta Hospital; (780)428-3246

LOCKYER, Joseph M; Health Sciences Centre, 300 Prince Philip Dr, St. John's NL A1B 3V6; Mem'04; FRCPC; IntMed; Respir. Staff, Health Sciences Centre; (709)777-2173

LOCKYER, Michelle A; South East Toronto Fam Health, 1871 Danforth Ave, Toronto ON M4C 1J3; Mem'08; CCFP; (416)699-7775

LOCZY, Katrin; Centre Med Orsainville, 14050 boul Henri-Bourassa, Quebec QC G1G 5S9; Laval'86; Langs: English; (418)622-8366; Fax. (418)622-8367.

LODEN, Stephen A; Meadow Lake Associate Clinic, PO Box 1510, Meadow Lake SK S9X 1Z1; Sask'09; CCFP; (306)236-5661

LODENQUAI, Gregory M; 3F-600 The East Mall, Etobicoke ON M9B 4B1; Ott'98; FRCPC; Psy (Child & Adolescent Psychiatry). Physician, George Hull Centre for Children & Families.

LODENQUAI, Jeffrey W; Bridle Trail Med Clinic, 102-9249 Kennedy Rd, Unionville ON L3R 6H8; West Indies (Jamaica)'63; (905)947-8933; Fax. (905)947-8245.

LODGE, Andrew M; Bella Coola General Hosp, PO Box 220 1027 Elcho St, Bella Coola BC V0T 1C0; Man'07; Staff, Bella Coola General Hospital; (250)799-5311

LODGE, Daniel J; Health Sciences Centre, 300 Prince Philip Dr, St. John's NL A1B 3V6; Mem'06; CardSurg. Staff, Health Sciences Centre; (709)737-6300

LODGE, Richard; Queen Elizabeth II HSC-Halifax, 2134-1796 Summer St, Halifax NS B3H 3A7; Edinburgh (Scotland)'69; MB ChB; DObstRCOG; MRCP(UK); FRCPC; IntMed (Cardiology). Assoc Prof Med, Queen Elizabeth II Health Sciences Centre - Halifax Infirmary Site; (902)473-7990; Fax. (902)473-2434.

LODHA, Abhay K; Foothills Med Centre, C211-1403 29 St NW, Calgary AB T2N 2T9; Rajasthan (India)'89; Staff, Foothills Medical Centre; (403)944-1087

LODHA, Vinay; Royal Ottawa Hlth Care Group, 1145 Carling Ave, Ottawa ON K1Z 7K4; Man'01; FRCPC; Psy. Staff, Royal Ottawa Mental Health Centre - Royal Ottawa Health Care Group; (613)722-6521 x7095

LODHEN, Tenzin; 50-470 Dundas St E, Belleville ON K8N 1G1; Delhi (India)'96; CCFP; (613)966-4045

LODHI, Abid M D; Gold Square Mall, 201-3988 Albert St, Regina SK S4S 3R1; Punjab (Pakistan)'00; FRCPC; Peds. (306)206-1290

LODHI, Gulshan; Woolwich Comm Health Centre, PO Box 370 10 Parkside Dr, St Jacobs ON N0B 2N0; Tor'74; Staff, St Mary's General Hospital; Physician, Sexual Health Clinic; Physician, Region of Waterloo Public Health Corporate Office; Langs: Swahili; Gujarati; (519)664-3794; Fax. (519)664-2182; glodi@wchc.on.ca.

LODHI, Shariq J; William Osler HC-Brampton, 2100 Bovaird Dr E, Brampton ON L6R 3J7; Qns'03; CCFP; Staff, William Osler Health System - Brampton Civic Hospital; (905)494-2120

LODYGENSKY, Gregory A; Hôpital Ste-Justine, 3175 ch Cote-Sainte-Catherine, Montreal QC H3T 1C5; Staff, Hôpital Ste-Justine.

LOE, Brian R; 141-31 Southridge Dr, Okotoks AB T1S 2N3; Alb'01; FRCPC; DiagRad. (403)995-2727

LOEB, Graham J; Lindsay Med Centre, 202-86 Angeline St S, Lindsay ON K9V 6C5; Tor'81; CCFP; FCFP; Ac Staff, Ross Memorial Hospital; Asst Prof DCFM, University of Toronto; (705)324-3344; Fax. (705)324-4737.

LOEB, Mark B; McMaster University HSC, MDCL 3200-1280 Main St W, Hamilton ON L8S 4K1; McG'90; FRCPC; IntMed; InfectDis; MedMicrobiol. Asst Prof Path & Molecular Med, McMaster University; (905)525-9140 x26679; loebm@mcmaster.ca.

LOEB, Robert S; Ville Marie MRI, 900-1538 rue Sherbrooke O, Montreal QC H3G 1L5; Tor'88; DiagRad.

LOEBACH, Paul M; Windsor Prof Centre, 101-2462 Howard Ave, Windsor ON N8X 3V6; Wes'83; CCFP; FCFP; Staff, Hôtel-Dieu Grace Hospital; (519)256-4949; Fax. (519)256-9280.

LOEFFLER, Kimberly N; Grey Nuns Family Med Centre, 2927 66 St NW, Edmonton AB T6K 4C1; Alb'04; CCFP; Clinical Asst Prof, University of Alberta; (780)342-1470; Fax. (780)490-0953.

LOEHR, Jane M; Alberta Prof Bldg, 303-320 23 Ave SW, Calgary AB T2S 0J2; Qns'98; CCFP; (403)686-2150

LOEMBA, Hugues D; Montfort Hosp, 713 ch Montreal, Ottawa ON K1K 0T2; Kiev (Ukraine)'86; CCFP; Staff, Montfort Hospital; (613)746-4621

LOEPP, M Christine; Concordia Health Associates, 102-1155 Concordia Ave, Winnipeg MB R2K 2M9; Man'82; CCFP; FCFP; Staff, Concordia General Hospital; Staff, Pembina Place Personal Care Home; Staff, Bethania Personal Care Home; Langs: German; (204)415-0322

LOERTSCHER, Rolf; Lakeshore Gen Hosp, 160 av Stillview, Pointe-Claire QC H9R 2Y2; Zurich (Switzerland)'75; Staff, Lakeshore General Hospital - Pointe Claire; Langs: German; Bilingual(French/English); (514)630-2225; rolf.loertscher@rogers.blackberry.net.

LOEWEN, A Waldemar; Lake of the Woods Dist Hosp, RR 1 21 Sylvan St, Kenora ON P9N 3W7; Man'68; Staff, Lake of the Woods District Hospital; (807)468-9861

LOEWEN, Andrea H S; Peter Lougheed Centre, 3500 26 Ave NE, Calgary AB T1Y 6J4; UBC'01; DABIM; FRCPC; IntMed (Sleep Medicine); Respir. Staff, Peter Lougheed Centre; Staff, Foothills Medical Centre; (403)943-5425

LOEWEN, Ann E; Red River Valley H D-Morris, PO Box 519, Morris MB R0G 1K0; McG'89; CCFP; FCFP; Staff Chief, Morris General Hospital; (204)746-2301; Fax. (204)746-2838; aloewen@rha-central.mb.ca.

LOEWEN, David A J; Gulf Canada Square, 370-401 9 Ave SW, Calgary AB T2P 3C5; UBC'01; CCFP; (403)221-4467; Fax. (403)221-4442.

LOEWEN, E Nadine; Simon Fraser Health Region, 300-4946 Canada Way, Burnaby BC V5G 4H7; Man'86; Med Officer of Hlth/Dir, City Of Burnaby; (604)918-7444; nadine.loewen@burnaby.ca.

LOEWEN, George; Capilano Med Clinic, 7905 106 Ave NW, Edmonton AB T6A 1H7; Alb'64; (780)465-0951; Fax. (780)465-6928; ghl@primus.ca.

LOEWEN, Mary L; 6668 Fraser St, Vancouver BC V5X 3T5; UBC'82; Vis Staff, Vancouver General Hospital - Centennial Pavillion; Langs: German; (604)321-6651; Fax. (604)325-3915.

LOEWEN, Shaun K; CancerCare Manitoba, 675 McDermot Ave, Winnipeg MB R3E 0V9; Alb'06; FRCPC; RadOncol.

LOEWEN, Sylvia R; Legacy Sports Med Clinic, 14-160 Meadowood Dr, Winnipeg MB R2M 5L6; Man'94; CCFP; Staff, Concordia General Hospital; (204)667-1560

LOEWEN, Theodore E; West End Prof Bldg, 302-9509 156 St NW, Edmonton AB T5P 4J5; Alb'79; BMedSci; Staff Non-Admitting, Covenant Health - Misericordia Community Hospital; (780)486-2060; Fax. (780)481-3273; drloewen@loewenco.com.

LOEWEN, Todd A; Rocky Mountain Health Centre, PO Box 2019, Fernie BC V0B 1M0; UBC'93; CCFP; (250)423-4718; Fax. (250)423-6463.

LOEWEN, Trenton D; 203-2051 McCallum Rd, Abbotsford BC V2S 3N5; Sask'95; CCFP; (604)855-0677

LOEWITH, Brenda B; 277 Wilson St E, Ancaster ON L9G 2B8; McM'87; Staff, Hamilton Health Sciences Centre - McMaster University Medical Centre; (905)648-7973

LOEWY, John A; Athabasca Place, 114-80 Chippewa Rd, Sherwood Park AB T8A 4W6; McM'78; FRCPC; DiagRad. (780)467-2773

LOFARO, Anthony D; Meadowlands Fam Health Centre, 20-888 Meadowlands Dr, Ottawa ON K2C 3R2; Tor'03; CCFP; Physician, Meadowlands Family Health Centre; (613)228-2882

LOFCHY, A Norman; Albany Med Clinic, Main Fl-807 Broadview Ave, Toronto ON M4K 2P8; Tor'54; (416)461-9471; Fax. (416)461-2710.

LOFCHY, Jodi S; Univ Hlth Network-Toronto Western Hosp, 9E 467D-399 Bathurst St, Toronto ON M5T 2S8; Tor'84; FRCPC; Psy (Emergency Psychiatry). Dir Psy Emerg Services, Toronto Western Hospital - University Health Network; (416)603-5500; Fax. (416)603-6289.

LOFFELMANN, Carol M; St Michael's Hosp, 30 Bond St, Toronto ON M5B 1W8; Tor'96; FRCPC; Anes. Staff Anes, St Michael's Hospital; (416)864-6060 x5071; Fax. (416)864-6014.

LOFGREN, Sandra R; Dauphin Med Clinic, 622 3rd St SW, Dauphin MB R7N 1R5; Man'83; BSc; CCFP; FCFP; Staff, Dauphin Regional Health Centre; University of Manitoba; (204)638-6445; Fax. (204)638-5670.

LOFSKY, Stanley; 28 Clovercrest Rd, North York ON M2J 1Z6; Tor'66; CCFP; FCFP; Ac Staff, North York General Hospital; Asst Prof Family & Commun Med, University of Toronto; (416)493-2639; Fax. (416)493-2125; slofsky@sympatico.ca.

LOFTERS, Aisha K; St Michael's Hosp, 30 Bond St, Toronto ON M5B 1W8; Baltimore(MA) (USA)'04; CCFP; Staff, St Michael's Hospital; (416)867-7428

LOGACHEV, Evgeny; Red Deer Reg Hosp Centre, 3942 50A Ave, Red Deer AB T4N 4E7; Staff, Red Deer Regional Hospital Centre; (403)343-4422

LOGAN, Alexander G; Mount Sinai Hosp, Mount Sinai Hospital 435-600 University Ave, Toronto ON M5G 1X5; Tor'66; FRCPC; IntMed (Hypertension). Ac Staff, Toronto General Hospital - UHN; Sr Scientist, Mount Sinai Hospital; (416)586-4800 x5187; Fax. (416)586-5039; alogan@mtsinai.on.ca.

LOGAN, Alison C; Manitoba Clinic, 790 Sherbrook St, Winnipeg MB R3A 1M3; Man'92; BSc; FRCSC; ObstGyn. (204)774-6541; Fax. (204)775-6373.

LOGAN, Cecile A M; CSSSG-Hop de Gatineau, 909 boul de la Verendrye O, Gatineau QC J8P 7H2; West Indies (Jamaica)'76; MB BS; FRCPC; AnatPath (Gastrointestinal Disorders). Staff, Hôpital de Gatineau; (819)966-6100

LOGAN, Charlotte A; Hotel-Dieu Grace Hosp, 1030 Ouellette Ave, Windsor ON N9A 1E1; Detroit (USA)'97; Staff, Hôtel-Dieu Grace Hospital.

LOGAN, David A; MD Health Med Centre, 186 Main St S, Brampton ON L6W 2E2; London (England)'57; MB; BSc; LMSSA; LMCC; (905)456-7774; Fax. (905)456-1158.

LOGAN, Diane M; London Reg Cancer Centre, 790 Commissioners Rd E, London ON N6A 4L6; Ott'79; FRCPC; IntMed; MedOncol. Dep Chief Div of Med Oncol, London Health Sciences Centre - University Hospital; Assoc Prof, University of Western Ontario; Langs: English; French; (519)685-8640; Fax. (519)685-8624.

LOGAN, Dolores A F; Regina Community Clinic, 1106 Winnipeg St, Regina SK S4R 1J6; Sask'84; CCFP; Clin Instructor, University of Saskatchewan; (306)543-7880; Fax. (306)543-6888; dlogan@reginacommunityclinic.ca.

LOGAN, Heather; Addiction Services, 65 Brunswick St, Fredericton NB E3B 1G5; Dal'01; Staff, Dr Everett Chalmers Regional Hospital; (506)452-5558

LOGAN, Karl John; IWK Health Centre, PO Box 9700 Rpo CSC 5850-5980 University Ave, Halifax NS B3K 6R8; Liverpool (England)'99; MB ChB; Staff, IWK Health Centre; (902)470-8888

LOGAN, Laurie A; Fairmont Medical Bldg, 510-750 Broadway W, Vancouver BC V5Z 1H4; Qns'82; CCFP; FCFP; Ad Staff, Vancouver General Hospital - Centennial Pavillion; Vis Staff Privil, BC Women's Hospital & Health Centre; Clin Instructor, University of British Columbia; Langs: Bilingual(English/French); (604)879-5385; Fax. (604)879-8568.

LOGAN, Louise C; Sudbury Reg Hosp-Laurentian, 41 Ramsey Lake Rd, Sudbury ON P3E 5J1; Mon'97; CCFP; CCFP(E.M.); Staff, Health Sciences North-Laurentian Site; (705)675-4700

LOGAN, Patrick A; PO Box 1750, New Liskeard ON P0J 1P0; Tor'84; Ac Staff, Temiskaming Hospital; (705)647-8133

LOGAN, R Brent; 403-400 Crowfoot Cres NW, Calgary AB T3G 5H6; Cal'75; (403)970-9008; Fax. (403)547-2029.

LOGAN, Renee C; LFCA TC Meaford, RR 1 31 CF HSves C det Meaford, Meaford ON N4L 1W5; Ott'93; CCFP; FCFP; (519)538-6748; Fax. (519)538-6689.

LOGAN, Vance H; Dartmouth Gen Hosp, 325 Pleasant St, Dartmouth NS B2Y 4G8; Dal'79; BSc; MSc; FRCPC; Anes. Staff, Dartmouth General Hospital; Lecturer Anes, Dalhousie University; (902)465-8316

LOGAN, Vance M; C102-219 St Clair Ave W, Toronto ON M4V 1R3; Qns'87; FRCPC; Psy. (416)968-0660; Fax. (416)968-0660.

LOGAN, William J; The Hosp for Sick Children, 555 University Ave, Toronto ON M5G 1X8; Chicago(IL) (USA)'63; DABPed; DABPN; FRCPC; Neur. Chief Div of Neurol, The Hospital For Sick Children; Prof Ped Neurol, University of Toronto; (416)813-6660; Fax. (416)813-6334; william.logan@sickkids.ca.

LOGANATHAN, Rajes Wary; Denison Family Med Centre, 8-7380 McCowan Rd, Markham ON L3S 3H8; Jaffna (Sri Lanka)'86; CCFP; (905)944-0100; Fax. (905)944-8599.

LOGARAKIS, Nick F; SGH Medical Hall, 316-3030 Lawrence Ave E, Scarborough ON M1P 2T7; Tor'95; FRCSC; Urol (Oncology). Consultant, Bridgepoint Health Centre; Staff Urol, The Scarborough Hospital - General Campus; Langs: Greek; French; (416)439-8897; Fax. (416)439-6128.

LOGARIDIS, Terry E; The Court, 316-2863 Ellesmere Rd, Scarborough ON M1E 5E9; Athens (Greece)'77; BSc(McG); FRCSC; ObstGyn (Colposcopy). Ac Staff, Rouge Valley Health System - Centenary Health Centre Site; University of Toronto; (416)283-8121; Fax. (416)283-8171.

LOGE, John M; 4610 50 Ave, Bonnyville AB T9N 1A4; Man'94; BSc; CCFP; (780)826-3346; Fax. (780)826-6362.

LOGSETTY, Giridhar; 2475 Bloor St W, Toronto ON M6S 1P7; Tor'96; FRCPC; IntMed; Cardiol. Staff, St Joseph's Health Centre; (416)352-7445; Fax. (416)352-7447.

LOGSETTY, Niraja; Glenmore Landing, A301-1600 90 Ave SW, Calgary AB T2V 5A8; Qns'00; CCFP; (403)246-0200

LOGSETTY, Sarvesh; Health Sciences Centre, GC401-820 Sherbrook St, Winnipeg MB R3A 1R9; Alb'90; FACS; FRCSC; GenSurg (Burns). Staff, Health Sciences Centre; (204)774-6511

LOGUE, Kenneth J M; Balmoral Med Arts Facility, 401-1366 Yonge St, Toronto ON M4T 3A7; Alb'84; BSc; Clin Associate Immunodeficiency Clinic, Toronto General Hospital - UHN; Clin Associate Med, University of Toronto; (416)966-0178; Fax. (416)929-0843; dr.logue@stclairmedical.com.

LOH, Alvin W H; Surrey Place Centre, 2 Surrey Pl, Toronto ON M5S 2C2; Tor'00; FRCPC; Peds (Developmental Pediatrics). Staff Peds, The Hospital For Sick Children; Staff, Holland Bloorview Kids Rehabilitation Hospital; (416)925-5141

LOH, Diana P Y; 300-5511 West Boulevard, Vancouver BC V6M 4H3; Malaya (Malaysia)'56; DCH(Lond); FRCPC; Psy. Staff, Grandview-Woodlands Mental Health Team; Langs: Mandarin; Cantonese; (604)264-9400

LOH, Eldon; St Joseph's HC-Parkwood Hosp, 4F-801 Commissioners Rd E, London ON N6C 5J1; Wes'05; FRCPC; PhysMed&Rehab. Staff, Parkwood Hospital - St Joseph's Health Care; (519)685-4080

LOH, George; 110 Keefer St, Vancouver BC V6A 1X4; Dal'58; Langs: Mandarin; Cantonese; (604)688-9968; Fax. (604)688-9795; lohgeorge@hotmail.com.

LOH, Karmen K M; 3770 Oak St, Vancouver BC V6H 2M3; UBC'86; Langs: Cantonese; Mandarin; (604)873-1838

LOH, Lawrence C; Main Street Med Centre, 9-10886 Hurontario St, Brampton ON L7A 3R9; Wes'06; FRCPC; Public Health & Preventive Med;CCFP; (905)846-7477

LOHLUN, Graham B; 101-6603 132 Ave NW, Edmonton AB T5C 2A4; S.Africa (South Africa)'94; (780)476-1388; Fax. (780)473-3530.

LOHMANN, Reinhard C; London HSC-Victoria Hosp, A2 401-800 Commissioners Rd E, London ON N6A 5W9; Kiel (Germany)'61; FACP; FRCPC; IntMed (Lymphoma); Hem. Consultant HemOncol, London Health Sciences Centre - Victoria Campus; Staff, St Joseph's Hospital - St Joseph's Health Care; Staff, St Thomas Elgin General Hospital; Staff, Stratford General Hospital - Huron Perth Healthcare Alliance; Consultant, London Regional Cancer Centre; Clin Assoc Prof, University of Western Ontario; (519)685-8479; Fax. (519)685-8294.

LOHMANN, Tara E; Peter Lougheed Centre, 3500 26 Ave NE, Calgary AB T1Y 6J4; Qns'06; FRCPC; IntMed; Respir. Staff, Peter Lougheed Centre; (403)943-4971; Fax. (403)943-5508.

LOHRASBE, Happy; Dr Harpreet Lohrasbe Inc, 212-1641 Hillside Ave, Victoria BC V8T 5G1; Mysore (India)'79; MB BS; FRCPC; Psy (Anxiety & Mood Disorders). (250)472-0381; Fax. (250)472-0382.

LOHRASBE, Shabehram S; PO Box 2010 Stn Main, Sidney BC V8L 3S3; Mysore (India)'77; MB BS; FRCPC; Psy (Forensic Psychiatry).

LOHRENZ, Keith S; 1125 Mayor Magrath Dr S, Lethbridge AB T1K 2P9; Sask'93; CCFP; FCFP; (403)942-3600

LOHRISCH, Caroline A; BC Cancer Agency-Vancouver CC, 600 10th Ave W, Vancouver BC V5Z 4E6; Wes'94; BSc; FRCPC; IntMed (Breast Cancer); MedOncol. Staff, BC Cancer Agency Vancouver Centre; Clin Assoc Prof, University of British Columbia; Langs: French; Spanish; (604)877-6000 x2740; Fax. (604)877-0585; clohrisch@bccancer.bc.ca.

LOHSER, Jens; 2449-910 10th Ave W, Vancouver BC V5Z 4E3; Tor'99; FRCPC; Anes (Thoracic Anesthesia). Clin Instructor, Vancouver General Hospital - Centennial Pavillion; Clin Instructor, Stanford University Hospital; Clin Instructor, University of British Columbia; Langs: German; (604)875-4304; Fax. (604)875-5209; jens.lohser@vch.ca.

LOIGNON, Caroline; CLSC de la Haute Yamaska, 294 rue Deragon, Granby QC J2G 5J5; Mon'90; Staff, Centre Hospitalier de Granby; Langs: English; (450)375-1442; Fax. (450)375-1304.

LOIGNON, Julie; CHUS-Hop Fleurimont, 3001 12e Av N, Sherbrooke QC J1H 5N4; Sher'84; FRCPC; Peds. Staff, Centre Hospitalier Universitaire de Sherbrooke-Hopital Fleurimont; (819)346-1110 x14644; Fax. (819)564-5398; julie.loignon@usherbrooke.ca.

LOIGNON, Marie-Josee; CHUS-Hop Fleurimont, 3001 12e av N, Sherbrooke QC J1H 5N4; Sher'03; FRCPC; Anes. Staff, Centre Hospitalier Universitaire de Sherbrooke-Hopital Fleurimont; (819)346-1110 x14403; Fax. (819)820-6413.

LOISEL, France; Ctr Hosp Affilie-Enfant-Jesus, 1401 18e rue, Quebec QC G1J 1Z4; Laval'95; FRCPC; Anes (Intensive Care); Critical Care Medicine (P.Q.). Staff, Centre Hospitalier Affilié Universitaire de Québec - Hôpital De L'Enfant Jésus; (418)649-0252

LOISEL, Suzanne; Inst U en Sante Mentale de QC, 2601 rue de la Canardiere, Quebec QC G1J 2G3; Laval'88; Staff, Institut Universitaire Sante; (418)663-5386

LOISEL, Yves; Ctr Hosp Affilie-St-Sacrement, 1050 ch Sainte-Foy, Quebec QC G1S 4L8; Laval'91; FRCPC; DiagRad. Staff, Centre Hospitalier Affilié Universitaire de Québec - Hôpital du St-Sacrement; (418)682-7511

LOISELLE, Andre; Havre Les Quatre Saisons, 6767 rue Cartier, Montreal QC H2G 3G2; Mon'77; (514)490-2429 x3100

LOISELLE, Denis; Direction de la Sante Publique, 1-205 boul de York O, Gaspe QC G4X 2W5; Mon'78; (418)368-4626; Fax. (418)368-1301; denis_loiselle@ssss.gouv.qc.ca.

LOISELLE, Francois; Clinique Med Chateauguay, 120 boul Saint-Jean-Baptiste, Chateauguay QC J6K 3A9; Mon'92; ObstGyn. (450)691-6104; Fax. (450)691-5235.

LOISELLE, Frederick B; 108-911 Island Hwy, Campbell River BC V9W 2C2; Cal'06; PlasSurg. (250)287-8077

LOISELLE, Joel A; St Boniface Gen Hosp, L2035-409 Tache Ave, Winnipeg MB R2H 2A6; Sask'97; FRCPC; Anes. Staff, St Boniface General Hospital; (204)233-8563

LOISELLE, Luc-Aurele; Hotel-Dieu de Levis, 143 rue Wolfe, Levis QC G6V 3Z1; Laval'95; Staff, Hôtel-Dieu de Lévis; (418)835-7121

LOISELLE, Maurice; CSST-Direction Regionale Montr, 1 Complexe Desjardins, Montreal QC H5B 1H1; Mon'78; (514)906-3135; Fax. (514)906-3133.

LOISELLE, Pierre; GMF Montee de la Baie, 3942 Ch Oka, St-Joseph-Du-Lac QC J0N 1M0; Mon'77; Langs: Bilingual(French/English); (450)473-3930; Fax. (450)473-2160.

LOISELLE, Rhea M; Allin Clinic, 10155 120 St NW, Edmonton AB T5K 2A2; Alb'92; BMedSci; CCFP; FCFP; (780)482-7551; Fax. (780)488-2056.

LOISKANDL, Barbara J; Downtown Med Centre, 527 Hugel Ave, Midland ON L4R 1V8; McM'86; BSc; Staff, Georgian Bay General Hospital - Midland; Clinical Asst Prof Family Med, McMaster University; (705)526-0721; Fax. (705)526-0943; dlc123@hotmail.ca.

LOISKANDL, Rainer H W; Downtown Med Centre, 527 Hugel Ave, Midland ON L4R 1V8; McM'84; Asst Prof, Georgian Bay General Hospital - Midland; Clinical Asst Prof Family Med, McMaster University; Asst Prof, Queen's University; (705)526-0721; Fax. (705)526-0943.

LOIZIDES, Photis; CSSS de Saint-Jerome, 290 rue de Montigny, Saint-Jerome QC J7Z 5T3; McG'04; FRCPC; PlasSurg. Staff, Hôtel-Dieu de Saint-Jérôme; (450)431-8200

LOK, Charmaine E; 8 North-844-200 Elizabeth St, Toronto ON M5G 2C4; McM'95; FRCPC; IntMed; Nephrol. Scientist, Toronto General Hospital - UHN; Consultant, Mount Sinai Hospital; (416)340-4140; charmaine.lok@uhn.on.ca.

LOK, Henry T C; William Osler HC-Etobicoke, 101 Humber College Blvd, Etobicoke ON M9V 1R8; (Taiwan)'68; MB; DA(McG); FRCPC; Anes (Intensive Care). Ac Staff Anes, William Osler Health System - Etobicoke General Hospital; Langs: Cantonese; Mandarin; (416)747-3400

LOK, Jennifer S; 402-1630 Pandosy St, Kelowna BC V1Y 1P7; Tor'99; BSc; FRCPC; Psy. (250)712-9807

LOK, Raymond T; 55 Park St, Inverness NS B0E 1N0; National Defense Med. Coll. (Taiwan)'77; CCFP; Staff, Inverness Consolidated Memorial Hospital; (902)258-3441; Fax. (902)258-3878.

LOK, San-Yu; Joseph Brant Mem Hosp, 1230 North Shore Blvd E, Burlington ON L7S 1W7; UBC'89; FRCPC; DiagRad. Staff, Joseph Brant Memorial Hospital; (905)632-3737 x5679

LOK, Winston A; Stapleford Med Clinic, 372 McCarthy Blvd N, Regina SK S4R 7M2; Witwatersrand (South Africa)'88; (306)545-3000; Fax. (306)545-5584.

LOKA, Safaa G T; St Mary Med Centre, 14-2120 North Park Dr, Brampton ON L6S 0C9; Baghdad (Iraq)'95; MB ChB; CCFP; (905)789-6279

LOKANATHAN, Ramesh; 1624 7th Ave, Prince George BC V2L 3P6; McG'91; VascSurg; GenSurg. Ac Staff, University Hospital of Northern British Columbia; Clin Assoc Prof, University of British Columbia; Langs: English; French; (250)561-2700; Fax. (250)561-2794.

LOKANATHAN, Vanita; 202-26 Hospital Dr, Peterborough ON K9J 7C3; McG'93; CCFP; (705)740-6867; Fax. (705)740-6881.

LOKE, Julian C P; William Osler HC-Etobicoke, 101 Humber College Blvd, Etobicoke ON M9V 1R8; Monash (Australia)'88; MB BS; BMedSci; FRCPC; Anes (Malignant Hyperthermia). Staff, William Osler Health System - Etobicoke General Hospital; Lecturer Anes, University of Toronto; (416)494-2120

LOKE, Mei Woei; King's Cross Med Centre, 120-7404 King George Blvd, Surrey BC V3W 0L4; Dal'06; CCFP; (604)594-7711

LOKEN, Jack D; Kelowna Gen Hosp, 2268 Pandosy St, Kelowna BC V1Y 1T2; Sask'65; Staff, Kelowna General Hospital; Asst Prof, University of British Columbia; (250)862-4000; jackloken@mac.com.

LOKEN, Steven D; Nanaimo Reg Gen Hosp, 1200 Dufferin Cres, Nanaimo BC V9S 2B7; Cal'01; FRCPC; AnatPath. Staff, Nanaimo Regional General Hospital; (250)755-7691 x2201

LOKHAT, M Hossen; Carlingwood Med Centre, 348 Woodroffe Ave, Ottawa ON K2A 3V5; Dublin (Ireland)'67; LRCPSI; LM; GenSurg (P.Q.) (Family Medicine). Langs: French; (613)728-4640; Fax. (613)728-4649; h.lokhat@gmail.com.

LOKOFF, Paul C; Markham Stouffville Hosp, PO Box 1800 Stn Main 381 Church St, Markham ON L3P 7P3; Tor'84; FRCPC; Anes. Staff/Chief Anes, Markham Stouffville Hospital; (905)472-7000

LOLAND, Peter; 577 5th Ave, Kamloops BC V2C 3R1; UBC'06; CCFP; (250)372-8568

LOMAGA, Mark; 102-333 Lakeshore Rd W, Mississauga ON L5H 1G9; Tor'04; FRCPC; Derm. Lecturer, Women's College Hospital; (905)274-9999; Fax. (905)274-9991.

LOMAX, Susan M; BC Women's Hosp & Health Ctre, 141-4500 Oak St, Vancouver BC V6H 3N1; UBC'82; FRCPC; Psy (Child & Adolescent Psychiatry). Clin Dir CAPE, BC Women's Hospital & Health Centre; Clinical Asst Prof, University of British Columbia; (604)875-2424

LOMBARD, Hermanus E; Yorkton Mental Health Centre, 270 Bradbrooke Dr, Yorkton SK S3N 2K6; Orange Free State (South Africa)'82; MB ChB; MMed(Psych); FFPsy(S.A.); FRCPC; Psy. Psychiatrist, Yorkton Mental Health & Addiction Centre; (306)786-0558; Fax. (306)786-0556; hermanus.lombard@shr.sk.ca.

LOMBARD, Jan H; Valley Med Clinic, PO Box 455, Fort Qu'Appelle SK S0G 1S0; Pretoria (South Africa)'86; MB ChB; LMCC; Staff, All Nations Healing Hospital; (306)332-4516; Fax. (306)332-5889.

LOMBARD, Jeane; Rhythm Health, 601 67 Ave SW, Calgary AB T2V 0M3; (South Africa)'98; MB ChB; (403)228-5866; Fax. (403)252-7442.

LOMBARD, Jennifer J; Western Mem Reg Hosp, PO Box 2005 Stn Main 1 Brookfield Ave, Corner Brook NL A2H 6J7; Mem'00; FRCPC; DiagRad. Staff, Western Memorial Regional Hospital; (709)637-5000

LOMBARD, Schalk J; South Hill Med Practice, 5-2685 2nd Ave W, Prince Albert SK S6V 5E3; Pretoria (South Africa)'85; MB ChB; Dip SportMed; MHSc(AvMed); DAvMed; CCFP; (306)922-9570; Fax. (306)922-2513.

LOMBARD, Theodore P; 184 No 6 School Rd RR 7, Brantford ON N3T 5L9; Witwatersrand (South Africa)'77; MB ChB; MMed(Anes.); FRCPC; Anes (Intensive Care Medicine). Staff Anes, The Brant Community Healthcare System - Brantford General Hospital Site; Langs: Afrikaans.

LOMBARD, Willem S J; Kitimat Gen Hosp & Health Ctr, 920 Lahakas Blvd S, Kitimat BC V8C 2S3; Stellenbosch (South Africa)'96; MB ChB; MMed; FRCSC; GenSurg. Staff General Surgeon, Kitimat Hospital & Health Centre; Langs: Afrikaans; (250)632-8671; Fax. (250)632-8670.

LOMBARDI, Luciano P; Victoria Health Centre, 521 Victoria Park Ave, Scarborough ON M4C 5H1; Tor'72; Med Staff Family Pract, Toronto East General Hospital Inc; Langs: Italian; Spanish; (416)690-8043; Fax. (416)690-8913.

LOMBARDI, Pietro; 4A-62 Overlea Blvd, Toronto ON M4H 1C4; Tor'92; CCFP; FCFP; Langs: Italian; (416)452-8800; Fax. (416)425-8801.

LOMBARDI, Rocco A; Lakeridge HC-Bowmanville Site, 47 Liberty St S, Bowmanville ON L1C 2N4; Tor'00; CCFP; CCFP(E.M.); Staff ER, The Scarborough Hospital - General Campus; Staff, Lakeridge Health - Bowmanville Site; Staff, Lakeridge Health - Port Perry Site; Langs: Italian; Spanish; French; (905)623-3331; rocco.lombardi@powergate.ca.

LONERGAN, Guy; Dir de la Sante Publique-Mtl, 1301 rue Sherbrooke E, Montreal QC H2L 1M3; Mon'85; Staff, Centre Hospitalier l'Université De Montréal (CHUM) - Hôpital Saint-luc; (514)528-2400 x3838

LONERGAN, Marc; Hop Du Sacre-Coeur De Mtl, 5400 boul Gouin O, Montreal QC H4J 1C5; McG'73; FRCPC; Psy (Consultation-Liaison). Staff Psychosomatic Med, Hôpital du Sacre-Coeur de Montréal; Clinical Asst Prof, Universite de Montreal; Langs: Bilingual(English/French); Bilingual(French/English); (514)338-2070; Fax. (514)338-3187; marc.lonergan@umontreal.ca.

LONEY, Elgin M; North Bruce Med Services, PO Box 88 2 Ferndale Rd, Lions Head ON N0H 1W0; Tor'78; MD; Ac Staff, Grey Bruce Health Services - Wiarton Site; Ac Staff, Grey Bruce Health Services - Owen Sound; Langs: French; (519)793-6100; Fax. (519)793-6101; emloney@eastlinnk.ca.

LONG, Adrian L H; Cargill Grain Bldg, 102-240 Graham Ave, Winnipeg MB R3C 0J7; Bristol (England)'65; MB ChB; DOphth; Langs: Portuguese; Polish; Chinese; Spanish; German; (204)925-9700; Fax. (204)947-2996.

LONG, Ann Marie E; Hys Med Centre, 604-11010 101 St NW, Edmonton AB T5H 4B9; Alb'96; BSc; MSc; FRCSC; ObstGyn. (780)421-4728; Fax. (780)426-6698.

LONG, Barry H; 404-235 Danforth Ave, Toronto ON M4K 1N2; Wes'74; FRCPC; IntMed; Derm. (416)465-2556; Fax. (416)465-3033.

LONG, Bradley F; Health Sciences North-Laurenti, 41 Ramsey Lake Rd, Sudbury ON P3E 5J1; Saba (Netherlands Antilles)'08; Staff, Health Sciences North-Laurentian Site.

LONG, Brenda M; Senior's Clinic-Edmonton Clini, 1A-1400 University Ave NW, Edmonton AB T6G 1Z1; Cal'92; CCFP; Staff, University of Alberta Hospital; (780)407-6947; Fax. (780)407-2006; blong@cha.ab.ca.

LONG, Briar A; U of Guelph-Student Hlth Serv, 158-50 Stone Rd E, Guelph ON N1G 2W1; McM'97; FRCPC; Psy. (519)824-4120 x52131

LONG, Cory S; Tantramar Health Centre, A-2 Main St, Sackville NB E4L 4A3; Dal'06; CCFP; (506)364-4734; Fax. (506)364-4737.

LONG, Edward G S; Oshawa Clinic, 117 King St E, Oshawa ON L1H 1B9; Alb'69; FRCPC; IntMed. Staff, Lakeridge Health - Oshawa Site; (905)723-8551; Fax. (905)723-6319.

LONG, G Richard; Aberhart Centre, 8334A-11402 University Ave NW, Edmonton AB T6G 2J3; Man'71; IntMed (Respirology). Staff, University of Alberta; (780)407-1427; Fax. (780)407-1429; richard.long@ualberta.ca.

LONG, Helene; Ctr Reg du Diabete Carl, 1515 boul Chomedey, Laval QC H7V 3Y7; Mon'89; FRCPC; IntMed (Diabetes); Endocrin&Metab; Endocrin (P.Q.). Coord Centre du Diabete Reg de Laval, Centre de Sante et de Services Sociaux; Langs: Bilingual(French/English); (450)978-8607

LONG, Jack A; Hotel-Dieu d'Arthabaska, 5 rue des Hospitalieres, Victoriaville QC G6P 6N2; Sher'03; ObstGyn. Staff, Hotel-Dieu d'Arthabaska; (819)357-2030

LONG, Jason A; Misericordia Community Hosp, 3F-16940 87 Ave NW, Edmonton AB T5R 4H5; Alb'95; LRCP; LMCC; MD; BMedSci; FRCPC; Psy. Staff Psy, Covenant Health - Misericordia Community Hospital; (780)735-2594; Fax. (780)735-2595; jasonlong@shaw.ca.

LONG, Lindsay C; Alberta Children's Hosp, 2888 Shaganappi Trail NW, Calgary AB T3B 6A8; Cal'05; FRCPC; Peds. Staff, Alberta Children's Hospital; (403)955-2953; Fax. (403)955-3055.

LONG, Malcolm J; University of Alberta Hosp, 8440 112 St NW, Edmonton AB T6G 2B7; Alb'86; CCFP; CCFP(E.M.); Medical Staff Emerg, University of Alberta Hospital; Asst Prof Emerg & Family Med, University of Alberta; (780)407-3229; Fax. (780)407-7215.

LONG, Michelle; Port Hope Med Centre, 202-249 Ontario St, Port Hope ON L1A 3Y9; Tor'90; (905)885-8371; Fax. (905)885-7695.

LONG, Rex; Delta Health Sciences Centre, 206-4515 Harvest Dr, Delta BC V4K 4L1; Man'86; Physician, Delta Health Sciences Centre; (604)946-7211; Fax. (604)946-8449.

LONG, S Ronald; Medical Clinic Associates, 200-3207 30 Ave, Vernon BC V1T 2C6; Wes'82; (250)549-1216; Fax. (250)549-3985.

LONG, Shane B; 406-2299 Dundas St W, Toronto ON M6R 1X7; Tor'86; (416)535-3511; Fax. (416)535-5993.

LONG, W John; St Joseph's Gen Hosp, 70 Spine Rd, Elliot Lake ON P5A 1X2; Melbourne (Australia)'61; MB BS; FRCS; Court Staff, Blind River District Health Centre; Chief Dept of Surg, St Joseph's General Hospital Elliot Lake; Med Examiner, Canadian Civil Air; Assoc Prof Gen Surg, Northern Ontario School of Medicine; (705)848-7181; Fax. (705)848-9006; johnlong37@msn.com.

LONG-INNES, Malcolm C; Eastport Shopping Centre, 3-200 52 St NE, Calgary AB T2A 4K8; (South Africa)'81; (403)569-7464; Fax. (403)248-6896.

LONGAIR, Terrence L; Bigelow Fowler Clinic West, 30 Jerry Potts Blvd W, Lethbridge AB T1K 5M5; Alb'79; CCFP; (403)381-8444; Fax. (403)381-8166.

LONGINO, Peter D; Univ of Calgary Sport Med Ctr, 330-2500 University Dr NW, Calgary AB T2N 1N4; Cal'00; FRCSC; OrthSurg. (403)210-8424; Fax. (403)282-6170; phartwic@ucalgary.ca.

LONGLAND, John W S; Atwood Med Clinic, 101-143 Fourth Ave S, Williams Lake BC V2G 1J8; Pretoria (South Africa)'06; MB ChB; Langs: Afrikaans; (250)398-5162

LONGLEY, Catherine D; St Michael's Hosp, 30 Bond St, Toronto ON M5B 1W8; Wes'96; BSc(Hons); CCFP; CCFP(E.M.); FCFP; Staff, St Michael's Hospital; (416)864-5095

LONGMAN, Shane A; 4-3855 9th Ave, Port Alberni BC V9Y 4T9; Wes'99; CCFP; (250)736-1900; Fax. (250)736-1902.

LONGPRE, Daniele; Clinique Med L'Actuel, 1130-1001 Boul De Maisonneuve, Montreal QC H2L 4P9; Sher'82; Médecin, Institut National de Sante Publique du Quebec; Langs: English; (514)524-1001; Fax. (514)524-3831.

LONGPRE, Denis; Hop Jean-Talon, 1385 rue Jean-Talon E, Montreal QC H2E 1S6; Mon'78; Staff Emerg Psy, CSSS du Coeur de l'Isle Hôpital Jean-Talon; (514)495-6767

LONGRIDGE, Neil S; Gordon & Leslie Diamond HCC, 4F-2775 Laurel St, Vancouver BC V5Z 1M9; Newcastle (England)'69; MB BS; MRCP; FRCS; BSc; FRCSC; Otol. Dir Neurotology Unit, Vancouver General Hospital - Centennial Pavillion; Clin Prof, University of British Columbia; (604)875-4645; Fax. (604)875-4644; nslongridge@hotmail.com.

LONGSTAFFE, Albert E; 304-400 Tache Ave, Winnipeg MB R2H 3C3; Man'71; FRCSC; OrthSurg. Staff, St Boniface General Hospital; Staff, Victoria General Hospital; University of Manitoba; (204)233-4710; Fax. (204)235-1654.

LONGSTAFFE, Sally E A; Pediatric Adolescent Clinic, 102-200 Goulet St, Winnipeg MB R2H 0R8; Man'71; FRCPC; Peds. Dir Child Development Clinic, Health Sciences Centre; Prof, University of Manitoba; slongstaffe@hsc.mb.ca.

LONGTIN, J D N Yves; Hôpital Laval, 2725 ch Sainte-Foy, Quebec QC G1V 4G5; Sher'00; FRCPC; MedMicrobiol; Microbio & Infect Dis (P.Q.). Staff, Hôpital Laval; (418)656-8711 x3078

LONGTIN, Jean; CHUQ-Ctr Hosp Univ Laval, 2705 boul Laurier, Quebec QC G1V 4G2; Laval'03; FRCPC; MedMicrobiol; Microbio & Infect Dis (P.Q.). Staff, Centre Hospitalier Universitaire de Quebec-CHUL; (418)656-4141 x47882

LONGTIN, Pierre; Clinique Med Ahuntsic, 115-241 rue Fleury O, Montreal QC H3L 1V2; Mon'64; FRCPC; Peds. Staff, Hôpital Ste-Justine; Staff, Centre Hospitalier l'Université De Montréal (CHUM) - Hôpital Saint-luc; Staff, Centre Hospitalier Fleury; (514)381-1862; Fax. (514)381-1088.

LONGTIN, Richard; Clinique Med Chemin St-Jean, 675 ch De Saint-Jean, La Prairie QC J5R 2L2; Mon'73; (450)444-2002; Fax. (450)444-4920.

LONGVAL, Michael; CHUS-Hotel-Dieu, 580 rue Bowen S, Sherbrooke QC J1G 2E8; Sher'89; CCFP; Staff, Centre Hospitalier Universitaire de Sherbrooke-Hôpital Hôtel-Dieu; (819)346-1110

LONN, Eva M; Hamilton HS-General Site, 237 Barton St E, Hamilton ON L8L 2X2; Hebrew (Israel)'84; MSc; FACC; ABCD; ABIM; LRCPS; FRC; FRCPC; FRCPC; Cardiol; IntMed (Adult Cardiology). Staff Cardiol, Hamilton Health Sciences Centre - Hamilton General Hospital; Prof Med, McMaster University; Langs: German; Hebrew; Romanian; (905)526-0970; Fax. (905)527-5380; lonnem@mcmaster.ca.

LOO, Karen M K; Halton HCS Corp-Oakville, 327 Reynolds St, Oakville ON L6J 3L7; McG'00; FRCPC; Anes. Staff, Halton Healthcare Services Corporation - Oakville Site; (905)845-2571

LOO, Tip Wah; Faculty of Medicine, 7342-1 King's College Cir, Toronto ON M5S 1A8; Tor'90.

LOO, Vivian G; MUHC-Royal Victoria Hosp, L5 06-687 av des Pins O, Montreal QC H3A 1A1; McG'85; FRCPC; IntMed; InfectDis; MedMicrobiol. Microbiologiste, McGill University Health Centre - Royal Victoria Hospital; (514)934-1934 x42818; Fax. (514)934-4476; vivian.loo@muhc.mcgill.ca.

LOO, Wei Jing; St Joseph's Health Care, PO Box 5777 Stn B A2 513-268 Grosvenor St, London ON N6A 4V2; New South Wales (Australia)'97; Derm. Staff, St Joseph's Hospital - St Joseph's Health Care; (519)646-6100

LOO, Wilson W S; 10A-30 Eglinton Ave W, Mississauga ON L5R 3E7; (Hong Kong)'74; MB BS; MPA; CCFP; FCFP; Court Staff, St Michael's Hospital; Langs: Cantonese; (905)712-2288; Fax. (905)712-8228; wilsonloo@sympatico.ca.

LOOCK, Christine A; BC Children's Hosp, 4480 Oak St, Vancouver BC V6H 3V4; Boston(MA) (USA)'81; FRCPC; Peds (Developmental Pediatrics). Staff, BC Children's Hospital; Consultant, Ministry of Health-British Columbia; Assoc Prof, University of British Columbia; (604)453-8383

LOOI-LYONS, C Lian; Trillium Hlth Ctr-Mississauga, 100 Queensway W, Mississauga ON L5B 1B8; Mem'89; FRCPC; Anes. Staff, Trillium Health Centre - Mississauga; (905)848-7628

LOOK, Didier S; Lakeshore Gen Hosp, 160 av Stillview, Pointe-Claire QC H9R 2Y2; Saba (Netherlands Antilles)'03; CCFP; Staff, Lakeshore General Hospital - Pointe Claire; (514)630-2225

LOOK, J Michael; Norburn Med Clinic, 200-4012 Hastings St, Burnaby BC V5C 2H9; UBC'87; Clinical Asst Prof Family Pract, University of British Columbia; (604)299-2677; Fax. (604)298-6656.

LOOK HONG, Nicole J; Sunnybrook Hlth Sciences Ctre, T2 102-2075 Bayview Ave, Toronto ON M4N 3M5; Tor'04; FRCSC; GenSurg. Staff, Sunnybrook Health Sciences Centre; (416)480-6002

LOOK HONG, William A; Southlake Reg Health Centre, 596 Davis Dr, Newmarket ON L3Y 2P9; West Indies (Jamaica)'73; MB BS; DABPN; FAPA; FRCPC; Psy (Neurology). Staff Psy, Southlake Regional Health Centre; (905)895-4521 x2904; Fax. (905)830-5977.

LOOK KIN, Karen T; Davisville Family Pract Unit, 600-1881 Yonge St, Toronto ON M4S 3C4; (Jamaica)'97; CCFP; (416)932-3172; Fax. (416)440-0238.

LOOMER, Richard L; 102-65 Richmond St, New Westminster BC V3L 5P5; Minneapolis(MN) (USA)'65; FRCSC; OrthSurg. Staff, Royal Columbian Hospital; Staff Orth. Surg., BC Sports Medicine Clinic; (604)526-7885; Fax. (604)525-4006.

LOONTJENS, Bernadette; CSSS du Nord de Lanaudière, 1000 boul Sainte-Anne, St-Charles-Brromee QC J6E 6J2; Louvain (Belgium)'90; Staff Geriatrie, Centre Hospitalier Régional de Lanaudière; Langs: English; Dutch; (450)759-8222

LOOPER, Karl J; SMBD Jewish Gen Hosp, 3755 ch Cote-Sainte-Catherine, Montreal QC H3T 1E2; Ott'95; FRCPC; Psy. Staff, Sir Mortimer B Davis Jewish General; Langs: English; French; (514)340-8222 x5890

LOOSLEY-MILLMAN, Margot E; Fontbonne Bldg, 4F-301 James St S, Hamilton ON L8P 3B6; McM'85; BSc; PhD; FRCSC; ObstGyn. Staff, St Joseph's Healthcare - Charlton Campus; Assoc Staff, Hamilton Health Sciences Centre - McMaster University Medical Centre; Assoc Prof, McMaster University; (905)572-1117

LOOTS, Leani; Meadow Lake Associate Clinic, PO Box 1510, Meadow Lake SK S9X 1Z1; Witwatersrand (South Africa)'01; MB ChB; (306)236-5661; Fax. (306)236-4355.

LOOVERE, Linda A; 4825 Dalhousie Dr NW, Calgary AB T3A 6K7; Qns'03; FRCPC; Peds. (403)239-9333; Fax. (403)208-1648.

LOPASCHUK, Catharine C; Workers' Comp Board, PO Box 2415 Stn Main 9912 107 St, Edmonton AB T5J 2S5; UBC'84; CCFP; (780)498-3999

LOPATKA, Joan E; 9803 34 Ave NW, Edmonton AB T6E 5X9; Alb'78; FRCPC; Peds. Ac Staff Privil Children's Health Centre, University of Alberta Hospital; Ac Staff Privil, Covenant Health - Grey Nuns Community Hospital; Clinical Asst Prof, University of Alberta; (780)461-9299; Fax. (780)465-7267.

LOPER, Raymond H; PO Box 23, Caronport SK S0H 0S0; (306)756-2262

LOPES, Laudelino M; London HSC-Victoria Hosp, PO Box 5010 Stn B B2 412-800 Commissioners Rd E, London ON N6A 5W9; Valencia (Spain)'77; FRCSC; ObstGyn. Staff, London Health Sciences Centre - Victoria Campus; (519)685-8500

LOPES, Paulo; Polyclinique Rosemont, 3377 boul Rosemont, Montreal QC H1X 1K4; Mon'00; (514)798-8688

LOPEZ, Carlos A; 102-65 Richmond St, New Westminster BC V3L 5P5; McM'06; OrthSurg. (604)526-7885

LOPEZ, Christopher J; 106-2425 Tecumseh Rd E, Windsor ON N8W 1E6; McM'06; OrthSurg.

LOPEZ, Elena; Sunny Hill Hlth Ctr for Childr, 3644 Slocan St, Vancouver BC V5M 3E8; Mexico (Mexico)'90; FRCPC; MedGenetics. Staff, Sunny Hill Health Centre for Children; Langs: Spanish; (604)453-8300; Fax. (604)453-8338.

LOPEZ, Isabelle; CSSS de Laval, D 0193-1755 boul René-Laennec, Laval QC H7M 3L9; Sher'93; FRCPC; Psy. Staff, Hopital de la Cite de la santé; Langs: Spanish; English; French; (450)668-1010 x2758

LOPEZ, Jose F; 103 Hospital Dr, Saskatoon SK S7N 0W8; Seville (Spain)'54; BSc; FACP; FACC; FRCPC; IntMed (Cardiology). Att Physician Hemodynamic Lab, Royal University Hospital; Emeritus Prof Med, University of Saskatchewan; Langs: English; Spanish; (306)655-6863; Fax. (306)655-6708; jflopez@shaw.ca.

LOPEZ, Mirtha I; Selkirk Mental Health Centre, PO Box 9600 Stn Main 825 Manitoba Ave, Selkirk MB R1A 2B5; Buenos Aires (Argentina)'84; Staff, Selkirk Mental Health Centre; (204)482-3810

LOPEZ, Pedro G; Northeastern On Reg Cancer Ctr, 41 Ramsey Lake Rd, Sudbury ON P3E 5J1; Qns'82; FRCPC; IntMed; Hem; MedOncol. Staff, Health Sciences North-Laurentian Site; Asst Prof, University of Ottawa; (705)522-6237 x2320; Fax. (705)523-7329.

LOPEZ, Roehl P F; Properties Med Clinic, 5102 Rundlehorn Dr NE, Calgary AB T1Y 1C1; Sask'92; BSc(Hon Biol); Staff, Properties Medical Clinic; (403)280-2700; Fax. (403)285-2641.

LOPEZ AGUDELO, Jose E; Clinique Med Racicot, 520 av d'Avaugour, Boucherville QC J4B 0G6; (Other Foreign)'01; (450)449-7525

LOPEZ-ALONSO, Jose O; Royal Victoria Hosp, 201 Georgian Dr, Barrie ON L4M 6M2; (Cuba)'01; CCFP; Staff, Royal Victoria Regional Health Centre; (705)728-9090

LOPEZ BLANCO, Alejandra V; Cape Breton Hlthcare Complex, 1482 George St, Sydney NS B1P 1P3; Bogota (Colombia)'96; Staff, Cape Breton Healthcare Complex; (902)567-8000

LOPEZ GARDNER, Leonora L; Dauphin Med Clinic, 622 3rd St SW, Dauphin MB R7N 1R5; Man'08; CCFP.

LOPEZ OSORIO, Isabel; CHSLD La Piniere, 4895 rue Saint-Joseph, Laval QC H7C 1H6; Man'94; CCFP; (450)661-3305

LOPEZ-VALLE, Carlos A; CSSS de Chicoutimi, 305 rue Saint-Vallier, Chicoutimi QC G7H 5H6; Niterol (Brazil)'77; PhD(Transplantation); PlasSurg (P.Q.). Staff, Complexe hospitalier de la Sagamie; (418)541-1000

LOPEZ-VALLE, Hilda R; St Mary's Hosp Centre, 3830 av Lacombe, Montreal QC H3T 1M5; San Luis Potosi (Mexico)'80; Staff, St Mary's Hospital Centre; (514)345-3511

LOPUSHINSKY, Steven R; Alberta Children's Hosp, 2888 Shaganappi Trail NW, Calgary AB T3B 6A8; Cal'02; FRCSC; GenSurg (Pediatric General Surgery). Staff, Alberta Children's Hospital; (403)955-2460; Fax. (403)955-7634.

LOR, Huy Sroy; Clin Opht Normand Isabelle Inc, 28 ch du Golf E, St-Charles-Brromee QC J6E 2B4; Laval'07; Ophth. (450)753-9293

LORANGER, Benoit; Centre Medical Des Generations, 200-465 rue Bibeau, Saint-Eustache QC J7R 0C8; Mon'84; Staff, Hôpital de Saint-Eustache; Langs: English; (450)472-1955; Fax. (450)472-1905.

LORANGER, Christian; Hop Charles LeMoyne, 3120 boul Taschereau, Greenfield Park QC J4V 2H1; Sher'96; FRCSC; OrthSurg. Staff, Hopital Charles LeMoyne; (450)466-5000

LORANGER, Louise; 212-731 rue Galt O, Sherbrooke QC J1H 1Z1; Sher'88; Derm. Staff, Centre Hospitalier Universitaire de Sherbrooke-Hopital Fleurimont; Langs: English; French; (819)564-8843; lloranger@videotron.ca.

LORANGER, Martin; Hop Charles Lemoyne, 3120 boul Taschereau, Greenfield Park QC J4V 2H1; Sher'98; CCFP; CCFP(E.M.); FCFP; Staff EmergMed, Hopital Charles LeMoyne; Clin Prof, Universite de Sherbrooke; (450)466-5000

LORBER, Estelle; Herzl Family Practice Centre, 5757 rue Legare, Montreal QC H3S 1X9; Laval'86; CCFP; (514)340-8213

LORBER, Eva; The Doctors Bldg, 504-208 Bloor St W, Toronto ON M5S 3B4; Tor'71; Ad Staff Privil, Mount Sinai Hospital; Langs: Slovak; Hungarian; (416)922-0983; Fax. (416)922-3882.

LORBERG, Gunter W; Central North Correctional Ctr, 1501 Fuller Ave, Penetanguishene ON L9M 2H4; Wes'98; BSc; MPhil; FRCPC; Psy (Forensic Psychiatry). Staff, Waypoint Centre for Mental Health Care; Consultant Psy, Central North Correctional Centre; (705)549-9470; gunter.lorberg@rogers.com.

LORD, Christine; Clinique Med de Roberval, 714 boul Marcotte, Roberval QC G8H 1Z6; Mon'94; Staff, Hotel-Dieu de Roberval; (418)275-3833; Fax. (418)275-6747.

LORD, Christopher J; Edmonton Gen Cont Care Centre, 5Y-11111 Jasper Ave NW, Edmonton AB T5K 0L4; Edinburgh (Scotland)'66; CCFP; FCFP; Physician, Covenant Health - Edmonton General Continuing Care Centre; Clin Assoc Prof, University of Alberta; (780)482-8225; Fax. (780)452-5900.

LORD, Claire; Centre Sante Rene-Richard, CP 1300 32 3e Av, Chapais QC G0W 1H0; Laval'92; CCFP; (418)745-2591; Fax. (418)745-3038.

LORD, Francois; CHUS-Hop Hotel-Dieu, 580 rue Bowen S, Sherbrooke QC J1G 2E8; Laval'93; Staff, Hôpital Laval; Staff, Centre Hospitalier Universitaire de Sherbrooke-Hôpital Hôtel-Dieu; (819)346-1110

LORD, Frank R; Dr Georges-L Dumont Reg Hosp, 330 av Universite, Moncton NB E1C 2Z3; Sher'85; Staff, Dr Georges-L-Dumont University Hospital Centre; (506)862-4113; Fax. (506)862-4256.

LORD, Frederic; 1503-625 av President-Kennedy, Montreal QC H3A 1K2; Mon'94; FRCSC; Ophth (Cataract). Staff, Centre Hospitalier l'Université de Montréal (CHUM) - Hôpital Notre-Dame; Universite de Montreal; (514)849-9215; Fax. (514)849-5115.

LORD, Guillaume; CSSS de la Haute-Cote-Nord, RR 1 4 rue de l'Hopital, Les Escoumins QC G0T 1K0; Laval'05; Staff, Centre de santé des Côté-Nord; (418)233-2931

LORD, Hugh L; 7 Kingswood Ave, Rothesay NB E2E 5R5; West Indies (Jamaica)'68; MB BS; ObstGyn (Colposcopy). Consultant ObstGyn, Saint John Regional Hospital; Consultant, St Joseph's Hospital; Consultant, Charlotte County Hospital; Asst Prof, Dalhousie University; (506)848-2110

LORD, Helene; Hop Maisonneuve-Rosemont, 5415 boul de l'Assomption, Montreal QC H1T 2M4; Mon'88; Nephrol; IntMed. Staff, Hopital Maisonneuve-Rosemont; (514)252-3400

LORD, Jacinthe; Clinique Med St-Sulpice, 12-1420 rue Legendre E, Montreal QC H2M 1H5; Mon'84; (514)382-0552; Fax. (514)382-4324.

LORD, Jason A; Peter Lougheed Centre, 24-3500 26 Ave NE, Calgary AB T1Y 6J4; Qns'98; FRCPC; EmergMed (Intensive Care); Critical Care Medicine. Staff, Peter Lougheed Centre; (403)954-5488; Fax. (403)291-1491; jasonlord@albertahealthservices.ca.

LORD, Julien; 100-235 boul Rene-Levesque E, Montreal QC H2X 1N8; Laval'63; MS(Ed.); CSPQ; FRCSC; ObstGyn (Infertility). Prof ObstGyn, Universite de Montreal; Langs: Bilingual(French/English); (514)866-2446

LORD, Marie-Josee; Hotel-Dieu du Sacre-Coeur, 1 av du Sacre-Coeur, Quebec QC G1N 2W1; Laval'92; FRCPC; Psy (Pedology Psychiatry). Staff, Hotel-Dieu du Sacre-Coeur de Jesus de Quebec; Langs: Spanish; English; (418)529-6851

LORD, Martin; CHUM-Hotel-Dieu, 3840 rue Saint-Urbain, Montreal QC H2W 1T8; Laval'98; FRCPC; NuclearMed. Staff, Centre Hospitalier l'Université de Montréal (CHUM) - Hôtel-Dieu; (514)890-8000

LORD, Patricia; Clinique Med Laval, 1110 boul Vanier, Laval QC H7C 2R8; Mon'02; Langs: Bilingual(French/English); (450)661-2521; patricialord@videotron.ca.

LORD, Rene; Clinique Med St-Pierre, 200-85 rue Saint-Pierre, Saint-Constant QC J5A 1G8; Mon'76; (450)845-4646

LORD, Sarah E; 309-2818 Main St W, Vancouver BC V5T 0C1; UBC'05; FRCSC; GenSurg. (604)639-5371

LORD, Veronique; CSSS de Chicoutimi, 305 rue Saint-Vallier, Chicoutimi QC G7H 5H6; Laval'05; DiagRad. Staff, Complexe hospitalier de la Sagamie; (418)541-1000

LORDE, Ingrid L A; Bloor Med Clinic, 844 Bathurst, Toronto ON M5R 3G1; Qns'07; CCFP; (416)534-4214

LOREE, Scott B; PO Box 89140 Mackenzie Rpo, Calgary AB T2Z 3W3; Cal'05; CCFP; (403)984-4877; Fax. (403)984-4877.

LOREFICE, Sylvia E; Toronto East Gen Hosp Inc, 825 Coxwell Ave, Toronto ON M4C 3E7; Alb'02; FRCPC; Psy. Staff, Toronto East General Hospital Inc; (416)461-8272

LORENZ, Darren A; Mt Ida Medical Clinic, PO Box 1870 200 Trans Canada Hwy SW, Salmon Arm BC V1E 4P9; Cal'05; CCFP.

LORENZ, Konstantin; Queen Elizabeth II HSC, 10W-1276 South Park St, Halifax NS B3H 2Y9; Duisberg-Essen (Germany)'99; Staff, Queen Elizabeth II Health Sciences Centre - Victoria General Site.

LORENZEN, David; 17 Allandale Dr, St Catharines ON L2T 1V9; Tor'62; Hon Consultant, Niagara Health System - St Catharines General Site; Med Examiner Aviation USA & Canada & FAA USA, Ministry Of Transportation; Med Examiner Aviation USA & Canada FAA, Transport Canada; (289)438-2275; Fax. (905)684-3034; doc@drlorenzen.ca.

LORENZO, Armando J; The Hosp For Sick Children, 299-555 University Ave, Toronto ON M5G 1X8; (Panama)'94; FRCSC; Urol. Staff Div of Ped Urol, The Hospital For Sick Children; Langs: Spanish; (416)813-6580; Fax. (416)813-6461.

LORENZO, Thomas; 2A-2379 Bevan Ave, Sidney BC V8L 4M9; Cape Town (South Africa)'82; Fax. (250)656-4133.

LORENZON, C Gabriella; 306-460 Nanaimo St, Vancouver BC V5L 4W3; Milan (Italy)'82; Staff, Providence Health Care - Mount Saint Joseph Hospital; Langs: Italian; French; (604)255-9819; Fax. (604)255-9808.

LORETO, Chris J; Timmins & Dist Hosp, 700 Ross Ave E, Timmins ON P4N 8P2; Qns'92; CCFP; CCFP(E.M.); Clin Chief Emerg Dept/Med Dir, Timmins & District Hospital; Med Dir Orange Air Ambulance, Northeast Land Base Hospital Program; Preceptor Northern Ontario Family Med, University of Ottawa; (705)268-2391; Fax. (705)268-4948; cloreto@tadh.com.

LORETO, Michael P; Univ of Toronto, 2F-500 University Ave, Toronto ON M5G 1V7; Tor'07; FRCPC; DiagRad.

LORETTE, Jason G; 26 CF Health Services Centre, PO Box 5000 Rpo Greenwood, Greenwood NS B0P 1N0; Dal'10; CCFP.

LORIMER, John W; The Ottawa Hosp-Gen Campus, K 11-501 Smyth Rd, Ottawa ON K1H 8L6; Dal'76; FACS; FRCSC; GenSurg; VascSurg. Ac Staff, The Ottawa Hospital - General Campus; Ac Staff, The Ottawa Hospital - Civic Campus; Ac Staff, The Ottawa Hospital - Riverside Campus; Assoc Prof Surg, University of Ottawa; Langs: English; French; (613)737-8428

LORIOT, Marie-Helene; Hop Charles LeMoyne, 3120 boul Taschereau, Greenfield Park QC J4V 2H1; Mon'03; FRCSC; GenSurg. Staff, Hopital Charles LeMoyne; (450)466-5000

LORITZ, Frank; Beaches Wellness Centre, 2277 Queen St E, Toronto ON M4E 1G5; McM'83; CASM; Dip SportMed(SportMed); (416)698-7070; Fax. (416)698-7928.

LORNE, Jennifer G W; King Edward Mall, PO Box 38112, Vancouver BC V5Z 4L9; UBC'05; CCFP; (604)879-3900

LORQUET, Annie; CSSS de la Haute-Yamaska, 205 boul Leclerc O, Granby QC J2G 1T7; Sher'94; Staff, Centre Hospitalier de Granby; (450)375-8000

LORQUET, Yvan; Clin Med Fam D'Edmundston, 50 Av Bateman, Edmundston NB E3V 4A4; Laval'82; Staff, Hôpital regional d'Edmundston; Physician, Fraser Papers; Physician, Boise Alljoist Ltd; Langs: Bilingual(French/English); (506)735-4433; Fax. (506)739-1008.

LORRAIN, Brandene L; Child & Adolescence Serv Assoc, 10645 63 Ave NW, Edmonton AB T6H 1P7; Sask'95; BSc; FRCPC; Psy (Child Psychiatry). (780)438-0011; Fax. (780)437-6133.

LORRAINE, Joanne; Eli Lilly Canada, 3650 Danforth Ave, Scarborough ON M1N 2E8; Tor'86; MEd; FRCPC; IntMed (Diabetology). Court Staff, Toronto Rehabilitation Institute - Rumsey Centre; Assoc Dir Research, Eli Lilly Canada Inc; (416)699-7310; Fax. (416)699-7352.

LORTIE, Anne; Hôpital Ste-Justine, 3175 ch Cote-Sainte-Catherine, Montreal QC H3T 1C5; Mon'84; FRCPC; Peds; Electroenceph (P.Q.); Neur. Staff, Hôpital Ste-Justine; (514)345-4653; anne_lortie@ssss.gouv.qc.ca.

LORTIE, Carole; 200-3030 boul Le carrefour, Laval QC H7T 2P5; Mon'82; (450)686-8899; Fax. (450)686-7466.

LORTIE, Elise; CSSS Pierre Boucher, 1333 boul Jacques-Cartier E, Longueuil QC J4M 2A5; Mon'04; FRCPC; Anes. Staff, Centre Hospitalier Pierre Boucher; (450)468-8111

LORTIE, Gilles; Hotel-Dieu de Levis, 143 rue Wolfe, Levis QC G6V 3Z1; Laval'90; FRCPC; EmergMed;CCFP; CCFP(E.M.); Staff, Hôtel-Dieu de Lévis; Head Family Med, Université Laval; (418)835-7121

LORTIE, Jocelyne; Hotel-Dieu Du Sacre-Coeur, 1 av Du Sacre-Coeur, Quebec QC G1N 2W1; Laval'77; Staff, Hotel-Dieu du Sacre-Coeur de Jesus de Quebec; (418)529-6851; Fax. (418)691-0750.

LORTIE, Karine J; 311-1919 Riverside Dr, Ottawa ON K1H 1A2; Ott'03; FRCSC; ObstGyn. (613)526-3480

LORTIE, Marcel; CSSS de Laval, 280 boul Du Roi-Du-Nord, Laval QC H7L 4L2; Laval'65; DiagRad. Diag Radiol, Hopital de la Cite de la santé; (450)622-5110

LORTIE, Marie-Noelle; Clinique Med Saint-Eugene, 397 rue Jacques-Cartier S, St-Jean-sur-Richel QC J3B 7T1; Mon'05; CCFP; (450)347-3748

LORTIE, Mélissa S; 100-2555 St. Joseph Blvd, Orleans ON K1C 1S6; Ott'08; CCFP; (613)830-1298

LORTIE, Richard; 215-1144 rue Saint-Laurent O, Longueuil QC J4K 1E2; Mon'74; Ac Staff, Hopital Charles LeMoyne; Asst Prof Family Med, Universite de Sherbrooke; (450)442-5044

LORTIE, Sylvie; Hop Louis-H Lafontaine, 7401 rue Hochelaga, Montreal QC H1N 3M5; Mon'85; FRCPC; Psy. Staff, Hopital Louis-H Lafontaine; Universite de Montreal; (514)251-4000

LORTIE FORGUES, Aude; Centre d'Urgence Salaberry, 2758 rue de Salaberry, Montreal QC H3M 1L3; Mon'07; CCFP; (514)337-4772

LOSA-VAZQUEZ, Jesus; Clin Med Place La Prairie, 200-170 Boul Taschereau, La Prairie QC J5R 5H6; (Mexico)'80; (450)444-5789; Fax. (450)444-6848.

LOSHAJ, Ryve; West End Med Centre, 510 Prince St, Truro NS B2N 1G1; Pristina (Albania)'95; CCFP; Staff, Colchester East Hants Health Centre; (902)893-7422; Fax. (902)893-1026.

LOSIE, Keith T; 313-877 Goldstream Ave, Victoria BC V9B 2X8; Cal'85; CCFP; FCFP; Clin Instructor, University of British Columbia; (250)478-4421; Fax. (250)474-6098.

LOSIER, Andrea M; Children's Hosp Eastern Ont, 401 Smyth Rd, Ottawa ON K1H 8L1; Dal'98; FRCPC; Peds. Staff EmergMed, Children's Hospital of Eastern Ontario (CHEO); (613)737-2328

LOSIER, Arthur J; Baie Ste Anne Med Clinic, 13 rue de l'Eglise, Baie-Sainte-Anne NB E9A 1A9; McM'84; (506)228-2004; Fax. (506)228-2008.

LOSIER, Christopher L; PO Box 607 Stn Main, Moncton NB E1C 8M7; Dal'89; CCFP; CCFP(E.M.); Staff, The Moncton Hospital.

LOSIER, Gerard B; 312-10 Hotel Dieu St, Miramichi NB E1N 3X7; Dal'81; (506)773-3293; Fax. (506)778-9918.

LOSIER, Juliana; Mayne Island Health Clinic, RR 2 210-526 Felix Jack Rd, Mayne BC V0N 2J2; (Macedonia)'92; CCFP; Clin Instructor, University of British Columbia; Langs: Macedonian; German; (250)539-2312; Fax. (250)539-3215.

LOSIER, Lise; Clinique Med Caron Dion Losier, PO Box 3603 Stn Main 1-3980 rue Principale, Tracadie-Sheila NB E1X 1G5; Mon'91; CCFP; Staff Family Med, Hôpital de Tracadie-Sheila; Langs: Bilingual(French/English); (506)395-2554; Fax. (506)395-2443; lisel@bellaliant.ca.

LOSLIER, Julie; DSP de la Monteregie, 1255 rue Beauregard, Longueuil QC J4K 2M3; Sher'00; CSPQ; FRCPC; CommunMed. (450)928-6777 x4284

LOSSING, Alan G; Bayview Business Centre, 101-16700 Bayview Ave, Newmarket ON L3X 1W1; Tor'78; FRCSC; VascSurg. Court Staff, St Joseph's Health Centre; Court Staff, Sunnybrook Health Sciences Centre; Staff Vascular Surg/Med Dir Telemedicine Program, St Michael's Hospital; Assoc Prof Surg, University of Toronto; (905)953-8787; alossing@yahoo.com.

LOSTRACCO, Robert; 222 Eramosa Rd, Guelph ON N1E 2M4; Tor'95; CCFP; Staff, Guelph General Hospital; (519)821-1507; Fax. (519)821-5058.

LOSZAK, Karl G; 505-1200 Bay St, Toronto ON M5R 2A5; Man'73; DPsy; DABPN; FRCPC; Psy (Psychoanalysis). (416)922-8131

LOTA, Shashi; Westbrook Walk-In Clinic, P57-1610 37 St SW, Calgary AB T3C 3P1; Dublin (Ireland)'68; DMRD; Langs: Punjabi; Gujarati; Hindi; (403)246-0887; Fax. (403)246-0422.

LOTFALLAH, Talaat K; 307-797 Princess St, Kingston ON K7L 1G1; Ain Shams (Egypt)'61; MB ChB; DS; DU; CCFP; Assoc Staff, Kingston General Hospital; Assoc Staff, Hotel-Dieu Hospital; (613)545-1158

LOTFI-SEYSAN, Lotfullah; CFB Petawawa, PO Box 9999 Stn Main, Petawawa ON K8H 2X3; Athens (Greece)'85; CCFP; Langs: Persian; Greek; (613)678-5511

LOTHIAN, James B; Royal University Hosp, 103 Hospital Dr, Saskatoon SK S7N 0W8; Cal'96; FRCPC; Peds; Critical Care Medicine; Respir. Staff Peds, Royal University Hospital; (306)966-8116; Fax. (306)966-8640.

LOTHIAN, Tara J; Southgate Med Clinic, 1-45905 Yale Rd, Chilliwack BC V2P 2M6; Loma Linda(CA) (USA)'05; CCFP; (604)795-7228

LOTHSTEIN, Daniel B; Grey Bruce Health Services, RR 5 201-369 Mary St, Wiarton ON N0H 2T0; Philadelphia (USA)'07; CCFP; Staff, Grey Bruce Health Services - Wiarton Site; (519)534-2411

LOTOCKA-REYSNER, Hanna; 209-6411 Nelson Ave, Burnaby BC V5H 4H3; Stettin (Poland)'87; FRCPC; Peds (Palliative Care). Langs: Polish; Russian; Spanish; (604)620-5247

LOTOCKI, Robert J; CancerCare Manitoba, 675 McDermot Ave, Winnipeg MB R3E 0V9; Man'75; FRCSC; ObstGyn (Colposcopy). Staff, Health Sciences Centre; Staff, St Boniface General Hospital; Med Dir, Manitoba Cervical Cancer Screening Program; Assoc Prof, University of Manitoba.

LOTT, Bettina; 10917 82 Ave PO Box 52069 Rpo Garneau, Edmonton AB T6G 2T5; Qns'09; CCFP; (780)910-1060; blott@ualberta.ca.

LOTT, Paula M; 202-595 Columbia St W, Kamloops BC V2C 1K7; Alb'00; FRCSC; ObstGyn. Clin Instructor, University of British Columbia; (250)434-4762; Fax. (250)434-4763.

LOTTER, Wian H; La Scie Med Clinic, PO Box 160, La Scie NL A0K 3M0; Pretoria (South Africa)'88; MB ChB; Langs: Afrikaans; (709)675-2429; Fax. (709)675-2039; wlotter@nf.sympatico.ca.

LOTTERING, Wilraad; Professional Bldg, 3100-222 King St E, Bowmanville ON L1C 1P6; Pretoria (South Africa)'87; CCFP; CCFP(E.M.); Staff, Lakeridge Health - Bowmanville Site; (905)623-2355

LOTZ, Albertus B; Stapleford Med Clinic, 372 McCarthy Blvd N, Regina SK S4R 7M2; Orange Free State (South Africa)'84; MB ChB; Langs: Afrikaans; (306)545-3000; Fax. (306)545-5584.

LOTZ, Christo; Prince Albert Med Clinic, 681 15th St W, Prince Albert SK S6V 7H9; (Other Foreign)'01; (306)764-1505

LOTZ, Heloise; Regina Qu'Appelle HR-Regina, 1440 14th Ave, Regina SK S4P 0W5; Pretoria (South Africa)'04; Staff, Regina General Hospital; Langs: Afrikaans; (306)766-4444

LOTZ, Petrus C; The Medical Clinic, 4634 Park Ave, Terrace BC V8G 1V7; Pretoria (South Africa)'83; Langs: Afrikaans; (250)975-0395

LOTZE, Tracey A; 1110 4th Ave, Prince George BC V2L 3J3; Cape Town (South Africa)'05; MB ChB; Langs: Afrikaans; (250)564-4422; traceylotze@yahoo.com.

LOU, Allison S; Sherbourne Health Centre, 333 Sherbourne St, Toronto ON M5A 2S5; Tor'04; CCFP; (416)324-4180; Fax. (416)324-4262.

LOU, Lawrence; 300-401 9 Ave SW, Calgary AB T2P 3C5; McM'03; FRCPC; DiagRad; NuclearMed. (403)284-0230

LOU, Samuel; 1A 102-11400 University Ave NW, Edmonton AB T6G 1Z1; Alb'09; CCFP; Staff, University of Alberta Hospital; (780)407-7755; Fax. (780)407-1828.

LOU, T Y Justin; Trillium Doctor's Office, 406-2299 Dundas St W, Toronto ON M6R 1X7; Tor'00; CCFP; Staff, Toronto Western Hospital - University Health Network; (416)535-3511

LOUAHLIA, Said; CSSS de Rimouski-Neigette, CP 3150 Succ A 150 av Rouleau, Rimouski QC G5L 5T1; Hassan II (Morocco)'86; Staff, Hôpital Regional Rimouski; (418)724-3000

LOUBANI, Eman M; London HSC-Victoria Hosp, PO Box 5010 Stn B 800 Commissioners Rd E, London ON N6A 5W9; Wes'04; FRCPC; Peds. Staff, London Health Sciences Centre - Victoria Campus; (519)685-8500

LOUBANI, Mahmoud M; Bathurst Shopping Mall, 206-1300 St. Peter Ave, Bathurst NB E2A 3A6; Cairo (Egypt)'74; Staff, Hospital Regional Chaleur; (506)546-5911; Fax. (506)546-5911.

LOUBANI, Mohammed M; London HSC-Victoria Hosp, PO Box 5010 Stn B 800 Commissioners Rd E, London ON N6A 5W9; Wes'06; CCFP; CCFP(E.M.); Staff, London Health Sciences Centre - Victoria Campus; (519)200-6468

LOUBANI, Sara A H; Hôpital régional Chaleur, 1750 Sunset Dr, Bathurst NB E2A 4L7; Cairo (Egypt)'78; MB ChB; DCH(Ire); Staff, Hopital Regional Chaleur; (506)548-8961; Fax. (506)547-9095.

LOUBANI, Tarek M; London HSC-Victoria Hosp, PO Box 5010 Stn B 800 Commissioners Rd E, London ON N6A 5W9; Wes'07; CCFP; CCFP(E.M.); Staff, London Health Sciences Centre - Victoria Campus; (519)685-8500

LOUBERT, Christian; Hop Maisonneuve-Rosemont, 5415 boul de l'Assomption, Montreal QC H1T 2M4; Mon'03; FRCPC; Anes. Staff, Hopital Maisonneuve-Rosemont; (514)252-3400

LOUBERT, Francois; Clinique Maisonneuve-Rosemont, RC60-5345 boul de l'Assomption, Montreal QC H1T 4B3; Mon'93; Staff, Centre Hospitalier Fleury; (514)257-7000; Fax. (514)257-7003.

LOUBERT, Lise E; Mid-Main Comm Health Centre, 3998 Main St, Vancouver BC V5V 3P2; Ott'87; (604)873-3666; Fax. (604)875-8790.

LOUCHI, Abdellatif; CSSS de Manicouagan, 635 boul Joliet, Baie-Comeau QC G5C 1P1; (Morocco)'90; Staff, Centre Hospitalier Régional Baie-Comeau; (418)589-3701

LOUCKS, Ellen J; Lake Country Family Practice, 1-9966 Pollard Rd, Winfield BC V4V 1Z4; Cal'81; (250)766-3938; Fax. (250)766-5231.

LOUCKS-GRAY, Teresa E; William Osler HC-Brampton, 2100 Bovaird Dr E, Brampton ON L6R 3J7; Ott'97; FRCPC; DiagRad. Staff Med Imaging, William Osler Health System - Brampton Civic Hospital; (905)494-2121

LOUDON, Michael; Michael Loudon Med Corp, PO Box 127 34 Main St, Teulon MB R0C 3B0; Stellenbosch (South Africa)'98; MB ChB; Staff, Teulon/Hunter Memorial Hospital; Langs: Afrikaans; (204)886-2131; Fax. (204)886-8304.

LOUGH, David D; 203-3825 Sunset St, Burnaby BC V5G 1T4; Qns'68; Ac Staff, Royal Columbian Hospital; (604)434-9515; Fax. (604)434-5984.

LOUGH, Rod D; St Joseph's Mountain H Serv, PO Box 585 Stn Lcd 1 100 West 5th St, Hamilton ON L8N 3K7; Dal'92; BSc; Psy (Forensic Psychiatry). Staff, St Joseph's Healthcare Hamilton - West 5th Campus; PT-Time Prof, McMaster University; (905)522-1155 x36775; Fax. (905)381-5620; rlough@stjosham.on.ca.

LOUGHEAD, Garth T; Weld Street Clinic, PO Box 1060 Stn Main 168 Weld St, Parksville BC V9P 2H1; Cal'84; BSc; CCFP; (250)248-5677; Fax. (250)248-4287.

LOUGHEED, Brenda L; Royal University Hosp, 103 Hospital Dr, Saskatoon SK S7N 0W8; Sask'06; FRCPC; Anes. Staff Anes, Royal University Hospital; (306)655-1183; Fax. (306)655-1279.

LOUGHEED, Daryl B; Markham Family Health Team, 101-377 Church St, Markham ON L6B 1A1; Man'06; CCFP; (905)471-9999; Fax. (905)471-3627.

LOUGHEED, Donna C; Royal Ottawa Hlth Care Group, 1145 Carling Ave, Ottawa ON K1Z 7K4; Cal'81; MSc; FRCPC; Psy (Diagnosis). Head Dual Diagnosis Consultation Outreach & Psy Outreach Team, Royal Ottawa Mental Health Centre - Royal Ottawa Health Care Group; Asst Prof, University of Ottawa; Langs: French; (613)722-6521 x7010; Fax. (613)233-8664; donna-lougheed@rohcg.on.ca.

LOUGHEED, Eileen M; Markham Family Health Team, 101-377 Church St, Markham ON L6B 1A1; Tor'73; AB; CCFP; FCFP; Assoc Staff, North York General Hospital; Physician Palliative Care, Markham Stouffville Hospital; Med Advisor, South East York Region; Med Dir, Woodhaven LTC Hospital; Fellow Ian Anderson, University of Toronto; (905)471-9999; Fax. (905)471-3627.

LOUGHEED, George E; Georgian Radiology Consultants, 115-121 Wellington St W, Barrie ON L4N 1L2; Wes'81; FRCPC; DiagRad. Staff, Georgian Bay General Hospital - Midland; Staff, Royal Victoria Regional Health Centre; Staff, Collingwood General & Marine Hospital; (705)726-4531

LOUGHEED, Jane; Children's Hosp Eastern Ont, 401 Smyth Rd, Ottawa ON K1H 8L1; Qns'93; BA; MD; FRCPC; FRCPC; Cardiol; Peds (Pediatric Cardiology). Staff Cardiol, Children's Hospital of Eastern Ontario (CHEO); Asst Prof Peds, University of Ottawa; (613)737-2389; Fax. (613)738-4835; jlougheed@cheo.on.ca.

LOUGHEED, M Diane; 102 Stuart St, Kingston ON K7L 2V6; McM'86; FRCPC; IntMed; Respir. Staff, Providence Care - St Mary's of the Lake Hospital Site; Kingston General Hospital; Staff, Hotel-Dieu Hospital; Assoc Prof Med, Queen's University; (613)548-2348; Fax. (613)549-1459; mdl@queensu.ca.

LOUGHLIN, Kevin F; Reddendale Family Health Ctre, 125 Lakeview Ave, Kingston ON K7M 3T6; Wes'97; CCFP.

LOUIE, Andrew J; 234 Hastings St E, Vancouver BC V6A 1P1; Cal'77; Staff, Providence Health Care - Mount Saint Joseph Hospital; Langs: Cantonese; (604)688-0351; alo@qltinc.com.

LOUIE, Donald F; 313-2083 Alma St, Vancouver BC V6R 4N6; UBC'71; MD; FRCPC; Psy (Child & Adolescent Psychiatry). Ac Staff, BC Children's Hospital; Staff Consultant, Vancouver General Hospital - Centennial Pavillion; Staff, BC Women's Hospital & Health Centre; Clin Prof Psy, University of British Columbia; (604)222-2083; Fax. (604)222-2045; almadoctor@uniserve.ca.

LOUIE, Donald L; Westbrook Prof Bldg, 205-1610 37 St SW, Calgary AB T3C 3P1; Alb'76; (403)242-7788

LOUIE, Gorman; Garneau Prof Centre, 201-11044 82 Ave NW, Edmonton AB T6G 0T2; Alb'80; BMedSci; FRCSC; PlasSurg (Cosmetics). Ac Staff, Covenant Health - Grey Nuns Community Hospital; Ac Staff, Covenant Health - Misericordia Community Hospital; Ac Staff Surg, University of Alberta Hospital; Clinical Asst Prof Surg, University of Alberta; (780)433-4225; Fax. (780)439-6732; glouie@ualberta.ca.

LOUIE, Heather M; Richmond Health Science Ctre, 290-6091 Gilbert Rd, Richmond BC V7C 5L9; Man'76; DAA; FRCPC; Peds. Staff, BC Children's Hospital; Asst Prof, University of British Columbia; (604)273-8360; Fax. (604)270-0462.

LOUIE, Karen D; Links Clinic, 104-11910 111 Ave NW, Edmonton AB T5G 3G6; Alb'95; CCFP; FCFP; (780)454-0351; Fax. (780)452-6767.

LOUIE, Marie; Provincial Laboratory, 3030 Hospital Dr NW, Calgary AB T2N 4W4; Man'81; FRCPC; IntMed; InfectDis; MedMicrobiol.

LOUIE, Peter; Fairmont Med Bldg, 1314-750 Broadway W, Vancouver BC V5Z 1J3; Alb'01; FRCPC; Peds. Clin Instructor, BC Children's Hospital; Langs: Cantonese; (604)879-4564

LOUIE, Richard A; BC Biomedical Laboratories, 7455 130 St, Surrey BC V3W 1H8; Alb'64; GenPath (Hematology Pathology). (604)507-5000

LOUIE, Thomas J; Foothills Med Centre, 1403 29 St NW, Calgary AB T2N 2T9; Alb'69; FRCPC; IntMed (Infectious Diseases). Staff, Foothills Medical Centre; Staff, Peter Lougheed Centre; Med Dir, Infection Prevention & Control, Calgary Health Region; Prof Med & InfectDis, University of Calgary; (403)943-4024; Fax. (403)291-2571; louie@ucalgary.ca.

LOUIE, William L; Riverside Med Clinic, 121-4411 16 Ave NW, Calgary AB T3B 0M3; Alb'59; CCFP; Langs: Cantonese; (403)247-6966; Fax. (403)247-6838.

LOUIS, Donald K; William Osler HC-Brampton, 2100 Bovaird Dr E, Brampton ON L6R 3J7; Mem'77; FRCSC; GenSurg; VascSurg. Staff, William Osler Health System - Brampton Civic Hospital; (905)455-5550; Fax. (905)455-5551.

LOUIS, Ihab K; Royal Victoria Hosp, 201 Georgian Dr, Barrie ON L4M 6M2; Ain Shams (Egypt)'95; FRCPC; Anes. Staff, Royal Victoria Regional Health Centre.

LOUIS, Lenus S; North Hamilton Comm Health Ctr, 438 Hugson St N, Hamilton ON L8L 4N5; Jaffna (Sri Lanka)'89; (905)523-6611

LOUIS, Luck J; Vancouver Gen Hosp, 855 12th Ave W, Vancouver BC V5Z 1M9; Cal'96; FRCPC; DiagRad. Staff Radiol, Vancouver General Hospital - Centennial Pavillion; (604)875-4111

LOUIS, Melissa A; 3835 rue Wellington, Verdun QC H4G 1V1; Sher'02; Ophth. (514)768-1250

LOUIS BAYLISS, Amy G; The Credit Valley Hosp, 2200 Eglinton Ave W, Mississauga ON L5M 2N1; McM'06; FRCPC; EmergMed. Staff, The Credit Valley Hospital; (905)813-2200

LOUIS-ZAHER, Amani; Clinique Med Mariam, 200-4531 boul des Sources, Roxboro QC H8Y 3C2; Assuit (Egypt)'72; (514)685-8840

LOUISE, Gina; Ridge Meadows Hosp & Hlth Ctr, 11666 Laity St, Maple Ridge BC V2X 5A3; UBC'98; CCFP; Staff, Ridge Meadows Hospital & Health Care Centre; (604)476-7117

LOUISY, Coventry L; Burlington X-Ray & Radiology, 2-760 Brant St, Burlington ON L7R 4B7; Bristol (England)'63; MB ChB; DMRD; FFR; FRCPC; DiagRad; NuclearMed. Consultant Radiol/Dir, Joseph Brant Memorial Hospital; (905)637-7606

LOUKIDES, Nicholas E; 501-294 Main St, Toronto ON M4C 4X5; Tor'74; Staff, Toronto East General Hospital Inc; (416)698-8788; Fax. (416)691-3641.

LOUKRAS, Lucinda; The Medical Centre, PO Box 4200 Stn Main 707 Charlotte St, Peterborough ON K9J 7B3; McM'83; FRCPC; Peds (Neuro Development Pediatrics). (705)876-4538; Fax. (705)876-4526; ljloukras@gmail.com.

LOULI, Sam; Eglinton Square Mall, 135-1 Eglinton Sq, Scarborough ON M1L 2K1; Tor'83; (416)752-6006; Fax. (416)751-4854.

LOUNG, Kenneth C; 2 Elfindale Cres, North York ON M2J 1B5; Dublin (Ireland)'64; MB ChB; BAO; Court Staff, Toronto Western Hospital - University Health Network; (416)497-5076

LOUNGNARATH, Rasmy; CHUM-Hop St-Luc, 1058 rue Saint-Denis, Montreal QC H2X 3J4; Mon'96; FASCRS; FRCSC; GenSurg (Colon & Rectal Surgery). Staff, Centre Hospitalier l'Université De Montréal (CHUM) - Hôpital Saint-luc; Langs: English; (514)890-8000 x35476; Fax. (514)412-7355; rasmy.loungnarath.chum@ssss.gouv.qc.ca.

LOUNGNARATH, Vilaysoun; CSSS d'Antoine-Labelle-Mt Laur, RR 1 2561 ch de la Lièvre S, Mont-Laurier QC J9L 3G3; Mon'62; GenSurg. Staff, CSSS d'Antoine-Labelle; (819)623-1234

LOUNGNARATH, Vilayvong; Ctr Hosp Affilie-Enfant-Jesus, 1401 18e rue, Quebec QC G1J 1Z4; Sher'86; FRCPC; MedMicrobiol; Microbio & Infect Dis (P.Q.). Staff, Centre Hospitalier Affilié Universitaire de Québec - Hôpital De L'Enfant Jésus; (418)649-0252; Fax. (418)649-5509.

LOUNSBURY, Catherine; Concordia Univ Health Services, GM200-1455 boul Maisonneuve O, Montreal QC H3G 1M8; Dal'83; ac Staff, St Mary's Hospital Centre; Dir Prof Serv, Catherine Booth Hospital; Consultant Health Services, Concordia University; (514)848-2424; Fax. (514)848-2834.

LOUNSBURY, David S; 1 Field Ambulance, PO Box 10500 Stn Forces, Edmonton AB T5J 4J5; Wes'08; CCFP; (780)973-4011; Fax. (780)973-1635.

LOURENS, M Elizabeth; Age Management Institute, 207-1205 Bow Valley Trail, Canmore AB T1W 1P5; (South Africa)'85; DA; CCFP; FCFP; (403)609-2196; Fax. (403)609-2194.

LOURENS, Marc; Medical Clinic, PO Box 730 Stn Main, Salmon Arm BC V1E 4N8; Cape Town (South Africa)'87; MB ChB; DA(SA); Staff, Shuswap Pain Management Clinic; Langs: Afrikaans; (250)832-6092; Fax. (250)832-5235.

LOUTFI, Antoine; MUHC-Royal Victoria Hosp, 30-687 av des Pins O, Montreal QC H3A 1A1; Beyrouth (Lebanon)'74; AB; FACS; FRCSC; GenSurg (Surgical Oncology). Ac Staff, McGill University Health Centre - Royal Victoria Hospital; assoc Prof, McGill University; (514)934-1934 x35611; Fax. (514)843-1454; antoine.loutfi@muhc.mcgill.ca.

LOUTFI, Joseph; Centre Med Pierrefonds, 12774 boul Gouin O, Pierrefonds QC H8Z 1W5; (Lebanon)'71; Gastroent (P.Q.). Staff, CSSS de Dorval-Lachine-Lasalle; (514)684-8460; Fax. (514)685-4756.

LOUTFY, Mona R; Maple Leaf Med Arts, 501-14 College St, Toronto ON M5G 1K2; Tor'95; FRCPC; IntMed; InfectDis. Physician, Maple Leaf Medical Clinic; Langs: Bilingual(English/French); (416)465-0856 x2444

LOUVARIS, James H; Vaughan Med Centre, H 26-9200 Weston Rd, Woodbridge ON L4H 2P8; McG'93; (905)417-2273; Fax. (905)417-7088.

LOUW, Adriaan P; Esterhazy District Med Clinic, PO Box 940, Esterhazy SK S0A 0X0; Stellenbosch (South Africa)'97; MB ChB; (306)745-6681; Fax. (306)745-2995.

LOUW, Alexander F; Moose Jaw Union Hosp, 455 Fairford St E, Moose Jaw SK S6H 1H3; Staff, Moose Jaw Union Hospital; (306)694-0200

LOUW, Alexander M; PO Box 1250, Grimshaw AB T0H 1W0; Pretoria (South Africa)'74; MB ChB; (780)332-4643

LOUW, Andre J; Midtown Med Centre, 5706 50 Ave, Vermilion AB T9X 1L4; (South Africa)'77; MB ChB; (780)853-2809; Fax. (780)853-2977.

LOUW, Andries P; Peter Lougheed Centre, 3500 26 Ave NE, Calgary AB T1Y 6J4; Orange Free State (South Africa)'95; MB ChB; CCFP; Staff, Peter Lougheed Centre; (403)943-5461

LOUW, Chrisman J; Tumbler Ridge Med Clinic, PO Box 1690, Tumbler Ridge BC V0C 2W0; Stellenbosch (South Africa)'74; MB ChB; (250)242-4251

LOUW, Deon F; Crowfoot Village Fam Practice, 340-600 Crowfoot Cres NW, Calgary AB T3G 0B4; Cape Town (South Africa)'83; FRCPC; Neursurg (Spine Surgery). Langs: Afrikaans.

LOUW, Hendrik B; 101-111 Kootenay St N, Cranbrook BC V1C 3T5; Pretoria (South Africa)'89; MB ChB; (250)426-7997

LOUW, Jacob A; Hotel-Dieu Hosp, 166 Brock St, Kingston ON K7L 5G2; Stellenbosch (South Africa)'80; FRCPC; Gastroent. Staff Gastroent, Hotel-Dieu Hospital; (613)544-3400 x2450

LOUW, Johannes; Surrey Mem Hosp, 13750 96 Ave, Surrey BC V3V 1Z2; Stellenbosch (South Africa)'93; Staff, Surrey Memorial Hospital; (604)581-2211

LOUW, Marina; 700 3rd St SS 3, Keremeos BC V0X 1N3; Orange Free State (South Africa)'87; MB ChB; (250)499-3000

LOUW, Perold J; Site 11 Comp 71 RR 1, Naramata BC V0H 1N0; Pretoria (South Africa)'92; MB ChB; CCFP; (250)496-5336; Fax. (250)496-5264.

LOUW, Wynand F; Chisel Peak Med Clinic, PO Box 2769 417 10th Ave, Invermere BC V0A 1K0; Pretoria (South Africa)'97; MB ChB; DA; CCFP; Staff, Invermere & District Hospital; Langs: Afrikaans; Dutch; Flemish; (250)341-6900; Fax. (250)341-3226.

LOUWRENS, Pierre J; Pierre Louwrens Med Prof Corp, PO Box 300, Climax SK S0N 0N0; (South Africa)'93; MB ChB; (306)293-2233

LOUZADA, Martha D L; London HSC-Victoria Campus, PO Box 5010 Stn B D6 212-800 Commissioners Rd E, London ON N6A 5W9; Souza Marques (Brazil)'99; Staff, London Health Sciences Centre - Victoria Campus; (519)685-8631

LOVAS, David A; IWK Health Centre, PO Box 9700 Rpo CSC 5980 University Ave, Halifax NS B3K 6R8; Dal'04; FRCPC; Psy. Staff, IWK Health Centre; (902)470-8087

LOVASCO, Salvatore; Polyclinique Cabrini, 109-5700 rue Saint-Zotique E, Montreal QC H1T 3Y7; Mon'78; pers Médecin, Hôpital Santa Cabrini Ospedale; Physician, Centre d'Accueil Dante; (514)254-4018

LOVATSIS, Danny; Hydro Place Bldg, 8 814-700 University Ave, Toronto ON M5G 1Z5; Qns'94; MSc; FRCSC; ObstGyn (Reconstructive Surgery). Ac Staff, Women's College Hospital; Ac Staff, Mount Sinai Hospital; Asst Prof, University of Toronto; (416)586-4566; Fax. (416)586-3152; dlovatsis@mtsinai.on.ca.

LOVE, Jonathan R; GI Clinic, A2-3330 Hospital Dr NW, Calgary AB T2N 4N1; Qns'85; FRCPC; IntMed (Therapeutic Endoscopy); Gastroent. Staff, Foothills Medical Centre; Clin Assoc Prof, University of Calgary; Langs: Bilingual(English/French); (403)592-5015; Fax. (403)592-5090.

LOVE, Michael P; Queen Elizabeth II HSC-Halifax, 6896K-1796 Summer St, Halifax NS B3H 3A7; Aberdeen (Scotland)'90; MB ChB; Staff Cardiol, Queen Elizabeth II Health Sciences Centre - Halifax Infirmary Site; (902)473-5572; Fax. (902)473-6293.

LOVE, Nancy E; Richmond Square Med Centre, 70-3915 51 St SW, Calgary AB T3E 6N1; Alb'83; CCFP; FCFP; (403)229-2273; Fax. (403)246-9688.

LOVE, Richa P; Thorncliffe Med Centre, 5618 4 St NW, Calgary AB T2K 1B2; Cal'98; CCFP; Langs: Hindi; Urdu; (403)295-7666; Fax. (403)295-8960; richalove@hotmail.com.

LOVE, Robert B; 206-99 Kakulu Rd, Kanata ON K2L 3C8; McG'70; FRCSC; Otol. Consultant Otol, Carleton Place & District Memorial Hospital; Staff, Queensway Carleton Hospital; Langs: English; French; (613)270-9720; Fax. (613)254-8618.

LOVE, Robert J; Victoria Square Med Centre, 5619 Victoria Dr, Vancouver BC V5P 3W2; Alb'76; BSc; (604)656-2090

LOVE, Robin R R; Medical Arts Centre, 103-650 Terminal Ave, Nanaimo BC V9R 5E2; UBC'86; CCFP; FCFP; (250)753-3431; Fax. (250)754-6897.

LOVE, William; 488 Locust St, Burlington ON L7S 1V2; Wes'77; FRCSC; Urol. Assoc Staff, Halton Healthcare Services Corporation - Oakville Site; Ac Staff, Joseph Brant Memorial Hospital; Ac Staff, West Lincoln Memorial Hospital; (905)632-3025; Fax. (905)632-2893.

LOVEDAY, Benjamin D; Regional Mental HC-London, PO Box 5532 Stn B 850 Highbury Ave, London ON N6A 4H1; Qns'04; Psy. Staff, Regional Mental Health Care-St Joseph's Health Care; (519)455-5110

LOVEGROVE, Michael A; Northtown Med Associates, 325 Thorold Rd, Welland ON L3C 3W4; McG'75; Ac Staff, Niagara Health System - Welland Hospital Site; (905)732-4777; Fax. (905)732-7262.

LOVELESS, Wendy J; 4313 Gallant Ave, North Vancouver BC V7G 2C1; (England)'86; LMCC; DRCOG; MRC; MCFP; CCFP; Clin Asst Residency Prog, University of British Columbia; (604)929-5029; Fax. (604)929-3256.

LOVELL, Richard E; Amherstburg Med Associates, 71 Sandwich St S, Amherstburg ON N9V 1Z5; Wes'77; Staff, Hôtel-Dieu Grace Hospital; (519)736-5444; Fax. (519)736-7687.

LOVELY, Donald S; 101-7784 East Saanich Rd, Saanichton BC V8M 2B3; McG'78; (250)652-9121; Fax. (250)652-0306.

LOVERIDGE, Peter L; RR 1, Glenwood NS B0W 1W0; London (England)'69; DMRD; Staff, Yarmouth Regional Hospital; Langs: English; French; (902)643-2665; Fax. (902)643-2665.

LOVESEY, Natalie J; Southdale Med Clinic, 395 Southdale Rd E, London ON N6E 1A2; Dal'07; CCFP; (519)691-0100

LOVETT, Audrey; MUHC-Montreal Children's Hosp, C 215-2300 rue Tupper, Montreal QC H3H 1P3; Mon'02; FRCPC; Derm. (514)412-4310

LOVETT, Katrin A; Vital Health Med & Aesthetic, 1855 4th Ave W, Vancouver BC V6J 1M5; UBC'07; CCFP; (604)558-4825

LOVEYS, Annabeth J; Kelligrews Med Clinic, PO Box 17160 Stn Kelligrews, Conception-Bay-S NL A1X 3H1; Mem'07; CCFP; (709)834-2171

LOVINSKY, Reena; Scarborough Hosp-General Div, 3050 Lawrence Ave E, Scarborough ON M1P 2V5; Tor'97; FRCPC; IntMed; InfectDis. Staff, The Scarborough Hospital - General Campus; (416)431-8120

LOVISI NETO, Bianca; CSSS de Chicoutimi, 305 rue Saint-Vallier, Chicoutimi QC G7H 5H6; Juiz de Fora (Brazil)'97; Staff, Complexe hospitalier de la Sagamie; (418)541-1234; Fax. (418)541-1108.

LOVO, Lana M; Alberta Prof Bldg, 303-320 23 Ave SW, Calgary AB T2S 0J2; Sask'98; CCFP; FCFP; (403)686-2150; Fax. (403)209-1299.

LOVRICS, Peter J; St Joseph's Healthcare, 8F-50 Charlton Ave E, Hamilton ON L8N 4A6; Qns'88; FRCSC; GenSurg (Critical Care Medicine). Staff, St Joseph's Healthcare - Charlton Campus; (905)521-6060; Fax. (905)521-6042; lovricsp@mcmaster.ca.

LOW, Aaron A L; 1256 Danforth Rd, Scarborough ON M1J 1E5; Wes'94; (416)261-3500

LOW, Anthony C L; Hazelwood Med Clinic, 201-16088 84 Ave, Surrey BC V4N 0V9; UBC'89; (604)572-6665; Fax. (604)572-8912.

LOW, Bligh K W; 4-13791 72 Ave, Surrey BC V3W 9Y9; UBC'76; FACEP; Staff, Surrey Memorial Hospital; (604)591-9404; Fax. (604)591-8108.

LOW, Catherine M; 16 Chatham St, Belleville ON K8N 3S3; McM'78; BSc(Med); (613)962-3353; Fax. (613)962-1154.

LOW, Charles T; Brockville Gen Hosp, 75 Charles St, Brockville ON K6V 1S8; Qns'79; CCFP; Ac Staff, Brockville General Hospital - Charles Street; Ac Staff, Providence Continuing Care Centre (PCCC) - St Vincent de Paul Hospital; Langs: English; French; (613)345-8323

LOW, D Brian; Cardston Clinic, PO Box 550 34 2 Ave, Cardston AB T0K 0K0; Alb'82; Staff, Cardston Hospital; (403)653-3311; Fax. (403)653-1098.

LOW, Donald E; Mount Sinai Hosp, 1487-600 University Ave, Toronto ON M5G 1X5; Man'72; FRCPC; IntMed; InfectDis; MedMicrobiol. Staff, Mount Sinai Hospital; Prof Lab Med & Pathobiol, University of Toronto; (416)586-4435; Fax. (416)586-8746.

LOW, Edmond C M; Hazelwood Med Clinic, 201-16088 84 Ave, Surrey BC V4N 0V9; UBC'84; Staff, Surrey Memorial Hospital; (604)572-6665; Fax. (604)572-8912.

LOW, Gavin W Y; Hys Med Centre, 202-11010 101 St NW, Edmonton AB T5H 4B9; (United Kingdom)'98; MB ChB; (780)426-1121; Fax. (780)425-5979.

LOW, George A; Scarborough Bone Analysis, 1101-3000 Lawrence Ave E, Scarborough ON M1P 2V1; Tor'46; IntMed (Bone Densitometry). (416)289-0029

LOW, Graeme L; MUHC-Montreal Gen Hosp, 1650 av Cedar, Montreal QC H3G 1A4; Ott'66; DPsy; DABPN(Psy); FRCPC; Psy (Consultant Liaison Psychiatry). Sr Staff Psy, McGill University Health Centre - Montreal General Campus; adj Prof, McGill University; (514)934-1934 x42069; Fax. (514)934-8237; graeme.low@muhc.mcgill.ca.

LOW, Jason D; 4904 48 St, Leduc AB T9E 6X4; Alb'09; CCFP; (780)986-2712

LOW, Ling Ling; Chilliwack Med Clinic, 45779 Luckakuck Way, Chilliwack BC V2R 4E8; UBC'89; (604)858-5544; Fax. (604)858-5566.

LOW, Louise J Y; 4-13791 72 Ave, Surrey BC V3W 9Y9; UBC'92; CCFP; (604)591-9404

LOW, Nancy; McGill University, 111-1033 av des Pins O, Montreal QC H3A 1A1; Sask'97; BSc; MSc; FRCPC; Psy (Epidemiology). adj Prof, McGill University; (514)934-1934 x31798; nancy.low@mcgill.ca.

LOW, Rhonda S; Copeman Helthcare Centre, 400-1128 Hornby St, Vancouver BC V6Z 2L4; UBC'82; CCFP; FCFP; Ac Staff, Providence Health Care - St Paul's Hospital; Clin Assoc Prof, University of British Columbia; (604)707-5523

LOW, Richard A; Professional Corp, 931 19 St S, Lethbridge AB T1J 3H5; Alb'06; FRCPC; IntMed. (403)328-0693; Fax. (403)328-0619.

LOW, Ronald R; 203-1410 Mayor Magrath Dr S, Lethbridge AB T1K 2R3; Alb'87; FRCPC; Derm. (403)328-3100; Fax. (403)328-3166.

LOW, Steven L; Campbell Clinic, PO Box 180 Stn Main, Coaldale AB T1M 1M3; Alb'87; CCFP; Sec Medical, Coaldale Health Centre; Med Dir, Coaldale Ambulance; Langs: French; (403)345-3072; Fax. (403)345-2141.

LOW, Susan E; Yellowbird Family Clinic, 3380 Gateway Blvd NW, Edmonton AB T6J 6V1; Alb'81; CCFP; FCFP; Staff, Covenant Health - Misericordia Community Hospital; Clinical Asst Prof Family Med, University of Alberta; (780)434-8293; Fax. (780)435-1057.

LOW, Thomas D P; CSSSG-Hop de Hull, 116 boul Lionel-Emond, Gatineau QC J8Y 1W7; Ott'06; FRCPC; EmergMed; Critical Care Medicine. Staff, Hull Hospital; (819)966-6200

LOW AH KEE, Julia; PO Box 163, Hagensborg BC V0T 1H0; UBC'05; CCFP.

LOW-BEER, Sophie C; Delta Hosp, 5800 Mountain View Blvd, Delta BC V4K 3V6; UBC'03; CCFP; CCFP(E.M.); Staff, Delta Hospital; (604)946-1121

LOWCOCK, Donald G; Avenue Med Centre, 1-221 Brant Ave, Brantford ON N3T 3J2; Tor'77; CCFP; FCFP; Ac Staff, The Brant Community Healthcare System - Brantford General Hospital Site; (519)753-8666; Fax. (519)753-6880.

LOWDEN, Bruce A; 101-4450 Chatterton Way, Victoria BC V8X 5J2; Tor'68; FAAO; FRCSC; Ophth (Cataract). Ac Staff, Royal Jubilee Hospital; Ac Staff, Victoria General Hospital; (250)384-2622

LOWDEN, Cameron S; Southwood Med Centre, 3/F-2385 Pembina Hwy, Winnipeg MB R3T 2H4; Man'95; CCFP; FCFP; Staff, Victoria General Hospital; (204)261-3037; Fax. (204)261-3046.

LOWDEN, Keith G; 13 24th Ave N, Cranbrook BC V1C 3H9; UBC'86; Staff Community Oncology Prog, East Kootenay Regional Hospital; (250)417-6228; Fax. (250)417-6226.

LOWE, Alan D; North York Gen Hosp-Branson, 2F-555 Finch Ave W, North York ON M2R 1N5; McM'89; BScPharm; FRCPC; Psy (Sleep Medicine). Staff, North York General Hospital - Branson Division; (416)632-8701 x6305; Fax. (416)632-8718.

LOWE, Aviva H; 100-1333 Neilson Rd, Scarborough ON M1B 4Y9; McG'99; FRCPC; Peds. (416)291-7719

LOWE, Catherine E; Hotel-Dieu Hosp, 166 Brock St, Kingston ON K7L 5G2; Dal'93; FRCPC; IntMed (Hepatology); Gastroent. Staff, Hotel-Dieu Hospital; Staff, Kingston General Hospital; Asst Prof, Queen's University; (613)544-3400 x2483; Fax. (613)544-3114.

LOWE, David A; U of Toronto-Health Services, 214 College St, Toronto ON M5T 2Z9; Tor'88; Dip SportMed; CCFP; (416)978-8030; Fax. (416)971-2089.

LOWE, David G; 2-460 Hume St, Collingwood ON L9Y 1W6; Tor'72; Ac Staff, Collingwood General & Marine Hospital; (705)444-7200; Fax. (705)444-7203.

LOWE, David W W; Bridlewood Prof Centre, 303-3443 Finch Ave E, Scarborough ON M1W 2S1; West Indies (Jamaica)'71; FRCPC; Psy. Court Staff, The Scarborough Hospital - Birchmount Campus; (416)494-8880; Fax. (416)494-7594.

LOWE, Derek W; Saunte Medical Clinic, 101-15850 26 Ave, Surrey BC V3S 2N6; UBC'93; CCFP; Staff Privil Palliative Care, Peace Arch Hospital; (604)542-7788

LOWE, Gregory J J T; 125 Welland Ave, St. Catharines ON L2R 2N5; National (Ireland)'90; IntMed. (905)814-0204

LOWE, Jeffrey K; PO Box 1260, Mayerthorpe AB T0E 1N0; Cal'84; (780)786-2412; Fax. (780)786-2249.

LOWE, Julia M; Sunnybrook Hlth Sciences Ctre, H1 45-2075 Bayview Ave, Toronto ON M4N 3M5; Dundee (Scotland)'73; Staff, Sunnybrook Health Sciences Centre; (416)480-6948; Fax. (416)480-4250.

LOWE, Sonya S; Cross Cancer Institute, 2001-11560 University Ave NW, Edmonton AB T6G 1Z2; Alb'03; CCFP; Staff, Cross Cancer Institute; (780)432-8318; Fax. (780)432-8419.

LOWE, William M; College of Phys & Surg of NS, 5005-7071 Bayers Rd, Halifax NS B3L 2C2; Mem'77; CCFP; FCFP; Ac Staff, Valley Regional Hospital; Member, College of Physicians & Surgeons of Nova Scotia; Preceptor, Dalhousie University; (902)422-5823; Fax. (902)422-5035; wlowe@cpsns.ns.ca.

LOWER, Darlene P; Mount Sinai Fam Hlth Team, 4F-60 Murray St, Toronto ON M5T 3L9; Qns'10; CCFP.

LOWER, Gary D; Northwest Walk-In Clinic, 300A-595 Arthur St W, Thunder Bay ON P7E 5R5; Ott'87; (807)623-7101

LOWEY, John; Queen Elizabeth Hosp, PO Box 6600 Stn Central, Charlottetown PE C1A 8T5; Staff, Queen Elizabeth Hospital.

LOWN, Peter W; Sioux Lookout Meno-Ya-Win H C, PO Box 1500 Stn Main, Sioux Lookout ON P8T 1C2; Alb'98; BSc(BioChem); CCFP; Staff, Sioux Lookout Meno-Ya-Win Health Centre; (807)737-5161

LOWNEY, Mark J; Medical Arts Bldg, 115 Hazen St, Saint John NB E2L 3L3; Dal'76; Staff Family Med, St Joseph's Hospital; Assoc Staff, Saint John Regional Hospital; Att Physician, Loch Lomond Villa Nursing Home; (506)634-1273; Fax. (506)642-2814.

LOWNIE, Stephen P M; London HSC-University Hosp, PO Box 5339 Stn B 339 Windermere Rd, London ON N6A 5A5; Dal'83; FRCSC; Neursurg (Neuro Surgery & Endovascular Therapy). Staff, London Health Sciences Centre - Victoria Campus; Staff, London Health Sciences Centre - University Hospital; Co-Chair/Prof DiagRad, University of Western Ontario; (519)663-2927; Fax. (519)663-3888.

LOWRY, Brigittie H; New Waterford Consilidated, 716 King St, New Waterford NS B1H 3Z5; St George (Grenada)'96; CCFP; (902)592-3404; Fax. (902)592-3405.

LOWRY, Helen A; Knox Manse, 505 4th Ave N, Saskatoon SK S7K 2M5; Sask'06; Psy. (306)668-0505

LOWRY, Josiah B; 200-100 Colborne St W, Orillia ON L3V 2Y9; McM'78; ATLS; ACLS; CCFP; FCFP; Ac Staff, Orillia Soldiers' Memorial Hospital; Assoc Prof Family Med, University of Toronto; (705)327-3330; Fax. (705)327-7675.

LOWRY, Noel J; Royal University Hosp, 103 Hospital Dr, Saskatoon SK S7N 0W8; Dublin (Ireland)'73; MB ChB; BAO; MRC; DCH; FRCPC; Peds (Child Neurology); Neur. Staff Div of Ped Neurol, Royal University Hospital; Prof Med, University of Saskatchewan; (306)966-8115; Fax. (306)975-3767.

LOWRY, Peter; North Bay Reg Health Centre, 50 College Dr, North Bay ON P1B 0A4; McG'70; Staff, North Bay Regional Health Centre - Regional Mental Health; (705)474-1200

LOWRY, R Brian; Alberta Children's Hosp, 2888 Shaganappi Trail NW, Calgary AB T3B 6A8; Queen's U Belfast (Ireland)'56; DCH; FCCMG; DSc; FRCPC; Peds (Surveillance); MedGenetics. Att Staff, Alberta Children's Hospital; Med Consultant, Alberta Health & Wellness; Emeritus Prof, University of Calgary; (403)955-7370; brian.lowry@albertahealthservices.ca.

LOWRY, Robin P; Phoenix Med Centre, 202-2155 10th Ave, Prince George BC V2M 5J6; McG'71; BSc; ABIM(Nephrol); FRCPC; IntMed (Dialysis); Nephrol (P.Q.). Consultant IntMed & Nephrol, University Hospital of Northern British Columbia; (250)564-4225; Fax. (250)564-4229.

LOWTHER, Glen M; Cowichan Dist Hosp, 3045 Gibbins Rd, Duncan BC V9L 1E5; Man'82; FACEP; Staff, Cowichan District Hospital; (250)746-4141

LOWTON, Shamira; Family Med Clinic, 4615 49 Ave, Lloydminster SK S9V 0T1; Witwatersrand (South Africa)'03; MB BCh; (306)825-8877; Fax. (306)825-5167; sham2187@yahoo.co.uk.

LOY, Frank Y; The Pain Management Centre, 200-50 Westmount Rd N, Waterloo ON N2L 2R5; Cape Town (South Africa)'64; MB ChB; FRCPC; Anes (Pain Management). (519)747-1118; Fax. (519)747-4047. Semi-Retired.

LOY SON, Glenn; 4 46-125 Delhi St, Guelph ON N1E 4J5; Cape Town (South Africa)'82; MB ChB; FRCPC; Peds (Endocrinology). Staff, Guelph General Hospital; (519)767-5163; Fax. (519)767-5167.

LOYER, Deborah M; 100-14770 Boul De Pierrefonds, Pierrefonds QC H9H 4Y6; McG'85; FRCPC; Peds (Primary Care). Clin Asst Neonatol, McGill University Health Centre - Montreal General Campus; assoc Prof, McGill University; Langs: French; (514)696-2442; Fax. (514)624-3099.

LOYER, Michel; Hôpital Anna-Laberge, 200 boul Brisebois, Chateauguay QC J6K 4W8; Mon'79; Staff, Hôpital Anna-Laberge; (450)699-2425

LOYOLA, Vicente; Kootenay-Boundary Reg Hosp, 1200 Hospital Bench, Trail BC V1R 4M1; (Mexico)'82; FRCPC; GenPath. Ac Staff, Kootenay Boundary Regional Hospital; (250)364-3475; Fax. (250)364-3457.

LOZANO, Andres M; Univ Hlth Network-Toronto Western Hosp, WW4 431-399 Bathurst St, Toronto ON M5T 2S8; Ott'83; BSc; BMedSci; PhD; AB; FRCSC; Neursurg. Sr Scientist, Toronto Western Hospital - University Health Network; Prof Surg, University of Toronto; Langs: French; Spanish; (416)603-6200; Fax. (416)603-5298.

LOZANO, Marina; Greenboro Family Med Centre, 25 Tapiola Cres, Ottawa ON K1T 2J7; Ott'08; CCFP; (613)738-0303

LOZINSKI, Ala Z; Health Sciences Bldg, 312-15 Mountain Ave S, Stoney Creek ON L8G 2V6; McM'82; DAB; FRCPC; Derm (Dermatology Surgery). Asst Prof, McMaster University; Langs: Polish; (905)664-5060; Fax. (905)664-9972.

LOZON, Alan M; Grey Bruce HS-Owen Sound, PO Box 1800 Stn Main 5104-1800 8th St E, Owen Sound ON N4K 6M9; Ott'95; FRCSC; GenSurg (Vascular Surgery). Staff, Grey Bruce Health Services - Owen Sound; (519)376-3662; Fax. (519)376-3920.

LU, Annie; Mount Forest Fam Health Team, 525 Dublin St, Mount Forest ON N0G 2L3; Tor'05; CCFP; Staff GP Anaesthesia, Groves Memorial Community Hospital; Langs: Cantonese; (519)323-0255

LU, Charles C; Malton Med Arts Bldg, 106-3530 Derry Rd E, Mississauga ON L4T 4E3; (Taiwan)'70; DAB; (905)671-1052; Fax. (905)671-8489.

LU, Christopher M; Georgetown Med Associates, 201-1A Princess Anne Dr, Georgetown ON L7G 4W4; Glasgow (Scotland)'02; FRCSC; OrthSurg. (289)831-1549

LU, Diane J; KFL & A Public Health Unit, 221 Portsmouth Ave, Kingston ON K7M 1V5; Tor'97; PhD; CCFP; FCFP; Teach Staff Family Med, Queen's University; (613)549-1232; Fax. (613)549-7896.

LU, Fang-I; Sunnybrook Hlth Sciences Ctre, E4 32-2075 Bayview Ave, Toronto ON M4N 3M5; McG'06; MDCM; FRCPC; AnatPath. Staff, Sunnybrook Health Sciences Centre; (416)480-4600

LU, Grant S T; Scarborough Hosp-Birchmount, 3030 Birchmount Rd, Scarborough ON M1W 3W3; Wes'92; FRCPC; Anes;CCFP; Staff, The Scarborough Hospital - Birchmount Campus; (416)495-2561

LU, James D; 8100 Granville Ave, Richmond BC V6Y 3T6; UBC'81; (604)244-5129

LU, Jian-Qiang; University of Alberta Hosp, 5B2.24-8440 112 St NW, Edmonton AB T6G 2B7; (China)'87; FRCPC; NeurPath. Staff, University of Alberta Hospital; Langs: Chinese; Japanese; (780)407-2117; Fax. (780)407-3009.

LU, Paul B; Family Matters Med Centre, X-730 St Anne's Rd, Winnipeg MB R2N 0A2; Man'92; BSc; CCFP; FCFP; (204)253-5320

LU, Shao-Hua; Gordon & Leslie Diamond HCC, 8157B-2775 Laurel St, Vancouver BC V5Z 1M9; UBC'93; FRCPC; Psy (Addiction Medicine). Staff, Vancouver General Hospital - Centennial Pavillion; Staff, Gordon & Leslie Diamond Health Care Centre; Langs: Cantonese; Mandarin; (604)875-4111 x66121; Fax. (604)875-5652.

LU, Thomas S; Richmond Health Science Ctre, 310-6091 Gilbert Rd, Richmond BC V7C 5L9; UBC'99; BSc; FRCSC; OrthSurg (Hip & Knee Reconstruction). Med Staff, Richmond Hospital; Vis Specialist, Bella Coola General Hospital; Vis Specialist, Queen Charlotte Islands General Hospital - Queen Charlotte Site; Medical Staff, Delta Hospital; Medical Staff, UBC Hospital - Koerner Pavillion; Langs: Mandarin; (604)273-6148; Fax. (604)273-3421.

LU, William H Y; Weston Road Med Clinic, 2549 Weston Rd, York ON M9N 2A7; Tor'88; (416)240-8282; Fax. (416)240-8870.

LU, Ying; 210-220 Duncan Mill Rd, North York ON M3B 3J5; Qns'94; FRCSC; Ophth. Staff, The Scarborough Hospital - General Campus; Staff, The Scarborough Hospital - Birchmount Campus; Staff, Kensington Eye Institute; Lecturer, University of Toronto; (416)444-7502; Fax. (416)444-0025; ying.lu@uhn.on.ca.

LU, Yvette C; 5633 177B St, Surrey BC V3S 4H9; UBC'05; CCFP; (604)576-2828

LUBA, Robert M A; 213-520 Ellesmere Rd, Scarborough ON M1R 0B1; Man'78; FRCSC; OrthSurg (Arthroscopic Knee Surgery). Staff OrthSurg, Rouge Valley Health System - Centenary Health Centre Site; (416)287-2123; Fax. (416)281-2605.

HUBERT, Elzbieta G; St Joseph's Healthcare, 50 Charlton Ave E, Hamilton ON L8N 4A6; Gdansk (Poland)'71; Anes (Obstetrics). Staff, St Joseph's Healthcare - Charlton Campus; McMaster University; (905)522-4941

LUBANSKI, Martin S; Windsor Cardiac Centre, 5-130 Ouellette Place, Windsor ON N8X 1L9; Poznan (Poland)'07; (519)250-4449

LUBARSKY, Robert; 3020-6900 Boul Decarie, Cote Saint-Luc QC H3X 2T8; Montpellier (France)'75; AB; Sr Physician, Sir Mortimer B Davis Jewish General; Asst Prof Family Med, McGill University; (514)737-6060; Fax. (514)737-5937.

LUBARSKY, Stuart E; MUHC-Montreal Gen Hosp, L7 409-1650 av Cedar, Montreal QC H3G 1A4; McG'03; FRCPC; Neur. Staff, McGill University Health Centre - Montreal General Campus; (514)934-8060

LUBBAD, Nibal; St Joseph's Med Clinic, 906 Brant St, Burlington ON L7R 2J5; Leningradskij (Russia (Federation))'94; MHSc; CCFP; Langs: Arabic; English; Russian; (905)631-8898; Fax. (905)631-8895.

LUBBE, Gerald W; Village Med Clinic, PO Box 1720, 100 Mile House BC V0K 2E0; Stellenbosch (South Africa)'86; MB ChB; CCFP; (250)395-3000; Fax. (250)395-3055.

LUBCZANSKI, Aron; Bluewater Health-Norman Site, 89 Norman St, Sarnia ON N7T 6S3; Pretoria (South Africa)'75; MB ChB; MMed(Psych)(Wit; FRCPC; Psy (Adult & Geriatric Psychiatry). Staff, Bluewater Health - Norman Site; (519)464-4500

LUBCZYNSKI, Celina M; Whitby Family Physicians, 6-701 Rossland Rd E, Whitby ON L1N 8Y9; Atlanta(GA) (USA)'85; CCFP; (905)493-3447

LUBELL, Richard F; Children's After Hours Clinic, 101 Fanshawe Park Rd E, London ON N5X 3V9; Wes'67; FRCPCH; ABPeds; FRCPC; Peds (Primary Care). Consultant, St Joseph's Hospital - St Joseph's Health Care; Consultant, Children's Hospital of Western Ontario; Clin Assoc Prof, University of Western Ontario; (519)850-3800; richard.lubell@sympatico.ca.

LUBELSKY, Bruce J; 209-1110 Sheppard Ave E, North York ON M2K 2W2; Tor'79; FRCPC; IntMed; Cardiol. Ac Staff, North York General Hospital; Court Staff, Sunnybrook Health Sciences Centre; Instructor, University of Toronto; (416)229-4941; Fax. (416)229-4940.

LUBELSKY, Sari M; Mackenzie Richmond Hill Hosp, 10 Trench St, Richmond Hill ON L4C 4Z3; Wes'01; FRCPC; AnatPath. Staff, Mackenzie Richmond Hill Hospital; (905)883-1212 x7139

LUBIANTORO, Elsa; Royal University Hosp, 103 Hospital Dr, Saskatoon SK S7N 0W8; Jakarta (Indonesia)'92; FRCPC; CCFP; IntMed. Staff, Royal University Hospital; (306)655-1000

LUBIN, Alexandre S; Miramichi Med Arts Centre, 1-679 King George Hwy, Miramichi NB E1V 1N9; Puebla (Mexico)'89; (506)627-7536

LUBIN, Stanley; The Doctors' Office, 103-777 Broadway W, Vancouver BC V5Z 4J7; McG'73; CCFP; FCFP; Ac Staff, Vancouver General Hospital - Centennial Pavillion; Court Staff, BC Women's Hospital & Health Centre; Dir Post Grad/Prof Family Pract, University of British Columbia; Langs: Bilingual(English/French); (604)734-8252

LUBITZ, Paul A; Canmore Gen Hosp, 1100 Hospital Pl, Canmore AB T1W 1N2; Qns'96; AAD; ACLS; ABD; ABCS; BSc; FRCPC; Derm (Cosmetic Surgery). Staff Canmore Dermatology Clinic, Canmore General Hospital; Langs: French; Fax. (403)678-1205.

LUBITZ, Rebecca J; Andrew Street Family Hlth Ctre, 16 Andrew St, Kitchener ON N2H 5R2; San Francisco(CA) (USA)'06; CCFP; (519)804-9234

LUBKIEWICZ, Krzysztof; 160 av Stillview, Pointe-Claire QC H9R 2Y2; Warsaw (Poland)'62; PhD(Liverpool); Peds (P.Q.). Staff, Lakeshore General Hospital - Pointe Claire; Langs: Polish; Russian; klubkiewicz@hotmail.com.

LUBYNSKI, Rosemary A; Bluewater Health-Norman Site, 89 Norman St, Sarnia ON N7T 6S3; Cape Town (South Africa)'73; MB ChB; FRCPC; AnatPath (General Pathology). Assoc Dir, Bluewater Health - Mitton Site; Court Staff, Strathroy Middlesex General Hospital - Middlesex Hospital Alliance; Staff, Bluewater Health - Norman Site; Aj Prof, University of Western Ontario.

LUC, Mario; MUHC-Montreal Gen Hosp, 19 317-1650 av Cedar, Montreal QC H3G 1A4; Laval'03; FRCSC; PlasSurg. Staff, McGill University Health Centre - Montreal General Campus; (514)934-1934 x48341

LUCA, Anne-Marie; CLSC Saint-Michel, 3355 rue Jarry E, Montreal QC H1Z 2E5; Sher'90; CCFP; FCFP; (514)374-8223; Fax. (514)374-3812; anne-marie.luca@ssss.gouv.qc.ca.

LUCA, Nadia J C; The Hosp for Sick Children, 555 University Ave, Toronto ON M5G 1X8; Tor'06; FRCPC; Peds; Rheum. Staff, The Hospital For Sick Children; (416)813-7654

LUCA, Virgil A; Centre De Read Lucie-Bruneau, 2275 av Laurier E, Montreal QC H2H 2N8; Mon'86; (514)527-4527; Fax. (514)527-6637.

LUCAS, Jan P; 191 Grandview Ave, Thornhill ON L3T 1J3; Amsterdam (Netherlands)'60; FRCPC; Anes. (905)889-9265

LUCAS, Nathalie; Hôpital Ste-Justine, 3175 ch Cote-Sainte-Catherine, Montreal QC H3T 1C5; Laval'94; ABPeds; FRCPC; Peds (Emergency Pediatrics). Staff, Hôpital Ste-Justine; Langs: Bilingual(English/French); Spanish; (514)345-4931 x5885; Fax. (514)345-4965; lucasnath@yahoo.com.

LUCAS, William J; Office Reg Supervising Coroner, 700-24 Queen St E, Brampton ON L6V 1A3; Tor'76; MD; (905)874-3972; Fax. (905)874-3976; William.Lucas@ontario.ca.

LUCE, John T; Medicine Professional Corp, 541 Glenridge Ave, St Catharines ON L2T 4C2; Man'66; BSc; Chief of Staff, Hôtel Dieu Shaver Health & Rehabilitation Centre; (905)734-2411; Fax. (905)687-3232; jluce3@cogeco.ca.

LUCE, Kiersten A; New Vision Family Health Team, 421 Greenbrook Dr, Kitchener ON N2M 4K1; Tor'91; BSc; CCFP; FCFP; Court Staff, Grand River Hospital - Kitchener/Waterloo Health Centre; Court Staff, St Mary's General Hospital; Staff, New Vision Family Health Team - Greenbrook; (519)570-1655; Fax. (519)570-3477.

LUCES, Kevin F; Medical Clinic, 460 King St W, Oshawa ON L1J 2K9; Tor'76; Staff, Lakeridge Health - Oshawa Site; (905)725-3523; Fax. (905)725-0702.

LUCEWICZ, Michael; Calgary Trail Medicentre, 1-10407 51 Ave NW, Edmonton AB T6H 0K4; (Poland)'77; Staff, Calgary Trail Medicentres; Langs: Polish; Ukrainian; Russian; (780)436-8071; Fax. (780)435-6034.

LUCEY, Michele D; Institut de Cardiologie de Mtl, 5000 rue Belanger, Montreal QC H1T 1C8; McG'00; CCFP; CCFP(E.M.); Staff, Institut de Cardiologie de Montréal; (514)376-3330

LUCEY, William F; 209-282 Linwell Rd, St Catharines ON L2N 6N5; National (Ireland)'72; (905)935-0770; Fax. (905)935-9147.

LUCIANI, Lee M; 186 Talbot St S, Essex ON N8M 1B6; Ott'98; CCFP; (519)776-1559; Fax. (519)776-9050.

LUCIDO, Barbara M; Sheldon Chumir Centre, 1213 4 St SW, Calgary AB T2R 0X7; Cal'04; FRCPC; Psy. (403)955-6679

LUCIUK, George H; Richmond Health Science Ctre, 850-6091 Gilbert Rd, Richmond BC V7C 5L9; Alb'76; FACP; FAAAI; FRCPC; Peds; ClinImmunol&Allergy. Ac Staff, BC Children's Hospital; Ac Staff, Vancouver General Hospital - Centennial Pavillion; Ac Staff, Richmond Hospital; Clin Instructor, University of British Columbia; (604)270-7801; Fax. (604)270-3283.

LUCK, Geoffrey M; Oshawa Clinic, 117 King St E, Oshawa ON L1H 1B9; West Indies (Jamaica)'72; CCFP; (905)721-4952; Fax. (905)721-4329.

LUCKHURST, Geoffrey W M; 2519 Estevan Ave, Victoria BC V8R 2S6; Man'70; CCFP; (250)598-7200; Fax. (250)598-7414.

LUCKOW, David; 180 av Cartier, Pointe-Claire QC H9S 4S1; McG'01; CCFP; (514)697-4110

LUCKY, Cindy-Ann; Gordon & Leslie Diamond HCC, 11F-2775 Laurel St, Vancouver BC V5Z 1M9; West Indies (Jamaica)'88; CCFP; CCFP(E.M.); FCFP; Clin Associate Prof Family & Emerg Med, University of British Columbia; (604)875-4500

LUCMAN, Lydia L; St Boniface Gen Hosp, 409 Tache Ave, Winnipeg MB R2H 2A6; Manila (Philippines)'63; FRCPC; GenPath. Staff, St Boniface General Hospital; (204)237-2490; Fax. (204)235-3423.

LUCMAN, Tahir S; Winnipeg Clinic, 425 St Mary Ave, Winnipeg MB R3C 0N2; Punjab (Pakistan)'63; MB BS; FRCPC; IntMed (Cardiology). Consultant, Victoria General Hospital; Langs: Urdu; Punjabi; (204)957-1900; Fax. (204)957-7410.

LUCO, Gerald G; Richmond Med Bldg, 203-2020 Richmond Rd, Victoria BC V8R 6R5; Alb'80; (250)595-4252

LUCY, Simon J; St Boniface Gen Hosp, 409 Tache Ave, Winnipeg MB R2H 2A6; Man'80; FRCPC; Anes. Staff Obstertical Anes, St Boniface General Hospital; Asst Prof, University of Manitoba; Langs: French; (204)237-2580; Fax. (204)231-0425.

LUCYK, Chad M; PO Box 71134 Rpo North Town Ma, Edmonton AB T5E 6J8; Sask'05; CCFP; CCFP(E.M.).

LUCYK, Scott; University of Alberta Hosp, 8440 112 St NW, Edmonton AB T6G 2B7; Alb'08; Staff, University of Alberta Hospital; (780)407-8822

LUCZAK, L Alexander; 408 1-49 High St, Barrie ON L4N 5J4; Ott'82; FRCPC; Psy. Consultant, Waypoint Centre for Mental Health Care; (705)721-7813; Fax. (705)721-9217.

LUDEMANN, Jeffrey P; Children's & Women's HC of BC, K2 183-4480 Oak St, Vancouver BC V6H 3V4; McG'92; FRCSC; Otol (Pediatric Otolaryngology). Att Staff Otol, BC Children's Hospital; Asst Prof Otol, University of British Columbia; (604)875-2113

LUDGATE, Charles M; BC Cancer Agency-Vanc Isl Ctr, 2410 Lee Ave, Victoria BC V8R 6V5; Edinburgh (Scotland)'70; MB ChB; MD; DMRT; FRCS; FRCPC; RadOncol. Staff, BC Cancer Agency Vancouver Island Centre; (250)519-5576

LUDMAN, Ronald B; 420-245 Av Victoria, Westmount QC H3Z 2M6; McG'77; PhD; CCFP; Att Staff Family Med, Sir Mortimer B Davis Jewish General; Dir-svcs prof, CH Richardson; Asst Prof Family Med, McGill University; (514)939-9633; Fax. (514)939-7382; ronald.ludman.chr@ssss.gouv.qc.ca.

LUDWICK, Catherine L; Great West Life Company, 60 Osborne St N, Winnipeg MB R3C 1V3; Man'96; FRCPC; AnatPath.

LUDWIG, John J; Omemee Med Centre, PO Box 310 23 Wellington St, Omemee ON K0L 2W0; Qns'72; Staff Family Pract, Peterborough Regional Health Centre - Hospital Drive; Dist Dir, Ontario Medical Association; (705)799-0000; Fax. (705)799-0271.

LUDWIG, Louis W; Psychealth Centre, PZ275-771 Bannatyne Ave, Winnipeg MB R3E 0W3; Man'73; FRCPC; EmergMed; Psy. Assoc Prof, University of Manitoba; (204)787-3806; Fax. (204)787-7480.

LUDWIG, Mara S; MUHC-Royal Victoria Hosp, 687 av des Pins O, Montreal QC H3A 1A1; Man'79; Respir; IntMed. Assoc Physician, McGill University Health Centre - Royal Victoria Hospital; Att Physician, McGill University Health Centre - Montreal Chest Institute; Assoc Dean Faculty Affairs, McGill University; Langs: English; French; (514)934-1934; mara.ludwig@mcgill.ca.

LUDWIG, Sora M; St Boniface Gen Hosp, 409 Tache Ave, Winnipeg MB R2H 2A6; Man'77; FRCPC; IntMed; Endocrin&Metab. Ac Staff Section of Endocrin & Metabolism, St Boniface General Hospital; Med Advisor, Manitoba Provincial Program in Diabetes Education; Asst Prof Med, University of Manitoba; (204)237-2908; Fax. (204)233-7154.

LUDWIN, David; St Joseph's Healthcare, 50 Charlton Ave E, Hamilton ON L8N 4A6; Witwatersrand (South Africa)'72; MB ChB; FRCP(Lond); FACP; FRCPC; IntMed (Transplantation); Nephrol. Ac Staff Transplantation, St Joseph's Healthcare - Charlton Campus; Staff, Hamilton Health Sciences Centre - McMaster University Medical Centre; Staff, The Brant Community Healthcare System - Brantford General Hospital Site; Prof Med, McMaster University; (905)521-6049; Fax. (905)521-6088.

LUEDTKE, Chad C; Peter Lougheed Centre, 3500 26 Ave NE, Calgary AB T1Y 6J4; McG'04; FRCPC; AnatPath. Staff, Peter Lougheed Centre; (403)943-2549

LUELO, Christine A; McKenzie Family Practice, 71 High St SE, Calgary AB T2Z 3T9; Alb'97; BSc; CCFP; Board of Directors, South Calgary Primary Care Network; (403)257-0500; Fax. (403)257-3186.

LUER, Andrew Z; Western Mem Reg Hosp, PO Box 2005 Stn Main 1 Brookfield Ave, Corner Brook NL A2H 6J7; Gdansk (Poland)'76; Staff, Western Memorial Regional Hospital; (709)637-5000

LUETKEHOELTER, Jonathan; St Michal's Hosp Academic-FHT, 940-790 Bay St, Toronto ON M5G 1N8; McM'92; Court Staff/Med Dir Casey House Hospice, St Michael's Hospital; Physician, Toronto HIV Primary Care Physicians Group; (416)926-0101; Fax. (416)926-1910; jonathanl@ca.inter.net.

LUEY, Lai-Lane; U of Toronto-Health Services, 214 College St, Toronto ON M5T 2Z9; Tor'86; (416)978-8030; Fax. (416)971-2089.

LUFT, Wendy A; 169-4625 Varsity Dr NW, Calgary AB T3A 0Z9; Cal'06; CCFP.

LUFTSPRING, Lawrence; 1-2085 Weston Rd, Toronto ON M9N 1X7; Tor'86; Staff, William Osler Health System - Etobicoke General Hospital; Staff, Humber River Regional Hospital - Church Street Site; (416)244-1150; Fax. (416)245-1546.

LUGER, Sherry; 3020-6900 boul Decarie, Cote Saint-Luc QC H3X 2T8; McG'83; BSc; MDCM; (514)737-6060; Fax. (514)737-5937.

LUGINBUEHL, Igor A; The Hosp for Sick Children, 555 University Ave, Toronto ON M5G 1X8; Basel (Switzerland)'92; Staff, The Hospital For Sick Children; (416)813-7445; Fax. (416)813-7543.

LUHNING, Allan H; Hammond Bldg, 407-310 Main St N, Moose Jaw SK S6H 3K1; Sask'76; Ac Staff, Moose Jaw Union Hospital; (306)694-0707; Fax. (306)693-1677.

LUI, Albert K H; Norburn Med Centre, 200-4012 Hastings St, Burnaby BC V5C 2H9; UBC'91; (604)299-2677

LUI, Alwin; Olive Med Clinic, 101-117 17 Ave NE, Calgary AB T2E 1L7; Sask'03; CCFP; (403)276-8866

LUI, Andrew B; St Joseph's Health Centre, 30 The Queensway, Toronto ON M6R 1B5; Tor'08; CCFP; CCFP(E.M.); Staff, St Joseph's Health Centre; (416)530-6000

LUI, Anne C P; The Ottawa Hosp-Civic Campus, 1053 Carling Ave, Ottawa ON K1Y 4E9; UBC'83; BSc; MSc; FRCPC; Anes (Acute Pain Management). Att Staff, The Ottawa Hospital - Civic Campus; Asst Prof, University of Ottawa; (613)761-4169

LUI, Bosco T M; 101-7155 Woodbine Ave, Markham ON L3R 1A3; McM'05; FRCSC; Otol. (416)628-4020; Fax. (416)628-4021.

LUI, Charlene L; Burnaby Hosp, 3935 Kincaid St, Burnaby BC V5G 2X6; UBC'94; Staff, Burnaby Hospital; (604)431-2822

LUI, Clementine J P M; The Ottawa Hosp-Gen Campus, L2248-501 Smyth Rd, Ottawa ON K1H 8L6; Alb'08; FRCPC; IntMed. Staff, The Ottawa Hospital - General Campus; (613)737-8899

LUI, Derek P K; 369 Hunter St, Woodstock ON N4S 4G3; Mem'87; FRCSC; Ophth (Cataract). Staff Surg, Woodstock General Hospital; Langs: Chinese; (519)421-1851; Fax. (519)421-9234.

LUI, Frederick C C; Queen Square Doctors FHT, 201-366 Main St N, Brampton ON L6V 1P8; London (England)'71; MB BS; Staff, William Osler Health System - Brampton Civic Hospital; (905)455-1331; Fax. (905)455-5498.

LUI, Harvey; Skin Care Centre, 835 10th Ave W, Vancouver BC V5Z 4E8; UBC'86; ABD; FAAD; FRCPC; Derm (Laser Surgery). Ac Staff, Vancouver General Hospital - Centennial Pavillion; Prof/Chair/Dept Head & School Dir Derm & Skin Science, University of British Columbia; Langs: Cantonese; (604)875-4747; Fax. (604)873-9919.

LUI, Jaime; Bridgepoint Family Health Team, 430 Broadview Ave, Toronto ON M4K 2N1; Tor'06; CCFP; (416)470-6690; jlui@mtsinai.on.ca.

LUI, Kim C; C-12-8380 Kennedy Rd, Unionville ON L3R 0W4; (Hong Kong)'87; MB BS; MRCP(UK); DCH(Glas); Langs: Cantonese; Mandarin; (905)946-0882; Fax. (905)946-0436.

LUI, Robert C; Market Mall Bldg, 316-4935 40 Ave NW, Calgary AB T3A 2N1; McG'77; FRCSC; GenSurg (Biliary Surgery). Clinical Asst Prof Surg, University of Calgary; Langs: Cantonese; (403)247-3855

LUI, Spenser M Y; 218-7031 Westminster Hwy, Richmond BC V6X 1A3; Tor'77; FRCSC; OrthSurg. Langs: Chinese; Cantonese; Mandarin; (604)276-8818; Fax. (604)276-8123.

LUI, Alexander; Oakville Health Centre, 214-1060 Speers Rd, Oakville ON L6L 2X4; Wes'81; Ac Staff, Halton Healthcare Services Corporation - Oakville Site; Langs: Chinese; Cantonese; (905)842-6922; Fax. (905)842-5561; dralexlui@gmail.com.

LUI, Yuk Ming; Chinatown X-Ray/Ultrasound Cli, 205-618 Quebec St, Vancouver BC V6A 4E7; Man'67; FRCPC; DiagRad. (604)688-9428

LUIS, Christine; CSSS de Sept-Iles, 45 rue du Pere-Divet, Sept-Iles QC G4R 3N7; Mon'09; CCFP; Staff, Centre Hospitalier Regional de Sept-Iles; (418)962-9761

LUISON, Fabio; Four Corners Med Bldg, 402-2009 Long Lake Rd, Sudbury ON P3E 6C3; Ott'92; BMedSci; FRCSC; GenSurg; Critical Care Medicine; ThorSurg. Staff ThorSurg & Critical Care Med, Health Sciences North - Memorial Site; Asst Prof, Northern Ontario School of Medicine; (705)523-5626; Fax. (705)523-0827.

LUITINGH, Ursula; Golden Ears Fam Practice, 140-20395 Lougheed Hwy, Maple Ridge BC V2X 2P9; Pretoria (South Africa)'92; MB ChB; Staff, Ridge Meadows Hospital & Health Care Centre; Langs: Afrikaans; (604)465-1066; info@goldenearsclinic.ca.

LUJIC-THEBAUD, Jelka-Maria; Univ of Alberta, 8 120-152 University Campus NW, Edmonton AB T6G 2G3; (France)'95; Staff, University of Alberta Hospital; Langs: French; German; Croatian; (780)407-8861; Fax. (780)407-3200.

LUK, Adriana C; University of Toronto, 602-500 University Ave, Toronto ON M5G 1V7; Ott'08; IntMed.

LUK, Alan L; 204-240 Alton Towers Circle, Scarborough ON M1V 4P3; Loma Linda(CA) (USA)'84; CCFP; Ac Staff, The Scarborough Hospital - Birchmount Campus; Ac Staff, The Scarborough Hospital - General Campus; Court Staff, North York General Hospital - Branson Division; (416)292-1200

LUK, Cynthia S Y; Stronach Reg Cancer Centre, 596 Davis Dr, Newmarket ON L3Y 2P9; Qns'96; FRCPC; IntMed; MedOncol; Hem. Staff, Southlake Regional Health Centre; Staff, Stronach Regional Cancer Centre; (905)895-4521 x6091; Fax. (905)952-3053.

LUK, Cynthia T; St Michael's Hosp, 7F-61 Queen St E, Toronto ON M5C 2T2; Alb'06; FRCPC; IntMed; Endocrin&Metab. Staff, St Michael's Hospital; (416)867-7424

LUK, Kenneth D; Trillium Health Centre, 100 Queensway W, Mississauga ON L5B 1B8; Wes'03; FRCSC; Anes. Staff, Trillium Health Centre - Mississauga.

LUK, Tracy C C; William Osler HC-Brampton, 2100 Bovaird Dr E, Brampton ON L6R 3J7; Wes'05; FRCPC; IntMed; Critical Care Medicine. Staff, William Osler Health System - Brampton Civic Hospital; (905)494-2120

LUK, Tse Li; Linden Ridge Med Centre, E-123 Scurfield Blvd, Winnipeg MB R3Y 1L6; Cardiff (Wales)'84; MB ChB; Staff, Misericordia Health Centre; Langs: Cantonese; (204)488-9988

LUK, David W T; Guildford Med Dental Centre, 23-15300 105 Ave, Surrey BC V3R 6A7; UBC'76; Staff, Surrey Memorial Hospital; (604)588-2882

LUKARIS, Andrew D; 200-1440 2nd Ave, Prince George BC V2L 3B6; (Wales)'96; Ophth. Langs: Greek; (250)596-3011

LUKASIK, Mark H; Greystone Office Centre, 106-345 8th St E, Owen Sound ON N4K 1L3; Wes'84; CCFP; CCFP(E.M.); FCFP; Staff, Grey Bruce Health Services - Owen Sound; (519)371-1700; Fax. (519)371-8684.

LUKASZEWSKA-ANDZIAK, Bozenna; 207-14 Prince Arthur Ave, Toronto ON M5R 1A9; Warsaw (Poland)'70; FRCPC; Psy. Staff, Centre for Addiction & Mental Health (CAMH) - Queen Site; (416)927-9595

LUKE, Edward C H; Oakridge Centre South Tower, 360-650 41st Ave W, Vancouver BC V5Z 2M9; McG'94; CCFP; CCFP(E.M.); FCFP; Langs: Taiwanese; Mandarin; Cantonese; (604)261-6000; Fax. (604)261-6667; eluke94@yahoo.com.

LUKE, Koon-Hung; Children's Hosp Eastern Ont, 401 Smyth Rd, Ottawa ON K1H 8L1; (Hong Kong)'59; MB BS; DAB; Peds. Ac Staff Peds, Children's Hospital of Eastern Ontario (CHEO); University of Ottawa; Langs: Chinese; (613)737-7600 x2210; luke@cheo.on.ca.

LUKE, Patrick P W; London HSC-University Hosp, PO Box 5339 Stn B 339 Windermere Rd, London ON N6A 5A5; Tor'93; FRCSC; Urol. Staff, London Health Sciences Centre - University Hospital; (519)663-3180

LUKE, Philip B; St Joseph's Gen Hosp, 2137 Comox Ave, Comox BC V9M 1P2; UBC'89; CCFP; CCFP(E.M.); Staff, St Joseph's General Hospital; (250)339-1557

LUKE, Seema; Thames Valley FHT-Whitehills M, 1225 Wonderland Rd N, London ON N6G 2V9; Wes'93; BSc; CCFP; (519)472-0040; Fax. (519)472-7732; seema.luke@gmail.com.

LUKENDA, Michael A; 500-340 College St, Toronto ON M5T 3A9; St Maarten (Netherlands Antilles)'99; CCFP; (416)324-8677; Fax. (416)324-9490.

LUKEY, Judith G T; PO Box 21083 Rpo Terwillegar, Edmonton AB T6R 2V4; Alb'77.

LUKIC, Dusan; St Joseph's Healthcare, 50 Charlton Ave E, Hamilton ON L8N 4A6; Belgrade (Serbia)'82; MD; Staff, St Joseph's Healthcare - Charlton Campus; Asst Prof, McMaster University; Langs: Serbian; Croatian; (905)522-1155 x35007; Fax. (905)521-6192; lukic@hhsc.ca.

LUKIE, Brian; Pan Am Sports Med Centre, 75 Poseidon Bay, Winnipeg MB R3M 3E4; Man'80; (204)927-2699; Fax. (204)452-5362.

LUKIN, Svitlana; North Med Medical Centre, 102-7131 Bathurst St, Thornhill ON L4J 7Z1; Danylo Halytsky Lviv (Ukraine)'99.

LUKKA, Himanshu R; The Juravinski Cancer Centre, 3-699 Concession St, Hamilton ON L8V 5C2; Manchester (England)'78; MRCP; FRCR; FRCPC; RadOncol. Staff, Hamilton Health Sciences Centre-Juravinski Site; Staff, Hamilton Regional Cancer Centre; Assoc Prof, McMaster University; (905)387-9495; Fax. (905)575-6326.

LUKOMSKA, Katarzyna E; 202-1950 Algonquin Ave, North Bay ON P1B 4Z2; Warsaw (Poland)'82; CCFP; FCFP; Ac Staff (All Sites), North Bay Regional Health Centre - Regional Mental Health; Langs: Polish; (705)476-0086; Fax. (705)476-7850.

LUKOWSKA, Irena; 7667 Nanaimo St, Vancouver BC V5P 4M6; Szczecin (Poland)'72; (604)324-3900

LUKSUN, Warren J; Univ Hlth Network-Toronto Gen, 200 Elizabeth St, Toronto ON M5G 2C4; UBC'07; Anes. Staff, Toronto General Hospital - UHN; (416)340-4800

LUKUBISA, Alexander; Albert Park Med Clinic, 3992 Albert St, Regina SK S4S 3R1; (306)584-3833

LUKWINSKI, Angelina T; Charles Clark Med Centre, 201-303 9 Ave SW, High River AB T1V 0H2; (Poland)'05; LMCC; FRCSC; ObstGyn. (403)652-2929

LULASHNYK, Ben J; Dauphin Med Clinic, 622 3rd St SW, Dauphin MB R7N 1R5; Man'09; CCFP.

LULIC-HRVOJIC, Ana; High Park Health Centre, 200-2333 Dundas St W, Toronto ON M6R 3A6; Zagreb (Croatia)'63; FRCPC; Psy (Adult Psychiatry). Langs: Croatian; (416)531-2660

LULJA, Nevila; York Med Health Centre, C-17215 Leslie St, Newmarket ON L3Y 8E4; Tiranes (Albania)'99; CCFP; (905)853-0404

LUM, Cheemun; The Ottawa Hosp-Civic Campus, 1053 Carling Ave, Ottawa ON K1Y 4E9; Ott'92; FRCPC; DiagRad (Neuro Radiology). Staff, The Ottawa Hospital - Civic Campus; (613)737-8844

LUM, David W K; St Thomas-Elgin Gen Hosp, PO Box 2007 Stn Main 189 Elm St, St Thomas ON N5P 3W2; McG'84; CCFP; Staff, St Thomas Elgin General Hospital; Langs: Cantonese; French; (519)631-2030

LUM, Derek W; Kootenay Boundary Reg Hosp, 1200 Hospital Bench, Trail BC V1R 4M1; Cal'97; CCFP; Staff, Kootenay Boundary Regional Hospital; (250)368-3311

LUM, Edward; 5688 Victoria Dr, Vancouver BC V5P 3W4; UBC'94; BSc; Langs: Toishan; Cantonese; Mandarin; (604)323-8723

LUM, Grant; Athletic Edge Sports Med, PO Box 33 1100-121 King St W, Toronto ON M5H 3T9; Tor'92; Dip SportMed; CCFP; Staff Family & Commun Med, Toronto Western Hospital - University Health Network; Aj Prof, York University; Consultant, National Hockey League Player's Association; Lecturer, University of Toronto; (416)800-0800; Fax. (416)800-0802; info@aesm.ca.

LUM, Jeffrey H; Terra Nova Health Services, 160-3675 Westminster Hwy, Richmond BC V7C 5V2; Qns'91; CCFP; CCFP(E.M.); FCFP; (604)278-9525

LUM, Julie K; Niagara Med Group Fam Hlth Team, 4421 Queen St, Niagara Falls ON L2E 2L2; Ott'90; CCFP; FCFP; (905)356-2236; Fax. (905)356-2568.

LUM, P Andrea; London HSC-Victoria Hosp, PO Box 5010 Stn B 800 Commissioners Rd E, London ON N6A 5W9; Ott'83; FRCPC; DiagRad (Gastrointestinal Radiology). Staff, London Health Sciences Centre - Victoria Campus; Dept Chair Diagnostic Radiol & Nuclear Med, University of Western Ontario; (519)685-8500 x55003; Fax. (519)667-6771.

LUM MIN, Suyin A; Health Sciences Centre, 820 Sherbrook St, Winnipeg MB R3A 1R9; Cal'99; FRCSC; GenSurg; PedGenSurg. Staff Surg, Health Sciences Centre; (204)774-6511

LUMB, Barry J; Hamilton HS-Juravinski Site, 711 Concession St, Hamilton ON L8V 1C3; McM'79; FRCPC; IntMed; Gastroent. Staff, Hamilton Health Sciences Centre-Juravinski Site; Prof, McMaster University; (905)527-4322; blumb@mcmaster.ca.

LUMB, Kathleen J; Associate Med Clinic, 400-20 14th St W, Prince Albert SK S6V 3K8; Cal'07; FRCSC; GenSurg. (306)764-1513

LUMB, Kevin A; 202-100 Humber College Blvd, Etobicoke ON M9V 5G4; Tor'05; FRCPC; IntMed; Respir. Staff, William Osler Health System - Etobicoke General Hospital; (416)746-1011

LUMBY, Pollie S; Copeman Health Care Centre, 400-628 12 Ave SW, Calgary AB T2R 0H6; Cal'90; CCFP; FCFP; (403)270-2273; Fax. (403)521-2250.

LUMMACK, Keith F; 236 Parkdale Ave N, Hamilton ON L8H 5X5; Ott'70; (905)545-7711; Fax. (905)545-9282.

LUMMER, Charles R; Hys Med Centre, 202-11010 101 St NW, Edmonton AB T5H 4B9; Alb'85; FRCPC; DiagRad. Staff Radiol & Diag Imaging, Covenant Health - Grey Nuns Community Hospital; (780)426-1121

LUN, Victor M Y; Sports Med Centre, 2500 University Dr NW, Calgary AB T2N 1N4; UBC'95; CCFP; (403)220-8161; Fax. (403)282-6170; vmylun@ucalgary.ca.

LUNA, Alberto; Inuulitsivik Health Centre, GD, Puvirnituq QC J0M 1P0; McG'05; CCFP; Staff, Inuulitsivik Health Centre; (819)988-2957

LUNA, Fernando A; 325 Boul Greber, Gatineau QC J8T 8J3; (Mexico)'79; Physician, Adolescent Clinic & CLSC le Moulin-Gatineau; Langs: Spanish; French; (819)561-5862; Fax. (819)561-8998.

LUNACZEK-MOTYKA, Ewa M; Victoria Gen Hosp, 1 Hospital Way, Victoria BC V8Z 6R5; Cal'02; BSc; FRCPC; Peds (Pediatric Hematology Oncology). Staff, Victoria General Hospital; (250)727-4212

LUND, Adam; Royal Columbian Hosp, 330 Columbia St E, New Westminster BC V3L 3W7; UBC'98; FRCPC; EmergMed. Staff Emerg, Royal Columbian Hospital; (604)520-4283

LUND, Chad R; BC Cancer Agency-Fraser Valley, 13750 96 Ave, Surrey BC V3V 1Z2; Ott'03; FRCPC; RadOncol. Staff, BC Cancer Agency Fraser Valley Centre; (604)930-2098

LUND, Charles R; 401-3320 Richter St, Kelowna BC V1W 4V5; Cape Town (South Africa)'75; MB ChB; FRCPC; Anes. (250)868-9799

LUND, Christine L; Beaumont Med Clinic, 4-5102 49 Ave, Beaumont AB T4X 1E4; Alb'91; CCFP; (780)929-5400; Fax. (780)929-2126.

LUND, Christopher U; PO Box 244 Stn Main, Fergus ON N1M 2W8; Massachusetts (USA)'86; AB; MD; CCFP; FCFP; Clinical Asst Prof, McMaster School of Medicine; (519)323-7331; Fax. (519)787-0941.

LUND, Mark A; Alder Med Centre, 277 Evergreen Rd, Campbell River BC V9W 5Y4; UBC'93; FRCPC; Peds (Diabetology). Staff Peds, Campbell River & District General Hospital; Vis Staff, Port Hardy Hospital; Vis Staff, Port McNeill & District Hospital; (250)287-7454

LUND, R Daryl; 9th Avenue Med Centre, 6-3855 9th Ave, Port Alberni BC V9Y 4T9; UBC'90; (250)724-4492; Fax. (250)724-5033.

LUNDALL, Evan; Red Deer Reg Hosp Centre, PO Box 5030 Stn Postal Box Ctr, Red Deer AB T4N 6R2; Durban (South Africa)'83; MB ChB; Staff, Red Deer Regional Hospital Centre; (403)343-4519; Fax. (403)309-2809; evan.lundall@impacthealth.ca.

LUNDEEN, Richard C; Cedars Prof Park, 2931 66 St NW, Edmonton AB T6K 4C1; Alb'73; FRCPC; Psy. Ac Staff, Covenant Health - Grey Nuns Community Hospital; Asst Prof, University of Alberta; (780)461-1729; Fax. (780)461-1155.

LUNDERVILLE, Peggy R; Crest Med Clinic, 8695 10th Ave, Burnaby BC V3N 2S9; UBC'76; (604)525-3828; Fax. (604)525-3829.

LUNDGARD, Karen A H; Associate Med Clinic, PO Box 7590 Stn Main, Peace River AB T8S 1T2; Alb'77; CCFP; FCFP; Ac Staff, Peace River Community Health Centre; Clin Lecturer Family Med, University of Alberta; (780)624-2581; Fax. (780)624-4015.

LUNDGREN, A Christin; The Doctor's Office at Nosehil, 137-1829 Ranchlands Blvd NW, Calgary AB T3G 2A7; Goteborg (Sweden)'78; LMCC; CCFP; Langs: Swedish; (403)239-8888; Fax. (403)241-1506.

LUNDINE, Kristopher M; 305-1120 Yates St, Victoria BC V8V 3M9; Cal'03; FRCSC; OrthSurg. (250)381-5424

LUNDY, Stephen E; Dr Stephen Lundy Med Clinic, 225-1900 Richmond Rd, Victoria BC V8R 4R2; Wes'80; FRCPC; IntMed. Staff Respirol, Vancouver Island Health Authority; (250)339-1625; Fax. (250)339-1628.

LUNEAU, Colette P; CHUS-Hop Fleurimont, 3001 12e Av N, Sherbrooke QC J1H 5N4; Bordeaux (France)'74; Neursurg (Trauma). Staff, Centre Hospitalier Universitaire de Sherbrooke-Hopital Fleurimont; Langs: Bilingual(French/English); (819)346-1110 x6451; Fax. (819)820-6424.

LUNEAU, Katie; CHUM-Hop Notre-Dame, 1560 rue Sherbrooke E, Montreal QC H2L 4M1; Laval'02; FRCPC; Ophth. Staff, Centre Hospitalier l'Université de Montréal (CHUM) - Hôpital Notre-Dame; Langs: Bilingual(French/English); (514)890-8000 x27103; Fax. (514)412-7663.

LUNEAU, Mance; CSSS de Thérèse de Blainville, 100 Chanoine Lionel-Giroulx, Sainte-Therese QC J7E 5E1; Sher'99; Staff, CSSS de Thérèse de Blainville; (450)437-4267

LUNEAU, Micheline; Clinique Fam De St-Hyacinthe, 2955 boul Laframboise, Saint-Hyacinthe QC J2S 4Z3; Toulouse (France)'79; Consultant Geriatrics, Centre d hebergement de l Hôtel-Dieu de Saint-Hyacinthe; Staff Continuing Prof Training, Universite de Montreal; (450)774-4611; Fax. (450)773-9913; mluneau@sympatico.ca.

LUNG, Gilbert G; Royal Alexandra Hosp, 541-10240 Kingsway NW, Edmonton AB T5H 3V9; Alb'01; CCFP; CCFP(E.M.); Staff Kingsway Emergency Agency, Royal Alexandra Hospital; (780)735-4442; Fax. (780)735-4916.

LUNGE, Ryan J; Kimberley Med Clinic, PO Box 160, Kimberley BC V1A 2Y6; Cal'08; CCFP; (250)427-4861

LUNN, H R Darlene; The Medical Centre FHT, PO Box 4200 Stn Main 707 Charlotte St, Peterborough ON K9J 7B3; Tor'87; BSc(Psychol); (705)876-4556; Fax. (705)742-7076.

LUNNEY, James L; The Westend Family Care Clinic, 80 Michael Cowpland Dr, Kanata ON K2M 1P6; Ott'77; CCFP; CCFP(E.M.); Staff, Westend Family Care Clinic Family Health Team; (613)596-3321

LUNNEY, M Claire; 304-1407 Yonge St, Toronto ON M4T 1Y7; Tor'80; CCFP; FCFP; Staff, St Michael's Hospital; (416)964-8989; Fax. (416)487-8743.

LUNTAO, Yuri M A; Fredericton Med Clinic, 502-1015 Regent St, Fredericton NB E3B 6H5; MD; FCCP; Staff Pulmonary & Critical Care Med, Dr Everett Chalmers Regional Hospital; (506)447-4747; Fax. (506)447-4166.

LUNTLEY, Jeremy B; Alberta Children's Hosp, 2888 Shaganappi Trail NW, Calgary AB T3B 6A8; (England)'87; MB BS; Staff Anes, Alberta Children's Hospital; (403)955-7810; Fax. (403)229-7606.

LUO, Yigang; Royal University Hosp, 161-103 Hospital Dr, Saskatoon SK S7N 0W8; (China)'82; PhD; FRCSC; GenSurg (Surgical Oncology). Staff Surg, Royal University Hospital; Langs: Chinese; (306)966-1848

LUOMA, Andrew A; 201-2903 Pandosy St, Kelowna BC V1Y 1W1; Qns'82; FRCSC; GenSurg; ThorSurg. Ac Staff, Kelowna General Hospital; (250)763-7660

LUONG, Angela; Toronto East Gen Hosp Inc, 825 Coxwell Ave, Toronto ON M4C 3E7; Tor'96; FRCP; DABR; FRCPC; DiagRad (Radiology). Staff Radiol, Toronto East General Hospital Inc; (416)469-6075; aluon@tegh.on.ca.

LUONG, Dien Hung; Institut de Physiatrie Quebec, 2049 rue Sherbrooke E, Montreal QC H2K 1C1; Mon'06; FRCPC; PhysMed&Rehab. (514)527-4155

LUONG, Diep T; CLSC Saint-Henri, 3833 rue Notre-Dame O, Montreal QC H4C 1P8; Saigon (Vietnam)'75; Langs: English; Vietnamese; (514)933-7541; Fax. (514)933-1740.

LUONG, Loan T; 2671 Concession Rd PO Box 2113, Kemptville ON K0G 1J0; Tor'04; CCFP; Langs: Vietnamese; (613)258-0100

LUONG, Me-Linh; CHUM-Hop St-Luc, 1058 rue Saint-Denis, Montreal QC H2X 3J4; Sher'03; FRCPC; IntMed; MedMicrobiol; InfectDis. Staff, McGill University Health Centre - Montreal General Campus; (514)890-8305 x36210

LUONG, Tinh-Nhan; Hop Maisonneuve-Rosemont, 5415 boul de l'Assomption, Montreal QC H1T 2M4; Laval'97; FRCPC; Peds (Tropical Medicine). Staff, Hopital Maisonneuve-Rosemont; Langs: Bilingual(French/English); (514)252-3400 x1900; Fax. (514)373-8101.

LUONGO, Rolfe M; 200-3825 Sunset St, Burnaby BC V5G 1T4; UBC'96; FRCPC; IntMed; Rheum. (604)431-8884; Fax. (604)431-8841.

LUPE, Krystine K; The Ottawa Hosp-Gen Campus, 501 Smyth Rd, Ottawa ON K1H 8L6; Ott'03; FRCPC; RadOncol. Staff, The Ottawa Hospital - General Campus; (613)737-6111

LUPICHUK, Sasha M; 1331 29 St NW, Calgary AB T2N 4N2; UBC'98; BSc; FRCPC; IntMed; MedOncol. Staff, Tom Baker Cancer Centre; (403)521-3093; Fax. (403)283-1651.

LUPIEN, Christine A; CSSS de Saint-Jerome, 290 rue de Montigny, Saint-Jerome QC J7Z 5T3; Sher'79; DiagRad. Staff, Hôtel-Dieu de Saint-Jérôme; (450)431-8300; Fax. (450)431-8244.

LUPIEN, J R Guy; Anson Gen Hosp, 58 Anson Dr, Iroquois Falls ON P0K 1E0; Mon'81; CCFP; CCFP(E.M.); Staff, Anson General Hospital; Langs: English; French; (705)258-3911; Fax. (705)298-4159.

LUPIEN, Jacques; CHUQ-St-Francois D'Assise, 10 rue de l'Espinay, Quebec QC G1L 3L5; Laval'85; Anes. Staff, Centre Hospitalier Universitaire De Québec - Pavillon De St-françois-d'assise; (418)525-4444; Fax. (418)525-4434.

LUPIEN, Luc; 1300 boul du Mi-Valon CP 5016 Succ Rock Forest, Sherbrooke QC J1N 3B9; Sher'82; (819)565-3272

LUPIEN, Melanie; Clinique Med Mascouche, 1025 Montee Masson, Mascouche QC J7K 2L9; Mon'09; (450)474-6000

LUPIEN, Nicolas; Ctr Hosp St-Joseph de la Malba, CP 340 Succ Bureau-Chef 303 rue Saint-Etienne, La Malbaie QC G5A 1T8; Mon'03; CCFP; Staff, Hôpital de la Malbaie; (418)665-1700

LUPIEN-ST PIERRE, Mariline; CSSS-IUGS, 8 rue Speid, Sherbrooke QC J1M 1R6; Sher'04; CCFP; (819)780-2222

LUPIN, Mark H; 207-1990 Fort St, Victoria BC V8R 6V4; Tor'88; FRCPC; Derm. (250)598-3320; Fax. (250)598-3360; cosmedica@telus.net.

LUPOVICI, Ninia M; 1001-123 Edward St, Toronto ON M5G 1E2; Tor'84.

LUPTON, Brian A; BC Women's Hosp & Health Ctre, 1R47-4500 Oak St, Vancouver BC V6H 3N1; Belfast (Ireland)'77; DCH; MRCP(UK); FRCPC; Peds (Neonatology). Med Dir Neonatal Intensive Care Unit, BC Women's Hospital & Health Centre; Clin Assoc Prof, University of British Columbia; (604)875-2135; Fax. (604)875-3106.

LUPTON, P Lauren; St Joseph's Gen Hosp, 2137 Comox Ave, Comox BC V9M 1P2; UBC'86; FRCPC; Psy. Staff, St Joseph's General Hospital; (250)890-3060

LUPTON, Richard D; Lions Gate Hosp, 231 15th St E, North Vancouver BC V7L 2L7; Liverpool (England)'71; MB ChB; DRCOG; MRCGPract; Ac Staff/Sr Med Dir, Lions Gate Hospital; Med Dir, Vancouver Coastal Health; (604)987-3383; Fax. (604)987-3382.

LUPU, G Harvey; 114-5450 ch de la Cote-des-Nei, Montreal QC H3T 1Y6; McG'59; FAAP; Peds. Asst Staff, Sir Mortimer B Davis Jewish General; Asst Staff, St Mary's Hospital Centre; Asst Staff, McGill University Health Centre - Montreal Children's Hospital; McGill University; Langs: English; French; Spanish; Hebrew; (514)487-8826

LUPU, Ioana; Airport Way Med Clinic, PO Box 2000 5216 Aiport Dr, Fort Nelson BC V0C 1R0; UBC'05; CCFP; (250)774-7838

LUPUL, Sheri; Airdrie Med Clinic, 10-620 1 Ave NW, Airdrie AB T4B 2R3; Cal'03; MD; BSc(Hon); CCFP; (403)948-3109; Fax. (403)948-6284.

LUQMAN, Zubair; Queen Elizabeth II HSC-Halifax, 1796 Summer St, Halifax NS B3H 3A7; Punjab (India)'98; MB BS; Staff, Queen Elizabeth II Health Sciences Centre - Halifax Infirmary Site; (902)473-3808

LURIE, Arnold; Courtice Health Centre, 1450 Highway 2, Courtice ON L1E 3C3; Witwatersrand (South Africa)'78; Court Staff Privil, North York General Hospital - Branson Division; (905)721-4366; Fax. (905)723-6319.

LUSCOMBE, Kristopher D; Killick Health Services Inc, 54 Union St, Grnd-Falls-Windsor NL A2A 2E2; Mem'99; FRCPC; Psy. (709)292-8400

LUSCOMBE, Sandra J; Dr Charles A Janeway Child HC, 300 Prince Philip Dr, St. John's NL A1B 3V6; Mem'95; Staff, Janeway Children's Health & Rehabilitation Centre; Clinical Asst Prof, Memorial University Of Newfoundland; (709)777-4641; Fax. (709)777-4955; sandra.luscombe@easternhealth.ca.

LUSCOTT, Kathleen S J; Wellesley Township Commun HC, PO Box 187 1180 Queen's Bush Rd, Wellesley ON N0B 2T0; Tor'76; CCFP; (519)656-9025; Fax. (519)656-9027.

LUSH, Jennifer D; 106-4480 West Saanich Rd, Victoria BC V8Z 3E9; UBC'00; CCFP; (250)213-7992

LUSH, Richard B; Central Health Consultants, 129 Lincoln Rd, Grnd-Falls-Windsor NL A2A 1P3; Mem'99; FRCPC; IntMed. (709)489-2700

LUSHER, Brandon E; Oak Ridges Med Centre, 13291 Yonge St, Richmond Hill ON L4E 4L6; (Other Foreign)'10; CCFP.

LUSIGNAN, Daniel E; Ctr de Sante Comm de l'Estrie, 2081 Laval St, Bourget ON K0A 1E0; Ott'88; CCFP; FCFP; Physician Family Med, Hamilton Health Sciences Centre - McMaster Children's Hospital; Langs: Bilingual(English/French); (613)487-1802

LUSINA, Jillian B; UBC Family Practice Centre, F326-4500 Oak St, Vancouver BC V6H 3N1; UBC'03; CCFP; Staff, BC Women's Hospital & Health Centre; (604)875-2029

LUSIS, Janis G; 100-178 John St, Brampton ON L6W 2A4; Tor'72; Ac Staff, William Osler Health System - Brampton Civic Hospital; Langs: Latvian; (905)457-4840; Fax. (905)457-3936.

LUSKEY, Gary W; Centre Medical Cardiogenix, 100-8250 boul Decarie, Montreal QC H4P 2P5; McG'75; FRCSC; ObstGyn. Staff High Risk Obst, Sir Mortimer B Davis Jewish General; Staff, St Mary's Hospital Centre; adj Prof, McGill University; (514)731-1253

LUSSIER, Anne; Hôpital Ste-Justine, 3175 ch Cote-Sainte-Catherine, Montreal QC H3T 1C5; Mon'06; Peds. Staff, Hôpital Ste-Justine; (514)345-4931

LUSSIER, Bruno; 101-2984 Boul Taschereau, Greenfield Park QC J4V 2G9; Mon'75; Chief Dept of Med, Hopital Charles LeMoyne; (450)466-4333; Fax. (450)466-0716.

LUSSIER, Catherine; Hop Charles Lemoyne, 3120 boul Taschereau, Greenfield Park QC J4V 2H1; McG'07; MDCM; AnatPath. Staff, Hopital Charles LeMoyne; (450)466-5000

LUSSIER, Christian; Hop Du Sacre-Coeur De Mtl, 5400 boul Gouin O, Montreal QC H4J 1C5; Mon'93; AnatPath. Staff, Hôpital du Sacre-Coeur de Montréal; (514)338-2222

LUSSIER, David; MUHC-Montreal Gen Hosp, 4565 chemin Queen-Mary, Montreal QC H3W 1W5; Mon'95; FRCP; FRCPC; IntMed (Pain Management); GeriatricMed. Staff, McGill University Health Centre - Montreal General Campus; adj Prof, Universite de Montreal; adj Prof, McGill University; Langs: Bilingual(French/English); (514)340-3515; Fax. (514)340-2832; david.lussier@mcgill.ca.

LUSSIER, Dominique; Tottenham Med Centre, PO Box 2000 119 Queen St N, Tottenham ON L0G 1W0; Ott'79; (905)936-4211; Fax. (905)936-3493.

LUSSIER, France; DSPE de Lanaudiere, 245 rue du Curé-Majeau, Joliette QC J6E 8S8; Sher'82; Med Consultant Commun Health, Centre Hospitalier Régional de Lanaudière; Langs: English; (450)759-1157 x4442; Fax. (450)759-5149; france_lussier@ssss.gouv.qc.ca.

LUSSIER, J R Yves; Les Aliments Ultima Inc, 2177 boul Fernand-Lafontaine, Longueuil QC J4G 2V2; Mon'83; Langs: Bilingual(French/English); (450)651-3737 x3309; Fax. (450)651-4408; yves.lussier@yoplait.ca.

LUSSIER, Marie-Therese; CSSS de Laval, 1755 boul Rene-Laennec, Laval QC H7M 3L9; Mon'83; CCFP; FCFP; Staff, Hopital de la Cite de la santé; Clin Teach Staff Family Med, Universite de Montreal; Langs: English; (450)975-5444; Fax. (450)975-5497.

LUSSIER, Marielle; 900 Boul Saint-Joseph E, Montreal QC H2J 1K6; Mon'78; IntMed (Vascular Medicine). (514)521-0442; Fax. (514)521-4665.

LUSSIER, Nathalie; Hop Charles Lemoyne, 3120 boul Taschereau, Greenfield Park QC J4V 2H1; Mon'94; FRCPC; MedMicrobiol; Microbio & Infect Dis (P.Q.). Staff, Hopital Charles LeMoyne; (450)466-5000

LUSSIER, Normand; Clinique Metro Cote-Vertu, 3-1077 rue Decarie, Saint-Laurent QC H4L 3M8; Sher'75; (514)747-0432; Fax. (514)747-6304.

LUSSIER, Richard; CSSS du Suroît, 150 rue Saint-Thomas, Salaber-de-Valleyf QC J6T 6C1; Mon'07; CCFP; Staff, Centre Hospitalier Régional du Suroît; (450)371-9920

LUSSIER, Robert; 403-2555 St. Joseph Blvd, Orleans ON K1C 1S6; Sher'77; FRCSC; ObstGyn. Staff, Montfort Hospital; Vis Staff, The Ottawa Hospital - General Campus; Asst Prof, University of Ottawa; Langs: Bilingual(French/English); (613)837-8396; Fax. (613)837-8398.

LUSSIER, Sebastien; Hotel-Dieu de Sorel, 400 av de l'Hotel-Dieu, Sorel-Tracy QC J3P 1N5; McG'03; FRCPC; AnatPath. Staff, Hôtel-Dieu de Sorel; (418)746-6000

LUSSIER, Sylvain; Clinique Physiatrie Rive Sud, 3725 rue Mont-Royal, Saint-Hubert QC J4T 2G9; Mon'77; ABPMR; FRCPC; PhysMed&Rehab (Electromyography). Staff, Hopital Charles LeMoyne; (450)678-1980; Fax. (450)678-0538.

LUSSIER, Timothy; Barrie Mem Hosp, 28 rue Gale, Ormstown QC J0S 1K0; McG'09; CCFP; Staff, Barrie Memorial Hospital; (450)829-3582

LUSSIER, Veronique; CHUS-Hop Hotel-Dieu, 580 rue Bowen S, Sherbrooke QC J1G 2E8; Sher'03; FRCPC; IntMed; Gastroent. Staff, Centre Hospitalier Universitaire de Sherbrooke-Hôpital Hôtel-Dieu; (819)346-1110

LUSSIER, Yvan; CLSC d'Hebergement Valcourt, GD 1150 rue Champlain, Valcourt QC J0E 2L0; Laval'88; Staff, Centre Hospitalier l'Université de Montréal (CHUM) - Hôpital Notre-Dame; (450)532-3191

LUSSIER-LAZAROFF, Jeannette; Centre De Radiol Hochelaga, 101-8695 rue Hochelaga, Montreal QC H1L 6J5; Ott'65; DiagRad (P.Q.). (514)353-5730; Fax. (514)353-4729.

LUSSIER-MONTPLAISIR, M; Curateur Public Du Quebec, 1000-600 boul René-Lévesque O, Montreal QC H3B 4W9; Mon'71; (514)873-0281; Fax. (514)864-8951.

LUSSIER-PLOURDE, Yolande; CSST-Dir Reg de Valleyfield, 9 rue Nicholson, Salaber-de-Valleyf QC J6T 4M4; Mon'71; ac Staff, Centre Hospitalier Régional du Suroît; (450)377-6200

LUSTIG, Andrew J M; Addiction & Mental Hlth-Clarke, 501-250 College St, Toronto ON M5T 1R8; Tor'00; FRCPC; Psy. Staff, Centre for Addiction & Mental Health (CAMH) - College Street Site; (416)535-8501

LUTCHMAN, Carla N R; Lawrence Curlew Med Centre, 1260 Lawrence Ave E, North York ON M3A 1C4; Qns'05; FRCSC; Ophth. (416)289-4000

LUTCHMEDIAL, Sohrab R A; Saint John Reg Hosp, PO Box 2100 Stn Main, Saint John NB E2L 4L2; McG'93; FRCPC; IntMed (Interventional Cardiology); Cardiol. Staff, Saint John Regional Hospital; (506)648-6000

LUTERMAN, Leonard; St Mary's Hosp Centre, B348-3830 av Lacombe, Montreal QC H3T 1M5; McG'77; FRCPC; IntMed; Gastroent. Dir Dept of Gastroent, St Mary's Hospital Centre; Ac Staff Gastroent, McGill University Health Centre - Montreal General Campus; adj Prof Med, McGill University; (514)345-3511 x3040

LUTERMAN, Maynard; Niagara H System-Welland Site, 65 Third St, Welland ON L3B 4W6; McG'85; MSc; CCFP; Staff, Niagara Health System - Welland Hospital Site; (905)738-4647

LUTERMAN, Rosalind A; Family Med Centre, 202-3400 rue Du Marche, Dollard-D-Ormeaux QC H9B 2Y1; Wes'91; CCFP; FCFP; (514)683-0414

LUTHER, John K; Normanview Med Clinic, 330 McCarthy Blvd N, Regina SK S4R 7M2; Sask'76; Langs: French; (306)924-6200; Fax. (306)924-6201.

LUTHRA, Atul; 217 Terrace Hill St, Brantford ON N3R 1G8; New Delhi (India)'86; FRCPC; Psy (Adult & Geriatric Psychiatry). Physician-in-Charge Mental Health Program & Med Dir, The Brant Community Healthcare System - Brantford General Hospital Site; Clinical Asst Prof, McMaster University.

LUTHRA, Meera; St Joseph's Healthcare, 5F-50 Charlton Ave E, Hamilton ON L8N 4A6; Tor'01; FRCPC; IntMed (Pregnancy Medical Complications); Endocrin&Metab. Staff, St Joseph's Healthcare - Charlton Campus; Langs: Hindi; Punjabi; (905)522-1155 x32739; tlaporte@stjoes.ca.

LUTHRA, Sanjeev S; Main Street Med Centre, 9-10866 Hurontario St, Brampton ON L7A 3R9; Tor'03; FRCPC; Peds. Staff, The Hospital For Sick Children; Staff, William Osler Health System - Etobicoke General Hospital; Langs: Punjabi; Hindi; Urdu; (905)846-9911

LUTON, Robert G; 109-205 Oxford St E, London ON N6A 5G6; Wes'72; (519)645-2467; Fax. (519)645-0492.

LUTSCH, Albrecht P; Kelowna Gen Hosp, 2268 Pandosy St, Kelowna BC V1Y 1T2; Pretoria (South Africa)'79; FRCPC; Anes. Staff, Kelowna General Hospital; (250)862-4022; Fax. (250)862-4020.

LUTSKY, Peter M; Broadway Med Centre, 810-943 Broadway W, Vancouver BC V5Z 4E1; UBC'88; CCFP; FCFP; Assoc Staff, Vancouver General Hospital - Centennial Pavillion; (604)734-1213; Fax. (604)734-5751.

LUTTERODT, Alfred; Cardiometabolic Evaluation Ris, 210-1016 68 Ave SW, Calgary AB T2V 4J2; Accra (Ghana)'71; MB ChB; MSc; DABIM; FACP; FRCPC; IntMed (Clinical Pharmacology). Staff, Cardiometabolic Evaluation & Risk Assessment Centre; Clin Prof Med, University of Saskatchewan; (403)541-0033; Fax. (403)541-0032; alutterodt@nbnet.nb.ca.

LUTTFY, Ghyda; 223 ch Madawaska, Grand Falls NB E3Y 1A5; (Algeria)'92; Staff, Hôpital Général de Grand-Falls; (506)473-6435; Fax. (506)473-6866.

LUTTRELL, Kerry S S; 199 Seagull Lane, Nanaimo BC V9S 3G9; UBC'78; BSc.

LUTWICK, Renee E; Soma Vein Clinic, 204-1475 Bedford Hwy, Bedford NS B4A 3Z5; Dal'85; CCFP; CCFP(E.M.); FCFP; Staff, Cobequid Multiservice Centre; (902)835-2266; info@somaveinclinic.ca.

LUTYNSKI, Andrzej; Univ Hlth Network-Princess M, 5 211-610 University Ave, Toronto ON M5G 2M9; Warsaw (Poland)'70; Staff Ontario Cancer Inst, Princess Margaret Hospital - University Health Network; (416)946-2000 x4788

LUTZAK, Gregory D; Hys Med Centre, 310-11010 101 St NW, Edmonton AB T5H 4B9; Alb'05; FRCPC; IntMed; Gastroent. (780)421-1029

LUU, Chinh-Duc; Clinique Med Mercier, 101-464 boul Saint-Jean-Baptis, Mercier QC J6R 2B1; Sher'93; Langs: Vietnamese; English; (450)699-0539

LUU, Huu Ni; Ctr Hosp Fleury, 2180 rue Fleury E, Montreal QC H2B 1K3; Saigon (Vietnam)'81; CCFP; Staff, Centre Hospitalier Fleury; Staff, CHSLD Lucille-Teasdale; (514)383-5050

LUU, Kelly; The Richmond Hosp, 7000 Westminster Hwy, Richmond BC V6X 1A2; McM'08; Peds. Staff, Richmond Hospital; (604)233-3222

LUU, Kiet-Quan; Clinique Med Carron, 995 Boul Saint-Laurent, Montreal QC H2Z 1J4; Sher'87; (514)861-9154

LUU, Lien Ngoc; Main Street Med Centre, 9-10886 Hurontario St, Brampton ON L7A 3R9; Tor'03; CCFP; (905)846-9911

LUU, Thanh; Reach Community Health Ctre, 1145 Commercial Dr, Vancouver BC V5L 3X3; Sask'00; CCFP; (604)254-1354; Fax. (604)258-9190.

LUU, Yen; CSSS de Saint-Jerome, 290 rue de Montigny, Saint-Jerome QC J7Z 5T3; Mon'94; FRCSC; GenSurg; VascSurg. Staff, Hôtel-Dieu de Saint-Jérôme; Langs: Bilingual(French/English); (450)431-8200; Fax. (450)431-8303.

LUU, Thanh-Phi; Clinique Med Mistral, 751 rue Mistral, Montreal QC H2P 1R7; Saigon (Vietnam)'72; (514)387-4932; Fax. (514)387-1941.

LUU, Thuy Mai; Hôpital Ste-Justine, 3175 ch Cote-Sainte-Catherine, Montreal QC H3T 1C5; McG'01; CSPQ; FRCPC; Peds. Staff, Hôpital Ste-Justine; (514)345-4931

LUVISOTTO, Terri L; 304-840 Coxwell Ave, Toronto ON M4C 5T2; Cal'92; CCFP; FCFP; (416)461-4761

LUYCKX, Valerie; Heritage Medical Research Ctre, 260-107 University Campus NW, Edmonton AB T6G 2S2; (South Africa)'90; Staff, University of Alberta Hospital; Asst Prof, University of Alberta; (780)407-6069; Fax. (780)407-8488.

LUYELA, Asunta; Hôpital de CSC de Lamèque, 29 rue de l'Hopital, Lameque NB E8T 1C5; (Congo (Democratic Republic))'89; Staff, Hôpital de CSC de Lamèque; (506)344-2261

LUYET, Joseph-Andre; Hop Louis-H Lafontaine, 7401 rue Hochelaga, Montreal QC H1N 3M5; Mon'85; MBA; FRCPC; Psy (Hospital Psychiatry). Staff, Hopital Louis-H Lafontaine; Clin Staff, Universite de Montreal; Langs: English; (514)251-4000 x2935; Fax. (514)251-2498.

LUYKENAAR, Vincent J; Campbell Clinic, PO Box 180 Stn Main, Coaldale AB T1M 1M3; Erasmus (Netherlands)'72; Staff, Chinook Regional Hospital; Staff, Coaldale Health Centre; Staff, Covenant Health - St Michael's Health Centre; (403)345-3072; Fax. (403)345-2141.

LUYT, Nathan J R; Norfolk Gen Hosp, 365 West St, Simcoe ON N3Y 1T7; Qns'07; CCFP; Staff, Norfolk General Hospital; (519)426-0130

LWANGA, Steven K; Transcona Med Clinic, 4936 4th Ave, Regina SK S4T 0J3; Makerere (Uganda)'75; FRCPC; IntMed. (306)565-8820; slwanga@sasktel.net.

LWU, Shelly H; Queen Elizabeth II HSC-Halifax, 3809-1796 Summer St, Halifax NS B3H 3A7; UBC'04; FRCSC; Neursurg. Staff, Queen Elizabeth II Health Sciences Centre - Halifax Infirmary Site; (902)473-2656

LY, Joseph P H; St Michael's Hosp, 30 Bond St, Toronto ON M5B 1W8; Tor'02; FRCPC; IntMed; Nephrol. Staff IntMed, St Michael's Hospital; (416)864-6060

LY, Quoc Hung; Institut de Cardiologie de Mtl, 5000 rue Belanger, Montreal QC H1T 1C8; Mon'97; FRCPC; IntMed; Cardiol. Staff, Institut de Cardiologie de Montréal; (514)376-3330 x3800

LY, T Nhu-Khue; MUHC-Montreal Gen Hosp, 1650 av Cedar, Montreal QC H3G 1A4; Laval'06; IntMed. Staff, McGill University Health Centre - Montreal General Campus; (514)934-1934

LY, Thai Yen; Dr Everett Chalmers Hosp, PO Box 9000 Stn A, Fredericton NB E3B 5N5; Tor'05; FRCPC; AnatPath. Staff, Dr Everett Chalmers Regional Hospital; (506)452-5400

LY, Thien-Hong; CSSS Haut-Richelieu-Rouville, 920 boul du Seminaire N, St-Jean-sur-Richel QC J3A 1B7; Laval'99; DiagRad. Staff, Hôpital du Haut-Richelieu; (450)359-5000

LYCHACZ, Bohdan I; St Joseph's Health Centre, 30 The Queensway, Toronto ON M6R 1B5; Tor'79; FRCPC; DiagRad (Diagnostic Imaging). Staff, St Joseph's Health Centre; (416)530-6001; Fax. (416)530-6060; blych@hotmail.com.

LYCKA, Barry A S; First Edmonton Place, 780-10665 Jasper Ave NW, Edmonton AB T5J 3S9; Alb'83; BSc(Hons.); ABD; FRCPC; Derm (Cosmetic Surgery). Consultant, Royal Alexandra Hospital; Consultant, Covenant Health - Misericordia Community Hospital; Asst Clin Prof, University of Alberta; (780)425-1212; Fax. (780)425-1217.

LYDDELL, Christopher; Prairie Med Clinic, 10309 98 St, Grande Prairie AB T8V 2E7; University of Cape Town (South Africa)'81; MB ChB; (780)539-4010; Fax. (780)538-2290.

LYDELL, Carmen P; Foothills Med Centre, 87-1403 29 St NW, Calgary AB T2N 2T9; UBC'03; FRCPC; DiagRad (Cardiothoracic). Staff, Foothills Medical Centre; (403)994-1969

LYDON, Patrick; Medical-Dental Bldg, 404-1120 Yates St, Victoria BC V8V 3M9; Galway (Ireland)'69; BAO; DPM; MRCPsy; FRCPC; Psy (Attention Deficit Disorders). Consultant Psy, Royal Jubilee Hospital; (250)480-5100; Fax. (250)480-5140.

LYEN, Catherine L; Findlay Creek Med Centre, 4744 Bank St, Ottawa ON K1T 3W7; Ott'02; CCFP; (613)317-2584

LYEW, Warren J; Campbellton Reg Hosp, PO Box 880 Stn Main 189 Lily Lake Rd, Campbellton NB E3N 3H3; Qns'03; FRCPC; AnatPath. Staff, Hôpital Régional Campbellton; (506)789-5000

LYEW, Winston J; 61 Hyde Park Dr, Richmond Hill ON L4B 1X2; Wes'71; (905)731-9095

LYLE, Terrance C; Broadview Medical Bldg, B2-770 Broadview Ave, Ottawa ON K2A 3Z3; Ott'67; FRCPC; DiagRad. (613)729-1396; Fax. (613)729-7688.

LYMBURNER, Dana L; Dartmouth Gen Hosp, 325 Pleasant St, Dartmouth NS B2Y 4G8; UBC'09; Staff, Dartmouth General Hospital; (902)465-8300

LYN, Basil E; CancerCare Manitoba, 675 McDermot Ave, Winnipeg MB R3E 0V9; Cambridge (England)'82; FRCPC; RadOncol.

LYN, Sheldon A; Univ of Toronto, 2F-500 University Ave, Toronto ON M5G 1V7; Wes'07; FRCPC; Anes.

LYNAGH, Niall J; Woodbine Med Centre, 9-76 Arlington Dr, Keswick ON L4P 0A9; Alb'90; Staff, Southlake Regional Health Centre; (905)476-0308; Fax. (905)476-1079.

LYNCH, Anthony; Calgary Ctre-Fire Dept Wellnes, 271 Midpark Blvd SE, Calgary AB T2X 1S3; Sheffield (England)'84; MB ChB; PhD(Eng); DRCOG(Eng); DAvMed(NZ); Med Dir Occupational Environmental & Aviation, The Columbia Rehabilitation Centre; (403)873-2352

LYNCH, Ciara M R; Quest Community Health Centre, 145 Queenston St, St. Catharines ON L2R 2Z9; Cal'01; (905)688-2558

LYNCH, Erin C; 101-9006 Edward St, Chilliwack BC V2P 4E1; Qns'04; CCFP; (604)701-6866

LYNCH, Jennifer A; 102-145 Station St, Belleville ON K8N 2S9; Ott'08; CCFP; (613)771-1910

LYNCH, Joanna M; Northern Connection Med Ctre, 425 Elgin Ave, Winnipeg MB R3A 1P2; Man'92; BSc; CCFP; FCFP.

LYNCH, Mary E; Pain Management Unit, 4F-5820 University Ave, Halifax NS B3H 1V7; Dal'82; FRCPC; Psy (Pain Management). Dir Research Pain Mgmt Unit, Queen Elizabeth II Health Sciences Centre - Victoria General Site; Prof Psy Anes & Pharmacol, Dalhousie University; (902)473-4130; Fax. (902)473-4126.

LYNCH, Michel; Polyclinique D'Argenteuil, 551 rue Berry, Lachute QC J8H 1S4; Mon'84; Staff, Centre Hospitalier d'Argenteuil; Langs: Bilingual(French/English); (450)562-3751; Fax. (450)562-1852.

LYNCH, Sebastien; CSSS de Laval, 1755 boul Rene-Laennec, Laval QC H7M 3L9; Mon'03; CCFP; Staff, Hopital de la Cite de la santé; (450)668-1010

LYNCH, Sheila M P; Waterford Hosp, 306 Waterford Bridge Rd, St. John's NL A1E 4J8; Mem'79; BMedSci; BSc; LMCC; FRCPC; Psy (Forensic Psychiatry). Staff Psy Forensic Unit, Waterford Hospital; Asst Prof Psy/Asst Dean Student Affairs, Memorial University Of Newfoundland; (709)777-3311; Fax. (709)777-3993.

LYNCH, Timothy P; Children's Hosp Western Ont, 800 Commissioners Rd E, London ON N6C 2V5; Mem'94; FRCPC; Peds. Staff, Children's Hospital of Western Ontario; (519)685-8500; Fax. (519)685-8164; tim.lynch@lhsc.on.ca.

LYNDE, Charles W; Lynde Centre for Dermatology, 201-5762 Highway 7, Markham ON L3P 1A8; Tor'78; BSc; FRCPC; Derm (Clinical Trials). Assoc Staff, Toronto Western Hospital - University Health Network; Assoc Staff, Markham Stouffville Hospital; Assoc Staff, The Scarborough Hospital - Birchmount Campus; Asst Prof Med, University of Toronto; (905)471-5022; Fax. (905)471-1878; derma@lynderma.com.

LYNDON, Charlene A; Wentworth Medical & Dental, 6201-873 85 St SW, Calgary AB T3H 0J5; Tor'89; FACOG; FRCSC; ObstGyn. Staff, Rockyview General Hospital; (403)217-6453; Fax. (403)217-5235.

LYNETT, Christopher P; Tremont Med Clinic, 2A-2F Tremont Dr, St Catharines ON L2T 3B2; McM'95; CCFP; Staff, Niagara Health System - Ontario Street Site; Staff, Niagara Health System - St Catharines General Site; (905)687-8887

LYNK, Andrew D; Cape Breton Hlthcare Complex, 1482 George St, Sydney NS B1P 1P3; Dal'82; MSc(CTM); FRCPC; Peds. Staff, Cape Breton Healthcare Complex; (902)567-7700; Fax. (902)567-7997; alynk@ns.sympatico.ca.

LYNK, Mary E; PO Box 148 Stn Main, New Waterford NS B1H 4K4; Dal'72; Ac Staff, New Waterford Consolidated Hospital; (902)862-7711; Fax. (902)862-7349; mary.lynk@ns.sympatico.ca.

LYNN, Brian W; 11-60 Stanley Ave, Ottawa ON K1M 1P6; McM'88; (613)247-8880

LYNN, Hazel R; 101 17th St E, Owen Sound ON N4K 0A5; Tor'76; MHSc; CCFP; FCFP; Staff, Hanover & District Hospital; Staff, Grey Bruce Health Services - Owen Sound; Med Officer of Hlth, Grey Bruce Health Unit Corporate Office; (519)376-9420 x1242; Fax. (519)376-0605.

LYNSKEY, Jeffrey W; The Medical Clinic Associates, 4794 Joyce Ave, Powell River BC V8A 3B6; Cal'86; CCFP; (604)485-6261; Fax. (604)485-2820.

LYON, David C; Chinook Reg Hosp, 960 19 St S, Lethbridge AB T1J 1W5; Man'78; ABPath; FRCP; MSc; MCFP; FRCPC; AnatPath (Cytopath); GenPath. Staff, Chinook Regional Hospital; (403)388-6151; Fax. (403)388-6067.

LYON, Michael R; 1550 United Blvd, Coquitlam BC V2K 6Y2; Cal'85; (604)777-5500

LYON, Ronald G; PO Box 3248 Stn Main, Meaford ON N4L 1A5; McM'79; Staff Chief Med, Grey Bruce Health Services - Meaford Site; (519)538-3110; Fax. (519)538-3221.

LYON, W Kirk; Univ Hlth Network-Toronto Western Hosp, 2W404-399 Bathurst St, Toronto ON M5T 2S8; Tor'74; FCFP; CCFP; FCFP; Ac Staff, Toronto Western Hospital - University Health Network; Assoc Prof Family Med, University of Toronto; (416)603-5888 x3; Fax. (416)603-5821.

LYONNAIS, Jean; Ctr Hosp Affilie-Enfant-Jesus, 1401 18e rue, Quebec QC G1J 1Z4; Laval'68; Hem (P.Q.) (Oncology). Staff, Centre Hospitalier Affilié Universitaire de Québec - Hôpital De L'Enfant Jésus; Langs: English; (418)649-5726; Fax. (418)649-5553.

LYONS, Anthony W; Med-Emerg International Inc, 404-6711 Mississauga Rd, Mississauga ON L5N 2W3; Dal'95; CCFP; (905)858-1368

LYONS, Brian J; Yarmouth Reg Health Centre, 406-60 Vancouver St, Yarmouth NS B5A 2P5; Dal'89; Staff, Yarmouth Regional Hospital; (902)742-3541

LYONS, Christopher J; Children's & Women's HC of BC, A136-4480 Oak St, Vancouver BC V6H 3V4; London (England)'82; MB BS; FRCSC; Ophth (Pediatric Ophthalmology). Staff, Vancouver General Hospital - Centennial Pavillion; Staff, BC Children's Hospital; Prof, University of British Columbia; Langs: Bilingual(English/French); (604)875-3117; Fax. (604)875-3561; clyons@cw.bc.ca.

LYONS, David J; Sunridge Diagnostic Imaging, 2133 36 St NE, Calgary AB T1Y 5S3; Qns'77; FRCPC; DiagRad. (403)568-7676

LYONS, Edward A; Health Sciences Centre, GE342-820 Sherbrook St, Winnipeg MB R3A 1R9; Man'68; ABR; FACR; FRCPC; DiagRad (Ultrasound). Staff Sect of Ultrasound, Health Sciences Centre; Pres, Canadian Association of Radiologists; Prof Radiol Anatomy & ObstGyn, University of Manitoba; (204)787-3724; Fax. (204)787-3355.

LYONS, Elliott R; Hydro Place Bldg, 3F 3016-700 University Ave, Toronto ON M5G 1Z5; Tor'71; FRCSC; ObstGyn. Att Staff, Mount Sinai Hospital; Prof, University of Toronto; (416)586-5366; Fax. (416)586-4512.

LYONS, Jerome A; Dalecliff Med Clinic, 209 Ellesmere Rd, Scarborough ON M1R 4E2; McM'74; Court Staff Gen Med, The Scarborough Hospital - General Campus; (416)444-5600

LYONS, Jessica E; Sunridge Medical Gallery, 200-2580 32 St NE, Calgary AB T1Y 7M8; Cal'04; FRCPC; Psy. (403)944-9750

LYONS, Kristin J; University of Alberta Hosp, 2C2-8440 112 St NW, Edmonton AB T6G 2B7; McG'08; IntMed. Staff Cardiol, University of Alberta Hospital; (780)407-8822

LYONS, Laura M; St Joseph's Fam Med & Dental C, 346 Platt's Lane, London ON N6G 1J1; McM'03; CCFP; (519)672-9660

LYONS, Michael J; Concordia Gen Hosp, 1095 Concordia Ave, Winnipeg MB R2K 3S8; Cal'08; CCFP; Staff, Concordia General Hospital; (204)667-1560

LYONS, Paul H; Plantagenet Family Health Team, PO Box 305 179 Old Highway 17, Plantagenet ON K0B 1L0; McM'82; CCFP; FCFP; (613)673-4318; Fax. (613)673-4480; p.lyons@nursinghomeratings.ca.

LYPCHUK, Lauren C; Workers' Comp Board, 110-2045 Enterprise Way, Kelowna BC V1Y 9T5; UBC'92; CCFP; (250)979-4123

LYPOURLIS, Katherine; 1902 Richmond Ave, Victoria BC V8R 4R2; (Other Foreign)'99; MB BS; (250)389-0532

LYSACK, Allan M; Dauphin Reg Health Centre, 625 3rd St SW, Dauphin MB R7N 1R7; Man'60; DS; FRCSC; GenSurg (Gastroenterology). Ac Staff GenSurg, Dauphin Regional Health Centre; Asst Prof Surg, University of Manitoba; (204)638-3010; Fax. (204)638-1267.

LYSACK, David A; Brandon Reg Health Centre, 150 Mctavish Ave E, Brandon MB R7A 2B3; Qns'90; FRCPC; DiagRad. Staff, Brandon Regional Health Centre; (204)726-2155; Fax. (204)726-2396.

LYSACK, Elizabeth J; Foothills Med Centre, 1403 29 St NW, Calgary AB T2N 2T9; Man'10; CCFP; Staff, Foothills Medical Centre; (403)944-1110

LYSACK, John T; Foothills Med Centre, 1403 29 St NW, Calgary AB T2N 2T9; Qns'00; FRCPC; DiagRad (Neuro Radiology). Staff, Foothills Medical Centre; (403)944-1969

LYSAK, Pauline S; Grandin Park Plaza, 406-22 Sir Winston Churchill A, St. Albert AB T8N 1B4; Alb'99; FRCPC; Psy. Staff, Sturgeon Community Hospital; (780)800-5210; Fax. (780)800-5211.

LYSTER, Kish E; Pasqua Hosp, 4101 Dewdney Ave, Regina SK S4T 1A5; Sask'01; CCFP; CCFP(E.M.); Staff, Pasqua Hospital; (306)766-2222

LYSY, Paul; Hillside Med Centre, 100 av Metcalfe, Westmount QC H3Z 2H4; Tor'73; CCFP; FCFP; principale Médecin, McGill University Health Centre - Montreal General Campus; adj Prof Family Med, McGill University; Langs: French; (514)931-2162; Fax. (514)931-8436.

LYSYSHYN, Mark A; Univ of British Columbia, 2206 East Mall, Vancouver BC V6T 1Z3; Qns'00; FRCPC; IntMed. (604)822-2772

LYTE, Kristina; Canadian Forces Health Serv, PO Box 1000 31 Ortona Rd, Borden ON L0M 1C0; Ott'10; CCFP; (705)795-2299

LYTHGOE, Elizabeth S; 107-3215 49 Ave, Red Deer AB T4N 0M8; Alb'91; BSc; PhD; FRCSC; Ophth (Cataract). Staff, Red Deer Regional Hospital Centre; (403)340-1835; Fax. (403)340-2803.

LYTLE, Craig R; Lougheed Health Centre, 106-22838 Lougheed Hwy, Maple Ridge BC V2X 2V6; UBC'74; (604)463-8844; Fax. (604)463-9987.

LYTTLE, Brian D B; Children's Asthma Clinic, 239 Oxford St E, London ON N6A 1V2; Wes'80; ABPeds; FRCPC; Peds (Pediatric Respirology); Respir. Ac Staff Peds/Dir, London Health Sciences Centre - Victoria Campus; Ac Staff Peds, St Joseph's Hospital - St Joseph's Health Care; Teach Staff, University of Western Ontario; (519)433-2242; Fax. (519)645-7565.

LYTWYN, Alice; Hamilton HS-Henderson Site, 711 Concession St, Hamilton ON L8V 1C3; McG'82; FRCPC; AnatPath. Staff Path, Hamilton Health Sciences Centre-Juravinski Site; Asst Prof, University of Toronto; (905)389-4411 x43851; Fax. (905)389-1698.

LYUBETSKA, Valeria; Lifemark Health Institute, 154 Meadowlark Shopping Ctr NW, Edmonton AB T5R 5W9; Man'06; CCFP; (780)429-4761

LYWOOD, Allegra; Lakefront Clinics, 550 Queens Quay W, Toronto ON M5V 3M8; Dal'07; CCFP; (647)347-0576

LYWOOD, Colin J; Meadowlark Health Centre, 200 Meadowlark Shopping Ctr NW, Edmonton AB T5R 5W9; Sask'91; FRCPC; DiagRad. (780)489-5313; Fax. (780)486-5160.

LYZNYK, Roman G; Royal York Med Arts, 203-1436 Royal York Rd, Etobicoke ON M9P 3A9; Tor'84; (416)248-1300

M'CWABENI, Constantine T; 150 King St PO Box 1376 Stn Main, Peterborough ON K9J 7H6; Birmingham (England)'73; MB ChB; CCFP; CCFP(E.M.); FCFP; (705)749-9064; tmcwabeni@cogeco.ca.

M'SEFFAR, Abdelmajid; Polyclinique Cabrini, 105-5700 rue Saint-Zotique E, Montreal QC H1T 3Y7; Rabat (Morocco)'70; CSPQ; FRCPC; Rheum; IntMed. (514)494-7654

MA, Alan S; 5623 177B St, Surrey BC V3S 4H9; UBC'77; Ac Staff Family Med, Surrey Memorial Hospital; (604)576-8604; Fax. (604)576-9660.

MA, Eileen A; University Health Services, 370-2500 University Dr NW, Calgary AB T2N 1N4; Alb'00; CCFP; (403)210-9355

MA, Felix; SMBD Jewish Gen Hosp, A520-3755 Ch Cote-Sainte-Cathe, Montreal QC H3T 1E2; McG'89; FRCSC; Cardiovasc&ThorSurg (P.Q.); CardSurg. Staff, Sir Mortimer B Davis Jewish General; Langs: Cantonese; French; (514)340-8222; Fax. (514)340-7561; fma@surg.jgh.mcgill.ca.

MA, Gilbert; 103-329 Main St, Vancouver BC V6A 2S9; UBC'62; Ac Staff, Vancouver General Hospital - Centennial Pavillion; Langs: Chinese; Mandarin; (604)688-5822

MA, Grace C M; Univ Hlth Network-Princess M, 16F-610 University Ave, Toronto ON M5G 2M9; Qns'06; CCFP; Staff, Princess Margaret Hospital - University Health Network; (416)946-2135; Fax. (416)946-2866.

MA, Ian S; 3809 Main St, Vancouver BC V5V 3P1; UBC'75; Langs: Cantonese; Mandarin; (604)872-4025; Fax. (604)872-2252.

MA, Irene W Y; University of Calgary, 3330 Hospital Dr NW, Calgary AB T2N 4N1; UBC'98; MSc; FRCPC; IntMed; Nephrol. (403)210-7369

MA, Joanne L C; The Court, 417-2863 Ellesmere Rd, Scarborough ON M1E 5E9; Qns'99; FRCSC; ObstGyn. Staff, Rouge Valley Health System - Centenary Health Centre Site; Langs: Mandarin; Chinese; (416)282-4242; Fax. (416)282-3812.

MA, Joseph J K; 305-500 Sheppard Ave E, North York ON M2N 6H7; Tor'98; DABOph; FRCSC; Ophth (Cataract). Asst Prof, University of Toronto; Langs: Cantonese; Mandarin; (416)221-2093; Fax. (416)221-2097.

MA, Judy P; North Burlington Med Centre, 18-1960 Appleby Line, Burlington ON L7L 0B7; McM'90; BSc; (905)319-2000; Fax. (905)319-6292; judy@pol.net.

MA, Lai Man; Whitemud Crossing Med Clinic, 127-4211 106 St NW, Edmonton AB T6J 6L7; Alb'93; BSc; CCFP; FCFP; (780)435-7555; Fax. (780)436-0582.

MA, Ling Ling; 143-2515 90 Ave SW, Calgary AB T2V 0L8; (China)'94; FRCPC; IntMed. (403)251-6066

MA, Lingli; Toronto East Gen Hosp Inc, 825 Coxwell Ave, Toronto ON M4C 3E7; Tor'02; CCFP; CCFP(E.M.); Staff, Toronto East General Hospital Inc; (416)469-6580 x6435

MA, Mang-Ming; Zeidler Ledcor Centre, 130 University Campus NW, Edmonton AB T6G 2X8; Alb'87; FRCPC; IntMed (Hepatology); Gastroent. Staff, University of Alberta Hospital; Asst Prof, University of Alberta; Langs: Chinese; (780)492-8146; Fax. (780)492-1440.

MA, Marian C; PO Box 579, Elkford BC V0B 1H0; Ott'95; CCFP; FCFP; Langs: Mandarin.

MA, Martin T; Univ Hlth Network-Toronto Gen, 3EN-200 Elizabeth St, Toronto ON M5G 2C4; Dal'02; FRCPC; Anes. Staff, Toronto General Hospital - UHN; (416)340-3111

MA, Michael Z; Properties Med Clinic, 5102 Rundlehorn Dr NE, Calgary AB T1Y 1C1; (China)'82; FRCPC; IntMed; Gastroent. Staff Med, Peter Lougheed Centre; Staff, Properties Medical Clinic; (403)568-9789

MA, Mona K S; Aurora Med Centre, 200-15017 Yonge St, Aurora ON L4G 1M5; Tor'91; CCFP; Assoc Staff Family Med, Southlake Regional Health Centre; (905)727-9481; Fax. (905)727-6280.

MA, Patrick E; UBC Eye Care Centre, 2550 Willow St, Vancouver BC V5Z 3N9; Cal'86; AB; FRCSC; Ophth (Retina Vitreous Ophthalmology). Staff, Vancouver General Hospital - Centennial Pavillion; Staff, Providence Health Care - St Paul's Hospital; Staff, BC Children's Hospital; Clinical Asst Prof, University of British Columbia; (604)875-5500; Fax. (604)875-5501.

MA, Patrick; Bridgeland Med Bldg, 201-803 1 Ave NE, Calgary AB T2E 7C5; Dublin (Ireland)'80; MB ChB; FCCP; FACP; FACC; FRCPC; IntMed (Lipidology); Cardiol. Staff, Rockyview General Hospital; Staff, Foothills Medical Centre; Consultant Cardiol Clinic, Lipid, Hyperten & Research Clinic; Assoc Prof, University of Calgary; (403)571-8600; Fax. (403)215-2214; pma@cardiologyconsultants.ca.

MA, Raymond L T; 3140 Main St, Vancouver BC V5T 3G7; UBC'85; Staff, Providence Health Care - Mount Saint Joseph Hospital; Staff, BC Children's Hospital; Staff, Providence Health Care - St Vincent's Hospital-Heather Site; Teach Staff Family Pract, University of British Columbia; (604)879-4545; Fax. (604)879-4549.

MA, Roderick K C; Vancouver Gen Hosp, 855 12th Ave W, Vancouver BC V5Z 1M9; Tor'92; CCFP; FCFP; Staff, Vancouver General Hospital - Centennial Pavillion; (604)875-4754

MA, Roy M K; BC Cancer Agency-Vancouver CC, 600 10th Ave W, Vancouver BC V5Z 4E6; UBC'89; FRCPC; RadOncol. Staff, BC Cancer Agency Vancouver Centre; (604)877-6000 x2660; Fax. (604)708-2000; rma@bccancer.bc.ca.

MA, Steven S; 1-8948 202 St, Langley BC V1M 4A7; Tor'90; FRCSC; Ophth (General Ophthalmic Surgery). (604)881-4747

MA, Tze Y; 501-3461 Dixie Rd, Mississauga ON L4Y 3X4; (Hong Kong)'88; MB BS; MRCP(UK); FRCPC; Peds (Neonatology). Staff Ped, Trillium Health Centre - Mississauga; Langs: Cantonese; Mandarin; (905)212-9750; Fax. (905)212-9751; mickey4500@hotmail.com.

MA, Warren K; University of Alberta Hosp, 8440 112 St NW, Edmonton AB T6G 2B7; Alb'08; Staff, University of Alberta Hospital; (780)407-8822

MAAL-BARED, Haya; 211-101 Spadina Ave, Toronto ON M5V 2K2; Ott'03; FRCPC; Psy. (647)347-8186

MAALOUF-SFEIR, Nada; Ctr Hosp Anna-Laberge, 200 boul Brisebois, Chateauguay QC J6K 4W8; Beirut (Lebanon)'85; Staff, Hôpital Anna-Laberge; (450)699-2425; Fax. (450)699-2525.

MAAMAR-SAMET, Maamar; CSSS de Trois-Rivieres, 1991 boul du Carmel, Trois-Rivieres QC G8Z 3R9; Laval'01; Ophth. Staff, CSSS de Trois-Rivières; (819)697-3333

MAAMARI, Caroline; 300-3234 Boul Taschereau, Greenfield Park QC J4V 2H3; Mon'84; Langs: English; Greek; Arabic; (450)466-1125; Fax. (450)466-9646.

MAARI, Catherine; CHUM-Hop St-Luc, 1058 rue Saint-Denis, Montreal QC H2X 3J4; McG'97; Derm. Staff, Centre Hospitalier l'Université De Montréal (CHUM) - Hôpital Saint-luc; (514)890-8000 x34401

MAASKANT, Lori M; York Medical, 123-14800 Yonge St, Aurora ON L4G 1N3; McM'93; Staff, Southlake Regional Health Centre; (905)841-1882; Fax. (905)841-3385.

MAAZ, Umar; 210-5 Brockley Dr, Scarborough ON M1P 3J2; FRCSC; GenSurg. r.shaikh@sympatico.ca.

MABADEJE, Oladapo; Associate Med Clinic, 400-20 14th St W, Prince Albert SK S6V 3K8; (306)953-1653; Fax. (306)764-3091.

MABERLEY, Alan L; 614-2525 Willow St, Vancouver BC V5Z 3N8; Alb'64; BSc; FAAO; FRCSC; Ophth (Vitreo Retina). Staff, Vancouver General Hospital - Centennial Pavillion; Staff, BC Children's Hospital; Clin Prof Ophth, University of British Columbia; (604)875-9996; Fax. (604)875-9694; almvit@telus.net.

MABERLEY, David A L; UBC Eye Care Centre, 2550 Willow St, Vancouver BC V5Z 3N9; UBC'91; MSc(Epid); FRCSC; Ophth. Assoc Prof, University of British Columbia; (604)875-4599; Fax. (604)875-4699.

MABIFA, Olasunkanmi L; Grand River Hosp-KW Hlth Ctre, PO Box 9056 Stn C 835 King St W, Kitchener ON N2G 1G3; FRCPC; Psy. Staff, Grand River Hospital - Kitchener/Waterloo Health Centre; (519)749-4300

MABIN, Deborah; The Pas Health Complex, PO Box 240 Stn Main, The Pas MB R9A 1K4; Cape Town (South Africa)'83; FRCPC; DiagRad. Staff, St. Anthony General Hospital; (204)623-6431; Fax. (204)623-5372.

MABINI, Aimee J V; Oakville Med Arts Bldg, 7-358 Reynolds St, Oakville ON L6J 3L9; McM'00; BSc(Hon); FRCSC; Otol. Ac Staff, Halton Healthcare Services Corporation - Oakville Site; Ac Staff, Halton Healthcare Services Corporation - Milton District Hospital; Assoc Staff, Joseph Brant Memorial Hospital; Langs: Tagalog; (905)815-1704; Fax. (905)815-1706.

MABON, Lorraine M; Alberta Children's Hosp, 2888 Shaganappi Trail NW, Calgary AB T3B 6A8; Man'86; FRCPC; EmergMed (Flight Physician). Staff Emerg, Alberta Children's Hospital; Clin Lecturer Family Med, University of Calgary; Langs: English; French; (403)955-7070; Fax. (403)955-7398.

MABON, Michele; Hop Maisonneuve-Rosemont, 5415 boul de l'Assomption, Montreal QC H1T 2M4; Man'90; FRCSC; Ophth. Staff, Hopital Maisonneuve-Rosemont; Langs: English; French; Portuguese; Spanish; (514)252-3400 x4928; Fax. (514)252-3905.

MABUNDA, Nella G; 16642 McKenzie Lake Blvd SE, Calgary AB T2Z 1N4; Natal (South Africa)'97; (403)257-6669

MAC, Thien Bich; CSSS de Saint-Jerome, 290 rue de Montigny, Saint-Jerome QC J7Z 5T3; Mon'00; CSPQ; FRCPC; Anes. Staff, Hôtel-Dieu de Saint-Jérôme; (450)431-8266

MAC, Thien Hung; Polyclinique Rosemont, 3377 boul Rosemont, Montreal QC H1X 1K4; Mon'96; CCFP; (514)798-8688

MAC, Thien Vu; Clinique Chir Ortho C-Lemoyne, 126 rue Saint-Louis, Lemoyne QC J4R 2L5; Sher'93; FRCSC; OrthSurg. Staff, Hopital Charles LeMoyne; (450)672-1212; Fax. (450)622-9834.

MAC, Van Trong; Clinique Med MDM, 6955 boul Taschereau, Brossard QC J4Z 1A7; Saigon (Vietnam)'71; (450)656-2310

MAC-THIONG, Jean-Marc; Hop du Sacre-Coeur de Mtl, 5400 boul Gouin O, Montreal QC H4J 1C5; Mon'02; OrthSurg. Staff, Hôpital du Sacre-Coeur de Montréal; (514)338-2222

MAC VAN, Tin; Hop Louis-H Lafontaine, 7401 rue Hochelaga, Montreal QC H1N 3M5; Saigon (Vietnam)'71; Staff, Hopital Louis-H Lafontaine; (514)251-4000

MAC-WAY, Fabrice; CHUQ-Hotel-Dieu de Quebec, 11 Cote du Palais, Quebec QC G1R 2J6; Laval'02; FRCPC; IntMed; Nephrol. Staff, Centre Hospitalier Universitaire de Québec (CHUQ) - Siege Social; (418)525-4444

MACADAM, Christine M; North York Gen Hosp, 4001 Leslie St, North York ON M2K 1E1; Wes'78; FRCPC; DiagRad (Diagnostic Imaging). Staff Diag Imaging, North York General Hospital; (416)756-6184

MACADAM, Sheina A; 1000-777 Broadway W, Vancouver BC V5Z 4J7; UBC'02; FRCSC; PlasSurg. (604)876-1300

MACADAMS, Charles L; Foothills Med Centre, 1403 29 St NW, Calgary AB T2N 2T9; UBC'82; FRCPC; Anes. Staff Anes, Foothills Medical Centre; (403)944-1430; Fax. (403)944-2425.

MACALUSO, Salvatore E; 884 Concession St, Hamilton ON L8V 1E6; McM'77; CCFP; FCFP; (905)387-2612; Fax. (905)387-6313.

MACANOVIC, Mladen; Queen Elizabeth II HSC, 1276 South Park St, Halifax NS B3H 2Y9; London (England)'01; Staff, Queen Elizabeth II Health Sciences Centre - Victoria General Site; (902)473-5453

MACARTHUR, Alison J; Mount Sinai Hosp, 1514-600 University Ave, Toronto ON M5G 1X5; Alb'86; BMedSci; FRCPC; Anes. Staff Anes, Mount Sinai Hospital; (416)586-4800 x6632; Fax. (416)586-8664.

MACARTHUR, Angela M; Southwood Med Clinic, 80-10233 Elbow Dr SW, Calgary AB T2W 1E8; London (England)'81; FRCS(Edin); Staff Privil, Rockyview General Hospital; (403)252-1111

MACARTHUR, Roderick G G; University of Alberta Hosp, 3H2 11-8440 112 St NW, Edmonton AB T6G 2B7; Dal'96; FRCSC; CardSurg. Staff, University of Alberta Hospital; Langs: English; French; (780)407-2186; Fax. (780)407-2184.

MACASKILL, Kimberly R; The Westend Family Care Clinic, 80 Michael Cowpland Dr, Kanata ON K2M 1P6; Dal'95; BSc(Hons.); CCFP; Staff, Westend Family Care Clinic Family Health Team; Langs: English; French; (613)596-3321; Fax. (613)599-3366.

MACASKILL, Leslie; Royal University Hosp, 103 Hospital Dr, Saskatoon SK S7N 0W8; Pretoria (South Africa)'89; FRCPC; Anes. Staff, Royal University Hospital; (306)655-1183

MACAULAY, Alexander W; Mount Carmel Clinic, 886 Main St, Winnipeg MB R2W 5L4; Dal'92; MSc; CCFP; FCFP; Prog Coord, University of Manitoba; (204)582-2311; Fax. (204)582-1341; alecm@mts.net.

MACAULAY, Andria J; Village Family Physicians, 275 Pictou Rd, Truro NS B2N 2S7; Dal'01; CCFP; (902)895-1232

MACAULAY, Ann C; SMBD-Jewish Gen Hosp, 3755 ch Cote-Sainte-Catherine, Montreal QC H3T 1E2; St. Andrews (Scotland)'66; DObstRCOG; CCFP; FCFP; Staff, Sir Mortimer B Davis Jewish General; Prof Family Med/Dir Participating Research, McGill University; (514)340-8253

MACAULAY, Bruce D; IWK Health Centre, PO Box 9700 Rpo CSC 5850-5980 University Ave, Halifax NS B3K 6R8; Dal'94; FRCPC; Anes. Staff Anes, IWK Health Centre; (902)470-8888

MACAULAY, Christy J; Associate Clinic, 363-401 9 Ave SW, Calgary AB T2P 3C5; Dal'05; CCFP; (403)221-4428

MACAULAY, Peter M; Forest Hills Med Clinic, 4 Forest Hills Pky, Dartmouth NS B2W 5G7; Dal'86; CCFP; FCFP; Ac Staff Family Med, Dartmouth General Hospital; Physician Occup Med, Atlantic Offshore Medical Services; (902)435-5530; Fax. (902)462-6398.

MACAULAY, Robert J B; Mackenzie Bldg, 7F-5788 University Ave, Halifax NS B3H 1V8; Qns'88; FRCPC; NeurPath. Staff, Queen Elizabeth II Health Sciences Centre - Victoria General Site; (902)473-3156; Fax. (902)473-1049; robert.macaulay@cdha.nshealth.ca.

MACBEATH, Lyn S; Interior Health Mental Hlth Se, 311 Columbia St, Kamloops BC V2C 2T1; Dal'81; FRCPC; Psy (Consultation-Liaison). Staff Associate, Royal Inland Hospital; (250)314-2122

MACBRIDE, Ajana P; Carlington Comm Hlth Services, 900 Merivale Rd, Ottawa ON K1Z 5Z8; Wes'03; CCFP; CCFP(E.M.); Staff, South Huron Hospital Association; (613)722-2161; Fax. (613)761-1805.

MACCALLUM, Christie A; Davenport Perth Comm Hlth Ctr, 1892 Davenport Rd, Toronto ON M6N 1B7; McM'91; Staff Family Med, St Joseph's Health Centre; Lecturer Community & Family Med, University of Toronto; Langs: Spanish; (416)658-6812; Fax. (416)658-4611; cmaccallum@dpnc.ca.

MACCALLUM, Eoin D; Sudbury Med Centre, 309-65 Larch St, Sudbury ON P3E 1B8; Glasgow (Scotland)'71; DCH; Hon Staff, Health Sciences North-St Joseph's Health Centre; Hon Staff, Health Sciences North - Memorial Site; Hon Staff, Health Sciences North-Laurentian Site; (705)674-3509

MACCALLUM, G Calvin; Healt Sciences Centre, 300 Prince Philip Dr, St. John's NL A1B 3V6; Dal'71; FRCPC; IntMed; Cardiol. Ac Staff/Consultant, Health Sciences Centre; (709)777-6331

MACCALLUM, Johnstone S; St Joseph's Health Care, 100 Westmount Rd, Guelph ON N1H 5H8; Mem'75; ABIME; ABEDM; FRCPC; PhysMed&Rehab (Electromyography). Ac Member, Canadian Society of Medical Evaluators; Staff, St Joseph's Health Centre; (519)824-6000 x4290; Fax. (519)767-4165; johnstone.maccall@sjhcg.ca.

MACCALLUM, Margaret T; 3B-28 King St, Saint John NB E2L 1G3; Dal'88; CCFP; (506)634-7772; Fax. (506)634-7101.

MACCALLUM, Patricia L; Professional Arts Bldg, 401-100 Arden St, Moncton NB E1C 4B7; Wes'95; FRCSC; Otol. Staff, Dr Georges-L-Dumont University Hospital Centre; Langs: English; French; (506)855-9331; Fax. (506)855-9239.

MACCARA, A Shirley; 139 Water St PO Box 669, Pictou NS B0K 1H0; Dal'81; Assoc Staff, Sutherland-Harris Memorial Hospital; Ac Staff, Aberdeen Regional Hospital; (902)485-5377

MACCARA, Melanie L; Eastside Health Centre, 688 East River Rd, New Glasgow NS B2H 3S1; Dal'91; CCFP; FCFP; (902)752-3632; Fax. (902)755-5532.

MACCARI, Robert J; 202-180 McCarter St PO Box 1540 Stn Main, Parksville BC V9P 2H4; McG'82; Assoc Staff Priivl, Nanaimo Regional General Hospital; (250)954-1499; Fax. (250)954-1479.

MACCARTHY, Daniel D; BC Medical Association, 115-1665 Broadway W, Vancouver BC V6J 5A4; Cork (Ireland)'72; MB ChB; BAO; Dir Professional Relations, British Columbia Medical Association; (604)638-2830; Fax. (604)638-2918.

MACCARTHY, John A J; Royal City Med Bldg, 103-250 Keary St, New Westminster BC V3L 5E7; National (Ireland)'71; BAO; DCH; ABIM; FACP; FRCPC; IntMed; Respir. Staff Consultant, Eagle Ridge Hospital & Health Care Centre; Staff, Royal Columbian Hospital; Assoc Prof Med, University of British Columbia; (604)525-8822; Fax. (604)525-9470.

MACCAUSLAND, Owen; Prince County Hosp, PO Box 3000 Stn Main, Summerside PE C1N 2A9; Dal'81; Staff, Prince County Hospital; (902)438-4200

MACCHARLES, George R; Surrey Mem Hosp, 13750 96 Ave, Surrey BC V3V 1Z2; Mem'91; Staff, Surrey Memorial Hospital; (604)581-2211

MACCORDICK, Alexander; Ctr Hosp Pierre-Janet, 20 rue Pharand, Gatineau QC J9A 1K7; Strasbourg (France)'89; FRCPC; Psy (Geriatric Psychiatry). Staff, Hôpital de Gatineau; Staff, Hull Hospital; Staff, Centre Hospitalier Pierre-Janet; Langs: German; Spanish; French; (819)776-8028; Fax. (819)776-8006; alexander.maccordick@ssss.gouv.qc.ca.

MACCORMICK, Elizabeth C; 4 Jacob St, Sydney Mines NS B1V 3M4; Dal'81; (902)736-2840

MACCORMICK, Johnna A; Children's Hosp Eastern Ont, 401 Smyth Rd, Ottawa ON K1H 8L1; Dal'88; FRCSC; Otol. Staff, Children's Hospital of Eastern Ontario (CHEO); (613)737-7600 x2706; Fax. (613)738-4244.

MACCORMICK, Ronald E; Cape Breton Hlthcare Complex, 1482 George St, Sydney NS B1P 1P3; Dal'77; FRCPC; IntMed (Oncology); MedOncol. Staff, Cape Breton Healthcare Complex; Assoc Prof, Dalhousie University; (902)567-8072; maccormickr@cbdha.nshealth.ca.

MACCORMICK, Shaun A; Wagmatcook Health Centre, PO Box 3004 73A Humes Rear Rd, Wagmatcook NS B0E 3N0; Dal'83; CCFP; District Health Authority 4; (902)295-2725

MACCRIMMON, Duncan J; St Joseph's Mountain H Serv, PO Box 585 Stn Lcd 1 100 West 5th St, Hamilton ON L8N 3K7; McG'63; DPsy; FRCPC; Psy. Ac Staff, St Joseph's Healthcare Hamilton - West 5th Campus; Ac Staff, Hamilton Health Sciences Centre - McMaster University Medical Centre; Ac Staff, St Joseph's Healthcare - Charlton Campus; Assoc Prof, McMaster University; (905)388-2511

MACDIARMID, Andrew L; St Boniface Gen Hosp, C5008-409 Tache Ave, Winnipeg MB R2H 2A6; Man'93; BSc(Hons.Physics); FRCPC; IntMed (General Medicine). Staff Med, St Boniface General Hospital; Teach Staff, University of Manitoba; (204)258-1216; Fax. (204)233-7154; amacdiar@sbgh.mb.ca.

MACDONALD, A Ian; Royal Alexandra Hosp, 10240 Kingsway NW, Edmonton AB T5H 3V9; Alb'81; FRCPC; Anes. Ac Staff Anes, Royal Alexandra Hospital; Ac Staff, Alberta Hospital Edmonton; Clin Lecturer, University of Alberta; (780)735-4010; Fax. (780)735-4386.

MACDONALD, Alan L; 262B Main St N, Markham ON L3P 1Y7; Qns'69; MSc; FRCSC; Ophth. Staff, Sunnybrook Health Sciences Centre; University of Toronto; (905)294-1331

MACDONALD, Alison H; L4-30 Dupont St E, Waterloo ON N2J 2G9; McM'05; FRCSC; ObstGyn. (519)746-7878

MACDONALD, Allan S; Cumberland Reg Hlth Care Ctre, 19428 Highway 2, Amherst NS B4H 1N6; Dal'63; FRCSC; GenSurg (Transplantation). Consultant, IWK Health Centre; Staff, Cumberland Regional Health Care Center; Prof Surg, Dalhousie University; (902)667-5400; Fax. (902)667-1920.

MACDONALD, Angus; The Moncton Hosp, 135 MacBeath Ave, Moncton NB E1C 6Z8; Ott'08; CCFP; Staff, The Moncton Hospital; (506)857-5111

MACDONALD, Angus L; 3340A Yonge St, Toronto ON M4N 2M4; Wes'69; FRCSC; Ophth. (416)482-5352

MACDONALD, Anne-Marie H; Abbottsfield Shoppers Mall, 214-3210 118 Ave NW, Edmonton AB T5W 4W1; Alb'88; (780)471-2071; Fax. (780)474-8001.

MACDONALD, Avril M; 15 Grand Ave W, Chatham ON N7L 1B4; Tor'86; Ac Staff, Chatham-Kent Health Alliance; (519)436-1272

MACDONALD, Brian K; 716L Arlington Park Pl, Kingston ON K7M 8H9; Qns'82; LLB; MPA; FRCPC; Psy (Mood Disorders). (613)384-8222; Fax. (613)384-8221.

MACDONALD, Carla K; Woodlawn Med Clinic, 92 Main St, Dartmouth NS B2X 1R5; Dal'95; CCFP; (902)434-1500; Fax. (902)434-4368.

MACDONALD, Catherine A; 500 Raglan St N, Renfrew ON K7V 1P5; McM'91; CCFP; (613)432-8548; Fax. (613)432-8549.

MACDONALD, Catherine E; The Hosp for Sick Children, 555 University Ave, Toronto ON M5G 1X8; Tor'84; FRCPC; DiagRad. Staff Radiologist, The Hospital For Sick Children; University of Toronto; (416)813-6067; Fax. (416)813-7644; cathy.macdonald@sickkids.ca.

MACDONALD, Christine A; London HSC-Victoria Hosp, PO Box 5010 Stn B 800 Commissioners Rd E, London ON N6A 5W9; Tor'05; CCFP; CCFP(E.M.); Staff, London Health Sciences Centre - Victoria Campus; (519)685-8500

MACDONALD, Christopher; Selkirk Med Group, PO Box 590, Revelstoke BC V0E 2S0; Sask'95; CCFP; CCFP; Chief/Staff, Queen Victoria Hospital; (250)837-9321; Fax. (250)837-9444.

MACDONALD, Colin A W; 18 Manitou Cres W, Amherstview ON K7N 1S3; McM'79; FRCPC; IntMed (General Medicine). Staff, Kingston General Hospital; Staff, Hotel-Dieu Hospital; Med Consultant, The Empire Life Insurance Co; (613)634-1078

MACDONALD, Colin F; 205-9148 23 Ave NW, Edmonton AB T6N 1H9; Alb'95; BSc; FRCPC; IntMed (Diabetes). Staff, Covenant Health - Grey Nuns Community Hospital; Clin Assoc Prof, University of Alberta; (780)462-3010; Fax. (780)440-2911.

MACDONALD, D Blair; The Ottawa Hosp-Gen Campus, 501 Smyth Rd, Ottawa ON K1H 8L6; Qns'98; FRCPC; DiagRad. Staff, The Ottawa Hospital - General Campus; (613)798-5555

MACDONALD, D Christopher; 406-113 Roseberry St PO Box 367 Stn Main, Campbellton NB E3N 3G7; Dal'75; CCFP; Ac Staff, Hôpital Régional Campbellton; (506)753-2244; Fax. (506)759-7495.

MACDONALD, D James; Hanover & Dist Hosp, 90 7th Ave, Hanover ON N4N 1N1; Tor'59; DPsy; FRCPC; Psy (Community Psychiatry). Staff, Hanover & District Hospital; Consultant, Central Grey Bruce Community Mental Health Centre; (519)364-2340

MACDONALD, D Ross; 108-30 Springborough Blvd SW, Calgary AB T3H 0N9; RCSI (Ireland)'80; Ac Staff, Rockyview General Hospital; Clin Lecturer Family Practice, University of Calgary; (403)240-2221; Fax. (403)240-4670.

MACDONALD, D Scott; Providence Crosstown Clinic, 84 Hastings St W, Vancouver BC V6B 1G6; Dal'92; Staff, Providence Health Care - St Paul's Hospital; Physician, Mainland Medical Clinic; Physician, Vancouver Native Health Society; (604)689-8803; scott.maddonald@vch.ca.

MACDONALD, Damian A; Thunder Bay Reg HSC-T-Bay, 980 Oliver St, Thunder Bay ON P7B 6V4; Heidelberg (Germany)'01; FRCPC; EmergMed. Staff EmergMed, Thunder Bay Regional Health Sciences Centre; (807)684-6000

MACDONALD, Daniel J; 34 Maple Ave PO Box 250, Tatamagouche NS B0K 1V0; Dal'05; CCFP; (902)657-2910

MACDONALD, David A; Queen ELizabeth II HSC, 429-1276 South Park St, Halifax NS B3H 2Y9; Qns'99; FRCPC; IntMed; Hem. Staff, Queen Elizabeth II Health Sciences Centre - Victoria General Site; (902)473-2394; Fax. (902)473-4447.

MACDONALD, David R; London Reg Cancer Centre, 790 Commissioners Rd E, London ON N6A 4L6; Wes'75; DAB; FRCPC; Neur (Brain Tumors). Consultant, London Health Sciences Centre - University Hospital; Assoc Prof, University of Western Ontario; (519)685-8640; Fax. (519)685-8624.

MACDONALD, Denis F; North York Gen Hosp, 4SE 106-4001 Leslie St, North York ON M2K 1E1; Witwatersrand (South Africa)'74; DABPath; MBA(Tor); FRCPC; HemPath; AnatPath. Chief Lab, North York General Hospital; Assoc Prof, University of Toronto, Lab. Med. & Path.; (416)756-6517

MACDONALD, Derek J; Sudbury Reg Hosp-Mem Site, M 131-865 Regent St, Sudbury ON P3E 3Y9; Dal'99; FRCSC; CardSurg. Staff, Health Sciences North - Memorial Site; (705)671-5353

MACDONALD, Dianne D; 306-6155 North St, Halifax NS B3K 5R3; Dal'78; FRCPC; Psy. (902)423-7182; Fax. (902)453-2856; mgt@eastlink.ca.

MACDONALD, Donald C; St Paul's Hosp, 1081 Burrard St, Vancouver BC V6Z 1Y6; Tor'75; Staff, Providence Health Care - St Paul's Hospital; (604)806-8480; Fax. (604)806-8424.

MACDONALD, Donald G; PO Box 187, Sheet Harbour NS B0J 3B0; Tor'84; CCFP; (902)885-2200; Fax. (902)885-2706.

MACDONALD, E Anne; Landmark Prof Centre, 101-2731 Hewes Way NW, Edmonton AB T6L 6W6; Alb'81; FRCSC; Ophth. Medical Staff Capital Health, Royal Alexandra Hospital; Assoc Prof Ophth, University of Alberta; (780)450-3200; Fax. (780)450-9861.

MACDONALD, E Athen; Hotel-Dieu Hosp, 166 Brock St, Kingston ON K7L 5G2; Qns'75; FRCPC; Peds. Att Staff, Kingston General Hospital; Att Staff Children's Out-Patient Centre, Hotel-Dieu Hospital; Asst Prof, Queen's University; (613)544-3310 x3324

MACDONALD, Elizabeth A; 130 Bayard Dr, Saint John NB E2L 3L6; Dal'95; BSc; FRCPC; IntMed; GeriatricMed. Staff, St Joseph's Hospital; Asst Prof Med, Dalhousie University; Asst Prof Med, Memorial University Of Newfoundland; (506)632-5398; Fax. (506)632-5512; Elizabeth.MacDonald2@HorizonNB.ca.

MACDONALD, Faye; 1414 King St E, Oshawa ON L1E 2M6; Ott'76; (905)743-0090

MACDONALD, Francis; The Ob/Gyn Suite, 403-199 Grafton St, Charlottetown PE C1A 1L2; Dal'78; FRCSC; ObstGyn. Consultant, The Ob/Gyn Suite; (902)629-8801; Fax. (902)629-8826.

MACDONALD, Gerald R C; 201-44 Mapleton Rd, Moncton NB E1C 7W8; Dal'02; CCFP; (506)858-7859

MACDONALD, H Paul; PO Box 1374, Stellarton NS B0K 1S0; Dal'72; Staff, Aberdeen Regional Hospital.

MACDONALD, Helene E; Cambie Plaza Med Clinic, 180-11700 Cambie Rd, Richmond BC V6X 1L5; UBC'01; CCFP; (604)270-9833

MACDONALD, Ian A G; Sudbury Reg Hosp-Laurentian, 41 Ramsey Lake Rd, Sudbury ON P3E 5J1; Wes'00; FRCPC; IntMed (Hypertension); Nephrol. Staff, Health Sciences North-Laurentian Site; (705)523-7004; Fax. (705)523-7161.

MACDONALD, Ian L; Burrard Med Bldg, 310-1144 Burrard St, Vancouver BC V6Z 2A5; Qns'66; ABIM; FACC; FRCPC; IntMed (Adult Cardiology); Cardiol. Ac Staff Cardiol, Providence Health Care - St Paul's Hospital; Clin Assoc Prof, University of British Columbia; (604)669-1014; Fax. (604)683-7992.

MACDONALD, Ian M; Fredericton Med Clinic, 207-1015 Regent St, Fredericton NB E3B 6H5; Dal'72; CCFP; FCFP; Staff Family Med, Dr Everett Chalmers Regional Hospital; Teach Staff, Dalhousie University; (506)458-0251; Fax. (506)457-4799; macian@nb.sympatico.ca.

MACDONALD, Ian M; Royal Alexandra Hosp, 2319-10240 Kingsway NW, Edmonton AB T5H 3V9; McG'79; MSc; FCCMG; CM; FRCSC; Ophth (Electrophysiology). Staff, Royal Alexandra Hospital; Dept Chair Opht, University of Alberta; Langs: English; French; (780)735-5932

MACDONALD, Ian R; Alpine Med Clinic, PO Bag 4000 Stn Main 201A-211 Bear St, Banff AB T1L 1J8; Glasgow (Scotland)'79; MB ChB; FRCS(Glas); Ac Staff, Covenant Health - Banff Mineral Springs Hospital; (403)762-3155; Fax. (403)762-5797.

MACDONALD, Ildiko L; Millcove Plaza, 207-967 Bedford Hwy, Bedford NS B4A 1A9; McM'97; CCFP; (902)835-6444

MACDONALD, J Gerard; Cumberland Reg Hlth Care Ctre, 19428 Highway 2, Amherst NS B4H 1N6; Dal'79; FRCSC; Otol. Staff, Cumberland Regional Health Care Center; (902)667-3868

MACDONALD, J Kelly M; Lake of the Woods Dist Hosp, RR 1 21 Sylvain St, Kenora ON P9N 3W7; Man'82; FRCPC; AnatPath. Staff, Lake of the Woods District Hospital; (807)468-9861

MACDONALD, James A; Huntsville District Mem Hosp, 100 Frank Miller Dr, Huntsville ON P1H 1H7; Ott'85; CCFP; CCFP(E.M.); Huntsville District Memorial Hospital - Muskoka Algonquin Healthcare; (705)789-2311

MACDONALD, James K; Lake of the Woods Dist Hosp, RR 1 21 Sylvan St, Kenora ON P9N 3W7; Man'81; FRCPC; AnatPath; GenPath. Dir Lab/Chief Staff, Lake of the Woods District Hospital; (807)468-9861 x480

MACDONALD, Janeen M; Social Development Canada, 333 North River Rd, Ottawa ON K1A 0L1; Dal'75; (613)954-6415

MACDONALD, Jay R; Windsor Reg Hosp-Metropolitan, 1995 Lens Ave, Windsor ON N8W 1L9; Tor'05; FRCPC; EmergMed. Staff, Windsor Regional Hospital - Metropolitan Site; (519)254-5577

MACDONALD, Jennifer L; 201-255 Main St PO Box 819, Liverpool NS B0T 1K0; Dal'00; BSc; CCFP; Langs: English; French; (902)354-4964; Fax. (902)354-2680.

MACDONALD, Jennifer L; 2045 Enterprise Way, Kelowna BC V1Y 9T5; Tor'90; (250)979-4159

MACDONALD, Jillian A; The Ottawa Clinic, 200-343 Preston St, Ottawa ON K1S 1N4; Dal'05; FRCPC; Derm. Staff, The Ottawa Hospital - Civic Campus; (613)729-1616

MACDONALD, Joanne L; IWK Health Centre, PO Box 9700 Rpo CSC 5850-5980 University Ave, Halifax NS B3K 6R8; Dal'84; FRCPC; Psy. Staff, IWK Health Centre; Asst Prof, Dalhousie University; (902)470-8722; Fax. (902)470-6760.

MACDONALD, John C; Univ of Ottawa Heart Institute, 40 Ruskin St, Ottawa ON K1Y 4W7; Wes'94; BSc; FRCPC; Anes; Critical Care Medicine. Staff, University of Ottawa Heart Institute; (613)761-4379; Fax. (613)761-4925.

MACDONALD, John J; 27022 Fraser Hwy, Aldergrove BC V4W 3L6; McM'76; (604)856-7771; Fax. (604)856-6594.

MACDONALD, John W; Woodlawn Med Clinic, 92 Main St, Dartmouth NS B2X 1R5; Dal'70; CCFP; FCFP; Staff, Dartmouth General Hospital; Staff, IWK Health Centre; Lecturer, Dalhousie University; (902)434-1500 x213

MACDONALD, Jon K; Aberdeen Hosp, 835 East River Rd, New Glasgow NS B2H 3S6; Dal'77; FRCPC; Anes. Staff, Aberdeen Regional Hospital; (902)752-8311

MACDONALD, Judy; Sheldon Chumir Health Centre, 5F-1213 4 St SW, Calgary AB T2R 0X7; Cal'95; BSc; MSc; FRCPC; CommunMed (Communicable Diseases). Clinical Asst Prof Commun Health Sciences, University of Calgary; (403)955-6801; Fax. (403)955-6818; judy.macdonald@calgaryhealthregion.ca.

MACDONALD, K Anne; Queen Elizabeth Hosp, PO Box 6600 Stn Central, Charlottetown PE C1A 8T5; Mem'86; Staff, Queen Elizabeth Hospital; (902)894-2111

MACDONALD, K Yvonne; West Elgin Commun Health Ctr, SS 1 153 Main St, West Lorne ON N0L 2P0; Mem'01; CCFP; (519)768-1715; Fax. (519)768-2548.

MACDONALD, Karen A; PO Box 1591 Stn Main, Antigonish NS B2G 2L8; Dal'00; CCFP.

MACDONALD, Karen A; Public Service Occup Hlth Prog, 1817-1505 Barrington St, Halifax NS B3J 3Y6; Dal'84; DOHS(McM); CCBOM; Medical Officer Public Service Occupational Health Prog, Health Canada-Atlantic Region; (902)426-3998; Fax. (902)426-5375; karen_macdonald@hc-sc.gc.ca.

MACDONALD, Kathryn J; Six Nations Family Health Team, PO Box 5000 1745 Chiefswood Rd, Ohsweken ON N0A 1M0; McM'93; FRCPC; Psy (Adult & Child Psychiatry). Langs: English; French; (519)445-2143; Fax. (519)445-0504.

MACDONALD, Kelly S; Mount Sinai Hosp, 1484-600 University Ave, Toronto ON M5G 1X5; Man'87; BA; FRCPC; IntMed (AIDS/HIV); MedMicrobiol; InfectDis. Microbio/Infec Dis Consultant, Mount Sinai Hospital; Assoc Prof, University of Toronto; (416)586-8879; Fax. (416)586-8746.

MACDONALD, Kristian I; Parkdale Med Tower, G3-1081 Carling Ave, Ottawa ON K1Y 4G2; Dal'06; Otol (Head & Neck Surgery). (613)729-2834

MACDONALD, Leah M; Burnaby Home Health Care, 400-4946 Canada Way, Burnaby BC V5G 4H7; Ott'00; CCFP; Staff, Burnaby Hospital; (604)918-7447

MACDONALD, Linda A; Polyclinique Prof Centre Inc, 199 Grafton St, Charlottetown PE C1A 1L2; Dal'78; Ac Staff, Queen Elizabeth Hospital; (902)629-8816; Fax. (902)629-8897.

MACDONALD, Linda D; The U of Toronto-Mississauga, 3359 Mississauga Rd, Mississauga ON L5L 1C6; Tor'82; BSc; (905)828-5255; Fax. (905)828-3852.

MACDONALD, Lorraine A; CFB Borden, PO Box 1000, Borden ON L0M 1C0; UBC'09; CCFP; (705)424-1200

MACDONALD, Malcolm K; 110-3540 41st Ave W, Vancouver BC V6N 3E6; Cal'84; Assoc Staff, BC Women's Hospital & Health Centre; Assoc Staff, UBC Hospital - Koerner Pavillion; Vis Staff, Vancouver General Hospital - Centennial Pavillion; (604)261-6361; Fax. (604)261-1656.

MACDONALD, Maria J; London Reg Cancer Centre, 790 Commissioners Rd E, London ON N6A 4L6; McM'06; FRCPC; Neur. Staff, London Health Sciences Centre - Victoria Campus; (519)685-8640; Fax. (519)685-8624.

MACDONALD, Marion N; Stellarton Med Centre, PO Box 2170 10 Jubilee Ave, Stellarton NS B0K 1S0; Dal'74; (902)755-6263; Fax. (902)752-7126.

MACDONALD, Mary R A; Grandview Children's Centre, 600 Townline Rd S, Oshawa ON L1H 7K6; Qns'72; FRCPC; Peds (Developmental Pediatrics). Staff, Grandview Children's Centre Main Site; (905)728-1673 x230; Fax. (905)728-2961; mary.macdonald@grtc.ca.

MACDONALD, Mary Rose; Parkdale Comm Health Centre, 1229 Queen St W, Toronto ON M6K 1L2; Tor'84; BSc; Staff, Parkdale Community Health Centre; Physician, Clair Vaughan Medical Clinic; Lecturer, University of Toronto; (416)537-2455; Fax. (416)537-3526.

MACDONALD, Matthew H; Medical Clinic Person-Ctred Ps, 403-265 Yorkland Blvd, North York ON M2J 1S5; Dal'10; CCFP.

MACDONALD, Matthew J; Harbourfront Health & Wellness, 4-8 York St, Toronto ON M5J 2Y2; Wes'09; CCFP; (416)366-2273

MACDONALD, Michael; CFB Gagetown BMC, PO Box 17000 Stn Forces, Oromocto NB E2V 4J5; Mem'08; CCFP; (506)422-2000

MACDONALD, Myron K; 209-575 16th St, West Vancouver BC V7V 4Y1; UBC'68; (604)921-2624; dr.mkmacdonald@yahoo.ca.

MACDONALD, Nancy L; Queen Elizabeth II HSC-Halifax, 2109-1796 Summer St, Halifax NS B3H 3A7; Dal'77; FRCPC; IntMed (Cardiology). Consultant Privil, Queen Elizabeth II Health Sciences Centre - Halifax Infirmary Site; Asst Prof Med, Dalhousie University; (902)465-8716; Fax. (902)461-9967.

MACDONALD, Nora Noni E; IWK Health Centre, PO Box 9700 Rpo CSC 5850-5980 University Ave, Halifax NS B3K 6R8; Ott'75; BSc; MSc; FRCPC; Peds; InfectDis. Staff, IWK Health Centre; (902)470-8888

MACDONALD, Ophelia L; 202-1407 Yonge St, Toronto ON M4T 1Y7; Alb'74; FRCPC; Psy (Psychoanalysis). (416)485-9461; Fax. (416)485-9461.

MACDONALD, P Hugh; Kingston Gen Hosp, Burr 2 058-76 Stuart St, Kingston ON K7L 2V7; Qns'84; ATLS; BSc; FRCS; FRCSC; GenSurg (Colon & Rectal Surgery). Staff, Kingston General Hospital; Asst Prof, Queen's University; (613)549-6666 x7662; Fax. (613)548-2500; phm@post.queensu.ca.

MACDONALD, Patricia J; 201-250 Keary St, New Westminster BC V3L 5E7; Dal'98; FRCSC; PlasSurg (Cranio Facial Surgery). Staff, Royal Columbian Hospital; Staff, Eagle Ridge Hospital & Health Care Centre; Staff, Surrey Memorial Hospital; (604)288-8517; Fax. (604)909-4929; macdonaldplasticsurgery@yahoo.ca.

MACDONALD, Paul J; Cape Breton Hlthcare Complex, 1482 George St, Sydney NS B1P 1P3; Dal'88; FRCPC; IntMed; Cardiol. Staff, Cape Breton Healthcare Complex; (902)567-7979

MACDONALD, Penny A; London HSC-University Hosp, PO Box 5339 Stn B C7 002-339 Windermere Rd, London ON N6A 5A5; McM'03; FRCPC; Neur. Staff, London Health Sciences Centre - University Hospital; (519)663-3631

MACDONALD, Peter B; Pan Am Clinic, 75 Poseidon Bay, Winnipeg MB R3M 3E4; Man'83; FRCSC; OrthSurg (Knee Shoulder & Sports Injuries). Reg Leader Orthopaedic, Winnipeg Regional Health Authority; Staff Surg, University of Manitoba; (204)925-1546; Fax. (204)453-9032; pmacdonald@panamclinic.com.

MACDONALD, Peter S; St Paul's Hosp, 1081 Burrard St, Vancouver BC V6Z 1Y6; Tor'91; BSc; FRCSC; GenSurg; VascSurg. Staff, Providence Health Care - St Paul's Hospital; Clinical Asst Prof Surg, University of British Columbia; (604)806-8698; Fax. (604)806-8666; smacdonald@providencehealth.bc.ca.

MACDONALD, Randal J; University of Alberta Hosp, 8440 112 St NW, Edmonton AB T6G 2B7; Alb'00; CCFP; CCFP(E.M.); Staff EmergMed, University of Alberta Hospital; (780)407-8822

MACDONALD, Rhea C; Inverness Consolid Mem Hosp, PO Box 610 39 James St, Inverness NS B0E 1N0; Dal'04; CCFP; Staff, Inverness Consolidated Memorial Hospital; (902)258-2555; Fax. (902)258-2555.

MACDONALD, Richard J; Oakville Med Arts Bldg, 8-358 Reynolds St, Oakville ON L6J 3L9; Tor'85; FAAP; DAB; FRCPC; Peds (Neonatology). Ac Staff, Halton Healthcare Services Corporation - Oakville Site; Court Staff, Trillium Health Centre - Mississauga; Court Staff, Grey Bruce Health Services - Lion's Head; (905)845-6181; Fax. (905)845-5924; kidsdoc1@me.com.

MACDONALD, R Loch; 30 Bond St, Toronto ON M5B 1W8; UBC'85; FRCS; AddicMed; MRCS; DABNS; DPhil; FRCSC; Neursurg (Neuro Surgical Consultant). Head Div of Neurosurg, St Michael's Hospital; (416)864-5452; macdonaldlo@smh.ca.

MACDONALD, Russell D; Ornge Transport Medicine, 5310 Explorer Dr, Mississauga ON L4W 5H8; Qns'91; BSc; MPH; CCFP; FCFP; FRCPC; EmergMed (Public Health); Att Staff Emerg Services, Sunnybrook Health Sciences Centre; Med Dir, Ornge Transport Medicine; Assoc Prof Emerg Med, University of Toronto; Langs: French; (647)428-2005

MACDONALD, Sara E; Whitehorse Med Services Ltd, 406 Lambert St, Whitehorse YT Y1A 1Z7; McM'76; DTMH; Staff, Whitehorse General Hospital; Staff, Whitehorse Medical Services Ltd; (867)393-6633; Fax. (867)393-6601.

MACDONALD, Sara E; CSSSG-Hop de Hull, 116 boul Lionel-Emond, Gatineau QC J8Y 1W7; Dal'04; FRCPC; IntMed; Nephrol. Staff, Hull Hospital; (819)966-6200; Fax. (819)966-6325.

MACDONALD, Shannon L; 645-5991 Spring Garden Rd, Halifax NS B3H 1Y6; Dal'02; FRCPC; Psy. Staff, IWK Health Centre; (902)431-8442

MACDONALD, Sharon M; Univ of Manitoba, S113-750 Bannatyne Ave, Winnipeg MB R3E 0W2; Man'72; BSc(Med); FRCPC; CommunMed. Dept Head Community Health Sciences, University of Manitoba; Langs: English; French.

MACDONALD, Shavaun I; Royal Alexandra Hosp, 541-10240 Kingsway NW, Edmonton AB T5H 3V9; Ott'04; Critical Care Medicine; EmergMed. Staff, Royal Alexandra Hospital; (780)735-4442

MACDONALD, Stephen J H; The Doctor's Office, 101-777 Broadway W, Vancouver BC V5Z 4J7; (Poland)'05; CCFP; (604)734-8252

MACDONALD, Steven J; Shoppers World Med Centre, 106-499 Main St S, Brampton ON L6Y 1N7; Tor'87; (905)796-6570

MACDONALD, Steven J M; London HSC-University Hosp, PO Box 5339 Stn B 339 Windermere Rd, London ON N6A 5A5; Tor'89; FRCSC; OrthSurg (Adult Reconstructive Surgery). Staff, London Health Sciences Centre - University Hospital; (519)663-3689; Fax. (519)663-3096; steven.macdonald@lhsc.on.ca.

MACDONALD, Stuart D; FW Green Medical Centre, 1629 Baker St, Cranbrook BC V1C 1B4; Cape Town (South Africa)'98; MB ChB; (250)426-6601

MACDONALD, Susan C; 600-299 Victoria St, Prince George BC V2L 5B8; McG'80; CCFP; Langs: English; French; (250)565-5886; Fax. (250)562-0308.

MACDONALD, Susan E; Family Med Centre, PO Box 8888 Stn Main 220 Bagot St, Kingston ON K7L 5E9; Qns'83; CCFP; FCFP; (613)533-9303; Fax. (613)544-9899.

MACDONALD, Susan J; 635 James St N PO Box 1140, Lumsden SK S0G 3C0; Sask'78; (306)731-2116

MACDONALD, Susan M; Dr L A Miller Centre, 360-100 Forest Rd, St. John's NL A1A 1E5; McM'89; BScN; CCFP; FCFP; Staff, St Clare's Mercy Hospital; Med Dir Palliative Care/Staff, Health Sciences Centre; Assoc Prof Med & Joint Appt, Memorial University Of Newfoundland.

MACDONALD, Suzanne F; MUHC-Montreal pour Enfants, 2300 rue Tupper, Montreal QC H3H 1P3; McG'95; LMCC; FAAP; FRCPC; Peds (Adolescent Medicine). adj Prof Peds, McGill University Health Centre - Montreal Children's Hospital; Langs: Italian; French; (514)412-4400

MACDONALD, Theresa M; Canadian Forces Hlth Serv Ctr, PO Box 99000 Stn Forces, Halifax NS B3K 5X5; Dal'89; Staff, Canadian Forces Health Services Centre (Atlantic); (902)427-8700

MACDONALD, Timothy L; Thames Valley FHT-Strathroy Me, 74 Front St E, Strathroy ON N7G 1Y7; Wes'00; CCFP; Associate, Strathroy Middlesex General Hospital - Middlesex Hospital Alliance; (519)245-0430; Fax. (519)245-5870; tmacdonald@strathroymedicalclinic.com.

MACDONALD, Walter A C; 7-431 King St PO Box 1169, Petrolia ON N0N 1R0; Glasgow (Scotland)'65; MB ChB; Staff, Bluewater Health - Charlotte Eleanor Englehart Hospital; Prov Coroner, Canada & Aviation Examiner; (519)882-0140; Fax. (519)882-3807.

MACDONALD, Wendy A; MUHC-Montreal Children's Hosp, C429-2300 rue Tupper, Montreal QC H3H 1P3; McG'70; Peds (Medical Education). Staff, McGill University Health Centre - Montreal Children's Hospital; Assoc Prof Peds, McGill University; (514)412-4308; Fax. (514)412-4311; wendy.macdonald@muhc.mcgill.ca.

MACDONALD, William A; Qikiqtani Gen Hosp, PO Box 1000, Iqaluit NU X0A 0H0; Mem'86; CCFP; FCFP; Staff, Baffin Regional Hospital; Dir Health & Social Services, Gov't of Nunavut; Asst Prof Family Med, University of Ottawa; Langs: English; French; (867)979-7601; Fax. (867)979-7346.

MACDONALD, William M; 145 King St, North Sydney NS B2A 1S1; Dal'81; (902)794-3542; keremeos107@gmail.com.

MACDONELL, Stephannie M; 3192 Logan Farm Dr RR 1, Osgoode ON K0A 2W0; Ott'07; CCFP; Langs: Bilingual(English/French); (613)826-2502; Fax. (613)826-1681.

MACDONNELL, B Jean; Westmount Med Bldg, 345-5025 rue Sherbrooke O, Montreal QC H4A 1S9; McG'78; CCFP; FCFP; Staff, St Mary's Hospital Centre; Langs: English; French; (514)938-4975; Fax. (514)938-4772.

MACDONNELL, Heather M M; Children's Hosp Eastern Ont, 401 Smyth Rd, Ottawa ON K1H 8L1; Qns'99; LMCC; FRCPC; Peds. Staff Peds, Children's Hospital of Eastern Ontario (CHEO); (613)737-7600 x2571; Fax. (613)738-4878.

MACDOUGALL, Alexander D; 1110-5991 Spring Garden Rd, Halifax NS B3H 1Y6; Dal'78; FRCPC; Neur. (902)425-2960; Fax. (902)425-2069.

MACDOUGALL, Andrea; Curans Health Centre, 384 Fort William Rd, Thunder Bay ON P7B 2Z3; Alb'03; FRCPC; IntMed; Cardiol. Staff, Thunder Bay Regional Health Sciences Centre; (807)345-3355; Fax. (807)345-0099.

MACDOUGALL, Bradley; Westville Med Clinic, PO Box 930, Westville NS B0K 2A0; Dal'09; CCFP; (902)396-4142; Fax. (902)396-1707.

MACDOUGALL, Brendan K; St Boniface Gen Hosp, 5C114-409 Tache Ave, Winnipeg MB R2H 2A6; Man'71; FRCPC; IntMed. Ac Staff, St Boniface General Hospital; Prof, University of Manitoba; (204)237-2545; Fax. (204)233-7154; bmacdoug@sbgh.mb.ca.

MACDOUGALL, Catherine E; Public Gardens Med Clinic, 200-5675 Spring Garden Rd, Halifax NS B3J 1H1; Dal'84; CCFP; (902)425-5440

MACDOUGALL, Eleanor R E; Manitoba Clinic, 790 Sherbrook St, Winnipeg MB R3A 1M3; Man'83; FRCPC; Peds. Pediatric Program Dir-Peds & Child Health, University of Manitoba; (204)788-5745; Fax. (204)772-2537.

MACDOUGALL, Frances J K; Southside Med Clinic, A-640 Prospect St, Fredericton NB E3B 9M7; Mem'84; (506)450-7887

MACDOUGALL, Grant L; Manitoba Clinic, 790 Sherbrook St, Winnipeg MB R3A 1M3; Man'87; FRCPC; Peds. (204)788-5511; Fax. (204)772-2537.

MACDOUGALL, Ian A T; Halton HSC Corp-Oakville, 327 Reynolds St, Oakville ON L6J 3L7; McM'07; CCFP; Staff, Halton Healthcare Services Corporation - Oakville Site; (905)845-2571

MACDOUGALL, Joseph A; Harvey Community Hosp, 2019 Route 3, Harvey Station NB E6K 3E9; Ott'70; Staff, Harvey Health Centre; (506)366-5658; Fax. (506)366-6403.

MACDOUGALL, Keith; London HSC-University Hosp, PO Box 5339 Stn B 399 Windermere Rd, London ON N6A 5A5; Alb'02; FRCSC; Neursurg. Staff, London Health Sciences Centre - University Hospital; (519)663-3696

MACDOUGALL, Lorna J; 4318 County Rd 124 PO Box 208, Nottawa ON L0M 1P0; McG'86; Staff, Collingwood General & Marine Hospital.

MACDOUGALL, Paul J; Hamilton HS-General Site, 237 Barton St E, Hamilton ON L8L 2X2; Wes'93; CCFP; CCFP(E.M.); Staff, Hamilton Health Sciences Centre - Hamilton General Hospital; (905)527-4322 x46368

MACDOUGALL, Peter C; Queen Elizabeth II HSC-Halifax, 1796 Summer St, Halifax NS B3H 3A7; McM'93; FRCPC; Anes. Staff, Queen Elizabeth II Health Sciences Centre - Halifax Infirmary Site.

MACDOUGALL, Peter E; Harbour City Health Centre, 303-1125 Dufferin Cres, Nanaimo BC V9S 2B5; UBC'92; FRCPC; Peds. Staff Peds, BC Children's Hospital; (250)754-5458; Fax. (250)754-1211.

MACDOUGALL, Peter L R; Royal University Hosp, 103 Hospital Dr, Saskatoon SK S7N 0W8; Tor'82; FRCPC; Anes. Ac Staff Anes, Royal University Hospital; (306)655-1183; Fax. (306)655-1279.

MACDOUGALL, Ryan; Valley Reg Hosp, 150 Exhibition St, Kentville NS B4N 5E3; Dal'07; FRCPC; DiagRad. Staff, Valley Regional Hospital; (902)679-2657

MACDOUGALL, Steven G; Health Park, 308-45 Weatherbee Rd, Mira Road NS B1M 0A1; Dal'83; CCFP; (902)567-0660; Fax. (902)270-3236.

MACDOUGALL, W Gregory; Doctor's Med Clinic, 215-3066 Shelbourne St, Victoria BC V8R 6T9; Glasgow (Scotland)'71; MB ChB; MHA; MA; CCFP; FCFP; Langs: Bilingual(English/French); (250)388-4211; Fax. (250)383-4119.

MACDUFF, Blair A; St Martha's Reg Hosp, 25 Bay St, Antigonish NS B2G 2G5; Mem'01; FRCPC; DiagRad. Staff, St Martha's Regional Hospital; (902)863-2830

MACE, Frank J; 11-1155 North Service Rd W, Oakville ON L6M 3E3; McG'81; FRCPC; Psy. (289)291-3951; Fax. (289)291-3952.

MACE, Jeanne R; Glenmore Clinic, 1605 Gordon Dr, Kelowna BC V1Y 3G8; UBC'97; CCFP; FCFP; (250)861-8838

MACE, Sean R; 301-2130 Lawrence Ave E, Scarborough ON M1R 3A6; Cambridge (England)'87; FRCPC; IntMed; ClinImmunol&Allergy. (416)264-4443; dr.allergy@ymail.com.

MACEACHERN, Janet A; Grand River Hosp-KW Hlth Ctre, PO Box 9056 Stn C 835 King St, Kitchener ON N2G 1G3; Tor'95; FRCPC; IntMed; Hem. Staff, Grand River Hospital - Kitchener/Waterloo Health Centre; (519)749-4300 x3512; Fax. (519)749-4378; janet_maceachern@grhosp.on.ca.

MACEACHERN, John R; 236 Main St RR 3, Berwick NS B0P 1E0; Dal'78; Staff, Western Kings Memorial Health Centre; Staff, Valley Regional Hospital; (902)538-7226; Fax. (902)538-1642.

MACEACHERN, Lisa K; U of Ottawa Health Services, 300-100 Marie Curie Pvt, Ottawa ON K1N 1A2; Wes'05; CCFP; (613)564-3950

MACEACHERN, M Shauna; Active Care Med Group, A-1108 Klondike Ave, Kanata ON K2K 0G1; Dal'90; (613)254-9777; Fax. (613)254-9778.

MACEACHERN, Michael H; PO Box 849 Stn Main, Moncton NB E1C 8N6; Liege (Belgium)'80; BSc; FRCPC; Neur (Electroencephalography). Ac Staff, Dr Georges-L-Dumont University Hospital Centre; Consultant, The Moncton Hospital; Langs: English; French; (506)858-0662; Fax. (506)858-0664.

MACEACHERN, Neil H; Leduc General Surgery, 202-4721 47 Ave, Leduc AB T9E 7J4; Dundee (Scotland)'76; FRCS(Ed); FRCSC; GenSurg. Staff, Leduc Community Hospital; (780)980-0891; Fax. (780)980-0202.

MACEACHERN, Norman A; Winnipeg Clinic, 425 St Mary Ave, Winnipeg MB R3C 0N2; Man'80; FRCSC; GenSurg (Thoracic Surgery). Staff Cardiac Surg Assisting, St Boniface General Hospital; (204)957-3351; Fax. (204)942-2044.

MACEACHERN, Paul; University of Calgary, 3330 Hospital Dr NW, Calgary AB T2N 4N1; Qns'02; FRCPC; IntMed; Respir. Staff, Foothills Medical Centre; Teach Staff, University of Calgary; (403)220-6882

MACEACHERN, Ronald T; Aberdeen Hosp, 835 East River Rd, New Glasgow NS B2H 3S6; Mem'96; FRCPC; DiagRad;CCFP; Staff, Aberdeen Regional Hospital; (902)752-7600

MACEACHERN, William N; 200 King St S, Waterloo ON N2J 1P9; Tor'58; BScPharm; DAB; FRCPC; Derm. (519)886-3450; Fax. (519)886-3895.

MACEDO, B A Ben; Summit Centre, 209-200 Boudreau Rd, St. Albert AB T8N 6B9; Alb'93; CCFP; (780)458-7000; Fax. (780)458-8484.

MACEK, Adrian S; Clinique Med Cowansville, 1001-101 rue Albert, Cowansville QC J2K 2W4; McG'90; CCFP; ac Staff, Hôpital Brome-Missisquoi-Perkins; adj Prof Family Med, McGill University; (450)266-4060; Fax. (450)266-5335.

MACEK, Daniel B; Hop Brome-Missisquoi-Perkins, 950 rue Principale, Cowansville QC J2K 1K3; McG'92; BSc; FRCPC; IntMed. Staff, Hôpital Brome-Missisquoi-Perkins; Langs: English; French; (450)263-2220; Fax. (450)266-5335.

MACEK, Ralf K W; Salvation Army Grace Gen Hosp, 300 Booth Dr, Winnipeg MB R3J 3M7; Man'82; CCFP; CCFP(E.M.); Staff, The Salvation Army Grace Hospital; (204)837-8311

MACELWAIN, Dale A; Upper River Valley Hosp, 11300 130 Rte, Watervil-Carleton NB E7P 0A4; Dal'70; BSc(UNB); AAFPhys; CCFP; FCFP; Staff, Upper River Valley Hospital - Waterville; (506)328-9391; Fax. (506)328-8501; damacel@health.nb.ca.

MACEOIN, Colin; The Hoy Clinic, 202-2155 10th Ave, Prince George BC V2M 5J6; (Other Foreign)'00; (250)564-9845

MACEWAN, Elspeth; Lanark County Mental Health, 2A-88 Cornelia St W, Smiths Falls ON K7A 5K9; Man'82; FRCPC; Psy. (613)283-2170; Fax. (613)283-9018.

MACEWAN, Gordon W; Peace Arch Hosp, 15521 Russell Ave, White Rock BC V4B 2R4; UBC'82; FRCPC; Psy. Staff, Peace Arch Hospital; Clin Instructor, University of British Columbia; (604)541-7171; Fax. (604)538-8500.

MACEWAN, Robert N; Cross Cancer Institute, 1135-11560 University Ave NW, Edmonton AB T6G 1Z2; Sask'97; FRCPC; DiagRad; NuclearMed. Staff Oncologic Imaging, Cross Cancer Institute; (780)432-8643; Fax. (780)432-8483.

MACEWEN, Melissa D; Beamsville Med Centre, PO Box 430 4279 Hixon St, Beamsville ON L0R 1B0; McM'07; CCFP; (905)563-5315; Fax. (905)563-0933.

MACFADDEN, Douglas K; 79 Doncaster Ave, Toronto ON M4C 5S6; McG'79; PhD; FRCPC; IntMed; ClinImmunol&Allergy. (416)686-1696; Fax. (416)686-1735; dkmacfadden@rogers.com.

MACFADDEN, Megan E; BC Women's Hosp & Health Ctre, 4500 Oak St, Vancouver BC V6H 3N1; UBC'05; Psy. Staff, BC Women's Hospital & Health Centre; (604)875-2345 x4844

MACFADYEN, Donald R; Chilliwack Allergy & Resp Clin, 201-45625 Hodgins Ave, Chilliwack BC V2P 1P2; UBC'77; BSc; FRCPC; IntMed (Cardiology). (604)792-4128; Fax. (604)795-4853.

MACFADYEN, John C; 216 Colborne St W, Orillia ON L3V 2Z6; Wes'87; FRCPC; IntMed (Cardiology). Chief Med, Orillia Soldiers' Memorial Hospital; (705)325-1120; Fax. (705)325-1185.

MACFARLANE, Amy E; Fall River Family Practice, PO Box 2160 Rpo Fall River 3060 Highway 2, Fall River NS B2T 1K6; UBC'04; CCFP; (902)576-3332; Fax. (902)576-3311.

MACFARLANE, J Grant; 243 Hurontario St, Collingwood ON L9Y 2M1; McM'83; FRCPC; IntMed. Ac Staff, Collingwood General & Marine Hospital; (705)444-0700

MACFARLANE, Robyn J; Queen Elizabeth II HSC, 458-1276 South Park St, Halifax NS B3H 2Y9; Dal'05; FRCPC; IntMed; MedOncol. Staff, Queen Elizabeth II Health Sciences Centre - Victoria General Site; (902)473-3748

MACFARLANE, Sonia T; St Mary's Hosp Centre, 4114-3830 av Lacombe, Montreal QC H3T 1M5; McG'05; ObstGyn. Staff, St Mary's Hospital Centre; (514)345-3511 x3050

MACGEACHY, Fiona J; 202-3400 rue Du Marche, Dollard-D-Ormeaux QC H9B 2Y1; Edinburgh (Scotland)'76; MB ChB; BMedSci; (514)683-0414; Fax. (514)683-5528.

MACGILLIS, Diane R; Kingston Laser & Cosmetic Clin, 1-863 Norwest Rd, Kingston ON K7P 2N2; Qns'84; Staff, Brockville General Hospital - Charles Street; (613)531-5200

MACGILLIS, Murray J; Brockville Gen Hosp, 75 Charles St, Brockville ON K6V 1S8; Qns'79; FRCPC; Anes (Chronic Pain). Staff, Brockville General Hospital - Charles Street; (613)345-5645

MACGILLIVRAY, B Jean; St Martha's Doctor's Offices, 169-23 Bay St, Antigonish NS B2G 2G7; Dal'95; FRCSC; GenSurg. Staff, St Martha's Regional Hospital; (902)863-3542

MACGILLIVRAY, Patrick S; 7 St Francis Memorial Dr PO Box 129, Barrys Bay ON K0J 1B0; Ott'07; CCFP; (613)756-3044

MACGILLIVRAY, William; 74 King St, Miramichi NB E1N 2N6; Dal'74; (506)773-3114; Fax. (506)773-0111; william.macgillivray@mbsradio.com.

MACGOUGAN, Cameron K; Royal Alexandra Hosp, 541-10240 Kingsway NW, Edmonton AB T5H 3V9; Qns'01; FRCPC; EmergMed. Staff, Royal Alexandra Hospital; (780)735-4449; Fax. (780)735-4916.

MACGOUGAN, Donald D; Northland Professional Bldg, 306-4600 Crowchild Trail NW, Calgary AB T3A 2L6; Cal'79; FRCPC; Psy (Community Psychiatry). (403)286-2499; Fax. (403)286-8499.

MACGOWAN, Nori A; Vancouver Home Hospice, 300-999 Boradway W, Vancouver BC V5Z 1K5; UBC'04; (604)742-4010

MACGREGOR, Daune L; The Hosp For Sick Children, 6517-555 University Ave, Toronto ON M5G 1X8; Sask'71; DCH; FAAP; FAAN; FRCPC; Peds (Acquired Brain Injury); Neur. Ac Staff, The Hospital For Sick Children; Ac Staff, Women's College Hospital; Prof Peds, University of Toronto; (416)813-7721; Fax. (416)813-6334; daune.macgregor@sickkids.ca.

MACGREGOR, Donald G; 203-300 Brae Rd, Duncan BC V9L 3T8; Alb'73; DAB; FRCSC; Ophth. Staff, Cowichan District Hospital; Staff, Lady Minto Gulf Islands Hospital; (250)748-2922; Fax. (250)748-9647; dgmacgregor@shaw.ca.

MACGREGOR, Janice M; Hydrostone Med Centre, 5521 Duffus St, Halifax NS B3K 2M5; Dal'89; (902)482-2683

MACGREGOR, John H M; Foothills Med Centre, 1403 29 St NW, Calgary AB T2N 2T9; Dal'80; FRCPC; DiagRad. Staff Diag Imaging, Foothills Medical Centre; (403)944-1969

MACGREGOR, Katherine E; Sheddon Avenue Med Assoc, 308-331 Sheddon Ave, Oakville ON L6J 1X8; Tor'96; BSc; CCFP; FCFP; (905)845-8771; Fax. (905)845-8379.

MACGREGOR, Lynne S; The Ottawa Hosp-Rehab Ctr, 505 Smyth Rd, Ottawa ON K1H 8M2; McM'85; FRCPC; PhysMed&Rehab (Spinal Cord Injury). Consultant/Staff Physical Med & Rehab, The Ottawa Hospital Rehabilitation Centre; Consultant Sports Med Clinic, University of Ottawa; Langs: English; French; (613)737-7350 x75591; Fax. (613)737-9638.

MACGREGOR, Marguerite A; PO Box 34149 Rpo Kingsway Mall, Edmonton AB T5G 3G4; Alb'63; (780)452-8677; Fax. (780)482-5278.

MACGREGOR, Stephen A; 395 Greenbrook Dr, Kitchener ON N2M 4K1; Tor'87; Ac Staff, St Mary's General Hospital; Ac Staff, Grand River Hospital - Kitchener/Waterloo Health Centre; (519)578-5710; Fax. (519)578-6419.

MACGREGOR, Suilven R; Coleman Med Clinic, 186 Kenneth St, Duncan BC V9L 1N4; UBC'96; CCFP; (250)746-4102; Fax. (250)746-5960.

MACGREGOR, Todd M; 502-345 Lakeshore Rd E, Oakville ON L6J 1J5; Tor'96; BSc; MSc; FRCPC; Peds. Assoc Staff Peds, Halton Healthcare Services Corporation - Oakville Site; Clinical Asst Prof, McMaster University; (905)338-2311

MACGREGOR, William G; Thunder Bay Reg HSC-T-Bay, 980 Oliver Rd, Thunder Bay ON P7B 6V4; Dal'93; CCFP; CCFP(E.M.); Staff, Thunder Bay Regional Health Sciences Centre; Prog Dir Emergency Med, Northern Ontario School of Medicine; (807)684-7000

MACHADO, John; Clinique Med Le Plein Ciel, 475 boul de la Cote-Vertu, Saint-Laurent QC H4L 1X7; McG'04; CCFP; (514)337-3171

MACHADO CONTRERAS, A Ricardo; Groupe Sante Physimed, 6363 rte Transcanadienne, Saint-Laurent QC H4T 1Z9; Havana (Cuba)'93; CCFP; (514)747-8888

MACHAMER, Mary E; Taddle Creek Connection, B102-726 Bloor St W, Toronto ON M6G 4A1; Tor'87; MSc; AAFPhys; BA; Langs: French; (416)964-0800; Fax. (416)964-2935.

MACHAN, Lindsay S; UBC Hospital, 2211 Wesbrook Mall, Vancouver BC V6T 2B5; Alb'79; FRCPC; DiagRad. Staff, UBC Hospital - Koerner Pavillion; (604)822-7077; Fax. (604)822-9701.

MACHAT, Jeffrey J J; Ocular Esthetics, 202-1200 Bay St, Toronto ON M5R 2A5; Tor'86; FRCSC; Ophth (Excimer Laser Refractive Eye Surgery). (416)628-5778; Fax. (416)628-5779.

MACHEL, Teresa M; 208 King St PO Box 2407, Windsor NS B0N 2T0; Warsaw (Poland)'68; FRCPC; IntMed (Cardiology). Staff, Hants Community Hospital; Langs: Polish; (902)798-8544; Fax. (902)798-1028.

MACHEL, Wieslaw J; 208 King St PO Box 2407, Windsor NS B0N 2T0; Warsaw (Poland)'67; Court Staff, Hants Community Hospital; Langs: Polish; (902)798-0363; Fax. (902)798-1028.

MACHER, Ted W; Chatham-Kent Hlth Alliance, PO Box 2030 80 Grand Ave W, Chatham ON N7M 5L9; Tor'10; CCFP; Staff, Chatham-Kent Health Alliance; (519)437-6050

MACHIDA, Helen M; Alberta Children's Hosp, 2888 Shaganappi Trail NW, Calgary AB T3B 6A8; Cal'80; BGS; Dip Occupational Therapy; FRCPC; Peds (Pediatric Gastroenterology). Ac Staff, Alberta Children's Hospital; Clin Assoc Prof Peds, University of Calgary; (403)955-3071; Fax. (403)955-7321.

MACHIN, Jack F; Clinique Med Lac Megantic, 102-5256 rue Frontenac, Lac-Megantic QC G6B 1H3; Louvain (Belgium)'83; Langs: German; Bilingual(English/French); (819)583-0109; Fax. (819)583-1456; jackmachin@axion.ca.

MACIE, Christine M G; 209-725 Coronation Blvd, Cambridge ON N1R 7S9; Ott'99; FRCPC; IntMed; Critical Care Medicine; Respir. Staff, Cambridge Memorial Hospital; (519)623-2366

MACIEJEWSKI, Conrad C; Hys Med Centre, 400-11010 101 St NW, Edmonton AB T5H 4B9; Alb'07; Staff, University of Alberta Hospital; (780)401-0424

MACIEL, Estanislao; Prince Albert Med Clinic, 681 15th St W, Prince Albert SK S6V 7H9; (Mexico)'69; Chief Urol, Victoria Hospital; (306)764-6244

MACIEL-MIRANDA, Jesus A; Queen Elizabeth II HSC-Halifax, 4443-1796 Summer St, Halifax NS B3H 3A7; (Mexico)'04; Staff Plastic & Reconstructive Surg, Queen Elizabeth II Health Sciences Centre - Halifax Infirmary Site; (902)473-7054

MACINNES, Aaron I; Pain Management Clinic, 9750 140 St, Surrey BC V3T 0G9; UBC'05; FRCPC; Anes. (604)582-4587

MACINNES, Alison M; Fairmont Med Bldg, 414-750 Broadway W, Vancouver BC V5Z 1H3; UBC'97; CCFP; FCFP; (604)675-9433; Fax. (604)675-9434.

MACINNIS, Benjamin F; PO Box 74630 Rpo Kitsilano, Vancouver BC V6K 4P4; Qns'05; CCFP.

MACINNIS, Brent J; Centrepointe Med Centre, 202-1 Centrepointe Dr, Nepean ON K2G 6E2; Ott'77; FRCSC; Ophth. Staff, The Ottawa Hospital - Riverside Campus; Staff, The Ottawa Hospital - Civic Campus; Staff, Children's Hospital of Eastern Ontario (CHEO); University of Ottawa.

MACINNIS, Maude D; Antigonish Mall, 133 Church St, Antigonish NS B2G 2E3; Dal'08; CCFP; (902)863-0848

MACINTOSH, Bernard H W; Bartown Medical, 176 Commercial St, North Sydney NS B2A 1B4; (Ireland)'07; BSc; MB BS; BAO; CCFP; (902)794-3494; Fax. (902)794-3702.

MACINTOSH, Donald G; Queen Elizabeth II HSC, 915-1276 South Park St, Halifax NS B3H 2Y9; Mem'83; MSc; ABIM(IntMed); ABIM(Gastroent); FRCPC; IntMed; Gastroent. Ac Staff Div of Gastroent, Queen Elizabeth II Health Sciences Centre - Victoria General Site; Prof Gastroent, Dalhousie University; (902)473-3721; Fax. (902)473-4406.

MACINTOSH, Donald S L; Sault Area Hosp, 750 Great Northern Rd, Sault Ste. Marie ON P6B 0A8; Dal'97; CCFP; CCFP(E.M.); FCFP; Staff EmergMed, Sault Area Hospital - Sault Ste Marie; (705)759-3434

MACINTOSH, Ethel L; Health Sciences Centre, GF419-820 Sherbrook St, Winnipeg MB R3A 1R9; Man'86; FRCSC; GenSurg (Surgical Oncology). Assoc Staff, Health Sciences Centre; Assoc Staff, St Boniface General Hospital; Asst Prof, University of Manitoba; (204)787-2945; Fax. (204)787-4063; ethel.macintosh@cancercare.mb.ca.

MACINTOSH, F Douglas; The Peterborough Clinic, 26 Hospital Dr, Peterborough ON K9J 7C3; Tor'73; BSc; CCFP; (705)743-2040

MACINTOSH, Jocelyn M; Medical Bldg, 801-805 Broadway W, Vancouver BC V5Z 1K1; Qns'83; FRCSC; Ophth. (604)873-3909; Fax. (604)873-3974.

MACINTOSH, Lachlan M; 203-9123 Mary St, Chilliwack BC V2P 4H7; Glasgow (Scotland)'72; MB ChB; MRCGPract; CCFP; FCFP; Ac Staff, Chilliwack General Hospital; (604)795-9161

MACINTOSH, Rebecca F; Dept of Lab Medicine, 5788 University Ave, Halifax NS B3H 1V8; Dal'82; FRCPC; AnatPath. Staff, South Shore Regional Hospital; Staff Path & LaMed, Queen Elizabeth II Health Sciences Centre - Victoria General Site; (902)473-4334

MACINTOSH, Daniel W; Murrayville Family Practice, 204-22112 52 Ave, Langley BC V2Y 2M6; UBC'83; Staff, Langley Memorial Hospital; (604)533-1140; Fax. (604)533-1159.

MACINTYRE, D Joanne; Health Sciences Centre, 300 Prince Philip Dr, St. John's NL A1B 3V6; Mem'91; Clin Associate Hematol Oncol, Health Sciences Centre; Memorial University Of Newfoundland; (709)777-7288

MACINTYRE, Douglas W; 20865 Dalton Rd PO Box 40, Sutton West ON L0E 1R0; Tor'86; BSc; Ac Staff, Southlake Regional Health Centre; (905)722-4126; Fax. (905)722-4449.

MACINTYRE, Erika J; The Ottawa Hosp-Gen Campus, 1201-501 Smyth Rd, Ottawa ON K1H 8L6; Sask'08; IntMed. Staff, The Ottawa Hospital - General Campus; (613)737-8899

MACINTYRE, Janet K; Queen Elizabeth II HSC-Halifax, 355-1796 Summer St, Halifax NS B3H 3A7; Dal'00; FRCPC; EmergMed. Staff, Queen Elizabeth II Health Sciences Centre - Halifax Infirmary Site; (902)473-8769; Fax. (902)473-3617.

MACINTYRE, John D; Brant Community HC-Brantford, 200 Terrace Hill St, Brantford ON N3R 1G9; Tor'75; Staff, The Brant Community Healthcare System - Brantford General Hospital Site; Staff, The Brant Community Healthcare System - Willett Hospital Site; (519)752-7871; jemacint@rogers.com.

MACINTYRE, Lisa A; Fall River Fam Practice Assoc, PO Box 2160 3060 Highway 2, Fall River NS B2T 1K6; Dal'92; (902)861-2237

MACINTYRE, M Arlene; PO Box 1450, Brighton ON K0K 1H0; McM'79; CCFP; FCFP; (613)475-0600; Fax. (613)475-1940; themaple@maine.rr.com.

MACINTYRE, Margaret A; 201-556 Josephine St, Nelson BC V1L 1W6; McM'88; CCFP; FCFP; Ac Staff, Kootenay Lake General Hospital; (250)352-1867; Fax. (250)352-1859.

MACISAAC, Jennifer L; 601-333 Preston St, Ottawa ON K1S 5N4; Tor'06; CCFP; (613)235-8079

MACISAAC, Michael G; Stratford Gen Hosp, 46 General Hospital Dr, Stratford ON N5A 2Y6; Dal'94; CCFP; CCFP(E.M.); Staff Emerg, Stratford General Hospital - Huron Perth Healthcare Alliance; (519)272-8210

MACIVER, Allison H; University of Alberta Hosp, 8440 112 St NW, Edmonton AB T6G 2B7; Wes'07; Staff, University of Alberta Hospital; (780)407-8822

MACIVER, Angus G; Dr Angus G Maciver in Trust, 589 West Gore St, Stratford ON N5A 1L4; Wes'73; FACS; FRCSC; GenSurg (Endoscopy). Ac Staff, Stratford General Hospital - Huron Perth Healthcare Alliance; Consultant, St Marys Memorial Hospital - Huron Perth Healthcare Alliance; Consultant, Seaforth Community Hospital - Huron Perth Healthcare Alliance; (519)273-4100; Fax. (519)273-3208; amaciver@rogers.com.

MACIVER, Douglas W; Solace Med Clinic, 36 St Thomas St, St. Albert AB T8N 7J6; Alb'91; BSc; CCFP; Ad Staff Privil, Sturgeon Community Hospital; (780)419-3627; Fax. (780)419-3565.

MACIVER, Shaunalee J; Solace Med Clinic, 36 St Thomas St, St. Albert AB T8N 7J6; Alb'91; (780)419-3627; Fax. (780)419-3565.

MACIVER, Suzanne A; 2032 Kingsway, Vancouver BC V5N 2T3; Glasgow (United Kingdom)'88; CCFP; (604)874-5555

MACK, Benjamin J; Surrey Mem Hosp, 13750 96 Ave, Surrey BC V3V 1Z2; Alb'98; FRCPC; IntMed; MedMicrobiol; InfectDis. Staff, Surrey Memorial Hospital; (604)585-5666

MACK, David R; Children's Hosp Eastern Ont, 401 Smyth Rd, Ottawa ON K1H 8L1; Tor'83; FRCPC; Peds (Gastroenterology). Staff, Children's Hospital of Eastern Ontario (CHEO); Prof Peds, University of Ottawa; (613)737-7600 x2516; Fax. (613)738-4854.

MACK, Douglas P; North Burlington Med Centre, 18-1960 Appleby Line, Burlington ON L7L 0B7; Wes'04; FRCPC; Peds; ClinImmunol&Allergy. (905)319-2000

MACK, Lloyd A; Tom Baker Cancer Centre, 1331 29 St NW, Calgary AB T2N 4N2; Wes'97; FRCSC; GenSurg; General Surgical Oncology. Staff, Foothills Medical Centre; Staff, Tom Baker Cancer Centre; (403)521-3169; Fax. (403)944-3926.

MACK, Martin D; Health Sciences Centre, 300 Prince Philip Dr, St. John's NL A1B 3V6; Dal'87; CCFP; CCFP(E.M.); Staff, Health Sciences Centre; (709)777-6300

MACK, Peter H; London HSC-University Hosp, PO Box 5339 Stn B 339 Windermere Rd, London ON N6A 5A5; Wes'04; FRCPC; Anes. Staff, London Health Sciences Centre - University Hospital; (519)685-8500

MACK, Tyson L; Associated Radiologists, 300-140 Wall St, Saskatoon SK S7K 1N4; Sask'94; LMCC; FRCPC; DiagRad. Staff, Royal University Hospital; (306)244-1167

MACKALSKI, Barbara A M; The Brandon Clinic, 620 Dennis St, Brandon MB R7A 5E7; Man'88; BSc; ABIM; FRCPC; IntMed; Gastroent. (204)728-4440; Fax. (204)726-1765.

MACKAY, Alison R; Professional Corp, 931 19 St S, Lethbridge AB T1J 3H5; Dal'03; FRCPC; IntMed; Endocrin&Metab. (403)328-0693

MACKAY, Alward M; Queen Elizabeth Hosp, PO Box 6600 Stn Central, Charlottetown PE C1A 8T5; Dal'64; FRCPC; DiagRad. Ac Staff, Queen Elizabeth Hospital; (902)894-2111; Fax. (902)894-2146.

MACKAY, Charles; Clinique de l'Alternative, 2034 rue Saint-Hubert, Montreal QC H2L 3Z5; Mon'72; (514)281-9848

MACKAY, Elizabeth A; Peter Lougheed Centre, 3500 26 Ave NE, Calgary AB T1Y 6J4; Dal'91; MPH; FRCPC; IntMed. Chief Med Teaching Unit, Peter Lougheed Centre; Asst Prof, University of Calgary; (403)943-5526; Fax. (403)943-4908; elizabeth.mackay@calgaryhealthregion.ca.

MACKAY, F Charles; CSSS du Lac-des-Deux-Montagnes, 520 boul Arthur-Sauve, Saint-Eustache QC J7R 5B1; McG'81; Staff, Hôpital de Saint-Eustache; (450)473-6811

MACKAY, Faye D; 319 15 Ave N PO Box 969, Creston BC V0B 1G0; Alb'83; BSc; CCFP; Dir Diabetes Teaching Centre, Creston Valley Hospital & Health Centre; Associate Clinical Faculty, University of British Columbia; (250)428-8873; Fax. (250)428-3346.

MACKAY, Helen; Univ Hlth Network-Princess M, 221A-610 University Ave, Toronto ON M5G 2M9; Edinburgh (Scotland)'90; Staff, Princess Margaret Hospital - University Health Network; (416)946-2253

MACKAY, Ian E; St Joseph Island Med Clinic, 1186 Richards St, Richards Landing ON P0R 1J0; Dal'04; CCFP; (705)246-2477

MACKAY, Lee D M; The Medical Assoc Clinic, 806 Vernon St, Nelson BC V1L 4G5; UBC'08; CCFP; Staff, Kootenay Lake General Hospital; (250)352-6611

MACKAY, M Jane; 2712 Ashridge Pl, Oakville ON L6J 7K3; Tor'91; BSc; PhD; CCFP; (905)829-9908; Fax. (905)829-9464.

MACKAY, Maralyn J; Selkirk Med Centre, 353 Eveline St, Selkirk MB R1A 1N1; Sask'66; FRCPC; Psy. Asst Prof, University of Manitoba; Fax. (204)942-5027; mjmackay@mb.sympatico.ca.

MACKAY, Michael J; Legacy Sport Med Clinic, 14-160 Meadowood Dr, Winnipeg MB R2M 5L6; Mem'85; Dip SportMed; Corp Physician, Manitoba Hydro; Staff, Institute of Sports Medicine; Teach Staff, University of Manitoba; (204)667-1550

MACKAY, R Fraser; Segue Clinic, 61 James St, St Catharines ON L2R 5B9; McM'79; FACEP; MCFP(EM); Staff, Niagara Health System - Ontario Street Site; Partner, AccessMD Inc; (905)688-1827

MACKAY, Rebecca E; Saskatoon Cancer Centre, 20 Campus Dr, Saskatoon SK S7N 4H4; Sask'06; Hem; IntMed. (306)655-0655; Fax. (306)655-2278.

MACKAY, Rory C; Royal Columbian Hosp, 330 Columbia St E, New Westminster BC V3L 3W7; UBC'95; Staff Emerg, Eagle Ridge Hospital & Health Care Centre; Staff, Royal Columbian Hospital; (604)520-4219

MACKAY, Rose; Glace Bay Healthcare Complex, 300 South St, Glace Bay NS B1A 1W5; Dal'01; CCFP; Staff, Glace Bay Healthcare Facility; (902)849-5511

MACKAY, Thomas J; Queen Elizabeth II HSC-Halifax, 3705-1796 Summer St, Halifax NS B3H 3A7; Wes'70; BSc; LLB; FRCPC; Psy (Forensic Psychiatry). Staff, Queen Elizabeth II Health Sciences Centre - Halifax Infirmary Site; Asst Prof School of Med, Dalhousie University; Langs: English; French; (902)473-3104; tom.mackay@cdha.nshealth.ca.

MACKEAN, Gerald L; Queen Elizabeth II HSC-Halifax, 4719-1796 Summer St, Halifax NS B3H 3A7; Dal'76; FRCSC; GenSurg; VascSurg. Ac Staff, Queen Elizabeth II Health Sciences Centre - Halifax Infirmary Site; Dalhousie University; (902)473-8506; Fax. (902)473-8507.

MACKEAN, Lynne C; 113-662 Goldstream Ave, Victoria BC V9B 0N8; Cal'89; BSc(PT); CASM; FRCPC; PhysMed&Rehab (Sports Medicine). Consultant Privil, Vancouver Island Health Authority; Clinical Asst Prof Med, University of British Columbia; (250)478-2002; Fax. (250)478-3005.

MACKEAN, Peter R; Kensington Family Med Centre, PO Box 160, Kensington PE C0B 1M0; Dal'81; BSc(McG); CCFP; FCFP; Chief Medical Staff, Prince County Hospital; Teach Staff, Dalhousie University; (902)836-4470; Fax. (902)836-3758.

MACKENZIE, Alexander E; Children's Hosp Eastern Ont, 401 Smyth Rd, Ottawa ON K1H 8L1; Tor'83; Peds. Staff, Children's Hospital of Eastern Ontario (CHEO); Prof, University of Ottawa; (613)737-2772; Fax. (613)738-4833; mackenzie@cheo.on.ca.

MACKENZIE, Andrew J; 506 Seventh Ave, New Westminster BC V3L 1W9; Birmingham (England)'66; MB ChB; DTMH; Court Staff, Royal Columbian Hospital; (604)526-7871

MACKENZIE, Ross B; Ross MacKenzie Consulting, 2261 Constance Dr, Oakville ON L6J 5L8; Dal'66; FACC; FRCPC; IntMed (Cardiology). (905)338-3024

MACKENZIE, Brian M; Peterbrough Clinic, 327 Charlotte St, Peterborough ON K9J 0B2; Wes'82; FRCPC; IntMed; Cardiol. Staff, Peterborough Regional Health Centre - Hospital Drive; (705)775-6869

MACKENZIE, D Scott; 90 West St, Corner Brook NL A2H 2Z3; Alb'80; FACS; FRCSC; GenSurg. Ac Staff, Western Memorial Regional Hospital; Staff, Labrador Health Centre; Memorial University Of Newfoundland; (709)634-1005

MACKENZIE, David E; 199 Grafton St, Charlottetown PE C1A 1L2; Dal'85; BSc; Dip SportMed; (902)629-8841; Fax. (902)626-3489.

MACKENZIE, David P; 1477 Jasmine Cres, Oakville ON L6H 3H2; McM'75; DOHS; CCBOM; Mgr Pharmacy, Procter & Gamble Co.; Physician Occupational Health Clinic, McMaster University; (905)842-4143

MACKENZIE, Ewen J; 128 Ontario St, Kingston ON K7L 2Y4; Wes'78; (613)544-9121; Fax. (613)544-9793; emackenzie1@cogeco.ca.

MACKENZIE, G Scott; Physician Anes Services, 303-400 Tache Ave, Winnipeg MB R2H 3C3; Man'83; FRCPC; Anes. (204)233-3413; Fax. (204)233-9763.

MACKENZIE, Ian M; Port Alice Health Centre, 1090 Marine Dr, Port Alice BC V0N 2N0; Cal'02; CCFP; (250)284-3555

MACKENZIE, Ian R A; Vancouver Gen Hosp, 855 12th Ave W, Vancouver BC V5Z 1M9; Wes'84; FRCPC; NeurPath. Staff NeuroPath, Vancouver General Hospital - Centennial Pavillion; Prof, University of British Columbia; (604)875-4111 x61415

MACKENZIE, J Stephen; Royal Jubilee Hosp, 1952 Bay St, Victoria BC V8R 1J8; UBC'96; CCFP; Staff, Royal Jubilee Hospital; (250)370-0520

MACKENZIE, James C; PO Box 1231, Mackenzie BC V0J 2C0; Dal'08; CCFP.

MACKENZIE, James R; Gulf Canada Square, 335-401 9 Ave SW, Calgary AB T2P 3C5; Alb'85; FRCSC; OrthSurg (Adult Hip & Knee Reconstruction). Clin Lecturer, University of Calgary; (403)221-4361; Fax. (403)221-4387.

MACKENZIE, Jennifer J; Kingston Gen Hosp, 4-76 Stuart St, Kingston ON K7L 2V7; Tor'88; FRCPC; Peds; MedGenetics. Staff, Kingston General Hospital; Staff Privil, Hotel-Dieu Hospital; Asst Prof, Queen's University; (613)548-2467

MACKENZIE, Jonathan A; 100-6501 Campeau Dr, Kanata ON K2K 3E9; McM'81; Med Dir, Forest Hill Nursing Home; (613)591-6588

MACKENZIE, Kent S; MUHC-Royal Victoria Hosp, S10 18-687 av des Pins O, Montreal QC H3A 1A1; McG'93; FRCSC; GenSurg; VascSurg. Staff, McGill University Health Centre - Royal Victoria Hospital; (514)843-1524; Fax. (514)843-1730; kent.mackenzie@muhc.mcgill.ca.

MACKENZIE, Liliana; Westmount Med Bldg, 77 Westmount Rd, Guelph ON N1H 5J1; (Colombia)'02.

MACKENZIE, Louisa K; 3-271 Ingram St, Duncan BC V9L 1P3; UBC'01; FRCPC; Peds; InfectDis. (250)597-0366

MACKENZIE, Mark A; Royal Alexandra Hosp, 10240 Kingsway NW, Edmonton AB T5H 3V9; McM'98; CCFP; CCFP(E.M.); Staff Emerg, Royal Alexandra Hospital; (780)735-7443; Fax. (780)735-4916; markmackenzie@shaw.ca.

MACKENZIE, Mark S; 9146 Mary St, Chilliwack BC V2P 4J1; Mem'89; CCFP; CCFP(E.M.); (604)792-5966; Fax. (604)792-5961.

MACKENZIE, Mary J F; London Reg Cancer Centre, 790 Commissioners Rd E, London ON N6A 4L6; Dal'94; FRCPC; IntMed; MedOncol. (905)685-8640

MACKENZIE, Megan S; 9146 Mary St, Chilliwack BC V2P 4J1; UBC'94; CCFP.

MACKENZIE, Meredith A; Queen's Health Counselling, 146 Stuart St, Kingston ON K7L 3N6; UBC'98; BSc; MD; CCFP; FCFP; Clin Associate Allergy & Immunol, Kingston General Hospital; Staff, Weeneebayko General Hospital; Clin Instructor Family Med, Queen's University; (613)533-6000

MACKENZIE, Michael A; Antigonish Mall, 133 Church St, Antigonish NS B2G 2E3; Dal'80; (902)863-2455; Fax. (902)867-6336.

MACKENZIE, Paul J; 108-575 16th Ave, West Vancouver BC V7V 4Y1; UBC'02; FRCSC; Ophth. Staff, Ophthalmology & Visual Sciences; (604)926-5722

MACKENZIE, Richard B; 305-1100 Sheppard Ave E, North York ON M2K 2W1; Tor'73; CCFP; FCFP; Ac Staff, North York General Hospital; University of Toronto; (416)223-4806; Fax. (416)223-0070; rmackenzie@ca.ibm.com.

MACKENZIE, Robert G; Toronto Sunnybrook Reg Cancer, 2075 Bayview Ave, Toronto ON M4N 3M5; McM'76; FRCPC; IntMed; RadOncol. Staff RadOncol, Sunnybrook Health Sciences Centre; Assoc Prof RadOncol, University of Toronto; (416)480-4974; Fax. (416)480-6002; bob.mackenzie@sunnybrook.ca.

MACKENZIE, Robert J; Cape Breton Healthcare Complex, 1482 George St, Sydney NS B1P 1P3; Dal'06; CCFP; Staff, Cape Breton Healthcare Complex; (902)567-8000

MACKENZIE, Robert L; Toronto East Gen Hosp Inc, 825 Coxwell Ave, Toronto ON M4C 3E7; Tor'69; FACS; FRCSC; GenSurg (Hepatobiliary & Pancreatic Disorders). Staff Surg, Toronto East General Hospital Inc; Asst Prof Surg, University of Toronto; (416)461-8710; Fax. (416)461-1332; rmack@tegh.on.ca.

MACKENZIE, Roberta C F; 204-855 Broadview Ave, Toronto ON M4K 3Z1; Qns'01; FRCSC; ObstGyn. (416)519-5967

MACKENZIE, Roderick M; Market Mall Prof Bldg, 104-4935 40 Ave NW, Calgary AB T3A 2N1; London (England)'66; MRCS; LRCP; MRCP; DCH; FRCPC; Peds. (403)247-1012; Fax. (403)247-1012.

MACKENZIE, Shelagh K; Children's Hosp, 840 Sherbrook St, Winnipeg MB R3A 1S1; Man'82; FRCPC; Peds (Emergency Medicine). (204)787-4244; Fax. (204)787-1775.

MACKENZIE, Susan E; Addiction & Mental Hlth-ARF, 33 Russell St, Toronto ON M5S 2S1; Wes'04; FRCPC; Psy. Staff, Centre for Addiction & Mental Health (CAMH) - Russell Street Site; (416)535-8501

MACKENZIE-FEDER, Jessica M; 4115-2775 Laurel St, Vancouver BC V5Z 1M9; McG'07; MDCM; Endocrin&Metab; IntMed. (604)875-4111

MACKESY, J T Derek; Active Health Sports Med Ctr, 102-115 Bell Farm Rd, Barrie ON L4M 5G1; Qns'73; Dip SportMed; MSc; (705)725-1050; Fax. (705)725-1496.

MACKETT, Robert L; Bayview Med Arts Bldg, 200A-145 Queenston St, St Catharines ON L2R 2Z9; Ott'80; ABIM(CardiovascDisease); ABIM(IntMed); FRCPC; IntMed (Adult Cardiology); Cardiol. Staff Med, Niagara Health System - Ontario Street Site; Med Dir Pacemaker Clinic, Niagara Health System - St Catharines General Site; (905)688-4804; Fax. (905)688-4808.

MACKEY, Ariane; Ctr Hosp Affilie-Enfant-Jesus, 1401 18e rue, Quebec QC G1J 1Z4; Laval'86; FRCPC; Neur (Neuro Vascular). Staff, Centre Hospitalier Affilié Universitaire de Québec - Hôpital De L'Enfant Jésus; Consultant, Hôpital Laval; Consultant, Centre Hospitalier Universitaire de Quebec-CHUL; (418)649-5892; Fax. (418)649-5896.

MACKEY, Denise A; University Hosp of Northern BC, 1475 Edmonton St, Prince George BC V2M 1S2; Ott'06; OrthSurg. Staff, University Hospital of Northern British Columbia; (250)564-9233

MACKEY, Duncan S; Chinook Reg Hosp, 960 19 St S, Lethbridge AB T1J 1W5; Alb'91; CCFP; CCFP(E.M.); FCFP; Staff EmergMed, Chinook Regional Hospital; Clin Assoc Prof, University of Alberta; (403)388-6111

MACKEY, Jennifer E; Medpoint Childrens Walk-in, 1240 Commissioners Rd W, London ON N6K 4H7; Ross U (Dominica)'01.

MACKEY, John R; Cross Cancer Institute, 11560 University Ave NW, Edmonton AB T6G 1Z2; Alb'90; FRCPC; FRCPC; MedOncol; IntMed. Staff, Cross Cancer Institute; Prof Oncology, University of Alberta; (780)432-8221

MACKEY, Paul V; The Medical Clinic, 10011 96 St, Fort St. John BC V1J 3P3; Melbourne (Australia)'89; MB BS; CCFP; FCFP; Staff/Site Dir Peace Liard Site, Fort St John Hospital & Health Centre; (250)785-6677; Fax. (250)787-0109.

MACKEY, Thomas D; 4319 Cove Rd PO Box 58, Portland ON K0G 1V0; Ott'70; (613)272-3302

MACKIE, Aaron P; Foothills Med Centre, 1403 29 St NW, Calgary AB T2N 2T9; Cal'05; FRCPC; Psy. Staff, Foothills Medical Centre; (403)919-8467

MACKIE, Andrew S; Stollery Children's Hosp, 4C2-8440 112 St NW, Edmonton AB T6G 2B7; Qns'93; FRCPC; Peds (Pediatric Cardiology); Cardiol. Staff, Stollery Children's Hospital; (780)407-3964; Fax. (780)407-3954.

MACKIE, Carl C; Arbour Med Centre, 281 Stone Rd E, Guelph ON N1G 5J5; Wes'74; CCFP; FCFP; Staff, Guelph General Hospital; (519)823-5133; Fax. (519)827-0255.

MACKIE, Christopher A O; Public Health Services, 4F-1 Hughson St N, Hamilton ON L8R 3L5; Man'03; FRCPC; CommunMed;CCFP; (905)546-2424

MACKIE, Gordon F; 302-7031 Westminster Hwy, Richmond BC V6X 1A3; UBC'86; FRCPC; Neur. (604)279-0077; Fax. (604)279-0026.

MACKIE, Iain D F; VGH Internal Med Clinic, 7F-2775 Laurel St, Vancouver BC V5Z 1M9; Tor'79; FRCPC; IntMed (HIV/AIDS Clinical Care). Staff, Vancouver General Hospital - Centennial Pavillion; Staff, Providence Health Care - St Paul's Hospital; Prof Med, University of British Columbia; (604)875-5181; Fax. (604)875-5906.

MACKIE, J William; The Doctors' Office, 101-777 Broadway W, Vancouver BC V5Z 4J7; UBC'76; FACSM; Dip SportMed; CCFP; FCFP; Clin Assoc Prof Med, University of British Columbia; Langs: French; (604)734-8252; Fax. (604)945-6096.

MACKIE, Susan J; Simon Fraser University, 8888 University Dr, Burnaby BC V5A 1S6; UBC'89; (778)782-4615

MACKILLOP, James H; Health Park, 208-45 Weatherbee Rd, Mira Road NS B1M 0A1; Dal'81; CCFP; FCFP; (902)539-8566; Fax. (902)567-0635.

MACKILLOP, William J; Cancer Care of Southeastern On, 25 King St W, Kingston ON K7L 5P9; Glasgow (Scotland)'75; FRCPC; RadOncol. Staff, Kingston General Hospital; Head Commun Health & Epidemiol, Queen's University; (613)544-2630; Fax. (613)544-9708; william.mackillop@krcc.on.ca.

MACKINLAY, Duncan C; 185 Mitton St N, Sarnia ON N7T 6H3; Man'85; FRCSC; OrthSurg (Knee Shoulder & Sports Injuries). Staff Surgical Prog & Staff, Bluewater Health - Mitton Site; Board Member, Ontario Orthopaedic Association; (519)332-8040; Fax. (519)337-0522.

MACKINNON, Brian J; Nashwaaksis Med Clinic, 475 Brookside Dr, Fredericton NB E3A 8V4; Dal'77; (506)458-1331; Fax. (506)458-1326.

MACKINNON, David J; St Michael's Hosp, 30 Bond St, Toronto ON M5B 1W8; Wes'98; CCFP; CCFP(E.M.); Staff EmergMed, St Michael's Hospital; (416)360-4000

MACKINNON, Frederick N; Grand River Hosp-KW Hlth Ctre, PO Box 9056 Stn C 835 King St, Kitchener ON N2G 1G3; Wes'84; FRCPC; Anes; Critical Care Medicine. Staff, Grand River Hospital - Kitchener/Waterloo Health Centre; (519)749-4300

MACKINNON, Heather A; Public Gardens Med Clinic, 200-5675 Spring Garden Rd, Halifax NS B3J 1H1; Dal'88; Staff, Canadian Forces Health Services Centre (Atlantic); (902)425-5440

MACKINNON, James A; 2372 Dunwin Dr, Mississauga ON L5L 1J9; McM'83; FRCPC; Peds (Neonatology). Staff, The Credit Valley Hospital; (905)607-1600; Fax. (905)607-1603.

MACKINNON, Jennifer A; Chatham-Kent Family Health Team, 207-20 Emma St, Chatham ON N7L 5K5; McM'09; CCFP; (519)354-2172; jmackinnon@ckha.on.ca.

MACKINNON, John A; Tom Baker Cancer Centre, 1331 29 St NW, Calgary AB T2N 4N2; Tor'84; BSc; FRCPC; RadOncol. Staff Rad Oncol, Tom Baker Cancer Centre; Staff, Foothills Medical Centre; Ass't Clin Prof Med, University of Calgary; (403)521-3230; Fax. (403)283-1651.

MACKINNON, Judith A W; Stonechurch Family Health Ctre, 1475 Upper Ottawa St, Hamilton ON L8W 3J6; McM'98; CCFP; (905)575-1300; Fax. (905)575-1539; mackinjw@mcmaster.ca.

MACKINNON, Kevin M; Dixon Med Centre, 210-531 Davis Dr, Newmarket ON L3Y 6P5; Wes'87; (905)830-5551; Fax. (905)830-5597.

MACKINNON, Laura E; Amherstview Med Centre, 18 Manitou Crt W, Amherstview ON K7N 1S3; Tor'92; CCFP; (613)389-1604; Fax. (613)384-7359.

MACKINNON, Martin G; Saint John Reg Hosp, PO Box 2100 Stn Main 400 Universitiy Ave, Saint John NB E2L 4L2; Dal'00; FRCPC; IntMed; Nephrol. Staff, Saint John Regional Hospital; (506)648-6000

MACKINNON, Michael A; Lasalle Community Health Care, 2125 Front Rd, Windsor ON N9J 2C1; Dal'62; Honeywell Inc; (519)734-1234; Fax. (519)734-8674.

MACKINNON, Peter M; Lakeshore Health Centre, 330 Notre Dame St, Belle River ON N0R 1A0; Wes'84; (519)728-0777

MACKINNON, Randy J; Parkdale Med Centre, 3-30 Linden Ave, Charlottetown PE C1A 5Y9; Dal'93; BSc; CCFP; FCFP; (902)566-1229; Fax. (902)628-6337.

MACKINNON, Sarah J; 5 Park St PO Box 1059, Sundridge ON P0A 1Z0; Tor'97; CCFP; FCFP; Langs: French; (705)384-1277; Fax. (705)384-1279.

MACKINNON, Stephen M; Grey Bruce HS-Southampton, PO Box 310 340 High St, Southampton ON N0H 2L0; Ott'10; CCFP; Staff, Grey Bruce Health Services - Southampton Site.

MACKINTOSH, Alasdair J; Apple Hills Med Centre, 1221 Bloor St, Mississauga ON L4Y 2N8; Alb'84; CCFP; FCFP; Staff, Trillium Health Centre - Mississauga; (905)625-1241; Fax. (905)625-9514.

MACKLE, William R; Guisachan Family Medicine, 105-2395 Gordon Dr, Kelowna BC V1W 3X7; Dublin (Ireland)'78; MB BCh; BAO; DCH; DObst; Associate Privileges, Kelowna General Hospital; Med Advisor, Sutherland Hills Rest Home; Med Dir, Spring Valley Care Centre; Clin Instructor, University of British Columbia; Langs: Gaelic; (250)860-5888; Fax. (250)860-5880; docmackle@shaw.ca.

MACKLEM, Alan K; Portage Clinic Inc, 140 9th St SE, Portage La Prairie MB R1N 3V5; Man'75; CCFP; Staff, Portage District General Hospital; Lecturer Med, University of Manitoba; (204)857-3445; Fax. (204)239-1278; amacklem@shaw.ca.

MACKLEM, P Douglas; Campbellford Mem Hosp, PO Box 1027, Campbellford ON K0L 1L0; Cal'95; BSc; CCFP; CCFP(E.M.); Staff, Campbellford Memorial Hospital; (705)653-1140

MACKLER, Richard J; Seaforth Med Bldg, 230-3550 ch de la Cote-des-Nei, Montreal QC H3H 1V4; Columbia (USA)'67; FRCPC; IntMed (Diabetology); Endocrin (P.Q.). assoc Médecin, McGill University Health Centre - Montreal General Campus; assoc Prof, McGill University; Langs: French; German; Italian; (514)939-3751; Fax. (514)939-3752.

MACKLIN, G Elizabeth; Ottawa Children's Treatment, 395 Smyth Rd, Ottawa ON K1H 8L2; McM'87; MA; FRCPC; Peds (Developmental Pediatrics). (613)737-0871; Fax. (613)523-5167.

MACKNIGHT, Chris R; Camp Hill Veterans Memorial, 1308-5955 Veterans Memorial La, Halifax NS B3H 2E1; Dal'91; BSc; MSc; FRCPC; IntMed; GeriatricMed. Ac Staff, Queen Elizabeth II Health Sciences Centre - Victoria General Site; Asst Prof, Dalhousie University; (902)473-3888; Fax. (902)473-7133; chris.macknight@cdha.nshealth.ca.

MACKNIGHT, Roxanne E; Miramichi East Med Clinic, 4 Johnson Ave, Miramichi NB E1N 3B7; Tor'91; BPHE; CCFP; FCFP; (506)773-3333; Fax. (506)778-0035.

MACKOFF, Harley P; 260-8120 Cook Rd, Richmond BC V6Y 1T9; UBC'71; FRCSC; ObstGyn. Ac Staff, Richmond Hospital; (604)276-1666; Fax. (604)276-1655.

MACLACHLAN, A James; PO Box 520, Pictou NS B0K 1H0; Tor'68; Dip SportMed; Ac Staff, Aberdeen Regional Hospital; (902)485-5151; docmac@pchg.net.

MACLACHLAN, Diane; Glace Bay Healthcare Facility, 300 South St, Glace Bay NS B1A 1W5; Dublin (Ireland)'08; MB BCh; BAO; Staff, Glace Bay Healthcare Facility; (902)842-2820

MACLACHLAN, Donald A; 201-300 Veterans Blvd NE, Airdrie AB T4B 3P2; Cal'74; MCFP(EM); (403)948-4168

MACLACHLAN, Donna J; Youthdale Treatment Centre, 227 Victoria St, Toronto ON M5B 1T8; McM'94; FRCPC; Psy. (416)363-3751; Fax. (416)363-7945.

MACLACHLAN, Jean M; Inverness Consolid Mem Hosp, PO Box 610 39 James St, Inverness NS B0E 1N0; Dal'10; CCFP; Staff, Inverness Consolidated Memorial Hospital; (902)258-3210

MACLACHLAN, Richard A; Abbie J Lane Mem Bldg, 5909 Veterans Memorial Lane, Halifax NS B3H 2E2; Tor'74; CCFP; FCFP; Court Staff, IWK Health Centre; Ac Staff, Queen Elizabeth II Health Sciences Centre - Victoria General Site; Prof, Dalhousie University; (902)473-8042; Fax. (902)473-4760; richard.maclachlan@dal.ca.

MACLACHLAN, Shona M; 7803 119 St NW, Edmonton AB T6G 1W5; Alb'00; FRCPC; EmergMed. (780)238-4506; Fax. (780)482-6287; shona@ualberta.ca.

MACLAREN, Angela; Queen Elizabeth Hosp, PO Box 6600 Stn Central, Charlottetown PE C1A 8T5; Dal'09; CCFP; Staff, Queen Elizabeth Hospital; (902)894-2111

MACLAREN, Laura S; Kateri Memorial Hosp, CP 10, Kahnawake QC J0L 1B0; Alb'02; CCFP; CCFP(E.M.); Staff, Sir Mortimer B Davis Jewish General; Staff, Kateri Memorial Hospital Centre; Langs: Bilingual(English/French); (450)638-3930

MACLAREN, Susan I; Fiddlers Green Med Centre, 1065 Valetta St, London ON N6H 2Z9; Wes'83; BSc(Hon); (519)657-8118; Fax. (519)657-5547.

MACLAUGHLIN, Deirdre A; St Clare's Mercy Hosp, 154 Lemarchant Rd, St. John's NL A1C 5B8; Mem'79; FRCPC; Psy. Staff, St Clare's Mercy Hospital; (709)777-5278; Fax. (709)777-5490.

MACLE, Laurent; Institut de Cardiologie de Mtl, 5000 rue Belanger, Montreal QC H1T 1C8; Sher'93; FRCPC; IntMed (Electrophysiology); Cardiol. Staff, Institut de Cardiologie de Montréal; (514)376-3330

MACLEAN, A Vanessa M; Chinook Reg Hosp, 960 19 St S, Lethbridge AB T1J 1W5; Cal'85; Dip; CCFP; CCFP(E.M.); FCFP; Staff, Chinook Regional Hospital; (403)388-6135; Fax. (403)388-6708; rsvpb@telusplanet.net.

MACLEAN, Alan J; Seaforth Med Bldg, 640-3550 ch de la Cote-des-Nei, Montreal QC H3H 1V4; McG'70; ABIM; FRCPC; IntMed. adj Médecin, McGill University Health Centre - Montreal General Campus; McGill University; Langs: French; (514)931-3456; Fax. (514)931-7720.

MACLEAN, Anthony R; Foothills Med Centre, 1403 29 St NW, Calgary AB T2N 2T9; Dal'93; BSc; FACS; FRCSC; GenSurg (Colon & Rectal Surgery). Consultant Gen Surgeon, Foothills Medical Centre; Clin Assoc Prof Surg, University of Calgary; Langs: English; French; (403)944-2877; Fax. (403)944-1277; tony.maclean@calgaryhealthregion.ca.

MACLEAN, C Bernard; Inverness Med Clinic, PO Box 427, Inverness NS B0E 1N0; Dal'61; Staff, Inverness Consolidated Memorial Hospital; (902)258-2555; Fax. (902)258-2078.

MACLEAN, Catherine A; Health Sciences Centre, 300 Prince Philip Dr, St. John's NL A1B 3V6; Dal'85; BSc; MClSc; MBA; CCFP; FCFP; Staff, Health Sciences Centre; Chair of Clin Disciplines Family Med, Memorial University Of Newfoundland; (709)777-6300

MACLEAN, George W A; 220-1560 Yonge St, Toronto ON M4T 2S9; Sask'66; DPsy; CCST; FRCPC; Psy (Adult Psychiatry). Member, Canadian Psychoanalytic Society; Member, Toronto Psychoanalytic Society; Fellow, International Psychoanalytic Association; (416)929-9129; george.maclean@rogers.com.

MACLEAN, Glenda J; Southport, 110-10333 Southport Rd SW, Calgary AB T2W 3X6; Dal'04; CCFP; (403)403-2581

MACLEAN, Gregg L; 201-1 Magazine St, Saint John NB E2K 5S9; Dal'84; Neur. Assoc Staff Neurol, Saint John Regional Hospital; Consultant Neurol, St Joseph's Hospital; Pt-Time Lecturer, Dalhousie University; (506)634-0468; Fax. (506)632-6955; drgmaclean@nb.aibn.com.

MACLEAN, Gregor W; 201-810 East River Rd, New Glasgow NS B2H 3S3; Dal'86; BSc; Ac Staff Privil, Aberdeen Regional Hospital; (902)752-6266

MACLEAN, Heather J; The Ottawa Hosp-Gen Campus, 501 Smyth Rd, Ottawa ON K1H 8L6; Dal'95; BSc; FRCPC; Neur (Multiple Sclerosis). Staff Neurol, The Ottawa Hospital - General Campus; Asst Prof, University of Ottawa; (613)737-8532; Fax. (613)739-6631.

MACLEAN, Ian J; Chatham-Kent Hlth Alliance, PO Box 2030 Stn Main 80 Grand Ave W, Chatham ON N7M 5L9; Wes'76; Staff, Chatham-Kent Health Alliance; (519)352-6400

MACLEAN, James D C; Sterling Mall, 105-3 Sterling Rd, Glace Bay NS B1A 3X2; Dal'05; CCFP; (902)842-2130; Fax. (902)842-5309.

MACLEAN, James E W; 301-205 Dundas St E, Belleville ON K8N 5K6; Qns'81; (613)962-9511; Fax. (613)962-1722.

MACLEAN, James R L; West London Fam Health Clinic, 200-785 Wonderland Rd S, London ON N6K 1M6; Wes'80; (519)641-6712; Fax. (519)641-6189.

MACLEAN, Joanna E; Fraser Lake Health Centre, PO Box 98, Fraser Lake BC V0J 1S0; UBC'08; CCFP; (250)699-6225

MACLEAN, Joanna E; Edmonton Clinic Health Academy, 4 590-11405 87 Ave NW, Edmonton AB T6G 1C9; McM'00; FRCPC; Peds; Respir. Staff, University of Alberta Hospital; (780)248-5650; Fax. (780)248-5627.

MACLEAN, Jonathan A; Hamilton HS-McMaster Site, PO Box 2000 Stn Lcd 1 1200 Main St W, Hamilton ON L8N 3Z5; Dal'04; FRCSC; Otol (Head & Neck Surgery). Staff, Hamilton Health Sciences Centre - McMaster University Medical Centre; (905)521-2100

MACLEAN, Kenneth D; 621 Linden Ave PO Box 109, Kaleden BC V0H 1K0; Cal'85; BSc; MSc; Semi-Retired.

MACLEAN, Mary J; 524 Clarence St PO Box 880, Winchester ON K0C 2K0; McM'91; FRCPC; IntMed. Staff, Winchester District Memorial Hospital; (613)774-3452; Fax. (613)774-4321.

MACLEAN, Michele E; Kennetcook Med Centre, 6202 Highway 354, Kennetcook NS B0N 1P0; Dal'79; AAFP; CCFP; Langs: Spanish; (902)362-2021; Fax. (902)362-2186.

MACLEAN, Moira J; Hammonds Plains Fam Practice, 2120 Hammonds Plains Rd, Hammonds Plains NS B4B 1P3; Dal'96; CCFP; (902)832-9233

MACLEAN, Paul D; Middleton Med Clinic, PO Box 998, Middleton NS B0S 1P0; Dal'73; Staff, Soldiers Memorial Hospital; (902)825-2101; Fax. (902)825-6441.

MACLEAN, Rhonda A; Mayflower Med Clinic, 204-998 Parkland Dr, Halifax NS B3M 0A6; Dal'00; BSc; MSc; CCFP; (902)835-1628; Fax. (902)835-1151.

MACLEAN, Richard S; Nepean Med Centre, 404-1 Centrepointe Dr, Nepean ON K2G 6E2; McM'81; CCFP; (613)723-6690; Fax. (613)723-5697.

MACLEAN, Scott B A; Canadian Forces Base, PO Box 10500 Stn Forces, Edmonton AB T5J 4J5; Dal'10; CCFP; (780)973-4011

MACLEAN, Stephen W; VAC District Office, PO Box 8063 Rpo CSC 200-7105 Chebucto Rd, Halifax NS B3K 5L8; Dal'93; BSc(Hons); CCFP; FCFP; Staff Phys, Veterans Affairs Canada; Langs: English; French; (902)426-7992; stephen.maclean@vac-acc.gc.ca.

MACLEAN, Susan E; West London Fam Health Clinic, 200-785 Wonderland Rd S, London ON N6K 1M6; Wes'82; CCFP; FCFP; Med Advisor, Clindata Corporation; (519)641-6712; Fax. (519)641-6189; smaclean@uwo.ca.

MACLEAN, Tanya M; Barrie Med Clinics, 28-555 Essa Rd, Barrie ON L4N 6A9; Wes'97; CCFP; (705)792-5731; Fax. (705)792-5732.

MACLEAN-FRASER, Erin E; St Martha's Reg Hosp, 25 Bay St, Antigonish NS B2G 2G5; Dal'98; BSc; FRCSC; ObstGyn. Staff, St Martha's Regional Hospital; (902)863-1558; Fax. (902)863-4200.

MACLELLAN, Anne-Marie; College des Med du Quebec, 2170 boul Rene-Levesque O, Montreal QC H3H 2T8; McG'77; FRCPC; Peds. adj Sec/Dir Medical Education Division, College des Medecins du Quebec; Langs: French; Italian; (514)933-4441; Fax. (514)933-5167; amaclellan@cmq.org.

MACLELLAN, Dawn L; IWK Health Centre, PO Box 9700 Rpo Csc 5850-5980 University Ave, Halifax NS B3K 6R8; Dal'96; FRCSC; Urol (Pediatric Urology). Staff Urol, IWK Health Centre; Asst Prof, Dalhousie University; (902)470-8943; Fax. (902)470-8267; dawn.maclellan@iwk.nshealth.ca.

MACLELLAN, Keith A; Clinique Med de Shawville, CP 700 269 Main St, Shawville QC J0X 2Y0; McG'77; BSc; BA; Staff, Pontiac Hospital Centre; adj Prof Family Med, McGill University; Langs: Italian; (819)647-2924; Fax. (819)647-2845.

MACLELLAN, Rochelle; Queen Elizabeth II HSC, 1276 South Park St, Halifax NS B3H 2Y9; Dal'04; FRCPC; Anes. Staff, Queen Elizabeth II Health Sciences Centre - Victoria General Site; (902)473-7736

MACLELLAN, Steven J; Univ Hlth Network-Toronto Western Hosp, 8F-399 Bathurst St, Toronto ON M5T 2S8; Wes'06; GenSurg. Staff GenSurg, Toronto Western Hospital - University Health Network; (416)603-5224

MACLENNAN, Adam B; Muskoka Parry Sound Hlth Unit, 5 Pineridge Gate, Gravenhurst ON P1P 1Z3; Wes'06; CCFP; (705)687-2271

MACLENNAN, David J; Royal Columbian Hosp, 330 Columbia St E, New Westminster BC V3L 3W7; UBC'89; FRCPC; Anes. Staff, Royal Columbian Hospital; (604)520-4602; Fax. (604)520-4899.

MACLENNAN, Martin T; Dartmouth Gen Hosp, 325 Pleasant St, Dartmouth NS B2Y 4G8; Dal'96; CCFP; FCFP; Staff, Dartmouth General Hospital; (902)465-8300; Fax. (902)460-4142.

MACLENNAN, Virginia L; Ontario Shores Ctr Mental HS, 700 Gordon St, Whitby ON L1N 5S9; Tor'81; Staff, Ontario Shores Centre for Mental Health Sciences; (905)668-5881 x6321; maclennanv@ontarioshores.ca.

MACLEOD, A Cameron; Selkirk Med Group, PO Box 590, Revelstoke BC V0E 2S0; Qns'00; CCFP; (250)837-9321

MACLEOD, Alison D; 202-60 Aberdeen St, Kentville NS B4N 2N3; Wes'04; FRCPC; Peds.

MACLEOD, Andrew G; Montague Family Med Clinic, PO Box 877, Montague PE C0A 1R0; Dal'94; CCFP; (902)838-0830; Fax. (902)838-0834.

MACLEOD, Bruce A; Meadowood Med Centre, 1555 St Mary's Rd, Winnipeg MB R2M 5L9; Man'88; CCFP; FCFP; (204)256-4888; Fax. (204)254-0730; b.macleod@shaw.ca.

MACLEOD, Carol; Centre Med Chambly-Latour, B-5580 ch de Chambly, Saint-Hubert QC J3Y 3P5; Mon'84; (450)926-2236

MACLEOD, D Bruce; Foothills Med Centre, 1403 29 St NW, Calgary AB T2N 2T9; Cal'86; FRCPC; EmergMed. Staff EmergMed, Foothills Medical Centre; (403)944-1315; Fax. (403)944-2419.

MACLEOD, Eric C; 126 Hyland Dr, Sudbury ON P3E 1R6; Aberdeen (Scotland)'54; MB ChB; DPM; MRCPsy; FRCPC; Psy. Hon Staff, Health Sciences North-St Joseph's Health Centre; Member, Consent & Capacity Board; (705)674-0218

MACLEOD, G Stuart; 306-267 O'Connor St, Ottawa ON K2P 1V3; Qns'82; CCFP; FCFP; (613)521-7064; Fax. (613)233-0981.

MACLEOD, Heather C; Thunder Bay Reg HSC-T-Bay, 980 Oliver Rd, Thunder Bay ON P7B 6V4; Wes'07; GenSurg. Staff, Thunder Bay Regional Health Sciences Centre.

MACLEOD, Hugh M; Grand River Hosp-KW Hlth Ctre, PO Box 9056 Stn C 835 King St W, Kitchener ON N2G 1G3; UBC'94; CCFP; Staff, Cambridge Memorial Hospital; Staff EmergMed, Grand River Hospital - Kitchener/Waterloo Health Centre; (519)749-4300 x2631

MACLEOD, Jeanne Z; St Paul's Hosp, 1081 Burrard St, Vancouver BC V6Z 1Y6; UBC'96; CCFP; CCFP(E.M.); Staff, Providence Health Care - St Paul's Hospital; (604)682-2344

MACLEOD, John D; 940-790 Bay St PO Box 36, Toronto ON M5G 1N8; Dal'87; CCFP; FCFP; (416)926-0101

MACLEOD, John N; 203-300 Brae Road, Duncan BC V9L 3T8; Man'66; FRCSC; Ophth. Staff, Cowichan District Hospital; (250)748-2922; Fax. (250)733-2683; seaview9@telus.net.

MACLEOD, Kim S; 476 Dundas St W, Belleville ON K8P 1B7; Dal'89; CCFP; FCFP; (613)967-5852; Fax. (613)967-9981.

MACLEOD, Malcolm K; 1F-111 Huron St, Woodstock ON N4S 6Z6; McG'80; BSc; FACS; MS; FRCSC; GenSurg. Chief Medical Staff, Woodstock General Hospital; (519)539-4866; Fax. (519)539-4867.

MACLEOD, Mark D; London HSC-Victoria Hosp, PO Box 5010 Stn B E4 002-800 Commissioners Rd E, London ON N6A 5W9; Wes'88; FRCSC; OrthSurg (Orthopedic Trauma). Staff, London Health Sciences Centre - Victoria Campus; (519)685-8500 x53059; Fax. (519)685-8059.

MACLEOD, Michael D; 203-3040 Tutt St, Kelowna BC V1Y 2H5; Alb'84; FRCSC; GenSurg. (250)763-2226; Fax. (250)861-5937.

MACLEOD, N Wayne; Rockingham Ridge Plaza, 30 Farnham Gate Rd, Halifax NS B3M 3W8; Dal'98; CCFP; Att Physician Family Med, Queen Elizabeth II Health Sciences Centre - Victoria General Site; Langs: English; French; (902)443-8388; Fax. (902)443-9887.

MACLEOD, Neil F; Snow Lake Clinic, 100 Lakeshore Dr, Snow Lake MB R0B 1M0; Glasgow (Scotland)'69; MB ChB; DCH; FRCS; (204)358-2800; Fax. (204)358-7095.

MACLEOD, Patrick M J; Victoria Gen Hosp, 1 Hospital Way, Victoria BC V8Z 6R5; UBC'67; FCCMG; FABMG; FRCPC; Peds; MedGenetics. Staff Medical Genetics, Victoria General Hospital; Consultant, BC Mental Health & Addiction Service; Consultant, BC Children's Hospital; (250)727-4461; patrick.macleod@viha.ca.

MACLEOD, Roderick J; Hamilton HS-Chedoke Site, PO Box 2000 Stn Lcd 1 L2-1200 Main St W, Hamilton ON L8N 3Z5; Sask'64; DPsy(McGill); FRCPC; Psy (Child Psychiatry). Court Staff, St Joseph's Healthcare - Charlton Campus; Ac Staff Child & Family Centre, Hamilton Health Sciences Centre - McMaster University Medical Centre; Emeritus Prof Psy, McMaster University; (905)521-2100 x77294; Fax. (905)521-7968.

MACLEOD, Stuart M; A2 146-950 28th Ave W, Vancouver BC V5Z 4H4; Tor'67; PhD(McG)(Pharm); FRCPC; IntMed (Clinical Pharmacology). Staff, BC Children's Hospital; Exec Dir/Sr Scientist, Child & Family Research Institute; VP Research Coordination/Acad Liaison, Provincial Health Services Authority; Exec Dir, BC Research Institute for Children's & Women's Health; Assoc Dean Research/Prof Peds Faculty of Med, University of British Columbia; (604)875-2404; smacleod@cw.bc.ca.

MACLEOD, Susan E; Health Park, 308-45 Weatherbee Rd, Sydney NS B1M 0A1; Mem'00; CCFP; (902)567-0660; Fax. (902)270-3236.

MACLEOD, Tara Lee; 213-840 Coxwell Ave, East York ON M4C 5T2; Tor'83; FRCSC; ObstGyn. Staff ObstGyn, Toronto East General Hospital Inc; (416)690-6017

MACLEOD, Valerie A; Alexandra Marine & Gen Hosp, 120 Napier St, Goderich ON N7A 1W5; Dal'88; FRCPC; Psy (General Adult Psychiatry). Staff, Alexandra Marine & General Hospital; (519)524-8323

MACLEOD, Wendy; Royal Columbian Hosp, 330 Columbia St E, New Westminster BC V3L 3W7; Cape Town (South Africa)'82; MB ChB; LMCC; FRCPC; Anes. Staff Anes, Royal Columbian Hospital; Staff Med, University of British Columbia; (604)520-4602

MACLOGHLIN, Cynthia J; Queensway-Carleton Hosp, 3045 Baseline Rd, Nepean ON K2H 8P4; Tor'97; CCFP; CCFP(E.M.); Staff Emerg, Queensway Carleton Hospital; (613)721-4710; cmacloghlin@sympatico.ca.

MACLUSKY, Ian B; Children's Hosp Eastern Ont, 401 Smyth Rd, Ottawa ON K1H 8L1; London (England)'76; FRCPC; Peds; Respir. Staff, Children's Hospital of Eastern Ontario (CHEO); (613)737-7600

MACMAHON, Kristian P; Lakeshore Gen Hosp, 160 av Stillview, Pointe-Claire QC H9R 2Y2; Man'08; CCFP; CCFP(E.M.); Staff, Lakeshore General Hospital - Pointe Claire; (514)630-2225

MACMAHON, Ross G; 204-400 Tache Ave, Winnipeg MB R2H 3C3; Galway (Ireland)'72; MB ChB; BAO; FRCS(Ed); FRCSC; Urol. Staff, St Boniface General Hospital; Assoc Prof, University of Manitoba; rmacmaho@sbgh.mb.ca.

MACMANUS, Brian J; IWK Health Centre, PO Box 9700 Rpo CSC, Halifax NS B3K 6R8; Dublin (Ireland)'79; FRCPC; Anes (Pediatric Anesthesia). Assoc Chief PICU & Ped Anes, IWK Health Centre; Medical Control Phys, Dept of Health, NS; Assoc Prof, Dalhousie University; (902)470-8031; Fax. (902)470-7425; brian.macmanus@iwk.nshealth.ca.

MACMICHAEL, Gordon K; Great Northern Nursing Centre, 860 Great Northern Rd, Sault Ste. Marie ON P6A 5K7; Dal'71; (705)255-1459; Fax. (705)946-2857.

MACMILLAN, Andrew R; Huntsville Prof Bldg, 202-348 Muskoka Rd 3 N, Huntsville ON P1H 1H8; Qns'90; CCFP; FCFP; Ac Staff Privil, Huntsville District Memorial Hospital - Muskoka Algonquin Healthcare; Asst Prof, Northern Ontario School of Medicine; (705)788-3623; Fax. (705)788-3624.

MACMILLAN, Brent M; Ross Mem Hosp, 10 Angeline St N, Lindsay ON K9V 4M8; Wes'91; Staff, Ross Memorial Hospital; (705)324-6111; Fax. (705)876-9074.

MACMILLAN, Christina M; Mount Sinai Hosp, 6 500 11-600 University Ave, Toronto ON M5G 1X5; Tor'86; AB; FRCPC; AnatPath (Head & Neck). Staff Pathologist, Mount Sinai Hospital; Asst Prof Path, University of Toronto; (416)586-1575

MACMILLAN, David J; Carlingwood Family Med Centre, 35B-2121 Carling Ave, Ottawa ON K2A 1H2; Tor'91; CCFP; (613)761-6777; Fax. (613)761-7744.

MACMILLAN, David J; Sussex Family Med Centre, PO Box 5394 44 Lower Cove Rd, Sussex NB E4E 5L4; Dal'82; CCFP; Staff, Sussex Health Centre; (506)432-9055; mcmillan@nbnet.nb.ca.

MACMILLAN, Douglas G; 201-520 University Ave W, Waterloo ON N2T 2Z6; Wes'85; (519)578-3150; Fax. (519)745-3684; macmillandoug@yahoo.com.

MACMILLAN, J Barry; London HSC-Victoria Hosp, PO Box 5010 Stn B 800 Commissioners Rd E, London ON N6A 5W9; Wes'89; FRCSC; ObstGyn (Urogynecology). Consultant, London Health Sciences Centre - Victoria Campus; Consultant ObstGyn, St Joseph's Hospital - St Joseph's Health Care; Teach Staff ObstGyn, University of Western Ontario; (519)646-6247; Fax. (519)646-6039.

MACMILLAN, J Stewart; PO Box 9 Stn Main, Miramichi NB E1V 3M2; Dal'91; FRCPC; DiagRad. (506)623-3145; Fax. (506)623-6147.

MACMILLAN, James I; Niagara H System-Ontario Site, 356-155 Ontario St, St Catharines ON L2R 5K3; Tor'72; FRCSC; GenSurg (Thoracic Surgery). Staff, Niagara Health System - Ontario Street Site; Staff, Niagara Health System - St Catharines General Site; (905)687-3411; Fax. (905)687-9271.

MACMILLAN, James; Rosthern Med Clinic, PO Box 1089, Rosthern SK S0K 3R0; Sask'09; CCFP; (306)232-4894; Fax. (306)232-4970.

MACMILLAN, James R; Mel Lloyd Health Centre, 167 Centre St, Shelburne ON L0N 1S4; Edinburgh (Scotland)'63; FRCS(Ed); Gen Practice, Headwaters Health Care Centre - Shelburne Site; Gen Practice, Headwaters Health Care Centre - Orangeville Site; (519)925-0017; Fax. (519)925-6717; jmacmillan@cvh.on.ca.

MACMILLAN, Jennifer C; Huntsville Prof Bldg, 205-348 Muskoka Rd 3 N, Huntsville ON P1H 1H8; Tor'96; FRCSC; GenSurg. Staff, Huntsville District Memorial Hospital - Muskoka Algonquin Healthcare; (705)789-6510; Fax. (705)789-4734.

MACMILLAN, Kier L; Foul Bay Prof Centre, 212-1964 Fort St, Victoria BC V8R 6R3; Dal'88; Staff, Gorge Road Hospital; (250)592-5311; Fax. (250)592-5201; rocdok@shaw.ca.

MACMILLAN, Leslie G; Univ Hlth Network-Princess M, 610 University Ave, Toronto ON M5G 2M9; Tor'78; MHSc; FRCPC; IntMed; MedMicrobiol. Staff, Princess Margaret Hospital - University Health Network; (416)946-4501 x3469

MACMILLAN, Lindsay E; Family Practice Unit, 61 Queen St, Toronto ON M5C 2T2; Dal'04; CCFP; Staff, St Michael's Hospital; Asst Lecturer, University of Toronto; (416)867-7428; Fax. (416)867-7498; macmillanl@smh.ca.

MACMILLAN, Mark; Dr Everett Chalmers Reg Hosp, PO Box 9000 Stn A 700 Priestman St, Fredericton NB E3B 5N5; Dal'06; Gastroent; IntMed. Staff, Dr Everett Chalmers Regional Hospital; (506)454-6882

MACMILLAN, Michael B; Seven Oaks Med Centre, 205-1750 Main St, Winnipeg MB R2V 1Z7; Man'78; CCFP; FCFP; Staff Women's Centre, Health Sciences Centre; Staff, Seven Oaks General Hospital; (204)338-0384; Fax. (204)338-0386.

MACMILLAN, Suzanne M; 501-595 Montreal Rd, Ottawa ON K1K 4L2; Ott'83; FRCPC; IntMed (Rheumatoid Arthritis); Rheum. Langs: French; (613)741-2645; Fax. (613)741-6849.

MACMILLAN, Vona; 7-110 Plaza Blvd, Dalhousie NB E8C 2E2; (Hungary)'98; CCFP; Pres Restigouche Med Society/Sec-Treas General Med Staff, Hôpital Régional Campbellton; Langs: Bilingual(English/French); (506)684-2000; Fax. (506)684-3365.

MACMULLIN, Elwood C; Cape Breton Hlthcare Complex, 3F-1482 George St, Sydney NS B1P 1P3; Dal'76; FRCSC; GenSurg. Hd GenSurg, Cape Breton Healthcare Complex; (902)562-0031; Fax. (902)564-9492.

MACMULLIN, Sunita; Sussex Health Centre, 75 Leonard Dr, Sussex NB E4E 2P7; Alb'95; Staff, Sussex Health Centre; (506)432-3130

MACNAB, Andrew J; BC Women's Hosp & Health Ctre, C323-4500 Oak St, Vancouver BC V6H 3N1; London (England)'67; FRCPC; Peds. Staff, BC Women's Hospital & Health Centre; (604)875-2850

MACNAB, Jessica M; Royal Columbian Hosp, 330 Columbia St E, New Westminster BC V3L 3W7; Mem'89; MMed; FRCPC; CCFP; EmergMed. Staff Emerg Phys, Royal Columbian Hospital; Staff Emerg Phys, Eagle Ridge Hospital & Health Care Centre; Clin Staff Surg, University of British Columbia; (604)520-4253; Fax. (604)520-4722.

MACNAB, Timothy I; St Clair X-Ray, 1223 St Clair Ave W, Toronto ON M6E 1B5; Tor'86; FRCPC; Otol; DiagRad. (416)656-6034

MACNABB, Nancy J; 8-600 Hespeler Rd, Cambridge ON N1R 8H2; Tor'91; BSc; MSc; CCFP; Staff, Hanover & District Hospital; (519)624-9887; Fax. (519)624-6801.

MACNAIR, Tracy L; Boundary Trails Health Centre, PO Box 2000 Stn Main, Winkler MB R6W 1H8; Man'02; FRCPC; DiagRad. Staff, Boundary Trails Health Centre; (204)331-8800

MACNAMARA, Elizabeth M; SMBD Jewish Gen Hosp, 3755 ch Cote-Sainte-Catherine, Montreal QC H3T 1E2; Dublin (Ireland)'79; MRCPath(UK); MRCP(Ire.); FRCPC; MedBiochem (Internal Medicine). Staff Med Biochemistry, Sir Mortimer B Davis Jewish General; assoc Prof, McGill University; Langs: English; French; (514)340-8222 x5091; Fax. (514)340-7524; elizabeth.macnamara@mcgill.ca.

MACNAUGHTON, David J; Jubilee Med Clinic, 1902 Richmond Rd, Victoria BC V8R 4R2; Alb'71; Ac Staff, Royal Jubilee Hospital; Associate, Victoria General Hospital; (250)595-8231

MACNAUGHTON, Donald M; Hotel-Dieu Hosp, 166 Brock St, Kingston ON K7L 5G2; Qns'83; BSc(Hon); FRCSC; Otol. Staff, Kingston General Hospital; Consultant, Weeneebayko General Hospital; Staff, Hotel-Dieu Hospital; Asst Prof, Queen's University; (613)544-3400 x3620; Fax. (613)547-5654; dmm3@queensu.ca.

MACNAUGHTON, Heather P; Royal Columbian Hosp, 330 Columbia St E, New Westminster BC V3L 3W7; UBC'79; FRCPC; DiagRad. Staff, Royal Columbian Hospital; (604)520-4640

MACNAUGHTON, Jane M; 370 Select Dr, Kingston ON K7M 8T4; Qns'84; (613)536-3092; Fax. (613)536-3185.

MACNAUGHTON, Janet E; Mud Creek Med Co-Op Ltd, 12 Elm Ave, Wolfville NS B4P 1Z9; Dal'84; Ac Staff, Valley Regional Hospital; (902)542-3633; Fax. (902)542-2709.

MACNAUGHTON, Janis A; Stratford Gen Hosp, 46 General Hospital Dr, Stratford ON N5A 2Y6; Qns'81; FRCPC; IntMed. Ac Staff, Stratford General Hospital - Huron Perth Healthcare Alliance; (519)271-2120

MACNAY, Ramsay G; 604-25 Charlton Ave E, Hamilton ON L8N 1Y2; Wes'94; FRCPC; Peds. Clinical Asst Prof, McMaster University; (905)523-1209; Fax. (905)523-7526.

MACNEARNEY, P Christine; Kensington Family Med Centre, PO Box 160, Kensington PE C0B 1M0; Dal'84; BSc(Acadia); (902)836-4350

MACNEIL, Catherine M; Alberta Children's Hosp, 2888 Shaganappi Trail NW, Calgary AB T3B 6A8; Dal'00; FRCPC; Peds. Staff, Alberta Children's Hospital; (403)955-7211

MACNEIL, David R; 204-967 Bedford Hwy, Bedford NS B4A 1A9; Dal'86; (902)835-6200

MACNEIL, Donna M; St Joseph's Hosp, 130 Bayard Dr, Saint John NB E2L 3L6; Alb'97; FRCPC; IntMed; GeriatricMed. Staff, St Joseph's Hospital; (506)632-5556; Fax. (506)632-5512.

MACNEIL, Dorothy E; Well Women's Clinic, 102-336 Kings Rd, Sydney NS B1S 1A9; Dal'80.

MACNEIL, Gerard M; B1-2135 Dorchester Rd SS 2, Dorchester ON N0L 1G2; Wes'86; Assoc Staff, London Health Sciences Centre - Victoria Campus; (519)268-2011

MACNEIL, Hugh A K; Pinecrest-Queensway CHC, 2F-1365 Richmond Rd, Ottawa ON K2B 6R7; Dal'98; CCFP; Physician, Pinecrest-Queensway Community Health Centre; (613)820-4922; Fax. (613)820-2006.

MACNEIL, Iain P; Elmsdale Med Centre, 106 Elmsdale Rd, Elmsdale NS B2S 1K6; Dal'88; BSc; CCFP; FCFP; (902)883-2216; Fax. (902)883-1734.

MACNEIL, John P; The Credit Valley Hosp, 2200 Eglinton Ave W, Mississauga ON L5M 2N1; Dal'90; Anes. Staff, The Credit Valley Hospital; (905)813-4466

MACNEIL, M Graham; PO Box 4791, Rothesay NB E2E 5X5; Dal'95; BSc; CCFP; Staff Family Pract & Geriatric Med, Saint John Regional Hospital; (506)849-8510; Fax. (506)849-8777.

MACNEIL, M Lawrence; 2372 Highway 206 PO Box 3000, Arichat NS B0E 1A0; Dal'82; CCFP; Chief of Staff, St. Anne Centre; Preceptor, Dalhousie University; (902)226-1674; Fax. (902)226-9312; lmacneil66@yahoo.ca.

MACNEIL, Mary V; Queen Elizabeth II HSC, 453-1276 South Park St, Halifax NS B3H 2Y9; Dal'89; BSc; FRCPC; IntMed; MedOncol. Staff Med Oncol, Queen Elizabeth II Health Sciences Centre - Victoria General Site; (902)473-8317; Fax. (902)473-6186.

MACNEIL, Robert B; The Ottawa Hosp-Civic Campus, B312-1053 Carling Ave, Ottawa ON K1Y 4E9; Dal'86; Anes. Staff, The Ottawa Hospital - Civic Campus; Asst Prof, University of Ottawa; (613)761-4169

MACNEIL, S Danielle; Unviersity of Alberta Hosp, 1E4-8440 112 St NW, Edmonton AB T6G 2B7; Dal'06; FRCSC; Otol. Staff, University of Alberta Hospital; (780)407-7958

MACNEILL, Heather L; Bridgepoint Hosp, 227-14 St Matthews Rd, Toronto ON M4M 2B5; Qns'00; CSCN; FRCPC; PhysMed&Rehab (Neuro Rehabilitation). Staff, Bridgepoint Health Centre; Lecturer Med, University of Toronto; (416)461-8252; Fax. (416)470-6714.

MACNEILL, James R; 404-6389 Coburg Rd, Halifax NS B3H 2A5; Dal'72; FRCSC; Ophth. (902)420-9036; Fax. (902)490-0306.

MACNEILL, Judith L; Parkland Med Clinic, 203-998 Parkland Dr, Halifax NS B3M 0A6; Dal'92; CCFP; (902)404-7737

MACNEILL, Kara E; Cumberland Med Hlth Services, 33 Havelock St, Amherst NS B4H 4W1; Dal'02; FRCPC; Psy. Staff, Aberdeen Regional Hospital; (902)667-3879

MACNEILL, Karen N; Royal Victoria Hosp, 201 Georgian Dr, Barrie ON L4M 6M2; Dal'00; FRCPC; AnatPath. Staff, Royal Victoria Regional Health Centre; (705)728-9090

MACNEILL, Phillip; Alder Med Centre, 277 Evergreen Rd, Campbell River BC V9W 5Y4; UBC'67; BSc; Sr Medical Staff, Campbell River & District General Hospital; (250)287-7441; Fax. (250)287-4384.

MACNEILL, R Steven; Prince County Hosp, PO Box 3000 Stn Main 65 Roy Boates Ave, Summerside PE C1N 2A9; Dal'00; BSc; CCFP; CCFP(E.M.); Staff, Prince County Hospital; (902)432-2500

MACNEILL, Robert B; Cape Breton Hlthcare Complex, 1482 George St, Sydney NS B1P 1P3; Dal'81; FRCPC; Anes. Anesthetist, Cape Breton Healthcare Complex; (902)567-8000

MACNEILL, Susan J; The Ottawa Hosp-Gen Campus, 4306-501 Smyth Rd Box 400, Ottawa ON K1H 8L6; Ott'99; FRCPC; Psy. Staff Psy, The Ottawa Hospital - General Campus; (613)737-8010; Fax. (613)737-8115.

MACNEILY, Andrew E; Children's & Women's HC of BC, K0 134-4480 Oak St, Vancouver BC V6H 3V4; Qns'86; FRCSC; Urol (Adult Urology). Staff, Children's & Women's Health Centre of British, Ambulatory Care; (604)875-2734; Fax. (604)875-2721.

MACNICOL, Brent J; Royal Alexandra Hosp, 10240 Kingsway NW, Edmonton AB T5H 3V9; UBC'97; FRCPC; Anes. Staff Anes, Royal Alexandra Hospital; (780)735-4010

MACNICOL, Melanie L; Victoria Medical Bldg, 212-1669 Victoria St, Prince George BC V2L 2L5; UBC'08; CCFP; (250)614-2330

MACNICOL, Wayne M; Yukon ObstGyn Clinic, 5 Hospital Rd, Whitehorse YT Y1A 3H7; Alb'77; FRCSC; ObstGyn. Staff, Whitehorse General Hospital; (867)393-8915; Fax. (867)393-8909; wayne.macnicol@wgh.yk.ca.

MACPHADYEN, Norris B; Trillium Hlth Ctr-Mississauga, 100 Queensway W, Mississauga ON L5B 1B8; Ott'92; FRCPC; DiagRad. Staff, Trillium Health Centre - Mississauga; (905)848-7525

MACPHAIL, Gisela L P; Cups Community Health Centre, 1001 10 Ave SW, Calgary AB T2R 0B7; Cal'88; MPH; MD; FRCPC; IntMed (Hepatitis C); InfectDis. Langs: German; (403)221-8797; Fax. (403)221-8785.

MACPHAIL, Iain A; 260 Sherbrooke St, New Westminster BC V3L 3M2; Qns'87; MHSc; CCFP; CCFP(E.M.); Staff, Royal Columbian Hospital; (604)520-4320

MACPHEE, Ian J; 110-77 Westmount Rd, Guelph ON N1H 5J1; Dal'03; CCFP; (519)766-9559; Fax. (519)766-1709.

MACPHEE, Shannon P; IWK Health Centre, PO Box 9700 Rpo CSC 5850-5980 University Ave, Halifax NS B3K 6R8; Dal'99; FRCPC; Peds (Pediatric Emergency Medicine). Staff, IWK Health Centre; (902)470-8824

MACPHERSON, Andrew I; Victoria Emergency Phys Assoc, 327-1627 Fort St, Victoria BC V8R 1H8; UBC'97; CCFP; CCFP(E.M.); FCFP; (250)479-1442; Fax. (250)479-1472.

MACPHERSON, Bruce A; The Hosp for Sick Children, 555 University Ave, Toronto ON M5G 1X8; Wes'82; FRCPC; Anes. Staff Anes, The Hospital For Sick Children; (416)813-7445; Fax. (416)813-7543.

MACPHERSON, Colin A; Ottawa Valley Hlth & Wellness, 715 MacKay St, Pembroke ON K8A 0C6; Dal'84; Clin Lecturer Family Med, University of Ottawa; (613)735-1089

MACPHERSON, Colin J; Quinte HC Corp-Belleville Gen, 265 Dundas St E, Belleville ON K8N 5A9; Wes'02; FRCPC; Psy. Staff, QHC Belleville General; (613)969-7400

MACPHERSON, David A; Family Med Centre, PO Box 8888 Stn Main 220 Bagot St, Kingston ON K7L 5E9; Tor'70; CCFP; FCFP; (613)549-4480

MACPHERSON, Douglas W; Migration Hlth Consultants Inc, 14130 Creditview Rd, Cheltenham ON L7C 1Y4; McM'78; MSc(Clin.Trop.Med.); FRCPC; IntMed (Infectious Diseases); MedMicrobiol. Langs: English; French.

MACPHERSON, Gail L; 115-1060 Speers Rd, Oakville ON L6L 2X4; McM'83; BSc; CCFP; FCFP; Staff, Halton Healthcare Services Corporation - Oakville Site; (905)842-9735; Fax. (905)842-9731; gailmac@cogeco.ca.

MACPHERSON, Jeffrey D; Northumberland Hills Hosp, 1000 DePalma Dr, Cobourg ON K9A 5W6; Dublin (Ireland)'07; CCFP; CCFP(E.M.); Staff, Northumberland Hills Hospital; (905)372-6811

MACPHERSON, Jennifer R; 10-8180 MacLeod Trail SE, Calgary AB T2H 2B8; UBC'89; FRCPC; Peds. Staff, Alberta Children's Hospital; (403)252-6651; macphers@associateclinic.com.

MACPHERSON, John K F; Pennbridge Med Bldg, 200-4475 Viewmont Ave, Victoria BC V8Z 6L8; Ott'74; CCFP; Ac Staff, Royal Jubilee Hospital; Ac Staff, Victoria General Hospital; (250)727-3122; Fax. (250)727-3363.

MACPHERSON, Kathleen M; Dalhousie University, 418-5790 University Ave, Halifax NS B3H 1V7; Dal'81; MPH; Asst Prof, Dalhousie University; (902)494-2343

MACPHERSON, Margaret A; York-Med Medical Arts Centre, 308-250 Harding Blvd W, Richmond Hill ON L4C 9M7; Tor'81; FRCPC; Derm. (905)737-0420

MACPHERSON, Marilyn P; C-339 Willow St, Truro NS B2N 5A6; Qns'92; FRCPC; Peds. Hd Peds, Colchester East Hants Health Centre; (902)893-5505; Fax. (902)893-3444.

MACPHERSON, Nicol A; BC Cancer Agency-Vanc Isl Ctr, 2410 Lee Ave, Victoria BC V8R 6V5; Qns'91; PhD; BSc(Hon); FRCPC; IntMed (Breast Cancer); MedOncol. Staff, BC Cancer Agency Vancouver Island Centre; Clinical Asst Prof Med, University of British Columbia; (250)519-5500 x695572; nmacpher@bccancer.bc.ca.

MACPHERSON, Nicola; Ridge Meadows Hosp & Hlth CC, 11666 Laity St, Maple Ridge BC V2X 5A3; Ott'85; DABHPM; FRCPC; Anes (Palliative Medicine). Staff Tertiary Palliative Care Unit, Burnaby Hospital; Staff, Ridge Meadows Hospital & Health Care Centre; Physician, Tri-Cities & Ridge Meadows Home Hospice; (604)469-3185; Fax. (604)608-3179; nicola.macpherson@fraserhealth.ca.

MACPHERSON, Paul A; The Ottawa Hosp-Gen Campus, Module G-501 Smyth Rd, Ottawa ON K1H 8L6; McM'98; PhD; BSc; MD; LMCC; FRCP; FRCPC; IntMed (AIDS/HIV); InfectDis. Staff InfectDis, The Ottawa Hospital - General Campus; Asst Prof Med, University of Ottawa; (613)737-8899 x74184

MACPHERSON, Rayma D; Forest Hills Med Clinic, 4 Forest Hills Pky, Dartmouth NS B2W 5G7; Dal'81; Staff Family Pract, IWK Health Centre; (902)435-5530

MACQUARRIE, Donald C; Dartmouth Gen Hosp, 325 Pleasant St, Dartmouth NS B2Y 4G8; Dal'03; CCFP; CCFP(E.M.); Staff, Dartmouth General Hospital; Locum Tenens, Toronto East General Hospital Inc; (902)465-8491; Fax. (902)460-4148.

MACQUARRIE, Kirk J; Queen Elizabeth II HSC, 1276 South Park St, Halifax NS B3H 2Y9; Dal'93; FRCPC; Anes. Staff, Queen Elizabeth II Health Sciences Centre - Victoria General Site; (902)473-2331; Fax. (902)423-9454.

MACQUARRIE, Robyn M; Cumberland Reg Hlth Care Ctre, 19428 Highway 2, Amherst NS B4H 1N6; Dal'06; FRCSC; ObstGyn (Medical Genetics). Staff, Cumberland Regional Health Care Center; (902)667-5400

MACQUEEN, Allison J; Westbrook Prof Bldg, 211-1610 37 St SW, Calgary AB T3C 3P1; Alb'06; CCFP; Physician, Well Women Clinic; (403)246-2052; Fax. (403)246-2219.

MACQUEEN, Glenda M; 7F-3280 Hospital Dr NW, Calgary AB T2N 4Z6; McM'92; PhD; FRCPC; Psy (Mood Disorders). Staff, Foothills Medical Centre; Dept Head Psy, University of Calgary; (403)220-2587; Fax. (403)270-1828.

MACRAE, Donald K; Carlyle Med Clinic, PO Box 1090, Carlyle SK S0C 0R0; Sask'68; FRCPC; Psy (Psychotherapy). (306)453-6795; Fax. (306)453-6796.

MACRAE, Duncan L; London HSC-Victoria Hosp, PO Box 5010 Stn B 800 Commissioners Rd E, London ON N6A 5W9; Qns'72; FACS; FRCSC; Otol (Pediatric Otolaryngology). Ac Staff, London Health Sciences Centre - Victoria Campus; Prof, University of Western Ontario; (519)685-8126; Fax. (519)685-8185; duncan.macrae@lhsc.on.ca.

MACRAE, Emerson E; 223 Commissioners Rd E, London ON N6C 2S9; Dal'60; DAA; Otol (Trauma). Att Staff, London Health Sciences Centre - Victoria Campus; Att Staff, St Joseph's Hospital - St Joseph's Health Care; Consultant, Wingham & District Hospital - Listowel Wingham Hospitals Alliance; Asst Prof Otol, University of Western Ontario; (519)672-3910

MACRAE, Helen M; Mount Sinai Hosp, 451-600 University Ave, Toronto ON M5G 1X5; Alb'86; FACS; FRCSC; GenSurg (Colon & Rectal Surgery). Staff, Mount Sinai Hospital; Assoc Prof Surg, University of Toronto; (416)586-4800 x2836; Fax. (416)586-8644.

MACRAE, Jennifer M; Foothills Med Centre, C210-1403 29 St NW, Calgary AB T2N 2T9; Cal'97; FRCPC; IntMed; Nephrol. Staff, Peter Lougheed Centre; Staff, Rockyview General Hospital; Staff, Foothills Medical Centre; (403)944-8168; Fax. (403)944-2876.

MACRAE, John D C; 5-1435 Plains Rd E, Burlington ON L7R 3P9; Dublin (Ireland)'84; BSc; FRCSC; Otol. Staff, Joseph Brant Memorial Hospital; (905)639-2244; Fax. (905)639-2253.

MACRAE, Robert M; The Ottawa Hosp-Gen Campus, 501 Smyth Rd, Ottawa ON K1H 8L6; Ott'95; FRCPC; RadOncol. Staff Reginal Cancer Centre, The Ottawa Hospital - General Campus; Langs: English; French; (613)737-7700 x70206; Fax. (613)247-3511.

MACRAE, William G; 206-125 Bell Farm Rd, Barrie ON L4M 6L2; Tor'65; FRCSC; Ophth (Cataract Surgery). Staff, St Michael's Hospital; Asst Prof, University of Toronto; (705)725-5443; Fax. (705)725-5442; wgmacrae@bellnet.ca.

MACREDMOND, Ruth E; St Paul's Hosp, 1081 Burrard St, Vancouver BC V6Z 1Y6; Dublin (Ireland)'94; Critical Care Medicine; IntMed. Staff, Providence Health Care - St Paul's Hospital; (604)862-2344

MACRITCHIE, Donald M; University Hosp of Northern BC, 1475 Edmonton St, Prince George BC V2M 1S2; UBC'70; BSc; FRCPC; IntMed (Cardiology). Staff, University Hospital of Northern British Columbia; (250)565-2464

MACRITCHIE, Kenneth J; Sheppard Associates, 649 Sheppard Ave W, North York ON M3H 2S4; Aberdeen (Scotland)'60; DPM(Eng); FRCPsy(UK); FRCPC; Psy. Staff Psy, Toronto General Hospital - UHN; Staff Psy, The Credit Valley Hospital; Assoc Prof Psy, University of Toronto; Langs: Gaelic; (416)630-0610; kenmacritchie@hotmail.com.

MACRODIMITRIS, Angelo G; Winnipeg Clinic, 425 St Mary Ave, Winnipeg MB R3C 0N2; Alexandria (Egypt)'63; MB ChB; DOphth(Lond.); FAAO; FRCOphth(U.K.); FRCSC; Ophth (Cataract & Anterior Segment Surgery). Ac Staff, Misericordia Health Centre; Consultant, Health Sciences Centre; Asst Prof Ophth, University of Manitoba; Langs: Greek; Arabic; French; (204)957-3255

MACSWEEN, J Mark; Saint John Reg Hosp, PO Box 2100 Stn Main, Saint John NB E2L 4L2; Dal'95; FRCPC; DiagRad. Staff DiagRad, Saint John Regional Hospital; Lecturer Med, Dalhousie University; (506)648-7102; mmacsween@hotmail.com.

MACSWEEN, Margaret J; Royal Alexandra Hosp, 10240 Kingsway NW, Edmonton AB T5H 3V9; Dal'07; FRCPC; Psy. Staff, Royal Alexandra Hospital; (780)735-4111

MACSWEEN, Mary C; The Moncton Hosp, 135 MacBeath Ave, Moncton NB E1C 6Z8; Dal'87; FRCPC; IntMed (Diabetes). Staff Med, The Moncton Hospital; Lecturer, Dalhousie University; (506)857-5635; Fax. (506)857-5726.

MACSWEEN, Moira A; Chigamik Commun Health Centre, 845 King St, Midland ON L4R 0B7; Wes'01; CCFP; CCFP(E.M.); (705)527-4154

MACSWEEN, Ruth M; Limestone Dermatology, 163 Brock St, Kingston ON K7L 1S2; Cambridge (England)'89; BSc; MB BCh; FRCPC; Derm. Langs: English; French; (613)549-6660; Fax. (613)547-2079.

MACSWEENEY, Orla; Royal Jubilee Hosp, 1952 Bay St, Victoria BC V8R 1J8; McM'01; CCFP; CCFP(E.M.); Staff, Royal Jubilee Hospital; (250)516-6181

MACTAVISH, Alison J; Portage Prof Bldg, 603-5400 Portage Rd, Niagara Falls ON L2G 5X7; Cal'87; CCFP; FCFP; Assoc Staff Gen Pract, Niagara Health System - Greater Niagara General Site; Clin Assoc Prof, Queen's University; Clin Assoc Prof, McMaster University; (905)354-2323; Fax. (905)356-2210.

MACTAVISH, James C; Manitouwadge Med Clinic, 1 Clinic Crt, Manitouwadge ON P0T 2C0; McM'92; CCFP; CCFP(E.M.); FCFP.

MACTAVISH, James W E; Tiger Hills Health Centre, PO Box 191 64 Clark St, Treherne MB R0G 2V0; Man'10; CCFP.

MACVICAR, G Neil; Cape Breton Hlthcare Complex, 1482 George St, Sydney NS B1P 1P3; Dal'89; CCFP; CCFP(E.M.); Staff, Cape Breton Healthcare Complex; (902)567-8145; Fax. (902)842-2873.

MACYK-DAVEY, Andrea; Grey Nuns Community Hosp & HC, 1100 Youville Drive West NW, Edmonton AB T6L 5X8; Alb'06; FRCPC; GenPath. Staff, Covenant Health - Grey Nuns Community Hospital; (780)735-9627

MADALA, Kiran; Scarborough Gastroent Assoc, 208-1585 Markham Rd, Scarborough ON M1B 2W1; Ott'94; FRCPC; IntMed; Gastroent. (416)439-9253; Fax. (416)439-3875.

MADAN, Minakshi; Sunnybrook Hlth Sciences Ctre, D380-2075 Bayview Ave, Toronto ON M4N 3M5; McG'91; FRCPC; IntMed (Interventional Cardiology); Cardiol. Staff Cardiol, Sunnybrook Health Sciences Centre; Asst Prof Med, University of Toronto; (416)480-4119; Fax. (416)480-4657; mina.madan@sunnybrook.ca.

MADAN, Monika K; Roncesvalles Village Med Clini, 137 Roncesvalles Ave, Toronto ON M6R 2L2; Qns'03; CCFP; (416)534-6699; Fax. (416)534-0172.

MADAN, Nipun M L; Mango Tree Family Health Team, 35 Harvard Rd, Guelph ON N1G 3A2; Ott'93; CCFP; (519)837-5410; Fax. (519)837-4853.

MADAN, Pooja; Wise Elephant Fam Health Team, 280 Main St N, Brampton ON L6V 1P6; Bonaire (Netherlands Antilles)'08; (905)216-1065

MADAN, Robert I; Baycrest Ctre/Geriatric Care, 3560 Bathurst St, Toronto ON M6A 2E1; Wes'98; FRCPC; Psy. Staff, Baycrest Centre for Geriatric Care; (416)785-2500 x2457

MADAN, Suparna; Rockyview Gen Hosp, 7007 14 St SW, Calgary AB T2V 1P9; Cal'98; FRCPC; Psy. Staff Psy, Rockyview General Hospital; (403)943-3808; Fax. (403)212-1234.

MADANI, Daniel L; CSSS d'argenteuil, 145 av de la Providence, Lachute QC J8H 4C7; Staff, Centre Hospitalier d'Argenteuil; (450)562-3761

MADARNAS, Alexandre; CSSS de Laval, 1755 boul Rene-Laennec, Laval QC H7M 3L9; Laval'99; FRCPC; MedBiochem. Staff, Hopital de la Cite de la santé; (450)668-1010; Fax. (450)975-5044.

MADARNAS, Yolanda; Cancer Ctr for Southeastern On, 25 King St W, Kingston ON K7L 5P9; Mon'90; LMCC(IntMed); ABIM(MedOncol); FRC; FRCPC; IntMed (Breast Cancer); MedOncol. Att Staff, Hotel-Dieu Hospital; Att Staff, Kingston General Hospital; Teach Staff Oncology Medicine Pharmacology & Toxicology, Queen's University; Langs: Spanish; Bilingual(French/English); Italian; (613)544-2631 x4502; Fax. (613)546-8209; yolanda.madarnas@krcc.on.ca.

MADDEFORD, William R; London Medical-Dental Bldg, 309-450 Central Ave, London ON N6B 2E8; Wes'60; Court Staff, St Joseph's Hospital - St Joseph's Health Care; Physician, Sunoco Refinery-Sarnia, Ont.; (519)672-2260; Fax. (519)433-2154.

MADDEN, Joanne I; Sudbury Reg Hosp-Laurentian, 41 Ramsey Lake Rd, Sudbury ON P3E 5J1; Mem'94; BMedSci; FRCPC; Anes. Staff, Health Sciences North-Laurentian Site; Asst Prof, University of Ottawa; Reg/Prog Dir Anaes, Northern Ontario School of Medicine-Laurentian University; (705)523-7113; Fax. (705)523-7112; joanne.madden@normed.ca.

MADDEN, Joseph K; 400 McKeown Ave, North Bay ON P1B 0B2; Dublin (Ireland)'76; BAO; DObst(RCPI); MRC; DCH(RCSI); FRCPC; Peds. Staff, North Bay Regional Health Centre - Regional Mental Health; Vis Staff, Kirkland & District Hospital; Asst Prof Attached to Northern Family Practice Prog, University of Ottawa; (705)474-6655; Fax. (705)474-4853.

MADDEN, Kenneth M; Geriatric Assessment Clinic, 7F-2775 Laurel St, Vancouver BC V5Z 1M9; Qns'96; MSc; FRCPC; IntMed; GeriatricMed. Staff Geriatric Med, UBC Hospital - Koerner Pavillion; (604)875-5312; Fax. (604)875-5696.

MADDEN, Sharen N; The Hugh Allen Clinic, PO Box 489 79 Fifth Ave, Sioux Lookout ON P8T 1A8; McM'84; CCFP; FCFP; Staff, Sioux Lookout Meno-Ya-Win Health Centre; Staff, The Hugh Allen Clinic; (807)737-3803; Fax. (807)737-1771.

MADDEN-FITZSIMONS, Therese; 29 Willow Farm Lane, Aurora ON L4G 6K1; Dublin (Ireland)'84; FRCPC; Psy (Counselling). (905)841-2437

MADDIGAN, Barbara A; Hart Bldg, 202-15 Rowan St, St. John's NL A1B 2X2; Mem'90; FRCPC; Psy. Staff, Janeway Children's Health & Rehabilitation Centre; (709)579-6800

MADDISON, G David; Brant Community HC-Brantford, 200 Terrace Hill St, Brantford ON N3R 1G9; Dal'64; BSc; FACS; FRCSC; GenSurg; VascSurg. Ac Staff, The Brant Community Healthcare System - Brantford General Hospital Site; Consultant, The Brant Community Healthcare System - Willett Hospital Site; (519)752-7871; maddison@execulink.com.

MADDISON, Glen J; St Josephs Hospice, 475 Christina St N, Sarnia ON N7T 5W3; Ott'76; Clin Asst ICU, St Joseph's Healthcare - Charlton Campus; Staff Emerg, Bluewater Health - Mitton Site; Staff Emerg, Bluewater Health - Norman Site; (519)337-0537

MADER, Judith A; Halifax Prof Centre, 420-5991 Spring Garden Rd, Halifax NS B3H 1Y6; Dal'90; BSc; CCFP; (902)429-6958; Fax. (902)422-4996.

MADHANI, Kurban J; Medical Bldg, 1503-805 Broadway W, Vancouver BC V5Z 1K1; Kashmir (India)'79; FRCPC; Psy. (604)879-1503; Fax. (604)879-1594.

MADHVANI, Ashwin K; Yarmouth Reg Health Centre, 317-60 Vancouver St, Yarmouth NS B5A 2P5; Sheffield (England)'74; MB ChB; FRCOG; FACOG; FRCSC; ObstGyn. Consultant ObstGyn, Yarmouth Regional Hospital; (902)742-4044; Fax. (902)742-4044; madhvani@yar.eastlink.ca.

MADHVANI, Seema N; Halton HCS Corp-Oakville, 327 Reynolds St, Oakville ON L6J 3L7; Wes'02; CCFP; CCFP(E.M.); Staff, Halton Healthcare Services Corporation - Oakville Site; (905)845-2571

MADIGAN, Maureen A; Valley Reg Hosp, 150 Exhibition St, Kentville NS B4N 5E3; Dal'99; FRCPC; DiagRad. Staff, Valley Regional Hospital; (902)679-2657

MADIGANE, Joyce; Tyne Valley Med Clinic, PO Box 78, Tyne Valley PE C0B 2C0; Bristol (England)'70; MB ChB; BSc; DObstRCOG; MRCOG; Chief/Medical Staff, Stewart Memorial Hospital; Ac Staff, Prince County Hospital; (902)831-2659; Fax. (902)831-3074; jmadigane@canada.com.

MADIKIZA, Aggrey P; Woburn Med Dental Centre, 4129 Lawrence Ave E, Scarborough ON M1E 2S2; Natal (South Africa)'72; BSc; FAAP; FRCPC; Peds. Staff Peds, Rouge Valley Health System - Centenary Health Centre Site; Langs: Xhosa; Zulu; (416)439-1991; Fax. (416)439-3593; paksmadikiza@yahoo.com.

MADILL, David W; 2323 Hollyhill Pl, Victoria BC V8N 1V1; Qns'68; Ac Staff, Royal Jubilee Hospital; Ac Staff, Victoria General Hospital; (250)477-9867; david_madill@telus.net.

MADILL, Melanie L; Chilliwack Family Care Centre, 45779 Luckakuck Way, Chilliwack BC V2R 4E8; UBC'86; CCFP; FCFP; Asst Prof Family Med, University of British Columbia; (604)792-2266; Fax. (604)792-2494.

MADILL, Robert W; Bridlewood Med Centre, 64 Stonehaven Dr, Kanata ON K2M 2Y2; Belfast (Ireland)'70; (613)592-0805; Fax. (613)592-0961.

MADISON, Adena M; Manitoba Clinic, 790 Sherbrook St, Winnipeg MB R3A 1M3; Man'05; FRCPC; Peds.

MADISON, Vera V; 1-21 Imperial St, Toronto ON M5P 1B9; Belgrade (Serbia)'70; Staff, St Michael's Hospital; Dir, Madison Clinic; Langs: Spanish; German; (416)944-8296

MADON, Shilpa; Rebecca Med Clinic, 170 Rebecca St, Oakville ON L6K 1J6; Man'00; CCFP; (905)845-9293

MADONIK, Bonnie H; North York Gen Hosp-Branson, 122-555 Finch Ave W, North York ON M2R 1N5; McM'83; BSc; CASM; MD; FASAM; DABAM; Med Dir Addiction Program, North York General Hospital - Branson Division; Pres Medical Staff Association, North York General Hospital; Asst Prof, University of Toronto; (416)635-2506; Fax. (416)635-2441; bmadonik@nygh.on.ca.

MADONIK, Michael L; Bolton Med Centre, 205-12295 Highway 50, Bolton ON L7E 1M2; Tor'69; (416)388-4138

MADOR, David R; Hys Med Centre, 400-11010 101 St NW, Edmonton AB T5H 4B9; Tor'77; FRCSC; Urol. Ac Staff, Royal Alexandra Hospital; Assoc Clin Prof, University of Alberta; (780)990-7086

MADOR, Joseph A; 225-970 Burrard St, Vancouver BC V6Z 2C7; Tor'81; FRCPC; Psy (Adolescent Psychiatry). (604)724-5364; mador@telus.net.

MADORE, Francois; 5400 boul Gouin O, Montreal QC H4J 1C5; Mon'89; MSc; FRCPC; IntMed; Nephrol. Staff, Hôpital du Sacre-Coeur de Montréal; Prof Med, Universite de Montreal; Langs: English; (514)338-2222 x2491; Fax. (514)338-2694.

MADORE, Gervais; Hotel-Dieu de Levis, 143 rue Wolfe, Levis QC G6V 3Z1; Laval'79; Staff, Hôtel-Dieu de Lévis; (418)835-7122

MADORE, Stephanie; Hotel-Dieu de Quebec, 11 Cote du Palais, Quebec QC G1R 2J6; Sher'01; Staff, Hôpital Sainte-croix; Staff, Centre Hospitalier Universitaire de Québec (CHUQ) - Siege Social; (418)525-4444

MADRILEJOS, Jose C B; Oasis Med Centre, 405-9650 Harvest Hills Blvd NE, Calgary AB T3K 0B3; (Philippines)'85; (403)226-8647; Fax. (403)226-8645.

MADRONICH, J Robert; Gates of Maple Med Center, 5-2200 Rutherford Rd, Concord ON L4K 5V2; Wes'85; FRCSC; PlasSurg (Cosmetic Surgery). Staff, Mackenzie Richmond Hill Hospital; Court Staff, Southlake Regional Health Centre; Court Staff, Markham Stouffville Hospital; Langs: Italian; (905)508-1148; Fax. (905)303-6832; info@madronich.com.

MADSEN, Michael F P; Burrard Med Bldg, 450-1144 Burrard St, Vancouver BC V6Z 2A5; London (England)'70; MB BS; LRCP; CCFP; Ac Staff, Providence Health Care - St Paul's Hospital; Langs: Danish; (604)681-9229; Fax. (604)681-2421; madsen@interchg.ubc.ca.

MADU, Ikechukwu S; James Paton Mem Hosp, 125 Trans Canada Hwy, Gander NL A1V 1P7; (Nigeria)'87; MB BS; Staff, James Paton Memorial Hospital; (709)256-5454

MAEHLE, Waldemar M; Workplace Safety & Ins Board, 101-200 Front St W, Toronto ON M5V 3J1; Tor'62; (416)344-4789; Fax. (416)344-6965.

MAEROV, Perry H; 102-1111 Lonsdale Ave, North Vancouver BC V7M 2H4; Alb'69; FRCSC; Ophth (Comprehensive Ophthalmology). Ac Staff, Lions Gate Hospital; Med Dir, London Eye Centre; Clin Assoc Prof Ophth & Med, University of British Columbia; (604)988-1166; Fax. (604)988-0166; pmaerov@nseyes.ca.

MAEROV, Phillip J; Humber River Reg Hosp-Keele, 2175 Keele St, North York ON M6M 3Z4; UBC'96; FRCPC; Psy. Staff, Humber River Regional Hospital - Keele Street Site; (416)249-8111

MAESTRE MENDOZA, Mariam; CSSS Vallee-de-la-Gatineau, 309 boul Desjardins, Maniwaki QC J9E 2E7; Camaguey (Cuba)'95; CCFP; Staff, CSSS de la Vallée de la Gatineau; Langs: Spanish; (819)441-4690

MAGALHAES-GRAVE, Marc-Andre; CHUS-Hop Hotel-Dieu, 580 rue Bowen S, Sherbrooke QC J1G 2E8; Sher'02; FRCSC; OrthSurg. Staff, Centre Hospitalier Universitaire de Sherbrooke-Hôpital Hôtel-Dieu; (819)346-1110

MAGAR, Janice D; CFB Petawawa, 258 Somme Rd, Petawawa ON K8H 2X3; Ott'91; FRCPC; Psy. (613)687-5511

MAGDER, David M; Medical & Dental Centre, 306-586 Eglinton Ave E, Toronto ON M4P 1P2; McG'65; DABPN; FRCPC; Psy (Individual Therapy). Ac Staff Part Time, Centre for Addiction & Mental Health (CAMH) - College Street Site; Asst Prof, University of Toronto; (416)487-1805

MAGDER, Ilana; 114-250 Lawrence Ave W, Toronto ON M5M 1B2; Technion-Israel Institute (Israel)'04; FRCPC; Peds. Staff Ped, William Osler Health System - Etobicoke General Hospital; Langs: French; Hebrew; (416)899-6116; Fax. (416)590-1932; dr.ilanamagder@yahoo.ca.

MAGDER, Sheldon A; MUHC-Royal Victoria Hosp, 687 av des Pins O, Montreal QC H3A 1A1; Tor'74; Critical Care Medicine (P.Q.); Cardiol; IntMed. Dir Critical Care, McGill University Health Centre - Royal Victoria Hospital; Prof, McGill University; Langs: French; (514)843-1664; Fax. (514)843-1686; sheldon.magder@muhc.mcgill.ca.

MAGEAU, Andre; Clinique Medi-Val, 100-408 rue Jeanne-Mance, Salaber-de-Valleyf QC J6T 4G1; Mon'77; LMCC; Langs: English; (450)370-3387; Fax. (450)370-3395; andre.mageau@rrsss16.gouv.qc.ca.

MAGEE, C J Bruce; 170-5 Fairview Mall Dr, North York ON M2J 2Z1; Tor'90; Ac Staff, The Scarborough Hospital - General Campus; Court Staff, Rouge Valley Health System - Centenary Health Centre Site; (416)447-5531; Fax. (416)447-5691.

MAGEE, Gary L; Gary Magee Med Prof Corp, 8188 Yonge St, Thornhill ON L4J 1W5; Tor'65; CCFP; Staff, Mackenzie Richmond Hill Hospital; Staff Community, Markham Stouffville Hospital; Medical Officer Reg Aviation, Transport Canada; (905)889-2222; Fax. (905)889-8534; drmagee@mycybernet.net.

MAGEE, James F; Royal University Hosp, 103 Hospital Dr, Saskatoon SK S7N 0W8; Staff, Royal University Hospital; (306)655-1000

MAGEE, James Fergall; IWK Health Centre, PO Box 9700 Rpo CSC 5850-5980 University Ave, Halifax NS B3K 6R8; Dublin (Ireland)'77; MB ChB; BAO; MRCP(I); FRCPC; AnatPath (Pediatric Pathology). Staff/Assoc Prof Peds & Lab Med, IWK Health Centre; (902)470-8185

MAGEE, Kirk D; Queen Elizabeth II HSC-Halifax, 355-1796 Summer St, Halifax NS B3H 3A7; Dal'95; FRCPC; EmergMed. Staff Emerg, Queen Elizabeth II Health Sciences Centre - Halifax Infirmary Site; Asst Prof, Dalhousie University; (902)473-8564; Fax. (902)473-3617.

MAGEE, Laura A; BC Women's Hosp & Health Ctre, 2H30-4500 Oak St, Vancouver BC V6H 3N1; Tor'88; MSc(ClinEpidem); FRCPC; IntMed (Pregnancy Medical Complications). Staff, BC Women's Hospital & Health Centre; (604)875-3054; lmagee@cw.bc.ca.

MAGEE, Richard E L; Nelson Mental Health Centre, 2F-333 Victoria St, Nelson BC V1L 4K3; Tor'79; FRCPC; Psy. Staff, Kootenay Lake General Hospital; Staff, Kootenay Boundary Regional Hospital; Staff, Nelson Mental Health Centre; (250)505-7248

MAGEE, Robert A; Niagara H System-Welland Site, 65 Third St, Welland ON L3B 4W6; McM'79; RT; BSc; MSc; Staff, Niagara Health System - Welland Hospital Site; (905)732-6111

MAGEE-ADAMS, Kelly M A; Harbour View Med Clinic, 43 Court St N, Thunder Bay ON P7A 4T5; Ott'00; CCFP; (807)343-0300; Fax. (807)346-8687.

MAGENNIS, W Terrence; Kings County Med Centre, PO Box 817, Montague PE C0A 1R0; Dal'85; Staff, Kings County Memorial Hospital; (902)838-4673; Fax. (902)838-2758; terdor@eastlink.ca.

MAGERMAN, Eugene W A; 250-8730 Country Hills Blvd NW, Calgary AB T3G 0E2; (South Africa)'97; MB ChB; Lead Physician, Oasis Medical Clinics; Langs: Afrikaans; Zulu; (403)262-7787

MAGERMAN, Moira P Z; Oasis Med Clinic, 216-8338 18 St SE, Calgary AB T2C 4E4; (South Africa)'96; (403)236-2344

MAGGI, Julie D; St Michael's Hosp, 17 033-30 Bond St, Toronto ON M5B 1W8; McM'97; MSc; FRCPC; Psy (HIV Psychiatry). Staff, St Michael's Hospital; (416)864-3082; Fax. (416)864-3091.

MAGGIO, Frederick J; Workplace Hlth & Public Safety, 1817-1505 Barrington St, Halifax NS B3J 3K5; McM'81; LMCC; (902)426-3998; Fax. (902)426-5375; fred_maggio@hc-sc.gc.ca.

MAGGISANO, Robert; Sunnybrook Hlth Sciences Ctre, H185-2075 Bayview Ave, Toronto ON M4N 3M5; Tor'74; FACS; FRCSC; GenSurg; VascSurg. Staff VascSurg, Sunnybrook Health Sciences Centre; Assoc Prof, University of Toronto; (416)480-4737; Fax. (416)480-5815.

MAGGISANO, Stephanie N; 9-140 Woodbridge Ave, Woodbridge ON L4L 4K9; McM'09; CCFP; (905)850-0753

MAGHARIOUS, Lucy N; 201-4800 Leslie St, North York ON M2J 2K9; CCFP; Langs: Arabic; (416)491-2270

MAGI, Enzio; 102-7 Glenbrook Pl SW, Calgary AB T3E 6W4; Tor'71; FRCSC; PlasSurg (Hand & Wrist Surgery). Asst Prof, University of Calgary; (403)571-3130; Fax. (403)571-3133.

MAGIER, Michael G; Slocan Comm Health Center, 403 Galena Ave, New Denver BC V0G 1S0; Indiana(IN) (USA)'96; CCFP; GP, Slocan Community Health Centre; (250)358-7911; mmagier@cw.bc.ca.

MAGIL, Alexander B; St Paul's Hosp, 1081 Burrard St, Vancouver BC V6Z 1Y6; Qns'69; FRCPC; AnatPath (Nephropathology). Staff Lab, Providence Health Care - St Paul's Hospital; Prof Path, University of British Columbia; (604)806-8700; Fax. (604)806-8701; amagil@providencehealth.bc.ca.

MAGILL, Chandra A; 4018 rue Sainte-Catherine O, Westmount QC H3Z 1P2; Alb'00; FRCPC; Psy. Staff, McGill University Health Centre - Montreal Children's Hospital; (514)412-4449

MAGIN, Daniel; CSSS d'Argenteuil, 145 av de la Providence, Lachute QC J8H 4C7; McG'05; Anes. Staff, Centre Hospitalier d'Argenteuil; (450)562-3761 x4181

MAGLIOCCO, Anthony M; Tom Baker Cancer Centre, 1331 29 St NW, Calgary AB T2N 4N2; Alb'87; FRCPC; AnatPath. Dir Path, Tom Baker Cancer Centre; Assoc Prof, University of Calgary; (403)521-3073

MAGLIOCCO, Maria; The Medical Centre FHT, PO Box 4200 Stn Main 707 Charlotte St, Peterborough ON K9J 7B3; Tor'89; (705)740-0947; Fax. (705)740-8391.

MAGLOIRE, Patrick M; Hamilton HS-General Site, 520-237 Barton St E, Hamilton ON L8L 2K2; Univ La Salle Escuela (Mexico)'95; Staff, Hamilton Health Sciences Centre - Hamilton General Hospital; Asst Prof, McMaster University; Langs: Spanish; (905)527-4322 x44252; Fax. (905)577-1490; rosane.milliken@phri.ca.

MAGNAN, Anne; PAMQ-Prog Aide Med Quebec, 200-1 boul Rene-Levesque E, Montreal QC H2X 3Z5; Sher'86; (514)397-0888; Fax. (514)397-0654.

MAGNAN, Bernard; CHSLD de la MRC de Champlain, 831 av Notre-Dame, Saint-Lambert QC J4R 1S1; Mon'74; Staff, CHSLD de la MRC de Champlain-Centre Saint-Lambert; (450)672-3320; bernard.magnan@rrsss16.gouv.qc.ca.

MAGNAN, Francine; Clinique De Radiol Chomedey In, 610 boul Cure-Labelle, Laval QC H7V 2T7; Mon'75; DiagRad. Staff, Centre Hospitalier de Granby; (450)472-4250

MAGNAN, Johanne; CSSS de Laval, 1755 boul Rene-Laennec, Laval QC H7M 3L9; Mon'77; Staff, Hopital de la Cite de la santé; adj Prof, Universite de Montreal; (450)975-5444

MAGNAN, Michel C E; Worker's Compensation Board, PO Box 2145 Stn Main 9912 107 St NW, Edmonton AB T5J 2S5; Alb'85; Consultant, Workers' Comp Board of AB; (780)498-3999

MAGNAN, Michel; CSSS de la Region de Thetford, 1717 rue Notre-Dame E, Thetford Mines QC G6G 2V4; Laval'74; GenSurg. Staff, Hopital du CSS de la Region de Thetford; (418)338-7777; Fax. (418)338-7794.

MAGNAN, Pierre-Etienne; Clinique Med Fontainebleau, 102-10 boul des Chaôteaux, Sainte-Therese QC J7B 1Z5; Mon'99; CCFP; Staff, Hôpital de Saint-Eustache; (450)419-8811

MAGNAN, Renee; Bureau Dr Magnan, 1621 ch Chilerhouse, Dunham QC J0E 1M0; Mon'76; Staff, Hôpital Brome-Missisquoi-Perkins; (450)260-1936

MAGNANI, Lucia B; 17910 rue Antoine-Faucon, Pierrefonds QC H9K 1L2; McG'84; FRCPC; Peds (Neonatology). Langs: Italian; French; (514)624-2441; Fax. (514)624-0176.

MAGNAYE, Arturo D; Valley View Centre, PO Box 1300 Stn Main, Moose Jaw SK S6H 4R2; (Philippines)'64; (306)694-3122; Fax. (306)694-3003.

MAGNAYE, Joyce M; Town & Country Mall Med Clinic, 1235 Main St N, Moose Jaw SK S6H 6M4; Southwestern (Philippines)'64; MD; Staff, Moose Jaw Union Hospital; Langs: Tagalog; (306)693-4101; Fax. (306)692-6533.

MAGNER, Peter O; The Ottawa Hosp-Riverside, 511-1967 Riverside Dr, Ottawa ON K1H 7W9; Ott'78; FRACP; FRCPC; IntMed; Nephrol. Staff Nephrol, The Ottawa Hospital - Riverside Campus; Assoc Prof, University of Ottawa; (613)738-8400 x82512; Fax. (613)738-8337; pmagner@ottawahospital.on.ca.

MAGNOUX, Eric; Centre Medicale Roy, 281 rue Roy E, Montreal QC H2W 1M7; Mon'83; Langs: Bilingual(French/English); (514)499-0986; Fax. (514)499-9419.

MAGNUS, Kenneth G; Cross Cancer Institute, 11560 University Ave NW, Edmonton AB T6G 1Z2; Cape Town (South Africa)'70; MB ChB; Staff, Cross Cancer Institute; (780)432-8771

MAGNUSON, Paul H; 440 Comer St, Williams Lake BC V2G 1T7; UBC'88; Staff, Cariboo Memorial Hospital and Health Centre; Staff, Vancouver Island Health Authority; (250)398-8499; Fax. (250)398-8692; paul_magnuson@telus.net.

MAGNUSON, William H; Trillium Hlth Ctr-Mississauga, 100 Queensway W, Mississauga ON L5B 1B8; Tor'83; FRCPC; DiagRad. Staff Diag Imaging, Trillium Health Centre - Mississauga; (905)848-7529; Fax. (905)848-7676.

MAGNY, Jacqueline; CSSS de l'Hématite, GD 1 rue de l'Aquilon, Fermont QC G0G 1J0; Laval'86; Staff, CLSC de l'Hématite; (418)287-5461

MAGOR, Graeme F; 885 Sand Pines Dr, Comox BC V9M 3V3; McG'81; DOHS(McM); Langs: Bilingual(English/French); (855)778-8507; Fax. (855)778-8507.

MAGOWN, John D; CSSS Haut-Richelieu-Rouville, 920 boul Du Seminaire N, St-Jean-Sur-Richel QC J3A 1B7; Mon'71; AnatPath. ac Staff Path, Hôpital du Haut-Richelieu; (450)359-5000 x5200

MAGRABI, Hamdi H; Gander Med Clinic, 177 Elizabeth St, Gander NL A1V 1H6; Al-Fateh (Libya)'83; MB BCh; (709)256-7101

MAGSI, Noorullah; 204-10458 Mayfield Rd NW, Edmonton AB T5P 4P4; (Pakistan)'93; MB BS; (780)483-7115; Fax. (780)484-6531.

MAGUIRE, Anna-Marie L; 4739 Joyce Ave, Powell River BC V8A 3B5; Alb'86; BSc; Staff, Powell River General Hospital; (604)485-9866; Fax. (604)485-9836.

MAGUIRE, Anne-Marie D; 2923 66 St NW, Edmonton AB T6K 4C1; National (Ireland)'70; MB ChB; BAO; (780)482-1008

MAGUIRE, Conor G J; Health Sciences Centre, 300 Prince Phillip Dr, St. John's NL A1B 3V6; Mem'81; FRCPC; DiagRad; NuclearMed. Staff, Health Sciences Centre; (709)777-6300

MAGUIRE, Douglas S; Health Sciences Centre, 820 Sherbrook St, Winnipeg MB R3A 1R9; Man'82; FRCPC; Anes (Cardiac Anesthesia). Dir Pre-Admission Program, Health Sciences Centre; Asst Prof, University of Manitoba; (204)774-8511

MAGUIRE, Gerard H; Lakeridge Hlth Corp-Oshawa, 1 Hospital Crt, Oshawa ON L1G 2B9; McG'54; BSc; FRCPC; DiagRad; RadOncol. Staff Radiol, Lakeridge Health - Oshawa Site; (905)433-4305; Fax. (905)721-4770.

MAGUIRE, Hugh P; Colchester East Hants Hlth Ctr, 600 Abenaki Rd, Truro NS B2N 5A1; Mem'92; FRCPC; Psy. Staff, Colchester East Hants Health Centre; (902)893-5526

MAGUIRE, John A C; Vancouver Gen Hosp, 855 12th Ave W, Vancouver BC V5Z 1M9; National (Ireland)'82; MB ChB; BAO; FRCPC; AnatPath; NeurPath. Staff, Vancouver General Hospital - Centennial Pavillion; Langs: French; (604)875-4577; jmaguire@vanhosp.bc.ca.

MAGUIRE, Jonathon L; Paediatric Ambulatory Clinic, 2F-61 Queen St E, Toronto ON M5C 2T2; Tor'03; FRCPC; Peds. (416)867-3655

MAGUIRE, Nancy S; 1221 17 Ave NW, Calgary AB T2M 0P9; London (England)'52; MB BS; LRCP; MRCS(Eng); CCFP; FCFP; Ac Staff, Bethany Care Centre; Court Staff, Foothills Medical Centre; Ac Staff, Care West; (403)289-2501; Fax. (403)289-2508.

MAGUIRE, Robert; ASSS Bas-Saint-Laurent, 288 rue Pierre-Saindon, Rimouski QC G5L 9A8; Laval'71; CommunMed (P.Q.). Staff, Hôpital Regional Rimouski; Dir Public Health, Regie Regionale du Bas St-Laurent; (418)724-8138

MAGUIRE, Thomas; Pleasantview Prof Bldg, 206-11044 51 Ave NW, Edmonton AB T6H 5B4; Dublin (Ireland)'71; MB ChB; BAO; (780)434-7335; Fax. (780)434-0437.

MAGWOOD, Bryan D; Health Sciences Centre, AE404-820 Sherbrook St, Winnipeg MB R3A 1R9; McM'89; BSc(Hons.); FRCPC; Peds (Pediatric Intensive Care); Critical Care Medicine. Dir, Health Sciences Centre; Teach Staff, University of Manitoba; Langs: English; French; (204)774-6511

MAH, Catherine L; Addiction & Mental Hlth-ARF, 33 Russell St, Toronto ON M5S 2S1; Cal'98; FRCPC; Peds. Staff, Centre for Addiction & Mental Health (CAMH) - Russell Street Site; (416)535-8501; Fax. (416)595-6068.

MAH, Dean; 10565 124 St NW, Edmonton AB T5N 1R8; Ott'02; FRCSC; Ophth (Cornea). Clinical Asst Prof, University of Alberta; (780)432-1261; Fax. (780)433-2247.

MAH, Douglas W; First Med Place, 206-170 Queensway W, Mississauga ON L5B 3A8; Tor'92; Ac Staff Family Pract, Trillium Health Centre - Mississauga; (905)281-2642; Fax. (905)281-2539.

MAH, Elaine; Langley Obstetrics & Gyn, 21561 Old Yale Rd, Langley BC V3A 4M9; UBC'87; BSc; FRCSC; ObstGyn (Colposcopy). Clin Associate, BC Cancer Agency Vancouver Centre; Clin Instructor, University of British Columbia; Langs: Cantonese; (604)534-4441; Fax. (604)534-4491.

MAH, Franky; Exeter Clinic, PO Box 879, 100 Mile House BC V0K 2E0; UBC'98; BSc; CCFP; (250)395-2271; Fax. (250)395-2599.

MAH, Gordon K; 201-111 Main St W, North Bay ON P1B 2T6; Tor'95; CCFP; CCFP(E.M.); Staff, North Bay Regional Health Centre - Regional Mental Health; (705)475-1052

MAH, Jean K; Alberta Children's Hosp, 2888 Shaganappi Trail NW, Calgary AB T3B 6A8; Alb'86; FRCPC; Peds; Neur. Staff Ped Neurol, Alberta Children's Hospital; (403)955-7602; Fax. (403)955-7609; jean.mah@calgaryhealthregion.ca.

MAH, John F; Victoria Med Clinic, 204-1669 Victoria St, Prince George BC V2L 2L5; Alb'92; BScEngineering; CCFP; Staff Family Med, University Hospital of Northern British Columbia; Clin Associate, University of British Columbia; (250)562-2776

MAH, Johnny P; Chaparral Med Clinic, 216-10 Chaparral Dr SE, Calgary AB T2X 3R7; Sask'93; CCFP; (403)201-3003; Fax. (403)201-3009.

MAH, Jung Y; 674 Upper James St, Hamilton ON L9C 2Z6; Qns'75; FRCSC; OrthSurg (Pediatric Orthopedics). Staff, Hamilton Health Sciences Centre - McMaster Children's Hospital; Clin Prof OrthSurg, McMaster University; (905)575-3600; Fax. (905)575-1779.

MAH, K Bill; Mount Sinai Hosp, 9F-600 University Ave, Toronto ON M5G 1X5; UBC'98; FRCPC; Psy. Staff, Mount Sinai Hospital; Staff Psy, Centre for Addiction & Mental Health (CAMH) - College Street Site; (416)586-4800 x4549

MAH, Kevin A; Athabascan Place, 210-80 Chippewa Rd, Sherwood Park AB T8A 4W6; Alb'01; CCFP; (780)464-6300; Fax. (780)464-2120.

MAH, Larry K; Tillicum Med Clinic, 14-3170 Tillicum Rd, Victoria BC V9A 7C5; UBC'91; (250)381-8112

MAH, Leevin; 2951 Walker's Line, Burlington ON L7M 4Y1; Tor'99; CCFP; (905)336-9630; Fax. (905)336-9626.

MAH, Linda; Baycrest Ctre/Geriatric Care, 738-3560 Bathurst St, Toronto ON M6A 2E1; Cal'94; FRCPC; Psy. Staff Brain Health Complex, Baycrest Centre for Geriatric Care; (416)785-4230

MAH, Marian; 134-9450 137 Ave NW, Edmonton AB T5E 6C2; Alb'82; FRCPC; DiagRad. (780)478-7221

MAH, May Sue; 17703 98A Ave NW, Edmonton AB T5T 5W8; Alb'77; FRCSC; ObstGyn. (780)489-9730; Fax. (780)481-5086.

MAH, Michael; Milliken Finch X-Ray, LL-4040 Finch Ave E, Scarborough ON M1S 4V5; Tor'81; FRCPC; DiagRad. Staff, Rouge Valley Health System - Centenary Health Centre Site; Staff, The Scarborough Hospital - Birchmount Campus; (416)292-1505

MAH, Michael K; Riverside Med Clinic, 121-4411 16 Ave NW, Calgary AB T3B 0M3; Alb'94; BSc; CCFP; Langs: Cantonese; French; (403)247-6966; Fax. (403)247-6838.

MAH, Nancy E; Ermineskin Med Clinic, 301-2377 111 St NW, Edmonton AB T6J 5E5; Alb'89; (780)436-8731; Fax. (780)434-8732.

MAH, Norman A; Halton HCS Corp-Georgetown, 1 Princess Anne Dr, Georgetown ON L7G 2B8; Wes'00; BSc; CCFP; Staff, Halton Healthcare Services Corporation - Georgetown Hospital; (905)873-0111

MAH, Peter G; 203-475 Main St, Vancouver BC V6A 2T7; UBC'87; (604)251-4511

MAH, Peter; CSSSG-Hop de Hull, 116 boul. Lionel-Émond, Gatineau QC J8Y 1W7; McG'95; CCFP; FCFP; Staff, Hull Hospital; Langs: Bilingual(French/English); Spanish; (819)966-6200; mahpet@videotron.ca.

MAH, Peter; Piper Creek Med Clinic, 200-3215 49 Ave, Red Deer AB T4N 0M8; Alb'81; Physician, Associate Medical Group; (403)986-7265; Fax. (403)986-7604.

MAH, Phillip; 3A-747 Don Mills Rd, North York ON M3C 1T2; Tor'91; CCFP; (416)423-6000; Fax. (416)423-7000.

MAH, Richard; 1611 Bloor St W, Toronto ON M6P 1A6; Tor'74; (416)536-3750; Fax. (416)537-2688.

MAH, Rick H; St Mary's Hosp Centre, 3830 av Lacombe, Montreal QC H3T 1M5; Alb'92; CCFP; CCFP(E.M.); FCFP; Staff, St Mary's Hospital Centre; (514)345-3511; Fax. (514)934-8421.

MAH, Stanley M; Richard Smyth Med Serv Inc, 303-2963 Glen Dr, Coquitlam BC V3B 2P7; UBC'91; FRCSC; Otol. Staff, Eagle Ridge Hospital & Health Care Centre; (604)941-8474; Fax. (604)941-2455.

MAH, Stanley W; Grandview Heights Med Clinic, 12313 63 Ave NW, Edmonton AB T6H 1R4; Alb'87; CCFP; (780)437-1968; Fax. (780)438-4395.

MAH, Stephanie G; Shell Canada Ltd, PO Box 100 Stn M 400 4 Ave SW, Calgary AB T2P 2H5; Cal'88; CCFP; (403)691-2897; Fax. (403)691-3125.

MAH, Venetia S J; The Doctor's Office, 101-777 Broadway W, Vancouver BC V5Z 4J7; UBC'09; CCFP; (604)734-8252

MAH, Weiling G; 314-3980 Shelbourne St PO Box 31110, Victoria BC V8N 6J1; UBC'05; CCFP; (778)977-2307

MAH-POY, George L; Petro Canada Centre, 240-111 5 Ave SW, Calgary AB T2P 3Y6; Alb'66; DABD; FRCPC; Derm. (403)269-3300; Fax. (403)269-3305.

MAH-POY, Kimberly; St Michael's Health Centre, 7F-61 Queen St E, Toronto ON M5C 2T2; Tor'99; BSc; FRCPC; IntMed; Endocrin&Metab. Staff, St Michael's Hospital; (416)867-7424

MAHABIR, Vishwanath K; McMaster Univ Gilmour Hall, 20-1280 Main St W, Hamilton ON L8S 4K1; McM'08; IntMed.

MAHADEVA, Ranjith; Stirling Med Centre, RR 4 9C Tuftsville Rd, Stirling ON K0K 3E0; (Grenada)'94; BSc; CCFP; (613)395-5566; Fax. (613)395-3636.

MAHADEVAN, Varagunan; Toronto Street Med Centre, 202-29 Toronto St S, Uxbridge ON L9P 1V9; Chingleput (India)'91; CCFP; Langs: Sinhalese; Tamil; (905)852-3339; Fax. (905)852-9151.

MAHADOO, Jaysen; Lansdowne Med Centre, 120-1641 Hillside Ave, Victoria BC V8T 5G1; Sask'88; MSc; PhD(Physiol); Langs: English; French; (250)592-4212; Fax. (250)592-6060; drjm7@hotmail.com.

MAHAFFEY, Murray E; 198 Roxton Dr, Waterloo ON N2T 1N8; Tor'71; Anes. Staff, Grand River Hospital - Kitchener/Waterloo Health Centre; Staff, St Mary's General Hospital; (519)746-1192

MAHAJAN, Ashish; Univ of Toronto, 2F-500 University Ave, Toronto ON M5G 1V7; Alb'07; DiagRad.

MAHAJAN, Sushma; Westgrove Medicentre, 10232 142 St NW, Edmonton AB T5N 2N8; Meerut (India)'76; MB BS; LMCC; CCFP; Physician, Millcreek Medicentre; (780)452-0281

MAHALINGHAM, Aisling M; 144-1402 8 Ave NW, Calgary AB T2N 1B9; Alb'99; FRCSC; ObstGyn. Staff ObstGyn, Foothills Medical Centre; (403)289-8974; Fax. (403)289-8956.

MAHALLATI, Houman; EFW Radiology, 310-215 16 St SE, Calgary AB T2P 3C5; Cal'93; FRCPC; DiagRad. Staff Diag Imaging, Foothills Medical Centre; (403)284-0230; Fax. (403)210-8399.

MAHAM, Nava; Trillium Hlth Ctr-Mississauga, 100 Queensway W, Mississauga ON L5B 1B8; Tor'99; FRCPC; IntMed; Critical Care Medicine; Respir. Staff, Trillium Health Centre - Mississauga; (905)848-7663

MAHANEY JR., Gordon R; Rapha Med Centre, 8-50 Tacoma Dr, Dartmouth NS B2W 3E6; Dal'72; BSc; (902)465-3202; Fax. (902)465-3172.

MAHANT, Sanjay; The Hosp for Sick Children, 555 University Ave, Toronto ON M5G 1X8; Tor'95; FRCPC; Peds. Staff Peds, The Hospital For Sick Children; (416)813-5280; Fax. (416)813-8345; sanjay.mahant@sickkids.ca.

MAHAR, Robert K; Halifax Prof Centre, 585-5991 Spring Garden Rd, Halifax NS B3H 1Y6; Mem'77; FRCPC; PhysMed&Rehab (Musculoskeletal Injury). Court Staff, Queen Elizabeth II Health Sciences Centre - Victoria General Site; Assoc Staff, St Martha's Regional Hospital; (902)422-5884; Fax. (902)425-6388.

MAHARAJ, Ashwin R; 7750 Bayview Av, Thornhill ON L3T 4A3; Royal College of Surgeons (Ireland)'91; BSc; DABS; MD; FACS; Staff Surgeon, Shouldice Hospital; Staff Surgeon, Digestive Health Clinic; (905)707-5007; Fax. (905)707-5008; ashwinmaharaj@sympatico.ca.

MAHARAJ, Damien D; Abbotsford Reg Hosp & Cancer C, 32900 Marshall Rd, Abbotsford BC V2S 1K2; Wes'93; BSc; FRCPC; CCFP; NuclearMed. Staff, Abbotsford Regional Hospital & Cancer Centre; (604)851-4700 x64660

MAHARAJ, Deonarine; 925 Wonderland Rd S, London ON N6K 3R5; National (Ireland)'66; (519)641-6081

MAHARAJ, Gunness R; Crestview Med Clinic, 3004 Portage Ave, Winnipeg MB R3K 0X8; Dal'65; CCFP; FCFP; Med Advisor, Workers' Comp Board of MB; (204)888-0999; Fax. (204)831-7346.

MAHARAJ, Ian G; Crestview Medical Clinic, 3004 Portage Ave, Winnipeg MB R3K 0X8; Man'91; BSc(Med); Att Physician/Consultant, WRHA - Deer Lodge Centre; (204)888-0999; Fax. (204)831-7346.

MAHARAJ, Jaimala; Alpen Med Clinic, 346 Railway St W, Cochrane AB T4C 2E2; Andhra (India)'96; MB BS; (403)851-0091

MAHARAJ, Mandat; Cape Breton Hlthcare Complex, 1482 George St, Sydney NS B1P 1P3; West Indies (Jamaica)'78; MB BS; FRCPC; Neur. Staff, Cape Breton Healthcare Complex; (902)567-7917; Fax. (902)567-8053.

MAHARAJ, Mitra G; Dr MG Maharaj Inc, 206-22314 Fraser Hwy, Langley BC V3A 8M6; UBC'99; FRCSC; Otol. Pres/Medical Staff/Chief Surgery, Langley Memorial Hospital; (604)530-9802; Fax. (604)530-9807.

MAHARAJ, Neil; Sault Area Hosp, 750 Great Northern Rd, Sault Ste. Marie ON P6B 0A8; Ott'03; FRCPC; IntMed; Respir. Staff, Sault Area Hospital - Sault Ste Marie; (705)759-3434

MAHARAJ, Siobhan C; Westmount Med Walk-In Clinic, 925 Wonderland Rd S, London ON N6K 3R5; Wes'99; CCFP; (519)641-6081

MAHARAJ, Usha; Athabaska Place, 210-80 Chippewa Rd, Sherwood Park AB T8A 4W6; Alb'96; BSc; CCFP; Langs: English; French; (780)464-6300; Fax. (780)464-2120.

MAHARAJH, Gyaandeo S; Children's Hosp Eastern Ont, 3340-401 Smyth Rd, Ottawa ON K1H 8L1; McG'90; BSc; MSc; FRCSC; CardSurg (Adult Cardiac Surgery). Staff Cardiac Surg, University of Ottawa Heart Institute; A-Chief Cardiovascular Surg, Children's Hospital of Eastern Ontario (CHEO); Asst Prof, University of Ottawa; Langs: Hindi; Punjabi; Urdu; (613)738-3257; Fax. (613)738-4835; gmaharajh@cheo.on.ca.

MAHARAJH, Kamla; Royal Court Med Centre, 201-1 Quarry Ridge Rd, Barrie ON L4M 7G1; McM'94; FRCSC; GenSurg (Breasts). Ac Staff, Royal Victoria Regional Health Centre; (705)720-2003; Fax. (705)720-2109.

MAHARAJH, Sastri N; 103-2686 The Collegeway, Mississauga ON L5L 2M9; Tor'85; CCFP; FCFP; (905)569-2000; Fax. (905)569-2030.

MAHAY, Raj K; RKM Walk-In Clinic & Med Ctr, 14-1030 Keewatin St, Winnipeg MB R2R 2E2; Amritsar (India)'81; MB BS; Langs: Punjabi; Hindi; (204)697-0333; Fax. (204)697-0333; rkmjason@hotmail.com.

MAHDAVIAN, Fereydoun; 4255 av Papineau, Montreal QC H2H 2P6; Meched (Iran)'61; (514)526-4981

MAHDAVIFAR, Alireza; Prairie North Health Centre, 4806 50 St, Lloydminster SK S9V 0M9; (306)820-5997

MAHDI, Gamal E M; IWK Health Centre, PO Box 9700 Rpo CSC 5850-5980 University Ave, Halifax NS B3K 6R8; Ain Shams (Egypt)'74; MB BCh; Staff PEds, IWK Health Centre; (902)470-8888

MAHDI, Hayder T; 28-5353 Lakeshore Rd, Burlington ON L7L 1C8; Baghdad (Iraq)'87; CCFP; Langs: Arabic; (905)681-6640; Fax. (905)681-9213.

MAHDI, Rafid; Dr G B Cross Mem Hosp, 67 Manitoba Dr, Clarenville NL A5A 1K3; Al-Mustansiriyah (Iraq)'96; MB ChB; CCFP; Staff, The Dr G B Cross Memorial Hospital; (709)466-3411

MAHDI, Tahseen; Flin Flon Clinic, PO Box 340, Flin Flon MB R8A 1N2; Baghdad (Iraq)'95; Gen Practice, Flin Flon General Hospital Inc; (204)687-7591

MAHDY, Ibtihaj; Brookfield Bonnews HC Centre, PO Box 209 57 Main St, Brookfield NL A0G 1J0; Basra (Iraq)'83; MB ChB; Staff, Brookfield Bonnews Health Care Centre; (709)536-2405

MAHENDIRA, Chanmugam S S; 5560 McAdam Rd, Mississauga ON L4Z 1P1; Ceylon (Sri Lanka)'75; MB BS; LMSSA(Lond); LMCC; CCFP; (905)273-6895

MAHENDIRA, Dharini; St Michael's Hosp, 3 002B-30 Bond St, Toronto ON M5B 1W8; Tor'06; FRCPC; IntMed; Rheum. Staff, St Michael's Hospital; (416)864-5295

MAHENDRARAJAH, Ranjini; PO Box 260, Guysborough NS B0H 1N0; Jaffna (Sri Lanka)'88; MB BS; CCFP; Fam Med, Guysborough Memorial Hospital; (902)533-4040; Fax. (902)533-2040; justely7@hotmail.com.

MAHER, Daniel L; Royal Inland Hospital, 311 Columbia St, Kamloops BC V2C 2T1; UBC'81; Anes. Staff, Royal Inland Hospital; (250)314-2620

MAHER, Daniel T; 208-194 Main St, Ottawa ON K1S 1C2; McG'89; (613)233-7953

MAHER, Deviani; West Community Health Centre, 241-2121 Marine Dr, West Vancouver BC V7V 4Y2; Alb'94; BSc; BA; FRCPC; IntMed; GeriatricMed. Med Dir Transitional Care Unit, Lions Gate Hospital; Med Dir, Cedar View Lodge; Langs: Gujarati; (604)904-6200 x4112; deviani.maher@vch.ca.

MAHER, John; Atrium Prof Bldg, SS 103 304-190 Cundles Rd E, Barrie ON L4M 4S5; Dublin (Ireland)'84; MB ChB; BAO; MRC(1); FRCPC; Neur. Staff Neurol, Royal Victoria Regional Health Centre; (705)721-1060; Fax. (905)721-2442.

MAHER, John T; Outreach Service, 204-349A George St N, Peterborough ON K9H 3P9; McM'95; FRCPC; Psy. Staff, Ontario Shores Centre for Mental Health Sciences; Staff, Northumberland Hills Hospital; Langs: English; French; (705)742-9022; Fax. (705)742-1941.

MAHER, Lauren H; Yarmouth Reg Hosp, 60 Vancouver St, Yarmouth NS B5A 2P5; Dal'05; CCFP; Staff, Yarmouth Regional Hospital; (902)742-3541

MAHER, Neal P; Peter Lougheed Centre, 3500 26 Ave NE, Calgary AB T1Y 6J4; Sask'95; FRCPC; Anes. Med Staff, Peter Lougheed Centre; (403)943-5554; Fax. (403)943-4474.

MAHER, Terrence M; Deer Lake Clinic, 1-4 Clinic Dr, Deer Lake NL A8A 1E2; Mem'85; (709)635-5150

MAHER-LAPORTE, Valerie; 204B-860 Mountain Rd, Moncton NB E1C 2N7; Sher'10; CCFP; (506)853-5176

MAHESAN, Dhakshana; Grand River Hosp-KW Hlth Ctre, PO Box 9056 Stn C 835 King St W, Kitchener ON N2G 1G3; McM'90; Staff, Grand River Hospital - Kitchener/Waterloo Health Centre; (519)749-4242; Fax. (519)749-4285.

MAHESAN, Glory S; 203-3852 Finch Ave E, Scarborough ON M1T 3T9; Colombo (Sri Lanka)'79; MB BS; LRCP(Ed); CCFP; (416)321-6699; Fax. (416)321-1105.

MAHESAN, Sivagnanam; 203-3852 Finch Ave E, Scarborough ON M1T 3T9; Colombo (Sri Lanka)'79; MB BS; LRCP(Ed); LRCS(Edin); CCFP.

MAHESHWARI, Anil K; Grandview Med Ctr Fam Hlth Team, 167 Hespeler Rd, Cambridge ON N1R 3H7; New Jersey (USA)'97; (519)623-4200; Fax. (519)623-2546.

MAHESHWARI, Ekta; Mount Sinai Hosp, 568-600 University Ave, Toronto ON M5G 1X5; Jiwaji (India)'97; Staff, Mount Sinai Hospital; (416)586-4800

MAHESHWARI, Perkash; 5966 Mullen Way NW, Edmonton AB T6R 0S9; (Pakistan)'93; MB BS; CCFP; (780)801-1220

MAHESWARAN, Charuka V; Port McNeill Med Clinic, PO Box 14 2161 McNeill Rd, Port McNeill BC V0N 2R0; Newcastle-Upon-Tyne (England)'00; MB BS; (250)956-3377

MAHEU, Benoit; Clinique Med Lanaudiere, 222 rue Bernard, St-Charles-Brromee QC J6E 2C5; Laval'08; CCFP; (450)755-1033

MAHEU, Marie-Lise; CSSS de Saint-Jerome, 290 rue de Montigny, Saint-Jerome QC J7Z 5T3; Laval'84; FRCPC; Psy. Staff, Hôtel-Dieu de Saint-Jérôme; (450)431-8391; Fax. (450)431-8305.

MAHEU, Michel; CSSS du Sud de Lanaudière, 911 montee des Pionniers, Terrebonne QC J6V 2H2; Sher'74; FRCPC; IntMed; MedOncol (P.Q.); HemPath. ac Staff, Centre Hospitalier Pierre le Gardeur; (450)654-7525

MAHEUX, Brigitte; Univ De Montreal, CP 6128 Succ Centre Ville, Montreal QC H3C 3J7; Sher'72; PhD; MPH; Prof, Universite de Montreal; (514)343-6139

MAHEUX, Claude; Ctr Hosp Affilie-Enfant-Jesus, 1401 18e rue, Quebec QC G1J 1Z4; Laval'74; MSc; Staff, Centre Hospitalier Affilié Universitaire de Québec - Hôpital De L'Enfant Jésus; Université Laval; (418)649-0252; Fax. (418)649-5811.

MAHEUX, Pierre; CHUS-Hop Fleurimont, 3001 12e Av N, Sherbrooke QC J1H 5N4; Sher'86; FRCPC; IntMed (Diabetology); Endocrin (P.Q.); Endocrin&Metab. Staff, Centre Hospitalier Universitaire de Sherbrooke-Hopital Fleurimont; (819)564-5241; Fax. (819)564-5292.

MAHFOUD, Georges; Clinique Med Viau, 204-4750 rue Jarry E, Saint-Leonard QC H1R 1X8; St. Joseph (Lebanon)'69; LMCC; Langs: English; Arabic; (514)326-7203; Fax. (514)326-3656.

MAHFOUDI, Redha; PO Box 580 Stn Chatham, Miramichi NB E1N 3A8; (Algeria)'89; Psy. (506)623-3000

MAHFUD, Ahmed S; Northern Lights Health Region, 7 Hospital St, Fort McMurray AB T9H 1P2; Al Fateh (Libya)'93; FRCPC; DiagRad. Staff, Yorkton Regional Health Centre; (780)788-1723; Fax. (780)788-1362.

MAHIL, Neelam; Edmonton Oliver PCN, 10155 120 St NW, Edmonton AB T5K 2A2; Alb'00; FRCPC; Psy (Women's Mental Health). Staff, Royal Alexandra Hospital; Langs: Punjabi; (780)701-5545

MAHIM, Ardavan; The Medical Centre, PO Box 4200 Stn Main 707 Charlotte St, Peterborough ON K9J 7B3; (Montserrat)'95; MSc; FACC; FRCPC; IntMed; Cardiol. Staff Cardiologist, Peterborough Regional Health Centre - Hospital Drive; Staff Cardiologist, Campbellford Memorial Hospital; (705)876-4600

MAHINRAD-NATEGHI, Jinoos; CSSS Vallee-de-la-Gatineau, 309 boul Desjardins, Maniwaki QC J9E 2E7; Paris (France)'96; Staff, CSSS de la Vallée de la Gatineau; (819)449-4690

MAHLASE, Ephraim M; Everest Med Clinic, 121 14 St NW, Calgary AB T2N 1Z6; Medunsa (South Africa)'95; MB ChB.

MAHLER, Ronald H; Thunder Bay Med Centre, 320-63 Algoma St N, Thunder Bay ON P7A 4Z6; McG'81; FRCPC; Derm. Staff, St Joseph's Care Group - St Joseph's Hospital; Staff, Thunder Bay Regional Health Sciences Centre Port-Arthur; Staff, Thunder Bay Regional Health Sciences Centre; (807)343-9005

MAHMOOD, Adeel; 80 Catherine St, Trenton ON K8V 6N8; Wes'09; CCFP.

MAHMOOD, Arshad; Aspen Med Centre, 21-429 Tranquille Rd, Kamloops BC V2B 3G9; Punjabi (Pakistan)'94; MB BS; (250)376-7242

MAHMOOD, Bann N; Strait of Belle Isle Hlth Care, PO Box 59, Flowers Cove NL A0K 2N0; (Iraq)'97; MB ChB; Staff, Strait of Belle Isle Health Centre; (709)456-2401

MAHMOOD, Muhammad N; University of Alberta Hosp, 5B4. 55-8440 112 St NW, Edmonton AB T6G 2B7; Aga Khan (Pakistan)'98; MB BS; ABACPath; Staff, University of Alberta Hospital; (780)407-2145; Fax. (780)407-3009.

MAHMOOD, Nasir; Western Mem Reg Hosp, PO Box 2005 Stn Main 1 Brookfield Ave, Corner Brook NL A2H 6J7; Punjab (Pakistan)'83; MB BS; Staff, Western Memorial Regional Hospital; (709)637-5000

MAHMOOD, Nighat; 11-7750 Ranchview Dr NW, Calgary AB T3G 1Y9; (Other Foreign)'88; CCFP; (403)452-6240; Fax. (403)452-9626.

MAHMOOD, Shazia T; Allan Blair Cancer Centre, 300-4101 Dewdney Ave, Regina SK S4T 7T1; Lahore (Pakistan)'95; MB BS; Langs: Urdu; Punjabi; (306)766-2296

MAHMOOD, Tahir; Alpha Physical Rehabilitation, 2779 Avonhurst Dr, Regina SK S4R 3J3; Punjab (Pakistan)'88; OrthSurg. (306)522-5511

MAHMOOD, Tariq; 6-1577 Danforth Ave, Toronto ON M4C 1H7; King Edward Med. Coll. (Pakistan)'81; Assoc Staff, The Scarborough Hospital - General Campus; (416)461-0183; Fax. (416)461-4833.

MAHMOOD, Yasin; Spesmed Med Specialist Ctre, PO Box 1540 Stn Main 2591 99th St, North Battleford SK S9A 3W1; Punjab (Pakistan)'87; MB BS; MRCPsy(UK); DCP(Ire); DPM; FRCPC; Psy. Sr Staff Psy, Battlefords Union Hospital; Clin Assoc Prof, University of Saskatchewan; (306)446-5554; Fax. (306)446-5557; mahmood@sasktel.net.

MAHMOODI, Mahnaz; Southlake Med Centre, 201-581 Davis Dr, Newmarket ON L3Y 2P6; Ahwaz (Iran)'89; CCFP; OR Asst/FP Obstetrics, Southlake Regional Health Centre; Langs: Farsi; (905)853-3103; Fax. (905)853-2533.

MAHMOUD, Haidar A; Finch Midland Med Centre, 218-4190 Finch Ave E, Scarborough ON M1S 4T7; Al-Mustansiriah Baghdad (Iraq)'83; FRCSC; ObstGyn (Laparoscopic Surgery). Staff, The Scarborough Hospital - Birchmount Campus; Staff, Sunnybrook Health Sciences Centre; Langs: Arabic; (416)332-8128

MAHMOUD, Mohamed A S; London HSC-University Hosp, PO Box 5339 Stn B 339 Windermere Rd, London ON N6A 5A5; Cairo (Egypt)'90; CCFP; Staff, London Health Sciences Centre - University Hospital; (519)685-8300

MAHMOUD, Sarah; Health Centre @ 80 Bond, 80 Bond St, Toronto ON M5B 1X2; Tor'10; CCFP; (416)864-3011

MAHMOUD, Shireen F A H; Mount Sinai Hosp, 1514-600 University Ave, Toronto ON M5G 1X5; Cairo (Egypt)'95; Staff, Mount Sinai Hospital; (416)586-5270

MAHMOUD-AHMED, Ashraf S; Cape Breton Hlthcare Complex, 1482 George St, Sydney NS B1P 1P3; Ain Shams (Egypt)'90; MSc; MB BCh; MS; Staff Radiation Oncologist, Cape Breton Healthcare Complex; Asst Prof, Dalhousie University; (902)567-8081; Fax. (902)567-8075; mahmoud-ahmeda@cbdha.nshealth.ca.

MAHMOUDI, Ali; St Michael's Hosp, 30 Bond St, Toronto ON M5B 1W8; Ahwaz (Iran)'96; FRCSC; OrthSurg. Staff, St Michael's Hospital; (416)360-4000

MAHMOUDI, Nasim; 200-101 16th St W, North Vancouver BC V7M 1T3; Shiraz (Iran)'94; FRCPC; IntMed;CCFP; (604)904-0810

MAHMUD, Aamer; Kingston Reg Cancer Centre, 25 King St W, Kingston ON K7L 5P9; Punjab (Pakistan)'86; MB BS; FRCR(Lond); DMRT(Lond); MPhil(UK); FRCPC; RadOncol. (613)544-2631

MAHMUD, Farid H; THe Hosp for Sick Children, 555 University Ave, Toronto ON M5G 1X8; Alb'97; FRCPC; Peds; Endocrin&Metab. Staff, The Hospital For Sick Children; Assoc Prof, University of Toronto; (416)813-8159; Fax. (416)813-6304; farid.mahmud@sickkids.ca.

MAHMUD, Ghias U; Kingsland Med Clinic, 7712 Elbow Dr SW, Calgary AB T2V 1K2; Leeds (England)'64; DCH; Staff, Rockyview General Hospital; Physician, Calgary Board of Health; Langs: Urdu; (403)252-6681; Fax. (403)252-9741.

MAHMUD, M Hayat; Transcona Med Clinic, 4936 4th Ave, Regina SK S4T 0J3; (Other Foreign)'92; (306)775-2688

MAHMUD, Salaheddin M; Winnipeg Reg Health Authority, 490 Hargrave St, Winnipeg MB R3A 0X7; Al Arab (Libya)'93; FRCPC; CommunMed. (204)940-3610

MAHMUD, S Asad; 101 Cameron St, Moncton NB E1C 5Y7; Punjab (Pakistan)'67; MB BS; DPM(Lond); MRCPsy; FRCPC; Psy. Ac Staff, The Moncton Hospital; Consultant Psy, Dorchester Penitentiary; Langs: Urdu; Punjabi; (506)855-4141

MAHMUD-SULTAN, Farhat; 81 Albert St, Moncton NB E1C 1B3; Lahore (Pakistan)'66; MB BS; (506)856-2529; Fax. (506)856-2995.

MAHMUDI-AZER, Salahaddin; 203-1819 Beaufort Ave, Comox BC V9M 1R9; Cal'07; FRCPC; IntMed. (250)339-9500

MAHMUTOGLU, Saadet; 555 University Ave, Toronto ON M5G 1X8; Ege (Turkey)'92; FCCMG; Staff Clin Metabolic Genetics, The Hospital For Sick Children; Langs: German; Turkish; (416)813-7654 x1480; Fax. (416)813-4940; saadet.mahmutoglu@sickkids.ca.

MAHN, Joanna; Halton HSC Corp-Oakville, 327 Oakville St, Oakville ON L6J 3L7; Wes'08; CCFP; CCFP(E.M.); Staff, Halton Healthcare Services Corporation - Oakville Site; (905)845-2571

MAHOMED, Ahmed E; West Winds Med Clinic, 2130-4818 Westwinds Dr NE, Calgary AB T3J 3Z5; Mysore (India)'84; MB BS; (403)293-5454; Fax. (403)293-1511.

MAHOMED, Malini M; West Winds Med Clinic, 2130-4818 Westwinds Dr NE, Calgary AB T3J 3Z5; Mysore (India)'83; MB BS; (403)293-5454

MAHOMED, Nizar N; Univ Hlth Network-Toronto Western Hosp, EW 1 435-399 Bathurst St, Toronto ON M5T 2S8; Tor'88; MD; MPH; DSc(Harvard-PublicHealth); FRCSC; OrthSurg (Hip & Knee Replacement). Dir Arthritis Program/Head Div of OrthSurg/Chair Smith & Nephew Orthopaedic Surg/Chair Nicki & Bryce Douglas Orthopaedic Surg, Toronto Western Hospital - University Health Network; Mang Dir, Altum Health; Prof Surg, University of Toronto; Langs: Hindi; Urdu; (416)603-5328; Fax. (416)603-3437; nizar.mahomed@uhn.ca.

MAHON, Jeffrey L; St Joseph's Health Care, PO Box 5777 Stn B B5 025-268 Grosvenor St, London ON N6A 4V2; Alb'83; MSc; FRCPC; IntMed (Endocrinology). Staff, London Health Sciences Centre - University Hospital; Staff, St Joseph's Hospital - St Joseph's Health Care; University of Western Ontario; (519)646-6335

MAHONE, Michele; CHUM-Hop St-Luc, 1058 rue Saint-Denis, Montreal QC H2X 3J4; Mon'98; FRCPC; IntMed (Obstetrics). Staff, Centre Hospitalier l'Université De Montréal (CHUM) - Hôpital Saint-luc; Langs: English; (514)890-8000 x34444; Fax. (514)412-7308.

MAHONEY, Brian A; Lennox & Addington Gen Hosp, 8 Richmond Park Dr, Napanee ON K7R 2Z4; Dal'99; CCFP; Staff, Lennox & Addington County General Hospital; (613)354-3301; bmahoney@cogeco.ca.

MAHONEY, Charles J; Alder Med Centre, 277 Evergreen Rd, Campbell River BC V9W 5Y4; McM'79; ABIM; FRCPC; IntMed (Gastroenterology). Ac Staff, Campbell River & District General Hospital; (250)287-7454

MAHONEY, Daniel J; 555 Richmond St, Chatham ON N7M 1R2; McM'84; FRCSC; GenSurg. (519)352-9934; Fax. (519)352-0598.

MAHONEY, Donna G; 9-140 Woodbridge Ave, Woodbridge ON L4L 4K9; Ott'87; CCFP; Ac Staff, Humber River Regional Hospital - Finch Avenue Site; Ac Staff, William Osler Health System - Etobicoke General Hospital; (905)850-0753

MAHONEY, James L; St Michael's Hosp, 4 080Q-30 Bond St, Toronto ON M5B 1W8; McM'74; FACS; FRCSC; PlasSurg (Plastic & Reconstructive Surgery). Chief Div of PlasSurg, St Michael's Hospital; Prof Surg, University of Toronto; (416)864-5385; Fax. (416)864-5888.

MAHONEY, John E; The Ottawa Hosp-Gen Campus, 1667-501 Smyth Rd, Ottawa ON K1H 8L6; Tor'86; MSc(ClinEpidemiol.); DAB; FRCSC; Urol. Staff, The Ottawa Hospital - General Campus; Assoc Prof, University of Ottawa; (613)737-8030; Fax. (613)737-8982; jmahoney@ottawahospital.on.ca.

MAHONEY, Mary-Helen; North York Med Arts Bldg, 211-1333 Sheppard Ave E, North York ON M2J 1V1; Wes'06; FRCSC; PlasSurg. (416)554-9860

MAHONEY, Meagan E; Alberta Children's Hosp, 2888 Shaganappi Trail NW, Calgary AB T3B 6A8; McM'04; FRCPC; Peds (Critical Care Medicine). Staff Critical Care & PICU, Alberta Children's Hospital; (403)955-7931; Fax. (403)955-7081.

MAHONEY, Sean R; 9-2120 Regent St S, Sudbury ON P3E 3Z9; Tor'04; CCFP; CCFP(E.M.); Staff Family Med, Health Sciences North-St Joseph's Health Centre; (705)523-9199

MAHONEY, William J; McMaster University, 1-1280 Main St W, Hamilton ON L8S 4K1; McM'76; FRCPC; Peds (Developmental Pediatrics). Ac Staff, Hamilton Health Sciences Centre - McMaster University Medical Centre; Assoc Prof, McMaster University; (905)521-2100 x77605; Fax. (905)521-7953; mahoneyw@hhsc.ca.

MAHONY, Christopher J; Cedar Med Centre, 106-9648 128 St, Surrey BC V3T 2X9; Ott'80; FRCPC; IntMed. Ac Staff, Surrey Memorial Hospital; (604)585-5666 x3846

MAHOOD, J Mark; Central Alberta Prof Centre, 182-5201 43 St, Red Deer AB T4N 1C7; Alb'86; FRCPC; Peds. Staff/Chief Peds, Red Deer Regional Hospital Centre; (403)343-6404; Fax. (403)343-6215.

MAHOOD, James K; Orthopaedic Consultants, 10972 124 St NW, Edmonton AB T5M 0H8; Alb'82; FRCSC; OrthSurg (Spine). (780)453-6999; Fax. (780)451-1437.

MAHOOD, Robert F; CLSC Cote-des-Neiges, 5700 ch de la cote-des-Neiges, Montreal QC H3T 2A8; Sask'79; CCFP; FCFP; Médecin, CLSC Cote-des-Neiges; (514)731-8531; Fax. (514)731-0563.

MAHOOD, Sara S C; Academic Family Medicine, 172-1621 Albert St, Regina SK S4P 2S5; Sask'78; CCFP; FCFP; Staff Family Med, Regina General Hospital; (306)766-0444; Fax. (306)766-7137.

MAHOOD, Trudy L; Ridgeway Clinic, 1001 Ridgeway St, Thunder Bay ON P7E 5H8; McM'79; CCFP; FCFP; Staff, Thunder Bay Regional Health Sciences Centre; Assoc Prof Med, Northern Ontario School of Medicine; Langs: French; German; (807)622-0601

MAHROUCHE BELBACHIR, Lilia; Montfort Hosp, 713 Montreal Rd, Ottawa ON K1K 0T2; Ott'06; CCFP; Staff, Montfort Hospital; (613)746-4621

MAHROUS, Nevine A; MCI Medical Clinic, 800 Steeles Ave W, Thornhill ON L4J 7L2; CCFP; (905)738-6699; Fax. (905)738-6073.

MAHRUGH, Abdouraman A M; Western Memorial Reg Hosp, PO Box 2005 1 Brookfield Ave, Corner Brook NL A2H 6J7; Al Fateh (Libya)'03; MB BCh; Staff, Connaigre Peninsula Community Health Centre; (709)885-2401; abdouraman.mahrugh@easternhealth.ca.

MAHTANI, Ramona; Temmy Latner Centre, 60 Murray St, Toronto ON M5T 3L9; Tor'05; CCFP; (416)586-4800; Fax. (416)586-4804.

MAHUNGU LONGO-KITOKO, P; Grace Medical Clinic, 9655 137 St, Surrey BC V3T 4G8; (Congo (Democratic Republic))'82; (778)395-4434

MAHUTTE, Neal G; Centre de Fertile de Montreal, 220-5252 boul de Maisonneuve O, Montreal QC H4A 3S5; McG'95; FRCSC; ObstGyn (Infertility). (514)369-6116

MAHY, Jean-Noel; 107-6440 Royal Oak Ave, Burnaby BC V5H 3P2; Ott'98; BSc; FACS; FRCSC; GenSurg (Liver & Pancreas Surgery). Langs: Bilingual(English/French); (604)438-3361

MAI, Andrew D; 115A Leonard Ave, Ottawa ON K1S 4V8; Tor'87; CCFP; Staff, The Ottawa Hospital - General Campus; (613)737-7700

MAI, Daryl W; Cachet Family Physicians, 2-9255 Woodbine Ave, Markham ON L6C 1Y9; Tor'92; (905)887-2222; Fax. (905)887-3655.

MAI, David D; U of Ottawa Sport Med Clinic, N203-801 King Edward Ave, Ottawa ON K1N 6N5; Wes'98; Dip SportMed; CCFP; Staff, Renfrew Victoria Hospital; Langs: Vietnamese; French; (613)562-5970; Fax. (613)562-5608.

MAI, Francois M M; Human Resources of Canada, 5F-355 River Rd, Ottawa ON K1A 0L1; Cape Town (South Africa)'57; MB ChB; MD(Adel); FRCPsy; FRCP(Ed); FRCPC; Psy. (613)952-2755; Fax. (613)952-8466.

MAI, Joseph A; Thames Valley FHT-Windermere S, 301-460 Wellington St, St Thomas ON N5R 6H9; Wes'01; Ac Staff Privil, St Thomas Elgin General Hospital; (519)631-5670

MAI, Nghia Trung; Clinique Med L'Avenir, 200-1150 boul de l'Avenir, Laval QC H7N 6L2; Saigon (Vietnam)'73; (450)680-1150; Fax. (450)680-1151.

MAI, Ryan W; St Michael's Hosp, 1 026-30 Bond St, Toronto ON M5B 1W8; Tor'00; FRCPC; Anes. Staff Anes, St Michael's Hospital; (416)864-5071

MAI, Verna M; 802-35 Hollywood Ave, North York ON M2N 0A9; Alb'82; MHSc; MD; FRCPC; CommunMed (Public Health). Prov Lead Public Health, Cancer Care Ontario - Provincial Office; Chair Screening Portfolio, Canadian Partnership Against Cancer; Asst Prof Dalla Lana School of Public Health, University of Toronto; (416)217-1252; verna.mai@cancercare.on.ca.

MAI-TRUNG, Kien; The Ottawa Hosp-Gen Campus, 501 Smyth Rd, Ottawa ON K1H 8L6; Saigon (Vietnam)'70; FRCPC; AnatPath. Staff, The Ottawa Hospital - General Campus; Prof Path, University of Ottawa; (613)737-8292 x79033

MAIANSKI, Irit; IWK Health Centre, PO Box 9700 Rpo CSC 5980 University ave, Halifax NS B3K 6R8; Tel Aviv (Israel)'96; Staff, IWK Health Centre; (902)470-8888

MAIANSKI, Ziv; Queen Elizabeth II HSC, 6 019-1276 South Park St, Halifax NS B3H 2Y9; Tel Aviv (Israel)'94; Staff, Queen Elizabeth II Health Sciences Centre - Victoria General Site; (902)473-7624

MAICAS, Emmanuel; 330 Av Universite Pathologie, Hopital Dumont, Moncton NB E1C 2Z3; McG'93; BSc(Microbiol); PhD(Molecular Genetics); AnatPath. Staff Path, Dr Georges-L-Dumont University Hospital Centre; Langs: English; French; (506)862-4846; emmanuel.maicas@vitalitenb.ca.

MAIDA, Reem; MUHC-Montreal Gen Hosp, 1650 av Cedar, Montreal QC H3G 1A4; McG'08; IntMed. Staff, McGill University Health Centre - Montreal General Campus; (514)934-1934

MAIDA, Vincent; William Osler HS-Etobicoke, 101 Humber College Blvd, Toronto ON M9V 1R8; Tor'82; BSc; MSc(Wounds); ABHPM; CCFP; FCFP; Staff, William Osler Health System - Etobicoke General Hospital; Asst Prof Med, University of Toronto; Langs: Italian.

MAIDMENT, Julie L; 16-385 Frederick St, Kitchener ON N2H 2P2; McM'05; CCFP; (519)745-7482

MAIER, Fred; Prince Albert Med Clinic, 681 15th St W, Prince Albert SK S6V 7H9; Sask'73; Staff, Victoria Hospital; (306)764-1505; Fax. (306)764-7775.

MAIER, Joanne C; Western Med Clinic, 144 6th St, Brandon MB R7A 3N2; Man'84; CCFP; Ac Staff/Chief Family Pract, Brandon Regional Health Centre; Lecturer, University of Manitoba; (204)727-6451; Fax. (204)727-4150.

MAIER, Peter C; Toronto Headache & Pain Clinic, 801 York Mills Rd, North York ON M3B 1X7; (Hungary)'91; CCFP; FCFP; Staff, Rouge Valley Health System - Centenary Health Centre Site; Langs: German; Hungarian; (416)699-8843

MAIER, Ronald J C; Health Sciences Centre, 820 Sherbrook St, Winnipeg MB R3A 1R9; Man'89; Staff, Health Sciences Centre; University of Manitoba; (204)774-6511

MAIER, Vivian R; 620 Winnipeg St, Penticton BC V2A 5M9; Sask'83; (250)492-8802; Fax. (250)492-0610.

MAIER PHILLIPS, Laura; 310-1641 Hillside Avenue, Victoria BC V8T 5G1; UBC'01; BA; CCFP; (250)592-5312; Fax. (250)592-5910.

MAIETTA, Antonio; CHUM-Hop Notre-Dame, 1560 rue Sherbrooke E, Montreal QC H2L 4M1; Mon'04; FRCPC; AnatPath. Staff, Centre Hospitalier l'Université de Montréal (CHUM) - Hôpital Notre-Dame; (514)890-8000 x25765

MAIL, W John; BC Women's Hosp & Health Ctre, F326-4500 Oak St, Vancouver BC V6H 3N1; Tor'76; CCFP; FCFP; Staff, BC Women's Hospital & Health Centre; Staff, Vancouver General Hospital - Centennial Pavillion; Member, Therapeutics Initiative Committee; Clin Assoc Prof, University of British Columbia; (604)875-2029 x6644

MAILE, John K C; Holley Clinic, 348 Front St, Quesnel BC V2J 2K3; London (England)'61; MB BS; MRCS(Eng); LRCP(Lond); Staff, G R Baker Memorial Hospital; (250)992-2158; Fax. (250)992-9391.

MAILER, Colin M; London Hakim Talbot, 501 Talbot St, London ON N6A 2S4; Edinburgh (Scotland)'59; MB ChB(Ed); FRCSC; Ophth (Cataract). Consultant Ophth, St Joseph's Hospital - St Joseph's Health Care; Langs: Spanish; German; Bilingual(French/English); Latin; (519)434-9111; collin@rogers.com.

MAILHOT, Annie-Claude; CLSC Samuel de Champlain, 100-5811 boul Taschereau, Brossard QC J4Z 1A5; Mon'10; CCFP; (450)445-4452

MAILHOT, Emilie; Ctr Hosp Affilie-Enfant-Jesus, 1401 18e rue, Quebec QC G1J 1Z4; Laval'04; FRCSC; PlasSurg. Staff, Centre Hospitalier Affilié Universitaire de Québec - Hôpital De L'Enfant Jésus; (418)649-0252

MAILHOT, Jean; GMF de Grand-Mere, 200-1050 8e rue, Grand-Mere QC G9T 4L4; Laval'67; Endocrin (P.Q.) (Andropause). Staff Endocrin, Hopital de la Cite de la santé; Langs: English; (819)729-0178

MAILHOT, Marie-Christine; Hotel-Dieu-de-Levis, 143 rue Wolfe, Levis QC G6V 3Z1; Sher'03; CCFP; Staff, Hôtel-Dieu de Lévis; (418)835-7121

MAILHOT, Marie-Pierre; CSSS Pierre Boucher, 1333 boul Jacques-Cartier E, Longueuil QC J4M 2A5; Laval'06; FRCPC; Psy. Staff, Centre Hospitalier Pierre Boucher; (450)468-8111

MAILHOT, Melissa; CHSLD Cote-Jardins, 880 av Painchaud, Quebec QC G1S 0A3; Laval'00; (418)688-1221; Fax. (418)688-0105.

MAILHOT, Philippe; CSSSG-Hop de Hull, 116 boul Lionel-Emond, Gatineau QC J8Y 1W7; Mon'03; Staff, Hull Hospital; (819)966-6200

MAILHOT, Sylvain; CSSS De Rimouski-Neigette, CP 3150 Succ A 150 av Rouleau, Rimouski QC G5L 5T1; Mon'93; AnatPath (P.Q.). Staff, Hôpital Regional Rimouski; (418)724-8535

MAILHOT, Vincent; CSSS de Beauce-Etchemin, 1515 17e rue, Saint-Georges QC G5Y 4T8; Laval'00; DiagRad. Staff, Centre Hospitalier Beauce-Etchemin; (418)228-2031 x7201

MAILIS, Angela H; Univ Hlth Network-Toronto Western Hosp, 4F811-399 Bathurst St, Toronto ON M5T 2S8; Athens (Greece)'76; MSc; FRCPC; PhysMed&Rehab (Pain Management). Dir Comprehensive Pain Program, Toronto Western Hospital - University Health Network; Prof Med, University of Toronto; Langs: Greek; (416)603-5380; Fax. (416)603-5725; angela.mailis@uhn.on.ca.

MAILLETTE, Alain; CSSS de Trois-Rivières, 1991 boul du Carmel, Trois-Rivieres QC G8Z 3R9; Laval'95; FRCSC; Urol (Medical Oncology). Staff, CSSS de Trois-Rivières; Langs: Spanish; French; (819)697-3333; mayo222002@yahoo.ca.

MAILLETTE, Sylvie; CSSS Pierre Boucher, 1333 Boul Jacques-Cartier E, Longueuil QC J4M 2A5; Laval'82; FRCPC; IntMed; Cardiol. Cardiol/Internal Med, Centre Hospitalier Pierre Boucher; (450)468-8111

MAILLOUX, Caroline; Sudbury Reg Hosp-Laurentian, 3290-41 Ramsey Lake Rd, Sudbury ON P3E 5J1; Alb'03; CCFP; Staff, Health Sciences North-Laurentian Site; (705)523-7147

MAILLOUX, Cynthia; CHUQ-St-Francois D'Assise, 10 rue de l'Espinay, Quebec QC G1L 3L5; Laval'92; FRCPC; DiagRad. Staff, Centre Hospitalier Universitaire De Québec - Pavillon De St-françois-d'assise; (418)525-4444; Fax. (418)525-4498.

MAILLOUX, Jacques; CHUQ-Ctr Hosp Univ Laval, 2705 boul Laurier, Quebec QC G1V 4G2; Laval'81; FRCSC; ObstGyn. Staff, Centre Hospitalier Universitaire de Quebec-CHUL; Chef ObstGyn, Université Laval; (418)654-2738; Fax. (418)654-2714; jacques.mailloux@crchul.ulaval.ca.

MAILLOUX, Marie-Josee; CLSC Jacques Cartier, 1199A rue de l'Hopital, Quebec QC G2A 2T7; Mon'94; Staff, Centre Hospitalier Affilié Universitaire de Québec - Hôpital du St-Sacrement; Staff, Centre Hospitalier Chauveau; (418)843-2121

MAILLOUX, Martine; CSSS Pierre Boucher, 1333 boul Jacques-Cartier E, Longueuil QC J4M 2A5; Mon'93; Staff, Centre Hospitalier Pierre Boucher; (450)468-8111

MAILLOUX, Michel; Centre Med de Chambly, 205-1101 boul Brassard, Chambly QC J3L 5R4; Mon'72; Staff, Hôpital du Haut-Richelieu; (450)658-6601; Fax. (450)658-7849.

MAILLOUX, Pierre; Centre de Sante, 41 boul Comtois, Louiseville QC J5V 2H8; Laval'73; Psy. Staff, CSSS de Maskinongé; (819)228-2731

MAILLOUX, Stephanie; CHUS-Hop Fleurimont, 3001 12e av N, Sherbrooke QC J1H 5N4; Sher'02; FRCPC; Psy. Staff, Centre Hospitalier Universitaire de Sherbrooke-Hopital Fleurimont; (819)346-1110 x14000

MAILLY, Christian; CSSS de la Vallée de l'Or, 725 6e rue, Val-d'Or QC J9P 3Y1; Mon'10; CCFP; Staff, Centre Hospitalier de Val d'Or; (819)825-5858

MAILLY, Suzanne; Centre Ambulatoire de Laval, 1515 boul Chomedey, Laval QC H7V 3Y7; Mon'88; Staff Geriatric & Psychogeriatric, Hopital de la Cite de la santé; Langs: English; (450)978-8363; Fax. (450)978-2938.

MAILMAN, Timothy L; IWK Health Centre, PO Box 9700 Rpo CSC 5850-5980 University Ave, Halifax NS B3K 6R8; Dal'93; InfectDis; MedMicrobiol; Peds (Pediatric Infectious Diseases). Dir Clin Microbiology/Head Dept of Path & LabMed, IWK Health Centre; (902)470-7892; tim.mailman@iwk.nshealth.ca.

MAIMETS, Talvi C; Medical & Dental Bldg, 801-586 Eglinton Ave E, Toronto ON M4P 1P2; Tor'80; CCFP; FCFP; Langs: Estonian; Finnish; (416)486-4401; Fax. (416)486-6145.

MAIN, Alayne J M; Med-Team Clinic, 103-99 Kakulu Rd, Kanata ON K2L 3C8; Wes'89; BSc(Hons.); (613)592-1448

MAIN, Barbara A; Fairview Med Clinic, 101-1516 Fairview Rd, Penticton BC V2A 6A3; UBC'94; CCFP; Med Staff, Penticton Regional Hospital; Assoc Teacher, University of British Columbia; (250)493-7140; Fax. (250)493-8366.

MAIN, Blair F; Peach City Medical, 3090 Skaha Lake Rd, Penticton BC V2A 7H2; UBC'95; CCFP; (250)276-5050; drbmain@telus.net.

MAIN, Cheryl L; Hamilton HS-General Site, 1 114-237 Barton St E, Hamilton ON L8L 2X2; McM'98; FRCPC; IntMed; MedMicrobiol; InfectDis. Staff, Hamilton Health Sciences Centre - Hamilton General Hospital; (905)527-0271 x46182

MAIN, Christopher D; PO Box 897, Salmon Arm BC V1E 4N9; UBC'93; FRCPC; IntMed (Cardiology). Staff, Shuswap Lake General Hospital; Consultant, Queen Victoria Hospital; (250)832-6661

MAIN, James T D; Veterans Affairs Canada, 201-107 Shirreff Ave, North Bay ON P1B 7K8; Tor'69; (705)495-5910

MAIN, Jeffrey S; Grandview Med Ctr Fam Hlth Team, 167 Hespeler Rd, Cambridge ON N1R 3H7; Wes'94; CCFP; FCFP; (519)623-4200; Fax. (519)623-2546.

MAINDONALD, Kevin L; 81 Lakeshore Rd E PO Box 45031 Rpo Port Credit, Mississauga ON L5G 1C9; Tor'79; BSc; FRCPC; Psy (Psycho Geriatrics). (647)229-4111

MAINGI, Manish; Credit Valley Med Arts Centre, 412-2000 Credit Valley Rd, Mississauga ON L5M 4N4; Tor'91; BSc; FACC; FRCPC; IntMed; Cardiol. Med Dir Cardiol, The Credit Valley Hospital; Court Staff, Trillium Health Centre - Mississauga; Langs: Hindi; (905)828-4000; Fax. (905)828-7533.

MAINGOT-DOUKETIS, Maria J; Wardenwoods Health Centre Inc, 2361 Warden Ave, Scarborough ON M1T 1V7; McM'91; CCFP; Langs: English; French; (416)299-4999; Fax. (416)299-1322.

MAINGUY, Nicole; CSSS de Manicouagan, 635 boul Joliet, Baie-Comeau QC G5C 1P1; Laval'74; Psy (P.Q.). Staff, Centre Hospitalier Régional Baie-Comeau; (418)589-3701

MAINI, Bharat; Peterborough Reg HC-Hospital, 1 Hospital Dr, Peterborough ON K9J 7C6; London (England)'84; MB BS(Lond); FRCA(UK); DA(UK); MA(Cantab); FRCPC; Anes (Pediatric Anesthesia). Med Dir-Surg Servs, Peterborough Regional Health Centre - Hospital Drive; Langs: Hindi; Punjabi; (705)743-2121; bmaini@cogeco.ca.

MAINPRIZE, Thomas C; Royal University Hosp, 4544-103 Hospital Dr, Saskatoon SK S7N 0W8; Qns'81; FRCSC; ObstGyn (Urogynecology). Staff, Royal University Hospital; Dept Head ObstGyn & Reproductive Sciences, University of Saskatchewan; (306)966-8033; Fax. (306)966-8040; tom.mainprize@usask.ca.

MAINPRIZE, Todd G; Sunnybrook Hlth Sciences Ctre, A134-2075 Bayview Ave, Toronto ON M4N 3M5; Sask'96; FRCSC; Neursurg. Staff, Sunnybrook Health Sciences Centre; (416)480-6100

MAINRA, Rahul R; St Paul's Hosp, 1702 20th St W, Saskatoon SK S7M 0Z9; Sask'00; BScHons; MMedClinEpidemiol; FRCPC; IntMed (Transplant Nephrology); Nephrol. Staff, St Paul's Hospital (Grey Nuns) of Saskatoon; (306)655-5934

MAINRA, Rajesh R; 217-1433 Lonsdale Ave, North Vancouver BC V7M 2H9; Sask'92; FRCPC; IntMed (Pulmonary Medicine); Critical Care Medicine; Respir. Staff, Lions Gate Hospital; Langs: Hindi; (604)984-8480; Fax. (604)984-8481.

MAINVILLE, Barbara J; Hawkesbury Dist Gen Hosp, 1111 Ghislain St, Hawkesbury ON K6A 3G5; Ott'85; (613)632-1111; Fax. (613)636-6171; bjmbrook@cnwl.igs.net.

MAINVILLE, Christian; CSSS de la Cote-De-Gaspe, 215 boul De York O, Gaspe QC G4X 2W2; Laval'00; CCFP; CCFP(E.M.); Staff, Centre Hospitalier de Gaspe; (418)368-3301; Fax. (418)368-5358; christian.mainville.chgaspe@ssss.gouv.qc.ca.

MAINVILLE, Karine; CSSS du Sud de Lanaudière, 911 montee des Pionniers, Terrebonne QC J6V 2H2; Laval'00; DiagRad. Staff, Centre Hospitalier Pierre le Gardeur; (450)654-7525 x31195

MAINVILLE, Nathalie; CSSS de Coaticook, 138 rue Jeanne-Mance, Coaticook QC J1A 1W3; Sher'97; Staff, Centre Hospitalier de Coaticook; (819)849-4876

MAINVILLE, Norman P; Grey Bruce HS-Owen Sound, PO Box 1800 Stn Main 7220-1800 8th St E, Owen Sound ON N4K 6M9; McG'03; FRCSC; Ophth. Staff, Grey Bruce Health Services - Owen Sound; (519)376-2121 x2753

MAINVILLE, Pierre; CHUM-Hotel-Dieu, 3840 rue Saint-Urbain, Montreal QC H2W 1T8; Sher'73; Staff, Centre Hospitalier l'Université de Montréal (CHUM) - Hôtel-Dieu; (514)890-8000 x14240

MAIOLO, Giuseppe C; Westmount Med Bldg, 340-5025 rue Sherbrooke O, Montreal QC H4A 1S9; Florence (Italy)'81; Staff, McGill University Health Centre - Montreal General Campus; (514)485-3833; Fax. (514)485-8523.

MAIONE, Peter F; East Street Med Arts Centre, 302-170 East St, Sault Ste. Marie ON P6A 3C6; Ott'83; Staff, Sault Area Hospital - Sault Ste Marie; (705)759-1325

MAIR, Walter M J; Summit Centre Family Clinic, 209-200 Boudreau Rd, St. Albert AB T8N 6B9; Tor'77; Assoc Staff, Sturgeon Community Hospital; (780)458-7000; Fax. (780)458-8484.

MAIRE, Sebastien; Hotel-Dieu Levis, 143 rue Wolfe, Levis QC G6V 3Z1; Mon'01; FRCPC; EmergMed. Staff, Hôtel-Dieu de Lévis; (418)835-7122

MAISONNEUVE, Daryn T; East Kootenay Reg Hosp, 13 24th Ave N, Cranbrook BC V1C 3H9; Sask'85; FRCPC; DiagRad. Staff, East Kootenay Regional Hospital; (250)426-5281; Fax. (250)426-5610.

MAISONNEUVE, Denis; CSSS du Lac-des-Deux-Montagnes, CP 174 520 boul Arthur-Sauve, Saint-Eustache QC J7R 5B1; Sher'87; FRCPC; IntMed; Gastroent. Staff, Hôpital de Saint-Eustache; (450)473-6811; Fax. (450)473-0643.

MAISONNEUVE, Rachel J; Timmins Family Health Team, 3-227 Algonquin Blvd W, Timmins ON P4N 2R8; McM'89; BScN; CCFP; FCFP; Langs: English; French; (705)267-5511; Fax. (705)264-6373; rachel_maison@hotmail.com.

MAISTRELLI, Gianni; 307-2130 Lawrence Ave E, Scarborough ON M1R 3A6; Rome (Italy)'77; FRCSC; OrthSurg (Hip & Knee Replacement). Staff, Toronto East General Hospital Inc; Physician WCB, Non Economic Loss; Assoc Prof, University of Toronto; (416)751-6141

MAITER, Nasrin; Khatsalano Med Clinic, 2685 Broadway W, Vancouver BC V6K 2G2; (South Africa)'03; MB ChB; (604)731-9187

MAITI, Soubhik; Greencrest Pembina Clinic, B-2750 Pembina Hwy, Winnipeg MB R3T 2H8; Man'06; CCFP; (204)768-3821

MAITLAND, Alexander J M; 21 Mill St, Gananoque ON K7G 2L5; Qns'84; CCFP; FCFP; (613)382-2558

MAITLAND, Andrew; Foothills Med Centre, 1403 29 St NW, Calgary AB T2N 2T9; London (England)'77; FACS; FRCSC; GenSurg; Cardiovasc&ThorSurg. Att Staff Surg Oncol, Tom Baker Cancer Centre; Staff, Foothills Medical Centre; Assoc Prof, University of Calgary; (403)944-2499; Fax. (403)270-3715.

MAITRA, Rajat; Cedars Prof Park, 2923 66 St NW, Edmonton AB T6K 4C1; Calcutta (India)'63; LRCP; MRCS; DPM(Eng); FRCPC; Psy (Adult Psychiatry). Staff Psy, Covenant Health - Grey Nuns Community Hospital; Consultant Psy, Regional Mental Health Services-Edmonton; Ass't Clin Prof Psy, University of Alberta; (780)450-8810

MAIZLIN, Zeev V; McMaster University HSC, 1200 Main St W, Hamilton ON L8N 3Z5; Samara (Russia (Federation))'88; FRCPC; DiagRad. Teach Staff, McMaster University; (905)521-2100

MAJAESIC, Carina M; Edmonton Clinic Health Academy, 4 590-11405 87 Ave NW, Edmonton AB T6G 1C9; Alb'90; PhD(Immunol); FRCPC; Peds; Respir. Langs: Swedish; (780)248-5650

MAJAESS, George G; Halifax Prof Centre, 385-5991 Spring Garden Rd, Halifax NS B3H 1Y6; Dal'87; FRCPC; PhysMed&Rehab (Musculoskeletal). Staff, Nova Scotia Rehabilitation Centre; (902)492-6177; Fax. (902)492-2988.

MAJDA, Jolanta; CLSC Rene Cassin, 500-5800 boul Cavendish, Cote Saint-Luc QC H4W 2T5; Gdansk (Poland)'79; (514)484-7878; Fax. (514)485-2978.

MAJDAN, Agnieszka A; E 104 SMBD Jewish Gen Hosp, 3755 ch Cote-Sainte-Catherine, Montreal QC H3T 1E2; UBC'03; FRCPC; IntMed; Endocrin&Metab. Staff, Sir Mortimer B Davis Jewish General; (514)340-8222 x6770

MAJEAU, Luc; Clinique du Village, 200-382 rue Principale, St-Donat-de-Mtcalm QC J0T 2C0; Mon'74; MSc(Admin.Med.); (819)419-0123

MAJEED, Abeer A; 2660 Eglinton Ave E, Scarborough ON M1K 2S3; (Ireland)'07; CCFP; (416)642-9445; Fax. (416)284-1964.

MAJEED, Arshad; Lakeridge Hlth Corp-Oshawa, 1 Hospital Crt, Oshawa ON L1G 2B9; Punjab (Pakistan)'59; DPsy; DABPN; FRCPC; Psy (Mood Disorders). Dir CME, Lakeridge Health - Oshawa Site; Asst Prof, Queen's University; Langs: Urdu; Punjabi; (905)576-8711; Fax. (905)721-4742.

MAJEED, Faiza A; Davenport Perth Comm Hlth Ctr, 1892 Davenport Rd, Toronto ON M6N 1B7; Man'06; CCFP; (416)658-6812

MAJEED, Haseena; Mid-Main Comm Health Centre, 3998 Main St, Vancouver BC V5V 3P2; UBC'98; CCFP; (604)873-3666; Fax. (604)875-8790.

MAJEED, Sonilla; 201-222 King St E, Bowmanville ON L1C 1P6; Tor'10; CCFP; (905)440-3584

MAJEED, Yasmin T; 221-339 Aspen Glen Landing SW, Calgary AB T3H 0N6; (Pakistan)'83; CCFP; (403)263-7997; Fax. (403)263-7996.

MAJEED MOHAMMED, Asma'a; 4904 48 St, Leduc AB T9E 6X4; (Iraq)'90; MB ChB; CCFP; (780)986-2712

MAJEROVICH, Jo Ann; UNB Student Health Centre, PO Box 4400 Stn A, Fredericton NB E3B 5A3; Tor'92; MSc(Epidemiol.); MSc(Med.Biophysics); BSc(MolecularGenetics); CCFP; FCFP; Staff, Dr Everett Chalmers Regional Hospital; (506)453-4837; Fax. (506)452-6087; maverick@unb.ca.

MAJESKY, Ivan F; Vodden X-Ray & Ultrasound, 36 Vodden St E, Brampton ON L6V 4H4; Komensky (Slovakia)'62; FRCPC; DiagRad. (905)455-5455; Fax. (905)455-5154.

MAJEWSKI, Jakub; The Ottawa Hosp-Gen Campus, 501 Smyth Rd, Ottawa ON K1H 8L6; Ott'07; InfectDis; IntMed. Staff, The Ottawa Hospital - General Campus; (613)722-7000

MAJEWSKI, Zuzanna M; Woolwich Comm Health Centre, PO Box 370 10 Parkside Dr, St Jacobs ON N0B 2N0; Warsaw (Poland)'72; PhD; Court Staff, St Mary's General Hospital; Court Staff, Grand River Hospital - Kitchener/Waterloo Health Centre; Physician, Woolwich Community Health Centre - Woolwich Site; Langs: Polish; (519)664-3794; Fax. (519)664-2182.

MAJID, Falah S; Dr Falah Majid Med Prof Corp, 202-290 4th Ave NE, Moose Jaw SK S6H 0C6; Baghdad (Iraq), (United Kingdom)'83; MB ChB; MRCP; FRCP; Dir Diabetes Program/Ac Staff Member Internist, Five Hills Health Region; Langs: Arabic; (306)692-8229; fsmajidmed@sasktel.net.

MAJID, Nadine; Summerville Family Health Team, 5F-101 Queensway W, Mississauga ON L5B 2P7; McM'05; CCFP; (905)272-9700; Fax. (905)272-1416.

MAJKA, Marek; Kelowna Gen Hosp, 2268 Pandosy St, Kelowna BC V1Y 1T2; Sher'05; FRCPC; Anes. Staff, Kelowna General Hospital; (250)862-4309

MAJL, Lance B; 211-3420 Finch Ave E, Scarborough ON M1W 2R6; Mem'93; FRCPC; IntMed; Neur. Ac Staff, The Scarborough Hospital - Birchmount Campus; (416)498-6255; Fax. (416)498-9555.

MAJOR, Adrian C; St Clare's Mercy Hosp, 154 Lemarchant Rd, St. John's NL A1C 5B8; Mem'90; FRCPC; DiagRad. Staff, St Clare's Mercy Hospital; (709)777-5777

MAJOR, Andrew E; St Clare's Mercy Hosp, 154 Lemarchant Rd, St. John's NL A1C 5B8; Mem'83; FRCPC; Anes. Staff, St Clare's Mercy Hospital; (709)777-5520

MAJOR, Andrew F; 8630 120 St, Surrey BC V3W 3N6; Lublin (Poland)'73; CCFP; FCFP; (604)591-5505; Fax. (604)591-9053.

MAJOR, Bertrand; CSSS du Nord de Lanaudière, 1000 boul Sainte-Anne, St-Charles-Brromee QC J6E 6J2; Laval'86; Psy. Staff, Centre Hospitalier Régional de Lanaudière; (450)759-8222; Fax. (450)759-0011.

MAJOR, Brigitte; CSSS du Sud de Lanaudière, 911 montee des Pionniers, Terrebonne QC J6V 2H2; Laval'96; ObstGyn. Staff, Centre Hospitalier Pierre le Gardeur; (450)654-7525

MAJOR, M Gregory; M D M Medical Clinic, 80 Thickson Rd S, Whitby ON L1N 7T2; Wes'97; CCFP; (905)668-6448

MAJOR, Nathalie; Ctr Hosp Fleury, 2180 rue Fleury E, Montreal QC H2B 1K3; Mon'08; CCFP; CCFP(E.M.); Staff, Centre Hospitalier Fleury; (514)381-9311

MAJOR, Paul A; Medical Arts Bldg, 202-233 Kennedy St, Winnipeg MB R3C 3J5; Man'72; FRCPC; DiagRad. (204)942-6453; Fax. (204)944-8101.

MAJOR, Philippe; Hôpital Ste-Justine, 3175 ch Cote-Sainte-Catherine, Montreal QC H3T 1C5; Mon'01; FRCPC; Neur (Epilepsy). Staff, Hôpital Ste-Justine; Langs: Bilingual(French/English); (514)345-4931; Fax. (514)345-2372; philippe.major@umontreal.ca.

MAJOR, Pierre P; The Juravinski Cancer Centre, 699 Concession St, Hamilton ON L8V 5C2; Mon'74; FRCPC; IntMed (Gastrointestinal Cancer); MedOncol (P.Q.). Staff, Hamilton Health Sciences Centre - McMaster Children's Hospital; Staff Physician, St Joseph's Healthcare - Charlton Campus; Langs: English; French; (905)387-9495 x64602

MAJOR, Pierre; Centre Med St-Urbain, 209-3875 rue Saint-Urbain, Montreal QC H2W 1V1; Mon'86; FRCSC; OrthSurg. ac Staff, Centre Hospitalier l'Université de Montréal (CHUM) - Hôtel-Dieu; adj Prof, Universite de Montreal; (514)849-8391; Fax. (514)849-9313.

MAJOR, Sophie; Centre Med Laval, 1110 boul Vanier, Laval QC H7C 2R8; Mon'91; Staff Med, Hopital de la Cite de la santé; (450)661-2521; Fax. (450)661-7193.

MAJOR, Stephen R M; Campbell Med Group, 39 Campbell Ave, St. John's NL A1E 2Z3; Mem'93; CCFP; FCFP; (709)579-5001; Fax. (709)579-4499.

MAJUMDAR, Sumit R; University of Alberta Hosp, 2F1 24-8440 112 St NW, Edmonton AB T6G 2B7; Alb'92; MPH; FRCPC; IntMed (Osteoporosis). Prof, University of Alberta Hospital; (780)407-1399; Fax. (780)407-3132.

MAK, Anton; Hop Charles LeMoyne, 3120 boul Taschereau, Greenfield Park QC J4V 2H1; McG'02; FRCPC; IntMed; MedMicrobiol; InfectDis. Staff, Hopital Charles LeMoyne; (514)466-5000

MAK, Ellen N; 202-2494 Danforth Ave, Toronto ON M4C 1K9; Tor'76; Ac Staff, Toronto East General Hospital Inc; Langs: Chinese; (416)698-8411; Fax. (416)698-6244.

MAK, Ian; 1-2810 Major Mackenzie Dr, Maple ON L6A 3L2; Wes'08; CCFP; (905)832-3838

MAK, Janet; Senior Outreach Team, 2828 Nanaimo St, Victoria BC V8T 4W9; Tor'01; CCFP; (250)519-3566

MAK, Kam Kong; 404-1100 Sheppard Ave E, North York ON M2K 2W1; Wes'67; BSc; Court Staff Family & CommunMed, Toronto Western Hospital - University Health Network; Court Staff Family & CommunMed, Princess Margaret Hospital - University Health Network; Court Staff Family & CommunMed, Toronto General Hospital - UHN; Langs: Chinese; Cantonese; Mandarin; (416)222-0660; Fax. (416)222-9238.

MAK, Kelvin; North York Gen Hosp, 4001 Leslie St, North York ON M2K 1E1; Qns'91; FRCPC; DiagRad. Staff, North York General Hospital; (416)633-9420; Fax. (416)635-2401.

MAK, Mabel; The Medical Centre FHT, PO Box 4200 Stn Main 707 Charlotte St, Peterborough ON K9J 7B3; Alb'99; CCFP; Assoc Physician, Partners In Pregnancy Clinic; Langs: Chinese; Cantonese; (705)876-4598; Fax. (705)876-4599.

MAK, Manson M T; Brampton East Med Group, 200-300 Main St N, Brampton ON L6V 4H6; (Hong Kong)'85; MB BS; MRCP(UK); CCFP; CCFP(E.M.); FCFP; Langs: Chinese; Mandarin; (905)451-1937; Fax. (905)451-8272.

MAK, S C Ernie; Univ Hlth Network-Princess M, 16 757-610 University Ave, Toronto ON M5G 2M9; Wes'06; CCFP; Ac Staff Family & Comm Med, Princess Margaret Hospital - University Health Network; (416)946-4501

MAK, Susanna S S; Mount Sinai Hosp, 18 365-600 University Ave, Toronto ON M5G 1X5; Tor'91; FRCPC; IntMed; Cardiol. Staff, Mount Sinai Hospital; (416)586-4800 x5554; Fax. (416)586-4775.

MAK, Victor; 203-22 Richmond St, Richmond Hill ON L4C 3Y1; Tor'91; MSc; FRCSC; Urol (Andrology). Ac Staff, Mackenzie Richmond Hill Hospital; Langs: Chinese; Cantonese; (905)770-0087; Fax. (905)770-0047.

MAK, Vincent C W; 222-8787 Woodbine Ave, Markham ON L3R 9S2; (Hong Kong)'84; MRCP(UK); FRCPC; IntMed; Rheum. Ac Staff, Mackenzie Richmond Hill Hospital; (905)948-1717; Fax. (905)948-1714.

MAK, Walter H H; St Michael's Hosp, 30 Bond St, Toronto ON M5B 1W8; Wes'01; FRCPC; DiagRad. Staff, St Michael's Hospital; (416)864-5692

MAK, Wang-Cheong; 313-1650 Elgin Mills Rd E, Richmond Hill ON L4S 0B2; Sheffield (England)'84; Peds. Staff, Niagara Health System - Greater Niagara General Site; (905)237-8118; Fax. (905)809-3437.

MAKADIAMA-BANTSIMBA, Yvon; University Hosp of Northern BC, 1475 Edmonton St, Prince George BC V2M 1S2; (South Africa)'03; MB ChB; Staff, University Hospital of Northern British Columbia; (250)565-2000

MAKAN, Gopal; Markham Stouffville Hosp, PO Box 1800 Stn Main 381 Church St, Markham ON L3P 7P3; Natal (South Africa)'70; MB ChB; FRCPC; Anes. Staff, Markham Stouffville Hospital; (905)472-7074

MAKAN, Narendra K; Horizon Square Med Centre, 401-3508 32 Ave NE, Calgary AB T1Y 6J2; Shivaji (India)'89; CCFP; (403)291-5599; narendramakan@hotmail.com.

MAKANJEE, Bhavanesh; Scarborough Prof Centre, 406-1371 Neilson Rd, Scarborough ON M1B 4Z8; Natal (India)'94; FRCPC; IntMed; Cardiol. (416)281-9499; Fax. (416)283-5705.

MAKAR, Amany S H; Royal Oak Clinic, C2-2524 Third Line, Oakville ON L6M 0G8; Cairo (Egypt)'88; CCFP; (905)827-7000

MAKAR, Hossam S H; 107-330 Bronte St S, Milton ON L9T 7X1; Cairo (Egypt)'90; FRCSC; GenSurg. (905)693-1795; Fax. (905)693-0970.

MAKAR, Kami L; Univ of Lethbridge Hlth Ctre, 4401 University Dr W, Lethbridge AB T1K 3M4; Alb'98; BSc; CCFP; CCFP(E.M.); Staff, Chinook Regional Hospital; Langs: French; (403)329-2484

MAKAR, Magdy S I; 47 West St S, Orillia ON L3V 5G2; Cairo (Egypt)'81; MB ChB; FRCSEd.; FRCSC; GenSurg (Laparoscopy). Chief GenSurg, Orillia Soldiers' Memorial Hospital; Aj Asst Prof Gen Surg, Queen's University; Langs: Arabic; (705)325-1944; Fax. (705)325-7508.

MAKAR, Sherif S M; The Ottawa Hosp-Gen Campus, 501 Smyth Rd, Ottawa ON K1H 8L6; Alexandria (Egypt)'84; IntMed. Staff, The Ottawa Hospital - General Campus; (613)722-7000

MAKAR ABDEL MESSIH, Inas H; St Joseph's Health Care, PO Box 5777 Stn B 268 Grosvenor St, London ON N6A 4V2; Cairo (Egypt)'85; Staff, St Joseph's Hospital - St Joseph's Health Care; (519)685-8281

MAKAREWICZ, Pawel A; 6935 Harvie Ave, Powell River BC V8A 5H9; Warsaw (Poland)'75; FRCSC; GenSurg., Powell River General Hospital; Langs: Polish; (604)485-0152; Fax. (604)485-0158; pmakarew@shaw.ca.

MAKARLA, Prakash B; University of Alberta Hosp, 5B4 56 WCM-8440 112 St NW, Edmonton AB T6G 2B7; (India)'86; Staff, University of Alberta Hospital; (780)407-3441

MAKARY, David; Southlake Reg Health Centre, 596 Davis Dr, Newmarket ON L3Y 2P9; McM'10; CCFP; Staff, Southlake Regional Health Centre; (905)853-3103

MAKARY, Hala; Dr Everett Chalmers Reg Hosp, PO Box 9000 Stn A 700 Priestman St, Fredericton NB E3B 5N5; Ain Shams (Egypt)'93; Staff, Dr Everett Chalmers Regional Hospital; (506)452-5286

MAKER, Dara; Women's College Hosp, 76 Grenville St, Toronto ON M5S 1B2; Tor'03; CCFP; Staff, Women's College Hospital; (416)323-6060; Fax. (416)323-6135.

MAKEREWICH, Leonard A; Niagara ENT Consultants, 204-6453 Morrison St, Niagara Falls ON L2E 7H1; Tor'72; DABOT; DABSM; FRCSC; Otol (Sleep Medicine). Ac Staff, Niagara Health System - Greater Niagara General Site; Consultant, Niagara Health System - St Catharines General Site; Consultant, Niagara Health System - Welland Hospital Site; (905)374-2451; Fax. (905)374-9267; lmakerewich@hotmail.com.

MAKHAN, Bernard A; 440 Browns Line, Etobicoke ON M8W 3T9; Dal'63; CCFP; FCFP; Hon Staff Family Med, Trillium Health Centre - West Toronto; (416)251-8831; Fax. (416)251-7314.

MAKHAN, Winston M; PO Box 3030, Stellarton NS B0K 1S0; Dal'71.

MAKHANI, Naila; The Hosp for Sick Children, 555 University Ave, Toronto ON M5G 1X8; UBC'05; Neur (Pediatrics). Staff, The Hospital For Sick Children; (416)813-6332

MAKHDOOM, Safana A; Strathcona Med Dental Bldg, 8225 105 St NW, Edmonton AB T6E 4H2; (Dominica)'08; LMCC; DABFP; (780)432-0211

MAKHDOOM, Sarah; Charles Clark Med Centre, 201-303 9 Ave SW, High River AB T1V 0H2; Punjab (Pakistan)'97; MB BS; CCFP; Staff Physician, High River General Hospital; Staff, Low Risk Obstetrics Clinic; Langs: Urdu; Punjabi; Hindi; (403)652-2929; Fax. (403)652-1510.

MAKHDOOM, Sohail; Child & Parent Resource Inst, 600 Sanatorium Rd, London ON N6H 3W7; Karachi (Pakistan)'95; Psychiatrist, Child & Parent Resource Institute; (519)858-2774

MAKHENE, Edward; Trillium Hlth Ctr-Mississauga, 100 Queensway W, Mississauga ON L5B 1B8; Witwatersrand (South Africa)'57; MB ChB; BSc; DAB; FAAP; FRCPC; Peds (Consultant Pediatrics). Staff, Trillium Health Centre - Mississauga; (905)848-7580

MAKHIJA, Sapna; 32-1960 Appleby Line, Burlington ON L7L 0B7; Sask'02; FRCPC; IntMed; Gastroent. Staff Gastroent, St Michael's Hospital; (905)335-1888

MAKHLOUF, Samia M; 309-6633 Highway 7, Markham ON L3P 7P2; Cairo (Egypt)'83; CCFP; (905)294-5566

MAKHOULIAN, Natalie; Clinique du Dr Savaria, 75 boul des Chateaux, Blainville QC J7B 2A4; Sher'10; CCFP; (450)434-2009

MAKI, John D; Sudbury Med Centre, 300B-65 Larch St, Sudbury ON P3E 1B8; Tor'67; Ac Staff, Health Sciences North-St Joseph's Health Centre; Coroner, City of Sudbury District 19; (705)674-3502; Fax. (705)674-1729; maki@isys.ca.

MAKI, Ron S; Downtown Comm Health Centre, 569 Powell St, Vancouver BC V6A 1G8; UBC'88; Staff, Downtown Community Health Clinic; (604)255-3151; Fax. (604)255-0314.

MAKIN, G J Vance; 201-520 17th St, West Vancouver BC V7V 3S8; Cal'79; BSc(Hons); MSc; FRCPC; Neur (Electrodiagnosis). Staff, Lions Gate Hospital; Staff, Burnaby Hospital; (604)913-8183 x2788

MAKIN, Michael D; Omineca Clinic, RR 2 3348 Hospital Rd, Vanderhoof BC V0J 3A2; Cape Town (South Africa)'80; MB ChB; CCFP; Clin Assoc Prof Family Med, University of British Columbia; (250)567-2201; mmakin@telus.net.

MAKINDE, Olumide A; Ottawa Street Med Centre, 1535 Ottawa St, Windsor ON N8X 2G3; Lagos (Nigeria)'89; MB BS; CCFP; (519)969-1319; Fax. (519)969-5285.

MAKINDE, Oluwatomilola O; Hayyan Healthcare, 8-9301 Bathurst St, Richmond Hill ON L4C 9S2; Birmingham (USA)'07; CCFP; (905)237-7472

MAKINDE, Oluyele A; Victory Med Associates, 137 20th St W, Saskatoon SK S7M 0W7; (Other Foreign)'83; MB BS; MSc; MPH(UK); MRCGPract(UK); (306)249-2227; Fax. (306)249-2348.

MAKINEN, Patrice; CSSS de Saint-Jerome, 290 rue de Montigny, Saint-Jerome QC J7Z 5T3; Mon'00; FRCSC; OrthSurg. Staff, Hôtel-Dieu de Saint-Jérôme; (450)431-8200

MAKIS, Viliam; Brandon Reg Health Centre, 150 McTavish Ave E, Brandon MB R7A 2B3; McG'05; FRCPC; NuclearMed. Staff, Brandon Regional Health Centre.

MAKIWANE, Unati; Core Medicenter, 1635 11th Ave, Regina SK S4P 0H5; (South Africa)'05; MB ChB; (306)584-8880; Fax. (306)584-8865.

MAKKAR, Nina; Village Family Physicians, 275 Pictou Rd, Truro NS B2N 2S7; Wes'94; BSc(Biol.); CCFP; Assoc Staff Privil, Colchester East Hants Health Centre; (902)895-1232; Fax. (902)897-9749; makkar@eastlink.ca.

MAKKEN, Hilda A; 43 Hagey Ave, Fort Erie ON L2A 1W4; Groningen (Netherlands)'81; FRCPC; Peds. Consultant Peds, Haldimand War Memorial Hospital; Asst Prof Clinical Peds, McMaster University; Langs: Dutch; (905)871-9288; Fax. (905)871-9544; hilda.makken@sympatico.ca.

MAKKI, Mehdi; Rouge Valley-Centenary HC, 2867 Ellesmere Rd, Scarborough ON M1E 4B9; Luton (England)'06; Staff, Rouge Valley Health System - Centenary Health Centre Site.

MAKOKIS, James A; PO Box 1130, Siksika AB T0J 3W0; Ott'10; (403)734-5686; Fax. (403)734-3916.

MAKOWIECKA, Maria I; William Osler HC-Etobicoke, 101 Humber College Blvd, Etobicoke ON M9V 1R8; Warsaw (Poland)'74; FRCPC; Anes. Staff, William Osler Health System - Etobicoke General Hospital; (416)747-3554

MAKRETSOV, Nikita A; St Paul's Hosp, 1081 Burrard St, Vancouver BC V6Z 1Y6; Far-Eastern State (Russia (Federation))'93; CEd; PhD; DPath; FRCP; FRCPC; AnatPath (Breast Pathology). Staff AnatPath, St Clare's Mercy Hospital; Langs: Russian; (604)682-2344 x66038

MAKROPOULOS, Dimitri; Queensway-Carleton Hosp, 3045 Baseline Rd, Nepean ON K2H 8P4; Ott'02; FRCPC; EmergMed. Staff, Queensway Carleton Hospital; (613)721-2000

MAKSYMEC, Marta S; Bayridge Family Med Clinic, PO Box 20103 Taylor Kidd PO 775 Strand Blvd, Kingston ON K7P 2T6; McM'88; CCFP; (613)507-1212; Fax. (613)507-1213.

MAKSYMIUK, Andrew W; CancerCare Manitoba, 2057-675 McDermot Ave, Winnipeg MB R3E 0V9; Sask'72; FRCPC; IntMed; MedOncol. (204)787-2021; Fax. (204)787-1345; maksymiu@cc.umanitoba.ca.

MAKSYMOV, Volodymyr I; Grand River Hosp-KW Hlth Ctre, PO Box 956 Stn C 835 King St W, Kitchener ON N2G 1G3; Danylo Halytsky Lviv University (Poland)'80; FRCPC; AnatPath. Staff, Grand River Hospital - Kitchener/Waterloo Health Centre; (519)749-4300

MAKSYMOWYCH, Wolodymyr P; Heritage Med Research Centre, 562-107 University Campus NW, Edmonton AB T6G 2S2; Manchester (England)'81; MB ChB; ABIM(Rheum); FRCPC; IntMed; Rheum. Med Staff, University of Alberta Hospital; Assoc Prof Med, University of Alberta; (780)407-1964; Fax. (780)407-6055; walter.maksymowych@ualberta.ca.

MAKUCH, Patricia A; 307 Lakeshore Dr, North Bay ON P1A 2B9; Tor'93; BScChemEng.

MAKUS, Kenneth G; Dr Norbert J Witt Neuro Servic, 10816 124 St NW, Edmonton AB T5M 0H3; Alb'94; FRCPC; Neur. Staff Privil, Royal Alexandra Hospital; Privil., Walter C. McKenzie Health Centre; Langs: German; (780)454-3344; Fax. (780)455-7992; kmakus@telusplanet.net.

MAKUZA, Aimable; Clinique Med de Buckingham, 200-620 av de Buckingham, Mont-Tremblant QC J8E 2H5; (Burundi)'85; CCFP; (819)986-6006; Fax. (819)986-1616; aimablem@hotmail.com.

MALAAB, Suzanne; CSSS de la Vallée de l'Or, 725 6e rue, Val-d'Or QC J9P 3Y1; Beirut (Lebanon)'85; FRCPC; Peds. Staff, Centre Hospitalier de Val d'Or; Langs: French; Arabic; (819)825-6711; Fax. (819)825-5624.

MALABANAN, Edilberto A; 202-1385 Sargent Ave, Winnipeg MB R3E 3P8; (Philippines)'76; Staff, Seven Oaks General Hospital; Langs: Tagalog; (204)956-0988; eddie091500@aol.com.

MALACH, Jaye A; 1818 10 Ave S, Lethbridge AB T1K 0B6; Sask'92; FRCSC; ObstGyn;CCFP; (403)327-4637

MALAGON BARRERA, Maria F; Rockyview Gen Hosp, 7007 14 St SW, Calgary AB T2V 1P9; (Colombia)'98; CCFP; Staff, Rockyview General Hospital; (403)943-3597; Fax. (403)943-8411.

MALAGUTI, Santina M; 201-20 Corporate Park Dr, St Catharines ON L2S 3W2; Mysore (India)'84; Staff, Niagara Health System - St Catharines General Site; (905)684-7985; Fax. (905)684-6016.

MALAISE, Jacques; CHUM-Hop Notre-Dame, 1560 rue Sherbrooke E, Montreal QC H2L 4M1; Louvain (Belgium)'88; Staff, Centre Hospitalier l'Université de Montréal (CHUM) - Hôpital Notre-Dame; (514)890-8000

MALAK, Emad Y W; Montebello Med Clinic, 249 Waverley Rd, Dartmouth NS B2X 2C5; Ain Shams (Egypt)'87; CCFP; (902)406-4444

MALAK, M Nabil; CSSS de Papineau, 500 rue Belanger, Gatineau QC J8L 2M4; Tours (France)'69; FRCSC; GenSurg. Staff, CH-CHSLD de Papineau - Pavillon du centre hospitalier; (819)986-3341; Fax. (819)986-4118.

MALAK, Monzer; C S C Hamilton-Niagara, 810 East Main St, Welland ON L3B 3Y4; Montpellier (France)'77; CCFP; (905)734-1141

MALAK, Ramez; Hop Charles Lemoyne, 3120 boul Taschereau, Greenfield Park QC J4V 2H1; Mon'03; FRCSC; Neursurg. Staff, Hopital Charles LeMoyne; (450)466-5000

MALAK, Ziad; Quest Commun Health Centre, 100-145 Queenston St, St. Catharines ON L2R 2Z9; Beirut (Lebanon)'01; CCFP; (905)668-2558

MALAK DOSS, Sherlene S; St Mary's Clinic, PO Box 45 110 Roe Ave, Gander NL A1V 1W8; Ai Shams (Egypt)'92; CCFP.

MALAKIEH, Amira L; Greenbelt Family Health Team, 1C-3500 Fallowfield Rd, Nepean ON K2J 4A7; Qns'07; CCFP; Staff, Kemptville District Hospital; (613)843-1718

MALAKIEH, Nadia; Greenbelt Family Health Team, 1C-3500 Fallowfield Rd, Ottawa ON K2J 4A7; Ott'06; FRCPC; IntMed. Staff, The Ottawa Hospital - Riverside Campus; (613)843-1718

MALAM, Faiz G; William Osler HC-Brampton, 2100 Bovaird Dr E, Brampton ON L6R 3J7; McM'01; CCFP; Staff, William Osler Health System - Brampton Civic Hospital; (905)494-2120

MALAMED, Phillip J; Lakeridge Hlth Corp-Oshawa, 1 Hospital Crt, Oshawa ON L1G 2B9; Cape Town (South Africa)'60; MB ChB; DPM; MRCPsy; Psy. Assoc Staff Psy, Lakeridge Health - Oshawa Site; (905)576-8711 x4253; Fax. (905)721-4742.

MALAN, Albert J; Royal University Hosp, 103 Hospital Dr, Saskatoon SK S7N 0W8; Pretoria (South Africa)'91; MB ChB; FRCPC; Anes. Staff Anes, Royal University Hospital; (306)655-1183

MALAN, Catharina M; Saskatoon East Fam Physicians, 21-2105 8th St E, Saskatoon SK S7H 0T8; Pretoria (South Africa)'91; MB ChB; Staff, Royal University Hospital; (306)373-5520; Fax. (306)374-9414.

MALAN, Francois A; 414 13 St N, Lethbridge AB T1H 2S2; Pretoria (South Africa)'76; MB ChB; MMed(Psych); Staff, Chinook Regional Hospital; Langs: Afrikaans; (403)328-3121; Fax. (403)328-3133.

MALAN, Jacobus F; 102-1315 Summit Dr, Kamloops BC V2C 5R9; Stellenbosch (South Africa)'99; MB ChB; BScHons; MSc; (250)851-9413

MALAN, Jean E; Aberdeen Hosp, 835 East River Rd, New Glasgow NS B2H 3S6; Witwatersrand (South Africa)'77; Staff, Aberdeen Regional Hospital; (902)752-8311

MALAN, Johann H; Kenderdine Med Clinic, 110-1804 McOrmond Dr, Saskatoon SK S7S 0A6; Pretoria (South Africa)'87; MB ChB; DObst; LMCC; Langs: Afrikaans; German; (306)934-6606; Fax. (306)955-3180.

MALAN, Johannes J; Chaparral Corner Shopp Centre, 208-803 Chaparral Dr SE, Calgary AB T2X 0E5; Pretoria (South Africa)'85; MB ChB; Langs: Afrikaans; (403)873-7734; Fax. (403)873-7735; j.malan@sasktel.net.

MALAN, Maurice D; Peterborough Reg HC-Hospital, 1 Hospital Dr, Peterborough ON K9J 7C6; Cape Town (South Africa)'72; FRCPC; Anes. Staff, Peterborough Regional Health Centre - Hospital Drive; (705)743-2121

MALAN, Stephan P; Provost Med Centre, PO Box 90 Stn Main, Provost AB T0B 3S0; (South Africa)'83; MB ChB; Med Examiner, Province of Alberta; Langs: Afrikaans; (780)753-2271; Fax. (780)753-2371.

MALANOWSKA, Anna J; Allin Clinic, 10155 120 St NW, Edmonton AB T5K 2A2; Warsaw (Poland)'83; FRCPC; Peds (Pulmonary Medicine). Staff, University of Alberta Hospital; Staff, Royal Alexandra Hospital; Clin Assoc Prof, University of Alberta; Langs: Polish; (780)482-7551; Fax. (780)701-5397.

MALAT, Jan; E1 218-60 White Squirrel Way, Toronto ON M6J 1H4; Tor'94; FRCPC; Psy. Staff, Centre for Addiction & Mental Health (CAMH) - Russell Street Site; jan_malat@camh.net.

MALAVIARACHCHI, Krishangi; The Westend Family Care Clinic, 80 Michael Cowpland Dr, Kanata ON K2M 1P6; Dal'06; CCFP; Staff, Westend Family Care Clinic Family Health Team; (613)599-3321

MALAVIARACHCHI, Pushpa K; Eric Martin Pavillion, 2334 Trent St, Victoria BC V8R 4Z3; Ceylon (Sri Lanka)'72; DPM; MRCPsy(UK); MB BS; FRCPC; Psy (Affective Disorders). Staff Psychiatrist Affective Disorder Clinic, Royal Jubilee Hospital; (250)370-8155; Fax. (250)370-8199.

MALAYIL, Nina B; Unison Hlth & Commun Services, 12 Flemington Rd, North York ON M6A 2N4; Wes'93; CCFP; FCFP; (416)787-1661; Fax. (416)787-3761.

MALCHY, Brian A; Selkirk Mental Health Centre, PO Box 9600 Stn Main 825 Manitoba Ave, Selkirk MB R1A 2B5; Man'88; FRCPC; Psy. Staff, Selkirk Mental Health Centre; (204)482-3810

MALCOLM, Barry; Sunnybrook Holland Ortho Arthr, 317-43 Wellesley St E, Toronto ON M4Y 1H1; Tor'71; DAB; MBA; FRCSC; OrthSurg (Spine/Disability). Ac Staff, Sunnybrook Health Sciences Centre - Holland Orthopaedic & Arthritic Centre; Consultant Staff, Women's College Hospital; Asst Prof Surg, University of Toronto; (416)967-8783; Fax. (416)967-8785; barry.malcolm@sunnybrook.ca.

MALCOLM, Brendan P; Front-Frederick Health Service, 14F-365 Bloor St E, Toronto ON M4W 3L4; Tor'88; CCFP; FCFP; (416)362-8777; Fax. (416)362-7879.

MALCOLM, Christine E; 103-9815 97 St, Grande Prairie AB T8V 8B9; Alb'04; FRCPC; Derm. (780)513-2255

MALCOLM, Dennis; CSSS de Laval, 1755 boul Rene-Laennec, Laval QC H7M 3L9; Mon'86; Staff, Hopital de la Cite de la santé; (450)668-1010 x2001

MALCOLM, Gordon; 104-1240 Kensington Rd NW, Calgary AB T2N 3P7; Mem'99; CCFP; (403)837-7800; Fax. (403)837-7800.

MALCOLM, Ian D; MUHC-Royal Victoria Hosp, M 476-687 av des Pins O, Montreal QC H3A 1A1; McG'74; ABIM(Cardiol); FRCPC; IntMed; Cardiol. principale Médecin, McGill University Health Centre - Royal Victoria Hospital; assoc Prof, McGill University; (514)934-1934 x36151

MALCOLM, Jacqueline I; 202-10 Alcorn Ave, Toronto ON M4V 3A9; Qns'86; FRCPC; Psy. (416)927-7603

MALCOLM, Janine C; The Ottawa Hosp-Riverside, 4F-1967 Riverside Dr, Ottawa ON K1H 7W9; Qns'97; FRCPC; IntMed; Endocrin&Metab. Staff, The Ottawa Hospital - Riverside Campus; (613)738-8400 x81940

MALCOLM, Jennifer P; High Park Health Centre, 507-2333 Dundas St W, Toronto ON M6R 3A6; Qns'98; CCFP; (416)766-2718; Fax. (416)766-0196.

MALCOLM, Scott F; Dept of National Defense, PO Box 99000 Stn Forces, Halifax NS B3K 5X5; Dal'01; CCFP; Staff, Canadian Forces Health Services Centre (Atlantic); (902)427-7768; Fax. (902)427-0504.

MALCOLM, W Neil; Niagara H System-St Catharine, PO Box 3018 Stn Main 142 Queenston St, St Catharines ON L2R 7C6; Dundee (Scotland)'74; Anes. Staff, Niagara Health System - St Catharines General Site.

MALCOLMSON, Charles H; McMaster University, HSC 3A-1280 Main St W, Hamilton ON L8S 4K1; Qns'58; FRCPC; Peds (Critical Care Medicine). Staff, Hamilton Health Sciences Centre - McMaster Children's Hospital; Clin Assoc Prof Peds, McMaster University; (905)521-2100 x75702; Fax. (905)524-5707; malcolm@mcmaster.ca.

MALDONADO, Juan E; Women's College Hosp, 76 Grenville St, Toronto ON M5S 1B2; Central (Ecuador)'71; FRCPC; IntMed. Staff, Women's College Hospital; (416)323-6339; Fax. (416)323-6304.

MALDONADO GONZALEZ, David F; IWK Health Centre, PO Box 9700 Rpo CSC, Halifax NS B3K 6R8; (Ecuador)'03; Staff, IWK Health Centre; (902)470-8939

MALE, Ross S; Cobblestone Medicine & Rehab, 8-1084 Rest Acres Rd, Paris ON N3L 0B5; Cal'96; MSc; BSc(Hons); CCFP; FCFP; Staff Family Med, The Brant Community Healthcare System - Brantford General Hospital Site; Langs: English; French; (519)442-7674; Fax. (519)975-4364.

MALE, Roy A; Regent Park Comm Health Centre, 465 Dundas St E, Toronto ON M5A 2B2; McG'90; CCFP; FCFP; Langs: French; Spanish; (416)203-4507; Fax. (416)364-0822.

MALEC, Carolyn L; 206-470 Bronte St S, Milton ON L9T 2J4; Ott'98; CCFP; FCFP; (905)878-6793; Fax. (905)878-6711.

MALEC, Elizabeth A; Ormstown Med Centre, GD 24 rue Gale, Ormstown QC J0S 1K0; (Poland)'84; CCFP; Langs: Bilingual(French/English); (450)829-2331; Fax. (450)829-3636.

MALEC, Tadeusz S; Ctr Hosp Anna-Laberge, 200 boul Brisebois, Chateauguay QC J6K 4W8; N.Copernicus (Poland)'84; FRCPC; Psy. Staff, Hôpital Anna-Laberge; (450)699-2425; Fax. (450)699-2525.

MALEK, Anna M; 201-626 King St W, Toronto ON M5V 1M7; Wes'10; CCFP; (416)703-1313; Fax. (416)703-1310.

MALEK, Batu; 728 Anderson St, Whitby ON L1N 3V6; London (England)'59; MB BS; LMCC; LMSSA; (905)668-6851; Fax. (905)668-2609.

MALEK, Michael L; Civic Family Health Team, 210 Melrose Ave, Ottawa ON K1Y 4K7; Ott'95; CCFP; FCFP; Ac Staff, The Ottawa Hospital - Civic Campus; Physician, Hillel Lodge-Home for the Aged; (613)761-4334; mmalek@magma.ca.

MALEK, Rowja; 307-2130 Lawrence Ave E, Scarborough ON M1R 3A6; Islami Azad (Iran)'96; CCFP; Langs: Farsi; (416)751-6141

MALEK MARZBAN, Peiman; Winnipeg Clinic, 425 St Mary Ave, Winnipeg MB R3C 0N2; Tehran (Iran)'94; (204)957-1900; Fax. (204)957-7410.

MALEKALKALAMI, Azadeh; Norway House Indian Hosp, PO Box 730, Norway House MB R0B 1B0; (Iran)'93; Staff, Norway House Indian Hospital; (204)359-6731

MALEKI, Babak; Fenwick Med Centre, 315-5595 Fenwick St, Halifax NS B3H 4M2; McM'03; FRCSC; Ophth (Oculo Plastic Surgery). Staff, Queen Elizabeth II Health Sciences Centre - Victoria General Site; Langs: Bilingual(English/French); (902)405-8477; Fax. (902)405-8479.

MALEKI, Mohammad; MUHC-Montreal Gen Hosp, L7 516-1650 av Cedar, Montreal QC H3G 1A4; Shiraz (Iran)'75; FRCSC; Neursurg. Dir Neurotrauma, McGill University Health Centre - Montreal General Campus; (514)934-8061; Fax. (514)934-8227.

MALEKI-YAZDI, Mohammad R; 608-790 Bay St, Toronto ON M5G 1N8; Tehran (Iran)'77; FRCPC; IntMed; Respir. Coord Respirol, Women's College Hospital; Asst Prof Respirol & Med, University of Toronto; Langs: Farsi; (416)921-7704; Fax. (416)921-3277.

MALEMPATI, N Rao; 440 Giles Blvd E, Windsor ON N9A 4C6; Andhra (India)'74; MB BS; DPM(N.I.M.H.); FRCPC; Psy (Family Therapy). Chief Psy, Windsor Regional Hospital - Metropolitan Site; Langs: Telugu; (519)258-1282; Fax. (519)258-9758.

MALENFANT, Claude; Clinique Dr Claude Malenfant, 100-1731 3e av, Val-d'Or QC J9P 1W3; Mon'74; Physician/Coroner, CLSC le Minordet; (819)825-6678; Fax. (819)825-4288; drclaudemalenfant@cablevision.qc.ca.

MALENFANT, Dominic; Clinique Med Notre-Dame Inc, 147 rue Notre-Dame E, Victoriaville QC G6P 3Z8; Mon'98; Langs: English; (819)758-3165; Fax. (819)758-0745.

MALENFANT, Helene; CLSC Drummond, 350 rue Saint-Jean, Drummondville QC J2B 5L4; Laval'89; Staff, CHSLD Coeur-du-Québec; Langs: Bilingual(French/English); (819)474-2572 x227; Fax. (819)474-4937; clscdr@dr.cgocable.ca.

MALENFANT, Jean-Guy; CLSC Desjardins, 15 rue de l'Arsenal, Levis QC G6V 4P6; Laval'79; (418)835-3400 x3207; Fax. (418)835-6413.

MALENFANT, Julie; Hotel-Dieu de Montmagny-L'Isle, 350 boul Tache O, Montmagny QC G5V 3R8; Laval'05; Anes. Staff, CSSS de Montmagny-L'Islet; (418)248-0630

MALENFANT, Laurie; Clin de Med Interne d'Edmundst, 20 rue Carrier, Edmundston NB E3V 3Y1; Mon'04; FRCPC; IntMed. Staff, Hôpital regional d'Edmundston; Langs: Bilingual(French/English); (506)739-9511; Fax. (506)735-8118; clin.med.int@nb.aibn.com.

MALENFANT, Mario; Centre Oculaire de Quebec, 2480 ch Sainte-Foy, Quebec QC G1V 1T6; Laval'66; Ophth (Retina)., Université Laval; (418)780-6345; Fax. (418)780-3345.

MALENFANT, Michelle; CRSSS Baie-James-Chibougamau, 51 3e rue, Chibougamau QC G8P 1N1; Laval'99; CCFP; Staff, CRSSS de la Baie-James; Langs: English; (418)748-2676; Fax. (418)748-2549.

MALENFANT, Paul-Andre; CHUM-Hop St-Luc, 1058 rue Saint-Denis, Montreal QC H2X 3J4; Anes (P.Q.). Staff, Centre Hospitalier l'Université De Montréal (CHUM) - Hôpital Saint-luc; (514)890-8000

MALENFANT, Suzanne; Clinique Med de Lambton, 230A rue Du College, Lambton QC G0M 1H0; Laval'75; (418)486-7480

MALENFANT, Sylvain; Clinique Gyn De Trois-Rivieres, 2237 7e av, Trois-Rivieres QC G8Z 3E2; Laval'83; FRCSC; ObstGyn. Staff, Centre Hospitalier Affilié Universitaire de Québec - Hôpital du St-Sacrement; Staff, CSSS de Charlevoix; Staff, Hôpital de la Malbaie; Université Laval; (819)379-5353

MALETTE, Paul M J; 1679 Main St, Val Caron ON P3N 1R8; McM'84; Langs: English; French; (705)897-1018

MALEVICH, Victoria N; Stones Mill Family Health Ctr, 25 Mill St, Gananoque ON K7G 2L5; Minsk State (Belarus)'96; CCFP; (613)382-3974

MALEY, Garnet J M; 110-470 Bronte St S, Milton ON L9T 2J4; Tor'82; BSc; MSc; Ac Staff, Halton Healthcare Services Corporation - Milton District Hospital; Assoc Staff, Joseph Brant Memorial Hospital; Assoc Staff, Rouge Valley Health System - Centenary Health Centre Site; Langs: French; Italian; German; (905)878-0539; Fax. (905)878-0771.

MALEZA, Gerard; Centre Med Le Mesnil, 300-1300 boul Lebourgneuf, Quebec QC G2K 2N1; Laval'88; Staff, Jeffery Hale Hospital-Saint Brigid's; (418)624-1800; Fax. (418)624-1820.

MALFAIR, David M; Central Alberta Med Imaging, 4312 54 Ave, Red Deer AB T4N 4M1; Alb'00; FRCPC; DiagRad. (403)343-6172; Fax. (403)309-0092.

MALHERBE, David S; Children's & Women's HC of BC, B321-4480 Oak St, Vancouver BC V6H 3V4; (South Africa)'88; MB ChB; DA(SA); MMed(Anes); FRCPC; Anes. Staff, BC Children's Hospital; (604)875-2711

MALHERBE, Gerhardus J; Diamond Head Med Clinic, PO Box 9200 Stn Main 1365 Pemberton Ave, Squamish BC V8B 0C1; Orange Free State (South Africa)'94; MB ChB; CCFP; (604)892-3732

MALHERBE, Jan A; Ingram Family Physicians, 103-149 Ingram St, Duncan BC V9L 1N8; Stellenbosch (South Africa)'92; MB ChB; LMCC; CCFP; Physician Emerg Room/Staff GP Anaesthetist, Lady Minto Gulf Islands Hospital; (250)746-4401

MALHERBE, Stéphanie C; Montfort Hosp, 713 Montreal Rd, Ottawa ON K1K 0T2; Mon'99; LMCC; MCFP(EM); CCFP; CCFP(E.M.); Staff EmergMed, Children's Hospital of Eastern Ontario (CHEO); Staff EmergMed, Montfort Hospital; Langs: Spanish; English; (613)746-4621 x4212; stephmalherbe@hotmail.com.

MALHI, Arfan M; Concordia Joint Replacement Gr, 300-1155 Concordia Ave, Winnipeg MB R2K 2M9; London (England)'98.

MALHI, Rajvinder K; Cameron Med Centre, 240-9600 Cameron St, Burnaby BC V3J 7N3; Birmingham (England)'04; MB ChB; (604)421-1027

MALHOTRA, Birinder; Student Health Services, UCCR 1-1151 Richmond St, London ON N6A 3K7; Delhi (India)'75; MB BS; FRCPC; Psy (Telehealth). Asst Dir Outpatient Dept, Regional Mental Health Care-St Joseph's Health Care; University of Western Ontario; (519)661-3030; Fax. (519)661-3380.

MALHOTRA, Gaurav S; Unviersity of Alberta Hosp, 8440 112 St NW, Edmonton AB T6G 2B7; Alb'08; CCFP; Staff, University of Alberta Hospital; (780)407-8822

MALHOTRA, Gurpreet S; Fifth Avenue Walk-In Clinic, 14 Fifth Ave, Orangeville ON L9W 1G2; Gulbarga (India)'94; CCFP; (519)942-0040

MALHOTRA, Jana L; 309-1580 Merivale Rd, Nepean ON K2G 4B5; Wes'05; CCFP; (613)226-4030

MALHOTRA, Kenneth S; Digestive Health Clinic Inc, 1031 Brock Rd, Pickering ON L1W 3T7; Tor'96; BSc(Hons.); FRCPC; IntMed;CCFP; Gastroent (Gastrointestinal Disorders). Clin Asst, St Joseph's Health Centre; Staff IntMed, Lakeridge Health - Bowmanville Site; (905)683-1700

MALHOTRA, Lalita; Orpheum Plaza, 100-1316 Central Ave, Prince Albert SK S6V 6P5; Gwalior (India)'62; MB BS; MRC(Eng); LRCP(Lond); (306)763-7039; Fax. (306)763-7558.

MALHOTRA, Rohin T; McMaster University, 20-1280 Main St W, Hamilton ON L8S 4K1; Tor'03; FRCPC; DiagRad.

MALHOTRA, Samir; 103-250 Keary St, New Westminster BC V3L 5E7; UBC'02; FRCPC; IntMed; Respir. (604)525-8822

MALHOTRA, Sangita; 203-245 Columbia St E, New Westminster BC V3L 3W4; UBC'02; FRCPC; IntMed (HIV); InfectDis. Clin Instructor Med, University of British Columbia; (604)525-9666

MALHOTRA, Sanjay; Hillsborough Hsp & Special CC, PO Box 1929 Stn Central, Charlottetown PE C1A 7N5; Staff, Hillsborough Hospital & Special Care Centre; (902)368-5400

MALHOTRA, Sonia; Women's Hlth in Women's Hands, 500-2 Carlton St, Toronto ON M5B 1J3; McM'05; CCFP; Staff, St Joseph's Health Centre; (416)593-7655

MALHOTRA, Sonya; Foothills Med Centre, 1403 29 St NW, Calgary AB T2N 2T9; Ott'07; FRCPC; Psy. Staff, Foothills Medical Centre; (403)944-1271

MALHOTRA, Tilak R; Orpheum Plaza, 100-1316 Central Ave, Prince Albert SK S6V 6P5; Punjab (India)'63; MB BS; DCH(UK); DTMH(UK); MRCS(UK); MRCP(UK); LRCP; FRCPC; Peds (Asthma). Consultant Ped, Prince Albert Parkland Health Region; Vice Pres, Prince Albert Parkland Regional Medical Association; Chairman Sect of Prov Peds/RA Member, Saskatchewan Medical Association; Member Governing Council, College of Physicians & Surgeons of Saskatchewan; Langs: Hindi; Punjabi; Urdu; (306)764-2122; Fax. (306)763-7558; tmalhotra@paphr.sk.ca.

MALHOTRA, Unjali; Crossroads Clinic-Women's Hlth, 330-507 Broadway W, Vancouver BC V5Z 1E6; (Ireland)'03; MB ChB; CCFP; (604)872-5484

MALHOTRA, Verinder; Queen-Lynch Med Centre, 202-157 Queen St E, Brampton ON L6W 3X4; Christian Med. Coll. (India)'81; (905)457-0000; Fax. (905)456-9912.

MALHOTRA, Veronica; The Alex Seniors Comm Health, 630 9 Ave SE, Calgary AB T2G 4V9; Alb'94; BSc; CCFP; FCFP; (403)920-0011

MALHOTRA, Vikram K; CSSS du Lac-des-Deux-Montagnes, 520 boul Arthur-Sauve, Saint-Eustache QC J7R 5B1; McG'97; FRCSC; GenSurg. Staff, Hôpital de Saint-Eustache; Langs: English; French; (450)473-6811

MALI, Bahera; 1440 14th Ave, Regina SK S4P 0W5; Karachi (Pakistan)'77; MB BS; FRCPath(UK); FRCPC; MedBiochem. Staff Med Biochemist, Regina General Hospital; Langs: Farsi; (306)766-4493; Fax. (306)766-4772; bahera.mali@rqhealth.ca.

MALIAKKAL, Rita K; 2130-4818 Westwinds Dr NE, Calgary AB T3J 3Z5; Calicut (India)'92; MB BS; CCFP; Langs: Urdu; Hindi; (403)293-5454

MALICK, Arfa K; 208-597 Parliament St, Toronto ON M4X 1W3; Patna (India)'80; (416)515-1333; Fax. (416)927-8065.

MALICKI, Krzysztof W; City Centre Family Physicians, 500-71 King St W, Mississauga ON L5B 4A2; Tor'76; Affil Staff, Trillium Health Centre - Mississauga; Langs: Spanish; Polish; (905)273-3176; Fax. (905)848-1500.

MALIG, Lita L; Credit Valley Med Arts Centre, 416-2000 Credit Valley Rd, Mississauga ON L5M 4N4; Manila (Philippines)'93; CCFP; Langs: Tagalog; (905)569-8377; Fax. (905)569-8378.

MALIK, Aasim N; 214PL-9909 102 St, Grande Prairie AB T8V 2V4; Nishtar (Pakistan)'88; (780)532-9067

MALIK, Abdul; Chinguacousy & Sandalwood Med, 6-10671 Chinguacousy Rd, Brampton ON L7A 0N5; (Pakistan)'78; CCFP; Langs: Urdu; Punjabi; Sindhi; Kacchi; (905)840-4343; Fax. (905)840-4303.

MALIK, Abid I; Percy E Moore Hosp, PO Box 190, Hodgson MB R0C 1N0; (Other Foreign)'98; Staff, Percy E Moore Hospital; (204)372-8444

MALIK, Amrit A; St Boniface Gen Hosp, 409 Tache Ave, Winnipeg MB R2H 2A6; Man'99; FRCPC; IntMed; Cardiol. Staff, St Boniface General Hospital; (204)233-8563

MALIK, Anita C; North East Community Health Ct, 14007 50 St NW, Edmonton AB T5A 5E4; Sask'02; FRCPC; Peds. Staff/Clin Asst Prof, University of Alberta Hospital; (780)342-4168; Fax. (780)342-4196.

MALIK, Anjna A; 2-1907 Baseline Rd, Ottawa ON K2C 0C7; Delhi (India)'75; MB BS; MD; Langs: Hindi; (613)224-7381; Fax. (613)224-0105.

MALIK, Anupam; Westbram Family Physicians, 104-100 Pertosa Dr, Brampton ON L6X 0H9; Delhi (India)'77; Staff, William Osler Health System - Brampton Civic Hospital; Langs: Hindi; Punjabi; (905)451-1244

MALIK, Arinder K; 100A-3305 Harvester Rd, Burlington ON L7N 3N2; Punjab (India)'85; FRCPC; Peds (Neonatology). Clinical Asst Prof, Hamilton Health Sciences Centre - McMaster Children's Hospital; Consultant Ped, Joseph Brant Memorial Hospital; (289)337-2716; Fax. (289)337-8396.

MALIK, Azhar M; Queen Square Doctors, 305-36 Vodden St E, Brampton ON L6V 4H4; Cairo (Egypt)'84; FACS; FRCSC; GenSurg. Staff, William Osler Health System - Brampton Civic Hospital; (905)456-1256; Fax. (905)456-9411.

MALIK, Bittoo S; Dauphin Reg Health Centre, 625 3rd St SW, Dauphin MB R7N 1R7; Man'95; Staff, Dauphin Regional Health Centre; (204)638-3010

MALIK, Hatim G; Medical Arts Bldg, 110-336 Kings Rd, Sydney NS B1S 1A9; Jabalpur (India)'65; MB BS; DAB; Neursurg (Neuro Trauma). (902)539-1756

MALIK, Kartika; Univ of Toronto, 602-500 University Ave, Toronto ON M5G 1V7; Man'07; GeriatricMed; IntMed.

MALIK, Khalid S; Doctors Urgent Care & Fam Med, 1145 Morningside Ave, Scarborough ON M1B 0A7; Nishtar Medical College (Pakistan)'99; CCFP; Staff, Peterborough Regional Health Centre - Hospital Drive; (647)352-3621

MALIK, Nariman; Scarborough Hosp-Birchmount, 3030 Birchmount Rd, Scarborough ON M1W 3W3; Tor'01; FRCPC; Anes. Staff, The Scarborough Hospital - Birchmount Campus; (416)495-2561

MALIK, Nazir A; Royal Victoria Hosp, 201 Georgian Dr, Barrie ON L4M 6M2; Punjab (Pakistan)'69; MB BS; DPM; Staff, Royal Victoria Regional Health Centre; (705)728-9090

MALIK, Puja; Humber Health Centre, H206-3199 Lake Shore Blvd W, Etobicoke ON M8V 1K8; Tor'10; CCFP; (416)675-6622 x3234

MALIK, R Neesh; Dauphin Reg Health Centre, 625 3rd St SW, Dauphin MB R7N 1R7; Man'99; FRCPC; DiagRad. Staff Diag Imaging, Dauphin Regional Health Centre; (204)638-3010

MALIK, Rashid; Trans Canada Mall, 152-1440 52 St NE, Calgary AB T2A 4T8; Gulf Medical College Ajman (United Arab Emirates)'07; CCFP; (403)272-3627; Fax. (403)272-3647.

MALIK, Rizwan; Queen Elizabeth II HSC, 2035-1276 South Park St, Halifax NS B3H 2Y9; Dundee (Australia)'98; MB ChB; Staff, Queen Elizabeth II Health Sciences Centre - Victoria General Site; (902)473-4343

MALIK, Rubina; A I M Health Group, 320 Adelaide St S, London ON N5Z 3L2; Tor'91; CCFP; (519)438-4161

MALIK, Saeed A; Headwaters Health Care Centre, 100 Rolling Hills Dr, Orangeville ON L9W 4X9; Islamia (Pakistan)'88; CCFP; CCFP(E.M.); Staff Emerg, Headwaters Health Care Centre - Orangeville Site; (519)941-2410

MALIK, Saira; Portland Med Clinic, 67 Portland St, Dartmouth NS B2Y 1H1; Kashmir (India)'69; MB BS; Staff, IWK Health Centre; Langs: Urdu; (902)406-3434; Fax. (902)406-3465.

MALIK, Saira; Dawson Creek & Dist Hosp, 11100 13 St, Dawson Creek BC V1G 3W8; Cork (Ireland)'10; MB BCh; BAO; CCFP; Staff, Dawson Creek & District Hospital; (250)782-8501

MALIK, Saleem T; 204-1139 Alloy Dr, Thunder Bay ON P7B 6M8; Cambridge (England)'78; MA; PhD; MRC; FRCPC; IntMed (Diabetes); MedOncol. Staff, Thunder Bay Regional Health Sciences Centre; Assoc Prof/Section Leader Internal Med, Northern Ontario School of Medicine; (807)345-1170; Fax. (807)768-1580; smalik@tbaytel.net.

MALIK, Samaad M; Richmond Med Bldg, 302-2020 Richmond Rd, Victoria BC V8R 6R5; Sask'02; FRCSC; GenSurg. (250)592-4313

MALIK, Samreen S; Parkland Med Associates, 205-505 Queen St, Spruce Grove AB T7X 2V2; (Pakistan)'02; MB BS; CCFP; (780)962-2001

MALIK, Shiraz; London HSC-Victoria Hosp, PO Box 5010 Stn B 800 Commissioners Rd E, London ON N6A 5W9; Wes'07; CCFP; Staff, London Health Sciences Centre - Victoria Campus; (519)685-8500

MALIK, Vinod; Orleans Medical-Dental Centre, 400-2555 St. Joseph Blvd, Orleans ON K1C 1S6; Delhi (India)'75; MB BS; FRCPC; Psy. Consultant, Children's Hospital of Eastern Ontario (CHEO); Dir Training, University of Ottawa; (613)834-8913; Fax. (613)834-9121.

MALINOWSKI, Ann; Ontario Power Generation Bldg, 3F 3149-700 University Ave, Toronto ON M5G 1Z5; McM'04; FRCSC; ObstGyn (Maternal Fetal Medicine). Staff, Mount Sinai Hospital; (416)586-5309; Fax. (416)586-8740.

MALINOWSKI, Ben A; Allin Clinic, 10155 120 St NW, Edmonton AB T5K 2A2; Alb'69; FRCPC; Peds. Langs: Polish; (780)482-7551; Fax. (780)488-2056; bmalinowski@theallinclinic.net.

MALINOWSKI, Cindy E; Shuswap Family Practice, 102-571 6 St NE, Salmon Arm BC V1E 1R6; Sask'81.

MALINOWSKI, Danuta J; 2385 Burnhamthorpe Rd W, Mississauga ON L5L 6A4; Tor'73; BSc; Langs: Polish; (905)607-6661; Fax. (905)607-5552.

MALINOWSKI, Jason R J; St Francis Health Centre, PO Box 130 21 St Francis Memorial Dr, Barrys Bay ON K0J 1B0; Qns'99; CCFP; Staff, St Francis Memorial Hospital; (613)756-9888; Fax. (613)756-3180.

MALISH, Dean G; Kelowna Orthopedics, 303-3330 Richter St, Kelowna BC V1W 4V5; UBC'97; BSc; FRCSC; OrthSurg. (250)717-7990

MALISIC, Dragoljub; 900 Albion Rd, Etobicoke ON M9V 1A5; Wes'08; CCFP.

MALIZIA, Mario L; 1033 Dundas St, London ON N5W 3A4; Wes'69; Med Examiner, Civil Aviation Canada; Langs: Italian; (519)455-1990; Fax. (519)455-6812.

MALKIN, Aaron; Sheppard Associates, 649 Sheppard Ave W, North York ON M3H 2S4; Man'49; PhD(Biochem); IntMed. Hon Staff, Sunnybrook Health Sciences Centre; Emeritus Prof, University of Toronto; (416)630-0610; Fax. (416)398-5712.

MALKIN, David D; The Hosp for Sick Children, 555 University Ave, Toronto ON M5G 1X8; Tor'84; MD; FAAP; FRCPC; Peds (Pediatric Oncology). Staff Physician Hem/Oncol, The Hospital For Sick Children; Prof Peds, University of Toronto; (416)813-5348; Fax. (416)813-5327; david.malkin@sickkids.ca.

MALKIN, Lilia; Scarborough Hosp-General Div, 3050 Lawrence Ave E, Scarborough ON M1P 2V5; Tor'01; CCFP; CCFP(E.M.); Staff, The Scarborough Hospital - General Campus; (416)431-8181; l.malkin@utoronto.ca.

MALKIN, Mendl; Bridgepoint Hosp, 14 St Matthews Rd, Toronto ON M4M 2B5; Man'73; CCFP; FCFP; Staff, Bridgepoint Health Centre; (416)461-8251 x2002; Fax. (416)470-6722; mmalkin@bridgepointhealth.ca.

MALL, Austin; London HSC-University Hosp, PO Box 5339 Stn B 339 Windermere Rd, London ON N6A 5A5; Massachussetts (USA)'07; CCFP; Staff, London Health Sciences Centre - University Hospital; (519)685-8500

MALL, Omar; Royal Victoria Hosp, 3F-201 Georgian Dr, Barrie ON L4M 6M2; Man'10; CCFP; Staff, Royal Victoria Regional Health Centre; (705)792-3333

MALLA, Ashok K; Douglas Mental Hlth Univ Inst, 6875 Lasalle Blvd, Verdun QC H4H 1R3; Punjab (India)'71; DPM(Eng); MRCPsy; FRCPC; Psy (Other Psychosis). Staff, Douglas Mental Health University Institute; (514)761-6131 x3390; Fax. (514)888-4064; ashok.malla@douglas.mcgill.ca.

MALLAM, Paul W; PO Box 2250 Stn Sardis Main, Chilliwack BC V2R 1A6; Mem'79; BMedSci; CCFP; CCFP(E.M.); FCFP; Staff Emerg, Chilliwack General Hospital.

MALLAVARAPU, Harinath; Surrey Med Arts Bldg, 207-13710 94A Ave, Surrey BC V3V 1N1; Osmania (India)'65; MB BS; DABPN; FRCPC; Psy (Adult Psychiatry). Staff, Surrey Memorial Hospital; Langs: Telugu; Hindi; (604)581-0576; Fax. (604)581-9375.

MALLECK, Naseem; City Plaza Specialist Clinic, 3-330 Central Ave N, Swift Current SK S9H 0L4; (Other Foreign)'82; MB BS; FCOG(SA); FRCSC; ObstGyn (Endocrinology). Clin Chief ObstGyn, Cypress Regional Hospital; Langs: French; (306)778-3988; Fax. (306)778-3989; nmalleck@yahoo.com.

MALLEK, Noa K; Kerrisdale Prof Centre, 320-2025 42nd Ave W, Vancouver BC V6M 2B5; Cal'01; FRCSC; Ophth. (604)261-0811

MALLERY, Laurie H; 5955 Veterans Memorial Lane, Halifax NS B3H 2E1; Pennsylvania (USA)'85; FRCPC; IntMed; GeriatricMed. Staff Geriatric Med, Queen Elizabeth II Health Sciences Centre - Victoria General Site; (902)473-8603; laurie.mallery@cdha.nshealth.ca.

MALLESON, Roey M; Willow Women's Clinic, 1013-750 Broadway W, Vancouver BC V5Z 1H9; London (England)'77; MB BS; MHSc; Dir Education, BC Women's Hospital & Health Centre; Clinical Asst Prof Family Pract/Assoc Member, University of British Columbia; (604)709-5611

MALLET, Jacques L; 2B boul St-Pierre O, Caraquet NB E1W 1B6; Mon'92; CCFP; Ac Member, Hôpital de l'Enfant-Jésus RHSJ; (506)727-6591; Fax. (506)727-6570.

MALLET, Marcel; 247 av Universite, Moncton NB E1C 5K4; Laval'95; ABIM; FRCPC; IntMed; Respir. Staff Pneumol & IntMed, Dr Georges-L-Dumont University Hospital Centre; Langs: English; (506)382-1202; Fax. (506)855-2375; marcelmallet@vitalitenb.ca.

MALLET, Michele; Hôpital de CSC de Lamèque, 29 rue de l'Hopital, Lameque NB E8T 1C5; Sher'05; CCFP; Staff, Hôpital de CSC de Lamèque; Langs: Bilingual(French/English); (506)344-2261

MALLET, Veronique; CSSS Cleophas-Claveau, CP 38 succ La Baie 1000 rue du Docteur-Desgagne, La Baie QC G7B 3P9; Paris(Fr) (France)'03; Staff, CHSLD-CLSC Cleophas-Claveau; (418)544-3381

MALLETT, Aaron G; Royal Alexandra Hosp, 521-10240 Kingsway NW, Edmonton AB T5H 3V9; Alb'08; Staff, Royal Alexandra Hospital; (780)735-4443; Fax. (780)735-4916.

MALLETTE, Yvon; Clinique Med Richelieu, 200-500 Rte Marie-Victorin, Sorel-Tracy QC J3R 1K7; Sher'71; Staff, Hôtel-Dieu de Sorel; Langs: Bilingual(French/English); (450)742-5638; Fax. (450)742-0995.

MALLETTE-EDWARDS, Shelley A; Village Med Associates, 27-1077 North Service Rd, Mississauga ON L4Y 1A6; McM'91; CCFP; FCFP; (905)949-1700

MALLETTE-GRATTON, Veronique; CSSS Pierre Boucher, 1333 boul Jacques-Cartier E, Longueuil QC J4M 2A5; Mon'05; CCFP; Staff, Centre Hospitalier Pierre Boucher; (450)468-8111

MALLETTE-TETREAULT, Lise; Clinique Med MD Plus, 301-1100 av Beaumont, Mont-Royal QC H3P 3H5; Sher'75; LMCC; Langs: English; (514)738-4445

MALLEY, Laura K; Burke Mountain Med Clinic, 210-1465 Salisbury Ave, Port Coquitlam BC V3B 6J3; UBC'08; (604)941-8277

MALLIA, Salvatore; COSTI Family & Mental Hlth Ser, 105-1700 Wilson Ave, North York ON M3L 1B2; Palermo (Italy)'79; FRCPC; Psy. Staff, William Osler Health System - Etobicoke General Hospital; Physician, Schizophrenia Clinic/Psychogeriatric/Villa Colombo & Psychiatric Comm. Clinic-Costi; (416)244-7714

MALLICK, Kiron C; Kildonan Crossing Walk-In Clin, 640-1615 Regent Ave W, Winnipeg MB R2C 5C6; Dacca (Bangladesh)'60; MB BS; MRCS(Eng); LRCP(Lond); FRCS(Ed); Langs: Bengali; (204)663-1977; Fax. (204)663-2058.

MALLIN, A Rebecca; Hamilton HS-General Site, 237 Barton St E, Hamilton ON L8L 2X2; Dal'00; FRCPC; EmergMed. Staff EmergMed, Hamilton Health Sciences Centre - Hamilton General Hospital; (905)527-4322 x46368

MALLIN, Constantine; Grand Valley Med Clinic, PO Box 340 21 Main St N, Grand Valley ON L9W 5S6; Tor'74; CCFP; FCFP; Ac Staff, Headwaters Health Care Centre - Orangeville Site; Asst Prof, University of Toronto; Langs: Macedonian; (519)928-5666; Fax. (519)928-3260; cdan.mallin@utoronto.ca.

MALLON, Joseph S; Sunnybrook Hlth Sciences Ctre, 2075 Bayview Ave, Toronto ON M4N 3M5; Tor'79; Anes. Staff, Sunnybrook Health Sciences Centre; Staff, Mount Sinai Hospital; Staff, Princess Margaret Hospital - University Health Network; Asst Prof, University of Toronto; (416)480-4864

MALLORY, Amy E; Dalhousie Univ Health Services, 6230 Coburg Rd, Halifax NS B3H 4R2; Dal'05; CCFP; (902)494-2171

MALLORY, Jonathan G; Buckhorn Reg Health Centre, 865 William St, Buckhorn ON K0L 1J0; Ott'94; CCFP; (705)657-7933

MALLOUH, George E; Clinique Med Diamant, 5512 ch de la cote-des-Neiges, Montreal QC H3T 1Y9; Cairo (Egypt)'54; MB ChB; MD; FACOG; FRCSC; ObstGyn. Att Staff, St Mary's Hospital Centre; McGill University; (514)931-3275

MALLOUH, Suzy Z; Albany Med Clinic, 807 Broadview Ave, Toronto ON M4K 2P8; McM'99; CCFP; (416)461-9471

MALLOY, Susan J; Rockingham Ridge Plaza, 30 Farnham Gate Rd, Halifax NS B3M 3W8; Dal'86; CCFP; Staff, IWK Health Centre; (902)443-8388; Fax. (902)443-9887.

MALLOZZI, Angelina; MUHC-Royal Victoria Hosp, F4 29-687 av des Pins O, Montreal QC H3A 1A1; McG'84; FRCSC; ObstGyn. Staff, McGill University Health Centre - Royal Victoria Hospital; (514)934-1934

MALM, David N; False Creek Healthcare Centre, 555 8 Ave W, Vancouver BC V5Z 1C6; UBC'77; DABA; FRCPC; Anes (Adult Anesthesia). Staff, Vancouver General Hospital - Centennial Pavillion; Asst Prof, University of British Columbia; (604)739-9695

MALMBERG, James L; Edmonton Mental Health Clinic, 5-9942 108 St NW, Edmonton AB T5K 2J5; Alb'82; FRCPC; Psy. Clin Lecturer, University of Alberta; (780)342-7700; Fax. (780)422-0832.

MALMEDY, Natacha; Clinique Gyn De Trois-Rivieres, 2237 7e av, Trois-Rivieres QC G8Z 3E2; Mon'92; FRCSC; ObstGyn (Fertility). Staff ObstGyn, CSSS de Trois-Rivières; Langs: Bilingual(French/English); (819)379-5353

MALMSTROM, Jennifer K; Cartier Health Centre, PO Box 127, Elie MB R0H 0H0; Man'96; CCFP.

MALO, Celine; Polyclinique Med PAT, 101-12905 rue Sherbrooke E, Pte-aux-Trembles QC H1A 1B9; Sher'75; (514)498-4050

MALO, J Pierre C; 295 Eltham Rd, Victoria BC V9B 1K1; Ott'90; Staff, Vancouver Island Health Authority; (250)708-0102; Fax. (250)708-0177; drmalo@telus.net.

MALO, Jacques; Hop Du Sacre-Coeur De Mtl, 5e-5400 boul Gouin O, Montreal QC H4J 1C5; Mon'74; Respir (P.Q.). ac Staff, Hôpital du Sacre-Coeur de Montréal; (514)338-2162; Fax. (514)338-3699.

MALO, Jean; Clin De Med Fam Cowansville, 499 rue du Sud, Cowansville QC J2K 2X9; Mon'85; Staff, Hôpital Brome-Missisquoi-Perkins; (450)263-8890; Fax. (450)263-9737.

MALO, Jean-Luc; Hop Du Sacre-Coeur de Mtl, 5400 Boul Gouin O, Montreal QC H4J 1C5; Mon'70; Respir (P.Q.). Staff, Hôpital du Sacre-Coeur de Montréal; Langs: Bilingual(French/English); (514)338-2162; Fax. (514)338-3699.

MALO, Laurence G; Timmins Family Health Team, 250-123 Third Ave, Timmins ON P4N 1C6; Tor'85; CCFP; CCFP(E.M.); FCFP; Staff, Timmins & District Hospital; Teacher, University of Ottawa; Lecturer Family & Cummun Med, University of Toronto; Assoc Prof, Laurentian University; (705)264-9151; Fax. (705)268-7444; malowodd@gmail.com.

MALO, Michel; Hop Du Sacre-Coeur De Mtl, 5400 boul Gouin O, Montreal QC H4J 1C5; Mon'95; FRCSC; OrthSurg. Staff, Hôpital du Sacre-Coeur de Montréal; (514)338-2222; Fax. (514)338-3661.

MALO-POIRIER, Ann-Claude; CSSS De La Haute-Yamaska, 205 boul Leclerc O, Granby QC J2G 1T7; Sher'06; Staff, Centre Hospitalier de Granby; (450)375-8000

MALOKA, Nabil; The Doctor's Office, 207-8120 Beddington Blvd NW, Calgary AB T3K 2A8; (Egypt)'79; CCFP; (403)275-4611

MALOLEY, Jeffrey W; 609-267 O'Connor St, Ottawa ON K2P 1V3; Ott'76; Staff Privil OPD, Canadian Forces Health Services Centre; Ac Staff, The Ottawa Hospital - Civic Campus; Exec Med Examiner, E.B. Eddy & Med. Examiner, Bank of Canada; (613)594-2831; Fax. (613)594-5831.

MALON, Catherine R; 5-100 Highland Rd W, Kitchener ON N2M 3B5; McM'85; BSc; CCFP; FCFP; Supvr Commun & Family Med, McMaster University; (519)742-3600; Fax. (519)742-3386.

MALON, Paul A; Lions Gate Hosp, 231 15th St E, North Vancouver BC V7L 2L7; McG'89; BSc; Staff, Lions Gate Hospital; (604)988-3131

MALON, Peter H; St Mary's Gen Hosp, 911 Queens Blvd, Kitchener ON N2M 1B2; Tor'79.

MALONE, Danny; Empire Med Centre, 3-204 Freshwater Rd, St. John's NL A1C 2P5; Mem'88; (709)753-2055; Fax. (709)753-2056.

MALONE, Marilyn L; 1952 Bay St, Victoria BC V8R 1J8; UBC'94; BSc; MHSc; FRCPC; IntMed (Dementia); GeriatricMed. Staff, Royal Jubilee Hospital; (250)370-8509; Fax. (250)370-8285.

MALONE, Richard F; East Kootenay Reg Hosp, 13 24th Ave N, Cranbrook BC V1C 3H9; St. Louis(MO) (USA)'77; FRCPC; GenPath. Staff, East Kootenay Regional Hospital; (250)426-5281

MALONE, Robert D; Brockville Gen Hosp, 75 Charles St, Brockville ON K6V 1S8; Qns'93; FRCPC; Psy. Staff, Brockville General Hospital - Charles Street; (613)345-5645

MALONE, Shawn C; Ottawa Reg Cancer Centre, 501 Smyth Rd, Ottawa ON K1H 8L6; Ott'89; FRCPC; RadOncol. Assoc Prof, University of Ottawa; (613)737-7700 x70212; Fax. (613)247-3511; smalone@ottawahospital.on.ca.

MALONE, Sonya M; UWO Student Health Services, 11UCC-1151 Richmond St, London ON N6A 3K7; Ott'07; CCFP; (519)661-3030

MALONE, William C; Dufferin Orthopedic Clinic, 1135 Dufferin Cres, Nanaimo BC V9S 2B5; Wes'73; FRCSC; OrthSurg. (250)754-3727; Fax. (250)754-1447.

MALONEY, Amanda P; Business Bldg, 802-777 Broadway W, Vancouver BC V5Z 4J7; UBC'86; FRCSC; Otol. (604)685-0080; Fax. (604)688-5905.

MALONEY, Gerald P; St Martins Med Clinic, 1-73 Main St, St Martins NB E5R 1B4; Dal'77; Ac Staff, St Joseph's Hospital; Ac Staff, Saint John Regional Hospital; (506)833-2012

MALONEY, Justin P; The Ottawa Hosp-Gen Campus, 501 Smyth Rd, Ottawa ON K1H 8L6; Ott'71; FRCPC; CCFP; EmergMed;CCFP(E.M.); FCFP; Staff, The Ottawa Hospital - General Campus; Asst Prof, University of Ottawa; (613)737-8000; Fax. (613)737-8967.

MALONEY, Patrick; Rothesay Med Clinic, 11 Gondola Point Rd, Rothesay NB E2E 5J6; Dal'09; CCFP; (506)847-7592

MALONEY, Paul A; St Martha's Reg Hosp, 23 Bay St, Antigonish NS B2G 2G5; Dal'07; FRCPC; Peds. Staff, St Martha's Regional Hospital; (902)867-1417; Fax. (902)863-1186.

MALONEY, Robert J; Sault Area Hosp, 750 Gerat Northern Rd, Sault Ste. Marie ON P6B 0A8; McM'84; Ac Staff Gen Practice & Emerg, Sault Area Hospital - Sault Ste Marie; (705)759-3434

MALONEY, Tshai Nkasi; Appletree Med Group, 900 Albion Rd, Etobicoke ON M9V 1A5; (Other Foreign)'05.

MALONEY, William J; Queen Elizabeth II HSC-Halifax, 1796 Summer St, Halifax NS B3H 3A7; Mem'76; BSc; FRCPC; DiagRad (Neuro Radiology). Staff, Queen Elizabeth II Health Sciences Centre - Halifax Infirmary Site; Ac Staff Radiol, Queen Elizabeth II Health Sciences Centre - Victoria General Site; Asst Prof Med, Dalhousie University; (902)473-4910; Fax. (902)473-5323; wmaloney@accesscable.net.

MALOON, Stephen; Surrey Med Arts Bldg, 320-13710 94A Ave, Surrey BC V3V 1N1; Witwatersrand (South Africa)'79; MB BCh; FRCSC; OrthSurg (Spine Surgery). Ac Staff, Surrey Memorial Hospital; (604)585-8469; Fax. (604)585-8479.

MALOUF, Benoit; Hop Jean-Talon, 1385 rue Jean-Talon E, Montreal QC H2E 1S6; Mon'09; Staff, CSSS du Coeur de l'Isle Hôpital Jean-Talon; (514)495-6767

MALOWANY, Leo E R; Circle Square Prof Centre, 202-11808 St Albert Trail NW, Edmonton AB T5L 4G4; Alb'78; FACP; ABIM; FRCPC; IntMed. Staff Physician, Royal Alexandra Hospital; Asst Prof, University of Alberta; (780)479-3055; Fax. (780)474-9804.

MALPASS, Kristian G; Northern Health Authority, 904-299 Victoria St, Prince George BC V2L 5B8; UBC'00; FRCSC; PlasSurg. Staff, University Hospital of Northern British Columbia; (250)563-8568

MALPASS, Phillip B; Kootenay Lake Hosp, 426-3 View St, Nelson BC V1L 2V1; UBC'73; FRCPC; IntMed. Staff, Kootenay Lake General Hospital; (250)352-7295; Fax. (250)352-7066.

MALPICA VERA, Carlos; Haig Clinic, 601 6 Ave S, Lethbridge AB T1J 0Z2; (Other Foreign)'02; (403)328-6641; Fax. (403)328-6118.

MALTAIS, Catherine; GMF Maizerets, 2480 ch de la Canardiere, Quebec QC G1J 2G1; Laval'06; CCFP; Staff, Centre Hospitalier de Matane; Staff, Unite de Medecine familiale Maizerets; (418)661-1413

MALTAIS, Cathrine; Clinique Med Nepisiguit, 950 av Picot, Bathurst NB E2A 4Z9; Sher'06; CCFP; (506)546-1018

MALTAIS, Francois; Hôpital Laval, 2725 ch Sainte-Foy, Quebec QC G1V 4G5; Laval'84; FRCPC; IntMed; Respir. Staff, Hôpital Laval; (418)656-4747; Fax. (418)656-4762.

MALTAIS, Gerard; Centre De Med Familiale, 552 av Saint-Alphonse, St-Bruno-du-L-St-J QC G0W 2L0; Laval'76; (418)343-2444

MALTAIS, Lucie; CSSS de Rivière-de-Loup, 75 rue Saint-Henri, Riviere-du-Loup QC G5R 2A4; Laval'06; Staff, Centre Hospitalier Regional du Grand-Portage; (418)868-1000

MALTBY, C Christine; 99A Webster St, Kentville NS B4N 1H8; Dublin (Ireland)'82; MB BCh; BAO; FRCSC; Otol. Staff, Valley Regional Hospital; (902)678-4233; Fax. (902)678-4234.

MALTHANER, Richard A; London Health Sciences Centre, E2-124-800 Commissioners Rd E, London ON N6A 5W9; Tor'85; DABS; FACS; FCCP; MSc; FRCS; FRCSC; GenSurg (Surgical Oncology); ThorSurg. Consultant, St Joseph's Hospital - St Joseph's Health Care; Staff, London Health Sciences Centre - Victoria Campus; Consultant, London Regional Cancer Centre; Prof Surg, University of Western Ontario; (519)667-6835; Fax. (519)667-6517; richard.malthaner@lhsc.on.ca.

MALTHOUSE, Stephen C; 3646 D Denman Rd PO Box 80, Denman Island BC V0R 1T0; Wes'78; (250)335-2260

MALTMAN, Craig J; 201-170 Simcoe St, Peterborough ON K9H 2H7; Qns'87; CCFP; (705)748-2673

MALTMAN, Shirley A; Mediclinic, 101-3333 8th St E, Saskatoon SK S7H 4K1; Sask'85; BSc; Staff, St Paul's Hospital (Grey Nuns) of Saskatoon; Teacher Pt-Time, Royal University Hospital; (306)955-1530; Fax. (306)955-8811.

MALTSEVA, Ekatherena V; The Polyclinic, 5-4646 Dufferin St, North York ON M3H 5S4; Kharkov (Ukraine)'84; CCFP; Langs: Russian; (416)222-6160; Fax. (416)222-9604.

MALUS, Dale A; 52-7930 Bowness Rd NW, Calgary AB T3B 0H3; Man'78; CCFP; (403)247-1303; Fax. (403)288-6670.

MALUS, Eli; Hôtel-Dieu Grace Hosp, 1030 Ouellette Ave, Windsor ON N9A 1E1; McG'98; FRCPC; IntMed; Critical Care Medicine; Respir. Staff Intensive Care Unit, Hôtel-Dieu Grace Hospital; (519)973-4411

MALUS, Michael; 4726-SMBD Jewish Gen Hosp, 3755 ch Cote-Sainte-Catherine, Montreal QC H3T 1E2; McG'64; CCFP; FCFP; Staff Family Med, Sir Mortimer B Davis Jewish General; Consultant, Hôpital Ste-Justine; (514)340-8234; Fax. (514)340-8298; mmalus@her.jgh.mcgill.ca.

MAMALIAS, Nikolaos; Medcan Health Mgmt Inc, 1500-150 York St, Toronto ON M5H 3S5; Tor'05; CCFP; CCFP(E.M.); Staff, North York General Hospital; (416)350-5900

MAMALINGAS, Zoe; Statcare-Stillview Clinic, 104-175 av Stillview, Pointe-Claire QC H9R 4S3; Mon'09; CCFP; (514)694-9282

MAMAZZA, Joseph; The Ottawa Hosp-Civic Campus, CPC R327-1053 Carling Ave, Ottawa ON K1Y 4E9; McG'78; FACS; FRCSC; GenSurg (Laparoscopic Surgery). Chief GenSurg, The Ottawa Hospital - Civic Campus; Chairman Div of GenSurg, University of Ottawa; Langs: Italian; French; (613)798-5555 x13151; Fax. (613)761-4124; jmamazza@ottawahospital.on.ca.

MAMCHUR, Lori L; 21st Medical Clinic, 502-402 21st St E, Saskatoon SK S7K 0C3; Alb'01; FRCPC; IntMed. (306)956-3444; Fax. (306)956-3577.

MAMELAK, Joshua D; William Osler HC-Etobicoke, 101 Humber College Blvd, Etobicoke ON M9V 1R8; Tor'96; FRCPC; DiagRad. Staff, William Osler Health System - Etobicoke General Hospital; (416)747-3400

MAMELAK, Mortimer; 313-4800 Leslie St, North York ON M2J 2K9; McG'63; FRCPC; Psy (Head Injury). Staff, Baycrest Centre for Geriatric Care; University of Toronto; (416)785-2500; Fax. (416)785-2492; m.mamelak@utoronto.ca.

MAMEN, Natalie K; Toronto East Gen Hosp Inc, 825 Coxwell Ave, Toronto ON M4C 3E7; McM'99; CCFP; CCFP(E.M.); Staff, Toronto East General Hospital Inc; (416)469-6435

MAMET, Francoise G; CSSS Les Eskers de l'Abitibi, 622 4e rue O, Amos QC J9T 2S2; Mon'91; FRCPC; Peds. Staff, CH Hôtel-Dieu d'Amos; (819)732-3341 x137; fmamet@lino.com.

MAMI, Mustafa G A; All Well Primary Care Centre, 2835 Mill Woods Rd NW, Edmonton AB T6K 4A9; (Libya)'01; MB BCh; CCFP; (780)450-4550

MAMMEN, Cherry; Children's & Women's HC of BC, 4480 Oak St, Vancouver BC V6H 3V4; Mem'03; Nephrol; Peds. Staff, BC Children's Hospital; (604)875-2000 x5222

MAMMEN, Thomas; Health Sciences Centre, GA216-820 Sherbrook St, Winnipeg MB R3A 1R9; Ott'08; Staff, Health Sciences Centre.

MAMO, Andrew P T; Central Alberta Med Imaging, 4312 54 Ave, Red Deer AB T4N 4M1; Qns'94; FRCPC; DiagRad. (403)343-6172

MAMODE, Chemir; 210-1575 boul de l'Avenir, Laval QC H7S 2N5; Sher'91; FRCPC; Derm. (450)629-3376

MAMOGOBO, Charmaine M; Nanton Med Clinic, PO Box 940, Nanton AB T0L 1R0; S.Africa (South Africa)'00; (403)646-2218; Fax. (403)646-3046.

MAMPUYA, Warner M; CHUS-Hop Fleurimont, 3001 12e av N, Sherbrooke QC J1H 5N4; Peking (China)'93; FRCPC; IntMed; Cardiol. Staff, Centre Hospitalier Universitaire de Sherbrooke-Hopital Fleurimont; (819)346-1110

MAN, Denise I; Oakridge Centre South Tower, 350-650 41st Ave W, Vancouver BC V5Z 2M9; Caribbean (Montserrat)'07; CCFP; (604)261-6000

MAN, Emmeline L; Grey Nuns Community Hosp, 1100 Youville Drive West NW, Edmonton AB T6L 5X8; (Hong Kong)'72; FRCPC; Anes. Ac Staff Anes, Covenant Health - Grey Nuns Community Hospital; (780)735-7020; Fax. (780)735-7279.

MAN, Godfrey C W; University of Alberta Hosp, 2E4 26-8440 112 St NW, Edmonton AB T6G 2B7; (Hong Kong)'72; FACP; FRCPC; IntMed; Respir. Ac Staff, University of Alberta Hospital; Prof Med, University of Alberta; (780)407-6215; Fax. (780)407-6384.

MAN, Gregory C K; 206-10168 Yonge St, Richmond Hill ON L4C 1T6; (Hong Kong)'70; MB BS; FRCPC; Peds (Clinical Immunology & Allergy). Court Consultant, Mackenzie Richmond Hill Hospital; Langs: Chinese; (905)883-3042

MAN, Hon-Sum J; Dept of Adult Respirology, 11C 1170-585 University Ave, Toronto ON M5G 2N2; Alb'02; Respir; IntMed (Critical Care Medicine). (416)340-4485

MAN, Jeremy R; 11516 Jasper Ave NW, Edmonton AB T5K 0M8; Alb'04; FRCPC; Derm. (780)482-1548; Fax. (780)482-1317.

MAN, Kwok-Chu; 106 Mary St E, Whitby ON L1N 2P2; Mem'85; PhD; FRCPC; IntMed (Cardiology). Staff Consultant, Lakeridge Health - Oshawa Site; Langs: Cantonese; Mandarin; (905)430-6795

MAN, S F Paul; St Paul's Hosp, 548-1081 Burrard St, Vancouver BC V6Z 1Y6; Alb'70; DABIM; FACP; FCCP; FRCPC; IntMed; Respir. Head Med, Providence Health Care - St Paul's Hospital; Prof Med, University of British Columbia; (604)806-8495; Fax. (604)806-8870; phcdeptmedicine@providencehealth.bc.ca.

MAN, Christopher; Com-El Med Bldg, 102-2620 Commercial Dr, Vancouver BC V5N 4C4; Man'74; FRCSC; Otol. (604)872-2212; Fax. (604)872-4600.

MAN, Thomas M; Patient Networks, 157 Yonge St, Toronto ON M5C 1X7; New York (USA)'10; CCFP; (416)362-8822

MAN-SON-HING, Malcolm G; Campbell River & Dist Gen Hosp, 375 2nd Ave, Campbell River BC V9W 3V1; Cal'86; FRCPC; IntMed; GeriatricMed. Staff, Campbell River & District General Hospital; (250)287-7111

MANACKI, Leonard A; Finchlea Med Centre, 204-490 Bramalea Rd, Brampton ON L6T 0G1; Wes'84; BSc(Hon); CCFP; FCFP; Staff, William Osler Health System - Brampton Civic Hospital; Staff Physician, Peel Manor Nursing Home; Staff Physician, Tall Pines LTCC; (905)792-6500; Fax. (905)792-6853.

MANAFY, Chirina; Ctr Hosp Fleury, 2180 rue Fleury E, Montreal QC H2B 1K3; Antananarivo (Madagascar)'05; Staff, Centre Hospitalier Fleury; (514)384-2000

MANAK-MUHR, Mandy K; 401-321 Nicola St, Kamloops BC V2C 6G6; UBC'07; (778)471-5922

MANAREY, Casey R A; Kingsway Plaza Phase III, 611-4980 Kingsway, Burnaby BC V5H 4K7; UBC'97; BSc; FESBS; FRCSC; Otol (Rhinology). Asst Clin Instructor, University of British Columbia; (604)433-1599; sinusdocs@shaw.ca.

MANASSEH, Petrona M; Danforth Med Centre, 880 Danforth Rd, Scarborough ON M1K 1H8; Sint Eustatius (Netherlands Antilles)'07; (416)284-4848

MANASSIS, Katharina M; The Hosp for Sick Children, 555 University Ave, Toronto ON M5G 1X8; Tor'86; FRCPC; Psy (Child Psychiatry). Staff Psy, The Hospital For Sick Children; Prof Psy, University of Toronto; Langs: German; (416)813-7464; Fax. (416)813-5326.

MANAWADU, Gnanindra N; West Mississauga Medical, 3050 Argentia Rd, Mississauga ON L5N 8E1; Colombo (Sri Lanka)'92; CCFP; Langs: Sinhalese; (905)785-3627; Fax. (905)785-3628; henrymanawadu@sympatico.ca.

MANAX, Stanley J; 105-645 Commissioners Rd E, London ON N6C 2T9; Wes'64; FRCSC; GenSurg. (519)963-0232

MANCA, Donna P; Grey Nuns Family Med Centre, 2927 66 St NW, Edmonton AB T6K 4C1; Alb'81; MClSc; CCFP; FCFP; (780)342-1470; Fax. (780)490-0953.

MANCA, Georgina; Queensway-Carleton Hosp, 3045 Baseline Rd, Nepean ON K2H 8P4; Pretoria (South Africa)'96; CCFP; CCFP(E.M.); Staff, Queensway Carleton Hospital; (613)721-2000

MANCER, Jasdeep K; River East Health Access Ctre, 975 Henderson Hwy, Winnipeg MB R2K 4L7; Man'06; CCFP.

MANCHIA, Mirko; Abbie J Lane Memorial Bldg, 4081-5909 Veterans Memorial La, Halifax NS B3H 2E2; Cagliari (Italy)'04; (902)473-3574

MANCHANDA, Meera; 6-163 Commissioners Rd W, London ON N6J 1X9; Lucknow (India)'73; DCH(UK); FRCPC; Peds. Consultant, St Joseph's Hospital - St Joseph's Health Care; Pt-Time Lecturer, University of Western Ontario; (519)439-1431; Fax. (519)672-7888; mmanchan@uwo.ca.

MANCHANDA, Rahul; London HSC-Victoria Hosp, PO Box 5010 Stn B 800 Commissioners Rd E, London ON N6A 5W9; Lucknow (India)'73; MB BS; MRCPsy(UK); FRCPC; Psy. Staff, London Health Sciences Centre - Victoria Campus; Assoc Prof Psy, University of Western Ontario; (519)667-6866

MANCHANDA, Raman; Manchanda Med Clinic, 7550 King George Blvd, Surrey BC V3W 2T2; Wes'01; BSc(Hon); MSc; CCFP; Clin Instructor, University of British Columbia; Langs: Hindi; Punjabi; (604)598-9880; Fax. (604)598-2493.

MANCHIKANTI, Srinivasa M; Justik Med Clinic, 8225 105 St NW, Edmonton AB T6E 4H2; (India)'85; MB BS; CCFP; (780)432-0211; Fax. (780)439-9349.

MANCHUK, Derek R; Sudbury Reg Hosp-Laurentian, 41 Ramsey Lake Rd, Sudbury ON P3E 5J1; Tor'95; FRCPC; Anes; Critical Care Medicine. Staff, Health Sciences North-Laurentian Site; (705)522-2200

MANCHUL, Lee A; Univ Hlth Network-Princess M, 610 University Ave, Toronto ON M5G 2M9; Tor'83; BSc; FRCPC; RadOncol (Breast Cancer). Radiation Oncologist, Princess Margaret Hospital - University Health Network; Asst Prof, University of Toronto; (416)946-4501 x2963; Fax. (416)946-2111.

MANCINI, Catherine L; Fontbonne Bldg, 4F-301 James St S, Hamilton ON L8P 3B6; Wes'82; FRCPC; Psy (Anxiety Disorder). Court Staff, Hamilton Health Sciences Centre - McMaster Children's Hospital; Ac Staff, St Joseph's Healthcare - Charlton Campus; Assoc Prof, McMaster University; (905)522-1155 x35379; Fax. (905)540-6533.

MANCINI, Enrico V; Legacy Sport Med Clinic, 14-160 Meadowood Dr, Winnipeg MB R2M 5L6; Man'09; CCFP.

MANCINI, G B John; Gordon & Leslie Diamond HCC, 9F-2775 Laurel St, Vancouver BC V5Z 1M9; Tor'77; FACC; FRCPC; IntMed; Cardiol. Consultant, Providence Health Care - St Paul's Hospital; Staff Med/Cardiol/Internal Med, Vancouver General Hospital - Centennial Pavillion; Teach Staff Med, University of British Columbia; (604)875-5092; mancini@interchange.ubc.ca.

MAND, Gurpal S; 202-1625 Albion Rd, Etobicoke ON M9V 5H8; (India)'74; (416)748-5556; Fax. (416)748-9692.

MAND, Gurpreet T; Southlake Family Health Team, 201-581 Davis Dr, Newmarket ON L3Y 2P6; Davangere (India)'03; CCFP; (905)853-3103

MAND, Ravinder P; Portage Dist Gen Hosp, 524 5th St SE, Portage la Prairie MB R1N 3A8; (Other Foreign)'09; CCFP; CCFP(E.M.); Staff, Portage District General Hospital; (204)239-2280; rmand@shaw.ca.

MANDAL, Amal B; Windsor Health Centre, 362-1720 Howard Ave, Windsor ON N8X 5A6; Calcutta (India)'63; FACP; MB BS; FRCP(UK); FACC; FRCPC; IntMed (Cardiology). Ac Staff, Windsor Regional Hospital - Metropolitan Site; Teacher, South Western Ontario Medical Education Network; Aj Prof Med, University of Western Ontario; (519)254-1296

MANDALENAKIS, Andrew; SMBD Jewish Gen Hosp, 3755 ch Cote-Sainte-Catherine, Montreal QC H3T 1E2; McG'96; DiagRad. Staff, Sir Mortimer B Davis Jewish General; (514)340-8222

MANDALFINO, Patricia; 723 King St W, Kitchener ON N2G 1E3; McM'92; FRCPC; Neur (Multiple Sclerosis). (519)745-2366; Fax. (519)745-9035.

MANDEL, Drue H; 8A-9019 Bayview Ave, Richmond Hill ON L4B 3M6; Tor'86; CCFP; FCFP; Staff, Markham Stouffville Hospital; Staff, Sunnybrook Health Sciences Centre; Staff, North York General Hospital; Physician, Talk Shop-Teen Health Clinic; Instructor, University of Toronto; (905)886-9660; d.mandel@utoronto.ca.

MANDEL, Howard; Mandel Medicine Prof Corp, 305-27 Roncesvalles Ave, Toronto ON M6R 3B2; Tor'74; CCFP; FCFP; Staff, Hamilton Health Sciences Centre - McMaster University Medical Centre; (416)532-1939; Fax. (416)532-4860; howard.mandel@sickkids.ca.

MANDEL, Jonathan I; 104-450 Central Ave, London ON N6B 2E8; Tor'04; FRCPC; DiagRad; NuclearMed. (519)672-5270

MANDEL, Karen M; 401 Smyth Rd Division of Heme/Oncology, Ottawa ON K1H 8L1; Wes'91; FRCPC; Peds (Pediatric Hematology Oncology); Hem. Staff Div of Hem/Oncol, Children's Hospital of Eastern Ontario (CHEO); (613)737-7600; kmandel@cheo.on.ca.

MANDEL, Lisa F; Family Physicians, 1-390 Steeles Ave W, Thornhill ON L4J 6X2; Tor'90; BSc; CCFP; FCFP; Court Staff Privil, Mackenzie Richmond Hill Hospital; (905)881-3984; Fax. (905)881-3198.

MANDEL, O Jack; Jane-Finch Family Health Team, 136A-1 Yorkgate Blvd, North York ON M3N 3A1; Tor'72; CCFP; FCFP; Staff, North York General Hospital - Branson Division; Staff, North York General Hospital; Staff, Humber River Regional Hospital - Finch Avenue Site; (416)745-4555; Fax. (416)745-0786.

MANDEL, Romain; MUHC-Royal Victoria Hosp, 687 av des Pins O, Montreal QC H3A 1A1; Lille(Fr) (France)'95; MSc; Staff, McGill University Health Centre - Royal Victoria Hospital; Langs: Bilingual(French/English); (514)934-1934

MANDEL, Ronald M; 101-40 Westmore Dr, Etobicoke ON M9V 4C2; Tor'69; CCFP; FCFP; Staff, William Osler Health System - Etobicoke General Hospital; (416)745-0100; Fax. (416)745-6604.

MANDEL, Ruth J; St Mary's Hosp Centre, 3830 av Lacombe, Montreal QC H3T 1M5; McG'96; Peds. Staff, St Mary's Hospital Centre; (514)345-3511

MANDELBAUM, Saul H; SGH Medical Mall, 204-3030 Lawrence Ave E, Scarborough ON M1P 2T7; Tor'95; FRCSC; GenSurg. Staff Clinician Investigator Program, North York General Hospital; (416)431-1242

MANDELCORN, Efrem D; Univ Hlth Network-Toronto Western Hosp, 6E 415-399 Bathurst St, Toronto ON M5T 2S8; Tor'03; FRCSC; Ophth (Retina). Staff, Toronto Western Hospital - University Health Network; (416)603-5418

MANDELCORN, Jeffrey N; Toronto East Gen Hosp Inc, 825 Coxwell Ave, Toronto ON M4C 3E7; Tor'03; FRCPC; DiagRad; NuclearMed. Staff, Toronto East General Hospital Inc; (416)561-6703

MANDELCORN, Mark S; Univ Hlth Network-Toronto Western Hosp, 6E- 416-399 Bathurst St, Toronto ON M5T 2S8; McG'67; BSc; FAAOO; FRCSC; Ophth (Retina). Ac Staff, Toronto Western Hospital - University Health Network; Assoc Prof, University of Toronto; (416)603-5800 x2249; Fax. (416)603-5834; mark.mandelcorn@uhn.on.ca.

MANDELL, Daniel M; Univ Hlth Network-Toronto Western Hosp, 399 Bathurst St, Toronto ON M5T 2S8; McM'03; FRCPC; DiagRad (Neuro Radiology). Staff, Toronto Western Hospital - University Health Network; (416)603-5800 x4933

MANDELL, Howard B; Rouge Valley-Centenary HC, 2867 Ellesmere Rd, Scarborough ON M1E 4B9; Ott'62; FRCPC; Anes. Staff, Rouge Valley Health System - Centenary Health Centre Site; (416)284-8131 x4054

MANDELL, Lionel; One-Stop Med Centre, 1A-3585 Lawrence Ave E, Scarborough ON M1G 1P4; Tor'70; FRCPC; IntMed (Infectious Diseases). Prof, McMaster University.

MANDELL, Mark A; 100-385 The West Mall, Etobicoke ON M9C 1E7; Tor'06; FRCSC; Ophth. (416)622-1864; Fax. (416)622-1215.

MANDELMAN, Krystyna; 205-4430 Bathurst St, North York ON M3H 3S3; Warsaw (Poland)'63; MD; FRCPC; Psy. Langs: Polish; (416)398-8387

MANDER, Charanjeet; Burlington Prof Centre, 206-3155 Harvester Rd, Burlington ON L7N 3V2; Punjab (India)'65; (905)335-4616; Fax. (905)335-0513.

MANDER, Jatinder S; Medical Arts Centre, 103-650 Terminal Ave, Nanaimo BC V9R 5E2; Sheffield (England)'99; MB ChB; CCFP; (250)753-3431

MANDERS, David C; St Paul's Hosp, 1081 Burrard St, Vancouver BC V6Z 1Y6; UBC'06; FRCPC; DiagRad. Staff, Providence Health Care - St Paul's Hospital; (604)806-8008

MANDERS, Terence P; 12601 Lakeshore Dr S, Summerland BC V0H 1Z1; UBC'74; Staff, Penticton Regional Hospital; Staff, Summerland Memorial Health Centre; (250)494-2011

MANDERSON, Robert W; Braeside Med Centre Ltd, 111-1919 Southland Dr SW, Calgary AB T2W 0K1; Dundee (Scotland)'77; MB ChB; (403)258-2133; Fax. (403)258-2162.

MANDERVILLE, Eugene A; Bayview Med Clinic, 274 Dundas St E, Belleville ON K8N 1E6; Dal'62; CCFP; (613)968-5709

MANDEVILLE, Dominique; Clin Esthetique Lafond-Mandevi, 208-620 boul Saint-Jean, Pointe-Claire QC H9R 3K2; Mon'87; Staff, Centre Hospitalier de Verdun; (514)693-0009

MANDEVILLE, Helene; 103-10302 rue Chambord, Montreal QC H2C 2R5; Mon'81; Langs: Bilingual(French/English); Deaf-mute; (514)383-6646; Fax. (514)383-7686.

MANDHANE, Piushkumar J; 4 590-11405 87 Ave NW, Edmonton AB T6G 1C9; Tor'97; FRCPC; Peds; Respir. (780)248-5650

MANDICH, George H; 257 rue Saint-Jacques, Lachine QC H8R 1E4; McG'77; FAAP; FRCPC; Peds. ac Staff, McGill University Health Centre - Montreal Children's Hospital; adj Prof, McGill University; (514)367-1913; Fax. (450)671-7795.

MANDL, Michael A J; 200-1847 Broadway W, Vancouver BC V6J 1Y9; Sydney (Australia)'63; MB BS; IntMed. (604)878-2221

MANDOFF, Nedka; 21 Queensway W, Mississauga ON L5B 1B6; Sofia (Bulgaria)'71; FAAP; FRCPC; Peds. (905)897-0788

MANDRECK, Larrie H; 206-3203 30 St, Vernon BC V1T 9G9; Alb'75; BMedSci; Assoc Staff, Vernon Jubilee Hospital; (250)503-2205; Fax. (250)503-2206.

MANDRYK, Eugene W; Medicine Professional Corp, 38 David Wilson Trail, Sharon ON L0G 1V0; Tor'63; DPsy; FRCPC; Psy (Forensic Psychiatry). (905)478-2900

MANERKAR, Avdhut R; Miramichi Reg Hosp, 500 Water St, Miramichi NB E1V 3G5; Bombay (India)'75; MB BS; DA; Staff Cons Anes, Miramichi Regional Hospital; Langs: Konkani; Marathi; Hindi; (506)623-3450; armanerkar@hotmail.com.

MANES, Arturo S; 810-943 Broadway W, Vancouver BC V5Z 4E2; UBC'74; CCFP; FCFP; Ac Staff, Vancouver General Hospital - Centennial Pavillion; Ac Staff, BC Women's Hospital & Health Centre; (604)734-1213; Fax. (604)734-5751.

MANESHGAR, Mahnaz; Justik Med Clinic, 8225 105 St NW, Edmonton AB T6E 4H2; (Iran)'99; CCFP; Langs: Farsi; (780)432-0211

MANFREDI, Victoria E; Brock Community Health Centre, PO Box 69 64 Cameron St, Cannington ON L0E 1E0; Dal'91; BA; CCFP; FCFP; Staff, Princess Margaret Hospital - University Health Network; (705)432-3388

MANG, Annabelle L; Regina Qu'Appelle HR-Regina, 1440 14th Ave, Regina SK S4P 0W5; Sask'97; FRCPC; Anes. Staff, Regina General Hospital; (306)766-4444

MANG, Fan-Wah; Mississauga Med Centre, 205-1420 Burnhamthorpe Rd E, Mississauga ON L4X 2Z9; Tor'95; CCFP; FCFP; Staff Family Med, Trillium Health Centre - Mississauga; (905)625-4016; Fax. (905)625-7721; fanwah.mang@utoronto.ca.

MANGA, Ashok; Lark Med Services, 8679 120 St, Delta BC V4C 6R4; Guru Nanak Dev (India)'77; MB BS; CCFP; Langs: Punjabi; Hindi; Urdu; (604)591-5858; Fax. (604)591-5878.

MANGAL, Anil; Lifelabs Med Laboratory Serv, 3680 Gilmore Way, Burnaby BC V5G 4V8; Suva (Fiji)'73; ABIM; MBA; FRCPC; Hem (Hematology Pathology). Clinical Asst Prof, University of British Columbia; (604)431-5005

MANGAL, Sunil K; St Paul's Hosp, 1081 Burrard St, Vancouver BC V6Z 1Y6; Alb'94; CCFP; CCFP(E.M.); Staff Emerg, Providence Health Care - St Paul's Hospital; (604)682-2344

MANGALOGLU, Leyla F; Burlington Prof Centre, 309-3155 Harvester Rd, Burlington ON L7N 3V2; McM'04; FRCSC; ObstGyn. Staff, Hamilton Health Sciences Centre - McMaster Children's Hospital; (289)337-1663; Fax. (289)337-4407.

MANGAN, Kevin J; Sturgeon Community Hosp, 201 Boudreau Rd, St. Albert AB T8N 6C4; Alb'89; CCFP; CCFP(E.M.); Physician Emerg, Sturgeon Community Hospital; Clin Lecturer Family Med, University of Alberta; (780)418-8229

MANGANAS, Athena; CSSS Jeanne-Mance, 100-15 av du Mont-Royal O, Montreal QC H2T 2R9; Qns'03; CCFP; (514)286-9657

MANGANAS, Helene; CHUM-Hop Notre-Dame, 1560 rue Sherbrooke E, Montreal QC H2L 4M1; Mon'00; FRCPC; IntMed; Respir. Staff, Centre Hospitalier l'Université de Montréal (CHUM) - Hôpital Notre-Dame; (514)890-8000

MANGANAS, Therese; 380-1575 boul Henri-Bourassa O, Montreal QC H3M 3A9; Athens (Greece)'71; Langs: English; Greek; (514)953-4536; tessou4@yahoo.ca.

MANGAR, Mohini; North Halton Mental Hlth Clini, 217 Main St E, Milton ON L9T 1N9; Man'88; FRCPC; Psy. Staff, Halton Healthcare Services Corporation - Oakville Site; (905)693-4240

MANGAT, Amardeep S; North York Gen Hosp, 4001 Leslie St, Toronto ON M2K 1E1; California (USA)'06; Staff, North York General Hospital; (416)756-6000

MANGAT, Birender S; Placentia Health Centre, PO Box 480 1 Corrigan Place, Placentia NL A0B 2Y0; Punjabi (India)'84; MB BS; MS(ENT); CCFP; Sr Medical Officer, Placentia Health Centre; (709)227-2013; Fax. (709)227-4111; bsmangat@hotmail.com.

MANGAT, Iqwal S; St Michael's Hosp, 6 050 QW-30 Bond St, Toronto ON M5B 1W8; Tor'93; FRCPC; IntMed; Cardiol. Dir Arrhythmia Services, St Michael's Hospital; Asst Prof Med, University of Toronto; (416)864-5104; Fax. (416)864-5283.

MANGAT, Rajeev; 1545 Johnston Rd, White Rock BC V4B 3Z6; Saba (Netherlands Antilles)'09; CCFP; (604)560-6161

MANGAT, Ramanjot K; Abbotsford Mental Health Ctre, 11-32700 George Ferguson Way, Abbotsford BC V2T 4V6; UBC'02; CCFP; Staff, George Pearson Centre; (604)870-7800

MANGAT, Rupinder K; Sunridge Prof Centre, 401-2675 36 St NE, Calgary AB T1Y 6H6; Cal'96; CCFP; (403)717-0812; newomensclinic@gmail.com.

MANGAT, Sandeep; Placentia Health Centre, PO Box 480, Placentia NL A0B 2Y0; (Pakistan)'86; CCFP; Physician, Placentia Health Centre; Asst Medical Officer, Eastern Health Corporate Office; Langs: Hindi; Punjabi; (709)227-2013; Fax. (709)227-4111; mangatsandeep@yahoo.com.

MANGATAL, Moira C; Fort William Fam Health Team, 117 McKellar St S, Thunder Bay ON P7E 1H5; Dal'02; CCFP; (807)626-1234

MANGEL, Joy E; LHSC-Westminster Campus, A2 401-800 Commissioners Rd E, London ON N6A 4G5; McG'94; FRCPC; IntMed; Hem. Staff Hematologist, London Health Sciences Centre - Victoria Campus; Asst Prof, University of Western Ontario; Langs: French; (519)685-8479

MANGEL, Roman; MUHC-Montreal Gen Hosp, 1650 av Cedar, Montreal QC H3G 1A4; McG'63; FRCPC; IntMed; Nephrol (P.Q.). Staff, McGill University Health Centre - Montreal General Campus; adj Prof, McGill University; (514)934-1934 x44033

MANGEL, Ryan; Bluewater Health - Norman Site, 89 Norman St, Sarnia ON N7T 6S3; American Univ of the Caribbean (Netherlands Antilles)'05; CCFP; Staff, Bluewater Health - Norman Site; (519)464-4400

MANGIN, James E; Central Alberta Med Imaging, 4312 54 Ave, Red Deer AB T4N 4M1; Wes'98; FRCPC; DiagRad. (403)343-6172; Fax. (403)309-3063.

MANHAS, Deepak; Children's & Women's HC of BC, 4480 Oak St, Vancouver BC V6H 3V4; UBC'07; Peds. Staff, BC Children's Hospital; (604)875-2345 x7360

MANHAS, Prithpal S; Chemainus Med Clinic, RR 1 9892 Esplanade St, Chemainus BC V0R 1K1; UBC'94; CCFP; FCFP; (250)246-3261; Fax. (250)246-9144.

MANHAS, Surender S; Cartwright Plaza, 7 Cartwright St, Grnd-Falls-Wi NL A2A 1L7; Punjab (India)'68; MB BS; FRCPC; Psy. Staff, Central Newfoundland Regional Health Centre; (709)489-2233

MANHES, Gilles; CSSS de Quebec Nord, 3666 ch Royal, Quebec QC G1E 1X5; Laval'85; LMCC; BSc(BioChem); Langs: English; (418)663-2572; Fax. (418)663-2939; gilles.manhes@ssss.gouv.qc.ca.

MANIATE, Jerry M; St Joseph's Health Centre, 30 The Queensway, Toronto ON M6R 1B5; Man'01; MEd; FRCPC; IntMed (Medical Oncology). Staff, St Joseph's Health Centre; (416)530-6235; Fax. (416)530-6656.

MANIATIS, Thomas; MUHC-Royal Victoria Hosp, M10 02-687 av des Pins O, Montreal QC H3A 1A1; McG'96; MSc; FRCPC; IntMed (Biomedical Ethics). Staff, McGill University Health Centre - Royal Victoria Hospital; Langs: French; Greek; (514)843-1506; Fax. (514)843-1725; thomas.maniatis@mcgill.ca.

MANICATIDE, Mihai A; The Doctors Bldg, 901-208 Bloor St W, Toronto ON M5S 3B4; Bucharest (Romania)'61; Member, St Joseph's Health Centre; Langs: Romanian; (416)922-2554; Fax. (416)922-2858.

MANIERE, Thibault; Hop Charles Lemoyne, 3120 boul Taschereau, Greenfield Park QC J4V 2H1; (France)'04; Staff, Hopital Charles LeMoyne; (450)466-5000

MANIS, Danielle; 704-240 Duncan Mill Rd, North York ON M3B 3S6; Tor'01; BSc; CCFP; Ac Staff, North York General Hospital; (416)497-0880

MANISHEN, Wayne J; 405-400 Tache Ave, Winnipeg MB R2H 3C3; Man'83; FRCPC; IntMed (Gastroenterology). Staff, Victoria General Hospital; (204)943-9108; Fax. (204)947-0781.

MANJANATHA, Channagiri P; Chinook Reg Hosp, 960 19 St S, Lethbridge AB T1J 1W5; Mysore (India)'60; MD; DAB(USA); DA(McG); FRCPC; Anes (Chronic Pain Management). Staff Specialist Pain Management & Anes, Chinook Regional Hospital; Staff Specialist Pain Management & Anes, Taber Health Centre; Staff Specialist Pain Management & Anes, Fort MacLeod Health Centre; (403)388-6111 x6205; Fax. (403)388-6226.

MANJI, Aisha; Willow Clinic, 1-3801 28A St, Vernon BC V1T 9T6; UBC'04; CCFP; (250)542-9950; aisha.manji@gmail.com.

MANJI, Alaudin E; 7347A 120 St, Delta BC V4C 6P5; Sheffield (England)'71; MB ChB; CCFP; FCFP; Staff, Surrey Memorial Hospital; Asst Prof, University of British Columbia; Langs: Punjabi; Swahili; French; (604)590-2323; Fax. (604)590-0286; moodymd@hotmail.com.

MANJI, Arif; The Hosp for Sick Children, 9402 BW-555 University Ave, Toronto ON M5G 1X8; Wes'06; PedHemaOncol; Peds. Staff, The Hospital For Sick Children; (416)813-1500

MANJI, Mohamed; BC Cancer Agency, 399 Royal Ave, Kelowna BC V1Y 5L3; Makerere (Uganda)'71; MB ChB; DMRT; DABR; FRCPC; RadOncol. Staff, BC Cancer Agency Sindi Ahluwalia Hawkins Centre for the Southern Interior; (250)712-3979

MANJI, Rahimali; Surrey Mem Hosp, 13750 96 Ave, Surrey BC V3V 1Z2; Wes'09; CCFP; Staff, Surrey Memorial Hospital; (604)581-2211

MANJI, Rizwan A S; I H Asper Clin Research Inst, CR3014-369 Tache Ave, Winnipeg MB R2H 2A6; Alb'95; FRCSC; CardSurg; Critical Care Medicine.

MANJI, Salim A; Meadowlark Health Centre, 200 Meadowlark Shopping Ctr NW, Edmonton AB T5R 5W9; Alb'90; FRCPC; DiagRad. (780)489-7851; Fax. (780)486-5160.

MANJOO, Ajay; Upper Appleby Clinic, 22-1960 Appleby Line, Burlington ON L7L 0B7; (Jamaica)'98; FRCSC; OrthSurg. Staff, London Health Sciences Centre - Victoria Campus; (905)635-5606; Fax. (905)635-5516; ajay.manjoo@lhsc.on.ca.

MANJOO, Prija S; 601A Discovery St, Victoria BC V8T 5G4; (Jamaica)'97; Endocrin&Metab; IntMed. Staff, Victoria General Hospital.

MANJOS, Michael A; Jordan Med Centre, RR 1 3951 19th St, Jordan Station ON L0R 1S0; Tor'81; BSc(Hons.); (905)562-5221; Fax. (905)562-7699.

MANKAEVA, Soussa; Waterford Hosp, 306 Waterford Bridge Rd, St. John's NL A1E 4J8; North Ossetian State (Russia (Federation))'89; CCFP; Staff, Waterford Hospital; (709)777-3300

MANKAL, Fawzi A; Rideau Family Health Team, 5-3635 Rivergate Way, Ottawa ON K1V 2A4; Ott'02; MSc; BSc; CCFP; Langs: Arabic; (613)739-3700; Fax. (613)739-7043.

MANKARIOUS, Mervat F; 6675 Falconer Dr, Mississauga ON L5N 0C3; (Egypt)'87; MB ChB; CCFP; Langs: English; French; Arabic; (905)567-0008; Fax. (905)567-0009.

MANKAVIL KOVIL VEETIL, Aneesh K; Queen Elizabeth II HSC, 845-1276 South Park St, Halifax NS B3H 2Y9; Calicut (India)'95; MB BS; Staff, Queen Elizabeth II Health Sciences Centre - Victoria General Site; (902)473-7015

MANKLOW, Jennifer K; PO Box 35032 Rpo Hillside, Victoria BC V8T 5G2; UBC'04; CCFP.

MANLEY, W Arnold; 186-10654 82 Ave NW, Edmonton AB T6E 2A7; Cape Town (South Africa)'84; (780)498-7962

MANN, A Douglas; Northwest Prof Centre, 305-1640 16 Ave NW, Calgary AB T2M 0L6; Tor'60; FRCPC; Psy (Consultation-Liaison). Clinical Asst Prof, University of Calgary; (403)269-2000; Fax. (403)266-0787.

MANN, Baljinder; Sunridge Prof Centre, 7-2681 36 St NE, Calgary AB T1Y 5S3; (India)'76; MB BS; CCFP; Langs: Hindi; Punjabi; Urdu; (403)250-3010; Fax. (403)250-3065.

MANN, Catherine D; The Ottawa Hosp-Gen Campus, 501 Smyth Rd, Ottawa ON K1H 8L6; Tor'96; MSc; BSc(Hon); FRCPC; Psy. Staff Psy, The Ottawa Hospital - General Campus; Asst Prof, University of Ottawa; (613)737-8010; Fax. (613)737-8115; cmann@ottawahospital.on.ca.

MANN, Catherine L; 206 Lemarchant Rd, St. John's NL A1C 2H6; Dal'92; BSc(Hon); FRCSC; GenSurg; ThorSurg. Ac Staff, St Clare's Mercy Hospital; Ac Staff, Health Sciences Centre; (709)739-5515; Fax. (709)739-5530.

MANN, Clifford I; 204-10 Unionville Gate, Markham ON L3R 0W7; McG'84; FRCPC; DiagRad. (905)479-3945; Fax. (905)479-3945.

MANN, Colin G; South Shore Med Arts, 307-42 Glen Allan Dr, Bridgewater NS B4V 3N2; Dal'85; FRCSC; Ophth (Medical & Surgical Ophthalmology). Ac Staff, South Shore Regional Hospital; (902)543-3421; Fax. (902)543-9273; c.mann@ns.sympatico.ca.

MANN, David L; 106-7373 Duncan St, Powell River BC V8A 1W6; Cal'84; CCFP; CCFP(E.M.); FCFP; Staff EmergMed, Powell River General Hospital; (604)485-4660

MANN, Elizabeth; Queen Elizabeth II HSC, 405-1276 South Park St, Halifax NS B3H 2Y9; Dal'76; FRCPC; IntMed. Ac Staff, Queen Elizabeth II Health Sciences Centre - Victoria General Site; Consultant, IWK Health Centre; Prof Med, Dalhousie University; (902)473-3961; Fax. (902)473-8430.

MANN, Erika H; The Hosp for Sick Children, 555 University Ave, Toronto ON M5G 1X8; Qns'98; FRCPC; DiagRad. Staff, The Hospital For Sick Children; Asst Prof, University of Toronto; (416)813-6038; erika.mann@sickkids.ca.

MANN, Rick; West Region London Office, 303-235 North Centre Rd, London ON N5X 4E7; Qns'81; CCFP; FCFP; Reg Coroner Supervizing, Ontario Southwestern Region; (519)661-6624 x205; rick.mann@ontario.ca.

MANN, Gary M; 376 Flamingo Rd, Thornhill ON L4J 8L4; Louisville (USA)'79; BSc; Emerg Phys Lead, Central East LHIN; Langs: Hebrew; French; (416)823-4417; Fax. (905)731-4535.

MANN, George H; 306-2170 Lakeshore Rd, Burlington ON L7R 1A6; London (England)'63; MB BS; DA; DObstRCOG; Ac Staff Emerg & Family Med, Joseph Brant Memorial Hospital.

MANN, John R; Primary Medical Clinic, 5001 Anderson Way, Vernon BC V1T 9V1; Sask'76; Staff, Vernon Jubilee Hospital; (250)545-8338 Semi-Retired.

MANN, Jotinder S; 101-12827 76th Ave, Surrey BC V3W 2V3; Man'97; CCFP; (604)590-0443

MANN, Karen; Div of Medical Education, 205C-5849 University Ave, Halifax NS B3H 4H7.

MANN, Keith D; 215 King St W, Dundas ON L9H 1V6; Tor'77; FRCSC; Ophth. Ac Staff, St Joseph's Healthcare - Charlton Campus; (905)627-4975; Fax. (905)627-7553.

MANN, Kenneth F; Caledonian Med Clinic, 340 Campbell St, Nanaimo BC V9R 3G7; Glasgow (Scotland)'70; MB ChB; DObstRCOG; DCH; Ac Staff, Nanaimo Regional General Hospital; (250)753-3202; Fax. (250)753-1039.

MANN, Manjeet; Richmond Med Bldg, 206-2020 Richmond Rd, Victoria BC V8R 6R5; UBC'90; FRCPC; IntMed (Valvular Heart Disease); Cardiol. (250)595-3111; Fax. (250)595-4277.

MANN, Miriam E S; Stratford Gen Hosp, 46 General Hospital Dr, Stratford ON N5A 2Y6; Wes'88; FACEP; Dip SportMed; FRCPC; EmergMed (Sports Medicine). Chief Dept of EmergMed/Med Prog Dir ER Med, Stratford General Hospital - Huron Perth Healthcare Alliance; (519)272-8210; Fax. (519)271-7137; miriam.mann@hpha.ca.

MANN, Nooreen; St Joseph's Healthcare, 50 Charlton Ave E, Hamilton ON L8N 4A6; Wes'08; IntMed. Staff, St Joseph's Healthcare - Charlton Campus.

MANN, Otto; King Med Clinic, 380 Portland St, Dartmouth NS B2Y 1K8; Dal'73; (902)463-1525; Fax. (902)463-2945.

MANN, R Renwick; 315-869 Clonsilla Ave, Peterborough ON K9J 0B7; Qns'75; FRCPC; Anes. (705)930-7627; Fax. (705)745-0400; ren.mann@sympatico.ca.

MANN, Ramandeep; 9655 137 St, Surrey BC V3T 4G8; (Other Foreign)'08; CCFP; (778)395-0085

MANN, Ranbir S; 7255 Fraser St, Vancouver BC V5X 3V8; Man'85; (604)325-4907; Fax. (604)325-0070.

MANN, Rick R S; Cambridge Mem Hosp, 700 Coronation Blvd, Cambridge ON N1R 3G2; Wes'09; CCFP; Staff, Cambridge Memorial Hospital; (519)621-2330

MANN, Satish K; Phoenix Med Centre, 308-2155 10th Ave, Prince George BC V2M 5J6; Punjabi (India)'93; MB BS; CCFP; Staff, University Hospital of Northern British Columbia; Langs: Punjabi; Hindi; (250)564-6211; Fax. (250)564-2488.

MANN, Suba S; Regina Qu'Appelle HR-Regina, 1440 14th Ave, Regina SK S4P 0W5; Rohtak (India)'76; ABIM(Endo&Metab); FRCPC; IntMed. Med Dir Metabolic & Diabetes Out-Patient Centre, Regina General Hospital; Clin Assoc Prof, University of Saskatchewan; (306)766-4540; Fax. (306)766-4178.

MANN, Tejinder K; Care Point Med Centre, 140-555 Sixth St, New Westminster BC V3L 5H1; Ranchi (India)'76; Langs: Punjabi; Hindi; (604)523-1166

MANN HOSFORD, Lorraine E; Athabascan Place, 222-80 Chippewa Rd, Sherwood Park AB T8A 4W6; Cal'86; CCFP; FCFP; (780)464-9661; Fax. (780)417-0656.

MANNA, Jonaki; Royal Jubilee Hosp, DT5828-1952 Bay St, Victoria BC V8R 1J8; UBC'01; FRCPC; HemPath. Staff, Royal Jubilee Hospital; (250)519-1833

MANNARD, Allan C; Lakeshore Gen Hosp, 160 av Stillview, Pointe-Claire QC H9R 2Y2; McG'77; PhD(Physiol); DAB; FACEP; FRCPC; EmergMed. Staff Emerg, Lakeshore General Hospital - Pointe Claire; (514)630-2166; Fax. (514)694-0886.

MANNARINO, Marco G; North Edmonton Health Centre, 14007 50 St NW, Edmonton AB T5A 5E4; Alb'08; CCFP; (780)342-4038; Fax. (780)342-4192.

MANNESS, Robert C; Morris Clinic, PO Box 252, Morris MB R0G 1K0; Man'77; (204)746-2351; Fax. (204)746-6172.

MANNETHU, Anne E; Hamilton Commun Health Centre, M1B-414 Victoria Ave N, Hamilton ON L8L 5G8; McM'07; CCFP; (905)529-5221

MANNHEIMER, Gareth J; Invermere Med Clinic, PO Box 8000 937 7 Ave, Invermere BC V0A 1K0; Cape Town (South Africa)'06; MB ChB; (250)342-9206

MANNINEN, Pirjo H; Univ Hlth Network-Toronto Western Hosp, 399 Bathurst St, Toronto ON M5T 2S8; Tor'73; FRCPC; Anes. Staff Anes, Toronto Western Hospital - University Health Network; Assoc Prof, University of Toronto; (416)603-5118; Fax. (416)603-6494; pirjo.manninen@uhn.on.ca.

MANNING, A Eric; 104-8425 120 St, Delta BC V4C 6R2; UBC'69; FRCPC; DiagRad. (604)590-2211

MANNING, E David; 2768 Broadway W PO Box 74685 Rpo Kitsilano, Vancouver BC V6K 4P4; Cal'06; CCFP; (778)386-0105

MANNING, Fiona F; Health Point Care Centre, 1454 Hillside Ave, Victoria BC V8T 2B7; Cal'96; BSc; MSc; CCFP; (250)370-5637

MANNING, Hubert; Bramalea Med Centre, 301-18 Kensington Rd, Brampton ON L6T 4S5; Dublin (Ireland)'69; MB ChB; BAO; Staff, William Osler Health System - Brampton Civic Hospital; (905)791-5822

MANNING, J David; Queen Elizabeth II HSC, 440-1276 South Park St, Halifax NS B3H 2Y9; Mem'84; DTMH; FRCPC; IntMed. Staff, Queen Elizabeth II Health Sciences Centre - Victoria General Site; (902)473-3961; Fax. (902)473-8430; david.manning@cdha.nshealth.ca.

MANNING, Jeff A; St Joseph's Lifecare Centre, 4F-99 Wayne Gretzky Pky, Brantford ON N3S 6T6; McM'88; CCFP; FCFP; Staff, The Brant Community Healthcare System - Brantford General Hospital Site; Court Staff, The Brant Community Healthcare System - Willett Hospital Site; (519)756-6400; Fax. (519)756-7343; spfmc@bellnet.ca.

MANNING, Pamella A M; Foothills Med Centre, 1403 29 St NW, Calgary AB T2N 2T9; (Jamaica)'75; FRCPC; Psy. Staff Psy, Foothills Medical Centre; (403)944-4547; Fax. (403)270-3451.

MANNION, Vincent L; Glendon Med Clinic, PO Box 178, Glendon AB T0A 1P0; Galway (Ireland)'82; MRC; CCFP; FCFP; Staff, Glendon Community Health Clinic; (780)635-4086; Fax. (780)635-2624; vmannion@telusplanet.net.

MANNIX, Sharyn E; MUHC-Montreal Chest Institute, 3650 rue Saint-Urbain, Montreal QC H2X 2P4; Cornell (USA)'77; Respir; IntMed. Staff, McGill University Health Centre - Montreal Chest Institute; (514)934-1934; Fax. (514)843-2070.

MANNO, Maria P; 401-627 Lyons Lane, Oakville ON L6J 5Z7; McM'83; CCFP; Langs: Italian; (905)338-0813; Fax. (905)338-5747.

MANNS, Braden J; Foothills Med Centre, 1403 29 St NW, Calgary AB T2N 2T9; Tor'94; MSc; BSc; FRCPC; IntMed (Dialysis); Nephrol. Staff Nephrol, Foothills Medical Centre; Assoc Prof, University of Calgary; (403)944-2595; braden.manns@calgaryhealthregion.ca.

MANNY, Emmanuelle; CLSC Lamater, 1317 boul des Seigneurs, Terrebonne QC J6W 5B1; Mon'87; (450)471-2881; Fax. (450)471-6763.

MANOCHA, Anoop; Foothills Med Centre, C231-1403 29 St NW, Calgary AB T2N 2T9; Mem'01; CCFP; CCFP(E.M.); Staff, Foothills Medical Centre; (403)944-1635

MANOCHA, Sanjay; Humber River Reg Hosp, 200 Church St, Toronto ON M9N 1N8; Mem'96; MD; BMedSci; FRCPC; IntMed (Research); Critical Care Medicine; Respir. Staff IntMed Respitology & Critical Care Med, Humber River Regional Hospital - Church Street Site; (416)243-4103; smanocha71@hotmail.com.

MANOGARAN, Mansula; Rouge Valley-Centenary HC, 303-2863 Ellesmere Rd, Scarborough ON M1E 4B9; Bergen (Norway)'95; FRCPC; IntMed; Nephrol. Staff, Rouge Valley Health System - Centenary Health Centre Site; (647)436-3397; Fax. (647)436-3403.

MANOHAR, Prethima; First Med Place, 106-170 Queensway W, Mississauga ON L5B 3A8; Madras (India)'77; MB; BSc; DPM(India); MRCPsy; FRCPC; Psy. Court Staff, Trillium Health Centre - Mississauga; (905)272-3899

MANOHAR, Savalai V; First Med Place, 106-170 Queensway W, Mississauga ON L5B 3A8; Mysore (India)'77; MRC(Psy); DPM(Madras); FRCPC; Psy. (905)272-3899

MANOHARAN, Sathiyapooma; 6065 Steeles Ave E, Scarborough ON M1X 0A8; Madras (India)'91; CCFP; Langs: Tamil; (416)754-0003; Fax. (416)754-0005.

MANOKARA, Kamini; 303-1371 Neilson Rd, Scarborough ON M1B 4Z8; Jaffna (Sri Lanka)'96; (647)347-2401; Fax. (647)347-2801.

MANOLI, Sabrine; CLSC de Cote-des-Neiges, 5700 ch Cote-des-Neiges, Montreal QC H3T 2A8; Laval'06; CCFP; Staff, CLSC Cote-des-Neiges; (514)731-8531

MANOLOPOULOS, Vaselios; Credit Valley Prof Bldg, 410-2300 Eglinton Ave W, Mississauga ON L5M 2V8; Wes'94; FRCSC; OrthSurg. Staff, The Credit Valley Hospital; (905)608-1444

MANONYANE, Jacob M; Minor Emergency Clinic, 3110 Laurier Dr, Saskatoon SK S7L 5J7; (306)978-2200; Fax. (306)978-8750.

MANOS, Daria K C; Queen Elizabeth II HSC, 1276 South Park St, Halifax NS B3H 2Y9; Dal'00; FRCPC; DiagRad. Staff, Queen Elizabeth II Health Sciences Centre - Victoria General Site; (902)473-7770

MANOS, Sarah H; IWK Health Centre, PO Box 9700 Rpo CSC 5850-5980 University Ave, Halifax NS B3K 6R8; Dal'02; FRCPC; Peds. Staff, IWK Health Centre; (902)470-8888

MANOUCHEHRI, Namdar; University of Alberta Hosp, 8440 112 St NW, Edmonton AB T6G 2B7; Alb'06; Staff, University of Alberta Hospital; (780)407-8822

MANOUKIAN, John J V; CUSM-Montreal Children's Hosp, B240-2300 rue Tupper, Montreal QC H3H 1P3; Alexandria (Egypt)'75; MB ChB; FRCS; ABOtol; FRCSC; Otol (Pediatrics). Staff, McGill University Health Centre - Montreal Children's Hospital; Staff, Sir Mortimer B Davis Jewish General; Staff, Hôpital Santa Cabrini Ospedale; Assoc Prof Otol, McGill University; Langs: French; Arabic; Armenian; (514)412-4304; Fax. (514)412-4342; john.manoukian@muhc.mcgill.ca.

MANOWSKI, Zbigniew J; Trillium Hlth Ctr-Mississauga, 100 Queensway W, Mississauga ON L5B 1B8; Warsaw (Poland)'81; FRCPC; AnatPath. Staff Lab Med, Trillium Health Centre - Mississauga; Langs: Polish; (905)848-7299

MANRAJ, Lea H; Victoria Med Bldg, 105-1669 Victoria St, Prince George BC V2L 2L5; London (England)'72; (250)562-7416; Fax. (250)562-2979.

MANRIQUE BELLO, Hermes M; CHUQ-St-Francois D'Assise, 10 rue de l'Espinay, Quebec QC G1L 3L5; (Colombia)'95; CCFP; Staff, Centre Hospitalier Universitaire De Québec - Pavillon De St-françois-d'assise; (418)525-4444; Fax. (418)915-4681.

MANS, Pierre L G; PO Box 1299 Stn Main, Kamloops BC V2C 6H3; Stellenbosch (South Africa)'92; MB ChB; FRCPC; Anes. (250)426-5281

MANSARAY, Helene; CSSS de Jonquiere, CP 1200 Succ Pdf Jonquiere 2230 rue de l'Hopital, Jonquiere QC G7X 7X2; Montpellier (France)'00; Staff, Centre Hospitalier Jonquiere; (418)695-7707

MANSEAU, Danielle I M; CLSC Grande Riviere, 425 rue Leguerrier, Gatineau QC J9H 6N8; Ott'78; CCFP; FCFP; (819)684-2251

MANSEAU, Serge; Centre Medical Le Mesnil, 300-1300 boul Lebourgneuf, Quebec QC G2K 2N1; Laval'96; (418)624-1800; Fax. (418)624-1820.

MANSELL, Graham L; Synergy Wellness Centre, 221-501 Bethel Dr, Sherwood Park AB T8H 0N2; Alb'98; CCFP; (780)464-0123; Fax. (780)449-5609.

MANSER, Courtney A; 1882 Niagara Stone Rd PO Box 10, Virgil ON L0S 1T0; McM'09; CCFP; (905)468-3275

MANSFIELD, Joanna K; Sunnybrook Hlth Sciences Ctre, 2075 Bayview Ave, Toronto ON M4N 3M5; Tor'06; Psy. Staff, Sunnybrook Health Sciences Centre; (416)480-6100

MANSFIELD, John F; Salvation Army Grace Gen Hosp, 300 Booth Dr, Winnipeg MB R3J 3M7; Manchester (England)'67; MB ChB; FRCPC; Anes (Administrative). Staff, The Salvation Army Grace Hospital; (204)837-0391

MANSFIELD, Pamela; The Moncton Hosp, 135 MacBeath Ave, Moncton NB E1C 6Z8; Dal'03; CCFP; Staff, The Moncton Hospital; (506)857-5001

MANSFIELD, Robert W; Humber River Reg Hosp, 200 Church St, Toronto ON M9N 1N8; Tor'07; CCFP; Staff, Humber River Regional Hospital - Church Street Site; (416)249-8111

MANSINGH, Sohan; Mission Oaks Med Centre, 32136 Lougheed Hwy, Mission BC V2V 1A4; (South Africa)'04; MB ChB; (604)826-7111

MANSON, David E S; The Hosp for Sick Children, 555 University Ave, Toronto ON M5G 1X8; Pennsylvania (USA)'81; FRCPC; DiagRad. Staff Diagnostic Imaging, The Hospital For Sick Children; (416)813-6031; david.manson@sickkids.ca.

MANSON, Henry J; Windsor Reg Hosp-Metropolitan, 1995 Lens Ave, Windsor ON N8W 1L9; Aberdeen (Scotland)'70; MB ChB; FFARCS(Eng); Anes (Hyperbaric Medicine). Staff Anes, Windsor Regional Hospital - Metropolitan Site; (519)254-5577; Fax. (519)736-0214.

MANSON, Nadine E F; 200-300 Main St N, Brampton ON L6V 4H6; Qns'91; FABM; CCFP; Staff, William Osler Health System - Brampton Civic Hospital; Clinical Asst Prof, McMaster University; (905)451-1937; Fax. (905)451-8272.

MANSON, Neil A; Saint John Reg Hosp, PO Box 2100 Stn Main, Saint John NB E2L 4L2; Dal'99; FRCSC; OrthSurg. Staff, Saint John Regional Hospital; Asst Prof, Dalhousie University; Asst Prof, Memorial University Of Newfoundland; (506)649-2667; Fax. (506)649-2769.

MANSON, Peter; Queensway Prof Centre, 209-190 Sherway Dr, Etobicoke ON M9C 5N2; Dublin (Ireland)'75; MB ChB; BAO; DCH; FRCPC; Peds. Court Consultant Peds, Trillium Health Centre - West Toronto; (416)695-4153; Fax. (416)695-3451; pmanson@thc.on.ca.

MANSOOR, Dana R; U of Toronto-Health Services, 214 College St, Toronto ON M5T 2Z9; McM'04; CCFP.

MANSOOR, Fenar A; Milner Health Centre, 2-857 Milner Ave, Scarborough ON M1B 5N6; (Iraq)'86; MB ChB; CCFP; Langs: Arabic; (416)287-3611

MANSOOR, Samina; Cape Breton Hlthcare Complex, 1482 George St, Sydney NS B1P 1P3; Fatima Jinnah (Pakistan)'84; MB BS; Staff Path, Cape Breton Healthcare Complex; (902)567-8000

MANSOUR, Ahmed M; William Osler HC-Brampton, 2100 Bovaird Dr E, Brampton ON L6R 3J7; Al Arab (Libya)'90; FRCPC; Psy. Staff, William Osler Health System - Brampton Civic Hospital; (905)494-6695

MANSOUR, Anne-Marie; Hop Du Sacre-Coeur De Mtl, 5400 boul Gouin O, Montreal QC H4J 1C5; Mon'96; FRCPC; IntMed. Staff, Hôpital du Sacre-Coeur de Montréal; (514)338-2222; Fax. (514)338-2424.

MANSOUR, Fadi; CHUM-Hotel-Dieu, 3840 rue Saint-Urbain, Montreal QC H2W 1T8; Mon'00; Cardiol; IntMed. Staff, Centre Hospitalier l'Université de Montréal (CHUM) - Hôtel-Dieu; (514)890-8000

MANSOUR, Fady W; MUHC-Royal Victoria Hosp, F4 46-687 av des Pins O, Montreal QC H3A 1A1; McG'04; FRCSC; ObstGyn (Fibroid). Staff, McGill University Health Centre - Royal Victoria Hospital; (514)934-1934 x44287

MANSOUR, Firas; Phoenix Med Centre, 309-2155 10th Ave, Prince George BC V2M 5J6; Damascus (Syria)'92; FRCPC; IntMed. Staff, University Hospital of Northern British Columbia; (250)562-7014

MANSOUR, H Mansour S; Agassiz Med Centre, 130-30 Stephen St, Morden MB R6M 2G3; (Other Foreign)'96; (204)822-4474

MANSOUR, Michael; Inst Philippe Pinel de Mtl, 10905 boul Henri-Bourassa E, Montreal QC H1C 1H1; Mon'83; Ac Staff, Institut Philippe-Pinel de Montreal; Langs: Arabic; English; (514)648-8461

MANSOUR, Nabil; 200-2944 Boul Taschereau, Greenfield Park QC J4V 2G8; Beirut (Lebanon)'68; FRCSC; ObstGyn. (450)671-6189; Fax. (450)671-5486.

MANSOUR, Raafat A E; 275-5 Fairview Mall Dr, North York ON M2J 2Z1; Alexandria (Egypt)'80; MB ChB; CCFP; Langs: Arabic; (416)494-0377; Fax. (416)494-3633.

MANSOUR, Riad A; Smyth Med Centre, 306-1929 Russell Rd, Ottawa ON K1G 4G3; 85Cairo (Egypt)'83; CCFP; Staff Physician Med/Oncol, The Ottawa Hospital - General Campus; Physician Designated Immigration Practitioner, Citizenship & Immigration Canada; Clin Asst, Ottawa Regional Cancer Centre; (613)731-6247

MANSOUR, Samer; CHUM-Hotel-Dieu, 3840 rue Saint-Urbain, Montreal QC H2W 1T8; (Lebanon)'98; CSPQ; Staff, Centre Hospitalier l'Université de Montréal (CHUM) - Hôtel-Dieu; Langs: English; Arabic; (514)890-8000 x15233; Fax. (514)412-7212.

MANSOUR, Samir; Seven Regions Health Centre, PO Box 1000 24 Mill St, Gladstone MB R0J 0T0; (Other Foreign)'89; Staff, Seven Regions Health Centre; (204)385-2968

MANSOUR, Yasser M A; C107-3885 Duke of York Blvd, Mississauga ON L5B 0E4; Alexandria (Egypt)'92; FRCPC; Peds. Staff Peds, St Joseph's Health Centre; (905)366-4441

MANSOURI, Shireen M; PO Box 2697 Stn Main, Yellowknife NT X1A 2R1; Qns'92; CCFP; CCFP(E.M.); FCFP; (867)873-3515

MANSUKHANI, Tarun; Wardenwood Health Centre, 2361 Warden Ave, Scarborough ON M1T 1V7; (416)299-4999; Fax. (416)299-1322.

MANSWORTH, Colman; Brockville Family Med Ctre, 203-309 Park St, Brockville ON K6V 6E5; Cork (Ireland)'72; Med Dir, Levi Canada (Cornwall); Examiner, Queen's University; (613)345-0918; Fax. (613)345-0865.

MANSY, Diaa A Y; 10125 157 St NW, Edmonton AB T5P 2T9; (Egypt)'86; (780)486-6664

MANT, Michael J; Clinical Sciences Bldg, 4 112-152 University Campus NW, Edmonton AB T6G 2G3; Otago (New Zealand)'64; FRACP; FACP; FRCPC; IntMed (Thromboembolism); Hem. Ac Staff Med, University of Alberta Hospital; Prof, University of Alberta; (780)407-6232; Fax. (780)407-2680.

MANTAY, Erica M E; Newmarket Med Place, 303-712 Davis Dr, Newmarket ON L3Y 8C3; Tor'89; FRCSC; ObstGyn. Staff Obst & Gyn, Southlake Regional Health Centre; (905)898-6575; Fax. (905)898-6676.

MANTHA, Gaston; Clinique Med D'Alma, 935 av Du Pont S, Alma QC G8B 2V5; Laval'84; (418)668-6121; Fax. (418)668-5298.

MANTHA, Jean; 2635 boul Rosemont, Montreal QC H1Y 1L1; Mon'75; (514)722-5664; cliniquejeanmantha@videotron.ca.

MANTHORNE, Janice L A; Helmcken Pediatric Associates, 212-284 Helmcken Rd, Victoria BC V9B 1T2; Mem'00; FRCPC; Peds. Staff, Victoria General Hospital; (250)881-7347

MANTLE, Edward R; Hamilton HS-Henderson Site, 711 Concession St, Hamilton ON L8V 1C3; McM'90; CCFP; Staff, Hamilton Health Sciences Centre-Juravinski Site; (905)527-4322

MANTLE, Nancy G; North Bay Reg Health Centre, PO Box 2500 Stn Main 50 College Dr, North Bay ON P1B 5A4; McM'92; Staff, North Bay Regional Health Centre - Regional Mental Health; (705)474-1200 x2082; Fax. (705)495-7814.

MANTLE, Ross E; Four Corners Med Bldg, 201-2009 Long Lake Rd, Sudbury ON P3E 6C3; Wes'95; FRCSC; Neursurg. Staff, Health Sciences North-Laurentian Site; Asst Prof, Northern Ontario School of Medicine; (705)522-0292

MANTLE, Valerie I; 1-2120 Regent St, Sudbury ON P3E 3Z9; Ott'97; CCFP; Langs: French; German; (705)671-3011

MANTRO, Kiran B; 312-3850 Finch Ave E, Scarborough ON M1T 3T6; Punjab (India)'75; MB BS; FRCPC; Psy. Staff Psy, The Scarborough Hospital - Birchmount Campus; (416)298-6342; Fax. (416)298-6342.

MANTYNEN, Philip R; 200 Franklin Blvd, Cambridge ON N1R 8N8; Ott'83; FRCPC; Peds. Chief Serv-Peds, Cambridge Memorial Hospital; Clinical Asst Prof, McMaster University; (519)620-3600; Fax. (519)620-3602; philip.mantynen@rogers.com.

MANUCHA, Shalini; 2160 Weston Rd, North York ON M9N 1X6; New Delhi (India)'82; MB BS; Staff, Humber River Regional Hospital - Church Street Site; Langs: Hindi; (416)249-3313; Fax. (416)248-9482.

MANUEL, Douglas G; Ottawa Hosp Research Inst, 725 Parkdale Ave, Ottawa ON K1Y 4E9; Dal'89; MSc; BSc; FRCPC; CommunMed (Industrial Occupational Medicine). (613)798-5555 x19108

MANUEL, Mogamat A; York-Med Medical Arts Centre, 205-250 Harding Blvd W, Richmond Hill ON L4C 9M7; Cape Town (South Africa)'63; MB ChB; FACP; MEd; FRCPC; IntMed (Nephrology). Staff, Mackenzie Richmond Hill Hospital; (905)508-5911; Fax. (905)508-2972.

MANUEL, Paul L; Portage Clinic, 140 9th St SE, Portage la Prairie MB R1N 3V5; Man'03; FRCSC; GenSurg. (204)857-3445

MANUSOW, David N; Manitoba Clinic, 790 Sherbrook St, Winnipeg MB R3A 1M3; Man'75; ABOph; FRCSC; Ophth (Glaucoma). Consultant Staff, Misericordia Health Centre; Lecturer Ophth, University of Manitoba; (204)788-5764; Fax. (204)783-3805.

MANVILLE, Margaret L; St Joseph's Gen Hosp, E-2137 Comox Ave, Comox BC V9M 1P2; UBC'97; CCFP; FCFP; Med Coord Upper Island Geriatric Outreach Program, St Joseph's General Hospital; Med Dir, Glacier View Lodge; Langs: Bilingual(English/French); (250)339-1440

MANWELL, Stuart E E; Grey Bruce HS-Owen Sound, PO Box 1800 Stn Main 5110-1800 8th St E, Owen Sound ON N4K 6M9; Wes'98; FRCSC; OrthSurg (Arthroplasty). Staff Orthopedic Surg, Grey Bruce Health Services - Owen Sound; (519)376-2023; Fax. (519)376-1145.

MANYANDE, Tekesai T P; City Medical Centre, 398 Broadway St W, Yorkton SK S3N 0P1; Staff, Yorkton Regional Health Centre; (306)782-1122; Fax. (306)782-1155.

MANYARI, Dante E; Surrey Med Arts Bldg, 312-13710 94A Ave, Surrey BC V3V 1N1; Lima (Peru)'71; FACC; FAHA; LMCC; FRCPC; Cardiol (Heart Failure). Consultant Cardiol, Surrey Memorial Hospital; Langs: Spanish; (604)588-5600; Fax. (604)588-5688.

MANZAR, Asma; Pinawa Primary Hlth Care Ctr, PO Box 400, Pinawa MB R0E 1L0; (Pakistan)'86.

MANZAR, Khalid; Fredericton Med Clinic, 502-1015 Regent St, Fredericton NB E3B 6H5; Banaras Hindu (India)'88; Staff, Dr Everett Chalmers Regional Hospital.

MANZIG, Gloria B I; Parkdale Med Centre, 507-1081 Carling Ave, Ottawa ON K1Y 4G2; Cal'94; CCFP; (613)728-4605; Fax. (613)728-3083.

MANZIG, Loraine A; Yonge-Eglinton Med Centre, 210-2401 Yonge St, Toronto ON M4P 3H1; Ott'90; BSc(Hon); CCFP; FCFP; (416)485-9044; Fax. (416)485-8525.

MANZINI, Nicolas; CSSS des Basques, RR 1 550 rue Notre-Dame E, Trois-Pistoles QC G0L 4K0; Joseph Fourier (France)'98; Staff, Centre Hospitalier Trois-Pistoles; (418)851-3700; Fax. (418)851-2944.

MANZINI, Prince C; Saskatchewan Med Association, 402-321A 21st St E, Saskatoon SK S7K 0C1; (Other Foreign)'92; MB ChB; DipHIV; (306)244-2196

MAO, C Russell; Oakville Cardiologists, 302 5-690 Dorval Dr, Oakville ON L6K 3W7; Tor'99; BSc; FRCPC; IntMed; Cardiol. Staff Cardiol, Halton Healthcare Services Corporation - Oakville Site; (905)849-4567 x5

MAPE, Avelino M; 1319 Hall Ave, Windsor ON N8X 4R2; Manila (Philippines)'58; FRCPC; Psy (Adult Psychiatry). (519)977-9733; Fax. (519)977-7718.

MAPESO, Gabriel V; 1-1077 Golf Links Rd, Thunder Bay ON P7B 7A3; Cebu (Philippines)'81; FRCSC; GenSurg. Staff Surg/Pres Med Staff, Thunder Bay Regional Health Sciences Centre; (807)622-3995; Fax. (807)622-3430.

MAPLES, Gail A; Windsor-Essex Country Hlth Uni, 1005 Ouellette Ave, Windsor ON N9A 4J8; Tor'89; CCFP; FCFP; (519)258-2146; gmaples@wechealthunit.org.

MAR, Colin R; BC Cancer Agency-Vancouver CC, 600 10th Ave W, Vancouver BC V5Z 4E6; McM'98; FRCPC; DiagRad. Staff, BC Cancer Agency Vancouver Centre; (604)877-6000

MAR, Melanie C; Huntsville Prof Bldg, 102-348 Muskoka Rd 3 N, Huntsville ON P1H 1H8; McM'03; CCFP; Physician, Fairvern Nursing Home; (705)789-4377

MAR, Serena G; Links Clinic, 104-11910 111 Ave NW, Edmonton AB T5G 3G6; Alb'89; Ac Staff, Royal Alexandra Hospital; (780)454-0351; Fax. (780)452-6767.

MAR, Warren J; North Oshawa Med Centre, 205-1400 Ritson Rd N, Oshawa ON L1G 7W4; Cal'93; BSc; CCFP; (905)404-0372; Fax. (905)433-2108.

MARAGH, Dev K; Victoria Terrace Med Centre, 205-1448 Lawrence Ave E, North York ON M4A 2V6; West Indies (Jamaica)'85; MB BS; LMCC; CCFP; (416)444-8847

MARAGH, Haridath; Victoria Terrance Med Centre, 205-1448 Lawrence Ave E, North York ON M4A 2V6; London (England)'58; MB BS; FRCS(Ed); FRCSC; GenSurg (Proctology). (416)444-8847; Fax. (416)444-8816.

MARAGH, Krishna K; 300-4309 52 Ave, Red Deer AB T4N 6S4; (Trinidad & Tobago)'97; MB BS; FRCSC; OrthSurg. Staff, University of Alberta Hospital; (403)309-2001; Fax. (403)358-5808.

MARAGH, Vashti R; Red Deer Reg Hosp Centre, 3942 50A Ave, Red Deer AB T4N 4E7; (Trinidad & Tobago)'96; MB BS; FRCPC; Anes. Staff, Red Deer Regional Hospital Centre; (403)343-4639

MARAGHI, Elias R; Riverview Med Clinic, 2-8 Water St, Hastings ON K0L 1Y0; Tor'86; CDE; Head Team Phys, Belleville Bulls Hockey Club; Med Dir, Westgate Nursing Home; Med Dir, Crown Ridge Nursing Home; Langs: English; French; (705)696-2231; Fax. (705)696-2138; emaraghi@cogeco.ca.

MARAGHI, Kamal E; Groupe Sante Physimed, 121-6363 Rte Transcanadienne, Saint-Laurent QC H4T 1Z9; Cairo (Egypt)'64; ObstGyn. Staff, St Mary's Hospital Centre; Staff, Hôpital Santa Cabrini Ospedale; (514)747-8888

MARAH, Muhaned A; Dauphin Med Clinic, 622 3rd St SW, Dauphin MB R7N 1R5.

MARAIS, Abraham J; Yarmouth Reg Health Centre, 313-60 Vancouver St, Yarmouth NS B5A 2P5; Stellenbosch (South Africa)'93; MB ChB; Staff, Yarmouth Regional Hospital; (902)742-7598; Fax. (902)742-0072.

MARAIS, Andre; Melfort Union Hosp, PO Box 1480, Melfort SK S0E 1A0; Stellenbosch (South Africa)'77; MB ChB; LMCC; FRCPC; DiagRad. Staff, Melfort Hospital; (306)752-8727; Fax. (306)752-8711.

MARAIS, Cilliers; Mageta Med Centre, 110-20528 Lougheed Hwy, Maple Ridge BC V2X 2P8; Stellenbosch (South Africa)'84; MB ChB; LMCC; DObst; Langs: Afrikaans; (604)465-1100; cmarais@telus.net.

MARAIS, Francois; Dauphin Med Clinic, 622 3rd St SW, Dauphin MB R7N 1R5; Stellenbosch (South Africa)'98; Staff, Dauphin Regional Health Centre.

MARAIS, Ilke; 4808 Glentanna Rd PO Box 1142, Barriere BC V0E 1E0; (Other Foreign)'08; MB ChB; (250)672-9795

MARAIS, Nico F; Medical & Dental Bldg, 104-3939 50A Ave, Red Deer AB T4N 4E6; Orange Free State (South Africa)'82; MB ChB; MMed(ObstGyn); FRCSC; ObstGyn. Staff, Red Deer Regional Hospital Centre; (403)314-3420; Fax. (403)314-3480; nmarais@telus.net.

MARAJ, Ramsarran; 103-210 Dundas St E, Belleville ON K8N 5G8; Bristol (England)'68; (613)962-5966; Fax. (613)962-5230.

MARAJ, Reena; Synergy Wellness Centre, 221-501 Bethel Dr, Sherwood Park AB T8H 0N2; Natal (South Africa)'79; MB ChB; (780)464-0123; Fax. (780)449-5609.

MARAJ, Vikesh; 5565 Wyandotte St E, Windsor ON N8S 4T9; (South Africa)'99; MB ChB; CCFP.

MARANDA, Bruno; CHUS-Hop Fleurimont, 3001 12e av N, Sherbrooke QC J1H 5N4; Mon'01; FRCPC; MedGenetics. Staff, Centre Hospitalier Universitaire de Sherbrooke-Hopital Fleurimont; (819)345-1110 x13490

MARANDA, Claude R; 300-245 av Victoria, Westmount QC H3Z 2M6; Ott'71; FRCPC; IntMed; Cardiol. Staff, McGill University Health Centre - Royal Victoria Hospital; (514)938-2005

MARANDA, Francois; Hôpital Ste-Justine, 3175 ch Cote-Sainte-Catherine, Montreal QC H3T 1C5; Laval'78; FRCPC; Psy. Chief Adoles Psy, Hôpital Ste-Justine; (514)345-4931

MARANDA, Helene; CLSC Laurier-Station, RR 1 135 rue de la Station, Laurier-Station QC G0S 1N0; Laval'84; (418)728-3435; Fax. (418)728-2233.

MARANDA, Jacques; CSSS de Rivière-de-Loup, 75 rue Saint-Henri, Riviere-du-Loup QC G5R 2A4; Laval'65; Staff, Centre Hospitalier Regional du Grand-Portage; Langs: English; (418)862-6611

MARANDA, Julie P; Centre Med Ruby, 101-361 Main St E, Hawkesbury ON K6A 1A8; McG'98; MHSc; CCFP; Staff, Hawkesbury & District General Hospital; Asst Prof, University of Toronto; Asst Prof, University of Ottawa; Langs: English; French; (613)632-0605; Fax. (613)632-7073.

MARANDA, Robert C; 502-1355 Bank St, Ottawa ON K1H 8K7; McG'01; FRCPC; IntMed; Cardiol. (613)738-1584; Fax. (613)738-9097.

MARANDA, Sophie; CHUM-Hop St-Luc, 1058 rue Saint-Denis, Montreal QC H2X 3J4; Mon'09; CCFP; Staff, Centre Hospitalier l'Université De Montréal (CHUM) - Hôpital Saint-luc; (514)890-8000

MARANDO, Dominic; Medicine Familiale Lasalle, 6-2101 av Dollard, LaSalle QC H8N 1S2; Padova (Italy)'84; Langs: Italian; French; (514)595-8867; Fax. (514)363-9280.

MARANTZ, Jeffrey E; Medical Arts Bldg, 202-233 Kennedy St, Winnipeg MB R3C 3J5; Man'79; FRCPC; DiagRad (Body Computed Tomography). Assoc Staff, Health Sciences Centre; Assoc Staff, Seven Oaks General Hospital; Assoc Prof, University of Manitoba; (204)942-6453

MARANTZ, Susan G; RANA-Respiratory Care Group, 6-55 Henlow Bay, Winnipeg MB R3Y 1G4; Man'83; IntMed.

MARAZZI, Alex S; Cedar Care Clinic, 104-32423 Lougheed Hwy, Mission BC V2V 7B8; UBC'89; CCFP; CCFP(E.M.); Langs: Italian; (604)820-7676

MARBACK, Randolph M; Nanaimo Reg Gen Hosp, 1200 Dufferin Cres, Nanaimo BC V9S 2B7; UBC'90; Staff, Nanaimo Regional General Hospital; (250)716-7706

MARBURG, Lutz; Calgary Trail Medicentre, 1-10407 51 Ave NW, Edmonton AB T6H 0K4; Witwatersrand (South Africa)'55; Staff, Calgary Trail Medicentres; Langs: German; Afrikaans; (780)436-8071; Fax. (780)435-6034; ljmarburg@shaw.ca.

MARC, Maya; Ctr Hosp Anna-Laberge, 200 boul Brisebois, Chateauguay QC J6K 4W8; McG'95; Peds. Staff, Hôpital Anna-Laberge; Langs: Slovenian; French; (450)699-2425

MARC SERIES, Isabelle; CHUQ-Ctr Hosp Univ Laval, 1745-2705 boul Laurier, Quebec QC G1V 4G2; Paris (France)'83; Staff, Centre Hospitalier Universitaire de Quebec-CHUL; (418)654-2282

MARCACCIO, Michael J; Hamilton HS-Henderson Site, B3 158-711 Concession St, Hamilton ON L8V 1C3; McM'80; DABS; FACS; ERCP; SAGES; MD; FRCSC; GenSurg (Hepatobiliary & Pancreatic Surgery). Staff, Hamilton Health Sciences Centre-Juravinski Site; Ac Staff, Hamilton Health Sciences Centre - McMaster Children's Hospital; Prof Surg, McMaster University; (905)521-2622; Fax. (905)527-1700; marcacci@mcmaster.ca.

MARCARIAN, Berge; Scarborough North Med Arts, 209-4040 Finch Ave E, Scarborough ON M1S 4V5; Tor'89; FRCSC; Otol. Langs: Armenian; French; (416)293-5511; Fax. (416)293-5077.

MARCASSA, David A; Frontenac Med Associates, 201-791 Princess St, Kingston ON K7L 1E9; Qns'87; CCFP; FCFP; (613)544-2727; Fax. (613)544-7247.

MARCEAU, Annie; Clin Medico-Dentaire Pasteur, 770 1e av, Quebec QC G1L 3K2; Laval'85; (418)529-0042

MARCEAU, Daniele; CHUQ-Hotel-Dieu De Quebec, 11 Cote du Palais, Quebec QC G1R 2J6; Laval'80; MedOncol; Hem (P.Q.); IntMed (P.Q.). assoc Staff, CSSS de Quebec-Sud; ac Staff, Centre Hospitalier Universitaire de Québec (CHUQ) - Siege Social; Staff, Hôtel-Dieu de Lévis; (418)691-5225

MARCEAU, Danielle; Clinique Med Familiale de Hull, 202-15 boul Montclair, Gatineau QC J8Y 2E2; Laval'07; CCFP; (819)777-2752

MARCEAU, Jacinthe; CSSS Cleophas-Claveau, CP 38 succ La Baie 1000 av Dr Desgagne, La Baie QC G7B 3P9; Laval'94; Staff, CHSLD-CLSC Cleophas-Claveau; (418)544-3381

MARCEAU, Jean-Charles; CSSS de Jonquiere, CP 1200 Stn Pdf Jonquiere 2230 rue de l'Hopital, Jonquiere QC G7X 7X2; Laval'72; FRCPC; DiagRad (Mammography). ac Staff, Centre Hospitalier Jonquiere; (418)695-7700 x2324; Fax. (418)695-7742; jeanmarc49@videotron.ca.

MARCEAU, Julie; CHUQ-Hotel-Dieu de Quebec, 11 Cote du Palais, Quebec QC G1R 2J6; Laval'05; FRCPC; DiagRad. Staff, Centre Hospitalier Universitaire de Québec (CHUQ) - Siege Social; (418)525-4444

MARCEAU, Julie; Medi-Centre Chomedey, 610 boul Cure-Labelle, Laval QC H7V 2T7; Mon'00; (450)687-6452; Fax. (450)687-3243.

MARCEAU, Marie-Josee; Polyclinique Med Pierre LeGard, 300-1000 montee des Pionniers, Terrebonne QC J6V 1S8; Mon'96; Staff, Centre Hospitalier Pierre le Gardeur; Langs: Bilingual(French/English); (450)657-5799

MARCEAU, Michel; Centre de Surdite, 20-1657 rue Rachel E, Montreal QC H2J 2K6; Laval'62; Otol. (514)521-7720; Fax. (514)521-7761.

MARCEAU, Nicole; CLSC Metro, 1801 boul Maisonneuve O, Montreal QC H3H 1J9; Laval'76; (514)934-0354; Fax. (514)934-6155.

MARCEAU, Picard; Hôpital Laval, 2725 ch Sainte-Foy, Quebec QC G1V 4G5; Laval'58; MSc; PhD; FACS; FRCSC; GenSurg. Dir Dept of Surg, Hôpital Laval; Prof, Université Laval; (418)656-4810

MARCEAU, Pierre; CSSS du Lac-des-Deux-Montagnes, 520 boul Arthur-Sauve, Saint-Eustache QC J7R 5B1; Mon'84; FRCSC; GenSurg. Coord Bloc Opertoire, Hôpital de Saint-Eustache; (450)473-6811

MARCEAU, Simon; Hôpital Laval, 2725 ch Sainte-Foy, Quebec QC G1V 4G5; Laval'91; FRCSC; GenSurg (Bariatric Surgery). Staff, Hôpital Laval; (418)656-4810; Fax. (418)656-4825; simon.marceau@ssss.gouv.qc.ca.

MARCEAU, Stephane; Carrefour Med Vallee Richelieu, 665 boul Sir-Wilfrid-Laurier, Beloeil QC J3G 4J1; Mon'86; (450)467-0088; Fax. (450)467-6941.

MARCEAU-GAUVIN, Nathalie; Centre Med Christ-Roi, 102-40 rte du President-Kenned, Levis QC G6V 6C4; Mon'08.

MARCELLUS, Deborah C; The Juravinski Cancer Centre, 699 Concession St, Hamilton ON L8V 5C2; McM'81; FRCPC; IntMed; Hem. (905)575-9827

MARCELO-MACALINO, Magdalena; Battlefords Mental Health Ctr, 1092 107th St, North Battleford SK S9A 1Z1; Manila Central (Philippines)'64; Physician, Battlefords Health District; Langs: Tagalog; (306)446-6500 x6515; Fax. (306)446-6546.

MARCH, Gerard M J; 209-429 Exmouth St, Sarnia ON N7T 5P1; Wes'04; FRCSC; OrthSurg. (519)336-7860; Fax. (519)336-0020.

MARCH, Roderick J; Vancouver Gen Hosp, 855 12th Ave W, Vancouver BC V5Z 1M9; Mem'85; Staff, Providence Health Care - St Paul's Hospital; Staff, Vancouver General Hospital - Centennial Pavillion; (604)875-4111

MARCHADIER, Virginie; Sudbury Reg Hosp-Laurentian, 41 Ramsey Lake Rd, Sudbury ON P3E 5J1; Mon'05; CCFP; CCFP(E.M.); Staff, Health Sciences North-Laurentian Site; (705)523-7100

MARCHAK, Barbara E; Clinical Sciences Bldg, 8 120-152 University Campus NW, Edmonton AB T6G 2G3; Alb'76; FRCPC; Anes. Staff, University of Alberta Hospital; (780)407-8861; Fax. (780)407-3200.

MARCHAND, Audree; Clinique Med de Metabetchouan, 20 rue Saint-Basile, Metab-L-a-la-Croix QC G8G 1S9; Laval'06; CCFP; (418)349-8933

MARCHAND, Celine; Ctr Hosp Anna-Laberge, 200 boul Brisebois, Chateauguay QC J6K 4W8; Mon'89; ac Membre, Hôpital Anna-Laberge; Physician, Clinique Medicale Chateauguay; (450)699-2425

MARCHAND, Celine; Le Centre Medicale, 427-4 rue Taschereau, Gatineau QC J8Y 2V5; Sher'82; Peds. (819)771-9930

MARCHAND, Deborah J; 20-634 Reeves St, Port Hawkesbury NS B9A 2R7; McG'83; Staff, Strait Richmond Hospital; Langs: French; (902)625-1221; Fax. (902)625-0467.

MARCHAND, Eric; CHUQ-Ctr Hosp Univ Laval, 2705 boul Laurier, Quebec QC G1V 4G2; Laval'94; FRCPC; IntMed; GeriatricMed. Staff IntMed & Geriatric Med, Centre Hospitalier Universitaire de Quebec-CHUL; Langs: Bilingual(French/English); (418)654-2255

MARCHAND, Eve-Lyne; Sunnybrook Hlth Sciences Ctre, 2075 Bayview Ave, Toronto ON M4N 3M5; Mon'07; RadOncol. Staff, Sunnybrook Health Sciences Centre; (416)480-4974

MARCHAND, France; CSSS du Lac-des-Deux-Montagnes, 520 boul Arthur-Sauve, Saint-Eustache QC J7R 5B1; Sher'91; FRCPC; DiagRad. Staff, Hôpital de Saint-Eustache; (450)473-6811 x2211

MARCHAND, Francois; Clin Cardio Desilets, 200-1750 av de Vitré, Quebec QC G1J 1Z6; Laval'96; FRCPC; IntMed; Cardiol. Staff, Centre Hospitalier Affilié Universitaire de Québec - Hôpital De L'Enfant Jésus; (418)663-2858

MARCHAND, Francoise; Clin Med Marie-de-l'Incarnatio, 5A rue Marie-De-l'Incarnation, Quebec QC G1M 3J4; Laval'79; (418)687-6716; Fax. (418)687-9132.

MARCHAND, Guy-Ludovic; Centre Hosp Rég du Suroît, 150 rue Saint-Thomas, Salaber-de-Valleyf QC J6T 6C1; Mon'86; Staff, Centre Hospitalier Régional du Suroît; (450)371-9920

MARCHAND, Helene; Hotel-Dieu de Levis, 143 rue Wolfe, Levis QC G6V 3Z1; Mon'01; FRCPC; IntMed. Staff, Hôtel-Dieu de Lévis; (418)835-7121

MARCHAND, Ingrid; CHUM-Hop Notre-Dame, 1560 rue Sherbrooke E, Montreal QC H2L 4M1; Mon'03; CCFP; Staff, Centre Hospitalier l'Université de Montréal (CHUM) - Hôpital Notre-Dame; (514)890-8000

MARCHAND, Isabelle; CSSS Domaine du Roi, 450 rue Brassard, Roberval QC G8H 1B9; Mon'04; Staff, Hôpital de l'Archipel; Staff, Hotel-Dieu de Roberval; (418)275-0110

MARCHAND, Jacques; CHSLD Centreville, 66 boul Rene-Levesque E, Montreal QC H2X 1N3; Mon'63; ac Staff, CHSLD Centre-Ville de Montréal; (514)861-9331

MARCHAND, Julie; CSSS de Sept-Iles, 45 rue du Pere-Divet, Sept-Iles QC G4R 3N7; McG'02; FRCPC; Psy. Staff, Centre Hospitalier Regional de Sept-Iles; (418)962-9761

MARCHAND, Julie; CSSS de Manicouagan, 635 boul Jolliet, Baie-Comeau QC G5C 1P1; Laval'08; CCFP; Staff, Centre Hospitalier Régional Baie-Comeau; (418)589-3701

MARCHAND, Line; Clin Ped de Trois-Rivieres, 110-5725 Boul des Forges, Trois-Rivieres QC G8Y 5L5; Mon'90; FRCPC; Peds. Staff, CSSS de Trois-Rivières; (819)375-0504

MARCHAND, Luc; CHUM-Hop Notre-Dame, 1560 rue Sherbrooke E, Montreal QC H2L 4M1; Mon'71; FRCPC; Neur. Staff, Centre Hospitalier l'Université de Montréal (CHUM) - Hôpital Notre-Dame; adj Prof, Universite de Montreal; (514)890-8123; Fax. (514)412-7233.

MARCHAND, Luc; CSSS de Trois-Rivières, 1991 boul du Carmel, Trois-Rivieres QC G8Z 3R9; Laval'84; FRCSC; Urol. Staff, CSSS de Trois-Rivières; (819)697-3333; Fax. (819)372-3519.

MARCHAND, Luce; Clinique Med St-Etienne, 2-965 Rte Lagueux, St-Etienne-De-Lauz QC G6J 1T5; Laval'91; Staff Emerg, Hopital du CSS de la Region de Thetford; (418)831-9538; Fax. (418)831-8552.

MARCHAND, Lucie; Clinique Med Memphre, 200-323 rue Sherbrooke, Magog QC J1X 2R9; Sher'80; (819)847-1313; Fax. (819)847-3529.

MARCHAND, Marie-Hélène; CLSC Inukjuak, GD, Inukjuak QC J0M 1M0; Laval'09; (819)254-8416

MARCHAND, Marie-Josee; Hotel-Dieu de Saint-Hyacinthe, 1800 rue Dessaulles, Saint-Hyacinthe QC J2S 2T2; Mon'96; Staff, Hopital Charles LeMoyne; Staff, Centre d hebergement de l Hôtel-Dieu de Saint-Hyacinthe; (450)771-3333

MARCHAND, Michele; College des Med du Quebec, 2170 boul Rene-Levesque O, Montreal QC H3H 2T8; Mon'73; Consultant Ethics, College des Medecins du Quebec; (514)933-4441 x5376; Fax. (514)933-5374; mmarchand@cmq.org.

MARCHAND, Patricia; CSSS de Trois-Rivieres, 155 rue Toupin, Trois-Rivieres QC G8T 3Z8; Laval'07; Staff Family Med, Centre de santé Cloutier-du-Rivage; (819)370-2100; Fax. (819)370-2010.

MARCHAND, Pierre; Clinique Med Belvedere, 202-2235 rue Galt O, Sherbrooke QC J1K 1K6; Mon'73; Langs: English; (819)563-0536; Fax. (819)563-8924.

MARCHAND, Richard; Institut de Cardiologie de Mtl, 5000 rue Belanger, Montreal QC H1T 1C8; Mon'80; ABIM; Microbio & Infect Dis (P.Q.); MedMicrobiol (P.Q.); IntMed (P.Q.). Staff, Institut de Cardiologie de Montréal; assoc Prof Biomed, École Polytechnique; assoc Prof, Universite de Montreal; Langs: English; (514)376-3330

MARCHAND, Robert; GMF de Verdun au 55, 55 av de l'Eglise, Verdun QC H4G 3E7; Ott'79; CCFP; FCFP; Staff, Centre Hospitalier de Verdun; Teach Staff, Universite de Montreal; (514)766-8700

MARCHAND, Valerie; Hôpital Ste-Justine, 3175 ch Cote-Sainte-Catherine, Montreal QC H3T 1C5; Sher'90; FRCPC; Peds; Gastroent (P.Q.). Staff, Hôpital Ste-Justine; Langs: Bilingual(French/English); (514)345-4931 x3562; Fax. (514)345-4999.

MARCHAND, Valerie; Ctr Hosp du Centre la Mauricie, 50 119e rue, Shawinigan-Sud QC G9P 5K1; Laval'05; GenSurg. Staff, Centre Hospitalier du Centre la Mauricie; (819)536-7500

MARCHAND-ANTONIN, Benoit; CLSC Saint-Tite, 750 rue du Couvert, Saint-Tite QC G0X 3H0; Paris (France)'09; (418)365-7555; Fax. (418)365-6009.

MARCHAND-DROLET, Vincent; Centre Hosp Rouyn-Noranda, 4 9e rue, Rouyn-Noranda QC J9X 2B2; Laval'09; CCFP; CCFP(E.M.); Staff, Centre Hospitalier Rouyn-Noranda; Staff, Hôtel-Dieu de Lévis; (819)764-5131

MARCHANT, Rosemary E; 31 Doubletree Rd, North York ON M2J 3Z3; Dal'77; DECH; CCBOM; FRCPC; CommunMed (Environmental Medicine); OccupMed. Pres, Worksafe Inc; (416)491-5622

MARCHE, Janet E; Workers' Comp Board, PO Box 1150 Stn Central 5668 South St, Halifax NS B3J 2Y2; Qns'72; (902)491-8269; Fax. (902)491-8263.

MARCHESSAULT, Gilles; CLSC-CHSLD des Maskoutains, 2e-1225 rue des Cascades, Saint-Hyacinthe QC J2S 3H2; Laval'77; Staff, CLSC-CHSLD des Maskoutains; Fax. (450)773-1904.

MARCHETERRE, Louise; UMF Manicouagan, 340 rue Clement-Lavoie, Baie-Comeau QC G4Z 3B8; Mon'89; CCFP; Staff, Centre Hospitalier Régional Baie-Comeau; Langs: English; (418)296-2421; Fax. (418)295-2864.

MARCHETTI, Catherine A; Credit Valley Med Arts Centre, 206-2000 Credit Valley Rd, Mississauga ON L5M 4N4; Tor'87; CCFP; CCFP(E.M.); FCFP; Associate, The Credit Valley Hospital; Langs: Italian; (905)820-1046; Fax. (905)820-1899.

MARCHETTI, Paul J; 202-6990 Derry Rd, Milton ON L9T 7H3; Tor'90; FRCPC; Neur (Multiple Sclerosis). Staff, Halton Healthcare Services Corporation - Milton District Hospital; Court Staff, St Michael's Hospital; Langs: Italian; (905)878-4556; Fax. (905)878-4296.

MARCHI, Nicholas; Douglas Med Centre, 238 Bertie St, Fort Erie ON L2A 1Z3; Jagiellonian (Poland)'01; CCFP; Staff, Niagara Health System - Douglas Memorial Hospital Site; (905)871-1220; Fax. (905)871-1221.

MARCHIE, Anthony; Pinnacle Health Science Ctre, 9651 Yonge St, Richmond Hill ON L4C 1V7; Tor'04; MPhil; FRCSC; OrthSurg (Hip & Knee Reconstruction). Langs: Cantonese; French; (905)883-6614; Fax. (905)883-6904.

MARCHIE, Augustine; Stratford Gen Hospl, 46 General Hospital Dr, Stratford ON N5A 2Y6; Tor'08; Staff, Stratford General Hospital - Huron Perth Healthcare Alliance; (519)271-8120

MARCHINGTON, Katie L; SCOHS-Elizabeth Bruyere Hosp, 284 J-43 Bruyere St, Ottawa ON K1N 5C8; Tor'09; CCFP; Staff, SCO Health Service - Élisabeth Bruyère Hospital; (613)562-6262

MARCHOW, Leszek A; High Park Health Centre, 302-2333 Dundas St W, Toronto ON M6R 3A6; Poznan (Poland)'66; Ac Staff, St Joseph's Health Centre; Langs: Polish; (416)537-0724; Fax. (416)537-9329.

MARCHUK, Graeme G; 102-984 Oliver Rd, Thunder Bay ON P7B 7C7; Man'02; FRCSC; Neursurg. (877)701-5181

MARCHUK, Patricia M; 319 Pefferlaw Rd PO Box 158, Pefferlaw ON L0E 1N0; Tor'82; (705)437-2057; Fax. (705)437-2349.

MARCHUK, Yuri; Windsor Reg Hosp-Western Camp, 1453 Prince Rd, Windsor ON N9C 3Z4; '81; Staff, Windsor Regional Hospital - Tayfour Site; (519)257-5111

MARCIL, Brigitte; Hop Charles Lemoyne, 3120 boul Taschereau, Greenfield Park QC J4V 2H1; Sher'90; Staff, Hopital Charles LeMoyne; (450)466-5000

MARCIL, Dominique; Tribunal Administratif Du QC, 21e-500 boul Rene-Levesque O, Montreal QC H2Z 1W7; Mon'76; Staff, Pavillon Notre-Dame de la Merci; (514)873-7154; Fax. (514)864-3586.

MARCIL, Isabelle; CHUM-Hop St-Luc, 1058 rue Saint-Denis, Montreal QC H2X 3J4; Mon'93; FRCPC; Derm. Staff, Centre Hospitalier l'Université De Montréal (CHUM) - Hôpital Saint-luc; Langs: Bilingual(French/English); (514)890-8000; Fax. (514)412-7269.

MARCIL, J E Gilles; Hopital Charles LeMoyne, 1560 rue Sherbrooke E, Montreal QC H2L 4M1; Mon'65; FRCSC; Ophth. Staff, Centre Hospitalier l'Université de Montréal (CHUM) - Hôpital Notre-Dame; (514)890-8000

MARCIL, Josee; CSSS de la Baie-des-Chaleurs, RR 2 419 boul Perron, Maria QC G0C 1Y0; Mon'02; CCFP; Staff, CSSS de la Baie-des-Chaleurs; (418)759-3443; Fax. (418)759-1344.

MARCIL, Pierre; CSSS de Laval, 1755 boul Rene-Laennec, Laval QC H7M 3L9; Mon'89; DiagRad. Staff, Hopital de la Cite de la santé; (450)975-5406; Fax. (450)975-5096.

MARCILIO, Milton P; 300-200 St Clair Ave W, Toronto ON M4V 1R1; Bahia (Brazil)'60; FRCPC; Psy. (416)921-9631

MARCIN, Judi D; 347 Light St, Woodstock ON N4S 6J4; Wes'91; BSc(Zool); BScN; (519)539-9289

MARCINIAK, Zbigniew A; Sports Med & Rehab Clinic, 1539 Bloor St W, Toronto ON M6P 1A5; Poznan (Poland)'73; Langs: Polish; (416)539-0302; Fax. (416)539-0395.

MARCINIUK, Darcy D; Royal University Hosp, 103 Hospital Dr, Saskatoon SK S7N 0W8; Sask'84; ABIM; FCCP; FRCPC; IntMed; Respir. Staff Pulmonary Med, Royal University Hospital; Prof Med, University of Saskatchewan; (306)966-8298; Fax. (306)966-8694.

MARCINKOWSKI, Richard A; Bluewater Health-Norman Site, 89 Norman St, Sarnia ON N7T 6S3; Wes'80; FRCPC; DiagRad. Staff, Bluewater Health - Norman Site; Diagnostic-Radiology, Bluewater Health - Charlotte Eleanor Englehart Hospital; (519)464-4513; Fax. (519)383-8594; rmarcin@ebtech.net.

MARCK, Paul A; 307-11420 27 St SE, Calgary AB T2Z 3R6; Wes'85; Otol. (403)802-4040; Fax. (403)802-4020.

MARCO, Clayton V; Florenceville Med Clinic, 2-23 McCain St, Florenceville NB E7L 3J5; UBC'93; CCFP; (506)392-6267; Fax. (506)392-5501.

MARCON, Loretta; 919-300 rue Léo-Pariseau, Montreal QC H2X 4B3; McG'81; BSc; MSc; FRCSC; ObstGyn (Neurology). Att Staff, McGill University Health Centre - Montreal General Campus; Att Staff, McGill University Health Centre - Royal Victoria Hospital; adj Prof, McGill University; Langs: French; Italian; Spanish; (514)288-2700; Fax. (514)288-3218; lorettamarcon@hotmail.com.

MARCON, Margaret A; The Hosp for Sick Children, B 8409-555 University Ave, Toronto ON M5G 1X8; Louisiana (USA)'83; AB(Ped); FRCPC; Peds (P.Q.) (Gastroenterology). Staff Gastroenterol Hepatology & Nutrition, The Hospital For Sick Children; Asst Prof, University of Toronto; (416)813-7735; Fax. (416)813-6531; peggy.marcon@sickkids.ca.

MARCON, Norman E; St Michael's Hosp, 16 062VW-30 Bond St, Toronto ON M5B 1W8; Qns'62; FRCPC; IntMed (Gastroenterology). Staff, St Michael's Hospital; Prof Med, University of Toronto; (416)864-3092; Fax. (416)864-5993; norman.marcon@utoronto.ca.

MARCOTTE, Emile; Medisys, 11E-500 rue Sherbrooke O, Montreal QC H3A 3C6; Laval'58; FRCPC; IntMed; Cardiol (P.Q.). (514)845-1211; Fax. (514)845-4842.

MARCOTTE, Francois; Institut de Cardiologie de Mtl, 5000 rue Belanger, Montreal QC H1T 1C8; Mon'83; FRCPC; IntMed (Echocardiography); Cardiol. Staff, Institut de Cardiologie de Montréal; assoc Prof, Universite de Montreal; Langs: Bilingual(French/English); (514)593-2558; Fax. (514)593-2567.

MARCOTTE, Jacques E; Hôpital Ste-Justine, 3175 ch Cote-Sainte-Catherine, Montreal QC H3T 1C5; Laval'77; FRCPC; Peds; Respir (P.Q.). Dir C F Clinic/Chef Service Pulmonology, Hôpital Ste-Justine; adj Prof Ped, Universite de Montreal; (514)345-4654 x5409; Fax. (514)345-4804.

MARCOTTE, Jean; Ctr Hosp Affilie-Enfant-Jesus, 1401 18e rue, Quebec QC G1J 1Z4; Laval'99; CCFP; CCFP(E.M.); Staff Clinique des Medecins de l'Urgence, Centre Hospitalier Affilié Universitaire de Québec - Hôpital De L'Enfant Jésus; Langs: Bilingual(French/English); (418)649-5632

MARCOTTE, Jean; CHUQ-St-Francois d'Assise, 10 rue de l'Espinay, Quebec QC G1L 3L5; Sher'87; FRCPC; Anes. Staff, Centre Hospitalier Universitaire De Québec - Pavillon De St-françois-d'assise; (418)523-6445; Fax. (418)525-4434.

MARCOTTE, Jean; CSSS de Laval, CP 206 1755 boul Rene-Laennec, Laval QC H7M 3L9; Laval'90; Nephrol; IntMed (Dialysis). Staff, Hopital de la Cite de la santé; (450)668-1010; Fax. (450)975-5072.

MARCOTTE, Laura S; Quinte HC Corp-Belleville Gen, 265 Dundas St E, Belleville ON K8N 5A9; Qns'06; FRCPC; IntMed. Staff, QHC Belleville General; (613)969-7400

MARCOTTE, Marie-Eve; CHUQ-Ctr Hosp Univ Laval, 2705 boul Laurier, Quebec QC G1V 4G2; Mon'08; Peds. Staff, Centre Hospitalier Universitaire de Quebec-CHUL; (418)525-4444

MARCOTTE, Marie-Louise C; CSSS de Saint-Jerome, 290 rue de Montigny, Saint-Jerome QC J7Z 5T3; Sher'76; FRCPC; AnatPath. Staff, Hôtel-Dieu de Saint-Jérôme; (450)431-8200 x3006; Fax. (450)431-8206.

MARCOTTE, Patrick; Dr Georges-L Dumont Reg Hosp, 330 av Universite, Moncton NB E1C 2Z3; Laval'98; FRCPC; Psy. Staff Psychiatrist, Dr Georges-L-Dumont University Hospital Centre; Langs: English; (506)862-4177; Fax. (506)862-4325; crawfish@nb.sympatico.ca.

MARCOTTE, René; CSSS de Laval, U00 72A-1755 boul Rene-Laennec, Laval QC H7M 3L9; Laval'75; Staff, Hopital de la Cite de la santé; Langs: French; (450)668-1010

MARCOTTE, Yvan; CHSLD Saint-Anne, 411 rue de la Madone, Mont-Laurier QC J9L 1S1; Laval'55; Dir méd, CSSS d'Antoine-Labelle; (819)623-5940; Fax. (819)623-7347.

MARCOTTE LUPIEN, Lucie; CLSC De Charlevoix, 5 rue Boivin, Baie-Saint-Paul QC G3Z 1S6; Laval'92; CCFP; (418)435-5475; Fax. (418)435-5509.

MARCOU, John R; 31 Caradoc St N, Strathroy ON N7G 2M5; Tor'98; CCFP; CCFP(E.M.); (519)245-3590

MARCOUX, A William; Courtice Health Centre, 1450 Highway 2, Courtice ON L1E 3C3; Wes'92; CCFP; FCFP; (905)721-4942; Fax. (905)721-3526.

MARCOUX, Claude; CHUQ-Hotel-Dieu De Quebec, 11 Cote Du Palais, Quebec QC G1R 2J6; Laval'76; FRCPC; IntMed; Rheum. Staff, Centre Hospitalier Universitaire de Québec (CHUQ) - Siege Social; Langs: English; (418)691-5014; Fax. (418)691-5380.

MARCOUX, Danielle; Hôpital Ste-Justine, 3175 ch Cote-Sainte-Catherine, Montreal QC H3T 1C5; Mon'72; FAAD; FRCPC; Derm (Pediatric Dermatology). ac Staff, Hôpital Ste-Justine; Consultant, Hopital Maisonneuve-Rosemont; Clin Prof Peds, Universite de Montreal; Langs: English; Spanish; (514)345-4788; Fax. (514)345-4822.

MARCOUX, Diane; Hotel-Dieu de Levis, 143 rue Wolfe, Levis QC G6V 3Z1; Laval'89; Microbio & Infect Dis (P.Q.); MedMicrobiol. Staff, Hôtel-Dieu de Lévis; (418)835-7121 x3217

MARCOUX, Eugene S; Adult Comm Mental Health Serv, 4F-715 Queen St, Saskatoon SK S7K 4X4; Sask'84; FRCPC; Psy. Staff, Royal University Hospital; Clin Prof Psy, University of Saskatchewan; (306)655-8877; Fax. (306)655-8875.

MARCOUX, Francois; Ctr Hosp Laurentien, 234 rue Saint-Vincent, Ste-Agathe-des-Mts QC J8C 2B8; Sher'01; Staff, Centre Hospitalier Laurentien; (819)324-4000

MARCOUX, Hubert; Hop Jeffery Hale, 1250 ch Sainte-Foy, Quebec QC G1S 2M6; Laval'87; CCFP; FCFP; Staff, Jeffery Hale Hospital-Saint Brigid's; (418)683-4471; Fax. (418)684-2266; hubert.marcoux@mfa.ulaval.ca.

MARCOUX, Isabelle A; CSSS Aurores-Boreales, 679 2e rue E, La Sarre QC J9Z 2X7; Mon'05; CCFP; Staff, Centre Hospitalier La Sarre; (819)333-2311

MARCOUX, Judith; MUHC-Montreal Gen Hosp, L7 524-1650 av Cedar, Montreal QC H3G 1A4; Mon'97; MSc; FRCSC; Neursurg (Neuro Trauma). Staff Neurosurg, McGill University Health Centre - Montreal Neurological Hospital; Staff, McGill University Health Centre - Montreal General Campus; Langs: Bilingual(French/English); (514)934-1934; judith.marcoux@mcgill.ca.

MARCOUX, Laurent; CSSS du Nord de Lanaudière, 1000 boul Sainte-Anne, St-Charles-Brromee QC J6E 6J2; Laval'76; FRCPC; CommunMed; Public Health & Preventive Med. Physician Public Health, Centre Hospitalier Régional de Lanaudière; (450)759-1157 x4230; Fax. (450)759-0649; laurent_marcoux@ssss.gouv.qc.ca.

MARCOUX, Louis-Etienne; CHUQ-Ctr Hosp Univ Laval, 2705 boul Laurier, Quebec QC G1V 4G2; Laval'99; FRCSC; Ophth (Pediatrics). Staff, Centre Hospitalier Universitaire de Quebec-CHUL; Langs: English; (418)654-2119; Fax. (418)654-2188.

MARCOUX, Luc; Dir Des Services Medicaux-CSST, 6E-1199 rue de Bleury, Montreal QC H3B 3J1; Sher'83; OrthSurg (Industrial Occupational Medicine)., Direction des Services Medicaux-CSST; Langs: English; (514)906-3003 x2319; Fax. (514)906-3001; luc.marcoux@csst.qc.ca.

MARCOUX, Raymond; Hop Santa Cabrini Ospedale, 5655 rue Saint-Zotique E, Montreal QC H1T 1P7; Laval'62; GenSurg (P.Q.). Staff, Hôpital Santa Cabrini Ospedale; (514)252-6000 x6582

MARCOUX, Violaine; H325-5790 ch Cote-des-Neiges, Montreal QC H3S 1Y9; McG'01; FRCSC; ObstGyn. (514)340-8222; Fax. (514)340-7941.

MARCOVITZ, Leora; 201-960 Lawrence Ave W, North York ON M6A 3B5; Tor'81; Ac Staff Privil, Humber River Regional Hospital - Keele Street Site; Court Staff Privil, North York General Hospital - Branson Division; (416)781-7748

MARCOVITZ, Sorana; MUHC-Montreal Gen Hosp, C6 272-1650 av Cedar, Montreal QC H3G 1A4; McG'73; Endocrin (P.Q.); IntMed (Neuro Endocrinology). assoc Staff Endoctrin, McGill University Health Centre - Montreal General Campus; assoc Prof, McGill University; (514)934-8017; Fax. (514)934-8361.

MARCU, Maria; Salvus Family Med Clinic, 62-143 Liberton Dr, St. Albert AB T8N 6A7; (Romania)'84; CCFP; Staff, Royal Alexandra Hospital; Staff, Dominion Medical Centres Parsons Road; (780)460-4562; Fax. (780)460-4550.

MARCUS, Alexander T; St Mary's Hosp Centre, 3830 av Lacombe, Montreal QC H3T 1M5; McG'93; AnatPath. Staff, St Mary's Hospital Centre; (514)345-3511; alexander.marcus@ssss.gouv.qc.ca.

MARCUS, Harvey V; Medical Bldg, 1503-805 Broadway W, Vancouver BC V5Z 1K1; McG'70; FRCPC; Psy. (604)879-1503

MARCUS, Herbert I; Durham Reg Cancer Centre, C2 160G-1 Hospital Crt, Oshawa ON L1G 2B9; Tor'81; BSc; MSc; FRCSC; GenSurg; ThorSurg. Staff, Lakeridge Health - Oshawa Site; (905)576-8711 x4808; Fax. (905)433-4577.

MARCUS, Jonathan M; Royal Bank Med Centre, PO Box 134 Stn Royal Bank 200 Bay St, Toronto ON M5J 2J3; Tor'91; CCFP; (416)368-6787; Fax. (416)368-7632.

MARCUS, Lawrence A; Foothills Med Centre, 1403 29 St NW, Calgary AB T2N 2T9; Ibadan (Nigeria)'84; MB BS; MRCPsy; FRCPC; Psy. Staff Psy, Foothills Medical Centre; Langs: Yoruba; (403)944-8036; Fax. (403)270-3451; adejinka.marcus@calgaryhealthregion.ca.

MARCUS, Sandra A; 277 Scarboro Cres, Scarborough ON M1M 2J9; Tor'88; Ac Staff, Rouge Valley Health System - Centenary Health Centre Site; Ac Staff, The Scarborough Hospital - Birchmount Campus; Court Staff, The Scarborough Hospital - General Campus; (416)267-9551; Fax. (416)267-7029.

MARCUS, Victoria A; MUHC-Montreal Gen Hosp, 1650 av Cedar, Montreal QC H3G 1A4; McG'93; FRCPC; AnatPath. Staff Path, McGill University Health Centre - Montreal General Campus; Langs: English; French; (514)934-1934 x43860

MARCUS-MAND, Nufar; The Hosp for Sick Children, 555 University Ave, Toronto ON M5G 1X8; Ben Gurion (Israel)'99.

MARCUSHAMER, Samuel L; Grey Nuns Community Hosp & HC, 1100 Youville Drive West NW, Edmonton AB T6L 5X8; (Mexico)'79; FRCPC; IntMed (Intensive Care); Respir. Staff Physician, Royal Alexandra Hospital; Consultant, Cross Cancer Institute; Staff Physician Intensive Care & IntMed, University of Alberta Hospital; Staff, Covenant Health - Grey Nuns Community Hospital; Clin Assoc Prof Med, University of Alberta; (780)735-7399

MARCUZZI, Alfonso; Bloor-Jane Med Bldg, 501-2425 Bloor St W, Toronto ON M6S 4W4; Tor'77; FRCSC; Urol. Ac Staff Urol, St Joseph's Health Centre; Consultant, Toronto Rehabilitation Institute - University Centre; University of Toronto; (416)767-9396; Fax. (416)767-2403.

MARCUZZI, Danny W; St Michael's Hosp, 30 Bond St, Toronto ON M5B 1W8; Tor'84; FRCPC; DiagRad (Angiography/Interventional). Staff Radiol, St Michael's Hospital; Asst Prof, University of Toronto; (416)864-5681; Fax. (416)864-5380.

MARCZUK, Dorota; Spingbank Med Centre, 203-460 Springbank Dr, London ON N6J 0A8; Bialystok (Poland)'99; CCFP; (519)488-1951

MARDELL, Kevin; West Elgin Commun Health Ctr, PO Box 761 153 Main St, West Lorne ON N0L 2P0; McM'87; CCFP; FCFP; Staff, St Thomas Elgin General Hospital; (519)768-1715; Fax. (519)768-2548; kmardell@uwo.ca.

MARDIGYAN, Vartan; E206-SMBD Jewish Gen Hosp, 3755 ch Cote-Sainte-Catherine, Montreal QC H3T 1E2; McG'04; FRCPC; IntMed; Cardiol. Staff, Sir Mortimer B Davis Jewish General; (514)934-1934 x36151

MARDINI, Louay; MUHC-Royal Victoria Hosp, A4 21-687 av des Pins O, Montreal QC H3A 1A1; McG'08; IntMed. Staff, McGill University Health Centre - Royal Victoria Hospital; (514)934-1934 x34132

MARE, Abraham C W; Linden Ridge Med Centre, E-123 Scurfield Blvd, Winnipeg MB R3Y 1L6; Free State (South Africa)'80; MB ChB; (204)488-9988

MARE, Frans; Yarmouth Reg Hosp, 60 Vancouver St, Yarmouth NS B5A 2P5; Stellenbosch (South Africa)'02; MB ChB; Staff, Yarmouth Regional Hospital; (902)742-3541

MARE, Jean-Pierre; Associated Med Clinic, PO Box 510, Lac La Biche AB T0A 2C0; Pretoria (South Africa)'95; CCFP; Clin Lecturer, University of Alberta; Langs: Afrikaans; Zulu; (780)623-4421; Fax. (780)623-1920; jpmare@telusplanet.net.

MARE, Rulene; 4311 12 St NE, Calgary AB T2E 4P9; (South Africa)'05; MB ChB; (403)517-6000

MAREE, Gert; PO Box 63648 Rpo Capilano, North Vancouver BC V7P 3P1; Pretoria (South Africa)'87.

MAREE, Mattheus; Associate Clinic, 4620 50 AVE, Innisfail AB T4G 1A6; (South Africa)'92; MB ChB; (403)227-3301; Fax. (403)227-2856.

MAREE, Narinda; Kliniek on Main, 351 Main St N, Moose Jaw SK S6H 0W2; Orange Free State (South Africa)'93; MB ChB; Staff, Craik & District Health Centre; Staff, Davidson Health Centre; Langs: Afrikaans; (306)694-1440; Fax. (306)693-9990.

MAREE, Pieter J; Hudson Bay Med Group, PO Box 1170, Hudson Bay SK S0E 0Y0; Pretoria (South Africa)'99; MB ChB; CCFP; (306)865-2238; Fax. (306)865-2074; pmaree@kthr.sk.ca.

MAREE, Tamlyn; The Medical Clinic Associates, 4794 Joyce ave, Powell River BC V8A 3B6; Witwatersrand (South Africa)'06; MB BS; (604)485-3927

MARELLI, Ariane J; MUHC-Royal Victoria Hosp, H4 33-687 av des Pins O, Montreal QC H3A 1A1; Mon'85; FRCPC; IntMed; Cardiol. Staff, McGill University Health Centre - Royal Victoria Hospital; (514)934-1934 x43153

MARESCHAL, Veronique; CSSS de Chicoutimi, 305 rue Saint-Vallier, Chicoutimi QC G7H 5H6; Laval'00; FRCSC; ObstGyn. Staff, Complexe hospitalier de la Sagamie; (418)541-1000

MARESKY, David C; Medical & Dental Bldg, 605-586 Eglinton Ave E, Toronto ON M4P 1P2; Witwatersrand (South Africa)'76; MB ChB; FRCPC; Peds. Ad Staff Peds, The Hospital For Sick Children; Court Staff Newborn Care, Women's College Hospital; Court Staff, Mount Sinai Hospital; Asst Prof, University of Toronto; Langs: Hebrew; Afrikaans; (416)481-2191

MARFO, Elijah A; High Level Med Clinic, SS 1 10201 105 Ave, High Level AB T0H 1Z0; (Ghana)'84; MB BS; (780)926-2286; Fax. (780)926-3550.

MARGALIOT, Adit; The Credit Valley Hosp, 2200 Eglinton Ave W, Mississauga ON L5M 2N1; McM'98; FRCPC; Neur. Staff, The Credit Valley Hospital; (905)813-4466; Fax. (905)813-4046.

MARGALIOT, Zvi; 310-101 Queensway W, Mississauga ON L5B 2P7; Wes'95; FRCSC; PlasSurg (Hand & Wrist Surgery). Staff Clinician Investigator Program, Trillium Health Centre - Mississauga; (905)281-3482; Fax. (905)281-9916.

MARGARIDO, Clarita; Women's College Hosp, 253E-76 Grenville St, Toronto ON M5S 1B2; Sao Paulo (Brazil)'98; Staff, Women's College Hospital; (416)323-6269

MARGARIT, Marius L; Clinique Med de Coaticook, 206-18 rue du Manege, Coaticook QC J1A 3B3; Sher'03; CCFP; Staff, Clinique Medicale de Manege; (819)849-4808

MARGAU, Ryan; North York Gen Hosp, 4001 Leslie St, North York ON M2K 1E1; Tor'01; FRCPC; DiagRad. Staff, North York General Hospital; (416)756-6000; Fax. (416)756-6095.

MARGETTS, David J; St Joseph's Gen Hosp, 70 Spine Rd, Elliot Lake ON P5A 1X2; London (England)'63; MB BS; LRCP; MRCS; DObstRCOG; Chief Dept of Obst, St Joseph's General Hospital Elliot Lake; Med Dir, St Joseph's Manor; (705)848-5402; Fax. (705)848-8985.

MARGETTS, Peter J; St Joseph's Healthcare, 50 Charlton Ave E, Hamilton ON L8N 4A6; McM'94; PhD; FRCPC; IntMed; Nephrol. Staff, St Joseph's Healthcare - Charlton Campus; Assoc Prof, McMaster University; (905)522-1155 x32299; Fax. (905)540-6589; margetts@mcmaster.ca.

MARGINEAN, Esmeralda C; The Ottawa Hosp-Gen Campus, 4251-501 Smyth Rd, Ottawa ON K1H 8L6; Timisoara (Romania)'93; FRCPC; AnatPath. Staff Path, The Ottawa Hospital - Civic Campus; Staff, The Ottawa Hospital - General Campus; (613)737-8899 x79081

MARGITTAI, Katalin J; 909-2200 Yonge St, Toronto ON M4S 2C6; Ott'83; FRCPC; Psy (Consultant Liaison Psychiatry). Consultant Staff, North York General Hospital; Asst Prof, University of Toronto; (416)322-5662

MARGOLESE, Ellen A; Mount Sinai Hosp, 9F-600 University Ave, Toronto ON M5G 1X5; Ott'99; FRCPC; Psy (Consultation-Liaison). Staff, Mount Sinai Hospital; Lecturer, University of Toronto; (416)586-4800 x4560; emargolese@mtsinai.on.ca.

MARGOLESE, Howard C; 1025 Av des Pins O, Montreal QC H3A 1A1; McG'95; LMCC; FRCPC; Psy (Clinical Pharmacology). Att Staff Psy, McGill University Health Centre - Royal Victoria Hospital; adj Prof Psy/prog Dir McGill Clinical Pharmacology Residensy Program, McGill University; Langs: Bilingual(French/English); Hebrew; Yiddish; French; (514)843-1672; Fax. (514)843-2898; psychopharm.unit@mcgill.ca.

MARGOLESE, Richard G; SMBD Jewish Gen Hosp, E719-3755 ch Cote-Sainte-Cathe, Montreal QC H3T 1E2; McG'60; FRCSC; GenSurg. Dir Dept of MedOncol, Sir Mortimer B Davis Jewish General; Chaire Herbert Black in SurgOncol, McGill University; (514)342-3504; Fax. (514)340-8302.

MARGOLIN, Edward; Dept of Ophthalmology Visual S, 301-801 Eglinton Ave W, Toronto ON M5N 1E3; West Virginia(WV) (USA)'01; FRCSC; Ophth (Neuro Ophthalmology). Staff, Toronto Western Hospital - University Health Network; Langs: Russian; (647)748-8377

MARGOLIS, Ivor J; William Osler HC-Brampton, 2100 Bovaird Dr E, Brampton ON L6R 3J7; Cape Town (South Africa)'86; FRCPC; Peds (Hospitalist). Staff/Chief Peds, William Osler Health System - Brampton Civic Hospital; Langs: Afrikaans; Hebrew; (905)494-6519; Fax. (905)494-6508.

MARGOLIS, Myles; Mount Sinai Hosp, 600 University Ave, Toronto ON M5G 1X5; Man'85; FRCPC; DiagRad. Staff Radiol, Mount Sinai Hospital; (416)586-4800 x5277; Fax. (416)586-8695.

MARGOLIS, Neil; Manitoba Clinic, 790 Sherbrook St, Winnipeg MB R3A 1M3; Man'60; Peds. Ac Staff Children's Hosp, Health Sciences Centre; Ac Staff, St Boniface General Hospital; Asst Prof, University of Manitoba; (204)788-5797; Fax. (204)772-2537.

MARGULIES, Alfred I; 200-45 St Clair Ave W, Toronto ON M4V 1K9; Tor'59; DPsy; FAPA; FRCPC; Psy (Psychiatry Sequelae Of Trauma). Med Assessor, Workplace Safety & Insurance Board; Aj Prof, University of Toronto; (416)925-9822; Fax. (416)925-9387.

MARGULIES, Niculina M; Upper Canada Lower Bowel Clin, 301-1366 Yonge St, Toronto ON M4T 3A7; Craiova (Romania)'82; FRCPC; IntMed; Gastroent. Langs: Romanian; (416)926-0262 x221; Fax. (416)926-0936.

MARHIN, Wilson W; Children's & Women's HC of BC, F326-4500 Oak St, Vancouver BC V6H 3N1; Tor'03; CCFP; Staff, BC Women's Hospital & Health Centre; (604)875-2029

MARIAMPILLAI, Grace I; York-Finch Med Centre, 202-2115 Finch Ave W, North York ON M3N 2V6; Ceylon (Sri Lanka)'74; MB BS; MRCOG; FACOG; FRCSC; ObstGyn. Ac Staff, Humber River Regional Hospital - Finch Avenue Site; Langs: Tamil; (416)223-9114; Fax. (416)223-5067.

MARIAS-RADU, Ana; CSSS du Granit, 3569 rue Laval, Lac-Megantic QC G6B 1A5; Timisoara (Romania)'77; LMCC; CCFP; Staff, Carrefour Sante Granit; Langs: Romanian; Hungarian; (819)583-0330; Fax. (819)583-5664; ioan.radu@sympatico.ca.

MARIC, Peter; Grand River Hosp-KW Hlth Ctre, PO Box 9056 Stn C 835 King St W, Kitchener ON N2G 1G3; New South Wales (Australia)'05; Staff, Grand River Hospital - Kitchener/Waterloo Health Centre; (519)749-4316

MARIC-PLAVSIC, Jelena; 304-888 8th Ave W, Vancouver BC V5Z 3Y1; UBC'05; CCFP; (604)874-0261

MARIE, Julianne; Denison Armoury, 1 Yukon Lane, North York ON M3K 0A1; McM'09; CCFP; (416)633-6200; Fax. (416)631-5350.

MARIE, Simona G; West Coast Gen Hosp, 3949 Port Alberni Hwy, Port Alberni BC V9Y 4S1; Cluj-Napoca (Romania)'95; Staff, West Coast General Hospital; (250)723-2135

MARIEN, Leslie R; Fifth Avenue Med Centre, 500-14 Fifth Ave, Orangeville ON L9W 1G2; McM'78; (519)941-5250

MARIEN, Robert J; MUHC-Montreal Gen Hosp, 1650 av Cedar, Montreal QC H3G 1A4; McG'79; FRCSC; OrthSurg (Sports Medicine). Staff, McGill University Health Centre - Royal Victoria Hospital; Staff, McGill University Health Centre - Montreal General Campus; adj Prof, McGill University; (514)934-1934 x42976

MARIER, Gisele; 102-26 North St, Bridgewater NS B4V 2V6; Dal'92; BSc; CCFP; Att Staff, South Shore Regional Hospital; Langs: English; French; (902)543-2733; Fax. (902)543-1678.

MARIER, Jean-Jacques; Hôpital Ste-Justine, 3175 ch Cote-Sainte-Catherine, Montreal QC H3T 1C5; Sher'80; FRCPC; Psy. Staff, Hôpital Ste-Justine; (514)345-4931; Fax. (514)345-4679.

MARIER, Sylvie; Centre d'urgence Saint-Laurent, 200-1605 boul Marcel-Laurin, Saint-Laurent QC H4R 0B7; Laval'87; (514)747-2555; Fax. (514)747-7624.

MARIGNANI, Marilena; 272 Oxford St W, London ON N6H 1S9; Wes'90; BScPT(PhysTher); BSc; FRCSC; PlasSurg (Cosmetic Surgery). Staff, Strathroy Middlesex General Hospital - Middlesex Hospital Alliance; Langs: Italian; (519)438-1130; Fax. (519)438-0861; marilena.marignani@mha.tvh.ca.

MARILLIER, Justin R; Associate Med Clinic, PO Box 510, Slave Lake AB T0G 2A0; (South Africa)'03; MB ChB; DObst; DA; Langs: Afrikaans; (780)849-4155

MARIN, Alexandra; Misericordia Community Hosp, 16940 87 Ave NW, Edmonton AB T5R 4H5; Lviv (Ukraine)'93; CCFP; Staff, Covenant Health - Misericordia Community Hospital; (780)735-2609

MARIN, Alina; Hotel Dieu Hosp, 166 Brock St, Kingston ON K7L 5G2; Timisoara (Romania)'98; Staff, Hotel-Dieu Hospital; Langs: German; French; Romanian; (613)544-3310; Fax. (613)544-9666.

MARIN, Louis; Clinique Med D'Iberville, 120-383 boul du Seminaire N, St-Jean-sur-Richel QC J3B 8C5; Mon'69; Physician, Centre Medicale Medi-Soleil; Langs: English; (450)347-7557; Fax. (450)347-3099; mimi.marin@sympatico.ca.

MARIN, Patrick; CHUQ-St-Francois d'Assise, 10 rue de l'Espinay, Quebec QC G1L 3L5; Laval'07; FRCPC; Otol. Staff, Centre Hospitalier Universitaire De Québec - Pavillon De St-françois-d'assise; (418)525-4444

MARIN, Pierre; MUHC-Montreal Children's Hosp, 2300 rue Tupper, Montreal QC H3H 1P3; Mon'66; FRCPC; Peds. Staff, McGill University Health Centre - Montreal Children's Hospital; (514)412-4400

MARIN, Scott; Lennox & Addington Gen Hosp, 8 Richmond Park Dr, Napanee ON K7R 2Z4; McM'10; CCFP; Staff, Lennox & Addington County General Hospital; (613)354-3301

MARIN ARELLANO, Alejandra I; East Wellington Family Hlth Team, A-175 Alma St Box 51, Rockwood ON N0B 2K0; Pontificia Bolivariana (Colombia)'03; CCFP; Langs: Spanish; (519)856-4611

MARINEAU, Gilles; Clinique Med Du Boise, 6-275A rue Paradis, Repentigny QC J6A 8H2; Mon'80; Staff, Centre Hospitalier Pierre le Gardeur; Langs: English; French; (450)470-1300; cliniqueduboise@qc.aira.com.

MARINEAU, Luc; Clinique Med Havre Sante, 521 boul Du Havre, Salaber-de-Valleyf QC J6S 4Z5; Sher'85; (450)371-6444; Fax. (450)371-5315.

MARINEAU, Yves; Clinique Med Waterloo, CP 760 100-4900 rue Foster, Waterloo QC J0E 2N0; Sher'89; (450)539-1102

MARINESCU, Mihaela; Juravinski Cancer Centre, 328 Mountain Park Ave, Hamilton ON L8V 4X2; (Romania)'96; FRCPC; AnatPath.

MARINIER, Helene; Ctr Hosp de Verdun, 4000 boul Lasalle, Verdun QC H4G 2A3; Sher'88; FRCPC; DiagRad. Staff, Centre Hospitalier de Verdun; (514)362-1000 x2171

MARINIER, Pascale; Ctr de Derm et de Psoriasis, 202-2125 rue Jean-Talon E, Montreal QC H2E 1V4; Mon'91; Derm (Psoriasis). Staff, Hopital de la Cite de la santé; Langs: Bilingual(French/English); (514)728-9203; Fax. (514)728-1621; drmarinier@bellnet.ca.

MARINO, Nalini; Hopital Reg D'Edmundston, 275 boul Hebert, Edmundston NB E3V 4E4; Cork (Ireland)'99; Staff, Hôpital regional d'Edmundston; (506)739-2200

MARINOSYAN, Mari H; 101-13025 Yonge St, Richmond Hill ON L4E 1A6; Plovdiv (Bulgaria)'95; CCFP; (905)773-3342

MARINOV, Anton; Univ Hlth Network-Toronto Gen, 405-200 Elizabeth St, Toronto ON M5G 2C4; Qns'03; FRCPC; Anes. Staff, Toronto General Hospital - UHN; Staff, Sunnybrook Health Sciences Centre; (416)340-4800

MARINOVA, Evguenia L; Glazier Med Centre, 11 Gibb St, Oshawa ON L1H 2J9; Sofia (Bulgaria)'88; CCFP; Langs: Bulgarian; (905)579-1212; Fax. (905)579-1583.

MARION, Alain; CSSS de Laval, 1755 boul Rene-Laennec, Laval QC H7M 3L9; Mon'81; AnatPath. Staff, Hopital de la Cite de la santé; (450)668-1010; Fax. (450)975-5061.

MARION, Andre; Clinique D'Orl Rimouski, 306-176 av Rouleau, Rimouski QC G5L 8W1; Mon'68; Otol (Allergy). Staff, Hôpital Regional Rimouski; (418)723-4520; Fax. (418)723-4550.

MARION, Chantal; CHUM-Hop Notre-Dame, 1560 rue Sherbrooke E, Montreal QC H2L 4M1; Mon'94; Staff, Centre Hospitalier l'Université de Montréal (CHUM) - Hôpital Notre-Dame; (514)890-8000 x26767

MARION, Dennis A; Misericordia Community Hosp, 16940 87 Ave NW, Edmonton AB T5R 4H5; Man'02; FRCPC; IntMed. Staff, Covenant Health - Misericordia Community Hospital; (780)735-2000; Fax. (780)735-2268.

MARION, Marc H; Centennial Med Centre, 299 Lake Ave E, Carleton Place ON K7C 1J3; Ott'86; Ac Staff, Carleton Place & District Memorial Hospital; Langs: Bilingual(English/French); (613)257-2311; Fax. (613)253-0044.

MARION, Stephen A; James Mather Bldg-UBC, 5804 Fairview Cres, Vancouver BC V6T 1Z3; Tor'77; FRCPC; CommunMed. (604)822-2886

MARIOTTI, Carlo U A; Queen Elizabeth II HSC, 1276 South Park St, Halifax NS B3H 2Y9; Dal'97; FRCPC; Anes. Staff Anes, Queen Elizabeth II Health Sciences Centre - Victoria General Site; (902)473-2700

MARISETTE, Stephen R; Gibson Health Clinic, PO Box 9000 Stn A, Fredericton NB E3B 5N5; Tor'05; CCFP; (506)447-4444

MARITZ, Johann; 2010 129 St PO Box 500, Blairmore AB T0K 0E0; Stellenbosch (South Africa)'85; MB ChB; (403)562-2292; Fax. (403)562-2293.

MARITZ, Jaco J; James Paton Mem Hosp, 125 Trans Canada Hwy, Gander NL A1V 1P7; Saba (Netherlands Antilles)'00; ABPN; Staff, James Paton Memorial Hospital; (709)256-5423; Fax. (709)256-5727.

MARITZ, Jacobus C; Town Square Eye Clinic, 86 Elizabeth Dr, Gander NL A1V 1J8; Pretoria (South Africa)'63; MB ChB; MMed(Ophth).

MARITZ, Leonie; 105-2231 Louie Dr, Kelowna BC V4T 3K3; Orange Free State (South Africa)'85; MB ChB; (250)768-6985

MARK, David A; Kingston Gen Hosp, 76 Stuart St, Kingston ON K7L 2V7; Ott'88; FRCPC; Anes. Staff Anes, Kingston General Hospital; Staff, Hotel-Dieu Hospital; Asst Prof, Queen's University; (613)548-7827; Fax. (613)548-1375.

MARK, Dennis C P; Port Union Med Centre, 7-5550 Lawrence Ave E, Scarborough ON M1C 3B2; Tor'90; Ac Staff, Rouge Valley Health System - Centenary Health Centre Site; Langs: Cantonese; (416)283-3700; Fax. (416)283-1453.

MARK, Douglas J; 302-2330 Kennedy Rd, Scarborough ON M1T 0A2; Tor'85; Ac Staff Family Pract, The Scarborough Hospital - Birchmount Campus; Pres, Coalition of Family Physicians (COFP); (416)298-1303; Fax. (416)298-4872; drdjmark@aol.com.

MARK, Helmut W; The Family Practice Clinic, 2778A 104th St, Nanaimo BC V9T 2E4; Tor'73; (250)758-1711; Fax. (250)758-2802.

MARK, Larry K W; Dixon Med Centre, 301-531 Davis Dr, Newmarket ON L3Y 6P5; Tor'77; (905)895-4161; Fax. (905)895-5461.

MARK, M Kit; Student Hlth & Counselling Ser, 1 Campus Dr, Saskatoon SK S7N 5A3; Sask'06; CCFP; (306)966-5768

MARK, Pamela A; 202-2772 Danforth Ave, Toronto ON M4C 1L7; Tor'84; CCFP; FCFP; Staff, Toronto East General Hospital Inc; (416)699-8105; Fax. (416)699-3273.

MARK, Patricia H; Sow's Ear Med Clinic, PO Box 190 7186 Lantzville Rd, Lantzville BC V0R 2H0; Dublin (Ireland)'64; MB ChB; BAO; DCH; (250)390-4542; Fax. (250)390-4561.

MARK, Patrick W S; Toronto East Gen Hosp Inc, 825 Coxwell Ave, Toronto ON M4C 3E7; Tor'91; FRCPC; Anes. Med Staff, Toronto East General Hospital Inc; Asst Prof Anes, University of Toronto; (416)469-6212; Fax. (416)469-6874; patrick.mark@utoronto.ca.

MARK, Siobhan E V; Credit Valley Med Arts Centre, 502-2000 Credit Valley Rd, Mississauga ON L5M 4N4; Qns'07; ObstGyn. (905)820-8885

MARK, Suzanne C; Dept of Veteran's Affairs, PO Box 7700 Stn Central, Charlottetown PE C1A 8M9; Dal'85; (902)566-8888

MARK, Trisha M; Southlake Reg Health Centre, 596 Davis Dr, Newmarket ON L3Y 2P9; Tor'98; FRCPC; Anes. Staff Anes, Southlake Regional Health Centre; (905)853-2256

MARKANDAY, Anurag; Abbotsford Reg Hosp & Cancer C, 32900 Marshall Rd, Abbotsford BC V2S 0C2; Delhi (India)'93; MB BS; ABIM; FRCPC; IntMed (Infectious Diseases). Staff, Abbotsford Regional Hospital & Cancer Centre; (604)851-4700

MARKE, Charles J; Kamloops Mental Health Centre, 235 Lansdowne St, Kamloops BC V2C 1X8; Port Harcourt (Nigeria)'91; (250)377-6500

MARKEL, Kenneth N; Urgent Care Centre UBC, 2211 Wesbrook Mall, Vancouver BC V6T 2B5; McG'76; FRCPC; EmergMed. (604)822-7662

MARKENTIN, Morris; Saskatoon Commun Clinic, 455 2nd Ave N, Saskatoon SK S7K 2C2; Sask'96; CCFP; FCFP; (306)652-0300; Fax. (306)934-2506; mmarkentin@communityclinic.ca.

MARKEY, Scott T; 203-9123 Mary St, Chilliwack BC V2P 4H7; UBC'94; CCFP; (604)795-9161; Fax. (604)795-9937.

MARKHAM, Ray J; Valemount Health Centre, PO Box 697 1445 Fifth Ave, Valemount BC V0E 2Z0; Capetown (South Africa)'90; MB ChB; MRCGPract; CCFP; (250)566-9138 x231; Fax. (250)566-4319.

MARKLAND, Brenda A; Caledonia Clinic, 340 Campbell St, Nanaimo BC V9R 3G7; McG'85; FRCSC; OrthSurg (Upper Limb Surgery). Clin Prof, University of British Columbia; Langs: Bilingual(English/French); (250)753-3202

MARKLAND, Darren M; Kingsway Nephrology Assoc, 303-10611 Kingsway NW, Edmonton AB T5G 3C8; Cal'98; FRCPC; IntMed; Critical Care Medicine; Nephrol. Staff/Dir Education for Critical Care, Royal Alexandra Hospital; (780)496-9350

MARKLAND, Janet J; Markland Med Prof Corp, 302-39 23rd St E, Saskatoon SK S7K 0H6; Sask'75; FRCPC; IntMed (Rheumatology). Clin Prof Rheumatic Diseases Unit, Royal University Hospital; Med Staff, St Paul's Hospital (Grey Nuns) of Saskatoon; Vis Consultant, Saskatoon City Hospital; Clin Prof, University of Saskatchewan; (306)244-1424; jmarkland@sasktel.net.

MARKLE, Craig D; Orillia Soldier's Mem Hosp, 170 Colborne St W, Orillia ON L3V 2Z3; Wes'93; CCFP; CCFP(E.M.); Chief FamilyMed(EM), Orillia Soldiers' Memorial Hospital; (705)325-2201 x3720; Fax. (705)327-9169; cdmarkle@osmh.on.ca.

MARKO, Jana; Mississauga Med Centre, 340-1420 Burnhamthorpe Rd E, Mississauga ON L4X 2Z9; Prague (Czech Republic)'66; Staff, St Joseph's Health Centre; (905)625-6813; Fax. (905)625-9752.

MARKOSE, George; Hamilton HS-Henderson Site, 711 Concession St, Hamilton ON L8V 1C3; Charing Cross Hospital Medical School (Other Foreign)'94; Staff, Hamilton Health Sciences Centre-Juravinski Site; (905)527-4322

MARKOVIC, Ruth E; 9833 Tecumseh Rd E, Windsor ON N8R 1A5; Melbourne (Australia)'66; Assoc Staff, Hôtel-Dieu Grace Hospital; Ac Staff, Windsor Regional Hospital - Metropolitan Site; Assoc Staff, Windsor Regional Hospital - Tayfour Site; (519)735-6844; Fax. (519)735-5473.

MARKOVIC, Saira; 501-960 Lawrence Ave W, North York ON M6A 3B5; Belgrade (Serbia)'74; Ac Member, North York General Hospital - Branson Division; Ac Member, Humber River Regional Hospital - Finch Avenue Site; (416)256-7149

MARKOVSKI, Milena; Academic Family Medicine, 172-1621 Albert St, Regina SK S4P 2S5; CCFP; Staff, Regina General Hospital; (306)766-0444

MARKOWITZ, Samuel N; 300-1370 Dundas St E, Mississauga ON L4Y 4G4; Hebrew U. (Israel)'73; DOphth(Tor); FRCSC; Ophth. Staff, Trillium Health Centre - Mississauga; (905)279-1800

MARKOWSKI, Michael P; Spence Family Med Centre, 400 Spence Ave, Hawkesbury ON K6A 2Y3; Qns'90; Staff, Hawkesbury & District General Hospital; (613)632-0997; Fax. (613)632-9297.

MARKOWSKY, Donald G; Temple Med Clinic, 208-5401 Temple Dr NE, Calgary AB T1Y 3R7; Lagos (Nigeria)'69; FRCPC; Peds. Staff, Alberta Children's Hospital; University of Calgary; (403)291-0335; Fax. (403)219-0922.

MARKS, Alexander; 18 Connable Dr, Toronto ON M5R 1Z8; Tor'62; Langs: Polish; French; (416)921-6677

MARKS, Catherine; 7-2010 Trim Rd, Orleans ON K4A 0G4; Cairo (Egypt)'94; MB ChB; CCFP; Langs: Arabic; (613)590-1433

MARKS, Cyril P; 115 Doris Ave, North York ON M2N 4T2; Tor'58; Court Staff, North York General Hospital; (416)226-6884; Fax. (416)512-6872.

MARKS, Jennifer; London HSC-Victoria Campus, PO Box 5010 Stn B 800 Commissioners Rd E, London ON N6A 5W9; Wes'06; FRCSC; ObstGyn. Staff, London Health Sciences Centre - Victoria Campus; (519)685-8500

MARKS, Meridith B; The Ottawa Hosp-Rehab Ctr, 1200-505 Smyth Rd, Ottawa ON K1H 8M2; Mem'87; FRCPC; PhysMed&Rehab. Ac Staff Physical Med & Rehab, The Ottawa Hospital Rehabilitation Centre; Consultant, The Ottawa Hospital - General Campus; Consultant, The Ottawa Hospital - Civic Campus; Asst Dean Academy For Innovation in Med Educ/Asst Prof, University of Ottawa; (613)737-7350 x5595; Fax. (613)737-9638.

MARKS, Paul H; Sunnybrook Hlth Sciences Ctre, MG 350-2075 Bayview Ave, Toronto ON M4N 3M5; Tor'86; FRCSC; OrthSurg (Sports Medicine). Staff, Sunnybrook Health Sciences Centre; Teach Staff, University of Toronto; (416)480-6838; Fax. (416)480-6840; paul.marks@sunnybrook.ca.

MARKS, Richard; Vernon Jubilee Hosp, 2101 32 St, Vernon BC V1T 5L2; Otago (New Zealand)'73; FRCPC; Anes. Staff Anes/Chief Anes, Vernon Jubilee Hospital; (250)545-2211

MARKS, Saul I; North York Gen Hosp, 807-4001 Leslie St, North York ON M2K 1E1; Qns'90; FRCPC; Psy. Staff, North York General Hospital; (416)756-6655

MARKS, Seth D; Children's Hosp, FE307-685 William Ave, Winnipeg MB R3E 0Z2; Man'97; BSc; FRCPC; Peds (Clinician Investigator Program); Endocrin&Metab.

MARKS DE CHABRIS, Lionel; 10-450 Notre Dame Ave, Sudbury ON P3C 5K8; McG'88; CCFP; CCFP(E.M.); FCFP; Staff, Health Sciences North-St Joseph's Health Centre; (705)673-1116; Fax. (705)673-7267.

MARKSON, Lisa A; All In One Med Clinic, 202-10083 Keele St, Maple ON L6A 3Y8; Stony Brook(NY) (USA)'90; DABIM(Neurol); FRCPC; Neur. Staff, Mackenzie Richmond Hill Hospital; (905)832-6546; Fax. (905)832-6548.

MARKUS, Arthur J; MUHC-Royal Victoria Hosp, 687 av des Pins O, Montreal QC H3A 1A1; McG'52; BSc; Peds (Neonatology). Staff, McGill University Health Centre - Royal Victoria Hospital; Langs: English; French; (514)935-4311

MARKUS, Frank; Sport Injury& Rehab Centre, 7601 Martin Grove Rd, Woodbridge ON L4L 9E4; Budapest (Hungary)'50; FACS; FICS; Hon Member, North York General Hospital; Court Staff, Humber River Regional Hospital - Finch Avenue Site; Langs: Hungarian; (905)264-0631

MARKUS, Jurgita R; Rouge Valley-Centenary HC, 2867 Ellesmere Rd, Scarborough ON M1E 4B9; Kaunas (Lithuania)'92; FRCPC; Anes. Staff, Rouge Valley Health System - Centenary Health Centre Site; (416)854-5611

MARKUS, Newton; 410-340 College St, Toronto ON M5T 3A9; Tor'56; DABR; DiagRad. Hon Staff, Toronto General Hospital - UHN; (416)962-3203; Fax. (416)962-9653.

MARKUS, Yaacov M; William Osler HC-Brampton, 2100 Bovaird Dr E, Brampton ON L6R 3J7; Tor'01; FRCPC; OccupMed. Staff, William Osler Health System - Brampton Civic Hospital; (905)597-2722

MARLATT, Wanda J; Tamarack Med Clinic, 191-1500 Cranbrook St N, Cranbrook BC V1C 3S8; Man'95; BSc; CCFP; (250)426-7724

MARLEAU, Alain; Asclepios Med Clinic, 2-750 Taylor Creek Dr, Orleans ON K1C 1T1; Ott'04; FRCSC; ObstGyn. (613)830-2880; Fax. (613)830-8588.

MARLEAU, Daniel J; Medecins de Famille Marleau, 3 9e rue, Rouyn-Noranda QC J9X 2A9; Ott'79; CCFP; FCFP; Chef méd fam, Centre Hospitalier Rouyn-Noranda; Universite de Sherbrooke; (819)797-4535; Fax. (819)797-4665.

MARLEAU, Denis; CHUM-Hop St-Luc, 1058 rue Saint-Denis, Montreal QC H2X 3J4; Mon'65; Gastroent (P.Q.); IntMed. Staff, Centre Hospitalier l'Université De Montréal (CHUM) - Hôpital Saint-luc; Universite de Montreal; (514)890-8000; Fax. (514)412-7314; hepato.saint-luc@sympatico.ca.

MARLEAU, Ghislain; Glengarry Mem Hosp, PO Box 910 Highway 43, Alexandria ON K0C 1A0; Ott'82; Staff, Glengarry Memorial Hospital; (613)525-2378

MARLEAU, Michel; CSSS d'Argenteuil, 145 av de la Providence, Lachute QC J8H 4C7; Laval'03; CCFP; Staff, Centre Hospitalier d'Argenteuil; Langs: English; (450)562-3761

MARLES, Sandra L; Children's Hosp, FE229-685 William Ave, Winnipeg MB R3E 0Z2; Alb'84; FCCMG; FRCPC; Peds; MedGenetics. Staff Peds & Child Health/Asst Prof, Health Sciences Centre; Asst Prof Part-Time, University of Manitoba; (204)787-4945

MARLEY, Jaanus; Rosedale Med Centre, 510-600 Sherbourne St, Toronto ON M4X 1W4; Tor'76; BASc; Langs: Estonian; (416)323-1414; Fax. (416)323-1411.

MARLEY, Wayne F; Woodstock Gen Hosp, 310 Juliana Dr, Woodstock ON N4V 0A4; Tor'79; FRCPC; Anes. Staff Anes, Woodstock General Hospital; (519)537-0111

MARLINGA, Jazmin C; Peter Lougheed Centre, 3500 26 Ave NE, Calgary AB T1Y 6J4; Wes'07; CCFP; Staff, Peter Lougheed Centre; (403)943-4555

MARLISS, Errol B; Mcgill Nutr & Food Science, H6.91-687 av Des Pins O, Montreal QC H3A 1A1; Alb'64; FRCPC; IntMed (Diabetology). Dir, McGill University Health Centre - Royal Victoria Hospital; Chef Nutrition & Food Science Centre, McGill University; Langs: English; French; Fax. (514)843-1706.

MARLOW, Bernard A; Toronto Street Med Centre, 202-29 Toronto St S, Uxbridge ON L9P 1V9; Tor'71; CCFP; FCFP; Dir Cont Prof Development, College Of Family Physicians Of Canada-Ontario; Physician, Lake Shore Village Walk In Clinic; Asst Prof dept of Fam Comm Med, University of Toronto; (905)852-1999; Fax. (905)628-0893.

MARMAI, Kristine L; London HSC-University Hosp, PO Box 5339 Stn B 339 Windermere Rd, London ON N6A 5A5; Wes'05; FRCPC; Anes. Staff, London Health Sciences Centre - University Hospital; (519)685-8500

MARMEN, Yves; CSSS du Granit, 3569 rue Laval, Lac-Megantic QC G6B 1A5; Sher'76; DiagRad. Staff, Carrefour Sante Granit; (819)583-0330

MARMINA, Joseph E V; Dr Poon's Metabolic Clinic, 6-375 Kingston Rd, Pickering ON L1V 1A3; Tor'62; Langs: Italian; French; (905)509-6888; Fax. (905)509-0663.

MARMOR, Eric; 303-101 Queensway W, Mississauga ON L5B 2P7; McG'90; FRCSC; Neursurg (Brain Tumors). Ac Staff, Trillium Health Centre - Mississauga; (905)270-1104; Fax. (905)247-0359.

MARMOR, Goldie; MUHC-Montreal Gen Hosp, 1650 av Cedar, Montreal QC H3G 1A4; McG'07; MDCM; CCFP; Staff, McGill University Health Centre - Montreal General Campus; (514)934-1934 x46600

MARMOREO, Jean E; Wellpoint Family Practice, 9F-1240 Bay St, Toronto ON M5R 2A7; Tor'74; BScN; CCFP; Staff, Women's College Hospital; (416)971-7601; Fax. (416)971-7718.

MARNER, Paul A T; White Oaks Med Clinic, 116-12222 137 Ave NW, Edmonton AB T5L 4X5; London (England)'62; MB BS; LRCP; MRCS; Dip SportMed; Ac Staff, Royal Alexandra Hospital; Ac Staff, University of Alberta Hospital; Ac Staff, Long Term Care Facilities-Capital Care Group & Shepherd's Care Group; (780)473-9355; Fax. (780)473-2856.

MAROIS, Carlos; Bureau du Dr Carlos Marois, 300-3141 boul Taschereau, Longueuil QC J4V 2H2; Mon'93; FRCSC; Urol. Staff, Centre Hospitalier de Verdun; Staff, Hopital Charles LeMoyne; (450)812-2193

MAROIS, Denis; Ctr Hosp Affilie-Enfant-Jesus, 1401 18e rue, Quebec QC G1J 1Z4; Laval'72; ABS; VascSurg; GenSurg (Thoracic Surgery). pers Consultant, Centre Hospitalier Affilié Universitaire de Québec - Hôpital De L'Enfant Jésus; Université Laval; (418)649-5882; denis.marois@sympatico.ca.

MAROIS, Julie; Clinique Med Lacroix, 203-810 route Jean-Gauvin, Quebec QC G1X 0B6; Mon'94; CCFP; Staff, Hôpital Laval; (418)871-1911

MAROIS, Pierre; Ctr Readaptation Marie Enfant, 5200 rue Belanger, Montreal QC H1T 1C9; Mon'75; FRCPC; PhysMed&Rehab. Staff, Centre de Réadaptation Marie Enfant du CHU Sainte-Justine; Staff, Hôpital Ste-Justine; (514)374-1710

MARONEY, Roy T; Westside Med Associates, 3591 Elliott Rd, Westbank BC V4T 1N9; Cape Town (South Africa)'77; (250)768-6920

MAROO, Sanjay V; Children's & Women's HC of BC, 4480 Oak St, Vancouver BC V6H 3V4; Nairobi (Kenya)'83; Staff, BC Children's Hospital; (604)875-2502

MAROOF, Razawa F; Regina Community Clinic, 1106 Winnipeg St, Regina SK S4R 1J6; Salahaddin (Iraq)'86; MB ChB; CCFP; Staff Family Med, Regina General Hospital; Langs: Arabic; Kurdish; (306)543-7880; Fax. (306)543-6888.

MAROT, Jean-Paul; Hotel-Dieu de Levis, 143 rue Wolfe, Levis QC G6V 3Z1; Dijon (France)'85; Staff, Hôtel-Dieu de Lévis; (418)835-7121

MAROTTA, Giovanni C; Keele-Ingram Prof Centre, 311-2221 Keele St, North York ON M6M 3Z5; Tor'86; FRCPC; IntMed; GeriatricMed. Staff Physician, Baycrest Centre for Geriatric Care; Staff Physician, Humber River Regional Hospital - Keele Street Site; (416)663-4124

MAROTTA, Paul J; London HSC-University Hosp, PO Box 5339 Stn B 339 Windermere Rd, London ON N6A 5A5; Wes'91; FRCPC; IntMed (Hepatology); Gastroent. Staff, London Health Sciences Centre - University Hospital; Asst Prof Med, University of Western Ontario; (519)663-3406; Fax. (519)663-3858; paul.marotta@lhsc.on.ca.

MAROTTA, Robert W; Halton HCS Corp-Oakville, 327 Reynolds St, Oakville ON L6J 3L7; Wes'88; FRCPC; DiagRad (Radiology). Staff, Halton Healthcare Services Corporation - Oakville Site; (905)845-2571; Fax. (905)338-4636.

MAROTTA, Thomas R; St Michael's Hosp, 30 Bond St, Toronto ON M5B 1W8; Tor'84; FRCPC; DiagRad (Interventional Radiology). Staff, St Michael's Hospital; Staff, Toronto Western Hospital - University Health Network; Aj Prof Physics, Ryerson University; Assoc Prof, University of Toronto; (416)864-5675; Fax. (416)864-5380.

MAROTTE, Rachel; CLSC Samuel-de-Champlain, 100-5811 boul Taschereau, Brossard QC J4Z 1A5; Laval'77; (450)445-4452; Fax. (450)445-5535.

MAROUN, Falah B; Health Sciences Centre, 5202-300 Prince Philip Dr, St. John's NL A1B 3V6; Beirut (Lebanon)'60; FRCSC; Neursurg. Staff, Health Sciences Centre; Chairman Surg/Clin Prof, Memorial University Of Newfoundland; (709)777-6300; Fax. (709)777-8272.

MAROUN, Jean A; The Ottawa Hosp-Gen Campus, 501 Smyth Rd, Ottawa ON K1H 8L6; St. Joseph (Lebanon)'65; MRC(UK); FRCPC; IntMed; MedOncol. Staff, The Ottawa Hospital - General Campus; Prof, University of Ottawa; (613)737-8899 x72013; jmaroun@ottawahospital.on.ca.

MAROVAC, M Misha; Bank Respiratory Services, 217-1385 Bank St, Ottawa ON K1H 8N4; Ott'07; FRCPC; IntMed; Respir. Staff, Kingston General Hospital; (613)523-4444

MARPOLE, Derek G F; Greene Avenue Clinic, 210-1255 av Greene, Westmount QC H3Z 2A4; McG'63; FACC; FRCPC; Cardiol (P.Q.); IntMed. hon Staff Cardiol, St Mary's Hospital Centre; hon Staff, McGill University Health Centre - Royal Victoria Hospital; assoc Prof Med, McGill University; (514)484-4036

MARQUARDT, Hans R; Nipigon Med Centre, 125 Hogan Rd, Nipigon ON P0T 2J0; Wes'94; CCFP; Staff, Lady Dunn Health Centre; (807)887-1644; Fax. (807)887-1645.

MARQUES, Joseph R; 103-360 College St, Toronto ON M5T 1S6; Man'90; (416)975-0600; Fax. (416)975-0800.

MARQUES, Sylvia; E 0012-SMBD Jewish Gen Hosp, 3755 ch Cote-Sainte-Catherine, Montreal QC H3T 1E2; Paris (France)'74; Staff, Sir Mortimer B Davis Jewish General; (514)340-8221

MARQUETTE, Claude; 103-1333 rue de la Foret, Longueuil QC J4N 1S5; Mon'65; Psy (P.Q.). (450)448-6863; Fax. (450)677-4784.

MARQUETTE, Gerald; 1T61-4500 Oak St, Vancouver BC V6H 3N1; Mon'75; DABOG; FRCSC; ObstGyn (Fetal & Maternal Medicine). Staff ObstGyn, BC Women's Hospital & Health Centre; Med Dir, Perinatal Services of British Columbia; Clin Prof ObstGyn, University of British Columbia; Langs: French; (604)875-3174; Fax. (604)875-3099.

MARQUEZ AZALGARA, Vladimir; CSSS du Nord de Lanaudière, 1000 boul Sainte-Anne, Joliette QC J6E 6J2; McG'06; MDCM; Gastroent; IntMed. Staff, Centre Hospitalier Régional de Lanaudière; (450)759-7861

MARQUICIO DE THOMAS, Maria; CLSC Jardin du Quebec, 2 rue Ste-Famille, Saint-Remi QC J0L 2L0; (Other Foreign)'95; CCFP; (450)454-4671

MARQUIS, Annie; CSSS de la Matapedia, 135 av Gaetan-Archambault, Amqui QC G5J 2K5; Mon'94; CCFP; Staff, CSSS de la Matapedia; (418)629-2211; Fax. (418)629-4498.

MARQUIS, Catherine; Hotel-Dieu de Levis, 143 rue Wolfe, Levis QC G6V 3Z1; Laval'05; FRCSC; Ophth. Staff, Hôtel-Dieu de Lévis; (418)835-7121

MARQUIS, Chantal; CSSS de Rimouski-Neigette, CP 3150 Succ A 150 av Rouleau, Rimouski QC G5L 5T1; Laval'93; LMCC; CCFP; Staff, Hôpital Regional Rimouski; Langs: Bilingual(French/English); (418)724-8578; Fax. (418)724-8512.

MARQUIS, Edward J; Phoenix Med Centre, 406-2155 10th Ave, Prince George BC V2M 5J6; Alb'90; (250)564-7360; Fax. (250)564-1977.

MARQUIS, Elisabeth; CSSS de Rivière-de-Loup, 75 rue Saint-Henri, Riviere-Du-Loup QC G5R 2A4; Laval'85; FRCPC; Psy. Staff, Centre Hospitalier Regional du Grand-Portage; (418)868-1010; Fax. (418)868-1035.

MARQUIS, Etienne; 204-185 av Acadie, Dieppe NB E1A 1G6; Laval'95; FRCPC; Psy. Staff, Dr Georges-L-Dumont University Hospital Centre; Langs: Bilingual(French/English); (506)389-2200

MARQUIS, Francois; CHUQ-Hotel-Dieu de Quebec, 11 Cote Du Palais, Quebec QC G1R 2J6; Laval'81; FRCSC; OrthSurg (Joint Reconstruction). Staff, Centre Hospitalier Universitaire de Québec (CHUQ) - Siege Social; Physician, Sports Medicale Clinique de St-Louis; Prof, Université Laval; (418)691-5370; Fax. (418)691-5020.

MARQUIS, Francois; Hop Maisonneuve-Rosemont, 5415 boul de l'Assomption, Montreal QC H1T 2M4; Mon'99; FRCPC; IntMed; Critical Care Medicine (P.Q.). Staff, Hopital Maisonneuve-Rosemont; Langs: Bilingual(French/English); (514)252-3400

MARQUIS, Helene; CSSS de Laval, 1755 boul Rene-Laennec, Laval QC H7M 3L9; Mon'91; FRCSC; Ophth. Staff, Hopital de la Cite de la santé; (450)668-1010

MARQUIS, Isabelle; Clinique Sante Jacques-Cartier, 200-1815 rue King O, Sherbrooke QC J1J 2E3; Sher'95; Langs: Bilingual(French/English); (819)565-7446; Fax. (819)565-7780.

MARQUIS, Jean-Francois; Univ of Ottawa Heart Institute, H3410-40 Ruskin St, Ottawa ON K1Y 4W7; Laval'77; FRCPC; IntMed (Interventional Cardiology); Cardiol. Physician, University of Ottawa Heart Institute; Prof Med, University of Ottawa; Langs: English; (613)761-4919; Fax. (613)761-5215; jfmarquis@ottawaheart.ca.

MARQUIS, Josee; Univ De Sherbrooke, 2500 boul de l'Universite, Sherbrooke QC J1K 2R1; Laval'84; (819)821-7667; Fax. (819)821-7577.

MARQUIS, Katerine; CSSS de Rimouski-Neigette, CP 3150 succ A 150 av Rouleau, Rimouski QC G5L 5T1; Laval'03; FRCPC; IntMed; MedOncol; Hem. Staff, Hôpital Regional Rimouski; (418)724-3000

MARQUIS, Michel; CSSS de Manicouagan, 635 boul Jolliet, Baie-Comeau QC G5C 1P1; Sher'86; NuclearMed (P.Q.). Staff, Centre Hospitalier Régional Baie-Comeau; (418)589-3701 x2625; Fax. (418)295-3671; michel_marquis@ssss.gouv.qc.ca.

MARQUIS, Solange; Clinique Global Sante, 102-1107 boul du Cure-Labelle, Blainville QC J7C 2M2; Sher'78; Langs: Bilingual(French/English); (450)433-1748

MARQUS, Sami S; 410-325 Milner Ave, Scarborough ON M1B 5N1; Baghdad (Iraq)'81; MB ChB; FRCPC; IntMed (Diabetes). Staff, Rouge Valley Health System - Ajax & Pickering Health Centre Site; Langs: Arabic; Assyrian; (416)284-4744; Fax. (416)284-0141.

MARR, Alison J; Thames Valley FHT-Strathroy Me, 74 Front St E, Strathroy ON N7G 1Y7; Wes'79; Chief Obstetrical Serv, Strathroy Middlesex General Hospital - Middlesex Hospital Alliance; (519)245-0430; Fax. (519)245-5870; amarr@strathroymedicalclinic.com.

MARR, David R; Saint John Med Clinic, 299 Metcalf St, Saint John NB E2K 4P8; Dal'75; FRCPC; IntMed; Cardiol. Chief/Dir Coronary Care Unit, Saint John Regional Hospital; Consultant, Sussex Health Centre; Consultant, Charlotte County Hospital; Lecturer Med, Dalhousie University; (506)633-0479; Fax. (506)652-4426.

MARR, Douglas F; Northeast MHC-Sudbury Campus, 680 Kirkwood Dr, Sudbury ON P3E 1X3; Glasgow (Scotland)'76; MB ChB; FRCPC; Psy (Child & Adolescent Psychiatry). Prog Dir/Ac Staff, North Bay Regional Health Centre - Kirkwood; Asst Prof, Northern Ontario School of Medicine-Laurentian University; (705)675-9193 x8401; Fax. (705)675-5448.

MARR, Hubert K; 4016-3500 26 Ave NE, Calgary AB T1Y 6J4; Man'93; CCFP; Staff, Peter Lougheed Centre; Staff Palliative Care, Rockyview General Hospital; Langs: Cantonese; (403)943-4950; Fax. (403)943-4141; hubert.marr@calgaryhealthregion.ca.

MARR, Peter J; 200-1525 Robson St, Vancouver BC V6G 1C3; Ott'82; Staff Family Med, Providence Health Care - St Paul's Hospital; Teach Staff Family Med, University of British Columbia; (604)669-5669; Fax. (604)669-5689.

MARR, Sharon A; St Peter's Healty System, 88 Maplewood Ave, Hamilton ON L8M 1W9; McM'92; FRCPC; IntMed; GeriatricMed. Staff, Hamilton Health Sciences Centre - McMaster University Medical Centre; Staff, The Juravinski Cancer Centre; (905)777-3837; Fax. (905)525-2327.

MARRAS, Connie; Univ Hlth Network-Toronto Western Hosp, 7 MCL-399 Bathurst St, Toronto ON M5T 2S8; Qns'95; FRCPC; Neur (Movement Disorders). Staff Movement Disorders Centre, Toronto Western Hospital - University Health Network; (416)603-6422; Fax. (416)603-5004.

MARRAS, Theodore K; Univ Hlth Network-Toronto Western Hosp, 7E 452-399 Bathurst St, Toronto ON M5T 2S8; Qns'95; ABIM; FRCPC; IntMed (Clinician Investigator Program); Respir. Staff, Toronto Western Hospital - University Health Network; Staff, Mount Sinai Hospital; Langs: Greek; (416)603-5767; Fax. (416)603-5375; ted.marras@uhn.on.ca.

MARRAT, Saida; 302-1920 Ellesmere Rd, Scarborough ON M1H 2V6; (Morocco)'88; CCFP; Langs: Arabic; French; (416)913-0964; Fax. (416)913-0967.

MARRERO, Alier; Dr Georges-L Dumont Reg Hosp, 330 av Universite, Moncton NB E1C 2Z3; Pedro Henriques (Other Foreign)'00; Staff, Dr Georges-L-Dumont University Hospital Centre.

MARRIAGE, Keith J; Children's & Women's HC of BC, 141-4500 Oak St, Vancouver BC V6H 3N1; Melbourne (Australia)'68; MB BS; FRACP(Peds); FRANZCP; FRCPC; Peds (Child & Adolescent Psychiatry); Psy. Staff, BC Women's Hospital & Health Centre; Clin Prof Psy/Dir PG Child Psy Training, University of British Columbia; (604)875-2006; Fax. (604)875-2099; kmarriage@cw.bc.ca.

MARRIE, Thomas J J; Dalhousie University, C205-5849 University Ave, Halifax NS B3H 4H7; Dal'70; FRCPC; IntMed; InfectDis. Dean Faculty of Med/Prof, Dalhousie University; (902)494-8099; Fax. (902)494-7119; dean.medicine@dal.ca.

MARRIN, Andrea K; West Oak Med Clinic, 2495 Old Bronte Rd, Oakville ON L6M 4J2; Tor'99; FRCPC; Peds; ClinImmunol&Allergy. Affil Staff, Halton Healthcare Services Corporation - Oakville Site; Clin Asst Staff, Hamilton Health Sciences Centre - McMaster Children's Hospital; Langs: Bilingual(English/French); (905)582-7533

MARRIN, Michael L; Hamilton HSC-McMaster Site, PO Box 2000 Stn Lcd 1 4F1F-1200 Main St W, Hamilton ON L8N 3Z5; McM'80; BSc; FRCPC; Peds (Neonatology). Ac Staff, Hamilton Health Sciences Centre - McMaster Children's Hospital; Assoc Prof Peds, McMaster University; (905)521-2100 x76648; Fax. (905)521-5007; marrin@mcmaster.ca.

MARRIOTT, Anne E; Trillium Hlth Ctr-Mississauga, 100 Queensway W, Mississauga ON L5B 1B8; Alb'77; BMedSci; FRCPC; DiagRad. Staff, Trillium Health Centre - Mississauga; (905)848-7100

MARRIOTT, Christopher J C; Hamilton HSC-McMaster Site, PO Box 2000 Stn Lcd 1 1200 Main St W, Hamilton ON L8N 3Z5; Sher'94; PhD; FRCPC; NuclearMed. Staff Nuclear Med, Hamilton Health Sciences Centre - McMaster Children's Hospital; Langs: Bilingual(French/English); (905)521-2100 x73453; Fax. (905)546-1125; marric@mcmaster.ca.

MARRIOTT, James J; Health Sciences Centre, GF543-820 Sherbrook St, Winnipeg MB R3A 1R9; Qns'02; FRCPC; Neur. Staff, Health Sciences Centre; (204)774-8511

MARRIOTT, Jason J A; Sandy Hill Comm Health Centre, 221 Nelson St, Ottawa ON K1N 1C7; Ott'08; CCFP; (613)789-8458; Fax. (613)789-8710.

MARRIOTT, John A S; 392 Conc 6 Rd E RR 1, Millgrove ON L0R 1V0; Edinburgh (Scotland)'58; DPM; FRCPC; Psy (Geriatric Psychiatry). Court Staff, Grey Bruce Health Services - Southampton Site; Ac Staff, Joseph Brant Memorial Hospital; (905)690-1804; Fax. (905)690-1804.

MARRIOTT, M Lynne; Bear Street Family Physicians, PO Box 1048 Stn Main 302-220 Bear St, Banff AB T1L 1H6; Cal'86; CCFP; FCFP; Ac Staff, Covenant Health - Banff Mineral Springs Hospital; (403)762-4846; Fax. (403)762-2445.

MARRIOTT, Michael A; Dr Earl Health Centre, SS 3 786 Goderich St, Port Elgin ON N0H 2C3; Qns'90; CCFP; CCFP(E.M.); Staff, Grey Bruce Health Services - Southampton Site; Staff, South Bruce Grey Health Centre - Kincardine Site; (519)832-9600; Fax. (519)832-9602.

MARROCCO, Angela M P; Toronto East Gen Hosp Inc, 825 Coxwell Ave, Toronto ON M4C 3E7; Tor'03; CCFP; CCFP(E.M.); Staff, Toronto East General Hospital Inc; (416)461-8272

MARROCCO, Francis S; Northumberland Hills Hosp, 1000 Depalma Dr, Cobourg ON K9A 5W6; Tor'82; FRCPC; DiagRad. Staff, Northumberland Hills Hospital; (905)372-6811; Fax. (905)373-6922.

MARROCCO, Paul A D; Northumberland Hills Hosp, 1000 Depalma Dr, Cobourg ON K9A 5W6; Wes'78; CAB; CDD; DrMedCh; FRCP; FRCPC; DiagRad (Angiography/Interventional). Staff, Northumberland Hills Hospital; (905)372-6811; Fax. (905)373-6922.

MARRONE, Amanda D; Smithville Family Health Ctre, PO Box 218 230 Canboro Rd, Smithville ON L0R 2A0; McM'02; CCFP; (905)957-3328; Fax. (905)957-2475; amarrone@cogeco.ca.

MARSAN, Gilbert; Clinique Med Valmont, 101-783 rue Notre-Dame, Repentigny QC J5Y 1B4; Mon'84; Langs: English; (450)582-1260; Fax. (450)582-0677.

MARSAN, Joseph G; G-1081 Carling Ave, Ottawa ON K1Y 4G2; Mon'70; FRCSC; Otol (Rhinology). Asst Prof, University of Ottawa; Langs: French; Italian; (613)729-2834; Fax. (613)729-0909; joemarsan@hotmail.com.

MARSAN, Stephanie M; CHUM-Hop St-Luc, 1058 rue Saint-Denis, Montreal QC H2X 3J4; Ott'97; CCFP; Staff, Centre Hospitalier l'Université De Montréal (CHUM) - Hôpital Saint-luc; Langs: English; French; (514)890-8000

MARSCHALL, Jeffery G; Penticton Reg Hosp, 101-550 Carmi Ave, Penticton BC V2A 3G6; UBC'98; FRCSC; GenSurg. Staff, Penticton Regional Hospital; (250)493-7750

MARSDEN, John J; St Paul's Hosp, 1081 Burrard St, Vancouver BC V6Z 1Y6; Qns'87; CCFP; CCFP(E.M.); FCFP; Staff, Providence Health Care - St Paul's Hospital; Dept Head Emerg Med, University of British Columbia; (604)806-8984; Fax. (604)806-8488.

MARSDEN, Philip A; St Michael's Hosp, 30 Bond St, Toronto ON M5B 1W8; Wes'82; Staff, St Michael's Hospital; (416)847-1736

MARSDEN, Robert J; Owen Sound Med Associates, 2000-1415 1st Ave W, Owen Sound ON N4K 4K8; Wes'72; (519)470-3030; Fax. (519)470-3035.

MARSEU, Katherin L; Univ Hlth Network-Toronto Gen, 3F 437-200 Elizabeth St, Toronto ON M5G 2C4; McM'07; FRCPC; Anes. Staff, Toronto General Hospital - UHN; (416)340-5164

MARSH, Alexander S; Owen Sound Prof Centre, 216-945 3rd Ave E, Owen Sound ON N4K 2K8; Wes'79; DDS; DABOT; FRCSC; Otol (Audiology). Staff, Grey Bruce Health Services - Owen Sound; (519)376-6558; Fax. (519)376-7643.

MARSH, Ambrose A; 309-2453 Beacon Ave, Sidney BC V8L 1X7; Wes'79; Chief Staff, Saanich Peninsula Hospital; (250)656-0856; Fax. (250)656-0816.

MARSH, David C C; 10-450 Notre Dame Ave, Sudbury ON P3C 5K8; Mem'92; Assoc Dean Community Engagement, Northern Ontario School of Medicine; (705)673-1116; david.marsh@nosm.ca.

MARSH, David W; Transcona Med Clinic, 200-701 Regent Ave W, Winnipeg MB R2C 1S3; Durham (England)'61; (204)222-5221; Fax. (204)224-2053.

MARSH, Ian A; Quinsam Med Group, 280-1400 Dogwood St, Campbell River BC V9W 3A6; Trinity (Ireland)'79; FRCS(Ire); (250)286-0601

MARSH, J Ian; Vernon Jubilee Hosp, 2101 32 St, Vernon BC V1T 5L2; Sask'84; DiagRad. Staff Radiol, Vernon Jubilee Hospital; (250)558-1200

MARSH, Lorne A; Gladstone Prof Centre, 6155 North St, Halifax NS B3K 5R3; Dal'77; BSc; (902)453-3511; Fax. (902)454-9010.

MARSH-JOYAL, Melanie A; Royal Alexandra Hosp, 6408-10240 Kingsway NW, Edmonton AB T5H 3V9; Cal'04; BSc(Hon); FRCPC; Psy (Emergency Medicine). Consultant Psychiatrist, Royal Alexandra Hospital; Clin Lecturer, University of Alberta; (780)735-4567

MARSHALL, Andrew G; 202-595 Montreal Rd, Ottawa ON K1K 4L2; Ott'88; FRCSC; OrthSurg (Sports Medicine). (613)746-6745; Fax. (613)746-6008.

MARSHALL, Ann T; 31 Caradoc St N, Strathroy ON N7G 2M5; Queen's (Ireland)'52; MB ChB; CCFP; FCFP; Associate, Strathroy Middlesex General Hospital - Middlesex Hospital Alliance; (519)245-3590; Fax. (519)245-6032. Semi-Retired.

MARSHALL, Arthur D; South Shore Reg Hosp, 90 Glen Allan Dr, Bridgewater NS B4V 3S6; Dal'95; FRCPC; DiagRad. Staff, South Shore Regional Hospital; (902)543-4603

MARSHALL, Bonnie L; North Huron FHT-Wingham, PO Box 480 285 Catherine St, Wingham ON N0G 2W0; McM'89; BSc; CCFP; Ac Staff, Wingham & District Hospital - Listowel Wingham Hospitals Alliance; Adjunct Prof., University of Western Ontario; (519)357-1325; Fax. (519)357-1568.

MARSHALL, Bryan D; Stayner Med Centre, PO Box 220 7477 Highway 26, Stayner ON L0M 1S0; Tor'92; CCFP; FCFP; Staff, Collingwood General & Marine Hospital; (705)428-3246; Fax. (705)428-5652; marshall2@sympatico.ca.

MARSHALL, Carrie; Ucluelet Med Centre, PO Box 1090 1566 Peninsula Rd, Ucluelet BC V0R 3A0; Hawaii (USA)'09; (250)726-4443

MARSHALL, Cheryl P; 112 Queenston St, St Catharines ON L2R 2Z4; West Indies (Jamaica)'75; MB BS; DABIM; DAB; FRCPC; IntMed. Ac Staff, Niagara Health System - St Catharines General Site; (905)688-6072; Fax. (905)688-6073.

MARSHALL, Cindy L; Lockview Med Clinic, 204-159 Cobequid Rd, Lower Sackville NS B4C 2N1; Dal'92; CCFP; FCFP; Staff, Queen Elizabeth II Health Sciences Centre - Victoria General Site; Pt-Time Clin. Teach., Dalhousie University; (902)865-3335; Fax. (902)865-3331.

MARSHALL, Daniel R; 1-40 Mohawk Rd E, Hamilton ON L9A 2G7; McM'81; BSc; FAAP; FRCP; FRCPC; Peds (Developmental Pediatrics). (905)522-5522; Fax. (905)522-9339; drdan@drdanmarshall.com.

MARSHALL, David H; Nepean Med Centre, 202-1 Centrepointe Dr, Nepean ON K2G 6E2; Ott'92; FRCSC; Ophth. (613)226-8777; Fax. (613)226-5974.

MARSHALL, Denise I; West Lincoln Mem Hosp, 169 Main St E, Grimsby ON L3M 1P3; McM'86; BSc; CCFP; FCFP; Court Staff, St Joseph's Healthcare - Charlton Campus; Court Staff, West Lincoln Memorial Hospital; Ac Staff, Hamilton Health Sciences Centre - McMaster University Medical Centre; Dir Undergrad Med Studies, McMaster University; (905)945-7632; Fax. (905)945-4257; marshald@mcmaster.ca.

MARSHALL, Emmalee V; Sault Area Hosp, 750 Great Northern Rd, Sault Ste. Marie ON P6B 0A8; McM'99; FRCPC; Psy. Staff, Sault Area Hospital - Sault Ste Marie; (705)759-3434 x4615

MARSHALL, Gena M; Halifax Prof Centre, 820-5991 Spring Garden Rd, Halifax NS B3H 1Y6; Dal'95; CCFP; (902)422-3003; Fax. (902)429-3003.

MARSHALL, Geoffrey B; Associated Radiologist, 204-140 Wall St, Saskatoon SK S7K 1N4; Sask'01; FRCPC; DiagRad. Staff Medical Imaging, Saskatoon City Hospital; (306)244-1167

MARSHALL, Harvey P; 601A Discovery St, Victoria BC V8T 5G4; Sask'67; DAB; FRCPC; IntMed (Endocrinology). Att Physician, Royal Jubilee Hospital; Clinical Asst Prof Div of Endocrinology, University of British Columbia; (250)595-4441; Fax. (250)595-4100.

MARSHALL, Ian M; Dr Charles A Janeway Child Hc, 300 Prince Philip Dr, St. John's NL A1B 3V6; Mem'89; Staff, Janeway Children's Health & Rehabilitation Centre; Staff, Health Sciences Centre; Staff, St Clare's Mercy Hospital; (709)777-6300

MARSHALL, J Neil; 31 Caradoc St N, Strathroy ON N7G 2M5; Belfast (Ireland)'78; MB ChB; BAO; CCFP; FCFP; Ac Staff, Strathroy Middlesex General Hospital - Middlesex Hospital Alliance; Med Dir, Sprucedale Care Centre; Liaison Physician, Thames Valley Family Practice Research Unit; Asst Prof, University of Western Ontario; (519)245-3590; Fax. (519)245-6032.

MARSHALL, John C; St Michael's Hosp, BW4 007-30 Bond St, Toronto ON M5B 1W8; Tor'77; FRCSC; GenSurg (Critical Care Medicine). Staff, St Michael's Hospital; (416)864-5225; Fax. (416)864-5141; marshallj@smh.toronto.on.ca.

MARSHALL, John K; 2F59-1280 Main St W, Hamilton ON L8S 4K1; Qns'92; ABIM; FRCPC; IntMed; Gastroent. Staff Div of Gastroent, Hamilton Health Sciences Centre - McMaster Children's Hospital; Assoc Prof Med, McMaster University; (905)521-2100 x76782; Fax. (905)523-6048.

MARSHALL, Judith A; Toronto Rehab Institute, 520 Sutherland Dr, Toronto ON M4G 3V9; Tor'06; CCFP; Staff, Toronto Rehabilitation Institute - Lyndhurst Centre; (416)597-3422; Fax. (416)597-7046.

MARSHALL, Julia L; 11-6175 Dunn St, Niagara Falls ON L2G 2P4; Alb'99; CCFP; (905)356-0666

MARSHALL, K Wayne; Univ Hlth Network-Toronto Western Hosp, 1E 443-399 Bathurst St, Toronto ON M5T 2S8; Detroit(MI) (USA)'77; PhD; FRCSC; OrthSurg (Knee Arthroscopy). Staff, Toronto Western Hospital - University Health Network; Asst Prof, University of Toronto; (416)603-5171; Fax. (416)603-5542; kwm@uhnres.utoronto.ca.

MARSHALL, Karen L; The Malton Med Group, 22-7330 Goreway Dr, Mississauga ON L4T 4J2; McM'95; CCFP; FCFP; (905)677-4200; Fax. (905)677-0541.

MARSHALL, Kate M A; Unison Health & Comm Services, 1651 Keele St, York ON M6M 3W2; Qns'96; CCFP; FCFP; Langs: English; French; (416)653-5400; Fax. (416)657-3622.

MARSHALL, L Maureen; Townsite Med Clinic, 512 Campbell St, Nanaimo BC V9R 3H1; UBC'77.

MARSHALL, Laura; La Ronge Health Centre, PO Box 6000, La Ronge SK S0J 1L0; Sask'09; CCFP; Staff, La Ronge Health Centre; (306)425-2422; Fax. (306)425-8516.

MARSHALL, Luke A; CFB Borden, PO Box 1000 30 route Ortona Rd, Borden ON L0M 1C0; Man'10; CCFP.

MARSHALL, Lynn M; Women's College Hosp, 5F W-76 Grenville St, Toronto ON M5S 1B2; Qns'66; FRSM; Court Staff Environmental Hlth Clinic & Med Education Liaison, Women's College Hospital; Asst Prof Family Med, Northern Ontario School of Medicine-Lakehead University; Lecturer DFCM, University of Toronto; Aj Prof, Lakehead University / Library; (905)845-3462 x4991; Fax. (905)845-3794; lynn.marshall@utoronto.ca.

MARSHALL, Marilyn C; 117 Waterloo St S, Stratford ON N5A 4B3; McG'77; FRCPC; Psy (Anxiety & Mood Disorders). Langs: Bilingual(English/French); (519)271-0300; Fax. (519)273-2616.

MARSHALL, Michael T; Northmount Med Centre, 803-145 13th St E, North Vancouver BC V7L 2L4; UBC'76; BSc; (604)985-4177; Fax. (604)985-3442; mtmarshall@shaw.ca.

MARSHALL, Michelle T; St Joseph's Health Centre, 30 The Queensway, Toronto ON M6R 1B5; McM'93; BA; MA; FRCPC; Psy (Child & Adolescent Psychiatry). Staff, St Joseph's Health Centre; (416)530-6000; Fax. (416)530-6393.

MARSHALL, P Iris; 29 Gill Rd PO Box 159, Grand Bend ON N0M 1T0; Tor'76; BSc; Dip SportMed; MEd; (519)238-6888; Fax. (519)238-1317.

MARSHALL, Shaun A; North Huron FHT-Wingham, PO Box 480 285 Catherine St, Wingham ON N0G 2W0; Mem'96; BSc; BA; BEd; CCFP; FCFP; Staff, Wingham & District Hospital - Listowel Wingham Hospitals Alliance; Aj Prof, University of Western Ontario; (519)357-1325; Fax. (519)357-1568.

MARSHALL, Shawn C; 505 Smyth Rd, Ottawa ON K1H 8M2; Wes'89; MSc; FRCPC; PhysMed&Rehab (Traumatic Brain Injuries). Staff Physical Med & Rehab, The Ottawa Hospital Rehabilitation Centre; Assoc Prof, University of Ottawa; (613)737-7350 x75590; Fax. (613)739-6951; smarshall@ottawahospital.on.ca.

MARSHALL, Stuart A; Esquimalt Treatment Centre, 918 Esquimalt Rd, Victoria BC V9A 3M6; UBC'09; CCFP; (250)382-1213

MARSHALL, Thomas D; St Joseph's Healthcare, 50 Charlton Ave E, Hamilton ON L8N 4A6; Ott'93; FRCPC; EmergMed. Staff, St Joseph's Healthcare - Charlton Campus; (905)522-1155

MARSOLAIS, Anne-Sophie; CSSS de Laval, 1755 boul Rene-Laennec, Laval QC H7M 3L9; McG'96; Staff, Hopital de la Cite de la santé; (450)668-1010

MARSOLAIS, Marcel; Carrefour Med Vallee Richelieu, 665 boul Sir-Wilfrid-Laurier, Beloeil QC J3G 4J1; Mon'71; Consultant, Centre Hospitalier Honore-Mercier; (450)467-0088

MARSOLAIS, Pierre; Hop Du Sacre-Coeur De Mtl, 5400 boul Gouin O, Montreal QC H4J 1C5; Mon'90; FRCPC; IntMed (Intensive Care); Critical Care Medicine (P.Q.). Staff, Hôpital du Sacre-Coeur de Montréal; (514)338-2050

MARSTERS JR., David W; 1437 Belcher St PO Box 300, Port Williams NS B0P 1T0; Dal'77; FRCPC; IntMed. (902)542-0990; Fax. (902)542-1759.

MARSZAL, Maria M; 5E-210 Wilmott St, Cobourg ON K9A 0E9; Warsaw (Poland)'95; CCFP; Langs: Polish; (905)377-0728; Fax. (905)373-1482.

MARTA, Janet A; Psychiatric Service, 214 College St, Toronto ON M5T 2Z9; McM'85; Psy (Psychotherapy). Langs: Spanish; French.

MARTEL, Alain Y; CHUQ-Hop Laval, H 1353-2705 boul Laurier, Quebec QC G1V 4G2; Laval'76; RC; FRCPC; IntMed (P.Q.) (Infectiology); Microbio & Infect Dis (P.Q.); MedMicrobiol. ac Staff/adj Dir méd, Centre Hospitalier Universitaire de Quebec-CHUL; Clin Assoc Prof, Université Laval; Langs: Bilingual(French/English); (418)651-2485

MARTEL, Alison E; Westgrove Prof Bldg, 200-10230 142 St NW, Edmonton AB T5N 3Y6; Alb'91; CCFP; FCFP; (780)454-4242; Fax. (780)454-4224.

MARTEL, Andre; Clinique D'Anesthesie 5540, 145-100 ch Rockland, Mont-Royal QC H3P 2V9; Laval'67; AB; FRCPC; Anes. Langs: English; (514)955-6787; Fax. (514)955-6208; cliniqueag@videotron.ca.

MARTEL, Arold M; CHUS-Hop Hotel-Dieu, 580 rue Bowen S, Sherbrooke QC J1G 2E8; Mon'75; FRCSC; Urol. ac Staff, Centre Hospitalier Universitaire de Sherbrooke-Hôpital Hôtel-Dieu; Universite de Sherbrooke; (819)346-1110; armartel@videotron.ca.

MARTEL, Brent R; CSSS du Suroît, 150 rue Saint-Thomas, Salaber-de-Valleyf QC J6T 6C1; McG'92; FRCPC; Anes. Staff, Centre Hospitalier Régional du Suroît; (450)371-9920

MARTEL, Christiane; CLSC La Vallee des Patriotes, 300 boul Serge-Pepin, Beloeil QC J3G 0B8; Laval'95; Médecin Palliative Care, Maison Victor-Gadbois; (450)536-2572; Fax. (450)536-6367.

MARTEL, Colette; GMF de Saint-Donat, 377 rue Du Foyer CP 760, St-Donat-De-Mtcalm QC J0T 2C0; Mon'88; Staff, CLSC Joli-Mont de St-Donat; (819)424-1511; Fax. (819)424-4682.

MARTEL, Diane B; Clinique Mere-Enfant, 184 boul Leclerc O, Granby QC J2G 1T5; Sher'97; Langs: English; (450)776-6220; Fax. (450)776-7515.

MARTEL, Elaine; Residence Hotellerie Harmonie, 1024 rue Charcot, Longueuil QC J4B 8R5; Mon'86; Staff, Hopital Maisonneuve-Rosemont; Langs: English; (450)641-7501

MARTEL, Elise; Societe du Centre Chirurgical, 202-222 rue de la Visitation, St-Charles-Brromee QC J6E 4N5; Laval'93; FRCSC; GenSurg. Staff GenSurg, Centre Hospitalier Régional de Lanaudière; Langs: English; (450)753-7588; Fax. (450)756-6144.

MARTEL, France; CSSS du Lac-Temiscamingue, 22 rue Notre-Dame N, Ville-Marie QC J9V 1W8; Laval'05; CCFP; Staff, CSSS du Témiscamingue; (819)629-2420

MARTEL, Francois; Coop Sante La Prairie, 675 ch Saint-Jean, La Prairie QC J5R 2L2; Mon'90; CCFP; Staff, Hôpital du Haut-Richelieu; Staff, Clinique Medicale St-Jean; (450)444-2002

MARTEL, Gaetan; Unite de Medicine Familiale, 100-500 boul de l'Hopital, Gatineau QC J8V 2P5; Laval'85; ac Membre, Hôpital de Gatineau; Court Staff, The Ottawa Hospital - Civic Campus; Staff, Unite de Medicine Familiale; Clin Teacher, University of Ottawa; assoc Prof, McGill University; Langs: Bilingual(French/English); (819)966-6175

MARTEL, Gilles; CLSC La Region-Sherbrookoise, 1200 rue King E, Sherbrooke QC J1G 1E4; Sher'82; CCFP; FCFP; Staff, Centre Hospitalier Universitaire de Sherbrooke-Hopital Fleurimont; Assoc Prof Family Med, Universite de Sherbrooke; (819)563-2572; Fax. (819)563-9912.

MARTEL, Guillaume V D; The Ottawa Hosp-Civic Campus, 305-1053 Carling Ave, Ottawa ON K1Y 4E9; McG'05; FRCSC; GenSurg. Staff, The Ottawa Hospital - Civic Campus; (613)761-5015

MARTEL, Jacques; Centre Med St-Stanislas, 1380 rue Principale, St-Stanislas-D-Cha QC G0X 3E0; Laval'84; (418)328-8417; Fax. (418)328-8446.

MARTEL, Jean-Marie; Clinique Medicale 1746, 1746 ch De Chambly, Longueuil QC J4J 3X5; Besancon (France)'81; (450)646-2900; Fax. (450)651-8901; jmmartel@hotmail.com.

MARTEL, Jean-Pierre A; The Moncton Hosp, 135 MacBeath Ave, Moncton NB E1C 6Z8; Ott'03; FRCPC; DiagRad. Staff, The Moncton Hospital; (506)857-5520

MARTEL, Julie; Clinique Dermatologique, 1819 av Dollard, Lasalle QC H8N 1T9; Sher'94; FRCPC; Derm. Staff Derm, Centre Hospitalier Régional Baie-Comeau; Langs: English; (514)366-6666

MARTEL, Julie; CSSS Drummond, 350 rue Saint-Jean, Drummondville QC J2B 5L4; Mon'91; LMCC; FRCPC; Psy (Child Psychiatry). Staff, Hôpital Sainte-croix; Langs: Bilingual(French/English); (819)474-2572 x475; Fax. (819)474-2347; julie.martel@cgocable.ca.

MARTEL, Julien; CHUM-Hop Notre-Dame, 1560 rue Sherbrooke E, Montreal QC H2L 4M1; Mon'08; CCFP; CCFP(E.M.); Staff, Centre Hospitalier l'Université de Montréal (CHUM) - Hôpital Notre-Dame; (514)890-8000

MARTEL, Karine; CSSS de Saint-Jerome, 290 rue de Montigny, Saint-Jerome QC J7Z 5T3; Mon'02; FRCSC; GenSurg. Staff, Hôtel-Dieu de Saint-Jérôme; (450)431-8200

MARTEL, Laurent; Clinique Med 201, 104 rue Sainte-Agathe, Ste-Agathe-Des-Mts QC J8C 2K3; Mon'79; Staff, Centre Hospitalier Laurentien; (819)326-2020; Fax. (819)326-8801; martel@polyinter.com.

MARTEL, Louis; Clinique Med Sainte-Madeleine, 165 boul Sainte-Madeleine, Trois-Rivieres QC G8T 3L7; Mon'88; CCFP; Staff, Centre Hospitalier Regional de Trois-Rivieres; (819)379-8385

MARTEL, Marie-Jocelyne; Pacific Avenue Med Centre, 300-149 Pacific Ave, Saskatoon SK S7K 1N8; Sask'90; FRCSC; ObstGyn (Maternal Fetal Medicine). (306)653-5970; Fax. (306)653-5383.

MARTEL, Marie-Josee; CLSC de l'Erable, 1331 rue Saint-Calixte, Plessisville QC G6L 1P4; Laval'92; Staff, CLSC de l'Erable; (819)362-6301

MARTEL, Michel; Clinique Med Pierre-Boucher, 110-1615 boul Jacques-Cartier, Longueuil QC J4M 2X1; Mon'81; Staff, Centre Hospitalier Pierre Boucher; Langs: English; (450)468-6223; Fax. (450)468-5041.

MARTEL, Michelle; CSSS De Sept-Iles, 45 rue du Pere-Divet, Sept-Iles QC G4R 3N7; Sher'82; FRCSC; ObstGyn. Staff, Centre Hospitalier Regional de Sept-Iles; (418)962-9761

MARTEL, Nadine; CHUQ-Hotel-Dieu De Quebec, 11 Cote Du Palais, Quebec QC G1R 2J6; Sher'97; FRCPC; IntMed; MedOncol; Hem. Staff, Centre Hospitalier Universitaire de Québec (CHUQ) - Siege Social; (418)691-5280; Fax. (418)691-5383.

MARTEL, Patrick; Thunder Bay Reg HSC-T-Bay, 980 Oliver Rd, Thunder Bay ON P7B 6V4; Mon'97; CCFP; CCFP(E.M.); Staff, Thunder Bay Regional Health Sciences Centre; (807)684-6100

MARTEL, Pierre; CSSS de Montmagny-L'Islet, 350 boul Tache O RR 1, Montmagny QC G5V 3R8; Laval'07; Staff, CSSS de Montmagny-L'Islet; (418)248-0630; pierre.martel@gmf.gouv.qc.ca.

MARTEL, Pierre; Clinique Medicale 2200, 2200 ch de Chambly, Longueuil QC J4J 3Z3; Mon'78; Staff, CHSLD de la MRC de Champlain-Centre Saint-Lambert; (450)651-7331; pierre.martel@rrsss16.gouv.qc.ca.

MARTEL, Rodrigue; CSSS Haut-Richelieu-Rouville, 920 boul Du Seminaire N, St-Jean-Sur-Richel QC J3A 1B7; Sher'93; Staff, Hôpital du Haut-Richelieu; (450)359-5000; Fax. (450)359-5251.

MARTEL, Simon; Hôpital Laval, L3522-2725 ch Sainte-Foy, Quebec QC G1V 4G5; Mon'88; FRCPC; IntMed; Respir. Staff, Hôpital Laval; (418)656-4747; Fax. (418)656-4762; simon.martel@med.ulaval.ca.

MARTEL, Sonia; CSSS des Sources, 475 3e Av, Asbestos QC J1T 1X6; Mon'95; Staff, CSSS des Sources d'Asbestos; (418)879-7151; Fax. (418)879-7433.

MARTEL, Sophie; Centre Oculaire de Victoriavil, 340 rue Notre-Dame E, Victoriaville QC G6P 4A6; Sher'85; FRCSC; Ophth. Staff Ophth, Hotel-Dieu d'Arthabaska; (819)357-8227; Fax. (819)357-8228; smart@lino.com.

MARTEL, Sophie; Centre de Sante Cookshire, RR 5 1-160 rue Pope, Cookshire-Eaton QC J0B 1M0; Sher'08; CCFP; (819)875-5535

MARTEL, Yvan; Clinique Med Sainte-Dorothee, 102-1 boul Samson, Laval QC H7X 3S5; Mon'80; Staff, Hopital de la Cite de la santé; (450)689-6334; Fax. (450)689-6339.

MARTELL, David R; Lunenburg Med Clinic, PO Box 1450 42 High St, Lunenburg NS B0J 2C0; Wes'97; CCFP; (902)634-7000; Fax. (902)634-4982.

MARTELL, Rafael; 201-219 Oxford St W, London ON N6H 1S5; Brown(RI) (USA)'82; MD; FRCPC; IntMed (Cardiology). Ac Staff, Strathroy Middlesex General Hospital - Middlesex Hospital Alliance; Court Staff, South Bruce Grey Health Centre - Kincardine Site; Court Staff, London Health Sciences Centre - Victoria Campus; Med Dir, Diagnostics Consulting Associates; Langs: Spanish; (519)432-3771; Fax. (519)432-3814.

MARTEN, Dion M; Victoria Hosp, PO Box 3000 Stn Main 1200 24th St W, Prince Albert SK S6V 5T4; Sask'98; CCFP; Staff, Victoria Hospital; (306)765-6200; Fax. (306)765-6224.

MARTENS, Brian R; Queen Street Med Group, 502 Queen St, Saskatoon SK S7K 0M5; UBC'87; Staff, Saskatoon City Hospital; (306)652-9145; Fax. (306)652-1531.

MARTENS, Chandra G R; CSSSG-Hop de Gatineau, CP 2000 Succ Bureau-Chef 909 boul de la Verendrye O, Gatineau QC J8P 7H2; Qns'96; FRCPC; RadOncol. Staff, Hôpital de Gatineau; (819)966-6200

MARTENS, David B; Agassiz Med Centre, 130-30 Stephen St, Morden MB R6M 2G3; Man'07; CCFP.

MARTENS, David J; Adolescent Med Clinic, 1040 av Atwater, Montreal QC H3Z 1X3; Cal'06; FRCPC; Peds (Adolescent Medicine). Staff, McGill University Health Centre - Montreal Children's Hospital; (514)412-4481

MARTENS, Jay D; 106-15966 108th Ave, Surrey BC V4N 5V6; UBC'02; (604)582-8820

MARTENS, M Dawn; Medical Arts Bldg, 202-233 Kennedy St, Winnipeg MB R3C 3J5; Sask'92; FRCPC; DiagRad. (204)942-6453; Fax. (204)944-8101.

MARTENS, Mildred B; Royal Jubilee Hosp, DT 5811-1952 Bay St, Victoria BC V8R 1J8; Man'94; BSc; MD; FRCPC; AnatPath (Nephropathology). Staff, Royal Jubilee Hospital; (250)370-8208; Fax. (250)370-8069; mildred.martens@viha.ca.

MARTENS, Raymond L; Henderson Med Centre, 441 Henderson Hwy, Winnipeg MB R2K 2H5; Man'71; Staff, Concordia General Hospital; (204)667-8650; Fax. (204)668-1928.

MARTENS-BARNES, Carolyn; St James Street Med Clinic, 1600 Portage Ave, Winnipeg MB R3J 0C6; Man'82; (204)774-1868; Fax. (204)774-7303.

MARTENS-KMIOTEK, Ewa L; 24 Duncairn Rd, North York ON M3B 1C8; Warsaw (Poland)'73; FRCPC; Psy. (416)447-9398

MARTHYMAN, Azaria M; Admirals Walk Health Centre, 275 Island Hwy, Victoria BC V9B 1G4; UBC'92; Staff, Victoria General Hospital; Staff, Royal Jubilee Hospital; (250)380-9070

MARTI, Julien A; Sudbury Reg Hosp-Laurentian, 41 Ramsey Lake Rd, Sudbury ON P3E 5J1; Mon'96; FRCPC; Anes. Staff, Health Sciences North-Laurentian Site; (705)523-7100

MARTIAL, Jocelyne; Jocelyn Martial MD, 1889 rue de Toulouse, Sherbrooke QC J1J 3Z1; Mon'83; assoc Dir Professional Services, Centre Hospitalier Universitaire de Sherbrooke-Hôpital Hôtel-Dieu; assoc Dir Professional Services, Centre Hospitalier Universitaire de Sherbrooke-Hopital Fleurimont; Langs: English; (819)573-2102

MARTIAL, Johanne; Clinique Med Solumed Ltee, 1-8230 boul Taschereau, Brossard QC J4X 1C2; Mon'84; FRCPC; Psy (Affective Disorders). Staff, Douglas Mental Health University Institute; adj Prof, McGill University; Langs: Bilingual(French/English); (450)466-0003; Fax. (450)466-0022.

MARTIN, Alban; Univ Of New Brunswick, PO Box 4400 Stn A, Fredericton NB E3B 5A3; Mem'89; (506)453-4837; Fax. (506)452-6087.

MARTIN, Allison S; Associate Med Clinic, 400-20 14th St W, Prince Albert SK S6V 3K8; University of the West Indies (Other Foreign)'94; MB BS(UWI); MRCP; Staff, Victoria Hospital; (306)953-1681; Fax. (306)764-3091.

MARTIN, Andre-Guy; CHUQ-Hotel-Dieu de Quebec, 11 Cote Du Palais, Quebec QC G1R 2J6; Laval'96; FRC; Pharm; MSc; FRCPC; RadOncol (Gastrointestinal Cancer). Staff, Centre Hospitalier Universitaire de Québec (CHUQ) - Siege Social; Langs: Bilingual(English/French); (418)691-5264; Fax. (418)691-5268; andre-guy.martin@mail.chuq.qc.ca.

MARTIN, Andrew J; Thornhill Family Physicians, 35-7700 Bathurst St, Thornhill ON L4J 7Y3; Tor'89; BScPharm; CCFP; FCFP; Langs: English; French; (905)881-6510

MARTIN, Anne; Hop du Sacre-Coeur de Mtl, 5400 boul Gouin O, Montreal QC H4J 1C5; Mon'86; FRCPC; DiagRad. Staff, Hôpital du Sacre-Coeur de Montréal; (514)338-2130; Fax. (514)338-2384.

MARTIN, Anne J; Avon Family Med Centre, 511 Huron St, Stratford ON N5A 5T8; Wes'04; CCFP; (519)508-1255; Fax. (519)508-1240.

MARTIN, Anne-Marie; Polyclinique Isabell-sur-Mer, 8224 rue St-Paul, Bas-Caraquet NB E1W 6E2; Sher'08; CCFP; Staff, Hôpital de l'Enfant-Jésus RHSJ; (506)727-7549; Fax. (506)727-7320.

MARTIN, Barry A; Addiction & Mental Hlth-Clarke, 250 College St, Toronto ON M5T 1R8; Sask'70; FRCPC; Psy. Staff, Centre for Addiction & Mental Health (CAMH) - College Street Site; Assoc Prof, University of Toronto; (416)979-6808; Fax. (416)979-5679.

MARTIN, Barry M; Guelph Gen Hosp, 115 Delhi St, Guelph ON N1E 4J4; Tor'80; Dip SportMed; BSc; Staff, Guelph General Hospital; (519)822-5350; indskill@bserv.com.

MARTIN, Bosco C F; 514-5863 Leslie St, North York ON M2H 1J8; Tor'83; BSc; FRCPC; Anes. (416)410-0096

MARTIN, Brad W; Family Med Associates, 15-9701 84 Ave, Grande Prairie AB T8V 4Z8; Alb'89; (780)532-2280; Fax. (780)532-0037.

MARTIN, Brenda L; 6435 Erin Mills Pky, Mississauga ON L5N 4H4; McM'92; (905)821-1406

MARTIN, Brendan E; 102-5511 206 St, Langley BC V3A 2C6; Dublin (Ireland)'75; MB; DObst; CCFP; (604)534-6711; Fax. (604)534-2170.

MARTIN, Brian D; Lake Country Family Practice, 1-9966 Pollard Rd, Winfield BC V4V 1Z4; Alb'88; Court Staff Privil, Kelowna General Hospital; (250)766-3938; Fax. (250)766-5231.

MARTIN, Bruce D; Univ of Manitoba, 727 McDermot Ave, Winnipeg MB R3E 3P5; Qns'77; MSc; CCFP; FCFP; Dir J A Hildes Northern Med Unit/Assoc Dean Students, University of Manitoba.

MARTIN, Caroline I; CSSS de Chicoutimi, 305 rue Saint-Vallier, Chicoutimi QC G7H 5H6; McG'02; CCFP; CCFP(E.M.); Staff, Complexe hospitalier de la Sagamie; (418)541-1000

MARTIN, Catherine; Ctr de Sante Paul-Gilbert, 9330 du Centre-Hospitalier, Levis QC G6X 1L6; Laval'09; CCFP; Staff, Centre Hospitalier Paul-Gilbert; (418)380-8993

MARTIN, Charles; Unite de Medecine Familiale, 50 ch du Golf O, Joliette QC J6E 2B4; Mon'67; Peds. (450)759-3060

MARTIN, Christopher D; Royal Victoria Hosp, 201 Georgian Dr, Barrie ON L4M 6M2; Wes'05; FRCPC; EmergMed; Critical Care Medicine. Staff, Royal Victoria Regional Health Centre; (705)728-9802

MARTIN, Christopher G; Lincoln Med Centre, 4413 Ontario St, Beamsville ON L0R 1B5; Tor'93; BSc; CCFP; Ac Staff, West Lincoln Memorial Hospital; (905)563-1212; Fax. (905)563-4404.

MARTIN, Christopher J; 7-635 Water St, Miramichi NB E1N 4B9; Dal'10; CCFP; (506)352-3000

MARTIN, Claudio M; London HSC-Victoria Campus, PO Box 5010 Stn B D2 528-800 Commissioners Rd E, London ON N6A 5W9; Tor'84; FRCPC; IntMed (Critical Care Medicine). Staff, London Health Sciences Centre - Victoria Campus; Prof Med, University of Western Ontario; (519)685-8090; Fax. (519)685-8089.

MARTIN, Craig W; View Medical Inc, 1443 View Cres, Delta BC V4L 2K2; UBC'86; BSc(Hon); MHSc; Ac Staff/Co-Dir Clinical Rounds, Delta Hospital; Sr Advisor Medical, Workers' Comp Board of BC; (604)943-6999; Fax. (604)943-8344.

MARTIN, Daniel C; 108-2221 Keele St, North York ON M6M 3Z5; Tor'02; FRCSC; PlasSurg. Staff, St Michael's Hospital; (416)244-5506; Fax. (416)244-5507.

MARTIN, Daniel; CSSS Les Eskers de l'Abitibi, 622 4e rue O, Amos QC J9T 2S2; Sher'93; FRCPC; Anes. Staff, CH Hôtel-Dieu d'Amos; (819)732-3341

MARTIN, Danielle A S; Women's College Hosp, 76 Grenville St, Toronto ON M5S 1B2; Wes'03; CCFP; Staff, Women's College Hospital; Langs: Bilingual(English/French); (416)323-6400

MARTIN, David C; 102-93 Ontario St, St Catharines ON L2R 5J7; Witwatersrand (South Africa)'83; FRCSC; OrthSurg. Staff, Niagara Health System - St Catharines General Site; (905)984-3433; Fax. (905)984-4421.

MARTIN, David H; 101-730 Brant St, Burlington ON L7R 2H9; McM'80; FRCPC; IntMed; Respir. Staff, Joseph Brant Memorial Hospital; (905)632-5864

MARTIN, Deborah L; F-570 Bryne Dr, Barrie ON L4N 9P6; Qns'86; CCFP; CCFP(E.M.); Physician, Royal Victoria Regional Health Centre; Physician, Martin Vein Clinic; (705)735-0639; info@drmartinsclinic.com.

MARTIN, Diane C; West Coast Gen Hosp, 3949 Port Alberni Hwy, Port Alberni BC V9Y 4S1; Belfast (Ireland)'73; MB ChB; BAO; CCFP; FCFP; Staff, West Coast General Hospital; (250)731-1370

MARTIN, Douglas D; Hamilton HS-General Site, 237 Barton St E, Hamilton ON L8L 2X2; Qns'99; FRCPC; EmergMed. Staff, Hamilton Health Sciences Centre - Hamilton General Hospital; (905)527-4322

MARTIN, Edward S G; Anaesthesia Associates, 439 Park St, Kitchener ON N2G 1N4; Qns'95; FRCPC; Anes. (519)744-7361; Fax. (519)744-7363.

MARTIN, Elise J; CSSS Baie des Chaleurs, RR 2 419 boul Perron, Maria QC G0C 1Y0; Mon'85; CASM; FRCPC; Peds (Sports Medicine). Staff, CSSS de la Baie-des-Chaleurs; Langs: Italian; Bilingual(French/English); (418)759-3443

MARTIN, Eric; 33 Main St, Rexton NB E4W 0E5; Sher'02; CCFP; Langs: English; (506)523-2972; Fax. (506)523-2971.

MARTIN, Eva; 204-5293 Highway 7, Markham ON L3P 7M7; Tor'79; (905)294-2470; Fax. (905)294-2470.

MARTIN, Fabienne; Clinique Med Maskinonge, 147 A boul Est, Maskinonge QC J0K 1N0; Laval'80; Staff, CSSS de Maskinongé; (819)227-2228; Fax. (819)227-3737.

MARTIN, Francis; Corydon Primary Care Clinic, 102-1001 Corydon Ave, Winnipeg MB R3M 0B6; Man'75; BSc(Med); MClSc; MEd; CCFP; FCFP; Staff, Winnipeg Regional Health Authority; Assoc Prof Family Med, University of Manitoba; (204)940-2000; Fax. (204)477-5730.

MARTIN, Freda E; Silverman Bldg, 114 Maitland St, Toronto ON M4Y 1E1; Tor'56; DPM(Eng); FRCPsy(Lond); FRCPC; Psy (Child Psychiatry). Staff Psychiatrist, The Hincks-Dellcrest Centre - Toronto; Assoc Prof, University of Toronto; (416)972-1935; Fax. (416)924-9808.

MARTIN, Gerald; Clinique Med Dagenais, 2065 boul des Laurentides, Laval QC H7M 4M2; Mon'84; (450)975-1557; Fax. (450)975-1557.

MARTIN, Ginette; CHUM-Hop Notre-Dame, 1560 rue Sherbrooke E, Montreal QC H2L 4M1; Mon'89; FRCS; FRCP; ABS; MASc; FRCSC; GenSurg (Breast Cancer); General Surgical Oncology (P. Q.). Staff, Centre Hospitalier l'Université de Montréal (CHUM) - Hôpital Notre-Dame; Staff, Centre Hospitalier l'Université de Montréal (CHUM) - Hôtel-Dieu; assoc Prof, Universite de Montreal; (514)890-8000 x26607; Fax. (514)412-7821; ginette.martin.chum@ssss.gouv.qc.ca.

MARTIN, Glenn E; 675 Coronation Blvd, Cambridge ON N1R 3G4; Wes'80; FRCPC; IntMed. Staff, Cambridge Memorial Hospital; (519)740-8784; Fax. (519)740-2724; gmartin628@bellnet.ca.

MARTIN, Gregory J; Primary Health Care Unit, 82 Seventh Ave, Sioux Lookout ON P8T 1K2; Man'83; CCFP; FCFP; (807)737-1802

MARTIN, Guy; Ctr Hosp Laurentien, 234 rue Saint-Vincent, Ste-Agathe-Des-Mts QC J8C 2B8; Sher'93; FRCPC; Anes. Staff, Centre Hospitalier Laurentien; (819)324-4034

MARTIN, Heather S; Mill Creek Family Medicine, 101-1912 Enterprise Way, Kelowna BC V1Y 9S9; Sask'09; CCFP; (250)868-0700

MARTIN, Ian; Abbotsford Reg Hosp & Cancer C, 32900 Marshall Rd, Abbotsford BC V2S 0C2; Wes'98; CCFP; CCFP(E.M.); Staff, Abbotsford Regional Hospital & Cancer Centre; (604)851-4700

MARTIN, Isabel; Crowfoot Primary Care Centre, 201-60 Crowfoot Cres NW, Calgary AB T3G 3J9; Wes'00; CCFP; (403)374-0244; martin@cfpcn.ca.

MARTIN, Isabella L; Vancouver Gen Hosp, JPP2-855 12th Ave W, Vancouver BC V5Z 1M9; Mem'87; FRCPC; Anes. Staff, Vancouver General Hospital - Centennial Pavillion; Clinical Asst Prof, University of British Columbia; (604)875-4304

MARTIN, Isabelle M C; Clinique Med Plaza Gatineau, 381 boul Maloney E, Gatineau QC J8P 1E3; Sher'95; CCFP; Staff Palliative Care, Hôpital de Gatineau; Langs: English; (819)669-7393; Fax. (819)669-0077.

MARTIN, Jacques; CHSLD la Maree, 7015 boul Gouin E, Montreal QC H1E 5N2; Mon'59; (514)955-5229

MARTIN, Jacques; Clinique Med Boisbriand, 877 boul de la Grande-Allee, Boisbriand QC J7G 1W6; Mon'81; (450)437-4600; Fax. (450)437-7038.

MARTIN, Jacques; Clinique Dr Claude Malenfant, 100-1731 3e av, Val-d'Or QC J9P 1W3; Ott'75; (819)825-4560

MARTIN, James A; 88 Wentworth St S, Hamilton ON L8N 2Y9; Tor'77; FRCSC; Ophth (Vitreo Retinal Surgery). Ac Staff, St Joseph's Healthcare - Charlton Campus; (905)522-3563; Fax. (905)522-3564.

MARTIN, James G; Meakins Christie Labs, 3626 rue Saint-Urbain, Montreal QC H2X 2P2; Cork (Ireland)'73; Respir. Staff, McGill University Health Centre - Montreal Chest Institute; Respirology, McGill University Health Centre - Royal Victoria Hospital; Head Medicine(Interim), McGill University; Langs: French; (514)398-3864; Fax. (514)398-7483; james.martin@mcgill.ca.

MARTIN, James S B; Southern Ont Fertility Technol, 107-555 Southdale Rd E, London ON N6E 1A2; Wes'76; BSc(Hon); FRCSC; ObstGyn (Reproductive Endocrinology). Asst Prof, University of Western Ontario; (519)685-5559; Fax. (519)685-5519; drmartin@soft-infertility.com.

MARTIN, Jane E L; Grand River Hosp-Freeport HC, 3570 King St E, Kitchener ON N2A 2W1; Qns'95; CCFP; Staff, Grand River Hospital - Freeport Site; (519)749-4300

MARTIN, Jean; CSSS de la Matapedia, 135 av Gaetan-Archambault, Amqui QC G5J 2K5; Laval'92; MSc; BSc; Staff, CSSS de la Matapedia; (418)629-2211

MARTIN, Jennifer L; Saint John Reg Hosp, PO Box 2100 Stn Main, Saint John NB E2L 4L2; Dal'00; FRCPC; DiagRad; NuclearMed. Staff, Saint John Regional Hospital; (506)649-2648

MARTIN, Jocelyne; CHUM-Hop Notre-Dame, D 8051-1560 rue Sherbrooke E, Montreal QC H2L 4M1; Laval'92; FRCSC; GenSurg; ThorSurg. Staff, Centre Hospitalier l'Université de Montréal (CHUM) - Hôpital Notre-Dame; (514)890-8000 x26252; Fax. (514)412-7855.

MARTIN, John H; Dr Charles A Janeway Child HC, 4J378-300 Prince Philip Dr, St. John's NL A1B 3V6; Mem'04; Peds. Staff, Janeway Children's Health & Rehabilitation Centre; (709)777-4037

MARTIN, Joie C; 499 Oxford St E, London ON N5Y 3H8; Qns'95; CCFP; FCFP; (519)672-1495; Fax. (519)434-3048.

MARTIN, Josee; 160 rue Principale, Saint-Jacques NB E7B 1W4; Sher'03; CCFP; Staff, Hôpital regional d'Edmundston; Langs: Bilingual(French/English); (506)739-7708

MARTIN, Julie; Clinique Sante Jacques-Cartier, 200-1815 rue King O, Sherbrooke QC J1J 3M4; Sher'87; CCFP; FCFP; (819)565-7446; Fax. (819)565-7780.

MARTIN, Justin M E; Royal Jubilee Hosp, 1952 Bay St, Victoria BC V8R 1J8; Queen's (Ireland)'74; FRCPC; AnatPath. Staff Path, Royal Jubilee Hospital; (250)370-8739

MARTIN, Karen A; 253 James St, Bracebridge ON P1L 2C2; Wes'89; Staff, South Muskoka Memorial Hospital - Muskoka Algonquin Healthcare; (705)645-2281; Fax. (705)645-0057.

MARTIN, Keith L; Halton HCS Corp-Oakville, 327 Reynolds St, Oakville ON L6J 3L7; McG'89; CCFP; CCFP(E.M.); FCFP; Staff, Halton Healthcare Services Corporation - Oakville Site; (905)338-4618; Fax. (905)338-4616.

MARTIN, Keith O; Associate Med Clinic, PO Box 510, Slave Lake AB T0G 2A0; UBC'10; CCFP; (780)849-4155; Fax. (780)780-8494.

MARTIN, Kelly M; MUHC-Montreal Children's Hosp, 2300 rue Tupper, Montreal QC H3H 1P3; Tor'89; Staff, McGill University Health Centre - Montreal Children's Hospital; (514)421-4400

MARTIN, Kevin J F; Fern Tree Clinic, PO Box 550, Qualicum Beach BC V9K 1T1; Witwatersrand (South Africa)'02; MB BCh; (250)752-6568

MARTIN, Kim; Parkgate Med Centre, 220-3650 Mt Seymour Pky, North Vancouver BC V7H 2Y5; UBC'86; CCFP; FCFP; (604)929-8629; Fax. (604)929-7329.

MARTIN, Lawrence S; St Joseph's Mountain H Serv, PO Box 585 Stn Lcd 1 100 West 5th St, Hamilton ON L8N 3K7; McM'87; BA(Hon.); FRCPC; Psy (Anxiety Disorder). Clin Dir Head of Service Mood Disorder Prog, St Joseph's Healthcare Hamilton - West 5th Campus; V-Chair Education Dept of Psy & Behavioural Neurosciences, McMaster University; (905)575-6029

MARTIN, Lee Ann; BC Cancer Agency-Fraser Valley, 13750 96 Ave, Surrey BC V3V 1Z2; Ott'91; FRCPC; IntMed; MedOncol. Staff, BC Cancer Agency Fraser Valley Centre; (604)930-4064; Fax. (604)587-4312.

MARTIN, Lorne W; Halton HCS Corp-Oakville, 327 Reynolds St, Oakville ON L6J 3L7; Wes'82; CCFP; CCFP(E.M.); Med Dir Emerg Services/Chief of Staff, Halton Healthcare Services Corporation - Oakville Site; (905)338-4618; Fax. (905)338-4146.

MARTIN, Louise A; Diamond Head Med Clinic, PO Box 9200 Stn Main, Squamish BC V8B 0C1; Wes'76; CCFP; Staff, Squamish General Hospital / Hilltop House; (604)892-3544; Fax. (604)892-3542; adragon@telus.net.

MARTIN, Louise; Centre Med de Beauport, 737 av Royale, Quebec QC G1E 1Z1; Laval'76; Langs: English; (418)667-7114; Fax. (418)667-5843.

MARTIN, Luc P; Clin Gastroent Pierre-Boucher, 103-601 av Adoncour, Longueuil QC J4G 2M6; Sher'76; Gastroent (P.Q.). (450)647-2422

MARTIN, Lucie C; Montfort Hosp, 713 Montreal Rd, Ottawa ON K1K 0T2; Ott'99; BSc; FRCPC; DiagRad. Staff, Montfort Hospital; Langs: English; French; (613)746-4621

MARTIN, Lucile; Clinique Med La Pocatiere, 205-1200 6e Ave, La Pocatiere QC G0R 1Z0; Mon'72; Staff, Reseau Sante Kamouraska-Hôpital d'Anjou Inc; (418)856-4647; Fax. (418)856-3211.

MARTIN, Marcel; Saint John Regional Hosp, PO Box 2100 400 av Universite, Saint John NB E2L 4L2; Mon'67; GenSurg. Staff, Saint John Regional Hospital; (506)654-6724

MARTIN, Marie-Helene; MUHC-Montreal Gen Hosp, 1650 av Cedar, Montreal QC H3G 1A4; Laval'03; FRCPC; DiagRad. Staff, McGill University Health Centre - Montreal General Campus; (514)934-1934 x42566

MARTIN, Marina; Royal Alexandra Hosp, 10240 Kingsway NW, Edmonton AB T5H 3V9; Alb'73; Anes. Staff, Royal Alexandra Hospital; (780)735-4111

MARTIN, Markus C; Ellendale Med Bldg, 600-5845 ch de la Cote-des-Nei, Montreal QC H3S 1Z4; McG'74; FACOG; DAB; BSc(Hons Biochem); FRCSC; ObstGyn (Ambulatory General Gynecology). Consultant, Jewish Rehabilitation Hospital; Sr Staff Obst, Sir Mortimer B Davis Jewish General; Assoc Prof ObstGyn & Oncol, McGill University; Langs: English; French; (514)735-3122; Fax. (514)341-0588.

MARTIN, Martine; CSST Lanaudiere, CP 550 Succ Bureau-Chef 432 rue de Lanaudiere, Joliette QC J6E 7N2; Laval'88; (450)753-2600; Fax. (450)756-6832.

MARTIN, Mary M; 361 Waverley St, Ottawa ON K2P 0W4; Wes'64; FRCPC; Psy (Child & Adolescent Psychiatry). (613)233-7288

MARTIN, Matthew B; Lennox & Addington Gen Hosp, 8 Richmond Park Dr, Napanee ON K7R 2Z4; Ott'99; CCFP; Staff, Lennox & Addington County General Hospital; (613)354-3301

MARTIN, Michael L; St Paul's Hosp, 1081 Burrard St, Vancouver BC V6Z 1Y6; Alb'94; FRCPC; DiagRad. Staff, Providence Health Care - St Paul's Hospital; (604)806-8006

MARTIN, Michael; Glazier Med Centre, 11 Gibb St, Oshawa ON L1H 2J9; Tor'75; BASc; FAAOS; FRCSC; OrthSurg. Staff, Lakeridge Health - Bowmanville Site; Staff Section of OrthSurg, Lakeridge Health - Oshawa Site; Coroner, Durham Region; (905)579-1212; Fax. (905)579-1583.

MARTIN, Michel; Clinique Med Havre Sante, 521 boul Du Havre, Salaber-de-Valleyf QC J6S 4Z5; Mon'69; GenSurg. Staff, Centre Hospitalier Régional du Suroît; (450)371-6444; Fax. (450)371-8142.

MARTIN, Monique; COOP Sante TemiscaVie, 19 rue Dollard, Ville-Marie QC J9V 1L1; Laval'92; (819)622-2433

MARTIN, Montgomery A; BC Cancer Agency-Vancouver CC, 600 10th Ave W, Vancouver BC V5Z 4E6; Tor'83; FRCPC; DiagRad. Staff Radiol, BC Cancer Agency Vancouver Centre; (604)877-6000

MARTIN, Nancy M T; 100-5791 No. 3 Rd, Richmond BC V6X 2C9; UBC'06; DiagRad. (778)384-3907

MARTIN, Normand; Centre Med Sportive Laval, 3095 Autoroute Laval O, Laval QC H7P 4W5; Mon'88; Staff, Centre Hospitalier d'Argenteuil; Universite de Montreal; (450)688-5134

MARTIN, Paul B; 32 Collins Dr PO Box 642, Copper Cliff ON P0M 1N0; Tor'68; (705)682-0415

MARTIN, Perry M; Surrey Mem Hosp, 13750 96 Ave, Surrey BC V3V 1Z2; Xavier Univ (Aruba)'07; IntMed. Staff, Surrey Memorial Hospital; (604)581-2211

MARTIN, Pierre; Hopital Reg D'Edmundston, 275 Hebert Blvd, Edmundston NB E3V 4E4; Laval'70; Staff, Hôpital regional d'Edmundston; (506)739-2200 x2286; Fax. (506)735-4047.

MARTIN, Pierre; Ctr Hosp St-Joseph La Malbaie, PO Box 340 Succ Bureau-Chef 303 rue Saint-Etienne, La Malbaie QC G5A 1T8; Laval'63; Anes. Staff, Hôpital de la Malbaie; (418)665-1700

MARTIN, Pierre; Hotel-Dieu de Sorel, 400 av de l'Hotel-Dieu, Sorel-Tracy QC J3P 1N5; Mon'71; FICS; FACS; CSPQ; FRCS; FRCSC; GenSurg. Staff, Hôtel-Dieu de Sorel; Langs: Bilingual(English/French); (450)746-6000; pmartin012@sympatico.ca.

MARTIN, Pierre; Polyclinique Du Cap, 110-700 boul Thibeau, Trois-Rivieres QC G8T 7A1; Laval'83; Staff, CSSS de Maskinongé; Staff, Centre Hospitalier Regional de Trois-Rivieres; (819)373-4551; Fax. (819)373-6516.

MARTIN, Rachael D; 101-330 Festubert St, Duncan BC V9L 3S9; Cal'00; CCFP; (250)748-9000; Fax. (250)748-1299.

MARTIN, Rachel S C; St Michael's Hosp, 30 Bond St, Toronto ON M5B 1W8; Tor'05; FRCPC; Anes. Staff, St Michael's Hospital; (416)864-5071

MARTIN, Real; 8641 Av Chaumont, Anjou QC H1K 1N4; Mon'78; Staff, CSSS Saint-Leonard et Saint-Michel; (514)352-2482; Fax. (514)351-6866.

MARTIN, Rene F; Thames Valley FHT-Whitehills M, 1225 Wonderland Rd N, London ON N6G 2V9; Wes'87; CCFP; FCFP; Staff, St Joseph's Hospital - St Joseph's Health Care; (519)472-0040; Fax. (519)472-7732.

MARTIN, Rene; CHUS-Hop Fleurimont, 3001 12e Av N, Sherbrooke QC J1H 5N4; Sher'73; DABA; FRCPC; Anes (Pain Management). Staff, Centre Hospitalier Universitaire de Sherbrooke-Hopital Fleurimont; Chef Anes, Universite de Sherbrooke; Langs: English; (819)346-1110 x14403; Fax. (819)820-6413; rene.martin@usherbrooke.ca.

MARTIN, Richard A; Family Med Associates, 15-9701 84 Ave, Grande Prairie AB T8V 4Z8; Alb'91; CCFP; FCFP; (780)539-1193

MARTIN, Riley T; PO Box 21085 Rpo Co-Op Plaza, Grande Prairie AB T8V 6W7; Alb'10; CCFP.

MARTIN, Robert P; 698 7 Ave SW, Medicine Hat AB T1A 5C1; Dal'92; FRCSC; OrthSurg. Staff, Medicine Hat Regional Hospital; (403)526-0330; Fax. (403)526-9090.

MARTIN, Roderick D; 342 Pennywell Rd, St. John's NL A1E 1V9; Mem'88; FRCSC; OrthSurg (Adult Reconstructive Surgery). (709)726-4179

MARTIN, Rodney B; Radiology Associates, 1122 Scenic Dr S, Lethbridge AB T1K 7E5; Alb'77; FRCPC; DiagRad. (403)328-1122; Fax. (403)328-1218.

MARTIN, Ruth E; UBC School of Population & Pub, 157-2206 East Mall, Vancouver BC V6T 1Z3; UBC'79; CCFP; FCFP; Staff, BC Women's Hospital & Health Centre; Vis Staff, Vancouver General Hospital - Centennial Pavillion; (604)822-2496

MARTIN, Stephanie; UMF Charles Lemoyne, 201-299 boul Sir-Wilfrid-Lauri, Saint-Lambert QC J4R 2L1; Sher'98; LMCC; CCFP; Staff Geriatrics, Hopital Charles LeMoyne; (450)466-5630; Fax. (450)466-5631.

MARTIN, Stephen C; Roper Clinic, 4500 rue Sherbrooke O, Westmount QC H3Z 1E6; Tor'70; ABPM; MSc(Occup.Health); FCBOM; CCFP; ac Staff Family Med Group, McGill University Health Centre; adj Prof Biostatistics Epidemiol & Occup Health, McGill University; Langs: French; Italian; (514)937-8000; scmartin@sympatico.ca.

MARTIN, Steven A; Mayfair Place, 230-6707 Elbow Dr SW, Calgary AB T2V 0E4; Wes'87; FRCSC; GenSurg. (403)255-8744; Fax. (403)252-5773.

MARTIN, Steven E; Univ of Victoria Med Sciences, PO Box 1700 Stn CSC, Victoria BC V8W 2Y2; McM'87; MSc; FCBOM; LMCC; ABIME; BSc(Hon); Dip SportMed; Dir Clin Skills/Aj Associate Prof Div of Med Sciences Faculty of Educ & Faculty of Graduate Studies, University Of Victoria; Clin Assoc Prof, University Of British Columbia; (250)472-5500

MARTIN, Steven R; Alberta Children's Hosp, 2888 Shaganappi Trail NW, Calgary AB T3B 6A8; Cal'81; FRCPC; Peds (Pediatric Gastroenterology). Staff, Alberta Children's Hospital; (403)955-7721; Fax. (403)955-2922.

MARTIN, Stuart; 66 Charlton Ave W, Hamilton ON L8P 2C1; Qns'82; FRCSC; PlasSurg (Breasts). Ac Staff, Hamilton Health Sciences Centre - Hamilton General Hospital; Affil Staff, St Joseph's Healthcare - Charlton Campus; Clin Assoc Prof, McMaster University; Langs: French; Spanish; (905)572-6226; Fax. (905)572-6301.

MARTIN, Susanna M; Royal University Hosp, 103 Hospital Dr, Saskatoon SK S7N 0W8; McG'92; BSc; FAAP; FRCPC; Peds. Staff Peds, Royal University Hospital; Asst Prof, University of Saskatchewan; Langs: English; French; (306)966-8136; Fax. (306)966-8640.

MARTIN, Sylvie; AL 0701C-Sante Canada, 200 Tunney's Pasture Driveway, Ottawa ON K1A 0K9; Mon'83; Physician, Citizenship & Immigration Canada; (613)948-8524; sylvie.martin@cic.gc.ca.

MARTIN, Tara D; South Health Campus, 260180-4448 Front St SE, Calgary AB T3M 1M4; Alb'10; CCFP; (403)956-1111

MARTIN, Thomas C; Tsawwassen Med Clinic, 201-1077 56 St, Delta BC V4L 2A2; Sask'89; Staff, Richmond Hospital; Staff, Delta Hospital; (604)943-1131

MARTIN, Vickie J; Health Sciences Centre, 300 Prince Philip Dr, St. John's NL A1B 3V6; Mem'03; FRCSC; ObstGyn (Gynecologic Oncology). Staff, Health Sciences Centre; (709)777-6300

MARTIN, W R Wayne; Glenrose Rehabilitation Hosp, 10230 111 Ave NW, Edmonton AB T5G 0B7; Alb'75; FRCPC; Neur (Movement Disorders). Staff Movement Disorder Clinic, Glenrose Rehabilitation Hospital; Ac Staff, University of Alberta Hospital; Prof Neurol, University of Alberta; (780)735-8805; Fax. (780)735-8804.

MARTIN, William J; Miramichi Reg Hosp, 500 Water St, Miramichi NB E1V 3G5; Dal'80; CCFP; Staff, Miramichi Regional Hospital; (506)623-3348; Fax. (506)623-3347.

MARTIN, William O; HSC-Faculty of Med, 451A-3330 Hospital Dr NW, Calgary AB T2N 4N1; (Ireland)'75; MB ChB; BAO; FRCPC; IntMed; Rheum. Staff Rheumatologist, Foothills Medical Centre; Prof Med, University of Calgary; (403)220-7725; Fax. (403)283-5666.

MARTIN, Yolande; Dr Georges-L Dumont Reg Hosp, 330 av Universite, Moncton NB E1C 2Z3; Sher'01; CCFP; Staff, Dr Georges-L-Dumont University Hospital Centre; (506)862-4305

MARTIN-GODELIE, Robin S; Queensway Med Centre, 125 Queensway E, Simcoe ON N3Y 4M5; Wes'02; BSc; CCFP; Asst Clin Prof, McMaster University; (519)426-0911

MARTIN-SMITH, Paul; 2 Zina St, Orangeville ON L9W 1E1; Alb'75; ABIM; BSc; FRCPC; IntMed. Ac Staff, Headwaters Health Care Centre - Orangeville Site; (519)941-6659; Fax. (519)941-2503.

MARTIN WARD, Dawn-Marie L; Hôpital de CSC de Lamèque, 29 rue de l'Hopital, Lameque NB E8T 1C5; Mon'97; LMCC; CCFP; Staff, Hôpital de CSC de Lamèque; Langs: English; (506)344-2261; Fax. (506)344-3436; dmartin@reg6.health.nb.ca.

MARTINDALE, Michael E; Victoria Med Bldg, 304-1669 Victoria St, Prince George BC V2L 2L5; UBC'71; FRCPC; Derm. (250)562-8318; Fax. (250)562-5739.

MARTINEAU, Andre; Hôpital Laval, 2725 ch Sainte-Foy, Quebec QC G1V 4G5; Laval'75; FRCPC; Anes. Staff, Hôpital Laval; (418)656-4565; Fax. (418)656-4551.

MARTINEAU, Andre; Clinique privee, 227-655 prom du Centropolis, Laval QC H7T 0A3; Mon'88; Staff, Centre Hospitalier Laurentien; (514)316-1357

MARTINEAU, Bernard; CSSS-IUGS Sherbrooke, 1200 rue King E, Sherbrooke QC J1G 1E4; Laval'80; CCFP; FCFP; Staff, Centre Hospitalier Universitaire de Sherbrooke-Hopital Fleurimont; Langs: Bilingual(French/English); (819)780-2222

MARTINEAU, Catherine; UMF Charles Lemoyne, 201-299 boul Sir-Wilfrid-Lauri, Saint-Lambert QC J4R 2L1; Mon'06; CCFP; (450)466-5630; Fax. (450)466-5631.

MARTINEAU, France; CLSC de Disraeli, GD 245 rue Montcalm, Disraeli QC G0N 1E0; Laval'94; CCFP; Staff, Hôpital psychiatrique de Malartic; Physician, CLSC Malartic; Physician, CHSLD Villa St-Martin; (418)449-3513; france_martineau@ssss.gouv.qc.ca.

MARTINEAU, Francis; Hôpital régional Chaleur, 1750 Sunset Dr, Bathurst NB E2A 4L7; Laval'04; Staff, Hopital Regional Chaleur; (506)544-2316

MARTINEAU, Genevieve; Hotel-Dieu de Levis, 143 rue Wolfe, Levis QC G6V 3Z1; Laval'05; CCFP; CCFP(E.M.); Staff, Centre Hospitalier Beauce-Etchemin; Staff, Hôtel-Dieu de Lévis; (418)835-7121

MARTINEAU, Jean-Pierre; GMF de Lorraine, 99 boul De Gaulle, Lorraine QC J6Z 3Z9; Mon'78; CCFP; FCFP; Staff, Hopital de la Cite de la santé; (450)621-1444; Fax. (450)621-7193.

MARTINEAU, Louise; Institut ORL Montreal, 201-1361 av Beaumont, Mont-Royal QC H3P 2W3; Mon'76; CSPQ; Derm. (514)343-5244; Fax. (514)738-4668.

MARTINEAU, Marie E; Jeffery Hale Hosp-Saint Brigid, 1250 ch Sainte-Foy, Quebec QC G1S 2M6; Mon'88; Staff, Jeffery Hale Hospital-Saint Brigid's; (418)684-5333

MARTINEAU, Marie S; Centre Med Laval, 1110 boul Vanier, Laval QC H7C 2R8; Mon'87; Staff Obst, Hopital de la Cite de la santé; (450)661-2521; Fax. (450)661-7193.

MARTINEAU, Mario; Clinique Med Lavaltrie, 200-1400 rue Notre-Dame, Lavaltrie QC J5T 1M6; Sher'78; Staff, Centre Hospitalier Pierre le Gardeur; Langs: English; (450)586-2555; Fax. (450)586-4498.

MARTINEAU, Olivier; CSSS de la Haute-Yamaska, 205 boul Leclerc O, Granby QC J2G 1T7; Sher'98; FRCPC; Anes. Staff, Centre Hospitalier de Granby; (450)375-8000; Fax. (450)962-2701.

MARTINEAU, Paul A; MUHC-Montreal Gen Hosp, A5 175 1-1650 av Cedar, Montreal QC H3G 1A4; McG'00; FRCSC; OrthSurg (Sports Medicine). Staff, McGill University Health Centre - Montreal General Campus; Staff, Shriners Hospitals For Children - Canada; Langs: Bilingual(French/English); (514)934-1934 x42219

MARTINEAU CORBEIL, Elise; Institut Douglas, 6875 boul Lasalle, LaSalle QC H4H 1R2; McG'07; MDCM; (514)761-6131

MARTINEZ, Eddsel R; Sterling Lyon Health Centre, 401-1020 Lorimer Blvd, Winnipeg MB R3P 1C7; Man'03; FRCPC; Peds.

MARTINEZ, Jose A; Centre Hosp Pierre le Gardeur, 911 montee des Pionniers, Terrebonne QC J6V 2H2; Mon'99; FRCSC; Otol. Staff, Centre Hospitalier Pierre le Gardeur; Staff, Hôtel-Dieu de Saint-Jérôme; Langs: Spanish; French; (450)654-7525

MARTINEZ, Lionel G; 111-1525 Albion Rd, Etobicoke ON M9V 5G5; Tor'96; (416)783-2113

MARTINEZ, Luis A; 3201-4464 Markham St, Victoria BC V8Z 7X8; Bogota (Colombia)'65; MedMicrobiol. (250)881-3111 x2243

MARTINEZ, Raul R; Royal Oak Med Centre, 209-6440 Royal Oak Ave, Burnaby BC V5H 3P2; (Mexico)'74; Staff, Royal Columbian Hospital; (604)430-4144; Fax. (604)430-4155.

MARTINEZ, Ricardo L; Groupe Sante Physimed, 121-6363 Rte Transcanadienne, Saint-Laurent QC H4T 1Z9; Cuyo (Argentina)'73; (514)747-8888; Fax. (514)747-4705.

MARTINEZ-BELLART, Josette; CLSC Arthur-Buies, 430 rue Labelle, Saint-Jerome QC J7Z 5L3; Mon'76; (450)431-2221; Fax. (450)565-0133.

MARTINEZ CAJAS, Jorge L; Queen's University, 3007-94 Stuart St, Kingston ON K7L 3N6; Universidad Del Cauca (Colombia)'94; FRCPC; IntMed (Infectious Diseases). Asst Prof, Queen's University; (613)533-6000 x75471

MARTINEZ-GIRON, Fernando; Burntwood Comm Hlth Resource, 50 Selkirk Ave, Thompson MB R8N 0M7; (El Salvador)'82; (204)677-1769; Fax. (204)677-1758.

MARTINEZ MARIN, Jose Luis; Hôpital Ste-Justine, 3620-3175 Côte Sainte-Catherin, Montreal QC H3T 1C5; Antioquia(Colombia) (Colombia)'87; Staff, Hôpital Ste-Justine; Langs: English; Spanish; French; (514)345-4931

MARTINEZ MOTTA, Jose C; Coronation Med Centre, 3-695 Coronation Blvd, Cambridge ON N1R 7J9; Mexico (Mexico)'93; Staff Ped, Cambridge Memorial Hospital; Langs: Spanish; (519)624-9796

MARTINHO, Humberto; Citizenship & Immigration Cda, A304-365 Laurier Ave W, Ottawa ON K1A 1L1; Mem'88; CCFP; FCFP; Langs: Portuguese; French; (613)941-2625

MARTINHO, Valdemar; 401-595 Montreal Rd, Ottawa ON K1K 4L2; Ott'80; Langs: English; French; (613)741-1407; Fax. (613)741-7366.

MARTINIUK, Shauna O C; Mount Sinai Hosp, 206-600 University Ave, Toronto ON M5G 1X5; Tor'95; CCFP; CCFP(E.M.); Staff, Mount Sinai Hospital; (416)586-5058; Fax. (416)586-4719.

MARTINIUK KINGDON, Kris; The Sheddon Med Associates, 308-331 Sheddon Ave, Oakville ON L6J 1X8; Tor'93; BSc; CCFP; FCFP; Affil Staff, Halton Healthcare Services Corporation - Oakville Site; (905)845-8771; Fax. (905)845-8379.

MARTINKA, Grzegorz P; The Richmond Hosp, 7000 Westminster Hwy, Richmond BC V6X 1A2; Lublin (Poland)'86; FRCPC; IntMed; Critical Care Medicine. Staff, Richmond Hospital; Clin Researcher Critical Care Med Fellowship Prog, University of British Columbia; Langs: Polish; (604)244-4851; Fax. (604)278-5183.

MARTINKA, Magdalena; Vancouver Gen Hosp, 855 12th Ave W, Vancouver BC V5Z 1M9; Lublin (Poland)'86; FRCPC; AnatPath (Dermatological Pathology). Staff, Vancouver General Hospital - Centennial Pavillion; Clin Assoc Prof, University of British Columbia; Langs: Polish; (604)875-5555 x68227; Fax. (604)875-5707; magda.martinka@vch.ca.

MARTINO, Frank A; Queen Square Doctors FHT, 201-366 Main St N, Brampton ON L6V 1P8; Turin (Italy)'87; BSc; CCFP; CCFP(E.M.); FCFP; Dir Med Trainees/Chief Family Med, William Osler Health System - Brampton Civic Hospital; Asst Prof Family & Commun Med, University of Toronto; Clin Assoc Prof Family Med, McMaster University; Langs: Italian; (905)455-1331; Fax. (905)455-5498; dr.martino@sympatico.ca.

MARTINOVIC, Elaine C; Sunnybrook Hlth Sciences Ctre, MG 130B-2075 Bayview Ave, Toronto ON M4N 3M5; Cal'01; FRCPC; DiagRad. Staff, Sunnybrook Health Sciences Centre; (416)480-6100 x5862; Fax. (416)480-5855.

MARTINOVIC, Laurie A; Halton HCS Corp-Oakville, 327 Reynolds St, Oakville ON L6J 3L7; Qns'00; CCFP; Staff, Halton Healthcare Services Corporation - Oakville Site; (905)845-2571

MARTINS, Grace L; Avery Health Clinic, 31-665 Front St, Quesnel BC V2J 5J5; Man'95; BSc; MSc; CCFP; (250)992-8322; Fax. (250)992-1563.

MARTINS, Heidi; BC Cancer Agency-Vanc Isl Ctr, 2410 Lee Ave, Victoria BC V8R 6V5; Witwatersrand (South Africa)'76; MB ChB; FRCPC; IntMed (Lung Cancer); MedOncol. Staff, BC Cancer Agency Vancouver Island Centre; Staff, Vancouver Island Health Authority; Clin Instructor, University of British Columbia; (250)519-5570; Fax. (250)519-2017; hmartins@bccancer.bc.ca.

MARTINS, Isabel M; Leonard A Miller Centre, 712-100 Forest Rd, St. John's NL A1A 3Z9; Mem'84; FRCPC; Psy. (709)737-6717

MARTINS, Ivo P; 7040 Cheam Ave PO Box 159, Agassiz BC V0M 1A0; Pretoria (South Africa)'99; MB ChB; (604)703-2030

MARTINS, Rui F O; 203-565 College St, Toronto ON M6G 1B2; Tor'89; CCFP; FCFP; Staff, Women's College Hospital; University of Toronto; (416)538-6653; Fax. (416)538-9766.

MARTINS, Sandrew; Victoria Hosp, PO Box 3000 Stn Main 1200 24th St W, Prince Albert SK S6V 5T4; Pretoria (South Africa)'89; MB ChB; FRCSC; OrthSurg. Staff, Victoria Hospital; (306)953-8960

MARTINS GORRINDO, Anahi; 368 College St N PO Box 1260, Durham ON N0G 1R0; Buenos Aires (Argentina)'01; CCFP; (519)369-2510

MARTIQUET, Paul A; Vancouver Coastal Health, PO Box 78, Gibsons BC V0N 1V0; McG'85; MHSc; FRCPC; CommunMed. Staff Privil, St Mary's Hospital; Powell River General Hospital; Staff Privil, Squamish General Hospital / Hilltop House; Assoc Chief Med Health Officer, Vancouver Coastal Health; Clinical Asst Prof Med, University of British Columbia; (604)886-5620; Fax. (604)886-2250; paul.martiquet@vch.ca.

MARTOGLIO, Adelmo E; St Michael's Health Centre, 4F-61 Queen St E, Toronto ON M5C 2T2; Cordoba (Argentina)'66; FRCSC; ObstGyn. Staff, St Michael's Hospital; Asst Prof, University of Toronto; Langs: Spanish; Italian; (416)867-7480; Fax. (416)867-7478.

MARTON, Dominique; Radiologie Chomedey, 610 boul Cure Labelle, Laval QC H7V 2T7; Mon'64; DiagRad. (514)866-6622

MARTON, Monica E; PO Box 1282, Sechelt BC V0N 3A0; UBC'05; CCFP; (604)885-2384

MARTOSH, Anita M; Medical Clinic Bldg, 314-89 Humber College Blvd, Etobicoke ON M9V 4B8; Tor'89; Staff, William Osler Health System - Etobicoke General Hospital; (416)740-0255; Fax. (416)740-0655.

MARTOU, Glykerie; Sunnybrook Hlth Sciences Ctre, 2075 Bayview Ave, Toronto ON M4N 3M5; McM'03; FRCSC; PlasSurg. Staff, Sunnybrook Health Sciences Centre; (416)480-6868

MARTOW, Jeffrey; Markham Stouffville Health Ctr, 304-377 Church St, Markham ON L6B 1A1; McG'86; FRCSC; Ophth (Medical & Surgical Ophthalmology). Ac Staff, Markham Stouffville Hospital; Staff, North York General Hospital - Branson Division; Staff, St Michael's Hospital; (905)472-7360; Fax. (905)472-7148.

MARTUCCI, Giuseppe; MUHC-Royal Victoria Hosp, 4 38-687 av des Pins O, Montreal QC H3A 1A1; McG'97; FRCPC; IntMed; Cardiol. Staff, McGill University Health Centre - Royal Victoria Hospital; (514)934-1934

MARTYN, Lori E T; Oak Park Family Care Centre, 201 Oak Walk Dr, Oakville ON L6H 6M3; Qns'90.

MARTYN, Paul L; Foothills Med Centre, 1403 29 St NW, Calgary AB T2N 2T9; (Australia)'79; FRCOG; FRANZCOG; FRACS; ObstGyn (Endoscopic Surgery). Staff, Foothills Medical Centre; (403)944-1110; drmartynsoffice@telus.net.

MARTYNIAK, Dawid; London Intercommunity Hlth Ctr, 7-1355 Huron St, London ON N5V 1R9; Wes'10; CCFP; (519)659-6399

MARTZ, Laurie B; 1283 Nanaimo St, Vancouver BC V5L 4T5; Cal'84; Ac Staff, Vancouver General Hospital - Centennial Pavillion; (604)251-6313; Fax. (604)251-1311.

MARULLO, Carolle; Hop Louis-H Lafontaine, 118-7401 rue Hochelaga, Montreal QC H1N 3M5; Mon'91; FRCPC; Psy. Staff Psy, Hopital Louis-H Lafontaine; (514)251-4000; Fax. (514)251-4083.

MARUNCIC, Michael A; London HSC-Victoria Hosp, PO Box 5010 Stn B 800 Commissioners Rd E, London ON N6A 5W9; Wes'81; FRCSC; ObstGyn. Staff, St Joseph's Hospital - St Joseph's Health Care; Staff, London Health Sciences Centre - Victoria Campus; Asst Prof ObstGyn, University of Western Ontario; (519)685-8193

MARUSHAK, Karen L; Saskatoon East Fam Physicians, 21-2105 8th St E, Saskatoon SK S7H 0T8; Sask'80; (306)373-5500; Fax. (306)374-9414.

MARUSSI, Daphne R; 555 rue Murray, Sherbrooke QC J1G 2K8; (Brazil)'97; DPsy; adj Prof, Centre Hospitalier Universitaire de Sherbrooke-Hôpital Hôtel-Dieu; Langs: Portuguese; Bilingual(English/French); (819)346-1110 x25545; daphne.marussi@usherbrooke.ca.

MARVAL OSPINO, Heizer Jose; 255-5991 Spring Garden Rd, Halifax NS B3H 1Y6; Caracas (Venezuela)'03; FRCPC; Psy. (902)489-6752

MARWAHA, Avantika; 32-1960 Appleby Line, Burlington ON L7L 0B7; Ott'04; Gastroent; IntMed. Teach Staff, McMaster University; (905)335-1888

MARWAHA, Gulshan; St Thomas-Elgin Gen Hosp, PO Box 2007 Stn Main 189 Elm St, St Thomas ON N5P 3W2; North Bengal (India)'88; FRCPC; Anes. Staff, St Thomas Elgin General Hospital; (519)631-2020

MARWAHA, Seema; Univ Hlth Network-Toronto Gen, EN 4 214-200 Elizabeth St, Toronto ON M5G 2C4; Alb'08; FRCPC; IntMed. Staff, Toronto General Hospital - UHN; (416)340-4800

MARWOOD, Daniel C; Nanaimo Reg Gen Hosp, 1200 Dufferin Cres, Nanaimo BC V9S 2B7; UBC'90; Staff, Nanaimo Regional General Hospital; (250)754-2141

MARX, Theo; 900 Main St PO Box 1120, Swan River MB R0L 1Z0; Pretoria (South Africa)'77; Staff Chief, Swan River Valley Hospital; Langs: Afrikaans; (204)734-3812; Fax. (204)734-4597; theom@mts.net.

MARX, Yolanda; Kliniek on Main-PHC Team, 351 Main St N, Moose Jaw SK S6H 0W2; Pretoria (South Africa)'01; MB ChB; (306)694-1440; Fax. (306)693-9990; marxmedical@sasktel.net.

MARYNIARCZYK, Teresa P; Uptown Health Centre, 243 Eglinton Ave W, Toronto ON M4R 1B1; Lodz (Poland)'75; PhD(Poland); CCFP; Langs: Polish; (416)489-2106; Fax. (416)489-2981.

MARYNOWSKI, Bohdan; First Edmonton Place, 1295-10665 Jasper Ave NW, Edmonton AB T5J 3S9; Alb'65; FRCPC; Neur. Staff, Covenant Health - Misericordia Community Hospital; Staff, Covenant Health - Edmonton General Continuing Care Centre; Staff, University of Alberta Hospital; (780)424-6768; Fax. (780)426-6635.

MARZOUK, George; North York Gen Hosp, 4001 Leslie St, North York ON M2K 1E1; Sofia (Bulgaria)'74; Assoc Staff, North York General Hospital; (416)756-6002

MARZOUK, Nariman Z R; 229 1 St SW, Airdrie AB T4B 3L8; (Other Foreign)'02; CCFP; (403)948-3342

MARZOUK, Sherief E M; Univ Hlth Network-Toronto Western Hosp, 399 Bathurst St, Toronto ON M5T 2S8; Alexandria (Egypt)'99; Psy. Staff, Toronto Western Hospital - University Health Network; (416)603-5966

MARZOUKI, Monia S; Hôpital Ste-Justine, 3175 ch Cote-Dainte-Catherine, Montreal QC H3T 1C5; Staff, Hôpital Ste-Justine; (514)345-4931

MASANIC, Cheryl A; 550 University Ave, Toronto ON M5G 2A2; McM'93; FRCPC; PhysMed&Rehab. Staff, St Michael's Hospital; Staff, Toronto Rehabilitation Institute - University Centre; (416)597-3422 x3063; Fax. (416)597-3044.

MASATA, Hana S; Synergy Health Management, 106-3960 Quadra St, Victoria BC V8X 4A3; UBC'02; CCFP; (250)727-3737; Fax. (250)727-3732.

MASCAN, Lavinia M; Yorkdale Med Clinic, A103-11685 Yonge St, Richmond Hill ON L4E 0K7; Iasi (Romania)'00; CCFP; Langs: Romanian; (905)770-9057

MASCARENHAS, Lyndon; The Two Hundred, 101W-200 St Clair Ave W, Toronto ON M4V 1R1; Tor'84; ABIME; (416)960-1014

MASCARIN, Robert; Chamber of Commerce Bldg, 502-345 Lakeshore Rd E, Oakville ON L6J 1J5; Qns'80; CCFP; CCFP(E.M.); Ac Staff, Halton Healthcare Services Corporation - Oakville Site; (905)845-4511; Fax. (905)845-8133; rmascarin@cogeco.ca.

MASCHER, Karl H; Lillooet Med Clinic PO Box 850, Lillooet BC V0K 1V0; Innsbruck (Austria)'83; MD; Fam Med/Anesthesia, Lillooet District Hospital; Langs: German; (250)256-7505; Fax. (250)256-7591.

MASCIA, Anthony T; Humber River Reg Hosp-Church, 200 Church St, Toronto ON M9N 1N8; Tor'90; FRCPC; DiagRad. Staff, Humber River Regional Hospital - Church Street Site; (416)744-2500

MASE, Robert M; Burrard Health Bldg, 301-1160 Burrard St, Vancouver BC V6Z 2E8; UBC'80; FRCPC; IntMed; Endocrin&Metab. (604)681-3501; Fax. (604)681-4508.

MASEKA, Dereck; Drumheller Assoc Physicians, PO Box 5600 140 Riverside Drive E, Drumheller AB T0J 0Y0; Lusaka (Zambia)'86; MB ChB; FRACGP; BSc; CCFP; Clin Lecturer, University of Calgary; Langs: Lunda; Swazi; Zulu; (403)823-3345; Fax. (403)823-7823.

MASEKOAMENG, Ramatsiele; Hudson Bay Med Group, PO Box 1170, Hudson Bay SK S0E 0Y0; BSc; MB ChB; (306)865-2238; Fax. (306)865-2074.

MASELLIS, Antony; 201-5293 Highway 7, Markham ON L3P 7M7; Bologna (Italy)'75; Staff, The Scarborough Hospital - Birchmount Campus; Staff, Markham Stouffville Hospital; Staff, Rouge Valley Health System - Centenary Health Centre Site; Langs: Italian; (905)294-8011; Fax. (905)294-8153.

MASELLIS, Mario; Sunnybrook Hlth Sciences Ctre, A442-2075 Bayview Ave, Toronto ON M4N 3M5; Tor'01; FRCPC; Neur. Staff Neurol, Sunnybrook Health Sciences Centre; Langs: Italian; (416)480-4551

MASER, Joel E; Balmoral Med Arts Facility, 410-1366 Yonge St, Toronto ON M4T 3A7; Ott'70; FRCPC; IntMed (Geriatric Medicine). Ac Staff, Sunnybrook Health Sciences Centre - Holland Orthopaedic & Arthritic Centre; Ac Staff, Toronto Rehabilitation Institute - University Centre; Consultant, The Scarborough Hospital - General Campus; Consultant, The Scarborough Hospital - Birchmount Campus; Langs: English; French; (416)964-2220; Fax. (416)964-5649.

MASETTO, Ariel R; CHUS-Hopital Hotel-Dieu, 580 rue Bowen S, Sherbrooke QC J1G 2E8; Sao Paulo (Brazil)'96; Staff, Centre Hospitalier Universitaire de Sherbrooke-Hopital Fleurimont; Staff, Centre Hospitalier Universitaire de Sherbrooke-Hôpital Hôtel-Dieu; Langs: Bilingual(English/French); (819)346-1110 x15808

MASGORET, John C; 203-565 College St, Toronto ON M6G 1B2; Tor'94; CCFP; FCFP; Ac Staff, Toronto Rehabilitation Institute - University Centre; Court Staff, Toronto General Hospital - UHN; Langs: Spanish; Portuguese; (416)538-6653; Fax. (416)538-9766.

MASHAL, Orly H; Clinique Enfant-Medic, 3221 boul des Sources, Dollard-D-Ormeaux QC H9B 1Z6; McG'85; DCH; Langs: English; French; (514)685-0880; Fax. (514)685-6162.

MASHOUF-FARD, Mahsa; Yorkdale Med Clinic, A103-11685 Yonge St, Richmond Hill ON L4E 0K7; Tehran (Iran)'00; CCFP.

MASI, Ralph; 406-1017 Wilson Ave, North York ON M3K 1Z1; Man'74; CCFP; FCFP; Ac Staff, Humber River Regional Hospital - Church Street Site; Asst Prof Med, University of Toronto; Langs: Italian; (416)638-7288; Fax. (416)638-6076; ralph.masi@utoronto.ca.

MASIH, Robert J; Notre Dame Med Centre, 430 Notre Dame Ave, Sudbury ON P3C 5K7; Tor'85; Staff, Health Sciences North - Memorial Site; Staff, Health Sciences North-St Joseph's Health Centre; Staff, Health Sciences North-Laurentian Site; (705)671-9797; Fax. (705)671-2992.

MASIOWSKI, A Paul; 112-3502 Taylor St E, Saskatoon SK S7H 5H9; Qns'05; FRCPC; Neur. (306)244-8002; Fax. (306)244-8012.

MASKALL, Douglas D; Peace Arch Hosp, 15521 Russell Ave, White Rock BC V4B 2R4; UBC'91; FRCPC; Psy (Child & Adolescent Psychiatry). Consultant Psy, Peace Arch Hospital; Clinical Asst Prof, University of British Columbia; (604)541-7171; Fax. (604)538-8500.

MASKALYK, Milton J; St Michael's Hosp, 30 Bond St, Toronto ON M5B 1W8; Cal'99; FRCPC; EmergMed. Staff, St Michael's Hospital; (416)864-5095

MASKENS, Peter D; Alexander Prof Bldg, 205-849 Alexander Crt, Peterborough ON K9J 7H8; Tor'81; FRCSC; ObstGyn (Ultrasound). Chief ObstGyn, Peterborough Regional Health Centre - Hospital Drive; Queen's University; (705)741-5510; Fax. (705)741-0448.

MASKERINE, Courtney R; Queen's University, 70 Barrie St, Kingston ON K7L 3J7; Ott'09; CCFP.

MASKEY, Jean M; Royal Jubilee Hosp, 1952 Bay St, Victoria BC V8R 1J8; Dal'83; CCFP; FCFP; Staff, Royal Jubilee Hospital; (250)370-8111

MASLANY, Jurgen G; Regina Qu'Appelle HR-Regina, 1440 14th Ave, Regina SK S4P 0W5; Sask'01; FRCPC; Anes. Staff, Regina General Hospital; (306)766-4444

MASLIYAH, Tamara N; Queensway-Carleton Hosp, 3045 Baseline Rd, Ottawa ON K2H 8P4; Alb'05; FRCPC; Psy. Staff, Queensway Carleton Hospital; (613)721-2000

MASLO, Nestor E; Meadowlark Health Centre, 200 Meadowlark Shopping Ctr NW, Edmonton AB T5R 5W9; Alb'77; FRCPC; DiagRad. Staff, Covenant Health - Misericordia Community Hospital; University of Alberta; (780)489-5313; Fax. (780)489-5160.

MASLOVE, David M; Mackenzie Richmond Hill Hosp, 10 Trench St, Richmond Hill ON L4C 4Z3; Tor'04; FRCPC; IntMed; Critical Care Medicine. Staff, Mackenzie Richmond Hill Hospital; (905)883-1212

MASLOW, Kenny D; St Boniface Gen Hosp, 409 Tache Ave, Winnipeg MB R2H 2A6; Man'99; FRCSC; ObstGyn. Staff, St Boniface General Hospital; (204)233-8563

MASLOWSKI, Aleksander; Community Nursing Home, 1955 Valley Farm Rd, Pickering ON L1V 3R6; Bialystok (Poland)'75; CCFP; Staff, Lakeridge Health - Oshawa Site; Staff, Extendicare Oshawa; Langs: Polish; Russian; (905)831-2522

MASNYK, Robert D; Lakeshore Health Centre, 201-589 Lake St, St Catharines ON L2N 7L6; Tor'97; FRCSC; OrthSurg. (905)646-7650; Fax. (905)646-5671.

MASON, Alicia A J; PO Box 23115 Rpo Citadel, St. Albert AB T8N 6Z9; Cal'03; CCFP.

MASON, Andrew C; Ridge Meadows Hosp & Hlth CC, 11666 Laity St, Maple Ridge BC V2X 5A3; Cambridge (England)'83; MRCP(UK); FRCR; FRCPC; DiagRad. Staff Radiol, Ridge Meadows Hospital & Health Care Centre; (604)463-4111; Fax. (604)463-1879.

MASON, Andrew L; Katz-Rexall Centre, 7142J-1A University Campus NW, Edmonton AB T6G 2E1; (England)'83; MB BS; MRCP; (780)492-8176; andrew.mason@ualberta.ca.

MASON, Anna J; University Plaza Fam Practice, 200-3994 Shelbourne St, Victoria BC V8N 3E2; Tor'99; BSc(Hon); CCFP; (250)477-7100; Fax. (250)477-4135; anna.mason@utoronto.ca.

MASON, Cheryl R; 5277 224 St, Langley BC V2Y 2M2; UBC'84; (604)534-1421

MASON, Christa; Workers Comp Board of MB, 333 Broadway, Winnipeg MB R3C 4W3; Man'90; Staff, Workers' Comp Board of MB.

MASON, Christine R; 402-301 14 St NW, Calgary AB T2N 2A1; Tor'49; DABPN; FRCPC; Psy (Geriatric Psychiatry). (403)571-2480; christine.mason@calgaryhealthregion.ca.

MASON, Cindy A; Total Cardiology, 201-803 1 Ave NE, Calgary AB T2E 7C5; Dal'03; FRCPC; IntMed; Cardiol. Staff, Foothills Medical Centre; (403)571-8600; Fax. (403)215-2214.

MASON, James I A; 65 Dundas St E, Belleville ON K8N 1B9; Tor'80; CCFP; FCFP; Coroner, Province of Ontario; (613)966-7144; Fax. (613)966-3878.

MASON, Joan E; Centre Med Mira, 1560 boul de Rome, Brossard QC J4W 3A1; Ott'77; Physician Occup Health, CLSC des Faubourgs & CLSC des Seigneuries & Phys., Bank of Canada; Langs: English; French; (450)466-1880

MASON, Karen E; Murrayville Family Practice, 204-22112 52 Ave, Langley BC V2Y 2M6; Man'78; Ac Staff, Langley Memorial Hospital; (604)533-1140; Fax. (604)533-1159.

MASON, Lou E; Balmoral Med Arts Facility, 309-1366 Yonge St, Toronto ON M4T 3A7; Case Western(OH) (USA)'71; CCFP; FCFP; Ac Staff, Women's College Hospital; (416)966-3061; Fax. (416)966-3095.

MASON, Melanie P; Seymour Med Clinic, 200-1530 7th Ave W, Vancouver BC V6J 1S3; Ott'95; BSc; CCFP; FCFP; (604)739-5614

MASON, Robert B; Royal Victoria Hosp, 201 Georgian Dr, Barrie ON L4M 6M2; Tor'92; BASc; FRCPC; DiagRad (Interventional Radiology). Ac Staff, Royal Victoria Regional Health Centre; Court Staff, Georgian Bay General Hospital - Midland; (705)728-9802; Fax. (705)739-5629.

MASON, Robin L D; Acne Treatment Clinic, 412-4190 Finch Ave E, Scarborough ON M1S 4T7; Witwatersrand (South Africa)'72; (416)754-4545

MASON, Stephanie A; Copeman Health Care Centre, 440-628 12 Ave SW, Calgary AB T2R 0H6; Cal'82; FRCPC; Psy. Clin Instructor, University of Calgary; (403)270-2273; Fax. (403)521-2250.

MASON, Warren P; Univ Hlth Network-Princess M, 18 717-610 University Ave, Toronto ON M5G 2M9; Tor'87; FRCPC; IntMed (Neuro Oncology); Neur. Staff, Princess Margaret Hospital - University Health Network; University of Toronto; (416)946-2277; Fax. (416)946-2284; warren.mason@uhn.on.ca.

MASON, William F; 1664 Robie St, Halifax NS B3H 3E7; Dal'61; FACR; DiagRad. Staff Radiol, Miramichi Regional Hospital; Assoc Prof Radiol, Dalhousie University; (902)422-5256; Fax. (902)423-5679.

MASOOD, Ali K; Thunder Bay Reg HSC-T-Bay, 980 Oliver Rd, Thunder Bay ON P7B 6V4; St George's (Grenada)'03; Staff, Thunder Bay Regional Health Sciences Centre; (807)684-6000

MASOOD, Amna; Chatham-Kent Hlth Alliance, PO Box 2030 Stn Main 80 Grand Ave W, Chatham ON N7M 5L9; Punjab (Pakistan)'86; FRCPC; Anes. Staff, Chatham-Kent Health Alliance; (519)352-6400

MASOOD, Asim; William Osler HC-Brampton, 2100 Bovaird Dr E, Brampton ON L6R 3J7; UBC'97; Staff/Chief Staff, William Osler Health System - Etobicoke General Hospital; (905)494-2110

MASOOD, Khaja M; Thunder Bay Med Centre, 370-63 Algoma St N, Thunder Bay ON P7A 4Z6; Osmania (India)'61; FRCP; FRCPC; IntMed (Cardiology); NuclearMed. Langs: Urdu; (807)345-2113; Fax. (807)345-2114.

MASOOD, Mujaddid; Quinte HC Corp-Belleville Gen, 265 Dundas St E, Belleville ON K8N 5A9; Karachi (Pakistan)'85; MB; BSc; FRCPC; IntMed. Staff, QHC Belleville General; (613)969-7400

MASOOD, Syed F; 203-4383 Portage Rd, Niagara Falls ON L2E 6A6; Karachi (Pakistan)'03; MB BS; Staff, Niagara Health System - Greater Niagara General Site; (905)357-3988; Fax. (905)357-0968.

MASOOD, Zahida; Kingsbridge Med Centre, 5-20 Kingsbridge Garden Cir, Mississauga ON L5R 3K7; Osmania (India)'65; MB BS; CCFP; Langs: Urdu; Hindi; (905)507-1111; Fax. (905)890-7102; zama@sympatico.ca.

MASOUD, Ibtisam A R; Winnipeg Clinic, 425 St Mary Ave, Winnipeg MB R3C 0N2; Al Fateh (Libya)'99; ObstGyn.

MASOUDI, Hamid; St Paul's Hosp, 1081 Burrard St, Vancouver BC V6Z 1Y6; Isfahan (Iran)'92; FRCPC; GenPath. Staff, Providence Health Care - St Paul's Hospital; (604)682-2344 x63046

MASOUMI-RAVANDI, Mashallah; Hilden Med Clinic, RR 1 1174 Highway 2, Brookfield NS B0N 1C0; St George's (Grenada)'95; MB BS; CCFP.

MASRI, Bassam A; Gordon & Leslie Diamond HCC, 3F-2775 Laurel St, Vancouver BC V5Z 1M9; UBC'88; FRCSC; OrthSurg (Hip & Knee Reconstruction). Hd OrthSurg, Vancouver General Hospital - Centennial Pavillion; Prof/Dept Head & School Dir Orthopaedics, University of British Columbia; (604)875-5767

MASRI, Khalil; Polyclinique Med Concorde, 225-300 boul de la Concorde E, Laval QC H7G 2E6; Mon'86; FRCSC; OrthSurg (Knee Surgery). Ac Staff, Hopital de la Cite de la santé; (450)668-3840; Fax. (450)668-1157.

MASRI, Rogy O; Southlake Reg Health Centre, 596 Davis Dr, Newmarket ON L3Y 2P9; (Mexico)'03; CCFP; Staff, Southlake Regional Health Centre; Staff, Sunnybrook Health Sciences Centre; (905)954-3037

MASRI, Rola; 1100-1090 Pender St W, Vancouver BC V6E 2N7; Beirut (Lebanon)'91; (604)669-8188

MASRI, Sam; Oakland Associates, 6-315 Avenue Rd, Toronto ON M4V 2H2; San Pedro (Dominican Republic)'85; FRCPC; Psy. (416)972-9273

MASSA, Noah; 202-3607 31 St, Vernon BC V1T 5J4; UBC'99; FRCSC; Otol. (250)545-5433

MASSAAD, Viviane; Lakeridge Hlth Corp-Oshawa, 1 Hospital Crt, Oshawa ON L1G 2B9; Sher'94; FRCPC; DiagRad. Staff, Lakeridge Health - Oshawa Site; (905)433-4305; Fax. (905)721-4770.

MASSABKI, R Albert Y; Lakeridge Hlth Corp-Oshawa, 1 Hospital Court, Oshawa ON L1G 2B9; Cairo (Egypt)'84; FRCPC; Psy (Child & Adolescent Psychiatry). Staff Child & Youth Family Prog, Lakeridge Health - Oshawa Site; Langs: French; Arabic; (905)433-4345; Fax. (905)721-4881.

MASSAC, Charles-Henri; Clinique de Med Industrielle, 3-1665 rue Sainte-Catherine O, Montreal QC H3H 1L9; (Haiti)'57; FRCPC; Psy. (514)931-0801

MASSAD, Joseph; Ashdale Med Centre, 1566 Queen St E, Toronto ON M4L 1E9; Tor'88; CCFP; Langs: Bilingual(English/French); (416)469-5338; Fax. (416)469-1175.

MASSAM, Joanna L; Clairhurst Pediatrics, 201-1466 Bathurst St, Toronto ON M5R 3S3; McG'04; FRCPC; Peds; Respir. Staff, The Hospital For Sick Children; Langs: Bilingual(English/French); (416)531-3331; Fax. (416)531-1639.

MASSARELLA, Calum R; St Joseph's Healthcare, 50 Charlton Ave E, Hamilton ON L8N 4A6; Wes'90; FRCPC; EmergMed. Staff Emerg, St Joseph's Healthcare - Charlton Campus; (905)522-1155 x3112

MASSARELLI, Elizabeth A; Tantramar Commun Health Centre, l-2 Main St, Sackville NB E4L 4A3; Dal'85; CCFP; FCFP; Ac Staff GP Obstetrics, Cumberland Regional Health Care Center; Ac Staff, Sackville Memorial Hospital; Langs: English; French; (506)536-0210; Fax. (506)536-0761.

MASSE, Andre; 100-235 boul René-Lévesque E, Montreal QC H2X 1N8; Mon'74; FRCSC; ObstGyn. Chef obst & gynécol, Centre Hospitalier l'Université De Montréal (CHUM) - Hôpital Saint-luc; Clin Prof ObstGyn, Universite de Montreal; (514)866-2446; Fax. (514)866-4013; andre.masse@umontreal.ca.

MASSE, Andre P M; Hop Riviere-des-Prairies, 7070 boul Perras, Montreal QC H1E 1A4; Mon'66; Psy (P.Q.) (Autism). Dir-Clinic, Hôpital Riviere des Prairies; Universite de Montreal; Langs: English; (514)323-7260 x2667; Fax. (514)323-3286; massepm@videotron.ca.

MASSE, Caroline; Campbellton Reg Hosp, PO Box 880 Snt Main 189 Lily Lake Rd, Campbellton NB E3N 3H3; Sher'04; Staff, Hôpital Régional Campbellton; (506)789-5000

MASSE, Edith; CHUS-Hop Fleurimont, 3001 12e av N, Sherbrooke QC J1H 5N4; Laval'02; FRCPC; Peds (Neonatal & Perinatal Medicine). Staff, Centre Hospitalier Universitaire de Sherbrooke-Hopital Fleurimont; (819)346-1110 x14634

MASSE, Edith; CSSS de Chicoutimi, 305 rue Saint-Vallier, Chicoutimi QC G7H 5H6; Laval'93; FRCPC; Anes. Staff, Complexe hospitalier de la Sagamie; (418)541-1000

MASSE, Hugo; Ctr Hosp Laurentien, 234 rue Saint-Vincent, Ste-Agathe-Des-Mts QC J8C 2B8; Mon'93; Staff, Centre Hospitalier Laurentien; (819)324-4000; Fax. (514)843-2791.

MASSE, Isabelle; Clinique Med de l'Or, 228 2e rue E, La Sarre QC J9Z 2G9; Mon'03; Staff, Centre Hospitalier La Sarre; (819)339-5617

MASSE, Jacques; Ctr Hosp Affilie-Enfant-Jesus, 1401 18e rue, Quebec QC G1J 1Z4; Laval'85; MSc(ExpMed.); FRCPC; MedBiochem. assoc Membre, Centre de santé des Côté-Nord; Staff, Centre Hospitalier Affilié Universitaire de Québec - Hôpital De L'Enfant Jésus; Langs: English; (418)649-0252

MASSE, Janick; CSSS de Laval, 1755 boul Rene-Laennec, Laval QC H7M 3L9; Sher'92; FRCPC; AnatPath. Staff, Hopital de la Cite de la santé; (450)668-1010

MASSE, Julie; CSSS de la Vallée de l'Or, 725 6e rue, Val-d'Or QC J9P 3Y1; Mon'07; CCFP; Staff, Centre Hospitalier de Val d'Or; (819)825-6711; Fax. (819)825-7919.

MASSE, Lise; Clin Med du Faubourg de Mt-St-, 208-468 boul Sir-Wilfrid-Lauri, Mont-Saint-Hilaire QC J3H 6K3; Sher'00; Staff, Centre d hebergement de l Hôtel-Dieu de Saint-Hyacinthe; (450)813-9222

MASSE, Lyne; A-1490 rue Arthur-Forget, Carignan QC J3L 6X7; Mon'77; (450)658-0590

MASSE, Lyne; Centre Med Saint-Francois, 200-2125 boul Lemire, Drummondville QC J2B 8N8; Sher'88; assoc Staff, Hôpital Sainte-croix; (819)477-6793; Fax. (819)477-6962.

MASSE, Marie-Soleil; CHUM-Hop Notre-Dame, 1560 rue Sherbrooke E, Montreal QC H2L 4M1; Mon'03; FRCPC; IntMed; ClinImmunol&Allergy. Staff, Centre Hospitalier l'Université de Montréal (CHUM) - Hôpital Notre-Dame; (514)890-8231

MASSE, Melanie; CHUS-Hop Fleurimont, 3001 12e Av N, Sherbrooke QC J1H 5N4; Sher'94; Nephrol; IntMed (Hemodialysis). Staff Nephrol, Centre Hospitalier Universitaire de Sherbrooke-Hopital Fleurimont; Prof, Universite de Sherbrooke; (819)346-1110 x15221; Fax. (819)564-5269; melanie.masse@usherbrooke.ca.

MASSE, Michel; Clinique Med Sorel-Tracy, 330 av de l'Hotel-Dieu, Sorel-Tracy QC J3P 1N4; Ott'72; (450)742-9459; Fax. (450)742-9450.

MASSE, Michel; CSSS Antoine-Labelle, 757 rue de la Madone, Mont-Laurier QC J9L 1T3; Mon'77; Staff, CSSS d'Antoine-Labelle; (819)623-1228; Fax. (819)623-1311.

MASSE, Michele-Elaine; CSSS Pierre Boucher, 1333 boul Jacques-Cartier E, Longueuil QC J4M 2A5; Mon'07; FRCPC; Anes. Staff, Centre Hospitalier Pierre Boucher; (450)468-8111

MASSE, Nicholas; Clinique de Chirurgie du Litto, 111-822 boul Sainte-Anne, Rimouski QC G5M 1J5; Sher'96; FRCSC; OrthSurg. Staff, Hôpital Regional Rimouski; (418)723-0194

MASSE, Richard; Dir de la Sante Publique de Mt, 1301 rue Sherbrooke E, Montreal QC H2L 1M3; Sher'76; FRCPC; CommunMed. Staff, Hôpital Regional Rimouski; Pres, Institut National de Sante Publique du Quebec; Staff, Direction de la Sante Publique de Montreal; Langs: English; (514)528-2400

MASSE, Robert; CSSS de Mempremagog, 50 rue Saint-Patrice E, Magog QC J1X 3X3; Sher'74; Staff, Centre Hospitalier et CLSC de Memphremagog; (819)843-3381; Fax. (819)843-8902.

MASSE, Sylvain; 10 av Village PO Box 870 Stn Main, Campbellton NB E3N 3H3; Mon'81; Staff, Hôpital Régional Campbellton; Langs: Bilingual(French/English); (506)789-0991; Fax. (506)789-7641.

MASSE, Vincent; Hop Maisonneuve-Rosemont, 5415 boul de l'Assomption, Montreal QC H1T 2M4; Mon'04; FRCSC; OrthSurg. Staff, Hopital Maisonneuve-Rosemont; (514)835-2784; Fax. (514)373-5834.

MASSE, Yanick N R; Montfort Hosp, 713 Montreal Rd, Ottawa ON K1K 0T2; Ott'05; CCFP; CCFP(E.M.); Staff, Montfort Hospital; Langs: Bilingual(English/French); (613)748-4621

MASSE MARTEL, Felix; Hotel-Dieu de Levis, 143 rue Wolfe, Levis QC G6V 3Z1; Mon'07; Anes. Staff, Hôtel-Dieu de Lévis; (418)835-7121

MASSEL, David R; London HSC-University Hosp, PO Box 5339 Stn B C6 119-339 Windermere Rd, London ON N6A 5A5; Wes'83; FRCPC; IntMed; Cardiol. Staff, London Health Sciences Centre - University Hospital; (519)685-8500 x33482; Fax. (519)434-3278.

MASSELINK, William S; 38140 Behrner Dr, Squamish BC V8B 0J3; Dublin (Ireland)'06; (604)892-5211

MASSEY, Andrea; Crossroads Obstetrics & Gyn, 330-507 Broadway W, Vancouver BC V5Z 1E6; McG'07; MDCM; FRCPC; ObstGyn. Staff, Providence Health Care - St Paul's Hospital; (604)872-5484

MASSEY, Ephraim G; Clinique Med Priorite, 2111 av Northcliffe, Montreal QC H4A 3K6; McG'75; Langs: German; French; Spanish; (514)482-3311; Fax. (514)482-3492.

MASSEY, Simon R; Children's & Women's HC of BC, 4480 Oak St, Vancouver BC V6H 3V4; Wales (England)'84; MB BCh; FRCPC; Anes. Staff, BC Children's Hospital; (604)875-2158

MASSICOTTE, Caroline; Clinique Sante Jacques-Cartier, 200-1815 rue King O, Sherbrooke QC J1J 2E3; Sher'10; CCFP; (819)565-7446

MASSICOTTE, Claude J; 401-11 Rosemount Ave, Ottawa ON K1Y 4R8; Laval'72; FRCPC; IntMed; Gastroent (P.Q.). Ac Member, The Ottawa Hospital - General Campus; Langs: Bilingual(English/French); (613)728-6411; Fax. (613)728-7493.

MASSICOTTE, Eric M; Univ Hlth Network-Toronto Western Hosp, 4WW 447-399 Bathurst St, Toronto ON M5T 2S8; Ott'95; BSc; MSc; FRCSC; Neursurg. Staff, Toronto Western Hospital - University Health Network; Staff, The Hospital For Sick Children; University of Toronto; Langs: Bilingual(French/English); (416)603-5675; Fax. (416)603-5298; eric.massicotte@uhn.on.ca.

MASSICOTTE, Frederic; CHUM-Hopital Notre-Dame, 1560 rue Sherbrooke E, Montreal QC H2L 4M1; Mon'06; Rheum; IntMed. Staff, Centre Hospitalier l'Université de Montréal (CHUM) - Hôpital Notre-Dame; (514)890-8000

MASSICOTTE, Guy; CLSC Temiscouata, RR 1 101-33 rue Saint-Laurent, Cabano QC G0L 1E0; Mon'82; Staff, Centre Hospitalier Notre-Dame-du-Lac; (418)854-2572

MASSICOTTE, Josee; Direction de la Sante Publique, 1255 rue Beauregard, Longueuil QC J4K 2M3; Mon'86; (450)928-6777

MASSICOTTE, Luc; Chum-Hop St-Luc, 1058 rue Saint-Denis, Montreal QC H2X 3J4; Mon'81; Anes (P.Q.). Staff, Centre Hospitalier l'Université De Montréal (CHUM) - Hôpital Saint-luc; (514)890-8000

MASSICOTTE, Marie-Helene; Hop Du Sacre-Coeur De Mtl, 5400 boul Gouin O, Montreal QC H4J 1C5; Mon'05; FRCPC; IntMed; Endocrin&Metab. Staff, Hôpital du Sacre-Coeur de Montréal; (514)338-2222

MASSICOTTE, Mary P; Edmonton Clinic Health Academy, 3 539-11405 87 Ave NW, Edmonton AB T6G 1C9; McM'86; MSc; FRCPC; Peds (Thrombosis). Staff Peter Olley Endowed Chair, University of Alberta Hospital; Prof Peds, University of Alberta; (780)248-5595

MASSICOTTE, Nathalie; CHUM-Hop Notre-Dame, 1560 rue Sherbrooke E, Montreal QC H2L 4M1; Mon'97; FRCPC; Anes. Staff, Centre Hospitalier l'Université de Montréal (CHUM) - Hôpital Notre-Dame; (514)890-8000

MASSIE, Dani H; Ctr Hosp de Verdun, 4000 boul Lasalle, Verdun QC H4G 2A3; Sher'05; FRCSC; OrthSurg. Staff, Centre Hospitalier de Verdun; (514)362-1000

MASSIE, Rami; Hop du Sacre-Coeur de Mtl, 5400 boul Gouin O, Montreal QC H4J 1C5; McG'03; FRCPC; Neur. Staff, Hôpital du Sacre-Coeur de Montréal; (514)338-2222

MASSOEURS, Steven J; Professional Arts Bldg, 414-100 Arden St, Moncton NB E1C 4B7; Dal'91; FRCSC; OrthSurg. (506)857-3197; Fax. (506)857-0293.

MASSON, Claude; GMF Venta et Marees, 201-391 av Brochu, Sept-Iles QC G4R 4S7; Sher'79; Staff, Centre Hospitalier Regional de Sept-Iles; (418)962-6384; Fax. (418)962-4488.

MASSON, Edward C O; Orthopaedic Consultants, 10972 124 St NW, Edmonton AB T5M 0H8; Alb'92; BSc; FRCSC; OrthSurg (Trauma). Clin Assoc Prof Surg, University of Alberta; (780)732-3710; Fax. (780)451-1437.

MASSON, Guylaine; CLSC Du Vieux Lachine, 1900 rue Notre-Dame, Lachine QC H8S 2G2; Sher'88; (514)639-0650; Fax. (514)639-8593.

MASSON, Helene; CHUM-Hop Notre-Dame, 1560 rue Sherbrooke E, Montreal QC H2L 4M1; Mon'80; FRCPC; Neur (Dementia); Electroenceph (P.Q.). ac Staff, Centre Hospitalier l'Université de Montréal (CHUM) - Hôpital Notre-Dame; (514)890-8000 x25069; Fax. (514)412-7554.

MASSON, Isabelle; Clinique Med du College, GD 1396 rue Notre-Dame, Saint-Cesaire QC J0L 1T0; Mon'97; Staff, Hôpital du Haut-Richelieu; (450)469-0505

MASSON, Jacqueline E; 36 Madison Ave, Toronto ON M5R 2S1; McG'82; FRCPC; Psy (Neurology). (416)578-4645

MASSON, Jean-Bernard; CHUM-Hotel-Dieu, 3840 rue Saint-Urbain, Montreal QC H2W 1T8; Mon'00; Cardiol; IntMed. Staff, Centre Hospitalier l'Université de Montréal (CHUM) - Hôtel-Dieu; (514)890-8000 x15160

MASSON, Judith; Clin de Sante Jacques Cartier, 200-1815 rue King O, Sherbrooke QC J1J 2E3; Sher'05; CCFP; (819)565-7446

MASSON, Martine; CSSS de la Baie-des-Chaleurs, RR 2 419 boul Perron, Maria QC G0C 1Y0; Laval'94; Staff, CSSS de la Baie-des-Chaleurs; (418)759-3443

MASSON, Michel; Regie l'Assurance Maladie QC, Q044-1125 Grande Allée O, Quebec QC G1S 1E7; Laval'71; Peds (P.Q.) (Neonatology). Med Consultant, Regie de l'Assurance Maladie du Quebec; (418)682-5144 x4192; Fax. (418)643-3858; michel.masson@ramq.gouv.qc.ca.

MASSON, Pascale; Clinique Med Pierre-Boucher, 3e-1615 boul Jacques-Cartier E, Longueuil QC J4M 2X1; Mon'90; FRCPC; Psy (General Adult Psychiatry). Staff, Hopital Maisonneuve-Rosemont; (450)468-6223

MASSON, Pierre; CLSC et CHSLD Pommeraie, 660 rue Saint-Paul, Farnham QC J2N 3B9; Mon'70; Langs: Bilingual(French/English); (450)293-6742

MASSON, Robin K; 2685 36 St NE, Calgary AB T1Y 5S3; UBC'10; (403)943-5000; Fax. (403)476-8784.

MASSON, Sharonah R; St Clair Med Clinic, 50 St Clair Ave E, Toronto ON M4T 1M9; Tor'86; CCFP; FCFP; Court Staff, Women's College Hospital; University of Toronto; (416)921-1066; Fax. (416)921-8459.

MASSON, Suzanne; CSSS Drummond-Hop Sainte-Croix, 570 rue Heriot, Drummondville QC J2B 1C1; Laval'84; GenPath (P.Q.). Chef Dept of Path, Hôpital Sainte-croix; (819)478-6464 x22326; Fax. (819)478-6421.

MASSON-COTE, Laurence; CHUS-Hopital Fleurimont, 3001 12e av N, Sherbrooke QC J1H 5N4; Mon'05; FRCPC; RadOncol. Staff, Centre Hospitalier Universitaire de Sherbrooke-Hopital Fleurimont; Langs: Bilingual(French/English); (819)346-1110

MASSON-ROY, Marie-Helene; CSSS Haut-Richelieu-Rouville, 920 boul du Seminaire N, St-Jean-sur-Richel QC J3A 1B7; Sher'07; Staff, Hôpital du Haut-Richelieu; (450)359-5000

MASSOUD, Emad; Dickson Bldg, 3042-5820 University Ave, Halifax NS B3H 1V7; Cairo (Egypt)'79; MB ChB; MSc; DABOT; FRC; FRCSC; Otol (Rhinology). Staff Otol, Capital District Health Authority; Staff Consultant Otol, IWK Health Centre; Prof/Prog Dir Otol Head & Neck Surg, Dalhousie University; Langs: Arabic; French; (902)473-3905; Fax. (902)473-3854; emad.massoud@dal.ca.

MASSOUD, Fadi A; CHUM-Hop Notre-Dame, 1560 rue Sherbrooke E, Montreal QC H2L 4M1; Mon'92; FRCPC; IntMed; GeriatricMed. Staff Internist-Geriatric, Centre Hospitalier l'Université de Montréal (CHUM) - Hôpital Notre-Dame; adj Prof Med, Universite de Montreal; Langs: Arabic; English; (514)890-8000 x26769; Fax. (514)412-7506.

MASSOUD, Farid H; Halton HSC Corp-Oakville, 327 Reynolds St, Oakville ON L6J 3L7; Assiut (Egypt)'78; CCFP; Staff, Halton Healthcare Services Corporation - Oakville Site; (905)845-2571

MASSOUD, Reza; Arnprior & Dist Mem Hosp, 350 John St N, Arnprior ON K7S 2P6; Ott'91; Staff, Arnprior & District Memorial Hospital; Locum Tenens, Carleton Place & District Memorial Hospital; (613)623-3166

MASSY, Caroline; CSSS de Chicoutimi, 305 rue Saint-Vallier, Chicoutimi QC G7H 5H6; Sher'05; FRCPC; IntMed; Respir. Staff, Complexe hospitalier de la Sagamie; (418)541-1000

MASTALI, Kourosh; Collingwood Cardiol & IntMed, 300-393 First St, Collingwood ON L9Y 1B3; Shaheed Beheshti University (Other Foreign)'92; Langs: Persian; (705)444-1648; Fax. (705)444-1909.

MASTEL, Douglas G; 47 8 St NW, Medicine Hat AB T1A 6N9; Alb'87; CCFP; FCFP; (403)526-6982; Fax. (403)529-6535.

MASTER, Suketu; Bramalea Health Centre, 203-18 Kensington Rd, Brampton ON L6T 4S5; Dal'90; (905)791-2436

MASTER, Surya; Campbellton Reg Hosp, PO Box 880 Stn Main 189 Lily Lake Rd, Campbellton NB E3N 3H3; Bombay (India)'54; MB BS; FRCS(Ed & Eng); FACS; FRCSC; GenSurg. Staff, Regional Health Authority Region 5; Sr Staff Surgeon, Hôpital Régional Campbellton; Langs: English; Bilingual(English/French); French; Gujarati; Hindi; Kiswahili; (506)789-1519; smaster@nbnet.nb.ca.

MASTERS, Roy G; Univ of Ottawa Heart Institute, H3403B-40 Ruskin St, Ottawa ON K1Y 4W7; Mem'78; FACS; FRCSC; GenSurg (Cardiac Surgery & Transplantation); Cardiovasc&ThorSurg. Staff, University of Ottawa Heart Institute; Physician Cardiac Surg Program Dir, The Ottawa Hospital - Civic Campus; Prof Surg, University of Ottawa; (613)761-4233; Fax. (613)761-5367.

MASTERS, Susan A; North York Family Health Team, 701-240 Duncan Mill Rd, North York ON M3B 3S6; London (England)'80; MB BS; Staff, North York General Hospital; Clin Instructor Family Practice, University of Toronto; (416)229-6300; Fax. (416)229-6283.

MASTERSON, Grainne M; Brameast Family Health Org, 38-2130 North Park Dr, Brampton ON L6S 0C9; McM'02; CCFP; (905)792-2211; Fax. (905)792-2901.

MASTERSON, John S T; Children's & Women's HC of BC, K0 134-4480 Oak St, Vancouver BC V6H 3V4; UBC'77; BSc; DABU; FACS; FRCSC; Urol (Pediatric Urology). Staff, BC Children's Hospital; Clin Prof, University of British Columbia; (604)875-2734; Fax. (604)875-2721.

MASTERSON, Julia A; 304-1685 Main St W, Hamilton ON L8S 1G5; McM'90; MSc; FRCPC; Psy (Psycho Oncology). (905)308-0736; Fax. (905)522-0479.

MASTERSON, Mark F; Kelowna Gen Hosp, 2268 Pandosy St, Kelowna BC V1Y 1T2; Cal'07; FRCPC; Anes. Staff, Kelowna General Hospital; (250)862-4309

MASTERSON, Tami; Grey Nuns Community Hosp, 23-1100 Youville Drive West NW, Edmonton AB T6L 5X8; Alb'01; FRCPC; Peds. Staff, Glenrose Rehabilitation Hospital; Staff, Royal Alexandra Hospital; Staff, Covenant Health - Grey Nuns Community Hospital; Staff, University of Alberta; (780)735-7346; Fax. (780)735-7444.

MASTRANGELO, E Armando; Oak Park Med Clinic, 1-2530 Sixth Line, Oakville ON L6H 6W5; Wes'79; (905)257-1006

MASTROGIACOMO, Caterina; Scarborough Acad Fam Hlth Team, C 06-3000 Lawrence Ave E, Scarborough ON M1P 2V1; Tor'88; CCFP; FCFP; Court Staff, The Scarborough Hospital - General Campus; Court Staff, Toronto General Hospital - UHN; University of Toronto; Langs: Italian; (416)658-5228; Fax. (416)658-5585.

MASTROGIACOMO, Frank F; 200-658 Danforth Ave, Toronto ON M4J 5B9; Tor'99; BSc; PhD; FRCSC; OrthSurg (Lower Extremity Reconstruction). Staff Orth Surgeon/Coord Div of Orth, Toronto East General Hospital Inc; Lecturer, University of Toronto; Langs: Italian; (416)406-5666; Fax. (416)406-6667.

MASUCCI, Giuseppina L; CHUM-Hop Notre-Dame, 1560 rue Sherbrooke E, Montreal QC H2L 4M1; Mon'05; FRCPC; RadOncol. Staff, Centre Hospitalier l'Université de Montréal (CHUM) - Hôpital Notre-Dame; (514)890-8254

MASUCCI, Nicola; 200-72 Boul Saint-Jean-Baptist, Chateauguay QC J6K 4Y7; McG'85; ac Staff, Centre Hospitalier l'Université de Montréal (CHUM) - Hôpital Notre-Dame; Langs: English; French; (450)692-7282; Fax. (450)699-7788; masucci@videotron.ca.

MASUD, Chaudhry F; Peel Medical Walk-in-Clinic, 475 Charolais Blvd, Brampton ON L6Y 0M2; Pinjab (India)'87; MB BS; CCFP; Langs: Hindi; Punjabi; Urdu; (905)454-3347

MASUDA, Judith M; 101-9648 128 St, Surrey BC V3T 2X9; McM'75; (604)951-3351

MASUHARA, E Joy; North East Mental Health Team, 222-2750 Hastings St E, Vancouver BC V5K 1Z9; UBC'91; BScPharm; CCFP; Vis Staff, Vancouver General Hospital - Centennial Pavillion; (604)675-3890; masuhara@shaw.ca.

MASURKAR, Swapna; Marlborough Med Clinic, 160-495 36 St NE, Calgary AB T2A 6K3; Bombay (India)'95; CCFP; (403)514-6001

MATAND, Tshilay; Maximily Med Clinic, 3038 Dewdney Ave, Regina SK S4T 0Y2; Medunsa (South Africa)'96; MB ChB; LMCC; Langs: English; French; (306)522-3457; Fax. (306)522-0626.

MATANGI, Murray F; Kingston Heart Clinic, 460 Princess St, Kingston ON K7L 1C2; Otago (New Zealand)'75; FRACP; FACP; FACC; FRCPC; IntMed; Cardiol. Staff, Kingston Heart Clinic; (613)544-3242; Fax. (613)546-4487; matangikhc@king.igs.net.

MATANOVIC-TODOROVIC, Dragana; 1216 Upper Wentworth St, Hamilton ON L9A 4W2; Serbia (Croatia)'86; (905)389-5657

MATAR, Nadim; Hop Charles Lemoyne, 3120 boul Taschereau, Greenfield Park QC J4V 2H1; Beirut (Lebanon)'69; FRCPC; Respir. Staff, Hopital Charles LeMoyne; (450)466-5000 x2704

MATAR, Wadih Y; CSSS-Hopital De Hull, 116 boul Lionel-Emond, Gatineau QC J8Y 1W7; Ott'03; FRCSC; OrthSurg. Staff, Hull Hospital; (819)966-6200

MATAVA, Cliade T; The Hosp for Sick Children, 555 University Ave, Toronto ON M5G 1X8; (Zimbabwe)'02; Staff, The Hospital For Sick Children; (416)813-1500

MATAVA, Rachelle K; Headwaters Health Care Centre, 100 Rolling Hills Dr, Orangeville ON L9W 4X9; McM'07; CCFP; CCFP(E.M.); Staff, Headwaters Health Care Centre - Orangeville Site; (519)941-2410

MATCHETT, Michael; The Moncton Hosp, 135 MacBeath Ave, Moncton NB E1C 6Z8; Dal'09; CCFP; Staff, The Moncton Hospital.

DOWNER, Elizabeth A Mate; Leonard A Miller Centre, 712-100 Forest Rd, St. John's NL A1A 3Z9; Mem'91; CCFP; FCFP; (709)777-6301

MATE, Eva S; Rosedale Med Centre, 301-600 Sherbourne St, Toronto ON M4X 1W4; Santiago (Chile)'72; FCCP; ABIM; AB; FRCPC; Respir (Respiratory Disease). Asst Prof, University of Toronto; Langs: Spanish; Hungarian; (416)926-4940; Fax. (416)929-9906.

MATE, Gabor; 20 Hastings St W, Vancouver BC V6B 1G6; UBC'77; Ac Staff, Vancouver General Hospital - Centennial Pavillion; Ac Staff, BC Women's Hospital & Health Centre; Court Staff, Providence Health Care - Mount Saint Joseph Hospital; (604)683-0073 x233

MATEO-RODRIGUEZ, Patrocinio C; Royal Alexandra Hosp, 10240 Kingsway NW, Edmonton AB T5H 3V9; (Philippines)'96; Staff, Royal Alexandra Hospital; (780)735-4670

MATEOS-CORRAL, Dimas; IWK Health Centre, PO Box 9700 Rpo CSC 5850 University Ave, Halifax NS B3K 6R8; Baja California (Mexico)'00; Staff, IWK Health Centre; (902)470-8218; Fax. (902)470-7223.

MATER, Ahmed M A; Royal University Hosp, 103 Hospital Dr, Saskatoon SK S7N 0W8; Arabian Gulf University (Bahrain)'92; MB BS; FRCPC; Peds (Pediatric Emergency Medicine). Staff, Royal University Hospital; (306)655-1000; Fax. (306)655-2897; mater999@hotmail.com.

MATEREK, Lukasz A; Broadmead Village Med Clinic, 140-777 Royal Oak Dr, Victoria BC V8X 4V1; UBC'07; FRCPC; IntMed; Endocrin&Metab. Staff, Richmond Hospital; (250)479-7147

MATES, Mihaela; Cancer Ctr of Southern Ontario, 25 King St W, Kingston ON K7L 5P9; Romania (Romania)'95; FRCPC; IntMed. Staff, Cancer Centre of Southeastern Ontario; Staff, Kingston General Hospital; (613)544-2631

MATHAI, George; Cambridge Med Place, 5-695 Coronation Blvd, Cambridge ON N1R 7J9; Madras (India)'70; MB BS; FRCPC; IntMed (Respirology). Langs: Malayalam; (519)623-2830; Fax. (519)623-9569.

MATHAI, Shyla R; Cambridge Mem Hosp, 700 Coronation Blvd, Cambridge ON N1R 3G2; (Netherlands Antilles)'06; CCFP; Staff, Cambridge Memorial Hospital; (519)621-2330

MATHE, C Thomas; Glen Erin Med-Dental Centre, 11-2318 Dunwin Dr, Mississauga ON L5L 1C7; Wes'70; Ac Staff, Hamilton Health Sciences Centre - St Peter's Hospital; (905)828-1145; Fax. (905)828-1144.

MATHEN, Mathen K; Misericordia Health Centre, 271-99 Cornish Ave, Winnipeg MB R3C 1A2; National (Ireland)'80; FRCSC; Ophth. Staff, Misericordia Health Centre; Langs: Hindi; (204)788-8564; Fax. (204)788-0978; mmathen@miseri.winnipeg.mb.ca.

MATHER, J Frederick; 207-751 King St W, Kitchener ON N2G 1E5; Qns'79; CCFP; Staff, Grand River Hospital - Freeport Site; (519)578-3500; Fax. (519)741-0286.

MATHER, Mahomed S; Brant Community HC-Brantford, 200 Terrace Hill St, Brantford ON N3R 1G9; Dublin (Ireland)'60; LRCPS; FRCPC; Anes. Ac Staff Anes, The Brant Community Healthcare System - Brantford General Hospital Site; (519)752-7871

MATHER, Rookaya; St Joseph's Health Care, PO Box 5777 Stn B B2 057-268 Grosvenor Rd, London ON N6A 4V2; RCS (Ireland)'98; FRCSC; Ophth (Cataract). Staff, Ivey Eye Institute; University of Western Ontario; (519)646-6409; Fax. (519)646-6394.

MATHER, Susan A; Mather Medicine Prof Corp, RR 4 3958 Petrolia Line, Petrolia ON N0N 1R0; Wes'87; CCFP; FCFP; Staff, Wyoming Medical Centre; Med Dir, Lambton Meadowview Villa; (519)882-1678; Fax. (519)882-0533.

MATHER, William A D; Neilson-Ellesmere Med Centre, 2858 Ellesmere Rd, Scarborough ON M1E 4B8; Jaffna (Sri Lanka)'91; MB BS; LMCC; CCFP; Langs: Tamil; Sinhalese; (416)287-1500; Fax. (416)287-1275; dmather1@rogers.com.

MATHERS, Paul G; MUHC-Royal Victoria Hosp, 687 av des Pins O, Montreal QC H3A 1A1; Man'93; BSc; CCFP; CCFP(E.M.); Staff, McGill University Health Centre - Royal Victoria Hospital; Langs: Bilingual(English/French); (514)934-1934

MATHES, Edward J; Foul Bay Prof Centre, 314-1964 Fort St, Victoria BC V8R 6R3; Tor'64; BSc; Assoc Staff, Royal Jubilee Hospital; (250)598-9223; Fax. (250)598-9234.

MATHES, Sonja K; RebalanceMD, 104-3551 Blanshard St, Victoria BC V8Z 0B9; Qns'03; FRCSC; OrthSurg. (250)940-4444

MATHESON, A Grant; 24 Linden Ave, Charlottetown PE C1A 5Y8; Dal'91; BSc; Staff, Queen Elizabeth Hospital; (902)367-4250

MATHESON, David M; Elliot Lake Family Health Team, 2F-31 Nova Scotia Walk, Elliot Lake ON P5A 1Y9; Qns'80; Staff, St Joseph's General Hospital Elliot Lake; Langs: Bilingual(English/French); (705)848-3673; Fax. (705)848-3449.

MATHESON, Donald C; Metrotown Med Centre, 303-6411 Nelson Ave, Burnaby BC V5H 4H3; UBC'57; Ophth. Ac Staff, Burnaby Hospital; (604)433-1258; Fax. (604)433-6154.

MATHESON, Grant M; Collingwood Gen Marine Hosp, 459 Hume St, Collingwood ON L9Y 1W9; Dal'64; DiagRad. Staff, Collingwood General & Marine Hospital; (705)445-2550

MATHESON, Hugh B; Spryfield Med Centre, 205 Herring Cove Rd, Halifax NS B3P 1L1; Dal'82; Ad Staff Privil, IWK Health Centre; (902)477-5693; Fax. (902)477-0502.

MATHESON, J Douglas; Hys Med Centre, 601-11010 101 St NW, Edmonton AB T5H 4B9; Alb'84; FRCPC; IntMed; Critical Care Medicine; GenSurg. (780)424-3295; Fax. (780)426-2818.

MATHESON, Jeffrey R H; Aim Health Group, 9-6400 Millcreek Dr, Mississauga ON L5N 3E7; McG'91; BSc; MDCM; (905)288-1045

MATHESON, John A; 200-5503 206 St, Langley BC V3A 2C6; UBC'76; DObst(NZ); FRCPC; DiagRad. Staff, Langley Memorial Hospital; Staff, Abbotsford Regional Hospital & Cancer Centre; (604)534-4114

MATHESON, Leslie J; Orthopedic & Sports Med Clinic, 312-5595 Fenwick St, Halifax NS B3H 1R1; Dal'83; Staff Family Pract Newborn Care, IWK Health Centre; (902)421-7512

MATHESON, Timothy J; 206-27 Peakview Way, Halifax NS B3M 0G2; Saba (Netherlands Antilles)'06; CCFP; Att Staff, Hants Community Hospital; (902)444-8922

MATHEW, Baboo M; Burin Peninsula Hlth Care Ctr, PO Box 340, Burin NL A0E 1E0; Aligarh (India)'72; MB BS; FRCP(Lond & Edin); FACP; FACE; LMCC; MRCP; FRCPE; LRCPS; FRCPC; IntMed (Diabetes); Endocrin&Metab. Staff, Burin Peninsula Health Care Centre; Langs: Hindi; Malayalam; (709)891-1040; Fax. (709)891-3375.

MATHEW, Beena; Milton Urgent Care Clinic, 103-400 Bronte St S, Milton ON L9T 0H7; Calicut (India)'93; CCFP; (905)876-3843

MATHEW, Beena; Northeast Mental Hlth Centre, 680 Kirkwood Dr, Sudbury ON P3E 1X3; Calicut (India)'88; MB BS; MRCPsy; FRCPC; Psy. Staff, Health Sciences North-Laurentian Site; Staff, North Bay Regional Health Centre - Kirkwood; Langs: Malayalam; (705)675-9192; Fax. (705)671-3031.

MATHEW, Benjamin; Credit Valey Prof Bldg, 305-2300 Eglinton Ave W, Mississauga ON L5M 2V8; Man'00; FRCSC; Ophth. (905)820-5464; Fax. (905)569-2377.

MATHEW, Biju; Haney Health Associates, 22338 Selkirk Ave, Maple Ridge BC V2X 2X5; Karnatak (India)'80; FRCPC; Psy. Staff, Ridge Meadows Hospital & Health Care Centre; Langs: Hindi; Malayalam; (604)477-7202

MATHEW, Cizy; Four Corners Med Bldg, 410-2009 Long Lake Rd, Sudbury ON P3E 6C3; Calicut (India)'93; MB BS; MRCP(UK); FRCPC; Neur. Associate (All Sites), Health Sciences North-St Joseph's Health Centre; (705)523-5663; Fax. (705)523-1377.

MATHEW, George; Manitoba Clinic, 790 Sherbrook St, Winnipeg MB R3A 1M3; Sask'98; FRCPC; IntMed (Gastroenterology). (204)788-5754; Fax. (204)783-6558.

MATHEW, Jane M; CSSSG-Hop de Hull, 116 boul Lionel-Emond, Gatineau QC J8Y 1W7; McG'96; FRCSC; GenSurg; Critical Care Medicine (P.Q.). Staff, Hull Hospital; Staff, Centre Hospitalier de Gaspe; Staff, CSSS de la Vallée de la Gatineau; Langs: English; French; (819)595-6033; Fax. (819)595-6323.

MATHEW, Jinu J; Foremed Med Clinic, 420 Columbia St, New Westminster BC V3L 1B1; Manipal (India)'02; MB BS; CCFP; Surgical Ass't Cardiac Surg, Royal Columbian Hospital; (604)522-2206

MATHEW, Thomas M; The Group Health Centre, 240 McNabb St, Sault Ste. Marie ON P6B 1Y5; Madras (India)'70; FRCPC; IntMed; Cardiol. (705)759-1234

MATHEW, Paul K; B4D-350 Conestoga Blvd, Cambridge ON N1R 7L7; Mem'02; FRCSC; OrthSurg. (519)624-5999; Fax. (519)624-1117.

MATHEW, Roy K T; MD Health Med Centre, 186 Main St S, Brampton ON L6W 2E2; McG'00; CCFP; (905)456-7774

MATHEW, Silvy M; 202-179 Davie St, Vancouver BC V6Z 2Y1; Wes'05; CCFP; (604)669-7772

MATHEWS, John; Windsor Reg Cancer Centre, 2220 Kildare Rd, Windsor ON N8W 2X3; Bombay (India)'83; ABIM; FRCPC; IntMed (Hematology); MedOncol. Staff, Windsor Regional Hospital - Metropolitan Site; Staff, Hôtel-Dieu Grace Hospital; Medical Oncology, Windsor Regional Hospital - Windsor Regional Cancer Centre; Langs: Hindi; Malayalam; (519)253-5253; john_mathews@wrh.on.ca.

MATHEWS, Nicole M; 206-470 Bronte St S, Milton ON L9T 2J4; (Ireland)'01; BSc; CCFP; Staff, Halton Healthcare Services Corporation - Milton District Hospital; (905)878-6793; Fax. (905)878-6711.

MATHEWS, Sylvain; Hôpital Ste-Justine, 3175 ch Cote-Sainte-Catherine, Montreal QC H3T 1C5; Mon'81; FRCPC; Anes (Obstetrics)., Hôpital Ste-Justine; Langs: Bilingual(French/English); (514)345-4733; Fax. (514)345-4601; sylvain_mathews@ssss.gouv.qc.ca.

MATHIAS, Cathleen P; Laurel Med Centre Ltd, 215-888 8th Ave W, Vancouver BC V5Z 3Y1; UBC'90; BSc; CCFP; (604)873-6541; Fax. (604)873-6540.

MATHIAS, Michelle D; Royal Ottawa Hlth Care Group, 1145 Carling Ave, Ottawa ON K1Z 7K4; Ott'07; FRCPC; Psy. Staff, Royal Ottawa Mental Health Centre - Royal Ottawa Health Care Group; (613)722-6521

MATHIAS, Steven M; St Paul's Hosp, 2B 171-1081 Burrard St, Vancouver BC V6Z 1Y6; UBC'01; FRCPC; Psy. Staff, Providence Health Care - St Paul's Hospital; (604)806-8004

MATHIES, David J; Huntsville Prof Bldg, 104-348 Muskoka Rd 3 N, Huntsville ON P1H 1H8; Wes'79; CCFP; FCFP; Chief Staff, Huntsville District Memorial Hospital - Muskoka Algonquin Healthcare; (705)789-2355; Fax. (705)789-1051; david.mathies@mahc.ca.

MATHIESON, Alexander; Health Sciences Centre, 300 Prince Philip Dr, St. John's NL A1B 3V6; Mem'01; FRCSC; GenSurg; General Surgical Oncology. Staff, Health Sciences Centre; (709)777-6854; Fax. (709)777-6572.

MATHIESON, Angela L; Health Sciences Centre, 820 Sherbrook St, Winnipeg MB R3A 1R9; Man'91; FRCPC; Anes. Staff, Health Sciences Centre; (204)774-6511

MATHIESON, John R; Vancouver Island Hlth Authorit, 1952 Bay St, Victoria BC V8R 1J8; Cal'81; FRCPC; DiagRad. Med Dir/Dept Head Medical Imaging, Vancouver Island Health Authority; (250)370-8318

MATHIESON, Sarah; Health Sciences Centre, 300 Prince Philip Dr, St. John's NL A1B 3V6; Mem'08; CCFP; CCFP(E.M.); Staff, Health Sciences Centre.

MATHIEU, Andre; CSST Sherbrooke, M30-1650 rue King O, Sherbrooke QC J1J 2C3; Sher'75; ac Staff, Centre Hospitalier Universitaire de Sherbrooke-Hôpital Hôtel-Dieu; (819)822-4490

MATHIEU, Anne-Marie; 80 rue Saint-Louis, Quebec QC G1R 3Z5; Paris (France)'75; Ophth. Staff, Centre Hospitalier Universitaire de Québec (CHUQ) - Siege Social; (418)692-2130; Fax. (418)692-2130.

MATHIEU, Bernard; Hop Maisonneuve-Rosemont, 5415 boul de l'Assomption, Montreal QC H1T 2M4; Mon'84; Staff, Hopital Maisonneuve-Rosemont; Clin Teacher, Universite de Montreal; (514)252-3400 x4206; Fax. (514)252-3482; bmathieu.hmr@ssss.gouv.qc.ca.

MATHIEU, David; CHUS-Hop Fleurimont, 3001 12e av N, Sherbrooke QC J1H 5N4; Sher'99; FRCSC; Neursurg (Neuro Oncology). Staff, Centre Hospitalier Universitaire de Sherbrooke-Hopital Fleurimont; (819)346-1110 x13324; Fax. (819)820-6452; david.mathieu@usherbrooke.ca.

MATHIEU, Genevieve; Clinique Argyle, 32 rue Argyle, Longueuil QC J4P 2H4; Mon'95; FRCPC; IntMed (Diabetes). assoc Membre, Institut de Cardiologie de Montréal; Ac Member, Hopital Maisonneuve-Rosemont; Langs: Bilingual(French/English); (450)671-3179; Fax. (450)671-4796.

MATHIEU, Guy; Clinique Med Galt, 200-2235 rue Galt O, Sherbrooke QC J1K 1K6; Sher'82; Langs: Bilingual(French/English); (819)821-0088; Fax. (819)821-3901.

MATHIEU, Henri-Pierre; CSSS du Haut Saint Francis, 460 2e av, Weedon QC J0B 3J0; Staff, CSSS du Haut-Saint-François; (819)877-3434

MATHIEU, Isabelle; Hopital de Maria, 419 boul Perron, Maria QC G0C 1Y0; Laval'08; Staff, CSSS de la Baie-des-Chaleurs; (418)759-3443

MATHIEU, Jean; CSSS de Chicoutimi, 305 rue Saint-Vallier, Chicoutimi QC G7H 5H6; Mon'75; FRCPC; Neur. Staff, Complexe hospitalier de la Sagamie; (418)541-1000

MATHIEU, Jean-Francois; Ctr Hosp de Verdun, 4000 boul Lasalle, Verdun QC H4G 2A3; Mon'91; Staff, Centre Hospitalier de Verdun; Langs: Bilingual(French/English); (514)362-1000

MATHIEU, Jean-Luc; 205-2954 Boul Laframboise, Saint-Hyacinthe QC J2S 4Z2; Sher'77; FRCSC; ObstGyn. (450)771-4963

MATHIEU, Jean-Pierre; Hop Maisonneuve-Rosemont, 5415 boul de l'Assomption, Montreal QC H1T 2M4; Mon'71; CSPQ; FRCPC; Rheum. Ac Staff, Hopital Maisonneuve-Rosemont; adj Prof, Universite de Montreal; Langs: Bilingual(French/English); (514)252-3400; Fax. (514)252-3889.

MATHIEU, John F; 644A rue Jacques-Cartier E, Chicoutimi QC G7H 2A4; Laval'70; FRCSC; GenSurg; Cardiovasc&ThorSurg. Chef cardio/chirurgie thorac, Complexe hospitalier de la Sagamie; Langs: English; (418)545-4456; Fax. (418)545-1449.

MATHIEU, Josee; CLSC De Pierrefonds, 13800 boul Gouin O, Pierrefonds QC H8Z 3H6; Mon'91; (514)626-2572; Fax. (514)626-8857.

MATHIEU, Marie; CHUS-Hop Fleurimont, 3001 12e Av N, Sherbrooke QC J1H 5N4; Sher'87; Staff, Centre Hospitalier Universitaire de Sherbrooke-Hopital Fleurimont; (819)346-1110

MATHIEU, Michel A; Clinique Med Blainville, 519 boul du Cure-Labelle, Blainville QC J7C 2H6; Mon'80; Langs: Bilingual(French/English); (450)437-7337; Fax. (450)437-5129.

MATHIEU, Nicolas; CSSS d'Antoine-Labelle-l'Annon, 1525 rue l'Annonciation N, Riviere-Rouge QC J0T 1T0; Mon'87; Médecin, Centre de L'Annonciation; Physician, GMF de la Rouge; Langs: French; Spanish; (819)275-2118 x3334; Fax. (819)275-7218.

MATHIEU, Patrick; Hôpital Laval, 2725 ch Sainte-Foy, Quebec QC G1V 4G5; Mon'93; FRCSC; Cardiovasc&ThorSurg (P.Q.); CardSurg. Staff, Hôpital Laval; (418)656-4717

MATHIEU, R Brian; Place Notre-Dame, 101-711 boul Saint-Joseph, Roberval QC G8H 2L3; McG'88; FRCSC; Ophth. Langs: Bilingual(English/French); (418)275-7225; Fax. (418)275-7226.

MATHIEU, Virginie; CSSS de Beauce, 1515 17e rue, Saint-Georges QC G5Y 4T8; Sher'02; FRCPC; Anes. Staff, Centre Hospitalier Beauce-Etchemin; (418)228-2031 x5000

MATHIEU, Yvan; Clinique Medico-Sante, CP 62 1116 boul Vachon N, Sainte-Marie QC G6E 1N7; Laval'84; (418)387-2565

MATHIEU, Yves; Clinique Med Lyster, 2448 rue Becancour, Lyster QC G0S 1V0; Sher'75; Langs: English; (819)389-2000; Fax. (819)389-1187.

MATHIEU-MILLAIRE, Francine; Hop Maisonneuve-Rosemont, 5415 boul de l'Assomption, Montreal QC H1T 2M4; Mon'73; Ophth. Staff, Hopital Maisonneuve-Rosemont; Staff, Hôpital du Sacre-Coeur de Montréal; Assoc Staff, Hôpital Ste-Justine; (514)252-3400 x4956; Fax. (514)252-3905.

MATHIEU-SERRA, Andree; 1750-9405 rue Sherbrooke E, Montreal QC H1L 6P3; Mon'74; ABD; FRCPC; Derm (Alternative Medicine). Langs: Bilingual(French/English); (514)645-6453; Fax. (514)645-0004; info@dermatolaser.com.

MATHIS, Christel C; Hop Jean-Talon, 1385 rue Jean-Talon E, Montreal QC H2E 1S6; Alb'80; FRCPC; DiagRad. Staff, CSSS du Coeur de l'Isle Hôpital Jean-Talon; Langs: Bilingual(English/French); (514)495-6767 x6766

MATHISEN, Brit L; Medical Arts Bldg, 201-42 Glen Allan Dr, Bridgewater NS B4V 3N2; Dal'84; Ac Staff, South Shore Regional Hospital; (902)543-4446; Fax. (902)543-4446.

MATHISON, Trina L; Dauphin Med Clinic, 622 3rd St SW, Dauphin MB R7N 1R5; Man'99; BSc; CCFP; Med VP, Dauphin Regional Health Centre; Coord, Parkland Residency Program; (204)638-6445; Fax. (204)638-5670.

MATHIVANAN, Meena; McMaster University HSC, PO Box 2000 Stn Lcd 1 3W 10B-1200 Main St W, Hamilton ON L8N 3Z5; Sydney (Australia)'07; FRCPC; IntMed.

MATHOO, Julian; 240 James St S, Hamilton ON L8P 3B3; Tor'01; BSc(Hon); MSc; FRCPC; PhysMed&Rehab (Sports Medicine). Staff PhysMed, St Joseph's Healthcare - Charlton Campus; Staff Phys Med, Hamilton Health Sciences Centre - McMaster Children's Hospital; Clinical Asst Prof, McMaster University; (905)521-6376; Fax. (905)777-9399; julian.mathoo@utoronto.ca.

MATHUR, Arpana C; Halton Family Health Centre, 2951 Walker's Line, Burlington ON L7M 4Y1; Tor'97; BSc; CCFP; (905)336-3437 x3021

MATHUR, Arun K; Taunton Health Centre, SS 201 1290 Keith Ross Dr, Oshawa ON L1H 7K4; Dal'91; BSc; FRCSC; Urol. Staff, Lakeridge Health - Oshawa Site; Langs: Hindi; (905)721-3551; Fax. (905)721-4929.

MATHUR, Harshi; 7-3250 60 St NE, Calgary AB T1Y 3T5; (India)'80; CCFP; (403)293-5600; Fax. (403)285-6478.

MATHUR, Sanjiv; Sudbury Reg Hosp-Laurentian, 41 Ramsey Lake Rd, Sudbury ON P3E 5J1; Wes'94; Anes. Staff, Health Sciences North-Laurentian Site; (705)523-7100

MATHUR, Soania; Taunton Health Centre, SS 201 1290 Keith Ross Dr, Oshawa ON L1H 7K4; Dal'95; CCFP; (905)721-3551; Fax. (905)721-6697.

MATHUR, Vinod K; Doctors Bldg, 340-955 Queen St E, Sault Ste. Marie ON P6A 2C3; London (England)'67; MB BS; FRCS(Lond); FRCSC; Urol;CCFP; Staff, Sault Area Hospital - Sault Ste Marie; Langs: Hindi; (705)942-6646; Fax. (705)942-6614; vinkmathur@shaw.ca.

MATHURIN, Jean; CLSC Saint-Michel, 3355 rue Jarry E, Montreal QC H1Z 2E5; (Haiti)'69; Staff, CSSS Saint-Leonard et Saint-Michel; (514)374-8223; Fax. (514)374-3812.

MATHURIN, Johanne; Hotel-Dieu de Levis, 143 rue Wolfe, Levis QC G6V 3Z1; Laval'87; FRCPC; DiagRad. Staff, Hôtel-Dieu de Lévis; (418)835-7121 x7901

MATI, Neil M; Victoria Terrrace Med Centre, 202-1448 Lawrence Ave E, North York ON M4A 2V6; Baghdad (Iraq)'83; MB ChB; CCFP; Staff, The Scarborough Hospital - General Campus; (416)752-5426; Fax. (416)752-7332.

MATIC, Damir; London HSC-Victoria Hosp, PO Box 5010 Stn B E2 646-800 Commissioners Rd E, London ON N6A 5W9; Tor'95; FRCSC; PlasSurg (Cranio Maxillofacial Surgery). Staff, London Health Sciences Centre - Victoria Campus; Asst Prof, University of Western Ontario; (519)685-8557

MATIC, Kata; Hys Med Centre, 310-11010 101 St NW, Edmonton AB T5H 4B9; Alb'91; FRCPC; IntMed; Gastroent. Staff, Royal Alexandra Hospital; (780)421-1029; Fax. (780)425-5533.

MATIN, Roozbeh; Greenbelt Family Health Team, 1C-3500 Fallowfield Rd, Ottawa ON K2J 4A7; Ott'06; CCFP; (613)843-1718; Fax. (613)843-0201.

MATISHAK, Mark Z; 311-223 Nelson's Cres, New Westminster BC V3L 0E4; Alb'84; FRCSC; Neursurg. (604)526-6400; Fax. (604)526-5121.

MATISIC, Jasenka P; BC Cancer Agency-Vancouver CC, 600 10th Ave W, Vancouver BC V5Z 4E6; Zagreb (Croatia)'68; FRCPC; GenPath. Staff, BC Cancer Agency Vancouver Centre; Consultant, Vancouver General Hospital - Centennial Pavillion; (604)877-6000 x2073

MATLIS, Steven; 629 Markham Rd, Scarborough ON M1H 2A4; (Other Foreign)'07; CCFP; (416)642-9445

MATLOW, Anne G; Women's College Hosp, 76 Grenville St, Toronto ON M5S 1B2; Tor'77; MSc; FRCPC; MedMicrobiol; InfectDis; IntMed. Staff, Women's College Hospital; University of Toronto; (416)323-6400

MATOS, Aldina C S; Hamilton Harbour Comm Bldg, 102-605 James St N, Hamilton ON L8L 1J9; McM'90; Langs: Portuguese; (905)525-4900; Fax. (905)525-2295.

MATOSH, John; 500 Raglan St N, Renfrew ON K7V 1P5; UBC'87; Staff, Renfrew Victoria Hospital; (613)432-7855; Fax. (613)432-4722; dr.matosh@renfrewhosp.com.

MATOSSIAN, Sebouh M; Columbia Med Bldg, 406-301 Columbia St E, New Westminster BC V3L 3W5; Alb'95; FRCPC; IntMed. Staff, Eagle Ridge Hospital & Health Care Centre; (604)525-9177

MATOUK, Elias; 3830 av Lacombe, Montreal QC H3T 1M5; Alexandria (Egypt)'69; ABIM; FRCPC; Respir; IntMed. Staff, McGill University Health Centre - Montreal Chest Institute; Staff, St Mary's Hospital Centre; Langs: English; Arabic; French; (514)345-3511; Fax. (514)734-2704; elie.matouk@mcgill.ca.

MATOUK, Ivy; Clinique Med le Plein-Ciel, 475 boul de la Cote-Vertu, Saint-Laurent QC H4L 1X7; Alexandria (Egypt)'69; (514)337-3171

MATOUK, Karen; Hop Maisonneuve-Rosemont, 5415 boul de l'Assomption, Montreal QC H1T 2M4; McG'01; FRCPC; IntMed; Gastroent. Staff, Hopital Maisonneuve-Rosemont; (514)252-3400 x3367; Fax. (514)252-3486.

MATOUK, Zehra; Clinique de Pediatrie SENCRL, 218-383 boul du Seminaire N, St-Jean-sur-Richel QC J3B 8C5; (Algeria)'92; Staff, Hôpital du Haut-Richelieu; (450)348-4911; Fax. (450)348-6401.

MATOUS, J Stephen N; 559 6th St, Courtenay BC V9N 1M5; UBC'90; CCFP; (250)338-1391; Fax. (250)338-2385.

MATRICK, Lawrence E; 600-890 Pender St W, Vancouver BC V6C 1J9; Man'57; DPM; MRCPsy; FRCPC; Psy. Ac Staff, Vancouver General Hospital - Centennial Pavillion; Clin Assoc Prof, University of British Columbia; (604)681-5821

MATSELL, Douglas G; Children's & Women's HC of BC, K4 150-4480 Oak St, Vancouver BC V6H 3V4; McG'83; FRCPC; Peds (Pediatric Nephrology); Nephrol. Staff Nephrol, BC Children's Hospital; Langs: Bilingual(English/French); (604)875-2272; Fax. (604)875-3649.

MATSENKO, Oksana; Appleton Clinic, 685 Finch Ave W, North York ON M2R 1P2; (Ukraine)'97; (416)635-0909; Fax. (416)635-0300.

MATSHES, Evan V W; Calgary Lab Services, 9-3535 Research Rd NW, Calgary AB T2L 2K8; Sask'04; FRCPC; AnatPath (Forensic Pathology). Staff, Calgary Laboratory Services; (403)770-3569; Fax. (403)770-3788.

MATSOS, Mark; Charlton Med Centre, 708-25 Charlton Ave E, Hamilton ON L8N 1Y2; Wes'04; FRCPC; IntMed (Systemic Lupus Erythematosus); Rheum. Staff, St Joseph's Healthcare - Charlton Campus; (905)521-9034

MATSUBA, Carey A; Sunny Hill Hlth Ctr for Child, 3644 Slocan St, Vancouver BC V5M 3E8; McG'91; MHSc; FRCPC; Peds (Developmental Pediatrics). Staff, Sunny Hill Health Centre for Children; (604)453-8306

MATSUBARA, Timothy K; 343 Tache Ave, Winnipeg MB R2H 2A5; Man'84; FRCSC; GenSurg. (204)925-9594; Fax. (204)231-2283.

MATSUDA, Maria T; Preston Med Centre, 506 King St E, Cambridge ON N3H 3N2; Kansas (USA)'91; CCFP; (519)653-3321

MATSUDA-ABEDINI, Mina; Children's & Women's HC of BC, K4 150-4480 Oak St, Vancouver BC V6H 3V4; McG'99; FRCPC; Peds; Nephrol. Staff, BC Children's Hospital; (604)875-2272

MATSUI, Doreen M; LHSC-Children's Hosp, 800 Commissioners Rd E, London ON N6A 5W9; Qns'85; FRCPC; Peds (Clinical Pharmacology). Staff, London Health Sciences Centre - Victoria Campus; Assoc Prof Peds, University of Western Ontario; (519)685-8268; Fax. (519)685-8156.

MATSUI, Irene; 1075 Orser Dr, Bathurst NB E2A 4S3; Campinas State (Brazil)'88; Staff, Hopital Regional Chaleur.

MATSUMOTO, Edward D; St Joseph's Healthcare, G343-50 Charlton Ave E, Hamilton ON L8N 4A6; Tor'96; FRCSC; Urol. Staff, St Joseph's Healthcare - Charlton Campus; Staff, Hamilton Health Sciences Centre - Hamilton General Hospital; (905)521-6186; Fax. (905)308-7205.

MATSUO, Jill M; Alexandra Hosp, 29 Noxon St, Ingersoll ON N5C 1B8; Tor'96; CCFP; CCFP(E.M.); Staff Ingersoll Family Phys, Alexandra Hospital; (519)425-9000; Fax. (519)425-9020.

MATSUO, Kelly S A; Madrona Imaging Westhill Ctre, A-1804 Bowen Rd, Nanaimo BC V9S 5W4; UBC'95; FRCPC; DiagRad. Staff, Nanaimo Regional General Hospital; (250)753-4351; Fax. (250)753-0856.

MATSUSAKI, Dean I; Thamesview Family Health Team, 465 Grand Ave W, Chatham ON N7L 1C5; Wes'85; (519)351-9281

MATSUSAKI, Ronald; Digby Gen Hosp, PO Box 820 75 Warwick St, Digby NS B0V 1A0; Tor'73; Staff, Digby General Hospital; (902)245-2501; Fax. (902)245-2803; harleydoc_tx@yahoo.com.

MATSYK, Jacqueline B; 103-2025 Broadway W, Vancouver BC V6J 1Z6; Sask'85; (604)730-9769

MATTA, Ihab; 129-140 Great Lakes Dr, Brampton ON L6R 2K7; Tor'91; (905)790-6644; Fax. (905)790-6646.

MATTA, Roberto B; Flemingdon Park Shopp Centre, 3A-747 Don Mills Rd, North York ON M3C 1T2; (Philippines)'73; Ac Staff Family Pract, Toronto East General Hospital Inc; Langs: Tagalog; (416)421-6320; Fax. (416)421-5286.

MATTA, Vivian T Y; Crowfoot Village Prof Centre, 201-60 Crowfoot Cres NW, Calgary AB T3G 3J9; (Egypt)'94; CCFP; (403)374-0244; Fax. (403)374-0354.

MATTAR, Adel G; Chatham-Kent Health Alliance, PO Box 2030 Stn Main 80 Grand Ave W, Chatham ON N7M 5L9; Ain Shams (Egypt)'64; MB ChB; AB; FRCPC; NuclearMed. Staff, Chatham-Kent Health Alliance; Langs: Arabic; (519)352-6400

MATTAR, Kamal; 307-6453 Morrison St, Niagara Falls ON L2E 7H1; Tor'01; FRCSC; Urol (Uro Oncology). Staff Urologist, Niagara Health System - Ontario Street Site; Langs: Arabic; (905)356-7321; Fax. (289)296-0236; mattarmd@gmail.com.

MATTAR, Nabih; 310 West St, Simcoe ON N3Y 1T4; Cork (Ireland)'79; MB ChB; BAO; FACS; FRCSC; GenSurg. Staff Gen Surg, Norfolk General Hospital; Langs: Arabic; (519)426-2043; Fax. (519)426-2540; mattarn@kwic.com.

MATTAS, Shawn P; Parkdale Comm Health Centre, 1229 Queen St W, Toronto ON M6K 1L2; McM'00; CCFP; (416)537-2455

MATTATALL, Fiona M; Chrysalis Obst & Gyn Clinic, 21-10 Richard Way SW, Calgary AB T3E 7M9; Qns'00; BSc; MSc; FRCSC; ObstGyn. (403)242-0770

MATTE, Anouk; CSSS Jeanne-Mance, 100-15 av du Mont-Royal O, Montreal QC H2T 2R9; Mon'91; (514)286-9657; Fax. (514)940-3621.

MATTE, Claire; Hop Charles Lemoyne, 3120 boul Taschereau, Greenfield Park QC J4V 2H1; Laval'86; FRCPC; AnatPath. Staff, Hopital Charles LeMoyne; (450)466-5000

MATTE, Genevieve; CHUM-Hop Notre-Dame, 1560 rue Sherbrooke E, Montreal QC H2L 4M1; McG'03; FRCPC; Neur. Staff, Centre Hospitalier l'Université de Montréal (CHUM) - Hôpital Notre-Dame; (514)890-8237

MATTE, Gilbert; Clinique Psychiatrique, 1105 12e Av N, Sherbrooke QC J1E 2X4; Laval'70; FRCPC; Psy. Staff Psy, Centre Hospitalier et CLSC de Memphremagog; (819)563-5311; Fax. (819)563-9091.

MATTE, Hugues; Clinique d'Urologie, 2940 Boul Laframboise, Saint-Hyacinthe QC J2S 4Z2; Mon'94; FRCSC; Urol. Staff Urol, Centre Hospitalier Honore-Mercier; Langs: English; (450)250-8888; Fax. (450)250-8889.

MATTE, Lise; 965 boul Cure-Labelle CP 41525 Csp Ctr St-Martin, Laval QC H7V 4A3; Mon'74; (514)336-3809; Fax. (514)336-3809.

MATTE, Marie-Claude; Clinique de Med Familiale, 6e-2120 rue Sherbrooke E, Montreal QC H2K 1C3; Mon'03; CCFP; (514)527-1958; Fax. (514)527-1649.

MATTE, Pierre; Polyclinique Med Buckingham, 147 rue Joseph, Gatineau QC J8L 1G3; Mon'76; ac Staff, CH-CHSLD de Papineau - Pavillon du centre hospitalier; (819)986-1034; Fax. (819)986-3308.

MATTE, Raymond; Clinique Psychiatrique, CP 600 1105 12e Av N, Sherbrooke QC J1E 2X4; Laval'67; Psy. ac Staff, Hôpital Sainte-croix; Consultant, Centre Hospitalier Universitaire de Sherbrooke-Hôpital Hôtel-Dieu; Chef psychiatrie, Centre Hospitalier Universitaire de Sherbrooke-Hopital Fleurimont; Prof clin agrégé Psy, Universite de Sherbrooke; (819)563-5311; Fax. (819)563-9091.

MATTEAU, Sylvain; 203-140 Champlain St, Dieppe NB E1A 1N8; Mon'93; FACC; Cardiol (P.Q.); IntMed. Staff, Dr Georges-L-Dumont University Hospital Centre; (506)862-1098; Fax. (506)855-2324.

MATTER, Michele A; Selkirk & Dist Gen Hosp, PO Box 5000 Stn Main, Selkirk MB R1A 2M2; Cape Town (South Africa)'89; MB ChB; BSc(Hons); CCFP; FCFP; Chief Medical Staff, Selkirk & District General Hospital; Med Dir EMS, Interlake-Eastern Regional Health Authority Stonewall; Langs: Afrikaans; Swedish; French; (204)482-5800; Fax. (204)482-9464; mmatter@neha.mb.ca.

MATTHEIS, Kelly G; Three Bridges Comm Health Ctre, 1292 Hornby St, Vancouver BC V6Z 1W2; Alb'04; (604)633-4220

MATTHEW, James R; 101-13798 94A Ave, Surrey BC V3V 1N1; Mem'03; FRCSC; OrthSurg. (778)395-4232

MATTHEW, Keith A; Aurora Med Centre, 200-15017 Yonge St, Aurora ON L4G 1M5; Mem'81; Staff, Southlake Regional Health Centre; Staff, The Scarborough Hospital - Birchmount Campus; (905)727-9481; Fax. (905)727-6280.

MATTHEWS, Angela C; Complete Medical, 573 Torbay Rd, St. John's NL A1A 5G9; Mem'06; CCFP.

MATTHEWS, Barbara A; 185 Inkerman St E, Listowel ON N4W 2N1; McM'86; Med Dir Emerg, Listowel Memorial Hospital - Listowel Wingham Hospitals Alliance; (519)291-4200; Fax. (519)291-5947.

MATTHEWS, Christopher M; St Boniface Clinic, 343 Tache Ave, Winnipeg MB R2H 2A5; Man'08; CCFP.

MATTHEWS, Jill A; Health Canada, 2045 Broad St, Regina SK S4P 3T7; Sask'80; FCBOM; (306)780-7450; Fax. (306)789-8259; jmatthews@sasktel.net.

MATTHEWS, John H; Queen's Univ-Etherington Hall, 2025-94 Stuart St, Kingston ON K7L 3N6; Cambridge (England)'73; MB ChB; MRCP(UK); MA; MRCPath; FRCP; FRCPC; HemPath (Hematology)., Kingston General Hospital; Prof Med, Queen's University; (613)533-6803; matthewj@post.queensu.ca.

MATTHEWS, Keith L; St Mary's Hosp Centre, B270-3830 av Lacombe, Montreal QC H3T 1M5; McG'89; FRCSC; Urol. Staff, St Mary's Hospital Centre; Staff, McGill University Health Centre - Montreal General Campus; Langs: Bilingual(English/French); (514)345-3511; Fax. (514)735-0756.

MATTHEWS, Michael K; 541 Eglinton Ave E, Toronto ON M4P 1N7; Tor'75; CCFP; FCFP; Court Staff, North York General Hospital; Court Staff, Sunnybrook Health Sciences Centre; Lecturer Family Med, University of Toronto; (416)487-2442; Fax. (416)487-2508.

MATTHEWS, Nicola E; St Boniface Gen Hosp, C5119-409 Tache ave, Winnipeg MB R2H 2A6; Qns'05; FRCPC; IntMed. Staff, St Boniface General Hospital; (204)233-8563

MATTHEWS, Nicole; Campbellton Reg Hosp, PO Box 880 Stn Main 189 Lily Lake Rd, Campbellton NB E3N 3H3; St George's (Grenada)'99; Staff, Hôpital Régional Campbellton; (506)789-5417

MATTHEWS, Paul W; 725 Jane St Ground Floor, York ON M6N 4B3; Mem'90; (647)351-6429; Fax. (647)351-6439.

MATTHEWS, Peter J; Gander Med Clinic, 177 Elizabeth Dr, Gander NL A1V 1H6; Mem'82; (709)256-7101; Fax. (709)256-7109.

MATTHEWS, Rita; Halton HSC Corp-Oakville, 327 Reynolds St, Oakville ON L6J 3L7; Utkal (India)'91; CCFP; CCFP(E.M.); Staff, Halton Healthcare Services Corporation - Oakville Site; (905)845-2571

MATTHEWS, Ronald B; Glover Med Clinic, 101-5796 Glover Rd, Langley BC V3A 4H9; Qns'77; Staff, Langley Memorial Hospital; (604)530-3233

MATTHEWS, Sarah; Northtown Mall, 203-9450 137 Ave NW, Edmonton AB T5E 6C2; Tor'72; FRCPC; Psy (Child & Adolescent Psychiatry). (780)475-3472

MATTHEWS, Susan B; McKenzie Prof Centre, 201-1595 McKenzie Ave, Victoria BC V8N 1A4; McG'93; CCFP; (250)721-1188; Fax. (250)721-2292.

MATTHEWS, T Wayne; Foothills Med Centre, 602 ST-1403 29 St NW, Calgary AB T2N 2T9; Tor'84; FRCSC; Otol (Head & Neck Surgery). Staff Surg/Div Chief Otol-Head & Neck Surg, Foothills Medical Centre; Assoc Prof, University of Calgary; (403)944-4501; Fax. (403)210-9752.

MATTHEWS, Tina R; Lakeshore Med & Prof Bldg, 303-3170 Lake Shore Blvd W, Etobicoke ON M8V 3X8; Tor'86; BSc; CCFP; Staff, St Joseph's Health Centre; (416)251-3311; Fax. (416)251-8817.

MATTHEY, Peter W; Misericordia Community Hosp, 16940 87 Ave NW, Edmonton AB T5R 4H5; (Ireland)'92; MB ChB; FFARCS; FRCP; FRCPC; Anes. Staff, Covenant Health - Misericordia Community Hospital; (780)735-2000; pmatthey@ualberta.ca.

MATTI, Edward T; Cambridge Mem Hosp, 700 Coronation Blvd, Cambridge ON N1R 3G2; Mosul (Iraq)'71; MB ChB; FRCPC; Psy. Staff, Cambridge Memorial Hospital; Langs: Assyrian; Arabic; (519)621-2330; Fax. (519)740-4936.

MATTIMOE, Claire A; Hôpital Ste-Justine, 3175 Ch Cote-Sainte-Catherine, Montreal QC H3T 1C5; Dublin (Ireland)'79; FRCPC; Peds. Staff, Hôpital Ste-Justine; (514)345-4931

MATTMAN, Andre; Diamond Health Care Centre, 4F-2775 Laurel St, Vancouver BC V5Z 1M9; UBC'97; FRCPC; MedBiochem (Laboratory Medicine). Pathologist, BC Children's Hospital; (604)875-5965; andre.mattman@vch.ca.

MATTON, Jean P; Clinique Med Carleton, GD 197 rue du Quai, Carleton QC G0C 1J0; Mon'71; Langs: English; (418)364-3311; Fax. (418)364-6650; lavigie@globetrotter.net.

MATTON, Jean-Francois; 1652 rue Royale, Trois-Rivieres QC G9A 4K3; Laval'78; (819)376-1661; Fax. (819)376-9902.

MATTU, Gurdial S; Guildford Town Ctr Med Clinic, 1269-15170 104 Ave, Surrey BC V3R 1N3; Cardiff (Wales)'93; (604)588-8764

MATUK, Naeema B; 12 Amberly Crt, Gloucester ON K1J 8A3; Karachi (Pakistan)'58; (613)741-5573

MATUKAS, Larissa M; St Michael's Hosp, 2 040 CC-30 Bond St, Toronto ON M5B 1W8; Tor'01; MSc; FRCPC; IntMed; InfectDis; MedMicrobiol. Staff, St Michael's Hospital; Langs: Lithuanian; (416)864-6060 x2946; Fax. (416)864-5194.

MATVENKO, Jack; 101-4450 Chatterton Way, Victoria BC V8X 5J2; Tor'54; Ophth (Glaucoma). Staff, Royal Jubilee Hospital; Staff, Victoria General Hospital; (250)386-0312; Fax. (250)384-5660.

MATWIJECKY, Cornelius; CBI Health Centres, 605 Discovery St, Victoria BC V8T 5G4; Ott'75; FRCSC; Neursurg. (250)383-3638

MATYAS, Miklos; 501-1580 Merivale Rd, Nepean ON K2G 4B5; Cal'94; FRCSC; Otol. Staff, Queensway Carleton Hospital; Staff, Children's Hospital of Eastern Ontario (CHEO); (613)727-3132; Fax. (613)727-3075.

MATYS, Gail L; Kanata Prof Centre, 204-99 Kakulu Rd, Kanata ON K2L 3C8; Qns'82; CCFP; FCFP; (613)592-1269; Fax. (613)592-1141.

MATZ, Alexander; 203A-189 Kent St, Lindsay ON K9V 5G6; Kyrgyz State Medical Academy (Other Foreign)'89; DrMedCh; FRCSC; GenSurg (Laparoscopic Surgery). Langs: Hebrew; Russian; (705)880-1212; Fax. (705)880-1211; alex_matz@auracom.com.

MATZINGER, Dorothy J; Eau Claire Market, 182-200 Barclay Parade SW, Calgary AB T2P 4R5; Tor'84; FRCPC; NuclearMed; DiagRad. (403)261-0080; Fax. (403)261-0016.

MATZINGER, Frederick R; Pembroke Reg Hosp, 705 Mackay St, Pembroke ON K8A 1G8; Tor'83; FRCPC; DiagRad. Staff, Pembroke Regional Hospital Inc; Consultant, The Ottawa Hospital - General Campus; Consultant, Queensway Carleton Hospital; Assoc Prof, University of Ottawa; (613)732-2811 x8083; fmatzinger@ottawahospital.on.ca.

MATZINGER, Mary Ann E; Children's Hosp Eastern Ont, 401 Smyth Rd, Ottawa ON K1H 8L1; Tor'78; FRCPC; DiagRad (Nuclear Medicine). Staff, Children's Hospital of Eastern Ontario (CHEO); Assoc Prof, University of Ottawa; (613)737-7600 x2304; Fax. (613)737-2306; matzinger@cheo.on.ca.

MATZOV, Aviram; Headwaters Health Care Centre, 100 Rolling Hills Dr, Orangeville ON L9W 4X9; Qns'86; Staff, Headwaters Health Care Centre - Orangeville Site; (519)941-2410; Fax. (519)941-4707.

MAUCERI, Nella; Oak Ridges Med Centre, 100-13291 Yonge St, Richmond Hill ON L4E 4L6; Tor'90; CCFP; CCFP(E.M.); Staff Emerg, Mackenzie Richmond Hill Hospital; (905)773-7759; Fax. (905)773-1325.

MAUCOTEL, Jocelyne; CHUM-Hop Notre-Dame, 1560 rue Sherbrooke E, Montreal QC H2L 4M1; Mon'77; FRCPC; Anes. Staff, Centre Hospitalier l'Université de Montréal (CHUM) - Hôpital Notre-Dame; (514)890-8000 x26876

MAUER, Martin B; Humber River Reg Hosp-Finch, 2111 Finch Ave W, North York ON M3N 1N1; Tor'83; DABA; FRCPC; Anes. Court Staff, The Scarborough Hospital - General Campus; Court Staff, Southlake Regional Health Centre; Court Staff, Rouge Valley Health System - Centenary Health Centre Site; Court Staff, North York General Hospital; Assoc Staff, Humber River Regional Hospital - Finch Avenue Site; (416)747-3824; Fax. (416)747-3773.

MAUFFETTE, Andre A; 901-1851 rue Sherbrooke E, Montreal QC H2K 4L5; Mon'65; Psy. Langs: English; (514)524-3336; Fax. (514)524-3823.

MAUGUIN, Marc L P; Montfort Hosp, 713 Montreal Rd, Ottawa ON K1K 0T2; UBC'80; FRCPC; Psy (Psycho Geriatrics). Ac Staff, Montfort Hospital; Consultant, SCO Health Service - Élisabeth Bruyère Hospital; Consultant, Sensenbrenner Hospital; Physician Psy, Ontario Ministry of Health; Physician Psy, Northern Ontario Francophone Psychiatry Program; Clin Asst, University of Ottawa; Langs: English; French; (613)746-4621; Fax. (613)748-4938.

MAULUD, Awatef; Midtown Med Centre, 5706 50 Ave, Vermilion AB T9X 1L4; (Libya)'93; MB BCh; (780)853-2809; Fax. (780)853-2977.

MAUNDER, Robert G; Mount Sinai Hosp, 9F-600 University Ave, Toronto ON M5G 1X5; Tor'84; FRCPC; Psy. Staff Psy, Mount Sinai Hospital; Assoc Prof Psy, University of Toronto; (416)586-4800 x3200; Fax. (416)586-8654; rmaunder@mtsinai.on.ca.

MAUNDERS, John G; Ctr Hosp Laurentien, 234 rue Saint-Vincent, Ste-Agathe-Des-Mts QC J8C 2B8; McG'95; CCFP; Staff, Centre Hospitalier Laurentien; (819)324-4000

MAUNG, Raymond T A; Royal Inland Hosp, 311 Columbia St, Kamloops BC V2C 2T1; Rangoon (Burma)'76; MB BS; MBA; FRC; FRCPC; AnatPath. Staff Path, Royal Inland Hospital; Langs: Burmese; (250)314-2650; r_maung@yahoo.ca.

MAUNG, Tun Zan; 208-1945 McCallum Rd, Abbotsford BC V2S 3N2; Rangoon (Burma)'82; MB BS; LRCP(Lond); MRCS(Eng); ABIM; FRCPC; IntMed (Cardiology). Dir Diabetes Centre/Staff IntMed, Abbotsford Regional Hospital & Cancer Centre; Asst Prof Clinical Med, University of British Columbia; Langs: Burmese; (604)870-4800; Fax. (604)870-4804; tzmaung@telus.net.

MAUNSELL, Jonathan B; Elgin Med Centre, 101-2255 Elgin Ave, Port Coquitlam BC V3C 2B4; UBC'90; Assoc Staff, Royal Columbian Hospital; (604)942-7292

MAURAIS, Gilles; Centre Bois de Boulogne, 480-1575 boul Henri-Bourassa O, Montreal QC H3M 3A9; Laval'79; FRCSC; OrthSurg. Staff, Hôpital du Sacre-Coeur de Montréal; (514)332-6025; Fax. (514)332-4243.

MAURER, Deborah A; Royal University Hosp, 103 Hospital Dr, Saskatoon SK S7N 0W8; Man'97; BSc; FRCPC; Anes. Staff, Royal University Hospital; (306)655-1183; Fax. (306)655-1279; maurerd@shaw.ca.

MAURICE, Michael J; 302-749 King St W, Kitchener ON N2G 1E4; Tor'91; FRCSC; GenSurg. Staff Surgeon, St Mary's General Hospital; Staff, Grand River Hospital - Kitchener/Waterloo Health Centre; (519)584-0180; Fax. (519)584-0182.

MAURICE, Pascale; CHUS-Hop Fleurimont, 3001 12e Av N, Sherbrooke QC J1H 5N4; Sher'91; FRCPC; Peds. Staff, Centre Hospitalier Universitaire de Sherbrooke-Hopital Fleurimont; (819)346-1110 x14644

MAURICE, Pierre; Institut Nationale Sante Publi, 2400 av D'Estimauville, Quebec QC G1E 7G9; Laval'75; MBA; FRCPC; CommunMed. Chef D'Unite Scientifique, Centre Hospitalier Universitaire de Quebec-CHUL; Clin Prof, Université Laval; Langs: Spanish; Portuguese; English; (418)666-7000 x345; Fax. (418)666-2776.

MAURICE, Rachel; Royal Inland Hosp, 311 Columbia St, Kamloops BC V2C 2T1; UBC'97; FRCPC; Anes. Staff, Royal Inland Hospital; (250)374-5111

MAURICE, Stephane; Clinique Med Giffard, 210-3333 rue du Carrefour, Quebec QC G1C 5R9; Laval'90; (418)663-6345

MAURICE, William L; 1535 Broadway St W PO Box 29091 Rpo South Granvil, Vancouver BC V6J 5C2; McG'64; BA; FRCPC; Psy (Sexual Medicine). Member, Mental Health Review Board; maurice@mail.ubc.ca.

MAURO, Marina; Headwaters Specialist Clinic, 150 Rolling Hills Dr, Orangeville ON L9W 4X8; Univ of Buenos Aires (Argentina)'95; FRCPC; IntMed. Staff IntMed, Headwaters Health Care Centre - Orangeville Site; Langs: Spanish; (519)941-7117

MAUSOLF, Susanne; Abbottsfield Shoppers Mall, 214-3210 118 Ave NW, Edmonton AB T5W 4W1; Alb'82; BMedSci; (780)471-2071; Fax. (780)474-8001.

MAVRIPLIS, Cleo A; Primrose Family Med Centre, 35 Primrose Ave, Ottawa ON K1R 0A1; Mon'81; CCFP; FCFP; Asst Prof Family Med, University of Ottawa; Langs: French; Greek; (613)230-7788; Fax. (613)230-7778.

MAVROGIANNIS, Louie; 650 Church St, Toronto ON M4Y 2G5; Tor'02; DrSci; CCFP; Staff, The Salvation Army Toronto Grace Health Centre; Langs: Greek; (416)925-2251; Fax. (416)925-0939.

MAVROMICHALIS, Helen; CLSC Cote-des-Neiges, 500-5700 ch de la Cote-Des-Nei, Montreal QC H3T 2A8; Mon'06; CCFP; Médecin, CLSC Cote-des-Neiges; (514)731-8531; Fax. (514)731-0536.

MAWANI, Al-Karim; Family Health Plus, 5-6601 Main St, Stouffville ON L4A 6A9; Tor'91; BSc; CCFP; Langs: Gujarati; (905)642-9995; Fax. (905)642-9981.

MAWANI, Shiraz H L; C-22195 Dewdney Trunk Rd, Maple Ridge BC V2X 3H7; Sheffield (England)'71; Ac Staff, Ridge Meadows Hospital & Health Care Centre; (604)463-8877; Fax. (604)463-4514.

MAWDSLEY, Caitlin S; Riverview Med Clinic, 101-436 Lorne St, Kamloops BC V2C 1W3; Pretoria (South Africa)'04; MB ChB; (250)372-3828

MAWDSLEY, Michael G; Cook Medical Bldg, 202-1175 Cook St, Victoria BC V8V 4A1; Alb'80; CCFP; FCFP; (250)385-8754; Fax. (250)385-3627.

MAWDSLEY, Scott D; 105-35 Baker Dr, Dartmouth NS B2W 0H3; UBC'95; FRCSC; ObstGyn. Staff, IWK Health Centre; Staff, Dartmouth General Hospital; Dalhousie University; (902)463-1244; Fax. (902)466-4585; smawdsley@ns.sympatico.ca.

MAWHINNEY, Leah A; Victoria Family Med Centre, 60 Chelsey Ave, London ON N5Z 2C1; Tor'09; CCFP; Teach Staff, University of Western Ontario; (519)433-8424

MAWHINNEY, Shawn W; Southlake Reg Health Centre, 596 Davis Dr, Newmarket ON L3Y 2P9; Tor'98; FRCPC; Anes. Staff, Southlake Regional Health Centre; (905)895-4521

MAWJI, Altaf S J; 1-1695 Wonderland Rd N, London ON N6G 4W3; Wes'84; Assoc Staff, St Joseph's Hospital - St Joseph's Health Care; Physician, Mt Hope Nursing Home; Physician, Richmond Woods Retirement Home; (519)472-6464; Fax. (519)474-9779.

MAWJI, Yasmine; Mount Sinai Hosp, 206-600 University Ave, Toronto ON M5G 1X5; McG'95; CCFP; CCFP(E.M.); Staff, Mount Sinai Hospital; Langs: English; French; (416)586-5058; Fax. (416)586-4719.

MAWN, Steve; CSSS de Port-Cartier, 3 rue Shelterbay, Port-Cartier QC G5B 2W9; Mon'92; Staff, CLSC-CSSS de Port-Cartier; (418)766-2572

MAWSON, John B; Children's & Women's HC of BC, 1L57-4480 Oak St, Vancouver BC V6H 3V4; Auckland (New Zealand)'84; MB ChB; FRACR; FRCPC; DiagRad. Staff, BC Children's Hospital; (604)875-2131; Fax. (604)875-2367.

MAXAN, Emily E; Saint John Reg Hosp, PO Box 2100 Stn Main, Saint John NB E2L 4L2; Dal'06; FRCPC; Psy. Staff, Saint John Regional Hospital; (506)648-6000

MAXIMOUS, Emad F; Niagara H System-Ontario St, 155 Ontario St, St. Catharines ON L2R 5K3; Ain Shams (Egypt)'89; FRCPC; Anes. Staff, Niagara Health System - Ontario Street Site; (905)378-4647

MAXNER, Charles E; Queen Elizabeth II HSC-Halifax, 3819-1796 Summer St, Halifax NS B3H 3A7; Dal'79; FRCPC; Neur (Neuro Ophthalmology). Staff, Queen Elizabeth II Health Sciences Centre - Halifax Infirmary Site; Staff, Queen Elizabeth II Health Sciences Centre - Victoria General Site; Consultant, IWK Health Centre; Prof Neurol & Ophth, Dalhousie University; (902)473-2130; Fax. (902)473-4438.

MAXTED, Grant R; Humber River Reg Hosp-Finch, 2111 Finch Ave W, North York ON M3N 1N1; Otago (New Zealand)'76; FRCPC; Anes. Dep Chief Anes, Humber River Regional Hospital - Finch Avenue Site; (416)744-2500; Fax. (416)747-3773.

MAXTED, John M; Health For All Family Health T, 202-379 Church St, Markham ON L6B 0T1; Ott'74; MBA; CCFP; FCFP; Ac Staff, Markham Stouffville Hospital; Asst Prof DFCM, University of Toronto; (905)472-2200; Fax. (905)472-5662.

MAXWELL, Brenda S R; Gateway Primacy Med Clinic, 1035 Gateway Rd, Winnipeg MB R2K 4C1; Cal'86; MSc; BSc; CCFP; FCFP; Asst Prof, University of Manitoba.

MAXWELL, Cynthia V; Ontario Power Generation, OPG 3271-700 University Ave, Toronto ON M5G 1Z5; Boston(MA) (USA)'97; FRCSC; ObstGyn (Maternal Fetal Medicine). Staff Maternal Fetal Med, Mount Sinai Hospital; Langs: French; (416)586-4800 x3229; Fax. (416)586-5992.

MAXWELL, E Linda; Toronto North Med Arts Centre, 101-7155 Woodbine Ave, Markham ON L3R 1A3; Yale School of Medicine(CT) (USA)'00; FRCSC; Otol (Facial Plastic & Reconstructive Surgery). Langs: French; (416)628-4020; Fax. (416)628-4021.

MAXWELL, H Brent; London HSC-Victoria Hosp, PO Box 5010 Stn B 800 Commissioners Rd E, London ON N6A 5W9; Mem'82; FRCPC; EmergMed. Staff, London Health Sciences Centre - Victoria Campus; (519)667-6538

MAXWELL, Ian; Victoria Gen Hosp, 2340 Pembina Hwy, Winnipeg MB R3T 2E8; Glasgow (Scotland)'57; MB ChB; MRCP(UK); FRCPC; IntMed (Hematology). Dir Oncol, Victoria General Hospital; Consultant, Health Sciences Centre; Assoc Prof, University of Manitoba; (204)477-3329; Fax. (204)261-3045.

MAXWELL, Robert I; Royal Victoria Hosp, 201 Georgian Dr, Barrie ON L4M 6M2; (Ireland)'89; BSc; MSc; MB ChB; Staff Emerg, Royal Victoria Regional Health Centre; (705)728-9802

MAXWELL, Thomas E; Clinique de Med Familiale, 123-151 Main St E, Hawkesbury ON K6A 1A1; Ott'82; Staff, Hawkesbury & District General Hospital; (613)632-0151; Fax. (613)632-1073.

MAXWELL, Timothy J; Windsor Reg Hosp-Metropolitan, 1995 Lens Ave, Windsor ON N8W 1L9; Wes'06; FRCPC; Anes. Staff, Windsor Regional Hospital - Metropolitan Site; (519)254-5577

MAY, Andre B; Royal Victoria Hosp, 201 Georgian Dr, Barrie ON L4M 6M2; Mem'95; CCFP; CCFP(E.M.); Physician Emerg, Royal Victoria Regional Health Centre; (705)728-9090 x4121; andre.may2@sympatico.ca.

MAY, David J; 7019 Alberni St, Powell River BC V8A 2C2; London (England)'85; MB BS; MRCGPract; LMCC; Ac Staff, Powell River General Hospital; (604)485-9213; Fax. (604)485-9306; d.may@telus.net.

MAY, Donna L; Brampton Med Bldg, 307-164 Queen St E, Brampton ON L6V 1B4; Alb'88; FRCPC; IntMed; Endocrin&Metab. Staff, William Osler Health System - Brampton Civic Hospital; (905)457-3458; Fax. (905)450-0077.

MAY, Douglas C; Royal Inland Hosp, 311 Columbia St, Kamloops BC V2C 2T1; Alb'86; FRCSC; GenSurg. Staff, Royal Inland Hospital; (250)374-5111

MAY, Gary R; St Michael's Hosp, 16 058-30 Bond St, Toronto ON M5B 1W8; Alb'85; FRCPC; IntMed (Therapeutic Endoscopy); Gastroent. Staff Cardinal Carter Wing, St Michael's Hospital; (416)864-5345; Fax. (416)864-5749.

MAY, Janice L; Allin Clinic, 10155 120 St NW, Edmonton AB T5K 2A2; Alb'90; CCFP; FCFP; Med Staff, Royal Alexandra Hospital; (780)482-7551; Fax. (780)701-5396.

MAY, John D; Guelph Gen Hosp, 115 Delhi St, Guelph ON N1E 4J4; Tor'87; Staff, Cambridge Memorial Hospital; Staff, Guelph General Hospital; (519)822-5350

MAY, Michael J; Oakville Haelth Centre, 117-1060 Speers Rd, Oakville ON L6L 2X4; Mon'08; CCFP; (905)845-8884

MAY, Richard; MUHC-Montreal Chest Inst, 3650 rue Saint-Urbain, Montreal QC H2X 2P4; McG'80; Staff, McGill University Health Centre - Montreal Chest Institute; Langs: Bilingual(English/French); (514)934-1934

MAY, Terrence A; Peterborough Reg HC-Hospital, 1 Hospital Dr, Peterborough ON K9J 7C6; Cal'02; CCFP; CCFP(E.M.); Staff, Peterborough Regional Health Centre - Hospital Drive; (705)876-5022; Fax. (705)876-5096.

MAY, Tyler B; Associate Medical Clinic, 10018 101 St, Peace River AB T8S 2A5; (Other Foreign)'10; CCFP; (780)624-2581

MAYA, Nomtandazo P T; 114-2805 6th Ave E, Prince Albert SK S6V 6Z6; Natal (South Africa)'96; MB ChB; (306)763-2681; Fax. (306)953-1024; tandiemaya@hotmail.com.

MAYBA, Ihor I; Manitoba Clinic, 790 Sherbrook St, Winnipeg MB R3A 1M3; Man'57; DGS; DAB; FRCSC; GenSurg (Trauma); OrthSurg. Staff, Children's Hospital of Winnipeg; Staff, Health Sciences Centre; Langs: Ukrainian; (204)788-5757; Fax. (204)774-5772; knavitka@shaw.ca.

MAYBA, John I; Manitoba Clinic, 790 Sherbrook St, Winnipeg MB R3A 1M3; Man'89; Langs: Ukrainian; (204)774-6541; Fax. (204)775-6373.

MAYBAUM, Lloyd E M; Peter Lougheed Centre, 3675-3500 26 Ave NE, Calgary AB T1Y 6J4; Cal'97; FRCPC; Psy. Staff, Peter Lougheed Centre; (403)943-4904

MAYBEE, John D; Lakeridge Hlth Corp-Oshawa, 1 Hospital Crt, Oshawa ON L1G 2B9; Qns'85; FRCPC; Anes. Ac Staff, Lakeridge Health - Oshawa Site; (905)576-8711 x3312; Fax. (905)721-4337.

MAYBERRY, Thomas R; 483953 Sweaburg Rd RR 4, Ingersoll ON N5C 3J7; Wes'72; Ac Staff, Alexandra Hospital; (519)485-3908

MAYCHER, Bruce W; St Boniface Gen Hosp, 409 Tache Ave, Winnipeg MB R2H 2A6; Man'80; FRCPC; DiagRad. Ac Staff/Head Diag Imaging, St Boniface General Hospital; (204)233-8563

MAYER, Anna M; Stratford Gen Hosp, 46 General Hospital Dr, Stratford ON N5A 2Y6; Wes'03; CCFP; CCFP(E.M.); Staff, Clinton Public Hospital - Huron Perth Healthcare Alliance; Staff, St Marys Memorial Hospital - Huron Perth Healthcare Alliance; Staff, Stratford General Hospital - Huron Perth Healthcare Alliance; (519)272-2120; Fax. (519)271-7137.

MAYER, Chantal; Hop Du Sacre-Coeur De Mtl, 132-5400 boul Gouin O, Montreal QC H4J 1C5; Mon'80; ac Staff, Hôpital du Sacre-Coeur de Montréal; (514)338-2222 x2140

MAYER, Chantal M H; BC Women's Hosp & Health Ctre, 2H23A-4500 Oak St, Vancouver BC V6H 3N1; McG'99; BSc; FRCSC; ObstGyn (Maternal Fetal Medicine). Staff, BC Women's Hospital & Health Centre; Langs: Bilingual(French/English); (604)875-3108; cmayer@cw.bc.ca.

MAYER, J O Jean-Pierre; 14 rue Canvin, Kirkland QC H9H 4S4; Ott'70; FACC; ABIM(CVDisease); FRCPC; Cardiol (P.Q.); IntMed. Staff Cardiologist, Lakeshore General Hospital - Pointe Claire; Langs: English; (514)694-6950

MAYER, Jean; 400-28 ch du Golf E, St-Charles-Brromee QC J6E 2B4; Mon'80; Ophth (Cataract). Staff, Centre Hospitalier Régional de Lanaudière; (450)759-8499; Fax. (450)759-5796.

MAYER, Kailash K; 530-5450 Ch Cote-des-Neiges, Montreal QC H3T 1Y6; Punjab (India)'63; Staff, St Mary's Hospital Centre; (514)737-1669; Fax. (514)488-5064.

MAYER, Katalin E; Foothills Med Centre, 704-1403 29 St NW, Calgary AB T2N 2T9; Cal'04; FRCPC; Psy. Staff, Foothills Medical Centre; (403)944-5872; Fax. (403)944-2409.

MAYER, Kevin D; Yorkgate Mall, 136A-1 York Gate Blvd, North York ON M3N 3A1; Tor'10; CCFP; (416)745-4555; Fax. (416)745-0786.

MAYER, Kristine L; Riverside Prof Centre, 31 Riverside Dr, Sydney NS B1S 3N1; Man'96; BSc; FRCSC; Ophth. Staff, Cape Breton Healthcare Complex; (902)564-8580

MAYER, Perry V; The Mayer Institute, 20 Railway St, Hamilton ON L8R 2R3; RCS (Ireland)'90; BSc; MB BCh; CCFP; (905)523-1444; Fax. (905)523-6600; drpvmayer@themayerinstitute.ca.

MAYER, Pierre; CHUM-Hotel-Dieu, 3840 rue Saint-Urbain, Montreal QC H2W 1T8; Mon'88; FRCPC; IntMed (Sleep Disorders Medicine); Respir. Staff, Centre Hospitalier l'Université de Montréal (CHUM) - Hôtel-Dieu; Langs: English; Spanish; (514)890-8170; Fax. (514)412-7178; pierre.mayer@umontreal.ca.

MAYER, Sandeep K; CHUS-Hop Fleurimont, 3001 12e Av N, Sherbrooke QC J1H 5N4; McG'89; FRCSC; GenSurg; PedGenSurg. Staff, Centre Hospitalier Universitaire de Sherbrooke-Hopital Fleurimont; (819)346-1110; Fax. (819)820-6420.

MAYER, Stanley P; Rockyview Gen Hosp, 7007 14 St SW, Calgary AB T2V 1P9; Alb'86; CCFP; CCFP(E.M.); FCFP; Staff Emerg Med, Rockyview General Hospital; (403)943-3449

MAYER, Sudesh; 530-5450 Ch Cote-des-Neiges, Montreal QC H3T 1Y6; Gujarat (India)'63; (514)737-1669

MAYER, Sunita; 530-5450 ch de la Cote-des-Nei, Montreal QC H3T 1Y6; McG'96; CCFP; (514)737-1669

MAYERS, Alexandre; Clinique Access Md, 302-28 ch du Golf E, St-Charles-Brromee QC J6E 2B4; Laval'97; Staff, Centre Hospitalier Régional de Lanaudière; (450)756-2626

MAYERS, Irvin; College Plaza, 225-8215 112 St NW, Edmonton AB T6G 2C8; Man'77; FRCPC; IntMed; Respir. Staff, University of Alberta Hospital; Div Dir Pulmonary Med/Prof, University of Alberta; (780)407-1767; Fax. (780)407-3027; imayers@ualberta.ca.

MAYES, Adrienne A; Klondyke Med Clinic, 1-3089 3rd Ave, Whitehorse YT Y1A 5B3; Qns'06; CCFP; Staff, Klondyke Medical Clinic; (867)668-4046

MAYES, Camisha; Percy E Moore Hosp, PO Box 190, Hodgson MB R0C 1N0; (Other Foreign)'10; CCFP; Staff, Percy E Moore Hospital; (204)372-8444

MAYETTE, Michael; CHUS-Hop Hotel-Dieu, 580 rue Bowen S, Sherbrooke QC J1G 2E8; Mon'05; FRCPC; IntMed. Staff, Centre Hospitalier Universitaire de Sherbrooke-Hôpital Hôtel-Dieu; (819)346-1110

MAYETTE, Richard; Centre Medical Acton, GD 967 rue Boulay, Acton Vale QC J0H 1A0; Laval'71; (450)546-3245; jujumayette@hotmail.com.

MAYHEW, W James; Dalbrent Med Centre, 200-3604 52 Ave NW, Calgary AB T2L 1V9; Alb'68; CCFP; CCFP(E.M.); FCFP; Clin Assoc Prof, University of Calgary; (403)284-2261; Fax. (403)284-9434.

MAYICH, D Joshua; St Michael's Orthopaedic Assoc, 800-55 Queen St E, Toronto ON M5C 1R6; Wes'06; FRCSC; OrthSurg. (416)864-5392

MAYKUT, Andrew W; Guelph Gen Hosp, 115 Delhi St, Guelph ON N1E 4J4; Tor'79; FRCPC; Anes. Staff, Guelph General Hospital; (519)882-5350

MAYMAN, Barbara; Medisys, 500 rue Sherbrooke O, Montreal QC H3A 3C6; Laval'88; CCFP; FCFP; Staff Family Med, Sir Mortimer B Davis Jewish General; adj Prof Family Med, McGill University; (514)845-1211; Fax. (514)499-9536.

MAYNARD, John E; Lions Gate Hosp, 231 15th St E, North Vancouver BC V7L 2L7; Cal'74; Staff/Sr Med Dir, Lions Gate Hospital; (604)984-3894

MAYNARD, Judith A; Brameast Family Health Org, 38-2130 North Park Dr, Brampton ON L6S 0C9; McM'79; CCFP; FCFP; Ac Staff, William Osler Health System - Brampton Civic Hospital; (905)792-2211; Fax. (905)792-2901.

MAYNARD, Lucie; 471 car D'Effingham, Sainte-Therese QC J7E 3Y1; Mon'90; CCFP; Staff, CLSC Therese-de-Blainville; (450)971-6121; Fax. (450)971-4954.

MAYNARD, Olivier; CSSS De La Haute-Yamaska, 205 boul Leclerc O, Granby QC J2G 1T7; Mon'06; Staff, Centre Hospitalier de Granby; (450)375-3000; nalgene@hotmail.com.

MAYNARD, Sidney; Ctr Hosp Anna-Laberge, 200 boul Brisebois, Chateauguay QC J6K 4W8; Mon'94; Staff, Hôpital Anna-Laberge; (450)699-2425; Fax. (450)699-2525.

MAYNES, Douglas F; Community Mental Hlth Services, 109-7071 Bayers Rd, Halifax NS B3L 2C2; Dal'72; FRCPC; Psy. Consultant Psy, Queen Elizabeth II Health Sciences Centre - Victoria General Site; Asst Prof Psy, Dalhousie University; (902)454-1400

MAYNES, Jason T; The Hosp for Sick Children, 555 University Ave, Toronto ON M5G 1X8; Alb'06; Staff, The Hospital For Sick Children; (416)813-5934

MAYO, Edgar P; Burin Pharmacy Bldg, PO Box 250, Burin Bay Arm NL A0E 1G0; Mem'75; CCFP; FCFP; Ac Staff, Burin Peninsula Health Care Centre; (709)891-2260; Fax. (709)891-2725.

MAYO, John R; Dept of Radiology, G861-899 12th Ave W, Vancouver BC V5Z 1M9; Ott'81; FRCPC; DiagRad (Chest & Cardiac Radiology). Ac Staff, Vancouver General Hospital - Centennial Pavillion; Prof, University of British Columbia; (604)875-4111 x63193; Fax. (604)875-5195; john.mayo@vch.ca.

MAYO, Jorge P; Hys Med Centre, 510-11010 101 St NW, Edmonton AB T5H 4B9; San Marcos (Peru)'82; FRCSC; ObstGyn. Staff, Royal Alexandra Hospital; Staff, Sturgeon Community Hospital; (780)414-0782; Fax. (780)414-0784.

MAYO, Robert E; Chatham-Kent Health-Sydenham, 325 Margaret Ave, Wallaceburg ON N8A 2A7; Qns'83; BEng; CCFP; Ac Staff Privil Family Med, Chatham-Kent Health Alliance - Sydenham Hospital Campus; (519)359-0028; robertmayos50@gmail.com.

MAYO, Warren G; 401-1200 Lonsdale Ave, North Vancouver BC V7M 3H6; UBC'77; FRCPC; Anes (Intensive Care Medicine); IntMed. Staff, Lions Gate Hospital; (604)984-2406; Fax. (604)984-2279.

MAYR, Barbara J A; 601-475 13th St, West Vancouver BC V7T 2N7; Wes'76; Vis Staff, UBC Hospital - Koerner Pavillion; Physician Locum Privil, BC Mental Health & Addiction Service; Vis Staff, Vancouver General Hospital - Centennial Pavillion; Staff, Dr Bernstein Health & Diet Clinic; Langs: German; French; (604)767-4099

MAYR, Heinz George; 528 Dundas St, London ON N6B 1W6; Wes'75; Staff, St Joseph's Hospital - St Joseph's Health Care; Langs: German; (519)645-2227

MAYR, Michael S G; Norfolk Family Medical, 305-85 Norfolk St, Guelph ON N1H 4J4; Wes'75; DRCOG; CCFP; Ac Staff, Guelph General Hospital; Asst Prof Family Med, Queen's University; Asst Prof Family Med, McMaster University; (519)836-9440; Fax. (519)836-9530.

MAYR, Patricia J; Norfolk Family Medical, 305-85 Norfolk St, Guelph ON N1H 4J4; Wes'74; Court Staff, Guelph General Hospital; Langs: German; French; (519)836-9440; Fax. (519)836-9530.

MAYRAND, Dominic; SMBD Jewish Gen Hosp, 3755 ch Cote-Sainte-Catherine, Montreal QC H3T 1E2; Sher'90; FRCPC; Anes. Staff, Sir Mortimer B Davis Jewish General; (514)340-8222

MAYRAND, Helene; CSSS de Laval, 1755 boul Rene-Laennec, Laval QC H7M 3L9; Mon'93; FRCPC; IntMed; Cardiol. Staff, Hopital de la Cite de la santé; Langs: Bilingual(French/English); (450)668-1010; Fax. (450)975-5550.

MAYRAND, Isabel; GMF Centre Med du Parc, 101-84 rue Court, Granby QC J2G 4Y5; Laval'91; CCFP; FCFP; (450)375-1161; Fax. (450)375-7740.

MAYRAND, Luc; Clinique Med du Cuivre, 12 rue Gamble E, Rouyn-Noranda QC J9X 3B7; Sher'03; CCFP; Staff, Centre Hospitalier Rouyn-Noranda; (819)764-9441

MAYRAND, Luc P; 36 rue Guerrette, Edmundston NB E3V 1N8; Laval'83; Staff, Hôpital regional d'Edmundston; (506)739-8594; Fax. (506)735-7554.

MAYRAND, Marie-Helene; CHUM-Hop St-Luc, 1058 rue Saint-Denis, Montreal QC H2X 3J4; Mon'94; FRCSC; ObstGyn. Staff, Centre Hospitalier l'Université De Montréal (CHUM) - Hôpital Saint-luc; (514)890-8000; mhmayrand@videotron.ca.

MAYRAND, Martin; 4550 rue Principale, St-Felix-de-Valois QC J0K 2M0; Laval'53; (450)889-2679

MAYRAND, Serge; MUHC-Montreal Gen Hosp, D7 102-1650 av Cedar, Montreal QC H3G 1A4; Mon'84; FRCPC; IntMed (Esophageal Disorders); Gastroent. assoc Médecin, McGill University Health Centre - Montreal General Campus; adj Prof, McGill University; Langs: Bilingual(French/English); (514)934-1934 x43899; Fax. (514)934-8531.

MAYRAND, Sophie; CSSS de la Haute-Yamaska, 205 boul Leclerc O, Granby QC J2G 1T7; Laval'00; CCFP; CCFP(E.M.); Staff, Centre Hospitalier de Granby; (450)375-8000

MAYRHOFER, Ronald; Fish Creek Medical, 208-803 Chaparral Dr SE, Calgary AB T2X 0E5; Man'74; Clinical Asst Prof Med, University of Calgary; (403)873-7734

MAYSON, Kelly V; Dept of Anaes, 2449-899 12th Ave W, Vancouver BC V5Z 1M9; UBC'85; BSc; FRCPC; Anes. Ac Staff, Vancouver General Hospital - Centennial Pavillion; Clinical Asst Prof, University of British Columbia; (604)875-4304

MAYSON, Thomas A; Vancouver Gen Hosp, 3500-855 12th Ave W, Vancouver BC V5Z 1M9; Sask'82; FRCPC; Anes. Staff, Vancouver General Hospital - Centennial Pavillion; (604)822-7121

MAYTHAM, Colleen; Chisel Peak Med Clinic, PO Box 2769 417 10th Ave, Invermere BC V0A 1K0; Orange Free State (South Africa)'98; MB ChB; CCFP; Staff, Invermere & District Hospital; Langs: Afrikaans; German; (250)341-6900

MAYTOM, Peter A N; Kootenay Lake Hosp, 3 View St, Nelson BC V1L 2V1; Cape Town (South Africa)'79; MB ChB; FRCSC; Ophth. Staff, Kootenay Lake General Hospital; Langs: Afrikaans; (250)352-9984; Fax. (250)352-3489.

MAZAHERI, Arash; Islington at 401 Med Centre, 103-2257 Islington Ave, Etobicoke ON M9W 3W6; University of Medical Science & Hea (Iran)'94; CCFP; (416)746-0401; Fax. (416)746-3448.

MAZAMISA, Vusumzi M; Broadview Med Clinic, PO Box 39, Broadview SK S0G 0K0; (Other Foreign)'99; (306)696-2266; Fax. (306)696-2676.

MAZE, Aubrey H; Thornhill Square, 310-300 John St, Thornhill ON L3T 5W4; Cape Town (South Africa)'77; MB ChB; FRCPC; Peds. Staff, The Hospital For Sick Children; Court Staff, North York General Hospital; Court Staff, Mount Sinai Hospital; (905)881-9831; Fax. (905)886-5236.

MAZEK, Fawzi R E; Dr C W Wiebe Med Centre, 385 Main St, Winkler MB R6W 1J2; Al Arab Medical University (Saudi Arabia)'91; FRCSC; OrthSurg. (204)325-4312

MAZENGIA, Getachew; Lakeridge Hlth Corp-Bowmanvill, 47 Liberty St S, Bowmanville ON L1C 2N4; Jimma University (Other Foreign)'03; CCFP; Staff, Lakeridge Health - Bowmanville Site; (905)623-3331

MAZER, Bruce D; MUHC-Montreal Children's Hosp, C439-2300 rue Tupper, Montreal QC H3H 1P3; McG'84; ABPeds; ABAI; ClinImmunol&Allergy (P.Q.); Peds (Asthma). div Chef Allergy & Immunol, McGill University Health Centre - Montreal Children's Hospital; Dir recherche, Meakins-Christie Laboratories; assoc Prof Peds, McGill University; Langs: French; Hebrew; (514)412-4470

MAZER, C David; St Michael's Hosp, 30 Bond St, Toronto ON M5B 1W8; Sask'78; FRCPC; Anes (Critical Care Medicine). Staff, St Michael's Hospital; Assoc Prof, University of Toronto; (416)864-5071

MAZEROLLE, Eric; CHUS-Hop Hotel-Dieu, 580 rue Bowen S, Sherbrooke QC J1G 2E8; Sher'02; FRCSC; Ophth. Staff, Centre Hospitalier Universitaire de Sherbrooke-Hôpital Hôtel-Dieu; (819)346-1110

MAZEROLLE, Maryse F; Hespeler Med Clinic, 12-350 Conestoga Blvd, Cambridge ON N1R 7L7; McM'04; CCFP; Assoc Staff Family Health Centre, Toronto Western Hospital - University Health Network; (416)629-4630; Fax. (416)629-4615.

MAZEROLLE, Richard; Ctr Hosp Anna-Laberge, 200 boul Brisebois, Chateauguay QC J6K 4W8; Mon'92; FRCSC; GenSurg. Staff GenSurg, Hôpital Anna-Laberge; Langs: Spanish; English; (450)699-2425

MAZGANI, Mona; BC Cancer Agency, 2410 Lee Ave, Victoria BC V8R 6V5; Leiden (Netherlands)'97; Staff, BC Cancer Agency Vancouver Island Centre; (250)519-5578

MAZHAR, Mahmood M; Burlington Walk-In Clinic, 183-2025 Guelph Line, Burlington ON L7P 4M8; Bristol (England)'63; MB ChB; FRCS; Langs: Urdu; (905)681-7755; Fax. (905)333-1960.

MAZHAR, Mir Nadeem; Hotel-Dieu Hosp, J5-166 Brock St, Kingston ON K7L 5G2; Punjab (India)'96; FRCPC; Psy. Staff, Hotel-Dieu Hospital; (613)544-3400; Fax. (613)544-9666.

MAZHARI RAVESH, Amir H; Regent Med Centre, 208 Regent Ave W, Winnipeg MB R2C 1R2; (Other Foreign)'95; CCFP.

MAZIADE, Jean; CLSC Haute-Ville, 55 ch Sainte-Foy, Quebec QC G1R 1S9; Laval'84; CCFP; FCFP; Staff, Centre Hospitalier Affilié Universitaire de Québec - Hôpital du St-Sacrement; Clin Teach Staff Family Med, Université Laval; (418)641-2572; Fax. (418)522-5437; jean.maziade@ssss.gouv.qc.ca.

MAZIADE, Michel; Hotel-Dieu Du Sacre-Coeur, 1 av du Sacre-Coeur, Quebec QC G1N 2W1; Laval'72; FRCPC; Psy. Scientifique, Institut Universitaire Sante; Staff Child Psy, Hotel-Dieu du Sacre-Coeur de Jesus de Quebec; Researcher Representative, Sante au Quebec-Medicale Cons du Quebec; Prof Psy, Université Laval; (418)529-6851; Fax. (418)691-0750; michel.maziade@psa.ulaval.ca.

MAZIADE, Pierre-Jean; CSSS du Sud de Lanaudière, 911 montee des Pionniers, Terrebonne QC J6V 2H2; Sher'92; FRCPC; MedMicrobiol; Microbio & Infect Dis (P.Q.). Staff InfectDis, Centre Hospitalier Pierre le Gardeur; (450)654-7525; pierre-jean.maziade@ssss.gouv.qc.ca.

MAZIAK, Donna E; The Ottawa Hosp-Gen Campus, 6NW 6364-501 Smyth Rd, Ottawa ON K1H 8L6; McG'87; MSc(ClinEpidem); FACS; FRCSC; GenSurg (Esophageal Cancer); ThorSurg. Staff, The Ottawa Hospital - General Campus; Asst Prof, University of Ottawa; Langs: English; French; (613)737-8899 x74035; Fax. (613)737-8668.

MAZIARZ, Stanley T; 220-214 boul Cite-des-Jeunes, Gatineau QC J8Y 6S8; Lublin (Poland)'80; CCFP; Staff, CH-CHSLD de Papineau - Pavillon du centre hospitalier; Staff, Hull Hospital; Langs: Polish; Russian; Slovak; Ukrainian; French; (819)772-1118; ssandra@magma.ca.

MAZLOOM, Fereshteh; Rexdale Commun Health Centre, 8 Taber Rd, Etobicoke ON M9W 3A4; Barcelona (Spain)'81; CCFP; FCFP; Langs: Farsi; Persian; Spanish; (416)744-0066

MAZLOUM, Gloria M; Foothills Family Practice, 102-30 Crystalridge Dr, Okotoks AB T1S 2C3; Cal'01; BSc(PT); CCFP; (403)938-5455; Fax. (403)938-4749.

MAZMANIAN, Hagop K; Medical Arts Bldg, 3-165 Plymouth Rd, Welland ON L3B 3E1; Ain Shams (Egypt)'72; MB ChB; FACS; FRCSC; Urol (Prostate Cancer). Ac Staff, Niagara Health System - Welland Hospital Site; Assoc Staff, Niagara Health System - Port Colborne General Site; Assoc Staff, Niagara Health System - Douglas Memorial Hospital Site; Langs: Armenian; Arabic; French; (905)735-1375; Fax. (905)735-1696.

MAZOFF, Eric D; Statcare, 104-175 av Stillview, Pointe-Claire QC H9R 4S3; McG'76; NBME; LMCC; MCFP; BSc; CCFP; Langs: French; (514)694-9282; Fax. (514)697-0192.

MAZOWITA, Garey B M; St Paul's Hosp, 1081 Burrard St, Vancouver BC V6Z 1Y6; Man'79; BSc; FCFP; CCFP; FCFP; Head Family & Commun Med, Providence Health Care - St Paul's Hospital; Clin Prof Family Pract, University of British Columbia; (604)806-8444; Fax. (604)806-8556; gmazowita@providencehealth.bc.ca.

MAZUR, Sophie; Clinique Med St-Louis, 504 rue Saint-Louis, Joliette QC J6E 2Z2; Mon'94; (450)759-0581; Fax. (450)759-0584.

MAZUR-GEKAS, Severine; Centre Hosp Chauveau, 11999 rue de l'Hopital, Quebec QC G2A 2T7; Amiens (France)'97; Staff, Centre Hospitalier Chauveau; (418)840-0790

MAZUREK, Gordon G; Misericordia Community Hosp, 16940 87 Ave NW, Edmonton AB T5R 4H5; Alb'83; CCFP; CCFP(E.M.); FCFP; Staff Emerg, Covenant Health - Misericordia Community Hospital; (780)735-2819

MAZUREK, Karen A; Telus Plaza South, 2700-10020 100 St NW, Edmonton AB T5J 0N3; Alb'85; CCFP; FCFP; Asst Registrar, College of Physicians & Surgeons of Alberta; (780)423-4764; Fax. (780)420-0651.

MAZUREK, Michael F; McMaster University HSC, PO Box 2000 Stn Lcd 1 4U2-1200 Main St W, Hamilton ON L8N 3Z5; Tor'77; DAB; Neur. Consultant Neurol, Hamilton Health Sciences Centre - McMaster Children's Hospital; Prof, McMaster University; (905)521-2100 x76362; Fax. (905)521-2656.

MAZURIK, Laurel A; Sunnybrook Hlth Sciences Ctre, C753-2075 Bayview Ave, Toronto ON M4N 3M5; Sask'87; FRCPC; EmergMed. Staff Emerg Med, Sunnybrook Health Sciences Centre; (416)480-4037; Fax. (416)480-4704.

MAZURKA, John; The Juravinski Cancer Centre, 699 Concession St, Hamilton ON L8V 5C2; Qns'75; FRCSC; ObstGyn (Gynecologic Oncology). Head Gyn Oncol, Hamilton Health Sciences Centre-Juravinski Site; Court Staff, Joseph Brant Memorial Hospital; Court Staff, Health Sciences North-Laurentian Site; Staff, The Juravinski Cancer Centre; Assoc Prof ObstGyn, McMaster University; Langs: Hungarian; (905)389-5688; Fax. (905)575-6343; john.mazurka@jcc.hhsc.ca.

MAZURKA, Robert A; Anaesthesia Associates, 439 Park St, Kitchener ON N2G 1N4; Qns'75; FRCPC; Anes. Staff Anes, Grand River Hospital - Kitchener/Waterloo Health Centre; Staff Anes, St Mary's General Hospital; (519)744-7361; Fax. (519)744-7363.

MAZURSKI, Karen L; Dingwall Med Group, PO Box 3011 Stn Main, Dryden ON P8N 2Z6; Dal'81; BSc(Hon); CCFP; FCFP; (807)223-2258; Fax. (807)223-4733.

MAZZA, Christopher F; Sunnybrook Hlth Sciences Ctre, 2075 Bayview Ave, Toronto ON M4N 3M5; Tor'89; FRCPC; EmergMed. Staff, Sunnybrook Health Sciences Centre; (416)480-4207

MAZZA, Guiseppe; Clinique Force Medic, 1021 rue Jean-Talon St E, Montreal QC H2K 1V6; McG'86; Staff, Hôpital Santa Cabrini Ospedale; Langs: French; Italian; (514)787-1818; Fax. (514)787-1898.

MAZZA, Jorge A; London HSC-South Street, PO Box 5375 Stn B 2063-375 South St, London ON N6A 4G5; Buenos Aires (Argentina)'68; FRCPC; IntMed (Allergy). Consultant, St Joseph's Hospital - St Joseph's Health Care; Consultant, London Health Sciences Centre - University Hospital; Ac Staff Allergy Clinic, London Health Sciences Centre - South Street; Clin Assoc Prof, University of Western Ontario; Langs: Spanish; (519)685-8277; Fax. (519)685-8274.

MAZZA, Myriam; CLSC Saint-Hubert, 6800 boul Cousineau, Longueuil QC J3Y 8Z4; Mon'09; CCFP; (450)443-7400; Fax. (450)676-3488.

MAZZA-WHELAN, Angela M; Wentworth Limeridge Med Ctre, 205-849 Upper Wentworth St, Hamilton ON L9A 5H4; McM'81; CCFP; FCFP; (905)318-0303; Fax. (905)318-3050.

MAZZADI, Sergio; St Joseph's Health Centre, 50 Charlton Ave E, Hamilton ON L8N 4A6; Buenos Aires (Argentina)'87; Staff, St Joseph's Healthcare - Charlton Campus; Langs: Bulgarian; Italian; Spanish; Portuguese; (905)522-1155; Fax. (905)521-6068.

MAZZARELLA, Angelo A; Seymour Med Clinic, 200-1530 7th Ave W, Vancouver BC V6J 1S3; UBC'98; CCFP; (604)739-5615

MAZZARELLI, Mark; Medecine Familiale Lasalle, 6-2101 av Dollard, LaSalle QC H8N 1S2; McG'82; PhD(Physiol); Langs: French; Italian; (514)595-8867; Fax. (514)363-9280.

MAZZELLA-MAIOLO, Loraine; 5217 Av King-Edward, Montreal QC H4V 2J8; Florence (Italy)'81; Staff, McGill University Health Centre - Montreal General Campus; (514)489-3781

MAZZOLI, Paolo; Humber River Reg Hosp-Finch, 2111 Finch Ave W, North York ON M3N 1N1; Tor'92; CCFP; CCFP(E.M.); Humber River Regional Hospital - Finch Avenue Site; (416)747-3857

MAZZONE, Thomas; PromptDoc Urgent Care Clinic, 532 Lake St, St. Catharines ON L2N 4H4; New York (USA)'78; (905)646-0015

MAZZOTTA, Paolo; Sunnybrook Hlth Sciences Ctre, H 336-2075 Bayview Ave, Toronto ON M4N 3M5; Tor'04; CCFP; Staff, Sunnybrook Health Sciences Centre; Staff, St Joseph's Health Centre; (416)480-6100 x7255; Fax. (416)480-5146.

MAZZULLI, Tonino; Mount Sinai Hosp, 1485-600 University Ave, Toronto ON M5G 1X5; Tor'85; FACP; FRCPC; IntMed; InfectDis; MedMicrobiol. Staff Med, Mount Sinai Hospital; Toronto General Hospital - UHN; Prof, University of Toronto; (416)586-4695; Fax. (416)586-8746; tmazzulli@mtsinai.on.ca.

MBALA-KATANDA, Sylvie; Clinique Medicale, 157 Water St, Campbellton NB E3N 3L4; Kinshasa (Congo (Democratic Republic))'95; Staff, Hôpital Régional Campbellton; (506)753-7727; Fax. (506)753-7711.

MBANGI-BONTOLO, Faustin; CP 3670 Stn Main, Tracadie-Sheila NB E1X 1G5; Brussel (Belgium)'97.

MBANZA, Denis B; South End Med Clinic, 4661 Rae St, Regina SK S4S 6K6; Kinshasa (Congo (Democratic Republic))'87; BSc; MCFP(SA); Physician Long Term Care, Regina Nursing Homes; Langs: French; (306)352-9963; Fax. (306)522-0818.

MBAOGU, Michael N; PO Box 136, Edam SK S0M 0V0; MB ChB; DRCOG; CCFP; Staff, Lady Minto Health Care Center; Physician, Prairie North Health Region; (306)397-2334

MBAYE, Saliou D; Ungava Tulattavik Health Ctr, CP 149, Kuujjuaq QC J0M 1C0; (Senegal)'04; CCFP; Staff, Centre de sante Tulattavik de l'Ungava; (819)964-2905

MBENZA, Wenta L; Windermere Med Clinic, 204-32450 Simon Ave, Abbotsford BC V2T 4J2; Kinshasa (Congo (Democratic Republic))'88; (604)859-6774

MBONJO, Isaac B; CSSS de Papineau, 155 rue MacLaren E, Gatineau QC J8L 0C2; Paris (France)'03; CCFP; Staff, CH-CHSLD de Papineau - Pavillon du centre hospitalier; Staff, Hôpital de Papineau; Langs: Bilingual(French/English); (819)986-3341

MBUVA, Regina N; Englehart & District FHT, PO Box 1110 63 Fifth St, Englehart ON P0J 1H0; Nairobi (Kenya)'93; BSc; DTMH; MB ChB; CCFP; CCFP(E.M.); (705)544-2301 x5246

MBUYI, Felicien K M; 290-5255 Richmond Rd SW, Calgary AB T3E 7C4; Kinshasa (Congo (Democratic Republic))'89; BSc; MD; Langs: French; (403)240-1752; Fax. (403)249-3120; felicienmbuyi@yahoo.ca.

MCADAM, Donald W; Lansdowne Med Treatment Ctr, 120-1641 Hillside Ave, Victoria BC V8T 5G1; UBC'84; BSc; (250)592-4212; dw-king@shaw.ca.

MCADAM, Laura; Holland Bloorview Kids Rehab, 150 Kilgour Rd, Toronto ON M4G 1R8; Tor'01; FRCPC; Peds. Staff, Holland Bloorview Kids Rehabilitation Hospital; (416)753-6019; Fax. (416)494-6621.

MCADOO, Keri K; Birchwood Prof Centre, 24 Kentucky Crt, New Minas NS B4N 4N2; Dal'96; BSc; CCFP; FCFP; Assoc Member, Valley Regional Hospital; Teach Staff, Dalhousie University; (902)681-1080; Fax. (902)681-0600.

MCALDUFF, David E; 1436 Kensington Rd NW PO Box 61216 Rpo Kensington, Calgary AB T2N 4S6; Wes'04; BSc; MSc; CCFP; (403)399-4120

MCALEER, Dominic J; MacDonald Med Centre, 208-2786 16th Ave W, Vancouver BC V6K 4M1; Edinburgh (Scotland)'64; DPM(Lond); MRCPsy; FRCPC; Psy. Court Staff, Providence Health Care - St Paul's Hospital; Clin Instructor, University of British Columbia; (604)732-7525

MCALEER, Katherine A; St. James Cottage Hospice, 650 Penticton St N, Vancouver BC V6A 1G5; UBC'06; CCFP; Staff, Providence Health Care - St Paul's Hospital; (604)606-0440

MCALISTER, Edward D; Springdale Prof Bldg, 401-2250 Bovaird Dr E, Brampton ON L6R 0W3; Qns'05; General Surgical Oncology; GenSurg. (905)792-6222; Fax. (905)544-6388.

MCALISTER, Finlay A; Walter Mackenzie Hlth Science, 2F1 21-132 University Campus N, Edmonton AB T6G 2R7; Alb'90; MSc(Epidemiol); FRCPC; IntMed. Staff, University of Alberta Hospital; Prof, University of Alberta; (780)407-1399

MCALISTER, Kenneth R; Pegasus Med Centre, 201-1 Hesperus Rd, Thornhill ON L4J 0G9; Wes'82; Staff, Mackenzie Richmond Hill Hospital; (905)882-4949; Fax. (905)882-0560.

MCALISTER, Nazlin K; 6-1916 Dundas St E, Whitby ON L1N 2L6; Wes'76; CCFP; FCFP; Langs: Gujarati; (905)434-1662; Fax. (905)434-7448.

MCALISTER, Neil H; 6-1916 Dundas St E, Whitby ON L1N 2L6; Wes'75; MSc(ClinEpidem); PhD(MedSci); FRCPC; IntMed. Staff, Lakeridge Health - Port Perry Site; (905)434-1997; Fax. (905)434-7448; neilmac@durham.net.

MCALISTER, Vivian C; London HSC-University Hosp, PO Box 5339 Stn B C4 211-339 Windermere Rd, London ON N6A 5A5; (Ireland)'79; FRCSI; FRCSC; GenSurg (Hepatobiliary Surgery). Staff, London Health Sciences Centre - University Hospital; Prof Surg, University of Western Ontario; (519)663-2920; Fax. (519)663-3858.

MCALLISTER, Amy L; Bedford Waterfront Hlth Clinic, 207-967 Bedford Hwy, Bedford NS B4A 1A9; Dal'09; CCFP; Staff Primary Care Obst & Newborn Care, IWK Health Centre; (902)835-6444

MCALLISTER, Caroline D; Brooklin Med Centre, 5959 Anderson St, Brooklin ON L1M 2E9; Cal'01; CCFP; (905)655-3321

MCALLISTER, Debbie L; Alberta Children's Hosp, 2888 Shaganappi Trail NW, Calgary AB T3B 6A8; Cal'96; MSc; BSc; FRCPC; Anes (Pediatric Anesthesia). Staff Anes, Alberta Children's Hospital; (403)943-7810; Fax. (403)943-7606; debbie.mcallister@calgaryhealthregion.ca.

MCALLISTER, Elisabeth F A; Alberta Children Hosp, 2888 Shaganappi Trail NW, Calgary AB T3B 6A8; (Sweden)'96; Staff, Alberta Children's Hospital; (403)955-7810

MCALLISTER, G Rae; 8B 175-3110 8th St E, Saskatoon SK S7H 0W2; Sask'73; (306)655-2640; Fax. (306)655-2639; rae.mcallister@saskcancer.ca.

MCALLISTER, October E; Regina Qu'Appelle HR-Regina, 1440 14th Ave, Regina SK S4P 0W5; Sask'97; FRCPC; Anes. Staff Anes, Regina General Hospital; (306)766-4252

MCALLISTER, Patrick J; Rebalance MD, 104-3551 Blanshard St, Victoria BC V8Z 0B9; UBC'83; FRCSC; OrthSurg (Hip & Knee Reconstruction). Staff Orth Surg, Vancouver Island Health Authority; (250)381-5424; Fax. (250)385-8150.

MCALLISTER, Terrance B; Doctors Bldg, 310-955 Queen St E, Sault Ste. Marie ON P6A 2C3; Wes'87; FRCSC; OrthSurg (Sports Medicine). Ac Staff, Sault Area Hospital - Sault Ste Marie; (705)256-5702; Fax. (705)256-2614.

MCALPINE, Brian D; Forest Heights Med Clinic, 7461 101 Ave NW, Edmonton AB T6A 3Z5; Alb'76; Ac Staff, Royal Alexandra Hospital; (780)463-2323; Fax. (780)463-5514; bmcalpine@shaw.ca.

MCALPINE, Douglas G; Regina Qu'Appelle HR-Pasqua, 4101 Dewdney Ave, Regina SK S4T 1A5; Sask'82; FRCPC; Anes. Staff Anes, Pasqua Hospital; (306)766-2295; dmcalpine@sasktel.net.

MCALPINE, Jessica; Diamond Health Care Centre, 6F-2775 Laurel St, Vancouver BC V5Z 1M9; Baltimore(MD) (USA)'96; FRCSC; ObstGyn (Surgical Oncology). Staff GynOncol, BC Cancer Agency Vancouver Centre; Asst Prof, Vancouver General Hospital - Centennial Pavillion; (604)875-5608

MCALPINE, John C; Lions Gate Hosp, 231 15th St E, North Vancouver BC V7L 2L7; UBC'92; FRCPC; Anes. Staff, Lions Gate Hospital; (604)988-3131

MCANDIE, Catherine M; 2247 Rymal Rd E, Stoney Creek ON L8J 2V8; McM'92; BScN; CCFP; (905)578-7100

MCANULTY, Gregory J; 105-5512 Hastings St, Burnaby BC V5B 1R3; UBC'90; BSc; CCFP; FCFP; Staff, Burnaby Hospital; (604)291-1208

MCARDLE, Mary P; Westgrove Clinic, 101-505 Queen St, Spruce Grove AB T7X 2V2; (Ireland)'79; Ac Staff, Medicine Hat Regional Hospital; (780)960-9533; Fax. (780)960-9591.

MCARTHUR, Alastair; Valley Reg Hosp, 150 Exhibition St, Kentville NS B4N 5E3; London (England)'78; MB BS; MRC(UK); DA(Eng.); FRCPC; Anes. Staff, Valley Regional Hospital; (902)678-7381

MCARTHUR, Anne-Louise A; Owen Sound Med Centre, 2000-1415 1st Ave W, Owen Sound ON N4K 4K2; Qns'94; CCFP; Staff, Grey Bruce Health Services - Owen Sound; (519)470-3030; Fax. (519)370-4053.

MCARTHUR, H Susan; 21 McGivern St PO Box 1300, Walkerton ON N0G 2V0; Wes'92; CCFP; (519)881-4640; Fax. (519)881-4648.

MCARTHUR, James N; Medical Place, 360 Huron St, Stratford ON N5A 5T5; Tor'74; Ac Staff, Stratford General Hospital - Huron Perth Healthcare Alliance; (519)271-7141

MCARTHUR, Paul E; 21 McGivern St, Walkerton ON N0G 2V0; Wes'92; BSc; CCFP; Ac Staff, South Bruce Grey Health Centre - Walkerton Site; Aj Prof, Schulich School of Medicine-University of Western Ontario; (519)881-4640; Fax. (519)881-4648.

MCARTHUR, Peter D; Stanton Med Centre, PO Box 10 Stn Main 419 Bryne Rd, Yellowknife NT X1A 2N1; Alb'70; FRCSC; Otol.

MCASSEY, Karen L; Hamilton HS-McMaster Site, PO Box 2000 Stn Lcd 1 3A-1200 Main St W, Hamilton ON L8N 3Z5; Qns'94; FRCPC; Peds; Endocrin&Metab. Assoc Staff Peds, Hamilton Health Sciences Centre - McMaster Children's Hospital; (905)521-2100 x75702; Fax. (905)308-7548.

MCAULEY, Barbara C; 2772 Reginal Rd 81 PO Box 10, Jordan Station ON L0R 1S0; Tor'84; Court Staff, Niagara Health System - St Catharines General Site; Court Staff, Niagara Health System - Ontario Street Site; (905)562-4874

MCAULEY, David J; Ctr Hosp De Verdun, 4000 boul Lasalle, Verdun QC H4G 2A3; McG'88; FRCPC; DiagRad. Staff, Centre Hospitalier de Verdun; (514)286-6500

MCAULEY, Iain W; 200-1121 Yates St, Victoria BC V8V 3N1; UBC'92; FRCSC; Urol. (250)388-7334; Fax. (250)995-1201.

MCAULEY, James P; London HSC-University Hosp, PO Box 5339 Stn B B9006-339 Windermere Rd, London ON N6A 5A5; Dal'80; BSc; FRCSC; OrthSurg (Hip & Knee Arthroplasty). Staff, London Health Sciences Centre - University Hospital; Assoc Prof Ortho, University of Western Ontario; Langs: Bilingual(English/French); (519)663-3307; Fax. (519)663-3043.

MCAULEY, John T; Niagara H System-St Catharines, PO Box 3018 Stn Main 142 Queenston St, St Catharines ON L2R 7C6; Tor'83; CCFP; CCFP(E.M.); FCFP; Staff, Niagara Health System - St Catharines General Site; (905)684-7271

MCAULEY, Paul; PO Box 620, Mahone Bay NS B0J 2E0; Dal'86; Staff, Fishermen's Memorial Hospital; Staff, South Shore Regional Hospital; Teach Staff, Dalhousie University; (902)624-8331; Fax. (902)624-1524.

MCAULEY, Thomas J; Alexandra Marine & Gen Hosp, 120 Napier St, Goderich ON N7A 1W5; Ott'95; FRCPC; Psy. Staff Psy, Alexandra Marine & General Hospital; Teach Staff, University of Western Ontario; (519)524-8323 x288; Fax. (519)524-2745.

MCAULIFFE, D Noel; Office Of The Chief Coroner, 200-26 Grenville St, Toronto ON M7A 2G9; National (Ireland)'74.

MCAVINUE, Thomas; The Moncton Hosp, 135 MacBeath Ave, Moncton NB E1C 6Z8; Glasgow (Scotland)'79; MB ChB; FACP; FRCPC; IntMed (Cardiology). Staff, Miramichi Regional Hospital; Staff, The Moncton Hospital; (506)855-4589

MCBAIN, Adina M; 451 DeChauney Ave PO Box 160, Alhambra AB T0M 0C0; Cal'10; CCFP; (403)442-3814

MCBAIN, Daniel J; 2F-227 Second St S, Kenora ON P9N 1G1; McM'98; MA; CCFP; Langs: Spanish; Bilingual(French/English).

MCBAIN, Joelle H E; Regina Qu'Appelle HR-Regina, 1440 14th Ave, Regina SK S4P 0W5; Sask'03; FRCPC; Anes. Staff, Regina General Hospital; (306)766-4444

MCBEAN, Nora M; South-East Ottawa Centre, 600-1355 Bank St, Ottawa ON K1H 8K7; Ott'90; CCFP; (613)737-4809 x307; Fax. (613)739-3723; noram@seochc.on.ca.

MCBEATH, David J; Sparling East Med Centre, PO Box 820, Fernie BC V0B 1M0; UBC'94; CCFP; CCFP(E.M.); FCFP; (250)423-4442; Fax. (250)423-3424.

MCBEATH, Kim L; Royal Alexandra Hosp, 204-10240 Kingsway NW, Edmonton AB T5H 3V9; Alb'83; CCFP; FCFP; Staff, Royal Alexandra Hospital; (780)735-4512

MCBETH, Paul B; 2439-855 12th Ave W, Vancouver BC V5Z 1M9; Cal'07; FRCSC; GenSurg. (778)875-9309

MCBRIDE, Allen R; PO Box 1852 Kingston Main, Kingston ON K7L 5J7; Qns'72; BSc; CCFP; Assoc Staff, Kingston General Hospital; Assoc Staff, Providence Care - St Mary's of the Lake Hospital Site; Assoc Staff, Hotel-Dieu Hospital; Teach Staff Family Med, Queen's University; (613)544-7919; Fax. (613)544-8117.

MCBRIDE, David R; The Ottawa Hosp-Civic Campus, 1053 Carling Ave, Ottawa ON K1Y 4E9; UBC'97; FRCPC; Psy. Staff Psy, The Ottawa Hospital - Civic Campus; (613)761-4581

MCBRIDE, Eileen R A; Montfort Hosp, 713 Montreal Rd, Ottawa ON K1K 0T2; Ott'00; FRCPC; Peds; HemPath; Hem. Staff, Montfort Hospital; (613)746-4621

MCBRIDE, George A; Student Hlth & Counselling Ser, 1 Campus Dr, Saskatoon SK S7N 5A3; Sask'63; (306)966-5768; Fax. (306)966-5786.

MCBRIDE, Graeme N; Canadian Forces Hlth Serv Ctr, PO Box 99000 Stn Forces, Halifax NS B3K 5X5; Dal'09; CCFP; Staff, Canadian Forces Health Services Centre (Atlantic); (902)427-8700

MCBRIDE, Kathryn L; West Carleton Family Hlth Team, PO Box 218 119 Langstaff Dr, Carp ON K0A 1L0; UBC'97; CCFP; FCFP; (613)839-3271; Fax. (613)839-3273.

MCBRIDE, Michelle A; Kanata North Med Centre, 2-832 March Rd, Kanata ON K2W 0C9; McM'03; CCFP; (613)599-5599; Fax. (613)599-1005.

MCBRIDE, Simon; Ernest Walk-In Medical Clinic, 2-1101 Jalna Blvd, London ON N6E 3B3; McM'89; MCISc; Dir Laryngeal Endoscopy & Vocal Function Clinic, London Health Sciences Centre - Victoria Campus; Co-Dir, Spasmodic Dysphonia Clinic; Co-Dir, Vocal Health Clinic; Aj Prof Otol, University of Western Ontario; Langs: Spanish; French; (519)668-2208

MCBRIEN, Kerry; G230-3330 Hospital Dr NW, Calgary AB T2N 4N1; Tor'04; CCFP; Staff, Health Research Innovation Centre.

MCBROOM, Robert J; 410-101 Queensway W, Mississauga ON L5B 2P7; Qns'74; FRCSC; OrthSurg (Spine). Staff, Trillium Health Centre - Mississauga; Asst Prof, University of Toronto; (905)276-5829; Fax. (905)276-9677.

MCCABE, Amelia; St Thomas Elgin Gen Hosp, 189 Elm St, St Thomas ON N5R 5C4; Wes'09; CCFP; Staff, St Thomas Elgin General Hospital; (519)631-2020; Fax. (519)631-1825.

MCCABE, Gregory P; London HSC-Victoria Hosp, PO Box 5010 Stn B 800 Commissioners Rd E, London ON N6A 5W9; Wes'81; FRCPC; Anes (Cardiovascular Anesthesia). Ac Staff, London Health Sciences Centre - Victoria Campus; (519)685-8500 x58525

MCCABE, James B; Oliver Eye Centre, 11652 104 Ave NW, Edmonton AB T5K 2T7; Alb'01; ABOph; DPhil; FRCSC; Ophth. Staff, Royal Alexandra Hospital; (780)488-5600; Fax. (780)488-5682.

MCCABE, Jennifer L; St Michael's Hosp, 30 Bond St, Toronto ON M5B 1W8; Tor'96; CCFP; Staff, St Michael's Hospital; Asst Prof Family & Commun Med, University of Toronto; (416)867-7428; Fax. (416)867-7498.

MCCABE, P Kevin; Valley Ridge Family Physicians, 321-11245 Valley Ridge Dr NW, Calgary AB T3B 5V4; Cal'88; CCFP; (403)282-3806; Fax. (403)284-5601.

MCCABE, Philip C; SW Ont Aboriginal Access Ctr, 425-427 William St, London ON N6B 3E1; Ott'75; DOHS; CCBOM; MSc; CCFP; (519)672-4079; Fax. (519)672-7220.

MCCABE, Pierre; Ctr Hosp Anna Laberge, 200 boul Brisebois, Chateauguay QC J6K 4W8; Mon'01; CSPQ; FRCPC; IntMed. Staff, Hôpital Anna-Laberge; (450)699-2425

MCCABE, Richard D; PO Box 691 Stn Main, Grande Prairie AB T8V 3A8; Alb'80; FRCPC; DiagRad. (780)766-3584

MCCABE, Steven J; Univ Hlth Network-Toronto Western Hosp, 399 Bathurst St, Toronto ON M5T 2S8; Tor'80; FRCSC; PlasSurg. Staff, Toronto Western Hospital - University Health Network; (416)603-5455; Fax. (416)603-5392.

MCCAFFREY, Donald C; 1 Creek's End Lane, Nepean ON K2H 1C7; Ott'68; FRCPC; Anes. Staff Anes, Queensway Carleton Hospital; (613)829-8080

MCCAFFREY, Janis A; 3777 Southridge Ave, West Vancouver BC V7V 3H9; Cal'81; CAFCI; Ac Staff/Physician Palliative Care, Lions Gate Hospital; Med Dir Famil & Commun Health, North Shore Health Region; Clin Instructor, University of British Columbia; (604)773-5965

MCCAFFREY, Lindsay D; 101-4695 Hastings St, Burnaby BC V5C 2K6; Qns'09; CCFP; (604)298-7207

MCCAFFREY, Lisa M; St Clair Beach Health Centre, RR 1 6-500 Manning Rd, Windsor ON N8N 2L9; Ott'00; BSc; CCFP; (519)739-1550

MCCAFFREY, Michael C; North Walkerville Med Centre, 106-2425 Tecumseh Rd E, Windsor ON N8W 1E6; Ott'00; FRCSC; OrthSurg. Staff, Hôtel-Dieu Grace Hospital; Staff, Windsor Regional Hospital - Metropolitan Site; (519)254-5763

MCCAFFREY, Michael J; William Osler HC-Brampton, 2100 Bovaird Dr E, Brampton ON L6R 3J7; Tor'92; Staff, William Osler Health System - Brampton Civic Hospital.

MCCAHILL, John A; Villa Caritas, 16515 88 Ave NW, Edmonton AB T5R 0A4; Leicester (England)'90; MB ChB; MRCPsy; FRCPC; Psy (Geriatric Psychiatry). Staff, Alberta Hospital Edmonton; Clin Lecturer Psychiatry, University of Alberta; (780)342-6552

MCCAIN, W Gregory; North York Med Arts Bldg, 208-1333 Sheppard Ave E, North York ON M2J 1V1; Tor'68; BSc; FRCSC; PlasSurg. Staff, North York General Hospital; (416)491-5424; Fax. (416)491-7022.

MCCALDEN, Richard W; London HSC-University Hosp, PO Box 5339 Stn B 339 Windermere Rd, London ON N6A 5A5; Tor'86; MPhilEdin; FRCSC; OrthSurg (Adult Hip & Knee Reconstruction). Assoc Prof/Staff OrthSurg, London Health Sciences Centre - University Hospital; (519)663-3049; Fax. (519)663-3208; richard.mccalden@lhsc.on.ca.

MCCALL, Annette L; Lions Gate Integral Health Ctr, 503-145 13th St E, North Vancouver BC V7L 2L4; UBC'89; CCFP; CEO/Founder, Lions Gate Integral Health Centre; Langs: German; (604)985-8558; Fax. (604)985-8518; annette.mccall@lionsgatehealth.ca.

MCCALL, Joann C; 1-13 Nelson St W, Meaford ON N4L 1N1; Tor'77; DTMH; ABIM; FRCPC; IntMed (Geriatric Medicine). Staff, Grey Bruce Health Services - Meaford Site; (519)538-3101; Fax. (519)538-2788.

MCCALL, John G; Collingwood Health Centre, 205-186 Erie St, Collingwood ON L9Y 4T3; Glasgow (Scotland)'66; MB ChB; MS(Strathclyde); Dip SportMed; MSc; Consultant, Grey Bruce Health Services - Meaford Site; Consultant, Grey Bruce Health Services - Markdale; Ac Staff OrthSurg/Sports Injuries, Collingwood General & Marine Hospital; Staff OrthSurg, Collingwood Health Centre; Clinical Asst Prof OrthSurg, McMaster University; (705)445-5141; Fax. (705)445-9419; jmccall@bellnet.ca.

MCCALL, Margaret A; Maple Family Health Team, 325 University Ave, Kingston ON K7L 3R4; Wes'79; BSc; CCFP; FCFP; Att Staff, Kingston General Hospital; Asst Prof, Queen's University; (613)544-2902; Fax. (613)544-5768.

MCCALL, Maureen; Associate Med Group, 4705 48 Ave, Red Deer AB T4N 3T1; Alb'85; MPH(Harvard); Physician, Associate Medical Group; Aj Prof Family Med, University of Alberta; Aj Prof Commun & Family Med, University of Calgary; Langs: Spanish; (403)346-2057; Fax. (403)347-2989; mdmccall@yahoo.com.

MCCALL, Richard H; 517 McGill St, Hawkesbury ON K6A 1R1; Tor'99; BSc; MSc; CCFP; Staff, Hawkesbury & District General Hospital; Langs: English; French; (613)632-9500; Fax. (613)632-0747.

MCCALL, Simon O; 517 McGill St, Hawkesbury ON K6A 1R1; London (England)'66; LRCP; MRCS; DCH; GP/Anesthesia, Hawkesbury & District General Hospital; Langs: Bilingual(English/French); (613)632-9500; Fax. (613)632-0747.

MCCALLAGHAN, Johannes J; Tri-Cities Mental Health Centr, 2232 Elgin Ave, Port Coquitlam BC V3C 2B2; Stellenbosch (South Africa)'88; Langs: Afrikaans; (604)777-8400

MCCALLAN, Tara L; KDH Health Centre, PO Box 2113 2671 Concession Rd, Kemptville ON K0G 1J0; Dal'01; CCFP; Staff, Kemptville District Hospital; (613)258-0100

MCCALLION, Alexander; Queen-Lynch Med Centre, 209-157 Queen St E, Brampton ON L6W 3X4; Queen's (Ireland)'70; MB ChB; BAO; Staff, William Osler Health System - Brampton Civic Hospital; (905)457-7566; Fax. (905)457-7611.

MCCALLUM, Alison M; Public Gardens Med Clinic, 200-5675 Spring Garden Rd, Halifax NS B3J 1H1; Dal'82; (902)425-5440

MCCALLUM, Andrew L; Office of the Chief Coroner, 200-26 Grenville St, Toronto ON M7A 2G9; McM'80; FRCPC; EmergMed. Chief Coroner, Province of Ontario; Assoc Prof Emerg Med, Queen's University; (416)314-4000; Fax. (416)314-4030.

MCCALLUM, Annette H; Kingston Gen Hosp, 76 Stuart St, Kingston ON K7L 2V7; McM'91; MSc; FRCPC; DiagRad. Staff Diagnostic Services, Kingston General Hospital; Dept Head Diagnostic Radiol, Queen's University; (613)549-6666 x2865

MCCALLUM, Catherine L; Care Point Med Centres, 5138 Joyce St, Vancouver BC V5R 4H1; UBC'69; (604)436-0800

MCCALLUM, Grant; The Maple Tree Med Clinic, 1181 6 Ave NE, Salmon Arm BC V1E 2S5; Cape Town (South Africa)'88; MB ChB; Staff, Shuswap Lake General Hospital; (250)832-9361

MCCALLUM, Janis G; 450 Thompson Run, Bedford NS B4B 1W8; UBC'08; CCFP.

MCCALLUM, Kimberley C; 61 Wilson St W, Ancaster ON L9G 1N1; McM'88; BSc; CCFP; FCFP; Assoc Staff Privil, Hamilton Health Sciences Centre - McMaster Children's Hospital; (905)304-3080; Fax. (905)304-1768.

MCCALLUM, Nancy L; Women's College Hosp, 76 Grenville St, Toronto ON M5S 1B2; Tor'98; FRCPC; Psy. Staff, Women's College Hospital; (416)323-6400 x4937

MCCALLUM, Robert; Canamera Med Centre, B7B-350 Conestoga Blvd, Cambridge ON N1R 7L7; McG'88; CCFP; Langs: French; (519)620-4460; Fax. (519)620-8587.

MCCALLUM, Ryan C; 1 Field Ambulance, PO Box 10500 Stn Forces, Edmonton AB T5J 4J5; Dal'08; CCFP.

MCCALLUM, Theresa J; 22-5201 50 St, Leduc AB T9E 6T4; Cal'91; FRCSC; Urol (Male Infertility). (780)980-8200; Fax. (780)980-8207.

MCCAMMON, Richard J; 1600 Portage Ave, Winnipeg MB R3J 0C6; Man'75; CCFP; Langs: Other language.

MCCANN, D Burton; 301-6155 North St, Halifax NS B3K 5R3; Dal'88; LLB; CCFP; FCFP; Teach Staff, Dalhousie University; (902)426-7633; Fax. (902)426-6598.

MCCANN, John A; 21 Adams Ave, Miramichi NB E1V 3Y6; Mem'85; BMedSci; BSc; CCFP; FCFP; Ac Staff, Miramichi Regional Hospital; (506)623-3155; Fax. (506)623-3660.

MCCANN, Maureen; North Toronto Med Bldg, 110-250 Lawrence Ave W, Toronto ON M5M 1B2; Glasgow (Scotland)'60; DA; DRCOG; MB ChB; Court Staff, Women's College Hospital; Court Staff, Sunnybrook Health Sciences Centre; (416)256-4707; Fax. (416)256-4710.

MCCANN, Michael A; 4-8790 204 St, Langley BC V1M 2Y5; UBC'84; Staff, Langley Memorial Hospital; (604)888-3775

MCCANN, Shawn C; Dr Shawn McCann Inc, 301-3295 Lakeshore Rd, Kelowna BC V1W 3S9; McM'94; BSc; FRCPC; PhysMed&Rehab (Orthopedic Surgery). Staff, Kelowna General Hospital; (250)862-3421; Fax. (250)862-3470; scmccann@shaw.ca.

MCCANN, Thomas J; Bronte Medical Group, 78 Jones St, Oakville ON L6L 6C5; Glasgow (Scotland)'67; MB ChB; CHE; Physician, Halton Healthcare Services Corporation - Oakville Site; (905)827-9865; Fax. (905)827-3583.

MCCANN, Vernal L; Dynacare Kasper Med Labs, 200-10150 102 St NW, Edmonton AB T5J 5E2; Alb'76; FRCPC; GenPath (Cytology). Med Consultant, Covenant Health - Grey Nuns Community Hospital; Consultant, Sturgeon Community Hospital; Med Staff, Royal Alexandra Hospital; Medical Staff, Caritas Health Care Group; Asst Prof Clinical, University of Alberta; (780)451-3702 x8153

MCCANN, William G; South Muskoka Mem Hosp, 75 Ann St, Bracebridge ON P1L 2E4; Dublin (Ireland)'73; MB ChB; BAO; DABR; FRCPC; DiagRad. Dir DiagRad/Diag Imag, South Muskoka Memorial Hospital - Muskoka Algonquin Healthcare; (705)645-4404 x116; Fax. (705)645-4594; mccannjk@muskoka.com.

MCCANS, John L; Queen's Univ-Etherington Hall, 3041-94 Stuart St, Kingston ON K7L 2V6; Qns'68; MSc(Physiol.); FRCPC; Cardiol. Med Dir, Kingston General Hospital; Prof, Queen's University; (613)533-6327; Fax. (613)533-6695.

MCCARROLL, Kathryn E; 1517 Poplar St RR 6, Golden BC V0A 1H6; Dal'08; CCFP; (250)231-1611

MCCARROLL, Kirk P; PO Box 1449, Rossland BC V0G 1Y0; Dal'02; CCFP; Staff Anes, Prince Rupert Regional Hospital; (250)362-5977; kirkmccarroll@hotmail.com.

MCCARRON, Bonnie I; Grand River Reg Cancer Centre, PO Box 9056 Stn C 835 King St W, Kitchener ON N2G 1G3; McM'89; FRCPC; IntMed; Hem. (519)749-4370

MCCARRON, M Janet; Canadian Forces Hlth Serv Ctr, PO Box 99000 Stn Forces, Halifax NS B3K 5X5; Mem'97; CCFP; Staff, Canadian Forces Health Services Centre (Atlantic); (902)427-3652

MCCART, Judith A; Mount Sinai Hosp, 1225-600 University Ave, Toronto ON M5G 1X5; Wes'90; FRCSC; GenSurg. Affiliate Scientist, Mount Sinai Hospital; (416)586-4800 x4552; Fax. (416)586-8392; judith.mccart@utoronto.ca.

MCCARTER, Bryon; Lions Gate Hosp, 231 15th St E, North Vancouver BC V7L 2L7; Sask'97; FRCPC; Anes;CCFP; Staff, Lions Gate Hospital; (604)984-5709

MCCARTHY, Anne E; The Ottawa Hosp-Gen Campus, G12-501 Smyth Rd, Ottawa ON K1H 8L6; Mem'85; DTMH(Lond); FRCPC; IntMed (Tropical Medicine); InfectDis. Staff Div of InfectDis, The Ottawa Hospital - General Campus; Dir, Tropical Med. & Int'l. Health Clinic; Dir Global Health/Prof, University of Ottawa; Langs: Bilingual(English/French); (613)737-8184; Fax. (613)737-8164.

MCCARTHY, Annette M; Bay Bulls Family Practice, PO Box 10, Bay Bulls NL A0A 1C0; Mem'90; CCFP; Staff Women's Health Program, Health Care Corporation Of St John's; (709)334-2206; Fax. (709)334-2331.

MCCARTHY, Brendan G; Health Sciences Centre, GF441-820 Sherbrook St, Winnipeg MB R3A 1R9; Man'01; FRCSC; GenSurg; Critical Care Medicine. Staff, Health Sciences Centre.

MCCARTHY, F Paul; 104-1220 Place d'Orleans Dr, Orleans ON K1C 7K3; Mem'78; Assoc Staff Privil, The Ottawa Hospital - General Campus; (613)841-5397; Fax. (613)841-4274; droffice@bellnet.ca.

MCCARTHY, Gerard F; 305-400 Tache Ave, Winnipeg MB R2H 3C3; Queen's (Ireland)'64; MB ChB; MRCOG(Lond); FRCSC; ObstGyn. Ac Staff, St Boniface General Hospital; Clin. Tutor, University of Manitoba; (204)233-4224

MCCARTHY, Gregory; Regional Mental Health Centre, PO Box 5532 Stn B 850 Highbury Ave, London ON N6A 4H1; Cape Town (South Africa)'93; FRCPC; Psy. Staff, Regional Mental Health Care-St Joseph's Health Care; (519)455-5110; Fax. (519)452-4556.

MCCARTHY, J Martin; UBC Eye Care Centre, 2550 Willow St, Vancouver BC V5Z 3N9; Cal'83; FRCSC; Ophth. (604)875-4407; Fax. (604)875-5748; martin.mccarthy@vch.ca.

MCCARTHY, Jason J J; Leonard A Miller Centre, 1-100 Forest Rd, St. John's NL A1A 3Z9; Mem'99; CCFP.

MCCARTHY, Jeremiah; Burin Peninsula Hlth Care Ctr, PO Box 340, Burin NL A0E 1E0; National (Ireland)'72; MB ChB; LMCC; Staff, Burin Peninsula Health Care Centre; (709)891-3423; Fax. (709)891-3438; mccarthy99@hotmail.com.

MCCARTHY, John-Paul; Valley Prof Centre, 145-70 Exhibition St, Kentville NS B4N 4K9; Mem'05; FRCSC; Urol. Lecturer, Dalhousie University; (902)678-1130; Fax. (902)678-4020.

MCCARTHY, Joy S; Dr H Bliss Murphy Cancer Ctr, 300 Prince Philip Dr, St. John's NL A1B 3V6; Mem'96; FRCPC; IntMed; MedOncol. Staff, Dr H Bliss Murphy Cancer Centre; (709)777-8515

MCCARTHY, Kenneth G A; 24 Linden Ave, Charlottetown PE C1A 5Y8; (Jamaica)'73; DABIM; FRCPC; IntMed (Rheumatology). Staff, Queen Elizabeth Hospital; (902)367-3773; Fax. (902)367-3793.

MCCARTHY, Lauren O; Signal Road Med Clinic, 108 Wolverine Dr, Fort McMurray AB T9H 4Y7; UBC'92; CCFP; (780)790-9342

MCCARTHY, Leanne S; IWK Health Centre, PO Box 9700 Rpo CSC 5980 University Ave, Halifax NS B3K 6R8; Mem'05; FRCSC; ObstGyn. Staff, IWK Health Centre; (902)470-8888

MCCARTHY, Mairin; Hys Med Centre, 202-11010 101 St NW, Edmonton AB T5H 4B9; (Ireland)'90; (780)426-1121; Fax. (780)425-5979.

MCCARTHY, Martha A; Northside Med Group, 210-1465 Salisbury Ave, Port Coquitlam BC V3B 6J3; Dal'79; (604)941-8277; Fax. (604)941-5622.

MCCARTHY, Rodney P; Bay Bulls Family Practice, PO Box 10, Bay Bulls NL A0A 1C0; Mem'91; CCFP; (709)334-2206; Fax. (709)334-2331.

MCCARTHY, Stephen C P; Fundy Trail Med Centre, 68 Robie St, Truro NS B2N 1L2; Dal'80; CCFP; (902)893-0436; Fax. (902)893-0325.

MCCARTHY, Susanna M; 154-346 John St N, Arnprior ON K7S 2P6; McM'89; CCFP; Staff, Arnprior & District Memorial Hospital; (613)622-5869

MCCARTHY, Timothy G; Manitoba Clinic, 301-790 Sherbrook St, Winnipeg MB R3A 1M3; Man'86; ABIM; AB; FRCPC; IntMed; Rheum. Staff Pt-Time, Health Sciences Centre; Asst Prof Med, University of Manitoba; (204)788-5738; Fax. (204)784-4116.

MCCARTHY, Veronica J; The Ottawa Hosp-Gen Campus, 501 Smyth Rd, Ottawa ON K1H 8L6; Ott'00; FRCPC; Psy. Staff, The Ottawa Hospital - General Campus; (613)737-8955; Fax. (613)787-8010.

MCCARTHY, Vicky W K; St Joseph's Health Centre, 30 The Queensway, Toronto ON M6R 1B5; UBC'98; FRCPC; Anes. Staff, St Joseph's Health Centre; (416)530-6090

MCCARTNEY, Colin J L; Sunnybrook Hlth Sciences Ctre, 2075 Bayview Ave, Toronto ON M4N 3M5; Edinburgh (Scotland)'91; MB ChB; FRCA; FFARCS; FRCPC; Anes. Staff Anes, Sunnybrook Health Sciences Centre; Asst Prof Anes, University of Toronto; (416)480-6100 x4864

MCCARTNEY, Dawn M; Manitoba Adolescent Trmt Ctre, 228 Maryland St, Winnipeg MB R3G 1L6; FRCPC; Psy. Staff, St Boniface General Hospital.

MCCARTNEY, Eric D; 105 Park Dr, Rothesay NB E2H 1A9; McG'65; FRCSC; GenSurg. Consultant Surg, Worksafe-New Brunswick; (506)738-4012; Fax. (506)738-4050.

MCCARTY, David; London HSC-University Hosp, PO Box 5339 Stn B 339 Windermere Rd, London ON N6A 5A5; Queen's Belfast (Ireland)'97; Staff, London Health Sciences Centre - University Hospital; (519)663-3892

MCCARTY, Douglas M; Gateway Med Clinic, 950-3803 Calgary Trail NW, Edmonton AB T6J 5M8; Alb'79; Physician 1, Gateway Medical Clinic; (780)436-7240; Fax. (780)436-8142.

MCCARTY, Tara A; Centre Med Brunswick, 401-955 boul Saint-Jean, Pointe-Claire QC H9R 5K3; McG'09; CCFP; (514)426-6677; Fax. (514)459-0249.

MCCARTY, Tracey S; Family Med Centre, 101-155 James St S, Hamilton ON L8P 3A4; McM'93; MA; CCFP; FCFP; Assoc Staff, St Joseph's Healthcare - Charlton Campus; (905)528-8744; Fax. (905)528-5849.

MCCARVILL, Erin M; Bridgepoint Family Health Team, 430 Broadview Ave, Toronto ON M4K 2N1; Dal'08; CCFP; (416)470-6690; Fax. (416)470-6690.

MCCARVILLE, Clifford; 312-18 Acadia St, Dartmouth NS B2Y 4H3; Dal'93; FRCPC; IntMed. Staff, Dartmouth General Hospital; (902)444-8707; Fax. (902)444-8708.

MCCARVILLE, Donald J; Regina Qu'Appelle HR-Regina, 3F-1440 14th Ave, Regina SK S4P 0W5; Alb'88; FRCSC; GenSurg (Vascular Medicine); VascSurg. Head Section of Vascular Surg, Regina General Hospital; Exec Officer, Canadian Society for Vascular Surgery; Member Representative Assembly, Saskatchewan Medical Association; (306)766-6900; Fax. (306)766-6920.

MCCASKILL, Kenneth R; Kootenay-Boundary Reg Hosp, 1200 Hospital Bench, Trail BC V1R 4M1; Alb'87; BMedSci; FRCPC; Anes. Staff, Kootenay Boundary Regional Hospital; (250)368-3311

MCCAUGHEY, David F; Hop Charles LeMoyne, 3120 boul Taschereau, Greenfield Park QC J4V 2H1; McG'96; CCFP; CCFP(E.M.); Staff, Hopital Charles LeMoyne; (450)466-5000

MCCAUGHRY-CARDIGOS, David; CSSS Pierre-Boucher, 1333 boul Jacques-Cartier E, Longueuil QC J4M 2A5; Mon'98; FRCPC; Anes. Staff, Centre Hospitalier Pierre Boucher; (450)468-8111

MCCAULEY, Gordon F; 414-797 Princess St, Kingston ON K7L 1G1; Qns'75; BSc; DIH; CAFCI; CSAT; (613)548-7018; Fax. (613)548-7018.

MCCAULEY, Graeme; Kelowna Respiratory Clinic, 302-3975 Lakeshore Rd, Kelowna BC V1W 1V3; UBC'74; FRCPC; IntMed (Critical Care Medicine); Respir. Chairman Dept of Med, Kelowna General Hospital; Clin Instructor, University of British Columbia; (778)477-5805; Fax. (778)477-5807; kelownarespclinic@hotmail.com.

MCCAULEY, William A; London HSC-Victoria Hosp, PO Box 5010 Stn B 800 Commissioners Rd E, London ON N6A 5W9; Wes'87; FRCPC; EmergMed. Staff, London Health Sciences Centre - Victoria Campus; Medical Officer Physician Enhancement, College of Physicians & Surgeons of Ontario; (519)685-8500

MCCAW, Elizabeth; 220-500 Mapleton Rd, Moncton NB E1G 0N3; Dal'07; CCFP; (506)870-2938; Fax. (506)870-2978.

MCCAY, William A; Cedars Prof Park, 2915 66 St NW, Edmonton AB T6K 4C1; Alb'80; FRCPC; Psy. Psychiatrist, Covenant Health - Grey Nuns Community Hospital; Clin Associate Prof, University of Alberta; (780)450-9452; Fax. (780)461-6190.

MCCHESNEY, James; 202 Golf Links Rd, Ancaster ON L9G 3K6; Glasgow (Scotland)'76; MB ChB; FRCPC; Anes (Pain Management). Staff, St Joseph's Healthcare - Charlton Campus; Court Staff, Hamilton Health Sciences Centre - McMaster Children's Hospital; Clin Prof, McMaster University; (905)522-1155 x3853

MCCLARAN, Jacqueline; MUHC-Montreal Gen Hosp, D16-1650 av Cedar, Montreal QC H3G 1A4; Cincinnati (USA)'71; Staff, McGill University Health Centre - Montreal General Campus; Langs: English; French; (514)934-1934 x43960

MCCLARTY, Blake M; St Boniface Gen Hosp, 409 Tache Ave, Winnipeg MB R2H 2A6; Man'78; FRCPC; DiagRad. Clin Dir Support Srvcs, St Boniface General Hospital; Dept Head Radiol, University of Manitoba; (204)235-3610; Fax. (204)233-2777; bmcclarty@hsc.mb.ca.

MCCLEAN, Karen L; Royal University Hosp, 103 Hospital Dr, Saskatoon SK S7N 0W8; Alb'82; FRCPC; IntMed (AIDS/HIV); InfectDis. Staff InfectDis, Royal University Hospital; Assoc Prof Med, University of Saskatchewan; (306)655-1777

MCCLEAVE, John J; 33 Main St, Rexton NB E4W 0E5; Dal'77; Staff, Hôpital Stella-Maris-de-Kent; (506)523-7940; Fax. (506)523-7949; dr.john.mccleave@serha.ca.

MCCLELLAN, Kira; Haugen Med Group, 23C-3300 Smith Dr, Armstrong BC V0E 1B1; Mem'00; BSc; CCFP; Att Physician, Vernon Jubilee Hospital; (250)546-8115; Fax. (250)546-2553.

MCCLELLAND, Bruce; 231 Riverview Dr, Sydney river NS B1S 3R7; Cape Town (South Africa)'85; MB ChB; FRCPC; IntMed; Cardiol. Staff, Cape Breton Healthcare Complex; (902)270-9169; brucemcclelland42@hotmail.com.

MCCLELLAND, Janet M; Surrey Med Arts Bldg, 306-13798 94A Ave, Surrey BC V3V 1N1; London (England)'68; MB BS; MRCS; LRCP; Ac Staff, Surrey Memorial Hospital; (604)585-1677

MCCLENNAN, Sarah K; Trillium Hlth Ctr-Mississauga, 100 Queensway W, Mississauga ON L5B 1B8; McM'03; FRCPC; EmergMed. Staff, Trillium Health Centre - Mississauga; (905)848-7100

MCCLOSKEY, Deborah A; 103-100 Colborne St W, Orillia ON L3V 2Y9; McM'93; FRCPC; DiagRad. Staff Radiologist, Ontario Medical Imaging; (705)326-2244

MCCLOSKEY, Gregory T; 770 Bernard Ave, Kelowna BC V1Y 6P5; Ott'72; Ac Staff, Kelowna General Hospital; (250)762-2292

MCCLURE, Christine J; Region of Peel, 09-150 Central Park Dr, Brampton ON L6T 2T9; Belfast (Ireland)'69; MB ChB; BAO; DObstRCOG; (905)791-5905

MCCLURE, Donna J; St Paul's Hosp, 1081 Burrard St, Vancouver BC V6Z 1Y6; Wes'94; CCFP; Staff, Providence Health Care - St Paul's Hospital; Langs: English; French; (604)682-2344

MCCLURE, Douglas L; Springdale Prof Bldg, 108-2250 Bovaird Dr E, Brampton ON L6R 0W3; Wes'78; FRCSC; Otol. Court Staff, Halton Healthcare Services Corporation - Georgetown Hospital; Ac Staff, William Osler Health System - Brampton Civic Hospital; Court Staff, Trillium Health Centre - Mississauga; (905)792-7323; Fax. (905)792-1316.

MCCLURE, Lawrence H; Parksville Med Clinic, PO Box 250 Stn Main 154 Memorial Ave W, Parksville BC V9P 2G4; Cal'97; CCFP; (250)248-5757; Fax. (250)248-2128.

MCCLUSKEY, Stephen D; 102-984 Oliver Rd, Thunder Bay ON P7B 7C7; Ott'91; FRCSC; Neursurg. Staff, Thunder Bay Regional Health Sciences Centre; (807)766-3599; Fax. (807)766-3598.

MCCLUSKEY, Stuart A; Univ Hlth Network-Toronto Gen, 3 405-200 Elizabeth St, Toronto ON M5G 2C4; Tor'94; PhD; MSc; FRCPC; Anes. Staff Anes, Toronto General Hospital - UHN; University of Toronto; (416)340-4800 x8730; Fax. (416)340-3698; smccluskey@torhosp.toronto.on.ca.

MCCLUSKEY, Walter T P; Summit Injury Management, 605 Discovery St, Victoria BC V8T 5G4; UBC'05; CCFP; (250)370-6076

MCCOID, Elizabeth; Beaver Valley Clinic, PO Box 610, Fruitvale BC V0G 1L0; Mem'89; (250)367-9211; Fax. (250)367-7543.

MCCOLL, Christopher; Trillium Hlth Ctr-Mississauga, 100 Queensway W, Mississauga ON L5B 1B8; Tor'05; Critical Care Medicine; IntMed. Staff, Trillium Health Centre - Mississauga; Teach Staff, Queen's University; (905)848-7100

MCCOLL, Linda C P; Homewood Health Centre, 150 Delhi St, Guelph ON N1E 6K9; Ott'01; FRCPC; Psy. Staff, Homewood Health Centre; (519)824-1010

MCCOLL, Mary E; PO Box 2932 Stn Main, Strathmore AB T1P 1L5; Tor'68; CCFP; FCFP; (403)934-4444; Fax. (403)934-5218.

MCCOLL, Ryan J; 1921 10 Ave S, Lethbridge AB T1K 0B8; Alb'06; FRCSC; GenSurg. (403)380-4777

MCCOLLAM, Mary P; Weyburn Health Centre, 36 4th St, Weyburn SK S4H 0X7; Belfast (Ireland)'94; MB ChB; BAO; CCFP; Teacher Pt-Time-Family Med, University of Saskatchewan; (306)842-5444; Fax. (306)842-5449.

MCCOLLISTER, Christopher D; West Coast Gen Hosp, 3949 Port Alberni Hwy, Port Alberni BC V9Y 4S1; Cal'93; BSc; FRCPC; Peds. Staff, West Coast General Hospital; (250)724-9915; Fax. (250)724-9981; pipesdoc@yahoo.ca.

MCCOMB, Peter F; BC Women's Hosp & Health Ctre, D6-4500 Oak St, Vancouver BC V6H 3N1; Western (Australia)'73; MB BS; DRCOG; FRCSC; ObstGyn. Staff, BC Women's Hospital & Health Centre; Asst Prof, University of British Columbia; (604)875-2445

MCCOMB, Wendy M; Orillia Med/Dental Centre, 200-16 O'Brien St, Orillia ON L3V 5S2; Tor'93; BSc; CCFP; FCFP; Associate, Orillia Soldiers' Memorial Hospital; (705)325-2990

MCCOMBE, Jennifer A; University of Alberta Hosp, 2E3 WMC-8440 112 St NW, Edmonton AB T6G 2B7; Qns'04; FRCPC; Neur. Staff, University of Alberta Hospital; (780)407-8822

MCCOMBE, Padraic S C; 1B-200 Thickwood Blvd, Fort McMurray AB T9K 1X9; Dal'95; BSc; CCFP; FCFP; (780)790-9342; Fax. (780)791-0221.

MCCOMISKEY, Alan J; Stephenville Comm Med Clinic, 1 Washington Dr, Stephenville NL A2N 2V5; National (Ireland)'73; MB BCh; Chief of Staff, Sir Thomas Roddick Hospital; (709)643-5656; Fax. (709)643-5543; mccomiskey@nf.sympatico.ca.

MCCONACHIE, David R; Oakville Med Centre, 300 2-690 Dorval Dr, Oakville ON L6K 3W7; McM'88; BSc; MSc; FRCPC; IntMed; Cardiol. Staff, Halton Healthcare Services Corporation - Oakville Site; (905)849-4567 x4

MCCONACHIE, Ian W; St Joseph's Health Care, PO Box 5777 Stn B 268 Grosvenor Rd, London ON N6A 4V2; Aberdeen (Scotland)'82; FRCPC; Anes. Staff Anes, St Joseph's Hospital - St Joseph's Health Care; (519)646-6100

MCCONKEY, John P; 37979 Cleveland Ave PO Box 2417 Stn Main, Squamish BC V8B 0B6; UBC'69; FRCSC; OrthSurg (Sports Injuries). Consultant Staff, Squamish General Hospital / Hilltop House; Consultant Orth, UBC Hospital - Koerner Pavillion; Consultant Orthopaedics, Whistler Health Care Centre; Clin Prof, University of British Columbia; (604)815-4112; Fax. (604)815-4161; mcconkey0025@shaw.ca.

MCCONKEY, Mark O; 310-6091 Gilbert Rd, Richmond BC V7C 5L9; UBC'05; FRCSC; OrthSurg. (604)273-6148

MCCONNELL, Athena; Royal University Hosp, 103 Hospital Dr, Saskatoon SK S7N 0W8; Qns'00; FRCPC; Peds; InfectDis. Staff Peds, Royal University Hospital; (306)966-7927

MCCONNELL, C Maureen; Dahlstrom Clinic, 2-32442 George Ferguson Way, Abbotsford BC V2T 4Y4; Wes'80; CCFP; FCFP; Ac Staff, St Boniface General Hospital; (604)853-6667

MCCONNELL, Donald W; Meadowlark Prof Bldg, 270-8702 Meadowlark Rd NW, Edmonton AB T5R 5W5; Dal'93; FRCPC; Peds. Staff Ped, University of Alberta Hospital; (780)944-1840; Fax. (780)423-3961.

MCCONNELL, H Dianne; Medical Clinic Person-Ctred Ps, 403-265 Yorkland Blvd, North York ON M2J 1S5; McM'76; BSc; MSc; CCFP; FCFP; Staff, The Medical Clinic for Person-Centred Psychotherapy; (416)630-0610

MCCONNELL, Laura L; Harborn Med Associates, 510-89 Queensway W, Mississauga ON L5B 2V2; Tor'86; CCFP; FCFP; Ac Staff Family Pract, Trillium Health Centre - Mississauga; (905)273-4380; Fax. (905)273-4335.

MCCONNELL, Natalie R; West Street Health Centre, 206-216 West St, Simcoe ON N3Y 1S8; Qns'94; (519)428-3060; Fax. (519)428-1325.

MCCONNELL, Todd A; St Mary's Hosp Centre, B2 07-3830 av Lacombe, Montreal QC H3T 1M5; Wisconsin (USA)'73; IntMed. Chief IntMed, St Mary's Hospital Centre; assoc Prof, McGill University; Langs: French; (514)345-3511 x3112; Fax. (514)734-2641.

MCCONNELL, Yarrow J; PO Box 63004 Rpo Stadium, Calgary AB T2N 4S5; Dal'05; FRCSC; GenSurg.

MCCONNERY, Carol; CLSC de Hull, 85 rue Saint-Redempteur, Gatineau QC J8X 4E6; Ott'86; CCFP; FCFP; Staff DSC Immunization, Hull Hospital; Médecin, CLSC de Hull; (819)966-6510; Fax. (819)777-0271; carol_mcconnery@ssss.gouv.qc.ca.

MCCONVEY, Michael J; Wellington Med Arts Bldg, 121 Wellington St W, Barrie ON L4N 1L2; Qns'87; CCFP; (705)728-5536; Fax. (705)728-4885.

MCCONVILLE, Fiona C; Pickering Med Centre, 216-1885 Glenanna Rd, Pickering ON L1V 6R6; Cincinnati(OH) (USA)'98; FRCSC; ObstGyn. Langs: Bilingual(English/French); (905)420-5856

MCCONVILLE, James M; 202-2948 Baseline Rd, Nepean ON K2H 8T5; Dublin (Ireland)'79; DRCOG; FRCPC; Peds (Community Pediatrics). Ac Staff, Children's Hospital of Eastern Ontario (CHEO); Ac Staff, The Ottawa Hospital - Civic Campus; Ac Staff, Queensway Carleton Hospital; (613)828-4260; Fax. (613)828-1704; jmcconville4713@rogers.com.

MCCONVILLE, Raymond J; Care Point Med Centre, 1175 Denman St, Vancouver BC V6G 2N1; Glasgow (Scotland)'90; MB ChB; (604)681-5338

MCCOOK, Breanne T; Hys Med Centre, 505-11010 101 St NW, Edmonton AB T5H 4B9; McG'08; FRCPC; Peds. (780)414-6812; Fax. (780)428-0852.

MCCORD, Phyllis A; 288 Dundas St E PO Box 360, Waterdown ON L0R 2H0; McM'93; DC; CCFP; FCFP; Assoc Staff, Joseph Brant Memorial Hospital; Assoc Prof, Chiropractic & Post-Grad. Adjunct Prof., Canadian Mem. Chiropractic College; (905)689-8677; Fax. (905)689-8393.

MCCORDIC, D Frances; Beaverton Thorah Health Centre, 468 Main St E, Beaverton ON L0K 1A0; Tor'74; Med Dir, Lakeview Manor; (705)426-7331; Fax. (705)426-4272.

MCCORMACK, Brian C; Ontario Shores Ctr Mental HS, 613-700 Gordon St, Whitby ON L1N 5S9; Dublin (Ireland)'73; FRCPC; Psy. Sr Staff Psy/Med Dir, Ontario Shores Centre for Mental Health Sciences; (905)668-5881 x6310; Fax. (905)430-4032.

MCCORMACK, David G; London HSC-Victoria Hosp, PO Box 5010 Stn B 800 Commissioners Rd E, London ON N6A 5W9; Qns'80; FRCPC; IntMed; Respir. Staff, London Health Sciences Centre - Victoria Campus; Prog Dir Respirol/Prof, University of Western Ontario; (519)667-6767; Fax. (519)685-8406; david.mccormack@lhsc.on.ca.

MCCORMACK, Francis W; Nanaimo Reg Gen Hosp, 1200 Dufferin Cres, Nanaimo BC V9S 2B7; Sask'84; FRCPC; Anes. Staff, Nanaimo Regional General Hospital; (250)754-2141; Fax. (250)755-7633.

MCCORMACK, Grant S; Surrey Med Arts Bldg, 201-13798 94A Ave, Surrey BC V3V 1N1; UBC'78; FRCPC; IntMed; Respir. Staff, Surrey Memorial Hospital; Staff, Royal Columbian Hospital; (604)581-6727; Fax. (604)581-7692.

MCCORMACK, M Terry; CFB Winnipeg, PO Box 17000 Stn Forces 23 Health Services, Winnipeg MB R3J 3Y5; Ott'04; CCFP; (204)833-2500

MCCORMACK, Michael; Clinique 1851, 101-1851 rue Sherbrooke E, Montreal QC H2K 2W1; Mon'83; FRCSC; Urol. (514)524-7564; m.mccormack@umontreal.ca.

MCCORMACK, Noel C; PO Box 397 Stn Main, Guelph ON N1H 6K5; National (Ireland)'77; FRCPC; Anes. Staff, Guelph General Hospital; (519)826-9193

MCCORMACK, Paul A; Cowichan Dist Hosp, 3045 Gibbins Rd, Duncan BC V9L 1E5; Sask'83; FRCPC; DiagRad. Staff, Cowichan District Hospital; (250)709-3000 x4035

MCCORMACK, Philip C; Royal Oak Clinic, 103-10663 King George Hwy, Surrey BC V3T 2X6; London (England)'62; DObstRCOG; (604)438-6184; Fax. (604)438-6194.

MCCORMACK, Robert G; New West Ortho & Sports, 102-65 Richmond St, New Westminster BC V3L 5P5; Qns'79; Dip SportMed; FRCSC; OrthSurg (Sports Medicine). Staff, Royal Columbian Hospital; Assoc Prof, University of British Columbia; (604)526-7885; Fax. (604)525-4006.

MCCORMICK, Anna M; Children's Hosp Eastern Ont, 401 Smyth Rd, Ottawa ON K1H 8L1; Mem'88; FRCPCH; DPhysMed; FRCPC; Peds; PhysMed&Rehab. Staff Ottawa Rehab Centre, Children's Hospital of Eastern Ontario (CHEO); Asst Prof Peds & Med, University of Ottawa; (613)737-7600 x2831; Fax. (613)738-4893; amccormick@cheo.on.ca.

MCCORMICK, Brendan B; The Ottawa Hosp-Riverside, 527-1967 Riverside Dr, Ottawa ON K1H 7W9; Tor'98; FRCPC; IntMed; Nephrol. Staff Nephrol, The Ottawa Hospital - Riverside Campus; (613)738-8400 x82893; Fax. (613)738-8337.

MCCORMICK, Charles C K; Niagara H System-G Niagara, PO Box 1018 Stn Main 5546 Portage Rd, Niagara Falls ON L2E 6X2; Wes'82; FRCPC; Anes (Pain Management). Staff, Niagara Health System - Greater Niagara General Site; Staff, Niagara Health System - Welland Hospital Site; (905)358-0171 x3386

MCCORMICK, Iain A; Diamond Health Care Centre, 7F-2775 Laurel St, Vancouver BC V5Z 1M9; Qns'02; FRCPC; IntMed. (604)875-5181

MCCORMICK, John W; 53 Soudan Ave, Toronto ON M4S 1V5; Tor'72; DPsy; FRCPC; Psy. (416)481-3001; Fax. (416)481-9095; jwm@drjwm.ca.

MCCORMICK, Kathleen M; 52 Queen St, Dartmouth NS B2Y 1G1; Ott'86; CCFP; Staff, IWK Health Centre; (902)463-4311; Fax. (902)463-4315.

MCCORMICK, Myra J C; 262-1100 Memorial Ave, Thunder Bay ON P7B 4A3; McG'62; BSc; MSc; OrthSurg (Feet Seating & Mobility). Court Staff, St Joseph's Care Group - St Joseph's Hospital; Court Staff, Thunder Bay Regional Health Sciences Centre Port-Arthur; (807)628-6423

MCCORMICK, S Ashley; Soldier's Memorial Hosp, PO Box 730, Middleton NS B0S 1P0; Dal'07; CCFP; Staff, Soldiers Memorial Hospital; (902)825-3411

MCCORMICK, William D; 2C-2211 Wesbrook Mall, Vancouver BC V6T 2B5; Wes'06; FRCSC; OrthSurg. (604)875-4111 x66276

MCCORMICK, William O; Mental Health Services, 40 Freer Lane, Lower Sackville NS B4C 0A2; Cambridge (England)'53; FRCP; DPM; FRCPsy; FCPA; FRCPC; Psy. Emeritus Prof Psy, Dalhousie University; (902)865-3663; Fax. (902)865-2072; william.mccormick@cdha.nshealth.ca.

MCCOUBREY, David R; 200B-745 Montreal Rd, Ottawa ON K1K 0T1; McG'87; FACOG; MS; MD; FSOGC; FRCSC; ObstGyn. Staff, Montfort Hospital; Langs: Bilingual(English/French); (613)741-6767

MCCOURT, Catherine M; Place Vanier, 5A-333 North River Rd, Ottawa ON K1A 0L1; Ott'77; MHA; FRCPC; CommunMed; Public Health & Preventive Med. (613)952-2170; Fax. (613)952-8466; catherine.mccourt@phac-aspc.gc.ca.

MCCOURT, Francine D; Trafalgar Med Clinic, 200-1235 Trafalgar Rd, Oakville ON L6H 3P1; McM'01; CCFP; Staff, Halton Healthcare Services Corporation - Oakville Site; (905)844-3281

MCCOWAN, Conrad W; Market Mall Prof Bldg, 104-4935 40 Ave NW, Calgary AB T3A 2N1; Alb'59; (403)247-2253; Fax. (403)247-0669.

MCCOY, Stephen N; Family Medical Village, 207-197 Talbot St W, Leamington ON N8H 1N8; McG'82; (519)322-2522; Fax. (519)322-2514.

MCCRACKEN, James M; Sheep River Med Clinic, PO Box 1560 Stn Main 1-74 Elizabeth St, Okotoks AB T1S 1B5; Alb'83; Ac Staff, High River General Hospital; (403)938-4421; Fax. (403)938-5657.

MCCRACKEN, Jeffrey M; 201-1121 Yates St, Victoria BC V8V 3N1; UBC'02; FRCSC; Urol. (250)590-7422

MCCRACKEN, Peter; Glenrose Rehab Hosp, 1258-10230 111 Ave NW, Edmonton AB T5G 0B7; McG'70; GeriatricMed; IntMed. Staff, Glenrose Rehabilitation Hospital; Prof Med., University of Alberta; (780)735-8800; Fax. (780)735-8846; peter.mccracken@ualberta.ca.

MCCRACKEN, Rita K; 2F-1190 Hornby St, Vancouver BC V6Z 2K5; Cal'06; CCFP; (604)682-2344 x63745

MCCRANK, Ernest W T; Statesman Corporation, 102-7370 Sierra Morena Blvd SW, Calgary AB T3H 4H9; Qns'64; MD; FRCPC; Psy (Stress). Member, Alberta Mental Health Board; Emeritus Prof, University of Western Ontario; (403)217-2222

MCCREA, John C; Professional Arts Bldg, 527-100 Arden St, Moncton NB E1C 4B7; Mem'91; (506)855-6123; Fax. (506)855-6124.

MCCREA, Kristin E; Children's Hosp Eastern Ont, 401 Smyth Rd, Ottawa ON K1H 8L1; Man'07; Anes.

MCCREADY, David R; Univ Hlth Network-Princess M, 3 130-610 University Ave, Toronto ON M5G 2M9; Tor'80; FACS; FRCSC; GenSurg (Breast Cancer). Ac Staff, Mount Sinai Hospital; Ac Staff GenSurg (SurgOncol), Princess Margaret Hospital - University Health Network; Head Breast Prog, Toronto General Hospital - UHN; Prof Surg, University of Toronto; (416)946-6510; Fax. (416)946-4429; david.mccready@uhn.on.ca.

MCCREADY, Janine; Toronto East Gen Hosp Inc, 825 Coxwell Ave, Toronto ON M4C 3E7; Tor'07; FRCPC; IntMed; InfectDis. Staff, Toronto East General Hospital Inc; (416)469-6252

MCCREADY, John R; 387 St George St, London ON N6A 3A9; Wes'71; FRCPC; Psy. (519)438-1557; Fax. (519)439-1347; johnmccready@sympatico.ca.

MCCREADY, William G; Professional Bldg, 405-984 Oliver Rd, Thunder Bay ON P7B 7C7; Belfast (Ireland)'75; MB ChB; BAO; MRC(UK); FRCPC; IntMed (Nephrology). Staff Renal Serv, Thunder Bay Regional Health Sciences Centre; Assoc Dean Faculty Affairs, Northern Ontario School of Medicine; (807)345-8100; Fax. (807)345-5888.

MCCREARY, A James R; Medical Bldg, 120-6180 Blundell Rd, Richmond BC V7C 4W7; Qns'73; Ac Staff, Richmond Hospital; (604)271-4441; Fax. (604)241-8615; drajmccreary@gmail.com.

MCCREDIE, Victoria A; Sunnybrook Hlth Sciences Ctre, 2075 Bayview Ave, Toronto ON M4N 3M5; Manchester (England)'03; FRCPC; IntMed. Staff, Sunnybrook Health Sciences Centre; (416)480-6100

MCCRINDLE, Brian W; The Hosp For Sick Children, 555 University Ave, Toronto ON M5G 1X8; Alb'82; FRCPC; Peds; Cardiol. Staff Cardiol, The Hospital For Sick Children; Prof Peds, University of Toronto; (416)813-7610; Fax. (416)813-7547; brian.mccrindle@sickkids.ca.

MCCROSSIN, J Murray; Amherst Medical Associate, 200-158 Robert Angus Dr, Amherst NS B4H 4R7; Dal'90; CCFP; FCFP; Member Faculty/Preceptor, Dalhousie University; (902)667-3330; Fax. (902)667-4176.

MCCRUDEN, Jane E; Claresholm Addiction & Mental, PO Box 490 139 43 Ave W, Claresholm AB T0L 0T0; Cal'80; FRCPC; Psy. Staff, Rockyview General Hospital; Psychiatrist, Claresholm Centre for Mental Health and Addictions; Staff, Calgary Health Region; (403)682-3583; Fax. (403)625-8506.

MCCUAIG, Bradley M; Belmont Prof Centre, 209-564 Belmont Ave W, Kitchener ON N2M 5N6; Wes'92; FRCSC; Ophth. (519)579-5311; Fax. (519)579-2339.

MCCUAIG, Catherine C; Hôpital Ste-Justine, 3175 ch Cote-Sainte-Catherine, Montreal QC H3T 1C5; Qns'82; DABD; FRCPC; Derm (Pediatric Dermatology). Staff, Hôpital Ste-Justine; Pres, Societé de Dermatologie de Montréal; assoc Prof, Universite de Montreal; Langs: Italian; French; (514)345-4931; Fax. (514)345-2134; catherine_mccuaig@ssss.gouv.qc.ca.

MCCUAIG, Kenneth O; 2143 Russett Rd, Mississauga ON L4Y 1C2; Tor'57; (905)277-3029; kmccuaig1@rogers.com.

MCCUAIG, Randall E; Delta Hosp, 5800 Mountain View Blvd, Delta BC V4K 3V6; Sask'97; CCFP; FCFP; Staff, Delta Hospital; (604)946-1121

MCCUAIG, Wendy S; Medical Bldg, 400-18 Pine St, Kitchener ON N2H 5Z8; Wes'92; FRCSC; ObstGyn. (519)570-0090; Fax. (519)570-3202.

MCCUBBIN, Duncan; Dr Duncan J McCubbin Prof Corp, 108-770 6 St SW, Medicine Hat AB T1A 4J6; Alb'91; FRCSC; ObstGyn (Colposcopy). Staff Maternal Fetal Med, Medicine Hat Regional Hospital; (403)502-8935; Fax. (403)502-8962.

MCCUBBIN, Jacqueline M; Mill Woods Town Centre Prof, 314-6203 28 Ave NW, Edmonton AB T6L 6K3; Alb'91; FRCSC; ObstGyn. (780)430-2229; Fax. (780)468-2880.

MCCULLAGH, Scott R; Sunnybrook Hlth Sciences Ctre, FG10-2075 Bayview Ave, Toronto ON M4N 3M5; McM'90; FRCPC; Psy (Adult Psychiatry). Staff, Sunnybrook Health Sciences Centre; (416)480-4216; Fax. (416)480-4613.

MCCULLOCH, Donald F; 786 Goderich St GD, Port Elgin ON N0H 2C0; Wes'78; (519)832-2124; Fax. (519)389-5509.

MCCULLOCH, Donna M; Woodlawn Med Consultants, 92 Main St, Dartmouth NS B2X 1R5; Dal'85; FRCPC; Peds (Consultant Pediatrics). (902)434-1500

MCCULLOCH, Janet R; 916 Princess St, Kingston ON K7L 1H1; Qns'83; FRCPC; Psy. (613)531-6127; Fax. (613)507-6127.

MCCULLOUGH, Wendy M; J-6 Speers Blvd, Amherstview ON K7N 1Z6; Mem'93; Queen's University; (613)634-4354; Fax. (613)634-0320.

MCCULLY, E Kathleen; 15 Tower Lane, London ON N6A 2L9; Wes'75; CCFP; FCFP; Court Staff, Parkwood Hospital - St Joseph's Health Care; Med Staff Assoc, St Joseph's Hospital - St Joseph's Health Care; (519)432-7579; Fax. (519)433-8586.

MCCUNE, Marcie L; 589 West Gore St, Stratford ON N5A 1L4; Wes'96; FRCSC; GenSurg. (519)273-4100; Fax. (519)273-3208.

MCCUNN, P Donald; Riverside Prof Centre, 209-1919 Riverside Dr, Ottawa ON K1H 1A2; Ott'55; FRCSC; Ophth. Ac Staff, The Ottawa Hospital - General Campus; (613)233-4904; Fax. (613)236-6801.

MCCURDY, John; Queen Square Doctors FHT, 201-366 Main St N, Brampton ON L6V 1P8; Queen's (Ireland)'60; DObstRCOG; Hon Staff, William Osler Health System - Brampton Civic Hospital; Staff, Holland Christian Homes; (905)455-1455; Fax. (905)455-5498; jmccurdy@rogers.com.

MCCURLEY, Robert; Consent & Capacity Board of On, 151 Bloor St W, Toronto ON M5S 2T5; Belfast (Ireland)'66; MB ChB; BAO; DPM; MRCPsy; FRCPC; Psy. Staff, Centre for Addiction & Mental Health (CAMH) - Queen Site.

MCCURRACH, Anne E G; Medical Office, 212-840 Coxwell Ave, Toronto ON M4C 5T2; Edinburgh (Scotland)'66; (416)422-0899; Fax. (416)422-0666.

MCCUSKER, Christine T; MUHC-Montreal Children's Hosp, RMC510-2300 rue Tupper, Montreal QC H3H 1P3; McM'93; FRCPC; Peds; ClinImmunol&Allergy. Staff, McGill University Health Centre - Montreal Children's Hospital; adj Prof, McGill University; (514)412-4470; christine.mccusker@mcgill.ca.

MCCUSKER, Patricia J; Cancercare Manitoba, 2021-675 McDermot Ave, Winnipeg MB R3E 0V9; McM'86; FRCPC; IntMed; Hem. Physician, CancerCare Manitoba; (204)787-4135

MCCUTCHEON, N Larry; Huronia Med Centre, PO Box 790 Stn Main 240 Old Penetanguishene Rd, Midland ON L4R 4P4; Tor'75; Assoc Staff, North Simcoe Family Health Team; Assoc Staff, Georgian Bay General Hospital - Midland; (705)526-3734

MCCUTCHEON, Sharon; Health Services Complex, 7A-20 Kennedy Dr, Sussex NB E4E 2P1; McM'96; MB; CCFP; Staff, Sussex Health Centre; (506)432-4300; Fax. (506)432-4306; gumpy@nb.sympatico.ca.

MCDERMID, Brian J; 404-49 St Clair Ave W, Toronto ON M4V 1K6; McM'83; MES; (416)972-0691

MCDERMID, Cheryl E; 1202 Pender St W PO Box 17566, Vancouver BC V6E 2S8; UBC'78; (778)387-9080

MCDERMID, Jill C; Hys Med Centre, 310-11010 101 St NW, Edmonton AB T5H 4B9; Cal'98; FRCPC; IntMed; Gastroent. (780)421-1029; Fax. (780)425-5533.

MCDERMID, Kevin P; 201-22112 52 Ave, Langley BC V2Y 2M6; UBC'97; BSc; MSc; PhD; FRCPC; IntMed (Cardiology). (604)539-2022; Fax. (604)539-2023.

MCDERMID, Robert C; University of Alberta Hosp, 3C1 20 WCM-8440 112 St NW, Edmonton AB T6G 2B7; UBC'97; FRCPC; IntMed; Critical Care Medicine; Respir. Staff, University of Alberta Hospital; (780)407-6755

MCDERMOTT, Colleen; 308-55 Queen St E, Toronto ON M5C 1R6; Tor'02; FRCSC; ObstGyn. Staff, St Michael's Hospital; (416)864-6060

MCDERMOTT, John; 10155 120 St NW, Edmonton AB T5K 2A2; Sher'01; FRCPC; Neur (Epilepsy). Staff, Royal Alexandra Hospital; Langs: Bilingual(French/English); (780)482-7551; Fax. (780)488-2056.

MCDERMOTT, Pamela D; Huntsridge Park Bldg, 302-395 Centre St N, Huntsville ON P1H 2P5; McM'79; CCFP; FCFP; (705)789-2842

MCDERMOTT, Thomas M; Haileybury Family Health Team, PO Box 2010 95 Meridian Ave, Haileybury ON P0J 1K0; Qns'71; CCFP; FCFP; Ac Staff, Temiskaming Hospital; (705)672-3371; Fax. (705)672-5900.

MCDIARMID, Adam P; Lions Gate Hosp, 231 15th St E, North Vancouver BC V7L 2L7; UBC'01; FRCPC; Anes. Staff, Lions Gate Hospital; (604)988-3131

MCDONAGH, Mary; Regional Mental HC-London, PO Box 5532 Stn B 850 Highbury Rd N, London ON N6A 4H1; Dublin (Ireland)'77; LRCPSI; CCFP; FCFP; Staff, Regional Mental Health Care-St Joseph's Health Care; (519)455-5110; Fax. (519)455-9879; mary.mcdonagh@sjhc.london.on.ca.

MCDONAGH, Roderick J; 77 Hunter St E, Hamilton ON L8N 1M4; McM'95; MSc; FRCSC; ObstGyn. Staff, St Joseph's Healthcare - Charlton Campus; (905)521-8320; Fax. (905)521-1127.

MCDONAGH, Thomas H M; The Medical Centre, 1A-163 Commissioners Rd W, London ON N6J 1X9; Dublin (Ireland)'76; DCH; DObst; CCFP; FCFP; (519)660-8111; Fax. (519)660-4903.

MCDONALD, Allan A; Associate Med Clinic, 25 St. Michael St, St Albert AB T8N 1C7; Alb'95; CCFP; (780)458-1234; Fax. (780)460-7941.

MCDONALD, Andrea J; Duffus Health Centre, 708-7071 Bayers Rd, Halifax NS B3L 2C2; Dal'97; BSc; CCFP; FCFP; (902)453-4585; Fax. (902)453-5657.

MCDONALD, Andrew C; Sunnybrook Hlth Sciences Ctre, 2075 Bayview Ave, Toronto ON M4N 3M5; McG'85; MSc(Tor.); MHSc; FRCPC; EmergMed. Chief Emerg Services, Sunnybrook Health Sciences Centre; Asst Prof, University of Toronto; (416)480-6100; Fax. (416)480-4704.

MCDONALD, Andrew J; Canadian Forces Hlth Services, PO Box 17000 Stn Forces, Victoria BC V9A 7N2; Dal'07; CCFP; (250)363-4128

MCDONALD, Angus C; 101A-2099 152 St, Surrey BC V4A 4N7; UBC'83; CCFP; (604)538-5770; Fax. (604)536-5824.

MCDONALD, Anne J; 202-1280 Lasalle Blvd, Sudbury ON P3A 1Y8; NOSM'10; CCFP; (705)671-3002

MCDONALD, Barrie M; The Medical Clinic Associates, 4794 Joyce Ave, Powell River BC V8A 3B6; McG'91; MDCM; (604)485-6261; Fax. (604)485-2820.

MCDONALD, Bernard J; Univ of Ottawa Heart Institute, H2410-40 Ruskin St, Ottawa ON K1Y 4W7; Qns'95; FRCPC; Anes; Critical Care Medicine. Staff, University of Ottawa Heart Institute; Staff, The Ottawa Hospital - Civic Campus; (613)798-5555 x4379

MCDONALD, Bethany D; The Cove Clinic, 1608 Portugal Cove Rd, Port Cv-St Phil NL A1M 3H4; Mem'04; CCFP.

MCDONALD, Charles R J; Hamilton HS-General Site, 237 Barton St E, Hamilton ON L8L 2X2; Dal'07; GenSurg. Staff, Hamilton Health Sciences Centre - Hamilton General Hospital; (905)521-2100

MCDONALD, Charlotte G; St Joseph's Health Care, PO Box 5777 Stn B 268 Grosvenor St, London ON N6A 4V2; Wes'96; FRCPC; IntMed (Diabetes); Endocrin&Metab. Staff, St Joseph's Hospital - St Joseph's Health Care; Assoc Prof, University of Western Ontario; (519)646-6170; Fax. (519)646-6058.

MCDONALD, Clint A; Lakeside Med Clinic, 3919 8th St E, Saskatoon SK S7H 5M7; Durban (South Africa)'96; MB ChB; (306)374-6884

MCDONALD, D Angus; Addiction & Mental Hlth-Queen, 1001 Queen St W, Toronto ON M6J 1H4; McM'76; PhD; FRCPC; Psy (Forensic Psychiatry). Staff Psy, Ontario Shores Centre for Mental Health Sciences; Staff Psy Metro Toronto Forensic Service, Centre for Addiction & Mental Health (CAMH) - College Street Site; Staff METFORS, Centre for Addiction & Mental Health (CAMH) - Queen Site; Asst Prof, University of Toronto; (416)535-8501 x2950

MCDONALD, David I; Victoria Gen Hosp, 1 Hospital Way, Victoria BC V8Z 6R5; Man'71; FRACP; FRCPC; IntMed. Staff, Victoria General Hospital; Staff, Royal Jubilee Hospital; (250)727-4212 x5107; Fax. (250)595-3104.

MCDONALD, David S; Red Deer Med Centre, 210-3947 50A Ave, Red Deer AB T4N 6V7; Ott'07; PlasSurg. (403)357-5187

MCDONALD, Diana; Clinique Med St-Jerome, 102-450 boul Monseigneur-Duboi, Saint-Jerome QC J7Y 3L8; Mon'84; CCFP; (450)438-1518; Fax. (450)438-6119.

MCDONALD, Don G; 103-20644 Fraser Hwy, Langley BC V3A 4G5; UBC'86; (604)530-4979; Fax. (604)530-2975.

MCDONALD, Donald J; Kingsway Med Bldg, 21-2917 Bloor St W, Etobicoke ON M8X 1B4; Tor'56; FRCSC; Ophth. (416)239-3843; Fax. (416)239-3820.

MCDONALD, Gordon; Southside Med Clinic, 102-640 Prospect St, Fredericton NB E3B 9M7; Dal'05; CCFP; (506)458-1445; Fax. (506)458-1515.

MCDONALD, Heather D; Health Sciences Centre, 820 Sherbrook St, Winnipeg MB R3A 1R9; Man'98; FRCPC; Anes. Staff Anes, Health Sciences Centre; (204)774-6511

MCDONALD, Heather M W; Outreach Urban Health, 455 Leon Ave, Kelowna BC V1Y 6J4; Mem'91; CCFP; (250)868-2230

MCDONALD, Hector; 1655 Kilborn Ave, Ottawa ON K1H 6M7; Witwatersrand (South Africa)'82; MB ChB; BSc; FRCSC; Ophth (Cosmetic Eyelid Surgery)., University of Ottawa; (613)739-5437; hmcdonald@revisage.ca.

MCDONALD, J Christopher; Peterborough Clinic, 201-26 Hospital Dr, Peterborough ON K9J 7C3; West Indies (Jamaica)'75; DAB; FRCSC; Ophth. (705)743-2040; Fax. (705)743-4392.

MCDONALD, James; Medical Clinic Inglewood, 102-12418 118 Ave NW, Edmonton AB T5L 2K4; Dublin (Ireland)'80; MD; BAO; (780)452-1354

MCDONALD, Jane C; MUHC-Montreal Children's Hosp, C1242-2300 rue Tupper, Montreal QC H3H 1P3; McM'78; FRCPC; Peds; MedMicrobiol; InfectDis. Dir Dept of Med Microbiol/intérim, McGill University Health Centre - Montreal Children's Hospital; assoc Prof Peds, McGill University; (514)412-4313

MCDONALD, Jane E; 394 Guelph Line, Burlington ON L7R 3L4; McM'89; (905)333-1553; Fax. (905)333-1558.

MCDONALD, Jennifer K; Victoria Health Centre, 2F-521 Victoria Park Ave, Scarborough ON M4C 5H1; Tor'06; CCFP; (416)694-1400

MCDONALD, Joanna E; Newburgh Clinic, PO Box 129 5 Earl St, Newburgh ON K0K 2S0; Wes'91; CCFP; FCFP; (613)378-1754; Fax. (613)378-1776.

MCDONALD, Johannes V; Holley Clinic, 348 Front St, Quesnel BC V2J 2K3; Stellenbosch (South Africa)'03; MB ChB; Langs: Afrikaans; (250)992-2158

MCDONALD, John A; 2-90 King St GD, Picton ON K0K 2T0; Qns'85; (613)476-7882

MCDONALD, John W; Brant Community HC-Willet, 238 Grand River St N, Paris ON N3L 2N7; Wes'75; Ac Staff, The Brant Community Healthcare System - Willett Hospital Site; (519)442-3609; j.mcdonald@rogers.com.

MCDONALD, John W D; AIM Health and Wellness Centre, 458 Central Ave, London ON N6B 2E5; Wes'61; PhD; FACP; FRCP; LMCC; FRCPC; IntMed (Gastroenterology). Consultant, Alexandra Hospital; Physician, London Scoping Centre; Physician, Robarts Clinical Trials; Prof Med, University of Western Ontario; (519)432-1521; Fax. (519)679-9658; jmcdonald@robarts.ca.

MCDONALD, Kenneth O; St Paul's Hosp, 1081 Burrard St, Vancouver BC V6Z 1Y6; UBC'85; FRCPC; Anes; Critical Care Medicine. Staff, Providence Health Care - St Paul's Hospital; (604)628-2344

MCDONALD, Lois M; Quinte HC Corp-Belleville Gen, 265 Dundas St E, Belleville ON K8N 5A9; McM'90; CCFP; CCFP(E.M.); FCFP; Staff Emerg, QHC Belleville General; (613)969-5511 x2434; Fax. (613)969-0229.

MCDONALD, Lori J; Queen Elizabeth II HSC, 1276 South Park St, Halifax NS B3H 2Y9; Mem'01; FRCPC; DiagRad. Staff DiagRad, Queen Elizabeth II Health Sciences Centre - Victoria General Site; (902)473-2700

MCDONALD, Marguerite; Royal University Hosp, 103 Hospital Dr, Saskatoon SK S7N 0W8; Orange Free State (South Africa)'96; MB ChB; FRCPC; Anes. Staff, Royal University Hospital; (306)655-1183; Fax. (306)655-1279.

MCDONALD, Maureen M; The Medical Centre FHT, PO Box 4200 Stn Main 707 Charlotte St, Peterborough ON K9J 7B3; McG'84; BSc; CCFP; FCFP; Court Staff, Peterborough Regional Health Centre - Hospital Drive; (705)876-4554; Fax. (705)742-7076.

MCDONALD, Michael A; 11CSB 1188-585 University Ave, Toronto ON M5G 2N2; Ott'02; FRCPC; IntMed; Cardiol. Staff, Toronto General Hospital - UHN; (416)340-4800

MCDONALD, Norman A; Associate Med Clinic, 25 St Michael St, St Albert AB T8N 1C7; Alb'67; Ac Staff, Sturgeon Community Hospital; (780)458-1234; Fax. (780)460-7941.

MCDONALD, Patrick J; Health Sciences Centre, GB138-820 Sherbrook St, Winnipeg MB R3A 1R9; Tor'92; FRCSC; Neursurg (Pediatric Neuro Surgery). Staff NeuroSurg, Health Sciences Centre; (204)774-6511

MCDONALD, Ross M; Salmon Arm Med Clinic, PO Box 730 Stn Main, Salmon Arm BC V1E 4N8; UBC'92; CCFP; (250)832-2321

MCDONALD, Sandy I R; 50 Alliance Blvd, Barrie ON L4M 5K3; Qns'77; AB; FRCSC; GenSurg; Cardiovasc&ThorSurg. Staff, Orillia Soldiers' Memorial Hospital; Staff, Royal Victoria Regional Health Centre; (705)728-8778; Fax. (705)728-3053.

MCDONALD, Sarah D; McMaster University, 3N52B-1280 Main St W, Hamilton ON L8S 4K1; Tor'97; FRCSC; ObstGyn (Maternal Fetal Medicine). Langs: English; French; (905)525-9140 x26622

MCDONALD, Stacey L; SilverFern Clinic, 160 Jubilee St, Duncan BC V9L 1W7; Cal'91; BSc; CCFP; FCFP; (250)709-9600

MCDONALD, Susan E; 108-9123 Mary St, Chilliwack BC V2P 4H7; UBC'96; FRCSC; GenSurg. (604)795-0332

MCDONALD, Terrence J; Glen Sather Sports Med Clinic, L2-11400 University Ave NW, Edmonton AB T6G 1Z1; Mem'04; CCFP; (780)407-5160

MCDONALD, William N; St Paul's Hosp, 4B 437-1081 Burrard St, Vancouver BC V6Z 1Y6; UBC'75; FRCP; FRCPC; Anes (Pain Management); IntMed. Staff, Providence Health Care - St Paul's Hospital; Clin Prof, University of British Columbia; (604)682-2344 x62333; Fax. (604)806-9128; wnmcdonald@providencehealth.bc.ca.

MCDONALD, William R; Medical Bldg, 705-805 Broadway W, Vancouver BC V5Z 1K1; UBC'82; DMD; Ac Staff Oral & Maxillofacial Surg, UBC Hospital - Koerner Pavillion; Hd Oral & Maxillofacial Surg, BC Children's Hospital; Asst Prof, University of British Columbia; (604)873-0303; Fax. (604)873-0321.

MCDONALD BLUMER, M Heather; Joseph & Wolf Lebovic Bldg, 2 002-60 Murray St, Toronto ON M5T 3L9; McM'82; FRCPC; IntMed (Osteoporosis); Rheum. Assoc Dir Osteoporosis Prog, Toronto General Hospital - UHN; Ac Staff, Mount Sinai Hospital; Assoc Prof Med, University of Toronto; (416)586-4800 x4988; Fax. (416)586-8766; hmcdonald-blumer@mtsinai.on.ca.

MCDONNELL, Conor G; The Hosp For Sick Children, 555 University Ave, Toronto ON M5G 1X8; Ire. (Ireland)'94; (416)813-7500 x7240

MCDONNELL, Michael B; Sunnybrook Hlth Sciences Ctre, 2075 Bayview Ave, Toronto ON M4N 3M5; Ott'97; FRCPC; EmergMed. Staff Emerg Med, Sunnybrook Health Sciences Centre; (416)480-4037

MCDONOUGH, Erin T; 201-460 College St, Toronto ON M6G 1A1; Dal'00; FRCPC; Psy. (416)901-6690; Fax. (416)901-6693.

MCDOUGALL, Donald C; Carling-Broadview Med Bldg, 210-770 Broadview Ave, Ottawa ON K2A 3Z3; Ott'71; CCFP; FCFP; Att Staff, The Ottawa Hospital - Civic Campus; Asst Prof Family Med, University of Ottawa; (613)729-4811; Fax. (613)729-8906; dcmcdougall@sympatico.ca.

MCDOUGALL, Elspeth M; UBC Faculty of Medicine, 6F-2775 Laurel St, Vancouver BC V5Z 1M9; Cal'79; FRCSC; Urol. (604)875-4301

MCDOUGALL, J David; Viewpoint Med Assessment Servs, 1-9250 Macleod Trail SE, Calgary AB T2J 0P5; Tor'72; CCFP; Med Dir, Viewpoint Medical Assessment Services Inc; (403)253-4272; Fax. (403)253-7089.

MCDOUGALL, Jacqueline Y; 216 Stewart Green SW PO Box 75040 Rpo Westhills, Calgary AB T3H 3M1; Cal'90; CCFP; FCFP.

MCDOUGALL, Laura; Holy Cross Centre, 2210 2 St SW, Calgary AB T2S 3C3; Cal'87; FRCPC; CommunMed. Staff, Alberta Health Services; (403)607-9694

MCDOUGALL, Robert S; Cornwall Prof Bldg, 311-2125 11th Ave, Regina SK S4P 3X3; Sask'86; FRCPC; IntMed (Sports Medicine); Rheum (Sports Medicine). Clin Prof, University of Saskatchewan; (306)352-2130; Fax. (306)352-2117.

MCDOWALL, Moira L; 502 Oxford St E, London ON N5Y 3H7; London (England)'80; MB BS; LRCP; MRCS; (519)672-5878; Fax. (519)672-6450.

MCDOWELL, Anthony; Argus Med Centre, 300-581 Argus Rd, Oakville ON L6J 3J4; Qns'84; BSc(Hon)Biology; (905)338-9900; Fax. (905)338-9904.

MCDOWELL, Brenda J; Youhtdale Treatment Centres, 227 Victoria St, Toronto ON M5B 1T8; McM'75; CCFP; FCFP; Vice Chairman Research Ethics Board, St Michael's Hospital; Assoc Prof, University of Toronto; (416)363-3751; Fax. (416)363-7945; mcdowellb@smh.ca.

MCDOWELL, Timothy J; Trail Bay Clinic, PO Box 1760 5755 Cowrie St, Sechelt BC V0N 3A0; Man'95; CCFP; (604)885-5196; Fax. (604)885-5193.

MCEACHERN, Anita M; Royal Columbian Hosp, 330 Columbia St E, New Westminster BC V3L 3W7; UBC'90; FRCPC; DiagRad. Staff, Royal Columbian Hospital; (604)530-4640

MCEACHREN, Todd M; 31 Airport Rd, St. John's NL A1A 5A1; Dal'98; FRCSC; Ophth. Att Staff Ophthalmology, Health Sciences Centre; (709)726-8253; Fax. (709)746-0889; tmmceachren@yahoo.ca.

MCELGUNN, Dennis M; Victoria Emerg Phys Mgmt Ltd, 325-1627 Fort St, Victoria BC V8R 1H8; Alb'70; FRCPC; EmergMed. Ac Staff, Royal Jubilee Hospital; (250)479-1442; Fax. (250)479-1472.

MCELHANEY, Janet E; Sudbury Reg Hosp-Laurentian, 41 Ramsey Lake Rd, Sudbury ON P3E 5J1; Alb'86; FRCPC; IntMed; GeriatricMed. Staff, Health Sciences North-Laurentian Site; (705)523-7300

MCELLIGOTT, Michael A; 305 Nelson St, Wallaceburg ON N8A 4G7; National (Ireland)'70; MB ChB; BAO; CCFP; Ac Staff, Chatham-Kent Health Alliance - Sydenham Hospital Campus; Court Staff, Chatham-Kent Health Alliance; Coroner, Ontario Area 1; (519)627-1500; Fax. (519)627-2442.

MCELROY, Rosheen T; Humber River Reg Hosp-Church, 200 Church St, Toronto ON M9N 1N8; UBC'05; CCFP; CCFP(E.M.); Staff, Humber River Regional Hospital - Church Street Site; (416)249-8111

MCENERY, Peter J; 3 Cleak St PO Box 388, Bancroft ON K0L 1C0; Ott'72; CCFP; FCFP; Staff Family Med, QHC North Hastings; Court Staff Privil, Peterborough Regional Health Centre - Hospital Drive; Court Staff Privil, QHC Belleville General; (613)332-3305; Fax. (613)332-0425; pmcenery@bellnet.ca.

MCEVILLY, Rebecca; St Joseph Health Centre, 30 The Queensway, Toronto ON M6R 1B5; McM'07; FRCPC; Psy. Staff, St Joseph's Health Centre; (416)530-6060

MCEVOY, Patricia L; Grand Prairie Mental Health S, 600-10014 99 St, Grande Prairie AB T8V 3N4; Alb'94; BFA; (780)538-5160; Fax. (780)538-6279.

MCEWAN, Alexander J B; Cross Cancer Institute, 11560 University Ave NW, Edmonton AB T6G 1Z2; London (England)'75; MB BS; MSc; FRCPC; NuclearMed. Sr Specialist Nuclear Med/Oncologic Imaging/Med Dir, Cross Cancer Institute; Prof/Dept Chair Oncol, University of Alberta; (780)432-8524; Fax. (780)432-8483; sandymce@cancerboard.ab.ca.

MCEWAN, M M Patricia; Rosedale Med Centre, 309-600 Sherbourne St, Toronto ON M4X 1W4; Tor'72; FRCPC; IntMed (Nuclear Cardiology); Cardiol. Staff Outdoor Attending, Toronto General Hospital - UHN; Court Staff, St Michael's Hospital; Assoc Prof Med, University of Toronto; (416)926-1593; Fax. (416)926-8768; mcewanp@smh.ca.

MCEWEN, Jillene I; Vancouver Gen Hosp, 855 12th Ave W, Vancouver BC V5Z 1M9; Tor'82; FRCPC; EmergMed. Ac Staff, Vancouver General Hospital - Centennial Pavillion; Dir Undergrad Educ, University of British Columbia; (604)875-4995; Fax. (604)875-4872.

MCEWEN, Jonathan; JPP 2449-899 12th Ave W, Vancouver BC V5Z 1M9; Cal'02; FRCPC; Anes. (604)644-9714

MCEWEN, R Ross; Meadowlark Health Centre, 200 Meadowlark Shopping Ctr NW, Edmonton AB T5R 5W9; Man'90; FRCPC; DiagRad. (780)489-7851; Fax. (780)486-5160.

MCFADDEN, Andrew W J; Gordon & Leaslie Diamond H C, 5F-2775 Laurel St, Vancouver BC V5Z 1M9; Sask'86; FRCSC; GenSurg (Surgical Oncology). (604)875-5880

MCFADDEN, Caitlin; Hillside Med Centre, 360 2nd Ave, Campbell River BC V9W 3T9; Sask'85; CCFP; Staff, Campbell River & District General Hospital; Med Dir, Yucalta Longterm Care Facility; (250)287-7708; Fax. (250)287-3086.

MCFADDEN, D Murray; 201-20434 64 Ave, Langley BC V2Y 1N4; Alb'70; FAAO; FRCSC; Ophth (Cataract Surgery). Consultant, Vancouver General Hospital - Centennial Pavillion; Staff, Surrey Memorial Hospital; Ac Staff, Langley Memorial Hospital; Physician Webmaster, PRK & LASIK Today; Clin Assoc Prof, University of British Columbia; (604)530-3332; Fax. (604)530-5061; m2@prk.com.

MCFADDEN, Deborah E; Children's & Women's HC of BC, B321-4480 Oak St, Vancouver BC V6H 3V4; Cal'80; CCMG; FRCPC; AnatPath (Cytogenetics). Consultant, Vancouver General Hospital - Centennial Pavillion; Staff Path, BC Children's Hospital; Fax. (604)875-3529.

MCFADDEN, Erin L; Univ Hlth Network-Toronto Western Hosp, 2F WW-399 Bathurst St, Toronto ON M5T 2S8; Tor'10; CCFP; Staff, Toronto Western Hospital - University Health Network; (416)603-5888

MCFADDEN, Laura Lee; The Women's Clinic & Oshun H, 200-912 Idylwyld Dr N, Saskatoon SK S7L 0Z6; Man'93; BSc; CCFP; FCFP; (306)343-1799; Fax. (306)343-1383.

MCFADDEN, Nancy A; Courtenay Med Associates, 201-1350 England Ave, Courtenay BC V9N 8X6; UBC'93; CCFP; FCFP; (250)334-4411; Fax. (250)338-1245.

MCFADDEN, Nathalie; CHUS-Hopital Hotel-Dieu, 580 rue Bowen S, Sherbrooke QC J1G 2E8; Sher'94; FRCSC; GenSurg (Colorectal Surgery). Staff, Centre Hospitalier Universitaire de Sherbrooke-Hopital Fleurimont; Staff, Centre Hospitalier Universitaire de Sherbrooke-Hôpital Hôtel-Dieu; Langs: Bilingual(French/English); (819)346-1110

MCFADDEN, Robin G; St Joseph's Health Care, PO Box 5777 Stn B 268 Grosvenor St, London ON N6A 4V2; Wes'77; FRCPC; IntMed; Respir. Staff Med, St Joseph's Hospital - St Joseph's Health Care; Assoc Prof/Dept Chair Med, University of Western Ontario; (519)646-6065; Fax. (519)646-6064.

MCFADDEN, Sean D P; Foothills Med Centre, G33-1403 29 St NW, Calgary AB T2N 2T9; Cal'87; FRCSC; GenSurg; ThorSurg. Staff, Foothills Medical Centre; (403)944-4279; Fax. (403)270-8431; sean.mcfadden@crha-health.ab.ca.

MCFADDEN, Shelley; Clinique Dr Shelley McFadden, 300-30 Irving Blvd, Bouctouche NB E4S 3L2; Laval'01; CCFP; Langs: English; (506)955-1991; Fax. (506)955-1984.

MCFADYEN, Craig A; The Credit Valley Hosp, 2200 Eglinton Ave W, Mississauga ON L5M 2N1; Cal'82; FRCSC; GenSurg. Staff, The Credit Valley Hospital; (905)813-1100 x3153

MCFADYEN, Lorraine A; Red Deer Reg Hosp Centre, PO Box 5030 Stn Postal Box Ctr, Red Deer AB T4N 6R2; Cal'89; FRCSC; GenSurg. Staff, Red Deer Regional Hospital Centre; (403)343-4768

MCFADYEN, Roderick L; Victoria Emerg Phys Mgmt Ltd, 325-1627 Fort St, Victoria BC V8R 1H8; Man'78; FRCPC; EmergMed;CCFP; CCFP(E.M.); FCFP; (250)479-1442; Fax. (250)479-1472.

MCFADZEAN, I Laing; Tamworth Med Centre RR 1, Tamworth ON K0K 3G0; Qns'74; (613)379-2946; Fax. (613)379-5138; laingmcfadzean@gmail.com.

MCFARLAND, James D; Gibsons Med Clinic, 211-1100 Sunshine Coast Hwy, Gibsons BC V0N 1V7; McM'77; CCFP; FCFP; Staff, St Mary's Hospital; (604)886-2868; Fax. (604)886-9716.

MCFARLAND, Kathryn J E; 200-110 Bearbrook Rd, Gloucester ON K1B 5R2; Tor'90; Asst Surg, The Ottawa Hospital - Civic Campus; (613)824-6318; Fax. (613)824-0521.

MCFARLANE, Allan H; St Joseph's Healthcare, 3F-50 Charlton Ave E, Hamilton ON L8N 4A6; Qns'57; FRCPC; Psy (Cardiological Depression). Staff Comm Psy Services, St Joseph's Healthcare - Charlton Campus; Emeritus Prof, McMaster University; (905)522-1155 x35230; mcfarlan@mcmaster.ca.

MCFARLANE, Brian A E; 272 Church St PO Box 245, Pugwash NS B0K 1L0; Tor'74; CCFP; FCFP; (902)243-3350

MCFARLANE, Charles A; Tecumseh Manning Med Centre, 204-13278 Tecumseh Rd E, Windsor ON N8N 3T6; Glasgow (Scotland)'69; (519)979-5665; Fax. (519)979-5633.

MCFARLANE, Kari; Rockyview Gen Hosp, 7007 14 St SW, Calgary AB T2V 1P9; Wes'03; CCFP; CCFP(E.M.); Staff, Rockyview General Hospital; (403)943-3000; Fax. (403)212-1242.

MCFARLANE, Lisa A; 16-385 Frederick St, Kitchener ON N2H 2P2; Wes'95; CCFP; FCFP; (519)745-7482

MCFARLANE, Lori A; Courtenay Med Associates, 201-1350 England Ave, Courtenay BC V9N 8X6; Wes'91; CCFP; Staff, Providence Health Care - St Paul's Hospital; (250)334-4411

MCFARLANE, Martin H; Windsor Health Centre, 108-630 Tecumseh Rd E, Windsor ON N8X 4W2; Wes'95; FRCPC; IntMed (Cardiac Rehabilitation). (519)977-6850; Fax. (519)977-7722.

MCFARLANE, Nicholas A; Kitchener Urology Associates, 313-751 King St W, Kitchener ON N2G 1E5; Wes'95; FRCSC; Urol. (519)954-2370

MCFARLANE, Philip A; 9F-61 Queen St E, Toronto ON M5C 2T2; Wes'93; FRCPC; IntMed; Nephrol. (416)867-3702; Fax. (416)867-3709.

MCFARLANE, Ginny V J; 2F-2243 Queen St E, Toronto ON M4E 1G1; McM'88; BSc; CGPP; CCFP; (416)686-2138; Fax. (416)850-3749.

MCFAUL, Susan M; 201-1919 Riverside Dr, Ottawa ON K1H 1A2; Ott'84; FRCSC; ObstGyn. Ac Staff, The Ottawa Hospital - Civic Campus; Asst Prof, University of Ottawa; (613)722-5793; Fax. (613)728-4480.

MCFAYDEN, Ryan W C; 301-3320 Richter St, Kelowna BC V1W 4V5; Man'05; FRCPC; Psy. Staff, Victoria General Hospital; (250)763-1628

MCFEE, Colin D; Misericordia Health Centre, 99 Cornish Ave, Winnipeg MB R3C 1A2; (Other Foreign)'10; CCFP; Staff Misericordia Urgent Care, Misericordia Health Centre; (204)774-6581

MCFEE, Ingrid J; Chinook Centre, B8-6455 MacLeod Trail SW, Calgary AB T2H 0K8; UBC'09; BSc; MSc; CCFP; (403)444-0428; Fax. (403)537-0029.

MCFEELY, Neil H; Brockville Mental Health Ctr, PO Box 1050 Stn Main, Brockville ON K6V 5W7; Dublin (Ireland)'69; MB ChB; DPM; MRCPsy; Staff, Brockville Mental Health Centre - Royal Ottawa Health Care Group; Asst Prof Psy., University of Ottawa; Asst Prof Psy, Queen's University; (613)345-1461 x3103; Fax. (613)345-7276.

MCFETRIDGE, Gerald P; Avery Health Clinic, 31-665 Front St, Quesnel BC V2J 5J5; UBC'87; CCFP; (250)991-8136

MCGARRAGLE, James G; 277 Scarboro Cres, Scarborough ON M1M 2J9; Wes'85; Associate, The Scarborough Hospital - General Campus; (416)261-7212; Fax. (416)261-4812.

MCGARRY, Philip A; Millennium Trail Manor, 6861 Oakwood Dr, Niagara Falls ON L2E 6S5; Wes'78; Ac Staff, Niagara Health System - Greater Niagara General Site; Advisory Phys, Valley Park Lodge & Oakwood Park Lodge; (905)356-5005; Fax. (905)378-2815; pmcgarry6@cogeco.ca.

MCGARRY, Thomas G; Nurse Abernathy Clinic, PO Box 130, Trepassey NL A0A 4B0; Wes'77; (709)438-2828; Fax. (709)438-2264.

MCGARRY, Ursula M; Ottawa Valley Fam Health Team, 95 Spring St, Almonte ON K0A 1A0; McM'90; Staff, Almonte General Hospital; Staff, Kingston General Hospital; Staff, Hotel-Dieu Hospital; Assoc Prof Family Med/Clin Instructor, Queen's University; (613)256-9370; umcgarry@esphosp.on.ca.

MCGARVEY, Kathleen A; 101-283 11th Ave E, Vancouver BC V5T 2C4; UBC'86; BSc; FRCPC; Psy (Community Psychiatry). Staff Psy Emerg, Royal Columbian Hospital; Med Dir Commun Re-entry Program, BC Mental Health & Addiction Service; Clinical Asst Prof Academic, University of British Columbia; (604)675-2390; mcgarvey@interchange.ubc.ca.

MCGAW, W Timothy; Edmonton Clinic, 8D-11400 University Ave NW, Edmonton AB T6G 1Z1; Alb'91; Staff, University of Alberta Hospital; (780)492-5195; Fax. (780)492-7344.

MCGEE, Allison J; 9F-1240 Bay St, Toronto ON M5R 2A7; Tor'92; BSc; CCFP; CCFP(E.M.); FCFP; (416)971-7601; Fax. (416)971-7718.

MCGEE, Jacob D; London HSC-Victoria Hosp, PO Box 5010 Stn B 800 Commissioners Rd E, London ON N6A 5W9; Ott'03; GynOnco; ObstGyn. Staff, London Health Sciences Centre - Victoria Campus; (519)685-8500 x55645

MCGEE, Michel; Societe Ass Automobile du QC, CP 19600 Succ Terminus S2 1-333 boul Jean-Lesage, Quebec QC G1K 8J6; Laval'73; Med Evaluateur, Societe Assurance Automobile du Quebec; (418)528-3958; michel.mcgee@saaq.gouv.qc.ca.

MCGEE, Nancy; CSSS de la Vallée de l'Or, 725 6e rue, Val-d'Or QC J9P 3Y1; Mon'00; CCFP; Staff, Centre Hospitalier de Val d'Or; (819)825-6711

MCGEE, Neil J; Queensway-Carleton Hosp, 3045 Baseline Rd, Nepean ON K2H 8P4; Ott'85; CCFP; FCFP; CCFP(E.M.); Staff, Queensway Carleton Hospital; University of Ottawa; Langs: Bilingual(French/English); (613)721-4710; Fax. (613)721-4703.

MCGEER, Allison J; Mount Sinai Hosp, 210-600 University Ave, Toronto ON M5G 1X5; Tor'82; MSc(Biochem.); BSc(BioChem.); FRCPC; IntMed; InfectDis. Staff Microbiol, Mount Sinai Hospital; Prof Lab Med, University of Toronto; (416)586-4800 x3118; Fax. (416)586-8358; amcgeer@mtsinai.on.ca.

MCGEER, Patrick L; Kinsmen Laboratory, 2255 Wesbrook Mall, Vancouver BC V6T 1Z3; UBC'58; FRSC; FRCPC; MedScient(Med). (604)822-7377

MCGHEE, Donald J; Guelph Family Health Team, 19B-35 Harvard Rd, Guelph ON N1G 3A2; Tor'75; CCFP; FCFP; Court Staff, Guelph General Hospital; (519)837-8137; Fax. (519)822-8240.

MCGHEE, Irene D; Sunnybrook Hlth Sciences Ctre, 2075 Bayview Ave, Toronto ON M4N 3M5; Tor'79; FRCPC; Anes. Ac Staff, Sunnybrook Health Sciences Centre; Asst Prof, University of Toronto; (416)480-4864; Fax. (416)480-6039.

MCGHEE, Rachel A; PO Box 12016 Rpo Parkwood, Prince George BC V2L 0A8; UBC'06; CCFP; (250)552-2341

MCGHIE, John P; BC Cancer Agency-Vanc Isl Ctr, 2410 Lee Ave, Victoria BC V8R 6V5; UBC'05; FRCPC; IntMed; MedOncol. Staff, BC Cancer Agency Vancouver Island Centre; (250)519-5500

MCGIBBON, Angela M; 2F-340 Brunswick St, Fredericton NB E3B 1H1; Dal'98; FRCPC; IntMed (Diabetology); Endocrin&Metab. (506)447-4418; Fax. (506)447-4420.

MCGIBBON, Dianne L C; 207-603 Argus Rd, Oakville ON L6J 6G6; Tor'61; (905)849-8600

MCGIBNEY, Kieron D; Physicians Incorporated, 206-316 Willow St, Truro NS B2N 5A4; Qns'04; FRCSC; GenSurg. (902)893-9211

MCGILL, Sandra N; Dr Sandra McGill, 4459 rue Sherbrooke O, Westmount QC H3Z 1E7; Qns'99; CSPQ; FRCSC; PlasSurg. (514)508-3900; Fax. (514)508-3901.

MCGILLEN, Joseph E M; London Cardiac Institute, 302-256 Pall Mall St, London ON N6A 5P6; Tor'84; FACC; FCCP; FRCPC; IntMed (Cardiology). Staff, London Health Sciences Centre - University Hospital; Staff, Woodstock General Hospital; Staff, London Cardiac Institute; (519)645-0146

MCGILLIVRAY, Barbara C; BC Women's Hosp & Health Ctre, C234-4500 Oak St, Vancouver BC V6H 3N1; Cal'74; FCCMG; FRCPC; Peds; MedGenetics. Staff, BC Women's Hospital & Health Centre; Prof Med Genetics, University of British Columbia; (604)875-2157; Fax. (604)875-2376; bmcgillivray@cw.bc.ca.

MCGILLIVRAY, Cameron J; Thunder Bay Reg HSC-T-Bay, 980 Oliver Rd, Thunder Bay ON P7B 6V4; UBC'04; CCFP; CCFP(E.M.); Staff, Thunder Bay Regional Health Sciences Centre; (807)684-6115

MCGILLIVRAY, Colleen F; Toronto Rehab Inst-Lyndhurst, 520 Sutherland Dr, Toronto ON M4G 3V9; McM'87; FRCPC; PhysMed&Rehab (Spinal Cord Rehabilitation). Staff, Toronto Rehabilitation Institute - Lyndhurst Centre; (416)597-3422 x6133; Fax. (416)422-5402.

MCGILLIVRAY, Daniel L; LL100-720 Guelph Line, Burlington ON L7R 4E2; Cal'88; FRCSC; Ophth (Cornea & Refractive Surgery). Staff, Joseph Brant Memorial Hospital; Staff, Halton Healthcare Services Corporation - Oakville Site; (905)681-6809; Fax. (905)681-6207.

MCGILLIVRAY, James W; Notre Dame Hosp, PO Box 8000 1405 Edward St, Hearst ON P0L 1N0; Tor'53; FACS; FRCSC; GenSurg (Fractures). Staff, Sensenbrenner Hospital; Staff, Temiskaming Hospital; Staff, Hôpital Notre Dame Hospital - Hearst; Langs: Spanish; French; German; (705)362-4291; Fax. (705)372-2923; jwmcgillivray@live.com.

MCGILLIVRAY, Janis L; Burlington Prof Centre, 101-3155 Harvester Rd, Burlington ON L7N 3V2; Qns'81; (905)632-7501; Fax. (905)632-9624.

MCGILLIVRAY, Lee W; Copeman Healthcare Centre, 400-1128 Hornby St, Vancouver BC V6Z 2L4; Sask'81; BSc; CCFP; FCFP; Asst Staff Surg, Alberta Health Services; (604)707-2273

MCGILLIVRAY, Margaret J; Thunder Bay Reg HSC-T-Bay, 980 Oliver Rd, Thunder Bay ON P7B 6V4; UBC'02; CCFP; CCFP(E.M.); Staff, Thunder Bay Regional Health Sciences Centre; (807)684-6000

MCGILLIVRAY, William G; Project Skin MD, 1495 11th Ave W, Vancouver BC V6H 1K9; Sask'82; BSc; (604)732-0800

MCGILVRAY, Ian D; 11C 1250-585 University Ave, Toronto ON M5G 2N2; McG'93; FRCSC; GenSurg. Affil Scientist, Toronto General Hospital - UHN; (416)340-4800 x5230; Fax. (416)340-5242; ian.mcgilvray@uhn.on.ca.

MCGINLEY, Michael D; Niagara HS-St Catharines Gen, 142 Queenston St, St Catharines ON L2R 7C6; Wes'93; FRCPC; DiagRad; NuclearMed. Staff, Niagara Health System - St Catharines General Site; (905)684-7271

MCGINN, Gregory J; Manitoba X-Ray Clinic, 3263 Portage Ave, Winnipeg MB R3K 0W6; Man'84; FRCPC; DiagRad. (204)832-0273

MCGINN, M Joanne; Queen Elizabeth Hosp, PO Box 6600 Stn Central, Charlottetown PE C1A 8T5; Dal'93; Staff, Queen Elizabeth Hospital; (902)894-2111

MCGINN, Peter B; 2449 J-910 10th Ave W, Vancouver BC V5Z 1M9; UBC'72; FRCPC; Anes. Ac Staff, Vancouver General Hospital - Centennial Pavillion; Clinical Asst Prof, University of British Columbia; (604)875-4304

MCGINN, Rebecca; 309-1015 Regent St, Fredericton NB E3B 6H5; Dal'10; CCFP.

MCGINNESS, Clare A; 203-2689 Pandosy St, Kelowna BC V1Y 9V9; Edinburgh (Scotland)'87; MB ChB; DRCOG; MRCGPract; (250)762-9058

MCGINNIS, Randall P C; 1603 20 Ave NW, Calgary AB T2M 1G9; Cal'89; CCFP; FCFP; (403)210-3762; Fax. (403)289-8269.

MCGLYNN, James; Phoenix Med Centre, 402-2155 10th Ave, Prince George BC V2M 5J6; University Coll. (Ireland)'78; DRCOG; MRC; MB BCh; BAO; CCFP; (250)563-8878

MCGOEY, Brian V; Credit Valley Med Arts Centre, 102B-2000 Credit Valley Rd, Mississauga ON L5M 4N4; Tor'82; FRCSC; OrthSurg (General Orthopedics). Staff, The Credit Valley Hospital; (905)820-3416

MCGONIGAL, Donald J; Medical Clinic Bldg, 320-89 Humber College Blvd, Etobicoke ON M9V 4B8; Tor'73; DABOS; BSc; FRCSC; OrthSurg (Joint Replacement). Staff, William Osler Health System - Etobicoke General Hospital; (416)741-3404; Fax. (416)741-7850.

MCGONIGLE, Darcie; Natawihin/Nakasuwenik Clinic, GD, Ile-a-la-Crosse SK S0M 1C0; Sask'06; CCFP; Staff, St Joseph's Hospital; (306)833-2044; Fax. (306)833-2401; dmcgonigle@sasktel.net.

MCGONIGLE, Lyle F; 205-11044 82 Ave NW, Edmonton AB T6G 0T2; Alb'84; FRCPC; Peds. Clinical Asst Prof Peds, University of Alberta Hospital; Staff, University of Alberta; (780)432-0970; Fax. (780)432-1011.

MCGONIGLE, Reid M; Natawihin/Nakasuwenik Clinic, GD, Ile-a-la-Crosse SK S0M 1C0; Sask'06; CCFP; CCFP(E.M.); Staff, St Joseph's Hospital; (306)833-2044; Fax. (306)833-2401; rmcgonigle@sasktel.net.

MCGORMAN, James G; Peterborough Reg HC-Hospital, 1 Hospital Dr, Peterborough ON K9J 7C6; Tor'82; CCFP; CCFP(E.M.); Ac Staff, Peterborough Regional Health Centre - Hospital Drive; (705)743-2121; mcgorman@auracom.com.

MCGORY, Rodney W; Cape Breton Reg Hosp, 1482 George St, Sydney NS B1P 1P3; Mem'02; FRCSC; GenSurg; ThorSurg. Staff, Cape Breton Healthcare Complex; (902)567-6242

MCGOVERAN, Bruce M; Occupational Health Clinic, 4F-30 Bond St, Toronto ON M5B 1W8; Tor'97; FRCPC; OccupMed. Staff, St Michael's Hospital; (416)358-2905

MCGOVERN, Christine H; Foothills Med Centre, AC142-1403 29 St NW, Calgary AB T2N 2T9; Alb'86; FRCPC; PhysMed&Rehab. Staff, Foothills Medical Centre; Assoc Prof, University of Calgary; (403)944-4500; Fax. (403)283-2526.

MCGOVERN, Peter D A; 102-9814 97 St, Grande Prairie AB T8V 8H5; Dublin (Ireland)'73; (780)539-4770; Fax. (780)532-6997.

MCGOWAN, Allister J; Campbellton Reg Hosp, PO Box 880 Stn Main 189 Lily Lake Rd, Campbellton NB E3N 3H3; McG'91; FRCPC; DiagRad. Staff, Hôpital Régional Campbellton; (506)789-5407; Fax. (506)789-5025.

MCGOWAN, Brian J; 203-3825 Sunset St, Burnaby BC V5G 1T4; UBC'79; FRCPC; EmergMed. (604)434-9515; Fax. (604)434-5984.

MCGOWAN, Carolyn; Medcan Health Mgmt Inc, 1500-150 York St, Toronto ON M5H 3S5; Tor'95; BSc; CCFP; Staff, Medcan Health Management Inc; (416)350-5963

MCGOWAN, Hugh D; 408-1100 Sheppard Ave E, North York ON M2K 2W1; Tor'77; FRCS; FRCSC; Ophth (Ocular Oncology). Staff, North York General Hospital; Consultant, Princess Margaret Hospital - University Health Network; Assoc Prof Ophth, University of Toronto; (416)226-2999; Fax. (416)226-5829; hugh.mcgowan@uhn.on.ca.

MCGOWAN, Liam; Queen Elizabeth II Hosp, 10409 98 St, Grande Prairie AB T8V 2E8; Dal'88; FRCPC; Anes. Staff, Queen Elizabeth II Hospital; (780)538-7460

MCGOWAN, M Daniel; Foothills Med Centre, AC142-1403 29 St NW, Calgary AB T2N 2T9; Mem'85; FRCPC; PhysMed&Rehab (Amputee Rehabilitation). Staff Spinal Cord Injury Rehab. Prog., Foothills Medical Centre; Clin Assoc Prof, University of Calgary; (403)944-4224; Fax. (403)283-2526.

MCGOWAN, Thomas S; The Credit Valley Hosp, 4F-2200 Eglinton Ave W, Mississauga ON L5M 2N1; Qns'85; MBA; FRCPC; RadOncol. Staff, The Credit Valley Hospital; Staff, Princess Margaret Hospital - University Health Network; University of Toronto; (905)813-1100

MCGRAIL, J Simon; Montebello Medical, 249 Waverley Rd, Dartmouth NS B2X 2C5; Manchester (England)'55; MB ChB; DLO; MS; FRCSC; Otol (Facial Cosmetic). (902)406-4444; Fax. (902)406-4447.

MCGRATH, Colm R; 104-389 Connell St, Woodstock NB E7M 5G5; Cal'93; CCFP; Staff, Upper River Valley Hospital - Waterville; colm@nb.sympatico.ca.

MCGRATH, Fiona M M; St Mary's Univ Student HC, 431-923 Robie St, Halifax NS B3H 3C3; Dal'95; CCFP.

MCGRATH, Frances C; 102-8035 120 St, Delta BC V4C 6P8; McG'76; CCFP; FCFP; Staff, Surrey Memorial Hospital; (604)596-2263; Fax. (604)596-4263.

MCGRATH, Jerry S; Health Sciences Centre, 300 Prince Philip Dr, St. John's NL A1B 3V6; Mem'99; BSc; FRCPC; IntMed (Inflammatory Bowel Disease); Gastroent. Staff, Health Sciences Centre; Asst Prof Med, Memorial University Of Newfoundland; (709)777-6200; Fax. (709)777-7054; jmcgrath@mun.ca.

MCGRATH, Michael M J; Kingston Gen Hosp, V4-76 Stuart St, Kingston ON K7L 2V7; Qns'70; FACOG; FRCSC; ObstGyn (Maternal Fetal Medicine)., Kingston General Hospital; Att Staff, Hotel-Dieu Hospital; Dept Head ObstGyn, Queen's University; (613)548-6072; michael.mcgrath@queensu.ca.

MCGRATH, Sheilagh M; Primary Med Centre, 150 Old Placentia Rd, Mount Pearl NL A1N 4Y9; Mem'87; Staff, St Clare's Mercy Hospital.

MCGRAW, Elizabeth A; CSSS de Sorel-Tracy, 400 av de l'Hotel-Dieu, Sorel-Tracy QC J3P 1N5; Mon'80; Staff, Hôtel-Dieu de Sorel; Langs: Bilingual(French/English); (450)746-6062; emcgraw@emcgraw.com.

MCGRAW, Marie-Josee; The Moncton Hosp, 135 MacBeath Ave, Moncton NB E1C 6Z8; Laval'94; LMCC; CCFP; CCFP(E.M.); Staff, The Moncton Hospital; (506)859-5111

MCGRAW, Robert C; Kingston Gen Hosp, 76 Stuart St, Kingston ON K7L 2V7; UBC'88; FRCPC; EmergMed. Staff EmergMed, Kingston General Hospital; (613)549-6666 x3539; Fax. (613)548-2420.

MCGRAW, Robert W; 4-1864 1st Ave W, Vancouver BC V6J 1G5; UBC'60; DABOS; FRCSC; OrthSurg (Hips Surgery). Hon Staff, Vancouver General Hospital - Centennial Pavillion; Emeritus Prof, University of British Columbia; (604)731-1019

MCGRAW, Serge; 3526 rue Principale PO Box 3634 Stn Main, Tracadie-Sheila NB E1X 1G5; Sher'06; CCFP.

MCGREGOR, Alexander P; St Joseph's Health Centre, 30 The Queensway, Toronto ON M6R 1B5; St. Andrews (Scotland)'68; MB ChB; FFARCS; FRCPC; Anes. Ac Staff, St Joseph's Health Centre; (416)530-6000 x6090; Fax. (416)530-6093.

MCGREGOR, Caitlin T; Sunnybrook Hlth Sciences Ctre, MG130A-2075 Bayview Ave, Toronto ON M4N 3M5; Tor'96; BSc; FRCPC; DiagRad (Abdominal Imaging). Staff Radiol, Sunnybrook Health Sciences Centre; (416)480-4353; Fax. (416)480-5855; c.mcgregor@utoronto.ca.

MCGREGOR, Clare; West Lambton Community H C, 100-429 Exmouth St, Sarnia ON N7T 5P1; McM'03; CCFP; (519)344-3017; Fax. (519)344-6436.

MCGREGOR, David B; South Muskoka Mem Hosp, 75 Ann St, Bracebridge ON P1L 2E4; Wes'89; Staff, South Muskoka Memorial Hospital - Muskoka Algonquin Healthcare; (705)654-4404

MCGREGOR, Douglas M; Royal Jubilee Hosp, 3F-1952 Bay St, Victoria BC V8R 1J8; Glasgow (Scotland)'78; MB ChB; MRCP; MRCGPract; FRCP; Staff, Royal Jubilee Hospital; Langs: English; French; (250)370-8625

MCGREGOR, Fiona; Vernon Mental Health Centre, 1440 14 Ave, Vernon BC V1B 2T1; Dundee (Scotland)'78; MB ChB; MRCPsy(UK); FRCPC; Psy. Staff Psy, Vernon Mental Health Centre; (250)549-5737; Fax. (250)549-6358.

MCGREGOR, Gregor; Kildonan Med Centre, 2300 McPhillips St, Winnipeg MB R2V 3M3; St George's (Grenada)'06; CCFP; (204)632-3203

MCGREGOR, Gregor I; 5F-2775 Laurel St, Vancouver BC V5Z 1M9; Wes'71; FRCSC; GenSurg. Ac Staff, Vancouver General Hospital - Centennial Pavillion; (604)875-5770; Fax. (604)875-4315.

MCGREGOR, Jyoti M; Manitoba Clinic, 790 Sherbrook St, Winnipeg MB R3A 1M3.

MCGREGOR, Margaret; Mid-Main Comm Health Centre, 3998 Main St, Vancouver BC V5V 3P2; UBC'89; CCFP; (604)873-3666; Fax. (604)875-8790.

MCGREGOR, Penelope K; 28 St John St PO Box 70, Merrickville ON K0G 1N0; Ott'00; CCFP; Staff Locum, Kemptville District Hospital; Ac Staff, Perth & Smiths Falls District Hospital - Smiths Falls Site; (613)269-2970; Fax. (613)269-4194.

MCGREGOR, Robert D; PO Box 2000 Stn Main, Winkler MB R6W 1H8; Man'79; FRCPC; DiagRad (CT/X-Ray & Ultrasound). Staff, Boundary Trails Health Centre; Staff, St Boniface General Hospital; Staff, The Salvation Army Grace Hospital; University of Manitoba; (204)331-8811; rmcgreg4@yahoo.com.

MCGREGOR, Sumathi; 301-3001 Tutt St, Kelowna BC V1Y 2H4; Man'89; FACOG; FRCSC; ObstGyn. Ac Staff, Kelowna General Hospital; (250)762-0188

MCGREGOR, Thomas B; St Boniface Gen Hosp, Z3032-409 Tache Ave, Winnipeg MB R2H 2A6; Ott'04; FRCSC; Urol. Staff, St Boniface General Hospital; (204)233-8563

MCGREGOR-SHAW, Alyson M; Children's Hosp Eastern Ont, 401 Smyth Rd, Ottawa ON K1H 8L1; Dal'98; FRCPC; Peds. Staff, Children's Hospital of Eastern Ontario (CHEO); Asst Prof, University of Ottawa; Langs: French; (613)737-7600

MCGROGAN, Jonathan; Lions Gate Hosp, 231 15th St E, North Vancouver BC V7L 2L7; Qns'99; CCFP; CCFP(E.M.); Staff, Lions Gate Hospital; (604)984-5982

MCGUGAN, John A; Quinte Med Centre, 265 Dundas St E, Belleville ON K8N 5A9; Qns'93; FRCPC; Anes;CCFP; Staff, QHC Belleville General; Physician, Quinte Health Care; (613)969-7400

MCGUIRE, Abigail; The Ottawa Hosp-Gen Campus, 501 Smyth Rd, Ottawa ON K1H 8L6; Dal'10; CCFP; Staff, The Ottawa Hospital - General Campus; (613)798-5555

MCGUIRE, Caterina; Marpole Medical Clinic, 8675 Granville St, Vancouver BC V6P 5A3; UBC'98; MSc; BSc; CCFP; Langs: Italian; (604)263-2646; Fax. (604)263-2649.

MCGUIRE, Claudie; CSSS de Saint-Jerome, 290 rue de Montigny, Saint-Jerome QC J7Z 5T3; Mon'07; Neur. Staff, Hôtel-Dieu de Saint-Jérôme; (450)432-2777

MCGUIRE, Glenn P; Univ Hlth Network-Toronto Western Hosp, 399 Bathurst St, Toronto ON M5T 2S8; Dal'83; FRCPC; Anes (Critical Care Medicine). Staff, Toronto Western Hospital - University Health Network; Asst Prof, University of Toronto; (416)603-5118; Fax. (416)603-6494.

MCGUIRE, Jennifer J; PO Box 1331, Bragg Creek AB T0L 0K0; Cal'02; MSc; BSc; CCFP; Staff, South Calgary Urgent Care Centre; (403)949-4008

MCGUIRE, Kwesi C; Clarity Eye Institute, 105-880 Dufferin St, Vaughan ON L4K 0C5; West Indies (Other Foreign)'03; Ophth. (416)663-3937

MCGUIRE, Michael I; BC Cancer Agency, 2410 Lee Ave, Victoria BC V8R 6V5; UBC'82; Staff, BC Cancer Agency Vancouver Island Centre; (250)519-5520

MCGUIRE, Paul B; PO Box 160, Kingston NS B0P 1R0; Dal'74; (902)765-4044; Fax. (902)765-6668.

MCGUIRE, R Philip; Georgian Bay Gen Hosp-Midland, PO Box 760 Stn Main 1112 St Andrew's Dr, Midland ON L4R 4P4; Qns'85; CCFP; CCFP(E.M.); FCFP; Staff Emerg Med, Georgian Bay General Hospital - Midland; Langs: French; (705)526-1300 x1501; Fax. (705)526-3448; rpmcguire61@hotmail.com.

MCGUIRE, Shaun N; The Ottawa Hosp-Riverside, 1967 Riverside Dr, Ottawa ON K1H 7W9; Ott'87; CCFP; FCFP; Staff Family Med, The Ottawa Hospital - General Campus; Staff, The Ottawa Hospital - Riverside Campus; (613)738-8219; Fax. (613)738-8217.

MCHARDY, Paul G; Sunnybrook Hlth Sciences Ctre, M3200-2075 Bayview Ave, Toronto ON M4N 3M5; UBC'02; FRCPC; Anes. Staff, Sunnybrook Health Sciences Centre; (416)480-4864; Fax. (416)480-6039.

MCHATTIE, James D; Regina Internal Med Specialist, 1821 Rose St, Regina SK S4P 1Z7; Sask'67; FRCPC; IntMed; Gastroent. Clin Prof Med, University of Saskatchewan; Dir, Gastro Intestinal Investigation Unit; (306)522-6334; Fax. (306)359-1068.

MCHUGH, Sean M; Nanaimo Reg Gen Hosp, 1200 Dufferin Cres, Nanaimo BC V9S 2B7; McM'75; BSc; MBA; FRCPC; IntMed; Psy. Staff, Nanaimo Regional General Hospital; Co-Mgr, Nanaimo Commun Addictions & Mental Health Trmnt Team; (250)716-7791

MCILHARGEY, Trina L; Richmond Road Diag & Trmt Ctr, 1891-1820 Richmond Rd SW, Calgary AB T2T 5C7; UBC'07; FRCPC; IntMed; Endocrin&Metab. (403)955-8342

MCILQUHAM, W Ross; Maple Family Health Team, 71 Clergy St E, Kingston ON K7L 3J3; Qns'79; CCFP; FCFP; Assoc Staff, Kingston General Hospital; Assoc Staff, Hotel-Dieu Hospital; Physician, Invista of Canada & Kingston Works; Teach Staff, Queen's University; (613)542-7858; Fax. (613)544-9795.

MCILRAITH, Duncan M; Montfort Hosp, 713 Montreal Rd, Ottawa ON K1K 0T2; Ott'81; BSc; FRCPC; Neur. Staff, Montfort Hospital; Staff, Queensway Carleton Hospital; (613)746-4621; Fax. (613)748-4914.

MCILRAITH, Ian P; St Joseph's Health Care, PO Box 5777 Stn B 268 Grosvenor St, London ON N6A 4V2; Wes'00; FRCSC; Ophth (Glaucoma). Staff, St Joseph's Hospital - St Joseph's Health Care; (519)646-6208

MCILRATH, H Ruth; 702-1228 Marinaside Cres, Vancouver BC V6Z 2W4; Belfast (Ireland)'77; (604)263-2645

MCILREATH, Sean A; Quinte HC Corp-Belleville Gen, 359-265 Dundas St E, Belleville ON K8N 5A9; Alb'96; FRCSC; GenSurg (Gastroenterology). Staff, QHC Trenton Memorial; Staff, QHC Belleville General; Staff, QHC Prince Edward County Memorial; (613)961-0817; Fax. (613)961-0903.

MCILWAINE, Margaret C; Anchor Medical Clinic, 1450 Waddington Rd, Nanaimo BC V9S 4V9; UBC'86; (250)754-5545; Fax. (250)754-5954.

MCILWRICK, Joann G; 827-10 Discovery Ridge Hills S, Calgary AB T3H 5X2; Sask'98; BSc(Hon); MSc; FRCPC; Psy (Early Psychosis). Psychiatrist, Foothills Medical Centre; Fellow Psy/Asst Prof Med, University of Calgary; (403)452-6272; Fax. (403)452-6242; joann.mcilwrick@albertahealthservices.ca.

MCINNES, Craig M; 302-205 Dundas St E, Belleville ON K8N 5K6; Qns'88; FRCPC; PhysMed&Rehab. (613)967-4399; Fax. (613)967-8321.

MCINNES, J Gordon; Kelowna Gen Hosp, 2268 Pandosy Dr, Kelowna BC V1Y 1T2; UBC'97; FRCPC; EmergMed. Staff Emerg, Kelowna General Hospital; (250)862-4495

MCINNIS, James E R; 6-587 River Rd W, Hamilton ON L9A 2P2; Dal'04; CCFP; (705)422-0540; Fax. (705)422-0541.

MCINNIS, Joseph B; Eagle Ridge Hosp & Health C C, C2B-475 Guildford Way, Port Moody BC V3H 3W9; UBC'66; Staff, Eagle Ridge Hospital & Health Care Centre; Staff, Royal Columbian Hospital; (604)469-3185; Fax. (604)461-9972.

MCINROY, Gordon; Students Union Bldg, 2 200-66 University Campus NW, Edmonton AB T6G 2J7; Glasgow (Scotland)'68; MB ChB; DRCOG; Physician, University of Alberta; (780)492-2612; Fax. (780)492-0172; gordon.mcinroy@ualberta.ca.

MCINTOSH, Christopher A; Toronto East Gen Hosp Inc, 825 Coxwell Ave, Toronto ON M4C 3E7; Tor'01; BSc; MSc; Psy. Staff Psy, Toronto East General Hospital Inc; Staff Psy, Mount Sinai Hospital; (416)469-6580; Fax. (416)469-6805; cmcin@tegh.on.ca.

MCINTOSH, Diane M; 400-1128 Hornby St, Vancouver BC V6Z 2L4; Dal'93; BSc; FRCPC; Psy (Anxiety Disorder). Assoc Staff PTSD Clinic, Vancouver General Hospital - Centennial Pavillion; Clinical Asst Prof, University of British Columbia; (778)846-6381; drmcintosh@shaw.ca.

MCINTOSH, Donald B; Associated Radiologists, 300-140 Wall St, Saskatoon SK S7K 1N4; Sask'79; DABR; FRCPC; DiagRad. Ac Staff, Saskatoon City Hospital; Ac Staff, St Paul's Hospital (Grey Nuns) of Saskatoon; Clinical Asst Prof Med Imaging, University of Saskatchewan; (306)244-1167; Fax. (306)244-2911.

MCINTOSH, Douglas C; Hillsdale Estates, 590 Oshawa Blvd N, Oshawa ON L1G 5T9; Tor'75; CCFP; Staff, Lakeridge Health - Oshawa Site; (905)579-1777; Fax. (905)579-6243; doug.mcintosh@durham.ca.

MCINTOSH, Evan M; Mount Sinai Hosp, 206-600 University Ave, Toronto ON M5G 1X5; Tor'99; CCFP; CCFP(E.M.); Staff, Mount Sinai Hospital; (416)586-5058; Fax. (416)586-4719.

MCINTOSH, Frederick E A; King Dufferin Family Med Ctre, 5-1209 King St W, Toronto ON M6K 1G2; West Indies (Jamaica)'65; MB BS; FRCSC; Otol. Staff, Humber River Regional Hospital - Finch Avenue Site; Staff, Humber River Regional Hospital - Church Street Site; Staff, William Osler Health System - Etobicoke General Hospital; (416)536-2500; Fax. (416)532-7006.

MCINTOSH, Garfield G G; 406-2299 Dundas St W, Toronto ON M6R 1X7; Tor'80; (416)535-3511

MCINTOSH, Glenda J; Whitby Clinic, 200 Brock St N, Whitby ON L1N 4H5; Tor'76; BSc; CCFP; FCFP; (905)668-3378; Fax. (905)668-3807.

MCINTOSH, Jan K; 104-3040 Tutt St, Kelowna BC V1Y 2H5; Alb'73; CCFP; FCFP; Kelowna General Hospital; (250)763-6922; Fax. (250)763-6956; janmcintosh@shaw.ca.

MCINTOSH, Karen L; The Medical Centre, 607-1081 Carling Ave, Ottawa ON K1Y 4G2; Tor'78; CCFP; FCFP; (613)725-3237; Fax. (613)725-3237; kmcintosh@bellnet.ca.

MCINTOSH, Keith S; London HSC-Victoria Hosp, PO Box 5010 Stn B E1 317-800 Commissioners Rd E, London ON N6A 5W9; Tor'07; Gastroent; IntMed. Staff, London Health Sciences Centre - Victoria Campus; (519)685-8500

MCINTOSH, Kimberley A; Couchiching Family Health Team, 204-119 Memorial Ave, Orillia ON L3V 5X1; McM'99; CCFP; (705)323-9800; Fax. (705)323-9601.

MCINTOSH, Leslie A; Misericordia Health Centre, 99 Cornish Ave, Winnipeg MB R3C 1A2; Man'96; CCFP; FCFP; Staff, Misericordia Health Centre; (204)788-8364

MCINTOSH, Mary G; PO Box 428, Heriot Bay BC V0P 1H0; London (England)'63; MB BS; FRCPC; Psy (General Adult Psychiatry). (250)285-3133; Fax. (250)285-3122. Semi-Retired.

MCINTOSH, Robert E; 432 Ellis St, Penticton BC V2A 4M2; Alb'77; Assoc Staff, Penticton Regional Hospital; (250)493-3521; Fax. (250)492-2299.

MCINTOSH, Sandra L; South East Grey Community HC, PO Box 360 55 Victoria St, Markdale ON N0C 1H0; Alb'83; (519)986-2222; Fax. (519)986-3999.

MCINTOSH, Scott L A; Elmwood Family Health Centre, 3-204 First Ave, St Thomas ON N5R 4P5; Wes'07; CCFP; (519)631-3223; Fax. (519)286-0390.

MCINTOSH, Shiona M; Dr Everett Chalmers Reg Hosp, PO Box 9000 Stn A, Fredericton NB E3B 5N5; Mem'91; CCFP; FCFP; Staff, Dr Everett Chalmers Regional Hospital; (506)447-4444; Fax. (506)447-4221; dr.shiona.mcintosh@horizonb.ca.

MCINTYRE, Alexander W; Dr Alexander McIntyre Inc, 575 Ellis St, Penticton BC V2A 4M4; Pretoria (South Africa)'79; MMed(Psych); MB ChB; FRCPC; Psy. Staff Psy, Penticton Regional Hospital; (250)492-0053; Fax. (250)492-0020.

MCINTYRE, Allan J; The Landings Surg Ctr Anes, 7A-1477 Lower Water St, Halifax NS B3J 3Z2; Dal'76; FRCPC; Anes.

MCINTYRE, Brian G; Alberta Children's Hosp, 2888 Shaganappi Trail NW, Calgary AB T3B 6A8; Tor'82; DA; FRCPC; Anes (Pediatric Anesthesia). Staff, Alberta Children's Hospital; (403)955-7810; Fax. (403)955-7606.

MCINTYRE, Caroline M; Vancouver Gen Hosp, 855 12th Ave W, Vancouver BC V5Z 1M9; Ott'92; FRCPC; EmergMed. Staff Emerg, Vancouver General Hospital - Centennial Pavillion; (604)875-4700; Fax. (604)875-4872.

MCINTYRE, Grant; Abbotsford Reg Hosp & Cancer C, 32900 Marshall Rd, Abbotsford BC V2S 0C2; Cal'06; Critical Care Medicine; IntMed. Staff, Abbotsford Regional Hospital & Cancer Centre; (604)851-4700

MCINTYRE, Ian L; Chancellor Medical, 820 9th St, Brandon MB R7A 4B8; Man'87; FRCPC; Psy. (204)571-6876; Fax. (204)728-1987.

MCINTYRE, Ian W; Harry Medovy House, 2F-671 William Ave, Winnipeg MB R3E 0Z2; Man'06; FRCPC; Anes.

MCINTYRE, James A; Associate Med Group, 4705 48 Ave, Red Deer AB T4N 3T1; Sask'79; CCFP; FCFP; Physician, Associate Medical Group; (403)346-2057; Fax. (403)347-2989.

MCINTYRE, Julie J; 302-1835 Yonge St, Toronto ON M4S 1X8; Qns'81; CCFP; FCFP; Court Staff Newborn Nursery Priv, Women's College Hospital; Court Staff Newborn Nursery Priv, Mount Sinai Hospital; Lecturer Med, University of Toronto; (416)481-5453; Fax. (416)481-6949.

MCINTYRE, Karen L; Somenos Med Clinic, A-921 Canada Ave, Duncan BC V9L 1V2; UBC'99; CCFP; (250)709-9090; Fax. (250)709-9099.

MCINTYRE, Katherine V; Nelson Med Clinic, 806 Vernon St, Nelson BC V1L 4G5; Cal'10; CCFP; (250)352-6611

MCINTYRE, Keith R; Park Royal Plaza, 2425 Truscott Dr, Mississauga ON L5J 2B4; London (England)'70; MB BS; LRCP; MRCS; MRCP(UK); Ac Staff, Trillium Health Centre - Mississauga; (905)823-5020; Fax. (905)823-3443.

MCINTYRE, Kieran P D; 1011-123 Edward St, Toronto ON M5G 1E2; Wes'03; FRCPC; IntMed; Respir. (416)813-2277

MCINTYRE, L Lynn; TRW Bldg, 3E14-3280 Hospital Dr NW, Calgary AB T2N 4Z6; Tor'80; MHSc; FRCPC; CommunMed; Public Health & Preventive Med. Prof Commun Health Sciences, University of Calgary; Langs: Spanish; French; (403)220-8664; lmcintyr@ucalgary.ca.

MCINTYRE, Lauralyn A; The Ottawa Hosp-Gen Campus, 501 Smyth Rd Box 201, Ottawa ON K1H 8L6; McM'96; FRCPC; IntMed; Critical Care Medicine. Assoc Scientist, The Ottawa Hospital - General Campus; (613)737-8899 x73231; Fax. (613)739-6266.

MCINTYRE, Martin T J; 159 Brant Ave, Brantford ON N3T 3H6; Cork (Ireland)'70; MB ChB; BAO; FRCPC; Peds. Staff, The Brant Community Healthcare System - Brantford General Hospital Site; (519)756-1100; Fax. (519)756-1101.

MCINTYRE, Mary E; 128-75 Richmond St, Chatham ON N7M 1N8; McM'84; Langs: French; Spanish; (519)401-1699

MCINTYRE, Paul F; Queen Elizabeth II HSC, 307-1276 South Park St, Halifax NS B3H 2Y9; Ott'76; CCFP; FCFP; Staff, Queen Elizabeth II Health Sciences Centre - Victoria General Site; (902)473-4356; Fax. (902)473-6602.

MCINTYRE, R Alan; 109 Centre St S, Whitby ON L1N 4V6; Wes'81; FACOG; FRCSC; ObstGyn. Staff, Rouge Valley Health System - Ajax & Pickering Health Centre Site; (905)665-6886; Fax. (905)665-6355; dealan@bell.net.

MCINTYRE, Rebecca E; Alberta Children's Hosp, 2888 Shaganappi Trail NW, Calgary AB T3B 6A8; (Australia)'00; Staff Ped Anes, Alberta Children's Hospital; (403)955-7810; Fax. (403)955-7606.

MCINTYRE, Roger S; Univ Hlth Network-Toronto Western Hosp, MP9 325-399 Bathurst St, Toronto ON M5T 2S8; Dal'93; FRCPC; Psy (Pharmacology). Head Mood Disorders & Psychopharmacolgy Unit, Toronto Western Hospital - University Health Network; Assoc Prof Psy, University of Toronto; (416)603-5800 x6508; Fax. (416)603-5368.

MCINTYRE, Sigmund O; LAMP Community Health Centre, 185 Fifth St, Etobicoke ON M8V 2Z5; Ross University (USA)'00; AAFPhys; CCFP; (416)252-6475; Fax. (416)252-6395.

MCINTYRE-STEWART, Sarah M; St Joseph's Health Centre, 30 The Queensway, Toronto ON M6R 1B5; McM'09; Staff, St Joseph's Health Centre; (416)530-6000

MCISAAC, Gary P; King Street Med Arts Centre, 400-71 King St W, Mississauga ON L5B 4A2; Dublin (Ireland)'80; FRCSC; Urol. Consultant, Trillium Health Centre - Mississauga; Court Staff/Chief Surgical Health Care System, Trillium Health Centre - West Toronto; Court Staff, Halton Healthcare Services Corporation - Oakville Site; (905)896-3547; Fax. (905)272-0647.

MCISAAC, J Craig; Dr H Bliss Murphy Cancer Ctr, 300 Prince Philip Dr, St. John's NL A1B 3V6; (Ireland)'91; MB ChB; Staff, Dr H Bliss Murphy Cancer Centre; Staff, St Clare's Mercy Hospital; (709)777-7602

MCISAAC, J Hugh; Cleopatra LaserMed Clinic, 116-152 Cleopatra Dr, Nepean ON K2G 5X2; Ott'76; CCFP; Att Staff, The Ottawa Hospital - Civic Campus; (613)236-8182; Fax. (613)236-8154.

MCISAAC, Matthew C; Saskatoon Orth & Sports Med Ct, 104-311 Ludlow St, Saskatoon SK S7S 1N6; Sask'08; BSc(Hon); CCFP; (306)975-9889

MCISAAC, Warren J; Granovsky Gluskin Fam Med Ctre, PO Box 25 4F-60 Murray St, Toronto ON M5T 3L9; Wes'83; MSc; CCFP; Staff, Mount Sinai Hospital; Prin Investigator Cystitis Study, Canadian Institute of Health Research; Assoc Prof, University of Toronto; (416)586-3190; Fax. (416)586-3175; warren.mcisaac@usherbrooke.ca.

MCIVER, Colin H; Grey Bruce HS-Owen Sound, PO Box 1800 Stn Main 1800 8th St E, Owen Sound ON N4K 6M9; Qns'79; BSc; FRCPC; DiagRad. Staff, Grey Bruce Health Services - Owen Sound; (519)376-2121 x2283; Fax. (519)372-3954; cmciver@ghhs.on.ca.

MCIVER, D Keith; Penticton Reg Hosp, 101-550 Carmi Ave, Penticton BC V2A 3G6; Man'66; FRCSC; GenSurg (Endoscopy). Ac Staff, Penticton Regional Hospital; Consultant Surg, South Okanagan General Hospital; (250)493-0134; Fax. (250)493-9166; mciverk@shaw.ca.

MCIVER, Donald J L; RR 1, Ailsa Craig ON N0M 1A0; Otago (New Zealand)'73; (519)671-7711

MCIVER, Glen R; F W Green Med Centre, 1629 Baker St, Cranbrook BC V1C 1B4; Man'67; BScPharm; (250)426-6601

MCIVER, Ian Garth; 200-520 6th Ave W, Vancouver BC V5Z 4H5; Man'73; BSc; ASAM; Staff, Vancouver Coastal Health; (604)714-3753

MCIVER, Kevin R; F W Green Med Centre, 1629 Baker St, Cranbrook BC V1C 1B4; Alb'97; CCFP; FCFP; (250)426-6601; Fax. (250)426-6470; drkevinmciver@shaw.ca.

MCIVOR, Graeme W D; 117 Slimmon Rd, Saskatoon SK S7V 0B8; Sask'69; FRCSC; OrthSurg. Asst Surg, St Paul's Hospital (Grey Nuns) of Saskatoon; Asst Surg, Saskatoon City Hospital; (306)244-1247; Fax. (306)934-3330.

MCIVOR, John B; 123-11910 111 Ave NW, Edmonton AB T5G 0E5; Alb'77; FRCSC; OrthSurg (Pediatric Orthopedics). Ac Staff, University of Alberta Hospital; Clin Assoc Prof, University of Alberta; (780)453-8985; Fax. (780)447-4537.

MCIVOR, R Andrew; St Joseph's Healthcare, T2127-50 Charlton Ave E, Hamilton ON L8N 4A6; Queen's (Ireland)'84; MB ChB; BAO(Hons); DRCOG; MRC(UK); DCH; FRCPC; IntMed (Clinical Epidemiology); Respir. Staff Firestone Inst for Resp Health, St Joseph's Healthcare - Charlton Campus; Prof Medicine, McMaster University; (905)522-1155 x4330; Fax. (905)521-6183; amclvor@stjosham.on.ca.

MCKAGUE, Jeffrey; Sturgeon Community Hosp, 201 Boudreau Rd, St. Albert AB T8N 6C4; Alb'90; Staff, Sturgeon Community Hospital; (780)418-8229

MCKAGUE, Meredith; West Winds Primary Health Ctr, 3311 Fairlight Dr, Saskatoon SK S7M 3Y5; Sask'94; MSc; CCFP; FCFP; Staff, Royal University Hospital; Staff, Saskatoon City Hospital; Staff, St Paul's Hospital (Grey Nuns) of Saskatoon; Asst Prof, University of Saskatchewan; (306)655-4200; Fax. (306)655-4894.

MCKAIGNEY, Eimear P; East Edmonton Health Centre, 2F-7910 112 Ave NW, Edmonton AB T5B 0C2; (Ireland)'74; MB ChB; BAO; DPH; DRCOG; FRCPC; Psy. Asst Prof, University of Alberta; (780)342-4908

MCKAIGNEY, John P; Zeidler Ledcor Centre, 130 University Campus NW, Edmonton AB T6G 2X8; National (Ireland)'74; MB ChB; BAO; MRC(UK); DPH; FRCPC; IntMed; Gastroent. Staff Gastroent., University of Alberta Hospital; Clin Assoc Prof Med, University of Alberta; (780)492-8151; john.mckaigney@ualberta.ca.

MCKAY, A Robert; Medical Centre, 1428 Ouellette Ave, Windsor ON N8X 1K4; Wes'59; FRCSC; GenSurg. Court Staff, Hôtel-Dieu Grace Hospital; Hon Staff, Windsor Regional Hospital - Metropolitan Site; (519)252-8387; Fax. (519)252-8389.

MCKAY, Douglas R; Hotel-Dieu Hosp, B3 031-166 Brock St, Kingston ON K7L 5G2; Tor'02; FRCSC; PlasSurg (Cranio Facial Surgery). Staff, Hotel-Dieu Hospital; Asst Prof, Queen's University; (613)544-3400

MCKAY, James S; Northeastern Travel Clinic, B1-2009 Long Lake Rd, Sudbury ON P3E 6C3; Qns'89; CCFP; (705)586-3601; Fax. (705)586-3602.

MCKAY, Janet E; West Edge Med Clinic, 5-1634 Hyde Park Rd, London ON N6H 5L7; Wes'88; CCFP; CCFP(E.M.); FCFP; Associate, London Health Sciences Centre - Victoria Campus; (519)472-7795; Fax. (519)472-7816.

MCKAY, Laura-Lea M; Nackawic Med Clinic, 222-135 Otis Dr, Nackawic NB E6G 1H1; Dal'98; BSc; CCFP; FCFP; (506)575-8471; dr.laura-lea.mckay@horizonnb.ca.

MCKAY, M Andrew; Health Sciences Centre, GF 441-820 Sherbrook St, Winnipeg MB R3A 1R9; Man'99; BSc; MSc; FRCSC; GenSurg (Surgical Oncology). Staff General Surgeon, Health Sciences Centre; Asst Prof Surg, University of Manitoba; (204)787-1127; Fax. (204)787-4851.

MCKAY, Monica; Child Development Centre, 690 2nd Ave N, Williams Lake BC V2G 4C4; Witwatersrand (South Africa)'91; Langs: Dutch; Afrikaans; (250)392-4481

MCKAY, Rhonda J; St Paul's Hosp, 1081 Burrard St, Vancouver BC V6Z 1Y6; Sask'93; FRCPC; IntMed. Staff Eating Disorders Prog, Providence Health Care - St Paul's Hospital; (604)682-2344 x62595; Fax. (604)806-8631; jmckay@providencehealth.bc.ca.

MCKAY, Robert G R; South Windsor Med Centre, 2-3840 Howard Ave, Windsor ON N9E 3N9; Wes'84; CCFP; Staff, Hôtel-Dieu Grace Hospital; Staff, Windsor Regional Hospital - Tayfour Site; (519)969-3744

MCKAY, Roberta M; 2326 College Ave, Regina SK S4P 1C7; Sask'81; BScN; BAP(Hons.); FRCPC; Derm. Ac Staff, Regina General Hospital; Clin Prof, University of Saskatchewan; (306)546-4900; Fax. (306)546-4901.

MCKAY, Scott D; Byron Family Med Centre, 1228 Commissioners Rd W, London ON N6K 1C7; Wes'02; BSc; CCFP; Asst Prof, University of Western Ontario; (519)472-9670

MCKAY, Suzanne J; 33 Casey St PO Box 760, Barrys Bay ON K0J 1B0; Ott'85; FRCPC; Psy. Staff, Royal Ottawa Mental Health Centre - Royal Ottawa Health Care Group.

MCKAY, Timothy D; Dr Hugh Twomey Health Care Ctr, PO Box 250 25 Twomey Dr, Botwood NL A0H 1E0; (Other Foreign)'10; CCFP; Staff, Dr Hugh Twomey Health Care Centre.

MCKAY, Ross; 102-777 Blanshard St, Victoria BC V8W 2G9; UBC'78; Staff, Royal Jubilee Hospital; Staff, Victoria General Hospital; (250)388-5579; Fax. (250)388-5575.

MCKAY, William P S; Royal University Hosp, RUH-103 Hospital Dr, Saskatoon SK S7N 0W8; Tor'68; MCPS; BScAg; FRCPC; Anes. Staff Anes, Royal University Hospital; Prof, University of Saskatchewan; (306)655-1202; Fax. (306)655-1279; bill.mckay@usask.ca.

MCKEAN, John D S; University of Alberta Hosp, 2D102WCM-8440 112 St NW, Edmonton AB T6G 2B7; Otago (New Zealand)'70; MB ChB; DAB; FACS; FRCSC; Neursurg. Ac Staff, University of Alberta Hospital; Ac Staff, Royal Alexandra Hospital; Assoc Prof, University of Alberta; (780)407-6869; Fax. (780)407-8203.

MCKECHNIE, Catherine M; 6-701 Rossland Rd E, Whitby ON L1N 8Y9; Tor'07; CCFP; Staff, The Scarborough Hospital - General Campus; (905)493-3447; Fax. (905)493-4303.

MCKECHNIE, Kevin A; Nelson Med Clinic, 806 Vernon St, Nelson BC V1L 4G5; UBC'05; CCFP; (250)352-6611

MCKECHNIE, Kyle S; Sudbury Reg Hosp-Laurentian Si, 41 Ramsey Lake Rd, Sudbury ON P3E 5J1; Qns'04; Critical Care Medicine; Anes. Staff, Health Sciences North-Laurentian Site; (705)523-7100

MCKECHNIE, M Paula; Broadway & Burrard Med Clinic, 1816 Broadway W, Vancouver BC V6J 1Y9; Sask'77; (604)736-1888

MCKEE, Alexander C; 2-3635 Rivergate Way, Ottawa ON K1V 2A4; Qns'85; FRCPC; PhysMed&Rehab. (613)739-3459; Fax. (613)739-1471.

MCKEE, Alison M; Biggar Health Centre, PO Box 70, Biggar SK S0K 0M0; BScMed; MB ChB; DCH; MRCGPract; (306)948-3331; Fax. (306)948-5060; bhcone@sasktel.net.

MCKEE, David C; Thunder Bay Reg HSC-T-Bay, 980 Oliver Rd, Thunder Bay ON P7B 6V4; Qns'81; FRCPC; EmergMed. Staff, Thunder Bay Regional Health Sciences Centre; (807)684-6100

MCKEE, I Bruce F; Orchard Med Centre, 104-1990 Cooper Rd, Kelowna BC V1Y 8K5; Dal'90; (250)861-3235

MCKEE, John D; 303-190 Cundles Rd E SS 103, Barrie ON L4M 4S5; Tor'95; CCFP; (705)728-3722; Fax. (705)728-9449.

MCKEE, John D; Medical Bldg, B02-250 Harding Blvd W, Richmond Hill ON L4C 9M7; Dublin (Ireland)'76; MB ChB; FRCPC; DiagRad. Staff, Southlake Regional Health Centre; (905)737-0595

MCKEE, Kandice A; Spingbank Med Centre, 202-460 Springbank Dr, London ON N6J 0A8; Wes'80; CCFP; FCFP; Staff, St Joseph's Hospital - St Joseph's Health Care; Aj Prof, University of Western Ontario; (519)667-9554

MCKEE, Michael D; St Michael's Orthopaedic Assoc, 800-55 Queen St E, Toronto ON M5C 1R6; Tor'86; FRCSC; OrthSurg (Trauma). Staff Surg Orthopedics, St Michael's Hospital; Prof Orthopedics, University of Toronto; (416)864-5880; Fax. (416)359-1601.

MCKEE, Nancy H; Mount Sinai Hosp, 435-600 University Ave, Toronto ON M5G 1X5; Tor'70; FRCSC; PlasSurg. Assoc Staff, Mount Sinai Hospital; Assoc Staff, Toronto Western Hospital - University Health Network; Assoc Staff, Toronto General Hospital - UHN; Prof, University of Toronto; (416)586-4800 x5197; Fax. (416)586-8408; n.mckee@utoronto.ca.

MCKEE, Nora D; Academic Family Med, 3311 Fairlight Dr, Saskatoon SK S7M 3Y5; Sask'93; CCFP; FCFP; (306)655-4200; Fax. (306)655-4894.

MCKEE, Ryan W C; Centre for Family Medicine, 10B Victoria St S, Kitchener ON N2G 1C5; Qns'09; CCFP; (519)783-0020

MCKEE, Scott D; 370 Hudson St PO Box 88, Salmon Arm BC V1E 4N2; Duke (USA)'90; IntMed. (250)833-2429

MCKEE, W Hugh; Associated Family Physicians, 220-140 Wall St, Saskatoon SK S7K 1N4; Sask'71; CCFP; FCFP; Ac Staff, St Paul's Hospital (Grey Nuns) of Saskatoon; Ac Staff, Saskatoon City Hospital; Ac Staff, Royal University Hospital; (306)653-5522; Fax. (306)653-1723.

MCKEEN, Dolores M; IWK Health Centre, PO Box 9700 Rpo CSC, Halifax NS B3K 6R8; Mem'92; Anes. Staff, IWK Health Centre; (902)428-8888; Fax. (902)420-6626.

MCKEEN, Julie A; Gulf Canada Square, 352-401 9 Ave SW, Calgary AB T2P 3C5; Alb'93; FRCPC; IntMed; Endocrin&Metab. Staff, Foothills Medical Centre; Clinical Asst Prof, University of Calgary; (403)221-4476; Fax. (403)221-4418.

MCKEEN, Katharine I; Tillicum Med Clinic, 14-3170 Tillicum Rd, Victoria BC V9A 7C5; UBC'92; Dip SportMed; CCFP; FCFP; Fam Med, Canadian Forces Health Services - Pacific Centre; (250)381-5662

MCKELLAR, Robert G; Medical Office, 212-840 Coxwell Ave, Toronto ON M4C 5T2; Edinburgh (Scotland)'66; Staff, Toronto East General Hospital Inc; (416)422-0899; Fax. (416)422-0666.

MCKELVEY, J Roger; Dartmouth Med Centre, 504-46 Portland St, Dartmouth NS B2Y 1H4; Dal'78; FRCPC; Neur (Behavioural Neurology). Ac Staff, Queen Elizabeth II Health Sciences Centre - Victoria General Site; Asst Prof, Dalhousie University; Langs: English; French; (902)465-8723; Fax. (902)482-6959.

MCKELVIE, Robert S; Hamilton HS-General Site, 4 E-237 Barton St E, Hamilton ON L8L 2X2; Wes'79; MSc; PhD; FRCPC; IntMed (Heart Failure); Cardiol. Med Dir Heart Function Clinic & Rehab Program, Hamilton Health Sciences Centre - Hamilton General Hospital; Prof Med, McMaster University; (905)572-7155; Fax. (905)577-1480.

MCKENDRY, Robert J R; The Ottawa Hosp-Riverside, 6 29-1967 Riverside Dr, Ottawa ON K1H 7W9; Qns'68; FRCPC; IntMed; Rheum. Staff Rheum, The Ottawa Hospital - Riverside Campus; Prof Med, University of Ottawa; (613)738-8400 x81855; Fax. (613)738-8335.

MCKENNA, Anne M; St Michael's Hosp, 30 Bond St, Toronto ON M5B 1W8; Wes'08; IntMed. Staff, St Michael's Hospital; (416)360-4000

MCKENNA, Catherine; 4640 17 Ave NW, Calgary AB T3B 0P3; Wes'98; BSc(Hons); MSc; CCFP; Staff, Foothills Medical Centre; Dir, Dr McKenna Nutrition & Weight Management; Co-Founder, Calgary Well Woman Clinic; Clinical Asst Prof, University of Calgary; (403)202-2727; Fax. (403)202-2733.

MCKENNA, Christine J; Community Wellness Centre, 16 Dentith Rd, Halifax NS B3R 2H9; Mem'81; CCFP; FCFP; (902)473-1234

MCKENNA, Jocelyne M A; The Ottawa Hosp-Gen Campus, 501 Smyth Rd, Ottawa ON K1H 8L6; Ott'79; AB; FRCPC; Anes. Staff, The Ottawa Hospital - General Campus; Assoc Prof, University of Ottawa; Langs: Bilingual(French/English); (613)737-8187; Fax. (613)737-8189.

MCKENNA, Joseph M; 250 10th St E, Owen Sound ON N4K 1S4; McM'03; FRCSC; Otol.

MCKENNA, Joseph P; Rudd Clinic, 123 Edward St, Toronto ON M5G 1E2; Alb'63; FACS; FRCSC; GenSurg (Thoracic Surgery). (416)597-0997; Fax. (416)597-2912.

MCKENNA, Marianne M; 160-600 Main St, Saint John NB E2K 1J5; Mem'05; FRCPC; Peds. Staff, Saint John Regional Hospital; (506)648-7723; Fax. (506)648-7620.

MCKENNA, Patricia J; Antigonish Mall, 133 Church St, Antigonish NS B2G 2E3; Dal'73; Staff, St Martha's Regional Hospital; Physician, RK MacDonald Nursing Home; (902)863-4471; Fax. (902)863-2207.

MCKENNA, Paul G; The Moncton Hosp, 135 MacBeath Ave, Moncton NB E1C 6Z8; Dal'91; Staff, The Moncton Hospital; (506)857-5520

MCKENNA-BOOT, Patricia E; Workplace Safety & Ins Board, 101-200 Front St W, Toronto ON M5V 3J1; Dal'87; (416)344-3165

MCKENNEY, Roderick N; Arthur Street Med Clinic, 29 Arthur St, Truro NS B2N 1X7; Dal'84; FRCSC; GenSurg. Staff GenSurgeon, Colchester East Hants Health Centre; (902)897-1744; Fax. (902)897-0464; arthur@ns.sympatico.ca.

MCKENTY, Sylvie; CHUM-Hop Notre-Dame, 1560 rue Sherbrooke E, Montreal QC H2L 4M1; Sher'86; LMCC; FRCPC; Anes. Staff Anes, Centre Hospitalier l'Université de Montréal (CHUM) - Hôpital Notre-Dame; Clin Instructor, Universite de Montreal; (514)890-8000 x26876

MCKENZIE, Alvin H; Royal Alex Place, 106-10106 111 Ave NW, Edmonton AB T5G 0B4; Alb'52; MChOrth; FACS; FICS; FRCSC; OrthSurg (Spinal Injury). Sr Staff, Royal Alexandra Hospital; Clin Prof OrthSurg, University of Alberta; (780)479-6886; Fax. (780)474-9973.

MCKENZIE, C Ann; Concordia Gen Hosp, 1095 Concordia Ave, Winnipeg MB R2K 3S8; Man'81; Staff, Concordia General Hospital; (204)667-1560

MCKENZIE, Danica R; 2-32904 Ventura Ave, Abbotsford BC V2S 6J3; UBC'06; CCFP; (604)859-1211

MCKENZIE, Donald C; Allan McGavin Sports Med Ctr, 3055 Wesbrook Mall, Vancouver BC V6T 1Z3; UBC'77; PhD; Prof, University of British Columbia; (604)822-3614; Fax. (604)822-9058.

MCKENZIE, F Neil; London HSC-University Hosp, PO Box 5339 Stn B, London ON N6A 5A5; Aberdeen (Scotland)'68; MB ChB; FRCS(Ed); FRCSC; Cardiovasc&ThorSurg (Cardiac Surgery). Staff, London Health Sciences Centre - University Hospital; Prof Surg, University of Western Ontario; (519)663-3098; Fax. (519)663-8815; neil.mckenzie@lhsc.on.ca.

MCKENZIE, Gerard M; Burrard Med Bldg, 500-1144 Burrard St, Vancouver BC V6Z 2A5; UBC'77; FAAOS; FRCSC; OrthSurg. (604)683-3585; Fax. (604)683-3531.

MCKENZIE, J Scott; Royal Court Medical Bldg, LL2-1 Quarry Ridge Rd, Barrie ON L4M 7G1; McM'01; FRCSC; OrthSurg (Arthroplasty). (705)735-1479

MCKENZIE, John A; St Thomas-Elgin Gen Hosp, PO Box 2007 Stn Main 189 Elm St, St Thomas ON N5P 3W2; Alb'69; FRCSC; Urol. Staff, St Thomas Elgin General Hospital; (519)631-2020

MCKENZIE, Kenneth A; Wellington Ortho & Rehab, 3-86 Dawson Rd, Guelph ON N1H 1A8; Tor'85; FRCSC; OrthSurg. Staff, Guelph General Hospital; (519)837-2020; Fax. (519)763-9871.

MCKENZIE, Kim R; Wellington Med Arts Bldg, 214-121 Wellington St W, Barrie ON L4N 1L2; Cal'84; FRCPC; IntMed; GeriatricMed. IntMed & Geriatric Med, Royal Victoria Regional Health Centre; (705)733-4061; Fax. (705)733-4063.

MCKENZIE, Kwame J; 300-455 Spadina Ave, Toronto ON M5S 2G8; Southampton (England)'87; (416)538-8501

MCKENZIE, Kyle C; Central Alberta Prof Centre, 182-5201 43 St, Red Deer AB T4N 1C7; Alb'04; BSc; FRCPC; Peds. (403)343-6404; Fax. (403)343-6215.

MCKENZIE, Leanna S; 2888 Shaganappi Trail NW, Calgary AB T3B 6A8; Wes'97; BSc; MSc; FRCPC; Peds; Gastroent. Physician Ped Gastroenterol, Alberta Children's Hospital; Prog Dir Pediatric Gastroent/Asst Prof, University of Calgary; (403)955-7747; Fax. (403)955-7639.

MCKENZIE, Lynne M; Coronation Med Clinic, PO Box 430, Coronation AB T0C 1C0; Cal'78; CCFP; (403)578-3232

MCKENZIE, Mary A; Sheppard Med Bldg, 305-701 Sheppard Ave E, North York ON M2K 2Z3; Qns'75; FRCPC; IntMed (Melanoma); Derm. Ac Staff, North York General Hospital; Court Staff, Sunnybrook Health Sciences Centre; (416)590-9918; Fax. (416)590-9842.

MCKENZIE, Michael R; BC Cancer Agency, 600 10th Ave W, Vancouver BC V5Z 4E6; Qns'85; FRCPC; RadOncol (Genito Urinary Oncology). Staff, BC Cancer Agency Vancouver Centre; Staff, Vancouver General Hospital - Centennial Pavillion; Clin Assoc Prof, University of British Columbia; (604)877-6000; mmckenzi@bccancer.bc.ca.

MCKENZIE, Robert N; PO Box 187, Dwight ON P0A 1H0; Tor'71; FRCPC; Anes. Coroner, York Region.

MCKENZIE, Robert; 103-7031 Westminster Hwy, Richmond BC V6X 1A3; Sask'85; BSc; CCFP; (604)270-6004; Fax. (604)270-3215.

MCKENZIE, Stephen W; 103-101 Queensway W, Mississauga ON L5B 2P7; Ott'77; FRCPC; Neur (Neuro Oncology). Ac Staff, Trillium Health Centre - Mississauga; Assoc Staff, Toronto Western Hospital - University Health Network; University of Toronto; (905)273-6460; Fax. (905)273-6908; s.w.mckenzie@rogers.com.

MCKENZIE, Thomas; Eaton Place Med Centre, 81-333 St Mary Ave, Winnipeg MB R3C 4A5; National (Ireland)'58; MB ChB; CCFP; CCFP(E.M.); FCFP.

MCKENZIE, W G Mark; 418-2863 Ellesmere Rd, Scarborough ON M1E 5E9; Edinburgh (Scotland)'85; LMCC; MB BS; Member, American Board of Hair Restoration Surgery; (416)287-3733

MCKEOUGH, Michel F; 740 Main St PO Box 190 Stn Sydney Mines, Sydney Mines NS B1V 2Y5; RCS (Ireland)'81; CCFP; FCFP; (902)736-6259; Fax. (902)736-8192.

MCKEOUGH, Nancy; Thames Valley FHT-Byron Fam Me, 1228 Commissioners Rd W, London ON N6K 1C7; McM'86; CCFP; FCFP; Clin Teacher Pt-Time, University of Western Ontario; (519)472-9670; Fax. (519)657-1766.

MCKEOUGH, William P; Carling Heights Med Centre, 124 Barker St, London ON N5Y 1Y1; Tor'82; CCFP; FCFP; (519)451-6580; Fax. (519)451-1162.

MCKEOWN, Dave K; St Joseph's Gen Hosp, 2137 Comox Ave, Comox BC V9M 1P2; Alb'83; FRCPC; DiagRad (Diagnostic & Therapeutic Radiology). Staff, St Joseph's General Hospital; (250)339-2242; Fax. (250)339-1512.

MCKEOWN, David J; Toronto Public Health, 5F-277 Victoria St, Toronto ON M5B 1W2; McG'79; MHSc; FRCPC; CommunMed. Med Officer of Hlth, Toronto Public Health Corporate Office; Asst Prof, University of Toronto; (416)338-7820; Fax. (416)392-0713; dmckeown@toronto.ca.

MCKEOWN, Elizabeth M; Balmoral Med Arts Facility, 407-1366 Yonge St, Toronto ON M4T 3A7; Birmingham (England)'82; MB ChB; DRCOG; Court Staff, St Michael's Hospital; University of Toronto; (416)324-2242; Fax. (416)324-8330.

MCKEOWN, Emily J; St Joseph's Health Care, PO Box 5777 Stn B 268 Grosvenor St, London ON N6A 4V2; Tor'07; FRCPC; IntMed; Rheum. Staff, St Joseph's Hospital - St Joseph's Health Care; (519)685-8500

MCKEOWN, G Thomas; Associate Med Clinic, PO Box 7590 Stn Main 10011 101 St, Peace River AB T8S 1T2; Tor'75; Staff, Peace River Community Health Centre; (780)624-2581; Fax. (780)624-4015.

MCKEOWN, Iris; Misericordia Health Centre, 99 Cornish Ave, Winnipeg MB R3C 1A2; Man'99; CCFP; Staff, Misericordia Health Centre; (204)788-8364; imckeown@yahoo.com.

MCKEOWN, Janet C; UBC Health Clinic, 310-5950 University Blvd, Vancouver BC V6T 1Z3; Tor'90; Dip SportMed; Clinical Asst Prof UBC Health Clinic, University of British Columbia; (604)822-5431; Fax. (604)822-4089.

MCKEOWN, Kevin J; North York Gen Hosp, 4001 Leslie St, North York ON M2K 1E1; Tor'07; FRCPC; Anes. Staff, North York General Hospital; (416)756-6000

MCKEOWN, Martin J; UBC Hospital, M36-2221 Wesbrook Mall, Vancouver BC V6T 2B5; Tor'90; BEng; FRCPC; Neur (Movement Disorders). Staff, UBC Hospital - Koerner Pavillion; (604)827-5136; Fax. (604)822-7866.

MCKERCHER, Catherine D; Northland Professional Bldg, 400-4600 Crowchild Trail NW, Calgary AB T3A 2L6; Cal'87; FRCPC; Psy. (403)288-1944; Fax. (403)288-8240.

MCKERCHER, H Grant; Senior's Mental Health Program, 200-1164 Devonshire Ave, North Bay ON P1B 6X7; Ott'86; MD; CCFP; FCFP; Staff, North Bay Regional Health Centre - Regional Mental Health; (705)474-5885; Fax. (705)494-3097.

MCKERLIE, Ifeyinwa U; 10381 51 Ave NW, Edmonton AB T6H 0K4; Sask'98; FRCPC; DiagRad. (780)434-9270

MCKERNAN, Corinne G; Rockyview Gen Hosp, 7007 14 St SW, Calgary AB T2V 1P9; Alb'86; BSc; Staff, Rockyview General Hospital; (403)212-8223 x0270

MCKERNAN, Peter S; Crowsnest Med Clinic, PO Box 370, Bellevue AB T0K 0C0; (Australia)'87; Staff Chief, Crowsnest Pass Health Centre; (403)562-8804; Fax. (403)562-2905; peter@crowsnestpass.com.

MCKERRELL, Jeffrey G; Medical Arts Bldg, 508-750 Spadina Cres E, Saskatoon SK S7K 3H3; Sask'82; FRCSC; OrthSurg. Head Surgery/Ac Staff, Saskatoon City Hospital; Ac Staff, Royal University Hospital; Ac Staff, St Paul's Hospital (Grey Nuns) of Saskatoon; Chief OrthSurg, Saskatoon Health Region Corporate Office; Clin Assoc Prof, University of Saskatchewan; (306)244-5561; Fax. (306)934-4877; mckerrellj@shin.sk.ca.

MCKEVITT, Elaine C; Seymour Med Clinic, 200-1530 7th Ave W, Vancouver BC V6J 1S3; UBC'96; FRCSC; GenSurg. Staff, Providence Health Care - St Paul's Hospital; (604)739-5612

MCKIBBIN, Cecil S; Family Med Associates, 5021 51 St, Lacombe AB T4L 2A3; Belfast (Ireland)'78; (403)782-3351; Fax. (403)782-5879.

MCKIBBIN, R Douglas; Developm Disabilities Mental H, 207-2248 Elgin Ave, Port Coquitlam BC V3C 2B2; Man'88; BSc; BEng; FRCPC; Psy (Developmental Disability). Staff, Developmental Disabilities Mental Health Services; (604)477-8475

MCKIBBIN, Timothy G; Merivale Cardiovascular Cons, 201-1370 Clyde Ave, Nepean ON K2G 3H8; Ott'75; FRCPC; IntMed; Cardiol. Ac Staff, Queensway Carleton Hospital; Consultant Staff, Carleton Place & District Memorial Hospital; (613)722-8086; Fax. (613)761-1944.

MCKIBBON, Christopher D; 1935 Pari St, Sudbury ON P3E 3C6; McM'86; FRCPC; IntMed. Ac Staff, Health Sciences North-Laurentian Site; Ac Staff, Health Sciences North-St Joseph's Health Centre; Ac Staff, Health Sciences North - Memorial Site; (705)523-3322; Fax. (705)523-4343.

MCKIERNAN, Bernard; Brandon Reg Health Centre, 150 McTavish Ave E, Brandon MB R7A 2B3; Man'66; Anes. Staff, Brandon Regional Health Centre; (204)726-1122; bernardmckiernan@hotmail.com.

MCKIGGAN, John J; Gladstone Prof Centre, 200-6155 North St, Halifax NS B3K 5R3; Dal'60; FRCPC; IntMed. Staff, Queen Elizabeth II Health Sciences Centre - Victoria General Site; Asst Prof Med, Dalhousie University; (902)453-2891; Fax. (902)454-9010.

MCKILLOP, Graeme J; 95 Spring St SS 1, Almonte ON K0A 1A0; Cal'95; MSc; BSc; CCFP; FCFP; (613)256-9370

MCKILLOP, Sarah; Univ of Alberta Hosp, 4E2-8440 112 St NW, Edmonton AB T6G 2B7; McM'06; FRCPC; Peds. Staff, University of Alberta Hospital; (780)407-8821; Fax. (780)969-4857.

MCKILLOP, Scott D; London HSC-Victoria Hosp, PO Box 5010 Stn B 800 Commissioners Rd E, London ON N6A 5W9; Wes'99; FRCPC; DiagRad. Staff, London Health Sciences Centre - Victoria Campus; (519)685-8500

MCKIM, Aaron L; The Cove Clinic, 1608 Portugal Cove Rd, Port Cv-St Phil NL A1M 3H4; Mem'98; (709)895-7255

MCKIM, Douglas A; The Ottawa Hosp-Rehab Ctr, 505 Smyth Rd, Ottawa ON K1H 8M2; Wes'85; FRCPC; IntMed; Respir. Dir Respiratory Rehab/Staff IntMed, The Ottawa Hospital Rehabilitation Centre; (613)737-8899; Fax. (613)736-9054.

MCKIM, James C; Nashwaaksis Med Clinic, 475 Brookside Dr, Fredericton NB E3A 8V4; Dal'77; Staff, Dr Everett Chalmers Regional Hospital; (506)458-9450; Fax. (506)458-1326.

MCKIM, Susanne E D; Sandy Hill Comm Health Centre, 221 Nelson St, Ottawa ON K1N 1C7; Wes'85; CCFP; FCFP; (613)789-8458; Fax. (613)789-8710.

MCKINLEY, Craig A; Reimer Clinic, 385 Frederick St, Kitchener ON N2H 2P2; Tor'93; FRCPC; GenSurg. Staff, North Bay Regional Health Centre - Regional Mental Health; (519)957-9730; Fax. (519)957-9732.

MCKINLEY, Goldwin E; Aberfoyle Health Centre, 102-304 The East Mall, Etobicoke ON M9B 6E2; West Indies (Jamaica)'66; MB; BSc; FACEP; FRCPC; EmergMed. (416)231-7968

MCKINLEY, Marianne; Toronto East Gen Hosp Inc, 825 Coxwell Ave, Toronto ON M4C 3E7; Tor'91; CCFP; FCFP; Staff, Toronto East General Hospital Inc; (416)461-8272

MCKINNEY, James; Gordon & Leslie Diamond HCC, 9F-2775 Laurel St, Vancouver BC V5Z 1M9; Tor'08; IntMed. (604)875-4111 x69821

MCKINNEY, Katherine A; Churchill Court Bldg, 203-430 King St, London ON N6B 1S7; Wes'78; BSc; FRCPC; Psy (Child & Adolescent Psychiatry). (519)679-7310; Fax. (519)679-7310.

MCKINNEY, Kevin G; Appletree Med Group, 1770 Albion Rd, Etobicoke ON M9V 1C2; West Indies (Jamaica)'98; CCFP.

MCKINNEY, Martha L; Hôpital Ste-Justine, 3175 ch Cote-Sainte-Catherine, Montreal QC H3T 1C5; Bowman Gray(NC) (USA)'92; FRCPC; Peds; Respir. Staff, Hôpital Ste-Justine; (514)345-4931 x5409

MCKINNEY, Veronica R; Northern Medical Services, 404-333 25th St E, Saskatoon SK S7K 0L4; Sask'98; CCFP; (306)665-2898

MCKINNON, Danny; GMF-CLSC la Source, 190 76e rue E, Quebec QC G1H 7K4; Laval'82; Langs: Bilingual(French/English); (418)628-5630

MCKINNON, Genevieve M; Queen Elizabeth II HSC, 1276 South Park St, Halifax NS B3H 2Y9; Dal'05; FRCPC; Anes. Staff, Queen Elizabeth II Health Sciences Centre - Victoria General Site; (902)473-2331

MCKINNON, J Gregory; Tom Baker Cancer Centre, 1331 29 St NW, Calgary AB T2N 4N2; Dal'80; FRCSC; GenSurg. Staff, Tom Baker Cancer Centre; (403)521-3179; Fax. (403)944-3926.

MCKINNON, Jeffrey L; Headwaters Specialist Clinic, 133-150 Rolling Hills Dr, Orangeville ON L9W 4X8; Wes'88; FRCPC; IntMed (Gastroenterology). Ac Staff, Headwaters Health Care Centre; Lecturer, University of Toronto; (519)941-8357; Fax. (519)941-0027.

MCKINNON, John R; Lasalle Community Health Care, 2125 Front Rd, Windsor ON N9J 2C1; Dal'55; BSc; GenSurg. Hon Staff I O D E, Windsor Regional Hospital - Tayfour Site; (519)734-1234; Fax. (519)734-8674.

MCKINNON, Kent D L; Huron Business Centre, 8-31 McBrine Dr, Kitchener ON N2R 1J1; Qns'73; FACEP; FRCPC; EmergMed (Family Practice). Ac Staff, St Mary's General Hospital; Ac Staff, Grand River Hospital - Kitchener/Waterloo Health Centre; (519)893-5568; Fax. (519)893-5795; kentmckinnon@rogers.com.

MCKINNON, Maxine E; 3-47 Gore St E, Perth ON K7H 1H6; Qns'74; (613)812-0455; Fax. (613)267-2526.

MCKINNON, Michelle P; SCOHS-Elizabeth Bruyere Hosp, 270 J-43 Bruyere St, Ottawa ON K1N 5C8; Ott'08; CCFP; Staff Palliative Care, SCO Health Service - Élisabeth Bruyère Hospital; (613)562-6262

MCKINNON, Terry J; Centennial CMH & Brain Injury, PO Box 1000 Stn Main, Ponoka AB T4J 1R8; Alb'79; Staff, Centennial Centre for Mental Health & Brain Injury; (403)783-7600; Fax. (403)783-7790.

MCKINNY, Shari; Urology Associates, 537-750 Spadina Cres E, Saskatoon SK S7K 3H3; Sask'00; BSc; FRCSC; Urol. (306)653-3255

MCKINSTRY, John E; Guelph Gen Hosp, 115 Delhi St, Guelph ON N1E 4J4; Tor'68; FRCPC; DiagRad. Staff, Guelph General Hospital; (519)822-5350 x306; Fax. (519)766-9982.

MCKNEALLY, Martin F; Joint Centre for Bioethics, 211-100 College St, Toronto ON M5G 1L5; Cornell(NY) (USA)'61; PhD; Staff Surg, Toronto General Hospital - UHN; Member, Joint Centre for Bioethics; (416)978-8909

MCKNIGHT, Bruce E; Golden Med Clinic, PO Box 1170, Golden BC V0A 1H0; Cal'07; CCFP; (250)344-2211

MCKNIGHT, David J; St Michael's Hosp, 30 Bond St, Toronto ON M5B 1W8; Tor'75; FRCPC; Anes. Staff Anes, St Michael's Hospital; Assoc Dean Equity & Professionalism, University of Toronto; (416)978-2130; Fax. (416)978-1774; d.mcknight@utoronto.ca.

MCKNIGHT, David W G; Mid-Main Commun Health Centre, 3998 Main St, Vancouver BC V5V 3P2; UBC'01; CCFP; (604)873-3666

MCKNIGHT, J E Arlene; North Toronto Med Bldg, 110-250 Lawrence Ave W, Toronto ON M5M 1B2; Queen's (Ireland)'79; MB ChB; DCH; DRCOG; MRCGPract(UK); Court Staff, Sunnybrook Health Sciences Centre; Ac Staff Family Pract, North York General Hospital; (416)256-4707; Fax. (416)256-4710.

MCKNIGHT, Lisa C; Saint John Reg Hosp, PO Box 2100 Stn Main, Saint John NB E2L 4L2; Dal'04; FRCPC; IntMed; Gastroent. Staff, Saint John Regional Hospital; (506)648-6043

MCKNIGHT, Margaret J; 2902 29 Ave, Vernon BC V1T 1Y7; UBC'83; BSc; (250)541-1097; Fax. (250)541-1098.

MCKNIGHT, R Douglas; Vancouver Gen Hosp, 855 12th Ave W, Vancouver BC V5Z 1M9; Qns'73; FRCPC; IntMed; EmergMed. Ac Staff EmergMed, Vancouver General Hospital - Centennial Pavillion; (604)875-4995; Fax. (604)875-4700.

MCKNIGHT, Robyn C; George Street Family Practice, 1-1400 George St, White Rock BC V4B 4A3; Witwatersrand (South Africa)'86; MB BCh; (604)536-1686; Fax. (604)536-6440.

MCLACHLAN, Donna L; City View Family Practice, 2480 Heather St, Vancouver BC V5Z 3H9; UBC'94; CCFP; FCFP; (604)879-3900; Fax. (604)879-3969; dbchauvin@hotmail.com.

MCLACHLAN, Richard S; London HSC-University Hosp, PO Box 5339 Stn B 339 Windermere Rd, London ON N6A 5A5; Wes'72; FRCPC; Neur (Epilepsy). Staff, London Health Sciences Centre - University Hospital; Prof Dept. of Clinical Neurological Sciences, University of Western Ontario; (519)663-3293; Fax. (519)663-3294.

MCLACHLAN, Siobhan C; Northeast Mental Hlth Team, 2750 Hastings St E, Vancouver BC V5K 1Z9; UBC'92; FRCPC; Psy. Staff, UBC Hospital - Koerner Pavillion; (604)675-3890

MCLACHLIN, Catherine M; London HSC-University Hosp, PO Box 5339 Stn B 339 Windermere Rd, London ON N6A 5A5; Wes'87; FRCPC; AnatPath. Staff, London Health Sciences Centre - University Hospital; Assoc Prof Path & ObstGyn, University of Western Ontario; (519)685-8500 x36346; Fax. (519)663-2430; cm.mclachlin@lhsc.on.ca.

MCLACHLIN, Hugh A; The Surgeons Office, 236 Elm St, St Thomas ON N5R 1J5; McM'81; FRCSC; GenSurg; ThorSurg. Staff, St Thomas Elgin General Hospital; (519)631-0567; Fax. (519)631-0921.

MCLACHLIN, Lauren K; Collingwood Gen & Marine Hosp, 459 Hume St, Collingwood ON L9Y 1W9; McM'05; CCFP; Staff, Collingwood General & Marine Hospital; (705)445-2550; Fax. (705)444-6672.

MCLAREN, Andrew A; 1200 Dufferin Cres, Nanaimo BC V9S 2B7; UBC'00; FRCPC; IntMed (Trauma); Critical Care Medicine. Staff Consultant Intensive Care, Nanaimo Regional General Hospital; Dist Medical Staff, British Columbia Ambulance Services; (250)755-7606; andrew.mclaren@gov.bc.ca.

MCLAREN, David J; Mount Forest Fam Health Team, PO Box 129 50 Colborne St, Fenelon Falls ON K0M 1N0; Tor'95; BSc(Genetics); CCFP; (705)887-3535; davemclaren@yahoo.com.

MCLAREN, Drew H; Royal Inland Hosp, 311 Columbia St, Kamloops BC V2C 2T1; Qns'07; FRCPC; Anes. Staff, Royal Inland Hospital; (250)374-5111

MCLAREN, Jesse T T; The Credit Valley Hosp, 2200 Eglinton Ave W, Mississauga ON L5M 2N1; UBC'05; CCFP; CCFP(E.M.); Staff, The Credit Valley Hospital; (905)813-2200

MCLAREN, Meaghan E; Primrose Family Med Centre, 35 Primrose Ave, Ottawa ON K1R 0A1; McM'03; BSc; CCFP; Asst Prof Family Med, University of Ottawa; (613)230-7788; Fax. (613)230-7778.

MCLAREN, Roderick C; Brock Med Clinic, 204-1800 Tranquille Rd, Kamloops BC V2B 3L9; UBC'01; CCFP; Staff, Royal Inland Hospital; (250)554-7876

MCLAREN, Sherry L; Pleasantview Med Clinic, 11028 51 Ave NW, Edmonton AB T6H 0L4; Alb'84; Staff, Covenant Health - Edmonton General Continuing Care Centre; Assoc Staff, Covenant Health - Grey Nuns Community Hospital; (780)434-5129; Fax. (780)434-9992.

MCLAREN, Stephen T; McLaren Medicine Prof Corp, 1-122 Cornell Park Ave, Markham ON L6B 1B6; Tor'82; CCFP; FCFP; Staff, Markham Stouffville Hospital; (905)471-9999; Fax. (905)209-1501.

MCLAREN, Tyler L; Regina Gen Hosp, 1440 14th Ave, Regina SK S4P 0W5; Sask'05; FRCPC; Anes. Staff, Regina General Hospital; (306)766-4252; Fax. (306)766-4443.

MCLAUCHLAN, Gordon; Arbutus Med Centre, 1501 Boundary Cres, Nanaimo BC V9S 4P1; Glasgow (Scotland)'76; FRCSC; GenSurg. (250)754-4029; Fax. (250)754-4942.

MCLAUCHLIN, Lynn R; St Mary's Hosp Centre, 3777 av Lacombe, Montreal QC H3T 1M5; McG'79; CCFP; FCFP; Staff, St Mary's Hospital Centre; Asst Prof Family Med, McGill University; (514)734-2677; Fax. (514)734-2605.

MCLAUCHLIN, Michelle S; 208-3101 Bloor St W, Etobicoke ON M8X 2W2; Wes'96; BSc; ClinImmunol&Allergy (Asthma & Allergy); Peds. (416)233-0500; Fax. (416)233-0507.

MCLAUGHLIN, Janice A; Valley Care Med Clinic, E-310 8th St, Courtenay BC V9N 1N3; UBC'90; (250)331-0500

MCLAUGHLIN, Joseph H; 175 Old Hampton Hwy PO Box 4674 Stn Main, Rothesay NB E2E 5X4; Dal'82; Med Staff, Saint John Regional Hospital; (506)847-9920; Fax. (506)847-6716.

MCLAUGHLIN, Kevin J; Foothills Med Centre, 1403 29 St NW, Calgary AB T2N 2T9; Edinburgh (Scotland)'89; MB ChB; MRC; Staff Nephrol., Foothills Medical Centre; Asst Prof Med., University of Calgary; (403)944-2510; Fax. (403)944-3199; kevin.mclaughlin@calgaryhealthregion.ca.

MCLAUGHLIN, Kyle A; Canmore Gen Hosp, 1100 Hospital Place, Canmore AB T1W 1N2; Dal'03; BSc; CCFP; CCFP(E.M.); Staff, Canmore General Hospital; (403)678-5536; Fax. (403)678-5069.

MCLAUGHLIN, Lois Y; University Downs Fam Practice, 425 University Ave E, Waterloo ON N2K 4C9; McM'90; BSc(Hon); CCFP; FCFP; (519)569-8821; Fax. (519)569-8823.

MCLAUGHLIN, Mark F; Shelbourne Med Clinic, 150-3200 Shelbourne St, Victoria BC V8P 5G8; UBC'94; CCFP; (250)592-8485

MCLAUGHLIN, Nathalie; 104-140 Champlain St, Dieppe NB E1A 1N8; Mon'00; FRCSC; ObstGyn. Staff, Beausejour Reg Health Authority; Langs: Bilingual(French/English); (506)383-4201

MCLAUGHLIN, Peter R; Peterborough Reg HC-Hospital, 1 Hospital Dr, Peterborough ON K9J 7C6; Tor'70; FRCPC; IntMed; Cardiol. Chief-Med Staff/CMO, Peterborough Regional Health Centre - Hospital Drive; (705)743-2121; Fax. (705)876-5120.

MCLAUGHLIN, Robert J C; Cochrane Primary Care Centre, 103-100 Grande Blvd W, Cochrane AB T4C 0S4; Dublin (Ireland)'81; MB ChB; BAO; MRCGPract; CCFP; (403)932-2089; Fax. (403)932-1820; rmclaughlin@dthr.ab.ca.

MCLAUGHLIN, Robyn A; IWK Health Centre, PO Box 9700 Rpo CSC 5850-5980 University Ave, Halifax NS B3K 6R8; Mem'05; FRCPC; Peds; Nephrol. Staff, IWK Health Centre; (902)470-8888

MCLAUGHLIN, Sarah G; Broadway Family Physicians, 1801 Broadway Ave, Saskatoon SK S7H 2B6; Sask'04; CCFP; (306)652-2632

MCLEAN, Alan; Superior Family Health Team, 48-44 Great Northern Rd, Sault Ste. Marie ON P6B 4Y5; Wes'88; Chief Staff, Sault Area Hospital - Sault Ste Marie; (705)253-1313 x202; Fax. (705)253-8759.

MCLEAN, Anthony R; Bloor-Jane Med Bldg, 501-2425 Bloor St W, Toronto ON M6S 4W4; Wes'85; FRCSC; Urol (Minimal Invasive Surgery). Ac Staff, St Joseph's Health Centre; (416)767-8506; Fax. (416)767-2403.

MCLEAN, Astrid E; Sexual & Reproductive H Clinic, 5F-1213 4 St SW, Calgary AB T2R 0X7; CCFP; (403)217-6453; Fax. (403)217-5235.

MCLEAN, Carolyn A; University Hospital, PO Box 5339 Stn B A3 129-339 Windermere Rd, London ON N6A 5A5; Tor'80; FRCPC; AnatPath. Staff, London Health Sciences Centre - University Hospital; Assoc Prof, University of Western Ontario; (519)685-8500 x36344; Fax. (519)663-2930.

MCLEAN, Chris A; Gates Med Centre, 15-300 Kingston Rd, Pickering ON L1V 6Z9; Wes'03; CCFP; (905)509-4595; Fax. (905)509-4597.

MCLEAN, D Ross; Royal Alexandra Hosp, 10240 Kingsway NW, Edmonton AB T5H 3V9; Alb'82; FRCPC; AnatPath (Gastrointestinal Pathology); GenPath. Consultant, Cross Cancer Institute; Ac Staff Path., Royal Alexandra Hospital; Clinical Asst Prof, University of Alberta; (780)735-4703; Fax. (780)735-4715; rmclean@ualberta.ca.

MCLEAN, David A; Royal Ottawa Hlth Care Group, 1145 Carling Ave, Ottawa ON K1Z 7K4; Wes'76; FRCPC; Psy. Staff Psy, Royal Ottawa Mental Health Centre - Royal Ottawa Health Care Group; (613)722-6521 x6513; Fax. (613)724-6554.

MCLEAN, David I; Skin Care Centre, 835 10th Ave W, Vancouver BC V5Z 4E8; Man'71; DAB; FRCPC; Derm. Staff, Vancouver General Hospital - Centennial Pavillion; Staff, BC Cancer Agency Vancouver Centre; Prof Derm & Med, University of British Columbia; (604)875-5151; Fax. (604)873-9919.

MCLEAN, Deirdre E; 1-6220 Highway 2A, Lacombe AB T4L 2G5; Ott'88; BSc; FRCPC; PhysMed&Rehab (Sports Medicine). Physician Sports Med, Collegiate Sports Medicine Clinic; (403)782-6555; Fax. (403)782-6511.

MCLEAN, Gary D; 11 Stratford Rd, Stratford PE C1B 1T4; Dal'79; BSc; MRCS; FRCSC; PlasSurg. Chief PlasSurg, Queen Elizabeth Hospital; Staff, Prince County Hospital; (902)569-9133; Fax. (902)569-9188; twodocs@eastlink.ca.

MCLEAN, Heather L; 233 Van Norman St, Thunder Bay ON P7A 4B6; Dal'96; CCFP; (807)345-6064; Fax. (807)345-0366.

MCLEAN, Hugh A; McLean Clinic, 343-50 Burnhamthorpe Rd W, Mississauga ON L5B 3C2; Tor'75; FRCSC; PlasSurg (Cosmetic Surgery). Staff, Trillium Health Centre - Mississauga; (905)273-4888; Fax. (905)273-5581; info@mcleanclinic.com.

MCLEAN, J Lynda; York Prof Bldg, 101-679 Davis Dr, Newmarket ON L3Y 5G8; Tor'92; BSc; CCFP; Ac Staff, Southlake Regional Health Centre; (905)836-1150; Fax. (905)898-1121.

MCLEAN, James R B; Hubbards Med Clinic, PO Box 96, Hubbards NS B0J 1T0; Pretoria (South Africa)'84; MB ChB; CCFP; (902)857-3335; Fax. (902)857-3984.

MCLEAN, Jennifer L; Child & Parent Resource Inst, 600 Sanatorium Rd, London ON N6H 3W7; McM'84; FRCPC; Peds (Developmental Pediatrics). Staff, Child & Parent Resource Institute; (519)858-2774

MCLEAN, John J; PO Box 608 Stn Main, Yellowknife NT X1A 2N5; Glasgow (Scotland)'72; MB ChB; DObstRCOG; MRCGPract; CCFP; FCFP; (867)920-7777

MCLEAN, John S; St Michael's Hosp, 30 Bond St, Toronto ON M5B 1W8; Tor'69; FRCPC; Anes. Staff Anes, St Michael's Hospital; (416)864-5071; Fax. (416)864-6014.

MCLEAN, Joy E; Bear Street Family Physicians, PO Box 1048 220 Bear St, Banff AB T1L 1H6; (United Kingdom)'79; (403)762-4846; Fax. (403)762-2445.

MCLEAN, Laura E; Nanaimo Sleep Clinic, 130-2125 Bowen Rd, Nanaimo BC V9S 1H7; Sask'93; FRCPC; IntMed; Critical Care Medicine; Respir. Staff, Victoria General Hospital; (250)758-0060

MCLEAN, Laurie E; Kilborn Med Centre, 215-1385 Bank St, Ottawa ON K1H 8N4; Dal'96; ABOtol; MRCS; BSc(Hon); FRCSC; Otol (Hyperbaric Medicine). Ac Staff, The Ottawa Hospital - General Campus; Ac Staff, Children's Hospital of Eastern Ontario (CHEO); Asst Prof, University of Ottawa; (613)562-9000; Fax. (613)562-9898.

MCLEAN, Lynn E; PO Box 65072 Rpo North Hill, Calgary AB T2N 4T6; Alb'84; CCFP; FCFP.

MCLEAN, Margot L; Mission Med Clinic, 201-2303 4 St SW, Calgary AB T2S 2S7; Cal'88; (403)640-4320

MCLEAN, Mark E; Raven Song Comm Health Centre, 2450 Ontario St, Vancouver BC V5T 4T7; Wes'85; MSc(Epidem.); FRCPC; CommunMed (Population Health & Epidemiology); Public Health & Preventive Med. Staff, Vancouver General Hospital - Centennial Pavillion; Clin Instructor Health Care & Epidemiol, University of British Columbia; Langs: Bilingual(English/French); (604)709-6530

MCLEAN, Mary K; 209-170 The Donway W, North York ON M3C 2G3; Otago (New Zealand)'78; MB ChB; FRCPC; Psy (Psychoanalysis). (416)975-1544; Fax. (416)975-8341.

MCLEAN, Michael; Univ Hlth Network-Princess M, 610 University Ave, Toronto ON M5G 2M9; Belfast (Ireland)'69; MB ChB; FRCPC; RadOncol (Genito Urinary Oncology)., Princess Margaret Hospital - University Health Network; Asst Prof, University of Toronto; (416)946-2132; Fax. (416)946-6561.

MCLEAN, Nicola K; South Perth Endocrinol & Metab, RR 1 Box 881, Granton ON N0M 1V0; Wes'85; FRCPC; IntMed; Endocrin&Metab. (519)225-2035; Fax. (519)225-2700.

MCLEAN, Patrick R; Elliot Lake Family Health Team, 31 Nova Scotia Walk, Elliot Lake ON P5A 1Y9; Tor'76; Staff, St Joseph's General Hospital Elliot Lake; (705)461-8882; Fax. (705)848-3449.

MCLEAN, Pat L; Cachet Family Physicians, 2-9255 Woodbine Ave, Markham ON L6C 1Y9; Tor'91; BSc; (905)887-2222; Fax. (905)887-3655.

MCLEAN, Richard F; McMaster Univ Med Centre, 2E37-1200 Main St W, Hamilton ON L8N 3Z5; Tor'79; DABA; FRCPC; Anes. VP Medical Affairs & Quality, Hamilton Health Sciences Centre - Hamilton General Hospital; Assoc Prof, McMaster University; (905)527-4322 x42031; Fax. (905)521-5076; mcleanr@hhsc.ca.

MCLEAN, Robert H; Dr Everett Chalmers Reg Hosp, PO Box 9000 Stn A, Fredericton NB E3B 5N5; Dal'77; FRCPC; Anes. Staff, Dr Everett Chalmers Regional Hospital; (506)455-7683

MCLEAN, Ross R; Perth Med Clinic, 14 Isabella St, Perth ON K7H 2W6; Qns'70; CCFP; FCFP; Ac Staff, Perth & Smiths Falls District Hospital - Perth Site (Great War Memorial Site); Med Dir, Eastern Regional Med Educ Program; Staff Teacher, Queen's University; Staff Teacher, University of Ottawa; (613)267-5528; Fax. (613)264-8370.

MCLEAN, Shelley M; 700-1240 Bay St, Toronto ON M5R 2A7; Sask'79; CCFP; Physician, Osgoode Health Centre; (416)977-5427; Fax. (416)646-0205.

MCLEAN WIEST, Reid M; Crowfoot Village Fam Practice, 210-600 Crowfoot Cres NW, Calgary AB T3G 0B4; Cal'00; CCFP; Langs: Bilingual(English/French); (403)239-9733

MCLELLAN, Allan P; 730 Concession St, Hamilton ON L8V 1C1; McM'76; FRCPC; IntMed; Respir. Clin Assoc Prof, McMaster University; (905)387-5543; Fax. (905)387-3713; office@amclellan.ca.

MCLELLAN, Barry A; Sunnybrook Hlth Sciences Ctre, C104-2075 Bayview Ave, Toronto ON M4N 3M5; Tor'81; FRCPC; EmergMed. Pres/CEO, Sunnybrook Health Sciences Centre; Assoc Prof Surg, University of Toronto; (416)480-4112; barry.mclellan@sunnybrook.ca.

MCLELLAN, Catherine S; Kingston Gen Hosp, 76 Stuart St, Kingston ON K7L 2V7; Tor'95; FRCPC; IntMed; Cardiol. Staff, Kingston General Hospital; (613)548-1329; Fax. (613)548-2400.

MCLELLAN, Fiona J; Salmon Arm Med Clinic, PO Box 730 Stn Main 581 Hudson Ave NE, Salmon Arm BC V1E 4N8; Glasgow (Scotland)'85; MB ChB; (250)832-2321

MCLELLAN, James L; Foothills Med Centre, C231-1403 29 St NW, Calgary AB T2N 2T9; Cal'95; CCFP; CCFP(E.M.); Staff EmergMed., Foothills Medical Centre; (403)944-1315; Fax. (403)944-2419.

MCLELLAN, Kenneth C; 633 Colborne St, London ON N6B 2V3; Tor'98; MSc; BSc(Hon); CCFP; (519)433-8834; Fax. (519)433-8462.

MCLELLAN, Kenneth G; Morningside Crossing Med Ctr, H9-4525 Kingston Rd, Scarborough ON M1E 2P1; McG'78; CCFP; FCFP; Staff, Rouge Valley Health System - Centenary Health Centre Site; Staff, The Scarborough Hospital - General Campus; (416)284-0189; Fax. (416)284-1491.

MCLELLAN, Marie-Carolyne; Kelowna Gen Hosp, 2268 Pandosy St, Kelowna BC V1Y 1T2; Ott'90; CCFP; Staff, Kelowna General Hospital; (250)862-4000

MCLELLAN, Rowen A; Fredericton Med Clinic, 402-1015 Regent St, Fredericton NB E3B 6H5; Dal'00; BSc; FRCSC; Urol. Lecturer Urol, Dalhousie University; Langs: French; (506)458-0310; Fax. (506)457-4757.

MCLELLAND, Edwin N; Glazier Med Centre, 11 Gibb St, Oshawa ON L1H 2J9; Wes'77; (905)579-1212; Fax. (905)579-1583.

MCLELLAND, Hans; CSSS de Chicoutimi, 305 rue Saint-Vallier, Chicoutimi QC G7H 5H6; Sher'91; FRCSC; Neursurg. Staff, Complexe hospitalier de la Sagamie; (418)541-1000

MCLELLAND, Kirstie; University of Alberta Hosp, 1A7 19WCM-8440 112 St NW, Edmonton AB T6G 2B7; Qns'01; FRCPC; EmergMed. Staff, University of Alberta Hospital; (780)407-8433

MCLEMAN, Elizabeth R; Sheldon M Chumir Urgent Care, 1213 4 Ave SW, Calgary AB T2R 0X7; UBC'03; CCFP; CCFP(E.M.); (403)955-6011

MCLENNAN, James A; 101-600 Royal Ave, New Westminster BC V3M 1J3; Ott'57; (604)526-4277

MCLENNAN, John; Health Research Innovation Ctr, 3280 Hospital Dr NW, Calgary AB T2N 4Z6; Alb'91; PhD; MPH; BMedSci; FRCPC; Psy (Child Psychiatry). Consultant Psy, Alberta Children's Hospital; Staff, Health Research Innovation Centre; Asst Prof, University of Calgary; (403)210-8673; Fax. (403)270-7307.

MCLENNAN, Michael K; Markham Stouffville Hosp, PO Box 1800 Stn Main 381 Church St, Markham ON L3P 7P3; Tor'86; FRCPC; DiagRad. Staff Radiol, Markham Stouffville Hospital; Diag Radiol, Markham Stouffville Hospital - Uxbridge Site; (905)472-7093; Fax. (905)472-7078.

MCLEOD, Anne G; Sunnybrook Hlth Sciences Ctre, D677-2075 Bayview Ave, Toronto ON M4N 3M5; Tor'92; FRCPC; IntMed; Hem. Staff Hem, Sunnybrook Health Sciences Centre; (416)480-5376; Fax. (416)480-6753.

MCLEOD, B Daniel; Medical Clinic, 305-3330 Richter St, Kelowna BC V1W 4V5; Alb'73; FRCPC; IntMed (Soft Tissue Disorders); Rheum. Med Staff, Kelowna General Hospital; Consultant, Vernon Jubilee Hospital; (250)869-1445; Fax. (250)869-1475.

MCLEOD, D Ross; Alberta Children's Hosp, 2888 Shaganappi Trail NW, Calgary AB T3B 6A8; UBC'77; FCCMG; FRCPC; Peds; MedGenetics. Ac Staff, Alberta Children's Hospital; Consultant, Foothills Medical Centre; Assoc Prof Med Genetics, University of Calgary; (403)955-7246; ross.mcleod@albertahealthservices.ca.

MCLEOD, David S; McMaster University Campus, 49-1280 Main St W, Hamilton ON L8S 4S4; Wes'88; CCFP; (905)525-9140

MCLEOD, Denise; McLeod Medical Clinic, 229-100 Tabor Blvd, Prince George BC V2M 5T4; UBC'91; CCFP; Asst Dean Student Affairs, University of British Columbia; (250)562-5166

MCLEOD, Donald M; Nicola Valley Med Centre, PO Box 279 2087 Granite Ave, Merritt BC V1K 1B8; UBC'79; Chief/Staff, Nicola Valley Health Centre; (250)378-5115; Fax. (250)378-6424.

MCLEOD, Heather A; North Vancouver Med Clinic, 115 16th St W, North Vancouver BC V7M 1T3; Dal'90; CCFP; FCFP; Staff, Lions Gate Hospital; (604)904-8804

MCLEOD, Heather C; St Joseph's Healthcare, F536-50 Charlton Ave E, Hamilton ON L8N 4A6; McM'05; FRCPC; IntMed; GeriatricMed. Staff, St Joseph's Healthcare - Charlton Campus; (905)522-1155; Fax. (905)521-6068.

MCLEOD, Ian D; 1883 Turner Rd, Windsor ON N8W 3K2; Wes'72; (519)977-8216; Fax. (519)977-8216.

MCLEOD, Janet A; Central Algoma Health Centre, PO Box 398, Bruce Mines ON P0R 1C0; McM'85; CCFP; FCFP; Fax. (705)785-3672.

MCLEOD, Jaret K; AE305-671 William Ave, Winnipeg MB R3E 0Z2; Man'99; FRCPC; Peds. Staff, Health Sciences Centre; Staff Peds, St Boniface General Hospital.

MCLEOD, Joanne M; Allan Blair Cancer Centre, 300-4101 Dewdney Ave, Regina SK S4T 7T1; Sask'87; BSc; CCFP; Staff, Regina General Hospital; (306)766-2288; Fax. (306)766-2688.

MCLEOD, Kevin I; 200-101 16th St W, North Vancouver BC V7M 1T3; UBC'01; BSc; FRCPC; IntMed (Cardiology). Staff, Lions Gate Hospital; Staff, Whitehorse General Hospital; Clin Staff Faculty, University of British Columbia; (604)904-0810

MCLEOD, Laura J; 4143-10101 Southport Rd SW, Calgary AB T2W 3N2; Cal'78; FRCPC; CommunMed (Public Health). Med Officer of Hlth, Alberta Health Services; Staff, Health Research Innovation Centre; Clin Assoc Prof, University of Calgary; (403)943-1280

MCLEOD, Lindsay E C; North Shore Family Health Team, PO Box 819 20B Cartier Rd, Terrace Bay ON P0T 2W0; McM'04; CCFP; Fam Med, The McCausland Hospital; (807)825-3235; Fax. (807)825-3239.

MCLEOD, M Elizabeth; The Hosp for Sick Children, 555 University Ave, Toronto ON M5G 1X8; Tor'75; FRCPC; Anes. Staff Anes, The Hospital For Sick Children; (416)813-7445; Fax. (416)813-7543.

MCLEOD, N Lynne; IWK Health Centre, PO Box 9700 Rpo CSC 5850-5980 University Ave, Halifax NS B3K 6R8; Dal'96; FRCSC; ObstGyn (Maternal Fetal Medicine). Staff, IWK Health Centre; (902)470-8888

MCLEOD, Nancy J; 304-4420 Chatterton Way, Victoria BC V8X 5J2; Sask'88; (250)727-6336; Fax. (250)727-9445.

MCLEOD, R Bruce; Valley Reg Hosp, 150 Exhibition St, Kentville NS B4N 5E3; Mem'82; FRCPC; EmergMed. Ac Staff, Valley Regional Hospital; Asst Prof, Dalhousie University; (902)678-7381; Fax. (902)679-1206.

MCLEOD, Richard A; 303-321 Nicola St, Kamloops BC V2C 6G6; Alb'02; FRCPC; OrthSurg.

MCLEOD, Robert A H; Centre Med Brunswick, 203-955 boul Saint-Jean, Pointe-Claire QC H9R 5K3; McG'62; FRCSC; GenSurg. (514)426-9059; Fax. (514)697-9770.

MCLEOD, Robin S; Mount Sinai Hosp, 449-600 University Ave, Toronto ON M5G 1X5; Alb'75; FACS; ABS; DABCRS; FRCSC; GenSurg (Colon & Rectal Surgery). Prof Surg & Health Policy Management & Evaluation, University of Toronto; (416)586-4800 x8347; Fax. (416)586-8644.

MCLEOD, Ryan M; McMaster Family Practice, A-690 Main St W, Hamilton ON L8S 1A4; Wes'10; CCFP; (905)521-5015

MCLEOD, Valerie L; Kingston Gen Hosp, 76 Stuart St, Kingston ON K7L 2V7; Qns'06; CCFP; Staff, Kingston General Hospital; (613)549-6666

MCLEOD, W Alastair; Burrard Health Bldg, 302-1160 Burrard St, Vancouver BC V6Z 2E8; Alb'58; MSc; FRCPC; Derm (AIDS/HIV). Vis Consultant, Whitehorse General Hospital; Hon Staff, Providence Health Care - St Paul's Hospital; Hon Staff, Vancouver General Hospital - Centennial Pavillion; (604)688-1388; Fax. (604)688-9489.

MCLERNON, S Lynn; Colchester East Hants Hlth Ctr, 600 Abernaki Rd, Truro NS B2N 5A1; Cal'03; CCFP; CCFP(E.M.); Staff, Colchester East Hants Health Centre; (902)893-4321

MCLINDEN, David N; Huntsville Prof Bldg, 202-348 Muskoka Rd 3 N, Huntsville ON P1H 1H8; McM'91; CCFP; FCFP; Staff, Huntsville District Memorial Hospital - Muskoka Algonquin Healthcare; (705)788-3623; Fax. (705)788-3624.

MCLOONE, Mary B E; St Michael's Hosp, 30 Bond St, Toronto ON M5B 1W8; London (England)'96; FRCPC; Anes. Staff, St Michael's Hospital; (416)864-5071

MCLOUGHLIN, Diarmuid P; Sioux Lookout Meno-Ya-Win HC, PO Box 909 Stn Main, Sioux Lookout ON P8T 1B4; Dublin (Ireland)'58; MB ChB; BAO; DMRD; FRCPC; DiagRad. Staff Radiol, Sioux Lookout Meno-Ya-Win Health Centre; Clin Assoc Prof Radiol, McMaster University; Assoc Prof, Northern Ontario School of Medicine-Laurentian University; (807)737-3030; Fax. (807)737-4343; dmcloughlin@slmhc.on.ca.

MCLOUGHLIN, Martin G; Fairmont Med Bldg, 1216-750 Broadway W, Vancouver BC V5Z 1J2; UBC'68; FRCSC; Urol. Ac Staff, Vancouver General Hospital - Centennial Pavillion; Vis Staff, Providence Health Care - St Paul's Hospital; (604)873-9331; Fax. (604)873-9303.

MCLOUGHLIN, Ravana-Sue; 2280 Baron Rd, Kelowna BC V1X 7W3; UBC'85; (250)765-8565; Fax. (250)765-8590.

MCLUCKIE, Chantal A; Crowfoot West Business Ctr, 210-600 Crowfoot Cres NW, Calgary AB T3G 0B4; (South Africa)'06; MB BCh; (403)208-0722

MCLUCKIE, Duncan A; Bigelow Fowler Clinic East, 3515 Major Magrath Dr S, Lethbridge AB T1K 8A8; (South Africa)'06; MB BCh; (403)327-3977; Fax. (403)327-7878.

MCMAHEN, J Ivor; Cariboo Mem Hosp, 517 Sixth Ave N, Williams Lake BC V2G 2G8; UBC'83; Staff, Cariboo Memorial Hospital and Health Centre; (250)398-5162; ivor_mcmahen@telus.net.

MCMAHON, Alan W; University of Alberta Hosp, 11 107 CSB-8440 112 St NW, Edmonton AB T6G 2B7; Alb'91; FRCPC; IntMed; Nephrol. Staff, University of Alberta Hospital; Asst Prof Med, University of Alberta; (780)407-7717; Fax. (780)407-7771; alan.mcmahon@ualberta.ca.

MCMAHON, J Stephen; Markham Stouffville Health Ctr, 306-377 Church St, Markham ON L6B 1A1; Tor'82; FRCSC; OrthSurg. Orthopedic Surgery, Markham Stouffville Hospital - Uxbridge Site; Pres Med Staff Assoc, Markham Stouffville Hospital; Ac Staff, WCB Ont., N.E.L. Roster; (905)472-5375; Fax. (905)472-5651.

MCMAHON, James D R; Appletree Med Clinic, 368 Slater St, Ottawa ON K1R 5C1; Aberdeen (Scotland)'66; (613)236-9441; Fax. (613)236-9425.

MCMAHON, Lynne E; Dartmouth Gen Hosp, 325 Pleasant St, Dartmouth NS B2Y 4G8; Ott'99; CCFP; CCFP(E.M.); Staff, Dartmouth General Hospital; (902)465-8300

MCMAHON, Margaret A; Saskatoon Community Clinic, 455 2nd Ave N, Saskatoon SK S7K 2C2; Dublin (Ireland)'73; MB ChB; BAO; DCH; CCFP; Court Staff, Saskatoon City Hospital; Court Staff, St Paul's Hospital (Grey Nuns) of Saskatoon; Court Staff, Royal University Hospital; (306)652-0300; Fax. (306)652-0682.

MCMAHON, Patrick; Polyclinique Med de La Lievre, 536 rue de la Madone, Mont-Laurier QC J9L 1S7; Mon'00; CCFP; (819)440-2345; Fax. (819)440-2330.

MCMAHON, Robert G; 211-857 Grand Ave W, Chatham ON N7L 4T1; Qns'79; FRCOphth; FRCSC; Ophth. Ac Staff, Chatham-Kent Health Alliance; (519)354-4700; Fax. (519)354-2616; rmcmahon@ciaccess.com.

MCMAHON, Selma; Associated Family Physicians, 220-140 Wall St, Saskatoon SK S7K 1N4; Sask'86; CCFP; Staff, Saskatoon City Hospital; Staff, St Paul's Hospital (Grey Nuns) of Saskatoon; (306)653-5522; Fax. (306)653-1723.

MCMAIN, Peter B; Niagara H System-St Catharine, PO Box 3018 Stn Main 142 Queenston St, St Catharines ON L2R 7C6; Glasgow (Scotland)'53; MB ChB; FAAP; FRCPC; Peds. Ac Staff, Niagara Health System - St Catharines General Site; (905)684-7271; Fax. (905)682-9395; petermcmain@hotmail.com.

MCMANUS, Bruce M; St Paul's Hosp, 166-1081 Burrard St, Vancouver BC V6Z 1Y6; Sask'77; FRCPC; AnatPath. Staff Path/Acad Head, Providence Health Care - St Paul's Hospital; Scientist/Dir, Institute of Circulatory & Respiratory Health; Prof Path & LabMed/Dir UBC James Hogg Research Ctr, University of British Columbia; (604)806-8934; bruce.mcmanus@hli.ubc.ca.

MCMANUS, David J; Hys Med Centre, 300-11010 101 St NW, Edmonton AB T5H 4B9; Alb'95; PhD; FRCPC; Psy. Consultant Psy, Alberta Mental Health Board; Clin Lecturer, University of Alberta; (780)424-8383; Fax. (780)424-6404; mcmanus@telusplanet.net.

MCMANUS, Ruth M; St Joseph's Health Care, PO Box 5777 Stn B 268 Grosvenor St, London ON N6A 4V2; Wes'81; FRCPC; IntMed (Diabetes); Endocrin&Metab. Staff, St Joseph's Hospital - St Joseph's Health Care; Prof Med, University of Western Ontario; (519)646-6371; Fax. (519)646-6372; ruth.mcmanus@sjhc.london.on.ca.

MCMASTER, Jeffry J; Addiction & Mental Hlth-Queen, 3-4-1001 Queen St W, Toronto ON M6J 1H4; Man'94; FRCPC; Psy (Forensic Psychiatry). Staff Psy, Centre for Addiction & Mental Health (CAMH) - Queen Site; Lecturer Psy, University of Toronto; (416)535-8501 x2357; Fax. (416)583-4319; jeff_mcmaster@camh.net.

MCMASTER, Robert G; Ontario Shores Ctr Mental HS, 700 Gordon St, Whitby ON L1N 5S9; Wes'07; Staff, Ontario Shores Centre for Mental Health Sciences; (905)668-5881

MCMASTER, Robin D M; Regina Community Clinic, 1106 Winnipeg St, Regina SK S4R 1J6; Man'95; BSc; CCFP; Staff Family Pract, Regina General Hospital; Med Staff, Pasqua Hospital; (306)543-7880; Fax. (306)543-6888; rmcmaster@reginacommunityclinic.ca.

MCMEEKIN, Barbara L; Carlisle Med Centre, PO Box 311 1493 Centre Rd, Carlisle ON L0R 1H0; McM'78; CCFP; FCFP; Ac Staff, Hamilton Health Sciences Centre - McMaster University Medical Centre; (905)689-3301; Fax. (905)689-5772.

MCMEEKIN, James D; Foothills Med Centre, 880C-1403 29 St NW, Calgary AB T2N 2T9; Man'75; FRCPC; Cardiol (Angiography). Staff, Foothills Medical Centre; Staff, Rockyview General Hospital; Staff, Peter Lougheed Centre; (403)944-2561; Fax. (403)270-3715.

MCMEEKIN-DOWN, Nadine R; Hillsdale Med Clinic, 1380G 23rd Ave, Regina SK S4S 3S5; Sask'93; CCFP; FCFP; (306)584-1533; Fax. (306)584-1767.

MCMICHEN, Iain K S; Haldimand War Mem Hosp, 102-206 John St, Dunnville ON N1A 2P7; London (England)'76; MB BS; MRCS; LRCP; DRCOG; Chief Medical Staff, Haldimand War Memorial Hospital; (905)774-7415; Fax. (905)774-2512.

MCMILLAN, Alexandra E; Scarborough Hosp-General Div, 3050 Lawrence Ave E, Scarborough ON M1P 2V5; Mem'06; FRCPC; IntMed; Critical Care Medicine. Staff, The Scarborough Hospital - General Campus; (416)438-2911

MCMILLAN, Colin J; Parkdale Med Centre, 20 St. Peters Rd, Charlottetown PE C1A 5N1; McG'72; DABIM; FACP; FRCPC; IntMed (Adult Cardiology); Cardiol. Staff, Queen Elizabeth Hospital; Consultant, Kings County Memorial Hospital; Instructor, Dalhousie University; (902)368-7428; Fax. (902)368-7484; c.mcmillan@pei.aibn.com.

MCMILLAN, David R; Peterborough Clinic, LL03-26 Hospital Dr, Peterborough ON K9J 7C3; Wes'88; FRCPC; IntMed. Med Dir-ICU, Peterborough Regional Health Centre - Hospital Drive; (705)740-6868; Fax. (705)740-6898.

MCMILLAN, Douglas D; IWK Health Centre, PO Box 9700 Rpo CSC 5850-5980 University Ave, Halifax NS B3K 6R8; Alb'70; BSc; FAAP; FRCPC; Peds (Neonatology). Staff, IWK Health Centre; Emeritus Prof, University of Calgary; Prof, Dalhousie University; (902)470-8803; Fax. (902)470-6469; doug.mcmillan@dal.ca.

MCMILLAN, Duncan; 107-359 Riverside Dr, Sudbury ON P3E 1H5; McG'70; BSc; (705)671-1661; Fax. (705)671-0177.

MCMILLAN, Hugh J; Children's Hosp Eastern Ont, 401 Smyth Rd, Ottawa ON K1H 8L1; McM'00; MSc; FRCPC; Peds; Neur. Staff, Children's Hospital of Eastern Ontario (CHEO); (613)737-7600

MCMILLAN, J Stewart; Landmark Med Centre, 9-4150 Albert St, Regina SK S4S 3R8; Glasgow (Scotland)'72; MB ChB; CCFP; FCFP; Ac Staff, Wascana Rehabilitation Centre; Staff, Pasqua Hospital; Court Staff, Regina General Hospital; (306)352-9609; Fax. (306)781-7070.

MCMILLAN, James C D; Castor Med Clinic, GD 5402 47 St, Castor AB T0C 0X0; (United Kingdom)'99; MB ChB; Staff, Covenant Health - Our Lady of the Rosary Hospital; (403)882-2665; Fax. (403)882-3525.

MCMILLAN, James D; Dundas Valley Med Centre, 204-107 King St W, Dundas ON L9H 1V1; Qns'90; Member Med Staff, Hamilton Health Sciences Centre - McMaster Children's Hospital; (905)627-3505; Fax. (905)627-4193.

MCMILLAN, James F; 123-11910 111 Ave NW, Edmonton AB T5G 0E5; Alb'69; FRCSC; OrthSurg. Assoc Staff, Sturgeon Community Hospital; Ac Staff, Covenant Health - Misericordia Community Hospital; University of Alberta; (780)453-8985; Fax. (780)447-4537.

MCMILLAN, John K; Musicians Clinics of Canada, 201-565 Sanatorium Rd, Hamilton ON L9C 7N4; Qns'07; CCFP; (905)574-5444; Fax. (905)574-1119.

MCMILLAN, M Janette; 300-2902 Broadway W, Vancouver BC V6K 2G8; UBC'83; FRCPC; Psy. Staff, UBC Hospital - Koerner Pavillion; Clin Instructor, University of British Columbia; (604)730-8949

MCMILLAN, Merle K A; 201-100 Station Lane, Kentville NS B4N 0A3; UBC'86; CCFP; FCFP; (902)681-9410; Fax. (902)681-1058.

MCMILLAN, Morag J; Penticton Reg Hosp, 550 Carmi Ave, Penticton BC V2A 3G6; UBC'96; CCFP; CCFP(E.M.); Staff, Penticton Regional Hospital; (250)492-4000 x2401

MCMILLAN, Patricia M; SMBD Jewish Gen Hosp, 3755 ch Cote-Sainte-Catherine, Montreal QC H3T 1E2; Man'84; FRCPC; IntMed; Critical Care Medicine (P.Q.); Anes. Staff, Sir Mortimer B Davis Jewish General; (514)340-8222

MCMILLAN, Patrick R; PO Box 4396 Stn Main, Ponoka AB T4J 1R7; Cal'79; CCFP; Staff, Centennial Centre for Mental Health & Brain Injury; (403)783-7643; Fax. (403)783-7790.

MCMILLAN, Richard W; Niagara Rehab, 547 Glenridge Ave, St Catharines ON L2T 4C2; McM'95; BSc(Kinesiol); FRCPC; PhysMed&Rehab. Consultant, Niagara Health System - Greater Niagara General Site; Consultant, Niagara Health System - St Catharines General Site; Staff, Hôtel Dieu Shaver Health & Rehabilitation Centre; Consultant Privil, Niagara Health System - Welland Hospital Site; (905)685-1381 x85306; Fax. (905)687-3244.

MCMILLAN, Robert E; Quest Community Health Centre, 100-145 Queenston St, St Catharines ON L2R 2Z9; Qns'89; (905)688-2558

MCMILLAN, Ronald V; William Osler HC-Etobicoke, 101 Humber College Blvd, Etobicoke ON M9V 1R8; Ott'84; FRCPC; EmergMed. Staff, William Osler Health System - Etobicoke General Hospital; (416)494-2120

MCMILLAN, Sharon K; 326 Wilson St E, Ancaster ON L9G 2C2; McM'81; CCFP; FCFP; Staff, Hamilton Health Sciences Centre; (905)648-1517

MCMILLAN, Stephen J; College Care Walk-In Clinic, 351 College St, Toronto ON M5T 1S5; Tor'06; CCFP; (416)915-9285

MCMILLAN, Victor C S; Penticton Reg Hosp, 550 Carmi Ave, Penticton BC V2A 3G6; UBC'96; FRCPC; DiagRad. Staff, Penticton Regional Hospital; (250)492-4000

MCMILLAN, William G; The Juravinski Cancer Centre, 699 Concession St, Hamilton ON L8V 5C2; National (Ireland)'90; MB ChB; BAO; MSc; FRCPC; RadOncol. Asst Prof Oncology, McMaster University; (905)387-9495

MCMILLIN, Robert S; 4 King Street Cres, York ON M9N 1K6; Tor'54; BPHE; CCFP; Ac Staff, Humber River Regional Hospital - Church Street Site; (416)248-0283; Fax. (416)248-2977; rmcmillin@hrrh.on.ca.

MCMORRAN, John D R; Vancouver Family Health Centre, 100-2732 Hastings St E, Vancouver BC V5K 1Z9; McG'75; BSc(Hon)Zoo; Ac Staff, Providence Health Care - St Paul's Hospital; Asst Prof Family Med, University of British Columbia; Langs: English; French; (604)253-3166; Fax. (604)253-2048.

MCMULLEN, David H; Fredericton Med Clinic, 302-1015 Regent St, Fredericton NB E3B 6H5; Dal'71; FRCPC; IntMed. (506)458-0215; Fax. (506)458-0478.

MCMULLEN, David M; Riverside Psychiatric Consulta, 312-4411 16 Ave NW, Calgary AB T3B 0M3; Cal'90; FRCPC; Psy (Bipolar Disease). (403)571-5160; Fax. (403)571-5167.

MCMULLEN, Mark A; Dartmouth Gen Hosp, 325 Pleasant St, Dartmouth NS B2Y 4G8; Ott'98; CCFP; CCFP(E.M.); Staff, Dartmouth General Hospital; (902)465-8300

MCMULLEN, Michael C; Kingston Gen Hosp, 76 Stuart St, Kingston ON K7L 2V7; Qns'01; FRCPC; Anes. Staff, Kingston General Hospital; (613)548-3232

MCMULLEN, Sarah M; Queen Elizabeth II HSC, 376-1276 South Park St, Halifax NS B3H 2Y9; McM'05; FRCPC; IntMed (Critical Care Medicine). Staff, Queen Elizabeth II Health Sciences Centre - Victoria General Site; (902)473-3608; Fax. (902)473-3610.

MCMULLEN, Todd P; University of Alberta Hosp, 2D4 41WMC-8440 112 St NW, Edmonton AB T6G 2B7; Tor'02; FACS; FRCSC; GenSurg (Thyroid Diseases). Staff, University of Alberta Hospital; (780)407-1108; Fax. (780)407-2729.

MCMULLEN, William J M M; Sudbury Reg Hosp-SJHC, 700 Paris St, Sudbury ON P3E 3B5; McM'76; MSW; CCFP; CCFP(E.M.); FCFP; Court Staff, Espanola Regional Hospital and Health Centre; Court Staff, West Parry Sound Health Centre; Ac Staff, Health Sciences North-Laurentian Site; Staff, Health Sciences North-St Joseph's Health Centre; (705)674-3181

MCMULLEN, William R; 130-101 Queensway W, Mississauga ON L5B 2P7; Tor'76; FRCPC; IntMed; Gastroent., University of Toronto; (905)279-9397; Fax. (905)279-9401.

MCMULLIN, Joseph P; St Joseph's Healthcare, F533-50 Charlton Ave E, Hamilton ON L8N 4A6; McM'94; FRCPC; IntMed. Staff, St Joseph's Healthcare - Charlton Campus; Head Serv General IntMed/Asst Prof Med, McMaster University; (905)522-1155 x3134; Fax. (905)521-6068.

MCMURRAY, Lisa A; Royal Ottawa Hosp, 1145 Carling Ave, Ottawa ON K1Z 7K4; Tor'94; BSc; FRCPC; Psy (Geriatric Psychiatry). Staff, Royal Ottawa Mental Health Centre - Royal Ottawa Health Care Group; Langs: English; French; (613)722-6521 x6637; Fax. (613)798-2999.

MCMURRAY, Stephen J; 17 Central Ave E, Brockville ON K6V 1W5; Wes'81; CCFP; CCFP(E.M.); Staff, Brockville General Hospital - Charles Street; Staff, Providence Continuing Care Centre (PCCC) - St Vincent de Paul Hospital; (613)342-4386; Fax. (613)342-5410.

MCMURREN, Jaime L; Maternity Care Clinic, 109-178 96 Ave NE, Calgary AB T3K 6G4; Cal'03; CCFP; Staff, Maternity Care Clinic; (403)735-4922; Fax. (403)735-4901.

MCMURTRIE, Elissa J; BC Cancer Agency-Vanc Isl Ctr, 2410 Lee Ave, Victoria BC V8R 6V5; UBC'79; FRCSC; ObstGyn (Gynecologic Oncology). Ac Staff GynOncol, BC Cancer Agency Vancouver Island Centre; Ac Staff, Victoria General Hospital; Ac Staff, Vancouver Island Health Authority; Clin Instructor ObstGyn, University of British Columbia; (250)519-5571

MCMURTRY, Michael S; University of Alberta Hosp, 2C2-8440 112 St NW, Edmonton AB T6G 2B7; Dal'98; FRCPC; IntMed; Cardiol. Staff, University of Alberta Hospital; (780)407-2799

MCNAB, Brian D; Aberhart Centre 1, 8327-11402 University Ave NW, Edmonton AB T6G 2J3; Sask'90; BSc; DABSM; FRCPC; IntMed (Sleep Medicine); Respir. Staff, University of Alberta Hospital; (780)407-1348

MCNAB, Brian R; Tower B, 134-555 Legget Dr, Kanata ON K2K 2X3; Qns'76; FABMP; (613)599-9209

MCNAB, John W; Fall River Family Practice, PO Box 2160 Rpo Fall River 3060 Lake Thomas Dr, Fall River NS B2T 1K6; Tor'78; CCFP; FCFP; (902)861-2237; Fax. (902)861-1914.

MCNABB, Jamie A H M; 2-1 William St S, Lindsay ON K9V 3A3; Wes'95; BSc; FRCSC; GenSurg. Staff Surg, Ross Memorial Hospital; (705)324-8197; Fax. (705)324-8557.

MCNABB, Trudy C; Pine Seven Med Centre, 150-4600 Highway 7, Woodbridge ON L4L 4Y7; Tor'84; CCFP; FCFP; Staff, William Osler Health System - Etobicoke General Hospital; (905)856-1000; Fax. (905)851-9927.

MCNABB-BALTAR, Julia; Ctr Hosp Anna-Laberge, 200 boul Brisebois, Chateauguay QC J6K 4W8; Mon'07; FRCPC; IntMed; Gastroent. Staff, Hôpital Anna-Laberge; (450)699-2425

MCNAIR, David J; The Group Health Centre, 240 McNabb St, Sault Ste. Marie ON P6B 1Y5; Glasgow (Scotland)'62; MB ChB; DMRD; FRCPC; DiagRad (Diagnostic Imaging). Staff Diagnostic Imaging/Chief Dept, Group Health Centre; (705)759-5553; Fax. (705)759-7477.

MCNAIR, Nora L; Smith Clinic, 1-6601 48 Ave, Camrose AB T4V 3G8; Alb'96; CCFP; FCFP; (780)672-2425; Fax. (780)608-5895.

MCNAIR, Susan M; St Joseph's Family Med Centre, 346 Platt's Lane, London ON N6G 1J1; Tor'86; MClSc; CCFP; FCFP; Teach Staff Chair & Med/Dir Regional Sexual Assault & Domestic Violence Prog, St Joseph's Hospital - St Joseph's Health Care; Assoc Prof Family Med, University of Western Ontario; (519)672-9660; Fax. (519)672-7727.

MCNALLY, Catherine E; EKM Community Hlth Centre, 23 Earnscliffe Ave, Wolfville NS B4P 1X4; Tor'95; BA; FABHPM; CCFP; (902)542-2139; Fax. (902)542-6607; cmcnally@avdha.nshealth.ca.

MCNALLY, Catherine M; Balmoral Med Arts Facility, 305-1366 Yonge St, Toronto ON M4T 3A7; Qns'77; CCFP; (416)962-2273; Fax. (416)962-2526.

MCNALLY, Dermot M; Dept of Diagnostic Imaging, 132 University Campus NW, Edmonton AB T6G 2R7; (Ireland)'93; MB BCh; Staff, University of Alberta Hospital; (780)935-3749

MCNALLY, James D; Children's Hosp of Eastern Ont, 3002C-401 Smyth Rd, Ottawa ON K1H 8L1; Dal'05; FRCPC; Peds; Critical Care Medicine. Fellow, Children's Hospital of Eastern Ontario (CHEO); (613)737-7600

MCNALLY, James W; Downtown Toronto Doctors, 630-790 Bay St, Toronto ON M5G 1N8; Alb'78; (647)427-6001; Fax. (416)598-4659.

MCNALLY, Katherine; Queen Elizabeth Hosp, PO Box 6600 Stn Central 60 Riverside Dr, Charlottetown PE C1A 8T5; Dal'98; BSc; CCFP; FCFP; Staff, Queen Elizabeth Hospital; (902)367-3747

MCNALLY, Linda J; 71 Silver Maple Cres, Barrie ON L4N 8S8; McM'98; BSc; CCFP; Staff, Canadian Forces Health Services Centre; (705)792-6237

MCNAMA, Patricia M; Univ Hlth Network-Toronto Gen, 200 Elizabeth St, Toronto ON M5G 2C4; Tor'75; FRCPC; Anes. Staff Anes, Toronto General Hospital - UHN; (416)340-4800 x3242; Fax. (416)340-3698; patricia.mcnama@uhn.on.ca.

MCNAMARA, Brian T; St Mary's Gen Hosp, 911 Queens Blvd, Kitchener ON N2M 1B2; Dal'86; FRCPC; IntMed; Cardiol. Staff, St Mary's General Hospital; (519)744-3311

MCNAMARA, Daniel; Hop Charles LeMoyne, 3120 boul Taschereau, Greenfield Park QC J4V 2H1; Mon'83; NuclearMed. Staff, Hopital Charles LeMoyne; (450)466-5000

MCNAMARA, G Patrick; College of Phys & Surg of Ont, 80 College St, Toronto ON M5G 2E2; McM'74; CCFP; FCFP; Asst Prof Family Med, College of Physicians & Surgeons of Ontario; Asst Prof Family Med, University of Toronto; (416)967-2600 x380; Fax. (416)967-2616.

MCNAMARA, Jeffrey J; London HSC-University Hosp, PO Box 5339 Stn B 339 Windermere Rd, London ON N6A 5A5; McM'96; FRCPC; Anes. Staff, London Health Sciences Centre - University Hospital; (519)685-8500

MCNAMARA, Laura A; PO Box 1120, Wiarton ON N0H 2T0; Ott'91; CCFP; CCFP(E.M.); FCFP; Staff, Grand River Hospital - Kitchener/Waterloo Health Centre; (519)534-5253

MCNAMARA, Martin A J; Huronia District Hosp, PO Box 760 Stn Main 1112 St Andrew's Dr, Midland ON L4R 4P4; McM'95; CCFP; CCFP(E.M.); Chief Staff, Georgian Bay General Hospital - Midland; Langs: Bilingual(English/French); (705)528-4368; Fax. (705)549-0373.

MCNAMARA, Patrick J; The Hosp for Sick Children, 555 University Ave, Toronto ON M5G 1X8; Belfast (Ireland)'93; Staff Div of Neonatology, The Hospital For Sick Children; Assoc Prof Pediatrics, University of Toronto; (416)813-5773; Fax. (416)813-5245; patrick.mcnamara@sickkids.ca.

MCNAUGHT, Andrew F; Sunnybrook Hlth Sciences Ctre, 2075 Bayview Ave, Toronto ON M4N 3M5; London (England)'97; FRCPC; Anes. Staff, Sunnybrook Health Sciences Centre; (416)480-6100

MCNAUGHT, Jennifer L; Women's Hosp, WS029-735 Notre Dame Ave, Winnipeg MB R3E 0L8; Tor'99; BSc(HK); FRCSC; ObstGyn (Pediatric & Adolescent Gynecology). Asst Prof, University of Manitoba; (204)787-2995; Fax. (204)787-1692; jmcnaught@hsc.mb.ca.

MCNAUGHT, John J; London Med Arts Bldg, 406-746 Baseline Rd, London ON N6C 5Z2; Man'01; FRCSC; ObstGyn. Staff ObstGyn, St Thomas Elgin General Hospital; Staff, London Health Sciences Centre - Victoria Campus.

MCNAUGHTON, Jennifer L; 204-5 Quarry Ridge Rd, Barrie ON L4M 7G1; Cal'06; CCFP; Staff, Royal Victoria Regional Health Centre; (705)735-4944; Fax. (705)728-8583.

MCNAUGHTON-FILION, M Louise; Montfort Hosp, 713 Montreal Rd, Ottawa ON K1K 0T2; McG'87; CCFP; CCFP(E.M.); FCFP; Staff Emerg Med, Montfort Hospital; (613)748-4908; Fax. (613)748-4914.

MCNAULL, Benjamin B A; Couchiching Family Health Team, 104-119 Memorial Ave, Orillia ON L3V 5X1; Belfast (Ireland)'09; MB ChB; CCFP; (705)326-7727

MCNAULL, M Elizabeth; Couchiching Family Health Team, 104-119 Memorial Ave, Orillia ON L3V 5X1; Dal'09; CCFP; (705)326-7727; Fax. (705)329-0352.

MCNEELY, David J; Univ Hlth Network-Toronto Western Hosp, EW8 416-399 Bathurst St, Toronto ON M5T 2S8; Tor'71; FRCPC; IntMed (Infectious Diseases). Staff InfectDis, Toronto Western Hospital - University Health Network; Asst Prof Med & Microbiol, University of Toronto; (416)603-5282; Fax. (416)603-6495; david.mcneely@uhn.on.ca.

MCNEELY, Joni M; PO Box 279, Gleichen AB T0J 1N0; Cal'90; CCFP; (403)734-3434; Fax. (403)734-3389.

MCNEELY, Michael P; 272 Oxford St W, London ON N6H 1S9; Qns'02; FRCPC; Peds (Pediatric Dermatology). Aj Prof Peds, University of Western Ontario; (519)434-1112

MCNEELY, P Daniel; IWK Health Centre, PO Box 9700 Rpo CSC 5850-5980 University Ave, Halifax NS B3K 6R8; Ott'97; BMedSci; FRCSC; Neursurg (Pediatric Neuro Surgery). Staff, IWK Health Centre; Asst Prof, Dalhousie University; Langs: French; (902)470-7476; Fax. (902)470-7454; dmcneely@dal.ca.

MCNEELY, Patrick D; Surrey Mem Hosp, 13750 96 Ave, Surrey BC V3V 1Z2; McG'89; FRCPC; Anes (Ambulatory Anesthesia). Staff Anes, Surrey Memorial Hospital; Man Partner/Dir Anes., Valley Surgery Centre; (604)588-3367

MCNEELY, T Bruce D; Royal Inland Hosp, 311 Columbia St, Kamloops BC V2C 2T1; UBC'74; BSc; DABPath(AP,CP); AnatPath; GenPath. Ac Staff Path, Royal Inland Hospital; Langs: English; French; (250)314-3353

MCNEIL, Bernadette; St Paul Family Health Network, 99 Wayne Gretzky Pky, Brantford ON N3S 6T6; McM'95; Staff, The Brant Community Healthcare System - Brantford General Hospital Site; Staff, Cambridge Memorial Hospital; (519)756-6400; Fax. (519)756-7343.

MCNEIL, Ceara J; London HSC-Victoria Hosp, 800 Commissioners Rd E, London ON N6A 5W9; Qns'07; CCFP; CCFP(E.M.); Staff, London Health Sciences Centre - Victoria Campus; (519)685-8500

MCNEIL, Gordon; Foothills Med Centre, C231-1403 29 St NW, Calgary AB T2N 2T9; Alb'92; FRCPC; EmergMed. Staff, Foothills Medical Centre; (403)944-1635

MCNEIL, Karen A; Cowie Family Med Centre, 16 Dentith Rd, Halifax NS B3R 2H9; Dal'87; CCFP; FCFP; (902)473-1234; Fax. (902)473-4353.

MCNEIL, Kevin S; Bay Medical Clinic, 65 Minto St, Glace Bay NS B1A 5B5; Dal'80; FRCPC; IntMed. (902)849-5521; Fax. (902)849-5522.

MCNEIL, Marie-Sophie; CSSS de la Baie-des-Chaleurs, RR 2 419 boul Perron, Maria QC G0C 1Y0; Mon'94; Staff, CSSS de la Baie-des-Chaleurs; (418)759-3443

MCNEIL, Nancy L; Colchester East Hants Hlth Ctr, 600 Abenaki Rd, Truro NS B2N 5A1; Dal'96; DiagRad. Staff, Colchester East Hants Health Centre; (902)893-5508; Fax. (902)892-5534.

MCNEIL, Shelly A; Queen Elizabeth II HSC, 5014-1276 South Park Dr, Halifax NS B3H 2Y9; Dal'94; MD; InfectDis; IntMed (Vaccination). Staff, Queen Elizabeth II Health Sciences Centre - Victoria General Site; Asst Prof, Dalhousie University; (902)473-8477; Fax. (902)473-7394; shelly.mcneil@cdha.nshealth.ca.

MCNEIL, Stephen M; Foothills Med Centre, AC142-1403 29 St NW, Calgary AB T2N 2T9; McM'97; FRCPC; PhysMed&Rehab (Spasticity Management). Staff, Rockyview General Hospital; Staff, Foothills Medical Centre; (403)944-4226; Fax. (403)283-2526; stephen.mcneil@calgaryhealthregion.ca.

MCNEILL, Ann M; Health Sciences Ctr Gen Hosp, 700 William Ave, Winnipeg MB R3E 0Z3; Sask'77; DAB(Anes); FRCPC; Anes. Head Ped Anes, Health Sciences Centre; Assoc Prof, University of Manitoba; amcneill@hsc.mb.ca.

MCNEILL, Colin A; The Heights Med Centre, 4446 Hastings St, Burnaby BC V5C 2K2; London (England)'61; MB BS; DObstRCOG; Fam Med, Arrow Lakes Hospital; (604)298-4491

MCNEILL, David G; Canadian Mental Health Assn, 60 Bond St W, Oshawa ON L1G 1A5; Tor'90; Staff/Med Dir Integrated Hlth Servcs, Ontario Shores Centre for Mental Health Sciences; (905)436-8760; Fax. (905)436-9313.

MCNEILL, Jeanne M; 209-44 Mapleton Rd, Moncton NB E1C 7W8; Alb'85; Member, The Moncton Hospital; (506)853-5080; Fax. (506)857-1089.

MCNEILL, Laurie K; Dr Laurie McNeill Inc, PO Box 325 100 Hawthorn Rd, Mahone Bay NS B0J 2E0; Dal'65; FRCPC; Peds. (902)531-2181

MCNEILL, Michelle M; London HSC-Victoria Hosp, PO Box 5010 Stn B 800 Commissioners Rd E, London ON N6A 5W9; Ott'92; Peds. Staff General Academic, Children's Hospital of Western Ontario; Staff, London Health Sciences Centre - Victoria Campus; Teach Staff, University of Western Ontario; (519)685-8500; Fax. (519)685-8156.

MCNEILL, Monica L; Summerside Med Centre, 101-475 Granville St, Summerside PE C1N 3N9; Dal'78; Staff, Prince County Hospital; (902)432-8167; Fax. (902)436-9660.

MCNEILLY, Kenneth A; 10-137 Division St N, Kingsville ON N9Y 1E3; Belfast (Ireland)'63; MB ChB; BAO; Ac Staff, Leamington District Memorial Hospital.

MCNEILLY, Nancy E; PO Box 88004 Rpo Rabbit Hill, Edmonton AB T6R 0M5; Alb'94; Staff, Covenant Health - Misericordia Community Hospital.

MCNERN, John K; 105-2231 Louie Dr, Kelowna BC V4T 3K3; UBC'96; CCFP; (250)768-6985

MCNESTRY, Ailve M; College of Phys & Surg of BC, 300-669 Howe St, Vancouver BC V6C 0B4; Dublin (Ireland)'77; MB ChB; BAO; CCFP; (604)733-7758

MCNESTRY, Fergus G; Peterborough Reg HC-Hospital, 1 Hospital Dr, Peterborough ON K9J 7C6; Dublin (Ireland)'78; MB ChB; BAO; DCH; DObst; MRCPsy; FRCPC; Psy (Anxiety Disorder). Staff, Peterborough Regional Health Centre - Hospital Drive; Asst Prof, Queen's University; (705)876-5028; Fax. (705)876-5013.

MCNEVIN, Stephen H; Queen's University, 146 Stuart St, Kingston ON K7L 2V8; Qns'80; FRCPC; Psy. Att Staff, Providence Care - Mental Health Services; Assoc Staff, Hotel-Dieu Hospital; Assoc Staff, Kingston General Hospital; Dir Div of Psy Health Counselling & Disability Services, Queen's University; (613)533-2508; Fax. (613)533-2347; mcnevins@providence.ca.

MCNICHOL, Kim L; Humber River Reg Hosp-Keele, L1-2175 Keele St, York ON M6M 3Z4; Alb'95; FRCPC; Psy. Staff, Humber River Regional Hospital - Keele Street Site; (416)658-2022; Fax. (416)658-2074.

MCNICHOLAS, P John; Terrace On The Square, 8-10 Rowan St, St. John's NL A1B 2X1; National (Ireland)'77; MB ChB; BAO; FRCSC; Ophth (Anterior Segment).

MCNICHOLAS, Peter G; Penticton Reg Hosp, 550 Carmi Ave, Penticton BC V2A 3G6; Mem'84; FRCPC; DiagRad. (250)492-4000; Fax. (250)492-9094.

MCNICOL, Keith L; Queen Street Place, 201-505 Queen St, Spruce Grove AB T7X 2V2; UBC'85; (780)962-9888; Fax. (780)960-5298.

MCNICOLL, Annie; CSSS de l'Arhipel, 430 ch Principal, Cap-aux-Meules QC G4T 1R9; Sher'10; CCFP; Staff, Hôpital de l'Archipel; (418)986-2121

MCNICOLL, Johanne; 102-2854 rue Wilfrid-Legare, Quebec QC G1V 2H2; Laval'74; (418)659-3636; Fax. (418)659-7664.

MCNICOLL, Julie; Dept de Psychiatrie, 18 rue Saint-Omer, Levis QC G6V 5C2; Laval'03; FRCPC; Psy (Geriatric Psychiatry). (418)835-7155

MCNICOLL, Serge; CSSS de Saint-Jerome, 290 rue de Montigny, Saint-Jerome QC J7Z 5T3; Mon'93; Cardiol (P.Q.) (Echocardiography). Staff, Hôtel-Dieu de Saint-Jérôme; (450)431-8200 x2033; Fax. (450)431-8304.

MCNIE, R Scott; Caledonian Clinic, 340 Campbell St, Nanaimo BC V9R 3G7; Glasgow (Scotland)'74; (250)753-3202

MCNIECE, Lynne; 6 Grandor Crt, Scarborough ON M1E 1E1; McM'73; MSW; MHSc; (416)269-7570

MCPARLAND, Columba; Queen Elizabeth II HSC-Halifax, 4459-1796 Summer St, Halifax NS B3H 3A7; Dublin (Ireland)'82; MB ChB; BAO; FRCPC; IntMed (Chronic Obstructive Pulmonary Disease); Respir. Staff, Queen Elizabeth II Health Sciences Centre - Halifax Infirmary Site; Assoc Prof Med, Dalhousie University; (902)473-3698; Fax. (902)473-6202.

MCPEAK, Brian K; Dominion Health Centre, 2383 111 St NW, Edmonton AB T6J 5E5; Alb'93; BSc; CCFP; (780)436-0020

MCPHADEN, John; 118-1060 Speers Rd, Oakville ON L6L 2X4; Tor'84; FRCPC; IntMed; Hem (Thrombosis). Court Staff, The Credit Valley Hospital; Ac Staff, Halton Healthcare Services Corporation - Oakville Site; (905)815-8914; Fax. (905)815-8920; johnmcphaden@bellnet.ca.

MCPHAIL, Janice E; Loyalist Family Practice, 2A-150 Sidney St, Belleville ON K8P 5E2; Qns'81; (613)771-0008; Fax. (613)771-1861.

MCPHAIL, Marianne A; East Toronto Health Clinic, 1496 Danforth Ave, Toronto ON M4J 1N4; Tor'75; CCFP; (416)778-1496; Fax. (416)778-1400.

MCPHALEN, Donald F; Alberta Children's Hosp, 2888 Shaganappi Trail NW, Calgary AB T3B 6A8; Alb'82; FRCSC; PlasSurg (Pediatrics). Staff Ped Surg, Alberta Children's Hospital; Asst Prof, University of Calgary; (403)955-7570

MCPHEDRAN, Amy M; U of Guelph Student Hlth Serv, 158-50 Stone Rd E, Guelph ON N1G 2W1; Qns'01; CCFP; (519)824-4120 x52131

MCPHEDRAN, Margaret; Allin Clinic, 10155 120 St NW, Edmonton AB T5K 2A2; Alb'01; CCFP; (780)482-7551

MCPHEDRAN, Peter D; 70 Victoria St RR 5, Elora ON N0B 1S0; Cal'78; CCFP; FCFP; Ac Staff, Groves Memorial Community Hospital; Clinical Asst Prof Family Med, McMaster University; (519)846-5841; Fax. (519)846-8453.

MCPHEE, James S; 90 Baldry Bay, Winnipeg MB R3T 3C4; Man'73; FRC; BSc; LMCC; FCPA; DPsy; FRCPC; Psy (Community Psychiatry). Langs: Bilingual(French/English); (204)942-3813; jsemcphee@hotmail.com.

MCPHEE, Lisa C; Manitoba X-Ray Clinic, 3263 Portage Ave, Winnipeg MB R3K 0W6; Man'06; DiagRad.

MCPHEE, Michael; Cobequid Commun Health Centre, 40 Freer Lane, Lower Sackville NS B4C 0A2; Dal'91; FRCPC; DiagRad. Staff, Queen Elizabeth II Health Sciences Centre - Victoria General Site; Staff, Cobequid Community Health Centre; (902)869-6528; Fax. (902)869-6121.

MCPHEE, Nancy; Health Research Innovation Ctr, 402-3280 Hospital Dr NW, Calgary AB T2N 4Z6; Cal'93; CCFP; Physician, Health Research Innovation Centre.

MCPHERRIN, Lawrence; Cochrane Family Health Team, PO Box 2050 233 8th St, Cochrane ON P0L 1C0; McG'86; CCFP; FCFP; (705)272-4331; Fax. (705)272-2638.

MCPHERSON, Alan L; Bigelow Fowler Clinic West, 30 Jerry Potts Blvd W, Lethbridge AB T1K 5M5; McG'73; Ac Staff, Chinook Regional Hospital; Ac Staff, Covenant Health - St Michael's Health Centre; (403)381-8444; Fax. (403)381-8166.

MCPHERSON, Alexandra M C; Misericordia Community Hosp, 16940 87 Ave NW, Edmonton AB T5R 4H5; Cal'01; FRCPC; Psy. Staff, Covenant Health - Misericordia Community Hospital; (780)735-2594; Fax. (780)735-2595.

MCPHERSON, Brian K; Kirkland & Dis Hosp, PO Box 3000 Stn Main 145 Government Rd E, Kirkland Lake ON P2N 3P4; Univ of Queensland (Australia)'04; CCFP; Staff, Kirkland & District Hospital; (705)568-2203

MCPHERSON, Christa L; Ridgeview Med Centre, 212-1240 Railway Ave, Canmore AB T1W 1P4; UBC'07; BSc; CCFP; (403)609-8333; Fax. (403)609-3666.

MCPHERSON, David E; 48-4324 rue Sherbrooke O, Westmount QC H3Z 1E1; McG'76; FRCPC; Psy. Sr Staff Psy, McGill University Health Centre - Montreal General Campus; Asst Prof Psy, McGill University; Langs: English; French; (514)935-2425

MCPHERSON, Ewan C; 29 Brunel Rd, Huntsville ON P1H 1P4; St. Andrews (Scotland)'68; (705)784-2098; Fax. (705)787-5718.

MCPHERSON, Duncan; Laurel Med Centre, 308-888 8th Ave W, Vancouver BC V5Z 3Y1; Wes'56; MSc(UBC); AB; FRCSC; OrthSurg. Hon Staff, Vancouver General Hospital - Centennial Pavillion; (604)874-4717

MCPHERSON, Isla L; Glenrose Rehab Hosp, 10230 111 Ave NW, Edmonton AB T5G 0B7; McM'06; CCFP; Staff, Glenrose Rehabilitation Hospital; (780)735-7943; Fax. (780)735-8838.

MCPHERSON, John A M; Health Sciences Centre, AD415-820 Sherbrook St, Winnipeg MB R3A 1R9; Man'79; FRCSC; OrthSurg. Assoc Staff Ped Orth, Health Sciences Centre; Asst Prof Surg, University of Manitoba; (204)774-6511

MCPHERSON, John; Queen Elizabeth II HSC-Halifax, 4017-1796 Summer St, Halifax NS B3H 3A7; Alb'05; CCFP; Staff, Queen Elizabeth II Health Sciences Centre - Halifax Infirmary Site; (902)473-2220

MCPHERSON, Kathleen E; Nanaimo Mental Hlth & Addictio, 201-2000 Island Hwy N, Nanaimo BC V9S 5W3; Aberdeen (Scotland)'69; MB ChB; FRCPC; Psy. Staff, Nanaimo Regional General Hospital; Consultant, Nanaimo Mental Health Services; (250)739-5797; Fax. (250)739-5739.

MCPHERSON, P Ruth; Univ of Ottawa Heart Institute, H4203-40 Ruskin St, Ottawa ON K1Y 4W7; Tor'84; PhD; FACP; FRCPC; IntMed (Diabetes); Endocrin (P.Q.); Endocrin&Metab. Staff, University of Ottawa Heart Institute; Att Staff, The Ottawa Hospital - Civic Campus; Prof, University of Ottawa; Langs: English; French; (613)761-5257; Fax. (613)761-5281; rmcpherson@ottawaheart.ca.

MCPHERSON, Sarah; Foothills Med Centre, C231-1403 29 St NW, Calgary AB T2N 2T9; Cal'99; FRCPC; EmergMed. Staff, Foothills Medical Centre; (403)827-3053

MCPHERSON, Terrence P; Cardiology Consultants, 101-99 Airport Rd, St. John's NL A1A 4Y3; Mem'03; FRCPC; IntMed; Cardiol. Staff, Health Sciences Centre; (709)726-5311; Fax. (709)726-1028; cardiologyconsultants@nfld.net.

MCQUAID, Melanie A; Queen Elizabeth Hosp, PO Box 6600 Stn Central 60 Riverside Dr, Charlottetown PE C1A 8T5; McM'06; FRCPC; DiagRad. Staff, Queen Elizabeth Hospital; (902)894-2111

MCQUAID, Melissa C; Miramichi East Med Clinic, 4 Johnson Ave, Miramichi NB E1N 3B7; Mem'06; CCFP; Staff, The Moncton Hospital; Staff, Miramichi Regional Hospital; (506)773-3333; Fax. (506)778-8719.

MCQUARRIE, Lucinda J; Fort Family Practice Assoc, PO Box 99 stn Fort Langely 23148 96 Ave, Langley BC V1M 2R4; UBC'07; CCFP; (604)888-2433

MCQUARRIE, Shauna L; Nine Circles Comm Health Ctre, 705 Broadway, Winnipeg MB R3G 0X2; Man'94; BSc; CCFP; (204)940-6000; Fax. (204)940-6003.

MCQUEEN, Jodi L; Brant Comm HS-Brantford Gen, 200 Terrace Hill St, Brantford ON N3R 1G9; Qns'05; CCFP; CCFP(E.M.); Staff, The Brant Community Healthcare System - Brantford General Hospital Site; (519)752-7871

MCQUEEN, Keith R; McKenzie Prof Centre, 200-1595 McKenzie Ave, Victoria BC V8N 1A4; UBC'85; BSc; Staff, Vancouver Island Health Authority; (250)721-4105; Fax. (250)721-4213.

MCQUEEN, Matthew J; Hamilton HS-General Site, 1 60-237 Barton St E, Hamilton ON L8L 2X2; Glasgow (Scotland)'68; MB ChB; PhD; FRCPC; MedBiochem (Clinical Lipid Disorders). Staff, Hamilton Health Sciences Centre - Hamilton General Hospital; Prof, McMaster University; (905)527-4322 x46100; Fax. (905)577-8027.

MCQUIBBAN, George A; William Osler HC-Brampton, 2100 Bovaird Dr E, Brampton ON L6R 3J7; Tor'63; Staff, William Osler Health System - Brampton Civic Hospital; (905)494-2120

MCQUISTON, Terence; Donway Place, 8 The Donway E, North York ON M3C 3R7; Tor'76; Physician, Extendicare Scarborough; Physician, Christie Gardens Apts & Care; (416)445-7555

MCRAE, Andrew D; North Hill Centre, 1633-1632 14 Ave NW, Calgary AB T2N 1M7; Dal'02; FRCPC; EmergMed.

MCRAE, Harold P; Summerside Med Centre, 475 Granville St N, Summerside PE C1N 1N9; Dal'10.

MCRAE, Karen M; 585 University Ave, Toronto ON M5G 2N2; McG'88; Anes. Staff, Toronto General Hospital - UHN; (416)340-3242; Fax. (416)340-3698.

MCRAE, Shelagh M; 70 Meredith St PO Box 219, Gore Bay ON P0P 1H0; Alb'79; DObst(NZ); CCFP; FCFP; Coroner, City of Sudbury District 19; Asst Prof/Clin Teacher Family Med Program, Northern Ontario School of Medicine-Laurentian University; (705)282-2262; Fax. (705)282-2370.

MCREELIS, Kylen D; Peterborough Clinic, 26 Hospital Dr, Peterborough ON K9J 7C3; Tor'00; FRCSC; Ophth. (705)740-6879; Fax. (705)740-6865.

MCRITCHIE, Donna I; North York Gen Hosp, 102-4001 Leslie St, North York ON M2K 1E1; Tor'85; MD; BSc; MSc; ABS; FRCSC; GenSurg (Critical Care Medicine). Chief GenSurg/Med Dir Critical Care/Chair Med Advisory Committee, North York General Hospital; Asst Prof Surg, University of Toronto; (416)756-6906; Fax. (416)756-6909; donna.mcritchie@nygh.on.ca.

MCROBERT, Elizabeth A; Halifax Prof Centre, 425-5991 Spring Garden Rd, Halifax NS B3H 1Y6; Dublin (Ireland)'80; FRCPC; Peds. Staff, IWK Health Centre; Lecturer Ped, Dalhousie University; (902)422-5399; Fax. (902)422-6988.

MCSHANE, Lucy M; Lynn Valley Med & Travel Clin, 102-1200 Lynn Valley Rd, North Vancouver BC V7J 2A2; Dublin (Ireland)'82; MB ChB; BAO; LMCC; CCFP; (604)988-3747; Fax. (604)988-5339; lucymmcshane@hotmail.com.

MCSORLEY, John J; 201-836 1 Ave NW, Airdrie AB T4B 0V2; Dublin (Ireland)'83; MB ChB; BAO; DRCOG(UK); MRC; (403)948-6422; Fax. (403)948-4492.

MCSWEEN, Anne; Centre de Sante Carillon, 20 rue de Carillon, Sherbrooke QC J1J 2K8; Sher'84; Staff, International Board Certified Lactation Consultant; Staff, Registered Lactation Consultant; Langs: Bilingual(French/English); (819)564-1022; Fax. (819)564-0218.

MCSWEEN, Audrey; CSSS de Saint-Jerome, 290 rue de Montigny, Saint-Jerome QC J7Z 5T3; Mon'99; FRCPC; Anes. Staff, Hôtel-Dieu de Saint-Jérôme; (450)432-2777

MCSWEEN, Charles; Clinique Med Havre Sante, 521 boul du Havre, Salaber-de-Valleyf QC J6S 4Z5; Mon'78; (450)371-6444; Fax. (450)371-5315.

MCTAGGART, Dawn-Lynn M; Birchwood Med Clinic, 2416 Portage Ave, Winnipeg MB R3J 0M8; Man'95; CCFP; Staff, Teulon/Hunter Memorial Hospital.

MCTAGGART COWAN, Robert A; Foothills Med Centre, 1403 29 St NW, Calgary AB T2N 2T9; Mem'90; FRCPC; Anes. Staff Anes, Foothills Medical Centre; (403)944-1430

MCTAVISH, William G B; Heartland Fertility & Gyne Cli, 701-1661 Portage Ave, Winnipeg MB R3J 3T7; Man'85; FRCSC; ObstGyn. (204)779-8888

MCTAVISH, Wyatt; The Centre for Family Medicine, 10B Victoria St S, Kitchener ON N2G 1C5; (Ireland)'10; CCFP; (519)783-0021

MCTIMONEY, C A Michelle; IWK Health Centre, PO Box 9700 Rpo CSC 5850-5980 University Ave, Halifax NS B3K 6R8; Dal'96; FRCPC; Peds. Staff, IWK Health Centre; (902)428-8823

MCTURK, Bruce E; Grove Park Home, 234 Cook St, Barrie ON L4M 4H5; McM'85; Staff, Royal Victoria Regional Health Centre; Med Dir, Grove Park Home; Med Dir, Coleman Care Centre; (705)728-7135; Fax. (705)728-3770; bmcturk@groveparkhome.on.ca.

MCVEIGH, Sonja A; Nova Scotia Rehab Centre, 207-1341 Summer St, Halifax NS B3H 4K4; McM'01; FRCPC; PhysMed&Rehab (Spinal Cord Injury). Staff/Asst Prof, Nova Scotia Rehabilitation Centre; (902)473-1409; Fax. (902)473-3204.

MCVEY, J Terrence; Medical Clinic, PO Box 386 12 Alder Cres, Deep River ON K0J 1P0; Ott'85; Gen Practice, Deep River & District Hospital; (613)584-3398; Fax. (613)584-9340.

MCVEY, Jennifer J; Queen Elizabeth II HSC-Halifax, 3021-1796 Summer St, Halifax NS B3H 3A7; McM'01; MSc; BSc; FRCPC; EmergMed. Staff, Queen Elizabeth II Health Sciences Centre - Halifax Infirmary Site; (902)473-7070; Fax. (902)473-3617; mcveyj@dal.ca.

MCVICAR, Jason A J; Univ Hlth Network-Toronto Western Hosp, 399 Bathurst St, Toronto ON M5T 2S8; Man'07; FRCPC; Anes. Staff, Toronto Western Hospital - University Health Network; (416)603-2581

MCVICAR, Stephen F; 2197 Columbia Ave PO Box 789, Rossland BC V0G 1Y0; Dal'88; BSc; BMechEng; FRCSC; OrthSurg (Sports Medicine). Staff, Kootenay Boundary Regional Hospital; (250)362-7565; Fax. (250)362-7566.

MCVICKER, Charles R; Atlantic Offshore Med Services, 4 Henry St, St. John's NL A1C 1R5; Mem'89; CCBOM; MBA; CCFP; CCFP(E.M.); FCFP; (709)722-4074; cmcvicker@aoms.nf.net.

MCWATTERS, Dorothy L; Hycroft Med Bldg, 119-3195 Granville St, Vancouver BC V6H 3K2; Qns'66; FRCPC; Psy. Staff, Vancouver General Hospital - Centennial Pavillion; (604)267-2287

MCWHAE, John A; Script Med Bldg, 201-506 71 Ave SW, Calgary AB T2V 4V4; Alb'86; BMedSci; FRCSC; Ophth (Ocular Oncology). Court Staff, Canmore General Hospital; Consultant, Alberta Children's Hospital; Ac Staff Privil, Rockyview General Hospital; Clin Assoc Prof, University of Calgary; (403)640-1900; Fax. (403)640-4858.

MCWHINNEY, Murray A; 410-125 13th St E, North Vancouver BC V7L 2L3; Dal'93; BSc; (604)987-1414; Fax. (604)985-2779.

MCWHIRTER, Elaine; Juravinski Cancer Centre, 699 Concession St, Hamilton ON L8V 5C2; Tor'99; FRCPC; IntMed; MedOncol. (905)387-9411

MCWHIRTER, Jason R; Gulf Canada Square, 363-401 9 Ave SW, Calgary AB T2P 3C5; Alb'96; BSc; CCFP; (403)221-4428; Fax. (403)221-4483.

MCWILLIAM, Tina M; Dr Charles A Janeway Child HC, 300 Prince Philip Dr, St. John's NL A1B 3V6; Mem'94; FRCPC; Psy. Staff, Janeway Children's Health & Rehabilitation Centre; (709)777-4121

MDAWE, Isaac M; Hanna Med Clinic, PO Box 700, Hanna AB T0J 1P0; Cape Town (South Africa)'98; MB ChB; (403)854-3351; Fax. (403)854-4116.

MEA, Demetrio M; 86 boul St-Pierre E, Caraquet NB E1W 1B6; Manila (Philippines)'58; (506)727-4048

MEAD, Annabel J; Complex Pain & Addiction Servi, 8167-2775 Laurel St, Vancouver BC V5Z 1M9; Tasmania (Australia)'86; MB BS; Staff, Vancouver General Hospital - Centennial Pavillion; (604)875-4788

MEAD, Timothy G; Lions Med Clinic, PO Box 69, Fisherville ON N0A 1G0; Oxford (England)'70; (905)779-3436; Fax. (905)779-3022.

MEADE, Maureen O; McMaster University Med Ctre, 1280 Main St W, Hamilton ON L8S 4K1; McG'90; FRCPC; IntMed; Critical Care Medicine. (905)525-9140 x23162

MEADE, William M; Kawartha Urology Assoc, 101-380 Burnham St, Peterborough ON K9H 1T6; Tor'91; FRCSC; Urol. (705)743-6480; Fax. (705)585-4885.

MEADOR, Karine L; 10010 102A Ave NW, Edmonton AB T5J 0G5; Alb'05; CCFP; (780)422-1302; Fax. (780)427-0777.

MEADOWS, Terence F; PO Box 66 Stn Main, Saanichton BC V8M 2C3; UBC'85.

MEADOWS-YOUNGER, Malcolm D; West End Med Centre, 510 Prince St, Truro NS B2N 1G1; Dal'05; CCFP; (902)895-1556; Fax. (902)893-1026.

MEAGHER, Caroline; Ctr Hosp de Verdun, 4000 boul Lasalle, LaSalle QC H4G 2A3; Mon'08; CCFP; CCFP(E.M.); Staff, Centre Hospitalier de Verdun; (514)362-1000

MEAGHER, John M A; 120 Branch St, Moncton NB E1A 4Y1; National (Ireland)'70; MB ChB; BAO; Assoc Staff, The Moncton Hospital; (506)856-7843; Fax. (506)384-5389.

MEAGHER, Luc; Clinique Dr Luc Meagher, 611 boul Sainte-Anne, St-Charles-Brromee QC J6E 5A9; Mon'79; (450)759-1441; Fax. (450)759-6457.

MEAGHER, Suzy; Carrefour Medical, 200-3030 boul le Carrefour, Laval QC H7T 2P5; Mon'76; Staff, Hopital de la Cite de la santé; Langs: English; French; (450)686-8899; Fax. (450)686-7466.

MEAGHER, Timothy W; MUHC-Montreal Gen Hosp, D6 253-1650 av Cedar, Montreal QC H3G 1A4; Dublin (Ireland)'75; ABIM(IntMed); FRCP(Ire); FACP; FRCPC; IntMed. Staff, McGill University Health Centre - Montreal General Campus; assoc Prof, McGill University; Langs: French; Spanish; (514)398-3524

MEAKES, R Alan; Royal Jubilee Hosp, RB230-1952 Bay St, Victoria BC V8R 1J8; UBC'70; FRCPC; IntMed; Anes. Dir/Chief IntMed, Royal Jubilee Hospital; (250)361-5554

MEAKIN, Carmen R; CFB Petawawa, PO Box 9999 Station Main, Petawawa ON K8H 2X3; Sask'01; FRCPC; Psy. (613)687-5511 x4600; Fax. (613)588-4711.

MEAKINS, Diana M; University of Alberta Hosp, 1E1-8440 112 St NW, Edmonton AB T6G 2B7; Alb'05; FRCPC; Psy. Staff, University of Alberta Hospital; (780)407-6501; Fax. (780)407-6672.

MEAKINS, Douglas W; Cabrini Centre, 412-16811 88 Ave NW, Edmonton AB T5R 5Y6; Alb'75; FRCPC; Psy. Staff, Covenant Health - Misericordia Community Hospital; (780)735-9396; Fax. (780)735-9397.

MEANEY, Brandon F; Hamilton HS-McMaster Site, PO Box 2000 Stn Lcd 1 3A60-1200 Main St W, Hamilton ON L8N 3Z5; McG'92; FRCPC; Peds; Neur. Staff Peds, Hamilton Health Sciences Centre - McMaster Children's Hospital; (905)521-2100 x73392; Fax. (905)521-7914; meaneyb@mcmaster.ca.

MEARS, Paul A; Dartmouth Gen Hosp, 325 Pleasant St, Dartmouth NS B2Y 4G8; McM'02; FRCPC; Cardiol; IntMed. Staff, Dartmouth General Hospital; (902)460-4536; Fax. (902)460-4154.

MEASHAM, Toby J; CLSC Parc Extension, 204 11-7085 rue Hutchison, Montreal QC H3N 1Y9; McG'92; FRCPC; Psy. Staff, McGill University Health Centre - Montreal Children's Hospital; (514)273-3800; Fax. (514)380-8147.

MEATHERALL, Bonnie L; HSC Faculty of Med, 1007F-3330 Hospital Dr NW, Calgary AB T2N 4N1; Man'04; FRCPC; IntMed; InfectDis. (403)210-5442

MEATHREL, Karen A; 202-436 Cedar Ave, Kelowna BC V1Y 4X3; Wes'05; FRCSC; ObstGyn. (778)484-5611

MEATHREL, Kimberley E; Hotel-Dieu Hosp, 166 Brock St, Kingston ON K7L 5G2; Qns'00; FRCS; FRCSC; PlasSurg. Staff, Kingston General Hospital; Staff, Hotel-Dieu Hospital; Asst Prof, Queen's University; (613)544-3400 x2393; Fax. (613)547-4182; ucosmetic@gmail.com.

MEBREK, Nachida; CSSS du Nord de Lanaudière, 1000 boul Sainte-Anne, St-Charles-Brromee QC J6E 6J2; Laval'03; Staff, Centre Hospitalier Régional de Lanaudière; (450)759-8222

MECARBANE, Elie G; Clin Med Luso, 1 av Mont-Royal E, Montreal QC H2T 1N4; Cairo (Egypt)'51; (514)849-2391; Fax. (514)849-2394.

MECARBANE, Rose-Marie; CSSS Pierre Boucher, 1333 boul Jacques-Cartier E, Longueuil QC J4M 2A5; Mon'88; LMCC; Staff, Centre Hospitalier Pierre Boucher; (450)468-8111

MECH, Zdzislaw R; The Medical Place, 308-178 John St, Brampton ON L6W 2A4; Tor'56; DPsy; FRCPC; Psy. Court Staff, William Osler Health System - Brampton Civic Hospital; Langs: Polish; (905)451-2470

MECHALY-CHOKRON, Jeannine; Ctr Hosp de Lacine, 650 16e av, Lachine QC H8S 3N5; Paris (France)'70; ABOph; FRCSC; Ophth (Glaucoma). Staff, CSSS de Dorval-Lachine-Lasalle; Universite de Montreal; Langs: Spanish; (514)637-2351

MECHETIUC, Adriana E; Medica One, 1275 Rymal Rd E, Hamilton ON L8W 3N1; (Romania)'93; CCFP; Langs: Romanian; (905)387-0005; Fax. (905)387-0010.

MECHOR, Bradford D; Calgary Sinus Centre, 209-320 23 Ave SW, Calgary AB T2S 0J2; Sask'01; FRCSC; Otol (Rhinology). (403)270-8060; Fax. (403)252-8244.

MECKIN, Michael C; Alder Med Centre, 277 Evergreen Rd, Campbell River BC V9W 5Y4; Leeds (England)'77; MB ChB; LMCC; Preceptor Family Pract, University of British Columbia; (250)287-7441; Fax. (250)287-4384.

MECKLER, Garth D; Children's & Women's HC of BC, K4 226-4480 Oak St, Vancouver BC V6H 3V4; Harvard'97; Staff, BC Children's Hospital; (604)875-2345 x5216

MECKLING, Scott K; 204-3320 Richter St, Kelowna BC V1W 4V5; Alb'91; FRCPC; Neur. (250)763-2931; Fax. (250)763-2775; drmeckling@shaw.ca.

MEDA, Stephen J; Fairview Family Health Network, 144-1333 Sheppard Ave E, North York ON M2J 1V1; Detroit(MI) (USA)'64; Staff, North York General Hospital; (416)491-5900; Fax. (416)491-1149.

MEDAD, Ilan E; 505-3200 Dufferin St, North York ON M6A 3B2; Tor'00; FRCPC; IntMed (Hepatology); Gastroent. Ac Staff, Humber River Regional Hospital - Finch Avenue Site; (416)256-9500; Fax. (416)256-9522.

MEDANE, Nadia; CSSS de Rimouski-Neigette, CP 3150 Succ A 150 av Rouleau, Rimouski QC G5L 5T1; (Algeria)'88; FRCPC; MedBiochem. Staff, Hôpital Regional Rimouski; (418)724-3000

MEDD, Thomas M; The Pas Health Complex Inc, PO Box 240 Stn Main 61 1st St W, The Pas MB R9A 1K4; Man'82; FRCPC; Psy. Staff, St. Anthony General Hospital; (204)623-6431

MEDDINGS, Jonathan; Univ of Calgary Faculty of Med, 3330 Hospital Dr NW, Calgary AB T2N 4N1; Alb'79; FRCPC; IntMed (Gastroenterology). Med Staff, University of Alberta Hospital; Prof/Dept Chair Med, University of Alberta; Vice Dean, University of Calgary; (403)210-8182; jon.meddings@ualberta.ca.

MEDDOUN, Mamoun; Hopital Regional D'Edmundston, 275 boul Hebert, Edmundston NB E3V 4E4; Sousse (Tunisia)'92; Staff, Hôpital regional d'Edmundston; (506)739-2200

MEDELLIN-KOWALEWSKI, G Alexandra; Foothills Med Centre, 1403 29 St NW, Calgary AB T2N 2T9; Juan N Corpas Medical School (Colombia)'96; FRCPC; DiagRad. Staff, Foothills Medical Centre; Langs: Spanish; (403)282-2782; Fax. (403)210-0869.

MEDERSKI, Barbara D; North York Gen Hosp, GW 33-4001 Leslie St, North York ON M2K 1E1; Tor'76; BSc(Hon); ABIM(ID); FRCPC; IntMed (Infectious Diseases). Ac Staff, North York General Hospital; Staff, Bridgepoint Health Centre; Langs: Polish; French; Spanish; (416)756-6130; Fax. (416)756-6449; bmedersk@nygh.on.ca.

MEDHURST, Charles W; 130-180 Wilson St, Victoria BC V9A 7N6; UBC'82; (250)388-4341; Fax. (250)418-8879.

MEDINA, Damien R; McMaste University Med Ctre, 2U8-1280 Main St W, Hamilton ON L8S 4K1; (Ireland)'08; FRCPC; IntMed. (905)521-2100 x75180

MEDINA, Xavier V; Finch-Midland Med Centre, 301-4190 Finch Ave E, Scarborough ON M1S 4T7; Santo Tomas (Philippines)'74; Staff, The Scarborough Hospital - Birchmount Campus; (416)299-4463; Fax. (416)299-4560.

MEDING, Gerald C; Associate Clinic, A-4620 50 Ave, Innisfail AB T4G 1A6; Alb'75; Ac Staff, Innisfail Health Centre; (403)227-3301; Fax. (403)227-2856; gmeding@dthr.ab.ca.

MEDLICOTT, Shaun A C; Peter Lougheed Centre, 3500 26 Ave NE, Calgary AB T1Y 6J4; Cal'92; BSc; FRCPC; AnatPath. Staff, Peter Lougheed Centre; (403)943-4907; Fax. (403)291-2931.

MEDLINE, Alan; Humber River Reg Hosp-Finch, 2111 Finch Ave W, North York ON M3N 1N1; Wes'63; FRCPC; GenPath., Humber River Regional Hospital - Finch Avenue Site; Pathologist, Gamma-Dynacare Laboratories; (416)747-3080; Fax. (416)747-3743; amedline@hrrh.on.ca.

MEDLINE, Norton M; G1-250 Lawrence Ave W, Toronto ON M5M 1B2; Tor'60; FRCPC; GenPath (Dermatological Pathology); Derm. Staff, St Michael's Hospital; Staff, Humber River Regional Hospital - Keele Street Site; (416)787-3575; Fax. (416)787-8239; nmedline@hrrh.on.ca.

MEDLINE, Paul B; Gamma Dynacare Med Lab, 115 Midair Crt, Brampton ON L6T 5M3; Tor'90; FRCPC; AnatPath. Staff, William Osler Health System - Etobicoke General Hospital; (905)790-3000; Fax. (905)790-9659.

MEDNICK, Edward B; 385 The West Mall, Etobicoke ON M9C 1E7; Tor'69; FRCSC; Ophth;CCFP; FCFP; (416)622-1864; Fax. (416)622-1215.

MEDOFF, Elaine J; Hillside Pediatric Clinic, 65 av Hillside, Westmount QC H3Z 1W1; Mon'91; FRCPC; Peds; ClinImmunol&Allergy. Staff, McGill University Health Centre - Montreal Children's Hospital; (514)931-2524; elaine.medoff@muhc.mcgill.ca.

MEDOU-NTYAME, Leopold; CSSS de la Vallée de l'Or, 725 6e rue, Val-d'Or QC J9P 3Y1; Mon'73; FRCPC; Peds. Staff, Centre Hospitalier de Val d'Or; ac Staff, Hôpital Ste-Justine; (514)345-4931; lmedou@hotmail.com.

MEDVE, Paul W; Norfolk Gen Hosp, 365 West St, Simcoe ON N3Y 1T7; Wes'86; Staff, Norfolk General Hospital; (519)426-0130; Fax. (519)429-6945.

MEDVEDEV, Gueorgui A; 303-233 Nelson's Cres, New Westminster BC V3L 0E4; Moscow (Russia (Federation))'94; FRCPC; Neur. Staff, Royal Columbian Hospital; (604)759-2140

MEDVEDEV, Nadia; St Paul's Hosp, 1081 Burrard St, Vancouver BC V6Z 1Y6; Moscow (Russia (Federation))'94; Staff, Providence Health Care - St Paul's Hospital; (604)682-2344

MEDWIDSKY, Wolodymyr; C105-11 King St W, Toronto ON M5H 4C7; Wes'67; BA; FRCPC; Derm. Ac Staff, St Michael's Hospital; Ac Staff, Bridgepoint Health Centre; Consultant, Sunnybrook Health Sciences Centre - Holland Orthopaedic & Arthritic Centre; Langs: Ukrainian; (416)864-0732; Fax. (416)364-6278.

MEDYNSKI, Susan C; Mountain View Med Clinic, 201-1789 K.L. O. Rd, Kelowna BC V1W 3P3; McM'00; CCFP; (250)860-6799

MEE, David W; 2-210 Lorraine Ave, Kitchener ON N2B 3T4; Tor'86; Staff Privil, Grand River Hospital - Kitchener/Waterloo Health Centre; Staff Privil, St Mary's General Hospital; (519)570-1223; Fax. (519)570-9367.

MEEDER, Robert J J; Orillia Ped Teaching Assoc, 17 Dunedin St, Orillia ON L3V 5T3; McM'99; FRCPC; Peds. Staff Peds, Orillia Soldiers' Memorial Hospital; (705)327-9131; Fax. (705)327-9189.

MEEHAN, Anne R; 1-2530 St. Joseph Blvd, Orleans ON K1C 1G1; Alb'86; CCFP; FCFP; (613)830-5888; Fax. (613)830-1791.

MEEHAN, Catheryne; Mumford Professional Ctr, 2095-6960 Mumford Rd, Halifax NS B3L 4P1; UBC'81; CCFP; FCFP; Staff, Peace Arch Hospital; (902)453-5587; Fax. (902)455-3358.

MEEK, David C; 707 Millidge Ave, Saint John NB E2K 2N7; Cardiff (Wales)'74; MB ChB; FRCPC; Peds (Pediatric Neurology). Ac Staff, Saint John Regional Hospital; Consultant, Hopital Regional Chaleur; Consultant, Dr Everett Chalmers Regional Hospital; Asst Prof, Dalhousie University; Asst Prof, Memorial University Of Newfoundland; (506)648-7956; Fax. (506)648-7957.

MEEK, Douglas H; Polyclinic Prof Centre Inc, 199 Grafton St, Charlottetown PE C1A 1L2; Dal'73; CCFP; FCFP; Staff, Queen Elizabeth Hospital; (902)629-8839; Fax. (902)566-9251.

MEEK, Grant P; Panorama Village Med Clinic, 103-15157 56 Ave, Surrey BC V3S 9A5; Pretoria (South Africa)'04; CCFP; (604)574-0461

MEEK, Murray D; North Bay Reg Health Centre, 50 College Dr, North Bay ON P1B 0A4; Tor'03; CCFP; Staff, North Bay Regional Health Centre - Regional Mental Health; (705)474-8600

MEEN, Eric K; 601-400 Tache Ave, Winnipeg MB R2H 3C3; Alb'06; FRCSC; Otol.

MEEN, Richard; 2 Glenrose Ave, Toronto ON M4T 1K4; Wes'63; Psy (Forensic Psychiatry). Consultant, Catholic Children's Aid Society of Metro Toronto; Consultant, Covenant House Toronto; Clin Dir, Thistleton Reg Centre & Syl Apps Campus; Teach Staff, University of Toronto; (416)366-5708; kishniga@rogers.com.

MEENAN, John J; Heritage Park Shopping Centre, 9-200 Lorraine Ave, Kitchener ON N2B 3R3; Glasgow(SCot.) (Scotland)'69; (519)743-1041; Fax. (519)744-5472.

MEER, Ahmed; Sedgewick Med Centre, PO Box 159, Sedgewick AB T0B 4C0; RCS (Ireland)'62; LRCPSI; DCH; DObst; LM; Chief of Staff, Covenant Health - Killam Health Centre; (780)384-3842; Fax. (780)384-3802.

MEERE, Stephane B; La Clin de Sante Visuelle Mtl, 200-7355 boul Saint-Michel, Montreal QC H2A 2Z9; Mon'95; Ophth (Medical Ophthalmology). Staff Medical Ophthalmology, CSSS du Coeur de l'Isle Hôpital Jean-Talon; Langs: Bilingual(French/English); Spanish; Dutch; (514)593-6161; Fax. (514)593-3937; sbmeere@yahoo.com.

MEERHOLZ, Wilhelm A H C; PO Box 790 Stn Main, Cochrane AB T4C 1A9; Pretoria (South Africa)'71; MB ChB; Langs: Afrikaans.

MEETARBHAN, Bheemdev; Sunwood Medical, 3000 Lougheed Hwy, Coquitlam BC V3B 1C5; Glasgow (Scotland)'84; AACP; Langs: English; French; (604)464-0345

MEEUWISSE, Willem H; University of Calgary, 2500 University Dr NW, Calgary AB T2N 1N4; Wes'87; Dip SportMed; PhD; Court Staff, Foothills Medical Centre; Assoc Prof, University of Calgary; (403)220-8518; Fax. (403)282-6170; meeuwiss@ucalgary.ca.

MEEUWISSEN, Matthew J; Westview Hlth Ctr Stony Plain, 4405 South Park Dr, Stony Plain AB T7Z 2M7; UBC'98; CCFP; CCFP(E. M.); Staff, Westview Health Centre; (780)968-3600

MEFFE, Filippa; Enhanced Care Clinic, 3865 Lake Shore Blvd W, Etobicoke ON M8W 0A2; Tor'82; CCFP; FCFP; Court Staff, Women's College Hospital; (416)354-2640

MEFFE, Filomena M; Women's Health Care Centre, 5F-61 Queen St E, Toronto ON M5C 2T2; Tor'84; FRCSC; ObstGyn. Associate, St Michael's Hospital; (416)867-3653; Fax. (416)867-7478.

MEGAHED GHEIS, Mohamed A; Victoria Gen Hosp, 1 Hospital Way, Victoria BC V8Z 6R5; Cairo (Egypt)'90; MB ChB; MRCPsy; FRCPC; Psy. Staff, Victoria General Hospital; Langs: Arabic; (250)727-4090; mamgheis@hotmail.com.

MEGALLI BASALI, Sherif F; Wheat City Med Clinic, 1-1711C Kirkcaldy Dr, Brandon MB R7A 0B9; CCFP; (204)727-1711

MEGARBANE, Farid; CSSS Pierre Boucher, 1333 boul Jacques-Cartier E, Longueuil QC J4M 2A5; Beyrouth (Lebanon)'73; OrthSurg (P.Q.). Staff, Centre Hospitalier Pierre Boucher; (450)468-8111 x2723; Fax. (450)468-8284.

MEGGISON, Hillary E; The Ottawa Hosp-Civic Campus, 1053 Carling Ave, Ottawa ON K1Y 4E9; Sask'98; FRCPC; IntMed; Critical Care Medicine; Endocrin&Metab. Staff, The Ottawa Hospital - Civic Campus; (613)761-4516

MEGHANI, Hamidah K; Hassle Free Clinic, 2F-66 Gerrard St E, Toronto ON M5B 1G3; McM'07; FRCPC; Public Health & Preventive Med;CCFP; (416)922-0566; Fax. (416)922-2018.

MEGHJI, M Mohamed; Belmont Prof Centre, 309-564 Belmont Ave W, Kitchener ON N2M 5N6; Leeds (England)'71; MRCS; LRCP; DCH(Lond); DABIM; FRCPC; IntMed; Gastroent. Ac Staff, Grand River Hospital - Kitchener/Waterloo Health Centre; Ac Staff, St Mary's General Hospital; Court Staff, Hamilton Health Sciences Centre - McMaster Children's Hospital; (519)744-1167; Fax. (519)744-1168; gi-mo@rogers.com.

MEGHJI, Mohamed H; Hayyan Healthcare, 8-9301 Bathurst St, Richmond Hill ON L4C 9S2; Pradesh (India)'89; CCFP; (905)237-7472; Fax. (905)237-2854.

MEGHJI, Shahbegum A; 5706 19A Ave NW, Edmonton AB T6L 1L8; Bombay (India)'70; Langs: Gujarati; Hindi; Urdu; (780)450-1919; Fax. (780)450-1927.

MEGHORY, Yehiel C; Bolton Med Centre, 205-12295 Highway 50, Bolton ON L7E 1M2; Tor'71; BSc; MBA; CCFP; FCFP; Staff, Headwaters Health Care Centre - Orangeville Site; Langs: Hebrew; (905)857-3829; Fax. (905)857-7902.

MEGIE, Marie-Francoise; CLSC-CHSLD du Margot, 250 boul Cartier O, Laval QC H7N 5S5; (Haiti)'74; (450)668-1803; Fax. (450)972-6875; mmegie_marig@ssss.gouv.qc.ca.

MEGLIS, Gus; Marlee Med Centre, 249 Marlee Ave, North York ON M6B 4B8; Ott'94; CCFP; (416)780-9986; Fax. (416)780-1087.

MEGRAN, David W; Alberta Health Services, 120-10301 Southport Lane SW, Calgary AB T2W 1S7; McG'79; ABIM(InfectDis); FRCPC; IntMed; InfectDis. Staff, Peter Lougheed Centre; (403)943-1182; Fax. (403)943-1174; david.megran@albertahealthservices.ca.

MEGUERDITCHIAN, Ari N; MUHC-Royal Victoria Hosp, S7 30-687 av des Pins O, Montreal QC H3A 1A1; Mon'00; FRCSC; GenSurg; General Surgical Oncology (P.Q.). Staff, McGill University Health Centre - Royal Victoria Hospital; (514)934-1934 x34081

MEGURO, Kotoo; Royal University Hosp, 103 Hospital Dr, Saskatoon SK S7N 0W8; (Japan)'74; FRCSC; Neursurg (Cerebrovascular Disease). Staff, Royal University Hospital; (306)966-8161; Fax. (306)966-8140.

MEGYESI, Amy E; Salmon Arm Med Clinic, PO Box 730 Stn Main 581 Hudson Ave NE, Salmon Arm BC V1E 4N8; UBC'04; CCFP; (250)832-6094; Fax. (250)832-5235.

MEGYESI, Joseph F; London HSC-University Hosp, PO Box 5339 Stn B 10GE8-339 Windermere Rd, London ON N6A 5A5; Wes'85; FRCSC; Neursurg. Staff, London Health Sciences Centre - University Hospital; (519)663-3565; Fax. (519)663-3753.

MEHAN, Upender K; Centre for Family Medicine, 10B Victoria St S, Kitchener ON N2G 1C5; Wes'86; CCFP; FCFP; Ac Staff, Cambridge Memorial Hospital; (519)783-0020; Fax. (519)783-0033.

MEHARCHAND, Jacinta M; Toronto East Gen Hosp Inc, 825 Coxwell Ave, Toronto ON M4C 3E7; Natal (South Africa)'76; FRCPC; IntMed (Bone Marrow Transplant); Hem. Staff, Toronto East General Hospital Inc; Assoc Prof, University of Toronto; (416)469-3325

MEHARCHAND, Mervyn M; 1221 Bloor St E, Mississauga ON L4Y 2N8; Tor'88; Ac Staff, Trillium Health Centre - West Toronto; (905)625-1241

MEHAREB REDJAH, Nadia; CLSC Saint-Michel, 3355 rue Jarry E, Montreal QC H1Z 2E5; Oran Es-Senia (Algeria)'83; (514)374-8223

MEHBOOB, Mohammad; Battlefords Family Health Ctre, 103-1192 101st St, North Battleford SK S9A 0Z6; Lahore (Pakistan)'89; MB BS; CCFP; (306)937-6840; Fax. (306)445-4887.

MEHDI, Nadya B; Multi Specialty Clinic, 21 Queensway W, Mississauga ON L5B 1B6; Karachi (Pakistan)'94; FRCPC; IntMed. (905)897-8928

MEHDIAN, Hossein; 226-1333 Sheppard Ave E, North York ON M2J 1V1; Tehran (Iran)'92; FRCSC; OrthSurg. Staff, North York General Hospital; (416)850-4064; Fax. (416)850-6681.

MEHDIRATTA, Manu; 500-89 Queensway W, Mississauga ON L5B 2V2; McM'01; FRCPC; Neur. (905)848-0001; Fax. (905)848-6360.

MEHER, Abu F M A; 5973 Fraser St, Vancouver BC V5W 2Z6; Chittagong (Bangladesh)'89; MB BS; (604)324-1922

MEHIN, Ramin; 2080 McCallum Rd, Abbotsford BC V2S 3N4; Ott'96; FRCSC; OrthSurg. (604)853-6949; Fax. (604)852-3889.

MEHLING, Blair M; Meadowlark Health Centre, 218 Meadowlark Shopping Ctr NW, Edmonton AB T5R 5W9; Alb'93; BSc; FRCSC; PlasSurg (Aesthetic Surgery). Staff, Royal Alexandra Hospital; Staff, Covenant Health - Misericordia Community Hospital; Staff, WW Cross Cancer Institute; Clin Lecturer, University of Alberta; (780)438-0123; Fax. (780)438-0461.

MEHLOMAKULU, Mtimkulu; Kingston Med Arts Centre, 107-800 Princess St, Kingston ON K7L 5E4; Durban (South Africa)'60; MB ChB; BSc(Hyg.); FRCPC; Peds (Pediatrics & Adolescent Asthma). Staff Consultant, Ongwanada Resource Centre; Asst Prof, Queen's University; Langs: Zulu; Xhosa; Sotho; Afrikaans; (613)544-3939; Fax. (613)544-8390; zobozmehlo@live.com.

MEHMI, Sanghamitra A; Central Parkway Mall, 112-377 Burnhamthorpe Rd E, Mississauga ON L5A 3Y1; Baroda (India)'69; Court Staff, St Joseph's Health Centre; Staff, Trillium Health Centre - Mississauga; (905)896-3777

MEHMOOD, Rashid; Regina Qu'Appelle HR-Regina, 1440 14th Ave, Regina SK S4P 0W5; Punjab (India)'95; FRCPC; Anes. Staff, Regina General Hospital; (306)766-4444

MEHMOOD, Shehzad; Univ Hosp of Northern BC, 1475 Edmonton St, Prince George BC V2M 1S2; Punjab (Pakistan)'91; Staff, University Hospital of Northern British Columbia; (250)565-2000

MEHRA, Neeraj; Diamond Health Care Centre, 2775 Laurel St, Vancouver BC V5Z 1M9; Alb'05; FRCSC; ObstGyn. (604)875-4111 x62001

MEHRA, Sunil; Healthplex, 100-150 West Dr, Brampton ON L6T 4P9; Bhopal (India)'72; MB; BSc; DCH(Dublin&Delhi); FRCPC; Peds (Asthma & Allergy).

MEHRABIAN, Ali; CSSS de Saint-Jerome, 290 rue Montigny, Saint-Jerome QC J7Z 5T3; Kerman Univ (Iran)'98; FRCPC; NuclearMed. Staff, Hôtel-Dieu de Saint-Jérôme; (450)431-8200

MEHRAEIN, Nahid; 140-4977 Trenant St, Delta BC V4K 2K5; Tor'03; CCFP; CCFP(E.M.); (604)946-7661; Fax. (604)940-1743; nahid_mehraein@yahoo.ca.

MEHRAIN, Shirin; Stratford Gen Hosp, 46 General Hospital Dr, Stratford ON N5A 2Y6; Ott'00; CCFP; CCFP(E.M.); Staff, Stratford General Hospital - Huron Perth Healthcare Alliance; (519)272-8210

MEHRMANESH, Flora Z; 517-2250 Bovaird Dr E, Brampton ON L6R 0W3; Dal'73; FRCPC; Peds (Diabetes). Langs: Persian; (905)452-0015; Fax. (905)452-1309; flora.mehrmanesh@sympatico.ca.

MEHROTRA, Shruti; Children's Hosp of Western Ont, 800 Commissioners Rd E, London ON N6A 5W9; Qns'05; FRCPC; Peds; PedEmergMed. Staff, London Health Sciences Centre - Victoria Campus; (519)685-8500

MEHTA, Amit L; Niagara H System-St Catharines, PO Box 3018 Stn Main 142 Queenston St, St Catharines ON L2R 7C6; Mem'90; DABR; FRCPC; DiagRad. Staff, Niagara Health System - St Catharines General Site; (905)684-7271 x46319; Fax. (905)684-6990.

MEHTA, Arun K; Pickering Family Physicians, 6D-1450 Kingston Rd, Pickering ON L1V 1C1; Tor'82; Court Staff, Rouge Valley Health System - Centenary Health Centre Site; Court Staff, Markham Stouffville Hospital; Ac Staff, Rouge Valley Health System - Ajax & Pickering Health Centre Site; (905)420-6025; Fax. (905)837-1099.

MEHTA, Asita; Goulet Prof Centre, 300-200 Goulet St, Winnipeg MB R2H 0R8; London (England)'79; MB BS; (204)231-3232

MEHTA, Avnish C; 4002 Sheppard Ave E, Scarborough ON M1S 4R5; Ott'99; CCFP; Staff, Rouge Valley Health System - Ajax & Pickering Health Centre Site; (416)297-7490; Fax. (416)297-5371.

MEHTA, Bella; Rideau Family Health Team, 5-3635 Rivergate Way, Ottawa ON K1V 2A4; Ott'93; CCFP; FCFP; Ac Staff Family Med, The Ottawa Hospital - Civic Campus; (613)739-3700; Fax. (613)739-7043.

MEHTA, Chetan; Finchgate Medical Centre, 224-40 Finchgate Blvd, Brampton ON L6T 3J1; McM'06; CCFP; Staff, St Michael's Hospital; Physician, York Community Services Centre; (905)451-6959

MEHTA, Damini; A13-9600 Islington Ave, Woodbridge ON L4H 2T1; Ott'94; CCFP; FCFP; Langs: Gujarati; (905)893-8085; Fax. (905)893-8218.

MEHTA, Darshana J; Thunder Bay Reg HSC-T-Bay, 980 Oliver Rd, Thunder Bay ON P7B 6V4; Gujarat (India)'83; CCFP; Staff, Thunder Bay Regional Health Sciences Centre; (807)684-6030

MEHTA, Dilipkumar H; St Joseph's Health Centre, GW131-30 The Queensway, Toronto ON M6R 1B5; London (England)'75; MB BS; DCH(Lond); FRCPC; Peds (Neonatology). Staff Peds, St Joseph's Health Centre; Assoc Prof, University of Toronto; Langs: Gujarati; (416)530-6759; Fax. (416)530-6725; dilipmehta@rogers.com.

MEHTA, Hitesh; 101-3 Conestoga Blvd, Brampton ON L6Z 4N5; Tor'96; FRCPC; IntMed; Nephrol. Staff, William Osler Health System - Etobicoke General Hospital; Staff, William Osler Health System - Brampton Civic Hospital; (905)453-0715; Fax. (905)453-0972.

MEHTA, Karishma; Sheldon Chumir Centre, 1213 4 St SW, Calgary AB T2R 0X7; Qns'03; CCFP; (403)955-6600

MEHTA, Labhshanker S; Niagara Diagnostic Imaging, 589 Lake St, St Catharines ON L2N 7L6; London (England)'60; MB BS; DMRD(Liverpool); FRCPC; DiagRad. Staff Diag Imaging, Niagara Health System - St Catharines General Site; Langs: Gujarati; Hindi; (905)937-2255

MEHTA, Mahendra H; Kennedy & Sheppard Diagnostic, 304-4002 Sheppard Ave E, Scarborough ON M1S 4R5; Leeds (England)'67; LRCP(Lond); MRCS(Eng); DABR; DMRD(Eng); FRCPC; DiagRad (Angiography). Court Staff MRI Diag Imaging, St Michael's Hospital; Dir C T Studies, St Joseph's Health Centre; Asst Prof, University of Toronto; (416)299-9895; Fax. (416)299-9221.

MEHTA, Mitesh; Markham Stouffville Hosp, PO Box 1800 Stn Main 381 Church St, Markham ON L3P 7P3; Tor'91; FRCPC; DiagRad. Staff, Markham Stouffville Hospital; (905)472-7000

MEHTA, Navdeep; Sudbury Reg Hosp-Laurentian, 41 Ramsey Lake Rd, Sudbury ON P3E 5J1; Ott'90; BSc; FRCPC; IntMed (Critical Care Medicine); Nephrol. Ac Staff, Health Sciences North-Laurentian Site; (705)522-2200 x3948; Fax. (705)523-7008; nmehta@hrsrh.on.ca.

MEHTA, Paras B; 38001-968 King Edward Ave E, Vancouver BC V5Z 4L9; Alb'09; CCFP; (604)278-6838

MEHTA, Pravinsagar G; Laxmi Centre, 3F-200 Goulet St, Winnipeg MB R2H 0R8; Sheffield (England)'70; MB ChB; DObstRCOG; CCFP; FCFP; Staff, Concordia General Hospital; Staff, Riverview Health Centre; Asst Site Manager, St Boniface General Hospital; Med Advisor, Foyer Valade & Bettania Special Care Unit & Med. Dir., West Park Manor-Winnipeg; Asst Prof, University of Manitoba; Langs: Gujarati; (204)237-8479

MEHTA, Rajin; Sunnybrook Hlth Sciences Ctre, L101D-2075 Bayview Ave, Toronto ON M4N 3M5; Tor'86; FRCPC; IntMed; GeriatricMed. Staff, Sunnybrook Health Sciences Centre; (416)480-4076; Fax. (416)480-4778; rajin.mehta@sw.ca.

MEHTA, Rashi J; Southwood Medical Clinic, 1-3950 Dougall Ave, Windsor ON N9G 1X2; Man'99; BSc; CCFP; (519)966-6777; Fax. (519)966-7701.

MEHTA, Sangeeta; Mount Sinai Hosp, 18 216-600 University Ave, Toronto ON M5G 1X5; McG'90; FRCPC; IntMed (Critical Care Medicine); Respir. Dir-Research ICU & Staff Phys, Mount Sinai Hospital; Asst Prof Med, University of Toronto; (416)586-4800 x4604; Fax. (416)586-8480; geeta.mehta@utoronto.ca.

MEHTA, Sanjay; London HSC-Victoria Hosp, PO Box 5010 Stn B E1 325-800 Commissioners Rd E, London ON N6A 5W9; McG'88; ABIM; FRCPC; IntMed; Respir (Pulmonary Hypertention). Consultant Respirol, London Health Sciences Centre - Victoria Campus; Prof, University of Western Ontario; Langs: English; French; (519)667-6723; Fax. (519)685-8406; sanjay.mehta@lhsc.on.ca.

MEHTA, Sanjay V; 1201-525 University Ave, Toronto ON M5G 2L3; Cal'97; MEd; FRCPC; Peds; PedEmergMed. Staff, The Hospital For Sick Children; Staff, Trillium Health Centre - West Toronto; Asst Prof, University of Toronto; Langs: Gujarati; (416)813-7654 x2386; Fax. (416)813-5043; sanjay.mehta@sickkids.ca.

MEHTA, Shamir; Hamilton HS-General Site, DBCVSRI C3-237 Barton St E, Hamilton ON L8L 2X2; Tor'91; FRCPC; IntMed (Interventional Cardiology); Cardiol. Staff Cardiol, Hamilton Health Sciences Centre - McMaster Children's Hospital; Staff Cardiol, Hamilton Health Sciences Centre - Hamilton General Hospital; Dir Interventional Cardiology, Hamilton Health Sciences Centre; Assoc Prof Med, McMaster University; (905)521-2631; Fax. (905)296-0086.

MEHTA, Sowmil K; 404-1368 Ouellette Ave, Windsor ON N8X 1J9; Qns'96; FRCSC; GenSurg; VascSurg. Staff, Hôtel-Dieu Grace Hospital; Consultant, Windsor Regional Hospital - Metropolitan Site; (519)258-6504; Fax. (519)258-6098; dr.smehta@evlt.ca.

MEHTA, Sunil L; The Credit Valley Hosp, 2200 Eglinton Ave W, Mississauga ON L5M 2N1; Tor'94; FRCPC; DiagRad. Staff, The Credit Valley Hospital; (905)813-2200

MEHTA, Sunil P; Grey Bruce HS-Owen Sound, PO Box 1800 Stn Main 1800 8th St E, Owen Sound ON N4K 6M9; Wes'06; CCFP; CCFP(E.M.); Staff, Grey Bruce Health Services - Owen Sound; (519)280-5085

MEHTA, Suryakant D; 208-815 College St, Toronto ON M6G 1C9; Baroda (India)'69; MB BS; Langs: Gujarati; Hindi; Swahili; (416)536-5847; Fax. (416)536-5847; suryakant_mehta@hotmail.com.

MEHTA, Susan E; Oak Ridge Med Centre, 100-13291 Yonge St, Richmond Hill ON L4E 4L6; Tor'90; (905)773-7759; Fax. (905)773-1325.

MEHTA, Tushar; Wise Elephant Family Hlth Team, 247 Main St N, Brampton ON L6X 1N3; Tor'99; CCFP; Staff, William Osler Health System - Brampton Civic Hospital; Staff Emergency Med, Halton Healthcare Services Corporation - Georgetown Hospital; Langs: Gujarati; (905)459-4385; Fax. (905)459-6373; tmehta@ahealingplace.ca.

MEHTA, Viraj; Regional Mental HC-London, PO Box 5532 Stn B 850 Highbury Ave, London ON N6A 4H1; Wes'05; FRCPC; Psy. Staff, Regional Mental Health Care-St Joseph's Health Care; (519)685-8300

MEHTA, Vivek; University of Alberta Hosp, 21-8440 112 St NW, Edmonton AB T6G 2B7; Qns'92; MSc; FRCSC; Neursurg (Epidemiology). Staff Mackenzie Health Sciences Ctre, University of Alberta Hospital; (780)407-8346; Fax. (780)407-8435.

MEHTA, Yatin B; Rouge Valley-Ajax & Pickering, 580 Harwood Ave S, Ajax ON L1S 2J4; Tor'06; FRCPC; Anes. Staff, Rouge Valley Health System - Ajax & Pickering Health Centre Site.

MEHTAR, Maryam; St Mary Paediatric Clinic, 327 Avenue NS, Saskatoon SK S7M 2N2; Witwatersrand (South Africa)'89; MB ChB; FRCPC; Peds. Staff, Royal University Hospital; (306)359-7837; Fax. (306)659-2022.

MEIER, Courtney C L; City Centre Family Physicians, 100-514 Queen St, Saskatoon SK S7K 0M5; Sask'05; CCFP; Assoc Staff Family Med, University of Saskatchewan; (306)244-3016; Fax. (306)244-4737.

MEIER, Donald D; Town Centre Prof Bldg, 103-6203 28 Ave NW, Edmonton AB T6L 6K3; Sask'77; Ac Staff, Royal Alexandra Hospital; (780)462-9316; Fax. (780)462-9306.

MEIER, H M Rosemary; St Joseph's Health Centre, 4 S 33A-30 The Queensway, Toronto ON M6R 1B5; Aberdeen (Scotland)'67; DPM; MB ChB; FRCPsy; MSc; FRCPC; Psy (Geriatric Psychiatry). Staff, St Joseph's Health Centre; Asst Prof, University of Toronto; Langs: German; (416)530-6000 x4018; Fax. (416)530-6076.

MEIER, Kathleen R; Misericordia Community Hosp, 16940 87 Ave NW, Edmonton AB T5R 4H5; Cal'79; BSc; MSc; Staff, Covenant Health - Misericordia Community Hospital; Teach Staff Peds, University of Alberta; (780)735-2731; Fax. (780)735-2794.

MEIER, Lucja U; Calgary Lab Services, 9-3535 Research Rd NW, Calgary AB T2L 2K8; Gdansk (Poland)'63; FRCPC; AnatPath (Cytopath). Staff, Calgary Laboratory Services; Clinical Asst Prof Anatomical Path, University of Calgary; Langs: Polish; (403)770-3206; lucja.meier@cls.ab.ca.

MEIER, Michael A; University of Alberta Hosp, 3C1.12-8440 112 St NW, Edmonton AB T6G 2B7; Alb'84; FRCSC; GenSurg; Critical Care Medicine. Assoc Dir Children's Stollery Hosp Gen System ICU, University of Alberta Hospital; Staff Surg, Covenant Health - Grey Nuns Community Hospital; Asst Prof, University of Alberta; (780)407-6755

MEIERS, Pamela J; 222-750 Spadina Cres E, Saskatoon SK S7K 3H3; Sask'04; FRCSC; GenSurg. (306)653-3366; Fax. (306)653-8832.

MEIERS, Suzanne L; Regina Qu'Appelle HR-Regina, 1440 14th Ave, Regina SK S4P 0W5; Sask'97; FRCSC; GenSurg. Ac Staff, Regina General Hospital; Clin Assoc Prof, University of Saskatchewan; (306)766-6911; Fax. (306)766-6917.

MEIKLE, Andrew T J; JPP2N 2449-910 10th Ave W, Vancouver BC V5Z 1M9; Qns'95; FRCPC; Anes. (604)875-4304; Fax. (604)875-5209.

MEIKLE, Ben G; 400-920 1st Ave W, Owen Sound ON N4K 4K5; Tor'97; FRCPC; PhysMed&Rehab. Staff, Grey Bruce Health Services - Owen Sound; (519)371-5858; Fax. (519)371-4853.

MEIKLE, Gregg M; Red Deer Reg Hosp Centre, PO Box 5030 Stn Postal Box Ctr 3942 50A Ave, Red Deer AB T4N 6R2; Sask'04; CCFP; CCFP(E.M.); Staff, Red Deer Regional Hospital Centre; (403)343-4444; Fax. (403)986-3599.

MEIKLEHAM, Simone A; PO Box 549, Little Current ON P0P 1K0; Wes'94; CCFP; CCFP(E.M.); FCFP; Ac Staff, Manitoulin Health Centre - Little Current; Asst Prof, Northern Ontario School of Medicine; Langs: English; French; (705)368-2450; Fax. (705)368-2480.

MEILI, Ryan D; West Side Community Clinic, 1528 20th St W, Saskatoon SK S7M 0Z6; Sask'04; CCFP; (306)664-4310; Fax. (306)934-2506.

MEILLEUR, Carole; Clin Med Chutes-de-la-Chaudier, 170-1310 1re av, Saint-Redempteur QC G6K 1A5; Laval'82; (418)831-6226; Fax. (418)831-7698.

MEILLEUR, Christopher J M; 1-105 Progress Cres, Kapuskasing ON P5N 3J4; Ott'98; CCFP; CCFP(E.M.); Asst Prof, Northern Ontario School of Medicine-Laurentian University; Langs: Bilingual(French/English); (705)335-6012; Fax. (705)337-6296.

MEINDOK, Harry; Oakville Nuclear Medicine, B1-1235 Trafalgar Rd, Oakville ON L6H 3P1; London (England)'58; MB BS; MRCP(Lond); FRCPC; IntMed; NuclearMed. Assoc Prof IntMed & Radiol/Consultant, University of Toronto; Fax. (416)323-3961.

MEINDOK, James R; Markham Stouffville Hosp, PO Box 1800 Stn Main 381 Church St, Markham ON L3P 7P3; Tor'96; FRCPC; DiagRad. Staff, Markham Stouffville Hospital; (905)472-7000

MEINERI, Massimiliano; Univ Hlth Network-Toronto Gen, 3EN 442-200 Elizabeth St, Toronto ON M5G 2C4; Turin (Italy)'99; Staff, Toronto General Hospital - UHN; (416)340-3242

MEINERT, Paul C; Rouge Valley-Ajax & Pickering, 580 Harwood Ave S, Ajax ON L1S 2J4; McG'91; Peds. Staff, Rouge Valley Health System - Ajax & Pickering Health Centre Site; (905)683-2320 x4780

MEINIG, Elaine M; Markham Med Centre, 214-6633 Highway 7, Markham ON L3P 7P2; Wes'86; Ac Staff Surg & Preventive Oncol, Sunnybrook Health Sciences Centre; Ac Staff Family Pract, Markham Stouffville Hospital; (905)294-2290; Fax. (905)294-0029.

MEIR, David; 340-1641 Hillside Ave, Victoria BC V8T 5G1; Manchester (England)'69; MB ChB; DCH(Eng); Staff, Royal Jubilee Hospital; Staff, Victoria General Hospital; (250)595-6255; Fax. (250)265-3643.

MEIRING, Gert J; Broadway Med Clinic, 200-41 Broadway St W, Yorkton SK S3N 0L6; Stellenbosch (South Africa)'74; MB ChB; (306)783-2555; Fax. (306)783-2557.

MEIRING, Madeleine E; Southridge Prof Centre, 5-1224 Strachan Rd SE, Medicine Hat AB T1B 4R2; Pretoria (South Africa)'89; MB ChB; CCFP; FCFP; Langs: Afrikaans; (403)580-3888; Fax. (403)504-1220.

MEIRING, Peter de Vos; Gulf Canada Square, 330-401 9 Ave SW, Calgary AB T2P 3C5; (South Africa)'51; MB BCh; FRCP(Lond); FRCP(Edin); (403)221-4447; Fax. (403)221-4419; pameiring@shaw.ca.

MEISELS, Monica; Centre de Sante Valcartier, CP 1000 Bdp Succ Forces, Courcelette QC G0A 4Z0; Laval'94; CCFP; FCFP; Instructor, Université Laval; Langs: Spanish; English; (418)844-5000 x8245; Fax. (418)844-5000.

MEISSNER, Les A; St Mary's Hosp Centre, B207-3830 av Lacombe, Montreal QC H3T 1M5; McG'79; Endocrin (P.Q.); Endocrin&Metab; IntMed. Chief Endocrin/Metab, St Mary's Hospital Centre; Staff, McGill University Health Centre - Montreal General Campus; adj Prof, McGill University; (514)345-3511 x3112

MEISTER, Ashley; Royal University Hosp, 103 Hospital Dr, Saskatoon SK S7N 0W8; Sask'04; FRCPC; Anes. Staff, Royal University Hospital; (306)655-1183; Fax. (306)655-1279.

MEISTER, Mark G; 3970 156B St, Surrey BC V3S 0K8; Cape Town (South Africa)'98; FRCPC; DiagRad. (604)859-8998

MEITIN, Joan M; 77 MacLaren St, Ottawa ON K2P 0K5; McG'73; FRCPC; Psy. Langs: English; French; (613)230-5550

MEIWALD, Allison; London HSC-Victoria Hosp, PO Box 5010 Stn B 800 Commissioners Rd E, London ON N6A 5W9; Mem'07; EmergMed. Staff, London Health Sciences Centre - Victoria Campus; (519)685-8500

MEJIA, Jose H; Regional Mental HC-London, PO Box 5532 Stn B T276-850 Higbury Ave, London ON N6A 4H1; (Mexico)'90; PhD; FRCPC; Psy (Forensic Psychiatry). Staff Concurrent Discord, Regional Mental Health Care-St Joseph's Health Care; Staff Forensics, Regional Mental Health Care-St Joseph's Health Care; Consultant Psy Sex Behaviour Clinic, Child & Parent Resource Institute; Langs: Spanish; French; Bilingual(English/French); (519)631-8510 x49402; Fax. (519)204-0317; jmejia4@uwo.ca.

MEJRI, Abdelwaheb; CSSS du Nord de Lanaudière, 1000 boul Sainte-Anne, St-Charles-Brromee QC J6E 6J2; Tunis (Tunisia)'03; Staff, Centre Hospitalier Régional de Lanaudière; (450)759-8222 x2702; Fax. (450)756-7973.

MEKAEL, Hany R R; 51 Gerry Fitzgerald Dr, North York ON M3J 3N4; Cairo (Egypt)'87; MB ChB; CCFP; (416)739-1562; Fax. (416)739-6671.

MEKAWY, Mohamed; Health Sciences Centre, 300 Prince Philip Dr, St. John's NL A1B 3V6; Alexandria (Egypt)'95; MB ChB; Staff, Health Sciences Centre; (709)777-7297

MEKHAEIL, Nermin M E; Commissioners Walk-In Clinic, 111-1 Commissioners Rd E, London ON N6C 5Z3; (Egypt)'88; CCFP; Staff, Regional Mental Health Care-St Joseph's Health Care; (519)668-2400

MEKHAEL, Saly; Walk-In Med Center, 3-180 Steeles Ave W, Thornhill ON L4J 2L1; Tanta (Egypt)'92; CCFP; Langs: Arabic; (289)597-1071; Fax. (289)597-1073.

MEKHAIL, Ashraf S H; River West Med Centre, 5-6500 Roblin Blvd, Winnipeg MB R3R 3P9; Cairo (Egypt)'83; CCFP.

MEKONNEN TIZAZU, Girma; Oshawa Commun Health Centre, 115 Grassmere Ave, Oshawa ON L1H 3X7; Addis Ababa Univ (Ethiopia)'94; CCFP; (905)723-0036; Fax. (905)723-3391.

MEKWAN, Jayanand; Saint John Reg Hosp, PO Box 2100 Stn Main 400 University Ave, Saint John NB E2L 4L2; London (England)'98; Staff, Saint John Regional Hospital; (506)648-6000

MELA, Mansfield A; Royal University Hosp, 103 Hospital Dr, Saskatoon SK S7N 0W8; Zaria (Nigeria)'89; MB BS; FRCPC; Psy. Staff, Royal University Hospital; Clin. Tutor, University of Saskatchewan; (306)966-8232; Fax. (306)966-8177.

MELADY, Donald L; Mount Sinai Hosp, 206-600 University Ave, Toronto ON M5G 1X5; Wes'88; CCFP; CCFP(E.M.); FCFP; Staff, Mount Sinai Hospital; (416)586-5058; Fax. (416)586-4719.

MELAMED, Jennifer B; Alliance Clinic Ltd, 10085 Whalley Blvd, Surrey BC V3T 4G1; Witwatersrand (South Africa)'84; MB ChB; BSc(Med); (604)582-5826; Fax. (604)582-5827.

MELAMED, Penina; 5-2202 Jane St, North York ON M3M 1A4; Tor'06; CCFP; (416)249-8000; Fax. (416)249-4594.

MELAMEDOV, Daniel; Thornhill Endoscopy Centre, 11-390 Steeles Ave W, Thornhill ON L4J 6X2; Tor'98; FACS; BSc; FRCSC; GenSurg (Gastroenterology). Staff Surg, Village East Med Centre; Langs: Hebrew; Russian; (905)882-6566; Fax. (905)882-6567.

MELAMETH, Regine; Club Tiny Tots Med Centre, 3550-6900 boul Decarie, Cote Saint-Luc QC H3X 2T8; Mon'07; CCFP; (514)342-9911; Fax. (514)342-2911.

MELANCON, Denis; MUHC-Montreal Neurology Inst, 3801 rue University, Montreal QC H3A 2B4; Mon'60; CSPQ; DiagRad (P.Q.) (Neuro Radiology). Staff, McGill University Health Centre - Montreal Neurological Hospital; assoc Prof, McGill University; Langs: English; (514)398-1910; d.melan@hotmail.com.

MELANCON, Eric; Clinique Med Familiale de Malb, 515 rue Saint-Etienne, La Malbaie QC G5A 1W7; Laval'98; Staff Emerg, Hôpital de la Malbaie; Langs: English; (418)665-2366 x33; Fax. (418)665-7766.

MELANCON, Francois; Ctr de Sante Base Valcartier, CP 1000 Bdp Succ Forces, Courcelette QC G0A 4Z0; Sher'81; Staff, CSSS des Sources d'Asbestos; Langs: English; (418)844-5000 x6472

MELANCON, Genevieve; Clinique Med de l'Outaouais, 25 ch de la Savane, Gatineau QC J8T 8A4; Mon'03; CCFP; (819)561-6611

MELANCON, Geoffroy; Clinique Psyche, 400-400 av Laurier O, Montreal QC H2V 2K7; Mon'90; FRCPC; Psy. Staff Psy, Hopital Louis-H Lafontaine; Staff Psy, Institut Universitaire de Gériatrie de Montréal; Clin Teach Staff Psy, Universite de Montreal; (514)279-4141; Fax. (514)279-4101.

MELANCON, Karine; CSSS de Saint-Jerome, 290 rue de Montigny, Saint-Jerome QC J7Z 5T3; Sher'97; CSPQ; FRCPC; Anes. Staff Anes, Hôtel-Dieu de Saint-Jérôme; (450)431-8200; kmel@videotron.ca.

MELANCON, Marie-Lise; CLSC Jean Olivier Chenier, 29 ch d'Oka, Saint-Eustache QC J7N 1K6; Laval'08; (450)491-1233

MELANCON, Serge B; MUHC-Montreal Children's Hosp, A608-2300 rue Tupper, Montreal QC H3H 1P3; Mon'65; FRCPC; Peds (Biochemical Genetics); MedGenetics (P.Q.). Staff, McGill University Health Centre - Montreal Children's Hospital; Assoc Member, Hôpital Ste-Justine; Hon Prof Peds, Universite de Montreal; Langs: Bilingual(French/English); (514)412-4427; serge.melancon@muhc.mcgill.ca.

MELANSON, Adrien L; 38 rue Otho, Neguac NB E9G 4H3; Mon'89; (506)776-3876; Fax. (506)776-3877.

MELANSON, Claude; Clin Med Urgence Mont-Royal, 101-4689 rue Papineau, Montreal QC H2H 1V4; Mon'75; (514)521-5555; Fax. (514)521-0951.

MELANSON, Gilles G J; Great-West Assurance-Vie-DSMO, 300-11 Holland Ave, Ottawa ON K1Y 4T2; Dal'76; AB; FRCPC; Psy (P.Q.). Staff, Timmins & District Hospital; Langs: French; (613)241-4047; Fax. (613)482-4606; ggjm@ca.inter.net.

MELANSON, Karen A; 103-185 av Acadie, Dieppe NB E1A 1G6; Laval'95; CCFP; Prof Med, Universite de Sherbrooke; Assoc Prof, Universite de Moncton; Langs: Bilingual(French/English); (506)388-0808; Fax. (506)388-0801; drkarenm@nb.sympatico.ca.

MELANSON, Michel; 76 Stuart St, Kingston ON K7L 2V7; Mon'91; FRCPC; Neur (Neuromuscular Diseases). Assoc Prof Neurol, Kingston General Hospital; Assoc Prof, Queen's University; (613)549-6666 x2601; Fax. (613)548-1341.

MELANSON, Patrick R P; MUHC-Royal Victoria Hosp, L3 06-687 av des Pins O, Montreal QC H3A 1A1; Dal'85; FRCPC; EmergMed; Critical Care Medicine (P.Q.). Staff, McGill University Health Centre - Royal Victoria Hospital; (514)934-1934; Fax. (514)843-1638; patrick.melanson@muhc.mcgill.ca.

MELANSON, Stephanie; Dr Georges-L Dumont Reg Hosp, 330 av Universite, Moncton NB E1C 2Z3; Sher'06; CCFP; Staff, Dr Georges-L-Dumont University Hospital Centre; (506)862-4000

MELANSON, Vincent; 202-123 rue Champlain, Dieppe NB E1A 1N5; Mon'83; Staff, Dr Georges-L-Dumont University Hospital Centre; (506)857-0378; Fax. (506)852-9891.

MELANSON-CANDELA, Denise; Dr Georges-L Dumont Reg Hosp, 330 av Universite, Moncton NB E1C 2Z3; Laval'79; Staff, Dr Georges-L-Dumont University Hospital Centre; (506)862-4234; Fax. (506)862-4135.

MELBOURNE, Byron A; Jane Medical Clinic, LL2-2780 Jane St, North York ON M3N 2J2; (Jamaica)'67; Ac Staff, Humber River Regional Hospital - Finch Avenue Site; Ac Staff, Humber River Regional Hospital - Keele Street Site; (416)744-2000; Fax. (416)744-3133.

MELCHIOR, Maria F; Islington Med Clinic, 604-1243 Islington Ave, Etobicoke ON M8X 1Y9; Qns'96; FRCSC; ObstGyn (Laparoscopy). Ac Staff, St Joseph's Health Centre; Court Staff, Women's College Hospital; Langs: Italian; (416)207-1998; Fax. (416)207-9501.

MELCK, Adrienne L; St Paul's Hosp, C303-1081 Burrard St, Vancouver BC V6Z 1Y6; UBC'03; FRCSC; GenSurg. Staff, Providence Health Care - St Paul's Hospital; (604)806-9108

MELCK, Cyril I; Robson Professional Bldg, 322-1525 Robson St, Vancouver BC V6G 1C3; Natal (South Africa)'74; FRCPC; Psy (Adult ADHD). (604)687-0654; Fax. (604)687-0657.

MELCUK, Ekaterina; Clin Pediatrique Cote-St-Luc, 201-6164 ch de la Cote-Saint-L, Montreal QC H3X 2H1; McG'89; FRCPC; Peds (Adolescent Medicine). Staff, McGill University Health Centre - Montreal Children's Hospital; Langs: Russian; French; (514)369-9999; Fax. (514)369-6016.

MELDRUM, Donald; Bridgeland Med Bldg, 3F-803 1 Ave NE, Calgary AB T2E 7C5; McG'66; FACC; FRCPC; IntMed (Medico Legal Issues); Cardiol. Ac Staff, Foothills Medical Centre; Ac Staff, Rockyview General Hospital; Physician, Calgary Cardiology Consultants; Assoc Prof, University of Calgary; Langs: French; (403)571-8600; Fax. (403)571-8659.

MELDRUM, Joan M; Foothills Breastfeeding Clinic, 101-1318 Centre St NE, Calgary AB T2E 2R7; Sask'76; CCFP; Clinical Asst Prof, University of Calgary; (403)266-2622; Fax. (403)266-2692.

MELDRUM, Lee Anne H; Forensic Psychiatric Hosp, 3-70 Colony Farm Rd, Coquitlam BC V3C 5X9; Sask'84; FRCPC; Psy (Forensic Psychiatry). Staff, Forensic Psychiatric Hospital; Consultant, Kitsilano Fairview Mental Health Team; (604)524-7700; Fax. (604)660-1206; lmeldrum@forensic.bc.ca.

MELE, Tina S; London HSC-University Hosp, PO Box 5339 Stn B 339 Windermere Rd, London ON N6A 5A5; Tor'96; FRCSC; GenSurg. Staff, London Health Sciences Centre - University Hospital; (519)685-8500

MELE, Victor L; Pleasantview Med Centre, 2754 Victoria Park Ave, North York ON M2J 4A8; Wes'62; BA; Langs: Italian; (416)491-3910; Fax. (416)491-3919.

MELEGA, Douglas E; Grand River Hosp-KW Hlth Ctre, PO Box 9056 Stn C 835 King St W, Kitchener ON N2G 1G3; Wes'91; BComm; FRCPC; AnatPath. Staff Path, Grand River Hospital - Kitchener/Waterloo Health Centre; Staff Pathology, St Mary's General Hospital; (519)749-4300 x2158; Fax. (519)749-4221.

MELEMIS, Steven M; 601-160 Eglinton Ave E, Toronto ON M4P 3B5; Tor'86; (416)920-2982; Fax. (416)920-8259.

MELEN, Veronique C; CSSS de Rivière-du-Loup, 75 rue Saint-Henri, Riviere-Du-Loup QC G5R 2A4; Mon'96; FRCPC; Psy. Staff, Centre Hospitalier Regional du Grand-Portage; (418)868-1010; Fax. (418)868-0530.

MELENCHUK, Ron S; 82-4307 130 Ave SE, Calgary AB T2Z 3V8; Sask'83; CCFP; (403)259-3256; Fax. (403)253-2673.

MELENKA, Lyle S; First Edmonton Place, 1370-10665 Jasper Ave NW, Edmonton AB T5J 3S9; Alb'81; MSc(Epidemiol.); FRCPC; IntMed; Respir. Staff, Covenant Health - Grey Nuns Community Hospital; Asst Prof, University of Alberta; (780)702-3866; Fax. (780)702-3882; lsmmd@telus.net.

MELESHKO, Sarah A; Royal Alexandra Hosp, 10240 Kingsway NW, Edmonton AB T5H 3V9; Alb'07; CCFP; CCFP(E.M.); Staff, Royal Alexandra Hospital; (780)735-4442; Fax. (780)735-4916.

MELICHARKOVA, Andrea; The Medical Centre, 707 Charlotte St, Peterborough ON K9J 7B3; Buenos Aires (Argentina)'95; FRCPC; IntMed; Gastroent. Teach Staff, Queen's University; Langs: Czech; Spanish; (705)876-4539; Fax. (705)876-4557.

MELIGRANA, Peter D; Sault Area Hosp, 750 Great Northern Rd, Sault Ste. Marie ON P6B 0A8; (Ireland)'91; Staff, Sault Area Hospital - Sault Ste Marie; (705)759-3434 x5529

MELIJI, Zineb; Clinique Med Saint-Alexandre, 200-2310 rue Saint-Louis, Gatineau QC J8T 5L7; CCFP; Staff, Hôpital de Gatineau; (819)243-4500

MELITI, Abdelrazak; St Paul's Hosp, 1702 20th St W, Saskatoon SK S7M 0Z9; Al-Fateh (Libya)'99; FRCPC; AnatPath. Staff, St Paul's Hospital (Grey Nuns) of Saskatoon; (306)655-5176; Fax. (306)655-5123.

MELLE, Jesse R; Rosthern Med Clinic, PO Box 1089, Rosthern SK S0K 3R0; Sask'07; CCFP; (306)232-4894; Fax. (306)232-4970.

MELLER, David F; Bigelow Fowler Clinic, 1605 9 Ave S, Lethbridge AB T1J 1W2; Cal'77; CCFP; FCFP; (403)327-3121; Fax. (403)320-5593.

MELLER, Jack B; Selkirk Mental Health Centre, PO Box 9600 Stn Main 825 Manitoba Ave, Selkirk MB R1A 2B5; Man'73; Staff Psy, Selkirk Mental Health Centre; (204)482-1653; Fax. (204)482-3203; jmeller2@shaw.ca.

MELLICK, Zohra H; Cumberland Med Clinic, 11-900 Watters Rd, Orleans ON K4A 0B4; Alb'88; BSc; (613)830-3837

MELLING, Gordon W; Southwood Med Clinic, 80-10233 Elbow Dr SW, Calgary AB T2W 1E8; Alb'78; Ac Staff, Rockyview General Hospital; (403)252-1111; mellinggw@shaw.ca.

MELLING, James N; St Anthony's Med Centre, 203-582 Goldstream Ave, Victoria BC V9B 2W7; Mem'83; BSc; BMedSci; Staff Family Pract, Vancouver Island Health Authority; (250)478-4821; Fax. (250)478-7912.

MELLING, Michael T; Northside Med Clinic, 414 13 St N, Lethbridge AB T1H 2S2; Glasgow (Scotland)'57; MB ChB; FRCS(Glas); FACS; FRCSC; GenSurg. Staff, Chinook Regional Hospital; Staff, Covenant Health - St Michael's Health Centre; (403)394-1234; Fax. (403)320-9215; drmelling@nsmclinic.com.

MELLON, Aaron M; Manitoba Clinic, 790 Sherbrook St, Winnipeg MB R3A 1M3; Man'01; CCFP; (204)896-9678

MELLOR, Jeffrey; 109-4616 Valiant Dr NW, Calgary AB T3A 0X9; UBC'70; FACP; FRCPC; IntMed (Sleep Medicine). Ac Staff, Foothills Medical Centre; Ac Staff, Rockyview General Hospital; Consultant, Central Zone David Thompson Health Region; (403)250-5674; Fax. (403)202-0266.

MELMED, Calvin A; SMBD Jewish Gen Hosp, 3755 ch Cote-Sainte-Catherine, Montreal QC H3T 1E2; Man'68; FRCPC; Neur. Ac Staff, Sir Mortimer B Davis Jewish General; Langs: Yiddish; French; (514)340-8222 x4622; Fax. (514)340-7567; calvin.melmed@mcgill.ca.

MELNIK, Howard; CSSS du Sud de Lanaudière, 911 montee des Pionniers, Terrebonne QC J6V 2H2; McG'94; CSPQ; FRCPC; Anes. Assoc Member Anes, Centre Hospitalier Régional de Lanaudière; Staff, Centre Hospitalier Pierre le Gardeur; (450)654-7525 x32214; Fax. (450)654-7296.

MELNITZER, Melissa D; 411-401 Richmond St, Toronto ON M5V 3A8; McM'97; CCFP; (416)533-0172

MELNYCHUK, David A N; SMBD Jewish Gen Hosp, 3755 ch Cote-Sainte-Catherine, Montreal QC H3T 1E2; Alb'79; Staff, Sir Mortimer B Davis Jewish General; (514)340-8248; Fax. (514)340-8302.

MELNYK, Lydia C; Wee Care Clinic, 6624 av Somerled, Montreal QC H4V 1T2; McG'04; CCFP; Langs: Ukrainian; French; (514)486-6656; Fax. (514)486-0309.

MELNYK, Tatiana C; Univ Hlth Network-Princess M, 610 University Ave, Toronto ON M5G 2M9; McG'94; FRCPC; Psy. Staff, Princess Margaret Hospital - University Health Network; (416)946-4501 x5451

MELOCHE, Eryn N; PO Box 71134 Rpo Silver Spring, Calgary AB T3B 5K2; Qns'09; CCFP.

MELOCHE, Helene; Clinique Med l'Acadie, GD 1B rue Marion, Saint-Jacques QC J0K 2R0; Mon'94; (450)839-7851

MELOCHE, Judith; Hôpital Ste-Justine, 3175 ch Cote-Sainte-Catherine, Montreal QC H3T 1C5; Mon'86; Peds. Staff, Hôpital Ste-Justine; (514)345-4788

MELOCHE, Leslie N; 103-3374 Marshall Rd, Abbotsford BC V2S 1L1; Alb'10; CCFP; (604)853-5424

MELOCHE, R Mark; 5153-2775 Laurel St, Vancouver BC V5Z 1M9; Wes'80; FRCSC; GenSurg. Consultant, Vancouver General Hospital - Centennial Pavillion; Vis Staff, Providence Health Care - St Paul's Hospital; Head Surg, UBC Hospital - Koerner Pavillion; (604)875-5287; Fax. (604)875-5447.

MELOFF, Keith L; Baycrest Ctre/Geriatric Care, 3560 Bathurst St, Toronto ON M6A 2E1; Man'66; DABPed; Peds; Neur (Pediatric Neurology). Consultant, Toronto General Hospital - UHN; Staff, Baycrest Centre for Geriatric Care; Consultant, Bayview Centre for Geriatric Care; Consultant Neurol., Underserviced Area Prog., Min. of Health, Ontario; Aj Prof, University of Western Ontario; (416)784-3600; Fax. (416)784-5600; kmeloff@rogers.com.

MELOSKY, Barbara L; BC Cancer Agency-Vancouver CC, 600 10th Ave W, Vancouver BC V5Z 4E6; Man'87; FRCPC; IntMed; MedOncol. Staff, BC Cancer Agency Vancouver Centre; (604)877-6000

MELTON, Ellen; Curans Health Centre, 384 Fort William Rd, Thunder Bay ON P7B 2Z3; Novosibirsk (Russia (Federation))'87; FRCPC; IntMed (Cardiology). Staff Internist, Thunder Bay Regional Health Sciences Centre; Asst Prof, Lakehead University / Library; Langs: Russian; (807)345-3355; Fax. (807)345-0099.

MELTZER, Sara J; M922-687 av des Pins O, Montreal QC H3A 1A1; Alb'72; FRCP; CSPQ; FACP; FRCPC; IntMed (Diabetes); Endocrin (P.Q.). Staff Physician, McGill University Health Centre - Royal Victoria Hospital; Assoc Prof Med & ObstGyn, McGill University; Langs: Bilingual(English/French); (514)934-1934 x35576; sara.meltzer@mcgill.ca.

MELUN, Jean-Pierre G; Hop Louis-H Lafontaine, 7401 rue Hochelaga, Montreal QC H1N 3M5; Paris (France)'77; Psy (P.Q.). Staff, Hopital Louis-H Lafontaine; (514)251-4000

MELVILLE, Karen A; Peterborough Reg HC-Hospital, 1 Hospital Dr, Peterborough ON K9J 7C6; Dal'99; FRCPC; AnatPath. Staff, Peterborough Regional Health Centre - Hospital Drive; (705)743-2121 x3717

MELVILLE, Rhona D S; Southdale Med Clinic, 357 Southdale Rd E, London ON N6E 1A2; Wes'83; Ac Staff, London Health Sciences Centre - Victoria Campus; (519)685-9743; Fax. (519)685-9743.

MELVIN, Kenneth R; 220-340 College St, Toronto ON M5T 3A9; Tor'77; FRCPC; IntMed (Cardiac Rehabilitation); Cardiol. Staff Cardiol, Toronto Western Hospital - University Health Network; Assoc Prof Med, University of Toronto; (416)323-9440 x222; Fax. (416)323-9545; kenneth.melvin@uhn.on.ca.

MELVIN, Kevin N; 206 Lemarchant Rd, St. John's NL A1C 2H6; Dal'74; AB; FCCP; FACS; FICS; FRCSC; GenSurg; Cardiovasc&ThorSurg. Vascular Surgery, St Clare's Mercy Hospital; Asst Prof, Memorial University Of Newfoundland; (709)579-0542; Fax. (709)579-0613; kevinmelvin@nl.rogers.com.

MEMA, Briseida; The Hosp for Sick Children, 555 University Ave, Toronto ON M5G 1X8; Tirana (Albania)'97; FRCPC; Peds (Critical Care Medicine). Staff, The Hospital For Sick Children; Langs: Italian; Albanian; (416)813-1500

MEMARPOUR, Mahdi; Southlake Reg Health Centre, 5883-596 Davis Dr, Newmarket ON L3Y 2P9; Bucharest (Romania)'92; FRCPC; Psy. Staff, Southlake Regional Health Centre; (905)895-4521; Fax. (905)830-5977.

MEMAURI, Brett F; St Boniface Gen Hosp, 409 Tache Ave, Winnipeg MB R2H 2A6; Sask'02; FRCPC; DiagRad (Thoracic Radiology). Prog Dir Ungergraduate, St Boniface General Hospital; (204)233-8563; menetek@yahoo.com.

MEMICHE, Nejat; Vanier Med Centre, 7-325 Vanier Blvd, Bathurst NB E2A 3N1; Istanbul (Turkey)'82; FRCPC; Peds; Gastroent (P.Q.). Staff, Dr Georges-L-Dumont University Hospital Centre; Staff, Hopital Regional Chaleur; Staff, Hôpital de l'Enfant-Jésus RHSJ; Langs: Turkish; French; (506)546-3588; Fax. (506)547-1888.

MEMICHE, Reshat; Vanier Med Centre, 7-325 Vanier Blvd, Bathurst NB E2A 3N1; Istanbul (Turkey)'80; FRCPC; IntMed; Gastroent (P.Q.). Chief, Nor'East Health Network Regional Hospital Centre, IntMed. & GI Lab.; Staff, Hôpital de l'Enfant-Jésus RHSJ; Staff, Dr Georges-L-Dumont University Hospital Centre; Pres, Glouchester Medical Society; Langs: Turkish; French; (506)546-3588; Fax. (506)547-1888.

MEMON, Abdulaziz; Centennial CMH & Brain Injury, PO Box 1000 Stn Main, Ponoka AB T4J 1R8; Karachi (Pakistan)'81; Staff Psy, Centennial Centre for Mental Health & Brain Injury; (403)783-7600; Fax. (403)783-7790.

MEMON, Ghulam F; Carman Med Clinic, PO Box 728, Carman MB R0G 0J0; Liaquat (Pakistan)'92.

MEMON, Rukhsana F; Carman Med Group, PO Box 728, Carman MB R0G 0J0; Sind (Pakistan)'92; CCFP.

MENA, Chantal; Hotel-Dieu de Sorel, 400 av de l'Hotel-Dieu, Sorel-Tracy QC J3P 1N5; Nantes (France)'89; Staff, Hôtel-Dieu de Sorel; Gen Practice, CHSLD du Bas-Richelieu; (450)746-6000; Fax. (450)746-6227; cmena000@sympatico.ca.

MENARD, Alain L; Medico Dental Centre, 204-2555 St. Joseph Blvd, Orleans ON K1C 1S6; Ott'73; Ac Staff, Montfort Hospital; (613)824-8023; Fax. (613)824-7781.

MENARD, Alexandre S; Kingston Gen Hosp, 76 Stuart St, Kingston ON K7L 2V7; Ott'03; FRCPC; DiagRad. Staff, Kingston General Hospital; (613)549-6666

MENARD, Andre; Clinique Med le Gardeurois, 250-155 boul Lacombe, Repentigny QC J5Z 3C4; Mon'75; Médecin, Centre Hospitalier Pierre le Gardeur; Médecin, CHSLD Vigi Our Lady of Lourdes; Médecin, CHSLD Bourget Inc; Langs: English; (450)585-3683; Fax. (450)585-2107; docmenard@videotron.ca.

MENARD, Andre; Clinique Med Fabreville, 109-380 boul Curé-Labelle, Laval QC H7P 5L3; Mon'68; FRCPC; Derm. ac Staff, Centre Hospitalier l'Université de Montréal (CHUM) - Hôpital Notre-Dame; (450)628-5800; Fax. (450)628-0217.

MENARD, Carole; Clinique Fam d'Arthabaska, 2-39 rue Laurier E, Victoriaville QC G6P 6P6; Sher'81; (819)357-9322; Fax. (819)357-7926.

MENARD, Charles; CHUS-Hop Hotel-Dieu, 580 rue Bowen S, Sherbrooke QC J1G 2E8; Mon'01; Gastroent; IntMed (Endoscopy). Staff, Centre Hospitalier Universitaire de Sherbrooke-Hôpital Hôtel-Dieu; Langs: Bilingual(French/English); (819)346-1110 x23553; charle.menard@usherbrooke.ca.

MENARD, Christian; CSSS Maria-Chapdelaine, 2000 boul du Sacré-Coeur, Dolbeau-Mistassini QC G8L 2R5; Laval'92; GenSurg. Staff, Centre Maria-Chapdelaine - CH de Dolbeau-Mistassini; (418)276-1234

MENARD, Claude; 240-214 boul de la Cite-des-Je, Gatineau QC J8Y 6S8; Sher'82; FRCSC; Ophth (Cataract). Staff, CH-CHSLD de Papineau - Pavillon du centre hospitalier; Chef, Hull Hospital; Consultant, Focus Eye Centre; Langs: English; (819)775-2900; Fax. (819)775-2557; centre.ophtalmologie@bellnet.ca.

MENARD, Claude; Clin Med St-Pierre de Sorel, 338 boul Gagne, Sorel-Tracy QC J3P 5V8; Sher'77; Langs: English; (450)742-0415; Fax. (450)742-0417.

MENARD, Claude E; Clinique Med Cite des Jeunes, 220-214 boul de la Cite-des-Je, Gatineau QC J8Y 6S8; Laval'64; FRCPC; Psy. (819)243-0955 x220; Fax. (819)243-7972.

MENARD, Cynthia M M; Univ Hlth Network-Princess M, 5 809-610 University Ave, Toronto ON M5G 2M9; Cal'96; FRCPC; RadOncol. Staff, Princess Margaret Hospital - University Health Network; (416)946-6513; Fax. (416)946-2227.

MENARD, Daniel B; 200-1815 rue King O, Sherbrooke QC J1J 2E3; Sher'73; Gastroent (Hepatology). Staff, Centre Hospitalier Universitaire de Sherbrooke-Hôpital Hôtel-Dieu; Langs: English; (819)565-1921; Fax. (819)565-7780; daniel.b.menard@usherbrooke.ca.

MENARD, Daniel; Polyclinique Medical P A T, 103-12905 rue Sherbrooke E, Pte-Aux-Trembles QC H1A 1B9; Mon'74; LMCC; (514)498-4050

MENARD, Danielle; Clinique Med Soleil, 64 1re av O, Amos QC J9T 1T8; Sher'91; Staff, Centre de sante Tulattavik de l'Ungava; (819)732-8341; Fax. (819)732-1642; danielle.menard@ssss.gouv.qc.ca.

MENARD, Darrell C; 37 Parklands Ave, Russell ON K4R 1A2; Qns'88; Dip SportMed; (613)445-0201; Fax. (613)445-1544.

MENARD, Ginette; 215-1144 rue Saint-Laurent O, Longueuil QC J4K 1E2; Mon'81; Langs: Bilingual(French/English); (450)674-6281; Fax. (450)651-4271.

MENARD, Henri A; MUHC-Montreal Gen Hosp, A6 162-1650 av Cedar, Montreal QC H3G 1A4; Mon'67; CSPQ; Rheum. Ac Member, McGill University Health Centre - Montreal General Campus; Ac Member, McGill University Health Centre - Royal Victoria Hospital; Prof Med, McGill University; Langs: Bilingual(English/French); (514)934-1934 x44177; henri.a.menard@muhc.mcgill.ca.

MENARD, Jacinthe; Clinique Fam de St-Hyacinthe, 2955 boul Laframboise, Saint-Hyacinthe QC J2S 4Z3; Sher'81; Staff, Centre Hospitalier Honore-Mercier; (450)774-2428; Fax. (450)774-8986.

MENARD, Jacques G; 202-492 boul de l'Hopital, Gatineau QC J8V 2P4; Ott'85; Staff Privil, Centre Hospitalier Gatineau Mémorial; Langs: English; French.

MENARD, Keith M; Wesley Street Clinic, 360 Wesley St, Nanaimo BC V9R 2T6; Man'94; BSc; FRCPC; Peds. (250)951-2115

MENARD, Lucie L; Hop Charles LeMoyne, 3120 boul Taschereau, Greenfield Park QC J4V 2H1; Mon'81; CSPQ; Anes. Staff, Hopital Charles LeMoyne; (450)466-5000 x2680; Fax. (450)466-5007.

MENARD, Lyne; CSSS de la Baie-des-Chaleurs, RR 2 419 boul Perron, Maria QC G0C 1Y0; Mon'91; CCFP; FCFP; Staff, CSSS de la Baie-des-Chaleurs; (418)392-7373; Fax. (418)392-7378.

MENARD, Marc; Hôpital Ste-Justine, 3175 ch Cote-Sainte-Catherine, Montreal QC H3T 1C5; Mon'80; Peds. Staff, Hôpital Ste-Justine; (514)345-4919

MENARD, Marie-Chantal; Clin Familiale du Boulevard, 21 rue Moreau, St-Jean-Sur-Richel QC J2W 1J1; Mon'88; Langs: English; (450)349-7070 x1; Fax. (450)349-7070; mcmenard@videotron.ca.

MENARD, Nathalie; Ctr Hosp Laurentien, 234 rue Saint-Vincent, Ste-Agathe-Des-Mts QC J8C 2B8; Mon'93; Staff, Centre Hospitalier Laurentien; (819)324-4000; Fax. (819)324-4010.

MENARD, Nathalie P; Medical Centre, 201-171 Montreal Rd, Cornwall ON K6H 1B2; Ott'99; CCFP; Langs: Bilingual(French/English); (613)933-2686; Fax. (613)933-5789.

MENARD, Patricia; Antigonish Med Assoc, 40 Church St, Antigonish NS B2G 2C7; Dal'91; Staff, St Martha's Regional Hospital; (902)863-4558; Fax. (902)867-5665.

MENARD, Rejean; Ctr de Med Familiale de Granby, 48 rue Denison E, Granby QC J2G 4C6; Mon'70; CCFP; FCFP; (450)372-3996; Fax. (450)372-0430.

MENARD, Shaunna L; 2133 36 St NE, Calgary AB T1Y 5S3; Man'91; FRCPC; DiagRad. (403)568-7676; Fax. (403)568-7677.

MENARD, Sheila M; 622 3rd St SW, Dauphin MB R7N 1R5; Man'06.

MENARD, Sophie; Clinique Med l'Ouest Inc, 4475 rue Bannantyne, Verdun QC H4G 1E2; Laval'89; Staff, Centre Hospitalier de LaSalle; (450)765-3600

MENARD, Stephanie; CHUM-Hop Notre-Dame, 1560 rue Sherbrooke E, Montreal QC H2L 4M1; Mon'04; FRCPC; NuclearMed. Staff, Centre Hospitalier l'Université de Montréal (CHUM) - Hôpital Notre-Dame; (514)890-8000

MENARD, Suzanne; ASSS de l'Estrie, 300-300 rue King E, Sherbrooke QC J1G 1B1; Sher'82; Assoc Staff, Centre Hospitalier Universitaire de Sherbrooke-Hopital Fleurimont; (819)829-3400 x42484; Fax. (819)564-5435.

MENARD, Sylvain; CHUM-Hop St-Luc, 1058 rue Saint-Denis, Montreal QC H2X 3J4; Sher'04; ObstGyn (Gynecological Reproductive Endocrinology). Staff, Centre Hospitalier l'Université De Montréal (CHUM) - Hôpital Saint-luc; (514)890-8000

MENARD, Sylvain; Clinique Med St-Sauveur, 70 rue Principale, Saint-Sauveur QC J0R 1R6; Mon'79; Langs: Bilingual(French/English); (450)227-8436; Fax. (450)227-7222.

MENARD, Yves; Ctr Hosp Affilie-St-Sacrement, 1050 ch Sainte-Foy, Quebec QC G1S 4L8; Laval'93; Staff, Centre Hospitalier Affilié Universitaire de Québec - Hôpital du St-Sacrement; Staff, Centre Hospitalier Portneuf; (418)682-4511

MENARD, Yvon; Clinique Med Berger, 2200 ch de Chambly, Longueuil QC J4J 3Z3; Mon'64; Ac Staff, Hopital Charles LeMoyne; (450)674-7401; Fax. (450)677-8027; yvon.m@videotron.ca.

MENARD-BUTEAU, Carole; 200-4 Beechwood Ave, Vanier ON K1L 8L9; Mon'87; FRCPC; Psy. Physician, University of Ottawa Health Services; Asst Prof, University of Ottawa; (613)741-7174; Fax. (613)741-0176.

MENASRIA, Ali; Dr Georges-L Dumont Reg Hosp, 330 av Universite, Moncton NB E1C 2Z3; (Algeria)'76; Endocrinology & Metabolism, Dr Georges-L-Dumont University Hospital Centre; (506)869-2023; Fax. (506)869-2734.

MENASSA, Johanne; Hop Charles LeMoyne, 3120 boul Taschereau, Greenfield Park QC J4V 2H1; Mon'00; FRCSC; Ophth. Staff, Hopital Charles LeMoyne; Langs: English; (450)466-5000; Fax. (450)466-5403.

MENCHIONS, C W Bruce; Royal Bank Plaza, PO Box 83 Stn Royal Bank 200 Bay St, Toronto ON M5J 2J2; Tor'83; MSc; MBA; FRCPC; Psy (Psychosis). Staff, St Joseph's Healthcare Hamilton - West 5th Campus; Staff, Trillium Health Centre - West Toronto; Staff Psy, Workers' Comp Board of ON; Asst Clin Prof, McMaster University; (416)363-8850; Fax. (416)363-9466.

MENDELL, Lawrence M; The Ottawa Hosp-Riverside, 1967 Riverside Dr, Ottawa ON K1H 7W9; McG'73; CSPQ; FRCPC; DiagRad. Staff, The Ottawa Hospital - Riverside Campus; (613)738-8400 x82327; Fax. (613)738-8538; lmendell@ottawahospital.on.ca.

MENDELSOHN, Jeffrey D; First Med Place, 107-170 Queensway W, Mississauga ON L5B 3A8; Cape Town (South Africa)'78; ABOtol; FRCSC; Otol. Staff, William Osler Health System - Brampton Civic Hospital; Staff, Trillium Health Centre - Mississauga; Staff, The Credit Valley Hospital; (905)273-3140; Fax. (905)273-3049; jmendelsohn@thc.on.ca.

MENDELSON, Jack; SMBD Jewish Gen Hosp, 3755 ch Cote-Sainte-Catherine, Montreal QC H3T 1E2; McG'60; MSc; FRCPC; MedMicrobiol (Medical Microbiology & Infectious Diseases); InfectDis., Sir Mortimer B Davis Jewish General Hospital, Research Ethics office; Head Research Ethics Office, Sir Mortimer B Davis Jewish General; Prof Med & Microbiol, McGill University; Langs: English; French; (514)340-7940; Fax. (514)340-7951; jack.mendelson@mcgill.ca.

MENDELSON, Michael; The Hosp for Sick Children, 555 University Ave, Toronto ON M5G 1X8; Man'06; FRCPC; Peds; Cardiol. Staff, The Hospital For Sick Children; (416)813-7500

MENDELSON, Mitchell N; 101-1001 Broadway W, Vancouver BC V6H 4E4; Tor'78; (604)916-6786

MENDELSSOHN, David C; Humber River Reg Hosp-Church, 2024-200 Church St, Toronto ON M9N 1N8; Dal'83; FRCPC; IntMed; Nephrol. Head Nephrol, Humber River Regional Hospital - Church Street Site; Assoc Prof Med, University of Toronto; (416)243-4368; Fax. (416)243-4421; dmendelssohn@hrrh.on.ca.

MENDELSSOHN, Krisanne E; The Court, 312-2863 Ellesmere Rd, Scarborough ON M1E 5E9; Dal'83; CCFP; FCFP; Staff, Rouge Valley Health System - Centenary Health Centre Site; (416)281-9055; Fax. (416)281-9006.

MENDES, John M; 306-726 Bloor St W, Toronto ON M6G 4A1; Tor'83; FRCPC; Peds. Langs: Portuguese; (416)534-1159; Fax. (416)572-0083.

MENDEZ, Ivar M; Queen Elizabeth II HSC-Halifax, 3806-1796 Summer St, Halifax NS B3H 3A7; Wes'86; FACS; PhD; FRCSC; Neursurg. Staff, Queen Elizabeth II Health Sciences Centre - Halifax Infirmary Site; Chair Brain Repair Centre, Dalhousie University; (902)473-7046; Fax. (902)473-3343; mendez@dal.ca.

MENDEZ-FERNANDEZ, Anselmo; Hanover Med Clinic, 90-118 7th Ave, Hanover ON N4N 2G9; Jagiellonian University (Poland)'09; CCFP; Langs: Spanish; (519)364-2340

MENDEZ TEJADA, Hector; 701-1280 Finch Ave W, North York ON M3J 3K6; (El Salvador)'79; Langs: Spanish; (416)663-7077; Fax. (416)663-6529; hectormtmd@hotmail.com.

MENDIS, M M D Calista; 106-10055 120 Ave, Grande Prairie AB T8V 8H8; (Sri Lanka)'91; CCFP; (780)532-4415; Fax. (780)532-4559.

MENDIS, Maleen R; Workers' Comp Board of MB, 333 Broadway, Winnipeg MB R3C 4W3; Man'06; CCFP.

MENDIS, Tilak; Smyth Med Centre, 226-1929 Russell Rd, Ottawa ON K1G 4G3; London (England)'72; MB BS; ABPN; FACP; LMCC; FRCP; FRCPC; Neur (P.Q.); Psy (P.Q.) (Movement Disorders). Dir Parkinson's Dis. & Neurodegenerative Disorders Clinic/Staff Neurologist, The Ottawa Hospital - General Campus; Neurologist Movement Disorders Clinic, Kingston General Hospital; Asst Prof, University of Ottawa; Asst Prof, Queen's University; Langs: Sinhalese; French; (613)562-4235

MENDONCA, Janet A; Whitby Med Arts Centre, 202-1615 Dundas St E, Whitby ON L1N 2L1; Goa (India)'99; MB BS; CCFP; (289)240-7710; Fax. (289)240-8832.

MENDONCA, Paul V; 110-77 Westmount Rd, Guelph ON N1H 5J1; Debrecen (Hungary)'02; CCFP; (519)829-1212

MENDOZA, Maribel B; 1B-6941 Derry Rd, Milton ON L9T 7H5; (Philippines)'99; CCFP; Langs: Tagalog; (905)875-9999

MENDOZA, Patricia M; 1102-1633 10th Ave W, Vancouver BC V6J 2A2; Manila (Philippines)'82; FRCPC; Peds. (604)345-5798

MENDOZA, Paul J; 201-6355 152 St, Surrey BC V3S 3K8; UBC'01; CCFP; (604)592-2242; Fax. (604)592-9262.

MENDOZA, Valentina I; St Paul's Hosp, 1081 Burrard St, Vancouver BC V6Z 1Y6; UBC'05; Psy. Staff, Providence Health Care - St Paul's Hospital; (604)806-8589

MENDOZA-LONDONO, Roberto; The Hosp for Sick Children, 555 University Ave, Toronto ON M5G 1X8; Bogota (Colombia)'94; Staff, The Hospital For Sick Children; Langs: Spanish; (416)813-6122; Fax. (416)813-5345; roberto.mendoza@sickkids.ca.

MENEGHETTI, Adam T; Gordon & Leslie Diamond H C, 5F-2775 Laurel St, Vancouver BC V5Z 1M9; UBC'96; MHSc; FRCSC; GenSurg (Laparoscopic Surgery). Staff, Vancouver General Hospital - Centennial Pavillion; Staff, UBC Hospital - Koerner Pavillion; Staff, Ambulatory Surgical Centre Vancouver; (604)875-4498; Fax. (604)875-5588.

MENEGHETTI, Victor A; Jim Pattison Pavillion, 899 12th Ave W, Vancouver BC V5Z 1M9; UBC'04; FRCPC; GenPath. (604)875-4111

MENEILLY, Graydon S; Gordon & Leslie Diamond HC, 2775 Laurel St, Vancouver BC V5Z 1M9; Sask'78; FRCPC; IntMed (Diabetology); GeriatricMed. Staff, Vancouver General Hospital - Centennial Pavillion; Dept Head & School Dir Med, University of British Columbia; (604)875-4107; Fax. (604)875-4886; deptmedhead@vch.ca.

MENES, Catharine E; The Sleep Disorders Clinic, 7-55 Frid St, Hamilton ON L8P 4M3; Qns'76; DAB; FRCPC; Psy (Sleep Medicine). (905)529-2259; Fax. (905)529-2262.

MENESES, Gayzelle A; Dr G B Cross Mem Hosp, 67 Manitoba Dr, Clarenville NL A5A 1K3; De La Salle Univ (Philippines)'89; Staff, The Dr G B Cross Memorial Hospital; (709)466-3411; Fax. (709)466-4262.

MENESES, Gloria S; 110-1920 Ellesmere Rd, Scarborough ON M1H 2V6; Manila (Philippines)'78; CCFP; Assoc Staff, The Scarborough Hospital - General Campus; Langs: Tagalog; (416)269-5144; Fax. (416)269-5809.

MENESI, Wisam A; 750 Brunswick St, Fredericton NB E3B 1H9; Al Arab Medical University (Libya)'01; FRCSC; PlasSurg.

MENEZES, Antonio A C; Red Deer Reg Hosp Centre, PO Box 5030 Stn Postal Box Ctr 3942 50A Ave, Red Deer AB T4N 6R2; (India)'85; Staff, Red Deer Regional Hospital Centre; (403)343-4422

MENEZES, Janice A; St Paul's Hosp, 1081 Burrard St, Vancouver BC V6Z 1Y6; Ott'91; FRCPC; IntMed; GeriatricMed. Staff, Providence Health Care - St Paul's Hospital; (604)806-8029; Fax. (604)806-8390.

MENEZES, Natasja M; 703-25 Charlton Ave E, Hamilton ON L8N 1Y2; McG'97; FRCPC; Psy. (416)535-8501 x6913; Fax. (416)979-4676.

MENG, Chen; South Shore Reg Hosp, 90 Glen Allan Dr, Bridgewater NS B4V 3S6; Dal'00; BSc; FRCPC; DiagRad. Staff, South Shore Regional Hospital; (902)527-5230; Fax. (902)543-9793.

MENG, Joanne; The Ottawa Hosp-Gen Campus, 501 Smyth Rd, Ottawa ON K1H 8L6; Mem'88; FRCPC; RadOncol. Staff, The Ottawa Hospital - General Campus; (613)737-7700 x70212; Fax. (613)247-3511.

MENGEL, Michael H; University of Alberta Hosp, 5B2.27-8440 112 St NW, Edmonton AB T6G 2B7; (Hungary)'95; Staff, University of Alberta Hospital; Assoc Prof/Dept Chair Laboratory Med & Pathology (Acting), University of Alberta; Langs: German; (780)407-3922; Fax. (780)407-3009; michael.mengel@albertahealthservices.ca.

MENGUAL, Rose; Health Sciences Centre, 300 Prince Philip Dr, St. John's NL A1B 3V6; Qns'06; EmergMed. Staff, Health Sciences Centre; (709)737-6300

MENHEM, Menhem-Jean; Clinique Med du Lac, 69 boul Seigneurial O, Saint-Bruno QC J3V 2G9; St. Joseph (Lebanon)'68; Ac Staff Med, Centre Hospitalier Pierre Boucher; Langs: English; (450)653-2433; Fax. (450)653-2434.

MENHEM, Zoulficar H; Forest Lawn Medicentre, 1814 33 St SE, Calgary AB T2B 0T4; (Romania)'92; Staff, Alberta Children's Hospital; (403)235-5651; Fax. (403)248-1741.

MENIKEFS, Peter N; St Joseph's Health Centre, 30 The Queensway, Toronto ON M6R 1B5; McG'95; FRCPC; Anes. Staff, St Joseph's Health Centre; (416)530-6090

MENKARIOS, Cathy; Hop Maisonneuve-Rosemont, 5415 boul de l'Assomption, Montreal QC H1T 2M4; Mon'01; FRCPC; RadOncol. Staff, Hopital Maisonneuve-Rosemont; Langs: Bilingual(French/English); (514)252-3425

MENKARIOS, Gamil N; Hamilton Commun Health Centre, M12-414 Victoria Ave N, Hamilton ON L8L 5G8; Ain Shams (Egypt)'63; DAB; FRCSC; Otol. Court Staff, St Joseph's Healthcare - Charlton Campus; Court Staff/Hon Staff, Hamilton Health Sciences Centre - McMaster Children's Hospital; Asst Prof Surg, McMaster University; (905)383-3468; Fax. (905)383-6284.

MENKIS, Alan H; St Boniface Gen Hosp, Z3047-409 Tache Ave, Winnipeg MB R2H 2A6; McM'77; FRCSC; Cardiovasc&ThorSurg (Cardiac Surgery). Med Dir Cardiac Sciences, St Boniface General Hospital; (204)258-1203

MENLOVE, James F; St Thomas-Elgin Gen Hosp, PO Box 2007 Stn Main 189 Elm St, St Thomas ON N5P 3W2; Tor'00; CCFP; CCFP(E.M.); Staff, St Thomas Elgin General Hospital; (519)631-2020

MENNIE, Mary K; The Hosp for Sick Children, 555 University Ave, Toronto ON M5G 1X8; McM'07; FRCPC; Peds. Staff, The Hospital For Sick Children; (416)813-1500

MENON, Anilkumar S; 201-100 Pertosa Dr, Brampton ON L6X 0H9; Tor'91; MEng; PhD; FRCPC; Peds (Pediatric Cardiology); Cardiol. Staff PedCardiol, The Hospital For Sick Children; Staff PedCardiol, William Osler Health System - Brampton Civic Hospital; Langs: Hindi; Malayalam; (905)456-9370; Fax. (905)453-8672.

MENON, Bijoy; Foothills Med Centre, 1079-1403 29 St NW, Calgary AB T2N 2T9; (India)'99; Staff, Foothills Medical Centre; Asst Prof Med, University of Calgary; (403)944-3458; Fax. (403)944-2611; bijoy.menon@albertahealthservices.ca.

MENON, Gopinath T; 668 Concession St, Hamilton ON L8V 4T9; Bombay (India)'63; MB BS; FRCS(E); FRCSC; GenSurg. Langs: Spanish; Hindi; (905)389-2275; Fax. (905)389-7642.

MENON, Krishna; Credit Valley Prof Bldg, 210-2300 Eglinton Ave W, Mississauga ON L5M 2V8; Tor'93; FRCPC; IntMed; Gastroent. (905)569-7789; Fax. (905)569-7702.

MENON, Kusum; Children's Hosp Eastern Ont, 3002D-401 Smyth Rd, Ottawa ON K1H 8L1; UBC'89; FRCPC; Peds; Critical Care Medicine. Staff, Children's Hospital of Eastern Ontario (CHEO); (613)737-7600 x2538; Fax. (613)738-4287; menon@cheo.on.ca.

MENON, Matthew R G; 10150 121 St NW, Edmonton AB T5N 1K4; Wes'00; FRCSC; OrthSurg. (780)434-3668; Fax. (780)434-4859.

MENON, Rajashree K; 2136 Concorde Ave, Cornwall ON K6H 7E2; Kerala (India)'88; MB BS; MSGenSurg; FRCSC; GenSurg (Oncology). Staff, Cornwall Community Hospital; Lecturer Surg, University of Ottawa; Langs: Hindi; Malayalam; (613)938-2832; Fax. (613)938-6421.

MENSAH, Cynthia; City Centre Fam Physicians, 100-514 Queen St, Saskatoon SK S7K 0M5; Sask'04; BSc(Micro); CCFP; (306)244-3016; Fax. (306)244-4737.

MENSAH KWESI, Albert; New Vision Family Health Team, 421 Greenbrook Dr, Kitchener ON N2M 4K1; McM'08; CCFP; Staff, New Vision Family Health Team - Greenbrook; (519)578-3510; Fax. (519)578-6040.

MENSINK, Fred J; Peter Lougheed Centre, 3500 26 Ave NE, Calgary AB T1Y 6J4; Man'80; FRCPC; Anes. Staff, Peter Lougheed Centre; (403)943-5554

MENSINKAI, Arun; Hamilton HS-General Site, 237 Barton St E, Hamilton ON L8L 2X2; Mem'04; FRCPC; DiagRad. Staff, Hamilton Health Sciences Centre - Hamilton General Hospital; (905)527-4322; Fax. (905)527-5781.

MENSINKAI, Suchitra; Baywood Med Centre, 303-95 Bayly St W, Ajax ON L1S 7K8; Mem'85; (905)683-6422

MENSOUR, M'Hamed; Meadows Med Clinic, 2362 24 St NW, Edmonton AB T6T 0G9; (780)465-7335; Fax. (780)465-7325.

MENSOUR, Mark S; Huntsville District Mem Hosp, 100 Frank Miller Dr, Huntsville ON P1H 1H7; Wes'94; CCFP; CCFP(E.M.); FCFP; Staff, Huntsville District Memorial Hospital - Muskoka Algonquin Healthcare; (705)789-0022; Fax. (705)789-0557.

MENTICOGLOU, Savas M; Women's Hosp, WR120-735 Notre Dame Ave, Winnipeg MB R3E 0L8; McG'77; FRCSC; ObstGyn (Maternal Fetal Medicine). (204)787-1984; Fax. (204)787-2899.

MENTZ, Helena J; Mayfair Place, 236-6707 Elbow Dr SW, Calgary AB T2V 0E3; Pretoria (South Africa)'84; MB ChB; BMedSci; LMCC; Langs: Afrikaans; (403)259-3300; Fax. (403)259-3355; drhelenamentz@shaw.ca.

MENTZ, Hendrik; Ridge Meadows Hosp & Hlth CC, 11666 Laity St, Maple Ridge BC V2X 5A3; (South Africa)'05; MB ChB; Staff, Ridge Meadows Hospital & Health Care Centre; (604)466-6905

MENTZ, Monica; Cook Medical Bldg, 326-1175 Cook St, Victoria BC V8V 4A1; Stellenbosch (South Africa)'84; MB ChB; CCFP; (250)386-2449

MENTZ, Ricardo A; Royal Alexandra Hosp, 10240 Kingsway NW, Edmonton AB T5H 3V9; Stellenbosch (South Africa)'02; CCFP; Staff, Royal Alexandra Hospital; (780)735-4111

MENUCK, Morton N; Barrie Chronic Pain Clinic, 480 Huronia Rd, Barrie ON L4N 6M2; Man'68; LMCC; FRCPC; Psy (Chronic Pain Management). (705)722-8278; Fax. (705)722-8202.

MENZIES, Didier P; CHUQ-Hotel-Dieu de Quebec, 11 Cote du Palais, Quebec QC G1R 2J6; Staff, Centre Hospitalier Universitaire de Québec (CHUQ) - Siege Social; (418)691-5233

MENZIES, Fiona V; McMaster University, 1280 Main St W, Hamilton ON L8S 4K1; Tor'08; FRCPC; IntMed.

MENZIES, John E; Pembroke Reg Hosp, 705 MacKay St, Pembroke ON K8A 1G8; Man'82; FRCPC; DiagRad. Staff/Chief DiagRad, Pembroke Regional Hospital Inc; (613)732-2811 x8081

MENZIES, Richard I; MUHC-Montreal Chest Institute, 3650 rue Saint-Urbain, Montreal QC H2X 2P4; McG'78; MSc(Biostat & Epidemiol; Respir; IntMed (Pneumology). Staff, McGill University Health Centre - Montreal Chest Institute; Asst Prof Med Epidemiol & Biostat, McGill University; (514)934-1934 x32128; Fax. (514)843-2083.

MENZIES, Robert D; Hycroft Med Bldg, 103-3195 Granville St, Vancouver BC V6H 3K2; UBC'74; CCFP; Ac Staff, Vancouver General Hospital - Centennial Pavillion; Clin Instructor, University of British Columbia; Langs: German; French; (604)739-8011

MENZIES, Robert J; Agassiz Med Centre, 130-30 Stephen St, Morden MB R6M 2G3; Man'76; CCFP; FCFP; Asst Prof, University of Manitoba; (204)822-4474; Fax. (204)822-6886.

MEOLA, Carlo; 110-21 Queensway W, Mississauga ON L5B 1B6; UBC'85; (905)897-0788

MEQUANENT, Tewodros G; 204-9814 97 St, Grande Prairie AB T8V 8H5; Addis Ababa (Ethiopia)'91; CCFP; Langs: Amharic; (780)539-3322; Fax. (780)539-7507; tewodros@telus.net.

MERAHI, Ourida; CSSS du Suroît, 150 rue Saint-Thomas, Salaber-de-Valleyf QC J6T 6C1; Staff, Centre Hospitalier Régional du Suroît; (450)371-9920

MERALI, Abbas M; McMaster University, MDCL 3101A-1280 Main St W, Hamilton ON L8S 4K1; UBC'08; FRCPC; IntMed. (905)521-2100

MERALI, Fatima S M; Medica One, 2079 Lakeshore Rd, Burlington ON L7R 1E2; McM'98; MSc; FRCPC; IntMed; Cardiol. Staff, William Osler Health System - Etobicoke General Hospital; (905)634-1625; Fax. (905)634-5332.

MERALI, Nazmuddin; Lansdowne Professional Ctr II, 365-3066 Shelbourne St, Victoria BC V8R 6T9; UBC'83; Ac Staff, Vancouver Island Health Authority; (250)595-0595

MERALI, Sara; Humber River Reg Hosp-Church, 200 Church St, Toronto ON M9N 1N8; Qns'05; CCFP; Staff, Humber River Regional Hospital - Church Street Site; (416)249-8111

MERALI, Shamsh Y; Holly Med Clinic, 103-611 Holly Ave, Milton ON L9T 0K4; Tor'74; CCFP; FCFP; Lecturer Family Med, University of Ottawa; Asst Prof Family Med, Northern Ontario School of Medicine-Laurentian University; Langs: Gujarati; Hindi; Kacchi; Swahili; Urdu; (905)878-0086; Fax. (905)878-1562; smerali@laurentian.ca.

MERANDA, Clara; Dufferin Family Care Centre, 51 Gerry Fitzgerald Dr, North York ON M3J 3N4; Tor'83; CCFP; (416)739-1562; Fax. (416)739-6671.

MERAT, Yves M; CHUS-Hop Fleurimont, 3001 12e av N, Sherbrooke QC J1H 5N4; Clermont-Ferrand (France)'71; Prof, Centre Hospitalier Universitaire de Sherbrooke-Hopital Fleurimont; (819)346-1110 x16528; Fax. (819)829-3245.

MERBAUM, Allyson M; 704-240 Duncan Mill Rd, North York ON M3B 3S6; Tor'99; CCFP; FCFP; (416)497-0880; Fax. (416)497-2650.

MERCADO, Ashley J; St Joseph's Healthcare, PO Box 5777 Stn B 268 Grosvenor St, London ON N6A 4V2; Ott'05; FRCPC; DiagRad. Staff, St Joseph's Hospital - St Joseph's Health Care; (519)646-6035; Fax. (519)646-6204.

MERCANTE, Nadia F; 723 Rymal Rd W, Hamilton ON L9B 2W2; McM'04; CCFP; (905)574-7300; Fax. (905)574-2283.

MERCER, C Dale; Hotel-Dieu-Hosp, 166 Brock St, Kingston ON K7L 5G2; Qns'78; FRCSC; GenSurg (Esophageal Surgery). Att Staff, Hotel-Dieu Hospital; Att Staff/Clin Head Surg, Kingston General Hospital; Head Surg, Queen's University; (613)544-3400 x2474; Fax. (613)546-4854.

MERCER, C Wade; Bay Bulls Family Practice, PO Box 10, Bay Bulls NL A0A 1C0; Mem'91; CCFP; (709)334-2206; Fax. (709)334-2331.

MERCER, Christina L; PO Box 578, Berwick NS B0P 1E0; Mem'97; BMedSci; CCFP; FCFP; (902)538-0163; Fax. (902)538-1803.

MERCER, Christopher M; Perth-Smiths Falls Dist Hosp, 60 Cornelia St W, Smiths Falls ON K7A 2H9; Wes'02; CCFP; Staff, Perth & Smiths Falls District Hospital - Smiths Falls Site; (613)719-1146

MERCER, Deanna M; The Ottawa Hosp-Civic Campus, 1053 Carling Ave, Ottawa ON K1Y 4E9; Wes'87; FRCPC; Psy. Staff, The Ottawa Hospital - Civic Campus; (613)761-4581

MERCER, Dennis F; 106B 3 Ave W PO Box 5249 Stn Main, High River AB T1V 1M4; Alb'67; (403)652-2044

MERCER, Edwin E; Western Mem Reg Hosp, PO Box 2005 Stn Main 1 Brookfield Ave, Corner Brook NL A2H 6J7; Mem'90; FRCPC; DiagRad. Diag Radiol, Western Memorial Regional Hospital; (709)637-5000

MERCER, Gordon R; Medical Assoc of Port Perry, 462 Paxton St, Port Perry ON L9L 1L9; Qns'85; CCFP; FCFP; Staff, Lakeridge Health - Port Perry Site; (905)985-2895; Fax. (905)985-5403.

MERCER, Gregory P; Lourdes Med Clinic, PO Box 119 80 Main St, Lourdes NL A0N 1R0; Mem'89; CCFP; Staff, Western Memorial Regional Hospital; Clin Lecturer, Memorial University Of Newfoundland; (709)642-5371

MERCER, I David; 72-156 Country Path PO Box 331, Holyrood NL A0A 2R0; Dal'67; (709)229-3526; Fax. (709)229-1070.

MERCER, Jay G; Bruyere Family Med Centre, 75 Bruyere St, Ottawa ON K1N 5C8; McM'93; CCFP; FCFP; Langs: English; French; (613)683-4357; Fax. (613)241-2755.

MERCER, Jean A; Morgan Creek Med Clinic, 106-15252 32 Ave, Surrey BC V3S 0R7; Mem'78; (604)542-5996

MERCER, Jennifer L; Central Nfld Reg Health Centre, 50 Union St, Grnd-Falls-Windsor NL A2A 2E1; Mem'05; FRCSC; ObstGyn. Staff, Central Newfoundland Regional Health Centre; (709)292-2500

MERCER, Nicola J; 100-474 Wellington Rd 18, Fergus ON N1M 0A1; Tor'87; MBA; FRCPC; Anes. Staff, Guelph General Hospital; Staff, Homewood Health Centre; (519)846-2715; dandniki@albedo.net.

MERCER, Shauna L; 2412 4 St SW PO Box 94023 Rpo Elbow River, Calgary AB T2S 0S4; Mem'08; CCFP; (403)918-6372

MERCEREAU, Donald A; Kingsway Oral Surgery, 14310 111 Ave NW, Edmonton AB T5M 3Z7; Alb'73; FRCPC; Anes. Staff, Royal Alexandra Hospital; (780)454-6565; Fax. (780)481-3426.

MERCEREAU, Paul; Vancouver Gen Hosp, 855 12th Ave W, Vancouver BC V5Z 1M9; Wes'08; Staff, Vancouver General Hospital - Centennial Pavillion; (604)875-4111

MERCHANT, Naeem; Foothills Med Centre, 1403 29 St NW, Calgary AB T2N 2T9; Wes'90; FRCPC; DiagRad. Staff, Foothills Medical Centre; (403)944-1969

MERCHANT, Pradeep; The Ottawa Hosp-Civic Campus, 1053 Carling Ave, Ottawa ON K1Y 4E9; Bombay (India)'84; MB BS; FRCPC; Peds (Neonatology). A-Chief Div of Neonatol, The Ottawa Hospital - Civic Campus; A-Chief Div of Neonatol, The Ottawa Hospital - General Campus; Asst Prof Peds, University of Ottawa; Langs: Gujarati; Hindi; Marathi; (613)761-4267; Fax. (613)761-5017; pmerchant@ottawahospital.on.ca.

MERCHANT, Richard N; Royal Columbian Hosp, 330 Columbia St E, New Westminster BC V3L 3W7; UBC'79; FRCPC; Anes. Staff, Royal Columbian Hospital; Clinical Asst Prof, University of British Columbia; (604)520-4602; Fax. (604)520-4899.

MERCHANT, Saba M; Maple Kidz Clinic, 215-955 Major MacKenzie Dr, Maple ON L6A 4P9; Amravati (India)'92; MB BS; FRCPC; Peds. Hon Lecturer Peds, The Hospital For Sick Children; Ac Staff, Mackenzie Richmond Hill Hospital; Hon Lecturer Peds, University of Toronto; Langs: Urdu; Hindi; Marathi; (905)303-0304; Fax. (905)303-3035; mmerchant@maplekidz.ca.

MERCHANT, Sameena; 250-8730 Country Hills Blvd NW, Calgary AB T3G 0E2; Wes'89; CCFP; (403)262-7787; Fax. (403)262-7786.

MERCHEA, M Mohan; Ivey Eye Institute, 268 Grosvenor St, London ON N6A 4V2; Vikram (India)'64; MB BS; DABOph; FAAO; FRCSC; Ophth (Cataract Surgery). Ac Staff, St Joseph's Hospital - St Joseph's Health Care; Ac Staff, London Health Sciences Centre - Victoria Campus; Assoc Prof Ophth, University of Western Ontario; Langs: Hindi; Punjabi; Urdu; (519)646-6284; Fax. (519)646-6150; dr.merchea@gmail.com.

MERCIER, Annie; CSSS de Montmagny-L'Islet, RR 1 350 boul Tache O, Montmagny QC G5V 3R8; Laval'94; Staff, CSSS de Montmagny-L'Islet; (418)248-0630; annie.mercier@gmf.gouv.qc.ca.

MERCIER, Caroline; CSSS de Montmagny-L'Islet, RR 1 350 boul Tache O, Montmagny QC G5V 3R8; Laval'09; CCFP; Staff, CSSS de Montmagny-L'Islet; (418)248-0630

MERCIER, Christian; CSSS de l'Hématite, GD 1 rue de l'Aquillon, Fermont QC G0G 1J0; Laval'80; Staff, CLSC de l'Hématite; (418)287-5461

MERCIER, Christian; Clinique Fam de Lambton, CP 339 203 rue Principale, Lambton QC G0M 1H0; Laval'84; (418)486-7408; Fax. (418)486-2238.

MERCIER, Claude; CLSC de Chandler, CP 1090 633 rue Daigneault, Chandler QC G0C 1K0; Sher'77; (418)689-2572; Fax. (418)689-2840.

MERCIER, Claude; Hotel-Dieu de Levis, 143 rue Wolfe, Levis QC G6V 3Z1; Laval'91; FRCPC; Psy. Staff, Hôtel-Dieu de Lévis; (418)835-7155

MERCIER, Claude; Hôpital Ste-Justine, 3175 ch Cote-Sainte-Catherine, Montreal QC H3T 1C5; Sher'76; FRCSC; Neursurg (Pediatric Neuro Surgery). Che neurochirg, Hôpital Ste-Justine; Staff, Centre Hospitalier l'Université de Montréal (CHUM) - Hôpital Notre-Dame; Consultant, Centre Hospitalier l'Université de Montréal (CHUM) - Hôtel-Dieu; Langs: Bilingual(English/French); (514)345-4931 x6000; Fax. (514)345-4964; claude_mercier@ssss.gouv.qc.ca.

MERCIER, David; CSSS de Manicouagan, 635 boul Jolliet, Baie-Comeau QC G5C 1P1; Laval'97; Ac Staff, Centre Hospitalier Régional Baie-Comeau; Langs: Spanish; English; (418)589-3701

MERCIER, David; Ctr Hosp Affilie-Enfant-Jesus, 1401 18e rue, Quebec QC G1J 1Z4; Laval'02; FRCSC; Neursurg. Staff, Centre Hospitalier Affilié Universitaire de Québec - Hôpital De L'Enfant Jésus; (418)649-0252; Fax. (418)649-5915.

MERCIER, Denis; Clinique d'Orthopedie de Levis, 6620 rue Saint-Georges, Levis QC G6V 4H1; Laval'75; OrthSurg. Staff, Hôtel-Dieu de Lévis; (418)837-8251; Fax. (418)837-2033.

MERCIER, Dominique; CLSC de la Region-Sherbrooke, 50 rue Camirand, Sherbrooke QC J1H 4J5; Sher'87; Staff, Centre Hospitalier Universitaire de Sherbrooke-Hopital Fleurimont; Langs: Spanish; English; (819)780-2222; Fax. (819)565-8196.

MERCIER, Francois; CHUM-Hop St-Luc, 1058 rue Saint-Denis, Montreal QC H2X 3J4; Laval'81; Staff, Centre Hospitalier l'Université De Montréal (CHUM) - Hôpital Saint-luc; (514)890-8000 x34862

MERCIER, Gaetane; Agence SSSS-Dir Sante Publique, 363 Rte Cameron, Sainte-Marie QC G6E 3E2; Laval'88; Staff, Centre d'hébergement de Beauceville; (418)389-1510; Fax. (418)389-1515.

MERCIER, Gilles G; 809-1 av Holiday, Pointe-Claire QC H9R 5N3; Laval'67; ObstGyn (Echography). Chef obst & gyn, Lakeshore General Hospital - Pointe Claire; Langs: English; (514)697-5781; Fax. (514)697-5787; mergg2000@videotron.ca.

MERCIER, Gilles; SAAQ, 333 boul Jean-Lesage, Quebec QC G1K 8Z2; Laval'78; (418)528-3859; gilles.mercier@saaq.gouv.qc.ca.

MERCIER, Guylaine; Clinique Med de Levis, 100-4975 boul de la Rive-Sud, Levis QC G6V 4Z5; Laval'91; Staff, Hôtel-Dieu de Lévis; (418)833-5810; Fax. (418)833-2720.

MERCIER, Helene; Clinique Horizon Performance, 228-2959 boul de l'Universite, Sherbrooke QC J1K 2X6; Laval'95; Staff, Centre Hospitalier et CLSC de Memphremagog; (819)416-0473

MERCIER, Isabelle; Clinique Medic IM, 805 boul Frontenac E, Thetford Mines QC G6G 6L5; Sher'05; Langs: Bilingual(French/English); (418)338-1558; Fax. (418)338-6990.

MERCIER, Isabelle; 305-5835 boul Leger, Montreal-Nord QC H1G 6E1; Mon'82; (514)324-3818; Fax. (514)324-4108.

MERCIER, Jean-Claude; CHUQ-Ctr Hosp Univ Laval, 2705 boul Laurier, Quebec QC G1V 4G2; Laval'75; Peds. Staff, Centre Hospitalier Universitaire de Quebec-CHUL; Ac Staff, Centre Hospitalier Universitaire De Québec - Pavillon De St-françois-d'assise; Teach Staff Peds, Université Laval; (418)525-4444 x47505

MERCIER, Jean-Francois; CSSSG-Hop de Hull, 116 boul Lionel-Emond, Gatineau QC J8Y 1W7; Laval'07; DiagRad. Staff, Hull Hospital; (819)966-6200

MERCIER, Jean-Francois; 204-235 boul Rene-Levesque E, Montreal QC H2X 1N8; McG'75; FACS; FRCSC; PlasSurg (Laser Surgery). (514)875-9936; Fax. (514)875-9937; jfmercier@bellnet.ca.

MERCIER, Karine; CSSS de Trois-Rivières, 1991 boul du Carmel, Trois-Rivieres QC G8Z 3R9; Mon'06; Staff, CSSS de Trois-Rivières; (819)697-3333

MERCIER, Lise-Andree; Institut de Cardiologie de Mtl, 5000 rue Belanger, Montreal QC H1T 1C8; Mon'72; CSPQ; Cardiol. Staff, Institut de Cardiologie de Montréal; (514)376-3330; Fax. (514)593-2158.

MERCIER, Marie-Josee; Hop Ste-Anne-De-Beaupre, 11000 rue des Montagnards, Beaupre QC G0A 1E0; Laval'06; Staff, Centre Hospitalier de Chandler; Staff, Hôpital Sainte Anne de Beaupré; (418)827-8215

MERCIER, Marie-Lise; CHUQ-St-Francois d'Assise, 10 rue de l'Espinay, Quebec QC G1L 3L5; Laval'03; CCFP; CCFP(E.M.); Staff, Centre Hospitalier Universitaire De Québec - Pavillon De St-françois-d'assise; (418)525-4444 x55107; Fax. (418)525-4439.

MERCIER, Maryse; Clinique Fam d'Arthabaska, 101-39 rue Laurier E, Victoriaville QC G6P 6P6; Sher'86; FRCPC; IntMed. Ac Staff, Hotel-Dieu d'Arthabaska; (819)357-3930; Fax. (819)357-4310.

MERCIER, Mathieu; Clinique Med de Montmagny, 100-83 av de la Fabrique, Montmagny QC G5V 2J3; Sher'05; (418)248-4933; Fax. (418)248-2778; mathieu.mercier@gmf.gouv.qc.ca.

MERCIER, Nicolas; CSSS du Sud de Lanaudière, 911 montee des Pionniers, Terrebonne QC J6V 2H2; Mon'10; CCFP; Staff, Centre Hospitalier Pierre le Gardeur; (450)654-7525

MERCIER, Nicole; Clinique Med Blainville, 519 boul du Cure-Labelle, Blainville QC J7C 2H6; Sher'83; Staff, Clinique Medicale Blainville; Physician, CSSS Therese de Blainville; (450)430-2222; Fax. (450)430-1274.

MERCIER, Nicole; Transcona Med Clinic, 200-701 Regent Ave W, Winnipeg MB R2C 1S3; Mon'82; (204)222-5221; Fax. (204)224-2053.

MERCIER, Pierre; 297-2600 boul Laurier, Quebec QC G1V 4T3; Laval'78; FRCSC; OrthSurg. Ac Staff, Centre Hospitalier Universitaire De Québec - Pavillon De St-françois-d'assise; (418)623-1610; Fax. (418)623-8926.

MERCIER, Remi; CSSS de la Haute-Cote-Nord, RR 1 4 rue de l'Hopital, Les Escoumins QC G0T 1K0; Laval'98; CCFP; Staff, Centre de santé des Côté-Nord; (418)233-2931; Fax. (418)233-2608.

MERCIER, Rheo; CSSS de la Region de Thetford, 1717 rue Notre-Dame E, Thetford Mines QC G6G 2V4; Laval'72; CSPQ; Anes (P.Q.). Staff, Hopital du CSS de la Region de Thetford; (418)338-7777

MERCIER, Simon; CSSS de la Baie-des-Chaleurs, RR 2 419 boul Perron, Maria QC G0C 1Y0; Mon'92; OrthSurg (P.Q.). Staff, CSSS de la Baie-des-Chaleurs; (418)759-3443; Fax. (418)759-5063.

MERCILLE, Genevieve; CSSS de Rimouski-Neigette, CP 3150 Succ A 150 av Rouleau, Rimouski QC G5L 5T1; Mon'03; FRCSC; Ophth. Staff, Hôpital Regional Rimouski; (418)724-3000

MERCILLE, Suzanne; Hop Maisonneuve-Rosemont, 5415 boul de l'Assomption, Montreal QC H1T 2M4; Mon'85; BSc; CSPQ; Rheum (P.Q.); IntMed (P.Q.). Staff, Hopital Maisonneuve-Rosemont; Langs: Bilingual(French/English); (514)252-3400; Fax. (514)252-3889.

MERCKY, Jocelyn; CSSS du Lac-des-Deux-Montagnes, 520 boul Arthur-Sauve, Saint-Eustache QC J7R 5B1; Strasbourg (France)'08; ObstGyn (P.Q.). Staff, Hôpital de Saint-Eustache; (450)473-6811; Fax. (450)473-6966.

MERCKY, Nicolas; CSSS Haut-Richelieu-Rouville, 920 boul du Seminaire N, St-Jean-sur-Richel QC J3A 1B7; Besancon (France)'07; DiagRad (P.Q.). Staff, Hôpital du Haut-Richelieu; (450)359-5000

MERCURE, Claude; College des Med du Quebec, 2170 boul Rene-Levesque O, Montreal QC H3H 2T8; Mon'61; CSPQ; FRCPC; Peds; CommunMed (P.Q.). (514)933-4441 x5373

MERCUUR, Lester G; Foothills Med Centre, 1403 29 St NW, Calgary AB T2N 2T9; Cape Town (South Africa)'86; CCFP; CCFP(E.M.); FCFP; Staff Emerg Med, Foothills Medical Centre; (403)944-1820; Fax. (403)944-2419.

MEREDITH, A Ray; Ilderton Med Clinic, GD 36 Heritage Pl, Ilderton ON N0M 2A0; Wes'58; Assoc Staff, St Joseph's Hospital - St Joseph's Health Care; Ac Staff, London Health Sciences Centre - Victoria Campus; (519)666-1610

MEREDITH, Melanie J; Brandon Health Reg Centre, 150 McTavish Ave E, Brandon MB R7A 2B3; McM'95; BScN; CCFP; Staff, Brandon Regional Health Centre; (204)578-4000

MEREDITH, Samantha J; Royal Inland Hosp, 311 Columbia St, Kamloops BC V2C 2T1; UBC'05; CCFP; Staff, Royal Inland Hospital; (250)374-5111

MEREDITH, Steven R; 300-546 St. Paul St, Kamloops BC V2C 5T1; UBC'04; FRCSC; PlasSurg. (778)471-5979

MERENIUK, Bohdan; Ctr Hosp de Verdun, 4000 boul Lasalle, Verdun QC H4G 2A3; Mon'82; Chef méd urgence, Centre Hospitalier de Verdun; Teach Staff, Universite de Montreal; (514)362-1000

MERETTE, Guy; Ctr Hosp de Verdun, 4000 boul Lasalle, Verdun QC H4G 2A3; Mon'81; CSPQ; FRCPC; DiagRad. Staff, Centre Hospitalier de Verdun; (514)362-1000

MEREU, Adriana-Iona; G F Strong Rehab Centre, 4255 Laurel St, Vancouver BC V5Z 2G9; Bucharest (Romania)'87; Staff, G F Strong Rehabilitation Centre; (604)734-1313

MEREU, Laurie E; Heritage Med Research Centre, 362-107 University Campus NW, Edmonton AB T6G 2S2; Wes'90; FRCPC; IntMed; Endocrin&Metab. Ad Staff Privil, University of Alberta Hospital; Assoc Prof, University of Alberta; (780)407-3636; Fax. (780)407-6702; laurie.mereu@ualberta.ca.

MERG, Anders R; Stanton Terr Health Authority, PO Box 10 550 Byrne Rd, Yellowknife NT X1A 2N1; Wisconsin (USA)'96; FRCSC; GenSurg. Staff, Stanton Territorial Health Authority; (867)669-4111

MERGENS, Joseph E; 103-7110 120 St, Surrey BC V3W 3M8; UBC'72; (604)591-8008; Fax. (604)591-8755.

MERGLER, Sandra G; Mineral Springs Hosp, PO Box 1050 Stn Main 301 Lynx St, Banff AB T1L 1H7; Tor'89; CCFP; CCFP(E.M.); FCFP; Ac Staff, Covenant Health - Banff Mineral Springs Hospital; (403)762-2222; Fax. (403)762-4193; smergler@shaw.ca.

MERIANO, Antonio L; Windsor Reg Hosp-Metropolitan, 1995 Lens Ave, Windsor ON N8W 1L9; Tor'96; CCFP; CCFP(E.M.); Staff, Windsor Regional Hospital - Metropolitan Site; (519)985-2606

MERIZZI, Marc; Ctr Medi Soleil St-Jean-Sur-Ri, 120-383 boul du Seminaire N, St-Jean-sur-Richel QC J3B 8C5; Mon'82; Langs: Bilingual(French/English); (450)347-7557; Fax. (450)347-3099; mmerizzi@hotmail.com.

MERKER, Darren L; Queen Square Doctors FHT, 201-366 Main St N, Brampton ON L6V 1P8; Tor'04; CCFP; (905)455-1455; Fax. (905)455-5498.

MERKER, Donald S; Bramalea Med Group, 500-18 Kensington Rd, Brampton ON L6T 4S5; Ott'69; BSc; Staff, William Osler Health System - Brampton Civic Hospital; (905)791-7575; Fax. (905)791-7532.

MERKLEY, Barry D; Maple Leaf Med Clinic, 501-14 College St, Toronto ON M5G 1K2; Tor'90; BSc; Physician, Maple Leaf Medical Clinic; (416)465-0756; Fax. (416)465-8344.

MERKLI, Kimberly A; Pender Community Health Centre, 59 Pender St W, Vancouver BC V6B 1R3; UBC'08; CCFP; Staff, Pender Community Health Centre; (604)669-9181

MERKUR, Andrew B; UBC Eye Care Centre, 2550 Willow St, Vancouver BC V5Z 3N9; Ott'01; FRCSC; Ophth (Adult & Pediatric Vitreoretinal Surgery). (604)875-4656; Fax. (604)875-4652; amerkur@yahoo.com.

MERNAGH, John R P; McMaster University HSC, 1200 Main St W, Hamilton ON L8S 4J9; Tor'86; PhD; DABR; FRCPC; DiagRad. Staff, Hamilton Health Sciences Centre - McMaster Children's Hospital; Assoc Prof, McMaster University; (905)521-2100 x75297; Fax. (905)521-1390.

MERONEK, Deborah M; Canmore Associate Med Clinic, 124-1151 Sidney St, Canmore AB T1W 3G1; Cal'82; BSc; (403)678-5585; Fax. (403)678-6262.

MEROTTO, Robert A; 44 Main St E GD, Chelmsford ON P0M 1L0; Tor'84; (705)855-5099

MEROUANI, Aicha; Hôpital Ste-Justine, 3175 ch Cote-Sainte-Catherine, Montreal QC H3T 1C5; (Algeria)'76; Staff, Hôpital Ste-Justine; (514)345-4737; Fax. (514)345-4838.

MEROVITZ, Lisa; St Mary's Hosp Centre, 3830 av Lacombe, Montreal QC H3T 1M5; Qns'01; FRCSC; ObstGyn. Staff, St Mary's Hospital Centre; (514)345-3511

MERRETT, Donald G; 8065 Victoria St PO Box 400, Metcalfe ON K0A 2P0; Ott'74; Staff, Winchester District Memorial Hospital; Langs: Bilingual(English/French); (613)821-1390; Fax. (613)821-4484.

MERRETT, Patrick; CSSS de Laval, 1755 boul Rene-Laennec, Laval QC H7M 3L9; McG'06; MDCM; CCFP; Staff, Hopital de la Cite de la santé; (450)668-1010

MERRICK, Bruce W; Etobicoke Med Centre, 400 The East Mall, Etobicoke ON M9B 3Z9; Tor'61; (416)621-2220; Fax. (416)621-2203.

MERRICK, Evan P; Yarmouth Reg Hosp, 301-60 Vancouver St, Yarmouth NS B5A 2P5; Dublin (Ireland)'05; Cardiol; IntMed. Staff, Yarmouth Regional Hospital; (902)742-0235; Fax. (902)742-9416.

MERRIMAN, Sarah L; 3029 Cambie St, Vancouver BC V5Z 4N2; UBC'06; CCFP; (604)875-8999

MERRIMEN, Jennifer L; Dept of Pathology, 744-5788 University Ave, Halifax NS B3H 1V8; Dal'02; FRCPC; AnatPath. (902)473-2931; Fax. (902)473-1049.

MERRITT, Keith E; Castlegar Med Clinic, 1101 3rd St, Castlegar BC V1N 2A1; Qns'75; CCFP; FCFP; Ac Staff, Kootenay Boundary Regional Hospital; Ac Staff, Castlegar & District Communnity Health Centre; (250)365-7717; Fax. (250)365-0347.

MERRITT, Kyle D; Prince George Reg Hosp, 1475 Edmonton St, Prince George BC V2M 1S2; UBC'09; CCFP; Staff, University Hospital of Northern British Columbia; (250)565-2000

MERRITT, Neil; London HSC-Victoria Campus, PO Box 5010 Stn B 800 Commissioners Rd E, London ON N6A 5W9; McM'01; FRCSC; GenSurg (Pediatric Trauma); PedGenSurg. Staff, London Health Sciences Centre - Victoria Campus; Asst Prof Surg, University of Western Ontario; (519)685-8454; Fax. (519)685-8465; neil-merritt@lhsc.on.ca.

MERRITT, Richard D; Stamford Med Centre, 305-4256 Portage Rd, Niagara Falls ON L2E 6A4; Wes'68; FRCSC; Ophth. Ac Staff, Niagara Health System - Greater Niagara General Site; (905)358-6844; Fax. (905)358-1626.

MERRITT, Robert B; 5081 Highway 7, Porters Lake NS B3E 1J3; Dal'89; Twin Oaks Memorial Hospital; Staff, IWK Health Centre; (902)827-4001; Fax. (902)827-3206.

MERROW, Nancy M; Southlake Reg Health Centre, 596 Davis Dr, Newmarket ON L3Y 2P9; Tor'83; CCFP; FCFP; Staff Chief, Southlake Regional Health Centre; Med Advisor, Community Care Access Centre; (905)895-4521 x2625

MERRY, David A; Christina Lake Med Clinic, PO Box 570, Christina Lake BC V0H 1E0; Cal'86; CCFP; (250)447-6262; Fax. (250)447-6277.

MERRY, Graham F; 101-190 Cundles Rd E SS 103, Barrie ON L4M 4S5; London (England)'82; (705)728-0800

MERRYWEATHER, Leslie E; City Centre Fam Physicians, 100-514 Queen St, Saskatoon SK S7K 0M5; Sask'03; CCFP; (306)244-3016

MERRYWEATHER, Rachel J; Valley Reg Hosp, 150 Exhibition St, Kentville NS B4N 5E3; Dal'00; FRCPC; IntMed; MedOncol. Staff, Valley Regional Hospital; (902)678-7381

MERSHATI, Abdelwahab K; The Nova Scotia Hosp, PO Box 1004 Stn Main, Dartmouth NS B2Y 3Z9; Libya (Libya)'87; MB ChB; CCFP; Staff, The Nova Scotia Hospital; (902)464-3111; Fax. (902)464-3357.

MERSKEY, Harold; 71 Logan Ave, London ON N5Y 2P9; Oxford (England)'53; MA; FRCP(Lond); FRCPsy; FRCPC; Psy (Chronic Pain). Consultant/Psychiatrist, Woodstock General Hospital; Emeritus Prof, University of Western Ontario; Langs: Hebrew; (519)679-1045

MERTENS, Donald J; 286 York Mills Rd, North York ON M2L 1L1; Durham (England)'63; MB BS; MSc; Assoc Staff, Rouge Valley Health System - Centenary Health Centre Site; Lecturer Med, University of Toronto; (416)449-7249; Fax. (416)391-4872; dmertens@rogers.com.

MERTENS, Luc L; The Hosp for Sick Children, 1725-555 University Ave, Toronto ON M5G 1X8; Leuven (Belgium)'92; Staff, The Hospital For Sick Children; Langs: Bilingual(English/French); (416)813-7418; Fax. (416)813-5857; luc.mertens@sickkids.ca.

MERTH, Kevin D M; 101-1032 Austin Ave, Coquitlam BC V3K 3P3; Sask'81; Staff, Royal Columbian Hospital; (604)939-2441; Fax. (604)939-2420.

MERTZ, Dominik; Hamilton HS-Henderson Site, 711 Concession St, Hamilton ON L8V 1C3; Basel (Switzerland)'02; Staff, Hamilton Health Sciences Centre-Juravinski Site; (905)527-4322; Fax. (905)577-1415.

MERVITZ, Deborah L; Children's Hosp Eastern Ont, 401 Smyth Rd, Ottawa ON K1H 8L1; Alb'03; FRCPC; Anes. Staff, Children's Hospital of Eastern Ontario (CHEO); (613)737-2431

MERVITZ, David; 3914 Dewdney Ave, Regina SK S4T 1A1; Witwatersrand (South Africa)'73; FRCSC; Ophth (Cataract). Staff, Pasqua Hospital; (306)352-7695; Fax. (306)525-2237; dr. mervitz.office@sasktel.net.

MES, Tom A; Bayshore Med Bldg, 201-3029 Carling Ave, Ottawa ON K2B 8E8; Ott'72; Ac Staff, Queensway Carleton Hospital; (613)829-7660; Fax. (613)829-7744.

MESANA, Thierry G; Univ of Ottawa Heart Institute, H3402-40 Ruskin St, Ottawa ON K1Y 4W7; D'Aiz-Marseille (France)'85; FRCSC; CardSurg. Staff, University of Ottawa Heart Institute; (613)761-4712

MESAROS, J Helen; Toronto East Gen Hosp Inc, 825 Coxwell Ave, Toronto ON M4C 3E7; Belgrade (Serbia)'63; FRCPC; Psy. Staff, Toronto East General Hospital Inc; (416)461-8272; Fax. (416)469-6805.

MESBAHI, Karim; Clinique Forcemedic, 1021 rue Jean-Talon E, Montreal QC H2R 1V6; Sher'09; (514)787-1818

MESCHINO, Alfio; Toronto East Gen Hosp Inc, 825 Coxwell Ave, Toronto ON M4C 3E7; Tor'83; FRCPC; Anes. Asst Prof Anes, University of Toronto; (416)469-6580 x6282; Fax. (416)469-6554.

MESCHINO, Diane D; Women's College Hosp, 952-76 Grenville St, Toronto ON M5S 1B2; Tor'85; BSc(Hons); FRCPC; Psy (Psycho Pharmacology & Psychotherapy). Staff Psy, Women's College Hospital; Staff, Sunnybrook Health Sciences Centre; Asst Prof, University of Toronto; (416)323-6230; Fax. (416)323-6356; diane.meschino@wchospital.ca.

MESCHINO, Wendy S; North York Gen Hosp, 3 SE-4001 Leslie St, North York ON M2K 1E1; Tor'79; FCCMG; FRCPC; Peds (Clinical Genetics). Chief Genetics, North York General Hospital; Advisor Genetics, Porcupine Health Unit Corporate Office; Asst Prof, University of Toronto; (416)756-6346; Fax. (416)756-6727.

MESENSKY, Ladislav; 102-190 Sherway Dr, Etobicoke ON M9C 5N2; Palacky (Czech Republic)'68; Court Staff, North York General Hospital; Court Staff, St Michael's Hospital; Langs: Czech; German; Russian; (416)622-4762

MESENSKY, Marcella; The Doctors Bldg, 501-208 Bloor St W, Toronto ON M5S 3B4; Palacky (Czech Republic)'66; Staff, Women's College Hospital; Langs: Czech; (416)968-9539; Fax. (416)968-1273.

MESHESHA, Belayneh; Foothills Med Centre, 1403 29 St NW, Calgary AB T2N 2T9; (Ethiopia)'85; Staff, Foothills Medical Centre; (403)944-1110

MESHKAT, Nazanin; Univ Hlth Network-Toronto Gen, 200 Elizabeth St, Toronto ON M5G 2C4; Wes'99; FRCPC; EmergMed. Staff, Toronto General Hospital - UHN; (416)340-3111

MESHRKI, Hanan S D; Scott Medical Clinic, 2-387 Scott St, St Catharines ON L2M 3W2; Assiut (Egypt)'96; MB ChB; CCFP; (905)646-2444; Fax. (905)646-9099.

MESSEKHER, Ferial-Lilya; Hop Jean-Talon, 1385 rue Jean-Talon E, Montreal QC H2E 1S6; Algiers (Algeria)'01; Gastroent; IntMed. Staff, CSSS du Coeur de l'Isle Hôpital Jean-Talon; (514)495-6767

MESSELY, Marie-Claude; Centre de Sante Pulbique, 2400 av d'Estimauville, Quebec QC G1E 7G9; Laval'80; CSPQ; Public Health & Preventive Med; CommunMed (P.Q.). Staff, Centre Hospitalier Affilié Universitaire de Québec - Hôpital du St-Sacrement; (418)666-7000; Fax. (418)666-2776; marie-claude.messely@ssss.gouv.qc.ca.

MESSENGER, David W; Kingston Gen Hosp, 76 Stuart St, Kingston ON K7L 2V7; Qns'02; FRCPC; EmergMed; Critical Care Medicine. Staff, Kingston General Hospital; (613)548-2368; Fax. (613)548-1374.

MESSENGER, Mark D; Fredericton Med Clinic, 403-1015 Regent St, Fredericton NB E3B 6H5; Wes'93; FRCPC; Peds. (506)458-0287; Fax. (506)458-0327.

MESSENGER, Megan E; Sudbury Reg Hosp-Laurentian, 41 Ramsey Lake Rd, Sudbury ON P3E 5J1; NOSM'09; CCFP; Staff, Health Sciences North-Laurentian Site; (705)522-7100

MESSER, Charles J; 1957 Elphinstone St, Regina SK S4T 3N3; Bombay (India)'61; MB BS; DPM(Eng); LMCC; FAPA; FRCPC; Psy (Child & Adolescent Psychiatry). Consultant Psy, Regina Health District; Clin Assoc Prof, University of Saskatchewan; (306)352-4674; Fax. (306)525-0686.

MESSERVEY, Elizabeth A; 555 George St N, Peterborough ON K9H 3S1; Qns'87; BASc; CCFP; FCFP; Court Staff Privil, Peterborough Regional Health Centre - Hospital Drive; (705)741-0311; Fax. (705)741-5374; brieliz2@sympatico.ca.

MESSIEH, Mary L; 301-2951 Walker's Line, Burlington ON L7M 4Y1; Dal'99; FRCPC; IntMed; ClinImmunol&Allergy. Staff, Hamilton Health Sciences Centre - McMaster Children's Hospital; (905)331-3101; Fax. (905)319-2499.

MESSIER, Alain; Hop Charles LeMoyne, 1255 rue Beauregard, Longueuil QC J4K 2M3; Mon'63; MSc(CommunHealth); CSPQ; CCFP; CommunMed (P.Q.). assoc Membre, Hôpital du Haut-Richelieu; Ac Member, Hopital Charles LeMoyne; (450)928-6777 x4215; Fax. (450)928-3783.

MESSIER, Alexandre; Hop du Sacre-Coeur de Mtl, 5400 boul Gouin O, Montreal QC H4J 1C5; Mon'99; CCFP; CCFP(E.M.); Staff, Hôpital du Sacre-Coeur de Montréal; (514)338-2222 x2002; Fax. (514)338-2384.

MESSIER, Helen M V; 600-555 12 St SW, Vancouver BC V5Z 3X7; Cal'97; PhD; CCFP; (403)283-2350; hmessier@shaw.ca.

MESSIER, Mario; Ctr de Med Familale de Granby, 48 rue Denison E, Granby QC J2G 4C6; Sher'79; (450)372-3996; Fax. (450)372-0430.

MESSIER, Maryse; CLSC et CHSLD Pommeraie, 660 rue Saint-Paul, Farnham QC J2N 3B9; Mon'78; CCFP; (450)293-3622; Fax. (450)293-4429.

MESSIER, Michel J; Douglas Mental Hlth Univ Inst, 6875 boul Lasalle, Verdun QC H4H 1R3; Mon'64; MBA; Psy (P.Q.) (Psychiatric Rehabilitation). assoc Staff, Inuulitsivik Health Centre; assoc Staff, CH Hôtel-Dieu d'Amos; Staff Psy, Douglas Mental Health University Institute; adj Prof, McGill University; Langs: Bilingual(French/English); (514)761-6131 x2910; Fax. (514)888-4476; mesmic@douglas.mcgill.ca.

MESSIER, Michele; CHSLD Manoir Cartierville, 12235 rue Grenet, Montreal QC H4J 2N9; Mon'80; (514)337-7300

MESSIER, Nadine; CSSS Haut-Richelieu-Rouville, 920 boul du Seminaire N, St-Jean-Sur-Richel QC J3A 1B7; Mon'03; Staff, Hôpital du Haut-Richelieu; (450)359-5000; Fax. (450)359-5064.

MESSIER, Pierre; CSSS de Laval, 1755 boul Rene-Laennec, Laval QC H7M 3L9; Mon'02; Staff, Hopital de la Cite de la santé; (450)668-1010

MESSIER, Rejean L; Pavillon Rosemont, 5689 boul Rosemont, Montreal QC H1T 2H1; Mon'77; FRCPC; Psy. Staff, Hopital Maisonneuve-Rosemont; Universite de Montreal; (514)252-3914

MESSIER-NEPVEU, Nicole; Ctr Hosp Fleury, 2180 rue Fleury E, Montreal QC H2B 1K3; Mon'72; CSPQ; FRCPC; DiagRad. Staff Diag Imag, Centre Hospitalier Fleury; (514)381-9311

MESSINA, Sarina; Brockville Mental Health Ctre, PO Box 1050 1804 Highway 2 E, Brockville ON K6V 5W7; Cal'91; FRCPC; Psy. Staff, Brockville Mental Health Centre - Royal Ottawa Health Care Group; (613)345-1461

MESSNER, Hans A; Univ Hlth Network-Princess M, 610 University Ave, Toronto ON M5G 2M9; Freiburg (Germany)'67; PhD; FRCPC; IntMed (Bone Marrow Transplant). Sr Scientist, Princess Margaret Hospital - University Health Network; Prof Med, University of Toronto; Langs: German; (416)946-2266; Fax. (416)946-6585; hans.messner@uhn.on.ca.

MESSNER, Sandra J; Toronto Sunnybrook Reg Cancer, 2075 Bayview Ave, Toronto ON M4N 3M5; McM'74; BSc(Genetics); MSc(MedBiophysics); CCFP; FCFP; Med Coord Clin Breast Services Preventive Oncol, Sunnybrook Health Sciences Centre; Ac Staff, Women's College Hospital; Lecturer, University of Toronto; (416)480-6835; Fax. (416)480-6002.

MESTELMAN, Bryan P; Royal Jubilee Hosp, 1952 Bay St, Victoria BC V8R 1J8; McM'95; FRCPC; Psy (Geriatric Psychiatry). Staff, Royal Jubilee Hospital; (250)370-8765

MESTERMAN, Ronit; McMaster University, HSC 3A56-1280 Main St W, Hamilton ON L8S 4K1; Munich (Germany)'90; FRCPC; Neur; Peds. Staff Peds, Hamilton Health Sciences Centre - McMaster Children's Hospital; Teach Staff, McMaster University; Langs: German; Hebrew; (905)521-2100 x73392; Fax. (905)521-7914; mesteron@mcmaster.ca.

MESUROLLE, Benoit; MUHC-Royal Victoria Hosp, 687 av des Pins O, Montreal QC H3A 1A1; Paris (France)'92; DiagRad (P.Q.). Staff, McGill University Health Centre - Royal Victoria Hospital; (514)934-1934 x37602

MESZAROS, C Michele; Active Care Med Group, 1108A Klondike Rd, Kanata ON K2K 0G1; Tor'97; CCFP; FCFP; (613)254-9777; Fax. (613)254-9778.

METAWEE, Mohamed L M; Southlake Reg Health Centre, 596 Davis Dr, Newmarket ON L3Y 2P9; Ain Shams (Egypt)'98; FRCPC; IntMed. Staff, Southlake Regional Health Centre; (905)895-4521

METCALF, Corey M; BC Cancer Agency-Vancoucer CC, 600 10th Ave W, Vancouver BC V5Z 4E6; Man'08; IntMed. Staff, BC Cancer Agency Vancouver Centre; (604)877-6000

METCALFE, Brian D; Health Sciences Centre, 300 Prince Philip Dr, St. John's NL A1B 3V6; Mem'08; CCFP; CCFP(E.M.); Staff, Health Sciences Centre; (709)777-6300

METCALFE, Charles G; Associate Med Group, 4705 48 Ave, Red Deer AB T4N 3T1; Man'93; Physician, Associate Medical Group; (403)346-2057; Fax. (403)347-2989.

METCALFE, Donald; Rockyview Gen Hosp, 6635-7007 14 St SW, Calgary AB T2V 1P9; Alb'79; FRCSC; Urol. Staff, Rockyview General Hospital; (403)943-8973; Fax. (403)943-8972.

METCALFE, Francine; 100A-299 boul Sir-Wilfrid-Laur, Saint-Lambert QC J4R 2L1; Mon'86; Langs: English; (450)465-6551; Fax. (450)465-9810.

METCALFE, Ian L; Main Medical, 700 Main St E, Hamilton ON L8M 1K7; Cal'84; BSc; MSc; Asst Prof Family Med, University of Western Ontario; (905)545-1376; Fax. (905)545-6793.

METCALFE, Peter D; University of Alberta Hosp, 2C3 79-8440 112 St NW, Edmonton AB T6G 2B7; Alb'99; FRCSC; Urol (Pediatric Urology). Staff, University of Alberta Hospital; (780)407-3867; Fax. (780)407-6520.

METCALFE, Shelley E; Forest Glen Plaza, 700 Strasburg Rd, Kitchener ON N2E 2M2; Wes'85; CCFP; FCFP; (519)578-4450; Fax. (519)579-1142.

METCALFE, Sonja J; 330-507 Broadway W, Vancouver BC V5Z 1E6; Cal'08; CCFP; (604)872-5484

METE, Ozgur; Univ Hlth Network-Toronto Gen, 200 Elizabeth St, Toronto ON M5G 2C4; Istanbul (Turkey)'01; Staff, Toronto General Hospital - UHN; Langs: Turkish; (416)340-3004; Fax. (416)340-5517.

METELITSA, Andrei; Institute for Skin Advancement, 206-4935 40 Ave NW, Calgary AB T3A 2N1; Alb'05; FRCPC; Derm. (403)286-2394; Fax. (403)284-5272.

METELITSA, Yuri L; Southern Alberta Forensic Psy, 11333 85 St NW, Calgary AB T3R 1J3; Moscow (Russia (Federation))'72; PhD(Psychol); DSc(Psy); Staff, Peter Lougheed Centre; Langs: Russian; (403)944-6800; Fax. (403)944-6852.

METERISSIAN, Gregory B; MUHC-Montreal Gen Hosp, B6 233-1650 av Cedar, Montreal QC H3G 1A4; Mon'84; DPsy; FRCPC; Psy (General Adult Psychiatry). Staff Psy, McGill University Health Centre - Montreal General Campus; Dir Undergrad Educ & Prof, McGill University; Langs: Armenian; French; (514)934-1934 x42611; Fax. (514)934-8237; gregory.meterissian@muhc.mcgill.ca.

METERISSIAN, Sarkis H; MUHC-Royal Victoria Hosp, S10 22-687 av des Pins O, Montreal QC H3A 1A1; McG'85; MSc; FRCSC; GenSurg (Breasts); General Surgical Oncology (P.Q.). Prof Surg & Oncol, McGill University Health Centre - Royal Victoria Hospital; Assoc Dean Postgraduate Med Educ & Professional Affairs, McGill University; Langs: Bilingual(English/French); (514)934-1934 x36631; Fax. (514)843-1454; sarkis.meterissian@muhc.mcgill.ca.

METHERELL, Leslie S; Bonavista Med Clinic, 739 Lake Bonavista Dr SE, Calgary AB T2J 0N2; Alb'90; Court Staff Privil, Rockyview General Hospital; (403)278-1440

METHOT, Francis; Hop Maisonneuve-Rosemont, 5415 boul de l'Assomption, Montreal QC H1T 2M4; Mon'78; CSPQ; RadOncol. Staff, Hopital Maisonneuve-Rosemont; (514)252-3425

METHOT, Mireille; The Ottawa Hosp-Civic Campus, 1053 Carling Ave, Ottawa ON K1Y 4E9; Laval'07; GenSurg. Fellow, The Ottawa Hospital - Civic Campus; (613)761-4766

METHOT, Renee; Centre Med Saint-Charles, 1740 ch Saint-Charles, Terrebonne QC J6W 3R3; Sher'85; Staff, Centre Hospitalier Pierre le Gardeur; (450)492-2277; Fax. (450)492-1030.

METHVEN, Peter G; 104-22112 52 Ave, Langley BC V2Y 2M6; Cape Town (South Africa)'82; Staff, Langley Memorial Hospital; (604)534-6515

METIVIER, Annie; Clinique Med de Lavaltrie, 1400 rue Notre-Dame, Lavaltrie QC J5T 1M6; Sher'97; (450)586-1033; Fax. (450)586-4498.

METIVIER, Denis; Clin Familiale Saint-Victor, 225 rue Principale, Saint-Victor QC G0M 2B0; Laval'71; Physician, Clinique Familiale St-Victor; Physician, Clinique Med East-Broughton; (418)588-6611; Fax. (418)588-7612; metik9@telvic.net.

METIVIER, Yves; Centre Med Jeffery Hale, 305-1248 ch Sainte-Foy, Quebec QC G1S 2M5; Laval'74; Staff, Jeffery Hale Hospital-Saint Brigid's; (418)681-7854; Fax. (418)681-6173.

METRAKOS, P Peter; MUHC-Royal Victoria Hosp, S1026-687 av des Pins O, Montreal QC H3A 1A1; McG'87; FACS; FRCSC; GenSurg (Hepatobiliary & Pancreatic Surgery). Dir Hepatic, McGill University Health Centre - Royal Victoria Hospital; Assoc Prof Surg, McGill University; Langs: Greek; French; (514)843-1600; Fax. (514)843-1503.

METRAKOS, Stephanie; Medicentre Kirkland, 2971 boul Saint-Charles, Kirkland QC H9H 3B5; McG'82; FRCPC; Peds. Staff, McGill University Health Centre - Montreal Children's Hospital; Langs: Bilingual(English/French); (514)426-4656; Fax. (514)697-3929.

METRAS, Jacques; Hôpital Laval, 2725 ch Sainte-Foy, Quebec QC G1V 4G5; Laval'67; CSPQ; Cardiovasc&ThorSurg (P.Q.). Staff, Hôpital Laval; Université Laval; (418)656-4717; Fax. (418)656-4707; jacques.metras@chg.ulaval.ca.

METRIE, Mamdouh A H; Twain Med Clinic, 14-735 Twain Ave, Mississauga ON L5W 1X1; Ain Shams (Egypt)'77; MB ChB; CCFP; Langs: Arabic; (905)670-8209; Fax. (905)670-0346.

METROWICH, Peter J; Nanaimo Reg Gen Hosp, 1200 Dufferin Cres, Nanaimo BC V9S 2B7; Witwatersrand (South Africa)'89; CCFP; CCFP(E.M.); Staff, Nanaimo Regional General Hospital; (250)754-5545

METSER, Ur; Univ Hlth Network-Princess M, 3 960-610 University Ave, Toronto ON M5G 2M9; Haifa (Israel)'93; Staff, Princess Margaret Hospital - University Health Network; (416)946-4501; Fax. (416)946-6564.

METTLE, Armstrong N A; Greystone Med Clinic, 2921B 8th St E, Saskatoon SK S7H 0V4; (Ghana)'72; MB ChB; MRCS(Eng); LRCP(Lond); FRCS(Eng); (306)373-3223; Fax. (306)955-8802; anam@sasktel.net.

METTLE, Valerie; Regina Community Clinic, 1106 Winnipeg St, Regina SK S4R 1J6; CCFP; (306)543-7880; Fax. (306)543-6888.

METZ, Gila S; Sexual Health Centre, 179 Clarence St, Ottawa ON K1N 5P7; Alb'02; CCFP; (613)234-4641; Fax. (613)560-6096.

METZ, Luanne M; Foothills Med Centre, 1403 29 St NW, Calgary AB T2N 2T9; Cal'83; FRCPC; Neur (Multiple Sclerosis). Staff, Foothills Medical Centre; Dir MS Clinic, Alberta Health Services; Physician, MS Clinic; Prof Clin Neurosciences, University of Calgary; (403)944-4241; Fax. (403)944-4245.

METZAK, Danny J; New Westminster Med Centre, 101-600 Royal Ave, New Westminster BC V3M 1J3; Man'68; (604)526-4277; Fax. (604)521-3644.

METZGER, Daniel L; Children's & Women's HC of BC, K4 213-4480 Oak St, Vancouver BC V6H 3V4; Cleveland(OH) (USA)'85; FAAP; FRCPC; Peds (Pediatric Endocrinology); Endocrin&Metab. Ac Staff Ped Endocrinologist, BC Children's Hospital; Clin Prof Peds, University of British Columbia; Langs: German; (604)875-2117; Fax. (604)875-3231; dmetzger@cw.bc.ca.

MEUNIER, Bethann D; Kingston Gen Hosp, 76 Stuart St, Kingston ON K7L 2V7; Dal'95; FRCPC; Anes;CCFP; Staff, Kingston General Hospital; (613)548-7827

MEUNIER, Caroline C; Hop Charles Lemoyne, 3120 boul Taschereau, Greenfield Park QC J4V 2H1; Mon'91; CSPQ; FRCPC; AnatPath (Hematology Pathology). Staff, Hopital Charles LeMoyne; (450)466-5000

MEUNIER, Catherine; Newmarket Long Term Care, 194 Eagle St, Newmarket ON L3Y 1J6; Mon'96; BSc; MSc; CCFP; Med Dir, York Region Long Term Care Facilities; Langs: Italian; English; (905)895-3628; Fax. (905)895-5368.

MEUNIER, Helene F; CSSS de Manicouagan, 635 boul Jolliet, Baie-Comeau QC G5C 1P1; Laval'97; CCFP; Ac Member, Centre Hospitalier Régional Baie-Comeau; Langs: Bilingual(French/English); (418)589-3701; Fax. (418)294-2862.

MEUNIER, Louise; CSSS de Sept-Iles, 405 av Brochu, Sept-Iles QC G4R 2W9; Mon'75; Staff, Centre Hospitalier Regional de Sept-Iles; (418)962-2572 x4130; Fax. (418)962-1858.

MEUNIER, Mathieu; Ctr Hosp de Verdun, 4000 boul Lasalle, LaSalle QC H4G 2A3; Sher'01; FRCSC; GenSurg. Staff, Centre Hospitalier de Verdun; (514)362-1000

MEUNIER, Michel; Groupe Sante Medisys, 1100-500 rue Sherbrooke O, Montreal QC H3A 3C6; Mon'73; (514)845-1211

MEUNIER, Nicole; 133 rue Bernard, St-Charles-Brromee QC J6E 2C4; Sher'71; Derm. Langs: Spanish; English; (450)759-3505; Fax. (450)756-8879.

MEUNIER, Philippe; Ctr Hosp Rouyn-Noranda, 4 9e rue, Rouyn-Noranda QC J9X 2B2; Sher'98; FRCPC; IntMed. Staff, Centre Hospitalier Rouyn-Noranda; (819)764-5131

MEUNIER, Pierre; 308-400 boul Saint-Martin O, Laval QC H7M 3Y8; Mon'73; FRCPC; Gastroent. Ac Staff, Hopital de la Cite de la santé; (450)967-9767

MEUNIER, Pierre; Centre Medical de Varennes, 201-2082 Rte Marie-Victorin, Varennes QC J3X 2C7; Mon'70; (450)652-2959; Fax. (450)652-3792.

MEUNIER, Rosalie-Selene; Hop du Sacre-Coeur de Mtl, 5400 boul Gouin O, Montreal QC H4J 1C5; Mon'04; FRCPC; IntMed. Staff, Hôpital du Sacre-Coeur de Montréal; (514)338-2050

MEUSER, James C; Temmy Latner Centre, 60 Murray St, Toronto ON M5T 3L9; Tor'80; CCFP; FCFP; (416)586-4800 x1538; Fax. (416)586-4804.

MEW, Daphne J Y; 1441 29 St NW, Calgary AB T2N 4J8; Cal'87; PhD; FRCSC; GenSurg (Surgical Oncology). Staff Med & Surgs, Foothills Medical Centre; Staff Med & Surgs, Tom Baker Cancer Centre; Staff, Medical/Surgical, Grace Women's Health Centre; Asst Prof, University of Calgary; (403)220-2859

MEW, Jenny S; Rockyview Gen Hosp, 7007 14 St SW, Calgary AB T2V 1P9; Cal'88; FRCPC; Psy (Geriatric Psychiatry). Staff, Rockyview General Hospital; (403)943-3503; Fax. (403)212-1230.

MEWA, Amirudin A M; 504-790 Bay St, Toronto ON M5G 1N8; Sask'76; MD(IntMed&Rheum); FRCPC; IntMed (Adult Rheumatology); Rheum. Ac Staff Rheum, Sunnybrook Health Sciences Centre - Holland Orthopaedic & Arthritic Centre; Langs: Gujarati; Swahili; (416)964-9214; Fax. (416)964-6847.

MEYBURG, Jan M; Park Avenue Med Clinic, 4634 Park Ave, Terrace BC V8G 1V7; Stellenbosch (South Africa)'79; MB ChB; LMCC; Staff, Mills Memorial Hospital; Langs: Afrikaans; (250)615-5030; Fax. (250)615-5035.

MEYER, Abraham P; Regina Qu'Appelle HR-Pasqua, 100-4101 Dewdney Ave, Regina SK S4T 1A5; Cape Town (South Africa)'88; MB ChB; LMCC; CCFP; CCFP(E.M.); Staff Emerg, Pasqua Hospital; (306)766-2238; Fax. (306)766-2770.

MEYER, Allan B; 225-2306 Highway 6, Vernon BC V1T 7E3; UBC'94; (250)260-3800; Fax. (250)260-3806; ab.meyer@shaw.ca.

MEYER, Anthon M; Amdocs, 77 Main St, Winnipeg MB R3C 1A3; Orange Free State (South Africa)'91; CCFP; (204)676-2011

MEYER, Caroline M; St Mary's Gen Hosp, 911 Queens Blvd, Kitchener ON N2M 1B2; Wes'92; CCFP; Staff, St Mary's General Hospital; (519)749-6410

MEYER, Catharina J; Carlyle Med Clinic, PO Box 1090, Carlyle SK S0C 0R0; Cape Town (South Africa)'90; MB ChB; CCFP; Langs: German; Dutch; Afrikaans; (306)453-6795; Fax. (306)453-6796.

MEYER, Dominique H; Institut Prive de Chirurgie, 180-801 Grande Allee O, Quebec QC G1S 1C1; Laval'85; MBA; FRCSC; Ophth (Oculo Plastic Surgery). ac Staff, Jeffery Hale Hospital-Saint Brigid's; Prés, Institut Prive de Chirurgie Laser & Esthetique; Langs: English; (418)687-7328; Fax. (418)687-6110; info@ipdc.com.

MEYER, Frederick J T; 3062 2nd Ave, Port Alberni BC V9Y 1Y9; Orange Free (South Africa)'98; Staff, Nanaimo Regional General Hospital; Langs: Afrikaans; (250)723-9422

MEYER, George R; Brooks Health Centre, PO Box 300 Stn Main 440 3rd St E, Brooks AB T1R 1B3; (South Africa)'86; Staff, Brooks Health Centre; (403)501-3232; Fax. (403)362-6039.

MEYER, Jeffrey H; Addiction & Mental Hlth-Clarke, 250 College St, Toronto ON M5T 1R8; Tor'93; FRCPC; Psy. Staff, Centre for Addiction & Mental Health (CAMH) - College Street Site; (416)535-8501 x4007; Fax. (416)979-4656.

MEYER, Johannes G; Campbell Clinic, PO Box 180 Stn Main 1915 17 St, Coaldale AB T1M 1M3; (South Africa)'93; MB ChB; CCFP; Langs: Afrikaans; (403)345-3072; Fax. (403)345-2141.

MEYER, John P; Alberni Med Bldg, 7-3855 9th Ave, Port Alberni BC V9Y 4T9; Stellenbosch (South Africa)'81; (250)723-9424; Fax. (250)723-9321.

MEYER, L Joanne; St Joseph's Health Centre, 30 The Queensway, Toronto ON M6R 1B5; Tor'94; FRCPC; IntMed (Intensive Care); Critical Care Medicine. Staff IntMed & Intensive Care, St Joseph's Health Centre; Instructor, University of Toronto; (416)530-6085; joanne.meyer@utoronto.ca.

MEYER, Marius G; Dawson Creek Med Centre, 816 103 Ave, Dawson Creek BC V1G 2G1; Stellenbosch (South Africa)'92; Staff, Dawson Creek & District Hospital; Langs: Afrikaans; (250)782-5271; Fax. (250)782-6360.

MEYER, Maxwell W; Western Med Clinic, 1757 Robson St, Vancouver BC V6G 1C9; Cal'95; BSc; CCFP; Clin Associate HIV, Providence Health Care - St Paul's Hospital; (604)689-1828; Fax. (604)689-1849.

MEYER, Melissa; The Medical Clinic Associates, 4794 Joyce Ave, Powell River BC V8A 3B6; (Other Foreign)'08; MB ChB; Langs: Afrikaans; (604)485-6261

MEYER, Peter B; 2644 Quadra St, Victoria BC V8T 4E4; McM'89; BSc; Staff, Vancouver Island Health Authority; (250)361-4454; Fax. (250)386-6900.

MEYER, Petrus S; 206-314 25 St, Cold Lake AB T9M 1G6; (South Africa)'95; MB ChB; LMCC; Chief Staff C. H. R., Milk River Health Centre; Staff, Cold Lake Healthcare Centre; Med Dir Emergency Services, Town of Warner; Med Dir Emergency Services, Town of Milk River; Med Dir Emergency Services, Town of Coutts; Langs: Afrikaans; (780)639-3001; pmeyer@milkriver.ca.

MEYER, Rachel A; St Michael's Hosp, 30 Bond St, Toronto ON M5B 1W8; Tor'06; FRCPC; Anes. Staff, St Michael's Hospital; (416)360-4000

MEYER, Ralph M; Clin Trials Div Cancer Res Ins, 10 Stuart St, Kingston ON K7L 2V5; McM'78; FRCPC; IntMed; Hem. Ac Staff, Kingston General Hospital; Prof Oncol & Med Community Hlth & Epidemiol, Queen's University; (613)533-6430

MEYER, Steven R; University of Alberta Hosp, 2D4.37-8440 112 St NW, Edmonton AB T6G 2B7; UBC'98; BSc; PhD; FRCSC; CardSurg. Staff Surg, University of Alberta Hospital; Asst Prof Cardiac Surg, University of Alberta; (780)407-1959; Fax. (780)407-3672.

MEYER, Ulrike; Dawson Creek & Dist Hosp, 11100 13 St, Dawson Creek BC V1G 3W8; (Germany)'89; CCFP; FCFP; Staff, Dawson Creek & District Hospital; Langs: German; (250)782-8501

MEYERS, Brandon M; Juravinski Cancer Centre, 699 Concession St, Hamilton ON L8V 5C2; Ott'06; FRCPC; IntMed; MedOncol. (905)387-9495; Fax. (905)575-6326.

MEYERS, Christine M; MUHC-Royal Victoria Hosp, C4.78-687 av des Pins O, Montreal QC H3A 1A1; McG'95; FRCPC; EmergMed. Staff, McGill University Health Centre - Royal Victoria Hospital; (514)934-1934 x34277; Fax. (514)843-1638; christinemeyers@hotmail.com.

MEYERS, Kimberly L; The Emo Clinic, PO Box 569 Stn Main, Emo ON P0W 1E0; Wes'89; CCFP; FCFP; (807)482-2323; Fax. (807)482-3089.

MEYERS, Michael P; Medical Arts Bldg, 202-233 Kennedy St, Winnipeg MB R3C 3J5; Man'84; FRCPC; DiagRad (Thoracic Radiology). Ac Staff Radiol, Seven Oaks General Hospital; Ac Staff Radiol, Health Sciences Centre; Asst Prof Radiol, University of Manitoba; (204)942-6453; Fax. (204)944-8101; meyers@shaw.ca.

MEYERSON, Jeffrey; Medical Arts Bldg, 777-1 Young St, Hamilton ON L8N 1T8; Cape Town (South Africa)'78; MB ChB; ABIM; FRCPC; IntMed (Lipid Disorders/Obesity); Endocrin&Metab. Staff, Hamilton Health Sciences Centre - Hamilton General Hospital; Staff, St Joseph's Healthcare - Charlton Campus; Asst Prof, McMaster University; Langs: Afrikaans; (905)577-1141; Fax. (905)577-1141.

MEYLER, Paula E; Royal Columbia Hosp, 104-330 Columbia St E, New Westminster BC V3L 3W7; Alb'07; FRCPC; Anes. (604)520-4602

MEYN, M Stephen; Genetics & Genomic Biology, 15 314-101 College St, Toronto ON M5G 1L7; New York(NY) (USA)'80; PhD; AB; AB; Staff Clin & Metabolic Genetics, The Hospital For Sick Children; Prof Molecular & Med Genetics & Peds, University of Toronto; meyn@sickkids.ca.

MEYROWITZ, David M; Salvation Army Grace Gen Hosp, 300 Booth Dr, Winnipeg MB R3J 3M7; Man'75; FRCPC; IntMed. Staff, The Salvation Army Grace Hospital; (204)837-8311

MEZA-JUNCO, Judith; Coss Cancer Institute, 11560 University Ave NW, Edmonton AB T6G 1Z2; (Mexico)'97; Staff, Cross Cancer Institute; (780)432-8458; Fax. (780)432-8888.

MEZA VARGAS, Maria S; Miesericordia Health Centre, 376-99 Cornish Ave, Winnipeg MB R3C 1A2; Staff, Misericordia Health Centre; (204)774-6581

MEZEI, Michelle M; Neuromuscular Disease Unit, 8F-2775 Laurel St, Vancouver BC V5Z 1M9; McG'89; FRCPC; Neur (Neuromuscular Diseases). Staff, Vancouver General Hospital - Centennial Pavillion; Langs: Hungarian; French; (604)875-4405; Fax. (604)875-5867.

MEZHERICHER-SHENDEREY, Inna; 103-7121 Bathurst St, Thornhill ON L4J 7Z1; (Ukraine)'89; CCFP; (905)763-6682

MEZIANE, Hyjr; GMF Clinique Med St-Laurent, 201-200 av Saint-Laurent, Louiseville QC J5V 1J9; Paris (France)'05; (819)228-7171

MEZIAT-BURDIN, Anne; CHUS-Hop Fleurimont, 3001 12e av N, Sherbrooke QC J1H 5N4; St-Etienne (France)'92; Staff, Centre Hospitalier Universitaire de Sherbrooke-Hopital Fleurimont; (819)346-1110

MEZODY, Melitta; Univ Hlth Network-Toronto Western Hosp, 5E 568-399 Bathurst St, Toronto ON M5T 2S8; (Hungary)'82; Staff, Toronto Western Hospital - University Health Network; Asst Prof, University of Toronto; Langs: Hungarian; German; (416)605-5800

MEZON, Bernard R J; London HSC-University Hosp, PO Box 5339 Stn B 339 Windermere Rd, London ON N6A 5A5; Man'74; FRCPC; Anes. Ac Staff, London Health Sciences Centre - University Hospital; (519)663-3270

MEZRAHI, Michel; CLSC du Ruisseau-Papineau, 1665 rue du Couvent, Laval QC H7W 3A8; Paris (France)'89; (450)687-5690; Fax. (450)687-5998.

MGBEMENA, Benjamin E; Lorraine Wing Tower C, 201 Deacon St, Pembroke ON K8A 2J6; Ibadan (Nigeria)'67; MB BS; FRCPC; IntMed. (613)732-2332; Fax. (613)735-2622.

MHANNI, Aizeddin A M; Health Sciences Centre, FE 229-820 Sherbrook St, Winnipeg MB R3A 1R9; Tripoli (Libya)'91; MB ChB; FCCMG; FAB; FRCPC; MedGenetics. Staff, Health Sciences Centre; (204)774-6511

MHIRI, Selma; Hop Charles Lemoyne, 3120 boul Taschereau, Greenfield Park QC J4V 2H1; (Tunisia)'93; FRCPC; RadOncol. Staff, Hopital Charles LeMoyne; (450)466-5000 x3976

MI, Lei; Crescent Heights Med Clinic, 49 8 St NW, Medicine Hat AB T1A 6N9; (China)'84; CCFP; Staff, Alberta Health Services; (403)526-7422; Fax. (403)526-3349.

MIA, Mahomed; St Paul's Hosp, B2 85-1702 20th St W, Saskatoon SK S7M 0Z9; Natal (South Africa)'87; FRCSC; Otol (Rhinology). Staff, St Paul's Hospital (Grey Nuns) of Saskatoon; Asst Clin Prof, University of Saskatchewan; (306)655-5904; Fax. (306)655-5892; shabirmia@hotmail.com.

MIA, Raziya; Abbotsford Reg Hosp & Cancer C, 32900 Marshall Rd, Abbotsford BC V2S 0C2; UBC'77; CCFP; FCFP; Staff, Royal Inland Hospital; Physician, Abbotsford Regional Hospital & Cancer Centre; (604)851-4710

MIA, Shabir M; Willowgrove Med Group, 2-527 Nelson Rd, Saskatoon SK S7S 1P4; Durban (South Africa)'87; Langs: Afrikaans; Zulu; (306)653-1543; Fax. (306)653-0422; smia@fhhr.ca.

MIAH, Mohammad; Miramichi Reg Hosp, 500 Water St, Miramichi NB E1V 3G5; Dhaka (Bangladesh)'89; Staff, Miramichi Regional Hospital; (506)623-3000

MIAKHIL, Mohsen; Northumberland Med Clinic, F2-924 Northumberland Ave, Saskatoon SK S7L 3W6; Russia (Russia (Federation))'84; (306)955-1820; Fax. (306)955-1823.

MIAN, A Nadeem; Links Clinic, 104-11910 111 Ave NW, Edmonton AB T5G 3G6; (Pakistan)'80; MB BS; BSc; DABPed; FAAP; FRCPC; Peds. Staff, University of Alberta Hospital; Staff, Royal Alexandra Hospital; Asst Clin Prof, University of Alberta; Langs: Urdu; Punjabi; Hindi; (780)453-9472; Fax. (780)453-9471.

MIAN, Ahmed R; Humber River Reg Hosp-Church, 200 Church St, Toronto ON M9N 1N8; Ott'09; CCFP; CCFP(E.M.); Staff, Humber River Regional Hospital - Church Street Site; Langs: Punjabi; (416)249-8111

MIAN, Irfan A; 80 Workman Way, Toronto ON M6J 1H4; Dal'95; BSc; FRCPC; Psy (Child Psychiatry). Staff, Centre for Addiction & Mental Health (CAMH) - College Street Site; (416)535-8501 x4001; Fax. (416)979-4685; irfan_mian@camh.net.

MIAN, M Tariq; 7-794 Sargent Ave, Winnipeg MB R3E 0B7; Lahore (Pakistan)'85.

MIAN, Mamta; Specialized Geriatric Clinic, 232 Ross Dr, New Westminster BC V3L 0B2; Dal'93; FRCPC; IntMed; GeriatricMed. Staff, Eagle Ridge Hospital & Health Care Centre; Staff, Royal Columbian Hospital; (604)519-8548; Fax. (604)519-8579.

MIAN, Rizwan A; Surrey Med Arts Bldg, 308-13710 94A Ave, Surrey BC V3V 1N1; Dal'93; MS(Surg.); FRCSC; PlasSurg (Microvascular Surgery). Staff, Royal Columbian Hospital; Staff, Eagle Ridge Hospital & Health Care Centre; Staff, Surrey Memorial Hospital; (604)585-6001; Fax. (604)589-6841; dmi@telus.net.

MIAN, Zafer; Health Sense Medical, 8-2983 Westoak Trails Blvd, Oakville ON L6M 5E4; Man'00; MD; CCFP; (905)901-1217; Fax. (905)825-0239; zafermian@gmail.com.

MICFLIKIER, Allan B; 110-203 Edmonton St, Winnipeg MB R3C 1R4; Man'71; FRCPC; IntMed (Endoscopy); Gastroent. Staff, St Boniface General Hospital; Staff, Victoria General Hospital; Asst Prof Med, University of Manitoba; (204)942-7703; Fax. (204)942-7706; amicflik@mts.net.

MICHAEL, Antoinette A; Family Care Med Centre, 104-3050 Garden St, Whitby ON L1R 2G7; Cairo (Egypt)'73; CCFP; Langs: Arabic; French; (905)430-5305; Fax. (905)430-6416.

MICHAEL, Essam S N; 210-12295 50 Hwy, Bolton ON L7E 1M1; Cairo (Egypt)'82; MB ChB; FRCSC; ObstGyn. (905)857-1988; Fax. (905)857-1882.

MICHAEL, George P; Yonge Davis Centre, C2B-17480 Yonge St, Newmarket ON L3Y 8A7; Ain Shams (Egypt)'78; MD; CCFP; Langs: Arabic; (905)898-3700; Fax. (905)898-3738.

MICHAEL, Kevin; Kingston Gen Hosp, 76 Stuart St, Kingston ON K7L 2V7; Natal (South Africa)'94; Staff, Kingston General Hospital; (613)549-6666

MICHAEL, Liliane F F; Scotia Med, 961 Bedford Hwy, Bedford NS B4A 1A9; Ain Shams (Egypt)'95; MB ChB; CCFP; (902)832-2380; Fax. (902)444-3074.

MICHAEL, Roger T; Halifax Prof Centre, 285-5991 Spring Garden Rd, Halifax NS B3H 1Y6; Dal'68; ABIM; FCCP; FRCPC; IntMed (Respirology). Consultant, IWK Health Centre; Consultant, Dartmouth General Hospital; Med Dir Adult Cystic Fibrosis Clin, Queen Elizabeth II Health Sciences Centre - Victoria General Site; Consultant, Nova Scotia Home Oxygen Program; Asst Prof, Dalhousie University; (902)422-1708; Fax. (902)425-8962.

MICHAEL, Samer; CSSS Les Eskers de l'Abitibi, 622 4e rue O, Amos QC J9T 2S2; Damas (Syria)'92; Staff, CH Hôtel-Dieu d'Amos; (819)732-3341; Fax. (819)732-7054.

MICHAEL AWAD, Roula; CSSS Les Eskers de l'Abitibi, 622 4e rue O, Amos QC J9T 2S2; Staff, CH Hôtel-Dieu d'Amos; (819)732-3341

MICHAELS, George; Clinique MDCM, 5515 rue Saint-Jacques, Montreal QC H4A 2E3; McG'86; CCFP; FCFP; Staff, St Mary's Hospital Centre; (514)483-9911; Fax. (514)483-9910.

MICHAIEL, Mary F S; Harvest Hills Med Clinic, 715-500 Country Hills Blvd NE, Calgary AB T3K 4Y7; (Egypt)'82; CCFP; Langs: Arabic; (403)226-8647; Fax. (403)226-8645.

MICHAILIDIS, Michael; Southlake Reg Health Centre, 596 Davis Dr, Newmarket ON L3Y 2P9; Tor'95; FRCPC; Anes. Staff, Southlake Regional Health Centre; Langs: Greek; (905)895-4521

MICHAL, Paul T; Sparling East Med Centre, PO Box 820, Fernie BC V0B 1M0; McG'93; CCFP; (250)423-4442; Fax. (250)423-3424.

MICHALCHUK, Andre S; Foothills Med Centre, C231-1403 29 St NW, Calgary AB T2N 2T9; Alb'87; FRCPC; EmergMed. Staff Emerg Med, Foothills Medical Centre; (403)944-1820

MICHALIK, Edward J; Tillsonburg Med Centre, 200 Broadway St, Tillsonburg ON N4G 5A7; Warsaw (Poland)'85; Staff, Tillsonburg District Memorial Hospital; (519)842-4231; Fax. (519)842-3793.

MICHALKOVA, Jana; 1525 rue l'Annociation N, Riviere-Rouge QC J0T 1T0; Karlova (Czech Republic)'81; Staff, Centre de L'Annociation; (819)275-2118; Fax. (819)275-2464.

MICHALSKA, Elzbieta; Heritage Village Medicentre, 2041 111 St NW, Edmonton AB T6J 4V9; Bialystok (Poland)'68; (780)438-2306

MICHALSKA, Magdalena A; Kingsway Prof Centre, 303-10611 Kingsway NW, Edmonton AB T5G 3C8; Warsaw (Poland)'03; Nephrol; IntMed. (780)496-9350; Fax. (780)425-8475.

MICHALSKI, Andrzej J; 19 Harcroft Rd, Toronto ON M6S 2V8; Gdansk (Poland)'69; Staff, St Joseph's Health Centre; Langs: Polish; (416)767-7468; Fax. (416)767-2784.

MICHALSKI, Kathleen A; Couchiching Family Health Team, 201A-119 Memorial Ave, Orillia ON L3V 5X1; Tor'88; BSc; CCFP; FCFP; Staff, Orillia Soldiers' Memorial Hospital; Lecturer, University of Toronto; Clinical Asst Prof, McMaster University; Langs: English; French; (705)325-0630; Fax. (705)325-9498.

MICHALSKI, Roman T; Saskatoon City Hosp, 701 Queen St, Saskatoon SK S7K 0M7; Warsaw (Poland)'68; PhD; FRCPC; AnatPath. Staff, Saskatoon City Hospital; Clinical Asst Prof, University of Saskatchewan; (306)655-8000

MICHALSKI, Warren C; Northumberland Hills Hosp, 1000 Depalma Dr, Cobourg ON K9A 5W6; Wes'09; CCFP; Staff, Northumberland Hills Hospital; (905)372-6811

MICHALUK, Audrey; CSSS du Sud de Lanaudière, 911 montee des Pionniers, Terrebonne QC J6V 2H2; Mon'07; FRCSC; ObstGyn. Staff, Centre Hospitalier Pierre le Gardeur; (450)654-7525

MICHALUK, Harvey D; Langley Mem Hosp, 22051 Fraser Hwy, Langley BC V3A 4H4; Man'76; FRCPC; Anes. Staff, Langley Memorial Hospital; (604)534-4121

MICHALYSHYN, John G; Canmore Associate Med Clinic, 124-1151 Sidney St, Canmore AB T1W 3G1; Alb'79; Staff, Canmore General Hospital; (403)678-5585; Fax. (403)678-6262.

MICHANO-STEWART, Tracy L; Dilico Family Health Team, 200 Anemki Pl, Thunder Bay ON P7J 1L6; NOSM'09; CCFP; (807)623-5200

MICHAUD, Alain; Hotel-Dieu de Roberval, 450 rue Brassard, Roberval QC G8H 1B9; Mon'80; CSPQ; FRCPC; Anes. Staff, Hotel-Dieu de Roberval; (418)275-0110; Fax. (418)275-8087.

MICHAUD, Carole; CLSC Beauce-Sartigan, RR 1 763 14e av, La Guadeloupe QC G0M 1G0; Laval'80; (418)459-3441; Fax. (418)459-3142.

MICHAUD, Christian; CLSC des Etchemins, RR 1 331 rue du Sanatorium, Lac-Etchemin QC G0R 1S0; Laval'99; Staff, CSSS des Etchemins; (418)625-8001; killermichaud@hotmail.com.

MICHAUD, Claudine; Montfort Hosp, 713 Montreal Rd, Ottawa ON K1K 0T2; Laval'86; CSPQ; FRCPC; DiagRad. Staff, Montfort Hospital; (613)746-4621 x4532; cmichaud@montforthospital.on.ca.

MICHAUD, Danielle; Clinique Med de l'Est Inc, 100-30 boul Saint-Joseph E, Montreal QC H2T 1G9; Mon'77; (514)845-4240

MICHAUD, Dominick A; Ctr Hosp Pierre-Janet, 20 rue Pharand, Gatineau QC J9A 1K7; Ott'05; FRCPC; Psy. Staff, Centre Hospitalier Pierre-Janet; (819)776-8055

MICHAUD, Francois; Clinique Med Pelletier, 300-8330 boul Taschereau, Brossard QC J4X 1C2; Laval'81; (450)465-5379; Fax. (450)465-5615; frmichaud@distributel.net.

MICHAUD, Gilles; Hop du Sacre-Coeur de Mtl, 5400 boul Gouin O, Montreal QC H4J 1C5; Mon'74; Gastroent (P.Q.). Staff, Hôpital du Sacre-Coeur de Montréal; (514)338-2050

MICHAUD, Ginette; Clinique Med du Boise Langevin, 130-288 rue Pierre-Saindon, Rimouski QC G5L 9A8; Laval'82; (418)724-4672; Fax. (418)724-4753.

MICHAUD, Guillaume; CSSS Haut-Richelieu-Rouville, 920 boul du Seminaire N, St-Jean-sur-Richel QC J3A 1B7; Mon'07; OrthSurg (P.Q.). Staff, Hôpital du Haut-Richelieu; (450)359-5000

MICHAUD, Guillaume; 3835 boul Harvey, Jonquiere QC G7X 2Z5; Mon'06; (418)542-7519

MICHAUD, Guy A; Centre Pediatrique Laval, 300-1150 boul de l'Avenir, Laval QC H7N 6L2; Laval'67; FRCPC; Peds. Membre Conseil, Hôpital Ste-Justine; (450)686-0822; Fax. (450)686-2388.

MICHAUD, Isabelle; CSSS Pierre Boucher, 1333 boul Jacques-Cartier E, Longueuil QC J4M 2A5; Sher'06; FRCPC; Psy. Staff, Centre Hospitalier Pierre Boucher; (450)468-8111

MICHAUD, Isabelle; CHUQ-Hotel-Dieu de Quebec, 11 Cote du Palais, Quebec QC G1R 2J6; Laval'97; FRCPC; IntMed; Critical Care Medicine (P.Q.). Staff, Centre Hospitalier Universitaire de Québec (CHUQ) - Siege Social; (418)691-5151

MICHAUD, Jacques; Hôpital Ste-Justine, 3175 ch Cote-Sainte-Catherine, Montreal QC H3T 1C5; Mon'88; FRCPC; Peds; MedGenetics. Staff, Hôpital Ste-Justine; (514)345-4727 x6342; jacques.michaud@recherche-ste-justine.qc.ca.

MICHAUD, Jean; Children's Hosp Eastern Ont, 401 Smyth Rd, Ottawa ON K1H 8L1; Laval'72; ABNPath; CSPQ; FRCPC; AnatPath (Neuropathology). Neuropathologist, Children's Hospital of Eastern Ontario (CHEO); Neuropathologist, The Ottawa Hospital - Civic Campus; Prof, University of Ottawa; Langs: Bilingual(French/English); (613)737-7600 x2630; Fax. (613)738-4837; jmichaud@cheo.on.ca.

MICHAUD, Johan; CHUM-Hop Notre-Dame, 1560 rue Sherbrooke E, Montreal QC H2L 4M1; Mon'99; FRCPC; PhysMed&Rehab. Staff, Centre Hospitalier l'Université de Montréal (CHUM) - Hôpital Notre-Dame; (514)890-8000

MICHAUD, Josee; 1-1500 Paris St, Sudbury ON P3E 3B8; Laval'92; FRCPC; IntMed; Cardiol. Staff, Health Sciences North-Laurentian Site; Langs: Italian; (705)222-9009; Fax. (705)222-3221.

MICHAUD, Julie; Clinique Med de Mont-Joli, 1385 boul Benoit-Gaboury, Mont-Joli QC G5H 4B1; Mon'03; Staff, CSSS de la Mitis; (418)775-5353; Fax. (418)775-6487.

MICHAUD, Julie; CSSS de Chicoutimi, 305 rue Saint-Vallier, Chicoutimi QC G7H 5H6; Laval'78; Staff, Complexe hospitalier de la Sagamie; (418)541-1000; julie.michaud@videotron.ca.

MICHAUD, Julie-Christine; CSSS Haut-Richelieu-Rouville, 920 boul du Seminaire N, St-Jean-sur-Richel QC J3A 1B7; Mon'08; CCFP; Staff, Hôpital du Haut-Richelieu; (450)359-5000; Fax. (450)359-5251.

MICHAUD, Karine; Ctr Hosp Affilie-Enfant-Jesus, 1401 18e rue, Quebec QC G1J 1Z4; Sher'01; FRCSC; Neursurg. Staff, Centre Hospitalier Affilié Universitaire de Québec - Hôpital De L'Enfant Jésus; (418)649-0252; Fax. (418)649-5974.

MICHAUD, Marie T; Royal Inland Hosp, 311 Columbia St, Kamloops BC V2C 2T1; Cal'02; FRCPC; Nephrol; IntMed. Staff, Royal Inland Hospital; (250)374-5111

MICHAUD, Marie-Noelle; CSSSG-Hop de Gatineau, CP 2000 Succ Bureau-Chef 909 boul de la Verendrye O, Gatineau QC J8P 7H2; Mon'01; Staff, Hôpital de Gatineau; (819)561-8100

MICHAUD, Michele D; Hopital Reg D'Edmundston, 275 boul Hebert, Edmundston NB E3V 4E4; Laval'08; CCFP; Staff, Hôpital regional d'Edmundston; (506)739-2200

MICHAUD, Nathalie; CSSS de Sept-Iles, 45 rue du Pere-Divet, Sept-Iles QC G4R 3N7; Laval'98; FRCSC; GenSurg. Staff, Centre Hospitalier Regional de Sept-Iles; (418)962-9761

MICHAUD, Nicolas; Hotel-Dieu de Levis, 143 rue Wolfe, Levis QC G6V 3Z1; Laval'03; Cardiol; IntMed. Staff, Hôtel-Dieu de Lévis; (418)835-7121

MICHAUD, Nicole; CSSS Rimouski-Neigette, 165 rue des Gouverneurs, Rimouski QC G5L 7R2; Laval'86; (418)724-7204; Fax. (418)727-5479.

MICHAUD, Odile; Clinique Med de la Rive, 169 av Prince Albert, Otterburn Park QC J3H 1L4; Mon'92; Physician, CLSC Vallee des Patriotes; (450)446-7333; Fax. (450)446-3420.

MICHAUD, Patricia; Ctr Hosp Affilie-St-Augustin, 3509A-2135 rue Terrasse-Cadieu, Quebec QC G1C 1Z2; Laval'82; Staff, Centre d'hebergement Saint-Augustin; (418)667-3910 x266

MICHAUD, Pierre; 644A rue Jacques-Cartier E, Chicoutimi QC G7H 2A4; Laval'73; FRCSC; GenSurg; VascSurg; ThorSurg. Staff, Complexe hospitalier de la Sagamie; (418)545-4456

MICHAUD, Pierrette; Ctr de Sante Publique du Quebe, 2400 av d'Estimauville, Quebec QC G1E 7G9; Laval'74; MSc(Epid.); Staff, Centre Hospitalier Universitaire de Quebec-CHUL; Teach Staff Preventive Med, Université Laval; (418)666-7000 x443; Fax. (418)666-2776; pierette.michaud@ssss.gouv.qc.ca.

MICHAUD, Raymonde; CHUM-Hop St-Luc, 1058 rue Saint-Denis, Montreal QC H2X 3J4; Mon'79; ObstGyn. Staff, Centre Hospitalier l'Université De Montréal (CHUM) - Hôpital Saint-luc; (514)890-8000

MICHAUD, Real; 460 boul Talbot, Chicoutimi QC G7H 4A2; Laval'73; Ac Staff, Complexe hospitalier de la Sagamie; (418)545-3460; Fax. (418)543-8148.

MICHAUD, Renee; CSSS de Trois-Rivières, 1991 boul du Carmel, Trois-Rivieres QC G8Z 3R9; Mon'00; CSSS de Trois-Rivières; (819)697-3333

MICHAUD, Sophie; Hop Brome-Missisquoi-Perkins, 950 rue Principale, Cowansville QC J2K 1K3; Sher'91; FRCPC; IntMed (Medical Microbiology & Infectious Diseases); InfectDis; MedMicrobiol., Hôpital Brome-Missisquoi-Perkins; (450)266-4342; sophie.michaud@usherbrooke.ca.

MICHAUD, Sylvie Y; CSSS de Sept-Iles, 45 rue du Pere-Divet, Sept-Iles QC G4R 3N7; Laval'90; FRCPC; Psy. Staff, Centre Hospitalier Regional de Sept-Iles; Staff, Hôtel-Dieu de Lévis; (418)877-9761

MICHAUD, Yzabel; Hop Charles-LeMoyne, 3120 boul Taschereau, Greenfield Park QC J4V 2H1; Mon'99; FRCSC; Neursurg. Staff, Hopital Charles LeMoyne; (450)466-5000

MICHAUD-MCGEE, Louise; CHUQ-St-Francois d'Assise, 10 rue de l'Espinay, Quebec QC G1L 3L5; Laval'73; Ac Staff, Centre Hospitalier Universitaire De Québec - Pavillon De St-françois-d'assise; (418)535-4303

MICHEA, Rodrigo; Ctr Traitement Le Fabourg St-J, 175 rue Saint-Jean, Quebec QC G1R 1N4; Laval'01; FRCPC; Psy. Staff, Hôtel-Dieu de Lévis; (418)648-6166; Fax. (418)648-6227.

MICHEL, Alison J; 204-1931 Mount Newton Cross Rd, Saanichton BC V8M 2A9; McM'01; CCFP; (250)652-9227; Fax. (250)652-9224.

MICHEL, Caroline M; SMBD Jewish Gen Hosp, 3755 ch Cote-Sainte-Catherine, Montreal QC H3T 1E2; Sask'90; CSPQ; FRCPC; IntMed; Cardiol. Staff, Sir Mortimer B Davis Jewish General; (514)340-8222; cmichel@cardio.jgh.mcgill.ca.

MICHEL, Ernest R; 700 University Ave, Toronto ON M5G 1Z5; Tor'65; FRCPC; Anes (Palliative Medicine). Staff, Mount Sinai Hospital; Asst Prof, University of Toronto; (416)586-4800 x6898; Fax. (416)586-4804; emichel@mtsinai.on.ca.

MICHEL, Florence; Clinique Med Le Frontenac, 202-5200 rue Frontenac, Lac-Megantic QC G6B 1H3; Sher'06; CCFP; Staff, Carrefour Sante Granit; (819)583-0157

MICHEL, Jean-Marie C; 116A 1re rue, Shippagan NB E8S 1A3; Strasbourg (France)'68; Langs: German; English; (506)336-8653; Fax. (506)336-1911; mymichel@nbnet.nb.ca.

MICHEL, Joseph G; Lakeshore Med Clinic, 1380 23rd Ave, Regina SK S4S 3S5; Sask'78; BSc(Hon); MSc; CCFP; FCFP; Staff, Regina General Hospital; Staff, Pasqua Hospital; (306)584-9333; Fax. (306)584-9788.

MICHEL, Julie; CHUS-Hop Fleurimont, 3001 12e av N, Sherbrooke QC J1H 5N4; Mon'07; Psy. Staff, Centre Hospitalier Universitaire de Sherbrooke-Hopital Fleurimont; (819)346-1110

MICHEL, Normand; CSSS Quebec-Sud, 1550 rue de la Pointe-aux-Liev, Quebec QC G1L 4M8; Laval'69; Ac Staff, Centre Hospitalier Universitaire De Québec - Pavillon De St-françois-d'assise; (418)829-0274; Fax. (418)829-0314.

MICHEL, Pierre; CLSC Samuel de Champlain, 100-5811 boul Taschereau, Brossard QC J4Z 1A5; Sher'72; (450)445-4452; Fax. (450)445-5535.

MICHEL, Rene P; Lyman-Duff Med Sciences Bldg, 210-3775 rue University, Montreal QC H3A 2B4; McG'71; CSPQ; FACP(Anat Path); FRCPC; AnatPath. Sr Staff Path, McGill University Health Centre - Royal Victoria Hospital; Prof Path, McGill University; Langs: English; French; (514)398-7192; Fax. (514)398-7446; rene.michel@mcgill.ca.

MICHEL, Shawkat S; Meadowlark Health Centre, 214 Meadowlark Shopping Ctr NW, Edmonton AB T5R 5W9; (Egypt)'72; FRCS; (780)489-6685; Fax. (780)489-6645.

MICHELAKIS, Evangelos; University of Alberta Hosp, WMC2C2-8440 112 St NW, Edmonton AB T6G 2B7; (Greece)'90; Staff, University of Alberta Hospital; (780)407-1576; Fax. (780)407-6452; emichela@cha.ab.ca.

MICHELL, Marcus J; Silverman Bldg, 114 Maitland St, Toronto ON M4Y 1E1; Tor'81; FRCSC; Otol (Psychotherapy); Psy. (416)972-1935 x3315; Fax. (416)924-9170.

MICHELS, Jorg E; BC Cancer Agency-Vanc Isl Ctr, 2410 Lee Ave, Victoria BC V8R 6V5; Saar (Germany)'91; MRCP(UK); PhD; Sr Scientist Deeley Research Centre/Staff, BC Cancer Agency Vancouver Island Centre; Langs: German; (250)519-5572; Fax. (250)519-2019.

MICHIELETTI, Pina; 2311 Pandosy St, Kelowna BC V1Y 1T4; McM'84; FRCPC; IntMed (Hepatology); Gastroent. Ac Staff, Kelowna General Hospital; (250)763-8110; gi.group@kelownagi.com.

MICHIELS, John F; 206 John St, Dunnville ON N1A 2P7; McM'85; MBA; CCFP; FCFP; (905)774-7431

MICHON, Alain; Montfort Hosp, 713 Montreal Rd, Ottawa ON K1K 0T2; Ott'04; CCFP; CCFP(E.M.); Staff, Montfort Hospital; (613)746-4621 x6019

MICHON, Andre L; Northestern Ontario Med Office, 2009 Long Lake Rd, Sudbury ON P3E 6C3; Ott'00; CCFP; Langs: English; French; (705)586-3601; Fax. (705)586-3602.

MICHON, Bertrand; 100-235 boul René-Lévesque E, Montreal QC H2X 1N8; Mon'58; FRCSC; ObstGyn. Staff, Centre Hospitalier l'Université De Montréal (CHUM) - Hôpital Saint-luc; (514)866-2446; Fax. (514)866-4013.

MICHON, Bruno; CHUQ-Ctr Hosp Univ Laval, 2705 boul Laurier, Quebec QC G1V 4G2; Sher'99; FRCPC; Hem; Peds. Hematologist, Centre Hospitalier Universitaire de Quebec-CHUL; Fax. (418)654-2223; bruno.michon@mail.chuq.qc.ca.

MICHON, Nicole; Hôpital Ste-Justine, 3175 ch Cote-Sainte-Catherine, Montreal QC H3T 1C5; Mon'77; Endocrin (P.Q.); IntMed (P.Q.). Staff, Hôpital Ste-Justine; (514)345-4931; Fax. (514)345-4878.

MICHOU, Laetitia N F; CHUQ-Ctr Hosp Univ Laval, 2705 boul Laurier, Quebec QC G1V 4G2; Paris (France)'05; Staff, Centre Hospitalier Universitaire de Quebec-CHUL; (418)654-2242; Fax. (418)654-2798.

MICK, Paul; Gordon & Leslie Diamond HCC, 2775 Laurel St, Vancouver BC V5Z 1M9; Alb'05; FRCSC; Otol. Staff, Gordon & Leslie Diamond Health Care Centre; (604)875-4126

MICKELSON, Allan S; PO Box 39005 Rpo James Bay, Victoria BC V8V 4X8; Tor'71.

MICKELSON, Elizabeth C R; Sunny Hill Hlth Ctr for Child, 3644 Slocan St, Vancouver BC V5M 3E8; McM'85; DAB; FRCPC; Peds (Developmental Pediatrics). Staff, Sunny Hill Health Centre for Children; Teach Staff Peds, University of British Columbia; (604)453-8306; Fax. (604)453-8338.

MICKELSON, Jennifer J; MetroVan Urology, 650-6091 Gilbert Rd, Richmond BC V7C 5L9; UBC'02; FRCSC; Urol. Staff, BC Children's Hospital; (604)875-2734

MICKELSON, Jon-Ivar; 103-8556 120 St, Surrey BC V3W 3N5; Cal'04; FRCSC; Otol (Head & Neck Surgery). (778)565-3239

MICKELSON, R Ross; 506-2197 Riverside Dr, Ottawa ON K1H 7X3; Sask'84; (613)523-0108; Fax. (613)523-0108.

MICKLE, Donald A G; Family Hlth Med Centre, 11-10035 Hurontario St, Brampton ON L6Z 0E6; Tor'67; MSc; FRCPC; MedBiochem (Family Medicine). A-Chief Clin Biochem, Toronto General Hospital - UHN; Prof, University of Toronto; (905)453-2441

MICKUS, V Alexander; 108 Raglan St S, Renfrew ON K7V 1P9; Tor'63; (613)432-7720

MICLETTE, Sylvie; Centre Med Acton, CP 1589 967 rue Boulay, Acton Vale QC J0H 1A0; Mon'87; (450)546-3245; Fax. (450)546-4720; sylvie@actonmedical.com.

MICLETTE MENARD, Philippe-Antoine; Centre Medi-Soleil, 120-383 boul du Seminaire N, St-Jean-sur-Richel QC J3B 8C5; Mon'08; Staff, Hôpital du Haut-Richelieu; (450)349-5555

MICOMONACO, Damian C; Group Health Centre, 240 McNabb St, Sault Ste. Marie ON P6B 1Y5; Qns'04; BSc; FRCSC; Otol (Head & Neck Surgery). (705)759-1234

MICROYS, Sherissa L; The Ottawa Hosp-Gen Campus, 501 Smyth Rd, Ottawa ON K1H 8L6; Ott'97; FRCPC; Anes (Critical Care Medicine). Staff, The Ottawa Hospital - General Campus; (613)737-7777 x78187

MIDDAUGH, Jeffrey A; Sudbury Reg Hosp-Laurentian Si, 41 Ramsey Lake Rd, Sudbury ON P3E 5J1; NOSM'09; CCFP; CCFP(E.M.); Staff, Health Sciences North-Laurentian Site; (705)675-4790

MIDDELKAMP, Graeme; Vernon Jubilee Hosp, 2101 32 St, Vernon BC V1T 5L2; UBC'00; FRCPC; DiagRad. Staff, Vernon Jubilee Hospital; (250)558-1200 x1303

MIDDELKAMP, Janel E; 100-5791 No. 3 Rd, Richmond BC V6X 2C9; UBC'02; FRCPC; DiagRad. (604)278-9152

MIDDELKAMP, Lydia; Vernon Jubilee Hosp, 2101 32 St, Vernon BC V1T 5L2; Sher'05; CCFP; Staff, Vernon Jubilee Hospital; (604)545-2211

MIDDLEBROOK, Paul F; Greystone Office & Med Centre, 205-345 8 St E, Owen Sound ON N4K 1L3; Ott'84; BSc; MD; FRCSC; Urol. Ac Staff, Grey Bruce Health Services - Owen Sound; Court Staff, South Bruce Grey Health Centre - Kincardine Site; (519)372-0755; Fax. (226)664-5555; pmiddlebrook@sympatico.ca.

MIDDLEBROOK, Shelia M; 501-503 Plains Rd E, Burlington ON L7T 2E2; McM'96; BSc; CCFP; (905)681-9200; Fax. (905)681-9404.

MIDDLESTADT, Laurie A; Maplehurst Detention Centre, PO Box 1040 Stn Main 655 Martin St, Milton ON L9T 5E6; Tor'75; MMed; Staff, Humber River Regional Hospital - Finch Avenue Site; (905)876-8300; longh0rn@hotmail.com.

MIDDLETON, Claire; Univ Hlth Network-Toronto Gen, 200 Elizabeth St, Toronto ON M5G 2C4; Edinburgh (Scotland)'89; MRC(UK); FRCPC; Anes. Staff, Toronto General Hospital - UHN; (416)340-4800 x5164

MIDDLETON, James C; Perth-Smiths Falls Dist Hosp, 33 Drummond St W, Perth ON K7H 2K1; Tor'76; FRCPC; Anes. Staff, Perth & Smiths Falls District Hospital - Perth Site (Great War Memorial Site); Clinical Asst Prof Family Med, McMaster University; Asst Prof Anes, Queen's University; (613)267-1500; Fax. (613)283-8990.

MIDDLETON, Joanna R; Saint John Reg Hosp, PO Box 2100 Stn Main 400 University Ave, Saint John NB E2L 4L2; Alb'07; CCFP; CCFP(E.M.); Staff, Saint John Regional Hospital; (506)648-6000

MIDDLETON, William G; Advanced Cosmetic Surgery Ctre, 120 Spadina Rd, Toronto ON M5R 2T8; Wes'79; FRCSC; Otol (Botox Injection). Ac Staff, St Michael's Hospital; Dir, Advanced Cosmetic Surgery Centre; Asst Prof, University of Toronto; (416)966-3223; Fax. (416)966-1994; drwgm@hotmail.com.

MIDDLETON, William J; Univ Hlth Network-Toronto Western Hosp, 399 Bathurst St, Toronto ON M5T 2S8; Wes'90; FRCPC; Anes. Staff Anaesthesia, Toronto Western Hospital - University Health Network; (416)603-5118

MIDGEN, Craig A; IWK Health Care Centre, 5850 University Ave, Halifax NS B3H 1V7; Texas (USA)'06; (902)470-7567; Fax. (902)470-7215.

MIDGLEY, Janet E; Queen Elizabeth Hosp, PO Box 6600 Stn Central 60 Riverside Dr, Charlottetown PE C1A 8T5; Dal'91; Anes. Staff, Queen Elizabeth Hospital; (902)894-2111

MIDGLEY, Julian P; Alberta Children's Hosp, 2888 Shaganappi Trail NW, Calgary AB T3B 6A8; Oxford (England)'82; MB; BCh; FRCPCH(UK); DCH; Staff, Alberta Children's Hospital; Assoc Prof Peds, University of Calgary; (403)955-7823; julian.midgley@calgaryhealthregion.ca.

MIDGLEY, Peter I; Queen Elizabeth II HSC-Halifax, 4721-1796 Summer St, Halifax NS B3H 3A7; Dal'00; FRCSC; GenSurg; VascSurg. Staff, Queen Elizabeth II Health Sciences Centre - Halifax Infirmary Site; (902)473-8506; Fax. (902)473-8507.

MIDHA, Rajiv; Foothills Med Centre, 1195-1403 29 St NW, Calgary AB T2N 2T9; Tor'87; FRCSC; Neursurg (Peripheral Nerve Surgery). Staff, Foothills Medical Centre; (403)944-1259; Fax. (403)270-7878; rajmihad@ucalgary.ca.

MIDHA, Vishal M; Brampton East Med Centre, 1-4525 Ebenezer Rd, Brampton ON L6P 2K8; Shivaji (India)'99; CCFP; Langs: Hindi; Punjabi; (905)794-2003; Fax. (905)794-2054.

MIDIA, Mehran; McMaster Med Centre, 1200 Main St W, Hamilton ON L8S 4J9; Ankara (Turkey)'91; FRCPC; DiagRad. Staff, Hamilton Health Sciences Centre - McMaster Children's Hospital; (905)521-2100

MIDRONI, Gyl; St Michael's Hosp, 3QW-30 Bond St, Toronto ON M5B 1W8; Tor'90; FRCPC; Neur (Peripheral Neuropathology). Dir Clinical Neurophysiology/Staff Neurologist, St Michael's Hospital; Assoc Prof, University of Toronto; (416)864-5193; Fax. (416)864-6095.

MIEDZINSKI, Lilly J; University of Alberta Hosp, 2E417WCM-8440 112 St NW, Edmonton AB T6G 2B7; Alb'76; FRCPC; IntMed (Infectious Diseases). Ac Staff, University of Alberta Hospital; Consultant, Royal Alexandra Hospital; Consultant, Cross Cancer Institute; Dir Career Development, University of Alberta; Langs: Ukrainian; (780)407-7313; Fax. (780)407-7137; lil.miedzinski@ualberta.ca.

MIELKE, Cornelia I; Harvard Square Mall, 202-801 Mohawk Rd W, Hamilton ON L9C 6C2; McM'85; CCFP; FCFP; Assoc Staff, Hamilton Health Sciences Centre - McMaster University Medical Centre; Langs: German; (905)388-2447; Fax. (905)387-3965.

MIELNICZUK, Lisa M; Univ of Ottawa Heart Institute, 40 Ruskin St, Ottawa ON K1Y 4W7; McM'98; FRCPC; IntMed; Cardiol. Staff, University of Ottawa Heart Institute; (613)761-4059

MIERINS, Egils; Health Canada, 5A-333 North River Rd, Ottawa ON K1A 0L1; Ott'67; FRCPC; IntMed (Rheumatology). Staff, Renfrew Victoria Hospital; Consultant, Pembroke Regional Hospital Inc; Ac Staff IntMed & Rheum, The Ottawa Hospital - General Campus; Asst Prof, University of Ottawa; Langs: Latvian; (613)954-4944

MIETTINEN, Donald A; 202-959 Dundas St, Woodstock ON N4S 1H2; Tor'81; Staff, Woodstock General Hospital; (519)539-7401; Fax. (519)539-6478.

MIETTUNEN, Paivi M H; Alberta Children's Hosp, 2888 Shaganappi Trail NW, Calgary AB T3B 6A8; McM'95; FRCPC; Peds; Rheum. Staff, Alberta Children's Hospital; Asst Prof, University of Calgary; Langs: Finnish; Swedish; German; (403)955-7771

MIGALLY, Samir E B; St Pierre Med Clinic, PO Box 569, St Pierre Jolys MB R0A 1V0; Alexandria (Egypt)'89; CCFP.

MIGAS, Maria; Family Practice Associates, 200-6155 North St, Halifax NS B3K 5R3; Dal'02; CCFP; (902)453-3511; Fax. (902)454-9010.

MIGAY, Andrew S; Fort William Clinic, 117 Mckellar St S, Thunder Bay ON P7E 1H5; Man'01; CCFP; (807)626-1234

MIGAY, Marcia M; 289 Munro St, Thunder Bay ON P7A 2N3; Man'03; CCFP; Staff, Lakehead Psychiatric Hospital - St. Joseph's Care Group; (807)683-4355

MIGICOVSKY, Valerie R; Bruyere Family Med Centre, 75 Bruyere St, Ottawa ON K1N 5C8; NOSM'10; CCFP; (613)241-3344

MIGNAULT, Chantal; CSSS de Trois-Rivières, 1991 boul du Carmel, Trois-Rivieres QC G8Z 3R9; Laval'93; FRCPC; IntMed; MedOncol (P.Q.); Hem. Staff, CSSS de Trois-Rivières; (819)697-3333 x63337

MIGNAULT, Charles; Clinique Med Memphre, 200-323 rue Sherbrooke, Magog QC J1X 2R9; Sher'78; (819)847-1313; Fax. (819)847-3529.

MIGNEAULT, Brigitte; CHUM-Hop St-Luc, 1058 rue Saint-Denis, Montreal QC H2X 3J4; Mon'00; CSPQ; FRCPC; Anes (Chronic Pain). Staff, Centre Hospitalier l'Université De Montréal (CHUM) - Hôpital Saint-luc; Langs: English; (514)890-8000 x36581; Fax. (514)412-7323.

MIHAILOVIC, Alexandra; General Surgery & Critical Car, 302-2020 Richmond Ave, Victoria BC V8R 6R5; McM'01; FRCSC; GenSurg; Critical Care Medicine. (250)592-4313

MIHALCHUK, Ainslie J; River East Health Access Ctre, 975 Henderson Hwy, Winnipeg MB R2K 4L7; Man'06; CCFP; (204)938-5000

MIHALCIOIU, Catalin; A304-687 av des Pins O, Montreal QC H3A 1A1; Bucharest (Romania)'80; FRCPC; IntMed; MedOncol (P.Q.). Staff, McGill University Health Centre - Royal Victoria Hospital; Langs: French; (514)934-1934 x35800; Fax. (514)843-1417; catalin.mihalcioiu@muhc.mcgill.ca.

MIHALICZ, Patrick A; Alberta Children's Hosp, 2888 Shaganappi Trail NW, Calgary AB T3B 6A8; Sask'94; FRCPC; Peds. Staff, Alberta Children's Hospital; (403)955-7070

MIHALOVITS, Helena; 120-151 Main St E, Hawkesbury ON K6A 1A1; Mon'82; FRCSC; Ophth (Anterior Segment). ac Staff, McGill University Health Centre - Montreal General Campus; Consultant, Hawkesbury & District General Hospital; McGill University; Langs: Hungarian; English; (613)632-4796

MIHALYNUK, Tracy M; 3491 Saanich Rd, Victoria BC V8X 1W8; Alb'93; BSc(Zool); MSc(Embryology); CCFP; Clin Asst Teach Staff Family Pract Residency Program, University of British Columbia; Clin Teacher/Preceptor Island Med Prog, University of Victoria; (250)475-2551; Fax. (250)475-3530.

MIHIC, Alan J; North Park Med Centre, D2-2355 Keele St, North York ON M6M 4A2; Ott'88; (416)244-4377; Fax. (416)244-1004.

MIHIC, Annette M C; Victoria Med Centre, 301-304 Victoria Ave N, Hamilton ON L8L 5G4; National (Ireland)'70; DAB; FRCSC; Ophth. (905)529-4610; Fax. (905)387-8307.

MIHIC, Niko; Centre Med Hochelaga, 9080 rue Hochelaga, Montreal QC H1L 2N9; Guadalajara (Mexico)'84; CCFP; ac Staff, Centre Hospitalier l'Université De Montréal (CHUM) - Hôpital Saint-luc; (514)353-8742

MIHU, Elena; Kinmount & Dist Med Centre, PO Box 118 31 County Rd 503, Kinmount ON K0M 2A0; McM'95; CCFP; Hon Staff Privil, Haliburton Highlands Health Services - Miden Site; Hon Staff Privil, Haliburton Highlands Health Services - Haliburton Site; Clinical Asst Prof, McMaster University; Langs: Hungarian; Romanian; French; (705)488-1105; Fax. (705)488-1119; elena@hhfht.com.

MIJANGOS-PELAEZ, Jose L; CSSS de la Vallée de l'Or, 725 6e rue, Val-d'Or QC J9P 3Y1; San Carlos (Guatemala)'77; FRCSC; GenSurg (Endoscopic Surgery). Staff GenSurg, Centre Hospitalier de Val d'Or; Conférencier Surg, McGill University; Langs: English; French; Spanish; (819)825-5858

MIJAVEC, Borislava; 207-210 Centrum Blvd, Orleans ON K1E 3V7; Novi Sad (Serbia)'91; CCFP; Langs: Croatian; Serbian; (613)834-0814

MIKAEL, Gaby G; The Moncton Hosp, 135 MacBeath Ave, Moncton NB E1C 6Z8; McG'01; Gastroent; IntMed. Staff, The Moncton Hospital; (506)851-8196; Fax. (506)851-1545.

MIKAIL, Azza M; A2-3980 Grand Park Dr, Mississauga ON L5B 4M6; Ain Shams (Egypt)'85; CCFP; Langs: Arabic; (905)615-0107; Fax. (905)615-1711.

MIKELBERG, Frederick S; UBC Eye Care Centre, 2550 Willow St, Vancouver BC V5Z 3N9; McG'78; DABOph; FRCSC; Ophth (Glaucoma). Ac Staff, Vancouver General Hospital - Centennial Pavillion; Dept Head & School Dir Ophth & Visual Sciences/Prof, University of British Columbia; (604)875-4365; Fax. (604)875-4606; fsm@interchange.ubc.ca.

MIKELOVA, Lynda K; MCI The Doctor's Office, 13-205 Maycroft Ave, Woodbridge ON L4L 5X8; Qns'01; CCFP; (416)265-2255; Fax. (416)265-6737; lmikelova@hotmail.com.

MIKHAEL, Dalia; 308-1081 Carling Ave, Ottawa ON K1Y 4G2; Ott'04; FRCPC; Derm. (613)722-8532

MIKHAIEL, Sameh A B; 3-900 Main St PO Box 1318, Swan River MB R0L 1Z0.

MIKHAIL, Antoinette; Wheat City Med Clinic, 920 Victoria Ave, Brandon MB R7A 1A9.

MIKHAIL, Ashraf S; 10063 Yonge St, Richmond Hill ON L4C 1T7; Ain Shams (Egypt)'83; MB ChB; CCFP; (905)508-0090; Fax. (905)508-0023; ashrafm@yours.com.

MIKHAIL, Boutros B; Chinguacousy & Sandalwood Med, 6-10671 Chinguacousy Rd, Brampton ON L7A 0N5; Cairo (Egypt)'96; CCFP; (905)840-4343; Fax. (905)840-4303.

MIKHAIL, Christine; Centre Saint-Lambert, 831 rue Notre-Dame, Saint-Lambert QC J4R 1S1; Mon'08; CCFP; (450)672-3320

MIKHAIL, G Pierre; Huntsville District Mem Hosp, 100 Frank Miller Dr, Huntsville ON P1H 1H7; Tor'95; CCFP; CCFP(E.M.); FCFP; Staff, Huntsville District Memorial Hospital - Muskoka Algonquin Healthcare; (705)789-2311

MIKHAIL, Genevieve; 7913 rue Nadeau, Brossard QC J4Y 1X8; Sher'10; CCFP.

MIKHAIL, Mamdouh T; Family Care Med Centre, 104-3050 Garden St, Whitby ON L1R 2G7; Ain Shams (Egypt)'92; CCFP; Langs: Arabic; (905)430-5305; Fax. (905)430-6416.

MIKHAIL, Mary Y D; Carson Med Clinic, 876 Montreal Rd, Ottawa ON K1K 4L3; Zagazig (Egypt)'92; (613)741-3660

MIKHAIL, Raouf E; Centre medical de Cowansville, 101-370 rue de la Riviere, Cowansville QC J2K 1N3; Ain Shams (Egypt)'82; CCFP; Staff, Hôpital Brome-Missisquoi-Perkins; Langs: Bilingual(French/English); (450)263-0774; Fax. (450)263-6457.

MIKHAIL, Roland G; 101-1368 Ouellette Ave, Windsor ON N8X 1J9; Mon'97; BSc; FRCPC; IntMed (Hemodynamics); Cardiol. (519)977-6643; Fax. (519)915-6326.

MIKHAIL, Samy N F; Trinity Med Clinic, 335 18th St, Brandon MB R7A 5A8; Alexandria (Egypt)'77; CCFP.

MIKI, Kenneth K; 2006 Eighth Ave, New Westminster BC V3M 2T5; UBC'75; (604)524-2281; Fax. (604)524-2121.

MIKI, Nancy P H; Early Psychosis Intervention, 3F-2750 Hastings St E, Vancouver BC V5K 1Z9; Tor'98; FRCPC; Psy. Physician, Bosman Hotel Community; (604)675-3875

MIKLEA, Jonel; McMaster Family Practice, A-690 Main St W, Hamilton ON L8S 1A4; Bucharest (Romania)'94; CCFP; Asst Prof Family Med, McMaster University; Langs: Romanian; Serbo-Croatian; (905)521-5015; Fax. (905)521-5010.

MIKROGIANAKIS, Angelo; Alberta Children's Hosp, 2888 Shaganappi Trail NW, Calgary AB T3B 6A8; Wes'97; FRCPC; Peds (Pediatric Emergency Medicine). Staff, Alberta Children's Hospital; (403)955-7211

MIKSA, Ray A; CFB Edmonton Field Ambulance C, PO Box 10500 Stn Forces, Edmonton AB T5J 4J5; Dal'07; CCFP; (780)973-4011

MIKULA, Lynn A; 302-272 Charlotte St, Peterborough ON K9J 2V4; McG'02; MDCM; MSc; FRCSC; GenSurg. (705)874-5222; Fax. (705)874-5224.

MIKULIS, David J; Univ Hlth Network-Toronto Western Hosp, 3MC 431-399 Bathurst St, Toronto ON M5T 2S8; Tufts(MA) (USA)'81; FRCPC; DiagRad (Magnetic Resonance). Sr Scientist, Toronto Western Hospital - University Health Network; Assoc Prof, University of Toronto; (416)603-5800 x5612; Fax. (416)603-4257; mikulis@mac.com.

MILAD, M Naguib; North-Med Walk In, 202-7131 Bathurst St, Thornhill ON L4J 7Z1; Cairo (Egypt)'72; (647)547-1218; Fax. (647)547-2077.

MILADINOVIC, Ljiljana; Rosedale Med Centre, 405-600 Sherbourne St, Toronto ON M4X 1W4; Belgrade (Serbia)'92; CCFP; Langs: Croatian; Serbian; (416)929-2173; Fax. (416)929-4906.

MILADINOVIC, Mirko; North York Gen Hospital, 4SE 110-4001 Leslie St, North York ON M2K 1E1; Belgrade (Serbia)'89; DrMedCh; FRCPC; AnatPath. Staff, North York General Hospital; Langs: Serbian; (416)756-6367; mmiladin@nygh.on.ca.

MILAMBILING, Ernesto M; Medical Arts Bldg, 1603-233 Kennedy St, Winnipeg MB R3C 3J5; Santo Tomas (Philippines)'71.

MILAMBILING, Ligaya C; Medical Arts Bldg, 1603-233 Kennedy St, Winnipeg MB R3C 3J5; Santo Tomas (Philippines)'71.

MILANI, Ali-Reza; Sheldon Chumir Health Centre, 1213 4 St SW, Calgary AB T2R 0X7; Meshed (Iran)'92; Consultant Psy, Cypress Regional Hospital; Langs: Farsi; (403)955-6566; Fax. (403)955-6577.

MILANKOV, Kosta; North Oshawa Med Centre, 101-1400 Ritson Rd N, Oshawa ON L1G 7W4; Tor'98; CCFP; (905)433-1640; Fax. (905)721-1366.

MILANSKA, Janina; Riverside Prof Centre, 205-1919 Riverside Dr, Ottawa ON K1H 1A2; Gdansk (Poland)'92; FRCPC; Peds. Staff, The Ottawa Hospital - General Campus; Langs: Polish; French; (613)737-5091; Fax. (613)737-6048.

MILBEO, Yann G; Hop Charles Lemoyne, 3120 boul Taschereau, Greenfield Park QC J4V 2H1; Bordeaux (France)'04; Staff, Hopital Maisonneuve-Rosemont; Staff, Hopital Charles LeMoyne; Langs: Bilingual(French/English); (450)466-5000

MILBRANDT, Kristopher G; Harry Medovy House, AE402-671 William Ave, Winnipeg MB R3E 0Z2; Sask'02; FRCSC; GenSurg; PedGenSurg.

MILBURN, Christopher R; Cape Breton Hlthcare Complex, 1482 George St, Sydney NS B1P 1P3; Dal'97; CCFP; Staff, Cape Breton Healthcare Complex; (902)567-8000

MILCZAREK, John J; Stan Cassidy Centre for Rehab, 800 Priestman St, Fredericton NB E3B 0C7; Ott'83; FRCPC; PhysMed&Rehab (Neurologic Rehab). Staff, Phys Med & Rehab, Stan Cassidy Centre for Rehabilitation; Asst Prof, Dalhousie University; Langs: English; French; (506)452-5302; Fax. (506)443-2600.

MILDE, Richard W; The Medical Assoc Clinic, 806 Vernon St, Nelson BC V1L 4G5; UBC'92; Ac Staff, Kootenay Lake General Hospital; Langs: German; (250)352-6611; Fax. (250)352-6624.

MILDENBERGER, Richard R; Richmond Med Bldg, 202-2020 Richmond Rd, Victoria BC V8R 6R5; McG'77; ABIM; FRCPC; IntMed; Cardiol. Staff, Royal Jubilee Hospital; Staff, Victoria General Hospital; (250)595-3111; Fax. (250)595-4278.

MILDENBERGER, Sheila J; 180-809 41st Ave W, Vancouver BC V5Z 2N6; UBC'90; FRCPC; Psy. Staff, BC Mental Health & Addiction Service; (604)263-2271

MILDON, C Anne; 615 Yonge St, Toronto ON M4Y 1Z8; Ott'69; DOHS; Assoc Staff, Mount Sinai Hospital; (416)463-2991; Fax. (416)469-0538.

MILENCOFF, G Scott; Grey Bruce HS-Owen Sound, PO Box 1800 Stn Main 7200-1800 8th St E, Owen Sound ON N4K 6M9; McM'92; FRCSC; GenSurg; Critical Care Medicine. Staff, Grey Bruce Health Services - Owen Sound; (519)371-2454; Fax. (519)371-7208; smilencoff@gbhs.on.ca.

MILENKOVIC, Svetlana; High Park Health Centre, 407-2333 Dundas St W, Toronto ON M6R 3A6; Belgrade (Serbia)'82; MSc; FRCPC; Psy (Mood Disorders). Langs: Serbian; (416)516-6337; Fax. (416)516-0073.

MILES, Brandt D; Burrard Med Bldg, 240-1144 Burrard St, Vancouver BC V6Z 2A5; Man'67; Assoc Staff, Providence Health Care - St Paul's Hospital; Vis Staff, Vancouver General Hospital - Centennial Pavillion; (604)689-7105; Fax. (604)689-5358.

MILES, Brendan; Sheldon Chumir Health Centre, 1213 4 St SW, Calgary AB T2R 0X7; Qns'10; (403)200-6606

MILES, Gary E; 10830 Dallain Pl, North Saanich BC V8L 5M7; Cape Town (South Africa)'88; MB ChB; (250)655-4569

MILES, Graham C; St Martha's Reg Hosp, 25 Bay St, Antigonish NS B2G 2G5; Dal'81; IntMed. Staff, St Martha's Regional Hospital; (902)863-1565; Fax. (902)863-0640.

MILES, Michael H; 103-777 Blanshard St, Victoria BC V8W 2G9; UBC'83; BSc; Staff, Royal Jubilee Hospital; Staff, Victoria General Hospital; (250)388-7123; Fax. (250)384-8490.

MILES, Peter J; 214 Med Place, 9909 102 St, Grande Prairie AB T8V 2V4; Witwatersrand (South Africa)'86; FRCSC; GenSurg (Family Medicine). Chief Dept of Surg, Queen Elizabeth II Hospital; (780)539-4545; Fax. (780)532-6743.

MILES, Susan L; 3635 Snake Rd, Smithers BC V0J 2N7; Dal'72; Ac Staff, Bulkley Valley District Hospital; (250)847-6212

MILETIN, Michael S; William Osler HC-Etobicoke, 101 Humber College Blvd, Etobicoke ON M9V 1R8; Tor'96; FRCPC; IntMed; Respir. Staff, William Osler Health System - Etobicoke General Hospital; (416)747-3500

MILETSKAIA, Galina N; Lindsay Prof Bldg, 6-65 Angeline St N, Lindsay ON K9V 5N7; Chelyabinsk (Russia (Federation))'84; ABIM; FRCPC; IntMed. (705)879-0005

MILETTE, David; Clinique Med Les Gres, 104-190 rue St Honore, St-Etienne-Ds-Gres QC G0X 2P0; Laval'95; CCFP; Staff Emerg, CSSS de Trois-Rivières; (819)535-6512 x3000; Fax. (819)535-1627.

MILETTE, Francois; CSSS Pierre Boucher, 1333 boul Jacques-Cartier E, Longueuil QC J4M 2A5; Mon'86; CSPQ; AnatPath. Staff Path, Centre Hospitalier Pierre Boucher; (450)468-8200; Fax. (450)468-8201.

MILETTE, Isabelle; Le Mediclub, 6100 av du Boise, Montreal QC H3S 2W1; Mon'88; (514)739-5646; Fax. (514)739-6773; i. milette@sympatico.ca.

MILETTE, Linda; Dir de la Sante Publique, 550 rue Bonaventure, Trois-Rivieres QC G9A 2B5; Sher'99; CSPQ; FRCPC; CommunMed (Family Medicine). (819)693-3661

MILETTE, Pierre-D.; 75 rue St-Francois RR 2, Saint-Pie QC J0H 1W0; Mon'68; Staff Emerg Serv, Centre Hospitalier Honore-Mercier; (450)772-2284

MILETTO, Giovanni J; Travel Med Vaccination Ctre, 106-4180 Lougheed Hwy, Burnaby BC V5C 6A7; London (England)'97; MB BS; CCFP.

MILEV, Roumen; Providence Care-Mental Health, PO Box 603 Stn Main 752 King St W, Kingston ON K7L 4X3; Sofia (Bulgaria)'83; PhD; FRCPsy(UK); MD; FRCPC; Psy (Academic Psychiatry). Hd Psy, Providence Care - Mental Health Services; Head Dept of Psy, Kingston General Hospital; Head Dept of Psy, Hotel-Dieu Hospital; Dept Head Psy, Queen's University; Langs: Bulgarian; Russian; (613)546-1101 x5823; Fax. (613)548-5580; roumen.milev@ queensu.ca.

MILEVA, Lili G; Frontenac Med Associates, 201-791 Princess St, Kingston ON K7L 1E9; (Bulgaria)'85; CCFP; FCFP; Langs: Bulgarian; (613)542-2727; Fax. (613)544-7247.

MILEWSKI, M Martin; C-22195 Dewdney Trunk Rd, Maple Ridge BC V2X 3H7; UBC'80; BSc(Hon); Ac Staff, Ridge Meadows Hospital & Health Care Centre; Clinical Asst Prof Family Practice, University of British Columbia; Langs: German; (604)463-8877; Fax. (604)463-4514; milewski@telus.net.

MILGRAM, Mark Z; Bridlewood Prof Centre, 204-3443 Finch Ave E, Scarborough ON M1W 2S1; Tor'69; Staff Pt-Time, The Scarborough Hospital - General Campus; Staff Pt-Time, The Scarborough Hospital - Birchmount Campus; (416)499-3622; Fax. (416)499-6952; markmilgram@yahoo.ca.

MILGROM, Michael; 140-555 Sixth St, New Westminster BC V3L 5H1; London (England)'72; Physician Narcotics, Royal Canadian Mounted Police; (604)523-1166; mmilgrom@rcmp-grc.gc.ca.

MILIN, Robert P; Royal Ottawa Hlth Care Group, 3308-1145 Carling Ave, Ottawa ON K1Z 7K4; Ott'84; DrMedCh; FRCPC; Psy (Addiction Psychiatry). Clin Dir Youth Psy Prog, Royal Ottawa Mental Health Centre - Royal Ottawa Health Care Group; Consultant Psy, Children's Hospital of Eastern Ontario (CHEO); Assoc Prof Psy, University of Ottawa; (613)722-6521 x6275; Fax. (613)798-2973.

MILIO, Hany S; 201-10 Westheights Dr, Kitchener ON N2N 2A8; Cairo (Egypt)'91; MB ChB; CCFP; (519)578-5555; Fax. (519)578-5551.

MILKOVIC, Heather J; Thamesview Family Health Team, 103-20 Emma St, Chatham ON N7L 5K5; Tor'86; BSc; Ac Staff, Chatham-Kent Health Alliance; (519)354-5290; Fax. (519)354-9011.

MILKOVIC, Joseph S; 135 Ontario St, St Catharines ON L2R 5J9; Ott'98; CCFP; (905)685-3403; jmilkovic@hotmail.com.

MILKOVIC, Zeke; Thamesview Family Health Team, 103-20 Emma St, Chatham ON N7L 5K5; Tor'90; MSc(Tor.); CCFP; Ac Staff Privil Obst & EmergMed, Chatham-Kent Health Alliance; Aj Prof Family Med Schulich School of Med & Dentistry, University of Western Ontario; (519)354-5290; Fax. (519)354-9011; zeke. milkovic@gmail.com.

MILKOVICH, Daniel J; MD Esthetics Laser Centre, 201-1910 Sooke Rd, Victoria BC V9B 1V7; UBC'92; Dir, MD Esthetics Laser Centre; (250)478-2336; Fax. (250)478-2339.

MILL, Elizabeth; Clinique Med Centre-Ville, 95 av Rouleau, Rimouski QC G5L 5S4; Laval'99; Staff, Hôpital Regional Rimouski; (418)722-6816; Fax. (418)721-3262.

MILLAIRE, Melanie; CSSS de Manicouagan, 635 boul Jolliet, Baie-Comeau QC G5C 1P1; Mon'01; FRCSC; ObstGyn. Staff, Centre Hospitalier Régional Baie-Comeau; (418)589-3701

MILLAN, Mario S; 346-10230 142 St NW, Edmonton AB T5N 3Y6; Alb'72; ABIM; FRCPC; IntMed; Gastroent. Ac Staff, Covenant Health - Misericordia Community Hospital; Associate Clin Prof, University of Alberta; (780)455-1382; Fax. (780)455-1379.

MILLAR, Adam C; 60 Murray St, Toronto ON M5T 3L9; Ott'06; FRCPC; IntMed; Endocrin&Metab. (416)586-4800; Fax. (416)619-5523.

MILLAR, Barabara-Ann M; Univ Hlth Network-Princess M, 610 University Ave, Toronto ON M5G 2M9; Sheffield (England)'92; FRCPC; RadOncol. Staff, Princess Margaret Hospital - University Health Network; (416)946-6522

MILLAR, Barbara J; North Bramalea Med Centre, 202-9780 Bramalea Rd, Brampton ON L6S 2P1; Tor'83; CCFP; Ac Staff, William Osler Health System - Brampton Civic Hospital; (905)791-2390; Fax. (905)791-8476; barbmillar25@hotmail. com.

MILLAR, Brenda J; 214 Med Place, 1234-9909 102 St, Grande Prairie AB T8V 2V4; Alb'89; CCFP; FCFP; (780)539-3022; Fax. (780)532-0949.

MILLAR, Cassandra B; 206-1717 10 St NW, Calgary AB T2M 4S2; Alb'07; BS; CCFP; (403)282-9865; Fax. (403)282-9893.

MILLAR, Catherine; MUHC-Montreal Children's Hosp, F1341-2300 rue Tupper, Montreal QC H3H 1P3; McG'88; FRCPC; Peds; Critical Care Medicine (P.Q.). Staff, McGill University Health Centre - Montreal Children's Hospital; (514)412-4400; Fax. (514)412-4205; catherine.millar@muhc.mcgill.ca.

MILLAR, David C S; North Bramalea Med Centre, 202-9780 Bramalea Rd, Brampton ON L6S 2P1; Belfast (Ireland)'50; DObstRCOG; Ac Staff, William Osler Health System - Brampton Civic Hospital; (905)791-2390; Fax. (905)791-8476.

MILLAR, David R; Fifth Avenue Court, 17-99 Fifth Ave, Ottawa ON K1S 5K4; Wes'97; CCFP; FCFP; Ac Staff, The Ottawa Hospital - Civic Campus; University of Ottawa; (613)563-3670; Fax. (613)563-4124.

MILLAR, Debra M; Broadway Med Centre, 230-943 Broadway W, Vancouver BC V5Z 4E1; UBC'83; BSc; FRCSC; ObstGyn (Pediatric & Adolescent Gynecology). Ac Staff, BC Children's Hospital; Ac Staff, Vancouver General Hospital - Centennial Pavillion; Ac Staff, BC Women's Hospital & Health Centre; Clin Assoc Prof, University of British Columbia; (604)734-2712; Fax. (604)734-8572.

MILLAR, Grant A; St Paul's Hosp, 1081 Burrard St, Vancouver BC V6Z 1Y6; Cal'05; FRCPC; Psy. Staff Eating Disorder Program, Providence Health Care - St Paul's Hospital; (604)682-2344

MILLAR, Hamish S; 3935 Kincaid St, Burnaby BC V5G 2X6; UBC'08; CCFP; CCFP(E.M.); Staff, Providence Health Care - St Paul's Hospital; (604)434-4211

MILLAR, Jeffrey H; Enderby Med Clinic, PO Box 369 1-802 George St, Enderby BC V0E 1V0; Sask'91; (250)838-9494; Fax. (250)838-9363.

MILLAR, Kelly R; Alberta Children's Hosp, 2888 Shaganappi Trail NW, Calgary AB T3B 6A8; Wes'97; FRCPC; Peds (Pediatric Emergency Medicine). Staff, Alberta Children's Hospital; (403)955-7070

MILLAR, Thomas; Brookdale Family Clinic, 304 Bellevue St, Peterborough ON K9H 5G1; Glasgow (Scotland)'68; MB ChB; Med Dir, St Joseph's At Fleming Nursing Home; Med Dir, Riverview Nursing Home; (705)743-7100; Fax. (705)743-7104.

MILLAR-BOOK, Wendy D; 23 Main St S PO Box 29, Waterford ON N0E 1Y0; McM'92; CCFP; (519)443-6694; Fax. (519)443-6829.

MILLARD, Debbie; 2316 96 St NW, Edmonton AB T6N 1J8; Alb'99; CCFP; Physician Geriatric Prog, Glenrose Rehabilitation Hospital; (780)468-5999; Fax. (780)468-5398.

MILLARD, Matthew J R; Canmore Gen Hosp, 1100 Hospital Pl, Canmore AB T1W 1N2; Wes'91; CCFP; CCFP(E.M.); Staff, Canmore General Hospital; (403)678-5536

MILLARD, Wanda; London HSC-Victoria Hosp, PO Box 5010 Stn B E1 102-800 Commissioners Rd E, London ON N6A 5W9; Cal'01; FRCPC; EmergMed. Staff, London Health Sciences Centre - Victoria Campus; (519)667-6538

MILLAUD, Frederic; Inst Philippe Pinel de Mtl, 10905 boul Henri-Bourassa E, Montreal QC H1C 1H1; Lyon (France)'81; FRCPC; Psy. Staff, Institut Philippe-Pinel de Montreal; (514)648-8461; Fax. (514)881-3706.

MILLER, Allan J; Ministry of Health, 3475 Albert St, Regina SK S4S 6X6; Sask'74; CCFP; FCFP; (306)798-1177; Fax. (306)798-1124.

MILLER, Andrea E J; St Joseph's Health Centre, 30 The Queensway, Toronto ON M6R 1B5; McM'96; FRCPC; DiagRad. Staff, St Joseph's Health Centre; (416)530-6000 x4319

MILLER, Annette F; Westway Children's Clinic, 4-1723 Kipling Ave, Etobicoke ON M9R 4E1; Tor'94; FRCPC; Peds. (416)244-8404; Fax. (416)244-0310.

MILLER, Anthony; St Boniface Gen Hosp, C5011-409 Tache Ave, Winnipeg MB R2H 2A6; Man'60; FRCPC; IntMed (Cardiology). Staff, St Boniface General Hospital; Assoc Prof, University of Manitoba; (204)237-2315; Fax. (204)235-3560; amiller@sbgh. mb.ca.

MILLER, Anton R; Sunny Hill Hlth Ctr For Child, 3644 Slocan St, Vancouver BC V5M 3E8; Cape Town (South Africa)'79; FRCPC; Peds (Developmental Pediatrics). Staff, Sunny Hill Health Centre for Children; (604)453-8306; Fax. (604)453-8338.

MILLER, Ashley P; BC Women's Hosp & Health Ctre, 4500 Oak St, Vancouver BC V6H 3N1; McG'01; FRCPC; Psy. Staff, BC Women's Hospital & Health Centre; Langs: Bilingual(French/English); (604)875-2801; Fax. (604)875-2099.

MILLER, Barbara C; The Ottawa Hosp-Civic Campus, 1053 Carling Ave, Ottawa ON K1Y 4E9; McM'98; BSc; MSc; CCFP; CCFP(E.M.); Staff, The Ottawa Hospital - Civic Campus; Staff, Children's Hospital of Eastern Ontario (CHEO); Staff, Carleton Place & District Memorial Hospital; (613)798-5555

MILLER, Barry A; Windsor Reg Hosp-Western Camp, CPH 2616-1453 Prince Rd, Windsor ON N9C 3Z4; Wes'75; DPsy; FRCPC; CommunMed; Psy. Staff, Windsor Regional Hospital - Tayfour Site; (519)254-5577 x72324; Fax. (519)257-5177.

MILLER, Brian J; Okanagan Plastic Surgery Centr, 401-3320 Richter St, Kelowna BC V1W 4V5; Sask'99; BSc; FRCSC; PlasSurg (Cosmetic Surgery). Med Staff, Kelowna General Hospital; Staff Surgical Floor, Okanagan Plastic Surgery Centre; Dir Skin Care Floor, Okanagan Skin Care Centre; Clin Instructor, University of British Columbia; (250)868-9290; Fax. (250)868-9704.

MILLER, Carol E; Royal Columbian Hosp, 330 Columbia St E, New Westminster BC V3L 3W7; UBC'70; DiagRad. Staff, Royal Columbian Hospital; (604)520-4640

MILLER, Charlotte D; Toronto Allergy Group, 404K-650 Sammon Ave, East York ON M4C 5M5; McG'97; FRCPC; Peds; ClinImmunol&Allergy. Staff, The Hospital For Sick Children; (416)465-7999; Fax. (416)461-8999.

MILLER, Christine; Queens Student Hlth Ontario, 146 Stuart St, Kingston ON K7L 3N6; McM'90; CCFP; FCFP; (613)533-2596

MILLER, Claire L M; 80 Grand Ave W, Chatham ON N7L 1B7; Wes'95; BScN; CCFP; (519)352-6401

MILLER, D Alexander; Niagara Health Centre, 308-180 Vine St S, St Catharines ON L2R 7P3; UBC'81; FRCPC; IntMed; Gastroent. Ac Staff, Niagara Health System - St Catharines General Site; (905)682-8693; Fax. (905)682-0311.

MILLER, D Lewis G; Brant Community HC-Brantford, 200 Terrace Hill St, Brantford ON N3R 1G9; McM'79; BSc; DiagRad. Staff Radiol, The Brant Community Healthcare System - Brantford General Hospital Site; (519)752-7871; Fax. (519)751-5573.

MILLER, David B; 402-3939 Quadra St, Victoria BC V8X 1J5; Wes'87; FRCPC; IntMed; Endocrin&Metab. (250)727-6621; Fax. (250)727-0478; dmiller.endocrinology@shaw.ca.

MILLER, David D; Drumheller Assoc Physicians, PO Box 5600, Drumheller AB T0J 0Y0; London (England)'49; MB BS; MRCS; LRCP; DARCS; (403)823-3345; Fax. (403)823-7823.

MILLER, David; Miramichi Reg Hosp, 500 Water St, Miramichi NB E1V 3G5; McG'03; FRCPC; DiagRad. Staff, Miramichi Regional Hospital; (506)623-3000

MILLER, David L; Four Rivers Med Clinic, 878 Main St, Winnipeg MB R2W 3P1; Man'95; Peds.

MILLER, David P; Beaverlodge Med Clinic, PO Box 209 1030 1st Ave, Beaverlodge AB T0H 0C0; Dublin (Ireland)'68; MB ChB; BAO; DCH; CCFP; Staff Chief, Beaverlodge Municipal Hospital; Asst Clin Prof, University of Alberta; (780)354-2646; Fax. (780)354-8181; bmedical@telus.net.

MILLER, Debra S; Health Care Centre, 715 12th Ave W, Vancouver BC V5Z 1M9; Tor'98; FRCPC; Psy. Staff, Vancouver General Hospital - Centennial Pavillion; (604)875-5720; Fax. (604)875-5721.

MILLER, Dianne M; Gordon & Leslie Diamond HCC, 6F-2775 Laurel St, Vancouver BC V5Z 1M9; UBC'80; MD; FRCSC; ObstGyn (Gynecologic Oncology). Ac Staff ObstGyn, Vancouver General Hospital - Centennial Pavillion; Staff, Gordon & Leslie Diamond Health Care Centre; Div Head Gynecologic Oncol, University of British Columbia; (604)875-4268; Fax. (604)875-4869; dmmiller@vanhosp.bc.ca.

MILLER, Donald D; University of Alberta Hosp, 2J2.01-8440 112 St NW, Edmonton AB T6G 2B7; McG'78; FRCPC; IntMed; Cardiol. Staff, University of Alberta Hospital; (780)492-9728; Fax. (780)492-7303.

MILLER, Donald M; 130-2200 McPhillips St, Winnipeg MB R2V 3P4; Man'75; Ac Staff, Seven Oaks General Hospital; (204)697-2960

MILLER, Donald R; The Ottawa Hosp-Gen Campus, 501 Smyth Rd, Ottawa ON K1H 8L6; Qns'80; FRCPC; Anes. Staff Anes, The Ottawa Hospital - General Campus; Ed in Chief, Canadian Journal of Anesthesia; Assoc Prof, University of Ottawa; (613)737-8187; Fax. (613)737-8189; dmiller@ottawahospital.on.ca.

MILLER, Duncan R; U6-601 Broadway W, Vancouver BC V5Z 4C2; UBC'91; BSc; (604)872-2558; Fax. (604)874-6222.

MILLER, Elka; Children's Hosp Eastern Ont, 401 Smyth Rd, Ottawa ON K1H 8L1; (Costa Rica)'95; Staff, Children's Hospital of Eastern Ontario (CHEO); (613)737-7600

MILLER, Fraser A; Queensway-Carleton Hosp, 3045 Baseline Rd, Nepean ON K2H 8P4; McG'84; FRCPC; IntMed; Cardiol; GeriatricMed. Consultant, Bruyère Continuing Care - Saint-Vincent Hospital; Ac Staff/Chief GeriatricMed, Queensway Carleton Hospital; (613)721-4700 x2515

MILLER, Garfield L A; University of Ottawa Eye Inst, 501 Smyth Rd, Ottawa ON K1H 8L6; Tor'05; FRCSC; Ophth. Physician, University of Ottawa Eye Institute; (613)737-8899; Fax. (613)739-6139.

MILLER, George B; The Village of Winston Park, 695 Blockline Rd, Kitchener ON N2E 3K1; Edinburgh (Scotland)'70; CCFP; FCFP; Court Staff Privil, St Mary's General Hospital; Court Staff Privil, Grand River Hospital - Kitchener/Waterloo Health Centre; Med Dir, Winston Park Nursing Home; (519)576-2430

MILLER, George B; Victoria Place, 503-111 Fairford St E, Moose Jaw SK S6H 7X5; Sask'79; FACS; BSc(Hon); FRCSC; GenSurg (Hyperbaric Medicine). Staff Surg, Moose Jaw Union Hospital; (306)693-3638; Fax. (306)693-3774.

MILLER, Gerald A; Medical Clinic, 5031 49 St, Innisfail AB T4G 1A4; Cal'76; (403)227-3356; Fax. (403)227-2702.

MILLER, Gilbert; Health Care Med Centre, 1 Promenade Cir, Thornhill ON L4J 4P8; Alb'81; BMedSci; FRCPC; Peds. Hon Staff, The Hospital For Sick Children; Humber River Regional Hospital - Finch Avenue Site; Asst Prof, University of Toronto; (905)889-1761; Fax. (905)889-0295.

MILLER, Grant G; Royal University Hosp, 103 Hospital Dr, Saskatoon SK S7N 0W8; Sask'87; FRCSC; GenSurg; PedGenSurg. Staff, Royal University Hospital; Assoc Prof, University of Saskatchewan; (306)966-8141; Fax. (306)966-7542.

MILLER, Harold B; Cambridge Mem Hosp, 700 Coronation Blvd, Cambridge ON N1R 3G2; Tor'66; Staff, Cambridge Memorial Hospital; (519)621-2330 x1

MILLER, Howard J; 36 Ormond St, Thorold ON L2V 1Y4; Philadelphia (USA)'80; Staff, Niagara Health System - St Catharines General Site; (905)680-9010; Fax. (905)680-9000.

MILLER, J Lance; Renfrew Victoria Hosp, 499 Raglan St N, Renfrew ON K7V 1P6; Dal'66; BSc; FACS; GenSurg (Gastroenterology). Consultant, Almonte General Hospital; Consultant, St Francis Memorial Hospital; Ac Staff, Renfrew Victoria Hospital; (613)432-3135; Fax. (613)432-8649; airedale1@sympatico.ca.

MILLER, James R; London Place Eye Centre, 918 Twelfth St, New Westminster BC V3M 6B1; Alb'62; DAB; FRCSC; Ophth (Refractive Surgery). Med Dir Refractive Surg, London Place Eye Centre; (604)526-2020

MILLER, Jean; Clinique Med Baie-St-Paul, 101-4 rue du Moulin, Baie-Saint-Paul QC G3Z 2R8; Laval'79; Langs: Bilingual(French/English); (418)435-5760; Fax. (418)435-4137.

MILLER, John A D; 4394 Emily Carr Dr, Victoria BC V8X 5B5; UBC'74; Med Coord, Mount St Mary Hospital; Langs: Japanese; (250)391-3952; jmiller@mtstmary.victoria.bc.ca.

MILLER, John D; St Joseph's Healthcare, 50 Charlton Ave E, Hamilton ON L8N 4A6; Dal'80; FRCSC; GenSurg; ThorSurg. Staff, St Joseph's Healthcare - Charlton Campus; Prof Surg, McMaster University; (905)521-6126; Fax. (905)521-6156; jmiller@mcmaster.ca.

MILLER, Judith A; 8N 846-585 University Ave, Toronto ON M5G 2N2; McM'83; MSc; MHA; FRCPC; IntMed; Nephrol. Dep Dir Nephrol, Toronto General Hospital - UHN; Clin Dir, Ontario Renal Network; Prof, University of Toronto; (416)340-4966; Fax. (416)340-4951; judith.miller@utoronto.ca.

MILLER, Katherine J; 96 Spring St, Almonte ON K0A 1A0; McM'96; CCFP; FCFP; Staff, Almonte General Hospital; Teach Staff Family Med, University of Western Ontario; (613)256-5656

MILLER, Kevin F; Thunder Bay Reg Cancer Ctre, 980 Oliver Rd, Thunder Bay ON P7B 6V4; McM'95; BSc; CCFP; Staff, Nipigon District Memorial Hospital; Staff, Thunder Bay Regional Health Sciences Centre; (807)684-7200; Fax. (807)684-5800; kmiller@ndmh.ca.

MILLER, Kimberley L; Univ Hlth Network-Princess M, 16 710-610 University Ave, Toronto ON M5G 2M9; Dal'94; BSc; FRCPC; Psy. Staff, Princess Margaret Hospital - University Health Network; (416)946-2897

MILLER, Kirsten K; 1003-299 Victoria St, Prince George BC V2L 5B8; Ott'00; FRCPC; Peds. Staff, University Hospital of Northern British Columbia; (250)563-2257

MILLER, Lisa J; Fairmont Med Bldg, 713-750 Broadway W, Vancouver BC V5Z 1H6; Dal'91; (604)873-4808; Fax. (604)876-7622.

MILLER, Lisa M; Health Sciences Centre, GE441B-820 Sherbrook St, Winnipeg MB R3A 1R9; Mem'00; BSc; FRCPC; IntMed; Nephrol. Staff Nephrol, Health Sciences Centre; Asst Prof, University of Manitoba; (204)787-1524; Fax. (204)787-7366.

MILLER, Luella M; Caledonian Med Clinic, 340 Campbell St, Nanaimo BC V9R 3G7; Dal'05; CCFP; (250)753-3202

MILLER, Marian R; Psychiatric Urgent Clinic, 2334 Trent St, Victoria BC V8R 4Z3; Wes'87; FRCPC; Psy. (250)370-8152

MILLER, Mark J; 208-2051 McCallum Rd, Abbotsford BC V2S 3N5; Sask'86; Otol. (604)864-0747

MILLER, Mark L; 121 Main St N PO Box 149, Jarvis ON N0A 1J0; Tor'86; (519)587-2268

MILLER, Mark W; Fort Langley Med Clinic, PO Box 99 Stn Fort Langley 23148 96 Ave, Langley BC V1M 2R4; Dal'75; (604)888-2433

MILLER, Matthew C; St Joseph's Healthcare, 50 Charlton Ave E, Hamilton ON L8N 4A6; Tor'08; FRCPC; IntMed. Staff, St Joseph's Healthcare - Charlton Campus; (905)522-1155

MILLER, Megan E; Queen Elizabeth Hosp, PO Box 6600 Stn Central 60 Riverside Dr, Charlottetown PE C1A 8T5; Dal'04; CCFP; Staff, Queen Elizabeth Hospital; (902)894-2111

MILLER, Mervyn D; Cape Breton Hlthcare Complex, 1482 George St, Sydney NS B1P 1P3; Wes'90; FRCSC; Urol. Staff, Cape Breton Healthcare Complex; (902)567-8031; Fax. (902)567-8034.

MILLER, Michael; Credit Valley Prof Bldg, 407-2300 Eglinton Ave W, Mississauga ON L5M 2V8; Tor'77; FRCSC; Ophth. Ac Staff, The Credit Valley Hospital; (905)820-3130; Fax. (905)820-8759.

MILLER, Michal; Victoria Gen Hosp, 2340 Pembina Hwy, Winnipeg MB R3T 2E8; Man'99; FRCPC; Anes. Staff, Victoria General Hospital; (204)269-3570

MILLER, Milton C; Fairmont Med Bldg, 1116-750 Broadway W, Vancouver BC V5Z 1H3; UBC'74; BSc; (604)878-1103; Fax. (604)872-7684.

MILLER, Murray H; Six Points Radiology Associate, 303-5353 Dundas St W, Etobicoke ON M9B 6H8; Man'82; FRCPC; DiagRad. Staff, Trillium Health Centre - West Toronto; (416)231-3369; Fax. (416)231-4103.

MILLER, Naomi A; Univ Hlth Network-Toronto Gen, 200 Elizabeth St, Toronto ON M5G 2C4; Tor'78; FRCPC; AnatPath (Breast Pathology). Staff, Toronto General Hospital - UHN; Assoc Prof, University of Toronto; (416)340-3738; Fax. (416)340-5517; naomi.miller@uhn.ca.

MILLER, Owen S; Victoria East Med Clinic, 2068 Prince of Wales Dr, Regina SK S4V 3A6; Sask'01; CCFP; (306)789-4677; Fax. (306)789-3422.

MILLER, Paul C; Perth-Smiths Falls Dist Hosp, 60 Cornelia St W, Smiths Falls ON K7A 2H9; Ott'98; Staff, Perth & Smiths Falls District Hospital - Smiths Falls Site; (613)283-2330

MILLER, Paul Q; Hamilton HS-General Site, 237 Barton St E, Hamilton ON L8L 2X2; McM'01; FRCPC; EmergMed. Staff, Hamilton Health Sciences Centre - Hamilton General Hospital; (905)527-4322 x49997; Fax. (905)527-7051.

MILLER, Philip Y; Lions Gate Hosp, 231 15th St E, North Vancouver BC V7L 2L7; UBC'07; CCFP; CCFP(E.M.); Staff, Lions Gate Hospital; (604)988-3131

MILLER, Rivian S; Mount Pleasant Family Practice, 245 Eglinton Ave E, Toronto ON M4P 3B7; Man'86; (416)485-7663; Fax. (416)485-2671.

MILLER, Robert A; Valley Reg Hosp, 150 Exhibition St, Kentville NS B4N 5E3; Dal'95; BSc; CCFP; CCFP(E.M.); Staff, Valley Regional Hospital; (902)678-7381

MILLER, Robert A W; Dermatology Associates, 6088 Coburg Rd, Halifax NS B3H 1Z4; Dal'74; FRCPC; Derm (Wound Care). Consultant, Queen Elizabeth II Health Sciences Centre - Victoria General Site; Assoc Prof, Dalhousie University; Langs: Bilingual(English/French); (902)425-8038; Fax. (902)421-1580.

MILLER, Robert B; North York Med Arts Bldg, 142-1333 Sheppard Ave E, North York ON M2J 1V1; Tor'77; Otol. (416)498-7874; Fax. (416)850-1138.

MILLER, Robert E W; PO Box 35010 Rpo Hillside, Victoria BC V8T 5G2; Bristol (England)'75; FRCPC; Psy (Forensic Psychiatry). Head Dept of Psy/Med Dir Mental Health & Addiction Services, Vancouver Island Health Authority; Med Reg Mgr BC Mental Health & Addiction Services, Forensic Psy Services-Vancouver Island Region; (250)387-1465; rmiller@forensic.bc.ca.

MILLER, Robert M; Queen Elizabeth II HSC-Halifax, 6896D-1796 Summer St, Halifax NS B3H 3A7; Dal'74; FRCPC; DiagRad (Cardiac Radiology). Staff, Queen Elizabeth II Health Sciences Centre - Halifax Infirmary Site; Prof, Dalhousie University; (902)473-6529; Fax. (902)473-6293; bmiller@eastlink.ca.

MILLER, Robert T; Health Sciences Centre, 300 Prince Philip Dr, St. John's NL A1B 3V6; Wes'72; CCFP; FCFP; Staff, Health Sciences Centre; Chair Clin Disciplines, Memorial University Of Newfoundland; (709)777-6742; Fax. (709)777-7913.

MILLER, Saul; University of Toronto, 500 Univresity Ave, Toronto ON M5G 1V7; Wes'06; FRCPC; IntMed; Cardiol. Staff, Toronto Western Hospital - University Health Network.

MILLER, Sebastian J; Appletree Medical Group, 150 Robertson Rd, Ottawa ON K2H 9S1; University of Aberdeen (Scotland)'96.

MILLER, Stacy; Ctr for the North Prince Georg, 1215 Lethbridge St, Prince George BC V2M 7E9; UBC'04; FRCPC; RadOncol. Staff, Abbotsford Regional Hospital & Cancer Centre; (250)645-7335

MILLER, Stephen D; Bone & Joint Clinic, 4448 Front St SE, Calgary AB T3M 1M4; Cal'80; BSc; FRCSC; OrthSurg (Joint Replacement). Staff Orthoped, Foothills Medical Centre; Med Dir, Health Resource Centre; Chief Medical Officer, Network Health Inc; Asst Clin Prof, University of Calgary; Langs: Portuguese; (403)956-3250; Fax. (403)956-3275.

MILLER, Stephen F; The Hosp for Sick Children, 555 University Ave, Toronto ON M5G 1X8; Nashville(TN) (USA)'87; FRCPC; DiagRad. Staff, The Hospital For Sick Children; (416)813-6026; Fax. (416)813-7591; stephen.miller@sickkids.ca.

MILLER, Stephen G; Queen Elizabeth II HSC-Halifax, 355-1796 Summer St, Halifax NS B3H 3A7; Dal'93; BSc; CCFP; CCFP(E.M.); FCFP; Staff, Cobequid Community Health Centre; Staff, Queen Elizabeth II Health Sciences Centre - Victoria General Site; Staff, Queen Elizabeth II Health Sciences Centre - Halifax Infirmary Site; Lecturer EmergMed, Dalhousie University; (902)473-4220; Fax. (902)473-3617; sgmiller@eastlink.ca.

MILLER, Stephen; Polyclinic Prof Centre Inc, 307-199 Grafton St, Charlottetown PE C1A 1L2; Dal'91; OrthSurg (Sports Medicine). Staff, Queen Elizabeth Hospital; Preceptor Family Resident, Dalhousie University; (902)629-8807; Fax. (902)368-1694; drsmilleroffice@mac.com.

MILLER, Steven P; Children's & Women's HC of BC, 180-4480 Oak St, Vancouver BC V6H 3V4; McG'95; FRCPC; Neur. Staff, BC Children's Hospital; (604)875-2345 x5948; Fax. (604)875-2285.

MILLER, Steven; CSSS Drummond-Hop Sainte-Croix, 570 rue Heriot, Drummondville QC J2B 1C1; Sher'86; FRCSC; GenSurg. Staff, Hôpital Sainte-croix; (819)478-6464

MILLER, Tamara L; St Boniface Gen Hosp, L2035-409 Tache Ave, Winnipeg MB R2H 2A6; Man'99; FRCPC; Anes. Staff, St Boniface General Hospital; (204)233-8563

MILLER, Terrence R; Lillooet Med Clinic, PO Box 850, Lillooet BC V0K 1V0; UBC'87; (250)256-7505; Fax. (250)256-7591.

MILLER, Thomas; Peterborough Reg HC-Hospital, 1 Hospital Dr, Peterborough ON K9J 7C6; McM'91; MSc; CCFP; Staff Physician/Chief Dept of Emerg Med/Med Dir Emerg Med Services, Peterborough Regional Health Centre - Hospital Drive; Teach Staff Family Med, Queen's University; (705)876-5022

MILLER, Thomas; St Mary's Hosp Campus, 21 Grosvenor St, London ON N6A 1Y6; Qns'89; FRCPC; PhysMed&Rehab (Nerve Injury). Staff, London Health Sciences Centre - University Hospital; Physical Medicine & Rehab, St Mary's Hospital - St Joseph's Health Care London; Staff, St Joseph's Hospital - St Joseph's Health Care; Staff, Parkwood Hospital - St Joseph's Health Care; Assoc Prof Schulich School of Med, University of Western Ontario; (519)646-6100 x65364; Fax. (519)646-6174; ann.varallo@sjhc.london.on.ca.

MILLER, William D; The Ottawa Hosp-Civic Campus, C158-1053 Carling Ave, Ottawa ON K1Y 4E9; Man'80; FRCPC; DiagRad (Neuro Radiology). Dep Chief Diagnostic Imaging, The Ottawa Hospital - Civic Campus; Dept Head Radiol, University of Ottawa; (613)761-4547; Fax. (613)761-4623; wmiller@ottawahospital.on.ca.

MILLER, William W J; Eden Mental Health Centre, 1500 Pembina Ave, Winkler MB R6W 1T4; Ott'02; FRCPC; Psy. Staff, Eden Mental Health Centre; (204)325-4325

MILLER, Wilson; SMBD Jewish Gen Hosp, 3755 ch Cote-Sainte-Catherine, Montreal QC H3T 1E2; New York (USA)'84; PhD; Dir Clinical Research Unit, Sir Mortimer B Davis Jewish General; Staff Hem, McGill University Health Centre - Montreal General Campus; Co- Dir MedOncol & Prof, McGill University; Langs: French; (514)340-8222 x4572; wmiller@ldi.jgh.mcgill.ca.

MILLER-SHEWCHUK, Allison; 1-4188 Spratt Rd, Gloucester ON K1V 0Z6; Alb'05; CCFP; (613)822-0171; Fax. (613)822-1838.

MILLERS, Anna; U of Toronto-Health Services, 214 College St, Toronto ON M5T 2Z9; Tor'75; CCFP; FCFP; (416)978-8030

MILLET, Richard F; Hôpital régional Chaleur, 1750 Sunset Dr, Bathurst NB E2A 4L7; Aix-Marseille II (France)'80; Staff, Hopital Regional Chaleur; (506)544-3000

MILLETTE, Alain; Canadian Med Protective Assoc, 875 Carling Ave, Ottawa ON K1S 5P1; Mon'81; Physician Family Med, Coop Sante Aylmer; Physician, Canadian Medical Protective Association; Langs: English.

MILLETTE, Bernard A; CSSS de Laval, 1755 boul Rene-Laennec, Laval QC H7M 3L9; Mon'69; MSc(Exp.Med); CCFP; FCFP; Staff, Hopital de la Cite de la santé; Prof Family Med, Universite de Montreal; (450)975-5444; Fax. (450)975-5497; bernard.millette@umontreal.ca.

MILLETTE, Julie; Centre medical de Cowansville, 101-370 rue de la Riviere, Cowansville QC J2K 1N3; Mon'97; CCFP; (450)263-0774

MILLETTE, Maude; MUHC-Montreal Children's Hosp, E 3158-2300 rue Tupper, Montreal QC H3H 1P3; Laval'06; Endocrin&Metab; Peds. Staff, McGill University Health Centre - Montreal Children's Hospital; (514)412-4400 x22663

MILLETTE, Pierre; Hop Maisonneuve-Rosemont, 5415 boul de l'Assomption, Montreal QC H1T 2M4; Mon'88; Ac Staff, Hopital Maisonneuve-Rosemont; (514)252-3400; Fax. (514)252-3566.

MILLETTE, Rebecca; Clinique Familiale Pas-A-Pas, 3650 boul Henri-Bourassa E, Montreal-Nord QC H1G 2V1; Sher'10; (514)328-9797

MILLETTE-FRANCOEUR, Laura-Lou; CSSS de Saint-Jerome, 290 rue de Montigny, Saint-Jerome QC J7Z 5T3; Mon'08; Staff, Hôtel-Dieu de Saint-Jérôme; (450)432-2777

MILLIGAN, Brian E; PO Box 70, Neepawa MB R0J 1H0; Man'08; CCFP; Staff, Concordia General Hospital.

MILLIGAN, James D; Centre for Family Medicine, 10B Victoria St S, Kitchener ON N2G 1C5; McM'07; CCFP; Aj Prof, University of Western Ontario; Assoc Prof, McMaster University; (519)783-0022; Fax. (519)783-0032.

MILLIGAN, Scott R; Cape Breton Hlthcare Complex, 1482 George St, Sydney NS B1P 1P3; Alb'98; FRCPC; Psy. Staff, Cape Breton Healthcare Complex; (902)567-8091; Fax. (902)567-7905; milligans@cbdha.nshealth.ca.

MILLIKEN, A Donald; Eric Martin Pavillon, 2334 Trent St, Victoria BC V8R 4Z3; Dublin (Ireland)'66; MB ChB; MHA; DABPN; FRCPC; Psy (Administrative Psychiatry). Consultant Psy, Victoria Mood Disorders Service; Pres, Canadian Psychiatric Association; Clin Dir, Psychiatry Day Hosp-Victoria; (250)370-8155; dmilliken@shaw.ca.

MILLIKEN, Douglas R F; Workers' Comp Board, 9912 107 St NW, Edmonton AB T5K 1G5; Sask'72; MD; (780)498-4534; douglas.milliken@wcb.ab.ca.

MILLIKEN, Heather I; Abbie J Lane Mem Bldg, 3F-5909 Veterans Memorial Lane, Halifax NS B3H 2E2; McG'76; FRCPC; Psy (Chronic Psychosis). Staff Psy, Queen Elizabeth II Health Sciences Centre - Victoria General Site; Staff Psy, The Nova Scotia Hospital; Dir, Nova Scotia Early Psychosis Program; Assoc Prof Psy/Dir, Dalhousie University; Langs: Bilingual(French/English); (902)473-4883; Fax. (902)473-4545; heather.milliken@dal.ca.

MILLIKEN, Jacqueline H J; Dawson Centre Level 2, 197 Dufferin St, Bridgewater NS B4V 2G9; Dublin (Ireland)'67; MB ChB; BAO; FRCPC; Psy (Adult General Psychiatry). Staff, South Shore Regional Hospital; Lecturer Psy, Dalhousie University; (902)527-5228; Fax. (902)543-3120.

MILLIKEN, Megan P E; Victoria Gen Hosp, 1 Hospital Way, Victoria BC V8Z 6R5; Wes'04; CCFP; Staff, Victoria General Hospital; (250)893-9167

MILLINGTON, Scott J; The Ottawa Hosp-Gen Campus, 501 Smyth Rd, Ottawa ON K1H 8L6; Wes'04; Critical Care Medicine; IntMed. Staff, The Ottawa Hospital - General Campus; (613)737-8899; Fax. (613)737-8890.

MILLITZ, Kip; Peterborough Reg HC-Hospital, 1 Hospital Dr, Peterborough ON K9J 7C6; Wes'91; DiagRad. Staff, Peterborough Regional Health Centre - Hospital Drive; (705)743-2121; Fax. (705)743-1713.

MILLMAN, Christine G; Glengarry Mem Hosp, PO Box 910 2-20260 County Rd 43, Alexandria ON K0C 1A0; McM'94; BSc; CCFP; Staff, Glengarry Memorial Hospital; (613)525-2324

MILLMAN, John M; 112 Woolwich St, Guelph ON N1H 3V2; Wes'68; CCBOM; CCFP; Ac Staff, Guelph General Hospital; Med Dir, Wellserve Healthcare Managemet; Chief Medical Officer, Toronto Police Service; (519)767-1721; Fax. (519)837-3974; john.millman@wellserve.on.ca.

MILLMAN, William L; Anaesthesia Associates-London, 100 Piccadilly St, London ON N6A 1R8; Wes'65; FRCPC; Anes. Consultant, London Health Sciences Centre - Victoria Campus; Ac Staff, St Joseph's Hospital - St Joseph's Health Care; Consultant, London Health Sciences Centre - University Hospital; Asst Prof, University of Western Ontario; (519)672-2130

MILLO, Noam Z; Health Sciences Centre, GE3-820 Sherbrook St, Winnipeg MB R3A 1R9; Man'07; FRCPC; DiagRad. Staff, Health Sciences Centre; (204)774-8511

MILLOY, Douglas R; Trafalgar Med Clinic, 200-1235 Trafalgar Rd, Oakville ON L6H 3P1; Tor'69; Staff, Halton Healthcare Services Corporation - Oakville Site; (905)844-3281; Fax. (905)849-1076.

MILLS, Anne; Urgence Sante, 3232 rue Bélanger, Montreal QC H1Y 3H5; Laval'85; FRCPC; EmergMed (Sports Medicine). (514)723-5744; anne007@sympatico.ca.

MILLS, Barry J; Westwood Clinic, 3220 Portage Ave, Winnipeg MB R3K 0Y8; Otago (New Zealand)'62; DObst(N.Z.); DA(Eng.); (204)832-1363; Fax. (204)896-3445.

MILLS, Carol E; Orangeville Family Med, M1-32 First St, Orangeville ON L9W 2E1; McM'06; CCFP; (519)938-8000

MILLS, Catherine A; Campbellton Reg Hosp, PO Box 880 Stn Main 189 Lily Lake Rd, Campbellton NB E3N 3H3; Dal'93; FRCPC; AnatPath. Staff, Hôpital Régional Campbellton; (506)789-5062; Fax. (506)789-5156.

MILLS, Geoffrey C R; St Thomas-Elgin Gen Hosp, PO Box 2007 Stn Main 189 Elm St, St Thomas ON N5P 3W2; Wes'99; CCFP; CCFP(E.M.); Staff Emerg Dept, St Thomas Elgin General Hospital; (519)631-2020 x2047

MILLS, Gerald P; Bonaventure Med Clinic, 101-12427 Bonaventure Dr SE, Calgary AB T2J 3N8; Ott'81; CCFP; (403)225-9499; Fax. (403)225-2572.

MILLS, Heather E; 201-770 Broadview Ave, Ottawa ON K2A 3Z3; McM'93; CCFP; CCFP(E.M.); FCFP; (613)216-6985; Fax. (613)216-6986.

MILLS, Howard J P; City Centre Med Clinic, 284 City Centre, Kitimat BC V8C 1T6; London (England)'76; MB BS; (250)632-6131; Fax. (250)632-2092.

MILLS, Jeffrey K; 101-491 Lawrence Ave W, North York ON M5M 1C7; Wes'85; Staff, Women's College Hospital; Clin Lecturer, University of Toronto; (416)787-0117; Fax. (416)787-8094.

MILLS, Jessica L A; Children's & Women's HC of BC, K0 123ACB-4480 Oak St, Vancouver BC V6H 3V4; UBC'03; FRCSC; GenSurg; PedGenSurg. Staff, BC Children's Hospital; (604)875-2813

MILLS, Karen C; West Parry Sound Health Ctre, 6 Albert St, Parry Sound ON P2A 3A4; Wes'06; BSc(Hon.); FRCPC; IntMed (Cardiology). Staff, West Parry Sound Health Centre; (705)746-4540; Fax. (705)773-7033; kmills@wpshc.com.

MILLS, Martha L; Fredericton Med Clinic, 304-1015 Regent St, Fredericton NB E3B 6H5; Dal'96; BSc; FRCSC; ObstGyn. (506)457-2113; Fax. (506)459-7073.

MILLS, Michael D; Credit Valley Eye Care, 1-3200 Erin Mills Pky, Mississauga ON L5L 1W8; Wes'96; FRCSC; Ophth (Retina Vitreous Surgery). Staff, Credit Valley Eye Care; (905)820-3937; Fax. (905)820-0111.

MILLS, Michael J; The Children's Aid Society, PO Box 1170 Stn Lcd 1 26 Arrowsmith Rd, Hamilton ON L8N 4B9; Wes'76; CCFP; FCFP; Ac Staff, Joseph Brant Memorial Hospital; Clin Assoc Prof, McMaster University; Clin Assoc Prof Family Med, University of Toronto; millsm@mcmaster.ca.

MILLS, Natalie S; Brittany Health Care Plus, PO Box 479 Stn Main 203-2246 Laurier St, Rockland ON K4K 1K5; McG'89; CCFP; (613)446-6401; Fax. (613)446-6951.

MILLS, Patricia B; 4255 Laurel St, Vancouver BC V5Z 2G9; Tor'06; FRCPC; PhysMed&Rehab. Langs: Portuguese; (604)734-1313

MILLS, Philip J; Dartmouth Comm Mental Hlth, 500-33 Alderney Dr, Dartmouth NS B2Y 2N4; Belfast (Ireland)'83; FRCPC; Psy (Adult & Individual Psychotherapy). (902)466-1830; Fax. (902)466-1851.

MILLS, Philip; Lemarchand Tower, 1-11503 100 Ave NW, Edmonton AB T5K 2K7; Manchester (England)'61; MB ChB; DPM; MRCPsy; FRCPC; Psy. Staff, Covenant Health - Grey Nuns Community Hospital; Asst Clin Prof, University of Alberta; (780)482-3424; Fax. (780)488-1037.

MILLS, Sian E; Children's Hosp Eastern Ont, 401 Smyth Rd, Ottawa ON K1H 8L1; Thomas Jefferson University (USA)'91; Staff, Children's Hospital of Eastern Ontario (CHEO); (613)737-7600

MILLS, Thomas P D; 201-128 Penetang St, Barrie ON L4M 1V6; Qns'92; Staff, Royal Victoria Regional Health Centre; (705)726-4681; Fax. (705)739-8404.

MILLS, William G; Orleans Radiology & Ultrasound, 2555 St. Joseph Blvd, Orleans ON K1C 1S6; Ott'69; FRCPC; DiagRad. Staff, The Ottawa Hospital - General Campus; Asst Prof, University of Ottawa; (613)824-3535; Fax. (613)824-6633.

MILLS-TETTEY, Diana B; 503-1110 Sheppard Ave E, North York ON M2K 2W2; (Ghana)'78; MB ChB; FRCPC; Peds (Community Medicine). Staff, North York General Hospital; Staff Pt-Time, The Hospital For Sick Children; Lecturer, University of Toronto; Langs: Ga; Twi; (416)226-4294; Fax. (416)226-1928.

MILLSON, Margaret E; Dept of Public Health Sciences, 582-155 College St, Toronto ON M5T 3M7; Tor'75; MHSc; FRCPC; CommunMed (Research). Assoc Prof Public Health Sciences, University of Toronto; (416)978-5253; Fax. (416)971-2704; p.millson@utoronto.ca.

MILLSON, Richard C; Providence Care-Mental Health, PO Box 603 Stn Main 752 King St W, Kingston ON K7L 4X3; Qns'76; DTMH; FRCPC; Psy. Staff, Providence Care - Mental Health Services; (613)217-7058; Fax. (613)548-5578; rcmillson@gmail.com.

MILLSTEIN, Lisa T; Bayview-Finch Med Clinic, 300-3292 Bayview Ave, North York ON M2M 4J5; Tor'00; BSc; CCFP; Assoc Staff, North York General Hospital; Langs: French; (416)646-4455; Fax. (416)222-5722.

MILLWARD, Steven; Peterborough Reg HC-Hospital, 1 Hospital Dr, Peterborough ON K9J 7C6; Leeds (England)'78; FRCR; FRCPC; DiagRad. Staff, Peterborough Regional Health Centre - Hospital Drive; (705)743-2121

MILMAN, Nataliya; The Ottawa Hosp-Riverside, 1967 Riverside Dr, Ottawa ON K1H 7W9; Ott'06; FRCPC; IntMed; Rheum. Staff, The Ottawa Hospital - Riverside Campus; (613)738-8400; Fax. (613)738-8228.

MILNE, Andrew D; Queen Elizabeth II HSC, 226 10W-1276 South Park St, Halifax NS B3H 2Y9; Dal'03; FRCPC; Anes. Staff, Queen Elizabeth II Health Sciences Centre - Victoria General Site; (902)473-7736

MILNE, Ardyth A; South Albert Med Centre, 5-4150 Albert St, Regina SK S4S 3R8; Sask'92; FRCPC; IntMed; Rheum. Staff Rheumatol, Royal University Hospital; (306)584-6230; Fax. (306)352-5395.

MILNE, Beatrice D; 7-87 Main St, Sackville NB E4L 4A9; Tor'82; BSc; CCFP; (506)536-0326

MILNE, Brian; Kingston Gen Hosp, 76 Stuart St, Kingston ON K7L 2V7; Qns'75; MSc(Pharm.); FRCPC; Anes. Staff, Kingston General Hospital; Prof, Queen's University; (613)548-3232; Fax. (613)548-1375.

MILNE, C Michelle; Clin Med l'Actuel, 1130-1001 boul de Maisonneuve, Montreal QC H3A 3C8; McG'98; BSc; Langs: English; French.

MILNE, Catherine A; MUHC-Royal Victoria Hosp, 532-687 av des Pins O, Montreal QC H3A 1A1; McG'70; BSc; MDCM; FRCSC; GenSurg (Breasts). Ac Staff, McGill University Health Centre - Royal Victoria Hospital; assoc Prof, McGill University; Langs: Bilingual(English/French); (514)934-1934 x35443; Fax. (514)843-1405.

MILNE, Daniel; 103-33774 Marshall Rd, Abbotsford BC V2S 1L1; (South Africa)'84; CCFP; (604)853-5424

MILNE, Darryl D; 170 University Ave W, Waterloo ON N2L 3E9; Tor'86; (519)725-1514; Fax. (519)725-5137.

MILNE, David G; Queen Elizabeth II HSC, 1276 South Park St, Halifax NS B3H 2Y9; Dal'89; Anes (Thoracic Anesthesia). Staff, Queen Elizabeth II Health Sciences Centre - Victoria General Site; (902)473-2311

MILNE, Janette A; 104-1300 Don Mills Rd, North York ON M3B 2W6; Dublin (Ireland)'67; LRCPSI; FRCPC; Peds. Hon Staff, The Hospital For Sick Children; Court Staff, North York General Hospital; Asst Prof, University of Toronto; (416)446-1575; Fax. (416)446-2919.

MILNE, J Kenneth; Salus Global Corporation, 200-717 Richmond St, London ON N6A 1S2; Wes'65; FSOGC; FACOG; FRCSC; ObstGyn (P.Q.) (Patient Health Care). Pres/CEO, Salus Global Corp; (519)640-7333; Fax. (519)640-5762; kmilne@salusgc.com.

MILNE, Laura A; Quinte HC Corp-Belleville Gen, 265 Dundas St E, Belleville ON K8N 5A9; Qns'08; FRCPC; IntMed. Staff, QHC Belleville General; (613)969-7400

MILNE, Lois A; MacEwan Student Centre, 370-2500 University Dr NW, Calgary AB T2N 1N4; Alb'80; BSc; CCFP; FCFP; Clin Lecturer, University of Calgary; (403)210-9355; Fax. (403)282-5218; lmilne@ucalgary.ca.

MILNE, P Ronald; 105-375 Pleasant St, Dartmouth NS B2Y 4N4; Dal'78; CCFP; FCFP; (902)469-2445

MILNE, Steven M; Sunwood Medical, 3000 Lougheed Hwy, New Westminster BC V3B 1C5; Cape Town (South Africa)'82; (604)464-0345

MILNE, William K; 27 Bruce St W, Goderich ON N7A 2M5; Cal'95; CCFP; CCFP(E.M.); FCFP; Staff, Alexandra Marine & General Hospital; (519)524-4121; Fax. (519)524-1314; monycon@hurontel.on.ca.

MILNE-EPP, Andrea M; Royal Alexandra Hosp, 10240 Kingsway NW, Edmonton AB T5H 3V9; Sask'98; CCFP; FCFP; Staff, Royal Alexandra Hospital; (780)735-4201; Fax. (780)735-4978.

MILNER, Curtis A; 601-2000 Regent St, Sudbury ON P3E 5T5; Qns'67; DiagRad. Section Leader Diagnostic Radiol, Northern Ontario School of Medicine; (705)522-1835

MILNER, John F; Assiniboine Clinic, 633 Lodge Ave, Winnipeg MB R3J 0S9; Alb'69; FRCSC; Urol. Ac Staff, The Salvation Army Grace Hospital.

MILNER, Maurice F J; Queen-Lynch Med Centre, 205-157 Queen St E, Brampton ON L6W 3X4; National (Ireland)'74; MB ChB; BAO; DRCOG; (905)459-1774; Fax. (905)459-1781.

MILNER, Richard G; Maple FHT-Reddendale Family HC, 125 Lakeview Ave, Kingston ON K7M 3T6; Qns'81; CCFP; FCFP; (613)384-4664; Fax. (613)384-4182.

MILNER, Thomas G; Victoria Hosp, PO Box 3000 Stn Main 1200 24th St W, Prince Albert SK S6V 5T4; Freiburg (Germany)'88; FRCPC; GenPath. Staff, Pasqua Hospital; Staff, Victoria Hospital; (306)765-6154; Fax. (306)765-6163.

MILNER GERO, Heidi O; 101-55 Drury Cove Rd, Saint John NB E2H 2Z8; Dal'08; CCFP; Staff, Saint John Regional Hospital; (506)652-3900; Fax. (506)652-7976.

MILO, Michael E; Regional Mental HC-London, PO Box 5532 Stn B 850 Highbury Ave, London ON N6A 4H1; Wes'75; FRCPC; Psy (Endocrinology). Staff, Regional Mental Health Care-St Joseph's Health Care; (519)455-5110; Fax. (519)438-3689.

MILO-MANSON, Golda; Holland Bloorview Kids Rehab, 150 Kilgour Rd, Toronto ON M4G 1R8; McM'89; FRCPC; Peds (Developmental Pediatrics). Staff, Holland Bloorview Kids Rehabilitation Hospital; Staff, The Hospital For Sick Children; Asst Prof, University of Toronto; (416)425-6220 x3801; Fax. (416)425-9332.

MILONE, Stephanie M L; Highlands Health Network, 140 Rolling Hills Dr, Orangeville ON L9W 4X8; Tor'02; BSc; MSc; CCFP; Lecturer, University of Toronto; Aj Prof, Queen's University; (519)941-7575

MILONE, Stephen; Highlands Health Network, 140 Rolling Hills Dr, Orangeville ON L9W 4X8; Tor'02; CCFP; (519)941-7575

MILORD, Francois; Direction de la Sante Publique, 1255 rue Beauregard, Longueuil QC J4K 2M3; Sher'83; CSPQ; FRCPC; CommunMed (Infectious Diseases). Consultant Public Health, Hopital Charles LeMoyne; assoc Prof Dept of Commun Hlth Sciences, Universite de Sherbrooke; Langs: Bilingual(French/English); (450)679-6772; Fax. (450)928-3023; francois.milord@usherbrooke.ca.

MILOSEVIC, Lawrence M; Trillium Hlth Ctr-Mississauga, 100 Queensway W, Mississauga ON L5B 1B8; Qns'91; FRCPC; IntMed; Critical Care Medicine. Dir Intensive Care Unit, Trillium Health Centre - Mississauga; (905)848-7663

MILOSEVIC, Michael F; Univ Hlth Network-Princess M, 610 University Ave, Toronto ON M5G 2M9; Qns'87; FRCPC; RadOncol. Radiation Oncology, Princess Margaret Hospital - University Health Network; Prof RadOncol, University of Toronto; (416)946-2932; Fax. (416)946-2777.

MILOSEVIC, Slobodan; CSSS de la Maskinonge, 450 2e rue, Louiseville QC J5V 1V3; Belgrade (Serbia)'83; Staff, CSSS de Maskinongé; Langs: English; French; Russian; Serbian; (819)268-2731; Fax. (819)228-2973.

MILOSEVIC, Vladimir; Credit Valley Prof Bldg, 510-2300 Eglinton Ave W, Mississauga ON L5M 2V8; Tor'00; FRCPC; IntMed; Endocrin&Metab. (905)820-9233; Fax. (905)820-1779.

MILOT, Alain; CHUQ-St-Francois d'Assise, 10 rue de l'Espinay, Quebec QC G1L 3L5; Laval'85; MSc(Pharm); FRCPC; IntMed (Pharmacology). Staff Ctr des Maladies Vasculaires, Centre Hospitalier Universitaire De Québec - Pavillon De St-françois-d'assise; Med Consultant, Direction de la Sante Publique de Quebec; Prof, Université Laval; (418)525-4465

MILOT, Diane; CLSC Ahuntsic, 1165 boul Henri-Bourassa E, Montreal QC H2C 3K2; Mon'79; Langs: English; (514)384-2000 x8379; Fax. (514)381-0814; diane.milot.csssamn@ssss.gouv.qc.ca.

MILOT, Genevieve; Ctr Hosp Affilie-Enfant-Jesus, 1401 18e rue, Quebec QC G1J 1Z4; Laval'91; FRCSC; Neursurg. Staff, Centre Hospitalier Affilié Universitaire de Québec - Hôpital De L'Enfant Jésus; (418)649-5734; Fax. (418)649-5915.

MILOT, Julie; Hôpital Laval, 2725 ch Sainte-Foy, Quebec QC G1V 4G5; Laval'96; FRCPC; IntMed; Respir. Staff, Hôpital Laval; Langs: English; (418)656-4747; Fax. (418)656-4762.

MILOT, Laurent; Sunnybrook Hlth Sciences Ctre, 2075 Bayview Ave, Toronto ON M4N 3M5; Lyon I (France)'06; Staff, Sunnybrook Health Sciences Centre; (416)480-6100

MILOT, Marcel; Clin Pediatrie de Chicoutimi, 475 boul Talbot, Chicoutimi QC G7H 4A3; McG'81; FRCPC; Peds (Teaching). Ac Staff, Complexe hospitalier de la Sagamie; Langs: English; (418)549-1034; Fax. (418)696-4673.

MILOT, Martin; Polyclinique de Trois-Rivieres, 310-1900 boul des Recollets, Trois-Rivieres QC G8Z 4K4; Sher'76; OrthSurg. Staff, CSSS de Trois-Rivières; Staff, Centre de santé Cloutier-du-Rivage; Langs: English; (819)373-3244; Fax. (819)373-5997.

MILOT, Yvon; 1652 rue Royale, Trois-Rivieres QC G9A 4K3; Laval'68; Staff, CSSS de Trois-Rivières; Physician, U.Q.T.P.; (819)379-0451; Fax. (819)379-4920.

MILOT-ROY, Valerie; CHUQ-Ctr Hosp Univ Laval, 2705 boul Laurier, Quebec QC G1V 4G2; Laval'98; CSPQ; Anes. Staff, Centre Hospitalier Universitaire de Quebec-CHUL; (418)656-4141

MILOVAN, Eduard; C H Anna-Laberge-Clin Externe, 200-237 Saint-Jean-Baptiste, Chateauguay QC J6K 3C3; Bucharest (Romania)'90; FRCPC; Psy. Staff, Hôpital Anna-Laberge; (450)692-0002; Fax. (450)692-0008.

MILROD, Elise G; 500 Manning Rd, Windsor ON N8N 5H3; Wes'98; CCFP; (519)979-8580

MILROY, Christopher M; The Ottawa Hosp-Gen Campus, 4244-501 Smyth Rd, Ottawa ON K1H 8L6; Liverpool (England)'83; FRCPC; AnatPath. Staff, The Ottawa Hospital - General Campus; (613)737-7777

MILROY, Connie L; Westmount Community Health Ctr, 800-723 Rymal Rd W, Hamilton ON L9B 2W2; Wes'81; CCFP; FCFP; Ac Member Family Med, Hamilton Health Sciences Centre - McMaster Children's Hospital; (905)575-5200; Fax. (905)575-5383.

MILROY, Thomas M; MUHC-Montreal Gen Hosp, 1650 av Cedar, Montreal QC H3G 1A4; Maryland (USA)'74; ABNP; FRCPC; Psy (Electroconvulsive Therapy). Staff Central Exec Council of Phys, McGill University Health Centre - Montreal General Campus; adj Prof, McGill University; Langs: English; French; (514)934-1934 x42059; Fax. (514)934-8237.

MILTON, John R; Woodstock Med Clinic, 3-110 Chapel St, Woodstock NB E7M 1H1; Dal'80; FRCPC; IntMed. Staff, Carleton Memorial Hospital; (506)328-9747; Fax. (506)328-9792.

MIMEAULT, Richard E; The Ottawa Hosp-Civic Campus, 300-1053 Carling Ave, Ottawa ON K1Y 4E9; McG'82; FRCSC; GenSurg. Ac Staff Surg, The Ottawa Hospital - Civic Campus; Teach. Assoc., University of Ottawa; Langs: English; French; (613)761-5015; Fax. (613)761-4029.

MIMRAN, Gracia; Tiny Tots Med Centre, 203-3400 rue du Marche, Dollard-D-Ormeaux QC H9B 2Y1; Mon'97; (514)685-3531; Fax. (514)685-7971.

MIN, Frank; Southlake Reg Health Centre, 596 Davis Dr, Newmarket ON L3Y 2P9; Wes'04; Critical Care Medicine; Anes. Staff, Southlake Regional Health Centre; (905)895-4521

MIN, Jason K; 400-2000 Place Veteran's NW, Calgary AB T3B 4N2; Alb'99; FRCSC; ObstGyn (Family Medicine). (403)284-5444; Fax. (403)284-9293.

MIN, Simon T; Abbotsford Reg Hosp & Cancer C, 32900 Marshall Rd, Abbotsford BC V2S 0C2; Tor'90; FRCPC; IntMed; Critical Care Medicine. Staff, Abbotsford Regional Hospital & Cancer Centre; (604)807-7621

MINA, Mina M F; Fort Street Clinic, 300 Fort St, Winnipeg MB R3C 1E5; Alexandria (Egypt)'69; MB ChB; FACS; FRCSC; Otol (Rhinology). Staff, Health Sciences Centre; Staff, Seven Oaks General Hospital; Consultant, Otol., Workers Compensation Board of Manitoba; Assoc Prof, University of Manitoba; Langs: Arabic.

MINARDI, John; Hotel-Dieu Grace Hosp, 1030 Ouellette Ave, Windsor ON N9A 1E1; Tor'81; Staff, Hôtel-Dieu Grace Hospital; (519)973-4400

MINASSIAN, Berge A; The Hosp for Sick Children, 555 University Ave, Toronto ON M5G 1X8; McG'92; FRCPC; Neur. Staff, The Hospital For Sick Children; (416)813-7721; Fax. (416)813-6334; berge.minassian@sickkids.ca.

MINASSIAN, Viken; 787 Place des Rapides, Laval QC H7Y 2E6; Sher'90; Staff, Centre Hospitalier Fleury; (514)337-4772

MINC, Paul H; Acton Med Clinic, 10 Eastern Ave, Acton ON L7J 0A5; London (England)'56; MB BS; LMCC; CCFP; FCFP; Staff, Campbellford Memorial Hospital; Staff, QHC Belleville General; Langs: German; French; Spanish; (519)853-9997

MINDE, Klaus K; 435-5025 rue Sherbrooke O, Montreal QC H4A 1S9; Munich (Germany)'57; FABPN; MA(Psychol); Psy (AIDS/HIV). Staff, McGill University Health Centre - Montreal Children's Hospital; Prof Psy & Peds, McGill University; Langs: German; French; (514)489-1011; Fax. (514)939-3359; klaus.minde@mcgill.ca.

MINDE, Thomas; Centre d'Heberg la Peche, CP 59 9 ch Passe-Partout, Ste-Cecile-de-Mash QC J0X 2W0; Qns'90; BA; CCFP; FCFP; Ac Member, Centre Hospitalier Gatineau Mémorial; Asst Prof Family Med, University of Ottawa; Asst Prof Family Med, McGill University; Langs: German; French; (819)459-1112 x6250; Fax. (819)456-1460.

MINDEL, Michael J; Radiologix Hochelaga, 101-8695 rue Hochelaga, Montreal QC H1L 6J5; McG'70; CSPQ; DiagRad., McGill University; Langs: Italian; (514)353-5730; Fax. (514)353-4729; michael@mindel.ca.

MINDEN, Mark D; Univ Hlth Network-Princess M, 610 University Ave, Toronto ON M5G 2M9; Tor'74; MD; FRCPC; IntMed (Leukemia). Sr Scientist/Staff Phys, Princess Margaret Hospital - University Health Network; (416)946-2015; Fax. (416)946-6546; mark.minden@uhn.ca.

MINDRU, Cristina S; MUHC-Montreal Neurology Inst, 3801 rue University, Montreal QC H3A 2B4; Bucharest (Romania)'89; FRCPC; IntMed. Staff, McGill University Health Centre - Montreal Neurological Hospital; Langs: Romanian; French; (514)406-4968; Fax. (514)398-6644.

MINDRUM, Christa R; 1833 Kidston Ave PO Box 393, Port Williams NS B0P 1T0; Mem'03; CCFP; (902)300-2980

MINDRUM, Michael; 1437 Belcher St RR 1, Port Williams NS B0P 1T0; Kentucky (USA)'03; IntMed. (902)542-0990

MINER, Louise; SMBD Jewish Gen Hosp, 3755 ch Cote-Sainte-Catherine, Montreal QC H3T 1E2; Mem'82; FRCSC; ObstGyn (Ultrasound). Staff, McGill University Health Centre - Montreal General Campus; Staff, Sir Mortimer B Davis Jewish General; Staff, McGill University Health Centre - Royal Victoria Hospital; Teach Staff Pt-Time, McGill University; (514)340-8222 x4800; Fax. (514)340-7941.

MINER, Steven E S; 641 Davis Dr, Newmarket ON L3Y 2R2; McG'93; FRCPC; IntMed; Cardiol. Staff, Southlake Regional Health Centre; (905)898-5800; Fax. (905)898-5808.

MINET, Wyatt W; 103-361 George St N, Peterborough ON K9H 3R2; McM'03; FRCSC; Otol (Facial Plastic Surgery). Staff, Peterborough Regional Health Centre - Hospital Drive; (705)749-9262; Fax. (705)743-4416.

MINEYKO, Aleksandra; Alberta Children's Hosp, 2888 Shaganappi Trail NW, Calgary AB T3B 6A8; Qns'05; FRCPC; Neur. Staff, Alberta Children's Hospital; (403)955-3189; Fax. (403)955-2922.

MING, Vivian H C; 124-174 Wilson St, Victoria BC V9A 7N7; Witwatersrand (South Africa)'89; MB ChB; LMCC; CCFP; (250)857-2383

MING FOK, Judy; 200-99 Sinclair Ave, Georgetown ON L7G 5G1; Witwatersrand (South Africa)'94; MB ChB; LMCC; CCFP; (905)873-1383; Fax. (905)873-2931; warren_tong@hotmail.com.

MING-FOK, Terence L; Regina Med Centre, 100-2550 12th Ave, Regina SK S4P 3X1; Witwatersrand (South Africa)'02; BPharm; MB BCh; (306)566-4120; Fax. (306)566-4150.

MING-LUM, Corey; 250-5780 Cambie St, Vancouver BC V5Z 3A7; UBC'00; FRCSC; GenSurg. (604)324-4849

MINGIARDI, Anne Marie; Conestoga College, 299 Doon Valley Dr, Kitchener ON N2G 4M4; McM'92; CCFP; FCFP; Physician Student Health, Conestoga College; (519)748-5220 x3679; Fax. (519)748-3509.

MINGIE, Lorraine O; Markham Family Health Team, 1-122 Cornell Park Ave, Markham ON L6B 1A1; Tor'85; Ac Staff Family Pract, Markham Stouffville Hospital; (905)471-9999; Fax. (905)209-1501; lmingie@msh.on.ca.

MINGO, Nancy S; Rosedale Med Centre, 212-600 Sherbourne St, Toronto ON M4X 1W4; Tor'91; CCFP; FCFP; (416)966-8918; Fax. (416)966-1729.

MINHAS, Avinder S; 310-7031 Westminster Hwy, Richmond BC V6X 1A3; Amritsar (India)'75; FRCPC; Psy; IntMed. (604)273-3336; Fax. (604)273-7630.

MINHAS, Gurmit S; Central Nfld Reg Hlth Centre, 50 Union St, Grnd-Falls-Wi NL A2A 2E1; Guru Nanak Dev (India)'75; MB BS; Staff, Central Newfoundland Regional Health Centre; (709)292-2500; Fax. (709)292-2249.

MINHAS, Kuldip S; North York Gen Hosp, 4001 Leslie St, North York ON M2K 1E1; Kerala (India)'78; MB BS; FRCPC; Anes. Staff, North York General Hospital; (416)756-6265

MINHAS, Kunal K S; St Boniface Gen Hosp, Y3541-409 Tache Ave, Winnipeg MB R2H 2A6; Sask'00; FRCPC; IntMed; Cardiol. Staff, St Boniface General Hospital; (204)258-1276; Fax. (204)235-3826.

MINHAS, Ripudaman S; The Hosp for Sick Children, 555 University Ave, Toronto ON M5G 1X8; Tor'08; Peds. Staff, The Hospital For Sick Children; (416)813-1500

MINHAS, Shikha; Surrey Mem Hosp, N52-13750 96 Ave, Surrey BC V3V 1Z2; Sask'00; CCFP; Staff, Surrey Memorial Hospital; (604)585-5532

MINIC, Sanja; 214 Med Place, 12-9909 102 St, Grande Prairie AB T8V 2V4; (Serbia)'95; CCFP; (780)532-9067; Fax. (780)532-0949.

MINICH, Peter J; 110-210 Memorial Ave, Orillia ON L3V 7V1; Qns'87; FRCSC; Urol. (705)325-3603; Fax. (705)325-5483.

MINIER, Daniel; Clinique Med Rock Forest, 1-4870 boul Bourque, Sherbrooke QC J1N 3S5; Sher'92; FRCPC; Derm. (819)820-2673; Fax. (819)820-2112.

MINION, Daurel; Students Union Bldg, 2 200-66 University Campus NW, Edmonton AB T6G 2J7; Alb'84; (780)492-2612; Fax. (780)492-0172.

MINION, Jessica L; Regina Qu'Appelle HR-Regina, 1440 14th Ave, Regina SK S4P 0W5; Cal'05; FRCPC; MedMicrobiol. Staff, Regina General Hospital; (306)766-4482

MINISH, Kelley L; Admirals Medical Clinic, 275 Island Hwy, Victoria BC V9B 1G4; Man'88; CCFP; CCFP(E.M.); (250)380-9070; Fax. (250)380-9090.

MINISH, Kimberley J; Healthpoint Pain & Injury Clin, 627 Dudley Ave, Winnipeg MB R3M 1P5; Man'85; CCFP; FCFP.

MINISH, Travis M; Health Sciences Centre, 820 Sherbrook St, Winnipeg MB R3A 1R9; Man'98; FRCPC; EmergMed. Staff, Health Sciences Centre; (204)774-6511

MINK, Steven N; Respiratory Unit, 810 Sherbrook St, Winnipeg MB R3A 1R8; Temple(PA) (USA)'72; ABIM; Staff, Health Sciences Centre; Staff, St Boniface General Hospital; Head Section of Respirology/Prof Med, University of Manitoba.

MINKARIOUS, Edmon F W; 11-277 Welland Ave, St Catharines ON L2R 2P7; Cairo (Egypt)'69; MB ChB; FRCPC; IntMed (Cardiology); Nephrol. Ac Staff, Niagara Health System - Welland Hospital Site; Ac Staff, Niagara Health System - Greater Niagara General Site; Ac Staff, Niagara Health System - Ontario Street Site; Ac Staff, Niagara Health System - St Catharines General Site; (905)937-4283; Fax. (905)937-8003.

MINKLEY, Aaron A D; PO Box 1000 Stn Main, Lazo BC V0R 2K0; Alb'05; BSc; CCFP; (250)339-8267; minkley.a@forces.gc.ca.

MINKOVICH, Leonid L; Univ Hlth Network-Toronto Gen, 3 410-200 Elizabeth St, Toronto ON M5G 2C4; Perm (Russia (Federation))'80; Staff, Toronto General Hospital - UHN; (416)340-3242

MINKOWITZ, Joseph; Markham Stouffville Cardiol As, 205-110 Copper Creek Dr, Markham ON L6B 0P9; McG'85; FACC; MDCM; FRCPC; IntMed (Cardiovascular Disease); Cardiol. Court Staff, Southlake Regional Health Centre; Staff, Markham Stouffville Hospital; Court Staff, Sunnybrook Health Sciences Centre; (905)472-7357; Fax. (905)472-8548; jmink@markhamcardiology.com.

MINNA, Roberta; Medical Clinic Bldg, 302-89 Humber College Blvd, Toronto ON M9V 4B8; Tor'94; FRCSC; GenSurg. (416)746-1905; Fax. (416)746-9437.

MINNAAR, Johannes C H; Steinbach Family Med Centre, 10-333 Loewen Blvd, Steinbach MB R5G 0C3; Free State (South Africa)'96; CCFP; CCFP(E.M.); (204)326-3401; Fax. (204)326-3899.

MINNAAR, Petrus A; Regina Qu'Appelle HR-Regina, 1440 14th Ave, Regina SK S4P 0W5; Staff, Regina General Hospital; (306)766-4444

MINNAAR, Roy J; 101-250 Dogwood St, Campbell River BC V9W 2X9; Witwatersrand (South Africa)'78; MB BCh; MMed(Surg); FRCSC; GenSurg (Endoscopy). Staff, Campbell River & District General Hospital; (250)850-1104; Fax. (250)850-1105.

MINNEMA, Brian J; North York Gen Hosp, GW33-4001 Leslie St, North York ON M2K 1E1; Tor'05; FRCPC; IntMed; Critical Care Medicine; InfectDis. Staff, North York General Hospital; (416)756-6130; Fax. (416)756-6449.

MINNES, Bruce G; The Hosp for Sick Children, 555 University Ave, Toronto ON M5G 1X8; Qns'86; BSc; FAAP; ABPeds(EmergMed.); FRCPC; Peds (Pediatric Emergency Medicine). Staff, The Hospital For Sick Children; Asst Prof Peds, University of Toronto; (416)813-5238; Fax. (416)813-5043; bruce.minnes@sickkids.ca.

MINNES, Shir; Thunder Bay Paediatrics, 588 Arthur St, Thunder Bay ON P7E 5R7; UBC'07; FRCPC; Peds. (807)766-3370

MINNES, Yoram; Oakmount Med Centre, 110-809 41st Ave W, Vancouver BC V5Z 2N6; Jerusalem (Israel)'84; FRCPC; Psy (Child & Family Psychiatry). Consultant Child Psy, Richmond Mental Health Team; Consultant Child Psy, Richmond School Program; Physician, Richmond Mental Health Child & Adolescent Program; Langs: Hebrew; (604)676-4395; Fax. (604)676-4396; drminnes@showbiz.ca.

MINNETT, Seana K; Glen Sather Sports Med Clinic, 11400 University Campus NW, Edmonton AB T6G 1Z1; Ott'98; CCFP; FCFP; (780)407-5160; Fax. (780)407-5667.

MINNIS, Shantel M; 2425 Bloor St W, Toronto ON M6S 4W4; (Jamaica)'98; FRCPC; DiagRad. (416)763-4331

MINODIN, Mike O; Medicine in Motion Med Clinic, 121 Ilsley Ave, Dartmouth NS B3B 1S4; (Philippines)'82; Staff, Medicine in Motion Medical Centre; (902)468-2774; Fax. (902)468-1359.

MINOR, Adrian A; 1819 Campbell Ave RR 3, Peterborough ON K9J 6X4; Tor'69; FRCSC; GenSurg. (705)741-5751

MINOR, Samuel F; Queen Elizabeth II HSC, 813-1276 South Park St, Halifax NS B3H 2Y9; Tor'00; BSc; FRCSC; GenSurg; Critical Care Medicine. Staff, Queen Elizabeth II Health Sciences Centre - Victoria General Site; (902)473-2700; samuel_miron@hotmail.com.

MINORGAN, Stephanie; Meadowlands Family Hlth Ctre, 888 Meadowlands Dr, Ottawa ON K2C 3R2; McG'01; CCFP; Langs: Bilingual(French/English); (613)228-2882; Fax. (613)228-2856.

MINOS, Nick; Ontario Health Clinics, 40 Shellington Pl, Brantford ON N3S 0C3; McM'09; CCFP; (519)753-9581

MINOVI, Moshkoo; 200-31205 Maclure Rd, Abbotsford BC V2T 5E5; Saba (Netherlands Antilles)'07; (604)746-4700

MINSOS, Jennifer R; Saint Thomas Comm Health Ctre, 9040 84 Ave NW, Edmonton AB T6C 1E4; Alb'04; CCFP; (780)434-2778; Fax. (780)466-8702.

MINSTER, Richard; 200-2800 14th Ave, Markham ON L3R 0E4; Tor'78; (905)305-9829; Fax. (905)305-0849.

MINTSIOULIS, George; The Ottawa Hosp-Gen Campus, 501 Smyth Rd, Ottawa ON K1H 8L6; Ott'72; FRCSC; Ophth. Staff, The Ottawa Hospital - General Campus; (613)737-8926; Fax. (613)737-8836; gmintsioulis@ottawahospital.on.ca.

MINTSIOULIS, Stephen J G; Sheldon Chumir Centre, 1213 4 St SW, Calgary AB T2R 0X7; Qns'05; CCFP; Clinical Asst Prof, University of Calgary; Langs: Bilingual(English/French); (403)955-9300; Fax. (403)476-8766.

MINTY, Evan; 138-3385 26 Ave NE, Calgary AB T1Y 6L4; Cal'08; FRCPC; IntMed. Staff, Foothills Medical Centre; (403)472-6468

MINTY, Robert; The Hugh Allen Clinic, PO Box 489 Stn Main, Sioux Lookout ON P8T 1A8; UBC'80; CCFP; FCFP; Staff, The Hugh Allen Clinic; Clinical Asst Prof, Northern Ontario School of Medicine; (807)737-3803; Fax. (807)737-1771; rminty@sourceline.ca.

MINTZ, Donald R; Laurel Med Centre Ltd, 212-888 8th Ave W, Vancouver BC V5Z 3Y1; Qns'76; FRCSC; Otol (Laser Surgery Snoring & Sleep Apnea). Ac Staff, Vancouver General Hospital - Centennial Pavillion; Clin Assoc Prof, University of British Columbia; (604)872-1231; Fax. (604)873-5951.

MINTZ, Marcy J; HSC Faculty of Med, 3330 Hospital Dr NW, Calgary AB T2N 4N1; Cal'94; FRCPC; IntMed. Clinical Asst Prof, Foothills Medical Centre; (403)220-8892; Fax. (403)283-6151; mjmintz@ucalgary.ca.

MINTZ, Randall R; Building N 109, PO Box 9999 Stn Main, Petawawa ON K8H 2X3; McM'07; CCFP; (613)687-5511; Fax. (613)588-6845.

MINTZ, Sharon; Brookfield Place, 3000-181 Bay St, Toronto ON M5J 2T3; McM'79; CCFP; FCFP; Asst Prof, University of Toronto; (416)507-6762; Fax. (416)507-6750.

MINTZ, Sheldon; Women's College Hosp, W651-76 Grenville St, Toronto ON M5S 1B2; Tor'63; ABIM; MEd; FCCP; RC; FRCPC; IntMed (Respirology). Dir Med Education Ctr for Evaluation of Hlth Prof Educ Abroad, Women's College Hospital; Prof Med, University of Toronto; (416)323-7557; Fax. (416)323-7558.

MINUK, Cheryl F; Edward Street X-Ray, 600-123 Edward St, Toronto ON M5G 1E2; Man'76; FRCPC; DiagRad. Lecturer, University of Toronto; (416)597-1016; Fax. (416)597-6610.

MINUK, Earl S; 932 Grosvenor Ave, Winnipeg MB R3M 0N5; Man'80; FRCPC; IntMed; Derm.

MINUK, Gerald Y; Medical Outpatient Dept, 700 William Ave, Winnipeg MB R3E 0Z3; Man'75; FRCPC; IntMed. Staff, Health Sciences Centre.

MINUK, Howard L; 104-726 Bloor St W, Toronto ON M6G 4A1; Man'74; ABIM; FRCPC; IntMed. Chief Med Dir, Swiss Re Life & Health; (416)535-2162; Fax. (416)535-6708; hminuk@rogers.com.

MINUK, Jeffrey; SMBD Jewish Gen Hosp, 3755 ch Cote-Sainte-Catherine, Montreal QC H3T 1E2; Man'85; FRCPC; Neur (Adult Neurology). Staff, Sir Mortimer B Davis Jewish General; (514)340-8222 x2399; Fax. (514)340-7567.

MINUK, Leonard; London HSC-Victoria Hosp, PO Box 5010 Stn B A2 401-800 Commissioners Rd E, London ON N6A 5W9; Man'04; FRCPC; IntMed; Hem. Staff, London Health Sciences Centre - Victoria Campus; (519)685-8500 x5216; Fax. (519)685-8477.

MINUK, Terry G; Hamilton HS-Henderson Site, 711 Concession St, Hamilton ON L8V 1C3; Man'78; FRCPC; DiagRad (Mammography). Chief Radiol, Hamilton Health Sciences Centre-Juravinski Site; Clin Assoc Prof Radiol, McMaster University; (905)527-4322 x42261; Fax. (905)575-2660; minuk@hhsc.ca.

MINVILLE, Caroline; Hôpital Laval, 2725 ch Sainte-Foy, Quebec QC G1V 4G5; Laval'04; Respir; IntMed. Staff, Hôpital Laval; (418)835-7121

MINVILLE, Genevieve; CSSS de Chicoutimi, 305 rue Saint-Vallier, Chicoutimi QC G7H 5H6; McG'97; Staff, Complexe hospitalier de la Sagamie; Langs: English; French; (418)541-1000; Fax. (418)541-1131.

MINVILLE, Luc; CSSS de Rimouski-Niegette, CP 3150 Succ A 150 av Rouleau, Rimouski QC G5L 5T1; Laval'00; CSPQ; FRCPC; DiagRad. Staff, Hôpital Regional Rimouski; (418)724-3000

MINVILLE, Nathalie; CSSS de Saint-Jerome, 290 rue Montigny, Saint-Jerome QC J7Z 5T3; Sher'03; FRCSC; GenSurg. Staff, Hôtel-Dieu de Saint-Jérôme; (450)431-8201

MINZ, Gabriel R; 384 ch Bord-du-Lac Lakeshore, Dorval QC H9S 2A6; Strasbourg (France)'81; CCFP; Staff, Lakeshore General Hospital - Pointe Claire; Staff, CSSS de Dorval-Lachine-Lasalle; Langs: French; (514)636-8860; Fax. (514)633-9561; gabrielminz@hotmail.com.

MINZ, Lorna B H; 202-1371 Neilson Rd, Scarborough ON M1B 4Z8; Tor'82; BSc; FRCSC; Otol. Staff, Rouge Valley Health System - Centenary Health Centre Site; (416)281-0412; Fax. (416)281-6309.

MIOR, Frederic; CHUS-Hop Fleurimont, 3001 12e av N, Sherbrooke QC J1H 5N4; Sher'03; FRCPC; Anes. Staff, Centre Hospitalier Universitaire de Sherbrooke-Hopital Fleurimont; (819)346-1110 x14403

MIOT, Robert C; Urgence Rive-Sud, 3200 boul Taschereau, Greenfield Park QC J4V 2H3; (Haiti)'78; (450)672-5577

MIQUELON, Marianne; 500 boul de l'Hopital, Gatineau QC J8V 2P5; Sher'09; CCFP; (819)966-6171

MIR, Asad; Avenida Bonavista Shopp Ctre, 315-12445 Lake Fraser Dr SE, Calgary AB T2J 7A4; (Pakistan)'86; (403)723-2453; Fax. (403)723-2463.

MIR, Bilal T; Victoria Gen Hosp, 1 Hospital Way, Victoria BC V8Z 6R5; (Pakistan)'94; MB BS; CCFP; CCFP(E.M.); Staff, Victoria General Hospital; Langs: Urdu; Punjabi; (250)727-4212

MIR, Josef; Saint John Reg Hosp, PO Box 2100 Stn Main 400 University Ave, Saint John NB E2L 4L2; Karlinska (Sweden)'00; FRCPC; Anes. Staff, Saint John Regional Hospital; (506)648-6000

MIR, Kamran; Mount Forest Family Hlth Team, SS 3 525 Dublin St, Mount Forest ON N0G 2L3; St George Univ of Grenada (Grenada)'07; CCFP; (519)829-0066

MIRAL, Henriette; B-1771 ch Saint-Angelique, Saint-Lazare QC J7T 2X7; Mon'73; (450)455-5773

MIRANDER, Lennox G; Dorval Med Assoc Fam Hlth Team, 465 Morden Rd, Oakville ON L6K 3W6; Washington DC (USA)'09; CCFP; (905)842-7154; Fax. (905)842-3604; lmirander@cogeco.ca.

MIRCEA, Carmen; 222-20 14th St W, Prince Albert SK S6V 3K8; Bucharest (Romania)'03; ObstGyn. (306)922-3284; Fax. (306)922-3285.

MIRCESCU, Hortensia S; 3840 rue Saint-Urbain, Montreal QC H2W 1T8; Mon'94; FRCPC; IntMed (Thyroid Diseases); Endocrin (P.Q.); Endocrin&Metab. Staff Endocrin, Centre Hospitalier l'Université de Montréal (CHUM) - Hôtel-Dieu; assoc Prof, Universite de Montreal; Langs: English; French; Romanian; (514)890-8444; Fax. (514)412-7128; hortensia.mircescu@umontreal.ca.

MIRCHANDANI, Deepu; BC Cancer Ctre-Southern Interi, 399 Royal Ave, Kelowna BC V1Y 5L3; Calcutta (India)'87; MSc; MB BS; Staff, BC Cancer Agency Sindi Ahluwalia Hawkins Centre for the Southern Interior; (250)712-3996; dmirchandani@bccancer.bc.ca.

MIRCHANDANI, Mukesh G; Dewdney East Med Clinic, 1689 E Dewdney Ave, Regina SK S4N 4N6; Mysore (India)'80; MRCPsy(Psy); FRCPC; Psy (Hospital Based). Psychiatrist, St Peter's Hospital; (306)789-8816; Fax. (306)789-8862; mukesh.mirchandani@shr.sk.ca.

MIRCHANDANI, Natasha; Univ Hlth Network-Toronto Western Hosp, 399 Bathurst St, Toronto ON M5T 2S8; McG'04; CCFP; Staff, Toronto Western Hospital - University Health Network; (416)603-5448; Fax. (416)603-6228.

MIREAU, John R; Saint John Reg Hosp, PO Box 2100 Stn Main 400 University Ave, Saint John NB E2L 4L2; Alb'03; FRCPC; Anes; Critical Care Medicine. Staff, Saint John Regional Hospital; (506)648-6000

MIREAULT, Gilles; CSSS du Nord de Lanaudière, 1000 boul Sainte-Anne, St-Charles-Brromee QC J6E 6J2; Mon'72; CSPQ; FRCPC; Psy. Ac Staff, Centre Hospitalier Régional de Lanaudière; Langs: English; (450)759-8222; Fax. (450)759-0011.

MIREMADI, Saman; Surrey Mem Hosp, 13750 96 Ave, Surrey BC V3V 1Z2; UBC'04; FRCPC; Psy. Staff, Vancouver General Hospital - Centennial Pavillion; Staff, Surrey Memorial Hospital; Langs: Farsi; (604)581-2211

MIRESCO, Marc J; Inst Comm Family Psychiatry, 4333 ch Cote-Sainte-Catherine, Montreal QC H3T 1E4; McG'01; FRCPC; Psy. (514)340-8210

MIRESKANDARI, Kamiar; The Hosp for Sick Children, 555 University Ave, Toronto ON M5G 1X8; Leeds (England)'94; Fellow, The Hospital For Sick Children; (416)813-7654 x2832; Fax. (416)813-8266; kamiar.mireskandari@sickkids.ca.

MIRHOSSEINI, Mehrnoush; Grey Nuns Community Hosp & HC, 1100 Youville Drive West NW, Edmonton AB T6L 5X8; (Iran)'84; CCFP; Staff, Covenant Health - Grey Nuns Community Hospital; Langs: Farsi; (780)735-7834

MIRKA, Theresa M; Brady Clinic, 1-359 Riverside Dr, Sudbury ON P3E 1H5; NOSM'09; CCFP; (705)688-8833

MIRMIRAN, S Jamaluddin; Cross Cultural Psychiatric Cli, 715 12th Ave W, Vancouver BC V5Z 1M9; Karachi (Pakistan)'79; MB BS; LMCC; FRCPC; Psy. Staff Psy/Med Mgr Vancouver Coastel Tertiary Care Hosp, Vancouver General Hospital - Centennial Pavillion; Clin Instructor Psy, University of British Columbia; Langs: Persian; Urdu; (604)875-4115; Fax. (604)875-5386; jamal.mirmiran@vch.ca.

MIRO, Joaquim A; Hôpital Ste-Justine, 3175 ch Cote-Sainte-Catherine, Montreal QC H3T 1C5; Mon'84; CSPQ; FRCPC; Peds (Cardiac Catheterization); Cardiol. Staff Cardiol Ped Service, Hôpital Ste-Justine; Asst Prof Ped, Universite de Montreal; Langs: Spanish; French; (514)345-4931 x5401; Fax. (514)345-4896; joaquim_miro@ssss.gouv.qc.ca.

MIRO, Santiago M P; MUHC-Montreal Gen Hosp, 1650 av Cedar, Montreal QC H3G 1A4; Mon'92; CSPQ; DiagRad. Staff, McGill University Health Centre - Montreal General Campus; (514)934-1934

MIROLO, Hugh; Waterford Hosp, 306 Waterford Bridge Rd, St. John's NL A1E 4J8; Cordoba (Argentina)'83; Staff, Waterford Hospital; (709)777-3300

MIRON, Cristiana-Octavia; London HSC-University Hosp, PO Box 5339 Stn B 339 Windermere Rd, London ON N6A 5A5; Mon'07; FRCPC; Anes. Staff, London Health Sciences Centre - University Hospital; (519)663-3283

MIRON, Diane; CLSC Jardin du Quebec, 509 rue Saint-Jacques RR 1, Napierville QC J0J 1L0; Mon'95; (450)245-3336; Fax. (450)245-0278.

MIRON, Eric; Clinique Med Sainte-Dorothee, 102-1 boul Samson, Laval QC H7X 3S5; Sher'93; Staff, Hopital de la Cite de la santé; (450)689-6334; Fax. (450)689-6339.

MIRON, M Michele; Quinte HC Corp-Belleville Gen, 265 Dundas St E, Belleville ON K8N 5A9; McM'95; BSc; CCFP; CCFP(E.M.); FCFP; Staff, QHC Belleville General; (613)696-7400; michelemiron@hotmail.com.

MIRON, Marie-Claude; Hôpital Ste-Justine, 3175 ch Cote-Sainte-Catherine, Montreal QC H3T 1C5; Mon'84; CSPQ; FRCPC; DiagRad (Gastrointestinal Disorders). Staff, Hôpital Ste-Justine; Universite de Montreal; (514)345-4637; Fax. (514)345-4816; marie-claude_miron@ssss.gouv.qc.ca.

MIRON, Marie-Jose F; CHUM-Hop Notre-Dame, 1560 rue Sherbrooke E, Montreal QC H2L 4M1; Mon'92; MSc; BSc; IntMed. Staff, Centre Hospitalier l'Université de Montréal (CHUM) - Hôpital Notre-Dame; Langs: Italian; (514)890-8000 x27049; Fax. (514)412-7646.

MIRON, Michel; CSSS de Chicoutimi, 305 rue Saint-Vallier, Chicoutimi QC G7H 5H6; Mon'76; CSPQ; MedBiochem (P.Q.). Staff, Complexe hospitalier de la Sagamie; (418)541-1035 x2452

MIRON, Michel; Clinique Med 3000 Inc, 3000 rue Belanger, Montreal QC H1Y 1A9; Mon'74; (514)376-7702; Fax. (514)376-2639.

MIRON, Pierre; Ctr de Procreation Fertilys, 320-1000 montee des Pionniers, Terrebonne QC J6V 1S8; Sher'80; FRCSC; ObstGyn. Staff, Hopital Maisonneuve-Rosemont; (450)657-1313 x2266; Fax. (450)657-1809.

MIRON-PICHET, Roseline; CSSS du Nord de Lanaudière, 1000 boul Sainte-Anne, St-Charles-Brromee QC J6E 6J2; Sher'05; CCFP; Staff, Centre Hospitalier Régional de Lanaudière; (450)759-8222

MIROPOLSKY, Vladislav; Cambridge Mem Hosp, 700 Coronation Blvd, Cambridge ON N1R 3G2; Tor'03; FRCPC; DiagRad. Staff, St Joseph's Hospital - St Joseph's Health Care; Staff, Cambridge Memorial Hospital; (519)621-2330

MIROSH, Melissa D; Royal University Hosp, 4509-103 Hospital Dr, Saskatoon SK S7N 0W8; Qns'00; FRCSC; ObstGyn (Contraception). Staff, Royal University Hospital; (306)966-8623; Fax. (306)966-8040; miroshm@shaw.ca.

MIRSATTARI, Seyed M; London HSC-University Hosp, PO Box 5339 Stn B B10 110-339 Windermere Rd, London ON N6A 5A5; Qns'95; ABPN; FRCPC; Neur (Epilepsy). Staff Privileges, St Joseph's Hospital - St Joseph's Health Care; Staff Clin Neurol, London Health Sciences Centre - University Hospital; (519)663-3348; Fax. (519)663-3440.

MIRSKY, Douglas J; Woodroffe South Med Bldg, 205-1637 Woodroffe Ave, Nepean ON K2G 1W2; McG'71; MDCM; BSc; FACS; FRCSC; GenSurg (Breast Disease). Ac Staff GenSurg, Queensway Carleton Hospital; Consultant, Carleton Place & District Memorial Hospital; (613)723-2323; Fax. (613)224-0262; dmirsky1@hotmail.com.

MIRTLE, Brian R; 407/408-11523 100 Ave NW, Edmonton AB T5K 0J8; Alb'83; FRCPC; Psy (General Psychiatry & Psychotherapy). Associate Clin Prof, University of Alberta; (780)482-4902; Fax. (780)453-1219; bmirtle@incentre.net.

MIRTORABI, Nima; Stouffville Med Centre, 2-34 Civic Ave, Stouffville ON L4A 1H2; Sydney (Australia)'05; CCFP; (905)640-3100; Fax. (905)640-5346.

MIRWALDT, Patricia A; UBC Hospital, M334-2211 Wesbrook Mall, Vancouver BC V6T 2B5; Man'80; BSc(Med.); CCFP; Staff, UBC Hospital - Koerner Pavillion; Langs: Farsi; Urdu; (604)822-7011; Fax. (604)822-7889.

MIRZA, Aisha; Grey Nuns Community Hosp & HC, 1100 Youville Drive West NW, Edmonton AB T6L 5X8; Cal'03; CCFP; CCFP(E.M.); Staff, Covenant Health - Grey Nuns Community Hospital; (780)735-7000

MIRZA, Asma S; CSSS de Trois-Rivieres, 155 rue Toupin, Trois-Rivieres QC G8T 3Z8; Sher'93; LMCC; Staff, Centre de santé Cloutier-du-Rivage; Langs: English; (819)370-2200 x2109; Fax. (819)370-2010; mirzaasma@hotmail.com.

MIRZA, Nazneen S; 302-310 King St E, Kitchener ON N2G 2L3; Chittagong (Bangladesh)'98; CCFP; (519)743-2142; Fax. (519)743-2405.

MIRZA, Rida K; Child & Parent Resource Inst, 600 Sanatorium Rd, London ON N6H 3W7; Karachi (Pakistan)'93; FRCPC; Psy. Staff, Child & Parent Resource Institute; Langs: Urdu; (519)667-6640; Fax. (519)667-6814.

MIRZA, Yousha K; 3640 Wells St, Windsor ON N9C 1T9; Aga Khan (Pakistan)'96; FRCPC; Psy. (519)258-0484

MIRZAEI, Ameneh; Royal Ottawa Hlth Care Group, 1145 Carling Ave, Ottawa ON K1Z 7K4; Ott'04; FRCPC; Psy. Staff, Royal Ottawa Mental Health Centre - Royal Ottawa Health Care Group; (613)722-6521

MIRZANEJAD, Yazdan; Surrey Mem Hosp, 13750 96 Ave, Surrey BC V3V 1Z2; Tehran (Iran)'85; ABIM; FACP; DTMH; FRCPC; IntMed (AIDS/HIV); InfectDis. Consultant/Med Leader InfectDis, Surrey Memorial Hospital; Physician, Yazdan Medical Corporation; Clinical Asst Prof Infectious Diseased Clinic, University of British Columbia; Langs: Farsi; Italian; (604)587-3842; yazdan.mirzanejad@fraserhealth.ca.

MIS, Andrew A; Manitoba Clinic, 104-790 Sherbrook St, Winnipeg MB R3A 1M3; Man'88; MD(Med.); BSc(Med); FRC(S); FRCSC; Ophth (Ocular Oncology). Consultant Ophth, Misericordia Health Centre; Asst Prof Ophth, University of Manitoba; Langs: Polish; French; (204)788-5729; Fax. (204)774-5772; aamis@allstream.net.

MISERI, Frederic J S; SMBD Jewish Gen Hosp, 3755 ch Cote-Sainte-Catherine, Montreal QC H3T 1E2; Paris (France)'94; Staff, Sir Mortimer B Davis Jewish General; (514)340-8222

MISFELDT, Marlys; Kenderdine Med Clinic, 110-1804 McOrmond Dr, Saskatoon SK S7S 0A6; Sask'81; CASM(DipSportMed); Dip SportMed; Staff Med, Saskatoon District Health Board; (306)934-6606; Fax. (306)955-3180.

MISH, Joanna; Glenmore Landing D275-1600 90 Ave SW, Calgary AB T2V 5A8; Cal'97; CCFP; FCFP; Langs: Polish; (403)259-2709; Fax. (403)259-6014.

MISHKIN, Seymour; 770-4060 rue Sainte-Catherine, Westmount QC H3Z 2Z3; McG'65; FRCP; FRCPC; IntMed (Irritable bowel Syndrome); Gastroent. Sr Physician, McGill University Health Centre - Royal Victoria Hospital; Consultant, McGill University Health Centre - Montreal Children's Hospital; Consultant, Sir Mortimer B Davis Jewish General; assoc Prof, McGill University; (514)932-2686; Fax. (514)932-5758.

MISHO, Rita R H; Tuscany Med Centre, 105-9100 Jane St, Concord ON L4K 0A4; Baghdad (Iraq)'89; CCFP; (905)760-1140; Fax. (905)760-5587.

MISHRA, Achal; Mental Hlth & Addiction Servic, 15 Chipman Dr, Kentville NS B4N 3V7; (India)'92; MB BS; (902)365-1701; Fax. (902)678-4917.

MISHRA, Aditya V; Queen Elizabeth II HSC, 2035-1276 South Park St, Halifax NS B3H 2Y9; Dal'84; FRCSC; Ophth. Staff, Queen Elizabeth II Health Sciences Centre - Victoria General Site; (902)473-7053

MISHRA, Harsh V; Rockingham Ridge Plaza, 30 Farnham Gate Rd, Halifax NS B3M 3W8; Dal'83; CCFP; (902)443-7593; Fax. (902)443-7800.

MISHRA, Sharmistha; St Michael's Hosp, 4179-30 Bond St, Toronto ON M5B 1W8; Tor'02; FRCPC; IntMed; InfectDis. Staff, St Michael's Hospital; (416)864-5746; Fax. (416)864-5310.

MISHRIKI, Nahed R; Royal Bank Plaza Med Centre, PO Box 134 Stn Royal Bank 200 Bay St, Toronto ON M5J 2P3; Cairo (Egypt)'72; MB ChB; CCFP; Langs: Arabic; French; (416)368-6787; Fax. (416)368-7632.

MISIASZEK, Brian; St Peter's Hosp, 88 Maplewood Ave, Hamilton ON L8M 1W9; Wes'97; BSc(Hon); FRCPC; IntMed; GeriatricMed. Staff, Hamilton Health Sciences Centre - St Peter's Hospital; Staff, Hamilton Health Sciences Centre - McMaster University Medical Centre; (905)777-3837; Fax. (905)526-2062.

MISIK, Karl K A; Canadian Blood Services, 405 University Ave, Saint John NB E2L 4G7; Dal'70.

MISIR, Amita T R; London HSC-Victoria Hosp, PO Box 5010 Stn B E1 105-800 Commissioners Rd E, London ON N6A 5W9; Wes'06; FRCPC; Peds; PedEmergMed. Staff, London Health Sciences Centre - Victoria Campus; (519)685-8134; Fax. (519)667-6769.

MISIR, Anil J; Bluewater Health-Mitton Site, 220 Mitton St N, Sarnia ON N7T 6H6; Tor'04; FRCPC; AnatPath. Staff, Bluewater Health - Mitton Site; (905)521-2100

MISKEW, Linda D; 1603 20 Ave NW, Calgary AB T2M 1G9; Alb'81; CCFP; FCFP; (403)270-8978; Fax. (403)289-8269.

MISKIEWICZ, Laura M; Rivergrove Med Clinic, 2-2605 Main St, Winnipeg MB R2V 4W3; Man'90; (204)632-0024; Fax. (204)697-2047.

MISKIN, Murray; C M L Health Care, 612-1881 Yonge St, Toronto ON M4S 3C4; Tor'63; FRCPC; DiagRad (Diagnostic Ultrasound). (416)487-2425; Fax. (416)487-0746.

MISRA, Manjula; Oshawa Clinic, 117 King St E, Oshawa ON L1H 1B9; McG'95; FRCSC; Ophth. (905)721-4914; Fax. (905)721-4918.

MISRA, Sabeena; Windsor Health Centre, 115-700 Tecumseh Rd E, Windsor ON N8X 4T2; Kathmandu Univ (Nepal)'00.

MISRA, Tarun; 415 14 St NW, Calgary AB T2N 2A1; Man'00; FRCPC; IntMed; Gastroent. Staff, Peter Lougheed Centre; Langs: Hindi; (403)270-9555

MISRI, Shaila; BC Women's Hosp & Health Ctre, H214-4500 Oak St, Vancouver BC V6H 3N1; Calcutta (India)'72; MB BS; FRCPC; Psy (Reproductive Psy). Staff, BC Women's Hospital & Health Centre; Dir Reproductive Psy Prog, Providence Health Care - St Paul's Hospital; Clin Prof ObsyGyn & Psy, University of British Columbia; Langs: Hindi; (604)875-2025

MISSIHA, Sharif B; Oshawa Health Centre, 301-247 Simcoe St N, Oshawa ON L1G 4T3; Tor'03; FRCPC; IntMed; Gastroent (Endoscopy). (905)725-1596; Fax. (905)725-3900.

MISSIUNA, Paul; 700 Main St E, Hamilton ON L8M 1K7; Wes'81; FRCSC; OrthSurg (General Surgery). Ac Staff, Hamilton Health Sciences Centre - McMaster University Medical Centre; (905)527-3014; Fax. (905)527-9149.

MISTERSKI, Jacek E; Dr J Misterski Med Prof, 201B-83 Dawson Rd, Guelph ON N1H 1B1; Wroclaw (Poland)'79; FRCPC; IntMed; Cardiol. Staff, Guelph General Hospital; Langs: Polish; (519)836-0409; Fax. (519)836-0064; drmisterskiprofessional@bellnet.ca.

MISTRY, Aneeta J; Grey Nuns Community Hosp & HC, 1100 Youville Drive West NW, Edmonton AB T6L 5X8; UBC'08; CCFP; CCFP(E.M.); Staff, Covenant Health - Grey Nuns Community Hospital; (780)735-7000

MISTRY, Bergez F; SMBD Jewish Gen Hosp, 3755 ch Cote-Sainte-Catherine, Montreal QC H3T 1E2; McG'95; CSPQ; FRCPC; Anes. Staff, Sir Mortimer B Davis Jewish General; (514)340-8222 x5701; Fax. (514)340-8108.

MISTRY, Dalpatbhai B; Lakeridge Hlth Corp-Oshawa, 1 Hospital Crt, Oshawa ON L1G 2B9; Baroda (India)'75; FRCPC; Psy. Staff Psy, Lakeridge Health - Oshawa Site; Langs: Gujarati; Hindi; (905)433-4411; Fax. (905)721-4742.

MISTRY, Dinesh J; PO Box 36, Golden BC V0A 1H0; Witwatersrand (South Africa)'76; MB ChB; CCFP; Langs: Gujarati; Hindi; Afrikaans; (250)344-3653; dineshmistry@hotmail.com.

MISTRY, Dipan N; 3037-5820 University Ave, Halifax NS B3H 1V7; Manchester (England)'99; MB ChB; (902)473-1986; Fax. (902)473-1260.

MISTRY, G Gavin; Royal York Med Arts Bldg, 108-1436 Royal York Rd, Etobicoke ON M9P 3A9; Cal'87; Staff, Humber River Regional Hospital - Church Street Site; (416)249-3471; Fax. (416)249-3648.

MISTRY, Niraj K; The Hosp for Sick Children, 10203-555 University Ave, Toronto ON M5G 1X8; Tor'07; FRCPC; Peds. Staff, The Hospital For Sick Children; (416)813-6933

MISTRY, Nisha; 210-1077 North Service Rd, Mississauga ON L4Y 1A6; Tor'06; FRCPC; Derm. (905)273-9009; Fax. (905)273-6409.

MISTRY, Prabhudas N; 106-22190 48 Ave, Langley BC V3A 3N5; South Gujarat (India)'76; MB BS; FRCPC; Psy. Consultant Psy, Langley Memorial Hospital; Langs: Hindi; Gujarati; (604)530-3213; Fax. (604)534-6192.

MISTRY, Ramesh V; B-796 Burnhamthorpe Rd W, Mississauga ON L5C 2R9; UBC'75; Ac Staff, Trillium Health Centre - Mississauga; (905)272-4770; Fax. (905)272-4733.

MISTRY, Ritesh K H; William Osler HC-Brampton, 2100 Bovaird Dr E, Brampton ON L6R 3J7; Tor'03; CCFP; Staff, William Osler Health System - Brampton Civic Hospital; (905)494-2120

MISTRY, Sheela B; Associates Medical Clinic, 123 10th Ave S, Cranbrook BC V1C 2N1; CCFP; (250)426-4231

MISTRY, Silloo B; Oakville Med Arts Bldg, 8-358 Reynolds St, Oakville ON L6J 3L9; Bombay (India)'62; MB BS; DABPed; FAAP; FRCPC; Peds. Affil Staff, Halton Healthcare Services Corporation - Oakville Site; (905)845-6181; Fax. (905)845-5924.

MISZKIEWICZ, Paul; 425 Marlborough Way NE, Calgary AB T2A 7E7; (Poland)'00; CCFP; (403)272-6422; Fax. (403)272-4297.

MISZTAL, Margaret; Scarborough Hosp-Birchmount, 3030 Birchmount Rd, Scarborough ON M1W 3W3; Lodz (Poland)'82; FRCPC; AnatPath. Staff, The Scarborough Hospital - Birchmount Campus; (416)495-2701 x5505

MITAL, Bernard; 100-2984 boul Taschereau, Greenfield Park QC J4V 2G9; Mon'66; Staff Emerg, Hopital Charles LeMoyne; (450)466-4333; Fax. (450)466-0716.

MITAL, Seema; The Hosp for Sick Children, 4514-555 University Ave, Toronto ON M5G 1X8; Bombay (India)'89; FACC; FAHA; Staff Cardiol, The Hospital For Sick Children; Assoc Prof Peds, University of Toronto; (416)813-7418; Fax. (416)813-5857; seema.mital@sickkids.ca.

MITCHELL, A Gregor; Polyclinique d'Argenteuil, 201-551 rue Berry, Lachute QC J8H 1S4; McG'79; CCFP; Staff, Centre Hospitalier d'Argenteuil; Langs: English; French; (450)562-3751; Fax. (450)562-1852.

MITCHELL, Alexander D; 310-18 Acadia St, Dartmouth NS B2Y 4H3; Dal'02; FRCSC; GenSurg. (902)405-4017; Fax. (902)405-4016.

MITCHELL, Andrea R; Cabrini Centre, 16811 88 Ave NW, Edmonton AB T5R 5Y6; Alb'06; FRCPC; Psy. (780)735-2934; Fax. (780)735-2973.

MITCHELL, Barry A; 5-500 Muskoka Rd 118 W, Bracebridge ON P1L 1T4; Tor'93; CCFP; (705)645-1677

MITCHELL, Barry A; PO Box 670, Claresholm AB T0L 0T0; Sask'69.

MITCHELL, Brian J; The Group Health Centre, 240 McNabb St, Sault Ste. Marie ON P6B 1Y5; Tor'88; FRCSC; Ophth. Assoc Staff, Sault Area Hospital - Sault Ste Marie; (705)759-1234; Fax. (705)541-2306.

MITCHELL, Catherine J; Thunder Bay Reg HSC-T-Bay, 3414-980 Oliver Rd, Thunder Bay ON P7B 6V4; McM'94; FRCPC; IntMed (Geriatric Medicine). Staff Hospitalist, Thunder Bay Regional Health Sciences Centre; (807)684-6030; Fax. (807)684-5894.

MITCHELL, Clare E; Child & Parent Resource Inst, 600 Sanatorium Rd, London ON N6H 3W7; Wes'87; MD; BSc; FRCPC; Peds (Child Development). Consultant, London Health Sciences Centre - University Hospital; Physician, Thame's Valley Children's Centre; Asst Prof, University of Western Ontario; (519)858-2774 x2360; Fax. (519)858-1390.

MITCHELL, Cynthia L; Copeman Healthcare Ctre, 400-628 12 Ave SW, Calgary AB T2R 0H6; UBC'87; CCFP; FCFP; (403)270-2273; Fax. (403)521-2250.

MITCHELL, David A; Scarborough Hosp-General Div, 3050 Lawrence Ave E, Scarborough ON M1P 2V5; Tor'67; CCFP; CCFP(E.M.); FCFP; Ac Staff, The Scarborough Hospital - General Campus; Ac Staff, North York General Hospital; (416)463-4037; Fax. (416)463-4031.

MITCHELL, David A; MUHC-Montreal Children's Hosp, B336-2300 rue Tupper, Montreal QC H3H 1P3; McG'85; Hem (P. Q.); Peds (Hematological Oncology). Staff, McGill University Health Centre - Montreal Children's Hospital; Langs: English; French; Fax. (514)412-4301; david.mitchell@muhc.mcgill.ca.

MITCHELL, Gerald O F; 102-1925 McCallum Rd, Abbotsford BC V2S 3N2; Stellenbosch (South Africa)'85; MB ChB; CCFP; (604)855-9455

MITCHELL, Grant A; Hôpital Ste-Justine, 3175 ch Cote-Sainte-Catherine, Montreal QC H3T 1C5; Sask'78; CCMG; AB; FRCPC; Peds (Biochemical Genetics); MedGenetics. Staff, Hôpital Ste-Justine; Prof Peds, Universite de Montreal; Langs: English; French; (514)345-4931 x3584; mitchell@justine.umontreal.ca.

MITCHELL, Hugh J; Dr Mitchell's Med Walk-In Clin, 6-660 Garrison Rd, Fort Erie ON L2A 6E2; Qns'84; (905)994-9417; Fax. (905)994-9625.

MITCHELL, Ian; Alberta Children's Hosp, C3 200-2888 Shaganappi Trail N, Calgary AB T3B 6A8; Edinburgh (Scotland)'68; MB ChB; DCH; FCCP; MA; FRCPC; Peds (Respirology). Ac Staff/Specialist, Alberta Children's Hospital; Prof, University of Calgary; (403)955-7818; Fax. (403)955-7059; ian.mitchell@calgaryhealthregion.ca.

MITCHELL, Ian L; 308-8425 120 St, Delta BC V4C 6R2; Cal'77; BAP; (604)596-2211; Fax. (604)596-2233; dr.ian.mitchell@shaw.ca.

MITCHELL, Ian V; Royal Inland Hosp, 311 Columbia St, Kamloops BC V2C 2T1; McG'90; FRCPC; EmergMed. Staff, Royal Inland Hospital; (250)374-5111

MITCHELL, Jacqueline R; North Bramalea Med Centre, 202-9780 Bramalea Rd, Brampton ON L6S 2P1; Tor'87; CCFP; FCFP; Ac Staff, William Osler Health System - Brampton Civic Hospital; (905)791-2390; Fax. (905)791-8476.

MITCHELL, Jessica S; Maple Family Health Team, D2-1036 Princess St, Kingston ON K7L 1H2; Leicester (England)'07; CCFP; (613)531-5888

MITCHELL, Joanne E; Ridgeview Med Centre, 212-1240 Railway Ave, Canmore AB T1W 1P4; Cal'81; CCFP; FCFP; (403)609-8333; Fax. (403)609-3666.

MITCHELL, John J; MUHC-Montreal Children's Hosp, A429-2300 rue Tupper, Montreal QC H3H 1P3; UBC'98; MSc; FRCP; MD; FRCPC; Peds; Endocrin (P.Q.); Endocrin&Metab. Staff, McGill University Health Centre - Montreal Children's Hospital; (514)412-4400 x22438; Fax. (514)412-4296; john.mitchell@muhc.mcgill.ca.

MITCHELL, Kathleen S; Gulf Canada Square, 340-401 9 Ave SW, Calgary AB T2P 3C5; Cal'84; BSc(Hon); LLB; FRCPC; Peds. Staff, Alberta Children's Hospital; Staff, Rockyview General Hospital; Clinical Asst Prof, University of Calgary; (403)221-4434; Fax. (403)221-4466.

MITCHELL, L Andrew; Nanaimo Reg Gen Hosp, 1200 Dufferin Cres, Nanaimo BC V9S 2B7; Cal'80; Staff, Nanaimo Regional General Hospital; (250)754-2141

MITCHELL, L Brent; Foothills Med Centre, C822A-1403 29 St NW, Calgary AB T2N 2T9; Cal'75; FRCPC; IntMed (Electrophysiology); Cardiol. Prof Cardiac Sciences, University of Calgary; (403)944-1110; Fax. (403)944-2906.

MITCHELL, Lesley A; City of Lakes Fam Hlth Team, C-960 Notre Dame Ave, Sudbury ON P3A 2T4; Ott'82; CCFP; FCFP; Staff, Health Sciences North-St Joseph's Health Centre; Staff, Health Sciences North - Memorial Site; Staff, Health Sciences North-Laurentian Site; (705)560-1018; Fax. (705)566-7617.

MITCHELL, Marianna K; Dundas Med Centre, 306-220 Dundas St W, Whitby ON L1N 8M7; McM'89; FAAP; BSc; FRCPC; Peds (Neonatology). (905)665-9001; Fax. (905)665-9335; drmarymitchell@bellnet.ca.

MITCHELL, Michael J; Queen Elizabeth II HSC-Halifax, 1796 Summer St, Halifax NS B3H 3A7; Dal'80; FRCPC; DiagRad. Staff Radiol, Queen Elizabeth II Health Sciences Centre - Victoria General Site; Staff, Nova Scotia Rehabilitation Centre; Staff, Queen Elizabeth II Health Sciences Centre - Halifax Infirmary Site; Assoc Prof, Dalhousie University; (902)473-2796; Fax. (902)473-2018.

MITCHELL, Nadine C; Stratford Gen Hosp, 46 General Hospital Dr, Stratford ON N5A 2Y6; Saba (Netherlands Antilles)'08; Peds. Staff, Stratford General Hospital - Huron Perth Healthcare Alliance; (519)271-8120

MITCHELL, Nicholas D; University of Alberta Hosp, 1E1-8440 112 St NW, Edmonton AB T6G 2B7; Alb'05; FRCPC; Psy. Staff, University of Alberta Hospital; (780)407-6501

MITCHELL, Patrick C; Mitchell Eye Center, 5340 1 St SW, Calgary AB T2H 0C8; Cal'00; FRCSC; Ophth. (403)258-1773; Fax. (403)258-2704.

MITCHELL, Patrick J; 22-1517 Dufferin Cres, Nanaimo BC V9S 5H6; Cal'85; FACOG; FRCSC; ObstGyn (Colposcopy). Staff, Nanaimo Regional General Hospital; (250)754-1258; Fax. (250)754-2582; pjm7@shaw.ca.

MITCHELL, Paul A; Orleans Medical-Dental Centre, 400H-2555 St. Joseph Blvd, Orleans ON K1C 1S6; Wes'81; (613)724-6987

MITCHELL, Philip C; Suitor House, 1004 8 Ave SE, Calgary AB T2G 0M4; Qns'83; FRCPC; GenSurg (Upper Gastrointestinal Surgery). Staff Surg, Peter Lougheed Centre; Dir, Upper GI Center of Excellence; Clinical Asst Prof, University of Calgary; (403)264-6720; Fax. (403)237-0167; philipmitchell@mac.com.

MITCHELL, Rebecca S; Heritage Med Research Ctre, 362-107 University Campus NW, Edmonton AB T6G 2S2; Sask'00; FRCPC; IntMed; Endocrin&Metab. Staff, University of Alberta Hospital; Langs: French; (780)407-3636; Fax. (780)407-6702; rebeccam@ualberta.ca.

MITCHELL, Robert J; Mitchell Eye Center, 100-5340 1 St SW, Calgary AB T2H 0C8; Alb'71; FRCSC; Ophth (Refractive Cataract Surgery). Staff, Alberta Children's Hospital; Staff, Foothills Medical Centre; Staff Ophth, Canadian Forces Health Services; Physician, Alberta Health Services Calgary; Teach Staff, University of Calgary; (403)640-2020; Fax. (403)258-2704.

MITCHELL, Ryan W K; 204-119 Memorial Ave, Orillia ON L3V 5X1; Wes'10; CCFP.

MITCHELL, Sheona M; St Paul's Hosp, 435-1081 Burrard St, Vancouver BC V6Z 1Y6; Cal'07; Staff, Providence Health Care - St Paul's Hospital; Langs: Spanish; Swahili; (604)682-2344 x66140

MITCHELL, Theodore W; West Haldimand Gen Hosp, 75 Parkview Rd, Hagersville ON N0A 1H0; Wes'94; Staff, West Haldimand General Hospital; (905)768-3311; Fax. (905)768-4133.

MITCHELL, Thomas; Mediclinic, 101-3333 8th St E, Saskatoon SK S7H 4K1; Lusaka (Zambia)'86; CCFP; (306)955-1530; Fax. (306)955-8811.

MITCHELL, Victoria P; Gladstone Prof Centre, 200-6155 North St, Halifax NS B3K 5R3; Dal'81; BSc(Hon.); CCFP; Court Staff, Queen Elizabeth II Health Sciences Centre - Victoria General Site; Court Staff, IWK Health Centre; (902)422-7431; Fax. (902)454-8603.

MITCHELL, W Murray; 1519 Parkwood Dr, North Bay ON P1B 4R1; Qns'65; FRCPC; PhysMed&Rehab (Electromyography). Vis Consultant, Kirkland & District Hospital; Vis Consultant, Temiskaming Hospital; Vis Consultant, Timmins & District Hospital; (705)476-1141; Fax. (705)476-8972.

MITCHELL, Wade R; Central Med Clinic, 102-150 Saint Paul St, Collingwood ON L9Y 3P2; UBC'99; BA(Hon); CCFP; Staff, Collingwood General & Marine Hospital; Assoc Prof, McMaster University; Langs: Spanish; (705)445-2827; Fax. (705)445-1671.

MITCHELL, Wallace M M; Niagara H System-G Niagara, PO Box 1018 Stn Main 5546 Portage Rd, Niagara Falls ON L2E 6X2; Qns'60; DABPN; Psy. Court Staff, Niagara Health System - Greater Niagara General Site; (905)358-0171; Fax. (905)358-4954.

MITCHELL-GILL, Michael; 3-300 Taunton Rd E, Oshawa ON L1G 7T4; London (England)'63; LRCP; MRCS; LMCC; FFARCS; FRCPC; Anes. (905)723-2144; Fax. (905)723-6953.

MITCHNER, Leslie K; 1317-750 Broadway W, Vancouver BC V5Z 1J3; Cal'91; CCFP; (604)876-0711

MITELMAN, Bernice; Markham Stouffvile Hosp, PO Box 1800 Stn Main 381 Church St, Markham ON L3P 7P3; Tor'00; CCFP; CCFP(E.M.); Staff, Markham Stouffville Hospital; (905)472-5342; berniceyona@hotmail.com.

MITENKO, Nancy L; 401-1338 Broadway W, Vancouver BC V6H 1H2; Cal'97; FRCSC; ObstGyn. (604)736-7131; Fax. (604)736-5403.

MITENKO, Paul A; Medical Centre, 24-1515 Dufferin Cres, Nanaimo BC V9S 2B8; Man'67; FRCPC; IntMed. Staff, Nanaimo Regional General Hospital; (250)753-2446; Fax. (250)753-9686.

MITHA, Alim; Foothills Med Centre, 1403 29 St NW, Calgary AB T2N 2T9; Alb'02; FRCSC; Neursurg. Staff, Foothills Medical Centre; (403)944-4550; Fax. (403)944-8712.

MITHA, Hamza; 152-15277 Castle Downs Rd NW, Edmonton AB T5X 3N5; Natal (South Africa)'97; MB ChB; DA(SA); CCFP; (780)472-2273

MITHA, Karime; Norburn Med Clinic, 200-4012 Hastings St, Burnaby BC V5C 2H9; UBC'90; Staff/Chair Dept of Ob/Gyn, Burnaby Hospital; Clin Instructor, University of British Columbia; (604)299-2677; Fax. (604)298-6656.

MITHA, Pyarali A; 1347 12 Ave SW, Calgary AB T3C 0P6; Glasgow (Scotland)'65; MB ChB; DCH(Ire); DTMH(Liverpool); DObstRCOG; Langs: Gujarati; (403)245-3381; Fax. (403)245-0593.

MITHANI, Akber H; PO Box 33836 Stn D, Vancouver BC V6J 4L6; Mem'88; Ac Staff, BC Mental Health & Addiction Service; Langs: Gujarati; Hindi; Kacchi; Kiswahili; Swahili; Urdu.

MITHOOWANI, Mohamed H A; 1-17 Frank St, Strathroy ON N7G 2R2; Wes'74; Ac Staff, Strathroy Middlesex General Hospital - Middlesex Hospital Alliance; (519)245-3370; Fax. (519)245-5533.

MITMAKER, Benjamin; 100-6000 ch de la Cote-des-Nei, Montreal QC H3S 1Z8; Geneva (Switzerland)'57; MSc; PhD; FRCSC; GenSurg. Staff, Sir Mortimer B Davis Jewish General; McGill University; (514)733-5691

MITMAKER, Elliot; MUHC-Montreal Gen Hosp, L9 417-1650 av Cedar, Montreal QC H3G 1A4; Thomas Jefferson University (USA)'03; FRCSC; GenSurg. Staff, McGill University Health Centre - Montreal General Campus; (514)934-1934

MITNICK, Howard J; Club Tiny Tots, 3550-6900 boul Decarie, Montreal QC H2X 3T8; McG'00; CCFP; (514)342-9911

MITOFF, Peter; Dept of Cardiology, 1188-585 University Ave, Toronto ON M5G 2N2; Tor'06; FRCPC; IntMed; Cardiol.

MITRANA, Irene; Grand River Hosp-KW Hlth Ctre, PO Box 9056 Stn C 835 King St W, Kitchener ON N2G 1G3; Tor'05; CCFP; CCFP(E.M.); Staff, Grand River Hospital - Kitchener/Waterloo Health Centre; (519)749-4300

MITRI, Mira; Dept of Family Med, 60 Murray St, Toronto ON M5T 3L9; Mon'10; CCFP; (416)586-4800

MITRI, Ragheed K; Hotel-Dieu Grace Hosp, 1030 Ouellette Ave, Windsor ON N9A 1E1; Qns'03; FRCPC; DiagRad. Staff, Hôtel-Dieu Grace Hospital; (519)973-4411

MITRICA, Mirela; Groupe Med Stillview, 245-175 av Stillview, Pointe-Claire QC H9R 4S3; Bucharest (Romania)'88; CCFP; (514)697-1529

MITTAL, Charu; Niagara H System-Welland Site, 65 Third St, Welland ON L3B 4W6; Wes'00; FRCPC; DiagRad. Staff, Niagara Health System - Welland Hospital Site; (905)378-4647

MITTAL, Richa; Guelph Gen Hosp, 115 Delhi St, Guelph ON N1E 4J4; McM'01; FRCPC; DiagRad. Staff, Guelph General Hospital; (519)822-5350; richa_mittal@yahoo.com.

MITTELSTEADT, Lyle B; AMA Physician Locum Services, 12230 106 Ave NW, Edmonton AB T5N 3Z1; Alb'75; BMedSci; (780)482-0300; Fax. (780)482-5445.

MITTERMAIER, Barbara M E; Workers' Comp Board, 100-5500 152 St, Surrey BC V3S 5J9; Cape Town (South Africa)'87; MB ChB; CCFP; (604)232-7041

MITTERMAIER, Michael E R; Surrey Mem Hosp, 13750 96 Ave, Surrey BC V3V 1Z2; Cape Town (South Africa)'87; MB ChB; CCFP; CCFP(E.M.); Staff, Surrey Memorial Hospital; (604)588-3369

MITTLER, Gerald R; Medical Bldg, 1503-805 Broadway W, Vancouver BC V5Z 1K1; Man'73; BSc; FRCPC; Psy. (604)879-1503; Fax. (604)879-1594.

MITTON, Gregory D; Windsor Reg Hosp-Metropolitan, 1995 Lens Ave, Windsor ON N8W 1L9; Dal'77; FRCPC; DiagRad. Staff, Windsor Regional Hospital - Metropolitan Site; (519)254-5577

MITTON, Jennifer M; GMF de Gatineau, 201-908 boul Maloney E, Gatineau QC J8P 1H5; Dal'10; CCFP; (819)663-9676

MITTON, Kenneth A; 203-1789 Mountain Rd, Moncton NB E1G 5C4; Dal'83; CCFP; (506)387-2905; Fax. (506)387-3921.

MITTOO, Shikha; L2 003-60 Murray St, Toronto ON M5T 3L9; McM'01; FRCPC; IntMed; Rheum. Staff, Mount Sinai Hospital; (416)586-4800; Fax. (416)586-3101.

MITTRA-MELROSE, Vidushi; 4699 Marine Ave, Powell River BC V8A 2L2; Alb'06; CCFP; Langs: Hindi; (604)485-9500

MITWALLY, Mohamed F M; Div of Reproductive Science, 210-150 Bloor St W, Toronto ON M5S 2X9; Minya (Egypt)'90; (416)972-0777; Fax. (416)972-0036.

MIU, Daniela I; Ermineskin Med Clinic, 301-2377 111 St NW, Edmonton AB T6J 5E5; (Romania)'92; (780)436-8731; Fax. (780)434-8732.

MIURA, Carlos; Royal Ottawa Hlth Care Group, 1145 Carling Ave, Ottawa ON K1Z 7K4; Buenos Aires (Argentina)'67; FRCPC; Psy (Schizophrenia). Staff Psy, Royal Ottawa Mental Health Centre - Royal Ottawa Health Care Group; Asst Prof, University of Ottawa; (613)722-6521 x6533; Fax. (613)798-2971.

MIVILLE-DESCHENES, Marc; CSSS de la Region de Thetford, 1717 rue Notre-Dame E, Thetford Mines QC G6G 2V4; Laval'93; OrthSurg (P.Q.). Staff, Hopital du CSS de la Region de Thetford; (418)338-7711; Fax. (418)338-7794.

MIYAGISHIMA, Robert T; Copeman Healthcare Centre, 400-1128 Hornby St, Vancouver BC V6Z 2L4; UBC'60; FACS; FRCSC; GenSurg; Cardiovasc&ThorSurg. Consultant, Vancouver General Hospital - Centennial Pavillion; Dir Surg & Research, Providence Health Care - St Paul's Hospital; Prof/Head Cardiovasc & ThorSurg, University of British Columbia; Langs: Japanese.

MIYANJI, Firoz; Children's & Women's HC of BC, A234-4480 Oak St, Vancouver BC V6H 3V4; Ott'99; FRCSC; OrthSurg. Staff, BC Children's Hospital; (604)875-2651

MIYASAKI, Janis M; Univ Hlth Network-Toronto Western Hosp, 7MCL-399 Bathurst St, Toronto ON M5T 2S8; Tor'88; FRCPC; Neur (Movement Disorders). Ac Staff, Toronto Western Hospital - University Health Network; (416)603-6422; Fax. (416)603-5004; miyasaki@uhnresearch.ca.

MIYATA, Kenji S; Headwaters Health Centre, 100 Rolling Hills Dr, Orangeville ON L9W 4X9; Tor'03; PhD; CCFP; Staff, Headwaters Health Care Centre - Orangeville Site; Staff, Dryden Regional Health Centre; (519)941-2410; Fax. (519)942-0483.

MIYAUCHI, David K; Foothills Med Centre, 1403 29 St NW, Calgary AB T2N 2T9; Alb'60; FRCPC; Psy. Coord Psy/Dep Head Dept of Psy Alberta Health Services Calgary Zone Site, Foothills Medical Centre; Consultant Psy, Covenant Health - Banff Mineral Springs Hospital; Clin Prof Psy, University of Calgary; (403)944-1297; Fax. (403)270-3451; david.miyauchi@albertahealthservices.ca.

MIZDRAK, Nikolina; Univ Hlth Network-Toronto Western Hosp, 2W404-399 Bathurst St, Toronto ON M5T 2S8; McM'02; CCFP; Staff, Toronto Western Hospital - University Health Network; Langs: Serbian; French; (416)603-5888 x2; Fax. (416)603-5448.

MIZERA, Ryszard; Hamilton HS-Henderson Site, 711 Concession St, Hamilton ON L8V 1C3; Crakow (Poland)'76; FRCPC; IntMed. Staff, Hamilton Health Sciences Centre-Juravinski Site; Asst Prof, McMaster University; (905)389-6898; Fax. (905)575-7320.

MIZGALA, Henry F; UBC Hospital, S 110-2211 Wesbrook Mall, Vancouver BC V6T 2B5; McG'57; FACC; FRCPC; IntMed; Cardiol (P.Q.) (Clinical Cardiology). Staff, UBC Hospital - Koerner Pavillion; Hon Staff, Vancouver General Hospital - Centennial Pavillion; Hon Consultant, BC Cancer Agency Vancouver Centre; Hon Consultant, G F Strong Rehabilitation Centre; Emeritus Prof, University of British Columbia; Langs: Polish; French; (604)822-1747; Fax. (604)822-7625.

MIZRAHI, Romina; Addiction & Mental Hlth-Clarke, 250 College St, Toronto ON M5T 1R8; Buenos Aires (Argentina)'98; Staff, Centre for Addiction & Mental Health (CAMH) - College Street Site; (416)535-8501 x4508

MIZZI, Trent D; The Hosp for Sick Children, 555 University Ave, Toronto ON M5G 1X8; Cal'96; FRCPC; Peds. Staff, The Hospital For Sick Children; (416)813-7500; Fax. (416)813-5043; trent.mizzi@sickkids.ca.

MKHABELA, Sikhumbuzo G; 2835 Mill Woods Rd NW, Edmonton AB T6K 4A9; Witwatersrand (South Africa)'99; MB ChB; (780)440-9100; Fax. (780)461-1985.

MLYNAREK, Marcin A; SMBD Jewish Gen Hosp, 3755 ch Cote-Sainte-Catherine, Montreal QC H3T 1E2; McG'02; FRCSC; Otol. Staff, Sir Mortimer B Davis Jewish General; (514)340-8222

MNYUSIWALLA, Anisa; Stratford Gen Hosp, 46 General Hospital Dr, Stratford ON N5A 2Y6; Tor'04; FRCPC; DiagRad. Staff, Stratford General Hospital - Huron Perth Healthcare Alliance; (519)271-8210

MNYUSIWALLA, Yusuf A; St Mary's Gen Hosp, 911 Queens Blvd, Kitchener ON N2M 1B2; Bristol (England)'73; MB ChB; DABR; FRCPC; DiagRad. Chief Dept of Radiol, St Mary's General Hospital; (519)749-6455

MO, Anita B; Scarborough Prof Centre, 208-1371 Neilson Rd, Scarborough ON M1B 4Z8; Tor'00; BA(Science); FRCSC; ObstGyn. Staff, Rouge Valley Health System - Centenary Health Centre Site; Langs: Cantonese; (416)286-3830; Fax. (416)286-3133.

MO, Fan D; 206-311 McArthur Ave, Ottawa ON K1L 8M3; Ott'09; CCFP; (613)740-0200

MO, Lup-Ho; 105-4245 Sheppard Ave E, Scarborough ON M1S 1T6; Tor'79; FRCPC; Peds. (416)292-3363; Fax. (416)292-3399.

MOALLI, Linda; Clinique d'Urgence Pincourt, 430 boul Don-Quichotte, N-D-D-l'ILe-Perrot QC J7V 0J9; Mon'80; (514)453-0884; Fax. (514)425-3968; lindamoalli@hotmail.com.

MOAMAI, Javad; Ctr Hosp Pierre-Janet, 20 rue Pharand, Gatineau QC J9A 1K7; National (Iran)'77; Staff, Centre Hospitalier Pierre-Janet; (819)776-8010; Fax. (819)776-8002.

MOAMMER, Gemah M A; 115-675 Queen St S, Kitchener ON N2M 1A1; (Libya)'96; FRCSC; OrthSurg. (519)603-0989; Fax. (519)603-0996.

MOAVENI, Azadeh; Univ Hlth Network-Toronto Western Hosp, 399 Bathurst St, Toronto ON M5T 2S8; Wes'03; CCFP; Staff, Toronto Western Hospital - University Health Network; (416)603-5888; Fax. (416)603-5448.

MOAWAD, Medhat M M G; Jacksons Arm Med Clinic, PO Box 119, Jackson's Arm NL A0K 3H0; Ain Shams (Egypt)'82; MB BCh; (709)459-3231

MOAWAD, Victor F F; Assiniboine Clinic, 633 Lodge Ave, Winnipeg MB R3J 0S9; Cairo (Egypt)'89; CCFP; Staff, Elizabeth M Crowe Memorial Hospital; (204)958-6709; Fax. (204)888-1750; vmoawad@irha.mb.ca.

MOAYYEDI, Paul; McMaster University HSC, 4W8-1280 Main St W, Hamilton ON L8S 4K1; Bristol (England)'88; FRCPC; IntMed; Gastroent. Staff, Hamilton Health Sciences Centre - McMaster Children's Hospital; (905)521-2100 x76764; Fax. (905)521-4958.

MOBAYED, Georges N E; 102-4275 Innes Rd, Orleans ON K1C 1T1; Alexandria (Egypt)'81; CCFP; (613)841-2011

MOBBS, Christopher J; 402-3210 25th Ave, Vernon BC V1T 1P1; Pretoria (South Africa)'76; MB ChB; MRCOG; FRCSC; ObstGyn. Staff, Vernon Jubilee Hospital; (250)542-0343; Fax. (250)503-3919.

MOBILOS, Sophia; 501-294 Main St, Toronto ON M4C 4X5; Wes'08; BSc; CCFP; Langs: Greek; French; (416)698-8788; Fax. (416)691-3641.

MOCANU, Adriana; Glenrose Rehab Hosp, 10230 111 Ave NW, Edmonton AB T5G 0B7; (Romania)'89; CCFP; Staff, Glenrose Rehabilitation Hospital; (780)735-7934; Fax. (780)735-8837.

MOCANU, Brindusa I; Cancer Ctr of Southeastern Ont, 25 King St W, Kingston ON K7L 5P9; (Romania)'96; IntMed. Fellow, Cancer Centre of Southeastern Ontario.

MOCANU, Maria; Clinique Med Belanger, 3871 rue Belanger, Montreal QC H1X 3M7; (Romania)'79; Staff, Centre Hospitalier Pierre le Gardeur; (514)722-1166

MOCARSKI, Eva J M; 202-55 Queen St E, Toronto ON M5C 1R6; Tor'85; FRFPS; FRCSC; ObstGyn (Colposcopy). Ac Staff, St Michael's Hospital; Asst Prof, University of Toronto; Langs: Polish; (416)864-5241

MOCCIA, Patrizia; 835 10th Ave W, Vancouver BC V5Z 4E8; UBC'08; (604)875-5151

MOCCIA, Rino P; Com El Med Bldg, 301-2620 Commercial Dr, Vancouver BC V5N 4C4; UBC'77; Langs: Italian; (604)873-6633

MODDEL, Garry; 206-360 College St, Toronto ON M5T 1S6; Tor'72; BSc; FRCPC; Neur (Head Injury). Ac Staff, The Scarborough Hospital - General Campus; (416)923-7524; Fax. (416)923-8067.

MODDEMANN, Diane M; Children's Hosp, CK267-840 Sherbrook St, Winnipeg MB R3A 1S1; Man'80; FRCPC; Peds (Developmental Pediatrics). Staff Child Development Clinic, Health Sciences Centre; Assoc Prof, University of Manitoba; (204)787-2424; Fax. (204)787-1138; moddema@cc.umanitoba.ca.

MODI, Amita V; PO Box 5203 Stn B, Victoria BC V8R 6N4; UBC'88; CCFP; FCFP.

MODI, Anjana; 2 1-555 Concession St, Hamilton ON L8V 1A8; Kanpur (India)'71; MB BS; DCH; FAAP; FRCPC; Peds. (905)387-0831

MODI, Deepshikha; 8675 Granville St, Vancouver BC V6P 5A3; Aligarh (India)'98; CCFP; Langs: Hindi; (604)263-2646

MODI, Eesh; BC Cancer Agency-Fraser Valley, 13750 96 Ave, Surrey BC V3V 1Z2; Alb'93; FRCPC; Anes. Staff, BC Cancer Agency Fraser Valley Centre; (604)585-5530

MODI, Monica; University of Alberta Hosp, 5F4.01-8440 112 St NW, Edmonton AB T6G 2B7; Alb'97; BMedSci; CCFP; Clin Associate Hematology, University of Alberta Hospital; (780)407-6132; Fax. (780)407-1136; docmodi@yahoo.ca.

MODI, Renuca; Weight Wise Adult Bariatric Cl, 472-10405 111 Ave NW, Edmonton AB T5G 0B8; Alb'00; CCFP; Staff, Royal Alexandra Hospital; (780)735-5620

MODI, Thankamma; Mountain Med Walk-In Clinic, 5A-880 Upper Wentworth Ave, Hamilton ON L9A 5H2; Cologne (Germany)'72; Langs: German; Malayalam; (905)575-0808; Fax. (905)574-3003.

MODRY, Dennis L; University of Alberta Hosp, 3H210-8440 112 St NW, Edmonton AB T6G 2B7; Alb'73; MSc(ExpSurg.); AB; AB; FACS; FRCSC; GenSurg; Cardiovasc&ThorSurg. Staff, University of Alberta Hospital; Associate Clin Prof, University of Alberta; (780)407-3048; Fax. (780)407-3056; dennis.modry@albertahealthservices.ca.

MODY, Ami N; Credit Valley Prof Bldg, 204-2300 Eglinton Ave W, Mississauga ON L5M 2V8; Bombay (India)'96; FRCPC; IntMed; Rheum. Staff, The Credit Valley Hospital; Langs: Hindi; (905)369-0092; Fax. (905)369-0117.

MODY, Anita; Halton Heart Centre, 34-1960 Appleby Line, Burlington ON L7L 0B7; Wes'03; Cardiol; IntMed. (905)332-9292; Fax. (905)332-9244.

MODY, Christopher H; HSC-Faculty of Med, HRIC4AA14-3330 Hospital Dr NW, Calgary AB T2N 4N1; Qns'81; FACP; FCCP; FRCPC; IntMed (Pulmonology); Respir. Staff, Foothills Medical Centre; Prof, University of Calgary; (403)220-8479; Fax. (403)270-2772; cmody@ucalgary.ca.

MOE, Gordon W; St Michael's Hosp, 30 Bond St, Toronto ON M5B 1W8; Tor'79; FACC; DABIM; FRCP(Cardiol); MSc; FRCPC; IntMed (Adult Cardiology); Cardiol. Staff Cardiologist, St Michael's Hospital; Prof Med, University of Toronto; Langs: Cantonese; Mandarin; (416)864-5319; Fax. (416)864-5941; moeg@smh.toronto.on.ca.

MOE, Jan Fredrik; PO Box 100, Kinistino SK S0J 1H0; RCS (Ireland)'72; LRCPS(Ire); LM; Staff, Kinistino Jubilee Lodge; Staff, Melfort Hospital; Langs: Norwegian; German; Swedish; Danish; Bilingual(French/English); (306)864-2212; Fax. (306)864-3102; jfmoe@hotmail.com.

MOECK, Lori S; Lorraine Wing Tower C, 201 Deacon St, Pembroke ON K8A 2J6; Qns'88; CCFP; FCFP; (613)732-5777; Fax. (613)732-5774.

MOELLENHOFF, Michael E; St Mary's Hosp Centre, 3830 av Lacombe, Montreal QC H3T 1M5; New York (USA)'94; FRCPC; Anes. Staff, St Mary's Hospital Centre; (514)345-3511

MOELLER, Jeremy J; Dartmouth Med Centre, 504-44 Portland St, Dartmouth NS B2Y 1H4; Dal'04; FRCPC; Neur. (902)420-1878; Fax. (902)420-1623.

MOENS, Francois O P; The Juravinski Cancer Centre, 699 Concession St, Hamilton ON L8V 5C2; Ghent (Belgium)'76; FRCSC; ObstGyn (Gynecologic Oncology). Staff, Hamilton Health Sciences Centre-Juravinski Site; Staff, Thunder Bay Regional Health Sciences Centre; Court Staff, St Joseph's Healthcare - Charlton Campus; Affil Staff, Joseph Brant Memorial Hospital; Court Staff, The Brant Community Healthcare System - Brantford General Hospital Site; Assoc Prof, McMaster University; Langs: Dutch; French; Flemish; (905)389-5688; Fax. (905)575-6343; francois.moens@jcc.hhsc.ca.

MOENS, Hilda; 2F-2951 Walker's Line, Burlington ON L7M 4Y1; Gent (Belgium)'77; Langs: Dutch; French; (905)336-9620 x1030; Fax. (905)336-9650.

MOFFAT, Grant S; Credit Valley Surgical Assoc, 2207 Dunwin Dr, Mississauga ON L5L 1X1; Wes'96; FRCSC; GenSurg. (905)820-3633; Fax. (905)820-3352.

MOFFAT, John G; 2863 Ellesmere Rd, Scarborough ON M1E 5E9; Tor'60; MSc; FICS; FRCSC; GenSurg (Breast Surgery). Locum Tenens, Southlake Regional Health Centre; (416)284-8131

MOFFAT, Murray J; 292 King St W, Oshawa ON L1J 2J9; Tor'67; (905)436-6163; Fax. (905)432-7099.

MOFFAT, Robert C; Canada Place Bldg, 206-107 Shirreff Ave, North Bay ON P1B 7K8; Wes'62; DAB; FACS; FRCSC; GenSurg; VascSurg. Staff, North Bay Regional Health Centre - Regional Mental Health; (705)482-1063

MOFFAT, Stephanie M; The Richmond Hosp, 7000 Westminster Hwy, Richmond BC V6X 1A2; Tor'95; CCFP; Staff, Richmond Hospital; (604)278-9711

MOFFATT, Alexander J; Providence Healthcare, 3276 St Clair Ave E, Scarborough ON M1L 1W1; Tor'62; Staff, Providence Healthcare; (416)285-3603

MOFFATT, Dana C H; St Boniface Gen Hosp, C5122-409 Tache Ave, Winnipeg MB R2H 2A6; Man'04; FRCPC; IntMed; Gastroent. Staff, St Boniface General Hospital; (204)233-8563

MOFFATT, Hayley W M; Children's Hosp, 840 Sherbrook St, Winnipeg MB R3A 1S1; Man'05; FRCPC; DiagRad.

MOFFATT, Josiah B; 8 Heintzman St, Toronto ON M6P 2J6; Tor'94; FRCPC; IntMed (Family Medicine). Staff Emerg, Women's College Hospital; (416)604-8004; Fax. (416)604-2947.

MOFFATT, Michael E K; Winnipeg Reg Health Authority, 4F-650 Main St, Winnipeg MB R3B 1E2; Tor'70; MSc; FRCPC; Peds. Staff Child Health Program, St Boniface General Hospital; Ac Staff Prof/Head, Health Sciences Centre; Med Dir, Winnipeg Regional Health Authority Corporate Office; Prof, University of Manitoba; (204)926-7000; mmoffatt@exchange.hsc.mb.ca.

MOFFATT, Michael H; St Joseph's Health Centre, 30 The Queensway, Toronto ON M6R 1B5; McG'93; Staff Emerg, St Joseph's Health Centre; (416)530-6584; Fax. (416)530-6370.

MOFFATT, Richard A; Piper Creek Med Clinic, 200-3215 49 Ave, Red Deer AB T4N 0M8; Sask'86; CCFP; FCFP; (403)986-7265; Fax. (403)986-7604.

MOFFATT, Scott M; Health Sciences Centre, 300 Prince Philip Dr, St. John's NL A1B 3V6; Mem'87; CCFP; FCFP; Staff, Health Sciences Centre; Asst Dean Student Affairs, Memorial Univ of Newfoundland; (709)777-7920; Fax. (709)777-7916.

MOFFATT, Susan L; Kingston Gen Hosp, 76 Stuart St, Kingston ON K7L 2V7; Qns'78; ABIM(Resp.& Critical Car; FRCPC; IntMed; Respir. Staff Intensivist, Kingston General Hospital; Consultant, Providence Care - St Mary's of the Lake Hospital Site; Att Staff, Hotel-Dieu Hospital; (613)548-2332; Fax. (613)549-1459; moffatts@post.queensu.ca.

MOFFETT, Stephane; The Ottawa Hosp-Gen Campus, 501 Smyth Rd, Ottawa ON K1H 8L6; Ott'02; FRCPC; Anes. Staff, The Ottawa Hospital - General Campus; (613)737-8899 x72827

MOFFITT, Julie; 105-185 av Acadie, Dieppe NB E1A 1G6; Sher'09; CCFP.

MOFFORD, Linda M; North Hill Professional Ctr, 258-1632 14 Ave NW, Calgary AB T2N 1M7; Cal'85; CCFP; CCFP(E.M.); FCFP; (403)291-3001; Fax. (403)291-3139.

MOGA, Rebecca A; Univ Hlth Network-Toronto Western Hosp, 399 Bathurst St, Toronto ON M5T 2S8; Ott'07; FRCPC; Anes. Staff, Toronto Western Hospital - University Health Network; (416)603-2581

MOGAN, Norah; PO Box 2159, Liverpool NS B0T 1K0; Dal'01; CCFP; (902)354-5017; Fax. (902)354-4054.

MOGENTALE, Tara L; Victoria Gen Hosp, 1 Hospital Way, Victoria BC V8Z 6R5; UBC'99; CCFP; Staff, Victoria General Hospital; (250)727-4212

MOGHADAM, Soraya; Montfort Hosp, 713 Montreal Rd, Ottawa ON K1K 0T2; Ott'97; BSc; FRCPC; IntMed; Nephrol. Staff, Montfort Hospital; (613)327-9454

MOGHADDAM-ABRISHAMI, K; Halton Family Health Centre, 2951 Walkers Line, Burlington ON L7M 4Y1; (Iran)'93; CCFP; Med Staff, Joseph Brant Memorial Hospital; (905)336-3437; Fax. (905)336-9650; kmabrishami@hotmail.com.

MOGHARRABI, Mehran; The Group Health Centre, 240 McNabb St, Sault Ste. Marie ON P6B 1Y5; Jundi Shapur (Iran)'75; Ac Staff, Sault Area Hospital - Sault Ste Marie; Langs: Persian; (705)759-1234 x644; Fax. (705)541-2215; mogharrabi_m@ghc.on.ca.

MOGHRABI, Albert; Ctr Hosp de Verdun, 4000 boul Lasalle, Verdun QC H4G 2A3; Mon'86; FRCPC; IntMed; MedOncol (P.Q.); Hem. Staff, Centre Hospitalier de Verdun; (514)362-1000 x2609; Fax. (514)345-4792.

MOGHRABI, Bashar S; The Moncton Hosp, 135 MacBeath Ave, Moncton NB E1C 6Z8; Jordan (Jordan)'95; MB BS; Staff, The Moncton Hospital; (506)870-2934

MOGUS, Tally M; 1001 10 Ave SW, Calgary AB T2R 0B7; Alb'07; CCFP; (403)221-8797

MOHABIR, Nadira N; 120-70 University Ave, Toronto ON M5J 2M4; Alb'07; CCFP; (416)977-7474; Fax. (416)977-7464.

MOHAJERANI, Seyed-Alireza; Burntwood Comm Hlth Resource C, 50 Selkirk Ave, Thompson MB R8N 0M7.

MOHAMAD, May J; Clarenville Med Arts Centre, 204-105 Manitoba Dr, Clarenville NL A5A 1K2; Univ of Al-Mustansiriyah (Iraq)'96; CCFP; Staff, The Dr G B Cross Memorial Hospital.

MOHAMDEE, John; Providence Med Clinic, 4B-408 Main St, Stonewall MB R0C 2Z0; Dublin (Ireland)'94; MB ChB; BAO; AB; CCFP; (204)467-7782; Fax. (204)467-7783.

MOHAMDEE, M N Hassan; Barrhaven Med Clinic, 1002-900 Greenbank Rd, Nepean ON K2J 1S8; Trinity Coll. (Ireland)'63; MB ChB; BAO; (613)825-0276; Fax. (613)825-7514.

MOHAMED, Adel A A; Mount Sinai Hosp, 600 University Ave, Toronto ON M5G 1X5; Zagazig (Egypt)'94; Staff, Mount Sinai Hospital; (416)586-4800; Fax. (416)586-8745.

MOHAMED, Adel; Anatomy & Cell Biology, A319 HSC-107 Wiggins Rd, Saskatoon SK S7N 5E5; (Libya)'86; (306)966-4085; Fax. (306)966-4298.

MOHAMED, Ahmed A R; Yarmouth Reg Hosp, 60 Vancouver St, Yarmouth NS B5A 2P5; Cairo (Egypt)'90; MB ChB; Staff, Yarmouth Regional Hospital; (902)742-3541

MOHAMED, Ataher S; North Edmonton Clinic, 225 North Town Mall NW, Edmonton AB T5E 6C1; Al Fateh (Libya)'98; CCFP; Langs: Arabic; (780)478-2986; Fax. (780)478-2988.

MOHAMED, Curtis R; Vernon Jubilee Hosp, 2101 32 St, Vernon BC V1T 5L2; Man'90; FRCPC; NuclearMed. Staff, Vernon Jubilee Hospital; (250)558-1264

MOHAMED, Ibrahim; Hôpital Ste-Justine, 3175 ch Cote-Sainte-Catherine, Montreal QC H3T 1C5; Ain Shams (Egypt)'96; Staff, Hôpital Ste-Justine; (514)345-4685; Fax. (514)345-4811.

MOHAMED, Iman D; Don Valley Med Centre, 301-855 Broadview Ave, Toronto ON M4K 3Z1; RCS (Ireland)'71; CCFP; Court Staff, Toronto Western Hospital - University Health Network; (416)466-9908; Fax. (416)466-1394.

MOHAMED, Islam G; BC Cancer Ctre-Southern Interi, 399 Royal Ave, Kelowna BC V1Y 5L3; Alb'95; FRCPC; RadOncol. Physician RadOncol, BC Cancer Agency Sindi Ahluwalia Hawkins Centre for the Southern Interior; Clin Instructor, University of British Columbia; (250)712-3979; Fax. (250)712-3911.

MOHAMED, Ismail S; IWK Health Centre, PO Box 9700 Rpo CSC 5850-5980 University Ave, Halifax NS B3K 6R8; Alexandria (Egypt)'89; FRCPC; Neur. Staff, IWK Health Centre; (902)470-3990; Fax. (902)470-8486.

MOHAMED, John K; 1064 Lake St, Sault Ste. Marie ON P6B 6B6; Man'57; DS; FACS; FRCSC; Urol (Surgical Assistant). Court Staff Urol, Sault Area Hospital - Sault Ste Marie; (705)253-1914

MOHAMED, Mahmod S; 43 Panatella Parade NW, Calgary AB T3K 0V6; (Libya)'01; CCFP.

MOHAMED, Mohamed A; Lloydminster Hosp, 3820 43rd Ave, Lloydminster SK S9V 1Y5; Garyounis (Libya)'98; FRCSC; Otol. Staff, Lloydminster Hospital; (306)820-6194; Fax. (306)825-5167.

MOHAMED, Mohamed F; Saskatoon Cancer Centre, 20 Campus Dr, Saskatoon SK S7N 4H4; (Sri Lanka)'69; MB BS; DMRT; FRCR(Eng); Ac Staff, Royal University Hospital; Staff RadOncol, Saskatoon Cancer Centre; Asst Prof, University of Saskatchewan; (306)655-2708; Fax. (306)655-2639.

MOHAMED, Muftah A; The Brandon Clinic, 620 Dennis St, Brandon MB R7A 5E7; Al-Fateh (Libya)'86; FRCSC; ThorSurg; GenSurg. (204)728-4440

MOHAMED, Nashila N; William Osler HC-Etobicoke, 101 Humber College Blvd, Etobicoke ON M9V 1R8; Agakhan (Pakistan)'89; MSc(Epidem&Biostat.); CCFP; FCFP; Staff, William Osler Health System - Etobicoke General Hospital; Langs: Gujarati; Hindi; Urdu; Swahili; (416)494-2120

MOHAMED, Rachid; TRW Bldg, 711-3031 Hospital Dr NW, Calgary AB T2N 2T8; Alb'05; Gastroent; IntMed. Staff, Health Research Innovation Centre; (403)457-6133; Fax. (403)457-6134.

MOHAMED, Riyaz S E; PO Box 1250, Picture Butte AB T0K 1V0; (Tanzania)'89; (403)732-5515; Fax. (403)732-5516.

MOHAMED, Roubiya S; Clinicare Med Centre, 3-2250 Markham Rd, Scarborough ON M1B 2W4; Jaffna (Sri Lanka)'96; MB BS; CCFP; Langs: Tamil; Sinhalese; (416)293-5454; Fax. (416)293-7454.

MOHAMED, Sarab H; Chatham-Kent Hlth Alliance, PO Box 2030 Stn Main 80 Grand Ave W, Chatham ON N7M 5L9; Univ of Baghdad (Iraq)'82; AnatPath. Staff, Chatham-Kent Health Alliance.

MOHAMED, Shiraz N; 205-22190 48 Ave, Langley BC V3A 3N5; Makerere (Uganda)'73; MB ChB; FRCPC; Psy (Pain Management). Clin Dir Mental Health & Addiction Interior Health, Royal Inland Hospital; Consultant Psy, Regional Mental Health Services-Edmonton; (604)534-8151

MOHAMED, Zahra; Foothills Med Centre, 704-1403 29 St NW, Calgary AB T2N 2T9; Nottingham (England)'04; FRCPC; Psy. Staff, Foothills Medical Centre; (403)944-5872; Fax. (403)944-2409.

MOHAMED, Zainool A; Astotin Med Clinic, 5216 53 St, Lamont AB T0B 2R0; Natal (South Africa)'91; MB ChB; CCFP; Chief of Staff, Lamont Health Care Centre; Clin Lecturer Family Med, University of Alberta; (780)895-7436; Fax. (780)895-7493.

MOHAMED ABDOU, Mohamed S; Hotel-Dieu de Sorel, 400 av de l'Hotel-Dieu, Sorel-Tracy QC J3P 1N5; Cairo (Egypt)'96; FRCPC; Psy. Staff, Hôtel-Dieu de Sorel; (450)746-6000

MOHAMED LAMINE, Mohamed H; 3-640 Eglinton Ave W, Mississauga ON L5R 3V2; Al Fateh (Libya)'01; (416)533-1145; Fax. (416)533-3918.

MOHAMEDALI, Feisal A H; Royal Columbian Hosp, 330 Columbia St E, New Westminster BC V3L 3W7; UBC'03; FRCPC; Anes. Staff, Royal Columbian Hospital; (604)520-4602

MOHAMEDALI, Zeid; 3540 Barkley St, Port Alberni BC V9Y 8C8; UBC'96; FRCS; FRCSC; Urol. Consultant, Victoria General Hospital; Staff, Tofino General Hospital; Head Urol, West Coast General Hospital; (250)720-2200; Fax. (888)720-0244; westcoasturology@shaw.ca.

MOHAMMAD, Naveed S; Etobicoke Urgent Care Clinic, 10-25 Woodbine Downs Blvd, Etobicoke ON M9W 6N5; Ott'90; BSc; Staff Emerg/Chief EmergMed, William Osler Health System - Etobicoke General Hospital; Langs: Urdu; Hindi; Punjabi; (416)741-2273; Fax. (416)741-3542.

MOHAMMADI, Ehsan; Sault Area Hosp, 750 Great Northern Rd, Sault Ste. Marie ON P6B 0A8; UBC'96; BSc; CCFP; CCFP(E.M.); Staff, Royal Victoria Regional Health Centre; Staff, Stevenson Memorial Hospital; Staff, Sault Area Hospital - Sault Ste Marie; Langs: Farsi; (705)759-3434

MOHAMMADI, Lida; Glazier Med Centre, 11 Gibb St, Oshawa ON L1H 2J9; Shiraz (Iran)'90; CCFP; (905)579-1212

MOHAMMADI, Siamak; Hopital Laval, 2725 ch Sainte-Foy, Quebec QC G1V 4G5; Shahid Beheshti University (Israel)'93; FRCSC; CardSurg (Critical Care Medicine). Staff, Hôpital Laval; Staff, McGill University Health Centre - Royal Victoria Hospital; (418)656-8711 x2323

MOHAMMADY, Maryam; Willowdale Med Clinic, 6023 Yonge St, North York ON M2M 3W2; Isfahan (Iran)'98; CCFP; Langs: Farsi; (416)916-2733; Fax. (416)916-2315.

MOHAMMADZADEH, Gelareh; Univ Hlth Network-Toronto Western Hosp, 4 439-399 Bathurst St, Toronto ON M5T 2S8; Man'96; Neursurg. Staff, Toronto Western Hospital - University Health Network; (416)603-5503

MOHAMMADZADEH YAGHCHI, Behrooz H; Guelph Gen Hosp, 115 Delhi St, Guelph ON N1E 4J4; (Azerbaijan)'85; FRCPC; Anes. Staff, Guelph General Hospital; Langs: Persian; (519)822-5350

MOHAMMED, Adam H; First Med Place, 202-170 Queensway W, Mississauga ON L5B 3A8; Mem'95; FRCSC; GenSurg; ThorSurg. (905)281-9873; Fax. (905)281-8253.

MOHAMMED, Afzal; 510 Southdale Rd E, London ON N6E 1A5; West Indies (Jamaica)'80; FAAP(Peds); FRCPC; Peds (Neonatology). Consultant, St Joseph's Hospital - St Joseph's Health Care; Consultant, Woodstock General Hospital; Consultant, Children's Hospital of Western Ontario; Asst Prof, University of Western Ontario; (519)690-2806; Fax. (519)690-2807; amohamme@uwo.ca.

MOHAMMED, El-Fellani A; Dr E A Mohammed Prof Corp, 2-4150 Albert St, Regina SK S4S 3R8; Al-Fateh (Libya)'81; MB ChB; FRCPC; IntMed; Endocrin&Metab. Staff, Regina General Hospital; Staff, Pasqua Hospital; Physician, The Landmark Medical Centre; Consultant Endorinol, Regina Health District; Asst Prof Med, University of Saskatchewan; Langs: Arabic; (306)757-5143; Fax. (306)522-5555.

MOHAMMED, Fateh; Grey Nuns Community Hosp & HC, 23-1100 Youville Drive West NW, Edmonton AB T6L 5X8; Chittagong (Bangladesh)'87; MB BS; Staff, Covenant Health - Grey Nuns Community Hospital; Physician, Child Health Clinic; (780)735-7346; Fax. (780)735-7444.

MOHAMMED, Isa K; Pickering Urgent Care, 1450 Kingston Rd, Pickering ON L1V 1C1; Zaria (Nigeria)'87; MB BS; MMed; CCFP; (905)831-8333; Fax. (905)831-8858.

MOHAMMED, Ismail; 7A-1530 Regent Ave W, Winnipeg MB R2C 4J5; Man'68; (204)661-6464; Fax. (204)668-6960.

MOHAMMED, Javed; The Hosp for Sick Children, 555 University Ave, Toronto ON M5G 1X8; Wes'07; Peds. Fellow, The Hospital For Sick Children; (416)813-8185; Fax. (416)813-7909.

MOHAMMED, Joseph; 104-1240 Kensington Rd NW, Calgary AB T2N 3P7; Man'94; BSc; (403)837-7800

MOHAMMED, Michelle J; Trillium Hlth Ctr-Queensway, 100 Queensway W, Mississauga ON L5B 1B8; McM'00; FRCPC; IntMed. Staff, Trillium Health Centre - Mississauga; (905)848-7100

MOHAMMED, Naufal; Dept of Medicine, 816-1280 Main St W, Hamilton ON L8S 4K1; Calicut (India)'84; FRCPC; IntMed. Staff, Hamilton Health Sciences Centre - Hamilton General Hospital; Langs: Hindi; Malayalam; (905)521-2100

MOHAMMED, Nurhull H; Medical Arts Centre, 3 Maple Ave N GD, Burford ON N0E 1A0; Washington(DC) (USA)'74; Ac Staff, The Brant Community Healthcare System - Brantford General Hospital Site; (519)449-2468; Fax. (519)449-5352.

MOHAMMED, Reem W A; The Hosp for Sick Children, 555 University Ave, Toronto ON M5G 1X8; King Faisal (Saudi Arabia)'05; FRCPC; Peds; ClinImmunol&Allergy. Fellow, The Hospital For Sick Children; (416)813-1500

MOHAMMED, Samah A; 102-1 Centrepointe Dr, Ottawa ON K2G 6E2; Baghdad (Iraq)'02; MB ChB; CCFP; Staff, Central Newfoundland Regional Health Centre; (613)596-1320

MOHAMMED, Sheeja B; Hope Med Clinic, A-3208 Eglinton Ave E, Scarborough ON M1J 2H6; Kasturba (India)'91; MB BS; (416)267-6700; Fax. (416)267-0189.

MOHAMMED, Shelliza N; Vancouver Native Hlth Med Clin, 449 Hastings St E, Vancouver BC V6A 1P5; Tor'98; CCFP; Staff, Providence Health Care - St Paul's Hospital; (604)255-9766

MOHAMMED, Solomon; Dr S Mohammed Med Clinic, 2-7398 Edmonds St, Burnaby BC V3N 1A8; UBC'60; DABD; LMCC; Assoc Staff, Royal Columbian Hospital; Langs: Punjabi; Urdu; (604)522-1711; Fax. (604)522-7124.

MOHAN, Franklin S C; Hotel-Dieu Grace Hosp, 1030 Ouellette Ave, Windsor ON N9A 1E1; West Indies (Jamaica)'80; MB BS; BA; BEd; CCFP; FCFP; Staff, Hôtel-Dieu Grace Hospital; (519)973-4411 x3223; Fax. (519)255-2145.

MOHAN, Kanayalal D; Albany Med Clinic, 807 Broadview Ave, Toronto ON M4K 2P8; Witwatersrand (South Africa)'69; Assoc Staff, Toronto East General Hospital Inc; (416)461-9471; Fax. (416)461-2710.

MOHAN, Naresh; Malvern Med Arts Bldg, 335-1333 Neilson Rd, Scarborough ON M1B 4Y9; (Jamaica)'82; MB BS; FRCSC; GenSurg (Endocrinology). (416)724-7774; Fax. (416)724-7752.

MOHAN, Rajesh; Islington Med Ctr & Travel Cli, 4 Burnhamthorpe Rd, Etobicoke ON M9A 5C9; Meerut (India)'79; Langs: Hindi; Urdu; Punjabi; (416)234-1987; Fax. (416)234-8631.

MOHAN, Ravi M; Univ Hlth Network-Toronto Gen, 200 Elizabeth St, Toronto ON M5G 2C4; Tor'06; FRCPC; DiagRad. Staff, Toronto General Hospital - UHN; (416)340-3111

MOHANDAS, Rajender N; St Martha's Reg Hosp, 25 Bay St, Antigonish NS B2G 2G5; Dal'87; FRCSC; Ophth. Staff Ophth, St Martha's Regional Hospital; Teacher, Queen Elizabeth II Health Sciences Centre - Victoria General Site; Teach Staff, Dalhousie University; (902)863-6016; Fax. (902)863-6406; rmohandas@ns.sympatico.ca.

MOHANNA, Samy Stephane Maurice; 104 rue Lois, Gatineau QC J8Y 3R7; Laval'72; DECH; FACPrevMed; CSPQ; FRCPC; CommunMed (Industrial Occupational Medicine). Asst Prof, University of Ottawa; Langs: Arabic; English; (819)776-7645; mohgood@rogers.com.

MOHANRAJ, Thomas M; 1-1036 7 St SW, Medicine Hat AB T1A 8V7; Alb'88; CCFP; FCFP; Staff, Medicine Hat Regional Hospital; (403)528-4141; Fax. (403)528-2162.

MOHAREB, Michael M; Univ Hlth Network-Toronto Western Hosp, EW5 559-399 Bathurst St, Toronto ON M5T 2S8; Tor'09; Staff, Toronto Western Hospital - University Health Network; (416)603-5815; Fax. (416)603-5398.

MOHAREB, Mona M; Cornwall Comm Hosp-McConnell, PO Box 100 Stn Main 840 McConnell Ave, Cornwall ON K6H 5S5; Cairo (Egypt)'78; MB ChB; Staff, Cornwall Community Hospital; Langs: Arabic; (613)938-4240

MOHARIB, Nabil S; 510-1110 Panatella Blvd NW, Calgary AB T3K 0S6; (Ukraine)'77; CCFP; (403)274-9712; Fax. (403)274-9714.

MOHARIR, Mahendranath D; The Hosp for Sick Children, 555 University Ave, Toronto ON M5G 1X8; Bombay (India)'96; Staff, The Hospital For Sick Children; Langs: Hindi; Marathi; (416)813-7500

MOHASEB, Kam; 413-125 13th St E, North Vancouver BC V7L 2L3; UBC'00; BSc(Hon); MHSc; FRCSC; Ophth. Langs: Farsi; (604)988-2221

MOHATAREM, Afshan; Dundas Family Med Group, 201-133 King St W, Hamilton ON L9H 1V3; Karachi (Pakistan)'88; CCFP; (905)628-6355; Fax. (905)628-0664.

MOHER, Kelly L B; Gateway Comm Health Ctre, PO Box 99, Tweed ON K0K 3J0; McM'90; CCFP; FCFP; (613)478-1211; Fax. (613)478-1220.

MOHER, Matthew J; Royal Jubilee Hosp, 1952 Bay St, Victoria BC V8R 1J8; Ott'09; CCFP; Staff, Royal Jubilee Hospital; (250)634-3877

MOHIDE, Patrick T; McMaster University HSC, 4D11-1280 Main St W, Hamilton ON L8S 4K1; Tor'69; MSc(DME); FRCSC; ObstGyn (Maternal Fetal Medicine). Ac Staff, Hamilton Health Sciences Centre - McMaster Children's Hospital; Dept Head ObstGyn/Prof, McMaster University; (905)521-2100 x76245; Fax. (905)577-0471; mohide@mcmaster.ca.

MOHILE, Sonali A; Uxbridge Family Health Clinic, B-2 Elgin Park Dr, Uxbridge ON L9P 0B1; Punjabi (India)'94; FRCPC; Peds. Langs: Punjabi; Hindi; Marathi; (905)852-1009

MOHINDRA, Ruchi N; Toronto East Gen Hosp Inc, 825 Coxwell Ave, Toronto ON M4C 3E7; Mem'05; CCFP; CCFP(E.M.); Staff, Toronto East General Hospital Inc; (416)461-8272

MOHIUDDIN, M D; Saint John Reg Hosp, PO Box 2100 Stn Main 400 University Ave, Saint John NB E2L 4L2; Chittagong (Bangladesh)'88; Staff, Saint John Regional Hospital; (506)648-6000

MOHL, Robert W; Lakeridge Hlth Corp-Oshawa, 1 Hospital Crt, Oshawa ON L1G 2B9; Wes'94; FRCPC; Anes. Staff, Lakeridge Health - Oshawa Site; (905)576-8711; rmohl@sympatico.ca.

MOHLER, Jeffrey A; Royal Alexandra Hosp, 10240 Kingsway NW, Edmonton AB T5H 3V9; Alb'86; Staff EmergMed, Royal Alexandra Hospital; Clin Lecturer, University of Alberta; (780)735-4443; Fax. (780)735-4916.

MOHOMED, Dave A; Norfolk Gen Hosp, 365 West St, Simcoe ON N3Y 1T7; Univ of the West Indies (Jamaica)'90; Staff, Norfolk General Hospital; (519)426-0750

MOHR, Bruce P; Whistler Health Care Centre, 4380 Lorimer Rd RR 4, Whistler BC V0N 1B4; Ott'84; BSc(Hons.Kinesiol); Dip SportMed; CCFP; CCFP(E.M.); (604)932-4911; Fax. (604)932-4992.

MOHR, Gerard; SMBD Jewish Gen Hosp, 3755 ch Cote-Sainte-Catherine, Montreal QC H3T 1E2; Strasbourg (France)'69; FRCSC; Neursurg (Skull Base Surgery). Prof NeuroSurg, Sir Mortimer B Davis Jewish General; assoc Membre, Hopital Maisonneuve-Rosemont; Prof, McGill University; Langs: German; English; (514)340-8222 x4290; Fax. (514)340-7924; gmohr@jgh.mcgill.ca.

MOHR, Karen L; Royal University Hosp, 103 Hospital Dr, Saskatoon SK S7N 0W8; Man'00; CCFP; CCFP(E.M.); Staff, Royal University Hospital; (306)655-1364

MOHR, Veronica R; Maple Family Health Team, 325 University Ave, Kingston ON K7L 3R4; Qns'77; CCFP; FCFP; Assoc Staff, Kingston General Hospital; Assoc Staff, Hotel-Dieu Hospital; (613)544-2902; Fax. (613)544-5768.

MOHSEN, Yosra M K M; 302-10725 83 Ave NW, Edmonton AB T6E 2E5; (Egypt)'02.

MOHSENIBOD, Hadi; The Hosp for Sick Children, 555 University Ave, Toronto ON M5G 1X8; Tehran (Iran)'90; Staff, The Hospital For Sick Children; Langs: Farsi; (416)813-6486

MOHSIN, Afshan; Headwaters Health Care Centre, 100 Rolling Hills Dr, Orangeville ON L9W 4X9; Karachi (Pakistan)'96; ABIM; FACP; FRCPC; IntMed. Ac Staff, Headwaters Health Care Centre - Orangeville Site; Langs: Hindi; Urdu; (519)941-7117; Fax. (519)941-5481.

MOHSIN, Hina; IWK Health Centre, PO Box 9700 RPO CSC 5850-5980 University Ave, Halifax NS B3K 6R8; Rawalpindi (Pakistan)'90; MB BS; Staff, IWK Health Centre; (902)470-8888

MOHTADI, Nicholas G H; University of Calgary, 2500 University Dr NW, Calgary AB T2N 1N4; Cal'81; FRCSC; OrthSurg (Sports Medicine). Staff, Peter Lougheed Centre; Associate Clin Prof, University of Calgary; (403)220-5077; Fax. (403)282-6170; mohtadi@ucalgary.ca.

MOHTASHAMI-GOZELLOU, Fariba; 21561 Old Yale Rd, Langley BC V3A 4M9; Tehran (Iran)'92; FRCSC; ObstGyn. (604)534-4462

MOHYDEEN, Shwan S; B109-566 MIllbourne Road East, Edmonton AB T6K 3N4.

MOID, Farah; St Joseph's Health Centre, 30 The Queensway, Toronto ON M6R 1B5; Punjab (Pakistan)'85; ABPath; FRCPC; GenPath (Hematology Pathology). Staff Path, St Joseph's Health Centre; (416)530-6283; moidfa@stjoe.on.ca.

MOIEN AFSHARI, Farzad; Royal University Hosp, 103 Hospital Dr, Saskatoon SK S7N 0W8; Meshed University (Iran)'96; FRCPC; Neur. Staff, Royal University Hospital; (306)966-9036; Fax. (306)966-8008.

MOIN-DARBARI, Djavad; Centre Sante Kirkland, 17000 boul Hymus, Kirkland QC H9J 2W2; Meshed (Iran)'62; Chief Med., CLSC Parc Extension; (514)426-5927; djavad.moin-darbari@mcgill.ca.

MOINEAU, Genevieve; Children's Hosp Eastern Ont, 401 Smyth Rd, Ottawa ON K1H 8L1; Ott'84; FRCPC; Peds (Pediatric Emergency Medicine). Staff Ped Emerg, Children's Hospital of Eastern Ontario (CHEO); Assoc Dean Undergraduate Med Education/Asst Prof, University of Ottawa; (613)737-2318

MOINI, John; Clinique Medical Moini, 32-55 rue de l'Eglise, Verdun QC H4G 3E7; Laval'93; LMCC; CCFP; Langs: French; Persian; Spanish; (514)769-5500; moini_clinics@sympatico.ca.

MOIR, Adam; Dingwall Med Group, 40 Goodall St, Dryden ON P8N 1V8; NOSM'09; CCFP; (807)223-2258

MOIR, Vivian M; 9-76 Arlington Dr, Keswick ON L4P 0A9; Tor'85; CCFP; FCFP; Ac Staff Family Practice, Southlake Regional Health Centre; Langs: German; French; (905)476-0308; Fax. (905)476-1079.

MOISAN, Andree-Anne; Centre Jean Patrice Chiasson, 1930 rue King O, Sherbrooke QC J1J 2E2; Sher'10; CCFP; (819)821-2500

MOISAN, Danielle; CSSS de Rivière-de-Loup, 75 rue Saint-Henri, Riviere-Du-Loup QC G5R 2A4; Laval'93; FRCPC; MedMicrobiol; Microbio & Infect Dis (P.Q.). Staff, Centre Hospitalier Regional du Grand-Portage; (418)868-1000; Fax. (418)868-1032.

MOISAN, Martin; 209-369 rue Adolphe-Chapleau, Bois-des-Filion QC J6Z 1H1; Mon'93; (514)554-2878

MOISAN, Serge; Direction de la Sante Publique, 1255 rue Beauregard, Longueuil QC J4K 2M3; Laval'72; MPH; CSPQ; CommunMed (P.Q.). Staff, Hopital Charles LeMoyne; (450)928-6777 x3030; Fax. (450)928-3694; s.moisan@rrsss16.gouv.qc.ca.

MOISE, John P; The Ottawa Hosp-Gen Campus, 501 Smyth Rd, Ottawa ON K1H 8L6; Qns'97; FRCPC; Psy. Staff Psy, The Ottawa Hospital - General Campus; (613)737-8899; Fax. (613)739-6667.

MOISE, Josiane; Soins Continus Bruyere-Residen, 879 Hiawatha Park Rd, Orleans ON K1C 2Z6; Port-au-Prince (Haiti)'76; (613)562-6262

MOISE, Paul; Ctr Hosp Anna-Laberge, 200 boul Brisebois, Chateauguay QC J6K 4W8; (Haiti)'81; FRCSC; OrthSurg., Hôpital Anna-Laberge; paul.moise@rrss16.gouv.qc.ca.

MOISE, Roger C; 101-1723 Comox Ave, Comox BC V9M 3N2; McM'93; FRCSC; GenSurg. Staff, Grey Bruce Health Services - Owen Sound; (250)339-1002; Fax. (250)339-5340.

MOISESCU, Razvan; Clinique Saint-Georges, 1000 rue Chabanel, Chicoutimi QC G7H 2R3; Mon'89; FRCSC; Otol. Staff, Complexe hospitalier de la Sagamie; (418)549-0292

MOISEY, Clarence G; Clare Moisey Med Clinic, PO Box 3777, Smithers BC V0J 2N0; Alb'73; FRCPC; Peds (Developmental Pediatrics). (250)847-4800; Fax. (250)847-5694; george@bulkley.net.

MOISIUK, Peter D; St Joseph's Healthcare, 50 Charlton Ave E, Hamilton ON L8N 4A6; Ott'00; FRCPC; Anes. Staff, St Joseph's Healthcare - Charlton Campus; (905)522-1155 x3853; pmoisiuk@yahoo.com.

MOISIUK, Sharon E; St Boniface Gen Hosp, A8039-409 Tache Ave, Winnipeg MB R2H 2A6; Sask'75; FRCPC; Peds (Neonatology). Staff Neonatol, St Boniface General Hospital; (204)237-2764; Fax. (204)231-0137; smoisiuk@sbgh.mb.ca.

MOIST, Louise M; London HSC-Victoria Hosp, PO Box 5010 Stn B A2 338-800 Commissioners Rd E, London ON N6A 5W9; McM'93; MSc; FRCPC; IntMed; Nephrol. Consultant Nephrol, London Health Sciences Centre - Victoria Campus; Assoc Prof, University of Western Ontario; (519)685-8211; Fax. (519)685-8449; louise.moist@lhsc.on.ca.

MOJAB, Hamid; 208-4800 Leslie St, North York ON M2J 2K9; Shiraz (Iran)'91; FRCPC; IntMed; Endocrin&Metab. Staff, North York General Hospital; (647)352-0162; Fax. (647)352-0262.

MOJDAMI, Fatemeh; 404-13291 Yonge St, Richmond Hill ON L4E 4L6; McM'07; FRCPC; IntMed; Endocrin&Metab. (905)773-4444; Fax. (905)773-1777.

MOJICA CORREA, Ludy; Clinique Med Plein Ciel, 475 boul de la Cote-Vertu, Saint-Laurent QC H4L 1X7; Nuestra Senora del Rosario (Colombia)'99; CCFP; Staff, Hopital Marie Clarac; (514)313-3171

MOJTAHEDZADEH, Aghdas; The Moncton Hosp, 135 MacBeath Ave, Moncton NB E1C 6Z8; Tehran (Iran)'90; FRCPC; AnatPath. Staff, The Moncton Hospital; (506)857-5111

MOK, Andrea H; 6C-163 Commissioners Rd W, London ON N6J 1X9; Tor'05; CCFP; (519)472-8253; Fax. (519)471-1094.

MOK, Andrew K C; Seaforth Med Bldg, 500-3550 ch de la Cote-des-Nei, Montreal QC H3H 1V4; McG'74; FRCSC; ObstGyn (Infertility). assoc Staff, McGill University Health Centre - Royal Victoria Hospital; assoc Staff, McGill University Health Centre - Montreal General Campus; adj Prof, McGill University; Langs: Cantonese; Mandarin; French; (514)932-2234; Fax. (514)935-4345.

MOK, C Albert; 6C-163 Commissioners Rd W, London ON N6J 1X9; Wes'75; MSc; Ac Staff Family Med, London Health Sciences Centre - Victoria Campus; Court Staff Family Med, St Joseph's Hospital - St Joseph's Health Care; (519)472-8253; Fax. (519)471-1094.

MOK, David; Hop Charles LeMoyne, 3120 boul Taschereau, Greenfield Park QC J4V 2H1; McG'04; FRCSC; PlasSurg. Staff, Hopital Charles LeMoyne; (450)466-5000

MOK, Dereck C; 214PL-9009 102 St, Grande Prairie AB T8V 2V4; Alb'03; FRCSC; GenSurg. (780)539-4545; Fax. (780)532-6743.

MOK, Gary T; 51-103 Parkway Forest Dr, North York ON M2J 1L8; Tor'86; Langs: Chinese; (416)491-4040; Fax. (416)491-4040.

MOK, Gloria M C; Meadowlark Health Centre, 140 Meadowlark Shopping Ctr NW, Edmonton AB T5R 5W9; Alb'74; (780)489-8470; Fax. (780)484-1620.

MOK, Hiram L H; 715 12th Ave W, Vancouver BC V5Z 1M9; Dublin (Ireland)'91; MA; MB ChB; BAO; LMCC; FRCPC; Psy (Academic Psychiatry). Staff, Vancouver General Hospital - Centennial Pavillion; Langs: Cantonese; Mandarin; (604)875-4111 x632

MOK, Lawrence M S; Alexander Prof Bldg, 110-849 Alexander Crt, Peterborough ON K9J 7H8; Wes'72; FRCSC; PlasSurg. (705)743-1048; Fax. (705)743-1902.

MOK, Lesley J; 6C-163 Commissioners Rd W, London ON N6J 1X9; Tor'09; CCFP; (519)472-8253

MOK, S Simon; Central Parkway Mall, 110-377 Burnhamthorpe Rd E, Mississauga ON L5A 3Y1; Tor'78; Staff, Trillium Health Centre - Mississauga; (905)896-2990

MOKASHI, Arati S; IWK Health Centre, PO Box 9700 Rpo CSC 5850-5980 University Ave, Halifax NS B3K 6R8; Alb'97; FRCPC; Peds; Endocrin&Metab. Staff, IWK Health Centre; Asst Prof Peds, Dalhousie University; (902)470-8707; Fax. (902)470-7264.

MOKATE, Lionel M; Bethesda Reg Health Centre, PO Box 939 Stn Main 316 Henry St, Steinbach MB R5G 1A3; Johannesburg (South Africa)'98; CCFP; Staff, Bethesda Hospital Steinbach; (204)326-6411; lmokate@sehealth.mb.ca.

MOKHTARI, Makan; William Osler HC-Etobicoke, 101 Humber College Blvd, Etobicoke ON M9V 1R8; Wes'99; CCFP; Staff, William Osler Health System - Etobicoke General Hospital; (416)747-3500

MOKONE, M Christina; Sioux Lookout Meno-Ya-Win H C, PO Box 1500 Stn Main 82 7th Ave N, Sioux Lookout ON P8T 1C2; Medunsa (South Africa)'92; MB ChB; CCFP; Staff, Sioux Lookout Meno-Ya-Win Health Centre; (807)737-5191

MOKRZANOWSKI, Andrew D; Belmont Medicentre, 2903 137 Ave NW, Edmonton AB T5A 5G8; Warszawa (Poland)'74; (780)475-7070; Fax. (780)472-2367.

MOKRZANOWSKI, Elizabeth; Belmont Medicentre, 2903 137 Ave NW, Edmonton AB T5A 5G8; Warsaw (Poland)'74; CCFP; (780)475-7070; Fax. (780)472-2367.

MOKTASSI, Aiden; Mount Sinai Hosp, 570-600 University Ave, Toronto ON M5G 1X5; Tor'04; FRCPC; DiagRad. Staff, Mount Sinai Hospital; (416)586-7937; Fax. (416)586-8695.

MOL, Adrianus; Medical Centre, PO Box 28, Athabasca AB T9S 2A2; Alb'71; Att Staff, Athabasca Healthcare Centre; (780)675-2211; Fax. (780)675-3368; admol@telusplanet.net.

MOLAVI, Massood; North Shore Med Clinic, 1-1881 Marine Dr, North Vancouver BC V7P 1V5; Teheran (Iran)'75; FRCPC; IntMed. Langs: Persian; (604)984-9641

MOLBERG, Carey R; Pediatric Consultants Assoc, 182-5201 43 St, Red Deer AB T4N 1C7; Sask'63; FRCPC; Peds. (403)343-6404; Fax. (403)343-6215.

MOLBERG, Warren R; Royal Alexandra Hosp, CSC541-10240 Kingsway NW, Edmonton AB T5H 3V9; Alb'91; CCFP; CCFP(E.M.); Staff, Royal Alexandra Hospital; (780)735-4443; Fax. (780)735-4916.

MOLCKOVSKY, Andrea; Grand River Hosp-KW Hlth Ctre, PO Box 9056 Stn C 835 King St W, Kitchener ON N2G 1G3; Tor'04; FRCPC; IntMed; MedOncol. Staff, Grand River Hospital - Kitchener/Waterloo Health Centre; (519)749-4300; Fax. (519)749-4378.

MOLCKOVSKY, Bohdan; 207-2021 Cliff Rd, Mississauga ON L5A 3N7; Bratislava (Slovakia)'65; DMRT; DABR; Ac Staff, Trillium Health Centre - Mississauga; Langs: Czech; Slovak; (905)270-1601; Fax. (905)270-1636.

MOLDER, Cameron J; Selkirk Med Group, PO Box 590, Revelstoke BC V0E 2S0; Sask'92; CCFP; (250)837-9321; Fax. (250)837-9444.

MOLDER, Susan V; Public Health-The Talk Shop, 5100 Yonge St, North York ON M2N 5V7; McG'77; BSc; MSc; MDCM; (416)338-7000; Fax. (416)338-7001.

MOLDES, Andrea P; Sports Medicine & Rehab Centre, 104-480 Huronia Rd, Barrie ON L4N 6M2; McM'05; CCFP; (705)734-3340; Fax. (705)734-9210.

MOLDOFSKY, Harvey; Sleep Disorders Clinic, 580-340 College St, Toronto ON M5T 3A9; Tor'59; DPsy; FRCPC; Psy (Sleep Medicine). Hon Staff, Toronto Western Hospital - University Health Network; Consultant Psy, Humber River Regional Hospital - Keele Street Site; Emeritus Prof Faculty of Med, University of Toronto; (416)603-9531; Fax. (416)603-2388; h.moldofsky@utoronto.ca.

MOLDOVEANU, Adina A; 130-7155 Woodbine Ave, Markham ON L3R 1A3; Bucharest (Romania)'66; Ac Staff, The Scarborough Hospital - Birchmount Campus; Langs: Romanian; (905)475-2353

MOLDOVEANU, Andrei I; 215-1900 Richmond Ave, Victoria BC V8R 4R2; Albany(NY) (USA)'03; FRCPC; IntMed; Endocrin&Metab. (250)595-5952

MOLEDINA, Mohamed T A; PO Box 82077 Rpo Yellowbird, Edmonton AB T6J 7E6; Germany (Germany)'74.

MOLESKI, Luc; CSSSG Hop de Gatineau, CP 2000 Succ Bureau-Chef 909 boul de la Verendrye O, Gatineau QC J8P 7H2; Sher'06; FRCPC; IntMed. Staff, Hôpital de Gatineau; (819)966-6100

MOLGAT, Carmen V; Royal Inland Hosp, 311 Columbia St, Kamloops BC V2C 2T1; Bucharest (Romania)'91; MSc; FRCPC; Psy. Staff Psy, Royal Inland Hospital; Langs: Romanian; (250)374-5111; Fax. (250)314-2410.

MOLGAT, Gilles F; Royal Inland Hosp, 311 Columbia St, Kamloops BC V2C 2T1; Man'94; BSc; MSc; FRCPC; AnatPath. Staff, Royal Inland Hospital; (250)314-2669; Fax. (250)314-2505.

MOLGAT, Yvonne M; Ctr Hosp Affilie-Enfant-Jesus, 1401 18e rue, Quebec QC G1J 1Z4; McG'84; FRCSC; Ophth (Orbital, Lacrimal & Eyelid Surgery). Ac Staff, Centre Hospitalier Affilié Universitaire de Québec - Hôpital De L'Enfant Jésus; (418)649-5816

MOLIN, Franck; Hôpital Laval, 2725 ch Sainte-Foy, Quebec QC G1V 4G5; (France)'91; CSPQ; Cardiol (P.Q.) (Electrophysiology). Staff, Hôpital Laval; Staff, Institut Universitaire Cardiologie & Pneumologie de Quebec; assoc Prof Med, Université Laval; Langs: Spanish; English; (418)656-4598; Fax. (418)656-4581; franck.molin@med.ulaval.ca.

MOLINA-NEGRO, Pedro; CHUM-Hop Notre-Dame, 1560 rue Sherbrooke E, Montreal QC H2L 4M1; Santiago de Compostela (Spain)'56; PhD(Spain); Neursurg (P.Q.). Staff, Centre Hospitalier l'Université de Montréal (CHUM) - Hôpital Notre-Dame; Prof, Universite de Montreal; (514)412-7726

MOLINARI, Michele; Queen Elizabeth II HSC, 6 302-1276 South Park St, Halifax NS B3H 2Y9; Milan (Italy)'92; MSc; Staff, Queen Elizabeth II Health Sciences Centre - Victoria General Site; Asst Prof Surgery, Dalhousie University; (902)473-7624; Fax. (902)473-5297.

MOLINARI, Raynald; 1550 rue Robinson, Laval QC H7W 2W2; McG'83; FRCPC; Derm. (450)688-6405; Fax. (450)688-0065.

MOLINER, Peter H R; CHUS-Hop Fleurimont, 3001 12e av N, Sherbrooke QC J1H 5N4; McM'90; CSPQ; FRCPC; Anes. Clinical Asst Prof Family Med, Sir Mortimer B Davis Jewish General; Staff, Centre Hospitalier Universitaire de Sherbrooke-Hopital Fleurimont; adj Prof, McGill University; (819)346-1110

MOLL, Alexander S G; Cowichan Med Centre, 3106 Gibbins Rd, Duncan BC V9L 1E8; Cape Town (South Africa)'73; MB ChB; FRCPC; Neur (Movement Disorders). Staff Consultant, Cowichan District Hospital; Aj Prof, University Of Victoria; (250)746-7711; Fax. (250)746-8809.

MOLL, Allan L; 101-7700 Bathurst St, Thornhill ON L4J 7Y3; Tor'93; BSc; CCFP; Langs: Spanish; Hebrew; (905)764-8242

MOLL, Gillian; Anaesthetic Services, 213-2186 Oak Bay Ave, Victoria BC V8R 1G3; Cape Town (South Africa)'74; MB ChB; FRCPC; Anes (Cardiac Anesthesia). Staff, Royal Jubilee Hospital; (250)595-7211; Fax. (250)595-7211.

MOLLANJI, Roland; North York Gen Hosp, 4001 Leslie St, North York ON M2K 1E1; Tirana (Albania)'88; CCFP; Staff, North York General Hospital; Langs: Albanian; (416)756-6410

MOLLEKEN, Lynda L; 304-1670 Bayview Ave, Toronto ON M4G 3C2; Ott'91; BScPharm(Pharm); FRCPC; Psy (Eating Disorders). Staff, Toronto General Hospital - UHN; Lecturer, University of Toronto; (416)488-2838

MOLLER, Erika; Western Manitoba Cancer Ctre, 300 McTavish Ave E, Brandon MB R7A 2B3; Pretoria (South Africa)'96; Staff, Brandon Regional Health Centre.

MOLLER, Henry J; Univ Hlth Network-Toronto Western Hosp, 7 432-399 Bathurst St, Toronto ON M5T 2S8; Tor'96; BSc; DABSM; MSc; FRCPC; Psy (Neurology & Psychiatry). Staff, Toronto Western Hospital - University Health Network; Asst Prof Faculty of Med, University of Toronto; Langs: German; French; (416)603-5667; Fax. (416)603-5292; henry.moller@uhn.on.ca.

MOLLER, Liesel; The Brandon Clinic, 620 Dennis St, Brandon MB R7A 5E7; Pretoria (South Africa)'00; (204)728-4440

MOLLER, Philip R; Brandon Reg Health Centre, 150 McTavish Ave E, Brandon MB R7A 2B3; Pretoria (South Africa)'98; FRCPC; Anes. Staff, Brandon Regional Health Centre; (204)726-1122

MOLLICA, Luigina; Hop Maisonneuve-Rosemont, 5415 boul de l'Assomption, Montreal QC H1T 2M4; Mon'96; PhD; FRCPC; IntMed; MedOncol; Hem. Staff, Hopital Maisonneuve-Rosemont; Langs: English; Italian; (514)252-3400 x3404; Fax. (514)254-5094.

MOLLISON, Heather L; Regina Qu'Appelle HR-Pasqua, 4101 Dewdney Ave, Regina SK S4T 1A5; Sask'01; FRCPC; Anes. Staff, Pasqua Hospital; (306)766-2222

MOLLOT, Kimberley D; Halton HSC-Oakville Site, 327 Reynolds St, Oakville ON L6J 3L7; McM'05; FRCPC; Psy. Staff, Halton Healthcare Services Corporation - Oakville Site; (905)845-2571

MOLLOY, Francine; Clinique Medi Centre, 8 rue du Terminus E, Rouyn-Noranda QC J9X 3B4; Laval'82; Staff, Centre Hospitalier Rouyn-Noranda; Langs: English; (819)762-6161; Fax. (819)762-0808.

MOLNAR, Christine P; Foothills Med Centre, 1403 29 St NW, Calgary AB T2N 2T9; Sask'76; FRCPC; DiagRad; NuclearMed. Ac Staff, Foothills Medical Centre; Asst Prof, University of Calgary; (403)944-1969; Fax. (403)944-1687.

MOLNAR, Frank J; The Ottawa Hosp-Civic Campus, 1053 Carling Ave, Ottawa ON K1Y 4E9; McG'91; MSc(Epidemiol.); FRCPC; IntMed; GeriatricMed. Staff, The Ottawa Hospital - Civic Campus; Langs: English; French; (613)798-5555 x16486; Fax. (613)761-5334.

MOLNAR, Geza B; Brampton Hlth & Wellness Ctre, 100-178 John St, Brampton ON L6W 2A4; Tor'78; Langs: Hungarian; (905)457-4772; Fax. (905)457-3936.

MOLNAR, Laura A; London Health Sciences Centre, A2 668-800 Commissioners Ave W, London ON N6A 4G5; McG'75; BA; DABPN; FRCPC; Psy;CCFP; Staff, London Health Sciences Centre - South Street; (519)667-6550; Fax. (519)667-6864.

MOLNAR, Paula C; Harborn Med Associates, 510-89 Queensway W, Mississauga ON L5B 2V2; Ott'94; CCFP; FCFP; Staff, Trillium Health Centre - Mississauga; (905)273-4380; Fax. (905)273-4335.

MOLNAR, Szilamer Z A; Queen Elizabeth II Hospital, 10409 98 St, Grande Prairie AB T8V 2E8; Alb'71; Ac Staff, Queen Elizabeth II Hospital; (780)538-7100

MOLONEY, Gregory T; Eye Care Centre, G-2550 Willow St, Vancouver BC V5Z 3N9; New South Wales (Australia)'01; MB BS; FRCSC; Ophth. (604)875-5870

MOLONEY, Michael A; St Michael's Hosp, 30 Bond St, Toronto ON M5B 1W8; (Ireland)'99; Staff Vascular Surg, St Michael's Hospital; Asst Prof Med, University of Toronto; (416)864-5459; Fax. (416)864-6012.

MOLOO, Husein; Civic Parkdale Clinic, 330-737 Parkdale Ave, Ottawa ON K1Y 1J8; Wes'00; FRCSC; GenSurg. Staff, The Ottawa Hospital - Civic Campus; (613)761-4000

MOLOT, John M; Bank Med Centre, 105-1935 Bank St, Ottawa ON K1V 8A3; Ott'71; CCFP; FCFP; (613)521-2391; Fax. (613)521-5443.

MOLOTIU, Nicolae; Strathroy Middlesex Gen Hosp, 395 Carrie St, Strathroy ON N7G 3C9; Cluj (Romania)'60; FRCPC; Anes. Staff, Strathroy Middlesex General Hospital - Middlesex Hospital Alliance; Langs: Romanian; French; (519)245-1550 x5548; Fax. (519)245-5438.

MOLOUGHNEY, Brent W P; Public Health Consultant, 419 Kelly Cres, Newmarket ON L3Y 7K4; Tor'86; MSc; FRCPC; CommunMed (Public Health & Preventive Medicine). Aj Prof Dalla Lana School of Public Health, University of Toronto; (905)953-0153; Fax. (905)953-0948.

MOLSON, Jenny L; Queen's University, 146 Stuart St, Kingston ON K7L 2V8; Qns'88; CCFP; FCFP; Med Examiner Marine & Civil Aviation/Consultant Diving Med, Civil Aviation Canada; Asst Prof, Queen's University; (613)533-2506

MOLTYANER, Yuri; 216-40 Finchgate Blvd, Brampton ON L6T 3J1; Ott'95; FRCPC; IntMed (Critical Care Medicine); Respir. Langs: Russian; (905)456-3699 x33; Fax. (905)456-8768.

MOLTZAN, Catherine J; St Boniface Gen Hosp, L1 101 20-409 Tache Ave, Winnipeg MB R2H 2A6; Alb'92; FRCP; BMedSci; FRCPC; IntMed; HemPath; Hem. Asst Prof Med, University of Manitoba; St Boniface General Hospital; Staff, Health Sciences Centre; Staff, Concordia General Hospital; (204)235-3141; Fax. (204)237-6048; catherine.moltzan@cancercare.mb.ca.

MOLYNEAUX, Harold W; 54 Central St, Summerside PE C1N 3L1; Dal'76; Staff, Prince County Hospital; (902)436-7206; Fax. (902)436-7207.

MOLYNEAUX, Lloyd J; Bedeque Clinic, PO Box 4005, Bedeque PE C0B 1C0; Dal'69; (902)877-2433

MOLYNEAUX, Shelly D; Dept of Veterans Affairs, PO Box 7700 Stn Central, Charlottetown PE C1A 8M9; Dal'96; CCFP.

MOMENKHAN, Ibrahim M M; Regina Qu'Appelle HR-Regina, 1440 14th Ave, Regina SK S4P 0W5; Jeddah (Saudi Arabia)'01; FRCPC; IntMed; Critical Care Medicine. Staff, Regina General Hospital; Langs: Arabic; (306)766-4234; Fax. (306)766-4345.

MOMI, Rajinder S; Peterborough Reg HC-Hospital, 1 Hospital Dr, Peterborough ON K9J 7C6; Punjab (India)'92; FRCPC; Psy. Staff, Peterborough Regional Health Centre - Hospital Drive; (705)876-5028

MOMIN, Rizwanali; Stevenson Mem Hosp, PO Box 4000 Stn Main 200 Fletcher Cres, Alliston ON L9R 1W7; Mem'07; CCFP; Staff, Stevenson Memorial Hospital; (705)435-6281

MOMOH, John T; Medical Arts Bldg, 906-233 Kennedy St, Winnipeg MB R3C 3J5; (Nigeria)'71; MB BS; FRCSC; GenSurg. Staff, Seven Oaks General Hospital; Staff, The Salvation Army Grace Hospital; (204)942-6174; Fax. (204)956-0496.

MONAGHAN, Anthony J T; 1902 9 Ave S, Lethbridge AB T1J 1W7; Alb'83; FRCSC; Otol (Maxillo Facial Surgery). Staff Surg, Chinook Regional Hospital; (403)320-1066; Fax. (403)328-1297.

MONAGHAN, Deborah; Hotel-Dieu d'Arthabaska, 5 rue des Hospitalieres, Victoriaville QC G6P 6N2; Laval'89; FRCPC; IntMed; GeriatricMed. Staff Palliative Care, Hotel-Dieu d'Arthabaska; (819)357-2030; Fax. (819)357-6030.

MONAGHAN, Elizabeth M; 400-628 12 Ave SW, Calgary AB T2R 0H6; Alb'92; CCFP; (403)270-2273; Fax. (403)251-2250.

MONAGHAN, Michael J; 716L Arlington Park Pl, Kingston ON K7M 8H9; Qns'89; FRCPC; Psy (General Adult Psychiatry). (613)384-8222; Fax. (613)384-8221.

MONAGHAN, Patrick N; Central Alberta Prof Centre, 268-5201 43 St, Red Deer AB T4N 1C7; Alb'89; FRCSC; Otol. (403)343-0044; Fax. (403)343-0555.

MONAGHAN, Ronald A; Riverside Prof Centre, 312-1919 Riverside Dr, Ottawa ON K1H 1A2; Ott'88; FRCSC; GenSurg. Ac Staff/Chief Surgeon, Queensway Carleton Hospital; Consultant, Kemptville District Hospital; Consultant, Arnprior & District Memorial Hospital; (613)733-0964; Fax. (613)733-3651.

MONAHAN, Barbara J; Forcemedic, 1021 rue Jean-Talon E, Montreal QC H2R 1V6; McG'87; CCFP; FCFP; (514)787-1818

MONAHAN, M Anne; 423Y-75 Bruyere St, Ottawa ON K1N 5C7; Tor'01; CCFP; Staff Geriatric Day Hosp, SCO Health Service - Élisabeth Bruyère Hospital; Langs: English; French; (613)562-6262; Fax. (613)562-4265; amonahan@bruyere.org.

MONAHAN, Michael P; 201-190 Wellington St, Kingston ON K7L 3E4; Qns'81; (613)549-1697; Fax. (613)547-0004.

MONAHAN, Sarah K; 200-7031 Westminster Hwy, Richmond BC V6X 1A3; Seattle(WA) (USA)'92; FRCSC; ObstGyn. (604)821-1960

MONARQUE, Guy; GMF des Seigneuries, 2220 boul Rene-Gaultier, Varennes QC J3X 1E3; Laval'82; (450)652-2917; Fax. (450)652-9902.

MONARQUE, Nathalie; Polyclinique St-Eustache, 75 rue Grignon, St-Eustache QC J7P 4J2; Sher'91; Langs: English; (450)473-6882; Fax. (450)473-1916.

MONAST, Julie; CHUS-Hop Fleurimont, 3001 12e av N, Sherbrooke QC J1H 5N4; Sher'97; Staff, Centre Hospitalier Universitaire de Sherbrooke-Hopital Fleurimont; (819)346-1110

MONAVVARI, Arsalan; 116-250 Lawrence Ave W, Toronto ON M5M 1B2; Ghazvin (Iran)'92; CCFP; Staff Palliative Care, Sunnybrook Health Sciences Centre; Staff, North York General Hospital; Coord IMG, University of Toronto; Langs: Farsi; French; (416)782-4447; Fax. (416)782-1284.

MONCEK, John A; Seven Oaks Gen Hosp, 2300 McPhillips St, Winnipeg MB R2V 3M3; Man'78; CCFP; FCFP; Ac Staff, St Boniface General Hospital; Staff, Seven Oaks General Hospital; (204)632-7133

MONCHESKY, Theodore C; Oshawa Clinic, 117 King St E, Oshawa ON L1H 1B9; Qns'68; FRCPC; IntMed (Endocrinology). Assoc Staff, Lakeridge Health - Oshawa Site; (905)723-8551 x5340; Fax. (905)723-2541; tmonchesky@sympatico.ca.

MONCUR, Ross; Leamington & Area Fam Hlth Team, 197 Talbot St W, Leamington ON N8H 1N8; McM'09; CCFP; (519)322-1100; Fax. (519)322-2055.

MONDAL, Tapas; McMaster University, HSC 3A-1280 Main St W, Hamilton ON L8S 4K1; Calcutta (India)'87; FRCPC; Cardiol; Peds. Staff, Hamilton Health Sciences Centre - McMaster Children's Hospital; Teach Staff, McMaster University; Langs: Bengali; Hindi; (905)521-2100 x75259; Fax. (905)521-7914.

MONDAY, Jacques; Hop du Sacre-Coeur de Mtl, 5400 boul Gouin O, Montreal QC H4J 1C5; Mon'66; FRCPC; Psy. Ac Staff Psy, Hôpital du Sacre-Coeur de Montréal; Prof, Universite de Montreal; Langs: English; French; (514)338-2070; Fax. (514)338-3187; vanmon_2@yahoo.com.

MONDAY, Patrick; CLSC Ste-Therese de Blainville, 55 rue Saint-Joseph, Sainte-Therese QC J7E 4Y5; Mon'98; (450)430-4553 x4011

MONDOR, Claire; Clinique Med Point-Levy, 215 rue Saint-Omer, Levis QC G6V 8N3; Laval'81; Peds. Staff, Hôtel-Dieu de Lévis; (418)835-1767

MONDOR, Frances L; The Richmond Hosp, 7000 Westminster Hwy, Richmond BC V6X 1A2; McG'86; CCFP; CCFP(E.M.); Staff, Richmond Hospital; (604)244-5151; Fax. (604)244-5194.

MONDOR, Marie-Eve; CSSS de Laval, 1755 boul Rene-Laennec, Laval QC H7M 3L9; Mon'04; FRCPC; Anes. Staff, Hopital de la Cite de la santé; (450)668-1010

MONDOR, Thomas; Clinique Med de Rawdon, RR 4 201-3240 1re av, Rawdon QC J0K 1S0; Mon'75; Langs: English; (450)834-2304; Fax. (450)834-3345.

MONDOU, Melanie; MUHC-Montreal Gen Hosp, 1650 av Cedar, Montreal QC H3G 1A4; McG'04; FRCSC; IntMed; GeriatricMed. Staff, McGill University Health Centre - Montreal General Campus; (514)934-1934 x48015

MONETA, Ilaria; 4569 rue Sherbrooke O, Westmount QC H3Z 1E9; Pisa (Italy)'95; FRCPC; Peds (Developmental Pediatrics). Staff, Hôpital Ste-Justine; Langs: Spanish; Italian; (514)933-8437; Fax. (514)933-6398.

MONETTE, Andre; 201-181 rue Victoria, Salaber-de-Valleyf QC J6T 1A7; Mon'67; Psy. Staff Psy, Centre Hospitalier Régional du Suroît; Langs: English; (450)373-6252; Fax. (450)371-4910; andre.monette@rrsss16.gouv.qc.ca.

MONETTE, Diane; Clin Sante Beaute de Montagne, 400-1538 rue Sherbrooke O, Montreal QC H3G 1L5; Mon'79; Langs: English; (514)286-5555 x227; Fax. (514)286-0707.

MONETTE, Jocelyne; CSSS de Chicoutimi, 305 rue Saint-Vallier, Chicoutimi QC G7H 5H6; Sher'81; Staff, Complexe hospitalier de la Sagamie; (418)541-1000

MONETTE, Johanne; SMBD Jewish Gen Hosp, 3755 ch Cote-Sainte-Catherine, Montreal QC H3T 1E2; Mon'86; FRCPC; IntMed; GeriatricMed. Staff, Sir Mortimer B Davis Jewish General; (514)340-7501; Fax. (514)340-7547.

MONETTE, Luc; 206-15 boul Montclair, Gatineau QC J8Y 2E2; Sher'93; FRCSC; Otol. Staff, Hôpital de Gatineau; (819)776-0163

MONETTE, Lydia; Clin Med Lydia Monette Inc, 201-300 rue Marie-Victorin, Saint-Jerome QC J7Y 2G8; Sher'96; (450)565-2882; Fax. (450)565-2332.

MONETTE, Marie-Jose; CSSS de Laval, 1755 boul Rene-Laennec, Laval QC H7M 3L9; Mon'78; CSPQ; Neur; IntMed (Electromyography). Staff, Hopital de la Cite de la santé; Staff, Hôpital du Sacre-Coeur de Montréal; Langs: Spanish; English; (450)668-1010; Fax. (450)975-5550.

MONETTE, Steven; Clin Familiale de Coaticook, 206-18 rue du Manege, Coaticook QC J1A 3B3; Sher'94; (819)849-4808; Fax. (819)849-7400.

MONETTE, Virginie; Centre Med Iberville, 101-235 2e av, St-Jean-sur-Richel QC J2X 2B2; Sher'06; (450)347-5548

MONETTE, Yvan; Hotel-Dieu de Roberval, 450 rue Brassard, Roberval QC G8H 1B9; Mon'86; FRCPC; Psy. Staff, Hotel-Dieu de Roberval; (418)275-0110; Fax. (418)275-4829.

MONEY, Deborah M; BC Women's Hosp & Health Ctre, B327-4500 Oak St, Vancouver BC V6H 3N1; UBC'85; BSc; FRCSC; ObstGyn (Infectious Diseases). VP, BC Women's Hospital & Health Centre; Exec Dir, Health Research Institute; Prof ObstGyn, University of British Columbia; (604)875-3459; Fax. (604)875-3954.

MONEY, Phyllis M F; BC Women's Hosp & Health Ctre, 4500 Oak St, Vancouver BC V6H 3N1; UBC'91; BSc; FRCPC; Anes. Staff, BC Women's Hospital & Health Centre; (604)351-5876; Fax. (604)266-1480.

MONFETTE, Benoit; CSSS de la Haute-Yamaska, 205 boul Leclerc O, Granby QC J2G 1T7; Mon'98; Staff, Centre Hospitalier de Granby; (450)375-8000

MONFETTE, Claude D; CSSS de Trois-Rivières, 1991 boul du Carmel, Trois-Rivieres QC G8Z 3R9; Laval'84; CSPQ; Anes. ac Staff, CSSS de Trois-Rivières; (819)697-3333; Fax. (819)536-4360.

MONFETTE, Denis; CLSC Laurier-Station, 135 rue de la Station SS 1, Laurier-Station QC G0S 1N0; Laval'86; CCFP; Langs: Bilingual(French/English); (418)728-3435; Fax. (418)728-2233.

MONFETTE, Pascale; Ctr de Sante Vallee-Gatineau, 309 boul Desjardins, Maniwaki QC J9E 2E7; Mon'89; CCFP; Staff, CSSS de la Vallée de la Gatineau; Staff, CLSC Maniwaki; Langs: English; (819)449-4900; Fax. (819)449-6137.

MONFORTON, Anne-Marie; Aim Health Group, 1051 Wonderland Rd S, London ON N6K 3X4; Wes'87; CCFP; FCFP; Court Staff, St Joseph's Hospital - St Joseph's Health Care; (519)472-2060; Fax. (519)471-7299.

MONFRAIS, Jean-Luc; CSSS du Lac des deux Montagnes, 520 boul Arthur-Sauve, Saint-Eustache QC J7R 5B1; Paris (France)'75; CSPQ; Anes (P.Q.). Staff, Hôpital de Saint-Eustache; (450)473-6811 x2170

MONG, Irene E; Bedford Basin Women's Hlth Cli, 208B-967 Bedford Hwy, Bedford NS B4A 1A9; (South Africa)'99; MB ChB; (902)444-8726; Fax. (902)444-8722.

MONG, Kam W; Health Sciences Centre, 300 Prince Philip Dr, St. John's NL A1B 3V6; Alb'84; BMedSci; FRCSC; GenSurg; CardiothorSurg. Staff, Health Sciences Centre; Langs: Chinese; (709)777-6300

MONGA, Suneeta; The Hosp for Sick Children, 555 University Ave, Toronto ON M5G 1X8; Alb'89; FRCPC; Psy. Staff, The Hospital For Sick Children; (416)813-7531; Fax. (416)813-5326; suneeta.monga@sickkids.ca.

MONGE, Juan C; St Michael's Hosp, 6-041 Q-30 Bond St, Toronto ON M5B 1W8; (Costa Rica)'80; ABIM(Cardiol); ABIM(IntMed); FRCPC; Cardiol; IntMed. Staff Cardiologist, St Michael's Hospital; Assoc Prof Med, University of Toronto; Langs: Spanish; (416)864-5462; mongej@smh.toronto.on.ca.

MONGEAU, C Jacques; CHUS-Hop Hotel-Dieu, 580 rue Bowen S, Sherbrooke QC J1G 2E8; Sher'73; CSPQ; AnatPath (P.Q.). Staff, Centre Hospitalier Universitaire de Sherbrooke-Hopital Fleurimont; Staff, Centre Hospitalier Universitaire de Sherbrooke-Hôpital Hôtel-Dieu; assoc Prof, Universite de Sherbrooke; (819)346-1110 x14414; cjmongeau.chus@ssss.gouv.qc.ca.

MONGEAU, Frederic; CSSS de Saint-Jerome, 290 rue de Montigny, Saint-Jerome QC J7Z 5T3; Sher'07; Nephrol; IntMed. Staff, Hôtel-Dieu de Saint-Jérôme; (450)432-2777

MONGEAU, Laurent; Centre de Sante Carillon, 20 rue de Carillon, Sherbrooke QC J1J 2K8; Sher'78; AAFP; CCFP; Consultant, Centre Hospitalier Universitaire de Sherbrooke-Hôpital Hôtel-Dieu; (819)564-1022; Fax. (819)564-0218.

MONGEON, Anne; CSSS Haut-Richelieu-Rouville, 920 boul du Seminaire N, St-Jean-Sur-Richel QC J3A 1B7; Laval'97; Staff, Hôpital du Haut-Richelieu; (450)359-5000

MONGEON, Francois-Pierre; Institut de Cardiologie de Mtl, 5000 rue Belanger, Montreal QC H1T 1C8; Mon'02; FRCPC; IntMed; Cardiol. Staff, Institut de Cardiologie de Montréal; (514)376-3330

MONGEON, Guy J P; Notre Dame Med Centre, 430 Notre Dame Ave, Sudbury ON P3C 5K7; Mon'97; BSc; CCFP; Staff Family Med, Health Sciences North-St Joseph's Health Centre; Teach Staff Northern Ontario Family Med, University of Ottawa; Asst Prof, Northern Ontario School of Medicine-Laurentian University; Langs: Bilingual(French/English); (705)671-9797; Fax. (705)671-2992.

MONGEON, Mikael; CSSS du Nord de Lanaudiere, 1000 boul Sainte-Anne, Joliette QC J6E 6J2; Sher'08; Staff, Centre Hospitalier Régional de Lanaudière; (450)759-8222

MONGIARDI, Christopher N; Halton HCS Corp-Oakville, 327 Reynolds St, Oakville ON L6J 3L7; Ott'04; FRCPC; DiagRad. Staff, Halton Healthcare Services Corporation - Oakville Site; (905)845-2571

MONGRAIN, Eric; Ctre Dermatologique du Quebec, 105-2280 ch Quatre-Bourgeois, Quebec QC G1V 4X7; Laval'88; FRCPC; Derm.

MONGRAIN, Karine; Clinique Medival, 100-408 rue Jeanne-Mance, Salaber-de-Valleyf QC J6T 4G1; Mon'03; CCFP; Staff, Centre Hospitalier Régional du Suroît; (450)370-3387; Fax. (450)370-3395.

MONIER, Danielle; Hop Maisonneuve-Rosemont, 5415 boul de l'Assomption, Montreal QC H1T 2M4; Mon'66; Endocrin (P.Q.). Ac Staff, Hopital Maisonneuve-Rosemont; Med Consultant, Institut de Cardiologie de Montréal; (514)252-3400 x3723; monierd@sympatico.ca.

MONIUSZKO, Monika B; 10738 124 St NW, Edmonton AB T5M 0H1; Katowice (Poland)'66; (780)453-9800; Fax. (780)761-2915.

MONIWA, Emiko; St Paul's Hosp, 2B-1081 Burrard St, Vancouver BC V6Z 1Y6; UBC'04; FRCPC; Psy. Staff, Providence Health Care - St Paul's Hospital; (604)682-2344

MONIZ, Faustino P; Charlton Med Centre, 305-25 Charlton Ave E, Hamilton ON L8N 1Y2; McM'76; FRCP; FRCPC; IntMed; Cardiol. Ac Staff Cardiol, St Joseph's Healthcare - Charlton Campus; Asst Clin Prof Med, McMaster University; (905)522-5231; Fax. (905)522-1145.

MONK, Charles M; 103-704 Mara St, Point Edward ON N7V 1X4; Wes'77; (519)344-8283; Fax. (519)336-0459.

MONK, Tracy L; Lougheed Plaza, 260-9600 Cameron St, Burnaby BC V3J 7N3; McG'87; Staff, Royal Columbian Hospital; (604)420-9252

MONKEWICH, Gregory J; 200-3825 Sunset St, Burnaby BC V5G 1T4; Ott'96; FRCPC; IntMed; Gastroent. Physician, North Shore Medical Associates; Langs: Bilingual(English/French); (604)677-1624; Fax. (604)677-5883; gmonkewich@providencehealth.bc.ca.

MONKHOUSE, Alan K; Grandview Med Ctr Fam Hlth Team, 167 Hespeler Rd, Cambridge ON N1R 3H7; Tor'73; CCFP; FCFP; Staff, Cambridge Memorial Hospital; (519)623-9215; Fax. (519)623-2546.

MONKMAN, Lisa M; Dauphin Clinic, 622 3rd St SW, Dauphin MB R7N 1R5; Man'04; CCFP; (204)227-1818; Fax. (204)638-5670.

MONKMAN, Norman D; Foothills Med Centre, 1403 29 St NW, Calgary AB T2N 2T9; Man'97; Staff, Red Deer Regional Hospital Centre; (403)944-8741; Fax. (403)250-2093.

MONKS, Brian J; 9526 Erickson Dr, Burnaby BC V3J 1M9; National (Ireland)'67; MB ChB; Ac Staff, Royal Columbian Hospital; Ac Staff, Eagle Ridge Hospital & Health Care Centre; (604)421-1821; Fax. (604)421-0524.

MONNIER, Audrey; CSSS de la Minganie, CP 190 Bdp 1035 Prom des Anciens, Havre-Saint-Pierre QC G0G 1P0; Laval'08; CCFP; Staff, CSSS de la Minganie; (418)538-2212; Fax. (418)538-2365.

MONNIER, Patricia; MUHC-Royal Victoria Hosp, 687 av des Pins O, Montreal QC H3A 1A1; Nancy (France)'90; ObstGyn (P.Q.). Staff, McGill University Health Centre - Royal Victoria Hospital; (514)843-1650; Fax. (514)843-1496.

MONPREMIER, Pierre; 303-311 McArthur Ave, Vanier ON K1L 8M3; Port-au-Prince (Haiti)'69; DPM; LMCC; CSPQ; FRCPC; Psy (Mood Disorders). Langs: Creole; English; (613)746-4845; Fax. (613)746-7017.

MONROSE, Brigitte M A E; 208-9889 Highway 48, Markham ON L6E 0B7; Wes'83; CCFP; Langs: English; French; (905)294-4467

MONROY-CUADROS, Felix M; Foothills Med Centre, 725-1403 29 St NW, Calgary AB T2N 2T9; (Colombia)'93; FACS; TraSurg; Staff, Foothills Medical Centre; Asst Prof, University of Calgary; Langs: Spanish; (403)944-4266; mauricio.monroy@calgaryhealthregion.ca.

MONSON, Rochelle L; Victoria Terrace Med Centre, 302-1448 Lawrence Ave E, North York ON M4A 2V6; Tor'96; FRCPC; IntMed; Derm. (416)750-1066; Fax. (416)750-1091.

MONSON, Ronald C; 101-790 Sherbrook St, Winnipeg MB R3A 1M3; Man'67; FRCSC; OrthSurg (Pediatric Orthopedic Surgery). Ac Staff, Health Sciences Centre; (204)788-5758; Fax. (204)789-9220.

MONT, Erik; Nova Scotia Med Examiner Serv, 51 Garland Ave, Dartmouth NS B3B 0J2; New Jersey (USA)'97; (902)424-2722; Fax. (902)424-0607.

MONTAG, Randy J J; Hanover Med Associates, 118 7th Ave, Hanover ON N4N 2G9; Wes'01; CCFP; (519)364-2820; Fax. (519)364-3965.

MONTAGNE, Gerard; CHUM-Hop Notre-Dame, K.7-1560 rue Sherbrooke E, Montreal QC H2L 4M1; Mon'89; MSc; FRCPC; Psy (Consultant Holistic Medicine). Staff, Centre Hospitalier l'Université de Montréal (CHUM) - Hôtel-Dieu; Staff, Centre Hospitalier l'Université de Montréal (CHUM) - Hôpital Notre-Dame; Clin Prof, Universite de Montreal; (514)890-8000 x25678; gerard.montagne@sympatico.ca.

MONTAGUE, Michael; Montfort Hosp, 713 Montreal Rd, Ottawa ON K1K 0T2; Ott'08; CCFP; Staff, Montfort Hospital; (613)945-1140; Fax. (613)945-1347.

MONTALBETTI, David J; Lancer Bldg, 201-321 Lower Ganges Rd, Salt Spring Island BC V8K 2V4; Cal'84; FRCPC; Psy. Staff, Lady Minto Gulf Islands Hospital; (250)537-4432

MONTALBETTI, Kraig C; 1966 Harrison Way, Kamloops BC V1S 1M9; UBC'06; CCFP; (250)372-1004

MONTALIN, Livia; Clin Chir Plastique & Esthetiq, 425 Grande Allee E, Quebec QC G1R 2J5; Laval'99; FRCSC; PlasSurg (Esthetic Plastic Surgery). ac Membre, Centre Hospitalier Affilié Universitaire de Québec - Hôpital De L'Enfant Jésus; Langs: Bilingual(French/English); (418)682-8102; Fax. (418)681-2930.

MONTALVO, Max; Kingston Gen Hosp, 76 Stuart St, Kingston ON K7L 2V7; Qns'97; FRCPC; EmergMed. Staff EmergMed, Kingston General Hospital; (613)548-3232

MONTAMBAULT, Louis; I R D P Q-Site Francois-Charon, 525 boul Wilfrid-Hamel, Quebec QC G1M 2S8; Mon'70; FRCPC; IntMed. (418)529-9141 x6298; Fax. (418)649-3703.

MONTAMBAULT, Paul A; CHUS-Hop Fleurimont, 3001 12e av N, Sherbrooke QC J1H 5N4; Sher'70; Nephrol (P.Q.); IntMed. adj Prof, Centre Hospitalier Universitaire de Sherbrooke-Hopital Fleurimont; (819)346-1110

MONTANER, Julio S G; St Paul's Hosp, B667-1081 Burrard St, Vancouver BC V6Z 1Y6; Buenos Aires (Argentina)'79; FCCP; FRCPC; IntMed (AIDS/HIV). Ac Staff, Providence Health Care - St Paul's Hospital; Dir, AIDS Research Program & The John Ruedy Immunodeficiency Clinic & Chair, AIDS Research; Prof Med, University of British Columbia; Langs: French; Spanish; (604)806-8316; Fax. (604)806-8527.

MONTANERA, Walter J; St Michael's Hosp, CC3 075-30 Bond St, Toronto ON M5B 1W8; Tor'79; FRCPC; DiagRad (Neuro Radiology). Court Staff, Mount Sinai Hospital; Court Staff, Toronto General Hospital - UHN; Diag Therap Neuro Radiologist, St Michael's Hospital; Teach Staff Med, University of Toronto; Langs: Italian; (416)864-5671 x6495; Fax. (416)864-5380; montaneraw@smh.toronto.on.ca.

MONTANO-LOZA, Aldo J; Ziedler Ledcor Centre, 1 20B-130 University Campus NW, Edmonton AB T6G 2X8; (Mexico)'97; (780)248-1892; Fax. (780)248-1895.

MONTAS, Lys B; Centre Med Jean-Talon, 1392 rue Jean-Talon E, Montreal QC H2E 1S4; Paris (France)'67; FRCSC; Ophth. Ac Staff Ophth, CSSS du Coeur de l'Isle Hôpital Jean-Talon; (514)526-5536; Fax. (514)526-8484.

MONTBAZET, A X Anne; Ctr Hosp de Verdun, 4000 boul Lasalle, LaSalle QC H4G 2A3; Mon'09; CCFP; Staff, Centre Hospitalier de Verdun; (514)362-1000

MONTBRIAND, Michael W; Lakeshore Med Clinic, 1380 23rd Ave, Regina SK S4S 3S5; Sask'76; CCFP; (306)584-9333; Fax. (306)584-9788.

MONTE, Myrna M; Ramblewood Med Clinic, 101-14 Ramblewood Dr, Wasaga Beach ON L9Z 0C4; Qns'93; CCFP; Staff, Collingwood General & Marine Hospital; (705)429-1595; Fax. (705)429-6730.

MONTEIRO, Gerard E; Vista Med Centre, 1633B St Mary's Rd, Winnipeg MB R2N 1Z3; London (England)'63; MB BS.

MONTEL, Catherine; CSSS de la Haute-Yamaska, 205 boul Leclerc O, Granby QC J2G 1T7; Mon'97; LMCC; Staff, Centre Hospitalier de Granby; (450)375-8000

MONTELEONE, Bradley J; 104-1634 Harvey Ave, Kelowna BC V1Y 6G2; UBC'97; BSc; MSc; Dip SportMed; CCFP; (250)860-4122

MONTEMURO, Paul T; Lonsdale Med Dental Bldg, 217A-1940 Lonsdale Ave, North Vancouver BC V7M 2K2; Tor'83; Staff, Royal Columbian Hospital; Staff Privil, Lions Gate Hospital; (604)985-7104; Fax. (604)985-7128; montemuro@shaw.ca.

MONTEMURO, Suzanne M; Cook Street Village Med Clinic, 101A-230 Cook St, Victoria BC V8V 3X3; Qns'73; (250)220-9999

MONTEMURRO, Trina C; St Paul's Hosp, 1081 Burrard St, Vancouver BC V6Z 1Y6; Cal'99; BSc; FRCPC; Anes;CCFP; Staff, Providence Health Care - St Paul's Hospital; (604)682-2344

MONTERO ODASSO, Manuel M; St Joseph's HC-Parkwood Hosp, A 280-801 Commissioners Rd E, London ON N6C 5J1; Buenos Aires (Argentina)'90; FRCPC; IntMed; GeriatricMed. Staff, Parkwood Hospital - St Joseph's Health Care; Langs: Italian; French; (519)685-4021

MONTERROSA, Luis; Saint John Reg Hosp, PO Box 2100 Stn Main 400 University Ave, Saint John NB E2L 4L2; Del Norte (Colombia)'82; Staff, Saint John Regional Hospital; (506)639-9536; Fax. (506)648-6250.

MONTES, Jose; MUHC-Montreal Children's Hosp, C1137-2300 rue Tupper, Montreal QC H3H 1P3; San Luis Potosi (Mexico)'73; BSc; Neursurg (P.Q.) (Pediatric Neuro Surgery). Staff, McGill University Health Centre - Montreal General Campus; Staff, Shriners Hospitals For Children - Canada; Dir NeuroSurg Services, McGill University Health Centre - Montreal Children's Hospital; assoc Prof, McGill University; Langs: Spanish; (514)412-4400 x25224; Fax. (514)412-4368; jose.montes@muhc.mcgill.ca.

MONTESSORI, Valentina C; St Paul's Hosp, 520B-1081 Burrard St, Vancouver BC V6Z 1Y6; UBC'90; FRCPC; IntMed; InfectDis., Providence Health Care - St Paul's Hospital; Assoc Prof, University of British Columbia; Langs: Italian; French; (604)806-8644

MONTGOMERIE, H Stewart; Elmsdale Med Centre, 106 Elmsdale Rd, Elmsdale NS B2S 1K6; Dal'70; (902)883-2216; Fax. (902)883-1734.

MONTGOMERY, Alison G; McMaster Clinic, 506-1280 Main St W, Hamilton ON L8S 4K1; McM'91; BSc; FRCPC; IntMed (Echo & Nuclear Cardiology); Cardiol. Staff, Hamilton Health Sciences Centre - Hamilton General Hospital; Assoc Prof Med Div of Cardiol/Dir Residency Prog Cardiol, McMaster University; (905)521-2100 x73958; Fax. (905)577-8034.

MONTGOMERY, Angela B; 630-101 Queensway Blvd W, Mississauga ON L5B 2P7; Tor'01; FRCPC; IntMed; Rheum. (905)848-2444; Fax. (905)848-2447.

MONTGOMERY, Barbara A; Courtice Health Centre, 1450 Highway 2, Courtice ON L1E 3C3; McG'86; BSc(Hon); MDCM; CCFP; FCFP; Assoc Staff, Lakeridge Health - Oshawa Site; Langs: English; French; (905)721-4343; Fax. (905)721-6183.

MONTGOMERY, Brian F; Mainland Med Clinic, 1061 Hamilton St, Vancouver BC V6B 5T4; UBC'92; (604)683-3973; Fax. (604)683-3809.

MONTGOMERY, Carla M; Breast Cancer Supportive Care, 414-301 14 St NW, Calgary AB T2N 2A1; Alb'92; BSc; CCFP; (403)270-2242; Fax. (403)270-2251.

MONTGOMERY, Carolyne J; Children's & Women's HC of BC, 4480 Oak St, Vancouver BC V6H 3V4; Tor'80; FRCPC; Anes. Staff, BC Children's Hospital; Asst Prof, University of British Columbia; Langs: Bilingual(English/French); (604)875-2711

MONTGOMERY, Christopher W; North Oshawa Med Centre, 205-1400 Ritson Rd N, Oshawa ON L1G 7W4; McG'93; BSc; MSc; FRCPC; Peds. Assoc Staff, Lakeridge Health - Oshawa Site; Langs: English; French; (905)433-1721; Fax. (905)433-2108.

MONTGOMERY, G Bruce E; Elmsdale Med Centre, 106 Elmsdale Rd, Elmsdale NS B2S 1K6; Dal'81; BSc; (902)883-2216; Fax. (902)883-1734.

MONTGOMERY, George D; Montfort Hosp, 713 Montreal Rd, Ottawa ON K1K 0T2; Ott'07; FRCPC; EmergMed. Staff, Montfort Hospital; (613)746-4621; Fax. (613)748-4914.

MONTGOMERY, Gregory P J; Foothills Med Centre, 1403 29 St NW, Calgary AB T2N 2T9; Cal'06; FRCPC; Psy. Staff, Foothills Medical Centre; (403)944-1271; Fax. (403)270-3451.

MONTGOMERY, Helen F; Signal Hill Centre, 2-5986 Signal Hill Ctr SW, Calgary AB T3H 3P8; Alb'81; BMedSci; CCFP; (403)240-2660; Fax. (403)242-8390.

MONTGOMERY, Hugh J; 2660 Marchurst Rd RR 2, Dunrobin ON K0A 1T0; Ott'72; Assoc Staff Emerg, Queensway Carleton Hospital; (613)832-2515

MONTGOMERY, Ian D; Medical Arts Centre, 103-650 Terminal Ave, Nanaimo BC V9R 5E2; UBC'86; Staff, Nanaimo Regional General Hospital; (250)753-3431; Fax. (250)754-6897.

MONTGOMERY, Katherine P; Mount St Vincent University, 1-166 Bedford Hwy, Halifax NS B3M 2J6; Dal'83; (902)457-6354; Fax. (902)457-0828.

MONTGOMERY, Lori S; Calgary Chronic Pain Centre, 160-2210 2 St SW, Calgary AB T2S 3C3; Cal'03; CCFP; (403)943-9900; Fax. (403)209-2954.

MONTGOMERY, Mark D; Foothills Professional Bldg, 150-1620 29 St NW, Calgary AB T2N 4L7; Alb'81; FRCPC; Peds; Respir. Staff, Alberta Children's Hospital; Clin Assoc Prof, University of Calgary; (403)284-1333; Fax. (403)282-3223; mark.montgomery@albertahealthservices.ca.

MONTGOMERY, Matthew R; Edmonton Clinic Health Academy, 11405 87 Ave NW, Edmonton AB T6G 1C9; Dal'03; FRCPC; Peds; PedEmergMed. Staff, University of Alberta Hospital; (780)248-5575; Fax. (780)248-5625.

MONTGOMERY, Patrick R; Royal Jubilee Hosp, 106-1952 Bay St, Victoria BC V8R 1J8; Man'74; FRCPC; IntMed; GeriatricMed. Staff, Royal Jubilee Hospital; (250)370-8000

MONTGOMERY, Scott B; Royal Inland Hosp, 311 Columbia St, Kamloops BC V2C 2T1; UBC'88; Staff, Royal Inland Hospital; (250)374-5111

MONTGOMERY, W Roy; Tyne Valley Med Centre, PO Box 78, Tyne Valley PE C0B 2C0; Dal'77; Gen Practice, Stewart Memorial Hospital; Physician Emerg, Community Hospital Inc; Med Examiner Medical Aviation, Ministry of Transportation; (902)831-2659; rmontgomery@canada.com.

MONTGRAIN, Noel-H.; 2737 ch Saint-Louis, Quebec QC G1W 1N8; Laval'59; FRCPC; Psy. Ac Staff Psy, Centre Hospitalier Universitaire de Quebec-CHUL; Member, Canadian Psychoanalytic Society; (418)658-1785

MONTHROPE, Yvette; Women's College Hosp, 76 Grenville St, Toronto ON M5S 1B2; Tor'05; FRCPC; Derm. Staff, Women's College Hospital; (416)323-7546; Fax. (416)323-6236.

MONTI, Liliana L; 838 Fennell Ave E, Hamilton ON L8V 1V6; Tor'69; FRCPC; Psy (Individual Psychotherapy). Clinical Asst Prof Psychiatry, McMaster University; Langs: Italian; (905)389-6336; Fax. (905)389-6657.

MONTI DE FLORES, Silvia; Institut Allan Memorial, 1025 av des Pins O, Montreal QC H3A 1A1; San Salvador (El Salvador)'70; FRCPC; Psy (Psycho Geriatrics). Staff, McGill University Health Centre - Royal Victoria Hospital; Chef, Douglas Mental Health University Institute; Allan Memorial Institute; Teach Staff Psy, McGill University; Universite de Montreal; Langs: Spanish; French; (514)888-4455; Fax. (514)888-4057; defsil@douglas.mcgill.ca.

MONTIGNY, Martine; CSSS de Laval, 1755 boul Rene-Laennec, Laval QC H7M 3L9; Louvain (Belgium)'80; Cardiol (P.Q.) (Clinical Cardiology). Staff, Hopital de la Cite de la santé; (450)668-1010; Fax. (450)975-5550.

MONTINI, Alexandre; Clinique Med des Sommets, 1070 rue Principale, Ste-Agathe-des-Mts QC J8C 1L6; Mon'99; (819)321-1212; Fax. (819)321-3232.

MONTIVEROS, Carolina; The Jenny Trout Centre, 113-342 Erie St, Stratford ON N5A 2N4; Cordoba (Argentina)'91; FRCPC; Peds. Staff, Children's Hospital of Eastern Ontario (CHEO); (519)272-2040; Fax. (519)272-2323.

MONTMINY, Alphonse; Hop Charles LeMoyne, 190-3120 boul Taschereau, Greenfield Park QC J4V 2H1; Mon'85; EmergMed (P. Q.) (AIDS). Staff, Hopital Charles LeMoyne; (450)466-5000 x2552; Fax. (450)465-5795.

MONTMINY, Gilles; 450A rue Heriot, Drummondville QC J2B 1B5; Mon'77; (819)477-8898; Fax. (819)447-8081.

MONTMINY, Marie-Eve; CSSS de Rimouski-Neigette, CP 3150 succ A 150 av Rouleau, Rimouski QC G5L 5T1; Sher'03; FRCPC; IntMed; Endocrin&Metab. Staff, Hôpital Regional Rimouski; (418)723-7851

MONTMINY, Patrice; 150-1165 boul Lebourgneuf, Quebec QC G2K 2C9; Laval'79; FRCSC; OrthSurg (Spine Surgery). Ac Staff, Centre Hospitalier Universitaire De Québec - Pavillon De St-françois-d'assise; Langs: English; (418)627-3330; Fax. (418)627-5313.

MONTMINY-METIVIER, Stephane; CSSS de Saint-Jerome, 290 rue de Montigny, Saint-Jerome QC J7Z 5T3; Mon'95; FRCPC; IntMed (Hematological Oncology); MedOncol; Hem. Staff HematoOncol, Centre Hospitalier Laurentien; Staff HematoOncol, Centre Hospitalier d'Argenteuil; Staff HematoOncol, Hôtel-Dieu de Saint-Jérôme; Langs: English; (450)431-8200 x8366; Fax. (450)431-8302.

MONTOEDI, Jacqueline I; Selkirk & Dist Gen Hosp, PO Box 5000 Stn Main 100 Easton Dr, Selkirk MB R1A 2M2; Medunsa (South Africa)'99; CCFP; CCFP(E.M.); Staff, Selkirk & District General Hospital; (204)482-5800; jimontoedi@yahoo.com.

MONTON, Luis R; Clinique Medic Elle, 500 rue Sherbrooke O, Montreal QC H3A 3C6; McG'81; FRCSC; ObstGyn. Ac Staff, Sir Mortimer B Davis Jewish General; (514)939-3099; Fax. (514)939-5946.

MONTORO, Richard; MUHC-Montreal Gen Hosp, 1650 av Cedar, Montreal QC H3G 1A4; McG'91; FRCPC; Psy (Consultation-Liaison). Asst Psy, McGill University Health Centre - Montreal General Campus; Langs: Spanish; French; (514)934-8010; Fax. (514)934-8237.

MONTOUR, Laura; Avenue Med Centre, 221 Brant Ave, Brantford ON N3T 3J2; McM'06; CCFP; (519)753-8666; Fax. (519)753-6880.

MONTOYA, David R; Centretown Comm Health Centre, 420 Cooper St, Ottawa ON K2P 2N6; Mem'80; BMedSci; MBA; FRCPC; EmergMed (Family Medicine). Langs: Spanish; French; (613)233-4697; Fax. (613)233-4541.

MONTPETIT, Guy; Clinique Medicale, 2065 boul des Laurentides, Laval QC H7M 4M2; Mon'87; Staff, Centre Hospitalier Régional du Suroît; (450)975-1557

MONTPETIT, Madeleine R; The Ottawa Hosp-Riverside, 1967 Riverside Dr, Ottawa ON K1H 7W9; Ott'89; CCFP; FCFP; Staff Family Health Team, The Ottawa Hospital - Riverside Campus; Clin Staff Family Med, The Ottawa Hospital - Civic Campus; Langs: English; French; (613)738-8219; Fax. (613)738-8217.

MONTPETIT, Patrick; CSSS de Laval, 1755 boul Rene-Laennec, Laval QC H7M 3L9; Mon'00; FRCSC; GenSurg. Staff, Hopital de la Cite de la santé; (450)668-1010

MONTPETIT, Pierre; CSSS Bordeaux-Cartierville-St-, 555 boul Gouin O, Montreal QC H3L 1K5; Mon'62; Staff, Pavillon Notre-Dame de la Merci; (514)331-3025

MONTPLAISIR, Isabelle; Hop du Sacre-Coeur de Mtl, 5400 boul Gouin O, Montreal QC H4J 1C5; Laval'95; CCFP; CCFP(E.M.); FCFP; Ac Member Emerg, Centre Hospitalier Universitaire de Quebec-CHUL; Staff, Hôpital du Sacré-Coeur de Montréal; (514)335-1252; isabelle.montplaisir@videotron.ca.

MONTPLAISIR, Jacques Y; Hop du Sacre-Coeur de Mtl, 5400 boul Gouin O, Montreal QC H4J 1C5; Mon'66; PhD; CRCP; Electroenceph (P.Q.); Psy. Ac Staff, Hôpital du Sacre-Coeur de Montréal; Dir, Sleep Disorders Clinic; (514)338-2693; Fax. (514)338-2531.

MONTPLAISIR, Serge; Univ de Montreal, CP 6128 Succ Centre Ville, Montreal QC H3C 3J7; Mon'66; MSc; Microbio & Infect Dis (P.Q.); MedMicrobiol (P.Q.) (Immunology). Ac Member, Hôpital Ste-Justine; Assoc Member, Institut de Cardiologie de Montréal; Prof, Universite de Montreal; Langs: English; French; (514)343-6376; Fax. (514)397-1344; serge.montplaisir@umontreal.ca.

MONTPLAISIR, Sylvie; CSSS de Saint-Jerome, 290 rue de Montigny, Saint-Jerome QC J7Z 5T3; Mon'80; Ophth (Medical Retina). Staff, Hôtel-Dieu de Saint-Jérôme; (450)431-8290; smopht@videotron.ca.

MONTPLAISIR-GAUMONT, Antoine; CSSS de Beauce-Etchemin, 1515 17e rue, Saint-Georges QC G5Y 4T8; Laval'05; DiagRad. Staff, Centre Hospitalier Beauce-Etchemin; (418)228-2031

MONTREUIL, Ann; CHUQ-St-Francois D'Assise, 10 rue de l'Espinay, Quebec QC G1L 3L5; Laval'83; LMCC; CCFP; FCFP; Staff, Centre Hospitalier Universitaire De Québec - Pavillon De St-françois-d'assise; (418)525-4425; Fax. (418)525-4322.

MONTREUIL, Bernard; Hop Maisonneuve-Rosemont, 5415 boul de l'Assomption, Montreal QC H1T 2M4; Mon'90; FRCSC; GenSurg; VascSurg. Staff, Hopital Maisonneuve-Rosemont; (514)252-3400

MONTREUIL, Jean P; Ctr Hosp Affilie-Enfant-Jesus, 1401 18e rue, Quebec QC G1J 1Z4; Laval'81; CSPQ; FRCPC; Anes. Ac Staff, Centre Hospitalier Affilié Universitaire de Québec - Hôpital De L'Enfant Jésus; Vis Physician, Oregon Health Sciences University; Staff Teacher, Université Laval; (418)649-0252 x5803; Fax. (418)649-5918.

MONTREUIL, Jean-Francois; CHUQ-Ctr Hosp Univ Laval, 2705 boul Laurier, Quebec QC G1V 4G2; Laval'94; FRCPC; Psy. Staff, Centre Hospitalier Universitaire de Quebec-CHUL; (418)656-4141

MONTSION, Claude; 200 boul Greber, Gatineau QC J8T 6K2; Laval'69; Assoc Staff, Hôpital de Gatineau; Langs: Bilingual(French/English); (819)568-0444; Fax. (819)568-1356.

MONTULET, Evelyne C; CSSS du Sud de Lanaudière, 911 montee des Pionniers, Terrebonne QC J6V 2H2; Laval'89; FRCPC; Peds (Emergency Clinic). Staff, Centre Hospitalier Pierre le Gardeur; (450)654-7525 x12107

MONTY, Anne; Centre Med Pour Enfants, 1791 av Dollard, LaSalle QC H8N 1T9; Mon'92; Staff, Hôpital de Saint-Eustache; (514)368-0441; anne.monty@sympatico.ca.

MONUMENT, Michael J; HSC-Faculty of Med, G207-3330 Hospital Dr NW, Calgary AB T2N 4N1; Cal'05; FRCSC; OrthSurg. (403)220-3366

MONY, Marc F; Commission des Lesions Prof, 510-2 rue Saint-Germain E, Rimouski QC G5L 8T7; Laval'80; IntMed. Physician, Commission Sante Securite Travail; (418)727-4212; Fax. (418)727-4274; marc.mony@csst.qc.ca.

MONZON, Jose G; Tom Baker Cancer Centre, 1331 29 St NW, Calgary AB T2N 4N2; Tor'05; FRCPC; IntMed; MedOncol. Staff, Tom Baker Cancer Centre; (403)521-3723

MOOALLEM, Ronit; Tiny Tots Med Centre, 203-3400 rue du Marche, Dollard-D-Ormeaux QC H9B 2Y1; McG'89; CCFP; Langs: French; Hebrew; (514)685-3531 x6662; Fax. (514)685-7971.

MOODIE, Rosemary G; 303-89 Humber College Blvd, Etobicoke ON M9V 4B8; (Jamaica)'82; MB BS; FRCPC; Peds (Neonatology). Staff, The Hospital For Sick Children; Asst Prof, University of Toronto; (416)743-6063; Fax. (416)743-0101; rmoodie@rougevalley.ca.

MOODIE, Sarah M; Sechelt Medical Associates, 5531 Inlet Ave, Sechelt BC V0N 3A0; Qns'09; CCFP; (604)885-2257

MOODLEY, Anithadevi; Surrey Mem Hosp, 13750 96 Ave, Surrey BC V3V 1Z2; Cape Town (South Africa)'93; FRCPC; Peds (Neonatal & Perinatal Medicine). Staff, Surrey Memorial Hospital; (778)384-4437

MOODLEY, Clifford; 204-2825 Clearbrook Rd, Abbotsford BC V2T 6S3; Pretoria (South Africa)'05; Staff, Abbotsford Regional Hospital & Cancer Centre; (604)859-5449

MOODLEY, Deshinee; Border City Clinic, 2707 50th Ave, Lloydminster SK S9V 2A8; University of Natal (South Africa)'00; MB ChB; Physician ER, Lloydminster Hospital; (306)825-4427; Fax. (306)825-2028.

MOODLEY, Logan G; 400-871 Ottawa St, Windsor ON N8X 2C9; Natal (South Africa)'88; MB ChB; FCP (SA); FRCPC; Neur. Aj Prof Clinical, University of Western Ontario; (519)253-7067; Fax. (519)253-7312.

MOODLEY, Mathaven; Windsor Prof Centre, 130-2462 Howard Ave, Windsor ON N8X 3V6; Natal (South Africa)'79; MB ChB; FRCSC; GenSurg. (519)258-7207; Fax. (519)258-7208.

MOODLEY, Nateeran P; 204-2825 Clearbrook Rd, Abbotsford BC V2T 6S3; Pretoria (South Africa)'02; MB ChB; (604)853-8641

MOODLEY, Prabashnee; Milton Family Care Centre, 820 Main St E, Milton ON L9T 0J4; (South Africa)'00; MB BCh; BSc(Mathematics); CCFP; (905)864-9898; Fax. (905)864-9393.

MOODLEY, Santhiran; Victoria Hosp, PO Box 3000 Stn Main 1200 24th St W, Prince Albert SK S6V 5T4; Staff, Victoria Hospital; (306)953-8970; Fax. (306)953-8976.

MOODLEY, Shreya; Children's & Women's HC of BC, 4800 Oak St, Vancouver BC V6H 3V4; Sask'07; FRCPC; Peds. Staff, BC Children's Hospital; (604)875-2120

MOODLEY, Suseelan H; Guelph Family Health Team, 302-21 Surrey St W, Guelph ON N1H 3R3; RCS (Ireland)'87; MB ChB; BAO; LRCP; CCFP; FCFP; Ac Staff Privil, Guelph General Hospital; Med Dir, Cambridge Country Manor; (519)763-4338; Fax. (519)763-3696.

MOODLEY, U Otto; Royal University Hosp, 103 Hospital Dr, Saskatoon SK S7N 0W8; Sask'98; FRCPC; IntMed; Hem. Staff, Royal University Hospital; (306)655-1690; Fax. (306)655-1809.

MOODLEY, Vasse T; Medical Associates, 1212 The Queensway, Etobicoke ON M8Z 1R8; RCS (Ireland)'65; MB ChB; LM; LRCPS; Ac Staff, Trillium Health Centre - West Toronto; Ac Staff, Trillium Health Centre - Mississauga; (416)251-8257; Fax. (416)252-8870.

MOODLEY, Zenobia; 203-2825 Clearbrook Rd, Abbotsford BC V2T 6S3; Pretoria (South Africa)'02; MB ChB; Staff, Abbotsford Regional Hospital & Cancer Centre; (604)852-1567

MOODLIAR, Romashnee; Associate Med Clinic, 400-20 14th St W, Prince Albert SK S6V 3K8; (306)953-1688

MOODLIAR, Santhosian; Associate Med Clinic, 400-20 14th St W, Prince Albert SK S6V 3K8; Pretoria (South Africa)'98; FRCSC; ObstGyn. (306)953-1651; Fax. (306)764-3091.

MOODY, Alan R; Sunnybrook Hlth Sciences Ctre, AG57-2075 Bayview Ave, Toronto ON M4N 3M5; (England)'83; FRCPC; DiagRad. Staff, Sunnybrook Health Sciences Centre; Dept Chair Medical Imaging, University of Toronto; (416)480-4341; Fax. (416)480-5855.

MOODY, Frederick J; 205-2494 Danforth Ave, Toronto ON M4C 1K9; Tor'55; Assoc Staff, Toronto East General Hospital Inc; (416)693-1689; Fax. (416)693-1690.

MOODY, Helene; Clin Med St Felix de Valois, 610 ch Joliette RR 1, St-Felix-de-Valois QC J0K 2M0; Mon'94; Staff, Centre Hospitalier Régional de Lanaudière; (450)889-5577; Fax. (450)889-4239.

MOODY, Jane K; St Boniface Gen Hosp, M5020-409 Tache Ave, Winnipeg MB R2H 2A6; Man'00; FRCPC; Psy. Staff, St Boniface General Hospital; (204)233-8563

MOODY, Jeremy W; Queen Square Doctors FHT, 201-366 Main St N, Brampton ON L6V 1P8; RCS (Ireland)'78; MB ChB; BAO; LRCPS(Ire); (905)455-1331; Fax. (905)455-5498; jeremy.moody@bell.net.

MOODY, Richard G; The Medical Clinic, 10011 96 St, Fort St. John BC V1J 3P3; Newcastle (United Kingdom)'72; MB BS; DRCOG; CCFP; FCFP; (250)785-6677; Fax. (250)787-0109; rmoody@fsjmedicalclinic.com.

MOODY, Sandra; North York Gen Hosp, 4001 Leslie St, North York ON M2K 1E1; Tor'72; Ac Staff, North York General Hospital; (416)756-6000

MOOLA, Ashraf; Humboldt Med Clinic, PO Box 220, Humboldt SK S0K 2A0; Cape Town (South Africa)'08; MB BCh; (306)682-2618; Fax. (306)682-4499.

MOOLA, Cassim; St Mary's Gen Hosp, 911 Queens Blvd, Kitchener ON N2M 1B2; Natal (South Africa)'71; FRCPC; DiagRad. Med Dir-Radiol Serv, St Mary's General Hospital; (519)749-6455; Fax. (519)749-6513.

MOOLA, Dawood; Cypress Reg Health Centre, 2004 Saskatchewan Dr, Swift Current SK S9H 5M8; RCS (Ireland)'72; LRCS; LRCP; Head Diagnostic Imaging, Cypress Regional Health Authority Corporate Office; (306)778-9457; Fax. (306)778-9588; damoola@gmail.com.

MOOLA, Farhad O; 403-233 Nelson's Cres, New Westminster BC V3L 0E4; Sask'97; FRCSC; OrthSurg (Upper Extremity Surgery). (604)526-4646; Fax. (604)526-4664.

MOOLA, Shiraz; Kootenay Lake Hosp, 410-3 View St, Nelson BC V1L 2V1; Qns'97; BSc; FRCSC; ObstGyn (Laparoscopy). Staff, Kootenay Lake General Hospital; (250)352-1122; Fax. (250)352-1183.

MOOLLA, Hasan M; Battleford Med Clinic, PO Box 1540, Battleford SK S0M 0E0; Rangoon (Burma)'64; MB BS; LRCP(Lond); MRCS(Eng); LMCC; CISAM; CCFP; (306)937-7705; Fax. (306)937-2202.

MOOLLA, Mohamed; Golden Mile Medi Clinic, 50-3806 Albert St, Regina SK S4S 3R2; Madras (India)'91; MB BS; BSc; Ac Staff, Regina General Hospital; Ac Staff, Pasqua Hospital; Clinical Asst Prof Family Med, University of Saskatchewan; Langs: Afrikaans; Urdu; Hindi; (306)584-3701; Fax. (306)584-3721; drmoolla_md@hotmail.com.

MOOLLA, Riaz; Professional Bldg, 301-222 King St E, Bowmanville ON L1C 1P6; Natal (South Africa)'94; MB ChB; CCFP; Staff, Lakeridge Health - Bowmanville Site; (905)697-3607; Fax. (905)697-3645.

MOOLLA, Yunus E; Associate Clinic, 5215A 49 AVE, Wetaskiwin AB T9A 0R1; (India)'00; (780)352-7157; Fax. (780)352-2273.

MOOLMAN, Andre; Grand River Hosp-KW Hlth Ctre, PO Box 9056 Stn C 835 King St W, Kitchener ON N2G 1G3; Pretoria (South Africa)'87; LMCC; ACLS; ATLS; CCFP; Staff, Grand River Hospital - Kitchener/Waterloo Health Centre; Clinical Asst Prof Family Med, McMaster University; Langs: Afrikaans; Dutch; German; (519)749-4370; Fax. (519)749-4378.

MOOLMAN, Johannes Z; South Shore Med Clinic, 620 Cassils Rd E, Brooks AB T1R 1M6; (South Africa)'01; MB BS; (403)793-8111; Fax. (403)793-8118.

MOOLMAN, Johnathan; Park Avenue Med Centre, 4634 Park Ave, Terrace BC V8G 1V7; Orange Free State (South Africa)'89; MB ChB; DA; Langs: Afrikaans; Zulu; (250)615-5040; Fax. (250)615-5049.

MOON, Byung-Choo; 625 Davis Dr, Newmarket ON L3Y 2R2; Qns'82; FRCSC; GenSurg (Adult Cardiac Surgery); Cardiovasc&ThorSurg. Med Dir/Chief Div of Cardiac Surg, Southlake Regional Health Centre; (905)868-8386; Fax. (905)830-9931.

MOON, Michael C; St Boniface Gen Hosp, 3537-409 Tache Ave, Winnipeg MB R2H 2A6; Man'97; CardSurg. Staff, St Boniface General Hospital; (204)233-8563

MOONEY, Kevin K; Merrickville District CHC, PO Box 550 354 Read St, Merrickville ON K0G 1N0; Ott'68; CCFP; FCFP; (613)269-3400; Fax. (613)269-4958.

MOONJE, Vijay B; Riverside Prof Centre, 404-1919 Riverside Dr, Ottawa ON K1H 1A2; Nagpur (India)'61; FACS; FRCSC; GenSurg (Endocrinology Surgery). Staff, The Ottawa Hospital - General Campus; Staff, The Ottawa Hospital - Civic Campus; Staff, The Ottawa Hospital - Riverside Campus; Lecturer Surg, University of Ottawa; (613)521-4961; Fax. (613)521-5321.

MOONSAMY, Chrisen; Caledonian Clinic Ltd, 340 Campbell St, Nanaimo BC V9R 3G7; Mysore (India)'00; (250)753-3202; Fax. (250)753-1039.

MOONSAMY, Prunella; Caledonian Med Clinic, 340 Campbell St, Nanaimo BC V9R 3G7; Witwatersrand (South Africa)'05; (250)753-3202

MOORE, Aideen M A; The Hosp for Sick Children, 555 University Ave, Toronto ON M5G 1X8; National (Ireland)'76; FRCPC; Peds (Neonatology). Staff Neonatologist, The Hospital For Sick Children; Assoc Prof, University of Toronto; (416)813-6345; Fax. (416)813-5245; aideen.moore@sickkids.ca.

MOORE, Ainsley E; Stonechurch Family Health Ctre, 1475 Upper Ottawa St, Hamilton ON L8W 3J6; McM'96; BSc; MSc; CCFP; Staff, Hamilton Health Sciences Centre - Hamilton General Hospital; (905)975-1300

MOORE, Alan W; Cannon Clinic, 4-2151 McCallum Rd, Abbotsford BC V2S 3N9; Ott'75; Staff, Abbotsford Regional Hospital & Cancer Centre; (604)853-3314; Fax. (604)853-2171.

MOORE, Albert R; MUHC-Royal Victoria Hosp, 687 av des Pins O, Montreal QC H3A 1A1; Man'99; CSPQ; FRCPC; Anes. Staff, McGill University Health Centre - Royal Victoria Hospital; (514)934-1934

MOORE, Alison J; Alberta Children's Hosp, C4-335-2888 Shaganappi Trail N, Calgary AB T3B 6A8; Cal'98; FRCPC; Neur. Staff, Alberta Children's Hospital; (403)955-7211; alison.moore@muhc.mcgill.ca.

MOORE, Andrea M L; Hotel-Dieu Hosp, 166 Brock St, Kingston ON K7L 5G2; Wes'95; FRCPC; Peds. Staff Peds, Kingston General Hospital; Staff Peds, Hotel-Dieu Hospital; Asst Prof, Queen's University; (613)544-3400 x3359; Fax. (613)544-3559.

MOORE, Andrew D; 200-2984 boul Taschereau, Greenfield Park QC J4V 2G9; McG'94; FRCPC; IntMed; ClinImmunol&Allergy. Staff Allergy & Immunol, Hopital Charles LeMoyne; Langs: Bilingual(French/English); (450)465-9789

MOORE, Anne K; Queen Elizabeth Hosp, PO Box 6600 Stn Central 60 Riverside Dr, Charlottetown PE C1A 8T5; Wes'81; CSPQ; FRCPC; Anes. Staff, Queen Elizabeth Hospital; (902)894-2111

MOORE, April E; Headwaters Health Care Centre, 100 Rolling Hills Dr, Orangeville ON L9W 4X9; McM'96; FRCPC; DiagRad. Staff, Headwaters Health Care Centre - Orangeville Site; (519)941-2410

MOORE, Beryl M; Fairview Med Arts Centre, 208-2200 Fairview St, Burlington ON L7R 4H9; McM'82; CCFP; Clinical Asst Prof Family Med, McMaster University; (905)333-5245; Fax. (905)632-2617.

MOORE, Britt; Grey Bruce HS-Owen Sound, PO Box 1800 Stn Main 8236-1800 8th St E, Owen Sound ON N4K 6M9; Mem'01; FRCSC; ObstGyn. Staff, Grey Bruce Health Services - Owen Sound; (519)372-2100; Fax. (519)372-2109; gestewart@gbhs.on.ca.

MOORE, Charlotte; 555 University Ave, Toronto ON M5G 1X8; Baltimore(MD) (USA)'01; BA; ABPeds; FAAP; FRCPC; Peds. Staff/Teach Staff, The Hospital For Sick Children; (416)813-7654; Fax. (416)813-5663; charlotte.moore@sickkids.ca.

MOORE, Corey C; St Joseph's Health Care, PO Box 5777 Stn B 2F-268 Grosvenor St, London ON N6A 4V2; Man'96; ABOtol; MSc; BSc; ABFPS; FACS; FRCSC; Otol (Facial Plastic Surgery). Staff Otol, St Joseph's Hospital - St Joseph's Health Care; Staff, London Regional Cancer Center; Staff, Victoria Health Sciences Centre; Assoc Prof, University of Western Ontario; (519)646-6383; Fax. (519)646-6173; cmoore22@uwo.ca.

MOORE, Jeffrey; Fredericton Med Clinic, 302-1015 Regent St, Fredericton NB E3B 6H5; Dal'99; BSc(Biology); FRCPC; IntMed. Staff, Dr Everett Chalmers Regional Hospital; (506)447-4041; Fax. (506)457-4758.

MOORE, Dana L; London Medical-Dental Bldg, 301-450 Central Ave, London ON N6B 2E8; Wes'98; CCFP; FCFP; (519)439-0346

MOORE, David M; St Paul's Hosp, 608-1081 Burrard St, Vancouver BC V6Z 1Y6; McG'92; FRCPC; CommunMed. Staff, Providence Health Care - St Paul's Hospital; (604)806-8060

MOORE, David W; Care Point Med Centre, 1060-2929 Barnet Hwy, Coquitlam BC V3B 5R5; New South Wales (Australia)'72; (604)468-1202

MOORE, Deborah C; Ridge Meadows Hosp & Hlth CC, 11666 Laity St, Maple Ridge BC V2X 5A3; (Other Foreign)'99; MB ChB; Staff, Ridge Meadows Hospital & Health Care Centre; (604)463-4111

MOORE, Derrick D; Nanaimo Reg Gen Hosp, 1200 Dufferin Cres, Nanaimo BC V9S 2B7; Alb'88; CCFP; CCFP(E.M.); Staff, Nanaimo Regional General Hospital; (250)754-2141

MOORE, Dorothy L; MUHC-Montreal Children's Hosp, C1242-2300 rue Tupper, Montreal QC H3H 1P3; Mem'77; FRCPC; Peds; InfectDis. Staff, McGill University Health Centre - Montreal Children's Hospital; assoc Prof, McGill University; (514)412-4485; dorothy.moore@muhc.mcgill.ca.

MOORE, Doug; Charlottetown Area Hlth Ctre, 1 Rochford St, Charlottetown PE C1A 9L2; Dal'72; FRCPC; Psy (Adult Outpatient Psychiatry). (902)368-9355

MOORE, Eva M; 227-950 28th Ave W, Vancouver BC V5Z 4H4; Johns Hopkins (USA)'04; (604)875-2000 x7923

MOORE, Fraser G A; SMBD Jewish Gen Hosp, E005-3755 ch Cote-Sainte-Cathe, Montreal QC H3T 1E2; Alb'97; FRCPC; Neur. Staff, Sir Mortimer B Davis Jewish General; (514)340-8222 x3969

MOORE, G R Wayne; Vancouver Gen Hosp, 855 12th Ave W, Vancouver BC V5Z 1M9; McG'72; FRCPC; Neur; NeurPath. Staff Path & LabMed, Vancouver General Hospital - Centennial Pavillion; Staff, UBC Hospital - Koerner Pavillion; Clin Prof, University of British Columbia; (604)875-4480; Fax. (604)875-4797.

MOORE, Gerald D; Pender Island Med Clinic, 5715 Canal Rd RR 1, Pender Island BC V0N 2M1; Cal'85; CCFP; Assoc Staff, Saanich Peninsula Hospital; (250)629-3233; Fax. (250)629-3234.

MOORE, Grant E; The Credit Valley Hosp, 2200 Eglinton Ave W, Mississauga ON L5M 2N1; Ott'92; CCFP; CCFP(E.M.); Staff Emerg, The Credit Valley Hospital; (905)813-4141; Fax. (905)813-4477.

MOORE, Gregory P; The Ottawa Hosp-Gen Campus, 501 Smyth Rd, Ottawa ON K1H 8L6; Wes'02; FRCPC; Peds (Neonatal & Perinatal Medicine). Staff, The Ottawa Hospital - General Campus; (613)737-8561

MOORE, Irene T; Soldier's Mem Hosp, PO Box 730, Middleton NS B0S 1P0; Tor'77; Med Pres/Sec Med Staff, Soldiers Memorial Hospital; (902)825-3411

MOORE, James W; Sheridan Med Associates, 1-1960 Dundas St W, Mississauga ON L5K 2R9; Wes'72; (905)822-3993; Fax. (905)822-5522.

MOORE, Jennifer E; Capitol Hill Medical, 101-4695 Hastings St, Burnaby BC V5C 2K6; Dal'86; Ac Staff, Burnaby Hospital; Clin Instructor, University of British Columbia; (604)298-7201; Fax. (604)291-6176.

MOORE, Jennifer; Sunnybrook Hlth Sciences Ctre, 2075 Bayview Ave, Toronto ON M4N 3M5; Chicago (USA)'97; Staff, Sunnybrook Health Sciences Centre - Edmond Odette Cancer Centre; (416)480-6100; Fax. (416)480-5146.

MOORE, Joanna D; Civic Family Med Centre, 210 Melrose Ave, Ottawa ON K1Y 4K7; Tor'10; CCFP.

MOORE, Julie B; Alexandra Marine & Gen Hosp, 120 Napier St, Goderich ON N7A 1W5; Indiana(IN) (USA)'92; FRCSC; ObstGyn. Staff, Alexandra Marine & General Hospital; (519)524-8323 x407; Fax. (519)524-5865.

MOORE, Katherine; CHUQ-Ctr Hosp Univ Laval, 2705 boul Laurier, Quebec QC G1V 4G2; Laval'02; FRCSC; Urol (Pediatric Urology). Staff, Centre Hospitalier Universitaire de Quebec-CHUL; Langs: Bilingual(French/English); (418)654-2282

MOORE, Kathryn; Bayridge Family Med Clinic, 775 Strand Blvd, Kingston ON K7P 2S7; McM'91; CCFP; FCFP; (613)507-1212; Fax. (613)507-1213.

MOORE, Kieran M; KFLA Public Health, 221 Portsmouth Ave, Kingston ON K7M 1V5; Ott'86; DTMH; MMedSci; FRCPC; Public Health & Preventive Med;CCFP; CCFP(E.M.); FCFP; Att Physician Emerg Family Med, Kingston General Hospital; Assoc Prof Emerg Family Med, Queen's University; Langs: English; French; (613)549-1232; Fax. (613)549-1209; kmoore@kflapublichealth.ca.

MOORE, Kimberly; Centre for Family Medicine, GD 3742 Nafziger Rd, Wellesley ON N0B 2T0; Wes'03; (519)656-2220; Fax. (519)656-3173.

MOORE, Laurel E; STAR Family Health Team, RR 5 Stn Main 700 O'Loane Ave, Stratford ON N5A 6S6; McM'81; BA; BScN; CCFP; FCFP; Ac Staff Family Med/Chief Staff/Chief HPHA, Stratford General Hospital - Huron Perth Healthcare Alliance; (519)273-1060; Fax. (519)273-0371.

MOORE, Leonard J; O A S I S, 221 Nelson St, Ottawa ON K1N 1C7; Tor'96; BSc; CCFP; FCFP; (613)569-3488; Fax. (613)569-3484.

MOORE, Lisa J; Riverside Court Med Clinic, 5-3635 Rivergate Way, Ottawa ON K1V 2A4; McM'89; CCFP; FCFP; Asst Prof C F T, University of Ottawa; (613)739-3700; Fax. (613)739-7043; dr.moore@riversidecourt.ca.

MOORE, Lori A; Lakeridge Hlth Corp-Oshawa, 1 Hospital Crt, Oshawa ON L1G 2B9; Tor'84; FRCPC; DiagRad. Staff, Lakeridge Health - Oshawa Site; (905)433-4305; Fax. (905)721-4770.

MOORE, Malcolm J; Univ Hlth Network-Princess M, 5 708-610 University Ave, Toronto ON M5G 2M9; Wes'80; MedOncol; IntMed (Clinical Pharmacology). Sr Scientist Div AMO/OCI, Princess Margaret Hospital - University Health Network; Prof Med & Pharmacology, University of Toronto; (416)946-4501 x2263; Fax. (416)946-2082.

MOORE, Nathalie; Clinique medicale Waterloo, CP 760 100-4900 rue Foster, Waterloo QC J0E 2N0; Sher'88; (450)539-1102

MOORE, Nicholas J; One Med Place, 322-20 Wynford Dr, North York ON M3C 1J4; Tor'66; Court Staff, Toronto East General Hospital Inc; Physician, Chevron Oil; (416)445-9673; Fax. (416)445-9388.

MOORE, P Mary; 375 South St PO Box 5375 Stn B, London ON N6A 4G5; Wes'80; ABIM; FRCPC; IntMed. Staff, London Health Sciences Centre - South Street; Ac Staff, London Health Sciences Centre - Victoria Campus; Asst Prof, University of Western Ontario; (519)667-6676; Fax. (519)472-4614.

MOORE, Peter G B; Perth Med Clinic, 1-500 East Riverside Dr, Perth-Andover NB E7H 1Z1; McG'75; CCFP; FCFP; Att Staff, Hôtel-Dieu of St Joseph Hospital; Medical Officer, Victoria Glen Manor; (506)273-9529; Fax. (506)273-9560.

MOORE, Pierre; CSSS de la Minganie, CP 190 1035 Prom des Anciens, Havre-Saint-Pierre QC G0G 1P0; Sher'86; Staff, CSSS de la Minganie; (418)538-2212

MOORE, Randall W; 4-22932 Lougheed Hwy, Maple Ridge BC V2X 2W3; McM'83; CCFP; FCFP; Staff, Ridge Meadows Hospital & Health Care Centre; (604)466-5767

MOORE, Randell L; St Paul's Hosp, 1081 Burrard St, Vancouver BC V6Z 1Y6; Cal'80; FRCPC; Anes. Staff, Providence Health Care - St Paul's Hospital; (604)682-2344

MOORE, Randy D; Peter Lougheed Centre, 3601-3500 26 Ave NE, Calgary AB T1Y 6J4; Sask'90; BSc(Hons.); MSc; FRCSC; GenSurg (Aortic Aneurysm Surg); VascSurg. Chief Regional Clin Div, Peter Lougheed Centre; Pres Vascular Surg Section, Alberta Medical Association; Assoc Prof Cross Appt, University of Calgary; (403)943-5467; Fax. (403)943-4235; randyd.moore@albertahealthservices.ca.

MOORE, Ronald B; University of Alberta Hosp, 2D216-8440 112 St NW, Edmonton AB T6G 2B7; Alb'86; PhD; FACS; FRCSC; Urol (Transplantation). Ac Staff, University of Alberta Hospital; Ac Staff, Cross Cancer Institute; Clin Investigator, Alberta Heritage Foundation for Medical Research; Prof Surg & Oncol, University of Alberta; (780)407-6330; Fax. (780)407-6331; ron.moore@albertahealthsevices.ca.

MOORE, Sean W; The Ottawa Hosp-Civic Campus, 1053 Carling Ave, Ottawa ON K1Y 4E9; McG'93; FRCPC; EmergMed (Pre-Hospital Emergency Care). Staff, The Ottawa Hospital - Civic Campus; (613)722-7000

MOORE, Simon G D; Gordon & Leslie Diamond H C C, 2775 Laurel St, Vancouver BC V5Z 1M9; UBC'10; CCFP; (604)875-4834

MOORE, Stephen B; 91 Cornelia St W, Smiths Falls ON K7A 5L3; Wes'69; ABIM; FRCPC; IntMed. (613)283-1166; Fax. (613)283-2665; drsmoore@bellnet.ca.

MOORE, Terrence L; St Michael's Hosp, 30 Bond St, Toronto ON M5B 1W8; Wes'65; FRCPC; IntMed (Gastroenterology). Staff, St Michael's Hospital; Assoc Prof, University of Toronto; (416)864-5847; Fax. (416)864-5993; mooret@smh.toronto.on.ca.

MOORE, Wendy A L; St Joseph's Health Centre, 30 The Queensway, Toronto ON M6R 1B5; McM'93; FRCPC; Psy. Staff Psy, St Joseph's Health Centre; (416)530-6000 x3041; Fax. (416)530-6076.

MOORE, W Hanna; 303-4610 Highway 7, Woodbridge ON L4L 4Y7; Warsaw (Poland)'78; Langs: Polish; Russian; (905)850-6050

MOOREHEAD, Paul C; Richardson Labratory, 88 Stuart St, Kingston ON K7L 3N6; Man'04; FRCPC; Peds; PedHemaOncol. (613)533-2822

MOORES, Carl D; Health Sciences Centre, 300 Prince Philip Dr, St. John's NL A1B 3V6; Mem'06; FRCSC; OrthSurg. Staff, Health Sciences Centre; (709)737-6300

MOORES, Daisy E; Fifth Avenue Court, 17-99 Fifth Ave, Ottawa ON K1S 5K4; Ott'08; CCFP; Staff, SCO Health Service - Élisabeth Bruyère Hospital; (613)563-3670; Fax. (613)563-4124.

MOORES, David G; Royal Alexandra Hosp, 10240 Kingsway NW, Edmonton AB T5H 3V9; Mem'73; MSc; CCFP; FCFP; Staff, Royal Alexandra Hospital; Physician, Family Medicine Centre; Prof Family Med, University of Alberta; (780)735-4201; Fax. (780)735-4978.

MOORES, Mark S; North Huron FHT-Wingham, PO Box 480 285 Catherine St, Wingham ON N0G 2W0; Tor'92; BSc; CCFP; Staff, Wingham & District Hospital - Listowel Wingham Hospitals Alliance; Langs: Spanish; (519)357-1325; Fax. (519)357-1568.

MOORHOUSE, Cameron W; 100-240 First St E, Fort Frances ON P9A 1K5; Cal'81; CCFP; (807)274-2479; Fax. (807)274-6972.

MOORHOUSE, Paige A; Veterans Memorial Bldg, 1421-5595 Veterans Memorial La, Halifax NS B3H 2E1; Dal'02; FRCPC; IntMed; GeriatricMed. (902)473-3888; Fax. (902)473-7133.

MOORHOUSE-HERX, Leonie; Foothills Med Centre, 710-1403 29 St NW, Calgary AB T2N 2T9; Cal'04; CCFP; Staff, Foothills Medical Centre; (403)212-8223; Fax. (403)270-9652.

MOORJANI, Anoo; CLSC Rivieres Et Marees, 22 rue Saint-Laurent, Riviere-du-Loup QC G5R 4W5; Laval'97; (418)867-2642; Fax. (418)868-1350.

MOORJANI, Mira; CSSS de Papineau, 155 rue MacLaren E, Gatineau QC J8L 0C2; Laval'98; Staff, CH-CHSLD de Papineau - Pavillon du centre hospitalier; Staff, Hôpital de Papineau; (819)986-4115 x4006; Fax. (819)961-8018.

MOORJANI, Vijay; Alberta Children's Hosp, 2888 Shaganappi Trail NW, Calgary AB T3B 6A8; (India)'88; MB BS; Staff, Alberta Children's Hospital; (403)955-7985; Fax. (403)955-7656.

MOOROSI, Setsoana L; Albert Park Family Med Centre, 3992 Albert St, Regina SK S4S 3R1; (306)584-3833; Fax. (306)585-3833.

MOORSOM, David M; Northumberland Hills Hosp, 1000 Depalma Dr, Cobourg ON K9A 5W6; London (England)'68; MB; BSc; MRC; FRCPC; IntMed. Staff, Northumberland Hills Hospital; (905)372-6811

MOORTHY, Ramachandra N; 210-8120 Cook Rd, Richmond BC V6Y 1T9; Mysore (India)'59; FRCPC; Psy (Family Medicine). Court Staff, Richmond Hospital; Langs: Kanarese; (604)270-4220

MOORTHY, Sathasivam W; Homewood Health Centre, 150 Delhi St, Guelph ON N1E 6K9; Ceylon (Sri Lanka)'71; MRCPsy(UK); FRCPC; Psy. Staff Psy, Homewood Health Centre; (519)824-1010 x2196; Fax. (519)824-1827.

MOOSA, Alisha B; Family Matters Med Centre, X-730 St Anne's Rd, Winnipeg MB R2N 0A2.

MOOSA, Malek B; 117-7130 120th St, Surrey BC V3W 3M8; Punjab (India)'74; CCFP; Langs: Hindi; Punjabi; Urdu; (604)590-6905

MOOSA, Naseeba; Humboldt Med Clinic, PO Box 220, Humboldt SK S0K 2A0; (306)682-2618; Fax. (306)682-4499.

MOOSAVI, Homayoon; Grand River Hosp-KW Hlth Ctre, PO Box 9056 Stn C 835 King St W, Kitchener ON N2G 1G3; Shiraz (Iran)'85; DR; Staff/Consultant Neuroradiologist, Grand River Hospital - Kitchener/Waterloo Health Centre; Langs: Persian; (519)749-4300 x2981; Fax. (519)749-4296; moosavih@gmail.com.

MOOSAVIAN, Mona; Scarborough Hosp-Birchmount, 3030 Birchmount Rd, Scarborough ON M1W 3W3; Tor'08; FRCPC; IntMed. Staff, The Scarborough Hospital - Birchmount Campus; (416)431-8101

MOOSBRUGGER, Karen A; 103-300 St. Ann's Rd, Campbell River BC V9W 4C6; Mem'03; FRCSC; Ophth. (250)287-7980

MOOSBRUGGER, Peter; St Joseph's Gen Hosp, 2137 Comox Ave, Comox BC V9M 1P2; Innsbruck (Austria)'88; CCFP; FCFP; Staff, St Joseph's General Hospital; Langs: German; Spanish; French; (250)339-2242

MOOTE, D William; St Joseph's Health Care, PO Box 5777 Stn B B3 110-268 Grosvenor St, London ON N6A 4V2; Wes'79; FRCPC; ClinImmunol&Allergy (Asthma); IntMed. Consultant, St Joseph's Hospital - St Joseph's Health Care; Consultant, London Health Sciences Centre - University Hospital; Staff Med, London Health Sciences Centre - Victoria Campus; Staff, London Health Sciences Centre - South Street; Dir Training Prog, University of Western Ontario; (519)685-8167; Fax. (519)685-8274.

MOOZAR, Kouros; Taunton Health Centre, SS 201 1290 Keith Ross Dr, Oshawa ON L1H 7K4; McG'99; FRCSC; GenSurg (Clinician Investigator Program); General Surgical Oncology.

MOQUIN, Daniel H; Parry Sound Family Health Team, 57 James St, Parry Sound ON P2A 1T6; Man'88; CCFP; FCFP; Ac Staff, West Parry Sound Health Centre; Lecturer, Northern Ontario School of Medicine; Langs: English; French; (705)746-2181; Fax. (705)746-4753.

MOQUIN, Jean-Pierre; Hop du Sacre-Coeur de Mtl, 5400 boul Gouin O, Montreal QC H4J 1C5; Mon'80; CSPQ; FRCPC; IntMed; MedOncol (P.Q.); Hem. Staff, Hôpital du Sacre-Coeur de Montréal; Staff, Centre Hospitalier Fleury; assoc Prof, Universite de Montreal; Langs: English; (514)338-2150

MOQUIN, Kathleen M; Parry Sound Family Health Team, 57 James St, Parry Sound ON P2A 1T6; Man'89; BSc(Med); CCFP; Med Staff, West Parry Sound Health Centre; Teach Staff, University of Toronto; Lecturer, Northern Ontario School of Medicine; (705)746-2181; Fax. (705)746-4753.

MORADHASSEL, Fariedeh P; The Peterborough Clinic, 103-26 Hospital Dr, Peterborough ON K9J 7C3; Teheran (Iran)'70; FRCPC; Peds (Neonatology). Staff, Peterborough Regional Health Centre - Hospital Drive; (705)740-6843; Fax. (705)740-6897.

MORAES, Theo J; The Hosp for Sick Children, 4534-555 University Ave, Toronto ON M5G 1X8; Tor'97; FRCPC; Peds (Physiology); Respir. Staff, The Hospital For Sick Children; (416)813-6168; Fax. (416)813-6246.

MORAIS, J Alfred; Parkdale Med Center, 30 Linden Ave, Charlottetown PE C1A 5Y9; Dal'85; BSc; CCFP; FCFP; Staff, Queen Elizabeth Hospital; Med Dir Queen's Network, PEI Dept of Health; Teach Staff Med, Dalhousie University; (902)368-1991; Fax. (902)569-1563.

MORAIS, Jacques; Cite de la Sante de Laval, 1755 boul Rene-Laennec, Laval QC H7M 3L9; Mon'85; NuclearMed. Staff, Hopital de la Cite de la santé; (450)668-1010; Fax. (450)975-5545.

MORAIS, Jose A; MUHC-Royal Victoria Hosp, H661-687 av des Pins O, Montreal QC H3A 1A1; Mon'87; CSPQ; FRCPC; IntMed (Nutrition); GeriatricMed. assoc Médecin, McGill University Health Centre - Royal Victoria Hospital; assoc Prof, McGill University; Langs: Portuguese; English; (514)843-1665; Fax. (514)843-1706.

MORAIS, Michelle L; McMaster University, MDCL 3101A-1280 Main St W, Hamilton ON L8S 4K1; Mem'06; FRCSC; ObstGyn.

MORALEJO, Richard V; 5300 ch de la Cote-des-Neiges, Montreal QC H3T 1Y3; McG'49; GenSurg. Staff Surg, St Mary's Hospital Centre; (514)344-2000

MORALES, Alvaro; 59 Lakeshore Blvd., Kingston ON K7M 6R4; Bogota (Colombia)'64; FACS; FRCSC; Urol. Staff, Kingston General Hospital; Staff, Centre for Urological Research; Prof Dept of Urol, Queen's University; Langs: Spanish; (613)389-9275; moralesa@queensu.ca.

MORALES, Carmen M; Health Sciences Centre, MS5-820 Sherbrook St, Winnipeg MB R3A 1R9; Madrid (Spain)'81; MSc; AB; FRCPC; GenPath (Hematology Pathology). Staff HemPath, CancerCare Manitoba; Staff HemPath Diagnostic Services of Manitoba/Assoc Prof Path, University of Manitoba; Langs: Spanish; (204)787-4682

MORALES, Dora; Hotel-Dieu de Saint-Joseph, 10 Woodland Hill, Perth-Andover NB E7H 5H5; (El Salvador)'82; CCFP; Staff, Hôtel-Dieu of St Joseph Hospital; Langs: Spanish; (506)273-7100

MORALES, Eduardo; Miramichi Reg Hosp, 500 Water St, Miramichi NB E1V 3G5; (Colombia)'81; Staff, Miramichi Regional Hospital; (506)623-3000

MORALES, Fraulein; University of Alberta Hosp, 8440 112 St NW, Edmonton AB T6G 2B7; Quezon (Philippines)'98; BScBiology; FRCPC; IntMed. Staff, University of Alberta Hospital; (780)407-3856; Fax. (780)407-3132.

MORALES, Hilda A; Creekside Med Clinic, 4-12192 Symons Valley Rd NW, Calgary AB T3P 0A3; Cal'06; CCFP; (403)275-6606; Fax. (403)730-0941.

MORALES, Jose J; Hotel-Dieu de Saint-Joseph, 10 Woodland Hill, Perth-Andover NB E7H 5H5; (El Salvador)'74; PhD; FRCSC; GenSurg. Staff, Hôtel-Dieu of St Joseph Hospital; Langs: Spanish; (506)273-7100

MORAN, Andrew; Trillium Doctors Office, 406-2299 Dundas St W, Toronto ON M6R 1X7; Dublin (Ireland)'85; Assoc Staff, Ontario Shores Centre for Mental Health Sciences; (416)535-3511; Fax. (416)535-5993.

MORAN, Bryan C; St Michael's Hosp, 8-30 Bond St, Toronto ON M5B 1W8; Tor'87; CCFP; Staff, Toronto General Hospital - UHN; Teach Staff, Toronto Western Hospital - University Health Network; Staff, St Michael's Hospital; (416)692-7660

MORAN, Catherine T; 344 Hume St, Collingwood ON L9Y 1W3; McM'83; BSc(Hons.); MScPath; Pres Medical Staff, Collingwood General & Marine Hospital; (705)445-9044; Fax. (705)445-8017; ctmoran@hotmail.com.

MORAN, Geoffrey; 344 Hume St, Collingwood ON L9Y 1W3; McM'83; BPE; CCFP; Staff, Collingwood General & Marine Hospital; Assoc Prof, University of Toronto; Assoc Prof, McMaster University; (705)445-9044; Fax. (705)445-8017.

MORAN, Jane M; Victoria Emerg Phys Mgmt Ltd, 325-1627 Fort St, Victoria BC V8R 1H8; Qns'82; Dip SportMed; FRCPC; EmergMed. Physician Emerg, Victoria General Hospital; Physician Emerg, Royal Jubilee Hospital; Med Advisor, International Skating Union; Assoc Med Dir, Summit Injury Management; (250)479-1442

MORAN, Judith C; Hamilton HS-General Site, 237 Barton St E, Hamilton ON L8L 2X2; Man'68; BSc; BSc(Med.); CCFP; CCFP(E.M.); Court Staff Emerg, St Joseph's Healthcare - Charlton Campus; Ac Staff Emerg, Hamilton Health Sciences Centre - Hamilton General Hospital; Chair, Disaster Committee CAEP; Asst Prof, McMaster University; (905)521-2100 x46368; moran@hhsc.ca.

MORAN, Keith W V; 169 Hiram St, Bracebridge ON P1L 2B8; Tor'90; DABIM; NBEchoTestamur; FRCPC; IntMed. Ac Staff, South Muskoka Memorial Hospital - Muskoka Algonquin Healthcare; (705)646-1221; Fax. (705)646-1271.

MORAN, Kevin C; Rouge Valley-Centenary HC, 2867 Ellesmere Rd, Scarborough ON M1E 4B9; Wes'87; Staff, Rouge Valley Health System - Centenary Health Centre Site; Staff Gen Pract, The Scarborough Hospital - General Campus; (416)281-7270; Fax. (416)284-9229.

MORAN, Martin B; Glenrose Rehab Hosp, 1248-10230 111 Ave NW, Edmonton AB T5G 0B7; (Ireland)'85; CCFP; Staff, Glenrose Rehabilitation Hospital; (780)735-8845; Fax. (780)735-8846.

MORAN, Michael M; 1624 7th Ave, Prince George BC V2L 3P6; London (England)'87; BSc; MA; MB BS; FRCSC; OrthSurg. Att Surgeon, University Hospital of Northern British Columbia; Head Div of Comprehensive Ortho, University of British Columbia; (250)564-8800; Fax. (250)564-7580; mmoran@heritagemed.ca.

MORAN, Nancy I; St Michael's Hosp, 30 Bond St, Toronto ON M5B 1W8; Wes'93; FRCPC; Anes. Staff, St Michael's Hospital; (416)686-9021

MORAN, P Bruce; Ottawa Cardiovascular Centre, 502-1355 Bank St, Ottawa ON K1H 8K7; Tor'84; FRCPC; IntMed; Cardiol. Clin Assoc Staff, The Ottawa Hospital - Civic Campus; Assoc Staff, Montfort Hospital; (613)738-1584; Fax. (613)738-9097.

MORAN, Peter D; Central North Correctional Ctr, 1501 Fuller Ave, Penetanguishene ON L9M 2H4; Dublin (Ireland)'75; MB BCh; BAO; CCFP; FCFP; Physician, Central North Correctional Centre; (705)549-9480 x2814; Fax. (705)549-5124.

MORAN, Peter I M; Credit Valley Med Arts Centre, 409-2000 Credit Valley Rd, Mississauga ON L5M 4N4; (Ireland)'81; MB; MRCGPract; DCH; DObst; FRCPC; Psy (Geriatric Psychiatry). Consultant Psy, The Credit Valley Hospital; Consultant Psy, Mount Sinai Hospital; Consultant/Psychiatrist Seniors Mental Health Prog, Trillium Health Centre - Mississauga; Consultant Psy, Homes for Special Care, Ministry of Health-ON; Asst Prof Psy, University of Toronto; Langs: Irish; (905)607-9779; Fax. (905)607-7704; peter@drpetermoran.ca.

MORAN, Philip A; Markham Stouffville Hosp, PO Box 1800 Stn Main 381 Church St, Markham ON L3P 7P3; Wes'96; FRCPC; EmergMed. Staff, Markham Stouffville Hospital; (905)472-7000

MORAN DE MULLER, Karen M; Markham Prof Centre, 307-2265 Pembina Hwy, Winnipeg MB R3T 5J3; (Mexico)'85; Staff Obst & Newborn Care, Health Sciences Centre; Staff Obst & Newborn Care, St Boniface General Hospital; Staff Emerg Psy, The Salvation Army Grace Hospital; Staff Geriatrics, Personal Care Homes Inc; Langs: Spanish; (204)275-3769; Fax. (204)269-6574.

MORAN-MENDOZA, A Onofre; Richardson House, 211-102 Stuart St, Kingston ON K7L 2V6; (Mexico)'86; FRCPC; IntMed; Respir.

MORANA, Corrado G; Surrey Med Centre, 307-2130 Lawrence Ave E, Scarborough ON M1R 3A6; Tor'76; CCFP; Court Staff, The Scarborough Hospital - Birchmount Campus; Staff, Toronto East General Hospital Inc; Staff, Markham Stouffville Hospital; Staff, The Scarborough Hospital - General Campus; Langs: Italian; (416)751-6141; Fax. (416)751-5270.

MORAND, Allison R; Chatham-Kent Family Health Team, 209-20 Emma St, Chatham ON N7L 5K5; Tor'05; CCFP; CCFP(E.M.); Staff Emerg, Chatham-Kent Health Alliance; (519)354-2172

MORAND, Claudine; Clinique GMF Quatre-Bourgeois, 300-979 av de Bourgogne, Quebec QC G1W 2L4; Laval'87; MSc(HealthAdmin.); FRCPC; PhysMed&Rehab (Pain Management). (418)653-4050; Fax. (418)653-4475.

MORANTZ, Jesse; 103-5631 Inlet Ave PO Box 799, Sechelt BC V0N 3A0; Ben Gurion (Israel)'06; FRCPC; IntMed. (604)885-7103

MORANTZ-ORNSTEIN, Gillian; MUHC-Montreal Children's Hosp, 2300 rue Tupper, Montreal QC H3H 1P3; McG'05; Peds. Staff, McGill University Health Centre - Montreal Children's Hospital; (514)412-4400

MORANVILLE, Guy; La Cite Medicale, 295-2600 boul Laurier, Quebec QC G1V 4T3; Laval'95; Ac Staff, CHSLD St Augustin; Ac Staff, CHSLD St-Antoine; Langs: English; (418)781-0480; guy.moranville@irdpq.qc.ca.

MORAR, Champaklal; 3-246 Dundas St S, Cambridge ON N1R 8A8; Natal (South Africa)'67; CCFP; FCFP; Staff Emerg, Hamilton Health Sciences Centre - McMaster University Medical Centre; Staff, Cambridge Memorial Hospital; (519)622-5100; Fax. (519)622-2977.

MORAR, Parbhoo; Ellesmere Health Care Centre, 1-2060 Elesmere Rd, Scarborough ON M1H 2V6; Witwatersrand (South Africa)'57; MB ChB; Court Staff, Humber River Regional Hospital - Church Street Site; Court Staff, William Osler Health System - Etobicoke General Hospital; Langs: Gujarati; (416)439-2273

MORAR, Shaheen; 3-246 Dundas St S, Cambridge ON N1R 8A8; Glasgow (Scotland)'94; CCFP; (519)622-5100

MORASH, Angela H; 100-65 Prestwick Close, Halifax NS B3S 0C1; Dal'06; CCFP; (902)429-2722; Fax. (902)446-3038.

MORASH, Christopher G L; The Ottawa Hosp-Civic Campus, B3-1053 Carling Ave, Ottawa ON K1Y 4E9; Dal'88; FRCSC; Urol. Att Staff Urol, The Ottawa Hospital - Civic Campus; Consultant Urol, The Ottawa Hospital - General Campus; Asst Prof, University of Ottawa; (613)761-4500; Fax. (613)761-5305.

MORASH, Garry W; Dr Garry Morash Med Clinic, PO Box 790 157 Schoal St, Liverpool NS B0T 1K0; Dal'77; Staff, Queens General Hospital; (902)354-5204; Fax. (902)354-3749.

MORASSE, Charles; UMF Laval, 2690 ch des Quatre-Bourgeois, Quebec QC G1V 0B7; Laval'00; CCFP; (418)656-8711; Fax. (418)656-4503.

MORASSE, Daniel; Centre Med de la Montagne, 457 boul Laurier, Mont-Saint-Hilaire QC J3H 3P2; Sher'78; (450)464-1777; Fax. (450)464-1779.

MORASSUT, Patricia A; Nepean Med Centre, 404-1 Centrepointe Dr, Nepean ON K2G 6E2; Wes'81; BSc; FRCPC; IntMed; Rheum. Att Staff, The Ottawa Hospital - Civic Campus; Asst Prof, University of Ottawa; (613)723-5729; Fax. (613)723-5697.

MORASSUTTI, Dante J; 205-1106 Ouellette Ave, Windsor ON N9A 1C9; Tor'83; FRCSC; Neursurg. (519)973-8771

MORAUD, Edouard; Clinique Med Val-Belair, 202-1147 boul Pie-XI N, Quebec QC G3K 2P8; Laval'90; Staff, CSSS de la Minganie; (418)843-2473; edouard_moraud@ssss.gouv.qc.ca.

MORAVA-PROTZNER, Izabella; Calgary Laboratory Services, 3500 26 Ave NE, Calgary AB T1Y 6J4; Semmelweis (Hungary)'67; PhD(Physiol); ABPath; FRCPC; AnatPath (Breast Pathology). Clin Assoc Prof Path, University of Calgary; Langs: Hungarian; (403)943-5628

MORAWSKA-JABLONSKA, Joanna; 37 Thorncliff Pl, Nepean ON K2H 6L5; Cracow (Poland)'73; FRCPC; Peds. Staff, The Ottawa Hospital - Civic Campus; Staff, Queensway Carleton Hospital; Staff, Children's Hospital of Eastern Ontario (CHEO); Staff, The Ottawa Hospital - General Campus; Langs: Polish; (613)596-1993; Fax. (613)596-6764.

MORAZAIN, Louis; 320-900 boul du Seminaire N, St-Jean-Sur-Richel QC J3A 1C3; Mon'66; OrthSurg. (450)348-6966; Fax. (450)348-0664; louismorazain@videotron.ca.

MORCH, S Ellen; 110-200 St Clair Ave W, Toronto ON M4V 1R1; UBC'95; BScChemEng; CCFP; (416)928-9343; Fax. (416)928-9368.

MORCOM, Richard; Albert County Hlth & Welness C, 8 Forestdale Rd, Riverside-Albert NB E4H 3Y7; Witwatersrand (South Africa)'81; Staff, Albert County Health and Wellness Centre; (506)882-3100; Fax. (506)882-3101.

MORCOS, Leila; CHUQ-Ctr Hosp Univ Laval, 2705 boul Laurier, Quebec QC G1V 4G2; Sher'95; CSPQ; DiagRad. Staff, Centre Hospitalier Universitaire de Quebec-CHUL; (418)656-4141

MORCOS, Mohib; Ctr Hosp Affilie-St-Sacrement, 1050 ch Sainte-Foy, Quebec QC G1S 4L8; Cairo (Egypt)'92; Staff, Centre Hospitalier Affilié Universitaire de Québec - Hôpital du St-Sacrement; Langs: Arabic; Bilingual(English/French); (418)682-7511 x2085; Fax. (418)682-7383; mohib-w.morcos.cha@ssss.gouv.qc.ca.

MORCOS, Rami; Clinique Neurologique Laennec, 210-1100 av Beaumont, Mont-Royal QC H3P 3H5; Sher'79; FABPN; CSPQ; FRCPC; Neur (Electromyography); Electroenceph (P.Q.). Langs: Bilingual(English/French); (514)739-7740; Fax. (514)739-4882.

MORCOS, Roger; CHUS-Hop Hotel-Dieu, 580 rue Bowen S, Sherbrooke QC J1G 2E8; Damascus (Syria)'67; DABOS; FRCSC; OrthSurg (Arthroplasty). Staff, Centre Hospitalier Universitaire de Sherbrooke-Hôpital Hôtel-Dieu; Staff Orth, Centre Hospitalier Universitaire de Sherbrooke-Hopital Fleurimont; Clin Assoc Prof, Universite de Sherbrooke; Langs: Arabic; English; (819)346-1110

MORDASIEWICZ, Merunka A; Academic Family Medicine, 172-1621 Albert St, Regina SK S4P 2S5; Sask'04; CCFP; Staff, Regina General Hospital; Teach Staff College of Med, University of Saskatchewan; (306)766-0444; Fax. (306)766-4071.

MORDEN, Carla R; Alexandra Comm Health Centre, 101-1318 Centre St NE, Calgary AB T2E 2R7; Alb'02; CCFP; (403)266-2622; Fax. (403)266-2692.

MORE, Philippe; CSSS Haut-Richelieu-Rouville, 920 boul du Seminaire N, St-Jean-Sur-Richel QC J3A 1B7; Sher'99; CCFP; CCFP(E.M.); Staff, Hôpital du Haut-Richelieu; (450)359-5000; Fax. (450)359-5251.

MORE, Susan G; St Paul's Hosp, 1081 Burrard St, Vancouver BC V6Z 1Y6; Alb'93; FRCPC; Psy. Staff, Providence Health Care - St Paul's Hospital; (604)682-2344

MOREAU, Andre G; CSSS-Hop de Hull, 116 boul Lionel-Emond, Gatineau QC J8Y 1W7; Ott'79; Ac Staff, Hull Hospital; (819)966-6104

MOREAU, Anne; GMF-UMF Laval-Quebec, 2690 ch des Quatre-Bourgeois, Quebec QC G1V 0B7; Laval'79; CCFP; FCFP; ac Staff, Hôpital Laval; Prof, Université Laval; Langs: English; French; (418)656-4795; Fax. (418)656-4503.

MOREAU, Anne; CSSS de Laval, 1755 boul Rene-Laennec, Laval QC H7M 3L9; Mon'00; Staff, Hopital de la Cite de la santé; (450)668-1010

MOREAU, Arja E; Vancouver Gen Hosp, 855 12th Ave W, Vancouver BC V5Z 1M9; UBC'83; CCFP; Staff STAT Centre & Home VIVE, Vancouver General Hospital - Centennial Pavillion; Clin Instructor Family Med, University of British Columbia; (604)345-9143

MOREAU, Caroline; CSSS Drummond-Hop Sainte-Croix, 570 rue Heriot, Drummondville QC J2B 1C1; Sher'04; Staff, Hôpital Sainte-croix; (819)478-6464; Fax. (819)478-6410.

MOREAU, Chantal M M; University of Alberta Hosp, 1E714-8440 112 St NW, Edmonton AB T6G 2B7; Sask'95; BSc; FRCPC; Psy (Electroconvulsive Therapy). Staff Psy, University of Alberta Hospital; (780)407-6597; Fax. (780)407-6672.

MOREAU, Daniel; Orleans Medical-Dental Centre, 403-2555 St. Joseph Blvd, Orleans ON K1C 1S6; Sher'77; FRCS; FRCSC; ObstGyn (Gynecological Surgery). Staff, The Ottawa Hospital - General Campus; Staff, Canadian Forces Health Services Centre; Teach Staff, University of Ottawa; Langs: Bilingual(English/French); (613)837-8396; Fax. (613)837-8398; d.moreau@rogers.com.

MOREAU, Daphne; Clinique Med de Mont-Joli, 1385 boul Benoit-Gaboury, Mont-Joli QC G5H 4B1; Laval'07; CCFP; Staff, CSSS de la Mitis; (418)775-5353

MOREAU, Francois P; CHUS-Hop Fleurimont, 3001 12e av N, Sherbrooke QC J1H 5N4; Sher'03; Neur. Staff, Centre Hospitalier Universitaire de Sherbrooke-Hopital Fleurimont; (819)346-1110

MOREAU, Guy; 202-595 Montreal Rd, Ottawa ON K1K 4L2; Sher'85; FRCSC; OrthSurg (Arthroplasty). Chief of Staff, Montfort Hospital; (613)746-6745; Fax. (613)746-6008.

MOREAU, Jan P; 201-190 Cundles Rd E SS 103, Barrie ON L4M 4S5; McM'89; FRCSC; ObstGyn. Staff, Royal Victoria Regional Health Centre; (705)737-2450; Fax. (705)737-4250.

MOREAU, Judith; 101-1111 ch des Patriotes, Richelieu QC J3L 4W6; Sher'84; (450)658-0909; Fax. (450)658-7057.

MOREAU, Julie; Hop du Sacre-Coeur de Mtl, 5400 boul Gouin O, Montreal QC H4J 1C5; Mon'00; CCFP; Staff, Hôpital du Sacre-Coeur de Montréal; (514)338-2222

MOREAU, Kristina; 24 CF H Svcs CFB Trenton, PO Box 1000 PO Stn Forces, Astra ON K0K 3W0; McM'06; CCFP; (613)372-2811

MOREAU, Linda; MUHC-Royal Victoria Hosp, 687 av des Pins O, Montreal QC H3A 1A1; McG'94; BSc(BioChem); FRCPC; Derm. Staff, McGill University Health Centre - Royal Victoria Hospital; (514)934-1934 x34648; lmoreau@cyberglobe.net.

MOREAU, Louise; Centre Med Brunswick, 401-955 boul-Saint-Jean, Pointe-Claire QC H9R 5K3; Mon'01; CCFP; (514)426-6677 x355; Fax. (514)426-3323.

MOREAU, Marc J; University of Alberta Hosp, 2C3.77-8440 112 St NW, Edmonton AB T6G 2B7; Alb'73; FRCSC; OrthSurg. Staff Surg, University of Alberta Hospital; Asst Dean Admissions, University of Alberta; Langs: English; French; (780)407-3317; Fax. (780)407-3320; mmoreau@ualberta.ca.

MOREAU, Marc-Andre; Cooperative Med de Frampton, CP 1029 152 Principale, Frampton QC G0R 1M0; Laval'69; Staff, Centre Hospitalier Paul-Gilbert; (418)479-2660; marc-andre_moreau@ssss.gouv.qc.ca.

MOREAU, Marcel F; 1-706 Rte Begin GD, Saint-Anselme QC G0R 2N0; Laval'77; Langs: Bilingual(French/English); (418)885-9625; Fax. (418)885-9826.

MOREAU, Marie A; Grande Prairie Cancer Centre, 10409 98 St, Grande Prairie AB T8V 2E8; Alb'86; FRCPC; IntMed (Medical Oncology). Staff, Grande Prairie Cancer Centre - Queen Elizabeth II Hospital; Physician, Associate Cancer Clinic; (780)538-7588; Fax. (780)532-9120.

MOREAU, Mathieu; Ctr Hosp Fleury, 2180 rue Fleury E, Montreal QC H2B 1K3; Mon'10; CCFP; Staff, Centre Hospitalier Fleury; (514)384-2000

MOREAU, Michele; 5554 rue Saint-Zotique E, Montreal QC H1T 1P6; Mon'72; Staff Family Med Clin & Menopause, Centre Hospitalier l'Université de Montréal (CHUM) - Hôpital Notre-Dame; Pres, Montreal Clinical Study Center Inc; Clin Teach Staff Family Med, Universite de Montreal; Langs: English; (514)899-0922; Fax. (514)257-9109; michelemoreaumd@yahoo.ca.

MOREAU, Monique F; 2-180 Parsons Rd, Alliston ON L9R 1E8; Laval'82; CCFP; FCFP; Langs: English; French; (705)435-0058; Fax. (705)435-0062.

MOREAU, Natalie; Greenbelt Family Health Team, 1C-3500 Fallowfield Rd, Ottawa ON K2J 4A7; NOSM'09; CCFP; (613)843-1718

MOREAU, Paul G; 4-389 Collett Rd, Kelowna BC V1W 3A3; Alb'73; FRCSC; OrthSurg. (250)545-6177; Fax. (250)545-3074.

MOREAU, Vincent; Polyclinique de Trois-Rivieres, 365-1900 boul des Recollets, Trois-Rivieres QC G8Z 4K4; Laval'89; Nephrol; IntMed (Dialysis). Staff, Centre Hospitalier Regional de Trois-Rivieres; (819)373-1202; Fax. (819)693-1845.

MOREAU-BUSSIERE, Francois; CSSS de Lac-Saint Jean-Est, CP 1300 Succ Bureau-Chef 300 boul Champlain S, Alma QC G8B 5W3; Sher'05; FRCPC; Anes. Staff, CSSS de Lac-Saint Jean-Est; (418)669-2000

MOREAU-RICHARD, Rosalie; CSSS des Iles, 430 ch Principal, Cap-aux-Meules QC G4T 1R9; Mon'99; Staff, Hôpital de l'Archipel; (418)986-2121; Fax. (418)986-7001.

MOREAULT, Louise; Centre de Sante Publique, 2400 av d'Estimauville, Quebec QC G1E 7G9; Laval'81; MSc(Epidemiol); CSPQ; FRCPC; CommunMed (P.Q.) (Family Medicine); Public Health & Preventive Med. Staff, Centre Hospitalier Universitaire de Quebec-CHUL; (418)666-7000 x242; Fax. (418)666-2776.

MOREHOUSE, Douglas D; MUHC-Royal Victoria Hosp, 687 av des Pins O, Montreal QC H3A 1A1; McG'58; FICS; FACS; CSPQ; FRCSC; Urol. Staff, McGill University Health Centre - Royal Victoria Hospital; (514)843-1530; doris.giatras@muhc.mcgill.ca.

MOREHOUSE, Rachel L; Saint John Reg Hosp, PO Box 2100 Stn Main 400 University Ave, Saint John NB E2L 4L2; Dal'81; ABIM; FRCPC; Psy (Sleep Medicine). Dir Atlantic Sleep Ctre/Clin Head Dept of Psy, Saint John Regional Hospital; Prof Psy, Memorial University Of Newfoundland; Prof Psy, Dalhousie University; (506)648-6174; Fax. (506)648-6171; rachel.morehouse@horizonnb.ca.

MOREHOUSE, Scott P; 106-3417 Derry Rd E, Mississauga ON L4T 1A8; Tor'88; (905)673-3220; Fax. (905)673-2151.

MOREIRA BACHA, Omar; Hop Charles LeMoyne, 3120 boul Taschereau, Greenfield Park QC J4V 2H1; Staff, Hopital Charles LeMoyne; (450)466-5750

MOREL, Annie; CSSS de Lac-Saint Jean-Est, CP 1300 succ Bureau-Chef 300 boul Champlain S, Alma QC G8B 5W3; Laval'01; Staff, CSSS de Lac-Saint Jean-Est; (418)669-2000

MOREL, Chantal F J; 400-60 Murray St, Toronto ON M5T 3L9; Ott'00; FRCPC; MedGenetics. Staff, The Hospital For Sick Children; (416)813-1500

MOREL, Claude; CSST Lanaudiere, CP 550 Succ Bureau-Chef 432 rue de Lanaudiere, Joliette QC J6E 7N2; Mon'77; Langs: English; (450)753-2600 x2656; Fax. (450)753-3007; claude.morel@csst.qc.ca.

MOREL, Johanne; MUHC-Montreal Children's Hosp, 2300 rue Tupper, Montreal QC H3H 1P3; Mon'80; Peds. Staff, McGill University Health Centre - Montreal Children's Hospital; (514)412-4400 x22582; johanne.morel@muhc.mcgill.ca.

MOREL, Johanne; Clinique Med Monteuil, 200-4650 boul des Laurentides, Laval QC H7K 2J4; Mon'84; (450)628-8717; Fax. (450)628-5305.

MOREL, Linda D; Community Health Clinic, PO Box 484 50 Lorne St, Markdale ON N0C 1H0; McM'77; (519)986-1873

MOREL, Marie-Lou; Ctr Hosp Affilie-St-Sacrement, 1050 ch Sainte-Foy, Quebec QC G1S 4L8; Mon'01; CCFP; Staff, Centre Hospitalier Affilié Universitaire de Québec - Hôpital du St-Sacrement; (418)682-7511

MOREL, Rene; Clin Med Maisonneuve-Rosemont, 5345 boul de l'Assomption, Montreal QC H1T 4B3; Mon'85; (514)252-3400 x6270

MOREL, Richard F; 200-4 Beechwood Ave, Vanier ON K1L 8L9; UBC'88; AB(Psy); Psy. Langs: English; French; (613)741-7174; Fax. (613)741-0176.

MOREL, Stephanie; St Mary's Hosp Centre, 3830 av Lacombe, Montreal QC H3T 1M5; Laval'08; CCFP; Staff, St Mary's Hospital Centre; (514)734-2677; Fax. (514)734-2605.

MORELL, Thomas P; 13 Gore St W, Perth ON K7H 2L7; McM'84; FACS; FRCSC; GenSurg. Staff GenSurg/Pres Med Staff, Perth & Smiths Falls District Hospital - Smiths Falls Site; Staff GenSurg, Perth & Smiths Falls District Hospital - Perth Site (Great War Memorial Site); (613)264-1155

MORELLI, Gaetano; 300-245 av Victoria, Westmount QC H3Z 2M6; Mon'83; ABIM; FRCPC; IntMed; Gastroent (P.Q.). Staff, McGill University Health Centre - Royal Victoria Hospital; Staff, St Mary's Hospital Centre; adj Prof, McGill University; (514)938-3810; Fax. (514)938-4894.

MORELLI, Moreno; Concordia Physio Sport, 6530 rue Sherbrooke W, Montreal QC H4B 1N5; Mon'95; FRCSC; OrthSurg. (514)848-3317; Fax. (514)848-3316.

MORENCY, Anne-Maude; Mount Sinai Hosp, 600 University SAve, Toronto ON M5G 1X5; Mon'05; ObstGyn. Fellow, Mount Sinai Hospital; (416)596-4200

MORENCY, Chantale; Ctr Hosp Affilie-Enfant-Jesus, 1401 18e rue, Quebec QC G1J 1Z4; Mon'94; Staff, Centre Hospitalier Affilié Universitaire de Québec - Hôpital De L'Enfant Jésus; (418)649-0252

MORENCY, Elizabeth; 620-2954 boul Laurier, Quebec QC G1V 4T2; Laval'82; Staff, Centre Medico Esthetique; Langs: English; (418)650-6652; Fax. (418)650-6165.

MORENCY, Gilles; CSSS du Nord de Lanaudière, 1000 boul Sainte-Anne, St-Charles-Brromee QC J6E 6J2; Mon'83; CSPQ; FRCPC; DiagRad. Staff Diag Imaging, Centre Hospitalier Régional de Lanaudière; (450)759-8222 x2844; Fax. (450)759-2133.

MORENCY, Isabelle; CSSS du Nord de Lanaudiere, 264-1000 boul Sainte-Anne, St-Charles-Brromee QC J6E 6J2; Laval'75; GenSurg (Digestive Surgery). Staff GenSurg, Centre Hospitalier Régional de Lanaudière; Langs: Spanish; English; (450)759-8222 x2150

MORENCY, Jacques; Clin de Gynecologique de Levis, 400-4975 boul de la Rive-Sud, Levis QC G6V 4Z5; Laval'82; FRCSC; ObstGyn. (418)833-1522; Fax. (418)833-1526.

MORENCY, Jean-Pierre; Clin Chir Plast et Esth Grande, 425 Grande-Allee E, Quebec QC G1R 2J5; Laval'71; CSPQ; FRCPC; Anes. Ac Staff, Hôtel-Dieu de Lévis; (418)682-0182; Fax. (418)681-2930; cliniquegrandeallee@videotron.ca.

MORENCY, Johanne; Clinique d'Ophtalmologie, 100-2875 boul Laurier, Quebec QC G1V 2M2; Laval'75; FABO; FRCSC; Ophth. Staff, Centre Hospitalier Affilié Universitaire de Québec - Hôpital du St-Sacrement; Consultant, Centre Hospitalier Affilié Universitaire de Québec - Hôpital De L'Enfant Jésus; Dir Programme de Res en Ophtalmologie, Université Laval; Langs: English; (418)658-2010; Fax. (418)658-8310.

MORENCY, Mario B; 63 rue Girouard, Victoriaville QC G6P 5T3; Sher'91; LMCC; FRCPC; Psy (Family Therapy). Chef Pedopsychiatrie, Hotel-Dieu d'Arthabaska; Langs: Bilingual(French/English); (819)260-3363; Fax. (819)260-3373.

MORENCY, Nathalie; Hop du Sacre-Coeur de Montreal, 5400 boul Gouin O, Montreal QC H4J 1C5; Sher'03; Rheum; IntMed. Staff, Hôpital du Sacre-Coeur de Montréal; (514)338-2222

MORENCY, Patrick; Dir de la Sante Publique-Mtl, 1301 rue Sherbrooke E, Montreal QC H2L 1M3; Sher'94; CSPQ; FRCPC; CommunMed. (514)528-2400 x3327

MORENCY, Pierre; Clinique Med de Pierre Morency, 6825 av 1Re, Quebec QC G1H 2X1; Laval'65; Langs: Bilingual(French/English); (418)628-1642; Fax. (418)628-5484; morenvez@videotron.ca.

MORENCY, Renald; CHUQ-Hotel-Dieu de Quebec, 11 Cote du Palais, Quebec QC G1R 2J6; Laval'67; CSPQ; AnatPath (Otolaryngology). Staff, Centre Hospitalier Universitaire de Québec (CHUQ) - Siege Social; Langs: English; (418)691-5233; Fax. (418)691-5226.

MORENCY, Rene-Louis; 220-8100 Rock Island Hwy, Trail BC V1R 4N7; Laval'80; Ophth (Anterior Segment). Langs: English; French; (250)368-8585; Fax. (250)368-8584.

MORENO, Agustin A; Red Lake Med Associates, PO Box 311, Red Lake ON P0V 2M0; Wes'08; CCFP; (807)727-2617; Fax. (807)727-3122.

MORENO, Juan C; Royal Alexandra Hosp, 10240 Kingsway NW, Edmonton AB T5H 3V9; McM'04; FRCPC; AnatPath. Staff, Royal Alexandra Hospital; (780)735-5281; Fax. (780)735-4715.

MORENO MERLO, Fernando D; Medicine Hat Reg Hosp, 666 5 St SW, Medicine Hat AB T1A 4H6; Leon (Nicaragua)'88; FRCPC; AnatPath. Staff, Medicine Hat Regional Hospital; (403)529-8830

MORETTI, Eric; CSSS Haut-Richelieu-Rouville, 920 boul du Seminaire N, St-Jean-Sur-Richel QC J3A 1B7; Mon'95; CCFP; Staff, Hôpital du Haut-Richelieu; (450)359-5234; Fax. (450)359-5251.

MORETTI, Felipe M; The Ottawa Hosp-Gen Campus, 8472-501 Smyth Rd, Ottawa ON K1H 8L6; (Brazil)'95; Staff, The Ottawa Hospital - General Campus; (613)737-5506; Fax. (613)737-8070.

MORETTI, Justin S; Central Nfld Reg Hlth Centre, 50 Union St, Grnd-Falls-Windsor NL A2A 2E1; Flinders Univ (Australia)'96; Staff, Central Newfoundland Regional Health Centre; (709)292-2500

MORGAN, Aida E; 333-5 Fairview Mall Dr, North York ON M2J 2Z1; Ain Shams (Egypt)'80; CCFP; Staff, The Scarborough Hospital - General Campus; Staff, The Scarborough Hospital - Birchmount Campus; Langs: Arabic; (416)492-6700; Fax. (416)492-5460.

MORGAN, Andrew W; Addiction & Mental Hlth-Queen, 3-1001 Queen St W, Toronto ON M6J 1H4; UBC'07; FRCPC; Psy. Staff, Centre for Addiction & Mental Health (CAMH) - Queen Site; (416)535-8501; Fax. (416)583-4327.

MORGAN, Anwar V K; Women's College Hosp, 76 Grenville St, Toronto ON M5S 1B2; Cairo (Egypt)'79; MD; FRCPC; Anes (Chronic Pain). Staff, Women's College Hospital; Langs: Arabic; (416)323-6008; Fax. (416)323-6307; anwar.morgan@sw.ca.

MORGAN, Brian J; Four Oaks Med Centre, 5500 206 St, Langley BC V3A 8R3; Cape Town (South Africa)'89; MB ChB; DCH; PharmD; CCFP; FCFP; (604)534-4214; Fax. (604)534-6616.

MORGAN, Catherine J; Edmonton Clinic Health Academy, 4 5557-11405 87 Ave NW, Edmonton AB T6G 1C9; Alb'00; FRCPC; Peds; Nephrol. Staff, University of Alberta Hospital; Staff, Edmonton Clinic Health Academy; (780)248-5560; cmorgan@ualberta.ca.

MORGAN, Christopher D; Sunnybrook Hlth Sciences Ctre, E203-2075 Bayview Ave, Toronto ON M4N 3M5; Tor'73; FRCPC; IntMed; Cardiol. Ac Staff, Sunnybrook Health Sciences Centre; Assoc Prof, University of Toronto; (416)480-4822; Fax. (416)480-4722; chris.morgan@sunnybrook.ca.

MORGAN, David C; McKenzie Prof Centre, 205-1595 McKenzie Ave, Victoria BC V8N 1A4; UBC'71; Staff, Victoria General Hospital; Staff, Royal Jubilee Hospital; (250)721-4141; Fax. (250)721-4195.

MORGAN, David; St Joseph's Healthcare, 50 Charlton Ave E, Hamilton ON L8N 4A6; McM'85; BSc; MSc; FRCPC; IntMed (Gastrointestinal Cancer). Court Staff, Hamilton Health Sciences Centre; Ac Staff, St Joseph's Healthcare - Charlton Campus; Assoc Prof Gastroent, McMaster University; (905)574-7721; Fax. (905)308-7201.

MORGAN, David; Souris Hosp Inc, PO Box 640, Souris PE C0A 2B0; London (England)'78; Staff, Souris Hospital Inc; (902)687-7150

MORGAN, David W; Health Sciences Centre, 300 Prince Philip Dr, St. John's NL A1B 3V6; Mem'82; CCFP; CCFP(E.M.); Staff, Health Sciences Centre; Asst Prof Med/Prog Dir Emerg Med Residency & Discipline of FamMed, Memorial University Of Newfoundland; (709)777-6300

MORGAN, David W; Prince George Adult Forensic C, 2F-1584 7th Ave, Prince George BC V2L 3P4; Wales (United Kingdom)'98; (250)561-8060

MORGAN, Dennis E; Western Cardiology Associates, 335-1900 Richmond Ave, Victoria BC V8R 4R2; Mem'80; BMedSci; FACC; FRCPC; IntMed; Cardiol. Consultant Cardiol, Royal Jubilee Hospital; Consultant Cardiol, Victoria General Hospital; (250)595-1551; Fax. (250)595-6793.

MORGAN, Jane A; 213 Wilson St E, Ancaster ON L9G 2B8; McM'93; FRCPC; Psy. Staff Chedoke Child & Family Centre, Hamilton Health Sciences Centre - McMaster University Medical Centre; (905)304-0177; Fax. (905)304-6703.

MORGAN, Jonathon; The Hugh Allen Clinic, PO Box 489 Stn Main, Sioux Lookout ON P8T 1A8; Tor'83; CCFP; CCFP(E.M.); FCFP; Staff, The Hugh Allen Clinic; (807)737-3803; Fax. (807)737-3885.

MORGAN, Kathryn R; Healthlink, 10-350 Conestoga Blvd, Cambridge ON N1R 7L7; Qns'09; CCFP; Staff, Southlake Regional Health Centre; (519)740-5010; Fax. (519)740-6010.

MORGAN, Kenneth P; Queen Elizabeth II HSC-Halifax, 1796 Summer St, Halifax NS B3H 3A7; Edinburgh (Scotland)'96; MB ChB; Staff, Queen Elizabeth II Health Sciences Centre - Halifax Infirmary Site; (902)473-2184; Fax. (902)473-6293.

MORGAN, Lenna M; 218-2425 Tecumseh Rd E, Windsor ON N8W 1E6; Wes'88; FRCPC; Peds. Chief Peds, Windsor Regional Hospital - Metropolitan Site; Aj Prof, University of Western Ontario; (519)944-9924; Fax. (519)944-7282.

MORGAN, Magid; Grand River Hosp-KW Hlth Ctre, PO Box 9056 Stn C 835 King St W, Kitchener ON N2G 1G3; Cairo (Egypt)'97; FRCPC; Anes. Staff, Grand River Hospital - Kitchener/Waterloo Health Centre; (519)749-4300 x2242

MORGAN, Marianne N; Tutt Street Med Clinic, 314-3001 Tutt St, Kelowna BC V1Y 2H4; UBC'92; (250)763-0101

MORGAN, Matthew; Cobequid Commun Health Centre, 40 Freer Lane, Lower Sackville NS B4C 0A2; Cal'01; FRCPC; Psy. Staff, Cobequid Community Health Centre; (902)869-6100

MORGAN, Matthew W; Mount Sinai Hosp, 333a-600 University Ave, Toronto ON M5G 1X5; Dal'91; FRCPC; IntMed. Ac Staff, Toronto General Hospital - UHN; Ac Staff/VP Patient Experience & Outcomes, Mount Sinai Hospital; Dir Per-Se Technologies, Healthcare Informatics; Asst Prof Medicine, University of Toronto; (416)340-4800

MORGAN, Melanie M M; 2604 Kensington Rd NW PO Box 63126 Rpo Stadium, Calgary AB T2N 4S5; Cal'98; CCFP; (403)973-2844; Fax. (403)202-2733.

MORGAN, Moheb; Strathroy Middlesex Gen Hosp, 395 Carrie St, Strathroy ON N7G 3J4; McG'05; CCFP; Staff, Strathroy Middlesex General Hospital - Middlesex Hospital Alliance; (519)245-1550

MORGAN, Nancy; Hamilton HS-General Site, 237 Barton St E, Hamilton ON L8L 2X2; McM'03; Staff, Hamilton Health Sciences Centre - Hamilton General Hospital; (905)522-9017

MORGAN, Neal A; South Shore Reg Hosp, 90 Glen Allan Dr, Bridgewater NS B4V 3S6; (Ireland)'03; FRCPC; Psy. Staff, South Shore Regional Hospital; (902)527-5228; Fax. (902)527-5297.

MORGAN, Pamela J; Women's College Hosp, 76 Grenville St, Toronto ON M5S 1B2; Tor'79; FRCPC; Anes (Obstetrics Anesthesia). Staff, Women's College Hospital; Prof, University of Toronto; (416)323-6400 x4087; pam.morgan@utoronto.ca.

MORGAN, Paul F; Medical Clinic 14 Wing, PO Box 5000, Greenwood NS B0P 1N0; Cal'90; (902)765-1494

MORGAN, Robert B; Medical-Surgical Eye Bldg, 879 Shefford Rd, Gloucester ON K1J 8H9; Ott'73; FRCSC; Ophth (Cataract). Court Staff, Children's Hospital of Eastern Ontario (CHEO); Court Staff (All Sites), The Ottawa Hospital - General Campus; Ac Staff, Montfort Hospital; (613)741-0737; Fax. (613)741-7338.

MORGAN, Roderick A; Peoples Trust Plaza, 400-10216 124 St NW, Edmonton AB T5N 4A3; Alb'61; DAB; FRCSC; Ophth (Anterior Segment Surgery). Ac Staff, Royal Alexandra Hospital; Consultant, Glenrose Rehabilitation Hospital; Consultant, Cross Cancer Institute; Surgeon Ophth, Alberta Health Services; Clin Prof, University of Alberta; (780)428-6842; Fax. (780)428-6968.

MORGAN, Scott C; The Ottawa Hosp-Gen Campus, 501 Smyth Rd, Ottawa ON K1H 8L6; Qns'03; FRCPC; RadOncol (Prostate Cancer). Staff, The Ottawa Hospital - General Campus; Asst Prof, University of Ottawa; Langs: Bilingual(English/French); (613)737-7700; Fax. (613)247-3511.

MORGAN, Stephen R; 264 boul Rene-Levesque E, Montreal QC H2L 4M1; Mon'69; FRCSC; GenSurg (Proctology). Staff, Centre Hospitalier l'Université De Montréal (CHUM) - Hôpital Saint-luc; Langs: Bilingual(French/English); (514)890-8000; sm@procto.ca.

MORGAN, Stephen; Timmins & Dist Hosp, 700 Ross Ave E, Timmins ON P4N 8P2; (Australia)'09; CCFP; Staff, Timmins & District Hospital; (705)267-2131

MORGAN, Susan G M; 202-117 Murray St, Ottawa ON K1N 5M5; Cal'78; FRCPC; Peds. Staff, Children's Hospital of Eastern Ontario (CHEO).

MORGAN-PARKES, Jacqueline H; General Medical Imaging, 200-1144 Burrard St, Vancouver BC V6Z 2A5; Sask'73; FRCPC; DiagRad. (604)937-5588

MORGENSTERN, Justin; Markham Stouffville Hosp, PO Box 1800 Stn Main 381 Church St, Markham ON L3P 7P3; Wes'09; CCFP; CCFP(E.M.); Staff, Markham Stouffville Hospital; (905)472-7000

MORGENSTERN, Katherine V; PO Box 75537 Rpo Edgemont Vill, North Vancouver BC V7R 4X1; UBC'00; CCFP; Staff Hopitalist Program, Providence Health Care - St Paul's Hospital; (604)520-4001

MORGENTALER, Henry; 727 Hillsdale Ave E, Toronto ON M4S 1V4; Mon'53; Med Dir, Morgentaler Clinics; Langs: Polish; German; Italian; (416)932-0446; Fax. (416)932-0837.

MORGENTHAU, David R; 205-2221 Keele St, North York ON M6M 3Z5; Tor'79; FRCPC; IntMed; Neur. Ac Staff, Humber River Regional Hospital - Church Street Site; Att Staff, St Michael's Hospital; (416)256-9115; Fax. (416)256-9400.

MORHALIEK, Cameron S; 2F-10443 85 Ave NW, Edmonton AB T6E 2K2; Alb'93; MD; FRCP; BMedSci; ABNP; FRCPC; Psy (Adult & Child Psychiatry). Consultant Child Psychiatrist, Alberta Mental Hlth Clin.-Leduc; (780)431-1777; Fax. (780)439-0699.

MORHAM, Anthony R; South Sherbrook Health Centre, B-88 Sherbrook St, Winnipeg MB R3C 2B3; Ott'91; CCFP; morham@mts.net.

MORHART, Michael J; 303 East Tower, 14310 111 Ave NW, Edmonton AB T5M 3Z7; Sask'94; MSc; BSc; FRCSC; PlasSurg (Cosmetics). Staff, University of Alberta Hospital; Staff, Royal Alexandra Hospital; Staff, Covenant Health - Misericordia Community Hospital; (780)437-0404; Fax. (780)437-7882.

MORI, Michael K; 24 First St, Orangeville ON L9W 2C7; Man'00; BSc; CCFP; (519)943-0712; Fax. (519)943-0284; mikemori77@yahoo.ca.

MORI, Richard Y; 14116 Tamarack Dr, Vernon BC V1B 2E1; UBC'72; Staff Temporary, Vernon Jubilee Hospital; rmori@shaw.ca.

MORI, Tyler Y H; 103-8556 120th St, Surrey BC V3W 3N6; UBC'03; FRCSC; Otol. (778)565-3239

MORI-TORRES, Elisea M; Glenrose Rehab Hosp, 10230 111 Ave NW, Edmonton AB T5G 0B7; Lima (Peru)'79; CCFP; Staff, Glenrose Rehabilitation Hospital; (780)735-7934; Fax. (780)735-8837.

MORIARITY, Tracey A T; Dundas Family Med Group, 2F-133 King St W, Hamilton ON L9H 1V3; Wes'88; BSc(Hon); CCFP; FCFP.

MORIARTEY, Robert R; Tawa Centre, 219-3017 66 St NW, Edmonton AB T6K 4B2; Cal'73; BSc(Zool); FRCPC; Peds. Ac Staff, Covenant Health - Grey Nuns Community Hospital; Ac Staff, University of Alberta Hospital; Clin Prof, University of Alberta; (780)461-9284; Fax. (780)450-0360; rmoriart@telusplanet.net.

MORIARTY, Mary F; Pleasant Med Group, 105-375 Pleasant St, Dartmouth NS B2Y 4N4; Dal'77; CCFP; FCFP; (902)469-2447; Fax. (902)469-2449.

MORIC, Jakov; Women's College Hosp, 76 Grenville St, Toronto ON M5S 1B2; Tor'03; FRCPC; IntMed; Respir. Staff, Women's College Hospital; (416)323-6137; Fax. (416)323-6132.

MORIC, Aileen G; St Georges Med Clinic, 1315 St. Georges Ave, North Vancouver BC V7L 3J2; UBC'91; (604)984-9213; Fax. (604)986-1390.

MORICONI, Claudette; Polyclinique Masson, 200-3425 rue Masson, Montreal QC H1X 1R6; Mon'88; CCFP; Staff EmergMed, Centre Hospitalier l'Université de Montréal (CHUM) - Hôpital Notre-Dame; Physician, Polyclinique Massons; (514)376-9961; Fax. (514)376-8100.

MORICONI, Ronaldo; Centre Med Chambly, 205-1101 boul Brassard, Chambly QC J3L 5R4; Mon'73; Langs: Italian; English; (450)658-6601; Fax. (450)658-7849.

MORIER, Gisele S L; Psychealth Centre, PZ273-771 Bannatyne Ave, Winnipeg MB R3E 3N4; Man'81; BScPharm; ABPN; FCPA; LRCPS; FRCPC; Psy (Mood Disorders). Ac Staff, Health Sciences Centre; Assoc Prof, University of Manitoba; Langs: Bilingual(French/English); (204)787-7253; Fax. (204)787-7480.

MORIER, Marie-Josee; Clinique Med du Cuivre, 12 rue Gamble E, Rouyn-Noranda QC J9X 3B7; Mon'93; Staff, Centre Hospitalier Rouyn-Noranda; Langs: Spanish; (819)764-5131; Fax. (819)764-5792.

MORILLO, Carlos A; 237 Barton St E, Hamilton ON L8L 2X2; Pontificia Universidad Javeriana (Colombia)'83; Staff Cardiol, Hamilton Health Sciences Centre - Hamilton General Hospital; Langs: Spanish; (905)527-4322 x40311; Fax. (905)521-8820.

MORILLO, Luis E; Hamilton HS-General Site, 237 Barton St E, Hamilton ON L8L 2X2; Bogota (Colombia)'78; FRCPC; Neur. Staff, Hamilton Health Sciences Centre - Hamilton General Hospital; Langs: Spanish; (905)527-0271; Fax. (905)523-8352.

MORIN, Alain; Ctr Hosp Chauveau, 11999 rue de l'Hopital, Quebec QC G2A 2T7; Laval'92; Staff, Centre Hospitalier Chauveau; (418)842-3651

MORIN, Andre; CSSS Drummond-Hop Sainte-Croix, 570 rue Heriot, Drummondville QC J2B 1C1; Sher'88; Psy. Staff, Hôpital Sainte-croix; (819)478-6464

MORIN, Andre J; CSSS-Hop de Hull, 116 boul Lionel-Emond, Gatineau QC J8Y 1W7; Ott'67; FRCSC; OrthSurg. Staff, Hull Hospital; (819)595-6022

MORIN, Anne-Marie; CSSS Drummond-Hop Sainte-Croix, 570 rue Heriot, Drummondville QC J2B 1C1; Sher'05; CCFP; Staff, Hôpital Sainte-croix; (819)478-6464; Fax. (819)478-6410.

MORIN, Annie; CSSS du Haut Saint-Maurice, 885 boul Ducharme, La Tuque QC G9X 3C1; Laval'01; Staff, Centre Hospitalier Saint-Joseph de la Turque; (819)573-4581

MORIN, Annie; Ctr Hosp Affilie-Enfant-Jesus, 1401 18e rue, Quebec QC G1J 1Z4; Laval'05; Cardiol; IntMed. Staff, Centre Hospitalier Affilié Universitaire de Québec - Hôpital De L'Enfant Jésus; (418)649-0252

MORIN, Annie; CLSC Haute-Ville, 55 ch Sainte-Foy, Quebec QC G1R 1S9; Laval'00; Teacher, Université Laval; (418)641-2572; Fax. (418)522-5437; anmorin@hotmail.ca.

MORIN, Audree; CSSS de Montmagny-L'Islet, 350 boul Tache O, Montmagny QC G5V 3R8; Sher'06; Psy. Staff, CSSS de Montmagny-L'Islet; (418)248-0630

MORIN, Bernard; Clinique Med Neufchatel, 101-2425 boul Bastien, Quebec QC G2B 1B3; Laval'86; LMCC; Langs: Bilingual(English/French); Bilingual(French/English); (418)843-3771; Fax. (418)843-3865; bermor@videotron.ca.

MORIN, Brent D; Royal Victoria Hosp, 201 Georgian Dr, Barrie ON L4M 6M2; NOSM'10; CCFP; Staff, Royal Victoria Regional Health Centre; (705)792-3333

MORIN, Bruno; CSSS de Laval, 1755 boul Rene-Laennec, Laval QC H7M 3L9; Laval'91; CSPQ; FRCPC; DiagRad (Echography). Staff, Hopital de la Cite de la santé; (450)668-1010 x2016; Fax. (450)975-5545.

MORIN, Carl G; PO Box 392 Stn A, Ottawa ON K1N 8V4; Ott'72.

MORIN, Caroline; Ctr Hosp de Verdun, 4000 boul Lasalle, Verdun QC H4G 2A3; Mon'08; CCFP; Staff, Centre Hospitalier de Verdun; (514)362-1000

MORIN, Catherine; CSSS de Chicoutimi, 305 rue Saint-Vallier, Chicoutimi QC G7H 5H6; Sher'98; FRCPC; Psy. Staff, Complexe hospitalier de la Sagamie; (418)549-5474

MORIN, Charles; Clin Pediatrie de Chicoutimi, 475 boul Talbot, Chicoutimi QC G7H 4A3; Laval'83; Peds. Ac Staff, Complexe hospitalier de la Sagamie; (418)549-1034; Fax. (418)696-4673.

MORIN, Christian; Hop du Sacre-Coeur de Mtl, 5400 boul Gouin O, Montreal QC H4J 1C5; Mon'82; CSPQ; FRCPC; DiagRad. adj Prof, Universite de Montreal; (514)338-2130

MORIN, Christian G; 401-3030 boul Le carrefour, Laval QC H7T 2P5; Sher'83; FRCSC; Otol. Staff, Hôpital du Sacre-Coeur de Montréal; Staff, Hopital de la Cite de la santé; Physician, Centre d'ORL de Cartierville; (450)687-1750; Fax. (450)687-7797.

MORIN, Claude; Clinique Med St-Laurent, 202-500 Rte Marie-Victorin, Sorel-Tracy QC J3R 1K7; Mon'79; Med Coord Palliative Care, Hôtel-Dieu de Sorel; (450)742-9818; Fax. (450)742-9795.

MORIN, Claude; CHUQ-St-Francois d'Assise, 10 rue de l'Espinay, Quebec QC G1L 3L5; Laval'85; CCFP; CCFP(E.M.); Staff, Centre Hospitalier Universitaire De Québec - Pavillon De St-françois-d'assise; Langs: English; (418)525-4388; claudemorin@hotmail.com.

MORIN, Claude M; Millstream Med Centre, 107-2349 Millstream Rd, Victoria BC V9B 3R5; Laval'65; (250)391-7554

MORIN, Clement; Clinique Med Chaudiere, 102 18E rue, Saint-Georges QC G5Y 4T9; Laval'73; (418)228-6820; Fax. (418)226-0358.

MORIN, Cybele; Clinique Med St-Augustin, 220-334 Rte 138, Quebec QC G3A 1G8; Laval'93; (418)878-3590

MORIN, Diane; Clinique des Promenades, A222-3333 rue du carrefour, Quebec QC G1C 5R9; Laval'80; Staff, Centre d'hebergement Saint-Augustin; (418)663-6345

MORIN, Diane; Agence SSSS-Dir Sante Publique, 363 Rte Cameron, Sainte-Marie QC G6E 3E2; Laval'82; Staff, Hôtel-Dieu de Lévis; ac Staff, Direction de la Sante Publique de Montreal; (418)389-1510; Fax. (418)389-1515.

MORIN, Dominique; Inuulitsivik Health Centre, GD, Povungnituq QC J0M 1P0; Laval'10; CCFP; Staff, Inuulitsivik Health Centre; (819)988-2957

MORIN, Elodie; CSSS de la Minganie, CP 190 Bdp 1035 Prom des Anciens, Hvre-Saint-Pierre QC G0G 1P0; Laval'08; CCFP; Staff, CSSS de la Minganie; (418)538-2212; Fax. (418)538-3066.

MORIN, Emilie; CHUM-Hop Notre-Dame, 1560 rue Sherbrooke E, Montreal QC H2L 4M1; Laval'05; FRCPC; IntMed; Endocrin&Metab. Staff, Centre Hospitalier l'Université de Montréal (CHUM) - Hôpital Notre-Dame; (514)890-8000

MORIN, Eric; Clinique Med Blainville, 519 boul du Curé-Labelle, Blainville QC J7C 2H6; Mon'92; MSc; Staff, Hôpital de Saint-Eustache; Ac Member, CSSS Therese de Blainville; (450)430-2222; Fax. (450)430-1274.

MORIN, Evelyn; CSSS de la Pointe de l'Ile, 201-7905 boul Louis-H.-Lafonta, Anjou QC H1K 4E4; Mon'88; Langs: English; (514)356-2572; Fax. (514)493-0083.

MORIN, France; GMF des Seigneuries, 2220 boul Rene-Gaultier, Varennes QC J3X 1E3; Mon'90; (450)652-2917; Fax. (450)652-9902.

MORIN, France; CLSC-CHSLD la Pommeraie, CP 1140 34 boul St-Joseph, Bedford QC J0J 1A0; Laval'97; Gen Practice, CLSC-CHSLD La Pommeraie - Centre hospitalier de Bedford; (450)248-4321 x308; Fax. (450)248-3717; france_morin@rrsss16.gouv.qc.ca.

MORIN, Francine N; Hôpital Ste-Justine, 3175 ch Cote-Sainte-Catherine, Montreal QC H3T 1C5; McG'86; IntMed. Staff, Hôpital Ste-Justine; (514)345-4705; Fax. (514)345-4878.

MORIN, Francine P; Pavillon Louis-Charles-Simard, 2065 rue Alexandre-Deseve, Montreal QC H2L 2W5; Mon'91; FRCPC; Psy. Staff, Centre Hospitalier l'Université De Montréal (CHUM) - Hôpital Saint-luc; (514)890-8000

MORIN, Francis; CHUQ-Hotel-Dieu de Quebec, 11 Cote du Palais, Quebec QC G1R 2J6; Laval'92; MSc; BSc; NuclearMed (P.Q.). Staff, Centre Hospitalier Universitaire de Québec (CHUQ) - Siege Social; (418)691-5151; Fax. (418)691-5394.

MORIN, Francois D; CSSS de Rivière-de-Loup, 75 rue Saint-Henri, Riviere-du-Loup QC G5R 2A4; Sher'76; CSPQ; FRCPC; DiagRad. Staff, Centre Hospitalier Regional du Grand-Portage; (418)868-1010 x2381

MORIN, Francois; CHUQ-Ctr Hosp Univ Laval, 2705 boul Laurier, Quebec QC G1V 4G2; Laval'81; FRCSC; OrthSurg (Hip & Knee Replacement). Staff, Centre Hospitalier Paul-Gilbert; Staff, Centre Hospitalier Universitaire de Quebec-CHUL; Langs: Bilingual(French/English); (418)654-2102; Fax. (418)654-2288.

MORIN, Francois R; Echo Medic, 110-1575 boul de l'Avenir, Laval QC H7S 2N5; Sher'70; CSPQ; DiagRad. Staff, Hopital de la Cite de la santé; (450)688-3246

MORIN, Frederic; Clin Rhumatologie Ctre Quebec, 1119 rue Sainte-Marguerite, Trois-Rivieres QC G8Z 1Y2; Laval'90; CSPQ; Rheum (P.Q.); IntMed. (819)370-8106; Fax. (819)370-8120.

MORIN, Genevieve; CSSS Pierre Boucher, 1333 boul Jacques-Cartier E, Longueuil QC J4M 2A5; Mon'97; Staff, Centre Hospitalier Pierre Boucher; (450)468-8111; genmorin@videotron.ca.

MORIN, Gertrude; Clinique Argyle, 32 av Argyle, Saint-Lambert QC J4P 2H4; Mon'95; Staff, CSSS Champlain; Staff, Hopital Charles LeMoyne; Staff, CHSLD de la MRC de Champlain-Centre Saint-Lambert; Langs: Bilingual(French/English); (450)671-3179; Fax. (450)671-4796.

MORIN, Gilbert; Clinique Med En Route, F5-895 rue de la Gauchetiere O, Montreal QC H3B 4G1; Laval'79; CCFP; (514)954-1444; Fax. (514)954-1619.

MORIN, Gilles; 103-605 boul Simoneau, Asbestos QC J1T 4G7; Laval'66; Staff, CSSS des Sources d'Asbestos; Physician, Mine Jeffrey Inc; Langs: Bilingual(French/English); (819)879-7277; Fax. (819)879-7881.

MORIN, Guy; Polyclinique de Trois-Rivieres, 100-1900 boul des Recollets, Trois-Rivieres QC G8Z 4K4; Laval'73; CRCP; LMCC; Gastroent. Langs: Bilingual(French/English); French; (819)373-1538; Fax. (819)372-3516; guy.morin2@tr.cgocable.ca.

MORIN, Heather A; Canadian Forces Base St-Jean, PO Box 100 1 ch Grand Bernier, Richelain QC J0J 1R0; Ott'07; CCFP; (450)358-7099 x7680

MORIN, Helene; CLSC du Grand Chicoutimi, 411 rue de l'Hotel-Dieu, Chicoutimi QC G7H 7Z5; Laval'90; Staff Psy Pavillon Roland-Saucier, Complexe hospitalier de la Sagamie; (418)543-2221 x3757; Fax. (418)543-9512; helene.morin.sgc@ssss.gouv.qc.ca.

MORIN, Jacques; CSSS de Montmagny-L'Islet, RR 1 350 boul Tache O, Montmagny QC G5V 3R8; Laval'59; FRCPC; Psy. Staff, CSSS de Montmagny-L'Islet; Langs: German; English; (418)248-0630; jacques017@sympatico.ca.

MORIN, Jacques; Ctr Hosp Affilie-St-Sacrement, 1050 ch Sainte-Foy, Quebec QC G1S 4L8; Laval'72; GenSurg (Breast Cancer). Ac Staff, Centre Hospitalier Universitaire De Québec - Pavillon De St-françois-d'assise; Ac Staff, Centre Hospitalier Affilié Universitaire de Québec - Hôpital du St-Sacrement; (418)682-7511; Fax. (418)628-1041.

MORIN, Jacques; Ctr Hosp Affilie-Enfant-Jesus, 1401 18e rue, Quebec QC G1J 1Z4; Laval'78; MSc(Epidem.); FRCPC; IntMed; GeriatricMed. Dep Chief, Centre Hospitalier Affilié Universitaire de Québec - Hôpital De L'Enfant Jésus; Chef gériatrie, Centre Hospitalier Affilié Universitaire de Québec - Hôpital du St-Sacrement; Prof Med, Université Laval; (418)649-0252 x5521; Fax. (418)649-5507; jacques.morin.cha@ssss.gouv.qc.ca.

MORIN, Jason M; Niagara Med Group Fam Hlth Team, 4421 Queen St, Niagara Falls ON L2E 2L2; Dal'97; CCFP; FCFP; Physician Family Med, Niagara Health System - Greater Niagara General Site; (905)356-2236; Fax. (905)356-2568.

MORIN, Jean; Clinique Fam de lac St-Charles, 1514 rue Jacques-Bedard, Quebec QC G3G 3C1; Laval'84; (418)849-7171

MORIN, Jean R; Commission des Lesions Prof, 249-500 boul des Laurentides, Saint-Jerome QC J7Z 4M2; Mon'65; (450)569-7617

MORIN, Jean-Francois; SMBD Jewish Gen Hosp, 3755 ch Cote-Sainte-Catherine, Montreal QC H3T 1E2; Mon'79; FRCSC; GenSurg; VascSurg; Cardiovasc&ThorSurg. Staff, Sir Mortimer B Davis Jewish General; Staff Teacher, McGill University; (514)340-8222 x5598; Fax. (514)340-7561.

MORIN, Jean-Pierre; CHUQ-St-Francois d'Assise, 10 rue de l'Espinay, Quebec QC G1L 3L5; Laval'83; CSPQ; Anes. Ac Staff, Centre Hospitalier Universitaire De Québec - Pavillon De St-françois-d'assise; Staff Teacher, Université Laval; (418)525-4340; Fax. (418)525-4434.

MORIN, Jocelyn; UMF Rimouski, 165 rue des Gouverneurs, Rimouski QC G5L 7R2; Mon'09; (418)727-5493; Fax. (418)727-5480.

MORIN, Johanne; Hotel-Dieu de Sorel, 400 av de l'Hotel-Dieu, Sorel-Tracy QC J3P 1N5; Sher'84; FRCPC; Psy. Staff, Hôtel-Dieu de Sorel; (450)746-6150; Fax. (450)746-6082.

MORIN, Johanne; CSSS Pierre Boucher, 1333 boul Jacques-Cartier E, Longueuil QC J4M 2A5; Sher'81; AB; FRCPC; EmergMed. Staff, Centre Hospitalier Pierre Boucher; adj Dir méd Services Medicaux, Merck Frosst Canada Ltd; Langs: English; (450)468-8111

MORIN, Josee; Clin Cardio Desilets, 200-1750 av de Vitre, Quebec QC G1J 1Z6; Mon'97; FRCPC; IntMed; Cardiol. Staff Cardiol, Centre Hospitalier Affilié Universitaire de Québec - Hôpital De L'Enfant Jésus; (418)663-2858; Fax. (418)663-2352.

MORIN, Jovette; Ctr Hosp Affilie-Enfant-Jesus, 1401 18e rue, Quebec QC G1J 1Z4; Laval'96; FRCPC; IntMed. Staff IntMed, Centre Hospitalier Affilié Universitaire de Québec - Hôpital De L'Enfant Jésus; (418)649-0252; Fax. (418)649-5913; jovettemorin@videotron.ca.

MORIN, Julie; Centre Hosp Honore-Mercier, 2750 boul Laframboise, Saint-Hyacinthe QC J2S 4Y8; Mon'87; Peds. Staff, Centre Hospitalier Honore-Mercier; (450)771-3333

MORIN, Kevin W; Alberta Hosp Edmonton, PO Box 307 Stn Main 17480 Fort Rd, Edmonton AB T5J 2J7; Alb'01; FRCPC; Psy. Staff, Alberta Hospital Edmonton; (780)342-5473; Fax. (780)342-5411.

MORIN, Lise; CSSS Pierre Boucher, 1333 boul Jacques-Cartier E, Longueuil QC J4M 2A5; Mon'76; CSPQ; FRCPC; Anes. Staff Anes, Centre Hospitalier Pierre Boucher; (450)468-8111; lisemorin@hotmail.com.

MORIN, Louis-Philippe; CSSS de Rimouski-Neigette, CP 3150 succ A 150 av Rouleau, Rimouski QC G5L 5T1; Laval'02; FRCPC; DiagRad. Staff, Hôpital Regional Rimouski; (418)723-7851

MORIN, Louise; Centre De L'Osteoporose, 100-1200 av de Germain-des-Pre, Quebec QC G1V 3M7; Laval'74; LMCC; Médecin, Centre Hospitalier Affilié Universitaire de Québec - Hôpital du St-Sacrement; Physician/Investigator, Groupe de Recherche En Rhumatologie Et Maladies Osseuses QC; (418)650-2661; Fax. (418)650-6574.

MORIN, Luc; 1381 rue Simard, Sherbrooke QC J1J 3K5; Laval'65; DPM; DABPN; FAPA; FRCPC; Psy (Child & Adolescent Psychiatry). Consultant Pedopsychiatrie, Centre de Sante Isle-Dieu Matagami; Consultant, Institut Raymond Dewar; Langs: Bilingual(French/English); (819)569-1293; Fax. (819)563-6273; lucmorin@abacom.com.

MORIN, Lucie; Hôpital Ste-Justine, 3175 ch Cote-Sainte-Catherine, Montreal QC H3T 1C5; Sher'87; FRCSC; ObstGyn (Fetal & Maternal Medicine). Staff, Hôpital Ste-Justine; assoc Prof, McGill University; (514)345-4931 x4788

MORIN, M T Caroline; Sheldon Chumir Centre, 1213 4 St SW, Calgary AB T2R 0X7; Mon'95; ABNP; FRCPC; Psy. Staff, Hopital Louis-H Lafontaine; Langs: English; (403)955-9300

MORIN, Madeleine; Clin Med Colombus, 1140 rue Jean-Talon E, Montreal QC H2R 1V9; Mon'78; (514)270-2141; Fax. (514)270-6920.

MORIN, Marie-Eve; Clinique Medicale GMF-1851, 101-1851 rue Sherbrooke E, Montreal QC H2K 4L5; Sher'01; CCFP; Médecin, Clinique Medicale GMF-1851; Langs: Spanish; English; (514)524-7564; Fax. (514)527-5251; puce135@hotmail.com.

MORIN, Marie-Josee; Ctr de Med Familiale de Granby, 48 rue Denison E, Granby QC J2G 4C6; Sher'86; CCFP; (450)372-3996; Fax. (450)372-0430.

MORIN, Marie-Lise; Arcola Family Health Clinic, PO Box 479, Arcola SK S0C 0G0; Sask'98; LMCC; (306)455-2287; Fax. (306)455-2296.

MORIN, Marie-Paule; Hopital Ste-Justine, 3175 ch Cote-Sainte-Catherine, Montreal QC H3T 1C5; Sher'04; FRCPC; Peds; Rheum. Staff, Hôpital Ste-Justine; (514)345-4713

MORIN, Mario Y; 3402-219 Fort York Blvd, Toronto ON M5V 1B1; Ott'10.

MORIN, Martine; CSSS IUGS, 50 rue Camirand, Sherbrooke QC J1H 4J5; Sher'81; CCFP; Staff Obst & Family Planning Clin, Centre Hospitalier Universitaire de Sherbrooke-Hopital Fleurimont; Prof, Universite de Sherbrooke; Langs: English; Spanish; (819)563-2572; Fax. (819)565-8196.

MORIN, Maryse; 196 rue Veteran, Grand Falls NB E3Y 1C8; Sher'10; CCFP.

MORIN, Michel; 5824 boul Monk, Montreal QC H4E 3H3; Mon'76; (514)767-5307; Fax. (514)767-0217.

MORIN, Michel; Hop Maisonneuve-Rosemont, 5415 boul de l'Assomption, Montreal QC H1T 2M4; Mon'80; FRCSC; GenSurg. Clin Asst, Hopital Maisonneuve-Rosemont; (514)252-3822

MORIN, Michele; Ctr Hosp Affilie-St-Sacrement, 1050 ch Sainte-Foy, Quebec QC G1S 4L8; Laval'87; FRCPC; IntMed; GeriatricMed. Staff, Centre Hospitalier Affilié Universitaire de Québec - Hôpital De L'Enfant Jésus; Staff, Centre Hospitalier Affilié Universitaire de Québec - Hôpital du St-Sacrement; (418)682-7881

MORIN, Mireille; Clinique Medi-Val, 100-408 rue Jeanne-Mance, Salaber-de-Valleyf QC J6T 4G1; Mon'03; CCFP; (450)370-3395

MORIN, Nadine; CHUQ-Ctr Hosp Univ Laval, 2705 boul Laurier, Quebec QC G1V 4G2; Laval'04; CCFP; Staff, Centre Hospitalier Universitaire de Quebec-CHUL; (418)525-4444

MORIN, Nancy A; SMBD Jewish Gen Hosp, 3755 ch Cote-Sainte-Catherine, Montreal QC H3T 1E2; McG'95; FACS; FRCSC; GenSurg (Colon & Rectal Surgery). Asst Prof Surg, Sir Mortimer B Davis Jewish General; Staff Teacher, McGill University; (514)340-8422

MORIN, Nive; CSSS du Nord de Lanaudière, 1000 boul Saint-Anne, St-Charles-Brromee QC J6E 6J2; Mon'07; Psy (P.Q.). Staff, Centre Hospitalier Régional de Lanaudière; (450)759-8222

MORIN, Pascal; Clin ORL, 101-867 boul Saint-Joseph, Roberval QC G8H 2L8; Laval'97; FRCSC; Otol. (418)275-3266; Fax. (418)275-9152.

MORIN, Pierre; Clinique Med Saint-Vincent, 250 rue King E, Sherbrooke QC J1G 1A9; Laval'69; (819)563-0510; Fax. (819)564-6889.

MORIN, Raymond; CSSS de Beauce-Etchemin, 1515 71e rue, Saint-Georges QC G5Y 4T8; Laval'65; Staff, Centre d'hébergement de Beauceville; Staff, Centre Hospitalier Beauce-Etchemin; (418)228-3463; Fax. (418)226-0457.

MORIN, Real; Inst Nat'l de Sante Publique, 5F-945 av Wolfe, Quebec QC G1V 5B3; Laval'80; MSc; MBA; CSPQ; FRCPC; CommunMed (Health Promotion). Staff, Centre Hospitalier Affilié Universitaire de Québec - Hôpital du St-Sacrement; Med Consultant, Centre Hospitalier Affilié Universitaire de Québec - Hôpital De L'Enfant Jésus; Asst Med Cons, Institut National de Sante Publique du Quebec; (418)650-5115 x5500; real.morin@inspq.qc.ca.

MORIN, Renee; CSSS de Quebec Nord, 3666 ch Royal, Quebec QC G1E 1X5; Laval'81; LMCC; (418)663-2572; Fax. (418)663-2939; renee.morin@ssss.gouv.qc.ca.

MORIN, Richard H; 31 Cdn Health Svcs Unit Borden, PO Box 1000 Stn Main 30 Ortona Rd, Borden ON L0M 1C0; Ott'07; CCFP; (705)424-1200

MORIN, Serge; Centre Med Racine, 201-900 boul Raymond, Quebec QC G1B 3G3; Laval'78; (418)667-8066

MORIN, Simon; 105-534 St Francois O, St-Franc-Mont QC G0R 3A0; Laval'76; Staff, CSSS de Montmagny-L'Islet; (418)259-7317

MORIN, Stanislas; CHUQ-St-Francois d'Assise, 10 rue de l'Espinay, Quebec QC G1L 3L5; Laval'01; CSPQ; FRCPC; DiagRad. Staff, Centre Hospitalier Universitaire De Québec - Pavillon De St-françois-d'assise; (418)525-4444

MORIN, Stephane P; CSSS de Montmagny-L'Islet, RR 1 350 boul Tache O, Montmagny QC G5V 3R8; Laval'87; FRCSC; Ophth. Staff, CSSS de Montmagny-L'Islet; (418)248-0630; Fax. (418)248-0820.

MORIN, Stephanie; Photoderma, 202-11 boul Samson, Laval QC H7X 3S5; Mon'97; (450)314-3200

MORIN, Suzanne N; MUHC-Montreal Gen Hosp, B2 118-1650 av Cedar, Montreal QC H3G 1A4; Laval'87; FRCPC; IntMed. Staff, McGill University Health Centre - Montreal General Campus; Langs: English; French; (514)934-1934 x48053; Fax. (514)937-0803.

MORIN, Suzanne T; St Mary's Hosp Centre, 3830 av Lacombe, Montreal QC H3T 1M5; McM'96; FRCPC; IntMed. Staff, St Mary's Hospital Centre; (514)345-3511

MORIN, Valerie; CHUQ-Ctr Hosp Univ Laval, 2705 boul Laurier, Quebec QC G1V 4G2; Laval'92; FRCPC; ObstGyn (Maternal Fetal Medicine). Staff, Centre Hospitalier Universitaire de Quebec-CHUL; (418)525-4444; Fax. (418)577-2058.

MORIN, Yan; Hôpital Laval, 2725 ch Sainte-Foy, Quebec QC G1V 4G5; Laval'04; CCFP; Staff, Centre de santé des Côté-Nord; Staff, Hôpital Laval; Langs: English; (418)656-8711; raggaeman@hotmail.com.

MORIN-BIENVENU, Louise; 500-235 boul René-Lévesque E, Montreal QC H2X 1N8; Sher'72; Langs: English; (514)395-9090; Fax. (514)395-8877.

MORINIS, Julia B S; The Hosp for Sick Children, 10223-555 Unviersity Ave, Toronto ON M5G 1X8; McM'07; FRCPC; Peds. Staff, The Hospital For Sick Children; (416)813-7769; Fax. (416)813-5663.

MORINVILLE, Veronique D; MUHC-Montreal Children's Hosp, D562-2300 rue Tupper, Montreal QC H3H 1P3; McG'99; FRCPC; Peds; Gastroent. Staff, McGill University Health Centre - Montreal Children's Hospital; (514)412-4400

MORISHITA, Kimberley A; Children's & Women's HC of BC, K4 120-4480 Oak St, Vancouver BC V6H 3V4; UBC'03; FRCPC; Peds; Rheum. Staff Redident Education, BC Children's Hospital; (604)875-2437

MORISON, Jay W; Kingston Med Arts Centre, 213-800 Princess St, Kingston ON K7L 5E4; Qns'80; BSc; CCFP; FCFP; (613)548-4555; Fax. (613)548-4554.

MORISON, Nicholas J; Liberton Med Centre, 114-31 Liberton Dr, St. Albert AB T8N 3X6; London (England)'76; Clin Lecturer Family Med/Preceptor, University of Alberta; (780)459-7769; Fax. (780)459-9147.

MORISSET, Anne; CSSS de la Haute-Yamaska, 205 boul Leclerc O, Granby QC J2G 1T7; Laval'96; FRCPC; IntMed. Staff, Centre Hospitalier de Granby; (450)375-8000

MORISSET, Julie; CSSS du Nord de Lanaudière, 1000 boul Sainte-Anne Blvd, Joliette QC J6E 6J2; Sher'08; IntMed. Staff, Centre Hospitalier Régional de Lanaudière; (450)759-8222

MORISSET, Julie; CSSS de Trois-Rivières, 1991 boul du Carmel, Trois-Rivieres QC G8Z 3R9; Laval'88; CSPQ; FRCSC; Urol. Staff, CSSS de Trois-Rivières; (819)697-3333; Fax. (819)372-3519.

MORISSET, Marie-Eve; CSSS de Manicouagan, 635 boul Jolliet, Baie-Comeau QC G5C 1P1; Mon'93; BSc; MSc; CCFP; Staff, Centre Hospitalier Régional Baie-Comeau; Med Coord, Breast Cancer Detection Program; Langs: English; French; (418)589-3701; Fax. (418)589-5292.

MORISSET, Richard; CHUM-Hotel-Dieu, 3840 rue Saint-Urbain, Montreal QC H2W 1T8; Mon'64; MSc(Microbiol.); Microbio & Infect Dis (P.Q.); MedMicrobiol (P.Q.) (AIDS/HIV). ac Staff InfectDis & Microbiol Dept, Centre Hospitalier l'Université de Montréal (CHUM) - Hôtel-Dieu; Researcher Clinician, Research Ctre & Dir., International Proj.-Madagascar; Prof, Universite de Montreal; (514)890-8100 x14354

MORISSETTE, Alain; SAAQ, 333 boul Jean-Lesage, Quebec QC G1K 8J6; Laval'80; (418)528-4312; alain.morissette@saaq.gouv.qc.ca.

MORISSETTE, Carole; Dir de la Sante Publique-Mtl, 1301 rue Sherbrooke E, Montreal QC H2L 1M3; Mon'82; CSPQ; FRCPC; CommunMed. (514)528-2400 x3603; Fax. (514)528-2452; cmorisse@santepub-mtl.qc.ca.

MORISSETTE, Celine; 2A boul St-Pierre E, Caraquet NB E1W 1B6; Laval'83; Staff, Hôpital de l'Enfant-Jésus RHSJ; (506)727-6524; Fax. (506)727-1187.

MORISSETTE, Chantale; Centre Med Fusion, 200-2035 av Sainte-Anne, Saint-Hyacinthe QC J2S 5H3; Sher'90; CCFP; (450)773-6023

MORISSETTE, Diane; Centre Royal Comtois, 101-444 rue McGill, Hawkesbury ON K6A 1R2; Sher'01; FRCPC; Psy. Langs: Bilingual(French/English); (613)632-0139; Fax. (613)632-4791.

MORISSETTE, Guy; Agence de SSS de l'Outaouais, 104 rue Lois, Gatineau QC J8Y 3R7; Ott'79; Staff Emerg Room, Hull Hospital; (819)770-7747; Fax. (819)771-8632.

MORISSETTE, Isabelle; CSSS Haut-Richelieu-Rouville, 920 boul du Seminaire N, St-Jean-Sur-Richel QC J3A 1B7; Laval'86; FRCPC; MedMicrobiol; Microbio & Infect Dis (P.Q.). Staff Microbiol, Hôpital du Haut-Richelieu; (450)359-5000; Fax. (450)359-5237.

MORISSETTE, Jacqueline; CLSC de Cabano, 101-33 rue Saint-Laurent, Cabano QC G0L 1E0; Mon'81; (418)854-2572

MORISSETTE, Jean J; Ctr Hosp Affilie-Enfant-Jesus, 1401 18e rue, Quebec QC G1J 1Z4; Laval'64; CSPQ; DiagRad. Radiologist, Centre Hospitalier Affilié Universitaire de Québec - Hôpital De L'Enfant Jésus; Langs: Spanish; English; (418)649-5782; Fax. (418)649-5972.

MORISSETTE, Louis G; LL-100 Argyle Ave, Ottawa ON K2P 1B6; Ott'70; CCFP; FCFP; Langs: English; (613)232-8543; Fax. (613)232-2469.

MORISSETTE, Louis; Inst Philippe Pinel de Mtl, 10905 boul Henri-Bourassa E, Montreal QC H1C 1H1; Laval'78; LMCC; NBME; FRCPC; Psy (Adolescent Psychiatry). Staff, Institut Philippe-Pinel de Montreal; adj Prof, Universite de Montreal; Langs: English; (514)648-8461 x491; Fax. (514)494-4406.

MORISSETTE, Lucie; Ctr Hosp Affilie-Enfant-Jesus, 1401 18e rue, Quebec QC G1J 1Z4; Sher'89; CSPQ; LMCC; FRCPC; DiagRad (Echography). Staff Echo-IRM, Centre Hospitalier Affilié Universitaire de Québec - Hôpital De L'Enfant Jésus; Prof AMCEL, Université Laval; Langs: Bilingual(French/English); (418)649-0252 x5782; Fax. (418)649-5903; marks+laurent@videotron.ca.

MORISSETTE, Lucie; Ctr Medico Prof de Brosssard, 101-2424 boul Lapiniere, Brossard QC J4Z 2K9; Mon'81; Staff, Centre Hospitalier l'Université De Montréal (CHUM) - Hôpital Saint-luc; Langs: English; (450)678-9033; Fax. (450)678-8274.

MORISSETTE, Martin M; Centre Med Pierrefonds, 12774 boul Gouin O, Pierrefonds QC H8Z 1W5; Laval'67; Cardiol (P.Q.). ac Staff, Centre Hospitalier l'Université de Montréal (CHUM) - Hôpital Notre-Dame; Researcher, McGill University; (514)684-8460

MORISSETTE, Michel; Clinique Med St-Agapit, RR 1 105-1125 rue Principale, Saint-Agapit QC G0S 1Z0; Laval'74; Staff, Centre Hospitalier Universitaire De Québec - Pavillon De St-françois-d'assise; (418)888-3951; Fax. (418)888-3952.

MORISSETTE, Nadesh; CHUQ-Hotel-Dieu de Quebec, 11 Cote du Palais, Quebec QC G1R 2J6; Laval'07; IntMed. (418)691-5266

MORISSETTE, Nancy; Hop Maisonneuve-Rosemont, 5415 boul de l'Assomption, Montreal QC H1T 2M4; Mon'03; CCFP; Staff, Hopital Maisonneuve-Rosemont; (514)252-3400

MORISSETTE, Nathalie; Hop Charles LeMoyne, 3120 boul Taschereau, Greenfield Park QC J4V 2H1; McG'99; FRCPC; IntMed; Critical Care Medicine (P.Q.). Staff, Hopital Charles LeMoyne; Staff Critical Care, Centre Hospitalier l'Université de Montréal (CHUM) - Hôtel-Dieu; (450)466-5000 x2880; Fax. (450)466-5768.

MORISSETTE, Pierre; 29 boul Gerard-D-Levesque E GD, Paspebiac QC G0C 2K0; Laval'66; (418)752-6900; Fax. (418)752-6515.

MORISSETTE, Raymond; Hop Louis-H Lafontaine, 7401 rue Hochelaga, Montreal QC H1N 3M5; Laval'63; FRCPC; Psy. Staff, Hopital Louis-H Lafontaine; (514)251-4000; Fax. (514)251-8474.

MORISSETTE, Sebastien; Hotel-Dieu d'Arthabaska, 5 rue des Hospitalieres, Victoriaville QC G6P 6N2; Sher'07; DiagRad. Staff, Hotel-Dieu d'Arthabaska; (819)357-2030

MORKEL, Floris J; PO Box 670, Houston BC V0J 1Z0; Orange Free State (South Africa)'00.

MORLEY, Charlotte M; Medical Arts Bldg, 407-5880 Spring Garden Rd, Halifax NS B3H 1Y1; Dal'84; FRCPC; Peds. (902)422-6421; Fax. (902)423-5485.

MORLEY, Daniel; Montfort Hosp, 713 Montreal Rd, Ottawa ON K1K 0T2; Tor'92; BSc; CCFP; Staff, Montfort Hospital; (613)945-1474; Fax. (613)945-1472.

MORLEY, Ellise C; Lakeside Clinic, 202-15379 Castle Downs Rd NW, Edmonton AB T5X 3Y7; Alb'97; CCFP; (780)472-7575; Fax. (780)472-7404; emorley@shaw.ca.

MORLEY, John E; Waterford Hosp, 306 Waterford Bridge Rd, St. John's NL A1E 4J8; National (Ireland)'84; MB ChB; BAO; CCFP; FCFP; Med Staff, Waterford Hospital; (709)777-3300

MORLEY, Julia C; Eagle Ridge Hosp & Health CC, 475 Guildford Way, Port Moody BC V3H 3W9; Witwatersrand (South Africa)'99; Staff, Eagle Ridge Hospital & Health Care Centre; (604)461-2022

MORLEY, Rebecca E; Lansdowne Professional Ctr II, 305-3066 Shelbourne St, Victoria BC V8R 6T9; UBC'02; FRCSC; PlasSurg. (250)592-5510

MORLEY-FORSTER, Patricia K; B3-626-268 Grosvenor St PO Box 5777 Stn B, London ON N6A 4V2; Tor'77; BSc; FRCPC; Anes (Chronic Pain). Staff, St Joseph's Hospital - St Joseph's Health Care; Staff, London Health Sciences Centre - University Hospital; Dir Ontario Interdisciplinary Pain Prog, University of Western Ontario; (519)646-6000 x65065; Fax. (519)646-6376; pat.morley-forster@sjhc.london.on.ca.

MORLOCK, J Scott; Elmira Med Centre, 2 Park Ave W, Elmira ON N3B 1L1; Wes'82; CCFP; CCFP(E.M.); FCFP; Court Staff, Grand River Hospital - Kitchener/Waterloo Health Centre; Court Staff, St Mary's General Hospital; (519)669-5493; Fax. (519)669-5901.

MORNEAU, Colombe; 100-1144 rue Saint-Laurent O, Longueuil QC J4K 1E2; Mon'82; Physician, Walk-In Clinic; Langs: English; Spanish; (450)679-4333; Fax. (450)679-1672.

MORNEAU, Jean; Ctr Hosp Affilie-Enfant-Jesus, 1401 18e rue, Quebec QC G1J 1Z4; Laval'83; ACLS; ATLS; Ac Staff, Centre Hospitalier Affilié Universitaire de Québec - Hôpital De L'Enfant Jésus; Université Laval; (418)649-5632; Fax. (418)649-5975.

MORNEAU, Joanne; Clinique Familiale la Providen, 16405 av Bourdages S, Saint-Hyacinthe QC J2T 4G9; Laval'84; BSc; CCFP; Ac Medical Staff, CSSSRY, Saint-Hyacinthe; Prof, Universite de Sherbrooke; (450)773-6734; Fax. (450)773-9909.

MORNEAU, Kathryn A; Findlay Creek Med Centre, 3-4744 Bank St, Ottawa ON K1T 3W7; Tor'85; CCFP; FCFP; (613)822-2775

MORNEAU, Lucie; Polyclinique Med des Ponts, 120-1100 boul de la Rive-Sud, Saint-Romuald QC G6W 5M6; Laval'86; Staff Palliative Care & Geriatrics, Centre Hospitalier Paul-Gilbert; Langs: Bilingual(French/English); (418)834-1177; Fax. (418)834-9275.

MORNEAU, Micheline; Ctr de Dermatologie Maizerets, 2094 boul Sainte-Anne, Quebec QC G1J 1X7; Laval'72; FRCPC; Derm. Ac Staff, Centre Hospitalier Universitaire De Québec - Pavillon De St-françois-d'assise; (418)663-3000; Fax. (418)663-3018; mmorneau@bellnet.ca.

MORNINGSTAR, Beverly A; Sunnybrook Hlth Sciences Ctre, M3 200-2075 Bayview Ave, Toronto ON M4N 3M5; Tor'76; AB; FRCPC; Anes. Staff, Sunnybrook Health Sciences Centre; (416)480-4864; Fax. (416)480-6039.

MORNINGSTAR, Gary L; Dixie Road Med Associates, 2200 Dixie Rd, Mississauga ON L4Y 1Z4; Tor'75; CCFP; FCFP; Ac Staff, Trillium Health Centre - Mississauga; Lecturer Family & Commun Med, University of Toronto; (905)279-1700; Fax. (905)897-9167.

MORO, Elena; Univ Hlth Network-Toronto Western Hosp, MCL7 402-399 Bathurst St, Toronto ON M5T 2S8; Trieste (Italy)'89; Staff, Toronto Western Hospital - University Health Network; (416)603-6422

MORO, Jaydeep K; Medical Arts Bldg, 505-1 Young St, Hamilton ON L8N 1T8; Tor'93; FRCSC; OrthSurg (Sports Injuries). Court Staff, Toronto Western Hospital - University Health Network; Staff, St Joseph's Healthcare - Charlton Campus; Court Staff, Hamilton Health Sciences Centre - McMaster Children's Hospital; (905)540-8448; Fax. (905)540-8414.

MORO, Luciano F; Malton Med Arts Bldg, 102-3530 Derry Rd E, Malton ON L4T 4E3; Padova (Italy)'75; Langs: Italian; (905)678-6195

MORONG, Sharon E; U of Toronto Postgrad Med Educ, 500 University Ave, Toronto ON M5G 1V7; Tor'07; Otol.

MOROTTI, Linda; Clinique Le Medical, 285-1750 boul Marie-Victorin, Longueuil QC J4G 1A5; Mon'87; (450)442-9531; Fax. (450)442-1553.

MOROZ, Brenda E; MUHC-Montreal Children's Hosp, C215-2300 rue Tupper, Montreal QC H3H 1P3; Tor'64; BA; Derm. Associé, McGill University Health Centre - Royal Victoria Hospital; Dir Derm, McGill University Health Centre - Montreal Children's Hospital; assoc Prof Med & Peds, McGill University; Langs: Bilingual(English/French); (514)412-4310; Fax. (514)412-4202; brenda.moroz@mcgill.ca.

MOROZ, Leonard A; MUHC-Royal Victoria Hosp, 687 av des Pins O, Montreal QC H3A 1A1; Man'59; AB; CSPQ; Rheum (P.Q.); IntMed (Clinical Immunology & Allergy). Staff, McGill University Health Centre - Royal Victoria Hospital.

MOROZ, Paul J; Children's Hosp Eastern Ont, 401 Smyth Rd, Ottawa ON K1H 8L1; Cal'89; MSc(Med); FAAOS; FRCSC; OrthSurg (Pediatric Spinal Deformity). Staff, Children's Hospital of Eastern Ontario (CHEO); Member Non-Economic Loss Roster, Workers' Comp Board of ON; Coroner Investigative, Province of Ontario; Asst Prof Surg, University of Ottawa; Langs: Ukrainian; (613)737-7600 x3257; Fax. (613)738-4840; pmoroz@cheo.on.ca.

MORRA, Antonella; 1-1146 Birchview Dr, Mississauga ON L5H 3C8; Plymouth (Montserrat)'96; DABPed; FAAP; FRCPC; Peds. Staff, Trillium Health Centre - Mississauga; (905)271-7500; Fax. (905)271-6800.

MORRA, Dante J; Univ Hlth Network-Toronto Gen, 14 218-200 Elizabeth St, Toronto ON M5G 2C4; Tor'00; FRCPC; IntMed. Staff, Toronto General Hospital - UHN; (416)340-3111

MORRA, Pasqualino; 004-1400 Ritson Rd N, Oshawa ON L1G 7W4; Ott'88; FRCPC; IntMed. Staff Internist, Lakeridge Health - Oshawa Site; Langs: Italian; (905)404-2900; Fax. (905)404-0992; pmorramd@gmail.com.

MORRELL, Bobbi J; London HSC-Victoria Campus, PO Box 5010 Stn B D314-800 Commissioners Rd E, London ON N6A 5W9; Alb'02; Anes. Staff, London Health Sciences Centre - Victoria Campus; (519)685-8500

MORRELL, John D; 207-100 Humber College Blvd, Etobicoke ON M9V 5G4; Qns'01; FRCSC; Urol. (416)747-1591

MORRELL, Rachel A; 22 CF Health Services Centre, PO Box 6550 Stn Forces, Cold Lake AB T9M 2C6; Tor'03; CCFP; (780)840-8000; Fax. (780)840-4021.

MORRELL, Robert W; Richmond Health Science Ctre, 270-6091 Gilbert Rd, Richmond BC V7C 5L9; UBC'72; Staff, Richmond Hospital; Med Dir/Chairman FIS Med Educ Committe & Canadian Representative, Alpine Canada; Dir, YMCA Sports Medicine Clinic; (604)270-1998; Fax. (604)270-8584; rmorrel@telus.net.

MORRICE, Lora M; Family Med Centre, 103-7143 West Saanich Rd, Brentwood Bay BC V8M 1P7; UBC'94; BSc(Hons); PhD; CCFP; FCFP; (250)652-9191; Fax. (250)652-5576.

MORRIELLO, Florence F; Hamilton HS-General Site, 237 Barton St E, Hamilton ON L8L 2X2; Ferrara (Italy)'06; Staff, Hamilton Health Sciences Centre - Hamilton General Hospital.

MORRIN, Sharon M L; Queensway-Carleton Hosp, 3045 Baseline Rd, Nepean ON K2H 8P4; Mem'96; FRCPC; IntMed; Hem. Staff/Leader Hospitalist, Queensway Carleton Hospital; smorrin@qch.on.ca.

MORRIS, Adrian C B; Capri Medical Centre, 132-1835 Gordon Dr, Kelowna BC V1Y 3H4; Dal'96; CCFP; (250)717-3211; Fax. (250)717-3233.

MORRIS, Alison J; Labrador Grenfell Health, PO Box 7000 Stn C 227 Hamilton River Rd, Happy-Valley-Goose NL A0P 1C0; UBC'06; CCFP; Staff, Labrador Health Centre; (709)897-2000

MORRIS, Alyssa; Foothills Med Centre, 1403 29 St NW, Calgary AB T2N 2T9; Cal'07; EmergMed. Staff, Foothills Medical Centre; (403)944-1315

MORRIS, Andrew L; St Boniface Gen Hosp, 409 Tache Ave, Winnipeg MB R2H 2A6; Albert Einstein(NY) (USA)'67; ABIM(CV Diseases); FACP; FACC; Staff Cardiol, St Boniface General Hospital; Prof Cardiol, University of Manitoba; (204)235-3826; Fax. (204)233-2157; amorris@sbgh.mb.ca.

MORRIS, Andrew M; Mount Sinai Hosp, 415-600 University Ave, Toronto ON M5G 1X5; Tor'94; MSc; FRCPC; IntMed; InfectDis. Staff, Princess Margaret Hospital - University Health Network; Staff, Mount Sinai Hospital; Staff, Toronto Western Hospital - University Health Network; Staff, Toronto General Hospital - UHN; Assoc Prof Med, University of Toronto; (416)586-4800 x8102; amorris@mtsinai.on.ca.

MORRIS, Anna G; Cambridge Mem Hosp, 700 Coronation Blvd, Cambridge ON N1R 3G2; National (Ireland)'71; MB ChB; BAO; FRCPC; GenPath. Staff, Cambridge Memorial Hospital; (519)621-2330

MORRIS, Barbara D; Carling-Broadview Med Bldg, 305-770 Broadview Ave, Ottawa ON K2A 3Z3; McM'89; CCFP; FCFP; Court Staff, Bruyère Continuing Care - Saint-Vincent Hospital; Ac Staff, The Ottawa Hospital - Civic Campus; Court Staff, The Ottawa Hospital - General Campus; Asst Prof, University of Ottawa; (613)728-7700; Fax. (613)728-5848.

MORRIS, Brian A P; 303-190 Cundles Rd E SS 103, Barrie ON L4M 4S5; Tor'78; CCFP; FCFP; Staff, Royal Victoria Regional Health Centre; Coroner, Province of Ontario; (705)728-3722; Fax. (705)728-9449.

MORRIS, Brian M; Westmount Med Bldg, 455-5025 rue Sherbrooke O, Montreal QC H4A 1S9; Reims (France)'77; CSPQ; FRCSC; Urol. Staff, Hôpital Santa Cabrini Ospedale; Staff, St Mary's Hospital Centre; Langs: English; French; (514)485-1333; Fax. (514)485-8509; brianmorris@videotron.ca.

MORRIS, Catherine A W; St Joseph's Health Centre, 100 Westmount Rd, Guelph ON N1H 5H8; McM'81; BSc; MHSc; FRCPC; IntMed. Clin Assoc Prof Med, Hamilton Health Sciences Centre-Juravinski Site; Staff, St Joseph's Health Centre; Chief Staff/Hospitalist, Cambridge Memorial Hospital; (519)824-6000; cmorris@gghorg.ca.

MORRIS, Catherine; Wentworth Limeridge Med Ctre, 203-849 Upper Wentworth St, Hamilton ON L9A 5H4; Tor'81; BA; CCFP; FCFP; Assoc Staff, Hamilton Health Sciences Centre; (905)387-6897; Fax. (905)387-4899.

MORRIS, Chester N; 3949 Port Alberni Hwy, Port Alberni BC V9Y 4S1; UBC'90; (250)724-8800

MORRIS, Daniel C; Vancouver Gen Hosp, 855 12th Ave W, Vancouver BC V5Z 1M9; Dal'74; FRCPC; DiagRad. Ac Staff, Vancouver General Hospital - Centennial Pavillion; Asst Prof, University of British Columbia; (604)875-4366; Fax. (604)875-4319.

MORRIS, David; MUHC-Royal Victoria Hosp, M905-687 av des Pins O, Montreal QC H3A 1A1; Cambridge (England)'70; MRCP(UK); Endocrin (P.Q.) (Diabetes). Att Staff, McGill University Health Centre - Royal Victoria Hospital; assoc Prof Med, McGill University; Langs: Italian; German; French; (514)934-1934 x34050; Fax. (514)843-2838.

MORRIS, David P; Nova Scotia Cancer Centre, 3037-5820 University Ave, Halifax NS B3H 1V7; London (England)'91; MB BS; Staff, Queen Elizabeth II Health Sciences Centre - Victoria General Site; (902)473-1986; Fax. (902)473-1260.

MORRIS, Derrick G; Vernon Jubilee Hosp, 2101 32 St, Vernon BC V1T 5L2; Mem'80; FRCPC; Anes. Staff, Royal Inland Hospital; Staff, Vernon Jubilee Hospital; (250)374-5111; dmorris@shaw.ca.

MORRIS, Donald G; Tom Baker Cancer Centre, 1331 29 St NW, Calgary AB T2N 4N2; Cal'92; BSc; PhD; FRCPC; IntMed (Lung Cancer); MedOncol. Assoc Prof MedOncol, Tom Baker Cancer Centre; Dir Oncology Training/Assoc Prof Oncol, University of Calgary; (403)521-3447; Fax. (403)283-1651.

MORRIS, Dorian V; Seymour Med Clinic, 200-1530 7th Ave W, Vancouver BC V6J 1S3; UBC'69; Vis Staff, Vancouver General Hospital - Centennial Pavillion; Clin Instructor Med, University of British Columbia; (604)739-5613

MORRIS, Gail A; Boxgrove Family Practice, PH3-110 Copper Creek Dr, Markham ON L6B 0P9; Tor'84; CCFP; Staff, Markham Stouffville Hospital; (905)472-9400; Fax. (905)472-9409.

MORRIS, Gary F; Royal University Hosp, G525-103 Hospital Dr, Saskatoon SK S7N 0W8; Alb'82; FRCPC; Anes. Assoc Staff, St Paul's Hospital (Grey Nuns) of Saskatoon; Assoc Staff, Saskatoon City Hospital; Assoc Staff Anes, Royal University Hospital; Staff Med, Saskatoon District Health Board; Clin Assoc Prof Anes, University of Saskatchewan; (306)655-1183; Fax. (306)655-1279; gary.morris@saskatoonhealthregion.ca.

MORRIS, Gary L; Gulf Canada Sqaure, 330-401 9 Ave SW, Calgary AB T2P 3C5; Cal'96; PhD; FRCPC; IntMed; Rheum. Staff, Foothills Medical Centre; Staff, Peter Lougheed Centre; Staff, Rockyview General Hospital; (403)221-4465; Fax. (403)221-4419.

MORRIS, Geoffrey S; Trafalgar Med Group, 200-1235 Trafalgar Rd, Oakville ON L6H 3P1; Trinity Coll. (Ireland)'78; DCH; DObst; MRC; (905)844-3281

MORRIS, Glenn S; Pembina Village Walk-In Clinic, 2-2077 Pembina Hwy, Winnipeg MB R3T 5J9; Man'82; CCFP; (204)261-4691; Fax. (204)261-3012.

MORRIS, Ian R; Queen Elizabeth II HSC, 1276 South Park St, Halifax NS B3H 2Y9; Dal'76; DABA; FACEP; DABEM; FRCPC; Anes; EmergMed. Staff Anes, Queen Elizabeth II Health Sciences Centre - Victoria General Site; Assoc Prof Anes, Dalhousie University; (902)473-2331; Fax. (902)423-9454; ian.morris@ns.sympatico.ca.

MORRIS, John C B; Hillsdale Med Clinic, 1380G 23rd Ave, Regina SK S4S 3S5; (South Africa)'83; MB ChB; DCH(SA); (306)584-1533; Fax. (306)584-1767.

MORRIS, John E; Dr Everett Chalmers Reg Hosp, PO Box 9000 Stn A 700 Priestman St, Fredericton NB E3B 5N5; Dal'89; FRCPC; GenPath. Staff, Dr Everett Chalmers Regional Hospital; (506)452-5400 x5485

MORRIS, Judy; Hop du Sacre-Coeur de Mtl, 5400 boul Gouin O, Montreal QC H4J 1C5; McG'02; FRCPC; EmergMed (Family Medicine). Staff, Hôpital du Sacre-Coeur de Montréal; (514)338-2222 x3234

MORRIS, Kelly A; 200-158 Robert Angus Dr, Amherst NS B4H 4R7; Dal'08; CCFP; (902)667-3330; Fax. (902)667-4176.

MORRIS, Lauralee R; Region of Peel, 09-150 Central Park Dr, Brampton ON L6T 2T9; Tor'82; CCFP; (905)791-5905

MORRIS, Lawrence; Medical Arts Bldg, 803-1538 rue Sherbrooke O, Montreal QC H3G 1L5; McG'74; Att Staff Family Med, Sir Mortimer B Davis Jewish General; (514)931-1800; Fax. (514)931-1849.

MORRIS, Leigh J; Foothills Med Centre, C231-1403 29 St NW, Calgary AB T2N 2T9; Cal'91; CCFP; CCFP(E.M.); FCFP; Staff EmergMed, Foothills Medical Centre; (403)944-1635; Fax. (403)944-2419.

MORRIS, Leo C; McDermotts Med Clinic, 37 av Donegani, Pointe-Claire QC H9R 2V7; McG'58; FRCPC; IntMed (Allergy). (514)697-1410; lemorris@allstream.net.

MORRIS, Madeline; Lennox & Addington Gen Hosp, 8 Richmond Park Dr, Napanee ON K7R 2Z4; Dal'04; CCFP; Staff, Lennox & Addington County General Hospital; (613)354-3301

MORRIS, Margaret L; Respiratory Unit, 4F-810 Sherbrook St, Winnipeg MB R3A 1R8; Sask'79; FRCSC; ObstGyn (Pediatric & Adolescent Gynecology). Ac Staff, St Boniface General Hospital; Dept Head ObstGyn & Reproductive Sciences/Assoc Prof, University of Manitoba; (204)787-1984; Fax. (204)787-2314.

MORRIS, Mark W; Parksville Med Clinic, PO Box 250 Stn Main, Parksville BC V9P 2G4; Man'05; CCFP; (250)248-5757

MORRIS, Melanie I; Children's Hospital, AE402-840 Sherbrook St, Winnipeg MB R3A 1S1; Alb'04; FRCSC; GenSurg; PedGenSurg.

MORRIS, Michael J; Nanaimo Reg Gen Hosp, 1200 Dufferin Cres, Nanaimo BC V9S 2B7; London (England)'73; MB BS; DCH; MRC; CCFP; Chief Hospitalist Central Vancouver Island, Nanaimo Regional General Hospital; (250)754-2141; michael.morris@viha.ca.

MORRIS, Monica K; Jane-Bloor Centre, 500-2 Jane St, York ON M6S 4W3; McM'82; FRCPC; Psy (Psycho Pharmacology).

MORRIS, Patricia E; Parkdale Med Tower, 407-1081 Carling Ave, Ottawa ON K1Y 4G2; Tor'77; CCFP; FCFP; Staff, The Ottawa Hospital - Civic Campus; University of Ottawa; (613)722-3755; Fax. (613)722-8617.

MORRIS, Paul S; 102-304 The East Mall, Etobicoke ON M9B 6E2; McM'84; FRCPC; Psy. (416)231-7968; Fax. (416)231-7982.

MORRIS, Philip J; Murray Clinic, 1 Mount Bernard Ave, Corner Brook NL A2H 6Y5; Mem'85; (709)785-5211; Fax. (709)785-5705.

MORRIS, Randi E; SMBD Jewish Gen Hosp, 3755 ch Cote-Sainte-Catherine, Montreal QC H3T 1E2; McG'94; CCFP; Staff, Sir Mortimer B Davis Jewish General; (514)340-8278; Fax. (514)340-8298.

MORRIS, Richard D; Foothills Med Centre, 1403 29 St NW, Calgary AB T2N 2T9; McM'98; CCFP; CCFP(E.M.); Staff EmergMed, Foothills Medical Centre; (403)944-1635; Fax. (403)944-2419; rdmorris@hotmail.com.

MORRIS, Robert F; Dr Charles A Janeway Child HC, 300 Prince Philip Dr, St. John's NL A1B 3V6; Mem'76; FRCPC; Peds (Childhood Protection). Staff, Janeway Children's Health & Rehabilitation Centre; Assoc Prof Peds, Memorial University Of Newfoundland; (709)777-4150; Fax. (709)778-4333.

MORRIS, Rolf D T; Continuum Med Care, 202-520 17th St, West Vancouver BC V7V 3S8; Cambridge (England)'78; MScPharm; BA; PlasSurg (Cosmetic Surgery). Staff, Lions Gate Hospital; Pres, BC Section of Plastic Surgeons; (604)913-8183

MORRIS, S Anthony; Red Deer Reg Hosp Centre, PO Box 5030 Stn Postal Box Ctr 3942 50A Ave, Red Deer AB T4N 6R2; Cal'78; FRCPC; GenPath. Staff, Red Deer Regional Hospital Centre; Langs: English; French; (403)343-4515; tmorris@dthr.ab.ca.

MORRIS, Sandra; St Mary's Hosp Centre, 3830 av Lacombe, Montreal QC H3T 1M5; McG'05; CCFP; Staff, St Mary's Hospital Centre; (514)345-3511

MORRIS, Shaun K; The Hosp for Sick Children, 555 University Ave, Toronto ON M5G 1X8; Qns'03; FRCPC; Peds; InfectDis. Staff, The Hospital For Sick Children; (416)813-7500

MORRIS, Sheldon R; Cook Road Med Clinic, 100-8171 Cook Rd, Richmond BC V6Y 3T8; UBC'90; CCFP; FCFP; (604)270-7781

MORRIS, Steven; Queen Elizabeth II HSC-Halifax, 4443-1796 Summer St, Halifax NS B3H 3A7; Ott'83; MSc; FRCSC; PlasSurg (Reconstructive Surgery). Staff, Queen Elizabeth II Health Sciences Centre - Halifax Infirmary Site; Ac Staff, IWK Health Centre; Ac Staff, Queen Elizabeth II Health Sciences Centre - Victoria General Site; Prof Surg, Dalhousie University; Langs: English; French; (902)473-7054; Fax. (902)473-8773; sfmorris@dal.ca.

MORRIS, Sylvia; The Two Hundred, 401B-200 St Clair Ave W, Toronto ON M4V 1R1; Glasgow (Scotland)'49; MB ChB; Hon Staff, Humber River Regional Hospital - Keele Street Site; (416)923-5905 Semi-Retired.

MORRIS, Tanis G W; Chemainus Med Clinic, RR 1 9892 Esplanade St, Chemainus BC V0R 1K1; CCFP; (250)246-3261; Fax. (250)246-9144.

MORRIS, Thomas J; Westmount Med Bldg, 205-77 Westmount Rd, Guelph ON N1H 5J1; McM'80; FRCSC; Urol. Ac Staff, Guelph General Hospital; (519)824-7272; Fax. (519)824-0833.

MORRIS, Tracey M; St Paul's Hosp, 1081 Burrard St, Vancouver BC V6Z 1Y6; Dal'02; CCFP; Staff, Providence Health Care - St Paul's Hospital; (604)682-2344

MORRIS, Walter G; Scarborough Comm Mental Hlth, 12-2425 Eglinton Ave E, Scarborough ON M1K 5G8; Tor'63; (416)755-8301; Fax. (416)755-9220.

MORRIS, William F; Caremedics Hunt Club Clinic, 201-2446 Bank St, Ottawa ON K1V 1A4; Mem'91; (613)739-0998; Fax. (613)739-1485.

MORRIS, William J; BC Cancer Agency-Vancouver CC, 600 10th Ave W, Vancouver BC V5Z 4E6; UBC'85; FRCPC; RadOncol. Staff, BC Cancer Agency Vancouver Centre; (604)877-6000; Fax. (604)708-2000.

MORRIS-LARKIN, Carolyn; Health Sciences Centre, 300 Prince Philip Dr, St. John's NL A1B 3V6; Mem'84; GenPath. Staff, Health Sciences Centre; Asst Prof, Memorial University Of Newfoundland; (709)777-7298; Fax. (709)777-6395.

MORRISH, Donald W; Heritage Med Research Centre, 362B-107 University Campus NW, Edmonton AB T6G 2S2; Alb'74; PhD; FRCPC; IntMed (Endocrinology). Staff, Cross Cancer Institute; Staff Med, University of Alberta Hospital; Prof, University of Alberta; (780)407-3636; Fax. (780)407-6702.

MORRISH, William F; Foothills Med Centre, 1403 29 St NW, Calgary AB T2N 2T9; McG'88; FRCPC; DiagRad (Neuro Radiology). Staff Radiol, Foothills Medical Centre; Clinical Asst Prof, University of Calgary; (403)944-1969; Fax. (403)944-1687.

MORRISON, A Bruce; Vancouver Gen Hosp, 855 12th Ave W, Vancouver BC V5Z 1M9; London (England)'71; PhD; FACEP; FRCPC; CCFP; EmergMed;CCFP(E.M.); Staff Emerg, Vancouver General Hospital - Centennial Pavillion; Clin Assoc Prof, University of British Columbia; (604)875-4995

MORRISON, Allan F; South Kent Family Network, 65 Ellen St, Blenheim ON N0P 1A0; Ross University (Dominica)'07; (519)676-5592

MORRISON, Andree Y; 172 Ethel St, Sturgeon Falls ON P2B 1V9; Ott'93; CCFP; Staff, West Nipissing General Hospital; Langs: Bilingual(English/French); (705)753-5205; Fax. (705)753-5236.

MORRISON, Andrew B; Children's & Women's HC of BC, 4480 Oak St, Vancouver BC V6H 3V4; Aberdeen (Scotland)'91; Staff, BC Children's Hospital; (604)875-2711

MORRISON, Anne B; Alder Med Centre, 277 Evergreen Rd, Campbell River BC V9W 5Y4; UBC'06; CCFP; (250)287-7441

MORRISON, Catherine E; Royal Victoria Hosp, 201 Georgian Dr, Barrie ON L4M 6M2; McM'89; FRCPC; DiagRad. Staff, Royal Victoria Regional Health Centre; (705)728-9090 x43481

MORRISON, Clare; Lions Gate Hosp, 231 15th St E, North Vancouver BC V7L 2L7; UBC'00; FRCPC; Anes. Staff, Lions Gate Hospital; (604)984-5709

MORRISON, Cynthia M; 21-346 John St N, Arnprior ON K7S 2P6; Wes'83; CCFP; Ac Staff, Arnprior & District Memorial Hospital; (613)623-0311; Fax. (613)623-4095.

MORRISON, David E; Grey Bruce HS-Owen Sound, PO Box 1800 Stn Main 1800 8th St E, Owen Sound ON N4K 6M9; Wes'78; FRCPC; Psy. Ac Staff, Grey Bruce Health Services - Owen Sound; (519)376-2121 x2107; Fax. (519)372-3945.

MORRISON, Debra L; Abbie J Lane Mem Bldg, 4008-5909 Veterans Memorial La, Halifax NS B3H 2E2; Tor'85; FRCPC; IntMed (Sleep Medicine); Respir. Clin Dir Sleep Disorders Clinic & Lab, Queen Elizabeth II Health Sciences Centre - Victoria General Site; Assoc Prof Med, Dalhousie University; (902)473-6222; Fax. (902)473-7158.

MORRISON, Dennis; Sunridge Prof Bldg, R201-2675 36 St NE, Calgary AB T1Y 6H6; Mon'74; FAB; FRCPC; Psy (Forensic Psychiatry). Staff, Peter Lougheed Centre; Clin Assoc Prof Psy, University of Calgary; Langs: English; French; (403)943-5656; Fax. (403)219-3524; denis.morrison@calgaryhealthregion.ca.

MORRISON, Deric J; St Joseph's Health Care, PO Box 5777 Stn B B5 107-268 Grosvenor St, London ON N6A 4V2; Wes'05; FRCPC; IntMed; Endocrin&Metab. Staff, St Joseph's Hospital - St Joseph's Health Care; Staff, London Health Sciences Centre - University Hospital; (519)646-6296; Fax. (519)646-6372.

MORRISON, Douglas; Beamsville Med Ctr Fam Hlth Team, PO Box 430 4279 Hixon St, Beamsville ON L0R 1B0; Wes'75; DOHS; (905)563-5315; Fax. (905)563-0933.

MORRISON, Douglas M; Royal Columbian Hosp, 330 Columbia St E, New Westminster BC V3L 3W7; Cal'81; BSc; FRCPC; HemPath. Staff, Royal Columbian Hospital; (604)520-4273; Fax. (604)520-4769.

MORRISON, Earl G; Cape Breton Hlthcare Complex, 1482 George St, Sydney NS B1P 1P3; Dal'88; FRCPC; Anes. Assoc Member, Cape Breton Healthcare Complex; (902)567-8000

MORRISON, Elivia; 207-350 St. George St, Moncton NB E1C 1X1; Dal'84; BSc; (506)859-1011

MORRISON, Gavin C; Children's Hosp of Western Ont, 800 Commissioners Rd E, London ON N6A 5W9; Belfast (Ireland)'87; (519)685-8129

MORRISON, George H; 980 Oliver Rd, Thunder Bay ON P7B 6V4; Tor'52; AACP; FAGS; FRCPC; IntMed (Geriatric Medicine). Ac Staff Dementia Care, Lakehead Psychiatric Hospital - St. Joseph's Care Group; Staff, Thunder Bay Regional Health Sciences Centre; Ac Staff, St Joseph's Care Group - St Joseph's Hospital; (807)624-8899; morrisog@tbh.net.

MORRISON, Heather; Queen Elizabeth Hosp, PO Box 6600 Stn Central 60 Riverside Dr, Charlottetown PE C1A 8T5; Dal'99; CCFP; CCFP(E.M.); Staff, Queen Elizabeth Hospital; (902)894-2111

MORRISON, Heather M D; Kerrisdale Station Med Clinic, 2077 42nd Ave W, Vancouver BC V6M 2B4; Dal'74; Vis Staff, BC Women's Hospital & Health Centre; Vis Staff, Vancouver General Hospital - Centennial Pavillion; (604)261-9494

MORRISON, Ian R; Cannon Clinic, 4-2151 McCallum Rd, Abbotsford BC V2S 3N9; Tor'81; (604)853-3314; Fax. (604)853-2171.

MORRISON, James C; London Life, 255 Dufferin Ave, London ON N6A 4K1; Tor'92; (519)435-4990; Fax. (519)435-7057.

MORRISON, Jason M; Abbie J Lane Memorial Bldg, 3046-5909 Veterans Memorial La, Halifax NS B3H 2E2; Qns'01; FRCPC; Psy. (902)473-3417; Fax. (902)473-3456.

MORRISON, Jessica A; Hopital Ste-Justine, 3175 ch Cote-Sainte-Catherine, Montreal QC H3T 1C5; McG'05; FRCPC; Peds. Staff, Hôpital Ste-Justine; (514)345-4931

MORRISON, John A; 78 Victoria Ave, Chatham ON N7L 3A1; RCS (Ireland)'73; LRCPS(Ire); FICS; FACS; FRCSC; GenSurg. (519)352-0501; Fax. (519)352-0541.

MORRISON, Katherine M; HSC 2G Pediatric Lipid Clinic, 1280 Main St W, Hamilton ON L8S 4K1; Cal'85; FRCPC; Peds; Endocrin&Metab. (905)521-2100; Fax. (905)385-5033; kmorrison@mcmaster.ca.

MORRISON, Kathryn S; Queen Elizabeth Hosp, PO Box 6600 Stn Central 60 Riverside Dr, Charlottetown PE C1A 8T5; Dal'96; BSc; FRCPC; Peds. Staff, Queen Elizabeth Hospital; (902)894-2440; Fax. (902)894-2477.

MORRISON, Kenneth P; 109-230 First Ave, St Thomas ON N5R 4P5; Wes'80; BSc; Staff, St Thomas Elgin General Hospital; (519)633-7433; Fax. (519)633-0163.

MORRISON, Kevin B; 19-1527 Dufferin Cres, Nanaimo BC V9S 5H6; McG'97; MSc; FRCSC; Urol. Staff, Nanaimo Regional General Hospital; (250)753-6844

MORRISON, Kimberley; Thomas Street Clinic, C01 A-310 Bridge St W, Napanee ON K7R 0A4; Qns'93; CCFP; FCFP; Staff, Lennox & Addington County General Hospital; Assoc Prof, Queen's University; (613)354-2858; Fax. (613)354-6495.

MORRISON, Kristin R; Upper Country Clinic, RR 7 5529 Hwy 62, Belleville ON K8N 4Z7; Cal'92; FRCPC; Peds.

MORRISON, Laurie J; Rescu Keenan Research Ctre, 193 Yonge St, Toronto ON M5B 1M8; McM'81; FRCPC; EmergMed. Staff Emerg, Sunnybrook Health Sciences Centre; Staff, St Michael's Hospital; Assoc Prof, University of Toronto; (416)864-6060; Fax. (416)864-5934; l.morrison@utoronto.ca.

MORRISON, Lisa D; Foothills Prof Bldg, 245-1620 29 St NW, Calgary AB T2N 4L7; Alb'89; CCFP; (403)289-0069; Fax. (403)289-0533.

MORRISON, M Grace; 301-77 Westmount Rd, Guelph ON N1H 5J1; UBC'88; Ac Staff, St Joseph's Health Centre; Ac Staff, Guelph General Hospital; (519)836-1133; Fax. (519)836-7469.

MORRISON, Matthew K; Grove Med Centre, 115-187 Highway 16A, Spruce Grove AB T7X 4P9; Alb'85; Staff, Westview Health Centre; (780)962-4455; Fax. (780)962-4461.

MORRISON, Murray D; Gordon & Leslie Diamond HCC, 4F-2775 Laurel St, Vancouver BC V5Z 1M9; Sask'66; FRCSC; Otol (Laryngology). Ac Staff, Vancouver General Hospital - Centennial Pavillion; Staff, Gordon & Leslie Diamond Health Care Centre; Dir, Pacific Voice Clinic Inc; Prof, University of British Columbia; (604)875-4640; Fax. (604)875-5382.

MORRISON, Nancy J; Queen Elizabeth II HSC-Halifax, 4448-1796 Summer St, Halifax NS B3H 3A7; Dal'81; ABIM; FRCPC; FRCPC; Respir; IntMed (Cystic Fibrosis). Staff, Queen Elizabeth II Health Sciences Centre - Halifax Infirmary Site; Prof, Dalhousie University; (902)473-4024; Fax. (902)473-6202.

MORRISON, Robert G; Peterborough Reg HC-Hospital, 1 Hospital Dr, Peterborough ON K9J 7C6; Tor'73; Staff, Peterborough Regional Health Centre - Hospital Drive; (705)743-2121

MORRISON, Sandra L; Airdrie Med Clinic, 10-620 1 Ave NW, Airdrie AB T4B 2R3; UBC'95; BSc(Biol.&Physiol.); CCFP; FCFP; Staff Admitting, Peter Lougheed Centre; (403)948-3109; Fax. (403)948-6284.

MORRISON, Scott P; Quinte HC Corp-Belleville Gen, 265 Dundas St E, Belleville ON K8N 5A9; Tor'93; FRCPC; Anes. Chief Anes, QHC Belleville General; (613)696-7400

MORRISSETTE, Hugo; Hotel-Dieu de Levis, 143 rue Wolfe, Levis QC G6V 3Z1; Laval'01; FRCPC; IntMed; Gastroent. Staff, Hôtel-Dieu de Lévis; Langs: Bilingual(French/English); (418)835-7121; Fax. (418)835-7218.

MORRISSETTE, Roger; CSSS de la Baie-des-Chaleurs, RR 2 419 boul Perron, Maria QC G0C 1Y0; Laval'88; FRCSC; Ophth. Staff, CSSS de la Baie-des-Chaleurs; Langs: Bilingual(French/English); (418)759-3443; Fax. (418)759-1574; roger.morrissette@gmail.com.

MORRISSEY, Andrew T; Alberta ENT Consultants, 10130 111 St NW, Edmonton AB T5K 1K6; Alb'05; FRCSC; Otol. (587)521-1071; Fax. (587)521-1072.

MORRISSEY, Jean-Pierre P; 301-292 Montreal Rd, Vanier ON K1L 6B7; Ott'89; Langs: English; (613)745-5651; Fax. (613)745-7947.

MORRISSON, Heather; Queen Elizabeth Hosp, PO Box 6600 Stn Central 60 Riverside Dr, Charlottetown PE C1A 8T5; Staff, Queen Elizabeth Hospital; (902)894-2111

MORRISSY, Sean R; 1-10 Coakley Lane, Minto NB E4B 3K3; Mem'94; CCFP; Staff Family Pract Administrative Committee Phys Representative, Queens North Community Health Centre; Med Dir, WG Bishop Nursing Home; Langs: English; French; (506)327-3309; Fax. (506)327-4261.

MORROS, Michelle P; Misericordia Community Hosp, 16940 87 Ave NW, Edmonton AB T5R 4H5; Cal'07; CCFP; Staff, Covenant Health - Misericordia Community Hospital; (780)735-7800; Fax. (780)735-2857.

MORROW, A Meyer; 212 Blythwood Rd, Toronto ON M4N 1A6; Tor'56; Court Staff, Rouge Valley Health System - Centenary Health Centre Site; Court Staff, The Scarborough Hospital - General Campus; (416)485-7199; Fax. (416)485-7805; morrow@rogers.com.

MORROW, Adrienne; 1005-277 Wellington Cres, Winnipeg MB R3M 3V7; Man'10; CCFP.

MORROW, Christopher C; Royal Jubilee Hosp, 1952 Bay St, Victoria BC V8R 1J8; UBC'95; CCFP; CCFP(E.M.); Staff, Royal Jubilee Hospital; Staff, Saanich Peninsula Hospital; (250)370-8000

MORROW, David; Guelph Gen Hosp, 115 Delhi St, Guelph ON N1E 4J4; Qns'86; FRCPC; EmergMed. Staff, Guelph General Hospital; (519)837-6440; Fax. (519)837-0133.

MORROW, Donna M; St Mary's Hosp, 4607 53 St, Camrose AB T4V 1Y5; Alb'09; CCFP; Staff, Covenant Health - St Mary's Hospital; (780)679-6100

MORROW, Farrah L; Royal Inland Hosp, 311 Columbia St, Kamloops BC V2C 2T1; McM'00; FRCPC; Anes. Staff, Royal Inland Hospital; (250)314-2620

MORROW, Gary L; Medical Office, 204-840 Coxwell Ave, East York ON M4C 5T2; Tor'89; DABOph; FRCSC; Ophth (Cataract). Staff Ophth, Toronto East General Hospital Inc; Court Staff, Mount Sinai Hospital; Lecturer, University of Toronto; (416)461-0123; Fax. (416)462-2857.

MORROW, Nathan J; York-Finch Med Centre, 414-2115 Finch Ave W, North York ON M3N 2V6; Tor'60; FACS; DABOT; FRCSC; Otol. Ac Staff Otol, Humber River Regional Hospital - Finch Avenue Site; Ac Staff, North York General Hospital - Branson Division; Clin Teacher Otol, University of Toronto; (416)745-8440; Fax. (416)745-3268.

MORROW, Robert J; Oakville Med Arts Bldg, 12-358 Reynolds St, Oakville ON L6J 3L9; Belfast (Ireland)'81; MB ChB; BAO; FRCOG; FRCSC; ObstGyn. (905)339-0414; Fax. (905)339-0412.

MORROW, Sarah A; London HSC-University Hosp, PO Box 5339 Stn B 339 Windermere Rd, London ON N6A 5A5; Cal'02; FRCPC; Neur. Staff, London Health Sciences Centre - University Hospital; (519)663-2993; Fax. (519)663-3498.

MORROW, Walter G; Sudbury Reg Hosp-Laurentian, 41 Ramsey Lake Rd, Sudbury ON P3E 5J1; Queen's (Ireland)'62; MB ChB; BAO; FFARCS; Ac Staff, Health Sciences North-St Joseph's Health Centre; Ac Staff, Health Sciences North-Laurentian Site; (705)523-7100; Fax. (705)671-5458.

MORRY, Peter J; Blackmarsh Family Care Centre, 260 Blackmarsh Rd, St. John's NL A1E 1T2; Mem'75; (250)845-2515; Fax. (250)845-2504.

MORSE, Amy L; Hys Med Centre, 310-11010 101 St NW, Edmonton AB T5H 4B9; Sask'05; FRCPC; IntMed; Gastroent. (780)421-1029; Fax. (780)425-5533.

MORSE, Christopher R; Caleo Health, 340-600 Crowfoot Cres NW, Calgary AB T3G 0B4; Alb'98; CCFP; (403)452-0999; Fax. (403)452-0995.

MORSE, David W; Pelham Med Bldg, PO Box 1244 120 Pelham St, Lunenburg NS B0J 2C0; Dal'72; (902)634-4454; Fax. (902)634-3655.

MORSE, Ewart A; Medical Arts Bldg, 202-42 Glen Allan Dr, Bridgewater NS B4V 3N2; Dal'73; CCFP; FCFP; Ac Staff, South Shore Regional Hospital; Ac Staff, Fishermen's Memorial Hospital; (902)543-8801

MORSE, Janet L; Thornhill Village Fam Hlth Net, 18 Centre St, Thornhill ON L4J 1E9; Qns'91; CCFP; FCFP; Court Staff, Mackenzie Richmond Hill Hospital; (905)889-3634; Fax. (905)889-3986.

MORSE, John W I; Kings Lane Med Clinic, 101-164 Kings Lane, Salt Spring Island BC V8K 2P7; Dal'74; FRCPC; IntMed. Staff, Lady Minto Gulf Islands Hospital; (250)537-1828; Fax. (250)537-1848; john.morse@gmail.com.

MORSE, Linda A; 302-436 Gilmour St, Ottawa ON K2P 0R8; Wes'69; DPM; MRCPsy; FRCPC; Psy. Psychiatrist, Psychotherapy & Psychoanalysis Clinic; University of Ottawa; (613)238-3909; Fax. (613)234-6476.

MORSE, Michael J; Saint John Reg Hosp, PO Box 2100 Stn Main 400 University Ave, Saint John NB E2L 4L2; Dal'74; Urol (Oncology). Staff, Saint John Regional Hospital; (506)648-7935; Fax. (506)648-7937.

MORSI, A Ahmed; 101-1368 Ouellette Ave, Windsor ON N8X 1J9; Tor'94; FRCPC; IntMed; Cardiol. (519)977-6643; Fax. (519)915-6326.

MORSON, B Elizabeth; 104-1220 Place d'Orleans Dr, Orleans ON K1C 7K3; Qns'90; CCFP; FCFP; (613)841-5397; Fax. (613)841-4272.

MORTAZAVI, Amir A; 302-500 Sheppard Ave E, North York ON M2N 6H7; Mon'96; FACC; FRCPC; IntMed (Echocardiography); Cardiol. Langs: Farsi; French; Turkish; (416)221-2772; Fax. (416)221-3464.

MORTELLARO, Lia M; Medical Bldg, 207-250 Harding Blvd W, Richmond Hill ON L4C 9M7; Padua (Italy)'87; CCFP; Staff, Mackenzie Richmond Hill Hospital; Langs: Italian; (905)770-8817; Fax. (905)770-8862.

MORTEZAI, Berenice; MUHC-Montreal Chest Institute, 3650 rue Saint-Urbain, Montreal QC H2X 2P4; Laval'88; Staff, McGill University Health Centre - Montreal Chest Institute; (514)934-1934; Fax. (514)843-2070.

MORTIL, Nanette; Wilson Centre Family Practice, 1-2185 Wilson Ave, Port Coquitlam BC V3C 6C1; UBC'93; (604)942-7227

MORTIMER, Shane T; 1811 9 Ave S, Lethbridge AB T1J 1W6; Alb'96; BSc; MSc; LMCC; FACS; FRCSC; GenSurg. Teach Staff Surg, University of Alberta; (403)317-1890

MORTIS, Garth P; Country Hills Village, 234-5149 Country Hills Blvd NW, Calgary AB T3A 5K8; Cal'95; Nephrol; IntMed. Staff, Foothills Medical Centre; Clinical Asst Prof, University of Calgary; (403)241-5308; Fax. (403)241-5038.

MORTON, A Ross; Kingston Gen Hosp, 76 Stuart St, Kingston ON K7L 2V7; Manchester (England)'80; BSc(MedSci); MB ChB(Manchester); MRC(UK); FRCPC; IntMed; Nephrol. Staff Nephrol, Kingston General Hospital; Asst Prof Med, Queen's University; (613)548-1360; Fax. (613)548-2524.

MORTON, Charles E; 314-888 8th Ave W, Vancouver BC V5Z 3Y1; Qns'71; Derm; IntMed. (604)731-5353; Fax. (604)731-6166; mortonc@unixg.ubc.ca.

MORTON, Dann; Huntsville Prof Bldg, 104-348 Muskoka Rd 3 N, Huntsville ON P1H 1H8; McM'85; Ac Staff, Huntsville District Memorial Hospital - Muskoka Algonquin Healthcare; (705)789-2355; Fax. (705)789-1051.

MORTON, David H; Family Med Centre, 103-7143 West Saanich Rd, Brentwood Bay BC V8M 1P7; UBC'80; Staff, Saanich Peninsula Hospital; (250)652-9191; Fax. (250)652-5576.

MORTON, David N; North Battleford Med Clinic, 102-11427 Railway Ave E, North Battleford SK S9A 3G8; London (England)'70; MB BS; LRCP; MRCS; (306)445-4415; Fax. (306)445-5145.

MORTON, Gerard C; Toronto Odette Cancer Centre, T2 146-2075 Bayview Ave, Toronto ON M4N 3M5; Cork (Ireland)'85; FRCPC; RadOncol (Medical Education). Staff, Sunnybrook Health Sciences Centre; Asst Prof, University of Toronto; (416)480-6165; Fax. (416)480-6002; gerard.morton@sunnybrook.ca.

MORTON, Grazyna; Royal Ottawa Hlth Care Group, 1145 Carling Ave, Ottawa ON K1Z 7K4; Lublin (Poland)'79; FRCPC; Psy (Mood Disorders). Staff Psy, Royal Ottawa Mental Health Centre - Royal Ottawa Health Care Group; Asst Prof Psy, University of Ottawa; Langs: Polish; (613)722-6521

MORTON, Matthew L; Hydro Place Bldg, 3F-700 University Ave, Toronto ON M5G 1Z5; McG'02; FRCSC; ObstGyn (Minimal Invasive Surgery). Langs: Hebrew; French; Yiddish; (416)586-4479; Fax. (416)586-4650.

MORTON, Philip L; 307-650 Sammon Ave, East York ON M4C 5M5; Tor'54; FRCSC; Ophth. Sr Staff, Toronto East General Hospital Inc; Assoc Staff, Toronto General Hospital - UHN; Asst Prof, University of Toronto; (416)465-9198; Fax. (416)465-9873.

MORTON, Pol G D; South Vancouver Med Clinic, 2F-350 Marine Dr SE, Vancouver BC V5X 2S5; Dublin (Ireland)'84; MRCGPract(Lond); DObst; CCFP; (604)323-0077

MORTON, Richard I; Petitcodiac Health Centre, PO Box 2501 Stn Main, Petitcodiac NB E4Z 6H4; Mem'76; BSc; BMedSci; Ac Staff, The Moncton Hospital; Med Dir, Blue Cross Life of Canada & Dir., Jordan Life Care Ctr; (506)756-3400; Fax. (506)756-3406.

MORTON, Roy H; Fraser Health Authority, 260 Sherbrooke St, New Westminster BC V3L 3M2; UBC'82; FRCPC; Anes. (604)520-4662; Fax. (604)520-4992.

MORTON, Thomas J; Taunton Health Centre, SS 201 1290 Keith Ross Dr, Oshawa ON L1H 7K4; Qns'92; FRCSC; Urol. (905)721-4160

MORTON, Tracy L; Queen Charlotte Med Clinic, PO Box 9 3209 Oceanview Dr, Queen Charlotte BC V0T 1S0; Alb'97; CCFP; (250)559-4447; Fax. (250)559-8037; tracymorton@canada.com.

MORTON, William D; 4-66 Avenue Rd, Toronto ON M5R 3N8; McM'81; FRCPC; Anes. (416)922-2868

MORUM, Guy; Diamond Head Med Clinic, PO Box 9200 Stn Main, Squamish BC V8B 0C1; Witwatersrand (South Africa)'89; MB ChB; (604)892-3544; Fax. (604)892-3542.

MORVAL, Marie-Helene; CHSLD de la MRC de Champlain, 831 av Notre-Dame, Saint-Lambert QC J4R 1S1; Mon'90; Staff, CHSLD de la MRC de Champlain-Centre Saint-Lambert; Staff, Centre Hospitalier Pierre Boucher; (450)672-3328; marie-helene.morval@rrsss16.gouv.qc.ca.

MORVAY, Leslie C; Lasalle Med Associates, 2125 Front Rd, Windsor ON N9J 2C1; Wes'04; CCFP; (519)734-1234; Fax. (519)734-8674.

MORWEN-SMITH, Jennifer A; St Paul's Hosp, 1081 Burrard St, Vancouver BC V6Z 1Y6; UBC'85; MCFP; Consultant Complex Pain Service, Vancouver General Hospital - Centennial Pavillion; Clin Assoc Prof Med, UBC Hospital - Koerner Pavillion; Consultant Palliative Care, Providence Health Care - St Paul's Hospital; (604)682-2344; jennifer.morwen-smith@vch.ca.

MORWOOD, Christopher D C; 7019 Alberni St, Powell River BC V8A 2C2; UBC'00; CCFP; (604)485-9213

MORYS, Stephen J; Valley Ridge Family Physicians, 321-11245 Valley Ridge Dr NW, Calgary AB T3B 5V4; Cal'87; CCFP; Court Staff Family Med, Foothills Medical Centre; (403)282-3806; Fax. (403)284-5601; valleyridgemds@nucleus.com.

MORZARIA, Rasik N; 204-1920 Ellesmere Rd, Scarborough ON M1H 2V6; Bristol (England)'68; FRCPC; Peds (Consultant Pediatrics). Staff, The Scarborough Hospital - General Campus; (416)289-1999

MORZARIA, Sanjay; 103-8556 120th St, Surrey BC V3W 3N5; McM'98; MHSc; FRCSC; Otol. (778)565-3239

MORZYCKI, Wojciech; Queen Elizabeth II HSC, 462-1276 South Park St, Halifax NS B3H 2Y9; Pomeranian (Poland)'86; FRCPC; IntMed (Lung Cancer); MedOncol. Staff MedOncol, Queen Elizabeth II Health Sciences Centre - Victoria General Site; Langs: German; Russian; Polish; (902)473-8317; Fax. (902)473-6186; wojciech.morzycki@cdha.nshealth.ca.

MOSAAD, Sonia; CPM, 1118-123 Edward St, Toronto ON M5G 1E4; Cairo (Egypt)'95; CCFP; Langs: Arabic; (416)593-7700; Fax. (416)593-7702.

MOSAICO, Francesco; Boyle McCauley Health Centre, 10628 96 St NW, Edmonton AB T5H 2J2; Alb'05; CCFP; (780)422-7333; Fax. (780)422-7343.

MOSAKOSKI, Joan; 105-206 James St S, Hamilton ON L8P 3A9; Tor'77; BSc; FACS; FRCSC; GenSurg (Cardiac Pacing); Cardiovasc&ThorSurg. Chief Pacemaker Service/Staff Vascular Surg, St Joseph's Healthcare - Charlton Campus; Staff, Hamilton Health Sciences Centre - McMaster Children's Hospital; Clin Assoc Prof Surg, McMaster University; (905)524-1125; Fax. (905)524-1195.

MOSAM, Bashir A; 113-1055 Canadian Place, Mississauga ON L4W 0C2; RCS (Ireland)'66; Court Staff, Trillium Health Centre - Mississauga; (905)949-1940; Fax. (905)949-1940.

MOSAWE, Mothafar A; Port Aux Basques Med Centre, PO Box 68, Channel-Pab NL A0M 1C0; Mosul (Iraq)'84; MB ChB.

MOSCARELLO, Mario A; The Hosp for Sick Children, 555 University Ave, Toronto ON M5G 1X8; Tor'55; PhD(Biochem); Staff, The Hospital For Sick Children; Prof Biochem, University of Toronto; Langs: Italian; (416)813-5920; Fax. (416)813-5022; mam@sickkids.on.ca.

MOSCHONA, Penelope; Ctr Hosp Reg Chisasibi, CP 250, Chisasibi QC J0M 1E0; Mon'05; CCFP; Staff, Cree Board of Health & Social Services James Bay; (819)855-2844

MOSCOVITCH, Adam; 203-491 Lawrence Ave W, North York ON M5M 1C7; Cal'83; DABSM; DABPN; DABEM; FRCPC; Psy (Sleep Medicine). Clin Assoc Prof Psy, University of Calgary; Langs: Hungarian; Hebrew; (416)784-1430; Fax. (416)784-1590; drmoscovitch@somnisleep.com.

MOSCOVITZ, Walter; Southland Court Med Clinic, 300-10601 Southport Rd SW, Calgary AB T2W 3M6; McG'66; MDCM; FRCSC; ObstGyn. Ac Staff, Rockyview General Hospital; Assoc Prof, University of Calgary; Langs: Bilingual(English/French); (403)262-1410; Fax. (403)266-4159.

MOSDOSSY, Gregory J; London HSC-Victoria Hosp, PO Box 5010 Stn B E1 102-800 Commissioners Rd E, London ON N6A 5W9; McM'86; FRCPC; EmergMed. Staff, London Health Sciences Centre - Victoria Campus; Asst Prof, University of Western Ontario; Langs: Hungarian; French; (519)667-6538; Fax. (519)667-6769.

MOSELEY, Douglas M; 203-3825 Sunset St, Burnaby BC V5G 1T4; UBC'77; Staff, Burnaby Hospital; (604)434-9515; Fax. (604)434-5984.

MOSER, Andrea L; Baycrest Ctre/Geriatric Care, 3560 Bathurst St, Toronto ON M6A 2E1; Ott'91; CCFP; FCFP; Staff, Baycrest Centre for Geriatric Care; (416)785-2500

MOSER, Edith K; Royal Oak Clinic, 103-1638 Broadway E, Vancouver BC V5N 1W1; McG'85; CCFP; Langs: German; French; (604)438-6184

MOSER, Josef E; Clinique 900, 210-900 boul du Seminaire N, St-Jean-sur-Richel QC J3A 1C3; McG'93; (450)348-1118

MOSER, Meite S; Emergency Dept, 910 10th Ave W, Vancouver BC V5Z 1M9; Man'85; FRCPC; EmergMed. (604)875-4700

MOSER, Michael A J; Royal University Hosp, 103 Hospital Dr, Saskatoon SK S7N 0W8; Alb'93; BSc; MSc; FRCSC; GenSurg (Endoscopy). (306)966-1848; Fax. (306)966-7988.

MOSER, Nancy M; The Medical Centre, 12-163 Commissioners Rd W, London ON N6J 1X9; Wes'69; (519)433-0099

MOSER, Thomas P; CHUM-Hop Notre-Dame, 1560 rue Sherbrooke E, Montreal QC H2L 4M1; Strasbourg (France)'05; Staff, Centre Hospitalier l'Université de Montréal (CHUM) - Hôpital Notre-Dame; (514)890-8000 x23760

MOSES, Brian G; Yarmouth Reg Health Centre, 400-60 Vancouver St, Yarmouth NS B5A 2P5; Dal'04; FRCPC; IntMed (Vascular Disease). Chief IntMed, Yarmouth Regional Hospital; Staff, Digby General Hospital; Langs: Bilingual(English/French); (902)742-9128; Fax. (902)742-9781.

MOSES, Kathleen; South Bank Med Centre, 2430 Bank St, Ottawa ON K1V 0T7; Tor'63; FRCPC; Derm. Staff, SCO Health Service - Élisabeth Bruyère Hospital; Consultant Derm, The Ottawa Hospital - Civic Campus; Asst Prof Derm, University of Ottawa; (613)736-6946

MOSES, Ruth M; Toronto Women's Fertility Ctre, 810-56 Aberfoyle Cres, Etobicoke ON M8X 2W4; Tor'73; MSc; PhD; Pres., Toronto Women's Fertility Centre; (416)231-9919; Fax. (416)231-4748; rmoses202@rogers.com.

MOSEWICH, Russell K; Nicola Med Dental Bldg, 203-321 Nicola St, Kamloops BC V2C 6G6; Alb'89; FRCPC; Neur. (250)372-1731; Fax. (250)372-1381.

MOSHARRAF, Syed; Diagnostic Imaging Dept, PO Box 9000 Rpo CSC, Halifax NS B3K 6A3; Karachi (Pakistan)'97.

MOSHAVER, Ali; 103-1301 Main St, Penticton BC V2A 5E9; UBC'00; FRCSC; Otol. (778)476-5960

MOSHER, Dianne P; Health Research Innovation Ctr, 3AA18-3280 Hospital Dr NW, Calgary AB T2N 4Z6; Dal'83; BSc; FRCPC; IntMed; Rheum. Ac Staff, Queen Elizabeth II Health Sciences Centre - Victoria General Site; Assoc Prof, Dalhousie University; Langs: English; French; (403)210-7363; Fax. (403)210-7367.

MOSHER, Emily R; Toronto East Gen Hosp Inc, 825 Coxwell Ave, Toronto ON M4C 3E7; Tor'81; FRCPC; Anes. Staff, Toronto East General Hospital Inc; Lecturer, University of Toronto; (416)469-6588

MOSHER, Mathew C; 301-8837 201 St, Langley BC V2Y 0C8; UBC'88; BSc; FRCSC; PlasSurg. Ac Staff, Langley Memorial Hospital; Vis Consultant, Surrey Memorial Hospital; (604)888-9378; info@drmosher.com.

MOSHER, Pamela J; IWK Health Centre, PO Box 9700 Rpo Csc 5850-5980 University Ave, Halifax NS B3K 6R8; Stanford (USA)'06; Staff, IWK Health Centre; (902)470-8888

MOSHKIN, Olga M; Peterborough Reg HC-Hospital, 1 Hospital Dr, Peterborough ON K9J 7C6; (Russia (Federation))'80; FRCPC; AnatPath. Staff, Peterborough Regional Health Centre - Hospital Drive; (705)743-2121 x5014

MOSHOOD, Ibrahim A; Drumheller Assoc Physicians, PO Box 5600 140 Riverside Dr E, Drumheller AB T0J 0Y0; (Nigeria)'91; MB ChB; CCFP; (403)823-3345; Fax. (403)823-7823.

MOSHURCHAK, Kim M; Links Clinic, 104-11910 111 Ave NW, Edmonton AB T5G 3G6; Alb'89; CCFP; FCFP; (780)454-0351; Fax. (780)452-6767.

MOSIMANN, Francois; CHUS-Hop Fleurimont, 3001 12e av N, Sherbrooke QC J1H 5N4; Lausanne (Switzerland)'72; FRCSC; GenSurg. Chef chir gén, Centre Hospitalier Universitaire de Sherbrooke-Hopital Fleurimont; Prof, Universite de Sherbrooke; Langs: German; English; (819)346-1110 x14483

MOSKALYK, Tara M; 4-2120 Regent St S, Sudbury ON P3E 3Z9; Ott'99; FRCSC; Urol. (705)522-0006; Fax. (705)522-0018.

MOSKO, Jeffrey D; University of Toronto, 500 University Ave, Toronto ON M5G 1V7; Wes'08; FRCPC; IntMed.

MOSKOVITZ, David N; 505-3200 Dufferin St, North York ON M6A 3B2; Tor'00; FRCPC; IntMed; Gastroent. Staff, Humber River Regional Hospital - Church Street Site; Langs: Spanish; (416)256-9500; Fax. (416)256-9522.

MOSS, Christopher J; PO Box 280, Tatamagouche NS B0K 1V0; London (England)'81; Gen Practice, Lillian Fraser Memorial Hospital / Primary Health Care Centre; (902)657-2610; Fax. (902)657-2778; chris@drmoss.ca.

MOSS, Farley D; Rouge Valley-Centenary HC, 2867 Ellesmere Rd, Scarborough ON M1E 4B9; Tor'90; CCFP; Staff, Rouge Valley Health System - Centenary Health Centre Site; (416)480-4693

MOSS, Genevieve; Services Ext de Psychiatrie, 230-383 boul du Seminaire N, St-Jean-sur-Richel QC J3B 8C5; Mon'98; Psy. Psychiatrist, Hôpital du Haut-Richelieu; Psychiatre, Centre Hospitalier de Granby; Langs: English; (450)346-2222

MOSS, Jay J H; Sunnybrook Hlth Sciences Ctre, FG19-2075 Bayview Ave, Toronto ON M4N 3M5; Tor'82; FRCPC; Psy (Consultation-Liaison). Staff, Sunnybrook Health Sciences Centre; (416)480-4693; Fax. (416)480-6878.

MOSS, Judy M; Orleans Family Health Clinic, 101-210 Centrum Blvd, Orleans ON K1E 3V7; Man'81; BSc(Pharm); CCFP; FCFP; (613)837-5454; Fax. (613)837-3781.

MOSS, Margaret E M; Seymour Med Clinic, 1530 7th Ave W, Vancouver BC V6J 1S3; Dublin (Ireland)'72; (604)739-5611; Fax. (604)738-2102.

MOSS, Michael A; MDS Metro Lab Services, 3680 Gilmore Way, Burnaby BC V5G 4V8; London (England)'75; MB BS; MSc(Dal); FRCPC; MedBiochem (Pathology Administration). (604)412-4426; mike.moss@dal.ca.

MOSS, Michele A; 100-20 Heritage Meadows Rd SE, Calgary AB T2H 3C1; Cape Town (South Africa)'82; MB ChB; Physician Thoracic Surgical Assa, Calgary Osteoporosis Centre; Physician, Citizenship & Immigration Canada; Langs: Afrikaans; (403)252-8851; Fax. (403)252-1765; michelemoss@shaw.ca.

MOSS, Miriam A; 302-2330 Kennedy Rd, Scarborough ON M1T 0A2; Tor'89; CCFP; Staff Emerg, Rouge Valley Health System - Centenary Health Centre Site; Staff Emerg, The Scarborough Hospital - Birchmount Campus; Lecturer, University of Toronto; (416)298-1303; Fax. (416)298-4872.

MOSS, Morton G; Lake Beaumaris Prof Bldg, 202-15379 Castle Downs Rd NW, Edmonton AB T5X 3Y7; Cal'80; CCFP; CCFP(E.M.); Staff, Sturgeon Community Hospital; (780)472-7575; Fax. (780)472-7404.

MOSS, Philippa A; Cumberland Mental Hlth Clinic, 33 Havelock St, Amherst NS B4H 4W1; London (England)'82; FRCPC; Psy (Child & Adolescent Psychiatry). (902)667-3879; Fax. (902)667-5959; forensic@drmoss.ca.

MOSS, Robert R; St Paul's Hosp, 474-1081 Burrard St, Vancouver BC V6Z 1Y6; Sydney (Australia)'79; FRCPC; IntMed. Staff, Providence Health Care - St Paul's Hospital; (604)806-9410

MOSS, Steven M; Leslie Med Centre, 310-4800 Leslie St, North York ON M2J 2K9; Tor'87; FAAP; FRCPC; Peds (Pediatric Emergency Medicine). Staff, North York General Hospital; Chair Educ, The Hospital For Sick Children; Assoc Prof, University of Toronto; (416)492-5888; Fax. (416)492-6569.

MOSSANDA CHABIKULI, Kenyabu C; North Simcoe Family Hlth Team, PO Box 790 Stn Main 240 Penetanguishene Rd, Midland ON L4R 4P4; Medunsa (South Africa)'98; CCFP; Staff, O'Leary Health Centre; (705)527-7575; clarachabikuli@hotmail.com.

MOSSANEN, Ayoob; Pain & Diasbility Assessment, 10-4646 Dufferin St, North York ON M3H 5S4; Leeds (England)'63; FRCPC; Neur (Chronic Pain). Staff/Consultant, Toronto East General Hospital Inc; Langs: Persian.

MOSSDORF, Philipp; Children's Hosp Eastern Ont, 401 Smyth Rd, Ottawa ON K1H 8L1; Gottingen (Germany)'94; FRCPC; Anes. Staff, Children's Hospital of Eastern Ontario (CHEO); (613)737-2431

MOSSING, Morley S; East Street Med Arts Centre, 203-170 East St, Sault Ste. Marie ON P6A 3C6; Wes'70; FACS; FRCSC; GenSurg. Staff GenSurg, Sault Area Hospital - Sault Ste Marie; (705)759-3388; Fax. (705)759-3380.

MOSSMAN, Andrea L; Mud Creek Med Co-op Ltd, 12E Elm Ave, Wolfville NS B4P 1Z9; Dal'10; CCFP; (902)542-3633; Fax. (902)542-2709.

MOSSMAN, Hilary R L; Sandy Hill Comm Health Centre, 221 Nelson St, Ottawa ON K1N 1C7; Man'07; CCFP; (613)789-8458

MOSSMAN, Kerstin; Barrie Community Health Centre, 490 Huronia Rd, Barrie ON L4N 6M2; McM'02; CCFP; (705)503-9245; Fax. (705)503-5982.

MOST, Carole; BC Cancer Agency-Vanc Isl Ctr, 2410 Lee Ave, Victoria BC V8R 6V5; Dallas (USA)'80; Staff, BC Cancer Agency Vancouver Island Centre; (250)519-5572

MOSTACHFI, Omid; 101-4430 Chatterton Way, Victoria BC V8X 5J2; Tor'98; FRCSC; Otol. (250)592-4141

MOSTEFAI, Ahmed Y; Hotel-Dieu de Sorel, 400 av de l'Hotel-Dieu, Sorel-Tracy QC J3P 1N5; (Algeria)'90; Staff, Hôtel-Dieu de Sorel; (450)746-6000

MOSTERT, Andreas W; Selkirk Med Group, PO Box 590 101 1st St W, Revelstoke BC V0E 2S0; Orange Free State (South Africa)'89; MB ChB; CCFP; Langs: Afrikaans; (250)837-9321; Fax. (250)837-9444.

MOSTERT, Francois D P; Dr C W Wiebe Med Centre, 385 Main St, Winkler MB R6W 1J2; Stellenbosch (South Africa)'79; MB ChB; Langs: Afrikaans; (204)325-4312; fmostert@mts.net.

MOSTERT, Marius; Airport Way Med Clinic, PO Box 2000, Fort Nelson BC V0C 1R0; Pretoria (South Africa)'84; MB ChB; CCFP; (250)774-7838; Fax. (250)774-7038.

MOSTOWY, Stephan C; Mission View Medical, 205-616 K L O Rd, Kelowna BC V1Y 4X4; Tor'96; FRCSC; GenSurg; VascSurg. (250)762-7731; Fax. (250)762-7502.

MOSTRENKO, Michael S; Royal Columbian Hosp, 330 Columbia St E, New Westminster BC V3L 3W7; UBC'93; FRCPC; EmergMed. Staff, Royal Columbian Hospital; (604)520-4000

MOTA, Ihor R; 305-1160 Burrard St, Vancouver BC V6Z 2E8; L'viv (Ukraine)'81; PhD; ATLS; ACLS; LMCC; MD; CCFP; Staff, Vancouver General Hospital - Centennial Pavillion; Staff, Delta Hospital; Langs: Ukrainian; Polish; Russian; (604)974-0008; Fax. (604)974-1122.

MOTA, Jodi E; PO Box 47025 Rpo Edmonton Ctre, Edmonton AB T5J 4N1; McG'95; CCFP; Staff, Royal Alexandra Hospital.

MOTA, Jorge A R; Stratford Gen Hosp, 46 General Hospital Dr, Stratford ON N5A 2Y6; Bahia (Brazil)'79; FRCPC; Anes. Staff, Stratford General Hospital - Huron Perth Healthcare Alliance; (519)271-2120

MOTAKIS, Dimitrios; Toronto Dermatology Centre, 400-4256 Bathurst St, North York ON M3H 5Y8; McG'04; FRCSC; PlasSurg. Staff, Toronto Dermatology Centre; (416)633-0001; Fax. (416)633-0002.

MOTALA, Rasheda; Dr R Motala Ranchlands, 12-7750 Ranchview Dr NW, Calgary AB T3G 1Y9; RCS (Ireland)'77; MB ChB; BAO; LMCC; CCFP; Langs: Urdu; Afrikaans; Gujarati; (403)239-5822; Fax. (403)241-3530.

MOTAMEDI, Farhad; Family Med Centre, 210 Melrose Ave, Ottawa ON K1Y 4K7; Ott'01; CCFP; (613)761-4334; Fax. (613)761-4200.

MOTAN, Tarek; Royal Alexandra Hosp, 250-10240 Kingsway NW, Edmonton AB T5H 3V9; Cape Town (South Africa)'90; MB ChB; FRCSC; ObstGyn (Gynecological Reproductive Endocrinology);CCFP; Staff, Royal Alexandra Hospital; (780)735-5609

MOTARD, Alexandre; GMF Cote-des-Neiges, 500-5700 ch de la Cote-des-Nei, Montreal QC H3T 2A8; Mon'03; CCFP; (514)731-8531; Fax. (514)731-0563.

MOTAYNE, Gregory G; Royal Ottawa Hlth Care Group, 1145 Carling Ave, Ottawa ON K1Z 7K4; (Jamaica)'80; MB BS; FRCPC; Psy (Adolescent Forensics). Staff Psy, Royal Ottawa Mental Health Centre - Royal Ottawa Health Care Group; Asst Prof Psy, University of Ottawa; (613)722-6521 x6400; Fax. (613)724-6554.

MOTHELESI, Ronald R; 501 McBride St, Prince Rupert BC V8J 3G5; Cape Town (South Africa)'07; MB ChB; (250)622-6340

MOTHERON, Christine; Unite Med Familiale Maizerets, 2480 ch de la Canardiere, Quebec QC G1J 2G1; Laval'96; CCFP; ac Membre, Centre Hospitalier Universitaire De Québec - Pavillon De St-françois-d'assise; ac Membre, CSSS de Quebec Nord Pharmacie; Langs: English; French; (418)661-1413; Fax. (418)661-7504; cmotheron@videotron.ca.

MOTLAGH, Bahareh; 205-110 Copper Creek Dr, Markham ON L6B 0P9; McM'04; FRCPC; IntMed; Cardiol. Staff, Markham Stouffville Hospital; (905)472-9200; Fax. (905)472-9206.

MOTLANI, Faisal; Rothbart Centre for Pain Care, 9-4646 Dufferin St, North York ON M3H 5S4; Saba Univ School of Medicine (Netherlands Antilles)'05; (416)512-6407

MOTOLKO, Michael A; Ivey Eye Institute, 268 Grosvenor St, London ON N6A 4V2; Ott'76; DAB; FACS; FRCSC; Ophth (Glaucoma). Staff Ivey Eye Inst, London Health Sciences Centre - Victoria Campus; Ac Staff, St Joseph's Hospital - St Joseph's Health Care; Assoc Prof Ophth, University of Western Ontario; Assoc Prof Ophth Ivey Eye Inst, University of Toronto; (519)685-8131; Fax. (519)685-8173.

MOTT, Daniel D; Stratford Gen Hosp, 46 General Hospital Dr, Stratford ON N5A 2Y6; Ott'02; FRCPC; DiagRad. Staff, Stratford General Hospital - Huron Perth Healthcare Alliance; (519)272-8210

MOTT-TRILLE, Helen R; Centennial CMH & Brain Injury, PO Box 1000 Stn Main, Ponoka AB T4J 1R8; Tor'87; FRCPC; Psy. Staff, Canmore General Hospital; Staff, Centennial Centre for Mental Health & Brain Injury; (403)783-7600

MOTTA, James A T; PO Box 65058 Rpo North Hill, Calgary AB T2N 4T6; Man'59; FSOGC; FRCSC; ObstGyn (Colposcopy). Staff, Peter Lougheed Centre.

MOTTAGHIAN, Mojgan; York Central Hosp, 10 Trench St, Richmond Hill ON L4C 4Z3; Islami Azad University (Iran)'97; Psy. (905)883-1212

MOTTAHEDI, Roksana; The Westend Family Care Clinic, 80 Michael Cowpland Dr, Kanata ON K2M 1P6; Ott'06; CCFP; Staff, Westend Family Care Clinic Family Health Team; Langs: Farsi; (613)599-3321; Fax. (613)599-3366.

MOTTARD, Audrey; CSSS de Portneuf, 700 rue Saint-Cyrille, Saint-Raymond QC G3L 1W1; Laval'07; CCFP; Staff, Centre Hospitalier Portneuf; (418)337-4611; Fax. (418)337-4808.

MOTTARD, Jean-Pierre; Inst Albert Prevost, 6555 boul Gouin O, Montreal QC H4K 1B3; Laval'73; FRCPC; Psy. Staff, Hôpital du Sacre-Coeur de Montréal; (514)338-4246; Fax. (514)338-4391.

MOTTARD, Sophie; Hop Maisonneuve-Rosemont, 5415 boul de l'Assomption, Montreal QC H1T 2M4; Mon'03; FRCSC; OrthSurg (Oncology). Staff, Hopital Maisonneuve-Rosemont; Langs: Bilingual(French/English); (514)252-3400

MOTTIAR, Farouk; Pembroke Reg Hosp, 705 Mackay St, Pembroke ON K8A 1G8; RCS (Ireland)'69; Assoc Staff, Pembroke Regional Hospital Inc; (613)732-2811

MOTTIAR, Nasima S; Centre de Sante Communautaire, 2F-460 Main St E, Hamilton ON L8N 1K4; Belfast (Ireland)'95; CCFP; Langs: French; (905)528-0163; Fax. (905)528-9001.

MOTTIAR, Yousuff; Upper Grand Family Health Team, 350 St Andrew St W, Fergus ON N1M 1N9; Witwatersrand (South Africa)'54; MRC; (519)843-2770; Fax. (519)843-4451.

MOTTOLA, Jeffrey C; Radiol Consultants of Winnipeg, 202-233 Kennedy St, Winnipeg MB R3C 3J5; Man'04; FRCPC; DiagRad. (204)942-6453

MOTTRON, Laurent; Hop Riviere-des-Prairies, 7070 boul Perras, Montreal QC H1E 1A4; Tours (France)'81; PhD; Staff, Hôpital Riviere des Prairies; Prof, Universite de Montreal; (514)323-7260 x2189; Fax. (514)328-3502.

MOTYER, Michael I S; Chemong Region Med Centre, PO Box 330, Bridgenorth ON K0L 1H0; Mem'83; BSc; CCFP; (705)292-8844; Fax. (705)292-8929.

MOTZ, Catherine M; Kanata Prof Centre, 103-99 Kakulu Rd, Kanata ON K2L 3C8; Wes'94; CCFP; FCFP; Clin Associate, The Ottawa Hospital - Civic Campus; (613)592-1448

MOUAIKEL, Elie; Hop Santa Cabrini Ospedale, 5655 rue Saint-Zotique E, Montreal QC H1T 1P7; Beirut (Lebanon)'71; CSPQ; MedOncol (P.Q.); Peds; Hem (P.Q.) (Hematological Oncology). Staff Hem Oncol, Hôpital Santa Cabrini Ospedale; Langs: Arabic; English; (514)966-2535; Fax. (514)252-6114; toubibeliemouaikel@videotron.ca.

MOUAIKEL, Patricia; Bells Corners Medical Group, 103-1956 Robertson Rd, Nepean ON K2H 5B9; Ott'96; BSc(Biology); CCFP; FCFP; Langs: Arabic; Armenian; French; (613)596-0911; Fax. (613)596-3162.

MOUDGIL, Rohit; Univ of Ottawa Heart Institute, 3411-40 Ruskin St, Ottawa ON K1Y 4W7; Alb'08; IntMed. Staff, University of Ottawa Heart Institute; (613)761-5000

MOUFARREGE, Richard; Clin Richard Moufarrege Inc, 106-1111 rue Saint-Urbain, Montreal QC H2Z 1Y6; Mon'79; FRCS; FRCSC; PlasSurg (Cosmetic Surgery). Staff, Centre Hospitalier l'Université de Montréal (CHUM) - Hôpital Notre-Dame; Ac Staff, Clinique de Chirurgie Esthetique St-Urbain; assoc Prof, Universite de Montreal; Langs: Spanish; Portuguese; English; Lebanese; (514)393-9999; admin@plasticsurgery-canada.com.

MOUHAMMED, Samir I; Hampton Med Clinic, 6274 199 St NW, Edmonton AB T5T 2K4; (Egypt)'91; MB ChB; CCFP; (780)486-7370; Fax. (780)786-7335.

MOUKHEIBER, Alain; Ctr Hosp Rouyn-Noranda, 4 9E rue, Rouyn-Noranda QC J9X 2B2; (Lebanon)'95; Otol (P.Q.). Staff, Centre Hospitalier Rouyn-Noranda; Langs: French; Lebanese; (819)764-5131 x42107; Fax. (819)764-2900; almoukheiber@yahoo.com.

MOUKHORTOVA-VON LIPINSKI, Olga; 4085 41st Ave W, Vancouver BC V6N 3G3; Msocow (Russia (Federation))'91; FRCSC; ObstGyn. Physician, Southern Health Centre; Langs: German; Russian; (778)863-6542

MOUKHTAR, Clara F; UMF Notre-Dame, 2120 rue Sherbrooke E, Montreal QC H2K 1C3; Mon'09; CCFP; (514)527-1958

MOULAISON, William G; Shawnigan Village Fam Practice, PO Box 240 2749 Dundas Rd, Shawnigan Lake BC V0R 2W0; Tor'88; Assoc Staff, Vancouver Island Health Authority; (250)743-0793; Fax. (250)743-0754.

MOULAND, Sylvia P; Elizabeth Ave Family Practice, 116-100 Elizabeth Ave, St. John's NL A1B 1S1; Wes'01; CCFP; (709)579-5005; Fax. (709)579-5278.

MOULDEY, Peter G; Southdown Med Centre, 6-1375 Southdown Rd, Mississauga ON L5J 2Z1; Tor'90; Staff, Humber River Regional Hospital - Church Street Site; (905)822-2900; Fax. (905)822-2001.

MOULDEY, R Gordon; Children's Hosp Eastern Ont, 401 Smyth Rd, Ottawa ON K1H 8L1; Qns'58; MCPS; FRCPC; Psy (Child Psychiatry). Ac Staff, Children's Hospital of Eastern Ontario (CHEO); Pt-Time Faculty, University of Ottawa; (613)737-7600 x3411; Fax. (613)260-1890; gmouldey@cheo.on.ca.

MOULIN, Dwight E; London Reg Cancer Centre, 790 Commissioners Rd E, London ON N6A 4L6; Wes'73; FRCPC; Neur (Pain Medicine). Staff, London Health Sciences Centre - Victoria Campus; Prof, University of Western Ontario; (519)685-8661; Fax. (519)685-8636.

MOULIN, Jacinthe; Clinique Med Le Campanile, 104-3730 rue du Campanile, Quebec QC G1X 4G6; Laval'79; CCFP; Langs: Bilingual(French/English); (418)652-0030

MOULIN, Jana M; London Medicentre, 611 Wonderland Rd N, London ON N6H 4V6; McM'08; CCFP; (519)471-6686; Fax. (519)471-2801.

MOULSON, Brian C; 815 Baker St, Nelson BC V1L 4J8; UBC'79; Staff, East Shore Community Health Centre; (250)354-4861; Fax. (250)354-4865; 815baker@telus.net.

MOULSON, Robert A L; Ridgeway Clinic, 1001 Ridgeway St E, Thunder Bay ON P7E 5H8; Tor'61; CCFP; FCFP; Court Staff, Thunder Bay Regional Health Sciences Centre; Court Staff, St Joseph's Care Group - St Joseph's Hospital.

MOULT, Michael D; 899 12th Ave W, Vancouver BC V5Z 1M9; UBC'81; FRCPC; Anes. Staff, Vancouver General Hospital - Centennial Pavillion; (604)875-4304

MOULTON, Carol-Anne E; Univ Hlth Network-Toronto Gen, 10EN 212-200 Elizabeth St, Toronto ON M5G 2C4; Melbourne (Australia)'92; Staff, Toronto General Hospital - UHN; (416)340-4800 x5336; Fax. (416)340-3808.

MOULTON, Dagmar T; The Hosp for Sick Children, 555 University Ave, Toronto ON M5G 1X8; Dal'07; Anes. Staff, The Hospital For Sick Children; (416)813-7445

MOULTON, Richard J; The Ottawa Hosp-Civic Campus, C2 2202-1053 Carling Ave, Ottawa ON K1Y 4E9; Cal'79; FRCSC; Neursurg. Chair Div of Neurosurg, University of Ottawa; (613)798-5555 x19885; Fax. (613)761-5436; rimoulton@ottawahospital.on.ca.

MOULTON, William B; Pharamchoice Bldg, PO Box 460, Marystown NL A0E 2M0; Mem'84.

MOUMDJIAN, Robert A; CHUM-Hop Notre-Dame, 1560 rue Sherbrooke E, Montreal QC H2L 4M1; Beirut (Lebanon)'84; BSc(BioChem.); MSc(Neurol.Immunol.); FRCSC; Neursurg (Skull Base & Neurological Oncology). Consultant, Centre Hospitalier l'Université de Montréal (CHUM) - Hôtel-Dieu; ac Staff NeurSurg, Centre Hospitalier l'Université de Montréal (CHUM) - Hôpital Notre-Dame; Asst Prof Surg & Div of NeurSurg, Universite de Montreal; (514)890-8000 x24444

MOUNSEY, Robert A; SGH Medical Mall, 207-3030 Lawrence Ave E, Scarborough ON M1P 2T7; Tor'88; FRCSC; Otol. (416)438-8110; Fax. (416)438-6373.

MOUNSTEPHEN, William J; The Hosp for Sick Children, 555 University Ave, Toronto ON M5G 1X8; McM'77; FAAP; FRCPC; Peds (Pediatric Emergency Medicine). Dir Div of Emerg Med, The Hospital For Sick Children; Asst Prof, University of Toronto; (416)813-5810; Fax. (416)813-5043; bill.mounstephen@sickkids.ca.

MOUNT, John H; 1201 Oxford St W PO Box 28017 Oakridge Rpo, London ON N6H 5E1; McG'67; BSc; MD; FRCPC; Psy (Personal Injury). (519)438-6699; Fax. (519)472-6010.

BASTIANELLI, Heather L; Ottawa Reg Cancer Centre, 503 Smyth Rd, Ottawa ON K1H 1C4; Ott'84; Clin Asst, The Ottawa Hospital - Civic Campus; (613)737-7700

MOUNTAIN, Anita D; Nova Scotia Rehab Centre, 214-1341 Summer St, Halifax NS B3H 4K4; Dal'04; FRCPC; PhysMed&Rehab. Staff, Nova Scotia Rehabilitation Centre; (902)473-1409; Fax. (902)473-3204.

MOUNTAIN, G Brett; 118 Victoria St N, Sarnia ON N7T 5W9; Ott'99; CCFP; CCFP(E.M.); Staff, Bluewater Health - Norman Site.

MOUNTAIN, Mark A; Langley Mem Hosp, 22051 Fraser Hwy, Langley BC V3A 4H4; UBC'71; Anes. Staff, Langley Memorial Hospital; Staff, Vancouver General Hospital - Centennial Pavillion; (604)533-4121

MOUNTAIN, Scott A; Kootenay-Boundary Reg Hosp, 1200 Hospital Bench, Trail BC V1R 4M1; UBC'98; FRCPC; IntMed;CCFP; Critical Care Medicine. Staff, Kootenay Boundary Regional Hospital; (250)368-3311

MOUNTFORD, Catherine; DND, RR 1 935 Woodville Rd, Newport NS B0N 2A0; Dal'02; CCFP; Staff, Canadian Forces Health Services Centre (Atlantic); (902)757-0444

MOUNTJOY, Margo L; McMaster Medical School, 10B Victoria St S, Kitchener ON N2G 1C5; McM'86; Dip SportMed; CCFP; FCFP; Staff, Guelph General Hospital; Physician, FINA-International Aquatic Sports Med Committee; mmountjoy@ewfht.ca.

MOURABIT AMARI, Karim; Ctr Hosp Affilie-Enfant-Jesus, 1401 18e rue, Quebec QC G1J 1Z4; Laval'06; MedBiochem. Staff, Centre Hospitalier Affilié Universitaire de Québec - Hôpital De L'Enfant Jésus; (418)649-0252

MOURAD, Mustapha; CSSSG-Hop de Gatineau, CP 2000 Succ Bureau-Chef 909 boul de la Verendrye O, Gatineau QC J8P 7H2; (Lebanon)'95; Staff, Hôpital de Gatineau; (819)561-8100

MOURAD, Nathalie; Ctr Hosp Affilie-St-Sacrement, 1050 ch Sainte-Foy, Quebec QC G1S 4L8; (Lebanon)'99; Staff, Centre Hospitalier Affilié Universitaire de Québec - Hôpital du St-Sacrement; (418)682-7805

MOURAD, Ophyr; St Michael's Hosp, 4 151-30 Bond St, Toronto ON M5B 1W8; Tor'96; FRCPC; IntMed. Langs: Hebrew; (416)864-6060; Fax. (416)864-5714; mourado@smh.toronto.on.ca.

MOURAD, Walid A A; Calgary Lab Services, C412-3535 Research Rd NW, Calgary AB T2L 2K8; Ain-Shams (Egypt)'79; MB ChB; AB; FRCPC; AnatPath. Staff, Calgary Laboratory Services; (403)770-3467; Fax. (403)770-3292.

MOURCOS, Ashraf F Z; Westheight Med Clinic, 203-10 Westheights Dr, Kitchener ON N2N 2A8; Ain Shams (Egypt)'89; MB BS; MB BCh; CCFP; Staff, Grand River Hospital - Kitchener/Waterloo Health Centre; Staff, St Mary's General Hospital; (519)954-7742; Fax. (519)954-7743; mourcos@hotmail.com.

MOUREY, Sophie; Clinique Forcemedic, 1021 rue Jean-Talon E, Montreal QC H2R 1V6; Besancon (France)'02; Staff, CSSS de Maskinongé; (514)787-1818

MOURSY, Asmat; Carrefour Med Vallee Richelieu, 665 boul Sir-Wilfrid-Laurier, Beloeil QC J3G 4J1; Cairo (Egypt)'82; CCFP; Staff, Centre de santé Cloutier-du-Rivage; (450)467-9319

MOUSA, Anushi T; Southdale Med Clinic, 395 Southdale Rd E, London ON N6E 1A2; Moscow (Russia (Federation))'01; CCFP; Langs: Russian; Sinhalese; (519)691-0100; Fax. (519)691-1172.

MOUSA AHMADI, Elaheh; Dominion Med Centres Ltd, 9122 23 Ave NW, Edmonton AB T6N 1H9; (Iran)'94; (780)801-3360; Fax. (780)801-3366.

MOUSAVI, Negareh; University Hosp of Northern BC, 1475 Edmonton St, Prince George BC V2M 1S2; Tehran (Iran)'99; FRCPC; IntMed; Cardiol. Staff, University Hospital of Northern British Columbia; (250)565-2000

MOUSAVINEJAD, Kiarash; Prairie North Health Centre, 4806 50th St, Lloydminster SK S9V 0M9; (306)820-5997; Fax. (306)820-5978.

MOUSMANIS, Patricia A; Mackenzie Richmond Hill Hosp, 10 Trench St, Richmond Hill ON L4C 4Z3; Tor'83; CCFP; FCFP; Staff Physician, Markham Stouffville Hospital; Staff Physician, Mackenzie Richmond Hill Hospital; Physician Representative, York Region Advisory Forum on Children Youth & Families; Langs: Greek; (416)918-1837; Fax. (905)737-4989; drpat@rogers.com.

MOUSSA, Ahmed; Hôpital Ste-Justine, 3175 ch Cote-Sainte-Catherine, Montreal QC H3T 1C5; Mon'04; FRCPC; Peds (Neonatal & Perinatal Medicine). Staff, Hôpital Ste-Justine; (514)345-4931

MOUSSA, Bassem G F; Rouge Valley-Ajax & Pickering, 580 Harwood Ave S, Ajax ON L1S 2J4; Cairo (Egypt)'87; FRCPC; AnatPath. Staff, Rouge Valley Health System - Ajax & Pickering Health Centre Site; (905)683-2320

MOUSSA, Fuad; Sunnybrook Hlth Sciences Ctre, H429-2075 Bayview Ave, Toronto ON M4N 3M5; McG'97; FRCSC; CardSurg (Thoracic Surgery). Staff, Sunnybrook Health Sciences Centre; (416)480-6100; Fax. (416)480-6072.

MOUSSA, Madeleine; London HSC-University Hosp, PO Box 5339 Stn B 339 Windermere Rd, London ON N6A 5A5; Ain Shams (Egypt)'81; MB ChB; FRCPC; AnatPath (Genito Urinary Pathology). Staff, London Health Sciences Centre - University Hospital; (519)685-8500 x36356

MOUSSA, Raffy; Community Med Centre, A-3000 Lawrence Ave E, Scarborough ON M1P 2V1; Ott'06; MSc; BSc; CCFP; (416)431-8224; Fax. (416)439-8625.

MOUSSA, Sahar; Hampton Med Clinic, 6274 199 St NW, Edmonton AB T5T 2K4; (Egypt)'94; CCFP; (780)486-7370; Fax. (780)486-7335.

MOUSSA, Wasseem M I; McConnell Med Centre, 820 McConnell Ave, Cornwall ON K6H 4M4; Cairo (Egypt)'67; MB ChB; FRCS(Ed); FICS; DS; FRCSC; GenSurg (Urology). Staff GenSurg, Cornwall Community Hospital; Staff GenSurg, Cornwall Community Hospital - Second Street Site; Langs: Arabic; (613)938-0497; Fax. (613)938-9878.

MOUSSA FALTAS, Assanassios; Ste Marie Clinic, 7-2010 Trim Rd, Orleans ON K4A 0G4; Cairo (Egypt)'94; MB BS; CCFP; Langs: Arabic; (613)590-1433; Fax. (613)590-1563.

MOUSSADJI, Jack S; Maple Med Centre, 208-955 Major Mackenzie W, Vaughan ON L6A 4P9; Tor'98; CCFP; Staff Surgical Assist, Mackenzie Richmond Hill Hospital; (289)553-7711; Fax. (289)553-7722.

MOUSSADJI, Yael; Foothills Med Centre, C231-1403 29 St NW, Calgary AB T2N 2T9; McM'04; FRCPC; EmergMed. Staff, Foothills Medical Centre; (403)944-1110

MOUSSAOUI, Chloe; Hop du Sacre-Coeur de Mtl, 5400 boul Gouin O, Montreal QC H4J 1C5; Laval'05; CCFP; CCFP(E.M.); Staff, Hôpital du Sacre-Coeur de Montréal; (514)338-2222

MOUSSEAU, Roger; Hop Maisonneuve-Rosemont, 5415 boul de l'Assomption, Montreal QC H1T 2M4; Mon'68; CSPQ; Gastroent (P.Q.) (Hepatology). Ac Staff Gastroent, Hopital Maisonneuve-Rosemont; Clinical Asst Prof, Universite de Montreal; Langs: Bilingual(French/English); (514)252-3822; Fax. (514)252-3885.

MOUSSETTE, Normand; Centre Bois de Boulogne, 350-1575 boul Henri-Bourassa O, Montreal QC H3M 3A9; Mon'73; Neur (P. Q.). Ac Staff, Hôpital du Sacre-Coeur de Montréal; (514)337-1242; Fax. (514)337-8422; normand.moussette@videotron.ca.

MOUSSETTE, Patricia A; Winchester Dist Mem Hosp, 566 Louise St, Winchester ON K0C 2K0; McG'96; CCFP; FCFP; Staff, Winchester District Memorial Hospital; Langs: English; French; (613)774-2420; Fax. (613)774-2941; trish_moussette@hotmail.com.

MOUSTAPHA, Ahmad; Regina Qu'Appelle HR-Regina, 1440 14th Ave, Regina SK S4P 0W5; Reinish (Germany)'89; FRCSC; GenSurg; CardSurg. Staff, Regina General Hospital; Clinical Asst Prof Surg, University of Saskatchewan; (306)766-6900; Fax. (306)766-6920.

MOUSTARAH, Fady; Hop Laval, 2725 ch Sainte-Foy, Quebec QC G1V 4G5; Alb'97; FRCSC; GenSurg (Endoscopy). Staff, Hôpital Laval; (418)656-8711 x5978; Fax. (418)656-4825.

MOUT, Julie; Centre medical de Cowansville, 101-370 rue de la Riviere, Cowansville QC J2K 1N3; UBC'82; ac Staff, Hôpital Brome-Missisquoi-Perkins; (450)263-0774

MOUTIER, Antoine M; Ctr Hosp Trois-Riv-St-Joseph, 731 rue Sainte-Julie, Trois-Rivieres QC G9A 1Y1; Rouen (France)'79; Staff, Centre Hospitalier Regional de Trois-Rivieres; (819)697-3333; Fax. (819)372-3535.

MOUTON, Abraham J; Watrous Med Clinic, PO Box 1059, Watrous SK S0K 4T0; Pretoria (South Africa)'76; BSc(BioChem); DIH; MB ChB; (306)946-2075; Fax. (306)946-2072; mouton99@yahoo.com.

MOUTON, Godwin P; PO Box 940, Redwater AB T0A 2W0; Stellenbosch (South Africa)'88; MB ChB; CCFP; Langs: Afrikaans; drmouton@telus.net.

MOUTON, Robert W; Winnipeg Clinic, 425 St Mary Ave, Winnipeg MB R3C 0N2; Stellenbosch (South Africa)'90; MB ChB(SA); MMed(Derm); MSc(Derm); Physician, Winnipeg Clinic; (204)957-3247; Fax. (204)957-3248.

MOUTQUIN, Jean-Marie; INESSS, 10.083-2021 av Union, Montreal QC H3A 2S9; Mon'68; MSc(Epidem.); LMCC; FRCSC; ObstGyn (Fetal & Maternal Medicine). Prof, Universite de Sherbrooke; Langs: English; (514)873-3719; Fax. (514)873-1369; jean-marie.moutquin@inesss.qc.ca.

MOUTRAN, Joseph; CSSS de Argenteuil, 145 av de la Providence, Lachute QC J8H 4C7; Mon'04; Staff, Centre Hospitalier d'Argenteuil; (450)562-3761

MOUZAKI, Marialena; The Hosp for Sick Children, 555 University Ave, Toronto ON M5G 1X8; Athens (Greece)'05; Staff, The Hospital For Sick Children; (416)813-1500

MOVSESYAN, Arakel; Wilson Medical Centre, 130 Wilson St, Hamilton ON L8R 1E2; Xavier Univ School of Medicine (Aruba)'06; Langs: Armenian; Russian; (905)526-6250

MOWAT, David L; 7120 Hurontario St PO Box 667 RPO Streetsville, Mississauga ON L5M 2C2; Edinburgh (Scotland)'72; MPH; FRCPC; CommunMed; Public Health & Preventive Med. Assoc Prof Community Health & Epidemiol, Queen's University; Teach Staff Epidemiol & Community Med, University of Ottawa; (905)791-7800 x2566; david.mowat@peelregion.ca.

MOWAT, Gordon; Edmonton Mental Health Clinic, 9942 108 St NW, Edmonton AB T5K 2J5; Glasgow (Scotland)'73; MB ChB; MRCPsy; Ac Staff, Alberta Hospital Edmonton; Consultant Psy, Inuvik Regional Hospital; Consultant Psy, Regional Mental Health Services-Edmonton; Clin Lecturer Dept of Psy, University of Alberta; (780)342-7700; Fax. (780)422-0832.

MOWAT, Grenville S; St Boniface Gen Hosp, 409 Tache Ave, Winnipeg MB R2H 2A6; Man'84; CCFP; CCFP(E.M.); Staff, St Boniface General Hospital; Assoc Teacher Family Practice, University of Manitoba; (204)237-2260; Fax. (204)237-0779; mowatgs@cc.umanitoba.ca.

MOWAT, Jeffrey J; The Moncton Hosp, 135 MacBeath Ave, Moncton NB E1C 6Z8; UBC'99; FRCPC; DiagRad. Staff, The Moncton Hospital; (506)857-5520

MOWATT, James I; Saint John Reg Hosp, PO Box 2100 Stn Main 400 University Ave, Saint John NB E2L 4L2; Dal'88; FRCSC; GenSurg. Staff, Saint John Regional Hospital; (506)649-2501; Fax. (506)648-7925.

MOWATT, John A; Saint John Reg Hosp, PO Box 2100 Stn Main 400 University Ave, Saint John NB E2L 4L2; Dal'93; BSc; FRCSC; GenSurg (Critical Care Medicine). Med Dir I C U, Saint John Regional Hospital; Asst Prof, Dalhousie University; (506)648-7960; Fax. (506)648-6490.

MOWCHUN, Leon; Psychealth Centre, PX161-771 Bannatyne Ave, Winnipeg MB R3E 3N4; Man'79; FRCPC; Psy. Staff Psy, Health Sciences Centre; Dir, Short Term Assessment & Treatment Prog.; Assoc Prof Postgraduate Educ, University of Manitoba; (204)787-3986; Fax. (204)787-3206.

MOWCHUN, Neil; 1601-233 Kennedy St, Winnipeg MB R3C 3J5; Man'72; BSc(Med.); FRCPC; Psy. Staff, St Boniface General Hospital; Dir Consultation-Liason Serv/Assoc Prof, Health Sciences Centre.

MOXHAM, John P; BC Women's Hosp & Health Ctre, 4500 Oak St, Vancouver BC V6H 3N1; Alb'92; BMedSci; FRCSC; Otol (Pediatric Otolaryngology). Staff Otolaryngology Clinic, BC Women's Hospital & Health Centre; Staff, BC Children's Hospital; Clin Asst Prof/Prog Dir Otolaryngology, University of British Columbia; (604)875-2113

MOXON, Richard D; Perth Med Clinic, 14 Isabella St, Perth ON K7H 2W6; Qns'73; Staff, Perth & Smiths Falls District Hospital - Perth Site (Great War Memorial Site); Assoc Staff, Perth & Smiths Falls District Hospital - Smiths Falls Site; (613)267-1762; Fax. (613)264-8370.

MOYAL, Yoel; Ctr Hosp de Lachine, 650 16e av, Lachine QC H8S 3N5; Laval'98; CCFP; CCFP(E.M.); Staff, Centre Hospitalier de Lachine; (514)934-1934; yoel.moyal@mail.mcgill.ca.

MOYANA, Terence N; The Ottawa Hosp-Gen Campus, 501 Smyth Rd, Ottawa ON K1H 8L6; Harare (Zimbabwe)'80; MD; ABPath; LRCPS; FRCPC; AnatPath. Staff Path, The Ottawa Hospital - General Campus; Prof Path, University of Ottawa; (613)737-8290; tmoyana@ottawahospital.on.ca.

MOYEN, Eric J; CHUQ-Hotel-Dieu de Quebec, 11 Cote du Palais, Quebec QC G1R 2J6; Laval'02; Critical Care Medicine (P.Q.); Anes. Staff, Centre Hospitalier Universitaire de Québec (CHUQ) - Siege Social; (418)525-4444

MOYO, Jabulani; Clinical Sciences Bldg, 8 120-152 University Campus NW, Edmonton AB T6G 2G3; (Zimbabwe)'93; Staff, University of Alberta Hospital; (780)407-8887

MOYO, Margaret S; 204B-725 Coronation Blvd, Cambridge ON N1R 7S9; Nairobi (Kenya)'81; MRC(Ire); DCH; DC; FRCPC; Peds. (519)620-9444; Fax. (519)620-9444.

MOYSE, Cyril A; Summerside Med Centre, 1-475 Granville St, Summerside PE C1N 3N9; Dal'72; CCFP; FCFP; Ac Staff, Prince County Hospital; Coroner, Province Of Prince Edward Isand; Registrar, College of Physicians & Surgeons of Prince Edward Island; Lecturer, Dalhousie University; (902)432-8136; Fax. (902)436-9660.

MOZAFFARI, Babak; 5-201 Hurst Dr, Barrie ON L4N 8K8; Sask'91; CCFP; FCFP; (705)726-0966; Fax. (705)726-1056.

MOZAROWSKI, Paul T; Sault Area Hosp, 750 Great Northern Rd, Sault Ste. Marie ON P6B 0A8; Tor'81; FRCPC; GenPath. Staff, Sault Area Hospital - Sault Ste Marie; (705)759-3434 x3680; Fax. (705)759-3846.

MOZEG, Dan; Headwaters Health Care Centre, 100 Rolling Hills Dr, Orangeville ON L9W 4X9; Tor'00; FRCPC; DiagRad. Staff, Headwaters Health Care Centre - Orangeville Site; (519)941-2410

MOZES, Rami S; Yonge-Eglinton Med Centre, 200-2401 Yonge St, Toronto ON M4P 3H1; McG'82; Langs: Hebrew; Romanian; (416)486-9600; Fax. (416)486-9227.

MOZZON, Jeremy B; Dartmouth Gen Hosp, 325 Pleasant St, Dartmouth NS B2Y 4G8; Wes'07; CCFP; Staff, Dartmouth General Hospital; (902)465-8300

MPIANA, Pinos M; 842 Conception Bay Hwy PO Box 17009 Stn Main, Conception-Bay-S NL A1X 3H1; Kinshasa (Congo (Democratic Republic))'87; Langs: Bilingual(English/French); p.mpiana@nf.sympatico.ca.

MPISI, Bulelwa; Kelvington Med Clinic, PO Box 130, Kelvington SK S0A 1W0; (306)327-4661; Fax. (306)327-5353.

MPOFU, Christopher; Saskatoon Cancer Centre, 20 Campus Dr, Saskatoon SK S7N 4H4; Manchester (England)'84; MB ChB; FRCPC; Peds (Pediatric Oncology). Staff, Saskatoon Cancer Centre; Staff, Royal University Hospital; Clin Assoc Prof, University of Saskatchewan; Langs: French; Shona; (306)655-2744; Fax. (306)655-6382.

MRAD, Mohamed A A M; Sunnybrook Hlth Sciences Ctre, M1 525-2075 Bayview Ave, Toronto ON M4N 3M5; (Saudi Arabia)'03; FRCSC; PlasSurg. Staff, Sunnybrook Health Sciences Centre; (416)480-4868

MRKOBRADA, Marko; London HSC-University Hosp, PO Box 5339 Stn B 339 Windermere Rd, London ON N6A 5A5; Wes'05; FRCPC; IntMed. Staff, London Health Sciences Centre - University Hospital; (519)685-8500

MRKONJIC, Linda A; Foothills Med Centre, 1403 29 St NW, Calgary AB T2N 2T9; Alb'90; FRCSC; OrthSurg. Staff, Foothills Medical Centre; (403)944-2237; Fax. (403)270-8004.

MROCHUK, May; Royal Alexandra Hosp, 551-10240 Kingsway NW, Edmonton AB T5H 3V9; Alb'97; CCFP; CCFP(E.M.); Staff, Royal Alexandra Hospital; (780)735-4442

MROZ, Krzysztof S M; Cornwall Comm Hosp-McConnell, PO Box 100 Stn Main 840 McConnell Ave, Cornwall ON K6H 5S5; Slaska (Poland)'67; Anes. Staff, Cornwall Community Hospital; (613)938-4240

MSHIU, Merlyn E; The Brandon Clinic, 620 Dennis St, Brandon MB R7A 5E7; Dar Es Salaam (Tanzania)'89; FRCPC; IntMed. (204)728-4440

MTSHALI, Raphael T; Outlook Med Clinic, PO Box 1160, Outlook SK S0L 2N0; (306)867-8626; Fax. (306)867-8988.

MU, Lisa J; Coast Med Clinic, 1018 Seymour St, Vancouver BC V6B 3M6; Wes'07; CCFP; Public Health & Preventive Med. (604)569-3622

MUALLIM, Carol; Agincourt Med Centre, 2020 Brimley Rd, Scarborough ON M1S 4R7; Wes'99; CCFP; (416)293-2404

MUAMBI-KABONGO, Jean-Thadee; Saint John Med Clinic, 299 Melcalf St, Saint John NB E2K 4P8; (Congo (Democratic Republic))'83; Langs: French; (506)652-5250; Fax. (506)652-5259.

MUANZA, Thierry M; SMBD Jewish Gen Hosp, 3755 ch Cote-Sainte-Catherine, Montreal QC H3T 1E2; Sher'97; CSPQ; FRCPC; Psy; RadOncol (P.Q.). Staff, Sir Mortimer B Davis Jewish General; adj Prof, McGill University; Langs: French; (514)340-8222; thierry.muanza@muhc.mcgill.ca.

MUAYQIL, Taim A; Glenrose Rehabilitation Hosp, E223-10230 111 Ave NW, Edmonton AB T5G 0B7; Riyadh (Saudi Arabia)'99; MB BS; FRCPC; Neur (Cognitive Neurol). Staff, Glenrose Rehabilitation Hospital; Langs: Arabic; (780)735-8840; Fax. (780)735-6117.

MUBAREKA, Samira; Sunnybrook Hlth Sciences Ctre, B1 03-2075 Bayview Ave, Toronto ON M4N 3M5; Dal'99; FRCPC; MedMicrobiol; InfectDis; IntMed. Staff, Microbiologist, Sunnybrook Health Sciences Centre; (416)480-4549

MUBOYAYI, T Romain; Orleans Medical-Dental Centre, 204A-2555 St. Joseph Blvd, Orleans ON K1C 1S6; (Belgium)'93; CCFP; Staff, Montfort Hospital; Langs: Lingala; English; (613)834-8500; Fax. (613)824-7838.

MUCALOV, Peter; 12-204 Simcoe Ave, Keswick ON L4P 3S6; Tor'75; Staff Member, Southlake Regional Health Centre; Langs: German; (905)476-9300; Fax. (905)476-8753; mucalov@interhop.net.

MUCCIARONE, Antonio; Bashaw Health Centre, PO Box 159 3503 57 St, Bashaw AB T0B 0H0; Alb'86; Staff, Bassano Health Centre; (780)372-3740; Fax. (780)372-3741.

MUCHA, Mary Ann J; B22-550 Terminal Ave, Ottawa ON K1G 0Z3; Ott'69; CCFP.

MUCKLOW, Michael G; Scarborough Hosp -General Div, 3050 Lawrence Ave E, Scarborough ON M1P 2V5; Birmingham (England)'62; MedMicrobiol. Staff, The Scarborough Hospital - General Campus; (416)438-2911

MUCSI, Istvan; MUHC-Royal Victoria Hosp, R2.38-687 av des Pins O, Montreal QC H3A 1A1; Semmelweis (Hungary)'88; PhD; Nephrol (P.Q.). Staff, McGill University Health Centre - Royal Victoria Hospital; Langs: Hungarian; (514)843-1586; Fax. (514)843-2815; istvan.mucsi@mcgill.ca.

MUDALIAR, Adi K M; 6438 Fraser St, Vancouver BC V5W 3A4; UBC'81; CCFP; (604)324-5655

MUDIE, Dayna L; Columbia Med Bldg, 211-301 Columbia St E, New Westminster BC V3L 3W5; UBC'99; CCFP; (604)520-6263

MUDIE, Reidunn A; Surrey Mem Hosp, 13750 96 Ave, Surrey BC V3V 1Z2; UBC'82; FRCPC; Anes. Staff, Surrey Memorial Hospital; (604)588-3367

MUDINGAYI, Kabuya; Maple Creek Primary Hlth Care, PO Box 517 515 Hwy 21 S, Maple Creek SK S0N 1N0; (306)662-2829; Fax. (306)662-2332.

MUDRIK, Kevin P; Markham Stouffville Hosp, PO Box 1800 Stn Main 381 Church St, Markham ON L3P 7P3; Qns'92; CCFP; CCFP; CCFP(E.M.); Staff, Markham Stouffville Hospital; (905)472-7000

MUECKE, Cristin; Fredericton Regional Centre, PO Box 5001 1400-300 St Marys St, Fredericton NB E3B 5H1; Dal'99; FRCP; MSc; MB; FRCPC; CommunMed. Langs: Bilingual(French/English); (506)453-2830; Fax. (506)453-2848.

MUEHLENBERG, Bernd A; Orchard Medical Clinic, 3819 9th Ave, Port Alberni BC V9Y 4T8; Qns'75; BA; Staff, West Coast General Hospital; (250)723-8141; Fax. (250)723-4318.

MUELLER, Carmen L; University of Toronto, 602-500 University Ave, Toronto ON M5G 1V7; Tor'07; FRCSC; GenSurg. (416)802-6465

MUELLER, Caroline P; 186-8120 No. 2 Rd, Richmond BC V7C 5J8; Alb'91; FRCSC; ObstGyn. Staff, BC Women's Hospital & Health Centre; Clinical Asst Prof, University of British Columbia; Langs: German; (604)447-1107

MUELLER, Dagmar L; 45 St Thomas St, St. Albert AB T8N 6Z1; Alb'79; AB; DiagRad (Child Abuse). (780)470-5551

MUELLER, Daniel J; Addiction & Mental Hlth-Clarke, R30-250 College St, Toronto ON M5T 1R8; Bonn (Germany)'96; Staff/Head Pharmacogenetics Research Clin, Centre for Addiction & Mental Health (CAMH) - College Street Site; Asst Prof Psychiatry, University of Toronto; Langs: German; French; Italian; (416)535-8501

MUELLER, Edrise M; Cross Cancer Institute, 11560 University Ave NW, Edmonton AB T6G 1Z2; Minas Gerais (Brazil)'92; Staff, Cross Cancer Institute; (780)432-8846

MUELLER, Elizabeth K; 3-11 George St S, Cambridge ON N1S 2N3; Wes'77; CCFP; FCFP; Physician, Stirling Heights Long Term Care Facility; Langs: German; French; (519)740-5060; Fax. (519)740-0035; drekmueller1@live.com.

MUELLER, Eric M; Chinook Reg Hosp, 960 19 St S, Lethbridge AB T1J 1W5; UBC'94; CCFP; CCFP(E.M.); FCFP; Staff Emerg, Chinook Regional Hospital; (403)388-6304; Fax. (403)388-6183.

MUELLER, Harry D; 37 2 Ave SE, High River AB T1V 1G4; Alb'84; FRCSC; ObstGyn. (403)652-4505; Fax. (403)652-4724.

MUELLER, Jennifer L; Welland McMaster Family Hlth Team, 555 Prince Charles Dr, Welland ON L3C 6B5; McM'98; CCFP; (905)734-9699; Fax. (905)734-3947.

MUELLER, Thomas F; Heritage Med Research Centre, 260-107 University Campus NW, Edmonton AB T6G 2S2; (Germany)'84; (780)407-1571; Fax. (780)407-3417.

MUELLER, Valerie M L; 115 Delhi St, Guelph ON N1E 4J4; McM'94; FRCSC; ObstGyn (Maternal Fetal Medicine). (519)837-6444; Fax. (519)837-6426.

MUELLER, William; 403-855 Broadview Ave, Toronto ON M4K 3Z1; Tor'74; (416)961-9884; Fax. (416)961-5097.

MUELLER-WILM, Ingrid; 43 Quinan Dr, Toronto ON M6L 1E8; Heidelberg (Germany)'51; Associate, Humber River Regional Hospital - Keele Street Site; Associate, Humber River Regional Hospital - Church Street Site; Associate, Humber River Regional Hospital - Finch Avenue Site; Langs: German; (416)244-7391; Fax. (416)248-4016.

MUENDEL, Hans-Christoph; Westside Med Clinic, 3591 Elliott Rd, Westbank BC V4T 1N9; UBC'66; Staff, Royal Inland Hospital; (250)768-7656

MUFTAH, Abdalla G; Broad Med Specialists, 2275 Broad St, Regina SK S4P 1Y7; (Libya)'89; MB ChB; FRCPC; IntMed; Respir. Langs: Arabic; (306)757-2472; Fax. (306)757-2483.

MUFTAH, Anwar S A; Landmark Med Centre, 6-4150 Albert St, Regina SK S4S 3R8; Al Fateh (Libya)'90; MD; FRCPC; IntMed (Hematology). Staff, Regina General Hospital; Staff, Pasqua Hospital; Langs: Arabic; (306)352-5335; Fax. (306)352-4858.

MUFTEE, Naqsh; 11-7750 Ranchview Dr NW, Calgary AB T3G 1Y9; Punjab (Pakistan)'85; CCFP; (403)452-6240; Fax. (403)452-9626.

MUGARAB-SAMEDI, Veronica; Peter Lougheed Centre, 3500 26 AVE NE, Calgary AB T1Y 6J4; (Azerbaijan)'87; Staff, Peter Lougheed Centre; (403)943-4555; Fax. (403)252-8575.

MUGERWA, Abimanyi S J; Rochdale Med Clinic, 4936 4th Ave, Regina SK S4T 0J3; (306)775-2688; Fax. (306)543-4633.

MUGFORD, Johanna L; Davisville Fam Practice, 600-1881 Yonge St, Toronto ON M4S 3C4; Tor'93; CCFP; FCFP; Assoc Staff Family Med, Mount Sinai Hospital; Assoc Staff, Toronto General Hospital - UHN; Staff, Toronto Western Hospital - University Health Network; Lecturer, University of Toronto; (416)932-3172; Fax. (416)440-0238.

MUGGABERG, Sheri G; CFB Shilo, PO Box 5000, Shilo MB R0K 2A0; Man'09; CCFP.

MUGGAH, Elizabeth A; Bruyere Family Med Ctre, 75 Bruyere St, Ottawa ON K1N 5C7; McM'97; CCFP.

MUGGAH, J Jean; 1437 Belcher St PO Box 448, Port Williams NS B0P 1T0; Dal'79; Staff, Valley Regional Hospital; Langs: English; French; (902)542-0779; Fax. (902)542-0530.

MUGGLI, Jessica B; 11700 Sarcee Tr NW PO Box 80009 Rpo Beacon Hill, Calgary AB T3R 0B2; Sask'03; CCFP; (403)221-4467; Fax. (403)221-4442; gijess@hotmail.com.

MUGHAL, Jawaid I; King Street Med Arts Centre, 307-71 King St W, Mississauga ON L5B 4A2; Glasgow (Scotland)'74; Langs: Urdu; Punjabi; (905)279-1660; Fax. (905)279-9666.

MUGHAL, Maqbool A; Malton Med Arts Bldg, 207-3530 Derry Rd E, Mississauga ON L4T 4E3; Makerere (Uganda)'73; MB ChB; Court Staff, The Scarborough Hospital - General Campus; Langs: Swahili; Urdu; Punjabi; (905)673-7377; Fax. (905)673-9832.

MUGISHA, James K; Hazelwood Med Clinic, 201-16088 84 Ave, Surrey BC V4N 0V9; Makerere (Uganda)'73; DPH; DIH; Assoc Staff, Surrey Memorial Hospital; (604)572-6665; Fax. (604)572-8912.

MUHAMEDAGIC, Tatjana; Halton Health Care Services, 6F-700 Dorval Dr, Oakville ON L6K 3V3; Univ of Sarajevo (Bosnia-Herzegovina)'84; FRCPC; Psy. Langs: Croatian; (905)815-5140; Fax. (905)845-6419.

MUHAMMAD, Afzal; Notre Dame Clinic, PO Box 190, Notre-Dame-Lourdes MB R0G 1M0; Moscow (Russia (Federation))'99; CCFP; (204)248-2252

MUHAMMAD, Amin A; Trillium Hlth Ctr-Mississauga, 100 Queensway W, Mississauga ON L5B 1B8; Karachi (Pakistan)'84; DPM(Ire); DCPsy(Ire); MRCPsy; FRCPI(Ire); PhD; MB BS; FRCPC; Psy (Adult Psychiatry). Staff, Trillium Health Centre - Mississauga; Langs: Urdu; (905)848-7585; Fax. (905)848-7368; amin.muhammad@med.mun.ca.

MUHAMMAD, Iffat A; 217-3806 Albert St, Regina SK S4S 3R2; Lahore (Pakistan) MB BS; MRCGPract; Langs: Urdu; Punjabi; (306)545-6093; Fax. (306)545-6094.

MUHAMMAD, Ishtiaq; Harbourside Clinic, 243 Harbourside Dr, Summerside PE C1N 5R1; Punjab (India)'92; MB BS; (902)432-2600

MUHAMMAD, Mustafa; 102-16703 82 St NW, Edmonton AB T5Z 0H5; (Syria)'05; CCFP; (780)457-7142

MUHAMMAD, Naeem H; 201-240 Wharncliffe Rd N, London ON N6H 4P2; Punjab (Pakistan)'85; CCFP; Langs: Hindi; Punjabi; (519)435-0111

MUHAMMED, Khalid A E; Vita Med Centre, PO Box 208 217 First St W, Vita MB R0A 2K0; (204)425-3372; Fax. (204)425-3379.

MUHAMMED, Talib; 101-4015 17 Ave SE, Calgary AB T2A 0S8; Baghdad (Iraq)'89; Physician, Mosaic Primary Care Network; Staff, University of Manitoba; Langs: Arabic; (403)457-5900; Fax. (403)457-4433; talib_muhammed@hc-sc.gc.ca.

MUHLSTOCK, Joshua P; UL-2250 Fairview St, Burlington ON L7R 4C7; McM'02; FRCPC; PhysMed&Rehab. (905)333-5100; Fax. (905)333-5107.

MUHN, Channy Y; Dermetics, 8&9-3305 Harvester Rd, Burlington ON L7N 3N2; McM'97; BSc(Hons); FRCPC; Derm (Acne Treatment). Ac Staff, Hamilton Health Sciences Centre - Hamilton General Hospital; Surg Consultant, The Juravinski Cancer Centre; Asst Prof Med, McMaster University; Langs: English; French; (905)336-9624; Fax. (905)336-9625.

MUHN, Narry Y; St Joseph's Healthcare, 50 Charlton St E, Hamilton ON L8N 4A6; McM'03; FRCPC; DiagRad. Staff, St Joseph's Healthcare - Charlton Campus; (905)522-1155

MUHSEN, Jafaar; Univ Hlth Network-Princess M, 610 University Ave, Toronto ON M5G 2M9; Baghdad (Iraq)'89; BMedSci; CCFP; Staff, Princess Margaret Hospital - University Health Network; Vis Physician, The Wellington Retirement Home; Langs: Arabic; (416)946-2000

MUHSIN, Munir K; Norfolk Gen Hosp, 365 West St, Simcoe ON N3Y 1T7; Baghdad (Iraq)'91; CCFP; Staff, Norfolk General Hospital; (519)426-0750

MUHTADIE, Lina; Lakeshore Gen Hosp, 160 av Stillview, Pointe-Claire QC H9R 2Y2; McG'03; Nephrol; IntMed. Staff, Lakeshore General Hospital - Pointe Claire; (514)630-2225

MUHUNTHAN, Arumairajah; 140 Cameron St, Sarnia ON N7T 4A8; (Sri Lanka)'76; MB BS; FRCSC; GenSurg. Langs: Sinhalese; Tamil; (519)383-7594; Fax. (519)383-8741.

MUHUNTHAN, Jothimalar; Bluewater Health-Norman Site, 89 Norman St, Sarnia ON N7T 6S3; Colombo (Sri Lanka)'72; MB BS; MRCP(Ire.); FRCPC; Neur (Multiple Sclerosis). Staff, Bluewater Health - Norman Site; Langs: Sinhalese; Tamil; (519)383-6918; Fax. (519)383-7233.

MUI, Jimmy K Y; Durham Reg Cancer Centre, 1 Hospital Crt, Oshawa ON L1G 2B9; Dundee (Scotland)'90; MB ChB; BSc(Hons.); FRCPC; RadOncol. Staff, Lakeridge Health - Oshawa Site; Langs: Cantonese; Mandarin; (905)576-8711 x3625

MUIA, Frank V; Welkare Med Office, 268 Clarence St, London ON N6B 2K1; Wes'86; BSc; Langs: Italian; (519)672-9898; Fax. (519)858-5775.

MUINUDDIN, Ahmad; Univ of Western Ontario, 4-1151 Richmond St, London ON N6A 5C1; Tor'08; FRCPC; IntMed. (519)661-2019; Fax. (519)850-2492.

MUIR, Ava J F; The Nova Scotia Hosp, PO Box 1004 Stn Main 300 Pleasant St, Dartmouth NS B2Y 3Z9; McM'06; FRCPC; Psy. Staff, The Nova Scotia Hospital; (902)464-3322

MUIR, Brian P; 208-9815 97 St, Grande Prairie AB T8V 8B9; Sask'88; FRCSC; ObstGyn. Staff, Queen Elizabeth II Hospital; (780)538-2190; Fax. (780)538-2191.

MUIR, Craig F; City of Sudbury-Northern Regio, 199 Larch St, Sudbury ON P3E 5P9; McM'82; BSc; DAB; FACS; FRCSC; GenSurg (Endoscopy). Staff Regional Supervising Coroner, City of Sudbury District 19; (705)564-6149; Fax. (705)564-6155.

MUIR, Darcy G; Sunridge Adult Mental Health, 200-2580 32 St NE, Calgary AB T1Y 7M8; Sask'03; FRCPC; Psy. Staff, Foothills Medical Centre; (403)944-9749

MUIR, Erin E A; Mackenzie Richmond Hill Hosp, 10 Trench St, Richmond Hill ON L4C 4Z3; Dal'07; FRCPC; IntMed; Hem. Staff, Mackenzie Richmond Hill Hospital; (905)883-1212

MUIR, Jennifer C; 3809 Sunset St, Burnaby BC V5G 1T4; UBC'99; FRCSC; ObstGyn. (604)565-9447; Fax. (604)565-9448.

MUIR, John G; IWK Health Centre, PO Box 9700 Rpo CSC 5850-5980 University Ave, Halifax NS B3K 6R8; Aberdeen (Scotland)'76; MB ChB; FRCA; FRCPC; Anes (Pediatric Anesthesia). Staff, IWK Health Centre; Consultant, Queen Elizabeth II Health Sciences Centre - Victoria General Site; Assoc Prof/Assoc Chief Paramedic Anes, Dalhousie University; (902)470-8251; Fax. (902)470-7911.

MUIR, Karen Y; Omineca Med Clinic, RR 2 3348 Hospital Rd, Vanderhoof BC V0J 3A2; Orange Free State (South Africa)'77; (250)567-2201; Fax. (250)567-2105.

MUIR, Sarah A; Atlantic Med Clinic, PO Box 29119 Rpo Hal Shop Ctre, Halifax NS B3L 4T8; Dal'90; CCFP; (902)455-4333

MUIR, Sylvia K; KGW 55-60-2075 Bayview Ave, Toronto ON M4N 3M5; Tor'76; ABNEM; CSCN; FRCPC; CCFP; PhysMed&Rehab. Sr District Medical Officer, Veterans Affairs Canada; Langs: English; Fax. (416)973-6814.

MUIRHEAD, Brian D; St Paul's Hosp, 3F-1081 Burrard St, Vancouver BC V6Z 1Y6; Man'79; FRCPC; Anes. Staff, Providence Health Care - St Paul's Hospital; (604)806-8337

MUIRHEAD, Margaret A; West Haldimand Gen Hosp, 75 Parkview Rd, Hagersville ON N0A 1H0; UBC'87; CCFP; CCFP(E.M.); Staff, West Haldimand General Hospital; (905)768-3311; mmuirhead1@cogeco.ca.

MUIRHEAD, Norman; London HSC-University Hosp, PO Box 5339 Stn B 339 Windermere Rd, London ON N6A 5A5; Aberdeen (Scotland)'76; MB ChB; MRC(UK); FRCP(Edin); FRCPC; IntMed (Nephrology). Staff Nephrol & Dir, London Health Sciences Centre - University Hospital; Prof Med, University of Western Ontario; (519)663-3350; Fax. (519)663-8808; norman.muirhead@lhsc.on.ca.

MUIRHEAD, Matthew; Medical & Dental Bldg, 400-3939 50A Ave, Red Deer AB T4N 4E6; Dal'98; BSc; FRCSC; GenSurg. (403)347-9037

MUIRHEAD, William M; MF-125 Erb St W, Waterloo ON N2L 1T6; Wes'82; CCFP; FCFP; (519)746-4697; Fax. (519)746-2485.

MUISE, Aleixo M; The Hosp for Sick Children, 555 University Ave, Toronto ON M5G 1X8; Tor'01; FRCPC; Peds. Fellow, The Hospital For Sick Children; (416)813-1500; Fax. (416)813-4972; aleixo.muise@sickkids.ca.

MUISE, Roland J; Harbour South Med Clinic, 235 Main St, Yarmouth NS B5A 1E1; Dal'76; BSc; Member Med Advisory, Yarmouth Regional Hospital; Langs: Bilingual(English/French); (902)742-8333; Fax. (902)742-8355.

MUISE, Suzanne L; James Paton Mem Hosp, 125 Trans Canada Hwy, Gander NL A1V 1P7; Dal'01; FRCSC; ObstGyn. Staff, James Paton Memorial Hospital; (709)256-2500

MUISE, Thomas A; Yarmouth Reg Health Ctre, 301C-60 Vancouver St, Yarmouth NS B5A 2P5; Dal'85; Staff, Yarmouth Regional Hospital; (902)742-9149; Fax. (902)742-2501.

MUJOOMDAR, Amol; London HSC-Victoria Hosp, PO Box 5010 Stn B C2 200-800 Commissioners Rd E, London ON N6A 5W9; Sask'02; FRCPC; DiagRad. Staff, London Health Sciences Centre - Victoria Campus; (519)685-8500

MUJOOMDAR, Aneil A; The Moncton Hosp, 135 MacBeath Ave, Moncton NB E1C 6Z8; Dal'99; FRCSC; GenSurg; ThorSurg. Staff, The Moncton Hospital; (506)857-5520

MUKERJI, Amit; The Hosp for Sick Children, 555 University Ave, Toronto ON M5G 1X8; McM'08; Peds. Fellow, The Hospital For Sick Children; (416)813-1500

MUKERJI, Geetha; Univ Hlth Network-Toronto Gen, 12N 243-200 Elizabeth St, Toronto ON M5G 2C4; McM'08; FRCPC; IntMed. Staff, Toronto General Hospital - UHN; (416)340-3111

MUKHEIBIR, Peter; Surrey Med Arts Bldg, 104-13798 94A Ave, Surrey BC V3V 1N1; Pretoria (South Africa)'89; MB ChB; CCFP; (604)581-9333; Fax. (604)581-3837.

MUKHERJEE, Ashok; Corcare Inc, 410-325 Milner Ave, Scarborough ON M1B 5N1; Tor'87; Cardiol; IntMed. Staff Cardiol, Rouge Valley Health System - Centenary Health Centre Site; (416)284-4744; Fax. (416)284-0141; info@corcare.net.

MUKHERJEE, Diana; The Moncton Hosp, 135 MacBeath Ave, Moncton NB E1C 6Z8; Tor'86; Staff, The Moncton Hospital; Langs: Italian; Bengali; (506)857-5201

MUKHERJEE, Sanjib K; 6-160 The West Way, Etobicoke ON M9P 2C1; Calcutta University (India)'55; FRCPC; IntMed (Cardiology). (416)242-2062; Fax. (416)242-4347; cardiolog1@bellnet.ca.

MUKHERJEE, Siddhartha; Lorrain Med Clinic, C328-201 Deacon St, Pembroke ON K8A 2J6; Burdwan (India)'87; MB BS; BSc; FRCSC; ObstGyn. (613)635-7900

MUKHERJEE, Som D; The Juravinski Cancer Centre, 699 Concession St, Hamilton ON L8V 5C2; Mem'99; FRCPC; IntMed; MedOncol. (905)387-9711

MUKHERJEE, Sutapa; Women's College Hosp, W649-76 Grenville St, Toronto ON M5S 1B2; University of Adelaide (Australia)'89; Staff, Women's College Hospital; (416)323-6137

MUKHERJI, Atreyi; Hamilton HS-General Site, 237 Barton St E, Hamilton ON L8L 2X2; Dal'92; BSc(Biology); FRCPC; IntMed. Staff, Hamilton Health Sciences Centre - Hamilton General Hospital; Langs: Hindi; (905)527-0271

MUKIIBI, Herbert K; 290-5255 Richmondd Rd SW, Calgary AB T3E 7C4; (Uganda)'90; MB ChB; MSc; MMed; (403)249-3165; Fax. (403)249-3120.

MUKTY, Mahmuda A; 1578 Regent Ave W, Winnipeg MB R2C 3B4; CCFP.

MULA, David E; Toronto Poly Clinic, 204-5460 Yonge St, North York ON M2N 6K7; Wes'04; CCFP; Physician, Toronto Poly Clinic; (416)250-7171; Fax. (416)250-0323.

MULAISHO, Chilango; Stamford Med Centre, 203-4256 Portage Rd, Niagara Falls ON L2E 6A4; London (England)'70; MB BS; DABIM; DAB; FRCPC; IntMed (Endocrinology - Diabetes). (905)356-2062; Fax. (905)356-6290.

MULAJA WA MULAJA, Aubin; CSSS de Papineau, 155 rue Maclaren E, Gatineau QC J8L 0C2; Lubumbashi (Congo (Democratic Republic))'89; CCFP; Staff, Hôpital de Papineau; (819)986-3341

MULCASTER, Julian T; Hamilton HS-General Campus, 237 Barton St E, Hamilton ON L8L 2X2; Dal'94; FRCPC; Anes. Staff, Hamilton Health Sciences Centre - Hamilton General Hospital; (905)527-4322; Fax. (905)577-8022.

MULCHEY, Kimberley D; University of Alberta Hosp, 8440 112 St NW, Edmonton AB T6G 2B7; Man'07; Respir; IntMed. Staff, University of Alberta Hospital; (780)407-8822

MULDER, David S; MUHC-Montreal Gen Hosp, L9.512-1650 av Cedar, Montreal QC H3G 1A4; Sask'62; MSc(McG); FACS; FRCSC; GenSurg (Sports Medicine); Cardiovasc&ThorSurg. Staff, Sir Mortimer B Davis Jewish General; Dir CardioThoracic Surg, McGill University Health Centre - Montreal General Campus; Staff, McGill University Health Centre - Royal Victoria Hospital; Dir CardioThoracic Surg, McGill University; Langs: English; French; (514)935-4888; Fax. (514)937-5522.

MULDER, Eric M; Royal Victoria Hosp, 201 Georgian Dr, Barrie ON L4M 6M2; McM'04; FRCPC; Psy. Staff, Royal Victoria Regional Health Centre; (705)728-9090; Fax. (705)739-5631.

MULDER, Erik W; Riverwood Place, 205-49 Emma St, Guelph ON N1E 6X1; Qns'82; FRCPC; Psy. (519)836-5992; Fax. (519)836-5251.

MULDER, Jeffrey D; Associate Med Group, 4705 48 Ave, Red Deer AB T4N 3T1; Alb'92; CCFP; Physician, Associate Medical Group; (403)346-2057; Fax. (403)347-2989.

MULDER, John-Derek; Associate Med Clinic, 25 St Michael St, St Albert AB T8N 1C7; Pretoria (South Africa)'87; MB ChB; (780)458-1234; Fax. (780)460-7941.

MULDER, J Stefan; 195-4750 Rutherford Rd, Nanaimo BC V9T 4K6; Pretoria (South Africa)'85; MB ChB; Staff, Central Newfoundland Regional Health Centre; Langs: Afrikaans; (250)585-7100

MULDER, Karen E; Cross Cancer Institute, 11560 University Ave NW, Edmonton AB T6G 1Z2; Alb'97; BSc; MSc; FRCPC; IntMed (Gastrointestinal Cancer); MedOncol. Staff, Cross Cancer Institute; Asst Prof, University of Alberta; (780)432-8248; Fax. (780)432-8888; karenmul@cancerboard.ab.ca.

MULDER, Robert J; Associate Med Group, 4705 48 Ave, Red Deer AB T4N 3T1; Sask'67; Ac Staff, Red Deer Regional Hospital Centre; Physician, Associate Medical Group; (403)346-2057; Fax. (403)347-2989.

MULDOON, Laura K; Somerset West Comm Health Ctre, 55 Eccles St, Ottawa ON K1R 6S3; Qns'85; CCFP; FCFP; CommunMed. (613)238-1220; Fax. (613)235-2982; lmuldoon@swchc.on.ca.

MULDOWNEY, Siobhan M; 91 Cornelia St W, Smiths Falls ON K7A 5L3; Alb'90; BMedSci; CCFP; FCFP; Ac Staff, Perth & Smiths Falls District Hospital - Smiths Falls Site; Teach Staff Family Med, University of Ottawa; Langs: English; French; (613)283-0710; Fax. (613)284-8331.

MULE, Francesco; Northumberland Hills Hosp, 1000 DePalma Dr, Cobourg ON K9A 5W6; Mem'02; Staff, Northumberland Hills Hospital; (905)372-6811

MULERA, Muniini K; Medical Arts Bldg, 205-581 Davis Dr, Newmarket ON L3Y 2P6; Makerere (Uganda)'77; FRCPC; Peds (Neonatology). Staff, Southlake Regional Health Centre; (905)868-9800; Fax. (905)868-9900.

MULGUND, Manisha M; 34-1960 Appleby Line, Burlington ON L7L 0B7; Mumbai (India)'98; ABIM; FRCPC; IntMed; Rheum. Langs: Hindi; Gujarati; Marathi; (905)332-9292

MULHALL, David R; Valley Reg Hosp, 150 Exhibition St, Kentville NS B4N 5E3; Dublin (Ireland)'79; MB BCh; BAO; MRCPsy; FRCPC; Psy (Adult Psychiatry). Staff, Valley Regional Hospital; Med Dir, Mental Health & Addiction Services; Lecturer Psy, Dalhousie University; (902)678-7381 x2870; Fax. (902)679-2473; david.mulhall@saskatoonhealthregion.ca.

MULHERIN, Michael T; PO Box 532, Port Mouton NS B0T 1T0; Dal'95; CCFP; (902)542-0537; Fax. (902)542-0530.

MULHOLLAND, Michael G; PO Box 8973 Stn Main, Sylvan Lake AB T4S 1S6; U.K. (United Kingdom)'89; MB ChB; BAO.

MULJI, Amin S; Victoria Med Centre, 501-304 Victoria Ave N, Hamilton ON L8L 5G4; McM'80; FRCPC; IntMed; Cardiol. Staff, Hamilton Health Sciences Centre - Hamilton General Hospital; Clin Assoc Prof, McMaster University; (905)529-0793; Fax. (905)527-1941.

MULL, John D; 15330 Weston Rd, King City ON L7B 1K4; Tor'57; FRCPC; GenPath. Med Staff, Trillium Health Centre - West Toronto; Med Dir/Pathologist, Canadian Med. Labs. Ltd.; (905)751-0085; lab@canmedlab.com.

MULLA, Amith A; Central Med Clinic, 6-1061 Central Ave N, Swift Current SK S9H 4Y9; Staff/Surgeon, Cypress Regional Hospital; (306)773-5855; Fax. (306)778-3799; amithmulla@yahoo.com.

MULLALY, Christa L; 304-1015 Regent St, Fredericton NB E3B 6H5; McM'00; ObstGyn (Family Medicine). (506)457-2113

MULLAN, Michael J; Appletree Med Group, 4-150 Robertson Rd, Ottawa ON K2H 9S1; London (England)'70; MB BS; MRCS; LRCP; MRCP(UK); (613)482-0118; Fax. (613)680-6420.

MULLAN, Robert D; Centennial Prof Centre, 81 Exhibition St, Kentville NS B4N 1C2; Dal'81; BSc; CCFP; FCFP; Med Dir, Kings Regional Rehabilitation Centre; (902)678-4113; Fax. (902)678-1977; mullan@ns.sympatico.ca.

MULLAN, Terence J G; Bedford Family Care Assoc, 204-967 Bedford Hwy, Bedford NS B4A 1A9; Dal'87; Staff Family Med, IWK Health Centre; Physician, Cobequid Health Service Centre; Preceptor Family Med, Dalhousie University; (902)835-6200; Fax. (902)832-7100.

MULLARD, David P; Delta Mental Health Team, 129-6345 120 St, Delta BC V4E 2A6; London (England)'70; MB; BSc; (604)592-3700

MULLEN, Glen E; 209-155 Main St E, Grimsby ON L3M 1P2; Tor'76; Gen Practice, West Lincoln Memorial Hospital; (905)945-4811; Fax. (905)945-4491.

MULLEN, J Brendan M; Mount Sinai Hosp, 600 University Ave, Toronto ON M5G 1X5; Ott'77; FRCPC; AnatPath. Staff Path, Mount Sinai Hospital; Assoc Prof Path, University of Toronto; (416)586-4800 x4553; bmullen@mtsinai.on.ca.

MULLEN, John C; University of Alberta Hosp, 2D218-8440 112 St NW, Edmonton AB T6G 2B7; Tor'83; ABS; AB; MSc(Tor.); FRCSC; GenSurg (Cardiac Surgery); Cardiovasc&ThorSurg. Dir Heart Transplant Prog, University of Alberta Hospital; Clin Prof Surg, University of Alberta; (780)407-6327; Fax. (780)407-6752; jmullen@ualberta.ca.

MULLEN, Timothy J; Queen Elizabeth II HSC, 1276 South Park St, Halifax NS B3H 2Y9; Qns'06; Anes. Staff, Queen Elizabeth II Health Sciences Centre - Victoria General Site; (902)473-2700; Fax. (902)423-9454.

MULLENS, Jean L; 576 Main St E, Hamilton ON L8M 1J2; McM'82; CCFP; FCFP; Staff, St Joseph's Healthcare - Charlton Campus; Court Staff, Hamilton Health Sciences Centre - McMaster Children's Hospital; (905)528-5292; Fax. (905)528-7753.

MULLER, Andries J; West Winds Primary Hlth Ctr, 3311 Fairlight Dr, Saskatoon SK S7M 3Y5; Pretoria (South Africa)'91; MMed; MB ChB; CCFP; Staff, Royal University Hospital; Assoc Prof Family Med, University of Saskatchewan; Langs: Afrikaans; (306)655-4200; Fax. (306)655-4894.

MULLER, Anton M; Biggar & Dist Health Centre, PO Box 70, Biggar SK S0K 0M0; Pretoria (South Africa)'88; MB ChB; CCFP; (306)948-3331; Fax. (306)948-5060; anton@diamondresorts.com.

MULLER, Diederik J; Shoal Lake-Strathclair H Ctr, PO Box 490 524 Mary St, Shoal Lake MB R0J 1Z0; Pretoria (South Africa)'84; MB ChB; CCFP; FCFP; Fam Med, Shoal Lake/Strathclair Health Centre; Langs: Afrikaans; (204)759-2755; Fax. (204)759-2264; diederikmuller@hotmail.com.

MULLER, Florian L; Homewood Health Centre, 150 Delhi St, Guelph ON N1E 6K9; Wes'05; CCFP; Staff, Homewood Health Centre; (519)824-1010

MULLER, Francois; Downtown Med Centre, 622 Courtney St, Victoria BC V8W 1C1; Orange Free State (South Africa)'96; MB ChB; (250)380-2210

MULLER, Jacobus M; Bonnyville Med Clinic, PO Box 1007 Stn Main, Bonnyville AB T9N 2J7; (South Africa)'92; CCFP; (780)826-3346; Fax. (780)826-6362; jmuller@mcsnet.ca.

MULLER, Marlene; Downtown Med Centre, 622 Courtney St, Victoria BC V8W 1C1; Orange Free State (South Africa)'96; MB ChB; (250)380-2210

MULLER, Matthew P; St Michael's Hosp, 4 179-30 Bond St, Toronto ON M5B 1W8; Tor'97; FRCPC; IntMed; InfectDis. Staff, St Michael's Hospital; (416)864-5568

MULLER, Nestor L; 3350-950 10th Ave W, Vancouver BC V5Z 1M9; Porto Alegre (Brazil)'72; PhD; FRCPC; DiagRad. Ac Staff, Vancouver General Hospital - Centennial Pavillion; Prof/Dept Head Radiol, University of British Columbia; (604)875-4165; Fax. (604)875-4319; nmuller@vanhosp.bc.ca.

MULLER, Paul J; St Michael's Hosp, 3086-30 Bond St, Toronto ON M5B 1W8; Tor'69; MSc; FRCSC; Neursurg (Neuro Oncology). Staff Neurosurg, St Michael's Hospital; Prof Surg, University of Toronto; (416)864-5590; Fax. (416)864-5017.

MULLER, Petra; 312 3 St E PO Box 487, Oyen AB T0J 2J0; (South Africa)'04; MB ChB; (403)664-3577; Fax. (403)664-3323.

MULLER, Pieter E; Regina Qu'Appelle HR-Regina, 1440 14th Ave, Regina SK S4P 0W5; Stellenbosch (South Africa)'86; MB ChB; Staff, Pasqua Hospital; Staff, Regina General Hospital; (306)766-4444

MULLER, Samuel J; Strathmore Med Clinic, 216 Fourth Ave, Strathmore AB T1P 1B9; (South Africa)'89; MB ChB; CCFP; Staff Obstetrical, Lougheed Maternity Group; (403)361-2422; Fax. (403)361-2420.

MULLER, Thian; 316 8th Ave W PO Box 700 Stn Main, Brooks AB T1R 1B6; (South Africa)'98; (403)793-8883; Fax. (403)793-8890.

MULLER DELGADO, Hellmuth A; Manitoba Clinic, 790 Sherbrook St, Winnipeg MB R3A 1M3; (El Salvador)'80; FRCSC; OrthSurg. Langs: French; Spanish; Fax. (204)783-6558.

MULLIE, Marc A; Centre Med Rene-Laennec, 201-1100 av Beaumont, Mont-Royal QC H3P 3H5; Tor'78; FRCSC; Ophth (Refractive Surgery). Langs: Bilingual(English/French); (514)738-6666; Fax. (514)738-1769.

MULLIGAN, Anna M; Univ Hlth Network-Toronto Gen, 200 Elizabeth St, Toronto ON M5G 2C4; Dublin (Ireland)'96; Staff, Toronto General Hospital - UHN; (416)360-4000

MULLIGAN, John M; Polyclinic Prof Centre Inc, 308-199 Grafton St, Charlottetown PE C1A 1L2; Dal'89; FRCSC; Urol. (902)629-8862; Fax. (902)629-8863.

MULLIGAN, Matthew D; Montfort Hosp, 713 Montreal Rd, Ottawa ON K1K 0T2; Ott'02; FRCPC; IntMed. Staff, Montfort Hospital; Langs: Bilingual(English/French); (613)746-4621; Fax. (613)748-4995.

MULLIGAN, Patrick K; Thunder Bay Med Centre, 410-63 Algoma St N, Thunder Bay ON P7A 4Z6; Tor'01; CCFP; (807)343-0443; Fax. (807)343-0812.

MULLIN, James G; 315 Stewart St, Ottawa ON K1N 6K5; Ott'71; FRCPC; Psy. (613)789-8282

MULLIN, Roger A; Lakeridge Hlth Corp-Oshawa, 1 Hospital Crt, Oshawa ON L1G 2B9; Tor'71; Ac Staff Anes, Lakeridge Health - Oshawa Site; (905)576-8711; roger.mullin@sympatico.ca.

MULLIN, Stephanie E; Southland Sports Medicine, 2000 Southland Dr SW, Calgary AB T2V 4S4; Alb'08; CCFP; (403)251-9535; Fax. (403)252-9021.

MULLINS, Eugene; Topsail Road Med Clinic, 644 Topsail Rd, St. John's NL A1E 2E2; Mem'86; (709)368-2101; Fax. (709)368-6686.

MULLINS, Rosalind; 1802-45 Alderney Dr, Dartmouth NS B2Y 2N6; McM'04; CCFP; Physician, Orthopaedic & Sport Med Clinic of NS; (902)405-3200; Fax. (902)446-6886.

MULLOY, John V; New Sudbury Med Clinic, 105-1122 Lasalle Blvd, Sudbury ON P3A 1Y4; Wes'79; MCFP(EM); FCFP; Ac Staff, Health Sciences North - Memorial Site; Asst Prof, University of Ottawa; (705)566-5151

MULLOY, Robert H; Suitor House, 1004 8 Ave SE, Calgary AB T2G 0M4; Cal'82; FRCSC; GenSurg (Laparoscopic Surgery). Clin Assoc Prof, University of Calgary; (403)264-6720; Fax. (403)237-0167.

MULPURI, Udaya K K; Children's & Women's HC of BC, A207 A-4480 Oak St, Vancouver BC V6H 3V4; Kasturba (India)'95; Staff, BC Children's Hospital; Langs: Hindi; Telugu; (604)875-2054

MULPURU, Sunita S; The Ottawa Hosp-Civic Campus, 1053 Carling Ave, Ottawa ON K1Y 4E9; McM'06; FRCPC; IntMed; Respir. Staff, The Ottawa Hospital - General Campus; Staff, The Ottawa Hospital - Civic Campus; (613)737-8899; Fax. (613)761-4152.

MULROY, Brendan J; Grey Bruce HS-Owen Sound, PO Box 1800 Stn Main 1800 8th St E, Owen Sound ON N4K 6M9; McM'84; CCFP; FCFP; Ac Staff, Grey Bruce Health Services - Owen Sound; (519)376-2121; Fax. (519)376-9970.

MULROY, Liam A; Nova Scotia Cancer Centre, 2026-5820 University Ave, Halifax NS B3H 1V7; Wes'86; FRCPC; RadOncol. Med Staff, Queen Elizabeth II Health Sciences Centre - Victoria General Site; Dalhousie University; (902)473-6096; Fax. (902)473-7205.

MULSANT, Benoit H; Addiction & Mental Hlth-Queen, 1001 Queen St W, Toronto ON M6J 1H4; Laval'84; FRCPC; Psy. Staff, Centre for Addiction & Mental Health (CAMH) - Queen Site; (416)535-8501; Fax. (416)260-4189.

MULVEY, Jamin M; Alberta Children's Hosp, 2888 Shaganappi Trail NW, Calgary AB T3B 6A8; (Austria)'03; MB BS; Staff, Alberta Children's Hospital; (403)955-7211; Fax. (403)955-7606.

MULVEY, Michael R; The Electra Health, MZ1-970 Burrard St, Vancouver BC V6Z 2R4; Ponce (Puerto Rico)'00; BSc; FRCPC; Psy. (604)685-4325

MULZER, Paul G G; Sister Margaret Smith Centre, 301 Lillie St N, Thunder Bay ON P7C 0A6; McM'88; CSAM; FRCPC; Psy (Addiction Psychiatry). Staff, Thunder Bay Regional Health Sciences Centre; Physician, St Joseph Care Group; Physician, Sister Margaret Smith Centre; (807)684-5100; Fax. (807)622-1779.

MULZET, Darlana L; 178 101-1001 Broadway W, Vancouver BC V6H 4E4; UBC'99; CCFP; (604)874-5555

MUMERT, Donna J; IMJ Med Clinic, 106-10055 120 Ave, Grande Prairie AB T8V 8H8; Alb'92; CCFP; (780)532-4415; Fax. (780)532-4559.

MUMFORD, David A; First Med Place, 201-170 Queensway W, Mississauga ON L5B 3A8; McM'88; FRCSC; GenSurg (Laparoscopic Surgery). Consultant GenSurg, Trillium Health Centre - Mississauga; (905)276-7211; Fax. (905)276-6486.

MUMMERY, Martin R; Chilliwack Gen Hosp, 45600 Menholm Rd, Chilliwack BC V2P 1P7; Man'84; CCFP; CCFP(E.M.); Staff, Chilliwack General Hospital; (604)795-4141 x4283

MUMTAZ, Shariq; Health Sciences Centre, 4102-300 Prince Philip Dr, St. John's NL A1B 3V6; Karachi (Pakistan)'89; MB BS; Staff, Health Sciences Centre; (709)777-6300

MUNCEY, Joy A; Care Place Med Centre, 306-9014 152 St, Surrey BC V3R 4E7; Alb'91; CCFP; (604)581-3550; Fax. (604)581-4478.

MUNCNER, Amira; Castledowns Medicentre, 120-15277 Castle Downs Rd NW, Edmonton AB T5X 3N5; Palacky (Czech Republic)'80; Langs: Czech; Slovak; Serbo-Croatian; (780)457-5511; Fax. (780)456-4004; amiramuncner@hotmail.com.

MUNCNER, Peter; 2520 Tudor Glen, St. Albert AB T8N 3V3; Palacky (Czech Republic)'80; (780)458-5776; Fax. (780)460-1908.

MUNDENCHIRA, Amitha J; Postmaster Med Clinic, 2540 Postmaster Dr, Oakville ON L6M 0N2; Tor'02; BSc; CCFP; Langs: Hindi; Malayalam; (905)844-1700; Fax. (905)844-1705.

MUNDI, Christina; Montfort Hosp, 713 Montreal Rd, Ottawa ON K1K 0T2; Ott'97; CCFP; FCFP; Staff, Montfort Hospital; Langs: Hungarian; French; (613)945-1456

MUNDLE, R Murray; Queen Elizabeth Hosp, PO Box 6600 Stn Central 60 Riverside Dr, Charlottetown PE C1A 8T5; McG'59; MA; Urol., Queen Elizabeth Hospital; (902)894-2111

MUNDLE, William R; Windsor Reg Hosp-Metropolitan, 1995 Lens Ave, Windsor ON N8W 1L9; Mem'92; BSc; BMedSci; FRCSC; ObstGyn (Maternal Fetal Medicine). Med Dir Div of Maternal Fetal Med, Windsor Regional Hospital - Metropolitan Site; (519)254-5577 x52231; Fax. (519)256-6127; wrmundle@wrh.on.ca.

MUNDY, Ron; 108-4330 Sunshine Coast Hwy RR 1, Sechelt BC V0N 3A1; UBC'82; Staff, St Mary's Hospital; (604)485-6400; Fax. (604)885-6411.

MUNG, Dennis G; Gateway Village, 236-2 Hebert Rd, St. Albert AB T8N 5T8; Alb'84; (780)459-2997; Fax. (780)459-2998.

MUNGARA, Sunil K; 245 Eglinton Ave E, Toronto ON M4P 3B7; St. Maarten (Netherlands Antilles)'04; CCFP; (416)488-1455

MUNGER, Andre; CLSC de Sherbrooke, 50 rue Camirand, Sherbrooke QC J1H 4J5; Sher'76; (819)565-1330

MUNI, Rajeev H; 801-61 Queen St E, Toronto ON M5C 2T2; McM'02; FRCSC; Ophth (Retina Vitreous Surgery). Staff Retina Service, St Michael's Hospital; Staff Retina Service, The Hospital For Sick Children; Asst Prof Opht & Vision Screnes, University of Toronto; Langs: Gujarati; Hindi; French; (416)867-7411; Fax. (416)867-7491.

MUNISWAMAPPA SAMPATH, Nagendra; 203-3939 Quadra St, Victoria BC V8X 1J5; Mysore (India)'02; MB BS; (450)479-7005

MUNIZ RODRIGUEZ, Flor M; Hamilton HS-General Site, 237 Barton St E, Hamilton ON L8L 2X2; Santo Domingo (Dominican Republic)'93; FRCPC; PhysMed&Rehab (Acquired Brain Injury Rehabilitation). Staff, Hamilton Health Sciences Centre - Hamilton General Hospital; Staff, Hamilton Health Sciences Centre - McMaster Children's Hospital; Langs: Spanish; (905)521-2100; Fax. (905)577-8233.

MUNK, Marla R; Yonge-Eglinton Med Centre, 202-2401 Yonge St, Toronto ON M4P 3H1; Tor'01; CCFP; Assoc Staff, Toronto Western Hospital - University Health Network; (416)322-3700; Fax. (416)322-3707; m.munk@utoronto.ca.

MUNK, Paul; Medical & Dental Bldg, 202-1849 Yonge St, Toronto ON M4S 1Y2; Tor'70; FRCPC; Peds. Staff, The Hospital For Sick Children; Asst Prof, University of Toronto; Langs: Hungarian; (416)483-3105; Fax. (416)488-3969; paul.munk@utoronto.ca.

MUNK, Peter L; 899 12th Ave W, Vancouver BC V5Z 1M9; McG'83; FRCPC; DiagRad (Interventional Radiology). Staff, Vancouver General Hospital - Centennial Pavillion; Staff, BC Children's Hospital; Prof Diag Rad & OrthSurg, University of British Columbia; (604)875-4111 x63711; Fax. (604)875-5195.

MUNKLEY, Douglas P; 6453 Morrison St, Niagara Falls ON L2E 7H1; Tor'78; MCFP(EM); Staff, Niagara Health System - Greater Niagara General Site; (905)374-2966

MUNN, Catharine J; McMaster Univ Health Centre, 1280 Main St W, Hamilton ON L8S 4K1; McM'95; Psy. (905)525-9140

MUNN, Matthew B; Foothills Med Centre, C231-1403 29 St NW, Calgary AB T2N 2T9; Qns'07; CCFP; CCFP(E.M.); Staff, Foothills Medical Centre; (403)944-1110

MUNN, Robert I; 201-1100 Sheppard Ave E, North York ON M2K 2W1; Wes'84; FRCPC; Peds (Child Neurology); Neur. Staff, William Osler Health System - Etobicoke General Hospital; Staff, North York General Hospital; Asst Prof Peds, University of Toronto; (416)225-1531; Fax. (416)225-3728; robmunn@sympatico.ca.

MUNNINGS, Donald B; First Med Place, 201-170 Queensway W, Mississauga ON L5B 3A8; Tor'74; AB; FACS; FRCSC; GenSurg. Staff, Trillium Health Centre - Mississauga; (905)276-7211; Fax. (905)276-6486.

MUNNOCH, Katherine M; B-640 Ross Ave E, Timmins ON P4N 8P2; Qns'04; FRCSC; ObstGyn. (705)268-0966; Fax. (705)268-0964.

MUNOZ, Carlos; 885 38e av, Lachine QC H8T 2C4; Moscow (Russia (Federation))'71; Staff, Lakeshore General Hospital - Pointe Claire; (514)634-6322; Fax. (514)634-6322.

MUNOZ, David G; St Michael's Hosp, 30 Bond St, Toronto ON M5B 1W8; Navarra (Spain)'76; MSc(Path,Qns); FRCPC; NeurPath (Brain Tumors). Staff, St Michael's Hospital; (416)864-5858

MUNOZ, Gabriel; CHUM-Hop St-Luc, 1058 rue Saint-Denis, Montreal QC H2X 1J4; (Cuba)'80; Staff, Centre Hospitalier l'Université De Montréal (CHUM) - Hôpital Saint-luc; (514)890-8000

MUNOZ, Juan E; McMaster Family Practice, A-690 Main St W, Hamilton ON L8S 1A4; (Spain)'72; PhD; MClSc(FamMed); CCFP; FCFP; Ac Staff, Hamilton Health Sciences Centre - McMaster Children's Hospital; Prof Family Med, McMaster University; Langs: Spanish; Portuguese; (905)521-5015; Fax. (905)521-5010; munozj@mcmaster.ca.

MUNOZ, Marie; Clinique l'Actuel, 1001 boul de Maisonneuve E, Montreal QC H2L 4P9; Mon'96; Langs: Spanish; Italian; (514)524-1001; mariemunoz@sympatico.ca.

MUNOZ, Michael A; 150 Strickland Rd, Lakefield ON K0L 2H0; McG'89; BSc; CCFP; Ac Staff EmergMed, QHC North Hastings; Teach Staff Family Med, University of Ottawa; (705)651-0222; mmunoz@bancroftfht.com.

MUNRO, A Ian; Laurel Med Centre, 308-888 8th Ave W, Vancouver BC V5Z 3Y1; London (England)'55; MB BS(Eng); FRCS; FRCSC; Cardiovasc&ThorSurg (Medico Legal Surg). (604)876-7821

MUNRO, Camille; The Ottawa Hosp-Gen Campus, 501 Smyth Rd, Ottawa ON K1H 8L6; Dal'91; CCFP; Staff, The Ottawa Hospital - General Campus; (613)737-8940; Fax. (613)739-6182.

MUNRO, David; 216 Wharncliffe Rd N, London ON N6H 2B4; Wes'73; Court Staff, St Joseph's Hospital - St Joseph's Health Care; Court Staff, London Health Sciences Centre - Victoria Campus; (519)438-2464

MUNRO, Diane E; 5-23 Dairy Lane, Huntsville ON P1H 1T4; Tor'80; (705)788-3565; Fax. (705)788-1858.

MUNRO, Shane M; Greenbank Med Centre, 102-139 Greenbank Rd, Nepean ON K2H 9A5; Dal'91; FRCSC; Ophth. (613)829-2031; Fax. (613)829-2274.

MUNRO, Susan L; Thamesview Family Health Team, 465 Grand Ave W, Chatham ON N7L 1C5; McM'76; CCFP; Medical Staff, Chatham-Kent Health Alliance; (519)354-5540; Fax. (519)354-6120.

MUNROE, Alan R; 202-1789 Mountain Rd, Moncton NB E1G 5C4; Dal'84; CCFP; FCFP; (506)387-7787; Fax. (506)387-3921.

MUNROE, Tanya M; Fundy Trail Med Centre, 68 Robie St, Truro NS B2N 1L2; Dal'97; CCFP; CCFP(E.M.); FCFP; (902)895-7973; Fax. (902)895-3784.

MUNSAMY, Gonasagran K; Victoria Gen Hosp, 2340 Pembina Hwy, Winnipeg MB R3T 2E8; Natal (South Africa)'95; CCFP; Staff, Victoria General Hospital; (204)269-3570; gmunsamy@rha-central.mb.ca.

MUNSHI, Alpna; Addiction & Mental Hlth-Clarke, 833-250 College St, Toronto ON M5T 1R8; Dal'06; FRCPC; Psy. Staff, Centre for Addiction & Mental Health (CAMH) - College Street Site; (416)535-8501; Fax. (416)979-6815.

MUNSHI, Autar K; 303-319 Charlotte St, Sydney NS B1P 1E1; Jammu-Kashmir (India)'70; MB BS; DPM(Lond); MRCPsy(UK); FRCPC; Psy (Psychotherapy). Langs: Hindi; Urdu; Kashmiri; (902)562-2323; Fax. (902)562-5147.

MUNSHI, Laveena; Transplant Office, NCSB 11C-585 University Ave, Toronto ON M5G 2N2; Dal'07; IntMed. (416)340-4800

MUNSHI, Muhammad; Trillium Hlth Ctr-Mississauga, 100 Queensway W, Mississauga ON L5B 1B8; Tor'96; FRCPC; DiagRad. Staff, Trillium Health Centre - Mississauga; (905)848-7100 x3991

MUNSHI, Tariq A; Frontenac Clin Services Dept, 385 Princess St, Kingston ON K7L 1B9; Karachi (Pakistan)'92; (613)544-1356; Fax. (613)544-2346.

MUNT, Bradley I; St Paul's Hosp, W5C-1081 Burrard St, Vancouver BC V6Z 1Y6; UBC'86; BSc; FACC; FRC; ACLS; FRCPC; IntMed (Coronary Care); Cardiol. Staff, Providence Health Care - St Paul's Hospital; Clin Instructor, University of British Columbia; (604)806-8018; Fax. (604)806-8410; bmunt@providencehealth.bc.ca.

MUNZ, Diane L; 4569 rue Sherbrooke O, Westmount QC H3Z 1E9; McG'76; ABPeds; FRCPC; Peds (Adolescent Medicine). Att Staff Emerg Room, McGill University Health Centre - Montreal Children's Hospital; Physician, Philip Layton School for the Blind; Consultant, MacKay Rehabilitation Centre; adj Prof, McGill University; Langs: Bilingual(English/French); (514)933-8437; Fax. (514)933-6398.

MUNZAR, Michael R; 104-175 av Stillview, Pointe-Claire QC H9R 4S3; McG'79; (514)694-9282; Fax. (514)697-0192.

MUOTOH, Ikegwuonu C; 806-19369 Sheriff King St SW, Calgary AB T2X 0T9; (Nigeria)'94; CCFP; (403)873-7300

MURA, Marco; London HSC-South Street, PO Box 5375 Stn B 375 South St, London ON N6A 4G5; Bologna (Italy)'01; Staff, London Health Sciences Centre - South Street; Staff, London Health Sciences Centre - Victoria Campus; (519)667-6744; Fax. (519)667-6552.

MURABIT, Amera; University of Alberta Hosp, 8440 112 St NW, Edmonton AB T6G 2B7; Sask'06; FRCSC; PlasSurg. Staff, University of Alberta Hospital; (780)945-0560

MURACA, Maria; North York Family Health Team, 701-240 Duncan Mill Rd, North York ON M3B 3S6; Tor'03; MSc; CCFP; Staff, North York General Hospital; Assoc Prof, University of Toronto; Langs: Italian; (416)229-6300

MURAD, Khulood J; 150 Rolling Hills Dr, Orangeville ON L9W 4X8; Basra (Iraq)'91; FRCSC; ObstGyn. (519)938-5648; Fax. (519)938-5667.

MURAD, Moazzam; Cape Breton Hlthcare Complex, 1482 George St, Sydney NS B1P 1P3; Karachi (Pakistan)'91; MB BS; FRCPC; DiagRad. Staff, Cape Breton Healthcare Complex; (902)567-8000

MURAD, Nazar J; University Hosp of Northern BC, 1475 Edmonton St, Prince George BC V2M 1S2; Basra (Iraq)'94; Staff, University Hospital of Northern British Columbia; (250)565-2000

MURADALI, Derek; St Michael's Hosp, 30 Bond St, Toronto ON M5B 1W8; McG'88; FRCPC; DiagRad. Staff Med Imaging, St Michael's Hospital; (416)864-5652; Fax. (416)864-5380.

MURALEETHARAN, Nageswary; Good Steth Med Clinic, 112-6055 Steeles Ave E, Scarborough ON M1X 0A7; Jaffna (Sri Lanka)'93; MB BS; CCFP; Langs: Tamil; (416)626-6161

MURAM, Bhanu P; Family Wellness Place, 48 Commonwealth Ave, Mount Pearl NL A1N 5B6; Madras (India)'80; MB BS; FRCPC; Peds (Allergic Disorders). Physician, Regional Advisory Board of Glaxo; Clin Associate Prof Peds, Memorial University Of Newfoundland; (709)364-6650

MURAT, Brian W; Huntsville Prof Bldg, 206-348 Muskoka Rd 3 N, Huntsville ON P1H 1H8; Qns'85; ABIM; FRCPC; IntMed; Gastroent. Staff, Huntsville District Memorial Hospital - Muskoka Algonquin Healthcare; Consultant, South Muskoka Memorial Hospital - Muskoka Algonquin Healthcare; (705)789-3900; Fax. (705)787-1808.

MURATA, Ariana M A; Univ of Toronto, 263 McCaul St, Toronto ON M5T 1W7; Ott'05; CCFP; CCFP(E.M.).

MURATOGLU, Mikael S; Grey Nuns Community Hosp, 1100 Youville Drive West NW, Edmonton AB T6L 5X8; (Turkey)'82; ABPN; Staff, University of Alberta Hospital; Staff, Covenant Health - Grey Nuns Community Hospital; (780)735-9626; Fax. (780)735-9631.

MURCHISON, Sylvia A; 233-355 Wellington St, London ON N6A 3N7; Wes'00; CCFP; (519)432-1919; Fax. (519)432-2566.

MURDOCH, Jason E E; Caroline Family Hlth Team-BFMG, 205-3155 Harvester Rd, Burlington ON L7N 3V2; McM'00; (905)639-9717; Fax. (905)639-6132.

MURDOCH, John A C; Kingston Gen Hosp, 76 Stuart St, Kingston ON K7L 2V7; Glasgow (Scotland)'91; FRCPC; Anes. Staff Anes, Kingston General Hospital; (613)533-2952; Fax. (613)548-1375.

MURDOCH, John L; Cole Harbour Family Med Centre, 203-240 Baker St, Dartmouth NS B2W 6L4; Dal'84; BSc; FACS; FRCSC; GenSurg (Laparoscopic Surgery). Consultant Surgeon, Canadian Forces Base-Stadacona Hosp; (902)435-6312; Fax. (902)434-7920.

MURDOCH, Stuart A; Royal Victoria Hosp, 201 Georgian Dr, Barrie ON L4M 6M2; McM'88; CCFP; FCFP; Staff, Royal Victoria Regional Health Centre; (705)792-3333; Fax. (705)728-4120.

MURDOCK, Alan I; 3 Bellevue Cres, St. Albert AB T8N 0A5; McG'63; PhD; FRCPC; Peds (Neuro Development Pediatrics). Ac Staff, Glenrose Rehabilitation Hospital; Ac Staff, Royal Alexandra Hospital; Ac Staff, Sturgeon Community Hospital; Member Faculty Neurodevelopement Div, University of Alberta; (780)460-3059; Fax. (780)460-3058.

MURDOCK, H Ward; Fredericton Med Clinic, 304-1015 Regent St, Fredericton NB E3B 6H5; Dal'82; FRCSC; ObstGyn. (506)457-2113; Fax. (506)459-7073.

MURESAN, Letitia V; Centre Medical, 104-3400 rue du Marche, Dollard-D-Ormeaux QC H9B 2Y1; Mon'88; FRCPC; Neur (Alzheimer's Disease); Electroenceph (P.Q.). Staff, Lakeshore General Hospital - Pointe Claire; Langs: Italian; French; Spanish; Romanian; (514)685-4189; Fax. (514)685-3127.

MURFIN, Lynne; Heritage Hill Med Centre, 110-8180 Macleod Trail SE, Calgary AB T2H 2B8; Cape Town (South Africa)'88; MB ChB; CCFP; (403)259-3256; Fax. (403)253-2673.

MURJI, Ally; Hamilton HS-McMaster Site, PO Box 2000 Stn Lcd 1 2F 39-1200 Main St W, Hamilton ON L8N 3Z5; Tor'06; FRCSC; ObstGyn. Staff, Hamilton Health Sciences Centre - McMaster University Medical Centre; (905)521-2100

MURJI, Amin; K-W Urgent Care Clinic, 385 Fairway Rd S, Kitchener ON N2C 2N9; Wes'93; CCFP; (519)748-2327

MURJI, Salma B; Justik Med Centre, 8225 105 St NW, Edmonton AB T6E 4H2; Alb'88; CCFP; FCFP; Physician Family Med, Covenant Health - Grey Nuns Community Hospital; (780)432-0211; Fax. (780)439-9349.

MURJI-MERALI, Karim S; East York Med Health Centre, 27E-45 Overlea Blvd, Toronto ON M4H 1C3; Tor'85; (416)696-9836 x501; Fax. (416)696-8080.

MURKIN, John M; London HSC-University Hosp, PO Box 5339 Stn B 339 Windermere Rd, London ON N6A 5A5; Man'78; FRCPC; Anes. Staff, London Health Sciences Centre - University Hospital; (519)663-3384; Fax. (519)663-3260.

MURLEY, Vanessa R; 210 Melrose Ave, Ottawa ON K1Y 4K7; Ott'01; CCFP; (613)761-4334; Fax. (613)761-4200.

MURNAGHAN, John J; Sunnybrook Holland Ortho Arthr, 319-43 Wellesley St E, Toronto ON M4Y 1H1; Tor'81; BSc; MSc; MA; FRCSC; OrthSurg (Knee Surgery). Ac Staff, Sunnybrook Health Sciences Centre - Holland Orthopaedic & Arthritic Centre; Assoc Prof Surg, University of Toronto; (416)967-8778; Fax. (416)967-8780.

MURNAGHAN, Marion A; Children's Hosp Eastern Ont, 401 Smyth Rd, Ottawa ON K1H 8L1; Mem'07; FRCPC; EmergMed. Staff, Children's Hospital of Eastern Ontario (CHEO); (613)737-7600; Fax. (613)738-3216.

MURNAGHAN, Michael L; The Hosp for Sick Children, 555 University Ave, Toronto ON M5G 1X8; Qns'01; FRCSC; OrthSurg. Staff, The Hospital For Sick Children; (416)813-6414; Fax. (416)813-6414; lucas.murnaghan@sickkids.ca.

MURPHY, Alan S; 12863 54A Ave, Surrey BC V3X 3E1; Sask'74; Staff, Surrey Memorial Hospital; (604)970-3414

MURPHY, Anne M; Saint John Reg Hosp, PO Box 2100 Stn Main 400 University Ave, Saint John NB E2L 4L2; Ott'98; FRCPC; Peds. Staff, Saint John Regional Hospital; (506)648-6141

MURPHY, Bernadine S; 31 Frederick St, Orillia ON L3V 5W5; Tor'85; CCFP; Staff, Orillia Soldiers' Memorial Hospital; (705)327-5225; Fax. (705)327-5226.

MURPHY, Bradley D; Paton Med Centre, 16-1 Paton St, St. John's NL A1B 4S8; Mem'96; FRCSC; Ophth. (709)726-4784

MURPHY, Carol M; Spectrum Health, 702-1080 Howe St, Vancouver BC V6Z 2T1; McG'81; (604)681-1080; Fax. (604)681-0244.

MURPHY, Carole; Hop Louis-H Lafontaine, 7401 rue Hochelaga, Montreal QC H1N 3M5; Mon'87; FRCPC; Psy. Staff, Hopital Louis-H Lafontaine; (514)251-4000 x3060; Fax. (514)251-1604.

MURPHY, Charles W; South East Grey Community HC, PO Box360 55 Victoria St, Markdale ON N0C 1H0; Tor'73; Physician, South East Grey Community Health Centre; (519)986-2222; Fax. (519)986-3999.

MURPHY, Cheryl L; Abbie J Lane Mem Bldg, 6512-5909 Veterans Memorial La, Halifax NS B3H 2E2; Dal'99; BSc; MEd; FRCPC; Psy (Geriatric Psychiatry). (902)473-1422; Fax. (902)473-5713.

MURPHY, Christopher A; Yarmouth Reg Hosp, 403-60 Vancouver St, Yarmouth NS B5A 2P5; Dal'03; FRCSC; GenSurg. Staff, Yarmouth Regional Hospital; (902)881-3232; tracie.ckmurphy@eastlink.ca.

MURPHY, Colleen B; Gordon & Leslie Diamond HCC, 8209-2775 Laurel St, Vancouver BC V5Z 1M9; UBC'98; BSc; FRCPC; Neur. Staff, Gordon & Leslie Diamond Health Care Centre; (604)875-5301

MURPHY, Colm J; CSSS de Laval, 1755 boul Rene-Laennec, Laval QC H7M 3L9; Tor'05; FRCPC; IntMed; Cardiol. Staff, Hopital de la Cite de la santé; (514)245-4939

MURPHY, Daniel B; Ctr Hosp de Verdun, 4000 boul Lasalle, Verdun QC H4G 2A3; McG'98; CCFP; FCFP; Staff, Centre Hospitalier de Verdun; (514)362-1000

MURPHY, David A; 205A-190 Cundles Rd E, Barrie ON L4M 4S5; Manchester (England)'73; MB ChB; DABA; FRCPC; Anes (Pain Management). (705)739-4000; Fax. (705)739-3591.

MURPHY, David G; London HSC-Victoria Hosp, PO Box 5010 Stn B 800 Commissioners Rd E, London ON N6A 5W9; Mem'87; DAB; FRCPC; EmergMed. Staff EmergMed, London Health Sciences Centre - Victoria Campus; Clinical Asst Prof Emerg, University of Western Ontario; (519)667-6538; Fax. (519)667-6769.

MURPHY, Deanna M; Nfld & Labrador Fertility Serv, 103-35 Major's Path, St. John's NL A1A 4Z9; Mem'05; ObstGyn (Gynecological Reproductive Endocrinology). Staff, Central Newfoundland Regional Health Centre.

MURPHY, Emlene M; Youth Forensic Psychiatric Ser, 7900 Fraser Park Dr, Burnaby BC V5J 5H1; Mem'78; FRCPC; Psy (Forensic Psychiatry). Staff, Forensic Psychiatric Hospital; Physician, Youth Forensic Psychiatric Services; Clin Prof Dept of Psy, University of British Columbia; (778)452-2200; emurphy@forensic.bc.ca.

MURPHY, Francis A; 30 Clyde St, Almonte ON K0A 1A0; Belfast (Ireland)'69; MB ChB; BAO; Staff, Almonte General Hospital; Med Dir, Broadview Nursing Home; Med Dir, Almonte Country Haven; (613)256-2323; Fax. (613)256-2692.

MURPHY, Frank R; Dermatology Centre, 132 Young St, Hamilton ON L8N 1V6; McM'77; MSc; DAB; FRCPC; Derm (Psoriasis & Pediatric Dermatology). Hon Staff, Hamilton Health Sciences Centre - McMaster Children's Hospital; Hon Staff, St Joseph's Healthcare - Charlton Campus; (905)524-2048; Fax. (289)375-9073.

MURPHY, George F; Cobequid Commun Health Centre, 40 Freer Lane, Lower Sackville NS B4C 0A2; Dal'82; FRCPC; DiagRad. Ac Staff Radiol, Queen Elizabeth II Health Sciences Centre - Victoria General Site; Staff, Cobequid Community Health Centre; Lecturer, Dalhousie University; (902)869-6532; Fax. (902)869-6121.

MURPHY, Gregory N; K O P I, 500-797 Princess St, Kingston ON K7L 1G1; Qns'90; FRCPC; Anes (Pediatric Anesthesia). (613)344-1202

MURPHY, James J; Children's & Women's HC of BC, ACB K0134-4480 Oak St, Vancouver BC V6H 3V4; New Jersey (USA)'84; AB; FRCSC; GenSurg. Clin Staff, BC Children's Hospital; Asst Prof, University of British Columbia; (604)875-2667; Fax. (604)875-2721.

MURPHY, Jeffrey B; Canadian Forces Supp Unit HCC, 2A-1745 Alta Vista Dr, Ottawa ON K1A 0K6; Ott'95; CCFP; Staff, Canadian Forces Health Services Centre; (613)945-5897; Fax. (613)945-6745.

MURPHY, Joanne S; Dartmouth Gen Hosp, 325 Pleasant St, Dartmouth NS B2Y 4G8; Dal'89; BSc; FRCPC; AnatPath. Staff, Dartmouth General Hospital; Med Examiner, Province of Nova Scotia; Lecturer, Dalhousie University; (902)465-8458

MURPHY, Johanna M; Queen's Univ Etherington Hall, 1008-94 Stuart St, Kingston ON K7L 3N6; Tor'97; FRCPC; IntMed. Staff, Kingston General Hospital; Asst Prof/Prog Dir Internal Med Fellowship, Queen's University; (613)533-2780; Fax. (613)533-6654.

MURPHY, John D; PO Box 8178 Stn Main, Bonnyville AB T9N 2J5; Cork (Ireland)'80; Physician, Bonnyville Healthcare Centre; Clin Teacher, University of Alberta Hospital.

MURPHY, John L; Professional Arts Bldg, 105-100 Arden St, Moncton NB E1C 4B7; Dal'82; FRCSC; GenSurg; VascSurg. Staff, The Moncton Hospital; Lecturer, Dalhousie University; (506)857-5813; Fax. (506)857-5820.

MURPHY, John P; Rouge Valley-Centenary HC, 2867 Ellesmere Rd, Scarborough ON M1E 4B9; (Ireland)'82; FRCR(UK); MRCP; FRCPC; DiagRad. Staff, Rouge Valley Health System - Centenary Health Centre Site; (416)284-8131

MURPHY, John P E; Granville Med Clinic, 2578 Granville St, Vancouver BC V6H 3G8; National (Ireland)'78; MB ChB; (604)733-4700

MURPHY, K Joan; Univ Hlth Network-Princess M, M 700-610 University Ave, Toronto ON M5G 2M9; Cal'76; FRCSC; ObstGyn (Gynecologic Oncology). Staff Gyn Oncologist, Princess Margaret Hospital - University Health Network; Assoc Prof, University of Toronto; (416)946-4043; Fax. (416)946-2288; joan.murphy@uhn.ca.

MURPHY, Karma N; 403-50 Vancouver St, Yarmouth NS B5A 2P4; Alb'03; CCFP; (902)881-3232; Fax. (902)881-3234.

MURPHY, Katie E; 1FD AMB Edmonton Clinic, PO Box 10500 Stn Forces, Edmonton AB T5J 4J5; Mem'06; CCFP; (780)973-4011

MURPHY, Kellie E; 3918-700 University Ave, Toronto ON M5G 1Z5; Wisconsin (USA)'91; FRCSC; ObstGyn. Staff Maternal Fetal Med, Mount Sinai Hospital; Asst Prof, University of Toronto; (416)586-5363; Fax. (416)586-4792.

MURPHY, Kieran P; Univ Hlth Network-Toronto Western Hosp, 432-399 Bathurst St, Toronto ON M5T 2S8; (Ireland)'86; FRCPC; DiagRad. Staff, Toronto Western Hospital - University Health Network; (416)603-5800

MURPHY, Kirk J; Vancouver Hosp-Outpatient Psy, 715 12 Ave W, Vancouver BC V5Z 1M9; Hahnermann University (USA)'87; Staff, Vancouver General Hospital - Centennial Pavillion; (604)875-4794

MURPHY, Leah C; CFB Petawawa, PO Box 9999 Stn Main, Petawawa ON K8H 2X3; Mem'06; CCFP; (613)687-5511

MURPHY, Lindy; South Tower FMC, 710-3031 Hospital Dr NW, Calgary AB T2N 2T8; (South Africa)'90; MB ChB; CCFP; FCFP; Staff, Foothills Medical Centre; (403)944-2304; Fax. (403)270-9652.

MURPHY, M Claire C; Medical & Dental Bldg, 712-586 Eglinton Ave E, Toronto ON M4P 1P2; Tor'92; MMed; CCFP; FCFP; Asst Prof, University of Toronto; (416)440-1880; Fax. (416)440-1106.

MURPHY, M Madeleine H; Medical-Surgical Eye Bldg, 879 Shefford Rd, Gloucester ON K1J 8H9; Ott'80; FRCSC; Ophth;CCFP; Langs: Spanish; (613)741-0960; Fax. (613)741-7338.

MURPHY, Magnus; Rockyview Professional Ctre, 218-1011 Glenmore Trail SW, Calgary AB T2V 4R6; Stellenbosch (South Africa)'87; MB ChB; MMed(ObstGyn); FRCSC; ObstGyn (Pelvic Floor Reconst). Physician, Foothills Medical Centre; Physician, Grace Women's Health Ctre.; Clin Prof, University of Calgary; Dept Chair Anes & Pain Med, University of Alberta; Langs: Afrikaans; (403)692-0440; Fax. (403)692-0442.

MURPHY, Mark E F; Headwaters Health Care Centre, 100 Rolling Hills Dr, Orangeville ON L9W 4X9; Wes'07; CCFP; (519)941-2410

MURPHY, Melanie J; Cottage Med Clinic, PO Box 2140 300 Miette Ave, Jasper AB T0E 1E0; Mem'04; BSc; CCFP; (780)852-4885; Fax. (780)852-2199.

MURPHY, Michael F; 8-120 Clinical Sciences Bldg, 152 University Campus NW, Edmonton AB T6G 2G3; Dal'78; FRCPC; EmergMed; Anes. (780)407-8861; Fax. (780)407-3200.

MURPHY, Michael J; Medical Clinic Associates, 200-3207 30 Ave, Vernon BC V1T 2C6; McG'87; CCFP; FCFP; (250)549-1216

MURPHY, Michael R; Towers Med Clinic, PO Box 480, Evansburg AB T0E 0T0; (Ireland)'78; MB; MRC; DCH; DObst; (780)542-3366; Fax. (780)542-6207.

MURPHY, Michele P G; Antigonish Mall, 133 Church St, Antigonish NS B2G 2E3; Dal'72; Ad Staff Privil, St Martha's Regional Hospital; (902)863-4488; Fax. (902)863-2207.

MURPHY, Nadia L; 125-70 Exhibition St, Kentville NS B4N 4K9; Dal'05; BSc; FRCSC; OrthSurg (Hip & Knee Reconstruction). (902)678-7447; Fax. (902)678-1177.

MURPHY, Nancy; IWK Health Centre, PO Box 9700 Rpo CSC 5850-5980 University Ave, Halifax NS B3K 6R8; McG'96; CCFP; CCFP(E.M.); Staff, Queen Elizabeth II Health Sciences Centre - Victoria General Site; Staff, IWK Health Centre; Langs: English; French; (902)470-8888

MURPHY, Patricia M; St Joseph's Healthcare, 50 Charlton Ave E, Hamilton ON L8N 4A6; McM'79; FRCPC; Psy (Affective Disorders). Staff, St Joseph's Healthcare - Charlton Campus; Asst Prof, McMaster University; (905)522-1155; Fax. (905)521-6059.

MURPHY, Patricia M; 103-1350 England Ave, Courtenay BC V9N 8X6; McM'97; CCFP; CCFP(E.M.); (250)338-1301

MURPHY, Patricia M; Univ Hlth Network-Toronto Gen, 200 Elizabeth St, Toronto ON M5G 2C4; Mem'84; FRCPC; Anes (Cardiac Anesthesia); Critical Care Medicine. Staff, Toronto General Hospital - UHN; Assoc Prof, University of Toronto; (416)340-3227; Fax. (416)340-3698; patricia.murphy@uhn.on.ca.

MURPHY, Patricia; CLSC-CHSLD du Marigot, 250 boul Cartier O, Laval QC H7N 5S5; Mon'90; Université Laval; (450)668-1803; Fax. (450)972-6875.

MURPHY, Patrick G; 296 Metcalfe St, Ottawa ON K2P 1S2; Ott'85; DAB; FACS; BSc; FRCSC; Otol (Sleep Apnea). Staff, The Ottawa Hospital - Riverside Campus; Staff, The Ottawa Hospital - General Campus; Staff, Children's Hospital of Eastern Ontario (CHEO); University of Ottawa; (613)235-0469; Fax. (613)235-1374.

MURPHY, Patti E; The Ottawa Hosp-Civic Campus, B309-1053 Carling Ave, Ottawa ON K1Y 4E9; Cal'89; FRCPC; Anes. Staff, The Ottawa Hospital - Civic Campus; (613)761-4169; Fax. (613)761-5209.

MURPHY, Paul E; Gibsons Med Clinic, 211-1100 Sunshine Coast Hwy, Gibsons BC V0N 1V7; Liverpool (England)'94; (604)886-2868

MURPHY, Paul F; Howie Center, 2372 Kings Rd, Sydney NS B1L 1C1; Dal'74; CCFP; Head Physiol & Biophysics, Dalhousie University; (902)539-8780; Fax. (902)539-8653.

MURPHY, Paul H; Medical Arts Bldg, 208-750 Spadina Cres E, Saskatoon SK S7K 3H3; Sask'85; FRCSC; Ophth (Glaucoma). Dir Glaucoma Unit, Saskatoon City Hospital; Clin Prof, University of Saskatchewan; (306)242-9990; Fax. (306)244-1909; hamiltonmurphy@sasktel.net.

MURPHY, Ronald G; M16-15 Elizabeth St, Orangeville ON L9W 3X3; Mem'82; FRCPC; Peds. (519)942-3501; Fax. (519)942-3502.

MURPHY, Ronald J; 88 Estey Lane, Fredericton NB E3A 5N3; Dal'75; (506)458-0247; Fax. (506)458-0264.

MURPHY, Ross W; The Moncton Hosp, 135 MacBeath Ave, Moncton NB E1C 6Z8; Wes'75; FRCSC; GenSurg. Ac Staff Surg, The Moncton Hospital; Consultant, Dr Georges-L-Dumont University Hospital Centre; Clin Instructor Surg, Dalhousie University; (506)857-5111; rwmurphy@nbnet.nb.ca.

MURPHY, Sean F; IWK Health Centre, PO Box 9700 Rpo CSC 5850-5980 University Ave, Halifax NS B3K 6R8; Mem'07; ObstGyn. Staff, IWK Health Centre; (902)470-8888

MURPHY, Sean W; Health Sciences Centre, 300 Prince Philip Dr, St. John's NL A1B 3V6; Mem'93; FRCPC; FRCPC; Nephrol; IntMed. Staff, Health Sciences Centre; Asst Prof Med, Memorial University Of Newfoundland; (709)777-7226; Fax. (709)777-6995.

MURPHY, Stephen T; West Coast Med Consultants, 304-2 Herald Ave, Corner Brook NL A2H 4B5; Mem'95; FRCPC; IntMed; Nephrol. (709)639-9181

MURPHY, Terence P; Anaesthetic Services, 213-2186 Oak Bay Ave, Victoria BC V8R 1G3; UBC'94; FRCPC; Anes. Staff Anes, Victoria General Hospital; (250)595-7211; Fax. (250)595-7211.

MURPHY, Timothy A; Lake Country Family Practice, 1-9966 Pollard Rd, Winfield BC V4V 1Z4; UBC'81; CCFP; FCFP; Ac Staff, Kelowna General Hospital; (250)766-3938; Fax. (250)766-5231.

MURPHY, William F; South Health Campus, 4448 Front St SE, Calgary AB T3M 1M4; Ott'73; FRCPC; Neur. Staff Neurosciences, Foothills Medical Centre; Clin Assoc Prof, University of Calgary; (403)956-2459; Fax. (403)956-2992.

MURPHY-KAULBECK, Lynn; The Moncton Hosp, 135 MacBeath Ave, Moncton NB E1C 6Z8; McM'96; MSc; FRCSC; ObstGyn (Maternal Fetal Medicine). Staff Maternal Fetal Med, The Moncton Hospital; Asst Prof, Dalhousie University; (506)870-2551; Fax. (506)870-2610; dr.lynn.murphy-kaulbeck@horizonnb.ca.

MURPHY-LAVALLEE, Jessica; CHUM-Hop Notre-Dame, 1560 rue Sherbrooke E, Montreal QC H2L 4M1; McG'98; CSPQ; FRCPC; DiagRad. Staff, Centre Hospitalier l'Université de Montréal (CHUM) - Hôpital Notre-Dame; (514)890-8000

MURPHY-LAVERDIERE, Valerie; CHUQ-Hotel-Dieu de Quebec, 11 Cote-du-Palais, Quebec QC G1R 2J6; Laval'06; CCFP; CCFP(E.M.); Staff, Centre Hospitalier Universitaire de Québec (CHUQ) - Siege Social; (418)525-4444

MURRAY, Alastair M; 4 Strath Humber Crt, Etobicoke ON M9A 4C7; Wes'64; Ac Staff Family Med, Humber River Regional Hospital - Church Street Site; Physician, Boxers & Kickerboxers, Ontario Athletics Commission; Physician, World Boxing Council; Physician, National Boxing & Karate Association of Ontario; (416)234-0333

MURRAY, Alison J; Foothills Med Centre, 47-1403 29 St NW, Calgary AB T2N 2T9; Ott'89; MPH; CCFP; FCFP; Staff, Foothills Medical Centre; Asst Prof, University of Calgary; (403)944-1147; amurray@ucalgary.ca.

MURRAY, Allan G; Heritage Med Research Centre, 260F-107 University Campus NW, Edmonton AB T6G 2S2; Man'84; ABIM(IntMed); ABIM(Nephrol); FRCPC; IntMed (Transplant Nephrology); Nephrol. Att Physician Nephrol & Immunol, University of Alberta Hospital; Assoc Prof Nephrol, University of Alberta; (780)407-8741; allan.murray@ualberta.ca.

MURRAY, Allen R; Royal Alexandra Hosp, 541-10240 Kingsway NW, Edmonton AB T5H 3V9; Cal'75; Ac Staff Emerg, Royal Alexandra Hospital; (780)735-4442

MURRAY, Andrew; Community First Med Clinic, 105-518 Lake St, Nelson BC V1L 4C6; Stellenbosch (South Africa)'74; MB ChB; MClSc; CCFP; FCFP; Chief Staff, Kootenay Lake General Hospital; Langs: Afrikaans; (250)352-5259; Fax. (250)352-0323; office@firstmedical.ca.

MURRAY, Andrew I S; Seymour Med Clinic, 200-1530 7th Ave W, Vancouver BC V6J 1S3; London (England)'59; MB BS; DObstRCOG; DPhysMed(Eng.); FRCPC; PhysMed&Rehab. (604)739-5612; Fax. (604)738-1587.

MURRAY, Ariane; Ctr Hosp de Verdun, 4000 boul Lasalle, Verdun QC H4G 2A3; Mon'05; CCFP; Staff, Centre Hospitalier de Verdun; (514)362-1000

MURRAY, Brian J; Sunnybrook Hlth Sciences Ctre, M1 600-2075 Bayview Ave, Toronto ON M4N 3M5; Tor'95; DAB; FRCPC; Neur (Sleep Medicine). Staff, Women's College Hospital; Asst Prof, University of Toronto; (416)323-6486

MURRAY, Bryan H; 105-911 Yates St, Victoria BC V8V 4X3; Wes'79; Staff, Royal Jubilee Hospital; Staff, Victoria General Hospital; (250)388-3080

MURRAY, C Louise; Children's Hosp Eastern Ont, 401 Smyth Rd, Ottawa ON K1H 8L1; Ott'01; FRCPC; Peds. Staff, Children's Hospital of Eastern Ontario (CHEO); (613)737-7600; Fax. (613)738-4878.

MURRAY, Carolyn; Queensway Med Centre, 300-5307 Canotek Rd, Ottawa ON K1J 9M2; Ott'09; CCFP; (613)746-6223

MURRAY, Cathy M; Health Sciences Centre, 300 Prince Philip Dr, St. John's NL A1B 3V6; Mem'05; FRCPC; IntMed; Endocrin&Metab. Staff, Health Sciences Centre; (709)737-6300

MURRAY, Christian A; Women's College Hosp, 841-76 Grenville St, Toronto ON M5S 1B2; Dal'98; FRCPC; Derm (Skin Cancer). Staff, Women's College Hospital; (416)323-7732; Fax. (416)323-6306.

MURRAY, Christopher B; St Paul's Hosp, 1081 Burrard St, Vancouver BC V6Z 1Y6; Alb'00; FRCPC; Psy. Staff, Providence Health Care - St Paul's Hospital; (604)682-2344 x62422

MURRAY, Craig S; PO Box 56020 Rpo First Ave, Vancouver BC V5L 5E2; McG'97; BSc; CCFP; CCFP(E.M.); Langs: Bilingual(English/French).

MURRAY, Eric J; 374 Emerald St, Kingston ON K7P 3E1; Wes'49; CCFP; FCFP; (613)544-9326; Fax. (613)544-7870.

MURRAY, Gail A; Work Safe BC, 400-224 Esplanade Ave W, North Vancouver BC V7M 1J1; Sask'79.

MURRAY, Gerald P; Health Sciences Centre, 300 Prince Philip Dr, St. John's NL A1B 3V6; Mem'84; FRCSC; Neursurg. Staff, Health Sciences Centre; (709)747-1850; Fax. (709)738-0928.

MURRAY, Gilles; CSSS du Sud de Lanaudière, 911 montee des Pionniers, Terrebonne QC J6V 2H2; Mon'67; Microbio & Infect Dis (P.Q.); MedMicrobiol (Hospitalist). Staff, Centre Hospitalier Pierre le Gardeur; Clin Prof, Universite de Montreal; Langs: Bilingual(English/French); (450)654-7525 x32282; gilles.murray@ssss.gouv.qc.ca.

MURRAY, Harold S; Aberdeen Hosp, 835 East River Rd, New Glasgow NS B2H 3S6; Dal'67; Gastroent. Staff, Aberdeen Regional Hospital; (902)752-4265

MURRAY, Heather E; Kingston Gen Hosp, 76 Stuart St, Kingston ON K7L 2V7; Wes'92; FRCPC; EmergMed. Physician Emerg, Kingston General Hospital; Physician Emerg, Hotel-Dieu Hospital; Assoc Prof EmergMed, Queen's University; (613)548-2368; Fax. (613)548-1374; heather.murray@queensu.ca.

MURRAY, Iain C; 205-8312 McCowan Rd, Unionville ON L3P 8E1; McG'90; MSc; FRCPC; IntMed; Gastroent. Staff, Markham Stouffville Hospital; (905)947-9437; Fax. (905)947-8532; gimurray@rogers.com.

MURRAY, J David; Deer Lodge Centre Inc, 2109 Portage Ave, Winnipeg MB R3J 0L3; Man'75; CCFP; Leader Medical, WRHA - Deer Lodge Centre; Consultant, The Salvation Army Grace Hospital; Asst Prof Section of Geriatric & Family Med, University of Manitoba; (204)831-2131; Fax. (204)889-0430; dmurray@deerlodge.mb.ca.

MURRAY, J Scott; Lorraine Wing Tower C, 201 Deacon St, Pembroke ON K8A 2J6; Ott'75; FRCSC; Urol. Langs: Bilingual(English/French); (613)732-3675 x6652; Fax. (613)732-6347.

MURRAY, Jock A G; Dalhousie Fam Med Spryfield Ct, 27-16 Dentith Rd, Halifax NS B3R 2H9; Dal'92; BSc; MSc; CCFP; CCFP(E.M.); Staff, Queen Elizabeth II Health Sciences Centre - Halifax Infirmary Site; (902)473-1234; Fax. (902)473-4353; jockmurray@yahoo.com.

MURRAY, Jodie; Carling-Broadview Med Bldg, B4-770 Broadview Ave, Ottawa ON K2A 3Z3; Ott'88; (613)725-6260; Fax. (613)725-6243.

MURRAY, Jody L; Ottawa Valley Family Health Te, 95 Spring St, Almonte ON K0A 1A0; Ott'06; CCFP; (613)256-9370; Fax. (613)256-0949.

MURRAY, John A; Lady Dunn Health Centre, PO Box 179 17 Government Rd, Wawa ON P0S 1K0; Ott'83; CCFP; FCFP; Staff, Lady Dunn Health Centre; (705)856-1313; Fax. (705)856-9550.

MURRAY, John D M; Children's After-Hours Clinic, 100-1100 Sheppard Ave E, North York ON M2K 2W1; Tor'60; FRCPC; Peds. Hon Physician, The Hospital For Sick Children; Hon Physician, North York General Hospital; (416)250-5000

MURRAY, John M; 59 Charles St, Sackville NB E4L 3S7; Dal'72; BSc; Staff, Sackville Memorial Hospital; (506)536-0490; Fax. (506)364-8910.

MURRAY, Jonathan; The Professional Centre, 4 Little Rd, Wolfville NS B4P 1P4; Edinburgh (Scotland)'74; BSc; MB ChB; (902)542-1720; Fax. (902)542-1742; jlmurray@xcountry.tv.

MURRAY, Kenneth A; 240-444 St Mary Ave, Winnipeg MB R3C 3T1; Dal'76; DAB; FACS; AB; FRCSC; PlasSurg (Breasts). Staff PlasSurg, St Boniface General Hospital; Prof PlasSurg, University of Manitoba; Staff PlasSurg, Winnipeg Regional Health Authority; (204)944-9982; Fax. (204)956-0595; info@plasticsurgeryassociates.ca.

MURRAY, Kenneth R; Highlands Med Clinic, GD Stn Main, Neils Harbour NS B0C 1N0; Dal'72; CCFP; FCFP; Preceptor, Dalhousie University; (902)336-2200; Fax. (902)336-2228.

MURRAY, Kim P; Albro Lake Med Centre, 6 Primrose St, Dartmouth NS B3A 4C5; Dal'83; (902)465-4444; Fax. (902)463-2717.

MURRAY, Maureen A; Carewest-Sarcee, 3504 Sarcee Rd SW, Calgary AB T3E 2L3; Cal'97; CCFP; FCFP; Staff, Carewest Sarcee Hospice; (403)686-6145; Fax. (403)686-8127.

MURRAY, Maureen E; Anaesthetic Services, 213-2186 Oak Bay Ave, Victoria BC V8R 1G3; Ott'78; FRCPC; Anes. (250)595-7211; Fax. (250)595-7211.

MURRAY, Melanie C M; BC Women's Hosp & Health Ctre, E600B-4500 Oak St, Vancouver BC V6H 3N1; Man'04; BSc; FRCPC; IntMed (HIV); InfectDis. Staff Oak Tree Clinic, BC Women's Hospital & Health Centre; (604)875-2212; Fax. (604)875-3063.

MURRAY, Michael J; Tertiary Services Med Admin, 220-1815 Kirschener St, Kelowna BC V1Y 4N7; Wes'83; CCFP; CCFP(E.M.); (250)862-4008

MURRAY, Michael R; Village Family Physicians, 275 Pictou Rd, Truro NS B2N 2S7; Dal'83; CCFP; FCFP; (902)895-1232; Fax. (902)897-9749.

MURRAY, Michael R; 72 Brant Ave, Brantford ON N3T 5Z8; Dal'96; CCFP; (519)756-4310; Fax. (519)756-7553.

MURRAY, Michele L; Miramichi Reg Hosp, 500 Water St, Miramichi NB E1V 3G5; Dal'04; CCFP; CCFP(E.M.); Staff, Miramichi Regional Hospital; (506)623-3000

MURRAY, Paul M; Phoenix Med Centre, 106-2155 10th Ave, Prince George BC V2M 5J6; Dublin (Ireland)'78; MB BCh; BAO; MRCGPract; DRCOG; Staff, University Hospital of Northern British Columbia; (250)563-5111; Fax. (250)563-3649.

MURRAY, R David; Chinook Reg Hosp, 960 19 St S, Lethbridge AB T1J 1W5; Dal'93; CCFP; CCFP(E.M.); Staff EmergMed, Chinook Regional Hospital; (403)388-6111; Fax. (403)388-6183.

MURRAY, Robert B; Prairie North Health Region, 1092 107th St, North Battleford SK S9A 1Z1; Sask'75; FRCPC; GenPath. Staff Lab, Saskatoon City Hospital; A-Head Dept of Path, University of Saskatchewan; (306)446-7337; Fax. (306)446-4114; murrayr@sdh.sk.ca.

MURRAY, Robert C N; BC Cancer Agency-Vancouver CC, 600 10th Ave W, Vancouver BC V5Z 4E6; Sask'73; FRCPC; IntMed (Lung Cancer). Staff, BC Cancer Agency Vancouver Centre; Staff, Vancouver General Hospital - Centennial Pavillion; (604)877-6000; Fax. (604)877-0585; nmurray@bccancer.bc.ca.

MURRAY, Roya R; Village Family Physicians, 275 Pictou Rd, Truro NS B2N 2S7; Dal'83; CCFP; Ac Staff, Colchester East Hants Health Centre; Teach Staff, Dalhousie University; (902)895-1232; Fax. (902)897-9749.

MURRAY, Sandy J; Central Alberta Prof Centre, 240-5201 43 St, Red Deer AB T4N 1C7; Alb'77; BSc; CCFP; FCFP; (403)342-5400

MURRAY, Scott J; 5743 University Ave, Halifax NS B3H 0A2; Dal'80; FRCPC; Derm (Laser Surgery). Dir Res Training, Queen Elizabeth II Health Sciences Centre - Victoria General Site; Assoc Prof, Dalhousie University; (902)425-8038; Fax. (902)421-1580.

MURRAY, Sean R; 1485 Bancroft Dr, Sudbury ON P3B 1R6; Tor'96; FRCPC; Peds. Staff, Health Sciences North-St Joseph's Health Centre; (705)523-7120; Fax. (705)560-0977.

MURRAY, Shawn K; DJ Mackenzie Bldg, 736-5788 University Ave, Halifax NS B3H 1V8; Dal'94; FRCPC; AnatPath (Gynecological Pathology). Assoc Prof, Dalhousie University; (902)473-3172; shawn.murray@cdha.nshealth.ca.

MURRAY, Shirley Y; Brampton Nuclear Services, 28-470 Chrysler Dr, Brampton ON L6S 0C1; McG'61; DAB; NuclearMed; IntMed. Head Div of Nuclear Med/Staff Phys, Women's College Hospital; Asst Prof, University of Toronto; (905)791-3458; Fax. (905)791-3460.

MURRAY, Timothy I; Port Health Clinic, 7-600 Ontario St, St Catharines ON L2N 7H8; London (England)'76; MB BS; DRCOG; Court Staff, Niagara Health System - St Catharines General Site; (905)934-1666; Fax. (905)934-2595.

MURRAY, Yvonne A A; Royal Victoria Hosp, 201 Georgian Dr, Barrie ON L4M 6M2; McM'93; FRCPC; Anes. Staff, Royal Victoria Regional Health Centre; (705)728-9090 x4207; Fax. (705)739-5613.

MURSCHELL, Warren D; Oakridge Centre South Tower, 203-650 41st Ave W, Vancouver BC V5Z 2M9; Alb'76; BSc; CCFP; CCFP(E.M.); FCFP; Clin Assoc Prof, University of British Columbia; (604)263-3518; Fax. (604)263-9297; wdmurschell@telus.net.

MURSELL, Charlotte H; Saanich Plaza Med Clinic, 3544 Blanshard St, Victoria BC V8X 1W3; Ott'99; CCFP; (250)475-1101

MURTADA DITE AL-SAYED, Sukayna; Glazier Med Centre, 11 Gibb St, Oshawa ON L1H 2J9; Beirut (Lebanon)'00; CCFP; Langs: Arabic; (905)579-1212; Fax. (905)579-1583.

MURTAUGH, Karen E; 102-1100 Walker's Line, Burlington ON L7N 2G3; Qns'04; CCFP; (905)336-3340

MURTAZA, Atif; South Nepean Satellite CHC, 201-4100 Strandherd Dr, Ottawa ON K2J 0V2; Ott'05; CCFP; (613)288-2820; Fax. (613)288-3690.

MURTHA, Albert D; Cross Cancer Institute, 11560 University Ave NW, Edmonton AB T6G 1Z2; Alb'87; FRCPC; RadOncol. Staff, Cross Cancer Institute; (780)432-8517; Fax. (780)432-8380.

MURTHA, William J; Royal Alexandra Hosp, 10240 Kingsway NW, Edmonton AB T5H 3V9; (Australia)'78; Staff, Royal Alexandra Hospital; Asst Prof, University of Alberta; (780)735-4266; Fax. (780)491-5078; wmurtha@ualberta.ca.

MURTHY, Anant N; Trillium Hlth Ctr-Mississauga, 100 Queensway W, Mississauga ON L5B 1B8; Alb'92; FRCPC; IntMed; Critical Care Medicine. Staff Intensive, Trillium Health Centre - Mississauga; (905)848-7663; Fax. (905)804-7744; anantmurthy@pol.net.

MURTHY, Dakshina; Regina Internal Med Specialist, 1821 Rose St, Regina SK S4P 1Z7; Rajiv Gandhi University (India)'85; FRCPC; IntMed; Cardiol. (306)525-6455; Fax. (306)359-1068.

MURTHY, Poornima S; Regina Qu'Appelle HR-Regina, 1440 14th Ave, Regina SK S4P 0W5; (India)'85; MRCP(UK); FRCPC; Peds (Neonatology). Staff Neonatol, Regina General Hospital; (306)766-3485; Fax. (306)766-4149; poornima.murthy@rghealth.ca.

MURTHY, Prashanth; Hamilton HS-McMaster Site, PO Box 2000 Stn Lcd 1 4G37-1200 Main St W, Hamilton ON L8N 3Z5; Bangalore (India)'94; Staff, Hamilton Health Sciences Centre - McMaster University Medical Centre; (905)521-2100

MURTHY, Ravi; Humber Valley Med Centre, 2A-2630 Kipling Ave, Toronto ON M9V 4B9; Kashmir (India)'78; Ac Staff Family Pract & Surg Ass't/Asst, William Osler Health System - Etobicoke General Hospital; Langs: Hindi; Tamil; Punjabi; Urdu; (416)748-2000; Fax. (416)748-2001; ravimurthy54@hotmail.com.

MURTHY, Sanjay; Mount Sinai Hosp, 445-600 University Ave, Toronto ON M5G 1X5; Ott'04; FRCPC; IntMed; Gastroent. Staff, Mount Sinai Hospital; (416)586-5121; Fax. (416)586-3174.

MURTHY, Santhi K; Cove Med Clinic, 1608 Portugal Cove Rd, Port Cv-St Phil NL A1M 3H4; Mem'97; CCFP; (709)895-7255

MURTHY, Srinivas; The Hosp for Sick Children, 555 University Ave, Toronto ON M5G 1X8; McG'06; MDCM; FRCPC; Peds; InfectDis. Staff, The Hospital For Sick Children; (416)813-1500

MURTHY, Trisha R; Cedar Springs Prof Centre, F-960 Cumberland Ave, Burlington ON L7N 3J6; McM'06; FRCPC; Peds. Staff, Joseph Brant Memorial Hospital; (905)634-1311

MURTHY, Vaani V; The Ottawa Hosp-Riverside, 1967 Riverside Dr, Ottawa ON K1H 7W9; Saba (Netherlands Antilles)'10; CCFP; Staff, The Ottawa Hospital - Riverside Campus; (613)738-8400

MURTI, Mahdi; 1221 St Clair Ave W, Toronto ON M6E 1B5; Kiel (Germany)'70; Staff, St Joseph's Health Centre; Staff, Humber River Regional Hospital - Church Street Site; Langs: Chinese; Indonesian; German; (416)654-0124; Fax. (416)654-1627.

MURTI, Michelle; 1221 St Clair Ave W, Toronto ON M6E 1B5; Tor'06; FRCPC; Public Health & Preventive Med;CCFP; (416)654-0124

MURTO, Kimmo T T; Children's Hosp Eastern Ont, 401 Smyth Rd, Ottawa ON K1H 8L1; Ott'89; FRCPC; Anes. Staff Anes, Children's Hospital of Eastern Ontario (CHEO); Langs: Finnish; (613)737-2431

MURTON, Andrew G; Lakeshore Med Group, 502-345 Lakeshore Rd E, Oakville ON L6J 1J5; Tor'80; CCFP; CCFP(E.M.); Ac Staff, St Joseph's Healthcare - Charlton Campus; Assoc Staff, Halton Healthcare Services Corporation - Oakville Site; (905)845-4511; Fax. (905)845-8133.

MURTOZA, Golam; Woodsmere Shopping Centre, 15-630 Peter Robertson Blvd, Brampton ON L6R 1T4; Dhaka (Bangladesh)'92; MB BS; CCFP; Langs: Bengali; (905)793-8868; Fax. (905)793-8957.

MURTY, Hima T; Orleans Medical-Dental Centre, 406-2555 St. Joseph Blvd, Orleans ON K1C 1S6; McG'01; CCFP; (613)830-1771

MURTY, Manoranjan P; Appletree Med Centre, 2948 Baseline Rd, Ottawa ON K2H 8T5; Ott'76; CCFP; FCFP; (613)288-2059; Fax. (613)288-2060.

MURUVE, Daniel A; HSC-Faculty of Med, 3330 Hospital Dr NW, Calgary AB T2N 4N1; Man'89; FRCPC; IntMed; Nephrol. Staff, Calgary Regional Health Authority; Asst Prof, University of Calgary; Langs: English; French; (403)220-3908; Fax. (403)220-2418; dmuruve@ucalgary.ca.

MURUVE, Gabriel; Manitoba Clinic, 790 Sherbrook St, Winnipeg MB R3A 1M3; (Turkey)'55; FAAP; FRCPC; Peds. Staff, Health Sciences Centre; Staff, St Boniface General Hospital; Pt-Time Teach. Staff, University of Manitoba; Langs: Bilingual(English/French); (204)788-5746; Fax. (204)772-2537.

MURY, Muriel; CHUS-Hop Hotel-Dieu, 580 rue Bowen S, Sherbrooke QC J1G 2E8; Marseille (France)'89; FRCPC; Psy. Staff, Centre Hospitalier Universitaire de Sherbrooke-Hôpital Hôtel-Dieu; (819)346-1110 x26535

MURYNKA, Tania M; Signature Parke Plaza, 100-1919 Sirocco Dr SW, Calgary AB T3H 2Y3; Cal'09; CCFP; (403)242-0504; Fax. (403)398-9420.

MUSA, Ihsan M; Upper River Valley Hosp, 11300 130 Rte, Watervil-Carleton NB E7P 0A4; Baghdad (Iraq)'96; CCFP; CCFP(E.M.); Staff, Upper River Valley Hospital - Waterville; (506)357-2535

MUSA, Khalid M S K; GP Med Clinic, 12225 99 St, Grande Prairie AB T8V 6X9; Al Fateh (Libya)'03; CCFP; (780)533-4444; Fax. (780)533-4443.

MUSACCHIO, Mafalda S; Parkview Older Adult Supp Unit, 4950 Heather St, Vancouver BC V5Z 3L9; UBC'96; BSc; FRCPC; Psy (Geriatric Psychiatry). Staff, Providence Health Care-Youville Residence; Langs: Italian; (604)806-9565; mmusacchio@bcmhs.bc.ca.

MUSAH, Christopher A; Eaglesmed Clinic, 315-12445 Lake Fraser Dr SE, Calgary AB T2J 7A4; (Nigeria)'95; MB BS; DPH; DTMH; MMed; MPH; MCFP; CCFP; (403)723-2453; Fax. (403)723-2463.

MUSAJI, Shelina; Kootenay Lake Med Centre, 1140 Lakeside Dr, Nelson BC V1L 5Z3; Tor'95; CCFP; (250)352-4666

MUSANI, Rumina; Univ Hlth Network-Toronto Gen, 200 Elizabeth St, Toronto ON M5G 2C4; Karachi (Pakistan)'02; FRCPC; AnatPath. Staff, Toronto General Hospital - UHN; (416)340-3111

MUSAT, Laura; Oshawa Health Centre, 247 Simcoe St N, Oshawa ON L1G 4T3; (Romania)'98; CCFP; (905)728-7915

MUSAWIR, Amtul; Renfrew Victoria Hosp, 499 Raglan St N, Renfrew ON K7V 1P6; Karachi (Pakistan)'88; MB BS; ABIM; AB; FRCPC; IntMed. Staff, Renfrew Victoria Hospital; (613)432-4851 x201

MUSCA, Claudia E; 3201 Greenbank Rd, Nepean ON K2J 4H9; Ott'01; (613)825-1636; Fax. (613)825-5521.

MUSCAT, Anne H; Marmora Med Centre, PO Box 520 1 Madoc St, Marmora ON K0K 2M0; NOSM'09; CCFP; (613)472-6131; Fax. (613)472-6135.

MUSCAT, Colin J; Crowsnest Med Clinic, PO Box 370 2158 213 St, Alsike AB T0C 0C0; Alb'09; CCFP; (403)562-8804; Fax. (403)562-2905.

MUSCEDERE, Giulio; St Joseph's Health Care, PO Box 5777 Stn B 268 Grosvenor St, London ON N6A 4V2; Wes'93; FRCPC; DiagRad. Staff Radiol, St Joseph's Hospital - St Joseph's Health Care; (519)646-6035

MUSCEDERE, John G; Kingston Gen Hosp, 5 411-76 Stuart St, Kingston ON K7L 2V7; Wes'85; FRCPC; IntMed (Critical Care Medicine); Respir. Staff, Kingston General Hospital; Langs: Italian; (613)549-6666 x4642; jmuscede@wincom.net.

MUSELIUS, Brenda H; Sheldon Chumir Centre, 1213 4 St SW, Calgary AB T2R 0X7; Qns'79; CCFP; CCFP(E.M.); Physician, Sheldon M Chumir Urgent Care Physician Group; (403)955-6011; Fax. (403)955-6023; brenda.muselius@albertahealthservices.ca.

MUSEMBA, Justine; Hôpital de Tracadie-Sheila, CP 3180 Stn Main 400 rue des Hospitalieres, Tracadie-Sheila NB E1X 1G5; Kinshasa (Congo (Democratic Republic))'89; Staff, Hôpital de Tracadie-Sheila; (506)394-3000

MUSEWE, Norman N; Ashgrove Med Centre, 315-6633 Highway 7, Markham ON L3P 7P2; Birmingham (England)'75; Cardiol; Peds. Staff Cardiol, The Hospital For Sick Children; Court Consultant, Markham Stouffville Hospital; (905)471-3700; Fax. (905)471-3702; norman.musewe@sympatico.ca.

MUSGRAVE, Bruce L; 203-100 Station Lane, Kentville NS B4N 0A3; Dal'05; FRCPC; IntMed; Gastroent. (902)681-9126; Fax. (902)681-1058.

MUSGRAVE, David P; Courtenay Med Associates, 201-1350 England Ave, Courtenay BC V9N 8X6; Cal'74; Staff, St Joseph's General Hospital; (250)334-4411; Fax. (250)338-1245.

MUSGRAVE, John M; 35-3360 rue Notre-Dame, Lachine QC H8T 3E2; Belfast (Ireland)'66; BAO; BSc(Anat); (514)637-3078; Fax. (514)637-9920.

MUSGRAVE, Laurie; Brunswick Med Centre, 401-955 boul Saint-Jean, Pointe-Claire QC H9R 5K3; Mon'03; CCFP; (514)426-6677 x228

MUSGRAVE, Melinda A; St Michael's Hosp, Q 4077-30 Bond St, Toronto ON M5B 1W8; Tor'98; FRCS(Eng); FRCSC; PlasSurg (Plastic & Reconstructive Surgery). Staff, St Michael's Hospital; Teach Staff, University of Toronto; (416)864-5169; Fax. (416)864-5523.

MUSGRAVE, S Ian; Seven Oaks, 40-4575 Blenkinsop Rd, Victoria BC V8X 2C7; Qns'83; FRCPC; Psy. (250)479-7373

MUSGROVE, G Roy; Lasalle Community Health Care, 2125 Front Rd, Windsor ON N9J 2C1; Wes'70; CCFP; Ac Staff, Windsor Regional Hospital - Tayfour Site; Ac Staff, Hôtel-Dieu Grace Hospital; (519)734-1234; Fax. (519)734-8674.

MUSHI, Sophia; Varsity Plaza, P611-4515 Varsity Dr NW, Calgary AB T3A 0Z8.

MUSIAL, Alexander J; 4298 Dunbar St, Vancouver BC V6S 2E9; Wes'79; BSc(Hon); (604)731-3612; Fax. (604)731-2311.

MUSK, Mark C; Bigelow Fowler Clinic, 30 Jerry Potts Blvd W, Lethbridge AB T1K 5M5; Alb'88; CCFP; FCFP; Ac Staff, Chinook Regional Hospital; Ac Staff, Covenant Health - St Michael's Health Centre; (403)381-8444; Fax. (403)381-8166.

MUSLEMANI, Ali; CSSS de Jonquiere, CP 1200 Succ Pdf Jonquiere 2230 rue de l'Hopital, Jonquiere QC G7X 7X2; Zaporozhye (Ukraine)'90; CCFP; Staff, Centre Hospitalier Jonquiere; (418)695-7700; Fax. (418)699-1220.

MUSNGI, Cristina B; Summerville Family Health Team, 5F-101 Queensway W, Mississauga ON L5B 2P7; McM'05; BScN; CCFP; (905)272-9700; Fax. (905)272-1416.

MUSSANI, Yasmin; 23 Huron St W, Exeter ON N0M 1S2; Wes'75; Staff, South Huron Hospital Association; (519)235-3343; Fax. (519)235-3845; ymussani@uwo.ca.

MUSSARI, Benedetto; Kingston Gen Hosp, 76 Stuart St, Kingston ON K7L 2V7; Qns'92; FRCPC; DiagRad. Staff, Kingston General Hospital; (613)548-2301

MUSSELL, Broncyn; 7-7201 Vedder Rd, Chilliwack BC V2R 4G5; UBC'07; CCFP; (604)824-2490

MUSSELMAN, Laura J; Trillium Hlth Ctr-Mississauga, 100 Queensway W, Mississauga ON L5B 1B8; McM'99; FRCSC; GenSurg. Staff, Trillium Health Centre - Mississauga; (905)848-7100

MUSSETT, Steven A; 1371 Highway 2 PO Box 399, Maitland ON K0E 1P0; Cape Town (South Africa)'97; MB ChB; FRCSC; OrthSurg. Staff, Brockville General Hospital - Charles Street; stevemuss@canada.com.

MUSTAFA, Abdalhakim; North Walkerville Med Centre, 200-2425 Tecumseh Rd E, Windsor ON N8W 1E6; Al-Arab (Libya)'89; FRCPC; Neur. Associate, Windsor Regional Hospital - Metropolitan Site; Associate, Hôtel-Dieu Grace Hospital; Langs: Arabic; (519)256-4498; Fax. (519)256-3270.

MUSTAFA, Arjowan; Thompson Gen Hosp, 871 Thompson Dr, Thompson MB R8N 0C8; Univ of Mosul (Iraq)'81; FRCSC; ObstGyn. Staff, Thompson General Hospital; (204)677-2381

MUSTAFA, Hassan A; The Ottawa Hosp-Gen Campus, 501 Smyth Rd, Ottawa ON K1H 8L6; Benghazi (Libya)'92; FRCPC; IntMed; Nephrol. Staff, The Ottawa Hospital - General Campus; (613)854-0684

MUSTAPHA, Shareef F; St Boniface Gen Hosp, A8025-409 Tache Ave, Winnipeg MB R2H 2A6; Man'04; FRCPC; Peds. Staff, St Boniface General Hospital; (204)233-8563

MUSTARD, J Charles; Gateway Community Hlth Ctre, PO Box 99 41 McClellan St, Tweed ON K0K 3J0; Wes'83; CCFP; FCFP; CommunMed. (613)478-1211

MUSTARD, Janice E; North York Gen Hosp, 4001 Leslie St, North York ON M2K 1E1; Wes'77; FRCPC; Anes. Staff, North York General Hospital; Ac Staff, North York General Hospital - Branson Division; (416)756-6000 x6265

MUSTARD, Robert A; St Michael's Hosp, 30 Bond St, Toronto ON M5B 1W8; Wes'77; FACS; FRCSC; GenSurg (Family Medicine). Ac Staff, St Michael's Hospital; Assoc Prof, University of Toronto; (416)864-3046; Fax. (416)864-3049; mustardr@smh.toronto.on.ca.

MUSTATA, Stefan; Rockyview Gen Hosp, 7007 14 St SW, Calgary AB T2V 1P9; Bucharest (Romania)'89; FRCPC; IntMed; Nephrol. Staff, Rockyview General Hospital; Asst Prof, University of Calgary; (403)943-8896; Fax. (403)943-8666.

MUSTO, David J; 10-2168 McCallum Rd, Abbotsford BC V2S 6R6; UBC'99; FRCSC; PlasSurg. (604)854-5885

MUSTO, Richard J; Alberta Health Services, 120-10301 Southport Lane SW, Calgary AB T2W 1S7; Wes'78; FRCPC; CommunMed. Clin Assoc Prof, University of Calgary; (403)943-0215; Fax. (403)943-0200; richard.musto@albertahealthservices.ca.

MUSUKA, Charles; St Boniface Gen Hosp, L4006 7-409 Tache Ave, Winnipeg MB R2H 2A6; Harare(Zimbabwe) (Zimbabwe)'92; FRCPC; HemPath. Staff, St Boniface General Hospital; (204)787-8914

MUSYOKI, Francis; Chatham-Kent Health Alliance, PO Box 2030 Stn Main 80 Grand Ave W, Chatham ON N7M 5L9; McG'03; FRCPC; DiagRad. Staff, Chatham-Kent Health Alliance; (519)352-6400

MUTAT, Abdurrazag M; 165 15th St E, North Vancouver BC V7L 2P7; Tripoli (Libya)'84; ABPeds; FRCSC; Neursurg. Staff, Lions Gate Hospital; Langs: Arabic; (604)990-4624; Fax. (604)990-4607.

MUTCH, Cheryl L; Seymour Med Clinic, 1530 7th Ave W, Vancouver BC V6J 1S3; McG'88; FRCPC; Peds. Staff Peds, BC Children's Hospital; Clin Instructor Family Med, University of British Columbia; (604)738-2151; cmutch@telus.net.

MUTCH, David O; CSSS d'Argenteuil, 145 av de la Providence, Lachute QC J8H 4C7; McG'75; FRCSC; GenSurg. Staff, Centre Hospitalier d'Argenteuil; Assoc Staff, Centre Hospitalier Rouyn-Noranda; Assoc Staff, CH Hôtel-Dieu d'Amos; Asst Lecturer Surg, McGill University; (450)562-3761; Fax. (450)566-3325.

MUTCH, Linsey S; 400 McKeown Ave, North Bay ON P1B 0B2; Ott'03; FRCPC; Peds. Staff, North Bay Regional Health Centre - Regional Mental Health; (705)495-8135

MUTCH, W Alan C; Health Sciences Centre, GH611-820 Sherbrook St, Winnipeg MB R3A 1R9; Qns'77; FRCPC; Anes (Cardiology & Pulmonary Medicine). Staff, Health Sciences Centre; Co-Founder, Biovar Life Support Inc; Prof Anes, University of Manitoba; (204)789-3731

MUTCHMORE, Lucie; Clinique Med de Campbell's Bay, CP 250 35 Patterson, Campbell's Bay QC J0X 1K0; Ott'89; CCFP; CCFP(E.M.); ac Membre, Pontiac Hospital Centre; (819)648-2021; Fax. (819)648-2052; baymedclinic@personainternet.com.

MUTH, Brian H; 2718 39th Ave W, Vancouver BC V6N 2Z4; Tor'81; Langs: Arabic; (778)898-5221

MUTHALALY, Koshy; Rouge Valley-Centenary HC, 2867 Ellesmere Rd, Scarborough ON M1E 4B9; Kerala (India)'83; Staff Reg Newborn Child & Adolescent Prog, Rouge Valley Health System - Centenary Health Centre Site; (416)284-8131

MUTHAYAN, Dayananden V; Abbotsford Reg Hosp & Cancer C, 32900 Marshall Rd, Abbotsford BC V2S 0C2; Cape Town (South Africa)'86; MB ChB; BSc(Med.); Dip SportMed; CCFP; CCFP(E.M.); Staff, Mission Hills Medical Clinic; Physician, Abbotsford Regional Hospital & Cancer Centre; (604)851-4700

MUTHIAH, Karuppan C; Hotel-Dieu de Saint-Joseph, 10 Woodland Hill, Perth-Andover NB E7H 5H5; Madras (India)'78; MB BS; DA; Staff Anes, St Martha's Regional Hospital; Staff, Hôtel-Dieu of St Joseph Hospital; Langs: Tamil; (506)273-7100; muthiahk@hotmail.com.

MUTHIAH, Karuppan; The Winnipeg Clinic, 425 St. Mary Ave, Winnipeg MB R3C 0N2; Annamalai (India)'04; FRCPC; IntMed.

MUTHU, M Saravana; King Med Clinic, 380 Portland St, Dartmouth NS B2Y 1K8; Bangalore (India)'72; MB BS; MRCPsy(UK); Psy (Adult & Geriatric Psychiatry). Staff Psy, The Nova Scotia Hospital; Lecturer Psy, Dalhousie University; Langs: Tamil; (902)464-4646; Fax. (902)464-4647.

MUTHU, Sarasa; St Martha's Reg Hosp, 25 Bay St, Antigonish NS B2G 2G5; Bangalore (India)'70; MB BS; DTMH; FRCPC; AnatPath (Dermatology). Staff Path, St Martha's Regional Hospital; (902)867-4154; Fax. (902)863-3708.

MUTRIE, David E; PO Box 10204 Stn P, Thunder Bay ON P7B 6T7; Qns'77; CCFP; CCFP(E.M.); FCFP; Staff, Thunder Bay Regional Health Sciences Centre Port-Arthur; Section Leader Emergency Med, Northern Ontario School of Medicine-Laurentian University; Asst Prof, McMaster University; (807)683-6164; Fax. (807)683-6198.

MUTRIE, John H; 1187 Fischer Hallman Rd, Kitchener ON N2E 4H9; Wes'81; (519)570-1200; Fax. (519)570-1214.

MUTRIE, William M; Woodstock Med Clinic, 10-110 Chapel St, Woodstock NB E7M 1H1; Dal'75; Staff, Upper River Valley Hospital - Waterville; (506)328-9929; Fax. (506)325-1985.

MUTTER, Thomas C; Harry Medovy House, 671 William Ave, Winnipeg MB R3E 0Z2; Man'01; FRCPC; Anes. Staff, Health Sciences Centre.

MUTUKISTNA, Indren; Richpoint Med Centre, 10815 Yonge St, Richmond Hill ON L4C 3E3; Sask'87; (905)770-3004; Fax. (905)770-5663.

MUTZ, Shane D; Victoria Gen Hosp, 2340 Pembina Hwy, Winnipeg MB R3T 2E8; Man'04; FRCPC; EmergMed. Staff, Victoria General Hospital; (204)269-3570

MUWAIS, Osama W; Terwillegar Med Clinic, 101-121 Haddow Close NW, Edmonton AB T6R 3W3; Alb'97; CCFP.

MUWANGUZI, Michael M; Southwest Medi-Centre, 500-1 Springs Dr, Swift Current SK S9H 3X6; MB ChB; (306)773-4681; Fax. (306)778-3449.

MUWANGUZI, Stanley K; PO Box 1950 Stn Main, Camrose AB T4V 1X8; (Uganda)'81; DTMH; DPH; CCFP; MB BS; CCFP; CCFP(E.M.); Staff, Queen Elizabeth II Hospital; Staff, Peter Lougheed Centre; Associate Critical Care, Calgary Health Region; Langs: Swahili; Kiswahili; Luganda; Sotho; (780)679-6111; Fax. (780)679-6196.

MUWONGE, Stanley N M; 104-10055 120 Ave, Grande Prairie AB T8V 8H8; (Uganda)'94; MB ChB; CCFP; Langs: Swahili; (780)532-4415; Fax. (780)532-4559; lmj4559@telus.net.

MUZYKA, David L; Royal Alexandra Hosp, 10240 Kingsway NW, Edmonton AB T5H 3V9; Alb'86; BMedSci; FRCPC; Anes (Cardiology). Att Staff Stollery Children's & Gen Adult Systems ICU, University of Alberta Hospital; Ac Staff Coronary Care Unit/Consultant IntMed, Sturgeon Community Hospital; Chief Anes, Royal Alexandra Hospital; (780)735-4010; Fax. (780)735-4386; dmuzyka@compusmart.ab.ca.

MUZYKA, Raymond A; PO Box 4460 Stn South Cro, Edmonton AB T6E 4T5; Alb'92; CCFP.

MUZYKA, Timothy G; Misericordia Community Hosp, 16940 87 Ave NW, Edmonton AB T5R 4H5; Sask'85; FRCPC; IntMed (Interventional Cardiology); Cardiol. Med Staff, Covenant Health - Misericordia Community Hospital; Asst Prof Med, University of Alberta; (780)735-2255; Fax. (780)735-2257.

MUZYKA, William R; Terwillegar Med Clinic, 101-121 Haddow Close NW, Edmonton AB T6R 3W3; Alb'99; CCFP; (780)989-5300; Fax. (780)989-5301.

MVILONGO, Eding S; MUHC-Montreal Children's Hosp, 2300 rue Tupper, Montreal QC H3H 1P3; Laval'06; FRCPC; Anes. Staff, McGill University Health Centre - Montreal Children's Hospital; (514)934-1934

MWANA, N'siabar J; Prince Albert Commun Clinic, 110 8th St E, Prince Albert SK S6V 0V7; Physician, Prince Albert Community Clinic; (306)763-6464; Fax. (306)763-2101; mwana@shaw.ca.

MWANZ, K Joseph; Clinique Med Innes, 214-4275 Innes Rd, Orleans ON K1C 1T1; (Zambia)'91; CCFP; (613)424-6343

MWANZA, Jonathan; Family Practice Associates, PO Box 1260 4714 50 St, Mayerthorpe AB T0E 1N0; (Zambia)'88; (780)786-2412; Fax. (780)786-2249.

MWILAMBWE WA MWILAMBWE, Annick; CSSS du Sud de Lanaudiere, 911 montee des Pionniers, Terrebonne QC J6V 2H2; Kinshasa (Congo (Democratic Republic))'87; Ophth. Staff, Centre Hospitalier Pierre le Gardeur; (450)654-7525; Fax. (450)470-2602.

MYARA, Max N; Clinique Med Joliette, 3841 rue Ontario E, Montreal QC H1W 1S5; Louvain (Belgium)'71; Staff, Mount Sinai Hospital Center; Langs: Bilingual(French/English); (514)524-3731; Fax. (514)524-0675.

MYAT, Khin M; Northview Med Clinic, B6-10635 Creditview Rd, Brampton ON L7A 0T4; CCFP; (905)495-6555; Fax. (905)495-9145.

MYATT, Gerald L; 120-2751 Gladstone St, Halifax NS B3K 4W6; Dal'78; (902)835-5990

MYATT, Gregory A; Health Park, 210-45 Weatherbee Rd, Mira Road NS B1M 0A1; Mem'88; CCFP; CCFP(E.M.); FCFP; (902)564-8105

MYATT, Matthew; Alliston Family Health Team, 36 Victoria St W, Alliston ON L9R 1S8; (Grenada)'08; CCFP; (705)435-8887; Fax. (705)435-8867.

MYBURGH, Johannes L; Sylvan Med Centre, 5007 46 St, Sylvan Lake AB T4S 1C2; (South Africa)'85; MB ChB; Langs: Afrikaans; (403)887-2221; Fax. (403)887-3777.

MYBURGH, Johan; 3410 50 Ave, Red Deer AB T4N 3Y4; Bloemfontein (South Africa)'97; MB ChB; CCFP; (403)342-9444

MYBURGH, Willem M; Impala Med Clinic, 112-3722 57 Ave, Red Deer AB T4N 4R7; Stellenbosch (South Africa)'81; MB ChB; DA; CCFP; Med Staff, Dave Thompson Health Region; Langs: Afrikaans; (403)352-7425; Fax. (403)352-7428.

MYCKAN, Kerry A; 502-2000 Credit Valley Rd, Mississauga ON L5M 4N4; Tor'01; FRCSC; ObstGyn. (905)820-8748; Fax. (905)820-0255.

MYCKATYN, Michael M; 101-7380 Westminster Hwy, Richmond BC V6X 1A1; UBC'72; Staff, Richmond Hospital; Pres, Minoru Medical Education Society; Langs: Ukrainian; (604)273-9404; Fax. (604)273-3342.

MYCYK, Taras R; Royal University Hosp, 103 Hospital Dr, Saskatoon SK S7N 0W8; Ott'78; DABS; DABTS; FRCSC; GenSurg; Cardiovasc&ThorSurg. Ac Staff CardioVasc Surg, Royal University Hospital; (306)966-8167; Fax. (306)966-6932.

MYDEEN, M Firdaus M; Pembina Med Clinic, 104-10004 107 St, Westlock AB T7P 2K8; Dal'06; CCFP; Commun Med Dir/Coord Med Educ, Westlock Healthcare Centre; Langs: Tamil; Malay; (780)349-4425; Fax. (780)349-4478.

MYDEN, Curtis A; Kelowna Orthopedics, 303-3330 Richter St, Kelowna BC V1W 4V5; Cal'06; FRCSC; OrthSurg. Staff, Foothills Medical Centre.

MYDLARSKI, Marc B; SMBD Jewish Gen Hosp, 3755 ch Cote-Sainte-Catherine, Montreal QC H3T 1E2; Alb'99; FRCSC; Ophth. Staff, Sir Mortimer B Davis Jewish General; (514)340-8280

MYDLARSKI, P Regine; Richmond Road Diag & Trmt Ctr, 1820 Richmond Rd SW, Calgary AB T2T 5C7; Cal'95; FAAD; FRCP; FRCPC; Derm (Immuno Dermatology). Consultant, Alberta Children's Hospital; Consultant, Foothills Medical Centre; Consultant, Peter Lougheed Centre; Consultant, Rockyview General Hospital; Langs: English; French; (403)955-8345; Fax. (403)955-8200.

MYERS, Andrew B; Lakeridge Hlth Corp-Oshawa, 1 Hospital Crt, Oshawa ON L1G 2B9; McG'89; AB; FRCPC; DiagRad (Abdominal Imaging). Staff, Lakeridge Health - Oshawa Site; (905)433-4305; Fax. (905)721-4770.

MYERS, Danny M; Victoria Gen Hosp, 1 Hospital Way, Victoria BC V8Z 6R5; Man'86; FRCPC; IntMed. Consultant, Shuswap Lake General Hospital; Consultant, Queen Victoria Hospital; Staff, Victoria General Hospital; University of British Columbia; (250)727-4212

MYERS, Jeffrey A; The Credit Valley Hosp, 2200 Eglinton Ave W, Mississauga ON L5M 2N1; Tor'00; FRCPC; IntMed; MedOncol. Staff, The Credit Valley Hospital; Court Staff, Dufferin Caledon Health Care Corporation; (905)813-1100 x5135

MYERS, Jeffrey W; Sunnybrook Hlth Sciences Ctre, H336-2075 Bayview Ave, Toronto ON M4N 3M5; Cal'95; CCFP; Staff, Sunnybrook Health Sciences Centre; (416)480-6100 x7093; Fax. (416)480-5146.

MYERS, Kathryn A; St Joseph's Health Care, PO Box 5777 Stn B 268 Grosvenor St, London ON N6A 4V2; Wes'87; FRCPC; IntMed (Hypertension). Staff, Kingston General Hospital; Staff, St Joseph's Hospital - St Joseph's Health Care; Staff, St Mary's of the Lake; Queen's University; (519)646-6227

MYERS, Kimberley A; Alberta Children's Hosp, 2888 Shaganappi Trail NW, Calgary AB T3B 6A8; UBC'02; FRCPC; Peds; Cardiol. Staff, Alberta Children's Hospital; (403)955-7858; Fax. (403)955-7621.

MYERS, Leslie A; Grey Bruce HS-Owen Sound, PO Box 1800 Stn Main 1800 8th St E, Owen Sound ON N4K 6M9; Cleveland(OH) (USA)'90; CCFP; CCFP(E.M.); FCFP; Staff, Grey Bruce Health Services - Owen Sound; (519)376-2121

MYERS, M Lee; London HSC-University Hosp, PO Box 5339 Stn B B6 114-339 Windermere Rd, London ON N6A 5A5; Wes'77; FRCSC; GenSurg (Cardiac Surgery); Cardiovasc&ThorSurg. Staff, London Health Sciences Centre - University Hospital; Chief Cardiovascular Surg, London Health Sciences Centre - Victoria Campus; Assoc Prof, University of Western Ontario; (519)663-3479; Fax. (519)663-3276.

MYERS, Martin G; Sunnybrook Hlth Sciences Ctre, A 202-2075 Bayview Ave, Toronto ON M4N 3M5; Tor'68; FRCPC; IntMed (Cardiology). Ac Staff Cardiol, Sunnybrook Health Sciences Centre; Prof Med, University of Toronto; (416)480-4749; Fax. (416)480-5404; martin.myers@sunnybrook.ca.

MYERS, Miriam; Markham Place Med Centre, 206-2900 Steeles Ave E, Thornhill ON L3T 4X1; Tor'82; Langs: Bilingual(English/French); (905)882-7575; Fax. (905)731-1298.

MYERS, Nicholas; Memorial Med Clinic, 10-5268 Memorial Dr NE, Calgary AB T2A 2R1; London (England)'82; MB BS; BSc; DRCOG; DCH; (403)235-6333; Fax. (403)235-6349.

MYERS, Nigel T B; Village Med Clinic, PO Box 130 Stn Fort Langley 1-9089 Glover Rd, Langley BC V1M 2R5; Cape Town (South Africa)'81; MB ChB; CCFP; FCFP; Staff, Langley Memorial Hospital; (604)888-8300

MYERS, Renelle L; Hlth Sciences Ctr Respiratory, RS330-810 Sherbrook St, Winnipeg MB R3A 1R8; Man'05; FRCPC; IntMed; Respir. Staff, Health Sciences Centre.

MYERS, Robert B H; Sunnybrook Hlth Sciences Ctre, A217-2075 Bayview Ave, Toronto ON M4N 3M5; Man'88; ABIM(IntMed&Cardiol); FACC; FRCPC; IntMed; Cardiol. Dir/Founder Congestive Heart Failure Clinic, Sunnybrook Health Sciences Centre; Asst Prof, University of Toronto; (416)480-4746; Fax. (416)480-5251.

MYERS, Robert E; The Credit Valley Hosp, 2200 Eglinton Ave W, Mississauga ON L5M 2N1; Tor'71; FRCPC; IntMed. Ac Staff, The Credit Valley Hospital; Assoc Prof, University of Toronto; (905)813-1100 x5135; Fax. (905)813-4024.

MYERS, Robert P; Univ of Calgary Med Clinic, 3330 Hospital Dr NW, Calgary AB T2N 4N1; Wes'96; MSc; FRCPC; IntMed (Hepatology). Physician, Health Research Innovation Centre; Dir Viral Hepatitis Clinic/Asst Prof, University of Calgary; (403)944-6555; Fax. (403)944-6545.

MYERS, William D; 6-1080 Adelaide St N, London ON N5Y 2N1; Wes'81; (519)850-6937; Fax. (519)601-0578.

MYERS, William E; Souris Health Centre, PO Box 10 155 Brindle St, Souris MB R0K 2C0; Man'71; DAB; FRCSC; GenSurg (Biliary Surgery)., Souris Health Centre; Lecturer Surg, University of Manitoba; (204)483-2121; wmyers@arha.ca.

MYETTE, T Larry; Healthy Horizons Corp Hlth, 5202 Beckton Rd, Victoria BC V8Y 2C1; UBC'80; MPH; (250)882-8065

MYHILL-JONES, Brian J; Sechelt Med Clinic, PO Box 638, Sechelt BC V0N 3A0; UBC'74; BSc; CCFP; FCFP; Ac Staff, St Mary's Hospital; Clinical Asst Prof, University of British Columbia; (604)885-2257; Fax. (604)885-4718; bmyhilljones@yahoo.ca.

MYHR, Gail A; Allan Mem Institute, 1025 av des Pins O, Montreal QC H3A 1A1; McG'80; MSc; DPsy; FRCPC; Psy (Cognitive Behaviour Therapy). Staff, McGill University Health Centre - Royal Victoria Hospital; Langs: English; French; (514)934-1934 x36988; Fax. (514)843-1643.

MYHRE, Douglas L; Sheldon Chumir Centre, 1213 4 St SW, Calgary AB T2R 0X7; Alb'80; CCFP; FCFP; Ac Staff, Chinook Regional Hospital; Assoc Dean Distributed Learning & Rural Initiatives, University of Calgary; (403)955-9300

MYINT, Khin M; Churchill Med Clinic, 6-3050 Artesian Dr, Mississauga ON L5M 7P5; Mandalay (Burma)'83; MB BS; CCFP; Langs: Burmese; (905)607-6495; Fax. (905)607-0881.

MYINT, Wunna A; Peterborough Reg HC-Hospital, 1 Hospital Dr, Peterborough ON K9J 7C6; Qns'94; FRCPC; DiagRad. Staff, Peterborough Regional Health Centre - Hospital Drive; (705)743-2121

MYKYTIUK, Patricia A; Health Sciences Centre, 820 Sherbrook St, Winnipeg MB R3A 1R9; Sask'02; FRCPC; Anes. Staff, Health Sciences Centre; (204)774-6511

MYLES, Jeremy D; Foothills Med Centre, 1403 29 St NW, Calgary AB T2N 2T9; Cal'01; CCFP; Staff, Foothills Medical Centre; (403)944-2800; Fax. (403)283-7365.

MYLES, S Terence; 3630 7 St SW, Calgary AB T2T 2Y1; Alb'65; MSc(McG); DAB; FRCSC; Neursurg (Spine Surgery). Ac Staff, Foothills Medical Centre; Emeritus Prof, University of Calgary; (403)243-7350; terry.myles@shaw.ca.

MYLES, Virginia J; Westmount Med Bldg, 660-5025 rue Sherbrooke O, Montreal QC H4A 1S9; McG'90; CCFP; FCFP; Assoc Staff, Mount Sinai Hospital Center; Langs: English; French; (514)932-6122; Fax. (514)933-8739.

MYLES, W Michael; Nepean Med Centre, 211-1 Centrepointe Dr, Nepean ON K2G 6E2; Ott'87; BA; FRCSC; Ophth (Cataract Surgery). Staff Privil, The Ottawa Hospital - General Campus; Staff, The Ottawa Hospital - Riverside Campus; Staff, The Ottawa Hospital - Civic Campus; (613)226-8872; Fax. (613)226-3557; idoc@rogers.com.

MYLES-FERGUSON, Joyce M; Devon Gen Hosp, F-101 Erie St S, Devon AB T9G 1A6; Manchester (England)'57; MB ChB; DCH; Staff, Devon General Hospital; (780)987-4151; Fax. (780)987-4177.

MYLONAS, Ilias; Bridgeland Med Bldg, 803 1 Ave NE, Calgary AB T2E 7C5; Cracow (Poland)'04; FRCPC; IntMed; Cardiol. Staff, Royal University Hospital; (403)571-8633; Fax. (403)571-6992.

MYLREA, Cynthia B; PO Box 8357 Stn Main, Canmore AB T1W 2V1; Cal'87; CCFP; FCFP; Staff, Canmore General Hospital.

MYLVAGANAM, Rock R X; 278 O'Connor St, Ottawa ON K2P 1V4; Colombo (Sri Lanka)'71; MB BS; MRCPsy; FRCPC; Psy (Depression & Anxiety). Cons. Psy. & Psychotherapist, Private Pract.; Langs: Sinhalese; Tamil; (613)233-1565; Fax. (613)233-1851.

MYMIN, David; Health Sciences Centre, MS773N-820 Sherbrook St, Winnipeg MB R3A 1R9; Witwatersrand (South Africa)'52; MB ChB; FRCP; Staff, Health Sciences Centre; Teach Staff, University of Manitoba; (204)774-6511

MYMKO, Morris; Thunder Bay Reg HSC-T-Bay, 980 Oliver Rd, Thunder Bay ON P7B 6V4; Man'71; BScPharm(Pharm); CCFP; FCFP; Ac Staff, Thunder Bay Regional Health Sciences Centre; (807)684-6000

MYNHARDT, Heinrich D; Outlook Med Clinic, PO Box 1160, Outlook SK S0L 2N0; Pretoria (South Africa)'87; MB ChB; LMCC; CCFP; Staff, Outlook Health Centre; Fam Med, Rosetown & District Health Centre; (306)867-8626; Fax. (306)867-8988; heinm@sasktel.net.

MYO-LWIN, Tony Ong; Chinatown X-Ray/Ultrasound Cli, 205-180 Keefer St, Vancouver BC V6A 4E9; (Taiwan)'71; DABR; DAB; FRCPC; DiagRad (Diagnostic Imaging). Chief, Providence Health Care - Holy Family Hospital; Chief Radiol, Providence Health Care - Mount Saint Joseph Hospital; Physician, Chinatown X-Ray & Ultrasound; (604)688-9428; tmyo-lwin@providencehealth.bc.ca.

MYRAN, David D; Baycrest Ctre/Geriatric Care, 307-3560 Bathurst St, North York ON M6A 2E1; Tor'79; FRCPC; Psy (Family Medicine). Staff, Baycrest Centre for Geriatric Care; Staff, Centre for Addiction & Mental Health (CAMH) - College Street Site; Staff, William Osler Health System - Etobicoke General Hospital; Asst Prof, University of Toronto; (416)785-2500 x2883; Fax. (416)785-2492.

MYRON, Kathleen S; Inst of Commun & Family Psy, 4333 ch Cote-Sainte-Catherine, Montreal QC H3T 1E4; McG'83; FRCPC; Psy. (514)340-8210

MYRON, Philip M B; 180-5 Fairview Mall Dr, North York ON M2J 2Z1; McG'89; BSc; FRCPC; IntMed (Cardiac Catheterization); Cardiol. Associate, Toronto Western Hospital - University Health Network; Ac Staff, North York General Hospital; Lecturer, University of Toronto; Langs: English; French; (416)493-7571; Fax. (416)493-0851.

MYRONUK, Lonn D S; Nanaimo Reg Gen Hosp, G001-1200 Dufferin Cres, Nanaimo BC V9S 2B7; UBC'90; BSc; FRCPC; Psy (Geriatric Psychiatry). Ac Staff, Nanaimo Regional General Hospital; (250)716-7791; referrals@geripsych.com.

MYSLEK, Margaret A; 2-915 348th Ave PO Box 820, Oliver BC V0H 1T0; Katowice (Poland)'88; (250)498-2232

MYSORE, Munithanamma J; Salvation Army Grace Gen Hosp, 300 Booth Dr, Winnipeg MB R3J 3M7; Mysore (India)'83; FRCPC; Psy (Geriatric Psychiatry). Staff, The Salvation Army Grace Hospital; Langs: Kanarese; (204)837-0465; Fax. (204)885-3064; suresh@escape.ca.

MYSORE, Navya M; Clinic MDCM, 203-5515 rue Saint-Jacques, Montreal QC H3A 2E3; McG'09; CCFP; (514)483-9911

MYSORE, Suresh M; Victoria Gen Hosp, 2340 Pembina Hwy, Winnipeg MB R3T 2E8; Mysore (India)'83; ABACPath; FRCPC; AnatPath. Staff, Victoria General Hospital; (204)477-3181; Fax. (204)940-2260; smysore@vgh.mb.ca.

MYTOPHER, Kristine D; 300-149 Pacific Ave, Saskatoon SK S7K 1N8; Sask'02; FRCSC; ObstGyn. (306)653-5970; Fax. (306)653-5383.

NAAMAN, Saad; Windsor Reg Hosp-Western Camp, 1453 Prince Rd, Windsor ON N9C 3Z4; Baghdad (Iraq)'77; Staff, Windsor Regional Hospital - Tayfour Site; (519)257-5184; Fax. (519)257-5137.

NAAS, Abdulbasitt M; 1 Oak St, Simcoe ON N3Y 3J4; Tripoli (Libya)'95; FRCPC; IntMed; Cardiol. Staff, Thunder Bay Regional Health Sciences Centre; (519)426-6262

NAASSAN, Anthony E; Durham Regional Cancer Centre, 1 Hospital Crt, Oshawa ON L1G 2B9; McM'06; FRCPC; IntMed; Hem. Staff, Durham Regional Cancer Centre; (905)576-8711 x3625; Fax. (905)721-6103; anaassan@lakeridgehealth.on.ca.

NAASSAN, Natalie C; MCI The Doctor's Office-Whitby, 80 Thickson Rd, Whitby ON L1N 7T2; Wes'05; CCFP; (905)668-6448; Fax. (905)668-4023.

NAAYKENS, William E; Jubilee Med Clinic, 1902 Richmond Rd, Victoria BC V8R 4R2; UBC'89; CCFP; FCFP; Staff, Royal Jubilee Hospital; (250)595-8231; Fax. (250)385-3628.

NABATA, Elaine S; 200-372 Hollandview Trail, Aurora ON L4G 0A5; UBC'81; (905)727-3335; Fax. (905)726-9171.

NABAVI, Mitra; Univ Hlth Network-Toronto Gen, 444-200 Elizabeth St, Toronto ON M5G 2C4; Teheran (Iran)'95; FRCPC; AnatPath. Staff, Toronto General Hospital - UHN; (416)340-3111

NABI, Naeem U; IWK Health Centre, PO Box 9700 Rpo CSC 5850-5980 University Ave, Halifax NS B3K 6R8; Nishtar Medical College (Pakistan)'84; Staff, IWK Health Centre; (902)470-3929

NABI, Shahin; 200-6091 Gilbert Rd, Richmond BC V7C 5L9; UBC'07; FRCSC; Otol.

NABI, Waqar; 13-3355 Hurontario St, Mississauga ON L5A 4E7; Lahore (Pakistan)'88; LMCC; MB BS; CCFP; Langs: Urdu; (905)281-0115; Fax. (905)290-0256; wqari@yahoo.com.

NABID, Abdenour; CHUS-Hop Fleurimont, 3001 12e av N, Sherbrooke QC J1H 5N4; (Algeria)'76; CSPQ; FRCPC; RadOncol. Staff, Centre Hospitalier Universitaire de Sherbrooke-Hopital Fleurimont; (819)346-1110

NACCACHE, Lamia; CHUQ-Ctr Hosp Univ Laval, 2705 boul Laurier, Quebec QC G1V 4G2; Laval'04; FRCPC; Peds; PedHemaOncol (P.Q.). Staff, Centre Hospitalier Universitaire de Quebec-CHUL; (418)525-4444

NACCACHE, Maya; CHUQ-St-Francois d'Assise, 10 rue de l'Espinay, Quebec QC G1L 3L5; Laval'07; CCFP; CCFP(E.M.); Staff, Centre Hospitalier Universitaire De Québec - Pavillon De St-françois-d'assise; (418)525-4444

NACCARATO, Saverio; Strathcona Mental Health Team, 330 Heatley Ave, Vancouver BC V6A 3G3; Alb'86; BSc; Langs: Italian; (604)253-4401

NACHABE, Mahmoud; Service d'Urologie Rive-Sud, 304-3234 boul Taschereau, Greenfield Park QC J4V 2H3; St. Joseph (Lebanon)'81; CSPQ; FRCSC; Urol. Staff, Hopital Charles LeMoyne; Staff, Centre Hospitalier de Verdun; (450)671-2945; Fax. (450)671-8045; nacma@bigfoot.com.

NACHED, Adnan; Hop Santa Cabrini Ospedale, 5655 rue Saint-Zotique E, Montreal QC H1T 1P7; Paris (France)'62; LMCC; Staff, Hôpital Santa Cabrini Ospedale; Langs: Arabic; English; (514)252-6582

NACHIM, Ilan; 610 Major Mackenzie Dr E, Richmond Hill ON L4C 1J9; (Israel)'09; CCFP; (905)770-7500; Fax. (905)737-2383.

NACHT, Irwin J L; 560-1144 Burrard St, Vancouver BC V6Z 2A5; UBC'74; (604)806-9691

NACIUK, Mary E; 3024 Bridge St, South Mountain ON K0E 1W0; Ott'06; CCFP; (613)989-2205

NACUA, Judith B; Lapsley Family Doctors, 13 Lapsley Rd, Scarborough ON M1B 1K1; Cebu (Philippines)'71; (416)754-9593; Fax. (416)754-3946.

NADA-RAJAH, Shantha S; Dixie-Bloor Medical Centre, 3415 Dixie Rd, Mississauga ON L4Y 2B1; Sheffield (England)'76; LRCP; MRCS; CCFP; (905)629-8887; Fax. (905)629-2226.

NADALINI, Mary G; Thistlewood Prof Centre, 204-8077 Islington Ave, Woodbridge ON L4L 7X7; Tor'73; BSc(Hon); CCFP; Ac Staff, William Osler Health System - Etobicoke General Hospital; (905)851-3311; Fax. (905)851-8620.

NADARAJAH, Jeya T; Mount Sinai Hosp, 600 University Ave, Toronto ON M5G 1X5; McM'05; FRCPC; IntMed; MedMicrobiol; InfectDis. Staff, Mount Sinai Hospital; (416)586-4695

NADARAJAH, Senthilraj; Headwaters Health Care Centre, 100 Rolling Hills Dr, Orangeville ON L9W 4X9; Univ of Jaffna (Sri Lanka)'92; Staff, Headwaters Health Care Centre - Orangeville Site.

NADARAJAH, Sumathi; Credit Valley Med Arts Centre, 110-2000 Credit Valley Rd, Mississauga ON L5M 4N4; Tor'89; BSc(Biology); MSc(Anatomy); FAAP; FRCPC; Peds (Clinical Immunology & Allergy). Langs: Tamil; (905)569-8100; Fax. (905)607-3384.

NADASDI, Miklos; 6227 Bathurst St, North York ON M2R 2A5; Budapest (Hungary)'56; PhD; Emeritus Staff, North York General Hospital; Langs: Hungarian; French; (416)222-7044; Fax. (416)222-6840.

NADEAU, Alain; CSSS Therese de Blainville, 125 rue Duquet, Sainte-Therese QC J7E 0A5; Mon'95; MSc; (450)430-4553 x5500; Fax. (450)437-3209.

NADEAU, Amelie; CSSS de Laval, 251-1755 boul Rene-Laennec, Laval QC H7M 3L9; Sher'99; FRCPC; Neur. Staff, Hopital de la Cite de la santé; (450)668-1010

NADEAU, Andre; Hotel-Dieu d'Arthabaska, 5 rue des Hospitalieres, Victoriaville QC G6P 6N2; Laval'98; Staff Emerg, Hotel-Dieu d'Arthabaska; (819)357-2030 x2059; Fax. (819)357-6040; audrenad01@hotmail.com.

NADEAU, Aubert; CSSS de Rivière-de-Loup, 75 rue Saint-Henri, Riviere-du-Loup QC G5R 2A4; Laval'68; Staff, Centre Hospitalier Regional du Grand-Portage; (418)868-1000 x2394; Fax. (418)868-1033.

NADEAU, Caroline; Clinique Med de l'Atelier, 77 boul Seigneurial O, Saint-Bruno QC J3V 2G9; Laval'98; (450)461-1751; carnadeau@hotmail.com.

NADEAU, Caroline; CHUS-Hop Fleurimont, 3001 12e av N, Sherbrooke QC J1H 5N4; Mon'06; FRCPC; Anes. Staff, Centre Hospitalier Universitaire de Sherbrooke-Hopital Fleurimont; (819)346-1110

NADEAU, Chantal; Clin Familiale du Boulevard, 19-300 boul Saint-Luc, St-Jean-Sur-Richel QC J2W 2A3; Mon'91; Staff, Hôpital du Haut-Richelieu; (450)349-3333; Fax. (450)349-1155.

NADEAU, Claude; Clinique Fam de St-Hyacinthe, 2955 boul Laframboise, Saint-Hyacinthe QC J2S 4Z3; Mon'81; (450)774-4611; Fax. (450)773-9913.

NADEAU, Claude; Polyclinique de Trois-Rivieres, 385-1900 boul des Recollets, Trois-Rivieres QC G8Z 4K4; Laval'61; Otol (P.Q.) (Hearing Loss). assoc Staff, Centre Hospitalier Regional de Trois-Rivieres; assoc Staff, CSSS de Trois-Rivières; Otolaryngology, Hôpital de Christ-Roi; Langs: English; French; (819)379-2444; Fax. (819)691-9750.

NADEAU, Daniel; Clinique de Med Familiale, 101 rue Lavoie, Rimouski QC G5L 5Y2; Laval'81; Staff, Hôpital Regional Rimouski; (418)723-5272; Fax. (418)725-2030.

NADEAU, Denise; Centre Med Ste-Foy Inc, 802 av du Chanoine-Scott, Quebec QC G1V 3N4; Mon'93; Staff, Centre Hospitalier Universitaire de Quebec-CHUL.

NADEAU, Diane; CSSS Cleophas-Claveau, CP 38 succ La Baie 1000 rue du Docteur-Desgagne, La Baie QC G7B 3P9; Laval'72; CSPQ; DiagRad (Echography). Staff, CHSLD-CLSC Cleophas-Claveau; (418)544-3381 x290; Fax. (418)544-0414; dianenadeau1@videotron.ca.

NADEAU, Etienne; CSSS de Laval, 1755 boul Rene-Laennec, Laval QC H7M 3L9; Mon'00; Gastroent; IntMed. Staff, Hopital de la Cite de la santé; (450)668-1010; Fax. (450)372-3516.

NADEAU, Gaetan; Clinique la Cite Medicale, 295-2600 boul Laurier, Quebec QC G1V 4T3; Laval'75; Staff, Centre Hospitalier Chauveau; ac Staff, CSSS de Quebec-Sud; (418)781-0480

NADEAU, Gary J M; Niagara H System-G Niagara, PO Box 1018 Stn Main 5546 Portage Rd, Niagara Falls ON L2E 6X2; Tor'87; CCFP; Staff, Niagara Health System - Greater Niagara General Site; (905)378-4647

NADEAU, Genevieve; Sunnybrook Hlth Sciences Ctre, MG408-2075 Bayview Ave, Toronto ON M4N 3M5; Laval'06; Urol. Staff, Sunnybrook Health Sciences Centre; (416)480-4733

NADEAU, Jacques E; Shriners Hosp for Children, 1529 av Cedar, Montreal QC H3G 1A6; Laval'68; Staff, Shriners Hospitals For Children - Canada; (514)282-7209; Fax. (514)842-8664; jnadeau@shrinenet.org.

NADEAU, Jean-Claude; A-106 Commerciale Ave RR 1, Tring-Jonction QC G0N 1X0; Laval'79; Staff, Centre Hospitalier Beauce-Etchemin; Staff, Centre d'hébergement de Beauceville; Physician, Occupational Health & Safety; (418)426-2282; jean-claude_nadeau@ssss.gouv.qc.ca.

NADEAU, Johane M; Royal Ottawa Hlth Care Group, 1145 Carling Ave, Ottawa ON K1Z 7K4; Ott'02; FRCPC; Psy. Staff, Royal Ottawa Mental Health Centre - Royal Ottawa Health Care Group; (613)722-6521 x6507

NADEAU, John G; Royal Victoria Hosp, 201 Georgian Dr, Barrie ON L4M 6M2; Wes'87; FRCPC; DiagRad. Staff, Royal Victoria Regional Health Centre; (705)728-9802 x43486; Fax. (705)739-5629.

NADEAU, Julie; Clinique Medi-Val, 100-408 rue Jeanne-Mance, Salaber-de-Valleyf QC J6T 4G1; Sher'92; (450)370-3387; Fax. (450)370-3395.

NADEAU, Karine; CSSSG-Hop De Gatineau, CP 2000 Succ Bureau-Chef 909 boul de la Verendrye O, Gatineau QC J8P 7H2; Mon'02; FRCSC; ObstGyn. Staff, Hôpital de Gatineau; (819)561-8100

NADEAU, Linda; Ctr Hosp Affilie-Enfant-Jesus, 1401 18e rue, Quebec QC G1J 1Z4; Laval'81; CSPQ; FRCPC; MedBiochem. Medical Biochemistry, Centre Hospitalier Affilié Universitaire de Québec - Hôpital De L'Enfant Jésus; Assoc Prof Biochem, Université Laval; (418)649-0252 x3309

NADEAU, Louis; Misericordia Community Hosp, 16940 87 Ave NW, Edmonton AB T5R 4H5; Laval'82; FRCPC; Anes. Staff, Covenant Health - Misericordia Community Hospital; (780)735-2863; Fax. (780)735-2967.

NADEAU, Luc; Centre Med de St-Felicien, 1013 boul Sacre-Coeur, Saint-Felicien QC G8K 1R5; Laval'94; CCFP; Member Med, Centre Hospitalier Regional de Sept-Iles; (418)679-0943; Fax. (418)679-4066.

NADEAU, Lucie; CLSC Parc Extension, 204 10-7085 rue Hutchison, Montreal QC H3N 1Y9; Mon'94; FRCPC; Psy. Staff Psy, McGill University Health Centre - Montreal Children's Hospital; (514)273-3800 x6423; Fax. (514)380-8147.

NADEAU, Lynne; CSSS de Laval, 1755 boul Rene-Laennec, Laval QC H7M 3L9; Laval'94; Staff, Hopital de la Cite de la santé; (450)975-5444; Fax. (450)975-5497.

NADEAU, Marc; Clinique Med Desy, 5636 boul Henri-Bourassa E, Montreal-Nord QC H1G 2T2; Mon'79; (514)326-9060; Fax. (514)326-0919.

NADEAU, Marie-Claude; Clin Ped de Trois-Rivieres, 110-5725 boul des Forges, Trois-Rivieres QC G8Y 5L5; Laval'96; LMCC; FRCPC; Peds. Staff, Hôpital Sainte-croix; (819)375-0504; Fax. (819)375-8362.

NADEAU, Marie-Eve; CSSS de la Haute-Gaspésie, 50 rue du Belvedere, Ste-Anne-des-Monts QC G4V 1X4; Mon'99; FRCSC; GenSurg. Staff, Centre Hospitalier des Monts; Langs: Bilingual(French/English); (418)763-2261

NADEAU, Marie-Josee; Ctr Hosp Affilie-Enfant-Jesus, 1401 18e rue, Quebec QC G1J 1Z4; Laval'98; CSPQ; Anes. Staff, Centre Hospitalier Affilié Universitaire de Québec - Hôpital De L'Enfant Jésus; (418)649-5807; Fax. (418)649-5918.

NADEAU, Marie-Josee; Centre Hosp Honore-Mercier, 2750 boul Laframboise, Saint-Hyacinthe QC J2S 4Y8; Mon'92; CSPQ; Anes. Staff, Centre Hospitalier Honore-Mercier; (450)771-3333

NADEAU, Marie-Josee; 105-185 Acadie Ave, Dieppe NB E1A 1G6; Sher'07; CCFP; Staff, Dr Georges-L-Dumont University Hospital Centre; (506)862-4182; Fax. (506)862-4179.

NADEAU, Martine; Clinique Med des 21, 101-171 6e rue, La Baie QC G7B 0A3; Laval'82; Staff, CHSLD-CLSC Cleophas-Claveau; (418)544-3331; Fax. (418)544-7571.

NADEAU, Maryse; CLSC Bedford, GD 34 rue Saint-Joseph, Bedford QC J0J 1A0; Laval'89; MSc; CCFP; Staff, Hôpital Brome-Missisquoi-Perkins; Physician, Unite de Medicine Familiale; (450)248-4321

NADEAU, Melissa M T A; 3114-910 10th Ave W, Vancouver BC V5Z 1M9; McG'07; MDCM; OrthSurg. (604)875-4111 x66276

NADEAU, Michel; Centre Med de Riviere-du-Loup, 242 rue Lafontaine, Riviere-du-Loup QC G5R 3A7; Laval'71; Ac Staff, Centre Hospitalier Regional du Grand-Portage; (418)862-3110; Fax. (418)862-9656.

NADEAU, Michel; Ctr de Sante Paul-Gilbert, 9330 du Centre-Hospitalier, Charny QC G6X 1L6; Mon'95; Staff, Centre Hospitalier Paul-Gilbert; (418)380-8993; nadom1@hotmail.com.

NADEAU, Michel; Hop de Readaptation Lindsay, 6363 ch Hudson, Montreal QC H3S 1M9; Laval'65; Staff, Institut de Réadaptation Gingras-Lindsay de Montréal; (514)737-3661

NADEAU, Michel; CSSS de Beauce-Etchemin, 1515 17e rue, Saint-Georges QC G5Y 4T8; Laval'79; CSPQ; FRCPC; AnatPath (Surgical Pathology). Staff, Centre Hospitalier Regional de Sept-Iles; Staff, Centre Hospitalier Beauce-Etchemin; (418)228-2031; micnad@hotmail.com.

NADEAU, Nancy; CLSC Saint-Hubert, 6800 boul Cousineau, Saint-Hubert QC J3Y 8Z4; McG'99; CCFP; (450)443-7407

NADEAU, Nicole; Hopital Ste-Justine, 3175 ch Cote-Sainte-Catherine, Montreal QC H3T 1C5; Laval'79; FRCPC; Psy. Ac Staff, Hôpital Ste-Justine; (514)345-4695; Fax. (514)345-4679.

NADEAU, Patrick; CSSS Kamouraska Hop-Notre-Dame, 1201 6e av, La Pocatiere QC G0R 1Z0; Sher'94; FRCSC; GenSurg (Surgical Oncology). Staff, CSSS de Kamouraska; (418)856-7000

NADEAU, Paul O; 150-930 ch Sainte-Foy, Quebec QC G1S 2L4; Laval'70; FACS; ATLS; FAAOS; FRCSC; OrthSurg (Hand Surgery). Staff, Centre Hospitalier Affilié Universitaire de Québec - Hôpital du St-Sacrement; Lecturer, Université Laval; Langs: French; (418)527-0036; Fax. (418)527-0053.

NADEAU, Pierre-Olivier; Hopital Ste-Justine, 1816-3175 ch Cote-Sainte-Cathe, Montreal QC H3T 1C5; Laval'02; FRCPC; Psy (P.Q.). Staff, Hôpital Ste-Justine; (514)345-4931

NADEAU, Reginald A; 5400 boul Gouin O, Montreal QC H4J 1C5; Mon'57; FACC; FRCPC; IntMed; Cardiol (P.Q.). Staff, Hôpital du Sacre-Coeur de Montréal; Prof, Universite de Montreal; Langs: German; English; Spanish; (514)338-2216; Fax. (514)338-2566; r-nadeau@crhsc.rtss.qc.ca.

NADEAU, Richard; CSSS de Manicouagan, 635 boul Jolliet, Baie-Comeau QC G5C 1P1; Laval'67; GenSurg. Chief Dept of Surg, Centre Hospitalier Régional Baie-Comeau; (418)589-3701; Fax. (418)296-5217.

NADEAU, Robert; GMF Polyclinique des Ponts, SS 90 120-1100 boul de la Rive-Sud, Saint-Romuald QC G6W 5M6; Laval'86; VP CMDP/Chef, Centre Hospitalier Paul-Gilbert; (418)834-1177

NADEAU, Serge; GMF Polyclinique des Ponts, 120-1100 boul de la Rive-Sud, Saint-Romuald QC G6W 5M6; Laval'76; LMCC; Staff Equipe Soins Palliatifs, CSSS du Grand Littoral; (418)834-1177; Fax. (418)834-9275.

NADEAU, Simon; Centre Med Sillery, 1270 av William, Quebec QC G1S 4G1; Laval'72; ac Staff, Jeffery Hale Hospital-Saint Brigid's; (418)688-0664; Fax. (418)688-4601.

NADEAU, Sophie M; CHUQ-Hotel-Dieu de Quebec, 11 Cote du Palais, Quebec QC G1R 2J6; Laval'82; CSPQ; Anes. Ac Staff, Centre Hospitalier Universitaire de Québec (CHUQ) - Siege Social; (418)691-5323; Fax. (418)691-5728.

NADEAU, Sophie; CHUQ-Ctr Hosp Univ Laval, 2705 boul Laurier, Quebec QC G1V 4G2; Sher'97; FRCPC; Peds (Neonatal & Perinatal). Staff, McGill University Health Centre - Montreal Children's Hospital; Staff, Centre Hospitalier Universitaire de Quebec-CHUL; Asst Prof Geographic Full-Time, McGill University; Langs: English; (418)656-4141; sophie.nadeau@muhc.mcgill.ca.

NADEAU, Sylvie; 110-2880 ch des Quatre-Bourgeo, Quebec QC G1V 4X7; Laval'01; FRCSC; Otol. Staff Otol, Centre Hospitalier Affilié Universitaire de Québec - Hôpital De L'Enfant Jésus; Staff Otol, Centre Hospitalier Affilié Universitaire de Québec - Hôpital du St-Sacrement; (418)653-8717; Fax. (418)653-7199.

NADEAU, Sylvie; 104-140 Champlain St, Dieppe NB E1A 1N8; Laval'91; FRCSC; ObstGyn. Staff, Dr Georges-L-Dumont University Hospital Centre; (506)383-4205; Fax. (506)855-2189.

NADEAU, Yannick; Ctr Hosp Rouyn-Noranda, 4 9e rue, Rouyn-Noranda QC J9X 2B2; Laval'04; FRCPC; Neur. Staff, Centre Hospitalier Rouyn-Noranda; (819)764-5131

NADEAU, Yves; CSSS de Rivière-de-Loup, 75 rue Saint-Henri, Riviere-Du-Loup QC G5R 2A4; Laval'88; LMCC; FACOG; FRCSC; ObstGyn (Colposcopy). Staff, Centre Hospitalier Regional du Grand-Portage; (418)868-1000; Fax. (418)868-1075.

NADEAU, Yvon-A.; 9330 boul du Centre-Hospitalie, Levis QC G6X 1L6; Laval'72; LMCC; Staff, Centre Hospitalier Paul-Gilbert; Médecin, CSSS Alphonse-Desjardins; Physician, CHSLD Charny; Clin Instructor, Université Laval; Langs: English; (418)380-8993 x2276; yyan11@me.com.

NADEAU-FREDETTE, Annie C; Univ of Toronto, 602-500 University Ave, Toronto ON M5G 1V7; Mon'07; Nephrol; IntMed.

NADEEM, Muhammad B; 102-1669 Victoria St, Prince George BC V2L 2L5; Punjab (Pakistan)'91; MB BS; CCFP; (250)564-3133; Fax. (250)562-6840.

NADEEM, Syed M N A; Queen Elizabeth II HSC-Halifax, 6896B-1796 Summer St, Halifax NS B3H 3A7; Karachi (Pakistan)'93; Staff, Queen Elizabeth II Health Sciences Centre - Halifax Infirmary Site; (902)473-5769; Fax. (902)473-6293.

NADEEM, Taj G; Fletcher Healthcare, 10794 Chinguacousy Rd, Brampton ON L7A 0G9; Punjab (India)'89; CCFP; (905)970-8925; Fax. (905)970-8923.

NADEEM, Yasmin N; Access Transcona, 845 Regent Ave W, Winnipeg MB R2C 3A9; Man'05; CCFP; Teach Staff, University of Manitoba; (204)938-5700; Fax. (204)938-5510.

NADEL, Helen R; Children's & Women's HC of BC, 1K19-4480 Oak St, Vancouver BC V6H 3V4; Man'77; DABR; DAB; FRCPC; DiagRad (Pediatric Radiology); NuclearMed. Staff, BC Children's Hospital; Asst Prof, University of British Columbia; (604)875-3034; Fax. (604)875-2367.

NADEL, Mendel R; Oakdale Med Bldg, 104-2065 Finch Ave W, North York ON M3N 2V7; Tor'72; FRCSC; ObstGyn. Staff, Humber River Regional Hospital - Finch Avenue Site; Staff, Princess Margaret Hospital - University Health Network; (416)746-1955; Fax. (416)746-2878.

NADEL, Orli Y; 702-240 Duncan Mill Rd, North York ON M3B 3S6; Tor'07; CCFP; (416)494-7435

NADELLA, Rajasree; Ridge Meadows Hosp & Hlth CC, 11666 Laity St, Maple Ridge BC V2X 5A3; Vijayawada-Guntur (India)'95; Staff, Ridge Meadows Hospital & Health Care Centre; (604)463-4111

NADER, Nabil; Cumberland Health Authority, 34 Prince Arthur St, Amherst NS B4H 1V6; St. Joseph (Lebanon)'78; FRCSC; GenSurg. (902)667-2186

NADJAFI, Maral; University of Toronto, 500 University Ave, Toronto ON M5G 1V7; Tor'08; IntMed.

NADKARNI, Ashok B; Glengarry Mem Hosp, Highway 43, Alexandria ON K0C 1A0; Poona (India)'71; Staff, Glengarry Memorial Hospital; (613)525-2111

NADKARNI, Dipti A; Commercial Street Med Centre, 208-311 Commercial St, Milton ON L9T 3Z9; Sher'01; FRCSC; ObstGyn. (905)875-2280; Fax. (905)875-9172.

NADKARNI, Gauri; CSSSG-Hop de Gatineau, CP 2000 Succ Bureau-Chef 909 boul de la Verendrye O, Gatineau QC J8P 7H2; Sher'99; FRCSC; GenSurg. Staff, Hôpital de Gatineau; Langs: English; (819)561-8100

NADKARNI, Pallavi S; Kingston Gen Hosp, 76 Stuart St, Kingston ON K7L 2V7; Mumbai (India)'98; Staff, Kingston General Hospital; (613)548-7839

NADLER, Norman J; 1455 rue Peel, Montreal QC H3A 1T5; McG'51; PhD; IntMed (P.Q.) (Endocrinology). Assoc Staff, Sir Mortimer B Davis Jewish General; assoc Prof, McGill University; Langs: French; (514)933-1166; Fax. (514)933-1166; norman.nadler@mail.mcgill.ca.

NADLER, Steven P; The Ottawa Hosp-Riverside, 5 11-1967 Riverside Dr, Ottawa ON K1H 7W9; McG'77; FRCPC; IntMed; Nephrol. Ac Staff, The Ottawa Hospital - Riverside Campus; Assoc Prof, University of Ottawa; Langs: Bilingual(English/French); (613)738-8400 x82568; Fax. (613)738-8337.

NADOLNY, Laurie J; Woodroffe South Med Bldg, 202-1637 Woodroffe Ave, Nepean ON K2G 1W2; Tor'87; CCFP; Langs: English; French; (613)723-5635; Fax. (613)723-5918.

NADON, Dominique J; U of Ottawa Health Services, 100-100 Marie Curie Pvt, Ottawa ON K1N 1A2; Ott'86; FRCPC; Psy. Staff, Montfort Hospital; (613)564-3950 x225

NADON, F Vincent G; U of Ottawa Health Services, 300-100 Marie Curie Pvt, Ottawa ON K1N 1A2; Ott'84; Staff, Montfort Hospital; Consultant, Canadian Red Cross for Overseas Missions; (613)564-3930; Fax. (613)564-6627.

NADON, J W Grant; Bellwood Health Services Inc, 1020 McNicoll Ave, Scarborough ON M1W 2J6; Tor'61; FRCPC; IntMed (Geriatric Medicine). Physician Extended Care Dept, Sunnybrook Health Sciences Centre; Teach Staff Family & Community Med, University of Toronto; (416)495-0926 x103

NADON, Joel; CSSS de Papineau, 155 rue Maclaren E, Gatineau QC J8L 0C2; Ott'02; CCFP; Staff, Hôpital de Papineau; Staff, CH-CHSLD de Papineau - Pavillon du centre hospitalier; (819)986-3341; Fax. (819)986-4000.

NADON, Michel; Clinique Med Douville, 5460 boul Laurier O, Saint-Hyacinthe QC J2S 3V7; Mon'81; Centre Hospitalier Honore-Mercier; Fax. (450)771-7530; michel.delisle@rrsss16.gouv.qc.ca.

NADON, Philippe C; Child & Adolescence Serv Assoc, 10645 63 Ave NW, Edmonton AB T6H 1P7; Alb'99; BSc; FRCPC; Psy (Child & Adolescent Psychiatry). (780)438-0011; Fax. (780)437-6133; pnadon@casaservices.org.

NADOR, Roland G; Vancouver Gen Hosp, 855 12th Ave W, Vancouver BC V5Z 1M9; (Hungary)'92; Staff, Vancouver General Hospital - Centennial Pavillion; Langs: Hungarian; French; (604)875-4111

NADORI, Attila B; Glenbrook Med Center, 111-4306 Richmond Rd SW, Calgary AB T3E 4P6; (South Africa)'88; BSc; CCFP; (403)685-5480; Fax. (403)685-5482.

NADOUR, Jalaa; Bank of Montreal Bldg, 210-35 Commercial St, Truro NS B2N 3H9; (Syria)'95; Staff, Colchester East Hants Health Centre; (902)897-9395; Fax. (902)897-0873.

NADRA, Imad J; 202-2020 Richmond Ave, Victoria BC V8R 6R5; Edinburgh (Scotland)'97; (250)595-3111

NADWIDNY, Laurie A; Royal Alexandra Hosp, 10240 Kingsway NW, Edmonton AB T5H 3V9; Alb'89; Anes. Staff, Royal Alexandra Hospital; (780)735-4010

NAEEM, Mehmooda; Cape Breton Hlthcare Complex, 1A-1482 George St, Sydney NS B1P 1P3; Peshawar (Pakistan)'86; CCFP; Staff, Cape Breton Healthcare Complex; Staff, Northside General Hospital; (902)567-7703; Fax. (902)567-3310.

NAEEM, Nauman; Humber River Reg Hosp-Church, 200 Church St, Toronto ON M9N 1N8; Santo Domingo (Dominican Republic)'97; FRCPC; IntMed; Critical Care Medicine. Staff, Humber River Regional Hospital - Church Street Site; (416)249-8111

NAESSENS, Veronique; Univ Hlth Network-Toronto Gen, 200 Elizabeth St, Toronto ON M5G 2C4; McG'07; MDCM; Hem; IntMed. Staff, Toronto General Hospital - UHN; (416)340-5233

NAFIS, Anjum S; Alberta Hosp Edmonton, PO Box 307 Stn Main 17480 Fort Rd, Edmonton AB T5J 2J7; (New Zealand)'97; Staff, Alberta Hospital Edmonton; (780)342-5465

NAFISI, Sepideh; Wedgewood Med Centre, 202-12 Gleneyre St, St. John's NL A1A 2M7; Tehran (Iran)'96; CCFP; (709)722-9000

NAG, Sanjita; Baywood Med Centre, 200-95 Bayly St W, Ajax ON L1S 7K8; Qns'01; BScBiology; CCFP; (905)686-3900; Fax. (905)686-9222.

NAG, Shudeshna; The Rusholme Clinic, 1465 Dundas St W, Toronto ON M6J 1Y7; Qns'04; FRCPC; Peds. Staff, Toronto East General Hospital Inc; (416)534-1150; Fax. (416)534-9630.

NAGAHARA, Brian M; 9625 Yonge St, Richmond Hill ON L4C 5T2; Tor'89; (905)508-4114; Fax. (905)508-4116.

NAGAI, Gordon R; Corporate Med Centre, 10-78 Corporate Dr, Scarborough ON M1H 3G4; Wes'78; ABIM; ABNM; NBME; FRCPC; NuclearMed (Nephrology); IntMed. Staff, The Scarborough Hospital - General Campus; Court Staff Diagnostic Imaging, Lakeridge Health - Oshawa Site; Court Staff, Bridgepoint Health Centre; (416)279-0855 x245; Fax. (416)279-0857; gordonnagai@yahoo.ca.

NAGAI, Ryuta; Nagai Med Professional Corp, 6-100 Martindale Rd, St Catharines ON L2S 2Y3; Wes'86; FACP; FRCPC; IntMed; Nephrol. Staff, Niagara Health System - Ontario Street Site; Staff, Niagara Health System - St Catharines General Site; Teach Staff, McMaster University; (905)684-6529; Fax. (905)684-5577; niagnephs@bellnet.ca.

NAGAIAH, Theepa S; Mineville Health Centre, 4 Peter Crt, Mineville NS B2Z 1K2; Jaffna (Sri Lanka)'00; (902)829-3278; Fax. (902)829-2549.

NAGAMUTTU, Sivakumar; 8-9889 Highway 48, Markham ON L6E 0B7; Jaffna (Sri Lanka)'99; CCFP; Langs: Sinhalese; Tamil; (905)554-9400; Fax. (905)554-9401; drsiva@hotmail.com.

NAGARAJAN, Naveen P; Hamilton HS-Henderson Site, 711 Concession St, Hamilton ON L8V 1C3; Tamil Nadu (India)'97; FRCPC; DiagRad. Staff, Hamilton Health Sciences Centre-Juravinski Site; (905)527-4322

NAGARIA, Mohammad H; 107-301 Columbia St E, New Westminster BC V3L 3W5; Karachi (Pakistan)'87; (604)523-2085

NAGARIA, Neelam; 10153 King George Blvd, Surrey BC V3T 2W1; Karachi (Pakistan)'99; MB BS; IntMed. (604)951-0885

NAGASE, Daniel Y; Squamish Gen Hosp, 38140 Behrner Dr, Squamish BC V8B 0J3; Dal'04; CCFP; CCFP(E.M.); Staff, Squamish General Hospital / Hilltop House; (604)892-5211

NAGDEE, Muhammed Z; 203-9123 Mary St, Chilliwack BC V2P 4H7; Cape Town (South Africa)'09; MB ChB; (604)795-9161

NAGEL, Daniel P; Whitby Medical, 4-3910 Brock St N, Whitby ON L1R 3E1; Tor'95; BSc(Psychol); CCFP; Langs: Spanish; (905)444-9493; Fax. (905)444-9174.

NAGEL, Michael G; Niagara Med Group Fam Hlth Team, 4421 Queen St, Niagara Falls ON L2E 2L2; (Antigua & Barbuda)'05; CCFP; (905)356-2236

NAGENDRAN, Jayan; University of Alberta Hosp, 8440 112 St NW, Edmonton AB T6G 2B7; Alb'01; FRCSC; CardSurg. Staff, University of Alberta Hospital; (780)407-8822; Fax. (780)407-6752.

NAGHDI, Lili; The Health Centre of Maple, 2810 Major Mackenzie Dr, Maple ON L6A 3L2; Tehran (Iran)'97; CCFP; Langs: Farsi; (905)832-3838; Fax. (905)832-9097; naghdil@yahoo.com.

NAGHI, Alexandru; Main Square Med Centre, 2575 Danforth Ave, Toronto ON M4C 1L5; Iassy (Romania)'71; (416)694-0500; Fax. (416)694-9767.

NAGHIBI, Sam; 106-531 Davis Dr, Newmarket ON L3Y 6P5; Karachi (Pakistan)'79; MB BS; CCFP; Langs: Persian; Urdu; (905)235-8878; Fax. (905)235-8890.

NAGHIBI TORBATI, Bibi A; Kelowna Gen Hosp, 2268 Pandosy St, Kelowna BC V1Y 1T2; Karachi (Pakistan)'83; FRCPC; AnatPath. Staff, Kelowna General Hospital; (250)862-4300; Fax. (250)862-4051.

NAGHIU, Marius C; South Western Med Ctr, 813 Richmond St, London ON N6A 3H6; Cluj-Napoca (Romania)'97; MD; CCFP; Staff Emerg Room, Strathroy Middlesex General Hospital - Middlesex Hospital Alliance; Langs: Romanian; (519)433-4330; Fax. (519)433-4332.

NAGI, Harpinder S; Gordon & Leslie Diamond HCC, 2775 Laurel St, Vancouver BC V5Z 1M9; UBC'06; FRCPC; IntMed. Langs: Punjabi; (604)875-4111

NAGI, Kirandeep S; 409-2300 Eglinton Ave W, Mississauga ON L5M 2V8; Wes'92; FRCPC; IntMed (Cardiac Catheterization); Cardiol. Staff, Rouge Valley Health System - Ajax & Pickering Health Centre Site; (289)997-3264; Fax. (289)997-3265.

NAGI, Mohamed M; VM Med, 1000-1538 rue Sherbrooke O, Montreal QC H3G 1L5; McG'01; FRCSC; Otol. (514)933-2778

NAGIAH, Theepa S; Mineville Health Centre, 4 Peter Crt, Dartmouth NS B2W 1K2; (Sri Lanka)'00; CCFP; (902)829-3278; Fax. (902)829-2549; drtheepa@hotmail.com.

NAGJI, Ashnoor; Raven Song Commun Hlth Ctre, 2450 Ontario St, Vancouver BC V5T 4T7; Ott'05; CCFP; Langs: Gujarati; Hindi; Urdu; (604)709-6400

NAGJI, Noor; 343 Coxwell Ave, Toronto ON M4L 3B5; Karachi (Pakistan)'75; (416)469-0002; Fax. (416)469-2227.

NAGLE, Cheryl Y; 201-3811 Chatham St, Richmond BC V7E 2Z4; UBC'85; Assoc Medical Staff, Richmond Hospital; (604)274-6644; Fax. (604)274-2931.

NAGLIE, I Gary; Baycrest Geriatric Hlth Care C, 278-3560 Bathurst St, Toronto ON M6A 2E1; McG'83; FRCPC; IntMed; GeriatricMed. Staff, Baycrest Centre for Geriatric Care; (416)785-2500; Fax. (416)788-1199.

NAGPAL, Anil K; Belmont Prof Centre, 305-564 Belmont Ave W, Kitchener ON N2M 5N6; Nairobi (Kenya)'86; MB ChB; FACP; ABIM; FCCP; FRCPC; IntMed (Sleep Medicine); Respir. Langs: Hindi; Punjabi; (519)576-8080; Fax. (519)576-8619.

NAGPAL, Atul D; London HSC-University Hosp, PO Box 5339 Stn B B6 102-339 Windermere Rd, London ON N6A 5A5; Wes'04; FRCSC; CardSurg; Critical Care Medicine. Staff, London Health Sciences Centre - University Hospital; (519)685-8500

NAGPAL, Rohit S; 45-2130 North Park Dr, Brampton ON L6S 0C9; Baroda (India)'93; MB BS; CCFP; Langs: Hindi; Punjabi; Gujarati; (905)792-9419; Fax. (905)792-9049.

NAGPAL, Sandeep K; 201-16 Green St, Nepean ON K2J 3R2; Dal'90; BSc; (613)825-8405

NAGPAL, Sudhir K; The Ottawa Hosp-Civic Campus, A280-1053 Carling Ave, Ottawa ON K1Y 4E9; Dal'89; FRCSC; GenSurg (EndovascularSurg); VascSurg. Staff, The Ottawa Hospital - Civic Campus; (613)761-4766; Fax. (613)761-5362; snagpal@ottawahospital.on.ca.

NAGPURKAR, Ranjana; Child & Adolescent Clinic, 200-30A Kennedy Rd S, Brampton ON L6W 3E2; Poona (India)'72; MB BS; FRCPC; Psy (Child & Adolescent Psychiatry). Consultant Psy, William Osler Health System - Brampton Civic Hospital; Consultant Psy, Trillium Health Centre - Mississauga; Langs: Hindi; (905)453-1160; Fax. (905)453-8971; ranjana.nagpurkar@williamoslerhs.ca.

NAGRA, M Saleem; Medical Clinic, 1114-7318 137 St, Surrey BC V3W 1A3; Sind (Pakistan)'64; LRCP; MRCS; FRCS(Ed); FACS; FRCSC; GenSurg. (604)572-8812; Fax. (604)572-8819; nagra7@shaw.ca.

NAGRA, Riffat Saleem; Medical Clinic, 1114-7318 137 St, Surrey BC V3W 1A3; Punjab (Pakistan)'75; MB BS; (604)572-8812; Fax. (604)572-8819.

NAGRANI, Pritam-Lala; West Street Health Centre, 216 West St, Simcoe ON N3Y 1S8; Birmingham (England)'72; MB ChB; MRCP(UK); LMCC; FRCP(Ed); Consultant, Tillsonburg District Memorial Hospital; (519)428-0432; Fax. (519)428-9903; nags@kwic.com.

NAGY, Alexander G; Fairmont Med Bldg, 906-750 Broadway W, Vancouver BC V5Z 1H8; Ott'69; BSc; FRCSC; GenSurg (Laparoscopic Surgery). Ac Staff, Vancouver General Hospital - Centennial Pavillion; Assoc Staff, BC Cancer Agency Vancouver Centre; Langs: Hungarian; Italian; French; (604)873-1885; Fax. (604)873-1899.

NAGY, Francine; Clinique Med Rosemont, 1969 boul Rosemont, Montreal QC H2G 1S9; Montpellier (France)'78; Langs: Bilingual(French/English); (514)274-7344; Fax. (514)274-1165.

NAGY, Joan C; 2F-187 James St S, Hamilton ON L8P 3A8; McM'80; FRCPC; Psy (Psychotherapy). Psychiatrist, Niagara ACT Team; Psychiatrist, Hamilton Family Health Team; (905)521-1952; Fax. (905)521-9058; joan.nagy@niagararegion.ca.

NAGY, Maria; Forest Hill Family Health, 491 Eglinton Ave W, Toronto ON M5N 1A8; Budapest (Hungary)'64; Langs: Hungarian; (416)782-6111; Fax. (416)782-5515.

NAGY, Thomas; Park Avenue Med Centre, 101-4634 Park Ave, Terrace BC V8G 1V7; Cal'91; MSc; FRCSC; Ophth. (250)615-5002; Fax. (250)615-5004.

NAHAB, Reem; 5966 Mullen Way NW, Edmonton AB T6R 0S9; (Iraq)'04; Staff, Covenant Health - Grey Nuns Community Hospital; (780)801-1220; Fax. (780)801-1225.

NAHAL, Ayoub; MUHC-Montreal Gen Hosp, 1650 av Cedar, Montreal QC H3G 1A4; Aleppo (Syria)'93; CSPQ; AnatPath (P.Q.). Staff, McGill University Health Centre - Montreal General Campus; Langs: Arabic; (514)934-1934 x43839; ayoub.nahal@muhc.mcgill.ca.

NAHAS, Mirna; Sheldon Chumir Centre, 1213 4 St SW, Calgary AB T2R 0X7; Cal'00; CCFP; (403)955-6200; nahas_m@hotmail.com.

NAHAS, Richard; 942 Merivale Rd, Ottawa ON K1Z 5Z9; Tor'98; CCFP; (613)727-7246; Fax. (613)727-7247.

NAHAS, Samar H A; The Credit Valley Hosp, 2200 Eglinton Ave E, Mississauga ON L5M 2N1; King Faisal (Saudi Arabia)'02; ObstGyn. Staff, The Credit Valley Hospital; (905)813-2200

NAHER, Monzur; 1657 Dundas St, London ON N5W 3C6; Dhaka (Bangladesh)'94; CCFP; Langs: Bengali; (519)951-0061; Fax. (519)455-7103.

NAHIRNEY, David B; Glenrose Rehab Hosp, 335-10230 111 Ave NW, Edmonton AB T5G 0B7; Alb'82; FRCPC; Psy (Child & Adolescent Psychiatry). Staff, Royal Alexandra Hospital; Staff, Glenrose Rehabilitation Hospital; (780)735-7911; Fax. (780)735-8246.

NAHIRNIAK, Susan N; University of Alberta Hosp, 4B1. 23WMC-8440 112 St NW, Edmonton AB T6G 2B7; Alb'97; FRCPC; HemPath (Transfusion Medicine). Staff Hematology, University of Alberta Hospital; (780)407-2012; Fax. (780)407-8599; susan.nahirniak@albertahealthservices.ca.

NAHIRNY, Taras; Trafalgar Prof Centre, 300-1235 Trafalgar Rd, Oakville ON L6H 3P1; (Poland)'10; CCFP; (905)842-0071; Fax. (905)844-3811.

NAHON, Dahlia R; Doctor's Office, 101-491 Lawrence Ave W, North York ON M5M 1C7; Ott'04; (416)787-9796; Fax. (416)787-8094.

NAHORNICK, Boris; Drumheller Assoc Physicians, PO Box 5600, Drumheller AB T0J 0Y0; Alb'56; BSc; LMCC; Chairman, Drumheller Area Health Foundation; Langs: Ukrainian; (403)823-3345; Fax. (403)823-7823.

NAHRI, Dolly T; Access Med Centre, 1395 Bank St, Ottawa ON K1H 8N1; Dal'92; BSc; Langs: Arabic; Creole; (613)731-1114; Fax. (613)731-1116.

NAHVI, Shahab; The Pas Health Complex Inc, PO Box 240 Stn Main, The Pas MB R9A 1K4; CCFP; Staff, St. Anthony General Hospital; (204)623-6431

NAIB, Ravinder; 6143B 28 Ave NW, Edmonton AB T6L 6N5; Delhi (India)'79; MB BS; (780)490-7770

NAIBERG, David; SGH Medical Mall, 515-3030 Lawrence Ave E, Scarborough ON M1P 2T7; Tor'62; FACO; AAFP; FRCSC; Otol (Facial & Cosmetic Surgery). Court Staff, Rouge Valley Health System - Centenary Health Centre Site; Emeritus Chief Dept of Otol, The Scarborough Hospital - General Campus; (416)438-6285; Fax. (416)438-9161; drnaiberg@facial-cosmetics.com.

NAIBERG, Jerry B; Southlake Med Centre, 104-581 Davis Dr, Newmarket ON L3Y 2P6; Tor'83; FRCSC; Otol. Staff, Southlake Regional Health Centre; (905)898-2444; Fax. (905)898-5558; jerrynaiberg@rogers.com.

NAICKER, Sharman M; Trail Mental Hlth & Addiction, 3-1500 Columbia Ave, Trail BC V1R 1J9; Natal (South Africa)'82; MB ChB; MMed(Psych); FRCPC; Psy (Group Therapy). Staff, Kootenay Boundary Regional Hospital; (250)364-6262

NAICKER, Sivalingam S; Family Practice Associates, PO Box 1260, Mayerthorpe AB T0E 1N0; (India)'89; MB BS; (780)786-2412; Fax. (780)786-2249.

NAIDOO, Balakrishna P; Old Quebec Street Mall, 202-55 Wyndham St N, Guelph ON N1H 7T8; Cape Town (South Africa)'61; MB ChB; FRCPC; Peds. Hon Staff, Guelph General Hospital; (519)822-5751; Fax. (519)822-4181; bpnaidoo@gmail.com.

NAIDOO, Chitraleka; Scenic Acres Med Clinic, 8555 Scurfield Dr NW, Calgary AB T3L 1Z6; Durban (South Africa)'79; MB ChB; CCFP; (403)547-2255; Fax. (403)547-2254.

NAIDOO, Dadi B; Smyth Associate Clinic, 4904 48 St, Leduc AB T9E 6X4; Cape Town (South Africa)'69; MB ChB; Med Pres, Leduc Community Hospital; (780)986-3432; Fax. (780)986-0356.

NAIDOO, Denisha; Guelph Family Health Team, 101-21 Surrey St W, Guelph ON N1H 3R3; Tor'96; BSc; MSc; CCFP; (519)822-2188; Fax. (519)822-1223.

NAIDOO, Erin C; Clayton Heights Medical, 204-18730 Fraser Hwy, Surrey BC V3S 8E7; Witwatersrand (South Africa)'98; MB ChB; BSc; (604)575-0501

NAIDOO, Jayabalan A; CML Healthcare, 6560 Kennedy Rd, Mississauga ON L5T 2X4; Natal (South Africa)'79; MB ChB; FRCPC; GenPath (Cytology). Ac Staff, Trillium Health Centre - West Toronto; Ac Staff Lab Med, Trillium Health Centre - Mississauga; (905)565-1776

NAIDOO, Jenisa; Central Med Laboratories, 212-388 Portage Ave, Winnipeg MB R3C 0C8; Natal (South Africa)'87; (204)944-0757

NAIDOO, Karunagaran; Lloydminster Specialist Clinic, 1723 51 Ave, Lloydminster AB T9V 2J6; (South Africa)'92; FRCSC; GenSurg. Langs: Afrikaans; (780)874-1106; Fax. (780)874-1196; arny1naidoo@gmail.com.

NAIDOO, Kouslai; Windsor Prof Centre, 130-2462 Howard Ave, Windsor ON N8X 3V6; Natal (South Africa)'87; MB ChB; CCFP; FCFP; Teach Staff, Schulich School of Medicine-University of Western Ontario; (519)258-7865; Fax. (519)258-7208.

NAIDOO, Neelandran; Maple Creek Primary Hlth Care, PO Box 517 36A Pacific Ave, Maple Creek SK S0N 1N0; (306)662-2829; Fax. (306)662-2332.

NAIDOO, Niren; Hotel-Dieu Grace Hosp, 1030 Ouellette Ave, Windsor ON N9A 1E1; Medunsa (South Africa)'98; MB ChB; DObst; Staff, Hôtel-Dieu Grace Hospital; (519)973-4401

NAIDOO, Oshadhesa; Urban Med Clinic, 5619 23 Ave NW, Edmonton AB T6L 7B9; (South Africa)'97; MB ChB; DA; CCFP; (780)757-9545; Fax. (780)757-5337; onaidoo@cablerocket.com.

NAIDOO, Radhakrishnan P; 302-2238 Dundas St W, Toronto ON M6R 3A9; (Zimbabwe)'83; Staff, St Joseph's Health Centre; (416)534-6379

NAIDOO, Salendra D; C-22195 Dewdney Trunk Rd, Maple Ridge BC V2X 3H7; Kwazulu-Natal (South Africa)'84; MB ChB; (604)463-8877

NAIDOO, Sharmilla; Foothills Med Centre, 1403 29 St NW, Calgary AB T2N 2T9; (South Africa)'84; MB ChB; CCFP; FCFP; Staff, Foothills Medical Centre; (403)944-2800

NAIDOO, Shireen P; Salvation Army Grace Gen Hosp, 300 Booth Dr, Winnipeg MB R3J 3M7; Natal (South Africa)'74; DABPath; FCAP; FASCP; Staff Pathol, The Salvation Army Grace Hospital; Med Dir-Lab Serv, Misericordia Health Centre; Dir Labs, Riverview Health Centre; Med Dir/Head Lab Serv, Unicity Laboratory Services; (204)837-0131; Fax. (204)837-0552.

NAIDOO, Soobramani; 102-809 Brant St, Burlington ON L7R 2J4; Natal (South Africa)'68; BSc; MB ChB; LMCC; Ac Staff, Joseph Brant Memorial Hospital; (905)639-1521; Fax. (905)639-9382.

NAIDOO, Suryakumari; 300B-2085 Hurontario St, Mississauga ON L5A 4G1; Natal (South Africa)'84; FRCPC; Psy. Consultant Child & Adolescent Mental Health Prog, Trillium Health Centre - Mississauga; (905)848-7484; Fax. (905)804-7912.

NAIDOO, Therusha; Quance East Med Clinic, 49-2223 E Victoria Ave, Regina SK S4N 6E4; MB BCh; Physician, Quance East Medical Clinic; (306)522-2278; Fax. (306)522-2281.

NAIDOO, Vernon; Alta Sask Wellness Inc, 3-5202 12 St, Lloydminster AB T9V 0W1; (780)875-5200; vernonn@gmail.com.

NAIDU, Dhiren J; 710-11010 101 St NW, Edmonton AB T5H 4B9; Sask'99; FRCPC; PhysMed&Rehab (Sports Medicine). Asst Prof Physical Med & Rehab, University of Alberta; (780)453-5255; Fax. (780)453-9099.

NAIDU, Di; Saskatchewan Med Assoc, 402-321A 21st St E, Saskatoon SK S7K 0C1; Natal (South Africa)'84; MB ChB; DA(SA); (306)244-2196; Fax. (306)653-1631.

NAIDU, Kumar; Bluewater Health-Norman Site, 89 Norman St, Sarnia ON N7T 6S3; Madras (India)'78; MB BS; MD(Physiol); MRCPsy; FRCPC; Psy (General Adult Psychiatry). Consultant Psy, London Health Sciences Centre - Victoria Campus; Staff, Bluewater Health - Norman Site; Staff, Bluewater Health - Mitton Site; Assoc Prof Psy, University of Western Ontario; (519)464-4400

NAIDU, Mary; 403-265 Yorkland Blvd, North York ON M2J 5C7; Bangalore (India)'79; MB BS; MRCPsy; DPM; FRCP; FRCPC; Psy. Consultant Psy, Ontario Shores Centre for Mental Health Sciences.

NAIDU, P R Paul; 202 Rosemount Ave, York ON M9N 3C3; Dublin (Ireland)'56; DCH; (416)245-3122; Fax. (416)245-3122.

NAIDU, Padmaja R; 101-3335 Dougall Ave, Windsor ON N9E 1S8; Baroda (India)'99; (519)948-8000

NAIDU, Phnendren; Edson Med Centre, PO Box 6660 Stn Main 615 50 St, Edson AB T7E 1V1; (South Africa)'05; (780)723-3366; Fax. (780)723-3437.

NAIDU, Prenilla; University of Alberta Hosp, 2B4.01-8440 112 St NW, Edmonton AB T6G 2B7; Natal (South Africa)'93; Staff, Alberta Hospital Edmonton; Resd Staff, University of Alberta Hospital; Staff, Royal Alexandra Hospital; Langs: Afrikaans; Zulu; (780)407-7031

NAIDU, Rajgopaul; Pape Med Cente, 751 Pape Ave, Toronto ON M4K 3T1; Tor'89; FACC; FRCPC; IntMed; Cardiol. (416)778-0101; Fax. (416)778-4752.

NAIDU, Renuka S; Bluewater Health-Norman Site, 89 Norman St, Sarnia ON N7T 6S3; Nagpur (India)'92; FRCPC; IntMed; Critical Care Medicine. Staff, Bluewater Health - Norman Site; Langs: Hindi; Telugu; (519)464-4506

NAIDU, Veyantiz J; 200-10230 142 St NW, Edmonton AB T5N 3Y6; Sask'96; CCFP; (780)454-4242; Fax. (780)454-4224.

NAIK, Anjana T; 201-481 London Rd, Sarnia ON N7T 4X3; Kerala (India)'82; MB BS; BSc; (519)491-1119

NAIK, Latha D; Medical Arts Bldg, 641-750 Spadina Cres E, Saskatoon SK S7K 3H3; Mysore (India)'85; FACP; FRCPC; IntMed (Rheumatology). Staff, Royal University Hospital; Langs: Hindi; (306)384-1500; Fax. (306)384-9990.

NAIK, Sandeep S; University of Alberta Hosp, 8440 112 St NW, Edmonton AB T6G 2B7; Alb'94; FRCPC; DiagRad (Neuro Radiology). Staff, University of Alberta Hospital; (780)407-8822; Fax. (780)407-1202.

NAIK, Viren; The Ottawa Hosp-Civic Campus, 1053 Carling Ave, Ottawa ON K1Y 4E9; Tor'97; FRCPC; Anes. Staff, The Ottawa Hospital - Civic Campus; (613)722-7000

NAIKER, Erushka; 100B-504 Cottonwood Ave, Coquitlam BC V3J 2R4; Witwatersrand (South Africa)'05; (604)939-8831

NAIKER, Randy; Meadowlark Health Centre, 180 Meadowlark Shopping Ctr NW, Edmonton AB T5R 5W9; Alb'02; CCFP; (780)484-7574

NAIM, Maurice; Clinique Med de l'Ile, 182 rue Montcalm, Gatineau QC J8Y 3B5; Nancy (France)'69; Staff, Hull Hospital; (819)770-6564; Fax. (819)777-5437; mnaim@sympatico.ca.

NAIMAN, Alisa B; Doctor's Office, 101-491 Lawrence Ave W, North York ON M5M 1C7; Tor'04; CCFP; (416)787-9796; Fax. (416)787-8094.

NAIMAN, Lada; Hop du Scare-Coeur de Mtl, 5400 boul Gouin O, Montreal QC H4J 1C5; Saratov Medical Institute (Other Foreign)'91; FRCPC; IntMed; Rheum. Staff, Hôpital du Sacre-Coeur de Montréal; (514)338-2050

NAIMARK, Arnold; 230-745 Bannatyne Ave, Winnipeg MB R3E 0J9; Man'57; BSc(Med); MSc(Man); FRSC; FRCPC; IntMed (Respirology). Consultant, Health Sciences Centre; Consultant, St Boniface General Hospital; Dir Ctre for the Advancement of Med/Prof, University of Manitoba; (204)789-3826; Fax. (204)789-3904; arnold_naimark@umanitoba.ca.

NAIMARK, David M J; Sunnybrook Hlth Sciences Ctre, A139-2075 Bayview Ave, Toronto ON M4N 3M5; Man'87; BSc(Med); MSc; FRCPC; IntMed (Dialysis); Nephrol. Assoc Staff, Sunnybrook Health Sciences Centre; Asst Prof, University of Toronto; (416)480-4773; Fax. (416)480-5755.

NAIMER, Michelle S; 4F-60 Murray St, Toronto ON M5T 3L9; McM'98; MHSc; BSc; CCFP; Staff, Mount Sinai Hospital; Asst Prof Family Med, University of Toronto; (416)586-4800; Fax. (416)586-3175; mnaimer@mtsinai.on.ca.

NAIMI, Houshang; 1B-50 boul Saint-Charles, Beaconsfield QC H9W 2X3; Teheran (Iran)'60; LMCC; Staff, Lakeshore General Hospital - Pointe Claire; Langs: Persian; (514)695-1290; Fax. (514)695-1249.

NAINAR, Shamsia M; Queenston Walk-In Clinic, 103-631 Queenston Rd, Hamilton ON L8K 6R5; McG'95; AB; CCFP; Langs: Urdu; Hindi; French; (905)578-9255

NAIR, Asha; Children's Hosp Eastern Ont, 401 Smyth Rd, Ottawa ON K1H 8L1; UBC'96; FRCPC; Peds. Staff, Children's Hospital of Eastern Ontario (CHEO); (613)737-7600; Fax. (613)738-4878.

NAIR, Bina V; Peace Hills Trust Tower, 406-10011 109 St NW, Edmonton AB T5J 3S8; Sask'01; FRCPC; Psy. (780)415-6684; Fax. (780)415-6050.

NAIR, Bindu V; Royal University Hosp, 103 Hospital Dr, Saskatoon SK S7N 0W8; Sask'94; FRCPC; IntMed; Rheum. Staff Rheumatol, Royal University Hospital; (306)966-8267; Fax. (306)966-8381.

NAIR, Gangadharan N; 100-22190 48 Ave, Langley BC V3A 3N5; Kerala (India)'62; MSc; DAB; FRCPC; Psy (General Psychiatry). Consultant Psy, Langley Memorial Hospital; Consultant Psy, Langley Mental Health Centre; (604)534-8151; Fax. (604)534-6192.

NAIR, Girish M; Univ of Ottawa Heart Institute, H1285B-40 Ruskin St, Ottawa ON K1Y 4W7; Jawaharial (India)'96; MB BS; FRCPC; IntMed; Cardiol. Staff, University of Ottawa Heart Institute; Langs: Hindi; Malayalam; Tamil; (613)761-4914; Fax. (613)761-4407.

NAIR, Govindan K; 214-11044 51 Ave NW, Edmonton AB T6H 5B4; Mysore (India)'79; MB BS; LRCPS(Ed); LRCPS(Glas); FRCS(Ire); Ac Staff, Wetaskiwin Hospital & Care Centre; (780)436-8671

NAIR, Kieran; Eagle Ridge Hosp & Health C C, 475 Guildford Way, Port Moody BC V3H 3W9; Man'07; CCFP; Staff, Eagle Ridge Hospital & Health Care Centre; (604)469-2022

NAIR, Krishnakumar; Univ Hlth Network-Toronto Gen, GW3 522-200 Elizabeth St, Toronto ON M5G 2C4; Kerala (India)'94; Staff, Toronto General Hospital - UHN; (416)340-4442

NAIR, N P Vasavan; Douglas Mental Hlth Univ Inst, 6875 boul Lasalle, Verdun QC H4H 1R3; Kerala (India)'59; MB BS; DPM; FRCPsy; FRCP(Glas); FRCPC; Psy (Psycho Pharmacology). Dir Human Psychopharmacology, Douglas Mental Health University Institute; Prof, McGill Centre for Studies in Aging & Brain Bank; Prof Psy, McGill University; Langs: English; French; (514)762-3035; Fax. (514)762-3020; vasavan.nair@uhn.ca.

NAIR, Parameswaran K; St Joseph's Healthcare, 50 Charlton Ave E, Hamilton ON L8N 4A6; Kerala (India)'88; FRCPC; Respir. Staff, St Joseph's Healthcare - Charlton Campus; (905)522-1155 x5044

NAIR, Parvathy; Leslie & Gordon Diamond HCC, 9F-2775 Laurel St, Vancouver BC V5Z 1M9; Qns'97; FRCPC; IntMed; Cardiol. Staff, Gordon & Leslie Diamond Health Care Centre; (604)875-5092

NAIR, Ratheesh S; Family Med Clinic, 357 Albert St, Regina SK S4R 2N6; CCFP; (306)949-8840; Fax. (306)924-9355.

NAIR, Shona; The Ottawa Hosp-Gen Campus, 501 Smyth Rd, Ottawa ON K1H 8L6; Man'05; FRCPC; Anes. Staff, The Ottawa Hospital - General Campus.

NAIR, Suresh R; 1-436 Lorne St, Kamloops BC V2C 1W3; Kerala (India)'88; Staff, Royal Inland Hospital; (250)372-8622; Fax. (250)372-8665.

NAIR, Unni K; Salvation Army Grace Gen Hosp, 300 Booth Dr, Winnipeg MB R3J 3M7; Glasgow (Scotland)'76; MB ChB; FRCA; Ac Staff Anes, The Salvation Army Grace Hospital; (204)837-8311; Fax. (204)831-0029.

NAIR, Vidhya; Hamilton HS-General Site, 237 Barton St E, Hamilton ON L8L 2X2; Annamalai University (India)'96; FRCPC; AnatPath. Staff, Hamilton Health Sciences Centre - Hamilton General Hospital; (905)527-4322 x46170

NAIR, Vineet K; The Core Family Health Centre, 825 Richmond St, London ON N6A 3H7; UBC'00; CCFP; (519)963-1875; nvineet@hotmail.com.

NAIR, Vinod K; Grey Bruce HS-Owen Sound, PO Box 1800 Stn Main 1800 8th St E, Owen Sound ON N4K 6M9; Mem'96; FRCPC; Anes. Staff, Grey Bruce Health Services - Owen Sound; (519)376-2121

NAIRN, Janet C; Guelph Family Health Team, 101-83 Dawson Rd, Guelph ON N1H 1B1; Tor'87; Staff, Guelph General Hospital; (519)766-1360

NAIRN, Travis K; Grey Bruc HS-Owen Sound, PO Box 1800 Stn Main 1800 8th St E, Owen Sound ON N4K 6M9; Alb'98; BSc(Hon); Dip SportMed; FRCPC; Anes;CCFP; CCFP(E.M.); Staff, Grey Bruce Health Services - Owen Sound; (519)376-2121

NAISMITH, Amanda E; 203-9775 Fourth St, Sidney BC V8L 2Z8; Newcastle-upon-Tyne (England)'77; (250)656-4114; Fax. (250)656-7118; thedrsoffice@gmail.com.

NAISMITH, Angela D; University of Alberta Hosp, 8440 112 St NW, Edmonton AB T6G 2B7; UBC'04; CCFP; CCFP(E.M.); Staff, University of Alberta Hospital; (780)407-8822

NAISMITH, James R A; Workers' Comp Board, 4514 Chatterton Way, Victoria BC V8X 5H2; Newcastle-upon-Tyne (England)'77; (250)881-7292; Fax. (250)881-3435.

NAJAFI, Roya; Ocean Walk Med Centre, 1884 Marine Dr, West Vancouver BC V7V 1J6; (Iran)'95; CCFP; Staff, Ocean Walk Medical Centre; Physician, Bridge Community Health Clinic; Clinical Asst Prof Family Practice, University of British Columbia; Langs: Farsi; (604)925-1884; Fax. (604)925-1830; oceanmedical@ymail.com.

NAJARALI, A Ali; 100-178 John St, Brampton ON L6W 2A4; Bristol (England)'72; MB ChB; LMCC; Ac Staff, William Osler Health System - Brampton Civic Hospital; Langs: Portuguese; Gujarati; Urdu; (905)457-4772; Fax. (905)796-5241.

NAJARALI, Shamim G; William Osler HC-Brampton, 2100 Bovaird Dr E, Brampton ON L6R 3J7; Punjab (Pakistan)'71; MB BS; LMCC; FRCPC; Anes. Staff, William Osler Health System - Brampton Civic Hospital; Langs: Gujarati; Urdu; (905)494-2120; anajarali@rogers.com.

NAJEEB, Umberin; Sunnybrook Hlth Sciences Ctre, D45C-2075 Bayview Ave, Toronto ON M4N 3M5; Peshawar (Pakistan)'94; FRCPC; IntMed. Staff, Sunnybrook Health Sciences Centre; (416)480-6100; Fax. (416)480-6191.

NAJFI, Syed M; James Paton Mem Hosp, 125 Trans Canada Hwy, Gander NL A1V 1P7; (Pakistan)'85; MB BS; FRCSI; FRCSC; GenSurg. Staff GenSurg, James Paton Memorial Hospital; Langs: Urdu; Punjabi; (709)256-2500; smnajfi@hotmail.com.

NAJGEBAUER, Edward J; Sudbury Med Centre, 208-65 Larch St, Sudbury ON P3E 1B8; Tor'75; Ac Staff, Health Sciences North-St Joseph's Health Centre; (705)674-0770; Fax. (705)674-3603.

NAJM-TEHRANI, Nasrin; The Hosp for Sick Children, 555 University Ave, Toronto ON M5G 1X8; University of Wales (England)'87; MB ChB; FRCSC; Ophth. Staff, The Hospital For Sick Children; (416)813-7374; Fax. (416)813-6261.

NAKAI, Harumi; 13750 96 Ave, Surrey BC V3V 1Z2; UBC'86; MSc; Staff, Surrey Memorial Hospital; (604)220-7107

NAKAJIMA, Amy K; Wabano Aboriginal Health Ctre, 299 Montreal Rd, Ottawa ON K1L 6B8; Alb'94; FRCSC; ObstGyn. Staff, Almonte General Hospital; (613)748-5999

NAKAMURA, Liane S; Family Health Centre, C10-1410 Major Mackenzie Dr W, Vaughan ON L6A 4H6; Tor'91; Staff, North York General Hospital - Branson Division; (905)303-2700; Fax. (905)303-2780.

NAKAMURA, Richard M; 2523 St Johns St, Port Moody BC V3H 2B3; UBC'71; Langs: Japanese; (604)936-7277; Fax. (604)936-7112.

NAKASHIMA, Brenda; PO Box 74131Rpo Strathcona, Calgary AB T3H 3B6; Alb'08; CCFP.

NAKATSUI, Thomas C; Groot Dermasurgery Centre, 200-9670 142 St NW, Edmonton AB T5N 4B2; Alb'94; FRCPC; Derm (Hair Transplantation). Clin Lecturer Med & Pharmacy, University of Alberta; (780)482-1414; Fax. (780)482-7097; info@drnakatsui.com.

NAKATSUKA, Nao; 409-301 Columbia St E, New Westminster BC V3L 3W5; UBC'07; FRCSC; ObstGyn. (604)522-8272

NAKHLA, Adel L C; Brittany Glen Med Centre, 102-5602 Tenth Line W, Mississauga ON L5M 7L9; Cairo (Egypt)'91; CCFP; Langs: Arabic; French; (905)858-9393; Fax. (905)858-8960.

NAKHLA, Meranda M; MUHC-Montreal Children's Hosp, C518-2300 rue Tupper, Montreal QC H3H 1P3; McM'00; FRCPC; Endocrin&Metab; Peds. Staff, McGill University Health Centre - Montreal Children's Hospital; (514)412-4400

NAKHLE, Elias; Hotel-Dieu de Sorel, 400 av de l'Hotel-Dieu, Sorel-Tracy QC J3P 1N5; Staff, Hôtel-Dieu de Sorel; (450)746-6000

NAKHOST, Arash; Douglas Mental Hlth Univ Inst, 6875 boul Lasalle, Verdun QC H4H 1R3; McG'07; MDCM; FRCPC; Psy. Staff, Douglas Mental Health University Institute; (514)761-6131

NAKHOSTINE, Nabil; CSSS de la Vallée de l'Or, 725 6e rue, Val-d'Or QC J9P 3Y1; Mon'01; CCFP; Staff, Centre Hospitalier de Val d'Or; (819)825-5858

NAKHUDA, Gary S; Genesis Fertility Centre, 300-1367 Broadway W, Vancouver BC V6H 4A7; New York (USA)'99; Langs: Polish; (604)873-3032

NAKIELNA, Edina M; St Paul's Hosp, 1081 Burrard St, Vancouver BC V6Z 1Y6; Liverpool (England)'67; MB ChB; MRCP(UK); DCH(Lond); FRCPC; IntMed (Respirology). Ac Staff, Providence Health Care - St Paul's Hospital; Clin Assoc Prof Med, University of British Columbia; (604)806-8818

NAKONECHNY, Quentin B; Abbotsford Reg Hosp & Cancer C, C2 030-32900 Marshall Rd, Abbotsford BC V2S 0C2; Sask'01; FRCPC; GenPath. (604)851-4700

NALDER, Byron K; Chinook Reg Hosp, 960 19 St S, Lethbridge AB T1J 1W5; Alb'82; FRCPC; Anes. Staff, Chinook Regional Hospital; (403)388-6131

NALEZNY, Stephan J; 132 Parkdale Ave S, Hamilton ON L8K 3P3; Krakow (Poland)'06; CCFP; (905)547-3484

NALLA, Bhanu P; Sudbury Reg Hosp-Laurentian Si, 41 Ramsey Lake Rd, Sudbury ON P3E 5J1; London (England)'97; FRCPC; Anes. Staff, Health Sciences North-Laurentian Site; (705)523-7100

NALLAPANENI, Sailaja P; 202-3251 Sheppard Ave E, Scarborough ON M1T 3W5; Alb'03; FRCSC; GenSurg. Staff, Hamilton Health Sciences Centre - McMaster Children's Hospital; (416)773-1900; Fax. (416)773-1902.

NALLY, Colm; Elk Valley Hosp, PO Box 670 1501 5th Ave, Fernie BC V0B 1M0; (Ireland)'73; MCh; FRCS; FRCS(Eng); FRCSC; GenSurg. Staff, Elk Valley Hospital; (250)423-4453; Fax. (250)423-3732; colm.nally@interiorhealth.ca.

NALLY, Veronique; CSSS Jeanne-Mance, 100-15 av du Mont-Royal O, Montreal QC H2T 2R9; Geneva (Switzerland)'76; Langs: Bilingual(French/English); (514)286-9657 x4358

NAM, Diane; Sunnybrook Hlth Sciences Ctre, MG 301-2075 Bayview Ave, Toronto ON M4N 3M5; Tor'01; FRCSC; OrthSurg. Staff, Sunnybrook Health Sciences Centre; (416)480-5641; Fax. (416)480-5886.

NAM, Robert; Sunnybrook Hlth Sciences Ctre, MG 406-2075 Bayview Ave, Toronto ON M4N 3M5; Tor'95; FRCSC; Urol (Urological Oncology). Staff Surg, Sunnybrook Health Sciences Centre; Asst Prof, University of Toronto; (416)480-5075; Fax. (416)480-6121.

NAMAN, Nazem; La Clinique Med Du 2101, 2101 boul Edouard-Montpetit, Montreal QC H3T 1J3; Liege (Belgium)'91; CCFP; Staff, Hopital Marie Clarac; (514)343-6452; Fax. (514)343-7236.

NAMARUISH, Osama A A; 115 Millbourne Shopping Centre, Edmonton AB T6K 3L6; (Libya)'02; CCFP; (587)521-2022; Fax. (587)521-2023.

NAMAZI, Mojgan; George Pearson Centre, 700 57th Ave W, Vancouver BC V6P 1S1; UBC'90; BSc; (604)322-8350

NAMAZIE, Ali M; Brant Community HC-Brantford, 200 Terrace Hill St, Brantford ON N3R 1G9; Wes'05; Anes. Staff, The Brant Community Healthcare System - Brantford General Hospital Site; (519)752-7871

NAMBIAR, Sindhu; William Osler HC-Etobicoke, 101 Humber College Blvd, Etobicoke ON M9V 1R8; (India)'96; Staff, William Osler Health System - Etobicoke General Hospital; (416)494-2120

NAMBURI, Sriranjinee S; Meadowlands Family Health Ctre, 5-35 Stone Church Rd, Ancaster ON L9K 1S5; Colombo (Sri Lanka)'81; MB BS; CCFP; Langs: Tamil; (905)648-8999; Fax. (905)648-8969.

NAMEN, Samia; Hop Charles Lemoyne, 3120 boul Taschereau, Greenfield Park QC J4V 2H1; Sher'09; CCFP; Staff, Hopital Charles LeMoyne; (450)466-5000

NAMIS, Nabil N; Guelph Comm Hlth Med Bldg, 35-125 Delhi St, Guelph ON N1E 4J5; Ain Shams (Egypt)'71; MRC(UK); FRCSC; ObstGyn. Staff, Guelph General Hospital; (519)824-8730

NAMIT, Jaime W; Lamont Health Care Centre, PO Box 10 5216 53rd St, Lamont AB T0B 2R0; (Philippines)'69; Staff, Lamont Health Care Centre; (780)895-5910; Fax. (780)895-5913.

NAMUSUUBO-KACHOPE, Jane P; Zoe Med Centre, 8115 160 Av NW, Edmonton AB T5Z 0G3; Makerere (Uganda)'90; (780)475-9636; Fax. (780)478-9635.

NANAR, Bikramjit S; 201-7125 Goreway Dr, Mississauga ON L4T 4H3; Tor'89; Langs: Punjabi; (905)405-8393

NANAYA, Neil P; Surrey Mem Hosp, 13750 96 Ave, New Westminster BC V3B 1Z2; Dublin (Ireland)'04; FRCPC; Anes;CCFP; CCFP(E.M.); Staff, Surrey Memorial Hospital; (604)581-2211

NANAYA, Ponnettira K; Hotel-Dieu Grace Hosp, 1030 Ouellette Ave, Windsor ON N9A 1E1; Karnatak (India)'71; MB BS; FRCPC; Anes. Staff, Hôtel-Dieu Grace Hospital; (519)973-4411

NANCEKIEVILL, Elizabeth A; 8-389 Main St GD, Picton ON K0K 2T0; Wes'88; BSc(Hon); CCFP; FCFP; Ac Member Family Med, QHC Prince Edward County Memorial; (613)476-8323; Fax. (613)476-8211.

NANCEKIEVILL, Garry W; 11162 Ilderton Rd RR 2, Ilderton ON N0M 2A0; Wes'75; Assoc Staff Family Med, St Joseph's Hospital - St Joseph's Health Care; (519)666-2177; Fax. (519)666-1421.

NANCEKIEVILL, Ivan W; Ross Mem Hosp, 10 Angeline St N, Lindsay ON K9V 4M8; Wes'61; Staff, Ross Memorial Hospital; (705)324-6111

NANCI, Vanessa; MUHC-Royal Victoria Hosp, M4 76-687 av des Pins O, Montreal QC H3A 1A1; McG'08; IntMed. Staff, McGill University Health Centre - Royal Victoria Hospital; (514)406-3233

NANDA, Arvind; 407-2863 Ellesmere Rd, Scarborough ON M1E 5E9; Tor'98; FRCSC; GenSurg. Staff, Rouge Valley Health System - Centenary Health Centre Site; (416)283-7956

NANDA, Atul K; Ridge Meadows Hosp & Hlth CC, 11666 Laity St, Maple Ridge BC V2X 5A3; Nagpur (India)'78; MB BS; FRCPC; Psy (Geriatric Psychiatry). Staff, Ridge Meadows Hospital & Health Care Centre; Staff, South Delta Mental Health; (604)463-1814

NANDA, Meenakshi; MCI The Doctor's Office, 32-4604 37 St SW, Calgary AB T3E 3C9; (India)'93; MB BS; CCFP; Langs: Hindi; Punjabi; (403)269-9488; Fax. (403)269-9409.

NANDA, Sunit K; 185 Commissioners Rd W, London ON N6J 1X9; Kashmir (India)'71; MB BS; FRCPC; Peds. (519)438-3296

NANDAGOPAL, Meena; Hamilton HS-McMaster Site, PO Box 2000 Stn Lcd 1 1200 Main St W, Hamilton ON L8N 3Z5; Madras (India)'78; Staff, Hamilton Health Sciences Centre - McMaster Children's Hospital; (905)521-2100 x75171; Fax. (905)523-1224.

NANDAGOPAL, Narayanan; SGH Medical Mall, 211-3030 Lawrence Ave E, Scarborough ON M1P 2T7; Madras (India)'78; FRCSC; PlasSurg. Staff Plastic Surg, The Scarborough Hospital - General Campus; Langs: Tamil; (416)439-5775; Fax. (416)439-2526.

NANDAL, Vijay; Markham Stouffville Hosp, PO Box 1800 Stn Main 381 Church St, Markham ON L3P 7P3; Man'88; FRCPC; Anes. Staff, Markham Stouffville Hospital; (905)472-7074; Fax. (905)472-7398.

NANDI, Dilip K; Mission Med Clinic, 2303 4 St SW, Calgary AB T2S 2S7; Chittagong (Bangladesh)'88; MB BS; (403)229-1700; Fax. (403)229-1875.

NANDI, Jayashri K; Mission Med Clinic, 2303 4 St SW, Calgary AB T2S 2S7; Dhaka (Bangladesh)'97; LMCC; MB BS; (403)229-1700; Fax. (403)229-1875; nandicl@shaw.ca.

NANDRA, Sukhjeen K; Halton HCS Corp-Georgetown, 1 Princess Anne Dr, Georgetown ON L7G 2B8; Wes'09; CCFP; Staff, Halton Healthcare Services Corporation - Georgetown Hospital; (905)873-0111

NANDY, Ranendu; Etobicoke Med Centre, 400 The East Mall, Etobicoke ON M9B 3Z9; Patna (India)'67; Ac Staff, Trillium Health Centre - West Toronto; (416)621-2220 x242; Fax. (416)621-2203.

NANDY, Saibal; 101-1424 Southview Dr SE, Medicine Hat AB T1B 4E7; Calcutta (India)'74; MB BS; MRCPsy; FRCPC; Psy (General Psychiatry). (403)527-0400; Fax. (403)527-4884.

NANDY, Sunita; Scarborough Prof Centre, 217-1371 Neilson Rd, Scarborough ON M1B 4Z8; Patna (India)'67; Ac Staff, Rouge Valley Health System - Centenary Health Centre Site; Langs: Hindi; (416)284-0239

NANHOU DJOMO, Alice; CLSC Chateauguay, 95 av de la Verdure, Chateauguay QC J6K 0E8; Heidelberg (Germany)'99; CCFP; (450)699-3333

NANINI, Bianca; Centre Med de Chambly, 205-1101 boul Brassard, Chambly QC J3L 5R4; Laval'99; (450)658-6601; Fax. (450)658-7849.

NANJI, Alykhan; Cardiometabolic Evaluation Ris, 210-1016 68 Ave SW, Calgary AB T2V 4J2; McM'94; MPH; FRCPC; IntMed. Staff, Cardiometabolic Evaluation & Risk Assessment Centre; (403)541-0033; Fax. (403)541-0032.

NANJI, Amin A; Pathology Laboratory, 616-5788 University Ave, Halifax NS B3H 1V8; Nairobi (Kenya)'77; MB ChB; FRCPath; FRCPC; MedBiochem (Toxicology). Prof Path & LabMed, Dalhousie University; (902)473-6867; Fax. (902)473-2123; amin.nanji@cdha.nshealth.ca.

NANJI, Amirali M; McConnell Med Centre, 128-820 McConnell Ave, Cornwall ON K6H 4M4; Qns'74; CCFP; FCFP; Staff, Cornwall Community Hospital; Staff, Cornwall Community Hospital - Second Street Site; Lecturer/Examiner, Acupuncture Foundation of Canada Institute; (613)936-1564

NANJI, Gulammohamed G V; Riverview Surgical Centre, 3125 Bowwood Dr NW, Calgary AB T3B 2E7; Nairobi (Kenya)'77; MB ChB; DAB; FRCPC; Anes. Ac Staff, Foothills Medical Centre; Ac Staff, Alberta Children's Hospital; Ac Staff, Tom Baker Cancer Centre; Pres/CEO, Surgical Centres Inc; Asst Clin Prof, University of Calgary; Langs: Gujarati; Kiswahili; (403)640-1188; Fax. (403)640-4217.

NANJI, Sulaiman; Kingston Gen Hosp, 76 Stuart St, Kingston ON K7L 2V7; UBC'99; FRCSC; GenSurg. Staff, Kingston General Hospital; (613)549-6666; Fax. (613)548-2406.

NANKISSOOR, Basdeo; Medical & Foot Clinic, 2544 Guardian Rd NW, Edmonton AB T5T 1K8; Peoples Friendship Univ (Russia (Federation))'87; CCFP; Consultant Wound Clinics, Covenant Health - Misericordia Community Hospital; Physician, Good Samaritan Seniors Clinic; Langs: Russian; Spanish; (780)444-2252; Fax. (780)444-2210.

NANTAIS, Michel; CSSS de Sept-Iles, 45 rue du Pere-Divet, Sept-Iles QC G4R 3N7; Sher'87; FRCSC; GenSurg. Staff, Centre Hospitalier Regional de Sept-Iles; (418)962-9761

NANTEL, A J Albert; INSPQ, 1 27-190 boul Cremazie E, Montreal QC H2P 1E2; Mon'64; MSc(Pharm); AB; (514)864-1600 x3227; Fax. (514)864-7646; albert.nantel@inspq.qc.ca.

NANTEL, Andre; Inst Philippe Pinel de Mtl, 10905 boul Henri-Bourassa E, Montreal QC H1C 1H1; Mon'80; FRCPC; Psy. Ac Staff, Institut Philippe-Pinel de Montreal; (514)648-8461; Fax. (514)494-4406.

NANTEL, Claire; 417A rue Principale, St-Patr-Beaur QC G0S 1B0; Mon'78; Langs: English; (418)596-2213; Fax. (418)596-2024.

NANTEL, Stephen; Gordon & Leslie Diamond HCC, 10F-2775 Laurel St, Vancouver BC V5Z 1M9; Cal'83; ABIM; FRCPC; IntMed (Stem Cell Transplantation); Hem. Staff Hem, BC Cancer Agency Vancouver Centre; Ac Staff, Vancouver General Hospital - Centennial Pavillion; Member, Leukemia/Bone Marrow Transplantation Prog of BC; Staff, Gordon & Leslie Diamond Health Care Centre; Clin Prof Med, University of British Columbia; (604)875-4863; snantel@bccancer.bc.ca.

NANTES, Stephen H; 395 Greenbrook Dr, Kitchener ON N2M 4K1; McG'78; CCFP; FCFP; Staff, St Mary's General Hospital; Staff, Grand River Hospital - Kitchener/Waterloo Health Centre; Med Examiner, Ministry Of Transport Ontario; (519)570-3333; Fax. (519)578-6572; snantes@canada.com.

NANTHA-AREE, Manyart; Hamilton HS-General Site, 237 Barton St E, Hamilton ON L8L 2X2; Chiang Mai (Thailand)'95; Staff, Hamilton Health Sciences Centre - Hamilton General Hospital; (905)521-2100 x75171

NANTHAKUMAR, Kumaraswamy; Univ Hlth Network-Toronto Gen, GW3 522B-200 Elizabeth St, Toronto ON M5G 2C4; Tor'95; FRCPC; IntMed (Electrophysiology); Cardiol. Staff Cliniccian Scientist, Toronto General Hospital - UHN; Scientist, Toronto General Research Institute; Assoc Prof Med, University of Toronto; (416)340-4442; Fax. (416)340-4457.

NANTHAKUMAR, S Selvi; St Paul's Hosp, 1081 Burrard St, Vancouver BC V6Z 1Y6; (Sri Lanka)'72; MB BS; FRCPC; GenPath. Staff, Providence Health Care - St Paul's Hospital; Langs: Tamil; (604)806-8215; Fax. (604)806-8158.

NANTHEESWARAR, Chithakan; Oshawa Commun Health Centre, 115 Grassmere Ave, Oshawa ON L1H 3X7; McM'06; CCFP; (905)723-0036; Fax. (905)723-3391.

NANTON, Ertha A; Murakami Med Clinic, PO Box 1000 735 4th Ave, Hope BC V0X 1L0; St Augustine (Trinidad & Tobago)'97; BScChem & Biochem; MB BSMed & Surg; CCFP; (604)869-5648

NAOM, Nashwan A I; Leamington Dist Mem Hosp, 194 Talbot St W, Leamington ON N8H 1N9; Baghdad (Iraq)'88; FRCPC; IntMed. Staff, Leamington District Memorial Hospital; (519)326-2373

NAOUM, Serge; Cumberland Clinic, 25 Cumberland St, Cornwall ON K6J 4G8; Mon'02; FRCSC; GenSurg (Trauma). Chief Surgery, Cornwall Community Hospital; Langs: Bilingual(French/English); (613)938-2552; Fax. (613)938-2559.

NAOUM, Susanne; Etherington Hall, 94 Stuart St, Kingston ON K7L 3N6; McM'09; CCFP.

NAPIER, Jolene M; Jubilee Centre, 1823 Fort St, Victoria BC V8R 1J6; Natal (South Africa)'05; (250)595-6636

NAPIER, Lee B; 207-9808 King George Blvd, Surrey BC V3T 2V6; Cape Town (South Africa)'72; MB ChB; FRCS(Ed); FRCSC; Ophth. Staff, Surrey Memorial Hospital; (604)588-3811

NAPIER, Robert L; Burnaby Ctr for Mental Hlth &, 3405 Willingdon Ave, Burnaby BC V5G 3H4; Dal'89; FRCPC; Psy. (604)675-3950

NAPOLITANO, Giuseppe; CSSS du Lac-des-Deux-Montagnes, 520 boul Arthur-Sauve, Saint-Eustache QC J7R 5B1; Mon'02; FRCPC; DiagRad. Staff, Hôpital de Saint-Eustache; (450)473-6811 x2152

NAPPERT, Catherine; CSSS Drummond-Hop Sainte-Croix, 570 rue Heriot, Drummondville QC J2B 1C1; Mon'91; FRCSC; Otol (Maxillo Facial Surgery). Chief ORL Service, Hôpital Sainte-croix; (819)478-6464; drouin.nappert@sympatico.ca.

NAPPERT, Rejean A; Clinique Med de Touraine, 2B-520 boul de l'Hopital, Gatineau QC J8V 2P5; Laval'83; (819)568-4310

NAQI, Hadia; 194 Court St N, Thunder Bay ON P7A 4V7; Punjab (Pakistan)'96; CCFP; (807)346-1000

NAQVI, Arif; 2622 Eglinton Ave E, Scarborough ON M1K 2S3; Tor'91; Cardiol; IntMed. Langs: Urdu; Hindi; (416)755-7755; Fax. (416)755-7509.

NAQVI, Asghar H; St Joseph's Health Centre, 30 The Queensway, Toronto ON M6R 1B5; (India)'97; FRCPC; AnatPath. Staff, St Joseph's Health Centre; (416)530-6486; Fax. (416)530-6284.

NAQVI, Damian D N; Clin Signature, 100-1545 boul de l'Avenir, Laval QC H7S 2N5; McG'01; St Mary's Hospital Centre; (450)629-1818

NAQVI, Imran H; Niagara H System-G Niagara, PO Box 1018 Stn Main 5546 Portage Rd, Niagara Falls ON L2E 6X2; Karachi (Pakistan)'90; MB BS; FRCPC; Psy. Staff, Niagara Health System - Greater Niagara General Site; (905)358-0171

NAQVI, Khadija; Transcanada Med Centre, 152-1440 52 St NE, Calgary AB T2A 4T8; (Pakistan)'98; CCFP.

NAQVI, Mahmood A; Cape Breton Hlthcare Complex, 1482 George St, Sydney NS B1P 1P3; Karachi (Pakistan)'58; FACS; FRCSC; GenSurg; VascSurg. Med Dir Dist & Health Authority, Cape Breton Healthcare Complex; (902)567-7806; Fax. (902)567-7255; naqvim@cbdha.nshealth.ca.

NAQVI, Raza M; Sunnybrook Hlth Sciences Ctre, H478-2075 Bayview Ave, Toronto ON M4N 3M5; Wes'09; Staff, Sunnybrook Health Sciences Centre; (416)480-6100

NAQVI, Syed E; Western Hosp Corp, PO Box 10 148 Poplar St, Alberton PE C0B 1B0; Punjab (Pakistan)'95; MB BS; Staff, Western Hospital - Health PEI; (902)853-8650

NAQVI, Syed M A; The Hosp for Sick Children, 555 University Ave, Toronto ON M5G 1X8; Karachi (Pakistan)'77; DCH; MB BS; MRCP(UK); MCPS; Staff, The Hospital For Sick Children; (416)813-5872; Fax. (416)813-5327; ahmed.naqvi@sickkids.ca.

NARAGHI, Ali M F; Univ Hlth Network-Toronto Western Hosp, 3MC421-399 Bathurst St, Toronto ON M5T 2S8; London (England)'94; Radiologist, Toronto Western Hospital - University Health Network; (416)603-5800 x2898

NARAINE, Nadira D; The Ottawa Hosp-Gen Campus, 501 Smyth Rd, Ottawa ON K1H 8L6; Qns'89; FRCPC; Anes. Staff, The Ottawa Hospital - General Campus; (613)737-8187; Fax. (613)737-8189.

NARAINE, Virjanand; 216-40 Finchgate Blvd, Brampton ON L6T 3J1; Tor'00; FRCPC; IntMed (Sleep Medicine); Respir. Staff, William Osler Health System - Brampton Civic Hospital; (905)456-3699; Fax. (905)456-8768.

NARAN, Mineshbhai; 206A-145 15th St W, North Vancouver BC V7M 1R9; Natal (South Africa)'87; MB ChB; CAFCI; Staff, Lions Gate Hospital; (604)986-4214; Fax. (604)980-4208.

NARANG, Chander K; Walk-In Med Clinic, 21 Queensway W, Mississauga ON L5B 1B8; New Delhi (India)'64; (905)897-0788

NARANG, Gurpreet K; Children's & Women's HC of BC, 4480 Oak St, Vancouver BC V6H 3N1; Baroda (India)'00; MB BS; Staff, BC Children's Hospital; (604)875-2345

NARANG, Indra; The Hosp for Sick Children, 555 University Ave, Toronto ON M5G 1X8; (Wales)'93; Staff, The Hospital For Sick Children; (416)813-6167; Fax. (416)813-6246; indra.narang@sickkids.ca.

NARANG, Kapila; Deer Valley Centre, 26-1221 Canyon Meadows Dr SE, Calgary AB T2J 6G2; Ott'73; (403)278-2164; Fax. (403)278-3192.

NARANG, Rajendra; Liberton Med Centre, 205-31 Liberton Dr, St. Albert AB T8N 3X6; Indore (India)'65; FACS; FRCSC; OrthSurg. (780)458-8600; Fax. (780)460-9363.

NARANG, Satinder P S; Surrey Med Bldg, 301-9656 King George Blvd, Surrey BC V3T 2V5; Guru Nanak (India)'74; MRCPsy(UK); FRCPC; Psy. Langs: Punjabi; Hindi; Urdu; (604)581-2003; Fax. (604)581-2039.

NARANJO, Jose-E; Clinique Med Joliette, 3841 rue Ontario E, Montreal QC H1W 1S5; Louvain (Belgium)'74; (514)524-3731; Fax. (514)524-0675.

NARASIAH, Lavanya; CSSS de la Montagne, 5700 ch de la Cote-des-Neiges, Montreal QC H3T 2A8; Sher'96; Physician, CLSC Cote-des-Neiges; (514)731-8531; lavnarasiah@yahoo.com.

NARASIMHAN, Sowmya; Health Sciences Centre, 820 Sherbrook St, Winnipeg MB R3A 1R9; Staff, Health Sciences Centre; (204)774-8511

NARAYAN, Shanil V; The Jenny Trout Centre, 110-342 Erie St, Stratford ON N5A 2N4; Qns'99; FRCPC; IntMed. (519)273-1990; Fax. (519)273-0675.

NARAYANAN, Chitra; Huntingdale Med Centre, 3061 Pharmacy Ave, Scarborough ON M1W 2H1; Mysore (India)'81; MB BS; Med Dir, Yee Hong Centre For Geriatric Care; Langs: Hindi; Tamil; (416)502-0738; Fax. (416)502-1160; huntingdalemedctr@yahoo.com.

NARAYANAN, Gopalakrishnan; The Hosp for Sick Children, S 107-555 University Ave, Toronto ON M5G 1X8; Madras (India)'88; FRCSC; OrthSurg. Staff, The Hospital For Sick Children; (416)813-6432; Fax. (416)813-6414.

NARAYANAN, Kanna R S; Chatham-Kent Health Alliance, PO Box 2030 Stn Main 80 Grand Ave W, Chatham ON N7M 5L9; Alb'02; CCFP; Staff, Chatham-Kent Health Alliance; (519)352-6400; Fax. (519)436-2515.

NARAYANAN, Sujaatha; Gordon & Leslie Diamond HCC, 10F-2775 Laurel St, Vancouver BC V5Z 1M9; Chennai (India)'97; MB BS; Staff, Gordon & Leslie Diamond Health Care Centre; Langs: Tamil; (604)875-4863; Fax. (604)875-4763.

NARAYANSINGH, Marc J; Sunnybrook Hlth Sciences Ctre, 2075 Bayview Ave, Toronto ON M4N 3M5; Man'05; FRCPC; Neur. Staff, Sunnybrook Health Sciences Centre; (416)480-6100

NARBONNE, Claude; Clinique medicale Notre-Dame, 120-504 rue Notre-Dame, Repentigny QC J6A 2T8; Mon'75; ac Staff, Centre Hospitalier Pierre le Gardeur; (450)585-3232; Fax. (450)582-9763.

NARBONNE, Sabrina; St Mary's Hosp Centre, 3830 av Lacombe, Montreal QC H3T 1M5; Mon'06; CCFP; CCFP(E.M.); Staff, St Mary's Hospital Centre; (514)345-3511

NARDINI, Robert; 8224 rue St-Paul, Caraquet NB E1W 6E2; Laval'09; CCFP; (506)727-7549; Fax. (506)727-7320.

NARENDRAN, Aru Mugavadivel; Alberta Children's Hosp, 2888 Shaganappi Trail NW, Calgary AB T3B 6A8; McM'95; Staff, Alberta Children's Hospital; (403)955-7203; Fax. (403)955-7396.

NAREWAL, Mondeep; Hotel-Dieu Grace Hosp, 1030 Ouellette Ave, Windsor ON N9A 1E1; Wayne State(MI) (USA)'04; CCFP; Staff, Hôtel-Dieu Grace Hospital; (519)973-4411

NARIKUZHY, Annie; Credit Valley Med Arts Centre, E229A-5100 Erin Mills Pky, Mississauga ON L5M 4Z5; Louvain (Belgium)'68; Peds. (905)607-2600; Fax. (905)607-9292.

NARINE, Andy J; Stevenson Mem Hosp, PO Box 4000 Stn Main 200 Fletcher Cres, Alliston ON L9R 1W7; Dal'04; FRCSC; ObstGyn. Staff, Stevenson Memorial Hospital; (705)434-5144; Fax. (705)434-5131.

NARINE, Nyan K; Hop Santa-Cabrini Ospedale, 5655 rue Saint-Zotique E, Montreal QC H1T 1P7; Wes'02; FRCPC; IntMed. Staff, Hôpital Santa Cabrini Ospedale; (514)252-6000

NARINE, Rajkishan K; Foothills Med Centre, 1403 29 St NW, Calgary AB T2N 2T9; (Belgium)'89; Staff, Foothills Medical Centre; (403)944-1110

NARINE, Rishi A; 5A-880 Upper Wentworth St, Hamilton ON L9A 5H2; Wes'04; CCFP; (905)575-0808

NARINE, Tamara K; Port Arthur Health Centre, 194 Court St N, Thunder Bay ON P7A 4V7; Man'02; CCFP; (807)346-1000; Fax. (807)346-6251; tammynarine@hotmail.com.

NARINI, Philip P; Taunton Health Centre, SS 201 1290 Keith Ross Dr, Oshawa ON L1H 7K4; Tor'86; FRCSC; PlasSurg. (905)723-8551

NARNAWARE, Avisha; Queen Elizabeth II Hosp, 10409 98 St, Grande Prairie AB T8V 2E8; (India)'92; MB BS; Staff, Queen Elizabeth II Hospital; (780)538-7110

NAROD, Mairi M; Peace Arch Commun Med Clinic, 101-1790 152 St, Surrey BC V4A 7Z7; McG'54; (604)535-8496

NAROD, Steven A; Ctr for Research Women's Hlth, 714-790 Bay St, Toronto ON M5G 1N8; Wes'79; CommunMed (Prostate Brachytherapy). Staff Research, Women's College Hospital; Chair Breast Cancer Research/Prof, University of Toronto; Langs: English; French; (416)351-3765; Fax. (416)351-3767.

NAROTHUM, Paresh S; Associate Med Clinic, 400-20 14th St W, Prince Albert SK S6V 3K8; (306)953-1654

NARULA, Amarjit S; Dominion Med Centres Ltd, 9122 23 Ave NW, Edmonton AB T6N 1H9; India (India)'78; MB BS; CCFP; (780)801-3360; Fax. (780)801-3366.

NARULA, Archna; 661 Upper James St PO Box 60513, Cambridge ON N1T 1E2; McM'09; CCFP.

NARULA, Rajesh K; Chinook Reg Hosp, 960 19 St S, Lethbridge AB T1J 1W5; Staff, Chinook Regional Hospital; (403)388-6111

NARVAS, David E; Seymour Health Centre, 1530 7th Ave W, Vancouver BC V6J 1S3; Man'05; CCFP; (604)528-4677

NARVEY, Michael R; Health Sciences Centre, MS361J-820 Sherbrook St, Winnipeg MB R3A 1R9; Man'98; FRCPC; Peds (Neonatal & Perinatal Medicine).

NARWAL, A S; Guru Nanak Med Clinic, 103-9278 120 St, Surrey BC V3V 4B8; Delhi (India)'82; MB BS; (604)585-8020; Fax. (604)585-8019.

NASARULLAH, Fareeha; Lakeridge Hlth Corp-Oshawa, 1 Hospital Crt, Oshawa ON L1G 2B9; Karachi (Pakistan)'96; CCFP; Staff, Lakeridge Health - Oshawa Site; (905)576-8711; Fax. (905)721-7763.

NASCU, Camelia P; The Jenny Trout Centre, 120-342 Erie St, Stratford ON N5A 2N4; Timisoara (Romania)'99; FRCSC; ObstGyn. (519)275-3877

NASEEM, Iram; Cape Breton Hlthcare Complex, 1482 George St, Sydney NS B1P 1P3; Baluchistan (Pakistan)'94; DiagRad. Staff, Cape Breton Healthcare Complex; (902)567-8000

NASEEMUDDIN, Ather; Saint John Reg Hosp, PO Box 2100 Stn Main 400 University Ave, Saint John NB E2L 4L2; Jawaharlal (India)'02; Staff, Saint John Regional Hospital; (506)648-6000

NASEER, Muhammad A; Alberta Children's Hosp, 2888 Shaganappi Trail NW, Calgary AB T3B 6A8; Karachi (Pakistan)'87; MB BS; DABPN; Staff, Alberta Children's Hospital; Clin Lecturer Psy, University of Calgary; Langs: Urdu; (403)955-2956; Fax. (403)955-3105; manaseer99@hotmail.com.

NASELLO, Constance M; 211 St Clair St, Chatham ON N7L 3J4; Wes'91; BSc; DABOG; FRCSC; ObstGyn. Ac Staff, Chatham-Kent Health Alliance; Aj Prof ObstGyn/Acad Dir SWOMEN, University of Western Ontario; Langs: English; French; (519)351-0626; Fax. (519)351-6064.

NASER AL-MOBARAK, Basem I; The Hosp for Sick Children, 555 University Ave, Toronto ON M5G 1X8; King Faisal (Saudi Arabia)'86; MB BS; FRCPC; Anes. Staff, The Hospital For Sick Children; (416)813-7445

NASH, Carla L; 564 Leon Ave, Kelowna BC V1Y 6J6; Cal'96; FRCPC; IntMed (Endoscopic Ultrasound); Gastroent. (250)763-6433

NASH, E Lynn I; 326 Wilson St E, Ancaster ON L9G 2C2; McM'78; CCFP; FCFP; Ac Staff, Hamilton Health Sciences Centre - McMaster Children's Hospital; Court Staff, St Joseph's Healthcare - Charlton Campus; Pt-Time Faculty, McMaster University; (905)648-0770; Fax. (905)648-0777.

NASH, L W Sandy; Willow Park Shopping Ctre, 25-590 Highway 33 W, Kelowna BC V1X 6A8; UBC'70; (250)862-5915

NASH, Leslie A X; Fourth Avenue Med Centre, 411 Louth St, St Catharines ON L2S 4A2; Dal'74; FRCPC; Peds. Langs: Bilingual(English/French); (905)682-3692; Fax. (905)682-7549.

NASH, Michael B; Valley Women & Children H C, 202-60 Aberdeen St, Kentville NS B4N 2N3; Mem'02; FRCPC; Peds.

NASH, Ronald A; Kimberley Med Clinic, PO Box 160, Kimberley BC V1A 2Y6; UBC'92; (250)427-4861; Fax. (250)427-2082.

NASH, Stephen H; Humber River Reg Hosp-Finch, 2111 Finch Ave W, North York ON M3N 1N1; Tor'92; FRCPC; DiagRad. Staff, Humber River Regional Hospital - Finch Avenue Site; (416)744-2500

NASH, W Scott; 204-107 King St W, Dundas ON L9H 1V1; Wes'93; BSc; CCFP; FCFP; Ac Staff Family Med, Hamilton Health Sciences Centre - McMaster University Medical Centre; (905)627-3505; Fax. (905)627-4193.

NASH, Wesley A; Medical Arts Bldg, 302-1 Young St, Hamilton ON L8N 1T8; Wes'67; FRCSC; Ophth (Cataract Surgery). Staff, St Joseph's Healthcare - Charlton Campus; Clinical Asst Prof, Hamilton Health Sciences Centre - McMaster Children's Hospital; Asst Clin Prof, McMaster University; (905)527-5559; Fax. (905)527-3883.

NASHED, Maged S; Health Sciences Centre, 820 Sherbrook St, Winnipeg MB R3A 1R9; Cairo (Egypt)'93; FRCPC; RadOncol; DiagRad. Staff, Health Sciences Centre; (204)774-8511

NASHED, Yousery H; Providence Care-Mental Health, PO Box 603 Stn Main 752 King St W, Kingston ON K7L 4X3; Ain Shams (Egypt)'75; FRCPC; Psy (General Adult Psychiatry). Staff, Providence Care - Mental Health Services; Asst Prof Psy, Queen's University; (613)546-1101 x5932; Fax. (613)540-6120.

NASHI, Emil; MUHC-Montreal Gen Hosp, 1650 av Cedar, Montreal QC H3G 1A4; Alb'98; Rheum; ClinImmunol&Allergy; IntMed. Staff, McGill University Health Centre - Montreal General Campus; Langs: English; French; (514)934-8036; Fax. (514)934-8239; e_nashi@hotmail.com.

NASHI, Saad; Parkway Forest Med Centre, 40-105 Parkway Forest Dr, North York ON M2J 1L8; Baghdad (Iraq)'77; MB ChB; CCFP; (416)502-3404; Fax. (416)502-3017.

NASIR, Fareeha; Rockyview Gen Hosp, 7007 14 St SW, Calgary AB T2V 1P9; Staff, Rockyview General Hospital; (403)943-3000

NASIRZADEH, Ehsaneddin; Credit Valley Family Practice, 205-2300 Eglinton Ave W, Mississauga ON L5M 2V8; (Iran)'93; CCFP; Staff Family Med, The Credit Valley Hospital; Langs: Farsi; (905)820-8144; Fax. (905)820-1631.

NASMITH, James B; St Paul's Hosp, 477A-1081 Burrard St, Vancouver BC V6Z 1Y6; Tor'73; BSc(Hon); FRCPC; FRCPC; Cardiol; IntMed (Coronary Care). Staff, Providence Health Care - St Paul's Hospital; Langs: Bilingual(English/French); (604)682-2344

NASMITH, Louise L; UBC Health Clinic, 310-5950 University Ave, Vancouver BC V6T 1Z3; McG'78; CCFP; FCFP; A-Dept Head Family Practice, University of British Columbia; Langs: French; Spanish; (604)822-5431; louise.nasmith@ubc.ca.

NASON, Gregory M; 66 Broad Rd, Oromocto NB E2V 1C2; Mem'09; CCFP; (506)446-4626; Fax. (506)446-4483.

NASON, Richard W; 46-825 Sherbrook St, Winnipeg MB R3A 1M5; Dal'78; FRCSC; GenSurg (Surgical Oncology). Staff, Health Sciences Centre; Med Dir, Winnipeg Regional Health Authority; Asst Prof, University of Manitoba; (204)787-3125; Fax. (204)787-4851.

NASR, Ahmed L; Children Hosp of Eastern Ont, 401 Smyth Rd, Ottawa ON K1H 8L1; Cairo (Egypt)'94; FRCSC; GenSurg; PedGenSurg. Staff, Children's Hospital of Eastern Ontario (CHEO); (613)737-7600

NASR, Kamil; Centre Med Mira, 1560 boul de Rome, Brossard QC J4W 3A1; St. Joseph (Lebanon)'67; Ophth (P.Q.). Staff, McGill University Health Centre - Montreal General Campus; Lecturer, McGill University; Langs: Italian; French; Arabic; (450)466-1880; Fax. (450)466-4884.

NASR, Michel R; Health Sciences Centre, 820 Sherbrook St, Winnipeg MB R3A 1R9; Kursk (Russia (Federation))'98; Staff, Health Sciences Centre; (204)774-8511

NASR, Nagwa Y I; Trinity Med Clinic, 335 18th St, Brandon MB R7A 5A8; Alexandria (Egypt)'85; CCFP.

NASRALLA, George A T; Beautiful Plains Comm Med Clin, PO Box 70 499 Mountain Ave, Neepawa MB R0J 1H0; (Other Foreign)'91; CCFP; (204)476-3189

NASREDDINE, Ziad; 250-4896 boul Taschereau, Greenfield Park QC J4V 2J2; Sher'90; FRCPC; Neur. (514)672-1931; Fax. (514)672-3308.

NASREEN, Ruksana; Children' After Hours Clinic, 101 Fanshawe Park Rd E, London ON N5X 3V9; Dhaka (Bangladesh)'89; FRCPC; Peds. (519)850-3800

NASRI, Masood A; Grand River Hosp-KW Hlth Ctre, PO Box 9056 Stn C 835 King St W, Kitchener ON N2G 1G3; Karachi (Pakistan)'88; Staff, Grand River Hospital - Kitchener/Waterloo Health Centre; (519)749-4300

NASRI, Nabil; Douglas Mental Hlth Univ Inst, 6875 boul Lasalle, Verdun QC H4H 1R3; Ain Shams (Egypt)'78; Staff, Douglas Mental Health University Institute; (514)761-6131; nasnab@douglas.mcgill.ca.

NASRULLA, M Omar; Dixon Med Clinic, 101-531 Davis Dr, Newmarket ON L3Y 6P5; Panjab (Pakistan)'63; MB BS; MRCP(UK); Staff, Southlake Regional Health Centre; (905)830-9933

NASSAR, Bassam A; Mackenzie Bldg, 618-5788 University Ave, Halifax NS B3H 1V8; Cairo (Egypt)'80; MB ChB; PhDpon-Tyne,Eng.) - (Ne; BSc(Beirut,Leb.); FRCPC; MedBiochem. Staff, Queen Elizabeth II Health Sciences Centre - Victoria General Site; Prof, Dalhousie University; (902)473-2225; bassam.nassar@cdha.nshealth.ca.

NASSER, Ali M; 5486 Falsbridge Dr NE, Calgary AB T3J 5H4; Alb'99; CCFP; (403)280-2272; Fax. (403)280-2268.

NASSER, Hamid A; 202-73 Delhi St, Guelph ON N1E 6L9; St. Joseph (Lebanon)'84; FRCSC; GenSurg (Endovasc Aortic Surg); VascSurg. Ac Staff, Grand River Hospital - Kitchener/Waterloo Health Centre; Ac Staff, Guelph General Hospital; Consultant, Cambridge Memorial Hospital; Langs: Arabic; French; (519)836-9441; Fax. (519)836-1793; drnasseroffice@gmail.com.

NASSER, Joseph G; Dickson Centre, 3041-5820 University Ave, Halifax NS B3H 1V7; Dal'84; MRC(C); DDS; FRCSC; Otol. Staff, Queen Elizabeth II Health Sciences Centre - Victoria General Site; Teach Staff, Dalhousie University; (902)473-4323; Fax. (902)473-3879; jnasser@dal.ca.

NASSER, Kasim R; 102-1 Centre Point Dr, Ottawa ON K2G 6E2; Baghdad (Iraq)'96; CCFP; (613)596-1320; Fax. (613)596-1326.

NASSER-SHARIF, Farah J; Medical Assoc of Port Perry, 462 Paxton St, Port Perry ON L9L 1L9; Tor'98; BSc; FRCPC; IntMed. (905)985-5572; Fax. (905)985-8378.

NASSER-SHARIF, Susan B; Health Sciences Centre, AD401-820 Sherbrook St, Winnipeg MB R3A 1R9; McG'94; FRCSC; OrthSurg. Staff, Health Sciences Centre; (204)774-6511

NASSERI, Eiman; Women's College Hosp, 842-76 Grenville St, Toronto ON M5S 1B2; McG'07; MDCM; FRCPC; Derm. Staff, Women's College Hospital; (416)323-6400

NASSERI, Lili; 205-2773 Barnet Hwy, Coquitlam BC V3B 1C2; McG'02; CCFP; Staff, Eagle Ridge Hospital & Health Care Centre; Langs: Bilingual(French/English); (778)285-6088; Fax. (778)285-6081.

NASSIF, Edgard; CHUM-Hop Notre-Dame, 1560 rue Sherbrooke E, Montreal QC H2L 4M1; Mon'75; ABS; FRCSC; GenSurg; General Surgical Oncology (P.Q.). Staff, Centre Hospitalier l'Université de Montréal (CHUM) - Hôpital Notre-Dame; Clinical Asst Prof, Universite de Montreal; (514)890-8000

NASSIF, Mohammed; The Moncton Hosp, 135 MacBeath Ave, Moncton NB E1C 6Z8; King Abdul Aziz (Saudi Arabia)'04; FRCSC; GenSurg. Staff, The Moncton Hospital; (506)857-5111

NASSIF, Rachel; CSSS du Lac-des-Deux-Montagnes, 520 boul Arthur-Sauve, Saint-Eustache QC J7R 5B1; Mon'09; CCFP; Staff, Hôpital de Saint-Eustache; (450)473-6811

NASSIF, Raymond; Ctr Hosp Fleury, 2180 rue Fleury E, Montreal QC H2B 1K3; Mon'75; FRCSC; GenSurg. Ac Staff, Centre Hospitalier Fleury; (514)381-9311; Fax. (514)858-2435.

NASSIM, Mark; Greenboro Family Medicine, 25 Tapiola Cres, Ottawa ON K1T 2J7; Ott'05; CCFP; (613)738-0303

NASSIRI, Shirin; CSSS du Lac-des-Deux-Montagnes, 520 boul Arthur-Sauve, St-Eustache QC J7R 5B1; Mon'99; FRCPC; IntMed; Gastroent. Staff, Hôpital de Saint-Eustache; (450)473-6811

NASSO, Domenic; 212-1315 Finch Ave W, North York ON M3J 2G6; Tor'88; (416)630-7426; Fax. (416)630-2741.

NASSR, Donald G; The Canadian Mental Hlth Assoc, 1400 Windsor Ave, Windsor ON N8X 3L9; Wes'60; Psy (Psychotherapy). (519)971-0116; Fax. (519)252-5646.

NATALE, Renato; London HSC-Victoria Hosp, PO Box 5010 Stn B B2 412-800 Commissioners rd E, London ON N6A 5W9; Wes'73; FACOG; FRCSC; ObstGyn (Maternal Fetal Medicine). Assoc Chief, London Health Sciences Centre - University Hospital; Staff, London Health Sciences Centre - Victoria Campus; Prof ObstGyn, University of Western Ontario; Langs: Italian; (519)685-8500

NATARAJ, Andrew; University of Alberta Hosp, 2D102WCM-8440 112 St NW, Edmonton AB T6G 2B7; Sask'99; FRCSC; Neursurg. Staff Neurosurg, University of Alberta Hospital; (780)407-7179; Fax. (780)407-8203.

NATARAJ, Jonathon S Y; Midtown Med Centre, 200-39 23rd St E, Saskatoon SK S7K 0H6; Sask'06; BSc; CCFP; (306)242-0213; Fax. (306)683-0701.

NATARAJ, Yellepeddy; Midtown Med Centre, 200-39 23rd St E, Saskatoon SK S7K 0H6; Andhra (India)'67; MB BS; LRCP; LRCS(Ed); LRCPS(Glas); (306)242-0213; Fax. (306)683-0701.

NATARAJAN, Dhanapal; Regina Mental Health Clinic, 2110 Hamilton St, Regina SK S4P 2E3; Madras (India)'84; MB BS; MRCPsy(UK); DPM(Ire); FRCPC; Psy. Dept Head/Chief Psy, Regina Mental Health Clinic; Asst Prof, University of Saskatchewan; Langs: Tamil; (306)766-3601; Fax. (306)766-4953; d.natarajan@rqhealth.ca.

NATARAJAN, Madhu K; Hamilton HS-General Site, 237 Barton St E, Hamilton ON L8L 2X2; Tor'89; FRCPC; IntMed (Interventional Cardiology); Cardiol. Staff, Hamilton Health Sciences Centre - Hamilton General Hospital; Assoc Prof, McMaster University; (905)527-6241; Fax. (905)527-2337.

NATARAJAN, Meenakshi; St George Med Centre, 124 Main St, St George NB E5C 3S3; Dal'10; CCFP; (506)755-9020; Fax. (506)755-3440.

NATARAJAN, Monika N; Dalhousie Family Medicine, 265-6960 Mumford Rd, Halifax NS B3L 4P1; McM'94; CCFP; Staff Family Med, Queen Elizabeth II Health Sciences Centre - Halifax Infirmary Site; Assoc Prof, Dalhousie University; (902)473-4715; Fax. (902)473-8548; nandini.natarajan@dal.ca.

NATARAJAN, Nagamani C; 203-1370 Clyde Ave, Nepean ON K2G 3H8; (India)'72; (613)224-2258; Fax. (613)224-4519.

NATARAJAN-KAILLEY, Anita; 75 Tenth St, New Westminster BC V3M 3X4; UBC'98; CCFP; (604)526-3308; Fax. (604)526-2984.

NATAROS, Gary; 20595 Douglas Cres, Langley BC V3A 4B6; UBC'78; (604)534-0641; Fax. (604)530-4217.

NATEGHI, Vafa; Ctr de Sante Vallee-Gatineau, 309 boul Desjardins, Maniwaki QC J9E 2E7; Mon'00; Chef méd fam/Chef méd urgence, CSSS de la Vallée de la Gatineau; (819)449-4690; Fax. (819)449-6137.

NATES, Wayne; St Boniface Gen hosp, 409 Tache Ave, Winnipeg MB R2H 2A6; Staff, St Boniface General Hospital; (204)233-8563

NATH, Avik; The Ottawa Hosp-Gen Campus, 501 Smyth Rd, Ottawa ON K1H 8L6; Ott'04; CCFP; CCFP(E.M.); Staff, The Ottawa Hospital - General Campus; (613)737-8000

NATH, Rovindra R; CMH Med Centre, 111-1315 Finch Ave W, North York ON M3J 2G6; Tor'92; CCFP; FCFP; Court Staff, North York General Hospital; (416)631-6888; Fax. (416)631-6887.

NATHA, Dharmesh J; Lotus Integrative Med Ctre, 15551 Marine Dr, White Rock BC V4B 1C9; Witwatersrand (South Africa)'93; MB ChB; CCFP; FCFP; Langs: Gujarati; Afrikaans; (604)538-5993; Fax. (604)538-5441.

NATHA, Rajivkumar P C; 90-2525 Bridlecrest Way SW, Calgary AB T2Y 5J4; (South Africa)'88; (403)945-8216; Fax. (403)945-8276.

NATHAN, Howard J; The Ottawa Hosp-Gen Campus, 249B-501 Smyth Rd, Ottawa ON K1H 8L6; McG'72; FRCPC; Anes (Chronic Pain Management). Staff Pain Clinic, The Ottawa Hospital - General Campus; Staff, The Ottawa Hospital - Civic Campus; Prof Anes, University of Ottawa; (613)761-4775; Fax. (613)761-4895.

NATHAN, Nicole S; Don Valley Med Associates, 330-1333 Sheppard Ave E, North York ON M2J 1V1; Tor'04; CCFP; (416)494-7396; Fax. (416)497-4793; nnathan@baycrest.org.

NATHAN, Paul C; The Hosp for Sick Children, 555 University Ave, Toronto ON M5G 1X8; Tor'95; MSc; FRCPC; Peds (Pediatric Oncology). Staff, The Hospital For Sick Children; (416)813-8321 x28454; Fax. (416)813-5327.

NATHAN, Viji; 117 Wentworth Rd PO Box 3550, Windsor NS B0N 2T0; Madurai (India)'94; MB BS; CCFP; Physician, Dykeland Lodge; Physician, Windsor Elms Village; Langs: Tamil; (902)798-4652; Fax. (902)798-4110.

NATHANSON, Barbara A; Harvard Square Mall, 203-801 Mohawk Rd W, Hamilton ON L9C 6C2; McG'74; CCFP; FCFP; Ac Staff, Hamilton Health Sciences Centre - McMaster University Medical Centre; Court Staff, St Joseph's Healthcare - Charlton Campus; (905)318-5119; Fax. (905)318-2151.

NATHANSON, Barry N; Southlake Reg Health Centre, 596 Davis Dr, Newmarket ON L3Y 2P9; Tor'90; FRCPC; IntMed. Clin Assoc Staff, Mount Sinai Hospital; Staff Internist, Southlake Regional Health Centre; (905)895-4521 x2216

NATHANSON, Jay A; North York Gen Hosp, 4001 Leslie St, North York ON M2K 1E1; Wes'96; Psy. Staff, North York General Hospital; (416)756-6000; Fax. (416)756-6771.

NATHANSON, Martin M; Toronto East Gen Hosp Inc, 825 Coxwell Ave, Toronto ON M4C 3E7; McG'65; DABR; FRCPC; DiagRad. Chief Dept of Radiol, Toronto East General Hospital Inc; (416)469-6080; Fax. (416)469-6662; mnath@tegh.on.ca.

NATHANSON, Sheldon R; 103-5788 Birney Ave, Vancouver BC V6S 0A2; Detroit (USA)'74; Assoc Staff, Providence Health Care - St Paul's Hospital; Clin Instructor, University of British Columbia; (604)675-3975

NATHENS, Avery B; Sunnybrook Hlth Sciences Ctre, D574-2075 Bayview Ave, Toronto ON M4N 3M5; Qns'90; PhD; FRCSC; GenSurg. Head GenSurg, St Michael's Hospital; Staff, Sunnybrook Health Sciences Centre; (416)480-4711; Fax. (416)480-4712.

NATHENS, Marvin S; Ctr Radiologique Cote-des Neig, 600-5300 ch de la Cote-des-Nei, Montreal QC H3T 1Y3; Sask'60; CSPQ; FRCPC; DiagRad. Staff Radiol, St Mary's Hospital Centre; Lecturer, McGill University; (514)738-5306

NATHO, Lorraine R; Foothills Med Centre, 704-1403 29 St NW, Calgary AB T2N 2T9; McG'95; CCFP; Staff, Foothills Medical Centre; Langs: Bilingual(French/English); (403)944-5872; Fax. (403)944-2409.

NATHOO, Bharat C; York-Med Medical Arts Centre, 205-250 Harding Blvd W, Richmond Hill ON L4C 9M7; Natal (South Africa)'80; FACP; FRCPC; IntMed (Hypertension); Nephrol. Court Staff, Southlake Regional Health Centre; Med Dir York Region Dialysis Prog/Staff, Mackenzie Richmond Hill Hospital; Langs: Afrikaans; Gujarati; Hindi; (905)508-5911; Fax. (905)508-2972.

NATHOO, Munir F A; Family Care Med Centre, 104-3050 Garden St, Whitby ON L1R 2G7; Qns'94; BSc; (905)430-5305; Fax. (905)430-6416.

NATHOO, Sameer B; Medica One, 1275 Rymal Rd, Hamilton ON L8W 3N1; Cork (Ireland)'08; (905)599-1733

NATION, Jill G; Tom Baker Cancer Centre, 1331 29 St NW, Calgary AB T2N 4N2; Alb'77; FRCSC; ObstGyn (Gynecologic Oncology). Ac Staff Gyn, Tom Baker Cancer Centre; Ac Staff, Foothills Medical Centre; Prof, University of Calgary; (403)521-3721; Fax. (403)521-3573.

NATSHEH, Adam; 302-1448 Lawrence Ave E, North York ON M4A 2V6; Mem'02; FRCPC; Derm. (416)750-8400; Fax. (416)750-1091.

NATSHEH, Ishaq M; Goulds Med Centre, PO Box 70 Stn Main 355-367 Main Rd, Goulds NL A1S 1G3; Liverpool (England)'70; MB ChB; Court Staff, St Clare's Mercy Hospital; Langs: Arabic; (709)368-2591; Fax. (709)745-6029.

NATTEL, Celia A; Westmount Med Bldg, 415-5025 rue Sherbrooke O, Montreal QC H4A 1S9; McG'77; CCFP; FCFP; Staff, St Mary's Hospital Centre; (514)489-4014; Fax. (514)489-1955.

NATTEL, Stanley; Montreal Heart Institute, 5000 rue Belanger, Montreal QC H1T 1C8; McG'74; ABIM; BSc; DABIM; FACC; FRCP; FRSC; ABCD; FRCPC; Cardiol (Pharmacology) (Physiology) (Clinical Pharmacology); IntMed. Sr Scientist Research Centre, Institut de Cardiologie de Montréal; Chair Paul-David Cardiovasc & Electrophysiol, Universite de Montreal; Langs: Hebrew; Yiddish; Bilingual(French/English); German; (514)376-3330 x3990; Fax. (514)376-1355; stanley.nattel@icm-mhi.org.

NATUIK, Shannon A; Maitland Valley Med Centre, 180 Cambria Rd N, Goderich ON N7A 4N8; Man'08; CCFP; (519)524-6060

NAUD, Alain; Clinique d'Urologie Berger, 416-1000 ch Sainte-Foy, Quebec QC G1S 2L6; Laval'70; CSPQ; FRCSC; Urol. Ac Staff, Centre Hospitalier Universitaire de Québec (CHUQ) - Siege Social; (418)266-2876; Fax. (418)266-2879.

NAUD, Alain; CHUQ-St-Francois d'Assise, 10 rue de l'Espinay, Quebec QC G1L 3L5; Laval'84; LMCC; CCFP; FCFP; Ac Staff, Centre Hospitalier Universitaire De Québec - Pavillon De St-françois-d'assise; Prof Titulaire de Clinique, Université Laval; Langs: Spanish; English; (418)525-4351; Fax. (418)525-4322; alain.naud@mfa.ulaval.ca.

NAUD, Francoise; CHUQ-Hotel-Dieu de Quebec, 11 Côte du Palais, Quebec QC G1R 2J6; Laval'77; CSPQ; FRCPC; AnatPath. Staff, Centre Hospitalier Universitaire de Québec (CHUQ) - Siege Social; Teach Staff, Université Laval; Langs: Bilingual(English/French); (418)691-5233; francoise.naud@bm.ulaval.ca.

NAUD, Jean-Francois D; CSSS de Trois-Rivieres, 1991 boul du Carmel, Trois-Rivieres QC G8Z 3R9; McG'05; Critical Care Medicine; IntMed. Staff, CSSS de Trois-Rivières; (819)697-3333

NAUD, Jerome; CSSSG-Hop de Gatineau, CP 2000 Succ Bureau-Chef 909 boul de la Verendrye, Gatineau QC J8P 7H2; Laval'05; FRCPC; Anes. Staff, Hôpital de Gatineau; (819)966-6100

NAUD, Pierre G; CHUQ-Hotel-Dieu de Quebec, 11 Cote Du Palais, Quebec QC G1R 2J6; Sher'85; MSc; FRCPC; Neur; Electroenceph (P.Q.). Staff, Centre Hospitalier Universitaire de Québec (CHUQ) - Siege Social; Teach Staff, Université Laval; (418)691-5288; Fax. (418)691-5186.

NAUD, Simon; CSSS de Manicouagan, 635 boul Jolliet, Baie-Comeau QC G5C 1P1; Laval'06; CCFP; CCFP(E.M.); Staff, Centre Hospitalier Régional Baie-Comeau; (418)589-3701

NAUDE, Adel H; Lloydminster Clinic, 5120 46 St, Lloydminster AB T9V 2P7; Pretoria (South Africa)'89; MB ChB; Langs: Afrikaans; (780)875-2221; Fax. (780)875-0605.

NAUDE, David F; 403A-3210 25 Ave, Vernon BC V1T 1P1; Pretoria (South Africa)'83; MB ChB; MMed(Int); FRCPC; IntMed. Staff, Vernon Jubilee Hospital; (250)558-7755; Fax. (250)558-5899.

NAUDE, Francois P; Lloydminster Clinic, 5120 46 St, Lloydminster AB T9V 2P7; Pretoria (South Africa)'89; MB ChB; Med Staff, Lloydminster Hospital; Langs: Afrikaans; (780)875-2221; Fax. (780)875-0605.

NAUDE, Jan J S; The Medical Clinic Associates, 4794 Joyce Ave, Powell River BC V8A 3B6; Pretoria (South Africa)'98; MB ChB; DObst; Langs: Afrikaans; (604)485-6261; Fax. (604)485-2820.

NAUDE, Justin; 11-88 Duncan Ave W, Penticton BC V2A 7J7; Pretoria (South Africa)'82; MB ChB; Dip SportMed(Scot.); FRCSC; OrthSurg (Sports Medicine). Hd GenSurg, Penticton Regional Hospital; (250)492-6681; Fax. (250)492-8027.

NAUDIE, Douglas D R; London HSC-University Hosp, PO Box 5339 Stn B A9 028-339 Windermere Rd, London ON N6A 5A5; McG'97; FRCSC; OrthSurg (Hip & Knee Reconstruction). Asst Prof, London Health Sciences Centre - University Hospital; Langs: Bilingual(English/French); (519)663-3407; Fax. (519)663-3420.

NAUGHTON, Finola M; Univ Hlth Network-Toronto Gen, EN3 464-200 Elizabeth St, Toronto ON M5G 2C4; Dublin (Ireland)'95; Staff, Toronto General Hospital - UHN; (416)340-3567

NAUGLER, Christopher T; Calgary Lab Services, C414 9-3535 Research Rd NW, Calgary AB T2L 2K8; Dal'97; MSc; BScChemEng; FRCPC; GenPath;CCFP; FCFP; Staff, Calgary Laboratory Services; (403)770-3756

NAUGLER, R Gary; Erindale Health Centre, 2-50 Kenderdine Rd, Saskatoon SK S7N 3A1; Sask'81; Staff, St Paul's Hospital (Grey Nuns) of Saskatoon; (306)934-6601; Fax. (306)934-6615.

NAUGLER, Sharon M M; Women's Hosp, WR 120-735 Notre Dame Ave, Winnipeg MB R3E 0L8; Man'77; FRCSC; ObstGyn. Ac Staff, Health Sciences Centre.

NAULT, Isabelle; Hopital Laval, 2725 ch Sainte-Foy, Quebec QC G1V 4G5; Laval'01; FRCPC; IntMed; Cardiol. Staff, Hôpital Laval; (418)656-8711; Fax. (418)656-4581.

NAULT, Julie R; Montfort Hosp, 713 Montreal Rd, Ottawa ON K1K 0T2; Ott'98; FRCPC; Peds. Staff, Montfort Hospital; (613)746-4621

NAULT, Patrice; CSSSG-Hop de Hull, 116 boul Lionel-Emond, Gatineau QC J8Y 1W7; Mon'88; FRCSC; GenSurg; VascSurg. Staff, Hull Hospital; (819)595-6032; Fax. (819)595-6078; patrice_nault@ssss.gouv.qc.ca.

NAULT, Paul; Clin de Derm Esthetique de Mtl, 260-2040 rue Marcel-Laurin, Saint-Laurent QC H4R 1J9; Mon'78; DABD; FRCPC; Derm. Langs: Bilingual(French/English); (514)387-6433; Fax. (514)387-6041.

NAULT, Serge; CSSS Haut-Richelieu-Rouville, 920 boul du Seminaire N, St-Jean-Sur-Richel QC J3A 1B7; Mon'77; Staff, Hôpital du Haut-Richelieu; (450)359-5000; Fax. (450)359-5251.

NAULT, Theodore; Ctr Hosp de Matane, 333 rue Thibault, Matane QC G4W 2W5; Laval'72; OrthSurg. Staff, Centre Hospitalier de Matane; Langs: Bilingual(French/English); (418)562-0560; Fax. (418)562-9322; tednault@hotmail.com.

NAULT, Yvonne D M; 9976 Grenville St PO Box 403, St Peters NS B0E 3B0; Man'90; (902)535-2735; Fax. (902)535-3231; ynault@stpeterscable.com.

NAUMETZ, Victor A; Oakville Health Centre, 116-1060 Speers Rd, Oakville ON L6L 2X4; McG'71; FAAOS; FACS; Dip SportMed; FRCSC; OrthSurg (Trauma). Affil Staff, Joseph Brant Memorial Hospital; Consultant, Halton Healthcare Services Corporation - Milton District Hospital; Ac Staff, Halton Healthcare Services Corporation - Oakville Site; (905)844-9054; Fax. (905)844-5352.

NAUS, Gregory J; BC Cancer Agency-Vancouver CC, 600 10th Ave W, Vancouver BC V5Z 4E6; New York (USA)'80; Staff, BC Cancer Agency Vancouver Centre; (604)877-6000; Fax. (604)875-4596.

NAUS, Monika; BC Centre for Disease Control, 655 12th Ave W, Vancouver BC V5Z 4R4; Alb'83; MHSc; MD; ABPM; FRCPC; Public Health & Preventive Med., BC Centre For Disease Control; Assoc Prof, University of British Columbia; (604)707-2540; Fax. (604)707-2515; monika.naus@bccdc.ca.

NAUSE, Leanne N; Agassiz Med Centre, 130-30 Stephen St, Morden MB R6M 2G3; Man'03; BSc; CCFP; (204)822-4474; Fax. (204)822-6886.

NAUTH, Aaron; St Michael's Orthopaedic Assoc, 800-55 Queen St E, Toronto ON M5C 1R6; Qns'04; FRCSC; OrthSurg. (416)864-6003

NAUTH-MISIR, Dayanti; Promenade Village Hlth Centre, 3-7700 Bathurst St, Thornhill ON L4J 7Y3; Qns'93; CCFP; (905)660-9760

NAVAJAS, Eduardo V; St Michael's Health Centre, 801-61 Queen St E, Toronto ON M5C 2T2; Sao Paulo (Brazil)'99; FRCSC; Ophth. (416)867-7400

NAVANEELAN, G Christy; Queensway-Carleton Hosp, 3045 Baseline Rd, Nepean ON K2H 8P4; Ceylon (Sri Lanka)'76; MB BS; Anes (Anesthesia-ICU). Staff, Cornwall Community Hospital; Staff, Cornwall Community Hospital - Second Street Site; Staff, Queensway Carleton Hospital; (613)721-2000

NAVARATNAM, Srisaladevi; CancerCare Manitoba, 675 McDermot Ave, Winnipeg MB R3E 0V9; Ceylon (Sri Lanka)'84; FRCPC; IntMed. (204)787-2180

NAVARATNARAJAH, Prashanthini; West Vaughan Med Centre, 3900 Rutherford Rd, Woodbridge ON L4H 3G8; Transkei (South Africa)'04; CCFP; (905)417-5461; Fax. (905)417-5463.

NAVARATNARAJAH, Vaanathy; West Vaughan Med Centre, 3900 Rutherford Rd, Woodbridge ON L4H 3G8; Transkei (South Africa)'02; MB ChB; CCFP; (905)417-5461; Fax. (905)417-5463; navani@hotmail.com.

NAVARATNE, N K Pradeep; 101-2318 Lakeshore Blvd W, Etobicoke ON M8V 1B5; Colombo (Sri Lanka)'96; CCFP; (416)252-4440; Fax. (416)252-4433.

NAVARRE, Pierre; CSSS de l'Energie-Ste-Therese, 1705 av Georges, Shawinigan QC G9N 2N1; McG'07; MDCM; OrthSurg. Staff, CH du Centre-de-la-Mauricie (Ste-Thérèse de Shawinigan); (819)536-7500; pierre_navarre@ssss.gouv.qc.ca.

NAVARRO, Christine; 245 Eglinton Ave E, Toronto ON M4P 3B7; McM'10; CCFP; (416)488-1455

NAVARRO, Joaquin X R; 201-237 Argyle Ave, Ottawa ON K2P 1B8; Valencia (Spain)'63; DPsy; AB; FRCPC; Psy. Clinical Asst Prof Psy, University of Ottawa; Langs: Spanish; French; (613)238-7913; Fax. (613)238-7914; j.m.navarro@rogers.com.

NAVARRO, Margaret E; 201-237 Argyle Ave, Ottawa ON K2P 1B8; McG'68; DPsy; AB; FRCPC; Psy (Psychiatric Oncology). Clinical Asst Prof, University of Ottawa; (613)238-7913; Fax. (613)238-7914.

NAVARRO KUNSTMANN, Oscar M; The Hosp for Sick Children, 2133-555 University Ave, Toronto ON M5G 1X8; (Chile)'90; Staff Diagnostic Imaging, The Hospital For Sick Children; Langs: Spanish; (416)813-6939; Fax. (416)813-7591; oscar.navarro@sickkids.ca.

NAVE, Cynthia J; Lakeview Med Centre, 13-1945 McKercher Dr, Saskatoon SK S7J 4M4; Sask'97; CCFP; (306)244-5100; Fax. (306)244-5115.

NAVIDZADEH, Adel; St Mary's Hosp Centre, 3830 av Lacombe, Montreal QC H3T 1M5; Laval'04; FRCPC; Psy. Staff, St Mary's Hospital Centre; (514)345-3511 x3986

NAVIDZADEH, Niassa; Hop Jean-Talon, 1385 rue Jean-Talon E, Montreal QC H2E 1S6; Laval'05; FRCPC; Psy. Staff, CSSS du Coeur de l'Isle Hôpital Jean-Talon; (514)495-6767

NAVRATIL, Jan J; 611 Lansdowne St, Kamloops BC V2C 1Y6; Karlova (Czech Republic)'67; FARA; FRCPC; IntMed (Osteoporosis); Rheum. Ac Staff, Royal Inland Hospital; (250)374-2202; Fax. (250)374-2473.

NAVSARIKAR, Anup; The Richmond Hosp, 7000 Westminster Hwy, Richmond BC V6X 1A2; Tor'00; FRCPC; Anes. Staff, Richmond Hospital; (604)278-9711

NAWAB, Naveed A; Sherbourne Health Centre, 333 Sherbourne St, Toronto ON M5A 2S5; (Mexico)'99; CCFP; (416)324-4180; Fax. (416)324-4181.

NAWAR, Tewfik W; CHUS-Hop Fleurimont, 3001 12e av N, Sherbrooke QC J1H 5N4; Cairo (Egypt)'63; DABIM(Nephrol); MSc(McGill); FRCPC; IntMed; Nephrol. Staff, Centre Hospitalier Universitaire de Sherbrooke-Hopital Fleurimont; Prof, Universite de Sherbrooke; (819)346-1110

NAWAZ, Ahmad; PO Box 1145 Stn Main, Timmins ON P4N 7H9; Glasgow (Scotland)'58; DOphth(Eng.); FRCOphth; Ac Staff, Timmins & District Hospital; Langs: Urdu; (705)267-5959; Fax. (705)267-3131.

NAWAZ, Shah; 208 Caswell Dr, Sudbury ON P3E 2N8; Karachi (Pakistan)'71; FCCP; FRCPC; IntMed; Cardiol. Staff Cardiol, Health Sciences North - Memorial Site; Prin Investigator, Sudbury Cardiac Research; Langs: Hindi; Urdu; Malayalam; (705)522-2682; Fax. (705)522-3293; shah.nawaz1@sympatico.ca.

NAWROCKA, Dorothy; Regent Med Centre, 208 Regent Ave W, Winnipeg MB R2C 1R2; Warsaw (Poland)'84; Staff, Pembina-Manitou Health Centre.

NAWROCKA, Joanna; Children's Hosp Eastern Ont, 401 Smyth Rd, Ottawa ON K1H 8L1; Poznan (Poland)'77; Staff, Children's Hospital of Eastern Ontario (CHEO); (613)737-2431

NAWROT, Robin; PO Box 650, Rimbey AB T0C 2J0; Alb'82; Staff, Rimbey Hospital & Care Centre; (403)843-2256; Fax. (403)843-2255; mnawrot@telusplanet.net.

NAY, Derek W; Royal Victoria Hosp, 201 Georgian Dr, Barrie ON L4M 6M2; Alb'01; FRCPC; IntMed; MedOncol. Staff Cancer Care Program, Royal Victoria Regional Health Centre; (705)739-5661; Fax. (705)739-5619.

NAYAK, Lakhbir R; PO Box 2508 Stn Main, Petitcodiac NB E4Z 6H4; Bangalore (India)'72; (506)756-2831; Fax. (506)756-2207.

NAYAR, Anoop; Burlington Prof Centre, 201-3155 Harvester Rd, Burlington ON L7N 3V2; London (England)'82; MB BS; (905)632-4640; Fax. (905)632-2623.

NAYAR, Anuradha; 6430 Main St, Vancouver BC V5W 2V4; UBC'89; Langs: Kiswahili; Hindi; Punjabi; (604)321-4313; Fax. (604)321-4314.

NAYAR, Arun; Medical Arts Bldg, 125-750 Spadina Cres E, Saskatoon SK S7K 3H3; Mysore (India)'76; LRCP; MRCS; CCFP; FCFP; Staff, Saskatoon City Hospital; Staff, Royal University Hospital; Staff, St Paul's Hospital (Grey Nuns) of Saskatoon; (306)652-5414; Fax. (306)652-5554.

NAYAR, Kiran; South Community Birth Prog, 201-5838 Fraser St, Vancouver BC V5W 2Z5; McG'01; CCFP; (604)324-2201

NAYAR, M Jane; 22035 boul Gouin O, Pierrefonds QC H9K 1C1; UBC'73; hon Staff, Lakeshore General Hospital - Pointe Claire; (514)696-8787; Fax. (514)626-8904.

NAYAR, Shalini; Vancouver Gen Hosp, 855 12th Ave W, Vancouver BC V5Z 1M9; McM'05; Respir; IntMed. Staff, Vancouver General Hospital - Centennial Pavillion; (604)875-4715

NAYAR-KINGWELL, Sunita M; The Ottawa Hosp-Civic Campus, 1053 Carling Ave, Ottawa ON K1Y 4E9; Qns'02; FRCPC; Peds. Staff, The Ottawa Hospital - Civic Campus; (604)875-2345

NAYLOR, C David; Simcoe Hall Univ of Toronto, 206-27 King's College Circle, Toronto ON M5S 1A1; Tor'78; FRCPC; IntMed. Pres Faculty of Med, University of Toronto; (416)978-2121; president@utoronto.ca.

NAYLOR, John D; Forensic Adolescent Program, 5-2681 36 St NE, Calgary AB T1Y 5S3; Cal'90; FRCPC; Psy. Staff Forensic Psy, Peter Lougheed Centre; (403)297-7701; Fax. (403)297-7790.

NAYLOR, Margaret J; 245-1620 29 St NW, Calgary AB T2N 4L7; Cal'04; CCFP; (403)289-0069; Fax. (403)289-0523.

NAYLOR, Nancy L; Ilderton Med Clinic, PO Box 160 36 Heritage Dr, Ilderton ON N0M 2A0; Wes'75; CCFP; FCFP; Ac Staff, London Health Sciences Centre - University Hospital; Ac Staff, Strathroy Middlesex General Hospital - Middlesex Hospital Alliance; (519)666-1610

NAYLOR, Scott G; 302-1428 Ouellette Ave, Windsor ON N8X 1K4; Sask'78; (519)252-2757; Fax. (519)252-2758.

NAYMARK, Sharon I; St Joseph's Health Centre, 30 The Queensway, Toronto ON M6R 1B5; Tor'03; FRCPC; Peds. Staff, St Joseph's Health Centre; (416)530-6000

NAYSMITH, J David; Lansdowne Professional Ctr II, 305-3066 Shelbourne St, Victoria BC V8R 6T9; UBC'77; DMD; BSc; FRCSC; PlasSurg (Burns). Staff, Capital Health Region; (250)592-5510; Fax. (250)592-9601.

NAZ, Farah; Saint John Reg Hosp, PO Box 2100 Stn Main 400 University Ave, Saint John NB E2L 4L2; Dhaka (Bangladesh)'93; Staff, Saint John Regional Hospital; (506)648-6884; nazfa@reg2.health.nb.ca.

NAZAIR, Odette; Clinique Med Grand-Boulevard, 200-353 boul des Bois-Francs S, Victoriaville QC G6P 4T2; Laval'90; ac Membre, Hotel-Dieu d'Arthabaska; Langs: Bilingual(French/English); (819)751-3006; Fax. (819)751-6625.

NAZAIR, Pierre; CHUQ-Ctr Hosp Univ Laval, 2705 boul Laurier, Quebec QC G1V 4G2; Laval'84; Ac Staff Emerg, Centre Hospitalier Universitaire de Quebec-CHUL; (418)656-4141 x70553; Fax. (418)525-4564.

NAZAL, Faris A; Parkway Forest Med Centre, 40-105 Parkway Forest Dr, North York ON M2J 1L8; Basra (Iraq)'88; MB ChB; CCFP; (416)502-3404; Fax. (416)502-3017.

NAZAR, Dennis M; Linwell Xray, 116-282 Linwell Rd, St Catharines ON L2N 6N5; Ott'68; FRCPC; DiagRad. Staff, Niagara Health System - Ontario Street Site; Dir Radiology, Linwell X-Ray Centre; (905)935-0270; Fax. (905)935-8811.

NAZAR-UL-IMAN, Saiyed M; Manitoba Clinic, 790 Sherbrook St, Winnipeg MB R3A 1M3; Karachi (Pakistan)'86; Staff Neonatology, Health Sciences Centre; Physician, Manitoba Clinic; Teach Staff, University of Manitoba; Langs: Punjabi; Urdu; Hindi; (204)788-5510; Fax. (204)772-2537.

NAZARALI, Karim B; 102-2338 Hurontario St, Mississauga ON L5B 1N1; Tor'90; FACS; FRCSC; Otol (Head & Neck Surgery). Staff Consultant, Trillium Health Centre - Mississauga; Court Consultant, The Credit Valley Hospital; Court Consultant, William Osler Health System - Brampton Civic Hospital; Langs: Gujarati; (905)848-3130; Fax. (905)848-4343.

NAZARENO, Janice J Y; Scarborough Hosp-General Div, 3050 Lawrence Ave E, Scarborough ON M1P 2V5; Cal'02; FRCPC; DiagRad; NuclearMed. Staff, The Scarborough Hospital - General Campus; Staff, Scarborough Radiologists; (416)431-8200

NAZARENO, Jose V C; 335-1333 Neilson Rd, Scarborough ON M1B 4Y9; Cal'02; FRCPC; IntMed; Gastroent. (416)724-7774; Fax. (416)724-7752.

NAZARETH, A John; Markham College Med Clinic, 303-474 College St, Toronto ON M6G 1A4; Ranchi (India)'68; MB BS; MCFP(EM); (416)929-0616; Fax. (416)929-9072; john.nazareth@cic.gc.ca.

NAZEMI, Fariba; The Hosp for Sick Children, 555 University Ave, Toronto ON M5G 1X8; (Iran)'90; FRCSC; Ophth. Staff, The Hospital For Sick Children; (416)813-6838

NAZER, Rakan; St Michael's Hosp, 30 Bond St, Toronto ON M5B 1W8; Riyadh (Saudi Arabia)'02; FRCSC; CardSurg. Staff, St Michael's Hospital; (416)864-5110

NAZERALI, Latifa; Trillium Hlth Ctr-Mississauga, 100 Queensway W, Mississauga ON L5B 1B8; National (Ireland)'81; FRCPC; GenPath (Laboratory Medicine); AnatPath. Staff, Trillium Health Centre - Mississauga; (905)848-7657

NAZERALI-SUNDERJI, M Muni; Eagle Ridge Hosp & Health C C, 475 Guildford Way, New Westminster BC V3H 3W9; London (England)'78; MB BS; FRCPC; IntMed. Staff, Providence Health Care - Mount Saint Joseph Hospital; Staff, BC Mental Health & Addiction Service; Staff, Eagle Ridge Hospital & Health Care Centre; Langs: Kacchi; Swahili; (604)461-2022

NAZERALI-SUNDERJI, Najmi; Vancouver Gen Hosp, 855 12th Ave W, Vancouver BC V5Z 1M9; Qns'75; CCFP; FCFP; Staff, Vancouver General Hospital - Centennial Pavillion; Langs: Bilingual(English/French); (604)728-5994

NAZIF, A Aziz; 101-600 Royal Ave, New Westminster BC V3M 1J3; Cairo (Egypt)'57; DPsy; MSc(Psy); FRCPC; Psy. Staff, Royal Columbian Hospital; (604)526-6434

NAZIF, Anna S K; St Paul's Hosp, 2B 183-1081 Burrard St, Vancouver BC V6Z 1Y6; UBC'01; FRCPC; Psy. Staff, Providence Health Care - St Paul's Hospital; (604)682-2344; anna.nazif@gmail.com.

NAZIF, Omar A; Surrey Med Arts Bldg, 208-13710 94A Ave, Surrey BC V3V 1N1; UBC'01; FRCSC; Urol. Surgeon Urol, Surrey Memorial Hospital; Clin Instructor, University of British Columbia; (604)588-3400; Fax. (604)588-3440.

NAZIR, Talat M; Dynalife Dx, 200-10150 102 St NW, Edmonton AB T5J 5E2; (Pakistan)'92; (780)451-3702

NCHAMA, M Dokiso; McConnell Med Centre, 221-820 McConnell Ave, Cornwall ON K6H 4M4; RCS (Ireland)'71; LRCP; LRCS; FAAP; MPH(CA,USA); FRCPC; Peds (Child Abuse). Staff, Cornwall Community Hospital - Second Street Site; Chief Paediatric Services, Cornwall Community Hospital; Langs: Chichewa; (613)932-1810; Fax. (613)932-0558; hlokomd@hotmail.ca.

NDEKE, Issa A; Hoffer Med Clinic, 339 Hoffer Dr, Regina SK S4N 6E2; (306)206-0330; Fax. (306)206-0332.

NDOVI, Edwards D; Bonnyville Med Clinic, PO Box 1007 Stn Main 4610 50 St, Bonnyville AB T9N 2J7; Manchester (England)'81; MB ChB; MRCGPract; BSc; FRCP(Lond); FRCPC; IntMed. Staff, Bonnyville Healthcare Centre; Vis Staff, Cold Lake Healthcare Centre; Clin Assoc Prof Family Med, University of Alberta; Langs: Chichewa; (780)826-3346; Fax. (780)826-6362.

NDUBISI, Chukwulo C; Hotel-Dieu Grace Hosp, 1030 Ouellette Ave, Windsor ON N9A 1E1; (Nigeria)'99; Staff, Hôtel-Dieu Grace Hospital; (519)973-4411

NDUBISI, Ihuoma U; Hotel-Dieu Grace Hosp, 1030 Ouellette Ave, Windsor ON N9A 1E1; Lagos (Nigeria)'98; Psy. Staff, Hôtel-Dieu Grace Hospital; (519)973-4411

NDUR, Joshua D; 104-107 Edward St, St Thomas ON N5P 1Y8; Lagos (Nigeria)'72; MB BS; DABPed; FAAP; FRS(Med); Peds (Clinical Immunology & Allergy). Vis Consultant, Sensenbrenner Hospital; Chief Peds, St Thomas Elgin General Hospital; Vis Consultant, Hôpital Notre Dame Hospital - Hearst; Med Dir Long Term Care, Caressant Care Nursing Home; Aj Prof Peds, University of Western Ontario; (519)631-8778; Fax. (519)631-0080.

NEABLE, Barry W; 185 Inkerman St E, Listowel ON N4W 2N1; Wes'75; Chief/Staff, Listowel Memorial Hospital - Listowel Wingham Hospitals Alliance; (519)291-4200; neable@cyg.net.

NEAL, Donald O; Maitland Valley Family Hlth Team, 180 Cambria Rd N, Goderich ON N7A 4N8; Wes'79; CCFP; Ac Staff, Alexandra Marine & General Hospital; Aj Teach Staff, University of Western Ontario; (519)524-6060; Fax. (519)524-5225.

NEAL, Douglas; McKinney Med Centre, 207-510 Ingersoll Ave, Woodstock ON N4S 4X9; Wes'76; Ac Staff, Woodstock General Hospital; (519)539-5605; Fax. (519)539-4521.

NEAL, Ronald J; Orleans Medical-Dental Centre, 406-2555 St. Joseph Blvd, Orleans ON K1C 1S6; Sher'71; (613)830-1771; Fax. (613)830-2543.

NEAME, Peter Dion; Joseph Brant Mem Hosp, 1230 North Shore Blvd E, Burlington ON L7S 1W7; Dublin (Ireland)'91; MB ChB; FAAP; BSc; FRCPC; Peds (Vaccination). Chief Peds, Joseph Brant Memorial Hospital; Med Advisor, Meningitis Research Foundation of Canada; Med Dir, Emergency Responder Inc; Clinical Asst Prof, McMaster University; (905)632-3730

NEAMI, Khaldon A; Stevenson Mem Hosp, PO Box 4000 Stn Main 200 Fletcher Cres, Alliston ON L9R 1W7; Al-Fateh (Libya)'97; MB ChB; CCFP; Staff, Carbonear General Hospital; (705)435-6281

NEAMT, Elena; Medistat, 4965 rue Saint-Pierre, Pierrefonds QC H9H 5M9; CCFP; Staff, McGill University Health Centre - Montreal General Campus; (514)624-4774

NEAPOLE, Laurie A; Columbia Med Bldg, 302-301 Columbia St E, New Westminster BC V3L 3W5; McG'89; FRCSC; ObstGyn. Langs: English; French; (604)524-4441; Fax. (604)524-4425.

NEAR, E John A; 23 Jenson Blvd, Guelph ON N1L 1K9; Wes'68; CCFP; FCFP; Staff, Guelph General Hospital; Asst Prof, McMaster University; (519)837-8875; Fax. (519)836-3243.

NEARING, James P; 302-1005 Elgin St W Box 20, Cobourg ON K9A 5J4; McG'87; Staff, Northumberland Hills Hospital; (905)377-8544; Fax. (905)377-0125.

NEARY, Ann P; Victoria Med Bldg, 311-1669 Victoria St, Prince George BC V2L 2L5; Galway (Ireland)'86; MB ChB; BAO; LMCC; (250)562-9388

NEARY, Elizabeth L; New Creation MediCosmetic Ctr, 107 Lakeshore Rd, St. Catharines ON L2N 2T6; Mem'90; CCFP; (905)937-1100

NEARY, John D D; St Joseph Health Care, F514-50 Charlton Ave E, Hamilton ON L8N 4A6; Tor'06; FRCPC; IntMed. Staff, St Joseph's Healthcare - Charlton Campus; (905)522-1155; Fax. (905)521-6068.

NEARY, John M; 445 Beechwood Pl, Waterloo ON N2T 1Z2; Alb'95; CCFP; (519)772-0700; Fax. (519)772-0701.

NEARY, Peter A; 3-1032 17 Ave SW, Calgary AB T2T 0A5; Alb'97; (403)229-1771; Fax. (403)229-1812.

NEAULT, Daniel; Clinique Med d'Alma, 935 av du Pont S, Alma QC G8B 2V5; Laval'81; Staff, CSSS de Lac-Saint Jean-Est; (418)668-6121; Fax. (418)668-5298.

NEAULT, Robert; Centre Med de Mont-Laurier, 304 rue de la Madone, Mont-Laurier QC J9L 1R7; Laval'72; (819)623-1520; Fax. (819)623-9637.

NEBHWANI, Neetu V; Scarborough Hosp-General Div, 3050 Lawrence Ave E, Scarborough ON M1P 2V5; (India)'06; Staff, The Scarborough Hospital - General Campus; (416)438-2911

NECAS, Lucille M; 139 Boardwalk Dr, Toronto ON M4L 3X9; Tor'83; FRCPC; Psy. (416)690-1951

NECHALA, Patrik; Grey Bruce HS-Owen Sound, PO Box 1800 Stn Main 7105-1800 8th St E, Owen Sound ON N4K 6M9; Tor'99; FRCSC; GenSurg; ThorSurg. Staff, Grey Bruce Health Services - Owen Sound; (519)371-8311; Fax. (519)371-8365.

NECHIFOR, Roxana; Associate Med Group, 4705 48 Ave, Red Deer AB T4N 3T1; (Romania)'02; PhD; CCFP; Physician, Associate Medical Group; Langs: Romanian; (403)346-2057; Fax. (403)347-2989.

NECULAU, Madalina; Bridlewood Prof Centre, 310-3443 Finch Ave E, Scarborough ON M1W 2S1; Iasi (Romania)'95; FRCPC; IntMed; Endocrin&Metab. (416)773-0220; Fax. (416)771-1833.

NEDD, Kaiyo S; 1757 Robson St, Vancouver BC V6G 1C9; Washington(DC) (USA)'99; CCFP; (604)689-1828; Fax. (604)689-1849.

NEDD, Kenford W; 1757 Robson St, Vancouver BC V6G 1C9; Dal'70; Assoc Staff, Providence Health Care - St Paul's Hospital; (604)689-1828; Fax. (604)689-1849.

NEDELEC, Joelle; CSSS Jeanne-Mance, 2260 rue Parthenais, Montreal QC H2K 3T5; Mon'95; (514)527-2361 x2389; Fax. (514)527-6016.

NEDELEC, Laurence; CLSC de Sherbrooke, 1200 rue King E, Sherbrooke QC J1G 1E4; Mon'89; CCFP; Staff, Centre Hospitalier Universitaire de Sherbrooke-Hôpital Hôtel-Dieu; (819)563-2572; Fax. (819)563-9912.

NEDER SERAFINI, Jose A; Richardson House, 102 Stuart St, Kingston ON K7L 2V6; (Brazil)'89; (613)549-1379

NEDIC, Igor; 103-704 Mara St, Point Edward ON N7V 1X4; Wes'84; CCFP; FCFP; (519)344-8283; Fax. (519)336-0459.

NEDILSKI, Morris; 2406-1320 Islington Ave, Etobicoke ON M9A 5C6; Tor'54; FCCP; FRCPC; IntMed (Allergy). (416)234-5708

NEDIMOVIC, Ljubica; Highland Med Clinic, 40-875 Highland Rd W, Kitchener ON N2N 2Y2; Sarajevo (Bosnia-Herzegovina)'79; CCFP; (519)579-8181; Fax. (519)579-8180.

NEDZELSKI, Julian M; Sunnybrook Hlth Sciences Ctre, M1 102-2075 Bayview Ave, Toronto ON M4N 3M5; Ott'68; FRCSC; Otol. Head Dept of Otol, Sunnybrook Health Sciences Centre; Prof Otol, University of Toronto; (416)480-4141; Fax. (416)480-5761.

NEE, Lucy K Y; Evergreen Community Health Ctr, 3425 Crowley Dr, Vancouver BC V5R 6G3; UBC'93; BSc; CCFP; Langs: Burmese; (604)707-3639; Fax. (604)432-6632.

NEEDHAM-NETHERCOTT, Natalie; Grand River Hosp-KW Hlth Ctre, PO Box 9056 Stn C 835 King St W, Kitchener ON N2G 1G3; Wes'95; FRCPC; IntMed (Critical Care Medicine). Staff, Grand River Hospital - Kitchener/Waterloo Health Centre; (519)749-4300 x2631; nw.nethercott@sympatico.ca.

NEELAKANT, Harish K; Midtown Mental Health Team, 3-2450 Ontario St, Vancouver BC V5T 4T7; Vijayawada (India)'93; MB BS; FRCPC; Psy. Langs: Hindi; Telugu; (604)872-8441

NEELAM, Satbir S; 521 Greenpark Cres, Mississauga ON L5B 3P7; Tor'89; CCFP; (905)782-4402

NEELANDS, Patricia; 407-235 Danforth Ave, Toronto ON M4K 1N2; Tor'86; BASc; FRCPC; Peds. (416)465-7421; Fax. (416)465-6588.

NEEMEH, Jean A; Hop Santa Cabrini Ospedale, 5655 rue Saint-Zotique E, Montreal QC H1T 1P7; Alexandria (Egypt)'60; FRCPC; HemPath; MedOncol (P.Q.); Hem (P.Q.). Ac Staff, Hôpital Santa Cabrini Ospedale; Staff, Institut Universitaire de Gériatrie de Montréal; ac Staff Vascular Med, Centre Hospitalier l'Université de Montréal (CHUM) - Hôtel-Dieu; Clin Assoc Prof Med, Universite de Montreal; (514)252-6000

NEESON, George B; 5-4502 South Ave, Elizabethtown ON K6T 1A8; Tor'62; (613)498-1602

NEETHLING, Bertram L; La Ronge Med Clinic, PO Box 240, La Ronge SK S0J 1L0; (306)425-2174; Fax. (306)425-4199.

NEFFATI, Abdurrahman A L; Lakeridge Hlth Corp-Oshawa, 1 Hospital Crt, Oshawa ON L1G 2B9; Al Fateh (Libya)'99; Staff, Lakeridge Health - Oshawa Site; (905)576-8711

NEFFGEN, Joachim F; Drumheller Assoc Physicians, PO Box 5600, Drumheller AB T0J 0Y0; Ott'73; Langs: French; German; (403)823-3345; Fax. (403)823-7823.

NEGRAEFF, Mike D; 2449 JPPN2-910 10th Ave W, Vancouver BC V5Z 1M9; Sask'92; FRCPC; Anes (Neuropathic Pain). Staff, Vancouver General Hospital - Centennial Pavillion; (604)875-4304; michael.negraeff@vch.ca.

NEGRETE, Juan C; MUHC-Montreal Gen Hosp, G1 114-1650 av Cedar, Montreal QC H3G 1A4; (Argentina)'61; MD; DPsy; CSPQ; FRCPC; Psy (Addiction Psychiatry). principale Psychologue Griffith Edwards Addiction Centre, McGill University Health Centre - Montreal General Campus; Emeritus Prof, McGill University; Langs: Spanish; Portuguese; French; (514)934-1934 x42041; Fax. (514)934-8262; juan.negrete@mcgill.ca.

NEGRETE, Sebastian; Medicentre Lasalle, 1500 av Dollard, LaSalle QC H8N 1T5; McG'10; MDCM; CCFP; (514)366-4507

NEHME, Edgard W; Clinique Med Centrale, 2050 rue Regent, Saint-Hubert QC J4T 3R5; Beirut (Lebanon)'72; Peds. (450)678-9194

NEHRA, Lollita J; 2939 Bloor St W, Etobicoke ON M8X 1B3; Tor'74; (416)248-6810

NEHRA, Paul; 2587 Penrhyn St, Victoria BC V8N 1G4; Liverpool (England)'72; CCFP; FCFP; (250)592-6206

NEIDERT, Eric J; Bell Mews Shopp Centre, 205-2039 Robertson Rd, Nepean ON K2H 8R2; Ott'93; FRCSC; GenSurg (Critical Care Medicine). Staff, Queensway Carleton Hospital; Staff, Carleton Place & District Memorial Hospital; (613)828-0896; Fax. (613)828-4807.

NEIGHBOUR, Helen; St Joseph Health Care, T213-50 Charlton Ave E, Hamilton ON L8N 4A6; London (England)'97; Staff, St Joseph's Healthcare - Charlton Campus; (905)522-1155; Fax. (905)521-6183.

NEIL, Cynthia L; Beaver Valley Clinic, PO Box 610, Fruitvale BC V0G 1L0; UBC'87; (250)367-9211; Fax. (250)367-7543.

NEIL, Gordon F; Red Deer Reg Hosp Centre, PO Box 5030 Stn Postal Box Ctr 3942 50A Ave, Red Deer AB T4N 6R2; Alb'80; BSc; AB; Staff, Red Deer Regional Hospital Centre; Med Dir, City of Red Deer Fire Dept.; (403)343-4444; Fax. (403)343-4459; neilgabb@shaw.ca.

NEIL, Paul R; Western Mem Reg Hosp, PO Box 2005 Stn Main 1 Brookfield Ave, Corner Brook NL A2H 6J7; Mem'81; Western Memorial Regional Hospital; Fax. (709)634-9162.

NEIL, Stuart G; Alberta Children's Hosp, 2888 Shaganappi Trail NW, Calgary AB T3B 6A8; St. Andrews (Scotland)'69; MB ChB; DRCOG; Anes (Pain Management). Ac Staff Anes, Alberta Children's Hospital; Asst Prof, University of Calgary; (403)955-7810; Fax. (403)943-7606.

NEILIPOVITZ, Catherine J; 103-33774 Marshall Rd, Abbotsford BC V2S 1L1; Ott'90; CCFP; (604)853-5424

NEILIPOVITZ, David T; The Ottawa Hosp-Civic Campus, 1053 Carling Ave, Ottawa ON K1Y 4E9; Qns'94; FRCPC; Anes; Critical Care Medicine. Staff, The Ottawa Hospital - Civic Campus; Fellow Anes & Critical Care, University of Ottawa; (613)798-5555 x14940

NEILIPOVITZ, William A; Thunder Bay Reg HSC-T-Bay, 980 Oliver Rd, Thunder Bay ON P7B 6V4; Man'88; ATLS; ACLS; Staff, Thunder Bay Regional Health Sciences Centre; (807)684-6000; Fax. (807)622-1904.

NEILSEN, Philip D; Special Services Unit, 90 John St S, Stratford ON N5A 2Y8; Cal'94; FRCSC; ObstGyn; Psy. (519)272-8235

NEILSON, Andrea M; Hys Med Centre, 604-11010 101 St NW, Edmonton AB T5H 4B9; Alb'06; FRCSC; ObstGyn. (780)421-4728

NEILSON, Darren W; Misericordia Community Hosp, 16940 87 Ave NW, Edmonton AB T5R 4H5; Alb'87; Att Staff Emerg, Covenant Health - Misericordia Community Hospital; (780)735-2627; Fax. (780)963-4666.

NEILSON, Douglas J; Queen Elizabeth Hosp, PO Box 6600 Stn Central 60 Riverside Dr, Charlottetown PE C1A 8T5; Glasgow (Scotland)'83; MB ChB; BSc(Hons,Physiol); MRCP(UK); FRCR(UK); FRCPC; DiagRad. Staff, Queen Elizabeth Hospital; (902)894-2972; Fax. (902)894-2276.

NEILSON, Grainne E; East Coast Forensic Psy Hosp, 88 Gloria McCluskey Ave, Dartmouth NS B3B 2B8; Cal'85; MRCPsy; FRCPC; Psy. Staff, The East Coast Forensic Psychiatry Hospital; (902)460-7333; Fax. (902)460-7343; grainne.neilson@cdha.nshealth.ca.

NEILSON, Kevin D; University of Alberta Hosp, 8440 112 St NW, Edmonton AB T6G 2B7; Alb'82; Staff, University of Alberta Hospital; (780)407-8432

NEILSON, R Scott; Nanaimo Reg Gen Hosp, 1200 Dufferin Cres, Nanaimo BC V9S 2B7; UBC'83; FRCPC; Anes. Head Anes, Nanaimo Regional General Hospital; (250)755-7605

NEILSON, Shane D; JT Powell Bldg, 50 Stone Rd E, Guelph ON N1G 2W1; Dal'00; CCFP; (519)824-4120; Fax. (519)836-7431.

NEILY, Donald R; Sherwood Family Med Centre, 15 Brackley Point Rd, Charlottetown PE C1A 6Y1; Dal'88; BSc; Staff, Queen Elizabeth Hospital; (902)566-1540; Fax. (902)368-1142; carolann@sherwoodmedicalcentre.com.

NEILY, Lori L; 104 Winnebago St, Oromocto NB E2V 1C7; Dal'92; Staff, Dr Everett Chalmers Regional Hospital; Staff, Oromocto Public Hospital; Langs: French; (506)357-5553

NEIMA, David R S; Westminster Med Bldg, 204-625 Fifth Ave, New Westminster BC V3M 1X4; Dal'77; FRCSC; Ophth. (604)521-3232; Fax. (604)521-3824.

NEIMAN, Gregory; 403-4840 Cote-Saint Luc Rd, Montreal QC H3W 2H1; Dal'48; MSc(Med); DIM; CSPQ; FRCPC; IntMed. principale Médecin, Sir Mortimer B Davis Jewish General; Consultant, Elder Care; Langs: French; (514)482-3719

NEIMANIS, Ieva M; Harvard Square Mall, 204-801 Mohawk Rd W, Hamilton ON L9C 6C2; McM'77; CCFP; FCFP; Ac Staff, St Joseph's Healthcare - Charlton Campus; Clin Assoc Prof Family Med, McMaster University; (905)388-3541; Fax. (905)388-0477.

NEIRA, Rodrigo; Central Alberta Prof Centre, 145-5201 43 St, Red Deer AB T4N 1C7; (Colombia)'85; (403)343-0045; Fax. (403)352-0047.

NEIRA ARAGON, Victor M; Children's Hosp Eastern Ont, 3348-401 Smyth Rd, Ottawa ON K1H 8L1; Bogota (Colombia)'87; Staff, Children's Hospital of Eastern Ontario (CHEO); (613)737-2431

NEJAD GHAFFAR, Shahrokh; Avicenna Health Centre, 80 Finch Ave W, North York ON M2N 2H4; (Iran)'99; CCFP; (416)222-0909; Fax. (416)222-8292.

NEJAT, Amir M; Queen Elizabeth II HSC-Halifax, 2149-1796 Summer St, Halifax NS B3H 3A7; Shahid Beheshti (Iran)'92; Staff, Queen Elizabeth II Health Sciences Centre - Halifax Infirmary Site; (902)473-4153

NEJMEDDIN JALAL, Dleer; Queen Elizabeth II HSC-Halifax, 6896-1796 Summer St, Halifax NS B3H 3A7; Salahaddin (Iraq)'95; Staff, Queen Elizabeth II Health Sciences Centre - Halifax Infirmary Site; (902)473-4153

NEL, Andre J; Tiffin Med Clinic, 3-230 Aberdeen Blvd, Midland ON L4R 5N4; Pretoria (South Africa)'80; (705)526-4992

NEL, Anton J; Mokala Medical, 161A-31 Southridge Dr, Okotoks AB T1S 2N3; Pretoria (South Africa)'94; MB ChB; LMCC; (403)995-5740; Fax. (403)995-5743.

NEL, Gert; Dr A A Wilkinson Mem Hosp, PO Box 70 428-438 Station Dr, Old Perlican NL A0A 3G0; Orange Free State (South Africa)'91; MB ChB; Staff, Dr A A Wilkinson Memorial Health Centre; (709)587-2200; Fax. (709)587-2338.

NEL, Gert P; PO Box 3955 Stn Main, Olds AB T4H 1P6; (South Africa)'85; MB ChB; Langs: Afrikaans; (403)556-7130; Fax. (403)556-1944.

NEL, Izak B; 102-3949 Maple Way, Port Alberni BC V9Y 8H4; Stellenbosch (South Africa)'02; Langs: Afrikaans; (250)723-3211

NEL, Jacobus W A; 204-105 Manitoba Dr, Clarenville NL A5A 1K2; Stellenbosch (South Africa)'07.

NEL, J de la Rey; Regina Internal Med Specialist, 1821 Rose St, Regina SK S4P 1Z7; Stellenbosch (South Africa)'77; MB ChB; LMCC; FRCPC; IntMed; Gastroent. (306)522-2212; Fax. (306)359-1068.

NEL, Johann W; Esterhazy District Med Clinic, PO Box 940, Esterhazy SK S0A 0X0; (306)745-6681; Fax. (306)745-2995.

NEL, Joshka A; Associate Med Clinic, 400-20 14th St W, Prince Albert SK S6V 3K8; Orange Free State (South Africa)'97; MB ChB; MMed(Surg); GenSurg. Member Recruitment & Retention, Saskatchewan Medical Association; (306)953-1653; Fax. (306)764-3091.

NEL, Louis J; Bayside Med Centre, 3 Beck Blvd, Penetanguishene ON L9M 1B9; Orange Free State (South Africa)'98; CCFP; CCFP(E.M.); (705)549-3939; Fax. (705)549-0029; nell@neha.mb.ca.

NEL, Mandi; Esterhazy District Med Clinic, PO Box 940, Esterhazy SK S0A 0X0; Pretoria (South Africa)'01; MB ChB; (306)745-6681; Fax. (306)745-2995.

NEL, Philip N; Prince Rupert Reg Hosp, 1305 Summit Ave, Prince Rupert BC V8J 2A6; Cape Town (South Africa)'82; MB ChB; FRCSC; GenSurg. Staff, Prince Rupert Regional Hospital; Langs: Afrikaans; (250)622-6299; Fax. (250)622-6291; philip.nel@northernhealth.ca.

NEL, Pierre R; 102-1771 Comox Ave, Comox BC V9M 3L9; Cape Town (South Africa)'97; MB ChB; FRCPC; IntMed; Gastroent. (250)339-7300; nel_pierre@hotmail.com.

NEL, Stephan F; Kelowna Gen Hosp, 2268 Pandosy St, Kelowna BC V1Y 1T2; Pretoria (South Africa)'91; MB ChB; FRCPC; Anes. Staff, Kelowna General Hospital; (250)862-4309

NEL, Stephen O; Village Mall Med Clinic, 22-6320 50 Ave, Red Deer AB T4N 4C6; Orange Free State (South Africa)'94; CCFP; (403)314-5357

NEL, Wilhelmina E; Sylvan Med Centre, 5007 46 St, Sylvan Lake AB T4S 1C2; (South Africa)'82; (403)887-2221; Fax. (403)887-3777.

NELEMS, Bill; 201-2903 Pandosy St, Kelowna BC V1Y 1W1; Tor'66; BASc; MEd; FRCSC; GenSurg; ThorSurg. Staff, Kelowna General Hospital; Prof Surg, University of British Columbia; (250)763-7660

NELHAM, Mark W; South Huron Hosp, SS 2 Stn Main 24 Huron St W, Exeter ON N0M 1S2; Wes'83; MSc; Staff, South Huron Hospital Association; Langs: Portuguese; (519)235-2700; nelham@golden.net.

NELISSE, Nicolas; Clinique l'Alternative, 2034 rue Saint-Hubert, Montreal QC H2L 3Z5; Mon'96; (514)281-9848; Fax. (514)281-8057.

NELL, Antonie M; Boissevain Health Centre, PO Box 899, Boissevain MB R0K 0E0; Pretoria (South Africa)'93; Staff, Boissevain Health Centre; (204)534-3777; Fax. (204)534-6367.

NELL, Hermann S; Alberni Med Bldg, 8-3855 9th Ave, Port Alberni BC V9Y 4T9; Stellenbosch (South Africa)'81; MB ChB; DA; LMCC; Staff Anes, West Coast General Hospital; Langs: Afrikaans; (250)723-6213; Fax. (250)723-7739.

NELLES, C Ruth M; Heart Lake Med Centre, 101-10425 Kennedy Rd, Brampton ON L6Z 0A4; Wes'71; BSc; (905)846-7611; Fax. (905)846-7753.

NELLES, Sandra E; 502-89 Queensway W, Mississauga ON L5B 2V2; Tor'93; FRCPC; IntMed (Pancreatobiliary Endoscopy); Gastroent. Consultant, Trillium Health Centre - Mississauga; (905)275-5757; Fax. (905)275-3233.

NELSON, Charles A; Rebalance MD, 104-3551 Blanshard St, Victoria BC V8Z 0B9; Alb'94; FRCSC; OrthSurg (Sports Medicine). (250)384-4121; Fax. (250)385-9600; canelson@orthodocs.ca.

NELSON, Christopher G; PO Box 88064 Rpo Rabbit Hill, Edmonton AB T6R 0M5; Alb'10; CCFP.

NELSON, Colvin; Victoria Corneal Laser Centre, 201-3550 Saanich Rd, Victoria BC V8X 1X2; Queen's (Ireland)'64; MB ChB; BAO; FRCS(Ed); Dip Ortho; FRCSC; Ophth (Refractive Surgery). Ac Staff, Greater Victoria Hospital Group; Dir, Victoria Corneal Laser Centre; (250)360-2141; Fax. (250)360-1513; colin@see-better.com.

NELSON, Danielle L; Ladybug Pediatrics, 120-1620 29 St NW, Calgary AB T2N 4L7; Cal'02; FRCPC; Peds. Staff, Alberta Children's Hospital; (403)531-9757; Fax. (403)531-9752.

NELSON, David E; 205-1015 Austin Ave, New Westminster BC V3K 3N9; UBC'69; FRCSC; Ophth (Neuro Ophthalmology). Ac Staff, Langley Memorial Hospital; Clin Instructor NeuroOphth, University of British Columbia; (604)937-3211

NELSON, David R; 1624 7th Ave, Prince George BC V2L 3P6; UBC'98; FRCSC; OrthSurg (Orthopedic Trauma). Staff, University Hospital of Northern British Columbia; Staff, St John Hospital; Vis Specialist, Bulkley Valley District Hospital; (250)564-8800; Fax. (250)564-7580.

NELSON, Delene J; Fort William Clinic, 117 McKellar St S, Thunder Bay ON P7E 1H5; Ott'01; CCFP; Staff, Thunder Bay Regional Health Sciences Centre; (807)626-1257

NELSON, Dwight A; Sandlahey Med Corp, 2204-120 5 Ave W, Cochrane AB T4C 0A4; Alb'66; (403)981-6000; Fax. (403)981-6001.

NELSON, Elena; Care Place Med Centre, 7154 120 St, Surrey BC V3W 2M8; Chelyabinsk (Russia (Federation))'88; CCFP; (604)590-5811

NELSON, Gregg S; Tom Baker Cancer Centre, 1331 29 St NW, Calgary AB T2N 4N2; Cal'03; FRCSC; ObstGyn (Gynecologic Oncology). Staff, Tom Baker Cancer Centre; (403)521-3721; Fax. (403)521-3573; gregg.nelson@albertahealthservices.ca.

NELSON, James W; 244 Darcy St, Oshawa ON L1G 3B8; Tor'66; DMRD(Rad); FRCPC; DiagRad. (905)433-3859

NELSON, Jill D; Aboriginal Diabetes Wellness C, 204-10959 102 St NW, Edmonton AB T5H 2V1; Mem'77; FRCPC; IntMed (Diabetes); Endocrin&Metab. Staff, Royal Alexandra Hospital; (780)735-4512; Fax. (780)735-5878.

NELSON, John A; Bradley Med Centre, 595 Bradley Ave, London ON N6E 3Z8; Tor'97; PhD; MSc; CCFP; (519)680-1642; Fax. (519)680-0434.

NELSON, John C; 520 Caselton Pl, Victoria BC V8Z 7Y5; UBC'69; CCFP; (250)479-8420

NELSON, John; 311 Wilson St E, Ancaster ON L9G 2B8; Qns'78; BSc; Staff, Hamilton Health Sciences Centre; (905)648-1878; Fax. (905)648-1879.

NELSON, John N; Fort Frances Clinic, 301 Victoria Ave, Fort Frances ON P9A 2C1; Wes'85; CCFP; FCFP; (807)274-3287; Fax. (807)274-7875.

NELSON, Joseph F; Alder Med Clinic, 277 Evergreen Rd, Campbell River BC V9W 5Y4; UBC'97; CCFP; (250)287-7441; Fax. (250)287-4384; josephfnelson@yahoo.ca.

NELSON, Marna J; M334-2211 Wesbrook Mall, Vancouver BC V6T 2B5; UBC'80; CCFP; FCFP; Staff, UBC Hospital - Koerner Pavillion; Staff, Care Place Medical Centre; (604)822-7011; Fax. (604)822-7889.

NELSON, Michael G; Re Docs Pharm, 28 Langstaff Rd E, Thornhill ON L3T 3P8; Wes'95; BSc; CCFP; FCFP; (905)709-9955; Fax. (905)709-4138.

NELSON, Michelle L; Yates & Quadra Integrated H C, 105-911 Yates St, Victoria BC V8V 4Y9; Wiwatersrand (South Africa)'94; MB ChB; CCFP; (250)388-3080

NELSON, Rebecca A; 312-233 Nelson's Cres, New Westminster BC V3L 0E4; Cal'04; FRCSC; PlasSurg. (604)553-0315

NELSON, Robert F; Elisabeth Bruyere Health Ctre, 75 Bruyere St, Ottawa ON K1N 5C8; Dal'59; FRFPS; FAAN; FRCPC; Neur. Staff Neurol, The Ottawa Hospital - General Campus; Staff, SCO Health Service - Élisabeth Bruyère Hospital; Aj Prof Med, University of Ottawa; (613)562-6322; Fax. (613)562-6013; rnelson@ottawahospital.on.ca.

NELSON, Sarah L; Trillium Hlth Ctr-Queensway, 150 Sherway Dr, Etobicoke ON M9C 1A5; Wes'06; HBSc; FRCPC; IntMed; Respir. Staff, Trillium Health Centre - West Toronto; (416)521-4196; Fax. (416)521-4082.

NEMANI, Shantiprakash S; Renfrew Victoria Hosp, 3F-499 Raglan St N, Renfrew ON K7V 1P6; (India)'86; MB BS; FRCPC; IntMed. Staff, Renfrew Victoria Hospital; (613)432-8999; Fax. (613)432-9820.

NEMANISHEN, Gerald; Hillcrest Clinic, 7381 Hurd St, Mission BC V2V 3H8; Sask'75; CAFCI; CCFP; Staff, Mission Memorial Hospital; (604)826-8345; Fax. (604)826-1930.

NEMBO NOUANGUE, Joseph; 202-585 Mapleton Rd, Moncton NB E1G 2K5; Samara (Russia (Federation))'00; Staff, Dr Georges-L-Dumont University Hospital Centre.

NEMEC, Edith; Miramichi Reg Hosp, 500 Water St, Miramichi NB E1V 3G5; Bruxelles (Belgium)'90; Staff, Miramichi Regional Hospital; (506)623-3000

NEMES BRATIS, Roxana; CSSS Pierre Boucher, 1333 boul Jacques-Cartier E, Longueuil QC J4M 2A5; (Romania)'81; Staff, Centre Hospitalier Pierre Boucher; Langs: Romanian; French; (450)568-8111; Fax. (450)468-8403; rnbratis@aol.com.

NEMETH, Joe; MUHC-Montreal Gen Hosp, 1650 av Cedar, Montreal QC H3G 1A4; (Hungary)'94; CCFP; CCFP(E.M.); Staff, McGill University Health Centre - Montreal General Campus; Langs: French; Hungarian; German; (514)934-1934

NEMETH, Peter W; Pan Am Sports Med Centre, 75 Poseidon Bay, Winnipeg MB R3M 3E4; Man'85; (204)925-1550; Fax. (204)452-5362.

NEMETHY, Kevin M; St Paul's Hosp, 1081 Burrard St, Vancouver BC V6Z 1Y6; UBC'06; FRCPC; EmergMed. Staff, Providence Health Care - St Paul's Hospital; Staff Emerg Dept, Vancouver General Hospital - Centennial Pavillion; (604)806-8480

NEMNI, Jacqueline C; 207 Woolwich St, Guelph ON N1H 3V4; Mon'91; ABSleepMed; FRCPC; IntMed (Sleep Medicine); Respir. Staff, Guelph General Hospital; Preceptor, McMaster University; (519)341-3344; Fax. (519)341-4433.

NEMTEAN, David R; Clinique Med Viau, 4750 rue Jarry E, Saint-Leonard QC H1R 1X8; McG'79; Staff, Sir Mortimer B Davis Jewish General; Langs: English; French; (514)326-7203; Fax. (514)326-3656.

NEMTEAN, Theodore S; Summerville Family Health Team, 1221 Bloor St, Mississauga ON L4Y 2N8; McG'80; Staff, Trillium Health Centre - Mississauga; (905)625-1241; Fax. (905)625-9514.

NENSHI, Rahima N; Univ Hlth Network-Toronto Western Hosp, 325A-399 Bathurst St, Toronto ON M5T 1S8; McM'05; FRCSC; GenSurg. Staff, Toronto Western Hospital - University Health Network; (416)603-2581

NEPOMUCENO, Jean R; Northern Medical Unit, T162-770 Bannatyne Ave, Winnipeg MB R3E 0W3; Man'09; CCFP.

NEPON, Jack; Seven Oaks Med Centre, 102-1754 Main St, Winnipeg MB R2V 1Z7; Man'81; BSc; Att Staff Dept of Psy & Family Practice, Seven Oaks General Hospital; (204)334-4339; Fax. (204)338-2951.

NEPVEU, Francois; Hop Maisonneuve-Rosemont, 5415 boul de l'Assomption, Montreal QC H1T 2M4; Mon'72; Respir (P.Q.). Staff, Hopital Maisonneuve-Rosemont; (514)252-3400

NEPVEU, Marie-Eve; CSSS du Nord de Lanaudière, 1000 boul Sainte-Anne, St-Charles-Brromee QC J6E 6J2; Sher'01; FRCPC; Anes. Staff, Centre Hospitalier Régional de Lanaudière; (450)759-8222 x2960

NEPVEU, Marie-Helene; Ctr Hosp de Lasalle, 8585 Tsse Champlain, LaSalle QC H8P 1C1; McG'02; FRCPC; Gastroent; IntMed. Staff, Centre Hospitalier de LaSalle; (514)362-8000

NERENBERG, Kara A; Royal Alexandra Hosp, 331-10240 Kingsway NW, Edmonton AB T5H 3V9; McM'01; BScPT; ABIM; MSc; FRCPC; IntMed (Obstetrics). Staff, Royal Alexandra Hospital; Langs: Bilingual(English/French); (780)735-6827; Fax. (780)735-5313.

NERENBERG, Lucila; Vancouver Island Hlth Authorit, 1125 Pembroke St, Victoria BC V8T 1J3; Buenos Aires (Argentina)'86; FRCPC; Psy. Staff, USTAT/Group Mental Health Services; (250)213-4441

NERGA, Alicja B; Oasis Med Centre, 140-486 Advance Blvd, Windsor ON N8N 0B8; (519)727-3338

NERO, Brook A; Medical Arts Bldg, 270-1105 Pandora Ave, Victoria BC V8V 3P9; Man'88; BSc(Med.); (250)382-3322; Fax. (250)382-3322.

NERON, Anne C; Clinique Reseau Le Trait D'Uni, 38 boul Marie-Victorin, Delson QC J5B 1A9; Mon'06; CCFP; (450)633-0123

NERON, Raymond; Clinique de Med Familiale, 760A boul Vachon N, Sainte-Marie QC G6E 1M2; Laval'75; (418)387-4965; Fax. (418)386-1592.

NERON, Roxane; Centre Epic, 5055 rue Saint-Zotique E, Montreal QC H1T 1N6; Sher'83; Langs: Bilingual(French/English); (514)844-7818; Fax. (514)844-7819; roxaneron@hotmail.com.

NERON-VEILLEUX, Sebastien; CSSSG-Hop de Hull, 116 boul Lionel-Emond, Gatineau QC J8Y 1W7; Ott'06; FRCPC; Anes. Staff, Hull Hospital; (819)966-6200

NERY, Pablo B; Univ of Ottawa Heart Institute, H1285-40 Ruskin St, Ottawa ON K1Y 4W7; (Brazil)'01; Staff, University of Ottawa Heart Institute; (613)761-4820

NESATHURAI, Shanker; Hamilton HS-Juravinski Site, 711 Concession St, Hamilton ON L8V 1C3; McM'90; FRCPC; PhysMed&Rehab. Staff, Hamilton Health Sciences Centre-Juravinski Site; (905)574-8515

NESBITT, Gillian C; Mount Sinai Hosp, 600 University Ave, Toronto ON M5G 1X5; Ott'01; FRCPC; IntMed; Cardiol. Staff, Mount Sinai Hospital; (416)586-8495

NESBITT, John A; 417-1011 Glenmore Trail SW, Calgary AB T2V 4R6; Qns'83; MBA; Staff, Rockyview General Hospital; Med Dir, Calgary Foot & Ulcer Care Clinic; (403)228-5959; Fax. (403)228-6918; jnesbittmd@shaw.ca.

NESBITT, Patrick M; Caulfield Med Clinic, 220-5317 Headland Dr, West Vancouver BC V7W 3C5; UBC'83; BSc(Hons); Langs: Chinese; (604)922-1544; Fax. (604)922-1588; mafanxin@hotmail.com.

NESBITT, Raenelle E; Regina Qu'Appelle HR-Regina, 1440 14th Ave, Regina SK S4P 0W5; CCFP; Staff, Regina General Hospital; (306)766-4213

NESDOLY, Christine H; William Osler HC-Brampton, 2100 Bovaird Dr E, Brampton ON L6R 3J7; Sask'80; MD; FRCPC; IntMed; GeriatricMed. Staff, St Joseph's Health Centre; Staff Geriatrics, William Osler Health System - Brampton Civic Hospital; Staff Geriatrics, William Osler Health System - Etobicoke General Hospital; (905)494-6586

NESDOLY, Dennis R; Foothills Med Centre, C231-1403 29 St NW, Calgary AB T2N 2T9; Cal'81; FRCPC; EmergMed. Staff, Foothills Medical Centre; (403)944-8430; Fax. (403)944-2419.

NESDOLY, Derek S; 2372 Gill Rd RR 1, Midhurst ON L0L 1X0; Dal'82; (705)721-9388

NESKOVIC, Svetlana; Apple Tree Med Centre, 2948 Baseline Rd, Ottawa ON K2H 8T5; Belgrade (Serbia)'89; CCFP; Staff, Arnprior & District Memorial Hospital; (613)482-0118; Fax. (613)680-6420.

NESRALLAH, Gihad E; Humber River Reg Hosp-Church, 200 Church St, Toronto ON M9N 1N8; Wes'99; FRCPC; IntMed (Hypertension); Nephrol. Staff, Humber River Regional Hospital - Church Street Site; (416)658-2241

NESS, Larry M; Hillside Med Centre, 360 2nd Ave, Campbell River BC V9W 3T9; Sask'82; MD; CCFP; (250)287-7708; Fax. (250)287-3086.

NESS, Rhonda; Foothills Med Centre, 1403 29 St NW, Calgary AB T2N 2T9; Cal'96; FRCPC; EmergMed. Staff, Foothills Medical Centre; (403)944-1820

NESSIM, Carolyn; Mount Sinai Hosp, 600 University Ave, Toronto ON M5G 1X5; Mon'04; FRCSC; GenSurg; General Surgical Oncology. Staff, Mount Sinai Hospital; Staff, Princess Margaret Hospital - University Health Network; (647)539-4047

NESSIM, Sharon J; SMBD-Jewish Gen Hosp, 3755 ch Cote-Sainte-Catherine, Montreal QC H3T 1E2; McG'01; FRCPC; IntMed; Nephrol. Staff, Sir Mortimer B Davis Jewish General; (514)340-8229; Fax. (514)340-8147.

NESSIM, Sherif P; Enfield Place Med Centre, R208-265 Enfield Pl, Mississauga ON L5B 3Y7; Tor'89; Dip SportMed; BASc; MBA; Staff, Trillium Health Centre - Mississauga; Langs: Arabic; (905)949-4433; Fax. (905)949-4650.

NESTEL, Anthony W; PO Box 67 Stn Main, Bridgewater NS B4V 2W6; Pretoria (South Africa)'81; MB ChB; DTMH; FRCPC; IntMed (Gastroenterology). (902)527-0501; Fax. (902)541-1315.

NESTEL, Magdalena D; 105 Dawson St PO Box 67 Stn Main, Bridgewater NS B4V 2W6; Pretoria (South Africa)'81; MB ChB; FRCPC; IntMed (Intensive Care). (902)527-0501; Fax. (902)541-1315.

NESTERENKO, Maria; Uptown Health Centre, 9325 Yonge St, Richmond Hill ON L4C 0A8; (Ukraine)'97; CCFP; (905)508-8876

NETHIRASIGAMANI, Dinesh; Chatham-Kent Health Alliance, PO Box 2030 Stn Main 80 Grand Ave W, Chatham ON N7M 5L9; (India)'99; FRCPC; Anes. Staff, Chatham-Kent Health Alliance; (519)352-6400; Fax. (519)436-2535.

NETO, Gina M P; Children's Hosp Eastern Ont, 401 Smyth Rd, Ottawa ON K1H 8L1; Man'92; FRCPC; Peds. Staff Emerg, Children's Hospital of Eastern Ontario (CHEO); (613)737-7600 x2318

NETTE, Farrell; Valley Women's & Children's Ct, 60 Aberdeen St, Kentville NS B4N 2N3; Alb'04; BSc(Hons); FRCSC; ObstGyn. Staff Physician, Valley Regional Hospital; Physician, Valley Women's & Children's Centre; (902)678-4626; Fax. (902)678-6338.

NETTE, Hannah E; 116-555 12th Ave W, Vancouver BC V5Z 3X7; Dal'04; CCFP; (604)879-3900

NEU, Bernd R; One Med Place, 319-20 Wynford Dr, North York ON M3C 1J4; Dal'76; FRCSC; PlasSurg (Cosmetic Surgery). Ac Staff, North York General Hospital; Lecturer, University of Toronto; Langs: German; (416)447-6176; Fax. (416)447-5750; bneu@drneu.com.

NEU, Rolf-Dieter; 120-2751 Gladstone St, Halifax NS B3K 4W6; Dal'73; Court Staff, Queen Elizabeth II Health Sciences Centre - Victoria General Site; (902)423-8950; Fax. (902)423-6009.

NEU, S Randall; Forest Lawn Medicentre, 1814 33 St SE, Calgary AB T2B 0T4; Cal'73; (403)235-5651

NEUDORF, Cordell O; Sasktoon Health Region, 101-310 Idylwyld Dr N, Saskatoon SK S7L 0Z2; Sask'89; MHSc(Tor); FRCPC; CommunMed (Administrative). Staff, Royal University Hospital; Chief Med Officer of Hlth, Saskatoon Health Region Saskatoon Public Health; Asst Prof Community Hlth & Epidemiol, University of Saskatchewan; (306)655-4338; Fax. (306)655-4414; cory.neudorf@saskatoonhealthregion.ca.

NEUFELD, Allen V; B-22195 Dewdney Trunk Rd, Maple Ridge BC V2X 3H7; UBC'78; (604)463-4102; Fax. (604)463-4686.

NEUFELD, Dennis R; Lakeland Med Clinic, 1715 Ellis St, Kelowna BC V1Y 8M9; UBC'86; (778)478-0277; Fax. (778)478-0279.

NEUFELD, Gregory M; Western Surgical Centre, 189 Vaughan St, Winnipeg MB R3C 1T4; Man'04.

NEUFELD, Hertha; Concordia Health Associates, 102-1155 Concordia Ave, Winnipeg MB R2K 2M9; Man'77; CCFP; FCFP; Staff, St Boniface General Hospital; (204)415-0322; Fax. (204)415-3714.

NEUFELD, J Douglas; 402 Borland St, Williams Lake BC V2G 1R7; UBC'88.

NEUFELD, John D G; Rockyview Gen Hosp, 7007 14 St SW, Calgary AB T2V 1P9; Man'83; FRCPC; EmergMed. Staff, Rockyview General Hospital; (403)943-3000

NEUFELD, Keith T; Sudbury Reg Hosp-Laurentian Si, 41 Ramsey Lake Rd, Sudbury ON P3E 5J1; McM'91; FRCPC; DiagRad. Staff, Health Sciences North-Laurentian Site; (705)522-7100

NEUFELD, Kelsey M; The Richmond Hosp, 7000 Westminster Hwy, Richmond BC V6X 1A2; McM'06; FRCPC; Peds. Staff Child Health Centre, Richmond Hospital; (604)233-3222

NEUFELD, Mark V; 112-450 Speedvale Ave W, Guelph ON N1H 7Y6; Man'93; FRCSC; Ophth. (519)822-5501; Fax. (519)836-0783.

NEUFELD, Michael J; Comox Med Clinic, 100-1695 Comox Ave, Comox BC V9M 3M1; UBC'97; CCFP; (250)339-2266

NEUFELD, Peter R; Gordon & Leslie Diamond HCC, 5F-2775 Laurel St, Vancouver BC V5Z 1M9; UBC'97; MSc; BSc(Hon); LMCC; FRCPC; IntMed; Nephrol. Staff, Gordon & Leslie Diamond Health Care Centre; Clinical Asst Prof Nephrol, University of British Columbia; Langs: Bilingual(English/French); (604)875-5950; Fax. (604)875-5952.

NEUFELD, Ruth E; Kinsmen Children's Centre, 1319 Colony St, Saskatoon SK S7N 2Z1; Sask'03; FRCPC; Peds. (306)655-1070; Fax. (306)655-1449.

NEUFELD, Troy M; Maj Gen George R Pearkes Bldg, 101 Colonel By Dr, Ottawa ON K1A 0K2; McM'10; CCFP; (613)995-2534

NEUFELD, William P; Surrey Serv Delivery Location, 100-5500 152 St, Surrey BC V3S 5J9; Man'76; MD; Sr Advisor Medical, Workers' Comp Board of BC; (604)232-7042

NEULS, Rick A J; Allin Clinic, 10155 120 St NW, Edmonton AB T5K 2A2; Alb'95; CCFP; (780)482-7551; Fax. (780)488-2056.

NEUMAN, Glen D; Misericordia Community Hosp, 16940 87 Ave NW, Edmonton AB T5R 4H5; Alb'81; FRCPC; GenPath. Staff, Covenant Health - Misericordia Community Hospital; (780)735-2763

NEUMANN, Anna; Dalhousie Fam Med Spryfield Ct, 27-16 Dentith Rd, Halifax NS B3R 2H9; Warsaw (Poland)'05; CCFP; Staff, IWK Health Centre; Langs: Polish; (902)473-1234; Fax. (902)473-4353.

NEUMANN, Etela; Vancouver Nerve Block Clinic, 302-2620 Commercial Dr, Vancouver BC V5N 4C4; Komensky (Slovakia)'77; FRCPC; NeurPath (Interventional Pain Mgmt). Physician, Vancouver Nerve Block Clinic; Langs: Czech; Slovak; Croatian; Polish; German; Hungarian; (604)873-5561; neumann7@telus.net.

NEUMANN, Gary R; 111-1135 Adelaide St N, London ON N5Y 5K7; Wes'94; CCFP; (519)679-6000; Fax. (519)679-2736.

NEUMANN, Jeffrey L; SGH Medical Mall, 111-3030 Lawrence Ave E, Scarborough ON M1P 2T7; RCS (Ireland)'87; (416)438-4747; Fax. (416)438-7224.

NEUMANN, Laura V; Springbank Med Centre, 203-460 Springbank Dr, London ON N6J 0A8; (Ireland)'08; (519)432-2568

NEUMANN, Peter Z; Scarborough Medical Mall, 111-3030 Lawrence Ave E, Scarborough ON M1P 2T7; Szeged (Hungary)'56; FAAP; FRCPC; Peds. (416)438-4747; Fax. (416)438-7224.

NEUMANN, Timothy; GAMA Integrated Med Centre, PO Box 2060 102 Central St W, Warman SK S0K 4S0; Sask'08; CCFP; Staff, GAMA Integrated Medical Centre; (306)382-5554; Fax. (306)382-5567.

NEUMANN, Viktor; Oakmont Med Centre, 270-809 41st Ave W, Vancouver BC V5Z 2N6; Palacky (Czech Republic)'79; Langs: Czech; Slovak; (604)261-7521; Fax. (604)261-4527.

NEUMANN, William C; Worker's Comp Board, 150-4311 12 St NE, Calgary AB T2E 4P9; Alb'72; CCFP; (403)517-6023; Fax. (403)205-8042.

NEVELING, Christoffel H; Family Practice & Walk-In Clin, 10200 8 St, Dawson Creek BC V1G 3P8; Pretoria (South Africa)'97; MB ChB; FRCPC; Anes. Langs: Afrikaans; (250)782-1103

NEVEU, Alain; Constance-Lethbridge Rehab Ctr, 7005 boul de Maisonneuve O, Montreal QC H4B 1T3; Mon'73; LMCC; Med Consultant, Securimed; Langs: English; (514)487-1891 x384; Fax. (514)487-2197.

NEVEU, Francoise; Ctr Hosp Fleury, 2180 rue Fleury E, Montreal QC H2B 1K3; Mon'80; Staff, Centre Hospitalier Fleury; (514)381-9311

NEVEU, Marc; Ctr Hosp Rouyn-Noranda, 4 9e rue, Rouyn-Noranda QC J9X 2B2; Sher'96; LRCPS; FRCPC; Neur. Staff, Centre Hospitalier Rouyn-Noranda; Staff, Centre Hospitalier La Sarre; Staff, CSSS du Témiscamingue; Staff, Centre Hospitalier de Val d'Or; Langs: English; (819)764-5131 x43452

NEVEU, Nathalie A; Hop du Sacre-Coeur de Mtl, 5400 boul Gouin O, Montreal QC H4J 1C5; McG'98; FRCPC; IntMed (Reproductive Endocrinology); Endocrin (P.Q.); Endocrin&Metab. Staff, Hôpital du Sacre-Coeur de Montréal; Staff, PROCREA Cliniques; Langs: Spanish; English; (514)338-2222

NEVILL, Thomas J; L/BMT Program Diamond Centre, 10149-2775 Laurel St, Vancouver BC V5Z 1M9; Tor'83; FRCPC; IntMed (Bone Marrow Transplant); Hem. Ac Staff, Vancouver General Hospital - Centennial Pavillion; Ac Staff, BC Cancer Agency Vancouver Centre; Staff, Gordon & Leslie Diamond Health Care Centre; Clin Prof, University of British Columbia; (604)875-4863; tnevill@bccancer.bc.ca.

NEVILLE, Alan J; The Juravinski Cancer Centre, 699 Concession St, Hamilton ON L8V 5C2; Aberdeen (Scotland)'77; FRCPC; IntMed; MedOncol. Staff, Hamilton Health Sciences Centre-Juravinski Site; Chair Undergraduate Med Prog/Prof, McMaster University; (905)387-9495 x64605

NEVILLE, Amy A; MUHC-Royal Victoria Hosp, S6 24-687 av des Pins O, Montreal QC H3A 1A1; McG'05; FRCSC; GenSurg. Staff, McGill University Health Centre - Royal Victoria Hospital; (514)934-1934

NEVILLE, Christopher S; 205-2190 West Railway St, Abbotsford BC V2S 2E2; Ott'01; FRCSC; Urol. (604)853-9167; Fax. (604)853-9114.

NEVILLE, Jeffrey S; Brookdale Family Clinic, 304 Bellevue St, Peterborough ON K9H 5G1; Qns'91; CCFP; FCFP; (705)743-7100; Fax. (705)743-7104.

NEVILLE, Robert J; The Medical Centre FHT, PO Box 4200 Stn Main 707 Charlotte St, Peterborough ON K9J 7B3; Qns'84; CCFP; (705)743-6222; Fax. (705)743-5334.

NEVIN, Robert D; Lockwood Clinic, 108-790 Bay St, Toronto ON M5G 1N8; Tor'76; Member Peer Presenter, College Of Family Physicians Of Canada-Ontario; (416)921-2121; Fax. (416)921-0569.

NEVIN LAM, Alexandra C; 100-36 York Mills Rd, North York ON M2P 2E9; Tor'02; FRCSC; ObstGyn (Minimal Invasive Surgery). Staff, North York General Hospital; Staff, The Hospital For Sick Children; (416)644-1404; Fax. (416)644-1406.

NEVINS, Tara A; Weeneebayko Gen Hosp, PO Box 34, Moose Factory ON P0L 1W0; Ott'07; CCFP; Staff, Weeneebayko General Hospital; (705)658-4544

NEVO, Ori; Sunnybrook Hlth Sciences Ctre, M4 170-2075 Bayview Ave, Toronto ON M4N 3M5; Hebrew (Israel)'91; Staff, Sunnybrook Health Sciences Centre; (416)480-4920

NEWALL, John R; 12 Core Cres, Brampton ON L6W 2G7; Tor'64; FRCSC; OrthSurg (Independent Medical Evaluations). Aj Staff/Lecturer, Queen's University; (905)451-4010; Fax. (905)451-6097.

NEWBERY, Sarah-Lynn; Marathon Family Health Team, PO Box 399 22 Peninsula Rd, Marathon ON P0T 2E0; McM'93; CCFP; FCFP; Chief/Staff, Wilson Memorial General Hospital; (807)229-3243; Fax. (807)229-2672.

NEWBIGGING, Joseph L; Kingston Gen Hosp, 76 Stuart St, Kingston ON K7L 2V7; McM'96; CCFP; CCFP(E.M.); Staff, Kingston General Hospital; Chief EmergMed, Brockville General Hospital - Charles Street; Lecturer Family Med, Queen's University; (613)548-2368

NEWBIGGING, Peter D; William Osler HC-Etobicoke, 101 Humber College Blvd, Etobicoke ON M9V 1R8; Tor'64; FRCPC; IntMed. Ac Staff, William Osler Health System - Etobicoke General Hospital; (416)747-3400 x32388

NEWCOMB, Paulette; Sunnyside Wellness Family Med, 303B-1595 Bedford Hwy, Bedford NS B4A 3Y4; Dal'87; BSc; CCFP; FCFP; (902)407-9255; Fax. (902)407-4330.

NEWEDUK, Peter M; Riley Park Primary Care Clinic, 171-1402 8 Ave NW, Calgary AB T2N 1B9; Dublin (Ireland)'87; MB ChB; CCFP; Physician, CRHA, Auxiliary Hosp. & Nursing Homes; (403)228-0660; Fax. (403)228-6077.

NEWELL, Kendra N; 406-89 Queensway W, Mississauga ON L5B 2V2; Ott'05; FRCSC; ObstGyn. (905)268-9928; Fax. (905)268-9950.

NEWELL, Kenneth J; Grey Bruce HS-Owen Sound, PO Box 1800 Stn Main, Owen Sound ON N4K 6M9; McM'96; FRCPC; GenPath. Staff, Grey Bruce Health Services - Owen Sound; (519)376-2121; Fax. (519)376-1846.

NEWELL, Michael R; Chatham-Kent Health Alliance, PO Box 2030 Stn Main 80 Grand Ave W, Chatham ON N7M 5L9; Tor'90; CCFP; CCFP(E.M.); Staff/Chief EmergMed, Chatham-Kent Health Alliance; (519)437-6050; Fax. (519)436-2536.

NEWELL, Paul R; Windsor Health Centre, 1-700 Tecumseh Rd E, Windsor ON N8X 4T2; Qns'83; FRCPC; DiagRad. Reg Med Dir, DC Diagnosticare Inc; (519)258-4517; Fax. (519)258-6247; paul@cml.ca.

NEWELL, Geoff; 251 60 St SE, Salmon Arm BC V1E 1W4; Liverpool (England)'62; MB ChB; Assoc Staff, Shuswap Lake General Hospital; (250)832-4058

NEWHOOK, Leigh A; Dr Charles A Janeway Child HC, 300 Prince Philip Dr, St. John's NL A1B 3V6; Mem'93; FRCPC; Peds. Staff, Janeway Children's Health & Rehabilitation Centre; Asst Prof Peds, Memorial University Of Newfoundland; (709)778-4537

NEWKIRK, Lynda K; Centre de Sante Communautaire, 2F-460 Main St E, Hamilton ON L8N 1K4; Wes'00; CCFP; Langs: English; French; (905)528-0163

NEWMAN, Adam I S S; 235 Wellington St, Kingston ON K7K 0B5; McM'91; CCFP; FCFP; Staff, Kingston General Hospital; Lecturer, Queen's University; (613)549-1440; Fax. (613)549-7986.

NEWMAN, Alice A; Univ Hlth Network-Princess M, 610 University Ave, Toronto ON M5G 2M9; Tor'90; Staff, Princess Margaret Hospital - University Health Network; (416)946-4501 x3942; Fax. (416)946-2914.

NEWMAN, Alvin; Mount Sinai Hosp, 441-600 University Ave, Toronto ON M5G 1X5; Pittsburgh (USA)'64; FRCPC; Gastroent. Staff, Mount Sinai Hospital; Assoc Prof, University of Toronto; (416)586-5307; Fax. (416)586-4878; a.newman@mtsinai.on.ca.

NEWMAN, Barbara J; 303-343 Wilson Ave, North York ON M3H 1T1; Qns'85; MSc; CCFP; FCFP; Instructor Family & Community Med, Mount Sinai Hospital; (416)785-8412; Fax. (416)785-8324.

NEWMAN, Caroline G; Clinicare Med Centre, 3-2250 Markham Rd, Scarborough ON M1B 2W4; Wes'87; Staff, The Scarborough Hospital - General Campus; (416)293-5454; Fax. (416)293-7454.

NEWMAN, Christine J; The Hosp for Sick Children, 555 University Ave, Toronto ON M5G 1X8; Tor'82; Peds. Staff, The Hospital For Sick Children; Asst Prof Peds, University of Toronto; (416)813-6342; Fax. (416)813-5245; christine.newman@sickkids.ca.

NEWMAN, Colin D; Notre Dame Bay Mem Hlth Ctr, GD Hospital Lane, Twillingate NL A0G 4M0; Mem'10; CCFP; Staff, Notre Dame Bay Memorial Health Centre; (709)884-2131

NEWMAN, Dana E; St Joseph's Health Centre, 30 The Queensway, Toronto ON M6R 1B5; Ben Gurion (Israel)'09; CCFP; (416)530-6860

NEWMAN, David E; Burin Peninsula Hlth Care Ctr, PO Box 340 51-58 Main St, Burin NL A0E 1E0; Yeshiva Univ (USA)'81; Staff, Burin Peninsula Health Care Centre; (709)891-1040

NEWMAN, David G; Workers Rehabilitation Centre, 6951 Westminster Hwy, Richmond BC V7C 1C6; UBC'78; CCFP; Med Advisor, Workers' Comp Board of BC; (604)273-2266

NEWMAN, David M; 215-6633 Highway 7, Markham ON L3P 7P2; Dal'82; FACC; FRCPC; IntMed (Arrhythmias); Cardiol. Court Staff, Sunnybrook Health Sciences Centre; Court Staff Cardia & Arrhythmia Services, St Michael's Hospital; Assoc Prof Med, University of Toronto; (905)472-7127; Fax. (905)472-6534.

NEWMAN, Francis; Salvation Army Grace Gen Hosp, 300 Booth Dr, Winnipeg MB R3J 3M7; Man'83; BA; Psy (Research). Att Staff, The Salvation Army Grace Hospital; (204)837-0502; Fax. (204)885-3064.

NEWMAN, Harold J; Toronto East Gen Hosp Inc, 825 Coxwell Ave, Toronto ON M4C 3E7; Tor'71; FRCPC; DiagRad., Toronto East General Hospital Inc; (416)469-6556

NEWMAN, Helen B; The Bell Mews, 303-39 Robertson Rd, Nepean ON K2H 8R2; Manchester (England)'77; (613)829-6360

NEWMAN, Jack; 1255 Sheppard Ave E, North York ON M2K 1E2; Tor'70; FRCPC; Peds (Breast Feeding). Langs: French; Spanish; (416)498-0002; Fax. (416)498-0012.

NEWMAN, Jamie R; 200-101 Queensway W, Mississauga ON L5B 2P7; Tor'02; FRCPC; IntMed; Gastroent. Ac Staff, Trillium Health Centre - Mississauga; (905)624-5258; Fax. (905)624-6988.

NEWMAN, Leslie; 211-4415 boul Notre-Dame, Laval QC H7W 1T7; McG'73; (450)687-5510; Fax. (450)687-5511.

NEWMAN, Nicholas M; Centre Med St-Urbain, 209-3875 rue Saint-Urbain, Montreal QC H2W 1V1; Man'78; BSc(Med); FRCSC; OrthSurg (Arthroplasty). Clin Assoc Prof, Universite de Montreal; Langs: Bilingual(English/French); (514)849-8391; Fax. (514)849-9313.

NEWMAN, Peter R; Bayview North Med Clinic, 301-3292 Bayview Ave, North York ON M2M 4J5; Tor'68; CCFP; FCFP; Ac Staff Family Med, North York General Hospital; Asst Prof Family & Community Med, University of Toronto; (416)222-2200; Fax. (416)224-9880.

NEWMAN, Robert W; 7747 Kenyon Rd, Halfmoon Bay BC V0N 1Y1; UBC'79; Teacher Clin Clerkship Prog, University of British Columbia; (604)885-2667; rwnewman@pris.ca.

NEWMAN, S Lewis; Polyclinic, 199 Grafton St, Charlottetown PE C1A 1L2; Dal'69; (902)629-8810

NEWMAN, Stephen C; University of Alberta Hosp, 8440 112 St NW, Edmonton AB T6G 2B7; Tor'79; CCFP; Staff, University of Alberta Hospital; Staff, Covenant Health - Edmonton General Continuing Care Centre; Prof, University of Alberta; (780)492-5272; Fax. (780)492-0364; stephen.newman@ualberta.ca.

NEWMAN, S; Women's Health Clinic, C-419 Graham Ave, Winnipeg MB R3C 0M3; Man'92; CCFP; FCFP.

NEWMARCH, Bruce G; 203-474 Columbia St, Kamloops BC V2C 2T5; UBC'78; Staff Family Practice/Member, Royal Inland Hospital; (250)372-2377

NEWNHAM, Darlene J; CFB Borden, PO Box 1000, Borden ON L0M 1C0; Tor'93; CCFP; (705)424-1200 x2405

NEWNHAM, Peter J; 209-200 Boudreau Rd, St. Albert AB T8N 6B9; Alb'99; CCFP; (780)458-7000; Fax. (780)458-8484.

NEWPORT, David A; Peterborough Clinic FHT, LL02-26 Hospital Dr, Peterborough ON K9J 7C3; Ott'95; CCFP; Staff, Peterborough Regional Health Centre - Hospital Drive; (705)740-6889; Fax. (705)740-6847; dnewport@ptbclinic.com.

NEWSOME, William E; 25 12th Ave S, Cranbrook BC V1C 2R8; Oklahoma(OH) (USA)'75; FRCPC; IntMed. Staff, East Kootenay Regional Hospital; (250)426-1995

NEWSON, Kristy A; Boardwalk Prof Centre, 220 Water St, Charlottetown PE C1A 9M5; Dal'03; CCFP; (902)367-3705

NEWSTEAD, Freya J; Canora Med Clinic, PO Box 2040, Canora SK S0A 0L0; (306)563-5557; Fax. (306)563-4175.

NEWSTEAD-ANGEL, Jill C; Royal University Hosp, 103 Hospital Dr, Saskatoon SK S7N 0W8; Sask'01; BSc; FRCPC; IntMed (Obstetric Medicine). Staff, Royal University Hospital; (306)966-2180; Fax. (306)966-2383; jill.newsteadangel@saskatoonhealthregion.ca.

NEWTON, Arnold; 515-1385 Bank St, Ottawa ON K1H 8N4; Wes'73; FSOGC; FRCSC; ObstGyn. Clin Asst, The Ottawa Hospital - General Campus; (613)721-2907; Fax. (613)721-2908.

NEWTON, Barbara J; Healthcare, 3163 Winston Churchill Blvd, Mississauga ON L5L 2W1; Warsaw (Poland)'84; Court Staff, Trillium Health Centre - Mississauga; (905)607-2001; Fax. (905)607-1553.

NEWTON, Christie A; UBC Health Clinic, 320-5950 University Blvd, Vancouver BC V6T 1Z3; Qns'95; CCFP; FCFP; Physician, University of British Columbia; (604)822-5501; Fax. (604)822-4089.

NEWTON, Marcus F; Grey Bruce HS-Owen Sound, PO Box 1800 Stn Main 5101-1800 18th St E, Owen Sound ON N4K 6M9; Qns'95; FRCPC; IntMed; Respir. Staff, Grey Bruce Health Services - Owen Sound; (519)376-4888; Fax. (519)376-0024.

NEWTON, Gary E; Mount Sinai Hosp, 18 364-600 University Ave, Toronto ON M5G 1X5; Tor'88; FRCPC; IntMed; Cardiol. Staff, Mount Sinai Hospital; (416)586-4800 x4860; Fax. (416)586-4775; gary.newton@utoronto.ca.

NEWTON, Michael J; Clearbrook Family Practice, 101-2828 Cruickshank St, Abbotsford BC V2T 5M4; Stellenbosch (South Africa)'86; Ac Staff, Abbotsford Regional Hospital & Cancer Centre; Langs: Afrikaans; (604)852-8030; Fax. (604)852-4118; mjnewton@shaw.ca.

NEWTON, Paul X; PO Box 59 Stn Main, Bridgewater NS B4V 2W6; Dal'78; Ac Staff, South Shore Regional Hospital; (902)543-6948; pnewton@bwr.eastlink.ca.

NEWTON, Peter T; London HSC-Victoria Hosp, PO Box 5010 Stn B 800 Commissioners Rd E, London ON N6A 5W9; Wes'88; FRCPC; Anes. Staff, London Health Sciences Centre - Victoria Campus; Staff, London Health Sciences Centre - University Hospital; Lecturer Anes, University of Western Ontario; Langs: German.

NEWTON, Trevor M; Langley Mem Hosp, 22051 Fraser Hwy, Langley BC V3A 4H4; UBC'87; ACLS; ATLS; CCFP; CCFP(E.M.); Staff, Langley Memorial Hospital; Langs: English; French; (604)533-6402

NEWTON, William H; Markham Family Health Team, 101-377 Church St, Markham ON L6B 1A1; Tor'87; CCFP; FCFP; Ac Staff, Markham Stouffville Hospital; (905)471-9999; Fax. (905)471-3627.

NEWTON-MOORE, Allison M; Perth Med Clinic, 1-500 East Riverside Dr, Perth-Andover NB E7H 1Z1; Dal'03; CCFP; (506)273-3558

NEY, Patrick M B; Gold River Med Centre, PO Box 400, Gold River BC V0P 1G0; UBC'93; BSc; DTMH; CCFP; (250)283-2541

NEY, Philip G F; Mount Joy College, 1520 Connie Rd, Sooke BC V9Z 1C8; UBC'60; MA; FRCPC; Psy (Child & Family Psychiatry). (250)642-1848

NEYESTANI, Amir H; Surrey Mem Hosp, 13750 96 Ave, Surrey BC V3V 1Z2; Qns'00; FRCPC; DiagRad. Staff, Surrey Memorial Hospital; (604)588-3342

NEYLON, Norah; Centre de sante Queen Elizabet, 2100 av de Marlowe, Montreal QC H4A 3L5; London (England)'87; (514)485-5013

NEZARATI, Marjan; North York Gen Hosp, 4001 Leslie St, North York ON M2K 1E1; McM'94; MSc; FRCPC; MedGenetics. Staff, North York General Hospital; (416)756-6345

NEZIL, Frank A; Cool Aid Community Health Ctre, 713 Johnson St, Victoria BC V8W 1M8; UBC'93; Staff, Cormorant Island Health Centre; Physician, Cool Aid Community Health Centre; (250)385-1466; Fax. (250)383-1327.

NG, Albert; CSSS De Saint-Jerome, 290 rue de Montigny, Saint-Jerome QC J7Z 5T3; Mon'04; FRCPC; Psy. Staff, Hôtel-Dieu de Saint-Jérôme; (450)431-8200

NG, Albert P; 1460 Ouellette Ave, Windsor ON N8X 1K3; Wes'84; Chief Family Med, Windsor Regional Hospital - Metropolitan Site; Med Dir, Versa Care-Windsor Place; Med Dir, Regency Nursing Home; Langs: Cantonese; (519)258-2591; Fax. (519)258-6610; albertn6@hotmail.com.

NG, Ambrose C; Misericordia Comm Hosp & H C, 16940 87 Ave NW, Edmonton AB T5R 4H5; Alb'04; FRCPC; Anes. Staff, Covenant Health - Misericordia Community Hospital; (780)735-2000

NG, Anita D; Roncesvalles Village Med Clin, 137 Roncesvalles Ave, Toronto ON M6R 2L2; Tor'00; BSc; CCFP; (416)534-6699; Fax. (416)534-0172.

NG, Anthony T H; Mackenzie Richmond Hill Hosp, 10 Trench St, Richmond Hill ON L4C 4Z3; (Hong Kong)'67; DAB; FRCPC; Anes (Pain Management). Ac Staff, Mackenzie Richmond Hill Hospital; Langs: Cantonese; (905)883-1212

NG, Brian E; 4879 Kingsway, Burnaby BC V5H 4T6; Chicago (USA)'96; CCFP; (604)433-3341

NG, Rodney; Sheridan Med Associates, 1-1960 Dundas St W, Mississauga ON L5K 2R9; Tor'77; Ac Staff, The Credit Valley Hospital; (905)822-3993; Fax. (905)822-5522.

NG, Carol S C; Cook Medical Bldg, 326-1175 Cook St, Victoria BC V8V 4A1; UBC'00; CCFP; Staff Maternity Care, Victoria General Hospital; (250)386-2449; Fax. (250)386-2458.

NG, Chan-Poh; 101-13771 72A Ave, Surrey BC V3W 9C6; Man'78; Ac Staff, Surrey Memorial Hospital; (604)590-0162; Fax. (604)590-9049.

NG, Cindy K W; Northtown Med Clinic, 108-10 Northtown Way, North York ON M2N 7L4; Tor'05; CCFP; (416)270-8781; Fax. (416)912-8270.

NG, Danny G H; Foothills Med Centre, 1403 29 St NW, Calgary AB T2N 2T9; Tor'06; FRCPC; DiagRad. Staff, Foothills Medical Centre; (403)944-4530; Fax. (403)944-4577.

NG, David C; 202-236 Georgia St E, Vancouver BC V6A 1Z7; UBC'75; Ac Staff, Providence Health Care - Mount Saint Joseph Hospital; Vis Staff, Providence Health Care - St Paul's Hospital; Langs: Cantonese; (604)683-2053

NG, David C K; 2 Wootten Way N, Markham ON L3P 5T7; (Taiwan)'79; (905)294-4990

NG, David; 220 Main St W, Hamilton ON L8P 1J3; Wes'05; CCFP; CCFP(E.M.); (905)528-8088

NG, David; Hotel-Dieu Grace Hosp, 1030 Ouellette Ave, Windsor ON N9A 1E1; Qns'90; CCFP; Chief EmergMed, Hôtel-Dieu Grace Hospital; Ac Staff, Windsor Regional Hospital - Metropolitan Site; Langs: Cantonese; French; (519)973-4401

NG, David; Scarborough Comm Mental Hlth, 301-2425 Eglinton Ave E, Scarborough ON M1K 5G8; Tor'94; BSc; FRCPC; Psy (Child & Adolescent Psychiatry);CCFP; Staff Physician, The Scarborough Hospital - Birchmount Campus; Staff Child Psy, Markham Stouffville Hospital; Lecturer, University of Toronto; Langs: Chinese; (416)431-8135; Fax. (416)759-5162.

NG, David K K; 13506 127 St NW, Edmonton AB T5L 1B9; Alb'86; CCFP; (780)454-0738; Fax. (780)451-6702.

NG, Dawn M; Royal Victoria Hosp, 201 Georgian Dr, Barrie ON L4M 6M2; Tor'07; FRCPC; IntMed; MedOncol. Staff, Royal Victoria Regional Health Centre; (705)728-9090; Fax. (705)739-5619.

NG, Derek; Near North Med Clinic, 201-66 Josephine St, North Bay ON P1B 0A7; Cal'95; CCFP; CCFP(E.M.); FCFP; Ac Staff, North Bay Regional Health Centre - Regional Mental Health; Asst Prof, Northern Ontario School of Medicine; Langs: English; French; (705)495-2685; Fax. (705)495-4128.

NG, Dominic S K; St Michael's Hosp, 3 041-30 Bond St, Toronto ON M5B 1W8; Tor'88; PhD; FRCPC; IntMed; Endocrin&Metab. Ac Staff, St Michael's Hospital; Asst Prof, University of Toronto; Langs: Chinese; Cantonese; (416)864-5197; ngd@smh.toronto.on.ca.

NG, Douglas B G; 103-15122 72 Ave, Surrey BC V3S 2G2; Kaohsiung (Taiwan)'71; ACLS; Ad Staff Privil, Surrey Memorial Hospital; Langs: Mandarin; Cantonese; Taiwanese; Malay; (604)587-3228; Fax. (604)587-3223.

NG, Douglas S; St Michael's Hosp, 6F-30 Bond St, Toronto ON M5B 1W8; Tor'05; Cardiol; IntMed. Staff, St Michael's Hospital; (416)864-5431

NG, Eddy H C; Delta Med Clinic, 140-4977 Trenant St, Delta BC V4K 2K5; Alb'05; CCFP; (604)946-7661

NG, Edward H W; 1460 Ouellette Ave, Windsor ON N8X 1K3; Ott'60; BSc; Ac Staff, Windsor Regional Hospital - Metropolitan Site; Langs: Chinese; (519)258-2591; Fax. (519)258-2591.

NG, Elaine K Y; The Hosp for Sick Children, 555 University Ave, Toronto ON M5G 1X8; Tor'96; FRCPC; Anes. Staff Anes, The Hospital For Sick Children; (416)813-7445; Fax. (416)813-7543.

NG, Esther; 203-22 Richmond St, Richmond Hill ON L4C 3Y1; Tor'91; FRCSC; ObstGyn. Staff, Mackenzie Richmond Hill Hospital; Langs: Cantonese; (905)770-0087; Fax. (905)770-0047.

NG, Eugene H L; Sunnybrook Hlth Sciences Ctre, M4 230A-2075 Bayview Ave, Toronto ON M4N 3M5; Tor'94; FRCPC; Peds (Neonatal & Perinatal Medicine). Staff, Sunnybrook Health Sciences Centre; Staff, Women's College Hospital; Langs: Cantonese; Chinese; (416)480-6100; Fax. (416)480-5612; eugene.ng@swchsc.on.ca.

NG, Grace; 6408 Main St, Vancouver BC V5W 2V4; UBC'87; Vis Staff, Vancouver General Hospital - Centennial Pavillion; Langs: Chinese; (604)322-8881; Fax. (604)322-8690.

NG, Jane W Y; 200-233 16 Ave NW, Calgary AB T2M 0H5; McG'05; Peds. (403)230-3300; Fax. (403)230-3322.

NG, Jean S C; 45 St Thomas St, St. Albert AB T8N 6Z1; Ott'80; FRCPC; DiagRad. Consultant, Sturgeon Community Hospital; Staff, Westlock Healthcare Centre; Consultant, Covenant Health - St Mary's Hospital; Staff, Cross Cancer Institute; (780)470-5551

NG, John P Y; 1306-1333 Georgia St W, Vancouver BC V6E 4V3; (Hong Kong)'65; MB BS; Langs: Chinese; (604)558-2611

NG, Jonathan M; Westend Family Health Team, 80 Michael Cowpland Dr, Ottawa ON K2M 1P6; McM'07; CCFP; (613)599-3321; Fax. (613)599-3366.

NG, Kai-Ling; 172-17010 90 Ave NW, Edmonton AB T5T 1L6; UBC'02; FRCPC; DiagRad. (780)253-4666; Fax. (780)253-4669.

NG, Karen; Mount Sinai Hosp, 475-600 University Ave, Toronto ON M5G 1X5; Tor'06; AB; FRCPC; IntMed; GeriatricMed. Staff, Mount Sinai Hospital; (416)586-4800 x6355; Fax. (416)586-5113.

NG, Kathryn W; Clayton Gate Pediatrics, 215-6820 188th St, Surrey BC V4N 3G6; Man'05; FRCPC; Peds. (604)579-0270

NG, Kelvin K K; Main West Med Centre, 220 Main St W, Hamilton ON L8P 1J3; Tor'77; (905)528-8088; Fax. (905)528-8096.

NG, Ken H M; Heritage Med Centre, 2 Wootten Way N, Markham ON L3P 5T7; McG'80; Staff, The Scarborough Hospital - General Campus; Staff, The Scarborough Hospital - Birchmount Campus; Staff Family Practice, Markham Stouffville Hospital; Pres Scarborough Branch, Ontario Medical Association; Lecturer Family Practice, University of Toronto; Langs: Cantonese; (905)294-4990; Fax. (905)471-1916; drkenng@fccm.ca.

NG, Kenneth K-H; 20040 40A Ave, Langley BC V3A 2Y5; Adelaide (Australia)'77; MB BS; DObstRCOG(Edin.); Ac Staff, Langley Memorial Hospital; (604)530-8899

NG, Kwok Kuen; Henderson Centre Commercial, 2135A-1163 Pinetree Way, Coquitlam BC V3B 8A9; Glasgow (Scotland)'86; MB ChB; (604)464-1333; Fax. (604)464-1313.

NG, Liang; Ocean Walk Med Centre, 1884 Marine Dr, West Vancouver BC V7V 1J6; Glasgow (Scotland)'75; MB ChB; Staff Obst, Lions Gate Hospital; Staff, Ocean Walk Medical Centre; Langs: Fukinese; Mandarin; Teochew; Fookien; Malay; (604)925-1884; Fax. (604)922-3591; lianghmv@yahoo.com.

NG, Louis H S; 103-3325 Kingsway, Vancouver BC V5R 5K6; (Hong Kong)'80; MB BS; Langs: Cantonese; Mandarin; (604)431-5008; Fax. (604)431-5007.

NG, Lung K; 599 Broadway Ave, Toronto ON M4G 2S4; Hong Kong (Hong Kong)'78; (416)421-2282

NG, Matilda W; York-Med Medical Arts Centre, 408-250 Harding Blvd W, Richmond Hill ON L4C 9M7; Tor'79; FRCPC; IntMed (Oncology). Med Consultant, Mackenzie Richmond Hill Hospital; Langs: Chinese; (905)884-7858

NG, Matthew; Etobicoke Med Centre FHT, 400 The East Mall, Etobicoke ON M9B 3Z9; Wes'10; CCFP; (416)621-2220; Fax. (416)621-2203; matthew.ng@stjoe.on.ca.

NG, Nelly W; Scarborough North Med Arts, 208-4040 Finch Ave E, Scarborough ON M1S 4V5; McM'78; Staff, The Scarborough Hospital - Birchmount Campus; Langs: Chinese; (416)298-2277

NG, Paul S Y; Corporate Med Centre, 10-78 Corporate Dr, Scarborough ON M1H 3G4; (Taiwan)'64; FRCPC; IntMed (Nephrology). Court Staff IntMed, The Scarborough Hospital - General Campus; Consultant, Toronto Western Hospital - University Health Network; (416)279-0855 x245; Fax. (416)279-0857.

NG, Philip K; Westwood Med Centre, 3-2755 Lougheed Hwy, Port Coquitlam BC V3B 5Y9; Alb'85; PharmD; BScPharm; Langs: Cantonese; (604)944-1848; Fax. (604)944-6335.

NG, Raymond; 101-7155 Woodbine Ave, Markham ON L3R 1A3; Tor'88; BSc; PhD; FRCSC; Otol (Head & Neck Surgery). Assoc Staff, The Scarborough Hospital - General Campus; Langs: Chinese; (416)628-4020; Fax. (416)628-4021.

NG, Rose Ann L O; 1460 Ouellette Ave, Windsor ON N8X 1K3; Wes'88; DAB; Ac Staff, Windsor Regional Hospital - Tayfour Site; Ac Staff, Hôtel-Dieu Grace Hospital; (519)258-2591

NG, S Y Andrew; 230-3476 Glen Erin Dr, Mississauga ON L5L 3R4; Tor'81; CCFP; Ac Staff Family Practice, The Credit Valley Hospital; Langs: Chinese; (905)820-3822; Fax. (905)820-7623.

NG, Sai-Sun; North Scarborough Prof Bldg, 310-3420 Finch Ave E, Scarborough ON M1W 2R6; McG'82; Ac Staff, The Scarborough Hospital - Birchmount Campus; Court Staff, North York General Hospital; Langs: Chinese; (416)499-3500; Fax. (416)499-3500; saisun_ng@hotmail.com.

NG, Shang C; Kerrisdale Station Med Clinic, 2077 42nd Ave W, Vancouver BC V6M 2B4; Monash (Australia)'68; Ac Staff, Vancouver General Hospital - Centennial Pavillion; Langs: Chinese; (604)261-9494

NG, Sheau C; My Family Health, 205-1386 Topsail Rd, Paradise NL A1L 1P6; Mem'02; CCFP; (709)782-1110; sheauchian@yahoo.com.

NG, Simon; 376-1917 4th Ave W, Vancouver BC V6J 1M7; Alb'94; BSc; CCFP; (604)657-5989

NG, Stephen S; 6465 Victoria Dr, Vancouver BC V5P 3X5; UBC'82; BSc(Pharm); Staff, Providence Health Care - Mount Saint Joseph Hospital; Staff, BC Children's Hospital; Langs: Cantonese; (604)325-8300; Fax. (604)325-0150.

NG, Stephen; Runnymede Healthcare Centre, 625 Runnymede Rd, Toronto ON M6S 3A3; Tor'87; BScPharm; CCFP; FCFP; Runnymede Healthcare Centre; Fam Med, North York General Hospital - Branson Division; (416)762-7316

NG, Stephen; Market Village Health Centre, C13 B-4392 Steeles Ave E, Markham ON L3R 9V8; Tor'87; BSc; Langs: Cantonese; (905)477-7880

NG, Susanna N; 202-9808 King George Blvd, Surrey BC V3T 2V6; (Taiwan)'72; (604)585-1229; Fax. (604)585-6878.

NG, Victor K; Richmond Hill After Hours Clin, 301 High Tech Rd, Richmond Hill ON L4B 4R2; Wes'06; CCFP; (905)709-4274; Fax. (905)709-4985.

NG, Victor K H; Bluewater Health-CEE Site, 450 Blance St, Petrolia ON N0N 1R0; Man'09; CCFP; CCFP(E.M.); Staff, Bluewater Health - Charlotte Eleanor Englehart Hospital; (519)882-4325

NG, Vienna K Y; 4060-8171 Ackroyd Rd, Richmond BC V6X 3K1; Alb'03; CCFP; (778)297-1360; Fax. (778)297-1359.

NG, Wai-Pui; London HSC-University Hosp, PO Box 5339 Stn B 339 Windermere Rd, London ON N6A 5A5; Tor'90; MD; PhD; FRCSC; Neursurg (Spine Surgery). Staff Neurosurg, London Health Sciences Centre - University Hospital; Asst Prof, University of Western Ontario; (519)663-3048; Fax. (519)663-2987.

NG, Wing Hon; 201-475 Main St, Vancouver BC V6A 2T7; Tor'78; Langs: Cantonese; Mandarin; Toishan; (604)669-0058

NG-A-FOOK, Robert A; 6-105 Progress Cres, Kapuskasing ON P5N 3J4; Glasgow (Scotland)'72; MB ChB; Chief GenPract, Sensenbrenner Hospital; (705)337-1434; Fax. (705)337-1449.

NG CHENG HIN, Alan; Primrose Family Med Centre, 35 Primrose Ave, Ottawa ON K1R 0A1; Dundee (Scotland)'86; MB ChB; DObst(Otago); DCH(Lond); DTMH(Liverpool); MRCGPract; CCFP; FCFP; Asst Prof Dept of Family Med, University of Ottawa; Langs: English; French; (613)230-7788; Fax. (613)230-7778.

NG-CHENG-HIN, G Tommy; CLSC de la Petite-Nation, 14 rue St-Andre GD, St-Andre-Avellin QC J0V 1W0; Bordeaux (France)'89; (819)983-7341; Fax. (819)983-7708.

NG-CHENG-HIN, Raymond; 13 Garden St, Brockville ON K6V 2B8; Aberdeen (Scotland)'63; MB ChB; FRCOG(Eng); FSOGC; FACOG; FRCSC; ObstGyn. Chief ObstGyn, Providence Continuing Care Centre (PCCC) - St Vincent de Paul Hospital; Chief ObstGyn/Chairman Postgrad Med Education, Brockville General Hospital - Charles Street; (613)342-8048; Fax. (613)342-8787.

NG CHEONG, Caroline; Concordia University, 1455 boul de Maisonneuve O, Montreal QC H3G 1M8; McG'97; CCFP; Médecin, CLSC Lac St-Louis; Médecin, Concordia University; Langs: English; French; (514)848-2424 x3565

NG CHEONG, Nathalie; St Mary's Hosp Centre, 3830 av Lacombe, Montreal QC H3T 1M5; McG'00; FRCPC; IntMed; Nephrol. Staff, St Mary's Hospital Centre; (514)345-3511 x5528

NG FUK CHONG, Nicholas; Ctre Francophone de Toronto, 22 College St, Toronto ON M5G 1K2; Mon'10; CCFP; (416)922-2672

NG FUK CHONG, Raphael; MediCentre Ile Perrot, 401 Grand Blvd, L'Ile-Perrot QC J7V 4X3; Bordeaux (France)'82; Langs: English; (514)453-1100; Fax. (514)453-2339.

NG MAN SUN, Joanna; Hop Charles LeMoyne, 3120 boul Taschereau, Greenfield Park QC J4V 2H1; McG'06; MDCM; FRCPC; Anes. Staff, Hopital Charles LeMoyne; (450)466-5000

NG MING HING, Jackson; CSSS du Nord de Lanaudière, 1000 boul Sainte-Anne, St-Charles-Brromee QC J6E 6J2; Bordeaux (France)'93; Staff, Centre Hospitalier Régional de Lanaudière; (450)759-8222

NG-THOW HING, Roland; 240 MacKay St, Pembroke ON K8A 1C5; RCS (Ireland)'72; Ac Staff, Pembroke Regional Hospital Inc; Langs: English; French; (613)732-2611; Fax. (613)732-8914.

NG TUNG HING, Edward K K; Davis Drive Med Clinic, 5-291 Davis Dr, Newmarket ON L3Y 2N6; Tor'94; FRCPC; IntMed; Rheum. Staff, Southlake Regional Health Centre; Langs: French; Chinese; (905)836-6609; Fax. (905)836-5158.

NG WONG HING, France; 140 Brown St PO Box 160, Dresden ON N0P 1M0; RCS (Ireland)'66; (519)683-4023; Fax. (519)683-4646.

NGAE, Min Yi; Sudbury Reg Hosp-Laurentian, 1 179-41 Ramsey Lake Rd, Sudbury ON P3E 5J1; Cal'05; FRCPC; AnatPath. Staff, Health Sciences North-Laurentian Site; (705)522-7100

NGAI, Benjamin Y C; William Osler HC-Etobicoke, 101 Humber College Blvd, Etobicoke ON M9V 1R8; Tor'95; FRCPC; IntMed. Staff, William Osler Health System - Etobicoke General Hospital; (416)494-2120

NGAI, Henry C P; 150-8220 Lansdowne Rd, Richmond BC V6X 1B9; UBC'87; CCFP; (604)278-3322

NGAN, Bo-Yee; The Hosp for Sick Children, 3124-555 University Ave, Toronto ON M5G 1X8; Tor'82; MSc; ABPath; PhD; LMCC; FRCPC; AnatPath (Pediatric Pathology). Staff, The Hospital For Sick Children; Asst Prof, University of Toronto; (416)813-6409; bo-yee.ngan@sickkids.ca.

NGAN, Elizabeth M; Hys Med Centre, 202-11010 101 St NW, Edmonton AB T5H 4B9; Alb'03; FRCPC; DiagRad. Staff, University of Alberta Hospital; (780)426-1121; Fax. (780)425-5979.

NGAN, Elton T C; UBC-Dept of Psychiatry, 2N9-2255 Wesbrook Mall, Vancouver BC V6T 2A1; McG'86; FRCPC; Psy. (604)822-8047; Fax. (604)822-7756.

NGAN, Johnson C S; Queen Elizabeth II HSC-Halifax, 1796 Summer St, Halifax NS B3H 3A7; Dal'81; DABA; BSc; MSc; PhD; FRCPC; Anes. Staff Anes, Queen Elizabeth II Health Sciences Centre - Victoria General Site; Staff, Queen Elizabeth II Health Sciences Centre - Halifax Infirmary Site; Asst Prof Anes, Dalhousie University; (902)473-4326; Fax. (902)473-2380; jngan@ns.sympatico.ca.

NGAN, May; Mackenzie Richmond Hill Hosp, 10 Trench St, Richmond Hill ON L4C 4Z3; Tor'81; FRCPC; Anes. Staff, Mackenzie Richmond Hill Hospital; (905)883-2110

NGAN, Michael; The Doxx at Kingsway Med Clin, 303-1 Kingsway Garden Mall NW, Edmonton AB T5G 3A6; Alb'90; (780)479-3699; Fax. (780)479-3399; dr.ngan@thedoxx.com.

NGASSAM, Philippe; 203-3400 rue du Marche, Dollard-D-Ormeaux QC H9B 2Y1; Mon'71; FRCPC; Peds. (514)685-3531; Fax. (514)685-7971.

NGETH, Sereyrath; 65 Hewlett Park Landing, Sylvan Lake AB T4S 2J3; Alb'09; CCFP; (403)887-0510; Fax. (403)887-0520.

NGHIEM, Dung P; McDermot Med Clinic, 37 av Donegani, Pointe-Claire QC H9R 2V7; Mon'78; Langs: English; French; (514)697-1410; Fax. (514)697-1411.

NGO, Duc Sieu; Bathurst Shopping Mall, 210-1300 St. Peter Ave, Bathurst NB E2A 3A6; Sher'92; FRCSC; Urol. (506)546-3388; Fax. (506)546-0198.

NGO, Hieu-Hanh; Hop Maisonneuve-Rosemont, 5415 boul de l'Assomption, Montreal QC H1T 2M4; Sher'82; Otol. Staff, Hopital Maisonneuve-Rosemont; assoc Prof, Universite de Sherbrooke; (514)252-3400 x4270; Fax. (514)252-3458; hanh_ngo@hotmail.com.

NGO, Kenny Q P; 62 Colborne St E, Orillia ON L3V 1T6; Tor'01; FRCSC; Otol (Head & Neck). Staff, Orillia Soldiers' Memorial Hospital; (705)326-7779; Fax. (705)326-9969.

NGO, Michelle A; FEMAP, 860 Richmond St, London ON N6A 3H8; Wes'07; FRCPC; Psy. (519)685-8500

NGO, Quang; Hamilton HS-McMaster Site, PO Box 1200 Stn Lcd 1 1200 Main St W, Hamilton ON L8N 3Z5; Wes'06; PedEmergMed; Peds. Staff, Hamilton Health Sciences Centre - McMaster Children's Hospital; (905)521-2100

NGO, T K N Caroline; Lakeridge Health Corp-Oshawa, 1 Hospital Crt, Oshawa ON L1G 2B9; Tor'05; CCFP; Staff, Lakeridge Health - Oshawa Site; (905)576-8711

NGO, Thanh-Lan; Inst Albert Prevost, 6555 boul Gouin O, Montreal QC H4K 1B3; Mon'95; FRCPC; Psy. (514)338-2222

NGO, Thanh-Phuong; CLSC la Petite Patrie, 6520 rue de Saint-Vallier, Montreal QC H2S 2P7; Mon'97; (514)273-4508

NGO, Thi Minh H; CLSC Saint-Laurent, 1055 av Sainte-Croix, Saint-Laurent QC H4L 3Z2; Mon'98; Langs: Vietnamese; (514)748-6381; Fax. (514)748-6323.

NGO, Thi Ngoc T; 2233 Hurontario St, Mississauga ON L5A 2E9; Laval'88; CCFP; Physician, Multicultural Community Health Centre; (905)275-8226

NGO MINH, Cuong; Somerset West Comm Health Ctre, 55 Eccles St, Ottawa ON K1R 6S3; Mon'00; CCFP; Physician, The Perley & Rideau Veterans' Health Centre; Physician, Somerset West Community Health Centre; Langs: English; (613)238-1220; Fax. (613)238-7595.

NGO-MINH, Tin; Ctr Hosp Pierre-Janet, 20 rue Pharand, Gatineau QC J9A 1K7; Ott'06; FRCPC; Psy. Staff, Centre Hospitalier Pierre-Janet; (819)776-8085

NGODJOUM NITCHEU, Louis R; Ctr Hosp Gatineau Memorial, CP 160 101 ch Burnside, Wakefield QC J0X 3G0; Yaounde (Cameroon)'93; Staff, Centre Hospitalier Gatineau Mémorial; (819)459-1112; Fax. (819)459-3947.

NGUAN, Angela Y; Broadway Plaza Family Practice, U6-601 Broadway W, Vancouver BC V5Z 4C2; McM'05; CCFP; Langs: Korean; (604)872-2558

NGUAN, Christopher Y; Gordon & Leslie Diamond HCC, 6F-2775 Laurel St, Vancouver BC V5Z 1M9; Dal'99; FRCSC; Urol. Staff, Gordon & Leslie Diamond Health Care Centre; (604)875-5003

NGUAN, Oliver Y C; Rideau Family Health Team, 5-3635 Rivergate Way, Ottawa ON K1V 2A4; Dal'01; MBA; CCFP; Staff Family Med, The Ottawa Hospital - Civic Campus; (613)739-3700; Fax. (613)739-7043.

NGUEGNO, Anatole; Shellbrook Med Clinic, PO Box 504, Shellbrook SK S0J 2E0; Universite de Yaounde I (Cameroon)'96; (306)747-2171; Fax. (306)747-2173.

NGUETSOP, Martin; Northern Connection Med Ctre, 425 Elgin Ave, Winnipeg MB R3A 1P2; (Other Foreign)'99.

NGUI, Daniel K F; 102-5990 Fraser St, Vancouver BC V5W 2Z7; UBC'98; CCFP; FCFP; (604)322-3366

NGUI, Simon F P; 102-5990 Fraser St, Vancouver BC V5W 2Z7; Ott'71; Assoc Staff, Providence Health Care - Mount Saint Joseph Hospital; Court Staff, Providence Health Care - St Vincent's Hospital-Heather Site; Court Staff, BC Women's Hospital & Health Centre; (604)322-3366; Fax. (604)324-1118.

NGUIMFACK MBODIE, Pierre C; Hopital Regional D'Edmundston, 275 boul Hebert, Edmundston NB E3V 4E4; Yaounde (Cameroon)'96; MD; Staff, Hôpital regional d'Edmundston; Memb. Med. Staff, Reg. Health Authority 4 & Cons., Community Mental Health Centre-Edmundston; (506)739-2571; Fax. (506)739-2438.

NGUYEN, An-Huy; 101-4125 Lawrence Ave E, Scarborough ON M1E 2S2; Sher'90; (416)281-8088; Fax. (416)281-8081; xehoi@yahoo.com.

NGUYEN, Andre T H; 235-6655 ch Cote-des-Neiges, Montreal QC H3S 2B4; Saigon (Vietnam)'73; Med Consultant, Hôpital psychiatrique de Malartic; (514)735-8060; andre_nguyen@ssss.gouv.qc.ca.

NGUYEN, Anh Tu; CSSS de Laval, 1755 boul Rene-Laennec, Laval QC H7M 3L9; McG'96; FRCPC; IntMed; Critical Care Medicine; Respir. Staff, Centre Hospitalier Pierre Boucher; Staff, Hopital de la Cite de la santé; (450)668-1010

NGUYEN, Anh Tuan; 622 College St, Toronto ON M6G 1B6; Tor'89; Langs: Vietnamese; (416)531-1413; Fax. (416)531-2636.

NGUYEN, Augustin; 201-20 Hobson St, Cambridge ON N1S 2M6; Tor'03; MSc; FRCPC; IntMed; Gastroent. (519)740-8400; Fax. (519)740-8440.

NGUYEN, Ba-Long; Place Montreal Trust, C011-1500 av McGill College, Montreal QC H3A 3J5; Sher'94; Staff Emerg, CSSS de Dorval-Lachine-Lasalle; (514)845-1800; Fax. (514)845-1810.

NGUYEN, Bao Hoang; 104B-215 Highland Rd W, Kitchener ON N2M 3C1; Tor'91; (519)571-9893; Fax. (519)571-9893.

NGUYEN, Bao Thoai H; Monterey Med Centre, 750-2220 68 St NE, Calgary AB T1Y 6Y7; Alb'97; CCFP; Langs: Vietnamese; (403)280-0465; Fax. (403)280-0549; baothoai@hotmail.com.

NGUYEN, Bich Han; Inst De Readaptation De Mtl, 6300 av de Darlington, Montreal QC H3S 2J4; Laval'07; PhysMed&Rehab. Staff, Institut de Réadaptation Gingras-Lindsay de Montréal; (514)340-2085

NGUYEN, Bich Ngoc; Expertise Neurosciences, 101 av Laurier O, Montreal QC H2T 2N6; Mon'90; CSPQ; FRCPC; Psy (Adult General Psychiatry). Langs: Vietnamese; English; (514)526-1648; Fax. (514)526-2016.

NGUYEN, Bich-Hong; Hôpital Ste-Justine, 3175 ch Cote-Sainte-Catherine, Montreal QC H3T 1C5; Mon'92; FRCPC; Peds. Staff, Hôpital Ste-Justine; (514)345-4931

NGUYEN, Bich-Ngoc; CHUM-Hop St-Luc, 1058 rue Saint-Denis, Montreal QC H2X 3J4; Sher'91; CSPQ; FRCPC; AnatPath. Staff, Centre Hospitalier l'Université De Montréal (CHUM) - Hôpital Saint-luc; Staff, The Ottawa Hospital - General Campus; Langs: Vietnamese; English; (514)890-8000

NGUYEN, C L Remy; Hop du Sacre-Coeur de Mtl, 5400 boul Gouin O, Montreal QC H4J 1C5; Sher'93; LMCC; ABOtol; FRCSC; Otol (Facial Plastic & Reconstructive Surgery). Staff, Hôpital du Sacre-Coeur de Montréal; Langs: Spanish; Vietnamese; English; (514)338-2222

NGUYEN, Cam-Hanh; Esthemedica, 6584 rue Sherbrooke O, Montreal QC H4B 1N5; Ott'76; (514)482-2152; Fax. (514)482-0785.

NGUYEN, Can Dinh; Credit Valley Prof Bldg, 406-2300 Eglinton Ave W, Mississauga ON L5M 2V8; McG'83; FRCSC; OrthSurg. Ac Staff, The Credit Valley Hospital; (905)828-4482; Fax. (905)828-5136.

NGUYEN, Can Manh; Hôpital Laval, 2725 ch Sainte-Foy, Quebec QC G1V 4G5; McG'94; FRCPC; IntMed; Cardiol. Staff, Hôpital Laval; (418)656-4862; Fax. (418)656-4544.

NGUYEN, Chieu H T; The Hugh Allen Clinic, PO Box 489 Stn Main 79 5th Ave N, Sioux Lookout ON P8T 1A8; McM'08; CCFP; Physician, The Hugh Allen Clinic; (807)737-3803; Fax. (807)737-1771.

NGUYEN, Chinh; Norfinch Med Centre, 110-2100 Finch Ave W, North York ON M3N 2Z9; Ott'90; Staff, Humber River Regional Hospital - Finch Avenue Site; (416)667-0802; Fax. (416)667-0616.

NGUYEN, Chinh Nhan; Hop Santa Cabrini Ospedale, 5655 rue Saint-Zotique E, Montreal QC H1T 1P7; Mon'97; IntMed. Staff, Hôpital Santa Cabrini Ospedale; (514)252-6444; Fax. (514)252-6487.

NGUYEN, Cong L; Centre Med Metro Monk, 2351 rue Allard, Montreal QC H4E 2L1; Sher'87; DAB; FRCSC; Ophth (Cataract). Staff, Centre Hospitalier de Verdun; (514)769-3399; Fax. (514)769-9008.

NGUYEN, Cong Du; Ctr Hosp Anna-Laberge, 200 boul Brisebois, Chateauguay QC J6K 4W8; Laval'95; FRCPC; IntMed. Staff, Hôpital Anna-Laberge; (450)699-2425

NGUYEN, Cong-Nghiem; Westmount Med Bldg, 660-5025 rue Sherbrooke O, Montreal QC H4A 1S9; Dal'91; CCFP; Staff, Donald Berman Maimonides Geriatric Centre; (514)932-6122; Fax. (514)933-8739.

NGUYEN, Dang Khoa; CHUM-Hop Notre-Dame, 1560 rue Sherbrooke E, Montreal QC H2L 4M1; Mon'95; FRCPC; Neur. Staff, Centre Hospitalier l'Université de Montréal (CHUM) - Hôpital Notre-Dame; (514)890-8237; d.nguyen@umontreal.ca.

NGUYEN, Dang Minh; Trillium Hlth Ctr-Mississauga, 100 Queensway W, Mississauga ON L5B 1B8; McG'93; FRCPC; IntMed. Staff, Trillium Health Centre - Mississauga; (905)848-7100

NGUYEN, Dang Khoa; Hop Charles LeMoyne, 3120 boul Taschereau, Greenfield Park QC J4V 2H1; Sher'93; FRCPC; IntMed; Cardiol. Staff, Hopital Charles LeMoyne; (450)466-5000

NGUYEN, Daniel T; Ctr Hosp Fleury, 2180 rue Fleury E, Montreal QC H2B 1K3; Sher'09; Staff, Centre Hospitalier Fleury; (514)384-3000

NGUYEN, Dao; MUHC-Montreal Gen Hosp, L11 513-1650 av Cedar, Montreal QC H3G 1A4; McG'97; FRCPC; IntMed; Respir. Staff, McGill University Health Centre - Montreal General Campus; (514)934-1934 x48014

NGUYEN, Dao Q T; 201-2502 St John's St, Port Moody BC V3H 2B4; Ott'99; FRCSC; PlasSurg (Breast Reconstruction). (604)931-3312

NGUYEN, Dat Nhut; Ctr Hosp Rouyn-Noranda, 4 9e rue, Rouyn-Noranda QC J9X 2B2; Sher'84; CSPQ; Anes. Staff, Centre Hospitalier Rouyn-Noranda; (819)764-5131; Fax. (819)764-2909.

NGUYEN, David H A; Hop Maisonneuve-Rosemont, 5415 boul de l'Assomption, Montreal QC H1T 2M4; Mon'04; FRCPC; RadOncol. Staff, Hopital Maisonneuve-Rosemont; (514)252-3400

NGUYEN, De; 110-10924 107 Ave NW, Edmonton AB T5H 0X5; Saigon (Vietnam)'73; Langs: Vietnamese; (780)426-6277; Fax. (780)426-6278.

NGUYEN, Diem Hong; CSSS de Laval, 1755 boul Rene-Laennec, Laval QC H7M 3L9; Mon'91; Staff, Hopital de la Cite de la santé; (450)668-1010; Fax. (450)975-5545.

NGUYEN, Diem-Quyen; CHUM-Hop St-Luc, 1058 rue Saint-Denis, Montreal QC H2X 3J4; Mon'85; IntMed. Staff, Centre Hospitalier l'Université De Montréal (CHUM) - Hôpital Saint-luc; (514)890-8000 x34599

NGUYEN, Dinh Duc; Centre Medical de Varennes, 201-2082 Rte Marie-Victorin, Varennes QC J3X 2C7; Saigon (Vietnam)'75; (450)652-2959; Fax. (450)652-3792.

NGUYEN, Dinh Nam; Hop de Readaptation Lindsay, 6363 ch Hudson, Montreal QC H3S 1M9; Saigon (Vietnam)'71; Staff, Institut de Réadaptation Gingras-Lindsay de Montréal; (514)737-3661

NGUYEN, Dinh Tam; Hop Santa Cabrini Ospedale, 5655 rue Saint-Zotique E, Montreal QC H1T 1P7; Sher'98; CSPQ; FRCPC; Anes. Staff, Hôpital Santa Cabrini Ospedale; (514)252-6581

NGUYEN, Doan-Trang; Hop Maisonneuve-Rosemont, 5415 boul de l'Assomption, Montreal QC H1T 2M4; Mon'83; FRCPC; IntMed. Staff, Hopital Maisonneuve-Rosemont; Langs: English; Vietnamese; (514)252-3400

NGUYEN, Duc Truong; 7 Mollison Crt, Guelph ON N1C 1A7; Saigon (Vietnam)'78; DABPath; FRCPC; GenPath. Ac Staff, Groves Memorial Community Hospital.

NGUYEN, Duc Tung; 428 Broadway E, Vancouver BC V5T 1X2; Hue (Vietnam)'82; CCFP; (604)709-0100; Fax. (604)709-0885.

NGUYEN, Duong H; 102-2489 Bloor St W, Toronto ON M6S 1R6; Ott'01; MSc; DABOSSports Med; BSc; FRCSC; OrthSurg (Sports Medicine). (416)742-3736; Fax. (416)742-2818; dn@nguyensportsmedicine.com.

NGUYEN, Duy; CLSC Parc Extension, 7085 rue Hutchison, Montreal QC H3N 1Y9; Mon'84; Staff, Institut de Réadaptation Gingras-Lindsay de Montréal; Langs: Vietnamese; (514)273-9591

NGUYEN, Duy Don; Ctr Hosp Fleury, 2180 rue Fleury E, Montreal QC H2B 1K3; Sher'98; IntMed (P.Q.) (Gastroenterology). Staff, Centre Hospitalier Fleury; (514)384-2000; Fax. (514)381-9872; duydon@hotmail.com.

NGUYEN, Duy Quynh H; CSSS Pierre Boucher, 1333 boul Jacques-Cartier E, Longueuil QC J4M 2A5; Mon'96; FRCPC; IntMed. Staff, Centre Hospitalier Pierre Boucher; (450)468-8111

NGUYEN, Duy Toan; CLSC Riviere des Prairies, 8655 boul Perras, Montreal QC H1E 4M7; Saigon (Vietnam)'69; (514)494-4924

NGUYEN, Geoffrey C; Mount Sinai Hosp, 433-600 University Ave, Toronto ON M5G 1X5; Baltimore (USA)'00; FRCPC; IntMed; Gastroent. Staff, Mount Sinai Hospital; (416)586-4800 x8236

NGUYEN, Gia-Khanh; Centre Med Metro-Monk, 2376 rue Allard, Montreal QC H4E 2K9; Sher'92; CCFP; Staff, Centre Hospitalier de LaSalle; (514)769-9999; Fax. (514)769-9008.

NGUYEN, Giang Thuy; St Paul's Hosp, 1081 Burrard St, Vancouver BC V6Z 1Y6; Alb'00; FRCPC; DiagRad. Staff, Providence Health Care - St Paul's Hospital; Staff, Vancouver General Hospital - Centennial Pavillion; (604)682-2344

NGUYEN, Giao-Chi; Medicentre Chomedey, 610 boul Cure-Labelle, Laval QC H7V 2T7; Laval'99; (450)687-6452

NGUYEN, H Tuong Quan; CLSC Petite-Patrie, 6520 rue Saint-Vallier, Montreal QC H2S 2P7; Mon'96; Staff, Centre Hospitalier Régional du Suroît; Médecin, CLSC Seigneurie de Beauharnois; Langs: Bilingual(French/English); (514)273-4508

NGUYEN, Ha-Nam P; MUHC-Montreal Children's Hosp, B240-2300 rue Tupper, Montreal QC H3H 1P3; McG'99; MSc(Otol); FRCSC; Otol (Pediatric Otolaryngology). adj Prof, McGill University Health Centre - Montreal Children's Hospital; Dir Med Educ in Otol, McGill University; Langs: Vietnamese; Bilingual(French/English); (514)412-4304; lilynguyen1@yahoo.com.

NGUYEN, Hai; 126 rue Saint-Louis, Lemoyne QC J4R 2L5; Mon'00; FRCSC; OrthSurg. (450)672-1212; Fax. (450)672-9834.

NGUYEN, Hai Hac; Ctr Medi Soleil St-Jean-Sur-Ri, 120-383 boul du Seminaire N, St-Jean-sur-Richel QC J3B 8C5; Sher'86; Derm. Langs: English; Vietnamese; (450)347-7557; Fax. (450)347-3099.

NGUYEN, Hai Thong; Hop Ste-Anne, 305 boul des Anciens-Combattan, Ste-Anne-de-Bellev QC H9X 1Y9; Saigon (Vietnam)'78; Staff, Hopital Ste-Anne; (514)457-3440

NGUYEN, Hai-Nam; CSSS du Nord de Lanaudière, 1000 boul Sainte-Anne, St-Charles-Brromee QC J6E 6J2; Mon'99; Psy (Ethno Psychiatry). Staff, CSSS de Trois-Rivières; Staff, Centre Hospitalier Régional de Lanaudière; (450)759-8222

NGUYEN, Hanh T H; Stratford Gen Hosp, 46 General Hospital Dr, Stratford ON N5A 2Y6; Wes'99; Staff, Stratford General Hospital - Huron Perth Healthcare Alliance; (519)271-8120

NGUYEN, Hau; Clinique Med Viau, 204-4750 rue Jarry E, Saint-Leonard QC H1R 1X8; Saigon (Vietnam)'70; (514)326-0436

NGUYEN, Hiep Huu; Clin Med Masson, 3996 rue Masson, Montreal QC H1X 1T5; Saigon (Vietnam)'72; (514)728-2150; Fax. (514)728-0284.

NGUYEN, Hieu Dinh; Ctr Hosp Pierre-Janet, 20 rue Pharand, Gatineau QC J9A 1K7; Saigon (Vietnam)'69; LMCC; Staff, Centre Hospitalier Pierre-Janet; Langs: Vietnamese; (819)771-7761; Fax. (819)771-0887.

NGUYEN, Hoa Hieu; 1432 ch de Chambly, Longueuil QC J4J 3X3; Saigon (Vietnam)'62; LMCC; Langs: Vietnamese; English; (450)674-9937; Fax. (450)674-9957.

NGUYEN, Hoang Ngoc T; Hop Santa Cabrini Ospedale, 5655 rue Saint-Zotique E, Montreal QC H1T 1P7; Sher'96; Staff, Hôpital Santa Cabrini Ospedale; (514)252-6546

NGUYEN, Hoang-Thi; Clin Med Haut-Anjou, 45-7500 boul les Galeries d'An, Anjou QC H1M 3M4; Mon'84; (514)493-1999; Fax. (514)493-4428.

NGUYEN, Hoanh Khoi; 5085 McLaughlin Rd, Mississauga ON L5R 1B6; Tor'88; (905)896-0505; Fax. (905)896-4929.

NGUYEN, Hong Chau; Medical Associates, 462 Paxton St, Port Perry ON L9L 1L9; McG'08; CCFP; (905)985-2895

NGUYEN, Dinh Huan; 1066 Kingsway, Vancouver BC V5V 3C6; Saigon (Vietnam)'73; (604)875-1800

NGUYEN, Huan Truong; Clinique Med Urgence Brossard, 7601 boul Taschereau, Brossard QC J4Y 1A2; Saigon (Vietnam)'65; Physician, Clinique Urgence Brossard; (450)462-0863; Fax. (450)462-0174; htnguyen@videotron.ca.

NGUYEN, Hung Vuong; Ctr Hosp Jacques Viger, 1051 rue Saint-Hubert, Montreal QC H2L 3Y5; Saigon (Vietnam)'79; Staff, Centre Hospitalier Jacques Viger; (514)842-7181; Fax. (514)842-1212.

NGUYEN, Huu Nam; Clinique Med Urgence Rive-Sud, 3200 boul Taschereau, Greenfield Park QC J4V 2H3; Saigon (Vietnam)'59; Langs: English; French; (450)672-5577; Fax. (450)672-0535.

NGUYEN, Huu Tram Anh; Hop Maisonneuve-Rosemont, 5415 boul de l'Assomption, Montreal QC H1T 2M4; Sher'96; CSPQ; FRCPC; Anes. Staff Anes, Hopital Maisonneuve-Rosemont; (514)252-3426

NGUYEN, Huu Vi; Clinique Med Louis-Veuillot, 5840 rue Hochelaga, Montreal QC H1N 1W8; Saigon (Vietnam)'56; (514)252-0288

NGUYEN, Huy T S; 107-301 Columbia St E, New Westminster BC V3L 3W5; Ross (Dominica)'09; (604)522-7363

NGUYEN, Huy Thang; 1560 boul Saint-Jean-Baptiste, Pte-aux-Trembles QC H1B 4A4; Saigon (Vietnam)'75; (514)645-7551

NGUYEN, Huy Thanh V; Sherwood Med Centre, 15 Brackley Point Rd, Charlottetown PE C1A 6Y1; Tor'04; Cert Geront; MCFP; CCFP; Lecturer, Dalhousie University; Langs: Vietnamese; (902)367-4474; Fax. (902)892-4197.

NGUYEN, Jennifer; Ctr for Addiction & Mental Hlt, 80 Workman Way, Toronto ON M6J 1H4; Alb'05; Psy.

NGUYEN, Jennifer; Hop Brome-Missisquoi-Perkins, 950 rue Principale, Cowansville QC J2K 1K3; McG'05; FRCPC; IntMed. Staff, Hôpital Brome-Missisquoi-Perkins; (450)266-4342

NGUYEN, Jimmy; Lakeshore Gen Hosp, 160 av Stillview, Pointe-Claire QC H9R 2Y2; Sher'01; CSPQ; AnatPath. Staff, Lakeshore General Hospital - Pointe Claire; (514)630-2225

NGUYEN, John T; 2-1160 Beaverwood Rd, Manotick ON K4M 1L6; Cal'09; CCFP; (613)692-0244

NGUYEN, Khang Huu; Polyclinique CMI St-Laurent, 240-2040 boul Marcel-Laurin, Saint-Laurent QC H4R 1J9; Sher'95; (514)747-9936; Fax. (514)747-9331; khnguyen99@hotmail.com.

NGUYEN, Khiem Ngoc; CSSSG - Hop de Hull, 116 boul Lionel-Emond, Gatineau QC J8Y 1W7; McG'00; FRCPC; IntMed; Critical Care Medicine (P.Q.). Staff, Hull Hospital; (819)595-6000 x6099

NGUYEN, Khue Huu; MUHC-Royal Victoria Hosp, A462-687 av des Pins O, Montreal QC H3A 1A1; McG'87; DAB; FRCPC; Derm. Staff, McGill University Health Centre - Royal Victoria Hospital; Asst Staff, Sir Mortimer B Davis Jewish General; adj Prof, McGill University; Langs: Vietnamese; English; (514)934-1934 x34999; Fax. (450)466-4241.

NGUYEN, Kim Anh; Clinique Med de Castelnau, 785 rue de Castelnau E, Montreal QC H2R 3A3; Mon'02; CCFP; (514)277-4143

NGUYEN, Kim Anh; CLSC de Cote-des-neiges, 1271 av Van Horne, Montreal QC H2V 1K5; Mon'99; assoc Staff, Lakeshore General Hospital - Pointe Claire; Conférencier, McGill University; Langs: English; (514)270-1536 x1111; Fax. (514)270-8731.

NGUYEN, Kimberly; Esthemedica, 6584 rue Sherbrooke O, Montreal QC H4B 1N5; Sher'02; CCFP; Staff, CSSS du Coeur de l'Isle Hôpital Jean-Talon; (514)482-2152; Fax. (514)482-0785.

NGUYEN, Kinh-Tung T; 318-89 Humber College Blvd, Etobicoke ON M9V 4B8; Tor'00; FRCPC; IntMed; Endocrin&Metab.

NGUYEN, Lam Van; 215 Main St W, Hamilton ON L8P 1J4; 92Saigon (Vietnam)'65; Langs: Vietnamese; French; (905)525-4432; Fax. (905)525-4427.

NGUYEN, Lan Chau; Med Privee Notre-Dame, 597 av Notre-Dame, Saint-Lambert QC J4P 2K8; Mon'05; Langs: Bilingual(English/French); (450)766-0766; Fax. (450)766-0767.

NGUYEN, Lan-Anh; CSSS de la Vallée de l'Or, 725 6e rue, Val-d'Or QC J9P 3Y1; Laval'05; CCFP; Staff, Centre Hospitalier de Val d'Or; (819)825-6711; Fax. (819)825-7919.

NGUYEN, Lau K; Grey Nuns Community Hosp & HC, 1100 Youville Drive West NW, Edmonton AB T6L 5X8; Alb'98; CCFP; CCFP(E.M.); Staff, Covenant Health - Grey Nuns Community Hospital; (780)735-7180; Fax. (780)735-7498.

NGUYEN, Lien Hoang; 544 Ellice Ave, Winnipeg MB R3B 1Z4; Man'93; Physician, McMicken Medical Clinic; Langs: Vietnamese; (204)786-2496; Fax. (204)786-2511.

NGUYEN, Long Phan; Clin Med Diamant, 201-5885 ch de Cote-des-Neiges, Montreal QC H3S 2T2; McG'94; CCFP; (514)731-5994

NGUYEN, Lynda P; Magrath Med Clinic, 308-14127 23 Ave NW, Edmonton AB T6R 0G4; Alb'04; BSc; CCFP; Langs: Vietnamese; (780)430-8788; Fax. (780)435-3134.

NGUYEN, Manhluu; Clinique Med Luso Mtl Ltee, 1 av du Mont-Royal E, Montreal QC H2T 1N4; Saigon (Vietnam)'67; (514)849-2391; Fax. (514)849-2394.

NGUYEN, Marie-Therese H N; Echo Eco Nguyen Inc, 202-5675 ch de la Cote-des-Nei, Montreal QC H3T 1Y8; McG'00; CSPQ; FRCPC; DiagRad. (514)801-9912

NGUYEN, Martin M M; CSSS de Saint-Jerome, 290 rue de Montigny, Saint-Jerome QC J7Z 5T3; Sher'07; CCFP; CCFP(E.M.); Staff, Hôtel-Dieu de Saint-Jérôme; (450)432-2777

NGUYEN, Mau Hoang; 101-5900 boul Leger, Montreal-Nord QC H1G 1K9; Saigon (Vietnam)'61; Langs: English; French; (514)327-4200

NGUYEN, Mau Huan; CLSC Lamater, 1317 boul des Seigneurs, Terrebonne QC J6W 5B1; Mon'96; (450)471-2881 x4056; Fax. (450)471-6763; m_nguyen@videotron.ca.

NGUYEN, Melanie M L; Clinique Medicale, 101-2001 av Victoria, Saint-Lambert QC J4S 1H1; Mon'05; FRCPC; IntMed; ClinImmunol&Allergy. (450)465-9789

NGUYEN, Melody H H; 5-3477 Kennedy Rd, Scarborough ON M1V 3Z7; Tor'05; FRCPC; PhysMed&Rehab. (416)335-9700; Fax. (416)335-9800.

NGUYEN, Michel C K; CLSC Drummondville, 350 rue Saint-Jean, Drummondville QC J2B 5L4; Paris (France)'03; (819)474-2572

NGUYEN, Michel; 3001 12e av N, Sherbrooke QC J1H 5N4; Sher'84 Sherbrooke; FRCP; FRCPC; IntMed (Interventional Cardiology); Cardiol. Staff Interventional Cardiologie, Centre Hospitalier Universitaire de Sherbrooke-Hopital Fleurimont; Prof Med(Cardiology), Universite de Sherbrooke; Langs: Vietnamese; English; (819)346-1110 x74947; Fax. (819)564-5316; michel.nguyen@usherbrooke.ca.

NGUYEN, Micheline; CHUM-Hop St-Luc, 1058 rue Saint-Denis, Montreal QC H2X 3J4; Mon'05; FRCPC; Anes. Staff, Centre Hospitalier l'Université De Montréal (CHUM) - Hôpital Saint-luc; (514)890-8000

NGUYEN, Minh Hanh; Clinique Jeanne-Mance, 220-7895 av Papineau, Montreal QC H2E 2H4; Sher'94; Langs: Vietnamese; (514)439-3556; Fax. (514)439-9115.

NGUYEN, Minh Hien; Metro Health Clinic, 4879 Kingsway, Burnaby BC V5H 4T6; Qns'94; CCFP; Langs: Vietnamese; French; (604)433-3341; Fax. (604)433-8618.

NGUYEN, Minh Hung; Corner Med Centre, 11-794 Sargent Ave, Winnipeg MB R3E 0B7; Saigon (Vietnam)'75; (204)783-6430; Fax. (204)783-6493.

NGUYEN, Minh-Duc; Clin Med Legendre St-Michel, 6-8949 boul Saint-Michel, Montreal QC H1Z 3G3; Saigon (Vietnam)'72; Staff, Hopital Louis-H Lafontaine; (514)323-7435

NGUYEN, Mong Thuy; 5415 boul Grande-Allee, Brossard QC J4Z 3G9; Mon'80; Staff, Centre Hospitalier l'Université de Montréal (CHUM) - Hôpital Notre-Dame; (450)445-3600; Fax. (450)445-7140.

NGUYEN, My Chau; CLSC Parc Extension, 7085 rue Hutchison, Montreal QC H3N 1Y9; Sher'95; LMCC; CCFP; FCFP; (514)273-9591; Fax. (514)273-9113.

NGUYEN, My Lang; 204-6455 av Christophe-Colomb, Montreal QC H2S 2G5; Saigon (Vietnam)'74; (514)271-6033; Fax. (514)271-2424.

NGUYEN, M Anne-Marie; CLSC Saint-Michel, 3355 rue Jarry E, Montreal QC H1Z 2E5; McG'09; CCFP; (514)722-3000

NGUYEN, Myvan; CLSC Verdun/Cote-St-Paul, 400 rue de l'Eglise, Verdun QC H4G 2M4; Mon'83; Médecin, CLSC Verdun Cote St-Paul; Langs: English; (514)766-0546 x2316; Fax. (514)732-5103.

NGUYEN, N Vinh-Thuy; CSSS de la Region de Thetford, 1717 rue Notre-Dame E, Thetford Mines QC G6G 2V4; Laval'99; FRCSC; Otol. Staff, Hopital du CSS de la Region de Thetford; (418)338-7777

NGUYEN, N P Julie; Coast Med Clinic, 1018 Seymour St, Vancouver BC V6B 3M6; Mon'07; CCFP; Langs: Vietnamese; (604)569-3632

NGUYEN, Nadia; Centre Med Quatre-Bourgeois, 300-979 av de Bourgogne, Quebec QC G1W 2L4; Laval'94; CCFP; Staff, Centre Hospitalier Universitaire De Québec - Pavillon De St-françois-d'assise; (418)653-4050; Fax. (418)653-4475.

NGUYEN, Nam Anh; Pediatrics & Family Clinic, 1218 King St W, Toronto ON M6K 1G4; Saigon (Vietnam)'81; FCFP; DrMedCh; LMCC; CCFP; Langs: Vietnamese; (416)538-8833; Fax. (416)538-7685; namanh.nguyen@utoronto.ca.

NGUYEN, Nam Hoang; Crestwood Medical Dental, 207-6051 Gilbert Rd, Richmond BC V7C 3V3; UBC'91; FRCSC; GenSurg. Staff, Richmond Hospital; Asst Prof, University of British Columbia; (604)276-0952; Fax. (604)231-0583.

NGUYEN, Ngoc Bich; Hop du Sacre-Coeur de Mtl, 5400 boul Gouin O, Montreal QC H4J 1C5; Mon'99; FRCPC; IntMed; Respir. Staff Respiratory Med, Hôpital du Sacre-Coeur de Montréal; Langs: Vietnamese; English; (514)338-2222 x2162; Fax. (514)338-3699.

NGUYEN, Ngoc Chi; Clinique Medicale St-Zotique, RR 2 681 rue Principale, Saint-Zotique QC J0P 1Z0; Sher'94; (450)267-3536; Fax. (450)267-8632.

NGUYEN, Ngoc Quynh N; Clinique Med Pierre-Boucher, 110-1615 boul Jacques-Cartier, Longueuil QC J4M 2X1; Mon'87; Staff, Centre Hospitalier Pierre Boucher; (450)468-6223; Fax. (450)468-5041.

NGUYEN, Ngoc Thien; Inst de Readaptation de Mtl, 6300 av de Darlington, Montreal QC H3S 2J4; Saigon (Vietnam)'73; Staff, Institut de Réadaptation Gingras-Lindsay de Montréal; (514)340-2085; Fax. (514)340-2724.

NGUYEN, Ngoc Thuy; 407-5885 ch de la Cote-des-Nei, Montreal QC H3S 2T2; McG'96; FRCSC; ObstGyn. Staff, Hôpital Santa Cabrini Ospedale; (514)731-0554; Fax. (514)731-1726.

NGUYEN, Ngoc Toan; Clinique Millenia, 150 rue Sainte-Catherine O, Montreal QC H5B 1B2; Sher'96; (514)287-2683

NGUYEN, Ngoc Truong T; Extendicare Nursing Home, 82 Park Rd N, Oshawa ON L1J 4L1; Mon'93; CCFP; Staff, Lakeridge Health - Oshawa Site; Langs: Vietnamese; English; (905)579-0011; Fax. (905)579-1733.

NGUYEN, Ngoc-Huu; Hop Maisonneuve-Rosemont, 5415 boul de l'Assomption, Montreal QC H1T 2M4; Mon'93; LMCC; DABIM; FRCPC; Cardiol; IntMed (Hemodynamics). Staff, Hopital Maisonneuve-Rosemont; (514)252-3400

NGUYEN, Ngoc-Lang; Clinique Med Pie IX, 204-8131 boul Pie-IX, Montreal QC H1Z 3T5; Hue (Vietnam)'71; (514)326-3224; Fax. (514)326-0834.

NGUYEN, Ngoc-Tram; Centre Hosp Honore-Mercier, 2750 boul Laframboise, Saint-Hyacinthe QC J2S 4Y8; Mon'97; FRCPC; Psy. Staff, Centre Hospitalier Honore-Mercier; (450)771-3222; Fax. (450)771-3273.

NGUYEN, Ngoc-Van; Centre Med Chirurgical Lachine, 25-3360 rue Notre-Dame, Lachine QC H8T 3E2; McG'81; GenSurg (Colorectal Surgery). Staff, McGill University Health Centre; Langs: Bilingual(English/French); Vietnamese; (514)634-4973; Fax. (514)634-4150.

NGUYEN, Nhiem; 220-8120 Cook Rd, Richmond BC V6Y 1T9; Saigon (Vietnam)'67; FRCPC; Derm (Cosmetic & Laser Surgery). Consultant Derm, Richmond Hospital; Consultant Derm, Vancouver General Hospital - Centennial Pavillion; Hon Prof Derm, University of British Columbia; Langs: French; Vietnamese; Chinese; (604)278-8410; Fax. (604)278-8440.

NGUYEN, Oanh Thi; Centre Bois de Boulogne, 490-1575 boul Henri-Bourassa O, Montreal QC H3M 3A9; Saigon (Vietnam)'62; PhysMed&Rehab (P.Q.). Ac Staff, Hopital Charles LeMoyne; (514)337-5114

NGUYEN, Olivia K; Hop du Scare-Coeur de Mtl, 5400 boul Gouin O, Montreal QC H4J 1C5; Mon'06; CCFP; Staff, Hôpital du Sacre-Coeur de Montréal; (514)338-2222

NGUYEN, Phan Nha T; CSSS Pierre Boucher, 1333 boul Jacques-Cartier E, Longueuil QC J4M 2A5; Mon'98; Psy. Staff, Centre Hospitalier Pierre Boucher; (450)468-8111 x2425

NGUYEN, Phu-Cuong; Clinique Med Sherbrooke Est, 8687 rue Sherbrooke E, Montreal QC H1L 1C1; Saigon (Vietnam)'67; (514)354-3992; Fax. (514)354-9713.

NGUYEN, Phuoc Ngoc Diem; Ctr Hosp de Verdun, 4000 boul Lasalle, Verdun QC H4G 2A3; McG'97; FRCSC; GenSurg. Staff, Centre Hospitalier de Verdun; (514)362-1000

NGUYEN, Phuongbich; 103-1223 St Clair Ave W, Toronto ON M6E 1B5; Tor'90; Langs: Vietnamese; (416)653-7745; Fax. (416)915-0052.

NGUYEN, Quang D; CSSS de Manicouagan, 635 boul Jolliet, Baie-Comeau QC G5C 1P1; Sher'99; CCFP; Staff, CH du Centre-de-la-Mauricie (Ste-Thérèse de Shawinigan); Staff, Centre Hospitalier Régional Baie-Comeau; (418)589-3701; quang_nguyen@ssss.gouv.qc.ca.

NGUYEN, Quang V K; Sherbourne Family Health Team, 333 Sherbourne St, Toronto ON M5A 2S5; Wes'05; MPH; MBA; CCFP; Langs: Spanish; Vietnamese; French; (416)324-4100; Fax. (416)324-4262; qnguyen@sherbourne.on.ca.

NGUYEN, Quang Binh; 208-3369 Fraser St, Vancouver BC V5V 4C2; Laval'94; Clin Teach Staff, University of British Columbia; Langs: Bilingual(French/English); (604)876-5430; Fax. (604)876-5204; quangbinhnguyen@yahoo.com.

NGUYEN, Quang Hung; Clinique Med Saint-Henri, 3966 rue Notre-Dame O, Montreal QC H4C 1R1; Saigon (Vietnam)'79; (514)935-4330; Fax. (514)935-4292.

NGUYEN, Quang Thanh; Clinique Med Jeanne-Mance, 220-7895 av Papineau, Montreal QC H2E 2H4; Saigon (Vietnam)'65; (514)729-6371; Fax. (514)353-2351.

NGUYEN, Quoc Minh; Anesthesia Associates, 439 Park St, Kitchener ON N2G 1N4; Tor'03; FRCPC; Anes. (519)744-7361

NGUYEN, Quy Don; Ctr Hosp Anna-Laberge, 200 boul Brisebois, Chateauguay QC J6K 4W8; Mon'85; Cardiol (P.Q.) (Echocardiography). Staff, Hôpital Anna-Laberge; Langs: Vietnamese; (450)699-2425

NGUYEN, Quy Duong; West Nipissing Gen Hosp, 725 Coursol Rd, Sturgeon Falls ON P2B 2Y6; Sher'99; CCFP; Staff, West Nipissing General Hospital; (705)753-3110

NGUYEN, Quynh Nhu; Clinique Med Populaire, 1260 rue Sainte-Helene, Longueuil QC J4K 3S6; Laval'89; (450)670-7700; Fax. (450)928-0085.

NGUYEN, Quynh Nga; CH Jean la Lalande, 4255 av Papineau, Montreal QC H2H 2P6; Saigon (Vietnam)'74; (514)526-4981

NGUYEN, San Duy; 306-2238 Dundas St W, Toronto ON M6R 3A9; Saigon (Vietnam)'60; FRCPC; Psy. Dir, East-West Mental Health Clinic; Langs: Vietnamese; French; (416)588-3700; Fax. (416)588-6368.

NGUYEN, Sebastien; Ctr Hosp Affilie-St-Sacrement, 1050 ch Sainte-Foy, Quebec QC G1S 4L8; Mon'99; FRCSC; PlasSurg. Staff, Centre Hospitalier Universitaire de Québec (CHUQ) - Siege Social; Staff, Centre Hospitalier Affilié Universitaire de Québec - Hôpital du St-Sacrement; (418)682-7511

NGUYEN, Sy Hoang; 13-2437 Finch Ave W, Toronto ON M9M 2E7; McG'94; (416)740-0992; Fax. (416)740-2911.

NGUYEN, T Elsie; N C S B I C, 567-585 University Ave, Toronto ON M5G 2N2; Tor'00; FRCPC; DiagRad. (416)340-4800

NGUYEN, T Thanh Tra; Clin Med Fleury, 107-2157 rue Fleury E, Montreal QC H2B 1K1; Laval'94; CCFP; Staff, CSSS du Coeur de l'Isle Hôpital Jean-Talon; Langs: Vietnamese; (514)858-6110

NGUYEN, Tai Van; South Eastman Health Centre, 8-178 PTH 12 N, Steinbach MB R5G 1T7; Hue (Vietnam)'93.

NGUYEN, Tan-Ngoc; Ctr Hosp Jacques Viger, 1051 rue Saint-Hubert, Montreal QC H2L 3Y5; Saigon (Vietnam)'79; Staff, Centre Hospitalier Jacques Viger; (514)842-7181; Fax. (514)842-1212; tan-ngoc.nguyen@ssss.gouv.qc.ca.

NGUYEN, Tang-Dong; Clinique Med Pelletier, 300-8330 boul Taschereau, Brossard QC J4X 1C2; Sher'96; Ac Member, Hopital Charles LeMoyne; Langs: English; Vietnamese; (450)465-5379; Fax. (450)465-5615.

NGUYEN, Tang-Thong; CSSSG-Hop de Hull, 116 boul Lionel-Emond, Gatineau QC J8Y 1W7; Sher'98; CSPQ; Cardiol; IntMed (P.Q.) (Echocardiography). Staff, Hull Hospital; Langs: Vietnamese; English; (819)595-6000

NGUYEN, Thai Tong; Hop Louis-H Lafontaine, 7401 rue Hochelaga, Montreal QC H1N 3M5; Saigon (Vietnam)'77; LMCC; Staff, Hopital Louis-H Lafontaine; (514)251-4000

NGUYEN, Thang N; St Boniface Gen Hosp, Y3005-409 Tache Ave, Winnipeg MB R2H 2A6; Man'05; FRCPC; IntMed; Cardiol. Staff, St Boniface General Hospital; (204)233-8563

NGUYEN, Thanh; Polyclinique Med Pierre Le-Gar, 300-1000 montee des Pionniers, Terrebonne QC J6V 1S8; Mon'97; Staff, Centre Hospitalier Pierre le Gardeur; (450)657-5799; Fax. (450)657-1809; thanhnguyen57@hotmail.com.

NGUYEN, Thanh Binh; The Ottawa Hosp-Civic Campus, 1053 Carling Ave, Ottawa ON K1Y 4E9; McG'95; FRCPC; DiagRad (Neuro Radiology). Staff, The Ottawa Hospital - Civic Campus; University of Ottawa; (613)594-2490; Fax. (613)761-4529.

NGUYEN, Thanh Can; Centre Med Metro-Monk, 2376 rue Allard, Montreal QC H4E 2K9; Sher'98; CCFP; Staff, Centre Hospitalier de LaSalle; (514)769-9999; Fax. (514)769-9008.

NGUYEN, Thanh Long; Clinique Sante, 1260 rue Sainte-Helene, Longueuil QC J4K 3S6; Saigon (Vietnam)'67; (450)670-7700

NGUYEN, Thanh-Binh; Hop Santa Cabrini Ospedale, 5655 rue Saint-Zotique E, Montreal QC H1T 1P7; Saigon (Vietnam)'68; Gastroent (P.Q.). ac Staff, Hôpital Santa Cabrini Ospedale; (514)252-6000

NGUYEN, Thanh-Thao; Hop Maisonneuve-Rosemont, 5415 boul de l'Assomption, Montreal QC H1T 2M4; Mon'99; FRCPC; IntMed. Staff, Hopital Maisonneuve-Rosemont; (514)252-3400

NGUYEN, The Lac; 984 Colborne St, Brantford ON N3S 3T4; Saigon (Vietnam)'67; FRCSC; PlasSurg. Staff, The Brant Community Healthcare System - Brantford General Hospital Site; Staff, The Brant Community Healthcare System - Willett Hospital Site; (519)753-6477; Fax. (519)753-9472.

NGUYEN, The Thanh D; Hôpital Ste-Justine, 3175 ch Cote Sainte-Catherine, Montreal QC H3T 1C5; Mon'05; FRCPC; Peds; Respir. Staff, Hôpital Ste-Justine; (514)345-4931 x5409

NGUYEN, The-Huy; MD Health Med Centre, 186 Main St S, Brampton ON L6W 2E2; Saigon (Vietnam)'58; Langs: Vietnamese; French; (905)456-7774; Fax. (905)456-1158.

NGUYEN, The-Minh; Riverside Prof Centre, 205-1919 Riverside Dr, Ottawa ON K1H 1A2; McG'85; BSc; MDCM; FRCPC; Peds; Neur. Langs: Vietnamese; French; (613)737-3121; Fax. (613)737-6048.

NGUYEN, Therese N H M; 158-1 Place Laval, Laval QC H7N 1A1; Mon'01; CCFP; (450)668-7400; Fax. (450)668-5855.

NGUYEN, Thi Anh T; CSSSG-Hop de Hull, 116 boul Lionel-Emond, Gatineau QC J8Y 1W7; Sher'97; Staff, Hull Hospital; (819)595-6000

NGUYEN, Thao; Eye Health MD, 440-8000 boul Decarie, Montreal QC H4P 2S4; Mon'97; FRCSC; Ophth. Langs: Vietnamese; English; (514)340-2729; Fax. (514)340-3937; thao_100@yahoo.com.

NGUYEN, Thi Binh M; CSSS Pierre Boucher, 1333 boul Jacques-Cartier E, Longueuil QC J4M 2A5; Sher'93; Staff, Centre Hospitalier Pierre Boucher; (450)468-8111

NGUYEN, Thi Hong; Hop Santa Cabrini Ospedale, 5655 rue Saint-Zotique E, Montreal QC H1T 1P7; Saigon (Vietnam)'86; Staff, Hôpital Santa Cabrini Ospedale; (514)252-6000; Fax. (514)252-6501.

NGUYEN, Thi Ngoc L; Clinique Med Viau, 8465 boul Viau, Saint-Leonard QC H1R 2T6; Mon'97; LMCC; CCFP; Staff, Hôpital Santa Cabrini Ospedale; Langs: Vietnamese; (514)326-7203; Fax. (514)326-3656.

NGUYEN, Thi Ngoc Dang; 289 Frederick St, Kitchener ON N2H 2N3; (Vietnam)'87; CCFP; (519)742-0001; Fax. (519)742-2119.

NGUYEN, Thi Ngoc Diep; Clinique Ped des Mille-Iles, 203-233 rue Turgeon, Sainte-Therese QC J7E 3J8; Laval'99; FRCPC; Peds. Staff Peds, Hôpital de Saint-Eustache; (450)434-8006; Fax. (450)434-8007.

NGUYEN, Thi Phuong A; Place Montreal Trust, C11-1500 av McGill College, Montreal QC H3A 3J5; Mon'93; (514)845-1800; Fax. (514)845-1810.

NGUYEN, Thi Thanh T; CSSS de Laval, 1755 boul Rene-Laennec, Laval QC H7M 3L9; Sher'82; FRCPC; MedMicrobiol (Infectious Diseases); Microbio & Infect Dis (P.Q.). Staff Microbiol, Hopital de la Cite de la santé; Langs: Vietnamese; English; (450)668-1010 x23322; Fax. (450)975-5044.

NGUYEN, Thi Van Anh; CSSS de Laval, 1755 boul Rene-Laennec, Laval QC H7M 3L9; McG'98; CSPQ; FRCPC; DiagRad. Staff, Hopital de la Cite de la santé; Langs: Vietnamese; English; (450)668-1010 x2551; Fax. (450)975-5040.

NGUYEN, Thien Huong; Quinte HC Corp-Belleville Gen, 265 Dundas St E, Belleville ON K8N 5A9; Sher'92; FRCPC; NuclearMed. Chief NuclearMed, QHC Belleville General; Langs: English; (613)969-7400 x2741; Fax. (613)969-1307; eyee@kos.net.

NGUYEN, Thien-Hoa; CSSS Pierre Boucher, 1333 boul Jacques-Cartier E, Longueuil QC J4M 2A5; Mon'92; CCFP; Family Medicine, Centre Hospitalier Pierre Boucher; (450)468-8111; Fax. (450)647-5186.

NGUYEN, Thituong N; CLSC Bordeaux-Cartierville, 11822 av de Bois-de-Boulogne, Montreal QC H3M 2X6; Laval'90; (514)331-2572; Fax. (514)331-0137.

NGUYEN, Thuy-Khanh; Hop Maisonneuve-Rosemont, 5415 boul de l'Assomption, Montreal QC H1T 2M4; McG'95; CSPQ; DiagRad. Staff, Hopital Maisonneuve-Rosemont; (514)252-3400 x3535

NGUYEN, Tram T; University of Toronto, 602-500 University Ave, Toronto ON M5G 1V7; UBC'08; FRCPC; Peds.

NGUYEN, Tram Anh Thi; 102-1280 Finch Ave W, North York ON M3J 3K6; Medical and Pharmaceutical University (Other Foreign)'92; CCFP; (416)398-3738; Fax. (416)398-3733.

NGUYEN, Trung Khanh; Sault Area Hosp, 70 Great Northern Rd, Sault Ste. Marie ON P6B 0A8; Saigon (Vietnam)'73; FRCPC; DiagRad. Staff, Sault Area Hospital - Sault Ste Marie; (705)759-3610

NGUYEN, Trung Nghia; Hop Charles LeMoyne, 3120 boul Taschereau, Greenfield Park QC J4V 2H1; Mon'01; FRCPC; IntMed; MedOncol; Hem. Staff, Hopital Charles LeMoyne; (450)466-5000

NGUYEN, Truong V; 122-1315 Finch Ave W, North York ON M3J 2G6; Saigon (Vietnam)'74; CCFP; (416)398-0307; Fax. (416)398-0905.

NGUYEN, Tu Anh; Polyclinique Med Fabreville, 380 boul Cure-Labelle, Laval QC H7P 5L3; Mon'01; CCFP; (450)628-5800 x312; Fax. (450)628-0217.

NGUYEN, Tuan Khoat; CH Jean de la Lande, 4255 av Papineau, Montreal QC H2H 2P6; Saigon (Vietnam)'74; Gen Practice, Centre Hospitalier Jacques Viger; (514)526-4981; tuan.nguyen@ssss.gouv.qc.ca.

NGUYEN, Tuan Khoan; Clin Med Pie-IX, 204-8131 boul Pie-IX, Montreal QC H1Z 3T5; Saigon (Vietnam)'71; OrthSurg (P.Q.). (514)326-3224; Fax. (514)326-0834.

NGUYEN, Tuan Quynh T; Clinique O, 4845 rue Saint-Denis, Montreal QC H2J 2L7; Mon'99; Ophth (Oculo Plastic Surgery). Staff, Centre Hospitalier l'Université De Montréal (CHUM) - Hôpital Saint-luc; Universite de Montreal; Langs: Vietnamese; Spanish; (514)499-0101; Fax. (514)499-0108; eye_expert@yahoo.com.

NGUYEN, Tung Thanh C; The Ottawa Hosp-Civic Campus, 1053 Carling Ave, Ottawa ON K1Y 4E9; Wes'00; CCFP; Staff, The Ottawa Hospital - Civic Campus; (613)798-5555

NGUYEN, Tuong Minh; Clinique Med de Castelnau, 785 rue de Castelnau E, Montreal QC H2R 3A3; Sher'95; CCFP; Staff, CSSS du Coeur de l'Isle Hôpital Jean-Talon; Langs: Vietnamese; English; (514)277-4143; Fax. (514)277-4144.

NGUYEN, Tuong-Nam; Lakeshore Ophthalmology, 240-315 boul Brunswick, Pointe-Claire QC H9R 5M7; McG'98; DABOph; FRCSC; Ophth. Ac Member, Centre Hospitalier Pierre le Gardeur; Assoc Member, Sir Mortimer B Davis Jewish General; Assoc Member, St Mary's Hospital Centre; Langs: English; (514)694-2010; Fax. (514)694-0772.

NGUYEN, Tuyet Thi; 50-470 Dundas St E, Belleville ON K8N 1G1; Mon'84; FAAP; FRCPC; CCFP; Peds. Langs: English; French; Vietnamese; (613)966-4045; Fax. (613)966-0072.

NGUYEN, Uyen-Phuong; Hôpital Ste-Justine, 3175 ch Cote-Sainte-Catherine, Montreal QC H3T 1C5; Sher'82; Peds. Ac Staff, Hôpital Ste-Justine; Universite de Montreal; (514)345-4931; Fax. (514)345-4822.

NGUYEN, Van Dong; 8335 rue Notre-Dame E, Montreal QC H1L 3L2; Saigon (Vietnam)'75; (514)354-3330

NGUYEN, Van Hanh; 25-2300 Finch Ave W, York ON M9N 3Y3; (Vietnam)'79; CCFP; (647)748-4818

NGUYEN, Van Hoi; Clinique CMI, 240-2040 boul Marcel-Laurin, Saint-Laurent QC H4R 1J9; Saigon (Vietnam)'78; LMCC; CCFP; Langs: Vietnamese; English; (514)747-9936; vanhoi_nguyen@hotmail.com.

NGUYEN, Van Thanh; Ctr Hosp Fleury, 2180 rue Fleury E, Montreal QC H2B 1K3; Saigon (Vietnam)'75; Staff, Centre Hospitalier Fleury; (514)384-2000

NGUYEN, Van Thuy; 1001 10 Ave SW, Calgary AB T2R 0B7; Cal'05; CCFP; (403)221-8797; Fax. (403)221-8785.

NGUYEN, Van Tuong; 1450 Queen St W, Toronto ON M6K 1M2; Saigon (Vietnam)'71; Staff Family & Community Med, Toronto Western Hospital - University Health Network; Langs: Vietnamese; (647)436-8244; Fax. (647)436-8281.

NGUYEN, Van Vu; CSSS Pierre Boucher, 1333 boul Jacques-Cartier E, Longueuil QC J4M 2A5; Mon'90; FRCPC; IntMed; Gastroent. Staff, Centre Hospitalier Pierre Boucher; (450)647-2422

NGUYEN, Van-Hung; MUHC-Montreal Children's Hosp, D469-2300 rue Tupper, Montreal QC H3H 1P3; Mon'92; CSPQ; FRCPC; AnatPath (Pediatric Pathology). Staff, McGill University Health Centre - Montreal Children's Hospital; Langs: English; French; Vietnamese; (514)412-4400; van-hung.nguyen@muhc.mcgill.ca.

NGUYEN, Van-Phuc; 3-4298 rue Saint-Denis, Montreal QC H2J 2K8; Mon'78; (514)849-2261; Fax. (514)849-2262.

NGUYEN, Van-Tri; CLSC Riviere-des-Prairies, 8655 boul Perras, Montreal QC H1E 4M7; Lyon (France)'82; (514)494-4924

NGUYEN, Van-Tri; Clinique Med Viauville, 4639 rue Ontario E, Montreal QC H1V 1L1; Saigon (Vietnam)'70; (514)252-8778

NGUYEN, Vi Liet; 1019 Kingsway, Vancouver BC V5V 3C7; Saigon (Vietnam)'78; Langs: Vietnamese; (604)709-0859

NGUYEN, Viem Chung; 408-1160 Burrard St, Vancouver BC V6Z 2E8; Mon'02; FRCPC; PhysMed&Rehab. Staff, Providence Health Care - St Paul's Hospital; Staff, Providence Health Care - Holy Family Hospital; Langs: Vietnamese; French; (604)646-4637; vnguyen@providencehealth.bc.ca.

NGUYEN, Viet Huan; CHUM-Hotel-Dieu, 3840 rue Saint-Urbain, Montreal QC H2W 1T8; Mon'99; Staff, Centre Hospitalier l'Université de Montréal (CHUM) - Hôtel-Dieu; (514)890-8000

NGUYEN, Vinh-Kim; Clinique Med l'Actuel, 1001 boul de Maisonneuve E, Montreal QC H2L 4P9; Mon'90; Staff, McGill University Health Centre - Montreal General Campus; (514)524-1001; Fax. (514)524-3831.

NGUYEN, Viviane T Q; MUHC-Royal Victoria Hosp, M4.76-687 av des Pins O, Montreal QC H3A 1A1; McG'98; FRCPC; IntMed; Cardiol. Staff, McGill University Health Centre - Royal Victoria Hospital; (514)934-1934 x35737

NGUYEN, Xong Thi; Hotel-Dieu Grace Hosp, 1030 Ouellette Ave, Windsor ON N9A 1E1; (Vietnam)'78; FRCPC; AnatPath. Pathologist, Hôtel-Dieu Grace Hospital; Fax. (519)258-5421; xnguyen@hdgh.org.

NGUYEN, Xuan Trinh; CLSC Simonne-Monet-Chartrand, 1303 boul Jacques-Cartier E, Longueuil QC J4M 2Y8; Saigon (Vietnam)'65; (450)463-2850 x2208; Fax. (450)463-1879.

NGUYEN, Xuan-Tung; Riverview Health Centre, 1 Morley Ave, Winnipeg MB R3L 2P4; Man'87; Med Officer, Riverview Health Centre; (204)452-3411; Fax. (204)287-8718.

NGUYEN, Xuandieu T; 100-3633 Westwinds Dr NE, Calgary AB T3J 5K3; Alb'00; CCFP; Langs: Vietnamese; (403)266-8050; Fax. (403)663-8821.

NGUYEN BUU, Paul; CSSS du Sud de Lanaudière, 911 montee des Pionniers, Terrebonne QC J6V 2H2; Mon'95; GenSurg. Staff, Centre Hospitalier Pierre le Gardeur; (450)654-7525

NGUYEN-DANG, Thuy-Tien; CSSS de la Matapedia, 135 av Gaetan-Archambault, Amqui QC G5J 2K5; Laval'05; Staff, CSSS de la Matapedia; Langs: Vietnamese; English; Spanish; (418)629-2211

NGUYEN DO, Uyen Ly; CLSC Saint-Leonard, 5540 rue Jarry E, Saint-Leonard QC H1P 1T9; Laval'00; CCFP; Staff Med, Institut Universitaire de Gériatrie de Montréal; Langs: Vietnamese; (514)328-3460

NGUYEN DUONG, Y Nhu; Ctr Hosp Anna-Laberge, 200 boul Brisebois, Chateauguay QC J6K 4W8; Mon'04; CCFP; Staff, Hôpital Anna-Laberge; (450)699-2425

NGUYEN GIA, Le Thi; Hop Maisonneuve-Rosemont, 5415 boul de l'Assomption, Montreal QC H1T 2M4; Mon'97; Staff, Hopital Maisonneuve-Rosemont; (514)252-3400

NGUYEN-GIANG, Quynh-Lang; West Oak Med Clinic, 2495 Old Bronte Rd, Oakville ON L6M 4J2; Glasgow (Scotland)'06; BSc; MSc; CCFP; Surg Asst, St Joseph's Health Centre; Langs: Vietnamese; (905)582-7533; Fax. (905)582-0766.

NGUYEN-HO, Phong; Kawartha Cardiology Clinic, 327 Charlotte St, Peterborough ON K9J 0B2; Alb'96; BMedSci; Cardiol; IntMed (Interventional Cardiology). Langs: French; Vietnamese; (705)775-0145; Fax. (705)775-0128.

NGUYEN-HUYNH, Thu-Van; CHUM-Hop Notre-Dame, 1560 rue Sherbrooke E, Montreal QC H2L 4M1; Mon'91; CSPQ; FRCPC; RadOncol (Gynecology). Staff, Centre Hospitalier l'Université de Montréal (CHUM) - Hôpital Notre-Dame; (514)890-8254; Fax. (514)412-7537.

NGUYEN LUU, Nha-Uyen; CSSS de Laval, 1755 boul Rene-Laennec, Laval QC H7M 3L9; Mon'02; FRCPC; Peds; ClinImmunol&Allergy. Staff, Hopital de la Cite de la santé; (450)668-1010

NGUYEN-NGOC, Bao; Clin Med Papineau, 6930 av Papineau, Montreal QC H2G 2X7; Saigon (Vietnam)'67; Staff, Hopital Maisonneuve-Rosemont; (514)722-0000

NGUYEN-ONG, Thi Khanh Van; Inst U Geriatrie de Montreal, 4565 ch Queen-Mary, Montreal QC H3W 1W5; Mon'79; Staff, Institut Universitaire de Gériatrie de Montréal; (514)340-2800

NGUYEN-TAN, Felix Phuc; CHUM-Hop Notre-Dame, 1560 rue Sherbrooke E, Montreal QC H2L 4M1; McG'93; CSPQ; FRCPC; RadOncol. Staff, Centre Hospitalier l'Université de Montréal (CHUM) - Hôpital Notre-Dame; Langs: English; Vietnamese; (514)890-8254; Fax. (514)412-7537; felix.nguyen.chum@ssss.gouv.qc.ca.

NGUYEN THANH, Hien-Tu; CSSS de Laval, 1755 boul Rene-Laennec, Laval QC H7M 3L9; Sher'06; FRCPC; IntMed. Staff, Hopital de la Cite de la santé; (450)668-1010

NGUYEN THE, My; Clin de Med Familiale de Hull, 202-15 boul Montclair, Gatineau QC J8Y 2E2; Laval'81; Staff, Hull Hospital; (819)777-2752; Fax. (819)777-2269.

NGUYEN-TUONG, Phong; CHUM-Hotel-Dieu, 3840 rue Saint-Urbain, Montreal QC H2W 1T8; McG'96; FRCPC; IntMed (Echocardiography); Cardiol. Staff, Centre Hospitalier l'Université de Montréal (CHUM) - Hôtel-Dieu; (514)890-8000

NGUYEN VAN NGUYEN, Paul; CHUM-Hotel-Dieu, 3840 rue Saint-Urbain, Montreal QC H2W 1T8; Sher'80; FRCPC; IntMed (Clinical Pharmacology). Staff, Centre Hospitalier l'Université de Montréal (CHUM) - Hôtel-Dieu; adj Prof Med, Universite de Montreal; (514)890-8000 x12907; pnguyen920@aol.com.

NHAN, Toan D; Nhan Medicine Prof Corp, 506-800 Bathurst St, Toronto ON M5R 3M8; Saigon (Vietnam)'77; Staff, Toronto Western Hospital - University Health Network; Langs: Cantonese; Mandarin; Vietnamese; (416)535-2737; Fax. (416)531-7766.

NI, Hongyu; Calgary Lab Services, 9-3535 Research Rd NW, Calgary AB T2L 2K8; '82.

NIA, Ali; 1 Oak St, Simcoe ON N3Y 3J4; Tabriz (Iran)'73; ABIM; FRCPC; IntMed (Gastroenterology). Staff, Norfolk General Hospital; Langs: Persian; (519)426-1001; Fax. (519)426-1005.

NIA, Keon M; 2-125 Steamship Bay Rd, Gravenhurst ON P1P 1Z9; Tor'03; FRCSC; Ophth. (705)687-9520

NIAJKO, Anna; CLSC de Richelieu, 300 ch de Marieville, Richelieu QC J3L 3V8; Frankfurt (Germany)'98; Langs: German; English; Polish; (450)658-2264; Fax. (450)658-4390.

NIAKOSARI, Firouzeh; Bayview North Dermatology Clin, 205-3292 Bayview Ave, North York ON M2M 4J5; Shaheed Beheshti (Iran)'90; FRCPC; AnatPath (Dermatological Pathology); Derm. Staff, North York General Hospital; Langs: Farsi; Urdu; Arabic; (416)222-7546; Fax. (416)221-7546.

NIANIARIS, Nicholas; 200-245 Danforth Ave, Toronto ON M4K 1N2; Tor'88; FRCSC; Ophth. (416)462-0393; Fax. (416)462-3612.

NIAZ, Ayyan; Credit Valley Prof Bldg, 109-2300 Eglinton Ave W, Mississauga ON L5M 2V8; Tor'95; FRCSC; GenSurg. (905)607-6398

NIAZ, Majid; Moose Jaw Cardiac Centre, 361 Main St N, Moose Jaw SK S6H 0W2; (306)692-5066; Fax. (306)691-5966.

NIAZI, Ahtsham U; Univ Hlth Network-Toronto Western Hosp, MC2 405-399 Bathurst St, Toronto ON M5T 2S8; Karachi (Pakistan)'93; FRCPC; Anes. Staff, Toronto Western Hospital - University Health Network; (416)603-5118

NIAZI, Mohammad T; SMBD Jewish Gen Hosp, 3755 ch Cote-Sainte-Catherine, Montreal QC H3T 1E2; McG'01; FRCPC; RadOncol. Staff, Sir Mortimer B Davis Jewish General; Langs: Bilingual(French/English); (514)340-8288; Fax. (514)340-7548.

NIAZI, Nazia S; 103-8386 120 St, Surrey BC V3W 3N4; Punjab (Pakistan)'94; Langs: Punjabi; Hindi; Urdu; (604)592-9898; Fax. (604)592-9866.

NICA-DANES, Doina; Clinique de Med Industrielle, 1665 rue Sainte-Catherine O, Montreal QC H3H 1L9; Timisoara (Romania)'80; Staff, Providence Notre-Dame-de-Lourdes Inc; Médecin, Clinique de Medecin Industrielle; Langs: Italian; Romanian; English; (514)931-0801; Fax. (514)931-0437.

NICE, Charles A; Saint John Reg Hosp, PO Box 2100 Stn Main 400 University Ave, Saint John NB E2L 4L2; McG'01; CSPQ; FRCPC; Anes. Staff, Saint John Regional Hospital; (506)648-6861

NICHOL, Alan M; BC Cancer Agency-Vancouver CC, 600 10th Ave W, Vancouver BC V5Z 4E6; Cal'93; FRCPC; RadOncol (Brain Tumors);CCFP; Staff, BC Cancer Agency Vancouver Centre; Staff, Vancouver General Hospital - Centennial Pavillion; University of British Columbia; (604)877-6000 x2380; Fax. (604)877-0505; anichol@bccancer.bc.ca.

NICHOL, Christopher S; Smith Clinic, 1-6601 48 Ave, Camrose AB T4V 3G8; Cal'93; CCFP; (780)672-2425; Fax. (780)679-2668.

NICHOL, Erin J; Coast Med Clinic, 1018 Seymour St, Vancouver BC V6B 3M6; UBC'03; CCFP; (604)569-3632

NICHOL, Rowland T; Alberta Prof Bldg, 302-320 23 Ave SW, Calgary AB T2S 0J2; Man'79; CCFP; FCFP; Staff, Rockyview General Hospital; (403)228-9021; Fax. (403)228-7923.

NICHOLAS, Cynthia S; 203-10168 Yonge St, Richmond Hill ON L4C 1T6; UBC'80; BSc; FRCSC; ObstGyn (Menopause). Staff Ob/Gyn, Mackenzie Richmond Hill Hospital; (905)884-6119; Fax. (905)884-0528.

NICHOLAS, Garth A; The Ottawa Hosp-Gen Campus, 501 Smyth Rd, Ottawa ON K1H 8L6; Man'98; FRCPC; IntMed (Lung Tumors); MedOncol. Staff Regional Cancer Ctre, The Ottawa Hospital - General Campus; (613)737-7700

NICHOLAS, Paul R; Cambridge Mem Hosp, 800 Coronation Blvd, Cambridge ON N1R 3G2; Dal'74; FRCPC; Anes. Staff, Cambridge Memorial Hospital; (519)621-2330 x2100

NICHOLAS, R Everton S; 214-840 Coxwell Ave, Toronto ON M4C 5T2; University of theWest Indies (Jamaica)'85; MB BS; FRCPC; IntMed; Endocrin&Metab. Head Div of Endocrinology, Toronto East General Hospital Inc; (416)463-6280

NICHOLAS, Seetha D; Rouge Valley-Ajax & Pickering, 580 Harwood Ave S, Ajax ON L1S 2J4; Transkei (South Africa)'91; MB ChB; CCFP; FCFP; Staff, Rouge Valley Health System - Ajax & Pickering Health Centre Site; (905)683-2320 x3200

NICHOLAS, Timothy G; Aurora Med Centre, 201-15017 Yonge St, Aurora ON L4G 1M5; Tor'80; Staff, Southlake Regional Health Centre; (905)727-9447; Fax. (905)727-7938.

NICHOLLS, Eric; Thames Valley FHT-Whitehills M, 1225 Wonderland Rd N, London ON N6G 2V9; Wes'93; CCFP; FCFP; Staff, St Joseph's Hospital - St Joseph's Health Care; (519)472-0040; Fax. (519)472-7732.

NICHOLLS, Michael J; RCMP Training Depot, PO Box 6500 Stn Main, Regina SK S4P 3J7; Sask'90; BSc; Dip SportMed; CCFP; FCFP; Clin Assoc Prof, University of Saskatchewan; (306)780-3923

NICHOLLS, Pamela J H; Victoria Youth Clinic, 547 Michigan St, Victoria BC V8V 1S5; Cal'78; (250)388-7841

NICHOLLS, Vaughan; La Loche Health Centre, PO Box 1, La Loche SK S0M 1G0; London (England)'78; MB BS; MRCGPract; DA; DRCOG; Staff, La Loche Health Centre and Hospital; Clin Assoc Prof, University of Saskatchewan; Langs: English; French; (306)822-3201; Fax. (306)822-2798; v.nicholls@sasktel.net.

NICHOLS, Anthony; B3 431A-800 Commissioners Rd E, London ON N6A 5W9; Tor'03; BSc; FRCSC; Otol (Head & Neck Surgery). Asst Prof otol, University of Western Ontario; (519)685-8599; Fax. (519)685-8567; samantha.jones@lhsc.on.ca.

NICHOLS, Bruce; St Joseph's Health Care, PO Box 5777 Stn B 268 Grosvenor St, London ON N6A 4V2; McM'80; BSc; DAB; FACS; FRCSC; Ophth (Cornea). Consultant, London Health Sciences Centre - Victoria Campus; Consultant, St Joseph's Hospital - St Joseph's Health Care; Med Dir, TLC Laser Eye Center; Assoc Prof Ophth, University of Western Ontario; (519)646-6000

NICHOLS, Darren N; University of Alberta Hosp, 1G1.50WCM-8440 112 St NW, Edmonton AB T6G 2B7; Alb'00; CCFP; CCFP(E.M.); Staff, University of Alberta Hospital; (780)407-7047; Fax. (780)407-3314.

NICHOLS, Dorin; Hamilton HS-General Site, 237 Barton St E, Hamilton ON L8L 2X2; Cluj-Napoca (Romania)'82; FRCPC; Psy. Staff, St Joseph's Healthcare Hamilton - West 5th Campus; Staff, Hamilton Health Sciences Centre - Hamilton General Hospital; (905)527-4322; Fax. (905)527-3360.

NICHOLS, Erwin B; AIM Orleans Hlth & Wellness Cl, 3-1605 Orleans Blvd, Orleans ON K1C 7E2; Ott'57; Ac Staff, The Ottawa Hospital - General Campus; Ac Staff, Children's Hospital of Eastern Ontario (CHEO); (613)830-6890; Fax. (613)837-6312.

NICHOLS, J Bradley; 3-15 Elizabeth St E, Creemore ON L0M 1G0; Tor'83; CCFP; FCFP; Staff, Collingwood General & Marine Hospital; (705)466-2252; Fax. (705)466-2873.

NICHOLS, Jeffrey L; 729 Devonshire Ave, Woodstock ON N4S 5R3; McM'86; CCFP; FCFP; Assoc Staff, Woodstock General Hospital; (519)533-5321; Fax. (519)533-0499.

NICHOLS, Melinda; Penticton Reg Hosp, 550 Carmi Ave, Penticton BC V2A 3G6; Cluj-Nopoca (Romania)'82; FRCPC; Psy. Staff, Penticton Regional Hospital; Langs: Hungarian; Romanian; (250)492-4000

NICHOLS, Robert B; Queensway-Carleton Hosp, 3045 Baseline Rd, Ottawa ON K2H 8P4; Qns'08; FRCPC; IntMed. Staff, Queensway Carleton Hospital; (613)721-2000

NICHOLSON, Allan J B; Medical Clinic, 9815 Main St, Fort McMurray AB T9H 1T7; Alb'62; (780)743-2275; Fax. (780)743-5475.

NICHOLSON, Ashley; Ladner Family Practice, 204-4515 Harvest Dr, Delta BC V4K 4L1; (Czech Republic)'09; CCFP.

NICHOLSON, Brian M; St Martha's Reg Hosp, 25 Bay St, Antigonish NS B2G 2G5; Dal'97; FRCPC; DiagRad. Staff, St Martha's Regional Hospital; (902)863-2830

NICHOLSON, C David; Niagara Falls Med Centre, 103-6453 Morrison St, Niagara Falls ON L2E 7H1; Cambridge (England)'70; DObstRCOG; Ac Staff, Niagara Health System - Greater Niagara General Site; (905)356-4151; Fax. (905)356-7100.

NICHOLSON, Daniel J; Mineville Health Centre, 4 Peter Crt, Mineville NS B2Z 1K2; Dal'84; Ac Staff, Cape Breton Healthcare Complex; (902)829-3278; Fax. (902)829-2549.

NICHOLSON, Donna J; Univ of Ottawa Heart Institute, H213-40 Ruskin St, Ottawa ON K1Y 4W7; Man'95; FRCPC; Anes. Staff, University of Ottawa Heart Institute; (613)761-4379; Fax. (613)761-4925.

NICHOLSON, Elizabeth J; Maple Family Health Team, 325 University Ave, Kingston ON K7L 3R4; Dal'88; CCFP; (613)544-2902; Fax. (613)544-5768.

NICHOLSON, James K; 292 Main St, Toronto ON M4C 4X5; Tor'60; (416)694-4324; Fax. (416)694-4324.

NICHOLSON, Janis L; The Jenny Trout Centre, 110-342 Erie St, Stratford ON N5A 2N4; Dal'99; FRCPC; IntMed. Ac Staff, Stratford General Hospital - Huron Perth Healthcare Alliance; (519)273-0100; Fax. (519)273-0675.

NICHOLSON, Jennifer; 207-42 Glen Allan Dr, Bridgewater NS B4V 3N2; Cal'95; FRCSC; ObstGyn. Staff, South Shore Regional Hospital; (902)543-8788; Fax. (902)543-3334.

NICHOLSON, Joanne M; 172 Meadowlark Shopping Ctr NW, Edmonton AB T5R 5W9; Cal'01; FRCPC; IntMed. Staff, University of Alberta Hospital; (780)235-7511; Fax. (780)444-6936.

NICHOLSON, John D; Woodlawn Med Clinic, 92 Main St, Dartmouth NS B2X 1R5; Dal'91; CCFP; (902)434-1500; Fax. (902)434-7360.

NICHOLSON, Katrina M; Cochrane Primary Care Center, 103-100 Grande Blvd W, Cochrane AB T4C 0S4; (United Kingdom)'88; MB ChB; MRCGPract; LMCC; CCFP; Clin Lecturer Family Med, University of Calgary; (403)932-2089; Fax. (403)932-1820.

NICHOLSON, Marc D; 160-600 Main St, Saint John NB E2K 1J5; Dal'02; FRCPC; Peds. Staff, Saint John Regional Hospital; (506)648-7579; Fax. (506)648-7620.

NICHOLSON, Marcia A; Cachet Family Physicians, 2-9255 Woodbine Ave, Markham ON L6C 1Y9; Wes'02; CCFP; (905)887-2222; Fax. (905)887-3655.

NICHOLSON, Miriam L; Greenbank Med Centre, 206-139 Greenbank Rd, Nepean ON K2H 9A5; Dal'91; (613)680-8413; Fax. (613)680-8419.

NICHOLSON, Naomi L; 208-189 Kent St, Lindsay ON K9V 5G6; Wes'08; CCFP; (705)880-0501; Fax. (705)880-0505.

NICHOLSON, R Derek; Sheppard Med Bldg, 204-701 Sheppard Ave E, North York ON M2K 2Z3; Tor'69; FRCSC; ObstGyn (Obstetrics). Chair Practice Counsel Dept, North York General Hospital; Asst Prof, University of Toronto; (416)223-9505; Fax. (416)223-3243.

NICHOLSON, R Lawrence; Brant Community HC-Brantford, 200 Terrace Hill St, Brantford ON N3R 1G9; Dal'69; FRCPC; DiagRad; NuclearMed. Consultant, London Health Sciences Centre - University Hospital; Staff, The Brant Community Healthcare System - Brantford General Hospital Site; Assoc Staff, Woodstock General Hospital; Prof, University of Western Ontario; (519)752-7871

NICHOLSON, Raymond F; 1187 Fischer Hallman Rd, Kitchener ON N2E 4H9; Tor'81; Staff, St Mary's General Hospital; Staff, Grand River Hospital - Kitchener/Waterloo Health Centre; (519)570-1200; Fax. (519)570-1214.

NICHOLSON, Robert M; CSSS de la Haute-Yamaska, 205 boul Leclerc O, Granby QC J2G 1T7; McG'93; CSPQ; FRCPC; AnatPath. Staff, Centre Hospitalier de Granby; Langs: English; French; (450)375-8000 x2210

NICHOLSON, Ronald D; Summerside Med Centre, 101-475 Granville St, Summerside PE C1N 3N9; Dal'75; CCFP; Ac Staff, Prince County Hospital; (902)432-8181; Fax. (902)432-8166.

NICKEL, J Curtis; Kingston Gen Hosp, 76 Stuart St, Kingston ON K7L 2V7; Qns'78; FRCSC; Urol (Prostate Disorder). Staff, Kingston General Hospital; Staff, Hotel-Dieu Hospital; Staff, Weeneebayko General Hospital; Prof, Queen's University; (613)548-2497; Fax. (613)545-1970; marquesc@kgh.kari.net.

NICKEL, Krista H; Royal Columbian Hosp, 330 Columbia St E, New Westminster BC V3L 3W7; Sask'85; FRCPC; Anes. Staff Anes, Royal Columbian Hospital; (604)520-4602; Fax. (604)986-2243.

NICKEL, Lucy C; Packham Avenue Med Clinic, 104-335 Packham Ave, Saskatoon SK S7N 4S1; Sask'00; CCFP; (306)651-7091; Fax. (306)651-7092.

NICKEL, Murray; Abbotsford Reg Hosp & Cancer C, 32900 Marshall Rd, Abbotsford BC V2S 0C2; UBC'90; CCFP; CCFP(E.M.); FCFP; Staff, Ridge Meadows Hospital & Health Care Centre; (604)851-4700

NICKELL, Leslie A; Sunnybrook Hlth Sciences Ctre, A112-2075 Bayview Ave, Toronto ON M4N 3M5; McM'89; CCFP; Ac Staff Family & Community Med, Sunnybrook Health Sciences Centre; Assoc Dean Health Professions Student Affairs/Prof, University of Toronto; (416)480-4942; Fax. (416)480-6038.

NICKERSON, Duncan A; 101-7 Glenbrook Pl SW, Calgary AB T3E 6W4; Cal'95; FRCSC; PlasSurg. (403)282-6800; Fax. (403)282-6890; drnickerson@me.com.

NICKERSON, J Paul; Lake Country Family Practice, 1-9966 Pollard Rd, Winfield BC V4V 1Z4; UBC'98; CCFP; Staff, Kelowna General Hospital; (250)766-3938; Fax. (250)766-5231; pcnickerson@yahoo.com.

NICKERSON, Katelyn E; Arbour Family Medicine, 201-770 Broadview Ave, Ottawa ON K2A 3Z3; Dal'07; CCFP; (613)680-1065

NICKERSON, Kenneth R; Alberta Place, 1520 4 St SW, Calgary AB T2R 1H5; Dal'67; (403)297-8511; Fax. (403)297-6221; nickerson.ken@syncrude.com.

NICKERSON, Leigh; University of Alberta Hosp, 2D2.01-8440 112 St NW, Edmonton AB T6G 2B7; Mem'06; CCFP; Staff, University of Alberta Hospital; (780)407-6325; Fax. (780)407-3283.

NICKERSON, Peter W; Health Sciences Centre, GE421-820 Sherbrook St, Winnipeg MB R3A 1R9; Man'86; FRCPC; IntMed. Staff, Health Sciences Centre; Assoc Dean Research, University of Manitoba; (204)774-6511; sstokoloff@exchange.hsc.mb.ca.

NICKSON, Lisa; Airport Way Med Clinic, PO Box 2000 5216 Airport Dr, Fort Nelson BC V0C 1R0; Kharkov (Ukraine)'99; CCFP; (250)774-7838

NICLOUX, Nathalie; Clinique Privamed, 203-1052 rue Lionel-Daunais, Boucherville QC J4B 0B2; Mon'01; CCFP; (450)652-6222

NICOARA, Lucia V; Weeneebayko Gen Hosp, PO Box 34 19 Hospital Dr, Moose Factory ON P0L 1W0; (Romania)'81; CCFP; Staff, Weeneebayko General Hospital; (705)658-4544

NICOL, Julie A; East Kootenay Reg Hosp, 13 24th Ave N, Cranbrook BC V1C 3H9; Cal'01; FRCPC; DiagRad. Staff, East Kootenay Regional Hospital; (250)426-5281 x6366

NICOL, Odette; Centre Med Sainte-Foy Inc, 802 av du Chanoine-Scott, Quebec QC G1V 3N4; Laval'88; Physician, Clinique Medicale Universite Laval; (418)663-2572; Fax. (418)663-2624; odette.nicol@ssss.gouv.qc.ca.

NICOL, Olu-Kayode; 223 Lakeshore Rd E, Mississauga ON L5G 1G5; London (England)'82; MB BS; DOHS; Langs: French; (905)274-2779; Fax. (905)891-5697.

NICOLAIDIS, Stephen C; Clinique Contour, 4638 boul Saint-Laurent, Montreal QC H2T 1R3; McG'91; FRCSC; PlasSurg. (514)297-7768

NICOLAOU, Georghios; London HSC-Victoria Hosp, PO Box 5010 Stn B 2F-800 Commissioners Rd E, London ON N6A 5W9; Witwatersrand (South Africa)'88; FRCPC; Anes. Staff, London Health Sciences Centre - Victoria Campus; (519)685-8525; Fax. (519)685-8275.

NICOLAOU, Savvakis; 899 12th Ave W, Vancouver BC V5Z 1M9; Tor'92; FRCPC; DiagRad. Staff, Vancouver General Hospital - Centennial Pavillion; Staff, UBC Hospital - Koerner Pavillion; Staff, Ridge Meadows Hospital & Health Care Centre; Langs: Greek; (604)875-4111 x63659; Fax. (604)875-5195.

NICOLAS, Eric; Centre Hosp Honore-Mercier, 2750 boul Laframboise, Saint-Hyacinthe QC J2S 4Y8; Sher'81; CSPQ; FRCPC; DiagRad. Staff, Centre Hospitalier Honore-Mercier; (450)771-3377

NICOLAS, Hanna; Inst de MedSpecialisee de Lava, 1875 rue Maurice-Gauvin, Laval QC H7S 2M5; Laval'07; CCFP; (450)902-9985

NICOLAS, Isabelle; Hop Brome-Missiquoi-Perkins, 950 rue Principale, Cowansville QC J2K 1K3; Sher'99; CCFP; Staff, Hôpital Brome-Missisquoi-Perkins; (450)266-5500; Fax. (450)263-8669; isabelle_nicolas@hotmail.com.

NICOLAS, Marjolaine; CSSS de Rimouski-Neigette, CP 3150 Succ A 150 av Rouleau, Rimouski QC G5L 5T1; Laval'08; Staff, Hôpital Regional Rimouski; (418)724-3000; Fax. (418)724-8632.

NICOLE, Luc; Hop Louis-H Lafontaine, 304-7401 rue Hochelaga, Montreal QC H1N 3M5; Mon'86; FRCPC; Psy. Staff, Hopital Louis-H Lafontaine; (514)251-4000

NICOLE, Marie-Noelle; Montfort Hosp, 713 Montreal Rd, Ottawa ON K1K 0T2; Mon'98; CCFP; Staff, Montfort Hospital; Langs: English; (613)746-4621

NICOLE, Marjory; CSSS de Saint-Jerome, 290 rue de Montigny, Saint-Jerome QC J7Z 5T3; Mon'95; Staff, Hôtel-Dieu de Saint-Jérôme; Staff, Hôpital de Saint-Eustache; Staff, Carrefour Sante Granit; (450)432-2777

NICOLE, Patricia; CSSS Pierre Boucher, 1333 boul Jacques-Cartier E, Longueuil QC J4M 2A5; Mon'95; Staff, Centre Hospitalier Pierre Boucher; (450)468-8111

NICOLE, Pierre; Ctr Hosp Affilie-Enfant-Jesus, 1401 18e rue, Quebec QC G1J 1Z4; Laval'95; CSPQ; FRCPC; Anes. Staff, Centre Hospitalier Affilié Universitaire de Québec - Hôpital De L'Enfant Jésus; (418)649-5807; Fax. (418)649-5918.

NICOLE, Sophie; CSSSQS-Point de Serv Ste-Foy, 3108 ch Sainte-Foy, Quebec QC G1X 1P8; Laval'00; CCFP; (418)651-2572

NICOLELA, Marcelo T; Queen Elizabeth II HSC, 1276 South Park St, Halifax NS B3H 2Y9; Sao Paulo (Brazil)'89; FRCSC; Ophth (Glaucoma). Staff, Queen Elizabeth II Health Sciences Centre - Victoria General Site; Staff, IWK Health Centre; Dalhousie University; Langs: Portuguese; Spanish; (902)473-3622; Fax. (902)473-2839.

NICOLESCU-ZINCA, Alexandru; CLSC Cote-des-Neiges, 500-5700 ch de la Cote-des-Nei, Montreal QC H3T 2A8; Bucharest (Romania)'82; CCFP; Staff, Institut Universitaire de Gériatrie de Montréal; Langs: Romanian; English; (514)731-8531

NICOLET, Jannick M L; Cyclone Sante, 280A boul de la Seigneurie O, Blainville QC J7C 5A1; McG'87; CCFP; FCFP; Staff, St Mary's Hospital Centre; (450)979-1277

NICOLET, Viviane; CHUM-Hop Notre-Dame, 1560 rue Sherbrooke E, Montreal QC H2L 4M1; Sher'80; CSPQ; FRCPC; DiagRad. Staff, Centre Hospitalier l'Université de Montréal (CHUM) - Hôpital Notre-Dame; (514)890-8000 x28530

NICOLETTI, Bruno S; 16 Green St, Nepean ON K2J 3R2; Ott'01; CCFP; Langs: Italian; French; (613)825-9799

NICOLL, Robert D; 200-3994 Shelbourne St, Victoria BC V8N 3E2; Alb'75; (250)477-7100; Fax. (250)477-4135.

NICOLLE, David A; London HSC-University Hosp, PO Box 5339 Stn B 339 Windermere Rd, London ON N6A 5A5; Birmingham (England)'71; MB ChB; DOphth; FRCS(Ed); FRCSC; Ophth (Neuro Ophthalmology). Ac Staff, London Health Sciences Centre - University Hospital; Prof, University of Western Ontario; (519)663-3702; Fax. (519)663-3990.

NICOLLE, Lindsay E; Health Sciences Centre, GG443-820 Sherbrook St, Winnipeg MB R3A 1R9; Man'74; BScMed; FRCPC; IntMed; InfectDis. Consultant Infectious Diseases, Health Sciences Centre; Prof IntMed, University of Manitoba; (204)787-7029

NICOLLE, Michael W; London HSC-University Hosp, PO Box 5339 Stn B 339 Windermere Rd, London ON N6A 5A5; Wes'85; PhD(Oxford); FRCPC; Neur (Electromyography). Staff, London Health Sciences Centre - University Hospital; Staff, Neuromuscular Clinic; Asst Prof, University of Western Ontario; (519)663-3236; Fax. (519)663-3328.

NICOLSON, R Bruce; Exeter Clinic, PO Box 879, 100 Mile House BC V0K 2E0; UBC'76; (250)395-2271; Fax. (250)395-2599.

NICOLSON, Robert J; London HSC-Victoria Hosp, PO Box 5010 Stn B B8 026-800 Commissioners Rd, London ON N6A 5W9; Wes'93; FRCPC; Psy. Staff, London Health Sciences Centre - Victoria Campus; (519)685-8427; Fax. (519)685-8595.

NICULA, Mihaela; Lakeridge Hlth Corp-Oshawa, 1 Hospital Crt, Oshawa ON L1G 2B9; Bucharest (Romania)'96; FRCPC; IntMed; GeriatricMed. Staff, Lakeridge Health - Oshawa Site; Langs: Romanian; (905)576-8711

NICULAE, Natalia; Humber Valley Med Centre, 7-2630 Kipling Ave, Etobicoke ON M9V 4B9; Bucharest (Romania)'52; (416)746-0389

NIE, Robert G; 301-849 Alexander Crt, Peterborough ON K9J 7H8; Wes'97; BSc; MSc; FRCSC; GenSurg; VascSurg. Staff, Peterborough Regional Health Centre - Hospital Drive; (705)743-6760; Fax. (705)743-9912.

NIEC, Anne; 3N10B-1280 Main St W, Hamilton ON L8S 4K1; Tor'85; FRCPC; Peds (Child Abuse). Dir Child Advocacy & Assessment Prog, Hamilton Health Sciences Centre - McMaster Children's Hospital; Prof Peds & Psy, McMaster University; (905)521-2100 x73268; Fax. (905)522-7982; nieca@mcmaster.ca.

NIECE, Donald P; William Osler HC-Brampton, 2100 Bovaird Dr E, Brampton ON L6R 3J7; Tor'67; Staff, William Osler Health System - Brampton Civic Hospital; (905)494-2120

NIEDERMAYER, Robert W; F W Green Med Centre, 1629 Baker St, Cranbrook BC V1C 1B4; Sask'69; (250)426-6601; Fax. (250)426-6470.

NIEDOBA, Joseph E; Goodfellow Prof Bldg, 201-170 McEwan Dr E, Bolton ON L7E 4C8; Tor'77; Staff, Headwaters Health Care Centre - Orangeville Site; Staff, William Osler Health System - Etobicoke General Hospital; (905)857-2356; Fax. (905)857-6253.

NIEL, Ullanda; 629 Markham Rd, Scarborough ON M1H 2A4; Albany NY (USA)'09; CCFP; (416)642-9445; Fax. (416)284-1964.

NIELD, Antony S; Thistlewood Prof Centre, 301-8077 Islington Ave, Woodbridge ON L4L 7X7; Mem'85; (905)851-1449; Fax. (905)264-8847; nield.nieldmd@bellnet.ca.

NIELD, Gail L; Thistlewood Prof Centre, 301-8077 Islington Ave, Woodbridge ON L4L 7X7; Mem'84; FRCPC; Derm. Lecturer, University of Toronto; (905)851-1436

NIELD, Lynne E; The Hosp for Sick Children, 555 University Ave, Toronto ON M5G 1X8; Qns'94; FRCPC; Peds; Cardiol. Assoc Staff, The Hospital For Sick Children; Staff, North York General Hospital; Ac Staff, Toronto East General Hospital Inc; Langs: English; French; (416)813-6141; Fax. (416)813-5857.

NIELSEN, Anthony E; Doctor's Med Clinic, 215-3066 Shelbourne St, Victoria BC V8R 6T9; UBC'87; (250)388-4211; Fax. (250)383-4119.

NIELSEN, Darcy L; Lansdowne Professional Ctr II, 133-3066 Shelbourne St, Victoria BC V8R 6T9; UBC'91; (250)592-2219; Fax. (250)592-5398.

NIELSEN, Devin R; Canmore Gen Hosp, 1100 Hospital Pl, Canmore AB T1W 1N2; Cal'98; Dip SportMed; CCFP; FCFP; Staff, Canmore General Hospital; Langs: English; French; (403)678-5536; Fax. (403)678-1205.

NIELSEN, Gary K; Westside Integrated Health Ctr, 130-180 Wilson St, Victoria BC V9A 7N6; UBC'91; (250)388-4341

NIELSEN, Torsten; Vancouver Gen Hosp, JP1401-855 12th Ave W, Vancouver BC V5Z 1M9; McG'97; PhD; FRCPC; AnatPath. Staff, Vancouver General Hospital - Centennial Pavillion; Staff, Genetic Pathology Evaluation Centre; (604)875-4111 x66768; Fax. (604)875-4035.

NIELSEN, William R; Cowichan Med Centre, 3106 Gibbins Rd, Duncan BC V9L 1E8; Tor'84; FRCSC; Urol. (250)746-7711; Fax. (250)746-8809.

NIEMAN, Peter; 109-10333 Southport Rd SW, Calgary AB T2W 3X6; Stellenbosch (South Africa)'79; MB ChB; FRCPC; Peds. (403)253-2288; Fax. (403)255-9322.

NIEMAN, Riaan; Viking Med Clinic, PO Box 810 5301 51 St, Viking AB T0B 4N0; Pretoria (South Africa)'01; MB ChB; Langs: Afrikaans.

NIEMAN, Thomas E; East Kootenay Reg Hosp, 13 24th Ave N, Cranbrook BC V1C 3H9; Alb'69; BSc; FRCPC; Anes. Staff, East Kootenay Regional Hospital; (250)426-5281

NIEMAND, Rudolph E; Sylvan Med Centre, 5007 46 St, Sylvan Lake AB T4S 1C2; Stellenbosch (South Africa)'92; MB ChB; Langs: Afrikaans; (403)887-2221; Fax. (403)887-3777; rudiniemand@gmail.com.

NIEMANN, Andries J; Daysland Med Centre, PO Box 160 5120 50 St, Daysland AB T0B 1A0; Belleville (South Africa)'79; CCFP; (780)374-3944; Fax. (780)374-2433.

NIEMCZEWSKI, Pawel; 2685 36 St NE, Calgary AB T1Y 5S3; Cal'05; CCFP; (403)943-5000; Fax. (403)476-8784.

NIESNER, Claudia C F; 611 Wonderland Rd, London ON N6H 4V6; Saba (Netherlands Antilles)'08; CCFP; (519)471-6686; Fax. (519)471-2801.

NIESOBSKA, Violetta; The Doctor's Office, 387-25 Peel Centre Dr, Brampton ON L6T 3R5; Wes'89; CCFP; Ac Staff, William Osler Health System - Brampton Civic Hospital; Langs: Polish; (905)793-7077; Fax. (905)793-7506.

NIESSEN, Marcus P; 202-2224 Walker Rd, Windsor ON N8W 5L7; Wes'91; FRCSC; PlasSurg (Cosmetic Surgery). Ac Staff, Hôtel-Dieu Grace Hospital; Ac Staff, Windsor Regional Hospital - Metropolitan Site; (519)254-2676; Fax. (519)254-2659.

NIEUWOUDT, Stephanus; Family Med Associates, 5021 51 St, Lacombe AB T4L 2A3; (South Africa)'83; MB ChB; Langs: Afrikaans; (403)782-3351; Fax. (403)782-5879.

NIEUWSTRATEN, Paula; Taddle Creek Family Hlth Team, 302-790 Bay St, Toronto ON M5G 1N8; Amsterdam (Netherlands)'85; CCFP; FCFP; Court Staff, Women's College Hospital; Lecturer, University of Toronto; Langs: Dutch; German; (416)585-9555; Fax. (416)585-5815.

NIGAM, Anil; Institut de Cardiologie de Mtl, 5000 rue Belanger, Montreal QC H1T 1C8; Ott'93; FRCPC; IntMed; Cardiol. Staff Preventive Cardiol, Institut de Cardiologie de Montréal; assoc Prof Med, Universite de Montreal; Langs: English; French; (514)376-3330

NIGAM, Rashmi; 710 Pembina Hwy, Winnipeg MB R3M 2M6; Man'91; BSc; FRCSC; Ophth (Cataract Surgery). Staff, Misericordia Health Centre; Staff, Health Sciences Centre; Asst Prof, University of Manitoba; (204)956-0798; Fax. (204)949-1143.

NIGAM, Srishti P; D V Massey & Associates, 316-1 Kingsway Garden Mall NW, Edmonton AB T5G 3A6; Lucknow (India)'58; DTMH(Liverpool); FRCPC; GenPath (General Practice & Psychotherapy). Langs: Hindi; (780)471-1860; snigam@shaw.ca.

NIGAM, Tara; Smyth Med Centre, 326-1929 Russell Rd, Ottawa ON K1G 4G3; Sher'88; LMCC; FRCPC; Psy. Langs: English; French; (613)241-9494

NIGEN, Simon R J; 5415 boul de l'Assomption Service de dermatologie, Montreal QC H1T 2M4; Mon'97; PhmB; FAAD; FRCP; FRCPC; Derm (Allergy). Staff Derm, Hopital Maisonneuve-Rosemont; Langs: Breton; (514)252-3400 x1252; Fax. (514)768-9249; simonnigen@yahoo.com.

NIGHAT, Nazia; Killarney Medical Clinic, PO Box 1690, Killarney MB R0K 1G0; (Pakistan)'02; CCFP; (204)523-4609

NIGRIN, Jana; 200-10150 102 St NW, Edmonton AB T5J 5E2; Prague (Czech Republic)'66; FRCPC; MedMicrobiol (Bacteriology). Staff, Royal Alexandra Hospital; Staff, DynaLIFE Diagnostics; Clinical Asst Prof Med Microbiol & Immunol, University of Alberta; Langs: Slovak; Czech; (780)451-3702; Fax. (780)454-2845; jana.nigrin@albertahealthservices.ca.

NIGRO, Frank; Port Arthur Health Centre Inc, 194 Court St N, Thunder Bay ON P7A 4V7; Wes'91; FRCPC; IntMed (Cardiac Catheterization); Cardiol. Staff Invasive Cardiol/Dir Cardiol, Thunder Bay Regional Health Sciences Centre; Assoc Prof, Northern Ontario School of Medicine; Langs: Italian; (807)346-1000; Fax. (807)346-6206.

NIGRO, Mark K; Gordon & Leslie Diamond HCC, 6-2775 Laurel St, Vancouver BC V5Z 1M9; Alb'80; FRCSC; Urol. Staff, G F Strong Rehabilitation Centre; Staff, Vancouver General Hospital - Centennial Pavillion; Staff, Gordon & Leslie Diamond Health Care Centre; Clin Prof, University of British Columbia; (604)875-5003; Fax. (604)875-5604.

NIJHAWAN, Monica; Southlake Family Health Team, 201-581 Davis Dr, Newmarket ON L3Y 2P6; Wes'04; CCFP; (905)853-3103; Fax. (905)853-9136.

NIJHAWAN, Navdeep; Oshawa Clinic, 117 King St E, Oshawa ON L1H 1B9; Tor'95; FRCSC; Ophth. (905)721-4906; Fax. (905)721-3559.

NIJHAWAN, Pardeep K; Digestive Health Clinic, 510-330 Highway 7 E, Richmond Hill ON L4B 3P8; Ott'94; FRCPC; IntMed; Gastroent. Physician, Mackenzie Richmond Hill Hospital; (905)707-5007; Fax. (905)707-5008.

NIJHAWAN, Rajni; Toronto Rehab Institute, 347 Rumsey Rd, Toronto ON M4G 1R7; Moscow (Russia (Federation))'76; Staff, Sunnybrook Health Sciences Centre; Staff, Toronto Rehabilitation Institute - University Centre; (416)597-3422 x5200; Fax. (416)425-0301.

NIJJAR, Aman P; Internal Med Outpatient Clinic, 2775 Laurel St, Vancouver BC V5Z 1M9; California (USA)'04; FRCPC; IntMed. Staff, Providence Health Care - St Paul's Hospital; Staff, Gordon & Leslie Diamond Health Care Centre; (604)875-5181

NIJJAR, Pravjot K; PrimeCare Med Centre, 202-7315 Edmonds St, Burnaby BC V3N 1A7; UBC'97; BSc(Microbiol); CCFP; Locum Tenens, Royal Columbian Hospital; Langs: Punjabi; (604)526-2401; Fax. (604)526-1108.

NIJJAR, Satnam S; 1763 Portage Ave, Winnipeg MB R3J 0E7; Tor'03; FRCPC; Neur. Staff, Mount Sinai Hospital.

NIJJAR, Sundeep S; Associated Radiologists, 300-140 Wall St, Saskatoon SK S7K 1N4; Alb'03; FRCPC; NuclearMed. (306)244-1167; Fax. (306)244-2911.

NIJJAR, Tirath S; Cross Cancer Institute, 11560 University Ave NW, Edmonton AB T6G 1Z2; Man'81; FRCPC; IntMed; RadOncol; MedOncol. Staff, Cross Cancer Institute; (780)432-8516; Fax. (780)432-8380.

NIJMEH, Larry J; Lakeridge HC-Bowmanville Site, 47 Liberty St S, Bowmanville ON L1C 2N4; Tor'01; CCFP; Staff, Lakeridge Health - Bowmanville Site; (905)623-3331

NIJMEH, Paul; 302-2130 Lawrence Ave E, Scarborough ON M1R 3A6; Tor'87; CCFP; Staff, The Scarborough Hospital - Birchmount Campus; (416)443-9294

NIJSSEN-JORDAN, Cheri L D; South Health Campus, 4448 Front St SE, Calgary AB T3M 1M4; Sask'81; ABPeds; DTMH; MBA; FRCPC; Peds (Pediatric Emergency Medicine). Dir Emerg Services, Alberta Children's Hospital; Assoc Prof Faculty of Med, University of Calgary; Langs: English; French; (403)956-2472; Fax. (403)955-7398; cheri.nijssen-jordan@albertahealthservices.ca.

NIK-AKTHAR, Tanaz; Hop Charles LeMoyne, 3120 boul Taschereau, Greenfield Park QC J4V 2H1; Mon'99; Staff, Hopital Charles LeMoyne; (450)466-5000

NIKHILANANDHAN, Janarthan Y; 512-2000 Credit Valley Rd, Mississauga ON L5M 4N4; Tor'96; FRCPC; IntMed; Cardiol. (905)828-9441; Fax. (905)828-1690.

NIKKEL, Sarah M; Children's Hosp Eastern Ont, 401 Smyth Rd, Ottawa ON K1H 8L1; Alb'96; FRCPC; MedGenetics. Staff, Children's Hospital of Eastern Ontario (CHEO); (613)737-7600; snikkel@cheo.on.ca.

NIKOLAKIS, Michael A; Kamloops Neurosurgery, 210-300 Columbia St, Kamloops BC V2C 6L1; Alb'03; Neursurg. Staff, University of Alberta Hospital; (604)520-1120

NIKOLEYCHUK, Gerald; Queen Elizabeth II Hosp, 167-10409 98 St, Grande Prairie AB T8V 2E8; Alb'07; FRCPC; IntMed. Staff, Covenant Health - Misericordia Community Hospital; Staff, Queen Elizabeth II Hospital; (780)830-2844; Fax. (780)830-2843.

NIKOLIC, Ana; 5-65 University Ave E, Waterloo ON N2J 2V9; Tor'95; CCFP; FCFP; Langs: English; French; (519)342-1307; Fax. (519)342-0942.

NIKOLIS, Andreas; 1560 rue Sherbrooke E, Montreal QC H2L 4M1; Qns'96; MSc; FRCS; FRCSC; PlasSurg (Academic Surgery). Staff, Centre Hospitalier l'Université de Montréal (CHUM) - Hôpital Notre-Dame; Physician, Victoria Park MediSpa; Langs: French; Greek; (514)890-8000; anikolis@vicpark.com.

NIKOLSKY, Victor; Albany Med Clinic, 807 Broadview Ave, Toronto ON M4K 2P8; Ross University (USA)'08; CCFP; (416)461-9471

NIKON, Yaghoub; Newmarket Med Place, 308-712 Davis Dr, Newmarket ON L3Y 8C3; (Iran)'87; FRCPC; IntMed. (905)895-1090; Fax. (905)895-2680.

NIKORE, Veena; 484 West St, Brantford ON N3R 3W7; New Delhi (India)'71; Staff, The Brant Community Healthcare System - Brantford General Hospital Site; Staff, The Brant Community Healthcare System - Willett Hospital Site; Langs: Hindi; Punjabi; (519)751-3604

NIKORE, Vinay; Medical Arts Bldg, 353 St Paul Ave, Brantford ON N3R 4N3; New Delhi (India)'62; MB BS; FACP; DABIM; FRCPC; IntMed (Endocrinology). Att Staff, The Brant Community Healthcare System - Brantford General Hospital Site; (519)759-5971

NIKORE, Vineet; Humber River Reg Hosp-Church, 200 Church St, Toronto ON M9N 1N8; St. Maarten (Netherlands Antilles)'99; CCFP; CCFP(E.M.); Staff, Humber River Regional Hospital - Church Street Site; (416)249-8111

NILES, Clarence; Sow's Ear Clinic, GD 7186 Lantzville Rd, Lantzville BC V0R 2H0; Washington (USA)'81; CCFP; (250)390-4542; Fax. (250)390-4561.

NILSON, Linda Lee; Allan Blair Cancer Centre, 300-4101 Dewdney Ave, Regina SK S4T 7T1; UBC'78; BA; (306)766-2213; Fax. (306)766-2688.

NIMCHONOK, Punam M; 102-377 Church St, Markham ON L6B 1A1; Cal'02; Respir; IntMed. Staff, Markham Stouffville Hospital; (905)554-4686; Fax. (905)554-5727.

NIMETZ, Natalie A; Guelph Gen Hosp, 115 Delhi St, Guelph ON N1E 4J4; Wes'95; CCFP; CCFP(E.M.); FCFP; Staff, Guelph General Hospital; Physician, Guelph Emergency Medical Services; (519)837-6440

NIMIGAN, Andre S; The Medical Centre, PO Box 4200 Stn Main 707 Charlotte St, Peterborough ON K9J 7B3; Wes'05; FRCSC; PlasSurg. (705)876-4535; Fax. (705)743-7874.

NIMIGAN, Wayne R; 100-1220 Place D'Orleans Dr, Ottawa ON K1C 7K3; Tor'71; AB; EmergMed. (613)841-5389

NIMIR, Asim B; 1-2 Second Ave, St Thomas ON N5R 5S7; Khartoum (Sudan)'74; FRCPC; IntMed. (519)633-9555

NIMJEE, Tasleem M; Humber River Reg Hosp-Church, 200 Church St, Toronto ON M9N 1N8; Tor'07; CCFP; Staff, Humber River Regional Hospital - Church Street Site; (416)249-8111

NIMMO, Michael C; UBC Hospital, 2211 Wesbrook Mall, Vancouver BC V6T 2B5; UBC'95; LLB; BSc(Hon.); FRCPC; GenPath. Staff, UBC Hospital - Koerner Pavillion; (604)822-7202; michael.nimmo@vch.ca.

NIMNI, Gil B; Mackenzie Richmond Hill Hosp, 10 Trench St, Richmond Hill ON L4C 4Z3; Wes'97; DrMedCh; CCFP; CCFP(E.M.); Staff Emerg Med, Mackenzie Richmond Hill Hospital; Asst Clin Prof Family Med Div of Emerg Med, University of Toronto; Langs: Hebrew; (905)883-2041

NIMPAGARITSE, Rosalie; Clinique Med Masson-Angers, 1100 ch de Montreal O, Gatineau QC J8M 2A9; '95; (819)281-1509

NINAN, Abraham; Royal University Hosp, 103 Hospital Dr, Saskatoon SK S7N 0W8; Madras (India)'67; FRCPC; Peds (Neonatology). Staff, Royal University Hospital; Ac Staff, Regina General Hospital; Pres., Emmanuel Hospital Assoc.; University of Saskatchewan; Langs: Hindi; Malayalam; Fax. (306)975-3767; alninan@yahoo.com.

NINAN, Ajit T; Child & Parent Resource Inst, 600 Sanatorium Rd, London ON N6H 3W7; Ross (Dominica)'00; FRCPC; Psy. Staff, Child & Parent Resource Institute; (519)858-2774

NINAN, Vadakethu T; Peterborough Reg HC-Hospital, 1 Hospital Dr, Peterborough ON K9J 7C6; Madras (India)'77; FRCPC; IntMed. Staff, Peterborough Regional Health Centre - Hospital Drive; (705)743-2121

NING, Jean-Noel; AIM Health Group, B22-550 Terminal Ave, Ottawa ON K1G 0Z3; St. Etienne (France)'83; Langs: English; French; (613)731-4770; Fax. (613)731-4979.

NINIAN, Gregory M; Smith Clinic, 1-6601 48 Ave, Camrose AB T4V 3G8; Alb'75; (780)672-2424; Fax. (780)679-2668.

NINKOVIC, Svetlana; Hop Charles LeMoyne, 3120 boul Taschereau, Greenfield Park QC J4V 2H1; Paris (France)'70; Electroenceph (P.Q.); Neur (P.Q.); Peds. Staff, Hopital Charles LeMoyne; (450)466-5000

NINKOVICH, Snezana; Windsor Reg Hosp-Metropolitan, 1995 Lens Ave, Windsor ON N8W 1L9; McM'05; CCFP; CCFP(E.M.); Staff, Windsor Regional Hospital - Metropolitan Site; (519)254-5577

NINOS, Adam G; Trillium Hlth Ctr-Mississauga, 100 Queensway W, Mississauga ON L5B 1B8; Dal'00; FRCPC; HemPath. Staff, Trillium Health Centre - Mississauga; (905)848-7580

NIOU, Wayne P; Crystal Square Mall, 1612-4500 Kingsway, Burnaby BC V5H 2A9; Alb'97; CCFP; (604)436-1231

NIP, L Michael; Dufferin Family Care Centre, 51 Gerry Fitzgerald Dr, North York ON M3J 3N4; (Hong Kong)'80; MB BS; MRCP(UK); DCH(Glas); CCFP; FCFP; Langs: Chinese; (416)739-1562; Fax. (416)739-6671; michael_nip@hotmail.com.

NIRAULA, Saroj; CancerCare Manitoba, 2068-675 McDermot Ave, Winnipeg MB R3E 0V9; Henan (China)'03.

NIROUMAND-SARVESTANI, Mitra; Mount Sinai Hosp, 6 207-600 University Ave, Toronto ON M5G 1X5; Qns'92; DAB; FRCPC; IntMed (Sleep Disorders); Respir. Staff, Mount Sinai Hospital; (416)586-4800 x8394; Fax. (416)586-4736; mniroumand@mtsinai.on.ca.

NIRWAN, Amarjit S; Lansdowne Professional Ctr II, 375-3066 Shelbourne St, Victoria BC V8R 6T9; Cambridge (England)'80; BSc; MB ChB; CCFP; Staff, Vancouver Island Health Authority; Staff, Aberdeen Hospital; Physician, Victoria Med. Society; Langs: Hindi; Punjabi; Urdu; (250)595-1363; Fax. (250)595-2627; dranirwan@gmail.com.

NISBET, Colin G; Windsor Reg Hosp-Metropolitan, 1995 Lens Ave, Windsor ON N8W 1L9; Glasgow (Scotland)'71; Staff, Windsor Regional Hospital - Metropolitan Site; Staff, Selkirk & District General Hospital; (519)254-1661

NISBETT, Samuel; Mayfair Clinic, 33477A Mayfair Ave, Abbotsford BC V2S 1P6; West Indies (Jamaica)'79; MB BS; DABOph; FACS(Ophth); MBA; FRCSC; Ophth (Cataract & Glaucoma). Ac Staff, Chilliwack General Hospital; Ac Staff, Mission Memorial Hospital; Ac Staff, Fraser Canyon Hospital; Ac Staff, Abbotsford Regional Hospital & Cancer Centre; (604)853-6321; Fax. (604)853-7321; samuel.nisbett@fraserhealth.ca.

NISCHUK, Leighton L; Mainstreet Med Services, 4929 50 Ave, Lacombe AB T4L 1K3; Alb'80; Ac Staff, Lacombe Hospital & Care Centre; Court Staff, Red Deer Regional Hospital Centre; (403)782-6717; Fax. (403)782-4240.

NISHIKAWA, James A; 5230 Mitch Owens Rd PO Box 500, Manotick ON K4M 1A5; McM'81; FACP; FRCPC; IntMed (General). Staff Gen IntMed, The Ottawa Hospital - Civic Campus; Assoc Prof Med, University of Ottawa; (613)692-2571

NISHIKAWA, Richard A; Tottenham Med Centre, PO Box 2000 119 Queen St N, Tottenham ON L0G 1W0; Tor'85; BSc; CCFP; Staff, Southlake Regional Health Centre; (905)936-4211; Fax. (905)936-3493.

NISHIMURA, Brian K; Trillium Hlth Ctr-Mississauga, 100 Queensway W, Mississauga ON L5B 1B8; Qns'95; FRCPC; Anes. Staff, Trillium Health Centre - Mississauga; (905)848-7628

NISHIO, Karen R; 3199 Cliffe Ave, Courtenay BC V9N 2L9; Alb'84; (250)334-1512

NISHIWAKI, Maya; 2316 96 St NW, Edmonton AB T6N 1J8; Alb'99; CCFP; (780)468-5999; Fax. (780)468-5398.

NISKER, Jeffrey; London HSC-Victoria Hosp, PO Box 5010 Stn B E2 620E-800 Commissioners Rd E, London ON N6A 5W9; Tor'74; PhD; MD; FRCSC; ObstGyn (Reproductive Endocrinology). Staff, London Health Sciences Centre - Victoria Campus; Scientist, Children's Health Research Institute; Prof ObstGyn, University of Western Ontario; (519)685-8781; Fax. (519)685-8783; jeff.nisker@lhsc.on.ca.

NISKER, William A; 301-2951 Walker's Line, Burlington ON L7M 4Y1; Cal'81; FRCPC; IntMed; GeriatricMed. Ac Staff, Joseph Brant Memorial Hospital; (905)331-3101; Fax. (905)319-2499; info@jbnmedical.com.

NISSAIRE, Robert; Clinique Med Blainville, 519 boul du Curé-Labelle, Blainville QC J7C 2H6; Mon'77; ac Staff, Centre Hospitalier l'Université de Montréal (CHUM) - Hôpital Notre-Dame; (450)430-2222; Fax. (450)430-1274.

NISTICO, Amy R; Sudbury Reg Hosp-Laurentian, 41 Ramsey Lake Rd, Sudbury ON P3E 5J1; Qns'04; FRCPC; Nephrol; IntMed. Staff, Health Sciences North-Laurentian Site; (705)522-2200

NITKA, Monique; 209-85 rue de Bigarre, Victoriaville QC G6P 9P6; Mon'78; (819)751-0042

NITKIN, Robert S; Scarborough North Med Arts, 404-4040 Finch Ave E, Scarborough ON M1S 4V5; Tor'79; FACC; FRCPC; IntMed; Cardiol. Staff Cardiol, The Scarborough Hospital - Birchmount Campus; Assoc Staff, Mount Sinai Hospital; (416)297-7277

NITOIU, Daniela V; Lakeridge Hlth Corp-Oshawa, 1 Hospital Crt, Oshawa ON L1G 2B9; (Other Foreign)'90; CCFP; Staff, Lakeridge Health - Oshawa Site; (905)576-8711

NITSCH, Barbara A; West Eglinton Med Centre, 100-2010 Eglinton Ave W, Toronto ON M6E 2K3; McM'84; AB; FRCPC; DiagRad. (416)781-2050; Fax. (416)781-1910.

NITSCH, Romy; Kingston Gen Hosp, 76 Stuart St, Kingston ON K7L 2V7; Ott'00; FRCSC; ObstGyn (Minimal Invasive Surgery). Staff, Kingston General Hospital; (613)548-1327

NITTI, Nicole M; Access Alliance Multicultural, 340 College St, Toronto ON M5T 3A9; Ott'97; CCFP; CCFP(E.M.); FCFP; Staff, William Osler Health System - Etobicoke General Hospital; (416)324-9697; Fax. (416)324-9490.

NITZKIN, Steven; Oakdale Med Bldg, 305-2065 Finch Ave W, North York ON M3N 2V7; Tor'68; Ac Staff, Humber River Regional Hospital - Finch Avenue Site; Langs: Spanish; Italian; French; (416)744-6565; Fax. (416)744-1544.

NIVEN, Daniel J; Peter Lougheed Centre, 3500 26 Ave NE, Calgary AB T1Y 6J4; Cal'06; FRCPC; IntMed; Critical Care Medicine. Staff, Peter Lougheed Centre; (403)943-5488

NIXDORFF, M Faith; Chinook Prof Bldg, 405-6455 MacLeod Trail SW, Calgary AB T2H 0K9; Cal'81; DTMH(Eng); (403)252-4030; Fax. (403)253-0037.

NIXON, Alan J; Moog & Francis Hospice House, 1701 Government St, Penticton BC V2A 8J7; Belfast (Ireland)'74; MB ChB; BAO; CCFP; Staff, Burnaby Hospital; Staff, Richmond Hospital; (250)492-9071

NIXON, Donald R; 100C-190 Cundles Rd E, Barrie ON L4M 4S5; Qns'83; FRCSC; Ophth. Staff, Orillia Soldiers' Memorial Hospital; Staff, Royal Victoria Regional Health Centre; (705)737-3737

NIXON, Donald W; Westview Hlth Ctr Stony Plain, 4405 South Park Dr, Stony Plain AB T7Z 2M7; Alb'71; Med Officer, Westview Health Centre; (780)968-3674; Fax. (780)963-7192.

NIXON, G William H; 211-9764 Fifth St, Sidney BC V8L 2X2; Dublin (Ireland)'66; MB ChB; BAO; FRCPC; Psy (Psychotherapy). (250)652-2821; Fax. (250)652-6499.

NIXON, James A; Suitor House, 1004 8 Ave SE, Calgary AB T2G 0M4; Cal'76; BSc; FRCSC; GenSurg (Trauma). Chief Surg, Peter Lougheed Centre; (403)264-6720; Fax. (403)237-6646.

NIXON, Jane E M; 100-300 Main St N, Brampton ON L6V 4H6; Tor'89; Staff, William Osler Health System - Brampton Civic Hospital; (905)450-0151; Fax. (905)450-7152.

NIXON, Judith P; The Ottawa Hosp-Gen Campus, 501 Smyth Rd, Ottawa ON K1H 8L6; Dal'89; FRCPC; IntMed. Staff, The Ottawa Hospital - General Campus; (613)737-7700

NIXON, Lara L; 630 9 Ave SE, Calgary AB T2G 4V9; UBC'99; CCFP; (403)920-0011

NIXON, Mary K; Queen Alexandra Ctre Children, 2400 Arbutus Rd, Victoria BC V8N 1V7; Ott'86; FRCPC; Psy (Child Psychiatry). Staff, Queen Alexandra Centre for Children's Health; (250)477-1826

NIZALIK, C L Elizabeth; Children's Hosp Eastern Ont, 401 Smyth Rd, Ottawa ON K1H 8L1; Man'81; MD(PedPathol); FRCPC; GenPath (Pediatric Pathology). Staff AnatPath, Children's Hospital of Eastern Ontario (CHEO); Asst Prof Med, University of Ottawa; (613)737-7600 x3607; enizalik@cheo.on.ca.

NIZAM, Mahmood J; Heritage Lane Med Centre, 10835 23 Ave NW, Edmonton AB T6J 7B5; Kakatiya (India)'78; CCFP; Fort Saskatchewan Health Centre; Langs: Urdu; (780)424-6490; Fax. (780)425-4920.

NIZAMI, Tariq F; Springbank Med Centre, 204-460 Springbak Dr, London ON N6J 0A8; Pakistan (Pakistan)'92; MB BS; CCFP; (519)601-4766; Fax. (519)601-4866.

NIZARD, Jacques H V; Hop Charles LeMoyne, 3120 boul Taschereau, Greenfield Park QC J4V 2H1; Paris (France)'85; Staff, Hopital Charles LeMoyne; (450)466-5000; Fax. (450)466-5005.

NIZNICK, Joel M; Ottawa Cardiovascular Centre, 502-1355 Bank St, Ottawa ON K1H 8K7; Man'78; DABIM(IntMed&Cardiol); FRCPC; IntMed; Cardiol. Ac Staff, The Ottawa Hospital - Riverside Campus; Ac Staff, The Ottawa Hospital - General Campus; Consultant, The Ottawa Hospital - Civic Campus; (613)738-1584; Fax. (613)738-9097.

NIZZERO, Albert; Sudbury Reg Hosp-Laurentian, 41 Ramsey Lake Rd, Sudbury ON P3E 5J1; Tor'86; FRCPC; DiagRad (Diagnostic Imaging). Staff, Health Sciences North-Laurentian Site; (705)522-2200 x3520

NIZZERO, Christopher J L; Sudbury Reg Hosp-Laurentian, 41 Ramsey Lake Rd, Sudbury ON P3E 5J1; NOSM'10; CCFP; Staff, Health Sciences North-Laurentian Site; (705)523-7100

NJALSSON, Thorstein; North Nanaimo Med Clinic Ltd, 195-4750 Rutherford Rd, Nanaimo BC V9T 4K6; Iceland (Iceland)'84; CCFP; FCFP; (250)585-7100

NJIONHOU KEMENI, Marie M; Boyd Med Clinic, 392 Portage Ave, Winnipeg MB R3C 0C7; CCFP.

NJOKU, Anthony; Dr Everett Chalmers Reg Hosp, PO Box 9000 Stn A 700 Priestman St, Fredericton NB E3B 5N5; Ibadan (Nigeria)'87; Staff, Dr Everett Chalmers Regional Hospital; (506)452-5400

NJOO, Howard T H; Public Health Agency of Canada, PL6201 D-100 Colonnade Rd, Ottawa ON K1A 0K9; Tor'85; MHSc; FRCPC; CommunMed (Public Health). Staff TB Clinic, The Ottawa Hospital - General Campus; Dir-Research, Centre for Infectious Diseases Prevention & Control; Teach Staff Med, University of Ottawa; (613)948-6799; Fax. (613)954-4556.

NKANSAH, John; 318-220 Duncan Mill Rd, North York ON M3B 3J5; Tor'64; DPsy; FRCPC; Psy (Hospital Administration). Staff, The Scarborough Hospital - Birchmount Campus; Consultant, Toronto East General Hospital Inc; Asst Prof, University of Toronto; (416)391-5304; Fax. (416)391-5305; nkansah@arvotek.net.

NKEMDIRIM, Makela E; 100-20 Heritage Meadows Rd SE, Calgary AB T2H 3C1; Tor'01; CCFP; (403)252-8851; Fax. (403)252-1765.

NKOSI, Joel E; Health Sciences Centre, GC4-820 Sherbrook St, Winnipeg MB R3A 1R9; Medunsa (South Africa)'99; MB ChB; FRCPC; IntMed;CCFP; Staff, Health Sciences Centre; (204)774-8511

NKUNGU, B Mandisa; Toronto East Gen Hosp Inc, C423-825 Coxwell Ave, Toronto ON M4C 3E7; Natal (South Africa)'83; MB ChB; FRCPC; Psy. Staff, Toronto East General Hospital Inc; (416)461-8272

NKUT, Alfred; 2-2956 Highway 69 N, Val Caron ON P3N 1E3; Yaounde (Cameroon)'94; CCFP; (705)897-2345; Fax. (705)897-2344.

NNOROM, Onyenyechukwu; TAIBU Community Health Ctre, 1-27 Tapscott Rd, Scarborough ON M1B 4Y7; McG'07; MDCM; CCFP; Public Health & Preventive Med. (416)644-3536; Fax. (416)644-0102.

NOACK, Laura A; Downtown Health Access Ctre, 640 Main St, Winnipeg MB R3B 0L8; Ott'06; CCFP; (204)940-1626

NOAD, Donald V; King West Med Associates, 505 King St W, Hamilton ON L8P 1B9; Tor'77; Court Staff, St Joseph's Healthcare - Charlton Campus; Court Staff, Hamilton Health Sciences Centre - McMaster University Medical Centre; Med Dir, Idlewyld Manor, Hamilton; (905)525-3501; Fax. (905)528-5468.

NOAD, Garth; King West Med Associates, 505 King St W, Hamilton ON L8P 1B9; Qns'73; Court Staff, Hamilton Health Sciences Centre; Ac Staff, St Joseph's Healthcare - Charlton Campus; (905)525-3501; Fax. (905)528-5468; garth.noad@sympatico.ca.

NOAKES, Jeffrey E; 204-4430 Bathurst St, North York ON M3H 3S3; Tor'77; DAB; FRCSC; Urol. Ac Staff, North York General Hospital; (416)630-3174; Fax. (416)630-3070.

NOBECOURT, Philippe; CSSS de Beauce-Etchemin, 1515 17e rue, Saint-Georges QC G5Y 4T8; Laval'90; FRCPC; Psy. Staff, Centre Hospitalier Beauce-Etchemin; (418)228-2031; Fax. (418)227-1081.

NOBERT, Leo; Ctr Hosp de Lasalle, 8585 Tsse Champlain, LaSalle QC H8P 1C1; Mon'66; CSPQ; DiagRad. Staff, Centre Hospitalier de LaSalle; Staff, Centre Hospitalier de Verdun; (514)362-8000 x1549; Fax. (514)367-8631.

NOBERT-GAGNE, Suzanne; Polyclinique St-Martin, 307-1435 boul Saint-Martin O, Laval QC H7S 2C6; Laval'72; CSPQ; AnatPath. (450)667-2664

NOBLE, A Bruce; Seymour Med Clinic, 200-1530 7th Ave W, Vancouver BC V6J 1S3; Cal'78; (604)739-5623

NOBLE, Angela; Kingston Gen Hosp, 314-76 Stuart St, Kingston ON K7L 2V7; Mem'98; FRCPC; Peds; Gastroent. Staff, Kingston General Hospital; (613)549-6666

NOBLE, Colin J G; Royal Alexandra Hosp, 10240 Kingsway NW, Edmonton AB T5H 3V9; Tor'79; FRCPC; Anes. Staff, Royal Alexandra Hospital; (780)735-4010; Fax. (780)425-2634.

NOBLE, E Keith; Shoppers Drug Mart Bldg, 250 Lemarchant Rd, St. John's NL A1E 1P7; Dal'72; (709)722-6090

NOBLE, Stephen; Parksville Med Clinic, PO Box 250 Stn Main 154 Memorial Ave W, Parksville BC V9P 2G4; Cal'83; (250)248-5757; Fax. (250)248-2128.

NOBLE, Heather L; Student Health Services, 50 Stone Rd E, Guelph ON N1G 2W1; McM'86; CCFP; FCFP; (519)836-6392

NOBLE, Jason; 403-2130 Lawrence Ave E, Scarborough ON M1R 3A6; Tor'05; FRCSC; Ophth. (647)346-5222

NOBLE, John J R; Kelowna Medical Imaging, 101-3330 Richter St, Kelowna BC V1W 4V5; UBC'71; FRCPC; DiagRad. Staff, Kelowna General Hospital; (250)762-4420; Fax. (250)860-8348.

NOBLE, Jonathan C S; Northeastern ON Reg Cancer Ctr, 41 Ramsey Lake Rd, Sudbury ON P3E 5J1; Tor'92; BSc(Hons.); MSc; PhD; FRCPC; IntMed (Palliative Care); MedOncol. Staff, Health Sciences North-Laurentian Site; Asst Prof, University of Ottawa; (705)522-6237; Fax. (705)523-7348; jcnoble@hrsrh.on.ca.

NOBLE, Michael A; UBC Prog for Lab Quality Mgmt, 366-2733 Heather St, Vancouver BC V5Z 1M9; Wes'72; BA; FRC; FRCPC; IntMed; MedMicrobiol. Med Microbiologist/Med Dir Quality, UBC Program Office for Laboratory Quality Management; Prof Path & Lab Med/Chair Clin Microbiol Proficiency Testing/Chair Program Office for Lab Quality Management, University of British Columbia; (604)875-4685; Fax. (604)875-4100; mnoble@interchange.ubc.ca.

NOBLE, Peter C; Oshawa Clinic, 117 King St E, Oshawa ON L1H 1B9; Tor'70; CCFP; Ac Staff, Lakeridge Health - Oshawa Site; (905)721-3530; Fax. (905)721-3432.

NOBLE, Michael C; Westminster Med Bldg, 206-625 Fifth Ave, New Westminster BC V3M 1X4; Harvard (USA)'70; ABIM(Med); ABIM(Hem); FRCPC; IntMed (Hematological Oncology); Hem. Ac Staff, Royal Columbian Hospital; Ac Staff, Eagle Ridge Hospital & Health Care Centre; Clinical Asst Prof, University of British Columbia; (604)524-1414; Fax. (604)524-2285.

NOBLE, Sarah E; Waterford Hosp, 306 Waterford Bridge Rd, St. John's NL A1E 4J8; Qns'01; FRCPC; Psy. Staff, Waterford Hospital; (709)777-3300

NOBLE, Stewart J; Tsawwassen Med Clinic, 201-1077 56 St, Delta BC V4L 2A2; UBC'00; Staff, Delta Hospital; (604)943-1131

NOBLE, Vello K; Southgate Med Clinic, 1-45905 Yale Rd, Chilliwack BC V2P 2M6; UBC'78; (604)795-7228; Fax. (604)795-2535; vellonoble@shaw.ca.

NOBLE-WOHLGEMUT, Matthew; Smithville Family Health Ctre, PO Box 218 230 Canboro St, Smithville ON L0R 2A0; McM'03; CCFP; (905)957-3328; Fax. (905)957-2457; mnoble-wohlgemut@cogeco.ca.

NOCE, Emilia; 1083 The Parkway, London ON N6A 2W8; McM'83; FRCPC; Psy. (519)642-1252

NOCENT, Gregory L; Halton HSC Corp-Oakville, 327 Reynolds St, Oakville ON L6J 3L7; Tor'79; FRCPC; Anes. Staff, Halton Healthcare Services Corporation - Oakville Site; (905)845-2571

NODWELL, Allison C; 2029 Cassells St, North Bay ON P1B 4E1; Wes'98; BSc; BMath; CCFP; (705)474-2340; Fax. (705)474-2349.

NODWELL, S A Trefor; 200-343 Preston St, Ottawa ON K1S 1N4; McG'99; MDCM; FRCSC; PlasSurg (Aesthetic Surgery). Staff Plastic & Reconstructive Surg, Queensway Carleton Hospital; Langs: French; Fax. (613)567-0148; admin@nodwellplasticsurgery.com.

NOEL, Alain; Hop Ste-Croix, 570 rue Heriot, Drummondville QC J2B 1C1; Sher'88; IntMed (P.Q.). Staff, Hôpital Sainte-croix; (819)478-6464

NOEL, Ann; Hop Maisonneuve-Rosemont, 5415 boul de l'Assomption, Montreal QC H1T 2M4; Mon'05; ObstGyn. Staff, Hopital Maisonneuve-Rosemont; (514)252-3819; Fax. (514)251-7743.

NOEL, Audrey; Ctr Hosp Trois-Riv-St-Joseph, 731 rue Sainte-Julie, Trois-Rivieres QC G9A 1Y1; Laval'10; Staff, Centre Hospitalier Regional de Trois-Rivieres; (819)372-3536

NOEL, Bernard; Hôpital Laval, 2725 ch Sainte-Foy, Quebec QC G1V 4G5; Laval'97; FRCPC; IntMed; Cardiol. Staff, Hôpital Laval; (418)656-4767

NOEL, Bernard; CSSS de Saint-Jerome, 290 rue de Montigny, Saint-Jerome QC J7Z 5T3; McG'93; CSPQ; AnatPath; GenPath (P. Q.). Staff, Hôtel-Dieu de Saint-Jérôme; (450)431-8200 x22136

NOEL, Bernard C; CSSS de Chicoutimi, 305 rue Saint-Vallier, Chicoutimi QC G7H 5H6; Laval'93; LMCC; CCFP; CCFP(E.M.); FCFP; EmergMed. Staff, Complexe hospitalier de la Sagamie; Clin Prof, Universite de Sherbrooke; (418)541-1010

NOEL, Caroline; Ctr Hosp Fleury, 2180 rue Fleury E, Montreal QC H2B 1K3; Mon'10; CCFP; (514)384-2000

NOEL, Caroline P; Clin Externe de Pedopsychiatri, 200-2924 boul Taschereau, Greenfield Park QC J4V 2G8; Mon'04; FRCPC; Psy. (450)466-8486 x246

NOEL, Clement; Clinique Med Rosemont, 1969 boul Rosemont, Montreal QC H2G 1S9; Mon'65; Cardiol. Staff, Centre Hospitalier l'Université de Montréal (CHUM) - Hôpital Notre-Dame; (514)274-7344

NOEL, Colin T; C T Noel Med Clinic, PO Box 1140 320 Fisher Ave, The Pas MB R9A 1L1; Leeds (England)'73; MB ChB; MRC; CCFP; FCFP; Head Dept of Obst/Chief Medical Staff, St. Anthony General Hospital; Ass't. Lect., University of Manitoba; (204)623-4866; Fax. (204)623-4859; noelclinic@mts.net.

NOEL, Daniel A; Maitland Valley Family Hlth Team, 180 Cambria Rd N, Goderich ON N7A 4N8; McM'04; CCFP; (519)524-6060

NOEL, Daniel; Clinique Med Belvedere, 202-2235 rue Galt O, Sherbrooke QC J1K 1K6; Sher'75; AddicMed; CCFP; FCFP; Member CEMDP, Centre Hospitalier Universitaire de Sherbrooke-Hôpital Hôtel-Dieu; Clin Prof Family Med, Universite de Sherbrooke; (819)563-4244; Fax. (819)563-8924; danielnoel@sympatico.ca.

NOEL, Daniel R; CSSS du Sud de Lanaudière, 911 montee des Pionniers, Terrebonne QC J6V 2H2; Mon'71; FRCPC; HemPath; MedOncol (P.Q.); Hem (P.Q.) (Hematological Oncology). Hematology/Oncology, Centre Hospitalier Pierre le Gardeur; Clinical Asst Prof, Universite de Montreal; Langs: English; French; (450)654-7525 x21559; noeld@videotron.ca.

NOEL, Francis D; Health Sciences Centre, 300 Prince Philip Dr, St. John's NL A1B 3V6; Mem'77; FRCPC; Anes (Cardiovascular Anesthesia). Staff, Health Sciences Centre; (709)777-6540

NOEL, Francois; Hop Louis-H Lafontaine, 7401 rue Hochelaga, Montreal QC H1N 3M5; Mon'05; FRCPC; Psy. Staff, Hopital Louis-H Lafontaine; (514)251-4000

NOEL, Francoise; 3835 rue Wellington, Verdun QC H4G 1V1; Mon'74; FRCSC; Ophth. Ophthalmology, Centre Hospitalier de Verdun; Langs: English; (514)768-1250; Fax. (514)768-9240; francoisenoel@me.com.

NOEL, Fraser L; Yarrow Med Bldg, 409-645 Fort St, Victoria BC V8W 1G2; Mem'81; FACO(Neur); FRCSC; Otol (Neuro Otolaryngology). (250)920-5500; Fax. (250)920-5580.

NOEL, Gregoire E; CHUM-Hotel-Dieu, 5 206-3840 rue Saint-Urbain, Montreal QC H2W 1T8; U.N.A.M. (Mexico)'72; MSc; FACTM; CSPQ; FRCPC; MedMicrobiol (Infectious Diseases); Microbio & Infect Dis (P.Q.). ac Staff In Charge of Continuous Med Educ Infectious Dis, Centre Hospitalier l'Université de Montréal (CHUM) - Hôtel-Dieu; Clinical Asst Prof, Universite de Montreal; Langs: Spanish; Portuguese; English; (514)890-8000 x14816; gregoire.noel.chum@ssss.gouv.qc.ca.

NOEL, Guylaine; Hotel-Dieu de Roberval, 450 rue Brassard, Roberval QC G8H 1B9; Sher'07; FRCSC; GenSurg. Staff, Hotel-Dieu de Roberval; (418)275-0110

NOEL, Henri-Paul; CHUQ-St-Francois d'Assise, 10 rue de l'Espinay, Quebec QC G1L 3L5; Laval'65; GenSurg. Ac Staff, Centre Hospitalier Universitaire De Québec - Pavillon De St-françois-d'assise; (418)525-2279; Fax. (418)252-2264.

NOEL, Jean-Francois; CSSS des Iles, 430 ch Principal, Cap-aux-Meules QC G4T 1R9; Laval'99; Staff, Hôpital de l'Archipel; Langs: Bilingual(French/English); (418)986-2121; Fax. (418)986-7010; docjfnoel@gmail.com.

NOEL, Jean-Marc; Clinique Med de Labelle, 17 du Couvent, Labelle QC J0T 1H0; Laval'67; (819)686-2311; Fax. (819)686-9301.

NOEL, Kendall A; Clarence-Rockland Fam Hlth Team, 2741 rue Chamberland, Rockland ON K4K 0B4; McG'00; CCFP; (613)446-4565; Fax. (613)446-5737.

NOEL, Louis-Philippe; Clinique Med Fabreville, 380 boul Cure-Labelle, Laval QC H7P 5L3; Mon'68; Cardiol. Staff, Hôpital du Sacre-Coeur de Montréal; (450)963-1961; Fax. (450)963-1205.

NOEL, Luc; Clinique Med Frontenac, 24 rue Frontenac, Riviere-du-Loup QC G5R 1S5; Laval'97; Staff, Centre Hospitalier Regional du Grand-Portage; (418)868-1000; Fax. (418)868-1035.

NOEL, Marie L; Whitewater Clinic, PO Box 1530, The Pas MB R9A 1L4; Man'02; CCFP; (204)623-5899; bluems57@hotmail.com.

NOEL, Marie-France; CLSC Kateri, 90 boul Marie-Victorin, Candiac QC J5R 1C1; Laval'85; (450)659-7661; Fax. (450)444-6276.

NOEL, Marie-Frederique; Quinsam Med Clinic, 280-1400 Dogwood St, Campbell River BC V9W 3A6; Mon'04; CCFP; Langs: Bilingual(French/English); (250)286-3053; Fax. (250)286-0504.

NOEL, Melanie; Hôpital Ste-Justine, 3175 ch Cote-Sainte-Catherine, Montreal QC H3T 1C5; Mon'04; Peds. Staff, Hôpital Ste-Justine; (514)345-4931

NOEL, Melissandre; 103-1496 Cartwright St PO Box 14323 Rpo Granville Isl, Vancouver BC V6H 4J6; Mon'09; CCFP; Langs: Bilingual(English/French); (604)812-7422

NOEL, Patricia; CHUQ-Hotel-Dieu de Quebec, 11 Cote du Palais, Quebec QC G1R 2J6; Laval'99; CSPQ; FRCPC; DiagRad. Staff, Centre Hospitalier Universitaire de Québec (CHUQ) - Siege Social; (418)691-5453

NOEL, Peter J; Hillcrest Med Clinic, 83 Thorburn Rd, St. John's NL A1B 3M2; Mem'79; CCFP.

NOEL, Pierre; 347 rue Saint-Georges, Saint-Jerome QC J7Z 5A8; Mon'77; (450)436-8881; Fax. (450)436-8884.

NOEL, Real; CHUQ-Hotel-Dieu de Quebec, 11 Cote Du Palais, Quebec QC G1R 2J6; Laval'68; FRCPC; IntMed; Nephrol (P.Q.). Ac Staff, Centre Hospitalier Universitaire de Québec (CHUQ) - Siege Social; Staff, Hôtel-Dieu de Lévis; Clin Prof, Université Laval; (418)691-5151; Fax. (418)691-5757.

NOEL, Suzanne; CHUQ-Ctr Hosp Univ Laval, S 762-2705 boul Laurier, Quebec QC G1V 4G2; Sher'82; ObstGyn (P.Q.) (Colposcopy). Staff, Centre Hospitalier Universitaire de Quebec-CHUL; Staff Clin de Colposcopie, Centre Hospitalier Affilié Universitaire de Québec - Hôpital du St-Sacrement; (418)654-2738

NOEL BEAU, Noemie; CSSS Les Eskers de l'Abitibi, 622 4e rue O, Amos QC J9T 2S2; Mon'08; Staff, CH Hôtel-Dieu d'Amos; (819)732-3341

NOEL DE TILLY, France; Sunshine Clinic, 150 Montreal Rd, Ottawa ON K1L 8H2; Sher'90; Dip SportMed; (613)695-9001; Fax. (613)695-8002.

NOEL DE TILLY, Lyne; St Michael's Hosp, 30 Bond St, Toronto ON M5B 1W8; Laval'85; FRCPC; DiagRad (Neuro Radiology). Staff, St Michael's Hospital; (416)864-5674; Fax. (416)864-5380.

NOETZEL, Harry A; Port Arthur Health Centre Inc, 194 Court St N, Thunder Bay ON P7A 4V7; McG'83; (807)346-1000; Fax. (807)346-6206.

NOFECH-MOZES, Sharon; Sunnybrook Hlth Sciences Ctre, E4 32-2075 Bayview Ave, Toronto ON M4N 3M5; Tel Aviv (Israel)'92; Staff Breast Path, Sunnybrook Health Sciences Centre; (416)480-6100

NOFECH-MOZES, Yehuda; Rouge Valley-Centenary HC, 2867 Ellesmere Rd, Scarborough ON M1E 4B9; Tel-Aviv (Israel)'95; Staff, Rouge Valley Health System - Centenary Health Centre Site; (416)281-7234

NOFTALL, Francis E; 342 Pennywell Rd, St. John's NL A1E 1V9; Mem'82; FRCSC; OrthSurg. Ac Staff, St Clare's Mercy Hospital, OrthSurg.; Ac Staff, Health Sciences Centre; Clin Asst Prof Orthoped Surg, Memorial University Of Newfoundland; (709)579-5662; Fax. (709)753-2671.

NOFTALL, Lachelle; Fredericton Med Clinic, 510-1015 Regent St, Fredericton NB E3B 6H5; Mem'86; MD; FRCSC; Ophth (Ophthalmic Plastic & Reconstructive Surgery). (506)458-0271; Fax. (506)457-4720.

NOFTLE, Brooke M E; London Intercommunity Hlth Ctr, 659 Dundas St, London ON N5W 2Z1; Dal'88; BSc; BA; CCFP; FCFP; Staff Privil, St Joseph's Hospital - St Joseph's Health Care; Staff Privil, London Health Sciences Centre - University Hospital; Staff, London Intercommunity Health Centre - Dundas Street; Aj Prof Dept of Family Med, University of Western Ontario; Langs: German; Bilingual(French/English); (519)660-0874; Fax. (519)642-1532; bmnoftle@uwo.ca.

NOGA, Alexandra E; Family Med Associates, 15-9701 84 Ave, Grande Prairie AB T8V 4Z8; Alb'88; CCFP; (780)532-2205; Fax. (780)532-0037.

NOGA, Michelle L; University of Alberta Hosp, 41-8440 112 St NW, Edmonton AB T6G 2B7; Alb'90; FRCPC; DiagRad. Staff DiagRad, University of Alberta Hospital; (780)407-1260; Fax. (780)407-6176.

NOGA, Tom; University of Alberta Hosp, 4B1 04WMC-8440 112 St NW, Edmonton AB T6G 2B7; Alb'90; Staff, University of Alberta Hospital; (780)407-2012; Fax. (780)407-8599.

NOGAREDA, Jorge G; Red Deer Reg Hosp Centre, PO Box 5030 Stn Postal Box Ctr 3942 50A Ave, Red Deer AB T4N 6R2; La Plata(Argentina) (Argentina)'94; Staff, Red Deer Regional Hospital Centre; (403)356-4201; Fax. (403)358-4342.

NOGAREDE, Annick; Clin du Plateau Mont-Royal, 103-1374 av du Mont-Royal E, Montreal QC H2J 1Y7; Sher'03; FRCPC; Peds. (514)527-1032

NOGUE, Marc-Rene; Clinique Sante Famille, 3560 rue Laval, Lac-Megantic QC G6B 2X4; Laval'74; Staff, Carrefour Sante Granit; (819)583-5533; Fax. (819)583-2346.

NOHARA, Naomi J; 600-1881 Yonge St, Toronto ON M4S 3C4; Wes'04; CCFP; (416)932-3172; Fax. (416)440-0238.

NOHR, Carl W; 692 7 St SW, Medicine Hat AB T1A 4K8; McG'78; FACS(GenSurg); PhD; FRCSC; GenSurg. Staff, Medicine Hat Regional Hospital; (403)580-4610; Fax. (403)580-4612.

NOILES, James R; The Medical Assoc Clinic, 806 Vernon St, Nelson BC V1L 4G5; Qns'78; CCFP; FCFP; Ac Staff, Kootenay Lake General Hospital; (250)352-6611; Fax. (250)352-6624.

NOILES, Mary A; Glenmore Landing, D275-1600 90 Ave SW, Calgary AB T2V 5A8; McM'85; CCFP; FCFP; (403)259-2709; Fax. (403)259-6014.

NOISEUX, Daniel; Ctr d'Endocrin de Monteregie, 409 boul Saint-Luc, St-Jean-sur-Richel QC J2W 2A3; Mon'91; FRCPC; IntMed; Endocrin (P.Q.); Endocrin&Metab. Langs: English; (450)515-3688; Fax. (450)515-3689.

NOISEUX, Isabelle; Medi-Centre Chomedey, 610 boul Cure-Labelle, Laval QC H7V 2T7; Mon'95; LMCC; (450)687-6452; Fax. (450)687-3243.

NOISEUX, Jean-Marc; 201-2200 ch de Chambly, Longueuil QC J4J 3Z3; Mon'82; Langs: English; (450)646-3892

NOISEUX, Nicolas; CHUM-Hotel-Dieu, 3840 rue Saint-Urbain, Montreal QC H2W 1T8; Laval'96 Laval; MSc; BSc; FRCS; FRCSC; CardSurg. Staff, Centre Hospitalier l'Université de Montréal (CHUM) - Hôtel-Dieu; Langs: Bilingual(French/English); (514)890-8131; Fax. (514)412-7231; noiseuxn@videotron.ca.

NOISEUX, Pierre; Clinique Fam de St-Hyacinthe, 2955 boul Laframboise, Saint-Hyacinthe QC J2S 4Z3; Toulouse (France)'79; Langs: Bilingual(French/English); (450)774-4611; Fax. (450)773-9913; mluneau@sympatico.ca.

NOISEUX, Robert; Hotel-Dieu de Levis, 143 rue Wolfe, Levis QC G6V 3Z1; Laval'73; FRCPC; Psy (Geriatric Psychiatry). Dir Ctre de Psy, Hôtel-Dieu de Lévis; Teach Staff, Université Laval; Langs: English; French; (418)835-7155 x7141; Fax. (418)835-7199; robert_noiseux@ssss.gouv.qc.ca.

NOLAN, John F; 6668 Fraser St, Vancouver BC V5X 3T5; Glasgow (Scotland)'72; MB ChB; (604)321-6651; Fax. (604)325-3915.

NOLAN, John; Niagara H System-Niagara Lk, PO Box 1686 176 Wellington St, Niagara-Lake ON L0S 1J0; Wes'73; FRCPC; IntMed. Staff, Niagara Health System - Niagara-on-the-Lake Hospital Site; (905)468-0403; Fax. (905)468-4805.

NOLAN, Kathleen J; Mcmaster University, MDCL 3101A-1280 Main St W, Hamilton ON L8S 4K1; Dal'08; Peds.

NOLAN, Kevin J M; The Ottawa Hosp-Civic Campus, 1053 Carling Ave, Ottawa ON K1Y 4E9; Qns'74; FRCPC; Anes (Acute Pain Management). Att Staff, The Ottawa Hospital - Civic Campus; Assoc Staff, Royal Ottawa Mental Health Centre - Royal Ottawa Health Care Group; Asst Prof, University of Ottawa; Langs: English; French; (613)761-4169

NOLAN, Kevin R; 3237 Fraser St, Vancouver BC V5V 4B8; London (England)'69; MB BS; MRCS; FRCP; Vis Staff, UBC Hospital - Koerner Pavillion; (604)874-0252

NOLAN, Liana; Region Of Waterloo Public Hlth, PO Box 1633 Stn Waterloo 99 Regina St S, Waterloo ON N2J 4V3; Wes'89; MHSc; FRCPC; CommunMed. Commissioner/Med Officer of Hlth, Region of Waterloo Public Health Corporate Office; (519)883-2240; Fax. (519)883-2241; lnolan@regionofwaterloo.ca.

NOLAN, Maureen C; 5820 University Ave, Halifax NS B3H 1V7; Dal'88; FRCPC; RadOncol. Staff, Queen Elizabeth II Health Sciences Centre - Victoria General Site; Consultant, Cape Breton Healthcare Complex; Physician, Capital Health-Nova Scotia Cancer Centre; Asst Prof, Dalhousie University; (902)473-6081; Fax. (902)473-7205; maureen.nolan@cdha.nshealth.ca.

NOLAN, Robert L; 76 Stuart St, Kingston ON K7L 2V7; Dal'74; DABR; BSc; FRCPC; DiagRad (Thoracic & Body Imaging). Staff Radiol, Kingston General Hospital; Staff, Hotel-Dieu Hospital; Staff, Providence Care - St Mary's of the Lake Hospital Site; Prof Diagnostic Radiol, Queen's University; (613)548-2301 x3364; Fax. (613)548-2412; nolanr@queensu.ca.

NOLAN, Sean P; 370 Broadway E PO Box 95021, Vancouver BC V5T 4G5; UBC'99; FRCPC; Psy. Langs: Bilingual(English/French); (604)253-4401

NOLAN, Sheila M; Hycroft Med Bldg, 119-3195 Granville St, Vancouver BC V6H 3K2; Cal'76; ABIM; AB; FRCPC; IntMed; Psy. Ac Staff Psy, Vancouver General Hospital - Centennial Pavillion; Clin Assoc Prof Psy, University of British Columbia; (604)730-2481

NOLAN, Thomas J; Bayvalley Med Arts Bldg, 202-145 Queenston St, St Catharines ON L2R 2Z9; Wes'94; FRCPC; IntMed (Respirology); Respir. Staff, Niagara Health System - St Catharines General Site; Staff, Niagara Health System - Ontario Street Site; (905)641-1500; Fax. (905)641-1501.

NOLAN, William T; Ault Area Hosp, 750 Great Northern Rd, Sault Ste. Marie ON P6B 0A8; McM'84; FRCPC; Neur. Staff, Sault Area Hospital - Sault Ste Marie; (705)759-3434

NOLAND, Iris R; 56 Toronto Rd PO Box 339, Colborne ON K0K 1S0; McM'79; BSc; Staff Family Practice, QHC Trenton Memorial; (905)355-5355; Fax. (905)355-5929.

NOLET, Bernard; Centre Med Samson, 202-4599 boul Samson, Laval QC H7W 2H2; Mon'71; Assoc Staff, Hôpital du Sacre-Coeur de Montréal; (450)688-7170; Fax. (450)688-3335.

NOLET, Louise; Bureau du Coroner, 390-2875 boul Laurier, Quebec QC G1V 5B1; Laval'75; AnatPath. Chef Coroner, Gouvernement du Quebec; (418)643-1845 x20231; Fax. (418)644-4157; louise.nolet@msp.gouv.qc.ca.

NOLET, Mireille; Hop du Sacre-Coeur de Mtl, 5400 boul Gouin O, Montreal QC H4J 1C5; Sher'04; FRCPC; Anes. Staff, Hôpital du Sacre-Coeur de Montréal; (514)338-2222 x2680

NOLET-LEVESQUE, Philippe; CSSS de Trois-Rivieres, 1991 boul du Carmel, Trois-Rivieres QC G8Z 3R9; Laval'07; DiagRad. Staff, CSSS de Trois-Rivières; (819)697-3333

NOLIN, Clement; Clinique Med du Campanile, 104-3730 rue du Campanile, Quebec QC G1X 4G6; Laval'80; (418)652-0030; Fax. (418)652-9855.

NOLIN, Karine; Centre Med de Cowansville, 101-370 rue de la Riviere, Cowansville QC J2K 1N3; Sher'04; CCFP; Staff, Centre Maria-Chapdelaine - CH de Dolbeau-Mistassini; Staff, CHSLD-CLSC Cleophas-Claveau; (450)263-0774

NOLIN, Linda; Hop Maisonneuve-Rosemont, 5415 boul de l'Assomption, Montreal QC H1T 2M4; Sher'74; Nephrol (P.Q.) (Hemodialysis). Staff, Hopital Maisonneuve-Rosemont; Universite de Montreal; Langs: English; (514)252-3499; Fax. (514)255-3026.

NOLTE, Josephus J; Hilltop Med Clinic, 140-15321 16 Ave, Surrey BC V4A 1R6; Pretoria (South Africa)'79; MB ChB; LMCC; CCFP; Langs: Afrikaans; (604)531-5575; Fax. (604)535-0126.

NOLTEN, Audrey E; Vancouver Breast Centre, 505-750 Broadway W, Vancouver BC V5Z 1H4; Wisconsin (USA)'93; Staff, Vancouver Breast Centre; (604)879-4177

NOLZE, Christine; Clinique Dre Christine Nolze, CP 1820 5098 rue Foster, Waterloo QC J0E 2N0; Mon'83; Langs: Bilingual(French/English); (450)539-4171; Fax. (450)539-4661.

NONNENMAN, David K; Clin Chir Plastique David Nonn, 554 av Notre-Dame, Saint-Lambert QC J4P 2K7; McG'80; FRCSC; PlasSurg. Staff, Centre Hospitalier Pierre Boucher; Langs: Bilingual(French/English); (450)671-7366; Fax. (450)671-9938; dr.nonnenman@bellnet.ca.

NOONAN, Karen M; Downey Family Med Centre, 2-115 Downey Rd, Guelph ON N1C 1A2; McM'02; CCFP; (519)827-9779; Fax. (519)827-0255.

NOONAN, Liza M; Royal Alexandra Hosp, 10240 Kingsway NW, Edmonton AB T5H 3V9; Cal'04; FRCPC; Anes. Staff, Royal Alexandra Hospital; (780)735-4111

NOONAN, Peter G; Queen Elizabeth Hosp, PO Box 6600 Stn Central 60 Riverside Dr, Charlottetown PE C1A 8T5; Dal'85; FAAP; FRCPC; Peds. Med Staff, Queen Elizabeth Hospital; (902)844-2440

NOONE, Joseph A; 715 12th Ave W, Vancouver BC V5Z 1M9; Dublin (Ireland)'75; LRCPI&LM; LRCS; FAPA; FRCPC; Psy (Aggression Management). Staff, BC Mental Health & Addiction Service; Staff, Vancouver General Hospital - Centennial Pavillion; Aj Prof Psychology, Simon Fraser University; Clin Prof Psy, University of British Columbia; (604)224-1669; jnoone@telus.net.

NOOR, Amra; St Joseph's Health Centre, 100 Westmount Rd, Guelph ON N1H 5H8; Punjab (Pakistan)'95; FRCPC; IntMed; GeriatricMed. Staff, Guelph General Hospital; Staff, St Joseph's Health Centre; (519)837-6440

NOOR, Mounir H A; 14-10088 McLaughlin Rd, Brampton ON L7A 2X6; Cairo (Egypt)'74; MB ChB; LMCC; CCFP; Langs: Arabic; (905)495-9040; Fax. (905)459-0349.

NOORA, Joseph; 608-89 Queensway W, Mississauga ON L5B 2V2; McG'99; FRCSC; CardSurg. Staff, Hamilton Health Sciences Centre - Hamilton General Hospital; (905)848-7513; Fax. (905)848-7515.

NOORANI, Naushad A; William Osler HC-Brampton, 2100 Bovaird Dr E, Brampton ON L6R 3J7; Karachi (Pakistan)'90; MB BS; FRCPC; Psy. Staff, William Osler Health System - Brampton Civic Hospital; Langs: Urdu; Hindi; (705)728-9802

NOORANI, Shamidah; 312-450 Central Ave, London ON N6B 2E8; Karachi (Pakistan)'92; CCFP; (519)488-0208

NOORDIN, Nadia; West Winds Med Clinic, 2130-4818 Westwinds Dr NE, Calgary AB T3J 3Z5; Cal'06; (403)293-5454; Fax. (403)293-1511.

NOORDMAN, Annelies H; PO Box 540, Grande Cache AB T0E 0Y0; (Netherlands Antilles)'02; (780)827-2540; Fax. (780)827-5698.

NOORI, Mahir A; Iroquois Ridge Med Center, B5-360 Dundas St E, Oakville ON L6H 6Z9; Baghdad (Iraq)'79; MB ChB; CCFP; (905)257-8777; Fax. (905)257-0437.

NOORI LAHROUD, Marziyeh; 106-11420 27 St SE, Calgary AB T2Z 3R6; (Other Foreign)'94; (587)352-8718; Fax. (587)352-8728.

NOOROLAHI, Babak; CSSS de Trois-Rivières, 1991 boul du Carmel, Trois-Rivieres QC G8Z 3R9; Shahid Beheshti (Iran)'96; Respir (P.Q.). Staff, CSSS de Trois-Rivières; (819)697-3333

NOORY, Caroline; Centre de Sante de Rigaud, 1 rue Hotel de Ville, Rigaud QC J0P 1P0; Sher'84; CCFP; Teach Staff, Centre Hospitalier de Verdun; Universite de Montreal; Langs: Bilingual(French/English); (450)451-5336; Fax. (450)451-5214.

NOOTENS, Jean V; CHUS-Hop Hotel-Dieu, 580 rue Bowen S, Sherbrooke QC J1G 2E8; Louvain (Belgium)'64; PlasSurg (P.Q.) (Aesthetic Surgery). Staff, Centre Hospitalier Universitaire de Sherbrooke-Hopital Fleurimont; Staff, Centre Hospitalier Universitaire de Sherbrooke-Hôpital Hôtel-Dieu; Consultant, CSST-Chaudiere-Appalaches; (819)346-1110

NOPPERS, Willem H; CFB Wainwright, GD 12 CFHS Wainwright, Denwood AB T0B 1B0; Qns'08; CCFP; (780)842-1363; Fax. (780)842-1809.

NORBASH, Adrian A; 192-8888 Country Hills Blvd NW, Calgary AB T3G 5T4; Cal'02; FRCPC; Psy;CCFP; (403)239-3660

NORD, Peter W; Providence Healthcare, 3276 St Clair Ave E, Scarborough ON M1L 1W1; McM'87; CCFP; VP/Chief/Med Officer of Hlth, Providence Healthcare; (416)285-3666 x4100; Fax. (416)285-3670.

NORDAHL, Karen M; 202-5511 West Boulevard, Vancouver BC V6M 3W6; UBC'89; (604)266-3453

NORDAL, Robert A; Tom Baker Cancer Centre, 1331 29 St NW, Calgary AB T2N 4N2; Alb'92; FRCPC; RadOncol. Staff, Tom Baker Cancer Centre; (403)521-3077; Fax. (403)283-1651.

NORDIN, Christopher E; 709-1400 Blair Place, Gloucester ON K1J 9B8; Ott'77; (613)747-7711; Fax. (613)747-8414.

NORDLI, Charlene M; PO Box 88573 Rpo Newton, Surrey BC V3W 0X1; Cal'87; (604)596-6949

NORDLI, Tania C; 9917 87 St NW, Edmonton AB T5H 1N2; Alb'94; CCFP; FCFP; Staff, Centennial Centre for Mental Health & Brain Injury; (780)918-2451; Fax. (780)429-3913.

NORDSTROM, Scott; CSSSG-Hop de Hull, 116 boul Lionel-Emond, Gatineau QC J8Y 1W7; Alb'97; CSPQ; FRCPC; Anes. Staff, Hull Hospital; (819)966-6200

NORGROVE, Leah V A; Helmcken Cove Family Practice, 108-284 Helmcken Rd, Victoria BC V9B 1T2; McM'90; CCFP; FCFP; Staff Privil, Vancouver Island Health Authority; Assoc Physician, Victoria Hospice Society; Member Faculty of Med, University of British Columbia; (250)480-7333; Fax. (250)480-7335.

NORHEIM, Jennifer K; 103-309 9 Ave SW, High River AB T1V 0H2; Cal'96; BSc; CCFP; (403)652-1654; Fax. (403)652-1721.

NORIA, Dhun F; Scarborough Hosp-Birchmount, 3030 Birchmount Rd, Scarborough ON M1W 3W3; Osmania (India)'67; FRCPC; AnatPath. Dir Laboratory/Chief Path, The Scarborough Hospital - Birchmount Campus; (416)495-2476

NORIA, Sabrena; Univ Hlth Network-Toronto Gen, 200 Elizabeth St, Toronto ON M5G 2C4; Tor'05; FRCSC; GenSurg. Staff, Toronto General Hospital - UHN; (416)340-3111

NORIEGA, Eleazar H; 706-1881 Yonge St, Toronto ON M4S 3C4; (Mexico)'70; FRCPC; Peds. Langs: Spanish; (416)922-2657; Fax. (416)922-6082.

NORKUS, Daiva L; Islington Med Clinic, 1004-1243 Islington Ave, Etobicoke ON M8X 1Y9; Lithuania (Russia (Federation))'89; CCFP; Associate Family Practice Unit, St Joseph's Health Centre; Langs: Lithuanian; Russian; Polish; (416)767-7725; Fax. (416)767-9959.

NORMAN, Alia W; Dr H Bliss Murphy Cancer Ctre, 300 Prince Philip Dr, St. John's NL A1B 3V6; Man'01; FRCPC; RadOncol. Staff, Dr H Bliss Murphy Cancer Centre; (709)777-6480

NORMAN, Brian P; Dartmouth Gen Hosp, 325 Pleasant St, Dartmouth NS B2Y 4G8; Mem'03; FRCPC; Anes; Critical Care Medicine. Staff, Dartmouth General Hospital; (902)465-8355; Fax. (902)465-2550.

NORMAN, Charles; Brandon Reg Health Centre, 150 McTavish Ave E, Brandon MB R7A 2B3; Dundee (Scotland)'76; MB ChB; LMCC; Med Officer/Chief EmergMed, Brandon Regional Health Centre; (204)726-1122

NORMAN, David W; 107-151 Metcalfe St, Ottawa ON K2P 1N8; McG'50; Psy (General Adult Psychiatry). (613)235-6787

NORMAN, Gregory S; Burns Lake Med Clinic, PO Box 6000, Burns Lake BC V0J 1E0; Cal'83; BSc; CCFP; Staff, Lakes District Hospital & Health Centre; (250)692-3111; Fax. (250)692-7477.

NORMAN, Lawrence I; The Ottawa Hosp-Civic Campus, 1053 Carling Ave, Ottawa ON K1Y 4E9; Ott'02; CCFP; CCFP(E.M.); Staff, The Ottawa Hospital - Civic Campus; (613)761-5020

NORMAN, Lynne M; Halton HSC Corp-Oakville, 327 Reynolds St, Oakville ON L6J 3L7; Mem'92; CCFP; CCFP(E.M.); Staff, Halton Healthcare Services Corporation - Oakville Site; (905)338-4605

NORMAN, Nadine I E; SGH Medical Mall, 316-3030 Lawrence Ave E, Scarborough ON M1P 2T7; UBC'93; BSc; MSc; FRCSC; GenSurg (Breasts). Staff, The Scarborough Hospital - General Campus; Staff General Surgery, Albany Medical Clinic; (416)439-7779; Fax. (416)439-6128; nnorman@cheo.on.ca.

NORMAN, Richard W; 202-5110 St Margarets Bay Rd, Upper Tantallon NS B3Z 1E2; Dal'77; FRCSC; Urol (Stone Disorders). Ac Staff, Queen Elizabeth II Health Sciences Centre - Victoria General Site; Consultant, IWK Health Centre; Prof, Dalhousie University; (902)826-7200; Fax. (902)826-2887; richard.norman@dal.ca.

NORMAN, Tanya L; Minto-Mapleton Family Hlth Tea, 11 Andrews Dr W, Drayton ON N0G 1P0; McM'02; CCFP; (519)638-3088

NORMAN, Wendy V; BC Women's Hosp & Health Ctre, E202-4500 Oak St, Vancouver BC V6H 1N3; Qns'85; DTMH; MHSc; CCFP; FCFP; Med Dir CARE Prog, BC Children's Hospital; Staff CAER & WHRI, BC Women's Hospital & Health Centre; Clin Assoc Prof Family Pract, University of British Columbia; (604)875-2022; wvnorman@interchange.ubc.ca.

NORMAND, Jean-Pierre; CSSS de la Region de Thetford, 1717 rue Notre-Dame E, Thetford Mines QC G6G 2V4; Laval'85; CSPQ; DiagRad. Staff, Hopital du CSS de la Region de Thetford; (418)338-7777

NORMAND, Marie; Clinique Med Lauzon, 213 rue Saint-Joseph, Levis QC G6V 1C8; Laval'95; Staff, Centre Hospitalier l'Université De Montréal (CHUM) - Hôpital Saint-luc; Staff, Centre Hospitalier l'Université de Montréal (CHUM) - Hôpital Notre-Dame; (418)833-2473; Fax. (418)833-6954; carole.gagnon.chum@ssss.gouv.qc.ca.

NORMAND, Michel; CHUQ-Ctr Hosp Univ Laval, 2705 boul Laurier, Quebec QC G1V 4G2; Mon'86; FRCPC; IntMed. Staff, Centre Hospitalier Universitaire de Quebec-CHUL; (418)656-4141

NORMANDIN, Alexander; Clinique Access Med, 200-17001 rte Trans-Canada, Kirkland QC H9H 5J1; McG'10; MDCM; CCFP; (514)694-4644

NORMANDIN, Denyse; CHUS-Hop Fleurimont, 3001 12e av N, Sherbrooke QC J1H 5N4; Mon'74; FRCSC; GenSurg; Cardiovasc&ThorSurg. Staff, Centre Hospitalier Universitaire de Sherbrooke-Hopital Fleurimont; (819)346-1110

NORMANDIN, Diane M; Clin Prive de Med Familiale, GD 200-2871 boul des Promenades, Ste-Marthe-S-L-Lac QC J0N 1P0; McG'88; Langs: Bilingual(English/French); (450)472-7759; Fax. (450)472-2334.

NORMANDIN, Jean-Junior; 206-5125 boul Cousineau, Saint-Hubert QC J3Y 3K7; Mon'90; FAAD; CSPQ; LMCC; FRCPC; Derm. Chef Derm, Hopital Charles LeMoyne; Langs: English; (450)550-5566; Fax. (450)550-5567.

NORMANDIN, Louis; CHUM-Hote-Dieu, 2 2402-3840 rue Saint-Urbain, Montreal QC H2W 1T8; Mon'84; Cardiovasc&ThorSurg; GenSurg. Staff, Centre Hospitalier l'Université de Montréal (CHUM) - Hôtel-Dieu; (514)890-8000 x15808

NORMANDIN, Luc; Clinique Med St-Sulpice, 12-1420 rue Legendre E, Montreal QC H2M 1H5; Mon'76; Ac Staff, Centre Hospitalier Fleury; Langs: English; (514)382-0552; Fax. (514)382-4324.

NORMANDIN, Lucie; CLSC du Plateau Mont-Royal, 4625 av de Lorimier, Montreal QC H2H 2B4; Laval'79; (514)521-7663; Fax. (514)521-6426.

NORMANDIN, Olivier; Ctr Hosp Anna-Laberge, 200 boul Brisebois, Chateauguay QC J6K 4W8; Sher'05; Staff, Hôpital Anna-Laberge; (450)699-2425; Fax. (450)699-2525.

NORMANDIN, Pierre; Centre Med Iberville, 101-235 2e av, St-Jean-Sur-Richel QC J2X 2B2; Mon'77; ac Staff, Hôpital du Haut-Richelieu; (450)347-5548; Fax. (450)347-4091.

NORMANDIN-NOEL, Ginette; Polyclinique Pointe Aux Trembl, 103-12905 rue Sherbrooke E, Pte-aux-Trembles QC H1A 1B9; Mon'68; Médecin, Polyclinique Pointe Aux Trembles; Langs: English; (514)498-4050; Fax. (514)498-8239.

NORMANN, A Barbro; North Burlington Med Centre, 18-1960 Appleby Line, Burlington ON L7L 0B7; RCS (Ireland)'84; Langs: Norwegian; (905)319-2000; Fax. (905)319-6292.

NORMORE, Wayne J; Canadian Forces Hlth Serv Ctr, PO Box 99000 Stn Forces, Halifax NS B3K 5X5; Mem'84; FRCPC; DiagRad. Staff, Canadian Forces Health Services Centre (Atlantic); (902)427-0550 x8804; Fax. (902)427-8584.

NORONHA, Charles A; 203-86 Angeline St S, Lindsay ON K9V 6C5; Bangalore (India)'78; MB BS; FRCSC; OrthSurg. (705)878-5551; Fax. (705)878-8455.

NORONHA, Lionel J; Stirling Med Centre, 9C Tuftsville Rd RR 4, Stirling ON K0K 3E0; Tor'90; CCFP; FCFP; (613)395-5566; Fax. (613)395-3636.

NORONHA, Luis C E; 836 Bloor St W, Toronto ON M6G 1M2; Tor'94; BSc; FRCPC; IntMed (Cardiology). Consultant, Trillium Health Centre - Mississauga; Langs: Portuguese; Spanish; Italian; Cantonese; (416)924-5871; luis.noronha@utoronto.ca.

NORONHA, Marie G; Shakti Med Clinic, 1309 Main St W, Hamilton ON L8S 1C5; Madras (India)'65; Staff, Hamilton Health Sciences Centre - McMaster Children's Hospital; Court Staff Privil, St Joseph's Healthcare - Charlton Campus; (905)529-6560; Fax. (905)529-6573.

NORONHA, Osborne I; 2B-150 Sidney St, Belleville ON K8P 5E2; Tor'91; (613)968-3491

NOROOZI, Nastaran; McMaster University, MDCL 3101A-1200 Main St W, Hamilton ON L8N 3Z5; (Iran)'98; FRCPC; IntMed. (905)525-9140

NOROZI, Kambiz; London HSC-Victoria Hosp, PO Box 5010 Stn B 800 Commissioners Rd E, London ON N6A 5W9; Hanover (Germany)'92; FRCPC; Peds. Staff, London Health Sciences Centre - Victoria Campus; (519)685-8500 x57134; Fax. (519)685-8156.

NORRIE, Deborah L; 200-440 Boler Rd, London ON N6K 4L2; Wes'08; CCFP; (519)473-4394

NORRIE, Fraser R; Spectrum Health, 702-1080 Howe St, Vancouver BC V6Z 2T1; Man'87; CCFP; FCFP; Ac Staff, Providence Health Care - St Paul's Hospital; Staff, Three Bridges Community Health Centre; Clinical Asst Prof, University of British Columbia; (604)681-1080; Fax. (604)681-0244.

NORRIE, Robert G; Riverview Med Group, 205 Queen St E, Fergus ON N1M 1T2; McM'03; CCFP; (519)787-7418; Fax. (519)787-7421.

NORRIS, Barry K; Prairie Med Clinic, 10309 98 St, Grande Prairie AB T8V 2E7; Dal'72; CCFP; Staff, Queen Elizabeth II Hospital; (780)539-4010; Fax. (780)538-2290.

NORRIS, Desmond; Sault Area Hosp, 750 Great Northern Rd, Sault Ste. Marie ON P6B 0A8; Tor'76; FRCPC; Anes (Acute & Chronic Pain). Staff, Sault Area Hospital - Sault Ste Marie; (705)759-3630

NORRIS, Donald H; 2 Lyall Ave, Toronto ON M4E 1V8; Tor'67; Court Staff, Toronto East General Hospital Inc; Court Staff, St Michael's Hospital; (416)699-9823; Fax. (416)699-0459; nord@sympatico.ca.

NORRIS, Erin B; St Michael's Hosp, 3 002C-30 Bond St, Toronto ON M5B 1W8; Wes'03; FRCPC; IntMed; Rheum. Staff, St Michael's Hospital; (416)864-5295

NORRIS, I Michael; Elmira Med Centre, 2 Park Ave W, Elmira ON N3B 1L1; Tor'83; Ac Staff, Grand River Hospital - Kitchener/Waterloo Health Centre; Ac Staff, St Mary's General Hospital; (519)669-5493; Fax. (519)669-5901.

NORRIS, Jill R; Health Point Care Centre, 1454 Hillside Ave, Victoria BC V8T 2B7; Cal'04; CCFP; (250)370-5637

NORRIS, Mark L; Children's Hosp Eastern Ont, 401 Smyth Rd, Ottawa ON K1H 8L1; Mem'01; FRCPC; Peds. Staff, Children's Hospital of Eastern Ontario (CHEO); (613)737-7600

NORRIS, Mireille A; Sunnybrook Hlth Sciences Ctre, HG 69-2075 Bayview Ave, Toronto ON M4N 3M5; Mon'93; MHSc; BScPT; CSPQ; FRCPC; IntMed; GeriatricMed (Dementia). Staff, Sunnybrook Health Sciences Centre; Asst Prof Med, University of Toronto; Langs: Bilingual(French/English); (416)480-4076; Fax. (416)480-4778; mireille.norris@sunnybrook.ca.

NORRIS, Philip L; 12 Bushville Dr, Miramichi NB E1N 4R4; London (England)'58; MB BS; OrthSurg (Medico Legal Assessments). (506)622-7810

NORRIS, Phillip D; Regional Mental HC-St Thomas, PO Box 2004 Stn Main 467 Sunset Dr, St Thomas ON N5P 3V9; Leicester (England)'80; MRCPsy(UK); FRCPC; Psy (Forensic Psychiatry). Staff, Regional Mental Health Care-St Joseph's Health Care; Pt-Time Ass't. Prof., University of Western Ontario; (519)631-8510

NORRIS, Sandhaya; The Ottawa Hosp-Gen Campus, 400-501 Smyth Rd, Ottawa ON K1H 8L6; Mem'02; FRCPC; Psy. Staff, The Ottawa Hospital - General Campus; (613)737-7777

NORRIS, Sean A; 4 St Joseph St, St. Albert AB T8N 0B5; Alb'97; FRCSC; GenSurg; Critical Care Medicine. Staff, University of Alberta Hospital; (780)459-6633; Fax. (780)459-6609.

NORRIS, Stanley; CSSS du Haut Saint-Maurice, 885 boul Ducharme, La Tuque QC G9X 3C1; (Haiti)'62; Psy (Psychoanalysis). Staff, Centre Hospitalier Saint-Joseph de la Turque; Langs: Spanish; English; Creole; (819)523-4581; Fax. (819)523-4115.

NORTH, Robert H; Queen-Lynch Med Centre, 206-157 Queen St E, Brampton ON L6W 3X4; Wes'63; FRCSC; Otol. Ac Staff, Halton Healthcare Services Corporation - Georgetown Hospital; Ac Staff, Toronto Western Hospital - University Health Network; (905)459-5335

NORTH, Scott A; Cross Cancer Institute, 11560 University Ave NW, Edmonton AB T6G 1Z2; Ott'94; BSc; MD; LMCC; FRCPC; IntMed (Genito Urinary Oncology); MedOncol. Staff Med Oncol, Cross Cancer Institute; Assoc Prof Dept of Oncol, University of Alberta; Langs: English; French; (780)432-8762; Fax. (780)432-8888; scott.north@albertahealthservices.ca.

NORTHAN, Allan A; Algoma Public Health, 294 Willow Ave, Sault Ste. Marie ON P6B 0A9; Qns'72; FRCPC; Anes. A-Med Officer of Hlth, The District of Algoma Health Unit; (705)759-5421; Fax. (705)759-2540; allan_northan@ahu.on.ca.

NORTHCOTT, Colleen J; UBC-Dept of Psychiatry, 2C7-2255 Wesbrook Mall, Vancouver BC V6T 2A1; Man'92; FRCPC; Psy. (604)822-7512; Fax. (604)822-7922.

NORTHCOTT, Janet E; Maternal Child Clinic, 130-1402 8 Ave NW, Calgary AB T2N 1B8; UBC'93; CCFP; FCFP; (403)509-3080; Fax. (403)509-3082.

NORTHCOTT, Kimberly A; Vancouver Island Hlth Authorit, 2680 Richmond Rd, Victoria BC V8R 4S9; UBC'97; BSc(Hons); ABIM; FRCPC; IntMed; Rheum (Patient Health Care). Ac Staff Privil, Victoria General Hospital; Ac Staff Privil, Royal Jubilee Hospital; (250)519-4006; Fax. (250)598-7138.

NORTHCOTT, Michael G; Royal Victoria Hosp, 201 Georgian Dr, Barrie ON L4M 6M2; Wes'85; FRCPC; Anes. Staff, Royal Victoria Regional Health Centre; (705)728-9802 x4207; mnorthcott@sympatico.ca.

NORTHCOTT, Richard D; Medicine Hat Reg Hosp, 666 5 St SW, Medicine Hat AB T1A 4H6; Man'84; CCFP; Staff, Medicine Hat Regional Hospital; (403)529-8000; Fax. (403)529-8978.

NORTHCOTT, Rosemary D E; Royal Victoria Hosp, 201 Georgian Dr, Barrie ON L4M 6M2; Wes'89; CCFP; CCFP(E.M.); Staff, Royal Victoria Regional Health Centre; (705)728-9802; rdenorthcott@rogers.com.

NORTHCOTT, Sandra J; London HSC-Victoria Hosp, PO Box 5010 Stn B A2 632-800 Commissioners Rd E, London ON N6A 5W9; Mem'94; FRCPC; Psy. Staff, London Health Sciences Centre - Victoria Campus; Assoc Prof, University of Western Ontario; (519)667-6662; Fax. (519)667-6689.

NORTHEY, Angela J; Norfolk Med Centre, 302-85 Norfolk St, Guelph ON N1H 4J4; Ott'02; FRCPC; Anes. Staff, Guelph General Hospital.

NORTHEY, Karen; Cumberland Med Clinic, 11-900 Watters Rd, Orleans ON K4A 0B4; Tor'02; CCFP; (613)830-3837

NORTHEY, Robert A W; 33 Somerset St W, Ottawa ON K2P 0H3; Dal'93; BSc; Psy (Psychotherapy & Psychoanalysis)., University of Ottawa; Langs: German; (613)237-4452

NORTHGRAVE, Stacey A; Northgrave Med Inc, 110-336 Kings Rd, Sydney NS B1S 1A9; Dal'97; FRCPC; Derm. (902)539-3961

NORTHOFF, Georg F; Royal Ottawa Hlth Care Group, 1145 Carling Ave, Ottawa ON K1Z 7K4; (Germany)'89; Staff, Royal Ottawa Mental Health Centre - Royal Ottawa Health Care Group; (613)722-6521

NORTHORP, Sharon M E; 203-44 Mapleton Rd, Moncton NB E1C 7W8; Dal'86; CCFP; Staff, The Moncton Hospital; Pres, CFPC NB Chapter; (506)853-8983; Fax. (506)389-2529.

NORTON, Bryan; 306-125 13th St E, North Vancouver BC V7L 2L3; Cape Town (South Africa)'76; DA(SA); (604)988-6330; Fax. (604)987-3382.

NORTON, Seamus; Delhi Family Health Team, 105 Main Street of Delhi, Delhi ON N4B 2L8; Tor'98; FRCPC; Peds. Clinical Asst Prof, McMaster University; Langs: Bilingual(English/French); (519)582-2323; Fax. (519)582-3770.

NORUM, Joanne N; Royal Alexandra Hosp, 551 CSC-10240 Kingsway NW, Edmonton AB T5H 3V9; Sask'99; FRCPC; EmergMed. Staff, Royal Alexandra Hospital; (780)735-4442; Fax. (780)735-4916.

NORVAL, Ivan L; Associated Radiologist, 300-140 Wall St, Saskatoon SK S7K 1N4; Stellenbosch (South Africa)'96; MB ChB; FRCPC; DiagRad. (306)244-1167; Fax. (306)244-2911.

NORWICH, Kenneth H; 23 Peveril Hill S, Toronto ON M6C 3A7; Tor'63; BSc; MSc; PhD(Physics); Emeritus Prof, University of Toronto; (416)785-3611; Fax. (416)978-4317.

NOSAL, Robert M; Halton Reg Health Dept, 1151 Bronte Rd, Oakville ON L6M 3L1; Qns'78; FRCPC; CommunMed. Med Officer of Hlth, Halton Reg. Health Dept.; Lecturer, University of Toronto; (905)825-6000 x7806; Fax. (905)825-1444; bob.nosal@halton.ca.

NOSEWORTHY, A Lynn; H K P R Health Unit, 200 Roseglen Rd, Port Hope ON L1A 3V6; Mem'79; MHSc; FRCPC; CommunMed (Public Health). Aj Prof Commun Health & Epidemiol, Queen's University; Aj Teach Staff Dalla Lana School of Public Health, University of Toronto; (905)885-9100 x213; Fax. (905)885-9551.

NOSEWORTHY, Gordon W; Terrace Clinic, 204-35 Major's Path, St. John's NL A1A 4Z9; Mem'75; MHSc; FRCPC; Psy. Assoc Staff, St Clare's Mercy Hospital; Consultant Psy, St. John's Health Care Corp.; Clin Assoc Prof, Memorial University Of Newfoundland; (709)777-3450

NOSEWORTHY, Mary E; Alberta Children's Hosp, C3 202-2888 Shaganappi Trail N, Calgary AB T3B 6A8; Mem'93; BSc(Hon.); FRCPC; Peds (Asthma); Respir. Staff, Alberta Children's Hospital; (403)955-2952; Fax. (403)955-7059; mary.noseworthy@albertahealthservices.ca.

NOSEWORTHY, Melanie A; Cabot Square Med Clinic, 55 Stavanger Dr, St. John's NL A1A 5E8; Mem'04; CCFP; (709)576-7075

NOSEWORTHY, Robert F; Royal Columbian Hosp, 330 Columbia St E, New Westminster BC V3L 3W7; Mem'80; FRCPC; EmergMed. Staff, Royal Columbian Hospital; (604)520-4000; Fax. (604)520-4722.

NOSEWORTHY, Stephen; Children's Hosp Eastern Ont, 401 Smyth Rd, Ottawa ON K1H 8L1; Mem'01; FRCPC; Peds (Pediatric Emergency Medicine). Staff, Children's Hospital of Eastern Ontario (CHEO); (613)737-7600

NOSEWORTHY, Thomas W; HMRB-Commun Health Sciences, 3330 Hospital Dr NW, Calgary AB T2N 4N1; Mem'73; MSc(ExptMed); MPH(Harvard); FACP(IntMed); FCCP; IntMed. Dir, Centre for Health & Policy Studies; Dept Head Commun Health Sciences, University of Calgary; (403)220-2481; Fax. (403)270-7307; tnosewor@ucalgary.ca.

NOSIB, Shravankumar S; 502-402 21st St E, Saskatoon SK S7K 0C3; Gwalior (India)'87; MB BS; LMCC; FRCPC; IntMed; Cardiol. (306)956-3444; Fax. (306)956-3577.

NOSS, Mark B; Brockville Gen Hosp, 75 Charles St, Brockville ON K6V 1S8; Tor'92; MSc; FRCSC; Urol (Male Infertility). Staff, Providence Continuing Care Centre (PCCC) - St Vincent de Paul Hospital; Queen's University; (613)341-9333; Fax. (613)342-9009.

NOTARANDREA, Edoardo; Mackenzie Richmond Hill Hosp, 10 Trench St, Richmond Hill ON L4C 4Z3; Tor'91; CCFP; CCFP(E.M.); FCFP; Staff, Mackenzie Richmond Hill Hospital; (905)883-1212

NOTEBAERT, Eric; Hop du Sacre-Coeur de Mtl, 5400 boul Gouin O, Montreal QC H4J 1C5; Mon'87; Staff, Hôpital du Sacre-Coeur de Montréal; Staff, Hopital de la Cite de la santé; (514)338-2000

NOTICEWALA, Neelam N; Scarborough Hosp-Birchmount, 3030 Birchmount Rd, Scarborough ON M1W 3W3; Columbus(OH) (USA)'01; FRCPC; Peds. Staff, The Scarborough Hospital - Birchmount Campus; (416)495-2886

NOTKIN, Robert M; Psymed Inc, 200-5700 Yonge St, North York ON M2M 4K2; McG'82; FRCPC; Psy. (416)490-8347; Fax. (416)490-0953.

NOTMAN, Emily B H; 555 Barrydowne Rd, Sudbury ON P3A 3T2; Tor'10; CCFP; (705)524-7419

NOTTEBROCK, Douglas H; Kelowna Gen Hosp, 2268 Pandosy St, Kelowna BC V1Y 1T2; Sask'87; CCFP; Staff, Kelowna General Hospital; (250)862-4000

NOUCH, Susan L; Pender Community Health Centre, 59 Pender St W, Vancouver BC V6B 1R3; UBC'08; CCFP; Staff, Pender Community Health Centre; (604)669-9181

NOUH, Elias; CSSS Haut-Richelieu-Rouville, 920 boul du Seminaire N, St-Jean-Sur-Richel QC J3A 1B7; St. Joseph (Lebanon)'72; MedOncol (P.Q.); Hem (P.Q.). Ac Staff, Hôpital du Haut-Richelieu; (450)359-5000; Fax. (450)359-5237.

NOUH, Mohamed; 4713 48 Ave SS 3, St Paul AB T0A 3A3; Tanta (Egypt)'76; AddicMed; Staff, Moose Jaw Union Hospital; Langs: Arabic; French; (780)645-3331; mohamednouh@hotmail.com.

NOUH, Thamer A; MUHC-Montreal Gen Hosp, L94.24-1650 av Cedar, Montreal QC H3G 1A4; Riyadh (Saudi Arabia)'99; FRCSC; GenSurg; Critical Care Medicine. Staff, McGill University Health Centre - Montreal General Campus; (514)934-1934 x31532

NOULTY, Elizabeth J; Maple Lodge, PO Box 2018 115-54 Ridge Rd, Deep River ON K0J 1P0; Wes'86; CCFP; FCFP; Att Physician, Deep River & District Hospital; (613)584-3238; Fax. (613)584-3239.

NOUR, Emad I; Niagara H System-St Catharine, PO Box 3018 Stn Main 142 Queenston St, St Catharines ON L2R 7C6; Asyut (Egypt)'86; MB ChB; CCFP; CCFP(E.M.); Staff, Niagara Health System - St Catharines General Site; (905)684-7271 x45000

NOUR, Rabih; 104-2462 Howard Ave, Windsor ON N8X 3V6; Michigan (USA)'03; (519)946-2003; Fax. (519)946-2004.

NOURHOSSEINI, Seyed H; 214-250 Harding Blvd W, Richmond Hill ON L4C 9M7; (Iran)'89; FRCSC; OrthSurg (Hip & Knee Replacement). Staff, Mackenzie Richmond Hill Hospital; (905)237-4385; Fax. (905)237-4386.

NOURISSAT, Ghislain; CHUQ-St-Francois D'Assise, 10 rue de l'Espinay, Quebec QC G1L 3L5; Staff, Centre Hospitalier Universitaire De Québec - Pavillon De St-françois-d'assise; (418)525-4492

NOUSIAINEN, Markku T; Sunnybrook Holland Ortho Arthr, 621-43 Wellesley St E, Toronto ON M4Y 1H1; Tor'00; BAHons; MS; MEd; FRCSC; OrthSurg (Arthroplasty). Surgeon Orthopaedic, Sunnybrook Health Sciences Centre - Holland Orthopaedic & Arthritic Centre; Asst Prof, University of Toronto; (416)967-8639; Fax. (416)967-8781.

NOVA, Natalie; 477 King St, Welland ON L3B 3K4; Wes'07; CCFP; (905)378-4647; nnova@uwo.ca.

NOVAK, David J; 1302 Government St, Penticton BC V2A 4V8; Man'67; BSc; Neur (Stroke). Med Staff, Penticton Regional Hospital; Med Consultant, Kelowna General Hospital; (250)493-2981; Fax. (250)493-8381; djnovak@shawbiz.ca.

NOVAK, John J; 419 5 St S, Lethbridge AB T1J 2B6; Alb'82; FRCSC; Ophth. (403)329-8200; Fax. (403)328-0278.

NOVAK, Kerri L; Teaching Research & Wellness, 3280 Hospital Dr NW, Calgary AB T2N 4Z6; UBC'03; FRCPC; Gastroent; IntMed. Staff, Health Research Innovation Centre; (403)592-5025; Fax. (403)592-5050.

NOVAK, Marta; Univ Hlth Network-Toronto Gen, 200 Elizabeth St, Toronto ON M5G 2C4; Semmelweis (Hungary)'93; Staff, Toronto General Hospital - UHN; (416)340-3043

NOVAK, Michele Y L D; Canadian Sport Medicine, 2424 University Dr NW, Calgary AB T2N 3Y9; Alb'00; BSc; Dip SportMed; CCFP; (403)289-8959; Fax. (403)284-9139.

NOVAK, Paul G; Western Cardiology Associates, 335-1900 Richmond Ave, Victoria BC V8R 4R2; Wes'97; FRCPC; IntMed; Cardiol. (250)595-1551

NOVAK, Rudolf; 407-1265 Arthur St E, Thunder Bay ON P7E 6E7; Bratislava (Slovakia)'94; FRCSC; ObstGyn. rudolf@thunderbay.org.

NOVAK, Tomas; Mount Sinai Hosp, 206-600 University Ave, Toronto ON M5G 1X5; Qns'80; CCFP; CCFP(E.M.); FCFP; Staff Emerg, Lakeridge Health - Oshawa Site; Ac Staff, Mount Sinai Hospital; Court Staff, Sunnybrook Health Sciences Centre; Lecturer family & Community Med, University of Toronto; (416)586-5058; Fax. (416)586-4719.

NOVAKOVIC, Petar; Scarborough Hosp-General Div, 3050 Lawrence Ave E, Scarborough ON M1P 2V5; Tor'09; CCFP; CCFP(E.M.); Staff, The Scarborough Hospital - General Campus; (416)438-2911

NOVALES DIAZ, Javier; MUHC-Royal Victoria Hosp, 687 av des Pins O, Montreal QC H3A 1A1; Zaragoza (Spain)'71; CSPQ; FRCPC; DiagRad; NuclearMed (P.Q.). Staff, McGill University Health Centre - Royal Victoria Hospital; (514)843-1501; Fax. (514)843-1469.

NOVENA, Angela R; Windsor Reg Hosp-Metropolitan, 1995 Lens Ave, Windsor ON N8W 1L9; McM'06; CCFP; CCFP(E.M.); Staff, Windsor Regional Hospital - Metropolitan Site; (519)985-2606

NOVICE, Fred M; South Walkerville Med Centre, 198-2224 Walker Rd, Windsor ON N8W 5L7; Tor'83; FRCPC; Derm (Dermatological Pathology). Langs: English; French; (519)258-5020; Fax. (519)252-5368.

NOVICK, Jon S; 1-315 Avenue Rd, Toronto ON M4V 2H2; McG'97; FRCPC; Psy. Staff, St Michael's Hospital; (416)619-4994; Fax. (416)619-5984.

NOVICK, Richard; London HSC-University Hosp, PO Box 5339 Stn B B6 104-339 Windermere Rd, London ON N6A 5A5; McG'80; AB; MSc; FACS; FRCSC; GenSurg (Cardiac Surgery); Cardiovasc&ThorSurg. Consultant Cardiac Surg, London Health Sciences Centre - University Hospital; Chair Cardiac Surg Examination Board, Royal College Of Physicians &; Langs: Russian; Mandarin; Bilingual(French/English); Italian; German; (519)663-3159; Fax. (519)663-3081.

NOVICK, William H; Seaforth Med Bldg, 390-3550 ch de la Cote-des-Nei, Montreal QC H3H 1V4; Qns'54; FRCSC; Otol (Nasal & Sinus Surgery). Assoc Staff, McGill University Health Centre - Royal Victoria Hospital; Assoc Staff, McGill University Health Centre - Montreal General Campus; assoc Prof, McGill University; Langs: Bilingual(English/French); (514)935-3211; Fax. (514)935-2343.

NOVOSHINOV, Sergey; Mackenzie Richmond Hill Hosp, 10 Trench St, Richmond Hill ON L4C 4Z3; Moscow (Russia (Federation))'89; FRCPC; Anes. Staff, Mackenzie Richmond Hill Hospital; (905)883-1212

NOWACKI, Anna K; Univ Hlth Network-Toronto Gen, 200 Elizabeth St, Toronto ON M5G 2C4; Warsaw (Poland)'06; FRCPC; EmergMed. Staff, Toronto General Hospital - UHN; (416)340-3856

NOWACZYK, Malgorzata J M; McMaster University HSC, 3N16-1200 Main St W, Hamilton ON L8S 4J9; Tor'90; BSc; FCCMG; FRCPC; Peds (Medical Genetics). Staff, St Joseph's Healthcare - Charlton Campus; Staff, The Hospital For Sick Children; Staff, Hamilton Health Sciences Centre - McMaster Children's Hospital; Assoc Prof, McMaster University; Langs: Polish; French; Russian; (905)521-2100 x3042; Fax. (905)521-2651; nowaczyk@hhsc.ca.

NOWACZYNSKI, Mark J J; Senior People's Res in North T, 2F-140 Merton St, Toronto ON M4S 1A1; UBC'90; PhD(Physiol); BSc(Hons.); CCFP; Clin Dir Interdisciplinary Mobile Team Serving Frail Seniors, House Calls; Langs: French; Polish; (416)481-5099; Fax. (416)481-2590.

NOWAK, Agata M; Aspen Med Clinic, 221-339 Aspen Glen Landing SW, Calgary AB T3H 0N6; (Poland)'97; CCFP; Langs: Polish; (403)263-7997; Fax. (403)263-7996.

NOWAK, Jozef E; 102-519 Highway 33 W, Kelowna BC V1X 1Y2; Cracow (Poland)'72; FRCPC; PhysMed&Rehab (Chronic Pain Management). Staff, Kelowna General Hospital; Langs: Polish; (250)765-0145; Fax. (250)765-0146.

NOWAK, Justyna M M; Greenwood Med Centre, 10-496 Discovery Lane, Kingston ON K7K 7E9; Mem'97; CCFP; (613)507-7003; Fax. (613)507-7006.

NOWAK, Mary B; Unionville Family Physicians, 301-10 Unionville Gate, Unionville ON L3R 0W7; Tor'82; CCFP; Court Staff, Markham Stouffville Hospital; Asst Prof, University of Toronto; (905)475-3121; Fax. (905)475-4270.

NOWAK, Michael A; Markham Med Centre, 214-6633 Highway 7, Markham ON L3P 7P2; Tor'82; Dip SportMed; Ac Staff, Markham Stouffville Hospital; (905)294-2290; Fax. (905)294-0029.

NOWAK, Peter S; Heritage Hill Medicentre, 110-8180 MacLeod Trail SE, Calgary AB T2H 2B8; Cracow (Poland)'80; CCFP; (403)259-3256; Fax. (403)253-2673.

NOWAK, Zbigniew J; Miramichi Reg Hosp, 500 Water St, Miramichi NB E1V 3G5; Lublin (Poland)'72; Staff, Miramichi Regional Hospital; Langs: Polish; Russian; (506)623-3446; nowak@eastlink.ca.

NOWAK-HARIASZ, Daria J; 1450 King St, Courtice ON L1E 3C3; (Poland)'95; CCFP; (905)721-3520

NOWAKOWSKA, Dominika; CSSS Pierre Boucher, 1333 boul Jacques-Cartier E, Longueuil QC J4M 2A5; Mon'03; Cardiol; IntMed. Staff, Centre Hospitalier Pierre Boucher; (450)468-8136

NOWAKOWSKI, Christophe; 370 boul Saint-Joseph O, Montreal QC H2V 2N9; Mon'79; Psy (P.Q.). (514)656-3037; Fax. (514)656-3039.

NOWICKI, Aleksandra; Regional Mental HC-London, PO Box 5532 Stn B 850 Highbury Ave, London ON N6A 4H1; Ott'04; FRCPC; Psy. Staff, Regional Mental Health Care-St Joseph's Health Care; Teach Staff, University of Western Ontario; Langs: Polish; (519)455-5110

NOWICKI, Iwona M; Regional Mental HC-St-Thomas, PO Box 2004 Stn Main 467 Sunset Dr, St Thomas ON N5P 3V9; (Poland)'73; FRCPC; Psy. Staff, Regional Mental Health Care-St Joseph's Health Care; (519)631-8510 x49621; Fax. (519)631-2512.

NOWICKI, Robert D; 152 Ontario St, St Catharines ON L2R 5K5; Aberdeen (Scotland)'73; MB ChB; MRC; DAB; FRCSC; ObstGyn. Ac Staff, Niagara Health System - Ontario Street Site; Ac Staff, Niagara Health System - St Catharines General Site; (905)988-9600; Fax. (905)988-9518.

NOWLAN, Claire N; Ocean View Manor, PO Box 130 1909 Caldwell Rd, Eastern Passage NS B3G 1M4; Dal'97; BSc; CCFP; (902)465-6020; Fax. (902)465-4929; claire_nowlan@hotmail.com.

NOWLAN, Michael; 182 rue High, Gr-Sault/Gr-Falls NB E3Z 2T8; Mem'81; Med Dir, Hôpital Général de Grand-Falls; Langs: English; French; (506)473-3630; Fax. (506)473-4410; mnowlan@health.nb.ca.

NOWLAN, Ruth G; Phoenix Med Centre, 106-2155 10th Ave, Prince George BC V2M 5J6; National (Ireland)'76; MB ChB; BAO; MRCGPract(UK); DCH; Staff, University Hospital of Northern British Columbia; (250)563-5111; Fax. (250)563-3649.

NOWODWORSKI, Dorota J; Queensway-Carleton Hosp, 3045 Baseline Rd, Ottawa ON K2H 8P4; McG'08; CCFP; CCFP(E.M.); Staff, Queensway Carleton Hospital; Langs: Polish; (613)721-2000

NOWOSAD, Heather D; Rivers Med Clinic, PO Box 429 512 Quebec St, Rivers MB R0K 1X0; Man'08; CCFP.

NOWRY, Carolyn E; Glenmore Landing, 1600 90 Ave SW, Calgary AB T2V 5A8; Wes'09; CCFP; (403)470-0207

NOY, Janet L; Fort William Clinic, 117 McKellar St S, Thunder Bay ON P7E 1H5; Alb'97; CCFP; (807)626-1256; Fax. (807)623-2316.

NOYA, Francisco J D; MUHC-Montreal Children's Hosp, 2300 rue Tupper, Montreal QC H3H 1P3; Cayetano Heredia (Peru)'80; ABPeds; ABAI; ClinImmunol&Allergy (P.Q.); Peds (P.Q.) (Asthma). Dir Ashtma Centre, McGill University Health Centre - Montreal Children's Hospital; assoc Prof, McGill University; Langs: Spanish; (514)412-4485

NOYEK, Arnold M; Mount Sinai Hosp, 401-600 University Ave, Toronto ON M5G 1X5; Tor'61; FACS; DAB; FRCSC; Otol. Dir Peter A Silverman Centre for International Health, Mount Sinai Hospital; Chairman, Canada Int'l. Scientific Exchange Program; Prof Otol, University of Toronto; (416)586-4800 x8533; Fax. (416)586-8600.

NOZA, Assefa F; Medical Centre, 4-1723 Kipling Ave, Etobicoke ON M9R 4E1; McM'99; CCFP; (416)244-8404; Fax. (416)244-0350.

NRUSIMHADEVARA, Ravikrishna; Saskatoon Eye Surgeons, 704-201 1st Ave S, Saskatoon SK S7K 1J5; Utkal (India)'92; FRCSC; Ophth (Vitreo Retina). Staff, Saskatoon City Hospital; (306)974-4497; Fax. (306)974-4498; referral@retinafix.com.

NSAIR, Ali; 4-10625 85 Ave NW, Edmonton AB T6E 2K6; Alb'02; FRCPC; Cardiol; IntMed. Staff, University of Alberta Hospital; (780)695-9001; Fax. (780)433-6898.

NSEIR, Anas; Hop Santa Cabrini Ospedale, 5655 rue Saint-Zotique E, Montreal QC H1T 1P7; Mon'99; PhmB; CCFP; FCFP; Staff Emergency Med, Hôpital Santa Cabrini Ospedale; (514)252-6546; Fax. (514)252-6115; anas.nseir@sympatico.ca.

NSISI, Lazarus M; 414 13 St N, Lethbridge AB T1H 2S2; Kampala (Uganda)'80; MB ChB; (403)942-1505; Fax. (403)942-3220.

NSISI, Saturday N A; 414 13 St N, Lethbridge AB T1H 2S2; Kampala (Uganda)'76; MB ChB; Langs: Rutooro; Luganda; (403)942-1505; Fax. (403)942-3220; michael.anna@sasktel.net.

NSUNGU, Mandiangu; Sunrise Health Region, 150 Independent St, Yorkton SK S3N 0S7; Universite de Kinshasa (Congo (Democratic Republic))'84; MB BS; MPH; Med Officer of Hlth, Sunrise Health Region Yorkton Public Health Office; Langs: Bilingual(French/English); Kikongo; Lingala; (306)786-0600; Fax. (306)786-0630.

NTAMBAZI, Matthew; 406B-50 Vancouver St, Yarmouth NS B5A 2P4; Kampala (Uganda)'85; MB ChB; Staff, Yarmouth Regional Hospital; (902)881-3322; Fax. (902)881-3325.

NUAMAH, Francis N; Nanaimo Reg Gen Hosp, 1200 Dufferin Cres, Nanaimo BC V9S 2B7; (Ghana)'92; Staff, Nanaimo Regional General Hospital; (250)716-7791

NUDO, Carmine G; CSSS de Laval, 1755 boul Rene-Laennec, Laval QC H7M 3L9; McG'01; FRCPC; IntMed; Gastroent. Staff, Hopital de la Cite de la santé; (450)668-1010

NUECHTERLEIN, Barry; Queen Elizabeth Hosp, PO Box 6600 Stn Central 60 Riverside Dr, Charlottetown PE C1A 8T5; Loyola University Chicago (USA)'00; BA; MD; DABA; FRCPC; Anes. Staff, Queen Elizabeth II Health Sciences Centre - Victoria General Site; Staff Anesthetist, Queen Elizabeth Hospital; Langs: German; (902)894-2111; barry_nuechterlein@hotmail.com.

NUGENT, Kevin B; Kinark Child & Family Services, 275-380 Armour Rd, Peterborough ON K9H 7L7; Qns'81; DCPsy(Tor); FRCPC; Psy (Child & Adolescent Psychiatry). Clin Consultant, Lynx Early Psychosis Prevention Program; Clin Consultant, Fleming College; Clin Consultant Community Mental Health, Kinark Child & Family Services; Clin Consultant, Trent University; (705)742-3803; Fax. (705)743-4144; kevin.nugent@kinark.on.ca.

NUGENT, Linda M; Salvation Army Grace Gen Hosp, 300 Booth Dr, Winnipeg MB R3J 3M7; Man'74; FRCPC; Anes. Ac Staff, The Salvation Army Grace Hospital; Consultant, St Boniface General Hospital; Med Dir, Winnipeg Ambulance Service; Assoc Prof, University of Manitoba; (204)837-8311; Fax. (204)831-0029.

NUGENT, Robert W; Fort Frances Clinic, 301 Victoria Ave, Fort Frances ON P9A 2C1; Tor'93; CCFP; FCFP; Chief Anes, La Verendrye Hospital - Riverside Health Care Facility; Asst Prof Family Med, Northern Ontario School of Medicine; Langs: English; French; (807)274-3287; Fax. (807)274-7875.

NUICA, Alina D; C3-2501 Third Line, Oakville ON L6M 5A9; (Romania)'98; CCFP; (905)469-9934

NULLIAH, Shirdi; White Oak Square, 116-12222 137 Ave NW, Edmonton AB T5L 4X5; (India)'03; CCFP; (780)473-9355; Fax. (780)473-2856.

NULMAN, Irena; The Hosp for Sick Children, 555 University Ave, Toronto ON M5G 1X8; Ternopol (Russia (Federation))'67; MRCP; FRCPC; Neur (Clinical Pharmacology). Staff, The Hospital For Sick Children; (416)813-7887; Fax. (416)813-7562.

NUMAINVILLE, Louise; Polyclinique de Montreal, 410-12245 rue Grenet, Montreal QC H4J 2J6; Mon'76; CSPQ; FRCPC; IntMed; Rheum. Staff, Hôpital du Sacre-Coeur de Montréal; (514)334-9112; Fax. (514)334-2945.

NUMAIR, Huma N; Urgent Care Canada Halton, 2951 Walker's Line, Burlington ON L7M 4Y1; Punjab (India)'97; CCFP; (905)336-3437

NUMEROW, Leonard M; Foothills Med Centre, 1403 29 St NW, Calgary AB T2N 2T9; Man'87; FRCPC; DiagRad; NuclearMed. Staff, Foothills Medical Centre; (403)944-1969; Fax. (403)944-1687.

NUNAN-BARCLAY, Sarah J; Stouffville Med Centre, 2F-34 Civic Ave, Stouffville ON L4A 1H2; McM'01; CCFP; (905)640-3100

NUNES, Isabel M A; Welland McMaster Family Hlth Team, PO Box 920 2 Pancake Lane, Fonthill ON L0S 1E0; McM'81; Staff, Niagara Health System - Welland Hospital Site; Langs: Portuguese; (905)892-9705; Fax. (905)892-0394.

NUNES-VAZ, Claire M; Lawrence Park Med Centre, 116-250 Lawrence Ave W, Toronto ON M5M 1B2; Tor'71; CCFP; FCFP; Ac Staff, North York General Hospital; Court Staff, Sunnybrook Health Sciences Centre; Asst Prof, University of Toronto; Langs: Portuguese; French; (416)782-4447; Fax. (416)782-1284.

NUNEZ, Carlos E; St Paul's Hosp, 1081 Burrard St, Vancouver BC V6Z 1Y6; Arizona (USA)'06; Staff, Providence Health Care - St Paul's Hospital; (604)806-8320

NUNEZ, Desmond A; Gordon & Leslie Diamond HCC, 4F-2775 Laurel St, Vancouver BC V5Z 1M9; University of West Indies (Other Foreign)'82; FRCSC; Otol (Head & Neck Surgery). Staff, Vancouver General Hospital - Centennial Pavillion; Staff, Gordon & Leslie Diamond Health Care Centre; (604)875-4664

NUNN, David J; 202-100 Station Lane, Kentville NS B4N 0A3; Dal'87; CCFP; FCFP; (902)678-4140; Fax. (902)678-4143.

NUNN, Paul; Delhi Commun Health Centre, 105 Main Street of Delhi, Delhi ON N4B 2L8; Wes'90; Staff, Norfolk General Hospital; (519)582-3535; Fax. (519)582-3770.

NUNN, Robert T; IWK Health Centre, PO Box 9700 Rpo CSC 5850-5980 University Ave, Halifax NS B3K 6R8; Dal'86; FRCPC; Anes. Staff Anes, IWK Health Centre; Asst Prof Anes, Dalhousie University; (902)470-6627; Fax. (902)470-6626.

NUNWEILER, Donovan E S; 110-7 Strachan Bay SE, Medicine Hat AB T1B 4Y2; Alb'06; CCFP; (403)528-4490; Fax. (403)528-4481.

NURAE, Khalid A; 103B-3335 Dougall Ave, Windsor ON N9E 1S8; Jimma (Ethiopia)'94; CCFP; (519)250-6934; Fax. (519)250-6719.

NURI, Humayun; Royal University Hosp, 103 Hospital Dr, Saskatoon SK S7N 0W8; FRCPC; IntMed. Staff, Royal University Hospital; (306)655-1000

NURSE, William E; Grand River Hosp-Freeport HC, 3570 King St E, Kitchener ON N2A 2W1; RCS (Ireland)'62; LRCPS(Ire); FRCOG; Staff, Grand River Hospital - Freeport Site; (519)749-4300

NUSINOWITZ, Sidney; Doctor's Office, 101-491 Lawrence Ave W, North York ON M5M 1C7; Tor'78; CCFP; FCFP; Lecturer Family & Community Med, University of Toronto; (416)787-0323; Fax. (416)787-8094.

NUSSBAUM, Christopher J; The Ottawa Hosp-Civic Campus, 1053 Carling Ave, Ottawa ON K1Y 4E9; Qns'89; CCFP; CCFP(E.M.); Att Staff, The Ottawa Hospital - Civic Campus; Lecturer, University of Ottawa; (613)761-4773; cjnussbaum@hotmail.com.

NUSSBAUM, Earl B; 11-398 Steeles Ave W, Thornhill ON L4J 6X3; McG'86; FRCPC; IntMed; Cardiol. (905)881-0334; Fax. (905)881-1721.

NUSSBAUM, Marvin A; 204-46 King St, Welland ON L3B 3H9; Tor'65; Otol. Consultant, Niagara Health System - Welland Hospital Site; Consultant Otol, Niagara Health System - Douglas Memorial Hospital Site; (905)734-7911

NUSSBAUMER, Gary R; St Paul's Hosp, 6134 6B-1081 Burrard St, Vancouver BC V6Z 1Y6; Sask'90; Clin Associate Nephrol, Providence Health Care - St Paul's Hospital; (604)682-2344 x63132

NUTH, Janet E; Canadian Med Protective Assoc, 875 Carling Ave, Ottawa ON K1S 5P1; Ott'86; CCFP; CCFP(E.M.); Staff, The Ottawa Hospital - Civic Campus; Staff, Canadian Medical Protective Association; (613)725-2000

NUTH, Laura; 309-18 Acadia St, Dartmouth NS B2Y 4H3; Wes'84; FRCSC; GenSurg. Consultant, Dartmouth General Hospital; (902)463-0858; Fax. (902)463-9302; lauranuth@ns.aliantzinc.ca.

NUTIK, Melissa R; 4F-60 Murray St, Toronto ON M5T 3L9; Tor'97; BSc; CCFP; FCFP; Staff, Mount Sinai Hospital; Lecturer, University of Toronto; (416)586-4800 x5158; Fax. (416)586-3175.

NUTLEY, Mark T; Peter Lougheed Centre, 3601-3500 26 ave NE, Calgary AB T1Y 6J4; Tor'99; FRCSC; GenSurg; VascSurg. Staff, Peter Lougheed Centre; (403)943-4013; Fax. (403)291-2734.

NUTT, Samantha J; Family Practice Health Centre, 60 Grosvenor St, Toronto ON M5S 1B6; McM'94; FRCPC; CommunMed;CCFP; (416)323-6060; Fax. (416)323-6402.

NUTTALL, Richard N; 1284 Fairfield Rd, Victoria BC V8V 4W3; London (England)'74; MB BS; MPA(Harvard); MPH; MClSc; CCFP; FCFP; Med Coord, Mount St Mary Hospital; Staff, Royal Jubilee Hospital; Med Coord, The Lodge at Broadmead; (250)598-5158; Fax. (250)598-6066.

NUTTALL, S John; Quarry Family Med & Foot Clin, 409-797 Princess St, Kingston ON K7L 1G1; Manchester (England)'79; CCFP; FCFP; Ad Staff Privil, Kingston General Hospital; Ad Staff Privil, Hotel-Dieu Hospital; (613)541-3922; Fax. (613)541-0744.

NUTTING, Michael G; 224 Meadowlark Shopping Ctr NW, Edmonton AB T5R 5W9; London (England)'68; MB BS; MRC; FRCPC; IntMed (Breast Cancer). Staff, Covenant Health - Misericordia Community Hospital; Staff, Cross Cancer Institute; Clin Assoc Prof, University of Alberta; (780)484-8474; Fax. (780)489-3836; nutting88@gmail.com.

NUYT, Anne M; Hôpital Ste-Justine, 3175 ch Cote-Sainte-Catherine, Montreal QC H3T 1C5; Sher'88; FRCPC; Peds (Neonatology). Staff, Hôpital Ste-Justine; (514)345-4931 x3971; Fax. (514)345-4801; anne-monique.nuyt@recherche-ste-justine.qc.ca.

NWACHUKWU, Ikechukwu C; 569 5th Ave, Kamloops BC V2C 3R1; (Nigeria)'98; MB BS; MSc; MRCPsy; FRCPC; Psy. Staff, Royal Inland Hospital; (250)374-0375; Fax. (250)374-5021.

NWACHUKWU, Izunwanne U; Foothills Med Centre, 1403 29 St NW, Calgary AB T2N 2T9; (Nigeria)'99; MB BS; Staff, Foothills Medical Centre; (403)944-1296; Fax. (403)270-3451.

NWACHUKWU, Kingsley; Battlefords Mental Health Ctre, 1092 107th St, North Battleford SK S9A 1Z1; (306)446-6500; Fax. (306)446-6546.

NWADIARO, Nduka; Windsor Med Centre, 3-130 Ouellette Pl, Windsor ON N8X 1L9; Nsuka (Nigeria)'85; MB BS; FRCPC; IntMed. Staff, Windsor Regional Hospital - Tayfour Site; (519)254-9733; Fax. (519)254-7078.

NWAESEI, Chukwuma G; Windsor Reg Hosp-Metropolitan, 1995 Lens Ave, Windsor ON N8W 1L9; Leningrad (Russia (Federation))'73; MPH; FAAP; FRCPC; Peds (Neonatal & Perinatal Medicine). Staff, Windsor Regional Hospital - Metropolitan Site; Assoc Prof, Wayne State University (Detroit,Michigan-USA); (519)255-2467; Fax. (519)255-1735; chuks_nwaesei@wrh.on.ca.

NWAKA, Bernard C; Plaza 2 Shopping Ctr, 614-8600 Franklin Ave, Fort McMurray AB T9H 4G8; (Nigeria)'90; MB BS; CCFP; (780)715-4063; Fax. (780)715-4055.

NWAPA, Sylvia I; Harrow Health Centre Inc, PO Box 430 1480 Erie Rd S, Harrow ON N0R 1G0; (Nigeria)'94; (519)738-2000; Fax. (519)738-9944.

NWEBUBE, Anne O; Grimsby Children's Clinic, 361 South Service Rd, Grimsby ON L3M 4E8; Benin (Nigeria)'88; FRCPC; Peds. (905)945-2424; Fax. (905)945-0990.

NWEBUBE, Nkiruka I; Grey Bruce HS-Owen Sound, PO Box 1800 Stn Main 1800 8th St E, Owen Sound ON N4K 6M9; (Nigeria)'89; Staff, Grey Bruce Health Services - Owen Sound; (519)376-2121

NWEBUBE, Nwachukwu I; West Lincoln Mem Hosp, 169 Main St E, Grimsby ON L3M 1P3; University Nigeria (Nigeria)'86; MB BS; FRCSC; ObstGyn. Staff, West Lincoln Memorial Hospital; (905)309-1947

NWILATI, Hanad; CSSS de Saint-Jerome, 290 rue de Montigny, Saint-Jerome QC J7Z 5T3; Staff, CSSS St-Jerôme; (450)432-2777

NYACHWO, Caroline B; Crane Med Centre, 106-10055 120 Ave, Grande Prairie AB T8V 8H8; (Uganda)'94; MB ChB; CCFP; (780)532-4415; Fax. (780)532-4559.

NYATI, Lindiwe L; 108 Wolverine Dr, Fort McMurray AB T9H 4Y7; (South Africa)'94; (780)743-9008; Fax. (780)713-2489.

NYHOLT, Noranda; Belleville Queen's Univ-FMC, 103-145 Station St, Belleville ON K8N 2S9; Wes'08; CCFP; (613)771-1910

NYHUS, Nadine J; North Halton Mental Hlth Clin, 19 Willow St, Brampton ON L7A 1Z6; McM'92; FRCPC; Psy. Staff, Centre for Addiction & Mental Health (CAMH) - Queen Site.

NYIRENDA, Vera R; 102-9193 Main St, Chilliwack BC V2P 7S5; Lusaka (Zambia)'88; MB ChB; CCFP; (604)858-8343

NYKIFORUK, Edward M; 1-604 22nd St W, Saskatoon SK S7M 5W1; Sask'58; Ac Staff, St Paul's Hospital (Grey Nuns) of Saskatoon; Assoc Staff, Saskatoon City Hospital; Associate, Royal University Hospital; Med Examiner Family Practice Chelation Therapy & Alternative Med Aviation Med, Transport Canada; Langs: Ukrainian; Polish; (306)652-2620; Fax. (306)652-0626; dr.e.nykiforuk@shaw.ca.

NYNKOWSKI, Peter A; 101-2900 Yonge St, Toronto ON M4N 3N8; Warsaw (Poland)'73; FRCPC; Psy. Langs: Polish; (416)485-8711

NYOMBA, Bulangu L(Gregoire); Health Sciences Centre, GA2-820 Sherbrook St, Winnipeg MB R3A 1R9; (Congo (Democratic Republic))'74; Staff, Health Sciences Centre; Asst Prof, University of Manitoba; Langs: French; (204)787-3433; Fax. (204)787-4826.

NYUNHEIGN, Omer; Weyburn Health Centre, 36 4th St, Weyburn SK S4H 0X7; Yangon (Burma)'85; MB BS; LMCC; (306)842-5444; Fax. (306)842-5449.

NYVALL, Mary K; 2-32904 Ventura Ave, Abbotsford BC V2S 6J3; Ott'06; CCFP; (604)859-1211

NZAU, Duncun M M; Children's Hosp Eastern Ont, 401 Smyth Rd, Ottawa ON K1H 8L1; Russia (Russia (Federation))'87; Staff, Children's Hospital of Eastern Ontario (CHEO); (613)737-2316 x1

O'BEIRNE, Carole Patricia; 219-840 Coxwell Ave, Toronto ON M4C 5T2; Tor'97; FRFPS; MSc(Biochem); DrMedCh; FRCPC; Peds (Age-Related Macular Degeneration). Staff, Toronto East General Hospital Inc; Staff, The Hospital For Sick Children; Langs: French; (416)696-0003; Fax. (416)696-0022.

O'BEIRNE, Maeve; Low Risk Maternity Clinic, 130-1402 8 Ave NW, Calgary AB T2N 1B9; Cal'90; PhD(Physiol); CCFP; FCFP; Assoc Prof Family Med, University of Calgary; Staff Privil, Foothills Medical Centre; (403)509-3080; Fax. (403)509-3082; obeirne@ucalgary.ca.

O'BLENES, Stacy B; IWK Health Centre, PO Box 9700 Rpo CSC 5850-5980 University Ave, Halifax NS B3K 6R8; Dal'94; FRCSC; CardSurg (Pediatric Cardiac Surgery). Staff, IWK Health Centre; (902)470-8888

O'BLENIS CAINES, Shelley; Oromocto Public Hosp, 103 Winnebago St, Oromocto NB E2V 1C6; Dal'93; CCFP; CCFP(E.M.); FCFP; Staff, Oromocto Public Hospital; Langs: English; French; (506)357-4713; Fax. (506)422-1426.

O'BREASAIL, Aindrias; Nanaimo Mental Health, 528 Wentworth St, Nanaimo BC V9R 3E4; Galway (Ireland)'80; MRCPsy; FRCPC; Psy. (250)739-5868

O'BRIAIN, Barra F; 110-3540 41st Ave W, Vancouver BC V6N 3E6; McG'86; CCFP; FCFP; Vis Staff, Vancouver General Hospital - Centennial Pavillion; Langs: Spanish; French; (604)261-6361; Fax. (604)261-1656.

O'BRIEN, Anita M; University Hosp of Northern BC, 1475 Edmonton St, Prince George BC V2M 1S2; Dal'02; CCFP; Staff, University Hospital of Northern British Columbia; (250)565-2000

O'BRIEN, Ashley; Saint John Reg Hosp, PO Box 2100 Stn Main 400 University Ave, Saint John NB E2L 4L2; Dal'04; FRCPC; Anes. Staff, Saint John Regional Hospital; (506)648-6861

O'BRIEN, Brian J; PO Box 304 Stn Main, Glace Bay NS B1A 5V4; Dublin (Ireland)'69; MB ChB; BAO; Ac Staff, Glace Bay Healthcare Facility; (902)842-1121

O'BRIEN, Brian P; 405-2249 Carling Ave, Ottawa ON K2B 7E9; Dublin (Ireland)'76; MB ChB; BAO; FRCPC; Psy. Staff Psy, Queensway Carleton Hospital; (613)596-5623; Fax. (613)596-3250.

O'BRIEN, Catherine; Univ Hlth Network-Toronto Gen, 10EN 022-200 Elizabeth St, Toronto ON M5G 2C4; Qns'98; FRCSC; GenSurg; General Surgical Oncology. Staff, Toronto General Hospital - UHN; (416)340-4800

O'BRIEN, Catherine L; Banff Sport Medicine, 207-303 Lynx St, Banff AB T1L 1B3; Cal'07; FRCSC; OrthSurg. Staff, Foothills Medical Centre; (403)760-2897; Fax. (403)760-8234.

O'BRIEN, Christopher J M; Brant Community HC-Brantford, 200 Terrace Hill St, Brantford ON N3R 1G9; McG'88; FRCPC; NuclearMed. Staff, St Mary's General Hospital; Staff, Stratford General Hospital - Huron Perth Healthcare Alliance; (519)751-5544 x2455; Fax. (519)751-5582.

O'BRIEN, Christopher P; 102-1 Magazine St, Saint John NB E2K 5S9; Mem'83; CCFP; FCFP; Med Dir Palliative Care, Saint John Regional Hospital; Ac Staff, St Joseph's Hospital; (506)634-1272; Fax. (506)634-7215.

O'BRIEN, Clare E; Collingwood Gen & Marine Hosp, 459 Hume St, Collingwood ON L9Y 1W9; Mem'74; DiagRad (Mammography). Staff, Collingwood General & Marine Hospital; (705)445-2550; Fax. (705)444-2679.

O'BRIEN, Colleen M; Dr Charles A Janeway Child HC, 300 Prince Philip Dr, St. John's NL A1B 3V6; Mem'03; FRCPC; Peds (Adolescent Medicine). Staff, Janeway Children's Health & Rehabilitation Centre; (709)777-6300

O'BRIEN, Daniel M; 800-5991 Spring Garden Rd, Halifax NS B3H 1Y6; Dal'83; FRCSC; Ophth (Vitreo Retinal Surgery). Ac Staff, Queen Elizabeth II Health Sciences Centre - Victoria General Site; Assoc Prof Ophth, Dalhousie University; (902)429-2760; Fax. (902)425-0666.

O'BRIEN, David A L; 1802-45 Alderney Dr, Dartmouth NS B2Y 2N6; Dal'99; FRCSC; OrthSurg (Hip & Knee Arthroplasty). Clin Instructor, Dalhousie University; (902)405-3200; Fax. (902)469-4753.

O'BRIEN, David M; 118 Dundas St E, Belleville ON K8N 1C4; Qns'82; FAB; ObstGyn. Staff, QHC Belleville General; Staff/Chief ObstGyn, QHC Trenton Memorial; Clin Instructor, Queen's University; Langs: English; French; (613)967-9688; Fax. (613)967-2422.

O'BRIEN, Dennis F; Halton HC Serv Corp-Oakville, 327 Reynolds St, Oakville ON L6J 3L7; Tor'61; Staff, Halton Healthcare Services Corporation - Oakville Site; (905)845-2571

O'BRIEN, Dermot B; 8-25 Redmond Dr, Hamilton ON L8W 3K7; National (Ireland)'70; Ophth. Ac Staff, St Joseph's Healthcare - Charlton Campus; Langs: English; French; (905)387-6668; Fax. (905)318-8341.

O'BRIEN, Edward R M; Foothills Med Centre, 1403 29 St NW, Calgary AB T2N 2T9; Ott'85; BSc; FRCPC; IntMed (Interventional Cardiology); Cardiol. Staff, Foothills Medical Centre; (403)944-5918; Fax. (403)944-2906.

O'BRIEN, Elizabeth A; 103-3400 rue du Marche, Dollard-D-Ormeaux QC H9B 2Y1; Ott'75; ABD; FRCP; MD; CSPQ; FRCPC; Derm. Dermatology, CHSLD Bayview Inc; principale Staff Derm, McGill University Health Centre - Montreal General Campus; Dermatology Consultant, Lakeshore General Hospital - Pointe Claire; assoc Prof Derm, McGill University; (514)685-3850; Fax. (514)685-8050.

O'BRIEN, Elizabeth P; Medical Clinic Bldg, 225-89 Humber College Blvd, Etobicoke ON M9V 4B8; Cork (Ireland)'59; DPM; MRCPsy; FRCPC; Psy (Psychotherapy). Court Staff, William Osler Health System - Etobicoke General Hospital; (416)746-0386; Fax. (416)746-7977.

O'BRIEN, Fiona J; Hilltop Medical Clinic, 12894 16 Ave, Surrey BC V4A 1N7; Bristol (England)'89; MB ChB; CCFP; (604)531-7712

O'BRIEN, Gregory M; Dr H Bliss Murphy Cancer Ctr, 300 Prince Philip Dr, St. John's NL A1B 3V6; Mem'79; Anes. Staff, Dr H Bliss Murphy Cancer Centre; (709)777-8092

O'BRIEN, Heather V; Sault Area Hosp, 750 Great Northern Rd, Sault Ste. Marie ON P6B 0A8; Tor'86; MEd; FRCPC; Anes (Critical Care Medicine). Chief Dept of Anes, Sault Area Hospital - Sault Ste Marie; Langs: English; French; (705)759-3630; Fax. (705)759-3696.

O'BRIEN, James P; Saint John Reg Hosp, PO Box 2100 Stn Main 400 University Ave, Saint John NB E2L 4L2; Mem'80; FRCSC; PlasSurg (Plastic & Reconstructive Surgery). Ac Staff Plastic Surg, Saint John Regional Hospital; Assoc Prof Plastic Surg, Dalhousie University; (506)648-7933; Fax. (506)652-7573; obrja@reg2.health.nb.ca.

O'BRIEN, John A; Thunder Bay Reg HSC-T-Bay, 980 Oliver Rd, Thunder Bay ON P7B 6V4; Ott'82; FRCPC; DiagRad. Staff, Thunder Bay Regional Health Sciences Centre; Section Leader Diagnostic Radiol, Northern Ontario School of Medicine-Laurentian University; (807)684-6300

O'BRIEN, John I; Hilltop Med Clinic, 12894 16th Ave, Surrey BC V4A 1N7; Aberdeen (Scotland)'90; (604)531-7712

O'BRIEN, John M; Ucluelet Med Centre, PO Box 1090, Ucluelet BC V0R 3A0; Ott'84; CCFP; (250)726-4443; Fax. (250)726-7333.

O'BRIEN, Julie; Royal Columbian Hosp, 330 Columbia St E, New Westminster BC V3L 3W7; Dublin (Ireland)'00; Staff, Royal Columbian Hospital; (604)520-4253

O'BRIEN, Karel K E; Mount Sinai Hosp, 775-600 University Ave, Toronto ON M5G 1X5; National (Ireland)'83; MB ChB; BAO; DCH; FRCPC; Peds (Neonatal & Perinatal Medicine). Staff Neonatol & Dept of Peds, Mount Sinai Hospital; Staff Neonatology, The Hospital For Sick Children; Asst Prof Peds, University of Toronto; (416)586-4800 x8336; Fax. (416)586-8745; kobrien@mtsinai.on.ca.

O'BRIEN, Kristina G; Royal Alexandra Hosp, 10240 Kingsway NW, Edmonton AB T5H 3V9; Alb'09; CCFP; CCFP(E.M.); Staff, Royal Alexandra Hospital; (780)735-4443; Fax. (780)735-4916.

O'BRIEN, Lewis J; The Group Health Centre, 240 McNabb St, Sault Ste. Marie ON P6B 1Y5; Alb'78; CCFP; FCFP; Ac Staff, Sault Area Hospital - Sault Ste Marie; (705)759-1234 x604; Fax. (705)541-2302; obrien_l@ghc.on.ca.

O'BRIEN, M Kathleen; IWK Health Centre, PO Box 9700 Rpo CSC 5850-5980 University Ave, Halifax NS B3K 6R8; Dal'87; FRCPC; DiagRad (Pediatrics). Staff, IWK Health Centre; Asst Prof, Dalhousie University; (902)470-8060; Fax. (902)470-7463.

O'BRIEN, Mary H; 202-35 Major's Path, St. John's NL A1A 4Z9; National (Ireland)'86; BSc(Physiol); FRCPC; IntMed; Critical Care Medicine. Clin Staff ICU/Att Staff Intensivist, Eastern Health Authoriy; Clinical Asst Prof Med, Memorial University Of Newfoundland; Langs: Irish; (709)777-5151; obrienmaryh@gmail.com.

O'BRIEN, Maureen D; Gulf Canada Square, 335-401 9 Ave SW, Calgary AB T2P 3C5; Cal'83; BSc; MSc; MBA; FRCSC; OrthSurg (General Orthopedics). Staff, Rockyview General Hospital; (403)221-4367; Fax. (403)221-4387.

O'BRIEN, Meagan R; 104-460 Wellington St, St Thomas ON N5R 6H9; Ott'03; FRCSC; ObstGyn. (519)637-3987; Fax. (519)637-3980.

O'BRIEN, Melissa A; 137 O'Connell Dr, Corner Brook NL A2H 5M8; McM'09; CCFP.

O'BRIEN, Michael M; PO Box 477 Stn Fort Langley, Langley BC V1M 2R8; UBC'63; FRCPC; IntMed (Cardiology). Staff, Langley Memorial Hospital.

O'BRIEN, Paul F; Malvern Med Centre, 100-1333 Neilson Rd, Scarborough ON M1B 4Y9; Tor'86; (416)291-7719; Fax. (416)287-3775.

O'BRIEN, Paul G; Hotel-Dieu Hosp, 166 Brock St, Kingston ON K7L 5G2; Otago (New Zealand)'74; FRANZCR; MB ChB; FRCPC; DiagRad. Staff, Kingston General Hospital; Staff, Hotel-Dieu Hospital; Asst Prof Diagnostic Radiol, Queen's University; (613)544-3400 x3020; Fax. (613)544-6505.

O'BRIEN, Peter J; Ortho Trauma Clinic, 3F-2775 Laurel St, Vancouver BC V5Z 1M9; Alb'76; BMedSci; FRCSC; OrthSurg (Orthopedic Trauma). Ac Staff, Vancouver General Hospital - Centennial Pavillion; Assoc Prof, University of British Columbia; (604)875-5809; Fax. (604)875-5812; shelley@orthotrauma.ca.

O'BRIEN, R Jason; 104-3310 32 Ave, Vernon BC V1T 2M6; Ott'97; FRCSC; OrthSurg. (250)260-3344

O'BRIEN, Robert L; East Kootenay Reg Hosp, 13 24th Ave N, Cranbrook BC V1C 3H9; UBC'76; Staff, East Kootenay Regional Hospital; (250)426-5281 x6227

O'BRIEN, Robert P; Medisys, 500 rue Sherbrooke O, Montreal QC H3A 3C6; McG'92; CCFP; (514)845-1211; Fax. (514)845-4842.

O'BRIEN, Sharon R; 523-1200 Markham Rd, Scarborough ON M1H 3C3; Mem'88; BMedSci; FRCSC; ObstGyn (High Risk Obstetrics). Ac Staff, The Scarborough Hospital - General Campus; (416)439-2335; Fax. (416)439-3078.

O'BRIEN, Simon J; Providence Care-Mental Health, PO Box 603 Stn Main 752 King St W, Kingston ON K7L 4X3; Ott'93; FRCPC; Psy. Staff, Providence Care - Mental Health Services; (613)546-1101; Fax. (613)548-5585.

O'BRIEN, Stephen R; Worker's Comp Bd, PO Box 757 Stn Central, Charlottetown PE C1A 7L7; Dal'75; BSc; CCFP; FCFP; Staff, Hillsborough Hospital & Special Care Centre; Med Advisor, Worker's Comp Board of PEI; (902)368-5596; Fax. (902)368-5696; sobrien@wcb.pe.ca.

O'BRIEN, Tara E; Women's College Hosp, 76 Grenville St, Toronto ON M5S 1B2; Alb'95; FRCPC; IntMed. Staff, Women's College Hospital; (416)334-6046

O'BRIEN, Terrence O; Kingston Gen Hosp, 76 Stuart St, Kingston ON K7L 2V7; Cal'78; FRCPC; EmergMed. Att Staff, Hotel-Dieu Hospital; Co-Dir/Att Staff Trauma Serv, Kingston General Hospital; Asst Prof, Queen's University; (613)548-2368

O'BRIEN, Thomas H B; 323 Durie Street, Toronto ON M6S 3G2; Ott'78; FRCPC; Psy (Psychoanalysis). (416)928-0260

O'BRIEN, Thomas J; 421 Greenbrook Dr, Kitchener ON N2M 4K1; Tor'09; CCFP; (519)578-3510; Fax. (519)578-6040.

O'BRIEN, Wayne J; Kelligrews Med Clinic, PO Box 17160 Stn Main, Conception-Bay-S NL A1X 3H1; Dal'72; Ac Staff Emerg, St Clare's Mercy Hospital; Ac Staff, Escasoni Senior Citizen's Complex(St. John's); (709)834-2171; Fax. (709)834-1241.

O'BRIEN-BELL, John; 13354 56 Ave, Surrey BC V3X 2Z6; London (England)'56; MB BS; LRCP; MRCS; DRCOG; Med Pres, Surrey Memorial Hospital; (604)715-2702

O'BYRNE, Greg K; Victoria East Med Clinic, 2068 Prince of Wales Dr, Regina SK S4V 3A6; Sask'75; (306)789-4677; Fax. (306)789-3422.

O'BYRNE, Mary; Alberta Children's Hosp, 2888 Shaganappi Trail NW, Calgary AB T3B 6A8; Qns'87; FRCPC; Peds (Emergency Pediatrics). Staff, Alberta Children's Hospital; Langs: English; French; (403)955-7070

O'BYRNE, Paul M; McMaster Univ Med Centre, 1280 Main St W, Hamilton ON L8S 1K4; Dublin (Ireland)'75; MB ChB; BAO; FRCPC; IntMed (Asthma); Respir. Exec Dir Firestone Institute for Respiratory Health, St Joseph's Healthcare - Charlton Campus; Dept Head Medicine, McMaster University; (905)521-2100

O'BYRNE, Gray W L; 202-260 Dalhousie St, Ottawa ON K1N 7E4; Ott'78; CCFP; FCFP; (613)241-7400; Fax. (613)241-4308.

O'CALLAGHAN, Kieran P; 12620A 132 Ave NW, Edmonton AB T5L 3P9; Dublin (Ireland)'76; MB ChB; BAO; DCH; (780)990-1820; Fax. (780)488-0988.

O'CALLAHAN, Timothy S; Amherstburg Family Health Team, 681 Front Rd S, Amherstburg ON N9V 0B4; Ott'90; Ac Staff, Hôtel-Dieu Grace Hospital; (519)736-7770

O'CARROLL, Ruth F; General Surgery Group, 220-2345 10th Ave W, Prince Albert SK S6V 5T4; Sask'03; FRCSC; GenSurg. (306)922-8949; Fax. (306)922-3441.

O'CARROLL, Tiann F A; Regina Qu'Appelle HR-Regina, 1440 14th Ave, Regina SK S4P 0W5; Sask'02; CCFP; CCFP(E.M.); Staff, Regina General Hospital; (306)766-4213

O'CONNELL, Colleen M; Stan Cassidy Ctre for Rehab, 800 Priestman St, Fredericton NB E3B 0C7; Mem'95; BSc; BMedSci; FRCPC; PhysMed&Rehab (Neuro Rehabilitation). Staff, Phys Med & Rehab, Hopital Regional Chaleur; Staff, Phys Med & Rehab, Stan Cassidy Centre for Rehabilitation; Med Staff, Horizon Health Network Saint John Public Health; Med Staff, River Valley Health Authority; Lecturer Med, Dalhousie University; Associate Research, University of New Brunswick; Langs: English; French; (506)447-4294; Fax. (506)447-4749; brenda.casey@horizonnb.ca.

O'CONNELL, Daniel A; University of Alberta Hosp, 8440 112 St NW, Edmonton AB T6G 2B7; Alb'04; FRCSC; Otol (Head & Neck Surgery). Staff, University of Alberta Hospital; (780)407-8822

O'CONNELL, Daniel F; 969 Kangaroo Rd, Victoria BC V9C 4E1; Cal'87; (250)478-8776; Fax. (250)478-8748.

O'CONNELL, Jacqueline M; 206-7031 Westminster Hwy, Richmond BC V6X 1A3; UBC'05; FRCSC; ObstGyn. Langs: Bilingual(English/French); (604)821-0626

O'CONNELL, Jason C; 1966 Harrison Way, Kamloops BC V1S 1M9; Otago (New Zealand)'85; MB ChB; DipObst; Locum Tenens, Rural General Practitioner Service of British Columbia; Clin Instructor ObstGyn, University of British Columbia; (250)314-5344; Fax. (250)372-8331.

O'CONNELL, Jennifer; Crossroads Family Practice, 201-5110 St Margarets Bay Rd, Upper Tantallon NS B3Z 1E2; Dal'07; CCFP; (902)826-9096; Fax. (902)820-9399.

O'CONNELL, John X; Surrey Mem Hosp, 13750 96 Ave, Surrey BC V3V 1Z2; Dublin (Ireland)'86; MB ChB; BAO; FRCPC; AnatPath. Staff, Surrey Memorial Hospital; (604)585-5953; Fax. (604)585-5562.

O'CONNELL, Louis S; Greely Family Med Centre, 1399 Ellsworth Lane, Greely ON K4P 1N3; Ott'85; CCFP; FCFP; Ac Staff, The Ottawa Hospital - Riverside Campus; (613)821-3428

O'CONNOR, Brian A; Vancouver Coastal Hlth-North S, 5F-132 Esplanade W, North Vancouver BC V7M 1A2; Tor'70; MHSc; (604)983-6701; Fax. (604)983-6839; brian.o'connor@vch.ca.

O'CONNOR, Catherine S; Ottawa East Family Med Ctre, 216-1980 Ogilvie Rd, Gloucester ON K1J 9L3; McM'86; CCFP; Langs: Bilingual(English/French); (613)746-8559; Fax. (613)746-3640.

O'CONNOR, Daniel J; Rockyview Gen Hosp, 7007 14 St SW, Calgary AB T2V 1P9; Qns'90; CCFP; CCFP(E.M.); FCFP; Staff, Rockyview General Hospital; (403)943-3449

O'CONNOR, Deborah; Northeast Mental Hlth Centre, 318-680 Kirkwood Dr, Sudbury ON P3E 1X3; Qns'83; BSc; Staff, North Bay Regional Health Centre - Kirkwood; (705)675-9193; Fax. (705)675-5047.

O'CONNOR, Emily M; 1-106 Dryden Way PO Box 70, Seeleys Bay ON K0H 2N0; Wes'05; CCFP; (613)387-3120; Fax. (613)387-2842.

O'CONNOR, Gary D; 303-3330 Richter St, Kelowna BC V1W 4V5; Alb'78; BSc(Med.); FRCSC; OrthSurg. Staff Surg, Kelowna General Hospital; (250)763-8816; Fax. (250)862-5842.

O'CONNOR, Gregory J; Orthopaedic Consultants, 10972 124 St NW, Edmonton AB T5M 0H8; Alb'76; FRCSC; OrthSurg (Hips Surgery). Staff, Royal Alexandra Hospital; Clinical Asst Prof Surg, University of Alberta; (780)732-3714; Fax. (780)451-1437.

O'CONNOR, H Michael; Kingston Gen Hosp, E3 3 320-76 Stuart St, Kingston ON K7L 2V7; Qns'78; MEd; FRCPC; EmergMed. Staff Emerg, Kingston General Hospital; Head, Hotel-Dieu Hospital; Teach Staff, Queen's University; (613)548-2368; Fax. (613)548-1374; oconnorh@kgh.kari.net.

O'CONNOR, Helene L; Montfort Academic Family Hlth, 745 Montreal Rd, Ottawa ON K1K 0T1; Ott'07; CCFP; (613)749-4429; Fax. (613)749-7942.

O'CONNOR, J Patrick; UBC-Dept of Anaes, LP2 2449-910 10th Ave W, Vancouver BC V5Z 1M9; Dal'78; FRCPC; Anes. Ac Staff, Vancouver General Hospital - Centennial Pavillion; Vice Pres Clinical Quality & Safety, Vancouver Coastal Health; (604)875-4304

O'CONNOR, John A; PO Box 5360 Stn Main, Fort McMurray AB T9H 3G4; Galway (Ireland)'82; MB ChB; BAO; (780)799-1040; Fax. (780)828-2405.

O'CONNOR, John F; Dartmouth Med Centre, 203-46 Portland St, Dartmouth NS B2Y 1H4; Dal'69; CCFP; FCFP; (902)465-4543; Fax. (902)469-2400; jfoconnor@eastlink.ca.

O'CONNOR, Julia E; 14 West St, Corner Brook NL A2H 2Z1; Mem'88; BMedSci; BComm(Hons); (709)632-3464

O'CONNOR, Kathleen M; 5000-1200 Newlands Rd, Revelstoke BC V0E 2S1; McM'10; CCFP; (250)837-2131

O'CONNOR, Kevin P; Mindemoya Med Centre, PO Box 150 2120B Hwy 551, Mindemoya ON P0P 1S0; Ott'98; CCFP; Assoc Prof, Northern Ontario School of Medicine; (705)377-5371; Fax. (705)377-5372.

O'CONNOR, Kim; Hôpital Laval, 2725 ch Sainte-Foy, Quebec QC G1V 4G5; Laval'00; FRCPC; IntMed (Echocardiography); Cardiol. Staff, Hôpital Laval; Langs: Bilingual(French/English); (418)656-8711; Fax. (418)656-4581; kim.oconnor@criucpq.ulaval.ca.

O'CONNOR, Linda A; Queens Univ Student Hlth Serv, 146 Stuart St, Kingston ON K7L 3N6; Tor'86; (613)533-2506

O'CONNOR, M Peter; Specialized Geriatric Clinic, 232 Ross Dr, New Westminster BC V3L 0B2; Dublin (Ireland)'81; MB ChB; BAO; MRC; FRCPC; IntMed; GeriatricMed. Consultant Geriatric, Fraser Health Authority; Asst Clin Prof, University of British Columbia; (604)528-5031; geriatrician@doctor.com.

O'CONNOR, Madeline; Sandy Hill Community Hlth Ctre, 221 Nelson St, Ottawa ON K1N 1C7; McG'03; CCFP; (613)569-3488; Fax. (613)569-3484.

O'CONNOR, Mary E; 14 Bayswater Ave, Ottawa ON K1Y 2E4; Tor'71; BSc; (613)792-1751; Fax. (613)792-1751; meockg@aol.com.

O'CONNOR, Michael E; Medicine Hat Reg Hosp, 666 5 St SW, Medicine Hat AB T1A 4H6; National (Ireland)'79; FRCPC; AnatPath. Staff Path, Medicine Hat Regional Hospital; (403)529-8830; moconnor@palliserhealth.ca.

O'CONNOR, Paul W; St Michael's Hosp, 3 007-30 Bond St, Toronto ON M5B 1W8; Tor'79; MSc; AB; FRCPC; Neur (Multiple Sclerosis). Chief Div of Neurol/Dir MS Clinic & MS Research, St Michael's Hospital; Assoc Prof, University of Toronto; (416)864-5830; Fax. (416)864-5147; oconnorp@smh.toronto.on.ca.

O'CONNOR, Richard J A; Credit Valley Prof Bldg, 411-2300 Eglinton Ave W, Mississauga ON L5M 2V8; Dublin (Ireland)'69; FRCSC; GenSurg; VascSurg. Ac Staff, The Credit Valley Hospital; (905)820-2133; Fax. (905)820-7036; rjaoconnor@sympatico.ca.

O'CONNOR, Robert; Dept of Pathology, 910 10th Ave W, Vancouver BC V5Z 1M9; Trinity Coll. (Ireland)'78; MB ChB; BAO; DAB; FRCPC; AnatPath. Staff, Vancouver General Hospital - Centennial Pavillion; Clin Prof, University of British Columbia.

O'CONNOR, Russell J; Alder Med Clinic, 1211 8th Ave W, Vancouver BC V6H 1C7; Cal'98; BSc; MD; Dip SportMed; FRCPC; PhysMed&Rehab (Electromyography). Staff, G F Strong Rehabilitation Centre; Staff, Vancouver General Hospital - Centennial Pavillion; Clin Assoc Prof, University of British Columbia; (604)734-2553; Fax. (604)734-7148.

O'CONNOR, Thomas C; Trillium Hlth Ctr-Mississauga, 100 Queensway W, Mississauga ON L5B 1B8; Tor'89; FRCPC; IntMed (Critical Care Medicine); Respir. Staff, Trillium Health Centre - Mississauga; (905)848-7663; chrisoconnor@sympatico.ca.

O'CONNOR, Timothy M; Winchester Dist Mem Hosp, 566 Louise St, Winchester ON K0C 2K0; Ott'00; CCFP; Anes. Staff, Winchester District Memorial Hospital; (613)774-2420; Fax. (613)774-0453.

O'CONNOR, William F; 69 Main St E PO Box 101, Grand Bend ON N0M 1T0; Dublin (Ireland)'69; Ac Staff, South Huron Hospital Association; Coroner, Grand Bend Area; (519)238-2362; Fax. (519)238-6478.

O'CROININ, Feargus; Centennial CMH & Brain Injury, PO Box 1000 Stn Main, Ponoka AB T4J 1R8; National (Ireland)'81; Staff, Centennial Centre for Mental Health & Brain Injury; (403)783-7600; Fax. (403)783-7790.

O'DEA, Daneile F; Carbonear Gen Hosp, 86 Highroad South, Carbonear NL A1Y 1A4; Mem'00; FRCPC; DiagRad. Staff, Carbonear General Hospital; (709)945-5111

O'DEA, Dominic A; Rouge Valley-Centenary HC, 2867 Ellesmere Rd, Scarborough ON M1E 4B9; National (Ireland)'67; MB ChB; BAO; FRCPC; Psy. Staff, Rouge Valley Health System - Centenary Health Centre Site; (416)281-7318 x4535; Fax. (416)281-7320.

O'DEA, Francis J; Health Sciences Centre, 300 Prince Philip Dr, St. John's NL A1B 3V6; Mem'96; FRCSC; OrthSurg (Orthopedic Oncology). Staff, Health Sciences Centre; (709)777-6300

O'DEA, Jennifer; Dr Charles A Janeway Child HC, 300 Prince Philip Dr, St. John's NL A1B 3V6; Mem'96; FRCPC; Peds. Staff, Health Sciences Centre; (709)777-4520; jennifer.odea@easternhealth.ca.

O'DEA, Marie T F; Towers Med Clinic, 120-100 Elizabeth Ave, St. John's NL A1B 1S1; Mem'83; (709)753-9900; Fax. (709)753-6716.

O'DEA, Mary J; Family Med Centre, A2-150 Main St E, Grimsby ON L3M 1P1; Galway (Ireland)'77; MB ChB; (905)945-5424; Fax. (905)945-4772; grimsbyfmc@cogeco.net.

O'DOHERTY, Brian M J; 400-920 1st Ave W, Owen Sound ON N4K 4K5; Qns'94; FRCPC; PhysMed&Rehab. Aj Prof PhysMed & Rehab, University of Western Ontario; Aj Prof Rehab Med, Queen's University; (519)371-5858; Fax. (519)371-4853.

O'DOHERTY, James J; Grand River Hosp-KW Hlth Ctre, PO Box 9056 Stn C 835 King St W, Kitchener ON N2G 1G3; RCS (Ireland)'78; MRCPsy(U.K.); DABPN; DCH; DObst; FRCPC; Psy (General Adult Psychiatry). Staff, Grand River Hospital - Freeport Site; Staff Psy, Grand River Hospital - Kitchener/Waterloo Health Centre; Staff, Cambridge Memorial Hospital; Asst Prof psy, McMaster University; (519)749-4213; Fax. (519)745-1550.

O'DOHERTY, Michael; Hop Charles LeMoyne, 3120 boul Taschereau, Greenfield Park QC J4V 2H1; Laval'02; CCFP; CCFP(E.M.); Staff, Hopital Charles LeMoyne; (450)466-5000

O'DONNELL, David A; 302-717 Richmond St, London ON N6A 1S2; Galway (Ireland)'78; MB ChB; DObst; DCH; FRCPC; Psy (Adult Psychiatry). Aj Prof, University of Western Ontario; (519)438-1128; Fax. (519)438-8187; psychiatryassociates@on.aibn.com.

O'DONNELL, Denis E M; Richardson House, 102 Stuart St, Kingston ON K7L 2V6; National (Ireland)'78; MB ChB; BAO; FRCPI(Ire); FRCPC; IntMed; Respir. Staff, Kingston General Hospital; Staff, Hotel-Dieu Hospital; Staff, Providence Care - St Mary's of the Lake Hospital Site; Prof Med & Physiol, Queen's University; (613)548-2339; Fax. (613)549-1459; odonnell@post.queensu.ca.

O'DONNELL, James P; CSSSG-Hop de Gatineau, CP 2000 Succ Bureau-Chef 909 boul de la Verendrye O, Gatineau QC J8P 7H2; Mon'06; FRCPC; Psy. Staff, Hôpital de Gatineau; (819)966-6246

O'DONNELL, John T; Medical Arts Bldg, 2-165 Plymouth Rd, Welland ON L3B 3E1; Dublin (Ireland)'69; MB ChB; Ac Staff, Niagara Health System - Welland Hospital Site; (905)735-2128; Fax. (905)735-2171.

O'DONNELL, Maureen E; Child Health BC, 305-4088 Cambie St, Vancouver BC V5Z 2X8; Sask'87; MSc; FRCPC; Peds (Developmental Pediatrics). Sr Med Dir Child Dev & Rehab Prog, Sunny Hill Health Centre for Children; Staff, BC Children's Hospital; Assoc Prof, University of British Columbia; (604)877-6418

O'DONNELL, Michael; Seafield Eye Clinic, 5-1179 Seafield Cres, Nanaimo BC V9S 4S1; National (Ireland)'80; MB ChB; BAO; LMCC; FRCSC; Ophth. (250)753-5361; Fax. (250)753-1165.

O'DONNELL, Patricia M E; Maple Family Health Team, 325 University Ave, Kingston ON K7L 3R4; (Ireland)'82; MB ChB; BAO; CCFP; FCFP; Clin Assoc Staff Kingston Reg Cancer Centre, Kingston General Hospital; Asst Prof Family Med, Queen's University; (613)544-2902; Fax. (613)544-5768.

O'DONNELL, Shannon; St Paul's Hosp, 1081 Burrard St, Vancouver BC V6Z 1Y6; McM'06; FRCPC; EmergMed. Staff, Providence Health Care - St Paul's Hospital; (604)806-8480

O'DONNELL, Shawn M; Findley Creek Med Centre, 4744 Bank St, Ottawa ON K1T 3W7; Dublin (Ireland)'92; MB ChB; BAO; LMCC; CCFP; (613)317-2584

O'DONNELL, Trishia J; Appletree Med Centre, 4700 Keele St, North York ON M3J 1P3; Tor'06; CCFP; (647)722-2370; Fax. (416)736-5523.

O'DONOGHUE, J Paul; Hotel-Dieu Grace Hosp, 1030 Ouellette Ave, Windsor ON N9A 1E1; Sask'87; FRCPC; NuclearMed. Ac Staff Nuclear Med, Hôtel-Dieu Grace Hospital; Ac Staff Nuclear Med, Leamington District Memorial Hospital; Aj Prof DiagRadiol & Nuclear Med, University of Western Ontario; (519)973-4417; Fax. (519)973-4667; podonoghue@hdgh.org.

O'DONOGHUE, Rory; Appletree Med Center, 1971 Queen St E, Toronto ON M4L 1H9; (Ireland)'05; CCFP; (647)722-2370; Fax. (416)367-4301.

O'DONOHOE, Peter F; Four Corners Med Bldg, 2009 Long Lake Rd, Sudbury ON P3E 6C3; National (Ireland)'64; Langs: Gaelic; (705)522-5447

O'DONOVAN, M Claire; Abbie J Lane Mem Bldg, 3085-5909 Veterans Mem Lane, Halifax NS B3H 2E2; Dublin (Ireland)'85; MB ChB; BAO; FRCPC; Psy (Bipolar Disease). Staff Psy, Queen Elizabeth II Health Sciences Centre - Victoria General Site; Assoc Prof, Dalhousie University; (902)473-2585; Fax. (902)473-4877; claire.odonovan@cdha.nshealth.ca.

O'DRISCOLL, John K; CHUM-Hop Notre-Dame, 1560 rue Sherbrooke E, Montreal QC H2L 4M1; Qns'85; CCFP; CCFP(E.M.); ac Membre, Centre Hospitalier l'Université de Montréal (CHUM) - Hôpital Notre-Dame; Universite de Montreal; Langs: English; French; (514)890-8000

O'DRISCOLL, Mark F; Central Health Consultants, 129 Lincoln Rd, Grnd-Falls-Windsor NL A2A 1P3; Mem'95; FRCSC; GenSurg. (709)489-2700

O'DRISCOLL, Martha A; Sunnybrook Hlth Sciences Ctre, 2075 Bayview Ave, Toronto ON M4N 3M5; Mem'82; FRCPC; Anes. Staff Anes, Sunnybrook Health Sciences Centre; (416)480-4864 x4797

O'DRISCOLL, Mary-Louise; Workers' Comp Board, PO Box 94460 Stn Main, Richmond BC V6X 8V6; RCS (Ireland)'82; CCFP; FCFP; Staff, Workers' Comp Board of BC; Staff, OT Consulting & Treatment Services; (604)232-1502

O'DRISCOLL, Robert P; Medical Centre, 12-14 West St, Corner Brook NL A2H 2Z1; Mem'84; CCFP; FCFP; (709)634-7107; Fax. (709)634-0682.

O'DRISCOLL, Teresa; The Hugh Allen Clinic, PO Box 489 Stn Main, Sioux Lookout ON P8T 1A8; McM'80; CCFP; FCFP; Ac Staff, Sioux Lookout Meno-Ya-Win Health Centre; Staff, The Hugh Allen Clinic; (807)737-3803; Fax. (807)737-1771; todriscoll@slmhc.on.ca.

O'DWYER, Helena M; BC Cancer Agency-Vancouver CC, 600 10th Ave W, Vancouver BC V5Z 4E6; (Ireland)'97; MB BCh; BAO; FRCPC; DiagRad. Staff, BC Cancer Agency Vancouver Centre; (604)877-6000 x2261

O'DWYER, Niall P; PO Box 74055 Rpo Fraser Height, Surrey BC V4N 5H9; Alb'94; CCFP; Staff, Forensic Psychiatric Hospital; (604)523-7802; nodwyer@forensic.bc.ca.

O'DWYER, Robert L; Alberni Internal Medicine Clin, 3949 Port Alberni Hwy, Port Alberni BC V9Y 4S1; National (Ireland)'78; MB ChB; BAO; MRCP(I); FRCPC; IntMed. Staff, West Coast General Hospital; Physician, Alberni Internal Medicine Clinic; (250)724-8800; Fax. (250)724-8860.

O'FARRELL, Jennifer A C; Medical Arts Centre, 30-650 Terminal Ave, Nanaimo BC V9R 5E2; UBC'96; BSc(Hon); CCFP; (250)753-3431; Fax. (250)754-6897.

O'FARRELL, Lisa; Clinique Med Giffard, 210-3333 rue du Carrefour, Quebec QC G1C 5R9; Laval'00; CCFP; Médecin, Centre Hospitalier Affilié Universitaire de Québec - Hôpital du St-Sacrement; Langs: Bilingual(French/English); (418)663-6345; Fax. (418)663-8621; lisa_ofarrell@yahoo.ca.

O'FARRELL, Terry A; 303-3330 Richter St, Kelowna BC V1W 4V5; Alb'71; BSc; FRCSC; OrthSurg (Arthroplasty). Ac Staff, Kelowna General Hospital; Clin Instructor, University of British Columbia; Langs: English; French; (250)763-2042; Fax. (250)862-5842.

O'FERRALL, Erin K; MUHC-Montreal Neurology Inst, 3801 rue University, Montreal QC H3A 2B4; Cal'03; FRCPC; Neur. Staff, McGill University Health Centre - Montreal Neurological Hospital; (514)398-8551

O'FLANAGAN, Brian; PO Box 196, Rossland BC V0G 1Y0; RCS (Ireland)'68; LRCPS(Ire).

O'GORMAN, Augustin M; MUHC-Montreal Children's Hosp, 2300 rue Tupper, Montreal QC H3H 1P3; National (Ireland)'66; MB ChB; CSPQ; DiagRad. Staff Radiol, Shriners Hospitals For Children - Canada; Staff, McGill University Health Centre - Montreal Children's Hospital; assoc Prof, McGill University; (514)412-4450; Fax. (514)412-4347; gus.ogorman@muhc.mcgill.ca.

O'GORMAN, Monica M; 201-1205 Bow Valley Trail, Canmore AB T1W 1P5; Cal'00; BSc(Kinesiol); CCFP; (403)609-2228

O'GRADY, John P; Hotel-Dieu de Levis, 143 rue Wolfe, Levis QC G6V 3Z1; Wes'00; FRCPC; EmergMed. Staff, Hôtel-Dieu de Lévis; (418)835-7121

O'GRADY, Kevin; 205-955 Major Mackenzie Dr, Vaughan ON L6A 4P9; Tor'99; BASc; MHSc; FRCSC; PlasSurg (Breast Surgery). Ac Staff, Mackenzie Richmond Hill Hospital; Court Staff, Southlake Regional Health Centre; Court Staff, Markham Stouffville Hospital; (905)417-3544; Fax. (905)417-6675; info@drkevinogrady.com.

O'GRADY, Melanie D; Near North Med Clinic, 202-66 Josephine St, North Bay ON P1B 0A7; NOSM'10; CCFP; (705)474-1441

O'GRADY, Patrick G; Northside Family Practice, 145 King St, North Sydney NS B2A 3S1; Dal'91; (902)794-4600; Fax. (902)794-2327.

O'GRADY, Teresa; Health Sciences Centre, 300 Prince Philip Dr, St. John's NL A1B 3V6; Mem'85; FRCSC; ObstGyn (Reproductive Endocrinology & Infertility). Staff, Health Sciences Centre; (709)777-6300

O'HAGAN, David B; East Parkland Med Group, PO Box 310, Ste Rose du Lac MB R0L 1S0; Cape Town (South Africa)'77; CCFP; FCFP; (204)447-2089; Fax. (204)447-3258.

O'HALLORAN, Elizabeth; 319 15th Ave GD, Creston BC V0B 1G0; Duke University (USA)'03; (250)428-8873

O'HALLORAN, Harry M; 189 Saint Marie St, Collingwood ON L9Y 3K4; Tor'85; Staff, Collingwood General & Marine Hospital; (705)444-6700; Fax. (705)444-6866.

O'HALLORAN, James A; 17 Cowichan Dr, Oromocto NB E2V 1Z5; McM'10; CCFP.

O'HALLORAN, Patrick J; 544 Hugel Ave, Midland ON L4R 1V9; National (Ireland)'67; MB ChB; FRCSC; ObstGyn. (705)527-1360; Fax. (705)527-0188.

O'HALLORAN, Richard G; 102-17770 56 Ave, Surrey BC V3S 1C7; Witwatersrand (South Africa)'80; MB ChB; (604)574-7883; Fax. (604)574-9601.

O'HALPIN, Helen; The Hincks-Dellcrest Centre, 440 Jarvis St, Toronto ON M4Y 2H4; Dublin (Ireland)'77; Med Staff, The Hincks-Dellcrest Centre - Toronto; (416)924-1164 x3231; Fax. (416)924-8208.

O'HANLEY, G Marie; Dept of Veteran's Affairs, PO Box 7700 Stn Central, Charlottetown PE C1A 8M9; Dal'81; Staff, Queen Elizabeth Hospital.

O'HANLEY, Gerald P; Parkdale Med Centre, 20 St. Peters Rd, Charlottetown PE C1A 5N4; Dal'77; FRCSC; Ophth (Retina). Staff, Queen Elizabeth Hospital; (902)894-4449

O'HANLEY, Peter H; PO Box 29088 Rpo North End, Moncton NB E1G 4R3; Dal'80; Dalhousie University; (506)384-0883

O'HANLON, Jacinta; 93 Dewbourne Ave, Toronto ON M6C 1Y4; RCS (Ireland)'74; MRCPsy; DPM; LRCPS; FRCPC; Psy (Psychoanalysis). (416)789-2806; Fax. (416)784-3352; jas@leyne.com.

O'HARA, Carolyn D; DynaLIFE Dx, 200-10150 102 St NW, Edmonton AB T5J 5E2; Man'96; BSc(Biol.); FAB; FRCPC; GenPath (Bone Joint Path). Consultant Pathologist, Cross Cancer Institute; Asst Prof, University of Alberta; (780)451-3702 x8171; carolynohara@yahoo.com.

O'HARA, Gilles E; Hôpital Laval, 2725 ch Sainte-Foy, Quebec QC G1V 4G5; Mon'83; FACC; Cardiol (P.Q.); IntMed. Staff, Hôpital Laval; (418)656-8711; Fax. (418)656-4581.

O'HARA, Kathleen E; Sault Area Hosp, 750 Great Northern Rd, Sault Ste. Marie ON P6B 0A8; Ott'69; FRCPC; GenPath. Consultant, Sault Area Hospital - Sault Ste Marie; (705)759-3434 x3679; Fax. (705)759-3846.

O'HARA, William J; 711-1265 Arthur St E, Thunder Bay ON P7E 6E7; Tor'76; ABIM; FRCPC; IntMed. (807)623-1202; Fax. (807)623-7028.

O'HARE, Turlough J; St Joseph's Healthcare, 50 Charlton Ave E, Hamilton ON L8N 4A6; UBC'03; Anes. Staff, St Joseph's Healthcare - Charlton Campus; (905)522-1155 x33853

O'HAYON, Bonnie B E; North York Gen Hosp, 4001 Leslie St, North York ON M2K 1E1; Tor'99; FRCPC; DiagRad. Staff, North York General Hospital; (416)756-6000

O'HEARN, Bruce M; Canadian Forces Hlth Serv Ctr, PO Box 99000 Stn Forces, Halifax NS B3K 5X5; Dal'74; Staff, Canadian Forces Health Services Centre (Atlantic); Ac Staff, Cobiquid Multiservice Centre; (902)427-0550; Fax. (902)865-6814.

O'HERLIHY, Patrick J B; Medscan X-ray/Ultrasound, 12A-8401 Weston Rd, Woodbridge ON L4L 1A6; National (Ireland)'68; MB ChB; BAO; FRCPC; DiagRad (Ultrasound). Staff Radiol, St Michael's Hospital; Med Dir, Medscan Group; Dir, MCDU Ultrasound; (905)850-3025; Fax. (905)850-2179.

O'KANE, Janine M; The Rainbow Med Group, 300-5511 West Boulevard, Vancouver BC V6M 4H3; London (England)'71; MB BS; FRCPC; Psy. (604)264-9400; Fax. (604)264-9420.

O'KEANE, Joseph A; Reginal Fertility Program, 400-2000 Place Veteran's NW, Calgary AB T3B 4N2; National (Ireland)'80; MB ChB; BAO; FRCSC; ObstGyn. (403)284-9103; Fax. (403)284-9293.

O'KEEFE, Danielle; Family Med Clinic, 141 Torbay Rd, St. John's NL A1A 2H1; Mem'05; CCFP; Asst Prog Dir Family Med/Asst Prof Family Med, Memorial University Of Newfoundland; (709)777-7795; Fax. (709)777-2911.

O'KEEFE, Deborah L; Civic Parkdale Clinic, 411-737 Parkdale Ave, Ottawa ON K1Y 1J8; McM'84; FRCPC; IntMed; Rheum. Staff, The Ottawa Hospital - Civic Campus; Assoc Prof, University of Ottawa; (613)798-5555 x16574

O'KEEFE, Dennis; Commonwealth Med Clinic, 77 Commonwealth Ave, Mount Pearl NL A1N 1W7; Mem'76; Physician, St. John's Health Care Corp; (709)364-7555; Fax. (709)364-7554.

O'KEEFE, Erin L; Health Sciences Centre, 300 Prince Philip Dr, St. John's NL A1B 3V6; Saba (Netherlands Antilles)'06; FRCPC; Psy; FamilyMed. Staff, Health Sciences Centre; (709)777-7444

O'KEEFE, John B; Health Sciences Centre, 300 Prince Philip Dr, St. John's NL A1B 3V6; Mem'85; FRCPC; DiagRad. Staff Radiol, Health Sciences Centre; (709)777-6300; Fax. (709)777-6792.

O'KEEFE, Mary G; PO Box 1011, St. Anthony NL A0K 4S0; Tor'69; CCFP; FCFP; Staff, Charles S Curtis Memorial Hospital; Memorial University Of Newfoundland; (709)454-2200; Fax. (709)454-2228.

O'KEEFE, Megan N; Strathcona Mental Health Team, 330 Heatley Ave, Vancouver BC V6A 3G3; UBC'92; Staff, BC Mental Health & Addiction Service; (604)253-4401

O'KEEFE, Stephen J; Riley Park Family Practice, 171-1402 8 Ave NW, Calgary AB T2N 1B8; Dal'91; CCFP; (403)248-7955

O'KEEFFE, David; Madrona Imaging Westhill Ctre, A-1804 Bowen Rd, Nanaimo BC V9S 5W4; Sask'83; FRCPC; DiagRad (Pediatric Radiology). Ac Staff Radiol, Nanaimo Regional General Hospital; (250)753-4351; Fax. (250)753-0856.

O'KEEFFE, Kieran M; St Boniface Gen Hosp, 409 Tache Ave, Winnipeg MB R2H 2A6; Sask'92; FRCPC; Psy. Staff Psy, St Boniface General Hospital; Asst Prof Psy, University of Manitoba; (204)237-2979; Fax. (204)237-6264.

O'KEEFFE, Margaret M; Hys Med Centre, 202-11010 101 St NW, Edmonton AB T5H 4B9; Sask'82; FRCPC; DiagRad. (780)426-1121; Fax. (780)425-5979.

O'KEEFFE, Patrick D; 181B 22nd St W PO Box 369, Battleford SK S0M 0E0; Sask'92; FRCSC; Ophth. (306)445-7070; Fax. (306)445-7071.

O'KEEFFE, Teresa; Associate Med Clinic, PO Box 510, Slave Lake AB T0G 2A0; (Ireland)'83; (780)849-4115 x5; Fax. (780)849-4574.

O'KELLY, Cian; University of Alberta Hosp, 2D2 01-8440 112 St NW, Edmonton AB T6G 2B7; Alb'01; BSc; MSc; FRCSC; Neursurg (Cerebrovascular Surgery). Staff, University of Alberta Hospital; (780)407-1440

O'KELLY, Fionnuala; Smyth Med Centre, 204-1929 Russell Rd, Ottawa ON K1G 4G3; Dublin (Ireland)'77; MB ChB; BAO; FRCPC; Peds. Ac Staff, Children's Hospital of Eastern Ontario (CHEO); Ac Staff, The Ottawa Hospital - Civic Campus; (613)736-8999

O'KELLY, John G; University of Alberta Hosp, 1E703-8440 112 St NW, Edmonton AB T6G 2B7; Galway (Ireland)'72; MB ChB; MRCPsy; FRCPC; Psy (Individual & Group Psychiatry). Clin Coord Evening Treatment Prog/Consultant Psy, University of Alberta Hospital; Clin Prof Psy, University of Alberta; Langs: Gaelic; French; (780)433-8330; Fax. (780)407-6470; lnelson@cha.ab.ca.

O'KELLY, Kevin F; The Ottawa Hosp-Civic Campus, 1053 Carling Ave, Ottawa ON K1Y 4E9; National (Ireland)'82; MB ChB; FRCPC; DiagRad. Staff, The Ottawa Hospital - Civic Campus; (613)761-4982; Fax. (613)761-4476.

O'LEARY, Brendan P; PO Box 2327 Stn Main, Sarnia ON N7T 7S6; University Coll.(Cork) (Ireland)'66; MB; DCH; DA; DObst; Med Dir Surgical Prog, Bluewater Health - Mitton Site; (519)464-4159; Fax. (519)542-2777.

O'LEARY, Debi G; 203-389 Connell St, Woodstock NB E7M 5G5; Qns'91; CCFP; (506)325-1999; Fax. (506)328-2461.

O'LEARY, Denis F; White Rock Med Associates, 101-15451 Russell Ave, White Rock BC V4B 2R5; National (Ireland)'75; (604)531-5595; Fax. (604)531-9818.

O'LEARY, Gerald M; Univ Hlth Network-Toronto Gen, EN3 460-200 Elizabeth St, Toronto ON M5G 2C4; Dublin (Ireland)'80; FFARCSI; FRCPC; Anes. Chief Anes, Toronto General Hospital - UHN; Chief Anes, Mount Sinai Hospital; Asst Prof Anes, University of Toronto; (416)340-4800 x4359; Fax. (416)340-3698.

O'LEARY, James D; The Hosp for Sick Children, 2212J-555 University Ave, Toronto ON M5G 1X8; (Ireland)'03; Staff, The Hospital For Sick Children; (416)813-7240

O'LEARY, Sean W; 193 Elizabeth Ave, St. John's NL A1B 1S9; Mem'87; FRCSC; Ophth (Medical & Surgical Ophthalmology). (709)726-4667; Fax. (709)739-8384; soleary@nfld.net.

O'LEARY, Susan D; St Clare's Mercy Hosp, 154 Lemarchant Rd, St. John's NL A1C 5B8; Mem'91; FRCPC; Anes. Staff, St Clare's Mercy Hospital; (709)777-5000

O'LEARY, Thomas A; Clinical Sciences Bldg, 8 120-152 University Campus NW, Edmonton AB T6G 2G3; Man'74; FRCPC; Anes. (780)407-8861

O'LEARY, Timothy J; The Ottawa Hosp-Riverside, 1967 Riverside Dr, Ottawa ON K1H 7W9; Qns'81; FRCPC; IntMed; Endocrin&Metab., The Ottawa Hospital - Riverside Campus; Staff, The Ottawa Hospital - Civic Campus; Asst Prof, University of Ottawa; (613)738-8333

O'MAHONY, John C; London Road Diagnostic Clinic, 481 London Rd, Sarnia ON N7T 4X3; (Ireland)'97; CCFP; (519)491-7965; Fax. (519)491-7494.

O'MAHONY, Michael F J; London Road Diagnostic Clinic, 481 London Rd, Sarnia ON N7T 4X3; Dublin (Ireland)'66; MB ChB; BAO; (519)344-7456; Fax. (519)332-8214.

O'MAHONY, Michael; Clairhurst Med Centre, 301A-1466 Bathurst St, Toronto ON M5R 3S3; Dublin (Ireland)'77; MB ChB; FRCPC; Psy. Staff, Baycrest Centre for Geriatric Care; (416)785-2500 x2453; Fax. (416)785-2450.

O'MAHONY, William F; 348 Lyndock St, Corunna ON N0N 1G0; National (Ireland)'73; MB ChB; BAO; Media Dir, Afton Nursing Home; Investigator, Corunna Medical Research Centre; (519)862-1471; Fax. (519)862-3686.

O'MALLEY, Brendan D; Cowichan Med Centre, 3106 Gibbins Rd, Duncan BC V9L 1E8; Cape Town (South Africa)'89; MB ChB; FRCPC; IntMed. (250)748-1323

O'MALLEY, Frances P; St Michael's Hosp, 30 Bond St, Toronto ON M5B 1W8; Trinity Coll. (Ireland)'85; MB ChB; FRCPC; AnatPath (Breast Pathology). Staff, St Michael's Hospital; (416)586-4800 x4548

O'MALLEY, Kathleen; 106-2155 10th Ave, Prince George BC V2M 5J6; UBC'08; CCFP; (250)563-5111

O'MALLEY, Martin E; Univ Hlth Network-Princess M, 3 956-610 University Ave, Toronto ON M5G 2M9; RCS (Ireland)'91; FRCPC; DiagRad (Abdominal Imaging). Staff, Princess Margaret Hospital - University Health Network; Staff, Toronto General Hospital - UHN; (416)340-4800 x3296; Fax. (416)593-0502.

O'MALLEY, Maureen P; 34 Stone Church Rd, Ancaster ON L9K 1S5; Wes'93; BSc; FRCPC; Derm. Staff Pt-Time, Hamilton Health Sciences Centre - McMaster University Medical Centre; Asst Prof, McMaster University; (905)304-1122; Fax. (905)304-3768.

O'MALLEY, Michael J; Phoenix Med Centre, 408-2155 10th Ave, Prince George BC V2M 5J6; Galway (Ireland)'74; FCFP; CCFP; FCFP; Langs: Gaelic; (250)563-7522; momalley@canada.com.

O'MALLEY, Peter J; 402-2155 10th Ave, Prince George BC V2M 5J6; Galway (Ireland)'73; MB ChB; BAO; CCFP; FCFP; Ac Staff, University Hospital of Northern British Columbia; Langs: Irish; (250)563-8878; Fax. (250)563-8838.

O'MALLEY, Vincent P; 203-49 Cornwallis St, Kentville NS B4N 2E3; Galway (Ireland)'74; MB ChB; BAO; MCh; FRCS; FRCSC; GenSurg. Staff GenSurg, Valley Regional Hospital; (902)678-2583; Fax. (902)678-2262; vomalley@ns.sympatico.ca.

O'MAONAIGH, Conleth E; Health Sciences Centre, 300 Prince Philip Dr, St. John's NL A1B 3V6; Dublin (Ireland)'77; MB ChB; MPH; CCFP; Staff, Health Sciences Centre; (709)777-6300

O'MARA, Meghan M; 144-1333 Sheppard Ave E, North York ON M2J 1V1; UBC'10; CCFP; (416)491-5900; Fax. (416)491-1149.

O'MEARA, Eileen; Institut de Cardiologie de Mtl, 5000 rue Belanger, Montreal QC H1T 1C8; Mon'97; FRCPC; IntMed; Cardiol. Staff, Institut de Cardiologie de Montréal; (514)376-3330; Fax. (514)593-2540; eileen.omeara@icm-mhi.org.

O'NEAL, Erica L; Richmond Mental Health Team, 200-6061 No 3 Rd, Richmond BC V6Y 2B2; Michigan (USA)'02; (604)273-9121

O'NEIL, Barbara A; Hants North Health Centre, PO Box 46 4539 Highway 215, Noel NS B0N 2C0; Dal'00; BSc; CCFP; Staff, Colchester East Hants Health Centre; Preceptor Family Med, Dalhousie University; (902)369-2080; Fax. (902)669-2220.

O'NEIL, Cathy; Kanata Prof Centre, 203-99 Kakulu Rd, Kanata ON K2L 3C8; Sask'87; BSc; MSc; (613)599-4301; Fax. (613)599-4298.

O'NEIL, D Joseph; Parkdale Med Tower, 405-1081 Carling Ave, Ottawa ON K1Y 4G2; Ott'75; BSc; FRCSC; OrthSurg (Spine Surgery). Staff, The Ottawa Hospital - Civic Campus; Physician, Ontario Cancer Foundation; Asst Prof, University of Ottawa; (613)722-1825; joneil@ottawahospital.on.ca.

O'NEIL, David; Sundance Med Clinic, 7-402 Railway St W, Cochrane AB T4C 2B6; Alb'72; BSc; CCFP; FCFP; (403)932-2255; Fax. (403)932-2254.

O'NEIL, John A; St Mary's Hosp Centre, 3830 av Lacombe, Montreal QC H3T 1M5; McG'78; FRCPC; Psy (Dissociative Disorders). Staff, St Mary's Hospital Centre; adj Prof, McGill University; Langs: English; French; (514)345-3511 x3463

O'NEIL, Leonard S; Spryfield Med Centre, 205 Herring Cove Rd, Halifax NS B3P 1L1; Dal'72; CCFP; FCFP; (902)477-5693; Fax. (902)477-0502.

O'NEIL, Michael B; Lions Gate Hosp, 231 15th St E, North Vancouver BC V7L 2L7; Tor'74; CCFP; CCFP(E.M.); Med Coord Emerg Health Services/Physician Emerg, Lions Gate Hospital; (604)984-5799; Fax. (604)266-7243.

O'NEIL, Ross L; 166-2111 Main St, Penticton BC V2A 6W6; UBC'01; Staff, Penticton Regional Hospital; (250)276-5050

O'NEIL, Steven D; Summerside Med Centre, 1-475 Granville St, Summerside PE C1N 3N9; Mem'92; BSc(Hons.); MSc; Ac Staff, Prince County Hospital; (902)432-8155; Fax. (902)436-9660; sdoneil@pei.eastlink.ca.

O'NEILL, Blair J; University of Alberta Hosp, 2C2.34-8440 112 St NW, Edmonton AB T6G 2B7; Dal'83; FACC; FRCP; FRCPC; IntMed (Interventional Cardiology); Cardiol (Cardiac Intensive Care Unit). Div Dir Cardiol, University of Alberta Hospital; Div Dir Cardiol, Mazankowski Alberta Heart Institute; VP, Canadian Cardiovascular Society; Prof Med, University of Alberta; (780)407-6353; Fax. (780)407-6032; blair.oneill@albertahealthservices.ca.

O'NEILL, Brendan D; The Ottawa Hosp-Gen Campus, 3041-501 Smyth Rd, Ottawa ON K1H 8L6; Dal'07; FRCSC; OrthSurg. Staff, The Ottawa Hospital - General Campus; (613)737-8785

O'NEILL, Brian; Health Services Complex, 10-20 Kennedy Dr, Sussex NB E4E 2P1; Mem'08; CCFP; Staff, Sussex Health Centre; (506)434-0528; Fax. (506)432-3460.

O'NEILL, Carmen A C; 204-26 North St, Bridgewater NS B4V 2V6; Dal'87; CCFP; Ac Member, South Shore Regional Hospital; (902)543-2242; Fax. (902)530-3146.

O'NEILL, Craig D; Stratford Gen Hosp, 46 General Hospital Dr, Stratford ON N5A 2Y6; (Australia)'05; FRCSC; GenSurg. Staff, Stratford General Hospital - Huron Perth Healthcare Alliance; (519)274-7904

O'NEILL, Donald L; Family Health Centre, 200-2462 Howard Ave, Windsor ON N8X 3V6; Wes'85; CCFP; (519)258-2700; Fax. (519)258-4456.

O'NEILL, J Peter; Kingston Gen Hosp, 76 Stuart St, Kingston ON K7L 2V7; Qns'85; FSOGC; FRCSC; ObstGyn. Asst Prof ObstGyn Radiology, Kingston General Hospital; Asst Prof, Queen's University; (613)548-7840; Fax. (613)548-1330.

O'NEILL, John M D; St Joseph's Healthcare, 50 Charlton Ave E, Hamilton ON L8N 4A6; National (Ireland)'92; Staff, St Joseph's Healthcare - Charlton Campus; (905)521-6009

O'NEILL, Karen A; O'Neill Cosmetic Dermatology, 306-71 King St W, Mississauga ON L5B 4A2; Tor'83; FRCPC; Derm (Cosmetic Dermatology). Court Staff, Women's College Hospital; (905)949-1461; Fax. (905)949-6662.

O'NEILL, Kevin B; Cook Medical Bldg, 329-1175 Cook St, Victoria BC V8V 4A1; Galway (Ireland)'82; MB ChB; BAO; FRCPC; Psy. (250)595-4211; Fax. (250)595-8939.

O'NEILL, Kiley J; Boardwalk Prof Centre, 220 Water St, Charlottetown PE C1A 9M5; Dal'00; CCFP.

O'NEILL, Laura A; 110-10333 Southport Rd SW, Calgary AB T2W 3X6; Alb'99; CCFP; (403)258-1960; Fax. (403)253-5735.

O'NEILL, Linda J; 16-1710 Ellis St, Kelowna BC V1Y 2B5; Tor'89; BSc(Hon); CCFP; CCFP(E.M.); FCFP; (250)763-4111

O'NEILL, Marie-Therese A; Halifax Prof Centre, 583-5991 Spring Garden Rd, Halifax NS B3H 1Y6; Dublin (Ireland)'82; MB ChB; BAO; MRCP(I); MRCPsy; FRCPC; Psy (Anxiety Disorder). (902)423-0794; Fax. (902)423-1451.

O'NEILL, Mary C; Family Practice Associates, 6155 North St, Halifax NS B3K 5R3; Dublin (Ireland)'87; MB ChB; BAO.

O'NEILL, Michael O; 104-3551 Blanshard St, Victoria BC V8Z 0B9; Alb'71; FRCSC; OrthSurg (Arthroplasty). (250)940-4444

O'NEILL, Michelle E; 35 Glenwood St, Sydney NS B1P 1V8; Dal'01; FRCSC; OrthSurg. Staff, Cape Breton Healthcare Complex; (902)270-3778; Fax. (902)270-3779.

O'NEILL, Patrick S; Bramalea Med Centre, 300-18 Kensington Rd, Brampton ON L6T 4S5; Trinity Coll. (Ireland)'71; MB ChB; BAO; (905)791-3133; Fax. (905)791-8441.

O'NEILL, Roger R; 41 Broadway St W, Yorkton SK S3N 3T9; Dublin (Ireland)'69; Ac Staff Ophth, Yorkton Regional Health Centre; (306)783-3216

O'NEILL, Ryan D; Royal University Hosp, 103 Hospital Dr, Saskatoon SK S7N 0W8; Sask'01; CCFP; CCFP(E.M.); Staff, Royal University Hospital; (306)655-1363; Fax. (306)655-1011.

O'NEILL, Thomas; Clinique Dr Thomas C O'Neill, CP 610 320 Main St, Shawville QC J0X 2Y0; Dublin (Ireland)'74; MB ChB; BAO; CCFP; FCFP; Chef Gen Care Service, CSSS du Pontiac; assoc Conférencier, McGill University; (819)647-2218; Fax. (819)647-2219.

O'REGAN, Noel B; St Clare's Mercy Hosp, 154 Lemarchant Rd, St. John's NL A1C 5B8; Dal'95; FRCPC; Anes. Staff, St Clare's Mercy Hospital; (709)777-5521

O'REILLY, Alan G; Clarenville Med Arts Clinic, 204-105 Manitoba Dr, Clarenville NL A5A 1K2; Mem'76; (709)466-2631; Fax. (709)466-3895.

O'REILLY, Elaine; Montebello Med Clinic, 118 Lake St, St Catharines ON L2R 5Y1; Dublin (Ireland)'02; CCFP; Staff, Hôtel Dieu Shaver Health & Rehabilitation Centre; Clin Teach Staff, McMaster University; (905)685-6555; Fax. (905)685-6558.

O'REILLY, Kenneth V; Edmonton Cardiology Consultant, 350-11010 101 St NW, Edmonton AB T5H 4B9; Alb'80; FRCPC; IntMed (Echocardiography); Cardiol. Staff, Royal Alexandra Hospital; (780)428-3246; Fax. (780)425-0487.

O'REILLY, Michael G; Kingston Gen Hosp, 76 Stuart St, Kingston ON K7L 2V7; Mem'79; Cardiol; IntMed (Acute Coronary Care)., Kingston General Hospital; (613)549-6666

O'REILLY, Michael L; St Joseph's Gen Hosp, 2137 Comox Ave, Comox BC V9M 1P2; Sask'83; FRCPC; DiagRad. Staff, St Joseph's General Hospital; (250)339-2242; Fax. (250)339-0197.

O'REILLY, Philip J; Tabor Manor Nursing Home, 1 Tabor Dr, St Catharines ON L2N 1V9; RCS (Ireland)'71; CCFP; Ac Staff, Niagara Health System - St Catharines General Site; Ac Staff, Hôtel Dieu Shaver Health & Rehabilitation Centre; (905)934-2548

O'REILLY, Richard; Regional Mental HC-London, PO Box 5532 Stn B 850 Highbury Ave N, London ON N6A 4H1; Dublin (Ireland)'79; MB ChB; BAO; MRCP(I); MRCPsy; FRCPC; Psy (Mental Health Law). Staff, Regional Mental Health Care-St Joseph's Health Care; Prof Psy, University of Western Ontario; Prof Mental Health, Northern Ontario School of Medicine; (519)455-5110 x47240; Fax. (519)455-5090.

O'REILLY, Susan E; BC Cancer Agency-Vancouver CC, 600 10th Ave W, Vancouver BC V5Z 4E6; Dublin (Ireland)'76; MB ChB; BAO; MRC(Ire.); FRCPC; IntMed (Medical Oncology). VP Cancer Care I, BC Cancer Agency Vancouver Centre; Ac Staff, Vancouver General Hospital - Centennial Pavillion; (604)707-5973; soreilly@bccancer.bc.ca.

O'RIORDAN, Ailbhe E; London HSC-University Hosp, PO Box 5339 Stn B 339 Windermere Rd, London ON N6A 5A5; Dublin (Ireland)'89; MB ChB; BAO; DCH; FRCPC; DiagRad. Staff Radiol, London Health Sciences Centre - University Hospital; Asst Prof, University of Western Ontario; Langs: Irish; French; German; (519)663-3648

O'RIORDAN, John; The Credit Valley Hosp, 2200 Eglinton Ave W, Mississauga ON L5M 2N1; Dublin (Ireland)'78; MB ChB; BAO; MRCPsy; Psy. Staff, The Credit Valley Hospital; (905)813-2398; joriordan@cvh.on.ca.

O'RIORDAN, John W; The Credit Valley Hosp, 2200 Eglinton Ave W, Mississauga ON L5M 2N1; Dublin (Ireland)'78; MB BCh; BAO; MRCPsy(Lond); FRCPC; Psy (Adult Psychiatry). Staff, The Credit Valley Hospital; (905)813-2398; Fax. (905)813-4284.

O'RIORDAN, Matthew; 825 Don Mills Rd, North York ON M3C 1V4; National (Ireland)'70; MB ChB; (416)383-1251

O'SHAUGHNESSY, Gael; CLSC Cotes-des-Neiges, 5700 ch Cote-des-Neiges, Montreal QC H3T 2A8; McG'04; CCFP; (514)731-8531 x2850

O'SHAUGHNESSY, P Martin; Cottage Country Fam Hlth Team, 1-5 Pineridge Gate, Gravenhurst ON P1P 1Z3; Ott'90; Staff, South Muskoka Memorial Hospital - Muskoka Algonquin Healthcare; Langs: English; French; (705)687-2794; Fax. (705)687-8652.

O'SHAUGHNESSY, Roy J; The Forensic Group, 305-1245 Broadway W, Vancouver BC V6H 1G7; Ott'74; FRCPC; Psy. Consultant, Vancouver General Hospital - Centennial Pavillion; (604)733-5722; Fax. (604)739-3734.

O'SHEA, A Mary; 191 Ingram St PO Box 573, Duncan BC V9L 3X6; Cal'80; BSc; FRCPC; IntMed. (250)715-7864

O'SHEA, Ciaran P; Atlantic Offshore Med Services, PO Box 2442 Stn C 4 Henry St, St. John's NL A1C 6E7; RCS (Ireland)'73; CCBOM; Staff, St Clare's Mercy Hospital; Staff, Health Sciences Centre; Clinical Asst Prof Occup Med, Memorial University Of Newfoundland; (709)722-4074; Fax. (709)722-6801.

O'SHEA, Eoghan B; Ottawa Hosp-Family Med Ctre, 210 Melrose Ave, Ottawa ON K1Y 4K7; Dublin (Ireland)'82; MB ChB; BAO; CCFP; FCFP; Asst Prof Family Med, University of Ottawa Heart Institute; Court Staff Privil, Perth & Smiths Falls District Hospital - Smiths Falls Site; Langs: French; Gaelic; (613)761-4334; Fax. (613)761-4200.

O'SHEA, Fiona; Dr H Bliss Murphy Cancer Ctr, 300 Prince Philip Dr, St. John's NL A1B 3V6; RCS (Ireland)'82; MB BCh; Staff, Dr H Bliss Murphy Cancer Centre; (709)777-7436

O'SHEA, Patrick M; Eleven Elizabeth Family Practi, 201-11 Elizabeth Ave, St. John's NL A1A 1W6; Qns'80; CCFP; FCFP; Ac Staff, St Clare's Mercy Hospital; Ac Staff Family Pract, Health Sciences Centre; Clin Assoc Prof Family Pract, Memorial University Of Newfoundland; (709)579-1106; Fax. (709)579-0347.

O'SHEA, Timothy M; Hamilton HS-Henderson Site, A366-711 Concession St, Hamilton ON L8V 1C3; McM'02; FRCPC; IntMed; InfectDis; MedMicrobiol. Staff, Hamilton Health Sciences Centre-Juravinski Site; (905)389-4411

O'SULLIVAN, Brian; Univ Hlth Network-Princess M, 610 University Ave, Toronto ON M5G 2M9; Dublin (Ireland)'76; FRCPC; RadOncol. Staff, Princess Margaret Hospital - University Health Network; Teach Staff, University of Toronto; (416)946-2125; Fax. (416)946-6556; brian.osullivan@rmp.uhn.on.ca.

O'SULLIVAN, Colleen M; Aberdeen Hosp, 835 East River Rd, New Glasgow NS B2H 3S6; Cal'06; Staff, Aberdeen Regional Hospital; (902)752-7600

O'SULLIVAN, Eoghan; Enterprise Square, PO Box 912 157 Water St, Shelburne NS B0T 1W0; Dublin (Ireland)'82; MB ChB; BAO; CCFP; (902)875-3787; Fax. (902)875-3702.

O'SULLIVAN, Fiona E; Dual Diagnosis Services, 53 Bond St, Oakville ON L6K 1L8; Wes'02; (905)844-7864; Fax. (905)844-3545.

O'SULLIVAN, John J; Royal Court Med Centre, LL2-1 Quarry Ridge Rd, Barrie ON L4M 7G1; Mem'98; FRCSC; OrthSurg. (705)719-3075; Fax. (705)728-0349.

O'SULLIVAN, Joseph P; The Ottawa Hosp-Gen Campus, 501 Smyth Rd, Ottawa ON K1H 8L6; Ott'82; FRCPC; DiagRad. Staff, The Ottawa Hospital - General Campus; (613)737-8504; Fax. (613)737-8957.

O'SULLIVAN, Katherine; 215 rue du Sud, Cowansville QC J2K 2X5; Mon'88; FRCSC; GenSurg. Langs: English; (450)263-8551

O'SULLIVAN, P Niall; 2-481 London Rd, Sarnia ON N7T 4X3; National (Ireland)'76; (519)332-0222; Fax. (519)332-8214.

O'SULLIVAN, Peter D; Peterborough Reg HC-Hospital, 1 Hospital Dr, Peterborough ON K9J 7C6; National (Ireland)'73; FRCPC; DiagRad. Staff, Peterborough Regional Health Centre - Hospital Drive; (705)743-2121

O'SULLIVAN, S Karl C B; Halton Healthcare Services, 6F-700 Dorval Dr, Oakville ON L6K 3V3; Dublin (Ireland)'66; DABPN; DPM; FRCPI(Ire); FRCPsy(UK); FRCPC; Psy (Mood Disorders). Staff, Halton Healthcare Services Corporation - Oakville Site; (905)338-4630; Fax. (905)845-6419.

O'SULLIVAN, Sean J; 25 Hyman St, Tillsonburg ON N4G 2C3; RCS (Ireland)'68; LRCPSI; Ac Staff, Tillsonburg District Memorial Hospital; (519)842-9429; Fax. (519)842-3430.

O'TOOLE, Danielle M; McMaster Family Practice, 690 Main St W, Hamilton ON L8S 1A4; McM'10; CCFP; (905)521-5016

O'TOOLE, Eamon A; 263 First Ave W, North Bay ON P1B 3C2; Galway (Ireland)'67; FRCPC; Psy. Consultant, North Bay Regional Health Centre - Regional Mental Health; (705)476-0555; Fax. (705)476-0309.

O'TOOLE, Francis J; 12-1300 Garth St, Hamilton ON L9C 4L7; McM'87; FAAP; FRCPC; Peds (Child Abuse). Assoc Staff, St Joseph's Healthcare - Charlton Campus; Assoc Staff, Hamilton Health Sciences Centre - McMaster University Medical Centre; Asst Prof, McMaster University; (905)575-0611; Fax. (905)575-7737; f_otoole@email.com.

O'TOOLE, John D; 1029 Ridgeway Ave PO Box 1102, Coquitlam BC V3J 6Z4; Dublin (Ireland)'76; MB ChB; BAO; MRC; FRCPC; Peds (Neonatology). Ac Staff, Royal Columbian Hospital; (778)928-0403

O'TOOLE, Susan A; Collingwood Gen & Marine Hosp, 459 Hume St, Collingwood ON L9Y 1W9; Qns'99; FRCSC; ObstGyn. Staff, Collingwood General & Marine Hospital; (705)444-5533

OAD, Lachman D; Wetaskiwin Hosp & Care Centre, 6910 47 St, Wetaskiwin AB T9A 3N3; Sindh (Pakistan)'82; MB BS; FRCS(Ire); FRCSC; GenSurg (Breast Surgery). Staff Gen Surg, Wetaskiwin Hospital & Care Centre; Langs: Urdu; Sindhi; Punjabi; (780)361-4069; Fax. (780)361-4315.

OAKE, J Stuart; The Ottawa Hosp-Gen Campus, 501 Smyth Rd, Ottawa ON K1H 8L6; Mem'88; DAB; FRCSC; Urol. Staff, The Ottawa Hospital - General Campus; (613)737-8899 x79264; Fax. (613)737-8694.

OAKES, Jennifer A; Royal Inland Hospital, 311 Columbia St, Kamloops BC V2C 2T1; New York (USA)'00; Staff, Royal Inland Hospital; (250)374-5111

OAKES, Jennifer; Broadway Obstetrics & Gyn, 401-1338 Broadway Ave W, Vancouver BC V6H 1H2; Qns'00; FRCSC; ObstGyn. (604)689-1400

OAKTON, Suzannah E; Homewood Health Centre, 150 Delhi St, Guelph ON N1E 6K9; CCFP; Staff, Homewood Health Centre; (519)824-1010

OANDASAN, Ivy F; Univ Hlth Network-Toronto Western Hosp, 2W404-399 Bathurst St, Toronto ON M5T 2S8; Man'91; MHSc; CCFP; FCFP; Assoc Staff, Toronto Western Hospital - University Health Network; Asst Prof, University of Toronto; (416)603-5888 x2; Fax. (416)603-5448; ivy.oandasan@utoronto.ca.

OATES, D Julian; North Lambton Comm Hlth Ctre, 59 King St W, Forest ON N0N 1J0; Wes'76; CCFP; FCFP; Staff, St Joseph's Hospital - St Joseph's Health Care; (519)786-4545; Fax. (519)786-3023.

OATES, Jennifer; London HSC-Victoria Hosp, PO Box 5010 Stn B 800 Commissioners Rd E, London ON N6A 5W9; UBC'03; MSc; FRCPC; Psy (Geriatric Medicine). Staff/Clin Leader Geriatric Mental Health Prog, London Health Sciences Centre - Victoria Campus; (519)685-8500; Fax. (519)667-6707.

OBAID, Haron R; Royal University Hosp, 103 Hospital Dr, Saskatoon SK S7N 0W8; (Iraq)'94; FRCPC; DiagRad. Staff, Royal University Hospital; (306)655-2371; Fax. (306)655-2370.

OBAID, Laila; Royal Alexandra Hosp, 5027-10240 Kingsway NW, Edmonton AB T5H 3V9; (Ireland)'88; FRCPC; Peds. Staff, Royal Alexandra Hospital; (780)735-4670; Fax. (780)735-4072.

OBAID, Mona; Glenrose Rehab Hosp, 0601-10230 111 Ave NW, Edmonton AB T5G 0B7; Riyadh (Saudi Arabia)'00; FRCPC; Neur. Staff, Glenrose Rehabilitation Hospital; (780)735-7999

OBAJI, Hind I A B; 304-474 College St, Toronto ON M6G 1A4; Baghdad (Iraq)'69; DCP; Staff, St Joseph's Health Centre; (416)588-6660; Fax. (416)588-5750.

OBAJI, James; 204-474 College St, Toronto ON M6G 1A4; CCFP; (416)967-9368; Fax. (416)967-7385.

OBAYAN, Aderonke O; Pediatric Clinic, 1631 20th St W, Saskatoon SK S7M 0Z7; (Nigeria)'88; MB BS; MPH; (306)384-9888; Fax. (306)384-1565.

OBAYASHI, Jeffery T; Omineca Med Clinic, 3348 Hospital Rd, Vanderhoof BC V0J 3A0; UBC'08; BSc; CCFP; Staff, St John Hospital; (250)567-2201; Fax. (250)567-2105.

OBEDKOFF, Daniel P; Group One Med Associates, 1111 Springfield Rd, Kelowna BC V1Y 8R7; UBC'85; CCFP; (250)762-4286; Fax. (250)762-4213.

OBEID, Issam S; Corner Brook Long Term Care, 40 University Dr, Corner Brook NL A2H 5G4; Medical Univ of Szeged (Hungary)'95; CCFP; (709)637-3999

OBEIDAT, Motaz A; Royal Alexandra Hosp, 10240 Kingsway NW, Edmonton AB T5H 3V9; (Jordan)'97; Staff, Royal Alexandra Hospital; (780)735-4111

OBENSON, Ken; Saint John Reg Hosp, PO Box 2100 Stn Main 400 University Ave, Saint John NB E2L 4L2; Lagos (Nigeria)'87; FRCPC; AnatPath (Forensic Pathology). Staff, Saint John Regional Hospital; Staff, Dalhousie University; (506)648-6501

OBERAI, Anjali; Wawa Family Health Team, PO Box 858 17 Government Rd, Wawa ON P0S 1K0; Ott'93; CCFP; FCFP; (705)856-1313; Fax. (705)856-1330.

OBERG, Colin E; Leduc Comm Hosp & Hlth Ctr, 4210 48 St, Leduc AB T9E 5Z3; Alb'01; CCFP; Staff, Leduc Community Hospital; (780)980-4470; colinoberg@yahoo.com.

OBERHOLSTER, Melissa; Townsite Med Clinic, 512 Campbell St, Nanaimo BC V9R 3H1; Stellenbosch (South Africa)'05; (250)753-5665

OBERHOLZER, Werner; Radville Marian Health Centre, PO Box 310, Radville SK S0C 2G0; Orange Free State (South Africa)'89; MB ChB; CCFP; Fam Med, Weyburn General Hospital; Staff, Radville Marian Health Centre; Langs: Afrikaans; (306)869-3111; Fax. (306)869-3256.

OBERLANDER, Timothy F A; Sunny Hill Health Ctre for Chi, 3644 Slocan St, Vancouver BC V5M 3E8; Qns'85; FRCPC; Peds (Developmental Pediatrics). Staff, Sunny Hill Health Centre for Children; Staff, BC Children's Hospital; Prof/Teach Staff, University of British Columbia; (604)453-8306; Fax. (604)453-8338.

OBERLEITNER, Barry H; Kindersley Med Clinic, PO Box 1390, Kindersley SK S0L 1S0; (306)463-2621; Fax. (306)463-4101.

OBERMAN, Saul S; Clinique MD Sante, 8127 boul Saint-Laurent, Montreal QC H2P 2M1; Man'03; CCFP; (514)687-4372

OBEROI, Malika; B-560 Main St PO Box 1148, Winchester ON K0C 2K0; Sher'06; FRCSC; GenSurg. (613)774-0990; Fax. (613)774-3144.

OBIAJULU, Anthony C; 106-10055 120 Ave, Grande Prairie AB T8V 8H8; (Nigeria)'98; (780)532-4415; Fax. (780)532-4559.

OBIANYOR, Florence; Dept of Family Med, 1213 4 St SW, Calgary AB T2R 0X9; CCFP; Staff, Foothills Medical Centre; (403)955-9300

OBIENU, Emeka; Prince Albert Community Clinic, 110 8th St E, Prince Albert SK S6V 0V7; (306)763-6464; Fax. (306)763-2101.

OBIKOYA, Olubankole; Saskatchewan Hosp-Battleford, PO Box 39 Stn Main 1 Jersey St, North Battleford SK S9A 2X8; (Nigeria)'78; MB ChB; Sr Staff Psy, Saskatchewan Hospital - North Battleford; (306)446-6800; oobikoya@pnrha.ca.

OBIOHA, Godwin E; Haney Prof Bldg, 105-11743 224 St, Maple Ridge BC V2X 6A4; Ibadan (Nigeria)'85; MB BS; MRCOG; FRCSC; ObstGyn. Staff, Ridge Meadows Hospital & Health Care Centre; (604)467-5110; Fax. (604)467-5118.

OBLE, Darryl D A; Univ of Manitoba, 401-727 McDermot Ave, Winnipeg MB R3E 3P5; Man'99.

OBNAMIA, Maira; Cane Family Health Team, 120-135 Queens Plate Dr, Etobicoke ON M9W 6V1; University of Santo Tomas (Philippines)'03; Langs: Tagalog; (416)342-5140; Fax. (416)342-5148.

OBNEY, Jeannette; 3 Ovida Blvd, Markham ON L3P 7N8; Tor'70; Staff, Lakeridge Health - Oshawa Site; Staff, Lakeridge Health - Whitby Site; (905)471-5022

OBRAND, Daniel; SMBD Jewish Gen Hosp, 3755 ch Cote-Sainte-Catherine, Montreal QC H3T 1E2; Miami(FL) (USA)'89; FRCSC; GenSurg; VascSurg. Staff Vascular Surg, Sir Mortimer B Davis Jewish General; Asst Prof Surg, McGill University; (514)340-8222 x3324; dobrand@surg.jgh.mcgill.ca.

OBRIGAVITCH, Gregory R; Prince Albert Commun Clinic, 110 8th St E, Prince Albert SK S6V 0V7; Alb'94; BSc; CCFP; FCFP; (306)763-6464; Fax. (306)763-2101.

OBST, Jennifer M; Glen Sather Sports Med Clinic, 11400 University Ave NW, Edmonton AB T6G 1Z1; Alb'07; CCFP; (780)407-5160; Fax. (780)407-5667.

OCAMPO, Erlinda S; 9157 boul Lacordaire, Saint-Leonard QC H1R 2B5; Far Eastern (Philippines)'58; Staff, Hôpital Santa Cabrini Ospedale; (514)324-2952

OCANA, Anthony M; Hollyburn Med Bldg, 201-520 17th St, West Vancouver BC V7V 3S8; Tor'91; MSc; ABAM; CCFP; Langs: Spanish; French; German; (604)913-8183 x2235; Fax. (604)913-8804.

OCANA, Michael A; Kelowna Gen Hosp, 2268 Pandosy St, Kelowna BC V1Y 1T2; Ott'97; FRCPC; Psy. Staff Adolescent Psy Unit, Kelowna General Hospital; (250)862-4300 x3532; Fax. (250)862-4347.

OCASIONES, Carmencita; Jewish Rehab Hosp, 3205 Place Alton-Goldbloom, Laval QC H7V 1R2; (Philippines)'57; Staff, Jewish Rehabilitation Hospital; (450)688-9550; Fax. (450)688-7535.

OCHOA PINZON, Juan C; CSSS du Lac-des-Deux-Montagnes, 520 boul Arthur-Sauve, Saint-Eustache QC J7R 5B1; (Colombia)'00; Staff, Hôpital de Saint-Eustache; (450)473-6811

OCHOCINSKI, Jerzy R; 210-89 Queensway W, Mississauga ON L5B 2V2; Bialystok (Poland)'68; Associate Neur, Trillium Health Centre - Mississauga; (905)949-1270; Fax. (905)949-1210.

OCHOCINSKI, Pawel P; 201-1370 Dundas St E, Mississauga ON L4Y 4G4; McM'86; Ac Staff, St Joseph's Health Centre; (905)897-1738

OCHONSKA, W Margaret; 218B Regent Ave W, Winnipeg MB R2C 1R2; (Poland)'84; Staff, Health Sciences Centre.

OCKBAZGHI, Russom; Humboldt Med Clinic, PO Box 220, Humboldt SK S0K 2A0; Sask'96; LMCC; CCFP; (306)682-2618; Fax. (306)682-4499; humboldtclinic@sasktel.net.

OCKLEY, Carla; 13893 Highway 7 PO Box 4100 Stn Main, Georgetown ON L7G 4Y4; Alb'77; BMedSci; CCFP; Ac Staff, Halton Healthcare Services Corporation - Georgetown Hospital; (905)873-4505; Fax. (905)873-4531.

OCZACHOWSKI, Caroline; Ukrainian Canadian Care Center, 60 Richview Rd, Etobicoke ON M9A 5E4; (Poland)'08; (416)243-7653

OCZKOWSKI, Wieslaw J; Hamilton HS-General Site, 237 Barton St E, Hamilton ON L8L 2X2; McM'81; FRCPC; Neur (Stroke). Staff, Hamilton Health Sciences Centre - Hamilton General Hospital; Clin Assoc Prof, McMaster University; Langs: Polish; (905)529-4100; Fax. (905)529-8008; office@oczkowski.ca.

ODA, Jenny W N; Victoria Terrace Med Centre, 202-1448 Lawrence Ave E, North York ON M4A 2V6; Baghdad (Iraq)'86; MB ChB; CCFP; Ac Staff, The Scarborough Hospital - General Campus; (416)752-5426; Fax. (416)752-7332.

ODA, Joanna J; UBC School of Population, 2206 East Mall, Vancouver BC V6T 1Z3; Ott'09; CCFP; (604)822-7646

ODA, Ninos M; Mount Sinai Hosp, 476-600 University Ave, Toronto ON M5G 1X5; Prague (Czech Republic)'99; FRCSC; OrthSurg. Staff, Mount Sinai Hospital; Langs: Arabic; Assyrian; (416)967-8500

ODA, Ronald G; Dr Ronald G Oda Med Prof Corp, 17-20 Fred Varley Dr, Unionville ON L3R 1S4; Tor'76; CCFP; FCFP; Staff Community, Markham Stouffville Hospital; (905)477-3378; Fax. (905)477-3390.

ODAIBO, Felix S; 107-9840 97 Ave, Grande Prairie AB T8V 7K2; Zaria (Nigeria)'76; MB BS; DCH(Lond); LMCC; FRCPI; FRCPC; Peds (Neonatal & Perinatal Medicine). Consultant Peds/Dir Neonatal/Peds, Queen Elizabeth II Hospital; Langs: Nigerian; Yoruba; (780)513-1991; Fax. (780)513-1955.

ODAME, Isaac; The Hosp for Sick Children, 9411-555 University Ave, Toronto ON M5G 1X8; Accra (Ghana)'82; MB ChB; MRC(UK); MRCPath; Staff, The Hospital For Sick Children; Assoc Prof, McMaster University; Langs: Akan; Ga; (416)813-6194; Fax. (416)813-5327.

ODASHIRO, Alexandre; Ctr Hosp Affilie-Enfant-Jesus, 1401 18e rue, Quebec QC G1J 1Z4; Parana (Brazil)'00; AnatPath (P.Q.). Staff, Centre Hospitalier Affilié Universitaire de Québec - Hôpital du St-Sacrement; Staff, Centre Hospitalier Affilié Universitaire de Québec - Hôpital De L'Enfant Jésus; (418)649-0252

ODEGAARD, Paul R; 181 Tecumseh Ave E, London ON N6C 1S3; Wes'72; (519)433-9541; Fax. (519)433-5258; paul@odegaard.ca.

ODEH, Shaker Y H; Lakeshore Gen Hosp, 160 av Stillview, Pointe-Claire QC H9R 2Y2; Alexandria (Egypt)'77; CSPQ; Anes (P. Q.). Staff, Lakeshore General Hospital - Pointe Claire; (514)630-2225

ODELL, Margaret R; Centre de Med Fam de Wakefield, CP 400, Wakefield QC J0X 3G0; McG'93; Staff, Cree Board of Health & Social Services James Bay; (819)459-2363; Fax. (819)459-2997.

ODELL, Michael J; The Ottawa Hosp-Gen Campus, 501 Smyth Rd, Ottawa ON K1H 8L6; Qns'98; BSc; FRCSC; Otol (Head & Neck Surgery & Oncology). Staff, The Ottawa Hospital - General Campus; (613)737-8899 x73287; Fax. (613)739-6831; moddell@toh.on.ca.

ODELL, Paul F; 1-1800 Bank St, Ottawa ON K1V 0W3; Tor'67; Otol (Head & Neck Surgery & Oncology). (613)627-4700; Fax. (613)627-4660.

ODENDAAL, Morne L; 111-3722 57 Ave, Red Deer AB T4N 4R7; Orange Free State (South Africa)'91; MB ChB; CCFP; FCFP; (403)352-7425

ODENDAL, Lisa T; Children's & Women's HC Of BC, 4480 Oak St, Vancouver BC V6H 3V4; Alb'99; FRCPC; Peds (Emergency Pediatrics); PedEmergMed. Fellow Ped EmergMed, BC Children's Hospital; (604)875-2045; ldyke@cw.bc.ca.

ODENIGBO, Chukwuemeka; First Consultant Physicians, 3125F Woodham Dr, Regina SK S4V 2R5; (306)522-3043; Fax. (306)522-3044.

ODHIAMBO, Raphael L S; 33 Church St S, Ajax ON L1S 6A6; Makerere (Uganda)'72; MB ChB; MPH; MMed; FRCPC; Peds (Neonatology). (905)427-1445; Fax. (905)427-3343; odhiambor@sympatico.ca.

ODIER, Celine; CHUM-Hop Notre-Dame, 1560 rue Sherbrooke E, Montreal QC H2L 4M1; Mon'02; FRCPC; Neur. Staff, Centre Hospitalier l'Université de Montréal (CHUM) - Hôpital Notre-Dame; (514)890-8000

ODLOZINSKI, Michael P; Couchiching Family Health Team, 204-119 Memorial Ave, Orillia ON L3V 5X1; Wes'99; CCFP; (705)323-9800; Fax. (705)323-9601.

ODRCICH, Mark J J; Windsor Reg Hosp-Metropolitan, 1995 Lens Ave, Windsor ON N8W 1L9; Qns'01; FRCPC; Anes. Staff, Windsor Regional Hospital - Metropolitan Site; (519)254-5577

ODUBANJO, Oladipo O; Airdrie Med Clinic, 10-620 1 Ave NW, Airdrie AB T4B 2R3; (Nigeria)'77; CCFP; (403)948-3109; Fax. (403)948-6284.

ODUBOTE, Oladele O; 604 Columbia St, Kamloops BC V2C 2V3; Ibadan (Nigeria)'00; (250)374-4478

ODUEKE, Adebayo W; Rouge Valley-Ajax & Pickering, 580 Harwood Ave S, Ajax ON L1S 2J4; Ibadan (Nigeria)'85; MB BS; MRCOG; FRCSC; ObstGyn. Staff, Rouge Valley Health System - Ajax & Pickering Health Centre Site; (905)683-2320

ODUGBEMI, Oluwole David; Meadowlark Professional Bldg, 8704C-8702 Meadowlark Rd NW, Edmonton AB T5R 5W5; (Nigeria)'89; MB ChB; MCFP(SA); CCFP; Langs: Zulu; Yoruba; (780)761-1292; Fax. (780)761-1293.

ODUGBEMI, Olabisi O; Meridian Med Clinic, 3-4402 37 St, Stony Plain AB T7Z 2A9; Ogun (Nigeria)'92; MB ChB; (780)963-7800; Fax. (780)963-0468.

ODULANA-OGUNDIMU, Adebola O; 1486 Regent St, Sudbury ON P3E 3Z6; Ibadan (Nigeria)'74; MB BS; FRCPC; Peds. Staff, Health Sciences North-St Joseph's Health Centre; Staff, Health Sciences North-Laurentian Site; Langs: Yoruba; (705)523-5211; Fax. (705)523-5240.

ODULIO, Maria J; Northern Health Authority, 820-299 Victoria St, Prince George BC V2L 5B8; UBC'98; FRCSC; ObstGyn. (250)561-7224

ODUMAH, Godwin; Paediatrics Urgent Care, 106-222 Dixon Rd, Etobicoke ON M9P 3S5; (Nigeria)'86; (416)850-8947

ODUNTAN, Oluwole O; City Med Centre, 398 Broadway St W, Yorkton SK S3N 0P1; Ibadan (Nigeria)'92; MB BS; MMed; LMCC; (306)782-1122; Fax. (306)782-1155.

ODUNZE, Salome C; 90-2525 Bridlecrest Way SW, Calgary AB T2Y 5J4; (Nigeria)'92; CCFP; (403)984-3193; Fax. (403)984-3206.

ODUWOLE, Olusegun; 202-1130 Austin Ave, Coquitlam BC V3K 3P5; Ibadan (Nigeria)'72; MB BS; MRCPsy; FRCPC; Psy. Clin Teacher, University of British Columbia; (604)939-8143

ODUWOLE, Olusesan O; Parkland Medical, 102A-505 Queen St, Spruce Grove AB T7X 2V2; Ilorin (Nigeria)'89; DA; (780)960-4102; Fax. (780)962-8176.

ODUWOLE, Queenette; Leamington Dist Mem Hosp, 194 Talbot St W, Leamington ON N8H 1N9; (Nigeria)'98; Staff, Leamington District Memorial Hospital; (519)326-2373

OECHSLIN, Erwin N; Congenital Cardiac Centre, 5N 519-585 University Ave, Toronto ON M5G 2N2; Zurich (Switzerland)'85; FRCPC; IntMed (Adult Congenital Heart Disease); Cardiol. Staff, Toronto General Hospital - UHN; Langs: German; (416)340-4871; Fax. (416)340-5014; erwin.oechslin@uhn.ca.

OEI, Ien T; Health Park, 205-45 Weatherbee Rd, Mira Road NS B1M 0A1; Ruprecht Karl (Germany)'72; Staff, New Waterford Consolidated Hospital; (902)539-3191; Fax. (902)567-1503.

OEI, Tjong-Leng; Montreal Chinese Hosp, 189 av Viger E, Montreal QC H2X 3Y9; (Taiwan)'64; CSPQ; DiagRad (P.Q.). Staff, Hôpital Chinois de Montréal; (514)871-0961; Fax. (514)871-0966.

OELOFSE, Wouter; Tremont Med Clinic, 5-2A Tremont Dr, St Catharines ON L2T 3B2; Pretoria (South Africa)'97; CCFP; (905)687-8887

OELSCHIG, Ana-Maria; Mokala Medical, 161A-31 Southridge Dr, Okotoks AB T1S 2N3; Pretoria (South Africa)'94; MB ChB; Physician, Foothills County Hospice; Physician Urgent Care, Okotoks Health & Wellness Centre; Langs: Afrikaans; Portuguese; (403)995-5740; Fax. (403)995-5743.

OEN, Kiem G; Children's Hosp, 840 Sherbrook St, Winnipeg MB R3A 1S1; New York(NY) (USA)'73; FRCPC; Peds. Head Section of Peds Rheum & Immunol, Health Sciences Centre; University of Manitoba.

OESTREICHER, James H; 309-1033 Bay St, Toronto ON M5S 3A5; McM'80; FRCSC; Ophth (Ophthalmology Plastic Surgery). Staff, Princess Margaret Hospital - University Health Network; Staff, Mount Sinai Hospital; Staff, St Michael's Hospital; Prof, University of Toronto; (416)962-5005; Fax. (416)962-5856.

OETTER, Heidi M; College of Phys & Surg of BC, 300-669 Howe St, Vancouver BC V6C 0B4; UBC'85; Registrar, College of Physicians & Surgeons of British Columbia; (604)733-7758; Fax. (604)733-3503.

OEY, Audrey; Preston Med Centre, 506 King St E, Cambridge ON N3H 3N2; McM'05; CCFP; (519)653-3321; Fax. (519)653-3498.

OFFER, Robert C; 1560 George St, White Rock BC V4B 4A5; UBC'69; FRCPC; IntMed (Rheumatology). Ac Staff, Penticton Regional Hospital; Clin Assoc Prof, University of British Columbia; (604)385-4449; Fax. (604)385-4949; roffer@live.ca.

OFFIAH, Francis O; Harbour Landing Med Clinic, 4500 Gordon Rd, Regina SK S4W 0B7; (Nigeria)'88; MB BS; CCFP; (306)545-2888; Fax. (306)545-2844.

OFFIERSKI, Chris M; 6453 Morrison St, Niagara Falls ON L2E 7H1; Qns'74; FRCP; FRCSC; OrthSurg. Ac Staff, Niagara Health System - Greater Niagara General Site; (905)357-2900; Fax. (905)357-2734.

OFFMAN, Hilary J; 121 Balmoral Ave, Toronto ON M4V 1J5; Tor'92; BSc; FRCPC; Psy (Psychotherapy). Lecturer, University of Toronto; (416)925-8330; Fax. (416)925-2752.

OFFMAN, Saul L; Mackenzie Bldg, 5788 University Ave, Halifax NS B3H 1V8; Dal'05; FRCPC; AnatPath. (902)473-7334; Fax. (902)473-7978.

OFFRINGA, Martin; The Hosp for Sick Children, 555 University Ave, Toronto ON M5G 1X8; Erasmus University (Netherlands)'85; Staff, The Hospital For Sick Children; (416)813-8894

OFIESH, John G; Richmond Med Bldg, 106-2020 Richmond Rd, Victoria BC V8R 6R5; McG'80; FRCSC; GenSurg; CardiothorSurg. Staff, Vancouver Island Health Authority; (250)595-1833; Fax. (250)595-1431; jofiesh@cvtsurgery.com.

OFOSU, Kofi E A; St Joseph's Mountain H Serv, PO Box 585 Stn Lcd 1 100 West 5th St, Hamilton ON L8N 3K7; Ott'98; FRCPC; Psy. Staff, Hamilton Health Sciences Centre - McMaster Children's Hospital; Staff, St Joseph's Healthcare Hamilton - West 5th Campus; (905)522-1155 x36400

OGAH, Oshiomeghe K; Cape Breton Hlthcare Complex, 1482 George St, Sydney NS B1P 1P3; Ibadan (Nigeria)'97; Staff, Cape Breton Healthcare Complex; (902)567-8000

OGALI, Emmanuel; Kamsack Med Clinic, PO Box 69, Kamsack SK S0A 1S0; (306)542-2623; Fax. (306)542-3782.

OGARANKO, Christopher P; Victoria Gen Hosp, 2340 Pembina Hwy, Winnipeg MB R3T 2E8; Man'95; CCFP; FCFP; Staff, Victoria General Hospital; (204)269-3570

OGBEIDE, Samuel O; 5203 49 Ave PO Box 40, Killam AB T0B 2L0; Ibadan (Nigeria)'86; MB BS; MSc(SurgSci); FRCS(Ed); Site Med Dir, Swan Hills Healthcare Centre; (780)385-3741; Fax. (780)385-3904; daddy_gums@yahoo.com.

OGBORN, Malcolm R; Children's & Women's HC of BC, K4-4480 Oak St, Vancouver BC V6H 3V4; Adelaide (Australia)'77; FRCPC; Peds (Nephrology). Ac Staff, Health Sciences Centre; Staff, BC Children's Hospital; (604)875-2272

OGER, Joel J; UBC Hospital, S159-2211 Wesbrook Mall, Vancouver BC V6T 2B5; Rennes (France)'70; FRCPC; Neur (Multiple Sclerosis). Staff, UBC Hospital - Koerner Pavillion; Consultant, Vancouver General Hospital - Centennial Pavillion; Prof, University of British Columbia; Langs: French; (604)822-7696; Fax. (604)822-0758.

OGIEGLO, Adam; Lakeside Med Clinic, 3919 8th St E, Saskatoon SK S7H 5M7; Sask'09; CCFP; (306)374-6884; Fax. (306)374-2552.

OGILVIE, Gina S; BC Centre for Disease Control, 655 12th Ave W, Vancouver BC V5Z 4R4; McM'92; MSc; CCFP; FCFP; Assoc Dir STD-AIDS Control, BC Centre For Disease Control; Clinical Asst Prof, University of British Columbia; (604)707-5619; Fax. (604)775-0808; gina.ogilvie@bccdc.ca.

OGILVIE, Kelly; The Ottawa Hosp-Civic Campus, M206-1053 Carling Ave, Ottawa ON K1Y 4E9; Tor'07; FRCPC; EmergMed. Staff, The Ottawa Hospital - Civic Campus; (613)798-5555

OGILVIE, R Travis; Foothills Med Centre, C1150F-1403 29 St NW, Calgary AB T2N 2T9; Sask'94; FRCPC; AnatPath. Staff, Foothills Medical Centre; Staff, Calgary Laboratory Services; (403)944-8505; Fax. (403)944-4748; ogilvie@ucalgary.ca.

OGILVIE, Richard I; Univ Hlth Network-Toronto Western Hosp, 7E 453-399 Bathurst St, Toronto ON M5T 2S8; Tor'60; MD; FRCPC; IntMed (Clinical Pharmacology). Staff, Toronto Western Hospital - University Health Network; Prof, University of Toronto; (416)603-5005; ri.ogilvie@utoronto.ca.

OGILVIE, Rick A; 203-323 Wilson St E, Ancaster ON L9G 4A8; Wes'78; FRCSC; OrthSurg (Knee Surgery). Staff Orth, Hamilton Health Sciences Centre; Clin Assoc Prof, McMaster University; (905)304-5816; Fax. (905)304-5818.

OGILVIE, Robert V; Norfinch Med Centre, 107-2100 Finch Ave W, North York ON M3N 2Z9; London (England)'64; MB BS; CRCP; FRCSC; Otol. Ac Staff, Humber River Regional Hospital - Finch Avenue Site; Ac Staff, North York General Hospital - Branson Division; Langs: Spanish; (416)739-7771; Fax. (416)739-7822.

OGILVIE-HARRIS, Darrell J; Univ Hlth Network-Toronto Western Hosp, 1E47-399 Bathurst St, Toronto ON M5T 2S8; Liverpool (England)'75; MB ChB(Hons.); BSc(MedSci); MMedSci; FRCSC; OrthSurg. Staff, Toronto Western Hospital - University Health Network; Teach Staff, University of Toronto; (416)603-5862; Fax. (416)603-4376.

OGILVY, Caroline G; 245-175 av Stillview, Pointe-Claire QC H9R 4S3; McG'66; BSc; MDCM; Staff, Lakeshore General Hospital - Pointe Claire; adj Prof, McGill University; (514)697-6770; Fax. (514)697-4418.

OGLAZA, Piotr P; Verona Med Clinic, PO Box 160 6582 Hwy 38, Verona ON K0H 2W0; (Poland)'00; CCFP; (613)374-2077

OGOKE, Valentine C; High River Med Clinic, PO Box 5055 106B 3rd Ave W, High River AB T1V 1M3; (Nigeria)'84; (403)652-2880; Fax. (403)652-2887.

OGRADY, Mark J; Dr M J Ogrady Med Prof Corp, 330-2550 15th Ave, Regina SK S4P 1A5; Sask'80; FRCSC; Otol. Dept Head Surg, Regina General Hospital; Member Lean Six Sigma Black Belt, American Society of Quality; Clin Assoc Lecturer, University of Saskatchewan; (306)359-3263; Fax. (306)525-1780; dr. ogrady@sasktel.net.

OGSTON, Nigel G; Thessalon Med Clinic, PO Box 538 240 Main St, Thessalon ON P0R 1L0; Tor'79; CAFCI; Staff, Huntsville District Memorial Hospital - Muskoka Algonquin Healthcare; (705)842-2905; Fax. (705)842-0038.

OGUERI, Emmanuel; Renforth Med Clinic, 9-460 Renforth Dr, Etobicoke ON M9C 2N2; CCFP; (416)622-2211; Fax. (416)622-0033.

OGUNBIYI, Ajibola; Yorkton Reg Health Centre, 270 Bradbrooke Dr, Yorkton SK S3N 2K6; Staff, Yorkton Regional Health Centre; (306)786-0558; Fax. (306)786-0556.

OGUNDIMU, Fadegbola; 1486 Regent St, Sudbury ON P3E 3Z6; Ibadan (Nigeria)'74; MB BS; FACS; FRCSC; Neursurg. Staff, Health Sciences North-St Joseph's Health Centre; Asst Prof, Northern Ontario School of Medicine-Laurentian University; (705)523-5211; Fax. (705)523-5240.

OGUNDIPE, Tony B; 130-4411 16 Ave NW, Calgary AB T3B 0M3; (Nigeria)'90; MB ChB; (403)288-6711; Fax. (403)288-9136.

OGUNDIYA, Ayodeji L; Blue Spruce Med Centre, 16729 100 St NW, Edmonton AB T5X 3Z9; (Nigeria)'91; MB BS; CCFP; (780)457-1351; Fax. (780)478-7796.

OGUNKEYE, Alarape; 105-140 Niagara St, St Catharines ON L2R 4L4; Ibadan (Nigeria)'99; FRCPC; Peds. Staff, London Health Sciences Centre - Victoria Campus.

OGUNLEWE, Obafemi A; Prairie North Specialists Clin, 107-4910 50th St, Lloydminster SK S9V 0Y5; (306)820-2599; Fax. (306)825-4774.

OGUNMODEDE, O David; 104-279 Wharncliffe Rd N, London ON N6H 2C2; Lagos (Nigeria)'90; MB BS; FRCSI; CCFP; (519)601-0095

OGUNSINA, Ayodeji O; Burin Peninsula Hlth Care Ctr, PO Box 340, Burin NL A0E 1E0; Lagos (Nigeria)'93; MB BS; Staff, Burin Peninsula Health Care Centre; (709)891-1040

OGUNSINA, Olurotimi O; Northern Lights Health Region, 7 Hospital St, Fort McMurray AB T9H 1P2; (Nigeria)'94; Staff, Northern Lights Regional Health Centre; (780)791-6161

OGUNSONA, Adeoluwa O; Aberdeen Hosp, 835 East River Rd, New Glasgow NS B2H 3S6; (Nigeria)'03; Staff, Aberdeen Regional Hospital; (902)752-7600; Fax. (902)752-6231.

OGUNTADE, John A; Yarmouth Reg Hosp, 60 Vancouver St, Yarmouth NS B5A 2P5; Lagos (Nigeria)'92; MB BS; Staff, Yarmouth Regional Hospital; (902)742-3542; Fax. (902)742-0369.

OGUNTOYINBO, Funmi A; 304-121 Willowdale Ave, North York ON M2N 6A3; Lagos (Nigeria)'75; MB BS(Hons.); MPH; FRCPC; Psy (Public Health). Teach Staff Psy, University of Toronto; Langs: Yoruba; (416)225-9092; Fax. (416)225-7730; ogun@bellnet.ca.

OGUNYEMI, Abayomi O; Health Sciences Centre, 300 Prince Philip Dr, St. John's NL A1B 3V6; (Nigeria)'75; MB BS; DAB(ClinNeuroPhys); FRCPC; Neur. Staff Epileptol Clin NeuroPhysiol, Health Sciences Centre; Assoc Prof Med(Neurol), Memorial University Of Newfoundland; (709)777-6948; Fax. (709)777-6656.

OH, Alfred Y G; Columbus Med Arts Bldg, 208-8333 Weston Rd, Woodbridge ON L4L 8E2; Wes'98; FRCSC; Otol. (905)265-2280; Fax. (905)265-2072.

OH, Charles S; Medical & Dental Bldg, 215-4900 Kingsway, Burnaby BC V5H 2E3; Alb'88; Vis Staff, Vancouver General Hospital - Centennial Pavillion; (604)436-1611; Fax. (604)436-1625.

OH, Clifford; Trillium Hlth Ctr-West Toronto, 150 Sherway Dr, Etobicoke ON M9C 1A5; Tor'98; FRCPC; IntMed. Staff, Trillium Health Centre - West Toronto; (416)259-6671

OH, Dennis E; Burquitlam Med Clinic, 100B-504 Cottonwood Ave, Coquitlam BC V3J 2R4; Sask'02; BSc; CCFP; Langs: Korean; (604)939-8831

OH, Eric J; Groves Mem Community Hosp, 235 Union St E, Fergus ON N1M 1W3; Ott'10; CCFP; Staff, Groves Memorial Community Hospital; (519)843-2010

OH, Jiwon; St Michael's Hosp, 30 Bond St, Toronto ON M5B 1W8; Qns'05; Neur. Staff, St Michael's Hospital; (416)864-6060

OH, Paul I T; The Rumsey Centre, 347 Rumsey Rd, Toronto ON M4G 1R7; Tor'88; FRCPC; IntMed (Clinical Pharmacology). Med Dir Cardiac Prog, Toronto Rehabilitation Institute - Rumsey Centre; Asst Prof Med, University of Toronto; (416)597-3422 x5263; Fax. (416)425-0301.

OHANJANIANS, Edward; Deer Park Mall, 69 Dunlop St, Red Deer AB T4R 2H6; (Iran)'88; (403)347-6811; Fax. (403)347-6899.

OHAYON-AFILALO, Catherine; CLSC le Minordet, 961 rue de la Clinique, Senneterre QC J0Y 2M0; Paris (France)'84; (819)737-2243

OHAYON, Jason A; 201-1685 Main St W, Hamilton ON L8S 1G5; McM'93; FRCPC; Peds (Allergic Disorders); ClinImmunol&Allergy. Asst Prof, Hamilton Health Sciences Centre - McMaster Children's Hospital; Langs: English; French; (905)777-0088; ohayonj@mcmaster.ca.

OHAYON, Michele; Clin de Derm Esthetique de Mtl, 260-2040 boul Marcel-Laurin, Saint-Laurent QC H4R 1J9; Mon'84; FRCPC; Derm. Staff, Hôpital Anna-Laberge; (514)387-6433

OHAYON-GABBAY, Huguette; Clin de Med Familiale Notre-Da, 2120 rue Sherbrooke E, Montreal QC H2K 1C3; Paris (France)'81; Staff, Centre Hospitalier l'Université de Montréal (CHUM) - Hôpital Notre-Dame; (514)527-1958

OHENE-DARKOH, Charles; William Osler HC-Brampton, 2100 Bovaird Dr E, Brampton ON L6R 3J7; (Ghana)'97; FRCPC; Psy. Staff, William Osler Health System - Brampton Civic Hospital; (905)494-2121

OHLHAUSER, Larry R; 304-9426 51 Ave NW, Edmonton AB T6E 5A6; Alb'71; Registrar, College of Physicians & Surgeons of Alberta; Ohlhauser & Associates; (780)423-9952; Fax. (780)423-1195; larry@ohlhauserassociates.com.

OHSON, Kamal K S; 59 Airport Rd, St. John's NL A1A 4Y3; Bombay (India)'94; MB BS; FRCPC; CCFP; Derm. Staff, Janeway Children's Health & Rehabilitation Centre; Clinical Asst Prof Derm & Med, Memorial University Of Newfoundland; Langs: Hindi; Punjabi; (709)739-7669; Fax. (709)739-9898.

OHSON, Ravinderpal S; Rymal Square Health Centre, 505 Rymal Rd E, Hamilton ON L8W 3X1; Delhi (India)'82; FCFP; CCFP; FCFP; Assoc Staff Family Med, Hamilton Health Sciences Centre - McMaster University Medical Centre; Assoc Staff, St Joseph's Healthcare - Charlton Campus; Clin Lecturer EmergMed, McMaster University; Langs: Punjabi; Hindi; (905)318-1444; Fax. (905)318-0062.

OIKNINE, Albert; CHUM-Hotel-Dieu, 3840 rue Saint-Urbain, Montreal QC H2W 1T8; Sher'80; FRCPC; Cardiol. Staff, Centre Hospitalier l'Université De Montréal (CHUM) - Hôpital Saint-luc; Staff, Centre Hospitalier l'Université de Montréal (CHUM) - Hôtel-Dieu; (514)890-8000 x34444

OINONEN, Ervin T; Court Street Clinic, 9 Court St, St Catharines ON L2R 4R3; Man'72; BSc; Ac Staff, Niagara Health System - St Catharines General Site; Ac Staff, Niagara Health System - Ontario Street Site; Langs: Finnish; (905)937-0000; Fax. (905)937-0030.

OISHI, Arlene S; Univ of Lethbridge Health Ctre, 4401 University Dr W, Lethbridge AB T1K 3M4; Alb'88; CCFP; FCFP; (403)329-2484; Fax. (403)329-2466.

OISHI, Cameron R; Caremedics Med Centre, 18-1910 St. Laurent Blvd, Ottawa ON K1G 1A4; Alb'95; BMedSci; CCFP; Langs: Bilingual(English/French); (613)749-1678; Fax. (613)749-9446; croishi@live.com.

OISHI, Roderick L; Edson Med Centre, PO Box 6660 Stn Main, Edson AB T7E 1V1; Alb'95; CCFP; Staff, Edson Healthcare Centre; (780)723-3366; Fax. (780)723-3437.

OJA, Conrad D; BC Cancer Agency-Fraser Valley, 13750 96 Ave, Surrey BC V3V 1Z2; UBC'01; FRCPC; IntMed; MedOncol. Staff, BC Cancer Agency Fraser Valley Centre; (604)930-4028

OJA, Mihkel A; 206-206 Rookwood Ave, Fredericton NB E3B 2M2; Dal'78; BSc(Hon)Physics; FRCSC; PlasSurg (Breasts). Staff PlasSurg, Dr Everett Chalmers Regional Hospital; Staff, Oromocto Public Hospital; (506)459-8126; Fax. (506)459-1774; maoja@rogers.com.

OJAGHI, Elham; 4041 200B St, Langley BC V3A 1P1; Paris (France)'02; CCFP; (604)530-1181

OJAH, Cecil R; Saint John Reg Hosp, PO Box 2100 Stn Main 400 University Ave, Saint John NB E2L 4L2; West Indies (Jamaica)'79; FRCPC; Peds. Staff Neonatol/Clin Head Dept of Pediatrics, Saint John Regional Hospital; Ac Staff, St Joseph's Hospital; Asst Prof, Dalhousie University; (506)648-6111

OJANGUREN, Andrea A; Hop du Sacre-Coeur de Mtl, 5400 boul Gouin O, Montreal QC H4J 1C5; Lausanne (Switzerland)'99; Staff, Hôpital du Sacre-Coeur de Montréal; (514)338-2222

OJEDOKUN, Jane O; PO Box 1076 Stn Main, Whitecourt AB T7S 1P9; (Nigeria)'01; MB BS; CCFP.

OJEDOKUN, Joseph O; PO Box 1076 Stn Main, Whitecourt AB T7S 1P9; (Nigeria)'99; (780)778-2224; Fax. (780)778-2127.

OJIEGBE, Chinyere C; Lakeridge Hlth Corp-Oshawa, 1 Hospital Crt, Oshawa ON L1G 2B9; Ibadan (Nigeria)'83; MB BS; MRC(Psy); LMCC; FRCPC; Psy. Staff, Lakeridge Health - Oshawa Site; (905)576-8711

OJO, Alaba; Cypress Reg Health Centre, 2004 Saskatchewan Dr, Swift Current SK S9H 5M8; (306)778-9584; Fax. (306)778-9588.

OJUAWO, Akinlolu B; Saint John Med Clinic, 299 Metcalf St, Saint John NB E2K 4P8; Ife (Nigeria)'89; MB ChB; FRCSC; ObstGyn. (506)652-7579; Fax. (506)652-9699.

OKADA, William T; 4-5431 43 St, Red Deer AB T4N 1C8; McG'81; FRCSC; Ophth. (403)340-3735; Fax. (403)343-2925.

OKAFO, Benjamin A; Orillia Urology Associates, 110-210 Memorial Ave, Orillia ON L3V 7V1; RCS (Ireland)'77; LRCPSI; FACS; FRCSC; Urol. (705)325-3603; Fax. (705)325-5483.

OKAFOR, Innocent C; Phoenix Med Clinic, 212-10095 Bramalea Rd, Brampton ON L6R 0K1; Benin (Nigeria)'90; CCFP; Staff Hospitalist, William Osler Health System - Brampton Civic Hospital; Langs: Ibo; Yoruba; (905)793-5700; Fax. (905)793-5709; drdokafor@gmail.com.

OKAFOR, Livinus; Aberdeen Hosp, 835 East River Rd, New Glasgow NS B2H 3S6; Lagos (Nigeria)'99; Staff, Aberdeen Regional Hospital; (902)752-7600

OKAFOR, Rosemary E I; Dr G B Cross Mem Hosp, 67 Manitoba Dr, Clarenville NL A5A 1K3; Ibadan (Nigeria)'99; CCFP; Staff, The Dr G B Cross Memorial Hospital; (709)466-3411; Fax. (709)466-6526; rosemary.okafor@easternhealth.ca.

OKAMURA, James Y; Kingsway Prof Centre, 710-4980 Kingsway, Burnaby BC V5H 4K7; Alb'89; FRCSC; GenSurg (Colon & Rectal Surgery). (604)433-8500; Fax. (604)433-8506.

OKAN, Denis; Concordia Health Services, 200-1455 boul de Maisonneuve O, Montreal QC H3G 1M8; Mem'08; CCFP; (514)848-2424

OKANO, Kyle S K; 240-546 St Paul St, Kamloops BC V2C 5T1; Man'94; BSc; FAAP; FRCPC; Peds (Allergy). Med Dir NICU/Med Consultant SCAN Team, Royal Inland Hospital; Clin Instructor, University of British Columbia; (250)374-7722; Fax. (250)374-0446.

OKAWARA, Gordon S; The Juravinski Cancer Centre, 699 Concession St, Hamilton ON L8V 5C2; Tor'84; MBA; BEng; MEng; FRCP; FRCPC; RadOncol (Breast Cancer). Staff, Hamilton Health Sciences Centre-Juravinski Site; Staff, Hamilton Regional Cancer Centre; Assoc Prof, McMaster University; (905)387-9495 x64705; Fax. (905)575-6326; gord.okawara@jcc.hhsc.ca.

OKEREKE, Sunday O; Nanaimo Mental Hlth & Addictio, 201-2000 Island Hwy N, Nanaimo BC V9S 5W3; (Nigeria)'98; FRCPC; Psy. Staff, Nanaimo Regional General Hospital; (250)739-5797

OKETCH, Consolata; Oshawa Commun Health Centre, 115 Grassmere Ave, Oshawa ON L1H 3X7; Nairobi (Kenya)'95; CCFP; (905)723-0036; Fax. (905)723-3391.

OKOLI, Chukwuemeka V; Headwaters Health Care Centre, 100 Rolling Hills Dr, Orangeville ON L9W 4X9; Man'08; CCFP; Staff, Headwaters Health Care Centre - Orangeville Site; (519)941-2410

OKOLO, Godwin O; Northgate Med Centre, 9535 135 Ave NW, Edmonton AB T5E 1N8; Dublin (Ireland)'71; LRCPSI; LM; Ac Staff, Capital Care - Grandview; Consultant, University of Alberta Hospital; Langs: Ibo; (780)476-3344; Fax. (780)478-5248; godwin.okolo@capitalhealth.ca.

OKON, Marquis M A; Medical Office, 6-261 Martindale Rd, St Catharines ON L2W 1A1; Ibadan (Nigeria)'84; MB BS; FRCSC; ObstGyn. Staff, Niagara Health System - St Catharines General Site; (905)682-4534; Fax. (905)682-6281.

OKONKWO, Cletus C; Kootenay Boundary Reg Hosp, 1200 Hospital Bench, Trail BC V1R 4M1; Lagos (Nigeria)'95; FRCPC; Psy. Staff, Kootenay Boundary Regional Hospital; (250)364-3484

OKONTA, Henry I; 106-10055 120 Ave, Grande Prairie AB T8V 8H8; (Romania)'84; (780)532-4415; Fax. (780)532-4559.

OKORIE, Chidimna I; Wilson Med Centre, 130 Wilson St, Hamilton ON L8R 1E2; Enugu (Nigeria)'83; CCFP; (905)526-6250; Fax. (905)526-9745.

OKORIE, Eugene; Mental Health & Addictions, 1308 Alward St, Prince George BC V2M 7B1; (Nigeria)'99; (250)612-4500

OKORO, Daniel C; South Health Campus, 4448 Front St SE, Calgary AB T3M 1M4; Lagos (Nigeria)'84; MB BS; FRCPC; Psy. Staff, Queen Elizabeth II Hospital; (587)228-6448

OKORONKWO, Elendu; Northeast Mental Hlth Centre, 680 Kirkwood Dr, Sudbury ON P3E 1X3; (Nigeria)'02; FRCPC; Psy. Staff, North Bay Regional Health Centre - Kirkwood; (705)675-9193

OKRAINEC, Allan E P P; Univ Hlth Network-Toronto Western Hosp, 8 325-399 Bathurst St, Toronto ON M5T 2S8; McG'00; FRCSC; GenSurg. Staff, Toronto Western Hospital - University Health Network; (416)603-5224

OKRAINEC, Karen; Sunnybrook Hlth Sciences Ctre, C4 10-2075 Bayview Ave, Toronto ON M4N 3M5; Ott'07; FRCPC; IntMed. Staff, Sunnybrook Health Sciences Centre; (416)480-4290

OKUN, Nanette B; Dept of Obst & Gynecology, 3276-700 University Ave, Toronto ON M5G 1Z5; UBC'83; FRCSC; ObstGyn (Maternal Fetal Medicine). Staff, Mount Sinai Hospital; (416)586-5363; Fax. (416)586-1551; nokun@mtsinai.on.ca.

OKUNOLA, Olubusola A; Victory Med Associates, 137 20th St W, Saskatoon SK S7M 0W8; Ibadan (Nigeria)'98; MB BS; FRCPC; Psy (General Adult Psychiatry). Clinical Asst Prof Psychiatry, University of Saskatchewan; (306)249-2227; Fax. (306)249-2348; busola.okunola@usask.ca.

OKUSANYA, Olanrewaju O; Toronto East Gen Hosp Inc, 825 Coxwell Ave, Toronto ON M4C 3E7; Ibadan (Nigeria)'99; FRCSC; OrthSurg. Staff, Toronto East General Hospital Inc; (416)461-8272

OKYERE, Ebenezer; Rouge Valley-Centenary HC, 2867 Ellesmere Rd, Scarborough ON M1E 4B9; (Ghana)'81; MB ChB; MRCPsy; FRCPC; Psy (General Adult Psychiatry). Staff Psy, Toronto East General Hospital Inc; Staff, Rouge Valley Health System - Centenary Health Centre Site; Aj Lecturer, University of Toronto; (416)281-7318; Fax. (416)281-7320.

OLA, Ebele I; Walking Mobility Clinics, 11-750 Dundas St W, Toronto ON M6J 3S3; Tor'00; CCFP; Med Dir, Ventana Clinical Research Corp; (416)929-1015; Fax. (416)929-9918.

OLA, Foluso A; Bioflax Med Centre, GD 6-121 Highway 20 E, Fonthill ON L0S 1E0; (Nigeria)'90; MB BS; CCFP; (905)892-7728; Fax. (905)892-7811.

OLABIYI, Bamidele O; 782 Seymour St, Kamloops BC V2C 2H3; Varna (Bulgaria)'94; Staff, Royal Inland Hospital; (778)471-5874

OLADELE, Oluseyi S; PO Box 4584 Stn South Cro, Edmonton AB T6E 5G4; Alb'03; CCFP.

OLADIPO, Paul O; Carlton Med Clinic, 8-595 Carlton St, St Catharines ON L2M 4Y2; (Nigeria)'90; MB BS; CCFP; Langs: Yoruba; Hausa; (905)646-0063; Fax. (905)646-0084.

OLADOYIN, A Ajike; The Pavilions of Rocky Ridge, 28-369 Rocky Vista PK NW, Calgary AB T3G 5K7; Lagos (Nigeria)'91; MB BS; CCFP; Langs: Yoruba.

OLAFSON, Kendiss P; Health Sciences Centre, GC201B-820 Sherbrook St, Winnipeg MB R3A 1R9; Man'97; FRCPC; IntMed; Critical Care Medicine. Staff, Health Sciences Centre; (204)774-6511

OLAH, Marketa; 6 Beamish Dr, Etobicoke ON M9B 3P3; Prague (Czech Republic)'94; CCFP; (416)231-2233; Fax. (416)231-2234.

OLAH, Michael J; 6 Beamish Dr, Etobicoke ON M9B 3P3; Prague (Czech Republic)'98; CCFP; (416)239-2305

OLAH, Michael; 6 Beamish Dr, Etobicoke ON M9B 3P3; Safarika (Slovakia)'60; Court Staff Surgical Asst, St Michael's Hospital; Court Staff, Trillium Health Centre - West Toronto; Langs: Slovak; (416)239-2305

OLAND, Ryan C; Westview Hlth Ctr Stony Plain, 4405 South Park Dr, Stony Plain AB T7Z 2M7; Alb'00; BSc; CCFP; CCFP(E.M.); Staff, Royal Alexandra Hospital; Staff, University of Alberta Hospital; Staff, Westview Health Centre; (780)968-3600

OLAOSUN, Oluremi T; Sheldon Chumir Health Centre, 1213 4 St SW, Calgary AB T2R 0X7; Lagos (Nigeria)'91; FRCPC; Psy.

OLARIU, Carmen; Clin Med Familiale de Hull, 202-15 boul Montclair, Gatineau QC J8Y 2E2; Cluj-Napoca (Romania)'93; CCFP; (819)777-2752

OLARTE, John; Sheridan Med Associates, 1-1960 Dundas St W, Mississauga ON L5K 2R9; Santander (Colombia)'98; CCFP; Langs: Spanish; (905)822-3993; Fax. (905)822-5522.

OLATUNBOSUN, Olufemi A; Royal University Hosp, 103 Hospital Dr, Saskatoon SK S7N 0W8; Lagos (Nigeria)'73; MB BS; FWACS; FACOG; FRCSC; ObstGyn (Reproductive Endocrinology & Infertility). Staff, Royal University Hospital; Staff, Saskatoon Health Region Saskatoon Public Health; Assoc Dean Faculty Affairs/Prof ObstGyn & Reproductive Sciences, University of Saskatchewan; (306)966-2522; Fax. (306)966-8040; femi.olatunbosun@usask.ca.

OLATUNDE, Oluwasayo; 208-44 Mapleton Rd, Moncton NB E1C 7W8; Ibadan (Nigeria)'95; CCFP; (506)389-8747

OLBERG, Bernhard J; The Ottawa Hosp-Gen Campus, 501 Smyth Rd, Ottawa ON K1H 8L6; Ott'79; FRCPC; AnatPath (Anatomical Pathology). Med Dir Lab, Hawkesbury & District General Hospital; Dir Blood Bank & Path, The Ottawa Hospital - General Campus; Asst Prof, University of Ottawa; Langs: Dutch; (613)737-8356; bolberg@ottawahospital.on.ca.

OLD, C Lee; Lenore Centre Med Clinic, 4-123 Lenore Dr, Saskatoon SK S7K 7H9; Sask'81; CCFP; FCFP; Assoc Staff ObstGyn, Royal University Hospital; Ac Staff, Saskatoon City Hospital; Clinical Asst Prof Family Med, University of Saskatchewan; (306)242-6700; Fax. (306)242-1168.

OLD, Jason A; Pan Am Sports Med Centre, 75 Poseidon Bay, Winnipeg MB R3M 3E4; Man'02; FRCSC; OrthSurg. (204)925-1550

OLDERS, Henry G; 369 av Lansdowne, Westmount QC H3Z 2L5; McG'81; FRCPC; Psy (Geriatric Psychiatry). Staff, Hopital Ste-Anne; adj Prof Psy, McGill University; Langs: French; (514)846-8464; henry.olders@mcgill.ca.

OLDFIELD, M Anne; Ottawa Valley Family Hlth Team, PO Box 460 95 Spring St, Almonte ON K0A 1A0; Wes'75; (613)256-9370; Fax. (613)256-0949.

OLDRIDGE, Stephen C; 85 Bolton St PO Box 28, Bobcaygeon ON K0M 1A0; Ott'90; CCFP; FCFP; Court Staff, Ross Memorial Hospital; (705)738-6136; Fax. (705)738-3771; steve.oldridge@specialty-care.com.

OLDRING, Brian W; Royal Columbian Hosp, 330 Columbia St E, New Westminster BC V3L 3W7; Alb'72; DAB; FRCPC; EmergMed. Staff, Royal Columbian Hospital; Staff, Eagle Ridge Hospital & Health Care Centre; Asst Prof, University of British Columbia; (604)910-6512

OLEARCZYK, Bohdan; 303-2150 Bloor St W, Toronto ON M6S 1M8; Szczecin (Poland)'86; Staff Family Pract & Emerg, St Joseph's Health Centre; Lecturer, University of Toronto; Langs: Polish; Ukrainian; Russian; (416)762-6346; Fax. (416)769-8659.

OLECH, Victoria M; 3-45 Grist Mill Rd, Holland Landing ON L9N 1M7; Tor'93; CCFP; FCFP; Staff Family Med, Southlake Regional Health Centre; (905)853-8966; Fax. (905)853-2953.

OLEJAROVA, Emilia; Brant Community HC-Brantford, 200 Terrace Hill St, Brantford ON N3R 1G9; Safarika (Slovakia)'96; FRCPC; Psy. Staff, The Brant Community Healthcare System - Brantford General Hospital Site; (519)751-5885

OLEKSHY, John A; Royal Columbian Hosp, 330 Columbia St E, New Westminster BC V3L 3W7; Alb'66; AB; GenPath. Assoc Staff Nuclear Med, Royal Columbian Hospital; (604)520-4436; Fax. (604)520-4444.

OLEKSINSKI, W Stanley; West Hill Med Clinic, 1A-2995 2nd Ave W, Prince Albert SK S6V 5V5; Sask'82; LMCC; CCFP; FCFP; Pres, Prince Albert Parkland Regional Medical Association; Speaker Representative Assembly, Saskatchewan Medical Association; (306)765-8500; Fax. (306)765-8501.

OLENIUK, Fredrick H; Queen Street Surgical Assoc, 202-610 Queen St, Saskatoon SK S7K 0M8; Tor'77; BSc(Hon); FACS; FRCSC; GenSurg (Critical Care Medicine). (306)244-6818; Fax. (306)664-3462.

OLESEN, Peter R; 108-911 Island Hwy, Campbell River BC V9W 2C2; Alb'87; BSc; FRCSC; PlasSurg (Cosmetic Surgery). Consultant, Campbell River & District General Hospital; Langs: English; French; Danish; Spanish; (250)287-8077 x222; Fax. (250)287-8097.

OLESEN, Sarah A H; Cochrane Primary Care Centre, 103-100 Grande Blvd W, Cochrane AB T4C 0S4; Cal'09; CCFP; (403)932-2089; Fax. (403)932-1820.

OLFERT, Lawrence A; Drumheller Assoc Physicians, PO Box 5600, Drumheller AB T0J 0Y0; Sask'73; CCFP; FCFP; Assoc VP Med, Central Zone David Thompson Health Region; (403)823-3345; Fax. (403)823-7823.

OLIAEI, Alireza; The Pas Health Complex Inc, PO Box 240 Stn Main, The Pas MB R9A 1K4; Shiraz (Iran)'93; CCFP; Staff, St. Anthony General Hospital; (204)623-6431

OLIGNY, Luc L; Hôpital Ste-Justine, 3175 ch Cote-Sainte-Catherine, Montreal QC H3T 1C5; McG'86; MSc; CSPQ; GenPath (P.Q.) (Molecular Biology). Chef Path, Centre Hospitalier l'Université de Montréal (CHUM) - Hôtel-Dieu; Chef patho gén, Hôpital Ste-Justine; assoc Prof, Universite de Montreal; adj Prof, McGill University; Langs: English; Spanish; Greek; (514)345-4649; luc_oligny@ssss.gouv.qc.ca.

OLIJNIK, Helen; 303 Kingsway Garden Mall, 1 Kingsway Garden Mall NW, Edmonton AB T5G 3A6; Alb'87; CCFP; Court Staff Privil, Covenant Health - Edmonton General Continuing Care Centre; (780)479-3667; Fax. (780)479-3399.

OLIPHANT, Lawrie D; Sudbury Reg Hosp-Laurentian, 3212-41 Ramsey Lake Rd, Sudbury ON P3E 5J1; Ott'82; FCCP; FRCPC; IntMed (Sleep Disorders); Respir. Ac Staff Med (Respirology), Health Sciences North-Laurentian Site; (705)523-7056; Fax. (705)523-7084.

OLISA, Obidike M; Bayside Med Centre, 3 Beck Blvd, Penetanguishene ON L9M 1B9; CCFP; (705)549-3939; Fax. (705)549-0029.

OLIVA, Jiri; Montfort Hosp, 713 Montreal Rd, Ottawa ON K1K 0T2; Purkyne (Czech Republic)'62; Staff, Montfort Hospital; (613)746-4621

OLIVA, Maria A; Edmonton Clinic Health Academy, 11405 87 Ave NW, Edmonton AB T6G 1C9; Santo Tomas (Philippines)'97; Staff, Stollery Children's Hospital; Staff, Edmonton Clinic Health Academy; (780)248-5575; Fax. (780)248-5626; moliva@ualberta.ca.

OLIVA, Rossella; CSSS du Sud de Lanaudière, 911 montee des Pionniers, Terrebonne QC J6V 2H2; Laval'07; Staff, CSSS Du Sud De Lanaudière; (450)654-7525

OLIVA, Teresa; Appletree Med Group, 2948 Baseline Rd, Nepean ON K2H 8T5; Purkyne (Czech Republic)'99; CCFP; Staff, CH-CHSLD de Papineau - Pavillon du centre hospitalier; Langs: Czech; French; (613)288-2059; Fax. (613)288-2060.

OLIVA, Vincent; CHUM-Hop Notre-Dame, 1560 rue Sherbrooke E, Montreal QC H2L 4M1; Sher'85; CSPQ; FRCPC; DiagRad. Staff, Centre Hospitalier l'Université de Montréal (CHUM) - Hôpital Notre-Dame; (514)890-8000 x28530; Fax. (514)412-7547.

OLIVE, Christopher M; 201-219 St Clair Ave W, Toronto ON M4V 1R3; Minneapolis(MN) (USA)'88; FRCPC; Psy (Psychoanalysis). Staff, Centre for Addiction & Mental Health (CAMH) - College Street Site; Lecturer, University of Toronto; (416)921-6023; Fax. (416)921-6652.

OLIVEIRA, Katia F; St Michael's Hosp, 30 Bond St, Toronto ON M5B 1W8; Sao Paulo (Brazil)'06; Staff, St Michael's Hospital; (416)864-6060

OLIVEIRA, Liliana M; Riverside Prof Centre, 206-1919 Riverside Dr, Ottawa ON K1H 1A2; Ott'04; FRCPC; IntMed; Gastroent.

OLIVENSTEIN, Ronald; MUHC-Montreal Chest Institute, 3650 rue Saint-Urbain, Montreal QC H2X 2P4; Brussels (Belgium)'83; FRCPC; IntMed (Allergy); Respir. Ac Staff, McGill University Health Centre - Montreal Chest Institute; adj Prof, McGill University; Langs: English; French; (514)934-1934; Fax. (514)843-2088.

OLIVER, Afsaneh; Klinic, 870 Portage Ave, Winnipeg MB R3G 0P1; Qns'95; CCFP; FCFP.

OLIVER, Catherine; Davenport Perth Comm Hlth Ctr, 1892 Davenport Rd, Toronto ON M6N 1B7; McG'73; (416)658-6812; Fax. (416)658-4611; coliver@dpnchc.ca.

OLIVER, Dijana; 130 Ontario St, Kingston ON K7L 2Y4; Sarajevo (Bosnia-Herzegovina)'85; FRCPC; Psy (Adult Psychiatry). Staff, Kingston General Hospital; Queen's University; Langs: Serbian; Croatian; (613)544-9121

OLIVER, Douglas M; McMaster Family Practice, A-690 Main St W, Hamilton ON L8S 1A4; McM'01; CCFP; (905)521-5016; Fax. (905)521-5010.

OLIVER, Enrique; CSSSG-Hop de Gatineau, CP 2000 Succ Bureau-Chef 909 boul de la Verendrye O, Gatineau QC J8P 7H2; Montevideo (Uruguay)'73; CSPQ; FRCPC; Anes. Staff, Hôpital de Gatineau; (819)561-8299

OLIVER, Gillian D; 7-920 King St W, Kitchener ON N2G 1G4; Wes'84; FACOG; FRCSC; ObstGyn (Pelvic Floor Reconst). Ac Staff Reproductive Med, Grand River Hospital - Kitchener/Waterloo Health Centre; (519)744-0800; Fax. (519)744-0180.

OLIVER, Ian C; Queensway-Carleton Hosp, 3045 Baseline Rd, Nepean ON K2H 8P4; Wes'89; CCFP; FCFP; Staff, Queensway Carleton Hospital; (613)721-2000

OLIVER, John H W; 303-3330 Richter St, Kelowna BC V1W 4V5; McG'73; FRCSC; OrthSurg. Staff, Kelowna General Hospital; (250)763-7988; Fax. (250)862-5842.

OLIVER, Karin; MUHC-Montreal Gen Hosp, 1650 av Cedar, Montreal QC H3G 1A4; Tor'04; FRCSC; Ophth. Staff, McGill University Health Centre - Montreal General Campus; (514)934-1934

OLIVER, Matthew J; Sunnybrook Hlth Sciences Ctre, A239-2075 Bayview Ave, Toronto ON M4N 3M5; Wes'93; FRCPC; IntMed; Nephrol. Staff, Sunnybrook Health Sciences Centre; (416)480-4755; Fax. (416)480-6940.

OLIVER, Robert A; Woodlawn Med Clinic, 92 Main St, Dartmouth NS B2X 1R5; McG'77; CCFP; FCFP; Preceptor, Dalhousie University; (902)434-1500; Fax. (902)462-4994.

OLIVER, Sarah J; U of Ottawa Health Services, 300-100 Marie Curie Pvt, Ottawa ON K1N 1A2; Cal'97; CCFP; FCFP; (613)564-3950; Fax. (613)564-6627.

OLIVER, Steven W; Barrhaven Sports Med Centre, 3-3570 Strandherd Dr, Nepean ON K2J 5L4; UBC'00; FRCSC; OrthSurg (Sports Medicine). Staff, Kemptville District Hospital; Staff, Brockville General Hospital - Charles Street; Physician, Barrhaven Sports Med Centre; (613)823-4991; Fax. (613)823-6221; soliver100@gmail.com.

OLIVER, Susan L; 302-2330 Kennedy Rd, Scarborough ON M1T 0A2; Tor'84; (416)298-1303; Fax. (416)298-4872.

OLIVER, Zoe J; Health Sciences Centre, GF 201-820 Sherbrook St, Winnipeg MB R3A 1R9; Wes'01; CCFP; CCFP(E.M.); Staff, Health Sciences Centre; (204)774-8511

OLIVER FERNANDEZ, Alejandro; F-640 Ross Ave E, Timmins ON P4N 0A2; Monterrey (Mexico)'00; FRCSC; Ophth. Staff, Timmins & District Hospital; (705)267-1744

OLIVERIO, Paolo; 7-20 Highway 20 E, Fonthill ON L0S 1E0; McM'97; (905)892-0008; Fax. (905)892-0065.

OLIVIE, Damien A R; CHUM-Hop St-Luc, 1058 rue Saint-Denis, Montreal QC H2X 3J4; Rennes (France)'00; Staff, Centre Hospitalier l'Université De Montréal (CHUM) - Hôpital Saint-luc; (514)890-8000

OLIVIER, Andre; MUHC-Montreal Neurology Inst, 109D-3801 rue University, Montreal QC H3A 2B4; Mon'64; PhD; CSPQ; FRCS; DABNS; Neursurg (Epilepsy). Che neurochirg, McGill University Health Centre - Montreal Neurological Hospital; Prof, McGill University; Langs: Bilingual(French/English); (514)398-1937; Fax. (514)398-2811.

OLIVIER, Andre D; Montfort Hosp, 713 Montreal Rd, Ottawa ON K1K 0T2; Ott'94; FRCPC; DiagRad. Staff, Montfort Hospital; (613)746-4621

OLIVIER, Antoinette; Main Street Med Services, 4929 50 Ave, Lacombe AB T4L 1K3; Stellenbosch (South Africa)'91; MB ChB; (403)782-6717; Fax. (403)782-4240.

OLIVIER, Barend G; Fox Creek Med Clinic, PO Box 640 600 3 St, Fox Creek AB T0H 1P0; Stellenbosch (South Africa)'72; MB ChB; (780)622-3010; Fax. (780)622-4169; bgo@telusplanet.net.

OLIVIER, Chantal; CLSC Samuel-de-Champlain, 100-5811 boul Taschereau, Brossard QC J4Z 1A5; Mon'00; Langs: English; (450)445-4452; Fax. (450)445-6751.

OLIVIER, David; CSSS de l'Energie-Ste-Therese, 1705 av Georges, Shawinigan QC G9N 2N1; Laval'00; Psy. Staff, CH du Centre-de-la-Mauricie (Ste-Thérèse de Shawinigan); Langs: Spanish; English; (819)536-7500 x4276; david_olivier@ssss.gouv.qc.ca.

OLIVIER, Erin P; Pritchard Farm Health Centre, 5-3014 Henderson Hwy, East St Paul MB R2E 0H9; Man'09; CCFP.

OLIVIER, Genevieve; CLSC de la Region-Sherbrooke, 50 rue Camirand, Sherbrooke QC J1H 4J5; Sher'94; (819)565-1330; Fax. (819)565-8196.

OLIVIER, Jean-Francois; SMBD Jewish Gen Hosp, 3755 ch Cote-Sainte-Catherine, Montreal QC H3T 1E2; Mon'01; CSPQ; FRCPC; Anes. Staff, Sir Mortimer B Davis Jewish General; (514)340-8222 x5701

OLIVIER, Jeremie; Ctr Hosp Fleury, 2180 rue Fleury E, Montreal QC H2B 1K3; Mon'09; Staff, Centre Hospitalier Fleury; (514)384-2000

OLIVIER, Jerome; CSSS du Nord de Lanaudière, 1000 boul Sainte-Anne, Joliette QC J6E 6J2; Sher'97; FRCPC; Psy. Staff, Centre Hospitalier Régional de Lanaudière; Staff, Centre Hospitalier La Sarre; (450)759-8222

OLIVIER, Johannes C; Caledonian Med Clinic, 340 Campbell St, Nanaimo BC V9R 3G7; Pretoria (South Africa)'77; MB ChB; MCFP; DipOccupational Health; (250)753-3202; Fax. (250)753-1039; johnolivier@shaw.ca.

OLIVIER, Kary G; 555 Barrydowne Rd, Sudbury ON P3A 3T4; Ott'96; BSc(Hons.); CCFP; FCFP; (705)524-7419; Fax. (705)524-9087.

OLIVIER, Marc-Andre P; CSSS du Sud de Lanaudière, 911 montee des Pionniers, Terrebonne QC J6V 2H2; Laval'96; Staff, Centre Hospitalier Pierre le Gardeur; (450)654-7525

OLIVIER, Marie-Jo; 5775 boul Leger, Montreal-Nord QC H1G 1K7; McG'94; FRCSC; Otol (Oncology). Staff, Hopital Maisonneuve-Rosemont; Clin Teacher Otol Maxillo Facial & Facial Plastic Surg, Universite de Montreal; (514)327-4040

OLIVIER, Marlene; Urgence Chauveau, 11999 rue de l'Hopital, Quebec QC G2A 2T7; Laval'98; LMCC; Staff, Centre Hospitalier Universitaire De Québec - Pavillon De St-françois-d'assise; Langs: English; Spanish; (418)683-1433

OLIVIER, Nathalie; Clinique Med Legendre, 201-1650 av Jules-Verne, Quebec QC G2G 2R1; Laval'89; (418)872-5600; Fax. (418)872-8408.

OLIVIER, Patricia; Hôpital Ste-Justine, 3175 ch Cote-Sainte-Catherine, Montreal QC H3T 1C5; Laval'03; FRCPC; Peds; Endocrin&Metab. Staff, Hôpital Ste-Justine; (514)345-4735

OLIVIER, Patrick; 2005 rue King O, Sherbrooke QC J1J 2E6; Sher'76; FRCSC; Ophth (Pediatric Ophthalmology & Strabismus). Langs: Spanish; English; (819)821-0064; Fax. (819)821-2289.

OLIVIER, Pierre; Clin Med Carleton-Sur-Mer, GD 197 rue du Quai, Carleton QC G0C 1J0; Laval'81; Langs: Bilingual(French/English); (418)364-3311; Fax. (418)364-6650.

OLIVIER, Sebastien; Hop Maisonneuve-Rosemont, 5415 boul de l'Assomption, Montreal QC H1T 2M4; Mon'97; FRCSC; Ophth. Staff, Hopital Maisonneuve-Rosemont; (514)252-3400 x4956

OLIVIER, Stephane; Carrefour Sante le St-Laurent, 140-5300 boul Saint-Laurent, Sainte-Catherine QC J5C 1A8; Mon'96; CCFP; (450)638-6383

OLIVIER, Stephane; CSSS de Beauce-Etchemin, 1515 17e rue, Saint-Georges QC G5Y 4T8; Laval'93; CSPQ; FRCPC; Anes. Staff, Centre Hospitalier Beauce-Etchemin; (418)228-2031; clovis2@globetrotter.qc.ca.

OLIVIER, Stephanie; Universite de Sherbrooke, 2500 boul de l'Universite, Sherbrooke QC J1K 2R1; Sher'01; FRCSC; PlasSurg. (819)346-1110 x27900

OLIVIERI, Loretta S; Hamilton HS-General Site, 237 Barton St E, Hamilton ON L8L 2X2; McM'01; FRCPC; Anes. Staff, Hamilton Health Sciences Centre - Hamilton General Hospital; (905)527-4322 x46698

OLIVIERI, Nancy F; Univ Hlth Network-Toronto Gen, EN10 225-200 Elizabeth St, Toronto ON M5G 2C4; McM'78; ABIM; AB; FRCPC; IntMed; Hem. Dir Haemoglogmopathy Prog, The Hospital For Sick Children; Staff Hem, Toronto General Hospital - UHN; Assoc Prof, University of Toronto; (416)340-3979

OLIVOTTO, Ivo A; BC Cancer Agency-Vanc Isl Ctr, 2410 Lee Ave, Victoria BC V8R 6V5; UBC'81; FRCPC; RadOncol (Breast Cancer). Staff, Vancouver Island Health Authority; Staff RadOncol, BC Cancer Agency Vancouver Island Centre; Prof RadOncol, University of British Columbia; (250)519-5577; Fax. (250)519-2018; iolivott@bccancer.bc.ca.

OLLEGASAGREM, Nirmaladevi; Greystone Med Clinic, 2921 8th St E, Saskatoon SK S7H 0V4; Jaffna (Sri Lanka)'86; MB BS; CCFP; Langs: Tamil; Sinhalese; (306)373-3223; Fax. (306)955-8802; nirmala_ollega@hotmail.com.

OLLENBERGER, Glenn P; Regina Qu'Appelle HR-Regina, 1440 14th Ave, Regina SK S4P 0W5; Sask'00; FRCPC; NuclearMed. Staff, Regina General Hospital; (306)766-3590; Fax. (306)766-4134.

OLLEWAGEN, Ferdinand J; Aurora Med Laser & Vein Ctre, 3617 50 Ave, Red Deer AB T4N 3Y5; Pretoria (South Africa)'89; (403)358-5818; Fax. (403)358-7797.

OLLIVER, Steven B; Sunnyhill Pediatric Clinic, 200-1632 14 Ave NW, Calgary AB T2N 1M7; Alb'98; FRCPC; Peds; Critical Care Medicine. (403)284-0001; Fax. (403)284-1593.

OLLSON, Gary L; Lennox & Addington Gen Hosp, 8 Richmond Park Dr, Napanee ON K7R 2Z4; Qns'80; Court Staff, Lennox & Addington County General Hospital; (613)354-3301 x225

OLMESDAHL, Arthur B; PO Box 775, Invermere BC V0A 1K0; Pretoria (South Africa)'09; MB ChB; (250)688-1645

OLMSTEAD, David; Harvey Community Hosp, 2019 Route 3, Harvey Station NB E6K 3E9; Dal'67; Staff, Harvey Health Centre; (506)366-5658; Fax. (506)366-6403.

OLNEY, Harold J; CHUM-Hop Notre-Dame, 1560 rue Sherbrooke E, Montreal QC H2L 4M1; McG'92; FRCPC; IntMed; MedOncol; Hem (P.Q.). Staff, Centre Hospitalier l'Université de Montréal (CHUM) - Hôpital Notre-Dame; (514)890-8000 x28228; Fax. (514)412-7572.

OLOKO, Saliu; 275 Bradbrooke Dr, Yorkton SK S3N 3L3; Lagos (Nigeria)'94; MB BS; MRCP; LMCC; (306)782-4363; Fax. (306)782-4364; drsaoloko@sasktel.net.

OLOKODANA, Femi A; 95 Meridian Ave, Haileybury ON P0J 1K0; CCFP; Staff, Englehart & District Hospital Inc; (705)672-3371; Fax. (705)672-5900.

OLORUNFEMI, Ayodele O; Mills Memorial Hosp, 4720 Haughland Ave, Terrace BC V8G 2W7; Obafemi Awolowo (Nigeria)'97; Staff, Mills Memorial Hospital; (250)635-2211

OLORUNSOLA, Kehinde; 3-204 First Ave, St Thomas ON N5R 4P5; Vienna (Austria)'98; CCFP; (519)631-3223; Fax. (519)282-0390.

OLOWU, Sunday; Westbrook Shopping Centre, 28-1200 37 St SW, Calgary AB T3C 1S2; Univ of Ilorin (Nigeria) MB BS; LMCC; (587)225-7535

OLSEN, Brian W; William Osler HC-Brampton, 2100 Bovaird Dr E, Brampton ON L6R 3J7; UBC'90; FRCPC; GenPath (Hematology Pathology). Staff, William Osler Health System - Brampton Civic Hospital; (905)494-2120

OLSEN, Ingrid; CLSC Gaston-Lessard, 8 rue Speid, Sherbrooke QC J1M 1R6; Sher'92; CCFP; Staff, Centre Hospitalier Universitaire de Sherbrooke-Hopital Fleurimont; (819)566-1906; Fax. (819)566-8059.

OLSEN, Jeanine; Dundas Med Centre, 404-220 Dundas St W, Whitby ON L1N 8M7; Cardiff (Wales)'55; MB ChB; DPM(Eng); MRCPsy; FRCPC; Psy. (905)668-5300; Fax. (905)668-5433.

OLSEN, Kristina L; Waterview Med & Chiro Centre, 464 Locust St, Burlington ON L7S 1V1; McM'96; CCFP; FCFP; (289)245-1071; Fax. (289)245-1486.

OLSEN, Monica M; Grey Bruce HS-Owen Sound, PO Box 1800 Stn Main 1800 8th St E, Owen Sound ON N4K 6M9; Alb'04; FRCPC; Anes. Staff, Grey Bruce Health Services - Owen Sound; (519)376-2121

OLSEN, Patricia N; 201-284 Helmcken Rd, Victoria BC V9B 1T2; Ott'90; BSc; CCFP; FCFP; (250)480-1401; Fax. (250)480-1422.

OLSEN, Sharla-Rae J; Heritage Med Clinic, 1624 7th Ave, Prince George BC V2L 3P6; Man'03; FRCPC; IntMed; Respir. (250)596-9180

OLSEN, Terry M; Misericordia Community Hosp, 16940 87 Ave NW, Edmonton AB T5R 4H5; Alb'94; CCFP; Staff, Covenant Health - Misericordia Community Hospital; (780)735-2769

OLSEN, Valerie P; PO Box 40 Stn Main, Prince Albert SK S6V 5R4; Sask'94; FRCSC; GenSurg. (306)763-5972; Fax. (306)763-5974.

OLSHESKI, Wayne; Albany Med Clinic, 807 Broadview Ave, Toronto ON M4K 2P8; Wroclaw (Poland)'85; Langs: Polish; Spanish; (416)461-9471; Fax. (416)461-2710.

OLSON, Cynthia I; Synergy Wellness Centre, 225-501 Bethel Dr, Sherwood Park AB T8H 0N2; Alb'92; (780)464-4506; Fax. (780)416-0957.

OLSON, David C; Meadowlark Health Centre, 200 Meadowlark Shopping Ctr NW, Edmonton AB T5R 5W9; Alb'05; FRCPC; DiagRad. (780)669-2233; Fax. (780)486-5160.

OLSON, David W; Meadowlark Health Centre, 184 Meadowlark Shopping Ctr NW, Edmonton AB T5R 5W9; Alb'97; MSc; FRCSC; GenSurg (Colorectal Surgery). Staff, Covenant Health - Misericordia Community Hospital; University of Alberta; (780)484-1122; Fax. (780)489-4121.

OLSON, James G; 3039 Armada St, Coquitlam BC V3C 3S4; Ott'96; BSc; LMCC; Consultant, Aerospace Medical Industries; Member, Tri-Cities Homeless Shelter Society; Member, Canadian Sport Parachuting Associaton; Dir, Preventive Medicine Clinics; (604)999-3626; Fax. (604)944-3626.

OLSON, Jaret L; University of Alberta Hosp, 2D382-8440 112 St NW, Edmonton AB T6G 2B7; Alb'96; FRCSC; PlasSurg. Staff, University of Alberta Hospital; Staff, Covenant Health - Misericordia Community Hospital; Asst Prof, University of Alberta; (780)407-8108; Fax. (780)407-8131.

OLSON, Joshua; Chilliwack Gen Hosp, 45600 Menholm Rd, Chilliwack BC V2P 1P7; UBC'02; CCFP; CCFP(E.M.); Staff, Chilliwack General Hospital; (604)795-4141

OLSON, Robert A; BC Cancer Agency-Vancouver CC, 600 10th Ave W, Vancouver BC V5Z 4E6; Cal'05; FRCPC; RadOncol. Staff, BC Cancer Agency Vancouver Centre; (604)877-6000

OLSON, Robyn L; Markham Prof Centre, 200-2265 Pembina Hwy, Winnipeg MB R3T 5J3; Man'89; BScPharm; CCFP; Staff, Victoria General Hospital; Teach Staff Med, University of Manitoba; (204)989-4200; Fax. (204)989-4205.

OLSON, Sarah E; South Community Birth Program, 5838 Fraser St, Vancouver BC V5W 2Z5; UBC'10; CCFP; (604)324-2201

OLSON, Shanna M; Dakota Med Centre, 17-845 Dakota St, Winnipeg MB R2M 5M3; Sask'02; CCFP.

OLSON, Stanley A; 12511 39A Ave NW, Edmonton AB T6J 0P4; Alb'67; FRCPC; Anes. Staff, Royal Alexandra Hospital; (780)435-7635; Fax. (780)436-0192.

OLSSON, Larry S M; Norfolk Gen Hosp, 365 West St, Simcoe ON N3Y 1T7; Wes'70; FACS; FRCSC; GenSurg. Staff, Norfolk General Hospital; (519)426-0130; olsn@kwic.com.

OLSZYNSKI, Ewa P; Saskatoon Community Clinic, 455 2nd Ave N, Saskatoon SK S7K 2C2; Warsaw (Poland)'74; CCFP; FCFP; Langs: Polish; (306)652-0300; Fax. (306)652-0682.

OLSZYNSKI, Paul A; Royal University Hosp, 103 Hospital Dr, Saskatoon SK S7N 0W8; Sask'05; CCFP; CCFP(E.M.); Staff, Royal University Hospital; (306)655-1000

OLSZYNSKI, Wojciech P; Midtown Med Centre, 103-39 23rd St E, Saskatoon SK S7K 0H6; Warsaw (Poland)'74; MD; PhD; CDD; FRCPC; IntMed (Rheumatology). Physician 1, Saskatoon Health Region Saskatoon Public Health; Dir, Saskatoon Osteoporosis Centre; Clin Prof, University of Saskatchewan; Langs: Polish; French; (306)244-2277; Fax. (306)244-6755.

OLUBAJO, Olabisi A; The Clinic, PO Box 190 115B 1st Ave E, Rosetown SK S0L 2V0; CCFP; (306)882-3664; Fax. (306)882-3670.

OLUBOKA, Oloruntoba J; Sheldon Chumir Centre, 1213 4 St SW, Calgary AB T2R 0X7; Ilorin (Nigeria)'86; FRCPC; Psy (Mood Disorders). Langs: Yoruba; (403)955-6566; Fax. (403)955-6585.

OLUFEMI, Ademola O; 308-3025 Hurontario St, Mississauga ON L5A 2H1; Lagos (Nigeria)'83; MB BS; CCFP; (905)279-1341

OLUFOWOBI, Olufemi O; 308-6453 Morrison St, Niagara Falls ON L2E 7H1; Lagos (Nigeria)'91; FRCSC; ObstGyn.

OLUGHOR, Jerome O; 15965 97 St NW, Edmonton AB T5X 0C7; (Nigeria)'88; (780)784-0895; Fax. (780)784-0896.

OLUJOHUNGBE, Adebayo B K; CancerCare Manitoba, ON2070-675 McDermot Ave, Winnipeg MB R3E 0V9; Ibadan (Nigeria)'85; Staff, Health Sciences Centre.

OLUMA, Elias T; Harbour Landing Med Clinic, 4500 Gordon Rd, Regina SK S4W 0B7; (Ethiopia)'94; (306)545-2888; Fax. (306)545-2844.

OLUPONA, Samuel M; 402-100 Colborne St W, Orillia ON L3V 2Y9; Ibadan (Nigeria)'76; FRCOG; FRCSC; ObstGyn. Staff ObstGyn, Orillia Soldiers' Memorial Hospital; (705)323-9776; Fax. (705)323-9778.

OLURIN, Olubunmi I; F1-7070 McLaughlin Rd, Mississauga ON L5W 1W7; Ibadan (Nigeria)'00; MB BS; CCFP.

OLUWADAIRO, Samuel A; Foothills Med Centre, 1403 29 St NW, Calgary AB T2N 2T9; Ibadan (Nigeria)'86; MSc(Addiction); DPM(Ire); MB BS; FRCPC; Psy (Addiction Medicine). Consultant Psy, Foothills Medical Centre; Clinical Asst Prof, University of Calgary; Langs: Yoruba; (403)944-8492; Fax. (403)270-3451; samuel.oluwadairo@calgaryhealthregion.ca.

OLUYEDE, Kehinde B; Mental Health & Addictions, 528 Wentworth St S, Nanaimo BC V9S 2B7; (Nigeria)'99; MB BS; (250)739-5868

OLUYEDE, Olumayokun; Mineville Health Centre, 4 Peter Crt, Mineville NS B2Z 1K2; Staff, Souris Hospital Inc; (902)829-3278; Fax. (902)829-2549.

OLYNYK, Fred; Rougeau Plaza Med Centre, N-1522 Regent Ave W, Winnipeg MB R2C 3B4; Man'81; BSc; (204)663-0827; Fax. (204)668-6870.

OLYNYK, Kimberley A; Royal Victoria Hosp, 201 Georgian Dr, Barrie ON L4M 6M2; McM'89; CCFP; FCFP; Staff, Royal Victoria Regional Health Centre; (705)739-5607

OMABOE, Narh; PO Box 22077 RPO Trenton Ctre, Trenton ON K8V 6S3; Geneva (Switzerland)'60; BSc; DABOG; FRCSC; ObstGyn (Allergy). Langs: English; French; (613)965-0710; Fax. (613)965-0711.

OMAH-MAHARAJH, Dave A; 3536 Roblin Blvd, Winnipeg MB R3R 0C9; West Indies (Jamaica)'80; MB BS.

OMAHEN, David A; 212-300 Columbia St, Kamloops BC V2C 6L1; Ott'99; FRCSC; Neursurg. (778)471-6477

OMAN-GANES, A Loraine; RBC Life Insurance Company, 6880 Financial Dr, Mississauga ON L5N 7Y5; Sask'83; CCMG; FACMG; FRCPC; Peds (Clinical Genetics). Chief Med Dir, RBC Life Insurance Company; (905)606-1189; Fax. (905)567-1217; loraine.oman.ganes@rbc.com.

OMAR, Assad B; 2039-8882 170 St NW, Edmonton AB T5T 3J7; Alb'07; CCFP; (780)444-1935; Fax. (780)444-3092.

OMELAN, Craig K; Health Sciences Ctr Gen Hosp, 700 William Ave, Winnipeg MB R3E 0Z3; Man'88; FRCPC; Psy (Geriatric Psychiatry). Staff, St Boniface General Hospital; Staff, Health Sciences Centre; Staff, Selkirk Mental Health Centre; Asst Prof Psy, University of Manitoba.

OMELCHENKO, Victor; 101-8927 152nd St, Surrey BC V3R 4E5; Danylo (Ukraine)'87; (604)588-4449; Fax. (604)588-4459.

OMELCHUK, Alex; Medi-Kel Family Clinic, 2280 Baron Rd, Kelowna BC V1X 7W3; Alb'62; CCFP; FCFP; (250)862-4996

OMER, Saeed A; William Osler HC-Brampton, 2100 Bovaird Dr E, Brampton ON L6R 3J7; Khartoum (Sudan)'89; FRCPC; IntMed. Staff, William Osler Health System - Brampton Civic Hospital; (905)494-2120

OMEROGLU, Attila-Orhan; 3775 rue University, Montreal QC H3A 2B4; Istanbul (Turkey)'94; CSPQ; AnatPath (P.Q.). (514)398-7192

OMEROGLU, Gulbeyaz; Duff Med Bldg, B18-3775 rue University, Montreal QC H3A 2B4; Istanbul (Turkey)'95.

OMICHINSKI, L Michael; Portage Clinic Inc, 140 9th St SE, Portage La Prairie MB R1N 3V5; Man'89; CCFP; FCFP; Staff, Portage District General Hospital; Lecturer Family Med/Assoc Lecturer CME, University of Manitoba; (204)857-3445; Fax. (204)239-1278; momichinski@shaw.ca.

OMIWOLE, Olufemi O; 196 King St, Bowmanville ON L1C 1P1; Obafemi Awolowo (Nigeria)'92; MCFP; MMed; DPH; MB BS; CCFP; Langs: Yoruba; (905)697-8300

OMORUYI, Enosakhare B; Rouge Valley-Ajax & Pickering, 580 Harwood Ave S, Ajax ON L1S 2J4; Univ of Benin (Nigeria)'88; FRCPC; Psy. Staff, Rouge Valley Health System - Ajax & Pickering Health Centre Site; (905)683-2320

OMOSENI, Olusegun B; 105-860 Tecumseh Rd E, Windsor ON N8X 2S5; Ibadan (Nigeria)'00; FRCPC; Psy.

OMOSIGHO, Osamudiamen C; St Joseph's Hosp, 600-1176 Nicholson Rd, Estevan SK S4A 2V6; University of Benin (Nigeria)'84; MB BS; MCFP; FRCP(UK); DCH; Staff, St Joseph's Hospital; Clin Lecturer, University of Saskatchewan; Langs: Edo; French; (306)637-2760; Fax. (306)637-2762; oomosigho@shalommedicalclinic.com.

OMOTANI, Sandra; Toronto Rehab Institute, 550 University Ave, Toronto ON M5G 2A2; Ott'82; Staff Occupational Health & Safety, Centre for Addiction & Mental Health (CAMH) - Queen Site; (416)597-3422 x3051

OMOTO, Daniel M; Royal York Med Arts Bldg, 311-1436 Royal York Rd, Etobicoke ON M9P 3A9; Guadalajara (Mexico)'04; CCFP; (416)241-4689

OMOTOSO, Patrick; 206-199 Chesley Dr, Saint John NB E2K 4S9; Ilorin (Nigeria)'88; Staff, Saint John Regional Hospital.

OMURA, John D; UBC School of Population, 2206 East Mall, Vancouver BC V6T 1Z3; Wes'07; CCFP; Staff, Pender Community Health Centre; (604)822-7646

OMYLANOWSKI, Diana; Carmen Vanderwater Med Centre, PO Box 790 Stn Main 33-180 Parsons Rd, Alliston ON L9R 1V9; Tor'73; (705)435-6225; Fax. (705)435-6062.

ONASANYA, Olanrewaju; 2046 Broad St, Regina SK S4P 1Y3; Ife (Nigeria)'83; MB ChB; FRCSC; ObstGyn (Infertility). Att Physician, Regina General Hospital; Pt-Time Teacher, University of Saskatchewan; (306)751-5151; Fax. (306)751-5155.

ONAYEMI, Adebusola O; Royal Victoria Hosp, 201 Georgian Dr, Barrie ON L4M 6M2; Ibadan (Nigeria)'74; MB BS; DA; FRCPC; Anes. Ac Staff Anes, Royal Victoria Regional Health Centre; Court Staff, Orillia Soldiers' Memorial Hospital; Court Staff, Stevenson Memorial Hospital; (705)728-9090; Fax. (705)728-0980; bonayemi@sympatico.ca.

ONDHIA, Manharlal V; Sunnybrook Hlth Sciences Ctre, 2075 Bayview Ave, Toronto ON M4N 3M5; Leeds (England)'65; LRCP; MRCS; DA(Eng.); AB; FRCPC; Anes. Staff Anes, Sunnybrook Health Sciences Centre; Asst Prof, University of Toronto; (416)480-4864; Fax. (416)480-6039.

ONDIVEERAN, Hari K; Saint John Reg Hosp, PO Box 2100 Stn Main 400 University Ave, Saint John NB E2L 4L2; (Malaysia)'87; MB BS(Malaya); FRCS(Ed); FRCSC; GenSurg (Trauma Surgery); Critical Care Medicine. Staff, Saint John Regional Hospital; Langs: Tamil; Malay; (506)648-6000

ONDRO, Milena; Pleasantview Prof Bldg, 204-11044 51 Ave NW, Edmonton AB T6H 5B4; Tor'76; (780)434-4130; Fax. (780)434-1872.

ONDRUS, Peter; Royal Alexandra Hosp, 10240 Kingsway NW, Edmonton AB T5H 3V9; (Slovakia)'79; Staff, Royal Alexandra Hospital; (780)735-4111

ONELL, Rodrigo I; Misericordia Community Hosp, 1N801-16940 87 Ave NW, Edmonton AB T5R 4H5; Alb'06; FRCPC; HemPath. Staff, Covenant Health - Misericordia Community Hospital; (780)735-2476

ONERHEIM, Ronald M; St Mary's Hosp Centre, 3830 av Lacombe, Montreal QC H3T 1M5; Alb'78; CSPQ; FRCPC; AnatPath. Chef Dept of Path, St Mary's Hospital Centre; assoc Prof, McGill University; Langs: English; French; (514)345-3511 x3182; ronald.onerheim@mcgill.ca.

ONESCHUK, Doreen M; Health Services Centre, 416-1090 Youville Drive West N, Edmonton AB T6L 5X8; Alb'87; CCFP; Staff, Covenant Health - Grey Nuns Community Hospital; (780)735-7834; Fax. (780)735-7302.

ONESCHUK, Gail P; The Ottawa Hosp-Riverside, 1967 Riverside Dr, Ottawa ON K1H 7W9; Tor'77; AB; FRCPC; Anes. Staff, The Ottawa Hospital - Riverside Campus; (613)738-8237

ONG, Alan P Y; Univ Hlth Network-Toronto Western Hosp, 7MP 431-399 Bathurst St, Toronto ON M5T 2S8; Tor'95; DABPN; DABSM; FRCPC; Neur (Sleep Medicine). Staff, Toronto Western Hospital - University Health Network; (416)603-5667; Fax. (416)603-5292.

ONG, Aldrich D T; CancerCare Manitoba, 675 McDermot Ave, Winnipeg MB R3E 0V9; Qns'03; FRCPC; RadOncol.

ONG, Bill Y; Harry Medovy House, 671 William Ave, Winnipeg MB R3E 0Z2; Man'74; BSc(Med); FRCPC; Anes. Dir Anes, Health Sciences Centre; Prof, University of Manitoba.

ONG, Dennis D; Royal University Hosp, 103 Hospital Dr, Saskatoon SK S7N 0W8; Phillipines (Philippines)'85; BSc; FRCPC; Anes. Staff, Royal University Hospital; Clinical Asst Prof, University of Saskatchewan; Langs: Fookien; Tagalog; (306)655-1183; Fax. (306)655-1279; dennis.ong@saskatoonhealthregion.ca.

ONG, George H E; Beautiful Plains Comm Med Clin, 499 Mountain Ave, Neepawa MB R0J 1H0; London (England)'72; MB BS; MRCP(UK); gong@arha.ca.

ONG, Geraldine; Centre Med Berger Inc, 1000 ch Sainte-Foy, Quebec QC G1S 2L6; Mon'08; IntMed. (418)650-2295

ONG, Hoang; Clinique Med Viau, 8465 boul Viau, Saint-Leonard QC H1R 2T6; Mon'84; (514)326-7203; Fax. (514)326-3656.

ONG, Larry S; Midtown Mental Health, 3F-2450 Ontario St, Vancouver BC V5T 4T7; UBC'94; FRCPC; Psy. Med Staff, Vancouver General Hospital - Centennial Pavillion; Clin Instructor Psy, University of British Columbia; Langs: Tagalog; (604)872-8441

ONG, Sharon Rose Y; Surrey Med Arts Bldg, 214-13710 94A Ave, Surrey BC V3V 1N1; Cal'99; MEd; FRCSC; GenSurg; ThorSurg. Staff, Surrey Memorial Hospital; Staff, Fraser Health Authority; Langs: Tagalog; Mandarin; (604)588-5634; Fax. (604)588-5638.

ONG-LAM, May C; Burrard Health Bldg, 502-1160 Burrard St, Vancouver BC V6Z 2E8; Tor'78; FRCPC; IntMed (Pain Management). Co-Dir/Staff Pain Management Prog, Providence Health Care - St Paul's Hospital; Assoc Prof Med, University of British Columbia; (604)688-2580; Fax. (604)688-2507.

ONG-TONE, Lindsay; Cornwall Prof Bldg, 215-2125 11th Ave, Regina SK S4P 3X3; Glasgow (Scotland)'79; FRCS(Ed); FRCOphth; FRCSC; Ophth (Cataract Surgery). Ac Staff, Regina General Hospital; Clinical Asst Prof, University of Saskatchewan; Langs: French; (306)565-3535; Fax. (306)565-0988; longtone@accesscomm.ca.

ONI, Oluwole; Campbellton Reg Hosp, PO Box 880 Stn Main 189 Lilly Lake Rd, Campbellton NB E3N 3H3; Ilorin (Nigeria)'99; Staff, Hôpital Régional Campbellton; (506)789-5000

ONISHENKO, Donna K; 192 Riddell St, Woodstock ON N4S 8M7; Wes'90; CCFP; (519)537-5044

ONLOCK, Stephen G; Royal Victoria Hosp, 201 Georgian Dr, Barrie ON L4M 6M2; Qns'88; CCFP; CCFP(E.M.); Staff, Royal Victoria Regional Health Centre; (705)728-9090

ONOCHIE, Lawrence M; 2016 Ogilvie Rd, Ottawa ON K1J 7N9; Ibadan (Nigeria)'71; MB BS; DA; DABOG; FACOG; FRCSC; ObstGyn. Ac Staff/Chief ObstGyn, Pembroke Regional Hospital Inc; (613)749-5549; Fax. (613)749-3105.

ONOFERSON, Brian K; RCMP Health Services Office, 1091 Portage Ave, Winnipeg MB R3C 3K2; Man'81.

ONORATO, Linda; Hamilton HS-General Site, 237 Barton St E, Hamilton ON L8L 2X2; McM'96; FRCPC; Anes; Critical Care Medicine. Staff, Hamilton Health Sciences Centre - Hamilton General Hospital; (905)527-0271

ONOTERA, Rodney T; Greencrest Med Clinic, 2750B Pembina Hwy, Winnipeg MB R3T 2H8; Man'82; FACS; FRCSC; GenSurg (Endoscopy). Ac Staff, Victoria General Hospital.

ONROT, John M; St Paul's Hosp, 5912B-1081 Burrard St, Vancouver BC V6Z 1Y6; Tor'75; FRCPC; IntMed (Hypertension). Ac Staff, Providence Health Care - St Paul's Hospital; Clin Prof Med, University of British Columbia; (604)806-8164; Fax. (604)806-8338.

ONSONGO, Foose M; White Rose Med Centre, PO Box 3955 Stn Main 4607 50 Ave, Olds AB T4H 1P6; (South Africa)'03; MB BCh; (403)556-7130; Fax. (403)556-1944.

ONUGHA, Edward C; South Health Campus, 4448 Front St SE, Calgary AB T3M 1M4; (Nigeria)'96; FRCPC; Psy. (403)956-1111

ONUORA, Abraham N; Hilyard Place Bldg A, 220-560 Main St, Saint John NB E2K 1J5; Ibadan (Nigeria)'76; MB BS; MRCPsy(UK); FRCPC; Psy. Staff Psy, Saint John Regional Hospital; (506)658-1766; Fax. (506)658-1833.

ONUSKA, Frank P; Elmira Med Centre, 2 Park Ave W, Elmira ON N3B 1L1; Wes'88; Staff, Joseph Brant Memorial Hospital; Staff, St Mary's General Hospital; Staff, Grand River Hospital - Kitchener/Waterloo Health Centre; (519)669-5493

ONWUDIWE, Herbert O; 216 4 Ave PO Box 2465 Stn Main, Strathmore AB T1P 1K3; Dublin (Ireland)'68; Langs: Ibo; (403)361-2422

ONWUKWE, Victor N; Access Med Clinic, 610B-8600 Franklin Ave, Fort McMurray AB T9H 4G8; (Nigeria)'90; MB BS; DTM&H; MPH; Langs: Portuguese; (780)743-4553; Fax. (780)750-4553.

ONYEGBULE, Henry O; Linden Med Clinic, 7-385 Broadway st E, Yorkton SK S3N 2W1; Staff, Yorkton Mental Health & Addiction Centre; (306)783-7926; Fax. (306)783-7932; henry.onyegbule@shr.sk.ca.

ONYEKWELU, Onyema A; CLSC Metro, 1801 boul de Maisonneuve O, Montreal QC H3H 1J9; McG'09; CCFP; (514)934-0505

ONYETT, Heather A; Kingston Gen Hosp, 76 Stuart St, Kingston ON K7L 2V7; Mem'74; DTM&H; MPH; FAAP; FRCPC; Peds (International Health); InfectDis. Staff, Kingston General Hospital; Staff, Hotel-Dieu Hospital; Assoc Prof Int'l Health School of Public Health, Boston University; Prof Peds Microbiology Immunology Comm Health & Epidemiol, Queen's University; Langs: English; French; (613)548-3232; onyetth@post.queensu.ca.

ONYETT-JEFFRIES, Katherine A G; West Park Health Centre, 82 Buttonwood Ave, York ON M6M 2J5; Ott'09; CCFP; Staff, West Park Healthcare Centre; (416)243-3706; Fax. (416)243-3645.

ONYSHKO, Daniel; Minnedosa Med Group, PO Box 810 129 2nd Ave SW, Minnedosa MB R0J 1E0; Man'91; Med Staff Member, Minnedosa Health Centre; Asst Prof, University of Manitoba; (204)867-2722; Fax. (204)867-2986.

OOI, Althea L; Maternal Child Clinic, 130-1402 8 Ave NW, Calgary AB T2N 1B8; Tor'01; CCFP; (403)509-3080; Fax. (403)509-3082.

OOI, Daylily; The Ottawa Hosp-Riverside, 1967 Riverside Dr, Ottawa ON K1H 7W9; (Singapore)'72; MB BS; FRCPC; MedBiochem. Staff, The Ottawa Hospital - Riverside Campus; Assoc Prof Path & LabMed, University of Ottawa; (613)738-8333; Fax. (613)738-8261; dsooi@toh.on.ca.

OOI, See Wei; Kirkland & District Hosp, PO Box 3000 Stn Main 145 Government Rd E, Kirkland Lake ON P2N 3P4; Dundee (Scotland)'00; CCFP; Staff, Kirkland & District Hospital; (705)567-5251

OOI, Teik Chye; The Ottawa Hosp-Riverside, 1967 Riverside Dr, Ottawa ON K1H 7W9; (Singapore)'72; MB BS; FRACP(Endocrin); FACE; FRCP; FRCPC; IntMed (Endocrinology). Head Div of Endocrin & Metabolism, The Ottawa Hospital - Riverside Campus; Prof Med Univ of Med, University of Ottawa; Langs: Cantonese; Hokkin; (613)738-8400 x81950; Fax. (613)738-8396; tcooi@toh.on.ca.

OOI, Teik Im; Albert Park Family Med Centre, 56-3992 Albert St, Regina SK S4S 3R1; Mysore (India)'80; Admin, Albert Park Family Medical Centres; (306)584-3833; Fax. (306)585-3833.

OOMMEN, Ashok; Cardiogenix Med Centre, 100-8250 boul Decarie, Montreal QC H4P 2P5; McG'93; CCFP; CCFP(E.M.); Staff, St Mary's Hospital Centre; Staff, McGill University Health Centre - Montreal General Campus.

OOMMEN, Samuel P; Sudbury Reg Hosp-Laurentian, 41 Ramsey Lake Rd, Sudbury ON P3E 5J1; Man'93; BSc; CCFP; CCFP(E.M.); Assoc Staff, Health Sciences North-St Joseph's Health Centre; Assoc Staff, Health Sciences North - Memorial Site; Assoc Staff, Health Sciences North-Laurentian Site; (705)688-3735

OOSMAN, Farook N; Hawkwood Village Med Clinic, 20-217 Hawksbrow Dr NW, Calgary AB T3G 3K2; Cardiff (Wales)'67; MB ChB; FFARCS; Langs: English; French; (403)777-2757; Fax. (403)777-2755; fno@shaw.ca.

OOSMAN, Jodie J; 451 Marsh Rd NE, Calgary AB T2E 5B2; Sask'96; BSc(Anatomy); FRCPC; Psy (General Adult Psychiatry). Consultant Psychiatrist, Mahoney, Coleman & Assoc; Consultant Psychiatrist, Citta Psychological Services; (403)264-6886; Fax. (403)264-6889.

OOSTENBRINK, Jacob; Chilliwack Gen Hosp, 45600 Menholm Rd, Chilliwack BC V2P 1P7; Orange Free State (South Africa)'95; MB ChB; Staff Emerg & Anes, Chilliwack General Hospital; (604)795-4141

OOSTERHOLT, Adrian; 201-6411 Nelson Ave, Burnaby BC V5H 4H3; Tor'81; (604)451-4100; Fax. (604)451-4101.

OOSTHUIZEN, Annelie; PO Box 174 Stn Del Centre, Yorkton SK S3N 2V7; Orange Free State (South Africa)'84; MB ChB; (306)782-2444; Fax. (306)783-2220.

OOSTHUIZEN, Jacobus F; 9805 103 St PO Box 130, Sexsmith AB T0H 3C0; (South Africa)'84; MB ChB; (780)568-2277; Fax. (780)568-2299.

OOSTHUIZEN, James H; Westend Med Clinic, 496 Topsail Rd, St. John's NL A1E 2C2; Pretoria (South Africa)'91; MB ChB; (709)747-1110

OOSTHUIZEN, Jean F M; Cariboo Mem Hosp, 401-517 Sixth Ave N, Williams Lake BC V2G 2G8; Pretoria (South Africa)'83; MB ChB; FRCSC; GenSurg. Staff, Cariboo Memorial Hospital and Health Centre; (250)392-4411; jean_oosthuizen@telus.net.

OOSTHUIZEN, Jean M; Appletree Clinic, 2573 Baseline Rd, Ottawa ON K2H 7B3; Pretoria (South Africa)'87; MB ChB; LMCC; CCFP; Langs: Afrikaans; (613)721-8630; Fax. (613)721-8643.

OOSTHUIZEN, Madeline; Tamarack Med Clinic, 191-1500 Cranbrook St N, Cranbrook BC V1C 3S8; Pretoria (South Africa)'97; (250)426-7724

OOSTHUIZEN, Petrus P E; St Paul Wellness Centre, PO Box 219 4909 50 Ave, St Paul AB T0A 3A0; (South Africa)'85; (780)645-4411

OOZEER, Yusuf; 1-1270 Walker Rd, Windsor ON N8Y 4T4; Wes'89; (519)977-9222; Fax. (519)977-9532.

OPALINSKI, Yvonne A V; Southlake Reg Hlth Centre, 596 Davis Dr, Newmarket ON L3Y 2P9; Tor'90; Staff, Southlake Regional Health Centre; Langs: Italian; Polish; (905)895-4521

OPATRNY, Lucie; St Mary's Hosp Centre, 3830 av Lacombe, Montreal QC H3T 1M5; McG'98; FRCPC; IntMed. Staff, St Mary's Hospital Centre; (514)345-3511

OPDAHL, Murray D; 109-294 Venture Cres, Saskatoon SK S7K 6M1; Sask'91; CCFP; (306)933-0755

OPENSHAW, David J; Carbonear Gen Hosp, 86 Highroad South, Carbonear NL A1Y 1A4; London (England)'59; MB BS; FRCA; DA; FRCPC; Anes (Anesthesia Surgery). Staff, Carbonear General Hospital; (709)945-5111; djopenshaw@yahoo.ca.

OPGENORTH, Andrea A; Heritage Med Research Centre, 362-107 University Campus NW, Edmonton AB T6G 2S2; Alb'95; PhD; FRCPC; IntMed (Endocrinology); Endocrin&Metab. Clinical Asst Prof, University of Alberta; (780)407-3636; Fax. (780)407-6702.

OPHEL, Judith M; Labrador Grenfell Health, PO Box 7000 Stn C 227 Hamilton River Rd, Happy-Valley-Goose NL A0P 1C0; Qns'79; CCFP; FCFP; Physician, Labrador Health Centre; Clinical Asst Prof Family Med, Memorial University Of Newfoundland; (709)897-2000; Fax. (709)896-4607.

OPIE, J Anthony; Rosedale Med Group, 280 Queenston Rd, Hamilton ON L8K 1H1; Wes'62; CCFP; FCFP; Court Staff, Hamilton Health Sciences Centre - McMaster University Medical Centre; Court Staff, St Joseph's Healthcare - Charlton Campus; Clin Assoc Prof Family Med & Commun Base Res Training Prog, McMaster University; (905)547-0508; Fax. (905)547-6865.

OPIE, John W; St Joseph's Healthcare, 50 Charlton Ave E, Hamilton ON L8N 4A6; Wes'92; BSc(Biol.); CCFP; CCFP(E.M.); Staff Emerg Care, Hamilton Health Sciences Centre - Hamilton General Hospital; Staff, Hamilton Health Sciences Centre-Juravinski Site; Staff, St Joseph's Healthcare - Charlton Campus; (905)522-1155; Fax. (905)521-6017.

OPITZ, Silke A; Valley Reg Hosp, 150 Exhibition St, Kentville NS B4N 5E3; (Germany)'92; Staff, Valley Regional Hospital; (902)678-7381

OPONDO, Johnmark O; Saskatoon Health Region, 101-310 Idylwyld Dr N, Saskatoon SK S7L 0Z2; Nairobi (Kenya)'89; MB ChB; MPH; Med Officer of Hlth, Saskatoon Health Region Saskatoon Public Health; (306)655-4338; Fax. (306)655-4414; johnmark.opondo@saskatoonhealthregion.ca.

OPPEL, Lloyd B; UBC Hospital, 2211 Wesbrook Mall, Vancouver BC V6T 2B5; UBC'88; CCFP; CCFP(E.M.); FCFP; Staff Urgent Care Centre, UBC Hospital - Koerner Pavillion; (604)822-7662; Fax. (604)822-7573.

OPPENHEIMER, Lawrence W; The Ottawa Hosp-Gen Campus, 8424-501 Smyth Rd, Ottawa ON K1H 8L6; London (England)'80; FRCS; FSOGC(Eng); MA(Oxon); FRCOG; FRCSC; ObstGyn (Maternal Fetal Medicine). Site Leader Obst, The Ottawa Hospital - General Campus; Prof/Head Div of Maternal Fetal Med, University of Ottawa; (613)737-8564 x8055; Fax. (613)737-8070; loppenheimer@ottawahospital.on.ca.

OPPENHEIMER, Luis; Winnipeg Reg Health Authority, 4F-650 Main St, Winnipeg MB R3B 1E2; Barcelona (Spain)'69; PhD; FRCSC; GenSurg (Critical Care Medicine). (204)926-7000; Fax. (204)926-7007; loppenheimer@wrha.mb.ca.

OPPER, David B; Brant Community HC-Brantford, 200 Terrace Hill St, Brantford ON N3R 1G9; Man'83; CCFP; FCFP; Ac Staff, The Brant Community Healthcare System - Brantford General Hospital Site; Ac Staff, The Brant Community Healthcare System - Willett Hospital Site; Examiner Civil Aviation, Rural Ontario Medical Program & Preceptor-ROMP; Clin Teacher, McMaster University; Langs: English; French; (519)751-5544 x2338; Fax. (519)751-5548.

OPPERMAN, Estelle M; Medicine Hat Reg Hosp, 666 5 St SW, Medicine Hat AB T1A 4H6; (South Africa)'94; Staff, Medicine Hat Regional Hospital; (403)529-8000; Fax. (403)529-8044.

OPREA, Petra; York Medical Green Lane, RR1 Lcd 1 18120 Yonge St, Newmarket ON L3Y 4V8; University of Medicine & Pharmacy (Other Foreign)'98; CCFP; (905)868-9243

OPRIS, Alexandru A F; 404-1240 Bay St, Toronto ON M5R 2A7; Cluj (Romania)'66; Ac Staff, St Joseph's Health Centre; Med Dir, Yorkville Vein Clinic; Langs: Romanian; Italian; French; (416)927-0533; Fax. (416)927-8897; yvc@live.ca.

OPRYSZCZKO, Krzysztof; The Group Health Centre, 240 McNabb St E, Sault Ste. Marie ON P6B 1Y5; (Poland)'00; CCFP; (705)759-1234

OPTHOF, Nick P; Annapolis Valley Health, 15 Chipman Dr, Kentville NS B4N 3V7; Dal'06; CCFP; nick.opthof@hotmail.com.

OPYR, Oksana; Winston Park Family Physicians, 104-2315 Bristol Cir, Oakville ON L6H 6P8; Danylo Halytsky Lviv State Med Univ (Ukraine)'97; CCFP; (905)829-2826; Fax. (905)829-2846.

ORAIF, Ayman M K; London HSC-University Hosp, PO Box 5339 Stn B 339 Windermere Rd, London ON N6A 5A5; Jeddah (Saudi Arabia)'03; FRCSC; ObstGyn. Staff, London Health Sciences Centre - University Hospital; (519)685-8500

ORAVEC, Michael; Medical Sciences Bldg, 372 King St W, Oshawa ON L1J 2J9; McG'75; FRCPC; Gastroent; IntMed. Staff Gastroent, Lakeridge Health - Oshawa Site; (905)721-1221; Fax. (905)721-8564.

ORBECK, Kenneth W; 200-1500 Bank St, Ottawa ON K1H 7Z2; Alb'64; LMCC; Ac Staff, Children's Hospital of Eastern Ontario (CHEO); Ac Staff, The Ottawa Hospital - Riverside Campus; (613)738-7660; Fax. (613)738-8614.

ORBINSKI, James J; St Michael's Hosp, 30 Bond St, Toronto ON M5B 1W8; McM'89; BSc(Hons.); Staff, St Michael's Hospital; (416)867-3712; Fax. (416)867-3739.

ORCHARD, Basil C L; Credit Valley Med Arts Centre, 514-2000 Credit Valley Rd, Mississauga ON L5M 4N4; Tor'61; DPsy; FRCPC; Psy (Genal Psychiatry). Ac Staff, The Credit Valley Hospital; (905)828-4333; Fax. (905)828-4333.

ORDEAN, Alice; St Joseph's Health Centre, 30 The Queensway, Toronto ON M6R 1B5; Tor'98; MHSc; CCFP; FCFP; Staff, St Joseph's Health Centre; (416)530-6860; Fax. (416)530-5160.

ORDON, Michael; 9103Q-61 Queen St E, Toronto ON M5C 2T2; Tor'05; FRCSC; Urol.

ORELLANA-JORDAN, Edwin R; Medicine Hat Reg Hosp, 666 5 St SW, Medicine Hat AB T1A 4H6; (Guatemala)'83; Staff, Medicine Hat Regional Hospital; Langs: Spanish; (403)529-8053

ORENSTEIN, Teddi L; Richmond Health Science Ctre, 750-6091 Gilbert Rd, Richmond BC V7C 5L9; Tor'86; FRCPC; IntMed; Cardiol. Staff, Richmond Hospital; (604)273-1555; Fax. (604)273-2969.

OREOPOULOS, George D; Univ Hlth Network-Toronto Gen, 6EN 214-200 Elizabeth St, Toronto ON M5G 2C4; Tor'96; MSc; FRCSC; GenSurg; VascSurg. Staff, Toronto General Hospital - UHN; (416)340-3275; Fax. (416)340-5029.

ORFALI, Charles G; Clin Chirurgie Plastique et Es, 260-437 rue King E, Sherbrooke QC J1G 1B7; Alexandria (Egypt)'68; CSPQ; FRCSC; PlasSurg (Aesthetic Surgery). adj Chef chir gén, Centre Hospitalier Universitaire de Sherbrooke-Hôpital Hôtel-Dieu; Prof Pastic Surg, Universite de Sherbrooke; Langs: English; French; Arabic; (819)563-9313; Fax. (819)563-9314.

ORFALY, Roland; Royal Columbian Hosp, 330 Columbia St E, New Westminster BC V3L 3W7; McG'96; FRCPC; Anes (Critical Care Medicine). Staff, Royal Columbian Hospital; Clin Instructor, University of British Columbia; (604)520-4602; rorfaly@shaw.ca.

ORFI, Ezel F; Chalmers Gate Med Bldg, 309-328 Highway 7 E, Richmond Hill ON L4B 3P7; Dublin (Ireland)'57; DMRD(Eng); LRCPSI; FRCPC; DiagRad. Langs: Turkish; (905)731-4001; Fax. (905)731-1458.

ORFI, Jan N E; Oakville Med Centre, 300 1-690 Dorval Dr, Oakville ON L6K 3W7; London (England)'88; MB BS; FRCPC; IntMed; Cardiol. Court Staff, Trillium Health Centre - West Toronto; Staff Cardiol, Halton Healthcare Services Corporation - Oakville Site; (905)849-4567 x6; Fax. (905)338-3607.

ORGAN SHIN, Jennifer L; 509-2000 Credit Valley Rd, Mississauga ON L5M 4N4; Tor'02; FRCPC; IntMed; Gastroent. (905)607-9926

ORGANEK, Andrew J; Scarborough Hosp-General Div, 3050 Lawrence Ave E, Scarborough ON M1P 2V5; Tor'06; CCFP; CCFP(E.M.); Staff, The Scarborough Hospital - General Campus; (416)431-8200

ORGANOWSKI, Slawomir; Foothills Med Centre, 1403 29 St NW, Calgary AB T2N 2T9; Wroclaw (Poland)'78; FRCPC; Anes. Staff, Foothills Medical Centre; (403)944-1430; Fax. (403)944-2425.

ORHADJE, Charles; Tisdale Med Clinic, PO Box 1510, Tisdale SK S0E 1T0; (306)873-4561; Fax. (306)873-4489.

ORIEE, Mandhira I; Prince Albert Community Clinic, 110 8th St E, Prince Albert SK S6V 0V7; (South Africa)'00; MB ChB; (306)763-6464; Fax. (306)763-2101; mandhira.orice@gmail.com.

ORKIN, Aaron M; Groves Mem Community Hosp, 235 Union St E, Fergus ON N1M 1W3; McM'07; CCFP; Staff, Groves Memorial Community Hospital.

ORLICKA, Katarzyna; CHUM-Hop Notre-Dame, 1560 rue Sherbrooke E, Montreal QC H2L 4M1; Mon'06; FRCPC; IntMed; Gastroent. Staff, Centre Hospitalier l'Université de Montréal (CHUM) - Hôpital Notre-Dame; (514)890-8000

ORLIK, Benjamin C; IWK Health Centre, PO Box 9700 Rpo Csc 5850-5980 University Ave, Halifax NS B3K 6R8; Dal'05; FRCSC; OrthSurg. Staff, IWK Health Centre; (902)470-7245; Fax. (902)470-7341.

ORLIK, Herbert; IWK Health Centre, PO Box 9700 Rpo CSC 5850-5980 University Ave, Halifax NS B3K 6R8; UBC'66; FRCPC; Psy (Child & Adolescent Psychiatry). Ac Staff, IWK Health Centre; Consultant, Cumberland Regional Health Care Center; Assoc Prof Psy, Dalhousie University; (902)470-8375; Fax. (902)470-8937.

ORLIK, Jason R; Dartmouth Gen Hosp, 325 Pleasant St, Dartmouth NS B2Y 4G8; Dal'09; CCFP; CCFP(E.M.); Staff, Dartmouth General Hospital; (902)465-8491; Fax. (902)460-4148.

ORLUP, Gerard; Clinique Bois-de-Boulogne, 1575 boul Henri-Bourassa O, Montreal QC H3M 3A9; McG'82; CCFP; FCFP; Staff, Hôpital du Sacre-Coeur de Montréal; (514)338-2383; Fax. (514)338-3155.

ORMISTON, John D; Transcona Med Clinic, 200-701 Regent Ave W, Winnipeg MB R2C 1S3; Man'88; BSc; Member Family Pract, Concordia General Hospital; (204)222-5221; Fax. (204)224-2053.

ORNER, Abraham I; Scarborough Hosp-General Div, 3050 Lawrence Ave E, Scarborough ON M1P 2V5; Tor'06; CCFP; Staff, The Scarborough Hospital - General Campus; (416)854-3435

ORNG, Kanitha; Integrated Wellness Med Centre, 4655 Central Blvd, Burnaby BC V5H 4J5; McG'10; MDCM; CCFP; (604)558-1175

ORNSTEIN, Amy E; IWK Health Centre, PO Box 9700 Rpo CSC 5850-5980 University Ave, Halifax NS B3K 6R8; McG'97; MDCM; FRCPC; Peds (Child Maltreatment). Staff, IWK Health Centre; Langs: French; (902)470-8222; Fax. (902)470-7761; amy.ornstein@iwk.nshealth.ca.

ORNSTEIN, David H; Six Point Radiology, 303-5353 Dundas St W, Etobicoke ON M9B 6H8; McG'71; AB; FRCPC; DiagRad. Staff, Trillium Health Centre - West Toronto; (416)231-3369

ORNSTEIN, Melanie P; 311-658 Danforth Ave, Toronto ON M4J 5B9; Tor'96; BSc; MA(Educ); FRCSC; ObstGyn (Pediatric Gynecology). Staff ObstGyn, Toronto East General Hospital Inc; Prof, University of Toronto; (416)466-2360; Fax. (416)466-5076.

OROVAN, William L; St Joseph's Healthcare, 839-50 Charlton Ave E, Hamilton ON L8N 4A6; McM'75; AB; FACS; FRCSC; Urol (Surgical Oncology). Staff Surg, St Joseph's Healthcare - Charlton Campus; Dept Head Surg, McMaster University; (905)529-3313; Fax. (905)540-6580; orovanw@mcmaster.ca.

OROVEC, Natalie M; 201-15 Mountain Ave S, Stoney Creek ON L8G 2V6; Ott'98; BSc; FRCPC; Peds. Ac Staff, Hamilton Health Sciences Centre - Hamilton General Hospital; Staff, St Joseph's Healthcare - Charlton Campus; Asst Prof, McMaster University; (905)664-9992; Fax. (905)664-9910; norovec@sympatico.ca.

OROZ, Budimka; Riverside South Med Ctre, C-665 Earl Armstrong Rd, Gloucester ON K1V 2G2; (Bosnia-Herzegovina)'89; CCFP; (613)822-0411; Fax. (613)822-1399.

ORQUIN, Jacqueline; Hôpital Ste-Justine, 3175 ch Cote-Sainte-Catherine, Montreal QC H3T 1C5; Paris (France)'67; AddicMed; Ophth (Electrodiagnostic). Chef opthal, Hôpital Ste-Justine; adj Prof, Universite de Montreal; Langs: Spanish; English; (514)345-4931 x5963; jacqueline_orquin@ssss.gouv.qc.ca.

ORR, Alexandra R; Ctr Hosp Reg Chisasibi, CP 250, Chisasibi QC J0M 1E0; McG'10; MDCM; CCFP; Staff, Cree Board of Health & Social Services James Bay; (819)855-2844

ORR, Andrew C; Queen Elizabeth II HSC, 2035-1276 South Park St, Halifax NS B3H 2Y9; Mem'86; FRCSC; Ophth. Staff Nova Scotia Eye Care Centre, Queen Elizabeth II Health Sciences Centre - Victoria General Site; (902)473-1483; Fax. (902)473-2839.

ORR, Darin C; 2931 20 Ave S, Lethbridge AB T1K 3M5; Man'10; CCFP; (403)328-2326; Fax. (403)327-0123.

ORR, James F; 206-1370 Dundas St E, Mississauga ON L4Y 4G4; Qns'71; FACS; FRCSC; GenSurg; VascSurg. Ac Staff, Trillium Health Centre - Mississauga; (905)949-0344; Fax. (905)803-9094.

ORR, Jessica N; Crowfoot Village Fam Practice, 210-600 Crowfoot Cres NW, Calgary AB T3G 0B4; Alb'04; CCFP; (403)239-9733; Fax. (403)241-8112.

ORR, Pamela H; Health Sciences Centre, GG443-820 Sherbrook St, Winnipeg MB R3A 1R9; Tor'78; MSc(CommunMed); FRCPC; IntMed; InfectDis. Att Physician, Health Sciences Centre; Prof, University of Manitoba; (204)787-7029; Fax. (204)787-3159; porr@hsc.mb.ca.

ORR, Richard J; 1360 20th St E RR 1 Stn Main, Owen Sound ON N4K 5N3; Wes'91; BSc; FRCSC; Ophth. Staff, Grey Bruce Health Services - Owen Sound; (519)371-8096; Fax. (519)371-5631.

ORR, Suzanne A; Mainstreet Med Services, 4929 50 Ave, Lacombe AB T4L 1K3; Queen's (Ireland)'79; MB ChB; BAO; Staff Emer Dept, Lacombe Hospital & Care Centre; (403)782-6717; Fax. (403)782-4240; msms@telusplanet.net.

ORR, Thomas; 10018 Fifth St, Sidney BC V8L 2X9; Glasgow (Scotland)'60; MB ChB; Med Advisor, Medical Services Branch BC; Med Advisor, Insured Health & Hearing Services YT; (250)655-4755; t.p.orr@telus.net.

ORR, W Malcolm; Medical-Dental Bldg, 403-1120 Yates St, Victoria BC V8V 3M9; Qns'78; FRCSC; Ophth. Staff, Vancouver Island Health Authority; (250)388-6404; Fax. (250)384-6813.

ORR, Wesley D L; Chinook Reg Hosp, 960 19 St S, Lethbridge AB T1J 1W5; Alb'00; CCFP; CCFP(E.M.); Staff, Chinook Regional Hospital; (403)388-6301

ORRANTIA, Eliseo; Marathon Family Health Team, PO Box 399 22 Peninsula Rd, Marathon ON P0T 2E0; McM'93; CCFP; FCFP; Langs: Spanish; (807)229-3243; Fax. (807)229-2672.

ORRELL, Kevin G S; Health Park, 301-45 Weatherbee Rd, Mira Road NS B1M 0A1; Dal'81; FRCSC; OrthSurg (Joint Arthroplasty). Associate OrthSurg, Cape Breton Healthcare Complex; (902)539-1188; Fax. (902)539-8330.

ORRELL, Liam F M; Sydney Family Practice, 196 Kings Rd, Sydney NS B1S 1A1; Dal'84; (902)567-0030; Fax. (902)539-9250.

ORROM, William J; Richmond Med Bldg, 302-2020 Richmond Rd, Victoria BC V8R 6R5; Qns'81; ABGenSurg; ABCRS; FRCSC; GenSurg (Colon & Rectal Surgery). (250)592-4313

ORSER, Beverley A; Sunnybrook Hlth Sciences Ctre, 2075 Bayview Ave, Toronto ON M4N 3M5; Qns'81; PhD; FRCPC; Anes. Staff Anes, Sunnybrook Health Sciences Centre; Member, Institute of Safe Medication Practices Canada; Prof Dept of Physiol, University of Toronto; (416)480-4864; Fax. (416)480-6039.

ORSINI, Silvia A; 1-1261 Beaverbrook Ave, London ON N6H 0G6; Ott'00; HBSc; CCFP; Aj Prof Family Med, University of Western Ontario; (519)432-4107; Fax. (519)432-6921.

ORSINO, Angelina; Holland Bloorview Kids Rehab, 150 Kilgour Rd, Toronto ON M4G 1R8; Tor'01; FRCPC; Peds (Developmental Pediatrics). Staff, Holland Bloorview Kids Rehabilitation Hospital; (416)425-6220 x3905; Fax. (416)424-3837.

ORTAASLAN, Sevan G; 201-17001 Rte Trans-Canada, Kirkland QC H9H 5J1; McG'92; FRCSC; OrthSurg. Langs: Armenian; English; (514)426-1000; Fax. (514)426-1135.

ORTEGA, Gustavo A; 116-11910 111 Ave NW, Edmonton AB T5G 3G6; Salamanca (Spain)'69; FRCPC; Peds. Ac Staff, University of Alberta Hospital; Asst Prof, University of Alberta; (780)453-3883; Fax. (780)452-3364.

ORTEGA, Sarah J; Mackenzie Richmond Hill Hosp, 10 Trench St, Richmond Hill ON L4C 4Z3; McM'01; FRCSC; GenSurg. Staff, Mackenzie Richmond Hill Hospital; (905)918-0960; Fax. (905)918-0961.

ORTENBERG, June; MUHC-Montreal Children's Hosp, F 134-2300 rue Tupper, Montreal QC H3H 1P3; McG'83; FRCPC; Peds (Medical Genetics). Staff, McGill University Health Centre - Montreal Children's Hospital; adj Prof, McGill University; (514)412-4400 x22811; Fax. (514)412-4329.

ORTH, Michael J; Leduc Comm Hosp & Health Ctr, 4210 48 St, Leduc AB T9E 5Z3; Alb'97; CCFP; CCFP(E.M.); (780)986-7711

ORTH, Peter M R; Red Lake Med Associates, PO Box 311, Red Lake ON P0V 2M0; UBC'10; CCFP.

ORTIZ-ALVAREZ, Oliva; St Martha's Reg Hosp, 25 Bay St, Antigonish NS B2G 2G5; (Mexico)'84; MSc; FRCPC; Peds (Pediatric Rheumatology). Staff, St Martha's Regional Hospital; Langs: Spanish; (902)867-1417; Fax. (902)803-1186.

ORTIZ BEDOYA, Clara L; Alberta Children's Hosp, 2888 Shaganappi Trail NW, Calgary AB T3B 6A8; Bogota (Colombia)'85; Staff, Alberta Children's Hospital; (403)955-7211

ORTIZ-DOMINGUEZ, Tania A; Abbie J Lane Bldg, 4031-5909 Veterans Memorial La, Halifax NS B3H 2E2; (Mexico)'01.

ORTIZ-SINGH, Janice; Bram Centre Med Clinic, 16-7910 Hurontario St, Brampton ON L6Y 0P6; (289)752-1571; Fax. (289)752-6439.

ORTON, Robert B; St Joseph's Health Care, PO Box 5777 Stn B 268 Grosvenor St, London ON N6A 4V2; Wes'69; FACS; FRCSC; Ophth (Pediatric Ophthalmology). Staff, St Joseph's Hospital - St Joseph's Health Care; (519)685-8300

ORTON, Tanya D; St Paul's Hosp, 1081 Burrard St, Vancouver BC V6Z 1Y6; UBC'02; FRCSC; Ophth. Staff, Providence Health Care - St Paul's Hospital; (604)806-8168

ORTYNSKY, Garry B; North Vancouver Med Clinic, 115 16th St W, North Vancouver BC V7M 1T3; Sask'76; CCFP; (604)904-8804; Fax. (604)904-0972.

ORVOLD, Jason N; Saskatoon Cardiol Consultants, 920-606 Spadina Cres E, Saskatoon SK S7K 3H1; Sask'00; BSP; FRCPC; IntMed; Cardiol. Staff, Royal University Hospital; (306)655-6603; Fax. (306)655-1347.

ORYEMA, John U; Kennedy-Eglinton Med Centre, 2F-2416 Eglinton Ave E, Scarborough ON M1K 2P3; McM'84; (416)750-1222; Fax. (416)750-0751.

ORYSCHAK, Allan F; Rockyview Gen Hosp, 7007 14 St SW, Calgary AB T2V 1P9; Sask'69; MSc; FRCPC; AnatPath. Ac Staff, Rockyview General Hospital; Ac Staff, Peter Lougheed Centre; Ac Staff, Foothills Medical Centre; (403)943-3578; Fax. (403)943-3333.

ORZESZYNA, Magdalena M; MUHC-Montreal Gen Hosp, D16. 108-1650 av Cedar, Montreal QC H3G 1A4; McG'99; CCFP; Staff, McGill University Health Centre - Montreal General Campus; (514)934-1934

OSAK, Roberta; Pine Seven Office Park, 302-4610 Highway 7, Woodbridge ON L4L 4Y7; McG'90; FRCSC; ObstGyn. Staff ObstGyn, Mackenzie Richmond Hill Hospital; (905)707-5678; Fax. (905)264-7310.

OSBERG, Peter E; 1104-160 14th St E, North Vancouver BC V7L 2N3; Qns'74; BA; FRCSC; PlasSurg (Orthopedic Surgery). Ac Staff/Hd GenSurg, Lions Gate Hospital; (604)980-1211; Fax. (604)980-1525.

OSBORN, David D; 363 Rd 4 E, Kingsville ON N9Y 2E5; Wes'79; (519)733-5929

OSBORN, Jill A; St Paul's Hosp, 1081 Burrard St, Vancouver BC V6Z 1Y9; UBC'99; FRCPC; Anes. Staff, Providence Health Care - St Paul's Hospital; (604)806-8337

OSBORNE, Cynthia A; Thames Valley FHT-W London FH, 200-785 Wonderland Rd S, London ON N6K 1M6; Mem'86; Staff Family Med, St Joseph's Hospital - St Joseph's Health Care; (519)641-6712; Fax. (519)641-6189; cosborne@uwo.ca.

OSBORNE, Edward J; Professional Bldg, 3100-222 King St E, Bowmanville ON L1C 1P6; Tor'93; MSc; CCFP; FCFP; Staff, Lakeridge Health - Bowmanville Site; (905)623-2355; Fax. (905)623-9607.

OSBORNE, Gary; Bayridge Family Med Clinic, PO Box 20103 Taylor Kidd PO 775 Strand Blvd, Kingston ON K7P 2T6; McM'92; CCFP; FCFP; (613)507-1212; Fax. (613)507-1213.

OSBORNE, Penelope J; JPP2N 2449-910 10th Ave W, Vancouver BC V5Z 1M9; UBC'81; FRCPC; Anes. Ac Staff Anes, Vancouver General Hospital - Centennial Pavillion; Clinical Asst Prof, University of British Columbia; (604)875-4304

OSBORNE, Perry; Baie Verte Peninsula Hlth Ctr, GD, Baie Verte NL A0K 1B0; Mem'06; Staff, Baie Verte Peninsula Health Centre.

OSBORNE, Raymond J; Toronto Sunnybrook Reg Cancer, 2075 Bayview Ave, Toronto ON M4N 3M5; Tor'70; MBA; ObstGyn (Gynecologic Oncology). Ac Staff, Sunnybrook Health Sciences Centre; Staff, Women's College Hospital; Staff, St Michael's Hospital; Asst Prof, University of Toronto; (416)480-4026; Fax. (416)480-6002.

OSEGBUE, Emmanuel U; River City Family Clinic, 606-8600 Franklin Ave, Fort McMurray AB T9H 4G8; (South Africa)'90; DObst; MB BS; Staff, Northern Lights Regional Health Centre; (780)743-0444; Fax. (780)743-0455.

OSEI, William D; 1600 3rd Ave, Prince George BC V2L 3G6; (Ghana)'74; MB ChB; MPH; FACE; (250)565-7461; Fax. (250)565-2144.

OSEI-BONSU, Adelaide; Boyd Med Clinic, 392 Portage Ave, Winnipeg MB R3C 0C7; (204)415-2740

OSEI-TUTU, Davida; Foothills Med Centre, 1403 29 St NW, Calgary AB T2N 2T9; Alb'06; CCFP; Staff, Foothills Medical Centre; (403)944-2800; Fax. (403)283-7365.

OSEI-TUTU, Francis K; 4626 Park Ave, Terrace BC V8G 1V7; Tor'68; FRCSC; Urol. Staff, Kitimat Hospital & Health Centre; (250)635-4370; Fax. (250)635-7667.

OSEI-TUTU, Kannin; Foothills Med Centre, 1403 29 St NW, Calgary AB T2N 2T9; Dal'04; CCFP; Staff, Foothills Medical Centre; (403)944-1110

OSHRY, Ronald; Glenmore Landing, D167-1600 90 Ave SW, Calgary AB T2V 5A8; Witwatersrand (South Africa)'76; CCFP; (403)517-6084; Fax. (403)475-4420; ronoshry@shaw.ca.

OSILI, Maed; CSSS Les Eskers de l'Abitibi, 622 4e rue O, Amos QC J9T 2S2; (Syria)'02; MedOncol (P.Q.). Staff, CH Hôtel-Dieu d'Amos; (819)732-3341; Fax. (819)732-7054.

OSINCHUK, James W; Royal Alexandra Hosp, 10240 Kingsway NW, Edmonton AB T5H 3V9; Alb'78; BMedSci; FRCPC; Psy (Mental Health Act). Ac Staff Mental Health Services, Royal Alexandra Hospital; Clin Prof, University of Alberta; (780)735-4564; Fax. (780)735-4797; james.osinchuk@albertahealthservices.ca.

OSINGA, Christopher J; Taunton Surgical Centre, SS 201 1290 Keith Ross Dr, Oshawa ON L1H 7K4; Qns'95; FRCSC; OrthSurg. (905)721-8551; Fax. (905)721-6679.

OSINOWO, Adegboyega O; Cumberland Mental Hlth Service, 33 Havelock St, Amherst NS B4H 4W1; Univ of Lagos (Nigeria)'97; MB BS; (902)667-3879; Fax. (902)667-5959.

OSIOVICH, Horacio C; Children's & Women's HC of BC, 1R47-4480 Oak St, Vancouver BC V6H 3V4; Buenos Aires (Argentina)'81; FRCPC; Peds (Neonatal & Perinatal Medicine). Staff, BC Children's Hospital; (604)875-2135

OSKIN, O Alec; 701-10242 105 St NW, Edmonton AB T5J 3L5; Alb'00; (780)428-4524; Fax. (780)428-8904.

OSKOUI, Ahmad; Hop Louis-H Lafontaine, 7401 rue Hochelaga, Montreal QC H1N 3M5; Teheran (Iran)'63; FRCPC; Psy. Staff, Hopital Louis-H Lafontaine; (514)251-4000 x3006

OSKOUI, Maryam; MUHC-Montreal Children's Hosp, A 512-2300 rue Tupper, Montreal QC H3H 1P3; McG'99; FRCPC; Neur. Staff, McGill University Health Centre - Montreal Children's Hospital; (514)412-4466; Fax. (514)412-4373.

OSLER, Flordeliz G; 601-400 Tache Ave, Winnipeg MB R2H 3C3; Man'92; FRCSC; Otol.

OSMAN, Ebtihal; 3236 82 St NW, Edmonton AB T6K 3Y3; (Sudan)'01; CCFP; (780)761-3335

OSMAN, Fahima A; North York Gen Hosp, 4001 Leslie St, North York ON M2K 1E1; McM'04; FRCSC; GenSurg. Staff, North York General Hospital; (416)756-6444

OSMAN, Maisoon A; Univ of Alberta Hosp-SCC/WCM, 8440 112 St NW, Edmonton AB T6G 2B7; (Sudan)'98; Nephrol; IntMed. Staff, University of Alberta Hospital; (780)407-8822

OSMAN, Said; St Joseph's Health Care, PO Box 57777 Stn B 268 Grosvenor St, London ON N6A 4V2; Wes'95; FRCPC; DiagRad. Staff, St Joseph's Hospital - St Joseph's Health Care; (519)646-6035; sidosman@hotmail.com.

OSMAN, Samir; Polyclinique, 103-12905 rue Sherbrooke E, Pte-aux-Trembles QC H1A 1B9; Cairo (Egypt)'68; (514)498-4050; Fax. (514)498-8239.

OSMOND, Colette; PO Box 30006 Rpo South Park, Stony Plain AB T7Z 2Y8; Mem'97; FRCPC; Anes. Staff, Royal Alexandra Hospital; (780)418-7310

OSMOND, Martin H; Children's Hosp Eastern Ont, 401 Smyth Rd, Ottawa ON K1H 8L1; McG'86; FRCPC; Peds. Staff, Children's Hospital of Eastern Ontario (CHEO); (613)737-7600 x2318; Fax. (613)738-4885.

OSMUN, William E; Thames Valley Family Hlth Team, RR 5 22262 Mill Rd, Mount Brydges ON N0L 1W0; Wes'79; MClSc; CCFP; FCFP; Staff Family Med, Strathroy Middlesex General Hospital - Middlesex Hospital Alliance; Assoc Prof Family Med, University of Western Ontario; (519)264-2800; Fax. (519)264-2742; williamo@smhc.net.

OSORO, Beatrice K; Georgina Family Med Centre, 417 The Queensway S, Keswick ON L4P 2C7; (Russia (Federation))'02; CCFP; Langs: Russian; Swahili; (905)989-7800; Fax. (905)463-2871.

OSPINA, Luis H; Hôpital Ste-Justine, 3175 ch Cote-Sainte-Catherine, Montreal QC H3T 1C5; Pontificia (Colombia)'95; MD; Staff, Hôpital Ste-Justine; Langs: Spanish; French; (514)345-4715

OSPINA-ORDONEZ, Julian A; Pacific Spirit Community Hlth, 2110 43rd Ave W, Vancouver BC V6M 2E1; Valle (Colombia)'95; CCFP; Langs: Spanish; (604)261-6366; julian.ospina@hotmail.com.

OSSA ALEMPARTE, Juan; The Hosp for Sick Children, 555 University Ave, Toronto ON M5G 1X8; (Chile)'03; Staff, The Hospital For Sick Children; (416)813-6182

OSSENI, Fadel; CSSS de Laval, 1755 boul Rene-Laennec, Laval QC H7M 3L9; Mon'04; IntMed (Critical Care Medicine). Staff, Hopital de la Cite de la santé; (450)668-1010

OSSIP, Marc G; William Osler HC-Etobicoke, 101 Humber College Blvd, Etobicoke ON M9V 1R8; Tor'98; FRCPC; DiagRad. Staff, William Osler Health System - Etobicoke General Hospital; (416)747-3400

OSSWALD, Ivana G; Royal Court Med Centre, 211-5 Quarry Ridge Rd, Barrie ON L4M 7G1; Wes'05; FRCPC; Peds. Staff, Kingston General Hospital; (705)797-0800; Fax. (705)797-0900.

OSTAPENKO, Elena; Stoney Creek Med Walk-In Clin, 2A-140 Centennial Pky N, Hamilton ON L8E 1H9; McM'00; CCFP; Staff, Westdale Walk-In Clinic; (905)561-9255; Fax. (905)561-4391.

OSTAPKOWICZ, Eugenia; 3237 Fraser St, Vancouver BC V5V 4B8; Gdansk (Poland)'60; Vis Staff Privil, Providence Health Care - Mount Saint Joseph Hospital; Vis Staff Privil, Vancouver General Hospital - Centennial Pavillion; Langs: Polish; (604)875-9633

OSTASHKO, Sergiy; Hôpital régional Chaleur, 1750 Sunset Dr, Bathurst NB E2A 4L7; Donetsk (Ukraine)'85; Staff, Hopital Regional Chaleur; (506)544-3000

OSTBY, Randi A; Shuswap Lake Gen Hosp, PO Box 520 Stn Main 601 10th St NE, Salmon Arm BC V1E 4N6; UBC'96; BSc; CCFP; CCFP(E.M.); FCFP; Staff, Shuswap Lake General Hospital; (250)833-3600

OSTEN, Mark D; Univ Hlth Network-Toronto Gen, 6EN 238-200 Elizabeth St, Toronto ON M5G 2C4; McM'00; BSc; FRCPC; IntMed (Interventional Cardiology); Cardiol. Ac Staff Cardiol, Toronto General Hospital - UHN; (416)340-4615; Fax. (416)340-4144; mark.osten@uhn.on.ca.

OSTER, Adam; 1403 21 St NW, Calgary AB T2N 2M1; Cal'01; FRCPC; EmergMed. Staff, Foothills Medical Centre; (403)270-4520

OSTER, Eric; Centre Hosp Honore-Mercier, 2750 boul Laframboise, Saint-Hyacinthe QC J2S 4Y8; Laval'96; IntMed. Staff Internal Med, Centre Hospitalier Honore-Mercier; (450)771-3333; Fax. (450)771-3501.

OSTERMAN, John W; Service de Sante au Travail, 1515 boul Chomedey, Laval QC H7V 3Y7; McG'78; DSc(Environmental Healt; CSPQ; FRCPC; CommunMed (Musculoskeletal); Public Health & Preventive Med; OccupMed (P.Q.). Staff, Shriners Hospitals For Children - Canada; Staff, Hopital de la Cite de la santé; Staff, McGill University Health Centre - Montreal General Campus; Med Dir, Harvard Santex Health Inc; Langs: English; French; (450)978-8300 x3318; Fax. (450)978-8627; johnwosterman@hotmail.com.

OSTIC, Heather A; Cancer Ctr of Southeastern Ont, 25 King St W, Kingston ON K7L 5P9; Dal'95; CCFP; Assoc Staff, Kingston General Hospital; Staff, Cancer Centre of Southeastern Ontario; Clin Associate, Kingston Regional Cancer Centre; (613)544-2631 x4505; heather.ostic@krcc.on.ca.

OSTIGUY, Gaston L; MUHC-Montreal Chest Institute, 3650 rue Saint-Urbain, Montreal QC H2X 2P4; Mon'61; MSc; LMCC; Respir (P.Q.); IntMed (Public Health). Staff, McGill University Health Centre - Montreal Chest Institute; Pres, Pulmonary Disease Committee, CSST-Quebec; assoc Prof, McGill University; Langs: English; (514)934-1934 x32490; Fax. (514)843-2096.

OSTIGUY, Genevieve; Clinique Rockland MD, 110-100 ch Rockland, Mont-Royal QC H3P 2V9; Mon'99; MCFP; LMCC; CCFP; Médecin, Hydro-Quebec; Prof adj clin, Universite de Montreal; Langs: English; (514)667-3383; Fax. (514)667-3834.

OSTIGUY, Mario; Centre Med Pierre Boucher, 1615 boul Jacques-Cartier E, Longueuil QC J4M 2X1; Mon'86; Staff, Hôpital Brome-Missisquoi-Perkins; (450)468-6223

OSTIGUY, Nadine P; Aim Health Group, 22B-550 Terminal Ave, Ottawa ON K1G 0Z3; McG'94; CCFP; (613)731-4770; Fax. (613)731-4979.

OSTIGUY, Richard; Ctr Hosp Fleury, 2180 rue Fleury E, Montreal QC H2B 1K3; Sher'80; FRCPC; Gastroent. Staff, Centre Hospitalier Fleury; Langs: Bilingual(French/English); (514)384-2000

OSTIGUY, Therese; CSSS de Memphremagog, 50 rue Saint-Patrice E, Magog QC J1X 3X3; Sher'80; Staff, Centre Hospitalier et CLSC de Memphremagog; (819)843-2572; Fax. (819)868-3248.

OSTOLOSKY, Lara J; University of Alberta Hosp, 1E7 26-8440 112 St NW, Edmonton AB T6G 2B7; Alb'98; FRCPC; Psy (Eating Disorders). Staff, University of Alberta Hospital; Clin Teacher Psy, University of Alberta; (780)407-1855; Fax. (780)407-6672.

OSTRANDER, John J; Grey Bruce HS-Owen Sound, PO Box 1800 Stn Main 1800 8th St E, Owen Sound ON N4K 6M9; Wes'68; FRCPC; IntMed (Neurology). Staff, Grey Bruce Health Services - Owen Sound; (519)371-2125; Fax. (519)371-2126.

OSTRO, Michael J; Credit Valley Prof Bldg, 414-2300 Eglinton Ave W, Mississauga ON L5M 2V8; Tor'79; FRCPC; IntMed; Gastroent. Staff, The Credit Valley Hospital; (905)828-9998; Fax. (905)820-6361; michael.ostro@sympatico.ca.

OSTRO, Michael; 101-160 Dundas St E, Mississauga ON L5A 1W4; Tor'76; Staff, Norfolk General Hospital; Ac Staff, Mount Sinai Hospital; Ac Staff, Trillium Health Centre - Mississauga; Langs: Hebrew; Yiddish; (905)273-3777; Fax. (905)277-9882.

OSTROFF, Shirley J; Oakdale Med Bldg, 403-2065 Finch Ave W, North York ON M3N 2V7; Tor'83; BSc; PhD; Ac Staff, Humber River Regional Hospital - Finch Avenue Site; (416)744-4242; Fax. (416)743-2858.

OSTROW, David N; Gordon & Leslie Diamond HCC, 2775 Laurel St, Vancouver BC V5Z 1M9; Man'68; FCCP; FACP; MA; FRCPC; IntMed (Respirology). Ac Staff, Vancouver General Hospital - Centennial Pavillion; Physician, The Lung Centre; Pres/CEO, Vancouver Coastal Health; Staff, Gordon & Leslie Diamond Health Care Centre; Prof Med, University of British Columbia; (604)875-4122; Fax. (604)875-4695; david.ostrow@vch.ca.

OSTROW, Olivia A; The Hosp for Sick Children, 555 Unviersity Ave, Toronto ON M5G 1X8; (USA)'02; Staff, The Hospital For Sick Children; (416)813-1500

OSTROWSKA, Krystyna I; Trillium Hlth Ctr-Mississauga, 100 Queensway W, Mississauga ON L5B 1B8; Wroclaw (Poland)'81; FRCPC; IntMed; MedMicrobiol; InfectDis. Staff Lab & InfectDis Specialist, Trillium Health Centre - Mississauga; Staff, The Credit Valley Hospital; Langs: Polish; (905)848-7472; Fax. (905)804-7995; kostrowska@thc.on.ca.

OSTROWSKI, John D; Portage Prof Bldg, 301-5400 Portage Rd, Niagara Falls ON L2G 5X7; Ott'90; BSc; OrthSurg. Staff OrthSurg, Niagara Health System - Greater Niagara General Site; Court Staff OrthSurg, Niagara Health System - Welland Hospital Site; (905)356-8333; Fax. (905)356-1702; jostrow@vaxxine.com.

OSTROWSKI, Leisha N; Highlands Health Network, 140 Rolling Hills Dr, Orangeville ON L9W 4X8; McM'02; CCFP; Physician, Headwaters Health Care Centre - Orangeville Site; (519)941-7575; Fax. (519)941-7060.

OSTROWSKI, Mario; St Michael's Hosp, 4CC 180-30 Bond St, Toronto ON M5B 1W8; Wes'84; FRCPC; AnatPath; InfectDis; IntMed. Staff, St Michael's Hospital; (416)864-5568; Fax. (416)864-5310; m.ostrowski@utoronto.ca.

OSTRY, Avrum J; St Paul's Hosp, 1081 Burrard St, Vancouver BC V6Z 1Y6; UBC'85; FRCPC; GenPath. Staff, Providence Health Care - St Paul's Hospital; (604)806-8216

OSTRY, Carol J; Sea Cove Med Clinic, 201-1757 Beaufort Ave, Comox BC V9M 1R8; Alb'87; (250)339-5335; Fax. (250)339-1898.

OSUCH, Elizabeth A; London HSC FEMAP, 860 Richmond St, London ON N6A 3H8; Michigan State(MI) (USA)'93; FRCPC; Psy. Staff, London Health Sciences Centre - University Hospital; (519)646-6000; Fax. (519)646-6211.

OSUNDWA, Vincent M; Associated Engineering Plaza, 101-10909 Jasper Ave NW, Edmonton AB T5J 3L9; Nairobi (Kenya)'76; MB ChB; DABPed; MPH; ClinImmunol&Allergy; Peds. Staff, Covenant Health - Grey Nuns Community Hospital; Staff, Covenant Health - Misericordia Community Hospital; Langs: Swahili; (780)425-3400; osundwa@telusplanet.net.

OSUSZEK, Andrew R; Whitby Med Arts Imaging, X17-1615 Dundas St E, Whitby ON L1N 2L1; Tor'73; FRCPC; DiagRad (Diagnostic Imaging). Ac Staff, Humber River Regional Hospital - Finch Avenue Site; Court Staff, Lakeridge Health - Whitby Site; (905)576-9729; Fax. (905)438-9729.

OSWALD, Angus; Amherstburg Walk In Clinic, 71 Sandwich St, Amherstburg ON N9V 1Z5; St. Andrews (Scotland)'63; MB ChB; DA; Staff, Hôtel-Dieu Grace Hospital; Staff, Windsor Regional Hospital - Tayfour Site; (519)736-8046

OSWALD, Anna E; Heritage Med Research Centre, 562-107 University Campus NW, Edmonton AB T6G 2S2; Alb'00; FRCPC; IntMed; Rheum. (780)407-7546; Fax. (780)407-6055.

OSWALD, Kevin M; Lake Country Family Practice, 1-9966 Pollard Rd, Winfield BC V4V 1Z4; Qns'84; CCFP; FCFP; (250)766-3938; Fax. (250)766-5231.

OSWALD, Ronald E; Edmonton Mental Health Clinic, 9942 108 St NW, Edmonton AB T5K 2J5; Alb'00; FRCPC; Psy. (780)427-4444; Fax. (780)425-9317.

OTA, Kaede; The Hosp for Sick Children, 555 University Ave, Toronto ON M5G 1X8; McM'01; FRCPC; Peds; MedMicrobiol; InfectDis. Staff, The Hospital For Sick Children; (416)442-8920

OTAKY, Naim F; Centre Med Ville-Marie, 1000-1538 rue Sherbrooke O, Montreal QC H3G 1L5; McG'98; FRCSC; GenSurg. (514)933-2778

OTANI, Christine M L; Packham Avenue Med Clinic, 104-335 Packham Ave, Saskatoon SK S7N 4S1; Alb'01; CCFP; Staff Family Med, Royal University Hospital; (306)651-7091; Fax. (306)651-7092.

OTANI, Robert K; Packham Avenue Med Clinic, 104-335 Packham Ave, Saskatoon SK S7N 4S1; Alb'00; BSc; FRCPC; DiagRad. Staff, Royal University Hospital; (306)651-7091; Fax. (306)717-4718; robert.otani@saskatoonhealthregion.ca.

OTERO FUENTES, Carmen G; Hamilton HS-McMaster Site, PO Box 2000 Stn Lcd 1 1200 Main St W, Hamilton ON L8N 3Z5; Chile (Chile)'92; Staff, Hamilton Health Sciences Centre - McMaster University Medical Centre; (905)521-2100

OTIS, Daniel; GMF Centre de sante, 3745 rue Georges Couture, Drummondville QC J2B 7P4; (819)477-2231; Fax. (819)477-1122.

OTIS, Gilles; GMF Centre de santé, 3745 rue Georges-Couture, Drummondville QC J2B 7P4; Sher'79; CCFP; FCFP; Boursier CMFC, Hôpital Sainte-croix; adj Prof, Universite de Sherbrooke; (819)477-2231; Fax. (819)477-1122.

OTITOJU, Chinyere; Avon Med Centre, 2781 Avonhurst Dr, Regina SK S4R 3J3; Saba (Netherlands Antilles)'05; (306)543-4955; Fax. (306)545-7006.

OTLEY, Anthony R; IWK Health Centre, PO Box 9700 Rpo CSC 5850-5980 University Ave, Halifax NS B3K 6R8; Tor'91; FRCPC; Peds (Gastroenterology). Staff, IWK Health Centre; Assoc Prof, Dalhousie University; (902)470-8746; Fax. (902)470-7249.

OTOO, Andrew A; 101-2346 Kingston Rd, Scarborough ON M1N 1V2; Birmingham (England)'65; MRCP; MRCS; LRCP; DCH; Med Dir, Craiglee Nursing Home; (416)264-3268; Fax. (416)264-4755.

OTREMBA, Mirek; Mount Sinai Hosp, 431-600 University Ave, Toronto ON M5G 1X5; Tor'96; BSc(Biol.); FRCPC; IntMed (Diabetes). Staff, Mount Sinai Hospital; Asst Prof, University of Toronto; Langs: Polish; (416)586-4800; Fax. (416)586-3186; motremba@mtsinai.on.ca.

OTRUBA, Zdenek; Penticton Reg Hosp, 550 Carmi Ave, Penticton BC V2A 3G6; Tor'86; FRCPC; Anes. Staff, Penticton Regional Hospital; (250)492-4000

OTT, Carol L B; Applewood Shopping Centre, 210-1077 North Service Rd, Mississauga ON L4Y 1E1; Man'04; FRCPC; IntMed; GeriatricMed. Staff, Women's College Hospital; Staff, Baycrest Centre for Geriatric Care; (905)273-9009

OTT, Michael C; London HSC-Victoria Hosp, PO Box 5010 Stn B 800 Commissioners Rd E, London ON N6A 5W9; Wes'01; FRCSC; GenSurg. Staff, London Health Sciences Centre - Victoria Campus; (519)685-8260

OTT, Monica S; Maj Gen George R Pearkes Bldg, 101 Colonel By Dr, Ottawa ON K1A 0K2; Mem'06; CCFP; CCFP(E.M.); (613)992-2481

OTT-BRASCHI, Sylvie; CHUM-Hotel-Dieu, 4 413-3840 rue St-Urbain, Montreal QC H2W 1T8; Nantes (France)'93; Staff, Hull Hospital; Staff, Centre Hospitalier l'Université de Montréal (CHUM) - Hôtel-Dieu; Teach Staff, University of Ottawa; Langs: English; (514)890-8000; sylvie.ott.braschi.chum@ssss.gouv.qc.ca.

OTTAWAY, Clifford; St Michael's Hosp, 30 Bond St, Toronto ON M5B 1W8; Tor'73; PhD; FRCPC; IntMed (Gastroenterology). Ac Staff Gastroent, St Michael's Hospital; Assoc Prof, University of Toronto; (416)864-5684; Fax. (416)864-5882; ottawayc@smh.toronto.on.ca.

OTTE, Jessica A; Medical Arts Centre, 103-650 Terminal Ave S, Nanaimo BC V9R 5E2; UBC'09; CCFP; (250)753-3431

OTTEM, Derek P; 410-175 Second Ave, Kamloops BC V2C 5W1; UBC'03; FRCSC; Urol. (250)851-4475

OTTLEY, Linda L; Lansdowne Prof Bldg, 310-1641 Hillside Ave, Victoria BC V8T 5G1; Alb'72; Staff, Vancouver Island Health Authority; Ac Staff, Victoria General Hospital; Ac Staff, Royal Jubilee Hospital; (250)592-5312; Fax. (250)592-5910.

OTTO, Anthony G; 3237 Fraser St, Vancouver BC V5V 4B8; Manchester (England)'70; MB ChB; MScHealth Informatics; Langs: Polish; (604)874-0252; Fax. (604)879-1502; aotto@drotto.net.

OTTO, Catherine E; 8425 83 St NW, Edmonton AB T6C 2Z2; Alb'98; CCFP; FCFP; (780)989-3289; Fax. (780)466-3043.

OTTO, David D; 200-8225 105 St NW, Edmonton AB T6E 4H2; Alb'88; FRCSC; OrthSurg (Knee Surgery). Staff, Covenant Health - Grey Nuns Community Hospital; Staff, Royal Alexandra Hospital; Dir Orth Surg, University of Alberta; (780)439-5858; Fax. (780)433-1344.

OTTO, George W; 3-2111 Jane St, North York ON M3M 1A2; McM'84; Langs: Swahili; (416)241-0515; Fax. (416)241-4318.

OTTO, Johan F; Smith Clinic, 1-6601 48 Ave, Camrose AB T4V 3G8; Pretoria (South Africa)'88.

OTTO, Patrick W; Upper Grand Family Health Team, LL-205 Queen St E, Fergus ON N1M 1T2; Cal'82; BSc; CCFP; FCFP; Chief Medical Staff, Groves Memorial Community Hospital; Asst Clin Prof, McMaster University; (519)787-1200; Fax. (519)787-1803.

OTUKOYA, Folorunsho; 277 Bradbrooke Dr, Yorkton SK S3N 3L3; (306)782-6333; Fax. (306)782-6335.

OU, Che-Wei R; Pinnacle Health Science Ctre, 9651 Yonge St, Richmond Hill ON L4C 1V7; (Taiwan)'89; MB; PhD; FRCSC; ObstGyn. Staff Obst, Mackenzie Richmond Hill Hospital; Langs: Mandarin; (905)918-0522

OU, Chuhua; Montfort Hosp, 713 Montreal Rd, Ottawa ON K1K 0T2; Hunan (China)'83; CCFP; Staff, Montfort Hospital; (613)746-4621

OU HINGWAN, Gilbert; 304-800 Bathurst St, Toronto ON M5R 3M8; Glasgow (Scotland)'63; DMRD(DiagRad); FRCPC; DiagRad. (416)531-1127; Fax. (416)531-1128.

OU TIM, David Ou; David Ou Tim Consultants Inc, 206-250 Keary St, New Westminster BC V3L 5E7; Cape Town (South Africa)'67; MB ChB; FRCPC; Peds (Neonatology). Chief Dept of Peds, Royal Columbian Hospital; (604)525-7301; Fax. (604)525-7302.

OUADI, Lydia-Amina; CSSS du Suroît, 150 rue Saint-Thomas, Salaber-de-Valleyf QC J6T 6C1; (Algeria)'95; Staff, Centre Hospitalier Régional du Suroît; (450)371-9920 x2092; Fax. (450)371-5275.

OUALLOUCHE, Karim; Ctr Hosp Fleury, 2180 rue Fleury E, Montreal QC H2B 1K3; Algiers (Algeria)'87; FRCPC; AnatPath. Staff, Centre Hospitalier Fleury; (514)384-2000 x4039

OUASTI, Abdessebar; CSSS Haut-Richelieu-Rouville, 920 boul du Seminaire N, St-Jean-Sur-Richel QC J3A 1B7; (Algeria)'87; FRCPC; Psy. Staff, Hôpital du Haut-Richelieu; Langs: Arabic; English; (450)359-5000 x5420

OUCHAREK, Jennifer J; Queen Street Surgical Assoc, 202-610 Queen St, Saskatoon SK S7K 0M8; Sask'03; BSc; FRCSC; GenSurg. (306)244-6818; Fax. (306)664-3462.

OUCHTERLONY, David P; Temmy Latner Centre, 1407-61 St Clair Ave W, Toronto ON M4V 2Y8; Tor'66; BPHE; FABHPM; FCFP; CCFP; FCFP; Staff Family & Commun Med, Mount Sinai Hospital; Att Physician Palliative Care Dept of Med & Family Med, North York General Hospital; Coroner, Province of Ontario; Asst Prof Family & Commun Med, University of Toronto; (416)922-9009; davidouchterlony@sympatico.ca.

OUCHTERLONY, M Donna; 55 Queen St E, Toronto ON M5C 1R6; Ott'67; CCFP; Dir Head Injury Clinic, St Michael's Hospital; Asst Prof Family & Commun Med, University of Toronto; (416)864-5520; Fax. (416)864-6098.

OUDAR, Valerie; Clinique Med St-Vallier, 201-205 rue Montmagny, Quebec QC G1N 4V3; Laval'92; Staff, Jeffery Hale Hospital-Saint Brigid's; Langs: Bilingual(French/English); (418)688-0872; Fax. (418)688-4951.

OUDIT, Gavin Y; University of Alberta Hosp, 2C236 WCM-8440 112 St NW, Edmonton AB T6G 2B7; Tor'98; FRCPC; IntMed; Cardiol. Staff, University of Alberta Hospital; (780)407-8569; Fax. (780)407-6452; gavin.oudit@ualberta.ca.

OUDJHANE, Kamaldine; The Hosp For Sick Children, 555 University Ave, Toronto ON M5G 1X8; Alger (Algeria)'75; MSc(PH); ABR; Consultant Radiologie Neonatale, Mount Sinai Hospital; Staff Radiol, The Hospital For Sick Children; Assoc Prof Diagnostic Radiol, University of Toronto; Langs: Arabic; Berber; Bilingual(English/French); (416)813-7014; Fax. (416)813-7591; kamaldine.oudjhane@sickkids.ca.

OUEDRAOGO, Eva; CSSS du Rocher-Perce, CP 3300 451 rue Mgr Ross E, Chandler QC G0C 1K0; Laval'10; CCFP; Staff, Centre Hospitalier de Chandler; (418)689-2261

OUEDRAOGO, Yacine B; CLSC de Gatineau, 777 boul de la Gappe, Gatineau QC J8T 8R2; Sher'04; CCFP; (819)966-6550

OUELLET, Alain; Clinique familiale de Thetford, 1001-926 rue Labbe, Thetford Mines QC G6G 2A8; Laval'78; ac Staff, Hopital du CSS de la Region de Thetford; (418)338-3521; Fax. (418)338-4580.

OUELLET, Alain C; 79 rue Leblanc O, Longueuil QC J4J 1K1; Mon'83; FRCPC; Derm. (450)463-3881; Fax. (450)463-0908.

OUELLET, Andre; Centre Med Dolbeau, 1530 rue des Erables, Dolbeau-Mistassini QC G8L 2W7; Laval'83; (418)276-2915; Fax. (418)276-6298.

OUELLET, Andre-Denis; Clinique Med Barrette, 152 boul Barrette, Chicoutimi QC G7H 7W8; Laval'78; Staff, Complexe hospitalier de la Sagamie; (418)543-3838; Fax. (418)543-3216.

OUELLET, Anne; Clinique Med Pelletier, 300-8330 boul Taschereau, Brossard QC J4X 1C2; Laval'90; (450)465-5379; Fax. (450)465-5615.

OUELLET, Annie; CHUS-Hop Fleurimont, 3001 12e av N, Sherbrooke QC J1H 5N4; Sher'96; FRCSC; ObstGyn. Staff, Centre Hospitalier Universitaire de Sherbrooke-Hopital Fleurimont; (819)346-1110

OUELLET, Annie; CSSS de Rivière-de-Loup, 75 rue Saint-Henri, Riviere-du-Loup QC G5R 2A4; Laval'01; CSPQ; FRCPC; DiagRad. Staff, Centre Hospitalier Regional du Grand-Portage; (418)868-1000

OUELLET, Bertrand; CSSS du Lac-des-Deux-Montagnes, 520 boul Arthur-Sauve, St-Eustache QC J7R 5B1; Mon'87; CSPQ; DiagRad. Staff, Hôpital de Saint-Eustache; (450)473-6811 x2211

OUELLET, C Anne; Viacar Rech Clin Inc, 170-1875 rue du Caribou, Longueuil QC J4N 0C9; Laval'79; CSPQ; Cardiol (Preventive Cardiology). Staff, Hôpital Anna-Laberge; Médecin, Institut de Cardiologie de Montréal; (450)448-2345; Fax. (450)448-1086; anneou@videotron.ca.

OUELLET, Caroline; Clinique Med St-Louis, 220-3165 ch Saint-Louis, Quebec QC G1W 4R4; Laval'93; Staff, Centre Hospitalier Beauce-Etchemin; (418)653-1970; Fax. (418)653-9956; cogauvin@hotmail.com.

OUELLET, Caroline; CHUM-Hotel-Dieu, 3840 rue Saint-Urbain, Montreal QC H2W 1T8; Sher'01; CSPQ; FRCPC; Anes; Critical Care Medicine (P.Q.). Staff, Centre Hospitalier l'Université de Montréal (CHUM) - Hôtel-Dieu; (514)890-8000 x14444

OUELLET, Caroline; MUHC-Montreal Children's Hosp, 2300 rue Tupper, Montreal QC H3H 1P3; Mon'01; FRCPC; Peds; PedEmergMed (P.Q.). Staff, Centre Hospitalier Pierre le Gardeur; Langs: Bilingual(French/English); (514)412-4400; caro.ouellet@gmail.com.

OUELLET, Chantal; CSSS Pierre Boucher, 1333 boul Jacques-Cartier E, Longueuil QC J4M 2A5; Mon'02; CCFP; Staff, Centre Hospitalier Pierre Boucher; Staff, CHSLD Manoir Trinite; (450)468-8111

OUELLET, Claudine; CSSS Kamouraska-Hop Notre-Dame, CP 460 1201 6e av, La Pocatiere QC G0R 1Z0; Mon'05; Staff, CSSS de Kamouraska; (418)856-7000; Fax. (418)856-5916.

OUELLET, Daniel; Ctr Hosp de Matane, 333 rue Thibault, Matane QC G4W 2W5; Laval'82; FRCSC; GenSurg. Staff, Centre Hospitalier de Matane; (418)562-4022; Fax. (418)562-8530.

OUELLET, Danielle; Centre Med de la Malbaie, 515 rue Saint-Etienne, La Malbaie QC G5A 1W7; Laval'82; Staff, Hôpital de la Malbaie; Langs: Bilingual(French/English); (418)665-2366; Fax. (418)665-7766.

OUELLET, Didier; Polyclinique de Parfondeval, 668 rue de Parfondeval, Baie-Comeau QC G5C 3R3; Laval'87; (418)589-2222

OUELLET, Eric; Clinique Med Val-Belair, 202-1147 boul Pie-XI N, Quebec QC G3K 2P8; Laval'76; (418)843-2473; Fax. (418)843-0224.

OUELLET, Eve-Marie; CLSC Lamater, 1317 boul des Seigneurs, Terrebonne QC J6W 5B1; Laval'00; Médecin, CLSC Lamater; Langs: Bilingual(French/English); (450)471-2881 x4056; Fax. (450)471-6763.

OUELLET, Francine; Clin de Pedopsy Irma-Levasseur, 107-291 rue Saint-Vallier E, Quebec QC G1K 3P5; Laval'91; CSPQ; FRCPC; CommunMed (P.Q.); Psy. (418)529-0555

OUELLET, Frederic; Centre Med des Generations, 200-465 rue Bibeau, Saint-Eustache QC J7R 0C8; Sher'91; FRCSC; GenSurg (Breast Cancer). Staff GenSurg, Hôpital de Saint-Eustache; (450)472-1955; Fax. (450)472-1905; fouellet@cm25.ca.

OUELLET, Georges; Hop Maisonneuve-Rosemont, 5415 boul de l'Assomption, Montreal QC H1T 2M4; Mon'04; FRCPC; IntMed; Nephrol. Staff, Hopital Maisonneuve-Rosemont; (514)252-3489

OUELLET, Gilles; Centre Med Robinson Inc, 4 rue Robinson N, Granby QC J2G 8Z9; Sher'78; Staff, Centre Hospitalier de Granby; (450)378-8435; Fax. (450)375-8832.

OUELLET, Gilles; Clinique Med Chateauguay, 120 boul Saint-Jean-Baptiste, Chateauguay QC J6K 3A9; Laval'72; Cardiol (P.Q.). Staff, Centre Hospitalier l'Université De Montréal (CHUM) - Hôpital Saint-luc; (450)691-8191

OUELLET, Gilles; Centre Med Drummond, 60 rue Loring, Drummondville QC J2C 7Y9; Mon'85; ac Staff, Hôpital Sainte-croix; (819)477-2500; Fax. (819)477-6249.

OUELLET, Henri; Clinique Med Fam des Recollets, 101-940 boul des Recollets, Trois-Rivieres QC G8Z 3W9; Laval'69; (819)373-0303; Fax. (819)373-8431.

OUELLET, Isabelle; CHUS-Hop Fleurimont, 3001 12e av N, Sherbrooke QC J1H 5N4; Sher'07; CCFP; CCFP(E.M.); Staff, Centre Hospitalier Universitaire de Sherbrooke-Hopital Fleurimont; (819)346-1110

OUELLET, Jacques; CSSS de Laval, 1755 boul Rene-Laennec, Laval QC H7M 3L9; Mon'83; NBME; EmergMed (P.Q.). Dir Emerg Dept, Hopital de la Cite de la santé; Clin Instructor, Universite de Montreal; (450)668-1010; Fax. (450)975-5353.

OUELLET, Jean; Unite Med Familiale Maizerets, 2480 ch de la Canardiere, Quebec QC G1J 2G1; Laval'86; CCFP; FCFP; Université Laval; (418)661-1413; Fax. (418)661-7504.

OUELLET, Jean-Albert; MUHC-Montreal Children's Hosp, C521-2300 rue Tupper, Montreal QC H3H 1P3; Ott'94; FRCSC; OrthSurg (Pediatric Orthopedics). Staff, McGill University Health Centre - Montreal Children's Hospital; McGill University; Langs: English; French; (514)934-4464

OUELLET, Jean-Francois; CHUQ-Hotel-Dieu de Quebec, 11 Cote du Palais, Quebec QC G1R 2J6; Laval'95; FRCSC; GenSurg; General Surgical Oncology (P.Q.). Staff, Centre Hospitalier Universitaire de Québec (CHUQ) - Siege Social; (418)691-5370

OUELLET, Jean-Francois; CHAUQ, 1401 18e rue, Quebec QC G1J 1Z4; Laval'05; FRCSC; GenSurg. Staff, Foothills Medical Centre; (418)649-0252

OUELLET, Jean-Marc; CHUQ-Hotel-Dieu de Quebec, 11 Cote du Palais, Quebec QC G1R 2J6; Laval'83; CSPQ; Anes. Staff, Centre Hospitalier Universitaire de Québec (CHUQ) - Siege Social; (418)525-4444 x5323

OUELLET, Jean-Pascal; Club Sante Estrie, 632 rue Bowen S, Sherbrooke QC J1G 2E9; Mon'80; LMCC; NBME; ABEM; EmergMed (Family Medicine). Langs: Bilingual(French/English); (819)822-1202; Fax. (819)822-2027.

OUELLET, Jean-Yves; CSSS Pierre Boucher, 1333 boul Jacques-Cartier E, Longueuil QC J4M 2A5; Mon'83; CSPQ; DiagRad. Staff, Centre Hospitalier Pierre Boucher; (450)468-8157

OUELLET, Jean-Yves; 1000 boul Sainte-Anne, St-Charles-Brromee QC J6E 6J2; Laval'71; CSPQ; FRCPC; DiagRad. Staff Radiol, Centre Hospitalier Régional de Lanaudière; Langs: French; (450)759-8222 x5733; Fax. (450)759-2133.

OUELLET, Joanie; CLSC de Pte-aux-Trembles Mtl-E, 13926 rue Notre-Dame E, Montreal QC H1A 1T5; Mon'09; (514)642-4050

OUELLET, Kim; CSSS d'Antoine-Labelle-Mt Laur, RR 1 2561 ch de la Lièvre S, Mont-Laurier QC J9L 3G3; Mon'97; FRCSC; GenSurg (Digestive Surgery). Chirurgien, CSSS d'Antoine-Labelle; (819)623-1234

OUELLET, Linda; CSSS de Rivière-de-Loup, 75 rue Saint-Henri, Riviere-du-Loup QC G5R 2A4; Sher'90; Peds. Staff, Centre Hospitalier Regional du Grand-Portage; Langs: English; (418)868-1000; Fax. (418)868-3338.

OUELLET, Louis-Olivier; CSSS de la Cote-de-Gaspe, 215 boul de York O, Gaspe QC G4X 2W2; Mon'05; CCFP; Staff, Centre Hospitalier de Gaspe; (418)368-3301; Fax. (418)368-6850.

OUELLET, Louise; Clinique Med Barrette, 152 boul Barrette, Chicoutimi QC G7H 7W8; Sher'88; Staff, Complexe hospitalier de la Sagamie; (418)543-3838; Fax. (418)543-3216.

OUELLET, Lucie; CSSS des Basques, 550 rue Notre-Dame E RR 1, Trois-Pistoles QC G0L 4K0; Laval'80; LMCC; Staff, Centre Hospitalier Trois-Pistoles; (418)851-1111; Fax. (418)851-2944.

OUELLET, Marie-Caroline; CSSS du Sud de Lanaudière, 911 montee des Pionniers, Terrebonne QC J6V 2H2; Mon'92; CSPQ; DiagRad. Staff, Centre Hospitalier Pierre le Gardeur; (450)654-7525 x21300

OUELLET, Marie-France; Centre médicale Centrale, 4-135 rue Saint-Antoine N, Granby QC J2G 5G7; Sher'08; (450)372-5401; Fax. (450)372-4174.

OUELLET, Mark; CHUQ-St-Francois d'Assise, 10 rue de l'Espinay, Quebec QC G1L 3L5; Laval'82; CSPQ; FRCPC; Anes. Ac Staff, Centre Hospitalier Universitaire De Québec - Pavillon De St-françois-d'assise; Université Laval; (418)525-4340; Fax. (418)525-4434.

OUELLET, Martin; 397 av Laurier O, Montreal QC H2V 2K3; Mon'79; (514)793-9771

OUELLET, Nathalie; CSSS du Lac-des-Deux-Montagnes, 520 boul Arthur-Sauve, St-Eustache QC J7R 5B1; Sher'89; FRCSC; ObstGyn. Staff, Hôpital de Saint-Eustache; (450)473-6811

OUELLET, Pascale; Hopital Ste-Justine, 3175 ch Cote-Sainte-Catherine, Montreal QC H3T 1C5; Laval'06; FRCPC; Anes. Staff, Hôpital Ste-Justine; (514)345-4931

OUELLET, Paul G; Inst U en Sante Mentale de QC, 2601 ch de la Canardiere, Quebec QC G1J 2G3; Laval'81; FRCPC; Psy (Affective Disorders). ac Staff, Institut Universitaire Sante; assoc Staff, Institut Philippe-Pinel de Montreal; Université Laval; (418)663-5321 x5551; Fax. (418)661-6891.

OUELLET, Pierre A; Centre Med Ste-Foy Inc, 802 av du Chanoine-Scott, Quebec QC G1V 3N4; Laval'73; Psy (Clinical Psychiatry). Clin Prof Psy, Université Laval; (418)653-4931; Fax. (418)653-4797.

OUELLET, Pierre; CHUQ-Hotel-Dieu de Quebec, 11 Cote du Palais, Quebec QC G1R 2J6; Laval'72; MedOncol (P.Q.); Hem (P. Q.). ac Staff, Centre Hospitalier Universitaire de Québec (CHUQ) - Siege Social; ac Staff, Hôtel-Dieu de Lévis; Langs: Bilingual(French/English); (418)691-5225

OUELLET, Pierre-Luc; Ctr Hosp Anna-Laberge, 200 boul Brisebois, Chateauguay QC J6K 4W8; Mon'05; IntMed. Staff, Hôpital Anna-Laberge; (450)699-2425

OUELLET, Robert; Radiologie Concorde, 300 boul de la Concorde E, Laval QC H7G 2E6; Mon'69; CSPQ; FRCPC; DiagRad. Staff Radiol, Hopital de la Cite de la santé; Dir, Tomo Concorde & Reso-Concorde; (450)667-8244; rouellet@videotron.ca.

OUELLET, Robin; Pav Albert Prevost, 6555 boul Gouin O, Montreal QC H4K 1B3; Ott'04; Psy. (514)338-4273; Fax. (514)338-4352.

OUELLET, Rodrigue; Clinique de Med Familiale, 101 rue Lavoie, Rimouski QC G5L 5Y2; Laval'74; (418)723-5272; Fax. (418)725-2030.

OUELLET, Ronald; Ctr Hosp Affilie-St-Sacrement, 1050 ch Sainte-Foy, Quebec QC G1S 4L8; Laval'81; FRCPC; Psy (Psychotherapy). Staff, Centre Hospitalier Affilié Universitaire de Québec - Hôpital du St-Sacrement; Teach Staff, Université Laval; (418)682-7898; Fax. (418)682-7959.

OUELLET, Sandie; CSSS de Sept-Iles, 45 rue du Pere-Divet, Sept-Iles QC G4R 3N7; McG'07; MDCM; CCFP; Staff, Centre Hospitalier Regional de Sept-Iles; (418)962-9761

OUELLET, Stephane; Les Gynecologues Associes, 100-235 boul Rene-Levesque E, Montreal QC H2X 1N8; Mon'96; FRCSC; ObstGyn. (514)866-2446; Fax. (514)866-4013.

OUELLET, Sylvie; CLSC la Petite Patrie, 6520 rue de Saint-Vallier, Montreal QC H2S 2P7; Laval'82; (514)273-4508; Fax. (514)272-6278.

OUELLET, Sylvie; Ctr Hosp Fleury, 2180 rue Fleury E, Montreal QC H2B 1K3; Mon'05; Staff, Centre Hospitalier Fleury; (514)381-9311

OUELLET, Tracy Lara; 1-1261 Beaverbrook Ave, London ON N6H 0G6; Wes'98; BSc; CCFP; FCFP; (519)672-2273; Fax. (519)672-2668.

OUELLET, Vianney; Centre Med Quatre-Bourgeois, 300-979 av de Bourgogne, Quebec QC G1W 2L4; Laval'90; CCFP; (418)653-4050; Fax. (418)653-4475.

OUELLET, Vincent; CSSS du Sud de Lanaudière, 911 montee des Pionniers, Terrebonne QC J6V 2H2; Laval'96; LMCC; Gastroent; IntMed. Staff, Centre Hospitalier Pierre le Gardeur; (450)654-7525

OUELLET, Yanick; Montfort Hosp, 713 Montreal Rd, Ottawa ON K1K 0T2; Ott'04; CCFP; CCFP(E.M.); Staff, Montfort Hospital; (613)746-4621

OUELLET, Yves; CSSS Drummond, 205-355 boul Bois-Francs S, Victoriaville QC G6P 4T2; Sher'77; FRCSC; Otol. Langs: English; (819)758-6488

OUELLET-PELLETIER, Julie; Ctr Hosp Affilie-Enfant-Jesus, 1401 18e rue, Quebec QC G1J 1Z4; Laval'08; Staff, Centre Hospitalier Affilié Universitaire de Québec - Hôpital De L'Enfant Jésus; (418)649-0252

OUELLET-PLAMONDON, Clairelaine; CHUM-Hop Notre-Dame, 1560 rue Sherbrooke E, Montreal QC H2L 4M1; Mon'07; Psy. Staff, Centre Hospitalier l'Université de Montréal (CHUM) - Hôpital Notre-Dame; (514)890-8000

OUELLETTE, Audrey; Clinique Med de Kingsley-Falls, 19 rue Comeau, Kingsey Falls QC J0A 1B0; Mon'08; (819)363-3030; Fax. (819)363-3030.

OUELLETTE, Chantal; Centre médicale Centrale, 135-4 rue Saint-Antoine N, Granby QC J2G 5G7; Sher'07; (450)372-5401; Fax. (450)372-4174.

OUELLETTE, David W; Dept of Emergency Med, E1 102-800 Commissioners Rd E, London ON N6A 5W9; Wes'04; Critical Care Medicine; EmergMed. (519)685-8500

OUELLETTE, Erik; Clinic of Orthopaedic Med, 206-2555 St. Joseph Blvd, Orleans ON K1C 1S6; Mon'97; CCFP; CCFP(E.M.); Staff, Hôtel-Dieu de Sorel; Langs: Bilingual(French/English); (613)824-4223; Fax. (613)824-2418.

OUELLETTE, Gilles; 8187 boul Viau, Saint-Leonard QC H1R 2T2; Mon'62; (514)376-2881; Fax. (514)376-0095.

OUELLETTE, Helene; 501A rte Principale RR 3, Ste-Anne-du-Sault QC G0Z 1C0; Sher'89; Staff, Hotel-Dieu d'Arthabaska; (819)367-2714; Fax. (819)367-2715.

OUELLETTE, Hugue A; Vancouver Gen Hosp, 855 12th Ave W, Vancouver BC V5Z 1M9; Ott'96; FRCPC; DiagRad. Staff, Vancouver General Hospital - Centennial Pavillion; Langs: Bilingual(English/French); (604)875-4111

OUELLETTE, Jean; 101-480 McGill St, Hawkesbury ON K6A 1R2; Ott'80; BA; FRCPC; Psy (Geriatric Psychiatry). Consultant, Service de Gerontopsychiatrie de Prescott-Russell; (613)632-7763; Fax. (613)632-0472; jouellette@montfort.on.ca.

OUELLETTE, Jean-Paul; Orleans Clin Orthopaedic Med, 206-2555 St. Joseph Blvd, Orleans ON K1C 1S6; Ott'70; CCFP; FCFP; Court Staff, The Ottawa Hospital - General Campus; Asst Prof, University of Ottawa; Langs: Bilingual(French/English); (613)824-4223; Fax. (613)824-2418; info@cproloc.ca.

OUELLETTE, Josiane; Polyclinique St-Eustache Inc, 75 rue Grignon, Saint-Eustache QC J7P 4J2; Mon'09; CCFP; (450)473-6777; Fax. (450)473-1916.

OUELLETTE, Denise M A; 5415 boul de l'Assomption, Montreal QC H1T 2M4; Ott'83; FRCSC; GenSurg; ThorSurg. Staff, Hopital Maisonneuve-Rosemont; Langs: English; French; Italian; (514)252-3400 x4420; Fax. (514)252-3894.

OUELLETTE, Marc; Clinique medicale de Fleurimon, 210-2140 rue King E, Sherbrooke QC J1G 5G6; Mon'75; ac Staff, Centre Hospitalier Universitaire de Sherbrooke-Hôpital Hôtel-Dieu; (819)563-4462; Fax. (819)563-4464.

OUELLETTE, Michael K; 20-1450 O'Connor Dr, East York ON M4B 2T8; Man'06; CCFP; Staff, Weeneebayko General Hospital; (416)285-1459; Fax. (416)285-8959.

OUELLETTE, Michele; Polyclinique Saint-Eustache, 75 rue Grignon, Saint-Eustache QC J7P 4J2; Mon'74; Langs: English; (450)473-6882

OUELLETTE, Nathalie; 100-14770 boul de Pierrefonds, Pierrefonds QC H9H 4Y6; McG'86; FRCPC; Peds. Staff, McGill University Health Centre - Montreal Children's Hospital; adj Prof, McGill University; Langs: English; French; (514)696-2442; Fax. (514)624-3099; ouellette.nat@hotmail.com.

OUELLETTE, Paul; Centre Med Robinson, 4 rue Robinson N, Granby QC J2G 8Z9; Sher'92; CSPQ; RC; Urol; Urol (Clinical Research). Staff, Centre Hospitalier de Granby; Langs: English; (450)372-1818; Fax. (450)770-8567; uropaul@videotron.ca.

OUELLETTE, Pierre; GMF de Lorraine, 99 boul de Gaulle, Lorraine QC J6Z 3Z9; Mon'76; (450)621-1444; Fax. (450)621-7193.

OUELLETTE, Rachel E; 403-1015 Regent St, Fredericton NB E3B 6H5; Mem'07; FRCPC; Peds. Langs: Bilingual(English/French).

OUELLETTE, Robert A; Hop Sainte-Anne, 305 boul des Anciens-Combattan, Ste-Anne-de-Bellev QC H9X 1Y9; Mon'69; FRCPC; Psy (Pedology Psychiatry). Staff, Hopital Ste-Anne; Langs: English; Spanish; (514)457-3440

OUELLETTE, Rodney J; Dr Georges-L Dumont Reg Hosp, 330 av Universite, Moncton NB E1C 2Z3; Laval'96; Staff, Dr Georges-L-Dumont University Hospital Centre; (506)862-4000

OUELLETTE, Sylvie A; The Moncton Hosp, 4502-135 MacBeath Ave, Moncton NB E1C 6Z8; Dal'93; BSc; FRCPC; IntMed; Rheum. Staff, The Moncton Hospital; Langs: Bilingual(English/French); (506)857-5111; jdowner@accesswave.ca.

OUERTANI, Sofiane; CSSS des Aurores Boreales, CP 6000 Succ Bureau-Chef 679 2e rue E, La Sarre QC J9Z 2X7; Tunis (Tunisia)'99; Staff, Centre Hospitalier La Sarre; (819)333-2311; Fax. (819)333-4316; sefever2003@yahoo.fr.

OUEZZANI, Salma; Hotel-Dieu de Levis, 143 rue Wolfe, Levis QC G6V 3Z1; (Morocco)'02; Staff, Hôtel-Dieu de Lévis; (418)835-7140

OUGHTON, Matthew T; SMBD Jewish Gen Hosp, 3755 ch Cote-Sainte-Catherine, Montreal QC H3T 1E2; Man'00; FRCPC; IntMed; Microbio & Infect Dis (P.Q.); MedMicrobiol; InfectDis. Staff, Sir Mortimer B Davis Jewish General; (514)340-8222 x2662; matthew.oughton@mcgill.ca.

OUHILAL, Sophia A; Montreal Fertility Centre, 220-5252 boul de Maisonneuve O, Montreal QC H4A 3S5; McG'95; FRCSC; ObstGyn. (514)369-6116; Fax. (514)369-2662.

OUIMET, Alain A; Hôpital Ste-Justine, 3175 ch Cote-Sainte-Catherine, Montreal QC H3T 1C5; Sher'71; FRCSC; GenSurg (Pediatric Surgery). ac Staff, Hôpital Ste-Justine; Langs: Bilingual(French/English); (514)345-4915; Fax. (514)345-4964.

OUIMET, Alain; Clinique Med Ste-Adele, 1150 rue du Bourg-Joli, Sainte-Adele QC J8B 1W8; Mon'75; LMCC; (450)229-6633; Fax. (450)229-5765.

OUIMET, Denis; Hop Maisonneuve-Rosemont, 5415 boul de l'Assomption, Montreal QC H1T 2M4; Sher'75; Nephrol (P.Q.) (Peritonial Dialysis). ac Staff, Hopital Maisonneuve-Rosemont; Prof clin agrégé, Universite de Montreal; Langs: Bilingual(French/English); (514)252-3489; Fax. (514)255-3026.

OUIMET, Denise; Ctr Hosp Rouyn-Noranda, 4 9e rue, Rouyn-Noranda QC J9X 2B2; Mon'56; LMCC; CSPQ; FRCPC; DiagRad (Breast Imaging); RadOncol. Staff, Centre Hospitalier Rouyn-Noranda; ac Staff/Prof Radiol, Centre Hospitalier l'Université de Montréal (CHUM) - Hôpital Notre-Dame; assoc Radiologiste RUM Radiologists, Universite de Montreal; Langs: Spanish; English; German; (819)764-5431; dlol@total.net.

OUIMET, Dominique; CSSS de Saint-Jerome, 290 rue de Montigny, Saint-Jerome QC J7Z 5T3; Mon'92; Cardiol; IntMed (Clinical Cardiology). Staff Cardiol, Hôtel-Dieu de Saint-Jérôme; Chef Cardiol Echography Lab, Centre Hospitalier d'Argenteuil; Langs: Spanish; English; (450)431-8201; Fax. (450)431-8331.

OUIMET, France; Clinique Med Chemin Chambly, 101-3090 ch de Chambly, Longueuil QC J4L 4N5; Mon'81; (450)670-5700; Fax. (450)670-8830.

OUIMET, Gilles; CSSS de Saint-Jerome, 290 rue de Montigny, Saint-Jerome QC J7Z 5T3; Mon'77; Respir. Staff, Hôtel-Dieu de Saint-Jérôme; (450)431-8200 x2182; Fax. (450)431-8209.

OUIMET, Helene; CSSS du Nord de Lanaudière, 1000 boul Sainte-Anne, St-Charles-Brromee QC J6E 6J2; Mon'82; Cardiol. Staff, Centre Hospitalier Régional de Lanaudière; (450)759-8222 x2892

OUIMET, Luc J; Ctr Medi Soleil St-Jean-Sur-Ri, 120-383 boul du Seminaire N, St-Jean-sur-Richel QC J3B 8C5; Mon'84; Staff, Hôpital du Haut-Richelieu; (450)347-7557; Fax. (450)347-3099.

OUIMET, Luc; CSSS de Chicoutimi, 305 rue Saint-Vallier, Chicoutimi QC G7H 5H6; Laval'82; Psy. Staff, Complexe hospitalier de la Sagamie; (418)549-5477; Fax. (418)549-7604.

OUIMET, Lucie; Clinique Med Pelletier, 300-8330 boul Taschereau, Brossard QC J4X 1C2; Sher'86; (450)465-5379; Fax. (450)465-5615.

OUIMET, Marie-Andree; St Mary's Hosp Centre, 3830 av Lacombe, Montreal QC H3T 1M5; Sher'96; Psy. Staff, St Mary's Hospital Centre; (514)345-3511 x5132; Fax. (514)734-2609.

OUIMET, Marie-Jo; Direction de la Sante Publique, 1301 rue Sherbrooke E, Montreal QC H2L 1M3; Mon'95; MSc; Staff, McGill University Health Centre - Montreal Chest Institute; Physician, PRAIDA-CLSC Cote des Neiges; Langs: Spanish; English; (514)528-2400

OUIMET, Myriam H; Hop Brome-Missisquoi-Perkins, 950 rue Principale, Cowansville QC J2K 1K3; Mon'10; CCFP; Staff, Hôpital Brome-Missisquoi-Perkins; (450)266-4342

OUIMET, Stephane; Hop Charles LeMoyne, 3120 boul Taschereau, Greenfield Park QC J4V 2H1; Mon'00; Psy. Staff, Hopital Charles LeMoyne; (450)466-5000

OUIMET, Veronique; CSSS de Manicouagan, 635 boul Jolliet, Baie-Comeau QC G5C 1P1; Mon'05; CCFP; Staff, Centre Hospitalier Régional Baie-Comeau; (418)589-3701

OUKACHBI, Salima; Thunder Bay Reg HSC-T-Bay, 980 Oliver Rd, Thunder Bay ON P7B 6V4; (Algeria)'95; CCFP; Staff, Thunder Bay Regional Health Sciences Centre; (807)684-6000

OULIANINE, Karen; Hop Maisonneuve-Rosemont, 5415 boul de l'Assomption, Montreal QC H1T 2M4; Sher'82; CCFP; CCFP(E.M.); Staff, Hopital Maisonneuve-Rosemont; Langs: Spanish; English; (514)252-3523; Fax. (514)252-3566.

OUNG, Christopher M; Woodstock Gen Hosp, 310 Juliana Dr, Woodstock ON N4V 0A4; Rangoon (Burma)'76; DABS; FACS; FRCSC; GenSurg (Family Medicine). Staff, Woodstock General Hospital; Dist Chief Surg, District Health Authority 5; Langs: Burmese; French; (519)421-4211

OURADOU, Jean-Luc; 380 Monseigneur Desmarais GD, Upton QC J0H 2E0; Mon'84; (450)549-5392; Fax. (450)549-6092.

OUSSEDIK, Youcef; Dr Georges-L Dumont Reg Hosp, 330 av Universite, Moncton NB E1C 2Z3; Algiers (Algeria)'75; DABPath; (506)862-4120; Fax. (506)862-4195.

OUTERBRIDGE, A Ross; Sage Sport Institute, 200-910 McGill Rd, Kamloops BC V2C 6N6; Cal'86; BSc; Dip SportMed; FRCSC; OrthSurg (Knee Arthroscopy). (250)314-5000; Fax. (250)314-5260; routerbridge@sagesportinstitute.com.

OUTRAM, Christopher P E; 202-616 K.L.O. Rd, Kelowna BC V1Y 4X4; Cape Town (South Africa)'94; MB ChB; Langs: Afrikaans; (250)763-4330; Fax. (250)763-7008.

OUZILLEAU, Christian; CHUS-Hop Hotel-Dieu, 580 rue Bowen S, Sherbrooke QC J1G 2E8; Sher'98; Staff, Centre Hospitalier Universitaire de Sherbrooke-Hôpital Hôtel-Dieu; (819)346-1110

OVAKIM, Daniel H; Royal Jubilee Hosp, 1952 Bay St, Victoria BC V8R 1J8; Tor'06; FRCPC; IntMed (Clinical Pharmacology); Critical Care Medicine. Staff, Royal Jubilee Hospital; (250)370-8111

OVAKPORAYE, Moses O I; 10-140 East Chestermere Dr, Chestermere AB T1X 1M1; (Nigeria)'86; CCFP; Staff, Queen Elizabeth II Hospital; (403)273-2215; Fax. (403)273-2213.

OVCHINNIKOV, Vladislav L; 833 Coxwell Ave, East York ON M4C 3E8; Moscow (Russia (Federation))'86; FRCPC; Cardiol; IntMed. Staff, Toronto East General Hospital Inc; Langs: Russian; (416)250-7474; Fax. (416)250-6784; ovchinnikovmed@gmail.com.

OVENS, Howard J; Mount Sinai Hosp, 206-600 University Ave, Toronto ON M5G 1X5; Tor'78; CCFP; CCFP(E.M.); FCFP; Dir Div of Emerg Services, Mount Sinai Hospital; Assoc Prof Family & Community Med, University of Toronto; (416)586-5058; Fax. (416)586-4719; howard.ovens@utoronto.ca.

OVER, Danielle M; Dorval Med Assoc Fam Hlth Team, 104-465 Morden Rd, Oakville ON L6K 3W6; Leiden (Netherlands)'70; Court Staff, Halton Healthcare Services Corporation - Oakville Site; Langs: Dutch; German; (905)842-7154; Fax. (905)842-3604.

OVERGAARD, Christopher B; Univ Hlth Network-Toronto Gen, 6EN 232-200 Elizabeth St, Toronto ON M5G 2C4; Tor'99; Cardiol; IntMed. Staff, Toronto General Hospital - UHN; (416)340-4800; Fax. (416)340-3390.

OVERHOLT, Todd M; Niagara Detention Centre, PO Box 1050 Stn Main 1355 Uppers Rd, Thorold ON L2V 4A6; Tor'87; (905)227-6321

OVERINGTON, Nancy L; Maple Family Health Team, 325 University Ave, Kingston ON K7L 3R4; Qns'77; CCFP; FCFP; Assoc Staff, Kingston General Hospital; Assoc Staff, Hotel-Dieu Hospital; (613)544-2902; Fax. (613)544-5768.

OVERLI-DOMES, Carmel L K; Avon Med Centre, 2781 Avonhurst Dr, Regina SK S4R 3J3; Sask'06; CCFP; (306)543-4955; Fax. (306)545-7006.

OVETCHKINE, Philippe; Hôpital Ste-Justine, 3175 ch Cote-Sainte-Catherine, Montreal QC H3T 1C5; Paris (France)'93; Staff, Hôpital Ste-Justine; (514)345-4931 x5566; philippe.ovetchkine@umontreal.ca.

OVIATT, Patrick L; 1903 9 Ave S, Lethbridge AB T1J 1W8; Alb'04; FRCPC; IntMed; Respir. (403)320-0633; Fax. (403)320-0353.

OVIEDO, Angelica; BC Women's Hosp & Health Ctre, 4500 Oak St, Vancouver BC V6H 3N1; Northwestern(IL) (USA)'94; Staff, BC Women's Hospital & Health Centre; (604)875-2137; Fax. (604)875-3529.

OVUENI, Efe M; Estevan Med Clinic, 110-1175 Nicholson Rd, Estevan SK S4A 2S7; (306)634-2661; Fax. (306)634-8821.

OW, Emily J; 1475 Upper Ottawa St, Hamilton ON L8W 3J6; Tor'09; CCFP; (905)575-1300

OWADALLY, Bilaal A; 106-10055 120 Ave, Grande Prairie AB T8V 8H8; (South Africa)'06; (780)532-4415; Fax. (780)532-4559.

OWATZ, Todd S; Riverside Med Clinic, 303-1101 Dewdney Ave, Trail BC V1R 4T1; Sask'96; FRCSC; GenSurg. Staff, Kootenay Boundary Regional Hospital; (250)364-1178; Fax. (250)364-1179.

OWEGA, Josef; McBride & Dist Hosp, PO Box 669 594 King St, McBride BC V0J 2E0; Qns'88; CCFP; FCFP; Fam Med, McBride & District Hospital; (250)569-2251; josef.owega@northernhealth.ca.

OWEN, Andrew J; MUHC-Montreal Gen Hosp, 1650 av Cedar, Montreal QC H3G 1A4; Sask'97; CSPQ; FRCPC; Anes. Staff, McGill University Health Centre - Montreal General Campus; (514)934-1934 x43261

OWEN, Carolyn J; Foothills Med Centre, 603-1403 29 St NW, Calgary AB T2N 2T9; Tor'01; FRCPC; IntMed; Hem. Staff, Foothills Medical Centre; Langs: Bilingual(English/French); (403)944-3265

OWEN, Catherine M; 210-1920 Ellesmere Rd, Scarborough ON M1H 2V6; McG'99; FRCSC; ObstGyn (Minimal Invasive Surgery). Langs: Bilingual(English/French); (416)289-2288; Fax. (416)289-1555.

OWEN, David A; 1436-910 10th Ave W, Vancouver BC V5Z 1M9; Cardiff (Wales)'67; FRCPath; FRCPC; AnatPath (Gastrointestinal Pathology). Head Anat Path, Vancouver General Hospital - Centennial Pavillion; Staff, Dr David A Owen Inc; Prof, University of British Columbia; (604)875-5555 x63974

OWEN, Dawn; BC Cancer Agency, 600 10th Ave W, Vancouver BC V5Z 4E6; Tor'07; FRCPC; RadOncol. Staff, BC Cancer Agency Vancouver Centre; (604)877-6000

OWEN, Diana C; Montfort Hosp, 713 Montreal Rd, Ottawa ON K1K 0T2; Ott'01; CCFP; CCFP(E.M.); Staff, Montfort Hospital; (613)748-4996

OWEN, James E L; Sault Area Hosp, 750 Great Northern Rd, Sault Ste. Marie ON P6B 0A8; Glasgow (Scotland)'71; MB ChB; Court Staff, Sault Area Hospital - Sault Ste Marie; Med Dir, Sault Ste Marie Sleep Laboratory; Dir, Pain & Sleep Disorder Clinic Group Health Centre; (705)759-3434

OWEN, James R M; Health Centre at 410, 410 Sherbourne St, Toronto ON M4X 1K2; Wes'10; CCFP; (416)867-3728; Fax. (416)867-3726.

OWEN, John S; 314 Lake Cres, Saskatoon SK S7H 3A2; Birmingham (England)'45; MB ChB; FFPH; DPH(Birm); DipHealthEd; FRIPH; (306)374-7913; jso195@mail.usask.ca.

OWEN, Julian J; Hamilton HS-General Site, 241A-237 Barton St E, Hamilton ON L8L 2X2; McM'08; Staff, Hamilton Health Sciences Centre - Hamilton General Hospital; (905)521-2100

OWEN, Michael L S; PO Box 23001 Rpo St Mike's, Lethbridge AB T1J 4P5; Alb'85; Psy. Staff, Chinook Regional Hospital; (403)388-6244; Fax. (403)388-6250.

OWEN, Richard J T; University of Alberta Hosp, 8440 112 St NW, Edmonton AB T6G 2B7; Cardiff (Wales)'87; MB BCh; FRCR; MRCP; Staff, Royal Alexandra Hospital; Staff, Covenant Health - Grey Nuns Community Hospital; Assoc Prof, University of Alberta; (780)407-1210; Fax. (780)407-6176.

OWEN, Richard John; London HSC-Victoria Hosp, PO Box 5010 Stn B 800 Commissioners Rd E, London ON N6A 5W9; Manchester (England)'91; Staff, London Health Sciences Centre - Victoria Campus; (519)667-6503; Fax. (519)667-6836.

OWEN, Scott; MUHC-Montreal Gen Hosp, 1650 av Cedar, Montreal QC H3G 1A4; McG'05; FRCPC; IntMed; MedOncol. Staff, McGill University Health Centre - Montreal General Campus; (514)934-1934

OWEN, Stephen M; Glen Allan Med Center, 207-42 Glen Allan Dr, Bridgewater NS B4V 3N2; Manchester (England)'72; MB ChB; FRCSC; ObstGyn. (902)543-8788; Fax. (902)543-3334.

OWEN, Timothy E; Cancer Ctr of Southeastern Ont, 25 King St W, Kingston ON K7L 5P9; Man'02; FRCPC; RadOncol. Staff, Cancer Centre of Southeastern Ontario; (613)544-2631; Fax. (613)548-1355.

OWENS, Erinn L; 20B-385 Frederick St, Kitchener ON N2H 2P2; McM'96; BSc(Kinesiol); CCFP; FCFP; (519)747-1200; Fax. (519)747-1560.

OWENS, Jennifer L; UWO Student Health Services, 11-1151 Richmond St, London ON N6K 3K7; Tor'00; CCFP; (519)661-3030; Fax. (519)661-3380.

OWENS, Mary C; 1712-2200 Yonge St, Toronto ON M4S 2C6; Otago (New Zealand)'78; MB ChB; FRCPC; Psy (Anxiety Disorder). Assoc Staff Psy, The Hospital For Sick Children; (416)488-8035; mary.owens@utoronto.ca.

OWENS, Thomas R; Lakeside Med Walk-In Clinic, 104-227 Lake St, Pembroke ON K8A 5M2; Qns'79; (613)732-3209

OWER, Katherine M; London HSC-Victoria Hosp, PO Box 5010 Stn B 800 Commissioners Rd E, London ON N6A 5W9; Alb'99; FRCPC; Anes. Staff, St Joseph's Hospital - St Joseph's Health Care; Staff, London Health Sciences Centre - Victoria Campus; (519)685-8525; Fax. (519)685-8275.

OWERS, David P; Coquitlam Vein Clinic, 308-1196 Lansdowne Dr, New Westminster BC V3E 1J7; Ott'92; CCFP; Langs: French; (604)945-7546

OWSIANIK, Walter D J; Hamilton Port Authority Bldg, 101-605 James St N, Hamilton ON L8L 1J9; Qns'76; BSc(Hons.); DTMH(Lond); CCFP; FCFP; Court Staff, St Joseph's Healthcare - Charlton Campus; Court Staff, Hamilton Health Sciences Centre - McMaster University Medical Centre; Medical Officer, Hamilton Port Authority; Asst Prof, McMaster University; (905)529-8558; Fax. (905)577-6306.

OWUSU-ANSAH, Kevin; BC Women's Hosp & Health Ctre, 4500 Oak St, Vancouver BC V6H 3N1; Leicester (England)'04; MB ChB; Staff, BC Women's Hospital & Health Centre; (604)875-2135

OXLEY, Paul J; Surrey Med Arts Bldg, 308-13710 94A Ave, Surrey BC V3V 1N1; UBC'98; FRCSC; PlasSurg. (604)580-0515; Fax. (604)589-6481.

OXNER, James H; Dartmouth Gen Hosp, 325 Pleasant St, Dartmouth NS B2Y 4G8; Dal'70; LRCP(Lond); FRCPC; DiagRad. Staff, Dartmouth General Hospital; (902)465-8318; Fax. (902)465-8360.

OXNER, William M; Queen Elizabeth II HSC-Halifax, 4881-1796 Summer St, Halifax NS B3H 3A7; Dal'94; BSc; FRCSC; OrthSurg (Spine Surgery). Staff, Queen Elizabeth II Health Sciences Centre - Victoria General Site; Staff, Queen Elizabeth II Health Sciences Centre - Halifax Infirmary Site; Asst Prof Surg, Dalhousie University; (902)473-3717; Fax. (902)473-4364.

OYAMA, Sonnie E; PO Box 86, Gibbons AB T0A 1N0; (Nigeria)'88; (780)923-2200; Fax. (780)923-3564; seoyamadr@yahoo.com.au.

OYEBANJI, Olubunmi B; PO Box 91012 Rpo Royal Oak, Calgary AB T3G 5W6; Nigeria (Nigeria)'94; CCFP.

OYEBODE, Ayobami O; 5334 50 Ave PO Box 10, Elk Point AB T0A 1A0; Ilorin (Nigeria)'94; MB BS; CCFP; (780)724-3500; Fax. (780)724-3504.

OYEBODE, Omoniyi O; Weyburn Mental Health Centre, PO Box 2003 Stn Main, Weyburn SK S4H 2Z9; Ilorin (Nigeria)'95; FRCPC; Psy. Psychiatrist, Weyburn Community Health Services (Mental Health); (306)842-8665; Fax. (306)842-8690.

OYEKANMI, Oyekunle A; Quarry Park Med, 120-109 Quarry Park Blvd SE, Calgary AB T2C 5E7; (Nigeria)'91; MB BS; DABIM; (403)930-7111; Fax. (403)930-7114.

OYELESE, Olutoyese O; Westside Med Associates, 3591 Elliott Rd, West Kelowna BC V4T 1N9; Ibadan (Nigeria)'85; MB BS; CCFP; FCFP; Staff, Didsbury Medical Clinic; Staff, Orion Health Calgary; Med Dir, Starpoint Health Corp; Langs: Yoruba; (250)768-6920; drtoye@shaw.ca.

OYENIRAN, Idowu; 91 Champlain St, North Bay ON P1B 7M3; Univ of Benin (Nigeria)'90; CCFP; (705)495-2323; Fax. (705)495-3281.

OYENUBI, Abimbola; 450 Lillooet St W, Moose Jaw SK S6H 7T1; (306)694-5508; Fax. (306)694-5419.

OYENUBI, Ademilola N; Markham Stouffville Hosp, PO Box 1800 Stn Main 381 Church St, Markham ON L3P 7P3; Lagos (Nigeria)'91; FRCPC; IntMed. Staff, Markham Stouffville Hospital; (905)472-7373

OYEWOLE, Olusegun; Spesmed Med Specialist Ctre, PO Box 1540 Stn Main 2951 99th St, North Battleford SK S9A 3W1; Ogun State Univ (Nigeria)'89; MB BS; MRCP(I); Staff ObstGyn, Battlefords Union Hospital; Langs: Yoruba; (306)446-5545; Fax. (306)446-5547.

OYEWUMI, L Kola; Markham Stouffville Hosp, PO Box 1800 Stn Main 381 Church St, Markham ON L3P 7P3; Ibadan (Nigeria)'73; BSc; MB BS; DABPN; DPsy; FRCPC; Psy (Psychosis). Consultant Heads Up Southeastern Ont Dist Early Intervention Prog, Hotel-Dieu Hospital; Staff, Markham Stouffville Hospital; Fellow, Canadian Psychiatric Association; Prof Psy, Biomedical & Molecular Sciences, Queen's University; Langs: Yoruba; (905)472-7000

OYEYE, Grant; 410-229 Victoria St, Prince George BC V2L 5B8; (Nigeria)'97; (250)564-8869

OYEYEMI, Joseph O; 3233-150 Millrise Blvd SW, Calgary AB T2Y 5G7; (Nigeria)'88; MB BS; CCFP; (403)256-4669

OYLER, Jeffrey R; 470-546 St Paul St, Kamloops BC V2C 5T1; UBC'96; FRCPC; Neur. (250)377-3133; Fax. (250)372-1025.

OYSTON, John P; 18 Whitehall Rd, Toronto ON M4W 2C6; Newcastle-Upon-Tyne (England)'80; BMedSci; FFARCS; Anes. Pres, Oyston Associates (Web Site Design E Internet Consulting); (416)972-1292

OZA, Amit M; Univ Hlth Network-Princess M, 5 717-610 University Ave, Toronto ON M5G 2M9; London (England)'83; MB BS; BSc; FRCP; FRCPC; IntMed (Medical Oncology)., Princess Margaret Hospital - University Health Network; Assoc Prof Med, University of Toronto; (416)946-2818; Fax. (416)946-4467; amit.oza@uhn.on.ca.

OZA, Pari U; Summerville Family Health Team, 211-190 Sherway Dr, Etobicoke ON M9C 5N2; Tor'05; CCFP; Staff Active Comprehensive MRP, Trillium Health Centre - West Toronto; (416)621-9700; Fax. (416)621-4438; poza@thc.on.ca.

OZA, Sangeeta A; MCI The Doctor's Office, 255 Morningside Ave, Scarborough ON M1E 3E6; London (England)'83; MRCGPract; CCFP; (416)284-1020; Fax. (416)284-1271.

OZARD, Ian D; Queensway-Carleton Hosp, 3045 Baseline Rd, Nepean ON K2H 8P4; Wes'01; FRCPC; Anes. Staff, Queensway Carleton Hospital; (613)721-2000 x2900

OZARD, Jennifer G; Manotick Med Centre, 5230 Mitch Owens Rd, Manotick ON K4M 1B2; Qns'04; CCFP; (613)692-2571; Fax. (613)692-0271.

OZELSEL, Timur J; Clinical Sciences Bldg, 8 120-152 University Campus NW, Edmonton AB T6G 2G3; (Germany)'98; (780)407-8861; Fax. (780)407-3200.

OZEN, Nilay; St Mary's Hosp Centre, 2339-3830 av Lacombe, Montreal QC H3T 1M5; McG'88; FRCPC; IntMed; Cardiol. Staff, St Mary's Hospital Centre; (514)734-2614; Fax. (514)734-2766.

OZERE, Chris; Albro Lake Med Centre, 6 Primrose St, Dartmouth NS B3A 4C5; Mem'88; (902)465-4444; Fax. (902)463-2717.

OZERKAN, Ebru; Paton Paediatric Centre, 008-1 Paton St, St. John's NL A1B 4S8; Staff, James Paton Memorial Hospital.

OZERSKY, Sam; 86 Glen Park Ave, North York ON M6B 2C4; Man'77; AB; FRCPC; Psy (Mood Disorders). Sr Consultant Mood Disorders Clinic, Toronto General Hospital - UHN; Pres/CEO, Mensante Corporation; Lecturer, University of Toronto; Langs: Hebrew; (416)928-9195; Fax. (416)783-6000.

OZIMOK, Daniel; Atrium Prof Bldg, SS 103 305-190 Cundles Rd E, Barrie ON L4M 4S5; McM'80; Staff, Royal Victoria Regional Health Centre; (705)728-5099; Fax. (705)726-8063; dozimok@rogers.com.

OZOG-BARTLETT, Joanne L; Medical Arts Centre, 3 Maple Ave N, Burford ON N0E 1A0; Ott'86; BSc; CCFP; (519)449-2468; Fax. (519)449-5352.

OZOLINS, Laura N; 106-15252 32 Ave, Surrey BC V3S 0R7; Tor'07; CCFP; (604)542-4885

OZOLS, Dina Y; St Clair Beach Hlth Ctr, 6-500 Manning Rd, Windsor ON N8N 2L9; McM'93; CCFP; (519)979-7314

OZON, Pierre J; Stevenson Mem Hosp, PO Box 4000 Stn Main 200 Fletcher Cres, Alliston ON L9R 1W7; Mem'97; CCFP; Staff, Stevenson Memorial Hospital; (705)435-6281

OZUMBA, Obioma; Dr Everett Chalmers Reg Hosp, PO Box 9000 Stn A 700 Priestman St, Fredericton NB E3B 5N5; (Nigeria)'03; Staff, Dr Everett Chalmers Regional Hospital; (506)452-5400

PABANI, Anizmohamed S; Surlang Med Clinic, 106-19475 Fraser Hwy, Surrey BC V3S 6K7; Tor'91; (604)533-5051; Fax. (604)533-8353.

PABANI, Shehnaz; Notre Dame Med Centre, 430 Notre Dame Ave, Sudbury ON P3C 5K7; Tor'80; CCFP; FCFP; (705)671-9188

PABBIES, Arone; 104-5010 43 St, Red Deer AB T4N 6H2; Wes'01; BSc; FRCSC; Otol. (403)340-3130; Fax. (403)340-3135.

PABBIES, Ashesh K; 125-1620 29 St NW, Calgary AB T2N 4L7; (Australia)'07; CCFP; (403)289-7223; Fax. (403)289-7523.

PABST, Henry F; Walter Mackenzie HSC, 132 University Campus NW, Edmonton AB T6G 2R7; Alb'62; FRCPC; Peds (Immunology). Staff Peds, University of Alberta Hospital; Emeritus Prof Peds/Researcher, University of Alberta; Langs: German; (780)735-2731

PACAUD, Daniele; Alberta Children's Hosp, 2888 Shaganappi Trail NW, Calgary AB T3B 6A8; Mon'89; FRCPC; Peds; Endocrin (P.Q.); Endocrin&Metab. Staff, Alberta Children's Hospital; (403)955-7819; Fax. (403)955-5001.

PACE, Beverly A; Lexitor Med Clinic, 205-1808 Bowen Rd, Nanaimo BC V9S 5W4; Dal'76; CCFP; Staff, Nanaimo Regional General Hospital; Clin Preceptor, University of British Columbia; (250)753-6646; Fax. (250)753-6174.

PACE, David E; Health Sciences Centre, 1832-300 Prince Philip Dr, St. John's NL A1B 3V6; Mem'94; FRCSC; GenSurg. Staff, Health Sciences Centre; (709)777-6300

PACE, Kenneth T; 9 106Q-61 Queen St E, Toronto ON M5C 2T2; Tor'94; MSc; FRCSC; Urol (Laparoscopy). Staff Surgeon, St Michael's Hospital; Assoc Prof, University of Toronto; (416)867-3695; Fax. (416)867-3675; kenneth.pace@utoronto.ca.

PACE, Peter-John; 421 Shepherdson Rd PO Box 2380, New Liskeard ON P0J 1P0; Qns'84; MDiv; BA; CCFP; (705)647-8414; Fax. (705)647-8414; ppace@temiskaming-hospital.com.

PACE, Ron F; 301-749 King St W, Kitchener ON N2G 1E4; Wes'79; FRCSC; GenSurg (Endoscopy). Staff, St Mary's General Hospital; Staff, Grand River Hospital - Kitchener/Waterloo Health Centre; (519)570-2833; Fax. (519)570-2865.

PACHAI, Indira; First Medical Place, 104-170 Queensway W, Mississauga ON L5B 3A8; Natal (South Africa)'79; MB ChB; FAAP; FRCPC; Peds. Ac Staff, Trillium Health Centre - Mississauga; (905)267-3104; Fax. (905)267-3106.

PACHAL, Cindy A; Plessis Med Centre, 12-801 Regent Ave W, Winnipeg MB R2C 3A7; Man'81; Ac Staff, Concordia General Hospital; (204)222-4200; Fax. (204)222-8181.

PACHAL, Richard G; Duncan Mental Health Centre, 3088 Gibbins Rd, Duncan BC V9L 1E8; UBC'94; FRCPC; Psy. (250)709-3040; Fax. (250)709-3045.

PACIN, Alojz; Victoria Gen Hosp, 2340 Pembina Hwy, Winnipeg MB R3T 2E8; Komenskeho (Czech Republic)'65; Staff, Victoria General Hospital; (204)269-3570

PACIN, Ondrej; Pan Am Sports Med Centre, 75 Poseidon Bay, Winnipeg MB R3M 3E4; Man'96; BSc; BScMed; CCFP; Langs: Czech; (204)927-2699; Fax. (204)452-5362.

PACIN, Stefan; 10-1200 Waverley St, Winnipeg MB R3T 0P4; Man'98; FRCPC; Neur.

PACIS, Ruth B; Forest Hills Med Clinic, 4 Forest Hills Pky, Dartmouth NS B2W 5G7; Manila (Philippines)'77; BSc; CCFP; Staff, Dartmouth General Hospital; Langs: Tagalog; Spanish; (902)435-5530; Fax. (902)462-6398.

PACKER, Karen E; 4640 17 Ave NW, Calgary AB T3B 0P3; McM'93; CCFP; FCFP; (403)202-2727; Fax. (403)202-2733.

PACKER, Richard T; 446 Concession St, Hamilton ON L9A 1C2; McM'86; CCFP; FCFP; (905)318-3877; Fax. (905)318-0016.

PACKER, Samuel; Humber River Reg Hosp-Keele, 2175 Keele St, York ON M6M 3Z4; Chicago(IL) (USA)'72; FRCPC; Psy (Community Psychiatry)., Humber River Regional Hospital - Keele Street Site; Assoc Prof, University of Toronto; (416)658-2061

PACKER, Tamar W; 446 Concession St, Hamilton ON L9A 1C2; McM'87; CCFP; FCFP; (905)318-3877; Fax. (905)318-0016.

PACKWOOD, Nadine; Hop Jeffery Hale, 1250 ch Sainte-Foy, Quebec QC G1S 2M6; Laval'94; Staff, Jeffery Hale Hospital-Saint Brigid's; Langs: English; (418)684-5333

PACO, Charles A; 825-123 Edward St, Toronto ON M5G 1E2; Liege (Belgium)'86; DABIM; FRCPC; IntMed (Gastroenterology). Staff, The Scarborough Hospital - General Campus; Langs: English; French; (416)597-0997; Fax. (416)597-2912.

PACURARU, Jean-Pierre; CLSC Mer et Montagnes, 71 boul St-Francois-Xavier E, Grande-Vallee QC G0E 1K0; Sher'92; CCFP; (418)393-2001; Fax. (418)393-2767; pacuraru@globetrotter.qc.ca.

PADAMADAN, Philsamma G; 217 Terrace Hill St, Brantford ON N3R 1G8; Kerala (India)'78; MB BS; FRCPC; Peds. Staff, The Brant Community Healthcare System - Brantford General Hospital Site; (519)752-7002; Fax. (519)752-8320.

PADAN, Callie; Centre Med Vaudreuil-Dorion, 600 boul Harwood, Vaudreuil-Dorion QC J7V 6A3; Mon'10; CCFP; (450)455-9301

PADANILATHU KUNJUMMAR, Shakkeela; 24-130 Davis Dr, Newmarket ON L3Y 2N1; Mysore (India)'93; MB BS; DCH; CCFP; Langs: Hindi; Malayalam; Tamil; (905)853-8525

PADAYACHEE, Vinogaran T; Saskatchewan Med Assoc, 402-321A 21st St E, Saskatoon SK S7K 0C1; Natal (South Africa)'82; MB ChB; DA(SA); Chief Staff, St Joseph's Hospital; Pres, Saskatchewan Medical Association; (306)244-2196; Fax. (306)653-1631; vino@sma.sk.ca.

PADDA, Jagdish S; Abbotsford Reg Hosp & Cancer C, 32900 Marshall Rd, Abbotsford BC V2S 0C2; UBC'94; FRCPC; Anes. (604)851-4873

PADDA, Roop-Preet K; 6438 Fraser St, Vancouver BC V5W 3A4; UBC'05; CCFP; (604)327-3330

PADDOCK, Vernon W; Saint John Reg Hosp, PO Box 2100 Stn Main 400 University Ave, Saint John NB E2L 4L2; Mem'84; FRCPC; IntMed; Cardiol. Staff, Saint John Regional Hospital; (506)648-6101

PADDON, Robert C; SRS Consultants Inc, 827 Richmond St, London ON N6A 3H7; Tor'87; CCFP; FCFP; (519)858-4694; Fax. (519)858-4692.

PADEANU, Florin; Prairie Trails Med Clinic, 100-1345 Taylor Ave, Winnipeg MB R3M 3Y9; Man'01; CCFP; (204)475-0088

PADGETT, Richard W W; F247-100 West 5th St PO Box 585 Stn Lcd 1, Hamilton ON L8N 3K7; Tor'77; FRCPC; Psy (Forensic Psychiatry). Court Staff, Hamilton Health Sciences Centre; Ac Staff, St Joseph's Healthcare Hamilton - West 5th Campus; Affil Staff, Joseph Brant Memorial Hospital; Clinical Asst Prof, McMaster University; (905)522-1155 x36263; Fax. (905)381-5605.

PADILLA, Julio R; 405-125 13th St E, North Vancouver BC V7L 2L3; (Guatemala)'75; FRCSC; Neursurg (Neuro Oncology). Court Staff Neurosurg, University Hospital of Northern British Columbia; Staff, Lions Gate Hospital; Langs: Spanish; (604)987-7085; jrpadilla@shaw.ca.

PADILLA-THORNTON, Amie E; Mount St Joseph Hosp, 3080 Prince Edward St, Vancouver BC V5T 3N4; UBC'04; FRCPC; DiagRad. Staff, Providence Health Care - Mount Saint Joseph Hospital; (604)877-8323

PADMORE, Dave E; 1019 Prince St, Truro NS B2N 1H7; Jamaica (Jamaica)'90; FRCSC; Urol. Staff, Colchester East Hants Health Centre; (902)897-0600; Fax. (902)897-2361.

PADMORE, Lloyd G; Woburn Med Dental Centre, 4129 Lawrence Ave E, Scarborough ON M1E 2S2; Aberdeen (Scotland)'63; FRCOG(Eng); FRCSC; ObstGyn. Court Staff ObstGyn, The Scarborough Hospital - General Campus; (416)439-1991; Fax. (416)439-3593.

PADMORE, Ruth F; The Ottawa Hosp-Gen Campus, 501 Smyth Rd, Ottawa ON K1H 8L6; Dal'80; PhD; FRCPC; AnatPath; HemPath. Staff HemPath, The Ottawa Hospital - General Campus; Consultant, Children's Hospital of Eastern Ontario (CHEO); Assoc Prof, University of Ottawa; (613)737-8355

PADMOS, M Andrew; Royal College of Physicians, 774 Echo Dr, Ottawa ON K1S 5N8; McM'72; ABIM; FACP; FRCPC; IntMed (Administration); Hem. CEO, Royal College Of Physicians &; Prof Med, Dalhousie University; (613)730-6205; Fax. (613)730-8250; apadmos@royalcollege.ca.

PADONOU, Michael K; 208-101 Queensway W, Mississauga ON L5B 2P7; Tor'85; FRCSC; GenSurg. Court Staff Surg, The Credit Valley Hospital; Consultant, Trillium Health Centre - Mississauga; (905)896-8996; Fax. (905)896-8199; mpadonou@thc.on.ca.

PADRON CASTILLO, Oswaldo E; 50 rue de Belvedere, Ste-Anne-des-Monts QC G4V 1X4; CCFP; (418)763-2261; oswapadron@yahoo.ca.

PADUA, Raymond R; PO Box 324, Bushell Park SK S0H 0N0; Cal'03; CCFP; (306)972-8562; Fax. (306)694-2875.

PADUA, Rodolfo N; Winnipeg Clinic, 425 St Mary Ave, Winnipeg MB R3C 0N2; (Philippines)'62; FRCPC; IntMed (Cardiology). Staff, Misericordia Health Centre; Internal Med, WRHA - Deer Lodge Centre; Teacher, University of Manitoba; (204)957-1900; Fax. (204)943-2164.

PADUREANU, Magdalena; Polyclinique Med Fabreville, 380 boul Cure-Labelle, Laval QC H7P 5L3; Mon'04; (450)628-5800 x312

PADWAL, Rajdeep S; University of Alberta Hosp, 2F1.26 WCM-8440 112 St NW, Edmonton AB T6G 2B7; Sask'95; FRCPC; IntMed (Clinical Pharmacology). Staff, University of Alberta Hospital; Asst Prof, University of Alberta; (780)407-2732; Fax. (780)407-3132.

PAEK, Wusun; Hydro Place Bldg, 8711-700 University Ave, Toronto ON M5G 1Z5; Tor'87; FRCSC; ObstGyn (Advanced Laparoscopic Surgery). Staff, Mount Sinai Hospital; Asst Prof ObstGyn, University of Toronto; (416)586-4800 x3120; Fax. (416)586-5331.

PAES, Bosco A; McMaster University, HSC 3A-1280 Main St W, Hamilton ON L8S 4K1; Dublin (Ireland)'72; MB ChB; BAO; DCH; FRCPI(Ire); FRCPC; Peds (Neonatology). Assoc Member Dept of Family Med, Hamilton Health Sciences Centre - McMaster Children's Hospital; Teach Staff, McMaster University; (905)521-2100; Fax. (905)521-5007; paes@mcmaster.ca.

PAETKAU, Carla; Gibsons Med Clinic, 211-1100 Sunshine Coast Hwy, Gibsons BC V0N 1V7; UBC'89; (604)886-2868; Fax. (604)886-9716.

PAETKAU, Donald J M; Health Sciences Ctr Gen Hosp, 700 William Ave, Winnipeg MB R3E 0Z3; Man'77; FRCPC; Anes. Staff, Health Sciences Centre; (204)787-3796; Fax. (204)787-3656.

PAETSCH, Paul R; Grey Nuns Community Hosp & HC, 1100 Youville Drive West NW, Edmonton AB T6L 5X8; Alb'96; FRCPC; Anes. Staff, Covenant Health - Grey Nuns Community Hospital; (780)735-7020

PAGACZ, Alexis A; Hawkesbury Dist Gen Hosp, 1111 Ghislain St, Hawkesbury ON K6A 3G5; Mon'64; CSPQ; FRCPC; DiagRad. Staff, Hawkesbury & District General Hospital; (613)632-1111

PAGANO, Joseph J P; University of Alberta Hosp, 4C2-8440 112 St NW, Edmonton AB T6G 2B7; Alb'04; FRCPC; Peds; Cardiol. Staff, University of Alberta Hospital; (780)407-8822

PAGDIN, Grant; Mission Med Centre, 102-3320 Richter St, Kelowna BC V1W 4V5; UBC'88; CCFP; Clin Instructor Southern Medical Program, University of British Columbia; (250)868-8222; Fax. (250)868-8269.

PAGE, Alain; CSSS de Trois-Rivières, 1991 boul du Carmel, Trois-Rivieres QC G8Z 3R9; Laval'95; OrthSurg. Staff, CSSS de Trois-Rivières; (819)697-3333; alain_page@hotmail.com.

PAGE, Andrea E; Sunnybrook Hlth Sciences Ctre, C703-2075 Bayview Ave, Toronto ON M4N 3M5; Wes'06; FRCSC; ObstGyn. Staff, Sunnybrook Health Sciences Centre; (416)480-4535; Fax. (416)480-4405.

PAGE, Andrea V; Mount Sinai Hosp, 436-600 University Ave, Toronto ON M5G 1X5; Wes'02; FRCPC; IntMed; InfectDis. Staff, Mount Sinai Hospital; (416)596-4200

PAGE, Anne-Marie J; UCMC North Hill, 258-1632 14 Ave NW, Calgary AB T2N 1M7; Mon'86; (403)291-3001

PAGE, Brian C; PO Box 95 Rpo, Lake Louise AB T0L 1E0; Alb'76.

PAGE, Christopher R W; Drivercheck Inc, PO Box 1186 1 Manley St, Ayr ON N0B 1E0; Qns'72; Pres, Drivercheck Inc; (519)632-9371; Fax. (519)632-9534.

PAGE, Crystal; PO Box 308, Smithers BC V0J 2N0; UBC'02; CCFP; (250)847-2240

PAGE, David A; Crossroads Family Practice, 201-45800 Promontory Rd, Chilliwack BC V2R 5Z5; Cape Town (South Africa)'86; MB ChB; DA(SA); CCFP; (604)858-3725; Fax. (604)858-8625.

PAGE, Douglas B; Lake Louise Med Clinic, PO Box 95, Lake Louise AB T0L 1E0; Qns'10; CCFP; (403)522-2451; Fax. (403)522-3807.

PAGE, Francine M G; 200-4 Beechwood Ave, Vanier ON K1L 8L9; Sher'77; Psy (Adult Psychiatry). Langs: Bilingual(French/English); (613)741-7431; Fax. (613)741-0176.

PAGE, Francoise; Centre Med Boucherville, 201-600 boul du Fort Saint-Lou, Bouchervulle QC J4B 1S7; Mon'75; (450)655-7321

PAGE, Kevin B; Fort St John Med Clinic, 10011 96 St, Fort St. John BC V1J 3P3; Cape Town (South Africa)'83; MB ChB; (250)785-6677; Fax. (250)787-0109.

PAGE, Michael S; Vancouver Gen Hosp, 2449-855 12th Ave W, Vancouver BC V5Z 1M9; UBC'75; FRCPC; Anes. Ac Staff Anes, Vancouver General Hospital - Centennial Pavillion; (604)875-4304

PAGE, Michel; 3881 boul Saint-Jean, Dollard-D-Ormeaux QC H9G 2V1; Mon'78; LMCC; Assoc Staff, Hôpital du Sacre-Coeur de Montréal; Langs: English; (514)624-0444; mpag1@videotron.ca.

PAGE, Paul D; Saint John Reg Hosp, PO Box 2100 Stn Main 400 University Ave, Saint John NB E2L 4L2; Mem'09; CCFP; CCFP(E.M.); Staff, Saint John Regional Hospital; (506)648-6000

PAGE, Pierre; Hop du Sacre-Coeur de Mtl, 5400 boul Gouin O, Montreal QC H4J 1C5; Mon'75; FACC; FACS; FRCSC; GenSurg; Cardiovasc&ThorSurg. Ac Staff Surg, Hôpital du Sacre-Coeur de Montréal; Ac Staff, Institut de Cardiologie de Montréal; Prof Surg, Universite de Montreal; (514)338-2222 x3246; Fax. (514)338-2694; pierre.page@umontreal.ca.

PAGE, Robert J; City Centre Health Care, 1400 Windsor Ave, Windsor ON N8X 3L9; Wes'71; CCFP; Staff, Canadian Mental Health Associaton; (519)971-0116; Fax. (519)252-5646.

PAGE, Shannon; Invermere Med Centre, PO Box 8000, Invermere BC V0A 1K0; Leeds (England)'99; MB ChB; BSc; DRCOG; Med Staff, Invermere & District Hospital; Instructor Rural Graduate, University of British Columbia; (250)342-9206; Fax. (250)342-6669; rockiesdoc@msn.com.

PAGE, Simon Y; CSSS de Sept-Iles, 45 rue du Pere-Divet, Sept-Iles QC G4R 3N7; Ott'06; FRCPC; Anes. Staff, Centre Hospitalier Regional de Sept-Iles; (418)962-9761

PAGE, Sylvain; Hopital Laval, 2725 ch Sainte-Foy, Quebec QC G1V 4G5; Laval'95; CSPQ; FRCPC; AnatPath. Staff, Hôpital Laval; (418)691-5233; Fax. (418)656-4571; sylvain.page@mail.chuq.qc.ca.

PAGE, Vesna; The Credit Valley Hosp, 2200 Eglinton Ave W, Mississauga ON L5M 2N1; McM'94; BScArts & Sci; FRCPC; IntMed; GeriatricMed. Staff, The Credit Valley Hospital; (905)813-1100 x5178; Fax. (905)813-4229; vpage@cvh.on.ca.

PAGEAU, Alain; CHUS-Hop Fleurimont, 3001 12e av N, Sherbrooke QC J1H 5N4; Mon'95; Staff, Centre Hospitalier Universitaire de Sherbrooke-Hopital Fleurimont; (819)346-1110; Fax. (819)820-6420.

PAGEAU, Paul G; The Ottawa Hosp-Civic Campus, 1053 Carling Ave, Ottawa ON K1Y 4E9; McM'99; CCFP; CCFP(E.M.); Staff, The Ottawa Hospital - Civic Campus; (905)813-2200

PAGENKOPF, Cort W; Canmore Gen Hosp, 1100 Hospital Pl, Canmore AB T1W 1N2; Alb'93; FRCSC; GenSurg. Staff, Canmore General Hospital; (403)678-7198; Fax. (403)678-7196; drcort@telusplanet.net.

PAGLIARELLO, Giuseppe; The Ottawa Hosp-Civic Campus, 260-1053 Carling Ave, Ottawa ON K1Y 4E9; Qns'79; FACS; FRCSC; GenSurg (Critical Care Medicine). Att Staff, The Ottawa Hospital - Civic Campus; Asst Prof, University of Ottawa; (613)761-5199; Fax. (613)761-5371.

PAGLIARULO, Giovanni; Polyclinique Med Pierre Le Gar, 300-1000 Montee des Pionniers, Terrebonne QC J6V 1S8; Mon'99; CCFP; Staff, Hopital Maisonneuve-Rosemont; (450)657-5799; Fax. (450)657-1809.

PAGNOUX, Christian; Div of Rheumatology, 2 220-60 Murray St, Toronto ON M5T 3L9; Paris (France)'02.

PAGTAKHAN, Arlene L; Parkdale Med Tower, 801-1081 Carling Ave, Ottawa ON K1Y 4G2; Man'87; CCFP; Clin Associate Cardiol, University of Ottawa Heart Institute; (613)725-2334

PAHIL, Rajbir S; Cape Breton Cancer Centre, 1482 George St, Sydney NS B1P 1P3; Punjab (India)'87; FACP; Staff MedOncol, Cape Breton Healthcare Complex; Asst Prof IntMed, Dalhousie University; Langs: Punjabi; Hindi; (902)567-7771; Fax. (902)567-8075; pahilr@cbdha.nshealth.ca.

PAHULJE, Bernadette F; West Village Mall, 160 Columbia Blvd W, Lethbridge AB T1K 4J4; Alb'85; CCFP; (403)381-7000; Fax. (403)381-8250.

PAHUTA, Zenon; 718 Annette St, Toronto ON M6S 2E2; Tor'69; Ac Staff, St Joseph's Health Centre; (416)769-8050

PAI, Emily; Lansdowne Professional Ctr II, 215-3066 Shelbourne St, Victoria BC V8R 6T9; UBC'99; CCFP; FCFP; (250)388-4211

PAI, Howard H; BC Cancer Agency-Vanc Isl Ctr, 2410 Lee Ave, Victoria BC V8R 6V5; Wes'93; FRCPC; RadOncol (Genito Urinary Oncology). Staff RadOncol, BC Cancer Agency Vancouver Island Centre; Med Staff, Royal Jubilee Hospital; Asst Prof Surg, University of British Columbia; Aj Asst Prof School of Health Info Science, University of Victoria; Langs: Chinese; Mandarin; (250)519-5575; Fax. (250)519-2018.

PAI, Menaka; Hamilton HS-General Site, 1 270A-237 Barton St E, Hamilton ON L8L 2X2; McM'03; FRCPC; IntMed (Thrombosis); Hem. Hematologist, Hamilton Health Sciences Centre - Hamilton General Hospital; Asst Prof Med, McMaster University; (905)527-0271 x46139

PAI, Rajeev N; Royal Jubilee Hosp, 1952 Bay St, Victoria BC V8R 1J8; Kerala (India)'77; MB BS; MRC(UK); ABIM; FRCPC; IntMed; GeriatricMed. Staff, Royal Jubilee Hospital; (250)370-8509; Fax. (250)370-8285.

PAICE, Naomi; Hillside Pediatric Clinic, 65 rue Hillside, Montreal QC H3V 1W1; McG'00; FRCPC; Peds. Staff, McGill University Health Centre - Montreal Children's Hospital; (514)931-2524

PAIDRA, Astrid; Sexual Health Centre, 179 Clarence St, Ottawa ON K1N 5P7; Qns'76; Physician, Sexual Health Centre-Ottawa Carleton Health Dept; (613)560-6099; Fax. (613)560-6096.

PAIDRA, Erik J; Lakeridge Hlth Corp-Oshawa, 1 Hospital Crt, Oshawa ON L1G 2B9; Tor'80; FACEP; Staff, Lakeridge Health - Oshawa Site; (905)576-8711; Fax. (905)721-4749.

PAIEMENT, Francois L; 624 Wilson St, Ottawa ON K1K 4S5; Ott'98; CCFP; (613)741-1257

PAIEMENT, Isabelle; Inst Philippe Pinel de Mtl, 10905 boul Henri-Bourassa E, Montreal QC H1C 1H1; Mon'92; FRCPC; Psy. Staff, Institut Philippe-Pinel de Montreal; (514)648-8461 x411; Fax. (514)881-3705.

PAIEMENT-LAMOTHE, Anie; Ctr Hosp Rouyn-Noranda, 4 9e rue, Rouyn-Noranda QC J9X 2B2; Mon'04; CCFP; Staff, Centre Hospitalier Rouyn-Noranda; (819)764-5131; aniepl@hotmail.com.

PAIKATT, Santosh C; 456 Dundas St, Cambridge ON N1R 5R4; Bangalore (India)'78; MB BS; FAAP; FRCPC; Peds (Neonatology). Consultant, Cambridge Memorial Hospital; (519)740-7205

PAIKIN, Jeremy; Hamilton HS-General Site, NW8N 01-237 Barton St E, Hamilton ON L8L 2X2; McM'07; FRCPC; IntMed. Staff, Hamilton Health Sciences Centre - Hamilton General Hospital; (905)521-2100

PAIKIN, Sarah; Earl Bales Med Clinic, 106-1333 Sheppard Ave E, North York ON M2J 1V1; McM'90; BSc; BEd; MPs; BA; Physician, Earl Bales Medical Clinic; Langs: Yiddish; French; (647)348-2688; Fax. (416)247-3463.

PAILLARD, Christian; Clinique de Med Interne, 20 rue Carrier, Edmundston NB E3V 3Y1; Mon'93; FRCPC; IntMed. Staff, Hôpital regional d'Edmundston; (506)739-9511; Fax. (506)735-8118; clin.med.int@nb.aibn.com.

PAILLARD, Jean-Francois; Clin Med Fam d'Edmundston, 52 av Bateman, Edmundston NB E3V 4A4; Sher'00; DSS; FRCSC; OrthSurg. Staff/Chief Orthopedics, Hôpital regional d'Edmundston; Langs: English; (506)735-8442; Fax. (506)739-6271.

PAILLE, Catherine; Centre Hosp Honore-Mercier, 2750 boul Laframboise, Saint-Hyacinthe QC J2S 4Y8; Laval'07; FRCPC; Psy. Staff, Centre Hospitalier Honore-Mercier; (450)771-3333 x4500

PAILLE, Fernand; Clinique Med Fam des Recollets, 101-940 boul des Recollets, Trois-Rivieres QC G8Z 3W9; Laval'74; (819)373-0303; Fax. (819)373-8431.

PAIN, Clare M; Mount Sinai Hosp, 600 University Ave, Toronto ON M5G 1X5; McM'85; BSc; MSc; FRCPC; Psy (Psychological Trauma). Staff, Mount Sinai Hospital; Asst Prof, University of Toronto; (416)586-4800 x8890; Fax. (416)586-8654.

PAIN, Tarun K; Lockwood Clinic, 320-790 Bay St, Toronto ON M5G 1N8; Calcutta (India)'59; MRC; DTMH; FRCPC; IntMed. (416)921-2121; Fax. (416)921-0569.

PAINCHAUD, Genevieve; Unite Med Familiale Maizerets, 2480 ch de la Canardiere, Quebec QC G1J 2G1; Mon'05; (418)661-1413; Fax. (418)661-7504.

PAINCHAUD, Guillaume; CLSC Haute Ville, 55 ch Sainte-Foy, Quebec QC G1R 1S9; Mon'98; CCFP; Staff, Centre Hospitalier Trois-Pistoles; Staff, Centre Hospitalier Universitaire De Québec - Pavillon De St-françois-d'assise; (418)641-2572

PAINCHAUD, Magalie; Hotel-Dieu de Levis, 143 rue Wolfe, Levis QC G6V 3Z1; Laval'97; FRCPC; Psy. Staff, Hôtel-Dieu de Lévis; (418)835-7121

PAINSON, Bossuet; CHSLD Jeanne le Ber, 7445 rue Hochelaga, Montreal QC H1N 3V2; (Haiti)'58; CSPQ; GenPath (P.Q.). Staff, CSSS Lucille Teasdale; Langs: Creole; English; (514)251-6000 x45080

PAINTER, Nigel A; West Hill Med Clinic, 1A-2995 2nd Ave W, Prince Albert SK S6V 5V5; Stellenbosch (South Africa)'99; MB ChB; Langs: Afrikaans; Xhosa; (306)765-8500; Fax. (306)765-8501; dr.painter@westhillmedical.com.

PAINTSIL, James E; Cypress Reg Health Centre, 2004 Saskatchewan Dr, Swift Current SK S9H 5M8; (Ghana)'92; FRCPC; Anes. Staff, Cypress Regional Health Authority Corporate Office; (306)778-9400; Fax. (306)774-3346; jpaintsil@shaw.ca.

PAIRAUDEAU, Nicholas V J; Nicholas Pairaudeau Prof Corp, 402-1100 Sheppard Ave E, North York ON M2K 2W1; London (England)'70; MB BS; FRCSC; ObstGyn (Infertility). Staff Consultant, North York General Hospital; Asst Prof, University of Toronto; Langs: Spanish; Italian; French; (416)226-1661; Fax. (416)222-2538; g2p@rogers.com.

PAISLEY, David M A; 587 Penticton Ave, Penticton BC V2A 2M5; Stellenbosch (South Africa)'84; MB ChB; DA(SA); LMCC; ACLS; Staff, Penticton Regional Hospital; Langs: Afrikaans; (250)492-5552; Fax. (250)492-6784.

PAISLEY, J Kenneth; Elginwood Long Term Care Ctre, 182 Yorkland St, Richmond Hill ON L4S 2M9; UBC'78; PhD; BSc; Att Physician, Sherwood Court LTC; Att Physician, Specialty Care Ontario; Att Physician, Eagle Terrace Long Term Care Facility; (905)737-0858; Fax. (905)737-1866; kpaisley@yorkmed.ca.

PAITICH, C Bruce; 48-2140 North Park Dr, Brampton ON L6S 0C9; Tor'87; BSc; FRCSC; OrthSurg (Spine Surgery). Staff, William Osler Health System - Brampton Civic Hospital; Staff, Halton Healthcare Services Corporation - Georgetown Hospital; (905)874-1759; Fax. (905)874-1652.

PAJER, Kathleen A; IWK Health Centre, PO Box 9700 Rpo Csc 5850-5980 University Ave, Halifax NS B3K 6R8; Univ of South Alabama (USA)'82; Staff, IWK Health Centre; (902)470-8087; Fax. (902)470-7937.

PAJOT, Denise M; Chelsea Court Health Centre, 779 Chelsea St, Brockville ON K6V 6J8; Ott'85; BSc; CCFP; (613)342-1199

PAKENHAM, Susan E; The Medical Centre, 707 Charlotte St, Peterborough ON K9J 2X5; Qns'07; FRCSC; ObstGyn. (705)743-6222

PAKES, Barry N; North York Med Arts Bldg, 242-1333 Sheppard Ave E, North York ON M2J 1V1; Tor'01; FRCPC; CommunMed;CCFP; Public Health & Preventive Med.

PAKES, Eddy H; North York Med Arts Bldg, 242-1333 Sheppard Ave E, North York ON M2J 1V1; Alb'61; DPsy; FAPA; FRCPC; Psy (Bereavement). Langs: Hebrew; (416)497-0447; Fax. (416)497-7365.

PAKES, Judith B; North York Med Arts Bldg, 242-1333 Sheppard Ave E, North York ON M2J 1V1; Tor'65; FRCPC; Psy. (416)756-2114

PAKHALE, Smita S; The Ottawa Hosp-Gen Campus, 501 Smyth Rd, Ottawa ON K1H 8L6; Nagpur (India)'88; FRCPC; IntMed; Critical Care Medicine; Respir. Staff, The Ottawa Hospital - General Campus; (613)737-8899; Fax. (613)739-6807.

PAKIJAVAN, Abdolreza P; Lakeridge Health Oshawa, 1 Hospital Crt, Oshawa ON L1G 2B9; Tehran (Iran)'91; CCFP; CCFP(E.M.); Staff, The Ottawa Hospital - General Campus; (905)576-8711

PAKULIS, Valdis; 204-857 Grand Ave W, Chatham ON N7L 4T1; Wes'69; FRCSC; Urol. Ac Staff, Chatham-Kent Health Alliance; (519)354-9300; Fax. (519)354-5035; pakulis@wincom.net.

PAL, Raveen S; Kingston Gen Hosp, 76 Stuart St, Kingston ON K7L 2V7; Tor'00; FRCPC; IntMed; Cardiol. Staff, Kingston General Hospital; Langs: Hindi; (613)548-3232

PALACIOS-BOIX, Jorge A; 1547 av des Pins O, Montreal QC H3G 1B3; (Mexico)'82; FRCPC; Psy (Addiction Psychiatry). Med Dir Addictions Unit, McGill University Health Centre - Montreal General Campus; adj Prof, McGill University; Langs: English; French; Spanish; (514)934-8311

PALAD, Catalino G; Malton Med Centre, 7330 Goreway Dr, Mississauga ON L4T 4J2; Manila (Philippines)'62; (905)677-4200; Fax. (905)677-0541.

PALAD, Marcella M S; Orangeville Family Med Centre M1-32 First St, Orangeville ON L9W 2E1; Qns'99; BSc; CCFP; FCFP; Langs: Bilingual(English/French); (519)938-8000; Fax. (519)938-8080.

PALAIC, Mladen; Kirkland Med Center, 100-17000 boul Hymus, Kirkland QC H9J 2W2; McG'89; FRCPC; IntMed; Cardiol. Staff, Lakeshore General Hospital - Pointe Claire; Staff, Sir Mortimer B Davis Jewish General; Teach Staff, McGill University; (514)426-1010; Fax. (514)426-4018; mladen.palaic@mcgill.ca.

PALANGI, Monga-N'Dimo; Leader Med Clinic, PO Box 638, Leader SK S0N 1H0; (306)628-4584; Fax. (306)628-3998.

PALAO, France A; Alliston Family Health Team, 36 Victoria St W, Alliston ON L9R 1S8; Cebu (Philippines)'91; CCFP; (705)435-8887

PALARDY, Jean; Clin Endorin-Metabolism de Lav, 305-3030 boul Le carrefour, Laval QC H7T 2P5; Mon'84; Endocrin (P.Q.); Endocrin&Metab; IntMed. Ac Member, Hopital de la Cite de la santé; (450)688-3132 x219

PALARDY, Maryse; CHUM-Hotel-Dieu, 3840 rue Saint-Urbain, Montreal QC H2W 1T8; Mon'01; FRCPC; Cardiol; IntMed. Staff, Centre Hospitalier l'Université de Montréal (CHUM) - Hôtel-Dieu; (514)890-8000

PALARDY, Sylvain; Ctr Hosp Univ Ste-Justine, 3175 ch Cote-Sainte-Catherine, Montreal QC H3T 1C5; Mon'81; FRCPC; Psy (Pediatric Psychiatry). Staff Ped Psy, Hôpital Ste-Justine; Langs: Bilingual(French/English); (514)345-4695; Fax. (514)345-4635.

PALATNICK, Carrie S; Manitoba Clinic, 790 Sherbrook St, Winnipeg MB R3A 1M3; Man'06; FRCSC; ObstGyn.

PALATNICK, Wesley B; Health Sciences Centre, GF201-820 Sherbrook St, Winnipeg MB R3A 1R9; Man'79; ABEM; ABMT; FRCPC; EmergMed (Toxicology). Assoc Prof Health Section of EmergMed, University of Manitoba; (204)787-2934; Fax. (204)787-2231; wpalatnick@wrha.mb.ca.

PALAYEW, Karen S; 505 O'Connor St, Ottawa ON K1S 3P6; McG'87; FRCPC; Peds. Langs: English; French; (613)230-5958

PALAYEW, Mark D; SMBD Jewish Gen Hosp, 3755 ch Cote-Sainte-Catherine, Montreal QC H3T 1E2; McG'85; FRCPC; IntMed; Respir. adj Prof, McGill University; Langs: English; French; (514)340-7900; mpalayew@pne.jgh.mcgill.ca.

PALAYEW, Max J; SMBD Jewish Gen Hosp, 3755 ch Cote-Sainte-Catherine, Montreal QC H3T 1E2; Montpellier (France)'56; FACR; CSPQ; FRCP; RadOncol (P.Q.); DiagRad (Chest Radiology). Sr Staff Radiol, Sir Mortimer B Davis Jewish General; Consultant, McGill University Health Centre - Royal Victoria Hospital; Emeritus Prof, McGill University; Langs: Bilingual(English/French); (514)340-8233 x5345; Fax. (514)340-7907; max.palayew@sympatico.ca.

PALCU, Sorin; 204-3251 Sheppard Ave E, Scarborough ON M1T 3W5; Timisoara (Romania)'95; CCFP; (416)297-1693

PALEKSIC, Sanja; Glenrose Rehab Hosp, 10230 111 Ave NW, Edmonton AB T5G 0B7; Tor'05; FRCPC; PhysMed&Rehab. Staff, Glenrose Rehabilitation Hospital; (780)735-8870

PALENCAR-FROST, Adriana; Lakeridge HC-Bowmanville Site, 47 Liberty St S, Bowmanville ON L1C 2N4; McM'97; CCFP; Staff, Lakeridge Health - Bowmanville Site; (905)623-3331

PALENCIA ANGULO, Joaquin A; Salveo Family Med Clinic, B8-6455 Macleod Trail SW, Calgary AB T2H 0K8; (Colombia)'97; CCFP; (403)444-0428; Fax. (403)537-0029.

PALEPU, Anita; St Paul's Hosp, 620B-1081 Burrard St, Vancouver BC V6Z 1Y6; McM'91; MPH; FRCPC; IntMed. Staff, Providence Health Care - St Paul's Hospital; Staff, Rapid Access Specialist Clinic; Asst Prof Gen IntMed, University of British Columbia; (604)682-2344 x63194; Fax. (604)806-8005; anita@hivnet.ubc.ca.

PALERME, Louis-Philippe; 305-1669 Victoria St, Prince George BC V2L 2L5; Ott'94; BSc; FRCSC; GenSurg; VascSurg. Staff, University Hospital of Northern British Columbia; Langs: English; French; (250)562-3396

PALERME, Stephanie; 403-2555 St Joseph Blvd, Orleans ON K1C 1S6; Ott'98; FRCSC; ObstGyn. Staff, Kingston General Hospital; (613)837-8396; Fax. (613)837-8398.

PALERMO, Eligio; South Lake Reg Health Centre, 596 Davis Dr, Newmarket ON L3Y 2P9; Tor'77; MBA; CCFP; CCFP(E.M.); FCFP; Staff, Southlake Regional Health Centre; (905)895-4521; Fax. (905)478-2840.

PALETA, John; 11 Highway 329 PO Box 31, Hubbards NS B0J 1T0; Cape Town (South Africa)'88; CCFP; Langs: Afrikaans; Czech; (902)857-1212; Fax. (902)857-1471; kimka94@yahoo.ca.

PALETTA, Michael J; Royal Columbian Hosp, 330 Columbia St E, New Westminster BC V3L 3W7; UBC'90; Staff Physician, Royal Columbian Hospital; (604)520-4001

PALETZ, Justin L; Queen Elizabeth II HSC-Halifax, 4445-1796 Summer St, Halifax NS B3H 3A7; Alb'79; BMedSci; FRCSC; PlasSurg (Hand Microsurgery). Staff, Queen Elizabeth II Health Sciences Centre - Halifax Infirmary Site; Chief Div of Plastic Surg, Queen Elizabeth II Health Sciences Centre - Victoria General Site; Ac Staff, IWK Health Centre; Assoc Prof Plastic & Reconstructive Surg, Dalhousie University; (902)473-6300; Fax. (902)473-7369; jpaletz@dal.ca.

PALEY, Paula M; Saskatoon East Fam Physicians, 21-2105 8th St E, Saskatoon SK S7H 0T8; Sask'92; BSc(Hon); CCFP; FCFP; Staff, Saskatoon City Hospital; Staff Saskatoon Dist Health Bd, Royal University Hospital; Staff, St Paul's Hospital (Grey Nuns) of Saskatoon; Langs: French; (306)373-5500; Fax. (306)374-9414.

PALFRAMAN, David S; Children's Hosp Eastern Ont, 401 Smyth Rd, Ottawa ON K1H 8L1; Tor'67; FRCPC; Psy. Dir Community Psy Prog, Children's Hospital of Eastern Ontario (CHEO); Assoc Prof, University of Ottawa; (613)737-2759

PALFREEMAN, Mark H; Ctr Hosp Laurentien, 234 rue Saint-Vincent, Ste-Agathe-des-Mts QC J8C 2B8; McG'84; CCFP; CCFP(E.M.); FCFP; Staff, Centre Hospitalier Laurentien; (819)324-4000

PALIGA, Andrzej H; Active Care Med Group, 1108A Klondike Rd, Kanata ON K2K 0G1; Cal'88; (613)254-9777; Fax. (613)254-9778.

PALINKA, Sandra J; Courtice Health Centre, 1450 Highway 2, Courtice ON L1E 3C3; Alb'91; CCFP; FCFP; (905)721-4310; Fax. (905)721-6185.

PALISAITIS, Donald; Hop du Sacre-Coeur de Mtl, 5400 boul Gouin O, Montreal QC H4J 1C5; Sher'82; FRCPC; IntMed; Cardiol. Staff, Hôpital du Sacre-Coeur de Montréal; (514)338-2200; Fax. (514)338-3699.

PALLANDI, Derek V; Addiction & Mental Hlth-Queen, 1001 Queen St W, Toronto ON M6J 1H4; McM'95; FRCPC; Psy (Forensic Psychiatry). Locum Tenens, Timmins & District Hospital; Consultant Oak Ridge Div, Waypoint Centre for Mental Health Care; Staff Forensic Psy, Centre for Addiction & Mental Health (CAMH) - Queen Site; Teach Staff, University of Toronto; (416)535-8501 x2545; Fax. (416)583-1324; derek_pallandi@camh.net.

PALLEN, Alphie; 3F-115 Maclean Pl, Welland ON L3B 5X9; Kerala (India)'75; MB BS; MRCPsy(UK); FRCPC; Psy. (905)714-7772; Fax. (905)788-1817.

PALLIE, Dudu A; 205-589 Lake St, St Catharines ON L2N 7L6; Tor'87; Langs: Turkish; (905)646-2282; Fax. (905)646-3251.

PALLIE, Sven; 205-589 Lake St, St Catharines ON L2N 7L6; Tor'88; BSc; MSc; FRCPC; IntMed; Cardiol. Staff, Niagara Health System - St Catharines General Site; Staff, Niagara Health System - Ontario Street Site; Clinical Asst Prof Med, McMaster University; (905)646-2525; Fax. (905)646-3251.

PALLISTER, Crystal; Markham Stouffville Health Ctr, 401-377 Church St, Markham ON L6B 1A1; McG'97; GenSurg. Staff, Markham Stouffville Hospital; (905)472-7122

PALLY, Elliott M; Royal University Hosp, 103 Hospital Dr, Saskatoon SK S7N 0W8; Sask'04; FRCSC; OrthSurg. Staff, Royal University Hospital; (306)655-1993; Fax. (306)655-1998.

PALMA, Alberto; 1618 9 Ave S, Lethbridge AB T1J 1W3; (Spain)'94; (403)328-3836; Fax. (403)328-3846.

PALMA, David A; London Reg Cancer Centre, 790 Commissioners Rd E, London ON N6A 4L6; Wes'04; FRCPC; RadOncol. (519)685-8600; Fax. (519)685-8614.

PALMA, Peter; Northern Lights Health Region, 7 Hospital St, Fort McMurray AB T9H 1P2; Alb'89; CCFP; CCFP(E.M.); FCFP; Staff, Northern Lights Regional Health Centre; Clin Lecturer Med, University of Alberta; Langs: Dutch; German; (780)791-6128

PALMAY, Christine A; Midtown Health & Wellness, 702-110 Eglinton Ave E, Toronto ON M4P 2Y1; Wes'06; CCFP; (416)486-3300; Fax. (416)486-9433.

PALME, Leif M; Canmore Associate Med Clinic, 124-1151 Sidney St, Canmore AB T1W 3G1; Cape Town (South Africa)'88; CCFP; (403)678-5585

PALMER, Bruce W; Valley Prof Centre, 145-70 Exhibition St, Kentville NS B4N 4K9; Dal'82; FRCSC; Urol. Staff, Valley Regional Hospital; (902)679-1223; Fax. (902)678-4020.

PALMER, Christopher R T; Abbotsford Reg Hosp & Cancer C, 32900 Marshall Rd, Abbotsford BC V2S 0C2; London (England)'69; DA; DObstRCOG; FRCPC; Anes (Clinical Anaesthesia). Staff, Abbotsford Regional Hospital & Cancer Centre; (604)851-4873; christopher.palmer@spchc.hnet.bc.ca.

PALMER, Dale P; Vodden Med Arts Centre, 303-36 Vodden St E, Brampton ON L6V 4H4; Tor'76; BSc; (905)450-0028; Fax. (905)450-0029.

PALMER, Darrell J; 10-8180 Macleod Trail SE, Calgary AB T2H 2B8; Alb'89; FRCPC; Peds. Ac Staff Privil, Rockyview General Hospital; Ac Staff Privil, Alberta Children's Hospital; (403)252-6651; Fax. (403)640-0710.

PALMER, David D; Streetsville Med Centre, 8-5425 Creditview Rd, Mississauga ON L5V 2P3; McM'99; CCFP; Ac Staff, The Credit Valley Hospital; (905)826-1164; Fax. (905)826-1214; palmer.david@rogers.com.

PALMER, Erin; Saint John Reg Hosp, PO Box 2100 Stn Main 400 University Ave, Saint John NB E2L 4L2; Dal'09; CCFP; Staff, Saint John Regional Hospital; (506)648-6000

PALMER, Geoffrey M; 19-1527 Dufferin Cres, Nanaimo BC V9S 5H6; UBC'97; FRCSC; Urol. (250)753-6844

PALMER, Janet M; Tudor Glen Medicentre, 2520 Tudor Glen Market, St. Albert AB T8N 3V3; Alb'72; BSc; (780)458-5776; Fax. (780)460-1908.

PALMER, Jessica L A; 1018 Jasper Ave PO Box 35054 Rpo Midtown, Edmonton AB T5J 0B7; UBC'08; CCFP; Physician, Dominion Medical Centre Century Park.

PALMER, John T; 5679 Main St, Niagara Falls ON L2G 5Z3; Qns'68; Staff, Niagara Health System - Greater Niagara General Site; (905)356-0434; Fax. (905)356-2777.

PALMER, Karen A; 1863 Oak Bay Ave, Victoria BC V8R 1C6; McM'00; FRCPC; Psy. (250)507-5292

PALMER, Robert D; Peter Lougheed Centre, 3500 26 Ave NE, Calgary AB T1Y 6J4; Cal'90; CCFP; CCFP(E.M.); FCFP; Staff, Peter Lougheed Centre; (403)943-4555

PALMER, Robert W; London Scoping Center, 310 Wellington Rd, London ON N6C 4P4; Tor'84; FRCSC; GenSurg. Staff, Shouldice Hospital; (519)433-4702

PALMERT, Mark R; The Hosp for Sick Children, 555 University Ave, Toronto ON M5G 1X8; Ohio (USA)'92; Staff, The Hospital For Sick Children; (416)813-6122; Fax. (416)813-6304; mark.palmert@sickkids.ca.

PALMGREN, Elisabeth; Don Mills Surgical Unit, 20 Wynford Dr, North York ON M3C 1J4; Karolinska (Sweden)'66; Anes. Staff, Toronto East General Hospital Inc; (416)441-2111

PALMIERI, Sandra; Dir de la Sante Publique-Mtl, 1301 rue Sherbrooke E, Montreal QC H2L 1M3; Mon'92; MSc(Public Health); CSPQ; Public Health & Preventive Med; CommunMed (P.Q.) (Environmental Medicine). (514)528-2400; Fax. (514)528-2459; spalmier@santepub-mtl.qc.ca.

PALOMBO, Alessandra D; Brameast Family Health Org, 38-2130 North Park Dr, Brampton ON L6S 0C9; Tor'07; CCFP; (905)792-2211; Fax. (905)792-2901.

PALOUX, Jean-Philippe; CHUQ-Ctr Hosp Univ Laval, 2705 boul Laurier, Quebec QC G1V 4G2; Laval'07; CCFP; CCFP(E.M.); Staff, Centre Hospitalier Universitaire de Quebec-CHUL; (418)525-4444

PALUDET, Paul P; Westgrove Professional Bldg, 200-10230 142 St NW, Edmonton AB T5N 3Y6; Alb'75; Ac Staff, Royal Alexandra Hospital; Fam Med, Capital Care - Norwood; Physician, Capital Care - Dickinsfield; Physician, Venta Nursing Home; Hon Clin Lecturer Family Med, University of Alberta; (780)454-4242

PALUMBO, Michel; SMBD Jewish Gen Hosp, 3755 ch Cote-Sainte-Catherine, Montreal QC H3T 1E2; McG'08; IntMed. Staff, Sir Mortimer B Davis Jewish General; (514)340-8222

PALUMBO, Nicole M; 1265 Clarkson Rd N, Mississauga ON L5J 2W4; McM'07; CCFP; (905)822-9171

PAMBRUN, Chantale A; IWK Health Centre, PO Box 9700 Rpo CSC 5850-5980 University Ave, Halifax NS B3K 6R8; Cal'07; FRCPC; HemPath. Staff, IWK Health Centre; (902)470-2797; Fax. (902)470-6974.

PAMIDI, Sushmita; MUHC-Royal Victoria Hosp, 687 av des Pins O, Montreal QC H3A 1A1; Tor'04; FRCPC; IntMed; Respir. Staff, McGill University Health Centre - Royal Victoria Hospital; (514)934-1934

PAMPALON, Federico; Hamilton HS-General Site, 237 Barton St E, Hamilton ON L8L 2X2; Florence (Italy)'95; Staff, Hamilton Health Sciences Centre - Hamilton General Hospital; (905)527-4322; Fax. (905)527-1941.

PAMPALONI, Federico; McMaster University, MDCL3101A-1280 Main St W, Hamilton ON L8S 4K1; Univ of Florence (Italy)'95; FRCSC; GenSurg.

PAMPE, J Robert; 39 Pleasant Blvd, Toronto ON M4T 1K2; Tor'69; Med Dir, Munich Reinsurance Co; (416)964-8015

PAMPHILE, Louis G; Hop Riviere-des-Prairies, 7070 boul Perras, Montreal QC H1E 1A4; (Haiti)'72; Staff, Hôpital Riviere des Prairies; (514)323-7260; Fax. (514)323-9801.

PAMULA, Andrea; Family Med Centre, 611 Wonderland Rd N, London ON N6H 4V6; McM'04; CCFP; (519)471-6686; Fax. (519)471-2801.

PAN, Janice M W; Workers Comp Board of MB, 333 Broadway, Winnipeg MB R3C 4W3; Man'97; CCFP; FCFP; Staff, Workers' Comp Board of MB; janice.pan@reveraliving.com.

PAN, Larry; Queen Elizabeth Hosp, PO Box 6600 Stn Central 60 Riverside Dr, Charlottetown PE C1A 8T5; Tor'04; FRCPC; RadOncol. Staff, Queen Elizabeth Hospital; (902)894-2111

PAN, Ming; Windsor Reg Cancer Centre, 2220 Kildare Rd, Windsor ON N8W 2X3; Tianjin Medical College (China)'96; FRCPC; RadOncol. (519)253-5253

PAN, Wen-Mei; Lorraine Med Clinic, 201 Deacon St, Pembroke ON K8A 2J6; (Taiwan)'59; FACA; FRCPC; Anes (Pain Management). Dir Pain Clin, Pembroke Regional Hospital Inc; Langs: Chinese; (613)732-2811; Fax. (613)732-6350.

PANABAKER, J Paul; 527 Causley St, Blind River ON P0R 1B0; Tor'60; Court Staff, Blind River District Health Centre; Court Staff, St Joseph's General Hospital Elliot Lake; Hon Staff, Halton Healthcare Services Corporation - Georgetown Hospital; (705)356-1666; ppanabaker@brdhc.on.ca.

PANABAKER, Robert D; 593 Deborah Cres, Burlington ON L7T 2N2; Tor'71; MD; BEng; Ac Staff, Hanover & District Hospital; (905)681-9234; bobpanabaker@hotmail.com.

PANACCIO, Francois; 1427 rue Fleury E, Montreal QC H2C 1R9; Mon'68; CSPQ; FRCPC; Derm. Staff Derm Clin, Hopital Louis-H Lafontaine; Langs: Bilingual(French/English); (514)728-3376; Fax. (514)728-9049.

PANACCIONE, Remo; Wellness Bldg, 6D28-3280 Hospital Dr NW, Calgary AB T2N 4N1; Wes'93; BSc; FRCPC; IntMed (Inflammatory Bowel Disease); Gastroent. Ad Staff Privil, Peter Lougheed Centre; Ad Staff Privil, Rockyview General Hospital; Ad Staff Privil, Foothills Medical Centre; Physician, Health Research Innovation Centre; Med Advisor, Crohn's Colitis Foundation of Canada; Dir Inflammatory Bowel Disease Clinic/Research GI Division/Assoc Gastroent Training Prog/Assoc Prof Med, University of Calgary; (403)592-5025; Fax. (403)592-5090; rpanacci@ucalgary.ca.

PANAGIOTOPOULOS, Constadina; Children's & Women's HC of BC, K4 213-4480 Oak St, Vancouver BC V6H 3V4; Qns'95; FRCPC; Peds; Endocrin&Metab. Staff, BC Children's Hospital; (604)875-2345 x5121; Fax. (604)875-3231.

PANAGIOTOPOULOS, Konstantino P; 213-145 15th St W, North Vancouver BC V7M 1R9; Tor'97; BSc; FRCSC; OrthSurg (Orthopedic Trauma). Staff, Lions Gate Hospital; Clin Instructor, University of British Columbia; Langs: Greek; (604)983-0699; Fax. (604)980-5750.

PANARO, Carlo D A; Meadowlark Health Centre, 172 Meadowlark Shopping Ctr NW, Edmonton AB T5R 5W9; Alb'03; FRCSC; OrthSurg. Staff, Covenant Health - Misericordia Community Hospital; Staff, Royal Alexandra Hospital; Staff, University of Alberta Hospital; (780)481-5650; Fax. (780)444-6936.

PANARO, Linda K; Correctional Service Canada, 340 Laurier Ave W, Ottawa ON K1A 0P9; McG'85; FRCPC; CommunMed (Communicable Diseases & Environmental Health); Public Health & Preventive Med. Langs: English; French; (613)943-9587; Fax. (613)943-9600.

PANASCI, Lawrence; SMBD Jewish Gen Hosp, 3755 ch Cote-Sainte-Catherine, Montreal QC H3T 1E2; Washington(DC) (USA)'72; MedOncol; IntMed (P.Q.). Ac Staff, Sir Mortimer B Davis Jewish General; Prof, McGill University; (514)340-8248; Fax. (514)340-8302; lpanasci@hotmail.com.

PANASKEVICH, Tatiana; Leila Med Clinic, 630 Leila Ave, Winnipeg MB R2V 3N7; (Ukraine)'84; CCFP; FCFP; (204)632-0024

PANAYIDES, Panayiotis; Medical & Dental Bldg, 400-3939 50A Ave, Red Deer AB T4N 4E6; Alb'02; FRCSC; GenSurg. Staff, Red Deer Regional Hospital Centre; Langs: Greek; (403)347-9037; Fax. (403)347-9038.

PANCARO, Luigia M; Dufferin Med Clinic, 102-2045 Dufferin St, York ON M6E 3R4; Rome (Italy)'60; Court Staff, Sunnybrook Health Sciences Centre; Langs: Italian; French; (416)656-7733; Fax. (416)656-6502.

PANCER, Larry B; Markham Pediatric Health Ctre, 207-5293 Highway 7, Markham ON L3P 7M7; Wes'83; MSc; FRCPC; Peds., Markham Stouffville Hospital; Staff, The Hospital For Sick Children; Clinical Asst Prof, McMaster University; Hon Staff, University of Toronto; (905)471-7787; Fax. (905)472-5148.

PANCHAM, Paul I; Oshawa Clinic, 117 King St E, Oshawa ON L1H 1B9; Qns'94; BComm; FRCSC; ObstGyn. Staff, Lakeridge Health - Oshawa Site; (905)721-4312; Fax. (905)721-3558.

PANCHAPAKESAN, Vivek; 316-89 Humber College Blvd, Etobicoke ON M9V 4B8; Qns'03; BSc; FRCSC; PlasSurg (Cranio Facial Surgery). (416)644-1840; Fax. (416)644-1841; dr. panchapakesan@gmail.com.

PANDE, Suniti; 3-39 Robertson Rd, Nepean ON K2H 8R2; New Delhi (India)'79; MB BS; FRCPC; Psy (Adult Psychiatry). Staff, Queensway Carleton Hospital; Langs: Hindi; (613)252-8107; Fax. (613)596-0233.

PANDES, Michael S; Medical Bldg, 205-250 Harding Blvd W, Richmond Hill ON L4C 9M7; Tor'00; FRCPC; IntMed; Nephrol. Langs: Armenian; (905)508-5911; Fax. (905)508-2972.

PANDEY, A Shekhar; Cambridge Cardiac Care Centre, 150 Hespeler Rd, Cambridge ON N1R 6V6; Tor'91; BSc; ABIM(IntMed&Cardiol); FRCPC; IntMed (Nuclear Cardiology); Cardiol. Staff Cardiol, Cambridge Memorial Hospital; Langs: Hindi; Punjabi; Urdu; (519)624-3511; Fax. (519)624-3411.

PANDEY, Anil K; Thompson Gen Hosp, 871 Thompson Dr, Thompson MB R8N 0C8; Patna (India)'85; FRFPS; MB BS; FRCPC; Psy. Staff, Thompson General Hospital; Langs: Hindi; (204)677-2381; Fax. (204)778-1456; apandey@shaw.ca.

PANDEY, Annada K; Forbes Park Med Centre, 26 Forbes St, Cambridge ON N3C 2E2; Patna (India)'64; MB BS; MS(GenSurg); LMCC; (519)658-4617; Fax. (519)658-4630.

PANDEYA, Sanjaya; 308-435 Reynolds St, Oakville ON L6J 3M5; Ott'95; FRCPC; FRCPC; Nephrol; IntMed. Staff, Halton Healthcare Services Corporation - Oakville Site; (905)815-9283; Fax. (905)815-9492.

PANDHER, Darshan S; Northgate Centre, 2018-9499 137 Ave NW, Edmonton AB T5E 5R8; Guru Nanak (India)'75; MB BS; FRCPC; DiagRad. (780)476-9729; Fax. (780)476-9732.

PANDHI, Hemant M; Malton Med Arts Bldg, 108-3530 Derry Rd E, Mississauga ON L4T 4E3; Gujarat (India)'72; MB BS; FRCS(Glas.); Langs: Hindi; Urdu; Punjabi; (905)678-7324; Fax. (905)678-7145; hphp2003@hotmail.com.

PANDIAN, A M Chelvi; Clinique Med Place du Centre, 200 Prom du Portage, Gatineau QC J8X 4B7; Madras (India)'80; MB BS; CCFP; Physician, Apple Tree Medical Group; Physician-in-Charge, Centre Medical du Portage; Langs: Tamil; French; Hindi; (819)778-0025

PANDIAN, Alagarsamy; St Boniface Gen Hosp, 409 Tache Ave, Winnipeg MB R2H 2A6; Staff, St Boniface General Hospital.

PANDIT, Rajani V; Guelph Gen Hosp, 115 Delhi St, Guelph ON N1E 4J4; Sri Venkatesvara (India)'85; FRCPC; AnatPath. Staff, Guelph General Hospital; (519)837-6440 x2571; Fax. (519)837-6461.

PANDITH, Vikas; 2079 Lakeshore Rd, Burlington ON L7R 1E2; Tor'91; DABIM; FRCPC; IntMed (Cardiology); Rheum. Ac Staff, Joseph Brant Memorial Hospital; Langs: Hindi; Urdu; (905)634-1625; Fax. (905)634-5322.

PANDYA, Ambrish R; Medical Clinic, 3-3315 26 Ave SW, Calgary AB T3E 0N2; Gujarat (India)'70; (403)246-3100; Fax. (403)246-1225.

PANDYA, Anand H; 103-1A Conestoga Dr, Brampton ON L6Z 4N5; Wes'01; FRCSC; GenSurg; Critical Care Medicine (Trauma). Staff, William Osler Health System - Brampton Civic Hospital; Langs: Hindi; Gujarati; (905)497-4708; Fax. (905)497-5709.

PANDYA, Rupang; Peter Lougheed Centre, 1926-3500 26 Ave NE, Calgary AB T1Y 6J4; Mem'00; FRCPC; Psy (Adult Psychiatry). Clin Asst Prof, Peter Lougheed Centre; (403)943-5694; Fax. (403)219-3568.

PANDYA, Seema R; Sunnybrook Hlth Sciences Ctre, M3 200-2075 Bayview Ave, Toronto ON M4N 3M5; Bombay (India)'96; Staff, Sunnybrook Health Sciences Centre; (416)480-6100; Fax. (416)480-6033.

PANDYA, Sudhir D; Foothills Med Centre, 1403 29 St NW, Calgary AB T2N 2T9; Man'79; FRCP; DABEM; FRCPC; EmergMed (Legal Consultation). Staff Emerg, Foothills Medical Centre; Physician, S T A R S; Sr Physician Emerg, Calgary Health Region; Asst Prof Med, University of Calgary; Langs: Gujarati; Hindi; Swahili; (403)944-1315; Fax. (403)944-1833; pandyas@shaw. ca.

PANDYA, Sudhir P; 412-700 Dorval Dr, Oakville ON L6K 3V3; Nairobi (Kenya)'84; ABIM; FRCPC; IntMed; Gastroent. Langs: Punjabi; Gujarati; Hindi; Kiswahili; (905)815-0755; Fax. (905)815-0757.

PANEK, Romuald; Dept of Med, 5099-5820 University Ave, Halifax NS B3H 1V7; Krakow (Poland)'80; FRCPC; IntMed; Nephrol. (902)473-4021; Fax. (902)473-2675; kbp@eastlink.ca.

PANENKA, William J; Detwiller Pavillion, 1852-2255 Westbrook Mall, Vancouver BC V6T 2A1; Cal'01; FRCPC; Psy; Neur. Staff Neuropsy Program, University of British Columbia; (604)377-5597; wpanenka@psych.ubc.ca.

PANESAR, Bhavlene K; Solace Med Clinic, 36 St Thomas St, St. Albert AB T8N 7J6; Alb'89; (780)419-3627; Fax. (780)419-3565.

PANESAR, Jarnail S; 8461 120 St, Delta BC V4C 6R2; Amritsar (India)'78; MB BS; (604)597-8088

PANET, Diane; Clinique medicale du Luc, 33 rue Saint-Patrice E, Magog QC J1X 5B7; Mon'85; (819)843-3353; Fax. (819)843-7217.

PANET-RAYMOND, Dominique; Hop Maisonneuve-Rosemont, 5415 boul de l'Assomption, Montreal QC H1T 2M4; Mon'92; FRCPC; Peds (Developmental). Staff Peds, Hopital Maisonneuve-Rosemont; Langs: Spanish; English; (514)252-3400 x4558; Fax. (514)374-8101.

PANET-RAYMOND, Valerie; MUHC-Montreal Gen Hosp, 1650 av Cedar, Montreal QC H3G 1A4; Tor'03; FRCPC; RadOncol. Staff, McGill University Health Centre - Montreal General Campus; (514)934-1934 x48040

PANG, Benjamin; Hamilton Med Walk-In Clinic Lt, 2247 Rymal Rd E, Hamilton ON L8J 2V8; New Jersey (USA)'08; CCFP; (905)578-7100

PANG, Eileen G; Riverwood Med Centre, 1295 Pembina Hwy, Winnipeg MB R3T 2B3; Man'92; CCFP; FCFP.

PANG, G Hannah; Forensic Psychiatric Hosp, 70 Colony Farm Rd, Coquitlam BC V3C 5X9; UBC'08; CCFP; Staff, Forensic Psychiatric Hospital; (604)523-7802; Fax. (604)524-7783; hpang@ forensic.bc.ca.

PANG, Jeffrey T W; Sunnybrook Hlth Sciences Ctre, A235-2075 Bayview Ave, Toronto ON M4N 3M5; Ott'94; ABIM; FRCPC; IntMed (Interventional Cardiology); Cardiol. Staff Cardiol, Sunnybrook Health Sciences Centre; Langs: Cantonese; (416)480-4752; Fax. (416)480-4912.

PANG, Natalie; One Care Med Clinic, 1755 Brimley Rd, Scarborough ON M1P 0A3; Wes'06; CCFP; (416)290-0361; Fax. (416)290-5986.

PANG, Patrick K K; Chippawa Med Dental Bldg, 3700 Main St, Niagara Falls ON L2G 6A8; Ott'76; CCFP; FCFP; Staff, Niagara Health System - Greater Niagara General Site; (905)295-4323

PANG, Peter H L; Clinique Med d'Urgence, 25 ch de la Savane, Gatineau QC J8T 8A4; Man'79; Langs: Bilingual(English/French); Hakka; Chinese; (819)561-6611; Fax. (819)561-7997.

PANG, Peter S; 219-3447 Kennedy Rd, Scarborough ON M1V 3S1; Mem'83; Court Staff, Trillium Health Centre - West Toronto; Court Staff, The Scarborough Hospital - Birchmount Campus; (416)297-8724; Fax. (416)253-1685.

PANG, Susan M W; Humber River Reg Hosp-Church, 200 Church St, Toronto ON M9N 1N8; (Hong Kong)'73; FRCPC; DiagRad. Staff, Humber River Regional Hospital - Church Street Site; (416)243-4158

PANG, Wei-Hsi; Courtice Health Centre, 1450 Highway 2, Courtice ON L1E 3C3; Wes'99; CCFP; (905)721-3520; Fax. (905)721-3581.

PANG, Wei-Mei; Village Square Med Centre, A202-3000 Highway 7, Markham ON L3R 6E1; Tor'99; CCFP; (905)480-1050; Fax. (905)480-0898.

PANGILINAN, Ben L; Bathurst Med Centre, LL58-7117 Bathurst St, Thornhill ON L4J 2J6; Manila (Philippines)'91; BSc; CCFP; Langs: Tagalog; (905)707-8707; Fax. (905)707-7018; benjopangilinan@hotmail.com.

PANIC, Stephane; 100-100 ch Rockland, Mont-Royal QC H3P 2V9; Sher'87; FACS; FRCSC; GenSurg (Intensive Care). Ac Member GenSurg & Intensive Care Traumatology, Hôpital du Sacre-Coeur de Montréal; Clin Teach Staff, Universite de Montreal; (514)331-7066; Fax. (514)331-8683.

PANICH, Nicole E; Maternity Care Clinic, 109-178 96 Ave NE, Calgary AB T3K 6G4; Cal'05; CCFP; Staff, Maternity Care Clinic; (403)735-4922; Fax. (403)735-4901.

PANIKIAN, Jean-Claude; Clinique Med Joliette, 3841 rue Ontario E, Montreal QC H1W 1S5; Beirut (Lebanon)'71; (514)524-3731 x32; Fax. (514)524-0675.

PANISKO, Daniel M; Univ Hlth Network-Toronto Western Hosp, EW8 421-399 Bathurst St, Toronto ON M5T 2S8; Man'84; BSc(Med.); DABIM; MPH(Johns Hopkins); FRCPC; IntMed (Tropical Medicine). Staff Gen IntMed, Toronto Western Hospital - University Health Network; Assoc Prof, University of Toronto; (416)603-5824; Fax. (416)603-6495.

PANISSET, Alain; 304-420 rue Jean-Talon E, Montreal QC H2R 1T5; Mon'65; Ophth. Staff, Centre Hospitalier l'Université de Montréal (CHUM) - Hôpital Notre-Dame; adj Prof, Universite de Montreal; (514)591-5189; Fax. (450)458-1143.

PANISSET, Michel; CHUM-Hop Notre-Dame, 1560 rue Sherbrooke E, Montreal QC H2L 4M1; Mon'86; FRCPC; Neur (Movement Disorders). Consultant, McGill University Health Centre - Montreal Neurological Hospital; Ac Member Neurol Serv, St Mary's Hospital Centre; Staff, Centre Hospitalier l'Université de Montréal (CHUM) - Hôpital Notre-Dame; Dir, Movement Disorder Research Centre; adj Prof, McGill University; (514)890-8123; michel.panisset@uhn.ca.

PANJU, Akbar A; Hamilton HS-Henderson Site, 11A-711 Concession St, Hamilton ON L8V 1C3; Liverpool (England)'74; MB ChB; FRCPC; IntMed (Cardiology). Staff, Hamilton Health Sciences Centre-Juravinski Site; Div Dir GIM, McMaster University; (905)527-4322 x42446; Fax. (905)389-9849; panjuaa@mcmaster.ca.

PANJU, Mohamed; Hamilton HS-General Site, 237 Barton St E, Hamilton ON L8L 2X2; Illinois (USA)'07; FRCPC; IntMed. Staff, Hamilton Health Sciences Centre - Hamilton General Hospital; (905)521-2100

PANJWANI, Dilip D; Abbotsford Reg Hosp & Cancer C, 32900 Marshall Rd, Abbotsford BC V2S 0C2; Bombay (India)'80; MB BS; FRCPC; RadOncol (Oncology) (Chemotherapy). Staff, Abbotsford Regional Hospital & Cancer Centre; (604)851-4742

PANJWANI, Dilkhush D; Queensway Prof Centre, 311-190 Sherway Dr, Etobicoke ON M9C 5N2; Poona (India)'75; MB BS; DPM; MRCPsy; FRCPC; Psy. Staff Psy, Trillium Health Centre - West Toronto; Langs: Hindi; Punjabi; Urdu; (416)622-1100; Fax. (416)622-0786.

PANJWANI, Gulshan D; 204-50 Westmount Rd N, Waterloo ON N2L 2R5; Saurashtra (India)'83; FRCPC; Psy. (519)342-6654; Fax. (519)342-6655.

PANKOWSKI, Dahlia K; 101-491 Lawrence Ave W, North York ON M5M 1C7; McM'06; CCFP; (416)787-0323; Fax. (416)787-8094.

PANKRATZ, Werner J; 303-1497 Marine Dr, West Vancouver BC V7T 1B8; UBC'62; ABPN; FRCPC; Psy (Clinical Psychiatry). (604)926-6211; Fax. (604)922-4823; pankratz-paragos@ hotmail.com.

PANNELL, Dylan G; Univ of Toronto Dept of Gen Su, 500 University Ave, Toronto ON M5G 1V7; Qns'07; CCFP; (416)978-6976; Fax. (416)978-7144.

PANNETIER, Evelyne; Clinique Med 24 Juin, 223-1055 12e av N, Sherbrooke QC J1E 2X4; Lyon (France)'76; Neur (P.Q.). assoc Membre Neurol, Centre Hospitalier Universitaire de Sherbrooke-Hopital Fleurimont; Prof adj clin Med, Universite de Sherbrooke; (819)823-6954; epannetier@qc.aira.com.

PANNETIER, Marie-France; CLSC Jean Olivier-Chenier, 29 ch d'Oka, St-Eustache QC J7R 1K6; Mon'84; (450)491-1233; Fax. (450)491-3424.

PANNETON, Isabelle; Ctr Hosp Affilie-Enfant-Jesus, 1401 18e rue, Quebec QC G1J 1Z4; Laval'07; FRCPC; Psy. Staff, Centre Hospitalier Affilié Universitaire de Québec - Hôpital De L'Enfant Jésus; (418)649-0252

PANNOZZO, Gino; 201-50 Westmount Rd N, Waterloo ON N2L 2R5; Tor'77; Staff, Grand River Hospital - Freeport Site; Staff, St Mary's General Hospital; (519)746-1820; Fax. (519)746-6969.

PANNU, Fazeelat A; Stonewall Med Group, GD 589 3rd Ave S, Stonewall MB R0C 2Z0; Punjab (Pakistan)'84; CCFP; Staff, Tri-Lake Health Centre.

PANNU, Neesh I; 11-107 Clinical Sciences Bldg, 152 University Campus NW, Edmonton AB T6G 2G3; Alb'95; FRCPC; IntMed (Critical Care Medicine); Nephrol. Staff, University of Alberta Hospital; Assoc Prof, University of Alberta; (780)407-8520; Fax. (780)407-7878.

PANOPALIS, Pantelis; MUHC-Montreal Gen Hosp, A6 162-1650 av Cedar, Montreal QC H3G 1A4; McG'99; CSPQ; Rheum; IntMed. Staff, McGill University Health Centre - Montreal General Campus; (514)934-1934 x44178

PANOS, Larry L; Scarborough Hosp-General Div, 3050 Lawrence Ave E, Scarborough ON M1P 2V5; Tor'83; FRCPC; Anes. Staff Anes, The Scarborough Hospital - General Campus; (416)431-8133

PANOWYK, Timothy J; North Oshawa Med Centre, 205-1400 Ritson Rd N, Oshawa ON L1G 7W4; Tor'83; CCFP; Staff, Lakeridge Health - Oshawa Site; (905)433-1721; Fax. (905)433-2108.

PANSEGRAU, Gary K; BC Cancer Agency-Fraser Valley, 13750 96 Ave, Surrey BC V3V 1Z2; Tor'99; FRCPC; IntMed; MedOncol. Staff, BC Cancer Agency Fraser Valley Centre; (604)930-4064

PANSEGROUW, Sandra; 166-2111 Main St, Penticton BC V2A 6W6; Orange Free State (South Africa)'85; MB ChB; CCFP; Langs: Afrikaans; (250)276-5050

PANTANO, Alfredo A; Southlake Reg Health Centre, 596 Davis Dr, Newmarket ON L3Y 2P9; Cordoba (Argentina)'93; Staff, Southlake Regional Health Centre; (905)895-4521

PANTAROTTO, Jason R; The Ottawa Hosp-Gen Campus, 501 Smyth Rd, Ottawa ON K1H 8L6; Wes'02; FRCPC; RadOncol. Chief Div of Radiation Oncology, The Ottawa Hospital - General Campus; Chair Div of Radiation Oncology, University of Ottawa; (613)737-7777; Fax. (613)247-3511.

PANTAZI, Sophia; Mount Sinai Hosp, 600 University Ave, Toronto ON M5G 1X5; Tor'86; FRCPC; DiagRad. Staff, Mount Sinai Hospital; (416)586-5279

PANTAZOPOULOS, Efrosini; Centre Med Brunswick, 401-955 boul Saint-Jean, Pointe-Claire QC H9R 5K3; Nottingham (England)'00; CCFP; (514)426-6677

PANTEL, Mitchell S; Occupational Hlth & Safety Ser, 1701 rue Parthenais, Montreal QC H2K 3S7; McG'98; CCFP; Staff Emerg Room, Sir Mortimer B Davis Jewish General; Langs: English; French; (514)598-4953; Fax. (514)598-4439.

PANTEL, Richard J; 415-1641 Lonsdale Ave, North Vancouver BC V7M 2J5; Cal'83; FRCPC; Anes. (604)960-0996

PANTON, Ormond; Gordon & Leslie Diamond HCC, 5F-2775 Laurel St, Vancouver BC V5Z 1M9; (Jamaica)'77; MB BS; FRCS; FRCSC; GenSurg (Laparoscopic Surgery). Head Div of GenSurg, Vancouver General Hospital - Centennial Pavillion; Staff, UBC Hospital - Koerner Pavillion; Staff, Gordon & Leslie Diamond Health Care Centre; (604)875-5790; Fax. (604)875-5869; Neely.Panton@vch.ca.

PANTURESCU, Michael J; Enhanced Care Clinic, 3857 Lake Shore Blvd W, Etobicoke ON M8W 0A2; Tor'74; Assoc Staff, Trillium Health Centre - West Toronto; (416)259-8441; Fax. (416)259-5442.

PANU, Neety; Thunder Bay Reg HSC, 980 Oliver Rd, Thunder Bay ON P7B 6V4; Tor'02; FRCPC; DiagRad. Staff, Thunder Bay Regional Health Sciences Centre; (807)684-6000

PANZINI, Benoit-Pierre; CHUM-Hop Notre-Dame, 1560 rue Sherbrooke E, Montreal QC H2L 4M1; Sher'81; FRCPC; IntMed. Staff, Centre Hospitalier l'Université de Montréal (CHUM) - Hôpital Notre-Dame; (514)281-6000 x27057

PANZINI, Henriette A; Credit Valley Med Arts Centre, 310-2000 Credit Valley Rd, Mississauga ON L5M 4N4; Sher'80; DAB; FRCPC; Derm. Langs: English; French; (905)828-0626; Fax. (905)828-1490.

PAO, Jin-Si; Centro Medical & Surgical Ctre, 4610 Main St, Vancouver BC V5V 3R7; Tor'04; FRCSC; GenSurg. Staff, Richmond Hospital; Langs: Cantonese; Mandarin; (604)559-9933

PAO, Peter S; 170A Rebecca St, Oakville ON L6K 1J6; Manchester (England)'72; MB ChB; Ac Staff, Halton Healthcare Services Corporation - Oakville Site; (905)845-9293

PAOLONE, John A; Pelham Group Health Centre, 108-245 Pelham Rd, St Catharines ON L2S 1X8; Ott'80; Assoc Staff Emerg & Family Med, Niagara Health System - Ontario Street Site; Assoc Staff, Niagara Health System - St Catharines General Site; (905)988-1223; Fax. (905)988-3783.

PAOLUCCI, Fulvio; Frontenac Med Associates, 201-791 Princess St, Kingston ON K7L 1E9; Qns'71; Assoc Staff, Providence Care - St Mary's of the Lake Hospital Site; Assoc Staff, Kingston General Hospital; Langs: Italian; (613)544-2727; Fax. (613)544-7247; paolucci@frontenacmedical.ca.

PAP, Genevieve; Hop Jeffery Hale, 1250 ch Sainte-Foy, Quebec QC G1S 2M6; Mon'83; GenSurg. Staff, Jeffery Hale Hospital-Saint Brigid's; (418)683-4471

PAPACOTSIA, Jean; Hop du Sacre-Coeur de Mtl, 5400 boul Gouin O, Montreal QC H4J 1C5; Laval'93; EmergMed. Staff, Hôpital du Sacre-Coeur de Montréal; (514)338-2000

PAPADATOS, Demetrios; The Ottawa Hosp-Civic Campus, 1053 Carling Ave, Ottawa ON K1Y 4E9; McG'93; FRCPC; DiagRad. Staff, The Ottawa Hospital - Civic Campus; Langs: English; French; (613)798-5555; Fax. (613)761-5268; dpapadatos@ottawahospital.on.ca.

PAPADOPOULOS, Anastasios S; Toronto Allergy Group, 404-650 Sammon Ave, East York ON M4C 5M5; Tor'07; FRCPC; Peds; ClinImmunol&Allergy.

PAPADOPOULOS, Faez; 405-658 Danforth Ave, Toronto ON M4J 5B9; Tor'79; Ac Staff, Providence Healthcare; Ac Staff Family Practice & Casualty Officer, Toronto East General Hospital Inc; (416)466-1188; Fax. (416)466-4310.

PAPADOPOULOS, Platon V K; Coop Sante Gatineau, 200 boul Greber, Gatineau QC J8T 6K2; Beirut (Lebanon)'77; FRCSC; OrthSurg. Ac Staff, Hôpital de Gatineau; (819)568-0444

PAPADOPOULOS, Yasmin A; Taunton Health Centre, SS 201 1290 Keith Ross Dr, Oshawa ON L1H 7K4; Palackeho (Czech Republic)'05; CCFP; (905)721-6884; Fax. (905)721-6690.

PAPADOPOULOS, Yousef G; Homewood Health Centre, 150 Delhi St, Guelph ON N1E 6K9; (Czech Republic)'05; FRCPC; Psy (Family Medicine). Staff, Homewood Health Centre; (519)824-1010

PAPADOURIS, Evangelia; The Doctors Bldg, 803-208 Bloor St W, Toronto ON M5S 3B4; Alexandria (Egypt)'66; FRCPC; Peds. Ac Staff, The Hospital For Sick Children; Ac Staff, Women's College Hospital; Asst Prof, University of Toronto; (416)923-6443; Fax. (416)923-2133.

PAPAGEORGAKOPOULOS, Pashalitsa; Clinique Access Med, 200-17001 rte Trans-Canada, Kirkland QC H9H 5J1; Laval'96; CCFP; (514)694-4644; Fax. (514)694-4646.

PAPAGEORGES, Jean; 48 boul Marie-Victorin, Delson QC J5B 1A9; Mon'82; (450)635-8480

PAPAGEORGIOU, Apostolos; SMBD Jewish Gen Hosp, 3755 ch Cote-Sainte-Catherine, Montreal QC H3T 1E2; Paris (France)'66; FAAP; ABPeds; FRCPC; Peds (Neonatology). Chief Dept of Peds, Sir Mortimer B Davis Jewish General; Chef pédiatrie, St Mary's Hospital Centre; Prof Peds & ObstGyn, McGill University; Langs: Greek; French; (514)340-7598; Fax. (514)340-7566.

PAPAIOANNOU, Alexandra; Hamilton HS-St Peter's Site, 88 Maplewood Ave, Hamilton ON L8M 1W9; McM'88; MSc; BN; FRCPC; IntMed (Rheumatology); GeriatricMed. Staff, Hamilton Health Sciences Centre - St Peter's Hospital; Staff, Hamilton Health Sciences Centre - McMaster University Medical Centre; Prof Med, McMaster University; Langs: Greek; (905)521-2100 x77717

PAPAMARKAKIS, Crystalia; Hop Louis-H Lafontaine, 7401 rue Hochelaga, Montreal QC H1N 3M5; Sher'95; FRCPC; Psy. Staff, Hopital Louis-H Lafontaine; (514)356-2336; Fax. (514)356-8491.

PAPANAGNU, Paraskevi-Eleni; Ctr Hosp Fleury, 2180 rue Fleury E, Montreal QC H2B 1K3; Mon'04; FRCSC; Ophth. Staff, Centre Hospitalier Fleury; (514)384-2000

PAPANASTASIOU, Vasilios W; Westmount Inst of Plastic Surg, 4131 rue Sherbrooke O, Westmount QC H3Z 1B7; McG'79; MSc; MDCM; FRCSC; PlasSurg (Cosmetic Surgery). Staff, St Mary's Hospital Centre; Clin Lecturer, McGill University; Langs: Greek; French; (514)933-3009; Fax. (514)933-7087.

PAPANIKOLAOU, Frank F; Credit Valley Med Arts Centre, 410-2000 Credit Valley Rd, Mississauga ON L5M 4N4; Ott'97; FRCSC; Urol. (905)607-3363; Fax. (905)607-3079.

PAPANOU, Alec; 80 Valleybrook Dr, Toronto ON M3B 2S9; Wes'95; (416)442-5600; Fax. (416)510-5175; apapanou@scottsinfo.com.

PAPAS, Konstantin; Institut de Cardiologie de Mtl, 5000 rue Belanger, Montreal QC H1T 1C8; Mon'02; FRCPC; DiagRad. Staff, Institut de Cardiologie de Montréal; (514)376-3330

PAPASTERGIOU, Derek L; 201-520 University Ave W, Waterloo ON N2T 2Z6; Ott'98; CCFP; (519)741-0115

PAPASTERGIOU, Thanos; 1824 Concession Dr, Newbury ON N0L 1Z0; Wes'96; CCFP; (519)693-4441

PAPATHEODOROU, George; Addiction & Mental Hlth-Clarke, 725-250 College St, Toronto ON M5T 1R8; McG'86; FRCPC; Psy (Adolescent Psychiatry). Staff, Centre for Addiction & Mental Health (CAMH) - College Street Site; Asst Prof, University of Toronto; Langs: Greek; French; (416)535-8501 x4925; Fax. (416)979-6936; george_papatheodorou@camh.net.

PAPAY, Karen D; Heartline Med Clinic, 110-2504 Skaha Lake Rd, Penticton BC V2A 6G1; Wes'04; FRCPC; IntMed; Gastroent. (250)492-3511

PAPAZIAN, Apkar; Clinique Med Jean-Talon-Pie IX, 4679 rue Jean-Talon E, Saint-Leonard QC H1S 1K3; Beirut (Lebanon)'72; CSPQ; FRCSC; Urol. Staff, Hôpital Santa Cabrini Ospedale; Staff, Hopital Louis-H Lafontaine; Langs: Armenian; Arabic; English; (514)374-5901; apapazian@videotron.ca.

PAPE, Gavin M; Scarborough Hosp-General Div, 3050 Lawrence Ave E, Scarborough ON M1P 2V5; Tor'81; Assoc Staff, Rouge Valley Health System - Centenary Health Centre Site; Assoc Staff, The Scarborough Hospital - General Campus; (416)431-8101

PAPE, Karen E; TASC Network Inc, 31 Alderbrook Dr, North York ON M3B 1E3; Tor'70; FRCPC; Peds (Neuro Rehabilitation). (416)928-0559; Fax. (416)928-6830.

PAPENBURG, Jesse; MUHC-Montreal Children's Hosp, C 1246-2300 rue Tupper, Montreal QC H3H 1P3; McG'02; FRCPC; Peds; Microbio & Infect Dis (P.Q.); MedMicrobiol; InfectDis. Staff, McGill University Health Centre - Montreal Children's Hospital; (514)412-4485

PAPENBURG, Robert R; 403-1625 boul de Maisonneuve O, Montreal QC H3H 2N4; McG'84; GenSurg (P.Q.). (514)935-4434; Fax. (514)935-7053.

PAPENFUS, William J; Royal University Hosp, 103 Hospital Dr, Saskatoon SK S7N 0W8; Stellenbosch (South Africa)'94; MB ChB; LMCC; CCFP; CCFP(E.M.); Staff, Royal University Hospital; (306)655-1000

PAPETTI, Selena J; Lac du Bonnet Dist Health Ctre, 89 McIntosh Ave, Lac du Bonnet MB R0E 1A0; Man'10; CCFP; Physician, Lac du Bonnet District Health Centre.

PAPIA, Giuseppe; Sunnybrook Hlth Sciences Ctre, H1 85-2075 Bayview Ave, Toronto ON M4N 3M5; Ott'99; FRCSC; GenSurg; Critical Care Medicine; VascSurg. Staff, Sunnybrook Health Sciences Centre; (416)480-6100

PAPIC, Ognjen; Lakeshore Gen Hosp, 160 av Stillview, Pointe-Claire QC H9R 2Y2; Tor'08; CCFP; CCFP(E.M.); Staff, Lakeshore General Hospital - Pointe Claire; (514)630-2225

PAPILLON, Daphne; Ctr Hosp de Verdun, 4000 boul Lasalle, LaSalle QC H4G 2A3; Mon'09; CCFP; Staff, Centre Hospitalier de Verdun; (514)362-1000

PAPILLON, Elise; MUHC-Montreal Gen Hosp, 1650 av Cedar, Montreal QC H3G 1A4; Mon'10; CCFP; Staff, McGill University Health Centre - Montreal General Campus; (514)934-1934

PAPILLON, Evelyne; CSSS de Trois-Rivières, 1991 boul du Carmel, Trois-Rivieres QC G8Z 3R9; Mon'06; CCFP; CCFP(E.M.); Staff, CSSS de Trois-Rivières; (819)697-3333

PAPILLON, Marianne; CSSS des Iles, 430 ch Principal, Cap-aux-Meules QC G4T 1R9; Mon'00; CCFP; Staff, Hôpital de l'Archipel; (418)986-2121

PAPIN, Lisanne; Clinique Med La Rose des Vents, 3498 boul Sainte-Rose, Laval QC H7P 4K7; Mon'83; LMCC; Langs: Spanish; English; (514)624-1844

PAPINEAU, Alain; CSSS de la Baie-des-Chaleurs, RR 2 419 boul Perron, Maria QC G0C 1Y0; Mon'91; CCFP; FCFP; Staff, CSSS de la Baie-des-Chaleurs; (418)759-1336

PAPINEAU, Cynthia; CSSS Haut-Richelieu-Rouville, 920 boul du Seminaire N, St-Jean-sur-Richel QC J3A 1B7; Mon'02; CCFP; CCFP(E.M.); Staff, Hôpital du Haut-Richelieu; (450)359-5000

PAPINEAU, Martin; NORD-ASKI Family Health Team, PO Box 130 1403 Edward St, Hearst ON P0L 1N0; Ott'98; CCFP; Pres/Medical Staff, Hôpital Notre Dame Hospital - Hearst; Langs: English; French; (705)362-7511; Fax. (705)372-2923.

PAPINI, Osvaldo; Columbus Med Arts Bldg, 408-8333 Weston Rd, Woodbridge ON L4L 8E2; Rome (Italy)'77; CCFP; FCFP; Langs: Italian; (905)266-1861; Fax. (905)266-1172.

PAPISH, Andriyka L M; Regina Mental Health Clinic, 2110 Hamilton St, Regina SK S4P 2E3; Cal'06; Psy. (306)766-7800; Fax. (306)766-7811.

PAPNEJA, Purti; Sunnybrook Hlth Sciences Ctre, A100-2075 Bayview Ave, Toronto ON M4N 3M5; McM'06; CCFP; Staff, Sunnybrook Health Sciences Centre; (416)480-6100

PAPNEJA, Sooraja P; Iona Doctors Clinic, 1585 Mississauga Valley Blvd, Mississauga ON L5A 3W9; Jabalpur (India)'83; MB BS; MD; Court Staff, Trillium Health Centre - Mississauga; Langs: Hindi; Urdu; Punjabi; (905)897-2000; Fax. (905)897-2953; ajanmaom@yahoo.ca.

PAPNEJA, Tripti; 314-40 Finchgate Blvd, Brampton ON L6T 3J1; Tor'06; FRCPC; IntMed; Rheum. Staff, University of Alberta Hospital; (905)799-1850

PAPO, Khomotso; Mid Island Med Clinic, PO Box 310 744 Memorial Ave, Qualicum Beach BC V9K 1S8; Limpopo (South Africa)'01; (250)594-2009

PAPP, A Jane; 201-284 Helmcken St, Victoria BC V9B 1T2; UBC'91; (250)480-1401

PAPP, Anthony A; Gordon & Leslie Diamond HCC, 3-2775 Laurel St, Vancouver BC V5Z 1M9; Kuopio (Finland)'89; FRCSC; PlasSurg. Staff, Vancouver General Hospital - Centennial Pavillion; Langs: Finnish; (604)875-5866

PAPP, Edward W; 7004 98 Ave NW, Edmonton AB T6A 0A5; Alb'71; MD; BMedSci; CCFP; FCFP; Ac Staff, Covenant Health - Grey Nuns Community Hospital; Fam Med, Covenant Health - St. Joseph's Auxilliary Hospital; Clin Assoc Prof, University of Alberta; (780)468-6035; Fax. (780)466-9132; edpapp@remote.net.

PAPP, Jamie D; Medical Arts Bldg, 430-1105 Pandora Ave, Victoria BC V8V 3P9; Cal'81; BSc; FRCPC; IntMed; Gastroent. Staff, Vancouver Island Health Authority; (250)361-1493; Fax. (250)360-2998.

PAPP, Kim A; 135 Union St E, Waterloo ON N2J 1C4; Cal'85; PhD; FRCPC; Derm. Consultant, St Mary's General Hospital; Consultant, Grand River Hospital - Kitchener/Waterloo Health Centre; Pres, Probity Medical Research; (519)579-9535; kalepapp@hotmail.com.

PAPP, Steven R; The Ottawa Hosp-Civic Campus, J157-1053 Carling Ave, Ottawa ON K1Y 4E9; McG'98; FRCSC; OrthSurg. Staff, The Ottawa Hospital - Civic Campus; (613)798-5555

PAPPACHAN, Michael J; Hys Med Centre, 710-11010 101 St NW, Edmonton AB T5H 4B9; Alb'07; PhysMed&Rehab. Staff, University of Alberta Hospital; (780)407-8822

PAPSIN, Blake C; The Hosp for Sick Children, 6117-555 University Ave, Toronto ON M5G 1X8; Tor'88; MSc; FACS; FAAP; FRCSC; Otol (Pediatric Otolaryngology). Staff, The Hospital For Sick Children; Prof, University of Toronto; (416)813-2190; Fax. (416)813-5036.

PAPUKNA, Vasiliki; Thames Valley FHT-Whitehills M, 1225 Wonderland Rd N, London ON N6G 2V9; Regele (Romania)'83; Langs: Greek; Romanian; French; (519)472-0040; Fax. (519)472-7732.

PAQUET, Benoit; Hop Maisonneuve-Rosemont, 5415 boul de l'Assomption, Montreal QC H1T 2M4; Mon'07; CCFP; CCFP(E.M.); Staff, Hopital Maisonneuve-Rosemont.

PAQUET, Carine; CLSC du Val St-Francois, 23 rue Ambroise-Dearden, Windsor QC J1S 1G8; Sher'00; (819)845-2751

PAQUET, Catherine; MUHC-Montreal Children's Hosp, C1118A-2300 rue Tupper, Montreal QC H3H 1P3; Laval'02; FRCPC; Anes. Staff, McGill University Health Centre - Montreal Children's Hospital; (514)934-1934 x22463

PAQUET, Christine; CSSS des Iles, 430 ch Principal, Cap-aux-Meules QC G4T 1R9; Laval'95; Staff, Hôpital de l'Archipel; (418)986-2121

PAQUET, Francois; Hotel-Dieu de Levis, 143 rue Wolfe, Levis QC G6V 3Z1; Laval'91; EmergMed. Staff, Hôtel-Dieu de Lévis; (418)835-7121 x6178; Fax. (418)838-9016.

PAQUET, Ghislain; Clinique Med Saint-Luc, 264 boul Saint-Luc, St-Jean-Sur-Richel QC J2W 1C3; Ott'76; Staff, Hôpital du Haut-Richelieu; Langs: Bilingual(French/English); (450)348-6124; Fax. (450)348-4163; ghislainkn@hotmail.com.

PAQUET, Guy; Clinique Med de Nemaska, 8 rue Badabin, Nemiscau QC J0Y 3B0; Mon'82; Staff, Hôpital de Saint-Eustache; (819)673-2311

PAQUET, Isabelle; CSSS du Sud de Lanaudière, 911 montee des Pionniers, Terrebonne QC J6V 2H2; Laval'99; Respir; IntMed. Staff, Centre Hospitalier Pierre le Gardeur; Langs: English; (450)654-7525; Fax. (450)654-4396.

PAQUET, J A Ronald; 209 rue Saint-Antoine, Gatineau QC J8T 3N1; Ott'65; (819)568-9222; Fax. (819)568-9222.

PAQUET, Jean-Claude; COOP de Solidarite Sante Lapra, 675 ch Saint-Jean, La Prairie QC J5R 2L2; Laval'67; ObstGyn (Gynecological Surgery). Staff, Hôtel-Dieu de Lévis; (450)444-2002; paquet.jclaude@videotron.ca.

PAQUET, Jean-Denis; Centre Med Fafard Enr, 201-975 boul Monseigneur-de La, Baie-Saint-Paul QC G3Z 2W3; Laval'69; (418)435-6310

PAQUET, Jean-Rene; Ctr Readaptation Ubald-Villene, 2525 ch de la Canardiere, Quebec QC G1J 2G2; Laval'68; (418)663-5008

PAQUET, Jerome; Ctr Hosp Affilie-Enfant-Jesus, 1401 18e rue, Quebec QC G1J 1Z4; Laval'98; FRCSC; Neursurg. Staff, Centre Hospitalier Affilié Universitaire de Québec - Hôpital De L'Enfant Jésus; Langs: Bilingual(French/English); (418)649-5882

PAQUET, Karine; Peace Arch Hosp, 15521 Russell Ave, White Rock BC V4B 2R4; Laval'03; FRCPC; Psy. Staff, Peace Arch Hospital; (604)531-5512

PAQUET, Louis F; CSSSG-Hop de Gatineau, CP 2000 Succ Bureau-Chef 909 boul de la Verendrye O, Gatineau QC J8P 7H2; Mon'87; Staff, Hôpital de Gatineau; (819)561-8100

PAQUET, Marc; CSSS de la Minganie, CP 190 1035 Prom des Anciens, Havre-Saint-Pierre QC G0G 1P0; Laval'89; CCFP; Staff, CSSS de la Minganie; (418)538-2212; marc_paquet@ssss.gouv.qc.ca.

PAQUET, Mariane; Ministere de la Sante, 165 St. Andrew St, Bathurst NB E2A 1C1; Sher'06; FRCPC; Public Health & Preventive Med.

PAQUET, Marie; Ctr Med Legendre, 201-1650 av Jules-Verne, Quebec QC G2G 2R1; Laval'90; CCFP; Staff Obstetrique-Perinatalite, Centre Hospitalier Universitaire De Québec - Pavillon De St-françois-d'assise; (418)872-5600; Fax. (418)872-8408.

PAQUET, Marie-Claude; CHUQ-St-Francois d'Assise, 10 rue de l'Espinay, Quebec QC G1L 3L5; Laval'06; FRCPC; Anes. Staff, Centre Hospitalier Universitaire De Québec - Pavillon De St-françois-d'assise; (418)525-4444

PAQUET, Martin; Clin Med Vingt Quatre Juin, 105-1055 12e av N, Sherbrooke QC J1E 2X4; Sher'83; MA; Langs: Spanish; English; (819)821-2142; Fax. (819)821-0248.

PAQUET, Michel R; CHUM-Hop Notre-Dame, 1560 rue Sherbrooke E, Montreal QC H2L 4M1; Sher'95; MSc; FRCPC; IntMed (Renal Transplant); Nephrol. assoc Prof, Universite de Montreal; Staff Nephrol, Centre Hospitalier l'Université de Montréal (CHUM) - Hôpital Notre-Dame; (514)890-8000 x25904; Fax. (514)412-7831.

PAQUET, Nadine; Clinique familiale des Hauts-B, 99 boul des Hauts-Bois, Sainte-Julie QC J3E 3J9; McG'95; Staff Emerg, Centre Hospitalier Pierre Boucher; Langs: Bilingual(French/English); (450)649-2490; Fax. (450)649-2218.

PAQUET, Nancy; 3001 12e av N, Sherbrooke QC J1H 5N4; Laval'92; ABNM; FRCP; FRCPC; NuclearMed (Positron Emission Tomography). Staff, Centre Hospitalier Universitaire de Sherbrooke-Hopital Fleurimont; Langs: Bilingual(French/English); (819)346-1110 x16146; Fax. (819)820-6462; nancy.paquet@usherbrooke.ca.

PAQUET, Nathalie; Clinique des Med d'Urgence, 632 rue Bowen S, Sherbrooke QC J1G 2E9; Laval'91; Staff Emerg, Centre Hospitalier Universitaire de Sherbrooke-Hôpital Hôtel-Dieu; (819)822-2700

PAQUET, Roger; CLSC Jean Olivier-Chenier, 29 ch d'Oka, St-Eustache QC J7R 1K6; Mon'77; (450)491-1233; Fax. (450)491-3424; roger_paquet@ssss.gouv.qc.ca.

PAQUET, Stephanie; CSSS du Sud de Lanaudière, 911 montee des Pionniers, Terrebonne QC J6V 2H2; Laval'99; Gastroent; IntMed. Staff, Centre Hospitalier Pierre le Gardeur; (450)654-7525 x21300

PAQUET, Stephanie; Clinique Med Grande Ourse, 534 3e rue, Chibougamau QC G8P 1N9; Laval'02; CCFP; Staff, CRSSS de la Baie-James; (418)748-3469

PAQUET, Suzanne; Hotel-Dieu de Levis, 143 rue Wolfe, Levis QC G6V 3Z1; Sher'89; CCFP; FCFP; Staff, Hôtel-Dieu de Lévis; Staff, Carrefour Sante Granit; (418)835-7121

PAQUETTE, Amelie; CSSS des Sources, 475 3e av, Asbestos QC J1T 1X6; Sher'03; Staff, CSSS des Sources d'Asbestos; (819)879-7151; Fax. (819)879-0075.

PAQUETTE, Anne; CLSC la Source-Point de Servic, 190 76e rue E, Quebec QC G1H 7K4; Mon'06; CCFP; Staff, Hôpital Regional Rimouski; (418)628-2572; Fax. (418)780-3631.

PAQUETTE, Camille; Dir Sante Publique de l'Outaou, 323-104 rue Lois, Gatineau QC J8Y 3R7; Laval'06; CSPQ; FRCPC; Public Health & Preventive Med; CommunMed (P.Q.). (819)776-7660

PAQUETTE, Celine; Ctre Med Prive St-Bruno, 1435 rue Roberval, Saint-Bruno QC J3V 3P7; Laval'85; (450)653-3636

PAQUETTE, Charles; Polyclinique Med de La Lievre, 536 rue de la Madone, Mont-Laurier QC J9L 1S7; Sher'85; Staff, Centre de L'Annonciation; (819)440-2345; Fax. (819)440-2330.

PAQUETTE, Claudie; Clin Med du Sud-Ouest, 4475 rue Bannantyne, Verdun QC H4G 1E2; Mon'93; BSc; MSc; CCFP; Staff, Centre Hospitalier de Verdun; (514)765-3600

PAQUETTE, Daniel; 1000-1440 rue Sainte-Catherine, Montreal QC H3G 1R8; Sher'83; ACLS; ATLS; CCFP; FCFP; ac Staff, Hôpital Sainte-croix; (514)878-1911

PAQUETTE, Daniel; Dir Reg Sante Publique Laval, 800 boul Chomedey, Laval QC H7V 3Y4; Mon'98; CSPQ; MSc; MBA; FRCPC; CommunMed. Staff, Hopital de la Cite de la santé; Langs: English; (450)978-2121 x2646; Fax. (450)978-2100.

PAQUETTE, Elaine; Centre Med Iberville, 101-235 2E av, St-Jean-Sur-Richel QC J2X 2B2; Sher'80; (450)347-5548; Fax. (450)347-4091.

PAQUETTE, Eric R; Timmins Family Health Team, 208-38 Pine St N, Timmins ON P4N 6K6; Ott'83; CCFP; FCFP; Timmins & District Hospital; Staff, White Pines Health Network; (705)267-3272; Fax. (705)267-4212.

PAQUETTE, Isabelle; 7401 rue Hochelaga, Montreal QC H1N 3M5; Mon'88; MSc; FRCPC; Psy (Geriatric Psychiatry). Staff Psy Geriatric Service, Hopital Louis-H Lafontaine; Clin Teach Staff Psy & Med, Universite de Montreal; Langs: English; (514)251-4000 x3060; Fax. (514)251-1604; isabelle.paquette@umontreal.ca.

PAQUETTE, Jean-Levy; Polyclinique Med de La Lievre, 536 rue de la Madone, Mont-Laurier QC J9L 1S7; Mon'78; Staff, CSSS d'Antoine-Labelle; Coroner, District of Labelle; (819)440-2345; Fax. (819)440-2330; polylieu@lino.com.

PAQUETTE, Jean-Pierre; Clinique Med Sainte-Dorothee, 102-1 boul Samson, Laval QC H7X 3S5; Mon'80; Staff, Hôpital du Sacre-Coeur de Montréal; (450)689-6334; Fax. (450)689-6339.

PAQUETTE, Jean-Sebastien; CSSS du Nord de Lanaudière, 1000 boul Sainte-Anne, St-Charles-Brromee QC J6E 6J2; Mon'02; LMCC; CCFP; Staff, Centre Hospitalier Régional de Lanaudière; (450)759-8222

PAQUETTE, Lise J; 408-1366 Yonge St, Toronto ON M4T 3A7; Tor'86; MSc; CCFP; FCFP; Langs: English; French; (416)924-7799; Fax. (416)924-8243.

PAQUETTE, Louis; Clinique Familiale, 13555 boul Lacroix, Saint-Georges QC G5Y 1P1; Mon'91; CCFP; CCFP(E.M.); Staff Obst, Centre Hospitalier Beauce-Etchemin; Langs: English; (418)228-8001

PAQUETTE, Manon; CLSC Saint-Hubert, 6800 boul Cousineau, Saint-Hubert QC J3Y 8Z4; Mon'86; (450)443-7407; Fax. (450)676-4645; manon.paquette@rrsss16.gouv.qc.ca.

PAQUETTE, Marc; Clinique Med de Verdun, 25-55 av de l'Eglise, Verdun QC H4G 3E7; Mon'74; (514)766-8511

PAQUETTE, Nicole; 205-12905 rue Sherbrooke E, Pte-aux-Trembles QC H1A 1B9; Mon'83; FRCPC; Derm. Langs: English; (514)640-4848; Fax. (514)640-4435.

PAQUETTE, Odile; CSSS Drummond-Hop Sainte-Croix, 570 rue Heriot, Drummondville QC J2B 1C1; Sher'04; FRCPC; IntMed. Staff, Hôpital Sainte-croix; (819)478-6464

PAQUETTE, Pierre; Centre Med Salaberry, 2758 rue de Salaberry, Montreal QC H3M 1L3; Mon'68; Staff, Hôpital du Sacre-Coeur de Montréal; (514)337-4772; Fax. (514)337-4923.

PAQUETTE, Ross N; Callingwood Crossing Med Clini, 6905 172 St NW, Edmonton AB T5T 5Y1; Alb'86; (780)444-0350; Fax. (780)444-0476.

PAQUETTE, Scott J; Blusson Spinal Cord Centre, 818 10th Ave W, Vancouver BC V5Z 1M9; Mem'97; FRCSC; Neursurg. Staff Combined Neurosurgical & Orthopedic Spine Program, Vancouver General Hospital - Centennial Pavillion; (604)875-5562

PAQUETTE, Serge; suite 649-1271 Boul. Jolibourg, Laval QC H7Y 1Z8; Mon'70; Langs: English; French; (450)689-2424; Fax. (450)689-9548.

PAQUETTE, Suzanne; Clin Externe de Psychiatrie, 203-100 rue Grenier, Charlemagne QC J5Z 4C6; Mon'95; LMCC; FRCPC; Psy (Adult Psychiatry). Teach Staff Adult Psy, Universite de Montreal; Langs: Bilingual(French/English); (450)585-9010; Fax. (450)585-2709.

PAQUETTE-L'ECUYER, Lucie; Clinique Med des 2 Tours, A-1001 rue University, Montreal QC H3B 4L4; Mon'76; (514)954-4444; Fax. (514)954-4446.

PAQUIN, Claude; 430-1265 rue Berri, Montreal QC H2L 4X4; Mon'80; (514)843-7904; Fax. (514)843-6706; femina@clinique-femina.com.

PAQUIN, Claude-Elene; CSSS du Lac-des-Deux-Montagnes, 520 boul Arthur-Sauve, St-Eustache QC J7R 5B1; Mon'99; Staff, Hôpital de Saint-Eustache; (450)473-6811

PAQUIN, Colette; Yonge-Eglinton Med Centre, 210-2401 Yonge St, Toronto ON M4P 3H1; McG'80; FRCPC; Derm. Langs: English; French; (416)485-0659; Fax. (416)485-8525.

PAQUIN, France; Centre Med Berger, 116-1000 ch Sainte-Foy, Quebec QC G1S 2L6; Mon'83; (418)688-1385; Fax. (418)688-3249.

PAQUIN, Francine; Ctr Hosp du Centre la Mauricie, 50 119e rue, Shawinigan-Sud QC G9P 5K1; Sher'88; CSPQ; DiagRad. Staff, Centre Hospitalier du Centre la Mauricie; (819)536-7523

PAQUIN, Francois J; CSSS Haut-Richelieu-Rouville, 920 boul du Seminaire N, St-Jean-sur-Richel QC J3A 1B7; Mon'70; CSPQ; AnatPath. Staff, Hôpital du Haut-Richelieu; Staff, Centre Hospitalier l'Université de Montréal (CHUM) - Hôpital Notre-Dame; assoc Prof, Universite de Montreal; (450)359-5000 x5205

PAQUIN, Isabelle; 23 CFH Svcs Centre Winnipeg, PO Box 17000 Stn Forces, Shilo MB R0K 2A0; Ott'05; CCFP.

PAQUIN, Isabelle; CLSC Longueuil-Ouest, 201 boul Cure-Poirier O, Longueuil QC J4J 2G4; Sher'01; (450)651-9831; Fax. (450)651-0924.

PAQUIN, Jean-Marie; College des Med du Quebec, 2170 boul Rene-Levesque O, Montreal QC H3H 2T8; Mon'67; CSPQ; FRCSC; Urol. Adj Syndic, College des Medecins du Quebec; (514)933-4441 x5295; Fax. (514)933-2291.

PAQUIN, Johanne; CLSC Haute-Ville-des-Rivieres, 2400 av d'Estimauville, Quebec QC G1E 7G9; Laval'77; CSPQ; GenPath (P. Q.). Staff, Centre Hospitalier Universitaire de Quebec-CHUL; (418)623-1010 x272; johanne.paquin@ssss.gouv.qc.ca.

PAQUIN, Marc; Clin Memoire Dr Marc Paquin, 30 av Byette, Ste-Agathe-des-Mts QC J8C 2R4; Mon'78; Langs: Bilingual(French/English); (819)323-7113; Fax. (819)323-3043.

PAQUIN, Marie-Josee; Ctr Hosp Rouyn-Noranda, 4 9E rue, Rouyn-Noranda QC J9X 2B2; Sher'92; Staff, Centre Hospitalier Rouyn-Noranda; (819)764-5131

PAQUIN, Michel; Inst Glaucome de Mtl, 4135 rue de Rouen, Montreal QC H1V 1G5; Mon'65; DABOph; Ophth (Glaucoma). (514)256-0007

PAQUIN, Michel; Clinique Med Havre Sante, 23-521 boul du Havre, Salaber-de-Valleyf QC J6S 4Z5; Sher'76; FRCSC; ObstGyn. assoc Staff, Centre Hospitalier Régional du Suroît; Langs: Bilingual(French/English); (450)370-1300; Fax. (450)370-1314.

PAQUIN, Michel; GMF Concorde, 300 boul de la Concorde E, Laval QC H7G 2E6; Laval'82; (450)667-5310

PAQUIN, Pierre; Ctr Hosp Laurentien, 234 rue Saint-Vincent, Ste-Agathe-des-Mts QC J8C 2B8; Mon'69; CSPQ; FRCP; FRCPC; Anes. Staff, Centre Hospitalier Laurentien; (819)324-4034; Fax. (819)324-4082.

PAQUIN, R Wayne; Radiology Cons of Winnipeg, 202-233 Kennedy St, Winnipeg MB R3C 3J5; Man'71; FRCSC; Urol; DiagRad. Staff, Victoria General Hospital.

PAQUIN, Raphael; Royal University Hosp, 103 Hospital Dr, Saskatoon SK S7N 0W8; Mon'05; FRCPC; Peds; PedEmergMed. Staff, Royal University Hospital; (306)966-8117; Fax. (306)975-3767.

PAQUIN, Sarto; CHUM-Hop Saint-Luc, 1058 rue Saint-Denis, Montreal QC H2X 3J4; Mon'98; FRCPC; IntMed; Gastroent. Staff, Centre Hospitalier l'Université De Montréal (CHUM) - Hôpital Saint-luc; (514)890-8000

PAQUIN, Sebastien; CHUQ-St-Francois d'Assise, 10 rue de l'Espinay, Quebec QC G1L 3L5; Laval'07; CCFP; CCFP(E.M.); Staff, Centre Hospitalier Universitaire De Québec - Pavillon De St-françois-d'assise; (418)525-4444

PAQUIN, Stephanie; CSSS de Montmagny-L'Islet, RR 1 430 rue Jean-Leclerc, St-Jean-Port-Joli QC G0R 3G0; Laval'10; CCFP; Staff, CSSS de Montmagny-l'Islet; (418)248-0630

PAQUIN, Yvon; Ctr Hosp du Centre la Mauricie, 50 119e rue, Shawinigan QC G9P 5K1; Laval'68; Chef chirg ortho, Centre Hospitalier du Centre la Mauricie; Langs: Bilingual(French/English); (819)536-7500; Fax. (819)536-7654; yvon_paquin@ssss.gouv.qc.ca.

PARACHA, Muhammad S; Percy E Moore Hosp, PO Box 190, Hodgson MB R0C 1N0; Staff, Percy E Moore Hospital; (204)372-8444

PARACHIN, Deborah C; Dofasco Med Department, PO Box 2460 Stn Lcd 1 1400 Burlington St, Hamilton ON L8N 3J5; McM'00; CCFP; (905)548-7152; Fax. (905)548-4345; deborah.parachin@arcelormittal.com.

PARADIS, Alain; Ctr Hosp Affilie-Enfant-Jesus, 1401 18e rue, Quebec QC G1J 1Z4; Laval'84; FRCPC; MedMicrobiol; Microbio & Infect Dis (P.Q.). Staff, Centre Hospitalier Affilié Universitaire de Québec - Hôpital De L'Enfant Jésus; (418)649-0252 x3693

PARADIS, Andre; Clin Sante-Voyager la Cite Med, 122-2600 boul Laurier, Quebec QC G1V 4T3; Laval'88; CCFP; Médecin Ergency Med, CSSS Alphonse-Desjardins; Langs: English; (418)651-8015

PARADIS, Bruno; Cite de la Sante de Laval, 1755 boul Rene-Laennec, Laval QC H7M 3L9; Mon'85; FRCPC; IntMed; Respir. Staff, Hopital de la Cite de la santé; (450)668-1010; Fax. (450)965-7181.

PARADIS, Chantal; CLSC Basse-Ville-Limoilou, 50 rue Saint-Joseph E, Quebec QC G1K 3A5; Laval'90; (418)529-6592; Fax. (418)529-1515.

PARADIS, Christian; Thames Valley FHT-Windermere S, 301-460 Wellington St, St Thomas ON N5R 6H9; Mon'98; CCFP; FCFP; Staff, Thames Valley Family Health Team - Windermere Site; Staff, St Thomas Elgin General Hospital; Langs: French; (519)631-5670

PARADIS, Clement; CSSS de Chicoutimi, 305 rue Saint-Vallier, Chicoutimi QC G7H 5H6; Sher'97; CCFP; CCFP(E.M.); Staff, Complexe hospitalier de la Sagamie; (418)541-1000

PARADIS, Denise; Clin Med Napierville, 343 rue Saint-Jacques, Napierville QC J0J 1L0; Mon'74; (450)245-0081; Fax. (450)245-0615.

PARADIS, Desmond; 1306-70 rue de la Barre, Longueuil QC J4K 5J3; Laval'61; FACOG; ObstGyn. (450)651-7767

PARADIS, Elisabeth; Ctr de Sante Basse Cote Nord, CP 130 1070 boul Dr Camille Marcou, Lourdes-D-Bl-Sabl QC G0G 1W0; Laval'85; Staff, CSSS de la Basse Côté-Nord; (418)461-2144; Fax. (418)461-2962.

PARADIS, Eric; CSSS Pierre Boucher, 1333 boul Jacques-Cartier E, Longueuil QC J4M 2A5; Mon'92; ObstGyn. Staff, Centre Hospitalier Pierre Boucher; (450)468-6121; Fax. (450)468-3309.

PARADIS, Eric; CSSS de Chicoutimi, 305 rue Saint-Vallier, Chicoutimi QC G7H 5H6; Mon'93; FRCPC; IntMed; Critical Care Medicine (P.Q.). Staff, Complexe hospitalier de la Sagamie; (418)541-1000

PARADIS, Eric; Clinique Med Frontenac, 24 rue Frontenac, Riviere-du-Loup QC G5R 1S5; Laval'85; Staff, Centre Hospitalier Regional du Grand-Portage; (418)862-0333; Fax. (418)868-0505.

PARADIS, France; Centre de Sante Publique, 2400 av d'Estimauville, Quebec QC G1E 7G9; Laval'74; MSc(CommunHealth); Ac Staff, Centre Hospitalier Universitaire de Quebec-CHUL; (418)666-7000 x241; Fax. (418)666-2776; france.paradis@ssss.gouv.qc.ca.

PARADIS, Francois; CHUS-Hop Hotel-Dieu, 580 rue Bowen S, Sherbrooke QC J1G 2E8; Mon'89; CCFP; CCFP(E.M.); FCFP; Staff, Centre Hospitalier Universitaire de Sherbrooke-Hôpital Hôtel-Dieu; (819)346-1110 x21000

PARADIS, Gaetan; Hotel-Dieu de Levis, 143 rue Wolfe, Levis QC G6V 3Z1; Laval'82; CSPQ; FRCSC; Urol. ac Staff Urol, Hôtel-Dieu de Lévis; Consultant, Centre Hospitalier Paul-Gilbert; Langs: Bilingual(English/French); (418)835-7121; gaetanpar@videotron.ca.

PARADIS, Gaston R; Ctr Hosp Affilie-Enfant-Jesus, 1401 18e rue, Quebec QC G1J 1Z4; Laval'67; FRCSC; OrthSurg. Ac Staff, Centre Hospitalier Affilié Universitaire de Québec - Hôpital De L'Enfant Jésus; Assoc Staff, Jeffery Hale Hospital-Saint Brigid's; Consultant, CSSS de Quebec-Sud; (418)649-0252

PARADIS, Gilles; Inst Nat'l Sante Publique Queb, 190 boul Cremazie E, Montreal QC H2P 1E2; Mon'80; CSPQ; MSc; FRCPC; CommunMed (Research); Public Health & Preventive Med. Sr Physician, McGill University Health Centre - Montreal General Campus; Chef Epidemiology Biostatistics & OccupHealth/adj Prof, McGill University; (514)864-1600; Fax. (514)864-1616; gparadis@santepub-mtl.qc.ca.

PARADIS, Isabelle; CLSC Riviere-des-Prairies, 8655 boul Perras, Montreal QC H1E 4M7; Mon'06; (514)494-4924; Fax. (514)494-8182.

PARADIS, Jacinthe; Ctr de Sante Vallee-Gatineau, 309 boul desjardins, Maniwaki QC J9E 2E7; Sher'91; Staff, CSSS de la Vallée de la Gatineau; (819)449-4690; Fax. (819)449-6137.

PARADIS, Jacques; Clin Med Industrielle Laurenti, 200-352 boul Curé-Labelle, Laval QC H7P 2P1; Mon'79; ac Staff, Hôpital Santa Cabrini Ospedale; (450)624-9990; Fax. (450)624-9991.

PARADIS, Jean; Clinique medicale GMF-1851, 101-1851 rue Sherbrooke E, Montreal QC H2K 4L5; Mon'84; FRCPC; IntMed; ClinImmunol&Allergy. (514)524-7564; Fax. (514)527-5251.

PARADIS, Jean-Benoit; CSSS de Chicoutimi, 305 rue Saint-Vallier, Chicoutimi QC G7H 5H6; Laval'93; CSPQ; Urol (P.Q.). Staff, Complexe hospitalier de la Sagamie; (418)541-1000

PARADIS, Jean-Francois; CSSS de Chicoutimi, 305 rue Saint-Vallier, Chicoutimi QC G7H 5H6; Laval'76; FRCPC; MedMicrobiol; Microbio & Infect Dis (P.Q.). Staff, Complexe hospitalier de la Sagamie; (418)541-1046; Fax. (418)541-1137.

PARADIS, Jean-Michel; CSSS de Jonquiere, CP 1200 Succ Pdf Jonquiere 2230 rue de l'Hopital, Jonquiere QC G7X 7X2; Laval'01; Staff, Centre Hospitalier Jonquiere; (418)695-7700

PARADIS, Joanne; Centre Med Quatre-Bourgeois, 300-979 av de Bourgogne, Quebec QC G1W 2L4; Laval'85; (418)653-4050; Fax. (418)653-4475.

PARADIS, Louis; Polyclinique St-Eustache, 75 rue Grignon, St-Eustache QC J7P 4J2; Laval'89; FRCPC; IntMed; ClinImmunol&Allergy. (450)473-6777; Fax. (450)491-7470.

PARADIS, Marie-Claude; CSSS de Rimouski-Neigette, CP 3150 Succ A 150 av Rouleau, Rimouski QC G5L 5T1; Laval'96; LMCC; CSPQ; FRCPC; Anes. Staff, Hôpital Regional Rimouski; (418)724-3000

PARADIS, Marie-Renee; Clinique Med Fam Montcalm, 309 rue Montcalm, Chicoutimi QC G7J 2V1; McG'02; (418)545-4211

PARADIS, Michel; CHUM-Hop Notre-Dame, 1560 rue Sherbrooke E, Montreal QC H2L 4M1; Laval'84; FRCPC; Psy (Brief Therapy). Staff Emerg Psy, Hôpital du Haut-Richelieu; Staff Emerg Psy, Centre Hospitalier l'Université de Montréal (CHUM) - Hôpital Notre-Dame; Teach Staff Psy, Universite de Montreal; (514)890-8000 x26791; Fax. (514)412-7647.

PARADIS, Paul E; CSSS du Granit, 3569 rue Laval, Lac-Megantic QC G6B 1A5; Mon'69; GenSurg. Staff, Carrefour Sante Granit; (819)583-0330

PARADIS, Pierre J; Centre Med de Mont-Laurier, 304 rue de la Madone, Mont-Laurier QC J9L 1R7; Mon'77; (819)623-1520; Fax. (819)623-9637; centre.medical.ml@tlb.sympatico.ca.

PARADIS, Pierre; Anapharm Inc, 2500 rue Einstein, Quebec QC G1P 0A2; Laval'82; (418)527-4000; Fax. (418)527-3456.

PARADIS, Rachelle L; Sudbury Med Centre, 401-65 Larch St, Sudbury ON P3E 1B8; Ott'82; FRCSC; GenSurg (Breasts). Staff, Health Sciences North-Laurentian Site; Langs: English; French; (705)673-8391; Fax. (705)673-7330.

PARADIS, Rejean; PO Box 489 Stn A, Ottawa ON K1N 8V5; Laval'70; MPH; CSPQ; FRCPC; CommunMed; Public Health & Preventive Med. Langs: English; Spanish.

PARADIS, Rodrigue; Inst U en Sante Mentale de QC, 2601 ch de la Canardiere, Quebec QC G1J 2G3; Mon'78; Staff, Institut Universitaire Sante; (418)663-5253

PARADIS, Sabrina; CSSS des Aurorés-Boréales, CP 6000 Succ Bureau-Chef 679 2e rue E, La Sarre QC J9Z 2X7; Laval'09; CCFP; Staff, Centre Hospitalier La Sarre; (819)333-2311

PARADIS, Serge J; Ctr Med Rock Forest, 4870 boul Bourque, Sherbrooke QC J1N 3S5; Mon'75; ABOtol; FRCSC; Otol (Laryngology). Consultant ORL, Centre Hospitalier et CLSC de Memphremagog; Clin Prof Otorhinolaryngology, Universite de Sherbrooke; (819)820-8980

PARADIS, Serge; CSSS Pierre Boucher, 1333 boul Jacques-Cartier E, Longueuil QC J4M 2A5; Sher'98; FRCPC; Psy. Staff, Centre Hospitalier Pierre Boucher; (450)468-8401

PARADIS, Serge; Clinique Fam d'Hebertville, 9 rue Commerciale, Hebertville QC G8N 1N3; Laval'76; (418)344-1018; Fax. (418)344-1846.

PARADIS, Yves; Clinique Med d'Amos, 641 4E rue O, Amos QC J9T 2S1; Mon'80; Staff, CH Hôtel-Dieu d'Amos; Langs: English; (819)732-1244; Fax. (819)732-4646; dryvesparadis@msn.com.

PARADIS-ROBERT, Nina; Clin Med Champlain, 103-195 rue de l'Atmosphere, Gatineau QC J9A 0A3; Sher'06; CCFP; (819)777-7270

PARADISO, Guillermo; Moncton Med Clinic, 402-860 Mountain Rd, Moncton NB E1C 2N7; Buenos Aires (Argentina)'73; Staff, The Moncton Hospital; (506)857-5520

PARAGAS, Pedro G; 303-1497 Marine Dr, West Vancouver BC V7T 1B8; (Philippines)'62; FRCPC; Psy. (604)926-1112; Fax. (604)922-4823; pankratzparagas1947@gmail.com.

PARAI, Jacqueline L; The Ottawa Hosp-Gen Campus, 501 Smyth Rd, Ottawa ON K1H 8L6; Ott'94; BSc(Chem.); MSc(Epidemiol.); FRCPC; AnatPath (Forensic Pathology). Staff Dept of AnatPath, The Ottawa Hospital - General Campus; (613)737-8899 x72691; Fax. (613)737-8619.

PARAI, Milton S; The Ottawa Hosp - Gen Camp, 3041-501 Smyth Rd, Ottawa ON K1H 8L6; Mem'04; FRCSC; OrthSurg. Staff, The Ottawa Hospital - General Campus; (613)722-7000

PARAI, Mira R; Red Deer Reg Hosp Centre, PO Box 5030 Stn Postal Box Ctr 3942 50A Ave, Red Deer AB T4N 6R2; Dacca (Bangladesh)'75; FRCPC; AnatPath. Staff, Red Deer Regional Hospital Centre; (403)343-4712

PARAI, Sushil K; Red Deer Reg Hosp Centre, PO Box 5030 Stn Postal Box Ctr 3942 50A Ave, Red Deer AB T4N 6R2; Dacca (Bangladesh)'73; MB BS; DABPath; FRCPC; AnatPath. Staff, Red Deer Regional Hospital Centre; (403)309-5890; Fax. (403)343-4877.

PARAMANATHAN, Thalayasingam; Finch-Warden Med Walk-In Clin, 6A-3430 Finch Ave E, Scarborough ON M1W 2R5; Ceylon (Sri Lanka)'71; MB BS; CCFP; (416)496-1990; Fax. (416)496-1984.

PARAMBIL, Sumitha; Chatham-Kent Family Health Team, 209-20 Emma St, Chatham ON N7L 5K5; Calicut (India)'98; CCFP; (519)354-2172; sparambil@ckha.on.ca.

PARAMESHWAR, Manoj; 125-725 Carmi Ave, Penticton BC V2A 3G8; (India)'89; MRCP; Staff, Penticton Regional Hospital; Langs: Hindi; (778)476-5788

PARAMESWARAN, Charmaine D; Edmonton Clinic, 1A. 102-11400 University Ave, Edmonton AB T5G 1Z1; (Sri Lanka)'79; MB BS; CCFP; Staff, University of Alberta Hospital; (780)407-7755; Fax. (780)407-1828.

PARAMESWARAN, Krishanthan; Halton HC Serv Corp-Oakville, 327 Reynolds St, Oakville ON L6J 3L7; Wes'07; FRCPC; Peds. Staff, Halton Healthcare Services Corporation - Oakville Site; (905)845-3721

PARAMESWARAN, Sandrasekeram; Cold Lake Health Centre, 203-314 25 St, Cold Lake AB T9M 1G6; Ceylon (Sri Lanka)'73; FRCSC; GenSurg. Staff, Cold Lake Healthcare Centre; (780)639-3322; Fax. (780)639-3631.

PARAMONOFF, Catherine E; G F Strong Rehabilitation Ctre, 4255 Laurel St, Vancouver BC V5Z 2G9; UBC'04; FRCPC; PhysMed&Rehab. Staff, G F Strong Rehabilitation Centre; (604)734-1313

PARAMSOTHY, Koushalya; Lakeridge Health Corp-Oshawa, 1 Hospital Crt, Oshawa ON L1G 2B9; Ott'01; FRCPC; IntMed; Hem. Staff, Lakeridge Health - Oshawa Site; (905)576-8711 x4519; Fax. (905)721-6100.

PARAMSOTHY, Rasiah; Dixon Med Centre, 402-531 Davis Dr, Newmarket ON L3Y 6P5; Colombo (Sri Lanka)'74; MRCPsy(UK); FRCPC; Psy. Staff Psy, Southlake Regional Health Centre; Consultant Psy., Long Term Care Facilities-Newmarket; (905)836-6733; Fax. (905)836-6733.

PARARAJASINGAM, Thevaki; Wardenwood Hlth Centre, 549 Bur Oak Ave, Markham ON L6C 3E5; Saba (Netherlands Antilles)'07; (905)554-0199

PARAS, Dwight J; Smyth Associate Clinic, 4904 48 St, Leduc AB T9E 6X4; Cal'89; (780)986-2712; Fax. (780)986-0356.

PARAS, Emilyos; 34 Dorchester St, Saint John NB E2L 3H8; Istanbul (Turkey)'66; FRCPC; Peds (Pediatric Oncology). Ac Staff, Saint John Regional Hospital; Ac Staff, St Joseph's Hospital; Asst Prof Peds, Memorial University Of Newfoundland; Lecturer, Dalhousie University; Langs: Greek; Turkish; (506)634-7560; Fax. (506)658-9078; emileparas@outlook.com.

PARASCAN, Oana S; Medisante Saint-Jean, 67 Ragged Point Rd, Saint John NB E2K 5C3; Bucharest (Romania)'95; CCFP.

PARASCANDALO, Richard J; St Joseph's Healthcare, 50 Charlton Ave E, Hamilton ON L8N 4A6; Tor'80; FRCPC; Anes. Staff, St Joseph's Healthcare - Charlton Campus; (905)522-1155 x33853; Fax. (905)521-6140.

PARASHAR, Rakesh K; 300 Giles Blvd E, Windsor ON N9A 4C4; Delhi (India)'79; MB BS; FRCS; FRCSC; GenSurg. (519)252-4049

PARASHAR, Sujata H; Venture Place, 302-2525 Rose Ville Garden Dr, Windsor ON N8T 3J8; Bhopal (India)'85; CCFP; Langs: Punjabi; Hindi; (519)948-7550; Fax. (519)944-1703.

PARASKEVAS, Steven; S1030-687 av des Pins O, Montreal QC H3A 1A1; McG'92; DrMedCh; FRCSC; GenSurg (Transplantation). Staff, McGill University Health Centre - Royal Victoria Hospital; Langs: French; Greek; (514)934-1934 x36522; Fax. (514)843-1434.

PARASKEVOPOULOS, Chryssi I; St Mary's Hosp Centre, 3830 av Lacombe, Montreal QC H3T 1M5; Ott'89; Staff, St Mary's Hospital Centre; Staff, Sir Mortimer B Davis Jewish General; adj Prof, McGill University; (514)345-3511

PARASKEVOPOULOS, Elena Z; Pender Community Health Centre, 59 Pender St W, Vancouver BC V6B 1R3; Wes'10; CCFP; (604)669-9181

PARAYRE, Michel; Medecins de Famille Marleau, 3 9E rue, Rouyn-Noranda QC J9X 2A9; Ott'79; CCFP; FCFP; Clin Assoc Prof UMF Horizon de Rouyn-Noranda, Universite de Sherbrooke; Langs: Bilingual(French/English); (819)797-4535; Fax. (819)797-4665.

PARBHAKAR, Meenakshi; Lifesource Health Centre, 130 Robertson Rd, Ottawa ON K2H 5Z1; Ott'03; CCFP; (613)828-3122; Fax. (613)828-2010.

PARBHAKAR, Samir R; William Osler HC-Brampton, 2100 Bovaird Dr E, Brampton ON L6R 3J7; Tor'03; Staff, William Osler Health System - Brampton Civic Hospital; (905)494-2120

PARBTANI, Anwar; Eagle Ridge Family Health Ctre, 203-480 Huronia Rd, Barrie ON L4N 6M2; Saba (Netherlands Antilles)'03; MSc; BSc(Hon); PhD; CCFP; Staff, Royal Victoria Regional Health Centre; Clinical Asst Prof, University of Toronto; Clinical Asst Prof, Queen's University; Clinical Asst Prof, McMaster University; (705)727-7688; Fax. (705)734-6284.

PARDHAN, Alim; Hamilton HS-General Site, 237 Barton St E, Hamilton ON L8L 2X2; Man'04; FRCPC; EmergMed. Staff, Hamilton Health Sciences Centre - Hamilton General Hospital; (905)527-0271

PARDIS, Bijan; 10171 Yonge St, Richmond Hill ON L4C 1T5; Bruxelles (Belgium)'88; CCFP; (905)883-8183; Fax. (905)918-0037.

PARE, Bruno; Clin Laser Esthetique Quebec, 1693 Rte de l'Aeroport, L'Ancienne-Lorette QC G2G 2P3; Sher'86; Staff, Centre Hospitalier Universitaire de Québec (CHUQ) - Siege Social; (418)871-3434; Fax. (418)844-6671.

PARE, Chantal; CSSS de Manicouagan, 635 boul Joliet, Baie-Comeau QC G5C 1P1; Laval'99; FRCPC; IntMed; GeriatricMed. Staff, Centre Hospitalier Régional Baie-Comeau; (418)589-3701

PARE, Daniel F; 920 Seymour St, Vancouver BC V6B 3L9; UBC'09; CCFP; (604)257-2630

PARE, Gilles; Clinique Med Galt, 200-2235 rue Galt O, Sherbrooke QC J1K 1K6; Laval'64; FAAP; Peds. (819)791-5455

PARE, Gregoire; GMF de l'Assomption, CP 3406 Succ Bureau-Chef 814 boul l'Ange-Gardien N, L'Assomption QC J5W 4M9; Mon'76; (450)589-5778; Fax. (450)589-5779.

PARE, Guillaume; Hamilton HS-McMaster Site, PO Box 2000 Stn Lcd 1 3206-1200 Main St W, Hamilton ON L8N 3Z5; Mon'02; FRCPC; MedBiochem. Staff, Hamilton Health Sciences Centre - McMaster University Medical Centre; (905)527-4322

PARE, Guylaine; Clinique Med St-Nicolas, 845 Rte Marie-Victorin, Saint-Nicolas QC G7A 3S8; Sher'97; ABNP; Staff, Centre De Sante Valcartier; Staff, CLSC Nouvelle-Beauce; (418)831-4141; Fax. (418)831-4141.

PARE, Jean-Louis; 201-404 St. George St, Moncton NB E1C 1X6; Laval'84; Langs: Bilingual(French/English); (506)204-7414

PARE, Louise; ASSS-Chaudiere Appalaches, 363 Rte Cameron, Sainte-Marie QC G6E 3E2; Mon'84; MSc(Lav); CSPQ; Public Health & Preventive Med; CommunMed (P.Q.). Staff, Centre de Readaptation en Toxicomanie; (418)389-1547; Fax. (418)389-1540.

PARE, Lyne; CLSC Saint-Pamphile, CP 580 103 rue du Foyer N, Saint-Pamphile QC G0R 3X0; Laval'76; Langs: Bilingual(French/English); (418)356-3393; Fax. (418)356-5535.

PARE, Maryse; Clin Externe de Psychiatrie, 7345 rue Garnier, Montreal QC H2E 2A1; Ott'92; FRCPC; Psy. Staff, CSSS du Coeur de l'Isle Hôpital Jean-Talon; Langs: Spanish; (514)729-3036; Fax. (514)332-6188.

PARE, Michael F; Medical Clinic Person-Ctred Psy, 403-265 Yorkland Blvd, North York ON M2J 1S5; Tor'88; MSc(NeuroScience); BSc(Psychol); Coord, The Medical Clinic for Person-Centred Psychotherapy; Aj Prof, Tyndale University College & Seminary; (416)229-2399 x120; Fax. (416)229-9771; michaelpare@rogers.com.

PARE, Peter D; St Paul's Hosp, 166-1081 Burrard St, Vancouver BC V6Z 1Y6; McG'69; BSc; Respir; IntMed. Assoc Dir Centre for Health Evaluation/Ac Staff, Providence Health Care - St Paul's Hospital; Prof Med, University of British Columbia; (604)682-2344 x62750; Fax. (604)631-5674.

PARE, Pierre; Ctr Hosp Affilie-St-Sacrement, 1050 ch Sainte-Foy, Quebec QC G1S 4L8; Laval'72; FRCPC; IntMed (Hepatology); Gastroent. Staff, Centre Hospitalier Affilié Universitaire de Québec - Hôpital du St-Sacrement; Prof Med, Université Laval; (418)682-7646; Fax. (418)682-7855.

PARE, Renee; Dir de Sante Publique-Mtl, 1301 rue Sherbrooke E, Montreal QC H2L 1M3; Mon'82; Staff General Med, Institut de Réadaptation Gingras-Lindsay de Montréal; Med Consultant, Direction de Sante Publique de Montreal; Med Consultant, CHSLD Champlain Manoir Verdun; (514)528-2400 x3649; Fax. (514)528-2452; rpare@santepub-mtl.qc.ca.

PARE, Robert; Centre Med Laval, 1110 boul Vanier, Laval QC H7C 2R8; Mon'82; Staff, Hopital de la Cite de la santé; Staff, Canadian Correctional Service; Staff, Universite de Montreal; Langs: English; (450)661-2521; Fax. (450)661-7193.

PAREDES, Jaime P; 201-3701 Hastings St E, Burnaby BC V5C 2H6; Santiago (Chile)'67; FRCPC; Psy. Langs: Spanish; (604)928-1397; Fax. (604)677-8238.

PAREKH, Jaintheelal M; Greenstone Clinic, 3F-5734 Yonge St, North York ON M2M 4E7; Dublin (Ireland)'61; FRCS(Lond); GenSurg. (416)222-5501; Fax. (416)222-1932.

PAREKH, Neal A; SGH Medical Mall, 505-3030 Lawrence Ave E, Scarborough ON M1P 2T7; Tor'05; FRCPC; Neur. (416)289-0185; Fax. (416)289-0187.

PAREKH, Praful K; 1102 Edmonton Trail NE, Calgary AB T2E 3K4; (Zimbabwe)'76; MB ChB; LRCP; LRCS; MRCP(UK); FRCPC; IntMed (Cardiology). Langs: Gujarati; (403)277-7047; Fax. (403)277-7098.

PAREKH, Ritesh; Chilliwack Gen Hosp, 45600 Menholm Rd, Chilliwack BC V2P 1P7; Sydney (Australia)'04; MB BS; Staff, Chilliwack General Hospital; (604)702-4704

PAREKH, Rulan S; The Hosp for Sick Children, 555 University Ave, Toronto ON M5G 1X8; Albany(NY) (USA)'91; FRCPC; Peds; Nephrol. Staff, The Hospital For Sick Children; Staff, University Health Network; (416)813-7654; Fax. (416)813-5979.

PAREKH, Shrenik P; Grand River Hosp-KW Hlth Ctre, PO Box 9056 Stn C 835 King St W, Kitchener ON N2G 1G3; Gujarat University (India)'05; Staff, Grand River Hospital - Kitchener/Waterloo Health Centre; (519)749-4300

PAREKH, Vipul Z; Prine Albert Community Clinic, 110 8th St E, Prince Albert SK S6V 0V7; CCFP; (306)763-6464; Fax. (306)763-2101.

PARENT, Alain; CHUQ-Hotel-Dieu de Quebec, 11 Cote du Palais, Quebec QC G1R 2J6; Ott'91; CCFP; Staff, Centre Hospitalier Universitaire de Québec (CHUQ) - Siege Social; (418)691-5042

PARENT, Andre; Clinique Med Saint-Isidore, 109 rue des Pinsons, Saint-Isidore QC G0S 2S0; Laval'71; LMCC; Staff, Hôtel-Dieu de Lévis; Langs: English; (418)882-5696; Fax. (418)882-1957.

PARENT, Andree-Anne; Inst U Geriatrie de Montreal, 4565 ch Queen-Mary, Montreal QC H3W 1W5; Mon'09; Staff, Institut Universitaire de Gériatrie de Montréal; (514)340-2800

PARENT, Bernard; CSSS de Chicoutimi, 305 rue Saint-Vallier, Chicoutimi QC G7H 5H6; Laval'70; Dir Services Professional, Complexe hospitalier de la Sagamie; (418)541-1091; Fax. (418)541-1131.

PARENT, Carole; Inst U en Sante Mentale de QC, 2601 ch de la Canardiere, Quebec QC G1J 2G3; Laval'77; FRCPC; Neur (Dementia). Staff, Institut Universitaire Sante; (418)663-5321; Fax. (418)661-6891.

PARENT, Christine M P; Montfort Hosp, 713 Montreal Rd, Ottawa ON K1K 0T2; Ott'97; FRCPC; Anes. Staff, Montfort Hospital; (613)746-4621 x3807

PARENT, Claude; Ctr Hosp Affilie-Enfant Jesus, 1401 18e rue, Quebec QC G1J 1Z4; Laval'80; FRCPC; IntMed; Gastroent. Ac Staff, Centre Hospitalier Affilié Universitaire de Québec - Hôpital De L'Enfant Jésus; (418)649-5732; Fax. (418)649-5570.

PARENT, Claude; Hydro-Quebec, 75 boul Rene-Levesque O, Montreal QC H2Z 1A4; McG'76; MSc; Med Consultant, Sunlife Financial; Med Consultant, Hydro-Quebec; (514)289-2211 x5165; Fax. (514)289-5049; parent.claude@hydro.ca.

PARENT, Daniel E; Institut de Cardiologie de Mtl, 5000 rue Belanger, Montreal QC H1T 1C8; Mon'81; Staff, Institut de Cardiologie de Montréal; (514)376-3330; Fax. (514)593-2540.

PARENT, Dominique; CLSC Jean Olivier-Chenier, 29 ch d'Oka, St-Eustache QC J7R 1K6; Sher'95; (450)491-1233; Fax. (450)491-3424.

PARENT, France; CLSC Dorval-Lachine, 1900 rue Notre-Dame, Lachine QC H8S 2G2; Mon'86; (514)639-0650 x333; Fax. (514)639-8593.

PARENT, Francois; CSSS de Trois-Rivières, 1991 boul du Carmel, Trois-Rivieres QC G8Z 3R9; Mon'89; CCFP; CCFP(E.M.); FCFP; Staff, CSSS de Trois-Rivières; (819)378-9868; francois_parent@cgocable.ca.

PARENT, Francois; CHUQ-Hotel-Dieu de Quebec, 11 Cote Du Palais, Quebec QC G1R 2J6; Laval'79; FRCSC; Otol. Staff, Centre Hospitalier Universitaire de Québec (CHUQ) - Siege Social; Staff, CSSS de Charlevoix; Staff, Hôpital de l'Archipel; Université Laval; (418)691-5490; Fax. (418)691-5018; orl.phdq@dechuq.ulaval.ca.

PARENT, Francois; Hôpital Laval, 2725 ch Sainte-Foy, Quebec QC G1V 4G5; Laval'87; CSPQ; FRCPC; Anes. Staff, Hôpital Laval; (418)656-8711 x4870; Fax. (418)656-4551; francois.parent@videotron.ca.

PARENT, Genevieve; CLSC Saint-Hubert, 6800 boul Cousineau, Saint-Hubert QC J3Y 8Z4; Mon'03; (450)443-7400

PARENT, Jean; Ctr Hosp Affilie-Enfant-Jesus, 1401 18e rue, Quebec QC G1J 1Z4; Laval'82; CSPQ; FRCPC; Anes. Staff, Centre Hospitalier Affilié Universitaire de Québec - Hôpital De L'Enfant Jésus; (418)649-5807

PARENT, Jean-Guy; CHUQ-St-Francois d'Assise, B2 526-10 rue de l'Espinay, Quebec QC G1L 3L5; Laval'71; LMCC; Respir (P.Q.) (Respiratory Disease). Ac Staff, Centre Hospitalier Universitaire De Québec - Pavillon De St-françois-d'assise; Physician, Commission Sante Securite Travail; Université Laval; Langs: English; (418)525-4312; Fax. (418)525-4318.

PARENT, Jean-Philippe; Ctr Hosp Anna-Laberge, 200 boul Brisebois, Chateauguay QC J6K 4W8; Mon'95; LMCC; CCFP; Staff, Hôpital Anna-Laberge; (450)699-2425; Fax. (450)699-2525.

PARENT, Jocelyne; 19 Whittaker Cres, North York ON M2K 1K7; Sher'80; FRCPC; Peds. Langs: English; French; (416)494-9616; Fax. (416)499-7440; jparent@rogers.com.

PARENT, Josee; CSSS de la Vallée de l'Or, 725 6e rue, Val-d'Or QC J9P 3Y1; Sher'92; FRCSC; ObstGyn. Staff, Centre Hospitalier de Val d'Or; (819)825-6711; Fax. (819)825-7909.

PARENT, Josee; MUHC-Montreal Gen Hosp, D7 344-1650 av Cedar, Montreal QC H3G 1A4; McG'90; DABIM; FRCPC; IntMed (Endoscopic Ultrasound); Gastroent. adj Prof, McGill University Health Centre - Montreal General Campus; Langs: English; Spanish; (514)934-8308; Fax. (514)934-8531.

PARENT, Josiane; Clinique Med Les Gres, RR 1 104-190 rue Saint-Honore, St-Etienne-de-Gres QC G0X 2P0; Sher'06; CCFP; (819)535-6512; Fax. (819)535-1627; josiane.parent@usherbrooke.ca.

PARENT, Lorne J; Sandy Hill Comm Health Centre, 221 Nelson St, Ottawa ON K1N 1C7; McG'81; CCFP; FCFP; Langs: French; (613)789-8458; Fax. (613)789-8710; loparent@sandyhillchc.on.ca.

PARENT, Marc C; CHUQ-Ctr Hosp Univ Laval, 2705 boul Laurier, Quebec QC G1V 4G2; Laval'95; FRCPC; EmergMed. Staff, Centre Hospitalier Universitaire de Quebec-CHUL; (418)656-4141 x70554

PARENT, Marc-Antoine; CSSS des Iles, 430 ch Principal, Cap-aux-Meules QC G4T 1R9; Sher'99; Staff, Hôpital de l'Archipel; (418)986-2121

PARENT, Marcel P F; Guelph Gen Hosp, 115 Delhi St, Guelph ON N1E 4J4; McM'08; CCFP; Staff, Guelph General Hospital; (519)822-5350

PARENT, Maria M; London Reg Cancer Centre, 790 Commissioner's Rd E, London ON N6A 4L6; Ott'02; CCFP; (519)685-8600

PARENT, Marie-Claude; CSSS Drummond-Hop Sainte-Croix, 570 rue Heriot, Drummondville QC J2B 1C1; Laval'93; FRCPC; Psy. Staff, Hôpital Sainte-croix; (819)478-6464 x3402; Fax. (418)478-6490.

PARENT, Marie-Claude; Hop du Sacre-Coeur de Mtl, 540 boul Gouin O, Montreal QC H4J 1C5; Mon'03; FRCPC; IntMed; Cardiol. Staff, Hôpital du Sacre-Coeur de Montréal; (514)338-2222

PARENT, Marie-Eve; CSSS Energie-UMF Shawinigan, 80 118e rue, Shawinigan-Sud QC G9P 3E4; Laval'04; CCFP; Staff, Centre Hospitalier du Centre la Mauricie; (819)536-7500 x7511

PARENT, Marie-Josee; 2400 av d'Estimauville, Quebec QC G1E 7G9; Laval'82; Langs: English; (418)623-1010 x241; Fax. (418)623-7513.

PARENT, Mariloue; Clinique Med des Trois Lacs, 160-585 av Saint-Charles, Vaudreuil-Dorion QC J7V 8P9; Sher'98; Staff Med, Centre Hospitalier Régional du Suroît; Langs: English; (450)455-3322; Fax. (450)455-0756.

PARENT, Michel; CHUS-Hop Fleurimont, 3001 12e av N, Sherbrooke QC J1H 5N4; Sher'83; CSPQ; FRCPC; Anes. Staff, Centre Hospitalier Universitaire de Sherbrooke-Hopital Fleurimont; (819)346-1110 x14403; Fax. (819)820-6420.

PARENT, Nancie; Westmount Med Bldg, 304-77 Westmount Rd, Guelph ON N1H 5J1; Ott'06; CCFP; (519)265-7025; Fax. (519)265-7154.

PARENT, Nathalie; CSSS de Beauce-Etchemin, 1515 17e rue, Saint-Georges QC G5Y 4T8; Sher'96; Staff, Centre Hospitalier Beauce-Etchemin; (418)228-2031

PARENT, Pierre; CHUS-Hop Fleurimont, 3001 12e av N, Sherbrooke QC J1H 5N4; Laval'83; CSPQ; FRCPC; Anes. Staff, Centre Hospitalier Universitaire de Sherbrooke-Hopital Fleurimont; (819)346-1000

PARENT, Rene; Ctr Hosp Affilie Enfant-Jesus, 1401 18e rue, Quebec QC G1J 1Z4; Laval'84; FRCPC; PhysMed&Rehab (Electromyography). Ac Staff, Centre Hospitalier Affilié Universitaire de Québec - Hôpital De L'Enfant Jésus; Langs: English; (418)649-5751; Fax. (418)649-5879.

PARENT, Robert; CLSC-CHSLD du Haut St-Francois, RR 1 700 rue Craig N, Cookshire QC J0B 1M0; Sher'78; Assoc Staff Community Health, Centre Hospitalier Universitaire de Sherbrooke-Hopital Fleurimont; (819)875-3373; Fax. (819)875-5565.

PARENT, Roch; CHUM-Hop St-Luc, 1058 rue Saint-Denis, Montreal QC H2X 3J4; Mon'78; IntMed. Staff, Centre Hospitalier l'Université De Montréal (CHUM) - Hôpital Saint-luc; (514)890-8000

PARENT, Roger; La Cite Medicale, 295-2600 boul Laurier, Quebec QC G1V 4T3; Sher'93; Langs: Bilingual(French/English); (418)781-0480

PARENT, Stefan; Hôpital Ste-Justine, 3175 ch Cote-Sainte-Catherine, Montreal QC H3T 1C5; McG'97; FRCSC; OrthSurg. Staff, Hôpital Ste-Justine; (514)345-4876; Fax. (514)345-4755; stefan.parent@umontreal.ca.

PARENT, Sylvie; Clinique Med Havre Sante, 521 boul du Havre, Salaber-de-Valleyf QC J6S 4Z5; Mon'86; (450)371-6444 x219; Fax. (450)371-5315.

PARENT, Sylvie; CSSS du Nord de Lanaudière, 1000 boul Sainte-Anne, St-Charles-Brromee QC J6E 6J2; Sher'91; Staff, Centre Hospitalier Régional de Lanaudière; (450)759-8222

PARENT, Veronique; CHUQ-St-Francois d'Assise, 10 rue de l'Espinay, Quebec QC G1L 3L5; Laval'05; CCFP; CCFP(E.M.); Staff, Centre Hospitalier Universitaire De Québec - Pavillon De St-françois-d'assise; (418)525-4444

PARENT, Yves; Clinique Med du Quartier Latin, 905 boul Rene-Levesque E, Montreal QC H2J 3B7; Mon'86; Staff, Centre Hospitalier l'Université De Montréal (CHUM) - Hôpital Saint-luc; Staff, Centre d'Accueil Lachine; Staff, Centre de Soins Longue Duree; Langs: English; French; Bilingual(French/English); (514)285-5500; Fax. (514)285-2226; yvep@videotron.ca.

PARENTE, Fabienne; MUHC-Montreal Children's Hosp, 2300 rue Tupper, Montreal QC H3H 1P3; Mon'04; FRCPC; MedBiochem. Staff, McGill University Health Centre - Montreal Children's Hospital; (514)412-4427

PARENTEAU, Chantal; Clin d'Endocrin Trois-Rivieres, 5050 boul des Forges, Trois-Rivieres QC G8Y 1X2; Sher'92; FRCPC; IntMed (Diabetology); Endocrin&Metab. Staff Endocrin, CSSS de Trois-Rivières; Langs: English; (819)379-1442; Fax. (819)379-9708.

PARENTEAU, Hugues; Clinique Med Notre-Dame Inc, 147 rue Notre-Dame E, Victoriaville QC G6P 3Z8; Laval'91; (819)758-3165; Fax. (819)758-0745.

PARENTEAU, Judith; Clinique Med Fleur de Lys, 8 rue du Terminus E, Rouyn-Noranda QC J9X 3B4; Sher'06; CCFP; (819)764-6185; Fax. (819)762-6079.

PARENTEAU, Pierre R; CFB Kingston, PO Box 17000 Stn Forces, Kingston ON K7K 7B4; Laval'71; FRCPC; Psy.

PARENTEAU, Rosaire; Hotel-Dieu d'Arthabaska, 5 rue des Hospitalieres, Victoriaville QC G6P 6N2; Laval'65; Psy (P.Q.). Staff, Hotel-Dieu d'Arthabaska; Prof, Universite de Sherbrooke; (819)357-2030 x2660; Fax. (819)357-6035.

PARENTEAU, Simon; Hop du Sacre-Coeur de Mtl, 5400 boul Gouin O, Montreal QC H4J 1C5; Mon'96; FRCPC; IntMed; Respir. Staff, Hôpital du Sacre-Coeur de Montréal; (514)338-2162; Fax. (514)338-3699.

PARFITT, Christopher J; 3403 32 Ave, Vernon BC V1T 2M9; Qns'78; FRCSC; OrthSurg (Arthroplasty). Staff, Shuswap Lake General Hospital; Staff, Vernon Jubilee Hospital; (250)545-2488; Fax. (250)545-6029.

PARFITT, Hugh L; 1776 Patricia Ave, Port Coquitlam BC V3B 2G7; London (England)'59; MB BS; DPsy(McG.); FRCPC; Psy (Geriatric Psychiatry). Member, Mental Health Review Board; Fellow, Canadian Psychiatric Association; Emeritus Prof, University of British Columbia; (604)464-8404; Fax. (604)475-0613; hugh_parfitt@telus.net.

PARFITT, Jeremy R; London HSC-University Hosp, PO Box 5339 Stn B 339 Windermere Rd, London ON N6A 5A5; Wes'02; FRCPC; AnatPath. Staff, London Health Sciences Centre - University Hospital; (519)685-8500

PARFITT, Kathleen P; 90 Jack Rd, Galiano BC V0N 1P0; London (England)'59; MB BS; FRCPC; Psy. (250)539-2822; Fax. (250)539-2825.

PARFREY, Brendan P; Kingston Gen Hosp, 76 Stuart St, Kingston ON K7L 2V7; Mem'04; FRCPC; IntMed; Cardiol. Staff, Kingston General Hospital; (613)548-3232

PARFREY, Patrick S; Health Sciences Centre, 300 Prince Philip Dr, St. John's NL A1B 3V6; National (Ireland)'75; FRCPC; IntMed. Staff Nephrol, Health Sciences Centre; Assoc Dean Clinical Research/Prof, Memorial University Of Newfoundland; (709)777-7261; Fax. (709)777-6995; pparfrey@mun.ca.

PARHAM, Shelley M; Salvation Army Grace Gen Hosp, 300 Booth Dr, Winnipeg MB R3J 3M7; Alb'88; FACS; FRCSC; GenSurg; ThorSurg. Staff ThoracicSurg, Health Sciences Centre; Staff, The Salvation Army Grace Hospital; Staff, St Boniface General Hospital; (204)837-0391

PARHAR, Gurdeep; 105-6602 Main St, Vancouver BC V5X 3H2; Cal'92; Ac Staff, Eagle Ridge Hospital & Health Care Centre; Ac Staff, Royal Columbian Hospital; Staff, CORE Occupational Health Centre; Clin Instructor Med/Assoc Dean Equity & Professionalism, University of British Columbia; Langs: Punjabi; (604)558-1803

PARHAR, Kuljit S; Foothills Med Centre, 1403 29 St NW, Calgary AB T2N 2T9; Qns'07; FRCPC; IntMed. Staff, Foothills Medical Centre; (403)944-1110

PARI, Giovanna; Kingston Gen Hosp, 76 Stuart St, Kingston ON K7L 2V7; Ott'93; FRCPC; Neur. Staff, Kingston General Hospital; (613)548-2519; Fax. (613)548-1341.

PARIAG, John K; 21 Queensway W, Mississauga ON L5B 1B6; West Indies (Jamaica)'78; GenSurg (Gastroenterology). Staff, Temiskaming Hospital; (905)897-9228

PARIBELLO, Carlo; 167 Queen St W, Brampton ON L6Y 1M5; Cebu (Philippines)'83; (905)453-9366; Fax. (905)452-0095.

PARIHAR, Sheela; Care Point Med Centre, 1175 Denman St, Vancouver BC V6G 2N1; Rajasthan (India)'75; MB BS; Langs: Hindi; (604)681-5338

PARIKH, Ameet; 10248 152 St, Surrey BC V3R 6N7; UBC'89; BSc; (604)588-4191; Fax. (604)588-4192.

PARIKH, Amish; Queensway Professional Ctre, 102-190 Sherway Dr, Etobicoke ON M9C 5N2; Tor'00; FRCPC; IntMed; Endocrin&Metab. Staff, Trillium Health Centre - Mississauga; (905)848-7100

PARIKH, Munjal S; Victoria Terrace Med Centre, 211-1448 Lawrence Ave E, North York ON M4A 2V6; Dal'82; Staff, North York General Hospital; Staff, The Scarborough Hospital - General Campus; (416)755-2285; Fax. (416)755-8786.

PARIKH, Nimish U; Perth-Smiths Falls Dist Hosp, 33 Drummond St W, Perth ON K7H 2K1; Pune (India)'92; FRCPC; DiagRad. Staff, Perth & Smiths Falls District Hospital - Perth Site (Great War Memorial Site); (613)267-1500

PARIKH, Sagar V; Univ Hlth Network-Toronto Western Hosp, 399 Bathurst St, Toronto ON M5T 2S8; McG'84; FRCPC; Psy. Staff, Centre for Addiction & Mental Health (CAMH) - College Street Site; Dep Chief Psy, Toronto Western Hospital - University Health Network; Dir CMHE, University of Toronto; (416)603-5734; Fax. (416)603-5039.

PARIKH, Samir S; Lakeshore Med Group, 502-345 Lakeshore Rd E, Oakville ON L6J 1J5; Tor'98; BSc; CCFP; (905)845-4551; Fax. (905)845-8133.

PARIMOO, Sabina A; 202-99 Sinclair Ave, Georgetown ON L7G 4L7; (India)'04; CCFP; (905)702-9988

PARIS, Catherine; CHUS-Hop Fleurimont, 3001 12e av N, Sherbrooke QC J1H 5N4; Sher'03; FRCSC; GenSurg; PedGenSurg (P.Q.). Staff, Centre Hospitalier Universitaire de Sherbrooke-Hopital Fleurimont; (819)346-1110

PARIS, Catherine; Clin Med Richelieu, 500 Rte Marie-Victorin, Sorel-Tracy QC J3R 1K7; Mon'03; CCFP; Staff, Centre Hospitalier Pierre Boucher; Physician, CHSLD Jeanne-Crevier; Langs: English; (450)742-5638

PARIS, Gaetan; CHUQ-Ctr Hosp Univ Laval, 2705 boul Laurier, Quebec QC G1V 4G2; Laval'73; FRCSC; ObstGyn (Coloscopy). Staff, Centre Hospitalier Affilié Universitaire de Québec - Hôpital du St-Sacrement; Staff, Centre Hospitalier Universitaire de Quebec-CHUL; Staff, Centre Hospitalier Universitaire de Québec (CHUQ) - Siege Social; (418)525-4444

PARIS, Joel F; Inst of Commun & Family Psy, 4333 ch Cote-Sainte-Catherine, Montreal QC H3T 1E4; McG'64; FRCPC; Psy. Sr Physician, Sir Mortimer B Davis Jewish General; Teach Staff, McGill University; (514)340-8210

PARIS, Marc R; Nanaimo Reg Gen Hosp, 1200 Dufferin Cres, Nanaimo BC V9S 2B7; UBC'94; BSc; Staff, Nanaimo Regional General Hospital; (250)751-8160

PARIS, Raphael; CSSS de Memphremagog, 50 rue Saint-Patrice E, Magog QC J1X 3X3; Sher'08; CCFP; Staff, Centre Hospitalier et CLSC de Memphremagog; (819)843-2572

PARISE, Patrick; CSSS de Laval, 1755 boul Rene-Laennec, Laval QC H7M 3L9; Mon'97; Staff, Hopital de la Cite de la santé; (450)668-1010

PARISER, Marc R; 81 Charles St W, Ingersoll ON N5C 2L7; Tor'80; CCFP; Ac Staff GP Anes, Alexandra Hospital; (519)485-3810; Fax. (519)485-0192; marc.pariser@bellnet.ca.

PARISER, Pauline C; 300-790 Bay St, Toronto ON M5G 1N8; McM'80; MAS; CCFP; FCFP; Asst Prof Family & Commun Med, University of Toronto; (416)960-1366; Fax. (416)960-1945.

PARISH, Barbara M; Fenwick Med Centre, 210-5595 Fenwick St, Halifax NS B3H 4M2; McM'86; FRCSC; ObstGyn (Colposcopy). Ac Staff, IWK Health Centre; Ac Staff, Queen Elizabeth II Health Sciences Centre - Victoria General Site; Assoc Prof, Dalhousie University; (902)423-4901; Fax. (902)423-2475.

PARISIEN, Gladys; Ctr Hosp du Centre la Mauricie, 50 119e rue, Shawinigan-Sud QC G9P 5K1; Louvain (Belgium)'72; DABPath; CSPQ; GenPath (P.Q.). Staff, Centre Hospitalier du Centre la Mauricie; Langs: English; (819)536-7500 x2506; Fax. (819)536-6162.

PARISSIER, Adrien; Clinique Med Bromont, C101-82 boul Bromont, Bromont QC J2L 2K3; Sher'10; Staff, Hôpital Brome-Missisquoi-Perkins; (450)534-5474

PARIZEAULT, Guy; Clinique Ped de Chicoutimi, 475 boul Talbot, Chicoutimi QC G7H 4A3; Laval'91; Peds. (418)549-1034; Fax. (418)696-4673.

PARK, Andrew J; Abbotsford Reg Hosp & Cancer C, 32900 Marshall Rd, Abbotsford BC V2S 0C2; Tor'05; CCFP; CCFP(E.M.); Staff, Abbotsford Regional Hospital & Cancer Centre; (604)851-4700; andrew.park@spchc.hnet.bc.ca.

PARK, Diane H; PO Box 33073 Rpo Quinpool Ctre, Halifax NS B3L 4T6; Wes'09; CCFP.

PARK, Donald; Medical Clinic, PO Box 1330 20 James St, Deep River ON K0J 1P0; Man'63; Staff, Deep River & District Hospital; (613)584-2344; Fax. (613)584-2344; donpark@magma.ca.

PARK, Esther M; 1-20 Edna Ave, Toronto ON M6P 1B5; Tor'93; FRCSC; ObstGyn. Ac Staff, St Joseph's Health Centre; Langs: Korean; (416)532-7612; Fax. (416)532-6577.

PARK, Grace H; 101A-2099 152 St, Surrey BC V4A 4N7; Cal'84; CCFP; Staff, Peace Arch Hospital; (604)538-5770; Fax. (604)536-5824.

PARK, Hae-Ryun; Regional Mental HC-London, PO Box 5532 Stn B 850 Highbury Ave, London ON N6A 4H1; Hanyang (Korea)'86; FRCPC; Psy. Staff, Regional Mental Health Care-St Joseph's Health Care; (519)455-5110

PARK, Hazel S; Lions Gate Hosp, 231 15th St E, North Vancouver BC V7L 2L7; Tor'87; CCFP; CCFP(E.M.); FCFP; Staff Emerg Dept, Lions Gate Hospital; Clin Instructor, University of British Columbia; (604)984-5799; Fax. (604)648-8606.

PARK, Ian R A; Trent Hills Family Health Team, RR 2 119 Isabella St, Campbellford ON K0L 1L0; Tor'90; PhD; Ac Staff, Campbellford Memorial Hospital; Langs: English; French; (705)653-1801; Fax. (705)653-5483.

PARK, Ingrid; Wilderman Med Clinic, 8054 Yonge St, Thornhill ON L4J 1W3; McG'05; Staff, Wilderman Medical Clinic; (905)886-0248; Fax. (905)886-1212.

PARK, James N; Tsawwassen Med Clinic, 201-1077 56 St, Delta BC V4L 2A2; UBC'84; Ac Staff, Delta Hospital; Assoc Staff, Richmond Hospital; (604)943-1131; Fax. (604)943-2617.

PARK, Jane; 8-5425 Creditview Rd, Mississauga ON L5V 2P3; McM'04; CCFP; Ac Physician, The Credit Valley Hospital; (905)826-1164; Fax. (905)826-1214.

PARK, Jason; St Boniface Gen Hosp, 409 Tache Ave, Winnipeg MB R2H 2A6; Tor'00; FRCSC; GenSurg (Surgical Oncology). Staff, St Boniface General Hospital; (204)233-8563

PARK, John C S; Mountain Road Med Clinic, 202-44 Mapleton Rd, Moncton NB E1C 7W8; Ott'79; (506)857-3171; Fax. (506)857-1776.

PARK, Jack J B; Stevenson Mem Hosp, PO Box 4000 Stn Main 200 Fletcher Cres, Alliston ON L9R 1W7; Wes'99; MHSc; BSc; CCFP; Staff, Stevenson Memorial Hospital; (705)435-6281

PARK, Joonseong; Dundas Med Centre, 801 Dundas St E, Mississauga ON L4Y 4G9; Man'88; Langs: Korean; (905)566-1501; Fax. (905)566-1895.

PARK, Joseph; 301-200 James St S, Hamilton ON L8P 3A9; Tor'86; FRCPC; Anes (Chronic Pain Management). Ac Staff, Hamilton Health Sciences Centre - McMaster Children's Hospital; Assoc Prof, McMaster University; Langs: Korean; (905)525-8607; Fax. (905)525-8459.

PARK, K Young; Bristol Family Physicians, 102-2315 Bristol Cir, Oakville ON L6H 6P8; UBC'07; Staff, William Osler Health System - Etobicoke General Hospital; (905)287-2035; Fax. (905)287-2036.

PARK, Kiriy; 24-1515 Dufferin Cres, Nanaimo BC V9S 2B8; Alb'07; FRCPC; IntMed; Respir. (250)753-2446

PARK, Myung I; Peel Med Arts Bldg, 505-145 Queen St E, Brampton ON L6W 3P8; Kyungpook Nat. (Korea)'72; FRCSC; GenSurg. (905)451-0196; Fax. (905)451-0228.

PARK, Phillip S; 45-4307 130 Ave SE, Calgary AB T2Z 3V8; Alb'86; BSc; FRCSC; Otol (Neuro Otolaryngology). Med Staff, Alberta Children's Hospital; Clinical Asst Prof, University of Calgary; (403)457-0063; Fax. (403)282-0075.

PARK, Rachel C; Leamington & Area Fam Hlth Team, 197 Talbot St W, Leamington ON N8H 1N8; Ott'84; CCFP; FCFP; Staff Emerg, Leamington District Memorial Hospital; Assoc Prof, Schulich School of Medicine-University of Western Ontario; (519)322-1100; Fax. (519)322-2055.

PARK, Randy; The Credit Valley Hosp, 2200 Eglinton Ave W, Mississauga ON L5M 2N1; Qns'02; CCFP; CCFP(E.M.); Staff, The Credit Valley Hospital; (905)813-4141

PARK, Roy Y; Foothills Med Centre, 1403 29 St NW, Calgary AB T2N 2T9; Alb'99; FRCPC; DiagRad. Staff, Foothills Medical Centre; (403)944-1969

PARK, Thomas J H; Thunderbird Family Practice, D114-20159 88 Ave, Langley BC V1M 0A4; Tor'92; CCFP; Ac Staff, Langley Memorial Hospital; (604)888-6220

PARK, Thomas R; 808 East River Rd, New Glasgow NS B2H 3S3; Dal'78; (902)752-9595

PARK, Vincent; Summerville Family Health Team, 5F-101 Queensway W, Mississauga ON L5B 2P7; Tor'90; CCFP; Ac Staff, Trillium Health Centre - Mississauga; Langs: Korean; (905)272-9700; Fax. (905)272-1416.

PARK, James Y; Lakeridge Hlth Corp-Oshawa, 1 Hospital Crt, Oshawa ON L1G 2B9; Tor'85; FRCPC; PhysMed&Rehab. Staff, Lakeridge Health - Oshawa Site; (905)576-8711 x3734

PARKASH, Rajender; Queen Elizabeth II HSC, 410-1276 South Park St, Halifax NS B3H 2Y9; Punjab (India)'59; MB BS; DTMH; MRCP(UK); FRCPC; IntMed (Cardiology). Staff, Queen Elizabeth II Health Sciences Centre - Victoria General Site; Lecturer IntMed, Dalhousie University; (902)473-2156; Fax. (902)473-8430; raj.parkash@cdha.nshealth.ca.

PARKASH, Ratika; Queen Elizabeth II HSC-Halifax, 2501D-1796 Summer St, Halifax NS B3H 3A7; Dal'96; FRCPC; IntMed; Cardiol. Staff, Queen Elizabeth II Health Sciences Centre - Halifax Infirmary Site; (902)473-2700

PARKASH, Ravi; Dartmouth Gen Hosp, 325 Pleasant St, Dartmouth NS B2Y 4G8; Dal'98; CCFP; CCFP(E.M.); FCFP; Staff, Dartmouth General Hospital; (902)465-8300

PARKASH, Sandhya; IWK Health Centre, PO Box 9700 Rpo CSC 5850-5980 University Ave, Halifax NS B3K 6R8; Dal'02; FRCPC; Peds. Staff, IWK Health Centre; (902)470-8888

PARKER, Alice E; 115 Woolwich St, Guelph ON N1H 3V1; Qns'84; Staff, Guelph General Hospital; (519)823-8543

PARKER, Anne M; 200-1892 Broadway W, Vancouver BC V6J 1Y9; Alb'85; FRCPC; Psy. (604)638-1673

PARKER, Barbara E; Kingston Family Health Team, 202-275 Bagot St, Kingston ON K7L 3G4; Qns'76; CCFP; FCFP; Assoc Staff, Kingston General Hospital; Assoc Staff, Hotel-Dieu Hospital; (613)549-7477; Fax. (613)549-4920.

PARKER, Christopher M; Richardson House, 20 201-102 Stuart St, Kingston ON K7L 2V6; Qns'00; MSc; FRCPC; IntMed; Critical Care Medicine; Respir. Staff, Kingston General Hospital; Asst Prof Med, Queen's University; (613)548-2384; Fax. (613)549-1459.

PARKER, John D; Mount Sinai Hosp, 1609-600 University Ave, Toronto ON M5G 1X5; Qns'84; FRCPC; IntMed; Cardiol. Staff, Mount Sinai Hospital; (416)586-4800 x4794; Fax. (416)586-8413.

PARKER, Deborah J R; Community Mental Health, 109-7071 Bayers Rd, Halifax NS B3L 2C2; Cal'06; FRCPC; Psy. (902)454-1400

PARKER, Elaine; 2958 Greenfield Rd, Ayr ON N0B 1E0; Tor'03; CCFP; (519)632-1229; Fax. (519)632-1253.

PARKER, Fred A; Guildwood Village Shopping Ctr, 5-123 Guildwood Pky, Scarborough ON M1E 4V2; Tor'88; Ac Staff, Rouge Valley Health System - Centenary Health Centre Site; (416)269-5088; Fax. (416)261-3112.

PARKER, Gavin G; The Associate Clinic, PO Box 549, Pincher Creek AB T0K 1W0; Alb'04; CCFP; (403)627-3321; Fax. (403)627-2280.

PARKER, Jacqueline M; The Ottawa Hosp-Civic Campus, 1053 Carling Ave, Ottawa ON K1Y 4E9; Newcastle (England)'81; CCFP; CCFP(E.M.); Staff, The Ottawa Hospital - Civic Campus; (613)761-4928

PARKER, Jennifer A; Fort St John Med Clinic, 10011 96 St, Fort St. John BC V1J 3P3; UBC'08; CCFP; (250)785-6677; Fax. (250)787-0109.

PARKER, John A; Yonge-Eglinton Med Centre, LL06-2401 Yonge St, Toronto ON M4P 3H1; Tor'61; FRCSC; Ophth. (416)483-1282; Fax. (416)483-1453.

PARKER, Julie L; Lakeshore Vein & Aesthetics Cl, 3293 Lakeshore Rd, Kelowna BC V1W 3S9; Cal'99; CCFP; Staff, Kelowna General Hospital; (250)860-9919

PARKER, Kenneth R; Portage Clinic Inc, 140 9th St SE, Portage La Prairie MB R1N 3V5; Man'95; CCFP; Att Staff, Portage District General Hospital; (204)857-3445; kparker@shaw.ca.

PARKER, Kerry J M; Glenn Allan Med Centre, 308-42 Glenn Allan Dr, Bridgewater NS B4V 3N2; Cal'99; CCFP; (902)530-3690; Fax. (902)530-3695.

PARKER, Kristy A; Children's Hosp Eastern Ont, 401 Smyth Rd, Ottawa ON K1H 8L1; Ott'08; FRCPC; Peds. Staff, Children's Hospital of Eastern Ontario (CHEO); (613)737-7600

PARKER, Melissa J; McMaster University, HSC 3A-1280 Main St W, Hamilton ON L8S 4K1; Wes'02; FRCPC; Peds; Critical Care Medicine; PedEmergMed. Teach Staff, McMaster University; (905)521-2100; Fax. (905)570-8973.

PARKER, Nur; 922 9 Ave SE, Calgary AB T2G 0S4; (South Africa)'03; MB ChB; (403)269-5588; Fax. (403)269-5868.

PARKER, Richard C; Red Lake Family Health Team, PO Box 311 51G Highway 105, Red Lake ON P0V 2M0; Cambridge (England)'75; MRC; DRCOG; DA; (807)727-2617; Fax. (807)727-3022; rparker@redlakehospital.ca.

PARKER, Robert A; Kelowna Mental Health Centre, 1340 Ellis St, Kelowna BC V1Y 9N1; Sask'87; FRCPC; CommunMed. Med Officer of Hlth/Dir, Maple Ridge Health Unit; (250)868-7832

PARKER, Robert D; Willowgrove Med Group, 2-527 Nelson Rd, Saskatoon SK S7S 1P4; Sask'85; BSc(Hon); MSc; (306)653-1543; Fax. (306)653-0422.

PARKER, Robin L; Abbotsford Reg Hosp & Cancer C, 32900 Marshall Rd, Abbotsford BC V2S 0C2; UBC'97; FRCPC; AnatPath (Gynecological Pathology). Staff, Abbotsford Regional Hospital & Cancer Centre; (604)851-4700; robin.parker@spchc.hnet.bc.ca.

PARKER, Salim; Burnaby Gen Hosp, 3935 Kincaid St, Burnaby BC V5G 2X6; Cape Town (South Africa)'96; MB ChB; CCFP; Staff, Burnaby Hospital; (604)434-4211

PARKER, Stuart M; Alexander Prof Bldg, 112-849 Alexander Crt, Peterborough ON K9J 7H8; Tor'69; BSc; FRCSC; OrthSurg (Arthroplasty). Staff, Peterborough Regional Health Centre - Hospital Drive; (705)743-8941; Fax. (705)743-7673.

PARKER, Susan E; 303-4430 Bathurst St, North York ON M3H 3S3; Qns'80; Assoc Staff, North York General Hospital; (416)638-6223; Fax. (416)638-8834.

PARKER, Thomas G; St Michael's Hosp, BW 2 027-30 Bond St, Toronto ON M5B 1W8; Wes'83; FRCPC; IntMed; Cardiol. Chief Physician Dept of Med, St Michael's Hospital; Prof Med, University of Toronto; (416)864-5271

PARKER, Vivien M; St Joseph's Health Centre, 30 The Queensway, Toronto ON M6R 1B5; Qns'95; DABPN; FRCPC; Psy. Staff, St Joseph's Health Centre; (416)530-6175 x4106; Fax. (416)530-6105.

PARKER, William R; Hys Med Centre, 202-11010 101 St NW, Edmonton AB T5H 4B9; Man'85; FRCPC; DiagRad. (780)426-1121; Fax. (780)425-5979.

PARKHILL, Nancy L; Therapeutic Prod Directorate, A/1 0202D2-101 Tunney's Pastur, Ottawa ON K1A 1B9; Tor'99; BA(Hons); CCFP; (613)941-3171; Fax. (613)941-1365.

PARKIN, Doriana M; Market Lane Med Dental Office, 9-140 Woodbridge Ave, Vaughan ON L4L 2S7; McM'05; CCFP; (905)850-0753

PARKIN, Henry N; 32740 Marshall Rd, Abbotsford BC V2S 1J7; Stellenbosch (South Africa)'86; MB ChB; (604)870-8717; Fax. (604)870-8792.

PARKIN, John A; St Joseph's Health Care, PO Box 5777 Stn B 268 Grosvenor St, London ON N6A 4V2; Wes'76; FRCPC; Anes. Chief, St Joseph's Hospital - St Joseph's Health Care; Clin Assoc Prof, University of Western Ontario; (519)646-6100 x66185; Fax. (519)646-6116.

PARKIN, Patricia C; The Hosp For Sick Children, 10221-555 University Ave, Toronto ON M5G 1X8; McM'82; FRCPC; Peds. Ac Staff Peds, The Hospital For Sick Children; Prof, University of Toronto; (416)813-6933; Fax. (416)813-5663.

PARKINS, Michael D; University of Calgary, 3330 University Drive NW, Calgary AB T2N 4N1; Cal'03; BSc(Hon); MSc; FRCPC; IntMed (AIDS); InfectDis. Staff, Foothills Medical Centre; Teach Staff, University of Calgary; (403)210-7913; Fax. (403)270-2772.

PARKINS, Vicky M; Richmond Road Diag & Trmt Ctr, 1886-1820 Richmond Rd SW, Calgary AB T2T 5C7; Cal'03; FRCPC; IntMed; Endocrin&Metab. (403)220-3908

PARKINSON, Bronwyn L; Peter Lougheed Centre, 3500 26 Ave NE, Calgary AB T1Y 6J4; Man'00; FRCPC; Anes. Staff, Peter Lougheed Centre; (403)943-5554

PARKINSON, Kevin M; Northside Med Group, 205-1015 Austin Ave, Coquitlam BC V3K 3N9; UBC'90; BSc; FRCSC; Ophth (Cataract & Glaucoma). Ac Staff, Ridge Meadows Hospital & Health Care Centre; (604)937-3211; Fax. (604)937-3231.

PARKINSON, Lillian M; Rouge Valley-Ajax & Pickering, 580 Harwood Ave S, Ajax ON L1S 2J4; Wes'88; Staff, Rouge Valley Health System - Ajax & Pickering Health Centre Site; (905)683-2320

PARKS, Paul; Medicine Hat Reg Hosp, 666 5 St SW, Medicine Hat AB T1A 4H6; Qns'00; FRCPC; EmergMed. Staff, Medicine Hat Regional Hospital; (403)529-8000; paulparks@gmail.com.

PARLAN, Gelasio F; Hurontario-Dundas Med Centre, 300-3024 Hurontario St, Mississauga ON L5B 4M4; Manila (Philippines)'72; Court Staff, Trillium Health Centre - Mississauga; Langs: Tagalog; (905)896-3303; Fax. (905)896-7956; dr_parlan@yahoo.ca.

PARLEA, Ileana C; 944 King St W, Kitchener ON N2G 1G4; Cluj (Romania)'78; CCFP; Langs: Romanian; (519)745-7363; Fax. (519)745-9132.

PARLEA, Luciana; 453 Park St, Kitchener ON N2G 1N5; Ott'04; FRCPC; IntMed; Endocrin&Metab. (226)772-0001

PARLEE, Katherine E; St Joseph's Healthcare, 50 Charlton Ave E, Hamilton ON L8N 4A6; Mem'77; Anes. Ac Staff, St Joseph's Healthcare - Charlton Campus; (905)522-4941 x3853

PARLIAMENT, Matthew B; Cross Cancer Institute, 11560 University Ave NW, Edmonton AB T6G 1Z2; Ott'84; FRCPC; RadOncol. Dir RadOncol, Cross Cancer Institute; Prof Oncol, University of Alberta; (780)432-8749; Fax. (780)432-8380.

PARLOW, Carol M; 505-700 Dorval Dr, Oakville ON L6K 3V3; Tor'82; FRCPC; Psy. Med Dir, RCG; (905)844-3600; Fax. (905)844-7179; office@psychability.com.

PARLOW, Joel L; Kingston Gen Hosp, 76 Stuart St, Kingston ON K7L 2V7; Tor'82; MSc(Pharmacol.); FRCPC; Anes (Cardiovascular Anesthesia). Staff, Kingston General Hospital; Dept Head Anesthesiology & Perioperative Med, Queen's University; Langs: English; French; (613)548-7827; Fax. (613)548-1375; parlowj@post.queensu.ca.

PARMAR, Gurpreet; St Boniface Gen Hosp, Y3515-409 Tache Ave, Winnipeg MB R2H 2A6; Wes'02; FRCPC; IntMed; Cardiol. Staff, St Boniface General Hospital; (204)233-8563

PARMAR, Jasneet K; Glenrose Rehab Hosp, 1259-10230 111 Ave NW, Edmonton AB T5G 0B7; Sgnd (India)'82; MB BS; Staff, Covenant Health - Misericordia Community Hospital; Staff, Glenrose Rehabilitation Hospital; Langs: Hindi; Punjabi; (780)735-8800; Fax. (780)735-8846; jasnet.parmar@albertahealthservices.ca.

PARMAR, Malvinder S; Medical Office Bldg, E-640 Ross Ave E, Timmins ON P4N 8P2; Meerut (India)'78; MB; ABIM(IntMed.); MS(Surg.); FACP; FRCPC; IntMed (Cardiology); Nephrol. Med Dir Int Med/Staff, Timmins & District Hospital; Staff, Anson General Hospital; Assoc Prof, Northern Ontario School of Medicine-Lakehead University; Langs: Hindi; Punjabi; (705)268-8067; Fax. (705)268-8066; atbeat@ntl.sympatico.ca.

PARMAR, Naaz; Station 2, 2775 Laurel St, Vancouver BC V5Z 1M9; UBC'07; FRCPC; IntMed. (778)828-7922

PARMAR, Varinderjit S; Ontario Shores Ctr Mental HS, 700 Gordon St, Whitby ON L1N 5S9; Kasturba (India)'04; Staff, Ontario Shores Centre for Mental Health Sciences; (905)668-5881

PARMINDER, Ranjit K; 1039 Kings Rd, Sydney NS B1S 1C6; New Delhi (India)'55; LMCC; (902)562-6900; Fax. (902)562-7970.

PARNA, Laura M H; Couchiching Family Health Team, 103-119 Memorial Ave, Orillia ON L3V 5X1; McM'91; CCFP; Staff, Orillia Soldiers' Memorial Hospital; (705)326-3549; Fax. (705)326-9529.

PARNANDI, Vandana N; 206-815 College St, Toronto ON M6G 1C9; Tor'08; CCFP; (416)923-5500; Fax. (416)923-2249.

PARNELL, Robert H A; Four Counties Med Clinic, RR 3 1824 Concession Dr, Newbury ON N0L 1Z0; Wes'83; CCFP; FCFP; Staff, Four Counties Health Services - Middlesex Hospital Alliance; Staff, Strathroy Middlesex General Hospital - Middlesex Hospital Alliance; (519)693-0350

PARNELL, Tracey A; 2017 8th St N, Cranbrook BC V1C 3N5; McM'94; (250)426-5266; Fax. (250)426-7855.

PARNES, Lorne; London HSC-University Hosp, PO Box 5339 Stn B B1 333-339 Windermere Rd, London ON N6A 5A5; Tor'80; ABOtol; FRCSC; Otol (Neuro Otology)., London Health Sciences Centre - University Hospital; Prof, University of Western Ontario; (519)663-3604; Fax. (519)663-3916; parnes@uwo.ca.

PARNES, Maria; Oakmont Med Centre, 210-809 41st Ave W, Vancouver BC V5Z 2N6; London (England)'77; MB BS; Court Staff, BC Women's Hospital & Health Centre; (604)266-2345; Fax. (604)266-2346.

PARNIANI, Sara; Clinique Force Medic, 200-1021 rue Jean-Talon E, Montreal QC H2R 1V6; McG'04; (514)787-1818; Fax. (514)787-1898.

PARPAL, Helene; Hop Maisonneuve-Rosemont, 5415 boul de l'Assomption, Montreal QC H1T 2M4; Sher'06; FRCPC; Neur. Staff, Hopital Maisonneuve-Rosemont; (514)252-3400

PARR, Jennifer L; Thames Valley Family Hlth Team, RR 5 22262 Mill Rd, Mount Brydges ON N0L 1W0; Dal'00; CCFP; Asst Prof Dept of Family Med, University of Western Ontario; (519)264-2800; Fax. (519)264-2742; jenniferp@smhc.net.

PARR, Mary G; Peace Arch Hosp, 15521 Russell Ave, White Rock BC V4B 2R4; Alb'03; CCFP; Staff, Peace Arch Hospital; (604)535-4577

PARRA, Dimitri A A; The Hosp for Sick Children, 555 University Ave, Toronto ON M5G 1X8; (Chile)'02; Staff, The Hospital For Sick Children; (416)813-6060; Fax. (416)813-2139; dimitri.parra@sickkids.ca.

PARRATT, David W; Stratford Gen Hosp, 46 General Hospital Dr, Stratford ON N5A 2Y6; Tor'79; Staff, Stratford General Hospital - Huron Perth Healthcare Alliance; (519)271-8120

PARRATTE, Jean; Cite de la Sante de laval, D0193-1755 boul Rene-Laennec, Laval QC H7M 3L9; Paris (France)'80; FRCPC; Psy (Psycho Geriatrics)., Universite de Montreal; (450)975-5589; Fax. (450)975-5090.

PARRAVANO, Joseph G; Northumberland Hills Hosp, 1000 Depalma Dr, Cobourg ON K9A 5W6; Tor'82; FRCPC; DiagRad. Pres, Northumberland Hills Hospital; (905)372-6811

PARRAY, Baynazir; Glazier Med Centre, 11 Gibb St, Oshawa ON L1H 2J9; Kashmir (India)'98; MB BS; CCFP; Langs: Hindi; Urdu; Kashmiri; (905)579-1212; Fax. (905)725-3110.

PARRENT, Andrew; London HSC-University Hosp, PO Box 5339 Stn B B10-134-339 Windermere Rd, London ON N6A 5A5; Tor'83; FRCSC; Neursurg (Epilepsy Surgery). Staff, London Health Sciences Centre - University Hospital; Consultant, St Joseph's Hospital - St Joseph's Health Care; Consultant, London Health Sciences Centre - Victoria Campus; Asst Prof, University of Western Ontario; (519)663-3707; Fax. (519)663-3753; andrew.parrent@lhsc.on.ca.

PARRINGTON, Barry D; Associate Med Group, 4705 48 Ave, Red Deer AB T4N 3T1; McM'76; Physician, Associate Medical Group; (403)346-2057; Fax. (403)347-2989.

PARRIS, Clark J; Jane Medical Clinic, 101-2780 Jane St, North York ON M3N 2J2; McG'95; Court Staff, Humber River Regional Hospital - Finch Avenue Site; (416)745-8500; Fax. (416)748-8730.

PARRISH, Adam A; Pleasantview Med Clinic, 11028 51 Ave NW, Edmonton AB T6H 0L4; Alb'86; Ac Staff, Covenant Health - Grey Nuns Community Hospital; Ac Staff, Capital Care - Grandview; Ac Staff, The Good Samaritan Society; (780)434-5129; Fax. (780)434-9992; adam.parrish@capitalhealth.ca.

PARRISH, James D; Bayview Med Centre, 2722 Bayview Ave, North York ON M2L 1B9; Tor'78; MASc; BASc; CCFP; Ac Staff, North York General Hospital; (416)730-1212; Fax. (416)730-1216.

PARRISH, Michael B; Hamilton HS-General Site, 237 Barton St E, Hamilton ON L8L 2X2; McM'95; FRCPC; Anes. Staff, Hamilton Health Sciences Centre - Hamilton General Hospital; (905)527-0271

PARROT, Benoit; Clinique Med des Promenades, A222-3333 rue du Carrefour, Quebec QC G1C 5R9; Laval'84; CCFP; Dir, Hôpital Regional Rimouski; (418)663-6345

PARRY, Debra J; Wilfrid Laurier Univ, 75 University Ave W, Waterloo ON N2L 3C5; Tor'92; CCFP; FCFP; Assoc Staff, Guelph General Hospital; (519)884-0710; Fax. (519)885-4865.

PARRY, Matthew T; 201-240 Wharncliffe Rd N, London ON N6H 4P2; UBC'01; CCFP; (519)435-0111

PARRY, Neil G; London HSC-Victoria Hosp, PO Box 5010 Stn B E2 217-800 Commissioners Rd E, London ON N6A 5W9; Wes'96; BSc(Hon)(Hon); TraSurg; FACS; FRCS; FRCSC; GenSurg (Critical Care Medicine). Staff, London Health Sciences Centre - Victoria Campus; Asst Prof, University of Western Ontario; (519)667-6583; Fax. (519)667-6546; neil.parry@lhsc.on.ca.

PARRY, Park W; 1-519 King St, Chatham ON N7M 1G8; Wes'70; Med Dir, Victoria Residence; (519)354-7778; Fax. (519)354-7779.

PARSHURAM, Christopher S; The Hosp For Sick Children, 555 University Ave, Toronto ON M5G 1X8; Otago (New Zealand)'90; Staff Critical Care Med, The Hospital For Sick Children; (416)813-6860; christopher.parshuram@sickkids.ca.

PARSONS, Arthur H; Family Practice Associates, 200-6155 North St, Halifax NS B3K 5R3; Dal'69; Méd légiste Marine, Transport Canada; Physician, Atlantic Offshore Medical Associates; (902)453-3511; Fax. (902)454-9010.

PARSONS, David G; Dept of Anaes, 2449-910 10th Ave W, Vancouver BC V5Z 1M9; UBC'74; FRCPC; Anes. Ac Staff, Vancouver General Hospital - Centennial Pavillion; (604)875-4304

PARSONS, David L; Alberta Children's Hosp, 2888 Shaganappi Trail NW, Calgary AB T3B 6A8; Mem'85; BSc(Hons); BMedSci; FRCSC; OrthSurg (Pediatric Orthopedic Surgery). Staff Ortho, Alberta Children's Hospital; Clinical Asst Prof, University of Calgary; (403)955-7730; Fax. (403)943-7634.

PARSONS, Ean J; Health Sciences Centre, 300 Prince Philip Dr, St. John's NL A1B 3V6; Mem'81; BMedSci; Dip SportMed; CCFP; FCFP; Staff Miller Centre, Health Sciences Centre; Assoc Prof Family Med, Memorial University Of Newfoundland; (709)777-6743; Fax. (709)777-7913.

PARSONS, Edwin L; Stephenville Crossing Med Clin, PO Box 370, Stphenvl-Xing NL A0N 2C0; Mem'74; (709)646-2301

PARSONS, Elizabeth P; Carleton Univ Health Services, 1125 Colonel By Dr, Ottawa ON K1S 5B6; Ott'97; CCFP; FCFP; (613)520-6674; Fax. (613)520-4059.

PARSONS, G Wayne; The Jenny Trout Centre, 205-342 Erie St, Stratford ON N5A 2N4; Tor'72; Staff Family Med, Stratford General Hospital - Huron Perth Healthcare Alliance; (519)271-7111; Fax. (519)271-5494.

PARSONS, Howard G; Children's & Women's HC of BC, K218-4800 Oak St, Vancouver BC V6H 3V4; Dal'72; FRCPC; Peds (Inborn Errors of Metabolism). Staff, BC Children's Hospital; (604)875-2345 x5113

PARSONS, Hugh M; 200-555 Sixth St, New Westminster BC V3L 5H1; Dal'82; FRCSC; Ophth. (604)521-4144; Fax. (604)521-4129.

PARSONS, J W Gerard; Dawson Med Clinic, PO Box 829, Dawson YT Y0B 1G0; Mem'82; BSc; CCFP; (867)993-5744

PARSONS, Jillian N; Nova Medical, 204-496 Topsail Rd, St. John's NL A1E 2C2; Mem'02; CCFP; Langs: French; (709)745-6682

PARSONS, John E; Montfort Health, 5-1968 Portobello Blvd, Orleans ON K4A 4E7; Qns'69; Langs: Bilingual(English/French); (613)837-7033; Fax. (613)837-5781.

PARSONS, Laurie M; Richmond Road Diag & Trmt Ctr, 1820 Richmond Rd SW, Calgary AB T2T 5C7; Mem'85; FRCPC; Derm (Wound Care). Staff, Foothills Medical Centre; Clinical Asst Prof Derm, University of Calgary; (403)955-8601; Fax. (403)955-8200.

PARSONS, Michael H; Health Sciences Centre, 300 Prince Philip Dr, St. John's NL A1B 3V6; Mem'04; CCFP; CCFP(E.M.); Staff, Health Sciences Centre; (709)777-6300

PARSONS, Mitchel B; Garneau Prof Centre, 407-11044 51 Ave NW, Edmonton AB T6H 5B4; Alb'80; FRCPC; Psy. Staff, Royal Alexandra Hospital; Staff, Glenrose Rehabilitation Hospital; Asst Prof, University of Alberta; (780)438-6181; Fax. (780)437-3499.

PARSONS, Patricia M; North York Family Health Team, PO Box 91130 Rpo Bayview Village 2901 Bayview Ave, North York ON M2K 2Y6; McM'09; CCFP; (416)221-3861

PARSONS, Robert W J; Atlantic Offshore Med Services, PO Box 2442 Stn C 4 Henry St, St. John's NL A1C 6E7; Mem'01.

PARSONS, Simon J; Alberta Children's Hosp, 2888 Shaganappi Trail NW, Calgary AB T3B 6A8; Australia (Australia)'83; MB BS; BMedSci; FRCPC; Peds (Critical Care Medicine). Staff Critical Care, Alberta Children's Hospital; (403)955-7461; Fax. (403)955-7081.

PARSONS, Steven M; Central Nfld Reg Hlth Centre, 50 Union St, Grnd-Falls-Windsor NL A2A 2E1; Mem'00; FRCSC; ObstGyn. Staff, Central Newfoundland Regional Health Centre; (709)292-2500

PARSONS, Susan G; Lake of the Woods Dist Hosp, RR 1 Stn Main 21 Sylvan St, Kenora ON P9N 3W7; Mem'88; Locum Tenens, Lake of the Woods District Hospital; (807)468-9861 x435; Fax. (807)468-3638.

PARSONS, Thomas David; Bear Creek Med Clinic, 110-13588 88th Ave, Surrey BC V3W 3K8; Qns'71; CCFP; (604)503-4947; tdparsons@shaw.ca.

PARSONS, Trent E; 205-1386 Topsail Rd, Paradise NL A1L 1P6; Mem'02; CCFP; (709)782-1110

PARSONS, Wanda L; Health Sciences Centre, 300 Prince Philip Dr, St. John's NL A1B 3V6; Mem'82; CCFP; FCFP; Staff Family Practice Unit, Health Sciences Centre; Asst Dean Admissions(Acting)/Assoc Prof Family Med, Memorial University Of Newfoundland; (709)777-7795; Fax. (709)777-7913; wparsons@mun.ca.

PARSONS, William D; Family Med Associates, 5-3360 rue Notre-Dame, Lachine QC H8T 3E2; Dal'70; CCFP; CCFP(E.M.); (514)634-7179; Fax. (514)634-4150.

PARSONS-SHELDRAKE, Jeffrey; Campbellford Mem Hosp, PO Box 1027 146 Oliver Rd, Campbellford ON K0L 1L0; Ott'00; CCFP; Staff, Campbellford Memorial Hospital; (705)653-1140

PARTAP, Nadine A; Psychealth Centre, PZ1-771 Bannatyne Ave, Winnipeg MB R3E 3N4; Man'96; FRCPC; Psy.

PARTAP, Vince A; Mackenzie Richmond Hill Hosp, 10 Trench St, Richmond Hill ON L4C 4Z3; Ott'96; FRCPC; DiagRad. Staff DiagRad, Mackenzie Richmond Hill Hospital; (905)883-2004; Fax. (905)883-0772.

PARTHAB, Omkar; N S S B, GS 433-190 Elizabeth St, Toronto ON M5G 2C4; Natal (South Africa)'90; CCFP; CCFP(E.M.); FCFP; (416)340-3856

PARTHASARATHI, Usha D; St Joseph's Healthcare, 50 Charlton St E, Hamilton ON L8N 4A6; Mangalore (India)'01; FRCPC; Psy. Staff, St Joseph's Healthcare - Charlton Campus; (905)522-4941

PARTLOW, Eric S; Foul Bay Prof Centre, 206-1964 Fort St, Victoria BC V8R 6R3; UBC'90; FRCPC; IntMed; InfectDis. (250)370-7717; epartlow@islandnet.com.

PARTON, David E; Medical Bldg, 403-1990 Fort St, Victoria BC V8R 6V4; Ott'77; FRCPC; Neur (Botox Injection). Staff, Vancouver Island Health Authority; (250)370-4300; Fax. (250)370-4398.

PARTRICK, Michael E; Kelowna Gen Hosp, 2268 Pandosy St, Kelowna BC V1Y 1T2; UBC'90; FRCPC; DiagRad. Staff, Kelowna General Hospital; (250)868-4454

PARTRIDGE, Bretta J; Rockyview Gen Hosp, 7007 14 St SW, Calgary AB T2V 1P9; Sask'02; FRCPC; Anes. Staff, Rockyview General Hospital; (403)943-3410

PARTRIDGE, Colin H; Admirals Med Centre, 275 Island Hwy, Victoria BC V9B 1G4; Cal'87; CCFP.

PARTRIDGE, Gerald W; South Similkameen HC-Keremeos, 700 3rd St, Keremeos BC V0X 1N3; Alb'71; Staff Emerg Fam Med, South Similkameen Health Centre; Physician, Keremeos Diagnostic & Treatment Centre; (250)499-3000; Fax. (250)499-3001.

PARTRIDGE, Jonathan A; Halton HC Serv Corp-Oakville, 327 Reynolds St, Oakville ON L6J 3L7; Tor'04; CCFP; CCFP(E.M.); Staff, Halton Healthcare Services Corporation - Oakville Site; (905)338-4690

PARTRIDGE, Lindsay A F; Happy Valley Family Hlth Team, PO Box 1120 Stn Main 268 Maiden Lane, St Marys ON N4X 1B7; Ott'09; CCFP; (519)284-3450

PARTRIDGE, Michael A C; Oak Ridge Med Centre, 100-13291 Yonge St, Richmond Hill ON L4E 4L6; Man'86; CCFP; CCFP(E.M.); Staff, Royal Victoria Regional Health Centre; (905)773-7759; rajpart@rogers.com.

PARTYKA, Joseph W; Beausejour Dist Hosp, PO Box 1178 151 1st St S, Beausejour MB R0E 0C0; Man'08; CCFP; Staff, Beausejour District Hospital; (204)268-1076

PARUK, Sameer; Erindale Health Centre, 2-50 Kenderdine Rd, Saskatoon SK S7N 3A1; (306)394-6601; Fax. (306)394-6615.

PARULEKAR, Wendy R; Cancer Ctr of Southeastern Ont, 25 King St W, Kingston ON K7L 5P9; Ott'88; FRCPC; IntMed; MedOncol. Staff, Cancer Centre of Southeastern Ontario; (613)544-2631; Fax. (613)546-8201.

PARVANOV, Tzvetan V; Fort Macleod Med Clinic, PO Box 820 744 26 St, Fort Macleod AB T0L 0Z0; (Bulgaria)'91; CCFP; (403)553-3351; Fax. (403)553-4549.

PARVEEN, Kazi S; Hamilton Medical Walk-In, 2B-1632 Upper James St, Hamilton ON L9B 1K4; Osmani (India)'92.

PARVEEN, Nighat; Grand River Hosp-KW Hlth Ctre, PO Box 9056 Stn C 835 King St W, Kitchener ON N2G 1G3; Sind (Pakistan)'82; FRCPC; Psy. Staff, Grand River Hospital - Kitchener/Waterloo Health Centre; (519)742-3611

PARVEZ, Boriana; The Hosp For Sick Children, 555 University Ave, Toronto ON M5G 1X8; Sofia (Bulgaria)'86; FRCPC; Peds. Staff, The Hospital For Sick Children; (416)813-5245

PARVEZ, Naeem; Regina Qu'Appelle HR-Regina, 1440 14th Ave, Regina SK S4P 0W5; Karachi (Pakistan)'85; FAAP; Staff, Regina General Hospital; Langs: Hindi; Urdu; Punjabi; (306)766-0702; Fax. (306)766-4149.

PARWEZ, Naumana A; Allied Health Centre, 3737 Wascana Pky, Regina SK S4S 0A2; MB BS; (306)337-2640; Fax. (306)585-4417.

PASCALI, Dante U; Harmony Med Centre, 106-152 Cleopatra Dr, Nepean ON K2G 5X2; Qns'98; BSc; FRCSC; ObstGyn (Urogynecology). Staff ObstGyn, The Ottawa Hospital - Civic Campus; Langs: Italian; French; (613)761-9292; Fax. (613)722-1310.

PASCOE, Lyn; 3-177 Fourth St, Duncan BC V9L 5J8; Otago (New Zealand)'78; (250)746-6557; Fax. (250)746-6575.

PASCOE, Michael I; 9 Shields Ave, Toronto ON M5N 2K1; Tor'71; Staff, Humber River Regional Hospital - Church Street Site; (416)482-9719; pascoe.mi@forces.gc.ca.

PASCOT, Agnes; CSSS de la Matapedia, 135 av Gaetan-Archambault, Amqui QC G5J 2K5; Laval'04; CCFP; Staff, CSSS de la Matapedia; (418)629-2211; Fax. (418)629-4498; apascot@gmail.com.

PASCUAL, Joan S; 407-1015 Regent St, Fredericton NB E3B 6H5; De La Salle (Philippines)'92; Staff, Hôpital Régional Campbellton; Langs: Tagalog; (506)458-0324

PASCUAL, Pierre-Gilbert; Ctr Hosp de Verdun, 4000 boul Lasalle, Verdun QC H4G 2A3; Montpellier (France)'82; Staff, Centre Hospitalier de Verdun; (514)362-1000 x2141

PASENAU, Allison M; Mill Creek Family Medicine, 101-1912 Enterprise Way, Kelowna BC V1Y 9S9; Cal'96; CCFP; (250)868-0700; Fax. (250)868-3003.

PASENAU, Jeffrey E H; Mission View Medical, 205-616 K L O Rd, Kelowna BC V1Y 4X4; Cal'96; FRCSC; GenSurg; VascSurg. (250)762-7731

PASH, Joel S; Mayfair Place, 225-6707 Elbow Dr SW, Calgary AB T2V 0E4; (USA)'06; FRCPC; Anes. (403)668-0877; Fax. (403)640-4685.

PASH, Michael P; Foothills Med Centre, 1403 29 St NW, Calgary AB T2N 2T9; Man'75; FRCPC; Anes. Ac Staff, Foothills Medical Centre; Asst Prof, University of Calgary; (403)944-1430; Fax. (403)253-9169.

PASHA, Tahir; Western Mem Reg Hosp, PO Box 2005 Stn Main 1 Brookfield Ave, Corner Brook NL A2H 6J7; Punjab (Pakistan)'85; MB BS; Staff, Western Memorial Regional Hospital; (709)637-5000

PASHBY, Robert C; One Med Place, 215-20 Wynford Dr, North York ON M3C 1J4; Tor'71; FRCSC; Ophth. Staff, The Hospital For Sick Children; Staff, Mount Sinai Hospital; Asst Prof, University of Toronto; (416)441-1313; Fax. (416)441-6138.

PASHNIAK, Paul A; Riley Park Primary Care Centre, 171-1402 8 Ave NW, Calgary AB T2N 1B9; Cal'93; CCFP; (403)284-3272; Fax. (403)265-5503.

PASIAN, Sergio G; Hôpital Laval, 2725 ch Sainte-Foy, Quebec QC G1V 4G5; (Brazil)'01; Staff Med Imaging, Hôpital Laval; Langs: French; Portuguese; (418)656-8711 x5147

PASIEKA, Janice L; Foothills Med Centre, NT-1403 29 St NW, Calgary AB T2N 2T9; Wes'83; FRCSC; GenSurg. Staff Surg, Foothills Medical Centre; Clin Prof Surg, University of Calgary; (403)944-2491; Fax. (403)283-4130; janice.pasieka@calgaryhealthregion.ca.

PASION, Stella R; 306-77 Westmount Rd, Guelph ON N1H 5J1; McM'97; CCFP; FCFP; (519)827-1399; Fax. (519)827-1858.

PASIOROWSKI, Michal P; Dominion Med Centre, 2383 111 St NW, Edmonton AB T6J 5E5; (Poland)'08; (780)436-0020; Fax. (780)436-0603.

PASK, Barbara E; Saskatoon City Hosp, 701 Queen St, Saskatoon SK S7K 0M7; Sask'77; FRCPC; Anes. Staff Anes, Saskatoon City Hospital; Asst Prof, University of Saskatchewan; (306)655-8371; Fax. (306)655-8817.

PASKAR, Lee S; Hys Med Centre, 202-11010 101 St NW, Edmonton AB T5H 4B9; Alb'92; FRCPC; DiagRad. (780)426-1121; Fax. (780)425-5979.

PASKVALIN, Mario; Riverview Health Centre, 1 Morley Ave, Winnipeg MB R3L 2P4; Sarajevo (Bosnia-Herzegovina)'85; Staff, Riverview Health Centre; (204)452-3411

PASLAWSKI, Doreen E; Rockyview Gen Hosp, 7007 14 St SW, Calgary AB T2V 1P9; Sask'89; BSc; FRCPC; AnatPath. Staff Med Lab, Rockyview General Hospital; Clinical Asst Prof, University of Calgary; (403)943-8759; Fax. (403)943-3333.

PASQUALUCCI, Renato; Bluewater Health-Norman Site, 89 Norman St, Sarnia ON N7T 6S3; Witwatersrand (South Africa)'89; MB ChB; CCFP; CCFP(E.M.); Staff, Bluewater Health - Mitton Site; (519)464-4400

PASQUASY, Veronique; CHUQ-Ctr Hosp Univ Laval, R1742-2705 boul Laurier, Quebec QC G1V 4G2; Staff, Centre Hospitalier Universitaire de Quebec-CHUL; (418)654-2282

PASQUET, Eric A; Queensway-Carleton Hosp, 3045 Baseline Rd, Nepean ON K2H 8P4; Dal'73; FAAP(C); BSc; FRCPC; Peds (Neonatology). Staff, Queensway Carleton Hospital; (613)721-2000

PASQUIER, Jean-Charles; CHUS-Hop Fleurimont, 3001 12e av N, Sherbrooke QC J1H 5N4; Grenoble (France)'96; Staff, Centre Hospitalier Universitaire de Sherbrooke-Hopital Fleurimont; (819)346-1110

PASQUINI, Filoteo; Lakeshore Gen Hosp, 160 av Stillview, Pointe-Claire QC H9R 2Y2; Tor'95; CCFP; Staff, Lakeshore General Hospital - Pointe Claire; (514)630-2225; Fax. (514)630-5144.

PASRICHA, Deepti; Markham Family Health Team, 1-122 Cornell Park Ave, Markham ON L6B 1B6; Wes'93; CCFP; Associate, Markham Stouffville Hospital; Langs: Hindi; (905)471-9999 x221; Fax. (905)471-3627; dpasricha@msh.on.ca.

PASRICHA, Suvercha; Addiction & Mental Hlth-Clarke, 938-250 College St, Toronto ON M5T 1R8; Baroda (India)'90; MB BS; FRCPC; Psy. Staff, Centre for Addiction & Mental Health (CAMH) - College Street Site; Asst Prof Psy, McMaster University; Langs: Hindi; (416)535-8501 x4119

PASSAPERUMA, Kavitha; Mackenzie Richmond Hill Hosp, 10 Trench St, Richmond Hill ON L4C 4Z3; Wes'07; MedOncol; IntMed. Staff, Mackenzie Richmond Hill Hospital; (905)883-1212; Fax. (905)883-2156.

PASSERIN, Orlando; 239 Lansdowne St, Kamloops BC V2C 1X8; '09; CCFP; (778)471-6488

PASSERINI, Louise; Hop Charles LeMoyne, 3120 boul Taschereau, Greenfield Park QC J4V 2H1; Mon'79; FRCP; FRCPC; IntMed; Critical Care Medicine (P.Q.); Respir. Ac Staff, Hopital Charles LeMoyne; ac Staff, Centre Hospitalier l'Université de Montréal (CHUM) - Hôtel-Dieu; Universite de Sherbrooke; Universite de Montreal; Langs: Bilingual(French/English); (450)466-5000 x2297; Fax. (450)466-5768; alain.poirpass@videotron.ca.

PASSEY, Greg; Medical Bldg, 1702-805 Broadway W, Vancouver BC V5Z 1K1; UBC'80; BSc(Kinesiol); FRCPC; Psy (Stress). (604)290-8482; Fax. (604)875-9056; gpassey@telus.net.

PASSI, William B; Vancouver Gen Hosp, 855 12th Ave W, Vancouver BC V5Z 1M9; Qns'04; FRCPC; EmergMed. Staff, Vancouver General Hospital - Centennial Pavillion; (604)875-4100

PASSMORE, Michael J; Mount St Joseph Hosp, 3080 Prince Edward St, Vancouver BC V5T 3N4; UBC'98; FRCPC; Psy. Staff, Providence Health Care - Mount Saint Joseph Hospital; (604)874-1141 x78230

PASTERKAMP, Hans; Children's Hosp, CS516-840 Sherbrook St, Winnipeg MB R3A 1S1; Lubeck (Germany)'76; LMCC; DrMedCh; FRCPC; Peds (Pediatric Respirology). Staff, Health Sciences Centre; Prof, University of Manitoba; Langs: German; (204)787-4753; Fax. (204)787-1944.

PASTERNAC, Andre; Westmount Square Hlth Group, 550-1 car Westmount, Westmount QC H3Z 2P9; Toulouse (France)'68; Cardiol (P.Q.). Staff Cardiol, Institut de Cardiologie de Montréal; Staff Cardiologist, Westmount Square Mental Centre; Clin Prof, Universite de Montreal; Langs: Spanish; Italian; English; (514)934-2334 x297; Fax. (514)931-2929.

PASTERNAK, Harvey S; 1302 Queen St E, Toronto ON M4L 1C4; Tor'73; Staff, Mount Sinai Hospital; (416)466-8640; Fax. (905)853-4406.

PASTERNAK, John L; 102-3215 Dunmore Rd SE, Medicine Hat AB T1B 2H2; Alb'79; Physician, Wittke Waste Equipment; (403)504-0450

PASTERNAK, Stephen H; St Joseph's Health Care, PO Box 5777 Stn B 268 Grosvenor St, London ON N6A 4V2; McG'95; FRCPC; Neur (Dementia). Staff Cognitive Neurology and Alzheimer Research Centre, St Joseph's Hospital - St Joseph's Health Care; Staff, London Health Sciences Centre - University Hospital; Assoc Scientist, The Robarts Research Institute; Asst Prof Clin Neurol Sciences, University of Western Ontario; (519)646-6032; Fax. (519)646-6226; spasternak@robarts.ca.

PASTERNAK, Sylvia; Pathology Laboratory, 5788 University Ave, Halifax NS B3H 1V8; Sao Paulo (Brazil)'91; FRCPC; AnatPath. (902)473-1459; Fax. (902)473-1049.

PASTIA, Cristina I; Toronto East Gen Hosp Inc, 825 Coxwell Ave, Toronto ON M4C 3E7; McG'07; MDCM; CCFP; CCFP(E.M.); Staff, Toronto East General Hospital Inc; (416)469-6435

PASTIEROVIC, Danielle E; Lansdowne Prof Bldg, 390-1641 Hillside Ave, Victoria BC V8T 5G1; McM'78; Assoc Staff, Royal Jubilee Hospital; Assoc Staff, Victoria General Hospital; Langs: French; Spanish; Czech; (250)598-6266

PASTOLERO, Gemma C; William Osler HC-Etobicoke, 101 Humber College Blvd, Etobicoke ON M9V 1R8; (Philippines)'79; FRCPC; AnatPath. Staff, William Osler Health System - Etobicoke General Hospital; (416)747-3400

PASTORE, Yves D; Hopital Ste-Justine, 3175 ch Cote-Sainte-Catherine, Montreal QC H3T 1C5; Geneva (Switzerland)'92; PedHemaOncol (P.Q.). Staff, Hôpital Ste-Justine; (514)345-4931 x5027; Fax. (514)345-4884.

PASTRE, Robert J; 1280 Lasalle Blvd, Sudbury ON P3A 1Y8; NOSM'09; CCFP; (705)222-1364

PASTUSZEWSKA, Natalia M; 30 William St, Brantford ON N3T 3K4; Warsaw (Poland)'89; ABIM; FRCPC; IntMed (Cardiac Surgery). Langs: Polish; French; (519)750-1450; Fax. (519)750-1308.

PASULA, Brian J; 107-2349 Millstream Rd, Victoria BC V9B 3R5; Alb'88; (250)391-7554

PASUT, George; Ontario Agency Hlth Protection, 300-480 University Ave, Toronto ON M5G 1V2; Tor'84; MHSc; FACPrevMed; FRCPC; CommunMed. A-Chief Med Officer of Hlth Public Health Div, Ontario Ministry of Health; Physician, Ontario Agency for Health; (416)260-7105; Fax. (416)260-7600; george.pasut@moh.gov.on.ca.

PASZAT, Lawrence F; Toronto Sunnybrook Reg Cancer, 2075 Bayview Ave, Toronto ON M4N 3M5; McM'80; AB(TherRad); FRCPC; RadOncol. Staff, Sunnybrook Health Sciences Centre; Teach Staff, University of Toronto; (416)480-5000; Fax. (416)480-6002.

PASZKIEWICZ, Mariusz T; Weyburn Med Clinic, 110 3rd St, Weyburn SK S4H 0W2; Lublin (Poland)'83; MB ChB; Langs: Polish; Russian; Ukrainian; (306)842-5404

PATAKI, Janos J; The Credit Valley Hosp, 2200 Eglinton Ave W, Mississauga ON L5M 2N1; Tor'93; FRCPC; IntMed. Staff Critical Care & IntMed/Dir, The Credit Valley Hospital; Langs: Hungarian; (905)813-4466; Fax. (905)813-4186; jpataki@cvh.on.ca.

PATASI, Beata; Smiths Falls Comm Hlth Ctr, 2 Gould St, Smiths Falls ON K7A 2S5; Univerzita Komenskeho (Slovakia)'91; CCFP; (613)283-1952

PATCAI, John T; St John's Rehab Hosp, 285 Cummer Ave, North York ON M2M 2G1; Tor'81; FRCPC; PhysMed&Rehab. Staff, St John's Rehabilitation Hospital; Staff, Princess Margaret Hospital - University Health Network; Staff, Toronto Rehabilitation Institute - University Centre; Lecturer, University of Toronto; (416)226-6780 x7240; Fax. (416)712-3622.

PATCH, J Randall; 444 Monarch Place, Kamloops BC V2E 2B2; UBC'77; BSc; DMD(Dental); CCFP; Ac Staff, Royal Inland Hospital; Clin Associate, University of British Columbia; (250)372-5425; Fax. (250)372-7779; docjr@kamloops.net.

PATE, Graham C; 102-65 Richmond St, New Westminster BC V3L 5P5; UBC'82; FRCSC; OrthSurg. (604)526-9138; Fax. (604)591-1050.

PATEK, Susan; Manitoba College of Fam Phys, 240-1695 Henderson Hwy, Winnipeg MB R2G 1P1; (204)668-3667; Fax. (204)668-3663.

PATEL, Aditi J; Medicine Hat Reg Hosp, 666 5 St SW, Medicine Hat AB T1A 4H6; (India)'93; FRCPC; Psy. Staff, Medicine Hat Regional Hospital; (403)529-8024; Fax. (403)529-8998.

PATEL, Alex; Hamilton HS-McMaster Site, PO Box 2000 Stn Lcd 1 MDCL3113-1200 Main St W, Hamilton ON L8N 3Z5; Tor'05; Critical Care Medicine; IntMed. Fellow, Hamilton Health Sciences Centre - McMaster University Medical Centre; (905)521-2100

PATEL, Anish; Compass Med Centre, 450-200 Wellington St W, Toronto ON M5V 3C7; Wes'09; CCFP; (416)593-5000; Fax. (416)593-5004.

PATEL, Bhasker M; Community Med Clinic, 5108 50 Ave, Wetaskiwin AB T9A 0S6; Makerere (Uganda)'68; MB BS; CCFP; Staff, Wetaskiwin Hospital & Care Centre; Langs: Gujarati; Hindi; (780)352-2511; Fax. (780)352-7599.

PATEL, Bhavin B; Hamilton HS-McMaster Site, PO Box 2000 Stn Lcd 1 1200 Main St W, Hamilton ON L8N 3Z5; Sydney (Australia)'01; CCFP; Staff, Hamilton Health Sciences Centre - McMaster Children's Hospital; (905)521-2100; bhavinpatel@hotmail.com.

PATEL, Bijal; Radiology Consultants Assoc, 120-6707 Elbow Dr SW, Calgary AB T2V 0E3; Alb'03; DiagRad. (403)777-3003; Fax. (403)777-3008.

PATEL, Daksha N; Strandherd Crossing Med Centre, 305-3161 Strandherd Dr, Nepean ON K2J 5N1; Gujarat (India)'79; CCFP; (613)823-7766; Fax. (613)823-0063.

PATEL, Deepen M; 100-1 Eva Rd, Etobicoke ON M9C 4Z5; Dal'89; CCFP; Staff, The Credit Valley Hospital; (647)722-2370

PATEL, Dharmendra; On Trac Clinic, 288 St. Paul St, St Catharines ON L2R 3M9; Man'90; Assoc Staff, Niagara Health System - Ontario Street Site; Assoc Staff, Niagara Health System - St Catharines General Site; (905)684-9339; Fax. (905)684-2098.

PATEL, Dinu G; Albert Park Family Med Centre, 3992 Albert St, Regina SK S4S 3R1; London (England)'57; MB BS; DObstRCOG; DGO; MRCOG; (306)584-3833; Fax. (306)585-3833.

PATEL, Dipak; Royal Alexandra Hosp, 10240 Kingsway NW, Edmonton AB T5H 3V9; Alb'88; CCFP; Staff, Royal Alexandra Hospital; (780)735-4111

PATEL, Divyesh M; 453 Park St, Kitchener ON N2G 1N5; Witwatersrand (South Africa)'98; (519)578-2680; Fax. (519)578-3967.

PATEL, Falguni; Appletree Med Center, 10-680 Rexdale Blvd, Etobicoke ON M9W 0B5; Tor'05; PhD; CCFP; (416)213-9577; Fax. (416)213-9588.

PATEL, Harilal B; 4309C boul Saint-Jean, Dollard-D-Ormeaux QC H9H 2A4; Witwatersrand (South Africa)'65; MRCP(Lond); Ac Staff, Lakeshore General Hospital - Pointe Claire; VP, Medical & Dental Council; (514)696-0707; Fax. (514)696-4958.

PATEL, Harshadrai M; CML Healthcare Diag Imag Ctr, H-17215 Leslie St, Newmarket ON L3Y 8E4; Birmingham (England)'61; MB ChB; LRCP; MRCS; DMRD; FRCPC; IntMed; DiagRad. (905)836-2626

PATEL, Harshna; Scarborough Hosp-Birchmount, 3030 Birchmount Rd, Scarborough ON M1W 3W3; Ott'06; Gastroent; IntMed. Staff, The Scarborough Hospital - Birchmount Campus; (416)495-2400

PATEL, Hasmukh G; Hotel-Dieu Grace Hosp, 1030 Ouellette Ave, Windsor ON N9A 1E1; Bombay (India)'74; MB; BSc; DAB; FAB; FRCPC; Anes (Pain Management). Staff, Hôtel-Dieu Grace Hospital; Langs: Gujarati; Hindi; Swahili; (519)973-4421

PATEL, Hasmukh J; 105-20 Sunpark Plaza SE, Calgary AB T2X 3T2; Aberdeen (Scotland)'82; DRCOG.

PATEL, Hema; MUHC-Montreal Children's Hosp, 2300 rue Tupper, Montreal QC H3H 1P3; Wes'90; FRCPC; Peds. Staff, McGill University Health Centre - Montreal Children's Hospital; (514)412-4400; Fax. (514)412-4424; hema.patel@muhc.mcgill.ca.

PATEL, Ila M; Parkway Medical, 39-325 Central Pky W, Mississauga ON L5B 3X9; Delhi (India)'74; CCFP; Court Staff Privil, Trillium Health Centre - Mississauga; Langs: Hindi; Punjabi; Gujarati; Swahili; (905)276-7077; Fax. (905)276-9589.

PATEL, Indravadan M; Glencairn Med Clinic, 1834 E Victoria Ave, Regina SK S4N 7K3; Liverpool (England)'76; MB ChB; (306)761-1466; Fax. (306)761-1467.

PATEL, J Susan; Thames Valley FHT-Whitehills M, 1225 Wonderland Rd N, London ON N6G 2V9; Wes'78; CCFP; FCFP; (519)472-0040; Fax. (519)472-7732.

PATEL, Jay; Foothills Med Centre, 1403 29 St NW, Calgary AB T2N 2T9; (USA)'06; Staff, Foothills Medical Centre; (403)944-1110; Fax. (403)944-8640.

PATEL, Jayanti B; York Lanes Health Centre, 28-4700 Keele St, North York ON M3J 1P3; Gujarat (India)'68; MB BS; Psy. (416)736-5525; Fax. (416)736-5523.

PATEL, Jayesh; Halton Healthcare Services, 412-700 Dorval Dr, Oakville ON L6K 3V3; Wes'06; FRCPC; IntMed; Gastroent. Staff, London Health Sciences Centre - University Hospital; (905)815-0755; Fax. (905)815-0756.

PATEL, Jayshree; Northgate Med Clinic, 3A-1353 McPhillips St, Winnipeg MB R2X 3A6; Banaras (India)'70; LRCP(Ed); MRCS(Ed); LRCPS(Glas); Staff, The Salvation Army Grace Hospital; (204)338-3155

PATEL, Kalavati B; Community Med Clinic, 5108 50 Ave, Wetaskiwin AB T9A 0S6; Bangalore (India)'71; MB BS; Staff, Wetaskiwin Hospital & Care Centre; Langs: Gujarati; Hindi; (780)352-2511; Fax. (780)352-7599.

PATEL, Kaleena; Surrey Mem Hosp, 13750 96 Ave, Surrey BC V3V 1Z2; Man'08; CCFP; CCFP(E.M.); Staff, Surrey Memorial Hospital; (604)588-3381

PATEL, Kalpana R; 2625 Dewdney Ave, Regina SK S4T 0X4; (India)'75; MB BS; Staff, Regina General Hospital; Staff, Pasqua Hospital; Physician, Park Plaza Medical Centre; (306)352-3454; Fax. (306)789-7924.

PATEL, Ketan N; 5-1385 North Routledge Park, London ON N6H 5N5; Tor'99; BSc; Staff, Hôtel-Dieu Grace Hospital; Staff, Stratford General Hospital - Huron Perth Healthcare Alliance; Staff, St Thomas Elgin General Hospital; Staff, Integrated Circle of Care Inc; Aj Prof, Schulich School of Medicine-University of Western Ontario; Langs: Gujarati; Bilingual(French/English); (519)472-8282; Fax. (519)472-8281.

PATEL, Kirit B; First Medical Place, 207-170 Queensway W, Mississauga ON L5B 3A8; Nairobi (Kenya)'77; FAAP; FRCPC; Peds. Consultant, Trillium Health Centre - Mississauga; Staff Peds, QHC Belleville General; (905)272-9993

PATEL, Kirit K; Patel Med Centre, 10 Elizabeth Ave, St. John's NL A1A 5L4; Dublin (Ireland)'72; LRCPS; LM; Ac Staff, Health Sciences Centre; Clin Asst Prof Family Pract, Memorial University Of Newfoundland; Langs: Gujarati; Swahili; (709)738-6060; Fax. (709)738-6060.

PATEL, Kirit M; Rouge Valley-Ajax & Pickering, 580 Harwood Ave S, Ajax ON L1S 2J4; Man'87; FRCPC; Anes. Staff, Rouge Valley Health System - Ajax & Pickering Health Centre Site; (905)428-5228; Fax. (905)428-5220.

PATEL, Leena R; Children's Hosp, 840 Sherbrook St, Winnipeg MB R3A 1S1; Bombay (India)'66; MB BS; FRCPC; Anes. Staff, Health Sciences Centre; (204)787-2595; Fax. (204)787-7391.

PATEL, M Ameen; Medicine JHCC, A3 69-1280 Main St W, Hamilton ON L8S 4K1; RCS (Ireland)'85; FRCPC; IntMed. Staff, Hamilton Health Sciences Centre - McMaster Children's Hospital; Staff, Hamilton Health Sciences Centre-Juravinski Site; Asst Prof, McMaster University; (905)521-2100

PATEL, Maltibehn P; The Juravinski Cancer Centre, 3-699 Concession St, Hamilton ON L8V 5C2; Natal (South Africa)'82; FRCPC; RadOncol (Obstetrics & Gynecology). Staff, Hamilton Health Sciences Centre-Juravinski Site; Assoc Prof, McMaster University; (905)387-9495 x64706; Fax. (905)575-6326.

PATEL, Meeta; North York Gen Hosp, 4001 Leslie St, North York ON M2K 1E1; McM'06; CCFP; CCFP(E.M.); Staff, North York General Hospital; (416)756-6165; Fax. (416)756-6735.

PATEL, Meeta; Burnside Family Med Clinic, 101 Burnside Rd W, Victoria BC V9A 1B7; Nottingham (England)'98; (250)381-4353

PATEL, Milan V; First Med Place, 105-170 Queensway W, Mississauga ON L5B 3A8; Wes'98; BSc; FRCPC; IntMed; Respir. Acad Staff, Trillium Health Centre - West Toronto; (905)848-6079

PATEL, Millan S; BC Women's Hosp & Health Ctre, C234-4500 Oak St, Vancouver BC V6H 3N1; Alb'94; FRCPC; MedGenetics., BC Women's Hospital & Health Centre; (604)875-2345 x6847; Fax. (604)875-2825; millan@interchange.ubc.ca.

PATEL, Mitesh; Addiction & Mental Hlth-Queen, 1001 Queen St W, Toronto ON M6J 1H4; Alb'07; Psy. Staff, Centre for Addiction & Mental Health (CAMH) - Queen Site; (416)535-8501

PATEL, Mohan C; Guelph Gen Hosp, 115 Delhi St, Guelph ON N1E 4J4; Mysore (India)'76; FRCPC; DiagRad. Staff, Guelph General Hospital; (519)822-5350 x2307

PATEL, Naresh R; Tilbury District Family Hlth Team, PO Box 760 22 Mill St W, Tilbury ON N0P 2L0; (India)'76; MB BS; DOHS; CCFP; Langs: Gujarati; Hindi; Swahili; (519)682-2307; Fax. (519)682-9979; nairobisimba@hotmail.com.

PATEL, Navin M; Louisbourg Med Clinic, 8-7527 Main St, Louisbourg NS B1C 1J3; Gwalior (India)'63; MB BS; (902)733-3111; Fax. (902)733-2740.

PATEL, Neesha; Prairie Trail Med Centre, 100-1345 Taylor Ave, Winnipeg MB R3M 3Y9; (South Africa)'06; CCFP; Staff, Foothills Medical Centre.

PATEL, Neeta; 405-1100 Sheppard Ave E, North York ON M2K 2W1; (Ireland)'91; FRCPC; Peds. (416)221-7865; Fax. (416)221-0637.

PATEL, Nirav; William Osler HC-Etobicoke, 101 Humber College Blvd, Etobicoke ON M9V 1R8; New York (USA)'04; FRCPC; DiagRad. Staff, William Osler Health System - Etobicoke General Hospital; (416)494-2120

PATEL, Parinkumar S; The Medical Group, 40-32243 Hurd St, Mission BC V2V 3J9; London (England)'95; MB BS; CCFP; (604)826-6231

PATEL, Paulum U; Highbury Med Clinic, 1345 Huron St, London ON N5V 2E3; Wes'95; FRCPC; IntMed. (519)659-2331; Fax. (519)659-4617.

PATEL, Piyush R; Credit Valley Med Arts Centre, 102-2000 Credit Valley Rd, Mississauga ON L5M 4N4; London (England)'82; MB BS; FAAP; FRCPC; Peds (Asthma); ClinImmunol&Allergy. (905)569-8100

PATEL, Praful C; Northgate Med Clinic, 3A-1353 McPhillips St, Winnipeg MB R2X 3A6; Makerere (Uganda)'70; MRCS(Eng); FRCS(Ed); CCFP; CCFP(E.M.); FCFP; Staff, Seven Oaks General Hospital; (204)338-3155; Fax. (204)338-3155.

PATEL, Prakash B R; 125-6700 ch de la Cote-des-Nei, Montreal QC H3S 2B2; Lusaka (Zambia)'77; BSc(BioChem.); (514)342-2941; Fax. (514)342-3976.

PATEL, Prakash C; Gold Square, 3970 Albert St, Regina SK S4S 3R1; Manchester (England)'83; MB ChB; DABIM; FRCPC; IntMed (Pulmonary Medicine). Assoc Prof Med, University of Saskatchewan; Langs: Gujarati; (306)522-9090; Fax. (306)522-9091.

PATEL, Pravin C; Victoria Gen Hosp, 2340 Pembina Hwy, Winnipeg MB R3T 2E8; Welsh National (Wales)'74; MB ChB; FRC(Eng); FRCPC; Anes. Ac Staff Anes, Victoria General Hospital; (204)269-3570

PATEL, Rajesh; Radiology Associates Of Regina, 6-2727 Parliament Ave, Regina SK S4S 6X5; Sask'01; FRCPC; DiagRad. Staff, Radiology Associates of Regina; (306)352-7653

PATEL, Rajnikant L; 2625 Dewdney Ave, Regina SK S4T 0X4; Mysore (India)'74; MB BS; LRCP(Lond); MRCS(Eng); Staff, Regina General Hospital; Staff, Pasqua Hospital; Med Advisor, Parkside Extendicare; Med Dir, Detox Centre; Physician, Park Plaza Med. Centre; Langs: Gujarati; (306)352-3454; Fax. (306)789-7924.

PATEL, Rakesh V; The Ottawa Hosp-Gen Campus, 1562-501 Smyth Rd, Ottawa ON K1H 8L6; McM'98; Critical Care Medicine; IntMed. Staff, The Ottawa Hospital - Civic Campus; Staff, The Ottawa Hospital - General Campus; (613)737-8701

PATEL, Ramanbhai C; 310 Sunset Dr PO Box 179, Gimli MB R0C 1B0; Gujarat (India)'61; MB BS; LRCP(Lond); MRCS(Eng); FRCOG(Lond); Ac Staff/Chief Staff, Gimli Community Health Centre (Johnson Memorial Hospital); (204)642-5540; Fax. (204)642-5540.

PATEL, Ramesh; Medical Centre, 106-2100 Ellesmere Rd, Scarborough ON M1H 3B7; Bombay (India)'70; Court Staff, St Joseph's Health Centre; (416)690-3533

PATEL, Rupa; Kingston Community Hlth Ctr, 400 Elliot Ave, Kingston ON K7K 6M9; Ott'93; CCFP; FCFP; Staff, Kingston General Hospital; Physician, Kingston Community Health Centres; Langs: Gujarati; (613)542-2949; Fax. (613)542-7657.

PATEL, Samir I; Cross Cancer Institute, 11560 University Ave NW, Edmonton AB T6G 1Z2; Alb'01; FRCPC; RadOncol. Staff, Cross Cancer Institute; (780)432-8518

PATEL, Samir; Guelph Gen Hosp, 115 Delhi St, Guelph ON N1E 4J4; Alb'98; FRCPC; DiagRad. Staff, Guelph General Hospital; (519)822-5350

PATEL, Santhya; Joseph Brant Mem Hosp, 1230 North Shore Blvd E, Burlington ON L7S 1W7; Mysore (India)'82; FRCPC; Anes. Staff, Joseph Brant Memorial Hospital; (905)336-4135

PATEL, Satyam R; 1771 Rose St, Regina SK S4P 1Z4; Sask'02; FRCSC; OrthSurg. Staff, Royal University Hospital; (306)522-7010; Fax. (306)522-7020.

PATEL, Sayera; 2479 McCallum Rd, Abbotsford BC V2S 3P8; Witwatersrand (South Africa)'03; (604)852-2279

PATEL, Serina V; Children's Hosp Eastern Ont, 2631-401 Smyth Rd, Ottawa ON K1H 8L1; Mem'05; FRCPC; Peds. (613)737-7600

PATEL, Shamir; Radiology Consultants Assoc, 120-6707 Elbow Dr SW, Calgary AB T2V 0E3; Sask'05; FRCPC; DiagRad. Fax. (403)777-3008.

PATEL, Shantilal M; Horizon Square Med Centre, 401-3508 32 Ave NE, Calgary AB T1Y 6J2; (India)'78; MB BS; CCFP; (403)291-5588

PATEL, Shashikant C; PO Box 5369 Stn Main, Westlock AB T7P 2P5; Birmingham (England)'63; MB ChB; FRCS(Eng & Ed); Staff, Westlock Healthcare Centre; (780)349-3578; Fax. (780)349-6686.

PATEL, Shobhana J; South Walkerville Med Centre, 165-2224 Walker Rd, Windsor ON N8W 5L7; Wes'94; FRCSC; ObstGyn. Staff, Windsor Regional Hospital - Metropolitan Site; (519)251-8629; Fax. (519)251-8631.

PATEL, Subhash C; 328 Second St W, Cornwall ON K6J 1G9; Makerere (Uganda)'73; MB ChB; CCFP; FCFP; Ac Staff, Cornwall Community Hospital; Med Dir, Glen Stor Dun Lodge; Med Dir, St Joseph's Villa; (613)938-1966; Fax. (613)938-5059; subhashpatel@mac.com.

PATEL, Subhash K; Niagara H System-G Niagara, PO Box 1018 Stn Main 5546 Portage Rd, Niagara Falls ON L2E 6X2; Bombay (India)'66; MB BS; MCPS; DABPath; FRCPC; GenPath. Ac Staff, Niagara Health System - Greater Niagara General Site; (905)378-4647 x53368; Fax. (905)358-4909; spatel@niagarahealth.on.ca.

PATEL, Sujay; Grand River Hosp Freeport, PO Box 9056 3750 King St E, Kitchener ON N2A 2W1; Dublin (Ireland)'03; FRCPC; Psy., Homewood Health Centre; Staff, Grand River Hospital - Freeport Site; (519)749-4300; Fax. (519)894-8308.

PATEL, Sunil P; Concordia Health Associates, 102-1155 Concordia Ave, Winnipeg MB R2K 2M9; Man'02; Cardiol; IntMed. Staff, Concordia General Hospital.

PATEL, Sunil T; Queen Elizabethh II HSC, 916-1276 South Park St, Halifax NS B3H 2Y9; Wes'93; FRCPC; IntMed; Gastroent. Staff, Queen Elizabeth II Health Sciences Centre - Victoria General Site; (902)473-3721; Fax. (902)473-4406.

PATEL, Sunilkumar V; Family Practice Associates, PO Box 1110, Gimli MB R0C 1B0; Sheffield (England)'72; MB ChB; LMCC; Med Dir, Seagram' Canada; Med Dir, Gimli Ford Ltd; Med Examiner D.O.T., Aviation & Marine; Dir, Manitoba Cancer Outreach Centre; (204)642-5152; Fax. (204)642-9164; patelsv@mts.net.

PATEL, Surekha G; 4210 Hastings St, Burnaby BC V5C 2J6; Aberdeen (Scotland)'78; (604)568-0762; Fax. (604)568-8736.

PATEL, Surendra K; 11664 223 St, Maple Ridge BC V2X 5X5; Newcastle-upon-Tyne (England)'72; MB ChB; FRCSC; OrthSurg (Hand Surgery). Consultant OrthSurg, Ridge Meadows Hospital & Health Care Centre; Staff, Mission Memorial Hospital; (604)467-0257; Fax. (604)467-0455.

PATEL, Surendra R; Riverside Prof Centre, 407-1919 Riverside Dr, Ottawa ON K1H 1A2; Baroda (India)'67; MB BS; FRCPC; Psy (Adult Psychiatry). (613)739-2875

PATEL, Tara J; 428-4190 Finch Ave E, Scarborough ON M1S 4T7; Baroda (India)'68; MB BS; (416)299-1893

PATEL, Tejal; HHS McMaster Family Practice, A-690 Main St W, Hamilton ON L8S 1A4; Qns'07; CCFP; (905)521-5016

PATEL, Umesh; Halton HSC Corp-Oakville, 327 Reynolds St, Oakville ON L6J 3L7; Wes'99; CCFP; CCFP(E.M.); Staff, Halton Healthcare Services Corporation - Oakville Site; (905)338-4618; umeshvpatel@hotmail.com.

PATEL, Vimal H; University of Alberta Hosp, 2H2WCM-8440 112 St NW, Edmonton AB T6G 2B7; (India)'84; Staff, University of Alberta Hospital; (780)407-1210; Fax. (780)407-1202.

PATEL, Vinod K; Patel Med Centre, 10 Elizabeth Ave, St. John's NL A1A 5L4; RCS (Ireland)'68; LRCP; LRCS; Cons. Phys., Nfld. Dept. of Health; Clin Assoc Prof, Memorial University Of Newfoundland; (709)754-9090; Fax. (709)738-6060.

PATEL, Vishal; North York Gen Hosp, 4001 Leslie St, North York ON M2K 1E1; Tor'05; Gastroent; IntMed. Staff, North York General Hospital; (416)756-6000

PATEL, Vishnu K; Orleans Urgent Care Clinic, 100-1220 Place D'Orleans Dr, Orleans ON K1C 7K3; Gujarat (India)'67; MB BS; Ac Staff, Orleans Urgent Care Centre; Coroner, Province of Ontario; Langs: Gujarati; Hindi; (613)841-2347; Fax. (613)841-5393; vpatel@rogers.com.

PATEL, Vivek R; The Ottawa Hosp-Gen Campus, W6287-501 Smyth Rd, Ottawa ON K1H 8L6; Sask'01; FRCSC; Ophth. Staff, The Ottawa Hospital - General Campus; (613)739-6805

PATEL, Yashesh; Mount Sinai Hosp, 429-600 University Ave, Toronto ON M5G 1X5; Man'90; FRCPC; IntMed. Staff IntMed, Mount Sinai Hospital; (416)596-4800 x3823

PATEL, Zeenat R; 8F-180 Queen St, Toronto ON M5V 3L7; Cal'02; FRCPC; CommunMed;CCFP; Public Health & Preventive Med. (416)952-7298

PATEL-CHRISTOPHER, Abha; 541 Queen St S, Kitchener ON N2G 1W9; Wes'88; BSc(Hon); (519)571-9127; Fax. (519)571-8313; abha@sympatico.ca.

PATELIS-SIOTIS, Irene; St Joseph's Mountain H Serv, PO Box 585 Stn Lcd 1 100 West 5th St, Hamilton ON L8N 3K7; Geneva (Switzerland)'83; FRCPC; Psy (Bipolar Disease). Ac Staff Mood Disorders Prog, St Joseph's Healthcare Hamilton - West 5th Campus; Affil Staff, St Joseph's Healthcare - Charlton Campus; Assoc Prof, McMaster University; Langs: Greek; (905)388-2511 x6372; Fax. (905)575-6029; siotisi@mcmaster.ca.

PATENAUDE, Amanda F; Pritchard Farm Health Centre, 5-3014 Henderson Hwy, East St Paul MB R2E 0H9.

PATENAUDE, Brian L; Clin d'Ophth de l'Outaouais, 29 rue Ducharme, Gatineau QC J8Y 3P7; Ott'74; FRCSC; Ophth (Cataract & Glaucoma). Ac Staff, Hull Hospital; Consultant, Pontiac Hospital Centre; Staff, The Ottawa Hospital - Civic Campus; Langs: English; French; (819)771-6015; Fax. (819)770-1066.

PATENAUDE, J J Francois; SMBD Jewish Gen Hosp, 3755 ch Cote-Sainte-Catherine, Montreal QC H3T 1E2; Mon'84; FRCPC; IntMed; Hem; MedOncol. Staff, Sir Mortimer B Davis Jewish General; Langs: Bilingual(French/English); (514)340-8222; Fax. (514)340-8733.

PATENAUDE, Jana R; Erindale Health Centre, 2-50 Kenderdine Rd, Saskatoon SK S7N 3A1; UBC'09; BSc; MSc; CCFP; (306)934-6601; Fax. (306)934-6615; jana.patenaude@gmail.com.

PATENAUDE, Jean-Victor; CHUM-Hop St-Luc, 1058 rue Saint-Denis, Montreal QC H2X 3J4; Mon'75; MSc(AdminMed); FRCPC; IntMed. Staff, Centre Hospitalier l'Université De Montréal (CHUM) - Hôpital Saint-luc; Member, Conseil du CRMCC; Prof, Universite de Montreal; (514)890-8000

PATENAUDE, Nathalie; Clinique Psy de St-Eustache, 111 rue Saint-Laurent, St-Eustache QC J7P 3Z5; Sher'92; FRCPC; Psy. (450)473-1720; Fax. (450)473-6369.

PATENAUDE, Nicolas; CHUS-Hop Hotel-Dieu, 580 rue Bowen S, Sherbrooke QC J1G 2E8; Mon'97; FRCSC; OrthSurg (Hand Surgery). Staff, Centre Hospitalier Universitaire de Sherbrooke-Hôpital Hôtel-Dieu; Langs: Bilingual(French/English); (819)346-1110 x28304; Fax. (819)822-6725.

PATENAUDE, Yves G; CHUS-Hop Fleurimont, 3001 12e av N, Sherbrooke QC J1H 5N4; Sher'87; CSPQ; FRCPC; DiagRad. Staff, Centre Hospitalier Universitaire de Sherbrooke-Hopital Fleurimont; (819)346-1110

PATENAUDE-CHAGNON, Sophie; Clinique Med du Village, 200-400 rue Meigs, Farnham QC J2N 2C8; Laval'01; CCFP; Staff, Hôpital Brome-Missisquoi-Perkins; (450)293-3681; Fax. (450)293-7463.

PATER, Elzbieta; Fraser Med Clinic, 108-22441 Dewdney Trunk Rd, Maple Ridge BC V2X 7X7; Wroclaw (Poland)'88; Staff Surgical Assists, Ridge Meadows Hospital & Health Care Centre; Langs: Polish; (604)463-1300; Fax. (604)463-1301.

PATER, Piotr C; 6935 Harvie Ave, Powell River BC V8A 5H9; Wroclaw (Poland)'87; Langs: Polish; (604)485-4156

PATERNITI, Sabrina; Royal Ottawa Hlth Care Group, 1145 Carling Ave, Ottawa ON K1Z 7K4; Trieste (Italy)'88; FRCPC; Psy. Staff, Royal Ottawa Mental Health Centre - Royal Ottawa Health Care Group; (613)722-6521; Fax. (613)761-3602.

PATERSON, Alexander H G; Tom Baker Cancer Centre, 1331 29 St NW, Calgary AB T2N 4N2; Edinburgh (Scotland)'69; MB ChB; FRCP(Ed); FACP; Ac Staff, Tom Baker Cancer Centre; Staff, Foothills Medical Centre; Consultant, Rockyview General Hospital; Prof, University of Calgary; Langs: Bilingual(French/English); (403)521-3688; Fax. (403)283-1651.

PATERSON, Corinne R S; 47 Marion St, Winnipeg MB R2H 0S8; Man'06; FRCSC; ObstGyn.

PATERSON, Craig J S; Dr Everett Chalmers Reg Hosp, PO Box 9000 Stn A 700 Priestman St, Fredericton NB E3B 5N5; Mem'04; FRCPC; DiagRad. Staff, Dr Everett Chalmers Regional Hospital; (506)452-5400

PATERSON, David I; University of Alberta Hosp, 2C243WCM-8440 112 St NW, Edmonton AB T6G 2B7; McG'95; FRCPC; IntMed; Cardiol. Staff, University of Alberta Hospital; (780)407-1857; Fax. (780)407-6452.

PATERSON, David J; South Windsor Med Centre, 2-3840 Howard Ave, Windsor ON N9E 3N9; Wes'74; CCFP; Staff, Windsor Regional Hospital - Metropolitan Site; (519)969-3744; Fax. (519)969-4478; paterson@mdirect.net.

PATERSON, Donald C; PO Box 160, Sorrento BC V0E 2W0; Man'66; (250)675-2322; Fax. (250)675-3441.

PATERSON, Guy S; 1569 6th Ave, Prince George BC V2L 3N4; Alb'02; FRCSC; Urol. (250)561-1503

PATERSON, Ian R; Kipps Lane Med Centre, 707 Kipps Lane, London ON N5Y 3C3; Wes'69; DPH(Tor); Court Staff, St Joseph's Hospital - St Joseph's Health Care; Court Staff, London Health Sciences Centre - University Hospital; Fam Med, St Mary's Hospital - St Joseph's Health Care London; (519)679-9970; Fax. (519)679-7315.

PATERSON, James G; 77 George Henry Blvd, North York ON M2J 1E8; Wes'73; MSc(Pharm.); FRCPC; Anes. Staff, North York General Hospital; Staff, The Scarborough Hospital - General Campus; Med Officer, Naval Reserve; (416)756-9830; Fax. (416)502-0264; paterson77@rogers.com.

PATERSON, Kimiko; Foothills Med Centre, 1403 29 St NW, Calgary AB T2N 2T9; UBC'00; FRCPC; DiagRad. Staff, Foothills Medical Centre; (403)944-4530

PATERSON, Robert A; PO Box 458 Stn Main, Dartmouth NS B2Y 3Y5; Dal'78; DAB; FRCPC; Anes (Pain Management). Consultant, Dartmouth General Hospital; Consultant, The Nova Scotia Hospital; (902)465-8316; Fax. (902)465-5579.

PATERSON, Ryan; Gordon & Leslie Diamond HCC, 6F-2775 Laurel St, Vancouver BC V5Z 1M9; UBC'95; FRCSC; Urol. Staff, Gordon & Leslie Diamond Health Care Centre; (604)875-5003; Fax. (604)875-5604.

PATERSON, Scott J G; Royal Alexandra Hosp, 10240 Kingsway NW, Edmonton AB T5H 3V9; Alb'90; Anes. Staff, Royal Alexandra Hospital; (780)735-4010

PATERSON, William G; Hotel-Dieu Hosp, 166 Brock St, Kingston ON K7L 5G2; Qns'79; FRCPC; IntMed (Esophageal Disorders); Gastroent. Att Staff, Hotel-Dieu Hospital; Att Staff, Kingston General Hospital; Prof, Queen's University; (613)544-3400 x2292; Fax. (613)544-3114; patersow@hdh.kari.net.

PATEY, Christopher P; Carbonear Gen Hosp, 86 Highroad South, Carbonear NL A1Y 1A4; Mem'00; CCFP; Staff, Carbonear General Hospital; (709)945-5111

PATEY, Gregory M; Frontenac Med Associates, 201-791 Princess St, Kingston ON K7L 1E9; Mem'79; BSc; BMedSci; CCFP; FCFP; Assoc Staff, Providence Care - St Mary's of the Lake Hospital Site; Assoc Staff, Kingston General Hospital; Assoc Staff, Hotel-Dieu Hospital; (613)544-2727; Fax. (613)544-7247; gmp@post.queensu.ca.

PATEY, Nathalie G; Hôpital Ste-Justine, 3175 ch Cote-Sainte-Catherine, Montreal QC H3T 1C5; Paris (France)'93; Staff, Hôpital Ste-Justine; (514)345-4931 x5348

PATGUNARAJAH, Anushi; 2-4000 Highway 7, Woodbridge ON L4L 8Z2; Ross University (Saint Kitts-Nevis)'08; (905)851-3777

PATHAK, Irvin K; Richmond Med Bldg, 403-2020 Richmond Rd, Victoria BC V8R 6R5; Wes'92; FRCSC; Otol. (250)595-5033; Fax. (250)595-5241.

PATHAK, Kumar A; Health Sciences Centre, GF440A-820 Sherbrook St, Winnipeg MB R3A 1R9; Banarus (India)'92; FRCSC; GenSurg. Staff, Health Sciences Centre; (204)774-8511

PATHAK, Parbeen K; 308-1990 Fort St, Victoria BC V8R 6V4; Ott'89; BSc; DABPN; FRCPC; Neur (Electroencephalography). (250)595-6210; Fax. (250)595-6240.

PATHAN, Aarif A; 15121 121 St NW, Edmonton AB T5X 3C8; Alb'01; BSc; CCFP; (780)472-7171; Fax. (780)478-9179.

PATHER, Adashnee Y; Dr CW Wiebe Med Centre, 385 Main St, Winkler MB R6W 1J2; MB ChB; (204)325-4312; Fax. (204)325-4594.

PATHER, Jhodipraghasen; Family Med Clinic, 4615 49 Ave, Lloydminster SK S9V 0T1; Kasturba (India)'88; MB BS; LMCC; Staff, Lloydminster Hospital; Langs: Afrikaans; (306)825-8877; Fax. (306)825-5167.

PATHER, Jhodipraghasen; Fraser Heights Med Clinic, 106-15966 108th Ave, Surrey BC V4N 5V7; Mangalore (India)'90; (604)582-8820

PATIDAR, Deepakkumar V; Fraser Med Clinic, 108-22441 Dewdney Trunk Rd, Maple Ridge BC V2X 7X7; Witwatersrand (South Africa)'81; MB ChB; (604)463-1300

PATIDAR, Jayprakash V; Misericordia Community Hosp, 3W-16940 87 Ave NW, Edmonton AB T5R 4H5; Witwatersrand (South Africa)'79; MB ChB; DCH; Leader Lab, Covenant Health - Misericordia Community Hospital; (780)735-2731; Fax. (780)735-2794.

PATIENT, Steven P; Monterey Med Centre, 750-2220 68 St NE, Calgary AB T1Y 6Y7; Alb'87; (403)280-0465; Fax. (403)280-0549.

PATIL, Dattu G; Eastport Medical Clinic, PO Box 130 113 Main St, Eastport NL A0G 1Z0; Marathwada (India)'91; MB BS; (709)677-2530; Fax. (709)677-2430.

PATIL, Deepali S; Clinical Sciences Bldg, 8 120-152 University Campus NW, Edmonton AB T6G 2G3; (India)'96; MB BS; FRCPC; Anes. (780)407-8887

PATIL, Nikhilesh G; Nova Scotia Cancer Centre, 2206-5820 University Ave, Halifax NS B3H 1V7; Mumbai (India)'01; (902)473-6185; Fax. (902)473-7205.

PATKAR, Shabari; 718-123 Edward St, Toronto ON M5G 1E2; Caribbean (Netherlands Antilles)'01; CCFP; (416)971-7730; Fax. (416)408-2802.

PATLAS, Michael; Hamilton HS-General Site, 237 Barton St E, Hamilton ON L8L 2X2; Hebrew (Israel)'95; FRCPC; DiagRad. Staff, Hamilton Health Sciences Centre - Hamilton General Hospital; (905)529-3732

PATMANIDIS, Stefanos; 5100 Rutherford Rd PO Box 12308 Rpo Rutherford, Woodbridge ON L4H 2T3; Alexandria (Egypt)'72; BMus; BCh; Psy (Affective Disorders). Staff, Humber River Regional Hospital - Finch Avenue Site; Langs: Greek; Arabic; French.

PATOCKA, Catherine; Ctr Hosp Gatineau Memorial, PO Box 160 101 ch Burnside, Wakefield QC J0X 3G0; McG'08; Staff, Centre Hospitalier Gatineau Mémorial; (819)459-1112

PATOCKA, Eva; Devon Gen Hosp, H-101 Erie St S, Devon AB T9G 1A6; Prague (Czech Republic)'73; Staff, Devon General Hospital; Langs: Czech; (780)987-4322; Fax. (780)987-4333.

PATOCSKAI, Erica J; CHUM-Hop Notre-Dame, 1560 rue Sherbrooke E, Montreal QC H2L 4M1; McG'94; FRCSC; GenSurg; General Surgical Oncology (P.Q.). Staff, Centre Hospitalier l'Université de Montréal (CHUM) - Hôpital Notre-Dame; (514)890-8000 x26607; Fax. (514)412-7821; erica.patocskai.chum@ssss.gouv.qc.ca.

PATODIA, Krishan K; Oakville Health Centre, 211-1060 Speers Rd, Oakville ON L6L 2X4; Qns'92; BSc; CCFP; (905)842-8163; Fax. (905)842-9059.

PATODIA, Murari L; 1298 Exmouth St, Sarnia ON N7S 1W6; Tor'88; BSc(Hon); FRCSC; Ophth. Staff, Bluewater Health - Mitton Site; (519)336-4448; Fax. (519)336-6981.

PATODIA, Sanjay K; The Medical Clinic, 403-265 Yorkland Blvd, North York ON M2J 5C7; Tor'92; CCFP; FCFP; (416)229-2399; Fax. (416)229-9771.

PATODIA, Shaila; 211-1060 Speers Rd, Oakville ON L6L 2X4; Wes'92; FRCPC; IntMed; Rheum. Langs: Hindi; (905)337-1107; Fax. (905)337-7361.

PATOINE, Claude; 211-810 av Champagneur, Outremont QC H2V 4S3; Mon'65; Psy (P.Q.). (514)279-4471

PATON, Katherine E; Regent Med Bldg, 210-2184 Broadway W, Vancouver BC V6K 2E1; Wes'83; FRCSC; Ophth (Cataract Surgery). Ac Staff Ophth, Vancouver General Hospital - Centennial Pavillion; Ac Staff, BC Children's Hospital; Staff, UBC Eye Care Centre; Clin Prof, University of British Columbia; Langs: Spanish; French; (604)732-8141; Fax. (604)732-7997.

PATON, Thomas J; Tudor Gen Medicentre, 2520 Tudor Glen Market, St. Albert AB T8N 3V3; Aberdeen (Scotland)'66; MB ChB; MPH; DTMH; DObstRCOG; FRCPC; Peds (Developmental). Ac Staff, Glenrose Rehabilitation Hospital; Consultant, University of Alberta Hospital; Assoc. Prof., Peds. & Ass't. Prof, University of Alberta; (780)458-5776; Fax. (780)460-1908; tpaton@telusplanet.net.

PATON, Walter M; White Rock Med Clinic, 101-15451 Russell Ave, White Rock BC V4B 2R5; UBC'66; Staff, Peace Arch Hospital; (604)531-5595; Fax. (604)531-9818.

PATON-GAY, John D; Royal Alexandra Hosp, 205 CSC-10240 Kingsway NW, Edmonton AB T5H 3V9; Alb'04; FRCSC; GenSurg (Trauma); Critical Care Medicine. Staff GenSurg, Internist, Royal Alexandra Hospital; Teach Staff, University of Alberta; Langs: Bilingual(English/French); (780)735-6924; Fax. (780)735-6925.

PATRICELLI, Charissa J; Maternity Clinics, 9750 140 St, Surrey BC V3T 0G9; UBC'02; CCFP; (604)582-4558

PATRICIO, Rodolfo V; Rosedale Med Centre, 506-600 Sherbourne St, Toronto ON M4X 1W4; Manila (Philippines)'60; (416)925-8181

PATRICK, Allan B; Kings Place, 604-440 King St, Fredericton NB E3B 5H8; Dal'84; FRCSC; Urol (Stress Incontinence). Staff, Dr Everett Chalmers Regional Hospital; Teach Staff Residency Teaching Prog/Asst Prof, Dalhousie University; (506)444-9020; Fax. (506)444-9021.

PATRICK, David G; Greene Stone Muskoka, 3571 Muskoka Rd 169, Bala ON P0C 1A0; Wes'05; CCFP; Staff, Homewood Health Centre.

PATRICK, David M; School of Population & Public, 2206 East Mall, Vancouver BC V6T 1Z3; Ott'86; MHSc; FRCPC; IntMed (Sexually Transmitted Diseases); InfectDis. Consultant, Vancouver General Hospital - Centennial Pavillion; Dir Epidemiol Services, BC Centre For Disease Control; Staff, School of Population & Public Health; Prof/Dept Head & School Dir Population & Public Hlth, University of British Columbia; (604)822-3910; david.patrick@bccdc.ca.

PATRICK, Lancelot L C; UBC Hospital, 2211 Wesbrook Mall, Vancouver BC V6T 2B5; UBC'80; FRCPC; Psy. Assoc Med Dir, UBC Hospital - Koerner Pavillion; Staff Psy, Vancouver General Hospital - Centennial Pavillion; Staff, Lions Gate Hospital; Assoc Prof, University of British Columbia; (604)822-7549

PATRICK, Lawrence; London HSC-Victoria Hosp, PO Box 5010 Stn B E1 313-800 Commissioners Rd E, London ON N6A 5W9; Wes'74; BSc; FACP; FRCPC; IntMed (Cardiology). Staff, St Joseph's Hospital - St Joseph's Health Care; Staff, London Health Sciences Centre - Victoria Campus; Aj Prof, University of Western Ontario; (519)685-8315; Fax. (519)685-8316.

PATRICK, Ward D; Queen Elizabeth II HSC, 346-1276 South Park St, Halifax NS B3H 2Y9; Mem'85; FRCPC; IntMed; Critical Care Medicine. Ac Staff, Queen Elizabeth II Health Sciences Centre - Victoria General Site; Prof, Dalhousie University; (902)473-3606; Fax. (902)473-3610; ward.patrick@cdha.nshealth.ca.

PATRIQUIN, Christopher J; McMaster Univ Med Centre, 3W11-1280 Main St W, Hamilton ON L8S 4K1; Wes'08; FRCPC; IntMed. (905)521-5030

PATRIQUIN, Maria J; Living Well Integrative Hlth C, 2176 Windsor St, Halifax NS B3K 5B6; McM'96; CCFP; (902)406-1500; Fax. (902)406-1501.

PATROI, Anca; Milton Family Care Centre, 820 Main St E, Milton ON L9T 0J4; Bucharest (Romania)'91; CCFP; (905)864-9898

PATRY, Claude; Ctr Med de Loretteville, 250-11000 boul de l'Ormiere, Quebec QC G2B 5S1; Sher'87; (418)842-3731; Fax. (418)842-3246; claude.patry@ssss.gouv.qc.ca.

PATRY, Danielle; Clinique de Varices, 101-8149 rue du Mistral, Charny QC G6X 1G5; Laval'73; Staff, South Health Campus; (418)832-7989

PATRY, David G; South Health Campus, 4448 Front St SE, Calgary AB T3M 1M4; Man'69; ABIM; FRCPC; IntMed; Neur (Multiple Sclerosis). Staff, Foothills Medical Centre; Consultant, Rockyview General Hospital; Consultant, Peter Lougheed Centre; Consultant, South Health Campus; Clin Assoc Prof, University of Calgary; Fax. (403)956-2992; dgpatry@gmail.com.

PATRY, Genevieve; Hotel-Dieu de Levis, 143 rue Wolfe, Levis QC G6V 3Z1; Laval'02; FRCSC; Urol. Staff, Hôtel-Dieu de Lévis; (418)835-7121

PATRY, Gilles; 100-441 rue Racine E, Chicoutimi QC G7H 1T5; Laval'70; FRCPC; Derm. Ac Member Derm, Complexe hospitalier de la Sagamie; (418)543-4473; patry.dermato@videotron.ca.

PATRY, Louis; Dir de la Sante Publique-Mtl, 1301 rue Sherbrooke E, Montreal QC H2L 1M3; Laval'72; FRCPC; OccupMed (Ergonomics). Consultant, Hopital Maisonneuve-Rosemont; McGill University; Université Laval; (514)528-2400 x3295; Fax. (514)528-2459; lpatry@santepub-mtl.qc.ca.

PATRY, Louise; Clinique Med Sainte-Dorothee, 102-1 boul Samson, Laval QC H7X 3S5; Sher'83; (450)689-6334; Fax. (450)689-6339.

PATRY, Luc; CSSS de Chicoutimi, 305 rue Saint-Vallier, Chicoutimi QC G7H 5H6; Mon'76; Consultant, Centre Hospitalier Jonquiere; Consultant, Complexe hospitalier de la Sagamie; (418)541-1000

PATRY, Manon; CLSC Simonne-Monet-Chartrand, 1303 boul Jacques-Cartier E, Longueuil QC J4M 2Y8; Mon'88; (450)463-2850 x2411; Fax. (450)463-1879.

PATRY, Michel; Clinique Gyn Obst Trois-Rivier, 2235 7e av, Trois-Rivieres QC G8Z 3E2; Sher'76; CSPQ; FRCPC; ObstGyn. Chef ObstGyn, CSSS de Trois-Rivières; Langs: English; (819)379-5353; Fax. (819)379-2893.

PATRY, Rose-Marie; CSSS Des Iles, 430 ch Principal, Cap-aux-Meules QC G4T 1R9; Sher'10; CCFP; Staff, Hôpital de l'Archipel; (418)986-2121

PATRY, Simon; Inst U en Sante Mentale de QC, J 1021-2601 ch de la Canardier, Quebec QC G1J 2G3; Laval'89; DFAPA; FRCPC; Psy (Psychotherapy). Staff Psy, Institut Universitaire Sante; Clin Prof Psy, Université Laval; Prof Psy, Universite de Montreal; Langs: English; (418)663-5020; Fax. (418)663-5758; simon.patry@institutsmq.qc.ca.

PATSIOS, Demetris A; Dept of Medical Imaging, 585 University Ave, Toronto ON M5G 2N2; Oxford (England)'94; (416)340-4800 x3372

PATT, Norman L; Oshawa Clinic, 117 King St E, Oshawa ON L1H 1B9; Tor'55; DABR; DMRD; FRCPC; DiagRad. (905)721-3522; Fax. (905)723-6319.

PATTEE, Carol L; Victoria Gen Hosp, 1 Hospital Way, Victoria BC V8Z 6R5; Qns'89; FRCPC; Anes. Staff, Victoria General Hospital; (250)727-4212

PATTEN, Scott B; Peter Lougheed Centre, 3500 26 Ave NE, Calgary AB T1Y 6J4; Alb'86; PhD(Epidemiol); FRCPC; Psy. Med Staff, Peter Lougheed Centre; Prof Dept Common Health Sciences, University of Calgary; (403)943-5694; Fax. (403)219-3568; patten@ucalgary.ca.

PATTERSON, Andrew J; 250 John St N, Arnprior ON K7S 2P6; McM'04; CCFP; (613)623-3166

PATTERSON, Andrew R; Stouffville Med Centre, 2F-34 Civic Ave, Stouffville ON L4A 1H2; McG'75; Staff, Markham Stouffville Hospital; Med Dir, Parkview Homes; Langs: Spanish; German; French; (905)640-3100; Fax. (905)640-5346.

PATTERSON, Bruce D; 10-3615 19th Ave W, Vancouver BC V6S 1C5; Alb'76; FRCPC; Psy. Asst Prof, University of British Columbia; (604)224-3394

PATTERSON, Bruce J; Sudbury Reg Hosp-Laurentian, 41 Ramsey Lake Rd, Sudbury ON P3E 5J1; McG'78; FRCPC; AnatPath (Hematology Pathology). Staff, Health Sciences North-Laurentian Site; Asst Prof Path, University of Toronto; (705)522-2200 x4779

PATTERSON, Christina J; Athabascan Place, 222-80 Chippewa Rd, Sherwood Park AB T8A 4W6; Alb'02; CCFP; (780)464-9661

PATTERSON, Christopher J; Hamilton HS-St Peter's Hosp, 88 Maplewood Ave, Hamilton ON L8M 1W9; London (England)'70; DABIM; MRCS; LRCP; FACP; FRCP(Glasg.); FRCPC; IntMed; GeriatricMed. Staff, Hamilton Health Sciences Centre - St Peter's Hospital; Prof Geriatric Med, McMaster University; (905)521-7939; Fax. (905)526-2062.

PATTERSON, Danielle E; Pemberton Med Clinic, PO Box 69, Pemberton BC V0N 2L0; Western Australia (Australia)'99; (604)894-6454

PATTERSON, David W; Clinique Med Diamant, 204-5512 ch de la Cote-des-Nei, Montreal QC H3T 1Y9; McM'05; CCFP; (514)737-3782

PATTERSON, Douglas S; Lansdowne Prof Bldg, 150-1641 Hillside Ave, Victoria BC V8T 5G1; McG'69; (250)370-9922

PATTERSON, Frederick; Albion Med Group, 101-1525 Albion Rd, Etobicoke ON M9V 5G5; Queen's (Ireland)'67; Staff Family Med, William Osler Health System - Etobicoke General Hospital; (416)741-1622; Fax. (416)741-2884.

PATTERSON, Harry S; PO Box 3400 Stn Main, Banff AB T1L 1E1; Cal'77; Ac Staff, Covenant Health - Banff Mineral Springs Hospital; (403)762-2222; Fax. (403)762-4193.

PATTERSON, Heather L; Foothills Med Centre, 1403 29 St NW, Calgary AB T2N 2T9; Qns'05; FRCPC; EmergMed. Staff, Foothills Medical Centre; (403)944-1110

PATTERSON, Janet A; 2-510 Concession St, Hamilton ON L9A 1C4; McM'82; FRCPC; Psy. (905)387-3561

PATTERSON, Jeffery M; Clinical Sciences Bldg, 4 112-11350 83 Ave NW, Edmonton AB T6G 2P4; Alb'07; FRCPC; IntMed; Hem. (780)407-1584

PATTERSON, Jeffrey D; Labrador Health Centre, PO Box 7000 Stn C 227 Hamilton River Rd, Happy-Valley-Goose NL A0P 1C0; Dal'05; CCFP; Staff, Labrador Health Centre; (709)897-2000

PATTERSON, Jennifer K; 48-44 Great Northern Rd, Sault Ste. Marie ON P6B 4Y5; NOSM'09; CCFP.

PATTERSON, Judy L; Canadian Forces Supp Unit HCC, 1745 Alta Vista Dr, Ottawa ON K1A 0K6; Wes'85; CCFP; FCFP; Staff, Canadian Forces Health Services Centre; Langs: English; French; (613)945-6600

PATTERSON, Leslie S; Saint John Reg Hosp, PO Box 2100 Stn Main 400 University Ave, Saint John NB E2L 4L2; Dal'97; FRCSC; ObstGyn. Staff, Saint John Regional Hospital; (506)648-6750; Fax. (506)648-6878.

PATTERSON, Lindsey J; Kingston Gen Hosp, 76 Stuart St, Kingston ON K7L 2V7; Leeds (England)'90; MB ChB; FRCA; FRCPC; Anes. Staff Anes, Kingston General Hospital; (613)548-7827; Fax. (613)548-1375; pattersl@kgh.kari.net.

PATTERSON, Margot; Bldg 633 CFB Wainwright, GD, Denwood AB T0B 1B0; Johannesburg (South Africa)'79; MB ChB; LMCC; Langs: Italian; Portuguese; Afrikaans; (780)842-1363; Fax. (780)842-1809.

PATTERSON, Robert S; 101-14 Duke St, Hamilton ON L8P 1X1; Wes'80; ABPS; FACS; FRCS; LMCC; MCPS; FRCSC; PlasSurg (Cosmetic Surgery). Affil Staff, Hamilton Health Sciences Centre; Ac Staff, St Joseph's Healthcare - Charlton Campus; Asst Prof, McMaster University; (905)572-1070; Fax. (905)572-1197; mail@plasticsurgerycan.com.

PATTERSON, Steven J; Peter Lougheed Centre, 3500 26 Ave NE, Calgary AB T1Y 6J4; Wes'83; FRCPC; Anes. Staff, Peter Lougheed Centre; (403)291-8555; Fax. (403)219-3574.

PATTERSON, Theresa M A; Nicola Med Dental Bldg, 300-321 Nicola St, Kamloops BC V2C 6G6; Sask'72; Ac Staff, Royal Inland Hospital; (250)372-1553

PATTERSON, William H; 102-1 Magazine St, Saint John NB E2K 5S9; Dal'70; Court Staff, Saint John Regional Hospital; (506)634-1272; Fax. (506)634-7215.

PATTINSON, Catherine S; Golden Ears Family Practice, 140-20395 Lougheed Hwy, Maple Ridge BC V2X 2P9; London (England)'82; MB BS; (604)465-1066; Fax. (604)465-7776.

PATTINSON, Howard A; 240-2224 Walker Rd, Windsor ON N8W 5L7; Liverpool (England)'76; MB BS; FRCOG; FRCSC; ObstGyn (Infertility). Chief ObstGyn, Windsor Regional Hospital - Metropolitan Site; (519)974-9991; Fax. (519)974-2718; mpattinson2@cogeco.ca.

PATTISON, Leslie D; 201-128 Penetang St, Barrie ON L4M 1V6; Tor'75; (705)726-4681; Fax. (705)739-8404.

PATTISON, Mark A; Early Psychosis Intervention P, 3F-2750 Hastings St E, Vancouver BC V5K 1Z9; UBC'02; FRCPC; Psy. Staff Child & Adolescent, BC Women's Hospital & Health Centre; (604)675-3875

PATTISON, Philip E; Radiology Consultants Assoc, 120-6707 Elbow Dr SW, Calgary AB T2V 0E3; Man'90; FRCPC; DiagRad. (403)777-3001; Fax. (403)777-3008.

PATTISON-BACON, James N; Westview Hlth Ctr Stony Plain, 4405 South Park Dr, Stony Plain AB T7Z 2M7; Stellenbosch (South Africa)'95; MB ChB; CCFP; CCFP(E.M.); Staff, Westview Health Centre; (780)968-3673

PATTISON-BACON, Manuela; Royal Alexandra Hosp, 10240 Kingsway NW, Edmonton AB T5H 3V9; Tor'98; CCFP; Staff, Royal Alexandra Hospital; (780)735-4670

PATTON, Daniel M; Kingston Gen Hosp, 76 Stuart St, Kingston ON K7L 2V7; Tor'08; IntMed. Staff, Kingston General Hospital; (613)549-6666

PATTON, David J; Alberta Children's Hosp, 2888 Shaganappi Trail NW, Calgary AB T3B 6A8; Cal'87; FRCPC; Peds (Pediatric Cardiology); Cardiol. Staff Cardiol, Alberta Children's Hospital; Teach Staff, University of Calgary; (403)955-7858; Fax. (403)955-7621.

PATTON, Marie B; 305-4625 Varsity Dr NW, Calgary AB T3A 0Z9; Cal'80; CCFP; (403)213-0700; Fax. (403)288-0038.

PATTON, Sheila W; The Forensic Group, 305-1245 Broadway W, Vancouver BC V6H 1G7; UBC'96; FRCPC; Psy. Staff, BC Women's Hospital & Health Centre; Clin Instructor, University of British Columbia; (604)733-5722

PATTON, William R; University of Alberta Hosp, 8440 112 St NW, Edmonton AB T6G 2B7; Alb'88; CCFP; CCFP(E.M.); FCFP; Staff, University of Alberta Hospital; (780)407-8822

PATTULLO, Andrew L S; 194-7007 14 St SW, Calgary AB T2V 1P9; Alb'85; FRCPC; IntMed (Infectious Diseases-HIV/AIDS); InfectDis. Staff, Rockyview General Hospital; (403)943-3897; Fax. (403)212-0972.

PATY, Breay W; Gordon & Leslie Diamond HCC, 8144-2775 Laurel St, Vancouver BC V5Z 1M9; UBC'93; FRCPC; IntMed (Diabetes); Endocrin&Metab. Staff, Gordon & Leslie Diamond Health Care Centre; (604)875-5990

PATZEV, Edi; Ctr de Sante Vallee-Gatineau, 309 boul Desjardins, Maniwaki QC J9E 2E7; Plovdiv (Bulgaria)'87; CCFP; Staff, CSSS de la Vallée de la Gatineau; (819)449-4690

PAUK, Tomas M; Medical Arts Bldg, 206-121 Wellington St W, Barrie ON L4N 1L2; Wes'87; CCFP; Staff, Royal Victoria Regional Health Centre; Langs: Czech; (705)722-5039; Fax. (705)722-8534; tomaspauk@hotmail.com.

PAUL, Adrien; CSSS Les Eskers de l'Abitibi, 622 4e rue O, Amos QC J9T 2S2; Mon'76; FRCPC; Peds. Chief Peds, CH Hôtel-Dieu d'Amos; Langs: English; (819)732-3341; Fax. (819)732-7054; amos@lino.sympatico.ca.

PAUL, Allister R; Bonavista Peninsula Comm HC, PO Box 1, Bonavista NL A0C 1B0; Mem'73; Staff, Bonavista Peninsula Health Centre.

PAUL, Ashalatha; 739 Lake Bonavista Dr SE, Calgary AB T2J 0N2; Kerala (India)'69; Langs: Malayalam; Hindi; (403)278-1440

PAUL, Ashis K; Broad Street Clinic, 2210 Broad St, Regina SK S4P 4V6; MB BS; MPH; (306)781-8080; Fax. (306)781-5644.

PAUL, James E; Hamilton HS-General Site, 237 Barton St E, Hamilton ON L8L 2X2; Cal'94; BSc; FRCPC; Anes. Staff, Hamilton Health Sciences Centre - Hamilton General Hospital; (905)527-4322

PAUL, John T; Oshawa Clinic, 117 King St E, Oshawa ON L1H 1B9; Washington (USA)'85; (905)721-4361

PAUL, Leslie V; Riverside Med Clinic, 307-1101 Dewdney Ave, Trail BC V1R 4T1; Chicago(IL) (USA)'96; (250)368-8802

PAUL, Margaret; 365 Elmwood Ave, North Bay ON P1B 9N4; Wes'73; FRCSC; GenSurg (Hand Surgery). Staff, North Bay Regional Health Centre - Regional Mental Health; Staff, West Nipissing General Hospital; Med Advisor, Community Care Access Centre; (705)495-2450; Fax. (705)495-6782; drpaul@bellnet.ca.

PAUL, Michael D; Health Sciences Centre, 4307-300 Prince Philip Dr, St. John's NL A1B 3V6; Tor'78; ABIM; FRCPC; IntMed; Nephrol. Staff Physician, Health Sciences Centre; Consultant, Janeway Children's Health & Rehabilitation Centre; Assoc Prof, Memorial University Of Newfoundland; Langs: French; (709)777-6548; Fax. (709)777-7054; mpaul@mun.ca.

PAUL, Myriam; CSSS Maria-Chapdelaine, 2000 boul du Sacré-Coeur, Dolbeau-Mistassini QC G8L 2R5; Laval'94; CSPQ; FRCPC; Anes. Staff, Centre Maria-Chapdelaine - CH de Dolbeau-Mistassini; (418)276-1234; Fax. (418)276-1153.

PAUL, Narinder S; Dept of Medical Imaging, NCSB 1C562-585 University Ave, Toronto ON M5G 2N2; Southampton (England)'87; MRC; FRCR; FRCPC; DiagRad. Head Cardio Thoracic Imaging, Mount Sinai Hospital; Head Cardio Thoracic Imaging, Princess Margaret Hospital - University Health Network; Div Head Rad/Asst Prof, University of Toronto; (416)340-4800; Fax. (416)340-3900.

PAUL, Niranjan C; Seven Regions Health Centre, PO Box 1000 24 Mill St, Gladstone MB R0J 0T0; (Russia (Federation))'94; Staff, Seven Regions Health Centre; (204)385-2968

PAUL, Partha; London Central Clinic, 458 Central Ave, London ON N6B 2E9; Wes'06; FRCPC; IntMed; Endocrin&Metab. (519)432-3595; Fax. (514)679-9658.

PAUL, Paulose J; Meadowlark Health Centre, 172 Meadowlark Shopping Ctr NW, Edmonton AB T5R 5W9; Cal'96; FRCSC; OrthSurg (Musculo Skeletal Oncology). (780)481-7151; Fax. (780)444-6936.

PAUL, Shefali; Broad Street Med Clinic, 2210 Broad St, Regina SK S4P 4V6; (306)781-8080; Fax. (306)781-5644.

PAUL, Stephane; CSSS Haut-Richelieu-Rouville, 920 boul du Seminaire N, St-Jean-Sur-Richel QC J3A 1B7; Laval'97; CSPQ; Anes. Staff, Hôpital du Haut-Richelieu; (450)359-5000

PAUL, T Gordon; Georgian Radiology Consultants, 121 Wellington St W, Barrie ON L4N 1L2; Wes'88; FRCPC; DiagRad; NuclearMed. Staff, Royal Victoria Regional Health Centre; (705)728-9090 x4266

PAUL, Tania; The Surrey Eye Care Centre, 13940 104th Ave, Surrey BC V3T 1V8; Tor'05; FRCSC; Ophth. (604)930-1010

PAUL, Terrance W; Cook Medical Bldg, 314-1175 Cook St, Victoria BC V8V 4A1; UBC'95; FRCPC; IntMed (Critical Care Medicine); Respir. (250)384-7377; Fax. (250)384-7372.

PAUL, Terri L; St Joseph's Health Care, PO Box 5777 Stn B B 109-268 Grosvenor St, London ON N6A 4V2; Ott'82; BSc; MSc; FRCPC; IntMed (Diabetes); Endocrin&Metab. Assoc Prof, St Joseph's Hospital - St Joseph's Health Care; Assoc Prof, London Health Sciences Centre - University Hospital; Assoc Prof Med/Assoc Dean Leamer Equity & Wellness Schulich School of Med & Dentistry, University of Western Ontario; (519)646-6245

PAUL, Vivian F; 200-2475 Bayswater St, Vancouver BC V6K 4N3; Man'76; CCFP; FCFP; Div Head Family Pract Obst, Providence Health Care - St Paul's Hospital; (604)731-0091

PAUL-HUS, Franck; Clinique Familiale St-Lambert, 201-209 rue Woodstock, Saint-Lambert QC J4P 1W7; Sher'79; Ac Staff, Centre Hospitalier Pierre Boucher; (450)466-8583; Fax. (450)466-4072.

PAUL-HUS, Myriam; CSSS de Montmagny-L'Islet, RR 1 350 boul Tache O, Montmagny QC G5V 3R8; Laval'99; CSPQ; Anes. Staff, CSSS de Montmagny-L'Islet; (418)248-0630 x5501; Fax. (418)248-3615.

PAULAITIS, Christina M M; 301-1223 St Clair Ave W, Toronto ON M6E 1B5; Tor'80; CCFP; (416)691-7385; Fax. (416)691-7099.

PAULGAARD, Tammy M; Doctors Plus Med Centre, 310-505 Main St SW, Airdrie AB T4B 3K3; Cal'02; CCFP; (403)945-0770; Fax. (403)945-8997.

PAULHUS-GOSSELIN, Eve; CSSS Pierre Boucher, 1333 boul Jacques-Cartier E, Longueuil QC J4M 2A5; Mon'06; CCFP; Staff, Centre Hospitalier Pierre Boucher; (450)468-8111

PAULICK, William C; Yarmouth Reg Health Centre, 60 Vancouver St, Yarmouth NS B5A 2P5; Man'77; AB; FRCPC; DiagRad. Staff Diag Imag/Radiol, Yarmouth Regional Hospital; Staff, Roseway Hospital; (902)742-3541; Fax. (902)742-1238.

PAULIN, Chantal; Clinique Med Plateau Marquette, 200-731 rue Galt O, Sherbrooke QC J1H 1Z1; Mon'94; FRCPC; IntMed; Cardiol. Langs: English; (819)564-8662; Fax. (819)564-1294.

PAULIN, Claude; 002-1321 rue Sherbrooke E, Montreal QC H3G 1J4; Laval'51; FCCP; FRCPC; IntMed. Consultant, Centre Hospitalier Jacques Viger; (514)287-9505; claude.paulin@ssss.gouv.qc.ca.

PAULIN, Frederic L; Health Sciences Centre, 300 Prince Philip Dr, St. John's NL A1B 3V6; Sher'03; FRCPC; IntMed; Cardiol. Staff, Health Sciences Centre; (709)737-6300

PAULIN, Jocelyne; Clinique Med Havre Sante, 521 boul du Havre, Salaber-de-Valleyf QC J6S 4Z5; Mon'83; Staff, Centre Hospitalier Régional du Suroît; (450)371-6444; Fax. (450)371-5315.

PAULIN, Mathieu; Centre Hosp Honore-Mercier, 2750 boul Laframboise, Saint-Hyacinthe QC J2S 4Y8; Sher'06; FRCPC; IntMed; Cardiol. Staff, Centre Hospitalier Honore-Mercier; (450)771-3333

PAULIN, Stephane; 66 Broad Rd, Oromocto NB E2V 1C2; Mon'02; CCFP; (506)357-3090

PAULOVIC, Robert P; Taunton Health Centre, SS 201 1290 Keith Ross Dr, Oshawa ON L1H 7K4; Tor'96; BSc; MSc; BEd; CCFP; FCFP; Associate Privileges, Lakeridge Health - Oshawa Site; Langs: Slovak; (905)721-4328; Fax. (905)721-6691.

PAULS, C John; 188 East Main St, Welland ON L3B 3W8; Mem'74; CCFP; Court Staff, Niagara Health System - Welland Hospital Site; (905)714-9364; Fax. (905)714-0438.

PAULS, Ernest J; 7-2168 McCallum Rd, Abbotsford BC V2S 6R6; Man'72; BA; CCFP; FCFP; Langs: German; (604)859-7121; Fax. (604)859-8090.

PAULS, Merril A; Health Sciences Centre, GF201-820 Sherbrook St, Winnipeg MB R3A 1R9; Man'91; MHSc; CCFP; CCFP(E.M.); Staff, Health Sciences Centre; (204)774-6511

PAULS, Roberta; 200-2475 Bayswater St, Vancouver BC V6K 4N3; UBC'90; (604)731-0091; Fax. (604)731-0081.

PAULS, Ryan J; Health Sciences Centre, AE2-820 Sherbrook St, Winnipeg MB R3A 1R9; Man'04; FRCPC; Anes. Staff, Health Sciences Centre; (204)774-8511

PAULSEN, Tennille D S; Halton HCS Corp-Milton, 7030 Derry Rd, Milton ON L9T 7H6; Tor'05; CCFP; Staff, Halton Healthcare Services Corporation - Milton District Hospital; (905)878-2383

PAULSETH, John E; Victoria Med Centre, 309-304 Victoria Ave N, Hamilton ON L8L 5G4; Wes'76; BMath; FRCPC; Neur. Ac Staff, Hamilton Health Sciences Centre - Hamilton General Hospital; Court Staff, St Joseph's Healthcare - Charlton Campus; Court Staff, Hamilton Health Sciences Centre - St Peter's Hospital; Clin Assoc Prof Med, McMaster University; (905)521-9774; Fax. (905)521-0825; jepaulseth@gmail.com.

PAULUS, Edmund M; Westminster Med Bldg, 305-625 Fifth Ave, New Westminster BC V3M 1X4; Mosul (Iraq)'72; MB ChB; FRCS(Eng); FRCSC; Urol. Staff, Surrey Memorial Hospital; Staff, Royal Columbian Hospital; Staff, Eagle Ridge Hospital & Health Care Centre; (604)521-8700; Fax. (604)521-7708; empaulus@shaw.ca.

PAULY, Robert P; 11-107 Clinical Sciences Bldg, 152 University Campus NW, Edmonton AB T6G 2G3; UBC'00; MSc(Epidemiol); FRCPC; IntMed; Nephrol. Staff, University of Alberta Hospital; Med Dir, Northern Alberta Renal Program; Med Dir, Home Hemodialysis Program; Asst Prof Med, University of Alberta; (780)407-3218; Fax. (780)407-7878; rpauly@ualberta.ca.

PAUN, Bogdan C; 311-751 King St W, Kitchener ON N2G 1E5; Wes'02; FRCSC; GenSurg (Colorectal Surgery). (519)741-5338; Fax. (519)741-9465.

PAUNOVIC, Bojan N; Salvation Army Grace Gen Hosp, 300 Booth Dr, Winnipeg MB R3J 3M7; Man'95; FRCPC; IntMed; Critical Care Medicine. Staff, The Salvation Army Grace Hospital; (204)837-0233

PAUPST, Elizabeth A; Timmins Family Health Team, 250-123 Third Ave, Timmins ON P4N 1C6; Rhode Island (USA)'05; CCFP; (705)264-9151; Fax. (705)268-7444.

PAUPST, James C; Key Personnel Med Examiners, 901-20 King St W, Toronto ON M5H 1C4; Tor'62; Staff, St Michael's Hospital; Med Dir, Marsh Canada & Quebecor; (416)363-3139; Fax. (416)363-7734.

PAUPST, Millie M M; North York Gen Hosp, 805J-4001 Leslie St, North York ON M2K 1E1; McM'90; DTM; DTMH; FRCPC; Psy. Staff, North York General Hospital; (416)756-6633

PAUSJENSSEN, Anne Marie; 502-402 21st St E, Saskatoon SK S7K 0C3; Sask'93; LMCC; FRCPC; IntMed. (306)956-3444; Fax. (306)956-3577.

PAUSJENSSEN, Elizabeth S; Royal University Hosp, 103 Hospital Dr, Saskatoon SK S7N 0W8; Sask'97; ABIM; FRCPC; IntMed; Respir. Staff, Royal University Hospital; (306)966-7951; Fax. (306)966-2383.

PAUSJENSSEN, Erik; Saskatoon Cardiol Consultants, 920-606 Spadina Cres E, Saskatoon SK S7K 3H1; Sask'96; ABIM; FRCPC; IntMed; Cardiol. (306)975-9000; Fax. (306)975-9888; epausjenssen@hotmail.com.

PAUTLER, Stephen E; St Joseph's Health Care, PO Box 5777 Stn B 268 Grosvenor St, London ON N6A 4V2; Cal'95; BSc; FRCSC; Urol (Minimal Invasive Urology). Att Physician, St Joseph's Hospital - St Joseph's Health Care; Asst Prof Surg, University of Western Ontario; (519)646-6384; Fax. (519)646-6037.

PAUYO, Eric; Douglas Mental Hlth Univ Inst, 6875 boul Lasalle, Verdun QC H4H 1R3; Louvain (Belgium)'74; Staff, Douglas Mental Health University Institute; (514)761-6131 x2890

PAUZE, Genevieve; Clinique Med Pauze Ferdais, 303-871 rue Shefford, Bromont QC J2L 1C4; Sher'94; Staff, Centre Hospitalier de Granby; (450)919-3911

PAVAN, Luigi A; Capri Med Centre, 132-1835 Gordon Dr, Kelowna BC V1Y 3H5; UBC'97; CCFP; (250)717-3211; Fax. (250)717-3233.

PAVANEL, M Ellen; Guelph Family Health Team, 109-83 Dawson Rd, Guelph ON N1H 1B1; Tor'80; (519)766-1360; Fax. (519)763-4315.

PAVENSKI, Katerina; St Michael's Hosp, 2 035CSC-30 Bond St, Toronto ON M5B 1W8; Tor'01; BSc(Hon); FRCPC; IntMed (Transfusion Medicine); Hem. Staff/Head Div of Transfusion Med, St Michael's Hospital; Langs: Ukrainian; Russian; (416)864-5058

PAVILANIS, Alan V; Family Medicine Centre, 3777 Jean Brillant St, Montreal QC H3T 1M5; McG'73; BA; MDCM; DipEpidemiol & Biostats; CCFP; FCFP; Family Physician-in-Chief, St Mary's Hospital Centre; assoc Prof, McGill University; Langs: Lithuanian; French; German; Spanish; (514)734-2648; Fax. (514)734-2732; alan.pavilanis@ssss.gouv.qc.ca.

PAVLIN, Charles J; Mount Sinai Hosp, 410-600 University Ave, Toronto ON M5G 1X5; Man'67; DAB; FRCSC; Ophth. Staff, Princess Margaret Hospital - University Health Network; Staff, Mount Sinai Hospital; Prof, University of Toronto; (416)586-3237; Fax. (416)586-5327.

PAVLIN, Jeanette E; 205-269 boul Saint-Jean, Pointe-Claire QC H9R 3J1; Man'78; FRCSC; PlasSurg. Staff, Lakeshore General Hospital - Pointe Claire; (514)697-0002

PAVLOSKY, William F; St Joseph's Health Care, PO Box 5777 Stn B 268 Grosvenor St, London ON N6A 4V2; Ott'79; FRCPC; DiagRad (Magnetic Resonance Imaging); NuclearMed. Assoc Prof Dept of DiagRad & Nuclear Med/Clin Dir PET/CT, St Joseph's Hospital - St Joseph's Health Care; Assoc Prof, University of Western Ontario; (519)646-6100 x64136; Fax. (519)646-6135; william.pavlosky@lawsonimaging.ca.

PAVLOV, Ivan; Ctr Hosp de Verdun, 4000 boul Lasalle, LaSalle QC H4G 2A3; Mon'09; CCFP; Staff, Centre Hospitalier de Verdun; (514)362-1000

PAVLOVA, Silvia; Carrefour Med Vallee Richelieu, 665 boul Sir-Wilfrid-Laurier, Beloeil QC J3G 4J1; Bucharest (Romania)'88; Langs: Romanian; Bulgarian; Russian; (450)467-0889; Fax. (450)467-4936.

PAVLOVA, Viktoria V; Ancaster Med Centre, 204-1144 Wilson St W, Ancaster ON L9G 3K9; (Russia (Federation))'98; FRCPC; IntMed; Rheum. (289)396-4442

PAVLOVICH, Peter; PO Box 45020 Rpo Dunbar, Vancouver BC V6S 2M8; UBC'04; CCFP; (604)936-7277

PAVONE, Elio; Oshawa Clinic, 117 King St E, Oshawa ON L1H 1B9; Tor'88; ABIM; FRCPC; IntMed (Hepatology); Gastroent. Staff, Lakeridge Health - Oshawa Site; Langs: Italian; French; (905)723-8551 x5312; Fax. (905)721-4978.

PAVRI, Daisy R; Daisy R Pavri Prof Med Corp, 301 Wellington Rd S, London ON N6C 4P1; Topiwala National (India)'79; MB BS; FRCPC; Peds (Developmental Pediatrics). Staff, London Health Sciences Centre - Victoria Campus; Consultant Ped, Norwich Med Centre; University of Western Ontario; Langs: Hindi; (519)673-6672; Fax. (519)673-6669.

PAWA, Baljit; 3525 4th Ave W, Vancouver BC V6R 1N9; Mem'88; BPharm; Staff, Westcoast Women's Clinic For Midlife Health; (604)738-9601; Fax. (604)738-9605.

PAWAROO, Patricia S R; 4-109 Old Kingston Rd, Ajax ON L1T 3A6; Qns'99; CCFP; Langs: Hindi; Urdu; (905)231-1988; Fax. (905)231-1989.

PAWELEC-BRZYCHCZY, Anna; Thames Valley FHT-Victoria Fam, 60 Chesley Ave, London ON N5Z 2C1; Wroclaw (Poland)'92; CCFP; (519)433-8424

PAWLAK, Jerzy; Corydon Family Practice Clinic, 894 Corydon Ave, Winnipeg MB R3M 0Y4; Lodz (Poland)'65; MSc; PhD; Langs: Polish.

PAWLEY, Amanda C; Med Associates of Port Perry, 462 Paxton St, Port Perry ON L9L 1L9; Qns'96; MSc; CCFP; (905)985-2895; pawleya@powergate.ca.

PAWLIK, Michal; ForeMed Cinics Inc, 420 Columbia St, New Westminster BC V3L 1B1; Jagiellonian (Poland)'03; CCFP; (604)522-2206

PAWLIK, Sara K; Foothills Med Centre, 1403 29 St NW, Calgary AB T2N 2T9; McM'09; CCFP; Staff, Foothills Medical Centre; (403)944-2304; Fax. (403)270-9652.

PAWLIUK, George K; 2334 Trent St, Victoria BC V8R 4Z3; UBC'95; FRCPC; Psy. (250)370-8152; Fax. (250)370-8199.

PAWLIWEC, Walter; Medical Arts Bldg, 353 St Paul Ave, Brantford ON N3R 4N3; McG'74; BSc; FRCSC; GenSurg (Surgical Oncology). Langs: Ukrainian; (519)751-2340; Fax. (519)751-1343; pawliwec@rogers.com.

PAWLOVICH, John P; Takla Landing Health Centre, GD, Takla Landing BC V0J 2T0; UBC'94; CCFP; FCFP; (250)996-7780; Fax. (250)996-7785.

PAWLOVICH, John P; Cannon Clinic, 4-2151 McCallum Rd, Abbotsford BC V2S 3N9; Sask'59; CCFP; FCFP; Ac Staff, Abbotsford Regional Hospital & Cancer Centre; (604)853-3314; Fax. (604)853-2171; john.pawlovich@spchc.hnet.bc.ca.

PAWLOVICH, Sarah L; Drs John & Sarah Pawlovich Inc, 30978 Polar Ave, Abbotsford BC V4X 1Y8; Wes'93; BSc; CCFP; FCFP; (604)853-6687

PAWLOWSKI, M Danuta; Univ Hlth Network-Toronto Western Hosp, 8E 471-399 Bathurst St, Toronto ON M5T 2S8; (Poland)'71; Staff Consultant Dermatol & Cross Appt, Toronto Western Hospital - University Health Network; (416)603-5721; Fax. (416)603-2782.

PAWLOWSKI, Susan M; Hollyburn Med Bldg, 202-520 17th St, West Vancouver BC V7V 3S8; UBC'90; Ad Staff Locum Hosp, Lions Gate Hospital; (604)913-8182

PAWLUCK, Larissa A; Saskatoon Community Clinic, 455 2nd Ave N, Saskatoon SK S7K 2C2; Sask'09; CCFP; (306)652-0300; Fax. (306)644-4120.

PAWLUK, Lawrence K; University of Alberta Hosp, 1E7. 17WMC-8440 112 St NW, Edmonton AB T6G 2B7; Alb'87; DABSM; FRCPC; Psy (Sleep Disorders Medicine). Dir Sleep Med Program, University of Alberta Hospital; Clin Prof Psy, University of Alberta; (780)407-6565; Fax. (780)407-6672; lpawluk@ualberta.ca.

PAWLUK, Randolph S; Meadowlark Health Centre, 200 Meadowlark Shopping Ctr NW, Edmonton AB T5R 5W9; Alb'90; FRCPC; DiagRad. (780)489-5313; Fax. (780)486-5160.

PAWLUSKI, Kerence P; Blatchford Field Med Clinic, 11541 Kingsway NW, Edmonton AB T5G 3E8; Alb'88; BSc; (780)809-1495; Fax. (780)809-1494.

PAYANDEH, Jubin B; 206-984 Oliver Rd, Thunder Bay ON P7B 7C7; Tor'01; FRCSC; OrthSurg.

PAYER, Pierre; Centre Med de l'Ile-Perrot, 6 boul Don-Quichotte, L'Ile-Perrot QC J7V 6N5; Mon'80; Physician, Centre D'Accueil; (514)453-7711; Fax. (514)453-3286.

PAYETTE, Clement; Clin Med St Felix de Valois, 610 ch Joliette RR 1, St-Felix-de-Valois QC J0K 2M0; Mon'77; Langs: English; (450)889-5577; Fax. (450)889-4239.

PAYETTE, Luc; Coop Serv Sante St-Barthelemy, GD S03-1980 rue Bonin, Saint-Barthelemy QC J0K 1X0; Mon'83; (450)885-1072; Fax. (450)885-1073.

PAYETTE, Mario; Clinique Med de l'Atelier, 77 boul Seigneurial O, Saint-Bruno QC J3V 2G9; Sher'78; Langs: Bilingual(French/English); (450)461-1751; Fax. (450)461-1602.

PAYEUR, B Jacques; Centre Hosp Honore-Mercier, 2750 boul Laframboise, Saint-Hyacinthe QC J2S 4Y8; Sher'72; FRCPC; Psy. Staff, Centre Hospitalier Honore-Mercier; (450)771-3333

PAYEUR, Helene; CLSC-CHSLD du Haut St-Francois, RR 1 700 rue Craig N, Cookshire-Eaton QC J0B 1M0; Sher'01; (819)875-3373

PAYEUR, Jean-Martin; CSSS du Sud de Lanaudière, 911 montee des Pionniers, Terrebonne QC J6V 2H2; Mon'10; CCFP; Staff, Centre Hospitalier Pierre le Gardeur; (450)654-7525

PAYEUR, Marie-Josee; CHSLD de Rimouski, 645 boul Saint-Germain, Rimouski QC G5L 3S2; Laval'90; Staff, Hôpital Regional Rimouski; Staff, Centre Hospitalier de Matane; (418)724-4111

PAYEUR, Richard; CSSSVG-CLSC-Sante Mentale, 149 rue Principale N, Maniwaki QC J9E 2B7; Mon'84; FRCPC; Psy (Depression & Anxiety). Staff, CSSS de la Vallée de la Gatineau; University of Ottawa; Lecturer Faculty, McGill University; Langs: English; (819)449-2513; Fax. (819)449-6316.

PAYLOR, Dascha L; Student Health Services-UCC, 1151 Richmond St, London ON N6A 3K7; Wes'88; (519)661-3771

PAYNE, Allen; 210-7895 av Papineau, Montreal QC H2E 2H4; Mon'83; Staff, CHSLD Lucille-Teasdale; Langs: English; (514)728-6622; Fax. (514)728-6154.

PAYNE, Arthur A; Sturgeon Community Hosp, 201 Boudreau Rd, St. Albert AB T8N 6C4; Mem'03; CCFP; CCFP(E.M.); Staff, Sturgeon Community Hospital; (780)418-8200

PAYNE, Daniel H; Slave Lake Family Clinic, 608 6 St SE SS 3, Slave Lake AB T0G 2A3; Alb'85; Chief/Medical Staff, Slave Lake Health Care Centre; (780)849-2860

PAYNE, Darrin; Kingston Gen Hosp, 76 Stuart St, Kingston ON K7L 2V7; Wes'03; FRCSC; CardSurg. Staff, Kingston General Hospital; (613)549-6666

PAYNE, David G; Univ Hlth Network-Princess M, 610 University Ave, Toronto ON M5G 2M9; McM'74; RadOncol; IntMed. Staff RadOncol, Princess Margaret Hospital - University Health Network; Assoc Prof RadOncol, University of Toronto; (416)946-2132; Fax. (416)946-6561; david.payne@rmp.uhn.on.ca.

PAYNE, Donald E; Rosedale Med Centre, 511-600 Sherbourne St, Toronto ON M4X 1W4; Tor'63; DPsy; FRCPC; Psy. (416)961-4678; Fax. (416)961-1418; payned@interlog.com.

PAYNE, Elizabeth E; Burke Mountain Medical, 210-1465 Salisbury Ave, Port Coquitlam BC V3B 6J3; McM'78; BScN; Staff Gen Pract & Hospitalist, Eagle Ridge Hospital & Health Care Centre; Staff Gen Pract, Royal Columbian Hospital; (604)941-8277; Fax. (604)941-5622.

PAYNE, Eric; The Hosp for Sick Children, 555 University Ave, Toronto ON M5G 1X8; Cal'06; FRCPC; Neur. Fellow, The Hospital For Sick Children; (416)813-6659

PAYNE, Irina E; 1777 Lonsdale Ave, North Vancouver BC V7M 2J6; (Russia (Federation))'01; CCFP; Langs: Russian; (604)628-6162

PAYNE, Jennifer R; 1425-1 car Westmount, Montreal QC H3Z 2P9; Cal'99; BSc; FRCPsy; MRCP; MRCPsy; FRCPC; Psy. (514)935-2470; Fax. (514)935-7261.

PAYNE, John C; 564 St George St PO Box 369, Dresden ON N0P 1M0; Wes'74; MCISc; FAAFP; CCFP; FCFP; Ac Staff, Chatham-Kent Health Alliance; (519)683-4479; Fax. (519)683-2763.

PAYNE, Kira L; Ontario Shores Ctr Mental HS, 700 Gordon St, Whitby ON L1N 5S9; McM'97; FRCPC; Psy;CCFP; FCFP; Staff, Ontario Shores Centre for Mental Health Sciences; (905)430-4055

PAYNE, Michael W C; St Joseph's HC-Parkwood Hosp, 801 Commissioners Rd E, London ON N6C 5J1; Wes'02; FRCPC; PhysMed&Rehab. Staff, Parkwood Hospital - St Joseph's Health Care; (519)685-4292

PAYNE, Richard J; SMBD Jewish Gen Hosp, 3755 ch Cote-Sainte-Catherine, Montreal QC H3T 1E2; McG'00; FRCSC; Otol. Staff, Sir Mortimer B Davis Jewish General; (514)340-8222 x8246

PAYNE, Rodney A; 4701 130 Ave SE, Calgary AB T2Z 4J2; Bristol (England)'69; MMed; MSc; MRCGPract; MRCP; (403)232-1000; Fax. (403)257-6353.

PAYNE, Wendy J; Ascot Heights, PO Box 3214 Stn Main, Wainwright AB T9W 1T2; Alb'05.

PAYNE, William L; 850 Waterloo St, London ON N6A 3W6; Wes'71; CCFP; Staff, Parkwood Hospital - St Joseph's Health Care; (519)681-6663; Fax. (519)681-2797; william.payne@sjhc.london.on.ca.

PAYOT, Antoine; Hôpital Ste-Justine, 3175 ch Cote-Sainte-Catherine, Montreal QC H3T 1C5; Geneva (Switzerland)'97; Peds; PhC; Staff Neonatologiste, Hôpital Ste-Justine; (514)345-4685; Fax. (514)345-4811; antoine.payot@umontreal.ca.

PAYOT, Isabelle; CHUM-Hop Saint-Luc, 1058 rue Saint-Denis, Montreal QC H2X 3J4; Geneva (Switzerland)'97; Staff, Centre Hospitalier l'Université De Montréal (CHUM) - Hôpital Saint-luc; (514)890-8000 x34980; Fax. (514)412-7376.

PAYRASTRE, Julien A O; Abbotsford Reg Hosp & Cancer C, 32900 Marshall Rd, Abbotsford BC V2S 0C2; Ott'06; FRCPC; EmergMed. Staff, Abbotsford Regional Hospital & Cancer Centre; (604)851-4700

PAYTEN, Susan A; Royal City Centre, 228B-610 Sixth St, New Westminster BC V3L 3C2; Cal'80; Staff, Royal Columbian Hospital; (604)521-2641; Fax. (604)521-4020.

PAYTON, Keith B; Dr Keith Payton Med Prof Corp, 409-450 Central Ave, London ON N6B 2E8; Qns'78; FRCPC; IntMed; ClinImmunol&Allergy. (519)936-0286; keithpayton@rogers.com.

PAYTON, Natasha A; Pacific Avenue Med Centre, 300-149 Pacific Ave, Saskatoon SK S7K 1N8; Sask'97; BScMed; FRCSC; ObstGyn. Clinical Asst Prof, University of Saskatchewan; (306)653-5970; Fax. (306)653-5383.

PAZIONIS, Greg; 102-304 The East Mall, Etobicoke ON M9B 6E2; McM'79; (416)231-7968; Fax. (416)231-7982.

PAZIRA, Hassibollah; CSSS de Beauce-Etchemin, 1515 17e rue, Saint-Georges QC G5Y 4T8; Sher'00; FRCSC; GenSurg. Staff, Centre Hospitalier Beauce-Etchemin; (418)228-2031; Fax. (418)227-3825.

PAZUKI, Kasra; Finch West Med Centre, 101-77 Finch Ave W, North York ON M2N 2H5; Tor'91; Assoc Staff, North York General Hospital; (416)225-2009; Fax. (416)225-5943; przcnz@gmail.com.

PAZUKI, Keyvan; Finch Med Centre, 78 Finch Ave E, North York ON M2N 7J5; Tor'88; Langs: Persian; Farsi; (416)222-3383; Fax. (416)222-8009.

PEACE, Janice L; Surrey Health Sciences, 204-13798 94A Ave, Surrey BC V3V 1N1; UBC'86; Clinical Asst Prof Med, University of British Columbia; (604)581-1119; Fax. (604)581-5952.

PEACH, Stephen C; Nordel Crossing Med Clinic, 115-12080 Nordel Way, Surrey BC V3W 1P6; Dal'95; BScChem; CCFP; (604)543-0888; Fax. (604)543-0231.

PEACHELL, John L; Kelowna Gen Hosp, 2268 Pandosy St, Kelowna BC V1Y 1T2; Alb'95; FRCSC; CardSurg. Staff, Kelowna General Hospital; (250)862-4000

PEACHELL, Milenija B; Canmore Gen Hosp, 1100 Hospital Pl, Canmore AB T1W 1N2; UBC'97; FRCPC; DiagRad. Staff, Canmore General Hospital; (403)678-7216; Fax. (403)678-1276.

PEACHEY, David K; Upper Village Walk-In Med Ctre, 901 Eglinton Ave W, York ON M6C 2C1; Wes'71; (416)781-8100; Fax. (416)781-8155.

PEACOCK, Edith M; Sherwood Med Centre, 15 Brackley Point Rd, Charlottetown PE C1A 6Y1; Mem'92; CCFP; (902)367-4025; Fax. (902)367-4035.

PEACOCK, Ingrid V; Eastern Med Clinic, PO Box 718 Stn Main 195 Water St, Carbonear NL A1Y 1C2; Ott'81; Staff, Carbonear General Hospital; Physician, Eastern Med. Clinic; (709)596-1006; Fax. (709)596-1506.

PEACOCK, Sandra C; 258-1011 Glenmore Trail SW, Calgary AB T2V 4R6; Cal'92; LMCC; CCFP; FCFP; (403)640-0388

PEALING, Robert D; William Kingston Mem Comm Clin, 90 School Rd, L'Ardoise NS B0E 1S0; (England)'77; MB ChB; (902)587-2800; Fax. (902)587-2813.

PEALING, Vivien; Dr Charles S Curtis Mem Hosp, 178-200 West St, St Anthony NL A0K 4S0; Leeds (England)'76; DA; Staff, Charles S Curtis Memorial Hospital; (709)454-3333

PEARCE, Andrew G; Sudbury Reg Hosp-Laurentian, 41 Ramsey Lake Rd, Sudbury ON P3E 5J1; Tor'04; FRCPC; RadOncol. Staff Regional Cancer Prog, Health Sciences North-Laurentian Site; (705)522-6237

PEARCE, Blaine F; Family Med Clinic, 111-246 Memorial Dr, Clarenville NL A5A 1N9; Mem'91; (709)466-5400

PEARCE, Colin B; Royal University Hosp, 3666-103 Hospital Dr, Saskatoon SK S7N 0W8; Sask'95; BScMicrobiology; BScPhysiol; FACC; FRCPC; IntMed (Interventional Cardiology); Cardiol. Clinical Asst Prof, Royal University Hospital; (306)655-1504; Fax. (306)655-1506; ptca@shaw.ca.

PEARCE, Craig R; 200-3555 North Service Rd E, Windsor ON N8W 5R7; (Ireland)'80; MB ChB; FRCSC; Cardiovasc&ThorSurg. (519)254-2897; Fax. (519)252-8128.

PEARCE, Dawn H; St Michael's Hosp, 30 Bond St, Toronto ON M5B 1W8; Wes'92; FRCPC; DiagRad. Staff, St Michael's Hospital; (416)864-6060 x6328; Fax. (416)864-5380; pearced@smh.toronto.on.ca.

PEARCE, Derek J; Cowichan Dist Hosp, 3045 Gibbins Rd, Duncan BC V9L 1E5; Ott'82; BSc; CCFP; CCFP(E.M.); FCFP; Ac Staff, Cowichan District Hospital; (250)737-2000 x4422

PEARCE, Llewellyn; Ste Marie Health Centre, 7-2010 Trim Rd, Orleans ON K4A 0G4; CCFP; (613)590-1433

PEARCE, Mark A; Addiction & Mental Hlth-Queen, 4-1001 Queen St W, Toronto ON M6J 1H4; UBC'02; FRCPC; Psy. Staff, Centre for Addiction & Mental Health (CAMH) - Queen Site; (416)535-8501; Fax. (416)583-4319.

PEARCE, Michelle M; Univ Hlth Network-Toronto Western Hosp, 3WW 402-399 Bathurst St, Toronto ON M5T 2S8; Tor'91; FRCPC; Psy (Tourette's Disorder). Staff, The Hincks-Dellcrest Centre - Toronto; Staff, Toronto Western Hospital - University Health Network; (416)603-5794; Fax. (416)603-5180.

PEARCE, Murray E; Belmont Prof Centre, 409-564 Belmont Ave W, Kitchener ON N2M 5N6; Tor'86; FRCPC; IntMed; Cardiol. Ac Staff, Hôtel-Dieu Grace Hospital; Ac Staff, Windsor Regional Hospital - Tayfour Site; (519)584-1104; Fax. (519)584-0959.

PEARCE, N Glenn; Belmont Family Medicine, 201-535 Belmont Ave W, Kitchener ON N2M 5E9; Mem'83; BEd; BSc; CCFP; (519)579-4870; Fax. (519)579-7903.

PEARCE, Neil J; Cardiology Consultants, 101-99 Airport Rd, St. John's NL A1A 4Y3; Mem'96; FRCPC; IntMed; Cardiol. Staff, Health Sciences Centre; (709)726-5311; Fax. (709)726-1028; cardiologyconsultants@nfld.net.

PEARCE, Nicolette S; Cowichan Dist Hosp, 220-3045 Gibbins Rd, Duncan BC V9L 1E5; Ott'81; BSc; CCFP; FCFP; Staff, Cowichan District Hospital; (250)737-2066

PEARCE, Patricia; Gladstone Prof Centre, 306-6155 North St, Halifax NS B3K 5R3; Dal'75; FRCPC; CCFP; FCFP; Psy (Reproductive Mental Health). Ac Staff, IWK Health Centre; Consultant, Queen Elizabeth II Health Sciences Centre - Victoria General Site; Asst Prof Psy & ObstGyn, Dalhousie University; (902)423-6463; Fax. (902)453-2598.

PEARCE, Paula A; Rockyview Gen Hosp, 7007 14 ST SW, Calgary AB T2V 1P9; (United Kingdom)'92; Staff, Rockyview General Hospital; (403)944-1536; Fax. (403)944-1095.

PEARCE, Stephen A; Surrey Med Arts Bldg, 117-13798 94A Ave, Surrey BC V3V 1N1; Tor'87; FRCPC; IntMed (Echocardiography); Cardiol. Staff Cardiol, Surrey Memorial Hospital; (604)588-3003; Fax. (604)588-3122; spearce@shaw.ca.

PEARCE, Timothy J; 300-4309 52 Ave, Red Deer AB T4N 6S4; Cal'93; FRCSC; OrthSurg. (403)309-2001; Fax. (403)358-5808.

PEARCE, William G; Workers' Compensation Board, PO Box 2415 Stn Main, Edmonton AB T5J 2S5; UBC'56; FCCMG; FRCS; Ophth. (780)498-4131

PEARCEY, Robert G; Cross Cancer Institute, 2117-11560 University Ave NW, Edmonton AB T6G 1Z2; London (England)'77; MB BS; FRCR; FRCPC; RadOncol (Gynecology). Staff RadOncol, Cross Cancer Institute; Prof Dept of Oncol, University of Alberta; (780)432-8518; Fax. (780)432-8380.

PEARL, Gerald J; Drummond Med Bldg, 1003-1414 rue Drummond, Montreal QC H3G 1W1; UBC'60; FRCSC; GenSurg. (514)845-6645; Fax. (514)738-3912.

PEARL, Monica C; Wellpoint Family Practice, 9F-1240 Bay St, Toronto ON M5R 2A7; Tor'88; CCFP; FCFP; Ac Staff, Women's College Hospital; Court Staff, Sunnybrook Health Sciences Centre; Lecturer, University of Toronto; (416)969-3240; Fax. (416)971-7718.

PEARL, Rachel J; William Osler HC-Brampton, 2100 Bovaird Dr E, Brampton ON L6R 3J7; Tor'97; FRCPC; Peds; Nephrol. Staff, The Hospital For Sick Children; Staff, William Osler Health System - Brampton Civic Hospital; Teacher, University of Toronto; (905)494-6593; Fax. (905)494-6594.

PEARL, Stephen; 20 Doctors Lane PO Box 370 Stn Main, King City ON L7B 1A6; Wes'70; Court Staff Family Practice, Mackenzie Richmond Hill Hospital; Court Staff, Southlake Regional Health Centre; (905)833-5381; Fax. (905)833-5649.

PEARLMAN, Jennifer B; 1650 Yonge St, Toronto ON M4T 2A2; Tor'01; CCFP; (416)644-1112; Fax. (416)479-0011.

PEARSALL, Donald F; Northeast Mental Hlth Centre, 680 Kirkwood Dr, Sudbury ON P3E 1X3; McM'81; MEd; FRCPC; Psy (Child Psychiatry). Staff, North Bay Regional Health Centre - Kirkwood; (705)675-9192; Fax. (705)675-5448.

PEARSE, Bryan F; Brockville Gen Hosp, 75 Charles St, Kingston ON K7M 6R5; McM'75; FRCPC; DiagRad. Staff, Brockville General Hospital - Charles Street; (613)354-5649

PEARSON, Brooke E; 379 St Paul Ave, Brantford ON N3R 4N5; Qns'75; BA; FRCPC; Peds. Langs: French; (519)512-0030; Fax. (519)512-0051.

PEARSON, D Mary; 19 Mack St, Kingston ON K7L 1N7; Qns'80; (613)549-3446

PEARSON, David C; 304-1964 Fort St, Victoria BC V8R 6R3; UBC'87; BSc; FRCPC; IntMed (Hepatology); Gastroent. Ac Staff, Victoria General Hospital; Ac Staff, Royal Jubilee Hospital; (250)595-3544; Fax. (250)595-3599.

PEARSON, Dawn M; South Health Campus, 4448 Front St SE, Calgary AB T3M 1M4; (USA)'93; Staff, Rockyview General Hospital; (403)956-2464

PEARSON, Derek S; Univ Hlth Network-Princess M, 610 University Ave, Toronto ON M5G 2M9; Sask'02; FRCPC; IntMed; Hem. Fellow, Princess Margaret Hospital - University Health Network; (416)946-2000

PEARSON, Eleena A; SMBD Jewish Gen Hosp, 3755 ch Cote-Sainte-Catherine, Montreal QC H3T 1E2; McG'98; FRCPC; CCFP; EmergMed. Staff, Sir Mortimer B Davis Jewish General; (514)340-8222 x5568

PEARSON, F Griffith; 796535 3rd Line E RR 3, Mansfield ON L0N 1M0; Tor'49; BSc(Med.); FACS; FRCSC; GenSurg (General & Thoracic Surgery). Staff, Stevenson Memorial Hospital; Emeritus Prof, University of Toronto; Langs: German; French; (519)925-6658; Fax. (519)925-6221.

PEARSON, H J; 203-120 Clarence St, Kingston ON K7L 1X4; Tor'81; FRCP; BSc(Hon); FRCPC; Psy (Pharmacotherapy). Att Staff Psy, Hotel-Dieu Hospital; Att Staff Psy, Kingston General Hospital; Asst Prof Psy, Queen's University; (613)545-2227; Fax. (613)235-5114; pearsonh@queensu.ca.

PEARSON, John C; Sault Area Hosp, 750 Great Northern Rd, Sault Ste. Marie ON P6B 0A8; Wes'70; Ac Staff, Sault Area Hospital - Sault Ste Marie; (705)759-3434

PEARSON, Margaret; CSSS de Laval, 280 boul du Roi-du-Nord, Laval QC H7L 4L2; Mon'85; CCFP; (450)622-5110; Fax. (450)622-4150.

PEARSON, W Dallas N; Royal University Hosp, 103 Hospital Dr, Saskatoon SK S7N 0W8; Sask'04; CCFP; CCFP(E.M.); Staff, Royal University Hospital; (306)655-1000

PEAT, Donald G S; Halton HSC Corp-Oakville, 327 Reynolds St, Oakville ON L6J 3L7; Tor'69; FACC; FRCPC; IntMed; Cardiol. Staff Heart Function Clinic/Med Dir Cardiac Rehab Prog, Halton Healthcare Services Corporation - Oakville Site; (905)845-2571 x5688

PEAT, Mary I; Westmount Specialty Clinic, 723 Rymal Rd W, Hamilton ON L9B 2W2; McM'80; FRCPC; IntMed; GeriatricMed. Asst Clin Prof Med, McMaster University; (905)627-9397; Fax. (905)574-2283.

PEBANE, Bright D; PO Box 579, Grenfell SK S0G 2B0; (306)697-3441; Fax. (306)697-3506.

PEBANE, Motlobeng D; 719 Grand Ave PO Box 580, Indian Head SK S0G 2K0; Natal (South Africa)'84; Langs: Sotho; Zulu; Swazi; Afrikaans; (306)695-2922; Fax. (306)695-2928.

PECHARSKY, Larry J; Avenida Bonavista Shopp Ctre, 315-12445 Lake Fraser Dr SE, Calgary AB T2J 7A4; Cal'78; (403)723-2453; Fax. (403)723-2463.

PECK, David J M; London HSC-University Hosp, PO Box 5339 Stn B 339 Windermere Rd, London ON N6A 5A5; Ott'92; FRCPC; DiagRad (Interventional Radiology). Staff Diagnostic Radiol, London Health Sciences Centre - University Hospital; Assoc Prof Diagnostic Radiol, University of Western Ontario; (519)663-3221; Fax. (519)663-8803.

PECK, Jared R; Mount Sinai Hosp, 600 University Ave, Toronto ON M5G 1X5; Tor'04; FRCPC; Psy. Staff, Mount Sinai Hospital; (416)586-4800

PECK, Jean-Philippe; Centre Med de Bedford, CP 140 1 Place d'Estrie, Bedford QC J0J 1A0; Mon'81; (450)248-3336; Fax. (450)248-7751; jean-philippe_peck@rrsss16.gouv.qc.ca.

PECK, Jonathan L; Queentario Med Centre, 4B-2325 Hurontario St, Mississauga ON L5A 4C7; Wes'93; BSc; CCFP; Langs: English; French; (905)270-8307; Fax. (905)270-6861.

PECK, Marcus J; Valley Reg Hosp, 150 Exhibition St, Kentville NS B4N 5E3; Cal'06; Anes. Staff, Valley Regional Hospital; (902)678-7381; Fax. (902)679-1904.

PECK, Ronnie; 1-2552 Finch Ave W, North York ON M9M 2G3; Tor'79; Ac Staff, William Osler Health System - Etobicoke General Hospital; (416)741-0601; Fax. (416)741-3326.

PECKAN, Catherine M; 108-450 Central Ave, London ON N6B 2E8; Wes'84; CCFP; FCFP; Ac Staff Family Med, St Joseph's Hospital - St Joseph's Health Care; Aj Prof Family Med, University of Western Ontario; (519)672-3020; Fax. (519)672-6090.

PECKAN, Karen M; E215-50 Westmount Rd N, Waterloo ON N2L 2R5; Wes'80; CCFP; FCFP; Court Staff, Grand River Hospital - Kitchener/Waterloo Health Centre; Court Staff, St Mary's General Hospital; Med Dir, Equitable Life of Canada; Med Dir, Faithlife Financial; (519)746-6762; Fax. (519)746-5965; kpeckan@faithlifefinancial.ca.

PECKHAM, Deborah C; St Clare's Mercy Hosp, 154 Lemarchant Rd, St. John's NL A1C 5B8; Mem'78; Staff, St Clare's Mercy Hospital; (709)777-5000

PECKHAM, Kenneth A; PO Box 40570 Rpo Six Points Pl, Etobicoke ON M9B 6K8; Tor'89.

PECKNOLD, John C; 323A av Grosvenor, Westmount QC H3Z 2M3; McG'66; DPM; FRCPC; Psy (Anxiety Disorder). Dir Community Psy Prog, Douglas Mental Health University Institute; assoc Prof, McGill University; Langs: Bilingual(English/French); (514)937-6355

PECKO, Krystyna; ASSSS Monteregie, 1255 rue Beauregard, Longueuil QC J4K 2M3; Sher'78; MSc; Staff, Hôpital Anna-Laberge; Staff, Hopital Louis-H Lafontaine; Dir Med Affairs, Regie Reg S2 SS Monteregie(Longueuil); (450)928-6777

PECORARI, Adriana I; Scarborough Hosp-Birchmount, 3030 Birchmount Rd, Scarborough ON M1W 3W3; Tor'81; FRCPC; DiagRad (Diagnostic Imaging). Staff Diagnostic Radiol, The Scarborough Hospital - Birchmount Campus; Staff Diagnostic Radiol, Rouge Valley Health System - Centenary Health Centre Site; (416)495-2480

PEDDER, Linda; McMaster University HSC, 1200 Main St W, Hamilton ON L8S 4J9; McM'86; FRCPC; Peds. (905)521-2100 x73086

PEDDIE, Elaine F; Children's & Women's HC of BC, A119-4480 Oak St, Vancouver BC V6H 3V4; Cape Town (South Africa)'82; MB ChB; DCH(SA); CCFP; Staff, BC Women's Hospital & Health Centre; Staff, BC Children's Hospital; Langs: Afrikaans; (604)875-2345

PEDDLE, Christopher J; Trinity Conception Health Ctre, PO Box 903 Stn Main 16 Goff Ave, Carbonear NL A1Y 1C4; Mem'90; (709)596-5135; Fax. (709)596-0212.

PEDDLE, Ronald C; Streetsville Med Centre, 8-5425 Creditview Rd, Mississauga ON L5V 2P3; Mem'84; (905)826-1164; Fax. (905)826-1214.

PEDDLE, Susan E; The Ottawa Hosp-Civic Campus, V259-1053 Carling Ave, Ottawa ON K1Y 4E9; Mem'00; FRCPC; DiagRad. Staff, The Ottawa Hospital - Civic Campus; (613)761-4982

PEDE, Leili; Brampton East Med Group, 200-300 Main St N, Brampton ON L6V 4H6; Tor'81; CCFP; FCFP; Ac Staff, William Osler Health System - Brampton Civic Hospital; Court Staff, North Wellington Health Care - Louise Marshall Hospital; Asst Clin Prof Family Med, McMaster University; Langs: Estonian; (905)451-1806; Fax. (905)451-8272.

PEDERSEN, Brian A; South Calgary Med Clinic, 118-40 Sunpark Plaza SE, Calgary AB T2X 3X7; Cal'02; CCFP; Asst Dir Family Med Residency Prog, University of Calgary; (403)254-4000; Fax. (403)254-1282.

PEDERSEN, John E; Cross Cancer Institute, 11560 University Ave NW, Edmonton AB T6G 1Z2; Alb'71; FRCPC; IntMed; RadOncol. Ac Staff, Cross Cancer Institute; Clin Prof, University of Alberta; (780)432-8755; Fax. (780)432-8380.

PEDERSEN, M Elizabeth; Orthopaedic Associates, 11202 76 Ave NW, Edmonton AB T6G 0K1; Tor'03; FRCSC; OrthSurg. (780)439-4945; Fax. (780)439-0396.

PEDERSEN, Sara A; Columbia Med Bldg, 409-301 Columbia St E, New Westminster BC V3L 3W5; Wes'92; BSc; FRCSC; ObstGyn (Colposcopy). Staff ObstGyn, Royal Columbian Hospital; (604)522-8272; Fax. (604)522-8273.

PEDERSEN, Susie D; C-ENDO Endocrinology Centre, 240-1016 68 Ave SW, Calgary AB T2V 4J2; Cal'00; FRCPC; IntMed (Diabetes); Endocrin&Metab. Langs: Danish; (403)705-3636; drsuepedersen@gmail.com.

PEDERSEN, Sven(Buzz) A; Paterson Med Centre, RR 1 Stn Main 45 Wolsley St, Kenora ON P9N 3W7; Man'93; BSc; CCFP; Ac Staff Privil, Lake of the Woods District Hospital; (807)468-3021; Fax. (807)468-5565; buzzrhonda68@gmail.com.

PEDERSON, D Troy; Peter Lougheed Centre, 3500 26 Ave NE, Calgary AB T1Y 6J4; Cal'94; BSc; FRCPC; IntMed. Staff, Peter Lougheed Centre; Clinical Asst Prof, University of Calgary; (403)943-4555

PEDERSON, Glen I; Woodstock Gen Hosp, 310 Juliana Dr, Woodstock ON N4V 0A4; Wes'93; CCFP; CCFP(E.M.); Staff, Woodstock General Hospital; (519)421-4211

PEDERSON, Karla J; College of Phys & Surg of BC, 300-669 Howe St, Vancouver BC V6C 0B4; Sask'00; CCFP; (604)733-7758

PEDERSON, Kristen L; Children's Hosp, FE009-840 Sherbrook St, Winnipeg MB R3A 1S1; Cal'97; FRCPC; Peds; Nephrol. Staff, Health Sciences Centre; (204)787-4947; Fax. (204)787-1075.

PEDNEAULT, Caroline; Clinique Med Pierre-Boucher, 1615 boul Jacques-Cartier E, Longueuil QC J4M 2X1; Sher'96; FRCPC; Peds (Transcultural Med). Staff, Hopital Maisonneuve-Rosemont; Langs: English; Spanish; (450)468-6223

PEDNEAULT, Janie; CSSS de Temiscouata, CP 310 58 rue de l'Eglise, Notre-Dame-du-Lac QC G0L 1X0; Laval'07; Staff, Centre Hospitalier Notre-Dame-du-Lac; (418)899-6751

PEDNEAULT, Josee; Clinique Med des Trois Lacs, 160-585 av Saint-Charles, Vaudreuil-Dorion QC J7V 8P9; Laval'98; CCFP; Staff, Centre Hospitalier Régional du Suroît; (450)455-3322

PEDNEAULT, Lisa; Clinique Med Fam de St-Nazaire, 210 rue Principale, St-Naz-Du-Lsj QC G0W 2V0; Laval'97; (418)668-8122; Fax. (418)668-5335.

PEDNEAULT, Melodie; CSSS de Jonquiere, CP 1200 Stn Pdf Jonquiere 2230 rue de l'Hopital, Jonquiere QC G7X 7X2; Laval'08; CCFP; CCFP(E.M.); Staff, Centre Hospitalier Jonquiere; (418)695-7700

PEDRETTI, Luigi T; Lakeridge Hlth Corp-Oshawa, 1 Hospital Crt, Oshawa ON L1G 2B9; Tor'91; CCFP; FCFP; Staff, Lakeridge Health - Oshawa Site; (905)576-8711

PEDRO, Maria E; Clinique MD Sante, 8127 boul Saint-Laurent, Montreal QC H2P 2M1; Mon'87; Staff, Centre Hospitalier Pierre le Gardeur; (514)687-4372

PEDVIS, Stacey R; 601-2200 Yonge St, Toronto ON M4S 2C6; Cal'95; BSc; FRCPC; IntMed; Rheum. Consultant, Sunnybrook Health Sciences Centre; (416)644-0984; Fax. (416)644-0985.

PEEBLES, Erin R; The Hosp for Sick Children, 555 University Ave, Toronto ON M5G 1X8; Ott'08; Peds.

PEEL, Cordell H; 2768 Broadway W PO Box 74685 Rpo Kitsilano, Vancouver BC V6K 4P4; Cal'06; CCFP.

PEENS, Erus J; Rocky Med Clinic, PO Box 99 Stn Main 5127 49 St, Rocky-Mtn-Hse AB T4T 1A1; (South Africa)'04; MB ChB; Langs: Afrikaans; (403)845-2315; Fax. (403)845-2177.

PEER, Brian R; The Health Centre, 1-108 Sophia St, St Andrews NB E5B 2B8; Wes'91; CCFP; FCFP; (506)529-9120; Fax. (506)529-9125.

PEER, Ihsaan C; 2479 McCallum Rd, Abbotsford BC V2S 3P8; Medunsa (South Africa)'03; MB BS; MB ChB; LMCC; CCFP; Langs: Afrikaans; (604)852-2279; Fax. (604)852-2863; ihsaanpeer@yahoo.com.

PEER, Ismail G H; South Walkerville Med Centre, 135-2224 Walker Rd, Windsor ON N8W 5L7; Johannesburg (South Africa)'66; FRCPC; IntMed (Gastroenterology). Ac Staff, Windsor Regional Hospital - Tayfour Site; Ac Staff, Windsor Regional Hospital - Metropolitan Site; (519)258-2261; Fax. (519)259-9239.

PEER, Ismail G M; Blind River Med Clinic, PO Box 1330, Blind River ON P0R 1B0; RCS (Ireland)'62; LRCS; LRCP; FRCSI; Ac Staff, Blind River District Health Centre; (705)356-1212; Fax. (705)356-0468.

PEER, Joseph; Charlton Med Centre, 807-25 Charlton Ave E, Hamilton ON L8N 1Y2; Brussels (Belgium)'65; FRCPC; Peds. Staff, St Joseph's Healthcare - Charlton Campus; Staff, Hamilton Health Sciences Centre - McMaster University Medical Centre; Asst Clin Prof, McMaster University; (905)528-7971; Fax. (905)528-8855.

PEER, Michael; Clairhurst Med Centre, 201-1466 Bathurst St, Toronto ON M5R 3S3; Wes'90; FRCPC; Peds. Staff, The Hospital For Sick Children; Asst Prof, University of Toronto; (416)531-3331; Fax. (416)531-1639.

PEER, Syed M A; Peel Med Clinic, 7070 Saint Barbara Blvd, Mississauga ON L5W 0E6; Bangalore (India)'78; MB BS; (905)565-9100

PEERA, Mohamed A; South Lake Reg Health Centre, 596 Davis Dr, Newmarket ON L3Y 2P9; McG'04; FRCPC; EmergMed. Staff, Southlake Regional Health Centre; (905)895-4521

PEERANI, Nargis; Quick Care Walk-In, 2F-4410 17 St NW, Edmonton AB T6T 0C1; London (England)'74; LRCP; MRCS; (780)468-1884; Fax. (780)468-1868.

PEERBAYE, G Hussein; Bendale Acres Nursing Home, 2920 Lawrence Ave E, Scarborough ON M1P 2T8; RCS (Ireland)'64; (416)397-7000; hussen.peerbaye@sympatico.ca.

PEERBAYE, Yousouf A; Sunnybrook Hlth Sciences Ctre, C7 53-2075 Bayview Ave, Toronto ON M4N 3M5; Tor'96; BSc; MSc; EmergMed (Pre-Hospital Emergency Care). Staff, Sunnybrook Health Sciences Centre; Langs: English; French; (416)480-4037

PEERIS, Sumithra A; 57 Church St E PO Box 489, Waterford ON N0E 1Y0; Dublin (Ireland)'64; LRCPSI(Ire); LM; LRCP; LRCS; Member Family Practice Hospital Foundation/Ac Staff, Norfolk General Hospital; Langs: Spanish; German; (519)443-7241; Fax. (519)443-4679; sumie@kwic.com.

PEERS, Glenn A; 1-497 Laurier Ave, Milton ON L9T 3K8; Tor'73; Ac Staff, Halton Healthcare Services Corporation - Milton District Hospital; (905)878-7619; Fax. (905)878-7660.

PEERS, Robert R; Royal Oak Med Centre, 106-6440 Royal Oak Ave, Burnaby BC V5H 3P2; UBC'73; MSc; FRCSC; PlasSurg (Cosmetic Surgery). Staff, Burnaby Hospital; Staff, Lions Gate Hospital; (604)435-2922; Fax. (604)435-6358.

PEET, Jonathan M; 104-445 Beechwood Pl, Waterloo ON N2T 1Z2; Tor'90; CCFP; FCFP; Ac Staff, St Mary's General Hospital; Ac Staff, Grand River Hospital - Kitchener/Waterloo Health Centre; (519)746-1540; Fax. (519)746-2350.

PEETS, Adam D; St Paul's Hosp, 239-1081 Burrard St, Vancouver BC V6Z 1Y6; Cal'00; FRCPC; IntMed; Critical Care Medicine. Staff, Providence Health Care - St Paul's Hospital; (604)682-2344

PEFANIS, John; Centre for Family Medicine, 10B Victoria St S, Kitchener ON N2G 1C5; Wes'96; CCFP; FCFP; (519)783-0023; Fax. (519)783-0033.

PEFFER, Dale V F; Nipawin Health Centre, PO Box 1925, Nipawin SK S0E 1E0; (306)862-3151; Fax. (306)862-2241.

PEGADO, V Vance; Burlington Prof Centre, 205-3155 Harvester Rd, Burlington ON L7N 3V2; CCFP; (905)632-1803; Fax. (905)632-3149.

PEGADO, Victor D; 206-1990 Fort St, Victoria BC V8R 6V4; Tor'00; BSc; FRCSC; Ophth (Pediatric Ophthalmology). Staff, Fort St John Hospital & Health Centre; Staff, Vancouver Island Health Authority; (250)590-5660; Fax. (250)590-5720.

PEGG, Anne-Marie; Fort Simpson Health Centre, 10101 100th Ave, Fort Simpson NT X0E 0N0; McM'04; CCFP; Staff, Fort Simpson Health Centre; (867)695-7000; anne-marie@fortsimpson.com.

PEGG, S Jane; Oceanview Paediatrics, 101-1650 Terminal Ave N, Nanaimo BC V9S 0A3; Tor'88; FRCPC; Peds. Consultant Peds, Nanaimo Regional General Hospital; (250)591-1906; Fax. (250)591-1913; ovpaeds@shaw.ca.

PEGG, William C; York Community Services Ctre, 1651 Keele St, York ON M6M 3W2; Cal'90; CCFP; FCFP; (416)653-5400; Fax. (416)657-3622.

PEGU, Satyaranjan; Children's Hosp Eastern Ont, 401 Smyth Rd, Ottawa ON K1H 8L1; Dibrugarh University (India)'96; Staff, Children's Hospital of Eastern Ontario (CHEO); (613)737-7600; Fax. (613)738-3216.

PEHLIVAN, Hakan; The Medical Centre, 2-137 King St, Estevan SK S4A 2T5; (306)634-6444; Fax. (306)634-9187.

PEHR, Kevin; 780-4060 rue Sainte-Catherine, Westmount QC H3Z 2Z3; New York(NY) (USA)'81; Derm (Cosmetic Dermatology). Staff, Sir Mortimer B Davis Jewish General; Asst Clin Prof, McGill University; Langs: English; French; (514)935-1051; Fax. (514)932-3793.

PEI, York P C; 8N838-585 University Ave, Toronto ON M5G 2N2; Wes'81; FASN; FACP; FRCPC; IntMed; Nephrol. Staff Nephrol, Toronto General Hospital - UHN; Prof Med, University of Toronto; Langs: Cantonese; Mandarin; (416)340-4257; Fax. (416)340-4999.

PEIMER, Jeffrey E; Cariboo Mem Hosp, 517 Sixth Ave N, Williams Lake BC V2G 2G8; Cape Town (South Africa)'89; MB ChB; Staff, Cariboo Memorial Hospital and Health Centre; Langs: Afrikaans; (250)305-4379

PEIN, Cho-Yee; 205-667 Sacville Dr, Lower Sackville NS B4C 2S4; Rangoon (Burma)'61; Staff, Queen Elizabeth II Health Sciences Centre - Victoria General Site; Staff, IWK Health Centre; (902)252-3884; Fax. (902)252-3988.

PEIRAVI, Haleh; East Calgary Health Centre, 4715 8 Ave SE, Calgary AB T2A 3N4; CCFP; (403)229-2273

PEIRCE, Karen L; Bolton Centre for Women's Hlth, 208-170 McEwan Dr E, Bolton ON L7E 4C8; McG'82; MSc; MDCM; CCFP; (905)951-0555; Fax. (905)880-0016; peircegauthier@gmail.com.

PEIRIS, Malwattage J P; Holly Med Clinic, 611 Holly Ave, Milton ON L9T 0K4; Colombo (Sri Lanka)'99; CCFP; (905)878-0086

PEIROVY, Javed; 400-1 Eglinton Ave E, Toronto ON M4P 3A1; Tehran (Iran)'96; Staff, Toronto Western Hospital - University Health Network.

PEIRSON, Mary C; Wellington Dufferin Guelph Pub, 600 Southgate Dr, Guelph ON N1G 4P6; Tor'90; CCFP; (519)846-2715; Fax. (519)836-7215; mcp@sentex.net.

PEK, Barbora M; Hamilton HS-General Site, 237 Barton St E, Hamilton ON L8L 2X2; Ott'05; CCFP; CCFP(E.M.); Staff, Hamilton Health Sciences Centre - McMaster Children's Hospital; Staff, Hamilton Health Sciences Centre - Hamilton General Hospital; (905)521-2100; Fax. (905)577-8247.

PEK, Bonavent; CSSS du Suroit, 150 rue Saint-Thomas, Salaber-de-Valleyf QC J6T 6C1; Sher'91; LMCC; CSPQ; FRCPC; Anes. Staff, Centre Hospitalier Régional du Suroît; (450)371-9920

PEK, Bonavuth; CSSS du Nord de Lanaudière, 1000 boul Sainte-Anne, St-Charles-Brromee QC J6E 6J2; Mon'94; FRCPC; IntMed; Respir. Staff, Centre Hospitalier Régional de Lanaudière; Langs: English; (450)759-8222; Fax. (450)759-0077.

PEKELES, Gary S; MUHC-Montreal Children's Hosp, R 379-2300 rue Tupper, Montreal QC H3H 1P3; Baylor(TX) (USA)'76; MSc(Epidemiol); FAB; FRCPC; Peds. Dir Inpatient Serv, McGill University Health Centre - Montreal Children's Hospital; Dir McGill Baffin Prog, McGill University; (514)412-4349; Fax. (514)412-4311; gary.pekeles@muhc.mcgill.ca.

PEKEZ, Jelena; Family MDS, 10134 111 Ave NW, Edmonton AB T5G 0B3; Novi Sad (Serbia)'97; CCFP; Physician, CHOICE Mental Health Program; Physician, St Michael's Nursing Home; Langs: Serbian; (780)474-3712; Fax. (780)474-7032.

PEKUSH, Robert D; 201-610 Queen St, Saskatoon SK S7K 0M8; Sask'97; BSc(Hons); FRCSC; Ophth (Cataract Surgery). Staff Med, Saskatoon Health Region Saskatoon Public Health; (306)244-1534; Fax. (306)244-5181.

PELAUSA, Ermelinda O; SMBD Jewish Gen Hosp, 3755 ch Cote-Sainte-Catherine, Montreal QC H3T 1E2; McG'80; FRCPC; Peds (Neonatology). Staff, Sir Mortimer B Davis Jewish General; adj Prof, McGill University; (514)340-8222 x4950; Fax. (514)340-7566.

PELCHAT, Suzanne; CLSC de la Jacques-Cartier, 043-11999 rue de l'Hopital, Quebec QC G2A 2T7; Laval'76; (418)843-2572 x7649; Fax. (418)843-3880.

PELCHAT, Veronique; CLSC Saint-Jean-Port-Joli, RR 1 430 rue Jean-Leclerc, St-Jean-Port-Joli QC G0R 3G0; Laval'05; (418)598-3355; Fax. (418)598-9800.

PELED, Elia; Children's Hosp, 840 Sherbrook St, Winnipeg MB R3A 1S1; Staff, Health Sciences Centre.

PELET, Stephane; Ctr Hosp Affilie-Enfant-Jesus, 1401 18e rue, Quebec QC G1J 1Z4; Lausanne (Switzerland)'94; Staff, Centre Hospitalier Affilié Universitaire de Québec - Hôpital De L'Enfant Jésus; Clin Prof Surg, Université Laval; Langs: German; English; (418)649-0252 x3169; Fax. (418)649-5567.

PELIOWSKI, Abraham; 5027 4-10240 Kingsway NW, Edmonton AB T5H 3V9; (Chile)'73; FRCP; ABPeds; FAAP; FRCPC; Peds (Neonatology). Ac Staff Div of Newborn Med, Royal Alexandra Hospital; Clin Prof Peds & Critical Care, University of Alberta; Langs: Spanish; Yiddish; (780)735-4670; Fax. (780)735-4072; abe.peliowski@albertahealthservices.ca.

PELIOWSKI, Arie; The Hospital for Sick Children, 555 University Ave, Toronto ON M5G 1X8; Alb'98; MD; BSc; FRCPC; Anes (Pediatric Anesthesia). Anesthetist, The Hospital For Sick Children; Staff, Princess Margaret Hospital - University Health Network; Staff Anes, Toronto General Hospital - UHN; Langs: Spanish; (416)813-7445; Fax. (416)813-7543; arie.peliowski@sickkids.ca.

PELIPYAGINA, Tetyana O; Core Family Health Centre, 825 Richmond St, London ON N6A 3H7; Kharkov (Ukraine)'95; CCFP; (519)963-1875; Fax. (519)963-1880.

PELISSIER, Lise; 205-492 boul de l'Hopital, Gatineau QC J8V 2P4; Laval'88; cmmp@qc.aira.com.

PELISSIER-SIMARD, Luce; UMF Charles Lemoyne, 201-299 boul Sir-Wilfrid-Lauri, Saint-Lambert QC J4R 2L1; Laval'88; MSc(Epidem.); CCFP; FCFP; Dir program Postgrad Family Med & Emergency Dept, Universite de Sherbrooke; (450)466-5630; Fax. (450)466-5631.

PELKEY, Michael C; Upper River Valley Hosp, 11300 130 Rte, Watervil-Carleton NB E7P 0A4; Mem'04; FRCPC; IntMed; Endocrin&Metab. Staff, Upper River Valley Hospital - Waterville; (506)375-8488

PELL, Tripler; 1001-2200 Yonge St, Toronto ON M4S 2C6; Rhode Island (USA)'05; CCFP; Langs: Bilingual(English/French); (416)481-1173; Fax. (416)481-7431.

PELLA, Tracy L; 202-1280 Lasalle Blvd, Sudbury ON P3A 1Y8; McM'00; MSc; BPE; CCFP; Staff Faculty Clinical Sciences Div, Northern Ontario School of Medicine; (705)671-3003; Fax. (705)671-3003.

PELLA FERNANDEZ, Denisse; Bank Med Centre, 1935 Bank St, Ottawa ON K1V 8A3; Havana (Cuba)'91; CCFP; Langs: Spanish; French; (613)521-2391; Fax. (613)521-5443.

PELLAND, Camille; Hop Charles LeMoyne, 3120 boul Taschereau, Greenfield Park QC J4V 2H1; Sher'04; FRCPC; Psy. Staff, Hopital Charles LeMoyne; (450)466-5020

PELLAND, Lynne; Polyclinique Med Concorde, 300 boul de la Concorde E, Laval QC H7G 2E6; Mon'95; CCFP; Staff, Centre Hospitalier Fleury; Staff, Centre Hospitalier Honore-Mercier; (450)667-5310

PELLAND, Marcel; B-5111 ch du Lac RR 1, St-Gabriel-d-Brand QC J0K 2N0; Mon'71; assoc Staff, Hôtel-Dieu de Sorel; Langs: English; (450)535-9990

PELLAND, Marie-France; CLSC Nord de l'Ile, 11822 av de Bois-de-Boulogne, Montreal QC H3M 2X6; Mon'96; CCFP; FCFP; Staff Fam Med & Obst, Hôpital du Sacre-Coeur de Montréal; Clin Staff, Universite de Montreal; (514)331-2572; Fax. (514)331-0137.

PELLAND, Yves; Hop Riviere-Des-Prairies, 7070 boul Perras, Montreal QC H1E 1A4; Mon'70; CSPQ; Anes. Staff, Hôpital Riviere des Prairies; (514)323-7260

PELLAR, Karen E; Wortley Village Med Centre, 215-190 Wortley Rd, London ON N6C 4Y7; Wes'83; Physician, Wortley Village Medical Centre; (519)438-7666; Fax. (519)438-7418.

PELLEMANS, Wilhelm B; Clin Chirurgicale St-Martin, 607-1435 boul Saint-Martin O, Laval QC H7S 2C6; Sher'74; CSPQ; FRCS; PlasSurg (General Surgery). Langs: Bilingual(French/English); (450)669-1344; Fax. (450)669-1901.

PELLER, Andrew A; Medcan Health Mgmt Inc, 1500-150 York St, Toronto ON M5H 3S5; Tor'80; Staff, Medcan Health Management Inc; (416)350-5971; Fax. (416)350-5927.

PELLER, Joseph A; Andre Peller Ltd, 697 South Service Rd, Grimsby ON L3M 4E8; Tor'48; AACP; FRCPC; IntMed. Chairman, Andre Peller Ltd; (905)643-4131; Fax. (905)643-8927; joe.peller@andrepeller.com.

PELLERIN, Charles; CSSS de Trois-Rivières, 1991 boul du Carmel, Trois-Rivieres QC G8Z 3R9; Laval'81; CSPQ; FRCPC; Anes. Staff, CSSS de Trois-Rivières; (819)378-9700

PELLERIN, Gabriel; Centre Med Robinson Inc, 4 rue Robinson N, Granby QC J2G 8Z9; Laval'69; Staff, Centre Hospitalier de Granby; (450)378-8435; Fax. (450)375-8832.

PELLERIN, Helene; Ctr Hosp Affilie-Enfant-Jesus, 1401 18e rue, Quebec QC G1J 1Z4; Laval'00; CSPQ; FRCPC; Anes. Staff, Centre Hospitalier Affilié Universitaire de Québec - Hôpital De L'Enfant Jésus; (418)649-5807

PELLERIN, Julie; 16405 av Bourdages S, Saint-Hyacinthe QC J2T 4G9; Mon'90; Staff, Centre Hospitalier Honore-Mercier; (450)773-6734; Fax. (450)773-9909.

PELLERIN, Michel; Institut de Cardiologie de Mtl, 5000 rue Belanger, Montreal QC H1T 1C8; Laval'86; MSc; FRCSC; GenSurg (Valve Surg); Cardiovasc&ThorSurg. Chief CardioThoracic Surg, Institut de Cardiologie de Montréal; Prof Surg, Universite de Montreal; Langs: English; French; (514)593-2511; Fax. (514)376-4766.

PELLERIN, Stephane; CSSS de Trois-Rivières, 1991 boul du Carmel, Trois-Rivieres QC G8Z 3R9; Laval'86; CSPQ; Anes. Staff, CSSS de Trois-Rivières; (819)697-3333

PELLETIER, Adrien; 4-396 William St, Dalhousie NB E8C 2X2; Mon'87; (506)684-5515

PELLETIER, Alain; CSSS de la Haute-Gaspésie, 50 rue du Belvedere, Ste-Anne-des-Monts QC G4V 1X4; Laval'92; CCFP; FCFP; Fam Med, Centre Hospitalier des Monts; (418)763-2261 x2064

PELLETIER, Anick; Polyclinique Isabell-sur-Mer, 8224 rue St-Paul, Bas-Caraquet NB E1W 6E2; Sher'05; CCFP; (506)727-7549; Fax. (506)727-7320.

PELLETIER, Anne-Marie; Centre Med Fontainebleau, 102-10 boul des Chateaux, Blainville QC J7B 1Z5; Mon'00; (450)419-8811; Fax. (450)419-7758.

PELLETIER, Anne-Marie; 262 Montreal Rd PO Box 79146 Rpo Carref Vanier, Vanier ON K1L 0A3; Qns'07; CCFP; (613)619-1247

PELLETIER, Annette M; 890 Mahoney Rd, Timmins ON P4N 7C3; McM'95; BA(Psych); CCFP; FCFP; Staff, Timmins & District Hospital; (705)365-7250; paleo@ntl.sympatico.ca.

PELLETIER, Bruno; Unite de Medecine Familiale, 5689 boul Rosemont, Montreal QC H1T 2H1; Mon'95; Staff, Hopital Maisonneuve-Rosemont; (514)252-3400 x4500

PELLETIER, Carole; 66 boul de la Concorde E, Laval QC H7G 4S4; Sher'84; (450)663-4014

PELLETIER, Caroline; CSSS de Portneuf, 700 rue Saint-Cyrille, Saint-Raymond QC G3L 1W1; Laval'99; Staff, CLSC-CSSS de Port-Cartier; Staff, Centre Hospitalier Portneuf; (418)337-4611; Fax. (418)337-8919.

PELLETIER, Christine; College Ahuntsic, 9155 rue Saint-Hubert, Montreal QC H2M 1Y8; Mon'83; Langs: Spanish; English; (514)389-5921 x2630; Fax. (514)381-8931.

PELLETIER, Clarence; Hotel-Dieu de Levis, 143 rue Wolfe, Levis QC G6V 3Z1; Laval'81; FRCPC; IntMed; Respir. Staff, Hôtel-Dieu de Lévis; (418)835-7171; Fax. (418)835-7215.

PELLETIER, Conrad R; Hop du Sacre-Coeur de Mtl, 5400 boul Gouin O, Montreal QC H4J 1C5; Mon'90; FRCSC; Ophth (Cataract). Staff, Hôpital du Sacre-Coeur de Montréal; (514)338-2679; Fax. (514)338-2614.

PELLETIER, Daniele; CLSC Jean Olivier-Chenier, 29 ch d'Oka, St-Eustache QC J7R 1K6; Mon'81; (450)491-1233; Fax. (450)491-3424.

PELLETIER, Danielle; CHUM-Hotel-Dieu, 3840 rue Saint-Urbain, Montreal QC H2W 1T8; Mon'73; CSPQ; FRCPC; Anes (Anesthesia & Reanimation). Staff, Centre Hospitalier l'Université de Montréal (CHUM) - Hôtel-Dieu; Clin Teach Staff, Universite de Montreal; (514)890-8000 x14570

PELLETIER, Denis; CSSS Kamouraska-Hop Notre-Dame, CP 460 1201 6e av, La Pocatiere QC G0R 1Z0; Mon'89; Staff, CSSS de Kamouraska; Langs: Italian; English; (418)856-7000

PELLETIER, Denis P; PO Box 576 Stn Main, Edmundston NB E3V 3L2; Mon'86; Staff, Hôpital regional d'Edmundston; Physician, Centre Medical D Leach; Langs: English; (506)739-1810; Fax. (506)739-7265.

PELLETIER, Diane; Centre Med Fontainebleau, 102-10 boul des Chateaux, Blainville QC J7B 1Z5; Sher'84; Staff, Hôpital de Saint-Eustache; (450)419-8811; Fax. (450)419-7758.

PELLETIER, Fabrice; Ctr Hosp Trois-Riv-St-Joseph, 731 rue Sainte-Julie, Trois-Rivieres QC G9A 1Y1; Laval'02; FRCPC; Psy. Staff, Centre Hospitalier Regional de Trois-Rivieres; (819)697-3333 x59849

PELLETIER, Francis; Clinique Med de Nicolet, 1691 boul Louis-Frechette, Nicolet QC J3T 1Z6; Laval'82; (819)293-2022; Fax. (819)293-2024.

PELLETIER, Garry; Hop Maisonneuve-Rosemont, 5415 boul de l'Assomption, Montreal QC H1T 2M4; Mon'99; Staff Emerg, Hopital Maisonneuve-Rosemont; (514)252-3400

PELLETIER, Gaston; CSSS de Memphremagog, 50 rue Saint-Patrice E, Magog QC J1X 3X3; Laval'69; Staff, Centre Hospitalier et CLSC de Memphremagog; (819)843-3381; Fax. (819)868-9318.

PELLETIER, Gilles; CSSS de la Baie-des-Chaleurs, RR 2 419 boul Perron, Maria QC G0C 1Y0; Mon'88; CCFP; Staff, CSSS de la Baie-des-Chaleurs; (418)759-3443

PELLETIER, Gilles; Ctr Hosp Affilie-Enfant-Jesus, 1401 18e rue, Quebec QC G1J 1Z4; Laval'98; FRCPC; MedMicrobiol; Microbio & Infect Dis (P.Q.). Staff, Centre Hospitalier Affilié Universitaire de Québec - Hôpital De L'Enfant Jésus; (418)649-0252

PELLETIER, Gilles; Hôpital Ste-Justine, 3175 ch Cote-Sainte-Catherine, Montreal QC H3T 1C5; Laval'78; MD(NeurolSciences); Psy (Child Psychiatry). Ac Staff, Hôpital Ste-Justine; (514)345-4931 x5596; Fax. (514)345-4880.

PELLETIER, Guy B; Institut de Cardiologie de Mtl, 5000 rue Belanger, Montreal QC H1T 1C8; McG'72; Cardiol (P.Q.); IntMed. Staff, Institut de Cardiologie de Montréal; (514)376-3330; Fax. (514)593-2540.

PELLETIER, Helene; Institut de Cardiologie de Mtl, 5000 rue Belanger, Montreal QC H1T 1C8; Mon'93; Staff, Institut de Cardiologie de Montréal; (514)376-3330

PELLETIER, Isabelle; CSSS Kamouraska-Hop Notre-Dame, CP 460 1201 6e av, La Pocatiere QC G0R 1Z0; Laval'97; Staff, CSSS de Kamouraska; (418)856-7000; Fax. (418)856-2265.

PELLETIER, J Steve N; Clarence-Rockland Fam Hlth Team, 2741 rue Chamberland, Rockland ON K4K 0B4; Ott'82; MBA; CCFP; FCFP; (613)446-7677; Fax. (613)446-5737; jnt@istar.ca.

PELLETIER, J E Claude; Ctr de Med Familiale de Granby, 48 rue Denison E, Granby QC J2G 4C6; Mon'79; (450)372-3996; Fax. (450)372-0430.

PELLETIER, Alain; Ctr Hosp du Centre la Mauricie, 50 119e rue, Shawinigan-Sud QC G9P 5K1; Mon'86; Staff, Centre Hospitalier du Centre la Mauricie; Langs: English; French; (819)536-7500; Fax. (819)536-7653.

PELLETIER, Jacques; 116 boul Gerard-D.-Levesque CP 940, Paspebiac QC G0C 2K0; Mon'83; CCFP; Staff, CLSC de Paspebiac; (418)752-6331; Fax. (418)752-6981.

PELLETIER, Jacques; CHUQ-St-Francois d'Assise, 10 rue de l'Espinay, Quebec QC G1L 3L5; Laval'78; CSPQ; FRCPC; Anes. ac Staff Anes, Centre Hospitalier Universitaire De Québec - Pavillon De St-françois-d'assise; (418)525-4340; Fax. (418)525-4434.

PELLETIER, Jean; CLSC la Petite Patrie, 6520 rue de Saint-Vallier, Montreal QC H2S 2P7; Laval'87; Staff, Institut Universitaire de Gériatrie de Montréal; (514)273-5600; Fax. (514)273-9288.

PELLETIER, Jean; Clinique de Med Familiale, 6F-2120 rue Sherbrooke E, Montreal QC H2K 1C3; Laval'86; CCFP; FCFP; Staff GenMed, Centre Hospitalier l'Université de Montréal (CHUM) - Hôtel-Dieu; dép Chef Family Med, Universite de Montreal; Langs: English; (514)527-1958; Fax. (514)527-1649; jean.pelletier@umontreal.ca.

PELLETIER, Jean-Philippe; MUHC-Royal Victoria Hosp, M4. 76-687 av des Pins O, Montreal QC H3A 1A1; McG'96; FRCPC; IntMed; Cardiol. Staff, McGill University Health Centre - Royal Victoria Hospital; (514)934-1934

PELLETIER, Jean-Pierre; CHUM-Hop Notre-Dame, 1560 rue Sherbrooke E, Montreal QC H2L 4M1; Mon'74; FACP; CSPQ; Rheum; IntMed. Staff Rheum, Centre Hospitalier l'Université de Montréal (CHUM) - Hôpital Notre-Dame; Prof, Universite de Montreal; (514)890-8000 x27216; Fax. (514)412-7582.

PELLETIER, Jean-Sebastien; University of Alberta Hosp, 2D3. 77-8440 112 St NW, Edmonton AB T6G 2B7; Ott'06; FRCSC; GenSurg. Staff, University of Alberta Hospital; (780)407-8822

PELLETIER, Jerry F; 277 Falshire Dr NE, Calgary AB T3J 1T9; Cal'79; BSc(Hons.); CCFP; FCFP; (403)293-7800

PELLETIER, Jocelyn; Dr Georges-L Dumont Reg Hosp, 330 av Universite, Moncton NB E1C 2Z3; Sher'01; FRCPC; Anes. Staff, Dr Georges-L-Dumont University Hospital Centre; (506)862-4000

PELLETIER, Jocelyne; Clin Dermatologique Longueuil, 501 rue Adoncour, Longueuil QC J4G 2M6; Sher'76; DABD; FRCPC; Derm. (450)651-8707

PELLETIER, Johanne; 207-235 boul René-Lévesque E, Montreal QC H2X 1N8; Laval'78; FRCSC; PlasSurg. Staff, Centre Hospitalier l'Université De Montréal (CHUM) - Hôpital Saint-luc; Teach Staff, Universite de Montreal; (514)393-4592

PELLETIER, Julie; CSSS de Rimouski-Neigette, CP 3150 Succ A 150 av Rouleau, Rimouski QC G5L 5T1; Sher'98; CSPQ; FRCPC; Anes. Staff, Hôpital Regional Rimouski; (418)723-7851

PELLETIER, Julien; CHUQ-Ctr Hosp Univ Laval, 2705 boul Laurier, Quebec QC G1V 4G2; Laval'99; FRCPC; Psy (Emergency Psychiatry). Staff, Centre Hospitalier Universitaire de Quebec-CHUL; Langs: Bilingual(English/French); (418)654-2121

PELLETIER, Kathleen; Dir de la Sante Publique, 930 rue Jacques-Cartier E, Chicoutimi QC G7H 7K9; Sher'90; Staff, Complexe hospitalier de la Sagamie; (418)545-4980 x431; Fax. (418)549-9710; kathleen.pelletier@ssss.gouv.qc.ca.

PELLETIER, Lorraine; CSSS Pierre Boucher, 1333 boul Jacques-Cartier E, Longueuil QC J4M 2A5; Sher'76; Microbio & Infect Dis (P.Q.); MedMicrobiol (P.Q.) (Infectious Diseases). Staff, Centre Hospitalier Pierre Boucher; (450)468-8111; lorraine.pelletier@rrsss16.gouv.qc.ca.

PELLETIER, Louis-Philippe; CSSS du Lac-des-Deux-Montagnes, 520 boul Arthur-Sauve, Saint-Eustache QC J7R 5B1; Laval'04; FRCPC; EmergMed. Staff, Hôpital de Saint-Eustache; (450)473-6811

PELLETIER, Louise; Agence Sante Publique Canada, AL6502G-785 Carling Ave, Ottawa ON K1S 5H4; Laval'87; FRCPC; CommunMed. Physician Hlth Promotion & Chronic Disease Prevention, Direction de la Sante Publique de l'Outaouais; (613)796-0672; Fax. (613)941-2057.

PELLETIER, Luc; CHUQ-Ctr Hosp Univ Laval, 2705 boul Laurier, Quebec QC G1V 4G2; Laval'83; FRCPC; Peds. Ac Staff, Centre Hospitalier Universitaire de Quebec-CHUL; (418)654-2282; Fax. (418)654-2137.

PELLETIER, Lysanne; CSSS de Rimouski-Neigette, CP 3150 Succ A 150 av Rouleau, Rimouski QC G5L 5T1; Sher'03; FRCPC; IntMed; Endocrin&Metab. Staff, Hôpital Regional Rimouski; Langs: Bilingual(French/English); (418)724-3000; Fax. (418)724-8573.

PELLETIER, Manon M A; Cross Lake Nursing Station, PO Box 160, Cross Lake MB R0B 0J0; Sher'10; CCFP; Staff, Cross Lake Nursing Station; (204)676-2011; Fax. (204)676-3179.

PELLETIER, Marc P; Saint John Reg Hosp, PO Box 2100 Stn Main 400 University Ave, Saint John NB E2L 4L2; Dal'94; MSc; BSc; FRCSC; CardSurg (Aortic Aneurysm Surg). Staff, Saint John Regional Hospital; (506)648-6000

PELLETIER, Marcel J; Clinique Medicale PL, 5-85 rue Saint-Charles O, Longueuil QC J4H 1C5; Laval'72; Physician, Centre Hospitalier Pierre Boucher; Langs: Bilingual(French/English); (450)674-9455; Fax. (450)674-9051; cliniquepl@qc.aira.com.

PELLETIER, Marie; Centre Med Christ-Roi, 102-40 rte du President-Kenned, Levis QC G6V 6C4; Laval'88; Staff, CSSS de Montmagny-l'Islet; Staff, CSSS de Montmagny-L'Islet; (418)833-4977

PELLETIER, Marie-Chantal; CHUM-Hop St-Luc, 1058 rue Saint-Denis, Montreal QC H2X 3J4; Mon'06; CCFP; Staff, Centre Hospitalier l'Université De Montréal (CHUM) - Hôpital Saint-luc; (514)890-8321

PELLETIER, Marie-Eve; CSSS de St-Jerome, 290 rue de Montigny, Saint-Jerome QC J7Z 5T3; Sher'05; Cardiol; IntMed. Staff, Hôtel-Dieu de Saint-Jérôme; (450)431-8200

PELLETIER, Marie-France; Ctr Hosp Anna-Laberge, 200 boul Brisebois, Chateauguay QC J6K 4W8; Laval'02; CCFP; Staff, Hôpital Anna-Laberge; (450)699-2425

PELLETIER, Marie-Josee; CHUQ-Hotel-Dieu de Quebec, 11 Cote-du-Palais, Quebec QC G1R 2J6; Sher'05; IntMed. Staff, Centre Hospitalier Universitaire de Québec (CHUQ) - Siege Social; (418)525-4444

PELLETIER, Marie-Josee; CHUQ-Ctr Hosp Univ Laval, 2705 boul Laurier, Quebec QC G1V 4G2; Laval'04; Cardiol; IntMed. Staff, Centre Hospitalier Universitaire de Quebec-CHUL; (418)525-4444

PELLETIER, Mario; CSSS de Trois-Rivières, 1991 boul du Carmel, Trois-Rivieres QC G8Z 3R9; Mon'98; FRCSC; Neursurg. Staff, CSSS de Trois-Rivières; (819)697-3333

PELLETIER, Martin; CSSS de Montmagny-L'Islet, RR 1 350 boul Tache O, Montmagny QC G5V 3R8; Laval'97; Staff, CSSS de Montmagny-L'Islet; (418)248-0630

PELLETIER, Mathieu; UMF du Nord de Lanaudiere, 50 ch du Golf E, St-Charles-Brromee QC J6E 2B4; Mon'01; CCFP; Staff Emerg, Centre Hospitalier Régional de Lanaudière; (450)759-3060; Fax. (450)759-7799.

PELLETIER, Michel; Institut de Physiatrie Quebec, 2049 rue Sherbrooke E, Montreal QC H2K 1C1; Mon'78; FRCPC; PhysMed&Rehab. Staff, Centre Hospitalier l'Université de Montréal (CHUM) - Hôpital Notre-Dame; (514)527-4155; Fax. (514)896-4708.

PELLETIER, Michele; AQESSS, 400-505 boul de Maisonneuve O, Montreal QC H3A 3C2; Mon'74; Dir, Raymond Chabot Grant Thornton; Langs: English; (514)282-4241

PELLETIER, Micheline; CHSLD Emilie-Gamelin, 1440 rue Dufresne, Montreal QC H2K 3J3; Mon'65; CSPQ; GenPath (P.Q.). (514)527-8921 x4600

PELLETIER, Pascal; CSSS de Trois-Rivières, 1991 boul du Carmel, Trois-Rivieres QC G8Z 3R9; Laval'03; FRCPC; MedBiochem. Staff, CSSS de Trois-Rivières; (819)697-3333

PELLETIER, Patricia; MUHC-Royal Victoria Hosp, 687 av des Pins O, Montreal QC H3A 1A1; McG'98; FRCPC; IntMed; Hem. Staff, McGill University Health Centre - Royal Victoria Hospital; (514)843-1558; Fax. (514)843-1418.

PELLETIER, Paul; CLSC des Faubourgs, 2260 rue Parthenais, Montreal QC H2K 3T5; Mon'96; Staff, Centre Hospitalier de Matane; (514)527-2361

PELLETIER, Pierre; 323 rue Sherbrooke CP 594 Csp Magog, Magog QC J1X 4W3; Sher'79; (819)847-1313; Fax. (819)847-3529.

PELLETIER, Pierre; Clinique Med Pierre-Bertrand, 212-303 boul Pierre-Bertrand, Quebec QC G1M 3L7; Laval'79; Ac Staff, CSSS de Quebec-Sud; (418)683-2721 x1433; Fax. (418)683-8861.

PELLETIER, Rene; CHUQ-Hotel-Dieu de Quebec, 11 Cote du Palais, Quebec QC G1R 2J6; Laval'77; FRCPC; MedMicrobiol (Infectiology); Microbio & Infect Dis (P.Q.). Staff, Centre Hospitalier Universitaire de Québec (CHUQ) - Siege Social; Langs: English; French; (418)691-5131; rene.pelletier@chuq.qc.ca.

PELLETIER, Renee; CLSC Cote-des-Neiges, 500-5700 ch de la Cote-des-Nei, Montreal QC H3T 2A8; Mon'76; (514)731-8531

PELLETIER, Stephan; CSSS Drummond-Hop Sainte-Croix, 570 rue Heriot, Drummondville QC J2B 1C1; Laval'93; CSPQ; FRCPC; Anes. Staff, Hôpital Sainte-croix; (819)478-6464; Fax. (819)478-6453.

PELLETIER, Stephanie; Clin Familiale du Boulevard, 19-300 boul Saint-Luc, St-Jean-sur-Richel QC J2W 2A3; Mon'01; (450)349-3333

PELLETIER, Suzanne; Clinique de l'Atelier, 77 boul Seigneurial O, Saint-Bruno QC J3V 2G9; Mon'92; FRCPC; Peds (Attention Deficit Hyperactivity Disorder). Langs: Bilingual(French/English); (450)461-1751; Fax. (450)461-1602.

PELLETIER, Sylvie; CSSS de Chicoutimi, 305 rue Saint-Vallier, Chicoutimi QC G7H 5H6; Sher'90; CCFP; CCFP(E.M.); FCFP; EmergMed (P.Q.). Staff, Complexe hospitalier de la Sagamie; Staff, Centre Hospitalier de Val d'Or; (418)541-1000; dre. pelletier@cablevision.qc.ca.

PELLETIER, Veronique Anne; Hôpital Ste-Justine, 3175 ch Cote-Sainte-Catherine, Montreal QC H3T 1C5; Laval'79; FRCPC; Peds (Nutrition). Ac Staff Peds, Hôpital Ste-Justine; adj Prof, Universite de Montreal; Langs: English; (514)345-4675; Fax. (514)345-4822; va.pelletier@umontreal.ca.

PELLETIER, Yvan; Inst Albert Prevost, 6555 boul Gouin O, Montreal QC H4K 1B3; Sher'83; Psy. Staff, Hôpital du Sacre-Coeur de Montréal; (514)338-2222 x4327

PELLEY, Lorraine V J; 2815 Main St PO Box 94, Shubenacadie NS B0N 2H0; Mem'91; BSc(Biol.); CCFP; FCFP; (902)758-2655; Fax. (902)758-3606.

PELLIGRA, Gustavo; Victoria Gen Hosp, 1 Hospital Way, Victoria BC V8Z 6R5; Buenos Aires (Argentina)'96; FRCPC; Peds. Staff, Victoria General Hospital; (250)727-4493

PELLISSIER, Janse V; Community Medi Centre, 2707 50 Ave, Lloydminster SK S9V 2A8; (306)825-4427; Fax. (306)825-2028.

PELLIZZARI, Michael P; The Jenny Trout Centre, 204-342 Erie St, Stratford ON N5A 2N4; (Australia)'08; CCFP; (519)271-3123; Fax. (519)271-6760.

PELLIZZARI, Rosana; Peterborough County Hlth Unit, 10 Hospital Dr, Peterborough ON K9J 8M1; McM'87; MSc; DOHS; FRCPC; CCFP; CommunMed; Public Health & Preventive Med. Staff, Stratford General Hospital - Huron Perth Healthcare Alliance; Staff, Listowel Memorial Hospital - Listowel Wingham Hospitals Alliance; Asst Prof Epidemiol & Biostatistics, University of Western Ontario; Asst Prof Community & Family Med, University of Toronto; Langs: Italian; Spanish; Nepali; (705)743-1000; rpellizzari@pcchu.ca.

PELLOW, M Robin; Medical Office, 2-8000 Bathurst St, Thornhill ON L4J 0B8; Qns'87; CCFP; CCFP(E.M.); Ac Staff Emerg & Family Med, Women's College Hospital; Instructor Family & Community Med, University of Toronto; (905)709-9709; Fax. (905)709-9701.

PELLOW, Tanya R; Abbie J Lane Mem Bldg, 5909 Veterans Memorial Lane, Halifax NS B3H 2E2; Dal'01; FRCPC; Psy. (902)473-6334

PELMAN, Aaron M; Dominion Med Centre, 2383 111 St NW, Edmonton AB T6J 5E5; UBC'10; CCFP; (780)436-0020; Fax. (780)436-0603.

PELOQUIN, Anne; CSSS de Laval, 1755 boul Rene-Laennec, Laval QC H7M 3L9; Sher'82; CSPQ; AnatPath; ObstGyn (Gynecology & Infertility). Staff, Hopital de la Cite de la santé; (450)975-5302; Fax. (450)975-5061.

PELOQUIN, Caroline; Clinique Fam de St-Hyacinthe, 2955 boul Laframboise, Saint-Hyacinthe QC J2S 4Z3; Sher'94; CCFP; Staff, Centre Hospitalier Honore-Mercier; Langs: Bilingual(French/English); (450)774-4611; Fax. (450)773-9913.

PELOQUIN, Francois A; CHUM-Hop St-Luc, 1058 rue Saint-Denis, Montreal QC H2L 4M1; Sher'84; MSc(ExperimentalSurg); CSPQ; FRCSC; Urol. Staff, Centre Hospitalier l'Université de Montréal (CHUM) - Hôpital Notre-Dame; Clinical Asst Prof, Universite de Montreal; Langs: English; (514)890-8000 x34444

PELOQUIN, Francois; CSSS de Lac-Saint Jean-Est, CP 1300 Succ Bureau-Chef 300 boul Champlain S, Alma QC G8B 5W3; Mon'09; Staff, CSSS de Lac-Saint Jean-Est; (418)669-2000

PELOQUIN, Jacques; GMF Montee de la Baie, RR 22 3942 ch d'Oka, St-Joseph-du-Lac QC J0N 1M0; Mon'90; Staff, Hôpital de Saint-Eustache; Langs: English; (450)473-3930; Fax. (450)473-2160.

PELOQUIN, Jean; Hop Charles Lemoyne, 3120 boul Taschereau, Greenfield Park QC J4V 2H1; Mon'77; FRCPC; Psy. ac Staff, Hopital Charles LeMoyne; Staff, Centre de Sante de la Haute-Gaspesie; Langs: English; (450)466-5020; Fax. (450)466-5015.

PELOQUIN, Jean; 2705 boul Laurier, Quebec QC G1V 4G2; Laval'73; FRCSC; GenSurg (Pediatric Surgery). Ac Staff, Centre Hospitalier Universitaire de Quebec-CHUL; Clin Prof Surg, Université Laval; Langs: English; French; Spanish; (418)654-2259; Fax. (418)654-2276; jean.peloquin@chg.ulaval. ca.

PELOQUIN, Laurence; CHUM-Hotel-Dieu, 3840 rue Saint-Urbain, Montreal QC H2W 1T8; McG'02; FRCPC; DiagRad. Staff, Centre Hospitalier l'Université de Montréal (CHUM) - Hôtel-Dieu; (514)890-8059

PELOQUIN, Louis; Hop Maisonneuve-Rosemont, 5415 boul de l'Assomption, Montreal QC H1T 2M4; Mon'89; ABOtol; FRCSC; Otol (Rhinology). Chief Dept of Surg, Hopital Maisonneuve-Rosemont; Prof, Universite de Montreal; (514)252-3400; Fax. (514)252-3458.

PELOQUIN, Lucie; Unite Med Familiale Maizerets, 2480 ch de la Canardiere, Quebec QC G1J 2G1; Sher'00; CCFP; Staff, Centre Hospitalier Affilié Universitaire de Québec - Hôpital De L'Enfant Jésus; Staff, Centre Hospitalier Universitaire De Québec - Pavillon De St-françois-d'assise; Physician EmergMed, Centre de Sante Orleans-Ste Anne de Beaupre; (418)661-1413; Fax. (418)661-7504.

PELOQUIN, Marie M; Clinique Jacques-Cartier, 200-1815 rue King O, Sherbrooke QC J1J 2E3; Sher'90; FRCPC; IntMed; GeriatricMed. Staff, Institut Universitaire de Geriatrie de Sherbrooke-Pavillon Argyll; (819)565-4446; mpeloquin.iugs@ssss.gouv.qc.ca.

PELOQUIN, Michel-Andre; Centre Med St-Charles, 357 rue de la Visitation, St-Charles-Brromee QC J6E 4N8; Sher'75; Staff Emerg, Centre Hospitalier Régional de Lanaudière; (450)759-5421; Fax. (450)759-5424.

PELOQUIN, Patrice; Clinique Med Warwick, 5A rue du Centre Sportif RR 3, Warwick QC J0A 1M0; Mon'94; BSc(Microbiol); MSc(Microbiol.); CCFP; (819)358-4600; Fax. (819)358-4620.

PELOQUIN, Robert; CSSS d'Antoine-Labelle-Mt Laur, RR 1 2561 ch de la Lièvre S, Mont-Laurier QC J9L 3G3; Mon'63; MedOncol (P.Q.); Hem (P.Q.). Staff, CSSS d'Antoine-Labelle; assoc Staff, Centre de L'Annociation; (819)623-1234 x4272

PELOQUIN, Sonia; CSSS Haut Richelieu-Rouville, 978 boul du Seminaire N, St-Jean-sur-Richel QC J3A 1E5; Sher'90; Médecin, CLSC-CHLSD Champagnat Vallee des Forts; (450)358-2572

PELOQUIN, Sophie; Coop Sante Contrecoeur, GD 4915 Rte Marie-Victorin, Contrecoeur QC J0L 1C0; Mon'94; LMCC; CCFP; Staff, CSSS Sorel-Tracy; (450)587-5998; Fax. (450)587-8866.

PELSER, Duane D; Welland McMaster Family Hlth Team, PO Box 920 2 Pancake Lane, Fonthill ON L0S 1E0; Pretoria (South Africa)'98; CCFP; (905)892-6333; Fax. (905)892-0394.

PELSER, Lorraine A; Fort St John Med Clinic, 10011 96 St, Fort St. John BC V1J 3P3; Pretoria (South Africa)'99; (250)785-6677; Fax. (250)787-0109.

PELSSER, Vincent; SMBD Jewish Gen Hosp, 3755 ch Cote-Sainte-Catherine, Montreal QC H3T 1E2; Mon'00; CSPQ; FRCPC; DiagRad. Staff, Sir Mortimer B Davis Jewish General; (514)340-8222

PELTEKIAN, Kevork Minas; Queen Elizabeth II HSC, 6-1276 South Park St, Halifax NS B3H 2Y9; Beirut (Lebanon)'85; DrMedCh; BSc; Gastroent; IntMed (Hepatology). Med Dir Atlantic Multi-Organ Transplant Prog/Ac Staff, Queen Elizabeth II Health Sciences Centre - Victoria General Site; Pres, Canadian Association for Study of Liver; Assoc Prof Med & Surg, Dalhousie University; Langs: Arabic; Armenian; English; French; (902)473-7833; Fax. (902)473-2783.

PELTZ, Julie E; Carlingwood Sport Medicine, 12-2121 Carling Ave, Ottawa ON K2A 1H2; Tor'88; (613)798-7277; Fax. (613)798-7273.

PELTZ, Lou; The Credit Valley Hosp, 2200 Eglinton Ave W, Mississauga ON L5M 2N1; McM'83; FRCPC; Psy. Med Staff Psy, The Credit Valley Hospital; Med Staff, The Hospital For Sick Children; Lecturer, University of Toronto; (905)813-4466; Fax. (905)813-1594.

PELUOLA, Akinlolu O; Victory Med Associates, 137 20th St W, Saskatoon SK S7M 0W7; Ibadan (Nigeria)'83; MB BS; DPM(Ire); FRCP; FRCPC; Psy. Consultant Psy, Royal University Hospital; Clinical Asst Prof, University of Saskatchewan; Langs: Yoruba; (306)249-2227; Fax. (306)249-2348.

PELZ, David M; London HSC-University Hosp, PO Box 5339 Stn B 339 Windermere Rd, London ON N6A 5A5; Wes'75; FRCPC; DiagRad (Neuro Radiology). Prof Dept of Diagnostic Rad/Nuclear Med & Clinical Neurological Sciences, London Health Sciences Centre - University Hospital; Assoc Prof Clin Neurol Sciences, University of Western Ontario; (519)685-8500 x32429; Fax. (519)663-8803; pelz@uwo.ca.

PELZ, Margaret A; 30-186 King St, London ON N6A 1C7; Wes'76; FRCPC; Psy. (519)642-3599

PEN, Visal; CSSS de Laval, 1755 boul Rene-Laennec, Laval QC H7M 3L9; Mon'00; CSPQ; FRCPC; DiagRad. Staff, Hopital de la Cite de la santé; (450)668-1010

PENA FERNANDEZ, Elena; The Ottawa Hosp-Gen Campus, 501 Smyth Rd, Ottawa ON K1H 8L6; Madrid (Spain)'02; Staff, The Ottawa Hospital - General Campus; (613)719-2775

PENAVA, Deborah A; St Joseph's Health Care, PO Box 5777 Stn B 268 Grosvenor St, London ON N6A 4V2; Wes'94; MPH; FRCSC; ObstGyn. Staff, St Joseph's Hospital - St Joseph's Health Care; Asst Prof, University of Western Ontario; (519)646-6326; Fax. (519)646-6360.

PENAVA, Laura M; Central Family Practice, 3955 Tecumseh Rd E, Windsor ON N8W 1J5; Wes'95; BSc; CCFP; FCFP; (519)948-3916; Fax. (519)948-0422.

PENCHARZ, James N; Credit Valley Family Hlth Team, 101-2300 Eglinton Ave W, Mississauga ON L5M 2V8; Tor'07; CCFP; (905)813-3850; Fax. (905)813-3853.

PENCHARZ, Paul B; The Hosp for Sick Children, 555 University Ave, Toronto ON M5G 1X8; Liverpool (England)'67; MB ChB; PhD; FRCPC; Peds (Gastroenterology). Staff Gastroent & Nutrition/Sr Scientist, The Hospital For Sick Children; Prof Peds & Nutritional Sciences, University of Toronto; (416)813-6171; Fax. (416)813-4972.

PENCINER, Richard D; North York Gen Hosp, 4001 Leslie St, North York ON M2K 1E1; Tor'91; FCFP; CCFP; CCFP(E.M.); FCFP; Ac Staff, North York General Hospital; Asst Prof, University of Toronto; (416)756-6165; rick.penciner@utoronto.ca.

PENCLE, Franz; Queen Elizabeth II HSC-Halifax, 1796 Summer St, Halifax NS B3H 3A7; West Indies (Jamaica)'00; Staff, Queen Elizabeth II Health Sciences Centre - Halifax Infirmary Site; (902)473-7214

PENDERELL, Adrienne D; Community Care Access Ctre, 310 Limeridge Rd W, Hamilton ON L9C 2V2; Dal'05; CCFP; (905)523-8600; Fax. (905)574-6335.

PENDERGAST, Amanda L; Shea Heights Community H C, PO Box 13122 57B Linegar Ave, St. John's NL A1B 4A4; Ott'99; CCFP.

PENDERGAST, Patrick J F; 205-8312 McCowan Rd, Unionville ON L3P 8E1; Tor'87; FRCSC; GenSurg. (905)947-9437; Fax. (905)947-8532.

PENDERGAST, Sara R; St Mary's Gen Hosp, 911 Queens Blvd, Kitchener ON N2M 1B2; Tor'92; CCFP; CCFP(E.M.); Staff, St Mary's General Hospital; (519)749-6910

PENDERGRAST, Jacob M; Univ Hlth Network-Toronto Gen, 3EC 306-200 Elizabeth St, Toronto ON M5G 2C4; Dal'99; FRCPC; IntMed (Transfusion Medicine); Hem. Staff Blood Transfusion Service Dept of Lab Hematol, Toronto General Hospital - UHN; (416)340-5390

PENDHARKAR, Raveendra B; Credit Valley Med Arts Centre, 403-2000 Credit Valley Rd, Mississauga ON L5M 4N4; Bombay (India)'68; MB BS; FRCPC; Psy (Adult Psychiatry). Ac Staff Psy, Trillium Health Centre - Mississauga; (905)412-3142; Fax. (905)412-3142.

PENDHARKAR, Sachin R; Rockyview Gen Hosp, 7007 14 St SW, Calgary AB T2V 1P9; Wes'02; FRCPC; IntMed (Sleep Medicine); Respir. Staff, Rockyview General Hospital; Langs: Marathi; (403)943-3475; Fax. (403)943-8666.

PENDHARKAR, Sushama R; Credit Valley Med Arts Centre, 403-2000 Credit Valley Rd, Mississauga ON L5M 4N4; Nagpur (India)'69; MB BS; FRCPC; Psy (Adult Psychiatry). Ac Staff Psy, Trillium Health Centre - Mississauga; Langs: Hindi; (905)412-3142; Fax. (905)412-3142.

PENES, Mihai C; CLSC des Mille-Iles, 4731 boul Levesque E, Laval QC H7C 1M9; (450)661-2572

PENFOLD, Jamie L; 135 MacBeath Ave, Moncton NB E1C 6Z8; UBC'87; BSc; FRCPC; Anes (Pain Management). Staff, The Moncton Hospital; (506)857-5258; Fax. (506)857-5261; jpenfold@nbnet.nb.ca.

PENFOLD, P Susan; BC Children's Hosp, H201-4480 Oak St, Vancouver BC V6H 3V4; London (England)'60; MB BS; MRCS; LRCP; FRCPC; Psy (Child & Adolescent Psychiatry). Staff Child & Family Clinic, BC Children's Hospital; Staff, Delta Child & Youth Mental Health; (604)875-2000 x5977; spenfold@cw.bc.ca.

PENG, Carol; 309-1920 Ellesmere Rd, Scarborough ON M1H 2V6; (Hong Kong)'88; MB BS; FRCSC; ObstGyn. Staff, The Scarborough Hospital - General Campus; Langs: Cantonese; (416)289-0519; Fax. (416)289-3910.

PENG, Judy; Glenrose Rehabilitation Hosp, 1259-10230 111 Ave NW, Edmonton AB T5G 0B7; (China)'91; DipCE; CCFP; Staff, Glenrose Rehabilitation Hospital; (780)735-8800; Fax. (780)735-8846.

PENG, Philip W; Univ Hlth Network-Toronto Western Hosp, MCL2 405-399 Bathurst St, Toronto ON M5T 2S8; (Hong Kong)'87; FRCPC; Anes. Staff Anes, Toronto Western Hospital - University Health Network; Asst Prof, University of Toronto; Langs: Chinese; (416)603-5118; Fax. (416)603-6494; philip.peng@uhn.on.ca.

PENGILLY, Christopher J; Tuscany Med Clinic, 102-1646 McKenzie Ave, Victoria BC V8N 0A3; Leeds (England)'69; MB ChB; CCFP; (250)818-0001; drpeng@telus.net.

PENHALL, John R H; Quinsam Med Clinic, 280-1400 Dogwood St, Campbell River BC V9W 3A6; Pretoria (South Africa)'94; MB ChB; CCFP; Langs: Afrikaans; Greek; (250)286-3053; Fax. (250)286-0504; jpenhall2002@yahoo.ca.

PENISTON, Charles M; 100-30 Prospect St, Newmarket ON L3Y 3S9; McG'81; DABS; DABTS; FACS; FRCSC; GenSurg (Cardiac Surgery); Cardiovasc&ThorSurg. Staff, Southlake Regional Health Centre; (905)868-8374; Fax. (905)868-8371; cmpeniston@gmail.com.

PENISTON, Neil T; Douglas Square Med Centre, 144-11520 24 St SE, Calgary AB T2Z 3E9; (South Africa)'78; (403)236-0211; Fax. (403)236-0261.

PENKMAN, Michael A; Oak Bay Med Centre, 159-2515 90 Ave SW, Calgary AB T2V 0L8; Cal'04; CCFP; (403)281-2020

PENMAN, John; Dept of Laboratory Med, 120 King George Terr, Victoria BC V8S 2K1; Cape Town (South Africa)'72; Staff, Victoria General Hospital; (250)589-9406

PENN, Andrew M W; Westside Integrated Health Ctr, 130-180 Wilson St, Victoria BC V9A 7N6; Cambridge (England)'80; FRCPC; Neur (Neuromuscular Diseases). (250)595-1551

PENN, Caroline M G; Eagle Ridge Hosp & Health C C, 475 Guildford Way, Port Moody BC V3H 3W9; UBC'82; CCFP; FCFP; Staff, Eagle Ridge Hospital & Health Care Centre; Staff, Travel Medicine & Vaccination Centre; (604)461-2022; cmpenn@sfu.ca.

PENN, Jeffrey R; 1-779 Prince St, Truro NS B2N 1G7; Massachusetts (USA)'77; ABNP; FRCPC; Psy (Psycho Pharmacology). Court Staff, Colchester East Hants Health Centre; Staff Psy, Nova Institution(CSC); (902)895-4055; Fax. (902)895-4344.

PENNELL, Mark L; 23-112 Front St, Wolfville NS B4P 1A4; Southampton (England)'82; MB(UK); MRCGPract; DRCOG; LMCC; (902)542-9343; Fax. (902)542-9558.

PENNER, Charles G; Brandon Reg Health Centre, 150 McTavish Ave E, Brandon MB R7A 2B3; Man'88; FRCPC; IntMed (Intensive Care); Critical Care Medicine; Respir. (204)578-4000

PENNER, Darrell A; Lindsay Park Sport Med Centre, 2225 Macleod Trail SE, Calgary AB T2G 5B6; Qns'78; FAAOS; DAB; FRCSC; OrthSurg (Knee Surgery). (403)221-8350; Fax. (403)221-8352.

PENNER, E Roseanne; Salveo Family Med Clinic, B8-6455 Macleod Trail SW, Calgary AB T2H 0K8; Cal'96; BSc; CCFP; Clin Assoc Prof, University of Calgary; (403)444-0428; Fax. (403)537-0029; erp@telusplanet.net.

PENNER, Jeremy; UBC Dept of Family Practice, 320-5950 University Ave, Vancouver BC V6T 1Z3; McM'01; CCFP; (604)827-4183

PENNER, Kristy J; PO Box 70, Coleman AB T0K 0M0; Alb'08; CCFP.

PENNER, Kurt; Victoria Gen Hosp, 2340 Pembina Hwy, Winnipeg MB R3T 2E8; Man'97; CCFP; CCFP(E.M.); Staff, Victoria General Hospital; (204)269-3570

PENNER, Layna R; St Boniface Gen Hosp, M4-409 Tache Ave, Winnipeg MB R2H 2A6; Man'90; FRCPC; Psy (Child & Adolescent Psychiatry). Staff, St Boniface General Hospital; (204)233-8563

PENNER, Lisa F; McKenzie Family Practice, 71 High St SE, Calgary AB T2Z 3T9; Man'91; CCFP; (403)257-0500; Fax. (403)257-3186.

PENNER, Lynnette E; Pacific Med Clinic, 2F-3185 Grandview Hwy, Vancouver BC V5M 2E9; UBC'96; CCFP; (604)434-2222; Fax. (604)434-2220.

PENNER, Melanie J; University of Toronto, 500 University Ave, Toronto ON M5G 1V7; Qns'08; Peds.

PENNER, Monica A; Kelowna Gen Hosp, 2268 Pandosy St, Kelowna BC V1Y 1T2; Alb'99; FRCPC; Anes. Staff, Kelowna General Hospital; (250)862-4309

PENNER, Murray J; 1000-1200 Burrard St, Vancouver BC V6Z 2C7; Cal'92; BSc(Mech.Eng); FRCSC; OrthSurg (Foot & Ankle Surgery). Staff, Royal Columbian Hospital; Physician Visiting Specialist, Workmen's Compensation Board; Teach Staff Orthopedics, University of British Columbia; (604)669-0101; Fax. (604)669-0104; murray.penner@worksafebc.com.

PENNER, Peter R; 1035 Cameron Ave, Kelowna BC V1Y 8V4; Man'87; (250)864-4488

PENNER, Ramona C; St Georges Med Clinic, 1315 St. Georges Ave, North Vancouver BC V7L 3J2; UBC'89; Staff, Lions Gate Hospital; (604)984-9213; Fax. (604)986-1390; ramocpener@sgmc.ca.

PENNER, Raymond C; St Georges Med Clinic, 1315 St. Georges Ave, North Vancouver BC V7L 3J2; Man'62; (604)984-9213; Fax. (604)986-1390.

PENNER, Robert J; Victoria Emerg Phys Mgmt Ltd, 325-1627 Fort St, Victoria BC V8R 1H8; Man'77; AB; FRCPC; EmergMed. Staff Emerg, Royal Jubilee Hospital; Staff Emerg, Victoria General Hospital; (250)479-1442

PENNER, Robert M; Kelowna Gastroent Associates, 564 Leon Ave, Kelowna BC V1Y 6J6; Alb'99; BSc; FRCPC; IntMed; Gastroent. Clinical Asst Prof, University of British Columbia; (250)763-6433; Fax. (250)763-3818; robpenner@kelownagi.com.

PENNER, S Brian; GG453-810 Sherbrook St, Winnipeg MB R3A 1R8; Man'74; FRCPC; IntMed (Hypertension). Prof Med Pharmacol & Therapeutics, University of Manitoba; (204)787-3633; Fax. (204)787-4826.

PENNER, Todd P; Univ Hlth Network-Toronto Western Hosp, 8MP 324-399 Bathurst St, Toronto ON M5T 2S8; Man'95; MCPS; ABS; MD; FRCS; SAGES; FACS; BSc; LMCC; FRCSC; GenSurg (Bariatric Surgery). Staff Laparascopic & Gen Surg, Toronto Western Hospital - University Health Network; (416)603-6220; Fax. (416)603-6221; todd.penner@uhn.on.ca.

PENNEY, Angela M; Waterford Hosp, 210-306 Waterford Bridge Rd, St. John's NL A1E 4J8; Mem'93; FRCPC; Psy. Staff, St Clare's Mercy Hospital; (709)777-5000

PENNEY, Brenda; Lewisporte Med Clinic, PO Box 1195 490 Main St, Lewisporte NL A0G 3A0; Mem'88; BSc; BEd; (709)535-8617; Fax. (709)535-0172.

PENNEY, Brian J; Smiths Falls Community H C, 2 Gould St, Smiths Falls ON K7A 2S5; London (England)'70; MB BS; LRCP; MRCS; DObstRCOG; (613)283-1952; Fax. (613)283-6322.

PENNEY, Catherine J; Dr Charles S Curtis Mem Hosp, 178-200 West St, St Anthony NL A0K 4S0; London (England)'72; MB BS; CCFP; Chief FamilyMed/Chief of Staff, Charles S Curtis Memorial Hospital; Physician Aviation Med, City of St John's; Clin Lecturer Family Med, Memorial University Of Newfoundland; (709)454-3333; Fax. (709)454-2194; dr.catherine.penney@lghealth.ca.

PENNEY, Christopher J; Health Sciences Centre, 3330 Hospital Dr NW, Calgary AB T2N 4N1; Dal'75; ABIME; ABIM; FRCPC; IntMed (Rheumatology); Rheum. Ac Staff, Foothills Medical Centre; Associate Clin Prof, University of Calgary; (403)210-8838; Fax. (403)283-6151; penney@ucalgary.ca.

PENNEY, H Ross; Placentia Med Clinic, PO Box 239, Placentia NL A0B 2Y0; Mem'73; (709)227-2081; Fax. (709)227-2837.

PENNEY, Lynette S; IWK Health Centre, PO Box 9700 Rpo CSC 5850-5980 University Ave, Halifax NS B3K 6R8; Mem'02; BSc; FCCMG; FRCPC; MedGenetics. Staff, IWK Health Centre; (902)470-8754; Fax. (902)470-8709.

PENNEY, Michael R; Lake Country Family Practice, 1-9966 Pollard Rd, Winfield BC V4V 1Z4; Cal'81; CCFP; Staff, Kelowna General Hospital; (250)766-3938; Fax. (250)766-5231.

PENNEY, Nicola J; Lawton's Med Clinic, PO Box 1052 L106-137 O'Connell Dr, Corner Brook NL A2H 5M8; McM'09; CCFP.

PENNEY, Vicki J; Sunpark Prof Centre, 40 Sunpark Plaza SE, Calgary AB T2X 3X7; Mem'93; CCFP; FCFP; (403)254-4004; Fax. (403)254-1282.

PENNIE, Ross A; Brant Community HC-Brantford, 200 Terrace Hill St, Brantford ON N3R 1G9; Qns'76; FRCPC; Peds; InfectDis. Prof, McMaster University; (519)752-7871

PENNING, John P; The Ottawa Hosp-Civic Campus, 1053 Carling Ave, Ottawa ON K1Y 4E9; Ott'80; FRCPC; Anes. Staff, Royal Ottawa Mental Health Centre - Royal Ottawa Health Care Group; Staff, The Ottawa Hospital - Civic Campus; (613)761-4169

PENNINGTON, Jason J; SGH Medical Mall, 308-3030 Lawrence Ave E, Scarborough ON M1P 2T7; Tor'00; FRCSC; GenSurg. (416)289-3899; Fax. (416)438-6503.

PENNOCK, Kevin; 1 Field Ambulance PO Box 10500 Stn Forces, Edmonton AB T5J 4J5; Dal'03; CCFP; (780)973-4931

PENNY, J Norgrove; RebalanceMD, 104-3551 Blanshard St, Victoria BC V8Z 0B9; Alb'73; BSc(Med); DABOS; FRCSC; OrthSurg (Pediatric Orthopedic Surgery). (250)940-4444; kidsortho@drpenny.ca.

PENROD, Tessa M; 5001A 50 Ave, Beaumont AB T4X 1E7; Alb'03; CCFP; Langs: French; (780)929-6050; Fax. (780)929-5848.

PENROSE, Michael; Dauphin Med Clinic, 622 3rd St SW, Dauphin MB R7N 1R5; Man'88; CCFP; FCFP; Ac Staff, Dauphin Regional Health Centre; College of Physicians & Surgeons of Manitoba; Asst Prof, University of Manitoba; (204)638-6445; Fax. (204)638-5670; penrose@inetlink.ca.

PENTELICHUK, Tanya K; Cadillac Fairview Tower 2, 960-321 6 Ave SW, Calgary AB T2P 3H3; Sask'96; CCFP; (403)232-6244

PENTLAND, Neomi; 228 Cobourg St, Ottawa ON K1N 8J1; Edinburgh (Scotland)'71; BSc; MB ChB(Edin); MRCPsy(Lond); FRCPC; Psy (Child & Adolescent Psychiatry). (613)233-9497; Fax. (613)233-1113.

PENTON, Mercedes D; Towers Med Clinic, 120-100 Elizabeth Ave, St. John's NL A1B 1S1; Mem'84; BSc; BMedSci; CCFP; FCFP; Staff Member, St Clare's Mercy Hospital; Staff MD Visiting, Tiffany Village Retirement Residence; Staff Member, St. Patrick's Mercy Home; (709)753-9900; Fax. (709)753-6716.

PENTZ, Daniel S S; PO Box 336 Stn Main, North Battleford SK S9A 2Y3; Pretoria (South Africa)'75; Staff, Battlefords Union Hospital; (306)446-6604

PENZ, Erika D; Rockyview Gen Hosp, 4A183-7007 14 St SW, Calgary AB T2V 1P9; McM'04; FRCPC; IntMed; Respir. Staff, Rockyview General Hospital; Staff, Foothills Medical Centre; (403)943-8660

PEOPLES, Brian J; 6-9025 Torbram Rd, Brampton ON L6S 3L2; Belfast (Ireland)'67; DObstRCOG; (905)792-3113; Fax. (905)792-9944.

PEPE, Carmela; SMBD Jewish Gen Hosp, 3755 ch Cote-Sainte-Catherine, Montreal QC H3T 1E2; Laval'99; FRCPC; IntMed; Respir. Staff, Sir Mortimer B Davis Jewish General; (514)340-8222

PEPELASSIS, Dionissios; Variety Children's Heart Centr, FE141-685 William Ave, Winnipeg MB R3E 0Z2; Thessaloniki (Greece)'89.

PEPELEA, Ancuta; Hop Ste-Anne, 305 boul Anciens-Combattants, Ste-Anne-de-Bellev QC H9X 1Y9; Mon'84; Staff, Hopital Ste-Anne; Langs: English; Romanian; (514)457-3440; Fax. (514)457-8466.

PEPIN, Annie; Med Privee Notre-Dame, 597 av Notre-Dame, Saint-Lambert QC J4P 2K8; Sher'96; Langs: Bilingual(French/English); (450)766-0766

PEPIN, Celine; CFB Kingston, PO Box 17000 Stn Forces, Kingston ON K7K 7B4; Laval'83; (613)541-5010 x3232

PEPIN, E Paul; Medi Centre Mascouche, 100-880 montee Masson, Mascouche QC J7K 2L7; Sher'80; AB; Neur (P.Q.). Langs: English; (450)474-2493; Fax. (450)966-0156; e_paul_pepil@canada.com.

PEPIN, Jacques; CHUS-Hop Fleurimont, 3001 12e av N, Sherbrooke QC J1H 5N4; Sher'79; FRCPC; IntMed. Staff, Centre Hospitalier Universitaire de Sherbrooke-Hopital Fleurimont; (819)346-1110; Fax. (819)820-6451; jacques.pepin@usherbrooke.ca.

PEPIN, Jean; Groupe Medisys, 500 rue Sherbrooke O, Montreal QC H3A 3C6; Mon'87; Staff, Centre Hospitalier d'Argenteuil; (514)499-2177; Fax. (514)747-4705.

PEPIN, Jean-Francois; Clinique Med Pierre Boucher, 1615 boul Jacques-Cartier E, Longueuil QC J4M 2X1; Mon'00; (450)468-6223

PEPIN, Jean-Pierre; Hop Jean-Talon, 1385 rue Jean-Talon E, Montreal QC H2E 1S6; Mon'73; Psy (P.Q.). Staff, CSSS du Coeur de l'Isle Hôpital Jean-Talon; Staff, Hôpital du Sacre-Coeur de Montréal; (514)495-6767

PEPIN, John W; 410 Giles Blvd E, Windsor ON N9A 4C6; Wes'75; DABOS; FRCSC; OrthSurg. Staff, Leamington District Memorial Hospital; Ac Staff, Windsor Regional Hospital - Metropolitan Site; Ac Staff, Hôtel-Dieu Grace Hospital; (519)256-1823; Fax. (519)254-3849.

PEPIN, Karine; CSSS du Sud de Lanaudière, 911 montee des Pionniers, Terrebonne QC J6V 2H2; Sher'05; Peds. Staff, Centre Hospitalier Pierre le Gardeur; (450)654-7525

PEPIN, Marie-Noelle; CHUM-Hop St-Luc, 1058 rue Saint-Denis, Montreal QC H2X 3J4; Mon'00; FRCPC; IntMed; Nephrol. Staff, Centre Hospitalier l'Université De Montréal (CHUM) - Hôpital Saint-luc; (514)890-8000

PEPIN, Marie-Pascale; Centre Hosp Honore-Mercier, 2750 boul Laframboise, Saint-Hyacinthe QC J2S 4Y8; Sher'96; Peds. Staff Peds, Centre Hospitalier Honore-Mercier; (450)771-3335; Fax. (450)771-3557.

PEPIN, Michele; Clinique Med Mont Ste-Anne, RR 1 100-10974 boul Ste-Anne, Beaupre QC G0A 1E0; Laval'91; (418)827-4022; Fax. (418)827-4964.

PEPIN, Michelle; MUHC-Montreal Children's Hosp, A611-2300 rue Tupper, Montreal QC H3H 1P3; Mon'81; FRCPC; Peds. Staff, McGill University Health Centre - Montreal Children's Hospital; (514)412-4302; Fax. (514)412-4367; michelle.pepin@muhc.mcgill.ca.

PEPIN, Nancy; Clinique Med Antoine-Labelle, 200-555 boul Saint-Antoine, Saint-Jerome QC J7Z 3B8; Sher'94; Staff, Hôtel-Dieu de Saint-Jérôme; (450)438-1252; Fax. (450)438-6441.

PEPIN, Paul; Centre Hosp de Verdun, 4000 boul Lasalle, Verdun QC H4G 2A3; McG'97; FRCPC; Anes. Staff, Centre Hospitalier de Verdun; Langs: French; (514)362-1000 x2829

PEPIN, Paul-Andre; Centre Med St-Leonard, 360 rue Beliveau, St-Leonard-d'Aston QC J0C 1M0; Laval'68; Staff, CHSLD Accueil CSSS Ste-Croix; (819)399-2030; Fax. (819)399-2343; paul-andre_pepin@gmf.gouv.qc.ca.

PEPIN, Sylvie; 2200 rue Principale, St-Jean-des-Piles QC G0X 2V0; Sher'81; Langs: English; (819)538-3992; sylvie_pepin@ssss.gouv.qc.ca.

PEPIN DUBOIS, Yanek; CHUS-Hop Fleurimont, 3001 12e av N, Sherbrooke QC J1H 5N4; Sher'08; FRCPC; IntMed. Staff, Centre Hospitalier Universitaire de Sherbrooke-Hopital Fleurimont; (819)346-1110

PEPLER, Pierre-Francois; Victoria Gen Hosp, 1 Hospital Way, Victoria BC V8Z 6R5; Stellenbosch (South Africa)'99; MB ChB; Staff, Victoria General Hospital; (250)727-4212

PEPPER, Dale J; Chatham-Kent Health-Sydenham, 325 Margaret Ave, Wallaceburg ON N8A 2A7; Wes'86; BSc; Staff Privil, Chatham-Kent Health Alliance; Staff, Chatham-Kent Health Alliance - Sydenham Hospital Campus; (519)628-4154

PEPPER, Erin R; 5-1060 Burnham St, Cobourg ON K9A 5V9; McM'05; CCFP; (905)373-9333; Fax. (905)373-8373.

PEPPER, Jonathan; CFB Valcartier, SS 481 100 rue Dube, Courcelette QC G0A 1R1; Mon'09; CCFP; (418)844-0111

PEPPIN, Andrew K; Peter Lougheed Centre, 3500 26 Ave NE, Calgary AB T1Y 6J4; Qns'03; FRCPC; DiagRad. Staff, Peter Lougheed Centre; (403)943-5554

PEPPLE, Kudirat F; 806-19369 Sheriff King St SW, Calgary AB T2X 0T9; (Nigeria)'98; MB BS; MRCGPract(UK); Langs: Yoruba; (403)873-7300; Fax. (403)873-8880.

PERACCHIA, Gabriele; Weston Road Med Centre, 1995A Weston Rd, York ON M9N 1X2; Tor'89; (416)242-2216; Fax. (416)242-9751.

PERAMAKI, Edwin R; Vancouver Gen Hosp, 855 112 Ave W, Vancouver BC V5Z 1M9; UBC'96; FRCPC; DiagRad. Staff, Vancouver General Hospital - Centennial Pavillion; (604)875-4111

PERANSON, Judith S; St Michael's Hosp, 30 Bond St, Toronto ON M5B 1W8; Ott'05; CCFP; Staff, St Michael's Hospital; (416)867-7428; Fax. (416)867-7498.

PERCHESON, Paul B; Janssen Ortho Inc, 19 Green Belt Dr, North York ON M3C 1L9; Cal'84; BSc; MSc; Dir/Med Advisor, Drug Safety & Surveillance; Langs: English; French; (416)382-4860; Fax. (416)382-5982.

PERCHIK, Robert Aslan; Aberdeen Hosp, 835 East River Rd, New Glasgow NS B2H 3S6; Dal'80; Staff, Aberdeen Regional Hospital; (902)752-7600

PERCHINSKY, Michael J; Richmond Med Bldg, 106-2020 Richmond Rd, Victoria BC V8R 6R5; Alb'89; FACS; FRCSC; CardiothorSurg (Cardiac Surgery). Staff Cardiac Surg, Royal Jubilee Hospital; (250)595-1833; Fax. (250)595-1889; cvtsurgery@cvtsurgery.com.

PERCIVAL, Heather A; Huron Commun Family Hlth Team, PO Box 460 32B-1 Centennial Dr, Seaforth ON N0K 1W0; Ott'90; CCFP; Ac Staff, Seaforth Community Hospital - Huron Perth Healthcare Alliance; (519)600-2273; Fax. (519)600-2501; hpercival@rogers.com.

PERCIVAL, Timothy A; Callander Lakeside Med Clinic, 299 Main St N, Callander ON P0H 1H0; Tor'06; Staff, North Bay Regional Health Centre - Regional Mental Health; (705)752-1004

PERCY, Glen H; Temiskaming Hosp, PO Box 4040 421 Shepherdson Rd, New Liskeard ON P0J 1P0; Wes'82; CCFP; FCFP; Sr Advisor Phys, Temiskaming Hospital; (705)647-8121

PERCY, Maria T; Riverbend Medicentre, 600 Riverbend Sq NW, Edmonton AB T6R 2E3; Poznan (Poland)'68; (780)434-7234; Fax. (780)988-8903; mariapercy@shaw.ca.

PERCY, William G; The Doctors Office, 80 Thickson Rd S, Whitby ON L1N 7T2; Wes'76; (905)668-6448; Fax. (905)668-4023.

PERDOMO, Jose R; Marlborough Mall, 560-433 Marlborough Way NE, Calgary AB T2A 5H5; (El Salvador)'80; Langs: Spanish; (403)204-2153; Fax. (403)204-2156.

PEREGOUDOV, Serguei; Bluewater Health-Norman Site, 89 Norman St, Sarnia ON N7T 6S3; Celjabinsk (Russia (Federation))'88; FRCPC; Anes. Staff, Bluewater Health - Norman Site; (519)464-4400; peregoudov@sympatico.ca.

PEREIRA, Christine; Credit Valley Family Hlth Team, 105-2300 Eglinton Ave W, Mississauga ON L5M 2V8; Tor'83; CCFP; Staff, The Credit Valley Hospital; Staff, Royal Canadian Mounted Police; Lecturer Family & Community Med, University of Toronto; (905)813-3850; Fax. (905)813-3853; christine.pereira@rcmp-grc.gc.ca.

PEREIRA, Derek J; William Osler HC-Etobicoke, 101 Humber College Blvd, Etobicoke ON M9V 1R8; Universidad Iberoamericana (Mexico)'04; Staff, William Osler Health System - Etobicoke General Hospital; (416)747-3400; Fax. (416)747-8608.

PEREIRA, Jaime M; South Huron Hosp, 24 Huron St W SS 2 Stn Main, Exeter ON N0M 1S2; Wes'99; CCFP; Staff, South Huron Hospital Association; (519)235-2700

PEREIRA, Jeffery; 208-7900 Hurontario St, Brampton ON L6Y 0P6; Karachi (Pakistan)'83; (905)450-9306; Fax. (905)450-9304.

PEREIRA, John X; Chronic Pain Centre, 160-2210 2 St SW, Calgary AB T2S 3C3; McG'03; CCFP; (403)943-9900; Fax. (403)209-2954.

PEREIRA, Jose L; SCOHS-Elisabeth Bruyere Hosp, 270J-43 Bruyere St, Ottawa ON K1N 5C8; Pretoria (South Africa)'87; DA(SA); MSc; CCFP; Med Chief Dept of Palliative Med, SCO Health Service - Élisabeth Bruyère Hospital; Head/Prof Div of Palliative Care, University of Ottawa; Langs: Portuguese; Afrikaans; French; (613)562-4262

PEREIRA, Leo V; St Martha's Doctor's Offices, 23 Bay St, Antigonish NS B2G 2G7; Dal'85; BSc(Hons.); MSc; FRCPC; IntMed (Endocrinology). Staff, St Martha's Regional Hospital; Consultant, Strait Richmond Hospital; (902)863-1565; Fax. (902)863-0640.

PEREIRA, Michelle M; Main & Marine Med Clinic, 235 Marine Dr SE, Vancouver BC V5X 2S4; UBC'91; CCFP; (604)322-3011; Fax. (604)322-2827.

PEREIRA, Miguel; 102-1629 Townsite Rd, Nanaimo BC V9S 1N3; Witwatersrand (South Africa)'89; MB ChB; (250)755-4031; Fax. (250)755-4081.

PEREIRA, Paul C; 680-1070 Douglas St, Victoria BC V8W 2C4; Tor'92; (250)383-0449

PEREIRA, Raoul S; Hys Med Centre, 11010 101 St NW, Edmonton AB T5H 4B9; Cal'02; FRCPC; DiagRad. (780)426-1121

PEREIRA, Robert B; Somerset Medical, 4-13791 72 Ave, Surrey BC V3W 9Y9; UBC'90; BSc; CCFP; Langs: English; (604)591-9404; robper@telus.net.

PEREIRA, W Malathi D; The Credit Valley Hosp, 2200 Eglinton Ave W, Mississauga ON L5M 2N1; (Sri Lanka)'75; ABIM; FRC; FRCPC; IntMed. Court Staff, The Credit Valley Hospital; Langs: Sinhalese; (905)813-2200; jivaka@hotmail.com.

PEREIRA-HONG, Natasha L; 105-21 Surrey St W, Guelph ON N1H 3R3; McG'98; FRCSC; GenSurg (Bariatric Surgery). (519)836-4830; Fax. (519)836-1341.

PERELES, Laurie; Alberta Prof Bldg, 302-320 23 Ave SW, Calgary AB T2S 0J2; Man'80; BSc(Med); MSc; CCFP; FCFP; Staff, Rockyview General Hospital; Teach Staff, University of Calgary; (403)228-4844; Fax. (403)228-7923.

PERELLO, Andrea S; CSSSG-Hop de Gatineau, CP 2000 Succ Bureau-chef 909 boul de la Verendrye O, Gatineau QC J8P 7H2; Staff, Hôpital de Gatineau; (819)966-6118 x3438

PERELMAN, Vsevolod S; Mount Sinai Hosp, 206-600 University Ave, Toronto ON M5G 1X5; Tor'97; BSc(Russia); MSc; CCFP; CCFP(E.M.); Staff Schwarts/Reisman Emerg Ctre, Mount Sinai Hospital; Lecturer Family & Community Med, University of Toronto; Langs: Russian; Ukrainian; (416)586-5058; Fax. (416)586-4719.

PERERA, Anoma K; 1139 Yates St, Victoria BC V8V 3N2; Hannover (Germany)'91; (250)590-3111

PERERA, Arjuna R A; Integrated Wellness Med Centre, 2-4665 Central Blvd, Burnaby BC V5H 4J5; Cal'10; CCFP; (604)558-1175

PERERA, Ethige S C; The Health Centre of Maple, 2810 Major Mackenzie Dr, Maple ON L6A 3L2; Colombo (Sri Lanka)'95; CCFP; (905)832-3838

PERERA, Francisco E; London Reg Cancer Centre, 790 Commissioners Rd E, London ON N6A 4L6; Tor'83; FRCPC; RadOncol. Asst Prof, University of Western Ontario; (519)685-8650; Fax. (519)685-8627.

PERERA, Jaspreet; Malton Medical Group, 22-7330 Goreway Dr, Mississauga ON L4T 4J2; Carribean (Montserrat)'04; (905)677-4200

PERERA, Ransri F; Quinte HC Corp-Trenton Mem, PO Box 1600 Stn Main 242 King St, Trenton ON K8V 5S6; Qns'07; CCFP; CCFP(E.M.); Staff, QHC Trenton Memorial; (613)392-2541

PERERA, Ruwan T; Malton Medical Group, 22-7330 Goreway Dr, Mississauga ON L4T 4J2; West Indies (Jamaica)'04; (905)677-4200

PERES, Amos; Woodlawn Med Clinic, 92 Main St, Dartmouth NS B2X 1R5; Tor'91; CCFP; FCFP; (902)434-1500; Fax. (902)462-4994.

PERESS, Leonard; Professional Place, 408-2901 Lawrence Ave E, Scarborough ON M1P 2T3; Cape Town (South Africa)'66; MB ChB; FRCPC; IntMed (Respirology). Ac Staff, The Scarborough Hospital - General Campus; (416)261-0710; Fax. (416)261-6414.

PERETZ, David; John Buhler Research Centre, 805B-715 McDermot Ave, Winnipeg MB R3E 3P4; (Israel)'05; FRCPC; IntMed; Gastroent.

PEREY, Bertrand H; Fraser Orthopaedic Institute, 403-233 Nelson's Cres, New Westminster BC V3L 0E4; Dal'86; FRCSC; OrthSurg (Hand Surgery). Staff, Royal Columbian Hospital; Staff, Eagle Ridge Hospital & Health Care Centre; Clin Instructor, University of British Columbia; (604)525-2640

PEREZ, Barbara; UMF de Gatineau, 500 boul de l'Hopital, Gatineau QC J8V 2P5; Ott'07; CCFP; (819)966-6100

PEREZ, Edgardo L; Niagara H System-St Catharines, PO Box 3018 Stn Main 142 Queenston St, St. Catharines ON L2R 7C6; New York (USA)'76; MPH; CHE; CPH; FRCPC; Psy. Staff, Niagara Health System - St Catharines General Site; Prof Psy, McMaster University; Prof Psy & Health Policy, University of Toronto; Langs: Spanish; (905)378-4647; Fax. (905)704-4406.

PEREZ, F Eduardo; Serenete Health Clinic, 888 The Queensway, Etobicoke ON M8Z 1P1; Quito (Ecuador)'74; Ac Staff, St Joseph's Health Centre; Langs: Spanish; (416)251-1919

PEREZ, G Alejandro; Royal Alexandra Hosp, 10240 Kingsway NW, Edmonton AB T5H 3V9; (Mexico)'75; FRCPC; Anes. Staff, Royal Alexandra Hospital; (780)735-4111

PEREZ, Gavino; Sir William Osler Health Inst, 202-565 Sanatorium Rd, Hamilton ON L9C 7N4; Napoli (Italy)'65; FRCPC; IntMed (Endocrinology). Staff, Hamilton Health Sciences Centre - McMaster Children's Hospital; Assoc Prof Med, McMaster University; Langs: Italian; Spanish; (905)575-5522; Fax. (905)575-9772.

PEREZ, Margarita J; Health Action Centre, 640 Main St, Winnipeg MB R3B 0L8; (El Salvador)'82; CCFP; FCFP; Staff, Health Sciences Centre; (204)940-1626

PEREZ, Prudencio G; Capilano Med Centre, 10143 50 St NW, Edmonton AB T6A 2C1; Manila (Philippines)'80; (780)468-2911

PEREZ, Yael; 312-89 Queensway W, Mississauga ON L5B 2V2; Tor'05; FRCPC; Neur. Langs: Bilingual(English/French); (905)281-9898; Fax. (905)281-9143.

PEREZ-DE-LEON, Adolfo J; CHUM-Hotel-Dieu, 3840 rue Saint-Urbain, Montreal QC H2W 1T8; Santiago (Spain)'64; AB; FRCPC; Neur; Electroenceph (P.Q.). Staff, Centre Hospitalier l'Université de Montréal (CHUM) - Hôtel-Dieu; (514)890-8000 x14117; Fax. (514)412-7133.

PEREZ-MARTINEZ, Jordi; MUHC-Montreal Gen Hosp, E19 128-1560 av Cedar, Montreal QC H3G 1A4; Staff, McGill University Health Centre - Montreal General Campus; (514)934-8222

PEREZ-ORDONEZ, Bayardo J; Univ Hlth Network-Toronto Gen, 11E226-200 Elizabeth St, Toronto ON M5G 2C4; Leon (Nicaragua)'85; FRCPC; AnatPath. Staff, Toronto General Hospital - UHN; (416)340-3852

PEREZ-PARADA, Jorge E; University of Alberta Hosp, 8440 112 St NW, Edmonton AB T6G 2B7; Alb'02; FRCPC; Psy. Staff, University of Alberta Hospital; (780)407-6566

PEREZ-YOUSSOUFIAN, Steven A; Mackenzie Richmond Hill Hosp, 10 Trench St, Richmond Hill ON L4C 4Z3; Wes'07; Psy. Staff, Mackenzie Richmond Hill Hospital; (905)883-1212

PERIGNY, Martine; CHUQ-Hotel-Dieu de Quebec, 11 Cote du Palais, Quebec QC G1R 2J6; Mon'01; FRCPC; AnatPath. Staff, Centre Hospitalier Universitaire de Québec (CHUQ) - Siege Social; (418)525-4444 x23610; Fax. (418)691-5226.

PERINI, Rafael F; Kelowna Gastroent Associates, 564 Leon Ave, Kelowna BC V1Y 6J6; (Brazil)'97; FRCPC; IntMed; Gastroent. (250)763-6433; Fax. (250)763-3818.

PERK, Masis; Colchester East Hants Hlth Ctr, 600 Abenaki Rd, Truro NS B2N 5A1; Istanbul (Turkey)'77; LMCC; FRCPC; IntMed (Cardiology). Staff Consultant, Colchester East Hants Health Centre; Supvr Community Residency Training, Dalhousie University; Langs: English; French; (902)893-4321; Fax. (902)895-0124; drmasios@ns.sympatico.ca.

PERKIN, Gary; Thames Valley FHT-Strathroy Me, 74 Front St E, Strathroy ON N7G 1Y7; Wes'74; Coroner, Province of Ontario; (519)245-0430; Fax. (519)245-5870; gperkin@strathroymedicalclinic.com.

PERKIN, Thomas R; 65 Ellen St, Blenheim ON N0P 1A0; Tor'79; CCFP; Ac Staff, Chatham-Kent Health Alliance; Court Staff, Chatham-Kent Health Alliance - Sydenham Hospital Campus; (519)676-5592; Fax. (519)676-2228.

PERKINS, Bruce J L A; Univ Hlth Network-Toronto Gen, 12EN 218-200 Elizabeth St, Toronto ON M5G 2C4; Tor'95; MPH; FRCPC; IntMed; Endocrin&Metab. Scientist, Toronto General Hospital - UHN; (416)340-4800; Fax. (416)340-3236.

PERKINS, C Suzanne; Railside Med Specialists, 4A-1306 Bow Valley Trail, Canmore AB T1W 1N6; McG'84; FRCPC; Psy. (403)678-4696; Fax. (403)678-9467.

PERKINS, D Garth; Queensway-Carleton Hosp, 3045 Baseline Rd, Nepean ON K2H 8P4; Man'73; FRCPC; GenPath (Anatomical Pathology). Staff, Queensway Carleton Hospital; Asst Prof, University of Ottawa; (613)721-2000 x1020; gperkins@qch.on.ca.

PERKINS, David N; 501-2300 Eglinton Ave W, Mississauga ON L5M 2V8; Qns'98; FRCPC; IntMed; Nephrol. Staff Internist & Nephrol, The Credit Valley Hospital; Court Staff Nephrol, Trillium Health Centre - Mississauga; Court Staff Nephrol, Headwaters Health Care Centre - Orangeville Site; (905)820-7203; Fax. (905)820-3703; umuzi@yahoo.com.

PERKINS, Laurie K; Stevenson Med Clinic, 210A-6640 Vedder Rd, Chilliwack BC V2R 0J2; Stellenbosch (South Africa)'85; MB ChB; LMCC; (604)858-2245

PERKINS, Philippe; Reseau de Sante Vitalite, A-144 rue Martin, Edmundston NB E3V 2N4; Laval'89; Chief Dept of Orthopedics, Hôpital regional d'Edmundston; (506)739-0892; Fax. (506)739-0897.

PERKS, Alexandra E; 201-5171 221A St, Langley BC V2Y 0A2; UBC'00; FRCSC; Urol. (604)514-8530

PERL, Avishay; Queensway Prof Centre, 413-190 Sherway Dr, Etobicoke ON M9C 5N2; Basel (Switzerland)'74; FRCPC; Respir (Sleep Medicine); IntMed. Court Staff, St Joseph's Health Centre; Ac Staff, Trillium Health Centre - West Toronto; (416)626-8416; Fax. (416)626-9286.

PERL, Jeffrey; St Michael's Hosp, 3 060-30 Bond St, Toronto ON M5B 1W8; Tor'03; FRCPC; IntMed; Nephrol. Staff, St Michael's Hospital; (416)864-6016; Fax. (416)864-3042.

PERLAS FONTANA, Anahi; Univ Hlth Network-Toronto Western Hosp, 399 Bathurst St, Toronto ON M5T 2S8; (Uruguay)'95; FRCPC; Anes (Regional Anesthesia). Consultant Anes, Toronto Western Hospital - University Health Network; Asst Prof, University of Toronto; Langs: Spanish; (416)603-5118; Fax. (416)603-6494.

PERLAU, Robert J R; 300-4309 52 Ave, Red Deer AB T4N 6S4; Alb'84; FRCSC; OrthSurg. Staff, Red Deer Regional Hospital Centre; (403)346-3315; Fax. (403)347-9657.

PERLER, Zelick; Burrard Med Bldg, 400-1144 Burrard St, Vancouver BC V6Z 2A5; Alb'59; FRCSC; Urol. Ac Staff, Providence Health Care - St Paul's Hospital; Vis Staff, BC Children's Hospital; Clin Instructor, University of British Columbia; (604)688-5116; Fax. (604)688-5608.

PERLEY, Michael P; 1 Maliseet Dr, Woodstock-Nat NB E7M 4J5; Dal'80; CCFP; FCFP; Staff, Upper River Valley Hospital - Waterville; Asst Prof Family Med, Dalhousie University; Asst Prof Family Med, Memorial University Of Newfoundland; (506)328-8813

PERLIN, Kimberley A; Espanola Reg Hosp & Hlth Ctre, 825 McKinnon Dr, Espanola ON P5E 1R4; NOSM'09; CCFP; Staff, Espanola Regional Hospital and Health Centre; (705)869-1420

PERLIN, Louise R B; 30 Bond St, Toronto ON M5B 1W8; McG'81; FRCPC; IntMed; Rheum. Staff, St Michael's Hospital; Teach Staff, University of Toronto; (416)864-5550; Fax. (416)864-5549; perlinl@smh.toronto.on.ca.

PERLIN, Shawna F; 502-1881 Yonge St, Toronto ON M4S 3C4; Dal'81; CCFP; FCFP; Court Staff, Women's College Hospital; Lecturer, University of Toronto; (416)539-9598; Fax. (416)539-0802.

PERLMAN, Isaac; 810-943 Broadway W, Vancouver BC V5Z 4E2; Sask'62; Hon Staff, Vancouver General Hospital - Centennial Pavillion; Langs: Hebrew; (604)734-1213; Fax. (604)734-5751.

PERLMAN, Kusiel; The Hosp For Sick Children, 5114-555 University Ave, Toronto ON M5G 1X8; Man'73; BSc(Med.); MD; FRCPC; Peds (Endocrinology). Staff Physician, The Hospital For Sick Children; Assoc Prof, University of Toronto; Langs: Hebrew; (416)813-5991; Fax. (416)813-6304; kusiel.perlman@sickkids.ca.

PERLMAN, Michael J; Surrey Mem Hosp, 13750 96 Ave, Surrey BC V3V 1Z2; UBC'83; IntMed. Staff, Peace Arch Hospital; Staff, Surrey Memorial Hospital; (604)587-3842

PERLMAN, Robert J; 120-1405 Rte Trans-Canada, Dorval QC H9P 2V9; McG'78; BSc; MDCM; Asst Physician, Sir Mortimer B Davis Jewish General; Med Dir, Mediservice McDonald's Restaurants Bombardier Aerospace; Sr Med Examiner Aviation, MOT, FAA, CAA-UK, EASA/SSA; Preceptor Family Med, McGill University; Langs: English; French; (514)683-7877; Fax. (514)683-0202; rperlman@mediservice.ca.

PERLMAN, Shelley D; Worksafe BC, 6951 Westminster Hwy, Richmond BC V7C 1C6; UBC'95; FRCPC; IntMed. (604)279-7519

PERLMUTAR, Marty; Danforth Pediatrics, 100-235 Danforth Ave, Toronto ON M4K 1N2; Paris (France)'81; FRCPC; Peds. Staff, Toronto East General Hospital Inc; Langs: Bilingual(English/French); (416)466-1311; Fax. (416)466-9629; mperl@tegh.on.ca.

PERLON, Paul; Oak Ridges Med & Urgent Care, 100-13291 Yonge St, Richmond Hill ON L4E 4L6; Tor'96; CCFP; CCFP(E.M.); Physician Emerg, Mackenzie Richmond Hill Hospital; Physician Emerg, Southlake Regional Health Centre; Langs: Russian; (905)773-7759; Fax. (905)773-1325; pperlon@toxpro.ca.

PERLOV, Jack; Psychealth Centre, 771 Bannatyne Ave, Winnipeg MB R3E 3N4; Man'73; DCPsy(Tor.); AB; FRCPC; Psy (Child & Adolescent Psychiatry). Staff, Health Sciences Centre; Assoc Prof, University of Manitoba; (204)787-7478; Fax. (204)787-4975.

PERMACK, Sheldon M; 5-871 Waverley St, Winnipeg MB R3T 5P4; Man'80; CCFP; Staff Family Med, Victoria General Hospital; (204)477-4862; Fax. (204)477-8925.

PERNA, Philip; Southlake Reg Health Centre, 596 Davis Dr, Newmarket ON L3Y 2P9; Tor'05; FRCPC; Anes. Staff, Southlake Regional Health Centre; (905)895-4521

PERNG, Jane; Humber River Reg Hosp-Church, 200 Church St, Toronto ON M9N 1N8; Dal'01; DiagRad. Staff, Humber River Regional Hospital - Church Street Site; (416)249-8111

PERNG, Richard J; Niagara H System-G Niagara, PO Box 1018 Stn Main 5546 Portage Rd, Niagara Falls ON L2E 6X2; Ott'99; FRCPC; DiagRad. Staff, Niagara Health System - Greater Niagara General Site; (905)358-0171

PERNICA, Jeffrey M; McMaster Children's Hosp, 1280 Main St W, Hamilton ON L8S 4K1; Dal'03; FRCPC; Peds; InfectDis. Langs: French; (905)521-2100 x76652

PERNISIE, Laurie D; Lansdowne Shopping Centre, 108-5124 122 St NW, Edmonton AB T6H 3S3; Alb'88; CCFP; FCFP; (780)435-3688

PERODIN, Farah; CSSSG-Hop de Gatineau, CP 2000 Succ Bureau-Chef 909 boul de la Verendrye O, Gatineau QC J8P 7H2; Mon'04; FRCSC; GenSurg. Staff, Hôpital de Gatineau; (819)961-6100

PEROLD, Jacobus A L; White Rock Med Associates, 101-15451 Russell Ave, White Rock BC V4B 2R5; Pretoria (South Africa)'90; MB ChB; CCFP; Physician, White Rock Medical Associates; Langs: Afrikaans; (604)531-5595; Fax. (604)531-9818; lp@wrma.ca.

PERPICK-BRETON, Marion L; Glenmore Landing, 271A-1600 90 Ave SW, Calgary AB T2V 5A8; Tor'93; BSc; MSc; PhD; FRCPC; Psy (Custody & Access). (403)571-5019; Fax. (403)571-5025.

PERPIGNAN, Frantz; CSSS de Saint-Jerome, 290 rue de Montigny, Saint-Jerome QC J7Z 5T3; Mon'08; FRCPC; IntMed. Staff, Hôtel-Dieu de Saint-Jérôme; (450)431-8200

PERRAS, Maurice B; CHUS-Hop Hotel-Dieu, 580 rue Bowen S, Sherbrooke QC J1G 2E8; Sher'73; ABR; CSPQ; FRCPC; DiagRad. Staff, Centre Hospitalier Universitaire de Sherbrooke-Hôpital Hôtel-Dieu; Staff, Centre Hospitalier Universitaire de Québec (CHUQ) - Siege Social; Clin Prof, Universite de Sherbrooke; (819)346-1110

PERRAS, Michel; Clinique Med Ahuntsic, 2-241 rue Fleury O, Montreal QC H3L 1V2; Mon'67; Derm. Prof adj clin Pediatric Derm, Hôpital Ste-Justine; Adj Clin Prof, Universite de Montreal; (514)387-6431

PERRATON-BRILLON, Melanie; Hop Maisonneuve-Rosemont, 5415 boul de l'Assomption, Montreal QC H1T 2M4; Mon'99; Respir; IntMed. Staff, Hopital Maisonneuve-Rosemont; (514)252-3400

PERRAULT, Jean L; CHUM-Hop Notre-Dame, 1560 rue Sherbrooke E, Montreal QC H2L 4M1; Mon'65; FCCP; Respir (P.Q.); IntMed. adj Prof, Centre Hospitalier l'Université de Montréal (CHUM) - Hôpital Notre-Dame; adj Prof, Universite de Montreal; (514)890-8000 x26617; Fax. (514)412-7687; jlperrault@videotron.ca.

PERRAULT, Louis P; Institut de Cardiologie de Mtl, 5000 rue Belanger, Montreal QC H1T 1C8; Mon'86; PhD(Pharm); FRCSC; GenSurg (Heart Transplantation); Cardiovasc&ThorSurg. Staff, Institut de Cardiologie de Montréal; Staff, Centre Hospitalier l'Université de Montréal (CHUM) - Hôpital Notre-Dame; Prof, Universite de Montreal; Langs: English; French; (514)376-3330 x3471; Fax. (514)376-1355; louis.perrault@icm-mhi.org.

PERRAULT, Michel-Antoine; CHUS-Hopital Fleurimont, 3001 12e av N, Sherbrooke QC J1H 5N4; Mon'98; CSPQ; FRCPC; Anes (Echography). Staff, Centre Hospitalier Universitaire de Sherbrooke-Hôpital Hôtel-Dieu; Staff, Centre Hospitalier Universitaire de Sherbrooke-Hopital Fleurimont; Langs: Bilingual(French/English); (819)346-1110

PERRAULT, Raymond; CSSS de Trois-Rivières, 1991 boul du Carmel, Trois-Rivieres QC G8Z 3R9; Laval'65; Peds (P.Q.). Staff, CSSS de Trois-Rivières; (819)697-3333

PERRAULT, Roger; Center Hosp Honore-Mercier, 2750 boul Laframboise, Saint-Hyacinthe QC J2S 4Y8; Sher'81; NuclearMed. Staff Nuclear Med, Centre Hospitalier Honore-Mercier; (450)771-3333 x3232; Fax. (450)771-3628.

PERREAULT, Alain; Centre Med Fusion, 200-2035 av Sainte-Anne, Saint-Hyacinthe QC J2S 5H3; Laval'74; ac Staff, Centre Hospitalier Honore-Mercier; (450)773-6023

PERREAULT, Andre; Clin Chir du Pied Montreal, 10-262 rue Saint-Jacques, Montreal QC H2Y 1N1; Mon'80; CSPQ; OrthSurg (Foot & Ankle Surgery). Langs: Bilingual(French/English); (514)387-3871; Fax. (514)387-6650; clinique@halluxvalgus.com.

PERREAULT, Caroline; CLSC de la Vallee des Forts, 978 boul du Seminaire N, St-Jean-sur-Richel QC J3A 1E5; Sher'88; Langs: Bilingual(French/English); (450)358-2578; Fax. (450)358-2034.

PERREAULT, Chantal; Ctr Hosp Anna-Laberge, 200 boul Brisebois, Chateauguay QC J6K 4W8; Mon'89; Staff, Hôpital Anna-Laberge; (450)699-2425; Fax. (450)699-2525.

PERREAULT, Christian; 350-1000 montee des Pionniers, Terrebonne QC J6V 1S8; Mon'84; DABOph; LMCC; CSPQ; Ophth (Refractive Cataract Surgery). Staff, Centre Hospitalier Pierre le Gardeur; Langs: Bilingual(French/English); (450)654-6049

PERREAULT, Christine M; Children's & Women's HC of BC, B321-4480 Oak St, Vancouver BC V6H 3V4; McG'88; FRCPC; Peds. Staff, BC Children's Hospital; Langs: Bilingual(English/French); (604)875-2000

PERREAULT, Claude; Hop Maisonneuve-Rosemont, 5415 boul de l'Assomption, Montreal QC H1T 2M4; Mon'74; HemPath; Hem (P.Q.). Staff, Hopital Maisonneuve-Rosemont; Prof, Universite de Montreal; (514)252-3557; cperreault.hmr@ssss.gouv.qc.ca.

PERREAULT, Claude; Hop du Sacre-Coeur de Mtl, 5400 boul Gouin O, Montreal QC H4J 1C5; McG'77; CSPQ; FRCPC; Anes. Staff, Hôpital du Sacre-Coeur de Montréal; Staff, Centre Hospitalier l'Université de Montréal (CHUM) - Hôpital Notre-Dame; (514)338-2222 x2680; cperrault@ssss.gouv.qc.ca.

PERREAULT, Danielle; Clin Voyage Saint-Luc, 1001 rue Saint-Denis, Montreal QC H2X 3H9; McG'82; Langs: Spanish; (514)890-8332; perreaultmd@videotron.ca.

PERREAULT, Eric; CSSS du Nord de Lanaudière, 1000 boul Sainte-Anne, St-Charles-Brromee QC J6E 6J2; Mon'85; Staff, Centre Hospitalier Régional de Lanaudière; (450)759-8222; Fax. (450)759-8289.

PERREAULT, Etienne; Hop Brome-Missisquoi-Perkins, 950 rue Principale, Cowansville QC J2K 1K3; Mon'03; Staff, Hôpital Brome-Missisquoi-Perkins; (450)266-4342

PERREAULT, Francois; Centre Hosp Honore-Mercier, 2750 boul Laframboise, Saint-Hyacinthe QC J2S 4Y8; Mon'88; Hem; IntMed. Staff, Centre Hospitalier Honore-Mercier; (450)771-3333; Fax. (450)771-3510.

PERREAULT, Francois; Centre Med Ste-Anne, 113 rue Sainte-Anne, Ste-Anne-De-Bellev QC H9X 1M2; Mon'79; Staff, Hopital Ste-Anne; Langs: English; (514)457-2772; Fax. (514)457-4397.

PERREAULT, Genevieve; DSP Laurentides, 1000 rue Labelle, Saint-Jerome QC J7Z 5N6; Sher'96; FRCPC; Public Health & Preventive Med.

PERREAULT, Gerard A; Hotel-Dieu d'Arthabaska, 5 rue des Hospitalieres, Victoriaville QC G6P 6N2; Laval'65; DPM(McG); Psy. Ac Staff Psy, Hotel-Dieu d'Arthabaska; (819)357-2030 x2660; Fax. (819)357-6035.

PERREAULT, Gilles; 630 boul du Seminaire N, St-Jean-Sur-Richel QC J3B 7X6; Laval'78; ObstGyn (P.Q.). (450)348-1171; Fax. (450)348-1172.

PERREAULT, Helene; Dispensaire Mistissini, GD, Mistissini QC G0W 1C0; Mon'90; (819)929-3307

PERREAULT, Isabelle; CHUM-Hotel-Dieu, 3840 rue Saint-Urbain, Montreal QC H2W 1T8; Mon'98; FRCSC; PlasSurg. Staff, Centre Hospitalier l'Université de Montréal (CHUM) - Hôtel-Dieu; (514)890-8000

PERREAULT, Isabelle; Clinique Specialisee CLAP, 122 rue Saint-Jean, Drummondville QC J2B 5K8; Laval'92; FRCPC; IntMed; Endocrin (P.Q.); Endocrin&Metab. (819)472-4823

PERREAULT, J J Daniel; Inst Albert Prevost, 6555 boul Gouin O, Montreal QC H4K 1B3; Mon'65; Psy. Staff, Hôpital du Sacre-Coeur de Montréal; (514)338-2100; Fax. (514)338-4402.

PERREAULT, Jacqueline; SAAQ, CP 19600 Succ Terminus 333 boul Jean-Lesage, Quebec QC G1K 8J6; Laval'79; (418)528-4943; jacqueline.perreault@saaq.gouv.qc.ca.

PERREAULT, Jean; Polyclinique St-Eustache, 75 rue Grignon, St-Eustache QC J7P 4J2; Mon'89; ASAM; Med Coord Drug & Alcohol Detox Prog, Centre Hospitalier Régional de Lanaudière; Pres, Groupe Toxpert; (450)473-6882; Fax. (450)473-1916.

PERREAULT, Jean-Paul; 301-235 boul René-Lévesque E, Montreal QC H2X 1N8; Mon'62; CSPQ; FRCSC; Urol (Oncology). Staff, Centre Hospitalier l'Université De Montréal (CHUM) - Hôpital Saint-luc; Langs: English; (514)861-0213; Fax. (514)861-3021.

PERREAULT, Josee; Clinique Med St-Louis, 220-3165 ch St-Louis, Quebec QC G1W 4R4; Mon'92; LMCC; Staff Psy, Hôtel-Dieu de Lévis; (418)653-1970; Fax. (418)653-9956.

PERREAULT, Julie; 203-1052 rue Lionel-Daunais, Boucherville QC J4B 0B2; Laval'10; (450)262-6222

PERREAULT, Line; Ctr des Service de Sante FC, 6560 rue Hochelaga, Montreal QC H1N 1X9; Mon'95; FRCPC; Psy. Staff, Centre Hospitalier Honore-Mercier; (514)252-2777

PERREAULT, Louis-Georges; Centre Med Montreal-Est, 201-11370 rue Notre-Dame E, Montreal-Est QC H1B 2W6; Mon'73; Med Consultant, Agence de santé et des services sociaux de la Montérégie; (514)645-7426; Fax. (514)645-7420.

PERREAULT, Louise; Ctr Hosp Rouyn-Noranda, 4 9e rue, Rouyn-Noranda QC J9X 2B2; Sher'84; FRCPC; Peds. Staff, Centre Hospitalier Rouyn-Noranda; (819)764-5131; lperreau@lino.com.

PERREAULT, Lyette; 140-950 Montee des Pionniers, Terrebonne QC J6V 1S8; Sher'80; CSPQ; FRCPC; DiagRad (Echography). Langs: English; French; (450)581-1424 x221; Fax. (450)581-9395; lyette@imageriedespionniers.com.

PERREAULT, Mariano; Clin Med Mirabel, CP 1059 Succ Saint-Janvier 13714 boul Cure-Labelle, Mirabel QC J7J 1A1; Laval'79; LMCC; (450)435-7630; Fax. (450)435-1716.

PERREAULT, Nathalie; Hop Brome-Missisquoi-Perkins, 950 rue Principale, Cowansville QC J2K 1K3; Mon'88; FRCPC; PhysMed&Rehab. Staff, Centre Hospitalier l'Université de Montréal (CHUM) - Hôpital Notre-Dame; Staff, Hôpital Brome-Missisquoi-Perkins; (450)266-4342

PERREAULT, Pierre; CHUM-Hop St-Luc, 1058 rue Saint-Denis, Montreal QC H2X 3J4; Sher'90; CSPQ; FRCPC; DiagRad (Interventional Radiology). Radiol, Centre Hospitalier l'Université De Montréal (CHUM) - Hôpital Saint-luc; assoc Prof, Universite de Montreal; Langs: English; (514)890-8350; Fax. (514)412-7359.

PERREAULT, Rene; CSSS de Rivière-de-Loup, 75 rue Saint-Henri, Riviere-du-Loup QC G5R 2A4; Laval'67; FRCSC; OrthSurg. Staff, Centre Hospitalier Regional du Grand-Portage; (418)868-1010

PERREAULT, Robert; Direction de la Sante Publique, 1301 rue Sherbrooke E, Montreal QC H2L 1M3; Mon'72; FRCPC; Psy. Staff, Hôpital du Sacre-Coeur de Montréal; (514)528-2400 x3564; Fax. (514)528-2423; rperreau@santepub-mtl.qc.ca.

PERREAULT, Stephanie; 261 boul Sir-Wilfred-Laurier, Mont-Saint-Hilaire QC J3H 3N8; Mon'05; CCFP; (450)464-5151

PERREAULT, Sylvie; Centre de Sante St-Elie, 5978 ch de Saint-Elie, Sherbrooke QC J1R 0L1; Sher'83; Langs: Bilingual(French/English); (819)564-1350; Fax. (819)564-1365; labperro@videotron.ca.

PERREAULT, Therese; MUHC-Montreal Children's Hosp, 2300 rue Tupper, Montreal QC H3H 1P3; Mon'79; FAAP; ABPeds; MCPS; FRCPC; Peds (Neonatology). Chef Newborn Med, McGill University Health Centre - Montreal Children's Hospital; Chef Newborn Med, McGill University Health Centre - Royal Victoria Hospital; assoc Prof Peds, McGill University; Langs: Spanish; Bilingual(English/French); (514)412-4452; Fax. (514)412-4356; therese.perreault@muhc.mcgill.ca.

PERREAULT, Yves; CSSS Haut-Richelieu-Rouville, 920 boul du Seminaire N, St-Jean-sur-Richel QC J3A 1B7; Mon'92; FRCSC; GenSurg. Staff, Hôpital du Haut-Richelieu; (450)359-5000

PERRI, Danny; St Joseph's Healthcare, F536-50 Charlton Ave E, Hamilton ON L8N 4A6; Tor'00; FRCPC; IntMed; Critical Care Medicine. Staff, St Joseph's Healthcare - Charlton Campus; (905)522-1155; Fax. (905)521-6068.

PERRI, Elizabeth M; 202-285 Aurora Cres, Kelowna BC V1X 7N6; UBC'88; (250)765-7756; Fax. (250)765-9015.

PERRI, Giulia-Anna; Baycrest Ctre/Geriatric Care, 3560 Bathurst St, Toronto ON M6A 2E1; McM'02; CCFP; Staff, Baycrest Centre for Geriatric Care; (416)785-2500

PERRIER, Alban; GMF Concorde, 300 boul de la Concorde E, Laval QC H7G 2E6; Mon'67; Langs: Bilingual(French/English); (450)667-5310; Fax. (450)667-5248.

PERRIER, Caroline; CLSC Rivieres et Marees, 22 rue Saint-Laurent, Riviere-du-Loup QC G5R 4W5; Laval'88; (418)867-2642

PERRIER, Guy; 400-671 2e rue E, La Sarre QC J9Z 3J7; Mon'76; LMCC; Staff, Centre Hospitalier La Sarre; Langs: English; (819)339-5661; Fax. (819)339-3015.

PERRIER, Jean; Centre Med St Basile, 101-275 boul Sir-Wilfrid-Lauri, St-Basile-Le-Grand QC J3N 1V6; Mon'77; (450)653-7323; Fax. (450)653-3021.

PERRIER, Kenneth R; 3591 31 St, Vernon BC V1T 5J4; UBC'93; BSc; CCFP; Staff, Vernon Jubilee Hospital; (778)475-7511; Fax. (250)542-0160.

PERRIER, Manuel; Ctr Hosp de Lachine, 650 16e av, Lachine QC H8S 3N5; Mon'99; FRCSC; Ophth. Staff, CSSS de Dorval-Lachine-Lasalle; (514)637-2351 x5256; Fax. (514)637-7954.

PERRIER, Marie-Pascale; CHUS-Hop Hotel-Dieu, 580 rue Bowen S, Sherbrooke QC J1G 2E8; Sher'94; FRCPC; Psy (Community Psychiatry). Clin Prof, Centre Hospitalier Universitaire de Sherbrooke-Hôpital Hôtel-Dieu; Langs: Spanish; English; (819)346-1110 x26546; Fax. (819)829-6259.

PERRIER, Renee L; Alberta Children's Hosp, 2888 Shaganappi Trail NW, Calgary AB T3B 6A8; Cal'02; FRCPC; MedGenetics. Staff, Alberta Children's Hospital; (403)955-7373; Fax. (403)955-2701.

PERRIGO, Bradley E; Couchiching Family Health Team, 204-119 Memorial Ave, Orillia ON L3V 5X1; McM'00; BHSc(Physiotherapy); BSc(Hons.)(Kinesiol); CCFP; Staff, Orillia Soldiers' Memorial Hospital; Associate Clin Prof, McMaster University; (705)323-9800; Fax. (705)323-9601.

PERRIN, Clifford; Pavillon Rosemont, 5689 boul Rosemont, Montreal QC H1T 2H1; Mon'77; FRCPC; Psy. Staff, Hopital Maisonneuve-Rosemont; (514)252-3914; cperrin@videotron.ca.

PERRIN, Hugh M; Mount Forest Fam Health Team, SS 3 525 Dublin St, Mount Forest ON N0G 2L3; Wes'81; Med Staff, North Wellington Health Care - Louise Marshall Hospital; Med Dir, Saugeen Valley Nursing Centre; (519)323-0255; Fax. (519)323-2113; svnc@wightman.ca.

PERRIN, Mark J; Univ of Ottawa Heart Institute, 40 Ruskin St, Ottawa ON K1Y 4W7; Sydney (Australia)'99; Staff, University of Ottawa Heart Institute.

PERRIN, Nadege; CSSS de Sept-Iles, 45 rue du Pere-Divet, Sept-Iles QC G4R 3N7; Sher'99; FRCSC; GenSurg. Staff, Centre Hospitalier Regional de Sept-Iles; (418)962-9761

PERRIN, Richard G; 948-55 Queen St E, Toronto ON M5C 1R6; Qns'68; MSc; MD; FRCSC; Neursurg (Spine). Staff, St Michael's Hospital; Assoc Staff, The Scarborough Hospital - General Campus; Assoc Prof Surg, University of Toronto; (416)864-5503; Fax. (416)864-5633; richard.perrin@utoronto.ca.

PERRON, Andre; Bureau d'Evaluation Medicale, 35 rue de Port-Royal E, Montreal QC H3L 3T1; Laval'77; (514)873-4214

PERRON, Denis; Clinique Centre-Ville, 929 3e av, Val-d'Or QC J9P 1T4; Sher'83; Staff, Hôpital psychiatrique de Malartic; (819)874-9111; Fax. (819)874-9191; denis_perron@ssss.gouv.qc.ca.

PERRON, Gino; Hotel-Dieu de Levis, 143 rue Wolfe, Levis QC G6V 3Z1; Laval'96; CSPQ; FRCPC; Anes. Staff, Hôtel-Dieu de Lévis; (418)835-7121 x3218; Fax. (418)835-3969; morphee@ssss.gouv.qc.ca.

PERRON, Jean; Hôpital Laval, 2725 ch Sainte-Foy, Quebec QC G1V 4G5; Laval'88; FRCSC; GenSurg (P.Q.); CardSurg; Cardiovasc&ThorSurg (P.Q.). Staff, Hôpital Laval; (418)656-4717

PERRON, Jean-Marc; Le Ctre de Read Lucie-Bruneau, 2275 av Laurier E, Montreal QC H2H 2N8; Mon'62; FRCP; FRCPC; Peds (Physical Medicine & Rehabilitation). Staff Neuro-Muscular Disease Prog & Deficit Cerebral Motors, Centre de Readaptation Lucie-Bruneau; (514)527-4527 x2308; jeanmarcperron@hotmail.com.

PERRON, Lina; Direction de la Sante Publique, 1255 rue Beauregard, Longueuil QC J4K 2M3; Laval'77 Laval; MSc; Med Consultant InfectDis &Community Health, Hopital Charles LeMoyne; (450)928-6777 x3107; Fax. (450)928-3023.

PERRON, Linda; Inst Nat'l de Sante Publique, 945 av Wolfe, Quebec QC G1V 5B3; Laval'91; CSPQ; FRCPC; CommunMed. Staff, Centre d'hébergement de Beauceville; Langs: Spanish; English; (418)650-5115 x5550

PERRON, Marie-Eve; CSSS de Laval, 1755 boul Rene-Laennec, Laval QC H7M 3L9; Laval'03; FRCPC; Anes. Staff, Hopital de la Cite de la santé; (450)668-1010

PERRON, Marie-Helene; Clinique Med Douville, 5460 boul Laurier O, Saint-Hyacinthe QC J2S 3V7; Mon'84; Staff, Centre Hospitalier Honore-Mercier; (450)773-8777; Fax. (450)771-7530.

PERRON, Mylene; CSSS de Jonquiere, CP 1200 Succ Pdf Jonquiere 2230 rue de l'Hopital, Jonquiere QC G7X 4H6; Laval'09; Staff, Centre Hospitalier Jonquiere; (418)695-7700

PERRON, Nancy C; CSSSG-Hop de Hull, 116 boul Lionel-Emond, Gatineau QC J8Y 1W7; Mon'82; CSPQ; AnatPath. Staff, Hull Hospital; (819)595-6038; nancy_perron@ssss.gouv.qc.ca.

PERRON, Odette; Ctr de Sante Vallee-Gatineau, 309 boul Desjardins, Maniwaki QC J9E 2E7; Sher'87; FRCSC; OrthSurg. Staff, CH-CHSLD de Papineau - Pavillon du centre hospitalier; Staff, CSSS de la Vallée de la Gatineau; Langs: Bilingual(English/French); (819)449-2301; cloper@videotron.ca.

PERRON, Patrice; CHUS-Hop Fleurimont, 3001 12e av N, Sherbrooke QC J1H 5N4; Sher'86; FRCPC; IntMed (Diabetology); Endocrin (P.Q.); Endocrin&Metab. Staff, Centre Hospitalier Universitaire de Sherbrooke-Hopital Fleurimont; Staff, Complexe hospitalier de la Sagamie; Chef Med, Universite de Sherbrooke; Langs: English; (819)564-5241; Fax. (819)820-6806; patrice.perron@usherbrooke.ca.

PERRON, Robert; CSSS de Trois-Rivières, 1991 boul du Carmel, Trois-Rivieres QC G8Z 3R9; Laval'77; CSPQ; FRCPC; AnatPath. Staff, CSSS de Trois-Rivières; (819)697-3333 x68208; robert_perron_chrtr@ssss.gouv.qc.ca.

PERRON, Robert; Societe P S M, 215-1600 boul Cure-Labelle, Laval QC H7V 2W2; Mon'70; Médecin, General Motors Canada Ltd; (450)688-9271; Fax. (450)688-4665; perrob20_siril@ssss.gouv.qc.ca.

PERRON, Roger J W; Guelph Med Place, 210-83 Dawson Rd, Guelph ON N1H 1B1; McM'86; FRCSC; ObstGyn. Staff, Guelph General Hospital; (519)821-2440; Fax. (519)821-2448.

PERRON, Sebastien; Ctr Hosp du Centre la Mauricie, 50 119e rue, Shawinigan-Sud QC G9P 5K1; Laval'02; FRCPC; IntMed. Staff, Centre Hospitalier du Centre la Mauricie; (819)536-7575

PERRON, Stephane; Dir de la Sante Publique de Mt, 1301 rue Sherbrooke E, Montreal QC H2L 1M2; Mon'99; CSPQ; FRCPC; CommunMed. (514)528-2400

PERRON, Stephanie; Ctr Hosp du Centre la Mauricie, 50 119e rue, Shawinigan-Sud QC G9P 5K1; Sher'97; CCFP; Staff, Centre Hospitalier du Centre la Mauricie; (819)536-7500 x8290

PERRON, Thierry; Hotel-Dieu de Sorel, 400 av de l'Hotel-Dieu, Sorel-Tracy QC J3P 1N5; Mon'98; FRCSC; GenSurg. Staff, Hôtel-Dieu de Sorel; Langs: English; (450)746-6000

PERRON, Wayne R; 300-333 24 Ave SW, Calgary AB T2S 3E6; Sask'74; FRCSC; PlasSurg (Aesthetic Surgery). (403)228-7076; Fax. (403)228-7077; drperron@drperron.com.

PERRON-COTE, Anne-Louise; CSSS de Chicoutimi, 305 rue Saint-Vallier, Chicoutimi QC G7H 5H6; Laval'07; CCFP; CCFP(E.M.); Staff, Complexe hospitalier de la Sagamie; (418)541-1000

PERRONE, Maria; CLSC Cote-des-Neiges, 1271 av Van Horne, Montreal QC H2V 1K5; McG'82; CCFP; FCFP; Staff Privil, Sir Mortimer B Davis Jewish General; adj Prof, McGill University; (514)270-1386; Fax. (514)270-8731.

PERROTTA, Rosalba; Clinique Medicale 910, 910 boul Saint-Joseph E, Montreal QC H2J 1K6; Mon'88; CCFP; Coord Family Med Ground Rounds, St Mary's Hospital Centre; (514)590-0910; Fax. (514)590-0448.

PERROTTE, Paul; Les Urologues Specialises, 200-235 boul Rene-Levesque E, Montreal QC H2X 1N8; Mon'91; BSc; CSPQ; BEngChem; FRCSC; Urol (Uro Oncology). assoc Prof Urol Service, Centre Hospitalier l'Université De Montréal (CHUM) - Hôpital Saint-luc; assoc Prof, Universite de Montreal; Langs: Bilingual(French/English); (514)393-1222; Fax. (514)393-3666; paul.perrotte@umontreal.ca.

PERRY, Anamrija M; Health Sciences Centre, 820 Sherbrook St, Winnipeg MB R3A 1R9; Staff, Health Sciences Centre; (204)774-8511

PERRY, Corinne A; 70 McLeod Ave, Spruce Grove AB T7X 3C7; Alb'00; CCFP; (780)962-9393; Fax. (780)962-4295.

PERRY, Daryl; Riverview Health Centre, PE309-1 Morley Ave, Winnipeg MB R3L 2P4; Man'01; FRCPC; PhysMed&Rehab. Staff, Riverview Health Centre; Staff, The Rehabilitation Centre; (204)452-3411; dperry@cc.umanitoba.ca.

PERRY, David A; 3089 Dufferin St, North York ON M6A 2S7; Tor'68; Court Staff, Humber River Regional Hospital - Church Street Site; (416)783-1417; Fax. (416)256-9638.

PERRY, Diane; CLSC Jean Olivier-Chenier, 29 ch d'Oka, St-Eustache QC J7R 1K6; Mon'98; MSc; Staff, Centre Hospitalier Rouyn-Noranda; (450)491-1233 x283; Fax. (450)491-6898.

PERRY, Douglas; Misericordia Community Hosp, 16940 87 Ave NW, Edmonton AB T5R 4H5; Alb'73; BSc; MCPS; MCFP; Staff, Covenant Health - Misericordia Community Hospital; Clin Assoc Prof, University of Alberta; (780)735-2819; Fax. (780)483-8059.

PERRY, Gad A; The Ottawa Hosp-Gen Campus, 501 Smyth Rd, Ottawa ON K1H 8L6; Ott'85; FRCPC; RadOncol (Lung Cancer). Ac Staff Ottawa Reg Cancer Centre, The Ottawa Hospital - General Campus; Asst Prof Radiol, University of Ottawa; (613)737-7700 x25395; Fax. (613)247-3511.

PERRY, Grace W K; PO Box 36518 Rpo McTaggart, Edmonton AB T6R 0T4; Alb'10; (780)969-4421

PERRY, J Christopher; SMBD Jewish Gen Hosp, 3755 ch Cote-Sainte-Catherine, Montreal QC H3T 1E2; Durham(NC) (USA)'74; MPH(Harvard); ABNP; Dir Psy Research & Staff, Sir Mortimer B Davis Jewish General; assoc Prof, McGill University; (514)340-8210

PERRY, James; Sunnybrook Hlth Sciences Ctre, A402-2075 Bayview Ave, Toronto ON M4N 3M5; Tor'89; BSc(Hons.); FRCPC; Neur (Neuro Oncology). Head Div of Neurol, Sunnybrook Health Sciences Centre; Consultant, Sunnybrook Health Sciences Centre - Edmond Odette Cancer Centre; Asst Prof, University of Toronto; (416)480-4766; Fax. (416)480-5054.

PERRY, Jeffrey J; The Ottawa Hosp-Civic Campus, 1053 Carling Ave, Ottawa ON K1Y 4E9; Ott'96; CCFP; CCFP(E.M.); Scientist, The Ottawa Hospital - Civic Campus; (613)761-4928; jperry@ohri.ca.

PERRY, Jowan M R; Lasalle Community Health Ctre, 2125 Front Rd, Windsor ON N9J 2C1; (Iraq)'85; CCFP; (519)734-1234; Fax. (519)734-8674.

PERRY, Judith A; Life Quest Thornhill, 218-7330 Yonge St, Thornhill ON L4J 7Y7; Ott'91; (905)731-5928; Fax. (905)731-4563.

PERRY, Katherine F; North East Mental Health Team, 2750 Hastings St E, Vancouver BC V5K 1Z9; UBC'84; FRCPC; Psy. Ac Staff, UBC Hospital - Koerner Pavillion; (604)675-3890

PERRY, Kyle D; Health Sciences Centre, 820 Sherbrook St, Winnipeg MB R3A 1R9; Staff, Health Sciences Centre; (204)774-8511

PERRY, Rebecca J; Alberta Children's Hosp, 2888 Shaganappi Trail NW, Calgary AB T3B 6A8; Staff, Alberta Children's Hospital; (403)955-7819; Fax. (403)955-5001.

PERRY, Scott R; Queensway Health Centre, 6-1750 The Queensway, Etobicoke ON M9C 5H5; McM'92; (647)722-2370

PERRY, Stephanie L; Miramichi Reg Hosp, 500 Water St, Miramichi NB E1V 3G5; Dal'93; FRCPC; Peds. Staff, Miramichi Regional Hospital; (506)623-3499; Fax. (506)623-3490; stephanie.perry@horizon.nb.ca.

PERRY, Theresa; B-22195 Dewdney Trunk Rd, Maple Ridge BC V2X 3H7; Witwatersrand (South Africa)'06; MB ChB; (604)463-4102

PERRY, Thomas L; UBC Hospital, 2211 Wesbrook Mall, Vancouver BC V6T 2B5; McG'78; BSc; DABIM; FRCPC; IntMed (Clinical Pharmacology). Staff, UBC Hospital - Koerner Pavillion; Staff, Vancouver General Hospital - Centennial Pavillion; Clinical Asst Prof, University of British Columbia; Langs: Spanish; French; (604)822-7134; Fax. (604)822-7897.

PERRY, Wayne J; 14-3170 Tillicum Rd, Victoria BC V9A 7C5; Dal'94; BSc; CCFP; FCFP; Staff, Canadian Forces Health Services - Pacific Centre; (250)381-8112

PERSAD, Atma; Family Practice Associates, PO Box 2010 223 16th Ave, Creston BC V0B 1G0; UBC'00; CCFP; Chief staff, Creston Valley Hospital & Health Centre; Clin Instructor, University of British Columbia; (250)428-9371; Fax. (250)428-9350.

PERSAD, Emmanuel; Markham Stouffville Hosp, PO Box 1800 Stn Main 381 Church St, Markham ON L3P 7P3; Durham (England)'64; MB BS; DPsy; FRCPC; Psy (Mood Disorders). Staff, Markham Stouffville Hospital; Staff, St Joseph's Hospital - St Joseph's Health Care; Emeritus Prof, University of Western Ontario; (905)472-7011; Fax. (905)472-7871; epersad@uwo.ca.

PERSAD, Karen N; Family Practice Associates, PO Box 2010 223 16th Ave, Creston BC V0B 1G0; UBC'00; CCFP; (250)428-9371; Fax. (250)428-9350.

PERSAD, Rabindranath; 4 594-11405 87 Ave NW, Edmonton AB T6G 1C9; (Jamaica)'87; MB BS; FRCPC; Peds. (780)248-5420

PERSAD, Vashti C; Streetsville Med Centre, 8-5425 Creditview Rd, Mississauga ON L5V 2P3; Univ of the West Indies (Trinidad & Tobago)'00; CCFP; (905)826-1164

PERSAD, Vidia L; Brampton Med Bldg, 100-164 Queen St E, Brampton ON L6V 1B4; West Indies (Jamaica)'87; MB BS; MRC; FRCSC; ObstGyn (Perinatology). Staff, William Osler Health System - Brampton Civic Hospital; (905)595-0552; Fax. (905)595-0557.

PERSADIE, Richard J; Fontbonne Bldg, 301 James St S, Hamilton ON L8N 4A6; McM'95; BSc; FRCSC; ObstGyn (Colposcopy). Staff ObstGyn, St Joseph's Healthcare - Charlton Campus; Asst Prof, McMaster University; (905)521-6041; Fax. (905)521-6089; richardpersadie@hotmail.com.

PERSAUD, Baneshwar; Halton HSC Corp-Oakville, 327 Reynolds St, Oakville ON L6J 3L7; Glasgow (Scotland)'67; MB ChB; Anes. Staff, Halton Healthcare Services Corporation - Oakville Site; (905)338-4647

PERSAUD, David H; PO Box 21059 Rpo University Ma, Windsor ON N9B 3T4; Tor'88.

PERSAUD, Desiree A; The Ottawa Hosp-Civic Campus B3-1053 Carling Ave, Ottawa ON K1Y 4E9; Dal'92; FRCPC; Anes. Staff, The Ottawa Hospital - Civic Campus; (613)761-4940; Fax. (613)761-5032.

PERSAUD, Ganeshwar; 103-279 Wharncliffe Rd N, London ON N6H 2C2; Wes'92; CCFP; FCFP; (519)645-0100; Fax. (519)645-0103.

PERSAUD, Jeeshan; Wise Elephant Family Hlth Team, 280 Main St N, Brampton ON L6V 1P6; McM'10; CCFP; (905)216-1065; jpersaud@ahealingplace.ca.

PERSAUD, Mitra M P; 104-2100 8th St E, Saskatoon SK S7H 0V1; (Jamaica)'75; MB BS; DCH; FRCPC; Peds; ClinImmunol&Allergy. Clinical Asst Prof Peds, University of Saskatchewan; (306)975-0220

PERSAUD, Navindra; Health Centre @ 80 Bond, 80 Bond St, Toronto ON M5B 1X2; Tor'09; CCFP; (416)864-3011; Fax. (416)864-3099.

PERSAUD, Rainer; Psychiatry Inpatients, E1-715 12th Ave W, Vancouver BC V5Z 1M9; Man'94; FRCPC; Psy. Staff, Vancouver General Hospital - Centennial Pavillion; (604)875-4139

PERSAUDE, Darshini D; 202-1885 Glenanna Rd, Pickering ON L1V 6R6; West Indies (Jamaica)'92; CCFP; (905)492-3376; Fax. (905)492-3379.

PERSON, Terri A; Spiritwood Primary Hlth Care C, PO Box 69, Spiritwood SK S0J 2M0; Sask'07; CCFP; (306)883-4400; Fax. (306)883-2140.

PERSSON, Enok D; Agassiz Med Centre, 130-30 Stephen St, Morden MB R6M 2G3; Johannesburg (South Africa)'89; CCFP; (204)822-4474

PERSSON, Erika B; Glen Sather Sports Med Clinic, 11400 University Ave, Edmonton AB T6G 1Z1; Alb'05; FRCPC; Peds. Staff, University of Alberta Hospital; (780)407-5160; Fax. (780)407-5667.

PERSSON, Megan A; MUHC-Montreal Gen Hosp, B2 117-1650 av Cedar, Montreal QC H3G 1A4; Sask'96; CCFP; CCFP(E.M.); Staff Emerg, McGill University Health Centre - Montreal General Campus; Langs: English; French; (514)934-1934

PERSYKO, Lucien; 42 Prospect St, Newmarket ON L3Y 3S9; Wes'64; FRCPC; IntMed (Gastroenterology). Ac Staff, Southlake Regional Health Centre; (905)895-3761

PERTMAN, Shea; Heritage Med Research Centre, 362-107 University Campus NW, Edmonton AB T6G 2S2; UBC'03; FRCPC; IntMed; Endocrin&Metab. (780)407-3636; Fax. (780)407-6702.

PERTTULA, Edward A; 226-250B Greenbank Rd, Ottawa ON K2H 8X4; Ott'74; DPsy; (613)723-3149

PERUSSE, Isabelle; CLSC Haute-Yamaska, 294 rue Deragon, Granby QC J2G 5J5; Laval'89; Staff, Centre Hospitalier de Granby; (450)375-1442; Fax. (450)373-1304.

PERUSSE, Richard; 4870 boul Bourque, Sherbrooke QC J1N 3S5; Laval'93; CCFP; Langs: French; (819)820-2673; Fax. (819)820-2112.

PERVAIZ, Khalid; Golden Mile Shopping Centre, 214-3806 Albert St, Regina SK S4S 3R2; Punjab (Pakistan)'92; MB BS; CCFP; Langs: Urdu; (306)205-5430; Fax. (306)205-5431.

PERVERSEFF, Robert A; Royal University Hosp, 103 Hospital Dr, Saskatoon SK S7N 0W8; Sask'88; FRCPC; Anes. Staff, Royal University Hospital; (306)655-1183; Fax. (306)655-1279.

PERVEZ, Nadeem; Cross Cancer Institute, 11560 University Ave NW, Edmonton AB T6G 1Z2; Karachi (Pakistan)'92; FFRCSI; MSc; FRCPC; RadOncol (Prostate Cancer). Staff/Asst Prof, Cross Cancer Institute; (780)432-8517; Fax. (780)432-8380.

PERVEZ, Yasmin; St Joseph's Health Centre, 100 Westmount Rd, Guelph ON N1H 5H8; Karachi (Pakistan)'80; Gen Practice, St Joseph's Health Centre; (519)824-6000; Fax. (519)763-0264; ypervez@gghorg.ca.

PERZOW, Sidney M; 940 20th Ave W, Vancouver BC V5Z 1Y5; Sask'66; MRCPsy; BSc; FRCPC; Psy (Psychoanalysis & Psychotherapy). Vice Chief Dept of Psy, Surrey Memorial Hospital; (604)738-9988; sperzow@telus.net.

PESANT, Caroline; CHUS-Hop Fleurimont, 3001 12e av N, Sherbrooke QC J1H 5N4; Sher'00; FRCPC; Peds (Adolescent Medicine). Staff, Centre Hospitalier Universitaire de Sherbrooke-Hopital Fleurimont; (819)346-1110

PESANT, Marie-Helene; CHUS-Hop Fleurimont, 3001 12e av N, Sherbrooke QC J1H 5N4; Sher'04; FRCPC; IntMed; Endocrin&Metab. Staff, Centre Hospitalier Universitaire de Sherbrooke-Hopital Fleurimont; (819)346-1110 x23599; Fax. (819)820-6899.

PESANT, Yves; CSSS de Saint-Jerome, 290 rue de Montigny, Saint-Jerome QC J7Z 5T3; Mon'76; FRCPC; IntMed (Cardiology). ac Staff, Hôtel-Dieu de Saint-Jérôme; (450)431-1020

PESCHISOLIDO, Vincenzo; 10-2917 Bloor St W, Etobicoke ON M8X 1B4; Dublin (Ireland)'85; Langs: Italian; (416)207-8800; Fax. (416)207-0363.

PESCHKEN, Christine A; The Rehabilitation Centre, RR149-800 Sherbrook St, Winnipeg MB R3A 1M4; Sask'89; MSc; FRCPC; IntMed; Rheum. Staff Physician, Health Sciences Centre; Staff Physician, St Boniface General Hospital; Staff, The Rehabilitation Centre; Asst Prof, University of Manitoba; (204)787-2209; Fax. (204)787-4594; peschken@cc.umanitoba.ca.

PESENTI, John G; St Paul's Hosp, 1702 20th St W, Saskatoon SK S7M 0Z9; Sask'01; CCFP; Staff, St Paul's Hospital (Grey Nuns) of Saskatoon; (306)655-5113; Fax. (306)655-5963; humboldtclinic@sasktel.net.

PESKUN, Christopher J; 225-1333 Sheppard Ave W, North York ON M2J 1V1; Tor'05; FRCSC; OrthSurg.

PESSOTTO, Daniele A; South River Med Centre, PO Box 579, South River ON P0A 1X0; Tor'93; CCFP; FCFP; (705)386-0512; Fax. (705)386-0716.

PESTELL, Deborah; Queen Elizabeth II HSC, 1033A-1276 South Park St, Halifax NS B3H 2Y9; McM'93; MPH; CCFP; Staff, Queen Elizabeth II Health Sciences Centre - Victoria General Site; Langs: German; (902)225-8214

PESTRIDGE, Andrew D; 3411 32 Ave, Vernon BC V1T 2M9; Southampton (England)'93; (250)542-3112

PETCHO, Yves G; Pegasus Medical, 201-1 Hesperus Rd, Thornhill ON L4J 0G9; Qns'06; CCFP; (905)882-4949

PETCONI, Anca V; Weeneebayko Gen Hosp, PO Box 34 19 Hospital Dr, Moose Factory ON P0L 1W0; Timisoara (Romania)'93; CCFP; Staff, Weeneebayko General Hospital; (705)658-4544

PETER, Chantelle A; Queen Elizabeth II Hosp, 10409 98 St, Grande Prairie AB T8V 2E8; Cal'06; FRCPC; Anes. Staff, Queen Elizabeth II Hospital; (780)538-7100

PETER, Elizabeth A; 1901 Ocean Park Rd, Surrey BC V4A 3M2; McM'80; FRCPC; Anes. Staff/Clin Assoc Prof Anes, BC Women's Hospital & Health Centre; (604)538-1848

PETER, Kevin K; 1-20654 Fraser Hwy, Langley BC V3A 4G5; UBC'78; DAB; FRCPC; Derm (Cutaneous Laser Surgery). Consultant, Vancouver General Hospital - Centennial Pavillion; Consultant, Langley Memorial Hospital; Clin Instructor Derm, University of British Columbia; (604)530-6111; Fax. (604)530-7943.

PETERDY, Anne E; St Boniface Gen Hosp, 409 Tache Ave, Winnipeg MB R2H 2A6; Man'76; FRCPC; DiagRad; NuclearMed. Consultant Radiol, Health Sciences Centre; Ac Staff Nuclear Med, St Boniface General Hospital; Ac Staff Nuclear Med, Victoria General Hospital; Assoc Prof Radiol, University of Manitoba; (204)237-2748; apeterdy@sbgh.mb.ca.

PETERKIN, Allan D; Mount Sinai Hosp, 965F-600 University Ave, Toronto ON M5G 1X5; Man'85; DPsy(McG.); BSc; FRCPC; Psy (Consultation-Liaison);CCFP; FCFP; Head Narrative & Healthcare Humanities Prog, Mount Sinai Hospital; Sr Fellow, Massey College; Assoc Prof Psy & Family Med, University of Toronto; Langs: Bilingual(English/French); (416)586-4800 x3204; Fax. (416)586-5970; apeterkin@mtsinai.on.ca.

PETERKIN, Christine E A; 11 Andrews Dr W, Drayton ON N0G 1P0; McG'01; CCFP; Physician, Palmerston & District Hospital; (519)638-3088; Fax. (519)638-3982.

PETERS, Ago; 1294 Weston Rd, York ON M6M 4R3; Wes'58; Court Staff, Humber River Regional Hospital - Church Street Site; Physician Health Services, Kodak Canada Inc; Langs: Estonian; (416)243-0700; Fax. (416)243-0624.

PETERS, Alexander P; Agincourt Med Centre, 2020 Brimley Rd, Scarborough ON M1S 4R7; Tor'65; Court Staff, The Scarborough Hospital - General Campus; Court Staff, Rouge Valley Health System - Centenary Health Centre Site; (416)293-2404

PETERS, Anthea C; Clinical Sciences Bldg, 4 112-152 University Campus NW, Edmonton AB T6G 2G3; Sask'06; FRCPC; IntMed; Hem. (780)407-1584; Fax. (780)407-2680.

PETERS, Brian G T; Health Sciences Centre, AD203-820 Sherbrook St, Winnipeg MB R3A 1R9; Man'04; FRCSC; Urol. Staff, Health Sciences Centre; (204)774-8511

PETERS, Calvin N; PO Box 20071, Vernon BC V1T 9L4; Cal'06; CCFP; Surgeon, Calian (DND).

PETERS, Carl W; South Okanagan Eye Surgery, 100-200 Marina Way, Penticton BC V2A 1H4; Alb'97; BSc; MD; DABOph; FAAO; FRCSC; Ophth (Cataract). Staff, Penticton Regional Hospital; Physician, Summerland Health Centre; Surg Dir, Front Street Laser & Skin Care; (250)770-3211; Fax. (250)770-3216; soes@shawbiz.ca.

PETERS, Catherine J; Dominion Med Centres Ltd, 9122 23 Ave NW, Edmonton AB T6N 1H9; Alb'06; CCFP; (780)801-3360; Fax. (780)801-3366.

PETERS, Christyne J; Markham Stouffville Health Ctr, 301-377 Church St, Markham ON L6B 1A1; Wes'83; BSc; FRCSC; ObstGyn (Colposcopy). Staff ObstGyn, Markham Stouffville Hospital; (905)472-7129; Fax. (905)472-1416; cpeters@msh.on.ca.

PETERS, Claire; CSSS de Trois-Rivières, 1991 boul du Carmel, Trois-Rivieres QC G8Z 3R9; Laval'84; FRCPC; IntMed (Oncology); Hem. Staff, CSSS de Trois-Rivières; (819)697-3333

PETERS, Curt S; 4-51 Forest Hills Pky, Dartmouth NS B2W 6C6; UBC'04; FRCPC; Psy. (902)434-3263; Fax. (902)434-0181.

PETERS, Daniel A; The Ottawa Hosp-Civic Campus, 1053 Carling Ave, Ottawa ON K1Y 4E9; Qns'02; FRCSC; PlasSurg. Staff, The Ottawa Hospital - Civic Campus; (613)798-5555

PETERS, Diana M; Gemini Health Centre, 2010-6708 48 Ave, Camrose AB T4V 4S3; Alb'99; (780)672-9850; Fax. (780)672-9104.

PETERS, Geoffrey A; St Lawrence Med Clinic, PO Box 501 214 Bridge St, Cardinal ON K0E 1E0; Tor'84; BSc; Staff, Winchester District Memorial Hospital; Staff, Kemptville District Hospital; (613)657-3197; Fax. (613)657-3195.

PETERS, Grant L; Bridgeland Med Bldg, 103-803A 1 Ave NE, Calgary AB T2E 7C5; Cal'99; BSc; FRCPC; IntMed (Echocardiography); Cardiol. (403)231-7968; Fax. (403)215-2213.

PETERS, Grant M; Peterborough Reg HC-Hospital, 1 Hospital Dr, Peterborough ON K9J 7C6; Wes'88; Staff, Peterborough Regional Health Centre - Hospital Drive; (705)876-5022

PETERS, H Thomas; Broadway-Burrard Med Clinic, 1816 Broadway W, Vancouver BC V6J 1Y9; Alb'84; NBME; Staff Occup Health, Vancouver General Hospital - Centennial Pavillion; Assoc Staff, Providence Health Care - St Paul's Hospital; Instructor Med, University of British Columbia; (604)736-1888; Fax. (604)736-5544.

PETERS, Harold O; Riverwood Med Centre, 1295 Pembina Hwy, Winnipeg MB R3T 2B3; Dublin (Ireland)'70; MB BCh; (204)452-3345; Fax. (204)452-5339.

PETERS, Hein; Pan Am Sports Med Centre, 75 Poseidon Bay, Winnipeg MB R3M 3E4; Universty of Pretoria (South Africa)'85; LMCC(SportMed); CCFP; Langs: Afrikaans; (204)927-2699; hlpeters@mts.net.

PETERS, Johannes; Rocky Med Clinic, PO Box 99 Stn Main, Rocky-Mtn-House AB T4T 1A1; Pretoria (South Africa)'70; MB ChB; LMCC; (403)845-2815; Fax. (403)845-2177.

PETERS, Karina M; Greenbelt Family Health Team, 1C-3500 Fallowfield Rd, Ottawa ON K2J 4A7; McM'07; CCFP; (613)843-1718; Fax. (613)843-0201.

PETERS, Laura M; Fall River Family Practice, 3254 Highway 2, Fall River NS B2T 1J5; Sask'87; (902)861-2237; Fax. (902)861-1914.

PETERS, Laurenna D; TB Control Clinic, 655 12th Ave W, Vancouver BC V5Z 4R4; Cal'03; FRCPC; IntMed; InfectDis. Staff, BC Centre For Disease Control; (604)707-2692

PETERS, Leanne M; Avon Family Med Centre, 511 Huron St, Stratford ON N5A 5T8; Wes'06; CCFP; Aj Prof Schulich School of Med, University of Western Ontario; (519)508-1212; Fax. (519)508-1240.

PETERS, Lynne S; McGill University, B 5500-3600 rue McTavish, Montreal QC H3A 0G3; Dal'99; FRCPC; Psy. Langs: French; (514)398-6019; Fax. (514)398-5529.

PETERS, Michael S; Moncton Med Clinic, 408-860 Mountain Rd, Moncton NB E1C 2N7; Dal'82; Staff, The Moncton Hospital; (506)857-0247; Fax. (506)857-2234.

PETERS, Myta; Appletree Med Clinic, 275 Dundas St W, Toronto ON M5T 3K1; Nagpur (India)'83; CCFP; Staff, North York General Hospital; (647)722-2370; Fax. (416)367-4301.

PETERS, Reginald L; Abbotsford Reg Hosp & Cancer C, 32900 Marshall Rd, Abbotsford BC V2S 0C2; UBC'94; CCFP; CCFP(E.M.); FCFP; Staff, Abbotsford Regional Hospital & Cancer Centre; (604)851-4700

PETERS, Richard J; Health Sciences Centre, 820 Sherbrook St, Winnipeg MB R3A 1R9; Man'89; Staff, Health Sciences Centre; (204)787-3167; Fax. (204)787-5134.

PETERS, Rudolf T; Justik Med Clinic, 8225 105 St NW, Edmonton AB T6E 4H2; Alb'66; Ac Staff, Covenant Health - Edmonton General Continuing Care Centre; (780)432-0211; Fax. (780)439-9349.

PETERS, Ruth E; Great West Life, PO Box 6000 Stn Main, Winnipeg MB R3C 3A5; Man'79.

PETERS, Sharon D; Health Sciences Centre, 2327-300 Prince Philip Dr, St. John's NL A1B 3V6; Mem'74; FRCPC; IntMed (Critical Care Medicine). Staff, Health Sciences Centre; Vice Dean Faculty of Med/Prof, Memorial University Of Newfoundland; (709)777-7090; Fax. (709)777-7569; speters@mun.ca.

PETERS, Sheila M; Health Sciences Centre, 820 Sherbrook St, Winnipeg MB R3A 1R9; Man'93; CCFP; CCFP(E.M.); Staff Emerg, Health Sciences Centre; (204)774-6511

PETERS, Thomas H; Fredericton Med Clinic, 507-1015 Regent St, Fredericton NB E3B 6H5; Dal'72; FRCSC; GenSurg; ThorSurg. (506)458-0297; Fax. (506)457-4730; tpeters@nb.aibn.com.

PETERS, Walter J; Rosedale Med Centre, 802-600 Sherbourne St, Toronto ON M4X 1W4; Tor'72; BSc; PhD; FRCSC; PlasSurg (Breast Surgery). Staff Plastic Surg, Mount Sinai Hospital; Staff Plastic Surg, St Michael's Hospital; Prof Surg, University of Toronto; (416)926-7790; Fax. (416)926-4997.

PETERS, William B; Beamsville Med Ctr Fam Hlth Team, PO Box 430 4279 Hixon St, Beamsville ON L0R 1B0; McM'80; CCFP; FCFP; Clin Prof Famil Med, McMaster University; (905)563-5315; Fax. (905)563-0933.

PETERS-MAINVILLE, Dagmar; Lakeshore Gen Hosp, 160 av Stillview, Pointe-Claire QC H9R 2Y2; (Germany)'99; CCFP; Staff, Lakeshore General Hospital - Pointe Claire; (514)630-2225

PETERSEN, Agnieszka; Cape Breton Hlthcare Complex, 1482 George St, Sydney NS B1P 1P3; Gdansk (Poland)'98; Staff, Cape Breton Healthcare Complex; (902)567-0559; Fax. (902)567-7259.

PETERSEN, Karin; Manitouwadge Med Clinic, GD 1 Clinic Crt, Manitouwadge ON P0T 2C0; Ott'00; CCFP; (807)826-3333

PETERSON, Brian D; Okanagan Plastic Surgery Centr, 401-3320 Richter St, Kelowna BC V1W 4V5; Sask'84; BSc(Anat.); FACS; FRCSC; PlasSurg (Aesthetic Surgery). Ac Staff, Kelowna General Hospital; Staff Surgical Floor, Okanagan Plastic Surgery Centre; Med Dir, Okanagan Health Surgical Centre; Dir Skin Care Floor, Okanagan Skin Care Centre; Assoc Prof, University of British Columbia; (250)868-9290; Fax. (258)868-9704.

PETERSON, Cameron G; Health Sciences Centre, 820 Sherbrook St, Winnipeg MB R3A 1R9; Man'92; BSc; CCFP; CCFP(E.M.); Staff, Health Sciences Centre; (204)787-2934; Fax. (204)787-2231.

PETERSON, Carly E; Univ Hlt Network-Toronto Gen, 3EN 461-200 Elizabeth St, Toronto ON M5G 2C4; UBC'05; Anes. Staff, Toronto General Hospital - UHN; (416)340-3111

PETERSON, Colin L; Royal Alexandra Hosp, 541-10240 Kingsway NW, Edmonton AB T5H 3V9; Sask'96; CCFP; CCFP(E. M.); Staff, Royal Alexandra Hospital; (780)735-4442; Fax. (780)735-4916.

PETERSON, Daniel R; Univ of Western Ontario, M106-1151 Richmond St, London ON N6A 5C1; Cal'08.

PETERSON, Darin C; Jackson Park Health Centre, 245-2475 McDougall St, Windsor ON N8X 3N9; Ott'96; CCFP; (519)250-5656

PETERSON, Devin C; McMaster University HSC, 4E11-1200 Main St W, Hamilton ON L8S 4J9; Dal'93; FRCSC; OrthSurg. (905)521-2100; Fax. (905)521-9992.

PETERSON, George; Clinique Med Payer Inc, 5975 boul Payer, Saint-Hubert QC J3Y 6W6; Mon'84; Langs: Spanish; English; (450)656-8221; Fax. (450)656-0515.

PETERSON, Jocelyn; Queen Elizabeth Hosp, PO Box 6600 Stn Central 60 Riverside Dr, Charlottetown PE C1A 8T5; Dal'10; CCFP; Staff, Queen Elizabeth Hospital; (902)894-2111

PETERSON, John C; 101-250 Lawrence Ave W, Toronto ON M5M 1B2; McM'93; FRCPC; IntMed; Cardiol. (416)256-7100; johncpeterson@hotmail.com.

PETERSON, John D; Windsor Park Med Centre, 159 St Anne's Rd, Winnipeg MB R2M 2Z5; Man'72; Staff, St Boniface General Hospital; (204)256-4343

PETERSON, Karina; Hôpital régional Chaleur, 1750 Sunset Blvd, Bathurst NB E2A 4L7; Hesse (Germany)'97; Staff, Hopital Regional Chaleur; (506)544-3000

PETERSON, Keir M; Royal Alexandra Hosp, 541CSC-10240 Kingsway NW, Edmonton AB T5H 3V9; Wes'03; CCFP; CCFP(E. M.); Staff, Royal Alexandra Hospital; (780)735-4442

PETERSON, Mark D; St Michael's Hosp, 30 Bond St, Toronto ON M5B 1W8; Man'98; BSc; PhD; FRCSC; CardSurg (EndovascularSurg). Staff Cardiovascular & Endovascular Surg/Asst Prof Surg, St Michael's Hospital; Aj Scientist, Li Ka Shing Knowledge Institute; (416)864-3086; Fax. (416)864-6096.

PETERSON, Michael; 280 Main St, Lucan ON N0M 2J0; Ott'06; BA; MSc; BSc; CCFP; Consultant, London Health Sciences Centre - University Hospital; Consultant, St Joseph's Hospital - St Joseph's Health Care; Aj Teacher, Schulich School of Medicine-University of Western Ontario; (519)227-4444; Fax. (519)227-4414.

PETERSON, Rebecca; 1053 Carling Ave, Ottawa ON K1Y 4E9; Sask'70; BSc; FRCPC; DiagRad (Chest & Cardiac Radiology). Chief Radiol, The Ottawa Hospital - Civic Campus; Assoc Prof, University of Ottawa; (613)798-5555 x14892; Fax. (613)761-4476; rpeterson@ottawahospital.on.ca.

PETERSON, Robert G; Children's & Women's HC of BC, 2H02-4480 Oak St, Vancouver BC V6H 3V4; Yale(CT) (USA)'74; AB; PhD; MPH; Staff, BC Children's Hospital; (604)875-2345 x5231; Fax. (604)875-2074.

PETERSON, Sean R D; Bluewater Health-Norman Site, 89 Norman St, Sarnia ON N7T 6S3; Wes'07; CCFP; CCFP(E.M.); Staff, Bluewater Health - Norman Site; (519)464-4400; Fax. (519)336-8780.

PETERSON, Todd M; Rockyview Gen Hosp, 7007 14 St SW, Calgary AB T2V 1P9; UBC'01; CCFP; CCFP(E.M.); Staff, Rockyview General Hospital; (403)943-3449

PETI, Charles A; Regina Qu'Appelle HR-Pasqua, 100-4101 Dewdney Ave, Regina SK S4T 1A5; UBC'81; Staff, Pasqua Hospital; Clin Instructor, University of Saskatchewan; (306)766-2238; Fax. (306)766-2770.

PETICCA, Patricia; Rideau Valley Health Services, 1221 Greenbank Rd, Ottawa ON K2J 5V7; Ott'05; IntMed. (613)258-8716; Fax. (613)440-3238.

PETIT, Bruno; Hop Maisonneuve-Rosemont, 5415 boul de l'Assomption, Montreal QC H1T 2M4; Sher'85; CSPQ; FRCPC; Anes. Staff, Hopital Maisonneuve-Rosemont; (514)252-3426

PETIT, Francine; Clinique Med Monchamp, 102-227 rue Sainte-Catherine, Saint-Constant QC J5A 2J5; Mon'82; ObstGyn. Staff, Hôpital Anna-Laberge; (450)632-2245

PETIT, Genevieve; ASSS de l'Estrie, 300-300 rue King E, Sherbrooke QC J1G 1B1; Sher'98; FRCPC; CommunMed (Family Medicine). (819)829-3400 x42019; Fax. (819)596-8894.

PETIT, Karine; CSSS Vallee de la Batiscan, 750 rue du Couvent, Saint-Tite QC G0X 3H0; Laval'06; CCFP; Teach Staff, Universite de Montreal; (418)365-7555; Fax. (418)365-3998; karine_petit@ssss.gouv.qc.ca.

PETIT, Lyndal C; The Ottawa Hosp-Gen Campus, 501 Smyth Rd, Ottawa ON K1H 8L6; Ott'04; FRCPC; Psy. Staff, The Ottawa Hospital - General Campus; (613)798-5555

PETIT, Michel; 202-144 ch de la Grande-cote, Rosemere QC J7A 1H3; Sher'77; (450)437-9911; m.petit@videotron.ca.

PETIT, Normand; CSSS de la Vallée de l'Or, 725 6e rue, Val-d'Or QC J9P 3Y1; Mon'86; FRCPC; Peds. Staff, Centre Hospitalier de Val d'Or; (819)825-6711; Fax. (819)825-5624.

PETITCLERC, Claude; CHUM-Hop Notre-Dame, 1560 rue Sherbrooke E, Montreal QC H2L 4M1; Mon'63; PhD(Biochem); CSPQ; FRCPC; MedBiochem (P.Q.); MedScient(Med). Chef Dept of Biochem, Centre Hospitalier l'Université de Montréal (CHUM) - Hôpital Notre-Dame; (514)890-8000 x25784; Fax. (514)412-7553.

PETITCLERC, Claude; Ctr Hosp Affilie-Enfant-Jesus, 1401 18e rue, Quebec QC G1J 1Z4; Laval'61; Hem (P.Q.) (Oncology). Staff, Centre Hospitalier Affilié Universitaire de Québec - Hôpital De L'Enfant Jésus; Consultant, Centre Hospitalier Universitaire De Québec - Pavillon De St-françois-d'assise; Clin Prof, Université Laval; Langs: Spanish; English; (418)649-0252

PETITCLERC, Luc; Ctr Hosp Affilie-Enfant-Jesus, 1401 18e rue, Quebec QC G1J 1Z4; Mon'93; FRCSC; OrthSurg (Trauma & Reconstructive Surgery). Staff OrthSurg, Centre Hospitalier Affilié Universitaire de Québec - Hôpital De L'Enfant Jésus; Teach Staff, Université Laval; (418)649-0252

PETITCLERC, Marc; Hotel-Dieu de Levis, 143 rue Wolfe, Levis QC G6V 3Z1; Mon'92; MSc; FRCPC; Neur; Electroenceph (P.Q.). Staff, Hôtel-Dieu de Lévis; Langs: English; (418)835-7121; Fax. (418)835-7212.

PETITCLERC, Michel; Centre Med Berger, 208-1000 ch Sainte-Foy, Quebec QC G1S 2L6; Laval'66; CSPQ; FRCPC; DiagRad. Ac Staff, Centre Hospitalier Affilié Universitaire de Québec - Hôpital du St-Sacrement; Assoc Staff, CSSS de Quebec-Sud; (418)681-2262; Fax. (418)681-0125.

PETITCLERC, Sophie; MUHC-Royal Victoria Hosp, 687 av des Pins O, Montreal QC H3A 1A1; Mon'02; FRCPC; DiagRad. Staff, McGill University Health Centre - Royal Victoria Hospital; (514)934-1934 x42927

PETITPAS, Anick; Clin externe de Psychiatrie, 279 rue de la Providence, Granby QC J2G 4S7; Sher'04; FRCPC; Psy. (450)375-8002

PETO, John J; The Court, 302-2863 Ellesmere Rd, Scarborough ON M1E 5E9; Tor'76; FRCPC; IntMed; GeriatricMed. (416)281-0025; Fax. (416)281-0026.

PETRAGLIA, Teresa; CLSC Nord de l'Ile, 11822 av de Bois-de-Boulogne, Montreal QC H3M 2X6; Mon'85; CCFP; Staff Teacher, Universite de Montreal; Langs: French; Italian; (514)331-2572; Fax. (514)331-0137.

PETRAKI, Nabil; CSSS de Memphremagog, 50 rue Saint-Patrice E, Magog QC J1X 3X3; Mon'73; FACS; GenSurg (P.Q.)., Universite de Sherbrooke; (819)843-3381

PETRAKOS, Andrew; Petrakos Med Professional Corp, 350-1720 Howard Ave, Windsor ON N8X 5A6; Wes'78; FRCSC; GenSurg. Ac Staff Surg, Windsor Regional Hospital - Metropolitan Site; (519)255-9616; Fax. (519)255-9908; a_petrakos@hotmail.com.

PETRAR, Steven D; St Paul's Hosp, 1081 Burrard St, Vancouver BC V6Z 1Y6; Cal'07; FRCPC; Anes. Staff, Providence Health Care - St Paul's Hospital; (604)682-2344

PETRASEK, Anthony J; Alexander Medical Bldg, 204-849 Alexander Crt, Peterborough ON K9J 7H8; Tor'89; FACS; DABS; FRCSC; GenSurg (Breast Oncology). Staff, Peterborough Regional Health Centre - Hospital Drive; (705)876-4544; Fax. (705)876-4548.

PETRASEK, John S; William Osler HC-Brampton, 2100 Bovaird Dr E, Brampton ON L6R 3J7; Tor'95; FRCPC; Anes. Staff, William Osler Health System - Brampton Civic Hospital; (905)494-2120; johnpetrasek@sympatico.ca.

PETRASEK, Paul F; Peter Lougheed Centre, 3500 26 Ave NE, Calgary AB T1Y 6J4; Tor'87; FRCSC; GenSurg; VascSurg. Staff, Peter Lougheed Centre; Staff, Foothills Medical Centre; Staff, Rockyview General Hospital; Assoc Prof, University of Calgary; (403)943-5507; Fax. (403)291-2734; paul.petrasek@calgaryhealthregion.ca.

PETRASZKO, Tanya R; Canadian Blood Services, 4750 Oak St, Vancouver BC V6H 2N9; Wes'93; FRCPC; IntMed; Hem. Staff Hem, Vancouver General Hospital - Centennial Pavillion; Med Consultant BC & Yukon Centre, Canadian Blood Services; Clin Assoc Prof, University of British Columbia; (604)470-3427; Fax. (604)875-8004; tanya.petraszko@blood.ca.

PETREA, Constantin; Trafalgar Prof Centre, 300-1235 Trafalgar Rd, Oakville ON L6H 3P1; Bucharest (Romania)'83; Ac Staff, Halton Healthcare Services Corporation - Oakville Site; (905)842-0071; Fax. (905)844-3811.

PETRECCA, Kevin; MUHC-Montreal Neurology Inst, 109-3801 rue University, Montreal QC H3A 2B4; McG'02; FRCSC; Neursurg. Staff, McGill University Health Centre - Montreal Neurological Hospital; (514)398-1933

PETRELLA, Nick J; 306-5993 rue Jean-Talon E, Saint-Leonard QC H1S 1M5; Ott'65; Langs: Italian; Bilingual(English/French); (514)252-9111; Fax. (514)252-7316; nicholaspetrella@bellnet.ca.

PETRELLA, Robert J; St Joseph's HC-Parkwood Hosp, B3002-801 Commissioners Rd E, London ON N6C 5J1; Cal'90; PhD; FACSM; CCFP; FCFP; Staff Aging Rehab & Geriatric Care Research Ctre, Parkwood Hospital - St Joseph's Health Care; Staff, London Health Sciences Centre - Victoria Campus; Staff Family Med, St Joseph's Hospital - St Joseph's Health Care; Med Dir, Centre for Activity & Ageing; Assoc Prof Family Med & Kinesiology, University of Western Ontario; (519)685-4292 x42983; Fax. (519)685-4071.

PETRELLA, Teresa M; Toronto Sunnybrook Reg Cancer, 2075 Bayview Ave, Toronto ON M4N 3M5; Qns'96; FRCPC; IntMed; MedOncol. Staff, Sunnybrook Health Sciences Centre; (416)480-5248; Fax. (416)480-6002.

PETRESCU, Claudia; 104-4430 Bathurst St, North York ON M3H 3S3; Bucharest (Romania)'66; Staff, North York General Hospital; Langs: Romanian; Hungarian; (416)633-6333; Fax. (416)633-2228.

PETRIE, Alison C R A; Owen Sound Med Centre, 2000-1415 1st Ave W, Owen Sound ON N4K 4K8; Wes'89; CCFP; FCFP; (519)470-3030; Fax. (519)370-4046.

PETRIE, Daniel W; Aberdeen Hosp, 835 East River Rd, New Glasgow NS B2H 3S6; Dal'07; FRCPC; DiagRad. Staff, Aberdeen Regional Hospital; (902)752-7600

PETRIE, David A; Queen Elizabeth II HSC-Halifax, 1796 Summer St, Halifax NS B3H 3A7; Dal'89; FRCPC; EmergMed. Staff, Queen Elizabeth II Health Sciences Centre - Halifax Infirmary Site; Staff, Queen Elizabeth II Health Sciences Centre - Victoria General Site; Head Emergency Med, Dalhousie University; (902)473-8959

PETRIE, Edward A; 224 Oxford St, Fredericton NB E3B 2W5; McG'59; FAB; BSc; MDCM; FRCPC; Anes. Court Staff Anes, Dr Everett Chalmers Regional Hospital; (506)454-5637

PETRIE, Ian B; 1415 1st Ave W, Owen Sound ON N4K 4K8; Edinburgh (Scotland)'62; Physician, Peel County Community Health Centre; (519)970-3030; Fax. (705)293-1067.

PETRIE, Matthew D; South Muskoka Mem Hosp, 75 Ann St, Bracebridge ON P1L 2E4; Qns'02; CCFP; CCFP(E.M.); Staff, South Muskoka Memorial Hospital - Muskoka Algonquin Healthcare; (705)645-4404

PETRIE, Neil M; Queen Elizabeth II HSC-Halifax, 1796 Summer St, Halifax NS B3H 3A7; Dal'06; FRCPC; EmergMed. Staff, Queen Elizabeth II Health Sciences Centre - Halifax Infirmary Site; (902)473-2700

PETRIK, David W; BC Cancer Ctre-Southern Interi, 399 Royal Ave, Kelowna BC V1Y 5L3; Alb'95; DABR; FRCPC; RadOncol. Staff, BC Cancer Agency Sindi Ahluwalia Hawkins Centre for the Southern Interior; (250)712-3958; Fax. (250)712-3911.

PETRINI, Mariano; Columbus Med Arts Bldg, 206-8333 Weston Rd, Woodbridge ON L4L 8E2; Rome (Italy)'80; Ac Staff, Humber River Regional Hospital - Finch Avenue Site; Ac Staff, William Osler Health System - Etobicoke General Hospital; (905)856-3433; Fax. (905)856-3390.

PETRINI, Michael J; 247 Bridge St PO Box 370, Eganville ON K0J 1T0; Davis(CA) (USA)'79; Ac Staff, Pembroke Regional Hospital Inc; (613)628-2523 x3477; Fax. (613)628-5088.

PETRISOR, Bradley A; McMaster University, 5N 529-1280 Main St W, Hamilton ON L8S 4K1; Tor'98; FRCSC; OrthSurg. Staff, Hamilton Health Sciences Centre - Hamilton General Hospital; (905)527-4322; Fax. (905)523-6776.

PETRIW, Boris Z; Royal Alexandra Hosp, 10240 Kingsway NW, Edmonton AB T5H 3V9; Alb'79; Anes. Staff, Royal Alexandra Hospital; (780)735-4010; Fax. (780)459-5190.

PETRLICH, Steve T; Bellwood Plaza, 14B-900 Oxford St E, London ON N5Y 5A1; Wes'91; CCFP; FCFP; Staff, London Health Sciences Centre - Victoria Campus; (519)451-0720; Fax. (519)451-4370.

PETROCCI, Michael C; Niagara H System-St Catharines, PO Box 3018 Stn Main 142 Queenston St, St Catharines ON L2R 7C6; McG'82; CCFP; CCFP(E.M.); Staff, Niagara Health System - St Catharines General Site; (905)684-7271 x5461

PETROF, Basil J; MUHC-Royal Victoria Hosp, L411-687 av des Pins O, Montreal QC H3A 1A1; Laval'83; FRCPC; IntMed; Respir. Staff, McGill University Health Centre - Royal Victoria Hospital; (514)934-1934 x35946; Fax. (514)843-1695; basil.petrof@mcgill.ca.

PETROF, Elaine O; Kingston Gen Hosp, 76 Stuart St, Kingston ON K7L 2V7; Tor'96; Staff, Kingston General Hospital; (613)549-6666

PETROFF, Howard L; Buliding E, 200B-1105 Kingston Rd, Pickering ON L1V 1B5; Tor'87; CCFP; CCFP(E.M.); FCFP; Ac Staff, Rouge Valley Health System - Ajax & Pickering Health Centre Site; Staff Emerg Dept, Mount Sinai Hospital; Lecturer Family & Commun Med, University of Toronto; (905)420-9999; Fax. (905)420-1090; h.petroff@utoronto.ca.

PETRONIENE, Rima; Barrie GI Associates, 301-5 Quarry Ridge Rd, Barrie ON L4M 7G1; Kaunas (Lithuania)'86; PhD; MD; FRCPC; IntMed (Gastroenterology). Staff, Royal Victoria Regional Health Centre; Staff, Stevenson Memorial Hospital; Langs: Lithuanian; Russian; (705)721-3344; Fax. (705)721-5522.

PETROPOLIS, Nicholas P; 303-301 Columbia st E, New Westminster BC V3L 3W5; Dal'07; CCFP; (604)525-5388

PETROPOLIS, Peter N; 6075 Lady Hammond Rd, Halifax NS B3K 2R8; Dal'84; (902)453-0161; Fax. (902)405-1503.

PETROPOULOS, Vivian; St Mary's Hosp Centre, 3830 av Lacombe, Montreal QC H3T 1M5; McG'92; FRCPC; IntMed; Cardiol. Staff, St Mary's Hospital Centre; (514)734-2614; Fax. (514)734-2766.

PETROSONIAK, Andrew M; Hamilton HS-General Campus, 237 Barton St E, Hamilton ON L8L 2X2; Ott'09; Staff, Hamilton Health Sciences Centre - Hamilton General Hospital; (905)522-9017

PETROSONIAK, Peter; Lindsay Prof Bldg, 9-65 Angeline St N, Lindsay ON K9V 5N7; Tor'75; Court Staff, Ross Memorial Hospital; Langs: Ukrainian; (705)324-8212; Fax. (705)324-8223.

PETROSSIAN, Caroline; Specialized Geriatric Clinic, 232 Ross Dr, New Westminster BC V3L 0B2; UBC'91; FRCPC; IntMed; GeriatricMed. (604)528-5031

PETROU, Constantine S; 210-3852 Finch Ave E, Scarborough ON M1T 3T9; Athens (Greece)'81; FAAP; FRCPC; Peds. Chief Peds, Toronto East General Hospital Inc; Langs: Greek; (416)297-5511

PETROV, Elena; Rockyview Gen Hosp, 7007 14 St SW, Calgary AB T2V 1P9; Moscow (Russia (Federation))'79; FRCPC; Psy. Clin Med Dir Unit 49, Rockyview General Hospital; Langs: Russian; (403)943-8704; Fax. (403)259-6289.

PETROV, Ivan; Medical Bldg, 206-1615 Dufferin St, Toronto ON M6H 4H4; Prague (Czech Republic)'80; Ac Staff, St Joseph's Health Centre; Facilitator Problem Based Small Grp Learning Prog, McMaster University; Clin Instructor Family & Community Med, University of Toronto; Langs: Czech; Slovak; Italian; (416)652-1070 x3771; Fax. (416)652-1070.

PETROV, Nicole M; Geddes Med Group, 143 Metcalfe St, Elora ON N0B 1S0; Qns'97; BSc; CCFP; (519)846-2224; Fax. (519)846-2005.

PETROVIC, Danica; Grandview Woodlands Mental HT, 1669 Broadway E, Vancouver BC V5N 1V9; UBC'92; Langs: Croatian; Serbian; (604)251-2264

PETROVIC, Sean; 3-1767 152 St, Surrey BC V4A 4N3; Man'88; BSc; Med Staff, Peace Arch Hospital; (604)535-3388; Fax. (604)542-2667.

PETROVIC, Vanja; Dept of Medicine, 10203-2775 Laurel St, Vancouver BC V5Z 1M9; UBC'07; IntMed. (604)716-2122

PETROVICH, Milenko; 212 ch Cote-Saint-Antoine, Westmount QC H3Y 2J3; Belgrade (Serbia)'84; IntMed (P.Q.) (Intensive Care).

PETROZ, Guy C; 555 University Ave, Toronto ON M5G 1X8; Geneva (Switzerland)'89; Staff, The Hospital For Sick Children; Langs: French; German; (416)813-7445; Fax. (416)813-7543.

PETRUCCELLI, Karen; The Credit Valley hosp, 2200 Eglinton Ave W, Mississauga ON L5M 2N1; Tor'03; FRCPC; Psy. Staff, The Credit Valley Hospital; (905)813-4426; Fax. (905)813-1594.

PETRUCCI, Martin; CSSS du Sud de Lanaudière, 911 montee des Pionniers, Terrebonne QC J6V 2H2; Laval'08; IntMed. Staff, Centre Hospitalier Pierre le Gardeur; (450)654-7525

PETRUK, Kenneth C; University of Alberta Hosp, 2D102-8440 112 St NW, Edmonton AB T6G 2B7; Alb'67; PhD; BSc; Neursurg (Neuro Oncology). Ac Staff, Royal Alexandra Hospital; Ac Staff, University of Alberta Hospital; Reg Prog Dir Neurosciences, Alberta Health Services; Dir Neuro Surg/Clin Prof, University of Alberta; (780)407-3029; Fax. (780)407-7465; kpetruk@ualberta.ca.

PETRUNIA, Denis M; Medical-Dental Bldg, 303-1120 Yates St, Victoria BC V8V 3M9; Cal'76; BSc; MSc; FRCPC; IntMed (Gastrointestinal Endoscopy); Gastroent. Consultant, BC Cancer Agency Vancouver Island Centre; Staff, Royal Jubilee Hospital; Staff, Victoria General Hospital; (250)381-9988; Fax. (250)381-9902.

PETRUT, Bianca; North York Gen Hosp, 4001 Leslie St, North York ON M2K 1E1; (Romania)'96; FRCPC; IntMed; GeriatricMed. Staff, North York General Hospital; (416)756-6000

PETRY, Thierry; CSSS de la Cote-de-Gaspe, 215 boul de York O, Gaspe QC G4X 2W2; Nancy (France)'77; CSPQ; Anes (P.Q.) (Pain Management). Anesthesiste, Centre Hospitalier de Gaspe; Staff Anes, CSSS Tulattavik; Langs: Bilingual(French/English); (418)368-3301; Fax. (418)368-6850.

PETRYK, Justin; Sturgeon Community Hosp, 201 Boudreau Rd, St. Albert AB T8N 6C4; Alb'06; FRCPC; Psy. Staff, Sturgeon Community Hospital; (780)418-7379; Fax. (780)418-8170.

PETRYK, Susan C; Wascana Rehab Centre, 2180 23rd Ave, Regina SK S4S 0A5; Alb'92; FRCPC; Peds (Neuro Development Pediatrics). Pediatrics, Wascana Rehabilitation Centre; Physician, Child & Youth Mental Health Services; Clin Assoc Prof, University of Saskatchewan; (306)766-5902; Fax. (306)766-5189.

PETSIKAS, Dimitri J; Richardson House, 102 Stuart St, Kingston ON K7L 2V6; McG'85; FRCSC; GenSurg; CardiothorSurg; Cardiovasc&ThorSurg (P.Q.); VascSurg. Staff, Kingston General Hospital; Staff, Hotel-Dieu Hospital; Asst Prof, Queen's University; (613)548-2383; Fax. (613)549-2902.

PETTAPIECE, Kenneth G; PO Box 391, Chemainus BC V0R 1K0; UBC'90; BSc(Zool); BA(Psychology); FRCPC; Anes.

PETTERSEN, Carl; 2-255 rue Collard, Alma QC G8B 1M8; Laval'86; GenSurg. Staff GenSurg, CSSS de Lac-Saint Jean-Est; (418)662-8221; Fax. (418)662-2125.

PETTERSEN, Geraldine; Hôpital Ste-Justine, 3175 ch Cote-Ste-Catherine, Montreal QC H3T 1C5; Sher'01; FRCPC; Peds; Critical Care Medicine (P.Q.). Staff, Hôpital Ste-Justine; (514)345-4931 x3315

PETTERSEN, Jacqueline A; University Hosp of Northern BC, 1475 Edmonton St, Prince George BC V2M 1S2; Tor'01; FRCPC; Neur. Staff, University Hospital of Northern British Columbia; (250)565-5770

PETTIGREW, Norman M; The Brodie Centre, 401-727 McDermot Ave, Winnipeg MB R3E 3P5; Glasgow (Scotland)'64; MB ChB; FRCPath; FRCS(Ed); FCAP; Prof Path, University of Manitoba.

PETTINGER, Cary S; Same Day Clinic, 100-1345 Taylor Ave, Winnipeg MB R3M 3Y9; Man'02; CCFP; (204)475-0088

PETTIS, Craig A; Amherstview Med Centre, 18 Manitou Cres W, Amherstview ON K7N 1S3; Qns'74; CCFP; FCFP; Court Staff, Kingston General Hospital; Court Staff, Hotel-Dieu Hospital; Physician, Invista Canada Co; (613)634-1813; Fax. (613)634-1253; craigpettis@gmail.com.

PETTLE, Alvin; Ruth Pettle Wellness Centre, 207-3910 Bathurst St, North York ON M3H 5Z3; Tor'69; ObstGyn (Bio-Identical Hormone Replacement). Med Dir, Ruth Pettle Wellness Centre; (416)633-4101; Fax. (416)633-9254; loracal@rogers.com.

PETTS, Leslie A; 2-38 Margaret St, Angus ON L0M 1B0; Alb'70; (705)424-7117; Fax. (705)424-1529.

PETTY, Ross E; Children's & Women's HC of BC, K4 121-4480 Oak St, Vancouver BC V6H 3V4; Sask'65; FRCPC; Peds; Rheum (Pediatric Rheumatology). Staff, BC Children's Hospital; (604)875-2437

PETZOLD, James E; Gibsons Med Clinic, 211-1100 Sunshine Coast Hwy, Gibsons BC V0N 1V7; UBC'79; Staff, St Mary's Hospital; (604)886-2868; Fax. (604)886-9716.

PEWARCHUK, Jesse A; Victoria Gen Hosp, 1 Hospital Way, Victoria BC V8Z 6R5; Alb'06; FRCPC; IntMed. Staff, Victoria General Hospital; (250)727-4212

PEWARCHUK, Willie J; Cowichan Med Centre, 3106 Gibbins Rd, Duncan BC V9L 1E8; Alb'84; FRCPC; IntMed (Hematological Oncology). Staff, Cowichan District Hospital; (250)748-1323

PEYSAR, Gerhard W; Orillia Soldiers' Mem Hosp, 170 Colborne St W, Orillia ON L3V 2Z3; Wes'04; CCFP; Staff, Orillia Soldiers' Memorial Hospital; (705)325-2201

PEYTON, Michael A; The Malone Med Clinic, 4955 41 Ave, Drayton Valley AB T7A 1V4; Queen's (Ireland)'77; MB ChB; BAO; (780)542-3366; Fax. (780)542-6207; malone@telusplanet.net.

PEYVANDI, Banafsheh; 7550 King George Blvd, Surrey BC V3W 2T2; Mashhad (Iran)'97; CCFP; (604)598-9880

PEZARRO, Christine E; 1504 15 Ave SW, Calgary AB T3C 0X9; Cal'83; BSc; CCFP; FCFP; (403)245-8008

PEZESHKI, Bijan; 9534 87 St NW, Edmonton AB T6C 3J1; (Iran)'92; CCFP; Staff, Glenrose Rehabilitation Hospital; (780)440-8274; Fax. (780)469-6495.

PEZIM, Michael E; Hycroft Med Bldg, 30-3195 Granville St, Vancouver BC V6H 3K2; Tor'79; DABS; DABCRS; FACS; FRCSC; GenSurg (Colon & Rectal Surgery). (604)730-5810; Fax. (604)730-5820.

PEZZOT, Donald E; 300-5511 West Boulevard, Vancouver BC V6M 3W6; Alb'75; BSc; FRCPC; Psy (Psychotherapy). (604)264-9400

PEZZUTTO, Donato; 1051 Wonderland Rd S, London ON N6K 3X4; Wes'83; Langs: Italian; (519)472-2060; Fax. (519)471-7299.

PEZZUTTO, Lucia; 1051 Wonderland Rd S, London ON N6K 3X4; Wes'85; CCFP; FCFP; Court Staff, London Health Sciences Centre - Victoria Campus; Court Staff, St Joseph's Hospital - St Joseph's Health Care; Langs: Italian; (519)472-2060; Fax. (519)471-7299.

PFAFF, James R; Transport Canada, 300-4900 Yonge St, North York ON M2N 6A5; Tor'74; BSc(RMC); MHSc; DAvMed(Lond); AFOM; LMCC; Med Consultant, Transport Canada; (416)952-0562; Fax. (416)952-0569; jim.pfaff@tc.gc.ca.

PFEFFER, Gerald; UBC Health Sciences Centre, 2211 Wesbrook Mall, Vancouver BC V6T 2B5; McG'05; FRCPC; Neur. (604)822-7121

PFEFFERKORN, Carol R; Northside Med Group, 102-1015 Austin Ave, Coquitlam BC V3K 3N9; UBC'86; (604)939-9251

PFEIFER, Joseph J T; Medical Arts Bldg, 222-750 Spadina Cres E, Saskatoon SK S7K 3H3; Sask'78; FRCSC; GenSurg. Member, College of Physicians & Surgeons of Saskatchewan; Clinical Asst Prof, University of Saskatchewan; (306)653-3366; Fax. (306)653-8832; pfeiferj@shin.sk.ca.

PFEIFER, Linda M; 9401 86 Ave, Fort Saskatchewan AB T8L 0C6; Sask'94; CCFP; Staff Privil, Fort Saskatchewan Health Centre; Staff Privil., Anes., Sturgeon Community Hospital; (780)998-2256; Fax. (780)992-7240.

PFEIFER, Sabine I; 16-385 Frederick St, Kitchener ON N2H 2P2; Ott'02; CCFP; Langs: German; (519)745-7932; Fax. (519)745-1881.

PFEIFFER, Any Z; 101-420 Bronte St S, Milton ON L9T 0H9; Sao Paulo (Brazil)'98; Staff, Halton Healthcare Services Corporation - Oakville Site; Staff, Halton Healthcare Services Corporation - Milton District Hospital; Langs: Portuguese; (905)878-9720; Fax. (905)878-3779.

PFEIFFER, David; Health Canada, 200 Tunney's Pasture Drwy, Ottawa ON K1A 0K9; Ott'78; CCFP; (613)948-3248; david_pfeiffer@carleton.ca.

PFEIFFER, Shannon L; PO Box 15085 Rpo Aspenwoods, Calgary AB T3H 0N8; Ott'05; CCFP.

PFEIFFER, Uta E; MUHC-Royal Victoria Hosp, 687 av des Pins O, Montreal QC H3A 1A1; Erlangen (Germany)'91; CSPQ; Anes (P.Q.). Staff, McGill University Health Centre - Royal Victoria Hospital; (514)834-1934

PFLUG, Michael; 7-3545 Kingston Rd, Scarborough ON M1M 1R6; Paris (France)'60; FRCPC; IntMed (Rheumatology). (416)264-2513; Fax. (416)264-2164.

PFLUGFELDER, Peter W; London HSC-University Hosp, 339 Windermere Rd, London ON N6A 5A5; Wes'78; FRCPC; IntMed (Cardiology). Ac Staff Cardiol, London Health Sciences Centre - University Hospital; (519)663-3809; Fax. (519)434-3278; ppflug@uwo.ca.

PHALA, Everard M; Niagara H System-G Niagara, PO Box 1018 Stn Main 5546 Portage Rd, Niagara Falls ON L2E 6X2; Ibadan (Nigeria)'74; DA(Anes); FRCPC; Anes (Intensive & Critical Care). Consultant Anes, Niagara Health System - Greater Niagara General Site; Consultant Anes, Niagara Health System - Welland Hospital Site; (905)358-0171 x3386

PHALPHER, Prashant; William Osler HC-Brampton, 2100 Bovaird St E, Brampton ON L6R 3J7; Qns'07; CCFP; CCFP(E.M.); Staff, William Osler Health System - Brampton Civic Hospital; (905)494-2120

PHAM, Alice Trang; 407-27 Roncesvalles Ave, Toronto ON M6R 3B2; Tor'05; FRCSC; ObstGyn. Staff, Sunnybrook Health Sciences Centre; (416)531-8671; Fax. (416)531-6039.

PHAM, Anne-Marie; South Common Med Centre, 3-2110 Burnhamthorpe Rd W, Mississauga ON L5L 5Z5; Mon'95; CCFP; Langs: Vietnamese; French; (905)820-3209; Fax. (905)820-2576.

PHAM, Christine Anh Ngoc; Radiology Consultants Assoc, 120-6707 Elbow Dr SW, Calgary AB T2V 0E3; Mon'89; CSPQ; FRCPC; DiagRad. Langs: French; Vietnamese; Spanish; (403)777-3003; Fax. (403)777-3008.

PHAM, Chau; St Boniface Gen Hosp, L1019-409 Tache Ave, Winnipeg MB R2H 2A6; Man'05; FRCPC; EmergMed. Staff, St Boniface General Hospital; (204)233-8563

PHAM, Chien; 2-796 Burnhamthorpe Rd W, Mississauga ON L5C 2R9; Tor'94; CCFP; Langs: Vietnamese; (905)270-6454; Fax. (905)270-6460.

PHAM, Cuong Duc; Clinique Medicale 1746, 1746 ch de Chambly, Longueuil QC J4J 3X5; McG'93; FRCPC; Derm. (450)646-2900; Fax. (450)651-8901.

PHAM, Dieu Huu; North York Gen Hosp, 4001 Leslie St, North York ON M2K 1E1; Saigon (Vietnam)'74; FRCPC; DiagRad (Nuclear Medicine). Staff, North York General Hospital; (416)756-6186; Fax. (416)756-6095.

PHAM, Dzu Quang; Doctor's Office at Birchmount, 202-3609 Sheppard Ave E, Scarborough ON M1T 3K8; Qns'00; CCFP; (416)321-2643; Fax. (416)321-5006; dzu_pham@yahoo.ca.

PHAM, Gia-Trong; Clinique Med Viau, 4750 rue Jarry E, Saint-Leonard QC H1R 1X8; Saigon (Vietnam)'75; (514)326-7203; Fax. (514)326-3656.

PHAM, H Nhat Tan; Centre de Med Integree, 240-2040 boul Marcel-Laurin, Saint-Laurent QC H4R 1J9; Sher'98; (514)747-9936; Fax. (514)747-9331.

PHAM, Hoa Cong; Ontario Shores Ctr Mental HS, 700 Gordon St, Whitby ON L1N 5S9; Ott'96; FRCPC; Psy. Staff, Ontario Shores Centre for Mental Health Sciences; (905)430-4055

PHAM, Huu-Trac; Centre Med Lacordaire, 201-5650 rue Jean-Talon E, Saint-Leonard QC H1S 1M1; Saigon (Vietnam)'66; (514)255-5595; Fax. (514)255-8550.

PHAM, Huy; 498 rue Saint-Jacques CP 789, Napierville QC J0J 1L0; Sher'83; (450)245-0032; Fax. (450)926-2236.

PHAM, Joe; 3-2125 Wyecroft Rd, Oakville ON L6L 5L7; Tor'00; FRCPC; IntMed; Gastroent. (905)849-7426; Fax. (905)849-9436.

PHAM, Luc Anh D; CSSS de Laval, 1755 boul Rene-Laennec, Laval QC H7M 3L9; McG'05; Cardiol; IntMed. Staff, Hopital de la Cite de la santé; (450)668-1010

PHAM, Mailan; CSSS Pierre Boucher, 1333 boul Jacques-Cartier E, Longueuil QC J4M 2A5; Sher'96; Staff, Centre Hospitalier Pierre Boucher; (450)468-8111

PHAM, Nam; 204-800 Bathurst St, Toronto ON M5R 3M8; McM'07; CCFP; (416)533-5882; Fax. (416)533-5943.

PHAM, Ngoc Huynh U; Centre Med Laval, 1110 boul Vanier, Laval QC H7C 2R8; Mon'08; (450)661-2521; Fax. (450)661-7193.

PHAM, Nhu-Ngoc; Centre de Med Integree, 240-2040 boul Marcel-Laurin, Saint-Laurent QC H4R 1J9; Sher'99; (514)747-9936

PHAM, Phuong-Vy; Ctr Hosp Fleury, 2180 rue Fleury E, Montreal QC H2B 1K3; Sher'02; Staff, Centre Hospitalier Fleury; (514)381-9311; pvpham@hotmail.com.

PHAM, Quynh N; Springdale Prof Bldg, 611-2250 Bovaird Dr E, Brampton ON L6R 0W3; Tor'89; FRCSC; GenSurg (Gastroenterology). Langs: Vietnamese; (905)866-6204; Fax. (647)799-0302.

PHAM, Thang; 240-2040 boul Marcel-Laurin, Saint-Laurent QC H4R 1J9; Louvain (Belgium)'72; (514)744-4922

PHAM, Thi Tam; Hop Charles LeMoyne, 3120 boul Taschereau, Greenfield Park QC J4V 2H1; Sher'85; CSPQ; DiagRad. Staff, Hopital Charles LeMoyne; (450)466-5000

PHAM, Thi Thanh D; CLSC Parc Extension, 7085 rue Hutchison, Montreal QC H3N 1Y9; Mon'05; CCFP; (514)273-9591; Fax. (514)273-8954.

PHAM, Thuy-Nga Tia; Family Health Centre, 105-840 Coxwell Ave, East York ON M4C 5T2; Tor'03; MSc; CCFP; Asst Prof Family & Community Med, University of Toronto; Langs: German; Vietnamese; (416)469-6464; Fax. (416)469-6164.

PHAM, Trai Ngoc; BL 67-3175 Rutherford Rd, Concord ON L4K 5Y6; Saigon (Vietnam)'87; CCFP; Langs: Vietnamese; (905)761-6082

PHAM, Tuong-Vi; CSSS de la Vallée de l'Or, 725 6e rue, Val-d'Or QC J9P 3Y1; Mon'88; CCFP; Staff, Centre Hospitalier de Val d'Or; Langs: Vietnamese; English; (819)825-5858; Fax. (819)825-1335.

PHAM, Van Dong H; Clinique Domus Medica, 5601 rue Belanger E, Montreal QC H1T 1G3; Sher'95; Staff, Hôpital Santa Cabrini Ospedale; (514)256-5011

PHAM, Van Duc; Normanview Med Clinic, 330 McCarthy Blvd N, Regina SK S4R 7M2; Saigon (Vietnam)'70; (306)924-6200; Fax. (306)924-6201.

PHAM, Vinh Phuc; Ctr Med Chambly-Latour, B-5580 ch de Chambly, Saint-Hubert QC J3Y 3P5; Sher'03; Staff, Centre Hospitalier Pierre Boucher; (450)926-2236

PHAM, Vu Hoang; Royal University Hosp, 119-103 Hospital Dr, Saskatoon SK S7N 0W8; Sask'04; FRCPC; Psy. Staff, Royal University Hospital; (306)655-1000

PHAM, Xuan H; The Ottawa Hosp-Gen Campus, 501 Smyth Rd, Ottawa ON K1H 8L6; Sher'88; FRCPC; NuclearMed. Staff, The Ottawa Hospital - General Campus; Langs: Vietnamese; English; (613)737-8528 x1; Fax. (613)737-8705.

PHAM-AN, Minh-Thy; CSSS de Saint-Jerome, 290 rue de Montigny, Saint-Jerome QC J7Z 5T3; Sher'02; FRCPC; Neur. Staff, Hôtel-Dieu de Saint-Jérôme; (450)431-8200; Fax. (450)431-8304.

PHAM-DANG, Huong; 202-5450 ch de la Cote-des-Nei, Montreal QC H3T 1Y6; Saigon (Vietnam)'73; Otol (P.Q.). Staff, McGill University Health Centre - Montreal General Campus; (514)733-8883; Fax. (514)733-4896.

PHAM-DINH, Martin; 909 boul de la Verendrye O CP 2000 Succ Bureau-Chef, Gatineau QC J8P 7H2; Sher'98; CCFP; CCFP(E.M.); Staff, Hôpital de Gatineau; Langs: English; French; (819)966-6333; martinphamdinh@gmail.com.

PHAM-HUY, Anne; Children's Hosp Eastern Ont, 3356-401 Smyth Rd, Ottawa ON K1H 8L1; Ott'03; FRCPC; Peds; InfectDis. Staff, Children's Hospital of Eastern Ontario (CHEO); (613)737-7600; Fax. (613)738-4832.

PHAM NHUT, Huong; Clinique Med Papineau, 6930 av Papineau, Montreal QC H2G 2X7; Saigon (Vietnam)'68; (514)722-0000

PHAN, Amelie; Ctr Hosp de Verdun, 4000 boul Lasalle, Verdun QC H4G 2A3; Sher'99; CCFP; Staff, Centre Hospitalier de Verdun; (514)362-1000

PHAN, Khai; Norburn Med Clinic, 200-4012 Hastings St, Burnaby BC V5C 2H9; Sask'97; CCFP; (604)299-2677

PHAN, Philippe T N; 202-595 Montreal Rd, Ottawa ON K1K 4L2; Ott'06; FRCSC; OrthSurg. Staff, Montfort Hospital; (613)746-4621

PHAN, Quynh Giao; CSSS de Laval, 1755 boul Rene-Laennec, Laval QC H7M 3L9; Mon'96; FRCPC; Peds. Staff, Hopital de la Cite de la santé; (450)688-1010

PHAN, T H I Dang; Clin Med Plateau Mont-Royal, 103-1374 av du Mont-Royal E, Montreal QC H2J 1Y7; Saigon (Vietnam)'81; CCFP; Staff, Centre de L'Annonciation; Langs: Vietnamese; French; (514)527-3997

PHAN, Tien Thi; Tom Baker Cancer Centre, 1331 29 St NW, Calgary AB T2N 4N2; Alb'03; FRCPC; RadOncol. Staff, Tom Baker Cancer Centre; (403)521-3077; Fax. (403)283-1651.

PHAN, Tuan X; CHSLD Jeanne Le Ber, 7445 rue Hochelaga, Montreal QC H1N 3V2; Saigon (Vietnam)'74; Staff, Hopital Louis-H Lafontaine; (514)251-6000

PHAN, Van Thanh; Clin Med Minh Chau, 235-6655 ch Cote-des-Neiges, Montreal QC H3S 2B4; Saigon (Vietnam)'67; (514)735-8060; Fax. (514)735-0698.

PHAN, Veronique; Hôpital Ste-Justine, 3175 ch Cote-Sainte-Catherine, Montreal QC H3T 1C5; McG'94; MSc; FRCPC; Peds (Pediatric Nephrology); Nephrol. Clinical Asst Prof, Hôpital Ste-Justine; Langs: Bilingual(French/English); (514)345-4737; Fax. (514)345-4838; veronique.phan.hsj@ssss.gouv.qc.ca.

PHAN, Xuan Khoa; CSSS Pierre Boucher, 1333 boul Jacques-Cartier E, Longueuil QC J4M 2A5; Sher'87; Electroenceph (P.Q.); Neur. Staff, Centre Hospitalier Pierre Boucher; (450)442-9967; Fax. (450)442-2785.

PHAN, Xuan Truong; Clinique Med Rosemont, 1969 boul Rosemont, Montreal QC H2G 1S9; Sher'81; Langs: Vietnamese; English; (514)274-7344; Fax. (514)274-1165.

PHAN CONG, Nicolas; Sunnybrook Hlth Sciences Ctre, B7 03-2075 Bayview Ave, Toronto ON M4N 3M5; McG'96; FRCSC; Neursurg. (416)480-5645; Fax. (416)480-6085.

PHANEUF, Claude; Clinique Med Boisbriand, 877 boul de la Grande-Allee, Boisbriand QC J7G 1W6; Mon'76; (450)437-4600; Fax. (450)437-7038.

PHANEUF, Denis C; CSSS du Sud de Lanaudière, 911 montee des Pionniers, Terrebonne QC J6V 2H2; Mon'74; FRCPC; Cardiol. Staff, Centre Hospitalier Pierre le Gardeur; assoc Prof, Universite de Montreal; Langs: Bilingual(French/English); (450)654-7525 x31285; denise.phaneuf@hotmail.com.

PHANEUF, Denis; CHUM-Hotel-Dieu, 3840 rue Saint-Urbain, Montreal QC H2W 1T8; Mon'72; FRCPC; MedMicrobiol (Infectious Diseases); Microbio & Infect Dis (P.Q.). ac Staff, Centre Hospitalier l'Université de Montréal (CHUM) - Hôtel-Dieu; Prof Microbiol & InfectDis, Universite de Montreal; Langs: English; (514)890-8175 x14816

PHANEUF, Jean-Luc; 212-8260 boul Maurice-Duplessi, Montreal QC H1E 3A3; Mon'82; (514)643-1113; Fax. (514)643-1767.

PHANEUF, Julie; Centre Hosp Honore-Mercier, 2750 boul Laframboise, Saint-Hyacinthe QC J2S 4Y8; Laval'98; FRCPC; Psy. Staff, Centre Hospitalier Honore-Mercier; (450)771-3222

PHANEUF, Louise; Clinique Med Sainte-Dorothee, 102-1 boul Samson, Laval QC H7X 3S5; Laval'89; CCFP; (450)689-6334; Fax. (450)689-6339.

PHANEUF, Simon; CSSS de la Cote-de-Gaspe, 215 boul de York O, Gaspe QC G4X 2W2; Mon'88; CCFP; CCFP(E.M.); Staff, Centre Hospitalier de Gaspe; Pres, Advanced Therapeutic Technologies; adj Prof, Universite de Sherbrooke; (418)368-3301

PHANEUF, Stella; Tribunal Admin du Quebec, RC10-575 rue Saint-Amable, Quebec QC G1R 5R4; Laval'77; (418)643-0355 x3087; Fax. (418)528-6881.

PHANEUF, Veronique; Clinique Med du College, GD 1396 rue Notre-Dame, Saint-Cesaire QC J0L 1T0; Sher'04; Physician, Clinique Medicale St-Cesaire; Langs: Bilingual(French/English); (450)469-0505; Fax. (450)469-4554.

PHANG, Min Sen; Fairmont Med Bldg, 1314-750 Broadway W, Vancouver BC V5Z 1J3; Aberdeen (Scotland)'81; MB ChB; MRCP(UK); FRCPC; Peds (Neonatology). Staff, BC Children's Hospital; Langs: Hakka; Hokkin; (604)879-4564; Fax. (604)879-5191.

PHANG, Paul T; St Paul's Hosp, C313-1081 Burrard St, Vancouver BC V6Z 1Y6; Tor'79; FRCSC; GenSurg. Ac Staff Surg, Providence Health Care - St Paul's Hospital; (604)806-8711

PHARAND, Annie; CSSS du Lac-des-Deux-Montagnes, 520 boul Arthur-Sauve, St-Eustache QC J7R 5B1; Mon'03; CSPQ; FRCPC; Anes. Staff, Hôpital de Saint-Eustache; (450)473-6811; annie_pharand@hotmail.com.

PHARAND, Daniel; CHUM-Hotel-Dieu, 3840 rue Saint-Urbain, Montreal QC H2W 1T8; Alb'86; CSPQ; FRCSC; Urol. ac Staff, Centre Hospitalier l'Université de Montréal (CHUM) - Hôtel-Dieu; (514)890-8106

PHARAND, Marielle R P; 13-20 Charlevoix St, Vanier ON K1L 8K5; Ott'61; Langs: English; (613)748-9855

PHARAND, Pierre; Clinique Med Havre Sante, 521 boul du Havre, Salaber-de-Valleyf QC J6S 4Z5; Mon'71; (450)371-6444 x262; Fax. (450)371-5315.

PHARIS, C Scott; Royal University Hosp, 103 Hospital Dr, Saskatoon SK S7N 0W8; Sask'03; FRCPC; Peds; Cardiol. Staff, Royal University Hospital; (306)966-7198; Fax. (306)966-8640.

PHATERPEKAR, Hem M; Fraser Health Authority, 260 Sherbrooke St, New Westminster BC V3L 3M2; Bombay (India)'86; MB BS; MRCPsy(UK); DPsy(UK); FRCPC; Psy (Geriatric Psychiatry). Consultant Psy, Royal Columbian Hospital; Consultant Psy, BC Mental Health & Addiction Service; Clin Instructor, University of British Columbia; (604)520-4662; Fax. (604)520-4871.

PHEGAN, Warren D; 117-747 Hyde Park Rd, London ON N6H 3S3; Sydney (Australia)'61; MB BS; DPsy; Psy. (519)473-3163; Fax. (519)473-3163; warrendphegan@on.aibn.com.

PHELAN, Cynthia C; Sandy Hill Community Hlth Ctr, 221 Nelson St, Ottawa ON K1N 1C7; McG'03; CCFP; (613)789-1500; Fax. (613)789-8710.

PHELAN, Patrick J; 115 Pacific Ave, Moncton NB E1E 2G2; Mem'81; CCFP; Ac Staff Family Med & Palliative Care, The Moncton Hospital; (506)857-1006; Fax. (506)855-0156; phelanp@nbnet.nb.ca.

PHELAN, Paul; Kensington Family Med Centre, PO Box 160 55 Victoria St, Kensington PE C0B 1M0; Dal'84; Staff, Prince County Hospital; (902)836-4450

PHELPS, Erica L; Langley Obstetrics & Gyn, 21561 Old Yale Rd, Langley BC V3A 4M9; UBC'01; FRCSC; ObstGyn. (604)534-4441; Fax. (604)534-4491.

PHELPS, Ian J; Medicine Hat Reg Hsop, 666 5 St SW, Medicine Hat AB T1A 4H6; Cal'01; CCFP; CCFP(E.M.); Staff, Medicine Hat Regional Hospital; (403)529-8800

PHELPS, James H; Guelph Gen Hosp, 115 Delhi St, Guelph ON N1E 4J4; Wes'86; CCFP; FCFP; Ac Staff, Guelph General Hospital; (519)822-5350; jphelps0128@rogers.com.

PHENIX, Pierre; DSP Sante au Travail, 1301 rue Sherbrooke E, Montreal QC H2L 1M3; Mon'77; (514)528-2400 x3706; Fax. (514)528-2459.

PHI, Chi-Minh; MUHC-Montreal Children's Hosp, 2300 rue Tupper, Montreal QC H3H 1P3; Dal'00; FRCPC; Peds. Staff, McGill University Health Centre - Montreal Children's Hospital; (514)412-4400 x23193

PHILBROOK, Paul S; Streetsville Med Centre, 5425 Creditview Rd, Mississauga ON L5V 2P3; McG'80; CCFP; Family Med, The Credit Valley Hospital; (905)826-1164; Fax. (905)826-1214.

PHILIBERT, Bruno; CSSS Haut-Richelieu-Rouville, 920 boul du Seminaire N, St-Jean-sur-Richel QC J3A 1B7; Mon'83; Staff, Hôpital du Haut-Richelieu; (450)359-5000

PHILIBERT, David; CHUQ-Hotel-Dieu de Quebec, 11 Cote du Palais, Quebec QC G1R 2J6; Mon'01; FRCPC; IntMed; Nephrol. Staff, Centre Hospitalier Universitaire de Québec (CHUQ) - Siege Social; (418)691-5464; Fax. (418)691-5757.

PHILIBERT, Jean-Claude; Clinique Saint-Joseph, 2283 av Saint-Marc, Shawinigan QC G9N 2J4; Mon'75; ac Staff, Centre Hospitalier du Centre la Mauricie; Physician, Employment & Immigration Canada; Langs: Bilingual(French/English); (819)536-5604; Fax. (819)536-2550.

PHILIBERT, Marie-Claude; CSSS Drummond-Hop Sainte-Croix, 570 rue Heriot, Drummondville QC J2B 1C1; Laval'96; LMCC; FRCSC; ObstGyn. Staff, Hôpital Sainte-croix; (819)478-6464; Fax. (819)478-6470.

PHILIE, Michel; Hop du Sacre-Coeur de Mtl, 5400 boul Gouin O, Montreal QC H4J 1C5; Mon'86; CSPQ; FRCPC; DiagRad. Staff, Hôpital du Sacre-Coeur de Montréal; Staff, Hôtel-Dieu de Saint-Jérôme; (514)338-2130; Fax. (514)338-3113.

PHILIPP, Diane A; The Hincks-Dellcrest Centre, 440 Jarvis St, Toronto ON M4Y 2H4; McM'90; FRCPC; Psy (Child & Adolescent Psychiatry)., The Hincks-Dellcrest Centre - Toronto; Asst Prof, University of Toronto; Langs: French; (416)972-1935 x3330; Fax. (416)924-8208.

PHILIPP, Roger K; Keary Centre, 103-245 Columbia St E, New Westminster BC V3L 3W4; Man'95; FRCPC; IntMed; Cardiol. Staff, St Boniface General Hospital; (604)522-1644

PHILIPPE, Johanne; 65 rue Uapakalu GD, Mashteuiatsh QC G0W 2H0; Mon'86; BSc(Physiol&Med); Staff Commun & Family Med, Centre de Sante de Mashteuiatsh; Langs: Bilingual(French/English); (418)275-5386; Fax. (418)275-4570; johanne.philippe@mashteviatsh.ca.

PHILIPPE, Pascal; Dr Georges L Dumont Reg Hosp, 330 av Universite, Moncton NB E1C 2Z3; Laval'00; FRCPC; Anes. Staff, Dr Georges-L-Dumont University Hospital Centre; (506)862-4000

PHILIPPON, Daniel; CHUQ-Ctr Hosp Univ Laval, 2705 boul Laurier, Quebec QC G1V 4G2; Laval'05; Otol. Staff, Centre Hospitalier Universitaire de Quebec-CHUL; (418)525-4444

PHILIPPON, Francois; Hôpital Laval, 2725 ch Sainte-Foy, Quebec QC G1V 4G5; Laval'86; FRCPC; IntMed (Electrophysiology); Cardiol. Chef cardio, Hôpital Laval; Chief Cardiology, Quebec Heart Institute; Langs: English; (418)656-8711; Fax. (418)656-4581; francois.philippon@med.ulaval.ca.

PHILIPPSON, Daniel O; Ingram Family Physicians, 103-149 Ingram St, Duncan BC V9L 1N8; UBC'80; (250)746-4401; Fax. (250)746-4473.

PHILIPS, Nabil A; Credit Valley Med Arts Centre, 413-2000 Credit Valley Rd, Mississauga ON L5M 4N4; Cairo (Egypt)'80; MB ChB; DABPN; FRCPC; Psy (Anxiety & Mood Disorders). Dir Adult Psy Services, The Credit Valley Hospital; (905)607-1262; Fax. (905)607-1263; n.philips@rogers.com.

PHILLIPOS, Ernest Z; University of Alberta Hosp, 3A3WCM-8440 112 St NW, Edmonton AB T6G 2B7; Khartoum (Sudan)'77; MB BS; MRCP(I); FRCPC; Peds (Congenital Heart Disease). Staff, University of Alberta Hospital; Langs: Arabic; (780)407-6297; Fax. (780)407-3030; ernest.phillipos@albertahealthservices.ca.

PHILLIPOWSKY, Michael A; Montfort Academic Family Hlth, 101B-745 Montreal Rd, Ottawa ON K1K 0T1; McG'80; Asst Prof Med, University of Ottawa; Langs: Bilingual(English/French); (613)749-4429; Fax. (613)749-7942.

PHILLIPS, Allen; Clinique Med Cowansville, 1001-101 rue Albert, Cowansville QC J2K 2W4; McG'76; CCFP; FCFP; Ac Member, Hôpital Brome-Missisquoi-Perkins; Ac Member, CLSC-CHSLD La Pommeraie - Centre hospitalier de Bedford; adj Prof, McGill University; (450)266-4060; Fax. (450)266-5335; allen_phillips@rrsss16.gouv.qc.ca.

PHILLIPS, Barrie L; Park Avenue Med Centre, 500-4634 Park Ave, Terrace BC V8G 1V7; Qns'64; BA; FRCPC; IntMed (Cardiology). Consultant IntMed, Mills Memorial Hospital; Consultant IntMed, Kitimat Hospital & Health Centre; Asst Prof, University of British Columbia; Asst Prof, University of Northern British Columbia; (250)615-5088; Fax. (250)615-5085; termed@northernhealthcare.ca.

PHILLIPS, Brian C M; Sussex Health Centre, 75 Leonard Dr, Sussex NB E4E 2P7; Tor'71; BSc; FRCSC; GenSurg. Staff, Sussex Health Centre; (506)432-3146; Fax. (506)432-3412; phillfam@nbnet.nb.ca.

PHILLIPS, Bruce A; Children's & Women's HC of BC, B321-4480 Oak St, Vancouver BC V6H 3V4; Natal (South Africa)'73; FRCPC; Peds (Emergency Medicine). Staff, BC Children's Hospital; Asst Prof, University of British Columbia; (604)875-2345; bphillips@cw.bc.ca.

PHILLIPS, Bruce A; Fundy Trail Med Centre, 68 Robie St, Truro NS B2N 1L2; Dal'91; CCFP; Ac Staff Family Med, Colchester East Hants Health Centre; (902)895-6364; Fax. (902)895-6365; brucephillips@eastlink.ca.

PHILLIPS, Callista M; Joseph Brant Mem Hosp, 1230 North Shore Blvd E, Burlington ON L7S 1W7; Pune (India)'89; MB BS; FRCPC; IntMed (Palliative Care); MedOncol. Staff Joseph Brant Cancer Clinic, Joseph Brant Memorial Hospital; Asst Clin Prof, McMaster University; (905)336-4103; Fax. (905)336-6492.

PHILLIPS, Catherine J; North Shore Med Imaging, 139 16th St W, North Vancouver BC V7M 1T3; Sask'86; FRCPC; DiagRad. Staff, Lions Gate Hospital; (604)987-9729

PHILLIPS, Catherine L; 240-14032 23 Ave NW, Edmonton AB T6R 3L6; Alb'82; FRCPC; Psy. (780)488-6585; Fax. (780)488-6535.

PHILLIPS, Danielle M; Kelligrews Med Clinic, PO Box 17160 Stn Main, Conception-Bay-S NL A1X 3H1; Mem'06; CCFP; (709)834-1241

PHILLIPS, David D; London HSC-Victoria Campus, PO Box 5010 Stn B 800 Commissioners Rd E, London ON N6A 5W9; Tor'10; CCFP; Staff, London Health Sciences Centre - Victoria Campus; (519)685-8500

PHILLIPS, Debbie J; 2102 32 Ave, Vernon BC V1T 2K1; UBC'93; CCFP; CCFP(E.M.); Ac Staff, Vernon Jubilee Hospital; Ac Staff, Shuswap Lake General Hospital; Langs: French; Spanish; (250)545-2211 x1401

PHILLIPS, Dianne K; PO Box 574 Stn Fort Langley, Langley BC V1M 2R9; Ott'82; Staff Surg, Langley Memorial Hospital; Staff Surg, Burnaby Hospital; Langs: Bilingual(English/French).

PHILLIPS, Elliott J; College of Phys & Surg of BC, 300-669 Howe St, Vancouver BC V6C 0B4; Tor'69; FRCSC; Urol (Administration). Dep Registrar, College of Physicians & Surgeons of British Columbia; (604)733-7758; Fax. (604)733-3503.

PHILLIPS, Gosia E; Abbie J Lane Mem Bldg, 4007-5909 Veterans Memorial La, Halifax NS B3H 2E2; Jagiellonski (Poland)'01; BSc; ABPN; Staff, Queen Elizabeth II Health Sciences Centre - Victoria General Site; Med Dir, Sleep Disorders Clinic & Lab; (902)473-6222; gosiaphillips@live.com.

PHILLIPS, Gregory L; 201-1555 Marine Dr, West Vancouver BC V7V 1H9; Alb'84; BMedSci; FCFP; Ad Staff, Lions Gate Hospital; (604)922-6595

PHILLIPS, Henry D; Formation Health Services Unit, PO Box 17000 Stn Forces 1200 Colville Rd, Victoria BC V9A 7N2; Man'88; BSc(Med); MSc; Staff, Canadian Forces Health Services - Pacific Centre; (250)363-4161; Fax. (250)363-4173.

PHILLIPS, Ian; 200-89 Dawson Rd, Guelph ON N1H 1R1; Tor'96; FRCSC; GenSurg (Laparoscopic Surgery). (519)824-0660; Fax. (519)824-2326; dr.ianphillips@sympatico.ca.

PHILLIPS, Jennifer M; PO Box 16066 Rpo Lynn Valley, North Vancouver BC V7J 3S9; UBC'08; CCFP.

PHILLIPS, John H; The Hosp for Sick Children, 5429-555 University Ave, Toronto ON M5G 1X8; Tor'80; MA; BSc; FRCSC; PlasSurg (Cranio Facial Surgery). Ac Staff Craniofacial Surg, The Hospital For Sick Children; Ac Staff, Sunnybrook Health Sciences Centre; Assoc Prof, University of Toronto; (416)813-6197; Fax. (416)813-6637; john.phillips@sickkids.ca.

PHILLIPS, Jonathan D; Care Place Med Centre, 306-9014 152 St, Surrey BC V3R 4E7; UBC'87; (604)581-3558

PHILLIPS, Karen A; Western Mem Reg Hosp, PO Box 2005 Stn Main 1 Brookfield Ave, Corner Brook NL A2H 6J7; Cape Town (South Africa)'95; Staff, Western Memorial Regional Hospital; (709)637-5000

PHILLIPS, Karen E; 326 Wilson St E, Ancaster ON L9G 2C2; McM'81; BSc; (905)648-0770; Fax. (905)648-0777.

PHILLIPS, Katherine G; Haldimand Family Health Team, 75 Parkview Rd, Hagersville ON N0A 1H0; McM'97; BSc; DDS; CCFP; FCFP; Staff, West Haldimand General Hospital; (905)768-9599; Fax. (905)768-2879; phillipskandr@sympatico.ca.

PHILLIPS, Kent M; Archdekin Med Group, PO Box 660 Stn Main 205 Hiram St, Bracebridge ON P1L 1T9; Wes'68; CCFP; FCFP; Staff, South Muskoka Memorial Hospital - Muskoka Algonquin Healthcare; Coroner, District of Bracebridge; (705)645-2223; Fax. (705)645-2342.

PHILLIPS, M Elizabeth; Health Services Complex, 20 Kennedy Dr, Sussex NB E4E 2P1; Mem'84; (506)433-4672; Fax. (506)432-5823.

PHILLIPS, Mark R; 18B-279 Kingston Rd E, Ajax ON L1Z 0K5; Tor'84; Ac Staff, Rouge Valley Health System - Ajax & Pickering Health Centre Site; (905)428-6131

PHILLIPS, Michael L; St Boniface Gen Hosp, 409 Tache Ave, Winnipeg MB R2H 2A6; Man'07; FRCPC; Psy. Staff, St Boniface General Hospital; (204)233-8563

PHILLIPS, Perry; 503-294 Main St, Toronto ON M4C 4X5; Montpellier (France)'74; BSc; FACS; FSOGC; FRCSC; ObstGyn (Infertility). Ac Staff, Toronto East General Hospital Inc; Dir, IVF Canada & Life Program; Langs: Italian; French; (416)694-8033; Fax. (416)694-8045.

PHILLIPS, Peter G; 27 Third St, Collingwood ON L9Y 1K4; Dal'75; ACLS; ATLS; CCFP; FCFP; Staff, Collingwood General & Marine Hospital; Med Dir, Bay Haven Nursing & Retirement Home; Physician, BM High Tech Industries; Langs: English; French; (705)445-4111; Fax. (705)445-8250; cmc@cois.on.ca.

PHILLIPS, Peter; St Paul's Hosp, B520-1081 Burrard St, Vancouver BC V6Z 1Y6; Tor'74; FRCPC; IntMed; InfectDis. Staff InfectDis, Providence Health Care - St Paul's Hospital; Clin Prof Med, University of British Columbia; (604)806-8317; Fax. (604)806-8527; pphillips@cfenet.ubc.ca.

PHILLIPS, R Keith; AVI Health Centre, 216-55 Victoria Rd, Nanaimo BC V9R 5N9; Alb'72; FCFP(Hons.); CCFP; FCFP; Ac Staff, Nanaimo Regional General Hospital; (250)754-9111; rkpmedarts@shaw.ca.

PHILLIPS, Randall N; MedPoint Med Centre, 233-355 Wellington St, London ON N6K 4Y4; Wes'73; FACEP; FRCPC; EmergMed. (519)432-1919

PHILLIPS, Richard A; 402-3939 Quadra St, Victoria BC V8X 1J5; Alb'90; FRCPC; IntMed; Endocrin&Metab. (250)727-6621; Fax. (250)727-0478.

PHILLIPS, Ross E; Whitehorse Med Services Ltd, 406 Lambert St, Whitehorse YT Y1A 1Z7; Cal'94; BSc(Hons.); CCFP; Staff, Whitehorse Medical Services Ltd; Langs: Finnish; French; (867)393-6626; Fax. (867)393-6601; wmsl@klondiker.com.

PHILLIPS, Rowland L; Columbia Family Medicine, 302-1101 Dewdney Ave, Trail BC V1R 4T1; Dal'77; Ac Staff, Kootenay Boundary Regional Hospital; (250)368-9394; Fax. (250)368-8281; columbiafamilymedicine@gmail.com.

PHILLIPS, Shauna D; 502-1881 Yonge St, Toronto ON M4S 3C4; Tor'10; CCFP; (416)539-9598; Fax. (416)539-0802.

PHILLIPS, Sheilagh J; Fairmont Med Bldg, 510-750 Broadway W, Vancouver BC V5Z 1H4; UBC'87; (604)879-5385

PHILLIPS, Stephanie E; Bayvalley Med Bldg, 204-145 Queenston St, St Catharines ON L2R 7C6; McM'04; FRCSC; GenSurg. Staff, Niagara Health System - St Catharines General Site; (905)641-5700

PHILLIPS, Stephen J; Queen Elizabeth II HSC-Halifax, 3831-1796 Summer St, Halifax NS B3H 3A7; London (England)'79; FRCPC; Neur (Cerebrovascular Disease). Staff, Queen Elizabeth II Health Sciences Centre - Halifax Infirmary Site; Ac Staff, Queen Elizabeth II Health Sciences Centre - Victoria General Site; Consultant, IWK Health Centre; Prof Med (Neurol), Dalhousie University; (902)473-5423; Fax. (902)473-4438; stephen.phillips@dal.ca.

PHILLIPS, Stephen V; Rockyview Gen Hosp, 7007 14 St SW, Calgary AB T2V 1P9; Cal'01; FRCPC; Anes. Staff, Rockyview General Hospital; (403)943-8720

PHILLIPS, Susan M; Health Sciences Centre, MS459-820 Sherbrook St, Winnipeg MB R3A 1R9; Man'83; FRCPC; AnatPath (Autopsy). Staff, Health Sciences Centre; Asst Prof, University of Manitoba; Fax. (204)787-4942.

PHILLIPS, Susan P; Family Med Centre, PO Box 8888 Stn Main 220 Bagot St, Kingston ON K7L 5E9; Qns'78; CCFP; Court Staff Family Med, Kingston General Hospital; Prof, Queen's University; (613)533-9303; Fax. (613)549-5403.

PHILLIPS, Thomas J; Central Peace Clinic, PO Box 608, Spirit River AB T0H 3G0; Alb'71; (780)864-3962; Fax. (780)864-4491.

PHILLIPS, Tim; Sage Med Clinic, 101-2210 Main St, Penticton BC V2A 5H8; UBC'97; (250)492-0990; Fax. (250)492-0992.

PHILLIPS, Vandana A; Calgary West Med Centre, LL-1107 37 St SW, Calgary AB T3C 1S5; (Australia)'02; BSc; MB BS; CCFP; (403)246-7788; Fax. (403)242-8850.

PHILLIPS, Wayne L; Wolfville Prof Centre, 1-4 Little Rd, Wolfville NS B4P 1P4; Dal'74; CCFP; Ac Staff Privil, Valley Regional Hospital; (902)542-2071; Fax. (902)542-4524.

PHILLIPS, William G B; St Paul's Hosp, 1081 Burrard St, Vancouver BC V6Z 1Y6; Qns'70; Anes. Staff, Providence Health Care - St Paul's Hospital; (604)682-2344

PHILLIPSON, Eliot A; Univ Hlth Network-Toronto Gen, 9N941-200 Elizabeth St, Toronto ON M5G 2C4; Alb'63; MSc; FRCPC; IntMed (Respirology). Staff, Toronto General Hospital - UHN; (416)340-4552; Fax. (416)340-4197; eliot.phillipson@utoronto.ca.

PHILLIPSON, Ronald A; B1-333 Wilson Ave, North York ON M3H 1T2; Man'02; CCFP; (647)317-1213

PHILLIPSON, Ryan T; Radiology Associates of Regina, 6-2727 Parliament Ave, Regina SK S4S 6X5; Sask'98; FRCPC; DiagRad. Staff, Radiology Associates of Regina; (306)352-7653; Fax. (306)522-4311; thephillipsons@accesscomm.ca.

PHILLIPSON, Wayne G; Guardian Med Arts Bldg, 302-1950 Algonquin Ave, North Bay ON P1B 4Z2; Tor'89; Staff, North Bay Regional Health Centre - Regional Mental Health; (705)495-6232

PHILLPOT, C Aimee; Piper Creek Med Clinic, 200-3215 49 Ave, Red Deer AB T4N 0M8; Alb'97; CCFP; FCFP; (403)986-7265; Fax. (403)986-7604.

PHILP, Ian J; Medical Clinic Associates, 200-3207 30 Ave, Vernon BC V1T 2C6; Sask'64; CCFP; FCFP; (250)542-8335

PHILP, Lorraine B; 700-1240 Bay St, Toronto ON M5R 2A7; Mem'90; MHSc; BEd; BSc(Hon); CCFP; (416)977-5427; Fax. (416)646-0205.

PHILPOTT, Jane P; Health For All Family Health T, 202-379 Church St, Markham ON L6B 0T1; Wes'84; CCFP; Staff Teaching Unit, Markham Stouffville Hospital; (905)472-2200; Fax. (905)472-5662.

PHILPOTT, John F; Women's College Hosp, 10-76 Grenville St, Toronto ON M5S 1B2; St. George's (Grenada)'87; FAAP; FRCPC; Peds (Sports Medicine). Consultant Ped, Toronto East General Hospital Inc; Staff Sport C A R E, Women's College Hospital; Asst Prof Section of Community Peds, University of Toronto; (416)323-6479; Fax. (416)323-6487.

PHILPOTT, Stephanie L; Shubenacadie Fam Practice Clin, PO Box 94, Shubenacadie NS B0N 2H0; Mem'93; CCFP; FCFP; (902)758-2655; Fax. (902)758-3606.

PHILTEOS, George S R; Ajax Med Arts Bldg, 205-601 Harwood Ave S, Ajax ON L1S 2J5; Ain Shams (Egypt)'83; DABSM; MB ChB; MSc; FRCPC; IntMed (Intensive Care); Respir. Staff, Rouge Valley Health System - Ajax & Pickering Health Centre Site; Assoc Staff, Lakeridge Health - Bowmanville Site; Langs: Arabic; (905)427-1419; Fax. (905)427-0346.

PHIMISTER, Wayne; Agassiz Community Hlth Ctre, PO Box 159 7040 Cheam Ave, Agassiz BC V0M 1A0; Aberdeen (Scotland)'95; MB ChB; CCFP; (604)703-2030; Fax. (604)796-0221.

PHIPPS, Lincoln R; Leamington Dist Mem Hosp, 194 Talbot St W, Leamington ON N8H 1N9; Guadalajara (Mexico)'80; FAAFP; Staff, Leamington District Memorial Hospital; Langs: Spanish; German; Bilingual(French/English); (519)322-2501

PHIPPS, Nigel M; Halton Hills Family Health Team, 204-99 Sinclair Ave, Georgetown ON L7G 5G1; Tor'85; Staff, Halton Healthcare Services Corporation - Georgetown Hospital; (905)873-3344; Fax. (905)873-8094.

PHIPPS, William H G; Alder Med Centre, 277 Evergreen Rd, Campbell River BC V9W 5Y4; UBC'72; BSc; Sr Staff, Campbell River & District General Hospital; Med Examiner Civil Aviation, Transport Canada; Asst Prof Family Med, University of British Columbia; (250)287-7441; Fax. (250)287-4384.

PHIRI, Young W; Plaza 2 Shopping Ctr, 607-8600 Franklin Ave, Fort McMurray AB T9H 4G8; Manchester (England)'77; MB ChB; FRCOG(UK); LMCC; (780)713-4001; Fax. (780)713-4002; ywphiri@shaw.ca.

PHO, Mark; Pacific Med Clinic, 6176 Fraser St, Vancouver BC V5W 3A1; Alb'08; CCFP; (604)301-9955

PHORD-TOY, Mark S; 5449 Victoria Dr, Vancouver BC V5P 3V9; UBC'93; BSc; (604)873-2661; Fax. (604)873-4865.

PHOTOPOULOS, George J; Avenue Bloor Med Group, 405-208 Bloor St W, Toronto ON M5S 3B4; Tor'90; CCFP; FCFP; (416)962-1200; Fax. (416)962-1223.

PHOTOPOULOS, Peter; Davisville Family Practice, 600-1881 Yonge St, Toronto ON M4S 3C4; Tor'90; CCFP; FCFP; Langs: Greek; (416)932-3172; Fax. (416)440-0238.

PHOTOPOULOS, Spiro; Solutions Family Med Clinic, 279 Herring Cove Rd, Halifax NS B3P 1M2; AUC (Jamaica)'91; (902)477-7656; Fax. (902)477-7434.

PHU, Tommy C; Royal Columbian Hosp, 330 Columbia St E, New Westminster BC V3L 3W7; Dal'02; FRCPC; Anes. Staff, Royal Columbian Hospital; (604)520-4253

PHUL, Rishi T; West Edmonton Mall, 2039-8882 170 St NW, Edmonton AB T5T 3J7; Alb'03; CCFP; (780)444-1935; Fax. (780)444-3092.

PHUNG, Thinh-Vinh; CSSS du Lac-des-Deux-Montagnes, 520 boul Arthur-Sauve, St-Eustache QC J7R 5B1; Laval'96; Staff, Hôpital de Saint-Eustache; (450)473-6811 x2100; Fax. (450)473-6307.

PI, David W; Vancouver Gen Hosp, 855 12th Ave W, Vancouver BC V5Z 1M9; (Hong Kong)'80; FRCPC; HemPath. Staff, Vancouver General Hospital - Centennial Pavillion; Langs: Cantonese; (604)875-4111 x66830

PIACENTINO, Angelo; First Med Place, 202-170 Queensway W, Mississauga ON L5B 3A8; Tor'89; CCFP; (905)275-3822; Fax. (905)275-4001.

PIANEZZA, Michael L; Northern Urology Centre, 101-845 Regent St, Sudbury ON P3E 4T3; Ott'02; FRCSC; Urol. (705)673-6836; Fax. (705)673-2304.

PIATEK, Dariusz P; 12-3615 Dixie Rd, Mississauga ON L4Y 4H4; Man'88; Langs: Polish; (905)238-1217; Fax. (905)238-1796; medexcorp@msn.com.

PIAZZA, Nicolo; MUHC-Royal Victoria Hosp, 687 av des Pins O, Montreal QC H3A 1A1; McG'01; FRCPC; IntMed; Cardiol. Staff, McGill University Health Centre - Royal Victoria Hospital; (514)934-1934 x33333

PICARD, Anne-C; CHUQ-St-Francois d'Assise, 10 rue de l'Espinay, Quebec QC G1L 3L5; Laval'76; FRCPC; MedMicrobiol; Microbio & Infect Dis (P.Q.). Ac Staff, Centre Hospitalier Universitaire De Québec - Pavillon De St-françois-d'assise; (418)525-4444 x53740

PICARD, Chantal; CSSS de la Cote-De-Gaspe, 215 boul de York O, Gaspe QC G4X 2W2; Mon'03; CCFP; Staff, Centre Hospitalier de Gaspe; (418)368-3301; Fax. (418)368-6850.

PICARD, Christian; Clinique Med Giffard, 210-3333 rue du Carrefour, Quebec QC G1C 5R9; Laval'89; CCFP; (418)663-6345; Fax. (418)663-8621.

PICARD, Claude; Ctr Hosp Affilie-Enfant-Jesus, 1401 18e rue, Quebec QC G1J 1Z4; Laval'75; FRCSC; Neursurg (Neuro Oncology). Staff, Centre Hospitalier Affilié Universitaire de Québec - Hôpital De L'Enfant Jésus; Assoc Staff, CSSS de Quebec-Sud; Consultant, Centre Hospitalier Universitaire De Québec - Pavillon De St-françois-d'assise; Langs: English; (418)649-5734; Fax. (418)649-5915.

PICARD, Claudette; Overbrook-Forbes Comm FHT, 120-225 Donald St, Ottawa ON K1K 1N1; Laval'85; CCFP; Langs: Bilingual(French/English); (613)745-2228

PICARD, Daniel; CSSS De Saint-Jerome, 290 rue de Montigny, Saint-Jerome QC J7Z 5T3; Mon'78; MSc; FRCPC; NuclearMed (Radiation Protection). Staff, Hôtel-Dieu de Saint-Jérôme; Consultant, Hôpital regional d'Edmundston; Staff, Centre Hospitalier l'Université De Montréal (CHUM) - Hôpital Saint-luc; Langs: English; (450)431-8200 x2297; Fax. (514)412-7340; daniel.picard@cdsj.org.

PICARD, Elizabeth; Clin Med de l'Or et des Bois, 1281 7e rue, Val-d'Or QC J9P 3S1; Mon'04; (819)825-0965

PICARD, France; CSSS Les Eskers de l'Abitibi, 622 4e rue O, Amos QC J9T 2S2; Mon'93; Staff, CH Hôtel-Dieu d'Amos; (819)732-3341; Fax. (819)732-4646.

PICARD, Georges; Urgence-Sante, 3232 rue Belanger, Montreal QC H1Y 3H5; Mon'77; (514)723-5740

PICARD, Jacques; Ctr Hosp Rouyn-Noranda, 4 9e rue, Rouyn-Noranda QC J9X 2B2; Laval'88; CSPQ; Anes. Staff, Centre Hospitalier Rouyn-Noranda; (819)764-5131

PICARD, Jean-Marc; Polyclinique Med des Ponts, 120-1100 boul de la Rive-Sud, Saint-Romuald QC G6W 5M6; Laval'71; Langs: Bilingual(French/English); (418)834-1177; Fax. (418)834-9275.

PICARD, Jean-Pierre; Clin Card du Bas Richelieu, 300 rue Paradis, Sorel-Tracy QC J3P 3G6; Mon'67; Cardiol. (450)743-3725; Fax. (450)743-5656.

PICARD, Jolene; Clinique Med du Centre, 15-2020 boul Rene-Gaultier, Varennes QC J3X 1N9; Mon'83; (450)652-2222; Fax. (450)652-3970.

PICARD, Josee; CSSS du Sud de Lanaudière, 911 montee des Pionniers, Terrebonne QC J6V 2H2; Laval'05; DiagRad. Staff, Centre Hospitalier Pierre le Gardeur; (450)654-7525

PICARD, Josee; Clinique Med Adoncour, 200-505 rue Adoncour, Longueuil QC J4G 2M6; Mon'94; Staff, Centre Hospitalier Pierre Boucher; (450)646-4445; Fax. (450)646-5526.

PICARD, Larry M; 306-360 College St, Toronto ON M5T 1S6; Tor'77; ABNP; FRCPC; Neur (Spinal Disorders). Staff, Mount Sinai Hospital; Staff, Toronto Western Hospital - University Health Network; Staff, Baycrest Centre for Geriatric Care; Instructor Med, University of Toronto; (416)324-8533; Fax. (416)324-9826; dr.lmpicard@rogers.com.

PICARD, Leo; 202-585 Mapleton Rd, Moncton NB E1G 2K5; Sher'88; FRCPC; IntMed; Rheum. Staff, Dr Georges-L-Dumont University Hospital Centre; Langs: Bilingual(French/English).

PICARD, Luce; CLSC Malauze, RR 1 107 132 Rte O, Matapedia QC G0J 1V0; Mon'89; CCFP; (418)364-2572

PICARD, Lyne; Clinique Med du Sud-Ouest, 103-4475 rue Bannatyne, Verdun QC H4G 1E2; Laval'94; FRCSC; Otol (Thyroid Diseases). Staff, Centre Hospitalier de Verdun; Langs: Bilingual(French/English); (514)765-3600

PICARD, Lyne; Ctr Hosp de Verdun, 4000 boul Lasalle, Verdun QC H4G 2A3; Sher'85; Staff, Centre Hospitalier de Verdun; (514)362-1000 x2525

PICARD, Maria-Elisa; Ctr Hosp Affilie-Enfant-Jesus, 1401 18e rue, Quebec QC G1J 1Z4; Laval'89; Staff, Centre Hospitalier Affilié Universitaire de Québec - Hôpital De L'Enfant Jésus; (418)649-0252

PICARD, Marie; CLSC de Forestville, 2 7e rue CP 790, Forestville QC G0T 1E0; Laval'90; (418)587-2212 x253

PICARD, Marie-Eve; CSSS Pierre Boucher, 1333 boul Jacques-Cartier E, Longueuil QC J4M 2A5; Sher'01; FRCPC; Psy. Staff, Centre Hospitalier Pierre Boucher; (450)468-8401

PICARD, Martine; CSSS de Saint-Jerome, 290 rue de Montigny, Saint-Jerome QC J7Z 5T3; Mon'91; PlasSurg. Staff Plastic Surg, Hôtel-Dieu de Saint-Jérôme; (450)431-8200

PICARD, Matthieu; Hop Maisonneuve-Rosemont, 5415 boul de l'Assomption, Montreal QC H1T 2M4; Mon'07; ClinImmunol&Allergy; IntMed. Staff, Hopital Maisonneuve-Rosemont; (514)252-3400

PICARD, Michel A; CHUM-Hop St-Luc, 3208-1058 rue Saint-Denis, Montreal QC H2X 3J4; Mon'81; FRCPC; NuclearMed. Staff, Centre Hospitalier l'Université De Montréal (CHUM) - Hôpital Saint-luc; (514)890-8000 x36230; Fax. (514)412-7340.

PICARD, Philippe; CSSS de Rimouski-Neigette, CP 3150 Succ A 150 av Rouleau, Rimouski QC G5L 5T1; Sher'01; CSPQ; FRCPC; Anes. Staff, Hôpital Regional Rimouski; (418)723-7851

PICARD, Pierre; Victoria Med Centre, 406-304 Victoria Ave N, Hamilton ON L8L 5G4; Ott'04; Neur. (905)538-0244

PICARD, Robert; Hotel-Dieu d'Arthabaska, 5 rue des Hospitalieres, Victoriaville QC G6P 6N2; Laval'72; Staff, Hotel-Dieu d'Arthabaska; (819)537-2030

PICARD, Sylvie; CHUQ-Ctr Hosp Univ Laval, 2705 boul Laurier, Quebec QC G1V 4G2; Laval'75; FRCPC; Psy. Staff, Centre Hospitalier Universitaire de Quebec-CHUL; (418)654-2177; Fax. (418)654-2132.

PICARD-TURCOT, Anae; CSSS du Nord de Lanaudière, 1000 boul Sainte-Anne, St-Charles-Brromee QC J6E 6J2; Mon'07; CCFP; Staff, Centre Hospitalier Régional de Lanaudière; (450)759-8222

PICCININ, Laura R; Sudbury Reg Hosp-Laurentian, 41 Ramsey Lake Rd, Sudbury ON P3E 5J1; McM'96; CCFP; CCFP(E.M.); Staff, Health Sciences North-Laurentian Site; Prog Dir Emergency Med, Northern Ontario School of Medicine; Langs: English; French; (705)523-7100

PICCININ, Susan S; Ancaster Sport Med Centre, 1015 Golf Links Rd, Ancaster ON L9K 1L6; McM'86; CCFP; FCFP; (905)304-4687

PICCININI, Helena; Dalhousie Family Med, 6960 Mumford Rd, Halifax NS B3L 4P1; Dal'90; BSc; MSc; CCFP; Ac Staff, Queen Elizabeth II Health Sciences Centre - Victoria General Site; Court Staff, IWK Health Centre; Langs: Portuguese; German; Italian; (902)473-4700; Fax. (902)473-8548.

PICCO, Bridget M; Health Sciences Centre, 300 Prince Philip Dr, St. John's NL A1B 3V6; Mem'84; CCFP; Staff, Health Sciences Centre; (709)777-6300

PICH, Bohdan O; Cloverdale Mall, 182-250 The East Mall, Etobicoke ON M9B 3Y8; Tor'85; PhD; Staff, Trillium Health Centre - West Toronto; Langs: Ukrainian; (416)239-6122; Fax. (416)239-4895.

PICH, Phay; Care Point Med Centres, 5138 Joyce St, Vancouver BC V5R 4H1; Phom Penh (Cambodia)'73; Langs: Bilingual(English/French); (604)436-0800

PICHE, Alain; CHUS-Hop Fleurimont, 3001 12e av N, Sherbrooke QC J1H 5N4; Laval'90; Microbio & Infect Dis (P.Q.); MedMicrobiol. Staff, Centre Hospitalier Universitaire de Sherbrooke-Hopital Fleurimont; (819)564-5321; alain.piche@usherbrooke.ca.

PICHE, Annie; Polyclinique Maisonneuve-Rosem, 360-5345 boul de l'Assomption, Montreal QC H1T 4B3; Mon'03; CCFP; (514)257-7000

PICHE, Daniele; Clinique Med St-Augustin, 220-334 Rte 138, St-Aug-D-Desm QC G3A 1G8; Sher'86; Langs: English; (418)878-3590; Fax. (418)878-4876.

PICHE, Jacqueline; Centre Medical 25, 135B 25e av, Saint-Eustache QC J7P 2V1; Sher'86; FRCSC; ObstGyn. Staff, Hôpital de Saint-Eustache; (450)491-3533; jpiche@cm25.ca.

PICHE, Janelle R M; William Osler HC-Brampton, 2100 Bovaird Dr E, Brampton ON L6R 3J7; Sask'07; CCFP; CCFP(E.M.); Staff, William Osler Health System - Brampton Civic Hospital; (905)494-2120

PICHE, Jean; CSSS Pierre Boucher, 1333 boul Jacques-Cartier E, Longueuil QC J4M 2A5; Mon'85; FRCPC; AnatPath. Anatomical Pathology, Centre Hospitalier Pierre Boucher; (450)468-8111 x82244; Fax. (450)468-8201.

PICHE, Karine; CLSC-CHSLD de l'Erable, 1331 rue Saint-Calixte, Plessisville QC G6L 1P4; Sher'90; CCFP; Staff, CLSC de l'Erable; (819)362-6301

PICHE, Lawrence C; 103A-1001 Adelaide St N, London ON N5Y 2M6; Wes'72; Staff, St Joseph's Hospital - St Joseph's Health Care; (519)433-7341

PICHE, Louise; Place Val des Arbres, 175-1600A boul Saint-Martin E, Laval QC H7G 4R8; McG'84; FRCPC; Peds. (450)669-6666; Fax. (450)669-5412.

PICHE, Marcel; 9 Place de Marsal, Lorraine QC J6Z 3R6; Ott'72; Ac Staff, Centres Drapeau Deschambault; Langs: Bilingual(French/English); (450)435-4190

PICHE, Marie-Chantal; CSSS de Vaudreuil-Soulanges, 490 boul Harwood, Vaudreuil-Dorion QC J7V 7H4; Mon'02; CCFP; Staff, CSSS de Vaudreuil-Soulanges; (450)455-9301; Fax. (450)455-8964; marie-chantal_piche@rrsss16.gouv.qc.ca.

PICHE, Robert; CLSC Metro, 312-1801 boul de Maisonneuve O, Montreal QC H3H 1J9; Ott'82; (514)934-0354; Fax. (514)934-6155.

PICHE, Stacey L; Penticton Reg Hosp, 550 Carmi Ave, Penticton BC V2A 3G6; UBC'01; FRCPC; DiagRad. Staff, Penticton Regional Hospital; (250)492-4000

PICHE, Yves; Les Gynecologues Ass De, 1299 boul de la Concorde O, Laval QC H7N 5T4; Mon'81; ObstGyn. (450)668-3250; Fax. (450)668-7595.

PICHER, Francois; 1 boul des Sources RR 1, Deschambault QC G0A 1S0; Laval'76; Consultant, Alcoa Canada; Langs: English; (418)286-5267; Fax. (418)286-5407.

PICHETTE, Carole; 304-895 boul du Seminaire N, St-Jean-Sur-Richel QC J3A 1J2; Mon'75; MSc; Nephrol (P.Q.). Chief Nephrol & Dialysis, Hôpital du Haut-Richelieu; (450)359-1357; Fax. (450)359-4569.

PICHETTE, Francois; Centre de Read Lucie-Bruneau, 2275 av Laurier E, Montreal QC H2H 2N8; Mon'86; Psy (P.Q.). (514)527-4527 x2327; Fax. (514)527-7968.

PICHETTE, Gilbert; Hop du Sacre-Coeur de Mtl, 5400 boul Gouin O, Montreal QC H4J 1C5; Mon'84; FRCPC; MedMicrobiol; Microbio & Infect Dis (P.Q.). Ac Staff, Hôpital du Sacre-Coeur de Montréal; (514)338-2222 x2157; Fax. (514)338-2909.

PICHETTE, Jeanne L; CHUQ-Ctr Hosp Univ Laval, 2705 boul Laurier, Quebec QC G1V 4G2; Laval'71; FRCPC; Peds. Ac Staff, Centre Hospitalier Universitaire De Québec - Pavillon De St-françois-d'assise; Ac Staff, Centre Hospitalier Universitaire de Quebec-CHUL; (418)654-2282 x48164; Fax. (418)654-2137.

PICHETTE, Maude; Hop Charles LeMoyne, 3120 boul Taschereau, Greenfield Park QC J4V 2H1; Sher'06; FRCSC; GenSurg. Staff, Hopital Charles LeMoyne; (450)466-5000

PICHETTE, Monique; Clinique Med Warwick, 5A rue du Centre Sportif RR 3, Warwick QC J0A 1M0; Sher'91; Staff, Hotel-Dieu d'Arthabaska; Langs: Bilingual(French/English); (819)358-4600; Fax. (819)358-4620.

PICHETTE, Nathalie; Polyclinique St-Eustache, 75 rue Grignon, Saint-Eustache QC J7P 4J2; Mon'01; CCFP; Staff, Hôpital de Saint-Eustache; (450)473-6882; Fax. (450)473-1916.

PICHETTE, Roxanne; Hop du Sacre-Coeur de Mtl, 5400 boul Gouin O, Montreal QC H4J 1C5; Mon'73; MedOncol (P.Q.); Hem (P.Q.) (Breast Oncology). Staff HemOncol, Hôpital du Sacre-Coeur de Montréal; Clin Staff, Universite de Montreal; (514)338-2050

PICHETTE, Vincent; Hop Maisonneuve-Rosemont, 5415 boul de l'Assomption, Montreal QC H1T 2M4; Mon'88; ABIM; PharmD; FRCPC; IntMed; Nephrol. Staff, Hopital Maisonneuve-Rosemont; (514)252-3489; vpichette.hmr@ssss.gouv.qc.ca.

PICHORA, David R; Kingston Gen Hosp, 9 311-76 Stuart St, Kingston ON K7L 2V7; Qns'78; FRCSC; OrthSurg (Upper Extremity Surgery). Staff, Kingston General Hospital; Staff, Hotel-Dieu Hospital; Prof, Queen's University; (613)545-6666 x3395; Fax. (613)548-2526; pichorad@kgh.kari.net.

PICK, Neora; BC Women's Hosp & Health Ctre, 4500 Oak St, Vancouver BC V6H 3N1; Ben Gurion (Israel)'89; FRCPC; IntMed. Staff, BC Women's Hospital & Health Centre; Langs: Hebrew; (604)875-2212

PICKARD, Kathleen; Tuxedo Fam Med Centre, 981 Corydon Ave, Winnipeg MB R3M 0X1; Man'77; CCFP; FCFP; Ac Staff, St Boniface General Hospital; (204)988-6040

PICKEN, Barbara R; Willow Clinic, 1-3801 28A St, Vernon BC V1T 9T6; Man'86; BSc; Staff Family Pract, Vernon Jubilee Hospital; (250)542-9950

PICKERING, Bryan G; Associated Anaes of Winnipeg, 849 Notre Dame Ave, Winnipeg MB R3E 0M4; Man'74; FRCPC; Anes. Staff, Health Sciences Centre; (204)775-6947

PICKERING, J Geoffrey; London HSC-University Hosp, PO Box 5339 Stn B 339 Windermere Rd, London ON N6A 5A5; Qns'83; MD; FAHA; FRCP; DPhil; FRCPC; IntMed; Cardiol. Staff, London Health Sciences Centre - South Street; Staff, London Health Sciences Centre - University Hospital; Prof, University of Western Ontario; (519)663-3973; Fax. (519)434-3278; gpickering@robarts.ca.

PICKERING, Joyce L; MUHC-Royal Victoria Hosp, A421-687 av des Pins O, Montreal QC H3A 1A1; McG'80; FRCPC; IntMed. assoc Médecin, McGill University Health Centre - Royal Victoria Hospital; Prof, McGill University; Langs: Japanese; French; (514)843-1515; Fax. (514)843-1676; joyce.pickering@muhc.mcgill.ca.

PICKERING, Tara L; Tom Baker Cancer Centre, 1331 29 St NW, Calgary AB T2N 4N2; Alb'94; BSc; CCFP; Staff, Tom Baker Cancer Centre; (403)521-3735; Fax. (403)283-1651.

PICKERSGILL, Heather M; Health & Counselling Services, 1125 Colonel By Dr, Ottawa ON K1S 5B6; Qns'00; CCFP; (613)520-6674

PICKERSGILL, Sara M; The Credit Valley Hosp, 2200 Eglinton Ave W, Mississauga ON L5M 2N1; McM'04; CCFP; CCFP(E.M.); Staff, The Credit Valley Hospital; (905)813-4530

PICKETT, Bryan M; Sunnyside Place CIBC Bldg, 209-967 Bedford Hwy, Bedford NS B4A 1A9; Dal'98; CCFP; (902)832-0527; Fax. (902)832-0673.

PICKETT, Gwynedd E; Queen Elizabeth II HSC-Halifax, 3812-1796 Summer St, Halifax NS B3H 3A7; Dal'98; FRCSC; Neursurg (Cerebrovascular Surgery). Staff, Queen Elizabeth II Health Sciences Centre - Halifax Infirmary Site; (902)473-1667; Fax. (902)425-4372.

PICKETT, Tracy A; St Paul's Hosp, 1081 Burrard St, Vancouver BC V6Z 1Y6; UBC'95; FRCPC; EmergMed. Staff, Providence Health Care - St Paul's Hospital; (604)806-8480

PICKETT, Wayne E; Scotia Med Clinic, 961 Bedford Hwy, Bedford NS B4A 1A9; Dal'91; CCFP; CCFP(E.M.); FCFP; (902)832-2380; Fax. (902)444-3074.

PICKETTS, Darrell K; 89 Lynden Rd PO Box 100, Lynden ON L0R 1T0; Qns'71; (519)647-3422; Fax. (519)647-2901.

PICKLE, Andrew R; 300-274 Dundas St E, Belleville ON K8N 1E6; Mem'98; FRCSC; OrthSurg (Sports Medicine). Staff, QHC Belleville General; (613)966-7522; Fax. (613)966-3997.

PICKLE, David A; 5970 Mullen Way PO Box 36565 Rpo McTaggart, Edmonton AB T6R 0T4; Alb'07; CCFP.

PICKLES, Angela M; Dr Charles A Janeway Child HC, 300 Prince Philip Dr, St. John's NL A1B 3V6; Mem'96; FRCPC; DiagRad. Staff, Janeway Children's Health & Rehabilitation Centre; (709)777-6300

PICKLES, Thomas A; BC Cancer Agency-Vancouver CC, 600 10th Ave W, Vancouver BC V5Z 4E6; London (England)'80; MB BS; MRCP(UK); FRCR; FRCPC; RadOncol. Ac Staff, Vancouver General Hospital - Centennial Pavillion; Ac Staff, BC Cancer Agency Vancouver Centre; Clin Prof, University of British Columbia; (604)877-6000 x2665; Fax. (604)877-0505.

PICKUP, Michael J; Prov Forensic Pathology Unit, 26 Grenville St, Toronto ON M7A 2G9; Tor'04; FRCPC; AnatPath (Forensic Pathology). (416)314-4040

PICOTTE, Frederic; Unite de Med Familiale, 80 118e rue, Shawinigan-Sud QC G9P 3E4; McG'08; CCFP; (819)536-7511

PICOTTE, Marie-Eve; CSSS Drummond-Hop Sainte-Croix, 570 rue Heriot, Drummondville QC J2B 1C1; Sher'03; CCFP; CCFP(E.M.); Staff, Hôpital Sainte-croix; Staff, Centre Hospitalier Honore-Mercier; (819)478-6464

PICOTTE, Rene-Paul; Clinique Med Fam des Recollets, 101-940 boul des Recollets, Trois-Rivieres QC G8Z 3W9; Laval'71; (819)373-0305

PICTON, Avis R; Orion Health Surrey, 120-16555 Fraser Hwy, Surrey BC V4N 0E9; UBC'89; CCFP; Staff, BC Cancer Agency Fraser Valley Centre; (604)802-8056

PICTON, Taralyn D; 405-275 Lansdowne St, Kamloops BC V2C 1X8; Alb'83; BMedSci; ABIM; FRCPC; IntMed; Gastroent. Staff, Royal Inland Hospital; (250)374-1898; Fax. (250)372-9983.

PIDDE, Richard J; 11807 Jasper Ave NW, Edmonton AB T5K 0N8; Alb'79; (780)488-1222

PIDGEON, Jean-Francois; CSSS de la Region de Thetford, 1717 rue Notre-Dame E, Thetford Mines QC G6G 2V4; Laval'90; FRCSC; GenSurg. Staff, Hopital du CSS de la Region de Thetford; Langs: English; French; (418)338-7777

PIDSADNY, Shelly; Hope Centre Health Care, 240 Powers St, Winnipeg MB R2W 5L1; Man'92; CCFP; FCFP; Staff, Hope Centre Health Care Inc; (204)589-8354

PIEBIAK-PATTERSON, Krista K; Westgrove Clinic, 201-505 Queen St, Spruce Grove AB T7X 2V2; Alb'09; BSc; CCFP; (780)962-9888; Fax. (780)960-5298.

PIECHOTA, Paul S; Clin AccesMed, 200-17001 Rte Trans-Canada, Kirkland QC H9H 5J1; Tor'88; CCFP; (514)694-4644; Fax. (514)694-4646.

PIECZONKA, Rosalind M; 502-1881 Yonge St, Toronto ON M4S 3C4; Tor'85; CCFP; (416)539-9598; Fax. (416)539-0802.

PIEDBOEUF, Bruno; CHUQ-Ctr Hosp Univ Laval, 2705 boul Laurier, Quebec QC G1V 4G2; Mon'85; FRCPC; Peds (Neonatology). Staff, Centre Hospitalier Universitaire de Quebec-CHUL; Prof, Université Laval; (418)654-2282; Fax. (418)654-2771; bruno.piedboeuf@crchul.ulaval.ca.

PIEKOS, Anna M; Univ Hlth Network-Toronto Western Hosp, 399 Bathurst St, Toronto ON M5T 2S8; Tor'10; CCFP; Staff, Toronto Western Hospital - University Health Network; (416)603-5397

PIEKOS, Lucyna M; Bluewater Health-Norman Site, 89 Norman St, Sarnia ON N7T 6S3; Warsaw (Poland)'87; FRCPC; DiagRad. Staff, Bluewater Health - Norman Site; (519)464-4400

PIEMONTESI, Roberto L G; Pacific Coast Eye Center, 1651 Boundary Ave, Nanaimo BC V9S 5R8; Cape Town (South Africa)'82; BSc; MB ChB; DA(SA); FRCSC; Ophth (Glaucoma). Langs: Italian; (250)753-8415; Fax. (250)753-5422.

PIENAAR, Christopher T; Kootenay Child Hlth & Dev't Ct, 16 12th Ave N, Cranbrook BC V1C 3V7; Stellenbosch (South Africa)'94; Staff, East Kootenay Regional Hospital; (250)426-9008

PIENAAR, Colette; 3680 Gilmore Way, Burnaby BC V5G 4V8; Stellenbosch (South Africa)'95; FCP (SA); MB ChB; DTMH; MMed; Langs: Afrikaans; (604)412-4409

PIENAAR, Johannes J; Grand River Hosp-KW Hlth Ctre, PO Box 9056 Stn C 835 King St W, Kitchener ON N2G 1G3; Stellenbosch (South Africa)'97; MB ChB; CCFP; Staff, Grand River Hospital - Kitchener/Waterloo Health Centre; (519)742-3611

PIENAAR, LeRoy C; Highland Park Med Clinic, 2B-6315 Horn St, Red Deer AB T4N 6H5; (South Africa)'88; MB ChB; (403)342-2040; Fax. (403)342-7390.

PIENAAR, Louise; Sow's Ear Med Clinic, PO Box 190 7186 Lantzville Rd, Lantzville BC V0R 2H0; Orange Free State (South Africa)'81; MB ChB; CCFP; Langs: Afrikaans; (250)390-4542

PIENAAR, Marius P; Prince Rupert Reg Hosp, 1305 Summit Ave, Prince Rupert BC V8J 2A6; Pretoria (South Africa)'83; FRCSC; ObstGyn. Staff, Prince Rupert Regional Hospital; Langs: Afrikaans; (250)624-0295; Fax. (250)624-0297.

PIENAAR, Petrus J; Burnaby Hosp, 3935 Kincaid St, Burnaby BC V5G 2X6; Pretoria (South Africa)'83; MB ChB; FRCPC; Anes. Staff Anes, Burnaby Hospital; (604)412-6311

PIENAAR, Sonja; Mayfair Place Med Centre, 313-6707 Elbow Dr SW, Calgary AB T2V 0E5; Pretoria (South Africa)'86; MB ChB; BMedSci; CCFP; Langs: Afrikaans; (403)252-6022; Fax. (403)253-1923; sonjapienaar@shaw.ca.

PIEPGRASS, Brent L; PO Box 22043 Rpo Southview, Grande Prairie AB T8V 6X1; Alb'78; Med Dir/Chief Medical Staff, Queen Elizabeth II Hospital.

PIEPRZAK, Patricia S; PO Box 39021 Rpo James Bay, Victoria BC V8V 4X8; McM'83; FRCSC; Otol. (250)382-5117

PIERCE, Cameron W; Royal University Hosp, 103 Hospital Dr, Saskatoon SK S7N 0W8; Man'04; FRCPC; IntMed; Respir. Staff, Royal University Hospital; (306)966-8274

PIERCE, Dawne E J; Broadway Family Physicians, 1801 Broadway Ave, Saskatoon SK S7H 2B6; UBC'96; BSc; CCFP; (306)652-2632; Fax. (306)652-2637.

PIERCE, Garvin W; Salvation Army Grace Gen Hosp, 300 Booth Dr, Winnipeg MB R3J 3M7; Man'73; FRCPC; DiagRad. Staff Radiologist, The Salvation Army Grace Hospital; Asst Dean, University of Manitoba; (204)837-8311

PIERCE, Glenn D; Orchardview Med Centre, 100-155 Main St E, Grimsby ON L3M 1P2; (Ireland)'90; DAB; CCFP; Staff Physician, West Lincoln Memorial Hospital; (905)945-5476; Fax. (905)945-7707.

PIERCE, Jennifer L; Wabano Ctr for Aboriginal Heal, 299 Montreal Rd, Ottawa ON K1L 6B8; Ott'07; CCFP; Staff, Arnprior & District Memorial Hospital; (613)748-5999; Fax. (613)748-0550.

PIERCE, Marianne; IWK Health Centre, PO Box 9700 Rpo Csc 5850-5980 University Ave, Halifax NS B3K 6R8; Dal'03; FRCSC; ObstGyn. Staff, IWK Health Centre; (902)470-7491; Fax. (902)425-1125.

PIERCEY, James R A; Medical Bldg, 405-1990 Fort St, Victoria BC V8R 6V4; Alb'70; BSc; ABIM; FRCPC; IntMed; Gastroent. Ac Staff, Royal Jubilee Hospital; Ac Staff, Victoria General Hospital; (250)370-9121; Fax. (250)370-0930.

PIERCEY, Karen-Lynne; Haig Clinic, 601 6 Ave S, Lethbridge AB T1J 0Z2; Mem'04; CCFP; (403)328-6641; Fax. (403)328-6118.

PIERCEY, Kevin R; St Joseph's Healthcare, 50 Charlton Ave E, Hamilton ON L8N 4A6; Qns'88; FRCSC; Urol. Court Staff, Hamilton Health Sciences Centre-Juravinski Site; Ac Staff, St Joseph's Healthcare - Charlton Campus; Asst Prof, McMaster University; (905)522-1155 x34987; Fax. (905)528-3043.

PIERCEY, Maureen L; College of Phys & Surg of BC, 300-669 Howe St, Vancouver BC V6C 0B4; Alb'69; Member, College of Physicians & Surgeons of British Columbia; (604)733-7758; Fax. (604)733-3503.

PIERCY, Gregory M; Brant Community HC-Willet, 238 Grand River St N, Paris ON N3L 2N7; Qns'83; MSc; Staff, The Brant Community Healthcare System - Willett Hospital Site; (519)442-7979; Fax. (519)442-2727; g.piercy@rogers.com.

PIERRAT, Audrey; Ctr de Perinatalite l'Autre Ma, 575 rue Saint-Charles E, Longueuil QC J4H 1B8; Mon'06; CCFP; (450)332-9833

PIERRATOS, Andreas; Humber River Reg Hosp-Church, 200 Church St, Toronto ON M9N 1N8; Athens (Greece)'73; FRCPC; IntMed (Dialysis); Nephrol. Staff, Humber River Regional Hospital - Church Street Site; Assoc Prof Med, University of Toronto; Langs: Greek; (416)657-2669; Fax. (416)657-2669; a.pierratos@utoronto.ca.

PIERRE, Andrew F; Univ Hlth Network-Toronto Gen, 9N 959-200 Elizabeth St, Toronto ON M5G 2C4; Tor'93; ABS; MSc; FRCSC; GenSurg (Gastroesophageal Reflux Dis); ThorSurg. Staff Thoracic Surg, The Hospital For Sick Children; Staff Thoracic Surg, Mount Sinai Hospital; Staff, Toronto General Hospital - UHN; Asst Prof, University of Toronto; (416)340-5354; Fax. (416)340-4556; andrew.pierre@uhn.on.ca.

PIERRE, Jean-Rene; Ctr de Sante Vallee-Gatineau, 309 boul Desjardins, Maniwaki QC J9E 2E7; Seville (Spain)'79; LMCC; Pres, CMDP; Physician, Domaine des Forestiers; Langs: English; Spanish; (819)449-4690 x172; Fax. (819)449-6136.

PIERRE, Sean A; Centrepointe Med Centre, 307-1 Centrepointe Dr, Nepean ON K2G 6E2; Wes'01; FRCSC; Urol (Endourology). Consultant, Queensway Carleton Hospital; Asst Prof, Queen's University; (613)221-9200; Fax. (613)221-9300.

PIERRE-LOUIS, Faudry; Montford-Ottawa French Team, 101-338 Montreal Rd, Vanier ON K1L 6B3; (Haiti)'63; FRCPC; Psy. Staff, Montfort Hospital; (613)688-1083; Fax. (613)688-1087.

PIERRE-LOUIS, Gerard; St Mary's Hosp Centre, 3830 av Lacombe, Montreal QC H3T 1M5; (Mexico)'69; FRCPC; Psy. Dir Psy Internal Services, St Mary's Hospital Centre; McGill University; (514)345-3349

PIERRE-LOUIS, Marie-Laurette; Ctr Hosp Pierre-Janet, 20 rue Pharand, Gatineau QC J9A 1K7; Lausanne (Switzerland)'71; FRCPC; Psy. Staff Psy, Centre Hospitalier Pierre-Janet; (819)776-8010; Fax. (819)776-8002.

PIERRE-LOUIS, Schiller; Hop du Sacre-Coeur de Mtl, 5400 boul Gouin O, Montreal QC H4J 1C5; Valencia (Spain)'70; FACP; LMCC; IntMed (P.Q.) (Vascular Medicine). Chef IntMed, Hôpital du Sacre-Coeur de Montréal; adj Prof, Universite de Montreal; (514)338-2050; Fax. (514)338-2384.

PIERSANTI, Monique; Credit Valley Prof Bldg, 403-2300 Eglinton Ave W, Mississauga ON L5M 2V8; Tor'98; FRCPC; IntMed; Endocrin&Metab. Langs: Italian; (905)828-6522; Fax. (905)828-6967.

PIERSCIANOWSKI, Tadeusz A; Hunt Club Med Centre, 103-3328 McCarthy Rd, Ottawa ON K1V 0H9; London (England)'73; MB BS; MRCPath(UK); FRCPC; IntMed; Derm. Consultant, The Ottawa Hospital - General Campus; Lecturer, University of Ottawa; Langs: Polish; (613)738-1064; Fax. (613)738-5328; drtad@bellnet.ca.

PIERSE, Michael P; Children's Hosp Eastern Ontari, 401 Smyth Rd, Ottawa ON K1H 8L1; Alb'05; FRCPC; Peds; PedEmergMed. Staff, Children's Hospital of Eastern Ontario (CHEO); (613)737-7600

PIERSE, Patrick M; Tawa Centre, 219-3017 66 St NW, Edmonton AB T6K 4B2; National (Ireland)'77; MB ChB; BAO; FRCPCH; FRCPC; Peds (Neonatal). Staff Peds, Covenant Health - Grey Nuns Community Hospital; Clin Assoc Prof, University of Alberta; (780)461-9343; Fax. (780)450-0360; ppierse@ualberta.ca.

PIERSON, Kathleen E; Foothills Med Centre, 1403 29 St NW, Calgary AB T2N 2T9; Dal'94; FRCPC; Psy (Mental Illness). Staff Psy, Foothills Medical Centre; Asst Prof Psy, University of Calgary; (403)944-2723; Fax. (403)270-3451; kathleen.pierson@calgaryhealthregion.ca.

PIESAS, David J; Strathmore Med Clinic, PO Box 2465 Stn Main, Strathmore AB T1P 1K3; Witwatersrand (South Africa)'86; MB ChB; CCFP; Staff, Strathmore District Health Services; (403)361-2422; Fax. (403)361-2420; drpies@shawbiz.ca.

PIESSENS, Eva A; Hamilton HS-Juravinski Site, 711 Concession St, Hamilton ON L8V 1C3; Columbia University (USA)'91; Staff, Hamilton Health Sciences Centre-Juravinski Site; (905)521-2100

PIETAK, Stanley P; 544 Armstrong Rd, Kingston ON K7M 7N8; Qns'67; Anes. Staff Anes, Kingston General Hospital; Staff, Hotel-Dieu Hospital; Assoc Prof, Queen's University; (613)546-4814

PIETERSE, Gert C S; Porcupine Plain Med Clinic, PO Box 520, Porcupine Plain SK S0E 1H0; Pretoria (South Africa)'77; MB ChB; (306)278-2151; Fax. (306)278-3102.

PIETERSE, Leonie; 214 Med Place, 9909 102 St, Grande Prairie AB T8V 2V4; Bloemfontein (South Africa)'92; MB ChB; Langs: Afrikaans; (780)814-5225; Fax. (780)402-2858; drleonie@telusplanet.net.

PIETERSE, Wickus; Russell Med Clinic, PO Box 549 117 Westbourne Ave, Virden MB R0M 2C0; Pretoria (South Africa)'99; CCFP; (204)773-2146

PIETERSE, Wilhelm S; Tamarack Med Clinic, 191-1500 Cranbrook St N, Cranbrook BC V1C 3S8; Pretoria (South Africa)'79; (250)426-7724

PIETRANGELO, Maria G; Hop Charles LeMoyne, 3120 boul Taschereau, Greenfield Park QC J4V 2H1; McG'93; FRCPC; IntMed. Staff, Hopital Charles LeMoyne; (450)466-5000 x2880; Fax. (450)466-5768; mgpietrangelo@sympatico.ca.

PIETRASZEK, Bogdan Z; 149 Roncesvalles Ave, Toronto ON M6R 2L3; Warsaw (Poland)'79; Ac Staff, St Joseph's Health Centre; (416)532-4317

PIETRASZEK, Mary D S; 669 The Queensway, Etobicoke ON M8Y 1K8; Warsaw (Poland)'79; Ac Staff, St Joseph's Health Centre; Langs: Polish; (416)604-0614; Fax. (416)604-2632.

PIETROBON, Gian F; Nepean Clinical Associates, 1437 Woodroffe Ave, Nepean ON K2G 1W1; Ott'88; (613)225-5532; Fax. (613)225-0540.

PIETRUS, Henryk C; Springbank Med Centre, 460 Springbank Dr, London ON N6J 1G8; Jagiellonian University (Poland)'84; (226)781-0859; Fax. (226)781-9809.

PIETRUS, Teresa; Springbank Med Centre, 207-460 Springbank Dr, London ON N6J 0A8; Jagiellonian University (Poland)'84; (226)781-0858; Fax. (226)781-9809.

PIETTE, Claude; Hop du Sacre-Coeur de Mtl, 5400 boul Gouin O, Montreal QC H4J 1C5; Mon'78; FRCPC; EmergMed. Staff, Hôpital du Sacre-Coeur de Montréal; (514)335-1252; Fax. (514)335-1753.

PIETTE, Eric; Hop du Sacre-Coeur de Mtl, 5400 boul Gouin O, Montreal QC H4J 1C5; Mon'05; FRCPC; EmergMed. Staff, Hôpital du Sacre-Coeur de Montréal; (514)338-2000

PIETUCHA, Przemyslaw A; Addiction & Mental Hlth-Clarke, 1235-250 College St, Toronto ON M5T 1R8; Cal'04; CCFP; Staff, Centre for Addiction & Mental Health (CAMH) - College Street Site; (416)535-8501

PIGEON, Amelie; Clinique Med Lanaudiere, 222 rue Bernard, St-Charles-Brromee QC J6E 2C5; Sher'03; CCFP; Staff Hosp & Emerg, Centre Hospitalier Régional de Lanaudière; (450)755-1033

PIGEON, Dany; Hotel-Dieu de Levis, 143 rue Wolfe, Levis QC G6V 3Z1; Laval'00; FRCPC; EmergMed. Staff, Hôtel-Dieu de Lévis; (418)835-7121 x6178

PIGEON, Edith; L'Omniclinique de l'Outaouais, 202-28 boul du Mont-Bleu, Gatineau QC J8Z 1J1; Mon'88; CCFP; FCFP; Langs: Bilingual(French/English); (819)777-2111; Fax. (819)771-6890.

PIGEON, Francois; Clinique Med le Gardeurois, 130-155 boul Lacombe, Repentigny QC J5Z 3C4; Mon'90; Staff, Hôtel-Dieu de Sorel; Médecin, Clinique Medicale Le Gardeurois; (450)582-5551

PIGEON, Julie; CLSC Malartic, GD 1141 rue Royale, Malartic QC J0Y 1Z0; Laval'03; Staff, Centre de Sante Vallee-de-l'Or; Staff, CSSSVO-Senneterre; (819)825-5858

PIGEON, Marie-Andree; Direction de la Sante Publique, U 2107-2400 av d'Estimauville, Quebec QC G1E 7G9; Mon'81; LMCC; (418)856-7000 x5100

PIGEON, Michel B J; Waypoint Centre for Mental H C, 500 Church St, Penetanguishene ON L9M 1G3; Wes'72; FRCSC; FRCPC; Psy; GenSurg (Borderline Personality Disorder). Staff/Consultant, Waypoint Centre for Mental Health Care; Court Staff/Consultant, Georgian Bay General Hospital - Midland; Staff, Penetanguishene Mental Health Centre; Langs: English; (705)549-3181 x2137; Fax. (705)549-1812; mpigeon@mhcp.on.ca.

PIGEON, Nicole; 232-1055 12e av N, Sherbrooke QC J1E 2X4; Sher'83; FRCPC; Peds (Cerebral Palsy). assoc Staff, Centre Hospitalier Universitaire de Sherbrooke-Hopital Fleurimont; Ac Staff, Centre de Readaptation de l'Estrie; Langs: Bilingual(French/English); (819)563-6232; Fax. (819)563-0159; nicole.pigeon@ssss.gouv.qc.ca.

PIGEON, Pierre D; CSSS du Lac-des-Deux-Montagnes, 520 boul Arthur-Sauve, St-Eustache QC J7R 5B1; Sher'85; FRCSC; GenSurg (Digestive Endoscopy). Staff, Hôpital de Saint-Eustache; Langs: Bilingual(French/English); (450)473-6811

PIGEON, Serge; Clinique Med de Rawdon, GD 201-3240 4e av, Rawdon QC J0K 1S0; Sher'74; assoc Staff Emerg, Manoir Heather Lodge; (450)834-2304

PIGGOTT, Zoe S; St Boniface Gen Hosp, 409 Tache Ave, Winnipeg MB R2H 2A6; Qns'07; FRCPC; EmergMed. Staff, St Boniface General Hospital; (204)233-8563

PIGNANELLI, Biaggio; Lasalle Community Health Care, 2125 Front Rd, Windsor ON N9J 2C1; Wes'87; (519)734-1234; Fax. (519)734-8674.

PIGNATIELLO, Antonio; The Hosp for Sick Children, 555 University Ave, Toronto ON M5G 1X8; Tor'87; FRCPC; Psy (Child & Adolescent Psychiatry). Staff, The Hospital For Sick Children; Court Staff, Trillium Health Centre - Mississauga; Asst Prof Psy, University of Toronto; Langs: Italian; (416)813-2188; Fax. (416)813-2189.

PIGNOL, Jean-Philippe; Sunnybrook Odette Reg Cancer, 2075 Bayview Ave, Toronto ON M4N 3M5; D'Aiz-Marseille (France)'87; FRCPC; RadOncol. Staff, Sunnybrook Health Sciences Centre; (416)480-5329; Fax. (416)480-6002.

PIGOTT, Tara G; Sparwood Primary Health Care, PO Box 1120 570 Pine Ave, Sparwood BC V0B 2G0; London (England)'91; MB BS; MRCGPract; CCFP; (250)425-4501; Fax. (250)425-4549.

PIKALUK, D Ryan; McMaster University, 1280 Main St W, Hamilton ON L8S 4K1; Sask'07; FRCPC; Anes.

PIKE, Cherry J; Eastgate Med Centre, 279 Portugal Cove Rd, St. John's NL A1B 2N8; Mem'83; FRCSC; ObstGyn. (709)753-9940; Fax. (709)753-9890.

PIKE, Eric J; St Clare's Mercy Hosp, 154 Lemarchant Rd, St. John's NL A1C 5B8; Mem'88; FRCPC; DiagRad. Staff, St Clare's Mercy Hospital; (709)777-5000

PIKE, Jeffrey H; The Moncton Hosp, 4520-135 MacBeath Ave, Moncton NB E1C 6Z8; Dal'98; FRCPC; PhysMed&Rehab (Sports Medicine). Staff, The Moncton Hospital; (506)870-2607; Fax. (506)870-2609.

PIKE, Jeffrey M; 590-1144 Burrard St, Vancouver BC V6Z 2A5; UBC'03; FRCSC; OrthSurg. (604)689-5144

PIKE, John G; Health Sciences Centre, 300 Prince Philip Dr, St. John's NL A1B 3V6; Mem'84; FRCSC; Urol (Pediatric Urology). Staff, Health Sciences Centre; (709)777-6300

PIKE, Judith A; BC Cancer Agency-Vancouver CC, 600 10the Ave W, Vancouver BC V5Z 4E6; Queen's (Ireland)'69; Ac Staff, BC Cancer Agency Vancouver Centre; (604)877-6000; jpike@bccancer.bc.ca.

PIKE, Malcolm J; Collins Barrow Place, 304-272 Charlotte St, Peterborough ON K9J 2V4; Tasminia (Australia)'71; FRACP(IntMed); FRCPC; IntMed (Endocrinology).

PIKE, Pamela A; Health Sciences Centre, 300 Prince Philip Dr, St. John's NL A1B 3V6; Mem'01; FRCPC; IntMed; Nephrol. Staff, Health Sciences Centre; (709)737-6300

PIKE AU, Krysta L; Eleven Elizabeth Family Practi, 201-11 Elizabeth Ave, St. John's NL A1A 1W6; Mem'02; CCFP.

PIKTEL, Henry M; University of Alberta Hosp, 1E712-8440 112 St NW, Edmonton AB T6G 2B7; Alb'74; FRCPC; Psy. Ac Staff Psy, University of Alberta Hospital; (780)407-6543; Fax. (780)407-6575.

PILAPIL-LEE, Rossali; 203-2620 Commercial Dr, Vancouver BC V5N 4C4; Cebu (Philippines)'98; CCFP; Langs: Tagalog; (604)876-0533

PILAR, Imelda S; Mississauga Med Centre, 360-1420 Burnhamthorpe Rd E, Mississauga ON L4X 2Z9; Manila (Philippines)'91; CCFP; Langs: Czech; (905)614-1944

PILAR, Saul; MacDonald Med Centre, 205-2786 16th Ave W, Vancouver BC V6K 4M1; Tor'76; BASc; (604)739-8858; Fax. (604)736-6424.

PILARSKI, Barbara A; Islington Med Clinic, 804-1243 Islington Ave, Etobicoke ON M8X 1Y9; Tor'89; CCFP; FCFP; Staff, St Joseph's Health Centre; Physician, Dom Lipa Nursing Home; Langs: Polish; (416)762-1233; Fax. (416)762-1236.

PILARSKI, Robert; Clinique du Quartier Latin, 905 boul Rene-Levesque E, Montreal QC H2L 5B1; Sher'09; CCFP; (514)285-5500; Fax. (514)285-2226.

PILAT, Edward J; Transcona Med Clinic, 200-701 Regent Ave W, Winnipeg MB R2C 1S3; Man'71; Dip SportMed; CCFP; Staff, St Boniface General Hospital; Staff, Concordia General Hospital; Lecturer Family Med, University of Manitoba; (204)222-5221; Fax. (204)224-2053.

PILAVDZIC, Dragana; SMBD Jewish Gen Hosp, 3755 ch Cote-Sainte-Catherine, Montreal QC H3T 1E2; Zagreb (Croatia)'80; CSPQ; FRCPC; AnatPath (Breast Pathology). Staff, Sir Mortimer B Davis Jewish General; adj Prof, McGill University; Langs: Serbo-Croatian; (514)340-8222 x5490; dpilavdzic@jgh.mcgill.ca.

PILECKI, Maciej W; Hotel-Dieu Hosp, 166 Brock St, Kingston ON K7L 5G2; Jagiellonian Univ (Poland)'94; Staff, Hotel-Dieu Hospital; (613)544-3310

PILEGGI, Lee A; Whitby Clinic, 200 Brock St N, Whitby ON L1N 4H5; Wes'82; (905)668-3378; Fax. (905)668-3807.

PILGRIM, Michael A; Dawson Creek Med Clinic, 2F-816 103 Ave, Dawson Creek BC V1G 2G1; Cal'94; BSc(Hons.); CCFP; Head Emerg Med, Dawson Creek & District Hospital; (250)782-5271; Fax. (250)782-6360.

PILGRIM, S Brent; Wedstern Mem Reg Hosp, PO Box 2005 Stn Main 1 Brookfield Ave, Corner Brook NL A2H 6J7; Mem'01; BSc; FRCPC; DiagRad (MRI). Staff, Western Memorial Regional Hospital; (709)637-5000

PILIOTIS, Eugenia; Odette Cancer Centre, 2075 Bayview Ave, Toronto ON M4N 3M5; Wes'97; BSc; MEd; FRCPC; IntMed; Hem. Staff, Sunnybrook Health Sciences Centre - Edmond Odette Cancer Centre; Langs: Greek; (416)480-4662; Fax. (416)480-6002.

PILKEY, Bradley D; Health Sciences Centre, 820 Sherbrook St, Winnipeg MB R3A 1R9; Sask'97; FRCSC; OrthSurg (Hip & Knee Reconstruction). Staff, Health Sciences Centre; (204)774-6511

PILKEY, Jana L; St Boniface Gen Hosp, 409 Tache Ave, Winnipeg MB R2H 2A6; Sask'97; FRCPC; IntMed. Staff, St Boniface General Hospital; (204)233-8563

PILLAI, Dylan R; Calgary Lab Services, 1W 416-3535 Research Rd NW, Calgary AB T2L 2K8; Tor'02; FRCPC; MedMicrobiol. Staff, Calgary Laboratory Services; (403)770-3338

PILLAI, Geetha; St Joseph's Healthcare, 50 Charlton Ave E, Hamilton ON L8N 4A6; Kerala (India)'95; FRCPC; IntMed. Staff, St Joseph's Healthcare - Charlton Campus; (905)521-2100

PILLAI, N Gopalakrishna; PO Box 456, Inverness NS B0E 1N0; Karnatak (India)'64; Assoc Staff, Inverness Consolidated Memorial Hospital; (902)258-2800; Fax. (902)258-3322.

PILLAY, Anandhan; 203-11001 13 St, Dawson Creek BC V1G 4Z8; Natal (South Africa)'95; MB ChB; (250)782-2827

PILLAY, Baven; Burnside Med Clinic, 2-101 Burnside Rd W, Victoria BC V9A 1B7; Alb'90; (250)381-4353

PILLAY, Intheran P; Larin Med Professional Corp, PO Box 150 619 Main St N, Gravelbourg SK S0H 1X0; Cape Town (South Africa)'88; MB ChB; LMCC(C); Chief Family Practice, Five Hills Health Region Corporate Office; Méd légiste Canadian Aviation, Transport Canada; Clin Lecturer, University of Saskatchewan; (306)648-4505; Fax. (306)648-2558; larin@sasktel.net.

PILLAY, Kumaravel K; Regina Qu'Appelle HR-Regina, 1440 14th Ave, Regina SK S4P 0W5; Natal (South Africa)'88; MB ChB; DA(SA); CCFP; CCFP(E.M.); Staff, Regina General Hospital; (306)766-4213; Fax. (306)766-4357.

PILLAY, Leanne; Caledonian Med Clinic, 340 Campbell St, Nanaimo BC V9R 3G7; Mysore (India)'00; MB BS; (250)753-3202; Fax. (250)753-1039.

PILLAY, Leveshen; 340 Campbell St, Nanaimo BC V9R 3G7; Witwatersrand (South Africa)'05; (250)753-3202

PILLAY, Nalini; 705-2125 11th Ave, Regina SK S4P 3X3; (306)352-4900; Fax. (306)352-6500.

PILLAY, Neelan; Foothills Med Centre, 1403 29 St NW, Calgary AB T2N 2T9; Natal (South Africa)'68; MRC(UK); FRCPC; Neur (Epilepsy). Staff/Clin Prof/Dir Epilepsy Prog, Foothills Medical Centre; Teach Staff, University of Calgary; (403)944-8087; pillay@ucalgary.ca.

PILLAY, Nemi N; 4274 Queen St PO Box 946, Beamsville ON L0R 1B0; Witwatersrand (South Africa)'67; MB ChB; CCFP; FCFP; Med Staff, Niagara Health System - St Catharines General Site; Asst Prof Family Med, McMaster University; (905)563-8216; Fax. (905)563-8747.

PILLAY, Paramesha; 205-9814 97 St, Grande Prairie AB T8V 8H5; (South Africa)'92; MB ChB; DCH; Staff Peds, Queen Elizabeth II Hospital; (780)513-1231; Fax. (780)513-1915.

PILLAY, Poogendren; Regina Qu'Appelle HR-Regina, 320-1440 14th Ave, Regina SK S4P 0W5; Durban (South Africa)'87; MB ChB; Staff, Regina General Hospital; (306)352-8555; Fax. (306)352-8556.

PILLAY, Pooventhran G; Teulon/Hunter Mem Hosp, PO Box 89, Teulon MB R0C 3B0; Natal (South Africa)'81; Staff, Teulon/Hunter Memorial Hospital; (204)886-2433

PILLAY, Shunmoogam W; 116-8434 120 St, Surrey BC V3W 7S2; RCS (Ireland)'68; LRCP; LRCS; LM(Ire.); FRCPC; IntMed (Dementia); GeriatricMed. Staff Geriatrics, Surrey Memorial Hospital; Clinical Asst Prof Med, University of British Columbia; Langs: Afrikaans; (604)597-0941; willie.pillay@fraserhealth.ca.

PILLAY, Thevanisha; Victoria Gen Hosp, 1 Hospital Way, Victoria BC V8Z 6R5; S.Africa (South Africa)'98; MB ChB; FRCPC; Peds. Staff, Victoria General Hospital; (250)727-4212

PILLAY, Vinesh; Regina Qu'Appelle HR-Regina, 1440 14th Ave, Regina SK S4P 0W5; Staff, Regina General Hospital; (306)525-8612; Fax. (306)525-8186.

PILLAY, Yagan; Associate Med Clinic, 400-20 14th St W, Prince Albert SK S6V 3K8; Manipal (India)'96; BSc; MB BS; (306)953-1653; Fax. (306)764-3091.

PILLISCH, Mary L; Durham Med Clinic, 368 College St N, Durham ON N0G 1R0; Man'87; CCFP; Staff, South Bruce Grey Health Centre - Durham Site; (519)369-2510; Fax. (519)369-3831.

PILLON, Sylvia M; London HSC-Victoria Campus, PO Box 5010 Stn B 800 Commissioners Rd E, London ON N6A 5W9; Wes'10; CCFP; Staff, London Health Sciences Centre - Victoria Campus; (519)685-8500

PILON, Claude; CHUM-Hotel-Dieu, 3840 rue Saint-Urbain, Montreal QC H2W 1T8; Mon'85; FRCPC; IntMed (Interventional Cardiology); Cardiol. Staff, Centre Hospitalier l'Université de Montréal (CHUM) - Hôtel-Dieu; adj Prof, Universite de Montreal; Langs: English; (514)890-8000; Fax. (514)412-7212.

PILON, Danielle; CHUS-Hop Fleurimont, 3001 12e av N, Sherbrooke QC J1H 5N4; Mon'93; FRCPC; IntMed (Clinical Pharmacology). Staff, Centre Hospitalier Universitaire de Sherbrooke-Hopital Fleurimont; (819)346-1110 x14948

PILON, Dominique; CLSC Bordeaux-Cartierville, 11822 av du Bois-de-Boulogne, Montreal QC H3M 2X6; Mon'96; CCFP; FCFP; Staff, Hôpital du Sacre-Coeur de Montréal; Universite de Montreal; (514)331-2572; Fax. (514)331-0137.

PILON, Edward W; St Joseph's Health Centre, 30 The Queensway, Toronto ON M6R 1B5; Tor'95; CCFP; CCFP(E.M.); Staff Phys, EmergMed, St Joseph's Health Centre; (416)530-6003

PILON, Jacques; CSSSG-Hop de Gatineau, CP 2000 Succ Bureau-Chef 909 boul de la Verendrye O, Gatineau QC J8P 7H2; Mon'86; CCFP; Staff, Hôpital de Gatineau; (819)561-8100

PILON, Jean-Claude; Pavillon Rosemont, 5689 boul Rosemont, Montreal QC H1T 2H1; Mon'82; FRCPC; Psy. Staff, Hopital Maisonneuve-Rosemont; (514)252-3914; Fax. (514)252-3810.

PILON, Josee L; NCR Occupational Health Clinic, PL 3712M-171 Slater St, Ottawa ON K1A 0K9; Ott'92; CCFP; FCFP; Med Officer, Occupational Health National Capital Region; Langs: English; French; (613)946-6583; Fax. (613)990-9397.

PILON, Liette; Clinique Med Monk, 6023 boul Monk, Montreal QC H4E 3H5; Mon'78; (514)761-5527

PILON, Line; CSSS du Nord de Lanaudière, 1000 boul Sainte-Anne, St-Charles-Brromee QC J6E 6J2; Mon'98; CSPQ; FRCPC; AnatPath. Pathologist, Centre Hospitalier Régional de Lanaudière.

PILON, Luc; CHUM-Hop Notre-Dame, 1560 rue Sherbrooke E, Montreal QC H2L 4M1; Mon'70; FRCSC; OrthSurg. Staff, Centre Hospitalier l'Université de Montréal (CHUM) - Hôpital Notre-Dame; (514)890-8000 x24444

PILON, M M Louise; Income Security Program Branch, 333 North River Rd, Ottawa ON K1A 0L1; Ott'74; (613)952-2166

PILON, Maurice M; GMF le Carrefour de Laval, 200-3030 boul Le Carrefour, Laval QC H7T 2P5; Ott'73; (450)686-8899; Fax. (450)686-7466.

PILON, Michel; CLSC-CHSLD Meilleur, 410 boul de l'Ange-Gardien, L'Assomption QC J5W 1S7; Mon'76; Assoc Staff Emerg, Centre Hospitalier Pierre le Gardeur; (450)589-2101

PILON, Normand; Externe Psychiatrique, 310-175 av Stillview, Pointe-Claire QC H9R 4S3; Mon'82; FRCPC; Psy. Staff, Lakeshore General Hospital - Pointe Claire; (514)630-2010

PILON, Pierre A; Dir de la Sante Publique-Mtl, 1301 rue Sherbrooke E, Montreal QC H2L 1M3; Mon'86; (514)528-2400 x3800; Fax. (514)528-2452; ppilon@santepub-mtl.qc.ca.

PILON, Pierre; Clinique Med de Saint-Jovite, CP 19069 Csp Place Ouimet 992 rue de Saint-Jovite, Mont-Tremblant QC J8E 3C1; Mon'70; (819)425-2728; Fax. (819)425-8012.

PILON, Raynald; Arcelor Mittal Mines Canada, GD 556 389 Rte, Fermont QC G0G 1J0; Mon'76; (418)287-4700

PILON, Richard A; Clin de Med Familiale de Hull, 202-15 boul Montclair, Gatineau QC J8Y 2E2; Ott'73; Staff, Hull Hospital; (819)777-2752; Fax. (819)777-2269.

PILON, Richard; Clinique Med le Gardeurois, 130-155 boul Lacombe, Repentigny QC J5Z 3C4; Mon'84; (450)582-5546; Fax. (450)582-2718.

PILORGE, Robert P; 302-5450 ch de la Cote-des-Nei, Montreal QC H3T 1Y6; Paris (France)'68; DABOG; CSPQ; ObstGyn (Echography). Staff, St Mary's Hospital Centre; adj Prof, McGill University; Langs: English; Spanish; German; (514)739-7555; Fax. (514)739-5599.

PILOT, Lorne R; Kenderdine Med Clinic, 110-1804 McOrmand Dr, Saskatoon SK S7S 0A6; Sask'76; Staff, Saskatoon City Hospital; Staff, Royal University Hospital; Staff, St Paul's Hospital (Grey Nuns) of Saskatoon; (306)934-6606; Fax. (306)955-3180.

PILOTE, Louise; MUHC-Montreal Gen Hosp, 1650 av Cedar, Montreal QC H3G 1A4; McG'85; MMed; MPH; FRCPC; IntMed (Epidemiology). Dir Int Med, McGill University Health Centre - Montreal General Campus; Langs: English; (514)934-1934 x44722; louise.pilote@mcgill.ca.

PILOTE, Nathalie; Hop Charles LeMoyne, 3120 boul Taschereau, Greenfield Park QC J4V 2H1; Mon'92; CCFP; Staff, Hopital Charles LeMoyne; (450)466-5000

PILOTE, Nicholas; 330 av Universite, Moncton NB E1C 2Z3; Sher'98; FRCPC; DiagRad. Staff, Dr Georges-L-Dumont University Hospital Centre; Langs: English; Bilingual(English/French); (506)862-4000 x4116

PILOTTE, Marie-Natacha; Clinique A L H P, 114-475 boul Talbot, Chicoutimi QC G7H 4A3; Laval'97; FRCSC; GenSurg. (418)549-5987

PILOTTE, Michele; CSSS Pierre Boucher, 1333 boul Jacques-Cartier E, Longueuil QC J4M 2A5; Mon'95; Emerg Med, Centre Hospitalier Pierre Boucher; Emergency Med, Centre Hospitalier Regional de Trois-Rivieres; Staff EmergMed, Hôpital Brome-Missisquoi-Perkins; (450)468-8111

PIM, Carolyn P; 100 Constellation Cres, Ottawa ON K2G 6J8; Cal'83; BSc; FRCPC; CommunMed; Public Health & Preventive Med. Staff, Tom Baker Cancer Centre; (613)580-6744

PIMLOTT, Nicholas J G; Women's College Fam Health Tea, 60 Grosvenor St, Toronto ON M5S 1B6; Tor'91; BSc(Hon); CCFP; Ac Staff, Women's College Hospital; Assoc Editor, College Of Family Physicians Of Canada-Ontario; Assoc Prof Family & Community Med, University of Toronto; (416)323-6065; nick.pimlott@utoronto.ca.

PIMM, Jeff R; Red Deer Reg Hosp Centre, PO Box 5030 Stn Postal Box Ctr SC3300 H10-3942 50A Ave, Red Deer AB T4N 6R2; Alb'96; FRCPC; IntMed. Staff, Red Deer Regional Hospital Centre; (403)356-4201; Fax. (403)358-4342.

PIMSTONE, Simon N; Xenon Genetics Inc, 200-3650 Gilmore Way, Burnaby BC V5G 4W8; Cape Town (South Africa)'91; MB ChB; PhD; FRCPC; IntMed (Cardiology). Pres. & C.E.O., Xenon Genetics Inc.; (604)484-3300 x602; Fax. (604)484-3450; spimstone@xenon-pharma.com.

PINARD, Anne-Marie; CHUQ-Ctr Hosp Univ Laval, 2705 boul Laurier, Quebec QC G1V 4G2; Mon'96; CSPQ; FRCPC; Anes. Staff, Centre Hospitalier Universitaire de Quebec-CHUL; (418)656-4141

PINARD, Georges-F.; Pavillon Rosemont, C 5309-5689 boul Rosemont, Montreal QC H1T 2H1; Mon'86; LMCC; FRCPC; Psy (Legal Psychiatry). Ac Staff, Hopital Louis-H Lafontaine; Universite de Montreal; (514)252-3400 x4765; Fax. (514)252-3810.

PINARD, Josiane; CSSS de l'Hématite, GD 1 rue de l'Aquilon, Fermont QC G0G 1J0; Sher'10; Staff, CLSC de l'Hématite; (418)287-5461

PINARD, Julie; CSSS de la Haute-Yamaska, 205 boul Leclerc O, Granby QC J2G 1T7; Laval'01; FRCPC; Psy. Staff, Centre Hospitalier de Granby; Staff, CSSS de la Baie-des-Chaleurs; (450)375-8000

PINARD, Louis G; CHUS-Hop Fleurimont, 3001 12e av, Sherbrooke QC J1H 5N4; Sher'08; CCFP; CCFP(E.M.); Staff, Centre Hospitalier Universitaire de Sherbrooke-Hopital Fleurimont; (819)346-1110

PINARD, Louis; MUHC-Montreal Gen Hosp, B6 152-1650 av Cedar, Montreal QC H3G 1A4; Mon'80; FRCPC; Psy. Staff, McGill University Health Centre - Montreal General Campus; (514)934-8010; Fax. (514)934-8237.

PINARD, Marie-Claude; CLSC Vallee de la Batiscan, RR 4 90 Rte Riviere-a-Veillette, Ste-Genev-D-Batisc QC G0X 2R0; Sher'89; (418)362-2728; Fax. (418)362-3130.

PINARD, Philippe; Renfrew Med Group, 510 Raglan St, Renfrew ON K7V 1P5; Sher'08; CCFP; (613)433-5712; Fax. (613)433-5727.

PINARD-SAINT-PIERRE, Vanessa; Ctr Hosp Anna-Laberge, 200 boul Brisebois, Chateauguay QC J6K 4W8; Sher'01; CCFP; CCFP(E.M.); Staff, Hôpital Anna-Laberge; (450)699-2425

PINARD-D'AMOUR, Catherine A; Clinique Neuro Rive-Sud, 250-4896 boul Taschereau, Greenfield Park QC J4V 2J2; Sher'04; FRCPC; Neur. (450)672-1931; Fax. (450)672-3308.

PINAULT, France; GMF Quatre-Bourgeois, 300-979 av de Bourgogne, Quebec QC G1W 2L4; Laval'94; Staff Emerg, Jeffery Hale Hospital-Saint Brigid's; Langs: Bilingual(English/French); (418)653-4050; Fax. (418)653-4475.

PINAULT, Jean-Jacques; Ctr Obstetrique et Gynecologie, 4250 av 1Re, Quebec QC G1H 2S5; Poitiers (France)'69; ObstGyn (Echography). (418)654-0555; Fax. (418)654-1898.

PINAULT, Marie; Clinique Med du Faubourg, 145-1160 boul Saint-Joseph, Gatineau QC J8Z 1T3; Sher'90; Staff, Hôpital de Gatineau; Langs: Spanish; English; (819)595-1991; Fax. (819)595-0486.

PINCHBECK, Melanie L; 408-8708 155 St NW, Edmonton AB T5R 1W2; Alb'07; Gastroent; IntMed. (780)930-1915

PINCHUK, Brian M; North York Med Arts Bldg, 336-1333 Sheppard Ave E, North York ON M2J 1V1; McG'03; FRCSC; GenSurg (Surgical Oncology). (416)492-1661

PINCHUK, David M; Victoria Gen Hosp, 2340 Pembina Hwy, Winnipeg MB R3T 2E8; Man'83; CCFP; CCFP(E.M.); FCFP; Ac Staff Emerg Med, Victoria General Hospital; (204)269-3570

PINCOCK, Robert J; Belleville Queen's U Fam Med, 104-145 Station St, Belleville ON K8N 2S9; Man'09; CCFP; (613)771-1910; Fax. (613)771-0689.

PINDER, Lesley J; F-21 River St, St Stephen NB E3L 3H2; Tor'76; MSc; Staff, Charlotte County Hospital; (506)466-4600; Fax. (506)465-8110.

PINDER, Michael; The Pinder Clinic, PO Box 2560 Stn Main, The Pas MB R9A 1M3; Manchester (England)'65; MB ChB; FRCS(Ed); Head, The Pas Health Complex, Surg.; Assoc Prof, University of Manitoba; (204)623-5443; Fax. (204)623-4648.

PINE, William E; Hamilton HS-General Site, 237 Barton St E, Hamilton ON L8L 2X2; McM'77; FRCPC; Anes. Staff, Hamilton Health Sciences Centre - Hamilton General Hospital; (905)527-0271

PINEAU, Christian A; MUHC-Montreal Gen Hosp, A6 163-1650 av Cedar, Montreal QC H3G 1A4; McG'95; CSPQ; BSc; FRCPC; IntMed; Rheum. Consultant, McGill University Health Centre - Montreal General Campus; Langs: English; French; (514)934-8037; Fax. (514)934-8402; christian.pineau@muhc.mcgill.ca.

PINEAU, F Edwin; PO Box 77, North Rustico PE C0A 1X0; Dal'81; (902)621-3050

PINEAU, Gilles; 10.083-2021 av Union, Montreal QC H3A 2S9; Mon'72; Consultant, Centre Hospitalier l'Université de Montréal (CHUM) - Hôtel-Dieu; (514)864-9124

PINEAU, Linda A; Belmont Prof Centre, 408-564 Belmont Ave W, Kitchener ON N2M 5N6; Qns'90; BA; FRCPC; Peds (Consultant Pediatrics). Dir Paediatric Cystic Fibrosis, Grand River Hospital - Kitchener/Waterloo Health Centre; (519)570-1492; Fax. (519)570-3387.

PINEAU, Michel; Ctr de Sante Basse Cote Nord, CP 130 1070 boul Dr Camille Marcou, Lourdes-D-Bl-Sabl QC G0G 1W0; Laval'97; CCFP; Staff, CSSS de la Basse Côté-Nord; Langs: English; French; (418)461-2144

PINEAU, Raymonde; Centre de Sante Publique, 2400 av d'Estimauville, Quebec QC G1E 7G9; Laval'76; Assoc Staff, Centre Hospitalier Affilié Universitaire de Québec - Hôpital du St-Sacrement; Ac Staff, Centre Hospitalier Universitaire de Quebec-CHUL; (418)666-7000 x270; Fax. (418)666-2776; raymonde.pineau@ssss.gouv.qc.ca.

PINEAU, Rene; Inst U en Sante Mentale de QC, 2601 ch de la Canardiere, Quebec QC G1J 2G3; Laval'72; Staff, Institut Universitaire Sante; (418)663-5321; Fax. (418)661-6891.

PINEAU, Robert W; Sudbury Reg Hosp-Laurentian, 41 Ramsey Lake Rd, Sudbury ON P3E 5J1; McM'02; CCFP; CCFP(E.M.); Staff, Health Sciences North-Laurentian Site; (705)675-4790

PINEAULT, Claude; CSSS de Lac-Saint Jean-Est, CP 1300 Succ Bureau-Chef 300 boul Champlain S, Alma QC G8B 5W3; Mon'88; CSPQ; FRCPC; DiagRad. Staff, CSSS de Lac-Saint Jean-Est; (418)669-2000 x6651; Fax. (418)668-9690.

PINEAULT, Daniel; Centre Med Fusion, 200-2035 av Sainte-Anne, Saint-Hyacinthe QC J2S 5H3; Mon'80; assoc Staff, Centre Hospitalier Honore-Mercier; Staff Admin, Pavillon Boisjoly; (450)773-6023; Fax. (450)773-5915.

PINEAULT, Jacinthe; Centre Hosp Honore-Mercier, 2750 boul Laframboise, Saint-Hyacinthe QC J2S 4Y8; Sher'87; FRCPC; Psy. Staff, Centre Hospitalier Honore-Mercier; (450)771-3333; Fax. (450)771-3273.

PINEAULT, Raynald; Dir de la Sante Publique-Mtl, 1301 rue Sherbrooke E, Montreal QC H2L 1M3; Laval'65; PhD; CSPQ; FRCPC; CommunMed. Staff, Centre Hospitalier l'Université de Montréal (CHUM) - Hôtel-Dieu; Staff, Hopital Maisonneuve-Rosemont; Prof, Universite de Montreal; (514)528-2400; Fax. (514)528-2512; rpineaul@santepub-mtl.qc.ca.

PINEDA, Maria D; Regina Qu'Appelle HR-Regina, 1440 14th Ave, Regina SK S4P 0W5; Wes'10; CCFP; Staff, Regina General Hospital; (306)766-1411; Fax. (306)766-4833.

PINEDA-SELVA, Ernesto; 70-3915 51 St SW, Calgary AB T3E 6N1; (Mexico)'69; AB; FAAP; Staff, Alberta Children's Hospital; Langs: Spanish; (403)229-2273; Fax. (403)246-9688.

PINEL-TREMBLAY, Diane; Clinique Med St-Redempteur, 266 rue Thibault, Matane QC G4W 2V9; Laval'77; ac Staff, Centre Hospitalier de Matane; (418)562-6133; Fax. (418)562-6947.

PINERO-MEDINA, Francisco; CHUS-Hop Hotel-Dieu, 580 rue Bowen S, Sherbrooke QC J1G 2E8; Madrid (Spain)'63; LMCC; Psy (P.Q.) (General & Forensic Psychiatry). Staff, Centre Hospitalier Universitaire de Sherbrooke-Hôpital Hôtel-Dieu; Clin Assoc Prof, Universite de Sherbrooke; Langs: Spanish; Bilingual(English/French); (819)346-1110 x25519; Fax. (819)564-0023; fjpinero@hotmail.com.

PINETTE, Gilles D; 2-875 Dakota St, Winnipeg MB R2M 5S5; Man'97; CCFP; FCFP; Assoc Dir Family Med/Lecturer, University of Manitoba; pinette@shaw.ca.

PING, Francis C; Lions Gate Hosp, 231 15th St E, North Vancouver BC V7L 2L7; Dublin (Ireland)'70; Anes. Staff Anes, Lions Gate Hospital; (604)984-5709; Fax. (604)984-5729.

PINHAS, Leora; The Hosp for Sick Children, 555 University Ave, Toronto ON M5G 1X8; Ott'89; FRCPC; Psy (Child & Adolescent Psychiatry). Staff, The Hospital For Sick Children; (416)813-7195

PINHO, Genevieve; Clinique Med Fleur-de-Lys, 8 rue du Terminus E, Rouyn-Noranda QC J9X 3B4; Sher'03; Staff, Centre Hospitalier Rouyn-Noranda; Langs: Bilingual(French/English); (819)764-6185; Fax. (819)762-6079.

PINILLA, J Vicente; Markham College Med Clinic, 206-474 College St, Toronto ON M6G 1A4; (Colombia)'60; Court Staff Gen Practice, Toronto Western Hospital - University Health Network; Langs: Spanish; Portuguese; (416)925-7434; Fax. (416)925-2368.

PINILLA, James F E; Tom Baker Cancer Centre, 1331 29 St NW, Calgary AB T2N 4N2; Sask'92; Staff, Tom Baker Cancer Centre; (403)521-3164; Fax. (403)270-8407.

PINKERTON, David H; Kingston Family Health Team, 500A Gardiners Rd, Kingston ON K7M 7W9; Qns'89; CCFP; FCFP; Assoc Staff, Kingston General Hospital; Assoc Staff Family Med, Hotel-Dieu Hospital; (613)389-5974; Fax. (613)389-0804; dpinkerton@kfhn.net.

PINKHASIK, Paul; Richmond Medical Spa Club, 6611 No. 2 Rd, Richmond BC V7C 3L5; UBC'86; Ac Staff, Richmond Hospital; (604)284-5501; Fax. (604)278-9529.

PINKSEN, Donald A; Guelph Comm Health Centre, 1-176 Wyndham St N, Guelph ON N1H 8N9; Mem'77; CCFP; FCFP; Court Staff, Guelph General Hospital; (519)821-6638; Fax. (519)821-5834; dpinksen@guelphchc.ca.

PINNEY, Stephen J; St Paul's Hosp, 323-1081 Burrard St, Vancouver BC V6Z 1Y6; McG'91; FRCSC; OrthSurg. Staff, Providence Health Care - St Paul's Hospital; (604)682-2344

PINNICK, Suzy A O; St Boniface Gen Hosp, A8024-409 Tache Ave, Winnipeg MB R2H 2A6; Staff, St Boniface General Hospital; (204)233-8563

PINNIGER, Gregory W; Stonewall Med Group, 589 3rd Ave S, Stonewall MB R0C 2Z0; Man'92; Chief Medical Staff, Stonewall & District Health Centre; (204)467-5509; Fax. (204)467-5576.

PINSK, Maury N; Edmonton Clinic Health Academy, 4 555-11405 87 Ave NW, Edmonton AB T6G 1C9; Tor'97; FRCPC; Peds; Nephrol. Staff, University of Alberta Hospital; Staff, Edmonton Clinic Health Academy; (780)248-5560

PINSKY, Merrille F; SMBD Jewish Gen Hosp, 3755 ch Cote-Sainte-Catherine, Montreal QC H3T 1E2; Philadelphia(PA)(USA)'64; CSPQ; FRCPC; DiagRad. Staff, Sir Mortimer B Davis Jewish General; Asst Prof DiagRad, McGill University; (514)340-8222; Fax. (514)340-7907; mpinsky@rad.jgh.mcgill.ca.

PINSONNEAULT, Celine; CSSS de Saint-Jerome, 290 rue de Montigny, Saint-Jerome QC J7Z 5T3; Sher'91; CSPQ; FRCPC; Anes (Thoracic Anesthesia). Staff, Hôtel-Dieu de Saint-Jérôme; (450)431-8200 x8599; kinase@videotron.ca.

PINSONNEAULT, Linda; AETMIS, 10.083-2021 av Union, Montreal QC H3A 2S9; Sher'86; CSPQ; FRCPC; CommunMed (Community Health). Staff, Hopital Charles LeMoyne; Langs: English; l.pinsonneault@rrsss16.gouv.qc.ca.

PINSONNEAULT, Monique; CSSS Pierre Boucher, 1333 boul Jacques-Cartier E, Longueuil QC J4M 2A5; Mon'94; FRCPC; IntMed; Respir. Specialist Lung, Centre Hospitalier Pierre Boucher; Specialist Lung, Centre Hospitalier Honore-Mercier; Langs: English; (450)468-8111; Fax. (450)468-8269.

PINSONNEAULT, Odette; CHUS-Hop Fleurimont, 3001 12e av N, Sherbrooke QC J1H 5N4; Sher'77; FRCSC; ObstGyn. Ac Staff, Centre Hospitalier Universitaire de Sherbrooke-Hopital Fleurimont; (819)346-1110; odette.pinsonneault@usherbrooke.ca.

PINSONNEAULT, Troy G; 1111 Fairview Rd, Penticton BC V2A 5Z3; Alb'94; FRCSC; OrthSurg. (250)492-3700; mcpinsonneault@hotmail.com.

PINTEA, Dana; Caroline Family Hlth Team-CMG, 15-3305 Harvester Rd, Burlington ON L7N 3N2; Bucharest (Romania)'87; CCFP; Staff, Joseph Brant Memorial Hospital; Langs: Romanian; French; (905)632-8007; Fax. (905)632-0375.

PINTER, Arnold; St Michael's Hosp, 30 Bond St, Toronto ON M5B 1W8; (Hungary)'91; Staff Electrophysiologist, St Michael's Hospital; Asst Prof Med, University of Toronto; (416)864-5431; pinter@smh.toronto.on.ca.

PINTHUS, Jehonathan H; Hamilton HS-Juravinski Site, 711 Concession St, Hamilton ON L8V 1C3; Hebrew (Israel)'95; Staff, Hamilton Health Sciences Centre-Juravinski Site; (905)387-9495 x64902

PINTIN-QUEZADA, Julio; Markham Professional Centre, 102-2265 Pembina Hwy, Winnipeg MB R3T 5J3; (El Salvador)'82; FACS; FRCSC; GenSurg. Staff, Victoria General Hospital; Langs: Spanish; (204)261-5513; Fax. (204)261-5605.

PINTO, Andrew; Health Centre at 410, 410 Sherbourne St, Toronto ON M4X 1K2; Tor'06; FRCPC; Public Health & Preventive Med;CCFP; (416)867-3728; Fax. (416)867-3726.

PINTO, Angelo; The Courtyards of Caledon, L8-18 King St E, Bolton ON L7E 1E8; Tor'88; BSc; DOHS; Staff, William Osler Health System - Etobicoke General Hospital; Langs: Italian; (905)857-9906; Fax. (905)857-9905.

PINTO, Anthony J; 203-360 College St, Toronto ON M5T 1S6; Bombay (India)'70; Ac Staff, St Joseph's Health Centre; (416)929-0615; Fax. (416)929-0615.

PINTO, Antonio; CLSC Villeray, 1425 rue Jarry E, Montreal QC H2E 1A7; Naples (Italy)'82; Staff, Sir Mortimer B Davis Jewish General; Langs: Italian; (514)376-4141; Fax. (514)376-7650.

PINTO, Artur C F; The Doctor's Office, 80 Thickson Rd S, Whitby ON L1N 7T2; (Portugal)'90; CCFP; (905)668-6448

PINTO, Barbara B; Meadowlands & Family Hlth Ctre, 5-35 Stonechurch Rd, Ancaster ON L9K 1S5; Karachi (Pakistan)'67; MB BS; FRCPC; Peds. Ac Staff, St Joseph's Healthcare - Charlton Campus; Affil. Member, McMaster University; (905)648-8999; Fax. (905)648-8969.

PINTO, Christopher; Islington Med Clinic, 800-1243 Islington Ave, Etobicoke ON M8X 1Y9; Tor'74; Assoc Staff, Humber River Regional Hospital - Church Street Site; (416)767-2525; Fax. (416)234-9128.

PINTO, Ivette R; 203-360 College St, Toronto ON M5T 1S6; Bombay (India)'71; Ac Staff, St Joseph's Health Centre; (416)929-0615

PINTO, Joyce F; Creditview Medical, B 14-1240 Eglinton Ave W, Mississauga ON L5V 1N3; Bombay (India)'92; CCFP; (905)567-4622

PINTO, Lucina M; 201-1263 St Clair Ave W, Toronto ON M6E 1B8; Bombay (India)'79; MB BS; Ac Staff, St Joseph's Health Centre; Langs: Italian; Portuguese; (416)653-3490; Fax. (416)653-2604.

PINTO, Martin; 808-367 Geneva St, St Catharines ON L2N 5S8; Howard University(USA)'97; Asst Clin Prof, Fam Med, McMaster University; pintomar66@yahoo.com

PINTO, Michael A; Queen-Lynch Med Centre, 209A-157 Queen St E, Brampton ON L6W 3X4; Bangalore (India)'79; FRCPC; IntMed; Rheum. (905)457-2877; Fax. (905)457-6259.

PINTO, Natasha; Georgian Bay Gen Hosp, PO Box 760 Stn Main 1112 St Andrews Dr, Midland ON L4R 4P4; Tor'09; CCFP; Staff, Georgian Bay General Hospital - Midland; (705)526-1300

PINTO, Nicholas; Ctr Hosp de Verdun, 4000 boul Lasalle, Verdun QC H4G 2A3; Laval'10; CCFP; Staff, Centre Hospitalier de Verdun; (514)765-7325

PINTO, Robin; 1333 Neilson Rd, Scarborough ON M1B 4Y9; Wes'09; CCFP; (416)291-7719

PINTO, Sarah R; 207-840 Coxwell Ave, East York ON M4C 5T2; Tor'03; FRCPC; Cardiol; IntMed. Staff, St Michael's Hospital; (416)463-1864

PINTO, Sebastian R; Peterborough Reg HC-Hospital, 1 Hospital Dr, Peterborough ON K9J 7C6; Bombay (India)'80; MB BS; FRCPC; Anes. Chief Anes, Peterborough Regional Health Centre - Hospital Drive; (705)876-5038

PINTO, Tanya R; Scarborough Hosp-General Div, 3050 Lawrence Ave E, Scarborough ON M1P 2V5; Qns'05; FRCPC; Psy. Staff, The Scarborough Hospital - General Campus; (416)431-8135

PINTO, Teresa; IWK Health Centre, PO Box 9700 Rpo CSC 5850-5890 University Ave, Halifax NS B3K 6R8; McG'02; FRCPC; Peds; Endocrin&Metab. Staff, IWK Health Centre; (902)470-8707; Fax. (902)470-7264.

PINTO, Victoria J M; 202-631 Queenston Rd, Hamilton ON L8K 6R5; Kasturba (India)'83; CCFP; (905)560-4600; Fax. (905)560-2644.

PINTO-ROJAS, Alfredo; Alberta Children's Hosp, 2888 Shaganappi Trail NW, Calgary AB T3B 6A8; Del Rosario (Colombia)'77; MB BS; FRCPC; AnatPath. Staff, Alberta Children's Hospital; (403)955-7983; Fax. (403)955-2321.

PINZON, Jorge L; 2888 Shaganappi Trail NW, Calgary AB T3B 6A8; (Colombia)'86; ABPeds; CRCP; FRCPC; Peds (Adolescent Medicine). Staff Adolescent Med, Alberta Children's Hospital; Clin Assoc Prof Peds, University of Calgary; Langs: Spanish; (403)955-7636; Fax. (403)955-7649; jorge.pinzon@albertahealthservices.ca.

PIO, Anton; Killarney Med Centre, PO Box 1690, Killarney MB R0K 1G0; Stellenbosch (South Africa)'80; CCFP.

PION, Kim; CSSS de Chicoutimi, 305 rue Saint-Vallier, Chicoutimi QC G7H 5H6; Sher'98; CCFP; CCFP(E.M.); Staff, Complexe hospitalier de la Sagamie; (418)541-1000

PIPE, Andrew L; Univ of Ottawa Heart Institute, 40 Ruskin St, Ottawa ON K1Y 4W7; Qns'74; LLD; DSc; FACSM; MCFP; Chief Div of Prevention & Rehabilitation, University of Ottawa Heart Institute; Prof, University of Ottawa; (613)761-4756; Fax. (613)729-8290; apipe@ottawaheart.ca.

PIPER, Dominique; Sunnybrook Hlth Sciences Ctre, HG 39-2075 Bayview Ave, Toronto ON M4N 3M5; Mon'09; CCFP; Staff, Sunnybrook Health Sciences Centre; (416)480-6100

PIPER, Hannah G; The Hosp for Sick Children, 555 University Ave, Toronto ON M5G 1X8; Boston (USA)'02; FRCSC; GenSurg (Pediatric Surgery). Staff, The Hospital For Sick Children; (416)813-1500

PIPER, Michael S; 102-65 Richmond St, New Westminster BC V3L 5P5; UBC'68; MSc; FAAOS; FACS; FRCSC; OrthSurg (Arthroplasty). Ac Staff, Royal Columbian Hospital; Clin Prof, University of British Columbia; (604)525-7666; Fax. (604)525-4006.

PIPHER, Bruce E; 309-1664 Richter St, Kelowna BC V1Y 8N3; Tor'86; FRCPC; Psy. (250)763-4899; Fax. (250)763-4809.

PIPPI-SALLE, Joao L P; The Hosp for Sick Children, M299-555 University Ave, Toronto ON M5G 1X8; Rio Grande (Brazil)'72; FRCSC; Urol (P.Q.). Div Head Urol, The Hospital For Sick Children; Langs: French; Portuguese; Spanish; (416)813-6460; Fax. (416)813-6461; pippi.salle@sickkids.ca.

PIPPY, Christine C; Saint John Reg Hosp, PO Box 2100 Stn Main 400 University Ave, Saint John NB E2L 4L2; Dal'96; MSc; FRCPC; IntMed; Nephrol. Staff, Saint John Regional Hospital; (506)648-6843; Fax. (506)648-7796; christine.pippy@rvh.nb.ca.

PIQUET-GAUTHIER, Blandine; Direction de la Sante Publique, 210-1000 rue Labelle, Saint-Jerome QC J7Z 5N6; Lyon (France)'75; CSPQ; FRCPC; CommunMed (Environmental Health). Staff, Hôtel-Dieu de Saint-Jérôme; (450)436-8622; Fax. (450)436-1761; blandine_piquet-gauthier@ssss.gouv.qc.ca.

PIQUETTE, Dominique; Sunnybrook Hlth Sciences Ctre, D 108-2075 Bayview Ave, Toronto ON M4N 3M5; Mon'00; FRCPC; IntMed; Critical Care Medicine. Staff, Sunnybrook Health Sciences Centre; (416)480-6100

PIRAN, Sanaz; Univ Hlth Network-Toronto Gen, 200 Elizabeth St, Toronto ON M5G 2C4; Ott'04; FRCPC; IntMed; Cardiol. Staff, Toronto General Hospital - UHN; (416)340-4800

PIRANI, Aminmohamed A; Westminster Med Bldg, B1-625 Fifth Ave, New Westminster BC V3M 1X4; Makerere (Uganda)'70; MB ChB; DiagRad. Med Dir, C M L Health Care; (604)522-6818

PIRANI, Asif; 199 Avenue Rd, Toronto ON M5R 2J3; Tor'06; FRCSC; PlasSurg. (416)925-7337

PIRANI, Mohamedraza J K; Joseph Brant Mem Hosp, 1230 North Shore Blvd E, Burlington ON L7S 1W7; (Ireland)'75; FRCPC; DiagRad. Staff, Joseph Brant Memorial Hospital; (905)632-3737

PIRANI, Shafique P; Keary Med Centre, 205-245 Columbia St E, New Westminster BC V3L 3W4; London (England)'82; MB BS; ABS; FAAOS; FRCSC; OrthSurg (Pediatric Orthopedic Surgery). Staff OrthSurg, Royal Columbian Hospital; Staff, BC Children's Hospital; Prof, University of British Columbia; (604)522-2332; Fax. (604)522-7686.

PIRBHAI, Adnan K; 1655 Kilborn Ave, Ottawa ON K1H 6M7; Wes'05; FRCSC; Ophth. (613)739-5437

PIRBHAI, Kalim H; Glenridge Med Bldg, 203-1 Belton Blvd, St Catharines ON L2T 3Y4; Makerere (Uganda)'70; DCH(Eng); DABPed; FRCPC; Peds (Allergy). (905)682-5611

PIRBHAI, Nureen; City Square Family Physicians, 116-555 12th Ave W, Vancouver BC V5Z 3X7; Cal'09; CCFP; (604)879-3917

PIRES, Arthur E; CHUQ-Hotel-Dieu de Quebec, 11 Cote du Palais, Quebec QC G1R 2J6; Coimbra (Portugal)'66; DCPsy; CRCP; CSPQ; MRCPsy; Psy. Staff, Centre Hospitalier Universitaire de Québec (CHUQ) - Siege Social; Prof Psy, Université Laval; Langs: French; Portuguese; (418)691-5151 x15808; artur_pires@hotmail.com.

PIRES, Jose M; 500 Old St. Patrick St, Ottawa ON K1N 9G4; McG'95; LMCC; DABS; FRCSC; GenSurg (Laparoscopy). Staff, Montfort Hospital; Langs: Portuguese; English; (613)241-3013; Fax. (613)241-4482.

PIRES, Serena; 2689 Broadway W, Vancouver BC V6K 2G2; UBC'04; CCFP; (604)731-9187

PIRIE, Jonathan R; The Hosp for Sick Children, 555 University Ave, Toronto ON M5G 1X8; UBC'88; BSc; MEd; FRCPC; Peds (Pediatric Emergency Medicine). Staff, The Hospital For Sick Children; Assoc Prof Peds, University of Toronto; (416)813-5277; Fax. (416)813-5043.

PIRLET, Martine J; CHUS-Hop Fleurimont, 3001 12e av N, Sherbrooke QC J1H 5N4; Liege (Belgium)'78; CSPQ; Anes (P.Q.) (Anesthesia & Reanimation). Staff, Centre Hospitalier Universitaire de Sherbrooke-Hopital Fleurimont; (819)346-1110 x14403; Fax. (819)820-6413; martine.pirlet@usherbrooke.ca.

PIRLOG, Tiberiu; Lakeshore Gen Hosp, 160 av Stillview, Pointe-Claire QC H9R 2Y2; (Romania)'96; CCFP; Staff, Lakeshore General Hospital - Pointe Claire; (514)630-2225

PIRLOT, Tyler S; Alberta Children's Hosp, 2888 Shaganappi Trail NW, Calgary AB T3B 6A8; Sask'00; FRCPC; Psy (Child Psychiatry). Staff, Alberta Children's Hospital; Clin Lecturer, University of Calgary; (403)955-7610; tyler.pirlot@calgaryhealthregion.ca.

PIROUZMAND, Farhad; Sunnybrook Hlth Sciences Ctre, A131-2075 Bayview Ave, Toronto ON M4N 3M5; Tehran (Iran)'90; FRCSC; Neursurg. Staff, Sunnybrook Health Sciences Centre; (416)480-5263; Fax. (416)480-6085.

PIRVU, Adriana M; Boissevain Health Centre, PO Box 899 305 Mill Rd, Boissevain MB R0K 0E0; Bucharest (Romania)'90; CCFP; Fam Med, Boissevain Health Centre; (204)534-3777

PIRWANY, Imran R; Med Arts Center, 103-770 6 St SW, Medicine Hat AB T1A 4J6; (Pakistan)'86; MB BS; (403)488-7799; Fax. (403)488-7797; ipirwany@yahoo.com.

PIRZADA, Amrah; Health Sciences Centre, 300 Prince Philip Dr, St. John's NL A1B 3V6; Karachi (Pakistan)'86; MB BS; DABPath; Staff Path, Health Sciences Centre; Asst Prof Med, Memorial University Of Newfoundland; Langs: Urdu; (709)777-6370

PIRZADA, Kashif S; William Osler HC-Brampton, 2100 Bovaird Dr E, Brampton ON L6R 3J7; Tor'04; CCFP; CCFP(E.M.); Staff, William Osler Health System - Brampton Civic Hospital; Physician, Toronto Poly Clinic; (905)494-2120; kpirzada@tpclinic.com.

PIRZADA, Munir A; Manitoba Clinic, 790 Sherbrook St, Winnipeg MB R3A 1M3; Karachi (Pakistan)'81; MB BS; Staff, Health Sciences Centre; Langs: Urdu; pirzada_munir@hotmail.com.

PISANI, Amin; Kingsway Prof Centre, 303-10611 Kingsway NW, Edmonton AB T5G 3C8; Alb'98; BSc; BScPharm; FRCPC; IntMed; Nephrol. (780)496-9350; Fax. (780)425-8475.

PISCIONE, Tino D; 555 University Ave, Toronto ON M5G 1X8; Qns'91; PhD; FRCPC; Peds (Nephrology). Staff/Physician, The Hospital For Sick Children; (416)813-2133; Fax. (416)813-6271.

PISESKY, Wayne A; PO Box 1879 Stn Main, Edmonton AB T5J 2P2; Alb'76; FRCSC; OrthSurg (Sports Medicine). Ac Staff, Kelowna General Hospital; (780)498-3999; Fax. (780)498-7807; bonespisesky@shawbiz.ca.

PISHE, Tushar; Saint John Reg Hosp, PO Box 2100 Stn Main 400 University Ave, Saint John NB E2L 4L2; Dal'99; CCFP; CCFP(E.M.); Staff, Saint John Regional Hospital; (506)648-6000

PISON, Cesar; CLSC Cote-des-Neiges, 6600 ch de la Cote-des-Neiges, Montreal QC H3T 2A8; Madrid (Spain)'65; MSc; DSc; FRCPC; NuclearMed; Endocrin (P.Q.). Langs: Spanish; English; (514)731-1386

PISTAWKA, Kevin J; 2606 Pandosy St, Kelowna BC V1Y 1V6; UBC'86; FRCPC; IntMed; Cardiol. Chief Cardiol, Kelowna General Hospital; (250)762-9211; Fax. (250)762-8337; cardiologyclinic@shaw.ca.

PISTONO, Andree-Anne; Hop Maisonneuve-Rosemont, 5415 boul de l'Assomption, Montreal QC H1T 2M4; Mon'01; CSPQ; FRCPC; DiagRad. Staff, Hopital Maisonneuve-Rosemont; (514)252-3400 x5876

PISTONO, Louis-Xavier; Hop du Sacre-Coeur de Mtl, 5400 boul Gouin O, Montreal QC H4J 1C5; Mon'03; FRCPC; DiagRad. Staff, Hôpital du Sacre-Coeur de Montréal; (514)338-2222; Fax. (514)338-2130.

PISTOR, Lino A; Sault Area Hosp, 750 Great Northern Rd, Sault Ste. Marie ON P6B 0A8; Ott'80; BSc; FRCPC; Psy (Forensic Psychiatry). Med Dir Mental Health Prog, Sault Area Hospital - Sault Ste Marie; Psychiatrist, Northern Treatment Center-Ministry of Corrections; Clin Dir, Ontario Addiction Treatment Centre; Langs: English; French; (705)759-3434 x4615; Fax. (705)256-3494.

PISZEL, Lloyd M; St Paul's Hosp, 1081 Burrard St, Vancouver BC V6Z 1Y6; Tor'91; Urol. Staff, Providence Health Care - St Paul's Hospital; (604)682-2344

PITCHER, Jeff; 3498 Shadow Creek Rd RR 3, Orillia ON L3V 6H3; McM'09; CCFP; (705)242-8085; Fax. (705)514-0770.

PITFIELD, Alexander F; Children's & Women's HC of BC, 2L5-4480 Oak St, Vancouver BC V6H 3V4; Qns'01; FRCPC; Peds (Critical Care Medicine). Staff, BC Children's Hospital; (604)875-2744

PITOUT, Johann D D; Calgary Lab Services, 9-3535 Research Rd NW, Calgary AB T2L 2K8; (South Africa)'85; MB ChB; Staff, Calgary Laboratory Services; Langs: Afrikaans; (403)770-3309; Fax. (403)770-3347; johann.pitout@cls.ab.ca.

PITRE, Jean-Marie; Clinique Med Bonaventure, 103 rue Nicolas-Denys GD, Bonaventure QC G0C 1E0; Laval'69; (418)534-2145; Fax. (418)534-2501.

PITRE, Lyne; Montfort Academic Family Hlth, 101B-745 Montreal Rd, Ottawa ON K1K 0T1; Ott'86; CCFP; FCFP; (613)749-4429; Fax. (613)749-7942.

PITRE, Theresa J; Univ of Waterloo Hlth Services, 200 University Ave W, Waterloo ON N2L 3G1; Wes'00; CCFP; (519)888-4096

PITT, Dennis F; The Ottawa Hosp-Gen Campus, W166 C-501 Smyth Rd, Ottawa ON K1H 8L6; Qns'72; MEd; FRCSC; GenSurg (Breast Cancer). Staff, The Ottawa Hospital - General Campus; Assoc Prof, University of Ottawa; (613)737-8899 x79622; Fax. (613)739-6644.

PITT, Paul L; Hillside Med Centre, 2867 Lawrence Ave E, Scarborough ON M1P 2T2; Tor'64; CCFP; FCFP; Ac Staff, The Scarborough Hospital - General Campus; Lecturer Commun & Family Med, University of Toronto; (416)261-7223; Fax. (416)261-6374.

PITT, Tracy J; FE125-685 William Ave, Winnipeg MB R3E 0Z2; Howard University (USA)'04; FRCPC; Peds; ClinImmunol&Allergy.

PITTER, Curt A; Peter Lougheed Centre, 3500 26 Ave NE, Calgary AB T1Y 6J4; Ott'95; FRCPC; Anes. Staff, Peter Lougheed Centre; (403)943-5554; Fax. (403)219-3574.

PITTERS, Carrol A; Children's Hosp Eastern Ont, 401 Smyth Rd, Ottawa ON K1H 8L1; West Indies (Jamaica)'79; MB BS; FRCPC; Peds (Emergency Medicine). Chief Div of EmergMed, Children's Hospital of Eastern Ontario (CHEO); Asst Prof, University of Ottawa; (613)737-7600 x2318; Fax. (613)738-4852; pitters@cheo.on.ca.

PITTINI, Richard J; Sunnybrook Hlth Sciences Ctre, C712-2075 Bayview Ave, Toronto ON M4N 3M5; Tor'93; MEd; FRCSC; ObstGyn (Endoscopic Surgery). Ac Staff, Women's College Hospital; Ac Staff, Sunnybrook Health Sciences Centre; Asst Prof, University of Toronto; (416)480-4579; Fax. (416)480-4588.

PITTMAN, C Dianne; Homewood Health Centre, 150 Delhi St, Guelph ON N1E 6K9; Mem'97; BSc; BSc(Hons); MSc; FRCPC; Psy. Asst Clin Prof, McMaster University; (519)824-1010 x2293; Fax. (519)824-1827.

PITTMAN, Carla E; Dartmouth Gen Hosp, 325 Pleasant St, Dartmouth NS B2Y 4G8; Mem'95; FRCPC; DiagRad. Staff, Dartmouth General Hospital; (902)465-8300; Fax. (902)465-8360.

PITTMAN, Jennifer M; Long Pond Med Clinic, PO Box 14097 Stn Main 88 Conception Bay Highway, Conception-Bay-S NL A1W 3J1; Saba (Netherlands)'10; CCFP.

PITTMAN, Patricia G; Manitoba Clinic, 101-790 Sherbrook St, Winnipeg MB R3A 1M3; Man'03; CCFP; (204)788-5756

PITZ, Marshall W; CancerCare Manitoba, 675 McDermot Ave, Winnipeg MB R3E 0V9; Man'02; FRCPC; IntMed; MedOncol.

PIUZE, Francois; Hop Jeffrey Hale, 1250 ch Sainte-Foy, Quebec QC G1S 2M6; Laval'98; CCFP; Staff Family Med, Centre Hospitalier Affilié Universitaire de Québec - Hôpital De L'Enfant Jésus; Staff Emergency Med, Hôpital Laval; Staff, Jeffery Hale Hospital-Saint Brigid's; (418)684-5333

PIUZE, Genevieve; Ctr d'Hebergement Le Faubourg, 925 av Turnbull, Quebec QC G1R 2X6; Laval'95; (418)534-2462

PIUZE, Genevieve-Helene; CHUQ-Ctr Hosp Univ Laval, 2705 boul Laurier, Quebec QC G1V 4G2; Laval'95; FRCPC; Peds (Neonatal & Perinatal Medicine). Staff, Centre Hospitalier Universitaire de Quebec-CHUL; (418)656-4141; Fax. (418)654-2137.

PIUZE, Jacques; Centre Med des Boulevards, 101-718 boul Frontenac E, Thetford Mines QC G6G 6H1; Laval'69; (418)335-7585; Fax. (418)335-7587.

PIVER, Andre; PO Box 24, Slocan Park BC V0G 2E0; Mon'82; CCFP; FCFP; Consultant, Kootenay Lake General Hospital; Staff, Nelson Mental Health Centre; Langs: Spanish; Polish; French; (250)226-7111

PIVNICK, Jeffrey S; 221-339 Aspen Glen Landing SW, Calgary AB T3H 0N6; Cal'79; CCFP; FCFP; Ac Staff, Rockyview General Hospital; (403)263-7997; Fax. (403)263-7996.

PIZZALE, Stephen; Hamilton HS-McMaster Site, PO Box 2000 Stn Lcd 1 1200 Main St W, Hamilton ON L8N 3Z5; Ott'09; Staff, Hamilton Health Sciences Centre - McMaster University Medical Centre; (905)521-2100

PIZZUTO, Michael; Columbus Med Arts Bldg, 404-8333 Weston Rd, Woodbridge ON L4L 8E2; Tor'85; Ac Staff, Humber River Regional Hospital - Finch Avenue Site; (905)856-6136; Fax. (905)856-6138.

PLACE, Christopher R; CSSS-Hop de Hull, 116 boul Lionel-Emond, Gatineau QC J8Y 1W7; Ott'81; CSPQ; FRCPC; DiagRad. Staff, Hull Hospital; (819)595-6028

PLACE, Rodney C; Dalbrent Med Centre, 110-3604 52 Ave NW, Calgary AB T2L 1V9; Cal'87; BSc(Hon); CCFP; Att Staff, Foothills Medical Centre; (403)282-9445; Fax. (403)284-0093.

PLACH, Nadia R; Joseph Brant Mem Hosp, 1230 North Shore Blvd E, Burlington ON L7S 1W7; McM'83; PhD; CCFP; FCFP; Ac Staff Palliative Care, Joseph Brant Memorial Hospital; Affil Staff, Hamilton Health Sciences Centre - Hamilton General Hospital; Assoc Prof, McMaster University; (905)632-3737 x4103; Fax. (905)336-6492.

PLACIDE, Joseph E; CLSC Bordeaux-Cartierville, 11844 av du Bois-de-Boulogne, Montreal QC H3M 2X7; (Haiti)'77; (514)331-2288 x6454

PLAGEMAN, Maxwell G; Workers' Comp Board, PO Box 2415 Stn Main, Edmonton AB T5J 2S5; Tor'72; (780)498-4482; Fax. (780)498-7855.

PLAISANCE, Yves; Ctr Hosp Affilie-St-Sacrement, 1050 ch Sainte-Foy, Quebec QC G1S 4L8; Laval'84; Staff, Centre Hospitalier Affilié Universitaire de Québec - Hôpital du St-Sacrement; Staff, Centre Hospitalier Universitaire De Québec - Pavillon De St-françois-d'assise; (418)682-7511

PLAMONDON, Catherine; Centre Med St-Francois, 200-2125 boul Lemire, Drummondville QC J2B 8N8; Mon'04; (819)477-6796

PLAMONDON, Gilles; Clinique Med Mont-Carmel, 933 boul Rene-Levesque E, Montreal QC H2L 4S4; Mon'79; Physician, CLSC du Marigot; Langs: English; (514)282-9197; Fax. (514)282-1973.

PLAMONDON, Isabelle; Hôpital Laval, 2725 ch Sainte-Foy, Quebec QC G1V 4G5; Laval'00; FRCPC; Nephrol (Intensive Care); Critical Care Medicine (P.Q.); IntMed. Staff, Hôpital Laval; Langs: Bilingual(French/English); (418)656-8711

PLAMONDON, Jacques; Clin TSO du CHUQ, 184 rue Racine, Quebec QC G2B 1E3; Laval'73; FRCPC; Psy (Trauma). Physician, Veterans Affairs Canada; Langs: Bilingual(French/English); (418)657-3696; Fax. (418)657-3697.

PLAMONDON, Lise; Clinique Med Les Saules, 100-2780 boul Masson, Quebec QC G1P 1J6; Laval'81; LMCC; (418)871-4492; Fax. (418)877-4478.

PLAMONDON, Marie-Jo; The Ottawa Hosp-Civic Campus, 1053 Carling Ave, Ottawa ON K1Y 4E9; McG'07; MDCM; Anes. Staff, The Ottawa Hospital - Civic Campus; (613)798-5555

PLAMONDON, Mireille; CHUM-Hotel-Dieu, 3840 rue Saint-Urbain, Montreal QC H2W 1T8; Laval'03; FRCPC; IntMed; Microbio & Infect Dis (P.Q.); MedMicrobiol; InfectDis. Staff, Centre Hospitalier l'Université de Montréal (CHUM) - Hôtel-Dieu; (514)890-8444

PLAMONDON, Nicole; CHUQ-Hotel-Dieu de Quebec, 11 Cote du Palais, Quebec QC G1R 2J6; Laval'80; CSPQ; DiagRad. Staff, Centre Hospitalier Universitaire de Québec (CHUQ) - Siege Social; (418)691-5453; Fax. (418)691-5394.

PLAMONDON, Sophie; CHUS-Hop Hotel-Dieu, 580 rue Bowen S, Sherbrooke QC J1G 2E8; Sher'00; FRCPC; IntMed; Gastroent. Staff, Centre Hospitalier Universitaire de Sherbrooke-Hôpital Hôtel-Dieu; (819)346-1110

PLAMONDON, Stephanie A; Foothills Med Centre, AC142-1403 29 St NW, Calgary AB T2N 2T9; McM'96; CSCN(EMG); FRCPC; PhysMed&Rehab (Brain Injury Rehabilitation). Staff, Foothills Medical Centre; Asst Prof Clinical Neurosciences, University of Calgary; (403)944-4224; Fax. (403)283-2526.

PLANET, Jean-Francois; 404B-595 Montreal Rd, Ottawa ON K1K 4L2; Sher'95; DAB; FRCSC; Otol. Staff, Montfort Hospital; Staff, Children's Hospital of Eastern Ontario (CHEO); Langs: English; (613)746-2235

PLANT, Howard M; 101-5818 Sheppard Ave E, Scarborough ON M1B 4Z6; McM'87; Ac Staff Family Practice, Rouge Valley Health System - Centenary Health Centre Site; Ac Staff, The Scarborough Hospital - Birchmount Campus; (416)321-9713

PLANT, Jeffery R; Penticton Reg Hosp, 550 Carmi Ave, Penticton BC V2A 3G6; Cal'95; FRCPC; EmergMed. Staff, Penticton Regional Hospital; (250)492-4000

PLANT, Louise A; Dr Everett Chalmers Reg Hosp, PO Box 9000 Stn A 700 Priestman St, Fredericton NB E3B 5N5; Ott'10; CCFP; Staff, Dr Everett Chalmers Regional Hospital; (506)452-5400

PLANT, Sandi L; North Woodlands Med Centre, 204-40 Shellington Pl, Brantford ON N3S 0C5; McM'02; CCFP; (519)759-6116; Fax. (519)759-7727.

PLANTE, Annick; GMF La Cigogne, 420-3141 boul Taschereau, Greenfield Park QC J4V 2H2; Mon'01; Staff Perinatal, Hopital Charles LeMoyne; Langs: Bilingual(French/English); (450)466-7892; Fax. (450)466-9602.

PLANTE, Bernard; Clinique Med Bernard Plante, 862 rue de Bellevue, Quebec QC G1V 2R5; Laval'83; LMCC; Staff, Centre Hospitalier Universitaire de Quebec-CHUL; (418)688-8118; Fax. (418)688-8198.

PLANTE, Christine; CSSS des Aurores Boreales, CP 6000 Succ Bureau-Chef 679 2e rue E, La Sarre QC J9Z 2X7; Sher'05; Staff, Centre Hospitalier La Sarre; (819)333-2311; Fax. (819)333-4316.

PLANTE, Daniel; Lorraine Wing Tower C, 2F-201 Deacon St, Pembroke ON K8A 2J6; McG'90; CCFP; Staff, Pembroke Regional Hospital Inc; Langs: Bilingual(French/English); (613)732-3422; Fax. (613)732-1082.

PLANTE, Danielle; Clinique Med de Lavaltrie, 200-1400 rue Notre-Dame, Lavaltrie QC J5T 1M6; Mon'84; (450)586-2555; Fax. (450)586-4498.

PLANTE, Denis; GMF Venta et Marees, 201-391 av Brochu, Sept-Iles QC G4R 4S7; Laval'86; Staff, Centre Hospitalier Regional de Sept-Iles; (418)968-1234; Fax. (418)962-4488; denis_plante@ssss.gouv.qc.ca.

PLANTE, Denis; Place Notre-Dame, 101-711 boul Saint-Joseph, Roberval QC G8H 2L3; Laval'67; Ophth (P.Q.). Staff, Hotel-Dieu de Roberval; (418)275-7225; Fax. (418)275-7226.

PLANTE, Diane; Clinique Sante Jacques-Cartier, 200-1815 rue King O, Sherbrooke QC J1J 2E3; Sher'75; Langs: English; (819)565-7446; Fax. (819)565-7780.

PLANTE, Francois; CHUM-Hop Notre-Dame, 1560 rue Sherbrooke E, Montreal QC H2L 4M1; Mon'86; CSPQ; Anes. Staff, Centre Hospitalier l'Université de Montréal (CHUM) - Hôpital Notre-Dame; (514)890-8000 x26876

PLANTE, Francois J; Clinique Med du Sud-Ouest, 4475 rue Bannantyne, Verdun QC H4G 1E2; Ott'71; LMCC; FRCPC; Respir (Internal Medicine). ac Membre, CSSS de Dorval-Lachine-Lasalle; Staff, Centre Hospitalier de Verdun; Universite de Montreal; Langs: Bilingual(French/English); (514)765-3600; Fax. (514)765-9625; francois.plante3@sympatico.ca.

PLANTE, Francois R; CHUS-Hop Fleurimont, 14985-3001 12e av N, Sherbrooke QC J1H 5N4; Sher'84; CSPQ; FRC; FRCPC; DiagRad (Thoracic Radiology). Ac Staff, Centre Hospitalier Universitaire de Sherbrooke-Hopital Fleurimont; (819)346-1110 x14985; Fax. (819)820-6423; francois.r.plante@usherbrooke.ca.

PLANTE, Gilles C; CLSC du Plateau Mont-Royal, 4625 av de Lorimier, Montreal QC H2H 2B4; Ott'59; FRCPC; Psy (Pediatric Psychiatry). Staff, Hôpital Ste-Justine; assoc Prof Psy, Universite de Montreal; (514)521-1320 x6134; Fax. (514)521-1886.

PLANTE, Isabelle; Hotel-Dieu de Levis, 143 rue Wolfe, Levis QC G6V 3Z1; Laval'96; FRCPC; Psy (Pedology Psychiatry). Staff, Hôtel-Dieu de Lévis; (418)835-7155

PLANTE, Jean-Francois; CSSS du Lac-des-Deux-Montagnes, 520 boul Arthur-Sauve, St-Eustache QC J7R 5B1; Mon'99; Staff, Hôpital de Saint-Eustache; (450)473-6811

PLANTE, Jean-Luc; 3e Escadre Bagotville CP 5000 Succ Bureau-chef, Alouette QC G0V 1A0; Sher'10; CCFP; (418)677-4000

PLANTE, Jeffrey L; 103-20644 Fraser Hwy, Langley BC V3A 4G5; UBC'08; CCFP; (604)530-4979

PLANTE, Jessica; Hotel-Dieu de Levis, 143 rue Wolfe, Levis QC G6V 3Z1; Laval'06; FRCPC; Peds. Staff, Hôtel-Dieu de Lévis; (418)835-7121

PLANTE, Johanne; CHSLD Marcelle-Ferron, 8600 boul Marie-Victorin, Brossard QC J4X 1A1; McG'85; DrMedCh; Physician Geriatrics, CHSLD St-Georges; Physician Geriatrics, CHSLD Marie-Rollet; Médecin, CHSLD d'Acceuil Marcelle Ferron; Physician Soins Palliatifs, Maison Source-Bleue; Langs: German; Bilingual(English/French); (450)923-1430; Fax. (450)923-1805; drjoplante@videotron.ca.

PLANTE, Judith C; Lorraine Wing Tower C, 2F-201 Deacon St, Pembroke ON K8A 2J6; McG'89; BSc; MDCM; CCFP; Ac Staff/Chief FamilyMed, Pembroke Regional Hospital Inc; Langs: English; French; (613)732-3422; Fax. (613)732-1082.

PLANTE, Julie; Hotel-Dieu de Levis, 143 rue Wolfe, Levis QC G6V 3Z1; Laval'95; FRCPC; Respir; IntMed (Sleep Apnea). Staff, Hôtel-Dieu de Lévis; (418)835-7121; Fax. (418)835-7215; julie_plante@yahoo.com.

PLANTE, Ludovic; 203-100 rue King E, Sherbrooke QC J1G 1A4; Sher'73; NBME; LMCC; Langs: Spanish; English; (819)563-7225; Fax. (819)563-7271.

PLANTE, Marie; CSSS de Manicouagan, 635 boul Jolliet, Baie-Comeau QC G5C 1P1; Laval'89; FRCPC; Psy. Staff, Centre Hospitalier Régional Baie-Comeau; Staff PedoPsy, Hotel-Dieu du Sacre-Coeur de Jesus de Quebec; Clin Teach Staff Psy, Université Laval; (418)589-3701 x2250

PLANTE, Marie-Carmen; CHUM-Hop Notre-Dame, 1560 rue Sherbrooke E, Montreal QC H2L 4M1; Mon'68; FRCPC; Psy (Clinical Psychiatry). Staff, Centre Hospitalier l'Université de Montréal (CHUM) - Hôpital Notre-Dame; Staff, Centre Hospitalier l'Université De Montréal (CHUM) - Hôpital Saint-luc; Researcher, Universite de Montreal; (514)890-8000 x22310; Fax. (514)412-7827; mariecarmenplante@hotmail.com.

PLANTE, Martin; Clinique Med Sainte-Julie, 286 rue de Normandie, Sainte-Julie QC J3E 1A7; Mon'08; Staff, Hôtel-Dieu de Sorel; (450)649-1593

PLANTE, Michel; Hydro-Quebec, 101-75 boul René-Lévesque O, Montreal QC H2Z 1A4; Mon'79; Staff, Centre Hospitalier Affilié Universitaire de Québec - Hôpital du St-Sacrement; Médecin, Hydro-Quebec; Langs: Spanish; English; (514)289-2211 x3039; Fax. (514)289-5049; plante.michel@hydro.qc.ca.

PLANTE, Monique; CHUQ-Ctr Hosp Univ Laval, 2705 boul Laurier, Quebec QC G1V 4G2; Laval'84; FRCPC; Peds. Staff Ped, Centre Hospitalier Universitaire de Quebec-CHUL; Staff Ped, Centre Hospitalier Universitaire De Québec - Pavillon De St-françois-d'assise; (418)654-2282; Fax. (418)654-2137; monique.plante@ped.ulaval.ca.

PLANTE, Pierre; Inst de Readaptation de Mtl, 6300 av de Darlington, Montreal QC H3S 2J4; Mon'81; PhysMed&Rehab. Staff, Institut de Réadaptation Gingras-Lindsay de Montréal; (514)340-2084; Fax. (514)340-2775.

PLANTE, Sylvain; 602-581 Davis Dr, Newmarket ON L3Y 2P6; Sher'83; FRCPC; IntMed; Cardiol (P.Q.). Staff, Southlake Regional Health Centre; (905)953-7917; Fax. (905)953-0046.

PLANTE, Valerie; CHUQ-Ctr Hosp Univ Laval, 2705 boul Laurier, Quebec QC G1V 4G2; Laval'97; GeriatricMed; IntMed. Staff, Centre Hospitalier Universitaire de Quebec-CHUL; (418)654-2255

PLANTE, Vicky; Unite Med Familiale Maizerets, 2480 ch de la Canardiere, Quebec QC G1J 2G1; Laval'98; CCFP; (418)661-1413; Fax. (418)661-7504.

PLANTE, Virginie; 1000 boul Sainte-Anne, St-Charles-Brromee QC J6E 6J2; Sher'05; CCFP; Staff, Centre Hospitalier Régional de Lanaudière; Langs: French; (450)759-8222 x2820

PLANTIVE, Richard; Montfort Hosp, 713 Montreal Rd, Ottawa ON K1K 0T2; Ott'02; FRCPC; EmergMed. Staff, Montfort Hospital; (613)746-4621

PLASKOS, Christina; 30-100 Fourth Ave, St Catharines ON L2S 3P1; Tor'90; BSc(Pharm); Ac Staff, Niagara Health System - St Catharines General Site; Physician, Contours MD Cosmetic Vein Laser Ctre; Langs: Greek; Macedonian; (905)704-1446; Fax. (905)704-0739.

PLASKOS, Nicholas; Guelph Gen Hosp, 115 Delhi St, Guelph ON N1E 4J4; Tor'04; FRCPC; DiagRad. Staff, Guelph General Hospital; (519)822-5350

PLASSE, Marylene; CHUM-Hop St-Luc, 9304B-1058 rue Saint-Denis, Montreal QC H2X 3J4; Laval'96; FRCSC; GenSurg. Staff, Centre Hospitalier l'Université De Montréal (CHUM) - Hôpital Saint-luc; Clinical Asst Prof, Universite de Montreal; (514)890-8000 x36146; Fax. (514)412-7380.

PLATERO MIRANDA, Hugo E; CSSSG-Hop de Hull, 116 boul Lionel-Emond, Gatineau QC J8Y 1W7; (El Salvador)'04; CCFP; Staff, Hull Hospital; (819)966-6222

PLATNICK, Howard A; 1008-2200 Yonge St, Toronto ON M4S 2C6; Tor'87; Staff, North York General Hospital; (416)482-8021

PLATONOV, Michael; 206-101 Queensway W, Mississauga ON L5B 2P7; Qns'99; FRCPC; IntMed (Electrophysiology); Cardiol. Staff, Trillium Health Centre - Mississauga; (905)848-7900; Fax. (905)615-8537.

PLATZKER, Daniel; The Doctor's Office, 595 Bay St, Toronto ON M5G 2C2; Wisconsin (USA)'05; CCFP; (416)515-0590

PLAUSINIS, Derek J A; Nicola Med Dental Bldg, 303-321 Nicola St, Kamloops BC V2C 6G6; Tor'98; BSc; MASc; FRCSC; OrthSurg (Shoulder & Elbow). Staff, Royal Inland Hospital; Asst Prof, University of British Columbia; (250)374-5141; Fax. (778)471-6021.

PLAXTON, E Kim; Dalhousie Univ Health Services, 6230 Coburg Rd, Halifax NS B3H 4J5; Tor'82; CCFP; FCFP; (902)494-2171; Fax. (902)494-6872; eplaxton@dal.ca.

PLAXTON, Patricia A; Chamber of Commerce Bldg, 502-345 Lakeshore Rd E, Oakville ON L6J 1J5; Tor'89; CCFP; FCFP; Ac Staff, Halton Healthcare Services Corporation - Oakville Site; (905)845-4511; Fax. (905)845-8133.

PLAXTON, William R; Grand River Hosp-KW Hlth Ctre, PO Box 9056 Stn C 835 King St W, Kitchener ON N2G 1G3; Wes'94; BSc(Hon); MSc(ClinEpid); MBA; FRCPC; IntMed; Critical Care Medicine. Staff, Grand River Hospital - Kitchener/Waterloo Health Centre; (519)749-4300

PLAYFAIR, David A; PO Box 247, Didsbury AB T0M 0W0; Cambridge (England)'70; MB ChB.

PLAYFAIR, David R; Cardston Clinic, PO Box 550, Cardston AB T0K 0K0; Cal'04; CCFP; Langs: Spanish; (403)653-3311; Fax. (403)653-1098; davidp@ualberta.ca.

PLECASH, B Gail; 208-440 Cascia Dr, Kelowna BC V1W 4Y4; Cal'75; CCFP; FCFP; (250)764-4677

PLEDGER, David J; Vancouver Gen Hosp, 855 12th Ave W, Vancouver BC V5Z 1M9; Dal'93; FRCPC; EmergMed. Staff, Vancouver General Hospital - Centennial Pavillion; (604)875-4111

PLENK, Katharina; Mackenzie Richmond Hill Hosp, 10 Trench St, Richmond Hill ON L4C 4Z3; Vienna (Austria)'96; FRCPC; IntMed. Staff, Mackenzie Richmond Hill Hospital; (905)883-2310

PLESS, Charles E; Clinique de Med Familiale, 6e-2120 rue Sherbrooke E, Montreal QC H2K 1C3; Mon'98; CCFP; Universite de Montreal; Langs: Spanish; (514)527-1958; Fax. (514)527-1649; plesscharles@hotmail.com.

PLESS, Robert P; Public Health Agency of Cda, AL6702B-120 Colonnade Rd, Ottawa ON K1A 0K9; McM'87; MSc(Epidemiol.); Langs: English; French; (613)948-6131

PLESSIS, Angela D; Salmon Arm Med Clinic, PO Box 730 Stn Main 581 Hudson Ave NE, Salmon Arm BC V1E 4N8; UBC'90; (250)832-6092

PLESU, Ioana; Hop de la Malbaie, 303 rue Saint-Etienne, La Malbaie QC G5A 1T1; Laval'08; CCFP; Staff, Hôpital de la Malbaie; (418)665-1700

PLESZEWSKI, Bartolomiej; Via Medica Imaging Services, 3943 boul Saint-Jean, Roxboro QC H9G 1X2; Mon'00; FRCPC; DiagRad. Staff, QHC Belleville General; (514)626-5888

PLEWES, E Arthur; Hys Med Centre, 303-11010 101 St NW, Edmonton AB T5H 4B9; UBC'84; BSc; FACS; FRCSC; GenSurg (Colon & Rectal Surgery). Associate Clin Prof of Surg, University of Alberta; (780)424-4405; Fax. (780)424-4467.

PLEWES, Katherine A; Gordon & Leslie Diamond HCC, 10-2775 Laurel Ave, Vancouver BC V5Z 1M9; Cal'06; FRCPC; IntMed; InfectDis. Staff, Vancouver General Hospital - Centennial Pavillion; Staff, Gordon & Leslie Diamond Health Care Centre; (604)840-5641

PLEWES, Michael E; Moosomin Family Practice Ctre, PO Box 1528, Moosomin SK S0G 3N0; Sask'95; CCFP; (306)435-3838; Fax. (306)435-2176.

PLEYDELL-PEARCE, Julian S; Chilliwack Gen Hosp, 45600 Menholm St, Chilliwack BC V2P 1P7; Bristol (England)'90; MRCS; MB ChB; MRCP; BA; FRCPCH; Staff, Chilliwack General Hospital; (604)793-4508; Fax. (604)795-6491; julian.pleydell-pearce@fraserhealth.ca.

PLIAMM, Lew; The Polyclinic, 5-4646 Dufferin St, North York ON M3H 5S4; Tor'92; CCFP; FCFP; Staff Consultant, Centre for Addiction & Mental Health (CAMH) - Russell Street Site; (416)222-6160; Fax. (416)222-9604.

PLIAMM, Naomi; 5-4646 Dufferin St, North York ON M3H 5S4; Tor'02; CCFP; (416)661-1838; Fax. (416)661-2831.

PLIAMM, Sara; 5-4646 Dufferin St, North York ON M3H 5S4; Kaunas (Lithuania)'65; Staff Physician, North York General Hospital - Branson Division; Langs: Russian; Lithuanian; (416)661-1838; Fax. (416)661-2831.

PLIMBLEY, W Roger; PO Box 159, Darwell AB T0E 0L0; Birmingham (England)'59; MB ChB; DA(Lond).

PLINT, Amy C; Children's Hosp Eastern Ont, 401 Smyth Rd, Ottawa ON K1H 8L1; McM'91; FRCPC; Peds. Staff, Children's Hospital of Eastern Ontario (CHEO); (613)738-7600 x3237

PLOESSER, Markus; St Paul's Hosp, 1081 Burrard St, Vancouver BC V6Z 1Y6; (Germany)'01; Staff, Providence Health Care - St Paul's Hospital; Langs: German; French; (604)682-2344; mploesser@forensic.bc.ca.

PLOTKIN, Anna; The Credit Valley Hosp, 2200 Eglinton Ave W, Mississauga ON L5M 2N1; (Russia (Federation))'94; FRCPC; AnatPath. Staff, The Credit Valley Hospital; (905)883-1100

PLOTNICK, Laurie H; MUHC-Montreal Children's Hosp, 103A-2300 rue Tupper, Montreal QC H3H 1P3; McG'91; FRCPC; Peds (Adolescent Medicine). Staff, McGill University Health Centre - Montreal Children's Hospital; (514)412-4400 x23039

PLOTNYK, Eugene; 1506 9th Ave S PO Box 5 Rpo St. Mike's, Lethbridge AB T1J 4P5; (Ukraine)'96; CCFP; Staff, Chinook Regional Hospital; (403)388-6111

PLOUFFE, Daniel T; Phoenix Med Centre, 402-2155 10th Ave, Prince George BC V2M 5J6; UBC'02; CCFP; (250)562-1961

PLOUFFE, Elyse; CSSS du Sud de Lanaudière, 911 montee des Pionniers, Terrebonne QC J6V 2H2; Laval'07; Gastroent (P.Q.); IntMed. Staff, Centre Hospitalier Pierre le Gardeur; (450)654-7525

PLOURDE, Andree-Anne; CSSS de Lac-Saint Jean-Est, CP 1300 Succ Bureau-Chef 300 boul Champlain S, Alma QC G8B 5W3; Laval'08; Staff, CSSS de Lac-Saint Jean-Est; (418)669-2000

PLOURDE, Claudia; CSSS de la Cote-de-Gaspe, 215 boul de York O, Gaspe QC G4X 2W2; Laval'02; CCFP; Staff, Centre Hospitalier de Gaspe; Langs: Bilingual(French/English); (418)368-6663; Fax. (418)368-5358.

PLOURDE, Diane; CSSS de Rivière-de-Loup, 75 rue Saint-Henri, Riviere-Du-Loup QC G5R 2A4; Laval'89; FRCSC; ObstGyn (Menopause). Ac Staff Gyn, Centre Hospitalier Regional du Grand-Portage; Langs: Bilingual(French/English); (418)868-1010; Fax. (418)868-1075.

PLOURDE, Isabelle; Clinique Med Frontenac, 24 rue Frontenac, Riviere-du-Loup QC G5R 1S5; Sher'06; Staff, Centre Hospitalier Regional du Grand-Portage; Langs: Bilingual(French/English); (418)862-0333

PLOURDE, Isabelle; CLSC Riviere-aux-Renards, 154 boul Renard E, Gaspe QC G4X 5R5; Laval'04; CCFP; (418)269-2572; Fax. (418)269-5294.

PLOURDE, J J Pierre; 490 Hargrave St, Winnipeg MB R3A 0X7; Ott'83; LMCC; FRCPC; IntMed (Public Health); InfectDis. Assoc Prof Community Health Sciences, University of Manitoba; Langs: Creole; French; (204)940-3607; Fax. (204)956-4494; pplourde@wrha.mb.ca.

PLOURDE, Madelaine; Queen Elizabeth II HSC, 7 008-1276 South Park St, Halifax NS B3H 2Y9; Ott'04; FRCSC; GenSurg; ThorSurg. Staff, Queen Elizabeth II Health Sciences Centre - Victoria General Site; (902)473-2281; Fax. (902)473-4426.

PLOURDE, Miville; CHUQ-St-Francois d'Assise, 10 rue de l'Espinay, Quebec QC G1L 3L5; Laval'05; FRCPC; EmergMed. Staff, Centre Hospitalier Universitaire De Québec - Pavillon De St-françois-d'assise; (418)525-4444

PLOURDE, Patrice; Clinique Med Hôp de Jonquière, 2230 rue de l'Hopital, Jonquiere QC G7X 7X2; Mon'91; FRCPC; IntMed. Staff, Centre Hospitalier Jonquiere; (418)695-7700; Fax. (418)695-7715; patrice.plourde@ssss.gouv.qc.ca.

PLOURDE, Pierre; CSSS du Suroit, 150 rue Saint-Thomas, Salaber-de-Valleyf QC J6T 6C1; Mon'71; IntMed (Neurology). Membre Med, Centre Hospitalier Régional du Suroît; Langs: English; French; (450)371-9925

PLOURDE, R Gilles; MUHC-Montreal Neurology Inst, 3801 rue University, Montreal QC H3A 2B4; Laval'78; MSc; CSPQ; FRCPC; Anes. Staff, McGill University Health Centre - Montreal Neurological Hospital; Prof, McGill University; (514)398-1917; Fax. (514)398-1352.

PLOURDE, Simon; Clinique Med Pierre-Bertand, 212-303 boul Pierre-Bertrand, Quebec QC G1M 3L7; Laval'92; CCFP; Fam Med, CH St-Sacrement Ltee; (418)683-2724; Fax. (418)683-8861; simon.plourde@orlo.ulaval.ca.

PLOURDE, Simon; Clinique Med Acces-Sante, 8 rue du Terminus E, Rouyn-Noranda QC J9X 3B4; Sher'94; Staff, Centre Hospitalier Rouyn-Noranda; (819)762-2130; Fax. (819)562-5130.

PLOURDE, Suzie; Ctr de Readaptation de l'Estri, 300 rue King E, Sherbrooke QC J1G 1B1; Mon'75; Langs: Bilingual(French/English); (819)346-8411 x43516; Fax. (819)780-8973; gouplou@hotmail.com.

PLOURDE, Victor; CSSS Pierre Boucher, 1333 boul Jacques-Cartier E, Longueuil QC J4M 2A5; Mon'88; FRCPC; Gastroent (Functional Bowel Disorder). Staff, Centre Hospitalier Pierre Boucher; (450)568-8111

PLOW-JARVIS, Lisa G; South Lake Reg Health Centre, 596 Davis Dr, Newmarket ON L3Y 2P9; McM'92; Staff, Southlake Regional Health Centre; (905)895-4521 x1384

PLOWMAN, Brian K; Northland Med Centre, 400-4600 Crowchild Trail NW, Calgary AB T3A 2L6; Man'74; FRCPC; Psy. Asst Clin Prof, University of Calgary; (403)288-8180

PLOWRIGHT, Linda R; Child & Parent Resource Inst, 600 Sanatorium Rd, London ON N6H 3W7; McM'06; FRCPC; Psy. Staff, Child & Parent Resource Institute; (519)858-2774 x2919

PLUCINSKA, Hanna M; East Edmonton Hlth Centre, 7910 112 Ave NW, Edmonton AB T5B 0C2; Alb'99; PhD; CCFP; (780)342-4740; Fax. (780)342-4745.

PLUE, Gordon F; 302-1005 Elgin St W, Cobourg ON K9A 5J4; McG'93; Att Staff, Northumberland Hills Hospital; (905)377-8544; Fax. (905)377-0125.

PLUMMER, A Gordon; Fredericton Med Clinic, 301B-1015 Regent St, Fredericton NB E3B 6H5; Dal'82; Ac Staff, Dr Everett Chalmers Regional Hospital; (506)458-0259; Fax. (506)457-4751.

PLUTA, Catherine J; Shkagamik-kwe Health Centre, 161 Applegrove St, Sudbury ON P3C 1N2; St George's (Grenada)'01; FRCPC; Peds. (705)675-1596; Fax. (705)675-8040.

PLUTA, Henryk; Gastroent & Hepatology Clinic, 205-2752 Allwood St, Abbotsford BC V2T 3R7; Krakow (Poland)'80; DABIM; FACG; FRCPC; IntMed (Gastroenterology). Staff, Abbotsford Regional Hospital & Cancer Centre; Ac Staff, Mission Memorial Hospital; Langs: Polish; Russian; (604)859-7176; Fax. (604)859-4814.

PLUTA, Paul L; 1-708 Reeves St, Port Hawkesbury NS B9A 2S1; Mem'89; Staff, Strait Richmond Hospital; (902)625-1452; Fax. (902)625-2320.

PLUVIOSE, William; Clin Med Beaubien-des-Erables, 2175 rue Beaubien E, Montreal QC H2G 1M5; (Mexico)'59; Peds (P.Q.). Staff, Hôpital Santa Cabrini Ospedale; Consultant, Hôpital Ste-Justine; (514)722-4625

PLUYE, Pierre; Universite McGill, 517 av des Pins O, Montreal QC H2W 1S4; Toulouse III (France)'92; (514)398-8483; Fax. (514)398-4202.

PNIAK, Ewa M; Fredericton Med Clinic, 506-1015 Regent St, Fredericton NB E3B 6H5; Krakow (Poland)'90; Neurologist, Dr Everett Chalmers Regional Hospital; Langs: Polish; (506)447-4224; Fax. (506)447-4226.

PO, Joseph L; The Ottawa Hosp-Civic Campus, F202-1053 Carling Ave, Ottawa ON K1Y 4E9; Tor'94; BSc; FRCPC; Anes; Critical Care Medicine. Staff, The Ottawa Hospital - Civic Campus; Langs: English; French; (613)798-5555

PO, Milton C; BC Cancer Agency-Fraser Valley, 13750 96 Ave, Surrey BC V3V 1Z2; (Philippines)'84; FRCP; FRCPC; RadOncol (Gastrointestinal Cancer). Staff, Surrey Memorial Hospital; Staff, BC Cancer Agency Fraser Valley Centre; Langs: Mandarin; Taiwanese; Fookien; (604)930-4036; Fax. (604)930-4065; mpo@bccancer.bc.ca.

POBLETE, Roel C; Allied Health Centre, 303-5673 North St, Niagara Falls ON L2G 1J4; Manila (Philippines)'76; FACC; ABIM(IntMed); FRCPC; IntMed; Cardiol. Court Staff IntMed, Niagara Health System - Greater Niagara General Site; Langs: Tagalog; (905)354-8354

POCE, Frank R M; Ministry of Health, 370 Select Dr, Kingston ON K7M 8T4; Qns'70; Physician, Greater Kingston After Hour Clinic; Physician Health Services Div Provider Services, Ontario Ministry of Health; (613)536-3165; Fax. (613)536-3184. Semi-Retired.

POCHINI, Craig M; Dr H Bliss Murphy Cancer Ctr, 300 Prince Philip Dr, St. John's NL A1B 3V6; Mem'04; FRCPC; DiagRad. Staff, Dr H Bliss Murphy Cancer Centre; (709)777-6480

POCOCK, Jeffrey L; West Coast Family Med Clinic, 1300-6660 Sooke Rd, Sooke BC V9Z 0A5; Sheffield (England)'82; MB ChB; DRCOG; CCFP; FCFP; Clinical Asst Prof Prof Family Med, University of British Columbia; (250)642-4233; Fax. (250)642-6032.

POCOCK, Rosemary F; Hillside Med Centre, 360 2nd Ave, Campbell River BC V9W 3T9; Cape Town (South Africa)'83; CCFP; (250)287-7708; Fax. (250)287-3086.

POCRNICH, Dante M; Belmont Prof Centre, 306-564 Belmont Ave W, Kitchener ON N2M 5N6; Wes'80; FRCSC; Ophth. Staff, St Mary's General Hospital; Staff, Grand River Hospital - Kitchener/Waterloo Health Centre; (519)742-2000; Fax. (519)579-0800.

PODARU, Elena-Ioana; Clinique Med Fabreville, 380 boul Cure-Labelle, Laval QC H7P 5L3; (450)628-5800

PODAVIN, Joey N; Lakeland Med Clinic, 1715 Ellis St, Kelowna BC V1Y 8M9; Sask'06; CCFP; (778)478-0277

PODELL, Marc J; Trillium Hlth Ctr-Mississauga, 100 Queensway W, Mississauga ON L5B 1B8; (Mexico)'77; Staff, Trillium Health Centre - Mississauga; (905)848-7100

PODER, Kulli; Community Mental Health, 65 Brunswick St, Fredericton NB E3B 1G5; Tartu (Estonia)'83; FRCPC; Psy. (506)453-2132

PODHRADSKY, Ludek; Orillia Soldiers' Mem Hosp, 170 Colborne St W, Orillia ON L3V 2Z3; Czech.Rep. (Czech Republic)'97; CCFP; Staff, Orillia Soldiers' Memorial Hospital; Langs: Czech; (705)325-2201

PODILSKY, Natalia M; Midtown Med Centre, 203-39 23rd St E, Saskatoon SK S7K 0H6; Sask'81; FACOG; FRCSC; ObstGyn. Staff, St Paul's Hospital (Grey Nuns) of Saskatoon; Staff, Saskatoon City Hospital; Staff, Royal University Hospital; Associate Clin Prof, University of Saskatchewan; (306)244-0220; Fax. (306)244-5411.

PODNIEKS, Mary Jane; Albany Med Clinic, 807 Broadview Ave, Toronto ON M4K 2P8; Sint Maarten (Netherlands Antilles)'08; (416)461-9471

PODTETENEV, Michel; 3835 rue Wellington, Verdun QC H4G 1V1; Mon'79; FRCSC; Ophth. Consultant, Centre Hospitalier l'Université de Montréal (CHUM) - Hôpital Notre-Dame; Staff, Hopital Maisonneuve-Rosemont; (514)768-1250; Fax. (514)768-9240.

PODYMOW, Tiina L; MUHC-Royal Victoria Hosp, R238-687 av des Pins O, Montreal QC H3A 1A1; McG'94; FRCPC; IntMed; Nephrol. Staff, McGill University Health Centre - Royal Victoria Hospital; (514)934-1934

POEL, Meg; 11-450 Westheights Dr, Kitchener ON N2N 2B9; McM'83; CCFP; FCFP; (519)725-4070; Fax. (519)725-4071.

POELMAN, Susan M; 45-4307 130 Ave SE, Calgary AB T2Z 3V8; Cal'04; FRCPC; Derm. (403)457-0063; Fax. (403)282-0075.

POELZER, Brian J; Royal Inland Hosp, 311 Columbia St, Kamloops BC V2C 2T1; UBC'82; Staff, Royal Inland Hospital; Staff Occupational Health Program, BC Health Services; (250)314-2782

POENARU, Dan; MUHC-Montreal Children's Hosp, 2300 rue Tupper, Montreal QC H3H 1P3; Tor'86; BSc; FACS; FRCSC; GenSurg; PedGenSurg. Staff, McGill University Health Centre - Montreal Children's Hospital; (514)412-4498

POENN, Dieter; Little Current Med Associates, PO Box 549, Little Current ON P0P 1K0; McM'86; Dip SportMed; CCFP; FCFP; Staff, Manitoulin Health Centre - Little Current; Coroner, Province of Ontario; Clin Associate, University of Ottawa; (705)368-2450; Fax. (705)368-2480; dpoenn@manitoulin.net.

POETTCKER, Robert J; Beautiful Plains Comm Med Clin, PO Box 70 449 Mountain Ave, Neepawa MB R0J 1H0; Man'97; CCFP.

POFFENROTH, Linda A; Health Branch of Health Canada, 300-391 York Ave, Winnipeg MB R3C 4W1; Man'80; FRCPC; CommunMed.

POGGEMILLER, Gertrude A; 201-3251 Sheppard Ave E, Scarborough ON M1T 3W5; Sask'82; Ac Staff, Rouge Valley Health System - Centenary Health Centre Site; Ac Staff, The Scarborough Hospital - Birchmount Campus; Ac Staff, The Scarborough Hospital - General Campus; Examiner, Ministry of Transportation; (416)491-7700; Fax. (416)491-7885.

POGOSYAN, Maryna; Colchester East Hants Hlth Ctr, 600 Abenaki Rd, Truro NS B2N 5A1; (Ukraine)'88; FRCPC; Psy. Staff, Colchester East Hants Health Centre; (902)625-1452

POHANI, Gina; North York Gen Hosp, 4001 Leslie St, North York ON M2K 1E1; Wes'05; CCFP; Staff, North York General Hospital; (416)756-6617

POHL, Andrea; CHUM-Hop St-Luc, 1058 rue Saint-Denis, Montreal QC H2X 3J4; University of Rostock (Other Foreign)'00; FRCPC; Anes. Staff, Centre Hospitalier l'Université De Montréal (CHUM) - Hôpital Saint-luc; (514)890-8000 x36581

POHL, Daniela; Children's Hosp Eastern Ont, 401 Smyth Rd, Ottawa ON K1H 8L1; Gottingen (Germany)'93; Staff, Children's Hospital of Eastern Ontario (CHEO); (613)737-7600 x3504; Fax. (613)736-4886.

POHLMANN-EDEN, Bernhard; Queen Elizabeth II HSC-Halifax, 3838-1796 Summer St, Halifax NS B3H 3A7; Heidelberg (Germany)'81; Dir Epilepsy Prog, Queen Elizabeth II Health Sciences Centre - Halifax Infirmary Site; Prof Neurology, Pharmacology & Psychology, Dalhousie University; Langs: German; (902)473-6501; Fax. (902)473-4438.

POHU, Andre; 380 boul Cartier O, Laval QC H7N 2K2; Mon'64; Cardiol (P.Q.). Staff Cardiol, Centre Hospitalier Fleury; (450)663-0012; Fax. (450)663-3228.

POILLY, Diane N F; Cornwall Comm Hosp-Mcconnell, 840 McConnell Ave, Cornwall ON K6H 5S5; Sher'90; CCFP; CCFP(E. M.); Staff, Glengarry Memorial Hospital; Staff, Cornwall Community Hospital; Langs: Bilingual(English/French); (613)938-4240; Fax. (613)347-1691.

POINTER, Rohan; CSSS du Nord de Lanaudière, 1000 boul Sainte-Anne, St-Charles-Brromee QC J6E 6J2; Mon'00; CCFP; Staff, Centre Hospitalier Régional de Lanaudière; (450)759-8222; Fax. (450)759-7969.

POIRIER, Alain; Min de la Sante Sociaux de QC, 1075 ch Sainte-Foy, Quebec QC G1S 2M1; Sher'81; MSc(CommunHealth); CSPQ; FRCPC; IntMed (Public Health); CommunMed. Médecin, Ministere de la sante et des services sociaux du Quebec; Prof Community Health, Universite de Montreal; (418)266-6701

POIRIER, André; CSSS de Trois-Rivières, 1991 boul du Carmel, Trois-Rivieres QC G8Z 3R9; Laval'84; Microbio & Infect Dis (P.Q.); MedMicrobiol. Staff, CSSS de Trois-Rivières; (819)697-3333 x68881; andre_poirier_chtr@ssss.gouv.qc.ca.

POIRIER, Angela M; Atlantic Med Clinic, PO Box 29119 Rpo Hal Shop Ctre, Halifax NS B3L 4T8; Dal'90; Staff Privil, IWK Health Centre; Staff Privil, Queen Elizabeth II Health Sciences Centre - Victoria General Site; Langs: Bilingual(English/French); (902)455-4333; Fax. (902)455-4034.

POIRIER, Annick; CSSS du Rocher-Perce, CP 3300 451 rue Mgr Ross E, Chandler QC G0C 1K0; Mon'04; FRCSC; ObstGyn. Staff, Centre Hospitalier de Chandler; (418)689-2261

POIRIER, Brigitte; Ctr Hosp Affilie-St-Sacrement, 1050 ch Sainte-Foy, Quebec QC G1S 4L8; Laval'97; FRCSC; GenSurg (Breast Cancer); General Surgical Oncology (P.Q.). Staff Med Specialist, Centre Hospitalier Affilié Universitaire de Québec - Hôpital du St-Sacrement; Langs: Bilingual(French/English); (418)682-7511

POIRIER, Carmen M; 217-1111 Olympic Way SE, Calgary AB T2G 0E6; Alb'86; CCFP; (403)538-8881; Fax. (403)262-6079.

POIRIER, Carole D; 105-185 av Acadie, Dieppe NB E1A 1G6; Sher'00; CCFP; (506)862-4182

POIRIER, Caroline; Centre Hosp Honore-Mercier, 2750 boul Laframboise, Saint-Hyacinthe QC J2S 4Y6; Sher'94; FRCSC; ObstGyn. Staff Gyn, Centre Hospitalier Honore-Mercier; (450)771-3333

POIRIER, Catherine; CSSS de la Matapedia, 135 av Gaetan-Archambault, Amqui QC G5J 2K5; Laval'07; Staff, CSSS de la Matapedia; (418)629-2211

POIRIER, Charles D; CHUM-Hop Notre-Dame, 1560 rue Sherbrooke E, Montreal QC H2L 4M1; Ott'90; FRCPC; IntMed (Epidemiology); Respir. Staff, McGill University Health Centre - Royal Victoria Hospital; Staff, Centre Hospitalier l'Université de Montréal (CHUM) - Hôpital Notre-Dame; assoc Prof, Universite de Montreal; assoc Prof, McGill University; Langs: English; French; (514)890-8000 x25151; Fax. (514)412-7516; charles.poirier.chum@ssss.gouv.qc.ca.

POIRIER, Claude; CHUM-Hotel-Dieu, 3840 rue Saint-Urbain, Montreal QC H2W 1T8; Sher'98; FRCPC; IntMed; Respir. Staff, Centre Hospitalier l'Université de Montréal (CHUM) - Hôtel-Dieu; (514)890-8000

POIRIER, Claude; 600-4975 boul de la Rive-Sud, Levis QC G6V 4Z5; Laval'70; Cardiol (P.Q.) (Insurance Medicine). ac Staff, Hôtel-Dieu de Lévis; Consultant, Centre Hospitalier Paul-Gilbert; Med Consultant, Desjardins Securite Financiere; Langs: English; (418)833-5750

POIRIER, David; Hotel-Dieu d'Arthabaska, 5 rue des Hospitalieres, Victoriaville QC G6P 6N2; Laval'98; LMCC; Staff Emerg Med, Hotel-Dieu d'Arthabaska; Physician, CLSC-CHSLD des Etchemins; (819)357-2030 x2059; Fax. (819)357-6040; poirierdavid@hotmail.com.

POIRIER, Denis; Clinique Med du Quartier Latin, 905 boul Rene-Levesque E, Montreal QC H2L 5B1; Sher'77; LMCC; Fam Med, Hôpital de réadaptation Villa Medica; (514)285-5500; Fax. (514)285-2226.

POIRIER, Denise; Clinique Medicale St-Zotique, RR 2 681 rue Principale, Saint-Zotique QC J0P 1Z0; Mon'78; (450)267-3535; Fax. (450)267-8632.

POIRIER, Diane; Clinique Externe Psychiatrie, 404-8000 boul Langelier, Saint-Leonard QC H1P 3K2; Sher'82; FRCPC; Psy. Staff, Hopital Louis-H Lafontaine; (514)527-3607; Fax. (514)527-9248.

POIRIER, Diane; CSSS Richelieu-Yamaska, 2750 boul Laframboise, Saint-Hyacinthe QC J2S 4Y8; Mon'87; Staff, Centre Hospitalier Honore-Mercier; (450)771-3334; Fax. (450)771-3552.

POIRIER, Dominique; CSSS de Montmagny-l'Islet, 350 boul Tache O, Montmagny QC G5V 3R8; Laval'03; Staff, CSSS de Montmagny-L'Islet; (418)248-0630; dominique.poirier@gmf.gouv.qc.ca.

POIRIER, Eric; Ctr Hosp Affilie-St-Sacrement, 1050 ch Sainte-Foy, Quebec QC G1S 4L8; Laval'01; FRCSC; GenSurg; General Surgical Oncology (P.Q.). Staff, Centre Hospitalier Affilié Universitaire de Québec - Hôpital du St-Sacrement; (418)682-7511

POIRIER, Eric; Polyclinique de l'Anse, 78 rue Lemaire, Sept-Iles QC G4S 1A3; Mon'90; CCFP; Staff, Centre Hospitalier Regional de Sept-Iles; (418)962-1212

POIRIER, Eve-Marie; CHUS-Hop Fleurimont, 3001 12e av N, Sherbrooke QC J1H 5N4; Sher'02; CCFP; CCFP(E.M.); Staff, Centre Hospitalier Universitaire de Sherbrooke-Hopital Fleurimont; (819)346-1110

POIRIER, Francine; Centre Hosp Honore-Mercier, 2750 boul Laframboise, Saint-Hyacinthe QC J2S 4Y8; Sher'10; CCFP; Staff, Centre Hospitalier Honore-Mercier; (450)771-3333

POIRIER, Francois; Hotel-Dieu de Levis, 143 rue Wolfe, Levis QC G6V 3Z1; Laval'86; FRCPC; Psy. Staff, Hôtel-Dieu de Lévis; (418)835-7155; Fax. (418)835-7199.

POIRIER, Gerald; Clinique Medicale GMF-1851, 101-1851 rue Sherbrooke E, Montreal QC H2K 4L5; Laval'73; (514)524-7564; Fax. (514)527-5251; gepoirier@videotron.ca.

POIRIER, Germain; Hop Charles LeMoyne, 3120 boul Taschereau, Greenfield Park QC J4V 2H1; McG'96; FRCPC; IntMed (Intensive Care); Critical Care Medicine (P.Q.). Staff, Hopital Charles LeMoyne; adj Prof, Universite de Sherbrooke; (450)466-5000; Fax. (450)466-5768.

POIRIER, Helene; Hop Maisonneuve-Rosemont, 5689 rue Rosemont, Montreal QC H1T 2H1; Mon'81; FRCPC; Psy (Hospital Psychiatry). Staff, Hôpital Regional Rimouski; Langs: English; (514)252-3400 x4727

POIRIER, Henri W; Centre Rouville, 300 rue du Docteur-Poulin, Marieville QC J3M 1L7; Mon'65; (450)460-4475

POIRIER, Hugues; CSSS des Iles, 430 ch Principal, Cap-aux-Meules QC G4T 1R9; Mon'93; FRCPC; Psy. Staff, Hôpital de l'Archipel; (418)986-2121; Fax. (416)986-3770.

POIRIER, Isabelle; CSSS de Rimouski-Neigette, CP 3150 Succ A 150 av Rouleau, Rimouski QC G5L 5T1; Laval'97; FRCSC; ObstGyn. Staff, Hôpital Regional Rimouski; (418)723-7851

POIRIER, Jacques; 288 boul Larochelle, Repentigny QC J6A 8K4; Mon'78; Staff, Centre Hospitalier Pierre le Gardeur; Langs: English; (450)581-2120; Fax. (450)581-2122.

POIRIER, Louise; Hop Maisonneuve-Rosemont, 5415 boul de l'Assomption, Montreal QC H1T 2M4; Mon'84; Microbio & Infect Dis (P.Q.); MedMicrobiol. Staff, Hopital Maisonneuve-Rosemont; (514)252-3400 x4524; Fax. (514)252-3898.

POIRIER, Lysane; Hop Santa Cabrini Ospedale, 5655 rue Saint-Zotique E, Montreal QC H1T 1P7; McG'89; FRCPC; IntMed; Endocrin (P.Q.); Endocrin&Metab. ac Membre, Hôpital Santa Cabrini Ospedale; adj Prof/ac Personnel, St Mary's Hospital Centre; Prof, McGill University; (514)252-6000

POIRIER, Madeleine; 5415 boul de l'Assomption, Montreal QC H1T 2M4; McG'98; ABS; FASCRS; FRCS; MCh; MPH; MSc; FRCSC; GenSurg (Colon & Rectal Surgery). Staff, Hopital Maisonneuve-Rosemont; Langs: English; (514)252-3822; Fax. (514)252-0896; madeleine.poirier@mail.mcgill.ca.

POIRIER, Manon; College des Medecins du Quebec, 2170 boul Rene-Levesque O, Montreal QC H3H 2T8; Sher'87; Staff, Pavillon Notre-Dame de la Merci; (514)933-4441; Fax. (514)933-4668.

POIRIER, Marc J; CSSS de Papineau, 155 rue Maclaren E, Gatineau QC J8L 0C2; Ott'89; Staff, CH-CHSLD de Papineau - Pavillon du centre hospitalier; Staff, Hôpital de Papineau; Langs: English; French; (819)986-4415

POIRIER, Marie-Andree; Polyclinique d'Argenteuil, 201-551 rue Berry, Lachute QC J8H 1S4; Laval'06; CCFP; (450)562-3751

POIRIER, Michel; CSSS de la Haute-Yamaska, 205 boul Leclerc O, Granby QC J2G 1T7; Laval'95; LMCC; Staff, Centre Hospitalier de Granby; Langs: English; (450)375-1161; Fax. (450)375-7740.

POIRIER, Mylene; Dr Georges-L Dumont Reg Hosp, 330 av Universite, Moncton NB E1C 2Z3; Sher'05; FRCPC; Psy. Staff, Dr Georges-L-Dumont University Hospital Centre; (506)862-4000

POIRIER, Nancy C; Hôpital Ste-Justine, 3175 ch Cote-Sainte-Catherine, Montreal QC H3T 1C5; Mon'92; FRCSC; Cardiovasc&ThorSurg (P.Q.) (Pediatric Cardiac Surgery); CardSurg. Staff, Hôpital Ste-Justine; Staff, Institut de Cardiologie de Montréal; Langs: Bilingual(French/English); (514)345-4676; Fax. (514)345-4917.

POIRIER, Paul; Hôpital Laval, 2725 ch Sainte-Foy, Quebec QC G1V 4G5; Laval'92; BHSc; PhD; FACC; FAHA; MMedSci; FRFPS; FRCPC; IntMed (Diabetology); Cardiol. Staff Cardiac Prevention & Rehab Program Inst de Cardiol et de Pneumologie IVCPQ, Hôpital Laval; Prof, Université Laval; (418)656-4767; Fax. (418)656-4562; paul.poirier@crhl.ulaval.ca.

POIRIER, Robert F; 600-157 Hampton Rd, Rothesay NB E2E 2R3; Dal'97; CCFP; (506)847-2141; Fax. (506)847-2147.

POIRIER, Roger M; CSSS de Memphremagog, 50 rue Saint-Patrice E, Magog QC J1X 3X3; Mon'84; FRCPC; Psy (Industrial Occupational Medicine). Staff, Centre Hospitalier et CLSC de Memphremagog; Chief Dept of Psy, Hopital Maisonneuve-Rosemont; Asst Prof Psychiatry, Universite de Montreal; (819)843-3381

POIRIER, Simon; CHUQ-Ctr Hosp Univ Laval, 2705 boul Laurier, Quebec QC G1V 4G2; Laval'06; FRCPC; Psy. Staff, Centre Hospitalier Universitaire de Quebec-CHUL; (418)525-4444

POIRIER, Steven F j; Kincardine Community Med Clin, 44 Queen St, Kincardine ON N2Z 3C1; NOSM'10; CCFP; (519)396-6747; Fax. (519)396-3810.

POIRIER, Suzanne; Terrasses Versailles, 107-6923 boul les Galeries d'A, Anjou QC H1M 3X6; Mon'69; Langs: Bilingual(French/English); (514)852-3898; Fax. (514)852-5843.

POIRIER, Vincent; MUHC-Montreal Gen Hosp, 1650 av Cedar, Montreal QC H3G 1A4; McG'96; FRCPC; EmergMed. Staff, McGill University Health Centre - Montreal General Campus; (514)934-1934 x42501; Fax. (514)934-8421.

POIRIER-GROULX, Lise C; Orleans Medical-Dental Centre, 400C-2555 St. Joseph Blvd, Orleans ON K1C 1S6; Ott'84; CCFP; FCFP; (613)830-7774; Fax. (613)835-7549.

POISSANT, Jean-Francois; Ctr Hosp du Centre la Mauricie, 50 119e rue, Shawinigan-Sud QC G9P 5K1; Mon'99; FRCSC; GenSurg. Staff, Centre Hospitalier du Centre la Mauricie; Langs: Bilingual(French/English); (819)536-7500

POISSON, Andre; Clinique Med de Mistassini, 148 boul Saint-Michel, Dolbeau-Mistassini QC G8L 5J8; Laval'85; Langs: English; (418)276-3161; Fax. (418)276-4581.

POISSON, Frederic; CSSS de Rimouski-Neigette, CP 3150 Succ A 150 av Rouleau, Rimouski QC G5L 5T1; NuclearMed (P.Q.). Staff, Hôpital Regional Rimouski; (418)724-3000

POISSON, Jacques; CSSS Haut Richelieu-Rouville, 978 boul du Seminaire N, St-Jean-sur-Richel QC J3A 1E5; Laval'67; AB; FRCSC; GenSurg. (450)358-2572

POISSON, Lucille J; U of Ottawa Hlth Services, 300-100 Marie Curie Pvt, Ottawa ON K1N 1A2; Wes'92; CCFP; Staff, University of Ottawa Health Services; Langs: Italian; French; (613)564-3950; Fax. (613)564-6627; lpjz@sympatico.ca.

POISSON, Marco; Hotel-Dieu d'Arthabaska, 5 rue des Hospitalieres, Victoriaville QC G6P 6N2; Mon'03; Staff, Hotel-Dieu d'Arthabaska; Langs: English; (819)357-2030

POISSON, Michel; CHUM-Hotel-Dieu, 3840 rue Saint-Urbain, Montreal QC H2W 1T8; Mon'75; FRCPC; MedMicrobiol; Microbio & Infect Dis (P.Q.). ac Staff, Centre Hospitalier l'Université de Montréal (CHUM) - Hôtel-Dieu; (514)890-8000 x14633; michel.poisson.chum@ssss.gouv.qc.ca.

POISSON, Mireille; Clin Med Riviere-du Moulin, 1388 boul du Saguenay E, Chicoutimi QC G7H 1G8; Sher'07; CCFP; (418)549-3564; Fax. (418)549-8463.

POITEVIN, Anne-Marie; CHUQ-St-Francois-d'Assise, 10 rue de l'Espinay, Quebec QC G1L 3L5; Laval'04; CCFP; Staff, Centre Hospitalier Universitaire De Québec - Pavillon De St-françois-d'assise; (418)525-4444 x53710; Fax. (418)525-4322.

POITEVIN, David G; 206-974 Queen St E, Sault Ste. Marie ON P6A 2C5; Tor'72; (705)759-1234 x2310

POITIER, Myles R; MCI The Doctors Office, 387-25 Peel Centre Dr, Brampton ON L6T 3R5; St Lucia (Dominican Republic)'92; CCFP; (905)793-7077

POITRAS, Anick; Dir Sante Publique de la Capit, 2400 rue d'Estimauville, Quebec QC G1E 7G9; Laval'95; CCFP; Staff, Centre Hospitalier Universitaire de Quebec-CHUL; (418)666-7000; anickpoitras@ssss.gouv.qc.ca.

POITRAS, Benoit P; Hôpital Ste-Justine, 7905-3175 ch Cote-Sainte-Cathe, Montreal QC H3T 1C5; Laval'65; FAAOS; FRCSC; OrthSurg (Pediatric Orthopedics). Chef, Hôpital Ste-Justine; Ac Staff, Shriners Hospitals For Children - Canada; Fellow, Paediatric Orthopaedic Society of America & Scoliosis Research Society; Langs: Bilingual(French/English); (514)345-4876; Fax. (514)345-4755; benoit_poitras@ssss.gouv.qc.ca.

POITRAS, Daniel; CLSC de Gatineau, 101-80 av Gatineau, Gatineau QC J8T 4J3; Ott'93; (819)966-6550 x1510

POITRAS, Daniel; 821 Tsse Lecavalier, Laval QC H7X 2C5; Mon'80; Staff, Hôpital de Saint-Eustache; Langs: English; French; (450)689-0128; Fax. (450)689-1010.

POITRAS, Francois; CSSS de Memphremagog, 50 rue Saint-Patrice E, Magog QC J1X 3X3; Sher'80; Ac Staff, Centre Hospitalier et CLSC de Memphremagog; (819)843-3381; Fax. (819)843-2786; francois.poitras@cgocable.ca.

POITRAS, Gaetan; Clinique Med Jean-Talon-Pie IX, 4679 rue Jean-Talon E, Saint-Leonard QC H1S 1K3; Mon'83; Langs: Spanish; English; (514)374-5901; Fax. (514)374-1668.

POITRAS, Guy; 285-1750 boul Marie-Victorin, Longueuil QC J4G 1A5; Mon'87; Staff, Centre Hospitalier Pierre Boucher; (450)442-9531

POITRAS, Jacqueline E H; 305-770 Broadview Ave, Ottawa ON K2A 3Z3; Tor'08; CCFP; (613)728-7700

POITRAS, Julien; Hotel-Dieu de Levis, 143 rue Wolfe, Levis QC G6V 3Z1; Laval'91; CCFP; CCFP(E.M.); EmergMed. Staff Emergency Med, Hôtel-Dieu de Lévis; Staff Emerg Med, CSSS de Montmagny-L'Islet; assoc Doyen Clinical Affairs, Université Laval; (418)835-7121

POITRAS, Liette; Clin Med Fam d'Edmundston, 52 av Bateman, Edmundston NB E3V 4A4; Sher'87; CCFP; Staff, Hôpital regional d'Edmundston; (506)735-8442; Fax. (506)739-6271.

POITRAS, Lucie; CIM, 1700-440 boul Rene-Levesque O, Montreal QC H2Z 1V7; Sher'84; Staff Prof Services, Hôpital Ste-Justine; (514)393-4563; Fax. (514)393-4598; lpoitras@cim-conseil.qc.ca.

POITRAS, Marie-Josee; 201-600 boul Dieppe, Dieppe NB E1A 9J8; Laval'99; CCFP; Staff, Dr Georges-L-Dumont University Hospital Centre; Physician, Clinique Medical Elmwood & Clinique Providence; Langs: English; (506)859-4772; Fax. (506)859-0587.

POITRAS, Michael P; Glenora Med Clinic, 310-10230 142 St NW, Edmonton AB T5N 3Y6; Alb'79; CCFP; Staff, Covenant Health - Misericordia Community Hospital; (780)455-3311; Fax. (780)451-4404.

POITRAS, Nathalie; Hopital Regional D'Edmundston, 275 boul Hebert, Edmundston NB E3V 4E4; Sher'05; CCFP; Staff, Hôpital regional d'Edmundston; (506)739-2200

POITRAS, Pierre; CSSS de Laval, 1755 boul Rene-Laennec, Laval QC H7M 3L9; Mon'70; Peds. Staff, Hopital de la Cite de la santé; Langs: English; (450)668-1010; ppoitras@videotron.ca.

POITRAS, Pierre; CHUM-Hop St-Luc, 1058 rue Saint-Denis, Montreal QC H2X 3J4; Laval'72; Gastroent. Staff, Centre Hospitalier l'Université De Montréal (CHUM) - Hôpital Saint-luc; assoc Prof, Universite de Montreal; (514)890-8000; Fax. (514)412-7314.

POITRAS, Rejean; CSSS de Laval, 280 boul du Roi-du-Nord, Laval QC H7L 4L2; Mon'75; Staff, Hopital de la Cite de la santé; (450)622-5110; Fax. (450)622-4150.

POKRANT, Colleen M; Thunder Bay Reg HSC-T-Bay, 980 Oliver Rd, Thunder Bay ON P7B 6V4; Man'85; FRCSC; ObstGyn. Staff, Thunder Bay Regional Health Sciences Centre; (807)684-6000

POKROY, Robert; 10816 124 St NW, Edmonton AB T5M 0H3; Pretoria (South Africa)'86; MB ChB; FRCPC; Neur. Staff, University of Alberta Hospital; Staff, Royal Alexandra Hospital; (780)413-6640; Fax. (780)455-7992.

POKRUPA, Ronald P; Kingston Gen Hosp, 3-76 Stuart St, Kingston ON K7L 2V7; Wes'75; DAB; FRCSC; Neursurg. Att Staff, Kingston General Hospital; Assoc Prof, Queen's University; Langs: English; French; (613)549-6666 x6282; Fax. (613)548-1346.

POLACK, Stanley S G; 203-300 Brae Rd, Duncan BC V9L 3T8; Wes'71; DAB; FRCSC; Ophth. Consultant, Cowichan District Hospital; Ophthalmology, Chemainus Health Care Centre; (250)748-2922; Fax. (250)748-9647.

POLACK, Zenith E; 101-73 Boulder Blvd, Stony Plain AB T7Z 1V6; Alb'71; Staff, Covenant Health - Misericordia Community Hospital; (780)963-3394; Fax. (780)963-6550.

POLAK, Patrick; Ctr Hosp de Verdun, 4000 boul Lasalle, Verdun QC H4G 2A3; Angers (France)'94; Staff, Centre Hospitalier de Verdun; (514)362-1000 x2489; Fax. (514)765-7314.

POLAK, Vivian A; Minto Mapleton Family Health T, 11 Andrews Dr W, Drayton ON N0G 1P0; Alb'00; FRCPC; Psy (Reproductive Psy). Staff, Wellington Reproductive Psychiatry Program; Langs: Italian; French; Spanish; (519)803-4718; Fax. (519)846-2097.

POLAK-FURIGAY, Yvetta M; Villa Caritas, 16515 88 Ave NW, Edmonton AB T5R 0A4; Alb'00; FRCPC; Psy. Staff, Alberta Hospital Edmonton; (780)342-6552; Fax. (780)342-6579.

POLAN, Kerstin M; 6497 Jeanne d'Arc Blvd N, Orleans ON K1C 2R1; Dublin (Ireland)'78; (613)841-8500; Fax. (613)841-5310.

POLAN, William F; 6497 Jeanne d'Arc Blvd N, Orleans ON K1C 2R1; Dublin (Ireland)'78; MB ChB; BAO; LRCPSI; Court Staff, Cornwall Community Hospital; Staff, Residence St-Louis-Sisters of Charity of Ottawa; (613)841-8500; Fax. (613)841-5310.

POLAND, George; Medistat Med Familiale, 4965 rue Saint-Pierre, Pierrefonds QC H9H 5M9; McG'68; (514)624-4774; Fax. (514)624-4704.

POLANSKI, Annette C; Quinte HC Corp-Belleville Gen, 265 Dundas St E, Belleville ON K8N 5A9; Alb'99; FRCPC; DiagRad. Staff, QHC Belleville General; (613)969-7400

POLASEK, Petr; Cardiology Associates, 2606 Pandosy St, Kelowna BC V1Y 1V6; Karlova (Czech Republic)'84; FACC; FRCPC; IntMed (Adult Cardiology); Cardiol. Consultant Cardiol, Cariboo Memorial Hospital and Health Centre; Clinical Asst Prof, University of British Columbia; Langs: Czech; Serbian; Croatian; (250)762-9211; Fax. (250)762-8337; petr_polasek@telus.net.

POLAY, Michael D; Care Point Med Centre, 1623 Commercial Dr, Vancouver BC V5L 3Y3; Cal'96; (604)254-5554; Fax. (604)254-9177.

POLDES, Anu; City Centre Med Clinic, 130-5 Park Home Ave, North York ON M2N 6L4; Tor'74; CCFP; FCFP; Court Staff Privil, North York General Hospital; (416)730-9588; Fax. (416)590-9371.

POLDRE, Peeter A; 2075 Bayview Ave, Toronto ON M4N 3M5; Tor'78; EdD; FRCPC; IntMed (Medical Education); Hem. Staff, Sunnybrook Health Sciences Centre; Physician, Sunnybrook Edmond Odette Cancer Ctre; Prof Med, University of Toronto; Langs: Estonian; (416)480-4757; peeter.poldre@sunnybrook.ca.

POLE, Chakrabarty L; 108-14914 104 Ave, Surrey BC V3R 1M7; Bombay (India)'76; MB BS; LMCC; FRCPC; Psy (Psycho Pharmacology). Dir CME, Fraser Valley Psychiatric Association; Langs: Hindi; Gujarati; Marathi; (604)589-2426; Fax. (604)589-3225; chakpole@shaw.ca.

POLE, Meena; University Park Med Clinic, 182 University Park Dr, Regina SK S4V 1A3; Bombay (India)'86; Physician, Regina General Hospital; Staff, Pasqua Hospital; (306)789-5802; Fax. (306)789-3443.

POLEMIDIOTIS, George J; West Vaughan Med Centre, 3900 Rutherford Rd, Woodbridge ON L4H 3G8; Ott'94; CCFP; (905)417-5461; Fax. (905)417-5463.

POLESKI, Steven A; Ottawa Eye Clinic, 680 Montreal Rd, Ottawa ON K1K 0T3; McG'80; DAB; FRCSC; Ophth (Cataract & Refractive). Ac Staff, The Ottawa Hospital - Riverside Campus; Ac Staff, Montfort Hospital; Court Staff, Children's Hospital of Eastern Ontario (CHEO); Asst Prof, University of Ottawa; Langs: English; French; (613)745-7844; Fax. (613)745-5957.

POLEVOY, Terry A; 903-570 University Ave E, Waterloo ON N2K 4P2; Wayne(MI) (USA)'70; Peds (Acne Treatment). (519)725-2263; Fax. (519)725-4953; drpolevoy@yahoo.com.

POLEY, Rachel; Kingston Gen Hosp, 76 Stuart St, Kingston ON K7L 2V7; Dal'07; FRCPC; EmergMed. Staff, Kingston General Hospital; (613)549-6666

POLIDOULIS, Irene; SGH Medical Mall, 309-3030 Lawrence Ave E, Scarborough ON M1P 2T7; Tor'84; FCFP; CCFP; FCFP; Asst Prof, University of Toronto; Langs: Greek; (416)439-2662; Fax. (416)439-0760.

POLIMENI, Christine J; Oakfield Med Clinic, 102-1021 Court Ave, Winnipeg MB R2P 1V7; Man'90; CCFP; (204)388-3062; Fax. (204)388-7660.

POLIMENI, Joseph O; 17 Wing Medical Clinic, PO Box 17000 Stn Forces, Winnipeg MB R3J 3Y5; Man'87; FRCPC; Psy (Schizophrenia). Assoc Prof Psy, University of Manitoba; Langs: Italian; (204)833-2500 x5086; Fax. (204)833-2667; jpolimeni@shaw.ca.

POLIQUIN, Denis; Ctr Med Soleil St-Jean Sur-Ric, 120-383 boul du Seminaire N, St-Jean-Sur-Richel QC J3B 8C5; Mon'68; LMCC; FRCSC; GenSurg. ac Staff, Hôpital du Haut-Richelieu; Langs: English; French; (450)347-7557

POLIQUIN, Marc; Ctr Hosp de Verdun, 4000 boul Lasalle, Verdun QC H4G 2A3; McG'85; FRCPC; IntMed; Gastroent (P.Q.). Staff, Centre Hospitalier de Verdun; (514)362-1000

POLIQUIN, Sophie A; McArthur Med Centre, 390 McArthur Ave, Vanier ON K1L 6N6; Ott'09; CCFP; (613)741-1134

POLIS, Ilona C; 301 Metcalfe St, Ottawa ON K2P 1R9; Lodz (Poland)'81; FRCPC; Psy. Langs: Polish; (613)565-3479; Fax. (613)565-8763.

POLIS, Tomasz; The Ottawa Hosp-Civic Campus, 1053 Carling Ave, Ottawa ON K1Y 4E9; Lodz (Poland)'81; FRCPC; Anes. Staff Anes, The Ottawa Hospital - Civic Campus; Asst Prof Anes, University of Ottawa; (613)761-4169; Fax. (613)761-5209.

POLJICAK, Mate; CHUM-Hop Notre-Dame, 1560 rue Sherbrooke E, Montreal QC H2L 4M1; Zagreb (Croatia)'71; FACS; MRCS; CSPQ; LMCC; FRCSC; GenSurg (Breast Surgery); General Surgical Oncology (P.Q.). ac Staff Surg, Centre Hospitalier l'Université de Montréal (CHUM) - Hôpital Notre-Dame; assoc Prof Surg, Universite de Montreal; Langs: English; Croatian; (514)890-8000 x26607; Fax. (514)412-7821; mpol@sympatico.ca.

POLLACK, Sheldon V; The Two Hundred, 218-200 St Clair Ave W, Toronto ON M4V 1R1; Tor'74; FAAD; MD; FRCPC; Derm (Cosmetic Dermatology). Court Staff Med, Women's College Hospital; Dir, Toronto Cosmetic Skin Surgery Centre; Assoc Prof Med(Derm), University of Toronto; (416)961-7731; Fax. (416)961-7673.

POLLAK, Michael N; SMBD Jewish Gen Hosp, 3755 ch Cote-Sainte-Catherine, Montreal QC H3T 1E2; McG'77; MedOncol; IntMed (Research). Staff, Sir Mortimer B Davis Jewish General; Scientist, Lady Davis Research Institue; Chair Alexandra-Goldfarb, McGill University; Langs: English; French; (514)340-8222 x5527; michael.pollak@mcgill.ca.

POLLAK, P Timothy; HSC-Faculty of Med, 1468-3330 Hospital Dr NW, Calgary AB T2N 4N1; Wes'80; PhD(Pharmacol); FACP; ABIM; FRCPC; IntMed (Clinical Pharmacology). (403)210-8694; Fax. (403)210-8723; pollak@dal.ca.

POLLANEN, Michael S; Office of the Chief Coroner, 200-26 Grenville St, Toronto ON M7A 2G9; Tor'99; PhD; BSc; FRCPC; AnatPath (Forensic Pathology). (416)314-4040

POLLARD, Alan; Mount Sinai Hosp, 1190-600 University Ave, Toronto ON M5G 1X5; Cambridge (England)'54; FRCP; FRCPath; LMCC; Staff, Mount Sinai Hospital; (416)586-5114

POLLARD, Brian A; St Michael's Hosp, 30 Bond St, Toronto ON M5B 1W8; Tor'96; BSc; MEd; FRCPC; Anes (Regional Anesthesia). Staff, St Michael's Hospital; Assoc Prof, University of Toronto; (416)864-5071; Fax. (416)864-6014.

POLLARD, Jeffrey K; Calgary Heart Centre, 100-3280 Hospital Dr NW, Calgary AB T2N 4Z6; Pennsylvania (USA)'88; FRCSC; ObstGyn. Staff, Foothills Medical Centre; Physician, Health Research Innovation Centre; (403)289-9269; jeffrey-pollard@calgaryhealthregion.ca.

POLLE, Mark R; Red Lake Family Health Team, PO Box 311, Red Lake ON P0V 2M0; Man'99; CCFP; FCFP; (807)727-2617; markpolle@yahoo.ca.

POLLET, Virginie; Health Sciences Centre, 820 Sherbrook St, Winnipeg MB R3A 1R9; Staff, Health Sciences Centre; (204)774-8511

POLLETT, Aaron F; Mount Sinai Hosp, 6 500 9-600 University Ave, Toronto ON M5G 1X5; Ott'95; FRCPC; AnatPath. Staff Path, Mount Sinai Hospital; Lecturer, University of Toronto; (416)586-4800 x6452

POLLETT, Harry F L; 517-520 Purves St, North Sydney NS B2A 1E3; Dal'66; DAB; FRCPC; Anes (Pain Management). Consultant, Cape Breton Healthcare Complex; Consultant, Northside General Hospital; Consultant, New Waterford Consolidated Hospital; (902)794-2369; Fax. (902)794-2369; polletth@cbdha.nshealth.ca.

POLLETT, J Anne W; Aim Health Group, 9-6400 Millcreek Dr, Mississauga ON L5N 3E7; Berlin (Germany)'69; DAB; FRCPC; Anes (Pain Management). Langs: German; (905)288-1045; Fax. (905)858-2144.

POLLETT, William G; St Clare's Mercy Hosp, 154 Lemarchant Rd, St. John's NL A1C 5B8; Dal'74; BSc; FRCSC; GenSurg (Colorectal Surgery). Ac Staff, St Clare's Mercy Hospital; Prof, Memorial University Of Newfoundland; (709)777-5611; Fax. (709)777-5929; wpollett@mun.ca.

POLLETTA, Sabrina; CLSC Saint-Hubert, 6800 boul Cousineau, Saint-Hubert QC J3Y 8Z4; Mon'03; CCFP; (450)443-7407

POLLOCK, A Patrice; Wall Street Med Bldg, 370-140 Wall St, Saskatoon SK S7K 1N4; Sask'89; FRCPC; IntMed (Rheumatology). Physician, Saskatoon District Health Board; Associate Clin Prof, University of Saskatchewan; (306)652-4704; Fax. (306)242-4855.

POLLOCK, Andrea E; BC Cancer Agency-Fraser Valley, 13750 96 Ave, Surrey BC V3V 1Z2; Ott'91; CCFP; FCFP; Staff, BC Cancer Agency Fraser Valley Centre; (604)930-4085

POLLOCK, Bradley J; Manitoba Clinic, 790 Sherbrook St, Winnipeg MB R3A 1M3; Man'83; FRCPC; Peds (Pediatric & Adolescent Medicine). Lecturer, University of Manitoba.

POLLOCK, Bruce G; T 109-33 Russell St, Toronto ON M5S 2S1; Tor'79; FRCPC; Psy (Geriatric Psychiatry). Staff, Centre for Addiction & Mental Health (CAMH) - Russell Street Site; Staff, Centre for Addiction & Mental Health (CAMH) - College Street Site; (416)979-6890; Fax. (416)260-4206; bruce.pollock@camh.ca.

POLLOCK, Cheryl; Health Sciences Centre, 300 Prince Philip Dr, St. John's NL A1B 3V6; Mem'01; CCFP; CCFP(E.M.); Staff, Health Sciences Centre; (709)777-6300

POLLOCK, Christopher S; Eye Care Center, H-2550 Willow St, Vancouver BC V5Z 3N9; Ott'07; FRCSC; Ophth. (604)874-4333

POLLOCK, Debbie; Greencrest Pembina Clinic, B-2750 Pembina Hwy, Winnipeg MB R3T 2H8; Man'87.

POLLOCK, I David; 941 O'Connor Dr, East York ON M4B 2S7; Tor'70; Staff Family Practice, Toronto East General Hospital Inc; Staff Family Practice, The Scarborough Hospital - General Campus; (416)751-0477; Fax. (416)750-3090; docpollock@gmail.com.

POLLOCK, J Whitcomb; The Ottawa Hosp-Gen Campus, 501 Smyth Rd Box 502, Ottawa ON K1H 8L6; Ott'01; BA; MScBioPhysics; FRCSC; OrthSurg (Shoulder & Elbow). Staff, The Ottawa Hospital - General Campus; Asst Prof, University of Ottawa; (613)737-8899 x73031; Fax. (613)737-8837.

POLLOCK, Jenni P; 307-615 Main St, Yarmouth NS B5A 1K1; Univ of Cape Town (South Africa)'02; (902)742-4528; Fax. (902)742-7216.

POLLOCK, Neil L; Westminster Med Bldg, 407-625 Fifth Ave, New Westminster BC V3M 1X4; Man'87; (604)717-6200; Fax. (604)526-8952.

POLLOCK, Sandy C; Queensway-Carleton Hosp, 3045 Baseline Rd, Nepean ON K2H 8P4; Ott'79; Staff, Queensway Carleton Hospital; (613)721-2000

POLLOCK, Susan L; Med Hlth Officer Interior Hlth, 1340 Ellis St, Kelowna BC V1Y 9N1; Cal'04; FRCPC; CommunMed. (250)868-7818

POLOMENO, Robert C; Gladstone Med Centre, 4095 rue Tupper, Westmount QC H3Z 3E5; Ott'66; FRCSC; Ophth (Pediatric Ophthalmology). Assoc Staff, Hôpital Ste-Justine; Staff, McGill University Health Centre - Montreal Children's Hospital; assoc Prof, Universite de Montreal; assoc Prof, McGill University; Langs: Italian; French; (514)935-0966; Fax. (514)935-0967.

POLSINELLI, Kristina; R 40-142 Fullarton St, London ON N6A 0A4; Wes'01; CCFP; Staff, Tillsonburg District Memorial Hospital; (519)438-2020; Fax. (519)438-2021.

POLSKY, Joshua N; 511 Erie St E, Windsor ON N9A 3X8; Tor'96; BSc; FRCSC; ObstGyn (Minimal Invasive Surgery). Clin Lecturer, University of Western Ontario; (519)253-6033; Fax. (519)253-6866; jnpolsky@cogeco.ca.

POLSON, Alasdair L; Richmond Med Bldg, 401-2020 Richmond Rd, Victoria BC V8R 6R5; McG'84; FRCPC; IntMed (Critical Care Medicine); Respir. Med TB Clinic/Co-Dir ICU, Vancouver Island Health Authority; (250)995-0211; Fax. (250)995-1443.

POLSON, George A; Hop Ste-Anne, 305 boul des Anciens-Combattan, Ste-Anne-de-Bellev QC H9X 1Y9; McG'82; Staff, Hopital Ste-Anne; (514)457-3440; Fax. (514)457-8466.

POLSON, Herbert A; 106-415 av Bourke, Dorval QC H9S 3W9; McG'76; FACS; BSc; FRCSC; GenSurg (Biliary Surgery). Ac Staff Surg, Lakeshore General Hospital - Pointe Claire; Langs: French; (514)636-9599; Fax. (514)636-3148.

POLSON, Ronald; York-Finch Med Centre, 101-2115 Finch Ave W, North York ON M3N 2V6; Man'85; FRCPC; DiagRad. (416)744-2655; Fax. (416)744-0581.

POLUSHIN, Margaret M; Pleasantview Med Clinic, 11028 51 Ave NW, Edmonton AB T6H 0L4; Alb'82; (780)434-5129; Fax. (780)434-9992.

POLYA, Daniel G; 606-133 Prince William St, Saint John NB E2L 2B5; Melbourne (Australia)'96; FRANZCO; MB BS; MPH; FRCSC; Ophth (Vitreo Retina). (506)642-3277; Fax. (506)642-8934.

POLYAKOV, Gregory M; East Van Med Bldg, 503-1750 10th Ave E, Vancouver BC V5N 5K4; Kharkov (Russia (Federation))'73; FRCSC; GenSurg (Colon & Rectal Surgery). Staff GenSurg, Providence Health Care - Mount Saint Joseph Hospital; Staff, Delta Health Sciences Centre; Langs: Russian; Ukrainian; Italian; (604)707-9171; Fax. (604)707-9181; drgpolyakov@telus.net.

POLYCHRONAKOS, Constantin; MUHC-Montreal Children's Hosp, C 244-2300 rue Tupper, Montreal QC H3H 1P3; Thessaloniki (Greece)'72; FRCPC; Peds; Endocrin (P.Q.). Dir Ped Endocrin, McGill University Health Centre - Montreal Children's Hospital; Staff, Research Inst.; Prof Dept of Peds, McGill University; Langs: Greek; English; (514)412-4315

POLYHRONOPOULOS, Gerry; Centre Med Brunswick, 203-955 rue Saint-Jean, Pointe-Claire QC H9R 5K3; McG'03; GenSurg. Staff, Lakeshore General Hospital - Pointe Claire; (519)459-0248; Fax. (519)426-9059.

POLYHRONOPOULOS, Spiro; Langley Mem Hosp, 22051 Fraser Hwy, Langley BC V3A 4H4; Alb'90; CCFP; CCFP(E.M.); FCFP; Staff, Langley Memorial Hospital; Langs: Greek; (604)514-6088

POMER, Edward S; 66B Wellesley St E, Toronto ON M4Y 1G2; Ott'72; Staff Family Practice, Toronto General Hospital - UHN; (416)964-7380; Fax. (416)964-3797.

POMERLEAU, Anne; Ctr Hosp Rouyn-Noranda, 4 9e rue, Rouyn-Noranda QC J9X 2B2; Sher'10; CCFP; Staff, Centre Hospitalier Rouyn-Noranda; (819)764-5131

POMERLEAU, Claude V; 999 17e rue, Saint-Georges QC G5Y 4W1; Laval'72; CSPQ; FRCSC; ObstGyn. (418)228-8311; Fax. (418)228-8317; cpomerleau@cgocable.ca.

POMERLEAU, Damien; Clinique Domus Medica, 110-5601 rue Belanger, Montreal QC H1T 1G3; Mon'63; Peds. Langs: English; Spanish; (514)256-5011; Fax. (514)254-9872.

POMERLEAU, Genevieve; Ctr de Readaptation Marie Enfa, 5200 rue Belanger E, Montreal QC H1T 1C9; Laval'05; FRCPC; Peds. Staff, Centre de Réadaptation Marie Enfant du CHU Sainte-Justine; (514)374-1710

POMERLEAU, Guy; CHUQ-Ctr Hosp Univ Laval, 2705 boul Laurier, Quebec QC G1V 4G2; Laval'65; FRCPC; Psy. Chef Psy Services, Centre Hospitalier Universitaire de Quebec-CHUL; Prof, Université Laval; (418)654-2177; Fax. (418)654-2716.

POMERLEAU, Marjorie; Centre Med St-Isidore, 4553 Ste-Catherine St, St Isidore ON K0C 2B0; Ott'08; CCFP; (613)524-3225

POMERLEAU, Robert; CSSS de Beauce-Etchemin, 1515 17e rue, Saint-Georges QC G5Y 4T8; Laval'04; CCFP; CCFP(E.M.); Staff, Centre Hospitalier Beauce-Etchemin; (418)228-2031 x7800; Fax. (418)227-3825.

POMERLEAU, Serge; CSSS de Beauce-Etchemin, 1515 17e rue, Saint-Georges QC G5Y 4T8; Laval'85; FRCSC; GenSurg. Staff, Centre Hospitalier Beauce-Etchemin; (418)228-2031

POMEROY, Carol A K; The Medical Group, 32243 Hurd St, Mission BC V2V 3J9; UBC'90; BSc; Staff, Mission Memorial Hospital; (604)826-6231; Fax. (604)820-1174.

POMIER LAYRARGUES, Gilles; CHUM-Hop Saint-Luc, 1058 rue Saint-Denis, Montreal QC H2X 3J4; Montpellier (France)'77; Gastroent (P.Q.). Staff, Centre Hospitalier l'Université De Montréal (CHUM) - Hôpital Saint-luc; Asst Researcher, Universite de Montreal; (514)890-8000

POMMERVILLE, John; Can-Med Clinical Research Inc, 230-1641 Hillside Ave, Victoria BC V8T 5G1; Ott'78; FRCSC; Urol (Erectile Dysfunction). Consultant Urol, Royal Jubilee Hospital; Physician, Victoria Surg. Clin./South Island Surg. Ctre-Cancer Agency of BC; Lecturer, University of Victoria; Langs: English; French; (250)370-2606; Fax. (250)370-2604; ppomm@pommerville-urology.com.

PON, Caroline; Valley Med Imaging, 102-32475 Simon Ave, Abbotsford BC V2T 5E3; Sask'88; FRCPC; DiagRad (Diagnostic Imaging). (604)859-4888; Fax. (604)859-3714.

PON, Darlene C; Hys Med Centre, 505-11010 101 St NW, Edmonton AB T5H 4B9; Cal'98; MSc; BSc; FRCPC; Peds. (780)414-6812; Fax. (780)428-0852; darlenepon@hotmail.com.

PON, Freddy A; Family Med Clinic, 236-2 Hebert Rd, St Albert AB T8N 5T8; Alb'84; (780)459-2997; Fax. (780)459-2998.

PON, Kucy; Sunnybrook Hlth Sciences Ctre, M1 700-2075 Bayview Ave, Toronto ON M4N 3M5; Sask'96; AAD; FRCPC; Derm (Cosmetic Dermatology). Staff, Sunnybrook Health Sciences Centre; Asst Prof, University of Toronto; (416)480-4908; Fax. (416)480-6897.

POND, Achla; Fredericton Med Clinic, 301-1015 Regent St, Fredericton NB E3B 6H5; Dal'85; Ac Staff, Dr Everett Chalmers Regional Hospital; (506)458-0262; Fax. (506)458-0202.

POND, Donald G; Timmins & Dist Hosp, 700 Ross Ave E, Timmins ON P4N 8P2; Dal'70; FACOG; FRCSC; ObstGyn (Perinatology). Staff, Timmins & District Hospital; (705)267-2131

POND, Stephen D; Fredericton Med Clinic, 301-1015 Regent St, Fredericton NB E3B 6H5; Dal'85; (506)458-0288; Fax. (506)458-0202.

PONESSE, David; 1309 Yonge St PO Box 968, Walkerton ON N0G 2V0; Tor'64; Staff Family Practice, South Bruce Grey Health Centre - Walkerton Site; (519)881-1200; Fax. (519)881-1201.

PONESSE, Jonathan S; Ottawa Children's Treatment, 395 Smyth Rd, Ottawa ON K1H 8L2; Qns'99; BSc(Hon); FRCP; LMCC; FRCPC; Neur (Behavioural Pediatrics). Neurologist Developmental Peds, Children's Hospital of Eastern Ontario (CHEO); Neurologist, Ottawa Children's Treatment Centre; Langs: Bilingual(French/English); (613)737-0871 x4327; jonathanponesse@hotmail.com.

PONETTE, Vincent B; MUHC-Royal Victoria Hosp, 687 av des Pins O, Montreal QC H3A 1A1; McG'02; ObstGyn (Maternal Fetal Medicine). Staff, McGill University Health Centre - Royal Victoria Hospital; (514)934-1934

PONICH, Terry; London HSC-Victoria Campus, PO Box 5010 Stn B 800 Commissioners Rd E, London ON N6A 5W9; McG'82; ABIM(IntMed&Gastroent); FRCPC; FRCPC; Gastroent; IntMed. Staff, London Health Sciences Centre - Victoria Campus; Assoc Prof, University of Western Ontario; (519)685-8500

PONKA, David; Family Med Centre, 75 Bruyere St, Ottawa ON K1N 5C7; McG'98; CCFP; CCFP(E.M.); FCFP; Asst Prof Dept of Family Med, University of Ottawa; Langs: Czech; French; (613)241-1154

PONKE, Jeffrey; 1 Cedar Dr, Caledon Village ON L7K 1H4; Qns'01; CCFP; (519)927-9516; Fax. (519)927-9518.

PONNAMBALAM, Chris; Rapha Med Centre, 114 Woodlawn Rd, Dartmouth NS B2W 2S7; Pereadeniya (Sri Lanka)'83; CCFP; Staff, Dartmouth General Hospital; Staff, IWK Health Centre; (902)465-4443; Fax. (902)466-8887.

PONNAMPALAM, Arjuna; St Boniface Gen Hosp, 409 Tache Ave, Winnipeg MB R2H 2A6; Man'06; FRCPC; IntMed; Hem. Staff, St Boniface General Hospital; (204)233-8563

PONNAMPALAM, Thurairajasingham; Maxum Prof Centre, 208-385 Silverstar Blvd, Scarborough ON M1V 0E3; Peradeniya (Sri Lanka)'73; MB BS; CCFP; Langs: Tamil; Sinhalese; (416)502-3787; Fax. (416)502-3789; tponn2004@yahoo.com.

PONNET, Natalie; Institut de Cardiologie de Mtl, 5000 rue Belanger, Montreal QC H1T 1C8; Mon'96; Staff, Hôpital de Saint-Eustache; Staff, Institut de Cardiologie de Montréal; (514)376-3300; Fax. (514)593-2540.

PONRAJAH, Sakunthala; Gates of Maple Med Center, 203-2200 Rutherford Rd, Concord ON L4K 5V2; Colombo (Sri Lanka)'92; CCFP; (905)303-7011; Fax. (905)303-7155.

PONSOT, Yves; CHUS-Hop Fleurimont, 3001 12e av N, Sherbrooke QC J1H 5N4; Paris (France)'76; CSPQ; FRCSC; Urol. Consultant Urol, Centre Hospitalier Universitaire de Sherbrooke-Hopital Fleurimont; (819)346-1110; Fax. (819)820-6420.

PONT, Karen; East Kootenay Reg Hosp, 13 24th Ave N, Cranbrook BC V1C 3H9; Stellenbosch (South Africa)'90; Staff, East Kootenay Regional Hospital; (250)426-5281

PONTARINI, Galdino E; First Med Place, 202-170 Queensway W, Mississauga ON L5B 3A8; Tor'77; Court Staff, Trillium Health Centre - Mississauga; Langs: Italian; (905)275-3822; Fax. (905)275-4001.

PONTBRIAND, Eric; Urgence Mineure de Windsor, 23 rue Ambroise-Dearden, Windsor QC J1S 1G8; Mon'02; Staff, Centre Hospitalier Universitaire de Sherbrooke-Hôpital Hôtel-Dieu; Langs: Spanish; English; (819)542-2777 x55245

PONTBRIAND, Robert; Med Sportive de Laval, 3095 Nord Laval A-440 O, Laval QC H7P 4W5; Ott'80; Dip SportMed; (450)682-2324; Fax. (450)688-8566.

PONTI-SGARGI, Michelle G; 1680 Oxford St E PO Box 7010 Stn Main, London ON N5Y 5R8; McM'95; FRCPC; Peds. Physician, Children's Aid Society of London & Middlesex; Langs: Italian; (519)455-9000 x451

PONTIFEX, Alison T; 3215 31 Ave, Vernon BC V1T 2H2; UBC'91; CCFP; (250)545-5034

PONTON, Anne-Marie; Hop Charles LeMoyne, 3120 boul Taschereau, Greenfield Park QC J4V 2H1; Sher'80; FRCPC; Psy (Community Psychiatry). Staff, Hopital Charles LeMoyne; Clin Teach Staff Psy, Universite de Sherbrooke; (450)466-5020; Fax. (450)466-5015; am.ponton@sympatico.ca.

PONTON-BELTRAN, Carlos M; 400-158 Robert Angus Dr, Amherst NS B4H 4R7; Habana (Cuba)'93; CCFP; CCFP(E.M.); Chief Emergency Dept, Cumberland Regional Health Care Center; Asst Prof, Dalhousie University; Langs: Spanish; (902)660-3131; Fax. (902)660-3132.

POOK, John J; St Marys Family Med Centre, PO Box 1288 Stn Main 268 Maiden Lane, St Marys ON N4X 1B8; Wes'74; Court Staff, St Marys Memorial Hospital - Huron Perth Healthcare Alliance; (519)284-3700; Fax. (519)284-1771.

POOLE, Alan; Central Alberta Med Imaging, 4312 54 Ave, Red Deer AB T4N 4M1; Alb'89; FRCPC; DiagRad. (403)343-6172; Fax. (403)346-5044.

POOLE, Alexander J; Whitehorse Gen Hosp, 5 Hospital Rd, Whitehorse YT Y1A 3H7; Cal'95; FACS; FRCSC; GenSurg. Staff, Whitehorse General Hospital; Langs: English; French; (867)393-8908; Fax. (867)667-6512.

POOLE, Angela M; Queen City Obst & Gyn, 3271 Quance St E, Regina SK S4V 3B7; Sask'03; FRCSC; ObstGyn. Physician, Queen City Obstetrics & Gynecology; (306)585-9565; Fax. (306)585-9209.

POOLE, Bruce J; Dr Everett Chalmers Reg Hosp, PO Box 9000 Stn A 700 Priestman St, Fredericton NB E3B 5N5; Qns'78; FRCPC; PhysMed&Rehab. Staff, Phys Med & Rehab, Stan Cassidy Centre for Rehabilitation; Ac Staff, Dr Everett Chalmers Regional Hospital; Ac Staff, Oromocto Public Hospital; Consultant, Carleton Memorial Hospital; (506)458-0227

POOLE, Colleen E; Clayton Gate Pediatrics, 215-6820 188 St, Surrey BC V4N 3G6; Cal'05; FRCPC; Peds. Staff, Foothills Medical Centre; (604)579-0270

POOLE, Richard F; Glengarry Mem Hosp, Hwy 43, Alexandria ON K0C 1A0; Manchester (England)'69; MB ChB; Staff Emerg, Glengarry Memorial Hospital; Langs: Bilingual(English/French); (613)525-2222; rf.poole@sympatico.ca.

POOLE, Robert T; Stroud Med Centre, 1-7869 Yonge St, Innisfil ON L9S 1K8; McM'07; CCFP; (705)436-2251

POOLE, Thomas E; Central Nfld Reg Hlth Centre, 50 Union St, Grnd-Falls-Wi NL A2A 2E1; Mem'76; Chief, Central Newfoundland Regional Health Centre; (709)292-2500; Fax. (709)292-2148.

POOLER, Stephen D; Regina Qu'Appelle HR-Regina, 1440 14th Ave, Regina SK S4P 0W5; Sask'03; BSc; FRCSC; GenSurg (Advanced Laparoscopic Surgery). Staff, Regina General Hospital; (306)766-6911; Fax. (306)766-6917.

POON, C C Terry; 233-8787 Woodbine Ave, Markham ON L3R 9S2; Alb'00; BSc; CCFP; Langs: Cantonese; (905)416-0800; Fax. (905)415-0801.

POON, Christina I; 102-123 15th St E, North Vancouver BC V7L 2P7; UBC'98; FRCSC; Urol. (604)987-8171

POON, Connie K H; Liberton Med Centre, 212-31 Liberton Dr, St. Albert AB T8N 3X6; Alb'85; (780)459-7760; Fax. (780)460-1799.

POON, Derek I; Cambridge Mem Hosp, 700 Coronation Blvd, Cambridge ON N1R 3G2; Tor'03; CCFP; CCFP(E.M.); Staff, Cambridge Memorial Hospital; (519)621-2330

POON, Ian D T; Odette Cancer Centre, 2075 Bayview Ave, Toronto ON M4N 3M5; Ott'95; FRCSC; RadOncol (Head & Neck). Staff, Sunnybrook Health Sciences Centre; Consultant, Toronto East General Hospital Inc; Asst Prof, University of Toronto; (416)480-4951; Fax. (416)480-6002; ian.poon@sunnybrook.ca.

POON, Jackson C; MD Health Med Centre, 186 Main St S, Brampton ON L6W 2E2; Wes'04; CCFP; (905)456-7774; Fax. (905)456-1158.

POON, Jason S Y; 203-2692 Clearbrook Rd, Abbotsford BC V2T 2Y8; UBC'00; FRCSC; ObstGyn. (604)746-0780

POON, Jimmy C M; 30-1675 The Chase, Mississauga ON L5M 5Y7; Tor'78; BSc; CCFP; FCFP; Langs: Cantonese; (905)820-1398; Fax. (905)607-6048; drjimmypoon@bellnet.ca.

POON, John C P; 1-6219 Centre St NW, Calgary AB T2K 0V2; Alb'91; CCFP; Langs: Chinese; (403)275-5300; Fax. (403)275-5301.

POON, Pat K C; 101-10 Royal Orchard Blvd, Thornhill ON L3T 3C3; Tor'87; BSc; PhD; Staff, Mackenzie Richmond Hill Hospital; (905)771-7600; Fax. (905)771-9600.

POON, Kea-Keu; Canora Hosp, PO Box 749, Canora SK S0A 0L0; Kumamoto (Japan)'61; Staff, Canora Hospital; (306)563-5621; Fax. (306)563-1257.

POON, Kenneth S; Richmond Health Science Ctre, 650-6091 Gilbert Rd, Richmond BC V7C 5L9; UBC'98; BSc; FRCSC; Urol (Male Infertility). Staff Urol, Richmond Hospital; Staff Urol, Delta Hospital; Clin Associate Div of Urol, University of British Columbia; (604)273-4320; Fax. (604)273-7599.

POON, Lorne; New Image Med Clinic, 10957 124 St NW, Edmonton AB T5M 0H9; Alb'79; BMedSci; CCFP; FCFP; Staff, Royal Alexandra Hospital; Pres, Chinese Canadian Medical Society of Edmonton; Langs: Cantonese; (780)756-3828; Fax. (780)756-8900.

POON, Man-Chiu; Foothills Med Centre, 1403 29 St NW, Calgary AB T2N 2T9; UBC'68; FRCP; ABIM(MedOncol); ABPath; FACP; FRCPC; IntMed (Hemostasis); Hem. Ac Staff, Foothills Medical Centre; Consultant, Alberta Children's Hospital; Consultant, Calgary Laboratory Services; Dir Comprehensive Care Prog, Southern Alberta Rare Blood & Bleeding Disorders; Prof Med, University of Calgary; (403)944-1564

POON, Mimi M L; 241-2906 Broadway W, Vancouver BC V6K 2G8; Dal'93; Langs: Cantonese; (604)588-2388

POON, Stephanie C; Univ Hlth Network-Toronto Gen, 200 Elizabeth St, Toronto ON M5G 2C4; Qns'06; FRCPC; IntMed; Cardiol. Fellow, Toronto General Hospital - UHN; (416)340-3111

POON, Susan; 216A Centre St SE, Calgary AB T2G 2B6; Cal'83; CCFP; FCFP; Staff, Rockyview General Hospital; (403)233-8899

POON, Vincent H K; Bayview-Finch Med Clinic, 201-3292 Bayview Ave, North York ON M2M 4J5; Man'72; DMin; DPsy; FCFP; CCFP; FCFP; Ac Staff Family & Community Med, St Joseph's Health Centre; Ac Staff, North York General Hospital; Asst Prof Family & Community Med, University of Toronto; (416)512-9908

POON, Wayne W C; Assiniboine Clinic, 633 Lodge Ave, Winnipeg MB R3J 0S9; Man'86; FRCPC; IntMed.

POON, Wendell Y C; 405-302 Spadina Ave, Toronto ON M5T 2E7; Indiana(IN) (USA)'70; (416)596-8529

POONAH, Muhammad F; 202-83 Mill St, Georgetown ON L7G 5E9; Univ of Sint Eustatius (Netherlands Antilles)'09; CCFP; (905)873-2402; Fax. (905)873-2411.

POONAI, Naveen P C; 84 Harris Rd, Delaware ON N0L 1E0; Tor'04; FRCP; FRCPC; Peds; PedEmergMed. Staff, London Health Sciences Centre - Victoria Campus; (519)685-8500 x52011; naveen.poonai@lhsc.on.ca.

POONJA, Zahir; Eagle Ridge Family Health Ctre, 203-480 Huronia Rd, Barrie ON L4N 6M2; Manchester (England)'85; CCFP; FCFP; Staff ER, Royal Victoria Regional Health Centre; (705)727-7688; Fax. (705)734-6284.

POOSTIZADEH, Ahmad; Dr Walter Anderson Bldg, 2551 Pandosy St, Kelowna BC V1Y 1T1; Tehran (Iran)'86; FRCSC; GenSurg; CardSurg. Staff, Vancouver General Hospital - Centennial Pavillion; Staff, Providence Health Care - St Paul's Hospital; Langs: Farsi; French; (250)862-4300 x2435

POOTHENCHERI, Sreeja N; Rockyview Gen Hosp, 7007 14 St SW, Calgary AB T2V 1P9; (India)'96; CCFP; Staff, Rockyview General Hospital; (403)680-7707; Fax. (403)943-8411.

POOYANIA, Sepideh; Riverview Health Centre, PE314-1 Morley Ave, Winnipeg MB R3L 2P4; Tehran (Iran)'94; FRCPC; PhysMed&Rehab. Staff, Riverview Health Centre; (204)478-6219; Fax. (204)478-5724.

POP, Aida M; CSSS de Vaudreuil-Soulanges, 490 boul Harwood, Vaudreuil-Dorion QC J7V 7H4; Craiova (Romania)'97; CCFP; Staff, CSSS de Vaudreuil-Soulanges; (450)455-6171; aida_pop@rrsss16.gouv.qc.ca.

POP, Anca; 304-240 Wharncliffe Rd N, London ON N6H 4P2; Carol Davila (Romania)'97; CCFP; (519)432-0400; Fax. (519)432-0401.

POP, Cristina A; Fairview Community Health, 55 Fairview Mall Dr, North York ON M2J 2Z1; McG'05; CCFP; Staff, Weeneebayko General Hospital; (416)640-5298; Fax. (416)642-2238.

POP, Mihai; 900-9001 boul de l'Acadie, Montreal QC H4N 3H5; Sher'75; Ophth (Cataract Surgery). Langs: Romanian; English; Italian; (514)381-2020; Fax. (514)381-2144; michelpop@cmpop.com.

POPA, Brindusa M; Family Practice Clinic, 103-15955 Airport Rd, Caledon East ON L7C 1H9; Iasi (Romania)'91; CCFP; Langs: Romanian; (905)584-9377; Fax. (905)584-5283.

POPA, Christina C; Markham Stouffville Hosp, PO Box 1800 Stn Main 381 Church St, Markham ON L3P 7P3; Bucharest (Romania)'92; CCFP; CCFP(E.M.); Staff, Toronto East General Hospital Inc; Staff, Markham Stouffville Hospital; (905)472-7000

POPA, Clara; 4 9e rue, Rouyn-Noranda QC J9X 2B2; Bucharest (Romania)'95; Staff Peds, Centre Hospitalier Rouyn-Noranda; Clin Dir, Fibrose Kystique Abitibi-Temiscamingue; Langs: Romanian; Bilingual(French/English); (819)764-5131; Fax. (819)764-2900.

POPA, Cornelia; Dawson Creek Med Clinic, 816 103 Ave, Dawson Creek BC V1G 2G1; Bucharest (Romania)'01; CCFP; Langs: Romanian; (250)782-5271; Fax. (250)782-6360.

POPA, Ion; Ctr Hosp Affilie-St-Sacrement, 1050 ch Sainte-Foy, Quebec QC G1S 4L8; (Romania)'96; AnatPath. Staff, Centre Hospitalier Affilié Universitaire de Québec - Hôpital du St-Sacrement.

POPADIUK, Catherine M; Health Sciences Centre, 300 Prince Philip Dr, St. John's NL A1B 3V6; Tor'91; MBA; FRCSC; ObstGyn (Gynecologic Oncology). Staff GynOncol, Health Sciences Centre; Assoc Prof ObstGyn, Memorial University Of Newfoundland; (709)777-6564

POPADYNEC, Ihor V; Medical Centre, 2H-1723 Kipling Ave, Etobicoke ON M9R 4E1; Ott'68; Staff, William Osler Health System - Etobicoke General Hospital; (416)244-8733

POPE, A James D; 10140 107 Ave, Grande Prairie AB T8V 1L9; Alb'73; CCFP; FCFP; Ac Staff/Chief Medical Staff, Queen Elizabeth II Hospital; (780)831-0135; Fax. (780)831-0132.

POPE, Elena; The Hosp for Sick Children, 555 University Ave, Toronto ON M5G 1X8; Bucharest (Romania)'90; MSc; FRCPC; Peds (Pediatric Dermatology). Head Section of Derm, The Hospital For Sick Children; Assoc Prof, University of Toronto; Langs: Romanian; (416)813-6883; Fax. (416)813-7909; elena.pope@sickkids.ca.

POPE, Janet E; St Joseph's Health Care, PO Box 5777 Stn B 268 Grosvenor St, London ON N6A 4V2; Wes'85; MPH; FRCPC; IntMed (Scleroderma & Inflammatory Arthritis); Rheum. Staff, St Joseph's Hospital - St Joseph's Health Care; (519)646-6332; Fax. (519)646-6334.

POPE, John D; New Vision Family Health Team, 421 Greenbrook Dr, Kitchener ON N2M 4K1; Tor'83; CCFP; FCFP; Clinical Asst Prof, McMaster University; (519)578-3510; Fax. (519)578-6040.

POPE, Marc; 500-89 Queensway W, Mississauga ON L5B 2V2; Wes'89; MSc; FRCSC; GenSurg; VascSurg. Staff VascSurg, Trillium Health Centre - West Toronto; Staff VascSurg, The Credit Valley Hospital; Langs: French; Romanian; (905)848-7777; Fax. (905)848-6360; mpope@thc.on.ca.

POPE, Octavian C; 309-1525 Albion Rd, Etobicoke ON M9V 5G5; Tor'91; (416)741-0410; Fax. (416)741-0310.

POPE, William D B; College of Phys & Surg of MB, 1000-1661 Portage Ave, Winnipeg MB R3J 3T7; Man'70; LLB; FRCPC; Anes (Administrative Medicine). Assoc Prof Dept of Anes/Asst Prof Dept of Community Hlth Sciences Faculty of Med, University of Manitoba; (204)774-4344; Fax. (204)774-0750; bpope@cpsm.mb.ca.

POPENCU, Madalina; Ungava Tulattavik Health Ctr, CP 149, Kuujjuaq QC J0M 1C0; Mon'10; CCFP; Staff, Centre de sante Tulattavik de l'Ungava; (819)964-2905

POPESCU, Ligia M; Woodroffe South Med Bldg, 202-1637 Woodroffe Ave, Nepean ON K2G 1W2; Cluj (Romania)'89; CCFP; FCFP; (613)723-5635; Fax. (613)723-5918; ligia_popescu@hotmail.com.

POPESCU, Adriana L; Wellserve Med Office, 110-112 Woolwich St, Guelph ON N1H 3V2; (Romania)'89; CCFP; Staff, Guelph General Hospital; Langs: Romanian; (519)767-1721

POPESCU, Oana-Eugenia; Children's & Women's HC of BC, L214-4480 Oak St, Vancouver BC V6H 3V4; Craiova (Other Foreign)'91; FRCPC; AnatPath. Staff, BC Children's Hospital; Langs: Romanian; (604)875-3422

POPESCU-CRAINIC, Sanda; SMBD Jewish Gen Hosp, 3755 ch Cote-Sainte-Catherine, Montreal QC H3T 1E2; CCFP; Staff, Sir Mortimer B Davis Jewish General; (514)340-8222; Fax. (514)340-7510.

POPESCU-DUMBRAVA, Laila; CSSS de Sept-Iles, 45 rue du Pere-Divet, Sept-Iles QC G4R 3N7; Bucharest (Romania)'75; CCFP; Staff, Centre Hospitalier Regional de Sept-Iles; Assoc Dir, Regie Formation Medicale Continue; Langs: English; Romanian; (418)962-9761; Fax. (418)962-4488; laila_popescu@ssss.gouv.qc.ca.

POPICK, Dallas; Herold Road Family Physicians, 1-325 Herold Rd, Saskatoon SK S7V 1J7; Sask'82; Staff, St Paul's Hospital (Grey Nuns) of Saskatoon; Staff Med, Saskatoon District Health Board; (306)374-2404; Fax. (306)477-0300.

POPIEL, Stephanie A; Perth Family Medicine, 39 Drummond St W, Perth ON K7H 2J9; Tor'98; BSc; MSc; CCFP; Staff, Perth & Smiths Falls District Hospital - Perth Site (Great War Memorial Site); Langs: French; Spanish; (613)264-2686; Fax. (613)264-0454.

POPKE, Manfred E; 9117 82 Ave NW, Edmonton AB T6C 0Z4; Alb'80; Langs: German; (780)822-6440; Fax. (780)468-1461.

POPLAK, Terence; Royal Victoria Hosp, 201 Georgian Dr, Barrie ON L4M 6M2; Witwatersrand (South Africa)'75; MB ChB; FRCPC; Anes. Staff, Royal Victoria Regional Health Centre; (705)728-9090 x4207

POPLAWSKI, Daniel H; 202-3400 rue du Marche, Dollard-D-Ormeaux QC H9B 2Y1; Mon'84; (514)683-0414; Fax. (514)683-5528.

POPLAWSKI, Stanley A; Grey Nuns Community Hosp & HC, 1100 Youville Drive West NW, Edmonton AB T6L 5X8; Alb'77; Head Dept of EmergMed, Covenant Health - Edmonton General Continuing Care Centre; Staff, Covenant Health - Grey Nuns Community Hospital; (780)735-7181

POPLAWSKI, Stephen R; Radiology Consultants Assoc, 120-6707 Elbow Dr SW, Calgary AB T2V 0E3; Alb'05; FRCPC; DiagRad. (403)777-3007; Fax. (403)777-3008.

POPLOVE, Steven H; Laurier Optical, 2121 Carling Ave, Ottawa ON K2A 1H2; Tor'92; (613)761-8080; Fax. (613)761-1527.

POPMA, Barbara H; Chinook Reg Hosp, 960 19 St S, Lethbridge AB T1J 1W5; Cal'73; BSc; FRCPC; AnatPath (Cytology). Staff, Chinook Regional Hospital; Staff Pathologist, Chinook Reg. Laboratory; (403)388-6153; Fax. (403)388-6067.

POPMA, Harold T; Sackville Mem Hosp, 8 Main St, Sackville NB E4L 4A3; UBC'69; CCFP; Ac Staff, Sackville Memorial Hospital; Court Staff, The Moncton Hospital; Med Advisor, United Church Home for Senior Citizens, District 2-New Brunswick; Langs: Dutch; (506)536-3052; Fax. (506)536-1620; popma@nbnet.nb.ca.

POPOFF, Jeffrey J; Royal Alexandra Hosp, 10240 Kingsway NW, Edmonton AB T5H 3V9; Man'00; FRCPC; Anes. Staff, Royal Alexandra Hospital; (780)735-4010; popofftercel@hotmail.com.

POPOOLA, Abraham J; Grand River Hosp-KW Hlth Ctre, PO Box 9056 Stn C 835 King st W, Kitchener ON N2G 1G3; Lagos (Nigeria)'95; FRCPC; Psy. Staff, Grand River Hospital - Kitchener/Waterloo Health Centre; (519)749-4300

POPOV, Serghei; 3-1032 17 Ave SW, Calgary AB T2T 0A5; (Moldova)'03; (403)229-1771; Fax. (403)229-1812.

POPOVA, Kalina; Anaesthetic Services, 213-2186 Oak Bay Ave, Victoria BC V8R 1G3; UBC'06; FRCPC; Anes. Staff, Vancouver General Hospital - Centennial Pavillion; Langs: Bulgarian; (250)595-7211

POPOVA, Margarita; CSSS de Manicouagan, 635 boul Jolliet, Baie-Comeau QC G5C 1P1; Sofia (Bulgaria)'97; CCFP; Staff, Centre Hospitalier Régional Baie-Comeau; (418)589-3701

POPOVEC, Bobbi J; MUHC-Montreal Neurology Inst, 548-3801 rue University, Montreal QC H3A 2B4; Ohio (USA)'83; CSPQ; Anes (P.Q.) (Pain Management). Staff, McGill University Health Centre - Montreal Neurological Hospital; (514)398-1917; Fax. (514)398-1352.

POPOVIC, Dina; 202-3825 Sunset St, Burnaby BC V5G 1T4; Wes'05; FRCSC; OrthSurg. (604)294-8209

POPOVIC, Ilija; Westbrook Shopping Centre, 28-1200 37 St SW, Calgary AB T3C 1S2; Belgrade (Serbia)'63; DGS(Hannover); PhD; Langs: Spanish; Romanian; German; Serbo-Croatian; French.

POPOVIC, Jelena; Toronto East Gen Hosp Inc, 825 Coxwell Ave, Toronto ON M4C 3E7; Belgrade (Serbia)'91; FRCPC; Peds (Neonatal & Perinatal Medicine). Dir Neonatology, Toronto East General Hospital Inc; Clin Asst Neonatology, Mount Sinai Hospital; Clin Asst Neonatology, The Hospital For Sick Children; Langs: Serbian; Serbo-Croatian; (416)469-6580 x6568; Fax. (416)469-6020; jpopo@tegh.on.ca.

POPOVIC, Stanislav; Group Practice, 711-600 Sherbourne St, Toronto ON M4X 1W4; Belgrade (Serbia)'60; IntMed(Yugoslavia); FRCPC; IntMed (Liver Disease). Langs: Serbian; (416)929-0929; Fax. (416)929-8084.

POPOVICI, Radu G; Lakeshore Gen Hosp, 160 av Stillview, Pointe-Claire QC H9R 2Y2; (Romania)'80; LMCC; CCFP; Staff E R, Lakeshore General Hospital - Pointe Claire; (514)630-2225; Fax. (514)630-5144.

POPOWICH, Kenneth R; Ligations Clinic, 2713 14 St SW, Calgary AB T2T 3V2; Cal'81; CCFP; FCFP; Assoc Staff Surg, Foothills Medical Centre; Staff, Rockyview General Hospital; Clinical Asst Prof, University of Calgary; (403)242-0499; Fax. (403)685-8012; vasman@telus.net.

POPOWICH, Shaundra L; St Boniface Gen Hosp, 2051-409 Tache Ave, Winnipeg MB R2H 2A6; Sask'96; FRCSC; ObstGyn; GynOnco. Staff, St Boniface General Hospital; (204)233-8563

POPPE, Alexandre Y; CHUM-Hop Notre-Dame, 1560 rue Sherbrooke E, Montreal QC H2L 4M1; McG'02; FRCPC; Neur. Staff, Centre Hospitalier l'Université de Montréal (CHUM) - Hôpital Notre-Dame; (514)890-8000 x26260

POPPEN, Jacquline; Greensborough Fam Med Ctre, 10-10 Greensborough Village Ci, Markham ON L6E 1M4; Calicut (India)'89; CCFP; (905)201-1143; Fax. (905)209-1172.

POPPLOW, James R; Manitoba Health, 70 Hagen Dr, Winnipeg MB R3K 1Y4; Qns'75; MSc; FACPrevMed; Med Advisor Occupational & Environmental Health Public Health Branch, Manitoba Health; Physician, Occupational Environmental & Aerospace Med Consulting; (204)831-7509; jpopplow@shaw.ca.

POPRADI, Gizelle A; MUHC-Royal Victoria Hosp, C6.82-687 av des Pins O, Montreal QC H3A 1A1; McG'01; FRCPC; IntMed (Stem Cell Transplantation); Hem. Staff, McGill University Health Centre - Royal Victoria Hospital; (514)934-1934 x34091

POPSOR, Emilia; Horizon Square Med Centre, 401-3508 32 Ave NE, Calgary AB T1Y 6J2; (Romania)'81; (403)291-5599

POPURI, Preeti; A-690 Main St W, Hamilton ON L8S 1A4; Kasturba (India)'01; CCFP; (905)521-5015

POPURI, Ramu; Cambridge Mem Hosp, 700 Coronation Blvd, Cambridge ON N1R 3G2; Liverpool (England)'95; FRCPC; DiagRad. Staff, Cambridge Memorial Hospital; (519)621-2330

POR-SOMFAI, Agnes; Dixie X-Ray Associates, B1-2065 Finch Ave W, North York ON M3N 2V7; Budapest (Hungary)'73; FRCPC; DiagRad. Langs: Hungarian; (416)745-8050; Fax. (416)745-1125; somfai@yahoo.com.

PORAY-WYBRANOWSKI, Jerzy; C A M U Longueuil, 100-1144 rue Saint-Laurent O, Longueuil QC J4K 1E2; McG'78; CCFP; Assoc Staff, Hopital Charles LeMoyne; Physician, City of Montreal; Langs: Polish; French; (450)651-5700; Fax. (450)651-9700.

PORAYKO, Lorne D; 213-2186 Oak Bay Ave, Victoria BC V8R 1G3; UBC'93; FRCPC; Anes; Critical Care Medicine. (250)595-7211

PORCHETTA, Simon; CSSS de Laval, 1755 boul Rene-Laennec, Laval QC H7M 3L9; Mon'09; CCFP; CCFP(E.M.); Staff, Hopital de la Cite de la santé; (450)668-1010

PORDAN, Eva; Clinique Med Joliette, 3841 rue Ontario E, Montreal QC H1W 1S5; (Hungary)'85; (514)524-3731

PORDELI, Peyvand; Real Time Radiology, 220 Superior Blvd, Mississauga ON L5T 2L2; Ghazvin (Iran)'92; FRCPC; DiagRad.

POREPA, Michelle E; 304-2115 Finch Ave W, North York ON M3N 2V6; Tor'04; FRCPC; Peds. Staff, The Hospital For Sick Children; (416)745-3411

POREPA, S Joseph; York Finch Med Centre, 304-2115 Finch Ave W, North York ON M3N 2V6; McG'74; FRCPC; Peds. Assoc Staff, The Hospital For Sick Children; Staff, Humber River Regional Hospital - Finch Avenue Site; Asst Prof Peds, University of Toronto; Langs: French; (416)745-3411

PORFIRIS, George S; 202-245 Danforth Ave, Toronto ON M4K 1N2; Tor'94; CCFP; CCFP(E.M.); FCFP; Ac Staff Family & Emergency Med, Toronto East General Hospital Inc; Asst Prof Family Med, University of Toronto; Langs: Greek; (416)461-1171; Fax. (416)461-1172.

PORHOWNIK, Nancy R; Health Sciences Centre, RS315-820 Sherbrook St, Winnipeg MB R3A 1R9; Man'04; FRCPC; IntMed; Respir. Staff, Health Sciences Centre; (204)774-8511

PORLIER, Caroline; CSSS de Sept-Iles, 45 rue du Pere-Divet, Sept-Iles QC G4R 3N7; Laval'07; CCFP; Staff, Centre Hospitalier Regional de Sept-Iles; (418)962-9761

PORLIER, Jean-Paul; CSSS de Sept-Iles, 45 rue du Père-Divet, Sept-Iles QC G4R 3N7; Laval'65; FRCSC; OrthSurg. Chief OrthSurg, Centre Hospitalier Regional de Sept-Iles; (418)962-9761

POROSTOCKY, Peter; 21st Medical Clinic, 502-402 21st St E, Saskatoon SK S7K 0C3; Alb'05; FRCPC; IntMed; Gastroent. (306)956-3444; Fax. (306)956-3444.

PORTE, Alexis N; The Ottawa Hosp-Civic Campus, 1053 Carling Ave, Ottawa ON K1Y 4E9; Qns'06; FRCSC; GenSurg. Staff, The Ottawa Hospital - Civic Campus; (613)798-5555; Fax. (613)761-4124.

PORTE, Arthur M; Medical Arts Bldg, 307-1 Young St, Hamilton ON L8N 1T8; West Indies (Jamaica)'79; FRCSC; OrthSurg (Orthopedics). Ac Staff, St Joseph's Healthcare - Charlton Campus; (905)529-2999; Fax. (905)528-8150.

PORTELANCE, Lorraine; MUHC-Montreal Gen Hosp, D5 400-1650 av Cedar, Montreal QC H3G 1A4; Mon'92; AB; CSPQ; FRCP; RadOncol. Staff, McGill University Health Centre - Montreal General Campus; (514)934-8040; Fax. (514)934-8220; lorraineportelance@yahoo.com.

PORTELANCE-HUOT, Marjolaine; CSSS du Lac-Temiscamingue, 22 rue Notre-Dame N, Ville-Marie QC J9V 1W8; Sher'05; Staff, CSSS du Témiscamingue; (819)629-2420; marjolaine_portelance-huot@ssss.gouv.qc.ca.

PORTEN, Wendy R; Kerrisdale Station Med Clinic, 2077 42nd Ave W, Vancouver BC V6M 2B4; UBC'71; Ac Staff, Vancouver General Hospital - Centennial Pavillion; (604)261-9494; Fax. (604)261-9405.

PORTER, Andrew D; Nicola Med Dental Bldg, 303-321 Nicola St, Kamloops BC V2C 6G6; Wes'88; FRCSC; OrthSurg (Spine). Staff, Royal Inland Hospital; (250)374-2153; Fax. (250)374-9232.

PORTER, Arthur; 14e-2155 rue Guy, Montreal QC H3H 2R9; Cambridge (England)'80; MBA; FRCPC; RadOncol (Brachy Therapy). (514)934-8328; Fax. (514)934-8200; arthur.porter@muhc.mcgill.ca.

PORTER, Barry J; St George's Med Clinic, PO Box 310, St Georges NL A0N 1Z0; Mem'92.

PORTER, Bonita M; Office of the Chief Coroner, 26 Grenville St, Toronto ON M7A 2G9; McM'78; BSc(Phm); MSc; CCFP; Dep Chief Inquests for Ontario, Province of Ontario; (416)314-4000; Fax. (416)314-4030.

PORTER, Ewan A; Grey Bruce HS-Owen Sound, PO Box 1800 Stn Main 1800 8th St E, Owen Sound ON N4K 6M9; Otago (New Zealand)'67; MB ChB; FRCPC; Peds. Assoc Staff, Grey Bruce Health Services - Owen Sound; (519)372-3920

PORTER, Gail S; Toronto Street Med Centre, 202-29 Toronto St S, Uxbridge ON L9P 1V9; Tor'71; (905)852-3339; Fax. (905)852-9151.

PORTER, Geoffrey A; Queen Elizabeth II HSC, 8 032-1276 South Park St, Halifax NS B3H 2Y9; Qns'92; MSc(Epid.); FACS; FRCSC; GenSurg (Surgical Oncology). Staff, Queen Elizabeth II Health Sciences Centre - Victoria General Site; Asst Prof Surg, Dalhousie University; Langs: English; French; (902)473-6499; Fax. (902)473-6496.

PORTER, George R; Victoria Professional Bldg, 405-1120 Yates St, Victoria BC V8V 3M9; Wes'70; DAB; FACS; FRCSC; GenSurg (Colon & Rectal Surgery). Staff, Royal Jubilee Hospital; Staff, Victoria General Hospital; (250)384-8154; Fax. (250)384-7571.

PORTER, Gordon A; Thunder Bay Reg HSC-T-Bay, 980 Oliver Rd, Thunder Bay ON P7B 6V4; Qns'80; ABIME; FRCSC; OrthSurg (Musculoskeletal). Staff Orthopedic Cons Dept Surg, Thunder Bay Regional Health Sciences Centre; (807)684-6024; Fax. (807)684-7405; porterg@tbh.net.

PORTER, Jean E; 404-3461 Dixie Rd, Mississauga ON L4Y 3X4; Tor'67; DPsy; FRCPC; Psy. Court Staff, Trillium Health Centre - Mississauga; (905)625-4745; Fax. (905)625-9533.

PORTER, John; Nortwestern Ontario Surg Prog, PO Box 22001 Rpo Strathcona 470 Hodder Ave, Thunder Bay ON P7A 8A8; Ott'72; FRCSC; OrthSurg (Knee Surgery). Surgeon Orthopedic, Dryden Regional Health Centre; Vis Specialist Orthopedic Surg, Lake of the Woods District Hospital; Surgeon Orthopedic, La Verendrye Hospital - Riverside Health Care Facility; (807)983-2118; Fax. (807)983-2327; j.porter@rhcf.on.ca.

PORTER, Justin M J; Couchiching Family Health Team, 104C-119 Memorial Ave, Orillia ON L3V 5X1; NOSM'09; CCFP; (705)327-6568

PORTER, Kathryn G; Kerrisdale Station Med Clinic, 2077 42nd Ave W, Vancouver BC V6M 2B4; UBC'96; CCFP; (604)261-9494

PORTER, Kenneth L; 1428 Shediac Rd, Moncton NB E1A 7A7; Mem'80; FRCPC; Anes;CCFP; (506)855-6030; Fax. (506)855-6003.

PORTER, M Anne; Carbonear Gen Hosp, 86 Highroad South, Carbonear NL A1Y 1A4; Mem'95; FRCPC; Psy. Staff, Carbonear General Hospital; (709)945-5111

PORTER, Mark C; Topsail Road Med Clinic, 644 Topsail Rd, St. John's NL A1E 2E2; Mem'06; CCFP; (709)368-2101; markpdg@nl.rogers.com.

PORTER, P Michael; Pelham Group Health Centre, 216-245 Pelham Rd, St Catharines ON L2S 1X8; McM'87; FRCPC; Psy. (905)687-8508

PORTER, Robert N; Dr Charles A Janeway Child HC, 300 Prince Philip Dr, St. John's NL A1B 3V6; Mem'91; CCFP; CCFP(E.M.); Staff Emerg, Janeway Children's Health & Rehabilitation Centre; Clinical Asst Prof Discipline of Peds, Memorial University Of Newfoundland; (709)777-4222 x4575; Robert.Porter@easternhealth.ca.

PORTER, Robin B A; Primacy Clinic, 8195 120 St, Delta BC V4C 6P7; UBC'86; BSc(Hons.); (604)596-1521; Fax. (877)845-2737.

PORTER, Sara L; Providence CCC-St Mary's, PO Box 3600 Stn Main 340 Union St, Kingston ON K7L 5A2; Qns'07; CCFP; Staff, Providence Care - St Mary's of the Lake Hospital Site; (613)544-5220

PORTER, Stephen C; The Hosp for Sick Children, 555 University Ave, Toronto ON M5G 1X8; Univ of Cincinnati (USA)'93; Staff, The Hospital For Sick Children; (416)813-5810

PORTER, W Ronald; Crown Med Clinic, 1116-123 Edward St, Toronto ON M5G 1E2; St. Andrews (Scotland)'60; MB ChB; LMCC; Med Examiner, Civil Aviation Canada; (416)595-2722; Fax. (416)595-2723.

PORTNER, Oliver T; 301-1919 Riverside Dr, Ottawa ON K1H 1A2; McG'66; FRCSC; OrthSurg. Ac Staff, The Ottawa Hospital - Riverside Campus; Ac Staff, Canadian Forces Health Services Centre; Asst Prof, University of Ottawa.

PORTNOI, Galina G; North Med Centre, 204-7131 Bathurst St, Thornhill ON L4J 7Z1; (Ukraine)'89; CCFP; Langs: Russian; Hebrew; Ukrainian; (905)764-7474; Fax. (905)695-0238.

PORTNOY, Aron; Sante Kildare, 14-7005 rue Kildare, Montreal QC H4W 1C1; Vermont (USA)'06; FRCPC; Psy. Staff, McGill University Health Centre - Royal Victoria Hospital; (514)397-0777

PORTNOY, David; MUHC-Montreal Gen Hosp, A5156-1650 av Cedar, Montreal QC H3G 1A4; Liege (Belgium)'73; FRCPC; MedMicrobiol; Microbio & Infect Dis (P.Q.). Ac Staff, McGill University Health Centre - Montreal General Campus; (514)934-8074; Fax. (514)934-8423.

PORTNOY, Joseph; SMBD Jewish Gen Hosp, 1401-3755 ch Cote-Sainte-Cathe, Montreal QC H3T 1E2; McG'66; MSc; MD; FRCPC; MedMicrobiol (AIDS/HIV); Microbio & Infect Dis (P.Q.). Dir Professional Services, Sir Mortimer B Davis Jewish General; Assoc Prof Microbiol & Med, McGill University; (514)340-8222 x5932; jportnoy@jgh.mcgill.ca.

PORTUGAL, Francisco S; 33 Howard St, Toronto ON M4X 1J6; Manila (Philippines)'75; (416)928-1197; Fax. (416)925-6093; fsportugal@msn.com.

PORTUGAL AIRES, Liana M; Queen Elizabeth II HSC, 1276 South Park St, Halifax NS B3H 2Y9; Dal'00; CCFP; Staff, Queen Elizabeth II Health Sciences Centre - Victoria General Site; (902)473-4341

PORTWIG, Georg H; Duggan Village Mall, 6601 48 Ave, Camrose AB T4V 3G8; (South Africa)'87; MB ChB; (780)672-2425; Fax. (780)679-2668.

PORTWINE, Carol Ann; McMaster University HSC, 3N27-1280 Main St W, Hamilton ON L8S 4K1; Tor'88; FRCPC; Peds; Hem. (905)521-2100 x73428; portwc@mcmaster.ca.

PORWAL, Hemraj R; Valley Park Lodge Nursing Home, 6400 Valley Way, Niagara Falls ON L2E 7E3; Karnataka (India)'85; MB BS; CCFP; Staff, Niagara Health System - Port Colborne General Site; Langs: Hindi; Marathi; Gujarati; (905)358-3277

PORWIT, Anna; Univ Hlth Network-Toronto Gen, 200 Elizabeth St, Toronto ON M5G 2C4; Warsaw (Poland)'77; Staff, Toronto General Hospital - UHN; (416)340-3294; Fax. (416)340-5517.

POSADAS CALLEJA, Juan G; Peter Lougheed Centre, 3500 26 Ave NE, Calgary AB T1Y 6J4; (Mexico)'97; Staff, Peter Lougheed Centre; (403)943-5548

POSEL, Clifford H; Sunnybrook Hlth Sciences Ctre, 2075 Bayview Ave, Toronto ON M4N 3M5; McG'93; FRCPC; Psy. Staff, Sunnybrook Health Sciences Centre; (416)480-6100; Fax. (416)480-6878.

POSEN, David B; Trafalgar Prof Centre, 406-1235 Trafalgar Rd, Oakville ON L6H 3P1; Tor'67; Court Staff, Halton Healthcare Services Corporation - Oakville Site; (905)844-0744; Fax. (905)844-4540; davidposen@iprimus.ca.

POSEN, David; Bayview-Finch Med Clinic, 202-3292 Bayview Ave, North York ON M2M 4J5; Tor'65; CCFP; FCFP; Staff, North York General Hospital; Staff, North York General Hospital - Branson Division; (416)222-9955

POSKITT, Kenneth J; 113-5788 Birney Ave, Vancouver BC V6S 0A2; McG'81; FRCPC; DiagRad. Staff Radiol, BC Children's Hospital; (604)263-1633

POSLOSKI, William G; Windsor Reg Hosp-Metropolitan, 1995 Lens Ave, Windsor ON N8W 1L9; Qns'84; Staff, Windsor Regional Hospital - Metropolitan Site; (519)254-1661

POSNER, Barry I; 360 av Wood, Westmount QC H3Z 1Z2; Man'61; OC; FACP; FRSC; Endocrin (P.Q.); IntMed (Diabetes). principale Médecin, McGill University Health Centre - Royal Victoria Hospital; Dir Polypeptide Hormone Research Lab, McGill University; Langs: Bilingual(English/French); (514)398-8094; Fax. (514)933-1235.

POSNER, Glenn D; 311-1919 Riverside Dr, Ottawa ON K1H 1A2; McG'99; BSc; FRCSC; ObstGyn. Ac Staff, The Ottawa Hospital - General Campus; Asst Prof, University of Ottawa; Langs: Bilingual(French/English); (613)526-0080; Fax. (613)526-9749.

POSNER, Paul L; Keele-Ingram Med Centre, 212-2221 Keele St, North York ON M6M 3Z5; Tor'86; FRCPC; Psy (Geriatric Psychiatry). Staff, Humber River Regional Hospital - Keele Street Site; (416)247-6175; Fax. (416)247-9936.

POSPISIL, Caroline S; Sunnybrook Hlth Sciences Ctre, C753-2075 Bayview Ave, Toronto ON M4N 3M5; (Ireland)'10; Staff, Sunnybrook Health Sciences Centre; (416)480-5959

POST, Ellen E; 202-170 Simcoe St, Peterborough ON K9H 2H7; Tor'85; CCFP; FCFP; Staff, Peterborough Regional Health Centre - Hospital Drive; (705)872-4353; Fax. (705)872-4357; epost@prhc.on.ca.

POST, Joel; 100-200 Marina Way, Penticton BC V2A 1H4; Sask'07; Ophth. (250)770-3211

POST, William D; East Kootenay Reg Hosp, 13 24th Ave N, Cranbrook BC V1C 3H9; Qns'75; FRCSC; ObstGyn. Staff, East Kootenay Regional Hospital.

POSTL, Brian; 260-727 McDermot Ave, Winnipeg MB R3E 3P5; Man'76; FRCPC; CommunMed; Peds. VP Clinical Services, Winnipeg Regional Health Authority; Dean Faculty of Med, University of Manitoba; bpostl@wrha.mb.ca.

POSTL, Lara A; The Hincks Dellcrest Centre, 114 Maitland St, Toronto ON M4Y 1E1; Man'07; FRCPC; Psy. (416)924-1164; Fax. (416)924-8208.

POSTNIKOFF, Ian M; Second Chance Recovery, 103-3716 61 Ave SE, Calgary AB T2C 1Z4; Tor'76; FRCPC; Psy (Addiction Psychiatry). Physician, Central Alberta Methadone Program-Second Chance Recovery; (403)232-6990; Fax. (403)232-6992.

POSTOLOW, Fabiana A; Women's Hospital, 735 Notre Dame Ave, Winnipeg MB R3E 0L8; Buenos Aires (Argentina)'90.

POSTUK, Peter C; 46 Stanley Rd PO Box 948, Lake Cowichan BC V0R 2G0; UBC'92; CCFP; (250)749-4114; Fax. (250)749-0120.

POSTUMA, Paul; St Joseph's Hosp, 130 Bayard Dr, Saint John NB E2L 3L6; McM'91; CCFP; CCFP(E.M.); FCFP; Staff, Saint John Regional Hospital; Asst Prof, Dalhousie University; Clinical Asst Prof, Memorial University Of Newfoundland; (506)632-5488; Fax. (506)632-5657.

POSTUMA, Ronald B; MUHC-Montreal Gen Hosp, L7 312-1650 av Cedar, Montreal QC H3G 1A4; Man'95; Neur. Staff, McGill University Health Centre - Montreal General Campus; Langs: Bilingual(English/French); (514)943-8026; Fax. (514)934-8265.

POTASHNER, Wayne J; 209-4430 Bathurst St, North York ON M3H 3S3; Tor'85; FRCPC; IntMed; Rheum. Court Staff, Sunnybrook Health Sciences Centre; Consultant, North York General Hospital; Lecturer, University of Toronto; Langs: Bilingual(English/French); (416)631-6090; Fax. (416)631-6535.

POTERYKO, Derek; Anchor Family Med, 1450 Waddington Rd, Nanaimo BC V9S 4V9; UBC'91; CCFP; FCFP; Dir, Central Island Smoking Intervention Clinic; (250)754-5545; Fax. (250)754-5954.

POTESTIO, Frank A; Port Arthur Health Centre Inc, 194 Court St N, Thunder Bay ON P7A 4V7; Tor'93; BHSc; MSc; FRCSC; ObstGyn. Staff ObstGyn, Thunder Bay Regional Health Sciences Centre; Asst Prof, Northern Ontario School of Medicine; Langs: Italian; (807)346-1000; Fax. (807)346-6206.

POTGIETER, Hermanus H J; Viking Med Clinic, PO Box 868 5301 51 St, Viking AB T0B 4N0; (South Africa)'99; MB ChB; DA; CCFP; (780)336-4780; Fax. (780)336-2020.

POTGIETER, Lucas-Martin; Regina Qu'Appelle HR-Regina, 1440 14th Ave, Regina SK S4P 0W5; Pretoria (South Africa)'99; MB ChB; CCFP; Staff, Regina General Hospital; (306)766-4444

POTGIETER, Petrus D; 9842 101 Ave, Fort St. John BC V1J 2B2; Orange Free State (South Africa)'04; Staff, Fort St John Hospital & Health Centre; (250)785-1220

POTGIETER, Stephanus D; Westview Hlth Ctr Stony Plain, 4405 South Park Dr, Stony Plain AB T7Z 2M7; Stellenbosch (South Africa)'85; MB ChB; DA(SA); CCFP; CCFP(E.M.); Ac Staff, Westview Health Centre; Langs: Afrikaans; (780)968-3674; Fax. (780)968-3774; s.potgieter515@gmail.com.

POTGIETER, Tania; Regina Qu'Appelle HR-Regina, 1440 14th Ave, Regina SK S4P 0W5; Pretoria (South Africa)'99; MB ChB; Staff, Regina General Hospital; (306)766-4444

POTHIER, Daniel; CLSC-CHSLD Champagnat, 978 boul du Seminaire N, St-Jean-Sur-Richel QC J3A 1E5; Mon'81; Staff Community Health, Hôpital du Haut-Richelieu; (450)358-2578 x8822; Fax. (450)349-0724.

POTHIER, David D; Univ Hlth Network-Toronto Gen, 200 Elizabeth St, Toronto ON M5G 2C4; Cape Town (South Africa)'97; Staff, Toronto General Hospital - UHN; (416)340-4630

POTHIER, Jacques; CHUQ-Hotel-Dieu de Quebec, 11 Cote du Palais, Quebec QC G1R 2J6; Laval'76; FRCPC; IntMed. Staff, Centre Hospitalier Universitaire de Québec (CHUQ) - Siege Social; Teach Staff, Université Laval; (418)691-5151; Fax. (418)691-5160.

POTHIER, Philippe; Clinique Med Sainte-Madeleine, 165 boul Sainte-Madeleine, Trois-Rivieres QC G8T 3L7; Laval'87; Physician, Region Maurice/Bois-Franc; (819)379-8385

POTHIER, Sylvie; OPMEDIC, 300-1565 boul de l'Avenir, Laval QC H7S 2N5; Mon'82; CSPQ; FRCPC; Anes. (450)662-9515

POTHOS, Mary; Children's Hosp Eastern Ont, 401 Smyth Rd, Ottawa ON K1H 8L1; Sher'86; FRCPC; Peds. Staff Peds, Children's Hospital of Eastern Ontario (CHEO); Assoc Prof, University of Ottawa; (613)737-7600 x2664; Fax. (613)738-4878.

POTIER, Elsa; CLSC Ste-Therese de Blainville, 55 rue Saint-Joseph, Sainte-Therese QC J7E 4Y5; Mon'98; (450)430-4553 x4011; Fax. (450)430-3859.

POTIUK, Dustin J; Oak Bay Family Physicians Ltd, 101-1640 Oak Bay Ave, Victoria BC V8R 1B2; Qns'01; Dip SportMed; CCFP; (250)598-6744; Fax. (250)598-6778.

POTOCZNY, Stefan; London X Ray Associates, 104-450 Central Ave, London ON N6B 2E8; Ott'06; FRCPC; DiagRad.

POTOCZNY, Walter M; Parkdale Med Tower, 304-1081 Carling Ave, Ottawa ON K1Y 4G2; Ott'78; FRCPC; Psy (Geriatric Psychiatry). (613)792-1694; Fax. (613)792-1695.

POTOKER, Steven D; Ellendale Med Bldg, 565-5845 ch Cote-des-Neiges, Montreal QC H3S 1Z4; McG'72; DABD; FRCPC; Derm. Clin Staff Derm, Sir Mortimer B Davis Jewish General; Consultant, Donald Berman Maimonides Geriatric Centre; Asst Lecturer, McGill University; Langs: English; French; (514)731-9161; Fax. (514)731-7256.

POTOPSINGH, Desmond M; Providence Care-Mental Health, PO Box 603 Stn Main 752 King St W, Kingston ON K7L 4X3; UCWI (Jamaica)'65; MB BS(Lond.-UK); DABPN; FRCPC; Psy. Staff Pt-Time Hospital/Clinic Practice, Providence Care - Mental Health Services; Asst Prof Psy, Queen's University; (613)540-6166 x4114; Fax. (613)540-6169.

POTOSKI, J Paul; The Potoski Med Clinic, 301 Main St N, Dauphin MB R7N 1C5; Man'68; Staff, Dauphin Regional Health Centre; (204)638-3366; Fax. (204)638-5761.

POTOTSCHNIK, Ralph; The Jenny Trout Centre, 115-342 Erie St, Stratford ON N5A 2N4; Tor'81; FRCSC; OrthSurg (Joint Arthroplasty). Consultant, Alexandra Marine & General Hospital; Staff, Stratford General Hospital - Huron Perth Healthcare Alliance; Consultant, Clinton Public Hospital - Huron Perth Healthcare Alliance; (519)272-2727; Fax. (519)272-2729.

POTTER, Brian J; CHUM-Hotel-Dieu, 3840 rue Saint-Urbain, Montreal QC H2W 1T9; McG'04; FRCPC; IntMed; Cardiol. Staff, Centre Hospitalier l'Université de Montréal (CHUM) - Hôtel-Dieu; (514)890-8000

POTTER, C Peter; Huron Med Centre, 1472 Huron St, London ON N5V 2E5; Wes'72; BA.

POTTER, Eleanor R A; West Durham Family Health Team, 200B-1105 Kingston Rd E, Pickering ON L1V 6B5; Cape Town (South Africa)'81; MB ChB; MRC(UK); CCFP; (905)420-9999; Fax. (905)420-6458.

POTTER, Geraldine D; Extendicare, 90 Chedmac Dr, Hamilton ON L9C 7W1; McM'87; (905)318-4472

POTTER, Jennifer A; East End Commun Health Centre, 1619 Queen St E, Toronto ON M4L 1G4; McM'99; CCFP; (416)778-5858; Fax. (416)778-5855.

POTTER, Jennifer L; Manitoba Clinic, 790 Sherbrook St, Winnipeg MB R3A 1M3; Man'03; CCFP; (204)786-8588

POTTER, Laurie A; Saint John Reg Hosp, PO Box 2100 Stn Main 400 University Ave, Saint John NB E2L 4L2; Mem'02; FRCPC; Psy. Staff, Saint John Regional Hospital; (506)648-6000

POTTER, Lynne M; Mission Mem Hosp, 7324 Hurd St, Mission BC V2V 3H5; UBC'73; Ac Staff, Mission Memorial Hospital; (604)826-6261

POTTER, Martin; MUHC-Montreal Chest Institute, J 803-3650 rue Saint-Urbain, Montreal QC H2X 2P4; Mon'00; CCFP; Staff, McGill University Health Centre - Montreal Chest Institute; (514)843-2090

POTTER, Miriam; Guelph Family Health Team, 305-85 Norfolk St, Guelph ON N1H 4J4; Qns'00; BSc; PhD; CCFP; Court Staff, Guelph General Hospital; (519)766-1490; Fax. (519)836-9530; mpotter@gbhs.on.ca.

POTTER, Murray A; McMaster University HSC, 3N17-1200 Main St W, Hamilton ON L8S 4J9; Man'95; FRCPC; MedBiochem (Biochemical Genetics). (905)521-2100 x73718; mpotter@hhsc.ca.

POTTER, Patrick J; St Joseph's HC-Parkwood Hosp, 801 Commissioners Rd E, London ON N6C 5J1; Dal'80; BSc; FRCPC; PhysMed&Rehab (Spinal Cord Injury). Ac Staff, Parkwood Hospital - St Joseph's Health Care; Assoc Prof, University of Western Ontario; (519)685-4080; Fax. (519)685-4081; patrick.potter@sjhc.london.on.ca.

POTTER, Terri; Alberta College of Family Phys, 370-10403 172 St NW, Edmonton AB T5S 1K9; (780)488-2395; Fax. (780)488-2396.

POTTER, Tracy; 101-9845 Resthaven Dr, Sidney BC V8L 3E7; Man'83; (250)656-4713

POTTER-COGAN, Rickard M; Comox Med Clinic, 100-1695 Comox Ave, Comox BC V9M 3M1; National (Ireland)'78; DCH; DObst; CCFP; Ac Staff, St Joseph's General Hospital; Clin Instructor Family Med, University of British Columbia; (250)339-2266; rickpc@shaw.ca.

POTTIE, Kevin C; Bruyere Academic Fam Hlth Team, 75 Bruyere St, Ottawa ON K1N 5C7; Dal'92; CCFP; FCFP; Langs: Spanish; French; (613)241-3344

POTTLE, M Kent; 250-5675 Spring Garden Rd, Halifax NS B3J 1H1; Dal'83; BSc; Dip SportMed; Staff, Queen Elizabeth II Health Sciences Centre - Victoria General Site; (902)420-9383; Fax. (902)425-7948.

POTTLE, Robert A; 88 Gloria McCluskey Ave, Dartmouth NS B3B 2B8; Dal'86; BSc(Hon); MSc; FRCPC; Psy (Forensic Psychiatry). Staff, The East Coast Forensic Psychiatry Hospital; Lecturer, Dalhousie University; (902)460-7300 x7349; Fax. (902)460-7343.

POTTS, Jayson M; Hamilton HS-General Site, 711 Concession St, Hamilton ON L8V 1C3; Qns'07; FRCPC; IntMed. Staff, Hamilton Health Sciences Centre-Juravinski Site; (905)521-2100

POTTS, John D; Ladysmith Family Practice Clin, PO Box 10 Stn Main 1111 4th Ave, Ladysmith BC V9G 1A1; UBC'77; DTMH(Liverpool); (250)739-5784; Fax. (250)245-9730.

POTTS, Lana R; Sheldon Chumir Centre, 1213 4 St SW, Calgary AB T2R 0X7; NOSM'09; CCFP; (403)955-6600

POTTS, Leslie A; Bluewater Health-Norman Site, 89 Norman St, Sarnia ON N7T 6S3; Cal'85; FRCPC; DiagRad. Staff, Bluewater Health - Norman Site; Staff, Bluewater Health - Mitton Site; (519)464-4513

POTTS, Peter G G; 202-475 Park St, Kitchener ON N2G 4V5; McM'86; FRCSC; ObstGyn. (519)744-8561; Fax. (519)744-3089.

POTVIN, Anne; CHUQ-Ctr Hosp Univ Laval, 2705 boul Laurier, Quebec QC G1V 4G2; Laval'84; FRCPC; Psy. Staff, Centre Hospitalier Universitaire de Quebec-CHUL; (418)654-2177; Fax. (418)654-2716.

POTVIN, Christelle; Clin de Med Familiale Montcalm, 309 rue Montcalm, Chicoutimi QC G7J 2V1; Laval'09; CCFP; (418)545-4211

POTVIN, Daniel; Hop Maisonneuve-Rosemont, 5415 boul de l'Assomption, Montreal QC H1T 2M4; Mon'93; LMCC; Staff Emerg, Hopital Maisonneuve-Rosemont; (514)252-3400 x4558

POTVIN, Earl G; Pontiac Health Centre, 200 rue Argue, Shawville QC J0X 2Y0; Ott'64; BSc; FRCSC; GenSurg. General Surgery, Pontiac Hospital Centre; Teach Staff Undergraduate, McGill University; (819)647-2211; Fax. (819)647-3275.

POTVIN, Frederic; CSSS du Sud de Lanaudière, 911 montee des Pionniers, Terrebonne QC J6V 2H2; Mon'05; Staff, Centre Hospitalier Pierre le Gardeur; (450)654-7525

POTVIN, Helene; Clinique Med Saint-Luc, 264 boul Saint-Luc, St-Jean-Sur-Richel QC J2W 1C3; Mon'77; (450)348-6124; Fax. (450)348-4163.

POTVIN, Jacques A; Action Sport Physio, 1451 rue Montarville, Saint-Bruno QC J3V 3T6; Laval'64; Neursurg (P.Q.) (Medico Legal Issues). Langs: English; (450)441-1451; Fax. (450)441-6749; jacquespotvinmd@yahoo.ca.

POTVIN, Jean; CSSS de Montmagny-L'Islet, RR 1 350 boul Tache O, Montmagny QC G5V 3R8; Laval'71; FRCSC; OrthSurg. Staff, CSSS de Montmagny-L'Islet; (418)248-0630 x545; Fax. (418)248-0820.

POTVIN, Jean-Guy; Clin Fam Basses-Laurentides, 2100 boul du Cure-Labelle, Saint-Jerome QC J7Y 1S8; Mon'65; Langs: English; (450)565-6493; Fax. (450)565-1099.

POTVIN, Jean-Michel; CHUQ-Hotel-Dieu de Quebec, 11 Cote du Palais, Quebec QC G1R 2J6; Laval'00; FRCPC; IntMed; Cardiol. Staff, Centre Hospitalier Universitaire de Québec (CHUQ) - Siege Social; (418)525-4444

POTVIN, Jeannot; CHUM-Hotel-Dieu, 3840 rue Saint-Urbain, Montreal QC H2W 1T8; Mon'02; FRCPC; IntMed; Cardiol. Staff, Centre Hospitalier l'Université de Montréal (CHUM) - Hôtel-Dieu; (514)890-8000

POTVIN, Johanne; CLSC du Grand Chicoutimi, 411 rue de l'Hotel-Dieu, Chicoutimi QC G7H 7Z5; Sher'83; Chief General Med, CLSC des Coteaux; (418)543-2221; Fax. (418)693-8663.

POTVIN, Julie; Clinique Med Saint-Prime, 581 rue Coulombe, Saint-Prime QC G8J 1P2; Sher'07; Staff, Hotel-Dieu de Roberval; (418)251-9080; Fax. (418)251-9073.

POTVIN, Kylea; London Reg Cancer Centre, A3917-790 Commissioners Rd E, London ON N6A 4L6; McM'00; MedOncol; IntMed (Breasts). Staff MedOncol, London Regional Cancer Center; Asst Prof Schulich School of Med & Dentistry, University of Western Ontario; (519)685-8640; Fax. (519)685-8624; kylea.potvin@lhsc.on.ca.

POTVIN, Marie-Eve; CSSS de Portneuf, 700 rue Saint-Cyrille, Saint-Raymond QC G3L 1W1; Laval'05; Fam Med, Centre Hospitalier Portneuf; (418)337-4611

POTVIN, Martin; Ctr Hosp de Charlevoix, 74 rue Ambroise-Fafard, Baie-Saint-Paul QC G3Z 2J6; Laval'72; FRCSC; GenSurg. Staff, CSSS de Charlevoix; (418)435-5150; Fax. (418)435-5874.

POTVIN, Michel; CHUQ-St-Francois d'Assise, 10 rue de l'Espinay, Quebec QC G1L 3L5; Laval'82; CCFP; FCFP; Ac Staff, Centre Hospitalier Universitaire De Québec - Pavillon De St-françois-d'assise; Clin Prof, Université Laval; (418)525-4351; Fax. (418)525-4322.

POTVIN, Nadine S; Peace River Assoc Med Clinic, PO Box 7590, Peace River AB T8S 1T2; Wes'09; CCFP; (780)814-5800; Fax. (780)538-4400.

POTVIN, Nathalie; GMF des Seigneuries, 2220 boul Rene-Gaultier, Varennes QC J3X 1E3; Mon'89; (450)652-2917; Fax. (450)652-9902.

POTVIN, Nicholas A; Associate Medical Clinic, 10018 101 St, Peace River AB T8S 2A5; Wes'09; CCFP; (780)624-2581

POTVIN, Pierre; CSSS de Lac-Saint Jean-Est, CP 1300 Succ Bureau-Chef 300 boul Champlain S, Alma QC G8B 5W3; Sher'87; CSPQ; Anes. Staff, CSSS de Lac-Saint Jean-Est; (418)669-2000 x2224

POTVIN, Richard; Hop Santa Cabrini Ospedale, 5655 rue Saint-Zotique E, Montreal QC H1T 1P7; Sher'81; Staff, Hôpital Santa Cabrini Ospedale; (514)252-6444; richardpotvin@sympatico.ca.

POTVIN, Sandra; Clinique Med des 21, 101-171 6e rue, La Baie QC G7B 0A3; Sher'10; CCFP; (418)544-3331

POTVIN, William R; 72 Bridge St, Carleton Place ON K7C 2V3; Tor'95; PhD; CCFP; Staff, Carleton Place & District Memorial Hospital; Staff, Almonte General Hospital; Assoc Prof, University of Ottawa; Assoc Prof, Queen's University; (613)253-8192; Fax. (613)253-2566.

POTVIN-GIRARD, Marie-Claude; Ctre Pedopsychiatrie de Quebec, 1 av du Sacre-Coeur, Quebec QC G1N 2W1; Laval'02; FRCPC; Psy.

POU, Vitiya; Centre Med Metro-Monk, 2376 rue Allard, Montreal QC H4E 2K9; Sher'87; CCFP; Staff, Centre Hospitalier de LaSalle; (514)769-9999; Fax. (514)769-9008.

POU-YOUTHOAN, Kimlay; 4689 rue Papineau, Montreal QC H2H 1V4; Phnom-Penh (Cambodia)'70; Consultant Med, Ctre Med d'Urgence Mont-Royal; (514)521-5555

POUBELLE, Patrice E E; 2705 boul Laurier, Quebec QC G1V 4G2; Montpellier (France)'79; CSPQ; Rheum (P.Q.). Ac Staff, Centre Hospitalier Universitaire de Quebec-CHUL; assoc Prof, Université Laval; Langs: English; (418)656-4141; Fax. (418)654-2765; patrice.poubelle@crchul.ulaval.ca.

POUDRIER, Samiha; Ctr Hosp du Centre la Mauricie, 50 119e rue, Shawinigan-Sud QC G9P 5K1; Laval'03; Staff, Centre Hospitalier du Centre la Mauricie; (819)536-7500

POUKHOVSKI, Andrei; Edmonton Mental Health Clinic, 3F-9942 108 St NW, Edmonton AB T5K 2J5; Moscow (Russia (Federation))'86; PhD; Staff Psy, Alberta Hospital Edmonton; (780)342-7700

POULIN, Anne; 420-900 boul du Seminaire N, St-Jean-Sur-Richel QC J3A 1C3; Laval'86; CSPQ; FRCPC; DiagRad. (450)348-1111; Fax. (450)348-8585.

POULIN, Brett W; The Centreville Clinic, 301-3210 25 Ave, Vernon BC V1T 1P1; Cal'08; CCFP; (250)549-1245

POULIN, Brigitte; CHUQ-Ctr Hosp Univ Laval, 2206-2705 boul Laurier, Quebec QC G1V 4G2; Laval'85; CSPQ; FRCPC; Anes. Staff, Centre Hospitalier Universitaire de Quebec-CHUL; (418)656-4141 x7565; Fax. (418)658-2710.

POULIN, Chantal; MUHC-Montreal Children's Hosp, A505-2300 rue Tupper, Montreal QC H3H 1P3; Laval'92; FRCPC; Neur (Electromyography); Electroenceph (P.Q.). Staff, McGill University Health Centre - Montreal Children's Hospital; Consultant, Shriners Hospitals For Children - Canada; Langs: English; (514)412-4484; Fax. (514)412-4373.

POULIN, Christiane C; Health Canada, 1505 Barrington St, Halifax NS B3J 3Y6; Laval'82; FRCPC; CommunMed (Public Health). Chair Canada Research, Population Health & Addictions; Prof, Dalhousie University; (902)426-4656; Fax. (902)426-8675.

POULIN, Claude; 213 13e av N, Sherbrooke QC J1E 2X8; Sher'74; Assoc Staff, Centre Hospitalier Universitaire de Sherbrooke-Hopital Fleurimont; Assoc Staff, CSSS des Sources d'Asbestos; (819)565-0767; Fax. (819)565-9377.

POULIN, Claude; Polyclinique d'Argenteuil, 201-551 rue Berry, Lachute QC J8H 1S4; Laval'67; (450)562-3751; Fax. (450)562-1852.

POULIN, Daniel; Clinique Med Monchamp, 102-227 rue Sainte-Catherine, Saint-Constant QC J5A 2J5; Mon'82; (450)632-2245; Fax. (450)632-2795.

POULIN, David N; College of Phys & Surg of SK, 500-321 A 21st St E, Saskatoon SK S7K 0C1; McG'79; CCFP; CCFP(E.M.); Dir Med Services, Royal Inland Hospital; Langs: French; (306)244-7355; Fax. (306)244-0090.

POULIN, Eric C; The Ottawa Hosp-Gen Campus, 501 Smyth Rd, Ottawa ON K1H 8L6; Laval'67; AB; FACS; FRCSC; GenSurg (Laparoscopic Surgery). Staff, The Ottawa Hospital - General Campus; Dept Head Surg, University of Ottawa; (613)737-8899 x71763; Fax. (613)739-6769.

POULIN, Eric; CSSS Pierre Boucher, 1333 boul Jacques-Cartier E, Longueuil QC J4M 2A5; Laval'89; IntMed. Staff, Centre Hospitalier Pierre Boucher; (450)468-8111 x2441; Fax. (450)468-8032.

POULIN, Eric S; Clinique Med St-Francois, RR 2 214 rue Saint-Francois, Saint-Pie QC J0H 1W0; Laval'95; Staff, Centre Hospitalier Honore-Mercier; (450)772-6526; Fax. (450)772-0827.

POULIN, Fernand; 1200 6e av, La Pocatiere QC G0R 1Z0; Laval'71; Staff, CSSS de Kamouraska; (418)856-4647; Fax. (418)856-3211.

POULIN, Frederic; Hop du Sacre-Coeur de Mtl, 5400 boul Gouin O, Montreal QC H4J 1C5; Mon'04; FRCPC; IntMed; Cardiol. Staff, Hôpital du Sacre-Coeur de Montréal; (514)338-2050

POULIN, Genevieve; Clinique Med de Mont-Joli, 1385 boul Benoit-Gaboury, Mont-Joli QC G5H 4B1; Laval'03; (418)775-5353

POULIN, Guy; Polyclinique Du Cap, 110-700 boul Thibeau, Trois-Rivieres QC G8T 7A1; Laval'72; (819)373-4551

POULIN, Jean-Francois; Ctr Hosp Affilie-St-Sacrement, 1050 ch Sainte-Foy, Quebec QC G1S 4L8; Mon'84; FRCPC; IntMed; Cardiol. Staff, Centre Hospitalier Affilié Universitaire de Québec - Hôpital De L'Enfant Jésus; ac Staff, Centre Hospitalier Affilié Universitaire de Québec - Hôpital du St-Sacrement; Langs: English; (418)649-5887; poulinjef@hotmail.com.

POULIN, Jean-Pierre; Carrefour Med Vallee du Richel, 665 boul Sir-Wilfrid-Laurier, Beloeil QC J3G 4J1; Laval'98; Staff, Centre Hospitalier Pierre Boucher; (450)467-0088

POULIN, Jose; Centre Med de Riviere-du-Loup, 242 rue Lafontaine, Riviere-du-Loup QC G5R 3A7; Laval'76; Staff, Centre Hospitalier Regional du Grand-Portage; (418)862-3110; Fax. (418)862-9656.

POULIN, Kathleen; CSSS d'Antoine-Labelle-Mt Laur, RR 1 2561 ch de la Lièvre S, Mont-Laurier QC J9L 3G3; Mon'00; CCFP; Staff, CSSS d'Antoine-Labelle; (819)623-1234

POULIN, Louis-Denis; CHUQ-Hotel-Dieu de Quebec, 11 Cote du Palais, Quebec QC G1R 2J6; Laval'81; FRCPC; IntMed; Nephrol. Staff Nephrol, Centre Hospitalier Universitaire de Québec (CHUQ) - Siege Social; Teach Staff, Université Laval; (418)691-5464; Fax. (418)691-5757.

POULIN, Marie-Claude; CHUQ-St-Francois d'Assise, 10 rue de l'Espinay, Quebec QC G1L 3L5; Laval'90; FRCPC; IntMed (Vascular Medicine). Physician, Centre Hospitalier Universitaire De Québec - Pavillon De St-françois-d'assise; Langs: Bilingual(French/English); (418)525-4444; Fax. (418)525-4467.

POULIN, Marie-Helene; Clinique Med de Montmagny, 100-83 av de la Fabrique, Montmagny QC G5V 2J3; Laval'97; (418)248-4933; marie-helene.poulin@gmf.gouv.qc.ca.

POULIN, Marie-Josee; Medi-Centre Chomedey, 610 boul Cure-Labelle, Laval QC H7V 2T7; Mon'89; (450)687-6452; Fax. (450)687-3243.

POULIN, Marie-Josee; Inst U en Sante Mentale de QC, 2601 ch de la Canardiere, Quebec QC G1J 2G3; Laval'81; LMCC; FRCPC; Psy (Perinatal Psychiatry). Dir Psychosis & Perinatal Psy Prog, Institut Universitaire Sante; Prof Psy, Université Laval; (418)663-5321

POULIN, Mark D; Seaforth Med Bldg, 390-3550 ch de la Cote-des-Nei, Montreal QC H3H 1V4; Burlington(VT) (USA)'88; Otol (P.Q.). (514)938-3933; Fax. (514)935-2343.

POULIN, Martine; CSSS de Beauce-Etchemin, 1515 17e rue, Saint-Georges QC G5Y 4T8; Laval'93; CSPQ; FRCPC; Anes. Staff, Centre Hospitalier Beauce-Etchemin; (418)228-2031 x5000; martipou@globetrotter.net.

POULIN, Maude; 166 Rte 132 E, St-Michel-de-Bell QC G0R 3S0; Laval'05; CCFP; (418)804-0556

POULIN, Maurice; Inst Nat'l de Sante Publique, 550 rue Bonaventure, Trois-Rivieres QC G9A 2B5; Laval'69; MPH; OccupMed (P.Q.) (Public Health). Langs: English; French; (819)693-3955; Fax. (819)373-1627; maurice.poulin@inspq.qc.ca.

POULIN, Michael; CSSS de la Cote-de-Gaspe, 215 boul de York O, Gaspe QC G4X 2W2; Mon'07; CCFP; Staff, Centre Hospitalier de Gaspe; (418)368-3301; Fax. (418)368-6850.

POULIN, Michael P; Vancouver Gen Hosp, 855 12th Ave W, Vancouver BC V5Z 1M9; UBC'80; FRCPC; GenPath. Staff, Vancouver General Hospital - Centennial Pavillion; (604)875-4111 x68397

POULIN, Michel; Clinique du Havre, 79A rue Jacques-Cartier, Gaspe QC G4X 1M5; Sher'83; (418)368-5609; Fax. (418)368-6498.

POULIN, Monic; CLSC Basse-Ville-Limoilou, 50 rue Saint-Joseph E, Quebec QC G1K 3A5; Laval'85; (418)529-6592; Fax. (418)529-1515.

POULIN, Pascale; CSSS de Laval, 421-1755 boul Renee Levesque, Laval QC H7M 3L9; Mon'05; Staff, Hopital de la Cite de la santé; (450)668-1010

POULIN, Pierre; Hop Charles LeMoyne, 3120 boul Taschereau, Greenfield Park QC J4V 2H1; Sher'92; FRCPC; Psy. Staff, Hopital Charles LeMoyne; (450)466-5020; Fax. (450)466-5015.

POULIN, Pierre-Claude; CSSS de Beauce-Etchemin, 1515 17e rue, Saint-Georges QC G5Y 4T8; Sher'75; Peds. Staff, Centre Hospitalier Beauce-Etchemin; (418)228-2031; Fax. (418)227-6246.

POULIN, Rejean; Clinique Med Vallee-Jonction, 315B rue Principale, Vallee-Jonction QC G0S 3J0; Laval'67; Staff, Centre Hospitalier Beauce-Etchemin; (418)253-5481; Fax. (418)253-5157.

POULIN, Renald M; 193 boul de Quen, Alma QC G8B 5N4; Laval'72; GenSurg (P.Q.). Ac Staff, CSSS de Lac-Saint Jean-Est; Langs: English; Spanish; (418)668-3008; Fax. (418)668-8452; renaldpoulin@bellnet.ca.

POULIN, Sacha; Clin de Psy Bois-de-Boulogne, 505-1575 boul Henri-Bourassa O, Montreal QC H3M 3A9; Laval'01; Psy (Mood Disorders). Staff Psy, Hôpital du Sacre-Coeur de Montréal; Langs: Bilingual(French/English); (514)338-4300; Fax. (514)338-4493.

POULIN, Sonya; Hôpital Laval, 2725 ch Sainte-Foy, Quebec QC G1V 4G5; Laval'97; FRCPC; IntMed; Nephrol. Staff, Hôpital Laval; Langs: English; (418)656-4511; Fax. (418)656-4587.

POULIN, Stephane; Ctr Hosp Laurentien, 234 rue Saint-Vincent, Ste-Agathe-Des-Mts QC J8C 2B8; Mon'89; Dip SportMed; Dir Service Professionel, Centre Hospitalier Laurentien; Physician Sports Med, Club Medico Sante Avantage; Langs: English; (819)324-4000; Fax. (819)324-4010; stephane.poulin.sommets@ssss.gouv.qc.ca.

POULIN, Stephane; Ctr Hosp Affilie-Enfant-Jesus, 1401 18e rue, Quebec QC G1J 1Z4; Mon'02; FRCPC; Psy. Staff, Centre Hospitalier Affilié Universitaire de Québec - Hôpital De L'Enfant Jésus; (418)649-0252

POULIN, Veronique; CSSS de Saint-Jerome, 290 rue de Montigny, Saint-Jerome QC J7Z 5T3; Staff, Hôtel-Dieu de Saint-Jérôme; (450)431-8200

POULIN, Veronique; CSSS de Beauce-Etchemin, 1515 17e rue, Saint-Georges QC G5Y 4T8; Laval'03; FRCPC; Anes. Staff, Centre Hospitalier Beauce-Etchemin; (418)228-2031

POULIN, Yannick; CHUS-Hop Fleurimont, 3001 12e av N, Sherbrooke QC J1H 5N4; Sher'03; FRCPC; IntMed; Respir. Staff, Centre Hospitalier Universitaire de Sherbrooke-Hopital Fleurimont; (819)346-1110

POULIN, Yves P; Ctr Dermatologique du Quebec, 105-2880 ch des Quatre-Bourgeo, Quebec QC G1V 4X7; Sher'78; CSPQ; FRCPC; Derm. Staff, Centre Hospitalier Universitaire de Québec (CHUQ) - Siege Social; Langs: English; (418)650-3555; Fax. (418)650-1260.

POULIN, Yves; CSSS de Rimouski-Neigette, CP 3150 Succ A 150 av Rouleau, Rimouski QC G5L 5T1; Sher'87; FRCPC; Psy (Assessment (Long Term)). Staff, Hôpital Regional Rimouski; Physician, Min. de la Securite Publique du Quebec; (418)724-8315; Fax. (418)724-8652.

POULIN DE COURVAL, Louise S; CLSC Cote-des-Neiges, 6600 ch Cote-des-Neiges, Montreal QC H3S 2A9; McG'71; DPH; CCFP; FCFP; Staff Dept of Family Med, Sir Mortimer B Davis Jewish General; Teach Staff, McGill University; (514)731-1386 x8219; Fax. (514)731-3532; lpoulind@ssss.gouv.qc.ca.

POULIN-TREPANIER, Evelyne; CSSS de Temiscouata, CP 310 58 rue de l'Eglise, Notre-Dame-du-Lac QC G0L 1X0; Laval'09; CCFP; Staff, Centre Hospitalier Notre-Dame-du-Lac; (418)899-6751

POULIOT, Bernard; CSSS de Rivière-de-Loup, 75 rue Saint-Henri, Riviere-Du-Loup QC G5R 2A4; Laval'73; CSPQ; MSc; Public Health & Preventive Med; CommunMed (P.Q.). Staff, Centre Hospitalier Regional du Grand-Portage; Langs: Bilingual(French/English); (418)868-1010 x2428; Fax. (418)868-1033; bernard.pouliot.asss01@ssss.gouv.qc.ca.

POULIOT, Catherine; Centre Hosp Honore-Mercier, 2750 boul Laframboise, Saint-Hyacinthe QC J2S 4Y8; Laval'96; FRCSC; OrthSurg. Staff, Centre Hospitalier Honore-Mercier; (450)771-3333 x3366; Fax. (450)771-3691.

POULIOT, Claude; Centre Med Laurier, 5661 boul Laurier, Terrebonne QC J7M 1T7; Laval'87; (450)477-5364; Fax. (450)477-5634.

POULIOT, Claudie; Clin Med du Vieux Limoilou, 755 3e av, Quebec QC G1L 2W7; Mon'96; Psy. (418)266-0500; Fax. (418)266-0501.

POULIOT, Denis; Ctr Hosp Affilie-Enfant-Jesus, 1401 18e rue, Quebec QC G1J 1Z4; Laval'71; FABOtolaryngology (Head; FRCSC; Otol (Otoneurology). assoc Staff, Hôpital de la Malbaie; assoc Staff, Hôpital Laval; ac Membre Dept of Otol, Centre Hospitalier Affilié Universitaire de Québec - Hôpital De L'Enfant Jésus; assoc Staff, Centre Hospitalier Chauveau; Langs: Bilingual(French/English); (418)649-0252; pouliotdenis@videotron.ca.

POULIOT, Frederic; CHUQ-Hotel-Dieu de Quebec, 11 Cote du Palais, Quebec QC G1R 2J6; Laval'03; Urol. Staff, Centre Hospitalier Universitaire de Québec (CHUQ) - Siege Social; (418)525-4444

POULIOT, Joel; CSSS de la Vallée de l'Or, 725 6e rue, Val-d'Or QC J9P 3Y1; Mon'88; Cardiol; IntMed. Staff, Centre Hospitalier de Val d'Or; (819)825-6711 x2238; Fax. (819)825-7975; joel_pouliot@ssss.gouv.qc.ca.

POULIOT, Johanne; Clinique Med Mascouche, 1025 Montee Masson, Mascouche QC J7K 2L9; Sher'91; Staff, Hopital de la Cite de la santé; Langs: English; (450)474-6000; Fax. (450)474-6666.

POULIOT, Kathleen; Clinique Med l'Avenir, 200-1150 boul de l'Avenir, Laval QC H7N 6L2; Laval'83; (450)680-1150; Fax. (450)680-1151; kpouliot@vl.videotron.ca.

POULIOT, Louis; Centre Med de Gentilly, 1775 boul Becancour, Becancour QC G9H 3V4; Laval'62; General Practice, Hôpital de Christ-Roi; Staff, Centre Hospitalier Regional de Trois-Rivieres; (819)298-3113

POULIOT, Marie-Christine; Clinique Med de Levis, 100-4975 boul de la Rive-Sud, Levis QC G6V 4Z5; Mon'96; Langs: Bilingual(French/English); (418)833-5810; Fax. (418)833-2720.

POULIOT, Martine; Clinique Med du Boise Langevin, 130-288 rue Pierre-Saindon, Rimouski QC G5L 9A8; Sher'82; Staff, Hôpital Regional Rimouski; (418)724-4672; Fax. (418)724-4753.

POULIOT, Michele; Ctr Hosp Laurentien, 234 rue Saint-Vincent, Ste-Agathe-Des-Mts QC J8C 2B8; Sher'92; FRCPC; Psy. Staff, Centre Hospitalier Laurentien; (819)324-4044; Fax. (819)324-4020.

POULIOT, Rene; Hôpital Laval, 2725 ch Sainte-Foy, Quebec QC G1V 4G5; Laval'71; IntMed; Nephrol (P.Q.). Asst Dir, Hôpital Laval; Langs: English; (418)656-4511; Fax. (418)656-4587.

POULOPOULOS, Vassilios; 303-100 Colborne St W, Orillia ON L3V 2Y9; Athens (Greece)'73; FRCPC; IntMed; Nephrol. Staff Nephrol, Orillia Soldiers' Memorial Hospital; Langs: Greek; (705)325-0077; Fax. (705)325-0677.

POULOS, Elena; Kingsway Derm & Cosmetic Ctr, 1000-1243 Islington Ave, Etobicoke ON M8X 1Y9; Ott'97; BSc; FRCPC; Derm. Langs: Greek; French; (416)231-0100; Fax. (416)231-0109.

POULOS, Robert K; Nova Scotia Rehabilitation Ctr, 0210-1341 Summer St, Halifax NS B3H 1K1; Dal'89; (902)473-1230; Fax. (902)473-3204.

POULSEN, P Dorothea; Drumheller Health Centre, PO Box 4500 351 9 St NW, Drumheller AB T0J 0Y0; Cal'82; CCFP; FCFP; Staff, Drumheller Health Centre; (403)823-6500; dpoulsen@dthr.ab.ca.

POUND, Brian S; 275-1555 McKenzie Ave, Victoria BC V8N 1A4; London (England)'65; MB BS; LRCP; MRCS; Ac Staff, Victoria General Hospital; Ac Staff, Royal Jubilee Hospital; Assoc Prof School of Nursing, University of Victoria; (250)477-9535; Fax. (250)477-2853; doctorpound@shawcable.com.

POUND, Catherine M; Children's Hosp Eastern Ont, 401 Smyth Rd, Ottawa ON K1H 8L1; McG'02; FRCPC; Peds (Hematology). Consultant Peds, Children's Hospital of Eastern Ontario (CHEO); Langs: Bilingual(English/French); (613)737-7600 x2571; Fax. (613)738-4878.

POUND, Jeremy I; Albany Med Clinic, 807 Broadview Ave, Toronto ON M4K 2P8; Tor'02; CCFP; (416)461-9471; Fax. (416)461-2710.

POUNDER, David R; Chinook Reg Hosp, 960 19 St S, Lethbridge AB T1J 1W5; Alb'81; FRCPC; Anes. Ac Staff Anes, Chinook Regional Hospital; (403)388-6131; Fax. (403)388-6154.

POUNGUI MOUNGONDO, Lionel A; CSSSG-Hop de Gatineau, CP 2000 Succ Bureau-Chef 909 boul de la Verendrye O, Gatineau QC J8P 7H2; Laval'04; FRCSC; ObstGyn. Staff, Hôpital de Gatineau; (819)966-6100

POUPART, Charles; CSSS Pierre Boucher, 1333 boul Jacques-Cartier E, Longueuil QC J4M 2A5; Mon'84; FRCPC; IntMed; Hem. Hematologist, Centre Hospitalier Pierre Boucher; Fax. (450)468-8201.

POUPART, Gilles; Tour A, 800 boul Chomedey, Laval QC H7V 3Y4; Mon'70; CSPQ; CommunMed (P.Q.). (450)978-2126; Fax. (450)978-2100.

POUPART, Helene; 11-56 boul Saint-Joseph O, Montreal QC H2T 2P4; Mon'78; MSc; (514)845-3229

POUPART, Normand; Clinique Med Sante du Village, D-294 du Village GD, Les Eboulements QC G0A 2M0; Mon'88; (418)635-1427

POUPART, Robert; Clin Pediatrique Laurentienne, 106-200 rue Durand, Saint-Jerome QC J7Z 7E2; Mon'89; FRCPC; Peds; Cardiol (P.Q.). Staff, Hôtel-Dieu de Saint-Jérôme; Langs: English; (450)438-1241; Fax. (450)438-3501; debbie.poupart@sympatico.ca.

POUR-AHMADI, Omid; Pacific Place Mall, 999 36 St NE, Calgary AB T2A 7X6; Santiago (Dominican Republic)'96; (403)387-3300

POURCHER, Emmanuelle; Clin Ste-Anne Memoire & Mouvem, 304-1248 ch Sainte-Foy, Quebec QC G1S 2M5; Lyon (France)'82; CRCP; FRFPS; MMed; FRCPC; Neur (Movement Disorders). Neurologue, Institut Universitaire Sante; Neurologue, Centre Hospitalier Affilié Universitaire de Québec - Hôpital De L'Enfant Jésus; Neurologist, Clinique Sainte-Anne Memoire et Mouvement; Teach Staff, Université Laval; Langs: Spanish; Russian; English; (418)692-2227; Fax. (418)692-3338; psa@riq.qc.ca.

POURDOWLAT, Afsaneh; 214-955 Major Mackenzie Dr W, Vaughan ON L6A 4P9; Ege (Turkey)'90; FRCPC; IntMed; Cardiol. (905)303-5701; Fax. (905)303-9813.

POURVALI, Reza; St Paul's Hosp, 1081 Burrard St, Vancouver BC V6Z 1Y6; UBC'08; CCFP; CCFP(E.M.); Staff, Providence Health Care - St Paul's Hospital; Langs: Farsi; (604)682-2344

POUTANEN, Susan M; Mount Sinai Hosp, 1470-600 University Ave, Toronto ON M5G 1X5; Tor'96; MPH; FRCPC; IntMed; MedMicrobiol; InfectDis. Assoc Staff, University Health Network; Ac Staff, Mount Sinai Hospital; Asst Prof Dept of Lab Med Path & Med, University of Toronto; (416)586-8423; spoutanen@mtsinai.on.ca.

POUTEAU, Dawn C; Ctr Hosp Reg Chisasibi, CP 250, Chisasibi QC J0M 1E0; McG'94; CCFP; Staff, Cree Board of Health & Social Services James Bay; (819)855-2844

POUTEAU, Kathleen M; Meno Ya Win Health Centre, PO Box 4000, Sioux Lookout ON P8T 1K2; Cal'03; CCFP; (807)737-5161; Fax. (807)737-5089.

POVAH, W Bruce; 202-3330 Richter St, Kelowna BC V1W 4V5; Man'75; FRCSC; Otol. (250)861-5578; Fax. (250)861-5979.

POVITZ, Marcus; Foothills Med Centre, 1403 29 St NW, Calgary AB T2N 2T9; McG'07; MDCM; FRCPC; IntMed; Respir. Staff, Foothills Medical Centre; (403)944-1110

POW, David G; Springborough Prof Centre, 221-30 Springborough Blvd SW, Calgary AB T3H 0N9; Cal'85; CCFP; Staff, Rockyview General Hospital; Staff Univ Health Services, University of Calgary; (403)240-0124; Fax. (403)240-0256.

POW, Randall F; 150-4625 Varsity Dr NW, Calgary AB T3A 0Z9; Cal'79.

POWALINSKY, Agnes C C; Kenderdine Med Clinic, 110-1804 McOrmond Dr, Saskatoon SK S7S 0A6; Sask'85; CCFP; FCFP; Clin Associate, Royal University Hospital; Staff Privil, St Paul's Hospital (Grey Nuns) of Saskatoon; Staff Privil, Saskatoon City Hospital; (306)934-6606; Fax. (306)955-3180; apowalinsky@yahoo.ca.

POWAR, Sukhbinderjit K; Winston Park Family Physicians, 104-2315 Bristol Cir, Oakville ON L6H 6P8; Glasgow (Scotland)'91; MB ChB; CCFP; Langs: Punjabi; (905)829-2826; Fax. (905)829-2846.

POWE, John E; Vancouver Gen Hosp, 855 12th Ave W, Vancouver BC V5Z 1M9; Wes'73; FRCPC; IntMed (Bone Densitometry); NuclearMed. Staff Radiol, Vancouver General Hospital - Centennial Pavillion; Assoc Prof, University of British Columbia; (604)875-4620; Fax. (604)875-5289; john.powe@vch.ca.

POWELL, Anne C; Avenue Med Centre, 221 Brant Ave, Brantford ON N3T 3J3; McM'02; FRCSC; ObstGyn. (519)753-8666

POWELL, Barbara M; PO Box 72099 Rpo Kanata North, Kanata ON K2K 2P4; Ott'77; CCFP; FCFP; Langs: German; (613)591-3942

POWELL, Calvin N; 286 Conception Bay Hwy PO Box 1017, Bay Roberts NL A0A 1G0; Mem'82; CCFP.

POWELL, Christopher C; 303 9th Ave SW PO Box 5550 Stn Main, High River AB T1V 0H2; Cal'96; CCFP; CCFP(E.M.); Clin Associate High River Community Cancer Clin, Alberta Cancer Board; (403)652-2929; Fax. (403)652-1510.

POWELL, Colin; Rockyview Gen Hosp, 7007 14 St SW, Calgary AB T2V 1P9; London (England)'65; FRCP; MB; Staff, Rockyview General Hospital; Staff Geriatric, Alberta Health Services-Calgary Zone; Board Member, Canadian Association of Retired Persons; Prof Med, University of Calgary; (403)943-8832; Fax. (403)943-8592; ccpowell@ucalgary.ca.

POWELL, D Gregory; STARS, 1441 Aviation Park NE, Calgary AB T2E 8M7; UBC'72; BSc; FRCPC; EmergMed (Travel Medicine). Ac Staff Emergency Med, Foothills Medical Centre; CEO/Pres, Shock Trauma Air Rescue Society; Prof, University of Calgary; (403)295-1811; Fax. (403)295-2426.

POWELL, Elizabeth; Peel Med Arts Bldg, 501-145 Queen St E, Brampton ON L6W 3P8; McG'75; FRCPC; IntMed (Asthma); Respir. Court Staff, Toronto General Hospital - UHN; Lecturer, University of Toronto; (905)456-2543

POWELL, Erin D; Dr H Bliss Murphy Cancer Ctr, 300 Prince Philip Dr, St. John's NL A1B 3V6; Mem'04; FRCPC; IntMed; MedOncol. Staff, Dr H Bliss Murphy Cancer Centre; (709)777-7802

POWELL, Garry W; Medical Arts Bldg, 507-180 Metcalfe St, Ottawa ON K2P 1P5; Alb'69; FRCPC; Psy (Psychotherapy & Psychoanalysis). (613)565-1484

POWELL, Gerald W; 339 Gilmour St, Ottawa ON K2P 0R1; Ott'84; BSc(Hon.); FRCPC; Psy.

POWELL, Gordon W W; Scott Clinic, 775 Monaghan Rd, Peterborough ON K9J 5K2; Tor'69; BSc; CCFP; FCFP; Ac Staff, Peterborough Regional Health Centre - Hospital Drive; Clin Prof Family Med, McMaster University; Clin Preceptor, Queen's University; (705)748-3933; Fax. (705)742-7661; gpowell@prhc.on.ca.

POWELL, James N; Bone & Joint Clinic, 0444-3134 Hospital Dr NW, Calgary AB T2N 5A1; Sask'80; FRCSC; OrthSurg. Ac Staff, Foothills Medical Centre; Associate Clin Prof, University of Calgary; (403)266-3494; Fax. (403)270-8004.

POWELL, Julie C; Hôpital Ste-Justine, 3175 ch Cote-Sainte-Catherine, Montreal QC H3T 1C5; Sher'76; ABD; FRCPC; Peds; Derm. Dir Derm Service, Hôpital Ste-Justine; Teach Staff, Universite de Montreal; (514)345-4675; Fax. (514)345-4822; julie_powell@ssss.gouv.qc.ca.

POWELL, Kara A; 213 3 Ave NE SS 2, Slave Lake AB T0G 2A2; Sask'06; CCFP; (780)849-4155; Fax. (780)849-4574.

POWELL, Mareli; South Common Med Clinic, 9711 23 Ave NW, Edmonton AB T6N 1K7; (South Africa)'95; (780)438-5920; Fax. (780)622-4169.

POWELL, Mark R; Mitchell Family Doctors, PO Box 790 7 Frances St, Mitchell ON N0K 1N0; Mem'04; CCFP; (519)348-8402

POWELL, Ruth; Dr Ruth M Powell Inc, 212-1669 Victoria St, Prince George BC V2L 2L5; Dal'82; BSc; CCFP; FCFP; Staff, University Hospital of Northern British Columbia; (250)614-2330; Fax. (250)614-2339; dr.rmpowell@gmail.com.

POWELL, Scott A; Royal Court Med Centre, 201-1 Quarry Ridge Rd, Barrie ON L4M 7G1; McM'94; FRCSC; GenSurg (Varicose Veins). Staff, Royal Victoria Regional Health Centre; (705)720-2003; Fax. (705)720-2109.

POWELL, T Lynette; Killick Health Services, 54 Union St, Grnd-Falls-Windsor NL A2A 2E2; Mem'01; CCFP; (709)489-5882

POWELL, Thomas; MUHC-Royal Victoria Hosp, 687 av des Pins O, Montreal QC H3A 1A1; Dublin (Ireland)'95; Staff, McGill University Health Centre - Royal Victoria Hospital; (514)934-1934 x43583; Fax. (514)843-1517.

POWELL, V Lynette; Rothbart Ctr for Pain Care Ltd, 9-4646 Dufferin St, North York ON M3H 5S4; Mem'81; FRCPC; Anes (Chronic Pain). (416)512-6407; Fax. (416)512-6375.

POWELL-FRANCIS, Kathryn A; Scarborough Pain Clinic, 425-1200 Markham Rd, Scarborough ON M1H 3C3; West Indies (Jamaica)'74; MB BS; FFARCS; DAAPM; Anes (Pain Management). Court Staff, Sensenbrenner Hospital; Langs: English; French; (416)438-7080; Fax. (416)438-7072.

POWER, Martina; 109-725 Coronation Blvd, Cambridge ON N1R 7S9; University Coll. (Ireland)'77; MB ChB; FRCPC; Psy (General Adult Psychiatry). Staff, Grand River Hospital - Kitchener/Waterloo Health Centre; (519)621-2828; Fax. (519)621-4904.

POWER, Adam H; London HSC-Victoria Hosp, PO Box 5010 Stn B E2 121-800 Commissioners Rd E, London ON N6A 5W9; Dal'04; VascSurg; GenSurg. Staff, London Health Sciences Centre - Victoria Campus; (519)667-6775

POWER, Alicia M; 201-284 Helmcken Rd, Victoria BC V9B 1T2; UBC'07; (250)480-1401

POWER, Alison; Moncton Med Clinic, 301-860 Mountain Rd, Moncton NB E1C 2N7; Flinders (Australia)'05; CCFP.

POWER, Barbara E; The Ottawa Hosp-Civic Campus, 1053 Carling Ave, Ottawa ON K1Y 4E9; Mem'83; FRCPC; IntMed; GeriatricMed. Staff, The Ottawa Hospital - Civic Campus; Asst Prof, University of Ottawa; (613)761-4795; Fax. (613)761-5334; bepower@ottawahospital.on.ca.

POWER, Brian M; 6 Alice St PO Box 220, Flesherton ON N0C 1E0; Tor'77; CCFP; FCFP; Ac Staff, Grey Bruce Health Services - Markdale; (519)924-2012; Fax. (519)924-3828; bmpower@bmts.com.

POWER, Christopher N; Heritage Med Research, 6 11-107 University Campus NW, Edmonton AB T6G 2S2; Ott'85; FRCPC; Neur (AIDS/HIV). Prof Dept of Med Microbiol & Immunol, University of Alberta; (780)407-1938; Fax. (780)407-3410; chris.power@ualberta.ca.

POWER, Daniel J; The Ottawa Hosp-Civic Campus, B309-1053 Carling Ave, Ottawa ON K1Y 4E9; Mem'95; FRCPC; Anes;CCFP; CCFP(E.M.); Staff, The Ottawa Hospital - Civic Campus; (613)737-8187

POWER, Ellen M; Glengarry Mem Hosp, Hwy 43, Alexandria ON K0C 1A0; Dal'86; Staff, Glengarry Memorial Hospital; (613)525-2222

POWER, Gerald A; Harbour Grace Med Centre, PO Box 280, Harbour Grace NL A0A 2M0; Dal'67; (709)596-6153; Fax. (709)596-6153.

POWER, Guy; Dr Georges-L Dumont Reg Hosp, 330 av Universite, Moncton NB E1C 2Z3; Mon'99; LMCC; CCFP; CCFP(E.M.); Staff, Dr Georges-L-Dumont University Hospital Centre; (506)862-4000

POWER, Kevin V; Nepean Med Centre, 401-1 Centrepointe Dr, Nepean ON K2G 6E2; Ott'96; FRCS; BA; Urol; FRCSC; Urol (Adult Urology). Att Staff Urol, Queensway Carleton Hospital; Lecturer Faculty of Med, Queen's University; Langs: Bilingual(French/English); (613)321-8213; Fax. (613)321-8369.

POWER, Lorena M; Western Memorial Health Clinic, 3 Herald Ave, Corner Brook NL A2H 4B8; Mem'06; CCFP; Staff, Bonne Bay Health Centre.

POWER, Lynette M; Burin Family Practice, PO Box 100 43-45 Main St, Burin Bay Arm NL A0E 1G0; Mem'96; CCFP; (709)891-5005

POWER, Maryse; Gordon & Leslie Diamond HCC, 2775 Laurel St, Vancouver BC V5Z 1M9; Cork (Ireland)'97; Staff, Vancouver General Hospital - Centennial Pavillion; Staff Leukemia/BMT Program, Gordon & Leslie Diamond Health Care Centre; Langs: Bilingual(English/French); (604)875-4863; Fax. (604)875-4763.

POWER, Michael G; 4-105 Progress Cres, Kapuskasing ON P5N 3J4; Mem'90; BSc; (705)335-6866; Fax. (705)335-8780.

POWER, Michael T; Lacewood Med Centre, 200-366 Lacewood Dr, Halifax NS B3S 1M7; Dal'96; CCFP; (902)445-9400; Fax. (902)445-7108.

POWER, Nicholas E; London HSC-Victoria Hosp, PO Box 5010 Stn B 800 Commissioners Rd E, London ON N6A 5W9; Dal'04; FRCSC; Urol. Staff, London Health Sciences Centre - Victoria Campus; (519)667-6787

POWER, R Patricia; Dr H Bliss Murphy Cancer Ctr, 300 Prince Philip Dr, St. John's NL A1B 3V6; Mem'97; BSc; MSc; FRCSC; ObstGyn; GynOnco. Staff, Dr H Bliss Murphy Cancer Centre; Asst Prof Dept of Women's Hlth, Memorial University Of Newfoundland; (709)777-6564; Fax. (709)777-8533.

POWER, Robert F; Royal Jubilee Hosp, 1952 Bay St, Victoria BC V8R 1J8; National (Ireland)'79; MRCPath(UK); FRCPC; AnatPath. Staff Lab Med, Royal Jubilee Hospital; (250)370-8832

POWER, Stephen G A; London HSC-Victoria Hosp, PO Box 5010 Stn B 800 Commissioners Rd E, London ON N6A 5W9; Wes'87; BSc; PhD; FRCSC; ObstGyn (Infertility). Consultant ObstGyn, London Health Sciences Centre - University Hospital; Staff, London Health Sciences Centre - Victoria Campus; Asst Prof Faculty of Med, University of Western Ontario; (519)685-8257; Fax. (519)685-8340; spower@uwo.ca.

POWER, Y Mark E; Western Mem Reg Hosp, PO Box 2005 Stn Main, Corner Brook NL A2H 6J7; Mem'02; FRCPC; Psy. Staff, Western Memorial Regional Hospital; (709)637-5000

POWERS, Bruce N; Burlington Prof Centre, 402-3155 Harvester Rd, Burlington ON L7N 3V2; McM'79; (905)632-3000; Fax. (905)632-7960.

POWERS, Peter J; St Joseph's Healthcare, 50 Charlton Ave E, Hamilton ON L8N 4A6; Sask'71; FRCPC; Hem; IntMed. Staff, St Joseph's Healthcare - Charlton Campus; Assoc Prof Path & Med, McMaster University; (905)521-6024; Fax. (905)540-6568.

POWIS, Jeff E; Toronto East Gen Hosp Inc, 825 Coxwell Ave, Toronto ON M4C 3E7; Ott'00; BSc; FRCP; FRCPC; IntMed (AIDS/HIV); InfectDis. Staff Dept of Med InfectDis, Toronto East General Hospital Inc; (416)469-6252; Fax. (416)469-6253; jpowi@tegh.on.ca.

POWLES, A C Peter; St Joseph's Healthcare, T2137-50 Charlton Ave E, Hamilton ON L8N 4A6; Otago (New Zealand)'66; MB ChB; FRACP; AB; FRCPC; IntMed (Sleep Disorders). Staff, St Joseph's Health Centre; Staff, St Joseph's Healthcare - Charlton Campus; Prof, University of Toronto; (905)522-1155 x4299; powlep@stjoe.on.ca.

POWLES, Kristina E; Granovsky Gluskin Fam Medicine, 4F-60 Murray St, Toronto ON M5T 3L9; Qns'09; CCFP; (416)586-4800; Fax. (416)586-3175.

POWLOWSKI, Marcus T; Thunder Bay Reg HSC-T-Bay, 980 Oliver Rd, Thunder Bay ON P7B 6V4; Tor'86; Staff, Thunder Bay Regional Health Sciences Centre; (807)684-6000

POYAH, Penelope; Dickson Bldg, 5095-5820 University Ave, Halifax NS B3H 1V8; UBC'03; FRCPC; IntMed; Nephrol. Staff, Queen Elizabeth II Health Sciences Centre - Victoria General Site; Staff Dialysis Unit, Dartmouth General Hospital; (902)473-5160; Fax. (902)473-2675.

POYNER, Matthew D; Collingwood Gen & Marine Hosp, 459 Hume St, Collingwood ON L9Y 1W9; McM'02; Staff, Collingwood General & Marine Hospital; (705)445-2550; Fax. (705)444-2679.

POYNTER, Aven J; 21765 48 Ave, Langley BC V3A 3N1; Dal'81; FRCPC; Peds. Consultant, Langley Memorial Hospital; (604)534-8707

POYNTER, Brittany A; Addiction & Mental Hlth-Clarke, 250 College St, Toronto ON M5T 1R8; Wes'05; FRCPC; Psy. Staff, Centre for Addiction & Mental Health (CAMH) - College Street Site; (416)535-8501

POZEG, Zlatko I; Southlake Reg Health Centre, 596 Davis Dr, Newmarket ON L3Y 2P9; Ott'99; CardSurg. Staff, Southlake Regional Health Centre; (905)895-4521

POZGAY, Anita M; The Ottawa Hosp-Civic Campus, 1053 Carling Ave, Ottawa ON K1Y 4E9; McM'95; Dip SportMed; DTM; FRCPC; EmergMed (Sports Medicine). Staff Emerg Dept, The Ottawa Hospital - Civic Campus; Teach Staff Sports Med Ctre, University of Ottawa; (613)761-4621; apozgay@rogers.com.

POZNAN, Zoltan; 105-1017 Wilson Ave, North York ON M3K 1Z1; Budapest (Hungary)'56; (416)630-7500

POZZI, Anthony C; Hotel-Dieu Grace Hosp, 1030 Ouellette Ave, Windsor ON N9A 1E1; Wes'98; CCFP; CCFP(E.M.); Staff, Hôtel-Dieu Grace Hospital; (519)973-4401

PRABHAKAR, Christopher P K; St Paul's Hosp, 1081 Burrard St, Vancouver BC V6Z 1Y6; Tor'05; CCFP; Anes. Staff, Providence Health Care - St Paul's Hospital; (604)806-8337 x62813

PRABHAKAR, Kristin; Pender Community Health Centre, 59 Pender St W, Vancouver BC V6B 1R3; Tor'05; CCFP; CCFP(E.M.); Staff, Richmond Hospital; Staff, Pender Community Health Centre; (604)669-9181

PRABHAKAR, Maneesh K; Toronto Dermatology Centre, 400-4256 Bathurst St, North York ON M3H 5Y8; Tor'02; FRCPC; IntMed. Staff, Timmins & District Hospital; (416)633-0001; Fax. (416)633-0002.

PRABHAKAR, Manu; P A C E Clinic, 581 Davis Dr, Newmarket ON L3Y 2P6; Wes'98; FRCPC; IntMed; Cardiol. Staff, Southlake Regional Health Centre; (905)953-7937; Fax. (855)215-4815.

PRABHAKARAN, Sivashankary Y; One Stop Med Centre, 1A-3585 Lawrence Ave E, Scarborough ON M1G 1P4; Tor'07; CCFP; Staff, The Scarborough Hospital - General Campus; (416)431-8641; Fax. (416)431-0648.

PRABHAKARAN, Varagur M; London HSC-South St, 3F-375 South St, London ON N6A 4G5; Bangalore (India)'67; MB BS; DLO(Lond); FRCPC; MedBiochem (Allergy & Immunology). Staff Discipline Leader, London Health Sciences Centre - Victoria Campus; Staff, London Health Sciences Centre - South Street; Langs: Tamil; (519)667-6615; prabhakv@lhsc.on.ca.

PRABHU, Atul J; Univ Hlth Network-Toronto Western Hosp, 2MCL 431-399 Bathurst St, Toronto ON M5T 2S8; Bangalore (India)'94; FRCPC; Anes. Staff, Toronto Western Hospital - University Health Network; (416)603-5118

PRABHU, Pooja D; North Med Centre, 206-7131 Bathurst St, Thornhill ON L4J 7Z1; (USA)'05; (905)731-7596

PRABHU, Umesh H; Yamouth Reg Hosp, 316-60 Vancouver St, Yarmouth NS B5A 2P5; Mysore (India)'74; MB BS; MRC(UK); FRCPC; IntMed (Gastroenterology). Staff Internist/IntMed, Yarmouth Regional Hospital; Langs: Bilingual(English/French); Kankani; (902)742-3541; uprabhu123@gmail.com.

PRABHU, Vijayalaxmi; Hotel-Dieu Hosp, 166 Brock St, Kingston ON K7L 5G2; Mysore (India)'66; MB BS; FRCPC; Psy. Staff Psy, Hotel-Dieu Hospital; (613)544-3310 x2550; Fax. (613)544-9666.

PRABHU, Vilas S; 847 Winnipeg St, Penticton BC V2A 5N4; Bombay (India)'74; MB BS; MS; FRCS(UK); FRCSC; Otol (Ear Nose & Throat Surgery). Staff Otol, Penticton Regional Hospital; Consultant, Summerland Memorial Health Centre; Langs: Hindi; Marathi; (250)493-0031; Fax. (250)492-6112; vilasprabhu@gmail.com.

PRABHUDESAI, Vikramaditya; St Michael's Hosp, 30 Bond St, Toronto ON M5B 1W8; Pune (India)'91; Staff, St Michael's Hospital; (416)864-5680

PRADHAN, Abhay M; South Country Med Clinic, PO Box 2106, Assiniboia SK S0H 0B0; (306)642-4454; Fax. (306)642-5949.

PRADHAN, Gautam N; Labrador Grenfell Health, PO Box 7000 Stn C 227 Hamilton River Rd, Happy-Valley-Goose NL A0P 1C0; Kiev (Russia (Federation))'72; FRCS; FRCSC; GenSurg. Staff, Labrador Health Centre; (709)897-2000; narsing85@hotmail.com.

PRADKO, Jacqueline A; Windsor River Walk-In Clinic, 500 Wyandotte St E, Windsor ON N9A 3H9; Wes'97; CCFP; (519)254-1594; Fax. (519)254-8355.

PRADKO, James F; Roseville Walk-In Clinic, 2525 Roseville Garden Dr, Windsor ON N8T 3J8; Alb'91; CCFP; (519)944-3393

PRADY, Catherine C; Hop Charles LeMoyne, E303-3120 boul Taschereau, Greenfield Park QC J4V 2H1; Paris (France)'90; Staff, Hopital Charles LeMoyne; (450)466-5024; Fax. (450)466-5025.

PRAGLOWSKI, Bozena; Kipling Heights Med Centre, 2291 Kipling Ave, Etobicoke ON M9W 4L6; Warsaw (Poland)'82; Ac Staff, Trillium Health Centre - Mississauga; Langs: Polish; (416)741-4545; Fax. (416)744-1484; no@sympatico.ca.

PRAKASH, Anil; 308-200 Boudreau Rd, St. Albert AB T8N 6B9; Lucknow (India)'58; MB BS; LRCP(Lond); MRCS(Eng); FRCS; FRCSC; GenSurg. Ac Staff, Sturgeon Community Hospital; (780)458-5330; Fax. (780)418-2157.

PRAKASH, Sankar N; Windsor Med Clinic, 1608 Tecumseh Rd W, Windsor ON N9B 1T8; Mysore (India)'66; Physician General IntMed., Electrocardiography-Travel & Verruca Clinic & Memb., A. C.P.(USA); Langs: Kanarese; (519)258-4400; Fax. (519)973-3914.

PRAKASH, Suma; 113-13798 94A Ave, Surrey BC V3V 1N1; Ott'99; FRCPC; IntMed; Nephrol. (604)582-6606

PRANGLEY, Kate A; 302-180 James St S, Hamilton ON L8P 4V1; McM'00; CCFP; (905)528-5553

PRANNO, Nicolas; Hop Maisonneuve-Rosemont, 5415 boul de l'Assomption, Montreal QC H1T 2M4; Mon'00; FRCPC; IntMed; Cardiol. Staff, Hopital Maisonneuve-Rosemont; (514)252-3400

PRASAD, Aduvala V; 102-2150 Bloor St W, Toronto ON M6S 1M8; Hyderabad (India)'64; DABPed; FRCPC; Peds. (416)516-8293

PRASAD, Asuri; Children's Hosp Western of Ont, B 174-800 Commissioners Rd E, London ON N6C 6B5; Delhi (India)'81; MB BS; FRCPC; Peds (Epilepsy); Neur. Assoc Prof Peds & Clin Neurosciences, University of Western Ontario; (519)685-8332; Fax. (519)685-8350.

PRASAD, Benjamin A A; St Boniface Gen Hosp, 409 Tache Ave, Winnipeg MB R2H 2A6; Man'95; FRCPC; Psy. Staff, St Boniface General Hospital; (204)233-8563

PRASAD, Chitra; Children's Hosp of Western Ont, 800 Commissioners Rd E, London ON N6C 2V5; Punjab (India)'82; MB BS; FRCPC; Peds. (519)685-8140; Fax. (519)685-8214.

PRASAD, G V Ramesh; 9F-61 Queen St E, Toronto ON M5C 2T2; Osmania (India)'90; MB BS; MSc; FRCPC; IntMed (Transplantation); Nephrol. Staff Physician, St Michael's Hospital; Assoc Prof Med, University of Toronto; (416)867-3722; Fax. (416)867-3709.

PRASAD, Kailash; Univ of Saskatchewan, 107 Wiggins Rd, Saskatoon SK S7N 5E5; (India)'57; PhD; FACC; FICAng; FIACS; MB BS; RN; FRCPC; MedScient(Med). Emeritus Prof Physiol/Aj Prof, University of Saskatchewan; (306)966-6539; Fax. (306)966-6532; k.prasad@usask.ca.

PRASAD, Lakshman; Rothbart Centre for Pain Care, 9-4646 Dufferin St, North York ON M3H 5S4; Patna (India)'58; Psy. (416)512-6407

PRASAD, Navin; Allan McGavin Sports Med Ctr, 3055 Wesbrook Mall, Vancouver BC V6T 1Z3; Alb'85; Clin Assoc Prof Family Pract, University of British Columbia; (604)822-3614; Fax. (604)822-9058; nprasad@interchange.ubc.ca.

PRASAD, Sadhana; St Mary's Gen Hosp, 911 Queens Blvd, Kitchener ON N2M 1B2; McM'81; FACP(Geriatrics); FRCPC; IntMed (Geriatric Medicine). Staff, St Mary's General Hospital; Staff, Grand River Hospital - Kitchener/Waterloo Health Centre; McMaster University; (519)749-6929; Fax. (519)749-6566.

PRASAD, Shailendra; The Burris Clinic, 300-275 Lansdowne St, Kamloops BC V2C 6J3; Jiwaji (India)'82; MB BS; FRCPC; IntMed. (250)377-3343; Fax. (250)372-5265.

PRASAD, Sharada; A-459 Dundas St W, Trenton ON K8V 3S4; Mysore (India)'68; (613)392-1084; Fax. (613)392-0977.

PRASAD, Vikash; The Moncton Hosp, 135 MacBeath Ave, Moncton NB E1C 6Z8; Dal'00; FRCPC; DiagRad. Staff, The Moncton Hospital; (506)857-5520

PRASEUTH, Billee; Clinique Med Ahuntsic, 117-241 rue Fleury O, Montreal QC H3L 1V2; Sher'09; CCFP.

PRASIL, Pascale; CHUQ-Ctr Hosp Univ Laval, 2211-2705 boul Laurier, Quebec QC G1V 4G2; Laval'93; FRCSC; GenSurg; PedGenSurg. Staff, Centre Hospitalier Universitaire de Quebec-CHUL; (418)656-4141

PRASLOSKI, P Bruce; St Paul's Hosp, 1081 Burrard St, Vancouver BC V6Z 1Y6; UBC'86; FRCPC; Anes. Staff, Providence Health Care - St Paul's Hospital; (604)682-2344; Fax. (604)806-8487.

PRAT, Alexandre; CHUM-Hop Notre-Dame, 1560 rue Sherbrooke E, Montreal QC H2L 4M1; Mon'95; FRCPC; Neur. Staff, Centre Hospitalier l'Université de Montréal (CHUM) - Hôpital Notre-Dame; Langs: German; English; (514)890-8212

PRAT, Franck G; Worker's Comp Board, 6951 Westminster Hwy, Richmond BC V7C 1C6; Ott'78; Staff, Worksafe BC (WCB) Review Division; Langs: Bilingual(English/French); (604)232-7154; Fax. (604)232-7728.

PRATT, Adele; Kootenay-Boundary Reg Hosp, 1200 Hospital Bench, Trail BC V1R 4M1; UBC'98; CCFP; Staff, Kootenay Boundary Regional Hospital; (250)368-3311

PRATT, Arthur W; Metrotown Med Centre, 303-6411 Nelson Ave, Burnaby BC V5H 4H3; McG'72; DAB; FRCSC; Ophth (Cataract). Att Staff, Burnaby Hospital; Asst Prof, University of British Columbia; (604)433-1258; Fax. (604)433-6154.

PRATT, Douglas R; Terrace Clinic, 204-35 Major's Path, St. John's NL A1A 4Z9; Mem'85; FRCPC; Psy. (709)777-3450

PRATT, J Graham; Clin Aux Petits Soins, 201-6624 av Somerled, Montreal QC H4V 1T2; Mon'04; (514)486-6656; Fax. (514)486-0309.

PRATT, Kathleen J; 201-429 Exmouth St, Sarnia ON N7T 5P1; Cal'90; BSc(BioChem.); BScN; FRCSC; GenSurg (Surgical Oncology). Staff, Bluewater Health - Norman Site; Staff, Bluewater Health - Mitton Site; Staff, Bluewater Health - Charlotte Eleanor Englehart Hospital; Clin Asst, McMaster University; (519)332-0612

PRATT, Marielle E; Liberton Med Centre, 212-31 Liberton Dr, St. Albert AB T8N 3X6; Alb'07; CCFP; (780)459-7760; Fax. (780)460-1799.

PRATT, Melanie; Central Med Bldg, 203-1105 Carling Ave, Ottawa ON K1Y 4G5; Ott'77; FRCPC; Derm (Contact Dermatitis). Consultant, The Ottawa Hospital - Civic Campus; Member Occupational Disease Speciality Unit, Workplace Safety & Insurance Board; Prof Med(Derm), University of Ottawa; (613)728-2711; Fax. (613)728-8699.

PRATT, S Lynn; Fort William Fam Hlth Network, 117 Mckellar St S, Thunder Bay ON P7E 1H5; Wes'78; Ac Staff (All Sites), Thunder Bay Regional Health Sciences Centre; Clinical Asst Prof, McMaster University; Clin Asst Prof, Northern Ontario School of Medicine; (807)626-1234; Fax. (807)622-2541.

PRAUD, Jean-Paul; CHUS-Hop Fleurimont, 3001 12e av N, Sherbrooke QC J1H 5N4; Paris (France)'84; PhD; Respir (P.Q.) (Pneumology). Staff PedResp, Centre Hospitalier Universitaire de Sherbrooke-Hopital Fleurimont; Prof Peds & Physiology, Universite de Sherbrooke; Langs: Bilingual(French/English); (819)346-1110 x14851; Fax. (819)564-5215; jean-paul.praud@usherbrooke.ca.

PRAUGHT, Jeffery C; CFB Petawawa, PO Box 9999 Stn Main, Petawawa ON K8H 2X3; Ott'10; CCFP; (613)687-5511

PRAY, Michael J; Hamilton Harbour Comm Bldg, 102-605 James St N, Hamilton ON L8L 1J9; Tor'79; Court Staff, St Joseph's Healthcare - Charlton Campus; Court Staff, Hamilton Health Sciences Centre - McMaster University Medical Centre; (905)525-4900

PRAYAGA, Rama S R; 225 St Paul Ave, Brantford ON N3R 5Z3; Andhra (India)'75; MB BS; FRCPC; Psy. Staff, The Brant Community Healthcare System - Brantford General Hospital Site; (519)770-4062; Fax. (519)770-4063.

PRAYAL-PRATTE, Marie-Eve; Centre Hosp Honore-Mercier, 2750 boul Laframboise, Saint-Hyacinthe QC J2S 4Y8; Mon'03; FRCPC; Psy. Staff, Centre Hospitalier Honore-Mercier; (450)771-3222

PRCHAL, David; 602-1160 Burrard St, Vancouver BC V6Z 2E8; McG'04; FRCPC; Nephrol; IntMed. Langs: Bilingual(English/French); (604)681-7191

PRCHAL, Jaroslav F; St Mary's Hosp Centre, 3830 av Lacombe, Montreal QC H3T 1M5; Charles (Czech Republic)'64; MD; FRCPC; Hem; MedOncol (P.Q.). Chief MedOncol, St Mary's Hospital Centre; Hematology, McGill University Health Centre - Royal Victoria Hospital; assoc Prof, McGill University; (514)345-3511; jaroslav.prchal@mcgill.ca.

PREACHUK, Christopher T J; Medical Arts Bldg, 202-233 Kennedy St, Winnipeg MB R3C 3J5; Man'95; FRCPC; DiagRad.

PREBBLE, Brenda L; South Georgian Bay CHC, 202-14 Ramblewood Dr, Wasaga Beach ON L9Z 0C4; McM'05; CCFP; (705)422-1888

PREBTANI, Ally K P H; Hamilton HS-General Site, 411-237 Barton St E, Hamilton ON L8L 2X2; McM'96; BScPharm; ABIM; FRCP; FRCPC; IntMed; Endocrin&Metab. Staff, Hamilton Health Sciences Centre - Hamilton General Hospital; Assoc Prof Med, McMaster University; Langs: Gujarati; (905)523-1714; Fax. (905)577-1418.

PRECOURT, Julie; Ctr Hosp Laurentien, 234 rue Saint-Vincent, Ste-Agathe-Des-Mts QC J8C 2B8; Mon'99; Staff, Centre Hospitalier Laurentien; (819)324-4000

PREDESCU, Dragos; McMaster University, 3A41-1200 Main St W, Hamilton ON L8S 4J9; (Romania)'94; (905)521-2100

PREDESCU, Oana; Sunnybrook Hlth Sciences Ctre, 3200-2075 Bayview Ave, Toronto ON M4N 3M5; Bucharest (Romania)'94; Anes. Staff, Sunnybrook Health Sciences Centre; (416)480-4864

PREDIGER, Lanette A; South Urgent Care Center, 31 Sunpark Plaza SE, Calgary AB T2X 3W5; Cal'05; CCFP; CCFP(E.M.); Staff, Foothills Medical Centre.

PREDY, Gerald N; Alberta Health Services, 104-14310 111 Ave NW, Edmonton AB T5M 3Z7; Alb'76; FAB; FRCPC; CommunMed. Sr Med Officer of Hlth, Alberta Health Services; (780)342-0186; Fax. (780)342-0249.

PREFONTAINE, Genevieve; 99-5764 av de Monkland, Montreal QC H4A 1E9; Mon'95; (514)483-6869

PREFONTAINE, J E J Michel; London HSC-Victoria Hosp, PO Box 5010 Stn B B2 461-800 Commissioners Rd E, London ON N6A 5W9; Mon'78; ABOG; FRCSC; ObstGyn (Gynecologic Oncology). Staff, London Health Sciences Centre - Victoria Campus; Langs: Spanish; French; (519)685-8088; Fax. (519)685-8176; michel.prefontaine@lhsc.on.ca.

PREFONTAINE, Odette; 1665 rue du Couvent, Laval QC H7W 3A8; Mon'96; (450)687-5690

PREFONTAINE, Patrick; 442 boul Sainte-Anne RR 3, Ste-Anne-Plai QC J0N 1H0; Mon'89; Staff, Hôtel-Dieu de Saint-Jérôme; Langs: English; (450)478-4737; Fax. (450)478-7508.

PREGENT, Ernest; Hop du Sacre-Coeur de Mtl, 5400 boul Gouin O, Montreal QC H4J 1C5; Mon'77; MCFP(EM); FCFP; EmergMed (P.Q.) (Emergency Family Medicine). Staff, Hôpital du Sacre-Coeur de Montréal; Dir, Services Medicaux de Recherche; Lecturer Hyperbaric Med, Universite de Montreal; (514)335-1252; Fax. (514)335-1753.

PREIKSAITIS, Jutta K; University of Alberta Hosp, WMC1B1 17-8440 112 St NW, Edmonton AB T6G 2B7; McM'76; FRCPC; IntMed (Infectious Diseases). Med Dir Provincial Lab for Public Health(Microbiol), University of Alberta Hospital; Aj Scientist, Canadian Blood Services; Prof Div of ID, University of Alberta; Langs: German; (780)407-8980; Fax. (780)407-7137; j.preiksaitis@provlab.ab.ca.

PREINER, John L; Bayview Business Centre, 216-16700 Bayview Ave, Newmarket ON L3X 1W1; Tor'93; FRCSC; Urol. Assoc Staff, Southlake Regional Health Centre; (905)954-0307; Fax. (905)836-9038.

PRELEVIC, Stanislav; Clinique Med Viau, 204-4750 rue Jarry E, Saint-Leonard QC H1R 1X8; Belgrade (Serbia)'61; CSPQ; Neur (Clinical Neurology). Ac Staff, Hôpital Santa Cabrini Ospedale; Affil Staff, McGill University Health Centre - Montreal General Campus; (514)326-7203; Fax. (514)326-3656.

PRELEVIC, Zorana; MUHC-Montreal Gen Hosp, 1650 av Cedar, Montreal QC H3G 1A4; Belgrade (Serbia)'71; FRCPC; Psy (Consultation-Liaison). Ac Staff, McGill University Health Centre - Montreal General Campus; Physician, Consultation Liaison Service; adj Prof, McGill University; Langs: Serbian; French; (514)934-8010; Fax. (514)934-8237.

PRELLER, Martelle; Wellpoint Health, 103-240 Midpark Way SE, Calgary AB T2X 1N4; (South Africa)'89; MB ChB; CCFP; Staff, Olds Hospital & Care Centre; Langs: Afrikaans; (403)256-8213

PRELYPCHAN, Christopher J; Royal Inland Hosp, 311 Columbia St, Kamloops BC V2C 2T1; UBC'97; CCFP; CCFP(E.M.); Staff, Royal Inland Hospital; (250)314-2425

PREM-SMITH, Melodie R; Pitt Meadows Prof Centre, 101-12195 Harris Rd, Pitt Meadows BC V3Y 2E9; Alb'98; DTMH; CCFP; (604)465-9977

PREMACHANDRA, Palliyage M; Community Health Centre, PO Box 213 3322 Hwy 3, Barrington Passage NS B0W 1G0; (Sri Lanka)'97; (902)637-1520; Fax. (902)637-3922.

PREMACHANDRA, Thusitha; Kilborn Med Centre, 100-1385 Bank St, Ottawa ON K1H 8N4; Peradeniya (Sri Lanka)'70; MB BS; Langs: Sinhalese; (613)523-7440; Fax. (613)523-7440.

PREMATILAKE, Suraj; Selkirk Med Clinic, 353 Eveline St, Selkirk MB R1A 1N1.

PREMI, Nora J; Family Med Centre, 101-155 James St S, Hamilton ON L8P 3A4; McM'93; CCFP; FCFP; Assoc Staff, St Joseph's Healthcare - Charlton Campus; (905)528-8744; Fax. (905)528-5849.

PREMJI, Kamila; 300-100 Marie Curie Pvt, Ottawa ON K1N 1A2; Wes'05; CCFP; (613)564-3950

PREMONT, Pierre; CSSS de Rimouski-Neigette, CP 3150 Succ A 150 av Rouleau, Rimouski QC G5L 5T1; Laval'88; FRCSC; ObstGyn. Staff, Hôpital Regional Rimouski; (418)723-7851

PREMSAGAR, Sarojadevi R; Family Focus Med Clinic, 3601 Joseph Howe Dr, Halifax NS B3L 4H8; Durban (South Africa)'87; MB ChB; CCFP; (902)433-2038; Fax. (902)443-2110.

PREMSAGAR, Vickesh; Hantz Community Hosp, 89 Payzant Dr, Windsor NS B0N 2T0; Durban (South Africa)'87; MB ChB; CCFP; CCFP(E.M.); Staff, Hants Community Hospital; (902)792-2000

PRENDERGAST, John A; Chipman Health Centre, 9 Civic Crt, Chipman NB E4A 2H8; Alb'99; CCFP; (506)339-7650

PRENDERGAST, Peter J; Addiction & Mental Hlth-Clarke, 250 College st, Toronto ON M5T 1R8; National (Ireland)'74; MB ChB; BAO; MRCPsy; FRCPC; Psy. Chief Psychiatrist, Ontario Shores Centre for Mental Health Sciences; Staff, Centre for Addiction & Mental Health (CAMH) - College Street Site; Asst Prof, University of Toronto; (416)979-6880; prendergastp@wmhc.ca.

PRENDERGAST, Philip R; Formation Hlth Services Unit, PO Box 17000 Stn Forces 1200 Colville Rd, Victoria BC V9A 7N2; Tor'91; MPH; Staff, Canadian Forces Health Services - Pacific Centre; (250)363-4161

PRENDIVILLE, Juliette S M; Children's & Women's HC of BC, K4 100-4480 Oak St, Vancouver BC V6H 3V4; Dublin (Ireland)'76; MB ChB; BAO; MRCP; DCH; FRCPC; Derm (Pediatric Dermatology). Ac Staff, BC Children's Hospital; Clin Prof, University of British Columbia; (604)875-2864; jprendiville@cw.bc.ca.

PRENDIVILLE, William G M; 105-704 Mara St, Point Edward ON N7V 1X4; Cork (Ireland)'72; (519)336-1788; Fax. (519)336-6150.

PRENOVAULT, Jean J M; 201-2265 Pembina Hwy, Winnipeg MB R3T 5J3; Man'87; CCFP; FCFP; Staff, Bethesda Hospital Steinbach; Coroner, Province of Manitoba; Lecturer, University of Manitoba; Langs: English; French; (204)269-2904; jprenovault@sehealth.mb.ca.

PRENOVAULT, Julie N; CHUM-Hop Notre-Dame, 1560 rue Sherbrooke E, Montreal QC H2L 4M1; Man'78; CSPQ; FRCPC; DiagRad. Staff Radiol, Centre Hospitalier l'Université de Montréal (CHUM) - Hôpital Notre-Dame; (514)890-8000 x28530; Fax. (514)412-7547.

PRENTICE, Bryan; 202-12894 16 Ave, Surrey BC V4A 1N7; UBC'80; Ac Staff, Peace Arch Hospital; (604)531-6433; Fax. (604)538-7360.

PRENTICE, James S; St Paul's Hosp, 1081 Burrard St, Vancouver BC V6Z 1Y6; UBC'90; FRCPC; Anes. Staff Anes, Providence Health Care - St Paul's Hospital; (604)806-8337; Fax. (604)806-8487.

PREOBRAZENSKI, Roman Z; McMaster University Campus, 1280 Main St W, Hamilton ON L8S 4S4; McM'80; CCFP; Court Staff, Trillium Health Centre - Mississauga; Court Staff, St Joseph's Health Centre; Langs: Polish; (905)525-9140 x27717

PRERADOVIC, Nikola; Rebecca Med Walk-In Clinic, 170A Rebecca St, Oakville ON L6K 1J6; Belgrade (Serbia)'61; CCFP; Affil Staff, Halton Healthcare Services Corporation - Oakville Site; Langs: Serbian; (905)849-0986; Fax. (905)845-0981.

PRESCOTT, Christopher R F; Elliot Lake Family Health Team, 2F-31 Nova Scotia Walk, Elliot Lake ON P5A 1Y9; Dal'90; Pres Medical Staff, St Joseph's General Hospital Elliot Lake; (705)461-8882; Fax. (705)848-3449; prescott@vianet.ca.

PRESCOTT, Lise; 41-55 av de l'Eglise, Verdun QC H4G 3E7; Mon'66; CSPQ; Neur (P.Q.). Neurology, Centre Hospitalier de Verdun; Langs: English; French; (514)768-6633; Fax. (514)769-0784.

PRESCOTT, Robert C; 1832 rue Sherbrooke O, Montreal QC H3H 1E4; Mon'67; (514)935-6616; Fax. (514)933-2104.

PRESS, Cyril I; 202-1939 Kennedy Rd, Scarborough ON M1P 2L9; Cape Town (South Africa)'63; FRCS(Ed); (416)298-2900; Fax. (416)299-9863.

PRESS, Joshua Z; SMBD Jewish Gen Hosp, 3755 ch Cote-Sainte-Catherine, Montreal QC H3T 1E2; Alb'01; FRCSC; ObstGyn; GynOnco. Staff, Sir Mortimer B Davis Jewish General; (514)340-8222

PRESS, Natasha M; St Paul's Hosp, 520B-1081 Burrard St, Vancouver BC V6Z 1Y6; Tor'95; FRCPC; IntMed; InfectDis. Staff, Providence Health Care - St Paul's Hospital; (604)806-8642; npress@cfenet.ubc.ca.

PRESSACCO, Josephine G; Institut de Cardiologie de Mtl, 5000 rue Belanger, Montreal QC H1T 1C8; Tor'98; CSPQ; PhD; FRCPC; DiagRad (Abdominal). Staff, Institut de Cardiologie de Montréal; (514)376-3330; Fax. (514)593-2580.

PRESSER, Baldomero; Allan Memorial Institute, 1025 av des Pins O, Montreal QC H3A 1A1; Santiago (Chile)'65; DPsy(McG); FRCPC; Psy. Associate Psy, McGill University Health Centre - Royal Victoria Hospital; adj Prof, McGill University; (514)934-1934 x35502

PRESSEY, David B; 316 George St, Sarnia ON N7T 4P4; Wes'79; FRCSC; ObstGyn. Ac Staff, Bluewater Health - Mitton Site; Ac Staff, Bluewater Health - Norman Site; (519)332-2709; Fax. (519)332-3341.

PRESSEY, Tracy L; BC Women's Hosp & Health Ctre, IU26-4500 Oak St, Vancouver BC V6H 3N1; Alb'99; FRCSC; ObstGyn. Staff, BC Women's Hospital & Health Centre; (604)875-3075

PRESSNAIL, Bryn L; Royal Victoria Health Centre, 201 Georgian Dr, Barrie ON L4M 6M2; Tor'77; BSc; FRCPC; IntMed (Medical Oncology). Ac Staff Cancer Care Program, Royal Victoria Regional Health Centre; Consultant, Stevenson Memorial Hospital; (705)737-3432; Fax. (705)737-3065.

PREST, Marcia E H; 4-13665 96 Ave, Surrey BC V3V 1Z1; Qns'79; FRCPC; IntMed; Gastroent. (604)584-2033; Fax. (604)584-5450.

PRESTAGE, Keith T; 200-500 West Ave, Kelowna BC V1Y 4Z4; Sask'82; FRCSC; Urol. (250)469-7763

PRESTIDGE, Timothy D; Children's & Women's HC of BC, 4480 Oak St, Vancouver BC V6H 3V4; Auckland (New Zealand)'99; Staff, BC Children's Hospital; (604)875-2345

PRESTON, Anthony J; Victoria Med Bldg, 311-1669 Victoria St, Prince George BC V2L 2L5; National (Ireland)'82; MB ChB; BAO; MRC; (250)562-9388

PRESTON, Gordon L; 204-190 Sherway Dr, Etobicoke ON M9C 5N2; Tor'74; Ac Staff, St Joseph's Health Centre; (416)251-5008

PRESTON, Helen A; The Two Hundred, 203W-200 St Clair Ave W, Toronto ON M4V 1R1; Tor'56; DPsy; FRCPC; Psy. (416)961-9740; Fax. (416)922-9981.

PRESTON, Leslie J; 201-5651 Riverbend Rd NW, Edmonton AB T6H 5K4; Alb'83; BSc; CCFP; (780)438-8844; Fax. (780)436-9511.

PRESTON, Paul R; 91 Champlain St, North Bay ON P1B 7M3; Tor'85; Ac Staff, North Bay Regional Health Centre - Regional Mental Health; (705)494-8733; Fax. (705)495-1162.

PRESTON, Roanne L; BC Women's Hosp & Health Ctre, 4500 Oak St, Vancouver BC V6H 3N1; Ott'88; FRCPC; Anes. Staff, BC Women's Hospital & Health Centre; (604)875-2158

PRETO, Adele F; Medical Clinic, PO Box 730 Stn Main, Salmon Arm BC V1E 4N8; UBC'68; Ac Staff, Shuswap Lake General Hospital; Langs: Italian; (250)832-6094; Fax. (250)832-5235.

PRETO, Antonio F; 412-125 13th St E, North Vancouver BC V7L 2L3; UBC'67; DABOS; FRCSC; OrthSurg (Total Joint). Staff Consultant, Lions Gate Hospital; Langs: Italian; (604)988-2032; Fax. (604)986-0653; afpreto@telus.net.

PRETO, Jodi; PO Box 3760, Smithers BC V0J 2N0; UBC'04; CCFP; (250)847-8761; Fax. (250)847-2814.

PRETORIUS, Alexander P; Health Sciences Centre, AE23-820 Sherbrook St, Winnipeg MB R3A 1R9; Pretoria (South Africa)'81; MB ChB; MMed; FRCPC; Anes. Staff, Health Sciences Centre; Lecturer Anes, University of Manitoba; Langs: Zulu; Afrikaans; (204)774-8511

PRETORIUS, Barbara A; Central Square Med Clinic, PO Box 3760, Smithers BC V0J 2N0; Stellenbosch (South Africa)'98; MB ChB; Langs: Afrikaans; (250)847-8761; Fax. (250)847-2814.

PRETORIUS, Francois; Vernon Mental Health & Addicti, 1440 14 Ave, Vernon BC V1B 2T1; Pretoria (South Africa)'96; MB ChB; (250)549-5737

PRETORIUS, Isaac G V; 1209 Main St PO Box 3760, Smithers BC V0J 2N0; Orange Free State (South Africa)'97; Staff, Bulkley Valley District Hospital; (250)847-8761; Fax. (250)847-2814; centralsquare@telus.net.

PRETORIUS, Juan M; Mission Oaks Med Ctr, 32136 Lougheed Hwy, Mission BC V2V 1A4; Stellenbosch (South Africa)'01; MB ChB; Langs: Afrikaans; (604)826-7111

PRETORIUS, Lennard; Thompson Rivers Med Clinic, 851 Seymour St, Kamloops BC V2C 2H6; Orange Free State (South Africa)'04; (250)374-3775

PRETORIUS, Luzelle; Steinbach Family Med Centre, 10-333 Loewen Blvd, Steinbach MB R5G 0C3; Orange Free State (South Africa)'96; MB ChB; Langs: Afrikaans; (204)326-3401; Fax. (204)326-3899.

PRETORIUS, Marina; Lindsay Prof Bldg, 14-65 Angeline St N, Lindsay ON K9V 5N7; Pretoria (South Africa)'90; MB ChB; CCFP; Langs: Afrikaans; (705)324-2420

PRETTY, J Alan; 12894 16 Ave, Surrey BC V4A 1N7; UBC'70; CCFP; (778)835-9201; alanpretty@shaw.ca.

PREUSS, Jeannette; Victoria CYMHC, 302-2955 Jutland Rd, Victoria BC V8Z 6R5; Texas (USA)'82; FRCPC; Psy. Staff, Victoria General Hospital; (250)356-1123

PREVILLE, Eric J; Meadowlark Health Centre, 200 Meadowlark Shopping Ctr NW, Edmonton AB T5R 5W9; Alb'75; FRCPC; DiagRad. Ac Staff, Covenant Health - Misericordia Community Hospital; (780)489-7851; Fax. (780)486-5160.

PREVILLE, Guy; 1565 rue de Maisonneuve, Val-David QC J0T 2N0; Mon'51; CSPQ; Anes (Obstetrics Anesthesia). hon Membre, Centre Hospitalier de Verdun; hon Membre, Centre Hospitalier Laurentien; hon Membre, Centre Hospitalier de LaSalle; Langs: Spanish; English; (819)322-7643

PREVILLE, Marie-Josee; Ctr Medi Soleil St-Jean-Sur-Ri, 120-383 boul du Seminaire N, St-Jean-sur-Richel QC J3B 8C5; Mon'83; Nephrol; IntMed. Staff, Hôpital du Haut-Richelieu; Staff Nephrol, Centre Hospitalier de Granby; (450)349-5555

PREVOST, Alexandra; CSSS de Laval, 1755 boul Rene-Laennec, Laval QC H7M 3L9; Mon'05; Psy. Staff, Hopital de la Cite de la santé.

PREVOST, Anne-Patricia; CSSS Pierre Boucher, 1333 boul Jacques-Cartier E, Longueuil QC J4M 2A5; Mon'06; CCFP; Staff, Centre Hospitalier Pierre Boucher; (450)468-8111

PREVOST, Catherine; Services Externe de Psychiatri, 230-383 boul du Seminaire N, St-Jean-sur-Richel QC J3B 8C5; Mon'99; FRCPC; Psy. (450)346-2222 x8428; Fax. (450)346-2311.

PREVOST, Claude; Dir de la Sante Publique, A-800 boul Chomedey, Laval QC H7V 3Y4; Sher'88; CSPQ; FRCPC; CommunMed (Environmental Medicine);CCFP; Public Health & Preventive Med. Staff, Hopital Charles LeMoyne; Clinical Asst Prof Community Health Prog, Universite de Sherbrooke; (450)978-2121 x2205; Fax. (450)978-2100; c.prevost@rrsss16.gouv.qc.ca.

PREVOST, Derek; Surrey Med Arts Bldg, 103-13710 94A Ave, Surrey BC V3V 1N1; UBC'94; BSc; FRCPC; Peds (Pediatric Hematology Oncology). Staff, BC Women's Hospital & Health Centre; Ac Staff, Surrey Memorial Hospital; Ac Staff Haem/Oncol, BC Children's Hospital; Clin Associate Peds, University of British Columbia; Langs: English; French; (604)583-7070; Fax. (604)582-5536.

PREVOST, Francois A; CLSC Inukjuak, GD, Inukjuak QC J0M 1M0; Mon'92; Langs: English; Spanish; (819)254-8154; Fax. (819)254-8577.

PREVOST, Francois-Yves; CLSC Mercier-Est/Anjou, 9503 rue Sherbrooke E, Montreal QC H1L 6P2; Laval'98; Staff, Centre Hospitalier d'Argenteuil; (514)356-2572; Fax. (514)356-1838; faius@hotmail.com.

PREVOST, Gilles; CSSS Montmagny-l'Islet, 214-848 rue Commerciale, St-J-Chrysostome QC G6Z 2L2; Laval'75; (418)839-2070 x2319

PREVOST, Guillaume; CSSS Haut-Richelieu-Rouville, 920 boul du Seminaire N, St-Jean-sur-Richel QC J3A 1B7; Mon'10; CCFP; Staff, Hôpital du Haut-Richelieu; (450)359-5251

PREVOST, Jason D; 2412 30 Ave SW, Calgary AB T2T 1R9; Qns'04; FRCPC; DiagRad. Staff, Chinook Regional Hospital; (403)328-1122; Fax. (403)328-1218.

PREVOST, Jay; Surrey Mem Hosp, 13750 96 Ave, Surrey BC V3V 1Z2; Cal'05; CCFP; Staff, Surrey Memorial Hospital; (604)581-2211

PREVOST, Jean F; Ctr Hosp Affilie-Enfant-Jesus, 1401 18e rue, Quebec QC G1J 1Z4; Laval'86; EmergMed (P.Q.). Staff, Centre Hospitalier Affilié Universitaire de Québec - Hôpital De L'Enfant Jésus; (418)649-5632

PREVOST, Julie; Clin Neurologie des Laurentide, 102-256 rue Montigny, Saint-Jerome QC J7Z 5P9; Sher'01; FRCPC; Neur (Electrophysiology). Staff, Hôtel-Dieu de Saint-Jérôme; (450)569-2987

PREVOST, Louis; College des Med du Quebec, 2170 boul Rene-Levesque O, Montreal QC H3H 2T8; Mon'88; (514)933-4441; Fax. (514)933-3112.

PREVOST, Michel; Clinique Med USS St-Jean, CP 100 Succ Bureau-Chef, St-Jean-sur-Richel QC J3B 6Z1; Mon'68; (450)358-7099 x7680

PREVOST, Michel R; Almonte Gen Hosp, PO Box 940 75 Spring St, Almonte ON K0A 1A0; Ott'94; FRCSC; ObstGyn. Hd ObstGyn, Almonte General Hospital; Langs: French; (613)256-0342; Fax. (613)256-7197.

PREVOST, Pierre; Carrefour Med Vallee Richelieu, 665 boul Sir-Wilfrid-Laurier, Beloeil QC J3G 4J1; Mon'78; (450)467-9319; Fax. (450)467-6941.

PREVOST, Simon; CSSS de la Baie-des-Chaleurs, RR 2 419 boul Perron, Maria QC G0C 1Y0; Laval'99; Staff, CSSS de la Baie-des-Chaleurs; (418)759-1336

PREVOST, Sylvain; CHUS-Hop Fleurimont, 3001 12e av N, Sherbrooke QC J1H 5N4; Laval'97; FRCPC; NuclearMed. Staff, Centre Hospitalier Universitaire de Sherbrooke-Hopital Fleurimont; Langs: English; (819)346-1110 x11865; Fax. (819)820-6490; s_prevost@hotmail.com.

PREVOST, Sylvie; Clinique Med Les Jardins, 200-72 boul Saint-Jean-Baptist, Chateauguay QC J6K 4Y7; Laval'96; CCFP; (450)692-7282; Fax. (450)699-7788.

PREVOST, Yvon M; 215-1144 rue Saint-Laurent O, Longueuil QC J4K 1E2; Laval'67; (450)679-6810

PREWAL, Hardeep K; Temmy Latner Centre, 4F-60 Murray St, Toronto ON M5T 3L9; Saba (Netherlands Antilles)'08; CCFP; (416)586-4800; Fax. (416)586-4804; hardeep.prewal@villagefht.ca.

PREYRA, Ian J R; 246-1500 Upper Middle Rd W, Oakville ON L6M 0C2; Qns'99; MBA; FRCPC; EmergMed (Trauma). Staff, William Osler Health System - Brampton Civic Hospital; Staff, Hamilton Health Sciences Centre - McMaster Children's Hospital; Staff, St Joseph's Healthcare - Charlton Campus; Asst Clin Prof Med, McMaster University.

PRICA, Anca; Sunnybrook Hlth Sciences Ctre, 2075 Bayview Ave, Toronto ON M4N 3M5; Tor'06; FRCPC; IntMed; Hem. Staff, Sunnybrook Health Sciences Centre; (416)480-6100

PRICE, April K; London HSC-Victoria Hosp, PO Box 5010 Stn B 800 Commissioners Rd E, London ON N6A 5W9; Wes'98; FRCPC; Peds (Pediatric Critical Care); Respir. Staff, London Health Sciences Centre - Victoria Campus; Staff Peds Resp PCCU, Children's Hospital of Western Ontario; Asst Prof, University of Western Ontario; (519)685-8500

PRICE, Brian T; Dr Everett Chalmers Reg Hosp, PO Box 9000 Stn A 700 Priestman St, Fredericton NB E3B 5N5; Mem'93; FRCPC; Anes. Staff, Dr Everett Chalmers Regional Hospital; (506)452-5400

PRICE, Carman S; 5-109 Old Kingston Rd, Ajax ON L1T 3A6; Dal'65; IntMed. Ac Staff, Rouge Valley Health System - Ajax & Pickering Health Centre Site; (905)686-2041

PRICE, Charles M; The Credit Valley Hosp, 2200 Eglinton Ave W, Mississauga ON L5M 2N1; McG'83; FRCPC; IntMed (Intensive Care); Respir. Staff, The Credit Valley Hospital; (905)813-4466; Fax. (905)813-4444.

PRICE, David H; Albion Finch Med Centre, 106-1620 Albion Rd, Etobicoke ON M9V 4B4; Wes'02; BSc(Hon); PhD; CCFP; (416)741-1500; Fax. (416)741-1506.

PRICE, David I; Dr Charles A Janeway Child HC, 300 Prince Philip Dr, St. John's NL A1B 3V6; Mem'80; FRCSC; GenSurg; PedGenSurg. Staff, Janeway Children's Health & Rehabilitation Centre; (709)777-6300

PRICE, David J; 1475 Upper Ottawa St, Hamilton ON L8W 3J6; UBC'87; CCFP; FCFP; Chief Dept of Family Med, Hamilton Health Sciences Centre - McMaster Children's Hospital; Dir, Maternity Centre of Hamilton; McMaster University; Langs: Bilingual(French/English); (905)575-1744; Fax. (905)575-0779; priced@mcmaster.ca.

PRICE, Duncan A; Surrey Med Arts Bldg, 307-13710 94A Ave, Surrey BC V3V 1N1; London (England)'68; MB BS; FRCSC; ObstGyn. Staff Consultant, Surrey Memorial Hospital; (604)589-1619; Fax. (604)589-5593.

PRICE, Howard L; Scarborough Prof Centre, 310-1371 Neilson Rd, Scarborough ON M1B 4Z8; Tor'72; FRCPC; IntMed (Gastroenterology). Court Staff, Sunnybrook Health Sciences Centre; Ac Staff, Rouge Valley Health System - Centenary Health Centre Site; (416)281-9552; Fax. (416)281-6242.

PRICE, Ira M; Hamilton HS-General Site, 237 Barton St E, Hamilton ON L8L 2X2; McM'05; FRCPC; EmergMed. Staff, Hamilton Health Sciences Centre - Hamilton General Hospital; (905)527-4322

PRICE, James B; Portage Clinic Inc, 140 9th St SE, Portage La Prairie MB R1N 3V5; Sheffield (England)'80; MB ChB; CCFP; (204)857-3445; Fax. (204)239-1278.

PRICE, James W; 3200-950 10th Ave W, Vancouver BC V5Z 4E3; UBC'04; FRCPC; Anes. Staff, Vancouver General Hospital - Centennial Pavillion.

PRICE, Jason W B; 2643 Yonge St, Toronto ON M4P 2J6; Tor'73; (416)222-8146

PRICE, Jeffrey J; Family Health Centre, 200-2462 Howard Ave, Windsor ON N8X 3V6; Wes'88; CCFP; Staff GP, Hôtel-Dieu Grace Hospital; Staff GP, Windsor Regional Hospital - Metropolitan Site; (519)258-4142; Fax. (519)258-4456.

PRICE, Joel E; Univ of Ottawa Heart Institute, H3401-40 Ruskin St, Ottawa ON K1Y 4W7; Wes'04; FRCSC; CardSurg. Staff, University of Ottawa Heart Institute; (613)761-4233

PRICE, Jonathan P M; Kelowna Gen Hosp, 2268 Pandosy Ave, Kelowna BC V1Y 1T2; (United Kingdom)'03; CCFP; Staff, BC Cancer Agency Sindi Ahluwalia Hawkins Centre for the Southern Interior; Staff, Kelowna General Hospital; (250)862-4438; jonathan.price@northernhealth.ca.

PRICE, Judy M; Hantsport Collaborative Practi, PO Box 395 27 Main St S, Hantsport NS B0P 1P0; Dal'02; CCFP; (902)684-3325; Fax. (902)684-0182.

PRICE, Laura A; E1 102-800 Commissioners Rd E, London ON N6A 5W9; Wes'99; FRCPC; EmergMed. (519)685-8500; Fax. (519)679-6969.

PRICE, Lawrence M; Foothills South Tower, 711-3031 Hospital Dr NW, Calgary AB T2N 2T8; Alb'71; FRCPC; IntMed; Gastroent. Ac Staff, Foothills Medical Centre; Clin Assoc Prof, University of Calgary; (403)283-6613; Fax. (403)270-7722.

PRICE, Morgan T; Cool Aid Community Health Ctre, 713 Johnson St, Victoria BC V8W 1M8; Cal'00; CCFP; Physician, Cool Aid Community Health Centre; (250)385-1466; Fax. (250)383-1327.

PRICE, Nancy A; Valley Reg Hosp, 150 Exhibition St, Kentville NS B4N 5E3; Mem'87; Staff, Valley Regional Hospital; (902)678-7381

PRICE, Paul A; Cornwall Med Centre, PO Box 69, Cornwall PE C0A 1H0; Dal'80; FRCSC; Ophth. (902)894-4852

PRICE, Russell G; Royal Victoria Hosp, 201 Georgian Dr, Barrie ON L4M 6M2; Ott'82; FCAP(AP/CP); FRCPC; GenPath. Chief Lab Med, Royal Victoria Regional Health Centre; Staff Path, Collingwood General & Marine Hospital; Staff, Georgian Bay General Hospital - Midland; (705)728-9802; pricer@rvh.on.ca.

PRICE, Shandis; Prairie Trail Med Centre, 100-1345 Taylor Ave, Winnipeg MB R3M 3Y9; Man'02; CCFP; (204)475-0088

PRICE, Susanne F G; Airport Heights Med Clinic, 40 Airport Heights Dr, St. John's NL A1A 4Z7; Mem'09; CCFP.

PRICE, Victoria E; IWK Health Centre, PO Box 9700 Rpo CSC 5850-5980 University Ave, Halifax NS B3K 6R8; Pretoria (South Africa)'94; MB ChB; MMed; Staff, IWK Health Centre; (902)470-8888

PRICE, William E H; Business Bldg, 325-1200 Burrard St, Vancouver BC V6Z 2C7; Man'72; FRCPC; Psy (Autism). (604)662-7755; Fax. (604)662-7215.

PRICE, William H F; Headwaters Health Care Centre, 100 Rolling Hills Dr, Orangeville ON L9W 4X9; Tor'74; BSc(Hon); Staff, Headwaters Health Care Centre - Orangeville Site; (519)941-2410

PRICE HILLER, Julie A; Cross Cancer Institute, 11560 University Ave NW, Edmonton AB T6G 1Z2; Ott'05; BSc; FRCPC; IntMed (Gastrointestinal Cancer); MedOncol. Staff Med Oncol, Cross Cancer Institute; (780)432-8514; Fax. (780)432-8888.

PRICE-JONES, R Greg; 62 Colborne St E, Orillia ON L3V 1T6; Qns'87; DAB; FRCSC; Otol. Staff, Orillia Soldiers' Memorial Hospital; Court Staff, Royal Victoria Regional Health Centre; (705)326-5852; Fax. (705)326-8401.

PRICHARD, Hugh L; Sudbury Reg Hosp-Laurentian, 41 Ramsey Lake Rd, Sudbury ON P3E 5J1; Sheffield (England)'75; MB ChB; MRCP(UK); DMRT; FRCR; BSc; FRCPC; RadOncol. Staff RadOncol Regional Cancer Program, Health Sciences North-Laurentian Site; Asst Prof Med, University of Ottawa; (705)522-6237 x2451; Fax. (705)523-7329.

PRIDDY, Richard E; Peter Lougheed Centre, 3500 26 Ave NE, Calgary AB T1Y 6J4; (Australia)'79; FRCPC; Anes. Ac Staff, Peter Lougheed Centre; (403)943-5554; Fax. (403)291-3574.

PRIDE, Sheila M; BC Women's Hosp & Health Ctre, D6-4500 Oak St, Vancouver BC V6H 3N1; Dal'73; FRCSC; ObstGyn. Staff, BC Women's Hospital & Health Centre; (604)875-2445 x5673

PRIDHAM, Cheryl J; 143 Metcalfe St PO Box 3000, Elora ON N0B 1S0; McM'09; CCFP.

PRIDHAM, Jeremy N; St Clare's Mercy Hosp, 154 Lemarchant Rd, St. John's NL A1C 5B8; Wes'84; FRCPC; Anes (Obstetrics). Assoc Staff, Health Sciences Centre; Staff, St Clare's Mercy Hospital; Chair of Clinical Disciplines Anes/Asst Prof, Memorial University Of Newfoundland; (709)777-5000; jpridham@mun.ca.

PRIE, Veronique; CLSC Charlevoix, 535 boul de Comporte, La Malbaie QC G5A 1S8; Laval'87; (418)665-6413 x3363; Fax. (418)665-7297; veronique.prie@ssss.gouv.qc.ca.

PRIEDITIS, J George P; MCI Clinics Six Points, 5230 Dundas St W, Etobicoke ON M9B 1A8; Tor'64; AB; FAAFP; FACEP; FRCPC; EmergMed;CCFP; Staff, QHC Belleville General; Asst Prof Surg, Queen's University; (416)234-8668; Fax. (416)234-8720.

PRIEDITIS, Markus P; Rouge Valley-Centenary HC, 2867 Ellesmere Rd, Scarborough ON M1E 4B9; Tor'91; BSc; FRCPC; DiagRad (Interventional Radiology). Assoc Staff, The Scarborough Hospital - Birchmount Campus; Assoc Staff, Rouge Valley Health System - Centenary Health Centre Site; Court Staff, Toronto East General Hospital Inc; (416)284-8131

PRIESNITZ, Alisha A; Maple Key Clinic Fam Hlth Team, D2-1036 Princess St, Kingston ON K7L 1H2; McM'05; CCFP; (613)546-9721

PRIEST, Vona G; 1373 Chimney Valley Rd, Williams Lake BC V2G 4W6; UBC'83; FRCPC; Psy. Staff, Cariboo Memorial Hospital and Health Centre; (250)398-2204; Fax. (250)398-9059; vona_priest@telus.net.

PRIESTLEY, Douglas W; Legacy Sports Med Clinic, 160 Meadowood Dr, Winnipeg MB R2M 5L6; Man'04; FRCPC; PhysMed&Rehab.

PRIESTMAN, B Anne; Columbia Med Bldg, 202-301 Columbia St E, New Westminster BC V3L 3W5; UBC'89; FRCPC; IntMed; Endocrin&Metab. (604)522-8399; Fax. (604)522-2635; wallprie@telus.net.

PRIESTNER, Ann Marie; Plainsview Med Centre, 501-503 Plains Rd E, Burlington ON L7T 2E2; McM'86; CCFP; FCFP; Chair Dept of Family Med, Joseph Brant Memorial Hospital; (905)681-9200; Fax. (905)681-9404.

PRIETO, Ignacio; CHUM-Hotel-Dieu, 3840 rue Saint-Urbain, Montreal QC H2W 1T8; Salamanca (Spain)'67; FRCS; FRCSC; Cardiovasc&ThorSurg. Chef cardiaque, Centre Hospitalier l'Université de Montréal (CHUM) - Hôtel-Dieu; Assoc Prof ClinSurg, Universite de Montreal; Langs: Spanish; Bilingual(English/French); (514)890-8131; ignacio.prieto.chum@ssss.gouv.qc.ca.

PRIEUR, Beverley J; Foothills Prof Bldg, 200-1620 29 St NW, Calgary AB T2N 4L7; Cal'78; BSc; FRCPC; Peds (Pediatric Neurology). Consultant Privil, Peter Lougheed Centre; Ac Staff Pediatric Neurol, Alberta Children's Hospital; Consultant, Foothills Medical Centre; Consultant Privil, Rockyview General Hospital; Clinical Asst Prof, University of Calgary; (403)215-6568; Fax. (403)289-5977.

PRIEUR, Timothy G; Bridgeland Med Bldg, 306-803A 1 Ave NE, Calgary AB T2E 7C5; Alb'78; FRCPC; IntMed; Cardiol. Ac Staff, Calgary Regional Health Authority; Clin Assoc Prof, University of Calgary; (403)571-8613; Fax. (403)571-8659.

PRIGMORE, Gerrard T; 1306 Central St E, Prince George BC V2M 3C1; Cardiff (Wales)'91; CCFP; (250)563-6417

PRIGOZHIKH, Viachislav; The Polyclinic, 5-4646 Dufferin St, North York ON M3H 5S4; Irkutsk (Russia (Federation))'85; Langs: Russian; (416)222-6160

PRIHAR, Rajiv K; Carling-Broadview Med Bldg, 208-770 Broadview Ave, Ottawa ON K2A 3Z3; Qns'93; FRCSC; OrthSurg. (613)798-5660; Fax. (613)725-9442.

PRIHODA, Marie B; Northside Med Group, 209-1015 Austin Ave, Coquitlam BC V3K 3N9; Alb'74; FRCPC; Derm. Staff, Royal Columbian Hospital; Consultant, Vancouver General Hospital - Centennial Pavillion; Asst Prof, University of British Columbia; Langs: Czech; (604)931-5811; Fax. (604)931-5811; prihoda@telus.net.

PRIMAVESI, Robert; MUHC-Montreal Gen Hosp, 1650 av Cedar, Montreal QC H3G 1A4; McG'85; CCFP; CCFP(E.M.); FCFP; assoc Médecin, McGill University Health Centre - Montreal General Campus; assoc Médecin, St Mary's Hospital Centre; assoc Médecin, McGill University Health Centre - Montreal Children's Hospital; assoc Doyen Undergrad Med Educ & Student Affairs, McGill University; (514)934-1934 x42501; Fax. (514)934-8421; robert.primavesi@muhc.mcgill.ca.

PRIMEAU, Alain W; 120 boul Saint-Jean-Baptiste, Chateauguay QC J6K 3A9; Mon'79; (450)691-8191; Fax. (450)691-8565.

PRIMEAU, Francois J; Hotel-Dieu de Levis, 143 rue Wolfe, Levis QC G6V 3Z1; Mon'83; DPsy; CSPQ; FRCPC; Psy (Geriatric Psychiatry). Staff, Hôtel-Dieu de Lévis; Pres, Societe de Psychogeriatrie du Quebec; Clin Prof Psy, Université Laval; Langs: Italian; English; (418)835-7155; Fax. (418)835-7199; francois.primeau@ssss.gouv.qc.ca.

PRIMEAU, Marie-Noel; MUHC-Montreal Children's Hosp, C 510-2300 rue Tupper, Montreal QC H3H 1P3; Sher'94; LMCC; FRCPC; Peds; ClinImmunol&Allergy. Staff, McGill University Health Centre - Montreal Children's Hospital; (514)412-4470

PRIMEAU, Robert E; Hop du Sacre-Coeur de Mtl, 5400 boul Gouin O, Montreal QC H4J 1C5; Mon'61; FACC; FRCPC; IntMed; Cardiol (P.Q.). Ac Staff Cardiol, Hôpital du Sacre-Coeur de Montréal; assoc Prof, Universite de Montreal; (514)338-2200; Fax. (514)338-2381.

PRIMEAU, Vanessa; Hop du Sacre-Coeur de Mtl, 5400 boul Gouin O, Montreal QC H4J 1C5; Mon'05; FRCPC; IntMed; Endocrin&Metab. Staff, Hôpital du Sacre-Coeur de Montréal; (514)338-2222

PRIMIANI, Nadia S; St Paul's Hosp, 1081 Burrard St, Vancouver BC V6Z 1Y6; McG'09; CCFP; CCFP(E.M.); Staff, Providence Health Care - St Paul's Hospital; (604)682-2344

PRIMMER, Janet J; Harbour View Med Clinic, 43 Court St N, Thunder Bay ON P7A 4T5; Tor'90; CCFP; FCFP; (807)343-4252; Fax. (807)346-8687.

PRINC, Michal; Devon Gen Hosp, H-101 Erie St S, Devon AB T9G 1A6; Prague (Czech Republic)'75; Staff, Devon General Hospital; Langs: Czech; (780)987-4322; Fax. (780)987-4333.

PRINCE, Douglas; Sudbury Med Centre, 307-65 Larch St, Sudbury ON P3E 1B8; Qns'62; BA; Ac Staff, Health Sciences North-St Joseph's Health Centre; Ac Staff, Health Sciences North-Laurentian Site; Ac Staff, Health Sciences North - Memorial Site; Consultant Psy Services, Ontario Correctional Institute; (705)675-1800; Fax. (705)675-5306.

PRINCE, Garry E; 201-1315 Lawrence Ave E, North York ON M3A 3R3; Tor'63; CRCP; DPsy; Psy. Court Staff, The Scarborough Hospital - Birchmount Campus; (416)444-7677; Fax. (416)444-3258.

PRINCE, Gerry D; Gershaw Prof Centre, 3-809 Bullivant Cres SW, Medicine Hat AB T1A 5G6; Alb'85; CCFP; FCFP; Staff, Medicine Hat Regional Hospital; Langs: Spanish; (403)529-2666; Fax. (403)529-5874.

PRINCE, Jennifer M; Surrey Med Arts Bldg, 319-13710 94A Ave, Surrey BC V3V 1N1; UBC'03; FRCSC; PlasSurg. (604)589-6021

PRINCE, Renee; Montfort Academic Family Hlth, 101B-745 Montreal Rd, Ottawa ON K1K 0T1; Mon'89; CCFP; Staff Family Med, Montfort Hospital; Staff, Bruyère Continuing Care - Saint-Vincent Hospital; Pres Med Staff, SCO Health Service - Élisabeth Bruyère Hospital; (613)749-4429; Fax. (613)749-7942.

PRINCE, Theodore A; Alberta Children's Hosp, 2888 Shaganappi Trail NW, Calgary AB T3B 6A8; Cal'74; FAAP; AB; FRCPC; Peds. Ac Staff, Alberta Children's Hospital; Clin Assoc Prof Peds, University of Calgary; (403)955-7515; Fax. (403)955-7649.

PRINCE, Timothy D P; Fourth Avenue Med Centre, 411 Louth St, St Catharines ON L2S 4A2; Dal'83; BSc; Dip SportMed; Dir, Niagara Sports Med Ctre; Dir Don Lorimer Sports Med Ctre, Brock Athletic Injury Clinic; Assoc Prof Family Med, McMaster University; (905)682-3692; Fax. (905)682-7549.

PRINCE, W Ross; Oakville Med Arts Bldg, 11-358 Reynolds St, Oakville ON L6J 3L9; Tor'59; FRCSC; Urol. Consultant, Trillium Health Centre - Mississauga; Ac Staff, Halton Healthcare Services Corporation - Oakville Site; Consultant, Joseph Brant Memorial Hospital; Consultant, The Credit Valley Hospital; (905)845-3272; Fax. (905)845-4742.

PRINCIPI, Tania; The Hosp for Sick Children, 555 University Ave, Toronto ON M5G 1X8; Wes'04; FRCPC; Peds; PedEmergMed. Fellow, The Hospital For Sick Children; (416)813-7500

PRINGLE, Allan C; 205-1920 Ellesmere Rd, Scarborough ON M1H 2V6; Qns'67; Staff, Rouge Valley Health System - Centenary Health Centre Site; (416)439-7122; Fax. (416)439-7141.

PRINGLE, C Elizabeth; The Ottawa Hosp-Gen Campus, 4125-501 Smyth Rd, Ottawa ON K1H 8L6; Alb'85; ABEDM; CSCN; LMCC; FRCP; DrMedCh; FRSM; BMedSci; FRCPC; Neur (Neuromuscular Diseases). Staff, The Ottawa Hospital - General Campus; Assoc Prof Neurol, University of Ottawa; (613)737-8689; Fax. (613)737-8857; epringle@ottawahospital.on.ca.

PRINGLE, Christopher; Queen Elizabeth II HSC, 1276 South Park St, Halifax NS B3H 2Y9; Dal'88; FRCPC; DiagRad. Staff, Queen Elizabeth II Health Sciences Centre - Victoria General Site; (902)473-2700

PRINGLE, Derrick J; London HSC-Victoria Hosp, PO Box 5010 Stn B 800 Commissioners Rd E, London ON N6A 5W9; Dal'94; FRCPC; EmergMed. Staff, London Health Sciences Centre - Victoria Campus; (519)667-6538

PRINGLE, Kerry B; Royal Jubilee Hosp, 1952 Bay St, Victoria BC V8R 1J8; Alb'79; FRCPC; GenPath. Staff Lab Med, Royal Jubilee Hospital; (250)370-8833; Fax. (250)370-8403.

PRINGLE, Peter S; Thorold Med Clinic, 60 Albert St W, Thorold ON L2V 2G7; Qns'71; Court Staff, Niagara Health System - St Catharines General Site; (905)227-5255; Fax. (905)227-2070.

PRINGSHEIM, Tamara M; Alberta Children's Hosp, C4 431-2888 Shaganappi Trail N, Calgary AB T3B 6A8; Qns'99; FRCPC; Neur. Staff, Alberta Children's Hospital; Asst Prof, University of Calgary; (403)955-5982; Fax. (403)955-5990.

PRINJA, Navin; Guardian Med Arts Bldg, 201-1950 Algonquin Ave, North Bay ON P1B 4Z2; McG'90; FRCSC; Otol (Facial Plastic & Reconstructive Surgery). Court Staff, West Nipissing General Hospital; Ac Staff, North Bay Regional Health Centre - Regional Mental Health; Langs: English; French; (705)472-2852; Fax. (705)472-0333.

PRINS, Claire A; Howard Mutual Med Centre, PO Box 250 20129 Erie St S, Ridgetown ON N0P 2C0; Tor'92; BSc; CCFP; FCFP; Staff/Med Dir Rehab/Continuing Care, Chatham-Kent Health Alliance; (519)674-2600; Fax. (519)674-2660.

PRINS, Henry B; Winchester Dist Mem Hosp, 566 Louise St, Winchester ON K0C 2K0; Ott'72; BSc(Hon); CCFP; FCFP; Ac Staff, Winchester District Memorial Hospital; (613)774-2420

PRINS, Johannes; Family Med Associates, 5021 51 St, Lacombe AB T4L 2A3; (South Africa)'94; MB ChB; Langs: Afrikaans; (403)782-3351; Fax. (403)782-5879.

PRINS, Leonard M; Howard Mutual Med Centre, PO Box 250 20129 Erie St S, Ridgetown ON N0P 2C0; Tor'92; CCFP; Staff, Chatham-Kent Health Alliance; (519)674-2600; Fax. (519)674-2660.

PRINS, Mark R; PO Box 393 Stn Main, Chilliwack BC V2P 6J7; Cal'06; CCFP; (604)798-4379

PRINS, Nicholas S; 400 Olive St, North Bay ON P1B 6J4; McM'86; (705)474-4250

PRINSLOO, Etienne; Cape Breton Hlthcare Complex, 1482 George St, Sydney NS B1P 1P3; Pretoria (South Africa)'86; MB ChB; Staff, Cape Breton Healthcare Complex; (902)567-8000

PRINSLOO, Gerrit C; 201-143 4th Ave S, Williams Lake BC V2G 1J8; Orange Free State (South Africa)'02; MB ChB; Langs: Afrikaans; (250)398-8102

PRINSLOO, Jochemus J; Altona Clinic, PO Box 999, Altona MB R0G 0B0; Stellenbosch (South Africa)'71.

PRINSLOO, Lodewyk; Royal Jubilee Hosp, 1952 Bay St, Victoria BC V8R 1J8; Stellenbosch (South Africa)'94; CCFP; CCFP(E.M.); Staff, Royal Jubilee Hospital; (250)370-8000

PRINSLOO, Willem N; Alder Med Centre, 277 Evergreen Rd, Campbell River BC V9W 5Y4; Orange Free State (South Africa)'98; MB ChB; CCFP; Langs: Afrikaans; willemrene@hotmail.com.

PRINSLOO, Yolanda; Cold Lake Health Centre, 206-314 25 St, Cold Lake AB T9M 1G6; (South Africa)'06; MB ChB; Staff, Cold Lake Healthcare Centre; (780)639-3001; Fax. (780)639-3009.

PRIOR, Donald F; 200 MacDonald St PO Box 23, Inglewood ON L7C 3L6; Tor'68; BSc; FRCSC; OrthSurg (Hip & Knee Arthroplasty). Assoc Staff Orthopaedic Surg, Halton Healthcare Services Corporation - Georgetown Hospital; Assoc Staff, Headwaters Health Care Centre - Orangeville Site; (905)456-2854; Fax. (905)453-0233.

PRIOR, Trevor I; Sheldon Chumir Centre, 1213 4 St SW, Calgary AB T2R 0X7; Cal'95; BSc(Hons.); PhD; FRCPC; Psy (General Adult Psychiatry). Staff Gen Adult Psy, Alberta Hospital Edmonton; Asst Prof Psy, University of Alberta; (403)955-6566

PRIPSTEIN, Laura P; Sherbourne Health Centre, 333 Sherbourne St, Toronto ON M5A 2S5; UBC'04; CCFP; Staff, St Michael's Hospital; (416)324-4180

PRISCIAK, Jared S; Lakeside Med Clinic, 3919 8th St E, Saskatoon SK S7H 5M7; Sask'05; BSc; CCFP; (306)374-6884; Fax. (306)374-2552.

PRISECARIU MOCANU, Daniela; CSSS Les Eskers de l'Abitibi, 622 4e rue O, Amos QC J9T 2S2; Iasi (Romania)'84; Staff, CH Hôtel-Dieu d'Amos; (819)732-3341

PRISMAN, Larraine D; City Square Pediatrics, 495-555 12th Ave W, Vancouver BC V5Z 3X7; Cape Town (South Africa)'87; MB ChB; FRCPC; Peds. Staff, BC Children's Hospital; Staff, BC Women's Hospital & Health Centre; Clin Associate, University of British Columbia; (604)709-6229; Fax. (604)875-6717.

PRITCHARD, Jennifer E; Royal Alexandra Hosp, 541-10240 Kingsway NW, Edmonton AB T5H 3V9; Alb'07; FRCPC; EmergMed. Staff, Royal Alexandra Hospital; (780)735-4442; Fax. (780)735-4916.

PRITCHARD, Kathleen I; Toronto Sunnybrook Reg Cancer, 2075 Bayview Ave, Toronto ON M4N 3M5; Qns'71; ABIM; FACP; FRCPC; IntMed (Breast Cancer); MedOncol. Ac Staff/Sr Scientist MedOncol Sunnybrook Odette Cancer Ctre, Sunnybrook Health Sciences Centre; Clin Dir, Ontario Clinical Oncology Group; Dir Departmental Div, Med Oncol Dept of Medicine/Prof, University of Toronto; (416)480-4616; Fax. (416)480-6002; kathy.pritchard@sunnybrook.ca.

PRITCHARD, Kenneth B; Kingston Family Health Team, 200-2437 Princess St, Kingston ON K7M 3G1; Ott'97; BSc; CCFP; FCFP; (613)546-6652; Fax. (613)546-5292; kpritchard@kfhn.net.

PRITCHARD, M Jane; Leaside Health Centre, 795 Eglinton Ave E, East York ON M4G 4E4; Qns'73; CCFP; FCFP; Staff, St Michael's Hospital; Staff, Toronto Western Hospital - University Health Network; Staff, Toronto East General Hospital Inc; Lecturer, University of Toronto; Langs: Spanish; (416)424-3145; Fax. (416)424-2611.

PRITCHARD, Neil G; 119 Isabella St RR 2, Campbellford ON K0L 1L0; Qns'87; (705)653-1801; Fax. (705)653-5483.

PRITCHARD, Sandy J; 1-66 Avenue Rd, Toronto ON M5R 3N8; Wes'77; FRCSC; PlasSurg (Cosmetic Surgery). (416)922-4513; Fax. (416)922-7942; info@sandypritchard.com.

PRITCHARD, Sheila L; Children's & Women's HC of BC, A119-4480 Oak St, Vancouver BC V6H 3V4; Nottingham (England)'77; MB BS; BSc; FRCPC; Peds (Bone Marrow Transplant). Clin Assoc Prof, BC Children's Hospital; Clin Assoc Prof Peds, University of British Columbia; (604)875-2294; spritchard@cw.bc.ca.

PRITCHETT, Lindsay B; 100-2917 28 Ave, Vernon BC V1T 8L1; London (England)'77; MB BS; MRCGPract; Physician, Vernon Jubilee Hospital; (250)503-1021

PRITCHETT, Sean B; 202-274 Dundas St E, Belleville ON K8N 1E6; Qns'04; FRCPC; IntMed; Gastroent. Staff, Toronto Western Hospital - University Health Network; (613)968-6969; Fax. (613)249-7017.

PRITZKER, Kenneth P H; Mount Sinai Hosp, 6 500-600 University Ave, Toronto ON M5G 1X5; Tor'67; BSc(Med); FRCPC; AnatPath. Pathologist Pathology & Lab Med, Mount Sinai Hospital; Fax. (416)586-8628; kpritzker@mtsinai.on.ca.

PRIVE, Annie-Claude; 220-874 boul de l'Universite E, Chicoutimi QC G7H 6B9; Sher'08; (418)545-2998

PRIVE, Myriam; CSSS de Chicoutimi, 305 rue Saint-Vallier, Chicoutimi QC G7H 5H6; Sher'81; CSPQ; GenPath (P.Q.). Staff, Complexe hospitalier de la Sagamie; (418)541-1234 x2571; myriam.prive@chs02.qc.ca.

PRIVITERA, Salvatore; York Thoracic Surgery Assoc, 56 Prospect St, Newmarket ON L3Y 3S9; Tor'02; FRCSC; GenSurg; ThorSurg. (905)853-5864; Fax. (905)853-5865.

PROBER, Mark A; A120-753 McDermot Ave, Winnipeg MB R3E 0T6; Man'67; BSc(Med); DABPN; FRCPC; Psy. Staff, Health Sciences Centre; Dir Counselling Services/Assoc Prof, University of Manitoba; (204)885-3917; Fax. (204)896-5885.

PROBIZANSKI, David C; Thunder Bay Med Centre, 410-63 Algoma St N, Thunder Bay ON P7A 4Z6; Ott'97; CCFP; Staff Privil, Thunder Bay Regional Health Sciences Centre Port-Arthur; (807)344-0105; Fax. (807)344-0135.

PROBST, Stephan; SMBD Jewish Gen Hosp, 3755 ch Cote-Sainte-Catherine, Montreal QC H3T 1E2; McG'04; NuclearMed. Staff, Sir Mortimer B Davis Jewish General; (514)340-8222 x5374; Fax. (514)340-7919.

PROBYN, Linda J; Sunnybrook Hlth Sciences Ctre, 2075 Bayview Ave, Toronto ON M4N 3M5; Wes'99; FRCPC; DiagRad. Staff, Sunnybrook Health Sciences Centre; (416)480-6100

PROCHETTE, Harry; UMF Legardeur, 135 boul Claude-David, Repentigny QC J6A 1N6; Port-au-Prince (Haiti)'82; Staff, Centre Hospitalier Pierre le Gardeur; Langs: Creole; English; (450)654-2911; Fax. (450)654-0359; hmaxp@videotron.ca.

PROCTER, Andrea M P; Woodstock Gen Hosp, 270 Ridell St, Woodstock ON N4S 6N6; UBC'03; FRCPC; Anes. Staff, Woodstock General Hospital; (519)421-4211

PROCTER, William C; 480 Guelph Line, Burlington ON L7R 3M1; Tor'59; (905)637-2340

PROCTOR, Bradley R; Royal Inland Hosp, 311 Columbia St, Kamloops BC V2C 2T1; Alb'03; FRCPC; IntMed; MedOncol. Staff, Royal Inland Hospital; (250)374-5111

PROCTOR, I Joan; Medical Arts Bldg, 302-42 Glen Allan Dr, Bridgewater NS B4V 3N2; Mem'83; FRCSC; GenSurg. (902)543-6882; Fax. (902)543-3765.

PROCTOR, James S; 203-2276 Island Hwy S, Campbell River BC V9W 1C3; UBC'89; CCFP; Med Staff, Campbell River & District General Hospital; (250)923-1189; Fax. (250)923-8897.

PROCTOR, Nicola J; Victoria Gen Hosp, 1 Hospital Way, Victoria BC V8Z 6R5; Qns'92; FRCPC; DiagRad. Staff Radiol, Victoria General Hospital; (250)727-4208

PROCTOR, Wendey R; MCI The Doctors Office, 4A-345 Bloor St E, Toronto ON M4W 3J6; McM'04; CCFP; (416)515-0590; Fax. (416)515-8853.

PRODAN, Orest; Winnipeg Clinic, 425 St Mary Ave, Winnipeg MB R3C 0N2; Man'84; (204)957-3235; Fax. (204)943-7921.

PRODGER, James D; 106-3305 Harvester Rd, Burlington ON L7N 3N2; McM'81; FRCSC; GenSurg. Asst Prof, McMaster University; (905)333-6245; Fax. (905)333-6266.

PROFETTO, Jason R; Health Sciences Bldg, 212-15 Mountain Ave S, Hamilton ON L8G 2V6; McM'09; CCFP; (905)662-9463

PROFETTO, Ralph; 102-980 Queenston Rd, Stoney Creek ON L8G 1B9; McM'83; CCFP; FCFP; Clin Assoc Prof Family Med, McMaster University; Langs: Italian; (905)662-4404; Fax. (905)662-1468.

PROFITI, Raffaela; 5-2125 Wyecroft Rd, Oakville ON L6L 5L7; Wes'03; FRCPC; Gastroent; IntMed.

PROFITT, Allen W; Polyclinic Prof Centre Inc, 199 Grafton St, Charlottetown PE C1A 1L2; Dal'80; FRCSC; OrthSurg. Staff, Queen Elizabeth Hospital; (902)629-8804; Fax. (902)566-9251.

PROKOPETZ, Robert D; Gamma Dynacare Laboratory, 750 Peter Morand Cres, Ottawa ON K1G 6S4; Alb'78; FRCPC; AnatPath (Clinical); Derm. Consultant DermPath, The Ottawa Hospital - General Campus; Consultant, The Ottawa Hospital - Civic Campus; Med Dir, Gamma-Dynacare Laboratories; Asst Prof IntMed & Derm Path, University of Ottawa; (613)728-5152; Fax. (613)728-8699; prokopetzr@gamma-dynacare.com.

PROKOPETZ, Sonia A; 407-190 Sherway Dr, Etobicoke ON M9C 5N2; Wisconsin (USA)'85; CCFP; FCFP; (416)626-1551; Fax. (416)626-1555.

PROKOPIAK, Allison B; Stittsville Med Centre, 1-1339 Stittsville Main St, Stittsville ON K2S 1C6; Qns'90; CCFP; FCFP; Langs: English; French; (613)836-5083; Fax. (613)836-2451.

PROLLIUS, Almereau; Spesmed Med Specialist Ctre, PO Box 1540 Stn Main 2591 99th St, North Battleford SK S9A 3W1; Bloemfontein (South Africa)'92; FCOG(SA); MMed; MB ChB; FRCSC; ObstGyn. (306)446-5550; Fax. (306)446-5055.

PROMNITZ, Michael; Old Quebec Street Mall, 204-55 Wyndham St N, Guelph ON N1H 7T8; Witwatersrand (South Africa)'83; MB ChB; FRCPC; Peds (Neonatology). Chief Peds, Guelph General Hospital; Clinical Asst Prof, McMaster University; promnitz@sentex.net.

PRONOVOST, Lyne; Ctr Med Giguere Pronovost, 1465 rue Roberval, Saint-Bruno QC J3V 3P8; Sher'90; FRCPC; Derm. (450)441-5222; Fax. (450)441-0938.

PRONOVOST, Marc E; Pine Med Clinic, 5110 5th Ave, Whitehorse YT Y1A 1L4; Laval'94; CCFP; CCFP(E.M.); Staff, Whitehorse General Hospital.

PRONOVOST, Martine; Clinique Saint-Marc, 1295 boul Saint-Sacrement, Shawinigan QC G9N 3M8; Laval'03; Staff Emerg, Centre Hospitalier du Centre la Mauricie; (819)539-2999

PRONOVOST, P Antoine; St Michael's Hosp, 30 Bond St, Toronto ON M5B 1W8; Ott'01; FRCPC; Anes; Critical Care Medicine. Staff, St Michael's Hospital; (416)864-6014

PRONOVOST, Robert; ASSS de l'Estrie, 300-300 rue King E, Sherbrooke QC J1G 1B1; Sher'79; CSPQ; FRCPC; CommunMed; Public Health & Preventive Med. Staff, Centre Hospitalier Universitaire de Sherbrooke-Hopital Fleurimont; Prevention-Promotion, Dir. Sante Publique de l'Estrie; (819)829-3400 x42503; Fax. (819)569-8894.

PRONOVOST NORMAND, Marie-Catherine; UMF Laval, 2690 ch des Quatres-Bourgeois, Quebec QC G1V 0B7; Sher'06; CCFP; Staff, Centre Hospitalier de Gaspe; (418)656-4795

PROPP, Donald J; Nanaimo Reg Gen Hosp, 1200 Dufferin Cres, Nanaimo BC V9S 2B7; Alb'91; CCFP; CCFP(E.M.); Staff, Nanaimo Regional General Hospital; (250)755-7627

PROPPER, Lukas; IWK Health Centre, PO Box 9700 Rpo CSC 5850-5980 University Ave, Halifax NS B3K 6R8; Prague (Czech Republic)'93; Staff, IWK Health Centre; Asst Prof, Dalhousie University; (902)470-8375; Fax. (902)470-8937.

PROPPEROVA, Iva; 200-5675 Spring Garden Rd, Halifax NS B3J 1H1; Charles (Czech Republic)'99; CCFP; (902)425-5730

PROPST, Arthur; Inst of Commun & Family Psy, 4333 ch Cote-Sainte-Catherine, Montreal QC H3T 1E4; McG'75; ABNP; FRCPC; Psy. Sr Staff Psy, Sir Mortimer B Davis Jewish General; Assoc Prof Psy, McGill University; (514)340-8210; arthur.propst@mcgill.ca.

PROPST, Evan J; The Hosp for Sick Children, 6F-555 University Ave, Toronto ON M5G 1X8; Tor'02; LRCPS; FRCSC; Otol (Airway Surgery). Staff, Hospital For Sick Children; Langs: French; (416)813-6532

PROPST, Lara G; North York Gen Hosp-Branson, 5F-555 Finch Ave W, North York ON M2R 1N5; Tor'98; FRCPC; Psy. Staff, North York General Hospital - Branson Division; (416)632-8740

PROSCHEK, Richard; 5-420 Erb St W, Waterloo ON N2L 6K6; Mon'80; (519)746-8118

PROSMANNE, Odile; CHUM-Hotel-Dieu, 3840 rue Saint-Urbain, Montreal QC H2W 1T8; Mon'81; CSPQ; FRCPC; DiagRad. ac Staff, Centre Hospitalier l'Université de Montréal (CHUM) - Hôtel-Dieu; (514)890-8150

PROSPER, J P Lionel; CLSC Saint-Michel, 3355 rue Jarry E, Montreal QC H1Z 2E5; (Haiti)'77; (514)374-8223

PROSSER, Robert G; 33 Loisville St, Oromocto NB E2V 1B9; Dal'64; Staff, Oromocto Public Hospital; (506)357-3316; Fax. (506)357-2080.

PROSSIN, Albert; Metro Medic Centreville, 100-1538 rue Sherbrooke O, Montreal QC H3G 1L5; Dal'55; FACOM; CCBOM; CCFP; Medical Officer, Citizenship & Immigration Canada; Langs: English; French; (514)932-2122

PROST, Eric W; Hotel-Dieu Hosp, 166 Brock St, Kingston ON K7L 5G2; McM'01; FRCPC; Psy. Staff, Hotel-Dieu Hospital; Staff, Kingston General Hospital; Asst Prof Psy, Queen's University; (613)544-3400

PROST, William J; 2 King St E, Stoney Creek ON L8G 1J8; Tor'68; DPM; (905)664-9498

PROTEAU, Caroline; Centre Med Saint-Francois, 200-2125 boul Lemire, Drummondville QC J2B 8N8; Sher'04; (819)477-6793

PROTEAU, Guylaine; E M I S, 150-930 ch Sainte-Foy, Quebec QC G1S 2L4; Laval'89; LMCC; FRCPC; Psy (Occupational Psychiatry). (418)688-7272

PROTZNER, Kalman; Saint John Reg Hosp, PO Box 2100 Stn Main 400 University Ave, Saint John NB E2L 4L2; Semmelweis (Hungary)'67; TraSurg(Hungary); DABPath; DPath; FRCPC; AnatPath (Forensic Pathology). Staff, Saint John Regional Hospital; Asst Prof, Dalhousie University; Langs: Hungarian; (506)648-6516; proka@reg2.health.nb.ca.

PROUDLOVE, Steven G; Centrepointe Med Centre, 303-1 Centrepointe Dr, Nepean ON K2G 6E2; Sask'96; BSc; FRCSC; Urol. Ac Staff, Queensway Carleton Hospital; (613)728-6660

PROULX, Alain A; St Joseph's Health Care, PO Box 5777 Stn B 268 Grosvenor St, London ON N6A 4V2; Wes'01; FRCSC; Ophth. Staff, St Joseph's Hospital - St Joseph's Health Care; (519)646-6315; Fax. (519)646-6193; aproulx6@uwo.ca.

PROULX, Alexandre; Hop Charles Lemoyne, 3120 boul Taschereau, Greenfield Park QC J4V 2H1; Sher'07; FRCPC; Psy. Staff, Hopital Charles LeMoyne; (450)466-5020

PROULX, Andre; CSSS de Laval, 1755 boul Rene-Laennec, Laval QC H7M 3L9; Mon'80; Staff, Hopital de la Cite de la santé; (450)668-1010

PROULX, Andree-Anne; Clin Externe de Psychiatrie, 250-2012 boul Rene-Laennec, Laval QC H7M 4J8; Mon'06; Psy. Staff, Hopital de la Cite de la santé; (450)662-3665

PROULX, Chantal; Ctr Hosp de Verdun, 4000 boul Lasalle, Verdun QC H4G 2A3; Mon'92; Staff, Centre Hospitalier de Verdun; (514)362-1000 x2141

PROULX, Christian A; 8-8 Hiscott St, St. Catharines ON L2R 1C6; Qns'01; BSc; CCFP; Asst Prof Family Med, McMaster University; Asst Prof Family Med, Queen's University; (905)834-2388; Fax. (905)834-2386; surferdoc77@hotmail.com.

PROULX, Cindy; CSSS du Nord de Lanaudière, 1000 boul Sainte-Anne, St-Charles-Brromee QC J6E 6J2; Mon'10; CCFP; Staff, Centre Hospitalier Régional de Lanaudière; (450)759-8222

PROULX, Claude; Rockland MD, 100-100 ch Rockland, Mont-Royal QC H3P 2V9; Mon'71; PlasSurg. Ac Staff, Hôpital du Sacre-Coeur de Montréal; Ac Staff, Hôpital Santa Cabrini Ospedale; (514)331-4322

PROULX, Clement; 8 ch des Pionniers O CP 808, Cap-Saint-Ignace QC G0R 1H0; Laval'77; (418)246-5071

PROULX, Danielle; Hotel-Dieu de Levis, 143 rue Wolfe, Levis QC G6V 3Z1; Laval'74; CSPQ; FRCPC; AnatPath. Staff, Anat Path, Hôtel-Dieu de Lévis; Instructor Med, Université Laval; (418)835-7121 x3267

PROULX, Denis; Carrefour Med Vallee Richelieu, 665 boul Sir-Wilfrid-Laurier, Beloeil QC J3G 4J1; Sher'71; Langs: Bilingual(French/English); (450)467-1230 x221; Fax. (450)467-4936; denisproulx47@hotmail.com.

PROULX, France; Inst Philippe Pinel de Mtl, 10905 boul Henri-Bourassa E, Montreal QC H1C 1H1; Mon'89; MSc; FRCPC; Psy (Adult General Psychiatry). Staff, Institut Philippe-Pinel de Montreal; adj Prof, Universite de Montreal; Langs: Bilingual(English/French); (514)648-8461 x467; Fax. (514)881-3706; proulxfra@hotmail.com.

PROULX, Francois; Surrey Mem Hosp, 13750 96 Ave, Surrey BC V3V 1Z2; Mon'07; FRCPC; Psy. Staff, Surrey Memorial Hospital; (604)587-3814

PROULX, Francois; Ctr Medi Soleil St-Jean-Sur-Ri, 120-383 boul du Seminaire N, St-Jean-sur-Richel QC J3B 8C5; Sher'81; (450)347-7557

PROULX, Francois; Hôpital Ste-Justine, 3175 ch Cote-Sainte-Catherine, Montreal QC H3T 1C5; Mon'87; Critical Care Medicine (P.Q.); Peds. Staff, Hôpital Ste-Justine; Langs: English; (514)345-4675; Fax. (514)345-4822.

PROULX, Genevieve C; Univ Hlth Network-Toronto Gen, EN8 219-200 Elizabeth St, Toronto ON M5G 2C4; Sher'07; Psy. Staff, Toronto General Hospital - UHN; (416)340-4445; Fax. (416)340-4896.

PROULX, Ginette; Carrefour Med Vallee Richelieu, 665 boul Sir-Wilfrid-Laurier, Beloeil QC J3G 4J1; Sher'82; LMCC; (450)467-1230 x225; Fax. (450)467-6941.

PROULX, Guy; Hôpital Laval, 2725 ch Sainte-Foy, Quebec QC G1V 4G5; Laval'78; Cardiol (P.Q.). Staff Cardiol, Hôpital Laval; (418)656-8711 x4657; Fax. (418)656-4544; guy.proulx@criucpq.ulaval.ca.

PROULX, Guylaine; UMF Gatineau, 100-500 boul de l'Hopital, Gatineau QC J8V 2P5; Sher'04; CCFP; Staff, Hôpital de Gatineau; Langs: Spanish; English; (819)561-8107

PROULX, Jacques; CSSS de Beauce-Etchemin, 1515 17e rue, Saint-Georges QC G5Y 4T8; Laval'60; CSPQ; GenPath (P.Q.). Staff, Centre Hospitalier Beauce-Etchemin; (418)228-2031

PROULX, Jean; Inst U en Sante Mentale de QC, 2601 ch de la Canardiere, Quebec QC G1J 2G3; Laval'81; Staff, Institut Universitaire Sante; (418)663-5253; Fax. (418)661-6891.

PROULX, Jean; Ctr Hosp Reg de Lanaudiere, 1000 boul Sainte-Anne, St-Charles-Brromee QC J6E 6J2; Sher'71; DrMedCh; Nephrol (P.Q.) (Hypertension). Staff, Centre Hospitalier Pierre le Gardeur; Staff, Centre Hospitalier Régional de Lanaudière; Langs: French; (450)759-8222 x2123; Fax. (450)759-1389.

PROULX, Jean-Francois; Centre de Sante Publique, 2400 av d'Estimauville, Quebec QC G1E 7G9; Laval'75; Ac Member, Centre Hospitalier Universitaire de Quebec-CHUL; (418)666-7000 x482; Fax. (418)666-3457; jean-francois.proulx@ssss.gouv.qc.ca.

PROULX, Joanne; 100A-299 boul Sir-Wilfrid-Laur, Saint-Lambert QC J4R 2L1; Mon'80; LMCC; (450)465-6551; Fax. (450)465-9810.

PROULX, M C Manon; Centre de Sante Rigaud, 1 rue Hotel de Ville, Rigaud QC J0P 1P0; Mon'80; CCFP; FCFP; (450)451-5336; Fax. (450)451-5214.

PROULX, Michele; 200-3030 boul Le carrefour, Laval QC H7T 2P5; Ott'78; (450)686-8899; Fax. (450)686-7466.

PROULX, Nicolas; Ctr Hosp Trois-Riv-St-Joseph, 731 rue Sainte-Julie, Trois-Rivieres QC G9A 1Y1; Laval'10; Staff, Centre Hospitalier Regional de Trois-Rivieres; (819)372-3536

PROULX, Normand L; CSSS-Hop de Hull, 116 boul Lionel-Emond, Gatineau QC J8Y 1W7; Ott'00; BSc; FRCPC; IntMed; Nephrol. Consultant, Hull Hospital; Langs: French; (819)595-6000 x5083; normand_proulx@hotmail.com.

PROULX, Pierre J L; 200-3030 boul Le carrefour, Laval QC H7T 2P5; Ott'79; (450)686-8899 x63; Fax. (450)686-7466.

PROULX, Pierre-Yvon; Clinique Med Notre-Dame Inc, 147 rue Notre-Dame E, Victoriaville QC G6P 3Z8; Laval'60; IntMed. assoc Staff, Hotel-Dieu d'Arthabaska; Langs: Bilingual(French/English); (819)758-8338; Fax. (819)752-5783.

PROULX, Pierrette; 120B rue Principale GD, St-Andre-Avellin QC J0V 1W0; Sher'74; (819)983-7919; Fax. (819)983-4477.

PROULX, Reno; ASSS de l'Estrie, 300-300 rue King E, Sherbrooke QC J1G 1B1; Sher'87; MBA; DECH; Staff, Centre Hospitalier Universitaire de Sherbrooke-Hopital Fleurimont; Langs: English; (819)829-3400 x42478; Fax. (819)566-2903; rproulx.agence05@ssss.gouv.qc.ca.

PROULX, Richard; Centre Med St-Leonard, 360 rue Beliveau, St-Leonard-d'Aston QC J0C 1M0; Laval'77; ac Staff, Hôpital Sainte-croix; (819)399-2030; Fax. (819)399-2343; richard_proulx@gmf.gouv.qc.ca.

PROULX, Sebastien; Inst U en Sante Mentale de QC, 2601 ch de la Canardiere, Quebec QC G1J 2G3; Laval'98; LLB; FRCPC; Psy (Legal Psychiatry). Staff, Institut Universitaire Sante; (418)663-5321; Fax. (418)661-6891.

PROULX, Simon-Pierre; Clinique Med Loretteville, 250-11000 boul de l'Ormiere, Quebec QC G2B 5S1; Laval'77; LMCC; Langs: English; (418)842-3731; Fax. (418)842-3246; simon-pierre.proulx@ssss.gouv.qc.ca.

PROULX, Stephane; Hop Maisonneuve-Rosemont, 5415 boul de l'Assomption, Montreal QC H1T 2M4; Mon'98; FRCPC; Psy. Staff, Hopital Maisonneuve-Rosemont; (514)252-3400; Fax. (514)252-3803.

PROULX, Stephane; Ctr Hosp de Verdun, 4000 boul Lasalle, Verdun QC H4G 2A3; Mon'91; Staff Emerg & I C U, Centre Hospitalier de Verdun; Clin Teach Staff, Universite de Montreal; (514)362-1000 x2141

PROULX, Sylvain; Centre Med Dolbeau, 1530 rue des Erables, Dolbeau-Mistassini QC G8L 2W7; McG'86; NBME; Staff Emerg, Centre Maria-Chapdelaine - CH de Dolbeau-Mistassini; (418)276-7196; Fax. (418)276-7489.

PROULX, Veronique; GMF La Cigogne, 420-3141 boul Taschereau, Greenfield Park QC J4V 2H2; Sher'97; Clin Prof, Universite de Sherbrooke; (450)466-7892; Fax. (450)466-9602.

PROULX, Yvan D; CSSS Kamouraska-Hop Notre-Dame, CP 460 1201 6e av, La Pocatiere QC G0R 1Z0; Laval'72; CSPQ; Anes. Staff Anes, Centre Hospitalier Paul-Gilbert; Staff, CSSS de Kamouraska; (418)856-7000

PROUSE, Kristy A; Institute for Hormonal Health, 128 Trafalgar Rd, Oakville ON L6J 3G5; Qns'97; BA; BSc; FRCSC; ObstGyn. Court Staff, Trillium Health Centre - Mississauga; (905)844-8884; Fax. (905)844-2009; info@hormonalhealth.ca.

PROUT, Alister J E; 419-1033 Davie St, Vancouver BC V6E 1M7; Cape Town (South Africa)'83; MB ChB; FRCP; FRCPC; Neur (Electromyography). Ac Staff, Providence Health Care - St Paul's Hospital; Consultant, Prince Rupert Regional Hospital; Clinical Asst Prof Neurol, University of British Columbia; (604)681-5440; Fax. (604)681-5644; prout@telus.net.

PROVAN, David C; Humber River Reg Hosp-Church, 200 Church St, Toronto ON M9N 1N8; Tor'08; CCFP; Staff, Humber River Regional Hospital - Church Street Site; (416)243-4191

PROVATOPOULOS, John; Sudbury Med Centre, 310-65 Larch St, Sudbury ON P3E 1B8; McG'87; FRCPC; ObstGyn. Langs: Greek; French; (705)675-8087; Fax. (705)675-8632.

PROVENCAL, Annie; CSSS du Suroît, 150 rue Saint-Thomas, Salaber-de-Valleyf QC J6T 6C1; Sher'98; GenSurg. Staff, Centre Hospitalier Régional du Suroît; (450)371-9920

PROVENCAL, Edith; Ctr Med Mercier-Chateauguay, 108-237 boul St-Jean-Baptiste, Chateauguay QC J6K 3C3; Mon'94; Langs: English; Spanish; (450)699-1888; Fax. (450)694-1458; mecier@sgi-medical.com.

PROVENCAL, Paul T; Hop Ste-Anne, 305 boul Anciens-Combattants, Ste-Anne-de-Bellev QC H9X 1Y9; Mon'79; Staff, Hopital Ste-Anne; (514)457-3440

PROVENCHER, Anne-Marie; Inst Albert Prevost, 6555 boul Gouin O, Montreal QC H4K 1B3; Mon'83; FRCPC; Psy. Staff, Hôpital du Sacre-Coeur de Montréal; (514)338-4356; Fax. (514)338-4357.

PROVENCHER, Claude A; CSSS du Nord de Lanaudière, 1000 boul Sainte-Anne, St-Charles-Brromee QC J6E 6J2; Laval'88; CCFP; Staff, Centre Hospitalier Régional de Lanaudière; (450)759-8222

PROVENCHER, Diane M; CHUM-Hop Notre-Dame, 1560 rue Sherbrooke E, Montreal QC H2L 4M1; Mon'79; FACOG; FRCSC; ObstGyn; GynOnco (P.Q.). Clin Chercheur, Centre Hospitalier l'Université de Montréal (CHUM) - Hôpital Notre-Dame; Clin Asst, Universite de Montreal; (514)890-8000 x27244

PROVENCHER, France; 200-3030 boul Le carrefour, Laval QC H7T 2P5; Mon'85; LMCC; Langs: English; French; (450)686-8899; Fax. (450)686-7466.

PROVENCHER, J J Denis; Polyclinique de la Capitale, 14-4225 4e av O, Quebec QC G1H 6P3; Laval'72; Derm. Ac Staff, Centre Hospitalier Universitaire De Québec - Pavillon De St-françois-d'assise; (418)628-9921; Fax. (418)628-3203.

PROVENCHER, Joanne; Hôpital Laval, 2725 ch Sainte-Foy, Quebec QC G1V 4G5; Sher'92; CCFP; CCFP(E.M.); Staff, Hôpital Laval; (418)656-4550; Fax. (418)656-4596.

PROVENCHER, Josee; Opmedic, 300-1565 boul de l'Avenir, Laval QC H7S 2N5; Mon'84; FRCSC; GenSurg (Breast Disease). Langs: Bilingual(English/French); (450)662-9393; Fax. (450)662-0676.

PROVENCHER, Louise; Ctr Hosp Affilie-St-Sacrement, 1050 ch Sainte-Foy, Quebec QC G1S 4L8; Laval'80; FRCSC; GenSurg (Breast Cancer); General Surgical Oncology (P.Q.). Ac Staff, Centre Hospitalier Affilié Universitaire de Québec - Hôpital du St-Sacrement; assoc Prof, Université Laval; (418)682-7511; Fax. (418)682-8046.

PROVENCHER, Robert; Clinique de l'Alternative, 2034 rue Saint-Hubert, Montreal QC H2L 3Z5; Sher'75; Langs: Bilingual(French/English); (514)281-9848; Fax. (514)281-8057.

PROVENCHER, Sawyna; CHUS-Hop Fleurimont, 3001 12e av N, Sherbrooke QC J1H 5N4; Laval'02; FRCPC; RadOncol. Staff, Centre Hospitalier Universitaire de Sherbrooke-Hopital Fleurimont; (819)346-1110

PROVENCHER, Simone; Dir de Sante Publique Montereg, 1255 rue Beauregard, Longueuil QC J4K 2M3; Laval'76; MSc(Epidemiol.); Staff Community Med, Hopital Charles LeMoyne; Langs: Bilingual(English/French); (450)928-6777 x4090; Fax. (450)928-3812; s.provencher@rrsss16.gouv.qc.ca.

PROVENCHER, Steeve; Hôpital Laval, 2725 ch Sainte-Foy, Quebec QC G1V 4G5; Laval'98; FRCPC; IntMed (Hypertension); Respir. Staff, Hôpital Laval; (418)656-8711

PROVENCHER, Yves; Centre de Read Lucie-Bruneau, 2275 av Laurier E, Montreal QC H2H 2N8; Mon'85; (514)527-4527; Fax. (514)527-0979; stemfan001@yahoo.ca.

PROVIAS, John P; Hamilton Health Sciences, 137 Barton St E, Hamilton ON L8L 8A8; McM'81; BSc(Tor); BSc(UWO); FRCPC; NeurPath. Staff, Hamilton Health Sciences Centre - Hamilton General Hospital; (905)527-0271; Fax. (905)524-2681.

PROVINCIALI, Beatrice; CLSC Kateri, 90 boul Marie-Victorin, Candiac QC J5R 1C1; Rome (Italy)'78; (450)659-7661; Fax. (450)444-6276.

PROVOST, Francine; 218-383 boul du Seminaire N, St-Jean-sur-Richel QC J3B 8C5; Sher'83; Peds. (450)348-4911; Fax. (450)348-6401.

PROVOST, Francois; CLSC du Ruisseau-Papineau, 200-800 boul Chomedey, Laval QC H7V 3Y4; Mon'89; (450)687-5691 x2009; Fax. (450)682-2475.

PROVOST, Marcel; Centre Marguerite Adam, 425 rue Hubert, Beloeil QC J3G 2T1; Mon'70; CCFP; CCFP(E.M.); FCFP; Dir L'Amelioration de l'Exercide, College des Medecins du Quebec; (450)467-1631 x5031; mprovost@cmq.org.

PROVOST, Nathalie; 264 boul Rene-Levesque E, Montreal QC H2X 1P1; Sher'91; Derm. Staff, Centre Hospitalier l'Université de Montréal (CHUM) - Hôtel-Dieu; (450)629-0222

PROVOST, Ninon M M; CSSS Pierre Boucher, 1333 boul Jacques-Cartier E, Longueuil QC J4M 2A5; McM'89; CSPQ; FRCPC; DiagRad. Staff, Centre Hospitalier Pierre Boucher; Staff, Hôpital de l'Archipel; (450)468-8111

PROVOST, Robert; Centre Med Saint-Hubert, 206-5125 boul Cousineau, Saint-Hubert QC J3Y 3K7; Sher'77; (450)678-8840; Fax. (450)678-5722.

PROVOST, Sylvie; Direction de la Sante Publique, 1301 rue Sherbrooke E, Montreal QC H2L 1M3; Mon'78; MPH; (514)528-2400 x3275; Fax. (514)528-2470; sprovost@santepub-mtl.qc.ca.

PROVOST, Valerie; Ctr Hosp du Centre la Mauricie, 50 119e rue, Shawinigan-Sud QC G9P 5K1; Mon'01; CSPQ; FRCPC; Anes. Staff, Centre Hospitalier du Centre la Mauricie; (819)536-7500

PROVOST, Viviane; Quest Community Health Ctre, 100-145 Queenston St, St. Catharines ON L2R 2Z9; Mon'85; CCFP; (905)688-2558

PROVOST, Yves L; CHUM-Hotel-Dieu, 3840 rue Saint-Urbain, Montreal QC H2W 1T8; Sher'85; FRCPC; DiagRad (Cardiac Radiology). Staff, Centre Hospitalier l'Université de Montréal (CHUM) - Hôtel-Dieu; Langs: English; (514)890-8000 x25200; yves.provost@uhn.on.ca.

PROVOST-MANSEAU, Suzanne; Polyclinique Med Fabreville, 217-380 boul Cure-Labelle, Laval QC H7P 5L3; Mon'74; Staff, Hôpital du Sacre-Coeur de Montréal; (450)628-5800 x368; Fax. (450)628-0217.

PROWSE, Arthur W H; 211-2453 Beacon Ave, Sidney BC V8L 1X7; Qns'76; FRCPC; Psy (Geriatric Psychiatry). Staff, Saanich Peninsula Hospital; Consultant Geriatric Psy., Elderly Outreach Service; (250)656-8866; Fax. (250)592-6960.

PROWSE, Gordon G; 3250 Eglinton Ave E, Scarborough ON M1J 2H6; Tor'58; CCFP; FCFP; Ac Staff, The Scarborough Hospital - General Campus; Lecturer Family & Commun Med, University of Toronto; (416)261-2111

PROWSE, Matthew T; Glenrose Rehabilitation Hosp, 10230 111 Ave NW, Edmonton AB T5G 0B7; Man'03; FRCPC; PhysMed&Rehab (Pediatric Rehabilitation). Staff, Glenrose Rehabilitation Hospital; Asst Prof Peds & Physical Med & Rehabilitation, University of Alberta; (780)735-6171; Fax. (780)735-8200.

PROWSE, Owen A; 103-1205 Amber Dr, Thunder Bay ON P7B 6M4; Tor'94; FRCSC; Urol. (807)346-1440

PROWSE, Sheryl; Terrace Hill Med Centre, 128-217 Terrace Hill St, Brantford ON N3R 1G8; McM'90; BSc; MSc; (519)756-4241; Fax. (519)756-0840.

PROZESKY, Benjamin V M; Centennial Health, PO Box 700 Stn Main, Brooks AB T1R 1B6; (South Africa)'06; (403)793-8883; Fax. (403)793-8890.

PRPIC, Jason C; Sudbury Reg Hosp-Laurentian, 41 Ramsey Lake Rd, Sudbury ON P3E 5J1; Ott'99; CCFP; CCFP(E.M.); Staff, Health Sciences North-St Joseph's Health Centre; Staff, Health Sciences North-Laurentian Site; (705)675-4700

PRSA, Milan; The Hosp for Sick Children, 555 University Ave, Toronto ON M5G 1X8; McG'03; Cardiol; Peds. Fellow, The Hospital For Sick Children; (416)813-7467

PRSALA, Jan; Formation Hlth Services Unit, PO Box 17000 Stn Forces 1200 Colville Rd, Victoria BC V9A 7N2; Dal'85; Staff, Canadian Forces Health Services - Pacific Centre; Staff, Vancouver Island Health Authority; Langs: Czech; (250)363-4120

PRUD'HOMME, Denis; Physio Outaouais, 382 boul Alexandre-Tache, Gatineau QC J9A 1M5; Laval'86; MSc; BSc; Dean Faculty of Health Sciences, University of Ottawa; Langs: English; (819)775-9515; Fax. (819)775-2743.

PRUD'HOMME, Gerald J; St Michael's Hosp, 2 013CC-30 Bond St, Toronto ON M5B 1W8; Ott'77; MD; CSPQ; FRCPC; AnatPath. Staff LabMed & Pathobiol/Clin Scientist, St Michael's Hospital; Prof LabMed & Pathobiol, University of Toronto; Langs: French; (416)864-6060 x3147; prudhommeg@smh.toronto.on.ca.

PRUD'HOMME, Henri; CSSS Portneuf-CLSC Donnacona, 400 138 Rte, Donnacona QC G3M 1C3; Laval'77; BSc; Ac Staff Employees Health Clin, Centre Hospitalier Universitaire de Quebec-CHUL; Physician Occupational Health, CSSS Nunavik/CSSS Terre Cree; Langs: Bilingual(French/English); (418)285-2626; Fax. (418)285-4589.

PRUD'HOMME, Jane M; The Ottawa Hosp-Gen Campus, 501 Smyth Rd, Ottawa ON K1H 8L6; Ott'89; FRCPC; Anes. Staff, The Ottawa Hospital - General Campus; (613)737-7777 x8187; Fax. (613)737-8189.

PRUD'HOMME, Louis; Cite de la Sante de Laval, 1755 boul Rene-Laennec, Laval QC H7M 3L9; Mon'89; FRCPC; IntMed; Nephrol. Staff, Hopital de la Cite de la santé; (450)668-1010; Fax. (450)975-5545.

PRUD'HOMME, Marie L P; CSSS du Val St-Francois, 23 rue Ambroise-Dearden, Windsor QC J1S 1G8; Mon'79; Langs: Bilingual(French/English); (819)542-2777 x55219

PRUD'HOMME, Michel; Ctr Hosp Affilie-Enfant-Jesus, 1401 18e rue, Quebec QC G1J 1Z4; Mon'96; PhD; MSc; BSc(Physiol); Neursurg (Neuromodulation). Staff, Centre Hospitalier Affilié Universitaire de Québec - Hôpital De L'Enfant Jésus; Teach Staff Research, Université Laval; (418)649-0252; Fax. (418)649-5915; m.prudhomme@videotron.ca.

PRUD'HOMME, Michel; CHUM-Hop Notre-Dame, 1560 rue Sherbrooke E, Montreal QC H2L 4M1; Mon'64; Nephrol (P.Q.); IntMed. Staff, Centre Hospitalier l'Université de Montréal (CHUM) - Hôpital Notre-Dame; (514)890-8000

PRUD'HOMME, Pierre T; Queensway-Carleton Hosp, 3045 Baseline Rd, Nepean ON K2H 8P4; Ott'98; FRCPC; DiagRad. Staff, Queensway Carleton Hospital; (613)721-2000

PRUD'HOMME, Rodrigue; Clin Med Gamelin, 3C-520 boul de l'Hopital, Gatineau QC J8V 2P5; Laval'68; Physician, Centre de Readaptation en Toxicomanie; Langs: English; (819)777-6664; Fax. (819)777-0138.

PRUD'HOMME, Veronique; Ctr Hosp Laurentien, 234 rue Saint-Vincent, Ste-Agathe-des-Mts QC J8C 2B8; Sher'03; LMCC; Staff, Centre Hospitalier Laurentien; Physician, Centre Medical du Lac; Physician, CLSC St-Felicien; (819)324-4000; veroprudhomme@hotmail.com.

PRUDENCIO, Jose A; 310-55 Erb St E, Waterloo ON N2J 4K8; Tor'95; BSc; FRCSC; Otol (Head & Neck). Staff, Grand River Hospital - Kitchener/Waterloo Health Centre; Staff, St Mary's General Hospital; Langs: Spanish; French; (519)576-6632; Fax. (519)576-6756.

PRUNEAU, Elaine; Ctr Hosp de Verdun, 4000 boul Lasalle, Verdun QC H4G 2A3; Mon'96; Staff, Centre Hospitalier de Verdun; (514)362-1000

PRUNEAU, Guylaine; CSSS de la Region de Thetford, 1717 rue Notre-Dame E, Thetford Mines QC G6G 2V4; Sher'87; FRCPC; IntMed. Staff, Hopital du CSS de la Region de Thetford; (418)338-7777; Fax. (418)338-7794.

PRUNEAU, Marc; Clinique Med Belvedere, 202-2235 rue Galt O, Sherbrooke QC J1K 1K6; Sher'95; CCFP; (819)563-4244

PRUPAS, David R; 13800 boul Gouin O, Pierrefonds QC H8Z 3H6; McG'86; Staff, Mount Sinai Hospital Center; Langs: French; (514)626-2572; Fax. (514)624-7486.

PRUSINKIEWICZ, Christopher; Foothills Med Centre, C229-1403 29 St NW, Calgary AB T2N 2T9; Cal'00; FRCPC; Anes. Staff, Foothills Medical Centre; (403)944-1430

PRUTIS-MISTERSKA, Krystyna; 303-960 Lawrence Ave W, North York ON M6A 3B5; (Poland)'73; PhD; FRCPC; PhysMed&Rehab. Physician, St. John's Med Centre; Langs: Polish; Italian; French; (416)785-0844; Fax. (416)785-8030.

PRUZANSKI, Waldemar; Rosedale Med Centre, 803-600 Sherbourne St, Toronto ON M4X 1W4; Jerusalem (Israel)'56; FACP; FACR; FRCPC; IntMed (Rheumatology & Clinical Immunology). Hon Consultant Staff, St Michael's Hospital; Emeritus Prof Med, University of Toronto; Langs: Russian; Polish; Hebrew; (416)972-9423; Fax. (416)972-0507.

PRYCHITKO, Jonathan T P; North Bay Reg Health Centre, 50 College Dr, North Bay ON P1B 0A4; Man'01; FRCPC; Anes. Staff, North Bay Regional Health Centre - Regional Mental Health; (705)474-8600

PRYSE-PHILLIPS, William E; 7 Monkstown Rd, St. John's NL A1C 3T1; London (England)'61; FRCP(London); FRCPC; Neur (Electromyography). Staff, Health Sciences Centre; Emeritus Prof Neurol, Memorial University Of Newfoundland; Langs: Bilingual(French/English); (709)726-9109; Fax. (709)726-0396; wpryse@mun.ca.

PRYSIAZNY, Brian K; Niagara Diagnostic Imaging Ctr, 589 Lake St, St Catharines ON L2N 7L6; Alb'78; FRCPC; DiagRad. (905)937-2255

PRYSTAI, Gregory D; Foothills Med Centre, C827-1403 29 St NW, Calgary AB T2N 2T9; Man'77; FRCSC; GenSurg; Cardiovasc&ThorSurg. Staff, Foothills Medical Centre; (403)944-1671; Fax. (403)944-2906.

PRYSTAJECKY, Maria S; Rockyview Gen Hosp, 7007 14 St SW, Calgary AB T2V 1P9; Alb'73; CCFP; CCFP(E.M.); Staff, Rockyview General Hospital; (403)943-3449; Fax. (403)943-3220.

PRYSTAWA, Barbara M; Kamloops Mental Health, 235 Lansdowne St, Kamloops BC V2C 1X8; Alb'88; FRCPC; Psy. (250)377-6500 x4032

PRYSTUPA, Aaron J; North Battleford Med Clinic, 102-11427 Railway Ave, North Battleford SK S9A 3G8; Sask'04; BScAnatomy; CCFP; (306)445-4415; Fax. (306)445-5145.

PRZYBOJEWSKI, Stefan J; Foothills Med Centre, 1403 29 St NW, Calgary AB T2N 2T9; Cape Town (South Africa)'98; MMedRad Diag; Staff, Foothills Medical Centre; (403)944-1110

PRZYSIEZNY, Janine M; 206-186 Albert St, London ON N6A 1M1; Cal'99; FRCPC; Psy (Psychotherapy). (519)858-9857; Fax. (519)858-3900.

PSARAKIS, Stella; 1418 Ontario St, Burlington ON L7S 1G4; Tor'86; BSc; MSc; FSOGC; FACOG; FRCSC; ObstGyn. Chief ObstGyn, Joseph Brant Memorial Hospital; Obstetrics & Gynecology, Hamilton Health Sciences Centre - McMaster University Medical Centre; Court Staff, Halton Healthcare Services Corporation - Oakville Site; Clin Assoc Prof ObstGyn, McMaster University; (905)681-2344; Fax. (905)681-2297.

PSARRAS, Thomas E; Montfort Hosp, 713 Montreal Rd, Ottawa ON K1K 0T2; Ott'01; FRCPC; IntMed; Critical Care Medicine. Staff, Montfort Hospital; (613)746-4621

PSOOY, Brian J; Queen Elizabeth II HSC, 1276 South Park St, Halifax NS B3H 2Y9; Man'97; FRCPC; DiagRad. Staff, Queen Elizabeth II Health Sciences Centre - Victoria General Site; (902)473-2700; Fax. (902)473-2018.

PSOOY, Karen J; Children's Hosp, AE301-840 Sherbrook St, Winnipeg MB R3A 1S1; Man'96; DABU; FRCSC; Urol (Pediatric Urology). Staff, Health Sciences Centre.

PTAK, Theadore W; York-Finch Med Centre, 310-2115 Finch Ave W, North York ON M3N 2V6; Ott'63; FRCPC; IntMed (Gastroenterology). Chief IntMed Dept of Med, Humber River Regional Hospital - Finch Avenue Site; (416)749-1139; Fax. (416)749-5467.

PTITO, Linda; 304-990 rue Notre-Dame O, Montreal QC H3C 1K1; Bordeaux (France)'77; (514)274-8001

PU, Qian; CSSS de Laval, 1755 boul Rene-Laennec, Laval QC H7M 3L9; (China)'85; MedBiochem (P.Q.). Staff, Hopital de la Cite de la santé; (450)668-1010

PU, Yunlong; 202-80 Finch Ave W, North York ON M2N 2H4; Alb'97; (416)218-0210

PUBBEN, Mary-Ann J; 202-1100 Sheppard Ave E, North York ON M2K 2W1; Wes'82; CCFP; Ac Staff, North York General Hospital; Langs: Dutch; (416)733-1500; Fax. (416)733-8267.

PUCAR, Frederic; 202-111 boul de l'Hopital, Gatineau QC J8T 7V1; Laval'94; FRCPC; IntMed; ClinImmunol&Allergy. (819)246-0500; Fax. (819)246-1043.

PUCELLA, Elisa; A-800 boul Chomedey, Laval QC H7V 3Y4; Mon'99; CCFP; (450)978-2121 x2037

PUCHALSKI, Stephen A; Hamilton HS-General Site, 237 Barton St E, Hamilton ON L8L 2X2; McM'85; FRCPC; Anes. Staff, Hamilton Health Sciences Centre - Hamilton General Hospital; Clin Assoc Prof, McMaster University; (905)527-4322; puchalsk@mcmaster.ca.

PUCHALSKI RITCHIE, Lisa M; Univ Hlth Network-Toronto Gen, 200 Elizabeth St, Toronto ON M5G 2C4; Tor'01; FRCPC; EmergMed. Staff, Toronto General Hospital - UHN; (416)340-4800

PUCHOLT, Vladimir; Jane Medical Clinic, 101-2780 Jane St, North York ON M3N 2J2; Sheffield (England)'74; MB ChB; MRCP(UK); FRCPC; Peds (Neonatology). Staff Ped(Neo-Natologist), Humber River Regional Hospital - Finch Avenue Site; Langs: Czech; (416)745-8500; Fax. (416)748-8730.

PUCHYR, Martina; Humber River Reg Hosp-Church, 200 Church St, Toronto ON M9N 1N8; Ott'04; FRCPC; IntMed; MedOncol. Staff, St Joseph's Health Centre; Staff, Humber River Regional Hospital - Church Street Site; Staff, Sunnybrook Health Sciences Centre; (416)243-4505; Fax. (416)243-4580.

PUCKRIN, Paul H; Medical Assoc of Port Perry, 462 Paxton St, Port Perry ON L9L 1L9; Tor'74; Ac Staff, Lakeridge Health - Port Perry Site; Med Examiner, Civil Aviation Canada; (905)985-2895; Fax. (905)985-3464.

PUDDESTER, Derek G; Children's Hosp Eastern Ont, 401 Smyth Rd, Ottawa ON K1H 8L1; Mem'95; BMedSci; FRCP; BA; MEd; FRCPC; Psy (Child & Adolescent Psychiatry). Ac Staff, Children's Hospital of Eastern Ontario (CHEO); Ac Staff, Royal Ottawa Mental Health Centre - Royal Ottawa Health Care Group; Dir Faculty of Wellness Prog/Assoc Prof Psy, University of Ottawa; (613)737-7600 x2703; Fax. (613)738-4202; puddester@cheo.on.ca.

PUDDICOMBE, Robert E; Northmount Med Centre, 704-145 13th St E, North Vancouver BC V7L 2L4; UBC'71; Ac Staff, Lions Gate Hospital; (604)985-4104; Fax. (604)985-9176.

PUDDU, Silvana; 187 James St S, Hamilton ON L8P 3A8; Rome (Italy)'84; Psy. (905)522-5778

PUDDY, Jennifer J; Foothills Med Centre, 231-1403 29 St NW, Calgary AB T2N 2T9; Tor'96; CCFP; CCFP(E.M.); Staff, Foothills Medical Centre; (403)944-1110

PUDUPAKKAM, Santosh R; Sudbury Vascular Lab Ltd, 345-2140 Regent St, Sudbury ON P3E 5S8; Wes'94; FRCSC; GenSurg; VascSurg. (705)522-4611; Fax. (705)522-4158; santoshpmd@hotmail.com.

PUENTE, Sara C; 31 Caradoc St N, Strathroy ON N7G 2M5; Wes'07; CCFP; (519)245-3590

PUETZ, Joel A; Univ Hlth Network-Toronto Gen, 200 Elizabeth St, Toronto ON M5G 2C4; Sask'06; CCFP; CCFP(E.M.); Staff, Toronto General Hospital - UHN; (416)340-3111

PUGACHEV, Alexander; R B White Clinic, 202-383 Ellis St, Penticton BC V2A 4L9; St Petersburg (Russia (Federation))'84; CCFP; (250)493-8484

PUGASH, Denise S; BC Women's Hosp & Health Ctre, 1T48-4500 Oak St, Vancouver BC V6H 3N1; McG'80; FRCPC; DiagRad. Staff, BC Women's Hospital & Health Centre; (604)875-2424 x6784; Fax. (604)875-3013.

PUGASH, Eric S; Columbia Med Bldg, 405-301 Columbia St E, New Westminster BC V3L 3W5; McG'79; FRCSC; PlasSurg (Aesthetic Surgery). Staff, Peace Arch Hospital; Staff, Royal Columbian Hospital; Staff, Eagle Ridge Hospital & Health Care Centre; Staff, Southern Health Centre; Langs: Bilingual(English/French); (604)522-5199; Fax. (604)522-5444; drpugash@telus.net.

PUGASH, Robyn A; Sunnybrook Hlth Sciences Ctre, MG 189-2075 Bayview Ave, Toronto ON M4N 3M5; Wes'84; FRCPC; DiagRad (Interventional Radiology). Ac Staff, Sunnybrook Health Sciences Centre; Asst Prof, University of Toronto; (416)480-6197; Fax. (416)480-5855; r.pugash@utoronto.ca.

PUGEN, Gregory L; 5-2930 Islington Ave, North York ON M9L 2K5; Tor'71; Staff, Humber River Regional Hospital - Finch Avenue Site; Staff, Humber River Regional Hospital - Church Street Site; Staff, The Scarborough Hospital - Birchmount Campus; Clin Prof Med, University of Toronto; (416)749-8911; Fax. (416)746-2875.

PUGH, Cheryl; 207-42 Glen Allan Dr, Bridgewater NS B4V 3N2; Mem'96; FRCSC; ObstGyn. Staff, South Shore Regional Hospital; (902)543-8788; Fax. (902)543-3334.

PUGH, David M W; Brant Community HC-Brantford, 200 Terrace Hill St, Brantford ON N3R 1G9; Wes'93; MD; BSc(Hon); FRCSC; OrthSurg (Upper Limb Surgery). Staff Surg, The Brant Community Healthcare System - Brantford General Hospital Site; Clinical Asst Prof, McMaster University; (519)751-5857; Fax. (519)751-5830; pugda@bchsys.org.

PUGH, Debra; The Ottawa Hosp-Gen Campus, 501 Smyth Rd, Ottawa ON K1H 8L6; Dal'01; FRCPC; IntMed. Staff, The Ottawa Hospital - General Campus; (613)737-8222

PUGH, E Denise; Dr Everett Chalmers Reg Hosp, PO Box 9000 Stn A 700 Priestman St, Fredericton NB E3B 5N5; Tor'89; BSc; FASCP; FCAP; FRCPC; AnatPath. Staff, Dr Everett Chalmers Regional Hospital; (506)452-5485; Fax. (506)443-2168; dr.denise.pugh@horizonnb.ca.

PUGH, J Christian; South Shore Reg Hosp, 90 Glen Allan Dr, Bridgewater NS B4V 3S6; Mem'96; CCFP; CCFP(E.M.); Staff, South Shore Regional Hospital; Staff, Health Sciences Centre; (902)527-5216

PUGH, James E V; The Hosp for Sick Children, 555 University Ave, Toronto ON M5G 1X8; London (England)'03; Peds (Neonatal & Perinatal Medicine). Staff, The Hospital For Sick Children; (416)813-7500

PUGH, Jeffrey A; University of Alberta Hosp, 2D1 02-8440 112 St NW, Edmonton AB T6G 2B7; UBC'00; BSc; MSc; FRCSC; Neursurg (Pediatric Neuro Surgery). Staff, University of Alberta Hospital; (780)407-1537; Fax. (780)407-7293; jeffrey.pugh@albertahealthservices.ca.

PUGLIA, Marco A; McMaster University, 2F51-1280 Main St W, Hamilton ON L8S 4K1; Ott'04; FRCPC; IntMed; Gastroent. Staff, Toronto General Hospital - UHN; (905)521-2100 x76733

PUGSLEY, Donald C G; Hilden Med Clinic, 1174 Highway 2 RR 1, Brookfield NS B0N 1C0; Dal'80; Ac Staff, Colchester East Hants Health Centre; (902)893-3157; Fax. (902)895-0588.

PUGSLEY, Stewart O; St Joseph's Healthcare, 50 Charlton Ave E, Hamilton ON L8N 4A6; Tor'67; FRCPC; IntMed (Respirology). Ac Staff Firestone Institute for Respiratory Health, St Joseph's Healthcare - Charlton Campus; Clin Assoc Prof, McMaster University; (905)521-6000; Fax. (905)521-6182.

PUHKY, Ronald S; 212-2187 Oak Bay Ave, Victoria BC V8R 1G1; McG'71; Co-Dir., Five Element Acupuncture for Physicians Training Program-San Diego, CA-USA; (250)595-7125

PUJARA, Bakulesh K P; Southwood Med Clinic, 80-10233 Elbow Dr SW, Calgary AB T2W 1E8; Manchester (England)'79; MB ChB; (403)252-1111; Fax. (403)252-8997.

PUKAY, Gregory; Northern Medical Unit, T162-770 Bannatyne Ave, Winnipeg MB R3E 0W3.

PUKSA, Serge; 730 Concession St, Hamilton ON L8V 1C1; Tor'78; FRCPC; IntMed (Lung Cancer); Respir. Staff Respirology, Hamilton Health Sciences Centre-Juravinski Site; Clin Assoc Prof Med, McMaster University; Langs: Ukrainian; (905)387-5543; Fax. (905)387-3713; office@puksa.ca.

PULEY, Geoffrey S; 206-101 Queensway W, Mississauga ON L5B 2P7; Tor'97; FRCPC; IntMed; Cardiol. Staff Interventional Cardiol, Trillium Health Centre - Mississauga; (905)615-9285

PULEY, Ronald J; Medical Bldg, 406-18 Pine St, Kitchener ON N2H 5Z8; Tor'68; FRCPC; IntMed (Cardiology). (519)741-5252; Fax. (519)576-8291.

PULFREY, Simon M; St Paul's Hosp, 1081 Burrard St, Vancouver BC V6Z 1Y6; UBC'00; CCFP; CCFP(E.M.); Staff, Providence Health Care - St Paul's Hospital; (604)806-8480; smpgompa@hotmail.com.

PULIDO, Analene F; East York Town Centre, B15-45 Overlea Blvd, Toronto ON M4H 1C3; FEU (Philippines)'86; CCFP; (416)421-1240; Fax. (416)421-9829.

PULIGANDLA, Pramod S; MUHC-Montreal Children's Hosp, C811-2300 rue Tupper, Montreal QC H3H 1P3; Wes'95; BSc(Hon); MSc(Physiol); FRCSC; GenSurg (Pediatric Intensive Care); Critical Care Medicine (P.Q.); PedGenSurg. Att Staff Ped Surg, McGill University Health Centre - Montreal Children's Hospital; Langs: English; French; (514)412-4438; Fax. (514)412-4341; pramod.puligandla@muhc.mcgill.ca.

PULIS, Randy P; Hinton Gen Hosp, 1280 Switzer Dr, Hinton AB T7V 1V2; Wes'93; FRCSC; GenSurg. Staff, Hinton Healthcare Centre; (780)865-1788; Fax. (780)865-1866; rpulis@shaw.ca.

PULLAN, Rhoda Z; Ingram Family Physicians, 103-149 Ingram St, Duncan BC V9L 1N8; Man'89; CCFP; FCFP; (250)746-4401; Fax. (250)746-4473.

PULLAN, Wendy M; Queensway Med Centre, 300-5307 Canotek Rd, Gloucester ON K1J 9M2; Tor'87; (613)746-6223; Fax. (613)746-6018.

PULLELA, Visweswara; Capt William Jackman Mem Hosp, 410 Booth St, Labrador City NL A2V 2K1; Patna (India)'77; MB BS; DA; FFARCSI; Staff, Captain William Jackman Memorial Hospital; (709)944-2632; rpullela@yahoo.com.

PULLMER, Lewis Z; 1110-750 Broadway W, Vancouver BC V5Z 1J1; Man'77; FRCPC; Psy. Ac Staff, Providence Health Care - St Paul's Hospital; Asst Prof, University of British Columbia; pullmer@unixg.ubc.ca.

PULMAN, Jonathan R; Canadian Forces Services Ctre, 101 Colonel by Drive, Ottawa ON K1A 0K2; Oxford (England)'71; MB ChB; FRCPC; Psy. Staff, Canadian Forces Health Services Centre; Staff, Canadian Forces Health Services Centre; Asst Prof Psy, University of Ottawa; (613)945-1082; Fax. (613)235-9199.

PULOSKI, Shannon K T; Foothills Med Centre, 1005-1403 29 St NW, Calgary AB T2N 2T9; Wes'98; FRCSC; OrthSurg. Staff, Foothills Medical Centre; (403)944-8634; Fax. (403)270-3587.

PUN, Christine W H; Sudbury Reg Hosp-Laurentian, 41 Ramsey Lake Rd, Sudbury ON P3E 5J1; Tor'99; CCFP; Staff, Health Sciences North-Laurentian Site; Ac Staff, St Joseph's General Hospital Elliot Lake; Asst Prof, Northern Ontario School of Medicine; Langs: Cantonese; (705)675-4700

PUN, Cynthia; Central Toronto CHC, 168 Bathurst St, Toronto ON M5V 2R4; Tor'07; CCFP; (416)703-8480; Fax. (416)703-8479.

PUN, Teresa W C; Health Sciences Centre, GC3-820 Sherbrook St, Winnipeg MB R3A 1R9; Tor'07; ClinImmunol&Allergy; IntMed. Staff, Health Sciences Centre; (204)787-3366

PUN, Yin Hun Ian; 302-4040 Finch Ave E, Scarborough ON M1S 4V5; Tor'90; Staff Family Pract, The Scarborough Hospital - General Campus; Staff, Toronto East General Hospital Inc; Pres, Med Logix Computer Systems; Langs: Cantonese; Mandarin; (416)848-7788; chinesemusic@rogers.com.

PUNAMBOLAM, Ryan J; 102-2216 McCallum Rd, Abbotsford BC V2S 3P3; Wes'05; FRCPC; Neur. (604)853-2390

PUNG, Carolyne H; 305-1062 Ghislain St, Hawkesbury ON K6A 3B2; Laval'00; (613)632-2779

PUNG, Evelyne H; MD Centropolis, 227-655 prom du Centropolis, Laval QC H7T 0A3; Laval'97; CCFP; Staff, Hopital de la Cite de la santé; (514)316-1357

PUNGUR, Judit; Mission Hills Med Clinic, 100-398 St Albert Rd, St Albert AB T8N 5J9; Mem'87; BSc(Hon.); (780)460-0424; Fax. (780)460-0524.

PUNGUR FARRELL, Erzsi; Mission Hills Med Clinic, 100-398 St Albert Rd, St Albert AB T8N 5J9; Mem'89; BSc; BMedSci; (780)460-0424; Fax. (780)460-0524.

PUNJA, Alim M; 101-240 Duncan Mill Rd, North York ON M3B 3S6; Cal'07; Anes. (416)840-5990

PUNJA, Karim G H; Mayfair Place, 250-6707 Elbow Dr SW, Calgary AB T2V 0E4; Qns'97; BScPT; FRCSC; Ophth (Oculo Facial Cosmetic Surgery). Clin Assoc Prof, University of Calgary; (403)255-5561; Fax. (403)255-7764.

PUNJANI, Yasmeen A B; Scarborough Hosp-General Div, 3050 Lawrence Ave E, Scarborough ON M1P 2V5; Karachi (Pakistan)'79; ABIM; FRCPC; IntMed (Geriatric Medicine). Staff, The Scarborough Hospital - Birchmount Campus; Staff, The Scarborough Hospital - General Campus; Langs: Hindi; Urdu; Gujarati; (416)495-2541; Fax. (416)431-8161.

PUNNA, Satish K; The Moncton Hosp, 135 MacBeath Ave, Moncton NB E1C 6Z8; Dal'00; FRCPC; DiagRad. Staff, The Moncton Hospital; (506)857-5520

PUNNEN, Chinnamma; Joseph Brant Mem Hosp, 1230 North Shore Blvd E, Burlington ON L7S 1W7; Kerala (India)'75; FFARCS; FRCPC; Anes. Staff Anes, Joseph Brant Memorial Hospital; Langs: Malayalam; (905)632-3730; Fax. (905)336-4821.

PUNNEN, Punnamkuzhil C; 404-960 Lawrence Ave W, North York ON M6A 3B5; Punjab (India)'68; MB BS; MS; FRCS(Ed); FRCSC; Urol (Impotence). Staff Urol, Halton Healthcare Services Corporation - Milton District Hospital; Staff Urol, Humber River Regional Hospital - Church Street Site; Langs: Hindi; Punjabi; Malayalam; (416)256-2737; Fax. (416)256-9098.

PUNNETT, Angela S; The Hosp for Sick Children, 9413-555 University Ave, Toronto ON M5G 1X8; Tor'96; BSc; FRCPC; Peds (Hematological Oncology). Assoc Staff, The Hospital For Sick Children; (416)813-7654 x1503; Fax. (416)813-5574.

PUNTHAKEE, Dinshaw K; Hamilton Commun Health Centre, M10-414 Victoria Ave N, Hamilton ON L8L 5G8; Tor'76; BScPT; FRCSC; OrthSurg (Hip & Knee Replacement). Gen Surgery, Hamilton Health Sciences Centre - Hamilton General Hospital; Staff Surgeon, McMaster University; Langs: Hindi; Gujarati; (905)577-6677; Fax. (905)522-5101.

PUNTHAKEE, Narsys; Hamilton Commun Health Centre, M10-414 Victoria Ave N, Hamilton ON L8L 5G8; Bombay (India)'68; FRCPC; Peds (Allergy). Staff, Hamilton Health Sciences Centre - McMaster Children's Hospital; (905)577-6338; Fax. (905)522-5101.

PUNTHAKEE, Xerxes D; 308-250 Lawrence Ave W, Toronto ON M5M 1B2; Tor'04; FRCSC; Otol (Head & Neck Surgery). (416)787-5511; Fax. (416)787-1592.

PUNTHAKEE, Zubin; McMaster University Med Centre, 3V51-1280 Main St W, Hamilton ON L8S 4K1; McM'98; FRCPC; IntMed (Endocrinology); Endocrin&Metab. Staff, Hamilton Health Sciences Centre - McMaster Children's Hospital; (905)521-2100; Fax. (905)521-4971.

PUNTI, Rosita; Hop Louis-H Lafontaine, 7401 rue Hochelaga, Montreal QC H1N 3M5; Sher'84; FRCPC; Psy (Geriatric Psychiatry). Staff, Hopital Louis-H Lafontaine; Universite de Montreal; Langs: Bilingual(French/English); (514)251-4000 x3060; Fax. (514)251-1604.

PUODZIUKAS, L Edward; Mobile Industrial Health Servi, 101-375 Finley Ave, Ajax ON L1S 2E2; Wes'71; (905)686-6000; Fax. (905)686-1491.

PUPKO, Harold; 400-4430 Bathurst St, North York ON M3H 3S3; Tor'83; (416)633-9152

PUPPALA, Venkata Karthik Rao; 558 Charlotte St, Sydney NS B1P 1E7; Osmania (India)'03; (902)539-7666; Fax. (902)567-1097.

PURANAM, Padma; Sudbury Reg Hosp-Laurentian, 41 Ramsey Lake Rd, Sudbury ON P3E 5J1; Sri Venkatesvara (India)'82; FRCPC; IntMed. Staff, Health Sciences North-Laurentian Site; (705)523-7147

PURCELL, Daniel M; Marathon Family Health Team, PO Box 399 22 Peninsula Rd, Marathon ON P0T 2E0; Wes'08; CCFP; (807)626-1234; Fax. (807)229-2672.

PURCELL, Jacqueline L; Broadway Med Centre, 230-943 Broadway W, Vancouver BC V5Z 4E1; UBC'90; BSc; MD; FSOGC; FRCSC; ObstGyn. Ac Staff, UBC Hospital - Koerner Pavillion; Ac Staff, BC Children's Hospital; Ac Staff, Vancouver General Hospital - Centennial Pavillion; (604)734-2712; Fax. (604)734-8572.

PURCELL, Laura K; David Braley Sport Med & Rehab, 1280 Main St W, Hamilton ON L8S 4K1; McM'95; Dip SportMed; FRCPC; Peds (Pediatric Sport Medicine). Physician Pediatric Sport Med, Elliott Sports Medicine Clinic; Clin Assoc Prof Peds, McMaster University; (905)525-9140; Fax. (905)526-7397.

PURCHASE, Janet E; C M L Healthcare, 102-150 Katimavik Rd, Kanata ON K2L 2N2; Ott'78; BSc; FRCPC; DiagRad. (613)592-0711; Fax. (613)592-1412; jep203@sympatico.ca.

PURDELL-LEWIS, J Geoffrey; Burlington Pain Centre, 24-1960 Appleby Line, Burlington ON L7L 0B7; London (England)'63; MB BS; MRCS; FAB; DA; FRCPC; Anes (Chronic Pain). Clin Assoc Prof Anes, McMaster University; (905)315-8802; Fax. (905)315-8433; purdell-lewis@sympatico.ca.

PURDON, Cameron J A; 108-21 Surrey St W, Guelph ON N1H 3R3; Wes'83; ABIM; FRCPC; IntMed; Endocrin&Metab. Staff, Guelph General Hospital; (519)763-6201

PURDON, Carey D; 55 John St PO Box 190, Cobden ON K0J 1K0; Tor'83; (613)646-2436

PURDON, Derek H; St Anthony's Med Centre, 303-582 Goldstream Ave, Victoria BC V9B 2W7; McG'64; (250)478-1744; Fax. (250)478-2751.

PURDON, Michael A J; Southern Interior Hlth Communi, 220-1815 Kirschner St, Kelowna BC V1Y 4N7; McG'92; BSc; DAB; (250)862-4294

PURDY, Anna C; Rockyview Gen Hosp, 7007 14 St SW, Calgary AB T2V 1P9; Qns'97; FRCPC; IntMed. Staff, Rockyview General Hospital; (403)943-3000

PURDY, Ceilidh L; Bruyere Family Med Centre, 75 Bruyere St, Ottawa ON K1N 5C8; McM'09; CCFP; (613)241-3344

PURDY, F Robert; BC Women's Hosp & Health Ctre, 1L7-4500 Oak St, Vancouver BC V6H 3N1; UBC'90; FRCPC; Anes. Staff, BC Women's Hospital & Health Centre; (604)875-3512

PURDY, Jennifer L; 2 Field Ambulance PO Box 9999 Stn Main, Petawawa ON K8H 2X3; Ott'08; CCFP; (613)687-5511; Fax. (613)588-4899.

PURDY, Kerri S; 401-6155 North St, Halifax NS B3K 5R2; Dal'05; FRCPC; IntMed; Derm. (902)455-7273; Fax. (902)453-1354.

PURDY, R Allan; Queen Elizabeth II HSC-Halifax, 3819-1796 Summer St, Halifax NS B3H 3A7; Dal'74; FRCPC; Neur. Staff, Queen Elizabeth II Health Sciences Centre - Halifax Infirmary Site; Prof Med, Dalhousie University; (902)473-2132; Fax. (902)473-4438; a.purdy@dal.ca.

PUREWAL, Bhupinder S; Village Square Med Centre, 103-2942 Finch Ave E, Scarborough ON M1W 2T4; Bihar (India)'79; Staff, The Scarborough Hospital - Birchmount Campus; Langs: Punjabi; Hindi; Urdu; (416)498-0070; Fax. (416)498-0075.

PURGINA, Bibianna M; The Ottawa Hosp-Gen Campus, 501 Smyth Rd, Ottawa ON K1H 8L6; Ott'05; FRCPC; AnatPath. Staff, The Ottawa Hospital - General Campus; (613)737-8899

PURI, Gaurav; St Joseph's Health Centre, 30 The Queensway, Toronto ON M6R 1B5; Wes'09; CCFP; CCFP(E.M.); Staff, St Joseph's Health Centre; (416)530-6000

PURI, Vinod; Brampton Gastroenterology, 11-470 Chrysler Dr, Brampton ON L6S 0C1; Qns'92; FRCPC; IntMed; Gastroent. (905)790-6362; Fax. (905)790-6612; vpuri@interlog.com.

PURI-ALANOLY, Lizy; Centre Med Dorion Vaudreuil, 600 boul Harwood, Vaudreuil-Dorion QC J7V 6A3; Louvain (Belgium)'71; DrMedCh; Langs: English; Malayalam; (450)455-9301; Fax. (450)455-8964; lizyalanoly@allstream.net.

PURKEY, Eva N; North Kingston Community HC, 400 Elliott Ave, Kingston ON K7K 6M9; Mon'02; CCFP; (613)542-2949; Fax. (613)542-3872.

PURKIS, Jeffrey W; White Rock Medical, 101-15451 Russell Ave, White Rock BC V4B 2R5; UBC'82; Staff, Peace Arch Hospital; Med Consultant, Back in Motion Rehabilitation Inc; Langs: Bilingual(English/French); (604)531-5595; Fax. (604)531-9818.

PURKISS, Susan E; BC Women's Hosp & Health Ctre, 4500 Oak St, Vancouver BC V6H 3N1; McM'88; FRCPC; IntMed (Obstetric Medicine). Staff, BC Women's Hospital & Health Centre; Staff, BC Children's Hospital; Clin Instructor, University of British Columbia; (604)875-3060

PURNELL, Roger A; 1624 7th Ave, Prince George BC V2L 3P6; Manchester (England)'86; MB ChB; FRCSC; OrthSurg. (250)564-8800

PUROHIT, Jigna R; 301-310 King St E, Kitchener ON N2G 2L3; (Zimbabwe)'89; CCFP; (519)745-5621; Fax. (519)745-5622.

PUROHIT, Nimishchandra N; Integrated Psychiatric Service, 306-672 Brant St, Burlington ON L7R 2H4; Baroda (India)'79; MRCPsy(UK); FRANZCP; FRCPC; Psy (General Adult Psychiatry). Staff Psy & Supervising Psy, Joseph Brant Memorial Hospital; Teach Staff Psy, University of Toronto; Langs: Gujarati; Urdu; Hindi; (905)637-2586 x11

PURSSELL, J Eileen; Monashee Med Clinic, PO Box 700 2067 Columbia Ave, Rossland BC V0G 1Y0; UBC'88; Staff, Kootenay Boundary Regional Hospital; (250)362-9040; Fax. (250)362-9032.

PURSSELL, Roy; BC Drug & Poison Info Centre, 655 12th Ave W, Vancouver BC V5Z 4R4; UBC'79; FRCPC; EmergMed. Ac Staff Emerg, Vancouver General Hospital - Centennial Pavillion; Staff, BC Centre For Disease Control; (604)707-2789

PURTZKI, Jacqueline S; Sunny Hill Hlth Ctr for Child, 3644 Slocan St, Vancouver BC V5M 3E8; UBC'91; FRCPC; PhysMed&Rehab (Brain Injury). Staff, Sunny Hill Health Centre for Children; Staff, G F Strong Rehabilitation Centre; Langs: German; (604)453-8300; Fax. (604)453-8338; jacqueline.purtzki@vch.ca.

PURVES, Sherrill J; Northmount Med Centre, 204-145 13th St E, North Vancouver BC V7L 2L4; UBC'71; BSc; FRCPC; Neur. Staff, Burnaby Hospital; Staff, Lions Gate Hospital; (604)924-4009; Fax. (604)924-4006; docpur@telus.net.

PURVIS, Alison; 1420 29th St E, North Vancouver BC V7J 1T1; UBC'89; BSc; MD; Staff, Lions Gate Hospital; Physician, Lynn Valley Medical & Travel Clinic; (604)984-2646; alison.cbo@shaw.ca.

PURVIS, Jane; 707 Charlotte St, Peterborough ON K9J 7B3; Ott'84; FRCPC; IntMed; Rheum. Staff, Peterborough Regional Health Centre - Hospital Drive; Staff, Campbellford Memorial Hospital; (705)876-4511; Fax. (705)743-3959; jpurvis@themedicalcentre.net.

PURYCH, Dale B; Royal Columbian Hosp, 330 Columbia St E, New Westminster BC V3L 3W7; Alb'92; FRCPC; MedMicrobiol;CCFP; FCFP; Staff, Royal Columbian Hospital; (604)520-4342

PURZNER, Andrew A; Elliot Lake Family Health Team, 31 Nova Scotia Walk, Elliot Lake ON P5A 1Y5; '07; CCFP; (705)461-8882

PUS, Jacqueline G; Kerrisdale Med Clinic, 2077 42nd Ave W, Vancouver BC V6M 2B4; Qns'10; CCFP; (604)261-9494; Fax. (604)261-9405.

PUSCA, Adrian; CSSS du Granit, 3569 rue Laval, Lac-Megantic QC G6B 1A5; Craiova (Romania)'87; IntMed (P.Q.) (Cardiology). Staff, Carrefour Sante Granit; Langs: Romanian; English; (819)583-0330 x271

PUSCA, Carina G; CSSS du Granit, 3569 rue Laval, Lac-Megantic QC G6B 1A5; Bucharest (Romania)'87; Staff, Carrefour Sante Granit; Staff, Centre Hospitalier Universitaire de Sherbrooke-Hopital Fleurimont; Langs: Romanian; (819)583-0330

PUSCAS, Radu; 3655 boul de Sainte-Adele, Sainte-Adele QC J8B 2N8; Mon'86; (450)229-7676; Fax. (450)229-8310.

PUSHIE, Harold D H; Queen-Spadina Med Centre, 455 Queen St W, Toronto ON M5V 2A9; Tor'75; BSc; MSc; (416)869-3627; Fax. (416)703-3962.

PUSHIE, Heather J; MUHC-Royal Victoria Hosp, 687 av des Pins O, Montreal QC H3A 1A1; McG'72; CCFP; FCFP; Att Staff, McGill University Health Centre - Royal Victoria Hospital; (514)934-1934

PUSHIE, Mary K; 4041 200B St, Langley BC V3A 1P1; Dal'81; Staff, Langley Memorial Hospital; (604)530-1181; Fax. (604)530-5609.

PUSHPANATHAN, Anita; Eleven Elizabeth Fam Practice, 201-11 Elizabeth Ave, St. John's NL A1A 1W6; Mem'09; CCFP.

PUSHPANATHAN, Chitra; Dr Charles A Janeway Child HC, 300 Prince Philip Dr, St. John's NL A1B 3V6; Madras (India)'74; MB BS; FRCPC; AnatPath. Staff, Janeway Children's Health & Rehabilitation Centre; Clin Assoc Prof, Memorial University Of Newfoundland; (709)778-4357; Fax. (709)778-4948.

PUSHPAPALAN, Jegathesan; Rouge Valley-Ajax & Pickering, 580 Harwood Ave S, Ajax ON L1S 2J4; Jaffna (Sri Lanka)'87; MB BS; ABIM; FRCPC; IntMed. Staff, Rouge Valley Health System - Ajax & Pickering Health Centre Site; Langs: Tamil; (905)683-2320

PUSKAS, David A; Big Thunder Orthopedic Assoc, 206-984 Oliver Rd, Thunder Bay ON P7B 7C7; Tor'91; FRCSC; OrthSurg (Arthroplasty). Staff, Thunder Bay Regional Health Sciences Centre; Prog Dir Orthopedic Surg, Northern Ontario School of Medicine-Laurentian University; (807)344-1123; Fax. (807)344-1166.

PUSZTAI, Edit Esther; 202-300 Columbia St, Kamloops BC V2C 6L1; Glasgow (Scotland)'88; MB ChB; MRCPsy; FRCPC; Psy (Developmental Disability). Staff Psy, Developmental Disabilities Mental Health Services; (250)372-9160; Fax. (250)372-9360.

PUTHENPARUMPIL, Jacob J; 1019 Prince St, Truro NS B2N 1H7; Gujarat (India)'92; FRCSC; Urol. Staff, Colchester East Hants Health Centre; (902)897-2541; Fax. (902)897-9105.

PUTLAND, Michael S; 310-777 Royal Oak Dr PO Box 53534 Rpo Broadmead, Victoria BC V8X 5K2; UBC'94; BSc; MSc; CCFP; (778)679-0440

PUTNAM, Debra C; Salveo Family Med Clinic, B8-6455 MacLeod Trail SW, Calgary AB T2H 0K8; Cal'89; CCFP; Staff, Foothills Medical Centre; (403)444-0428; Fax. (403)537-0029.

PUTNINS, Charles L; St Boniface Gen Hosp, 409 Tache Ave, Winnipeg MB R2H 2A6; Man'76; FRCPC; Anes. Staff, St Boniface General Hospital; (204)233-8563

PUTNINS, Rita E; Children's Hosp Eastern Ont, 401 Smyth Rd, Ottawa ON K1H 8L1; Man'79; FRCPC; DiagRad. Staff, Children's Hospital of Eastern Ontario (CHEO); (613)737-7600; Fax. (613)738-4811.

PUTS, Marc; West Coast Gen Hosp, 104-3949 Maple Way, Port Alberni BC V9Y 4S1; Louvain (Belgium)'83; Staff, West Coast General Hospital; Langs: Dutch; French; (250)724-8800

PUTTAGUNTA, Lakshmi; University of Alberta Hosp, 5B327-8440 112 St NW, Edmonton AB T6G 2B7; Alb'87; AnatPath. Assoc Prof, University of Alberta Hospital; (780)407-8922; Fax. (780)407-3009.

PUTTAPPA, Sandesh K; Hamilton HS-McMaster Site, PO Box 2000 Stn Lcd 1 4.F 1D-1200 Main St W, Hamilton ON L8N 3Z5; Mysore (India)'98; Staff, Hamilton Health Sciences Centre - McMaster Children's Hospital; (905)521-2100 x73489; Fax. (905)527-9808.

PUTTASWAMY, Shekar; Bonnyville Health Centre, PO Box 1008 Stn Main 5001 Lakeshore Dr, Bonnyville AB T9N 2J7; (India)'95; MB BS; FRCPC; GenPath. Staff, Bonnyville Healthcare Centre; (780)826-3311

PUTTER, J Dirk; Bluewater Health-Norman Site, 89 Norman St, Sarnia ON N7T 6S3; Orange Free State (South Africa)'96; MB ChB; CCFP; CCFP(E.M.); Staff, Bluewater Health - Norman Site; (519)464-4400

PUVENDRAN, Samuel N; Niagara H System-G Niagara, PO Box 1018 Stn Main 5546 Portage Rd, Niagara Falls ON L2E 6X2; Saba (Netherlands Antilles)'02; FRCPC; IntMed; GeriatricMed. Staff, Niagara Health System - Greater Niagara General Site; (905)378-4647

PUXTY, Gillian M; Ann Street Medical, PO Box 129 Stn Main 5528 Ann St, Manotick ON K4M 1A2; Leeds (England)'78; MB ChB; LMCC; (613)692-1764; Fax. (613)692-1766.

PUXTY, John A H; Providence CCC-St Mary's, PO Box 3600 Stn Main 340 Union St, Kingston ON K7L 5A2; Leeds (England)'76; MB ChB; FRCPC; IntMed; GeriatricMed. Head Geriatrics/Dir Reg Geriatric Prog, Providence Care - St Mary's of the Lake Hospital Site; Assoc Prof Med/Chief Geriatrics, Queen's University; (613)544-5220; Fax. (613)544-4017; puxtyj@post.queensu.ca.

PUYMIRAT, Jack; CHUQ-Ctr Hosp Univ Laval, 9300-2705 boul Laurier, Quebec QC G1V 4G2; Paris (France)'83; Staff, Centre Hospitalier Universitaire de Quebec-CHUL; Staff, Institut Readaptation Deficience Physique de Quebec; Prof Med, Université Laval; (418)654-2186; Fax. (418)654-2207; jack.puymirat@crchul.ulaval.ca.

PUZNAK, Kimbal N; Tawa Centre, 3017 66 St NW, Edmonton AB T6K 4B2; Sask'79; FRCPC; DiagRad. Staff, Covenant Health - Edmonton General Continuing Care Centre; (780)426-1121

PYE, Paula; Family Med Clinic, 111-246 Memorial Dr, Clarenville NL A5A 1N9; Mem'92; BSc; (709)466-5400; blaine.pearce@nf.sympatico.ca.

PYLE, Helen A; Oakville Health Centre, 117-1060 Speers Rd, Oakville ON L6L 2X4; Tor'73; Court Staff, Halton Healthcare Services Corporation - Oakville Site; (905)845-8884; Fax. (905)844-5537.

PYLYPCHUK, George B; Saskatoon Nephrology Group, 434-230 Avenue R S, Saskatoon SK S7M 2Z1; Sask'70; FRCPC; IntMed (Nephrology). Ac Staff, Royal University Hospital; Head Div of Nephrol, Saskatoon District Health Board; Clin Prof, University of Saskatchewan; Langs: Ukrainian; (306)934-3300; Fax. (306)934-3355.

PYLYPIAK, Daria C; William Osler HC-Etobicoke, 101 Humber College Blvd, Etobicoke ON M9V 1R8; Tor'10; CCFP; Staff, William Osler Health System - Etobicoke General Hospital; (416)747-3400

PYMAR, Helen C; Women's Hosp, WR125-735 Notre Dame Ave, Winnipeg MB R3E 0L8; Qns'94; MPH; FRCSC; ObstGyn (Contraception). Asst Prof, University of Manitoba; (204)787-4821; Fax. (204)787-2920.

PYPER, Anne M; Bayview Med Centre, 2722 Bayview Ave, North York ON M2L 1B9; Wes'80; Ac Staff, North York General Hospital; (416)730-1212; Fax. (416)730-1216.

PYPER, Elizabeth A H; St Joseph's Health Centre, 30 The Queensway, Toronto ON M6R 1B5; Glasgow (Scotland)'71; FRCPC; Anes. Ac Staff, St Joseph's Health Centre; (416)530-6090

PYPER, J Alexander; Fairview Med Arts Centre, 109-2200 Fairview St, Burlington ON L7R 4H9; Tor'82; BSc; FRCSC; OrthSurg. Head OrthSurg Dept, Joseph Brant Memorial Hospital; Staff, Halton Healthcare Services Corporation - Oakville Site; (905)681-6788; Fax. (905)333-9775.

PYPER, Sheelagh M; 576 Main St E, Hamilton ON L8M 1J2; McM'86; BSc; MHSc; CCFP; FCFP; Ac Staff, St Joseph's Healthcare - Charlton Campus; Assoc Staff, Hamilton Health Sciences Centre - McMaster Children's Hospital; (905)528-5292; Fax. (905)528-7753.

PYSELMAN, Colette R; Markham Stoffville Health Ctr, 305-377 Church St, Markham ON L6B 1A1; Tor'82; BSc; FRCSC; ObstGyn (Infertility). Ac Staff, Markham Stouffville Hospital; Physician, York Fertility Centre; (905)472-7130; Fax. (905)472-4130.

PYSKLYWEC, Michael W; Occupational Health Clinics, 848 Main St E, Hamilton ON L8M 1L9; Qns'97; BSc; CCFP; CCFP(E.M.); (905)549-2552

PYSYK, Christopher L; Foothills Med Centre, 1403 29 St NW, Calgary AB T2N 2T9; Alb'06; FRCPC; Anes. Staff, Foothills Medical Centre; (403)944-4309

PYTKA, Pauline S; Medical Arts Bldg, 706-1 Young St, Hamilton ON L8N 1T8; McM'80; FRCPC; Psy (Psychotherapy). (905)523-4146

PYTKA, Saul; Rockyview Gen Hosp, 7007 14 St SW, Calgary AB T2V 1P9; Tor'77; FRCPC; Anes (Acute Pain Management). Staff, Rockyview General Hospital; (403)943-8720; Fax. (403)252-2798.

PYTYCK, Jennifer M; Addiction & Mental Hlth-Queen, 1001 Main St W, Toronto ON M6J 1H4; Cal'07; Psy. Fellow, Centre for Addiction & Mental Health (CAMH) - Queen Site; (416)575-8501

QAADRI, M Shafiq; 103-15 Roncesvalles Ave, Toronto ON M6R 2K2; Tor'88; Langs: Hindi; French; Urdu; (416)536-9303; Fax. (416)537-4101.

QAADRI, Mussarrat K; 103-15 Roncesvalles Ave, Toronto ON M6R 2K2; Punjab (Pakistan)'58; MS; FACOG; FSOGC; FRCSC; ObstGyn. Staff, Women's College Hospital; Langs: Urdu; Punjabi; Hindi; (416)925-6726

QADEER, Shehla; Whitby Medical Arts Centre, 203-1615 Dundas St E, Whitby ON L1N 2L1; Karachi (Pakistan)'02; CCFP; Langs: Urdu; Hindi; (905)404-9666; Fax. (905)404-9135.

QADRY, Syed M S; CFB Edmonton, PO Box 10500 Stn Forces, Edmonton AB T5J 4J5; Cal'04; CCFP; CCFP(E.M.); (780)973-4011

QAISY, Yehia S; Main Street Med Centre, 9-10886 Hurontario St, Brampton ON L7A 3R9; (Iraq)'98; CCFP; (905)846-9911

QAMIRANI, Erion; University of Toronto, 2F-500 University Ave, Toronto ON M5G 1V7; Texas (USA)'07; OrthSurg.

QANUNGO, Muhammed T; Abbey Family Medicine, 2307 Khalsa Gate, Oakville ON L6M 4J2; Rajasthan (India)'84; CCFP; (905)847-1133; Fax. (905)847-9782; tariqqan@hotmail.com.

QARNI, Uwais; Clinical Sciences Bldg, 11 107F-152 University Campus, Edmonton AB T6G 2G3; Sind (Pakistan)'89; MB BS; FRCPC; IntMed; Nephrol. Staff, University of Alberta Hospital; University of Alberta; (780)407-6153; Fax. (780)407-7771.

QAWI, Huma; Grey Bruce HS-Owen Sound, PO Box 1800 Stn Main 1800 8th St E, Owen Sound ON N4K 6M9; Karachi (Pakistan)'95; MB BS; Staff, Grey Bruce Health Services - Owen Sound; (519)372-3922; Fax. (519)372-3940.

QAYUMI, Abdul K; Dept of Surgery, 3100-910 10th Ave W, Vancouver BC V5Z 1M9; Kiev (Ukraine)'76; (604)875-4499; Fax. (604)875-5832.

QAYYUM, Saba; Knox Manse, 505 4th Ave N, Saskatoon SK S7K 2M5; Sask'94; BSc; FRCPC; Psy (Anxiety & Mood Disorders). Consultant Psychiatrist Student Health Centre/Clinical Asst Prof College of Med, University of Saskatchewan; (306)668-0508; Fax. (306)668-0507.

QAZI, Khalida; Holly Med Clinic, 103-611 Holly Ave, Milton ON L9T 0K4; Peshawar (Pakistan)'83; MB BS; CCFP; Langs: Urdu; Punjabi; Hindi; Pashtu; (905)878-0086; Fax. (905)878-1562.

QI, Victoria Z; Regent Park Community Hlth Ctr, 465 Dundas St E, Toronto ON M5A 2B2; Tor'03; CCFP; (416)203-4507; Fax. (416)364-0822.

QIAN LEE, Ivy H; Markham Stouffville Hosp, PO Box 1800 Stn Main 381 Church St, Markham ON L3P 7P3; Dal'03; FRCPC; Psy. Staff, Markham Stouffville Hospital; (905)472-7000; Fax. (905)472-7371.

QING, Gefei; Health Sciences Centre, MS459-820 Sherbrook St, Winnipeg MB R3A 1R9; (China)'82; FRCPC; AnatPath. Pathologist, Health Sciences Centre; (204)787-4858; Fax. (204)787-4942; gqing@hsc.mb.ca.

QIU, Hongming; Health Sciences Centre, MS459-820 Sherbrook St, Winnipeg MB R3A 1R9; Anhui (China)'82; FRCPC; AnatPath. Staff, Health Sciences Centre; (204)774-6511

QIZILBASH, Ali H; Humber River Reg Hosp-Finch, 2111 Finch Ave W, North York ON M3N 1N1; Punjab (Pakistan)'60; MB BS; DTMH(Lond); FRCPC; GenPath (Laboratory Medicine). Staff, Humber River Regional Hospital - Finch Avenue Site; Consultant, Gamma-Dynacare Laboratories; Emeritus Prof, University of Toronto; (416)744-2500 x4139; Fax. (416)243-4296; drahq@hotmail.com.

QIZILBASH, Baqir A; Institut de Cardiologie de Mtl, 5000 rue Belanger, Montreal QC H1T 1C8; McG'95; CSPQ; FRCPC; Anes. Staff, Institut de Cardiologie de Montréal; Universite de Montreal; Langs: English; French; (514)376-3330 x3732

QUACH, Dieu Hoa; Family Practice 535, 535 Montreal Rd, Ottawa ON K1K 0V1; Tor'97; CCFP; FCFP; (613)746-5350; Fax. (613)746-5340.

QUACH, Huu-Nghi; Ctr de Sante Basse Cote Nord, CP 130 1070 boul Dr Camille-Marcoux, Lourdes-d-Bl-Sabl QC G0G 1W0; Sher'03; Fam Med, CSSS de la Basse Côté-Nord; (418)461-2144

QUACH, Sophie M; Hôpital Anna-Laberge, 200 boul Brisebois, Chateauguay QC J6K 4W8; Mon'10; Staff, Hôpital Anna-Laberge; (450)699-2425

QUACH, Thomas; Royal Victoria Hosp, 201 Georgian Dr, Barrie ON L4M 6M2; Tor'07; FRCPC; Anes. Staff, Royal Victoria Regional Health Centre; (705)728-9090

QUACH-THANH, Caroline; MUHC-Montreal Children's Hosp, C 1242-2300 rue Tupper, Montreal QC H3H 1P3; Mon'95; FRCPC; Peds (AIDS); Microbio & Infect Dis (P.Q.); MedMicrobiol; InfectDis. Staff, McGill University Health Centre - Montreal Children's Hospital; Langs: English; (514)412-4485; Fax. (514)412-4494; caroline.quach@mcgill.ca.

QUACKENBUSH, Benjamin R H; Little Current Med Associates, PO Box 549 15 Meredith St E, Little Current ON P0P 1K0; NOSM'09; CCFP.

QUACKENBUSH, Suzie J; 95 Spring St SS 1, Almonte ON K0A 1A0; Ott'95; CCFP; (613)256-9370

QUADIR, Ambereen; Lakeshore Woods Med Clinic, 7-3420 Rebecca St, Oakville ON L6L 6W2; Tor'95; CCFP; (905)847-2525

QUADIR, Shamima S; Bowmanville Prof Bldg, 222 King St E, Bowmanville ON L1C 1P6; CCFP; (905)697-8282

QUADRI, Syed M A; Royal Court Med Centre, 204-1 Quarry Ridge Rd, Barrie ON L4M 7G1; Osmania (India)'62; MB BS; FRCSC; Otol (Head & Neck Surgery). Staff, Royal Victoria Regional Health Centre; Staff, Orillia Soldiers' Memorial Hospital; (705)726-3071; Fax. (705)719-4622.

QUAGGIN, Susan E; St Michael's Hosp, 30 Bond St, Toronto ON M5B 1W8; Tor'88; Nephrol; IntMed. Staff, St Michael's Hospital; (416)864-5431

QUAIL, Patrick B; 67 Wing Bldg, 102-2210 2 St SW, Calgary AB T2S 3C3; Dublin (Ireland)'82; MB ChB; DCH; CCFP; FCFP; Med Dir Home Care Case, Calgary Health Region; Clinical Asst Prof Family Med, University of Calgary; (403)244-6500; Fax. (403)244-2622; quail@ucalgary.ca.

QUAN, Alyson D; Mission Mem Hosp, 7324 Hurd St, Mission BC V2V 3H5; UBC'95; Staff, Mission Memorial Hospital; (604)826-6261

QUAN, Corinna M; Tecumseh Byng Clinic, 2085 Tecumseh Rd E, Windsor ON N8W 1E3; Tor'85; BSc; MSc; FRCPC; IntMed (HIV); InfectDis. Staff, Windsor Regional Hospital - Metropolitan Site; Staff, Hôtel-Dieu Grace Hospital; Aj Prof Med, University of Western Ontario; (519)254-5577 x52539; Fax. (519)254-6861.

QUAN, Douglas; London HSC-University Hosp, PO Box 5339 Stn B 339 Windermere Rd, London ON N6A 5A5; Sask'89; FACS; FRCSC; GenSurg (Hepatobiliary Surgery). Staff, London Health Sciences Centre - University Hospital; Asst Prof Surg, University of Western Ontario; (519)663-3355; Fax. (519)663-3906; douglas.quan@lhsc.on.ca.

QUAN, Eric; Hop Charles LeMoyne, 3120 boul Taschereau, Greenfield Park QC J4V 2H1; Laval'99; FRCPC; IntMed; Cardiol. Staff, Hopital Charles LeMoyne; (450)466-5000

QUAN, F Wayne; Smyth Med Centre, 212-1929 Russell Rd, Ottawa ON K1G 4G3; Tor'72; DPsy; FRCPC; Psy. Consultant, Royal Ottawa Mental Health Centre - Royal Ottawa Health Care Group; Ac Staff, The Ottawa Hospital - General Campus; (613)521-3376

QUAN, James L; 217-3195 Granville St, Vancouver BC V6H 3K2; Alb'65; BSc(Zoology); FRCPC; Psy (Psychotherapy). Consultant Psy, Maples Adolescent Treatment Centre; Consultant Adolescent Psy & Psy Outreach, University of British Columbia; (604)730-0030; Fax. (604)730-0035; drjquan2@gmail.com.

QUAN, Jason K; Radiology Consultants Assoc, 120A-6707 Elbow Dr SW, Calgary AB T2V 0E5; Alb'95; FRCPC; DiagRad. (403)777-3003; Fax. (403)777-3008.

QUAN, Lan Phuong; 498 Kingsway, Vancouver BC V5T 3J9; Hochiminh (Vietnam)'82; CCFP; Staff, Providence Health Care - Mount Saint Joseph Hospital; (604)876-9907; Fax. (604)876-9927.

QUAN, May Lynn; Foothills Med Centre, 1403 29 St NW, Calgary AB T2N 2T9; McM'97; MSc; FRCSC; GenSurg (Surgical Oncology). Staff, Foothills Medical Centre; (403)944-0966; Fax. (403)944-1277.

QUAN, Minh Duc; Newin Centre, 31-2580 Shepard Ave, Mississauga ON L5A 4K3; Saigon (Vietnam)'80; CCFP; Staff, Trillium Health Centre - Mississauga; Langs: Vietnamese; (905)615-0468; Fax. (905)615-8495.

QUAN, T Diem-Mai; Medi-Centre Chomedey, 610 boul Cure-Labelle, Laval QC H7V 2T7; Mon'94; CCFP; Staff, Hopital de la Cite de la santé; (450)687-6452; Fax. (450)687-3242.

QUAN, Vu Hung; CHUM-Hotel-Dieu, 3840 rue Saint-Urbain, Montreal QC H2W 1T8; Sher'95; FRCPC; IntMed; Cardiol. Staff, Centre Hospitalier l'Université de Montréal (CHUM) - Hôtel-Dieu; (514)890-8000

QUANCE, Daniel R; SMBD Jewish Gen Hosp, 3755 ch Cote-Sainte-Catherine, Montreal QC H3T 1E2; Qns'82; FRCPC; Anes (Obstetrics Anesthesia). Ac Staff Anes, Sir Mortimer B Davis Jewish General; Langs: English; French; (514)340-8222 x5701

QUANSAH, Joseph S T; 303-540 College St, Toronto ON M6G 1A6; Liverpool (England)'70; MB ChB; DTMH; MRCP(UK); FRCPC; IntMed. Consultant Med, Sunnybrook Health Sciences Centre - Holland Orthopaedic & Arthritic Centre; (416)921-0059; Fax. (416)921-8420; jquansah@on.aibn.com.

QUANSAH, Samuel B; 260-6655 ch de la Cote-des-Nei, Montreal QC H3S 2B4; Leningrad (Russia (Federation))'68; DABPed; FRCPC; Peds (Neonatology). Staff, Sir Mortimer B Davis Jewish General; Staff, St Mary's Hospital Centre; Staff Teacher, McGill University Health Centre - Montreal Children's Hospital; McGill University; (514)341-6132; Fax. (514)341-0188.

QUANTZ, Mackenzie A; London HSC-University Hosp, PO Box 5339 Stn B 339 Windermere Rd, London ON N6A 5A5; McG'90; FRCSC; CardiothorSurg. Consultant Cardiothoracic Surg, London Health Sciences Centre - University Hospital; (519)663-3144; Fax. (519)663-3186.

QUANTZ, Marie C; Lakeridge Hlth Corp-Oshawa, 1 Hospital Crt, Oshawa ON L1G 2B9; Tor'65; FRCPC; GenPath (Clinical Pathology). Staff, Lakeridge Health - Oshawa Site; (905)576-8711 x3407

QUAO, Nii T; Westside Med Clinic, 240-4260 av Girouard, Montreal QC H4A 3C9; McG'68; BSc; MDCM; Physician, Concordia University Health Services; (514)489-5753; Fax. (514)489-1616; westsideclinic@primus.ca.

QUART, Reginald D J; Garden City Family Health Team, 22 Ontario St, St Catharines ON L2R 7M3; McG'81; CCFP; (905)984-3335

QUARTERMAIN, Melanie A; 16-385 Frederick St, Kitchener ON N2H 2P2; Tor'96; BSc; CCFP; (519)745-7482; Fax. (519)745-1881.

QUARTERO, Marsha A; South Calgary Med Clinic, 118-40 Sunpark Plaza SE, Calgary AB T2X 3X7; Alb'07; CCFP; (403)254-4000; Fax. (403)254-1282.

QUARTEY, Gilbert R C; 504-100 Arden St, Moncton NB E1C 4B7; Glasgow (Scotland)'71; MB ChB; FICS; FACS; FRCS; DABNS; LMCC; DABPainMed; FRCSC; Neursurg (Pain Management). Ac Staff, The Moncton Hospital; Consultant, Dr Georges-L-Dumont University Hospital Centre; Lecturer Surg, Dalhousie University; (506)857-5376; Fax. (506)857-5378; gilbert.quartey@horizonnb.ca.

QUARTLY, Caroline A; 180-1581H Hillside Ave, Victoria BC V8T 2C1; McM'81; BSc; FRCPC; PhysMed&Rehab. (250)391-8486

QUASTEL, Adam G; St Michael's Hosp, 30 Bond St, Toronto ON M5B 1W8; McG'94; FRCPC; Psy. Staff, St Michael's Hospital; (416)864-3090; Fax. (416)864-5480.

QUATEEN, Ahmed S; Royal Alexandra Hosp, 10240 Kingsway NW, Edmonton AB T5H 3V9; (Libya)'93; FRCPC; Neursurg. Staff, Royal Alexandra Hospital; (780)735-4111

QUAYE, Henry I; 3-4402 37 St, Stony Plain AB T7Z 2A9; Skopje (Macedonia)'81; BSc; MSc; Ac Staff Member, Westview Health Centre; Langs: Akan; Macedonian; Serbo-Croatian; (780)963-7800; Fax. (780)963-0468.

QUAYLE, Alandra N; 101-9006 Edward St, Chilliwack BC V2P 4E1; Cal'02; CCFP; (604)701-6866

QUAYYUM, Zahirul; Concession Wentworth Medical, 503 Concession St, Hamilton ON L9A 1C1; Dhaka (Bangladesh)'84; MB BS; CCFP; Langs: Bengali; Persian; (905)389-1295; Fax. (905)389-6568; arpa_q@yahoo.com.

QUEEN, Daniel S; Toronto East Gen Hosp Inc, 825 Coxwell Ave, Toronto ON M4C 3E7; Wes'06; CCFP; Staff, Toronto East General Hospital Inc; (416)469-6435

QUEEN, Martin; Sudbury Reg Hosp-Laurentian, 41 Ramsey Lake Rd, Sudbury ON P3E 5J1; Tor'81; BSc; ABForensic Pathology; FRCPC; AnatPath (Forensic Pathology). Dir Forensic Pathologist Northeastern Forensic Pathology Unit, Health Sciences North-Laurentian Site; Staff, Health Sciences North-St Joseph's Health Centre; (705)675-4779

QUEENTON, Marie-Josee; Clinique Med Galt, 2235 rue Galt O, Sherbrooke QC J1K 1K6; Sher'88; Physician, CSSS Windsor; (819)821-0088; Fax. (819)821-3901.

QUEH, Peter; 208-125 13th St E, North Vancouver BC V7L 2L3; Rangoon (Burma)'72; MB BS; FRCSC; GenSurg. Staff Surg, Lions Gate Hospital; (604)987-6940; Fax. (604)987-4239.

QUEJADA, Michael J; Univ Hlth Network-Toronto Western Hosp, 399 Bathurst St, Toronto ON M5T 2S8; Tor'10; CCFP; Staff, Toronto Western Hospital - University Health Network; (416)603-5800

QUEK, Kar Chi; West Edmonton Mall Clinic, 2-17303 Stony Plain Rd NW, Edmonton AB T5S 1B5; Alb'86; (780)484-0800; Fax. (780)484-0907.

QUELCH, Peter C; Steveston Med Group, 204-3811 Chatham St, Richmond BC V7E 2Z4; McG'70; Vis Staff, Richmond Hospital; (604)277-7166; Fax. (604)277-3811.

QUENNEVILLE, Louise A M; Saskatoon City Hosp, 701 Queen St, Saskatoon SK S7K 0M7; Sask'95; CSPQ; FRCPC; AnatPath. Staff, Saskatoon City Hospital; (306)655-7555

QUENNEVILLE, Michel L; 400-1 Main St E, Hawkesbury ON K6A 1A1; Laval'98; BScChemEng; (613)632-9967; Fax. (613)632-2417.

QUENNEVILLE, Nancy; Polyclinique St-Eustache, 75 rue Grignon, Saint-Eustache QC J7P 4J2; Mon'99; Staff Peds, Hôpital de Saint-Eustache; Staff, Hopital de la Cite de la santé; (450)473-2449

QUENNEVILLE, Robert; Ctr Hosp Laurentien, 234 rue Saint-Vincent, Ste-Agathe-Des-Mts QC J8C 2B8; Mon'87; FRCPC; Psy. Staff, Centre Hospitalier Laurentien; (819)324-4044; Fax. (819)324-4010.

QUENNEVILLE, Stephane P; Hop Jean-Talon, 1385 rue Jean-Talon E, Montreal QC H2E 1S6; McG'04; FRCPC; IntMed; Cardiol. Staff, McGill University Health Centre - Royal Victoria Hospital; Staff, CSSS du Coeur de l'Isle Hôpital Jean-Talon; (514)495-6767

QUENNEVILLE, Yves; CHUM-Hop Notre-Dame, 1560 rue Sherbrooke E, Montreal QC H2L 4M1; Laval'70; FRCPC; Psy. Staff, Centre Hospitalier l'Université de Montréal (CHUM) - Hôpital Notre-Dame; (514)890-8000 x25662

QUERESHY, Fayez A; Univ Hlth Network-Toronto Western Hosp, 320-399 Bathurst St, Toronto ON M5T 2S8; Tor'04; FRCSC; GenSurg; General Surgical Oncology. Staff, Toronto Western Hospital - University Health Network; (416)603-5224

QUERIN, Serge; Hop du Sacre-Coeur de Mtl, 5400 boul Gouin O, Montreal QC H4J 1C5; Mon'78; FRCPC; IntMed; Nephrol. Ac Staff Nephrol, Hôpital du Sacre-Coeur de Montréal; Prof, Universite de Montreal; Langs: Italian; Spanish; (514)338-2883; Fax. (514)338-2182; querins@videotron.ca.

QUERLEU, Denis; MUHC-Royal Victoria Hosp, 687 av des Pins O, Montreal QC H3A 1A1; Staff, McGill University Health Centre - Royal Victoria Hospital; Head ObsyGyn, McGill University; (514)934-1934

QUESADA, Ricardo; Portage Clinic Inc, 140 9th St SE, Portage La Prairie MB R1N 3V5; (El Salvador)'84; CCFP; Staff, Portage District General Hospital; Langs: Spanish; (204)857-3445; Fax. (204)239-1278; rquesada4@shaw.ca.

QUESNEL, Josee; CHUS-Hop Fleurimont, 3001 12e av N, Sherbrooke QC J1H 5N4; Sher'91; FRCPC; Peds. Staff, Centre Hospitalier Universitaire de Sherbrooke-Hopital Fleurimont; (819)346-1110; josee.quesnel@usherbrooke.ca.

QUESNEL, Louise; Centre Med Saint-Hubert, 206-5125 boul Cousineau, Saint-Hubert QC J3Y 3K7; Sher'79; (450)678-3500; Fax. (450)678-5722.

QUESNEL, Susan D; Addiction & Mental Hlth-ARF, 3034-33 Russell St, Toronto ON M5S 2S1; Tor'02; FRCPC; Psy. Staff, Centre for Addiction & Mental Health (CAMH) - Russell Street Site; (416)535-8501; Fax. (416)595-6399.

QUESNEL, Vanessa; CSSSG-Hop de Gatineau, CP 2000 Succ Bureau-Chef 909 boul de la Verendrye O, Gatineau QC J8P 7H2; Sher'10; CCFP; Staff, Hôpital de Gatineau; (819)966-6100

QUEVILLON, Andree; 5557 rue Belanger, Montreal QC H1T 1G2; Mon'74; Ophth (P.Q.). (514)256-5011 x250

QUEVILLON, J A Jean; 501-595 Montreal Rd, Ottawa ON K1K 4L2; Ott'71; FACC; FRCPC; IntMed (Clinical Cardiology); Cardiol. Ac Staff Ottawa Heart Inst, The Ottawa Hospital - General Campus; Court Staff, Montfort Hospital; Consultant, Hawkesbury & District General Hospital; Asst Prof, University of Ottawa; Langs: French; (613)741-9688; Fax. (613)741-9763.

QUEVILLON, Mathieu; Hotel-Dieu d'Arthabaska, 5 rue des Hospitalieres, Victoriaville QC G6P 6N2; Sher'04; FRCPC; DiagRad. Staff, Hotel-Dieu d'Arthabaska; (819)357-3020

QUEVILLON, Mylene; Clin Med Nicolet, 1691 boul Louis-Frechette, Nicolet QC J3T 1Z6; Sher'03; Staff GP, Hopital Maisonneuve-Rosemont; Staff, Hôpital de Christ-Roi; (819)293-2093; Fax. (819)293-2024; myquevillon@hotmail.com.

QUEVILLON, Nadine; Hop Charles LeMoyne, 3120 boul Taschereau, Greenfield Park QC J4V 2H1; Mon'06; CCFP; Staff, Hopital Charles LeMoyne; (450)466-5000

QUICKFALL, Jeremy P; Foothills Med Centre, 1403 29 St NW, Calgary AB T2N 2T9; Sask'01; FRCPC; Psy. Staff, Foothills Medical Centre; (403)944-3369

QUIDOZ, Amelie; Carrefour Med Vallee Richelieu, 665 rue Sir-Wilfrid Laurier, Beloeil QC J3G 4J1; Mon'05; (450)467-0088

QUIGG, Joseph M; Kingston Orthopaedic & Pain In, 500-797 Princess St, Kingston ON K7L 1G1; Wes'91; CCFP; CCFP(E.M.); (613)344-1202; Fax. (613)344-1203.

QUIGG, T Mark; Collingwood Health Centre, 204-186 Erie St, Collingwood ON L9Y 4T3; Tor'87; CCFP; FCFP; Staff, Collingwood General & Marine Hospital; Staff, Collingwood Health Centre; (705)445-5102; Fax. (705)445-1375.

QUIGLEY, Ciara J; LAMP Community Health Centre, 185 Fifth St, Etobicoke ON M8V 2Z5; Tor'95; CCFP; (416)252-6475; Fax. (416)252-6395.

QUIGLEY, John D; Brockville Gen Hosp, 75 Charles St, Brockville ON K6V 1S8; Dublin (Ireland)'65; MB ChB; BAO; FRCPC; DiagRad. Ac Staff, Brockville General Hospital - Charles Street; (613)345-5645 x1156

QUIGLEY, Mark J R; The Credit Valley Hosp, 2200 Eglinton Ave W, Mississauga ON L5M 2N1; McM'81; FRCPC; DiagRad (Angiography & Interventional Radiology). Staff, The Credit Valley Hospital; (905)813-3978; Fax. (905)813-3042.

QUIGLEY, Michael G; CHUM-Hop Notre-Dame, 1560 rue Sherbrooke E, Montreal QC H2L 4M1; Dal'79; AB; FRCSC; Ophth (Diabetic Retinopathy). Staff, Centre Hospitalier l'Université de Montréal (CHUM) - Hôpital Notre-Dame; Staff, Centre Hospitalier l'Université De Montréal (CHUM) - Hôpital Saint-luc; Staff, McGill University Health Centre - Royal Victoria Hospital; adj Prof, McGill University; Universite de Montreal; Langs: English; French; (514)890-8000 x34460; quigley.wilson@sympatico.ca.

QUILTER, Catherine M; Forest Hill Family Health Ctre, 491 Eglinton Ave E, Toronto ON M5N 1A8; Dublin (Ireland)'79; MB ChB; BAO; (416)782-6111; Fax. (416)782-5515.

QUINIOU, Alain-Andre; Polyclinique Med Concorde, 225-300 boul de la Concorde E, Laval QC H7G 2E6; Sher'88; FRCSC; OrthSurg. (450)668-3840; Fax. (450)668-1157.

QUINLAN, Christina W; Cancer Ctr of Southeastern Ont, 25 King St W, Kingston ON K7L 5P9; Qns'09; CCFP; Staff, Cancer Centre of Southeastern Ontario; (613)544-2631; Fax. (613)546-8201.

QUINLAN, David J; Foul Bay Prof Centre, 101-1964 Fort St, Victoria BC V8R 6R3; Witwatersrand (South Africa)'83; MB ChB; BSc; MRCOG; FRCSC; ObstGyn (Endoscopic Gynecology Surgery). Div Head Gyn, Vancouver Island Health Authority; Consultant, BC Cancer Agency Vancouver Island Centre; Clin Instructor, University of British Columbia; (250)595-1059; Fax. (250)595-1097; davidjquinlan@shaw.ca.

QUINLAN, Michael F; 1-9701 First St, Sidney BC V8L 3E1; Cape Town (South Africa)'83; MB ChB; FRCSC; Ophth. (250)656-4879; Fax. (250)656-5879; mfquinlan@shaw.ca.

QUINLAN, Michael W; 124-1151 Sidney St, Canmore AB T1W 3G1; McG'78; CCFP; FCFP; Ac Staff, Canmore General Hospital; Ac Staff, Covenant Health - Banff Mineral Springs Hospital; (403)678-5585; Fax. (403)678-6262; mike.quinlan2@gmail.com.

QUINLAN, Paul J; Brant Community HC-Brantford, 200 Terrace Hill St, Brantford ON N3R 1G9; Tor'75; Staff, The Brant Community Healthcare System - Brantford General Hospital Site; (519)752-7871

QUINLAN, Philip L; Medical Arts Centre, 3 Maple Ave N GD, Burford ON N0E 1A0; Wes'77; BA; Med Examiner Civil Aviation, Transport Canada; (519)449-2468; Fax. (519)449-5352; quinlanp@tc.gc.ca.

QUINN, Andrew P; 216-89 Humber College Blvd, Etobicoke ON M9V 4B8; Cal'03; FRCSC; OrthSurg. (416)749-7770; Fax. (416)749-9689.

QUINN, Andrew R; Tweed & Dist Comm Hlth Ctre, PO Box 99 41 McClellan St, Tweed ON K0K 3J0; McM'88; CCFP; FCFP; (613)478-1211; Fax. (613)478-1220.

QUINN, Brendan P; Ottawa Cardiovascular Centre, 502-1355 Bank St, Ottawa ON K1H 8K7; McG'81; FRCPC; IntMed; Cardiol. Chief Med/Staff, Montfort Hospital; Cardiol/Intl Med, The Ottawa Hospital - Civic Campus; Langs: English; French; (613)738-1584

QUINN, Bryan B; Cape Breton Hlthcare Complex, 1482 George St, Sydney NS B1P 1P3; Dal'73; AB; DiagRad. Staff Radiol, Cape Breton Healthcare Complex; (902)567-8000

QUINN, Dana L; Univ of Waterloo Hlth Services, 200 University Ave W, Waterloo ON N2L 3G1; Tor'00; CCFP; (519)888-4096; Fax. (519)746-5023.

QUINN, Danielle M; J E Stokes Med Centre, PO Box 760 415 Scotia St, Schreiber ON P0T 2S0; Tor'03; CCFP; Staff, The McCausland Hospital; (807)824-2934; Fax. (807)824-2758.

QUINN, Declan M P; Royal University Hosp, 241-103 Hospital Dr, Saskatoon SK S7N 0W8; Dublin (Ireland)'74; MB ChB; FRCPC; Psy (Child & Adolescent Psychiatry). Prof Child & Youth Psy, Royal University Hospital; Prof Psy, University of Saskatchewan; (306)966-7531; Fax. (306)966-8250.

QUINN, E Alan; 6162 Bradner Lane, Chilliwack BC V2R 5M7; UBC'72; BSc; Staff, Chilliwack General Hospital; Fax. (604)824-8740.

QUINN, Fiona S; Nanaimo Reg Gen Hosp, 1200 Dufferin Cres, Nanaimo BC V9S 2B7; UBC'08; CCFP; Staff, Nanaimo Regional General Hospital; (250)755-7691

QUINN, Francis R; Health Research Innovation Ctr, GAC 82-3280 Hospital Dr NW, Calgary AB T2N 4Z6; (United Kingdom)'95; Staff, Health Research Innovation Centre; (403)210-6152; Fax. (403)955-2068.

QUINN, Gerard; 94 Charing Cross St, Brantford ON N3R 2H6; Wes'87; CCFP; Coroner, Brant County; (519)752-0346; Fax. (519)752-7608; gerardquinn@rogers.com.

QUINN, Joan M; CFB Petawawa, PO Box 9999 Stn Main, Petawawa ON K8H 2X3; (Saint Lucia)'01; BSW; BScN; FRCPC; Psy. (613)678-5511; quinnjoan@nl.rogers.com.

QUINN, Leo P; Glazier Med Centre, 11 Gibb St, Oshawa ON L1H 2J9; Tor'67; (905)579-1212; Fax. (905)571-7548.

QUINN, Matthew T; 201-505 Queen St, Spruce Grove AB T7X 2V2; Alb'09; CCFP; (780)962-9888; Fax. (780)960-5298.

QUINN, Michael G; Royal Alexandra Hosp, 10240 Kingsway NW, Edmonton AB T5H 3V9; FRCPC; Anes. Staff, Royal Alexandra Hospital; (780)735-4111

QUINN, Robert R; Foothills Med Centre, C202C-1403 29 St NW, Calgary AB T2N 2T9; Wes'99; FRCPC; FRCPC; Nephrol; IntMed. Staff, Foothills Medical Centre; (403)944-5911; Fax. (403)944-5803.

QUINT, Avidor; Humber River Reg Hosp-Finch, 2111 Finch Ave W, North York ON M3N 1N1; Witwatersrand (South Africa)'73; MB ChB; FFARCS(Eng); FRCPC; Anes. Ac Staff, Humber River Regional Hospital - Finch Avenue Site; (416)744-2500

QUINT, Saul; Goodfellow Prof Bldg, 209-170 McEwan Dr E, Bolton ON L7E 4C8; Witwatersrand (South Africa)'79; (905)951-7525; Fax. (905)951-3419.

QUINTAL, Bernard; 29091 Route 134, Point La Nim NB E3N 6C6; Ott'79; CCFP; FCFP; Staff, Region 5 Health Authority; (506)684-5611; Fax. (506)684-5612.

QUINTAL, France; CLSC-CHSLD des Patriotes, 300 boul Serge-Pepin, Beloeil QC J3G 0B8; Sher'87; LMCC; Physician, CLSC-CHSLD des Patriotes; Langs: English; (450)536-2572

QUINTAL, Jean-Claude; 29091 Route 134, Point La Nim NB E3N 6C6; Ott'09; CCFP; (506)684-3031

QUINTAL, Louise; 4-544 av Notre-Dame, Saint-Lambert QC J4P 2K7; McG'83; CCFP; FCFP; (450)672-2456; Fax. (450)672-8766.

QUINTAL, M C Diane; 403-595 Montreal Rd, Ottawa ON K1K 4L2; Ott'79; FRCPC; Derm. Consultant, The Ottawa Hospital - Civic Campus; Consultant, The Ottawa Hospital - General Campus; Asst Prof, University of Ottawa; Langs: English; French; (613)744-4482

QUINTAL, Marie; 149B rue Principale, Gatineau QC J9H 3M7; Sher'83; FRCPC; Psy (Geriatric Psychiatry). Vis Staff, Montfort Hospital; Clin Staff, University of Ottawa; Clin Staff, McGill University; Langs: Spanish; English; (819)682-7952; Fax. (819)595-5132.

QUINTAL, Marie-Claude; Hôpital Ste-Justine, 3175 ch Cote-Sainte-Catherine, Montreal QC H3T 1C5; Sher'88; ABOtol; FRCSC; Otol (Pediatric Otolaryngology). Staff, Hôpital Ste-Justine; Universite de Montreal; (514)345-4931 x4857; Fax. (514)345-4791; quintalmc@videotron.ca.

QUINTAL, Marie-Luce; Inst U en Sante Mentale de QC, 2601 ch de la Canardiere, Quebec QC G1J 2G3; Laval'85; FRCPC; Psy. Staff, Institut Universitaire Sante; (418)663-5321

QUINTIN, Isabel; Hotel-Dieu d'Arthabaska, 5 rue des Hospitalieres, Victoriaville QC G6P 6N2; Sher'96; FRCPC; IntMed. Staff, Hotel-Dieu d'Arthabaska; (819)357-2030 x2300; Fax. (819)357-6016.

QUINTIN, Normand; CLSC la Petite Patrie, 6520 rue de Saint-Vallier, Montreal QC H2S 2P7; Mon'75; Staff Long Term Care Geriatric, Centre Hospitalier l'Université de Montréal (CHUM) - Hôpital Notre-Dame; (514)273-4508; Fax. (514)272-6278.

QUINTON, Jill A; North York Family Health Team, 702-240 Duncan Mill Rd, North York ON M3B 3S6; Man'07; CCFP; (416)494-7435; Fax. (416)494-4819.

QUINTON-GLADSTONE, Cindy; The Credit Valley Hosp, 2200 Eglinton Ave W, Mississauga ON L5M 2N1; McM'87; MHSc; FRCPC; IntMed; MedOncol. Staff, Sunnybrook Health Sciences Centre; Staff, The Credit Valley Hospital; (905)813-1100; Fax. (905)813-4024.

QUIRANTE-FLORA, Fe N; East York Town Centre, B9-45 Overlea Blvd, Toronto ON M4H 1C3; Manila (Philippines)'73; (416)421-1240; Fax. (416)421-9829.

QUIRING, David J; Chieftain Centre, PO Box 920 Stn Main, Squamish BC V8B 0A6; UBC'82; (604)892-5688; Fax. (604)892-9727.

QUIRION, Andre; GMF Centre Med du Parc, 101-84 rue Court, Granby QC J2G 4Y5; Mon'90; Staff, Centre Hospitalier de Granby; (450)375-1161; Fax. (450)375-7740.

QUIRION, Annie; CHUQ-Hotel-Dieu de Quebec, 11 Cote du Palais, Quebec QC G1R 2J6; Sher'97; FRCPC; Neur. Staff, Centre Hospitalier Universitaire de Québec (CHUQ) - Siege Social; (418)691-5288; Fax. (418)691-5186.

QUIRION, Charles-Antoine J; Pembroke Reg Hosp, 705 MacKay St, Pembroke ON K8A 1G8; Ott'07; CCFP; CCFP(E.M.); Staff, Pembroke Regional Hospital Inc; (613)732-2811

QUIRION, Karen; Clinique Med Soleil Enrg, 64 1re av O, Amos QC J9T 1T8; Mon'85; CCFP; (819)732-8341; Fax. (819)732-1642.

QUIRION, Marie-Andree A; Dr Georges-L Dumont Reg Hosp, 330 av Universite, Moncton NB E1C 2Z3; Mon'90; AnatPath (P.Q.). Chief Pathologist, Dr Georges-L-Dumont University Hospital Centre; (506)862-4314; Fax. (506)869-2895.

QUIRION, Melisa; CSSS Haut-Richelieu-Rouville, 920 boul du Seminaire N, St-Jean-sur-Richel QC J3A 1B7; Sher'05; CCFP; Staff, Hôpital du Haut-Richelieu; (450)359-5000

QUIRION, Sylvie; ASSS de Lanaudiere, 245 rue du Curé-Majeau, Joliette QC J6E 8S8; Mon'92; BSc; MSc; CommunMed (P.Q.) (Environmental Medicine). Med Consultant, Agence Sante Services Social Lanaudier; Langs: English; (450)759-1157 x4430; Fax. (450)759-0281; sylvie_quirion@ssss.gouv.qc.ca.

QUIRKE, David B; 301-1111 Lonsdale Ave, North Vancouver BC V7M 2H4; Cork (Ireland)'73; MB ChB; BAO; Staff, Vancouver General Hospital - Centennial Pavillion; (604)990-0008

QUIROS-CALINOIU, Elsa S; 202-5858 ch de la Cote-des-Nei, Montreal QC H3S 1Z1; San Marcos (Peru)'71; FRCSC; ObstGyn (Pediatric & Adolescent Gynecology). Dir Ped Adolescent Gyn Services, McGill University Health Centre - Montreal General Campus; Sr Staff, Sir Mortimer B Davis Jewish General; adj Prof, McGill University; Langs: French; Spanish; (514)731-3281; Fax. (514)731-5933.

QUIROUET, Adrienne; CSSSG-Hop de Gatineau, CP 2000 Succ Bureau-Chef 909 boul la Verendrye O, Gatineau QC J8P 7H2; Ott'07; Urol. Staff, Hôpital de Gatineau; (819)966-6333

QUIROZ MARTINEZ, Hector; CHUS-Hop Hotel-Dieu, 580 rue Bowen S, Sherbrooke QC J1G 2E8; (Mexico)'99; Critical Care Medicine (P.Q.). Staff, Centre Hospitalier Universitaire de Sherbrooke-Hôpital Hôtel-Dieu; (819)346-1110 x28303

QUMOSANI, Karim M Y; London HSC-University Hosp, PO Box 5339 Stn B 339 Windermere Rd, London ON N6A 5A5; Jeddah (Saudi Arabia)'03; MB BS; FRCPC; IntMed; Gastroent. Staff, London Health Sciences Centre - University Hospital; (519)663-3406

QUON, Bradley S; St Paul's Hosp, 8B-1081 Burrard St, Vancouver BC V6Z 1Y6; McG'05; FRCPC; IntMed; Respir. Staff, Providence Health Care - St Paul's Hospital; (604)806-8818

QUON, Deanna L; The Ottawa Hosp Rehab Ctre, 505 Smyth Rd, Ottawa ON K1H 8M2; Ott'06; FRCPC; PhysMed&Rehab. Staff, The Ottawa Hospital Rehabilitation Centre; (613)737-7350

QUON, Dick; Radiology Associates, 1122 Scenic Dr S, Lethbridge AB T1K 7E5; Alb'83; FRCPC; DiagRad. Chief Radiol, Chinook Regional Hospital; (403)328-1122; Fax. (403)328-1218.

QUON, Harvey C; CancerCare Manitoba, ON3247-675 McDermot Ave, Winnipeg MB R3E 0V9; Alb'04; FRCPC; RadOncol.

QUON, Leo; Anesthetic Services, 213-2186 Oak Bay Ave, Victoria BC V8R 1G3; UBC'97; FRCPC; Anes. Staff, Victoria General Hospital; (250)727-4152

QUONG, James K; Klondyke Med Clinic, 1-3089 3rd Ave, Whitehorse YT Y1A 5B3; UBC'87; CCFP; Staff, Klondyke Medical Clinic; (867)668-4065

QURAISHI, Ata-Ur-Rehman; Queen Elizabeth II HSC-Halifax, 6896-1796 Summer St, Halifax NS B3H 3A7; Karachi (Pakistan)'88; MB BS; FACC; Staff, Queen Elizabeth II Health Sciences Centre - Halifax Infirmary Site; Asst Prof Halifax Infirmary, Queen Elizabeth II Health Sciences Centre - Victoria General Site; Langs: Urdu; (902)473-3340; Fax. (902)473-6293; ata.quraishi@cdha.nshealth.ca.

QURAISHI, M Salim; 381 Clarke Side Rd, London ON N5W 5G5; Punjab (Pakistan)'65; Langs: Hindi; Punjabi; Urdu; (519)455-5060; Fax. (519)455-5224.

QURESHI, A Majid; Fairway X-Ray & Ultrasound, 385 Fairway Rd S, Kitchener ON N2C 1X2; Birmingham (England)'63; MB ChB; LRCP; MRCS; DABR; DiagRad (Bone Densitometry). (519)748-6844

QURESHI, A Quddus; 11718 Sarcee Trail NW, Calgary AB T3R 0A1; Karachi (Pakistan)'53; MB BS; LRCP; MRCS; FRCS(Ed); CCFP; Staff, Didsbury District Health Services; Langs: Urdu; Punjabi; Persian; (403)274-1864; Fax. (403)274-9093.

QURESHI, Alia P; 207-531 Davis Dr, Newmarket ON L3Y 6P5; Tor'04; FRCSC; GenSurg. (905)953-8838; Fax. (905)953-8521.

QURESHI, Amer S H; Sir Thomas Roddick Hosp, PO Box 5000 Stn Main 142 Minnesota Dr, Stephenville NL A2N 2V6; Punjab (India)'88; FRCPC; IntMed. Staff, Sir Thomas Roddick Hospital; (709)643-5111

QURESHI, Arif S; Listowel Clinic, 185 Inkerman St E, Listowel ON N4W 2N1; Tor'87; CCFP; FCFP; Court Staff, North Wellington Health Care - Palmerston & District Hospital; Listowel Memorial Hospital - Listowel Wingham Hospitals Alliance; Langs: German; (519)291-4200; Fax. (519)291-5947.

QURESHI, Azra; Medical Centre, 115-2100 Ellesmere Rd, Scarborough ON M1H 3B7; Karachi (Pakistan)'68; MB BS; Staff, The Scarborough Hospital - Birchmount Campus; Langs: Urdu; Hindi; Punjabi; (416)439-8497; Fax. (416)439-8574.

QURESHI, Bilquis; Mount Carmel Clinic, 886 Main St, Winnipeg MB R2W 5L4; CCFP.

QURESHI, Ehsan U; 103-3825 Sunset St, Burnaby BC V5G 1T4; Punjab (Pakistan)'58; MB BS; DABIM; FRCPC; IntMed. Consultant, Burnaby Hospital; (604)437-7034; Fax. (604)677-2013.

QURESHI, Irfan T; Morrison Centre, 211-9914 Morrison St, Fort McMurray AB T9H 4A4; Punjab (Pakistan)'88; MB BS; FRCSC; OrthSurg (Sports Injuries). Surgeon Orthopedic, Northern Lights Regional Health Centre; Langs: Urdu; Punjabi; Hindi; (780)791-3777; Fax. (780)791-6888.

QURESHI, Mosarrat J; Royal Alexandra Hosp, 10240 Kingsway NW, Edmonton AB T5H 3V9; Rajshahi Medical College (Bangladesh)'94; FAAP; FRCPC; Peds (Neonatology). Staff, Royal Alexandra Hospital; Clinical Asst Prof Peds, University of Alberta; (780)735-4670; Fax. (780)735-4072; mosarrat@yahoo.com.

QURESHI, Omar; Tauton Health Centre, SS 201 1290 Keith Ross Dr, Oshawa ON L1H 7K4; (Grenada)'06; CCFP; (905)721-3490

QURESHI, Rizwan; Westwood Clinic, 3320 Portage Ave, Winnipeg MB R3K 0Z1.

QURESHI, Roohi Y; St Michael's Hosp, 30 Bond St, Toronto ON M5B 1W8; Tor'99; FRCPC; OccupMed. Staff, St Michael's Hospital; (416)864-5074

QURESHI, Salman T; MUHC-Montreal Gen Hosp, L11-403 1650 av Cedar, Montreal QC H3G 1A4; Alb'87; FRCPC; IntMed; Critical Care Medicine (P.Q.); Respir; InfectDis. Staff, McGill University Health Centre - Montreal General Campus; Langs: English; French; (514)934-1934 x44654; isabelle.angers@hotmail.com.

QURESHI, Sameer; 101-178 96 Ave NE, Calgary AB T3K 6G4; Saba (Netherlands Antilles)'05; (403)693-1775

QURESHI, Shahab; Niagara H System-St Catharines, PO Box 3018 Stn Main 142 Queenston St, St Catharines ON L2R 7C6; Universita Palackeho (Czech Republic)'02; Staff, Niagara Health System - St Catharines General Site; (905)378-4647

QURESHI, Shahzad; Southlake Reg Health Centre, 596 Davis Dr, Newmarket ON L3Y 2P9; St George's Univ (Grenada)'01; FRCPC; IntMed. Staff, Southlake Regional Health Centre; (905)895-4521

QURESHI, Shujauddin; 912-700 Forest Hill Rd, Fredericton NB E3B 5X9; Karachi (Pakistan)'62; (506)454-3919

QURESHI, Tariq M; William Osler HC-Brampton, 2100 Bovaird Dr E, Brampton ON L6R 3J7; London (England)'95; MB BS; FRCPC; IntMed. Staff, William Osler Health System - Brampton Civic Hospital; (905)494-2120

QURESHI, Ziaur-Rehman T; Trans Canada Med Centre, 196-1440 52 St NE, Calgary AB T2A 4T8; Karachi (Pakistan)'77; MB BS; LRCP(Ed); LRCS(Edin); CCFP; Ac Staff, Peter Lougheed Centre; Langs: Urdu; Persian; Punjabi; (403)273-6566; Fax. (403)273-5757.

QURESHY, Bushra; Albany Med Clinic, 807 Broadview Ave, Toronto ON M4K 2P8; Punjab (Pakistan)'66; Staff, St Joseph's Health Centre; Staff Fam Med, Toronto East General Hospital Inc; Langs: Punjabi; Urdu; (416)461-9471 x264; Fax. (416)461-2710.

QURESHY, Kaiser A; Health Plus Med Centre, 1075 Autumnwood Dr, Winnipeg MB R2J 1C6; McM'07; Otol.

QURESHY, Kamran; Toronto East Gen Hosp Inc, 825 Coxwell Ave, Toronto ON M4C 3E7; Wes'97; FRCPC; IntMed; Endocrin&Metab. Staff, Toronto East General Hospital Inc; (416)461-8272

R RIOPEL, Marie Eve; The Hincks-Dellcrest Centre, 440 Jarvis St, Toronto ON M4Y 2H4; Laval'05; FRCPC; Psy (P.Q.). Staff, The Hincks-Dellcrest Centre - Toronto; (416)972-1935; Fax. (416)924-8208.

RA, Greta S; Univ Hlth Network-Toronto Western Hosp, 399 Bathurst St, Toronto ON M5T 2S8; Ott'08; IntMed. Fellow, Toronto Western Hospital - University Health Network; (416)603-5724

RA, Paul M U; 1995 Lens Ave, Windsor ON N8W 1L9; Chon-Nam (Korea)'72; DABPath; FRCPC; AnatPath (Hematology). Ac Staff, Windsor Regional Hospital - Metropolitan Site; Langs: Korean; (519)254-5577 x52493; Fax. (519)254-6861.

RAABE, Michael A; St Boniface Gen Hosp, Y3535-409 Tache Ave, Winnipeg MB R2H 2A6; Man'89; BSc; MSc; FRCSC; CardSurg (Aortic Surg). Staff Cardiac Surg, St Boniface General Hospital; Staff Manitoba Cardiac Sciences Prog, Health Sciences Centre; Asst Prof Cardiac Surg, University of Manitoba; Langs: German; (204)258-1213; Fax. (204)237-3429; mraabe@sbgh.mb.ca.

RAAD, Samar; Ctr de Sante Temiscaming, CP 760 180 rue Anvik, Temiscaming QC J0Z 3R0; Zaporozhye (Ukraine)'90; CCFP; Staff, Centre de santé de Témiscaming; Langs: Arabic; French; Russian; (819)627-3385; Fax. (819)627-9932; samar_raad@ssss.gouv.qc.ca.

RAAFAT, Sawsan; St Martha's Reg Hosp, 25 Bay St, Antigonish NS B2G 2G5; Cairo (Egypt)'78; Staff, St Martha's Regional Hospital; (902)867-4345; Fax. (902)864-7461.

RAATH, Abel H; Consort Med Centre, PO Box 58, Consort AB T0C 1B0; (South Africa)'78; CCFP; Langs: Afrikaans; Dutch; (403)577-3737; Fax. (403)577-3739.

RAATH, Annemie; St Joseph's Health Centre, PO Box 630, Ile-a-la-Crosse SK S0M 1C0; (306)833-2016; Fax. (306)833-3020.

RAATH, Johannes J; Royal Columbian Hosp, 330 Columbia St E, New Westminster BC V3L 3W7; Kansas (USA)'96; CCFP; Staff, Royal Columbian Hospital; Langs: Afrikaans; (604)520-4253

RAAZI, Mateen; Royal University Hosp, 103 Hospital Dr, Saskatoon SK S7N 0W8; Lahore (Pakistan)'87; MB BS; FRCPC; Anes. Staff, Royal University Hospital; (306)655-2501; Fax. (306)655-1279.

RABASA-LHORET, Remi; Inst de Recherches Clin de Mtl, 110 av des Pins O, Montreal QC H2W 1R7; Montpellier (France)'95; Staff Endocrin, Centre Hospitalier l'Université de Montréal (CHUM) - Hôtel-Dieu; Clin Prof Med, Universite de Montreal; (514)987-5666; Fax. (514)987-5670.

RABB, H Roderick; 6206 Perth St PO Box 370, Richmond ON K0A 2Z0; Ott'67; (613)838-2093; Fax. (613)838-2152.

RABB, Lucy M; 6206 Perth St PO Box 370, Richmond ON K0A 2Z0; Ott'65; Chief Family Med, Queensway Carleton Hospital; Coroner, Public Safety Canada; (613)838-2093; Fax. (613)838-2152.

RABBANI, F Nima; Vancouver Gen Hosp, 855 12th Ave W, Vancouver BC V5Z 1M9; Qns'98; Staff, Vancouver General Hospital - Centennial Pavillion; Chief Surgical Associate, Royal Columbian Hospital; (604)875-4472

RABBANI, Shahida N; 109-1400 boul Edouard, Saint-Hubert QC J4T 3T2; Punjab (Pakistan)'79; MB BS; FRCSC; ObstGyn (High Risk Obstetrics). Ac Member, Hopital Charles LeMoyne; Langs: Urdu; (450)923-5577; Fax. (450)923-4025.

RABBAT, Christian G; St Joseph's Health Care, M318-50 Charlton Ave E, Hamilton ON L8N 4A6; Qns'93; FRCPC; IntMed; Nephrol. Staff, St Joseph's Healthcare - Charlton Campus; Assoc Prof Med, McMaster University; (905)522-1155 x33542; Fax. (905)521-6153.

RABBAT, George R; Dryden Reg Health Centre, PO Box 3003 Stn Main 58 Goodall St, Dryden ON P8N 2Z6; Beirut (Lebanon)'02; FRCSC; GenSurg. Staff, Dryden Regional Health Centre; (807)223-8200

RABBATH, Patrick; CSSS de Saint-Jerome, 290 rue de Montigny, Saint-Jerome QC J7Z 5T3; Mon'92; LMCC; Cardiol; IntMed (Echocardiography). Staff Cardiol, Hôtel-Dieu de Saint-Jérôme; (450)431-8201; Fax. (450)431-8304.

RABEEH, Richard H; Pleasantview Prof Centre, 407-11044 51 Ave NW, Edmonton AB T6H 5B4; Alb'99; BSc; FRCPC; Psy (Child Psychiatry). Physician, Royal Alexandra Hospital; Physician, Glenrose Rehabilitation Hospital; Clin Lecturer, University of Alberta; (780)438-6181; Fax. (780)437-3499.

RABENECK, Linda; Cancer Care Ontario, 16F-620 University Ave, Toronto ON M5G 2L7; UBC'74; FRCPC; IntMed; Gastroent. Staff, Sunnybrook Health Sciences Centre; (416)217-1254

RABER, Earl L; Foothills Med Centre, 1403 29 St NW, Calgary AB T2N 2T9; Man'90; FRCPC; DiagRad. Staff, Foothills Medical Centre; (403)944-1969; Fax. (403)944-1687.

RABHERU, Kiran; 137Y-75 Bruyere St, Ottawa ON K1N 5C7; Wes'80; DABPN; FRCPC; Psy (Behavioural Problems/Dementia);CCFP; FCFP; Langs: Gujarati; (613)562-9777; kiran.rabheru@vch.ca.

RABHERU, Rita H; Middlesex London Health Unit, 101-50 King St, London ON N6A 5L7; Dal'78; CCFP; Ac Staff/Physician, Regional Mental Health Care-St Joseph's Health Care; Langs: Hindi; (519)663-5446; krabheru@sympatico.ca.

RABI, Doreen M; HSC-Faculty of Med, 3330 Hospital Dr NW, Calgary AB T2N 4N1; Wes'98; FRCPC; IntMed; Endocrin&Metab. Staff, Foothills Medical Centre; (403)220-8867; Fax. (403)270-0979.

RABI, Yacov; Foothills Med Centre, C211-1403 29 St NW, Calgary AB T2N 2T9; Wes'97; FRCPC; Peds (Neonatal). Staff, Foothills Medical Centre; Asst Prof, University of Calgary; (403)944-1615; Fax. (403)944-4892; jack.rabi@calgaryhealthregion.ca.

RABIA, Djamila; CLSC Saint-Leonard, 5540 rue Jarry E, Saint-Leonard QC H1P 1T9; (Algeria)'82; CCFP; (514)328-3460

RABIDEAU, Sparrow L; Westmount Community Health Ctr, 800-723 Rymal Rd W, Hamilton ON L9B 2W2; Tor'82; CCFP; FCFP; Court Staff, St Joseph's Healthcare - Charlton Campus; Ac Staff Family Med, Hamilton Health Sciences Centre - McMaster University Medical Centre; (905)575-5200; Fax. (905)575-5383.

RABIE, Christiaan S; South Calgary Med Clinic, 118-40 Sunpark Plaza SE, Calgary AB T2X 3X7; Pretoria (South Africa)'92; Langs: Afrikaans; (403)254-4000; Fax. (403)254-1282.

RABIE, Faten S; Kanata Prof Centre, 216-99 Kakulu Rd, Kanata ON K2L 3C8; Cairo (Egypt)'72; Langs: French; Arabic; (613)592-0994; Fax. (613)592-1137.

RABIE, Rania N; Medical Arts Bldg, 204B-581 Davis Dr, Newmarket ON L3Y 2P6; Wes'03; FRCPC; IntMed; Gastroent. Staff, Toronto General Hospital - UHN; Langs: Hindi; (905)853-4545

RABIEN, Anton; West Coast Family Med Clinic, 1300-6660 Sooke Rd, Sooke BC V9Z 0A5; UBC'02; BSc; CCFP; Clinical Asst Prof, University of British Columbia; (250)642-4233; Fax. (250)642-6032.

RABIN, David; 310-5655 av du Parc, Montreal QC H2V 4H2; Ott'68; FRCPC; Peds. Assoc Staff, McGill University Health Centre - Montreal Children's Hospital; Assoc Staff, Sir Mortimer B Davis Jewish General; Assoc Staff, McGill University Health Centre - Royal Victoria Hospital; (514)276-7273

RABIN, David G; 200-6061 No 3 Rd, Richmond BC V6Y 2B2; Witwatersrand (South Africa)'63; MB ChB; FRCPC; Psy. (604)786-9554

RABIN, Elijah Z; Niagara H System-Ontario Site, 2C-155 Ontario St, St Catharines ON L2R 5K3; Qns'61; PhD(McG); FACP; ABIM(Nephrol); FRCPC; IntMed (Nephrology). Staff, Niagara Health System - Ontario Street Site; (905)682-6411 x3513; Fax. (905)682-6996.

RABIN, Harvey R; HSC-Faculty of Med, 3330 Hospital Dr NW, Calgary AB T2N 4N1; Wes'65; FRCPC; IntMed; InfectDis. Ac Staff Med, Foothills Medical Centre; Prof Med, University of Calgary; (403)220-5951; Fax. (403)270-2772; rabin@ucalgary.ca.

RABIN, Irving; Centre Med de Place Brossard, 106-5635 boul Grande-Allee, Brossard QC J4Z 3G3; Qns'71; FRCPC; Peds. Associate, McGill University Health Centre - Montreal Children's Hospital; Langs: English; French; (450)676-0271; Fax. (450)676-0274.

RABIN, Michael; Royal University Hosp, 103 Hospital Dr, Saskatoon SK S7N 0W8; Witwatersrand (South Africa)'64; MB ChB; MMed(DiagRad.); Staff, Royal University Hospital; (306)655-2371; Fax. (306)655-2370.

RABINOVICH, Alexander; Brant Community HC-Brantford, 200 Terrace Hill St, Brantford ON N3R 1G9; McM'04; FRCSC; OrthSurg. Staff, The Brant Community Healthcare System - Brantford General Hospital Site; (519)751-5808

RABINOVICH, Solomon; Gamma-Dynacare Medical Lab, 115 Midair Crt, Brampton ON L6T 5M3; Tor'57; FRCPC; GenPath. (905)790-3000 x335

RABINOVITCH, Barry; MUHC-Montreal Chest Institute, 3650 rue Saint-Urbain, Montreal QC H2X 2P4; McG'77; Respir; IntMed. Staff, McGill University Health Centre - Montreal Chest Institute; Langs: Bilingual(English/French); (514)934-1934; Fax. (514)843-2070.

RABINOVITCH, Daniel E; CSSS de Laval, 1755 boul Rene-Laennec, Laval QC H7M 3L9; Wes'00; Neur. Staff, Hopital de la Cite de la santé; (450)668-1010

RABINOVITCH, Deborah L; Synergy Sports Medicine, 235 Wallace Ave, Toronto ON M6H 1V5; Ott'05; FRCPC; PhysMed&Rehab. Fax. (647)343-8073.

RABINOVITCH, Edward M; Misericordia Comm Hosp & H C, 16940 87 Ave NW, Edmonton AB T5R 4H5; Tor'63; FRCPC; Peds. Staff Child Health Clinic, Covenant Health - Misericordia Community Hospital; Clin Assoc Prof, University of Alberta; (780)735-2731; Fax. (780)735-2794.

RABINOVITCH, Eric A; 1425-1 car Westmount, Montreal QC H3Z 2P9; McG'97; FRCPC; Peds (P.Q.); Psy. (514)935-2470; Fax. (514)935-7261.

RABINOVITCH, Gerald I; 9-4400 Bathurst St, Toronto ON M3H 3R8; McG'73; DABPN; FRCPC; Psy (Dissociative Disorders). (416)638-0016; Fax. (416)638-0013.

RABINOVITCH, Hyman E; Nepean Med Centre, 406-1 Centrepointe Dr, Nepean ON K2G 6E2; McG'69; DAB; FRCPC; Neur. Ac Staff, Queensway Carleton Hospital; Consultant, Royal Ottawa Mental Health Centre - Royal Ottawa Health Care Group; Ac Staff, The Ottawa Hospital - General Campus; Asst Clin Prof, University of Ottawa; (613)228-4298; Fax. (613)228-9365.

RABINOVITCH, Jed; Scarborough North Med Arts, 309-4040 Finch Ave E, Scarborough ON M1S 4V5; McG'79; DAB; FRCSC; Ophth (Cornea External Disease & Anterior Segment Surgery). Ac Staff, The Scarborough Hospital - Birchmount Campus; Court Staff, Sunnybrook Health Sciences Centre; Clin Instructor, University of Toronto; Langs: Spanish; French; (416)754-7511; Fax. (416)754-7512; jed.rabinovitch@sympatico.ca.

RABINOVITCH, Mark A; The Greene Ave Clinic, 210-1255 av Greene, Westmount QC H3Z 2A4; McG'74; FRCPC; IntMed (Nuclear Cardiology); Cardiol. Staff, McGill University Health Centre - Montreal General Campus; assoc Prof, McGill University; Langs: English; French; (514)938-5535

RABINOVITCH, Mark H; Douglas Mental Hlth Univ Inst, 6875 boul Lasalle, Verdun QC H4H 1R3; Qns'00; CSPQ; FRCPC; Psy. Staff, Douglas Mental Health University Institute; (514)761-6131

RABINOVITCH, Samuel M; Scarborough North Med Arts, LL4-4040 Finch Ave E, Scarborough ON M1S 4V5; Strasbourg (France)'81; FRCPC; DiagRad. Ac Staff Radiol, The Scarborough Hospital - Birchmount Campus; Ac Staff Radiol, Rouge Valley Health System - Centenary Health Centre Site; Langs: English; French; (416)292-1505

RABINOVITCH, Theodore; North Toronto Eye Care, 407-2115 Finch Ave W, North York ON M3N 2V6; McG'83; FAAO; BSc; FRCSC; Ophth (Cataract). Court Staff, North York General Hospital - Branson Division; Staff Ophth, Humber River Regional Hospital - Finch Avenue Site; Asst Prof Ophth, University of Toronto; Langs: Bilingual(English/French); (416)748-2020; Fax. (416)748-8582; drrabinovitch@northtorontoeyecare.com.

RABINOWITZ, Alan N; St Paul's Hosp, 1081 Burrard St, Vancouver BC V6Z 1Y6; Cape Town (South Africa)'83; MB ChB; FRCPC; IntMed; Cardiol. Staff, Providence Health Care - St Paul's Hospital; (604)806-9625; Fax. (604)806-9629.

RABKIN, Simon; Gordon & Leslie Diamond HCC, 9119-2775 Laurel St, Vancouver BC V5Z 1M9; Man'67; FRCPC; IntMed; Cardiol. Consultant, Vancouver General Hospital - Centennial Pavillion; Staff Cardiology, Gordon & Leslie Diamond Health Care Centre; Prof Med, University of British Columbia; (604)875-5847; Fax. (604)875-5849.

RABOISSON, Marie-Josee; Hôpital Ste-Justine, 3175 ch Cote-Sainte-Catherine, Montreal QC H3T 1C5; Lyon (France)'98; Staff, Hôpital Ste-Justine; (514)345-4670; Fax. (514)345-4991.

RABSON, John L R; Medical Arts Bldg, 1217-233 Kennedy St, Winnipeg MB R3C 3J5; Man'73; BSc(Hon); FRCPC; Cardiol (Consulant Cardiologist). Att Staff CCU, Health Sciences Centre; Asst Prof, University of Manitoba; (204)943-4357; jrabson@mts.net.

RABUKA, Curtis E; University of Alberta Hosp, 1G162WCM-8440 112 St NW, Edmonton AB T6G 2B7; Sask'95; FRCPC; EmergMed. Staff, University of Alberta Hospital; (780)407-7047; Fax. (780)407-3314.

RABUKA, Shannon L; Clinical Sciences Bldg, 152 University Campus NW, Edmonton AB T6G 2G3; Sask'93; FRCPC; Anes. Staff, University of Alberta Hospital; (780)407-8861

RABY, Bruno; Hôpital Laval, 2725 ch Sainte-Foy, Quebec QC G1V 4G5; Laval'85; FRCPC; IntMed; Respir. Staff, Hôpital Laval; (418)656-4747; Fax. (418)656-4762.

RABY, France; CSSS de Rimouski-Neigette, CP 3150 Succ A 150 av Rouleau, Rimouski QC G5L 5T1; Laval'90; CCFP; Staff, Hôpital Regional Rimouski; (418)723-7851

RABY, Kathleen; Hôpital Laval, 2725 ch Sainte-Foy, Quebec QC G1V 4G5; Laval'91; FRCPC; IntMed. Internal Med, Hôpital Laval; (418)656-8711; kathleen.raby@videotron.ca.

RABY, Patricia M; 3-920 King St W, Kitchener ON N2G 1G4; McM'80; FRCSC; ObstGyn. (519)741-9939; Fax. (519)741-9388.

RABZEL, Martina; 309-2021 Cliff Rd, Mississauga ON L5A 3N7; McG'77; CCFP; Ac Staff, Trillium Health Centre - Mississauga; (905)276-8900; Fax. (905)276-8911.

RACANELLI, Sam; 7333 Mississauga Rd, Mississauga ON L5N 6L4; Tor'85; CCFP; FCFP; (905)814-3552

RACE, Karen J; Huron Square Med Centre, 2500 Hurontario St, Mississauga ON L5B 1N4; Cal'92; CCFP; (905)897-6160; Fax. (905)897-6729.

RACETTE, Francois; CSSS du Lac-des-Deux-Montagnes, 520 boul Arthur-Sauve, Saint-Eustache QC J7R 5B1; Mon'94; FRCPC; IntMed. Staff, Hôpital de Saint-Eustache; Langs: English; (450)473-6811; Fax. (450)473-2704.

RACETTE, Julie-Maude; CSSS de Saint-Jerome, 290 rue de Montigny, Saint-Jerome QC J7Z 5T3; Mon'06; Peds. Staff, Hôtel-Dieu de Saint-Jérôme; (450)431-8200

RACETTE, Nicole; Gordon & Leslie Diamond HCC, 6205-2775 Laurel St, Vancouver BC V5Z 1M9; Laval'82; FRCSC; ObstGyn (Infertility). Staff, Vancouver General Hospital - Centennial Pavillion; Staff Women's Health Centre, BC Women's Hospital & Health Centre; Staff, Gordon & Leslie Diamond Health Care Centre; Clinical Asst Prof, University of British Columbia; Langs: English; French; (604)875-5711; Fax. (604)875-4869; nicole.racette@vch.ca.

RACETTE, Richard; Ctr Hosp Laurentien, 234 rue Saint-Vincent, Ste-Agathe-Des-Mts QC J8C 2B8; Sher'93; CSPQ; FRCPC; DiagRad. Staff, Centre Hospitalier Laurentien; (819)324-4000

RACETTE-LE NEVEU, Therese J; Klinic, 870 Portage Ave, Winnipeg MB R3G 0P1; Alb'81; CCFP; Ac Staff, Selkirk & District General Hospital.

RACHAKONDA, Ramanamurthy V; Grand River Reg Cancer Ctre, PO Box 9056 Stn C 835 King St W, Kitchener ON N2G 1G3; Gujarat (India)'88; FRCPC; RadOncol. Staff, Grand River Hospital - Kitchener/Waterloo Health Centre; (519)749-4300; Fax. (519)749-4378.

RACHAPALLI, Satish M R; 2680 Richmond Rd, Victoria BC V8R 4S9; (India)'97; MB BS; (250)519-4007

RACHER, Laine; 101-5920 1A St SW, Calgary AB T2H 0G3; Alb'08; FRCPC; Peds. Staff, Foothills Medical Centre; (403)252-6651; Fax. (403)640-0710.

RACHIELE, Andre; Clinique Med Lamater, 2400-504 rue Notre-Dame, Repentigny QC J6A 2T8; Mon'83; CCFP; (450)582-3992

RACHINSKY, Irina V; London HSC-Victoria Hosp, PO Box 5010 Stn B 800 Commissioners Rd E, London ON N6A 5W9; (Russia (Federation))'88; FRCPC; NuclearMed. Staff, London Health Sciences Centre - Victoria Campus; (519)667-6570; Fax. (519)667-6734.

RACHINSKY, Maxim; St Joseph's Health Care, PO Box 5777 Stn B 268 Grosvenor St, London ON N6A 4V2; (Russia (Federation))'88; Anes. Staff, St Joseph's Hospital - St Joseph's Health Care; (519)646-6100

RACHLIS, Alisa C; University of Toronto, 500 University Ave, Toronto ON M5G 1V7; Tor'07; Peds.

RACHLIS, Anita R; Sunnybrook Hlth Sciences Ctre, A226-2075 Bayview Ave, Toronto ON M4N 3M5; Tor'72; FRCPC; IntMed; InfectDis. Staff, Sunnybrook Health Sciences Centre; Teach Staff, University of Toronto; Langs: English; French; (416)480-4689

RACHLIS, Michael M; 13 Langley Ave, Toronto ON M4K 1B4; Man'75; MSc(McMaster); FRCPC; CommunMed; Public Health & Preventive Med. Assoc Prof Health Policy Mgmt & Evaluation, University of Toronto; (416)466-0093; michaelrachlis@rogers.com.

RACHLIS, Val; 260-5 Fairview Mall Dr, North York ON M2J 2Z1; Tor'72; CCFP; FCFP; Court Staff, The Scarborough Hospital - General Campus; Court Staff, Mount Sinai Hospital; Staff Family Med, North York General Hospital; Assoc Prof Family Med, University of Toronto; (416)497-6363; Fax. (416)497-7610; vrachlis@aol.com.

RACIC, Anita R; Vancouver Native Hlth Society, 449 Hastings St E, Vancouver BC V6A 1P5; UBC'91; Staff, Surrey Mental Health & Addictions; (604)255-9766; aracic@shaw.ca.

RACICOT, Caroline; Centre Chirugical de Joliette, 202-222 rue de la Visitation, St-Charles-Brromee QC J6E 4N5; Mon'94; FRCSC; GenSurg. (450)753-7588

RACICOT, Jean; Ctr Hosp du Centre la Mauricie, 50 119e rue, Shawinigan-Sud QC G9P 5K1; Mon'75; CSPQ; DiagRad. Staff, Centre Hospitalier du Centre la Mauricie; (819)536-7523; Fax. (819)536-7557.

RACICOT, Jean-Mathieu; CSSS Les Eskers de l'Abitibi, 622 4e rue Ouest, Amos QC J9T 2S2; Laval'01; MCFP; FRCPC; Anes. Staff, CH Hôtel-Dieu d'Amos; Langs: Bilingual(English/French); (819)732-3341 x2356; Fax. (819)732-6423.

RACICOT, Marie-Helene; Hop Maisonneuve-Rosemont, 5415 boul de l'Assomption, Montreal QC H1T 2M4; Mon'04; FRCSC; ObstGyn. Staff, Centre Hospitalier l'Université De Montréal (CHUM) - Hôpital Saint-luc; (514)252-3400

RACICOT, Paolo; Clin Med Racicot Inc, 2000-520 rue d'Avaugour, Boucherville QC J4B 0G6; Mon'04; (450)449-7525; Fax. (450)655-0838.

RACICOT, Pierre; Hop Louis-H Lafontaine, 7401 rue Hochelaga, Montreal QC H1N 3M5; Mon'85; CSPQ; FRCPC; Psy. Staff, Hopital Louis-H Lafontaine; (514)251-4000

RACICOVSHI, Daria S; Lakeridge Hlth Corp-Oshawa, 1 Hospital Crt, Oshawa ON L1G 2B9; Bucharest (Romania)'85; Psy. Staff, Lakeridge Health - Oshawa Site; (905)576-8711

RACINE, Daniel; Hop Maisonneuve-Rosemont, 5415 boul de l'Assomption, Montreal QC H1T 2M4; Mon'76; Staff, Hopital Maisonneuve-Rosemont; (514)252-3859; Fax. (514)252-3573.

RACINE, Daniele; CSST DSM Montreal, 1199 rue de Bleury, Montreal QC H3B 3J1; Sher'80; Médecin, CSST-Direction Regionale Montreal; (514)906-3003 x2380

RACINE, Dominique M J; Canadian Med Protective Assn, PO Box 8225 Stn T CSC 875 Carling Ave, Ottawa ON K1G 3H7; Ott'79; CCFP; FCFP; Langs: Bilingual(French/English); (613)725-2000; dracine@cmpa.org.

RACINE, Elizabeth; Clinique Med Bromont, C101-82 boul de Bromont, Bromont QC J2L 2K3; Laval'87; Médecin, CSSS la Pommeraie; (450)534-5474; Fax. (450)534-1725.

RACINE, Francois R J; 404A-595 Montreal Rd, Ottawa ON K1K 4L2; Ott'71; FRCPC; PhysMed&Rehab. Teach Staff, University of Ottawa; Langs: Bilingual(French/English); (613)745-7399; Fax. (613)745-9875.

RACINE, Gilbert; CSSS du Sud de Lanaudière, 911 montee des Pionniers, Terrebonne QC J6V 2H2; Mon'86; CSPQ; DiagRad. Staff, Centre Hospitalier Pierre le Gardeur; (450)654-7525

RACINE, Louis; Clin Ophthalmology de l'Ouest, 1503-625 av du President-Kenne, Montreal QC H3A 1K2; Mon'98; FRCSC; Ophth (Cornea & Refractive Surgery). assoc Prof Ophth, Centre Hospitalier l'Université de Montréal (CHUM) - Hôpital Notre-Dame; Langs: Bilingual(French/English); (514)849-8215; Fax. (514)849-5115.

RACINE, Luc; Clinique Med l'Assomption, 320-5345 boul de l'Assomption, Montreal QC H1T 4B3; Mon'59; FICS; FRCSC; OrthSurg. Staff, Hopital Maisonneuve-Rosemont; Teach Staff, Universite de Montreal; (514)254-6161; Fax. (514)254-1585.

RACINE, Marie Lynn; Hop Charles LeMoyne, 3120 boul Taschereau, Greenfield Park QC J4V 2H1; Mon'02; RadOncol. Staff, Hopital Charles LeMoyne; (450)466-5000

RACINE, Marie-Claude; CSSS Kamouraska-Hop Notre-Dame, CP 460 1201 6e av, La Pocatiere QC G0R 1Z0; Laval'98; FRCPC; IntMed (Family Medicine). Staff, CSSS de Kamouraska; (418)856-7000; mcracine@hotmail.com.

RACINE, Marie-Claude; CLSC de Paspebiac, CP 7000 273 boul Gerard-D-Levesque, Paspebiac QC G0C 2K0; Mon'93; Staff, CLSC de Paspebiac; (418)752-2572; Fax. (418)752-6766.

RACINE, Michel; CSSS de Laval, 1755 boul Rene-Laennec, Laval QC H7M 3L9; Laval'69; CCFP; FCFP; Med Staff, CSSS de Trois-Rivières; Med Staff, Hopital de la Cite de la santé; Clinical Asst Prof, Universite de Montreal; Langs: English; (450)975-5444; Fax. (450)975-5497.

RACINE, Normand; Institut de Cardiologie de Mtl, 5000 rue Belanger, Montreal QC H1T 1C8; Mon'84; CSPQ; ABIM; ABCD; FRCP; FRCPC; IntMed (Academic Practice); Cardiol. Chief Dept of Med & Cardiol, Institut de Cardiologie de Montréal; assoc Prof, Universite de Montreal; Langs: English; (514)376-3330 x2192; normand.racine@icm-mhi.org.

RACINE, Pierre Y; 110-10302 rue Chambord, Montreal QC H2C 2R5; Mon'64; CSPQ; Urol. Staff, Centre Hospitalier Fleury; (514)382-0344

RACINE, Real; Clinique de Med Familiale, 1971 rue Bilodeau, Plessisville QC G6L 3J1; Laval'78; (819)362-6337; Fax. (819)362-9147.

RACINE, Simon; Inst U en Sante Mentale de QC, 2601 ch de la Canardiere, Quebec QC G1J 2G3; Laval'72; MSc(Admin.); LMCC; FRCPC; Public Health & Preventive Med; CommunMed (P.Q.) (Assessment & Program Planning). Chef dir, Institut Universitaire Sante; Langs: English; (418)663-5126; Fax. (418)663-9774; simon.racine@institutsmq.qc.ca.

RACINE, Stephanie; CSSS du Sud de Lanaudière, 911 montee des Pionniers, Terrebonne QC J6V 2H2; Mon'07; CCFP; Staff, Centre Hospitalier Pierre le Gardeur; (450)654-7525

RACINE, Suzanne; Inst de l'Oeil des Laurentides, 4800 rue Ambroise-Lafortune, Boisbriand QC J7H 1S6; Mon'76; FRCSC; Ophth. ac Staff, Hôtel-Dieu de Saint-Jérôme; (450)419-6345

RACKAL, Julia M; St Michael's Hosp, 30 Bond St, Toronto ON M5B 1W8; Qns'04; CCFP; Staff, St Michael's Hospital; (416)867-7426

RACO, Dominic L F; N2 918-2100 Bovaird Dr E, Brampton ON L6R 3J7; Tor'81; MD; FRCPC; IntMed (Interventional Cardiology); Cardiol. Staff, William Osler Health System - Brampton Civic Hospital; Langs: Italian; (905)494-6221; dominic.raco@williamoslerhs.ca.

RACO, Lina C; 20B-385 Frederick St, Kitchener ON N2H 2P2; Qns'93; CCFP; FCFP; Court Staff, Grand River Hospital - Kitchener/Waterloo Health Centre; Court Staff, St Mary's General Hospital; (519)747-1200; Fax. (519)747-1560.

RACZ, Elizabeth M; Drumheller Assoc Physicians, PO Box 5600, Drumheller AB T0J 0Y0; Cal'79; BSc; CCFP; FCFP; (403)823-3345; Fax. (403)823-7823.

RACZ, Heather N; 305-564 Belmont Ave W, Kitchener ON N2M 5N6; Qns'03; FRCPC; IntMed; Respir. Staff, London Health Sciences Centre - Victoria Campus; (519)954-6021

RACZYNSKA, Maria J; Credit Valley Med Arts Centre, 506-2000 Credit Valley Rd, Mississauga ON L5M 4N4; Stettin (Poland)'77; Staff, The Credit Valley Hospital; Langs: Polish; (905)828-4812; Fax. (905)828-6240.

RADAN, Aleksandar; Alexandria Marine & Gen Hosp, 120 Napier St, Goderich ON N7A 1W5; Ott'99; CCFP; Staff In-Patients Emerg Obst, Alexandra Marine & General Hospital; Staff In-Patients Emerg Obst, Clinton Public Hospital - Huron Perth Healthcare Alliance; (519)524-8323; Fax. (519)524-5579.

RADDATZ, Elaine; Harbourfront Health & Wellness, 4-8 York St, Toronto ON M5J 2Y2; Wes'06; CCFP; (416)366-2273; Fax. (416)366-5665.

RADDATZ, Eric; 4335 Bloor St W, Etobicoke ON M9C 2A5; Qns'08; CCFP; (416)695-8878; Fax. (416)695-2622.

RADER, Jeffrey J; PO Box 69005 Rpo Bridlewood, Calgary AB T2Y 4T9; Wes'05; CCFP.

RADERMAKER, Steve; Hôpital Laval, 2725 ch Sainte-Foy, Quebec QC G1V 4G5; Laval'07; Psy. Staff, Hôpital Laval; (418)656-8711 x4565

RADEVSKI, Ivelin; Southwest Medi-Centre, 500-1 Springs Dr, Swift Current SK S9H 3X6; Varna (Bulgaria)'91; CCFP; (306)773-4681; Fax. (306)773-9513.

RADFORD, Charles; Osler Eyecare, 210-164 Queen St E, Brampton ON L6V 1B4; Tor'59; Ophth. Court Staff, William Osler Health System - Brampton Civic Hospital; (905)456-3937; Fax. (905)459-5085.

RADHAKRISHNA, Mohan; MUHC-Montreal Gen Hosp, L7 510-1650 av Cedar, Montreal QC H3G 1A4; Qns'97; FRCPC; PhysMed&Rehab (Musculoskeletal Rehabilitation). Staff Physical Med & Rehab, McGill University Health Centre - Montreal General Campus; adj Prof, McGill University; Langs: English; French; (514)934-1934 x44185; Fax. (514)934-8265.

RADHAKRISHNAN, Arun K; 1118-123 Edward St, Toronto ON M5G 1E2; McG'98; CCFP; (416)593-7700; Fax. (416)593-7702.

RADHAKRISHNAN, Dhenuka K; London HSC-Victoria Hosp, PO Box 5010 Stn B B1 161C-800 Commissioners Rd E, London ON N6A 5W9; Tor'02; FRCPC; Peds; Respir. Staff, London Health Sciences Centre - Victoria Campus; (519)685-8379; Fax. (519)685-8156.

RADHAKRISHNAN, Seetha; The Hosp for Sick Children, 555 University Ave, Toronto ON M5G 1X8; McG'04; FRCPC; Peds; Nephrol. Staff, The Hospital For Sick Children; (416)530-3961

RADHAKRISHNAN, Shyam; Sunnybrook Hlth Sciences Ctre, A253-2075 Bayview Ave, Toronto ON M4N 3M5; Tor'93; FRCPC; IntMed (Interventional Cardiology); Cardiol. Leader Code STEMI Project, Sunnybrook Health Sciences Centre; Staff Interventional Cardiol, Schulich Heart Centre; (416)480-6100 x4777; Fax. (416)480-4745.

RADHI, Jasim M; Peterborough Reg HC-Hospital, 1 Hospital Dr, Peterborough ON K9J 7C6; Baghdad (Iraq)'76; MB ChB; FRCP(UK); FRCPC; AnatPath (Gastrointestinal & Liver Pathology). Staff, Peterborough Regional Health Centre - Hospital Drive; Prof Path & Molecular Med, McMaster University; Langs: Arabic; (705)743-2121

RADIN, Daniel A; 103A-13278 Tecumseh Rd E, Windsor ON N8N 1M2; Tor'99; FRCPC; Derm. (519)979-4000; Fax. (519)979-5777.

RADINSKAIA, Dina; 464F Woodbine Blvd SW, Calgary AB T2W 5H7; (Russia (Federation))'98; CCFP; Staff, Foothills Medical Centre.

RADISIC, Djordje G; Baker Clinic, 220-10405 Jasper Ave NW, Edmonton AB T5J 3N4; Belgrade (Serbia)'82; FRCPC; Peds. Staff, Sturgeon Community Hospital; Langs: Serbian; (780)421-1990; Fax. (780)944-9599.

RADKE, Steven; 510 Raglan St N, Renfrew ON K7V 1P5; Ott'02; CCFP; Staff, Renfrew Victoria Hospital; (613)433-9152

RADO, George; 600-285 Cummer Ave, North York ON M2M 2G1; Paris (France)'77; AB; FRCPC; PhysMed&Rehab. Consultant, Providence Healthcare; Langs: Hungarian; French; (416)226-6780

RADOMSKI, Sidney B; Univ Hlth Network-Toronto Western Hosp, MP8 304-399 Bathurst St, Toronto ON M5T 2S8; Tor'84; FRCSC; Urol (Impotence). Professor - Surgery, Toronto Western Hospital - University Health Network; Staff, Mount Sinai Hospital; Staff, Sunnybrook Health Sciences Centre; Prof, University of Toronto; (416)603-5713; Fax. (416)603-5391.

RADOS, Lawrence R; Misericordia Health Centre, 99 Cornish Ave, Winnipeg MB R3C 1A2; Man'89; CCFP; Staff, Misericordia Health Centre; (204)788-8364; Fax. (204)774-2075.

RADOUCO-THOMAS, Monelly; Inst U en Sante Mentale de QC, 2601 ch de la Canardiere, Quebec QC G1J 2G3; Laval'88; LMCC; CSPQ; FRCPC; Psy; Electroenceph (P.Q.). Staff, Institut Universitaire Sante; (418)663-5020; Fax. (418)661-6891.

RADOUX, Claude; Clinique Med St-Louis, 220-3165 ch Saint-Louis, Quebec QC G1W 4R4; Laval'71; Staff, Centre Hospitalier Universitaire de Québec (CHUQ) - Siege Social; (418)653-1970; Fax. (418)653-9956.

RADOUX, Victor; Centre Med Saint-Urbain, 409-3875 rue Saint-Urbain, Montreal QC H2W 1V1; McG'78; CSPQ; Rheum (P. Q.). Staff, Centre Hospitalier l'Université de Montréal (CHUM) - Hôtel-Dieu; Langs: English; (514)844-1105

RADOVIC, Tatjana; 3910 Hastings St E, Burnaby BC V5C 6C1; Bosnia-Hercegovina (Bosnia-Herzegovina)'90; CCFP; (604)299-4722

RADULOVIC, Dejana; St Boniface Gen Hosp, 409 Tache Ave, Winnipeg MB R2H 2A6; Man'03; FRCPC; DiagRad. Staff, St Boniface General Hospital; (204)233-8563

RADWAN, Farouk; CHUM-Hop Notre-Dame, 1560 rue Sherbrooke E, Montreal QC H2L 4M1; Laval'91; CSPQ; FRCPC; MedBiochem. Staff Nutritionist, Centre Hospitalier l'Université de Montréal (CHUM) - Hôtel-Dieu; Staff MedBiochem, Centre Hospitalier l'Université de Montréal (CHUM) - Hôpital Notre-Dame; Clinical Asst Prof Med, Universite de Montreal; Langs: English; Arabic; (514)890-8000 x27034; farouk.radwan.chum@ssss.gouv.qc.ca.

RADWAN, John S; The Credit Valley Hosp, 2200 Eglinton Ave W, Mississauga ON L5M 2N1; Warsaw (Poland)'79; FRCPC; RadOncol. Staff, The Credit Valley Hospital; Asst Prof, University of Western Ontario; Langs: Polish; (905)813-4532

RADWELL, Jyl; Royal Alexandra Hosp, 10240 Kingsway NW, Edmonton AB T5H 3V9; Sask'95; CCFP; CCFP(E.M.); Staff, Royal Alexandra Hospital; (780)735-4111

RADWI, Ghazala R H K; McMaster University, MDCL 3101A-1280 Main St W, Hamilton ON L8S 4K1; King Abdul Aziz Univ (Saudi Arabia)'02; IntMed.

RADZIMINSKI, Nicole A; PO Box 39034 Rpo Point Grey, Vancouver BC V6R 4P1; UBC'04; FRCPC; Peds. Langs: Spanish; (604)803-1575

RADZINSKI, Charles A; 404-960 Lawrence Ave W, North York ON M6A 3B5; Tor'85; FRCSC; Urol. Consultant, West Park Healthcare Centre; Staff Urol, Humber River Regional Hospital - Church Street Site; (416)256-2737; Fax. (416)256-9098.

RADZIUK, Jerry M; The Ottawa Hosp-Civic Campus, 1053 Carling Ave, Ottawa ON K1Y 4E9; McG'78; PhD; FRCPC; MedScient(Med). assoc Pers médical, McGill University Health Centre - Royal Victoria Hospital; Dir Clin Investigation Unit/Att Staff, The Ottawa Hospital - Civic Campus; Prof, University of Ottawa; Langs: Polish; French; (613)761-4112; jradziuk@ottawahospital.on.ca.

RAE, Christopher J; Lanark County Mental Health, 3-50 Bennett St, Carleton Place ON K7C 4J9; Qns'00; FRCPC; Psy. (613)283-8979; Fax. (613)257-8101.

RAE, Jennifer A; Queens University Health Centr, 146 Stuart St, Kingston ON K7L 3N6; McM'04; (613)533-2506; Fax. (613)533-6740.

RAE, Maureen P; The Westend Family Care Clinic, 80 Michael Cowpland Dr, Kanata ON K2M 1P6; McM'86; CCFP; FCFP; (613)599-3321

RAE, Randall J; Mount St Joseph Hosp, 3080 Prince Edward St, Vancouver BC V5T 3N4; Sask'86; FRCPC; Anes. Staff, Providence Health Care - Mount Saint Joseph Hospital; (604)877-8305

RAE, Robert E; 2024-400 Main St, Saint John NB E2K 4N5; Dal'77; FRCSC; Otol. Staff, Saint John Regional Hospital; Staff, St Joseph's Hospital; Assoc Lecturer, Dalhousie University; (506)658-1511; Fax. (506)658-1523; dr.rae.ent@gmail.com.

RAEDLER, Thomas Joseph; Health Research Innovation Ctr, 4D62-3280 Hospital Dr NW, Calgary AB T2N 4Z6; (Germany)'90; Staff, Foothills Medical Centre; (403)210-6899; Fax. (403)210-9114.

RAFAIL, Ehab A; Turnbull Diagnostic Imaging, 170 Simcoe St, Peterborough ON K9H 2H7; Cairo (Egypt)'67; MB ChB; FRCPC; DiagRad. Staff, Peterborough Regional Health Centre - Hospital Drive; Langs: Arabic; (705)742-3639; Fax. (705)742-8389.

RAFAT ZAND, Khashayar; MUHC-Montreal Gen Hosp, C5 118-1650 av Cedar, Montreal QC H3G 1A4; (Iran)'00; FRCPC; DiagRad. Staff, McGill University Health Centre - Montreal General Campus; (514)934-8084

RAFAY, Afshan; New Best Care Med Centre, 4-790 Burnhamthorpe Rd W, Mississauga ON L5C 4G3; Punjab (Pakistan)'90; MB BS; CCFP; Staff, New Best Care Medical Centre; Langs: Urdu; Punjabi; Hindi; (905)848-8686; arafay@sasktel.net.

RAFAY, Mubeen F; Health Sciences Centre, AE308-820 Sherbrook St, Winnipeg MB R3A 1R9; Sind (Pakistan)'87; Staff, Health Sciences Centre; Langs: Urdu; Punjabi.

RAFF, Errol; Baker Clinic, 290-10405 Jasper Ave NW, Edmonton AB T5J 1G5; Cape Town (South Africa)'84; FRCPC; IntMed. Staff, Sturgeon Community Hospital; Staff IntMed, Royal Alexandra Hospital; (780)944-9590; Fax. (780)944-1165.

RAFFA, Hacene; CSSS de Chicoutimi, 305 rue Saint-Vallier, Chicoutimi QC G7H 5H6; (Algeria)'76; Complexe hospitalier de la Sagamie; Staff, Institut Roland-Saucier; (418)549-5474; Fax. (418)549-8143.

RAFFARD, Skye; Cariboo Mem Hosp, 401-517 Sixth Ave N, Williams Lake BC V2G 2G8; UBC'93; BSc; FRCSC; ObstGyn (Gynecologic Oncology). Staff, Cariboo Memorial Hospital and Health Centre; Clin Instructor Dept of Obst & Gyn, University of British Columbia; (250)398-8280; Fax. (250)398-8287; skye_raffard@telus.net.

RAFFERTY, James L; North Queen's Health Centre, RR 1 Queens County, Caledonia NS B0T 1B0; Dal'74; BSc; CCFP; Assoc Medical Staff, Queens General Hospital; Chair, Southwest and Valley District Health Authorities; Chair, Services Review Advisory Committee Addictions South Shore; (902)682-2533; Fax. (902)682-3446.

RAFFLE, Valerie J; Windsor Square Shopp Centre, 240-1959 152 St, Surrey BC V4A 9E3; UBC'86; Staff, Peace Arch Hospital; (604)531-0888; Fax. (604)531-0881.

RAFFOUL, Joseph I; SMBD Jewish Gen Hosp, 3755 ch Cote-Sainte-Catherine, Montreal QC H3T 1E2; McG'89; FRCPC; IntMed. Staff, Sir Mortimer B Davis Jewish General; (514)340-8222 x7596

RAFI-ZADEH, Ebrahim; Lonsdale Med Dental Bldg, 105-1940 Lonsdale Ave, North Vancouver BC V7M 2K2; Tehran (Iran)'56; AACP; FRCPC; IntMed (Allergy & Immunology). (604)980-2478

RAFILOVICH, Seda S; Thunder Bay Reg HSC-T-Bay, 980 Oliver Rd, Thunder Bay ON P7B 6V4; Russian State Med Univ (Russia (Federation))'91; FRCPC; IntMed. Staff, Thunder Bay Regional Health Sciences Centre; (807)684-6030

RAFIQ, Arif; The Moncton Hosp, 135 MacBeath Ave, Moncton NB E1C 6Z8; Karachi (Pakistan)'96; FRCPC; Anes. Staff, The Moncton Hospital; (506)857-5520

RAFIQ, Fizza Z; Trans Canada Med Centre, 152-1440 52 St NE, Calgary AB T2A 4T8; (Pakistan)'96; MB BS; CCFP; Langs: Urdu; Punjabi; Hindi; (403)272-3627; Fax. (403)272-3647.

RAFIQ, Suraiya; Physicians Incorporated, 202-316 Willow St, Truro NS B2N 5A4; Madras (India)'88; MB BS; CCFP; Staff, Colchester East Hants Health Centre; (902)896-0550; Fax. (902)896-0551.

RAFIQ, Zahid; Trans Canada Med Centre, 152-1440 52 St NE, Calgary AB T2A 4T8; (Pakistan)'90; MB BS; CCFP; (403)272-3627; Fax. (403)272-3647.

RAFIQI, Wajahat H; 15 Allan Dr, Bolton ON L7E 2B5; Kashmir (India)'80; CCFP; (905)951-1234; Fax. (905)951-6090.

RAFLA, Miriam; Creditview Medical, B 14-1240 Eglinton Ave W, Mississauga ON L5V 1N3; Ain Shams (Egypt)'83; CCFP; (905)567-4622; Fax. (905)567-7545.

RAFUSE, Paul E; 208-6112 Quinpool Rd, Halifax NS B3L 1A3; Cal'88; PhD(Pharm); FRCSC; Ophth (Cataract). Consultant, IWK Health Centre; Ac Staff, Queen Elizabeth II Health Sciences Centre - Victoria General Site; Assoc Prof Ophth, Dalhousie University; (902)422-8353; Fax. (902)423-5069; prafuse@dal.ca.

RAGAN, Edward; 150 Billings Ave, Ottawa ON K1H 5K9; Wes'65; MPH(Johns Hopkins); BA; (613)737-3939; Fax. (613)737-0146.

RAGAZ, Joseph; 218-809 41st Ave W, Vancouver BC V5Z 2N6; London (England)'70; MB BS; LRCP; MRCS(Eng); IntMed (Breast Cancer). (604)569-2440; joseph.ragaz@muhc.mcgill.ca.

RAGAZ, Stephan C; Turnbull Med Bldg, 203-170 Simcoe St, Peterborough ON K9H 2H7; Berne (Switzerland)'76; CCFP; FCFP; Ac Staff, Peterborough Regional Health Centre - Hospital Drive; Langs: German; French; (705)743-3837; Fax. (705)740-7594; sragaz@prhc.on.ca.

RAGGI, Paolo; Mazankowski Alberta Heart Inst, 4A7.050-8440 112 St NW, Edmonton AB T6G 2B7; (Italy)'85; Staff, Mazankowski Alberta Heart Institute; (780)407-4575; Fax. (780)407-7834.

RAGHAVAN, Natya; Hamilton HS-General Site, 422-237 Barton St E, Hamilton ON L8L 2X2; McG'05; FRCPC; IntMed; Respir. Staff, St Joseph's Healthcare - Charlton Campus; Staff, Hamilton Health Sciences Centre - Hamilton General Hospital; (905)521-2100

RAGHAVAN, Prathapakumar T; PO Box 20017 Stn Sahali Mall, Kamloops BC V2C 6X1; Kerala (India)'88; FRCPC; PhysMed&Rehab. (250)374-5111

RAGHAVAN, Ramya; 303-13291 Yonge St, Richmond Hill ON L4E 4L6; McG'00; FRCPC; IntMed; Cardiol. (905)751-2941; Fax. (905)751-0107.

RAGHAVAN, Sai L; PO Box 69 Stn Main, Porters Lake NS B3E 1M1; Dal'89; CCFP; Staff, Twin Oaks Memorial Hospital; Staff, IWK Health Centre; Staff Privil, Cobequid Emergency Centre; (902)827-2255

RAGHAVENDRAN, Sreekrishna; University of Manitoba, 671 William Ave, Winnipeg MB R3E 0Z2; Dr M G R Medical University (India)'93; FRCPC; Anes.

RAGHAVJI, Allatif A; 1861 Meadowbrook Dr SE, Airdrie AB T4A 1V3; Nairobi (Kenya)'79; (403)948-3636; Fax. (403)948-3228.

RAGHEB, Bahaa G; Place Centrum Med Centre, 207-210 Centrum Blvd, Orleans ON K1E 3V7; Ain Shams (Egypt)'78; CCFP; Langs: Arabic; French; (613)830-5658; Fax. (613)834-3227.

RAGHEB, Salah R G; 6951 Westminster Hwy, Richmond BC V7C 1C6; Cairo (Egypt)'65; MRCS(Eng); LRCP(Lond); FRCS; Langs: Arabic; (604)279-7519; Fax. (604)279-7698; salahragheb@hotmail.com.

RAGHIG, Abdulhakim M; Univ of Regina Allied Hlth Ctr, 3737 Wascana Pky, Regina SK S4S 0A2; Al-Fateh (Libya)'00; FRCPC; Neur. (306)337-2646; Fax. (306)337-3192.

RAGHUBIR, Kushal V; 215-3447 Kennedy Rd, Scarborough ON M1V 3S1; West Indies (Jamaica)'88; MB BS; FRCPC; Peds (Neonatology). Staff, The Scarborough Hospital - Birchmount Campus; (416)335-9804; Fax. (416)335-9805.

RAGHURAMAN, Anusha; 649 Sheppard Ave W, North York ON M3H 2S4; Madras (India)'79; MB BS; MRCPsy(UK); FRCPC; Psy (Child & Adolescent Psychiatry). Staff, North York General Hospital - Branson Division; Staff, North York General Hospital; Langs: Bengali; (416)633-9420 x2042

RAGHURAMAN, Varadarajan; Sheppard Associates, 649 Sheppard Ave W, North York ON M3H 2S4; Madras (India)'78; MB BS; DPM; MRCPsy(UK); FRCPC; Psy (Adult Psychiatry). Staff, North York General Hospital - Branson Division; Langs: Tamil; (416)630-0610; Fax. (416)398-5712.

RAGNAUTH, D Reginald; Whitbourne Med Clinic, PO Box 179, Whitbourne NL A0B 3K0; RCS (Ireland)'70; LRCPS; (709)759-2800

RAGONETTI, Christopher H; Joseph Brant Mem Hosp, PO Box 93156 Rpo Headon 1230 North Shore Blvd E, Burlington ON L7S 1W7; McM'91; CCFP; FCFP; Staff, Joseph Brant Memorial Hospital; (905)632-3730

RAGOS, Glenn A; North York Gen Hosp, 4001 Leslie St, North York ON M2K 1E1; Qns'97; FRCPC; Anes. Staff, North York General Hospital; (416)756-6000

RAHA, Ronjon; The Credit Valley Hosp, 2200 Eglinton Ave W, Mississauga ON L5M 2N1; Tor'00; FRCPC; DiagRad. Staff, The Credit Valley Hospital; (905)813-4532

RAHAL, Akram; 5775 boul Leger, Montreal-Nord QC H1G 1K7; Mon'98; FRCSC; Otol. (514)327-4040; Fax. (514)327-9001.

RAHAL, Deric P; MUHC-Royal Victoria Hosp, 687 av des Pins O, Montreal QC H3A 1A1; McG'73; Cardiol; IntMed. Ac Staff, McGill University Health Centre - Royal Victoria Hospital; (514)843-1604

RAHAL, Hussain A; 1883 Bank St, Ottawa ON K1V 7Z9; Ott'89; (613)739-3044; Fax. (613)739-4995; hairdoc@gmail.com.

RAHAL, Kamaljit; West Oaks Med Centre, 310-32700 Fraser Way S, Abbotsford BC V2T 4M5; Sydney (Australia)'01; CCFP; (604)557-9938

RAHALKAR, Mangal R; 239 George St, Sarnia ON N7T 4P1; Pune (India)'75; MB BS; DA(Eng.); CCFP; FCFP; Staff, Bluewater Health - Mitton Site; Staff, Bluewater Health - Norman Site; (519)337-9931; Fax. (519)337-9936.

RAHAMAN, Omar S; Meadowalrk Health Centre, 154 Meadowlark Shopping Ctr NW, Edmonton AB T5R 5W9; Dom.Rep. (Dominican Republic)'98; CCFP; (780)429-4761; Fax. (780)425-4274.

RAHAMAN, Sheriff; Normanview Mall Med Clinic, 330 McCarthy Blvd N, Regina SK S4R 7M2; Dublin (Ireland)'64; MB ChB; BAO; DPH(Tor); (306)924-6200; Fax. (306)924-6201.

RAHBAOUI, Ahmed; Hopital Regional D'Edmundston, 275 boul Hebert, Edmundston NB E3V 4E4; Casablanca (Morocco)'96; Staff, Hôpital regional d'Edmundston; (506)739-2200

RAHEEL, Erum; North Oshawa Med Centre, 1400 Ritson Rd N, Oshawa ON L1G 7W4; Karachi (Pakistan)'97; CCFP; (905)433-1895

RAHEMTULLA, Amir; BC Cancer Agency-Vancouver CC, 600 10th Ave W, Vancouver BC V5Z 4E6; Cambridge (England)'90; Staff, BC Cancer Agency Vancouver Centre; (604)877-6000

RAHIL, Preetinder S; Arbour Med Centre, 281 Stone Rd E, Guelph ON N1G 5J5; Vellore (India)'03; CCFP; (519)823-5133; Fax. (519)827-0255.

RAHIM, Alya; Downtown Toronto Doctors, 630-790 Bay St, Toronto ON M5G 1N8; Tor'04; CCFP; (647)427-6001; Fax. (416)598-4659.

RAHIM, Sherali A; Oshawa Clinic, 117 King St E, Oshawa ON L1H 1B9; McM'02; FRCPC; IntMed; Cardiol. Staff, Lakeridge Health - Oshawa Site; Staff, St Michael's Hospital; (905)721-6151

RAHIM, Yasmin H; Southlake Reg Health Centre, 596 Davis Dr, Newmarket ON L3Y 2P9; Karachi (Pakistan)'81; FRCPC; IntMed; MedOncol; Hem. Staff Hematology, Sunnybrook Health Sciences Centre; Staff, Southlake Regional Health Centre; Staff HemOncol, Toronto East General Hospital Inc; Teach Staff, University of Toronto; Langs: Gujarati; (905)895-4521; Fax. (905)952-2818; yrahi@tegh.on.ca.

RAHIM, Zulficar K; Surrey Med Arts Bldg, 103-13798 94A Ave, Surrey BC V3V 1N1; Makerere (Uganda)'72; MB ChB; FRCPC; Derm. Staff, Surrey Memorial Hospital; Staff, Peace Arch Hospital; (604)581-0111

RAHIMI, Abdulwali S; Grand Family Health Organizati, 4-75 Parkview Rd, Hagersville ON N0A 1H0; Marathwada Univ (India)'02; (905)768-9540; Fax. (905)538-1274.

RAHIMI, Farid A; Mission Oaks Med Centre, 32136 Lougheed Hwy, Mission BC V2V 1A4; (Germany)'93; Langs: Farsi; Dari; German; (604)826-7996

RAHIMI, Kurosh; CHUM-Hop Notre-Dame, 1560 rue Sherbrooke E, Montreal QC H2L 4M1; Teheran (Iran)'94; FRCPC; AnatPath. Staff, Centre Hospitalier l'Université de Montréal (CHUM) - Hôpital Notre-Dame; (514)890-8000 x25765

RAHIMI-DARABAD, Mehdi; Southlake Reg Health Centre, 596 Davis Dr, Newmarket ON L3Y 2P9; Tehran (Iran)'02; FRCSC; GenSurg. Staff, Southlake Regional Health Centre; (905)895-4521

RAHIMI DARABAD, Parisa; Unicare Clinic, 401-1100 Sheppard Ave E, North York ON M2K 2W1; Teheran (Iran)'99; FRCPC; IntMed; Respir. Staff, Thunder Bay Regional Health Sciences Centre; Staff, Sunnybrook Health Sciences Centre; (416)548-9701; Fax. (416)548-9702.

RAHIMINEJAD, Farhad; Peace Arch Hosp, 15521 Russell Ave, White Rock BC V4B 2R4; (Iran)'86; CCFP; Staff, Peace Arch Hospital; (778)985-7260

RAHIMPOUR, Raoufeh; Halton Family Health Centre, 2951 Walker's Line, Burlington ON L7M 4Y1; McM'92.

RAHIMPOUR, Roya; Mississauga Med Centre, 418-1420 Burnhamthorpe Rd, Mississauga ON L4X 2Z9; McM'87; Langs: Persian; French; (905)629-1006

RAHMAN, Abdul; Richmond Road Diag & Trmt Ctr, 1820 Richmond Rd SW, Calgary AB T2T 5C7; Karachi (Pakistan)'81; MB BS; MRCPsy(Lond); LMCC; FRCPC; Psy. Staff, Alberta Children's Hospital; Consultant Psy/Head, Section of Child Psychiatry; Clinical Asst Prof, University of Calgary; Langs: Urdu; Punjabi; Hindi; (403)955-8344; kidsdoctor@hotmail.com.

RAHMAN, Adam N; St Joseph's Health Care, PO Box 577 Stn B 268 Grosvenor St, London ON N6A 4V2; Mem'04; FRCPC; IntMed; Gastroent. Staff, St Joseph's Hospital - St Joseph's Health Care; (905)684-7271

RAHMAN, Al-Amin M P; St Clare's Mercy Hosp, 1-154 Lemarchant Rd, St. John's NL A1C 5B8; Mem'90; MSc; Rheum; IntMed. Staff, St Clare's Mercy Hospital; Prof Med, Memorial University Of Newfoundland; (709)777-5736; Fax. (709)777-5212.

RAHMAN, Amaly; 7217A-11402 University Ave NW, Edmonton AB T6G 2J3; Maryland (USA)'03; FRCPC; Peds; PedEmergMed. (780)407-3667

RAHMAN, Diruba; South Shore Reg Hosp, 90 Glen Allan Dr, Bridgewater NS B4V 3S6; Dhaka (Bangladesh)'99; Staff, South Shore Regional Hospital; (902)543-4603; Fax. (902)527-5269.

RAHMAN, Faisal; St Martha's Reg Hosp, 25 Bay St, Antigonish NS B2G 2G5; Karachi (Pakistan)'91; MB; BSc; Staff, St Martha's Regional Hospital; (902)863-2830; Fax. (902)863-4496.

RAHMAN, Jennifer W; Tuxedo Park Shopping Centre, 221-2025 Corydon Ave, Winnipeg MB R3P 0N5; Man'97; FRCSC; Ophth.

RAHMAN, K M Anisur; North Woodlands Med Centre, 204-40 Shellington Pl, Brantford ON N3S 0C5; Dhaka (Bangladesh)'02; CCFP; (519)759-6116

RAHMAN, Mohammad M; Selkirk Mental Health Centre, PO Box 9600 Stn Main 825 Manitoba Ave, Selkirk MB R1A 2B5; Dhaka (Bangladesh)'59; MB BS; DTMH(Eng); FRCP; Staff, Elizabeth M Crowe Memorial Hospital; Staff, Selkirk Mental Health Centre; Langs: Bengali; Urdu; (204)482-3810; mrahman@irha.mb.ca.

RAHMAN, Muhammad Z; 5111 Northland Dr NW PO Box 67216 Rpo Northland Vlg, Calgary AB T2L 2L2; Punjab (Pakistan)'92; Staff, St. Paul (St. Therese) Healthcare Centre.

RAHMAN, Riffat Ur; Windsor Health Centre, 117-700 Tecumseh Rd E, Windsor ON N8X 4T2; Punjab (India)'84; FRCPC; Peds. (519)258-2553; Fax. (519)252-2857.

RAHMAN, Samina M; Saddletowne Med Clinic, 914 Saddletowne Cir NE, Calgary AB T3J 0H5; (India)'03; CCFP; (403)590-7710; Fax. (403)590-7113.

RAHMAN, Sana; Milliken Med Centre, 17-5651 Steeles Ave E, Scarborough ON M1V 5P6; Ott'09; CCFP; (416)291-6323; Fax. (416)291-0890.

RAHMAN, Shafiur; 1135 Adelaide St N, London ON N5Y 4J7; Chittagong (Bangladesh)'88.

RAHMAN, Zia U; Harbour South Med Clinic, 235 Main St, Yarmouth NS B5A 1E1; Dhaka (Bangladesh)'90; Staff, Roseway Hospital; (902)742-8333

RAHMANI, Armita; Kingston Gen Hosp, 76 Stuart St, Kingston ON K7L 2V7; Ott'99; CCFP; CCFP(E.M.); Staff, QHC Belleville General; Staff, Kingston General Hospital; (613)548-2368

RAHMANI, M Rose; 520-790 Bay St, Toronto ON M5G 1N8; Cape Town (South Africa)'78; DABR; FRCPC; DiagRad (Radiology Ultrasanol). Langs: English; French; (416)260-9739

RAHMANI, Mohammad F; Taylor Street Med Clinic, 3020 Taylor St E, Saskatoon SK S7H 4J2; Karachi (Pakistan)'85; FRCPC; Psy. (306)374-8082

RAHMANI GORJI, Anna P; St Paul's Hosp, 5912-1081 Burrard St, Vancouver BC V6Z 1Y6; UBC'05; FRCPC; IntMed. Staff, Providence Health Care - St Paul's Hospital; (604)806-8668

RAHMEH, Tarek; Saint John Reg Hosp, PO Box 2100 Stn Main 400 University Ave, Saint John NB E2L 4L2; Damascus (Syria)'97; Staff, Saint John Regional Hospital; (506)648-6000

RAHMILEVICH, Elena; CSSS de Portneuf, 700 rue Saint-Cyrille, Saint-Raymond QC G3L 1W1; Laval'09; CCFP; Staff, Centre Hospitalier Portneuf; (418)337-4611

RAHMOUNI, Dalia; Hop Charles LeMoyne, 3120 boul Taschereau, Greenfield Park QC J4V 2H1; Mon'95; CSPQ; DiagRad. Staff, Hopital Charles LeMoyne; (450)466-5000 x2030

RAHN, Andrea R; Hinton Med Clinic, 102 Allen Cove, Hinton AB T7V 2A6; McM'09; CCFP; (780)865-3338; Fax. (780)865-2024.

RAHN, Raymond J; Lennox & Addington Gen Hosp, 222-8 Richmond Park Dr, Napanee ON K7R 2Z4; Qns'80; GenSurg. Gen Surgeon, Lennox & Addington County General Hospital; (613)354-8240; Fax. (613)354-8241; raymondrahn@live.com.

RAHNAVARDI, Katayoun; Woodlawn Med Clinic, 92 Main St, Dartmouth NS B2X 1R5; (Iran)'94; CCFP; Langs: Persian; (902)434-1500; Fax. (902)462-8464.

RAHNEMA, Nazanine; 303-301 Columbia St E, New Westminster BC V3L 3W5; McG'04; CCFP; CCFP(E.M.); (604)525-5388

RAI, Amendeep S; AIM Health Group, 1657 Dundas St E, London ON N5W 3C6; Oakland (USA)'08; (519)455-8210

RAI, Avtar S; 8503 39A Ave NW, Edmonton AB T6K 3R8; Punjab (India)'75; (780)462-3008; Fax. (780)462-3008.

RAI, D Kimit; Columbia Med Bldg, 405-301 Columbia St E, New Westminster BC V3L 3W5; Madras (India)'65; MB BS; DAB; FRCSC; PlasSurg (Cosmetic Surgery). Ac Staff, Royal Columbian Hospital; Ac Staff, Eagle Ridge Hospital & Health Care Centre; (604)522-2925; Fax. (604)522-1422; kimit_rai@telus.net.

RAI, Gurinder S; Halton HCS Corp-Georgetown, 1 Princess Anne Dr, Georgetown ON L7G 2B8; West Indies (Trinidad & Tobago)'99; MB BS; CCFP; (905)873-0111

RAI, Inderpreet S; Queen Street Med Clinic, 505 Queen St, Spruce Grove AB T7X 2V2; West Indies (Jamaica)'06; CCFP; (780)962-2001

RAI, Jagtar S; 101-6905 120 St, Delta BC V4E 2A8; Glasgow (Scotland)'84; Staff, Surrey Memorial Hospital; (604)590-4966; Fax. (604)590-3855.

RAI, Kuljinder K; 101-6905 120 St, Delta BC V4E 2A8; Man'87; (604)590-4966; Fax. (604)590-3855.

RAI, Kulwant; 217-11433 Lonsdale Ave, North Vancouver BC V7M 2H9; Lucknow (India)'62; MB BS; MRCS; DPM; MRCPsy; LRCP; (604)984-8480; kulwantrai@shaw.ca.

RAI, Pardeep S; 7170 120 St, Surrey BC V3W 3M8; Saba (Netherlands Antilles)'08; (604)597-7770

RAI, Prem K K; Medical Bldg, 345-600 Tecumseh Rd E, Windsor ON N8X 4X9; Mysore (India)'73; MB BS; DA(UK); FRCPC; Psy. Consultant Psy, Hôtel-Dieu Grace Hospital; Consultant Psy, Windsor Regional Hospital - Metropolitan Site; (519)252-0555; Fax. (519)977-9503.

RAI, Santoch S; 26F-10004 104 Ave NW, Edmonton AB T5J 0K1; (England)'87; MB ChB; Staff, Alberta Hospital Edmonton; (780)342-6400; Fax. (780)426-7272.

RAI, Sharadindu; Hyde Park Med & Walk-In Clin, 4-640 Hyde Park Rd, London ON N6H 3S1; Qns'06; CCFP; (519)641-3627; Fax. (519)641-3628.

RAI, Sundeep; Canadian Place Endoscopy, 123-1065 Canadian Pl, Mississauga ON L4W 0C2; Qns'03; MSc; FRCSC; GenSurg; Critical Care Medicine. Surgeon, The Credit Valley Hospital; (416)626-2100; Fax. (416)620-7874; endoscopynow@gmail.com.

RAI, Vasanth; Miramichi Reg Hosp, 500 Water St, Miramichi NB E1V 3G5; Mangalore (India)'68; Staff, Miramichi Regional Hospital; (506)857-5520

RAI, Veena P K; Tecumseh Med Centre, 106-11811 Tecumseh Rd E, Windsor ON N8N 4M7; Mysore (India)'76; MB BS; (519)735-9844; Fax. (519)735-2132.

RAICHE, Evelyne; Clinique Med 24 Juin, 1055 12e av N, Sherbrooke QC J1E 2X4; Sher'06; ObstGyn. (819)563-2027

RAICHE, Isabelle M M; The Ottawa Hosp-Civic Campus, 327-1053 Carling Ave, Ottawa ON K1Y 4E9; Laval'05; FRCSC; GenSurg. (613)798-5555

RAICHE-MARSDEN, Michelle D; Woodlawn Med Clinic, 92 Main St, Dartmouth NS B2X 1R5; Dal'92; (902)434-1500; Fax. (902)434-4368.

RAICHURA, Kalpesh A; Marketplace Med Centre, 3201 Greenbank Rd, Nepean ON K2J 4H9; Man'92; Staff, Canadian Forces Health Services Centre; (613)825-1636; Fax. (613)825-5521.

RAIKHLIN, Anton; Univ of Toronto, 112A-150 College St, Toronto ON M5S 3E2; Tor'07; FRCPC; DiagRad. (416)978-8797

RAILTON, Craig J; London HSC-Victoria Hosp, PO Box 5010 Stn B D2 315-800 Commissioners Rd E, London ON N6A 5W9; Tor'00; BSc; FRCPC; Anes (Clinical Pharmacology). Staff, London Health Sciences Centre - Victoria Campus; Staff Consultant Anes, London Health Sciences Centre - South Street; (519)685-8500 x58525; Fax. (519)685-8275.

RAILTON, Karl T; Southlake Reg Health Cetnre, 596 Davis Dr, Newmarket ON L3Y 2P9; Ott'93; Anes. Staff, Southlake Regional Health Centre; (905)895-4521 x6783

RAILTON, Richard H; Medical Arts Bldg, E-165 Plymouth Rd, Welland ON L3B 3E1; Tor'55; FACS; FRCSC; GenSurg (Wound Care). (905)732-6181; Fax. (905)732-6182; rhrailton@live.ca.

RAIMAN, Julian A J; The Hosp for Sick Children, 555 University Ave, Toronto ON M5G 1X8; London (England)'92; MB BS; MSc; MRCP; Staff Metabolic Genetics, The Hospital For Sick Children; (416)813-5340; Fax. (416)813-4940.

RAIMONDI, Christina J; Prairie Trail Med Centre, 100-1345 Taylor Ave, Winnipeg MB R3M 3Y9; Man'04; CCFP; (204)475-0088

RAIMONDO, F Emilio; 2-100 Martindale Rd, St Catharines ON L2S 2Y3; Wes'81; FRCPC; IntMed (Cardiology). Consultant, Niagara Health System - St Catharines General Site; Teach Staff, McMaster University; Hon Lecturer, University of Western Ontario; Langs: Italian; (905)937-2011; Fax. (905)937-4520; reception@lakeshorecardiology.com.

RAINA, Raj Brinder S; Health Centre, 715 12th Ave W, Vancouver BC V5Z 1M9; Kashmir (India)'80; FRCPC; Psy. Dir Postgrad Educ Training, Vancouver General Hospital - Centennial Pavillion; (604)875-4111 x54104; Fax. (604)875-4708.

RAINBOW, Sandra M; 5909 Veterans Memorial Lane, Halifax NS B3H 2E2; Dal'10; CCFP; (902)473-4744

RAINE, Todd A; St Paul's Hosp, 1081 Burrard St, Vancouver BC V6Z 1Y6; Dal'01; CCFP; CCFP(E.M.); Staff, Providence Health Care - St Paul's Hospital; (604)682-2344

RAINHAM, David C; Northfield Family Health Ctre, 206-99 Northfield Dr E, Waterloo ON N2K 3P9; Cardiff (Wales)'68; Physician, Grand River Hospital - Freeport Site; Med Dir, Trinity Village Care Centre; Med Dir, Nithview Home for the Aged; Asst Prof Family Med, University of Western Ontario; (519)579-4612; Fax. (519)744-1197.

RAINIER-POPE, Nick; Royal Inland Hosp, 311 Columbia St, Kamloops BC V2C 2T1; Cape Town (South Africa)'92; MB BS; DCH; CCFP; CCFP(E.M.); FCFP; Staff Gen Practice & EmergMed, Royal Inland Hospital; (250)314-2425; nrpope@shaw.ca.

RAINKIE, Kristopher D; Ross Mem Hosp, 10 Angeline St N, Lindsay ON K9V 4M8; Wes'04; CCFP; Staff, Ross Memorial Hospital; (705)324-6111

RAINVILLE, Ginette D M; Real Med Corp, 101 Joseph St, Pembroke ON K8A 8C9; Ott'05; CCFP; (613)732-6662; Fax. (613)732-6666.

RAINVILLE, J C Bruno; Regie l'Assurance Maladie QC, 1125 Grande Allee O, Quebec QC G1S 1E7; Mon'91; FRCSC; GenSurg. Staff, Centre Hospitalier Jonquiere; Langs: Spanish; English; (418)682-5144 x4116

RAINVILLE, Josee; CHUM-Hop Notre-Dame, 1560 rue Sherbrooke E, Montreal QC H2L 4M1; Mon'00; CCFP; Staff, Centre Hospitalier l'Université de Montréal (CHUM) - Hôpital Notre-Dame; (514)890-8000

RAISON, Bradford W; 3550 Valleyview Rd, Penticton BC V2A 8W9; Alb'76; CCFP; CCFP(E.M.); (250)492-3621

RAISSI, Behirokh; Innovations Health Clinic, 106-11420 27 St SE, Calgary AB T2Z 3R6; (Iran)'98; CCFP; (587)352-8718; Fax. (587)352-8728.

RAIZEN, Marilyn; Children's Hosp, 840 Sherbrook St, Winnipeg MB R3A 1S1; Man'85; FRCPC; Peds. Staff, Health Sciences Centre.

RAIZMAN, Alla; Niagara H System-G Niagara, PO Box 1018 Stn Main 5546 Portage Rd, Niagara Falls ON L2E 6X2; (Uzbekistan)'84; (905)378-4647

RAJ, Sakina; 11-7750 Ranchview Dr NW, Calgary AB T3G 1Y9; (India)'85; MB BS; MScEpidemiol; CCFP; Langs: Urdu; Punjabi; Arabic; (403)452-6240; Fax. (403)452-9626; rajsakina@hotmail.com.

RAJA, Asim J; 200 Meadowlark Shopping Ctr NW, Edmonton AB T5R 5W9; Alb'05; FRCPC; DiagRad. (780)489-7851

RAJA, Faisal S; St Mary's Gen Hosp, 911 Queen Blvd, Kitchener ON N2M 1B2; Tor'00; FRCPC; DiagRad;CCFP; CCFP(E.M.); Staff, St Mary's General Hospital; Langs: Punjabi; French; Urdu; (519)749-6455

RAJA, Mohan K; 40 Shellington Pl, Brantford ON N3S 0C5; Wes'07; CCFP; (519)753-9581

RAJA, Sumaira Jamal; 2951 Walkers Line, Burlington ON L7M 4Y1; Karachi (Pakistan)'89; CCFP; (905)336-9615; Fax. (905)336-9650.

RAJAB, Khaled A M; R J A Medicentres Cnd Inc, 204-10458 Mayfield Rd NW, Edmonton AB T5P 4P4; Al Fateh (Libya)'01; MB BCh; CCFP; (780)483-7115

RAJABALE, Mahmud A; 41 Grand Ave W, Chatham ON N7L 1B4; Ain Shams (Egypt)'81; FRCPC; IntMed. (519)397-4753; Fax. (519)397-4518.

RAJABALI, Sultaneih S P; 214-624 Sixth St, New Westminster BC V3L 3C4; UBC'74; Assoc Staff, Royal Columbian Hospital; Langs: Hindi; Urdu; Gujarati; Swahili; (604)522-0688; Fax. (604)522-0522.

RAJABI-ASL, Akbar; 204 St Clair Ave W, Toronto ON M4V 1R2; Tabriz (Iran)'87; MD; FRCPC; Psy (Psychoanalysis). Staff, Rouge Valley Health System - Centenary Health Centre Site; Langs: Persian; Azeri; (416)921-1500; Fax. (416)921-1503.

RAJABIEH SHAYAN, Yasaman; Hôpital Ste-Justine, 3175 ch Cote-Sainte-Catherine, Montreal QC H3T 1C5; McG'08; Peds. Staff, Hôpital Ste-Justine; (514)345-4931

RAJADURAI, Sivaseelan; Avenida Bonavista Shopp Ctre, 315-12445 Lake Fraser Dr SE, Calgary AB T2J 7A4; New South Wales (Australia)'99; CCFP; (403)723-2453; Fax. (403)723-2463.

RAJAGOPA, Aarthi; London HSC-Victoria Hosp, PO Box 5010 Stn B 800 Commissioners Rd E, London ON N6A 5W9; Mumbai (India)'02; Staff, London Health Sciences Centre - Victoria Campus; (519)667-6778

RAJAGOPAL, Sudhashree; The Credit Valley Hosp, 2200 Eglinton Ave W, Mississauga ON L5M 2N1; McM'87; FRCPC; IntMed; MedOncol. Staff, The Credit Valley Hospital; (905)813-2200 x5135; Fax. (905)813-4024.

RAJAGOPALAN, Ashwyn; Office of the Chief Coroner, 26 Grenville St, Toronto ON M7A 2G9; Qns'07; FRCPC; AnatPath. Physician, Office of the Chief Coroner; (416)314-4040

RAJAGOPAUL, Kreasan; Niagara Falls Med Centre, 302-6453 Morrison St, Niagara Falls ON L2E 7H1; Natal (South Africa)'86; MB ChB; LMCC; FRCSC; GenSurg. (905)357-4800; Fax. (905)357-9800.

RAJAH, Rashid; Glazier Med Centre, 11 Gibb St, Oshawa ON L1H 2J9; Witwatersrand (South Africa)'77; MB ChB; FRCPC; Peds. Staff, Lakeridge Health - Oshawa Site; (905)579-1212; Fax. (905)579-7290.

RAJAKESARI, Meenalosany; Clinique Med Lanka, 107-5871 av Victoria, Montreal QC H3W 2R7; (Sri Lanka)'70; (514)344-2553

RAJAKUMAR, Alphonsus R J; Saskatchewan Heart Centre, 401 Packham Pl, Saskatoon SK S7N 2T7; Peradeniya (Sri Lanka)'71; MB BS; FACC; FRCPC; IntMed (Cardiovascular Medicine); Cardiol. Staff Cardiol, Royal University Hospital; (306)956-2500; Fax. (306)956-2501.

RAJAKUMAR, Derek D; Smyth Pediatrics Group, 220-1929 Russell Rd, Ottawa ON K1G 4G5; Sask'07; FRCPC; Peds. (613)737-7707; Fax. (613)737-4867.

RAJAKUMAR, Gwendoline S; Ellesmere Health Care Centre, 1-2060 Ellesmere Rd, Scarborough ON M1H 2V6; Colombo (Sri Lanka)'76; MB BS; CCFP; FCFP; (416)439-2273

RAJALA, Jennifer L; Gordon & Leslie Diamond HCC, 9F-2775 Laurel St, Vancouver BC V5Z 1M9; Alb'07; FRCPC; IntMed. Staff, Vancouver General Hospital - Centennial Pavillion; Staff, Gordon & Leslie Diamond Health Care Centre; (604)320-3712

RAJAMANICKAM, Sendhan; Univ Hlth Network-Toronto Western Hosp, 399 Bathurst St, Toronto ON M5T 2S8; (India)'98; Staff, Toronto Western Hospital - University Health Network; (416)603-2581; sendhan.rajamanickam@uhn.on.ca.

RAJAMOHAN, Chinniampalayam; St Boniface Gen Hosp, 409 Tache Ave, Winnipeg MB R2H 2A6; (India)'94; FRCPC; Anes. Staff, St Boniface General Hospital; (204)233-8563

RAJAN, Andrew I; 1760 Tecumseh Rd W, Windsor ON N9B 1V2; Wes'83; BSc(Hon); MSc(Biochem); Court Staff, Hôtel-Dieu Grace Hospital; Court Staff, Windsor Regional Hospital - Tayfour Site; (519)254-6457

RAJAN, Aziza A; Newmarket Med Place, 306-712 Davis Dr, Newmarket ON L3Y 8C3; Glasgow (Scotland)'79; MB ChB; FRCPC; Peds. (905)836-6721

RAJAN, Dheeraj K; N C S B, 1C 553-585 University Ave, Toronto ON M5G 2N2; Tor'94; FRCPC; DiagRad (Vascular & Interventional Radiology). Staff, Toronto General Hospital - UHN; Asst Prof, University of Toronto; (416)340-4911; Fax. (416)593-0502; dheeraj.rajan@uhn.on.ca.

RAJAN, Feroza; 192-8888 Country Hills Blvd NW, Calgary AB T3G 5T4; (Pakistan)'84; (403)568-0171

RAJAN, Gerald Leon; 80 Valleybrook Dr, North York ON M3B 2S9; UBC'83; (416)442-5600; Fax. (416)510-5175.

RAJAN, Idumban A; 1-1522 Ouellette Ave, Windsor ON N8X 1K7; Madras (India)'71; MB BS; DPM; MRCPsy; DPsy; FRCPC; Psy (Adult Psychiatry). Ac Staff, Windsor Regional Hospital - Metropolitan Site; Ac Staff, Hôtel-Dieu Grace Hospital; Consultant, PACT Team II Essex; Langs: Tamil; (519)258-3936; Fax. (519)258-6836.

RAJAN, Poonam; North York Med Arts Bldg, 319-1333 Sheppard Ave E, North York ON M2J 1V1; Tor'96; DABD; Derm (Cosmetic Dermatology). (416)502-1000; Fax. (416)502-1030.

RAJAN, Raghu D; MUHC-Montreal Gen Hosp, A7 130-1650 av Cedar, Montreal QC H3G 1A4; Man'86; MSc; FRCPC; IntMed (Clinical Epidemiology); MedOncol; Hem. Staff, McGill University Health Centre - Montreal General Campus; Assoc Prof Oncol, McGill University; (514)934-8007; Fax. (514)934-8379.

RAJAN, Yasmin A; Lions Gate Hosp, 231 15th St E, North Vancouver BC V7L 2L7; Nashville(TN) (USA)'80; FRCPC; Anes. Staff Anes, Lions Gate Hospital; (604)984-5709; Fax. (604)984-5749.

RAJANI, Hasmukhlal R; North Edmonton Health Centre, 14007 50 St NW, Edmonton AB T5A 5E4; London (England)'75; MB BS; FRCPC; Peds. Prof, University of Alberta; Langs: Gujarati; (780)342-4168; Fax. (780)342-4196.

RAJANI, Kantilal R; Manitoba Clinic, 790 Sherbrook St, Winnipeg MB R3A 1M3; London (England)'68; DCH; DObst; MRCP(UK); DTMH; FRCPC; Peds (Primary Care). Assoc Staff Children's Hosp, Health Sciences Centre; Assoc Prof, University of Manitoba; Langs: Gujarati; (204)788-5744; Fax. (204)789-9230.

RAJANI, Mohamed G V; Albany Med Clinic, 807 Broadview Ave, Toronto ON M4K 2P8; London (England)'67; MB BS; LRCP; MRCS; MRCP(UK); Langs: Gujarati; (416)461-9471; Fax. (416)461-2710.

RAJANI, Priya K; Appleby College Medical, 540 Lakeshore Rd W, Oakville ON L6K 3P1; Man'00; CCFP; Langs: Gujarati; (905)845-1544; Fax. (905)845-2024.

RAJANI, Shabnam S; Gamma-Dynacare Medical Lab, 115 Midair Crt, Brampton ON L6T 5M3; Delhi (India)'71; MB BS; FCAP; FRCPC; GenPath. Med Dir, Gamma-Dynacare Medical Lab; Langs: Hindi; Punjabi; (905)790-3000; Fax. (905)790-2990; rajanis@gamma-dynacare.com.

RAJAPPANNAIR, Lakshmi; Saint John Reg Hosp, PO Box 2100 Stn Main 400 University Ave, Saint John NB E2L 4L2; Trivandrum (India)'91; Staff, Saint John Regional Hospital; (506)648-6000

RAJARAM, Nikhil; Dalla Llana School of Public H, 155 College St, Toronto ON M5T 1P7; Wes'09; CCFP.

RAJARAMAN, Murali M; Nova Scotia Cancer Centre, 5820 University Ave, Halifax NS B3H 1V7; Dal'88; FRCPC; RadOncol. Med Staff, Queen Elizabeth II Health Sciences Centre - Victoria General Site; Asst Prof, Dalhousie University; (902)473-6018; Fax. (902)473-7205.

RAJARAMAN, Selva R; 165 Goyeau St, Windsor ON N9A 1G5; Dal'92; (519)258-1507; Fax. (519)258-8338.

RAJARATHNA, Mallika P A; 373 Steeles Ave W, Brampton ON L6Y 0P8; Colombo (Sri Lanka)'81; CCFP; (905)452-8881; Fax. (902)452-9997.

RAJARATNAM, Krishan; Hamilton Commun Health Centre, M5-414 Victoria Ave N, Hamilton ON L8L 5G8; Tor'95; FRCSC; OrthSurg. (905)526-8430

RAJASINGHAM, Melodye; Commercial Street Med Centre, 208-311 Commercial St, Milton ON L9T 3Z9; Wes'98; FRCSC; ObstGyn. Staff, Halton Healthcare Services Corporation - Milton District Hospital; (905)875-2280

RAJASINGHAM, Menaka; Markham Stouffville Hosp, PO Box 1800 Stn Main 381 Church St, Markham ON L3P 7P3; Ceylon (Sri Lanka)'77; MB BS; FRCPC; Anes. Staff, Markham Stouffville Hospital; (905)472-7000 x7074; Fax. (905)472-7386.

RAJASINGHAM, Rajanathan; Greystone Med Walk-In Clinic, CID-8 Greystone Walk Dr, Scarborough ON M1K 5J2; Colombo (Sri Lanka)'76; FRCS(E); CCFP; Staff, Sunnybrook Health Sciences Centre; (416)266-1818; Fax. (416)266-0800.

RAJCHGOT, Percy; Norfinch Med Centre, 202B-2100 Finch Ave W, North York ON M3N 2Z9; McG'75; FRCPC; Peds. Ac Staff, The Hospital For Sick Children; Asst Prof, University of Toronto; (416)665-8515; Fax. (416)661-9848.

RAJDA, Malgorzata; Abbie J Lane Memorial Bldg, 4008-5909 Veterans Memorial La, Halifax NS B3H 2E2; Silesia (Poland)'84; DABSM; FRCPC; Psy (Sleep Disorders). Ac Staff, Queen Elizabeth II Health Sciences Centre - Victoria General Site; Assoc Prof Psy, Dalhousie University; (902)473-4780; Fax. (902)473-7158; malgorzata.rajda@cdha.nshealth.ca.

RAJDA, Miroslaw; Queen Elizabeth II HSC-Halifax, 2261-1796 Summer St, Halifax NS B3H 3A7; Silesian (Poland)'84; FRCPC; IntMed (Echocardiography); Cardiol. Staff Cardiol/Asst Prof, Queen Elizabeth II Health Sciences Centre - Halifax Infirmary Site; Langs: Polish; (902)473-8913; Fax. (902)473-2434; dommr@cdha.nshealth.ca.

RAJENDRA, Jegapathy; Scarborough Hosp-Birchmount, 3030 Birchmount Rd, Scarborough ON M1W 3W3; (Sri Lanka)'71; MB BS; MRCPsy(UK); FRCPC; Psy. Staff, The Scarborough Hospital - Birchmount Campus; Langs: Tamil; (416)495-2701 x5376; Fax. (416)495-2426.

RAJENDRAN, Bahe; The Peterborough Clinic, 301-26 Hospital Dr, Peterborough ON K9J 7C3; Alb'02; FRCPC; IntMed. (705)740-6861; Fax. (705)740-6899.

RAJESAN, Ratheishan; Scarborough Acad Fam Hlth Team, 1125 Markham Rd, Scarborough ON M1H 2Y5; Wayne State (USA)'08; BSc(Hon); MSc; CCFP; (416)439-2273; Fax. (416)439-2244.

RAJESWARAN, Srirani; 1-3600 Ellesmere Rd, Scarborough ON M1C 4Y8; Peradeniya (Sri Lanka)'78; MB BS; CCFP; (416)283-0084; Fax. (416)283-0308.

RAJGOPAL, Chellappa; London HSC-University Hosp, PO Box 5339 Stn B C8 004-339 Windermere Rd, London ON N6A 5A5; Osmania (India)'70; FRCS(Eng); MS; FRCSC; GenSurg. Staff, London Health Sciences Centre - University Hospital; Assoc Prof Surg, University of Western Ontario; Langs: Hindi; Tamil; Telugu; (519)663-3460; Fax. (519)663-3459.

RAJGOPAL, Vaishnav; Strathroy Middlesex Gen Hosp, 332-395 Carrie St, Strathroy ON N7G 3C9; Wes'03; FRCSC; OrthSurg. Staff, Strathroy Middlesex General Hospital - Middlesex Hospital Alliance; (519)245-5775

RAJGURU, Manjulata; 7-695 Coronation Blvd, Cambridge ON N1R 7J9; Bhopal (India)'93; MB BS; FRCPC; Peds. Staff Ped, Cambridge Memorial Hospital; Langs: Hindi; (519)624-1551; Fax. (519)624-1581.

RAJJI, Tarek K; C A M H, 6312-80 Workman Way, Toronto ON M6J 1H4; Beirut (Lebanon)'99; FRCPC; Psy. Fellow, Centre for Addiction & Mental Health (CAMH) - Queen Site; (416)535-8501; Fax. (416)583-1307.

RAJKHOWA, Sudhir; Rajkhowa Med Prof Co, 46 Eugenia St, Barrie ON L4M 1P8; Gauhati (India)'71; MB BS; MRCPsy; FRCPC; Psy (Child & Adolescent Psychiatry). Consultant Psy, Barrie Community Services; (705)739-6245; Fax. (705)739-9575; srajkhowa@barrie.ca.

RAJKOTWALA, Victor A; William Osler HC-Etobicoke, 101 Humber College Blvd, Etobicoke ON M9V 1R8; Bombay (India)'79; FRCPC; IntMed. Staff, William Osler Health System - Brampton Civic Hospital; Staff, William Osler Health System - Etobicoke General Hospital; (416)494-2120

RAJKUMAR, Winston D; 150-1720 Howard Ave, Windsor ON N8X 5A6; West Indies (Jamaica)'76; ABIM; DABIM; FRCPC; IntMed; Respir. (519)255-7964; Fax. (519)255-9320.

RAJMOHAMED, Afzal E; North Park Med Centre, D2-2355 Keele St, North York ON M6M 4A2; Natal (South Africa)'93; MB ChB; CCFP; (416)244-4377; Fax. (416)244-1004.

RAJOO, S Nischal; 207-200 Boudreau Rd, St. Albert AB T8N 6B9; Alb'98; CCFP; FCFP; (780)569-5455

RAJORA, Manisha; Royal Columbian Hosp, 330 Columbia St E, New Westminster BC V3L 3W7; Alb'99; CCFP; Royal Columbian Hospital; (604)520-4253

RAJOTTE, Claude; CLSC des Faubourgs, 1705 rue de la Visitation, Montreal QC H2L 3C3; Mon'81; CCFP; Clin Prof, Universite de Montreal; (514)527-2361

RAJPAL, Anupma; Saskatoon East Fam Physicians, 21-2105 8th St E, Saskatoon SK S7H 0T8; Ott'92; LMCC; CCFP; (306)373-5500; Fax. (306)374-9414.

RAJPURA, Anjum; 50 Lorne Cres, Brantford ON N3T 4L7; Birmingham (England)'92; CCFP; (519)759-7233

RAJPUT, Alexander H; Royal University Hosp, 103 Hospital Dr, Saskatoon SK S7N 0W8; Sask'94; LMCC; FRCPC; Neur (Movement Disorders). Staff, Royal University Hospital; Prof, University of Saskatchewan; (306)966-8007; Fax. (306)966-8030; alex.rajput@usask.ca.

RAJPUT, Ali H; Royal University Hosp, 1663-103 Hospital Dr, Saskatoon SK S7N 0W8; Sind (Pakistan)'58; MB BS; MSc(Neurol.); FRCPC; Neur (Movement Disorders). Emeritus Prof Neurol, Royal University Hospital; Consultant Neurol, Saskatoon Health Region Saskatoon Public Health; Consultant Neurol, Regina Health District; Emeritus Prof Neurol, University of Saskatchewan; (306)966-8009; Fax. (306)966-8030; ali.rajput@saskatoonhealthregion.ca.

RAJPUT, Anshu; The Credit Valley Hosp, 2200 Eglinton Ave W, Mississauga ON L5M 2N1; Ott'04; FRCPC; DiagRad. Staff, The Credit Valley Hospital; (905)813-2200

RAJPUT, Romi; Millwoods Medicentre, 6426 28 Ave NW, Edmonton AB T6L 6N3; Cal'92; CCFP; (780)462-3491; Fax. (780)461-2650.

RAJPUT, Sobia I; 250-8730 Country Hills Blvd NW, Calgary AB T3G 0E2; (Pakistan)'99; CCFP; (403)262-7787; Fax. (403)262-7786.

RAJU, Dharmapaul L; Queensway-Carleton Hosp, 3045 Baseline Rd, Nepean ON K2H 8P4; Sask'98; FRCPC; IntMed; Nephrol. Staff, Queensway Carleton Hospital; (613)721-4842

RAJU, Mahesh; 60 Westmount Dr, Saint John NB E2K 5G2; Mysore (India)'82; FRCPC; IntMed (Intensive Care). Med Staff, Horizon Health Network Saint John Public Health; Asst Prof, Dalhousie University; Langs: Telugu; Hindi; (506)634-6111; Fax. (506)634-6112; mraju@rogers.com.

RAJU, Priyadarshani; The Hincks-Dellcrest Centre, 440 Jarvis St, Toronto ON M4Y 2H4; Tor'07; Psy. Staff, The Hincks-Dellcrest Centre - Toronto; (416)924-1164

RAJU, Shoba; 60 Westmount Dr, Saint John NB E2K 5G2; Andhra (India)'77; MB BS; DObst; Langs: Telugu; Hindi; (506)634-6111; Fax. (506)634-6112.

RAJVONG, Inthysone; CLSC St-Hubert, 6800 boul Cousineau, Saint-Hubert QC J3Y 8Z4; Mon'02; Staff, Hôpital Anna-Laberge; (450)443-7407

RAJWANI, Talib; Grey Nuns Community Hosp & HC, 1100 Youville Drive West NW, Edmonton AB T6L 5X8; Alb'06; FRCPC; Psy. Staff, Covenant Health - Grey Nuns Community Hospital; (780)735-7119

RAK, Janet; Bathurst Med Centre, LL56-7117 Bathurst St, Thornhill ON L4J 2J6; McG'84; CCFP; FCFP; Langs: English; French; (905)731-5662; Fax. (905)731-6841.

RAK, Viktoria; Ridge Meadows Hosp & Hlth CC, 11666 Laity St, Maple Ridge BC V2X 5A3; Rostov (Russia (Federation))'91; Staff, Royal Columbian Hospital; Staff, Ridge Meadows Hospital & Health Care Centre; Staff, Surrey Memorial Hospital; (604)463-4111

RAKEL, Agnes; CHUM-Hop St-Luc, 1058 rue Saint-Denis, Montreal QC H2X 3J4; Mon'00; FRCPC; IntMed; Endocrin (P.Q.); Endocrin&Metab. Staff, Centre Hospitalier l'Université De Montréal (CHUM) - Hôpital Saint-luc; (514)890-8000

RAKEM, Jamal A M H; 206-477 King St, Welland ON L3B 3K4; Tripoli (Libya)'91; FRCSC; OrthSurg. Staff, Niagara Health System - Welland Hospital Site; (905)732-4404; Fax. (905)732-4405.

RAKHRA, Kawanpreet S; The Ottawa Hosp-Gen Campus, 501 Smyth Rd, Ottawa ON K1H 8L6; Mem'98; FRCPC; DiagRad. Staff, The Ottawa Hospital - General Campus; (613)737-8899 x73249

RAKHRA, Ronbir S; Burnaby Square Fam Doctors, 105-7885 6th St, Burnaby BC V3N 3N4; UBC'02; CCFP; (604)526-8905

RAKHSHANI, Nasimeh; Univ Hlth Network-Toronto Western Hosp, 399 Bathurst St, Toronto ON M5T 2S8; Qns'10; CCFP; Staff, Toronto Western Hospital - University Health Network; (416)603-5800

RAKIC, Dubravka; Scenic Acres Med Clinic, 8555 Scurfield Dr NW, Calgary AB T3L 1Z6; Tuzla (Bosnia-Herzegovina)'85; CCFP; Langs: Serbian; (403)547-2255; Fax. (403)547-2255.

RAKOFF, David; 1712-2200 Yonge St, Toronto ON M4S 2C6; Cape Town (South Africa)'85; MB ChB; FRCPC; Psy (Child Psychiatry). (416)486-6368

RAKOFF, Vivian M; Addiction & Mental Hlth-Clarke, 250 College St, Toronto ON M5T 1R8; London (England)'57; MB BS; FACP; FAPA; DPsy(McG.); DSc(Hon); FRCPC; Psy (Adolescent Psychiatry). Staff Teacher, Centre for Addiction & Mental Health (CAMH) - College Street Site; Emeritus Prof, University of Toronto; (416)979-6848; Fax. (416)966-0290.

RAKOVICH, George; Hop Maisonneuve-Rosemont, 5415 boul de l'Assomption, Montreal QC H1T 2M4; Mon'98; FRCSC; GenSurg; ThorSurg. Staff, Hopital Maisonneuve-Rosemont; (514)252-3400

RAKOVITCH, Eileen; Sunnybrook Health Sciences Ctr, 2075 Bayview Ave, Toronto ON M4N 3M5; Tor'89; FRCPC; RadOncol. Head Breast Site/Chair L C Campbell Breast Cancer Reseaarch, Sunnybrook Health Sciences Centre - Edmond Odette Cancer Centre; (416)480-4806; Fax. (416)480-6002.

RAKOWSKI, Harry; Univ Hlth Network-Toronto Gen, 4N 504-200 Elizabeth St, Toronto ON M5G 2N2; Tor'72; FRCPC; Cardiol. Staff Cardiol, Toronto General Hospital - UHN; (416)340-4062; Fax. (416)591-0179.

RALEIGH, John P; PO Box 270, Sydenham ON K0H 2T0; Qns'84; CCFP; CCFP(E.M.); FCFP; Staff, Lennox & Addington County General Hospital; Assoc Staff, Kingston General Hospital; Assoc Staff, Hotel-Dieu Hospital; (613)376-3327; Fax. (613)376-9868.

RALH, Surender K; Ralh Med Clinic, 210-2365 Finch Ave W, North York ON M9M 2W8; Delhi (India)'78; Staff, William Osler Health System - Etobicoke General Hospital; Langs: Hindi; Punjabi; (416)740-1235; Fax. (416)740-6720.

RALHAN, Vikram; Georgian Bay Gen Hosp, PO Box 760 Stn Main 1112 St Andrews Dr, Midland ON L4R 4P4; Saba (Malaysia)'06; CCFP; Staff, Georgian Bay General Hospital - Midland; (705)526-1300

RALLEY, Fiona E; London HSC-University Hosp, PO Box 5339 Stn B C3 110-339 Windermere Rd, London ON N6A 5A5; Edinburgh (Scotland)'75; MB ChB; FFARCS; Consultant Anes, London Health Sciences Centre - University Hospital; Prof Anes, University of Western Ontario; (519)685-8500 x32832; Fax. (519)663-2957; fralley@uwo.ca.

RALLEY, Len; Albany Med Clinic, 807 Danforth Ave, Toronto ON M4K 2P8; Tor'56; DPsy; BA; FRCPC; Psy (Psychotherapy). Specialist, MCI Clinique; Langs: Bilingual(French/English); (416)461-9471; Fax. (416)461-2710.

RALPH, Douglas G; Pine Street Plaza, 32-9 Pine St N, Thorold ON L2V 3Z9; McM'76; Court Staff, Niagara Health System - St Catharines General Site; (905)227-7055; Fax. (905)227-9101.

RALPH, Edward D; London HSC-University Hosp, PO Box 5339 Stn B ALL 116-339 Windermere Rd, London ON N6A 5A5; Wes'70; FRCPC; IntMed (Infectious Diseases). Dir IDCP, St Joseph's Hospital - St Joseph's Health Care; Consultant InfectDis, London Health Sciences Centre - University Hospital; Prof Med, University of Western Ontario; (519)663-3452; Fax. (519)663-3062; edward.ralph@lhsc.on.ca.

RALPH, Samuel J; Killick Health Services Inc, 129 Lincoln Rd, Grnd-Falls-Windsor NL A2A 1P3; Mem'00; CCFP; (709)292-8400

RALPH-EDWARDS, Anthony C; 4N 449-585 University Ave, Toronto ON M5G 2N2; Qns'87; DAB; FRCSC; GenSurg (Cardiac Surgery); CardiothorSurg. Staff Cardiovascular Surg, Toronto General Hospital - UHN; Lecturer, University of Toronto; (416)340-4309; Fax. (416)340-3803.

RALSTON, Robert N; Alder Med Centre, 277 Evergreen Rd, Campbell River BC V9W 5Y4; Tor'76; (250)287-7441; Fax. (250)287-4384.

RALYEA, Evan P; 678 Colborne St, London ON N6A 3Z3; Detroit(MI) (USA)'73; FRCPC; Peds (Pediatric Psychiatry); Psy. Staff Psy, Family & Children's Services of St Thomas & Elgin; Staff Psy, Oxford-Elgin Child & Youth Centre; Staff Psy, West Elgin Comm Health Centre; (519)672-0420; eralyea@wechc.on.ca.

RAM, John R; Pickering Holistic Hlth Centre, 220-1101 Kingston Rd, Pickering ON L1V 1B5; McM'08; CCFP; (905)831-9797; Fax. (905)839-9984.

RAM, Katherine; The Credit Valley Hosp, 2200 Eglinton Ave W, Mississauga ON L5M 2N1; Qns'05; FRCPC; Psy. Staff, The Credit Valley Hospital; (905)813-4421; Fax. (905)813-1594.

RAM, Pawan K; 178-8138 128 St, Surrey BC V3W 1R1; Punjab (India)'80; MB BS; Langs: Punjabi; French; Hindi; (604)572-9191; Fax. (604)572-4111; pawan.ram@cic.gc.ca.

RAMACHANDRAN, Kizhake V; Saskatchewan Hosp-Battleford, PO Box 39 Stn Main 1 Jersey St, North Battleford SK S9A 2X8; Kerala (India)'70; MB BS; DPM; MRCPsy; Chief Psy, Saskatchewan Hospital - North Battleford; Staff Psy, Regional Psychiatric Centre - Prairies; (306)446-6878; Fax. (306)446-6867; kramachandran@pnrha.ca.

RAMACHANDRAN, N Rajesh; McMaster University, 1280 Main St W, Hamilton ON L8S 4K1; Kerala (India)'94; FRCPC; Peds; Neur. Staff, Hamilton Health Sciences Centre - McMaster Children's Hospital; (905)521-2100; Fax. (905)521-7914.

RAMACHANDRAN, Nirmala; Battlefords Union Hosp, 1092 107th St, North Battleford SK S9A 1Z1; Kerala (India)'77; MRCP(UK); Staff, Battlefords Union Hospital; (306)446-6500; Fax. (306)446-6546.

RAMACHANDRAN, Sanjay; Maple FHT-Reddendale Family HC, 125 Lakeview Ave, Kingston ON K7M 3T6; Wes'95; BSc; CCFP; CCFP(E.M.); FCFP; (613)384-4664

RAMADAN, Abdul-Nasser J; Thompson Gen Hosp, 871 Thompson Dr, Thompson MB R8N 0C8; Baghdad (Iraq)'82; FRCPC; IntMed. Staff, Thompson General Hospital; (204)677-2381

RAMADAN, Fauzi; Hammond Bldg, 310-310 Main St N, Moose Jaw SK S6H 3K1; Garyunis (Libya)'76; MB BS; MRCP(UK); MSc; Langs: Arabic; (306)693-2929; Fax. (306)693-4866.

RAMADAN, Khaled M A; Providence Hematology, 440-1144 Burrard St, Vancouver BC V6Z 2A5; Al Fateh (Libya)'96; MB BCh; MRCP; FRCPath; FRCP(Glas); FRCPC; HemPath (Hematology). Staff Hem Providence Hematology, Providence Health Care - St Paul's Hospital; Clinical Asst Prof, University of British Columbia; (604)684-5794; Fax. (604)684-5705.

RAMADAN, Said; Medicentres, 611 Wonderland Rd N, London ON N6H 4V6; Cairo (Egypt)'72; MB BS; DCH; MRCP(UK); FRCP; FRCPC; Peds. Staff, London Health Sciences Centre - University Hospital; Aj Prof Pediatrics, University of Western Ontario; Aj Prof Peds, Schulich School of Medicine-University of Western Ontario; Langs: Arabic; (519)471-6686 x29; Fax. (519)471-2801; said1948@hotmail.com.

RAMADAN, Samir I; Port Credit Med Clinic, 374 Lakeshore Rd E, Mississauga ON L5G 1H5; Al Fateh (Libya)'01; CCFP; (905)271-9000

RAMADAN, Ziad F B; 4243 118 Ave NW, Edmonton AB T5W 1A5; (Libya)'04; CCFP; (780)756-7700; Fax. (780)756-7788.

RAMADORI, Francesco; MUHC-Montreal Gen Hosp, D10 144-1650 av Cedar, Montreal QC H3G 1A4; McG'96; CSPQ; CCFP; Critical Care Medicine (P.Q.); Anes. Staff, McGill University Health Centre - Montreal General Campus; Langs: Italian; Spanish; (514)934-1934 x43261; Fax. (514)934-8249; francesco.ramadori@mcgill.ca.

RAMAKRISHNA, Veer; East Hamilton Walk-In-Clinic, 800 Queenston Rd, Hamilton ON L8G 1A7; Bangalore (India)'76; MB BS; BSc(Hons.); DLO; CCFP; Langs: Tamil; Telugu; Hindi; (905)662-4141

RAMAKRISHNAN, Srikanth; 308-16600 Bayview Ave, Newmarket ON L3X 1Z9; Bharathiar (India)'93; MB BS; FRCPC; IntMed (Sleep Disorders); Critical Care Medicine; Respir. Staff, Southlake Regional Health Centre; (905)235-8700; Fax. (905)235-8701.

RAMALHO, Denis C; Clin Med Pointe-du-Lac, CP 4099 Succ A 10300 ch Sainte-Marguerite, Trois-Rivieres QC G9B 7Y6; Laval'83; Langs: English; French; (819)377-5015; Fax. (819)377-5550.

RAMAN, Kalyanapuram R; Golf Links Community Clinic, 6-1077 Golf Links Rd, Thunder Bay ON P7B 7A3; Madras (India)'68; MB BS; MRC(UK); MRC(Ire.); FRCPC; IntMed (Nutrition); Gastroent. (807)622-9895

RAMAN, Mani; 312 Highway 7 E, Richmond Hill ON L4B 1A5; Tor'94; MSc; BSc; FRCPC; Derm (Cosmetic Dermatology). (905)889-2005; Fax. (905)889-2006; dermatology@canada.com.

RAMANATHAN, Krishnan; St Paul's Hosp, 475-1081 Burrard St, Vancouver BC V6Z 1Y6; Otago (New Zealand)'88; FRCPC; IntMed (Acute Coronary Care); Cardiol. Dir-Research, Providence Health Care - St Paul's Hospital; Staff, Gordon & Leslie Diamond Health Care Centre; Clinical Asst Prof/Asst Dir Postgrad Educ in Cardiol, University of British Columbia; Langs: Tamil; (604)806-9651

RAMANATHAN, Usha; SGH Medical Mall, 505-3030 Lawrence Ave E, Scarborough ON M1P 2T7; McM'06; FRCPC; Neur. (416)289-0185

RAMANAUSKAS, John V; Pelham Health Centre, 118-245 Pelham Rd, St Catharines ON L2S 1X8; McM'77; CCFP; FCFP; (905)688-9670; Fax. (905)688-6979.

RAMANI, Mathangi; Ctr Hosp de Lasalle, 8585 Tsse Champlain, Lasalle QC H8P 1C1; McG'92; CSPQ; FRCPC; DiagRad (Breast Imaging). Staff, Centre Hospitalier de LaSalle; Dir, Hôpital Anna-Laberge; Langs: English; French; (514)362-1000 x31549; mathangi.ramani.chl@ssss.gouv.qc.ca.

RAMANI, Nithyakalyani; Colebrook Family Practice, 107-15240 56 Ave, Surrey BC V3S 5K7; Madras (India)'83; CCFP; Langs: Hindi; Tamil; (778)574-1414

RAMANNA, Raj; Charlton Med Centre, 616-25 Charlton Ave E, Hamilton ON L8N 1Y2; Bangalore (India)'82; MB BS; FRCSC; ObstGyn (Infertility). Staff, St Joseph's Healthcare - Charlton Campus; Asst Prof, McMaster University; (905)972-0911; Fax. (905)972-0913.

RAMANNA, Venita; Market Mall Prof Bldg, 312-4935 40 Ave NW, Calgary AB T3A 2N1; Natal (South Africa)'82; MB ChB; CCFP; (403)247-2345; Fax. (403)247-6217.

RAMASUBBU, Rajamannar; Mental Hlth Ctr for Res & Educ, 4D64-3280 Hospital Dr NW, Calgary AB T2N 4Z6; Madurai-Kamaraj (India)'78; MB BS; DPM; MRCPsy(Lond); MSc; FRCPsy; FRCPC; Psy (Academic Psychiatry). Ac Staff, Foothills Medical Centre; Assoc Prof Psy Dept of Psy & Clin Neurosciences, University of Calgary; Langs: Tamil; (403)210-6890; Fax. (403)210-9114; rramasub@ucalgary.ca.

RAMAYA, Savitri; E-1700 Pacific Ave, Brandon MB R7A 7L9.

RAMBALDI, Antonio; 15-2020 boul René-Gaultier, Varennes QC J3X 1N9; McG'84; Langs: Italian; French; Spanish; (450)652-2222; Fax. (450)652-3970.

RAMBALDINI, Gloria M; LMC Endocrinology Centres Ltd, 17-531 Atkinson Ave, Thornhill ON L4J 8L7; Tor'00; BSc(Hon); FRCPC; IntMed; Endocrin&Metab. Staff, Mackenzie Richmond Hill Hospital; Endocrinologist, LMC Diabetes & Endocrinology Centres-Eglinton; Langs: Italian; (905)763-8660; Fax. (905)763-0708; gloria.rambaldini@lmc.ca.

RAMBARAN, Moses; Miramichi Med Arts Centre, 2-679 King George Hwy, Miramichi NB E1V 1N9; Carribean (Montserrat)'91; Staff, Miramichi Regional Hospital; (506)622-7490; Fax. (506)622-2705.

RAMBARANSINGH, Brian S; Hys Medical Centre, 710-11010 101 St NW, Edmonton AB T5H 4B9; Cal'06; FRCPC; PhysMed&Rehab. (780)453-5255; Fax. (780)453-9099.

RAMBERT, Julian J; 502-168 Charlotte St, Ottawa ON K1N 8K6; Jamaica (Jamaica)'68; (613)563-0320; Fax. (613)563-2211.

RAMBIHAR, Nadira; West Park Healthcare Centre, 92-82 Buttonwood Ave, York ON M6M 2J5; Wes'07; FRCPC; PhysMed&Rehab. Staff, West Park Healthcare Centre; (416)243-3680

RAMBIHAR, Sherryn P; Women's College Hosp, 76 Grenville St, Toronto ON M5S 1B2; Wes'05; FRCPC; IntMed; Cardiol. Staff, Mount Sinai Hospital; Staff, Women's College Hospital; (416)323-7726; Fax. (416)323-6304.

RAMBIHAR, Vivian S; Medical Centre, 3202-3000 Lawrence Ave E, Scarborough ON M1P 2V1; McM'75; BSc(Tor); FRCPC; IntMed (Echocardiography); Cardiol. Court Staff, The Scarborough Hospital - General Campus; (416)438-2100; Fax. (416)438-2106.

RAMCHANDAR, Kevin; TBRHSC Regional Cancer Care, 980 Oliver Rd, Thunder Bay ON P7B 6V4; Tor'04; FRCPC; RadOncol. (807)684-7200; Fax. (807)684-5801.

RAMDASS, Chitra; York Med Health Clinic, C-17215 Leslie St, Newmarket ON L3Y 8E4; (Cayman Islands)'08; CCFP; (905)853-0404; Fax. (905)853-3702.

RAMDHANI, Hemendra B; 306-17310 94A Ave, Surrey BC V3V 1N1; (South Africa)'92; FRCPC; Peds. (604)382-6555

RAMER, Sarah A; Queen Elizabeth II HSC-Halifax, 2111-1796 Summer St, Halifax NS B3H 3A7; Cal'00; FRCPC; IntMed; Cardiol. Staff, Queen Elizabeth II Health Sciences Centre - Halifax Infirmary Site; (902)473-2682; Fax. (902)473-2434.

RAMER, William D; 10028 164 St NW, Edmonton AB T5P 4Y3; Alb'69; BSc; (780)413-7218; Fax. (780)488-7253; wramer@telus.net.

RAMESH, Kuppuchipalayam K; Surrey Pediatrics Associates, 103-13710 94A Ave, Surrey BC V3V 1N1; Kilpauk (India)'92; MB BS; DCH(Dublin); MRCP(Dublin); FRCPC; Peds. Langs: Tamil; (604)583-7070; Fax. (604)582-5536.

RAMESH, Warren P; Edmonton Respiratory Consultan, 1370-10665 Jasper Ave NW, Edmonton AB T5J 3S9; Edinburgh (Scotland)'91; MB ChB; FCCP; ABIM; FRCPC; IntMed (Sleep Apnea); Respir. Staff, Royal Alexandra Hospital; University of Alberta; (780)702-3866; Fax. (780)702-3885.

RAMESSAR, Elena; Yarmouth Reg Health Centre, 60 Vancouver St, Yarmouth NS B5A 2P5; '82; Staff, Yarmouth Regional Hospital; (902)742-3541

RAMESSAR, John A S; Yarmouth Reg Health Centre, 60 Vancouver St, Yarmouth NS B5A 2P5; W.Indies (Jamaica)'77; MB BS; FRCR; Consultant Radiol, Yarmouth Regional Hospital; (902)742-3541; Fax. (902)742-1238.

RAMFUL, Droovnath; Elk Point Med Clinic, PO Box 480 5310 50 Ave, Elk Point AB T0A 1A0; Manchester (England)'80; MRCP; Langs: English; French; (780)724-4106; Fax. (780)724-4106; dramful@telus.net.

RAMGOOLAM, Rajendranath; Corydon Med Clinic, 894 Corydon Ave, Winnipeg MB R3M 0Y4; Dublin (Ireland)'67; LRCP; LRCS; Ac Staff Interim Care, Misericordia Health Centre; Med Dir, Golden Links Conval. Home/Lions Pembina/Mennonite & Vista Pk Personal Care, Active Staff-Tuxedo Villa PCH & Med. Exam.-Prov of MB; University of Manitoba; Langs: Hindi; French; (204)475-0876

RAMIN, Brodie; Univ of Ottawa Health Service, 300-100 Marie Curie Pvt, Ottawa ON K1N 1A2; Tor'09; CCFP; (613)564-3950; Fax. (613)564-6627.

RAMIREZ, Alvaro; London Diagnostic Centre, 481 London Rd, Sarnia ON N7T 4X3; Laval'02; FRCSC; Urol. (519)383-6427

RAMIREZ, Oswaldo C; Alliston Family Health Team, 36 Victoria St W, Alliston ON L9R 1S8; (Ecuador)'01; BSc; CCFP; Chief Emerg Dept, Stevenson Memorial Hospital; Langs: Spanish; French; Italian; (705)435-8887; Fax. (705)435-8867.

RAMIREZ MORENO, Saby E M; Powell River Gen Hosp, 5000 Joyce Ave, Powell River BC V8A 5R8; Lady of the Rosary (Colombia)'94; FRCPC; Psy. Staff, Powell River General Hospital; Langs: Spanish; (604)485-3245

RAMJATTAN, Brian R; First Line Medical, 203-496 Topsail Rd, St. John's NL A1E 2C2; Mem'91.

RAMJEESINGH, Ravi A; Cancer Ctr of Southeastern Ont, 25 King St W, Kingston ON K7L 5P9; Tor'08; FRCPC; IntMed. Fellow, Cancer Centre of Southeastern Ontario; (613)544-2630

RAMJI, Alnoor; Pacific Gastroenterology Assoc, 770-1190 Hornby St, Vancouver BC V6Z 2K5; UBC'98; BScPharm; FRCPC; IntMed (Hepatology); Gastroent. Staff, Providence Health Care - St Paul's Hospital; Clinical Asst Prof Prof, University of British Columbia; Langs: Swahili; French; (604)688-6332 x225

RAMJI, Ayaaz; Victoria Square Med Clinic, PO Box 5700 Stn Main 217-2345 10th Ave W, Prince Albert SK S6V 7V6; Dublin (Ireland)'89; MB ChB; DCH; FRCP; FRCPC; Peds. (306)953-5664; Fax. (306)922-9394; ayazramji@shaw.ca.

RAMJI, Farah; 710 Granville St PO Box 18466 Rpo West Georgia, Vancouver BC V6Z 0B3; UBC'10; CCFP; (778)838-7558

RAMJI, Moizali A; 113-47 Athabascan Ave, Sherwood Park AB T8A 4H3; Shiraz (Iran)'79; Langs: Persian; Gujarati; Swahili; (780)467-2255; Fax. (780)467-2256.

RAMJI, Munira M; 113-47 Athabascan Ave, Sherwood Park AB T8A 4H3; Shiraz (Iran)'79; FRCPC; Peds. (780)467-2255; Fax. (780)467-2256.

RAMJI, Nasreen; St James Town Health Ctr, 410 Sherbourne St, Toronto ON M4X 1K2; Wes'06; CCFP; (416)864-3096

RAMJI, Noor N W; 80 Bond Family Practice Unit, 80 Bond St, Toronto ON M5B 1X2; Cal'08; BSc(Hon); MSc; CCFP; Lecturer, University of Toronto; (416)864-3011; Fax. (416)864-3099.

RAMJI, Taheera; Health Sciences Bldg, 15 Mountain Ave S, Hamilton ON L8G 2V6; Alb'07; FRCPC; Peds. (905)664-9992

RAMJI, Zulfikar; 171 52 St SE, Calgary AB T2A 5H8; Makerere (Uganda)'72; MB BS; LRCP; MRC; (403)272-4218; Fax. (403)272-7406.

RAMJOHN, Zaid O A; Carbonear Gen Hosp, 86 Highroad South, Carbonear NL A1Y 1A4; Dublin (Ireland)'90; MB ChB; BAO; Staff, Carbonear General Hospital; (709)945-5111

RAMKISSOON, Sachin; Scarborough Hosp-General Div, 3050 Lawrence Ave E, Scarborough ON M1P 2V5; Tor'07; CCFP; CCFP(E.M.); Staff, The Scarborough Hospital - General Campus; (416)438-2911; sramkissoon@tsh.to.

RAMLAKHAN, Larita D; Gravelbourg Med Dental Clinic, PO Box 150 619 Main St N, Gravelbourg SK S0H 1X0; Natal (South Africa)'88; MB ChB; Staff, St Joseph's Hospital/Foyer d'Youville; (306)648-4505; Fax. (306)648-2558.

RAMLALL, A Kumar; 9136 23 Ave NW, Edmonton AB T6N 1H9; McM'91; FAAP; FRCPC; Peds (Asthma); Respir. (888)726-5255; Fax. (888)317-5502.

RAMLALL, Jacintha; 40 Elisabeth St PO Box 1560 Stn Main, Okotoks AB T1S 1B5; Natal (South Africa)'88; MB ChB; CCFP; Clin Lecturer Family Med, University of Alberta; (403)938-4421

RAMMOHAN, Gnanaprabha M; 102-140 Niagara St, St Catharines ON L2R 4L4; Madras (India)'82; CCFP; (905)688-4538; Fax. (905)688-1781.

RAMMOHAN, Surianarayanan; 106-4256 Portage Rd, Niagara Falls ON L2E 6A4; Madras (India)'82; MB BS; FRCS(Glas); PhD(UK); FACS; FRCSC; GenSurg; VascSurg. Consultant, Niagara Health System - Ontario Street Site; Consultant Vascular, Niagara Health System - St Catharines General Site; Clin Assoc Prof, McMaster University; Langs: Tamil; (905)357-3336; Fax. (905)357-3393.

RAMORASATA RANAIVONAR, David H; Exeter Clinic, PO Box 879, 100 Mile House BC V0K 2E0; (Madagascar)'95; 100 Mile House District General Hospital; (250)395-7600

RAMOS, Edna V; Argus Med Centre, 300-581 Argus Rd, Oakville ON L6J 3J4; Bombay (India)'91; CCFP; (905)338-9900; Fax. (905)338-9904.

RAMPERSAD, O'Hara E S; 120-1315 Finch Ave W, North York ON M3J 2G6; Ott'78; CCFP; Staff, North York General Hospital; Staff, The Scarborough Hospital - Birchmount Campus; (416)661-7000

RAMPERSAUD, Rai V S; Medical Clinic, 8195 120 St, Delta BC V4C 6P7; Wes'96; CCFP; Staff Family Pract, Surrey Memorial Hospital; (604)594-8451; Fax. (604)596-4819.

RAMPERSAUD, Yoga R; Univ Hlth Network-Toronto Western Hosp, 1 441-399 Bathurst St, Toronto ON M5T 2S8; Wes'92; FRCSC; OrthSurg (Spine Surgery). Spinal Surgeon, Toronto Western Hospital - University Health Network; Asst Prof Orthoped & Neurosurg, University of Toronto; (416)603-5399; Fax. (416)603-3437; raja.rampersaud@uhn.on.ca.

RAMPES, Hagen; Bell Gateway Bldg, 100 Stokes St, Toronto ON M6J 1H4; Staff, Centre for Addiction & Mental Health (CAMH) - College Street Site; (416)979-6027; Fax. (416)979-6864.

RAMPHAL, Premdath J; 209-4430 Bathurst St, North York ON M3H 3S3; West Indies (Jamaica)'62; MB BS; Ac Staff, North York General Hospital - Branson Division; Asst Editor, West Indian Medical Journal & Coroner, Ontario; (416)636-4815; Fax. (416)636-0471.

RAMPHAL, Raveena; Children's Hosp Eastern Ont, 2639-401 Smyth Rd, Ottawa ON K1H 8L1; Natal (South Africa)'94; Staff, Children's Hospital of Eastern Ontario (CHEO); (613)737-7600 x2210; Fax. (613)738-4828.

RAMPLING, Roger C; Lethbridge Centre Tower, 907-400 4 Ave S, Lethbridge AB T1J 4E1; Alb'75; DABPN; BMedSci; FRCPC; Psy (General Clinical Psychiatry). Ac Staff, Chinook Regional Hospital; Consultant, Covenant Health - St Michael's Health Centre; (403)329-0500; Fax. (403)329-1930.

RAMPRASAD, Harrinorine; 301-1017 Wilson Ave, North York ON M3K 1Z1; West Indies (Jamaica)'67; Court Staff Visiting, North York General Hospital - Branson Division; (416)631-6859

RAMPRASHAD, Claudius A; The Two Hundred, 114-200 St Clair Ave W, Toronto ON M4V 1R1; West Indies (Jamaica)'63; MB BS; FRCPC; DiagRad. (416)923-5148; Fax. (416)923-7462.

RAMPTON, Joey V; Royal Victoria Hosp, 201 Georgian Dr, Barrie ON L4M 6M2; Tor'91; CCFP; CCFP(E.M.); Staff, Royal Victoria Regional Health Centre; (705)728-9802 x4121

RAMRATTAN, Brian; Saint John Reg Hosp, PO Box 2100 Stn Main 400 University Ave, Saint John NB E2L 4L2; West Indies (Jamaica)'96; Staff, Saint John Regional Hospital; (506)648-6000

RAMROOPSINGH, Rickey B; King Dufferin Family Med Ctre, 5-1209 King St W, Toronto ON M6K 1G2; West Indies (Jamaica)'82; Court Staff, St Joseph's Health Centre; (416)536-2500

RAMSAHOYE, Max; PO Box 2903, Wainwright AB T9W 1S8; Alb'95; CCFP; Staff, Wainwright Health Centre; sandm@telusplanet.net.

RAMSAY, David A; London HSC-University Hosp, PO Box 5339 Stn B 339 Windermere Rd, London ON N6A 5A5; Glasgow (Scotland)'77; MB ChB; DPhil; BSc; FRCPath; MRCP(UK); FRCPC; NeurPath (Forensic & Neuro Pathology). Ac Staff Neuropath, London Health Sciences Centre - University Hospital; Associate Path, The Hospital For Sick Children; Assoc Prof, University of Western Ontario; (519)685-8500 x36354; Fax. (519)663-2930.

RAMSAY, Donald R; 200-3604 52 Ave NW, Calgary AB T2L 1V9; Sask'75; (403)284-2261; Fax. (403)284-9434.

RAMSAY, Gillian I; 205-9148 23 Ave NW, Edmonton AB T6N 1H9; Qns'02; FRCPC; IntMed. Staff, University of Alberta Hospital; (780)462-3010; Fax. (780)440-2911.

RAMSAY, Glenna L; Hawkstone Med Clinic, 204-18332 Lessard Rd NW, Edmonton AB T6M 2W8; Alb'87; CCFP; Staff, Covenant Health - Misericordia Community Hospital; University of Alberta; (780)486-3461

RAMSAY, J Douglas; 303 A-2181 Queen St E, Toronto ON M4E 1E5; Qns'74; FRCPC; Psy (Psychoanalysis). Ac Staff, St Michael's Hospital; Lecturer, University of Toronto; (416)231-3637; Fax. (416)231-4774; jdougramsay@rogers.com.

RAMSAY, Jacques; Commissaire la Sante et Bien-E, 11e étage-1701 rue Parthenais, Montreal QC H2K 3S7; Mon'87; FRACGP; Langs: English; French; (514)873-1845 x21227; Fax. (514)873-8943; jacques.ramsay@msp.gouv.qc.ca.

RAMSAY, Jennifer A; Hamilton HS-Henderson Site, 208-711 Concession St, Hamilton ON L8V 1C3; McG'82; BSc; FRCPC; AnatPath. Staff, Hamilton Health Sciences Centre-Juravinski Site; (905)521-2100; Fax. (905)389-1698.

RAMSAY, R Alec; Allan Memorial Institute, 1025 av des Pins O, Montreal QC H3A 1A1; McG'62; CSPQ; DPsy; FRCPC; Psy (Psychosomatic Medicine). Sr Staff Psy, McGill University Health Centre - Royal Victoria Hospital; assoc Prof, McGill University; Langs: English; French; (514)934-1934 x35321

RAMSAYWAK, Peggy C; Upper Appleby Med Assoc, 36-1960 Appleby Line, Burlington ON L7L 0B7; McM'06; CCFP.

RAMSDALE, E Helen; St Joseph's Healthcare, 50 Charlton Ave E, Hamilton ON L8N 4A6; Oxford (England)'73; MB BS; FRCPC; IntMed; Respir. Staff, St Joseph's Healthcare - Charlton Campus; Assoc Prof, McMaster University; (905)521-6000; Fax. (905)521-6183; ramsdale@mcmaster.ca.

RAMSDEN, John E; 1380 21st St, West Vancouver BC V7V 4B3; Wes'84; FRCPC; Anes. (604)922-8432

RAMSDEN, Michael F; Columbia Med Bldg, 403-301 Columbia St E, New Westminster BC V3L 3W5; UBC'78; MSc(Clin.Epidem.); FRCPC; IntMed; Rheum. Staff Physician, Royal Columbian Hospital; (604)526-2140; Fax. (604)526-2279; ramsden@jointdocs.ca.

RAMSEWAK, Ravi D; Listowel Mem Hosp, 255 Elizabeth St E, Listowel ON N4W 2P5; (Trinidad & Tobago)'94; BSc; MB BS; Staff, Listowel Memorial Hospital - Listowel Wingham Hospitals Alliance; (519)291-3125; Fax. (519)291-1528.

RAMSEWAK, Winston S; Winston Reg Hosp-Metropolitan, 1995 Lens Ave, Windsor ON N8W 1L9; West Indies (Jamaica)'77; MB BS; FRCPC; DiagRad. Med Dir Dept of Diag Imaging, Windsor Regional Hospital - Metropolitan Site; (519)254-5577 x52446

RAMSEY, Catherine O M V; Alder Med Centre, 277 Evergreen Rd, Campbell River BC V9W 5Y4; UBC'87; CCFP; (250)287-7441; Fax. (250)287-4384.

RAMSEY, Clare D; Respiratory Unit, RS320-810 Sherbrook St, Winnipeg MB R3A 1R8; Man'96; FRCPC; IntMed; Respir.

RAMSEY, Damon; 84 Hastings St W, Vancouver BC V6B 1G6; McM'09; CCFP; (604)689-8803

RAMSEY, Gillian D; Children's Hosp Eastern Ont, 401 Smyth Rd, Ottawa ON K1H 8L1; Qns'01; FRCPC; Anes. Staff, Children's Hospital of Eastern Ontario (CHEO); (613)737-2431

RAMSEY, Kevin M; 227-1634 Harvey Ave, Kelowna BC V1Y 6G2; Dal'01; FRCSC; Ophth (Retinal Disease). Staff, Kootenay Lake General Hospital; (250)979-2060; Fax. (250)979-2006.

RAMSEY, Michael S; Queen Elizabeth II HSC, 2035-1276 South Park St, Halifax NS B3H 2Y9; Belfast (Ireland)'61; FRCSC; Ophth. Ac Staff, Queen Elizabeth II Health Sciences Centre - Victoria General Site; Prof Ophth, Dalhousie University; (902)473-3226; Fax. (902)473-2839.

RAMSEY, N Bruce; Royal Alexandra Hosp, 10240 Kingsway NW, Edmonton AB T5H 3V9; Dal'96; PhD; MSc; BSc; FRCPC; Anes. Staff, University of Alberta Hospital; Staff, Royal Alexandra Hospital; (780)735-4010

RAMSEY, Patricia A; Queens North Hosp, PO Box 1004 Stn Main 1100 Pleasant Dr, Minto NB E4B 3Y6; Dal'94; Staff, Queens North Community Health Centre; (506)327-7888

RAMSEY, Robert T; Alder Med Centre, 277 Evergreen Rd, Campbell River BC V9W 5Y4; UBC'89; CCFP; (250)287-7441; Fax. (250)287-4384.

RAMSEY, Suzanne E; IWK Health Centre, PO Box 9700 Rpo CSC 2755-5850 University Ave, Halifax NS B3K 6R8; Ott'92; BSc; FRCPC; Peds (Pediatric Rheumatology); Rheum. Staff Ped Rheumatol, IWK Health Centre; Vis Consultant, Dr Everett Chalmers Regional Hospital; Consultant, Queen Elizabeth II Health Sciences Centre - Victoria General Site; Assoc Prof Peds, Dalhousie University; Langs: French; (902)470-8827; Fax. (902)470-7217.

RAMSEY, Una P; Bearspaw Med Associates, 1931 105 St NW, Edmonton AB T6J 5V9; Dal'99; CCFP; (780)438-3241; Fax. (780)435-2511.

RAMSEY, Wayne R; Grey Nun's Community Hosp & HC, 1100 Youville Drive West NW, Edmonton AB T6L 5X8; Alb'88; FRCPC; GenPath. Staff, Covenant Health - Grey Nuns Community Hospital; (780)735-7395

RAMSHAW, Lisa Anna Louise; Addiction & Mental Hlth-Queen, 3-1001 Queen St W, Toronto ON M6J 1H4; McM'95; BSc; PhD; FRCPC; Psy (Forensic Psychiatry). Staff, Centre for Addiction & Mental Health (CAMH) - College Street Site; Staff, Centre for Addiction & Mental Health (CAMH) - Queen Site; Lecturer, University of Toronto; (416)535-8501 x2471; Fax. (416)583-4319; lisa_ramshaw@camh.net.

RAMSHAW, Peter J; Shoniker Clinic, 2877A Ellesmere Rd, Scarborough ON M1E 4C1; Tor'86; FRCPC; Psy (Child & Adolescent Psychiatry). Staff, Rouge Valley Health System - Centenary Health Centre Site; Clin Dir, Shoniker Clinic; (416)281-7301; Fax. (416)281-7465.

RAMSINGH, Rosemarie; Porcupine Hlth Unit Corporate, PO Box 2012 Stn Main 169 Pine St S, Timmins ON P4N 8B7; Ott'93; FRCPC; CommunMed (Public Health & Preventive Medicine). Physician, Porcupine Health Unit Corporate Office; Langs: Spanish; French; (705)267-1181; Fax. (705)264-3980; rosemarie.ramsingh@porcupinehu.on.ca.

RAMSTEAD, Cory L; 200-300 Brae Rd, Duncan BC V9L 3T8; Sask'04; FRCSC; Ophth. (250)748-2922

RAMSTEAD, Margaret J; Royal Jubilee Hosp, 1952 Bay St, Victoria BC V8R 1J8; Sask'06; FRCPC; Psy. (250)370-8000

RAMSUNDHAR, Rohan; Tri Cities Mental Health, 1-2232 Elgin Ave, Port Coquitlam BC V3C 2B2; Natal (South Africa)'70; MB ChB; LMCC; FFPsy; FRCPC; Psy (Adult Psychiatry). Consultant, Community Mental Health Centre; (604)777-8400

RAMZY, Medhat N; Pro-Care Med Clinic, 3-3551 Sheppard Ave E, Scarborough ON M1T 3K8; Ain Shams (Egypt)'81; MB BCh; CCFP; Langs: Arabic; (416)298-1966; Fax. (416)298-1855.

RANA, Abdul Q; 305-1371 Neilson Rd, Scarborough ON M1B 4Z7; Punjab (Pakistan)'92; FRCPC; Neur.

RANA, Afshan N; Scarborough Hosp-Birchmount, 3030 Birchmount Rd, Scarborough ON M1W 3W3; Ott'94; FRCPC; IntMed; MedOncol. Staff, The Scarborough Hospital - Birchmount Campus; (416)495-2701 x5263; Fax. (416)495-2420.

RANA, Alia W; Rosedale Med Group, 280 Queenston Rd, Hamilton ON L8K 1H1; Punjab (Pakistan)'98; CCFP; (905)547-0508

RANA, Amira; Sunnybrook Odette Cancer Ctre, 2075 Bayview Ave, Toronto ON M4N 3M5; Punjab (India)'00; FRCPC; IntMed; MedOncol. Staff, Sunnybrook Health Sciences Centre - Edmond Odette Cancer Centre; (416)480-4617; Fax. (416)480-6002.

RANA, Amit M; Plains Med Centre, 141 Plains Rd W, Burlington ON L7T 1G1; McM'06; CCFP; (905)218-6444

RANA, Babra M; Kensington Med Clinic, 6546 Hastings St, Burnaby BC V5B 1S2; Punjab (Pakistan)'84; MB BS; FRCPC; Psy. Langs: Urdu; Hindi; Punjabi; (604)299-9769

RANA, Fakhara N; Healthplex, 2-452 Rathburn Rd, Etobicoke ON M9C 3S8; Alb'97; CCFP; (416)621-6161

RANA, Punam; Sunnybrook Hlth Sciences Ctre, 2075 Bayview Ave, Toronto ON M4N 3M5; McM'07; FRCPC; IntMed; MedOncol. Staff, Sunnybrook Health Sciences Centre; (416)480-6100

RANA, Ranjit S; A12-3300 McNicoll Ave, Scarborough ON M1V 5J6; Punjab (India)'80; Langs: Punjabi; Hindi; Urdu; (416)299-7711; Fax. (416)299-7226.

RANA, Shabana; Winston Park Med Centre, 2315 Bristol Cir, Oakville ON L6H 6P8; Punjab (Pakistan)'91; CCFP; (905)287-2035

RANA, Shreyas K; Medical Arts Bldg, 165 Plymouth Rd, Welland ON L3B 3E1; (Saint Lucia)'01; CCFP; (905)735-5627

RANALLI, Paul J; 403-2115 Finch Ave W, Toronto ON M3N 2V6; Tor'79; FRCPC; Neur (Neuro Ophthalmology). Staff Neurol, Humber River Regional Hospital - Finch Avenue Site; Lecturer, University of Toronto; (416)748-3002; Fax. (416)748-5967; pjranalli@aim.com.

RANAWAYA, Ranjit N; Movement Disorders Clinic, Area 3-3350 Hospital Dr NW, Calgary AB T2N 4N1; Southampton (England)'78; FRCP; MB; FRCPC; Neur (Movement Disorders). Staff Neurol, Calgary Regional Health Authority; Clin Assoc Prof Clin Neurosciences, University of Calgary; Langs: Gujarati; Hindi; (403)944-4364; Fax. (403)944-4063.

RANCHOD, Hetesh A; Mount St Joseph Hosp, 4284-3080 Prince Edward St, Vancouver BC V5T 3N4; Natal (South Africa)'80; MB ChB; LMCC; FRCPC; IntMed; GeriatricMed. Staff, Providence Health Care - Mount Saint Joseph Hospital; (604)877-8315

RANCHOD, Neelesh; 202-3001 Tutt St, Kelowna BC V1Y 2H4; Witwatersrand (South Africa)'95; FRCPC; Peds. (250)575-1281

RANCOURT, Agnes; CHSLD de la MRC de Champlain, 831 av Notre-Dame, Saint-Lambert QC J4R 1S1; Mon'04; Staff, CHSLD de la MRC de Champlain-Centre Saint-Lambert; (450)771-3333; agnes.rancourt@rrsss16.gouv.qc.ca.

RANCOURT, Claudine; CSSS Kamouraska-Hop-Notre Dame, CP 460 1201 6e av, La Pocatiere QC G0R 1Z0; Laval'10; CCFP; Staff, CSSS de Kamouraska; (418)856-7000

RANCOURT, Cynthia; Ctr Hosp Affilie-St-Sacrement, 1050 ch Sainte-Foy, Quebec QC G1S 4L8; Laval'06; Staff, Centre Hospitalier Affilié Universitaire de Québec - Hôpital du St-Sacrement; (418)682-7511

RANCOURT, Jean-Francois; Clinique Med de Montmagny, 100-83 av de la Fabrique, Montmagny QC G5V 2J3; Laval'84; Staff, CSSS de Montmagny-L'Islet; (418)248-4933; jean-francois.rancourt@gmf.gouv.qc.ca.

RANCOURT, Valerie; Hôpital Laval, 2725 ch Sainte-Foy, Quebec QC G1V 4G5; Laval'03; FRCPC; Anes. Staff, Hôpital Laval; Staff, Centre Hospitalier Universitaire de Quebec-CHUL; (418)656-8711

RAND, Juri; Time Square, 205-380 Armour Rd, Peterborough ON K9H 7L7; McM'80; Langs: Estonian; Swedish; (705)745-3215; jrand@prhc.on.ca.

RANDALL, James P; Carling-Broadview Med Bldg, 106-770 Broadview Ave, Ottawa ON K2A 3Z3; Mem'88; FRCS; FRCSC; OrthSurg (Arthroplasty). Staff, Queensway Carleton Hospital; (613)722-3987; Fax. (613)722-0902; ortho1@rogers.com.

RANDALL, Paul T; King City Medical Assoc, PO Box 370 Stn Main 20 Doctors Lane, King City ON L7B 1A6; Tor'72; CCFP; FCFP; Staff, Mackenzie Richmond Hill Hospital; (905)833-5381; Fax. (905)833-5649; staff-kcma@rogers.com.

RANDALL, Thomas E; Vancouver Gen Hosp, 855 12th Ave W, Vancouver BC V5Z 1M9; UBC'76; Anes. Staff, Vancouver General Hospital - Centennial Pavillion; (604)875-4575

RANDALL, Troy D; 34-435 Brookside Dr, Fredericton NB E3A 8V4; Dal'89; Assoc Staff, Dr Everett Chalmers Regional Hospital; tranda@nb.aibn.com.

RANDAZZO, Mary E; Norfolk Gen Hosp, 365 West St, Simcoe ON N3Y 1T7; McM'97; Staff, Norfolk General Hospital; (519)429-6975; mrandazzo@bancroftfht.com.

RANDELL, L Christopher; Yarmouth Reg Health Centre, 60 Vancouver St, Yarmouth NS B5A 2P5; Mem'81; CCFP; FCFP; Staff, Yarmouth Regional Hospital; (902)742-3541; chris.randell@nf.sympatico.ca.

RANDHAWA, Bawa S; Raspberry View Med Centre, 22 McCallum Rd, Abbotsford BC V2S 8A2; Sheffield (England)'74; MB ChB; Staff, Abbotsford Regional Hospital & Cancer Centre; (604)853-9521

RANDHAWA, Harkamal; The Hosp for Sick Children, 555 University Ave, Toronto ON M5G 1X8; Dal'98; FRCPC; Peds (Family Medicine). Staff, The Hospital For Sick Children; (416)813-1500; Fax. (416)813-7909.

RANDHAWA, Kavita; North York Total Rehab & Med C, 5292 Yonge St, North York ON M2N 5P9; Dublin (Ireland)'04; MB BCh; BAO; CCFP; Langs: Punjabi; Spanish; (416)223-6666; Fax. (416)223-5335; drkavitarandhawa@gmail.com.

RANDHAWA, Manjinder S; North Whitby Med Centre, 3975 Garden St, Whitby ON L1R 3A4; Tor'91; Staff, Lakeridge Health - Oshawa Site; Court Staff, Markham Stouffville Hospital; (905)430-2400; Fax. (905)430-1599.

RANDHAWA, Ramandeep S; UBC Hospital, M334-2211 Wesbrook Mall, Vancouver BC V6T 2B5; UBC'99; FRCPC; Psy. Staff, UBC Hospital - Koerner Pavillion; Dep Asst, Vancouver General Hospital - Centennial Pavillion; (604)733-2329

RANDHAWA, Roop S; UBC Faculty of Med, 3300-910 10th Ave W, Vancouver BC V5Z 1M9; UBC'08; (604)875-4575

RANDLE, John A; York Prof Bldg, 209-679 Davis Dr, Newmarket ON L3Y 5G8; Tor'92; FRCSC; OrthSurg. (905)967-1006; Fax. (905)967-1005.

RANDLETT, Mary Jane; 5-30 Thirteenth St E, Cornwall ON K6H 6V9; Dal'83; Staff, Cornwall Community Hospital; Med Dir, Carefor Cornwall Hospice; (613)933-2493; Fax. (613)932-2238.

RANDOIN, Michele-Anne; Tribunal Admin du Quebec, RC10-575 rue Saint-Amable, Quebec QC G1R 5R4; Laval'82; (418)643-3418

RANDUNNE, Avanthi; Winnipeg Reg Health Authority, 1001 Corydon Ave, Winnipeg MB R3M 0B6; (Sri Lanka)'95; CCFP; Staff, Winnipeg Regional Health Authority; (204)940-2000

RANDUNNE, Ayodya S; Selkirk Med Centre, 353 Eveline St, Selkirk MB R1A 1N1; Colombo (Sri Lanka)'98; CCFP.

RANEV, Dimitre; Clinique Med du Plateau, 300-195 rue de l'Atmosphere, Gatineau QC J9A 0A3; Tor'10; CCFP; (819)776-0001

RANG, Louise C F; Kingston Gen Hosp, 76 Stuart St, Kingston ON K7L 2V7; Wes'96; FRCPC; EmergMed. Staff, Kingston General Hospital; (613)549-6666 x2368

RANGANATHAN, Narasimhan; 415-2425 Bloor St W, Toronto ON M6S 4W4; Madras (India)'63; MB BS; DABIM; FACP; FACC; FRCPC; IntMed (Cardiology). Hon Consultant, St Michael's Hospital; Staff Cardiol, St Joseph's Health Centre; Assoc Prof Med, University of Toronto; Langs: Tamil; (416)762-0279; Fax. (416)762-0278.

RANGASWAMY, Satish; Urology Associates, 18A-450 Westheights Dr, Kitchener ON N2N 2B9; Dal'86; FRCSC; Urol. Assoc Staff Surg, Grand River Hospital - Kitchener/Waterloo Health Centre; Assoc Staff Surg, St Mary's General Hospital; (519)578-1282; Fax. (519)578-1362.

RANGER, Adrianna; London HSC-Victoria Hosp, PO Box 5010 Stn B B1 138C-800 Commissioners Rd E, London ON N6A 5W9; McM'93; FRCSC; Neursurg (Pediatric Neuro Surgery). Staff, London Health Sciences Centre - Victoria Campus; Assoc Prof NeuroSurg & Peds, University of Western Ontario; (519)685-8107; Fax. (519)685-8171; adriana.ranger@lhsc.on.ca.

RANGER, Jacques; CSSS de Laval, 280 boul du Roi-du-Nord, Laval QC H7L 4L2; Mon'84; (450)622-5110 x4251; Fax. (450)622-4150.

RANGER, Melissa; Hop Charles LeMoyne, 3120 boul Taschereau, Greenfield Park QC J4V 2H1; Mon'05; FRCPC; EmergMed. Staff, Hopital Charles LeMoyne; (450)466-5000

RANGER, Patrice A; Simon Fraser University, 300-515 Hastings St W, Vancouver BC V6B 5K3; Tor'90; CCFP; Staff, Simon Fraser University; Langs: English; French; (778)782-5200; pranger@sfu.ca.

RANGER, Pierre; Hop du Sacre-Coeur de Mtl, 5400 boul Gouin O, Montreal QC H4J 1C5; Mon'79; MSc; FRCSC; OrthSurg. Staff, Hôpital du Sacre-Coeur de Montréal; (514)338-2222

RANGWALA, Sohil; Primrose Family Med Centre, 35 Primrose Ave, Ottawa ON K1R 0A1; McG'06; MDCM; CCFP; (613)230-7788; Fax. (613)230-7778.

RANI, Ritu; Meadowlark Health Centre, 154 Meadowlark Shopping Ctr NW, Edmonton AB T5R 5W9; Punjabi University (India)'96; FRCPC; OccupMed. (780)429-4761

RANIERI, Thomas R; 200-10230 142 St NW, Edmonton AB T5N 3Y6; Alb'84; CCFP; FCFP; Staff, Covenant Health - Misericordia Community Hospital; (780)454-4242; Fax. (780)454-4224.

RANJI, Mostafa; Valley Reg Hosp, 150 Exhibition St S, Kentville NS B4N 5E3; Kashan (Iran)'95; Staff, Valley Regional Hospital; (902)679-2657

RANJIT, Ebenezer V; 4371 Walker Rd, Windsor ON N8W 3T6; Madras (India)'70; Ac Staff, Hôtel-Dieu Grace Hospital; Langs: Tamil; (519)254-6176; Fax. (519)253-6763.

RANJITH, Koshela; Stirling Med Centre, RR 4 9C Tuftsville Rd, Stirling ON K0K 3E0; (Grenada)'94; CCFP; Langs: Tamil; (613)395-5566; Fax. (613)395-3636.

RANKEN, Kersti A; 406-379 Church St, Markham ON L6B 0T1; McM'06; ObstGyn. (905)472-4553; Fax. (905)472-1877.

RANKIN, Aileen R; St Paul's Hosp, 1081 Burrard St, Vancouver BC V6Z 1Y6; Alb'06; FRCPC; DiagRad. Staff, Providence Health Care - St Paul's Hospital; (604)806-8006

RANKIN, Alastair S; Meadowlark Health Centre, 13651 St Albert Trail NW, Edmonton AB T5L 5E7; Alb'67; ABIME; CCFP; Langs: French; German; (780)732-0002

RANKIN, Allison A; Vernon Jubilee Hosp, 2101 32 St, Vernon BC V1T 5L2; McM'94; BSc(Hon); CCFP; FCFP; Staff Active Privileges, Vernon Jubilee Hospital; Teach Staff, University of British Columbia; (250)558-1235

RANKIN, Jason K; Smyth Clinic, 4904 48 St, Leduc AB T9E 6X4; Alb'04; BSc; CCFP; Staff, Leduc Community Hospital; (780)986-2712; Fax. (780)986-0356.

RANKIN, Linda; North Bay Reg Health Centre, 50 College Dr, North Bay ON P1B 0A4; Dal'06; CCFP; Staff, North Bay Regional Health Centre - Regional Mental Health; (705)474-8600

RANKIN, Richard N; London HSC-University Hosp, PO Box 5339 Stn B 339 Windermere Rd, London ON N6A 5A5; St Andrews (Scotland)'70; MB ChB; DMRD; FRCR; FRCPC; DiagRad (Interventional Radiology). Staff, London Health Sciences Centre - University Hospital; Prof Dept of DiagRad & Nuclear Med, University of Western Ontario; (519)663-2900; Fax. (519)663-8803; rankin@uwo.ca.

RANKIN, Wayne M; 6-940 Murphy Rd, Sarnia ON N7S 5C4; Sask'71; Langs: English; (519)542-7721; Fax. (519)542-7723.

RANSOM, Thomas; Queen Elizabeth II HSC, 7VGN-1276 South Park St, Halifax NS B3H 2Y9; Tor'98; FRCP; MD; MSc; FRCPC; IntMed; Endocrin&Metab. Staff, Queen Elizabeth II Health Sciences Centre - Victoria General Site; Asst Prof Med, Dalhousie University; (902)473-3727; Fax. (902)473-3726; thomas.ransom@cdha.nshealth.ca.

RANSON, Allan D; Hamiota Dist Health Centre, 177 Birch Ave, Hamiota MB R0M 0T0; Man'76; CCFP; FCFP; Staff, Hamiota District Health Centre; (204)764-4218; Fax. (204)764-2325; aranson@arha.ca.

RANSON, Marilyn D E; The Hosp for Sick Children, 555 University Ave, Toronto ON M5G 1X8; Man'88; BSc; FRCPC; DiagRad (Pediatric Radiology). Staff, The Hospital For Sick Children; (416)813-5530; Fax. (416)813-7591; marilyn.ranson@sickkids.ca.

RAO, Anita U; St Michael's Hosp, 30 Bond St, Toronto ON M5B 1W8; McG'95; CCFP; FCFP; Anes. Staff Family & Commun Med, Toronto General Hospital - UHN; Staff, Toronto East General Hospital Inc; Staff, St Michael's Hospital; Lecturer, University of Toronto; (416)360-4000

RAO, Chitra; Hamilton HS-General Site, 237 Barton St E, Hamilton ON L8L 2X2; Bihar (India)'66; MB BS; FRCPC; GenPath (Forensic Pathology). Head Reg Forensic Unit, Hamilton Health Sciences Centre - Hamilton General Hospital; Assoc Prof, McMaster University; Langs: Tamil; Hindi; Malayalam; (905)527-4322 x46150; raoc@hhsc.ca.

RAO, Geetha; Dr Langer & Associates, 180 Sandalwood Pky E, Brampton ON L6Z 1Y4; Tor'91; CCFP; FCFP; (905)846-9255; Fax. (905)846-2525.

RAO, Jagadish; Regina Qu'Appelle HR-Regina, 1440 14th Ave, Regina SK S4P 0W5; Wes'00; BScOrg Chem; MScEnv Chem; FRCSC; GenSurg (Critical Care Medicine). Staff, Regina General Hospital; (306)766-6925; Fax. (306)766-6920.

RAO, Jaggi; College Plaza 3, 1003-8215 112 St NW, Edmonton AB T6G 2C8; McM'98; FAAD; FRCPC; Derm (Cosmetic Dermatology). Clin Prof, University of Alberta; (780)437-7189; Fax. (780)437-2247; jrao@ualberta.ca.

RAO, Jayasimha M; Regional Mental HC-London, PO Box 5532 Stn B 850 Highbury Ave, London ON N6A 4H1; Mysore (India)'76; MB BS; MRCPsy(UK); DPM; FRCPC; Psy (Developmental Disability). Staff, Regional Mental Health Care-St Joseph's Health Care; Dir, Dual Diagnosis Research & Treatment Program; Assoc Prof, University of Western Ontario; Langs: Kanarese; (519)455-5110

RAO, Krishna B G; 67 Ontario St, Trenton ON K8V 2G8; Sask'96; FRCSC; Ophth (Glaucoma). (613)394-4545; Fax. (613)394-5048.

RAO, Myurathy; St Joseph's Health Centre, 332-30 The Queensway, Toronto ON M6R 1B5; Ott'98; BSc; FRCPC; IntMed; Nephrol. Staff Ambulatory Care Clinic Dept of Med & Nephrol, St Joseph's Health Centre; Langs: Tamil; French; (416)530-6000 x6227; Fax. (416)530-6233.

RAO, Namita; Glenrose Rehab Hosp, 10230 111 Ave NW, Edmonton AB T5G 0B7; Qns'95; CCFP; Staff, Sturgeon Community Hospital; Staff, Glenrose Rehabilitation Hospital; Clin Teacher Family Med, University of Alberta; (780)735-8800; Fax. (780)735-8846.

RAO, Nasa S K; Mental Hlth & Addiction Servic, 15 Chipman Dr, Kentville NS B4N 3V7; (India)'91; (902)365-1701; Fax. (902)679-1766.

RAO, Pramila; Thunder Bay Med Centre, 470-63 Algoma St N, Thunder Bay ON P7A 4Z6; Andhra (India)'76; MB BS; FRCPC; CCFP; PhysMed&Rehab. Advisor Rehab, St Joseph's Care Group - St Joseph's Hospital; (807)344-8475; Fax. (807)344-6323.

RAO, Rajeev V; McMaster University, 1280 Main St W, Hamilton ON L8S 4K1; Wes'06; FRCPC; IntMed; Cardiol. Staff, Hamilton Health Sciences Centre - McMaster University Medical Centre.

RAO, Sanjay C; BC Cancer Ctre-Southern Interi, 399 Royal Ave, Kelowna BC V1Y 5L3; Qns'98; FRCPC; IntMed; MedOncol. Staff, BC Cancer Agency Sindi Ahluwalia Hawkins Centre for the Southern Interior; (250)712-3996; Fax. (250)712-3911.

RAO, Shanti E; Hotel-Dieu Grace Hosp, 7F-1030 Ouellette Ave, Windsor ON N9A 1E1; Cal'99; CCFP; FCFP; Ac Staff Privil, Hôtel-Dieu Grace Hospital; Langs: Hindi; Kanarese; (519)973-4411

RAO, Sheshagiri A S; Delta Hosp, 5800 Mountain View Blvd, Delta BC V4K 3V6; Mysore (India)'65; MB BS; DABR; FRCPC; DiagRad (Diagnostic Imaging). Chief Med Imaging, Delta Hospital; Lecturer, University of British Columbia; (604)946-1121 x3228; Fax. (604)940-3974.

RAO, Venkat B; 7-900 King St W, Kitchener ON N2G 1G5; Osmania (India)'60; MS(Surg); FACS; FICS; FRCSC; GenSurg (Vascular Surgery). Ac Staff, St Mary's General Hospital; Ac Staff, Grand River Hospital - Kitchener/Waterloo Health Centre; (519)578-6960; Fax. (519)578-6969.

RAO, Vivek; Univ Hlth Network-Toronto Gen, 4N457-200 Elizabeth St, Toronto ON M5G 2C4; Tor'92; PhD; FRCSC; CardSurg (Heart Failure). Scientist, Toronto General Hospital - UHN; Court Staff, Peterborough Regional Health Centre - Hospital Drive; Consultant, Heartcare Clinic Oshawa; Consultant, Medcan Clinic Toronto; Assoc Prof Surg, University of Toronto; (416)340-3562; Fax. (416)340-3337; vivek.rao@uhn.on.ca.

RAOOF, Shariqa; Tri-Hospital Sleep Laboratory, 208-3024 Hurontario St, Mississauga ON L5B 4M4; Karachi (Pakistan)'00; ABIM; (905)566-1010; shariqa.raoof@sleeplab.ca.

RAOUF-ALKADHIMI, Ahmed; Acton Med & Urgent Care Clinic, 10 Eastern Ave, Acton ON L7J 0A5; Baghdad (Iraq)'96; CCFP; Langs: Arabic; (519)853-4449; Fax. (519)853-5242.

RAPANOS, Theodore; Hamilton HS-General Site, 237 Barton St E, Hamilton ON L8L 2X2; Tor'02; FRCSC; GenSurg; VascSurg. Staff, Hamilton Health Sciences Centre - Hamilton General Hospital; (905)527-4322

RAPHAEL, Frantz; CLSC Saint-Michel, 3355 rue Jarry E, Montreal QC H1Z 2E5; Port-au-Prince (Haiti)'68; Ac Staff, Hôpital Santa Cabrini Ospedale; (514)374-8223 x6352; Fax. (514)374-5753.

RAPHAEL, Julian M C; Campbell Clinic, 430 Major Magrath Dr S, Lethbridge AB T1J 3M1; Dublin (Ireland)'81; MB ChB; BAO; LRCPI&LM; LRCSI&LM; Ad Staff Privil, Chinook Regional Hospital; (403)328-8101

RAPHAEL, Malik; US Memorial Health Centre, PO Box 398, St Lawrence NL A0E 2V0; Baghdad (Iraq)'90; Staff, US Memorial Health Centre; (709)873-2330

RAPHAEL, Simon J; Sunnybrook Hlth Sciences Ctre, E 432-2075 Bayview Ave, Toronto ON M4N 3M5; Wes'84; FRCPC; AnatPath. Staff, Sunnybrook Health Sciences Centre; (416)480-6100

RAPHY, Pascale; Queensway-Carleton Hosp, 3045 Baseline Rd, Nepean ON K2H 8P4; Laval'99; CSPQ; FRCPC; DiagRad. Staff, Queensway Carleton Hospital; (613)721-2000

RAPOPORT, Adam L; The Hosp for Sick Children, 555 University Ave, Toronto ON M5G 1X8; Tor'02; FRCPC; Peds. Fellow, The Hospital For Sick Children; (416)813-1500

RAPOPORT, Daniel; 650-6091 Gilbert Rd, Richmond BC V7C 5L9; UBC'03; FRCSC; Urol. (604)273-4320

RAPOPORT, David; 303-4430 Bathurst St, North York ON M3H 3S3; Tor'67; CCFP; FCFP; Staff, North York General Hospital; (416)638-6223; Fax. (416)638-8834.

RAPOPORT, Mark J; Sunnybrook Hlth Sciences Ctre, FG 37-2075 Bayview Ave, Toronto ON M4N 3M5; McM'95; FRCPC; Psy (Brain Injury Psychiatry) (Geriatric Neuro Psychiatry). Staff, Sunnybrook Health Sciences Centre; Asst Prof, University of Toronto; (416)480-4085; Fax. (416)480-5318; mark.rapoport@sunnybrook.ca.

RAPOPORT-GLICK, Susan; North Med Centre, 201-7131 Bathurst St, Thornhill ON L4J 7Z1; Tor'81; CCFP; FCFP; Staff, North York General Hospital; Staff, North York General Hospital - Branson Division; (905)771-1778

RAPP, Morton S; 39 Elliotwood Crt, North York ON M2L 2P8; Tor'61; DPsy; Psy (Clinical Psychopharmacology). Court Staff, The Scarborough Hospital - General Campus; (416)449-0178; Fax. (416)449-0178.

RAPPAPORT, Jamie M; SMBD Jewish Gen Hosp, 3755 ch Cote-Sainte-Catherine, Montreal QC H3T 1E2; McG'89; FRCSC; Otol. Staff, Sir Mortimer B Davis Jewish General; assoc Prof, McGill University; Langs: Bilingual(English/French); (514)340-8246; Fax. (514)340-7581.

RAPPAPORT, Jerrold L; Decelles Med Centre, 555-5757 av Decelles, Montreal QC H3S 2C3; McG'81; Ac Staff Med, St Mary's Hospital Centre; Dir, Decelles Medical Centre; (514)739-7771; Fax. (514)739-8134.

RAPPAPORT, Maureen E; Dr B Russillo & M Rappaport Cl, 206-5450 ch de la Cote-des-Nei, Montreal QC H3T 1Y6; Sher'86; CCFP; FCFP; Staff, St Mary's Hospital Centre; assoc Prof, McGill University; (514)345-9121; Fax. (514)345-8844.

RAPPARD, Scott C; 103-277 Pleasant St, Dartmouth NS B2Y 4B7; McG'78; FRCPC; IntMed; Respir. Staff, Dartmouth General Hospital; Langs: French; (902)461-4576; Fax. (902)461-4877; scott.rappard@ns.sympatico.ca.

RAPSON, Dilys A; Kingston Gen Hosp, 76 Stuart St, Kingston ON K7L 2V7; Cape Town (South Africa)'66; MB ChB; DCH; FRCPC; HemPath (Medical Oncology). Staff Path, Kingston General Hospital; Asst Prof, Queen's University; (613)548-3232 x4166

RAPSON, Linda M; Rapson Pain Clinic, 207-600 Sherbourne St, Toronto ON M4X 1W4; Tor'65; CAFCI; Court Staff, Toronto General Hospital - UHN; Assoc Staff/Aj Scientist, Toronto Rehabilitation Institute - Lyndhurst Centre; Med Dir, Rapson Pain & Acupuncture Clinic; Exec Pres, Acupuncture Foundation of Canada Institute; (416)968-1366; Fax. (416)968-1367; rapsonclinic@rogers.com.

RAPSON, Valerie E; Atrium Prof Bldg, SS 103 307-190 Cundles Rd E, Barrie ON L4M 4S5; Tor'90; CCFP; FCFP; Court Staff, Royal Victoria Regional Health Centre; (705)739-1156; Fax. (705)739-9013.

RAPTIS, Stavros; Hop Santa Cabrini Ospedale, 5655 rue Saint-Zotique E, Montreal QC H1T 1P7; McG'88; CSPQ; FRCPC; AnatPath. Staff, Hôpital Santa Cabrini Ospedale; (514)252-6607

RASAIAH, Suvi B; 24-1515 Dufferin Cres, Nanaimo BC V9S 2B8; Qns'93; FRCPC; IntMed; Nephrol. (250)753-2446; Fax. (250)753-9686.

RASARATNAM, Asvini; 20-1450 O'Connor Dr, East York ON M4B 2T8; McG'09; CCFP; (416)285-4075

RASASINGHAM, Rajeevan; Humber River Reg Hosp-Keele, 2175 Keele St, York ON M6M 3Z4; Ross University (Dominica)'03; FRCPC; Psy. Staff, Humber River Regional Hospital - Keele Street Site; (416)658-2087

RASHED, Nashed; 104-704 Mara St, Point Edward ON N7V 1X4; Ain Shams (Egypt)'78; FRCPC; Peds (Consultant Pediatrics). Med Dir Maternal Infant Child Prog & Hd, Bluewater Health - Mitton Site; Staff, Bluewater Health - Norman Site; Langs: Arabic; (519)344-7819; Fax. (519)344-2599; nrashed@cogeco.ca.

RASHED, Selim; Hop Maisonneuve-Rosemont, 5415 boul de l'Assomption, Montreal QC H1T 2M4; Sher'80; Peds (P.Q.). Staff, Hopital Maisonneuve-Rosemont; (514)252-3400

RASHEED, Nida H; William Osler HC-Brampton, 2100 Bovaird Dr E, Brampton ON L6R 3J7; Baghdad (Iraq)'90; MB ChB; CCFP; Staff, William Osler Health System - Brampton Civic Hospital; (905)494-2120; Fax. (905)494-6563.

RASHID, M D Mizanur; Associate Med Clinic, 400-20 14th St W, Prince Albert SK S6V 3K8; Dhaka (Bangladesh)'85; MB BS; Staff Emerg Room, Victoria Hospital; (306)953-1687; Fax. (306)764-3091; rashidmizanur@yahoo.ca.

RASHID, Meb; Crossroads Clinic, 77 Grenville St, Toronto ON M5S 1B3; Tor'92; CCFP; FCFP; Staff, St Joseph's Health Centre; (413)323-6031; Fax. (416)323-6015.

RASHID, Mohsin; IWK Health Centre, PO Box 9700 Rpo CSC 5850 University Ave, Halifax NS B3K 6R8; Punjab (Pakistan)'83; DABPed; FRCPC; Peds (Pediatric Gastroenterology). Staff Peds & Gastroent, IWK Health Centre; Asst Prof Peds, Dalhousie University; Langs: Urdu; Punjabi; (902)470-8746; Fax. (902)470-7249; mohsin.rashid@iwk.nshealth.ca.

RASHID, Shahid; Toronto Poly Clinic, 204-5460 Yonge St, North York ON M2N 6K7; Pakistan (Pakistan)'84; (416)250-7171

RASHID, Yasmin; All Well Primary Care Centre, 2835 Mill Woods Rd NW, Edmonton AB T6K 4A9; Dar-es-Salaam (Tanzania)'74; (780)450-4550; Fax. (780)461-1985.

RASHID, Zaihan; Lakeridge Hlth Corp-Bowmanv, 47 Liberty St S, Bowmanville ON L1C 2N4; Karachi (Pakistan)'78; MB BS; FRCS(Edin); FRCS(Eng); FRCSC; GenSurg (Colorectal Surgery). Staff GenSurg, Pembroke Regional Hospital Inc; Staff, Lakeridge Health - Bowmanville Site; Langs: Urdu; (905)623-3331

RASHIDI, Farid; Royal University Hosp, 103 Hospital Dr, Saskatoon SK S7N 0W8; Shahid Beheshti (Iran)'93; FRCPC; DiagRad;CCFP; Staff, Royal University Hospital; (306)655-1000

RASHIQ, Saifudin; Clinical Sciences Bldg, 8 120-152 University Campus NW, Edmonton AB T6G 2G3; Nottingham (England)'87; MB BS; FRCPC; Anes. Staff, University of Alberta Hospital; Asst Prof Anes & Pain Med/Dir, University of Alberta; (780)407-8861; Fax. (780)407-3200.

RASHLEIGH, Dennis; Western Mem Reg Hosp, PO Box 2005 Stn Main 1 Brookfield Ave, Corner Brook NL A2H 6J7; Qns'98; CCFP; FCFP; Staff, Western Memorial Regional Hospital; (709)637-5000

RASIC, Nivez F; Alberta Children's Hosp, 2888 Shaganappi Trail NW, Calgary AB T3B 6A8; Man'02; FRCPC; Anes. Staff, Alberta Children's Hospital; (403)955-7810; Fax. (403)955-7606.

RASIO, Eugenio A; CHUM-Hop Notre-Dame, 1560 rue Sherbrooke E, Montreal QC H2L 4M1; Brussels (Belgium)'59; PhD(Physiol); Endocrin (P.Q.) (Endocrinology & Metabolism). assoc Dir Academic Affairs, Centre Hospitalier l'Université de Montréal (CHUM) - Hôpital Notre-Dame; Langs: French; Italian; (514)890-8000 x27282; Fax. (514)896-6237; eugenio.rasio@umontreal.ca.

RASK, Sara J; Royal Victoria Hosp, 201 Georgian Dr, Barrie ON L4M 6M2; Wes'05; FRCPC; IntMed; MedOncol. Staff, Royal Victoria Regional Health Centre; (705)728-9090; Fax. (705)739-5627.

RASKIN, Joel; Eli Lilly Canada, 3650 Danforth Ave, Toronto ON M1N 2E8; Tor'81; MD; NBME; FRCPC; Psy. Physician Clin Research Neurosciences, Eli Lilly Canada Inc; Aj Staff Psy, University of Toronto; (416)699-7260; Fax. (416)699-7352.

RASLAN, Tark M E; 12922 82 St NW, Edmonton AB T5E 2T2; (Egypt)'92; Staff, Alberta Hospital Edmonton; (587)521-3525; Fax. (587)521-3526.

RASMINSKY, Michael; MUHC-Montreal Gen Hosp, 1650 av Cedar, Montreal QC H3G 1A4; Harvard(MA) (USA)'64; PhD(Lond); Neur. Sr Physician, McGill University Health Centre - Montreal General Campus; Emeritus Prof, McGill University; Langs: French; (514)934-8059; Fax. (514)934-8265; michael.rasminsky@mcgill.ca.

RASMUSSEN, Derek J; Associate Med Centre, 5016 48 Ave, Taber AB T1G 1R8; (Netherlands Antilles)'06; CCFP; (403)223-3525; Fax. (403)223-9020.

RASMUSSEN, Lisa A; MUHC-Montreal Children's Hosp, A 501-2300 rue Tupper, Montreal QC H3H 1P3; Sask'06; FRCPC; Neur. Staff, McGill University Health Centre - Montreal Children's Hospital; (514)412-4400

RASMUSSEN, Ole S; Medical Prof Corporation, PO Box 37040 Rpo Landmark, Regina SK S4S 7K3; Sask'75; Ac Staff, Pasqua Hospital; Ac Staff, Regina General Hospital; Ac Staff, Wascana Rehabilitation Centre; Med Advisor, Extendicare/Sunset; Langs: Danish; (306)789-7600

RASMUSSEN, Steven L; Dept of Pathology & Lab Med, 910 10th Ave W, Vancouver BC V5Z 4E3; Denver (USA)'81; FRCPC; AnatPath. (604)875-4111 x63975

RASO, Dean A; Guelph Gen Hosp, 115 Delhi St, Guelph ON N1E 4J4; Qns'07; FRCPC; IntMed; Critical Care Medicine. Staff, Guelph General Hospital; (519)822-2170

RASOOL, Kashif G; Windsor Essex Community HC, 1585 Ouellette Ave, Windsor ON N8X 1K5; Karachi (Pakistan)'02; (519)258-6002; Fax. (519)258-7896.

RASOOL, Meenaz H A; 101-4430 Halifax St, Burnaby BC V5C 5R4; Man'76; (604)299-2411; Fax. (604)299-8709.

RASQUIN-WEBER, Andree; Hôpital Ste-Justine, 3175 ch Cote-Sainte-Catherine, Montreal QC H3T 1C5; Louvain (Belgium)'65; Peds (Gastroenterology). ac Staff Gastroent, Hôpital Ste-Justine; Prof Peds, Universite de Montreal; Langs: Bilingual(French/English); (514)345-4626; Fax. (514)345-4999.

RASSAM, Ammar F; Dr A A Wilkinson Mem Hosp, PO Box 70 428-438 Station Dr, Old Perlican NL A0A 3G0; Baghdad (Iraq)'97; Staff, Dr A A Wilkinson Memorial Health Centre; (709)587-2200

RASSEKH, Shahrad R; Children's & Women's HC of BC, A119-4480 Oak St, Vancouver BC V6H 3V4; UBC'00; FRCPC; Peds. Staff, BC Children's Hospital; (604)875-2161

RASSOULI-RASHTI, Mohammad; Royal Victoria Reg Health Cent, 201 Georgian Dr, Barrie ON L4M 6M2; Tor'98; FRCPC; IntMed; MedOncol. Staff, Royal Victoria Regional Health Centre; Langs: Farsi; (705)739-5661; Fax. (705)739-5619.

RASTIKERDAR, Ali; Woodlawn Med Clinic, 92 Main St, Dartmouth NS B2X 1R5; Isfahan (Iran)'01; CCFP; (902)434-1500; Fax. (902)462-8464.

RASTOGI, Aroop; Lakeridge Hlth Corp-Oshawa, 1 Hospital Crt, Oshawa ON L1G 2B9; Tor'94; FRCPC; DiagRad (Magnetic Resonance Imaging). Staff, Lakeridge Health - Oshawa Site; (905)576-8711; Fax. (905)721-4770.

RASTOGI, Nikhil K; The Ottawa Hosp-Gen Campus, 501 Smyth Rd, Ottawa ON K1H 8L6; Dal'88; BSc; FRCPC; Anes. Staff, The Ottawa Hospital - General Campus; (613)737-8187

RASTOGI, Sanjay; Health First Med Centre, 9625 Yonge St, Richmond Hill ON L4C 5T2; McM'92; CCFP; FCFP; (905)508-4114

RASTOGI, Shalini; Thornhill Family Practice, 35-7700 Bathurst St, Thornhill ON L4J 7Y3; Meerut (India)'97; MB BS; CCFP; Langs: Hindi; (905)881-6510; Fax. (905)881-6513.

RASTOGI, Swati; East Alberta Health Centre, 4715 8 Ave SE, Calgary AB T2N 3N4; (India)'01; FRCPC; Peds. (403)543-4090; Fax. (403)543-4093.

RASTY, Golnar; Univ Hlth Network-Toronto Gen, 200 Elizabeth St, Toronto ON M5G 2C4; (Iran)'87; AB; FRCPC; AnatPath (Cytopath). Staff, Toronto General Hospital - UHN; Asst Prof, University of Toronto; (416)480-4014

RASUL, Imran A; Credit Valley Med Arts Centre, 415-2000 Credit Valley Rd, Mississauga ON L5M 4N4; Tor'96; ABIM; FRCPC; IntMed; Gastroent. Staff Gastroent & IntMed, The Credit Valley Hospital; (905)607-8340; Fax. (905)607-7229; imranrasul@sympatico.ca.

RASUL, Zahara; Stouffville Med Centre, 2F-34 Civic Ave, Stouffville ON L4A 1H2; Chittagong (Bangladesh)'00; CCFP; (905)640-3100; Fax. (905)640-5346.

RASULI, Pasteur; The Ottawa Hosp-Gen Campus, 501 Smyth Rd, Ottawa ON K1H 8L6; Tehran (Iran)'75; AB; FRCPC; DiagRad (Interventional Radiology). Ac Staff Radiol, The Ottawa Hospital - General Campus; Consultant, Children's Hospital of Eastern Ontario (CHEO); Assoc Prof, University of Ottawa; Langs: Persian; Turkish; (613)737-8098; Fax. (613)737-8957.

RATANASEANGSUANG, Paul N; St Boniface Gen Hosp, L1019-409 Tache Ave, Winnipeg MB R2H 2A6; Cal'07; FRCPC; EmergMed. Staff, St Boniface General Hospital; (204)233-8563

RATCLIFFE, Elyanne M; McMaster University HSC, 3A27-1280 Main St W, Hamilton ON L8S 4K1; McM'98; FRCPC; Peds; Gastroent. (905)521-2100; Fax. (905)521-2655.

RATEB, George; CHUS- Hop Hotel-Dieu, 1816-580 rue Bowen S, Sherbrooke QC J1G 2E8; Cairo (Egypt)'94; Staff, Centre Hospitalier Universitaire de Sherbrooke-Hôpital Hôtel-Dieu; Langs: English; (819)346-1110 x25501

RATELLE, Richard; CHUM-Hop St-Luc, 1058 rue Saint-Denis, Montreal QC H2X 3J4; Mon'82; FRCSC; GenSurg (Colon & Rectal Surgery). Staff Surg, Centre Hospitalier l'Université de Montréal (CHUM) - Hôpital Notre-Dame; Staff, Centre Hospitalier l'Université De Montréal (CHUM) - Hôpital Saint-luc; Clin Assoc Prof Surg, Universite de Montreal; (514)890-8000 x34953; richard.ratelle.chum@ssss.gouv.qc.ca.

RATH, Michael B; Grove Med Centre, 401-21183 88 Ave, Langley BC V1M 2G5; McG'77; BSc; MDCM; CCFP; FCFP; Langs: English; French; (604)882-1250; Fax. (604)882-2194; grovemed@lightspeed.ca.

RATHBONE, Michel P; McMaster University, 1280 Main St W, Hamilton ON L8S 4K1; Liverpool (England)'66; MB ChB; PhD; FRCPC; Neur. Ac Staff/Staff Researcher, Hamilton Health Sciences Centre-Juravinski Site; Court Staff, St Joseph's Healthcare - Charlton Campus; Prof Med, McMaster University; (905)574-8630; Fax. (905)383-3958; mrathbon@mcmaster.ca.

RATHBUN, James B; B3306-3000 Lawrence Ave E, Scarborough ON M1P 2V1; Qns'66; BSc; OrthSurg. Staff, The Scarborough Hospital - General Campus; (416)267-2334; Fax. (416)267-2539.

RATHEE, Rajinder S; North York Eye Associates, 202-1333 Sheppard Ave E, North York ON M2J 1V1; Dal'96; BSc; FRCSC; Ophth (General Surgery). Assoc Staff, The Scarborough Hospital - Birchmount Campus; Clin Asst, North York General Hospital; Langs: Hindi; (416)494-7455

RATHEE, Seema R; 2533 Danforth Ave, Toronto ON M4C 1L1; Dal'90; CCFP; FCFP; Langs: Hindi; (416)698-5521

RATHGEBER, Lane A; Regina Qu'Appelle HR-Regina, 1440 14th Ave, Regina SK S4P 0W5; Sask'96; BSc(Med); CCFP; CCFP(E.M.); Staff Emerg/Physician, Regina General Hospital; Clinical Asst Prof College of Med, University of Saskatchewan; (306)766-4213; Fax. (306)766-4357; lane.r@sasktel.net.

RATHWELL, Jonathan M; 2671 Concession Rd PO Box 2113, Kemptville ON K0G 1J0; Qns'05; CCFP; (613)258-0100; Fax. (613)258-6171.

RATJEN, Felix; The Hosp for Sick Children, 555 University Ave, Toronto ON M5G 1X8; Frankfurt (Germany)'86; FRCPC; Peds. Staff, The Hospital For Sick Children; Langs: German; (416)813-1500; Fax. (416)813-6246; felix.ratjen@sickkids.ca.

RATNANATHER, Kingsley V J; 202-1575 Lawrence Ave W, North York ON M6L 1C3; (Sri Lanka)'58; MB BS; DPM; FRCPC; Psy (Psycho Pharmacology). Langs: Tamil; (416)781-2626; Fax. (416)781-7151.

RATNAPALAN, Savithiri; The Hosp for Sick Children, 555 University Ave, Toronto ON M5G 1X8; Colombo (Sri Lanka)'83; MRCP(UK); FAAP; MEd; FRCPC; Peds (Emergency Pediatrics). Staff, The Hospital For Sick Children; Assoc Prof, University of Toronto; Langs: Tamil; Sinhalese; (416)813-7532; Fax. (416)813-5043; savithiri.ratnapalan@sickkids.ca.

RATNASINGAM, Ranjith K; William Osler HC-Brampton, 2100 Bovaird Dr E, Brampton ON L6R 3J7; Prague (Czech Republic)'06; CCFP; (289)208-2045

RATNAYAKE, Aluthwala D V S P; Burntwood Comm Hlth Resource C, 50 Selkirk Ave, Thompson MB R8N 0M7; Colombo (Sri Lanka)'81; CCFP; (204)677-1777

RATNAYAKE, Quintine; 72 Brant Ave, Brantford ON N3T 5Z8; (Sri Lanka)'70; MB BS; DPM; MRCPsy; FRCPC; Psy (Depression). Ac Staff, Woodstock General Hospital; (519)751-1151; Fax. (519)751-1824.

RATNAYAKE, Wasantha P; Pembroke Reg Hosp, 705 Mackay St, Pembroke ON K8A 1G8; Peradeniya (Sri Lanka)'92; CCFP; Staff, Pembroke Regional Hospital Inc; (613)732-3675

RATNER, Jack T; Clin Med Sante Action, 220-5910 ch Cote-des-Neiges, Montreal QC H3S 1Z5; McG'54; BSc; DABIM; FRCPC; IntMed (Administration); GeriatricMed (P.Q.); Gastroent (P.Q.). Dir-svcs prof, Donald Berman Maimonides Geriatric Centre; assoc Prof, McGill University; Langs: English; French; (514)733-7381

RATTAN, Nav P S; Horizons Family Medicine, A-5016 51 Ave, Red Deer AB T4N 4H5; Cal'86; CASM; CCFP; Staff, Red Deer Regional Hospital Centre; (403)342-7270; Fax. (403)343-2677.

RATTAN, Nitasha; Forest Glade Med Centre, 3145 Forest Glade Dr, Windsor ON N8R 1W6; Medun (South Africa)'00; (519)739-2888

RATTAN, Simran K; Castlemore Family Med Centre, 2-9960 Airport Rd, Brampton ON L6S 0C5; Sask'06; CCFP; (905)799-2273; Fax. (905)799-2467.

RATTAN, Ukesha; St Paul's Hosp, 1702 20th St W, Saskatoon SK S7M 0Z9; Staff, St Paul's Hospital (Grey Nuns) of Saskatoon; Staff, Nipawin Hospital; (306)371-9752; ukesha@nipawin.com.

RATTE, Carole M R; CHUQ-Ctr Hosp Univ Laval, 2705 boul Laurier, Quebec QC G1V 4G2; Laval'75; CSPQ; FRCPC; Psy (Eating Disorders). Ac Staff, Centre Hospitalier Universitaire de Quebec-CHUL; Prof Psy, Université Laval; (418)654-2121; Fax. (418)654-2132; carole.ratte@fmed.ulaval.ca.

RATTE, Francois; Hotel-Dieu de Levis, 143 rue Wolfe, Levis QC G6V 3Z1; Laval'97; CCFP; CCFP(E.M.); Staff, Hôtel-Dieu de Lévis; (418)835-7121

RATTE, Richard R; Clinique Med de Touraine, 201-860 boul Saint-Rene O, Gatineau QC J8T 8M1; Laval'83; (819)243-2112; Fax. (819)243-0238.

RATTE, Sebastien; Hop Charles LeMoyne, 3120 boul Taschereau, Greenfield Park QC J4V 2H1; Sher'98; FRCSC; GenSurg. Staff, Hopital Charles LeMoyne; (450)466-5000

RATTE, Sonia; PAF, 350-9880 rue Clark, Montreal QC H3L 2R3; Mon'95; CCFP; (514)331-2929; Fax. (514)331-2965.

RATTI, Jillian M; PO Box 86026 Rpo Marda Loop, Calgary AB T2T 6B7; Cal'08; CCFP; Staff, Rockyview General Hospital; (403)943-3597; Fax. (403)943-8411.

RATTRAY, Bruce; Lakeshore Gen Hosp, 160 av Stillview, Pointe-Claire QC H9R 2Y2; Qns'90; Staff, Lakeshore General Hospital - Pointe Claire; (514)630-2225

RATTRAY, Darrien D; 100-2631 28th Ave, Regina SK S4S 6X3; Alb'07; FRCSC; ObstGyn. (306)586-1800; Fax. (306)586-3511.

RATTUE, Melissa; Ctr Hosp Laurentien, 234 rue Saint-Vincent, Ste-Agathe-des-Mts QC J8C 2B8; Mon'05; CCFP; Staff, Centre Hospitalier Laurentien; (819)324-4000 x4802

RATUSHNY, Jeffrey V; 203-26 North St, Bridgewater NS B4V 2V6; Saba (Netherlands Antilles)'07; FRCPC; IntMed. (902)530-3313; Fax. (902)530-3376.

RAU, Neil V; Infectious Diseases Consultant, 208-331 Sheddon Ave, Oakville ON L6J 1X8; Tor'91; DABIM; FRCPC; IntMed (AIDS/HIV); MedMicrobiol; InfectDis. Ac Staff, Halton Healthcare Services Corporation - Oakville Site; Court Staff, The Credit Valley Hospital; Instructor, University of Toronto; Langs: English; French; (905)844-5346; Fax. (905)849-6551.

RAU, Sabnavis M; Peninsula Youth Centre, RR 1 310 Cream St, Fenwick ON L0S 1C0; Mysore (India)'56; MB BS; BSc; MRCP(London); LMSSA(London); DCH(Eng); FRCPC; Peds (Dermatology). Court Staff, Niagara Health System - Welland Hospital Site; (905)892-9777; Fax. (905)735-9018; smrau@sympatico.ca.

RAUBENHEIMER, Anton M; 4212 55 Ave PO Box 1340, Smoky Lake AB T0A 3C0; (South Africa)'91; Langs: Afrikaans; (780)656-2505; Fax. (780)656-2507.

RAUBENHEIMER, Johannes P; Assiniboine Clinic, 633 Lodge Ave, Winnipeg MB R3J 0S9; CCFP.

RAUBENHEIMER, Stephan; 4212 55 Ave PO Box 1340, Smoky Lake AB T0A 3C0; (South Africa)'86; CCFP; Langs: Afrikaans; (780)656-2505; Fax. (780)656-2507; stephan.raubenheimer@aspenrha.ab.ca.

RAUCH, Frank T; Shriners Hosp for Children, 1529 av Cedar, Montreal QC H3G 1A6; Munich (Germany)'91; Staff, Shriners Hospitals For Children - Canada; Langs: German; (514)842-5964

RAUCH, Johan F; Dauphin Med Clinic, 622 3rd St SW, Dauphin MB R7N 1R5; (South Africa)'78.

RAUCH, Ralf; London HSC-Victoria Hosp, PO Box 5010 Stn B 800 Commissioners Rd E, London ON N6A 5W9; Munich (Germany)'93; Staff/Member Paed Cardiol, The Hospital For Sick Children; Staff, Windsor Regional Hospital - Metropolitan Site; Staff, London Health Sciences Centre - Victoria Campus; (519)685-8377; Fax. (519)685-8156.

RAUCHWERGER, David R; Mackenzie Richmond Hill Hosp, 10 Trench St, Richmond Hill ON L4C 4Z3; Qns'03; CCFP; CCFP(E.M.); Staff, Mackenzie Richmond Hill Hospital; (905)883-2041

RAUCHWERGER, Martin; Albany Med Clinic, 807 Broadview Ave, Toronto ON M4K 2P8; Qns'73; FRCPC; IntMed. Assoc Staff, Sunnybrook Health Sciences Centre; Lecturer, University of Toronto; (416)461-9471; Fax. (416)461-2710.

RAUDZUS, Dietmar E; Civil Aviation Med Pacific Reg, 620-800 Burrard St, Vancouver BC V6Z 2J8; UBC'68; CCFP; FCFP; Ac Staff, Providence Health Care - St Paul's Hospital; Civil Aviation Canada; Asst Prof, University of British Columbia; Langs: German; French; (604)666-5601; raudzus@direct.ca.

RAUDZUS, Julia A; St Paul's Hosp, 425 4-1081 Burrard St, Vancouver BC V6Z 1Y6; UBC'03; FRCPC; Psy. Staff, Providence Health Care - St Paul's Hospital; (604)682-2344

RAUH, Juergen R; 101-4695 Hastings St, Burnaby BC V5C 2K6; Alb'68; (604)298-7201; Fax. (604)291-6176.

RAUH, Michael J; Queen's U-Richardson Laborator, 88 Stuart St, Kingston ON K7L 3N6; UBC'07; FRCPC; HemPath. (613)533-2820; Fax. (613)533-2907.

RAUNIYAR, Pooja; 106-15252 32 Ave, Surrey BC V3S 0R7; Alb'09; CCFP; (604)542-4885

RAUPACH, Heinz D; 202-3005 30 St, Vernon BC V1T 9J5; UBC'87; CCFP; (250)542-1353

RAUSCHER, Christopher J; Three Birdges Comm Hlth Ctr, 1292 Hornby St, Vancouver BC V6Z 1W2; Man'81; FRCPC; IntMed; GeriatricMed. Langs: English; French; christopher.rauscher@ubc.ca.

RAUT, Abhishek; The Doctors Office, PO Box 134 Stn Royal Bank LR8-200 Bay St, Toronto ON M5J 2J3; McM'08; CCFP; (416)368-6787; Fax. (416)368-7637.

RAUT, Manisha; Clinique Medicale, 3060 boul Rome, Brossard QC J4Y 1V9; Bombay (India)'82; MB BS; LMCC; Langs: Hindi; French; (450)466-1052

RAUTENBACH, Derick A; Highland Park Med Clinic, 2-6315 Horn St, Red Deer AB T4N 6H5; (South Africa)'91; MB ChB; (403)342-2040; Fax. (403)342-7390.

RAUTH, Sarah J; The Credit Valley Hosp, 2200 Eglinton Ave W, Mississauga ON L5M 2N1; Qns'04; FRCPC; RadOncol. Staff, The Credit Valley Hospital; (905)813-2200

RAVAL, Manojkumar J; St Paul's Hosp, C313-1081 Burrard St, Vancouver BC V6Z 1Y6; UBC'98; MSc; ATLS; BSc; FRCSC; GenSurg (Colon & Rectal Surgery). Chair Colorectal Surgical Tumour Grp Surg Oncol Network, BC Cancer Agency Vancouver Centre; Staff Surg, Providence Health Care - St Paul's Hospital; Clinical Asst Prof, University of British Columbia; (604)806-8711; Fax. (604)806-9604.

RAVALIA, Mohamed I; PO Box 520, Twillingate NL A0G 4M0; (Zimbabwe)'80; LRCP(Ed); CCFP; FCFP; Staff, Notre Dame Bay Memorial Health Centre; Asst Dean Rural Clinical School Med Educ Network, Memorial University Of Newfoundland; (709)884-2131; Fax. (709)884-5159; ravalia@mun.ca.

RAVANDI, Amir; St Boniface Gen Hosp, 409 Tache Ave, Winnipeg MB R2H 2A6; Tor'03; FRCPC; IntMed; Cardiol. Staff, St Boniface General Hospital; (204)233-8563

RAVANI, Pietro; Foothills Med Centre, 1403 29 St NW, Calgary AB T2N 2T9; (Italy)'89; Staff, Foothills Medical Centre; (403)944-8168; Fax. (403)944-2876.

RAVEENDRAN, Arulanantham; St Bishoy Med Centre, C1-95 Times Ave, Thornhill ON L3T 0A2; Jaffna (Sri Lanka)'87; CCFP; (905)707-0666; Fax. (905)709-5666.

RAVEENDRAN, Arulpiragasam; B-640 Ross Ave E, Timmins ON P4N 8P2; Colombo (Sri Lanka)'82; MB BS; MRCOG; FRCSC; ObstGyn. Att Staff, Timmins & District Hospital; (705)268-0966; ravi@nt.net.

RAVEENDRAN, Manoranjitham R; Timmins & Dist Hosp, 700 Ross Ave E, Timmins ON P4N 8P2; Colombo (Sri Lanka)'82; MB BS; FRCPC; Psy (Adult General Psychiatry). Att Staff Psy/Med Dir Mental Hlth/LTC, Timmins & District Hospital; Assoc Prof Psychiatry, Northern Ontario School of Medicine; (705)360-6036; Fax. (705)264-6525.

RAVEENDRAN, Raviraj; Univ Hlth Network-Toronto Western Hosp, 399 Bathurst St, Toronto ON M5T 2S8; (India)'97; Staff Anes, Toronto Western Hospital - University Health Network; (416)603-5118

RAVI, Grama D; Four Corners Med Bldg, 205-2009 Long Lake Rd, Sudbury ON P3E 6C3; Mysore (India)'81; MB BS; DABIM; FRCPC; IntMed; Cardiol. Langs: Hindi; Kanarese; (705)674-8148; Fax. (705)674-8919.

RAVI, Tarsem S; A B C Med Clinic, 115-2985 Drew Rd, Mississauga ON L4T 0A4; McG'97; BSc; CCFP; Langs: Punjabi; French; Hindi; Urdu; (905)672-2800; Fax. (905)672-2805.

RAVICHANDER, Ann Meera; Medical Arts Bldg, 312-750 Spadina Cres E, Saskatoon SK S7K 3H3; Madras (India)'83; MB BS; DGO; FRCSC; ObstGyn. Langs: Tamil; (306)244-0177; Fax. (306)244-8705.

RAVID-EINY, Anat; 101-1106 Ouellette Ave, Windsor ON N9A 1C9; Hebrew (Israel)'91; FRCSC; GenSurg. Staff, Hôtel-Dieu Grace Hospital; (519)258-4433; Fax. (519)258-8793.

RAVIELE, Anelia K; Lakeridge Hlth Corp-Oshawa, 1 Hospital Crt, Oshawa ON L1G 2B9; (Bulgaria)'84; Staff Psy, Lakeridge Health - Oshawa Site; (905)576-8711

RAVINDRAN, Aravindhan; Valley Medical Imaging, 200-5503 206 St, Langley BC V3A 2C6; Kilpauk (India)'95; FRCPC; DiagRad. (604)534-4114

RAVINDRAN, Arun V; Ctr for Addiction & Mental Hlt, 100 Stokes St, Toronto ON M6J 1H4; Ceylon (Sri Lanka)'71; MSc; MB BS; FRCPsy; PhD; FRCPC; Psy (Psycho Pharmacology). Staff, Centre for Addiction & Mental Health (CAMH) - College Street Site; Prof Psy, University of Toronto; Prof Psy, University of Ottawa; (416)535-8501; Fax. (416)260-4171; arun_ravindran@camh.net.

RAVINDRAN, Girija; 11-175 George St N, Peterborough ON K9J 3G6; Madras (India)'69; MB BS; DPH; FRCPC; Psy (Adult Psychiatry). Court Staff, Ross Memorial Hospital; Court Staff, Northumberland Hills Hospital; Langs: Tamil; (705)743-5700

RAVINDRAN, Lakshmi N; Ctr for Addiction & Mental Hlt, 4217-100 Stokes St, Toronto ON M6J 1H4; Ott'01; Psy. Staff, Centre for Addiction & Mental Health (CAMH) - College Street Site; (416)535-8501

RAVINDRAN, Mathura P; Carlton Med Clinic, 16-595 Carlton St, St Catharines ON L2M 4Y2; Madras (India)'80; DCH; DTM; LMCC; MB BS; BSc; CCFP; (905)937-5000

RAVINDRAN, Nikila C; Univ Hlth Network-Toronto Gen, EN14 216-200 Elizabeth St, Toronto ON M5G 2C4; Tor'05; FRCPC; IntMed; Gastroent. Staff, Toronto General Hospital - UHN; (416)340-4800

RAVINDRAN, Nisha I; Partial Hospitalization Progra, 6 2-1001 Queen St W, Toronto ON M6J 1H4; (Ireland)'06; FRCPC; Psy.

RAVINDRAN, Vikram C; 216-40 Finchgate Blvd, Brampton ON L6T 3J1; McM'06; FRCPC; IntMed; Respir. Teach Staff, University of Toronto; (905)456-3699

RAVINDRANATH, Pathmanathan; Bur Oak Med Centre, 5B-20 Bur Oak Ave, Markham ON L6C 0A2; Jaffna (Sri Lanka)'88; CCFP; (905)887-0042; Fax. (905)887-0054.

RAVINSKY, Esther; 700 William Ave, Winnipeg MB R3E 0Z3; McG'71; FRCPC; AnatPath.

RAVINUTHALA, Saradadevi; Grand Falls Med Clinic, 164 Goodyear Ave, Grnd-Falls-Windsor NL A2A 1M4; (India)'82.

RAVITZ, Paula J; Mount Sinai Hosp, 600 University Ave, Toronto ON M5G 1X5; McM'95; FRCPC; Psy. Staff, Mount Sinai Hospital; Head of CE, Psy Outreach Prog, Centre for Addiction & Mental Health (CAMH) - College Street Site; Assoc Head Psychotherapy Prog/Head IPT Training Dept of Psy, University of Toronto; (416)586-4800

RAVULA, Niroop R; Harry Medovy House, 671 William Ave, Winnipeg MB R3E 0Z2.

RAWAL, Punam S; Sydney Family Practice, 196 Kings Rd, Sydney NS B1S 1A1; Leeds (England)'93; CCFP.

RAWAL, Sapna; Fitzgerald Bldg, 112-150 College St, Toronto ON M5S 3E2; McG'06; MDCM; FRCPC; DiagRad. (416)978-6801

RAWAL, Shail; St Michael's Hosp, 30 Bond St, Toronto ON M5B 1W8; Tor'09; Staff, St Michael's Hospital; (416)360-4000

RAWAL, Shashi K; Clinique Med Supra, 1160 av Victoria, Lemoyne QC J4R 1R1; Delhi (India)'69; Langs: French; Hindi; Urdu; (450)465-0655; Fax. (450)466-5898.

RAWANI, David A K; Glenrose Rehabilitation Hosp, 1259-10230 111 Ave NW, Edmonton AB T5G 0B7; Lahore (Pakistan)'86; MB BS; Staff, Glenrose Rehabilitation Hospital; (780)735-8800; Fax. (780)735-8846.

RAWAT, Brijendra K; Hys Med Centre, 202-11010 101 St NW, Edmonton AB T5H 4B9; Rajasthan (India)'79; MB BS; FRCPC; DiagRad. Staff, University of Alberta Hospital; Asst Prof, University of Alberta; Langs: Hindi; (780)426-1121

RAWJI, Anik; Trillium Hlth Ctr-Mississauga, 100 Queensway W, Mississauga ON L5B 1B8; Qns'03; CCFP; CCFP(E.M.); Staff, Trillium Health Centre - Mississauga; (905)848-7199

RAWKINS, Sian R; Mount Sinai Hosp, 932-600 University Ave, Toronto ON M5G 1X5; McM'01; FRCPC; Psy. Staff, Mount Sinai Hospital; (416)586-4800 x4554

RAWLEK, Peter J; Red Deer Reg Hosp Centre, PO Box 5030 Stn Postal Box Ctr 3942 50A Ave, Red Deer AB T4N 6R2; Alb'94; Staff, Red Deer Regional Hospital Centre; (403)343-4444

RAWLEK-STONE, Barbara M; PO Box 3087 Stn Main, Vernon BC V1B 3M1; UBC'83; BSc.

RAWLING, Edward G; PO Box 849, Erin ON N0B 1T0; Wes'57; FACS; FRCSC; GenSurg (Surgical Assistant). Surg Asst, Shouldice Hospital; Hon Staff, Trillium Health Centre - Mississauga; Court Staff, Halton Hill Georgetown; (519)833-2470; Fax. (519)833-2479; erawling@spectranet.ca.

RAWLING, Jean M; Valley View Family Practice, 350-1620 29 St NW, Calgary AB T2N 4L7; Cal'00; BSc; PhD; CCFP; (403)282-1269; Fax. (403)282-9545.

RAWLINGS, Nigel G; 400-10924 107 Ave NW, Edmonton AB T5H 0X5; Sask'05; FRCSC; Ophth. (780)448-1801; Fax. (780)448-1809.

RAWLINS, Jenna R; South Walkerville Med Ctre, 340-2224 Walker Rd, Windsor ON N8W 5L7; Tor'02; FRCSC; ObstGyn. Aj Prof, Schulich School of Medicine-Windsor Campus; (519)258-1592; Fax. (519)258-7350.

RAWLINSON, John; Joseph Brant Mem Hosp, 1230 North Shore Blvd E, Burlington ON L7S 1W7; Oxford (England)'80; FRCPC; DiagRad. Head Diag Raf/Staff, Joseph Brant Memorial Hospital; (905)632-3730

RAWLUK, Wieslaw M; Labrador Grenfell Health, PO Box 7000 Stn C 227 Hamilton River Rd, Happy-Valley-Goose NL A0P 1C0; Katowice (Poland)'68; CCFP; FCFP; Staff, Labrador Health Centre; (709)897-2000

RAWOF, Salma; Boxgrove Med Centre, 100-110 Copper Creek Dr, Markham ON L6B 0P9; McM'08; CCFP; (905)472-8911

RAWOOF, Ragad H; Lakeshore Health Centre, PO Box 110 1 Steenson Dr, Ashern MB R0C 0E0; Mosul (Iraq)'92; Staff, Lakeshore Health Centre; (204)768-2461

RAWOOT, Ashfaq; 207-200 Boudreau Rd, St. Albert AB T8N 6B9; Stellenbosch (South Africa)'03; MB ChB; Staff, Westview Health Centre; (780)569-5455; Fax. (780)569-5145; arawoot@gmail.com.

RAWSON, Claire G; Children's & Women's HC of BC, 3B-4480 Oak St, Vancouver BC V6H 3V4; Cape Town (South Africa)'03; Staff, BC Children's Hospital; (604)453-8300

RAWSTRON, Brock P; Chilliwack Gen Hosp, 45600 Menholm Rd, Chilliwack BC V2P 1P7; UBC'10; CCFP; Staff, Chilliwack General Hospital; (604)795-4141

RAY, A Andrew; 206-1 Quarry Ridge Rd, Barrie ON L4M 7G1; Dal'03; FRCSC; Urol. (705)728-9172; Fax. (705)728-8332; aray@wesdome.com.

RAY, Dalia; Bathurst Med Centre, 300-4256 Bathurst St, North York ON M3H 5Y8; Nagpur (India)'74; MB BS; FRCSC; ObstGyn. Ac Staff, Mackenzie Richmond Hill Hospital; Lecturer, University of Toronto; Langs: Hindi; Bengali; (416)631-7545; Fax. (416)631-6455.

RAY, Erin K; Royal Victoria Hosp, 201 Georgian Dr, Barrie ON L4M 6M2; Wes'96; FRCPC; Anes. Staff, Royal Victoria Regional Health Centre; (705)728-9802

RAY, Gary J; Foothills Family Med Centre, PO Box 460 114 1 St SW, Black Diamond AB T0L 0H0; UBC'98; BSc; CCFP; (403)933-4368; Fax. (403)933-2026; postmaster@ffmc.ca.

RAY, George M; 2-4337 Burnside Line, Orillia ON L3V 6H4; Qns'84; FRCPC; PhysMed&Rehab (Electrodiagnosis). (705)329-0253; Fax. (705)329-4733.

RAY, Janet E; Withdrawal Management Services, 5A-2334 Trent St, Victoria BC V8Y 1R4; McM'88; Assoc Staff, Vancouver Island Health Authority; Staff, University of Victoria Health Services; (250)519-7708

RAY, Joel G; St Michael's Hosp, 30 Bond St, Toronto ON M5B 1W8; McM'93; IntMed. Staff, St Michael's Hospital; (416)864-6060

RAY, Julie A; Geddes Med Group, GD 143 Metcalfe St, Elora ON N0B 1S0; Ott'07; CCFP; (519)846-2224; Fax. (519)846-2005.

RAY, Martin L; View Laser Skin Rejuvination, 1443 View Cres, Delta BC V4L 2K2; McM'81; BAP; LMCC; Dip SportMed; Staff, Delta Hospital; (604)943-6999; Fax. (604)943-8344; drray@viewlaser.com.

RAY, Morris N; Bridgepoint Hosp, 14 St Matthews Rd, Toronto ON M4M 2B5; Tor'68; CCFP; Staff, Bridgepoint Health Centre; (416)461-8251

RAY, Reema; 1190 Tecumseh Rd E, Windsor ON N8W 1B4; Calcutta (India)'99; CCFP; (519)255-9887; Fax. (519)255-9544.

RAYANI, Nargis A; Grey Nuns Community Hosp & HC, 1100 Youville Drive West NW, Edmonton AB T6L 5X8; Nairobi (Kenya)'74; MB ChB; FRCPC; AnatPath (Laboratory Medicine); GenPath. Hon Teacher, University of Alberta; (780)735-7395

RAYAR, Anusha D; Brameast Family Health Org, 38-2130 North Park Dr, Brampton ON L6S 0C9; Ott'08; CCFP; (905)792-2211; Fax. (905)792-2901.

RAYAR, Meera S; The Hosp for Sick Children, 555 University Ave, Toronto ON M5G 1X8; McM'08; FRCPC; Peds. Staff, The Hospital For Sick Children; (416)813-7742

RAYAR, Umesh; The Medical Place, 208-178 John St, Brampton ON L6W 2A4; Ceylon (Sri Lanka)'76; FAAP; FRCPC; Peds (Developmental/Behavioural Pediatrics). Corp Chief Peds(interim), William Osler Health System - Brampton Civic Hospital; Corp Chief Peds(interim), William Osler Health System - Etobicoke General Hospital; Asst Prof, University of Toronto; Asst Clin Prof, McMaster University; Langs: Sinhalese; Tamil; (905)450-0414; Fax. (905)450-0420.

RAYAVARAPU, Beaulah; 100-15129 100 Ave, Surrey BC V3R 9P4; Alb'95; BSc; CCFP; (604)583-3550

RAYBAUD, Charles A D; The Hosp For Sick Children, 2135-555 University Ave, Toronto ON M5G 1X8; Marseille (France)'71; FRCPC; DiagRad (Pediatric Neuro Radiology). Staff, The Hospital For Sick Children; Langs: Bilingual(English/French); (416)813-5171; Fax. (416)813-7591.

RAYCRAFT, Stephen W; 206-2223 Broadway W, Vancouver BC V6K 2E4; McM'87; MPs; FRCPC; Psy (Psychoanalytic & Psychotherapy). (604)731-4690; Fax. (604)251-1311.

RAYEL, Michael G; Dr G B Cross Mem Hosp, 67 Manitoba Dr, Clarenville NL A5A 1K3; Manila (Philippines)'88; DABPN; Staff, The Dr G B Cross Memorial Hospital; Langs: Tagalog; (709)466-3411; mrayel75@yahoo.com.

RAYES, Wagdy E A; Apsley Med Centre, PO Box 278, Apsley ON K0L 1A0; Cairo (Egypt)'65; Court Staff, Peterborough Regional Health Centre - Rogers St Site; Court Staff, Peterborough Regional Health Centre - Hospital Drive; Langs: Arabic; French; (705)656-4281

RAYMAN, Reiza; London HSC-University Hosp, PO Box 5339 Stn B 339 Windermere Rd, London ON N6A 5A5; Tor'90; MSc(Biophysics); Staff, London Health Sciences Centre - University Hospital; (519)685-8500

RAYMER, Karen E; Hamilton HS-General Site, 237 Barton St E, Hamilton ON L8L 2X2; Tor'90; FRCPC; Anes. Staff, Hamilton Health Sciences Centre - Hamilton General Hospital; Langs: English; French; (905)527-0271 x46698; Fax. (905)527-4322.

RAYMOND, Alain; Polyclinique de Trois-Rivieres, 305-1900 boul des Recollets, Trois-Rivieres QC G8Z 4K4; Laval'84; Cardiol (P.Q.); IntMed. Ac Staff, CSSS de Trois-Rivières; (819)378-8028; Fax. (819)378-7897.

RAYMOND, Barbara J; Public Health Agency of Canada, 130 Colonnade Rd, Ottawa ON K1A 0K9; Wes'91; BSc; Med Evaluator, Health Canada; (613)957-8685; dr.b.raymond@sympatico.ca.

RAYMOND, Bernard; Centre Med de Bedford, CP 140 1 Place de l'Estrie, Bedford QC J0J 1A0; McG'73; CCFP; FCFP; ac Staff, CLSC-CHSLD La Pommeraie - Centre hospitalier de Bedford; ac Staff, Hôpital Brome-Missisquoi-Perkins; (450)248-3336; Fax. (450)248-7751; bernard_raymond@rrsss16.gouv.qc.ca.

RAYMOND, Catherine; CSSS de Chicoutimi, 305 rue Saint-Vallier, Chicoutimi QC G7H 5H6; Mon'01; CSPQ; FRCPC; AnatPath. Staff, Complexe hospitalier de la Sagamie; (418)541-1000 x2288; Fax. (418)541-1143.

RAYMOND, Chantal; CSSS Drummond-Hop Sainte-Croix, 570 rue Heriot, Drummondville QC J2B 1C1; Mon'93; FRCSC; ObstGyn. Staff, Hôpital Sainte-croix; Clin Prof, Universite de Sherbrooke; (819)478-6464; Fax. (819)478-6470; gynrayc@hotmail.com.

RAYMOND, Daniel; CSSS de Rivière-de-Loup, 75 rue Saint-Henri, Riviere-du-Loup QC G5R 2A4; Mon'00; BScPT; FRCPC; IntMed. Staff/Chef Med Spec Dept, Centre Hospitalier Regional du Grand-Portage; Clin Prof, Université Laval; (418)868-1000; Fax. (418)868-1032.

RAYMOND, Denis; Inst de Physiatrie de Mtl, 2049 rue Sherbrooke E, Montreal QC H2K 1C1; Sher'78; FRCPC; PhysMed&Rehab. Staff, Institut de Réadaptation Gingras-Lindsay de Montréal; (514)527-4155; jnolet@ssss.gouv.qc.ca.

RAYMOND, Denis; Clinique Med St-Louis, 220-3165 ch Saint-Louis, Quebec QC G1W 4R4; Laval'87; Physician, CLSC Arthur-Caux; (418)653-1970

RAYMOND, Elin L; 311-658 Danforth Ave, Toronto ON M4J 5B9; Dal'97; FRCSC; ObstGyn. Staff, Toronto East General Hospital Inc; (416)466-2360; Fax. (416)466-5076.

RAYMOND, Francois; CSSS Haut-Richelieu-Rouville, 920 boul du Seminaire N, St-Jean-Sur-Richel QC J3A 1B7; Mon'84; Staff, Hôpital du Haut-Richelieu; (450)359-5000

RAYMOND, Francois; The Ottawa Hosp-Gen Campus, 501 Smyth Rd, Ottawa ON K1H 8L6; McG'88; ABNM; FRCPC; NuclearMed. Staff, The Ottawa Hospital - General Campus; Consultant, Children's Hospital of Eastern Ontario (CHEO); Asst Prof, University of Ottawa; (613)737-8528; Fax. (613)737-8705; fraymond@ottawahospital.on.ca.

RAYMOND, Francois; Clinique Med Adoncour, 200-505 rue Adoncour, Longueuil QC J4G 2M6; Mon'79; FRCPC; Peds. Staff, Centre Hospitalier Pierre Boucher; (450)646-4445; Fax. (450)646-5526.

RAYMOND, Giles P; Centre Med Pierrefonds, 208-12774 boul Gouin O, Pierrefonds QC H8Z 1W5; Mon'68; DABD; FAAD; FRCPC; Derm. Consultant, Lakeshore General Hospital - Pointe Claire; ac Staff, Centre Hospitalier l'Université De Montréal (CHUM) - Hôpital Saint-luc; Prof Derm, Universite de Montreal; Langs: English; (514)684-8460; Fax. (514)684-1348.

RAYMOND, Gregory S; 202-11010 101 St NW, Edmonton AB T5H 4B9; Dal'88; BSc; FRCP; ABR; FRCPC; DiagRad (Administration). Staff Radiol, University of Alberta Hospital; Staff Radiol, Sturgeon Community Hospital; Staff Radiol, Royal Alexandra Hospital; Member Diagnostic Imaging Committee, College of Physicians & Surgeons of Alberta; Clin Assoc Prof Fac of Med & Dentistry, University of Alberta; (780)426-1121; Fax. (780)425-5979; xrayfiles@shaw.ca.

RAYMOND, Jacques; 1895 boul Rene-Laennec, Laval QC H7M 5E2; Mon'88; CSPQ; Anes. (450)668-1010

RAYMOND, Jean; CHUM-Hop Notre-Dame, 1560 rue Sherbrooke E, Montreal QC H2L 4M1; Mon'81; CSPQ; FRCPC; DiagRad. Staff, Centre Hospitalier l'Université de Montréal (CHUM) - Hôpital Notre-Dame; Universite de Montreal; (514)890-8000 x25857; Fax. (514)876-5079.

RAYMOND, Jean-Marc; CHUM-Hotel-Dieu, 3840 rue Saint-Urbain, Montreal QC H2W 1T8; Mon'00; Cardiol; IntMed. Staff, Centre Hospitalier l'Université de Montréal (CHUM) - Hôtel-Dieu; (514)890-8000

RAYMOND, Louis-David; Clin Ortho Haut-Richelieu, 300-900 boul du Seminaire N, St-Jean-sur-Richel QC J3A 1C3; Mon'02; FRCSC; OrthSurg. Staff, Hôpital du Haut-Richelieu; (450)348-6966; Fax. (450)348-0664.

RAYMOND, Lynn A; UBC Hospital, 2211 Wesbrook Mall, Vancouver BC V6T 2B5; Bronx (USA)'86; FRCPC; Neur. Staff, UBC Hospital - Koerner Pavillion; Staff, Vancouver General Hospital - Centennial Pavillion; (604)822-7738; Fax. (604)822-7981.

RAYMOND, Marc R; Strathroy Middlesex Gen Hosp, 343-395 Carrie St, Strathroy ON N7G 3C9; Wes'98; BSc; FRCSC; Otol (Ear Nose & Throat Surgery). Staff, Strathroy Middlesex General Hospital - Middlesex Hospital Alliance; (519)245-3888; Fax. (519)245-3889.

RAYMOND, Margaret; CSSS du Suroît, 150 rue Saint-Thomas, Salaber-de-Valleyf QC J6T 6C1; McG'02; Staff, Centre Hospitalier Régional du Suroît; (450)371-9920

RAYMOND, Marie-Claude; Hop Maisonneuve Rosemont, 5415 boul de l'Assomption, Montreal QC H1T 2M4; Mon'89; MClSc(Wes); CCFP; FCFP; Staff, Hopital Maisonneuve-Rosemont; (514)252-3400 x3221; Fax. (514)252-3814.

RAYMOND, Mario; Clinique Med de Shawinigan-Sud, 200-2355 5e av, Shawinigan-Sud QC G9P 1P4; Sher'78; CCFP; (819)537-6205; Fax. (819)537-5596; mario.raymond@gmf.gouv.qc.ca.

RAYMOND, Martine; CSSS de Laval, 1755 boul Rene-Laennec, Laval QC H7M 3L9; Mon'91; FRCPC; IntMed (External Clinic); Nephrol. Staff, Hopital de la Cite de la santé; Langs: Bilingual(French/English); (450)668-1010; Fax. (450)975-5072.

RAYMOND, Michel; Centre Med d'Ormstown, GD 24 rue Gale, Ormstown QC J0S 1K0; Mon'06; CCFP; (450)829-2331; Fax. (450)829-3636.

RAYMOND, Michele; BCC-St Vincent Hospital, 60 Cambridge St N, Ottawa ON K1R 7A5; Ott'98; CCFP; Staff, Montfort Hospital; Staff, Bruyère Continuing Care - Saint-Vincent Hospital; Langs: French; Spanish; (613)562-6262

RAYMOND, Nicolas; CSSS de Laval, 1755 boul Rene-Laennec, Laval QC H7M 3L9; Mon'00; FRCPC; IntMed; MedOncol; Hem. Hematologist, Hopital de la Cite de la santé; nicolas.raymond@ssss.gouv.qc.ca.

RAYMOND, Paul-Emile; CSSS de Rimouski-Neigette, CP 3150 succ A 150 av Rouleau, Rimouski QC G5L 5T1; Laval'65; DMRT; CSPQ; FRCPC; RadOncol (Gynecologic Oncology). Consultant, Hôtel-Dieu de Lévis; Staff, Hôpital Regional Rimouski; Sr Staff RadOncol, Centre Hospitalier Universitaire de Québec (CHUQ) - Siege Social; Clin Prof, Université Laval; Langs: English; (418)834-7121

RAYMOND, Richard J; 2-1230 Alward St, Prince George BC V2M 7B1; Dal'73; CCFP; CCFP(E.M.); Staff, University Hospital of Northern British Columbia; (250)563-0414; Fax. (250)563-0278.

RAYMOND, Stephane; CLSC de Pohenegamook, RR 2 1922 rue Saint-Vallier, Pohenegamook QC G0L 1J0; Sher'95; CCFP; Staff, Centre Hospitalier de Granby; (418)859-2450; Fax. (418)859-1285.

RAYMOND, Vincent; CHUQ-Ctr Hosp Univ Laval, T2.39-2705 boul Laurier, Quebec QC G1V 4G2; Laval'79; NBME; DSc; MB; LMCC; MSc; Ac Staff Ctre de Recherche, Centre Hospitalier Universitaire de Quebec-CHUL; Langs: English; French; (418)654-2296; Fax. (418)654-2761; vincent.raymond@crchul.ulaval.ca.

RAYMOND, Yves L; Timmins Family Health Team, 4-227 Algonquin Blvd W, Timmins ON P4N 2R8; Ott'96; CCFP; Staff, Timmins & District Hospital; Langs: English; French; (705)360-5808; Fax. (705)360-8969.

RAYMOND, Yves; 254B boul Hotel-de-Ville CP 326, Riviere-du-Loup QC G5R 3Y9; Laval'82; (418)816-1216; Fax. (418)816-1218; yves.raymond2@videotron.ca.

RAYMOND-CARRIER, Stephanie; Hop du Sacre-Coeur de Mtl, 5400 boul Gouin O, Montreal QC H4J 1C5; Mon'99; FRCPC; IntMed; Nephrol. Staff, Hôpital du Sacre-Coeur de Montréal; (514)338-2222

RAYMOND-ROBICHAUD, Jean-Michel; Hotel-Dieu de Roberval, 450 rue Brassard, Roberval QC G8H 1B9; Mon'08; CCFP; Staff, Hotel-Dieu de Roberval; (418)275-0110

RAYMOND-TREMBLAY, Danielle; CHUM-Hop Notre-Dame, 1560 rue Sherbrooke E, Montreal QC H2L 4M1; Mon'62; CSPQ; DiagRad. ac Staff, Centre Hospitalier l'Université de Montréal (CHUM) - Hôpital Notre-Dame; Clinical Asst Prof, Universite de Montreal; (514)890-8000 x28530; d.rt@sympatico.ca.

RAYNAULD, Jean-Pierre; Institut Rhumatologie de Mtl, 1551 rue Ontario E, Montreal QC H2L 1S6; Mon'83; CSPQ; FRCPC; IntMed; Rheum. (514)523-3305; Fax. (514)523-5973; jp.raynauld@videotron.ca.

RAYNAULT, Marie-France; Dir de la Sante Publique-Mtl, 1301 rue Sherbrooke E, Montreal QC H2L 1M3; Mon'75; CSPQ; FRCPC; CommunMed. Dir Social & Preventive Med, Universite de Montreal; (514)528-2400 x3892

RAYNER, David C; 402-8440 112 St NW, Edmonton AB T6G 2B7; Man'77; BSc(Med); DAB; FRCPC; AnatPath (Surgical Pathology). Staff, University of Alberta Hospital; University of Alberta; (780)407-8822; Fax. (780)407-3009; david.rayner@ualberta.ca.

RAYNER, Sudesh; North Burlington Med Centre, 18-1960 Appleby Line, Burlington ON L7L 0B7; Dublin (Ireland)'64; Staff, Joseph Brant Memorial Hospital; Langs: Gujarati; Hindi; Urdu.

RAYNOR, Christopher F; U of Ottawa Sports Med, N203-801 King Edward Ave, Ottawa ON K1N 6N5; Wes'00; FRCSC; OrthSurg. (613)562-5970

RAYNOR, Lianne R; Wellington Med Clinic, 84C-3200 Island Hwy N, Nanaimo BC V9T 1W1; UBC'85; (250)740-2100; Fax. (250)740-2114; kraynor@island.net.

RAYSON, Daniel; Queen Elizabeth II HSC, 460-1276 South Park St, Halifax NS B3H 2Y9; Dal'89; FRC; FRCPC; IntMed (Breast Cancer); MedOncol. Att Staff IntMed & MedOncol, Queen Elizabeth II Health Sciences Centre - Victoria General Site; Prof Med, Dalhousie University; (902)473-6106; daniel.rayson@cdha.nshealth.ca.

RAYSON, Sandra; Allan Blair Cancer Centre, 4101 Dewdney Ave, Regina SK S4T 7T1; West Indies (Jamaica)'74; ABIM; FRCPC; IntMed (Medical Oncology). Staff, Regina Health District; Assoc Prof, University of Saskatchewan; (306)766-2278; Fax. (306)766-2688.

RAZA, Danyaal; Centretown Community HC, 420 Cooper St, Ottawa ON K2P 2N6; Wes'09; CCFP; (613)233-4443; Fax. (613)233-3987.

RAZA, Hammad; 104-15122 72 Ave, Surrey BC V3S 2G2; (Pakistan)'99; (604)593-5156

RAZA, Irfan; Oasis Med Centre, 184 Pth 12 N, Steinbach MB R5G 0Y5; Karachi (Pakistan)'91.

RAZA, Muhammad S; Dr Everett Chalmers Reg Hosp, PO Box 9000 Stn A 700 Priestman St, Fredericton NB E3B 5N5; Karachi (Pakistan)'89; Staff, Dr Everett Chalmers Regional Hospital; (506)452-5026

RAZA, Shaheen; Doctors Plus Med Centre, 310-505 Main St SW, Airdrie AB T4B 3K3; CCFP; (403)945-0770; Fax. (403)945-8997.

RAZA, Syed A; Cape Breton Healthcare Complex, 1482 George St, Sydney NS B1P 1P3; Dow Medical College (Pakistan)'01; Staff, Cape Breton Healthcare Complex; (902)567-8000

RAZACK, Jameel K I; Pape Danforth Echo Lab, 205-751 Pape Ave, Toronto ON M4K 3T1; West Indies (Jamaica)'73; MB BS; CCFP; (416)461-1822; Fax. (416)778-8779; jameel.razack@utoronto.ca.

RAZACK, Saleem I; MUHC-Montreal Children's Hosp, C807-2300 rue Tupper, Montreal QC H3H 1P3; Tor'90; FRCPC; Peds; Critical Care Medicine (P.Q.). Staff, McGill University Health Centre - Montreal Children's Hospital; adj Doyen Admissions, McGill University; (514)412-4475; Fax. (514)412-4211; saleem.razack@muhc.mcgill.ca.

RAZACK, Tamazadeene; Bingham Mem Hosp, PO Box 70 Stn Main 507 8th Ave, Matheson ON P0K 1N0; (Cuba)'89; CCFP; Staff, Bingham Memorial Hospital; (705)273-2333

RAZACK, Vanessa A; Paediatric Emergency Group, 1280 Main St W, Hamilton ON L8S 4K1; (Grenada)'05; (905)521-2100

RAZAK, Fahad; St Michael's Hosp, 14 077B-30 Bond St, Toronto ON M5B 1W8; Tor'09; Staff, Toronto General Hospital - UHN; Staff, St Michael's Hospital; (416)360-4000

RAZAVI, Amir H; Humber River Reg Hosp-Church, 200 Church St, Toronto ON M9N 1N8; Saba (Netherlands)'07; Staff, Humber River Regional Hospital - Church Street Site; (416)249-8111

RAZAVI, Aram; CHSLD Rousselot, 5655 rue Sherbrooke E, Montreal QC H1N 1A4; Montpellier (France)'69; (514)254-9421

RAZAVI, Jalees M S; Imperial Oil Resources Ltd, PO Box 2480 Stn M FAP 18039-237 4 Ave SW, Calgary AB T2P 0H6; Riyadh (Saudi Arabia)'89; DIH; FRCPC; OccupMed. Physician Occupational Med Specialist/Dir Occup Health, Imperial Oil Ltd; Langs: Arabic; Urdu; Punjabi; (403)237-4415; Fax. (403)237-2137.

RAZEK, Tarek S A; MUHC-Montreal Gen Hosp, L8.136-1650 av Cedar, Montreal QC H3G 1A4; McG'93; FRCSC; GenSurg; Critical Care Medicine (P.Q.). Staff, McGill University Health Centre - Montreal General Campus; (514)934-1934 x4334; Fax. (514)934-8210; tarek.razek@muhc.mcgill.ca.

RAZIAN, Ali; Mackenzie Richmond Hill Hosp, 10 Trench St, Richmond Hill ON L4C 4Z3; Teheran (Iran)'94; FRCPC; IntMed. Staff, Mackenzie Richmond Hill Hospital; (905)883-1212

RAZIK, Roshan A; Univ Hlth Network-Toronto Gen, 200 Elizabeth St, Toronto ON M5G 2C4; Tor'10; Staff, Toronto General Hospital - UHN; (416)586-5133

RAZMY, Ajmal; Addiction & Mental Hlth-Clarke, 535-250 College St, Toronto ON M5T 1R8; Tor'06; FRCPC; Psy. Staff, Centre for Addiction & Mental Health (CAMH) - College Street Site; (416)535-8501

RAZVI, Hassan A S; St Joseph's Health Care, PO Box 5777 Stn B B4 658-268 Grosvenor St, London ON N6A 4V2; Sask'88; FRCSC; Urol (Endourology). Chief Urol, London Health Sciences Centre - South Street; Chief Urol, St Joseph's Hospital - St Joseph's Health Care; Prof/Chairman Div of Urol, University of Western Ontario; (519)646-6259; Fax. (519)646-6037.

RAZVI, Nayyar K; Appletree Med Group, 402-53 Yonge St, Toronto ON M5E 1J3; Ott'98; CCFP; Langs: Hindi; Urdu; (416)367-4300

RAZVI, Yasar S; Georgetown Med Associates, 199 Princess Anne Dr, Georgetown ON L7G 0E3; Qns'00; CCFP; (905)873-3000; Fax. (905)873-0800.

RAZZAQ, Mahreen A; Pickering Urgent Care, 6B-1450 Kingston Rd, Pickering ON L1V 1C1; Karachi (Pakistan)'03.

RAZZAQUE, Asad; Battlefield Med Centre, 72 King St W, Stoney Creek ON L8G 1H8; McM'95; CCFP; (905)662-6959; Fax. (905)662-4100.

RE MARTINEZ, Felix C; Hyperbaric Oxygen Institute, 125 Welland Ave, St Catharines ON L2R 2N5; Madrid (Spain)'57; Langs: Italian; Spanish; French; (905)688-0560

REA, Elizabeth H; Toronto Public Health, 277 Victoria St, Toronto ON M5B 1W2; Man'88; MSc; FRCPC; CommunMed; Public Health & Preventive Med. Physician, Toronto Public Health Corporate Office; Teach Staff, University of Toronto; (416)525-3794; erea@toronto.ca.

REA, John C; Huntsville Prof Bldg, 104-348 Muskoka Rd 3 N, Huntsville ON P1H 1H8; Ott'84; CCFP; CCFP(E.M.); FCFP; Staff, Huntsville District Memorial Hospital - Muskoka Algonquin Healthcare; Supvr Northern Ontario Family Med Prog, University of Ottawa; (705)789-2355; Fax. (705)789-1051.

READ, Brandi L; Lions Gate Hosp, 231 15th St E, North Vancouver BC V7L 2L7; Dal'07; CCFP; CCFP(E.M.); Staff, Lions Gate Hospital; (604)988-3131

READ, Daniel L; Royal Alexandra Hosp, 10240 Kingsway NW, Edmonton AB T5H 3V9; Alb'06; FRCPC; Psy. Staff, Royal Alexandra Hospital; (780)735-4562

READ, Douglas E; Northside Med Group, 102-1015 Austin Ave, Coquitlam BC V3K 3N9; Sask'77; Staff, Royal Columbian Hospital; (604)939-9251; Fax. (604)939-2592.

READ, James A; Sherbourne Health Centre, 333 Sherbourne St, Toronto ON M5A 2S5; Cal'92; CCFP; CCFP(E.M.); Staff, Mount Sinai Hospital; (416)324-4180; Fax. (416)324-4181.

READ, James H; 102-9814 97 St, Grande Prairie AB T8V 8H5; Cambridge (England)'73; (780)539-4770

READ, Nancy E; London Reg Cancer Centre, 790 Commissioners Rd E, London ON N6A 4L6; Dal'90; FRCPC; RadOncol. Staff, London Health Sciences Centre - University Hospital; Asst Prof, University of Western Ontario; (519)685-8600; Fax. (519)685-8736.

READ, Robert M; Halifax Prof Centre, 1020-5991 Spring Garden Rd, Halifax NS B3H 1Y6; Dal'56; DABOph; LMCC; MDCM; FRCSC; Ophth (Glaucoma). (902)423-9222; Fax. (902)429-1388.

READ, Ronald R; 3500 26 Ave NE, Calgary AB T1Y 6J4; Cal'86; FRCPC; IntMed (Sexually Transmitted Diseases); InfectDis. Staff, Peter Lougheed Centre; Assoc Prof Med Microbiol & InfectDis, University of Calgary; (403)944-2325; ron.read@albertahealthservices.ca.

READ, Rua L; Squamish Med Clinic, PO Box 389 Stn Main 37979 Cleveland Ave, Squamish BC V8B 0A3; UBC'00; CCFP; (604)892-3535; Fax. (604)892-3545.

READ, Stanley E; The Hosp for Sick Children, 555 University Ave, Toronto ON M5G 1X8; Alb'65; FAAP; PhD; FRCPC; Peds (AIDS/HIV). Att Staff, The Hospital For Sick Children; University of Toronto; (416)813-6268; Fax. (416)813-8404; stanley.read@sickkids.ca.

READE, Clare J M; Univ Hlth Network-Princess M, M700-610 University Ave, Toronto ON M5G 2M9; McM'06; FRCSC; ObstGyn. Staff, Princess Margaret Hospital - University Health Network; (416)946-4043

READE, Elizabeth A; Homewood Health Centre, 150 Delhi St, Guelph ON N1E 6K9; Tor'82; FRCPC; Psy (Addiction Psychiatry). Staff, Homewood Health Centre; Clinical Asst Prof Psy & Behavioural Neurosciences, McMaster University; (519)824-1010 x2182; Fax. (519)767-3537; readbeth@homewood.org.

READE, Maurianne K; Mindemoya Med Clinic, PO Box 150 2120B Hwy 551, Mindemoya ON P0P 1S0; Alb'86; CCFP; CCFP(E.M.); FCFP; Asst Prof Family Practice, Northern Ontario School of Medicine-Laurentian University; (705)377-5371; Fax. (705)377-5372.

READER, Norman; CSSS de la Mitis, 800 av du Sanatorium, Mont-Joli QC G5H 3L6; Laval'62; CSPQ; DiagRad (P.Q.). Staff, CSSS de la Mitis; (418)775-7261

READY, Eric; City of Kawartha Lakes FHT, 101-86 Angeline St S, Lindsay ON K9V 6C5; Qns'84; CCFP; FCFP; Ac Staff Gen Pract & Anes, Ross Memorial Hospital; (705)324-3221; Fax. (705)324-1135; ericready@bellnet.ca.

READY, W Kirkby; North Bay Reg Health Centre, 50 College Dr, North Bay ON P1B 0A4; Sask'85; FRCP; FRCPC; GenPath. (905)474-8600

REARDON, Edward P; 235 Somerset St, Saint John NB E2K 2Y1; Dal'79; FRCSC; ObstGyn. Ac Staff, Saint John Regional Hospital; Ac Staff, St Joseph's Hospital; Asst Prof, Dalhousie University; (506)634-1848; Fax. (506)652-5977.

REARDON, Gerald; Queen Elizabeth II HSC-Halifax, 4865-1796 Summer St, Halifax NS B3H 3A7; Dal'74; FRCSC; OrthSurg. Staff, Queen Elizabeth II Health Sciences Centre - Halifax Infirmary Site; (902)473-5626; Fax. (902)473-5625.

REARDON, Mark L; The Ottawa Hosp-Gen Campus, 501 Smyth Rd, Ottawa ON K1H 8L6; Ott'78; FRCPC; EmergMed. Staff Emerg Dept, The Ottawa Hospital - General Campus; Asst Prof Family Med, University of Ottawa; Langs: English; French; (613)737-8000

REARDON, Mary-Lynne; Ottawa Reg Cancer Centre, 503 Smyth Rd, Ottawa ON K1H 8L6; Ott'77; Clin Asst MedOncol, The Ottawa Hospital - General Campus; Langs: French; (613)737-7700 x70100; mareardon@ottawahospital.on.ca.

REARDON, P Michael; Gladstone Prof Centre, 401-6155 North St, Halifax NS B3K 5R3; Dal'74; FRCPC; Derm. Asst Prof, Dalhousie University; (902)455-7273; Fax. (902)453-1354.

REAUME, John K; Mount Forest Fam Health Team, SS 3 525 Dublin St, Mount Forest ON N0G 2L3; Wes'88; CCFP; CCFP(E.M.); FCFP; Staff, North Wellington Health Care - Louise Marshall Hospital; Clinical Asst Prof, McMaster University; (519)323-0255; Fax. (519)323-2349.

REAUME, M Neil; The Ottawa Hosp Reg Cancer Ctr, 501 Smyth Rd, Ottawa ON K1H 8L6; Ott'94; FRCPC; IntMed; MedOncol. Staff, The Ottawa Hospital - General Campus; (613)737-7700 x70175; Fax. (613)247-3511.

REAVELY-DIAZ, Sheridan; 5-30 Thirteenth St E, Cornwall ON K6H 6V9; McG'79; (613)330-5914; Fax. (613)932-2238.

REBALKIN, Garry N; CN Towers, 901-201 1st Ave S, Saskatoon SK S7K 1J5; Sask'68; Ac Staff, St Paul's Hospital (Grey Nuns) of Saskatoon; Ac Staff, Saskatoon City Hospital; Ac Staff, Royal University Hospital; (306)653-1315; Fax. (306)664-1967.

REBANE, Ann K; Medical & Dental Bldg, 801-586 Eglinton Ave E, Toronto ON M4P 1P2; Tor'80; CCFP; FCFP; Court Staff, Mount Sinai Hospital; Langs: Estonian; (416)486-4401; Fax. (416)486-6145.

REBANE, Thomas M; King Street Med Arts Centre, 203-71 King St W, Mississauga ON L5B 4A2; Tor'80; FACC; FRCPC; IntMed; Cardiol. Chief Cardiac Health System, Trillium Health Centre - Mississauga; (905)279-0800; Fax. (905)279-2002.

REBBECK, Patricia M; College of Phys & Surg of BC, 400-858 Beatty St, Vancouver BC V6B 1C1; Edinburgh (Scotland)'59; MB ChB; FRCSC; GenSurg (Surgical Oncology). Dep Registrar, College of Physicians & Surgeons of British Columbia; Clin Assoc Prof Emer, University of British Columbia; (604)733-7758; Fax. (604)733-3503.

REBEL, Margaretha; London HSC-Victoria Hosp, PO Box 5010 Stn B 800 Commissioners Rd E, London ON N6A 5W9; McM'85; MEd; FRCSC; ObstGyn (Reprod Endocrin & Fertility). Staff, St Joseph's Hospital - St Joseph's Health Care; Staff, London Health Sciences Centre - Victoria Campus; Prof/Dept Chair ObstGyn, University of Western Ontario; Langs: English; French; (519)646-6103; maggie.rebel@schulich.uwo.ca.

REBELLO, Rosario; Queen Elizabeth II HSC, 410-1276 South Park St, Halifax NS B3H 2Y9; Manchester (England)'76; BSc; MB ChB; MRC(UK); FRCPC; IntMed. Staff, Queen Elizabeth II Health Sciences Centre - Victoria General Site; Asst Prof, Dalhousie University; (902)473-7788; Fax. (902)473-8430; rosario.rebello@cdha.nshealth.ca.

REBELLO, Ryan P; St Joseph's Healthcare, 50 Charlton Ave E, Hamilton ON L8N 4A6; Wes'97; FRCPC; DiagRad. Staff, St Joseph's Healthcare - Charlton Campus; (905)522-1155 x4984

REBELO, Raul A; PO Box 267 Glace Bay, Glace Bay NS B1A 5V4; Bombay (India)'64; FRCPC; IntMed. Att Staff, Glace Bay Healthcare Facility; Consultant, New Waterford Consolidated Hospital; (902)849-7663; Fax. (902)849-7707.

REBEYKA, Ivan M; University of Alberta Hosp, 3H2.04-8440 112 St NW, Edmonton AB T6G 2B7; Sask'79; FRCSC; GenSurg (Cardiac Surgery); Cardiovasc&ThorSurg. Staff, University of Alberta Hospital; (780)407-8033; Fax. (780)407-8052; ivan.rebeyka@albertahealthservices.ca.

REBEYKA, Walter P; 2006 Eighth Ave, New Westminster BC V3M 2T5; RCP&S (Ireland)'77; (604)524-2281; Fax. (604)524-2121.

REBICK, Gabriel; Univ Hlth Network-Toronto Gen, 200 Elizabeth St, Toronto ON M5G 2C4; McG'08; IntMed. Staff, Toronto General Hospital - UHN; (416)340-3505

REBOLLEDO, Lina; Clinique Med de l'Etoile, 16 rue Leblanc, L'Epiphanie QC J5X 4R9; Mon'91; CCFP; (450)588-7588; Fax. (450)588-7588.

REBOT, Morris T M; Queensway Prof Centre, 411-190 Sherway Dr, Etobicoke ON M9C 5N2; Wes'80; FRCSC; PlasSurg. (416)620-5070; Fax. (416)620-1564.

REBUS, Christopher D; Foothills Med Centre, 1403 29 St NW, Calgary AB T2N 2T9; (Australia)'06; CCFP; CCFP(E.M.); Staff, Foothills Medical Centre; (403)944-1110

REBUS, Lisa M; 13506 127 St NW, Edmonton AB T5L 1B9; Alb'90; CCFP.

RECEVEUR, Darryn S; Medical Imaging Consultants, 105-11010 101 St NW, Edmonton AB T5H 4B9; Sask'93; FRCPC; DiagRad (Body Imaging). Lecturer, University of Alberta; (780)426-1121

RECH, Eulalia; Terrace Office Tower, 888-4445 Calgary Trail NW, Edmonton AB T6H 5R7; (Brazil)'89; Langs: Portuguese; (780)454-4882; Fax. (780)401-3412; dr_rech@yahoo.ca.

RECHER, Martin O; CSSS du Lac-des-Deux-Montagnes, 520 boul Arthur-Sauve, Saint-Eustache QC J7R 5B1; Mon'03; CCFP; CCFP(E.M.); Staff, Hôpital de Saint-Eustache; (450)473-6811

RECHNER, Shelley J; Southwest Family Health Ctre, 204-200 James St S, Hamilton ON L8P 3A9; Alb'76; BSc; CCFP; FCFP; Ac Staff, St Joseph's Healthcare - Charlton Campus; Asst Clin Prof, McMaster University; (905)526-1606; Fax. (905)526-7692; rechner@mcmaster.ca.

RECK, Mona; Polyclinic, 199 Grafton St, Charlottetown PE C1A 1L2; Dal'84; CCFP; Ac Staff, Queen Elizabeth Hospital; (902)629-8810

RECOSKIE, Bryan; Stayner Med Centre, PO Box 220 7477 Highway 26, Stayner ON L0M 1S0; Ott'10; CCFP; (705)428-3246

RECOSKIE, Mary Jo; Hop Charles LeMoyne, 3120 boul Taschereau, Greenfield Park QC J4V 2H1; Mon'87; NuclearMed (P.Q.). Staff, Hopital Charles LeMoyne; Langs: Bilingual(French/English); (450)466-5000 x2578; Fax. (450)466-5071; mjrecoskie@hotmail.com.

RECTOR, Tara J; Health Sciences Centre, 300 Prince Philip Dr, St. John's NL A1B 3V6; Mem'05; CCFP; CCFP(E.M.); Staff, Health Sciences Centre; (709)777-6300

REDA, John E; Misericordia Health Centre, 99 Cornish Ave, Winnipeg MB R3C 1A2; Man'82; DABEM; FACEP; CCFP; Dir Urgent Care Centre, Misericordia Health Centre; Lecturer, University of Manitoba; (204)788-8144.

REDA, Margaret M; Concordia Hosp, 1095 Concordia Ave, Winnipeg MB R2K 3S8; Man'82; BSc(Med.); DABEM; ACLS; DrMedCh; Staff, Concordia General Hospital; (204)667-1560; Fax. (204)338-5645.

REDBURN, Alexandra; Ctr Hosp Reg de Lanaudiere, 1000 boul Sainte-Anne, St-Charles-Brromee QC J6E 6J2; Sher'98; CCFP; Staff, Centre Hospitalier Régional de Lanaudière; (450)759-8222

REDDEKOPP, Frieda J; Penticton Reg Hosp, 550 Carmi Ave, Penticton BC V2A 3G6; Tor'69; Anes. Staff, Penticton Regional Hospital; (250)492-8774

REDDI, Krishnavellie; Regina Mental Health Clinic, 2110 Hamilton St, Regina SK S4P 2E3; Durban (South Africa)'87; MB ChB; FRCPC; Psy. (306)766-7800; Fax. (306)766-7811.

REDDICK, D Susan; Toronto East Gen Hosp Inc, 825 Coxwell Ave, Toronto ON M4C 3E7; McM'93; FRCPC; Psy. Staff, Toronto East General Hospital Inc; (416)469-6580 x3098; Fax. (416)469-6179.

REDDICK, Richard D; McKinney Med Centre, 106-510 Ingersoll Ave, Woodstock ON N4S 4X9; Tor'75; Ac Staff, Woodstock General Hospital; (519)537-6501

REDDIN, Katharine P; The Moncton Hosp, 135 MacBeath Ave, Moncton NB E1C 6Z8; Ott'10; CCFP; Staff, The Moncton Hospital; (506)857-5111

REDDING, Keith G; Heritage Hill Prof Bldg, 308-8180 MacLeod Trail SE, Calgary AB T2H 2B8; Alb'69; DABD; FRCPC; Derm (Acne Treatment). Consultant, Foothills Medical Centre; Lecturer, University of Calgary; (403)252-1010; Fax. (403)255-9259.

REDDING, Rebecka G; 10738 124 St NW, Edmonton AB T5M 0H1; Alb'94; (780)453-9800; Fax. (780)761-2915.

REDDOCH, Allon; 401 Strickland St, Whitehorse YT Y1A 5N8; Wes'73; Ac Staff, Whitehorse General Hospital; Chief Med Cons, Yukon Workers Comp Health Safety Board & Phys., Klondyke Med Clinic; (867)667-8981; Fax. (867)667-8740; allon.reddoch@gov.yk.ca.

REDDOCH, Robert B; Cornwall Comm Hosp-McConnell, PO Box 100 Stn Main 840 McConnell Ave, Cornwall ON K6H 5S5; Wes'88; CCFP; CCFP(E.M.); FCFP; Staff, Cornwall Community Hospital; Staff, Hawkesbury & District General Hospital; Langs: English; French; (613)938-4080

REDDY, Desigen; McMaster University, 1280 Main St W, Hamilton ON L8S 4L8; Natal (South Africa)'85; MB ChB; FRCPC; Anes. Staff, Hamilton Health Sciences Centre - McMaster Children's Hospital.

REDDY, Devan; 202-1302 7th Ave, Prince George BC V2L 3P1; Witwatersrand (South Africa)'01; MB ChB; (250)563-9877

REDDY, Deven; Hamilton HS-General Site, 237 Barton St E, Hamilton ON L8L 2X2; (South Africa)'97; MB ChB; CCFP; Staff, Hamilton Health Sciences Centre - Hamilton General Hospital; Staff, Hamilton Health Sciences Centre - McMaster University Medical Centre; (905)521-2100

REDDY, Dhanasagren S; Lloydminster Specialist Clinic, 1723 51 Ave, Lloydminster AB T9V 2J6; Katsurba (India)'90; MB BS; BSc; LMCC; (780)875-6460; Fax. (780)875-6407.

REDDY, Dorothy; 213-1455 Bellevue Ave, West Vancouver BC V7T 1C3; Ross (Dominica)'99; FRCPC; Psy. Staff, BC Children's Hospital; (604)926-2250

REDDY, E Rajaram; Niagara H System-St Catharines, PO Box 3018 Stn Main 142 Queenston St, St Catharines ON L2R 7C6; Sri Venkateswara (India)'71; MB BS; DMRD; FRCR; FRCPC; DiagRad. Staff, Niagara Health System - St Catharines General Site; (905)684-7271 x6536; Fax. (905)684-6990.

REDDY, Esphiran; Martindale Med Clinic, 200-126 Martindale Dr NE, Calgary AB T3J 3G5; Natal (South Africa)'75; FRCSC; GenSurg. (403)293-7443; Fax. (403)293-7306.

REDDY, G Jagan Mohan; 435 Notre Dame Ave, Sudbury ON P3C 5K6; Sri Venkateswara (India)'81; MB BS; FRCPC; IntMed. Staff Gastroenterologist, Health Sciences North-Laurentian Site; (705)675-2100; Fax. (705)675-2101.

REDDY, Inbakumaran; 202-1302 7th Ave, Prince George BC V2L 3P1; Witwatersrand (South Africa)'94; MB BCh; Physician, Medical Clinic; (250)563-1306; Fax. (250)564-8945; inbakumaran.reddy@northernhealth.ca.

REDDY, Kesava K V; 644 Concession St, Hamilton ON L8V 1B5; Kurnool (India)'79; MB BS; FACS; FRCSC; Neursurg. Staff, St Joseph's Healthcare - Charlton Campus; Staff, Niagara Health System - Greater Niagara General Site; Staff, Hamilton Health Sciences Centre - McMaster Children's Hospital; Staff, Grand River Hospital - Kitchener/Waterloo Health Centre; Clin Prof, McMaster University; (905)521-0061; Fax. (905)521-9561.

REDDY, Kundavaram N; 5515 Portage Rd, Niagara Falls ON L2G 5Y2; Osmania (India)'60; DObstRCOG; FACS; FRCS(Ed); FRCSC; GenSurg; Urol. Consultant Urol, Niagara Health System - Greater Niagara General Site; Consultant Urol, Niagara Health System - Douglas Memorial Hospital Site; Consultant Urol, Niagara Health System - Niagara-on-the-Lake Hospital Site; (905)354-5007; Fax. (905)354-1474; dr.reddy@cogeco.net.

REDDY, M Rita; Innovations Health Clinic, 11420 27 St SE, Calgary AB T2Z 3R6; Natal (South Africa)'81; (587)352-8718; Fax. (587)352-8728.

REDDY, Nagaram J; Haldimand Family Health Team, 334 Broad St W, Dunnville ON N1A 1T1; Hyderabad (India)'69; CCFP; Staff, Haldimand Family Health Team; (905)774-7541; Fax. (905)774-4310.

REDDY, Natalie Y M; St Thomas-Elgin Gen Hosp, 189 Elm St, St Thomas ON N5R 5C4; Wes'06; FRCSC; ObstGyn. Staff, St Thomas Elgin General Hospital; (519)631-2020

REDDY, Nelini; Nipawin Med Group, PO Box 2135, Nipawin SK S0E 1E0; (306)862-4626; Fax. (306)862-3522.

REDDY, Neville; 106-11420 27 St SE, Calgary AB T2Z 3R6; Natal (South Africa)'88; MB ChB; FRCPC; Anes. (587)352-8718; Fax. (587)352-8728.

REDDY, Ramesh; London HSC-Victoria Hosp, PO Box 5010 Stn B 800 Commissioners Rd E, London ON N6A 5W9; Wes'06; CCFP; CCFP(E.M.); Staff, London Health Sciences Centre - Victoria Campus; (519)685-8500

REDDY, S Bharati; 301-49 Elizabeth Ave, St. John's NL A1A 1W9; Mem'81; FRCPC; IntMed; Gastroent. Gastroenterol, St Clare's Mercy Hospital; Clinical Asst Prof, Memorial University Of Newfoundland; (709)777-5858; Fax. (709)722-8706.

REDDY, Sudhakar D; Aberdeen Hosp, 835 East River Rd, New Glasgow NS B2H 3S6; Kasturba Medical College (India)'96; Staff, Aberdeen Regional Hospital; (902)752-7600

REDDY, Suresh P; PO Box 21113 Rpo Terwillegar, Edmonton AB T6R 2V4; Alb'99; FRCPC; IntMed; Nephrol.

REDDY, Suseela; MDS Metro Lab Services, 3680 Gilmore Way, Burnaby BC V5G 4V8; Kurnool (India)'61; MB BS; ABPath; FRCPC; GenPath. Langs: Telugu.

REDDY, U Stanislaus; Medical Complex, 1057 St. Peter Ave, Bathurst NB E2A 2Z6; Osmania (India)'70; Staff, GP, Hopital Regional Chaleur; Court Staff, Centre de santé Communitaire - St-Joseph; Staff, Jacquet River Health Centre; (506)546-9839; Fax. (506)548-2582.

REDEKOP, Gary J; 8115-2775 Laurel St, Vancouver BC V5Z 1M9; Wes'87; FRCSC; Neursurg. Staff, Vancouver General Hospital - Centennial Pavillion; Assoc Prof Surg/Dept Head & School Dir Surg, University of British Columbia; (604)875-5235; Fax. (604)875-5280.

REDEKOP, Theodore D; Occupational Health Branch, 200-401 York Ave, Winnipeg MB R3C 0P8; Man'67; BSc; FRCP; FRCPC; CommunMed (Occupational Medicine). Chief Occupational MO & Immigration, Province of Manitoba; Chief Medical Officer Occupational & Immigration, Workplace Safety & Health Divisions; Asst Prof Community Health Sciences, University of Manitoba; Langs: German; (204)945-3608; Fax. (204)945-4556; tredekop@shaw.ca.

REDEKOPP, Alan W; 105-309 Park St, Brockville ON K6V 6E5; Man'82; Staff, Brockville General Hospital - Charles Street; Staff, Providence Continuing Care Centre (PCCC) - St Vincent de Paul Hospital; (613)345-2841; Fax. (613)345-6963.

REDEL, Lioba; 4A-1306 Bow Valley Trail, Canmore AB T1W 1N6; (Germany)'98; FRCPC; Peds. (403)678-9600

REDELINGHUYS, Johannes N; Cambridge Mem Hosp, 700 Coronation Blvd, Cambridge ON N1R 3G2; Pretoria (South Africa)'91; MB ChB; CCFP; FCFP; Staff, Cambridge Memorial Hospital; Langs: Afrikaans; (519)621-2330

REDELINGHUYS, Tanja P; 301-3605 31st St, Vernon BC V1T 5J4; Pretoria (South Africa)'96; MB ChB; MMed; CCFP; (250)549-2444; tanja@sasktel.net.

REDELMEIER, Donald A; Sunnybrook Hlth Sciences Ctre, G 151-2075 Bayview Ave, Toronto ON M4N 3M5; Tor'84; FACP; FRCPC; IntMed. Staff, Sunnybrook Health Sciences Centre; Prof, University of Toronto; (416)480-6999; Fax. (416)480-6048.

REDENBACH, Zoe; 4-1230 Alward St, Prince George BC V2M 7B1; UBC'04; CCFP; CCFP(E.M.); (250)564-8513

REDFEARN, Damian P; Kingston Gen Hosp, 76 Stuart St, Kingston ON K7L 2V7; Leicester (England)'93; Cardiol; IntMed. Staff, Kingston General Hospital; (613)548-3232

REDGATE, Lauren M; Okotoks Health, 11 Cimarron Common, Okotoks AB T1S 2E9; Cal'08; FRCPC; Peds. (403)995-2670; Fax. (403)995-2671.

REDHEAD, Clint A; Mattawa Health Centre, PO Box 1190 Stn Main 150 Water St, Mattawa ON P0H 1V0; Wes'87; BSc(Hon); Dir-Lab Serv/Ac Staff, Mattawa Hospital; Court Staff Emerg, North Bay Regional Health Centre - Regional Mental Health; (705)744-2431; Fax. (705)744-0460.

REDINGTON, Andrew N; The Hosp for Sick Children, 555 University Ave, Toronto ON M5G 1X8; London (England)'81; Staff, The Hospital For Sick Children; (416)813-6135

REDLICK, Fara P; Kingsway Dermatology, 1000-1243 Islington Ave, Etobicoke ON M8X 1Y9; Tor'03; FRCPC; Derm. Staff, Women's College Hospital; (416)231-0103; Fax. (416)231-0109.

REDMAN, John A; Centric Health Seniors Centre, B-413 Linwell Rd, St Catharines ON L2M 7Y2; Edinburgh (Scotland)'59; MB ChB; Ac Staff, Niagara Health System - St Catharines General Site; Staff, Hôtel Dieu Shaver Health & Rehabilitation Centre; Staff, Niagara Health System - Ontario Street Site; Med Examiner, Marine & D. O. T. Aviation; (905)938-3533; Fax. (905)938-8318.

REDMAN, Kathryn H; 10015 98 St PO Box 900-8 Stn Main, Peace River AB T8S 1T4; (Australia)'88; FRANZCP; (780)624-6151; Fax. (780)624-6565.

REDMAN, Linda M; 505-200 Consumers Rd, Toronto ON M2J 4R4; Tor'87; FRCPC; Psy (Child & Adolescent Psychiatry). Langs: Bilingual(English/French); (416)493-8603

REDMOND, Carol A; Hannam Fertility Centre, 1103-655 Bay St, Toronto ON M5G 2K4; Tor'80; FRCSC; ObstGyn (Reproductive Biology). (416)595-1521; Fax. (416)506-0680; carol.redmond@hannamfertility.com.

REDMOND, Edwin B; Health Sciences Centre, 300 Prince Philip Dr, St. John's NL A1B 3V6; Mem'82; Anes (Cardiovascular Anesthesia). Staff, Health Sciences Centre; (709)777-6300

REDMOND, Mary L; 204-194 Main St, Ottawa ON K1S 1C2; Dal'79; BA; FRCSC; GenSurg (Chronic Pain Management); Cardiovasc&ThorSurg. (613)798-1113; Fax. (613)798-5227.

REDMOND, Michael P; Peace Arch Hosp, 15521 Russell Ave, White Rock BC V4B 2R4; Dal'87; FRCPC; Anes. Staff, Peace Arch Hospital; (604)531-5512

REDMOND, Timothy Y; West Parry Sound Health Ctre, 6 Albert St, Parry Sound ON P2A 3A4; McM'04; CCFP; CCFP(E.M.); Staff, West Parry Sound Health Centre; (705)746-9321

REDMOND, Wayne M; Paton Med Centre, 219-1 Paton St, St. John's NL A1B 4S8; Mem'84; FRCSC; Otol. Langs: English; French.

REDMOND, William C; 224 King St E, Brockville ON K6V 1C6; Qns'75; FRCSC; GenSurg. Chief Surg, Brockville General Hospital - Charles Street; (613)498-1700; Fax. (613)498-2670.

REDPATH, Calum J; Univ of Ottawa Heart Institute, 40 Ruskin St, Ottawa ON K1Y 4W7; Univ of Glasgow (Scotland)'97; Staff, University of Ottawa Heart Institute; (613)761-4708

REDPATH, Stephanie; Children's Hosp Eastern Ont, 401 Smyth Rd, Ottawa ON K1H 8L1; Univ of Glasgow (Scotland)'99; Staff, Children's Hospital of Eastern Ontario (CHEO); (613)737-7600

REDPATH, William L; Nanaimo Reg Gen Hosp, 1200 Dufferin Cres, Nanaimo BC V9S 2B7; Edinburgh (Scotland)'74; MB ChB; DRCOG; MRC(Eng); DCH(Lond); Staff, Nanaimo Regional General Hospital; (250)755-7691; william.redpath@viha.ca.

REDSTONE, Carol S; Mackenzie Richmond Hill Hosp, 10 Trench St, Richmond Hill ON L4C 4Z3; McM'96; FRCPC; IntMed; Critical Care Medicine. Staff, Mackenzie Richmond Hill Hospital; (905)883-2310

REDSTONE, Heather; 405-1015 Regent St, Fredericton NB E3B 6H5; Dal'01; FRCSC; GenSurg (Colorectal Surgery). Staff, Dr Everett Chalmers Regional Hospital; (506)458-8665; Fax. (506)458-8668; drredstone@nb.aibn.com.

REDUCKA, Kathryn G; Canadian Med Protective Assoc, 875 Carling Ave, Ottawa ON K1S 5P1; Alb'83; Physician, Canadian Medical Protective Association; (613)725-2000; kreducka@cmpa.org.

REDWAN, Hani A S; The Ottawa Hosp-Gen Campus, W1617-501 Smyth Rd, Ottawa ON K1H 8L6; King Abdul Aziz Univ (Saudi Arabia)'03; FRCSC; GenSurg. Staff, The Ottawa Hospital - General Campus; (613)890-0101

REDWOOD-CAMPBELL, Lynda; McMaster Family Practice, A-690 Main St W, Hamilton ON L8S 1A4; McM'92; DTMH; BSc; CCFP; FCFP; Staff, Hamilton Health Sciences Centre - McMaster Children's Hospital; Asst Prof Family Med, McMaster University; Langs: English; French; (905)521-5016; Fax. (905)521-5010; redwood@mcmaster.ca.

REEBYE, Nittin K; Royal City Med Bldg, 303-250 Keary St, New Westminster BC V3L 5E7; Bombay (India)'68; MB BS; FRCS(E); FRCPC; PhysMed&Rehab (Musculoskeletal). Staff Simon Fraser Health Region, Royal Columbian Hospital; Clin Instructor Med, University of British Columbia; Langs: English; French; (604)520-1013; Fax. (604)520-1413.

REEBYE, Pratibha N; BC Women's Hosp & Health Ctre, P4 218-4500 Oak St, Vancouver BC V6H 3N1; Bombay (India)'71; MB BS; LMCC; DPM(Leeds); MRCPsy(UK); FRCPC; Psy (Child Psychiatry). Staff, BC Women's Hospital & Health Centre; Consultant, Vancouver General Hospital - Centennial Pavillion; Clin Assoc Prof Psy, University of British Columbia; Langs: French; Hindi; (604)875-2206

REEBYE, Rajiv N; G F Strong Rehabilitation Cent, 4255 Laurel St, Vancouver BC V5Z 2G9; Nottingham (England)'00; FRCPC; PhysMed&Rehab. Staff, G F Strong Rehabilitation Centre; (604)734-1313

REECE, Cadi M; Summerville Family Health Team, 211-190 Sherway Dr, Etobicoke ON M9C 5N2; Wes'95; CCFP; Assoc Staff, St Joseph's Health Centre; (416)621-9700; Fax. (416)621-4438; creece@thc.on.ca.

REECE, Donna E; Univ Hlth Network-Princess M, 5 207-610 University Ave, Toronto ON M5G 2M9; Baylor(TX) (USA)'78; FRCPC; IntMed (Hematological Oncology). Dir Prog for Multiple Myeloma & Related Diseases, Princess Margaret Hospital - University Health Network; Prof, University of Toronto; (416)946-2824; Fax. (416)946-6546; donna.reece@uhn.ca.

REECE, Susan E; The Doctor's Office, 4099 Erin Mills Pky, Mississauga ON L5L 3P9; Tor'86; BSc; CCFP; Court Staff, Trillium Health Centre - Mississauga; (905)820-3310; Fax. (905)820-3312.

REECE-MILLS, Michelle N; The Hosp for Sick Children, 555 University Ave, Toronto ON M5G 1X8; West Indies (Jamaica)'99; Staff, The Hospital For Sick Children; (416)813-5320

REED, Andrew D; Kingston Gen Hosp, 76 Stuart St, Kingston ON K7L 2V7; McM'99; FRCPC; EmergMed. Staff, Kingston General Hospital; (613)548-3232

REED, Andrew R; Ridgeview Med Centre, 212-1240 Railway Ave, Canmore AB T1W 1P4; Newcastle (England)'94; MB BS; Dip Ortho; MRCGPract; CCFP; (403)609-8333; Fax. (403)609-3666; drreed@telus.net.

REED, Ann; Ctr Hosp de Charlevoix, 74 rue Ambroise-Fafard, Baie-Saint-Paul QC G3Z 2J6; Laval'89; Staff, CSSS de Charlevoix; (418)435-5150

REED, Brian; Oakwood Retirement Community, 3800 Brock St N, Whitby ON L1R 3A5; Wes'84; (905)666-3156

REED, Cari L; Beamsville Med Ctr Fam Hlth Team, PO Box 430 4279 Hixon St, Beamsville ON L0R 1B0; McM'98; CCFP; FCFP; Staff, West Lincoln Memorial Hospital; (905)563-5315; Fax. (905)563-0933.

REED, Charles E; 8 Kingsley Crt, Guelph ON N1E 1E3; Tor'51; LMCC; Staff Admin, Guelph General Hospital; Langs: English; French.

REED, J Kenneth; Guelph Family Health Team, 212-83 Dawson Rd, Guelph ON N1H 1B1; Tor'84; FRCSC; GenSurg. Staff, Guelph General Hospital; (519)763-8442; Fax. (519)763-1834.

REED, Jeremy G R; Aspen Med Centre, 225-3737 Wascana Pky, Regina SK S4S 0A2; Sask'01; FRCSC; OrthSurg (Arthroscopy). (306)337-2130; Fax. (306)337-3294; jeremy.reed@uregina.ca.

REED, Katherine M; Clinique Stat Care, 104-175 av Stillview, Pointe-Claire QC H9R 4S3; McG'77; Langs: English; French; (514)694-9282; Fax. (514)697-0192.

REED, Kathy E; Telus Plaza South, 2700-10020 100 St NW, Edmonton AB T5J 0N3; Cal'82; CCFP; FCFP; Asst Registrar, College of Physicians & Surgeons of Alberta; (780)969-4907; Fax. (780)420-0651.

REED, Martin H; Children's Hosp, 840 Sherbrook St, Winnipeg MB R3A 1S1; Man'67; FRCPC; DiagRad. Head Ped Radiol, Health Sciences Centre; (204)787-2603; Fax. (204)787-1402; mreed@exchange.hsc.mb.ca.

REED, Melanie J; BC Cancer Agency-Southern Int, 399 Royal Ave, Kelowna BC V1Y 5L3; Qns'84; FRCPC; RadOncol. Staff, BC Cancer Agency Sindi Ahluwalia Hawkins Centre for the Southern Interior; (250)712-3958; Fax. (250)712-3911.

REED, Stephen C; York-Finch Med Centre, 412-2115 Finch Ave W, North York ON M3N 2V6; Oxford (England)'85; BMus; BCh; MA(Oxon); MSc(Tor); FRCSC; OrthSurg (Knee Shoulder & Sports Injuries). Staff, Humber River Regional Hospital - Finch Avenue Site; Staff, North York General Hospital - Branson Division; Staff, Sunnybrook Health Sciences Centre - Holland Orthopaedic & Arthritic Centre; (416)744-4210; Fax. (416)744-9792.

REEDER, Bruce A; West Side Clinic, 1528 20th St W, Saskatoon SK S7M 0Z6; Sask'76; FRCPC; CommunMed (Family Medicine); Public Health & Preventive Med. Staff FamMed, Royal University Hospital; Prof, University of Saskatchewan; (306)664-4310; Fax. (306)934-2506; bruce.reeder@usask.ca.

REEDIJK, Michael J; Univ Hlth Network-Princess M, 3 130-610 University Ave, Toronto ON M5G 2M9; Tor'95; FRCSC; GenSurg (Surgical Oncology); General Surgical Oncology. Staff, Princess Margaret Hospital - University Health Network; Langs: Dutch; (416)946-2000

REEDYK, Martinus; Three Hills Med Clinic, PO Box 880 779 2nd St N, Three Hills AB T0M 2A0; Alb'69; Langs: Dutch; (403)443-5522; Fax. (403)443-5497.

REEMS, Hendrik W; Bayview Med Clinic, 102-1650 Terminal Ave N, Nanaimo BC V9S 0A3; Amsterdam (Netherlands)'78; Staff Family Pract, Nanaimo Regional General Hospital; Langs: Dutch; (250)591-3040; Fax. (250)591-3033.

REEN, Bajinder S; 101-3 Conestoga Dr, Brampton ON L6Z 4N5; Agra (India)'70; FRCPC; IntMed. Staff, William Osler Health System - Etobicoke General Hospital; Langs: Hindi; Punjabi; Urdu; (905)453-0715; Fax. (905)453-0972.

REEN, Mehar S; McConnell Med Centre, 110-820 McConnell Ave, Cornwall ON K6H 4M4; Kashmir (India)'72; MB BS; FRCPC; PhysMed&Rehab. Staff, Cornwall Community Hospital - Second Street Site; Staff, Cornwall Community Hospital; Consultant, Winchester District Memorial Hospital; Lecturer PhysMed & Rehab, Queen's University; Langs: Hindi; Punjabi; (613)933-8990; Fax. (613)933-8997.

REES, Henrike; Saskatoon City Hosp, 5510-701 Queen St, Saskatoon SK S7K 0M7; Muenster (Germany)'87; FRCPC; AnatPath (Breast Pathology). Staff Path, Saskatoon City Hospital; Clinical Asst Prof Path, University of Saskatchewan; Langs: German; (306)655-8283; henny.rees@saskatoonhealthregion.ca.

REES, Huw G; 203-610 Queen St, Saskatoon SK S7K 0M8; Sask'86; FRCSC; OrthSurg. (306)244-4433; Fax. (306)244-4464; rees.h@shaw.ca.

REES, John D; 505-8840 210 St, Langley BC V1M 2Y2; Pretoria (South Africa)'69; (604)850-1480

REES, Megan G; Medical Bldg, 803-805 Broadway W, Vancouver BC V5Z 1K1; Sask'86; DAB; FRCSC; Ophth (Adult Strabismus). Staff, BC Children's Hospital; Staff, Richmond Hospital; Clinical Asst Prof, University of British Columbia; (604)730-9192; Fax. (604)730-9190; kideyes@telus.net.

REES, Peter M; Royal Oak Med Centre, 102A-6440 Royal Oak Ave, Burnaby BC V5H 3P2; Oxford (England)'69; PhD; BSc(Eng.); MB ChB; MRCP(UK); FRCPC; Neur (Head & Neck). Staff Consultant, Burnaby Hospital; Consultant, Vancouver General Hospital - Centennial Pavillion; Consultant BC Rehab, G F Strong Rehabilitation Centre; (604)434-6232; Fax. (604)434-5733.

REES, Susan C; Associate Clinic, A-4620 50 Ave, Innisfail AB T4G 1A6; London (England)'81; MRCGPract; MB BS; (403)227-3301; Fax. (403)227-2856.

REES, Sylvia M; 22 CF Health Services Centre, PO Box 6550 Stn Forces, Cold Lake AB T9M 2C6; Mem'76; FRCPC; Psy. (780)840-8000; Fax. (780)840-4005.

REES, Walter J; Atwood Med Clinic, 101-143 Fourth Ave S, Williams Lake BC V2G 1J8; Alb'78; (250)398-5162; Fax. (250)398-5673.

REESE, Heather L; Yellowbird Family Clinic, 3380 Gateway Blvd NW, Edmonton AB T6J 6V1; Alb'82; BMedSci; (780)434-2893; Fax. (780)435-1057.

REESOR, David G; Headwaters Health Care Centre, 100 Rolling Hills Dr, Orangeville ON L9W 4X9; Wes'81; Ac Staff, Headwaters Health Care Centre - Orangeville Site; (519)941-2410

REESOR, John N; Kawartha Cardiology Clinic, 401-327 Charlotte St, Peterborough ON K9J 0B2; Wes'78; FRCPC; IntMed; Cardiol. Staff, Peterborough Regional Health Centre - Hospital Drive; Cardiology/Internal Med, Peterborough Regional Health Centre - Rogers St Site; (705)775-6870; Fax. (705)775-6868.

REEVE, Brenda K; Brant Community HC-Brantford, 200 Terrace Hill St, Brantford ON N3R 1G9; Tor'95; Critical Care Medicine; Anes. Staff, The Brant Community Healthcare System - Brantford General Hospital Site; Staff, St Joseph's Healthcare - Charlton Campus; (905)751-5508

REEVE, Kate C; Family Practice Health Centre, 77 Grenville St, Toronto ON M5S 1B3; McM'09; CCFP; (416)323-6060

REEVES, Francois; CHUM-Hotel-Dieu, 3840 rue Saint-Urbain, Montreal QC H2W 1T8; Mon'82; FRCPC; IntMed; Cardiol. Staff, Centre Hospitalier l'Université de Montréal (CHUM) - Hôtel-Dieu; (514)890-8000; francois.reeves.chum@ssss.gouv.qc.ca.

REEVES, Hien Nguyen; 200-1358 St Paul St, Kelowna BC V1Y 2E1; Texas (USA)'95; (250)762-0918; Fax. (250)762-7446.

REEVES, Terrence L; U6-601 Broadway W, Vancouver BC V5Z 4C2; Cal'83; CCFP; FCFP; (604)872-2558; Fax. (604)874-6222.

REFAT ZAKI, Maged S; Guelph Gen Hosp, 115 Delhi St, Guelph ON N1E 4J4; Ain Shams (Egypt)'89; FRCPC; Anes. Staff, Guelph General Hospital; (519)822-5350; Fax. (519)822-2170.

REGAN, Kelly A; London HSC-University Hosp, PO Box 5339 Stn B 339 Windermere Rd, London ON N6A 5A5; Wes'85; CCFP; CCFP(E.M.); FCFP; Staff, London Health Sciences Centre - University Hospital; (519)663-3200; Fax. (519)663-3013.

REGAN, William D; UBC Hospital, 2C-2211 Wesbrook Mall, Vancouver BC V6T 2B5; Tor'81; FRCSC; OrthSurg (Knee Reconstruction & Upper Extremity). Ac Staff, UBC Hospital - Koerner Pavillion; (604)822-9277; Fax. (604)822-1999; wregan@interchange.ubc.ca.

REGEHR, Jack C; PO Box 190, Magrath AB T0K 1J0; Alb'85; BSc; CCFP; Consultant, Chinook Regional Hospital; (403)758-3614; Fax. (403)758-3612.

REGEHR, Sonya M; Braeside Med Centre Ltd, 111-1919 Southland Dr SW, Calgary AB T2W 0K1; Cal'90; CCFP; FCFP; (403)258-2133; Fax. (403)258-2162; smregehr@gmail.com.

REGENSTREIF, Leonora J; St Peter's Hosp, 88 Maplewood Ave, Hamilton ON L8M 1W9; Tor'94; BSc; MSc; CCFP; Staff, Hamilton Health Sciences Centre - St Peter's Hospital; Assoc Med Dir, Shelter Hlth Network of Hamilton; Langs: English; French; (905)777-3837

REGGAD, Bouchra; 1000 boul Sainte-Anne, St-Charles-Brromee QC J6E 6J2; Hassan II (Morocco)'95; CCFP; CCFP(E.M.); Staff, Centre Hospitalier Régional de Lanaudière; Langs: French; (450)759-8222 x2820; Fax. (450)759-2994.

REGGLER, Jonathan G; Courtenay Med Associates, 201-1350 England Ave, Courtenay BC V9N 8X6; Cambridge (England)'84; MB BCh; CCFP; (250)334-4411; Fax. (250)338-1245.

REGIMBAL, Marc; Clinique Med de Touraine, 2B-520 boul de l'Hopital, Gatineau QC J8V 2P5; Mon'91; BSc; MSc; Staff, Hull Hospital; Physician, Residence Foyer du Bonheur; Langs: English; French; (819)568-0212

REGIMBAL, Sara M; Bells Corners Fam Med Centre, 103-3730 Richmond Rd, Nepean ON K2H 5B9; Ott'99; CCFP; (613)596-0911; Fax. (613)596-3162.

REGINALD, Arunun Y; The Hosp Sick Children, 555 University Ave, Toronto ON M5G 1X8; London (England)'98; Ophth. Staff, The Hospital For Sick Children; (416)813-8942

REGMI, Dybesh; Halton HCS Corp-Georgetown, 1 Princess Anne Dr, Georgetown ON L7G 2B8; Dal'05; CCFP; (905)873-0111

REGNAULT, R Scott; Peter Lougheed Centre, 3500 26 Ave NE, Calgary AB T1Y 6J4; Cal'88; BScN; CCFP; Staff, Peter Lougheed Centre; Court Staff Privil, Rockyview General Hospital; Ad Staff, Calgary Health Region Chronic Pain Centre; (403)943-5721

REGNIER, Laura R J; Ottawa Reg Cancer Centre, 503 Smyth Rd, Ottawa ON K1H 1C4; Ott'99; MSc; CCFP; Physician, Ottawa Regional Cancer Centre; Langs: English; French; (613)737-7700

REGUSH, Lexy C; Pacific Avenue Med Centre, 300-149 Pacific Ave N, Saskatoon SK S7K 1N8; Sask'02; BSc; FRCSC; ObstGyn. (306)653-5970; Fax. (306)653-5383.

REHAL, Ranjodh S; 1763 Portage Ave, Winnipeg MB R3J 0E7; RCS (Ireland)'80; MB ChB; LRCP; LRCS; LMCC; Langs: Punjabi; Hindi; Swahili; Gujarati.

REHALUK, Robert M; Humber River Reg Hosp-Keele, 2175 Keele St, North York ON M6M 3Z4; Noreste (Mexico)'89; FFPsy; FRCPC; Psy (Forensic Psychiatry). Staff, Ontario Shores Centre for Mental Health Sciences; Staff, Humber River Regional Hospital - Keele Street Site; Teach Staff Psy, University of Toronto; Langs: Spanish; (416)249-8111

REHAN, Fouzia Q; Musquodoboit Harbour Med Clin, PO Box 308 7907 Highway 7, Musquodoboit-Harbr NS B0J 2L0; Punjab (India)'88; CCFP; (902)889-2650; Fax. (902)889-2577.

REHANY, Mordechai; IRM Sud-Ouest, 200-5515 rue Saint-Jacques O, Montreal QC H4A 2E3; McG'90; CSPQ; DiagRad. (514)484-8484; Fax. (514)484-8400.

REHEL, Benoit; CSSS Energie-UMF Shawinigan, 80 118e rue, Shawinigan-Sud QC G9P 3E4; Laval'03; (819)536-7500

REHEL, Luc; CLSC-CHSLD Pabok, 98 Rte 132 CP 269, Perce QC G0C 2L0; Sher'79; (418)782-2572

REHEMTULA, Yasmin; Malton Med Arts Bldg, 206-3530 Derry Rd E, Mississauga ON L4T 4E3; Shiraz (Iran)'79; Ac Staff, William Osler Health System - Etobicoke General Hospital; Langs: Urdu; Hindi; Farsi; Gujarati; (905)672-3333

REHILL, Anjali; Springborough Prof Centre, 108-30 Springborough Blvd SW, Calgary AB T3H 0N9; Alb'04; CCFP; (403)240-2221; Fax. (403)240-4670.

REHMAN, Faisal; London HSC-University Hosp, PO Box 5339 Stn B ALL 139-339 Windermere Rd, London ON N6A 5A5; Qns'98; FRCPC; IntMed; Nephrol. Staff, London Health Sciences Centre - University Hospital; Langs: Urdu; (519)663-3285; Fax. (519)663-3232; faisalrehman@yahoo.com.

REHMAN, Habib; The Regina Med Centre, 100-2550 12th Ave, Regina SK S4P 3X1; University of Peshawar (Pakistan)'88; FACP; FRCPI; FRCP; FRCPC; IntMed (Endocrinology). Clinical Asst Prof, University of Saskatchewan; (306)566-4120; Fax. (306)566-4150; habib31@sasktel.net.

REHMAN, Mujeeb; Misericordia Community Hosp, 16940 87 Ave NW, Edmonton AB T5R 4H5; (Pakistan)'88; Staff, Covenant Health - Misericordia Community Hospital; (780)735-2000

REHMAN, Mujeeb U; The Credit Valley Hosp, 2200 Eglinton Ave W, Mississauga ON L5M 2N1; Karachi (Pakistan)'82; DABPN; ABCGP; FRCPC; Psy (Geriatric Psychiatry). Staff, The Credit Valley Hospital; Langs: Hindi; Punjabi; Urdu; (905)813-2200

REHMAN, Waseema; Glace Bay Family Practice Ctr, 35 Sterling Rd, Glace Bay NS B1A 3X6; Baluchistan (Pakistan)'97; MB BS; CCFP; Fam Med, Glace Bay Healthcare Facility; Langs: Hindi; Punjabi; Urdu; (902)842-1931; Fax. (902)842-1932.

REHMAN, Ziaur; Regina Qu'Appelle HR-Regina, 3F-1440 14th Ave, Regina SK S4P 0W5; Punjab (Pakistan)'90; MB BS; FRCPC; Neur. Staff, Regina General Hospital; Langs: Urdu; Punjabi; (306)790-1818; Fax. (306)790-1868.

REHMUS, Wingfield E; Children's & Women's HC of BC, K4 101-4480 Oak St, Vancouver BC V6H 3V4; Duke University (USA)'96; Staff, BC Children's Hospital; (604)875-2864

REHSIA, Davinder; 235-444 St Mary Ave, Winnipeg MB R3C 3T1; Punjab (India)'69; MB BS; DABOph; FRCSC; Ophth (Refractive Cataract Surgery). Staff, Misericordia Health Centre; Consultant/Staff, St Boniface General Hospital; Asst Prof, University of Manitoba; (204)957-1522; Fax. (204)943-8558.

REHSIA, Navneet; Percy E Moore Hosp, PO Box 190, Hodgson MB R0C 1N0; CCFP; Staff, Percy E Moore Hospital; (204)372-8444

REHSIA, Sabeer S; St Joseph's Healthcare, T2141-50 Charlton Ave, Hamilton ON L8N 4A6; Man'07; Urol. Staff, St Joseph's Healthcare - Charlton Campus; (905)928-5558

REHSIA, Sachdeep S; Halton HCS Corp-Oakville, 327 Reynolds St, Oakville ON L6J 3L7; Wes'07; FRCPC; IntMed; Critical Care Medicine. Staff, Halton Healthcare Services Corporation - Oakville Site; (905)845-2571

REIAL, Juri; Bloor-Jane Med Bldg, 504-2425 Bloor St W, Toronto ON M6S 4W4; Tor'68; FACC; FRCPC; IntMed; Cardiol. Ac Staff, St Joseph's Health Centre; Court Staff, St Michael's Hospital; Asst Prof, University of Toronto; (416)763-3239; Fax. (416)763-6953.

REICH, Dennis A G; Four Corners Med Bldg, 102-2009 Long Lake Rd, Sudbury ON P3E 6C3; Qns'96; CCFP; Langs: Italian; (705)522-5447; Fax. (705)839-1187.

REICH, Erin J; 473 Dupont St, Toronto ON M6G 1Y6; Wes'09; CCFP; (416)588-1888; Fax. (416)588-0388.

REICH, Heather N; Univ Hlth Network-Toronto Gen, 8N 849-200 Elizabeth St, Toronto ON M5G 2C4; McG'97; FRCPC; IntMed; Nephrol. Staff, Toronto General Hospital - UHN; Langs: English; French; (416)340-5093

REICH, Joseph A; The Group Health Centre, 240 McNabb St, Sault Ste. Marie ON P6B 1Y5; Qns'93; FRCSC; GenSurg. (705)759-1234; Fax. (705)759-7487.

REICH, Kurt D; Royal Columbian Hosp, 330 Columbia St E, New Westminster BC V3L 3W7; Cal'83; FRCPC; GenPath. Staff, Royal Columbian Hospital; (604)520-4365

REICH, M David; Hys Med Centre, 202-11010 101 St NW, Edmonton AB T5H 4B9; Sask'75; FRCPC; DiagRad. (780)428-1121; Fax. (780)425-5979.

REICHELD, Susan M; 180 Lesmill Rd, North York ON M3B 2T5; Tor'88; (416)441-7000

REICHER, Agnes E; North York Med Arts Bldg, 319-1333 Sheppard Ave E, North York ON M2J 1V1; Tor'62; FRCPC; Derm. Ac Staff, North York General Hospital; Ac Staff, Women's College Hospital; Court Staff, St Michael's Hospital; Asst Prof Med, University of Toronto; Langs: German; Hungarian; (416)494-7424; Fax. (416)494-7425.

REICHERT, Amber E; University of Alberta Hosp, 3A3.13-8440 112 St NW, Edmonton AB T6G 2B7; Cal'03; FRCPC; Peds (Neonatal & Perinatal Medicine). Staff, University of Alberta Hospital; (780)407-1305; Fax. (780)407-3030.

REICHERT, Clayton C; BC Women's Hosp & Health Ctre, 1L2-4500 Oak St, Vancouver BC V6H 3N1; UBC'86; FRCPC; Anes. Staff, BC Women's Hospital & Health Centre; (604)875-2345

REICHERT, Sonja-Maria; Primary Care Diabetes Support, 346 Platt's Lane, London ON N6G 1J1; McM'06; CCFP; (519)646-6000

REICHETZER, Barbara; CHUM-Hop St-Luc, 1058 rue Saint-Denis, Montreal QC H2X 3J4; Vienna (Austria)'99; FRCSC; ObstGyn. Staff, Centre Hospitalier l'Université De Montréal (CHUM) - Hôpital Saint-luc; (514)890-8000

REICHMAN, Peeter H; 28 Croxall Blvd, Whitby ON L1M 2E3; Tor'85.

REICHMAN, William; 3560 Bathurst St, North York ON M6A 2E1; Buffalo (USA)'84; Staff, Baycrest Centre for Geriatric Care; (416)785-2500 x2444; Fax. (416)785-2484.

REICHMANN, Jaak T; Centre for Inner Freedom, PO Box 20225 Rpo Bayfield North 560 Anne St N, Barrie ON L4M 6E9; Tor'81; FRCPC; Psy (Anxiety Disorder). Assoc Staff Psy, Toronto Western Hospital - University Health Network; Dir, Centre for Inner Freedom; Lecturer Psy, University of Toronto; Langs: Estonian; (705)722-7170; Fax. (705)722-6243.

REID, Alain; Clinique du Village, 102-1972 ch du Village, Mont-Tremblant QC J8E 1K4; Ott'75; (819)425-2741; Fax. (819)425-6529; clinique.village@cgocable.ca.

REID, Andre; Royal Alexandra Hosp, 10240 Kingsway NW, Edmonton AB T5H 3V9; Laval'97; CSPQ; FRCPC; AnatPath. Staff, Royal Alexandra Hospital; (780)735-5281; andre.reid@albertahealthservices.ca.

REID, Andrea S; Western Mem Reg Hosp, PO Box 2005 Stn Main 1 Brookfield Ave, Corner Brook NL A2H 6J7; Tor'99; Staff, Western Memorial Regional Hospital; (709)637-5000

REID, Andrew G; St Mary's Hosp Centre, 3830 av Lacombe, Montreal QC H3T 1M5; McG'06; MDCM; CCFP; CCFP(E.M.); Staff, St Mary's Hospital Centre; (514)345-3511

REID, Anna C; Stanton Terr Health Authority, PO Box 10 Stn Main 550 Byrne Rd, Yellowknife NT X1A 2N1; Ott'86; BSc(Biology); Staff, Stanton Territorial Health Authority; (867)669-4111

REID, Annick; Clinique Med Dr Annick Reid, 59 rue des Roseaux, Blainville QC J7C 6B6; Mon'96; MCFP; Langs: French; English; (450)818-1515; Fax. (450)818-0545.

REID, Anthony J; Orillia Soldiers Mem Hosp, 170 Colborne St W, Orillia ON L3V 2Z3; Tor'71; MSc; CCFP; FCFP; Staff, Orillia Soldiers' Memorial Hospital; (705)325-2201; Fax. (705)330-3220; tony@cfpc.ca.

REID, Barbara A; 510 Second St E, Cornwall ON K6H 1Z6; McG'77; CSPQ; FRCPC; AnatPath (Autopsy). Staff, Cornwall Community Hospital - Second Street Site; Staff Path, Cornwall Community Hospital; Langs: English; French; (613)932-3300

REID, Branden P; North East Med Centre, 7210 144 Ave NW, Edmonton AB T5C 2R7; Alb'07; Staff, University of Alberta Hospital; (780)478-2995; Fax. (780)472-0215.

REID, Brian J; 611-440 King St, Fredericton NB E3B 5H8; Mem'88; CCFP; Ac Staff Family Pract, Dr Everett Chalmers Regional Hospital; Ac Staff, Oromocto Public Hospital; (506)450-0270; Fax. (506)450-4389; drreid@health.nb.ca.

REID, Brian S; 104-186 Albert St, London ON N6A 1M1; Ott'88; BSc(Physiol.); FRCPC; Psy;CCFP; (519)663-8089

REID, Callum G; UBC IntMed Outpatient Clinic, 7F-2775 Laurel St, Vancouver BC V5Z 1M9; UBC'06; IntMed. Staff, Gordon & Leslie Diamond Health Care Centre; (604)875-4107

REID, Chantelle A; Dr Charles A Janeway Child HC, 300 Prince Philip Dr, St. John's NL A1B 3V6; Mem'01; FRCPC; Psy. Staff, Janeway Children's Health & Rehabilitation Centre; (709)777-6300

REID, Craig W; Queensway-Carleton Hosp, 3045 Baseline Rd, Nepean ON K2H 8P4; Ott'88; FRCPC; Anes. Staff, Queensway Carleton Hospital; Langs: English; French; (613)721-2000 x2651

REID, Daniel S; Woodlawn Med Clinic, 92 Main St, Dartmouth NS B2X 1R5; Dal'70; (902)434-1500; Fax. (902)434-4368.

REID, David A; Misericordia Community Hosp, 16940 87 Ave NW, Edmonton AB T5R 4H5; Tor'71; Ac Staff Emerg, Covenant Health - Misericordia Community Hospital; Clin Instructor Family Practice, University of Alberta; (780)735-2537; Fax. (780)735-2966.

REID, David B; Sherwood Family Med Centre, 15 Brackley Point Rd, Charlottetown PE C1A 6Y1; Dal'89; CCFP; FCFP; Ac Staff Family Med, Queen Elizabeth Hospital; (902)566-9730; Fax. (902)566-1061.

REID, David C; Glen Sather Sports Med Clinic, 11400 University Ave NW, Edmonton AB T6G 1Z1; Alb'74; MCh(Liverpool); CASM; FRCSC; OrthSurg (Arthroscopy). Ac Staff, University of Alberta Hospital; Assoc Staff, Covenant Health - Grey Nuns Community Hospital; Assoc Staff, Glenrose Rehabilitation Hospital; (780)407-6233; Fax. (780)407-6288; dcreid@ualberta.ca.

REID, David F; Foothills Med Centre, 1403 29 St NW, Calgary AB T2N 2T9; Man'77; FRCPC; DiagRad. Staff Radiological Science, Foothills Medical Centre; (403)944-1969; Fax. (403)944-2549.

REID, Dawn K; Ross Mem Hosp, 10 Angeline St N, Lindsay ON K9V 4M8; Wes'99; CCFP; CCFP(E.M.); Staff, Ross Memorial Hospital; (705)324-6111

REID, Debbie H R; Dr Charles A Janeway Child HC, 300 Prince Philip Dr, St. John's NL A1B 3V6; Mem'80; Critical Care Medicine; Peds (Pediatric Intensive Care). Staff, Janeway Children's Health & Rehabilitation Centre; (709)777-6300

REID, Dennis; The Ottawa Hosp-Gen Campus, 2600-501 Smyth Rd, Ottawa ON K1H 8L6; Aberdeen (Scotland)'67; MB ChB; DRCOG; FRCA(UK); FRCPC; Anes (Chronic Pain Management). Staff Chronic Pain Mgmt Unit, The Ottawa Hospital - General Campus; Prof, University of Ottawa; Langs: English; French; (613)737-8187; Fax. (613)737-8189; dereid@ottawahospital.on.ca.

REID, Diane E; McMaster University HSC, 1200 Main St W, Hamilton ON L8S 4J9; Sher'88; FRCSC; Otol (Laryngology). Assoc Staff, Hamilton Health Sciences Centre - McMaster Children's Hospital; Clinical Asst Prof, McMaster University; Langs: English; French; (905)521-2100 x73078; Fax. (905)521-8552.

REID, Douglas B; Towne Centre Medical, 19-2475 Dobbin Rd, West Kelowna BC V4T 2E9; St. Andrews (Scotland)'69; MB ChB; DLO(Lond); DRCOG; Staff, Princeton General Hospital; (250)768-8315

REID, Fiona; 212 6 Ave NE GD, Sundre AB T0M 1X0; (United Kingdom)'04; (403)638-4063; Fax. (403)638-4460.

REID, Genevieve; CSSS du Sud de Lanaudière, 911 Montee des Pionniers, Terrebonne QC J6V 2H2; Laval'05; Gastroent; IntMed. Staff, Centre Hospitalier Pierre le Gardeur; (514)418-9235

REID, Gordon N; Queensway-Carleton Hosp, 3045 Baseline Rd, Nepean ON K2H 8P4; Ott'81; FRCPC; Anes. Staff, Queensway Carleton Hospital; (613)721-2000 x2900

REID, Graham D; Laurel Med Centre Ltd, 306-888 8th Ave W, Vancouver BC V5Z 3Y1; Aberdeen (Scotland)'73; MB ChB; FRCPC; IntMed; Rheum. Staff, G F Strong Rehabilitation Centre; Ac Staff, Vancouver General Hospital - Centennial Pavillion; Asst Prof Med, University of British Columbia; (604)875-6815; Fax. (604)875-1670.

REID, Gregory J; Women's Hosp, WR-120-735 Notre Dame Ave, Winnipeg MB R3E 0L8; Qns'88; FACOG; FRCSC; ObstGyn (Maternal Fetal Medicine). Staff, Health Sciences Centre; Staff, St Boniface General Hospital; Asst Prof, University of Manitoba; (204)787-1984; Fax. (204)787-2899; gjreid@hsc.mb.ca.

REID, Iain C; Kootenay-Boundary Reg Hosp, 1200 Hospital Bench, Trail BC V1R 4M1; Otago (New Zealand)'86; MB ChB; FRCPC; Anes. Staff, Kootenay Boundary Regional Hospital; (250)368-3311

REID, James A; Port Arthur Health Centre Inc, 194 Court St N, Thunder Bay ON P7A 4V7; McM'75; BSc; (807)346-1000; Fax. (807)346-6206.

REID, James D; Allin Clinic, 10155 120 St NW, Edmonton AB T5K 2A2; UBC'08; CCFP; (780)482-7551

REID, James N; 476 Dundas St W, Belleville ON K8P 1B7; Qns'89; CCFP; FCFP; Med Dir, Hastings Manor Nursing Home; (613)967-5852; Fax. (613)967-9981.

REID, Jessica E; 9 Ann St, Bracebridge ON P1L 1S3; McM'06; FRCSC; GenSurg. Staff, South Muskoka Memorial Hospital - Muskoka Algonquin Healthcare; (705)646-1043

REID, John B; The Burris Clinic, 300-275 Lansdowne St, Kamloops BC V2C 6J3; Mem'74; Ac Staff, Royal Inland Hospital; (250)377-3347; Fax. (250)571-3361.

REID, John D S; St Paul's Hosp, C 318-1081 Burrard St, Vancouver BC V6Z 1Y6; Cal'80; FACS; FRCSC; GenSurg; VascSurg. Ac Staff, Providence Health Care - St Paul's Hospital; Clin Prof, University of British Columbia; (604)806-8698; Fax. (604)806-8666; jreid@providencehealth.bc.ca.

REID, John K; Royal University Hosp, 103 Hospital Dr, Saskatoon SK S7N 0W8; UBC'96; ABIM; DABSM; FRCPC; IntMed (Intensive Care); Critical Care Medicine; Respir. Staff/Dir Intensive Care Unit, Royal University Hospital; (306)966-8274; Fax. (306)966-8694.

REID, Katie; 709 1 StNE, Sundre AB T0M 1X0; (United Kingdom)'05; (403)638-2424; Fax. (403)638-3580.

REID, Kenneth R; Richardson House, 102 Stuart St, Kingston ON K7L 2V6; Ott'82; FRCSC; GenSurg; ThorSurg. Staff ThorSurg, Kingston General Hospital; Staff ThorSurg, Hotel-Dieu Hospital; Assoc Chief Thoracic Surg, Queen's University; Langs: English; French; (613)548-2383; Fax. (613)549-2902.

REID, Kristin S; Fort William Clinic, 117 McKellar St S, Thunder Bay ON P7E 1H5; Man'03; BSc; CCFP; (807)626-1222

REID, Linda M; 1864 Oak Bay Ave, Victoria BC V8R 1C5; Tor'84; CCFP; FCFP; Staff, Royal Jubilee Hospital; Staff, Victoria General Hospital; (250)380-1551; Fax. (250)380-2046.

REID, Lori; 181 Miller Park Ave, Bradford ON L3Z 2K3; Ott'07; FRCSC; IntMed; lthompson@bizinfogroup.ca

REID, Miles E; Northern Lights Health Region, 7 Hospital St, Fort McMurray AB T9H 1P2; McG'85; CSPQ; FRCPC; DiagRad. Staff, St Mary's Hospital Centre; Staff, Northern Lights Regional Health Centre; Langs: English; French; (514)345-3511

REID, Nancy C; Bagot Street Med Centre, 182 Bagot St, Kingston ON K7L 3G1; Qns'82; CCFP; (613)542-8783; Fax. (613)546-1321.

REID, Natisha D; The Allin Clinic, 10155 120 St NW, Edmonton AB T5K 2A2; Alb'08; BSc; CCFP; (780)482-7551; Fax. (780)488-2056.

REID, Owen G; Coastal Plastic Surgery, 201-6051 Gilbert Rd, Richmond BC V7C 3V3; UBC'03; FRCSC; PlasSurg. Staff, Foothills Medical Centre; (604)273-1034

REID, Philip H; PO Box 4817, Rothesay NB E2E 5X5; Dal'68; BSc; FRCPC; PhysMed&Rehab (Pain Management). Dir Rehab Unit, Saint John Regional Hospital; Consultant, St Joseph's Hospital; Consultant, Sussex Health Centre; Dalhousie University; Asst Prof, Memorial University Of Newfoundland; (506)847-0007; Fax. (506)634-8855; doctor@reidmd.com.

REID, R Ian; Polyclinic Prof Centre Inc, 303-199 Grafton St, Charlottetown PE C1A 1L2; Qns'81; FRCSC; Urol. Ac Staff Surg, Queen Elizabeth Hospital; (902)629-8808; Fax. (902)629-8830; dr_i_reid@hotmail.com.

REID, Richard A S; Summit Injury Management Inc, 605 Discovery St, Victoria BC V8T 5G4; Mem'91; BSc; FRCSC; Neursurg. (250)383-3638

REID, Robert H; London HSC-Victoria Hosp, PO Box 5010 Stn B 800 Commissioners Rd E, London ON N6A 5W9; Glasgow (Scotland)'77; MB ChB; FRCPC; NuclearMed. Ac Staff, London Health Sciences Centre - Victoria Campus; Assoc Prof, University of Western Ontario; (519)667-6566 x75365; Fax. (519)667-6734.

REID, Robert L; McKinney Med Centre, 107-510 Ingersoll Ave, Woodstock ON N4S 4X9; Tor'63; AB; FRCSC; OrthSurg (Arthritis Surgery). Consultant, Woodstock General Hospital; Consultant, Tillsonburg District Memorial Hospital; Consultant, Alexandra Hospital; (519)539-7444; Fax. (519)539-7445; robert.reid9@sympatico.ca.

REID, Robert L; Kingston Gen Hosp, V4-76 Stuart St, Kingston ON K7L 2V7; Qns'74; FRCS; FRCSC; ObstGyn (Reproductive Endocrinology & Infertility). Staff ObstGyn, Kingston General Hospital; Prof Repro Endocrin, Queen's University; (613)542-9473; Fax. (613)533-6779; robert.reid@queensu.ca.

REID, Ruth E; Campbell River & Dist Hosp, 375 2nd Ave, Campbell River BC V9W 3V1; Mem'75; FRCPC; DiagRad. Staff, Campbell River & District General Hospital; (250)287-7111

REID, Sarah J; Univ Hlth Network-Toronto Western Hosp, 2W404-399 Bathurst St, Toronto ON M5T 2S8; McM'02; CCFP; Staff, Toronto Western Hospital - University Health Network; (416)603-5888 x2

REID, Sarah M; Children's Hosp Eastern Ont, 401 Smyth Rd, Ottawa ON K1H 8L1; Ott'99; FRCPC; Peds. Staff, Children's Hospital of Eastern Ontario (CHEO); (613)737-7600 x2318; Fax. (613)738-3216.

REID, Stuart E; Kingston Gen Hosp, 76 Stuart St, Kingston ON K7L 2V7; Wes'00; FRCPC; Neur. Staff, Kingston General Hospital; (613)549-6666; Fax. (613)548-1341.

REID, Susan E; Hamilton HS-General Site, 606-237 Barton St E, Hamilton ON L8L 2X2; McM'87; FRCSC; GenSurg; Critical Care Medicine. Staff, St Joseph's Healthcare - Charlton Campus; Ac Staff, Hamilton Health Sciences Centre - Hamilton General Hospital; Assoc Prof Surg, McMaster University; (905)521-2617; Fax. (905)528-9388.

REID, Susan J; Grey Nuns Community Hosp & HC, 1100 Youville Drive West NW, Edmonton AB T6L 5X8; London (England)'80; MB BS; FRCPC; Anes. Staff, Covenant Health - Grey Nuns Community Hospital; University of Alberta; (780)735-7020

REID, Wilfrid; 55 av Willowdale, Outremont QC H3T 1G4; Mon'65; CSPQ; Psy. Staff, Hôpital du Sacre-Coeur de Montréal; (514)733-0974

REID-PERREAULT, Micheline; Inst Albert Prevost, 6555 boul Gouin O, Montreal QC H4K 1B3; Mon'67; CSPQ; Psy. Staff, Hôpital du Sacre-Coeur de Montréal; (514)338-4356

REID-RAFLA, Heather J; Guelph Family Health Team, 102-21 Surrey St W, Guelph ON N1H 3R3; McM'86; BScN; CCFP; FCFP; Staff, Guelph General Hospital; (519)837-3623; Fax. (519)837-5425.

REIKIE, W Roddick; Central Alberta Orthopaedics, 300-4309 52 Ave, Red Deer AB T4N 6S4; Cal'73; FRCSC; OrthSurg., B C Youth Development; (403)309-2001; Fax. (403)358-5808.

REILKOFF, Catherine R; Burrard Health Bldg, 307-1160 Burrard St, Vancouver BC V6Z 2E8; UBC'76; Assoc Staff, Providence Health Care - St Paul's Hospital; BC Youth Development; (604)687-7033; Fax. (604)602-0923.

REILLY, Christopher W; Children's & Women's HC of BC, A202-4480 Oak St, Vancouver BC V6H 3V4; UBC'88; FRCSC; OrthSurg. Staff, BC Children's Hospital; (604)875-3711

REILLY, Daniel R; Riverview Medical Group, 205 Queen St E, Fergus ON N1M 1T2; Qns'00; BSc; MHSc; FRCSC; ObstGyn. Staff, Groves Memorial Community Hospital; Consultant All Sites, North Wellington Health Care - Louise Marshall Hospital; (519)787-7418; Fax. (519)787-7421.

REILLY, James G; Forest Heights Med Clinic, 7461 101 Ave NW, Edmonton AB T6A 3Z5; Alb'73; CCFP; FCFP; Ac Staff, Royal Alexandra Hospital; Asst Prof Family Med, University of Alberta; (780)463-2323; Fax. (780)463-5514; jgreilly@shaw.ca.

REIMAN, Anthony J; Saint John Reg Hosp, PO Box 2100 Stn Main 400 University Ave, Saint John NB E2L 4L2; Tor'96; BSc; MSc; FRCPC; IntMed; MedOncol. Staff, Saint John Regional Hospital; (506)648-6000

REIMCHE, Leanne D; The Ottawa Hosp-Civic Campus, CPC406-1053 Carling Ave, Ottawa ON K1Y 4E9; UBC'91; BScPharm; FRCPC; IntMed. Staff, The Ottawa Hospital - Civic Campus; Staff, Queensway Carleton Hospital; (613)798-5555

REIMER, Cara L; Kingston Gen Hosp, 76 Stuart St, Kingston ON K7L 2V7; Sask'03; FRCPC; Anes. Staff, Kingston General Hospital; (613)548-3232

REIMER, Darren K; Steinbach Family Med Centre, 10-333 Loewen Blvd, Steinbach MB R5G 0C3; Man'93; BSc; CCFP; FCFP; Lecturer Family Med, University of Manitoba; Langs: German; (204)326-3401; Fax. (204)326-3899.

REIMER, David; Primary Health Centre, PO Box 1360 176 Wellington St, Niagara-Lk ON L0S 1J0; Tor'85; DTMH; CCFP; FCFP; Ac Staff, Niagara Health System - Niagara-on-the-Lake Hospital Site; Med Dir, Heritage Place Nursing Home; Clin Assoc Prof, McMaster University; (905)468-9961; Fax. (905)468-4947.

REIMER, David J; 703-400 Tache Ave, Winnipeg MB R2H 3C3; Man'95; FRCSC; GenSurg.

REIMER, Eleanor J; BC Women's Hosp & Health Ctre, 4500 Oak St, Vancouver BC V6H 3N1; Man'85; FRCPC; Anes. Staff, BC Women's Hospital & Health Centre; (604)875-2711

REIMER, Harwood L; 101-330 Festubert St, Duncan BC V9L 3S9; UBC'86; Dip SportMed; CCFP; Ac Staff, Cowichan District Hospital; (250)748-9000; Fax. (250)748-1299; dr.reimer@shaw.ca.

REIMER, Heinz; Children's Hosp, AE203-840 Sherbrook St, Winnipeg MB R3A 1S1; Man'83; FRCPC; Anes.

REIMER, Mark W; 6-385 Frederick St, Kitchener ON N2H 2P2; Wes'02; MBA; FRCSC; GenSurg. (519)957-9730; Fax. (519)957-9732.

REIMER, Murray B; Dr CW Wiebe Med Centre, 385 Main St, Winkler MB R6W 1J2; Man'78; CCFP; Staff, Boundary Trails Health Centre; Lecturer Med, University of Manitoba; (204)325-4312; Fax. (204)325-4594.

REIMER, Shirley A; Fairmont Med Bldg, 915-750 Broadway W, Vancouver BC V5Z 1H8; Ott'75; ObstGyn. Consultant, Vancouver General Hospital - Centennial Pavillion; Ac Staff, Providence Health Care - St Paul's Hospital; Ac Staff, BC Women's Hospital & Health Centre; Clinical Asst Prof, University of British Columbia; (604)872-2003

REIMER, Wendy J; 201-851 Fischer Hallman Rd, Kitchener ON N2M 5N8; Tor'91; Court Staff, St Mary's General Hospital; Court Staff, Grand River Hospital - Kitchener/Waterloo Health Centre; (519)743-1011; Fax. (519)743-0041.

REIMER, Wesley J; Joseph Brant Mem Hosp, 1230 North Shore Blvd E, Burlington ON L7S 1W7; Cal'95; CCFP; FCFP; Staff, Niagara Health System - St Catharines General Site; Staff, Joseph Brant Memorial Hospital; (905)632-3730

REINBLATT, Shauna L; MUHC-Royal Victoria Hosp, 687 av des Pins O, Montreal QC H3A 1A1; McG'03; FRCSC; ObstGyn. Staff, McGill University Health Centre - Royal Victoria Hospital; (514)934-1934

REINDERS, Francis X; St Mary's Gen Hosp, CVICU-911 Queens Blvd, Kitchener ON N2M 1B2; Tor'94; Anes. Staff, St Mary's General Hospital; (519)749-6690

REINDERS, Maarthen; 125-210 Memorial Ave, Orillia ON L3V 7V1; Tor'90; CCFP; Ac Staff, Orillia Soldiers' Memorial Hospital; (705)329-1223; Fax. (705)329-3255.

REINDERS, Sabrina M L; Two Rivers FHT-Healthlink, 10B-350 Conestoga Blvd, Cambridge ON N1R 7L7; Tor'04; CCFP; (519)740-5010; Fax. (519)740-6010.

REINDL, Rudolf; MUHC-Montreal Gen Hosp, B5 1592-1650 av Cedar, Montreal QC H3G 1A4; Tor'93; FRCSC; OrthSurg. Staff, McGill University Health Centre - Montreal General Campus; Langs: German; French; Czech; (514)934-1934 x42595; Fax. (514)934-8453; rudy.reindl@muhc.mcgill.ca.

REINECKE, Carolus J; Ancron Med Centre, 108-402 Baker St, Nelson BC V1L 4H8; Pretoria (South Africa)'06; Langs: Afrikaans; (250)352-9144

REINECKE, Marina; Health Sciences Centre, GB2-820 Sherbrook St, Winnipeg MB R3A 1R9; Orange Free State (South Africa)'00; CCFP; Staff, Health Sciences Centre; (204)774-8511

REINEKING, Samantha J; PO Box 75535 Rpo Edgemont Vill, North Vancouver BC V7R 4X1; UBC'09; CCFP.

REINER, Neil E; 452D-2733 Heather St, Vancouver BC V5Z 1M9; Cleveland(OH) (USA)'74; FRCPC; IntMed (Infectious Diseases). Ac Staff, Vancouver General Hospital - Centennial Pavillion; University of British Columbia; (604)875-4011; Fax. (604)875-4013.

REINGOLD, Morton J; 401-960 Lawrence Ave W, North York ON M6A 3B5; Tor'78; Ac Staff, Mount Sinai Hospital; Ac Staff, Humber River Regional Hospital - Keele Street Site; Langs: Italian; Spanish; (416)256-1150; Fax. (416)256-0742.

REINGOLD, Stephen M; William Osler HC-Brampton, 5N-2100 Bovaird Dr E, Brampton ON L6R 3J7; McM'84; MSc; FRCPC; IntMed (Hematology); MedOncol. Chief Clin MedOncol, William Osler Health System - Brampton Civic Hospital; Staff, The Oncology Group; (905)494-6542

REINGOLD, Terence M; 106-1575 Steeles Ave E, North York ON M2M 3Y7; Tor'75; (416)226-4565

REINHARDT, David J; 536 Frederick St, Kitchener ON N2B 2A6; Tor'67; CCFP; Chief Dept of Family Pract, St Mary's General Hospital; Staff, Grand River Hospital - Kitchener/Waterloo Health Centre; Langs: German; (519)579-0320

REINHARDT, Paul H; Rockyview Gen Hosp, 7007 14 St SW, Calgary AB T2V 1P9; Cal'03; FRCPC; Psy. Staff, Rockyview General Hospital; (403)943-3808; Fax. (403)212-1234.

REINHART, Steven J; 1-176 Wyndham St N, Guelph ON N1H 8N9; McM'81; CCFP; (519)821-8833 x314

REINHARTZ, Abraham D; 306-960 Lawrence Ave W, North York ON M6A 3B5; McM'82; Ac Staff, Humber River Regional Hospital - Finch Avenue Site; Physician, Occupational Health Clinic for Ontario Workers; (416)781-6199; Fax. (416)781-4515; abe_reinhartz@yahoo.ca.

REINHOLD, Caroline; MUHC-Montreal Gen Hosp, 1650 av Cedar, Montreal QC H3G 1A4; McG'84; CSPQ; FRCPC; DiagRad. Staff, McGill University Health Centre - Montreal General Campus; (514)934-1934 x42872; Fax. (514)934-8263; caroline.reinhold@muhc.mcgill.ca.

REINIGER, Rhonda M; Lakeside Med Clinic, 3919 8th St E, Saskatoon SK S7H 5M7; Sask'90; BSc; CCFP; (306)374-6884; Fax. (306)374-2552.

REIS, Marciano D; Sunnybrook Hlth Sciences Ctre, B204-2075 Bayview Ave, Toronto ON M4N 3M5; Parana (Brazil)'76; FRCPC; HemPath. Chief Dept of ClinPath, Sunnybrook Health Sciences Centre; Consultant, Sunnybrook Health Sciences Centre - Edmond Odette Cancer Centre; Assoc Prof LabMed & Pathobiol & Dept of Med, University of Toronto; Langs: Portuguese; Spanish; (416)480-4066

REISCH, Helga; Kensington Family Med Centre, PO Box 160, Kensington PE C0B 1M0; Alb'98; CCFP; FCFP; (902)836-3137

REISER, Wendy M; Burlington Prof Centre, 101-3155 Harvester Rd, Burlington ON L7N 3V2; Tor'84; Ac Staff, Joseph Brant Memorial Hospital; (905)639-1142; Fax. (905)632-9624.

REISLER, Hyman; Ellendale Med Bldg, 390-5845 ch de la Cote-des-Nei, Montreal QC H3S 1Z4; Melbourne (Australia)'56; MB BS; Cardiol (P.Q.); IntMed (Clinical Cardiology). Att Physician Cardiol, Sir Mortimer B Davis Jewish General; Med Dir, Wilmar Medical Services Ltd.; Teacher, McGill University; (514)739-6693; Fax. (514)739-5657.

REISMAN, John J; Children's Hosp Eastern Ont, W1530-401 Smyth Rd, Ottawa ON K1H 8L1; Tor'80; MBA; FRCPC; Peds (Pediatric Respirology); Respir. Prof, University of Ottawa; Langs: English; French; (613)737-7600 x2637; Fax. (613)738-4886.

REISNER, Debra M; The Clinic on 5th, 215 5th Ave N, Saskatoon SK S7K 2P2; Sask'81; FRCPC; Psy (Child & Adolescent Psychiatry). Staff, Royal University Hospital; (306)653-0002; Fax. (306)244-5362.

REISS, Dina; Univ of Toronto, 602-500 University Ave, Toronto ON M5G 1V7; Chicago (USA)'08; FRCPC; IntMed.

REISS, Jeffrey P; London HSC-Victoria Hosp, PO Box 5010 Stn B NT B8 142-800 Commissioners Rd, London ON N6A 5W9; Man'82; MSc(Psy); DABPN; FRCPC; Psy (General Adult Psychiatry). Staff, London Health Sciences Centre - Victoria Campus; Site Chief Psy, London Health Sciences Centre - South Street; Prof/Div Chair, University of Western Ontario; (519)685-8500

REITER, Harold I; The Juravinski Cancer Centre, 3F-699 Concession St, Hamilton ON L8V 5C2; Tor'86; FRCPC; RadOncol. Assoc Prof, McMaster University; Langs: Hebrew; (905)387-9495 x64704; Fax. (905)575-6326.

REITER, Sharon R; Sunnybrook Hlth Sciences Ctre, 2075 Bayview Ave, Toronto ON M4N 3M5; Tor'84; FRCPC; Psy. Head Div of Youth Psychiatry, Sunnybrook Health Sciences Centre; Teach Staff, University of Toronto; (416)480-4098; Fax. (416)480-6818.

REITER, Stephanie L; 306-2100 av de Marlowe, Montreal QC H4A 3L5; McG'94; Peds (Infectious Diseases). (514)482-3456; Fax. (514)485-1478.

REITSMA, Jeffrey J; University of Alberta Hosp, 8440 112 St NW, Edmonton AB T6G 2B7; Alb'07; FRCPC; EmergMed. Staff, University of Alberta Hospital; (780)407-8822; Fax. (780)407-3695.

REITZ, Francois; Saskatchewan Med Association, 402-321A 21st St E, Saskatoon SK S7K 0C1; (306)244-2196; Fax. (306)657-4587.

REIZGYS, Katerina L; Hespeler Med Clinic, 12-350 Conestoga Blvd, Cambridge ON N1R 7Z2; Wes'10; CCFP.

REKA, Altin; Urgent Care Niagara, 104-6150 Valley Way, Niagara Falls ON L2E 1Y3; Universiteti i Tiranes (Albania)'97; CCFP; (905)371-1881; Fax. (905)371-1888.

REKART, Michael L; School of Population & Public, 2206 Health Sciences Mall, Vancouver BC V6T 1Z3; Columbus(OH) (USA)'73; ABIM; DTMH; MHSc; FRCPC; IntMed. Dir STD.Aids Control, BC Centre For Disease Control; Clin Prof Med, University of British Columbia; (604)312-6555; michael.rekart@bccdc.ca.

REKIEH, Kassim M; 104-10004 107 St, Westlock AB T7P 2K8; Alb'10; CCFP; (780)349-4425; Fax. (780)349-4478.

RELJA, Malgorzata; Dr Everett Chalmers Reg Hosp, PO Box 9000 Stn A, Fredericton NB E3B 5N5; Warsaw (Poland)'94; Staff, Dr Everett Chalmers Regional Hospital; (506)444-5337

REMBEZ, Valentyna B; 748 Kingsway St, Vancouver BC V5V 3C1; Odessa (Ukraine)'88; CCFP; Langs: Russian; Ukrainian; (604)687-6871

REMER, Samuel T; 100-8171 Cook Rd, Richmond BC V6Y 3T8; Oklahoma (USA)'79; (604)297-1964

REMER, Zev; 100-1538 rue Sherbrooke, Montreal QC H3G 1L5; McG'89; CCFP; (514)932-2122

REMICK, Ronald A; St Paul's Hosp, 1081 Burrard St, Vancouver BC V6Z 1Y6; Washington(DC) (USA)'74; FRCPC; Psy (Mood Disorders). Consultant Psy, Providence Health Care - St Paul's Hospital; Staff, Mood Disorders Association of BC; (604)682-2344 x62121; Fax. (604)263-9334; rremick@shaw.ca.

REMILLARD, Elizabeth; 100-500 boul de l'Hopital, Gatineau QC J8V 2P5; Sher'05; (819)966-6380

REMILLARD, Francine; CSST Sherbrooke, 1650 rue King O, Sherbrooke QC J1J 2C3; Mon'68; Langs: English; (819)821-5000 x5072; Fax. (819)821-7029.

REMILLARD, Guy M; 10720 rue Tanguay, Montreal QC H3L 3H2; Ott'66; LMCC; CSPQ; Electroenceph (P.Q.); Neur (P.Q.) (Epilepsy). Consultant, Pavillon Notre-Dame de la Merci; Langs: English; (514)337-8310; Fax. (514)337-7564; guremillard@gmail.com.

REMILLARD, Jean; Ctr de Physiatrie Dorchester, 607-235 boul René-Lévesque E, Montreal QC H2X 1N8; Laval'76; FRCPC; PhysMed&Rehab (Electromyography). Langs: English; (514)861-9855; Fax. (514)861-9856.

REMILLARD, Marie-Anais; Institut de Rhumatologie, 155 rue Ontario E, Montreal QC H2L 1S6; Sher'02; Rheum; IntMed. Staff, Hopital Charles LeMoyne; (514)523-3305

REMILLARD, Stephanie; CSSS Haut-Richelieu-Rouville, 920 boul du Seminaire N, St-Jean-sur-Richel QC J3A 1B7; Mon'06; FRCPC; IntMed; Gastroent. Staff, Hôpital du Haut-Richelieu; (450)359-5000

REMILLARD, Timothy G; Blue Mountains Commun Hlth Ctr, PO Box 70 78 King St E, Thornbury ON N0H 2P0; McM'90; BSc; CCFP; FCFP; Staff, Grey Bruce Health Services - Meaford Site; Staff, Sault Area Hospital - Sault Ste Marie; Staff, Lady Dunn Health Centre; (519)599-2732; Fax. (519)599-5895; trem3161@rogers.com.

REMILLARD-LAMARRE, Denise; CSSS de Saint-Jerome, 290 rue de Montigny, Saint-Jerome QC J7Z 5T3; Laval'69; CSPQ; DiagRad. Ac Staff Radiol, Hôtel-Dieu de Saint-Jérôme; (450)431-8300; Fax. (450)431-8244.

REMINGTON, B Kent; 150-7220 Fisher St SE, Calgary AB T2H 2H8; Alb'66; DAB; FRCPC; Derm (Laser Surgery). Ac Staff, Foothills Medical Centre; Consultant, Rockyview General Hospital; (403)252-7784; Fax. (403)259-5245; inforemingtonlaser@shaw.ca.

REMINGTON, Gary J; Addiction & Mental Hlth-Clarke, 250 College St, Toronto ON M5T 1R8; McM'80; FRCPC; Psy (Schizophrenia). Staff Teacher, Centre for Addiction & Mental Health (CAMH) - College Street Site; Prof Psy, University of Toronto; (416)535-8501 x4750; Fax. (416)979-4292; gary_remington@camh.net.

REMINGTON, Jeffrey S; 340 Elgin St, Port Colborne ON L3K 6G9; McM'93; BSc(Hons.); CCFP; CCFP(E.M.); FCFP; Ac Staff, Niagara Health System - Port Colborne General Site; Court Staff, Niagara Health System - Welland Hospital Site; Clinical Asst Prof Family Med, McMaster University; (905)835-9817; Fax. (905)835-1647; jeffmd1@mac.com.

REMMERS, John E; HSC-Faculty of Med, 123-3330 Hospital Dr NW, Calgary AB T2N 4N1; Boston(MA) (USA)'63; Dir Centre for Advance Health, Foothills Medical Centre; Prof IntMed, University of Calgary; (403)210-8635; Fax. (403)270-8928; jeremmer@ucalgary.ca.

REMPEL, Brenda M; 206-245 Pelham Rd, St Catharines ON L2S 1X8; Man'02; FRCPC; IntMed. Staff, Niagara Health System - Ontario Street Site; (905)684-3111; Fax. (905)684-3112.

REMPEL, Elfrieda; Georgetown Med Associates, 199 Princess Anne Dr, Georgetown ON L7G 0E3; Man'84; Langs: German; (905)873-3000; Fax. (905)873-0800.

REMPEL, Jeremy L; Hys Med Centre, 105-11010 101 St NW, Edmonton AB T5H 4B9; Man'04; FRCPC; DiagRad. Staff, Health Sciences Centre; (780)426-1121; Fax. (780)425-5979.

REMPEL, Monika E; Whistler Health Care Centre, 4380 Lorimer Rd, Whistler BC V0N 1B4; UBC'92; BSc(Kinesiol); CCFP; CCFP(E.M.); (604)932-4911

REMPEL, Peter T; 11091 Tow Hill Rd PO Box 210, Masset BC V0T 1M0; Qns'84; Ac Staff, Northern Haida Gwaii Hospital and Health Centre; (250)626-3775; peter.rempel@northernhealth.ca.

REMPEL, Regina R; Rehabilitation for Children, 633 Wellington Cres, Winnipeg MB R3M 0A8; Man'79; FRCPC; Peds (Developmental Disability). Ac Staff Children's Hosp, Health Sciences Centre; Assoc Prof Peds & Child Health, University of Manitoba; Langs: German; (204)453-9854; Fax. (204)474-2387.

REMTULLA, Suleman S; Credit Valley Med Arts Centre, 508-2000 Credit Valley Rd, Mississauga ON L5M 4N4; Tor'83; MSc; DOHS; CCFP; FCFP; Ac Staff, The Credit Valley Hospital; Langs: Kacchi; (905)828-2837; Fax. (905)820-1738.

REMUS, John L; Ridgeway Clinic, 1001 Ridgeway St E, Thunder Bay ON P7E 5H8; Qns'61; FICS; AADEP; FRCSC; OrthSurg (Disability Assessment); GenSurg. Assoc Staff OrthSurg, Occupational Med Consultant, Thunder Bay Regional Health Sciences Centre; Asst Prof, Northern Ontario School of Medicine; (807)623-7252; Fax. (807)622-6427.

REMY, Joseph; Clinique Med Sainte-Anne, 11A boul Sainte-Anne E, Ste-Anne-des-Mts QC G4V 1M4; Port-au-Prince (Haiti)'77; Staff, Centre Hospitalier des Monts; (418)763-7741; Fax. (418)763-7742.

REMY, M E Huguette; MUHC-Montreal Gen Hosp, C5129-1650 av Cedar, Montreal QC H3G 1A4; Mon'65; CSPQ; DiagRad. Ac Staff, McGill University Health Centre - Montreal General Campus; (514)934-1934; Fax. (514)934-8263.

REN, Haifeng; Kingston Gen Hosp, 76 Stuart St, Kingston ON K7L 2V7; Shanghai (China)'91; Staff, Kingston General Hospital; (613)549-6666

REN, Jian Z; Scarborough Hosp-General Div, 3050 Lawrence Ave E, Scarborough ON M1P 2V5; Shanghai (China)'80; FRCPC; AnatPath. Staff, The Scarborough Hospital - General Campus; (416)438-2911

REN, Yubo; Pembroke Reg Hosp, 705 Mackay St, Pembroke ON K8A 1G8; Beijing (China)'86; CCFP; Staff, Pembroke Regional Hospital Inc; (613)732-2811

RENALD, Marie-Helene; Hotel-Dieu de Levis, 143 rue Wolfe, Levis QC G6V 3Z1; Laval'06; FRCSC; ObstGyn. Staff, Hôtel-Dieu de Lévis.

RENALD, Pierre; Place Levis, 116-50 Rte du President-Kenned, Levis QC G6V 6W8; Laval'72; Endocrin (P.Q.). Ac Staff, Hôtel-Dieu de Lévis; (418)835-1397; Fax. (418)835-1398.

RENARD, Pierre; CSSS de Trois-Rivieres, 155 rue Toupin, Trois-Rivieres QC G8T 3Z8; (France)'00; Staff, Centre de santé Cloutier-du-Rivage; (819)370-2100

RENAUD, Alain; UMF Shawinigan, 80 118e rue, Shawinigan-Sud QC G9P 3E4; Laval'83; CCFP; (819)537-8878; Fax. (819)537-3489.

RENAUD, Andre; Centre Med des Laurentides, 102-1100 rue Saint-Isidore, St-Lin-Laurentides QC J5M 2V6; Mon'74; Staff, Centre de L'Annonciation; (450)439-3870; Fax. (450)439-7849.

RENAUD, Andre; Hotel-Dieu de Levis, 143 rue Wolfe, Levis QC G6V 3Z1; Laval'86; CSPQ; FRCPC; DiagRad. Staff Radiol, Hôtel-Dieu de Lévis; (418)835-7101; Fax. (418)835-7169.

RENAUD, Christian; Hôpital Ste-Justine, 3175 ch Cote-Sainte-Catherine, Montreal QC H3T 1C5; Mon'04; FRCPC; MedMicrobiol; InfectDis (P.Q.). Staff, Hôpital Ste-Justine; (514)345-4931

RENAUD, Claude A; South Bank Med Centre, 3-2430 Bank St, Ottawa ON K1V 0T7; Ott'80; BSc; CCFP; FCFP; Assoc Sec General CMO & Prof Affairs, Canadian Medical Association; (613)736-6946; Fax. (613)736-6948.

RENAUD, Eric G; 2655 boul Daniel-Johnson, Laval QC H7P 5Y2; Mon'86; MSc; FRCSC; OrthSurg (Medico Legal Surg). Staff, Hôpital du Sacre-Coeur de Montréal; Langs: English; (450)688-4451; Fax. (450)688-5018; erenaud@medigestal.com.

RENAUD, Genevieve; Ctr Hosp Reg de Lanaudiere, 1000 boul Sainte-Anne, St-Charles-Brromee QC J6E 6J2; Mon'91; Gastroent (P.Q.); IntMed. Staff, Centre Hospitalier Régional de Lanaudière; (450)759-8222

RENAUD, Isabelle; Centre Med St-Jean, 202-1018 rue de la Prairie O, St-J-Chrysostome QC G6Z 0A7; Laval'00; Staff, Centre Hospitalier Universitaire de Quebec-CHUL; (418)839-4158; Fax. (418)839-3574.

RENAUD, Jacques; Centre Hosp Honore-Mercier, 2750 boul Laframboise, Saint-Hyacinthe QC J2S 4Y8; Mon'71; Peds. Staff, Centre Hospitalier Honore-Mercier; (450)771-3333 x3292; Fax. (450)774-4759.

RENAUD, Johanne; Douglas Mental Hlth Univ Inst, 6875 boul Lasalle, Verdun QC H4H 1R3; Mon'92; FRCP; CSPQ; FRCPC; Psy (Depressive Disorders). Staff, Douglas Mental Health University Institute; Staff, McGill Group for Suicide Studies; Langs: English; (514)761-6131 x3301; Fax. (514)888-4466; johanne.renaud@douglas.mcgill.ca.

RENAUD, Joseph A; Tecumseh Med Centre, 11811 Tecumsh Rd E, Windsor ON N8N 4M7; Tor'73; Staff, Windsor Regional Hospital - Metropolitan Site; Staff, Hôtel-Dieu Grace Hospital; (519)979-3355; Fax. (519)979-1429.

RENAUD, Leo P; 725 Parkdale Ave, Ottawa ON K1Y 4E9; Ott'65; PhD(Physiol); FRSC; FRCPC; MedScient(Med). Assoc Dir Ottawa Hosp Res Inst, The Ottawa Hospital - Civic Campus; Sr Scientist, Ottawa Hosp Research Institute; Prof, University of Ottawa; Langs: French; (613)761-5070; lprenaud@ohri.ca.

RENAUD, Marie-Claude; CHUQ-Hotel-Dieu de Quebec, 11 Cote du Palais, Quebec QC G1R 2J6; Laval'92; FRCSC; ObstGyn (Coloscopy); GynOnco (P.Q.). Staff, Centre Hospitalier Universitaire de Québec (CHUQ) - Siege Social; Langs: Bilingual(French/English); (418)691-5151; Fax. (418)691-5720; marieclaude.renaud@gmail.com.

RENAUD, Matthew J; Grand River Hosp-KW Hlth Ctre, PO Box 9056 Stn C 835 King St W, Kitchener ON N2G 1G3; Wes'06; CCFP; CCFP(E.M.); Staff, Grand River Hospital - Kitchener/Waterloo Health Centre; (519)749-4242

RENAUD, Monique M; Grand Bend Community Hlth Ctre, PO Box 1269 69 Main St E, Grand Bend ON N0M 1T0; Wes'08; CCFP; (519)238-2362; Fax. (519)238-6478.

RENAUD, Pascal; Ctr Hosp Affilie-Enfant-Jesus, 1401 18e rue, Quebec QC G1J 1Z4; Mon'99; CCFP; CCFP(E.M.); Staff, Centre Hospitalier Affilié Universitaire de Québec - Hôpital De L'Enfant Jésus; (418)649-5882; Fax. (418)649-5975.

RENAUD, Pierre; Orleans-Cumberland Comm FHT, 202-3095 St. Joseph Blvd, Orleans ON K1E 3W6; Ott'75; Ac Staff, Montfort Hospital; Langs: English; French; (613)590-0533; Fax. (613)590-7351.

RENAUD, Suzane M; Douglas Mental Hlth Univ Inst, 6875 boul Lasalle, Verdun QC H4H 1R3; Laval'76; CSPQ; DABPN; Psy (Personality Disorders). Staff, Centre Hospitalier l'Université De Montréal (CHUM) - Hôpital Saint-luc; Staff, Hôpital du Haut-Richelieu; Staff, Douglas Mental Health University Institute; Assoc Prof Psy, Universite de Montreal; Langs: English; (514)761-6131; suzanne.renaud.chum@ssss.gouv.qc.ca.

RENAUD, Sylvain; 550 rue Dufferin, Sherbrooke QC J1H 4N1; Sher'81; CSPQ; FRCPC; Psy. Staff, Centre Hospitalier Universitaire de Sherbrooke-Hôpital Hôtel-Dieu; (819)569-8403

RENAUD, Sylvie; CSST, CP 3 Succ Pl-Desjardins, Montreal QC H5B 1H1; Mon'91; LMCC; (514)906-3303

RENAULT, Paul S; 206A-7071 Bayers Rd, Halifax NS B3L 2C2; Dal'82; Court Staff, IWK Health Centre; Court Staff, Queen Elizabeth II Health Sciences Centre - Victoria General Site; (902)444-7072; Fax. (902)431-7071.

RENAULT, Paule; CLSC Kateri, 90 boul Marie-Victorin, Candiac QC J5R 1C1; Laval'77; Langs: English; (450)659-7661; Fax. (450)444-6276.

RENCHKO, Patrick A; 202-3716 61 Ave SE, Calgary AB T2C 1Z4; Alb'90; CCFP; (403)236-8400; Fax. (403)236-8806; parenchko@shaw.ca.

RENDAK, Ian; 400-300 John St, Thornhill ON L3T 5W4; Mon'83; CSPQ; NuclearMed; DiagRad (P.Q.).

RENDALL, Edward O; 335-401 9 Ave SW, Calgary AB T2P 5C3; Cal'97; FRCSC; OrthSurg. (403)265-4135; Fax. (403)221-4387.

RENDELL, M Jane; St Clares Mercy Hosp, 154 Lemarchant Rd, St. John's NL A1C 5B8; Mem'86; FRCPC; DiagRad. Staff, St Clare's Mercy Hospital; (709)777-5000; Fax. (709)777-5210.

RENDER, K Craig; Kelowna Gastroent Associates, 564 Leon Ave, Kelowna BC V1Y 6J6; Qns'80; FRCPC; IntMed (Endoscopy); Gastroent. Ac Staff, Kelowna General Hospital; (250)763-6433; Fax. (250)763-3818.

RENDER-TEIXEIRA, Caroline L; Etobicoke Med Centre, 400 The East Mall, Etobicoke ON M9B 3Z9; Tor'01; CCFP; (416)621-2220; Fax. (416)621-2203.

RENDON, Ricardo A; Urology Consultants, 620-5991 Spring Garden Rd, Halifax NS B3H 1Y6; Bogota (Colombia)'93; FRCSC; Urol (Urologic Oncology). Ac Staff Urol, Queen Elizabeth II Health Sciences Centre - Victoria General Site; Med Consultant, IWK Health Centre; Assoc Prof Dept of Urol, Dalhousie University; Langs: Spanish; (902)425-3940; Fax. (902)422-0033; rrendon@dal.ca.

RENE, Francois; 501A rue Principale CP 520, Daveluyville QC G0Z 1C0; Sher'89; assoc Staff, Hôpital Sainte-croix; (819)367-2714; Fax. (819)367-2715.

RENE, Philippe; CSSS de Saint-Jerome, 290 rue de Montigny, Saint-Jerome QC J7Z 5T3; Mon'91; CSPQ; FRCPC; DiagRad (Angioradiology). Staff, Hôtel-Dieu de Saint-Jérôme; (450)431-8300; Fax. (450)431-8750.

RENE, Pierre; MUHC-Royal Victoria Hosp, 687 av des Pins O, Montreal QC H3A 1A1; Sher'75; Microbio & Infect Dis (P.Q.); MedMicrobiol (P.Q.); IntMed (P.Q.). Staff, McGill University Health Centre - Royal Victoria Hospital; (514)934-1934 x35067; pierre.rene@muhc.mcgill.ca.

RENE, Sylvain A; Yonge-Eglinton Med Centre, 211-2401 Yonge St, Toronto ON M4P 3H1; Mon'87; (416)484-0069; Fax. (416)484-0037.

RENE DE COTRET, Paul; CHUQ-Hotel-Dieu de Quebec, 11 Cote du Palais, Quebec QC G1R 2J6; McG'77; FRCPC; IntMed; Nephrol. Staff, Centre Hospitalier Universitaire de Québec (CHUQ) - Siege Social; (418)691-5464

RENECKER, Glenn T; 1018-790 Bay St, Toronto ON M5G 1N8; Wes'60; DPsy; FRCPC; Psy. (416)960-3351; Fax. (416)944-2520.

RENEHAN, Elizabeth M; Pembroke Reg Hosp, 705 Mackay St, Pembroke ON K8A 1G8; Qns'98; FRCPC; Anes. Staff, Pembroke Regional Hospital Inc; (613)732-2811

RENFREE, Ian; Family Med Associates, 15-9701 84 Ave, Grande Prairie AB T8V 4Z8; Alb'91; CCFP; FCFP; (780)814-8857; Fax. (780)532-0037.

RENFREW, Paul D; 106A-1600 Main St, Moncton NB E1E 1G5; McM'88; MSc(Clin Epidemiol); FRCSC; GenSurg (Hepatobiliary & Pancreatic Surgery). Asst Prof Surgery, Dalhousie University; (506)857-5899; Fax. (506)857-5903.

RENGAN, Dhanakodi; Urban Med Clinic, 5619 23 Ave NW, Edmonton AB T6L 7B9; (India)'83; FRCS(UK); Langs: Tamil; (780)757-9545; Fax. (780)757-9546; drengan@telus.net.

RENNEBOHM, Robert M; Alberta Children's Hosp, C4 348-2888 Shaganappi Trail N, Calgary AB T3B 6A8; (USA)'72; Staff, Alberta Children's Hospital; (403)955-7771; Fax. (403)955-7649.

RENNER, David F; Preston Med Centre, 506 King St E, Cambridge ON N3H 3N2; Tor'74; Ac Staff, Cambridge Memorial Hospital; (519)653-3321; Fax. (519)653-3498.

RENNER, Eberhard L; N C S B 11C 1238, 585 University Ave, Toronto ON M5G 2N2; Basel (Switzerland)'79; FRCPC; Gastroent (Hepatology). Staff, Toronto General Hospital - UHN; Langs: German; (416)340-5221; Fax. (416)340-3126.

RENNER, Regina-Maria A K; 201-1801 Bowen Rd, Nanaimo BC V9S 1H1; Hannover Medical School (Germany)'01; FRCSC; ObstGyn. Staff, Penticton Regional Hospital; Langs: German; (250)714-1516

RENNER, Suzanne M; Belmont Prof Bldg, 402-564 Belmont Ave W, Kitchener ON N2M 5N6; Tor'93; FACC; FRCPC; IntMed; Cardiol (Interventional Cardiology). Assoc Staff, St Mary's General Hospital; (519)749-7911; Fax. (519)749-5644.

RENNIE, Courtney; Selkirk Med Group, PO Box 590, Revelstoke BC V0E 2S0; Ott'04; BSc; MSc; CCFP; Staff, Queen Victoria Hospital; (250)837-9321; Fax. (250)837-9444.

RENNIE, James S; 300 North Service Rd W, Oakville ON L6M 2S2; Tor'70; (905)338-3730; Fax. (905)338-3731.

RENOUF, Daniel J; BC Cancer Agency, 411-600 10th Ave W, Vancouver BC V5Z 4E6; Alb'04; FRCPC; IntMed; MedOncol. Staff, BC Cancer Agency Vancouver Centre; (604)877-6000

RENOUF, John J; Melfort Hosp, PO Box 1480 510 Broadway Ave N, Melfort SK S0E 1A0; Sask'80; Ac Staff, Melfort Hospital; Clin Associate Lect Family Med, University of Saskatchewan; (306)752-8700; Fax. (306)752-8711.

RENOUF, Tia; St Clare's Mercy Hosp, 154 Lemarchant Rd, St. John's NL A1C 5B8; Mem'84; CCFP; CCFP(E.M.); FCFP; Staff, St Clare's Mercy Hospital; (709)777-5000

RENOULT, Edith A; CHUM-Hop Notre-Dame, 1560 rue Sherbrooke E, Montreal QC H2L 4M1; Nantes (France)'83; Staff, Centre Hospitalier l'Université de Montréal (CHUM) - Hôpital Notre-Dame; (514)890-8000

RENUKA-PRASAD, Mysore S; Medical Arts Bldg, 104-750 Spadina Cres E, Saskatoon SK S7K 3H3; Mysore (India)'79; BSc; MRCPsy(UK); FRCPC; Psy (Geriatric Psychiatry). Staff, Royal University Hospital; Staff Med, Saskatoon District Health Board; Faculty Memb., University of Saskatchewan; (306)653-4843; Fax. (306)653-3190.

RENWICK, Robert B; North Bay Regional Health Ctre, 50 College Dr, North Bay ON P1B 0A4; Tor'06; FRCPC; Psy. (705)474-8600; Fax. (705)495-7890.

RENWICK, Sherri A; Little Current Med Associates, PO Box 549, Little Current ON P0P 1K0; Ott'97; CCFP; (705)368-2450; Fax. (705)368-2480.

RENY, Marcel; Clinique Med du Faubourg, 145-1160 boul Saint-Joseph, Gatineau QC J8Z 1T3; Ott'77; Chef General Med DRMG Outaouais, Hôpital de Gatineau; Langs: English; (819)595-1991; marcelreny@hotmail.com.

RENZ, Christine; Bowmont Med Clinic, 6535 Bowness Rd NW, Calgary AB T3B 0E8; Alb'00; Langs: German; (403)247-9797

RENZI, Gildo; CHUM-Hop Notre-Dame, 1560 rue Sherbrooke E, Montreal QC H2L 4M1; Mon'58; FCCP; Respir (P.Q.); IntMed. Staff, Centre Hospitalier l'Université de Montréal (CHUM) - Hôpital Notre-Dame; (514)890-8000 x25151

RENZI, Paolo; CHUM-Hop Notre-Dame, Z8905-1560 rue Sherbrooke E, Montreal QC H2L 4M1; Mon'81; FRCPC; IntMed (Pulmonary Diseases); Respir. Prof Research, Universite de Montreal; Médecin Pulmonary, Centre Hospitalier l'Université de Montréal (CHUM) - Hôpital Notre-Dame; Langs: Bilingual(English/French); (514)890-8000 x28031; Fax. (514)412-7579; renzip@earthlink.net.

RENZO, Alain; CHUQ-St-Francois d'Assise, 10 rue de l'Espinay, Quebec QC G1L 3L5; Sher'92; Staff, Centre Hospitalier de Chandler; Staff, Centre Hospitalier Universitaire De Québec - Pavillon De St-françois-d'assise; (418)525-4444

REPO-HENDSBEE, S Michele; 302-131 Wharncliffe Rd, London ON N6J 2K4; Qns'95; FRCPC; Psy. Staff, Homewood Health Centre; (519)824-1010

RERRI, Bernard; Brant Community HC-Brantford, 12-200 Terrace Hill St, Brantford ON N3R 1G9; Ibadan (Nigeria)'83; MB BS; FRCS; FRCSC; OrthSurg (Spine Surgery). Staff, The Brant Community Healthcare System - Brantford General Hospital Site; (519)751-5860; Fax. (519)751-5890.

RESCH, Lothar; Foothills Med Centre, C1123-1403 29 St NW, Calgary AB T2N 2T9; Dal'76; FRCPC; NeurPath. Staff, Foothills Medical Centre; (403)944-5808; Fax. (403)944-1460; lothar.resch@albertahealthservices.ca.

RESLEROVA, Martina; St Boniface Gen Hosp, BG007-409 Tache Ave, Winnipeg MB R2H 2A6; Prague (Czech Republic)'93; FRCPC; IntMed; Nephrol. Staff, St Boniface General Hospital; (204)233-8563; mreslerova@sbgh.mb.ca.

RESO, Artan M; Associate Clinic, 320-401 9 Ave SW, Calgary AB T2P 3C5; Tirana (Albania)'92; FRCSC; GenSurg (Minimal Invasive Surgery). (403)221-4489; Fax. (403)221-4420.

RESSL, Waqar-Un-Nissa; 7155 Kingsway PO Box 54605 Rpo Highgate, Burnaby BC V5E 4J6; UBC'10; CCFP; (604)421-1027

RESSLER, Ladislaus J; Univ of Ottawa Heart Institute, 40 Ruskin St, Ottawa ON K1Y 4W7; Semmelweis (Hungary)'88; Staff, University of Ottawa Heart Institute; (613)761-4220

RESTREPO, Alfonso; CSSS du Lac-des-Deux-Montagnes, 520 boul Arthur-Sauve, St-Eustache QC J7R 5B1; Mon'96; LMCC; Staff, Hôpital de Saint-Eustache; Langs: Spanish; English; (450)473-6811

RETALLACK, Jennifer E; Children's & Women's HC of BC, B321-4480 Oak St, Vancouver BC V6H 3V4; Alb'03; FRCPC; Peds. Staff, BC Children's Hospital; (604)875-2345 x2133

RETALLICK, Ricky D; Dr Everett Chalmers Reg Hosp, PO Box 9000 Stn A 700 Priestman St, Fredericton NB E3B 5M6; UBC'87; FRCPC; Anes. Staff, Dr Everett Chalmers Regional Hospital; (506)452-5166

RETIEF, Leon W; Moose Jaw Union Hosp, 455 Fairford St E, Moose Jaw SK S6H 1H3; Staff, Moose Jaw Union Hospital; (306)694-0200

RETIEF, Malcolm W; Spesmed Med Specialist Ctre, PO Box 1540 Stn Main 2591 99th St, North Battleford SK S9A 3W1; Pretoria (South Africa)'84; MB ChB; BMedSci; FRCSC; GenSurg. (306)446-5550; Fax. (306)446-5055.

RETIEF, PJ Petrus; PO Box 21021 Rpo Southgate, Chilliwack BC V2P 8A9; Pretoria (South Africa)'90; DA; MB ChB; CCFP; Anesthetist, Chilliwack General Hospital; Langs: Afrikaans; (604)795-4141; pjretief@sasktel.net.

RETNAKARAN, Ravi; Leadership Sinai Ctr for Diabe, L5 025-60 Murray St, Toronto ON M5T 3L9; Tor'99; FRCPC; IntMed; Endocrin&Metab. Staff, Mount Sinai Hospital; (416)586-4800 x3941; Fax. (416)586-8853.

RETSON, Jillie E M; Kenora Med Associates, RR 1 Stn Main 45 Wolsley St, Kenora ON P9N 3W7; Wes'06; CCFP; Staff, Lake of the Woods District Hospital; (807)468-3021

RETZER, Elisabeth C; Bridgeland Prof Centre, 306-1010 1 Ave NE, Calgary AB T2E 7W7; Cal'84; CCFP; CCFP(E.M.); FCFP; Teacher, University of Calgary; (403)263-5756; Fax. (403)263-9493.

REUBENI-ZALTZ, Renat; Univ Hlth Network-Toronto Western Hosp, 399 Bathurst St, Toronto ON M5T 2S8; Tor'92; CCFP; FCFP; Staff, Toronto Western Hospital - University Health Network; (416)603-5800

REV, Marianne; BC Women's Hosp & Health Ctre, 4500 Oak St, Vancouver BC V6H 3N1; McM'74; CCFP; FCFP; Ad Staff Privil, Vancouver General Hospital - Centennial Pavillion; Consultant Specialized Women's Health, BC Women's Hospital & Health Centre; Visiting Privil., Providence Group Hospitals; Asst Prof Family Prof, University of British Columbia; (604)875-2018

REVAH, Ayala; Oakdale Med Bldg, 311-2065 Finch Ave W, North York ON M3N 2V7; Tor'94; FRCSC; ObstGyn. Ac Staff, Humber River Regional Hospital - Finch Avenue Site; Langs: Hebrew; (416)743-2107; Fax. (416)743-6441.

REVAH, Giselle; University of Toronto, 500 University Ave, Toronto ON M5G 1V7; Tor'07; DiagRad.

REVEL, Lillian C; Trent Univ Student Health Serv, 1600 West Bank Dr, Peterborough ON K9J 7B8; Glasgow (Scotland)'76; MB ChB; (705)748-1481

REVITT, David R; Medical Clinic, 8195 120 St, Delta BC V4C 6P7; Alb'71; Staff, Surrey Memorial Hospital; (604)594-8451; Fax. (604)596-4819.

REWA, George; 211-688 Coxwell Ave, Toronto ON M4C 3B7; Tor'76; FACC; FACP; FRCPC; IntMed; Cardiol. Ac Staff, Toronto East General Hospital Inc; Asst Prof Family Med, University of Toronto; Langs: Ukrainian; (416)466-1700; grewa@sympatico.ca.

REWA, Oleksa G; Sunnybrook Hlth Sciences Ctre, D1 08-2075 Bayview Ave, Toronto ON M4N 3M5; Qns'08; FRCPC; IntMed. Staff, Sunnybrook Health Sciences Centre; (416)480-4522

REX, Gregory A; Park Lane Mall, 503-5657 Spring Garden Rd, Halifax NS B3J 3R4; Mem'97; FRCPC; Peds; ClinImmunol&Allergy. (902)425-3927

REY, Evelyne; Hôpital Ste-Justine, 3175 ch Cote-Sainte-Catherine, Montreal QC H3T 1C5; Mon'81; MSc; FRCPC; IntMed (Obstetrics). ac Staff, Hôpital Ste-Justine; Prof clin agrégé Med, Universite de Montreal; Langs: Bilingual(French/English); (514)345-4788; Fax. (514)345-4648.

REYBURN, Thomas H; 4631 rue Sherbrooke O, Westmount QC H3Z 1G2; Qns'68; DPsy; CSPQ; FRCPC; Psy. Clin Asst, Sir Mortimer B Davis Jewish General; (514)931-5314

REYES, Enrique G; 304-5 Quarry Ridge Rd, Barrie ON L4M 7G1; Montevideo (Uruguay)'78; FRCSC; ObstGyn (Infertility). Consultant, Royal Victoria Regional Health Centre; Langs: Spanish; (705)737-5038; Fax. (705)737-3547.

REYES, Romina C; Life Labs, 3680 Gilmore Way, Burnaby BC V5G 4V8; UBC'04; FRCPC; MedMicrobiol. (604)412-4451

REYES-SMITH, Larina M; 10085 Whalley Blvd, Surrey BC V3T 4G1; (Philippines)'87; CCFP; FCFP; Staff, Vancouver General Hospital - Centennial Pavillion; Langs: Tagalog; (604)582-5826

REYNEKE, Anna M E; Dr CW Wiebe Med Centre, 385 Main St, Winkler MB R6W 1J2; (204)325-4312

REYNOLDS, Clayton; 303-582 Goldstream Ave, Victoria BC V9B 2W7; McG'68; MMedSci; MDCM; FACP; ABMM; FRCPC; IntMed (Diabetology). Staff, Ladysmith Community Health Centre; Vis Specialist Endocrin, Prince Rupert Regional Hospital; Vis Specialist Endocrin, Mills Memorial Hospital; Vis Specialist Endocrin, Queen Charlotte Islands General Hospital - Queen Charlotte Site; Vis Specialist Endocrin, Kitimat Hospital & Health Centre; Physician, St Anthony's Medical Centre; Langs: Spanish; French; (250)478-1744; Fax. (250)478-5717; reynoldsclayton@msn.com.

REYNOLDS, David R; Trafalgar Prof Centre, 300-1235 Trafalgar Rd, Oakville ON L6H 3P1; Tor'76; Court Staff, Halton Healthcare Services Corporation - Oakville Site; (905)842-0071; Fax. (905)844-3811.

REYNOLDS, Donna L; 170-5 Fairview Mall Dr, North York ON M2J 2Z1; McM'94; BSc; MSc; FRCPC; CommunMed (Infectious Diseases);CCFP; FCFP; Asst Prof, University of Toronto; (416)447-5531; Fax. (416)447-5691.

REYNOLDS, James L; Women's Hosp, 735 Notre Dame Ave, Winnipeg MB R3E 0L8; Man'73; CCFP; FCFP; Staff, St Boniface General Hospital; Prof Family Med/Prof, University of Manitoba; reynolds@cc.umanitoba.ca.

REYNOLDS, Janet G G; Crowfoot Village Fam Practice, 210-600 Crowfoot Cres NW, Calgary AB T3G 0B4; Sask'97; BSc(Hon.); CCFP; FCFP; (403)239-9733; Fax. (403)241-8112.

REYNOLDS, Jason H; Sunnyside Mall, 302-1595 Bedford Hwy, Bedford NS B4A 3Y4; Dal'99; CCFP; (902)835-3361; Fax. (902)835-3363.

REYNOLDS, Jennifer L; 408-1160 Burrard St, Vancouver BC V6Z 2E8; Cal'01; FRCPC; IntMed; Rheum. (604)646-4637

REYNOLDS, Jody; Salvation Army Grace Gen Hosp, 300 Booth Dr, Winnipeg MB R3J 3M7; Man'06; FRCPC; DiagRad. Staff, The Salvation Army Grace Hospital; (204)837-0391

REYNOLDS, Julia C; 301-233 Nelson's Cres, New Westminster BC V3L 0E4; Sask'86; Assoc Staff, Royal Columbian Hospital; (604)524-9465

REYNOLDS, Kathleen A; Professional Bldg, 350-1620 29 St NW, Calgary AB T2N 4L7; Cal'98; CCFP; Staff, Alberta Children's Hospital; (403)282-1245; Fax. (403)282-9545.

REYNOLDS, Kenneth J; 101-100 Division St, Trenton ON K8V 4W8; Qns'71; Court Staff, QHC Trenton Memorial; (613)394-3338; Fax. (613)394-4613.

REYNOLDS, M Lynn; 19-1710 Ellis St, Kelowna BC V1Y 2B5; Cal'79; CCFP; FCFP; (250)763-5145; Fax. (250)763-3296.

REYNOLDS, Megan A; Toronto East Gen Hosp Inc, 825 Coxwell Ave, Toronto ON M4C 3E7; Tor'08; CCFP; CCFP(E.M.); Staff, Toronto East General Hospital Inc; (416)469-6435

REYNOLDS, Richard; St Joseph's Health Care, PO Box 5777 Stn B 268 Grosvenor St, London ON N6A 4V2; Qns'76; ABIM; FRCPC; IntMed; Gastroent. Teach Staff, St Joseph's Hospital - St Joseph's Health Care; Prof, University of Western Ontario; (519)646-6100 x64698

REYNOLDS, Robert B; 176 Centre St PO Box 409, Deseronto ON K0K 1X0; Qns'75; Ac Staff, Lennox & Addington County General Hospital; (613)396-3420; Fax. (613)396-5105.

REYNOLDS, Robert P; Div of Infectious Diseases, 452D-2733 Heather St, Vancouver BC V5Z 1M9; Tor'91; FRCPC; IntMed (AIDS/HIV); InfectDis. Staff, Vancouver General Hospital - Centennial Pavillion; Staff, BC Women's Hospital & Health Centre; Clin Associate, University of British Columbia; (604)875-4588; Fax. (604)875-4013; rprey@telus.net.

REYNOLDS, Steven C; Royal Columbia Hosp, 330 Columbia St E, New Westminster BC V3L 3W7; Cal'01; FRCPC; IntMed; Critical Care Medicine; InfectDis. Staff, Royal Columbian Hospital; (604)520-4576

REYNOLDS, Stuart F; University of Alberta Hosp, 3C1.12-8440 112 St NW, Edmonton AB T6G 2B7; Alb'96; CCFP; CCFP(E.M.); Staff, University of Alberta Hospital; (780)407-8822

REYNOLDS, Teresa B; Golden Plough Lodge, 983 Burnham St, Cobourg ON K9A 5J6; Dal'97; Staff, Northumberland Hills Hospital; (905)372-8759

REYNOLDS, Vernon L; Lions Gate Hosp Community Psy, 1350 St Andrews Ave, North Vancouver BC V7L 3L4; Otago (New Zealand)'95; MB ChB; Staff, Lions Gate Hospital; Staff, Surrey Memorial Hospital; (604)983-6020

REYNOLDS, Walter J F; Village Mall Med Clinic, 22-6320 50 Ave, Red Deer AB T4N 4C6; Pretoria (South Africa)'99; (403)314-5357; Fax. (403)314-5307.

REYNOLDS, William J; Mill Bay Med Centre, RR 1 230-2720 Mill Bay Rd, Mill Bay BC V0R 2P1; Cork (Ireland)'89; BSc; MB ChB; BAO; CCFP; (250)743-3211

REZAEIFAR, Parand; Hop du Sacre-Coeur de Mtl, 5400 boul Gouin O, Montreal QC H4J 1C5; Laval'02; CCFP; Staff, Hôpital du Sacre-Coeur de Montréal; (514)338-2222

REZAIE, Ali; 6D27-3280 Hospital Dr NW, Calgary AB T2N 4N1; Shahid Beheshti (Iran)'04; FRCPC; IntMed; Gastroent. (403)592-5020; Fax. (403)592-5090.

REZAIE, Raymond; Clinique Med Aplha Medic, 1253 rue Guy, Montreal QC H3H 2K5; (Mexico)'96; CCFP; (514)933-8383; Fax. (514)933-8303.

REZAIEFAR, Parisa; Bruyere Family Med Centre, 75 Bruyere St, Ottawa ON K1N 5C8; McM'01; CCFP; Langs: Persian; French; (613)241-3344; Fax. (613)241-1971.

REZANSOFF, Natalie A; Athabascan Place, 222-80 Chippewa Rd, Sherwood Park AB T8A 4W6; Alb'07; CCFP; (780)464-9661; Fax. (780)417-0656.

REZANSOFF, Walter E; Kamsack Med Clinic, PO Box 69, Kamsack SK S0A 1S0; Sask'72; (306)542-2623; Fax. (306)542-3782.

REZAZADAH, Fareidoon; 5-8948 202 St, Langley BC V1M 4A7; Avicenna (Afghanistan)'86; Staff, Burrard Health Centre; Langs: Dari; Farsi; (604)888-4472; Fax. (604)888-5472.

REZENDE, Flavio; Hop Maisonneuve-Rosemont, 5145 boul de l'Assomption, Montreal QC H1T 2M4; Staff, Hopital Maisonneuve-Rosemont; (514)252-3400 x4928

REZK, Emad; Roblin District Health Centre, PO Box 940 15 Hospital St, Roblin MB R0L 1P0; Ain Shams (Egypt)'90; Staff, Roblin & District Health Centre.

REZMOVITZ, Jeremy J; Sunnybrook Hlth Sciences Ctre, A120-2075 Bayview Ave, Toronto ON M4N 3M5; (Israel)'08; CCFP; Staff, Sunnybrook Health Sciences Centre; (416)480-4934

REZNEK, Lawrence R; Sunnybrook Hlth Sciences Ctre, FG41-2075 Bayview Ave, Toronto ON M4N 3M5; Cape Town (South Africa)'81; FRCPC; Psy. Staff Psy, Sunnybrook Health Sciences Centre; Assoc Prof, University of Toronto; (416)480-5836; Fax. (416)480-6878.

REZNEK, Stephen; Kingsway Plaza Phase III, 110-4980 Kingsway, Burnaby BC V5H 4K7; Cape Town (South Africa)'78; MB ChB; DCH; CCFP; FCFP; Staff, Burnaby Hospital; (604)435-5585

REZNICK, Richard K; Queen's University, 18 Barrie St, Kingston ON K7L 3J6; McG'77; AB; MEd; FACS; FRCSC; GenSurg (Colon & Rectal Surgery). Dean Faculty of Health Sciences/Dir School of Med, Queen's University; Langs: English; French; (613)533-2544; Fax. (613)533-6884.

INC, Ronald R Reznick; 2-306 Lower Ganges Rd, Salt Spring Island BC V8K 2V3; Sask'82; BSc; Ac Staff Privil, Vancouver Island Health Authority; Ac Staff Privil, Lady Minto Gulf Islands Hospital; (250)537-5321; Fax. (250)537-4838.

REZNICK, Simon; Upstream Family Medicine, 108-4330 Sunshine Coast Hwy, Sechelt BC V0N 3A1; UBC'04; CCFP; (604)885-6400; Fax. (604)885-6411.

REZONZEW, Rebeca; CSSS du Suroît, 150 rue Saint-Thomas, Salaber-de-Valleyf QC J6T 6C1; Antiqua (Colombia)'91; CSPQ; FRCPC; Anes. Staff, Centre Hospitalier Régional du Suroît; (450)371-9920 x2141

REZVANI, M Kazem; Pugwash Primary Health Care, 272 Church St, Pugwash NS B0K 1L0; (Iran)'93; (902)243-2527

REZVANI-KHORASSANI, Massoud; 170 Rebecca St, Oakville ON L6K 1J6; Teheran (Iran)'92; (905)842-1235

RGEI, Mahmoud; 15345 97 St NW, Edmonton AB T5X 5V3; (Libya)'99; (780)457-6060; Fax. (780)457-6111.

RHAINDS, Marc G; CHUQ-St-Francois d'Assise, D7 741-10 rue de l'Espinay, Quebec QC G1L 3L5; Laval'85; MSc(Epidemiol.); CSPQ; FRCPC; CommunMed (Environmental Medicine). Staff Aeronautical Med, Centre Hospitalier Affilié Universitaire de Québec - Hôpital De L'Enfant Jésus; Ac Staff Environmental Health, Centre Hospitalier Universitaire de Quebec-CHUL; Staff, Centre Hospitalier Universitaire De Québec - Pavillon De St-françois-d'assise; Clin Prof Preventive Med, Université Laval; (418)525-4444 x54683; marc.rhainds@crchul.ulaval.ca.

RHEAULT, Alain; Polyclinique de Trois-Rivieres, 305-1900 boul des Recollets, Trois-Rivieres QC G8Z 4K4; Laval'74; Cardiol (P.Q.). Staff, CSSS de Trois-Rivières; (819)375-4313; Fax. (819)378-7897.

RHEAULT, Christian; UMF Laurier, 2875 boul Laurier, Quebec QC G1V 2M2; Laval'81; ac Staff, Centre Hospitalier Universitaire de Quebec-CHUL; (418)654-2701; Fax. (418)654-2138.

RHEAULT, Diane; Clinique Med Sainte-Dorothee, 102-1 boul Samson, Laval QC H7X 3S5; Mon'85; Staff Geriatric Serv, Hopital de la Cite de la santé; (450)689-6334; Fax. (450)689-6339.

RHEAULT, Elise; Regie l'Assurance Maladie QC, Q044-1125 Grande Allée O, Quebec QC G1S 1E7; Laval'85; Staff, Regie de l'Assurance Maladie du Quebec; Langs: French; (418)682-5144 x4628; Fax. (418)643-3858.

RHEAULT, Isabelle; CSSS de la Cote-de-Gaspe, 215 boul de York O, Gaspe QC G4X 2W2; Laval'03; CCFP; Staff, Centre Hospitalier de Gaspe; (418)368-6663; Fax. (418)368-5354.

RHEAULT, Katherine M; 200-16 O'Brien St, Orillia ON L3V 5S2; McM'01; FRCSC; ObstGyn. (705)330-4061

RHEAULT, Louis-Serge; Polyclinique de Trois-Rivieres, 310-1900 boul des Recollets, Trois-Rivieres QC G8Z 4K4; Laval'71; OrthSurg. Staff, CSSS de Trois-Rivières; Staff, Centre de santé Cloutier-du-Rivage; (819)373-3244; Fax. (819)373-5997.

RHEAULT, Michel; Hôpital Laval, 2725 ch Sainte-Foy, Quebec QC G1V 4G5; Laval'01; CSPQ; FRCPC; Anes. Staff, Hôpital Laval; (418)656-8711; Fax. (418)656-4687.

RHEAULT, Michel; CSSS de Trois-Rivières, 1991 boul du Carmel, Trois-Rivieres QC G8Z 3R9; Laval'66; GenSurg. Staff, CSSS de Trois-Rivières; (819)697-3333

RHEAULT, Mylene; Hotel-Dieu de levis, 143 rue Wolfe, Levis QC G6V 3Z1; Laval'99; FRCPC; Peds. Staff, Hôtel-Dieu de Lévis; (418)835-7111

RHEAULT, Nathalie; CLSC Richelieu, 300 ch de Marieville, Chambly QC J3L 3V8; Laval'97; (450)658-7561; Fax. (450)658-4390.

RHEAULT, Paul L C; 202-1280 Lasalle Blvd, Sudbury ON P3A 1Y8; Ott'93; CCFP; Langs: English; French; (705)671-3001; Fax. (705)671-3003.

RHEAULT, Sylvie; CLSC Therese de Blainville, 125 rue Duquet, Sainte-Therese QC J7E 0A5; Mon'02; Staff, Institut Universitaire de Gériatrie de Montréal; (450)430-4553; Fax. (450)437-3209.

RHEAUME, Caroline; GMF-UMF Laval, 2690 ch des Quatre-Bourgeois, Quebec QC G1V 0B7; Laval'05; BSc; PhD; MSc; CCFP; Staff, Hôpital Laval; Langs: Bilingual(French/English); (418)656-4795; caroline.rheaume@criucpq.ulaval.ca.

RHEAUME, Caroline; Clinique Med de Courville, 1049 av Larue, Quebec QC G1C 1J5; Laval'87; (418)661-0097; Fax. (418)661-0307; crheaume@dr.com.

RHEAUME, Caroline I; CHUQ-Ctr Hosp Univ Laval, 2705 boul Laurier, Quebec QC G1V 4G2; Laval'95; FRCSC; ObstGyn. Staff, Centre Hospitalier Universitaire de Quebec-CHUL; Langs: English; (418)654-2738; Fax. (418)525-4281.

RHEAUME, Dorianne E; Nova Scotia Cancer Centre, 5820 University Ave, Halifax NS B3H 1V7; Tor'81; FRCPC; IntMed (Brain Tumors); RadOncol. Physician, Nova Scotia Cancer Center; (902)473-6096; Fax. (902)473-7205.

RHEAUME, Marc-Andre; CHUM-Hop Notre-Dame, 1560 rue Sherbrooke E, Montreal QC H2L 4M1; Mon'04; FRCSC; Ophth. Staff, Centre Hospitalier l'Université de Montréal (CHUM) - Hôpital Notre-Dame; (514)890-8000

RHEAUME, Marie-Claude; Clinique Med de la Capitale, 14-4225 4e av O, Quebec QC G1H 6P3; Laval'84; ac Staff, Centre Hospitalier Universitaire De Québec - Pavillon De St-françois-d'assise; (418)628-9921; Fax. (418)628-3203.

RHEAUME, Maxime; Hop du Sacre-Coeur de Mtl, 5400 boul Gouin O, Montreal QC H4J 1C5; Mon'08; IntMed. Staff, Hôpital du Sacre-Coeur de Montréal; (514)338-2222

RHEAUME, Nadia; Polyclinique Saint-Jerome, 102-200 rue Durand, Saint-Jerome QC J7Z 7E2; Sher'04; (450)431-7666

RHEAUME, Pascal; CHUQ-St-Francois d'Assise, 10 rue de l'Espinay, Quebec QC G1L 3L5; Laval'03; FRCSC; GenSurg; VascSurg. Staff, Centre Hospitalier Universitaire De Québec - Pavillon De St-françois-d'assise; (418)525-4444

RHEAUME, Pierre M; Centre Med Boucherville, 600 boul du Fort-Saint-Louis, Boucherville QC J4B 1S7; Mon'78; (450)655-7321; Fax. (450)655-6311.

RHEAUME, Sylvie; Ctr Hosp Fleury, 2180 rue Fleury E, Montreal QC H2B 1K3; Mon'96; Staff, Centre Hospitalier Fleury; (514)381-9311; Fax. (514)383-5086.

RHEAUME, Teresa A I; 20 Robertson Rd GD, Beachburg ON K0J 1C0; Ott'83; Court Staff, Wilson Memorial General Hospital; Court Staff, Wingham & District Hospital - Listowel Wingham Hospitals Alliance; Staff, Pembroke Regional Hospital Inc; Langs: English; French; (613)582-3685; Fax. (613)582-7095; trheaume@nrtco.net.

RHEAUME-LANOIE, Myriam; Centre Medical St-Jovite, 992 rue de Saint Jovite, Mont-Tremblant QC J8E 3J8; Mon'10; (819)425-2728

RHEE, Augustine Y; Lions Gate Hosp, 231 15th Ave E, North Vancouver BC V7L 2L7; Wes'06; FRCPC; Anes. Staff, Lions Gate Hospital; (604)984-5987

RHEE, Kunuk; Mackenzie Richmond Hill Hosp, 10 Trench St, Richmond Hill ON L4C 4Z3; Tor'99; CCFP; Staff, Mackenzie Richmond Hill Hospital; Staff, Humber River Regional Hospital - Church Street Site; (905)883-1212

RHEE, Steven J; St Joseph's Health Centre, 30 The Queensway, Toronto ON M6R 1B5; Tor'99; Staff, St Joseph's Health Centre; (416)530-6000

RHEIN, Anke; Klondyke Med Clinic, 1-3089 3rd Ave, Whitehorse YT Y1A 5B3; (Germany)'98; CCFP; Staff, Klondyke Medical Clinic; (867)668-4065

RHEIN, Stephane; Hop Charles LeMoyne, 3120 boul Taschereau, Greenfield Park QC J4V 2H1; Sher'04; CCFP; CCFP(E.M.); Staff, Hopital Charles LeMoyne; (450)466-5000

RHEMTULA, Haroun A; Associate Med Clinic, 2-8720 Franklin Ave, Fort McMurray AB T9H 3K8; (South Africa)'91; MB BCh(Rand); FCOG(SA); MMed(O&G); Staff, Northern Lights Regional Health Centre; (780)743-3252; Fax. (780)743-9586.

RHEMTULLA, El-Karim F J; Garden City Eyecare, 3-274 Fourth Ave, St Catharines ON L2R 6P9; Cambridge (England)'96; MB ChB; FRCSC; Ophth (Cataract Anterior Segment & Refractive Surgery). Staff, Niagara Health System - Ontario Street Site; Staff Ophth, Niagara Health System - St Catharines General Site; Langs: Gujarati; Hindi; Swahili; Urdu; (905)684-8521; Fax. (905)684-4996; erhemtulla@gmail.com.

RHINE, David J; Kelowna Gen Hosp, 2268 Pandosy St, Kelowna BC V1Y 1T2; Alb'77; BSc(Med.); FACEP; FRCPC; EmergMed. Staff Emerg Dept, Kelowna General Hospital; (250)862-4495; Fax. (250)717-1075.

RHO, Jong Min; Alberta Children's Hosp, 2888 Shaganappi I Trail NW, Calgary AB T3B 6A8; (USA)'87; Staff, Alberta Children's Hospital; (403)955-7803; Fax. (403)955-2922.

RHOADES, Elizabeth H; Ocean Pier Med Centre, 207-2537 Beacon Ave, Sidney BC V8L 1Y3; McG'83; Staff, Vancouver Island Health Authority; (250)656-4114

RHODES, Donald A; Belmont Family Medicine, 201-535 Belmont Ave W, Kitchener ON N2M 5E9; Wes'90; (519)579-4870; Fax. (519)579-7903.

RHODES, Ian N; 205-595 Montreal Rd, Ottawa ON K1K 4L2; Ott'84; FRCPC; IntMed; DiagRad. Langs: English; French; (613)749-3416

RHODES, Michael E; 100-175 av Stillview, Pointe-Claire QC H9R 4S3; McG'69; OrthSurg (P.Q.). Ac Staff, Lakeshore General Hospital - Pointe Claire; (514)426-2086; Fax. (514)694-3610.

RHOMA, Salahalden; Snow Lake Clinic, 100 Lakeshore Dr E, Snow Lake MB R0B 1M0; Al Fateh (Libya)'98.

RHONE, Stephanie A; 915-750 Broadway W, Vancouver BC V5Z 1H8; Emory(GA) (USA)'95; FRCSC; ObstGyn. Ac Staff, BC Women's Hospital & Health Centre; Ac Staff, Vancouver General Hospital - Centennial Pavillion; Clin Instructor, University of British Columbia; (604)730-1973; Fax. (604)877-8611.

RHYDDERCH, Gareth M; Hamilton HS-General Site, 237 Barton St E, Hamilton ON L8L 2X2; London (England)'68; MB BS; MRCS; LRCP; FRCPC; Anes (Chronic Pain). Ac Staff, Hamilton Health Sciences Centre - McMaster Children's Hospital; Staff, Hamilton Health Sciences Centre - Hamilton General Hospital; Associate Clin Prof Anes, McMaster University; (905)527-4322 x44621; Fax. (905)577-8022.

RHYNOLD, Elizabeth S; St Joseph's Hosp, 130 Bayard Dr, Saint John NB E2L 3L6; Sask'04; FRCPC; IntMed; GeriatricMed. Staff, St Joseph's Hospital; (506)632-5555

RIAHI, Mounir; CSSS du Nord de Lanaudière, 1000 boul Sainte-Anne Blvd, Joliette QC J6E 6J2; Mon'08; IntMed. Staff, Centre Hospitalier Régional de Lanaudière; (450)759-8222

RIANO ALVAREZ, Margarita R; Clinique Nazaret, 1771 av Dollard, LaSalle QC H8N 1T9; Bogota (Colombia)'96; CCFP; Langs: Spanish; English; (514)368-5500; Fax. (514)368-0056.

RIAR, Kulwant S; The Forensic Group, 305-1245 Broadway W, Vancouver BC V6H 1G7; Rajasthan (India)'82; MB BS; FRCPC; Psy. Staff, Maples Adolescent Treatment Centre; Langs: Hindi; Punjabi; Urdu; (604)733-5722

RIAZ, Asifa; Dominion Med Centre, 2383 111 St NW, Edmonton AB T6J 5E5; (Pakistan)'93; CCFP; (780)436-0020; Fax. (780)436-0603.

RIAZ, Salman; River Heights Prof Centre, 210-88 Valleyview Dr SW, Medicine Hat AB T1A 8N6; Punjab (Pakistan)'94; Staff, Medicine Hat Regional Hospital; (403)529-8034; Fax. (403)529-8935.

RIAZ, Sarah; PO Box 23022 Rpo Citadel, St. Albert AB T8N 6Z9; Tor'04; CCFP; (780)419-3627; Fax. (780)459-7860.

RIAZI, Sheila; Univ Hlth Network-Toronto Western Hosp, MCL2 427A-399 Bathurst St, Toronto ON M5T 2S8; Teheran (Iran)'99; FRCPC; Anes. Staff, Toronto Western Hospital - University Health Network; (416)603-5118; Fax. (416)603-6494.

RIBAS, Carlos S; St Joseph's Healthcare, F 403-50 Charlton Ave E, Hamilton ON L8N 4A6; Cordoba (Argentina)'96; Staff, St Joseph's Healthcare - Charlton Campus; Langs: Spanish; (905)522-1155 x32800; Fax. (905)521-6068.

RIBCHINSKY, Sofia; The Ottawa Hosp-Civic Campus, 1053 Carling Ave, Ottawa ON K1Y 4E9; Ott'10; CCFP; Staff, The Ottawa Hospital - Civic Campus; (613)761-4000

RIBEIRO, Luciana T; Hamilton HS-McMaster Site, PO Box 2000 Stn Lcd 1 1200 Main St W, Hamilton ON L8N 3Z5; (Brazil)'97; FRCPC; DiagRad. Staff, Hamilton Health Sciences Centre - McMaster Children's Hospital; (905)521-2100

RIBEIRO, Marcos; Univ Hlth Network-Toronto Western Hosp, EW7 449-399 Bathurst St, Toronto ON M5T 2S8; (Brazil)'87; Staff, Toronto Western Hospital - University Health Network; (416)603-5177

RIBEIRO, Ricardo A; Grey Nuns Community Hosp & HC, 1100 Youville Drive West NW, Edmonton AB T6L 5X8; CCFP; CCFP(E.M.); Staff, Covenant Health - Grey Nuns Community Hospital; (780)735-7000

RIBEIRO, Rona G; 2-140 Athabascan Ave, Sherwood Park AB T8A 4E3; CCFP; Langs: Spanish; Portuguese; (780)467-3244; rgh99rar@hotmail.com.

RIBEN, Celina M; Royal University Hosp, 103 Hospital Dr, Saskatoon SK S7N 0W8; Sask'98; BSc; LMCC; FRCPC; Anes. Staff, Royal University Hospital; (306)655-1183

RIBERDY, Jocelyne; Clinique de Ped de Rimouski, 301-161 av Rouleau, Rimouski QC G5L 5T3; Mon'83; FRCPC; Peds. Staff, Hôpital Regional Rimouski; (418)724-4221; Fax. (418)725-3025.

RIBERDY-ST PIERRE, Catherine; CSSS de Saint-Jerome, 290 rue de Montigny, Saint-Jerome QC J7Z 5T3; Mon'03; Microbio & Infect Dis (P.Q.); MedMicrobiol. Staff, Hôtel-Dieu de Saint-Jérôme; (450)431-8200 x2776

RIBEYRE, Jean-Marie; Royal Ottawa Hlth Care Group, 1145 Carling Ave, Ottawa ON K1Z 7K4; (France)'91; FRCPC; Psy. Staff, Royal Ottawa Mental Health Centre - Royal Ottawa Health Care Group; (613)722-6521

RIBIC, Christine M; St Joseph's Healthcare, 50 Charlton Ave E, Hamilton ON L8N 4A6; Tor'06; FRCPC; IntMed; Nephrol. Staff, St Joseph's Healthcare - Charlton Campus; (905)522-1155; Fax. (905)521-6088.

RICARD, Christian; CSSS de Lac-Saint Jean-Est, CP 1300 Succ Bureau-Chef 300 boul Champlain S, Alma QC G8B 5W3; Mon'86; CSPQ; Anes. Staff, CSSS de Lac-Saint Jean-Est; (418)669-2000

RICARD, Christyne; Medicentre Chomedey, 610 boul Cure-Labelle, Laval QC H7V 2T7; Mon'96; Staff, Hopital de la Cite de la santé; (450)687-6452

RICARD, Genevieve; Hotel-Dieu de Saint-Jerome, 290 rue de Montigny, Saint-Jerome QC J7Z 5T3; Sher'05; FRCPC; Neur. Staff, Hôtel-Dieu de Saint-Jérôme; Langs: Bilingual(French/English); (450)432-2777

RICARD, Genevieve; Inst U Geriatrie Sherbrooke, 375 rue Argyll, Sherbrooke QC J1J 3H5; Sher'06; GeriatricMed; IntMed. Staff, Institut Universitaire de Geriatrie de Sherbrooke-Pavillon Argyll; (819)780-2220

RICARD, Jacques; ASSS de la Monteregie, 1255 rue Beauregard, Longueuil QC J4K 2M3; Mon'80; Med Consultant, Ministere de la sante et des services sociaux du Quebec; (450)928-6777; jacques.ricard@sss.gouv.qc.ca.

RICARD, Jacques P J; Canadian Forces Supp Unit HCC, 1745 Alta Vista Dr, Ottawa ON K1A 0K6; Laval'83; Staff, Canadian Forces Health Services Centre; (613)945-6657; Fax. (613)945-6745.

RICARD, Jean-Francois; Hop Charles LeMoyne, 3120 boul Taschereau, Greenfield Park QC J4V 2H1; Mon'92; CSPQ; FRCPC; Psy. Staff, Hopital Charles LeMoyne; (450)466-5000

RICARD, Jean-Guy; CSSS de Rouyn-Noranda, 1 9e rue, Rouyn-Noranda QC J9X 2A9; Mon'89; CCFP; FCFP; Staff, Centre Hospitalier de Val d'Or; Physician, CLSC Le Minordet Point Service Malartic; (819)762-5599 x45038; jeanguy_ricard@ssss.gouv.qc.ca.

RICARD, Mario; Ctr Hosp Rouyn-Noranda, 4 9e rue, Rouyn-Noranda QC J9X 2B2; Sher'89; CSPQ; Anes. Staff, Centre Hospitalier Rouyn-Noranda; (819)764-5131

RICARD, Nadege; Ctr Jeunesse de Montreal IU, 12165 boul Saint-Jean-Baptiste, Montreal QC H1C 1S4; Mon'03; (514)858-3964

RICARD, Paul; GMF Clinique Med St-Laurent, 201-200 av Saint-Laurent, Louiseville QC J5V 1J9; Laval'83; Coord Geriatric Unit, CSSS de Maskinongé; (819)228-7171; Fax. (819)228-1480.

RICARD, Pauline; CSSS d'Antoine-Labelle-Mt Laur, RR 1 2561 ch de la Lièvre S, Mont-Laurier QC J9L 3G3; Mon'81; CSPQ; Anes. Staff, CSSS d'Antoine-Labelle; (819)623-1234; pauline.ricard@ssss.gouv.qc.ca.

RICARD, Stephane; CHUS-Hop Fleurimont, 4109-3001 12e av N, Sherbrooke QC J1H 5N4; Sher'91; LMCC; FRCSC; OrthSurg (Sports Medicine). Staff, Centre Hospitalier Universitaire de Sherbrooke-Hopital Fleurimont; Langs: English; (819)346-1110 x14233; Fax. (819)820-6410; stephane.ricard@usherbrooke.ca.

RICCI, Christopher J; Hamilton HS-General Site, 237 Barton St E, Hamilton ON L8L 2X2; Tor'80; FRCPC; Anes. Staff, Hamilton Health Sciences Centre - Hamilton General Hospital; (905)527-0271

RICCI, Donald R; Diamond Health Care Centre, L9-2775 Laurel St, Vancouver BC V5Z 1M9; UBC'72; FRCPC; IntMed; Cardiol. Ac Staff Med, Vancouver General Hospital - Centennial Pavillion; Clin Prof, University of British Columbia; (604)875-5487; Fax. (604)875-5504.

RICCI, Elio E; 588 Barton St E, Hamilton ON L8L 2Z5; Tor'51; Sr Staff, Hamilton Health Sciences Centre - McMaster University Medical Centre; St Joseph's Healthcare - Charlton Campus; Staff, Hamilton Health Sciences Centre-Juravinski Site; Langs: Italian; (905)529-6998; Fax. (905)529-9928.

RICCI, Joseph A; Corcare Inc, 410-325 Milner Ave, Scarborough ON M1B 5N1; Tor'79; ABIM; FACC; FRCPC; IntMed; Cardiol; InfectDis. Staff, Rouge Valley Health System - Centenary Health Centre Site; Lecturer Med(Pt-Time), University of Toronto; (416)284-4744; Fax. (416)284-0141.

RICCIARDI, Luigi T; Niagara Med Prof Centre, PO Box 10 1882 Niagara Stone Rd, Virgil ON L0S 1T0; Tor'90; CCFP; Staff, Sunnybrook Health Sciences Centre; Langs: Italian; Swahili; (905)468-3275; Fax. (905)468-7960; lricciardi@niagara.com.

RICCIUTI, Flora; 702-240 Duncan Mill Rd, North York ON M3B 3S6; McM'93; MSc; BSc; CCFP; Langs: Italian; French; (416)494-7435; Fax. (416)494-4819.

RICCIUTO, Daniel R; Lakeridge Hlth Corp-Oshawa, A6 24-1 Hospital Crt, Oshawa ON L1G 2B9; Tor'06; FRCPC; IntMed; InfectDis. Staff, Lakeridge Health - Oshawa Site; (905)721-7796

RICE, Brenda L; 201-849 Alexander Crt, Peterborough ON K9J 7H8; Dublin (Ireland)'05; MSc; Staff, Peterborough Regional Health Centre - Hospital Drive; (705)775-1017; Fax. (705)775-1019.

RICE, Clifford G; Prince Edward Family Hlth Team, SS 2 4-35 Bridge St, Picton ON K0K 2T0; Qns'79; CCFP; FCFP; Ac Staff, QHC Prince Edward County Memorial; (613)476-3008; Fax. (613)476-6301.

RICE, James H; Radiology Associates of Regina, 6-2727 Parliament Ave, Regina SK S4S 6X5; Sask'77; BSc; FRCPC; DiagRad. Ac Staff, Pasqua Hospital; Staff, Radiology Associates of Regina; University of Saskatchewan; (306)352-7653; Fax. (306)522-4311.

RICE, Jill L; SCOHS-Elizabeth Bruyere Hosp, 43 Bruyere St, Ottawa ON K1N 5C8; Ott'97; CCFP; Staff, SCO Health Service - Élisabeth Bruyère Hospital; (613)562-6262; Fax. (613)562-6371.

RICE, Leah L; St Joseph's Healthcare, 50 Charlton Ave E, Hamilton ON L8N 4A6; McM'81; GenSurg (Head & Neck Surgery & Oncology). Staff, St Joseph's Healthcare - Charlton Campus; (905)522-1255; Fax. (905)522-9460.

RICE, Maryanne; Riverside South Med Centre, 3-665 Earl Armstrong Rd, Gloucester ON K1V 2G2; Ott'87; (613)822-0411

RICE, Patrick O; Portage Clinic Inc, 140 9th St SE, Portage La Prairie MB R1N 3V5; Cork (Ireland)'75; MB BCh; BAO; DRCOG; DCH; CCFP; Staff, Portage District General Hospital; (204)857-3445; Fax. (204)239-1278; price@shaw.ca.

RICE, Sarah C; Somerset West Comm Health Ctre, 55 Eccles St, Ottawa ON K1R 6S3; McM'00; CCFP; (613)238-1220; Fax. (613)235-2982; srice@swchc.on.ca.

RICE, Sean B; North York Med Arts Bldg, 345-1333 Sheppard Ave E, North York ON M2J 1V1; McM'97; BA; MSc; FRCSC; PlasSurg. Court Staff, Sunnybrook Health Sciences Centre; (416)391-4048; Fax. (416)391-3979.

RICER, Michael W; Baywood Med Centre, 508-95 Bayly St W, Ajax ON L1S 7K8; Tor'86; FRCSC; GenSurg. (905)427-6111; Fax. (905)427-4482.

RICH, Alan D; Professional Bldg, 55 Selkirk Ave, Thompson MB R8N 0M5; Sask'71; (204)677-4521; Fax. (204)677-3909.

RICH, Barry W; 301B-6351 197 St, Langley BC V2Y 1X8; Man'78; (604)539-1915; Fax. (604)539-1983.

RICH, Eric; CHUM-Hop Notre-Dame, 1560 rue Sherbrooke E, Montreal QC H2L 4M1; Mon'88; CSPQ; FRCPC; IntMed; Rheum. Staff, Centre Hospitalier l'Université de Montréal (CHUM) - Hôpital Notre-Dame; adj Prof, Universite de Montreal; (514)890-8000 x28800; Fax. (514)412-7630.

RICH, Harold A; MUHC-Montreal Children's Hosp, 2300 rue Tupper, Montreal QC H3H 1P3; McG'69; MPH; Peds. Staff, McGill University Health Centre - Montreal Children's Hospital; assoc Prof, McGill University; (514)412-4400; harold.rich@muhc.mcgill.ca.

RICH, Kira E; St Paul's Hosp, 1081 Burrard St, Vancouver BC V6Z 1Y6; Dal'06; CCFP; CCFP(E.M.); Staff, Providence Health Care - St Paul's Hospital; (604)682-2344

RICH, Peter; Norfolk Gen Hosp, 365 West St, Simcoe ON N3Y 1T7; McM'80; Staff, Norfolk General Hospital; (519)426-0750 x2205

RICH, Thomas; C231-1403 29 St NW, Calgary AB T2N 2T9; UBC'91; ACLS; ATLS; FCFP; LMCC; AddicMed; CCFP; CCFP(E.M.); Staff, Foothills Medical Centre; Clinical Asst Prof, University of Calgary; (403)944-1596; Fax. (403)944-2419; tom.rich@albertahealthservices.ca.

RICHARD, Alex; Ctr Hosp Anna-Laberge, 200 boul Brisebois, Chateauguay QC J6K 4W8; Mon'03; Staff, Hôpital Anna-Laberge; (450)699-2436

RICHARD, Annette; 657 Central Ave, London ON N5W 3P7; McM'95; CCFP; Langs: Spanish; (519)667-2101; Fax. (519)667-0938.

RICHARD, Annie; Centre Med LeMesnil, 1300 boul Lebourgneuf, Quebec QC G2K 2N1; Mon'97; (418)624-1800; Fax. (418)624-1820.

RICHARD, Anouk; CSSS du Sud de Lanaudière, 911 montee des Pionniers, Terrebonne QC J6V 2H2; Laval'98; CSPQ; Anes. Staff, Centre Hospitalier Pierre le Gardeur; (450)654-7525

RICHARD, Bernard; Ctr Hosp Reg du Suroit, 150 rue Saint-Thomas, Salaber-de-Valleyf QC J6T 6C1; Sher'01; Staff, Centre Hospitalier Régional du Suroît; Chief Emerg Services, Centre Sante Service Sociaux Suroit; Langs: English; (450)371-9920; Fax. (450)377-1372.

RICHARD, Carole S; CHUM-Hop St-Luc, 6218-1058 rue Saint-Denis, Montreal QC H2X 3J4; Mon'88; FRCSC; GenSurg (Colon & Rectal Surgery). Ac Member Surg, Centre Hospitalier l'Université De Montréal (CHUM) - Hôpital Saint-luc; Clinical Asst Prof, Universite de Montreal; (514)890-8000 x34953; Fax. (514)412-7259; c.richard@umontreal.ca.

RICHARD, Caroline; CSSS Pierre Boucher, 1333 boul Jacques-Cartier E, Longueuil QC J4M 2A5; Laval'95; Staff, Centre Hospitalier Pierre Boucher; (450)468-8111 x2140

RICHARD, Christiane; CLSC Ahuntsic, 1165 boul Henri-Bourassa E, Montreal QC H2C 3K2; Mon'77; (514)384-2000; Fax. (514)381-0814.

RICHARD, Claude; 177 rue Manse, Gr-Sault/Gr-Falls NB E3Z 2X4; Mon'89; Staff Emerg Med, Hôpital Général de Grand-Falls; Langs: Bilingual(French/English); (506)473-1516; Fax. (506)473-4468.

RICHARD, Claude; Hotel-Dieu d'Arthabaska, 5 rue des Hospitalieres, Victoriaville QC G6P 6N2; Sher'73; DABIM; CSPQ; FRCPC; IntMed. ac Staff, Hotel-Dieu d'Arthabaska; Prof, Universite de Sherbrooke; Langs: English; (819)357-2030 x2300; Fax. (819)357-6016.

RICHARD, Elise; Hotel-Dieu d'Arthabaska, 5 rue des Hospitalieres, Victoriaville QC G6P 6N2; Sher'03; Staff, Hotel-Dieu d'Arthabaska; (819)357-2030 x2484; Fax. (819)357-6030.

RICHARD, Hugues J; 11 Royal Field Cres, Ottawa ON K2J 4G1; Laval'80; FRCPC; Psy. Consultant, Kirkland & District Hospital; Consultant, Timmins & District Hospital; (613)823-4748; hugues.richard@ontariomd.ca.

RICHARD, Jean-Paul; 16625 av Saint-Louis, Saint-Hyacinthe QC J2T 3E9; Mon'58; (450)773-3571

RICHARD, Jerry M; PO Box 1889 Stn Main, Cold Lake AB T9M 1P4; Sask'06.

RICHARD, Johanne; Inst de Readaptation de Mtl, 6300 av Darlington, Montreal QC H3S 2J4; Mon'92; CSPQ; FRCPC; Psy (Anxiety Disorder). Staff, Institut de Réadaptation Gingras-Lindsay de Montréal; (514)340-2111

RICHARD, Julie C; London HSC-Victoria Hosp, PO Box 5010 Stn B 800 Commissioners Rd E, London ON N6A 5W9; Ott'05; FRCPC; Psy. Staff, London Health Sciences Centre - Victoria Campus; (519)685-8102

RICHARD, Karine; 203-1052 rue Lionel-Daunais, Boucherville QC J4B 0B2; Sher'10; CCFP; (450)262-6222

RICHARD, Katayoun; St Joseph's Healthcare, 50 Charlton St E, Hamilton ON L8N 4A6; Tehran (Iran)'95; DiagRad. Fellow, St Joseph's Healthcare - Charlton Campus; (905)522-1155

RICHARD, Lise; 207-565 Elmwood Dr, Moncton NB E1A 2X4; Sher'08; CCFP; (506)856-9979; Fax. (506)856-5190.

RICHARD, Lorraine; Clinique Med Barrette, 152 boul Barrette, Chicoutimi QC G7H 7W8; Laval'88; Staff, Complexe hospitalier de la Sagamie; (418)543-3838; Fax. (418)543-3216.

RICHARD, Luc; CLSC de Forestville, CP 790 2 7e rue, Forestville QC G0T 1E0; Laval'83; Langs: Spanish; English; (418)587-2212; Fax. (418)587-6408.

RICHARD, Marie; GMF de Lorraine, 99 boul de Gaulle, Lorraine QC J6Z 3Z9; Mon'80; FRCPC; Derm. Staff, Centre Hospitalier l'Université De Montréal (CHUM) - Hôpital Saint-luc; (450)621-1444; Fax. (450)621-7193.

RICHARD, Marie-Claude; Clinique Med Havre Sante, 521 boul du Havre, Salaber-de-Valleyf QC J6S 4Z5; Laval'99; Staff, Centre Hospitalier Régional du Suroît; (450)371-6444

RICHARD, Mario; Dr Georges-L Dumont Reg Hosp, 330 av Universite, Moncton NB E1C 2Z3; Sher'01; FRCPC; DiagRad. Staff, Dr Georges-L-Dumont University Hospital Centre; (506)862-4000

RICHARD, Megan J; The Moncton Hosp, 135 MacBeath Ave, Moncton NB E1C 6Z8; Dal'07; CCFP; Staff, The Moncton Hospital; (506)857-5111

RICHARD, Michael T; The Ottawa Hosp-Gen Campus, 501 Smyth Rd, Ottawa ON K1H 8L6; Ott'60; FRCSC; Neursurg. Ac Staff Div of NeuroSurg, The Ottawa Hospital - General Campus; Ac Staff, The Ottawa Hospital - Civic Campus; Assoc Prof, University of Ottawa; Langs: English; French; (613)737-8107; Fax. (613)737-8398; mrichard@ottawahospital.on.ca.

RICHARD, Michel; CSSS de la Haute-Yamaska, 205 boul Leclerc O, Granby QC J2G 1T7; Sher'92; FRCSC; GenSurg. Staff, Centre Hospitalier de Granby; (450)372-5491

RICHARD, Norbert S; PO Box 456, Moncton NB E1C 8L9; Dal'74; Asst Med Dir/Ac Staff, Dr Georges-L-Dumont University Hospital Centre; Med Dir, Assumption Mutual Life Ins Co; Med Advisor, Noranda Smelter; Langs: English; French; (506)857-0015; Fax. (506)854-7874; maoc@nbnet.nb.ca.

RICHARD, Philippe F A; Ctr Hosp de Verdun, 24-4000 boul Lasalle, Verdun QC H4G 2A3; Brussels (Belgium)'64; FRCSC; GenSurg; Cardiovasc&ThorSurg (P.Q.). Staff, Centre Hospitalier de Verdun; Staff, Institut de Cardiologie de Montréal; (514)362-1000

RICHARD, Raymond; Vanier Med Centre, 11-325 Vanier Blvd, Bathurst NB E2A 3N1; Sher'76; (506)548-9788; Fax. (506)549-4259.

RICHARD, Sophie; Polyclinique St-Eustache, 75 rue Grignon, Saint-Eustache QC J7P 4J2; Mon'09; CCFP; (450)473-6882

RICHARD, Thomas C; The Medical Centre FHT, 707 Charlotte St, Peterborough ON K9J 2X5; Wes'87; CCFP; FCFP; (705)876-4500; Fax. (705)743-6288.

RICHARD-CHAPLEAU, Felix; CSSS de Manicouagan, 635 boul Jolliet, Baie-Comeau QC G5C 1P1; Sher'10; CCFP; Staff, Centre Hospitalier Régional Baie-Comeau; (418)589-3701

RICHARD-CHESNAY, Johanne; CHUM-Hotel-Dieu, 3840 rue Saint-Urbain, Montreal QC H2W 1T8; Mon'77; Staff, Centre Hospitalier l'Université de Montréal (CHUM) - Hôtel-Dieu; (514)890-8104

RICHARDS, Corey J; CSSS-Hop de Hull, 116 boul Lionel-Emond, Gatineau QC J8Y 1W7; McG'02; FRCSC; OrthSurg. Staff, Hull Hospital; (819)595-6022

RICHARDS, Crispen G; London HSC-Victoria Hosp, PO Box 5010 Stn B 2200-800 Commissioners Rd E, London ON N6A 5W9; Dal'02; FRCPC; EmergMed. Staff, London Health Sciences Centre - Victoria Campus; (519)685-8500

RICHARDS, Douglas L; Hamilton HS-General Site, 237 Barton St E, Hamilton ON L8L 2X2; McM'95; FRCPC; EmergMed. Staff, Hamilton Health Sciences Centre - Hamilton General Hospital; (905)527-4322

RICHARDS, Douglas W; David L MacIntosh Sport Med Cl, 55 Harbord St, Toronto ON M5S 2W6; Tor'79; Med Dir D L MacIntosh Sport Med Clin/Asst Prof, University of Toronto; Langs: English; French; (416)978-4678; Fax. (416)971-2846.

RICHARDS, Gail J E; Keele-Ingram Prof Centre, 208-2221 Keele St, North York ON M6M 3Z5; Tor'85; BSc; Staff, Humber River Regional Hospital - Keele Street Site; (416)244-3385; Fax. (416)244-4684.

RICHARDS, H Anne; 183 Glenrose Ave, Toronto ON M4T 1K7; Melbourne (Australia)'71; MB BS; FRCPC; Peds (Behavioural Pediatrics). Consultant, The Hospital For Sick Children; Asst Prof, University of Toronto; (416)754-8358

RICHARDS, J Gordon L; 110 Woolwich St, Guelph ON N1H 3V2; Wes'90; CCFP; (519)767-1721; Fax. (519)837-3974.

RICHARDS, James C; Bassano Health Centre, PO Box 120 608 5th Ave, Bassano AB T0J 0B0; Auckland (New Zealand)'99; BSc; CCFP; Staff, Bassano Health Centre; (403)641-6130; Fax. (403)641-6134.

RICHARDS, John B; SMBD Jewish Gen Hosp, 3755 ch Cote-Sainte-Catherine, Montreal QC H3T 1E2; Cal'00; Endocrin&Metab; IntMed. Staff, Sir Mortimer B Davis Jewish General; (514)340-8222

RICHARDS, John S F; UBC Eye Care Centre, 2550 Willow St, Vancouver BC V5Z 3N9; UBC'60; FRCOphth; FRCSC; Ophth (Cornea/External Disease). Emeritus Prof, University of British Columbia; (604)875-4435; Fax. (604)875-5748.

RICHARDS, Lisa K M; Winnipeg Reg Health Authority, 490 Hargrave St, Winnipeg MB R3A 0X7; Man'01; FRCPC; CommunMed. (204)940-3610; lrichards@wrha.mb.ca.

RICHARDS, Melinde; Royal Jubilee Hosp, 1952 Bay St, Victoria BC V8R 1J8; Stellenbosch (South Africa)'90; MB ChB; CCFP; Staff, Royal Jubilee Hospital; Langs: German; (250)514-3515; mkreye@shaw.ca.

RICHARDS, Peter V; 4313 Gallant Ave, North Vancouver BC V7G 2C1; Glasgow (Scotland)'72; Court Staff, Lions Gate Hospital; Clin Lecturer Family Practice, University of British Columbia; (604)929-7304; Fax. (604)929-3256; nrichards@telus.net.

RICHARDS, Richard L; Keele-Ingram Med Centre, 207-2221 Keele St, North York ON M6M 3Z5; Tor'68; BSc; Staff, Humber River Regional Hospital - Keele Street Site; Langs: Spanish; (416)592-0593; Fax. (416)536-0583; rrichards@look.ca.

RICHARDS, Robert N; Sheppard Med Bldg, 304-701 Sheppard Ave E, North York ON M2K 2Z3; Tor'62; DABD; FRCP; Derm (Hyperhidrosis). Staff, North York General Hospital; Lecturer, University of Toronto; (416)590-9918; Fax. (416)590-9842.

RICHARDS, Robert S; St Joseph's Health Care, PO Box 5777 Stn B 268 Grosvenor St, London ON N6A 4V2; Sask'83; FRCSC; PlasSurg (Cosmetic Surgery). Staff Div of Plastic Surg, St Joseph's Hospital - St Joseph's Health Care; Assoc Prof Div of Plastic Surg & OrthSurg, University of Western Ontario; (519)646-6046; Fax. (519)646-6049; rrichard@uwo.ca.

RICHARDS, Robin R; Sunnybrook Hlth Sciences Ctre, D574-2075 Bayview Ave, Toronto ON M4N 3M5; McM'76; FRCSC; OrthSurg (Upper Extremity Reconstruction). Chief Surgery, Sunnybrook Health Sciences Centre; Prof Surg, University of Toronto; (416)480-5051; Fax. (416)480-4925; robin.richards@sunnybrook.ca.

RICHARDS, Willem J; Golden Ears Family Practice, 140-20395 Lougheed Hwy, Maple Ridge BC V2X 2P9; Pretoria (South Africa)'99; MB ChB; LMCC; Staff, Ridge Meadows Hospital & Health Care Centre; (604)465-1066; Fax. (604)465-7776.

RICHARDSON, Alan J; 14104 Tamarack Dr, Vernon BC V1B 2C9; Alb'78; FRCSC; OrthSurg. (250)545-6151

RICHARDSON, Beverley J; Women's College Hosp, 76 Grenville St, Toronto ON M5S 1B2; Tor'72; FRCPC; IntMed. Ac Staff, Women's College Hospital; Asst Prof, University of Toronto; (416)967-4335; Fax. (416)323-6331.

RICHARDSON, Bonnie R; Regina Qu'Appelle HR-Regina, 1440 14th Ave, Regina SK S4P 0W5; Sask'06; FRCPC; IntMed; Nephrol. Staff, Regina General Hospital; (306)525-2404; Fax. (306)525-2553.

RICHARDSON, Bryan S; St Joseph's Health Care, PO Box 5777 Stn B 268 Grosvenor St, London ON N6A 4V2; Wes'74; FRCSC; ObstGyn (Maternal Fetal Medicine). Staff, St Joseph's Hospital - St Joseph's Health Care; Prof, University of Western Ontario; (519)646-6106; Fax. (519)646-6213.

RICHARDSON, C Glen; Queen Elizabeth II HSC-Halifax, 4561-1796 Summer St, Halifax NS B3H 3A7; Dal'96; BSc; FRCSC; OrthSurg (Adult Reconstructive Surgery). Staff, Queen Elizabeth II Health Sciences Centre - Halifax Infirmary Site; (902)473-1641; Fax. (902)429-2547.

RICHARDSON, Christine A; E1 102-800 Commissioners Rd E, London ON N6A 5W9; Wes'02; CCFP; CCFP(E.M.); (519)667-6538

RICHARDSON, Christopher W; South Muskoka Mem Hosp, 75 Ann St, Bracebridge ON P1L 2E4; Qns'08; CCFP; Staff, South Muskoka Memorial Hospital - Muskoka Algonquin Healthcare; (705)645-4400; Fax. (705)645-4594.

RICHARDSON, Cindy Jo; Winnipeg Clinic, 425 St Mary Ave, Winnipeg MB R3C 0N2; Alb'80; FRCPC; IntMed; Endocrin&Metab. Staff, Health Sciences Centre.

RICHARDSON, David C; William Osler HC-Brampton, 2100 Bovaird Dr E, Brampton ON L6R 3J7; Tor'96; FRCPC; IntMed; MedMicrobiol; InfectDis. Staff, William Osler Health System - Brampton Civic Hospital; (905)494-2120 x57658; david.richardson@williamoslerhs.ca.

RICHARDSON, David R; 103-20644 Fraser Hwy, Langley BC V3A 4G5; UBC'88; Staff, Langley Memorial Hospital; (604)530-4979; Fax. (604)530-2975.

RICHARDSON, Dellmari; 101-1912 Enterprise Way, Kelowna BC V1Y 9S9; Sask'99; CCFP; Staff, Kelowna General Hospital; (250)868-0700; Fax. (250)868-3003.

RICHARDSON, Denyse L; Toronto Rehab Inst-Univ Ctr, 550 University Ave, Toronto ON M5G 2A2; McM'92; BScPT; MEd; FRCPC; PhysMed&Rehab (Neuro Rehabilitation). Staff Physiatrist, Toronto Rehabilitation Institute - University Centre; Clin Educator/Assoc Prof, University of Toronto; (416)597-3422 x3865; Fax. (416)597-7107.

RICHARDSON, Donald B; 2-537 Frederick St, Kitchener ON N2B 2A7; Wes'82; (519)725-2641; Fax. (519)725-4064.

RICHARDSON, Donald W; 1313 Princess St, Kingston ON K7M 3E3; Tor'66; FRCPC; Peds (Adolescent Medicine). Staff, Kingston General Hospital; Att Staff, Hotel-Dieu Hospital; Assoc Prof, Queen's University; Langs: English; French; (613)549-1302; Fax. (613)549-1125.

RICHARDSON, Elizabeth A; 4F-1 Hughson St N, Hamilton ON L8R 3L5; Wes'89; MHSc(CommunHlth&Epidem); FRCPC; CommunMed. Med Officer of Hlth, City of Hamilton-Wentworth; Asst Prof Peds, McMaster University; (905)546-2424 x3501; Fax. (905)546-4075.

RICHARDSON, Gary; 2121 Boxwood Rd, Nanaimo BC V9S 4L2; Witwatersrand (South Africa)'89; MB ChB; CCFP; FCFP; Langs: Afrikaans; (250)751-0111; Fax. (250)751-2758.

RICHARDSON, George M J; Montreal Road Med Centre, 398 Montreal Rd, Ottawa ON K1K 0V4; Alb'87; GenPath (Family Medicine). (613)244-2005; Fax. (613)244-2004.

RICHARDSON, Ian D; Bruyere Continuing Care, 261 Y-75 Bruyere St, Ottawa ON K1N 5C7; Qns'74; CCFP; FCFP; (613)562-6322; Fax. (613)562-6013.

RICHARDSON, J Donald; St Joseph's HC-Parkwood Hosp, 801 Commissioners Rd E, London ON N6C 5J1; Qns'91; FRCPC; Psy. Consultant Psy, Parkwood Hospital - St Joseph's Health Care; Langs: French; (519)685-4992 x42399; Fax. (519)685-4585.

RICHARDSON, J Ian; Continuum Med Centre, 201-520 17th St, West Vancouver BC V7V 3S8; Alb'80; CAFCI; (604)913-8183

RICHARDSON, Janet A; Medcan Clinic, 1500-150 York St, Toronto ON M5H 3S5; Wes'91; CCFP; CCFP(E.M.); FCFP; Staff, William Osler Health System - Brampton Civic Hospital; (416)350-5900; Fax. (416)350-5981.

RICHARDSON, Jeannie L; 200-101 Queensway W, Mississauga ON L5B 2P7; Qns'01; FRCSC; GenSurg. (905)624-4531; Fax. (905)624-6988.

RICHARDSON, John B; MUHC-Montreal Neurology Inst, 3801 rue University, Montreal QC H3A 2B4; McG'62; CSPQ; NeurPath (P.Q.); AnatPath. Ac Staff, McGill University Health Centre - Montreal Neurological Hospital; Prof, McGill University; (514)398-5324

RICHARDSON, John D; Health Services Centre, 233 Sunbury Dr, Frederctn-Jct NB E5L 1S1; Dal'77; Assoc Staff, Dr Everett Chalmers Regional Hospital; Court Staff, Oromocto Public Hospital; (506)368-6501; Fax. (506)368-6502; ruth.richardson@rvh.nb.ca.

RICHARDSON, John W; Archdekin Med Group, PO Box 660 Stn Main, Bracebridge ON P1L 1T9; Belfast (Ireland)'67; MB ChB; DCH; CCFP; FCFP; Ac Staff, South Muskoka Memorial Hospital - Muskoka Algonquin Healthcare; Med Dir, Pines Home for the Aged; (705)645-2223; Fax. (705)645-2342.

RICHARDSON, Karyn P; Crowfoot Village Fam Practice, 210-600 Crowfoot Cres NW, Calgary AB T3G 0B4; Cal'07; CCFP; (403)239-9733

RICHARDSON, Katherine M; 25 Black Lake Rd, Lively ON P3Y 1J3; Ott'08; CCFP; (705)692-1018; Fax. (705)692-7156.

RICHARDSON, Keith; University of Alberta Hosp, 1E4.29-8440 112 St NW, Edmonton AB T6G 2B7; McG'07; MDCM; Otol. Staff, University of Alberta Hospital; (780)407-8397

RICHARDSON, Lisa A; Univ Hlth Network-Toronto Western Hosp, 399 Bathurst St, Toronto ON M5T 2S8; Cal'01; FRCPC; IntMed. Staff, Toronto Western Hospital - University Health Network; (416)603-5800; Fax. (416)603-5803.

RICHARDSON, Maria; The Four Villages CHC, 1700 Bloor St W, Toronto ON M6P 4C3; Ott'95; CCFP; Langs: Russian; (416)604-3361; Fax. (416)604-3367.

RICHARDSON, Martha V; 8-17310 Yonge St, Newmarket ON L3Y 7R8; Tor'91; BSc; CCFP; FCFP; Court Staff, Mackenzie Richmond Hill Hospital; (905)868-9966; Fax. (905)868-9495.

RICHARDSON, Robert M A; Univ Hlth Network-Toronto Gen, 8N 861-200 Elizabeth St, Toronto ON M5G 2C4; Tor'72; FRCPC; IntMed (Nephrology). Staff, Toronto General Hospital - UHN; Prof Med, University of Toronto; (416)340-3889; Fax. (416)340-4999.

RICHARDSON, Rosemarie T; Tisdale Med Clinic, PO Box 1510, Tisdale SK S0E 1T0; (306)873-4561; Fax. (306)873-4489.

RICHARDSON, Susan E; The Hosp for Sick Children, 3654-555 University Ave, Toronto ON M5G 1X8; McG'76; BSc; FRCPC; IntMed; MedMicrobiol; InfectDis. Head Div of Microbiol, The Hospital For Sick Children; Assoc Prof, University of Toronto; (416)813-5992

RICHARDSON, Wendy L; 13017 Rosedale Ave PO Box 69, Summerland BC V0H 1Z0; Cambridge (England)'85; MB BCh; (250)494-7376

RICHE, Barry R; The Brandon Clinic, 620 Dennis St, Brandon MB R7A 5E7; Mem'77; FRCPC; IntMed; Nephrol. Med Dir Hemodialysis Unit, Brandon Regional Health Centre; (204)571-7139; Fax. (204)726-8797.

RICHE, Cyril R; Pearlgate Med Clinic, 18 Gibson Dr, Mount Pearl NL A1N 5K8; Mem'78; (709)364-3909; Fax. (709)364-3944; candjriche@nl.rogers.com.

RICHER, Bernard; Ctr Hosp Laurentien, 234 rue Saint-Vincent, Ste-Agathe-des-Mts QC J8C 2B8; Man'64; FRCSC; GenSurg. Staff, Centre Hospitalier Laurentien; (819)324-4000

RICHER, Claude; Clinique Med Pierre-Boucher, 350-1615 boul Jacques-Cartier, Longueuil QC J4M 2X1; Sher'80; CSPQ; FRCPC; Psy. Staff, Hopital Maisonneuve-Rosemont; Clin Teacher, Universite de Montreal; (450)468-6223; Fax. (450)468-5041.

RICHER, Faisca; I N S P Q, 190 boul Cremazie E, Montreal QC H2P 1E2; Ott'95; CSPQ; FRCPC; CommunMed. (514)864-1600 x3732; Fax. (514)864-5180; faisca.richer@ssss.gouv.qc.ca.

RICHER, Genevieve; West Island Palliative Care, 265 rue Andre-Brunet, Kirkland QC H9H 3R4; Mon'90; Staff, Lakeshore General Hospital - Pointe Claire; Dir méd, West Island Palliative Care Residence; Langs: English; (514)693-1718; Fax. (514)693-0374; ghricher@hotmail.com.

RICHER, Jean-Claude; Clin Med Maisonneuve-Rosemont, 5345 boul de l'Assomption, Montreal QC H1T 4B3; Mon'93; Staff, Hopital Maisonneuve-Rosemont; (514)257-7000; Fax. (514)257-7003.

RICHER, Julie; Clinique Med Fleur de Lys, 8 rue du Terminus E, Rouyn-Noranda QC J9X 3B4; Laval'98; (819)764-6185; Fax. (819)762-6079.

RICHER, Julie; Children's Hosp Eastern Ont, 401 Smyth Rd, Ottawa ON K1H 8L1; Mon'03; FRCPC; MedGenetics. Staff, Children's Hospital of Eastern Ontario (CHEO); (613)737-7600 x2275

RICHER, Lawrence; Edmonton Clinic Health Academy, 4 588-11405 87 Ave NW, Edmonton AB T6G 1C9; Alb'96; BSc(Hon); FRCPC; Neur (Pediatric Neurology). Staff, University of Alberta Hospital; Staff, Glenrose Rehabilitation Hospital; Staff, Edmonton Clinic Health Academy; Assoc Prof, University of Alberta; Langs: English; French; (780)248-5568; Fax. (780)248-5627.

RICHER, Marc; Clinique Med En Route, F5-895 rue de la Gauchetiere O, Montreal QC H3B 4G1; Mon'70; (514)954-1444; Fax. (514)954-1619.

RICHER, Pierre; Ctr Metro Chirurgie, 999 rue de Salaberry, Montreal QC H3L 1L2; Mon'68; CSPQ; FRCPC; Anes (Pain Management). Staff Anes, Centre Metropolitan de Chirurgie Plastique; Physician, Clinique Orthopedique Duval; Langs: Bilingual(French/English); (514)332-7091 x215; Fax. (514)332-7095; biofeedback@videotron.ca.

RICHER, Suzanne; College des Med du Quebec, 2170 boul Rene-Levesque O, Montreal QC H3H 2T8; Sher'75; (514)933-4441 x5216; Fax. (514)933-2291.

RICHER-COMISSO, Adriana; CSSS de Laval, 280 boul Roi du Nord, Laval QC H7L 4L2; Mon'09; CCFP; Staff, Hopital de la Cite de la santé; (450)622-5110

RICHFORD, Carole M; St Paul's Hosp, 1081 Burrard St, Vancouver BC V6Z 1Y6; UBC'96; FRCPC; Psy. Staff, Providence Health Care - St Paul's Hospital; (604)682-2344 x63290; Fax. (604)806-8287.

RICHIE, Steven J; 84 Brant Ave, Brantford ON N3T 3H1; Tor'67; DABOS; FRCSC; OrthSurg (Adult Orthopaedics). Ac Staff, The Brant Community Healthcare System - Brantford General Hospital Site; (519)759-0911; Fax. (519)759-2304.

RICHLER, Michael E; 505 O'Connor St, Ottawa ON K1S 3P6; Mem'79; FRCPC; Peds. Att Staff, The Ottawa Hospital - Civic Campus; (613)237-5510; Fax. (613)237-8238.

RICHMAN, Jack; Assessmed Inc, 174-5945 Airport Rd, Mississauga ON L4V 1R9; Tor'67; DOHS; CCBOM(OccupMed); FAB; CCFP; Court Staff, Halton Healthcare Services Corporation - Oakville Site; Med Dir & Vice-Pres/VP, Assessmed Inc; Corp Consultant Med, The Woodbridge Group; (905)678-2924; Fax. (905)678-2939; jrichman@assessmed.com.

RICHMAN-EISENSTAT, Janice B Y; College Plaza 3, 225-8215 112 St NW, Edmonton AB T6G 2C8; Dal'84; FRCPC; IntMed. Staff, Health Sciences Centre; Physician, Manitoba Institute of Cell; (780)492-3996; Fax. (780)407-3027.

RICHMOND, Lara D; Sunnybrook Hlth Sciences Ctre, 2075 Bayview Ave, Toronto ON M4N 3M5; Tor'04; DiagRad. Staff, Sunnybrook Health Sciences Centre; (416)480-4336

RICHMOND, Les; 249 St Clair Ave W, Toronto ON M4V 1R3; Tor'73; (416)968-0828

RICHMOND, Martin I; 103-27 Major Mackenzie Dr E, Richmond Hill ON L4C 1G6; Tor'72; FRCP; FRCPC; IntMed. Staff, Mackenzie Richmond Hill Hospital; (905)884-0803; Fax. (905)884-8892.

RICHTER, Anne-Katrin; GMF Cote-des-Neiges, 5700 ch de la Cote-des-Neiges, Montreal QC H3T 2A8; McG'94; CCFP; Langs: German; French; Spanish; (514)731-8531; Fax. (514)731-0165.

RICHTER, Kenneth; Allan Memorial Institute, 1025 av des Pins O, Montreal QC H3A 1A1; McG'79; ABNP(Psy); CSPQ; FRCPC; Psy (General Adult Psychiatry). Psychiatre, McGill University Health Centre - Montreal General Campus; Staff Psy, Hawkesbury & District General Hospital; Lecturer Psy, McGill University; Langs: English; French; (514)934-1934 x31337

RICHTER, Margaret A; Sunnybrook Hlth Sciences Ctre, FG42-2075 Bayview Ave, Toronto ON M4N 3M5; Ott'85; MD; FRCP; FRCPC; Psy (Anxiety Disorder). Staff, Centre for Addiction & Mental Health (CAMH) - College Street Site; Dir Clin for OCD & Related Disorders Dept of Psy, Sunnybrook Health Sciences Centre; Assoc Prof Psy, University of Toronto; (416)480-6832; peggyrichter@sunnybrook.ca.

RICHTER, Suzanne C; Univ of Toronto, 500 University Ave, Toronto ON M5G 1V7; Wes'05; MedOncol; IntMed.

RICKARDS, Michael R; 111-9719 98 Ave, Grande Prairie AB T8V 8K6; McG'76; FRCPC; EmergMed. (780)539-7377

RICKARDS, Robin C; 2443 Christopherson Rd, Surrey BC V4A 3L2; Sher'78; OrthSurg. Staff, Langley Memorial Hospital; (604)538-9688

RICKETSON, Charles W; Victoria Emerg Phys Mgmt Ltd, 325-1627 Fort St, Victoria BC V8R 1H8; Qns'79; FRCPC; EmergMed. Ac Staff, Victoria General Hospital; Assoc Staff, Royal Jubilee Hospital; (250)479-1442; Fax. (250)475-1472.

RICKETSON, Ian M; Vancouver Gen Hosp, 855 12th Ave W, Vancouver BC V5Z 1M9; UBC'07; FRCPC; EmergMed. Staff, Vancouver General Hospital - Centennial Pavillion; (604)875-4111

RICKETSON, Jeffrey C; Campbell River& Dist Gen Hosp, 375 2nd Ave, Campbell River BC V9W 3V1; UBC'09; CCFP; CCFP(E.M.); Staff, Campbell River & District General Hospital; (250)850-2141

RICKETTS, John D; Kingston Gen Hosp, 76 Stuart St, Kingston ON K7L 2V7; Tor'93; FRCPC; DiagRad. Staff Radiol, Kingston General Hospital; (613)548-2301; Fax. (613)548-2412; rickettj@post.queensu.ca.

RICKHI, Badri G; B G Rickhi Prof Corp, 2020 18 St NW, Calgary AB T2M 3T1; West Indies (Jamaica)'74; MB BS; FRCPC; Psy (Alternative Medicine). Chair Research, Canadian Institute of Natural & Integrative Medicine; Clin Assoc Prof Med, University of Calgary; (403)220-0022; Fax. (403)210-2080; b.rickhi@cinim.org.

RICO, Michelle A; Royal Alexandra Hosp, 541-10240 Kingsway NW, Edmonton AB T5H 3V9; Cal'97; CCFP; CCFP(E.M.); Staff, Royal Alexandra Hospital; (780)735-4442; Fax. (780)735-4916.

RICO, Philippe; Hop du Sacre-Coeur de Mtl, 5400 boul Gouin O, Montreal QC H4J 1C5; McG'89; FRCPC; IntMed (Intensive Care); Critical Care Medicine (P.Q.). Staff, Hôpital du Sacre-Coeur de Montréal; (514)338-2050; Fax. (514)338-2424.

RICOT, Pierre-Jacques; Clin Ped Marie-Anne, 208-269 boul Saint-Jean, Pointe-Claire QC H9R 3J1; Laval'88; Peds (Pediatric Emergency Medicine). Staff, Hôpital Ste-Justine; Langs: English; French; (514)694-2983; Fax. (514)694-4640.

RIDAH, Dekrayat H; Linden Ridge Med Centre, E-123 Scurfield Blvd, Winnipeg MB R3Y 1L6; Baghdad (Iraq)'84; CCFP; Staff, Concordia General Hospital; (204)488-9988

RIDDELL, David; PO Box 1991 Stn Main, Cornwall ON K6H 6N7; McG'81; CSPQ; FRCPC; Anes. Staff, Cornwall Community Hospital; Staff Anes, Cornwall Community Hospital - Second Street Site; Langs: English; French; (613)936-4618

RIDDELL, D Alexander; 48 Church St, Orangeville ON L9W 1N8; Wes'82; Chief Medical Staff, Stevenson Memorial Hospital; Ac Staff, Headwaters Health Care Centre - Orangeville Site; (519)942-8022; Fax. (519)940-9817.

RIDDELL, Robert; 6 502-600 University Ave, Toronto ON M5G 1X5; London (England)'67; MB BS; FRCPath; FRCPC; AnatPath. Staff, Mount Sinai Hospital; (416)586-4800 x2296; rriddell@mtsinai.on.ca.

RIDDLE, Christopher; Niagara H System-St Catharines, PO Box 3018 Stn Main 142 Queenston St, St. Catharines ON L2R 7C6; Dal'09; CCFP; CCFP(E.M.); Staff, Niagara Health System - St Catharines General Site; (905)378-4647

RIDDLE, Gordon E; Archdekin Medical Group, PO Box 660 Stn Main 205 Hiram St, Bracebridge ON P1L 1T9; Ott'76; BSc; CCFP; FCFP; Ac Staff, South Muskoka Memorial Hospital - Muskoka Algonquin Healthcare; Asst Prof VPT Dept of Family Med, University of Ottawa; Asst Prof, Northern Ontario School of Medicine; (705)645-2223; Fax. (705)645-2342.

RIDDLE, Robert J; North York Gen Hosp, 4001 Leslie St, North York ON M2K 1E1; Tor'70; CCFP; CCFP(E.M.); FCFP; Ac Staff, St John's Rehabilitation Hospital; Ac Staff, North York General Hospital; Asst Prof, University of Toronto; (416)226-6790 x7111; Fax. (416)322-8312.

RIDDLER, Colin R; Royal Jubilee Hosp, 1952 Bay St, Victoria BC V8R 1J8; UBC'92; Staff, Vancouver Island Health Authority; Staff, Royal Jubilee Hospital; (250)370-8000; Fax. (250)592-2248.

RIDEOUT, Andrea N; North End Community Hlth Ctr, 2165 Gottingen St, Halifax NS B3K 3B5; Dal'96; CCFP; FCFP; (902)420-0303; Fax. (902)422-0859.

RIDEOUT, Arthur A; Dr Charles A Janeway Child HC, 2J743-300 Prince Philip Dr, St. John's NL A1B 3V6; Mem'88; FRCSC; PlasSurg (Cranio Facial Surgery). Staff, Janeway Children's Health & Rehabilitation Centre; Staff, Health Sciences Centre; Staff, St Clare's Mercy Hospital; Memorial University Of Newfoundland; (709)777-6300

RIDEOUT, Carolyn M; 5-227 Main St PO Box 1652 Stn Main, Antigonish NS B2G 2L8; Dal'72; DrMedCh; FRCPC; Psy (Child & Adolescent Psychiatry). Consultant Psychiatry, Aberdeen Regional Hospital; Staff Psy, St Martha's Regional Hospital; (902)863-9322; Fax. (902)867-1536; carolynrideout@hotmail.com.

RIDEOUT, David F; True North Imaging, 120-7330 Yonge St, Thornhill ON L4J 7Y7; London (England)'54; MB BS; LRCP; DMRD; FRCR; FRCPC; DiagRad. (905)707-1777

RIDEOUT, Debbie; Health Sciences centre, 2422-300 Prince Philip Dr, St. John's NL A1B 3V6; Staff, Health Sciences Centre; (709)744-3434; Fax. (709)744-3444.

RIDEOUT, Gary M; Pearl Gate Med Clinic, 18 Gibson Dr, Mount Pearl NL A1N 5K8; Mem'85; CCFP; Staff, St Clare's Mercy Hospital; (709)364-3909; Fax. (709)364-3944.

RIDEOUT, Gregory S; Churchill Square Med Clinic, 8-10 Rowan St, St. John's NL A1B 2X1; Mem'03; CCFP; (709)722-8561

RIDEOUT, John A; 101-4695 Hastings St, Burnaby BC V5C 2K6; McG'73; Ac Staff, Burnaby Hospital; (604)298-7201; Fax. (604)291-6176.

RIDEOUT-VIVIAN, Susan; Terrace On The Square, 8-10 Rowan St, St. John's NL A1B 2X1; Mem'86; BMedSci; CCFP; Examiner Designated Seafarers & Civil Aviation, City of St John's; Staff, Health Care Corporation Of St John's; sue.rideout@nf.sympatico.ca.

RIDGEWAY, Kimberly; Clinique GAIA, 106-195 boul de l'Atmosphere, Gatineau QC J9A 0A3; McG'09; CCFP; (819)770-1414

RIDHA, Mahmoud H; Lacewood Med Center, 200-366 Lacewood Dr, Halifax NS B3S 1M7; Al-Mustansiriyah (Iraq)'87; CCFP; Staff, Yarmouth Regional Hospital; (902)445-9400; Fax. (902)445-7108.

RIDI, Angela; St Clare's Mercy Hosp, 154 Lemarchant Rd, St. John's NL A1C 5B8; Dal'03; FRCPC; Anes. Staff, St Clare's Mercy Hospital; (709)777-5000

RIDI, Stacy; Kingston Gen Hosp, 76 Stuart St, Kingston ON K7L 2V7; Dal'06; FRCPC; Anes. Staff, Kingston General Hospital; (613)548-7827

RIDING, Timothy J; Medical Arts Bldg, 301-42 Glen Allan Dr, Bridgewater NS B4V 3N2; Dal'03; CCFP; (902)543-7124

RIDLEY, John A C; Vancouver Gen Hosp, 855 12th Ave W, Vancouver BC V5Z 1M9; UBC'98; BSc(Hon); MD; CCFP; Staff, Vancouver General Hospital - Centennial Pavillion; (604)317-7404; drjohnridley@hotmail.com.

RIDLEY, Julia Z; Univ Hlth Network-Princess M, 610 University Ave, Toronto ON M5G 2M9; UBC'05; CCFP; Staff, Princess Margaret Hospital - University Health Network; (416)946-4501

RIDLEY, Tracy S; Children's E R HSC, JL1-840 Sherbrook St, Winnipeg MB R3A 1S1; Alb'91; FRCPC; Peds. Staff, Health Sciences Centre; (204)787-4244; Fax. (204)487-3743.

RIDOUT, Rowena; WW1 442-399 Bathurst St, Toronto ON M5T 2S8; Tor'88; FRCPC; IntMed; Endocrin&Metab. Staff, Toronto Western Hospital - University Health Network; Asst Prof, University of Toronto; (416)603-6454; Fax. (416)603-5518.

RIEB, Launette M; Orion Health, 201-3150 54th Ave E, Vancouver BC V5S 1Z1; McM'92; MSc; CCFP; FCFP; Consultant, Providence Health Care - St Paul's Hospital; Consultant, Orion Health; Clin Assoc Prof, University of British Columbia; (604)263-4998

RIEBER, Joanna C; Hamilton HS-General Site, 237 Barton St E, Hamilton ON L8L 2X2; McM'01; FRCPC; Anes. Staff, Hamilton Health Sciences Centre - Hamilton General Hospital; (905)521-2100

RIECKENBERG, R Markus; Orillia Soldier's Mem Hosp, 170 Colborne St W, Orillia ON L3V 2Z3; Qns'88; FRCPC; AnatPath; GenPath. Dir Lab, Orillia Soldiers' Memorial Hospital; Langs: German; Spanish; French; (705)325-2201 x3525; Fax. (705)325-2870; mrieckenberg@osmh.on.ca.

RIEDEL, Kelly D; Sunnybrook Hlth Sciences Ctre, 2075 Bayview Ave, Toronto ON M4N 3M5; McM'03; FRCSC; OrthSurg. Staff, Sunnybrook Health Sciences Centre; (416)480-6100

RIEDER, Barry W; Royal University Hosp, 103 Hospital Dr, Saskatoon SK S7N 0W8; Sask'98; Staff, Royal University Hospital; (306)655-1363; Fax. (306)655-1011.

RIEDER, Michael J; Children's Hosp of Western Ont, 800 Commissioners Rd E, London ON N6C 2V5; Sask'80; PhD; ABPeds; FRCPC; Peds (Clinical Pharmacology). Staff, London Health Sciences Centre - Victoria Campus; Consultant, London Health Sciences Centre - University Hospital; Prof Peds/Assoc Dean Student Affairs, University of Western Ontario; Langs: Bilingual(French/English); (519)685-8293; Fax. (519)685-8156; mrieder@uwo.ca.

RIEDERER, Barbara; CHUQ-Ctr Hosp Univ Laval, 2705 boul Laurier, Quebec QC G1V 4G2; Lausanne (Switzerland)'79; CSPQ; FRCPC; DiagRad. Staff, Centre Hospitalier Universitaire de Quebec-CHUL; (418)654-2258; Fax. (418)654-2262; barbara.riederer@chuq.qc.ca.

RIEDL, Frank W; Wingfield Med Centre, 411 Wingfield St, Petrolia ON N0N 1R0; Wes'65; Dir Rural Health & Med, Bluewater Health - Charlotte Eleanor Englehart Hospital; (519)882-2110; Fax. (519)882-2111; friedel@bluewaterhealth.ca.

RIEGEL, Timothy M; University of Alberta Hosp, 2D3.83-8440 112 St NW, Edmonton AB T6G 2B7; Cal'97; FRCSC; PlasSurg (Burns). Staff, Covenant Health - Grey Nuns Community Hospital; Assoc Dir Firefighters Burn Treatment Unit, University of Alberta Hospital; (780)407-6322; Fax. (780)407-7097.

RIEGER, John; Nanaimo Reg Gen Hosp, 1200 Dufferin Cres, Nanaimo BC V9S 2B7; Wes'72; BSc; Anes (Family Medicine). Staff, Nanaimo Regional General Hospital; (250)937-9317

RIEGERT, Daniel G; Sunnybrook Hlth Sciences Ctre, M3-210-2075 Bayview Ave, Toronto ON M4N 3M5; Tor'76; FRCPC; Anes (Clinical Anaesthesia). Ac Staff, Sunnybrook Health Sciences Centre; Assoc Prof, University of Toronto; Langs: French; (416)480-4799

RIEKENBRAUCK, Neal W; Headwaters Health Care Centre, 100 Rolling Hills Dr, Orangeville ON L9W 4X9; Tor'91; CCFP; CCFP(E.M.); FCFP; Staff, Headwaters Health Care Centre - Orangeville Site; (519)941-2410; neal.riek@sympatico.ca.

RIEL, Sylvie; Ctr Hosp de Verdun, 4000 boul Lasalle, Verdun QC H4G 2A3; Sher'89; CSPQ; AnatPath. Staff, Centre Hospitalier de Verdun; (514)362-1000

RIENDEAU, Claudie; CLSC Ste-Therese de Blainville, 55 rue Saint-Joseph, Sainte-Therese QC J7E 4Y5; Mon'94; (450)430-4553 x6604; Fax. (450)430-3859.

RIENDEAU, Guy; Clin Med La Cite Place du Parc, 900-300 rue Léo-Pariseau, Montreal QC H2X 4B3; Mon'80; MSc; Staff Emerg, Centre Hospitalier l'Université de Montréal (CHUM) - Hôtel-Dieu; Staff, Air Canada; Médecin, Hydro-Quebec; Langs: Bilingual(French/English); (514)281-1722; Fax. (514)281-6697.

RIES, Craig R; JPP2N 2449-910 10th Ave W, Vancouver BC V5Z 1M9; Wes'79; PhD; FRCPC; Anes. Staff Anes, Vancouver General Hospital - Centennial Pavillion; Clin Assoc Prof Anes, University of British Columbia; (604)875-4304

RIES, Eugene F; Tamarack Med Clinic, 191-1500 Cranbrook St N, Cranbrook BC V1C 3S8; Stellenbosch (South Africa)'79; MB ChB; CAFCI; Staff, East Kootenay Regional Hospital; Langs: Afrikaans; (250)426-7724

RIESE, Nichole M M; Northern Medical Unit, T162-770 Bannatyne Ave, Winnipeg MB R3E 0W3; Man'84; BSc; MSc; CCFP; FCFP; Staff, Seven Oaks General Hospital; Assoc Dir, University of Manitoba; (204)789-3711

RIESLING, Micheal J; 302-8425 120 St, Delta BC V4C 6R2; UBC'97; CCFP; Clinical Asst Prof Med, University of British Columbia; (778)593-0155

RIESS, Jennifer A; Family Medicine Associates, 7004 98 Ave NW, Edmonton AB T6A 0A5; Alb'93; CCFP; (780)468-6035; Fax. (780)466-9132.

RIF, Maria; MUHC-Royal Victoria Hosp, C4 78-687 av des Pins O, Montreal QC H3A 1A1; Laval'05; CCFP; CCFP(E.M.); Staff, Sir Mortimer B Davis Jewish General; Staff, CSSS de Dorval-Lachine-Lasalle; Staff, McGill University Health Centre - Royal Victoria Hospital; (514)934-1934

RIFE, William J; Metrotown Med Centre, 305-6411 Nelson Ave, Burnaby BC V5H 4H3; Alb'75; CCFP; Vis Staff, Burnaby Hospital; (604)433-0009; Fax. (604)433-9527.

RIFF, Shena R; Queensway-Carleton Hosp, 3045 Baseline Rd, Ottawa ON K2H 8P4; Mem'98; BSc; BSc(Hons.); CCFP; CCFP(E.M.); Staff, Queensway Carleton Hospital; (613)721-4710

RIFKIND, Aaron W; 826 Main St E, Hamilton ON L8M 1L6; Edinburgh (Scotland)'67; DOMS(Lond); FAB; FRCSC; Ophth (Cataract). Affil Staff, Hamilton Health Sciences Centre - McMaster Children's Hospital; Ac Staff, St Joseph's Healthcare - Charlton Campus; (905)549-6123; Fax. (905)548-0770.

RIFKIND, Naomi D; Dufferin Family Care Centre, 51 Gerry Fitzgerald Dr, North York ON M3J 3N4; Ott'02; CCFP; (416)739-1562; Fax. (416)739-6671.

RIGAL, Wynne M; PO Box 4504 Stn South Cro, Edmonton AB T6E 4T7; Cape Town (South Africa)'55; MB ChB; DPhil(Oxon.); FRCS(Ed); FRCSC; OrthSurg (Trauma Surgery). Att Staff OrthSurg, Bonnyville Healthcare Centre; Att Staff OrthSurg, Cold Lake Healthcare Centre; Langs: Afrikaans.

RIGAMONT, Andrea; St Michael's Hosp, 30 Bond St, Toronto ON M5B 1W8; Milan (Italy)'99; Staff, St Michael's Hospital; (416)864-5071

RIGATTO, Claudio; Seven Oaks Gen Hosp, 2PD02-2300 McPhillips St, Winnipeg MB R2V 3M3; Man'93; FRCPC; IntMed; Nephrol. Staff, Seven Oaks General Hospital; Staff, St Boniface General Hospital; Langs: Portuguese; Italian; French; (204)632-7133

RIGAULT, Aude; Clinique Med Angus, 101-4101 rue Molson, Montreal QC H1Y 3L1; McG'95; Staff, McGill University Health Centre - Royal Victoria Hospital; (514)807-2333

RIGBY, Ian J; Foothills Med Centre, C231-1403 29 St NW, Calgary AB T2N 2T9; Cal'97; FRCPC; EmergMed. Staff, Foothills Medical Centre; (403)944-1820; Fax. (403)944-2419.

RIGBY, Mark E; Royal Columbian Hosp, 330 Columbia St E, New Westminster BC V3L 3W7; Man'96; FRCPC; DiagRad. Staff, Royal Columbian Hospital; (604)520-4253

RIGBY, Megan C; Sunningdale Medical Centre, 1-1695 Wonderland Rd N, London ON N6G 4W3; Wes'93; (519)641-3636

RIGBY, Ross S; South Calgary Med Clinic, 118-40 Sunpark Plaza SE, Calgary AB T2X 3X7; Man'70; CCFP; FCFP; (403)254-4000; Fax. (403)254-1282.

RIGHI, Roxanna V; Sudbury Med Centre, 400-65 Larch St, Sudbury ON P3E 1B8; Ott'92; FRCSC; ObstGyn. (705)670-9048; Fax. (705)670-9208.

RIGLEY, Joe; 7-635 Water St, Miramichi NB E1N 4B9; Mem'08; FRCPC; IntMed.

RIIVES, Mai Liis; The Nova Scotia Hosp, PO Box 1004 Stn Main, Dartmouth NS B2Y 3Z9; Dal'85; Staff, The Nova Scotia Hospital; Langs: Estonian; (902)464-3111

RIJO, Santos; 17-200 Whitmore Rd, Woodbridge ON L4L 7K4; Buenos Aires (Argentina)'75; Langs: Italian; Spanish; (905)265-1075; Fax. (905)265-1077.

RIKHYE, Rakesh K; Canes Family Health Team, 120-135 Queen's Plate Dr, Etobicoke ON M9W 6V1; Tor'79; Ac Staff, William Osler Health System - Etobicoke General Hospital; Langs: Hindi; Punjabi; (416)342-5140; Fax. (416)342-5148.

RILEY, G Terence; Halton HSC Corp-Oakville, 327 Reynolds St, Oakville ON L6J 3L7; Tor'60; BPHE; Member Family Med Obstetrics Group, Halton Healthcare Services Corporation - Oakville Site; (905)845-2571

RILEY, Jennifer F; St Michael's Hosp, 30 Bond St, Toronto ON M5B 1W8; Dal'96; FRCPC; EmergMed. Staff, St Michael's Hospital; (416)864-5095

RILEY, Mark E; 261 Carleton St PO Box 784, Shelburne NS B0T 1W0; Alb'81; (902)875-2868; Fax. (902)265-2048; mr@rosewaymanor.com.

RILEY, Mark P; Surrey Regional Forensic Clin, 10022 King George Blvd, Surrey BC V3T 2W4; Nottingham (England)'82; MB BS; BMedSci; MPhil; MRCPsy; FRCPC; Psy (Forensic Psychiatry). Staff/Psychiatrist, Forensic Psychiatric Hospital; Clin Instructor, University of British Columbia; (604)529-3300; mriley@forensic.bc.ca.

RILEY, Mark R; Northmount Med Centre, 303-145 13th St E, North Vancouver BC V7L 2L4; Dal'98; FRCPC; Peds (Pediatric Gastroenterology); Gastroent. Associate Pediatric Gastroenterology, BC Children's Hospital; Staff Peds, Lions Gate Hospital; (604)984-8880; Fax. (604)984-8887; ebbesonriley@hotmail.com.

RILEY, Sheilagh P; MUHC-Montreal Children's Hosp, A611-2300 rue Tupper, Montreal QC H3H 1P3; McG'72; FRCPC; Peds (Neonatology). Staff, McGill University Health Centre - Montreal Children's Hospital; Langs: Bilingual(French/English); (514)412-4302; Fax. (514)412-4356.

RILEY, Sheryl A; 299 Main St N PO Box 520, Callander ON P0H 1H0; Qns'98; Staff, North Bay Regional Health Centre - Regional Mental Health; (705)752-1004

RIMMER, Arthur T; A-921 Canada Ave, Duncan BC V9L 1V2; UBC'95; CCFP; FCFP; (250)709-9090

RIMMER, Emily K; CancerCare Manitoba, 675 McDermot Ave, Winnipeg MB R3E 0V9; Man'06; FRCPC; IntMed; Hem.

RIMMER, Isabel N; Cowichan District Hosp, 3045 Gibbins Rd, Duncan BC V9L 1E5; UBC'89; CCFP; CCFP(E.M.); Staff, Cowichan District Hospital; (250)746-1845

RIMMER, Karen P; Peter Lougheed Centre, 3500 26 Ave NE, Calgary AB T1Y 6J4; Cal'80; FRCPC; IntMed (Critical Care Medicine); Respir. Staff, Peter Lougheed Centre; Assoc Prof, University of Calgary; (403)943-5635; Fax. (403)943-4848.

RIMMER, Tara J; Misericordia Comm Hosp & H C, 16940 87 Ave NW, Edmonton AB T5R 4H5; Cal'05; FRCPC; Anes. Staff, Covenant Health - Misericordia Community Hospital; (780)735-2863; Fax. (780)437-1880.

RINALDI, Brent D; Carry Drive Med Centre, 116 Carry Dr SE, Medicine Hat AB T1B 3Z8; McG'84; FRCSC; Ophth. (403)502-8927; Fax. (403)504-4406.

RINALDI, Fredrykka D; 102-266 4 St SW, Medicine Hat AB T1A 4E5; Dal'89; CCFP; FCFP; (403)526-3400; Fax. (403)526-3496.

RINDLISBACHER, Timothy J; Brookfield Place, 3000-181 Bay St, Toronto ON M5J 2T3; Tor'92; BSc(PT); Dip SportMed; Staff, Sunnybrook Health Sciences Centre; (416)507-6600

RINFRET, Joanie; CLSC Lennox, 8 rue Speid, Sherbrooke QC J1M 1R6; Sher'08; CCFP; (819)780-2222

RINFRET, Stephane; Hôpital Laval, 2725 ch Sainte-Foy, Quebec QC G1V 4G5; Mon'92; FRCP; CSPQ; LMCC; MSc; FRCPC; IntMed (Epidemiology); Cardiol. Staff, Hôpital Laval; Prof, Université Laval; Langs: English; (418)656-8711; stephane.rinfret@criucpq.ulaval.ca.

RING, Heather L; 305-400 Tache Ave, Winnipeg MB R2H 3C3; Man'01; FRCSC; ObstGyn.

RING, Melanie S; 1278 Bedford Hwy, Bedford NS B4A 1C7; Dal'88; BSc; FRCPC; Psy (Adult Psychiatry). (902)444-7533; Fax. (902)444-7534.

RING, Roger D; Alder Med Centre, 277 Evergreen Rd, Campbell River BC V9W 5Y4; Alb'69; BSc; FRCSC; GenSurg. Ac Staff, Campbell River & District General Hospital; (250)287-7441; Fax. (250)287-4384.

RING, Todd J; Royal Inland Hosp, 311 Columbia st, Kamloops BC V2C 2T1; UBC'01; CCFP; CCFP(E.M.); Staff EmergMed, Royal Inland Hospital; (250)374-5111

RINGAERT, Kenneth R A; Health Sciences Ctr Gen Hosp, 700 William Ave, Winnipeg MB R3E 0Z3; Man'81; FRCPC; Anes. Staff, Health Sciences Centre; (204)787-3796; Fax. (204)787-3656.

RINGASH, Jolie G; Univ Hlth Network-Princess M, 610 University Ave, Toronto ON M5G 2M9; McM'93; MSc; BSc; FRCPC; RadOncol (Clinical Epidemiology). Staff RadOncol, Princess Margaret Hospital - University Health Network; Asst Prof RadOncol/Assoc Prof, University of Toronto; (416)946-2126; Fax. (416)946-2111.

RINGER, Kenneth; Carbonear Gen Hosp, 86 Highroad South, Carbonear NL A1Y 1A4; Mem'01; Staff, Carbonear General Hospital; (709)945-5111

RINGNALDA, Jacqueline; Victoria Health Centre, 521 Victoria Park Ave, Scarborough ON M4C 5H1; Tor'81; CCFP; FCFP; Ac Staff, The Scarborough Hospital - General Campus; Teach Staff, University of Toronto; (416)694-1400; Fax. (416)694-1985; ringnalda@rogers.com.

RINGROSE, Heather M; 200 Hospital Dr, Moose Factory ON P0L 1W0; Cal'07; CCFP; (705)658-4544

RINGROSE, Jennifer S; University of Alberta Hosp, 2F1 12-8440 112 St NW, Edmonton AB T6G 2B7; Cal'04; FRCPC; IntMed. Staff, University of Alberta Hospital; Staff, Covenant Health - Grey Nuns Community Hospital; (780)407-7055; Fax. (780)407-3132.

RINGUET, Jacques; MSSS-Dir Gen SS et Med Univ, 2400 av d'Estimauville, Quebec QC G1E 7G9; Laval'71; CSPQ; CommunMed (P.Q.) (Administrative Medicine). Staff, Centre Hospitalier Universitaire de Quebec-CHUL; Staff, Centre Hospitalier Universitaire de Québec (CHUQ) - Siege Social; (418)666-7000 x325; Fax. (418)666-2776; jacques.ringuet@ssss.gouv.qc.ca.

RINGUET, Jean; Ctr Hosp Affilie-Enfant-Jesus, 1401 18e rue, Quebec QC G1J 1Z4; Laval'81; Staff, Centre Hospitalier Affilié Universitaire de Québec - Hôpital De L'Enfant Jésus; (418)649-5632; Fax. (418)649-5975.

RINGUET, Serge; CLSC-CHSLD la Source, 190 76e rue E, Quebec QC G1H 7K4; Laval'78; (418)628-2572

RINGUETTE, Francois; CSSS de Sept-Iles, 45 rue du Pere-Divet, Sept-Iles QC G4R 3N7; Mon'08; CCFP; Staff, Centre Hospitalier Regional de Sept-Iles; (418)962-9761

RINGUETTE, Gaetan; CSSS de Laval, 1755 boul Rene-Laennec, Laval QC H7M 3L9; Mon'74; ABIM; AB; Cardiol; IntMed (P.Q.) (Adult Cardiology). Staff, Hopital de la Cite de la santé; (450)975-5307; Fax. (450)975-5550.

RINGUETTE, Julie; CSSS du Nord de Lanaudière, 1000 boul Sainte-Anne, St-Charles-Brromee QC J6E 6J2; Mon'92; ABR; LMCC; CSPQ; FRCPC; DiagRad. Staff, Centre Hospitalier Régional de Lanaudière; (450)759-8222; Fax. (450)759-2133.

RINGUETTE, Patricia; CSSS ded Rimouski-Niegette, CP 3150 Succ A 150 av Rouleau, Rimouski QC G5L 5T1; Laval'00; CSPQ; FRCPC; Anes. Staff, Hôpital Regional Rimouski; (418)723-7851

RINGWALD, Pierre; 148 Maclaren St, Ottawa ON K2P 0K9; Mon'68; DABD; FAAD; CSPQ; FRCPC; Derm. Staff Derm, The Ottawa Hospital - General Campus; Lecturer Med, University of Ottawa; Langs: English; French; (613)236-3126

RINHOLM, Larry E; Medicine Hat Reg Hosp, 666 5 St SW, Medicine Hat AB T1A 4H6; Sask'83; CCFP; Staff, Medicine Hat Regional Hospital; (403)529-8000

RININSLAND, H Volker; Stadacona Med Group, 202-53 Stadacona St W, Moose Jaw SK S6H 1Z2; Sask'81; CCFP; Assoc Prof Family Med, University of Saskatchewan; Langs: German; (306)693-0877; Fax. (306)693-3677; rossstclinic@sasktel.net.

RINN, Richard W; Southlake Reg Health Centre, 596 Davis Dr, Newmarket ON L3Y 2P9; Tor'77; FRCPC; AnatPath. Staff, Southlake Regional Health Centre; (905)895-4521 x2319; Fax. (905)952-2824; rrinn@southlakeregional.org.

RINNE, Claus H E; Medical Bldg, 202-18 Pine St, Kitchener ON N2H 5Z8; Qns'81; FRCPC; IntMed; Cardiol. Ac Staff, Grand River Hospital - Kitchener/Waterloo Health Centre; Med Dir Cardiac Care Prog, St Mary's General Hospital; (519)741-8660; Fax. (519)741-1657.

RIOLO, Giovanna; Kingston Gen Hosp, 76 Stuart St, Kingston ON K7L 2V7; McM'08; IntMed. Staff, Kingston General Hospital; (613)548-3232

RIOME-YORK, Sasha A; Northern Health Authority, 908-299 Victoria St, Prince George BC V2L 5B8; Sask'00; CCFP; (250)563-4706; Fax. (250)563-4549.

RIOPEL, Caroline; CHUQ-Hotel-Dieu de Quebec, 11 Cote du Palais, Quebec QC G1R 2J6; Laval'04; IntMed. Staff, Centre Hospitalier Universitaire de Québec (CHUQ) - Siege Social; (418)525-4444 x23652

RIOPEL, Jocelyn; 288 boul Larochelle, Repentigny QC J6A 8K4; Mon'77; Staff, Centre Hospitalier Pierre le Gardeur; (450)581-2120

RIOPEL, Julie; CHUQ-Hotel-Dieu de Quebec, 11 Cote du Palais, Quebec QC G1R 2J6; Sher'01; FRCPC; AnatPath (Nephropathology). Staff, Centre Hospitalier Universitaire de Québec (CHUQ) - Siege Social; Langs: Bilingual(French/English); (418)525-4444 x15233; Fax. (418)691-5226.

RIOPEL, M Eve; Cite de la Sante de Laval, 1755 boul Rene-Laennec, Laval QC H7M 3L9; Mon'04; FRCPC; Peds. Staff, Hopital de la Cite de la santé; (450)668-1010

RIOPEL, Mathieu; CSSS de Memphremagog, 50 rue Saint-Parice E, Magog QC J1X 3X3; Mon'08; CCFP; Staff, Centre Hospitalier et CLSC de Memphremagog; (819)843-2292; Fax. (819)868-3285.

RIOPELLE, Richard J; Kingston Gen Hosp, 76 Stuart St, Kingston ON K7L 2V7; Ott'68; FRCPC; IntMed (Movement Disorders); Neur. Staff, Kingston General Hospital; Langs: English; French; (613)548-3232; Fax. (613)548-2471.

RIORDON, Michele A; 47 West St S, Orillia ON L3V 5G2; Tor'06; FRCSC; GenSurg.

RIOU, Emilie; CHUS-Hop Fleurimont, 3001 12e av N, Sherbrooke QC J1H 5N4; Sher'02; FRCPC; Neur. Staff, Centre Hospitalier Universitaire de Sherbrooke-Hopital Fleurimont; (819)346-1110

RIOUX, Andre; GMF Concorde, 300 boul de la Concorde E, Laval QC H7G 2E6; Mon'73; Staff, Hopital de la Cite de la santé; (450)667-5310; Fax. (450)667-5248.

RIOUX, Caroline; CSSS de Temiscouata, CP 310 58 rue de l'Eglise, Notre-Dame-du-Lac QC G0L 1X0; Laval'07; Staff, Centre Hospitalier Notre-Dame-du-Lac; (418)899-6751

RIOUX, Celine; Centre de Sante Hydro-Quebec, 333 boul Jean-Paul-Hogue, Saint-Jerome QC J7Z 6Y3; Laval'73; (450)565-2210 x2075; Fax. (450)565-2184.

RIOUX, Dany; 5050 boul des Forges, Trois-Rivieres QC G8Y 1X2; Sher'88; Endocrin&Metab; Endocrin (P.Q.); IntMed. (819)379-1442

RIOUX, Denis; Centre Med Durocher, 140 rue Saint-Vallier O, Quebec QC G1K 1K1; Laval'78; (418)529-0291; Fax. (418)529-7405.

RIOUX, Germain; Clinique Med St-Laurent, 202-500 Rte Marie-Victorin, Sorel-Tracy QC J3R 1K7; Sher'77; Staff Palliative Care, Hôtel-Dieu de Sorel; (450)742-9818; Fax. (450)742-9795.

RIOUX, Gisele; CLSC de Saint-Jerome, 1000 rue Labelle, Saint-Jerome QC J7Z 5N6; Sher'87; Physician, Clinique Medicale de St-Hippolyte; Langs: Bilingual(French/English); (450)431-8001

RIOUX, Guylaine; Loto-Quebec, 500 rue Sherbrooke O, Montreal QC H3A 3G6; Laval'85; VP Partenariat et a l'Expertise-Conseil, Commission Sante Securite Travail; (514)499-8666; guylaine.rioux@csst.qc.ca.

RIOUX, Jean-Philippe; Hop du Sacre-Coeur de Mtl, 5400 boul Gouin O, Montreal QC H4J 1C5; Mon'03; FRCPC; IntMed; Nephrol. Staff, Hôpital du Sacre-Coeur de Montréal; (514)338-2883; Fax. (514)338-2182.

RIOUX, Johanne; Hop Charles LeMoyne, 3120 boul Taschereau, Greenfield Park QC J4V 2H1; Sher'90; CSPQ; FRCPC; Psy (External Clinic). Staff Psy, Hopital Charles LeMoyne; Langs: English; (450)466-5020; Fax. (450)466-5015.

RIOUX, Julie; CSSS de Laval, 1755 boul Rene-Laennec, Laval QC H7M 3L9; Laval'06; Staff, Hopital de la Cite de la santé; (450)975-5445

RIOUX, Kevin P; HSC-Faculty of Med, 1863-3330 Hospital Dr NW, Calgary AB T2N 4N1; Cal'99; PhD; FRCPC; IntMed (Inflammatory Bowel Disease); Gastroent. Asst Prof, University of Calgary; (403)220-8457; Fax. (403)270-0995.

RIOUX, Leon; CSSS de Rimouski-Neigette, CP 3150 Succ A 150 av Rouleau, Rimouski QC G5L 5T1; Laval'96; FRCPC; IntMed; Cardiol. Staff, Hôpital Regional Rimouski; (418)723-7851

RIOUX, Louis C; Hop Maisonneuve-Rosemont, 5415 boul de l'Assomption, Montreal QC H1T 2M4; Mon'86; ABIM; FRCPC; IntMed; Gastroent. Staff, Hopital Maisonneuve-Rosemont; (514)252-3400; Fax. (514)252-3486.

RIOUX, Marie-Claude; 203-3400 rue du Marche, Dollard-D-Ormeaux QC H9B 2Y1; Laval'92; Staff, Hôpital de Saint-Eustache; (514)685-3531; Fax. (514)685-7971.

RIOUX, Marie-Claude; Centre Med Montpellier, 4A rue du Bosquet, Montpellier QC J0V 1M0; Mon'92; CCFP; (819)428-2967; m-c_rioux@ssss.gouv.qc.ca.

RIOUX, Marie-France; CHUS-Hop Fleurimont, 3001 12e av N, Sherbrooke QC J1H 5N4; Sher'97; FRCPC; Neur (Neuro Genetics). Staff, Centre Hospitalier Universitaire de Sherbrooke-Hopital Fleurimont; Langs: English; (819)346-1110; Fax. (819)564-5395.

RIOUX, Martin; Hotel-Dieu de Roberval, 450 rue Brassard, Roberval QC G8H 1B9; Mon'92; Consultant Mortalite & Morbidite, Hotel-Dieu de Roberval; (418)275-0110

RIOUX, Michel; Ctr Hosp de Matane, 333 rue Thibault, Matane QC G4W 2W5; Laval'79; CSPQ; DiagRad. Staff, Centre Hospitalier de Matane; (418)562-3135

RIOUX, Samuel; CSSS de Trois-Rivières, 1991 boul du Carmel, Trois-Rivieres QC G8Z 3R9; Mon'06; CCFP; Staff, CSSS de Trois-Rivières; (819)697-3333

RIOUX, Stephane; UMF Laval CSSSVC, 2690 ch des Quatre-Bourgeois, Quebec QC G1V 0B7; Laval'90; Staff, Hôpital Laval; (418)656-4795; Fax. (418)656-4503.

RIOUX-MASSÉ, Benjamin; CHUM-Hop Notre-Dame, 1560 rue Sherbrooke E, Montreal QC H2L 4M1; Mon'03; FRCPC; IntMed; Hem. Staff, Centre Hospitalier l'Université de Montréal (CHUM) - Hôpital Notre-Dame; (514)890-8000

RIPLEY, Carl D; 1145 Carling Ave, Ottawa ON K1Z 7K4; Sask'76; FRCPC; Psy (Psychological Social Rehabilitation). Ac Staff Psy, Royal Ottawa Mental Health Centre - Royal Ottawa Health Care Group; (613)722-6521 x7050; Fax. (613)798-2988; carl.ripley@theroyal.ca.

RIPLEY, David K; Victoria Gen Hosp, 1 Hospital Way, Victoria BC V8Z 6R5; Sask'75; Staff, Victoria General Hospital; (250)727-4212

RIPLEY, Sharon A; White Hills Med Clinic, 262 Newfoundland Dr, St. John's NL A1A 3R5; Mem'78; BMedSci; Court Staff Privil Ambulatory Care Prog, Health Sciences Centre; Court Staff Privil Ambulatory Care Prog, St Clare's Mercy Hospital; Med Advisor, V.O.N., St. John's Branch; (709)753-1091; Fax. (709)753-1087.

RIPLEY, Susan M; Queen Elizabeth II HSC-Halifax, 1796 Summer St, Halifax NS B3H 3A7; Dal'08; CCFP; Staff, Queen Elizabeth II Health Sciences Centre - Halifax Infirmary Site; (902)473-6651

RIPLEY, Teresa M; Lions Gate Hosp, 231 15 St E, North Vancouver BC V7L 2L7; Cal'07; Anes. Staff, Lions Gate Hospital; (604)984-5987

RIPSTEIN, Ira T; St Boniface Gen Hosp, 409 Tache Ave, Winnipeg MB R2H 2A6; Man'80; MSc; Staff, St Boniface General Hospital; Assoc Dean Undergraduate Med Education, University of Manitoba; (204)237-2260; Fax. (204)237-2268.

RISDON, Catherine L; McMaster Family Practice, A-690 Main St W, Hamilton ON L8S 1A4; McM'92; CCFP; FCFP; Prof Family Med, McMaster University; (905)521-5016; Fax. (905)521-5010; risdonc@mcmaster.ca.

RISDON, James; NB College of Family Phys of C, 950 av Picot, Bathurst NB E2A 4Z9; (506)548-4707; Fax. (506)548-4761.

RISHI, B Jane; 314-3001 Tutt St, Kelowna BC V1Y 2H4; Alb'94; CCFP; (250)763-0101; Fax. (250)763-0114.

RISI, Catherine; Direction de la Sante Publique, 1255 rue Beauregard, Longueuil QC J4K 2M3; Laval'83; (450)928-6777 x3009

RISK, Paul J; Radiology Consultants Assoc, 120-6707 Elbow Dr SW, Calgary AB T2V 0E3; Dal'88; FRCPC; DiagRad. (403)777-3007; Fax. (403)777-3008.

RISKALLA, Frey F F; Jim Pattison Outpatient Care, 950 140 St, Surrey BC V3T 0G9; Ain Shams (Egypt)'98; MB ChB; CCFP; Staff, Surrey Memorial Hospital; (604)582-4585

RISKE, David M; Beaumont Family Med Associates, 4-5102 49 Ave, Beaumont AB T4X 1E4; Alb'84; (780)929-5400; Fax. (780)929-2126; d.riske@shaw.ca.

RISKIN, Ashley E; 205-2786 16th Ave W, Vancouver BC V6K 4M1; UBC'05; CCFP; (604)733-4400

RISLER, Marie-Claude; CSSS de la Haute-Yamaska, 205 boul Leclerc O, Granby QC J2G 1T7; Laval'95; Staff, Centre Hospitalier de Granby; (450)372-5491; Fax. (450)372-7197.

RISLING, Eva M; Kitsilano Mental Health Team, 400-1212 Broadway W, Vancouver BC V6H 3V1; Wes'86; FRCPC; Psy (Adult Psychiatry). (604)736-2881

RISMAN, Jared P; Mackenzie Richmond Hill Hosp, 10 Trench St, Richmond Hill ON L4C 4Z3; Wes'97; FRCPC; Psy. Staff, Mackenzie Richmond Hill Hospital; (905)832-1406

RISSANEN, John T; Royal Victoria Hosp, 201 Georgian Dr, Barrie ON L4M 6M2; McM'00; FRCPC; Anes. Staff, Royal Victoria Regional Health Centre; (705)728-9802

RISTEVSKI, Bill; Hamilton HS-General Site, 532-237 Barton St E, Hamilton ON L8L 2X2; Tor'04; MSc; FRCSC; OrthSurg (Trauma). Staff Orthopaedic Surg, Hamilton Health Sciences Centre - Hamilton General Hospital; Asst Prof, McMaster University; (905)527-4322 x44266; Fax. (905)577-8271.

RISTIC, Miodrag A; 4-500 Manning Rd, Windsor ON N8N 5H3; Belgrade (Serbia)'53; VascSurg; GenSurg. Ac Staff, Windsor Regional Hospital - Tayfour Site; Langs: Serbian; (519)979-2235; Fax. (519)979-4890.

RISTOSKI, Nikolce; Children's Hosp Eastern Ont, 401 Smyth Rd, Ottawa ON K1H 8L1; Wes'03; Peds. Staff, Children's Hospital of Eastern Ontario (CHEO); (613)737-7600

RITACCA, Frank V; Credit Valley Prof Bldg, 509-2300 Eglinton Ave W, Mississauga ON L5M 2V8; Tor'99; FRCPC; IntMed; Critical Care Medicine; Respir. (905)569-7600

RITCEY, Susan G; Health Park, 201-45 Weatherbee Rd, Mira Road NS B1M 0A1; Dal'90; Staff, Cape Breton Healthcare Complex.

RITCHIE, Alec H; Lions Gate Hosp, 231 15th St E, North Vancouver BC V7L 2L7; UBC'89; CCFP; CCFP(E.M.); FCFP; Staff Emerg, Lions Gate Hospital; (604)984-5799

RITCHIE, Andrew C; City Centre Family Physicians, 500-71 King St W, Mississauga ON L5B 4A2; Alb'84; Court Staff Family Med, Trillium Health Centre - Mississauga; (905)273-3176; Fax. (905)848-1500.

RITCHIE, Blair D; Foothills Med Centre, 1403 29 St NW, Calgary AB T2N 2T9; Qns'04; FRCPC; Psy. Staff, Foothills Medical Centre; (403)944-2489; Fax. (403)283-1563.

RITCHIE, Brian; Markham Professional Centre, 207-2265 Pembina Hwy, Winnipeg MB R3T 5J3; Alb'75; FRCSC; Urol. Staff, Victoria General Hospital; (204)233-8727; Fax. (204)233-3390.

RITCHIE, Brian D; Ermineskin Med Clinic, 301-2377 111 St NW, Edmonton AB T6J 5E5; Alb'79; CCFP; Ac Staff Family Med, Covenant Health - Grey Nuns Community Hospital; Clin Instructor Community Based, University of Alberta; (780)436-8731; Fax. (780)434-8732.

RITCHIE, D Bruce C; Medical Sciences Bldg, 4 71-131 University Campus NW, Edmonton AB T6G 2H7; Alb'78; FRCPC; IntMed; Hem; MedOncol. Staff, University of Alberta Hospital; (780)492-3550; Fax. (780)492-8767.

RITCHIE, Hendrica; Univ of Western Ontario, 1151 Richmond St, London ON N6A 3K7; McM'06; FRCPC; Psy. (519)661-3030; Fax. (519)661-3380.

RITCHIE, J W Knox; The Ontario Hydro Bldg, 3286-700 University Ave, Toronto ON M5G 1Z5; Belfast (Ireland)'68; FRCOG; FRCSC; ObstGyn (Maternal Fetal Medicine). Staff, Mount Sinai Hospital; Prof Obstetrics & Gyn, University of Toronto; (416)586-5309; Fax. (416)586-8740.

RITCHIE, Janet; Seaforth Med Bldg, 645-3550 ch de la Cote-des-Nei, Montreal QC H3H 1V4; McG'90; CSPQ; FRCPC; Psy. Langs: English; French; (514)937-6076

RITCHIE, Janet; St James Street Med Clinic, 1600 Portage Ave, Winnipeg MB R3J 0C6; Man'81; CCFP; (204)774-1868; Fax. (204)774-7303.

RITCHIE, John D; Telus Plaza South, 2700-10020 100 St NW, Edmonton AB T5J 0N3; Alb'77; Clin Teacher Family Med, University of Alberta; (780)969-4962

RITCHIE, Laura C; Hamilton HS-General Site, 237 Barton St E, Hamilton ON L8L 2X2; Qns'07; CCFP; Staff, Hamilton Health Sciences Centre - Hamilton General Hospital; (905)521-2100

RITCHIE, R Gordon; Merivale Med Imaging, 502-751 Parkdale Ave, Ottawa ON K1Y 1J7; Tor'83; FRCPC; DiagRad (Diagnostic Imaging). Radiologist (All Sites), The Ottawa Hospital - Civic Campus; Asst Prof Radiol, University of Ottawa; (613)798-5555; Fax. (613)761-4865; gritchie@ottawahospital.on.ca.

RITCHIE, William L; Hys Med Centre, 202-11010 101 St NW, Edmonton AB T5H 4B9; Man'74; FRCPC; DiagRad. Staff Radiol, Royal Alexandra Hospital; (780)426-1121; Fax. (780)425-5979.

RITENBURG, David L; Nicola Med Dental Bldg, 300-321 Nicola St, Kamloops BC V2C 6G6; Sask'72; Staff, Royal Inland Hospital; (250)372-2244; Fax. (250)372-8146.

RITENBURG, Hannelore; Nicola Med Dental Bldg, 301-321 Nicola St, Kamloops BC V2C 6G6; Sask'72; Ac Staff, Royal Inland Hospital; (250)374-5061; Fax. (250)374-1348.

RITENOUR, Rusty J; Victoria Bldg, 2035-1276 South Park St, Halifax NS B3H 2Y9; Cal'03; FRCPC; Ophth. (902)473-3764; Fax. (902)473-2839.

RITONJA, Laura M; Ocean Pier Med Centre, 207-2537 Beacon Ave, Sidney BC V8L 1Y3; Qns'96; CCFP; FCFP; (250)656-4114

RITSMA, Lindsay R; Civic Family Med Centre, 210 Melrose Ave, Ottawa ON K1Y 4K7; Wes'10; CCFP; (613)761-4334

RITTENBERG, David A; IWK Health Centre, PO Box 9700 Rpo CSC 5858-5980 University Ave, Halifax NS B3K 6R8; Wes'93; FRCSC; ObstGyn (Minimal Invasive Surgery). Staff, IWK Health Centre; Asst Prof, Dalhousie University; (902)470-7791; Fax. (902)470-8640; david.rittenberg@iwk.nshealth.ca.

RITTENBERG, Kevin M; 3-7700 Bathurst St, Thornhill ON L4J 7Y3; Tor'88; BSc; FCFP; CCFP; FCFP; Court Staff, North York General Hospital; Court Staff, Kirkland & District Hospital; Med Consultant, Toronto Star; Med Consultant, Sanofi Pasteur Ltd; (905)660-9760; Fax. (905)660-9762.

RITTENBERG, Paula V C; 5005-5820 University Ave, Halifax NS B3H 1V7; Wes'93; FRCSC; ObstGyn (Palliative Care); GynOnco. Asst Prof ObstGyn, Dalhousie University; (902)473-4029; Fax. (902)473-7765; paularittenberg@dal.ca.

RITTENHOUSE, Bryan R; Professional Artd Bldg, 2E-570 King St, Welland ON L3B 3L2; Alb'78; FRCSC; OrthSurg. (905)735-7079

RITTER, Douglas J; Carling-Broadview Med Bldg, 202-770 Broadview Ave, Ottawa ON K2A 3Z3; Qns'70; FRCSC; OrthSurg (Trauma/Joint Replacement). Chief Orthopedics, Queensway Carleton Hospital; Staff, Pembroke Regional Hospital Inc; Staff, Kemptville District Hospital; (613)728-8372; Fax. (613)728-8465.

RITTER, John A; Cape Breton Hlthcare Complex, 1482 George St, Sydney NS B1P 1P3; Cincinnati(OH) (USA)'89; CCFP; Staff, Cape Breton Healthcare Complex; (902)567-8000

RITTER, Kurt A; Cowichan Dist Hosp, 3045 Gibbins Rd, Duncan BC V9L 1E5; Cambridge (England)'96; MB ChB; BSc(Hons.); FRCPC; Anes. Staff, Cowichan District Hospital; (250)746-4141; Fax. (250)746-4247; ritterkurt@hotmail.com.

RIVAL, Richard A; 104-581 Davis Dr, Newmarket ON L3Y 2P6; Tor'89; ABFPS; FRCSC; Otol (Facial Plastic Surgery). Staff, Mackenzie Richmond Hill Hospital; Staff, Southlake Regional Health Centre; Staff, St Michael's Hospital; Clin Instructor, University of Toronto; (905)898-2444; Fax. (905)898-5558; rrival3@rogers.com.

RIVARD, Alain; CHUM-Hop Notre-Dame, 1560 rue Sherbrooke E, Montreal QC H2L 4M1; Mon'90; FRCPC; IntMed (Hemodynamics); Cardiol. Staff Cardiol, Centre Hospitalier l'Université de Montréal (CHUM) - Hôpital Notre-Dame; Prof adj clin, Universite de Montreal; (514)890-8000

RIVARD, Andre; 203-895 boul du Seminaire N, St-Jean-Sur-Richel QC J3A 1J2; Laval'69; (450)348-7744; Fax. (450)348-9722.

RIVARD, Andre; Ctr Cardiovasculaire Rive-Sud, 200-1615 boul Jacques-Cartier, Longueuil QC J4M 2X1; Mon'81; FRCPC; IntMed; Cardiol (P.Q.). (450)674-2345; Fax. (450)674-1622.

RIVARD, Chantal; Hop Maisonneuve-Rosemont, 5415 boul de l'Assomption, Montreal QC H1T 2M4; Mon'91; FRCSC; ObstGyn. Staff, Hopital Maisonneuve-Rosemont; (514)252-3400

RIVARD, Charles H; Hôpital Ste-Justine, 3175 ch Cote-Sainte-Catherine, Montreal QC H3T 1C5; Laval'69; FAAOS; FACS; FRCSC; OrthSurg (Scoliosis). Chef chirg ortho, Hôpital Ste-Justine; Scientist/Dir, Paradigm Spine; Prof Surg, Universite de Montreal; Langs: English; (514)345-4839; Fax. (514)345-2353; chrivard@gmail.com.

RIVARD, Claude; CSSS Pierre Boucher, 1333 boul Jacques-Cartier E, Longueuil QC J4M 2A5; Mon'93; CCFP; Chef Emerg Serv/Med Coord, Centre Hospitalier Pierre Boucher; (450)468-8111; clomi@videotron.ca.

RIVARD, Georges E; Hôpital Ste-Justine, 3175 ch Cote-Sainte-Catherine, Montreal QC H3T 1C5; Mon'67; MedOncol (P.Q.); Hem; Peds. Ac Staff, Hôpital Ste-Justine; Staff, McGill University Health Centre - Montreal General Campus; (514)345-4931 x6717

RIVARD, Lena I C; Intitut de Cardiologie de Mtl, 5000 rue Belanger, Montreal QC H1T 1C8; Claude Bernard(Lyon I) (France)'03; Cardiol (P.Q.). Staff, Institut de Cardiologie de Montréal; (514)376-3330

RIVARD, Louise-Isabelle; Institut de Cardiologie de Mtl, 5000 rue Belanger, Montreal QC H1T 1C8; Mon'99; ACLS; BSc; MSc; MB; MCFP; CCFP; Staff Emerg Med, Institut de Cardiologie de Montréal; Langs: Bilingual(English/French); (514)376-3330; l.i.rivard@videotron.ca.

RIVARD, Lyne; CHUS-Hop Fleurimont, 3001 12e av N, Sherbrooke QC J1H 5N4; Sher'84; FRCPC; Peds. Ac Staff, Centre Hospitalier Universitaire de Sherbrooke-Hopital Fleurimont; (819)346-1110; Fax. (819)564-5398.

RIVARD, Marc; Westmount Square Med Centre, 500-1 car Westmount, Westmount QC H3Z 2P9; Mon'92; (514)934-2334

RIVARD, Marc-Antoine; CSSS de la Haute-Yamaska, 205 boul Leclerc O, Granby QC J2G 1T7; Sher'06; FRCPC; IntMed. Staff, Centre Hospitalier de Granby; (450)375-8000

RIVARD, Marie; Clinique Familiale St-Lambert, 209 rue Woodstock, Saint-Lambert QC J4P 1W7; Mon'87; Staff, Centre Hospitalier Pierre Boucher; (450)466-8583; Fax. (450)466-4072.

RIVARD, Marie-Chantale; 227-655 Prom du Centropilis, Laval QC H7T 0A3; Mon'91; CCFP; (514)316-1357; Fax. (514)890-1135.

RIVARD, Paul; CSSS Rocher-Perce, GD 633 rue Daignault, Chandler QC G0C 1K0; Laval'87; CSPQ; FRCPC; Psy. Staff, Centre Hospitalier de Chandler; Langs: Bilingual(French/English); (418)689-2261

RIVARD, Sophie; Clin de Med Familiale Saguenay, 220-874 boul de l'Universite E, Chicoutimi QC G7H 6B9; Mon'98; Staff, Complexe hospitalier de la Sagamie; (418)545-1217; Fax. (418)545-4782.

RIVAS, Jose A; 300-900 boul du Seminaire N, St-Jean-sur-Richel QC J3A 1C3; Mexico (Mexico)'69; Staff, Hôpital du Haut-Richelieu; Langs: English; French; (450)348-2747

RIVAS HERNANDEZ, Juan-Hector; Sackville Sports Stadium, PO Box 625 Lcd Lower Sackville 409 Glendale Rd, Lower Sackville NS B4C 3J1; (El Salvador)'77; (902)864-0056; Fax. (902)484-7387.

RIVEN, Linda; 49-4324 rue Sherbrooke O, Westmount QC H3Z 1E1; McG'70; CSPQ; FRCPC; Psy. Langs: French; Italian; (514)932-2443; Fax. (514)935-4484.

RIVERA, Juan A; MUHC-Montrel Gen Hosp, C6.129-1650 av Cedar, Montreal QC H3G 1A4; Caracas (Venezuela)'92; CSPQ; FACE; LMCC; Endocrin&Metab (Tumor). Endocrinologue, McGill University Health Centre - Montreal General Campus; Staff Endocrinology, McGill University Health Centre - Royal Victoria Hospital; assoc Prof, McGill University; Langs: Spanish; (514)934-1934 x31510; Fax. (514)982-0825; juan.rivera@mcgill.ca.

RIVERA, Karen A; UBC Student Health Services, M334-2211 Wesbrook Mall, Vancouver BC V6T 2B5; McM'07; FRCPC; Psy. (604)822-7689

RIVERA, Loida R; 1195 Davie St, Vancouver BC V6E 1N2; UBC'05; FRCSC; ObstGyn. Staff, BC Women's Hospital & Health Centre; (604)875-2161

RIVERA, Raymond F; St Boniface Gen Hosp, 409 Tache Ave, Winnipeg MB R2H 2A6; Man'97; FRCPC; AnatPath. Staff, St Boniface General Hospital; (204)233-8563; riverar@brandonrha.mb.ca.

RIVERIN, Karine; CLSC Kateri, 90 boul Marie-Victorin, Candiac QC J5R 1C1; Laval'07; CCFP; (450)699-3333

RIVERIN, Sylvie; Hotel-Dieu de Levis, 143 rue Wolfe, Levis QC G6V 3Z1; Laval'82; CSPQ; Psy. Staff, Hôtel-Dieu de Lévis; (418)835-7155

RIVERO PINELO, Luis; Pontiac Health Centre, 200 rue Argue, Shawville QC J0X 2Y0; Tucuman (Argentina)'78; CCFP; FCFP; Staff, Pontiac Hospital Centre; Preceptor, University of Ottawa; Preceptor, McGill University; Langs: French; Spanish; (819)647-2271; luis.riveropinelo@mcgill.ca.

RIVEROS NEIRA, Luis G; 5-679 King George Hwy, Miramichi NB E1V 1N9; Bogota (Colombia)'93; Staff Ophth, Miramichi Regional Hospital; Langs: Spanish; (506)627-1919; Fax. (506)627-1798.

RIVERS, Angela S; Diamond Head Med Clinic, PO Box 9200 Stn Main, Squamish BC V8B 0C1; UBC'97; CCFP; (604)892-3544

RIVERS, Derek W; 340 Elgin St, Port Colborne ON L3K 6G9; Ott'97; BSc; CCFP; FCFP; Ac Staff, Niagara Health System - Port Colborne General Site; Court Staff, Niagara Health System - Welland Hospital Site; (905)835-9817; Fax. (905)835-1647; dwrivers@lastmilenet.ca.

RIVERS, Jason; Pacific Dermaesthetics Inc, 1790-1111 Georgia St W, Vancouver BC V6E 4M3; Ott'81; BSc; DABD; FAAD; FRCPC; Derm (Melanoma). Ac Staff, Providence Health Care - St Paul's Hospital; Clin Prof, University of British Columbia; Langs: English; French; (604)682-7546; Fax. (604)687-5462.

RIVEST, Annie; CSSS du Sud de Lanaudière, 911 montee des Pionniers, Terrebonne QC J6V 2H2; Sher'96; Staff, Centre Hospitalier Pierre le Gardeur; (450)654-7525

RIVEST, Candice D; UWO Clinical Skills Bldg, 1151 Richmond St, London ON N6A 5C1; McM'10; CCFP; (519)661-2111

RIVEST, Denis; Clinique médicale Le Norois, 201-641 4e rue O, Amos QC J9T 2S1; Sher'83; CCFP; FCFP; Médecin, CH Hôtel-Dieu d'Amos; Langs: English; (819)732-3368; Fax. (819)732-3442.

RIVEST, Donald; Hotel-Dieu de Levis, 143 rue Wolfe, Levis QC G6V 3Z1; Mon'91; FRCPC; Neur (Electromyography); Electroenceph (P.Q.). Staff Neurol, Hôtel-Dieu de Lévis; Langs: Spanish; English; (418)835-7158; Fax. (418)835-7212.

RIVEST, Genevieve; CSSS de Manicouagan, 635 boul Jolliet, Baie-Comeau QC G5C 1P1; Laval'05; Staff, Centre Hospitalier Régional Baie-Comeau; (418)589-3701

RIVEST, Genevieve; 340 rue Clement-Lavoie, Baie-Comeau QC G4Z 3B8; Mon'08; CCFP; (418)296-2421

RIVEST, Jacques; CSSS de Montmagny-L'Islet, RR 1 430 rue Jean-Leclerc, St-Jean-Port-Joli QC G0R 3G0; Laval'86; Staff, CSSS de Montmagny-l'Islet; (418)598-3355; Fax. (418)598-9794.

RIVEST, Jacynthe; CHUM-Hop St-Luc, 1058 rue Saint-Denis, Montreal QC H2X 3J4; Mon'03; FRCPC; Psy. Staff, Centre Hospitalier l'Université De Montréal (CHUM) - Hôpital Saint-luc; Staff, Centre Hospitalier l'Université de Montréal (CHUM) - Hôpital Notre-Dame; (514)890-8000 x25678

RIVEST, Jean; Clinique Med l'Envolee, 5025 rue de Salaberry, Montreal QC H4J 1J1; Mon'92; (514)331-2323

RIVEST, Jean; CHUS-Hop Fleurimont, 3001 12e av N, Sherbrooke QC J1H 5N4; Sher'80; FRCPC; Neur (Neuro Physiology); Electroenceph (P.Q.). Staff, Centre Hospitalier Universitaire de Sherbrooke-Hopital Fleurimont; Consultant, Hôpital Sainte-croix; (819)346-1110; Fax. (819)820-6420.

RIVEST, Jean-Francois; Lakeshore Gen Hosp, 160 av Stillview, Pointe-Claire QC H9R 2Y2; Sher'07; Psy. Staff, Lakeshore General Hospital - Pointe Claire; (514)630-2225

RIVEST, Louise; CSSS la Pommeraie, 200 rue Principale, Cowansville QC J2K 1J2; Mon'85; Staff, Centre Hospitalier et CLSC de Memphremagog; (450)266-4342

RIVEST, Marie-Christine; Ctr Hosp de Matane, 333 rue Thibault, Matane QC G4W 2W5; Mon'05; Staff, Centre Hospitalier de Matane; (418)562-3135

RIVEST, Martin; 300-1000 Montee des Pionniers, Terrebonne QC J6V 1S8; Sher'93; CCFP; CCFP(E.M.); FCFP; Staff, Centre Hospitalier Pierre le Gardeur; Langs: English; French; (450)657-5799; Fax. (450)657-1809.

RIVEST, Michele; 110-1615 boul Jacques-Cartier, Longueuil QC J4M 2X1; Sher'87; CCFP; Consultant, Centre Hospitalier Universitaire de Sherbrooke-Hopital Fleurimont; (450)468-6223; Fax. (450)468-5041.

RIVEST, Natalie; Cite de la Sante de Laval, 1755 boul Rene-Laennec, Laval QC H7M 3L9; Mon'84; FRCPC; MedMicrobiol; Microbio & Infect Dis (P.Q.). Staff, Hopital de la Cite de la santé; Langs: English; (450)975-5303; natalie_rivest@ssss.gouv.qc.ca.

RIVEST, Paul; Direction de la Sante Publique, 1301 rue Sherbrooke E, Montreal QC H2L 1M3; Mon'79; MSc; Med Consultant Public Health, McGill University Health Centre - Montreal General Campus; (514)528-2400; Fax. (514)524-2452; privest@santepub-mtl.qc.ca.

RIVET, Andre G; Medical & Dental Bldg, 405-1221 Algonquin Ave, North Bay ON P1B 4Y3; Tor'80; Staff, North Bay Regional Health Centre - Regional Mental Health; Langs: English; French; (705)474-2630; Fax. (705)474-2633.

RIVET, Caroline; Clinique Horizon Feminin, 200 rue Durand, Saint-Jerome QC J7Z 7E2; Mon'95; FRCSC; ObstGyn. (450)436-4228

RIVET, Christine C; Family Med Centre, 210 Melrose Ave, Ottawa ON K1Y 4K7; McG'75; CCFP; CCFP(E.M.); FCFP; (613)761-4334 x16512; Fax. (613)761-4200; crivet@ottawahospital.on.ca.

RIVET, Ghislain; 5300 ch de chambly, Saint-Hubert QC J3Y 3N7; Mon'03; PhysMed&Rehab (P.Q.). (450)676-7447

RIVET, Real J F; 10 rue Notre-Dame N, Ville-Marie QC J9V 1W7; Ott'67; Ac Staff, CSSS du Témiscamingue; Langs: English; (819)629-3301; Fax. (819)629-3139; realrivet@cablevision.qc.ca.

RIVET, Roxanne; Hop Charles LeMoyne, 3120 boul Taschereau, Greenfield Park QC J4V 2H1; Sher'98; IntMed. Staff, Hopital Charles LeMoyne; (450)466-5000

RIVETNA, Roxanna; Tecumseh Medical Center, 205-13278 Tecumseh Rd E, Tecumseh ON N8N 3T6; Saba Univ School of Medicine (Netherlands Antilles)'09.

RIVILIS, Jeffrey; 304-5655 av du parc, Montreal QC H2V 4H2; Liverpool (England)'58; MSc(McG); FRCS(Eng); FRCS(Ed); FRCSC; GenSurg. Staff Surg, Sir Mortimer B Davis Jewish General; (514)273-8080; Fax. (514)270-2121; jrivilis@sympatico.ca.

RIVINGTON, Elizabeth G; St Lawrence Med Clinic, PO Box 329, Ingleside ON K0C 1M0; Tor'87; MSc; Staff, Winchester District Memorial Hospital; (613)537-2044; Fax. (613)537-2693.

RIVINGTON, Jennifer H; Primary Health Care Centre, 54-346 John St N, Arnprior ON K7S 2P6; Qns'88; CCFP; Ac Staff, Arnprior & District Memorial Hospital; (613)623-7765; Fax. (613)623-0841.

RIVINGTON, Robert N; Canadian Med Protective Assn, PO Box 8225 Stn T CSC 875 Carling Ave, Ottawa ON K1G 3H7; Qns'74; FCCP; FACP; FRCPC; IntMed; Respir. Consultant, The Ottawa Hospital - Civic Campus; Assoc Prof Med, University of Ottawa; Langs: English; French; (613)725-2000; Fax. (613)725-1300.

RIVLIN, Alex S; 45-1170 Sheppard Ave W, North York ON M3K 2A3; Leningrad (Russia (Federation))'70; MD; Physician, Rivlin Hair Transplant Clinique; Langs: Russian; (416)827-1322; Fax. (416)650-9717.

RIVLIN, Leon; 312-89 Queensway W, Mississauga ON L5B 2V2; Tor'96; BA(Hon.); CCFP; CCFP(E.M.); FCFP; Staff Emerg, Markham Stouffville Hospital; Staff, Trillium Health Centre - Mississauga; (905)281-9898

RIYAT, Sharan; 3100-11666 Steveston Hwy, Richmond BC V7A 1N6; Bristol (England)'04; (604)448-9595; Fax. (604)304-9595.

RIYAZ, Rehan R; Lasik MD, 400-123 2nd Ave S, Saskatoon SK S7K 7E6; Qns'07; FRCSC; Ophth. (306)651-7243; Fax. (306)651-7246.

RIYAZ, Samreen H; Comstock Med Centre, 70 Charles St, Brockville ON K6V 1T3; (Pakistan)'98; CCFP; (613)345-1458; Fax. (613)345-5296.

RIZCALLAH, Edmond; CHUS-Hop Fleurimont, 3001 12e av N, Sherbrooke QC J1H 5N4; Kharkov (Russia (Federation))'94; CSPQ; AnatPath (P.Q.). Staff, Centre Hospitalier Universitaire de Sherbrooke-Hopital Fleurimont; Chef Pathology, Universite de Sherbrooke; (819)346-1110 x13984

RIZK, Abdalla M A; Portage Clinic, 140 9th St SE, Portage la Prairie MB R1N 3V5; Cairo (Egypt)'87; CCFP; (204)857-3445

RIZK, Dalia A S; 2951 Walker's Line, Burlington ON L7M 4Y1; Cairo (Egypt)'89; CCFP; (905)592-3951; Fax. (905)592-9632.

RIZK, Magdy G A; Cornwall Comm Hosp-Second St, 510 2nd St E, Cornwall ON K6H 1Z6; Cairo (Egypt)'81; Staff, Cornwall Community Hospital - Second Street Site; (613)932-3300

RIZK, Mounir; Hôpital Laval, 2725 ch Sainte-Foy, Quebec QC G1V 4G5; Beirut (Lebanon)'85; Staff, Hôpital Laval; (418)656-4717; Fax. (418)656-4707.

RIZK, Nabil M R; University of Alberta Hosp, 1E4.33-8440 112 St NW, Edmonton AB T6G 2B7; (Egypt)'88; Staff, University of Alberta Hospital; (780)407-3822; Fax. (780)407-6059.

RIZK, Nada N A; Oak Park Med Clinic, 2530 Sixth Line, Oakville ON L6H 6W5; Cairo (Egypt)'85; CCFP; (905)257-1006; Fax. (905)257-0661.

RIZK, Sarah Z Y Hanna; Goodfellow Prof Bldg, 210-170 McEwan Dr E, Bolton ON L7E 4C8; Cairo (Egypt)'68; Langs: Arabic; French; (905)951-6293

RIZK, Soha R; The Family Focus Med Clinic, 201-240 Baker Dr, Dartmouth NS B2W 6L4; CCFP; Langs: French; Arabic; (902)462-0893; Fax. (902)462-2015.

RIZKALLA, Hoda G; Lawrence-Victoria Park Med Ctr, 201-1719 Lawrence Ave E, Scarborough ON M1R 2X7; Ain Shams (Egypt)'79; CCFP; Langs: Arabic; (416)444-8404

RIZKALLA, Kamilia S; London HSC-University Hosp, PO Box 5339 Stn B 339 Windermere Rd, London ON N6A 5A5; Assiut (Egypt)'77; BMedSci; FRCPC; AnatPath (Hematology Pathology). Staff Path & Hematol, Anatomical Pathologist, London Health Sciences Centre - University Hospital; Prof, University of Western Ontario; Langs: Arabic; (519)658-8500 x36355; kamilia.rizkalla@lhsc.on.ca.

RIZKALLA, Michel; 12 Daleberry Pl, North York ON M3B 2A6; All Saints Univ of Medicine (Aruba)'09.

RIZKALLAH, Rizkallah; Clinique Med Chapleau, 101-431 boul Adolphe-Chapleau, Bois-des-Filion QC J6Z 1H9; Beyrouth (Lebanon)'70; FRCSC; OrthSurg. Staff, Hopital de la Cite de la santé; (450)965-2232; Fax. (450)965-7887.

RIZOLI, Sandro B; Sunnybrook Hlth Sciences Ctre, H1 71-2075 Bayview Ave, Toronto ON M4N 3M5; Campinas (Brazil)'84; FRCSC; GenSurg (Critical Care Medicine). Staff, Sunnybrook Health Sciences Centre; Langs: Portuguese; Spanish; (416)480-5255; Fax. (416)480-5499.

RIZOS, John D; The Credit Valley Hosp, 2200 Eglinton Ave W, Mississauga ON L5M 2N1; Tor'85; MCFP(EM); CCFP; CCFP(E.M.); Staff, The Credit Valley Hospital; Lecturer Family Med, University of Toronto; (905)813-4141; Fax. (905)813-4477; rizosj@rogers.com.

RIZOS, Nick; Centre Med Westmount Square, C180-1 car Westmount, Montreal QC H3Z 2P9; Tor'78; FRCSC; ObstGyn. (514)934-2334

RIZVI, Qaiser R; Castledowns Medicentre, 120-15277 Castle Downs Rd NW, Edmonton AB T5X 3N5; Alb'94; BMedSci; Dip SportMed; CCFP; Staff, Fort Saskatchewan Health Centre; (780)457-5511; Fax. (780)456-4004.

RIZVI, Shahbano H; 243 Dundas St E, Belleville ON K8N 1E2; Aga Khan (Pakistan)'91; FRCSC; GenSurg. Staff, QHC Belleville General; (613)968-9934; Fax. (613)968-9935.

RIZVI, Syed A; 210-44 Torbay Rd, St. John's NL A1A 2G4; Karachi (Pakistan)'92; Staff, Waterford Hospital; (709)726-0701

RIZVI, Syed M H; Windsor Health Centre, 110-700 Tecumseh Rd E, Windsor ON N8X 4T2; Karachi (Pakistan)'87; MB BS; Staff, Hôtel-Dieu Grace Hospital; Langs: Urdu; Hindi; Punjabi; (519)252-4500

RIZVI, Syed N A; London HSC-Victoria Hosp, PO Box 5010 Stn B E1 613-800 Commissioners Rd E, London ON N6A 5W9; Karachi (Pakistan)'86; FRCPC; Psy (Child & Adolescent Psychiatry). Staff, London Health Sciences Centre - Victoria Campus; (519)685-8500; syed.rizvi@lhsc.on.ca.

RIZWAN, Sara; 3945 17 Ave SW, Calgary AB T3E 0C3; (Pakistan)'91; (403)242-8633

RIZZI, Mario C; Hop Santa Cabrini Ospedale, 5655 rue Saint-Zotique E, Montreal QC H1T 1P7; McG'77; Respir. Affil Staff, McGill University Health Centre - Montreal General Campus; Ac Staff, Hôpital Santa Cabrini Ospedale; Ac Staff, Centre Hospitalier l'Université De Montréal (CHUM) - Hôpital Saint-luc; (514)252-6000 x6483; Fax. (514)252-6491.

RIZZO, Arturo J; Ellendale Med Bldg, 615-5845 ch de la Cote-des-Nei, Montreal QC H3S 1Z4; Sher'75; FRCPC; IntMed; Endocrin (P.Q.). Staff, Sir Mortimer B Davis Jewish General; (514)342-0535; Fax. (514)342-5276.

RIZZO, Daniel; CHUQ-St-Francois d'Assise, 10 rue de l'Espinay, Quebec QC G1L 3L5; Laval'88; CCFP; CCFP(E.M.); FCFP; ac Staff, Centre Hospitalier Universitaire De Québec - Pavillon De St-françois-d'assise; (418)525-4388

RIZZO, Nicholas A; Queenston Med & Dental Centre, 204-631 Queenston Rd, Hamilton ON L8K 6R5; Qns'58; CCFP; Ac Staff, St Joseph's Healthcare - Charlton Campus; Court Staff, Hamilton Health Sciences Centre - McMaster University Medical Centre; Staff, Joseph Brant Memorial Hospital; Clin Assoc Prof, McMaster University; Langs: Italian; (905)561-2932; Fax. (905)561-4882.

RIZZUTO, Anthony; CLSC Villeray, 1425 rue Jarry E, Montreal QC H2E 1A7; McG'10; MDCM; CCFP; (514)376-4141

RO, Athanasius S K; 201 King St W, Oshawa ON L1J 2J5; Qns'87; FRCSC; Ophth (Cataract Surgery). Ac Staff, Lakeridge Health - Whitby Site; Ac Staff, Lakeridge Health - Oshawa Site; Ac Staff, Lakeridge Health - Bowmanville Site; Langs: Korean; (905)434-1694; Fax. (905)434-6308.

ROA, Wilson H Y; Cross Cancer Institute, 11560 University Ave NW, Edmonton AB T6G 1Z2; Alb'87; FRCPC; RadOncol. Staff, Cross Cancer Institute; Langs: Chinese; (780)432-8783; Fax. (780)432-8380.

ROACH, Douglas W; Upper Grand Family Health Team, PO Box 460 70 Victoria St, Elora ON N0B 1S0; Cal'92; CCFP; FCFP; Ac Staff, Groves Memorial Community Hospital; Clin Assoc Prof, McMaster University; (519)846-5841; Fax. (519)846-8453.

ROACH, Muriel P; Queensway Prof Centre, 105-190 Sherway Dr, Etobicoke ON M9C 5N2; Tor'73; BSc; FRCSC; PlasSurg (Breast Surgery). Ac Staff, Trillium Health Centre - West Toronto; Ac Staff, Trillium Health Centre - Mississauga; (416)626-6076; Fax. (416)626-0076.

ROAD, Jeremy D; Leslie & Gordon Diamond H C C, 7F-2775 Laurel St, Vancouver BC V5Z 1M9; Sask'77; ABIM; FRCPC; IntMed; Respir. Staff, Vancouver General Hospital - Centennial Pavillion; Prof Med, University of British Columbia; (604)875-4241

ROBACK, Barbara R; Central Park Medical, 303-1711 Cook St, Victoria BC V8T 3P2; McM'87; CCFP; Langs: English; French; (250)388-0118; Fax. (250)385-4147.

ROBAEY, Philippe; Children's Hosp Eastern Ont, 401 Smyth Rd, Ottawa ON K1H 8L1; Bruxelles (Belgium)'78; FRCPC; Psy. Staff, Children's Hospital of Eastern Ontario (CHEO); (613)737-7600 x2088

ROBARTS, Simon T T; The Credit Valley Hosp, 2200 Eglinton Ave W, Mississauga ON L5M 2N1; Wes'90; CCFP; CCFP(E.M.); FCFP; Staff, The Credit Valley Hospital; (905)813-4141

ROBB, Clive B; Princeton Gen Hosp, PO Box 610, Princeton BC V0X 1W0; Sheffield (England)'80; MB ChB; DRCOG; MRC; CCFP; Staff, Princeton General Hospital; (250)295-3233

ROBB, George M M; Westminster Med Bldg, 701-625 Fifth Ave, New Westminster BC V3M 1X4; Aberdeen (Scotland)'53; FRCSC; GenSurg. (604)524-3133; Fax. (604)524-6716; veinclinic@telus.net.

ROBB, John A; Clin Sante Jacques-Cartier, 200-1815 rue King O, Sherbrooke QC J1J 2E3; McG'90; FRCPC; IntMed. (819)565-1921; Fax. (819)565-7880.

ROBB, Marjorie E; CHEO Outpatient Psychiatry, 311 McArthur Ave, Vanier ON K1L 8M3; Dal'87; FRCPC; Psy (Adolescent & Adult Medicine). marjrobb@rogers.com.

ROBBERTSE, Machiel J; Denman Place Med Clinic, 108-1030 Denman St, Vancouver BC V6G 2M6; Orange Free State (South Africa)'90; MB ChB; CCFP; (604)684-4412

ROBBINS, Anthony J; 1415 1st Ave W, Owen Sound ON N4K 4K8; St. George's (Grenada)'08; CCFP; (519)470-3030

ROBBINS, Megan; Complete Medical, 573 Torbay Rd, St. John's NL A1A 5G9; Mem'03; CCFP; Staff Eastern Health, Health Sciences Centre; (709)754-0050; Fax. (709)754-0212.

ROBBINS, Nicole; 401-517 Sixth Ave N, Williams Lake BC V2G 2G8; UBC'04; FRCSC; GenSurg. Staff, Vancouver General Hospital - Centennial Pavillion; (250)398-8280

ROBBINS, Peter S; Campbell Med Group, 39 Campbell Ave, St. John's NL A1E 2Z3; Mem'88; BSc; BMedSci; CCFP; FCFP; Staff, Health Sciences Centre.

ROBBINS, Sarah J; Hys Med Centre, 310-11010 101 St NW, Edmonton AB T5H 4B9; Cal'03; BSc(Hon); MSc; FRCPC; IntMed (Nutrition); Gastroent. Staff Gastroent, Royal Alexandra Hospital; (780)421-1029; Fax. (780)425-5533.

ROBBINS, Stephanie J; Fairview Med Arts Centre, 103-2200 Fairview St, Burlington ON L7R 4H9; Tor'80; FRCPC; IntMed. (905)639-5513; Fax. (905)639-0824.

ROBBINS, Steven E; 1540-800 boul René-Lévesque O, Montreal QC H3B 1X9; Boston(MA) (USA)'72; (514)392-0174; Fax. (514)392-0157.

ROBERECKI, Susan A; Manitoba Health, 4081-300 Carlton St, Winnipeg MB R3B 3M9; Man'89; FRCPC; CommunMed.

ROBERGE, Andre; CSSS du Rocher Perce, CP 269 98 Rte 132, Perce QC G0C 2L0; Laval'78; Ac Staff, Centre Hospitalier Universitaire De Québec - Pavillon De St-françois-d'assise; (418)782-2572; Fax. (418)782-5501.

ROBERGE, Anne-Marie; Hop Charles Lemoyne, 3120 boul Taschereau, Greenfield Park QC J4V 2H1; Laval'07; FRCPC; Psy. Staff, Hopital Charles LeMoyne; (450)466-5020

ROBERGE, Annie; CLSC Sherbrooke, 8 rue Speid, Sherbrooke QC J1M 1R6; Mon'91; Langs: English; (819)563-2572

ROBERGE, Celine; Place de la Cite-Tour Belcourt, 840-2590 boul Laurier, Quebec QC G1V 4M6; Laval'93; FRCSC; PlasSurg. Staff, Centre Hospitalier Universitaire de Quebec-CHUL; Université Laval; (418)780-8800; Fax. (418)780-8160.

ROBERGE, Claude A; Centre Bois de Boulogne, 365-1575 boul Henri-Bourassa O, Montreal QC H3M 3A9; Laval'65; Peds (Rehabilitation Medicine). Staff, Hôpital Ste-Justine; Staff Peds, Centre de Réadaptation Marie Enfant du CHU Sainte-Justine; Langs: English; (514)337-0306; Fax. (514)337-0307.

ROBERGE, Claude; Clinique Med Rock Forest, 1-4870 boul Bourque, Sherbrooke QC J1N 3S5; Sher'70; Assoc Staff, Centre Hospitalier Universitaire de Sherbrooke-Hôpital Hôtel-Dieu; (819)820-2673; Fax. (819)820-2112; isacherie@hotmail.com.

ROBERGE, Claude; Centre d'Urgence Salaberry, 2758 rue de Salaberry, Montreal QC H3M 1L3; Mon'71; Ac Staff, Hôpital du Sacre-Coeur de Montréal; (514)337-4772; Fax. (514)337-4923.

ROBERGE, Claude; Centre Med St-Stanislas, 1380 rue Principale, St-Stanislas-D-Cha QC G0X 3E0; Laval'76; (418)328-8417; Fax. (418)328-8446.

ROBERGE, Daniel; Tribunal Administratif du Queb, RC10-575 rue Saint-Amable, Quebec QC G1R 5R4; Laval'73; Adm Judge, Tribunal Administratif du Quebec; Langs: English; Spanish; (418)643-0355 x3097; daniel.roberge@taq.gouv.qc.ca.

ROBERGE, Danielle; CSSS de Saint-Jerome, 290 rue de Montigny, Saint-Jerome QC J7Z 5T3; Mon'94; Staff, Hôtel-Dieu de Saint-Jérôme; Langs: English; (450)431-8200; Fax. (450)431-8698.

ROBERGE, David; CHUM-Hop Notre-Dame, 1560 rue Sherbrooke E, Montreal QC H2L 4M1; Mon'97; CSPQ; FRCPC; RadOncol. Staff, Centre Hospitalier l'Université de Montréal (CHUM) - Hôpital Notre-Dame; (514)890-8254; Fax. (514)412-7537.

ROBERGE, Elise; CSSSG-Hop de Gatineau, CP 2000 Succ Bureau-Chef 909 boul de la Verendrye O, Gatineau QC J8P 7H2; Mon'02; CCFP; CCFP(E.M.); Staff, Hôpital de Gatineau; (819)966-6100

ROBERGE, Francois; Polyclinique Med Concorde, 300 boul de la Concorde E, Laval QC H7G 2E6; Laval'72; FRCSC; Ophth. Staff, Hopital de la Cite de la santé; (450)972-2476

ROBERGE, Genevieve; Hôpital Laval, 2725 ch Sainte-Foy, Quebec QC G1V 4G5; Laval'05; Staff, Hôpital Laval; (418)656-8711

ROBERGE, Ghislain; Place Saint-Nicolas, 845 Rte Marie-Victorin, Saint-Nicolas QC G7A 3S8; Laval'74; (418)831-4141; Fax. (418)831-4141.

ROBERGE, Guillaume; Ctr Hosp Reg de Lanaudiere, 1000 Sainte-Anne Blvd, Joliette QC J6E 6J2; Sher'08; IntMed. Staff, Centre Hospitalier Régional de Lanaudière; (450)759-8222

ROBERGE, Guy; 401-235 boul René-Lévesque E, Montreal QC H2X 1N8; Laval'63; FRCPC; Cardiol (P.Q.); IntMed. Chef cardio, Centre Hospitalier l'Université De Montréal (CHUM) - Hôpital Saint-luc; assoc Prof, Universite de Montreal; (514)861-2706; Fax. (514)861-6131.

ROBERGE, Guy; CLSC Haute-Ville-des-Rivieres, 2400 av d'Estimauville, Quebec QC G1E 7G9; Laval'81; CST; (418)623-1010 x253; Fax. (418)623-7513.

ROBERGE, Jean-Francois; 238 rue King O, Sherbrooke QC J1H 1P9; Laval'71; FRCSC; Ophth. Ac Staff, Centre Hospitalier Universitaire de Sherbrooke-Hôpital Hôtel-Dieu; Consultant, Centre Hospitalier Universitaire de Sherbrooke-Hopital Fleurimont; (819)566-4151; Fax. (819)566-4153.

ROBERGE, Jean-Guy R; Medical Centre, 305-1428 Ouellette Ave, Windsor ON N8X 1K4; Sher'73; FRCPC; Psy. (519)256-9292

ROBERGE, Johanne N; The Hosp for Sick Children, 555 University Ave, Toronto ON M5G 1X8; Tor'95; FRCPC; Psy. Staff, The Hospital For Sick Children; (416)813-8941; Fax. (416)813-7785.

ROBERGE, Julie; Cinique Med Ste-Therese, 101-233 rue Turgeon, Sainte-Therese QC J7E 3J8; Mon'99.

ROBERGE, Justine; Centre Med des Laurentides, 102-1100 rue Saint-Isidore, St-Lin-Laurentides QC J5M 2V6; Mon'06; CCFP; (450)439-3870

ROBERGE, Katerie; Clinique Med du Coteau, 100-440 boul Saint-Luc, St-Jean-Sur-Richel QC J2W 1C1; Mon'86; (450)359-6819; Fax. (450)359-3247.

ROBERGE, Kerryn L; Westbrook Prof Bldg, 211-1610 37 St SW, Calgary AB T3C 3P1; Cal'89; CCFP; FCFP; Staff, Foothills Medical Centre; Assoc Clin Lecturer, University of Calgary; Langs: Norwegian; French; German; (403)246-2052; Fax. (403)246-2219.

ROBERGE, Laurence; CSSS du Haut-Saint-Maurice, 885 boul Ducharme, La Tuque QC G9X 3C1; Laval'07; CCFP; Staff, Centre Hospitalier Saint-Joseph de la Turque; (819)523-4581

ROBERGE, Louise; Centre De L'Osteoporose, 100-1200 av de Germain-des-Pre, Quebec QC G1V 3M7; Laval'82; LMCC; Physician, Regie Assurance Maladie Quebec; (418)650-0698; Fax. (418)650-3916.

ROBERGE, Marcel; Polyclinique de Trois-Rivieres, 250-1900 boul des Recollets, Trois-Rivieres QC G8Z 4K4; Mon'74; Ophth. (819)374-6266

ROBERGE, Paul; 485 rue Dupuis RR 2, Chertsey QC J0K 3K0; Sher'80; (450)882-2488; Fax. (450)882-9072; sanrobpro@cogeco.ca.

ROBERGE, Rene R; Ctr Hosp de Charlevoix, 74 rue Ambroise-Fafard, Baie-Saint-Paul QC G3Z 2J6; Laval'66; CSPQ; Anes. Staff, CSSS de Charlevoix; Langs: English; Spanish; (418)435-5150

ROBERGE, Roger M J; Professional Arts Bldg, 221-100 Arden St, Moncton NB E1C 4B7; Laval'65; FACS; FICS; FRCSC; GenSurg (Breast Surgery). Langs: French; Spanish; (506)853-5178; Fax. (506)854-5952.

ROBERGE, Stephane; CSSS de Saint-Jerome, 290 rue de Montigny, Saint-Jerome QC J7Z 5T3; Sher'02; FRCSC; Otol. Staff, Hôtel-Dieu de Saint-Jérôme; (450)432-2777

ROBERGE, Suzanne; CSSS de Manicouagan, 635 boul Jolliet, Baie-Comeau QC G5C 1P1; Mon'89; FRCSC; ObstGyn. Staff, Centre Hospitalier Régional Baie-Comeau; (418)589-3701; Fax. (418)589-3659.

ROBERGE, Yolande; Clinique Externe Jean-Talon, 7345 rue Garnier, Montreal QC H2E 2A1; Laval'72; Med Staff, CSSS du Coeur de l'Isle Hôpital Jean-Talon; (514)729-3036 x7245; Fax. (514)495-6774; yolanderoberge@primus.ca.

ROBERN, Michael; Nepean Med Centre, 101-1 Centrepointe Dr, Nepean ON K2G 6E2; Tor'86; FRCPC; IntMed (Clinical Trials); Derm. Staff/Consultant, The Ottawa Hospital - Civic Campus; Consultant/Staff, The Ottawa Hospital - General Campus; Asst Prof, University of Ottawa; Langs: English; French; (613)224-6339; Fax. (613)224-2651; mrobern@primus.ca.

ROBERT, Benoit; CHSLD de la Cote Boisee, 4300 rue Angora, Terrebonne QC J6X 4P1; Sher'93; (450)471-5877

ROBERT, Bruno; CSSS Drummond-Hop Sainte-Croix, 570 rue Heriot, Drummondville QC J2B 1C1; Sher'95; CSPQ; FRCPC; Anes. Staff, Hôpital Sainte-croix; (819)478-6464

ROBERT, Bruno; Ctr Hosp du Centre la Mauricie, 50 119e rue, Shawinigan-Sud QC G9P 5K1; Laval'84; FRCPC; IntMed. Chef méd int, Centre Hospitalier du Centre la Mauricie; (819)536-7500; Fax. (819)536-7649.

ROBERT, Caroline; CSSS de la Haute-Yamaska, 205 boul Leclerc O, Granby QC J2G 1T7; Sher'05; FRCPC; IntMed (Echocardiography). Staff Internist, Centre Hospitalier de Granby; Langs: Bilingual(French/English); (450)375-8000; Fax. (450)375-8042.

ROBERT, Christopher E; 589 Lake St, St. Catharines ON L2N 7L6; Jagiellonian Univ (Poland)'06; OrthSurg. (905)684-4364; Fax. (905)624-4466.

ROBERT, Diane; CLSC La Source Nord, 791 rue de Sherwood, Quebec QC G2N 1X7; Laval'90; CCFP; (418)277-2256

ROBERT, Diane; GMF de Grand-Mere, 200-1050 8e rue, Grand-Mere QC G9T 4L4; Laval'77; (819)538-5870

ROBERT, Diane H; Clinique Med Napierville, RR 3 103-343 rue Saint Jacques, Napierville QC J0J 1L0; Mon'80; (450)245-0081; Fax. (450)245-0615.

ROBERT, Genevieve; CSSS du Sud de Lanaudière, 911 montee des Pionniers, Terrebonne QC J6V 2H2; Sher'03; CCFP; Staff, Centre Hospitalier Pierre le Gardeur; (450)654-7525

ROBERT, Ghislain; Hotel-Dieu d'Arthabaska, 5 rue des Hospitalieres, Victoriaville QC G6P 6N2; Sher'75; FRCPC; IntMed (Geriatric Medicine). Staff, Hotel-Dieu d'Arthabaska; (819)357-1151; Fax. (819)357-6030.

ROBERT, Guillaume; Ctr Hosp Fleury, 2180 rue Fleury E, Montreal QC H2B 1K3; Mon'86; Staff, Centre Hospitalier Fleury; (514)381-9311; Fax. (514)858-2435.

ROBERT, Jean G; Clinique de Gynecologie, 24 rue Melancon E, Alma QC G8B 6W3; Laval'80; FRCSC; Urol. Staff Urol, CSSS de Lac-Saint Jean-Est.

ROBERT, Jean; Ctr Sida Amitie des Laurentide, 707 14e av S, Saint-Jerome QC J7Z 4B8; Mon'63; CSPQ; FRCPC; MedMicrobiol (Infectiology); Microbio & Infect Dis (P.Q.); CommunMed (P.Q.). Staff, Hôtel-Dieu de Saint-Jérôme; Chef Dept of Community Hlth, Centre Hospitalier l'Université De Montréal (CHUM) - Hôpital Saint-luc; Clin Assoc Prof, Universite de Montreal; (450)432-9444

ROBERT, Johanne; 208-1062 Ghislain St, Hawkesbury ON K6A 3B2; Ott'95; CCFP; Staff, Hawkesbury & District General Hospital; (613)632-0399

ROBERT, Louis; Plexo Robert et Lizotte, RC-4205 4e av O, Quebec QC G1H 7A6; Laval'72; Médecin, Clinique Medicale Industrielle Robert & Lizotte; Dir méd, Clinique Plexo Mediclub; Langs: Bilingual(French/English); (418)624-3224; Fax. (418)624-0991; lrobert@plexo.ca.

ROBERT, Magali; Foothills Med Centre, 1403 29 St NW, Calgary AB T2N 2T9; Ott'91; BSc; FRCSC; ObstGyn (Pelvic Pain & Endometriosis). Staff, Foothills Medical Centre; Pelvic Dysfunction Clinic; Dir, Calgary Chronic Pain Clinic; Asst Prof, University of Calgary; Langs: Bilingual(English/French); (403)944-1636; Fax. (403)270-4249; magali.robert@calgaryhealthregion.ca.

ROBERT, Marie-Michelle; Hop du Sacre-Coeur de Mtl, 5400 boul Gouin O, Montreal QC H4J 1C5; Laval'97; CCFP; CCFP(E.M.); Staff, Hôpital du Sacre-Coeur de Montréal; (514)338-2000

ROBERT, Martin; CSSS du Lac-des-Deux-Montagnes, 520 boul Arthur-Sauve, St-Eustache QC J7R 5B1; Mon'95; Staff, Hôpital de Saint-Eustache; (450)473-6811

ROBERT, Melanie; CSSS Du Sud De Lanaudière, 911 montée des Pionniers, Terrebonne QC J6V 2H2; Laval'10; CCFP; Staff, Centre Hospitalier Pierre le Gardeur; (450)654-7525

ROBERT, Michel P; Ctr d'Hebergement Champlain, 1325 rue Crawford, Verdun QC H4H 2N6; Mon'71; ac Staff, Centre d'hébergement Champlain; ac Staff, Centre Hospitalier de Verdun; (514)765-8513

ROBERT, Monique; College des Medecins du Quebec, 2170 boul Rene-Levesque O, Montreal QC H3H 2T8; Sher'79; FRCPC; Peds. Ac Staff Ambulatory Peds, Hôpital Ste-Justine; Prof Agregee de Clinique/Clin Prof, Universite de Montreal; Langs: English; (514)933-4441; monique.robert.hsj@ssss.gouv.qc.ca.

ROBERT, Nicole; CSSS de Montmagny-L'Islet, RR 1 350 boul Tache O, Montmagny QC G5V 3R8; Sher'90; LMCC; CSPQ; FRCPC; Psy (Geriatric Psychiatry). Staff, CSSS de Montmagny-L'Islet; (418)248-0630; Fax. (418)248-8472; nicole.robert.csssml@ssss.gouv.qc.ca.

ROBERT, Paul F; Lake Street Med Clinic, 204-589 Lake St, St Catharines ON L2N 7L6; Ott'75; FACS; FRCSC; OrthSurg. Staff, Niagara Health System - Ontario Street Site; Staff, Niagara Health System - St Catharines General Site; Langs: English; French; (905)684-4364; Fax. (905)684-4466.

ROBERT, Yves; College des Med du Quebec, 2170 boul Rene-Levesque O, Montreal QC H3H 2T8; Mon'79; (514)933-4441; yrobert@cmq.org.

ROBERTS, A Edwin; Windsor Reg Hosp-Metropolitan, 1995 Lens Ave, Windsor ON N8W 1L9; McG'83; BSc(Hon); FRCPC; Anes. Staff, Windsor Regional Hospital - Metropolitan Site; Langs: Bilingual(French/English); (519)254-1661 x52201; Fax. (519)971-7924; eroberts@mnsi.net.

ROBERTS, Ashley D; Children's & Women's HC of BC, 2D5-4480 Oak St, Vancouver BC V6H 3V4; McM'02; FRCPC; Peds; InfectDis. Staff, Providence Health Care - St Paul's Hospital; Staff, BC Children's Hospital; (604)875-3465

ROBERTS, Bernard C; Medi Plus Plaza, PO Box 220, Marystown NL A0E 2M0; Madras (India)'73; (709)279-4500

ROBERTS, Carla D; The Moncton Hosp, 135 MacBeath Ave, Moncton NB E1C 6Z8; Alb'03; FRCSC; ObstGyn. Staff, The Moncton Hospital; (506)855-2414

ROBERTS, D Kenneth; Newmarket Med Place, 308-712 Davis Dr, Newmarket ON L3Y 8C3; Tor'78; FRCPC; IntMed (Critical Care Medicine); Respir. Chief Dept of Med/Staff IntMed & Respirology, Southlake Regional Health Centre; (905)895-1090; Fax. (905)895-2680.

ROBERTS, Daniel; Health Sciences Centre, GC430-820 Sherbrook St, Winnipeg MB R3A 1R9; Tor'78; FRCPC; IntMed (Critical Care Medicine). Staff IntMed/Dir Medical Intensive Care, Health Sciences Centre; Dir Medical Program, Winnipeg Regional Health Authority Carlton Street Office; Dept Head Med, University of Manitoba; (204)787-7772; Fax. (204)787-3159.

ROBERTS, Deanne M; 275-1555 McKenzie Ave, Victoria BC V8N 1A4; UBC'79; (250)384-8420

ROBERTS, Elizabeth A; Central Nfld Reg Hlth Centre, 50 Union St, Grnd-Falls-Windsor NL A2A 2E1; Mem'78; Staff, Central Newfoundland Regional Health Centre; (709)292-2559

ROBERTS, Evan W D; Sudbury Reg Hosp-Laurentian, 41 Ramsey Lake Rd, Sudbury ON P3E 5J1; Mem'91; FRCPC; DiagRad. Staff Radiol, Health Sciences North-Laurentian Site; (705)522-2200 x3125

ROBERTS, Eve A; The Hosp for Sick Children, 555 University Ave, Toronto ON M5G 1X8; Johns Hopkins(MD) (USA)'73; ABIM; FRCPC; IntMed (Hepatology); Gastroent. Assoc Staff Peds, The Hospital For Sick Children; Aj Prof Peds, Med & Pharmacol, University of Toronto; (416)813-7733; Fax. (416)813-4972; eve.roberts@sickkids.ca.

ROBERTS, Gerald K; White Rock Med Clinic, 101-15451 Russell Ave, White Rock BC V4B 2R5; McG'75; Ac Staff, Peace Arch Hospital; Teach Staff Family Med, University of British Columbia; (604)531-5595; Fax. (604)531-9818.

ROBERTS, Heidi C; Women's College Hosp, W2 72-76 Grenville St, Toronto ON M5S 1B2; Mainz (Germany)'88; FRCPC; DiagRad. Staff, Women's College Hospital; Langs: German; (416)323-6186

ROBERTS, James M; 10203-2775 Laurel St, Vancouver BC V5Z 1M9; California (USA)'83; FRCPC; IntMed. (604)875-5181; Fax. (604)875-5906.

ROBERTS, Janet R; 1555 St Mary's Rd, Winnipeg MB R2M 5L9; Tor'78; FRCP; FAAP; FRCPC; Peds (Allergy & Immunology); ClinImmunol&Allergy. Ac Staff, Health Sciences Centre; Asst Prof Peds, University of Manitoba; (204)255-8238; jroberts@meadowoodmedical.ca.

ROBERTS, Janice D; South Eastman Health, PO Box 2560 Stn Main 365 Reimer Ave, Steinbach MB R5G 1P1; Sydney (Australia)'71; Med Officer of Hlth, South Eastman Health Unit; jroberts@neha.mb.ca.

ROBERTS, Jeffrey E; Pacific Ctr for Reproductive M, 500-4601 Canada Way, Burnaby BC V5G 4X7; UBC'96; FRCSC; ObstGyn (Reproductive Endocrinology & Infertility). (604)422-7276; Fax. (604)434-5522; info@pacificfertility.ca.

ROBERTS, Kenneth F; 230-77 Westmorland St, Fredericton NB E3B 6Z3; Dal'07; Ophth.

ROBERTS, Kris A; CW Wiebe Clinic, 385 Main St, Winkler MB R6W 1J2; CCFP; (204)789-3711

ROBERTS, Kristine J; Kent Place Mall, 216-189 Kent St W, Lindsay ON K9V 5G6; Wes'90; CCFP; (705)878-1461; Fax. (705)878-1942.

ROBERTS, Lisa M; Sunnybrook Hlth Sciences Ctre, M3 200-2075 Bayview Ave, Toronto ON M4N 3M5; Tor'05; FRCPC; Anes. Staff, Sunnybrook Health Sciences Centre; (416)480-4864

ROBERTS, Mark A; 114 Queen St, St Catharines ON L2R 5H3; Tor'87; (905)688-3334; Fax. (905)688-6013.

ROBERTS, Mark S; Perth-Smiths Falls Dist Hosp, 33 Drummond St W, Perth ON K7H 2K1; London (England)'01; FRCSC; OrthSurg. Staff, Perth & Smiths Falls District Hospital - Perth Site (Great War Memorial Site); (613)267-3232

ROBERTS, Martyn J; Univ Hlth Network-Toronto Western Hosp, 399 Bathurst St, Toronto ON M5T 2S8; Cardiff (Wales)'70; MB BS; FFARCS; Anes. Ac Staff, Toronto Western Hospital - University Health Network; (416)603-5118; Fax. (416)603-6494.

ROBERTS, Matthew T; The Ottawa Hosp-Civic Campus, 1053 Carling Ave, Ottawa ON K1Y 4E9; Tor'03; FRCSC; Urol. Staff, The Ottawa Hospital - Civic Campus; (613)761-4500; Fax. (613)761-6305.

ROBERTS, Megan; Vancouver Gen Hosp, 855 12th Ave W, Vancouver BC V5Z 1M9; UBC'02; FRCPC; Psy. Staff, Vancouver General Hospital - Centennial Pavillion; (604)875-4111

ROBERTS, Michael C; 205-1466 Bathurst St, Toronto ON M5R 3S3; Tor'81; BEd; CCFP; FCFP; Court Staff, Humber River Regional Hospital - Keele Street Site; Court Staff, Mount Sinai Hospital; Asst Prof Family & Commun Med Dalla Lana School of Public Hlth, University of Toronto; Langs: English; French; (416)483-8111; Fax. (416)483-8182.

ROBERTS, Nasreen; Hotel-Dieu Hosp, 166 Brock St, Kingston ON K7L 5G2; Punjab (Pakistan)'71; FRCPC; Psy. Staff, Hotel-Dieu Hospital; Langs: Urdu; French; (613)544-3310 x3510

ROBERTS, R Avalon; 217-5809 Macleod Trail SW, Calgary AB T2H 0J9; Ott'72; FRCPC; Peds; Psy. (403)283-8291; Fax. (403)457-5845.

ROBERTS, R Neil; Westgrove Prof Bldg, 330-10230 142 St NW, Edmonton AB T5N 3Y6; Alb'70; FRCPC; IntMed; Neur. Ac Staff Neurol, Covenant Health - Misericordia Community Hospital; (780)451-6029; Fax. (780)451-6093; nroberts@shaw.ca.

ROBERTS, Richard D; 203A-263 boul Saint-Jean, Pointe-Claire QC H9R 3J1; Dal'95; FRCPC; Neur. Consultant Neurol, Sir Mortimer B Davis Jewish General; Teacher Faculty, McGill University; Langs: English; French; (514)695-8886; Fax. (514)695-9860.

ROBERTS, Robert; Univ of Ottawa Heart Institute, 40 Ruskin St, Ottawa ON K1Y 4W7; Dal'66; FRCPC; IntMed. Staff/Pres/CEO, University of Ottawa Heart Institute; (613)761-4779; robert@ottawaheart.ca.

ROBERTS, S Gwendoline; The Hosp for Sick Children, 555 University Ave, Toronto ON M5G 1X8; Tor'72; BSc; FRCPC; Peds (Autism). Co-Dir Autism Research Unit, The Hospital For Sick Children; Staff Developmental Ped, Holland Bloorview Kids Rehabilitation Hospital; Staff Developmental Peds, Surrey Place Centre; Prof Peds, University of Toronto; (416)813-7037; Fax. (416)813-5558.

ROBERTS, Stacey K; Beaumont Med Clinic, 5001A 50 Ave, Beaumont AB T4X 1E7; Alb'96; (780)929-6050; Fax. (780)929-5848.

ROBERTS, Stephen A; 4303 10th Ave W, Vancouver BC V6R 2H6; UBC'81; CCFP; FCFP; (604)224-1355; Fax. (604)224-0179.

ROBERTS, Steve A I; 102-11709 102 St, Grande Prairie AB T8V 7S6; McG'06; MDCM; DABOph; FRCSC; Ophth. Langs: Bilingual(French/English); (780)832-3937; Fax. (780)832-3999.

ROBERTS, Theodore E; University of Alberta Hosp, 2E3.26-8440 112 St NW, Edmonton AB T6G 2B7; Man'78; FRCPC; Neur (Movement Disorders). Dir Div of Neurol, University of Alberta Hospital; Assoc Prof, University of Alberta; (780)407-7456; Fax. (780)407-1325.

ROBERTSON, A Rocke; East Kootenay Reg Hosp, 13 24th Ave N, Cranbrook BC V1C 3H9; Dal'77; DABPath; FRCPC; GenPath. Staff, East Kootenay Regional Hospital; Fax. (250)426-5285.

ROBERTSON, Adrian F; Health Sciences Centre, 820 Sherbrook St, Winnipeg MB R3A 1R9; Man'97; FRCPC; EmergMed; Critical Care Medicine. Staff, Health Sciences Centre; (204)774-8511

ROBERTSON, Andrew P; OK Falls Med Clinic, PO Box 211 5205 9th Ave, Okanagan Falls BC V0H 1R0; Alb'06; CCFP; (250)497-8703

ROBERTSON, Barbara J; Peace Arch Hosp, 15521 Russell Ave, White Rock BC V4B 2R4; McG'77; FRCPC; Anes. Staff, Peace Arch Hospital; Langs: French; (604)531-5512

ROBERTSON, Carolyn J; 4 Shaftesbury Place, Toronto ON M4T 2A5; Tor'82; FRCPC; Psy (Adult & Individual Psychotherapy). (416)925-5543

ROBERTSON, Charlene M T; Glenrose Rehab Hosp, 10230 111 Ave NW, Edmonton AB T5G 0B7; Sask'65; FRCPC; Peds (Neuro Development Pediatrics). Consultant Peds, Glenrose Rehabilitation Hospital; Emeritus Prof Peds, University of Alberta; (780)735-6110; Fax. (780)735-7907; charlene.robertson@albertahealthservices.ca.

ROBERTSON, Christopher M; Forensic Psychiatric Hosp, 70 Colony Farm Rd, New Westminster BC V3C 5X9; Man'05; FRCPC; Psy. Staff, Forensic Psychiatric Hospital; (604)524-7700; crobertson@forensic.bc.ca.

ROBERTSON, Dale F; Railside Med Specialists, 4A-1306 Bow Valley Trail, Canmore AB T1W 1N6; McG'87; FRCPC; Peds (Pediatric Respirology); Respir. Staff, Covenant Health - Banff Mineral Springs Hospital; Staff, Canmore General Hospital; Clinical Asst Prof, University of Calgary; Langs: English; French; (403)678-9600; Fax. (403)678-9467.

ROBERTSON, Daniel K F; Baywood Med Centre, G02-95 Bayly St W, Ajax ON L1S 7K8; Tor'80; (905)427-3996

ROBERTSON, David I; Kingston Gen Hosp, 76 Stuart St, Kingston ON K7L 2V7; Qns'03; FRCSC; GenSurg. Staff, Kingston General Hospital; (613)549-6666

ROBERTSON, David W; St Michael's Hosp, 17 054-30 Bond St, Toronto ON M5B 1W8; Tor'01; FRCPC; Psy. Staff, St Michael's Hospital; Asst Prof, University of Toronto; (416)864-6060 x4007

ROBERTSON, Deborah G; 61 Queen St E, Toronto ON M5C 2T2; McG'00; FRCSC; ObstGyn. Staff, St Michael's Hospital; (416)867-7460; Fax. (416)867-3693.

ROBERTSON, Donald D; 508-1 Young St, Hamilton ON L8N 1T8; Qns'90; BSc(Hons.); FRCSC; Otol (Neuro Otology). (905)527-0123; Fax. (905)527-3192.

ROBERTSON, Duncan; AHS Seniors Hlth Strategic Cli, 200-10030 107 St NW, Edmonton AB T5J 3E4; Durham (England)'66; MB BS; FRCP(Lond); FACP; FRCPC; IntMed (Assessment) (Alzheimer's Disease); GeriatricMed. Staff Specilaized Geriatric Services, Red Deer Regional Hospital Centre; (780)735-0210; Fax. (780)735-0237; duncan.robertson@shaw.ca.

ROBERTSON, Glenn; 104-145 15th St W, North Vancouver BC V7M 1R9; UBC'01; FRCPC; Peds (Eating Disorders). Clinical Asst Prof, BC Children's Hospital; Staff, Lions Gate Hospital; (604)924-3133

ROBERTSON, Heather E; South Shore Reg Hosp, 90 Glen Allan Dr, Bridgewater NS B4V 3S6; UBC'85; Med Staff, Fishermen's Memorial Hospital; Med Staff, South Shore Regional Hospital; Med Dir, South Shore Drug Dep. Unit; (902)543-4603

ROBERTSON, Heather; Concurrent Disorders Unit, 715 12th Ave W, Vancouver BC V5Z 1M9; McM'93; FRCPC; Psy (Addiction Medicine). Consultant Psy, Vancouver General Hospital - Centennial Pavillion; Consultant Psy, Providence Health Care - St Paul's Hospital; Clinical Asst Prof Psy, University of British Columbia; (604)875-4139; Fax. (604)224-6865.

ROBERTSON, Helen M; Montfort Hosp, 713 Montreal Rd, Ottawa ON K1K 0T2; Glasgow (Scotland)'80; MB ChB; CCFP; FCFP; Staff, Canadian Forces Health Services Centre; Staff, Montfort Hospital; (613)945-1490

ROBERTSON, James G J; PO Box 211, Okanagan Falls BC V0H 1R0; Ott'74; Staff, Penticton Regional Hospital; (250)497-8703; Fax. (250)497-8766.

ROBERTSON, James M; The Hosp for Sick Children, 555 University Ave, Toronto ON M5G 1X8; Tor'97; FRCPC; Anes. Staff, The Hospital For Sick Children; (416)813-7445

ROBERTSON, Jeffery H; Canadian Med Protective Assn, PO Box 8225 Stn T CSC 875 Carling Ave, Ottawa ON K1G 3H7; Qns'78; FACC; FRCPC; IntMed; Cardiol. Sr Medical Officer, Canadian Medical Protective Association; (613)725-2000 x643; Fax. (613)725-1300; jhrobertson@cmpa.org.

ROBERTSON, Jennifer L; The Moncton Hosp, 135 MacBeath Ave, Moncton NB E1C 6Z8; Dal'07; CCFP; Staff, The Moncton Hospital; (506)857-5111

ROBERTSON, Jill D; Crossroads Family Practice, 201-5110 St Margarets Bay Rd, Upper Tantallon NS B3Z 1E2; Dal'07; CCFP; (902)826-9096; Fax. (902)826-9399.

ROBERTSON, John G M; Primacy Med Clinic, 45779 Luckakuck Way, Chilliwack BC V2R 4E8; UBC'88; BSc; FRCSC; ObstGyn., Chilliwack General Hospital; (604)846-4477; Fax. (604)846-4480.

ROBERTSON, John W; 19 Valhalla Pl, Sault Ste. Marie ON P6A 5Y9; Tor'70; IntMed (Cardiology). Ac Staff, Sault Area Hospital - Sault Ste Marie; (705)254-3252

ROBERTSON, Julia A; Sault Area Hosp, 750 Great Northern Rd, Sault Ste. Marie ON P6B 0A8; Ott'00; CCFP; Staff, Sault Area Hospital - Sault Ste Marie; (705)759-3434

ROBERTSON, Julia S; AL3105A Tower B, 5025-1600 Scott St, Ottawa ON K1A 0W9; Ott'79; (613)954-6494

ROBERTSON, Julie E; BC Women's Hosp & Health Ctre, 2H30-4500 Oak St, Vancouver BC V6H 3N1; Wes'03; FRCSC; ObstGyn (Maternal Fetal Medicine). (604)875-2665

ROBERTSON, Karen P; Haig Clinic, 601 6 Ave S, Lethbridge AB T1J 0Z2; Alb'98; BSc; CCFP; FCFP; (403)328-6641; Fax. (403)328-6118.

ROBERTSON, Kerri D; 204-135 Ormond St, Brockville ON K6V 5Y2; Alb'67; DAB; FRCSC; Otol. Ac Staff, Brockville General Hospital - Charles Street; Ac Staff, Providence Continuing Care Centre (PCCC) - St Vincent de Paul Hospital; Assoc Staff, Cornwall Community Hospital - Second Street Site; (613)342-5520

ROBERTSON, Lynne H; Richmond Road Diag & Trmt Ctre, 1820 Richmond Rd SW, Calgary AB T2T 5C7; Mem'87; BSc; FRCPC; IntMed; Derm. Staff, Foothills Medical Centre; Langs: English; French; (403)955-8601; Fax. (403)955-8200.

ROBERTSON, Marilyn S; Argyle Med Clinic, 3-245 Argyle St S, Caledonia ON N3W 1K7; Tor'90; CCFP; (905)765-5245; Fax. (905)765-1090.

ROBERTSON, Marli A; Alberta Children's Hosp, 2888 Shaganappi Trail NW, Calgary AB T3B 6A8; Auckland (New Zealand)'83; MB ChB; FRACP(Peds); FRCPC; Peds (Gastroenterology). Staff, Alberta Children's Hospital; Asst Prof, University of Calgary; (403)955-5507

ROBERTSON, Mary L; Lonsdale Med Dental Bldg, 110-1940 Lonsdale Ave, North Vancouver BC V7M 2K2; Tor'67; DPH; LLB; Ac Staff, Lions Gate Hospital; (604)985-6917; Fax. (604)985-8914.

ROBERTSON, Matthew A; Valley Care Med Clinic, E-310 8th St, Courtenay BC V9N 1N3; Alb'05; CCFP; (250)331-0500

ROBERTSON, Nadine L; Coleman Clinic, 186 Kenneth St, Duncan BC V9L 1N4; UBC'91; Ac Staff Privil, Cowichan District Hospital; (250)746-4102; Fax. (250)746-5960.

ROBERTSON, Nancy L; 209-967 Bedford Hwy, Bedford NS B4A 1A9; Dal'87; BSc(Hons.); MSc; Lecturer Psy, Dalhousie University; Langs: English; French; (902)832-0527; Fax. (902)832-0673.

ROBERTSON, R Scott; Fredericton Med Clinic, 204-1015 Regent St, Fredericton NB E3B 6H5; Dal'88; Physician, City of Fredericton; (506)458-0257

ROBERTSON, Sharman J; Royal Ottawa Hlth Care Group, 1145 Carling Ave, Ottawa ON K1Z 7K4; Ott'94; FRCPC; Psy. Staff Psy, Royal Ottawa Mental Health Centre - Royal Ottawa Health Care Group; (613)722-6521; Fax. (613)798-2971.

ROBERTSON, Susan J; The Ottawa Hosp-Gen Campus, 501 Smyth Rd, Ottawa ON K1H 8L6; Ott'75; FRCPC; AnatPath; GenPath. Staff, The Ottawa Hospital - General Campus; (613)737-8309

ROBERTSON, William D; Cowichan Dist Hosp, 3045 Gibbins Rd, Duncan BC V9L 1E5; Cambridge (England)'81; FRCPC; Anes. Staff, Cowichan District Hospital; Nanaimo Regional General Hospital; (250)709-3000

ROBERTSON MOORE, Rohan K; Comm Addictions & Mental H S, 103-216 West St, Simcoe ON N3Y 1S8; Tor'98; MSc; BSc; FRCPC; Psy. (519)426-8760; Fax. (519)426-3257.

ROBES, Reynaldo P; Boniface Park Med Centre, 6-700 Markham Rd, Scarborough ON M1H 2A7; Manila (Philippines)'92; FRCPC; IntMed (Cardiovascular Medicine). Langs: Tagalog; (416)431-7100; Fax. (416)431-7191.

ROBIBO, Daniel A; Delta Health Sciences Centre, 200-4515 Harvest Dr, Delta BC V4K 4L1; Qns'96; FRCSC; GenSurg. Staff, Delta Health Sciences Centre; (604)940-2177; Fax. (604)940-2180.

ROBICHAUD, Alfred; 31 rue Providence, Moncton NB E1C 8X3; Laval'73; ObstGyn. (506)857-3884

ROBICHAUD, Annie; CLSC Riviere aux Renard, 154 boul Renard E, Gaspe QC G4X 5R5; Laval'07; CCFP; Staff, Centre Hospitalier des Monts; (418)269-2572

ROBICHAUD, Delbe J; 100 Water St PO Box 384 Stn Main, Campbellton NB E3N 3G7; Dal'86; Ac Staff, Hôpital Régional Campbellton; Langs: English; French; (506)753-7575; Fax. (506)789-9305.

ROBICHAUD, Eric; Dr Georges-L Dumont Reg Hosp, 330 av Universite, Moncton NB E1C 2Z3; Sher'10; CCFP; Staff, Dr Georges-L-Dumont University Hospital Centre; (506)862-4000

ROBICHAUD, Helene; CSSS de Sept-Iles, 45 rue du Pere-Divet, Sept-Iles QC G4R 3N7; Mon'92; CCFP; Staff, Centre Hospitalier Regional de Sept-Iles; (418)962-9761

ROBICHAUD, J Victor; 105-185 av Acadie, Dieppe NB E1A 1G6; Laval'82; CCFP; FCFP; Ac Staff, Dr Georges-L-Dumont University Hospital Centre; Board Member, College of Family Physicians of Canada-New Brunswick; Physician, Centre de Sante Familiale; Prof Family Med, Universite de Sherbrooke; (506)862-4181; Fax. (506)862-4179; robichaudv@nbnet.nb.ca.

ROBICHAUD, Jean-Luc; CSSS du Suroît, 150 rue Saint-Thomas, Salaber-de-Valleyf QC J6T 6C1; Mon'82; Staff, Centre Hospitalier Régional du Suroît; Langs: Bilingual(French/English); (450)371-9920; Fax. (450)370-1257.

ROBICHAUD, Jeffrey M; Delta Med Arts Bldg, 104-105 Queenston St, St Catharines ON L2R 2Z5; Wes'96; BSc; FRCSC; Otol (Head & Neck Oncology). Staff, Niagara Health System - St Catharines General Site; Staff, Niagara Health System - Welland Hospital Site; Staff, Niagara Health System - Greater Niagara General Site; Asst Prof Surg, McMaster University; Langs: English; French; (905)685-0267; Fax. (905)685-0781.

ROBICHAUD, Johanne; Polyclinique Isabell-sur-Mer, 8224 rue St-Paul, Bas-Caraquet NB E1W 6E2; Mon'04; CCFP; Staff, Hôpital de l'Enfant-Jésus RHSJ; Staff, Hôpital de Tracadie-Sheila; (506)727-7549; Fax. (506)727-7320.

ROBICHAUD, Line; Hôpital régional Chaleur, 1750 Sunset Dr, Bathurst NB E2A 4L7; Laval'97; Staff, Hopital Regional Chaleur; Langs: Bilingual(French/English); (506)544-3000; Fax. (506)544-2532.

ROBICHAUD, Martin; Dr Georges-L Dumont Reg Hosp, 330 av Universite, Moncton NB E1C 2Z3; Mon'98; CCFP; Emerg Medicine, Dr Georges-L-Dumont University Hospital Centre; Langs: Bilingual(French/English); (506)862-4000

ROBICHAUD, Martine; Dr Georges-L Dumont Reg Hosp, 330 av Universite, Moncton NB E1C 2Z3; Sher'08; CCFP; Staff, Dr Georges-L-Dumont University Hospital Centre; (506)862-4000

ROBICHAUD, Michele; Base Militar de Bagotville, CP 5000 Csp, Alouette QC G0V 1A0; Laval'08; CCFP; (418)677-4000

ROBICHAUD, Monique; 201-123 rue Champlain, Dieppe NB E1A 1N5; Sher'08; CCFP; (506)383-7716

ROBICHAUD, Pascal; Hotel-Dieu de Levis, 143 rue wolfe, Levis QC G6V 3Z1; Sher'04; FRCPC; IntMed; Gastroent. Staff, Hôtel-Dieu de Lévis; (418)835-7121

ROBICHAUD, Philippe; CSSS de la Haute-Yamaska, 205 boul Leclerc O, Granby QC J2G 1T7; Mon'04; IntMed. Staff, Centre Hospitalier de Granby; (450)375-8000 x2549; Fax. (450)375-8042.

ROBICHAUD, Remi; CSSS de la Haute-Yamaska, 205 boul Leclerc O, Granby QC J2G 1T7; Sher'01; CSPQ; FRCPC; Anes. Staff, Centre Hospitalier de Granby; (450)375-8000; Fax. (450)375-8032.

ROBICHAUD, Rene; 9364 rue Main, Richibucto NB E4W 4C9; Sher'04; CCFP; (506)523-4868; Fax. (506)523-1374.

ROBICHAUD, Renee; Inst U en Sante Mentale de QC, 2601 ch de la Canardiere, Quebec QC G1J 2G3; Sher'03; FRCPC; Psy. Staff, Institut Universitaire Sante; (418)663-5000

ROBICHAUD, Ronald; 420 Champlain St, Dieppe NB E1A 1P3; Laval'92; FRCSC; Otol. Staff, Dr Georges-L-Dumont University Hospital Centre; (506)388-2083; Fax. (506)389-8588.

ROBICHAUD, Simon; CSSS de la Haute-Yamaska, 205 boul leclerc O, Granby QC J2G 1T7; Laval'07; DiagRad. Staff, Centre Hospitalier de Granby; (450)375-8000

ROBICHAUD, Sophie; Royal University Hosp, 103 Hospital Dr, Saskatoon SK S7N 0W8; Sher'97; FRCPC; Peds; MedMicrobiol; InfectDis. Staff, Royal University Hospital; (306)655-1104; Fax. (306)655-1726.

ROBICHAUD, Sylvie; Hôpital régional Chaleur, 1750 Sunset Dr, Bathurst NB E2A 4L7; Laval'96; FRCPC; IntMed; Nephrol. Staff Nephrol, Hopital Regional Chaleur; Langs: English; (506)544-3231; Fax. (506)544-2041.

ROBICHAUD, Veronique; 106 Main St, Sackville NB E4L 4A7; Sher'09; CCFP.

ROBICHAUD-GAUVIN, Nadia; CLSC la Petit-Patrie, 6520 rue de Saint-Vallier, Montreal QC H2S 2P7; Laval'00; Staff, Centre Hospitalier de Verdun; (514)273-4508

ROBICSEK, Leslie; 101 Tangreen Cir, Thornhill ON L4J 5C9; Tor'72; Court Staff, North York General Hospital; (905)707-8110; Fax. (905)886-4780; leslierobicsek@hotmail.com.

ROBIDAS, Francis; Dr Georges L-Dumont Reg Hosp, 330 av Universite, Moncton NB E1C 2Z3; Sher'05; Anes. Staff, Dr Georges-L-Dumont University Hospital Centre; (506)862-4000

ROBIDAS, Isabelle; Clin Pediatrique Laurentienne, 106-200 rue Durand, Saint-Jerome QC J7Z 7E2; Sher'02; FRCPC; Peds. Staff, Hôtel-Dieu de Saint-Jérôme; (450)438-1241; Fax. (450)438-3501.

ROBIDAS, Lorraine; Centre Med Mira, 1560 boul de Rome, Longueuil QC J4W 3A1; Sher'76; FAAO; FRCSC; Ophth (Cataract Surgery). Ac Staff, Hopital Charles LeMoyne; Assoc Staff, McGill University Health Centre - Montreal General Campus; McGill University; (450)466-1880

ROBIDOUX, Andre; CHUM-Hotel-Dieu, 3840 rue Saint-Urbain, Montreal QC H2W 1T8; Mon'72; FRCSC; GenSurg (Breast Cancer); General Surgical Oncology (P.Q.). ac Staff, Centre Hospitalier l'Université de Montréal (CHUM) - Hôtel-Dieu; Langs: Bilingual(French/English); (514)890-8000 x14191; Fax. (514)412-7158.

ROBIDOUX, Nathalie; Clinique Med Duberger, 2810 boul Pere-Lelievre, Quebec QC G1P 2Y1; Sher'92; CCFP; (418)688-8414; Fax. (418)688-4273; nanuk1818@hotmail.com.

ROBILLARD, Alain A; Hop Maisonneuve-Rosemont, 5415 boul de l'Assomption, Montreal QC H1T 2M4; Mon'78; BSc; Electroenceph (P.Q.); Neur (Dementia). adj Prof, Hopital Maisonneuve-Rosemont; adj Prof, Universite de Montreal; Langs: Bilingual(English/French); (514)252-3528; Fax. (514)252-3529; robillal@videotron.ca.

ROBILLARD, Andre; Ctr Sante des Femmes, 5180 boul Gouin O, Montreal QC H4J 1C3; Mon'69; ObstGyn. Staff, Centre Hospitalier Fleury; Staff, Hôpital du Sacre-Coeur de Montréal; (514)333-8105; Fax. (514)333-8150.

ROBILLARD, Andree; CSSS Bordeaux-Cartierville-St-, 555 boul Gouin O, Montreal QC H3L 1K5; Mon'85; CCFP; FCFP; Physician, Hôpital du Sacre-Coeur de Montréal; Physician, Pavillon Notre-Dame de la Merci; (514)331-3020 x1702; Fax. (514)338-4359.

ROBILLARD, Antoine; CSSS Pierre Boucher, 1333 boul Jacques-Cartier E, Longueuil QC J4M 2A5; Laval'01; CSPQ; FRCPC; DiagRad. Staff, Centre Hospitalier Pierre Boucher; (450)468-8111

ROBILLARD, Claude; CSSS des Basques, RR 1 550 rue Notre-Dame E, Trois-Pistoles QC G0L 4K0; Sher'74; Staff, Centre Hospitalier Trois-Pistoles; (418)851-1111; Fax. (418)851-2944.

ROBILLARD, Francine; CLSC St-Leonard, 5540 rue Jarry E, Saint-Leonard QC H1P 1T9; Mon'80; (514)328-3460 x6335; Fax. (514)328-1468.

ROBILLARD, Jean; CSSS de Rimouski-Neigette, CP 3150 Succ A 150 av Rouleau, Rimouski QC G5L 5T1; Mon'69; Gastroent; IntMed. Chef méd int, Hôpital Regional Rimouski; (418)723-7851

ROBILLARD, Joan L; South Community Birth Program, 201-5838 Fraser St, Vancouver BC V5W 2Z5; Man'85; Ac Staff/Ad Staff Privil, BC Women's Hospital & Health Centre; Ad Staff Family Pract, UBC Hospital - Koerner Pavillion; Clin Assoc Prof, University of British Columbia; Langs: French; (604)324-2201

ROBILLARD, Josee; CSSS du Lac-des-Deux-Montagnes, 520 boul Arthur-Sauve, St-Eustache QC J7R 5B1; Mon'93; Staff, Hôpital de Saint-Eustache; (450)473-6811

ROBILLARD, Lise-Anne; 201-2446 Bank St, Ottawa ON K1V 1A4; Tor'90; Langs: French; (613)739-0998; larobillard@sympatico.ca.

ROBILLARD, Matthew T; Baycrest Ctre/Geriatric Care, 3560 Bathurst St, North York ON M6A 2E1; Tor'83; FRCPC; Psy (Geriatric Psychiatry). Staff, Baycrest Centre for Geriatric Care; Asst Prof Med, University of Toronto; (416)785-2500 x2321; Fax. (416)785-2450; mrobillard@baycrest.org.

ROBILLARD, Michel; Centre Med St-Redempteur, 600 116 Rte, Saint-Nicholas QC G7A 4X8; Mon'82; (418)831-3677

ROBILLARD, Nicole; CHUM-Hop Notre-Dame, 1560 rue Sherbrooke E, Montreal QC H2L 4M1; Mon'80; FRCSC; Ophth. Staff, Centre Hospitalier l'Université de Montréal (CHUM) - Hôpital Notre-Dame; Langs: English; French; (514)890-8000 x27103

ROBILLARD, Pierre; 245 rue du Curé-Majeau, Joliette QC J6E 8S8; Mon'65; DPH; CSPQ; CommunMed (P.Q.); PH (P.Q.) (Environmental Health). Staff, Centre Hospitalier Régional de Lanaudière; Langs: French; (450)759-1157 x4455; Fax. (450)759-0281; pierre_robillard@ssss.gouv.qc.ca.

ROBILLARD, Pierre; CHUM-Hotel-Dieu, 3840 rue Saint-Urbain, Montreal QC H2W 1T8; Mon'75; ABR; CSPQ; FRCPC; DiagRad. Chef radiodiag, Centre Hospitalier l'Université de Montréal (CHUM) - Hôtel-Dieu; adj Prof, Universite de Montreal; (514)890-8150

ROBILLARD, Pierre; Hema-Quebec, 4045 boul de la Cote-Vertu, Saint-Laurent QC H4R 2W7; Mon'77; (514)832-5000

ROBILLARD, Susan C; Tuxedo Fam Med Centre, 981 Corydon Ave, Winnipeg MB R3M 0X1; Man'85; CCFP; FCFP; (204)988-6040

ROBILLARD-MCNULTY, Lucile C; The Ottawa Hosp-Gen Campus, 501 Smyth Rd, Ottawa ON K1H 8L6; Ott'78; Staff, The Ottawa Hospital - General Campus; Langs: Bilingual(French/English); (613)737-7700; Fax. (613)247-3511; lurobillard@ottawahospital.on.ca.

ROBIN, Roger; Clinique Med Les Saules, 100-2780 boul Masson, Quebec QC G1P 1J6; Laval'73; ac Staff, CSSS de Quebec-Sud; (418)871-4492; Fax. (418)877-4478.

ROBIN-BOUDREAU, Maxime; Ctr de Sante Basse Cote Nord, CP 130 1070 boul Dr Camille Marcoux, Lourdes-d-Bl-Sabl QC G0G 1W0; Laval'06; CCFP; Staff, CSSS de la Basse Côté-Nord; Langs: Bilingual(French/English); (418)461-2144; Fax. (418)461-2962.

ROBINEAULT, Antoine; CSSS de la Baie-des-Chaleurs, RR 2 419 boul Perron, Maria QC G0C 1Y0; McG'96; FRCPC; Peds. Staff, CSSS de la Baie-des-Chaleurs; Langs: English; (418)759-3443

ROBINETTE, Michael A; N C S B, 11 1264-585 University Ave, Toronto ON M5G 2N2; Tor'68; FRCSC; Urol (Benign Prostatic Hypertrophy). Staff, Toronto General Hospital - UHN; Asst Prof Surg, University of Toronto; (416)340-3855; Fax. (416)340-4500; m.robinette@utoronto.ca.

ROBINETTE, Mylene; CHUS-Hop Fleurimont, 3001 12 av N, Sherbrooke QC J1H 5N4; Sher'07; FRCPC; Peds. Staff, Centre Hospitalier Universitaire de Sherbrooke-Hopital Fleurimont; (819)346-1110

ROBINOW, R Oliver; Formation Helth Services Unit, PO Box 17000 Stn Forces 1200 Colville Rd, Victoria BC V9A 7N2; Wes'69; FRCPC; Psy (Sexual Medicine). Psychiatrist, Canadian Forces Health Services - Pacific Centre; Staff, Vancouver General Hospital - Centennial Pavillion; (250)363-4467

ROBINS, Ronald N; London HSC-Victoria Hosp, PO Box 5010 Stn B E5 126-800 Commissioners Rd E, London ON N6A 5W9; Wes'68; FACS; FACOG; DABOG; AB; FRCSC; ObstGyn. Staff, London Health Sciences Centre - Victoria Campus; Staff, St Joseph's Hospital - St Joseph's Health Care; Staff, London Health Sciences Centre - University Hospital; Asst Prof, University of Western Ontario; (519)432-7657; Fax. (519)432-9887.

ROBINS, Ronald N F; Woodstock Gen Hosp, 310 Juliana Dr, Woodstock ON N4V 0A4; Cal'04; CCFP; CCFP(E.M.); Staff, Woodstock General Hospital; (519)421-4211

ROBINSON, Andrew G; Sudbury Reg Hosp-Laurentian, 41 Ramsey Lake Rd, Sudbury ON P3E 5J1; Man'00; MedOncol; IntMed. Staff, Health Sciences North-Laurentian Site; (705)522-2200

ROBINSON, Andrew J; Foothills Med Centre, C231-1403 29 St NW, Calgary AB T2N 2T9; Qns'07; EmergMed. Staff, Foothills Medical Centre; (403)944-1635; Fax. (403)944-2419.

ROBINSON, Anna C; Uptown Med Clinic, 3460 Saanich Rd, Victoria BC V8Z 0B9; Edinburgh (Scotland)'01.

ROBINSON, Anne M; Primary Health Care Unit, PO Box 4000, Sioux Lookout ON P8T 1K2; Wes'00; BSc; CCFP; Staff, Thunder Bay Regional Health Sciences Centre; (807)737-5166; Fax. (807)285-3694.

ROBINSON, Anthony H; Oakridge Centre South Tower, 209-650 41st Ave W, Vancouver BC V5Z 2M9; London (England)'71; MB BS; Court Staff, BC Children's Hospital; Ac Staff, Vancouver General Hospital - Centennial Pavillion; Clinical Asst Prof, University of British Columbia; (604)261-5626; drrobinson@shawbiz.ca.

ROBINSON, Arthur; Saskatoon East Fam Physicians, 21-2105 8th St E, Saskatoon SK S7H 0T8; Pretoria (South Africa)'92; MB ChB; LMCC; CCFP; Reg Rep Saskatoon/Member Exexcutive Saskatoon Chapter, Saskatchewan Medical Association; Past Lecturer PreGrad, University of Saskatchewan; Langs: Afrikaans; (306)373-5500; Fax. (306)374-9414.

ROBINSON, Ashley J; Children's & Women's HC of BC, B321-4480 Oak St, Vancouver BC V6H 3V4; Leeds (England)'94; FRCPC; DiagRad. Staff, BC Children's Hospital; (604)875-2131; Fax. (604)875-2367.

ROBINSON, Bruce T; Trail Bay Doctors, PO Box 1760, Sechelt BC V0N 3A0; Dal'91; (604)885-5196; Fax. (604)885-5193.

ROBINSON, Catherine A; Kingston Family Health Team, 200-2437 Princess St, Kingston ON K7M 3G1; Qns'03; CCFP; (613)546-6652; Fax. (613)546-5292; crobinson@kfhn.net.

ROBINSON, Christopher A; Royal University Hosp, 103 Hospital Dr, Saskatoon SK S7N 0W8; Cal'94; BSc; MSc; FRCPC; NeurPath (Forensic & Neuro Pathology). Staff, Royal University Hospital; (306)655-2186; Fax. (306)655-2223.

ROBINSON, Claire E; St Georges Med Clinic, 1315 St. Georges Ave, North Vancouver BC V7L 3J2; UBC'07; CCFP; (604)984-9213

ROBINSON, Clifford L; Orillia Soldiers' Mem Hosp, 170 Colborne St W, Orillia ON L3V 2Z3; Man'71; FRCPC; Anes. Staff, Orillia Soldiers' Memorial Hospital; (705)325-9934

ROBINSON, Constance L; 140 Talbot St, Shedden ON N0L 2E0; Wes'88; (519)764-2245; Fax. (519)764-2244.

ROBINSON, Dale K; Markham Stouffville Health Ctr, 207-377 Church St, Markham ON L6B 1A1; Dal'85; FRCPC; Neur. Consultant Neurologist, Markham Stouffville Hospital; Langs: French; English; (905)554-8711; Fax. (905)554-8815; darobinson@msh.on.ca.

ROBINSON, Daphne; Ingram Family Physicians, 103-149 Ingram St, Duncan BC V9L 1N8; Edinburgh (Scotland)'77; BSc; MB ChB; DRCOG; CCFP; FCFP; (250)746-4401; Fax. (250)746-4473.

ROBINSON, David B; Arthritis Centre, RR149-800 Sherbrook St, Winnipeg MB R3A 1M4; Man'95; FRCPC; IntMed; Rheum. Staff, The Rehabilitation Centre; drobinson@cc.umanitoba.ca.

ROBINSON, David C G; David Braley Sport Med & Rehab, DBAC WB127-1280 Main St W, Hamilton ON L8S 4K1; McM'91; CCFP; (905)525-9140; Fax. (905)526-7397.

ROBINSON, David J; Bluewater Health-Norman Site, 89 Norman St, Sarnia ON N7T 6S3; Tor'87; DABPN; FRCPC; Psy (Consultation-Liaison). Staff, Bluewater Health - Norman Site; (519)464-4400; Fax. (519)464-4516.

ROBINSON, Debbie J; 305-400 Tache Ave, Winnipeg MB R2H 3C3; Man'97; FRCSC; ObstGyn. (204)237-4694; Fax. (204)233-6636.

ROBINSON, Deborah L; Guelph Gen Hosp, 115 Delhi St, Guelph ON N1E 4J4; Tor'99; CCFP; Staff, Guelph General Hospital; (519)837-6440 x2235

ROBINSON, Derek A; 107-2462 Howard Ave, Windsor ON N8X 3V6; Tor'86; CCFP; FCFP; Court Staff, Hôtel-Dieu Grace Hospital; Court Staff, Windsor Regional Hospital - Metropolitan Site; (519)258-8234; Fax. (519)258-4732.

ROBINSON, Donna L; 401-960 Lawrence Ave W, North York ON M6A 3B5; Wes'90; CCFP; CCFP(E.M.); FCFP; (416)256-1150; Fax. (416)256-0742.

ROBINSON, Elizabeth; CSSS Jeanne-Mance, 100-15 av du Mont-Royal O, Montreal QC H2T 2R9; McG'72; CSPQ; FRCPC; CommunMed;CCFP; ac Staff Med, Cree Board of Health & Social Services James Bay; Ac Staff Preventive Med, McGill University Health Centre - Montreal General Campus; Aj Prof Epidemiol, McGill University; Langs: English; French; (514)286-9657

ROBINSON, Elizabeth L; Alberta Children's Hosp, 2888 Shaganappi Trail NW, Calgary AB T3B 6A8; McM'88; FRCPC; Peds. Staff, Alberta Children's Hospital; (403)955-7211

ROBINSON, Emma; Quinte HC Corp-Belleville Gen, 265 Dundas St E, Belleville ON K8N 5A9; Tor'02; FRCPC; DiagRad. Staff, QHC Belleville General; (613)969-7400

ROBINSON, Eric J; Southside Hlth & Life Mgmt Ctr, 2-2120 Regent St, Sudbury ON P3E 3Z9; Ott'87; FRCSC; OrthSurg. Langs: English; French; (705)522-9101; Fax. (705)522-5744.

ROBINSON, G Gail E; Univ Hlth Network-Toronto Gen, 8231 EN-200 Elizabeth St, Toronto ON M5G 2C4; Tor'66; DPsy; FRCPC; Psy (Women's Mental Health). Consultant, Women's College Hospital; Consultant Psy, Sunnybrook Health Sciences Centre; Dir Women's Mental Health Prog/Sr Psychiatrist, Toronto General Hospital - UHN; Prof, University of Toronto; (416)340-3048; Fax. (416)340-4198.

ROBINSON, Glenn P; Coleman Clinic, 186 Kenneth St, Duncan BC V9L 1N4; UBC'81; (250)746-4102; Fax. (250)746-5960.

ROBINSON, Gregg; Rocky Med Clinic, PO Box 99 Stn Main, Rocky-Mtn-Hse AB T4T 1A1; Belfast (Ireland)'77; MB ChB; BAO; FRCSI; Staff, Rocky Mountain House Health Centre; (403)845-2815; Fax. (403)845-2177.

ROBINSON, Heather E; Hys Med Centre, 604-11010 101 St NW, Edmonton AB T5H 4B9; Sask'98; FRCSC; ObstGyn. (780)421-4728; Fax. (780)426-6698.

ROBINSON, Helena M; Welkare Med Office, 268 Clarence St, London ON N6B 2K1; Wes'84; CCFP; FCFP; Ac Staff, St Joseph's Hospital - St Joseph's Health Care; University of Western Ontario; (519)672-9898; Fax. (519)858-5775.

ROBINSON, Jacques; Bureau du Coroner, 11e-1701 rue Parthenais, Montreal QC H2K 3S7; Sher'73; (514)873-3284 x21203; Fax. (514)873-9843.

ROBINSON, James F; Assiniboine Clinic, 633 Lodge Ave, Winnipeg MB R3J 0S9; Man'83; FRCSC; GenSurg. (204)958-6725; Fax. (204)888-1750.

ROBINSON, Jeffery M; Misericordia Community Hosp, 1NW15-16940 87 Ave NW, Edmonton AB T5R 4H5; Cal'81; CCFP; FCFP; Staff, Covenant Health - Misericordia Community Hospital; Clin Instructor Family Med, University of Alberta; (780)735-2585; Fax. (780)735-2588.

ROBINSON, Jennifer M; 450-6450 Roberts St, Burnaby BC V5G 4E1; Witwatersrand (South Africa)'86; MB ChB; (604)232-5900

ROBINSON, Jennifer W; 305-1625 Oak Bay Ave, Victoria BC V8R 1B1; McM'04; FRCSC; PlasSurg. (250)590-7097

ROBINSON, Jo-Ann; Edson Med Centre, PO Box 6660 Stn Main, Edson AB T7E 1V1; Qns'04; CCFP; (780)723-3366; Fax. (780)723-3437.

ROBINSON, Joan; Edmonton Clinic Health Academy, 3 556-11405 87 Ave NW, Edmonton AB T6G 1C9; Alb'83; FRCPC; Peds; InfectDis. Staff, University of Alberta Hospital; Staff, Edmonton Clinic Health Academy; Assoc Prof, University of Alberta; (780)248-5528; jr3@uualberta.ca.

ROBINSON, John; Kerrisdale Station Med Clinic, 2077 42nd Ave W, Vancouver BC V6M 2B4; Belfast (Ireland)'57; MB ChB; BAO; Staff, Providence Health Care - St Vincent's Hospital-Heather Site; Staff, Providence Health Care - Holy Family Hospital; Staff, BC Women's Hospital & Health Centre; (604)261-9494; jrobinson@providencehealth.bc.ca.

ROBINSON, Juan; Queen Elizabeth II HSC-Halifax, 4875-1796 Summer St, Halifax NS B3H 3A7; London (England)'99; Staff, Queen Elizabeth II Health Sciences Centre - Halifax Infirmary Site; (902)473-4035; Fax. (902)473-4490.

ROBINSON, K Sue; 428-1276 South Park St, Halifax NS B3H 2Y9; Dal'82; FRCPC; IntMed; Hem. Staff, Queen Elizabeth II Health Sciences Centre - Victoria General Site; Assoc Prof, Dalhousie University; (902)473-2394; Fax. (902)473-4447; sue.robinson@cdha.nshealth.ca.

ROBINSON, Karen G; Northeastman Health Authority, PO Box 1690 646 James Ave, Beausejour MB R0E 0C0; Sask'99; FRCPC; CommunMed;CCFP.

ROBINSON, Karen M; PO Box 52028 Rpo Garneau, Edmonton AB T6G 2T5; Sask'93; CCFP.

ROBINSON, Katherine A B; Dalhousie Univ Health Services, PO Box 15000 Lcd 2 6230 Coburg Rd, Halifax NS B3H 4R2; Dal'88; CCFP; FCFP; (902)494-2171; Fax. (902)494-6872; krobinsonmd@hfx.eastlink.ca.

ROBINSON, Linda A; Central Med Bldg, 303-1105 Carling Ave, Ottawa ON K1Y 4G5; McG'79; AB; FRCPC; Anes (Chronic Pain). Dir Chronic Pain Clinic, The Ottawa Hospital - Civic Campus; Asst Prof, University of Ottawa; Langs: English; French; (613)866-2398

ROBINSON, Lisa A; The Hosp for Sick Children, 5265-555 University Ave, Toronto ON M5G 1X8; Tor'91; FRCPC; Peds. Staff, The Hospital For Sick Children; (416)813-7654 x1745; Fax. (416)813-6271; lisa.robinson@sickkids.ca.

ROBINSON, Lynne E; 201-6990 Derry Rd, Milton ON L9T 7H3; Ott'79; Ac Staff, Halton Healthcare Services Corporation - Milton District Hospital; Court Staff, Joseph Brant Memorial Hospital; (905)878-2043; Fax. (905)878-0945.

ROBINSON, Marie-Brigitte; Southside Hlth & Life Mgmt Ctr, 2-2120 Regent St, Sudbury ON P3E 3Z9; Ott'89; FRCSC; Otol. Langs: English; French; (705)522-9101; Fax. (705)522-5744.

ROBINSON, Martine; CSSS des Sources, 475 3e av, Asbestos QC J1T 1X6; (Haiti)'85; Staff, CSSS des Sources d'Asbestos; Langs: Bilingual(French/English); (819)879-7151

ROBINSON, Matthew G; Cedar Springs Prof Centre, D-960 Cumberland Ave, Burlington ON L7N 3J6; Tor'92; CCFP; Ac Staff, Joseph Brant Memorial Hospital; (905)639-3447; Fax. (905)639-3448.

ROBINSON, Matthew J; 405-1120 Yates St, Victoria BC V8V 3M9; Man'04; FRCSC; GenSurg; VascSurg. (250)384-8154

ROBINSON, Patrick N; Hop Charles LeMoyne, 3120 boul Taschereau, Greenfield Park QC J4V 2H1; Mon'96; GenSurg. Staff, Hopital Charles LeMoyne; (450)466-5000

ROBINSON, Paul; 100-84 rue Dumas, Gatineau QC J8Y 2N3; Sher'78; Langs: Bilingual(English/French); (819)778-6597; Fax. (819)778-0709.

ROBINSON, R Gordon; 8213-2775 Laurel St, Vancouver BC V5Z 1M9; UBC'73; FRCP; BSc; FRCPC; Neur (P.Q.) (Headache). Clin Prof Neurol, University of British Columbia; Staff/Med Dir Rehab Arthritis Spine & Neurosciences, Vancouver General Hospital - Centennial Pavillion; (604)875-5549; Fax. (604)269-3762; gordon.robinson@vch.ca.

ROBINSON, R Jane; E215-50 Westmount Rd N, Waterloo ON N2L 2R5; McM'81; CCFP; FCFP; Staff Supportive Care, Grand River Hospital - Kitchener/Waterloo Health Centre; Staff Supportive Care, St Mary's General Hospital; (519)746-3000; Fax. (519)746-5965.

ROBINSON, Richard G; Harbour City Health Centre, 201-1125 Dufferin Cres, Nanaimo BC V9S 2B5; UBC'85; FRCSC; PlasSurg. Ac Staff, Nanaimo Regional General Hospital; (250)753-1622; Fax. (250)753-8399; drrgrobinson@shaw.ca.

ROBINSON, Richard J S; MUHC-Montreal Gen Hosp, D8 132-1650 av Cedar, Montreal QC H3G 1A4; Cardiff (Wales)'73; MB ChB; CSPQ; FRCPC; Anes; Critical Care Medicine (P.Q.). Assoc Staff, McGill University Health Centre - Montreal General Campus; assoc Prof, McGill University; (514)934-1934 x43261

ROBINSON, Simon D; Richmond Med Bldg, 202-2020 Richmond Rd, Victoria BC V8R 6R5; Edinburgh (Scotland)'98; (250)595-3111

ROBINSON, Trevor I; St Michael's Hosp, 3 054CC-30 Bond St, Toronto ON M5B 1W8; Buffalo(NY) (USA)'67; Staff Cardiologist, St Michael's Hospital; Asst Prof Med, University of Toronto; (416)864-5331; Fax. (416)864-5571; robinsont@smh.toronto.on.ca.

ROBINSON, Virginia W; Elk Valley Hosp, PO Box 670 1501 5th Ave, Fernie BC V0B 1M0; Qns'94; CCFP; CCFP(E.M.); FCFP; Chief/Staff, Elk Valley Hospital; Langs: English; French; (250)423-4453

ROBINSON, Wesley K; Provencher Pediatrics, 103-147 Provencher Blvd, Winnipeg MB R2H 0G2; Man'75; FRCPC; Peds. Staff, St Boniface General Hospital; Staff, Victoria General Hospital; Staff, Health Sciences Centre.

ROBINSON, William E; 301-1466 Bathurst St, Toronto ON M5R 3S3; Qns'60; Psy (Psychoanalysis). (416)532-7207; Fax. (416)413-0519.

ROBINSON POWER, Alicia M; 201-284 Helmcken Rd, Victoria BC V9B 1T2; UBC'07; CCFP; (250)508-7752

ROBISON, E Jean; St Lawrence Health Services, 3-140 The Esplanade, Toronto ON M5A 4P5; Wes'82; CCFP; Staff Family & CommunMed, St Michael's Hospital; Physician, Fudger House Home for the Aged; Langs: English; French; (416)864-6000; Fax. (416)360-4902.

ROBISON, Gordon E A; Toronto East Gen Hosp Inc, 825 Coxwell Ave, Toronto ON M4C 3E7; Tor'88; FRCPC; Anes. Staff, Toronto East General Hospital Inc; Lecturer, University of Toronto; (416)469-6212; Fax. (416)469-6874.

ROBITAILLE, Andre; 116 rue du College, St-Aug-D-Desm QC G3A 1H4; Laval'72; (418)878-2795; Fax. (418)878-9510; andre.robitaille@videotron.ca.

ROBITAILLE, Arnaud; CHUM-Hop Notre-Dame, 1560 rue Sherbrooke E, Montreal QC H2L 4M1; McG'01; FRCPC; Anes. Staff, Centre Hospitalier l'Université de Montréal (CHUM) - Hôpital Notre-Dame; (514)890-8000

ROBITAILLE, Brigitte; CSSS des Pays-d'en-Haut, 707 boul de Sainte-Adele, Sainte-Adele QC J8B 2N1; Laval'93; (450)227-3447 x4368; Fax. (450)227-3467.

ROBITAILLE, Chantal; Clinique Med Lamater, 2400-504 rue Notre-Dame, Repentigny QC J6A 2T8; Laval'91; (450)582-3992

ROBITAILLE, Daniel; CSSS de Manicouagan, 635 boul Jolliet, Baie-Comeau QC G5C 1P1; Laval'92; CSPQ; FRCPC; MedBiochem (Clinical Lipid Disorders). Staff, Centre Hospitalier Régional Baie-Comeau; Langs: English; (418)589-3701 x2810; Fax. (418)589-1870.

ROBITAILLE, Danielle; Institut de Cardiologie de Mtl, 5000 rue Belanger, Montreal QC H1T 1C8; Sher'79; FRCPC; Hem. Staff, Institut de Cardiologie de Montréal; Chief Lab Med, Cirion Bio Pharma Research Inc; (514)376-3330

ROBITAILLE, David; CSSS Pierre Boucher, 1333 boul Jacques-Cartier E, Longueuil QC J4M 2A5; Mon'95; CSPQ; FRCPC; Psy (Primary Care). Staff Psychiatrist, Centre Hospitalier Pierre Boucher; Langs: Spanish; English; French; (450)468-8401; Fax. (450)468-8403; david.robitaille@rrsssspb.qc.ca.

ROBITAILLE, Diane; 123-70 rue O'Keefe, Salaber-de-Valleyf QC J6S 5C6; Mon'81; (450)371-5412

ROBITAILLE, Elisabeth; Clinique Medicale Mascouche, 100-1025 Montee Masson, Mascouche QC J7K 2L9; Mon'90; (450)474-6000

ROBITAILLE, Erik; CSSS de Laval, 1755 boul Rene-Laennec, Laval QC H7M 3L9; Mon'07; FRCPC; Psy. Staff, Hopital de la Cite de la santé; (450)668-1010

ROBITAILLE, Georges; Hop Charles LeMoyne, 3120 boul Taschereau, Greenfield Park QC J4V 2H1; Mon'89; CSPQ; Psy. Staff, Hopital Charles LeMoyne; (450)466-5000; Fax. (450)466-5015.

ROBITAILLE, Isabelle; CSSS Les Eskers de l'Abitibi, 622 4e rue O, Amos QC J9T 2S2; Laval'99; CCFP; Staff, CH Hôtel-Dieu d'Amos; (819)732-3341

ROBITAILLE, J Michel J P; 8 rue Cotnoir, Sorel-Tracy QC J3P 5R6; Mon'72; Peds. Staff, Hôtel-Dieu de Sorel; Consultant, Hôpital Ste-Justine; (450)743-0516

ROBITAILLE, Jean-Philippe; CSSS du Sud de Lanaudière, 911 montee des Pionniers, Terrebonne QC J6V 2H2; Laval'04; FRCPC; Anes. Staff, Centre Hospitalier Pierre le Gardeur; (450)654-7525

ROBITAILLE, Johane M; IWK Health Centre, PO Box 9700 Rpo CSC 5850-5980 University Ave, Halifax NS B3K 6R8; McG'89; FRCSC; Ophth (Pediatric Ophthalmology). Staff, IWK Health Centre; Langs: Bilingual(French/English); (902)470-8632; Fax. (902)470-7207.

ROBITAILLE, Josee; Hop Brome-Missisquoi-Perkins, 950 rue Principale, Cowansville QC J2K 1K3; Laval'92; FRCSC; GenSurg. Staff, Hôpital Brome-Missisquoi-Perkins; (450)266-4342; Fax. (450)263-8669.

ROBITAILLE, Julie; CHSLD St-Jean-Eudes Inc, 6000 3e av O, Quebec QC G1H 7J5; Laval'92; CCFP; (418)627-1124; Fax. (418)627-4995; julie.robitaille@videotron.ca.

ROBITAILLE, Julie; Centre Medical de l'Hetriere, 201-3520 rue de l'Hetriere, St-Augustin-D-Desm QC G3A 0B4; Laval'96; Staff, Centre Hospitalier du Centre la Mauricie; (418)651-3933; Fax. (418)651-0256.

ROBITAILLE, Manon; CSSS de Montmagny-L'Islet, RR 1 350 boul Tache O, Montmagny QC G5V 3R8; Laval'98; CSPQ; FRCPC; Psy (Personality Disorders). ac Staff Psy, CSSS de Montmagny-L'Islet; assoc Staff Psy, Hôpital de l'Archipel; Assoc Staff, Clinique le Faubourgs St-Jean; (418)248-0630 x5563; Fax. (418)248-8472; manonrobitaillecsssml@ssss.gouv.qc.ca.

ROBITAILLE, Manon; Centre Hosp Honore-Mercier, 2750 boul Laframboise, Saint-Hyacinthe QC J2S 4Y8; Laval'06; Gastroent; IntMed. Staff, Centre Hospitalier Honore-Mercier; (450)771-3333

ROBITAILLE, Marc; CSSS de Rouyn-Noranda, 1 9e rue, Rouyn-Noranda QC J9X 2A9; Laval'74; Staff, CSSS de Rouyn-Noranda; (819)764-3264 x49342; Fax. (819)797-1947; marc_robitaille@ssss.gouv.qc.ca.

ROBITAILLE, Michel; Clinique Med Giffard, A222-3333 rue du carrefour, Quebec QC G1C 5R9; Laval'79; (418)663-6345; Fax. (418)663-8621.

ROBITAILLE, Nancy; Hôpital Ste-Justine, 3175 ch Cote-Sainte-Catherine, Montreal QC H3T 1C5; Mon'98; FRCPC; Peds; Hem. Staff, Hôpital Ste-Justine; Langs: English; (514)345-4931; josee.robert.hsj@ssss.gouv.qc.ca.

ROBITAILLE, Nancy-Michelle; Hôpital Laval, 2725 ch Sainte-Foy, Quebec QC G1V 4G5; Laval'72; MPH; Cardiol (P.Q.) (Physical Medicine & Rehabilitation). Consultant Cardiol & Research, Hôpital Laval; Physician, Institute de Readaptation de Quebec; Langs: English; (418)656-8711 x4657; Fax. (418)656-4544; nancy-michelle.robitaille@med.ulaval.ca.

ROBITAILLE, Olivier; CSSS de Laval, 1755 boul Rene-Laennec, Laval QC H7M 3L9; Sher'99; CSPQ; Anes. Staff, Hopital de la Cite de la santé; (450)668-1010 x2477

ROBITAILLE, Pierre O; Hôpital Ste-Justine, 3175 ch Cote-Sainte-Catherine, Montreal QC H3T 1C5; Mon'65; MSc(McG); Nephrol (P.Q.) (Pediatrics). Dir Nephrol Div, Hôpital Ste-Justine; Prof Peds, Universite de Montreal; (514)345-4737; Fax. (514)345-4838; pierre_robitaille@ssss.gouv.qc.ca.

ROBITAILLE, Rejean; Inst U en Sante Mentale de QC, 2601 ch de la Canardiere, Quebec QC G1J 2G3; Laval'84; Staff, Institut Universitaire Sante; Assoc Staff, Centre Hospitalier Universitaire De Québec - Pavillon De St-françois-d'assise; (418)663-5321

ROBITAILLE, Sylvie A; CLSC des Mille-Iles, 4731 boul Levesque E, Laval QC H7C 1M9; Mon'85; (450)661-2572

ROBITAILLE, Sylvie; CSSS Maria-Chapdelaine, 2000 boul du Sacré-Coeur, Dolbeau-Mistassini QC G8L 2R5; Mon'83; Staff, Centre Maria-Chapdelaine - CH de Dolbeau-Mistassini; (418)276-1426; Fax. (418)276-7762.

ROBITAILLE, Yves; CSSS du Sud de Lanaudière, 911 montee des Pionniers, Terrebonne QC J6V 2H2; Mon'92; IntMed. Staff, Centre Hospitalier Pierre le Gardeur; (450)654-7525 x23000; Fax. (450)585-5939; robitaille.yves@me.com.

ROBITAILLE, Yves; Hôpital Ste-Justine, 3175 ch Cote-Sainte-Catherine, Montreal QC H3T 1C5; Mon'66; FCAP(AP&NP); DABPath; GenPath (P.Q.) (Neuropathology). ac Staff Path, Hôpital Ste-Justine; Prof, Universite de Montreal; Langs: English; French; (514)345-4649; Fax. (514)345-4819; yves.robitaille@umontreal.ca.

ROBLES, Harold I; McMaster University, MDCL 3101A-1280 Main St W, Hamilton ON L8S 4K1; UBC'07; FRCSC; OrthSurg.

ROBLES, Luis C; Sunnybrook Hlth Sciences Ctre, 2075 Bayview Ave, Toronto ON M4N 3M5; (Panama)'86; FRCPC; EmergMed. Staff, Sunnybrook Health Sciences Centre; (416)480-4037

ROBLES, Melanie A; Athabascan Place, 222-80 Chippewa Rd, Sherwood Park AB T8A 4W6; Alb'91; CCFP; FCFP; Staff, Hawkesbury & District General Hospital; (780)464-9661; Fax. (780)417-0656.

ROBSON, Alexander J; 9368 Southfort Dr, Fort Saskatchewan AB T8L 0C5; London (England)'63; MB BS; FRCS; GenSurg. (780)997-0177; Fax. (780)992-2065.

ROBSON, Daniel; 405-4800 Leslie St, North York ON M2J 2K9; Alb'02; FRCPC; IntMed; MedOncol. Staff MedOncol, North York General Hospital; (416)640-0892; Fax. (416)640-1243.

ROBSON, Helen J; 307-7031 Westminster Hwy, Richmond BC V6X 1A3; Man'86; FRCSC; ObstGyn. Staff Colposcopist, BC Cancer Agency Vancouver Centre; Staff, Richmond Hospital; Clin Teacher, University of British Columbia; (604)270-1434; Fax. (604)270-3431; helenrobson@telus.net.

ROBSON, Hugh G; MUHC-Royal Victoria Hosp, L505-687 av des Pins O, Montreal QC H3A 1A1; McG'60; BSc; FRCPC; IntMed (Infectious Diseases); Microbio & Infect Dis (P.Q.); MedMicrobiol (P.Q.). Staff Med & Microbiol, McGill University Health Centre - Royal Victoria Hospital; Prof Med, McGill University; Langs: English; French; (514)934-1934 x35066; Fax. (514)934-4476.

ROBSON, Kathleen E; B-22195 Dewdney Trunk Rd, Maple Ridge BC V2X 3H7; Pretoria (South Africa)'87; MB ChB; (604)463-4102; kerobson@hotmail.com.

ROBSON, Mark G; Primary Health Care Centre, 162-346 John St N, Arnprior ON K7S 2P6; McG'78; BSc; CCFP; (613)623-7939; Fax. (613)623-8334.

ROBSON, Michael; Tottenham Med Centre, PO Box 2000 119 Queen St N, Tottenham ON L0G 1W0; Manchester (England)'70; MB ChB; Ac Staff, Stevenson Memorial Hospital; (905)936-4211; Fax. (905)936-3493.

ROBSON, Nancy B A; University of Alberta Hosp, 8440 112 St NW, Edmonton AB T6G 2B7; Alb'99; CCFP; Staff, University of Alberta Hospital; (780)480-1550

ROBSON, Robert J; 116 York St E RR 5, Elora ON N0B 1S0; McG'72 Lund University (Sweden); ATLS; ACLS; FRCPC; EmergMed (Administrative Medicine). Langs: English; French; (519)846-2872; Fax. (519)846-9843; rrobson@mediatecalm.ca.

ROBSON, Scott M; 401-1366 Yonge St, Toronto ON M4T 3A7; Alb'67; CCFP; (416)966-0178; Fax. (416)929-0843.

ROBSON, W Lane M; The Childrens' Clinic, 111-4411 16 Ave NW, Calgary AB T3B 0M3; Cal'73; FRCPC; Peds (Pediatric Nephrology). Physician, The Childrens' Clinic; (403)202-2949; Fax. (403)202-2948.

ROCCA, Antonio S; Polyclinic Specialty Med, 5-4646 Dufferin St, North York ON M3H 5S4; Tor'02; FRCPC; IntMed; Cardiol. (416)222-6160; Fax. (416)645-1979.

ROCCA, Bruno A; Kelowna Gen Hosp, 2268 Pandosy St, Kelowna BC V1Y 1T2; McM'96; FRCPC; Anes. Staff, Kelowna General Hospital; (250)862-4309

ROCCI, Adriano; 1011 Upper Middle Rd E PO Box 86083 Rpo Upper Oakvill, Oakville ON L6H 5V6; Wes'83; CCFP; FCFP; Staff, Niagara Health System - St Catharines General Site; Staff, Niagara Health System - Ontario Street Site; Langs: Italian; (905)599-2675; Fax. (905)257-1084.

ROCH, J J C Andre; 310 York St, Sudbury ON P3E 2A6; Mon'83; Staff, Health Sciences North - Memorial Site; Staff, Health Sciences North-St Joseph's Health Centre; Ac Staff, North Bay Regional Health Centre - Kirkwood; Langs: English; French; (705)671-2768; Fax. (705)671-2757.

ROCHA, Guillermo; Medical Centre Bldg, 20-144 6th St, Brandon MB R7A 3N2; (Mexico)'89; FRCSC; Ophth (Cornea). Ophthalmology, Minnedosa Health Centre; Staff, Brandon Regional Health Centre; University of Manitoba; Aj Prof, University of Ottawa; Langs: English; French; Spanish; (204)727-1954; Fax. (204)728-5248.

ROCHA, Roland C; Toronto East Gen Hosp Inc, 825 Coxwell Ave, Toronto ON M4C 3E7; Wes'99; FRCPC; IntMed. Staff, Toronto East General Hospital Inc; (416)461-8272

ROCHA, Tristana M; St Clair Med Centre, 50 St Clair Ave E, Toronto ON M4T 1M9; Ott'99; CCFP; Staff, William Osler Health System - Etobicoke General Hospital; (416)921-1066; Fax. (416)921-8459.

ROCHA MICHAELS, Clara E; Academic Family Medicine, 172-1621 Albert St, Regina SK S4P 2S5; Staff, Regina General Hospital; (306)766-0444; Fax. (306)766-0471.

ROCHE, Anne L; Misericordia Community Hosp, 16940 87 Ave NW, Edmonton AB T5R 4H5; Mem'94; Staff, Covenant Health - Misericordia Community Hospital; (780)735-2819; Fax. (780)735-2966.

ROCHE, Gavin J; Minnedosa Med Group, PO Box 810, Minnedosa MB R0J 1E0; Cape Town (South Africa)'88; CCFP; Assoc Prof, University of Manitoba; (204)867-2722; Fax. (204)867-2986.

ROCHE, Mark J; Trillium Hlth Ctr-Mississauga, 100 Queensway W, Mississauga ON L5B 1B8; McM'87; FRCPC; Anes (Chronic Pain). Staff, Trillium Health Centre - Mississauga; (905)848-7628

ROCHE, Susan L; Toronto Congenital Cardiac Ctr, 585 University Ave, Toronto ON M5G 2N2; Leeds (England)'99; (416)340-4871

ROCHE-NAGLE, Michael G; Univ Hlth Network-Toronto Gen, 218-200 Elizabeth St, Toronto ON M5G 2C4; (Ireland)'98; Staff, Toronto General Hospital - UHN; (416)340-5332; Fax. (416)340-5029.

ROCHEFORT, Lucie; Pavillon Ferdinand-Landry, 4770-1050 av de la Medecine, Quebec QC G1V 0A6; Laval'89; CCFP; FCFP; Prog Dir, Université Laval; (418)656-2131 x7636

ROCHELEAU, France D; Centre Royal Comtois, 444 McGill St, Hawkesbury ON K6A 1R2; Mon'83; CSPQ; FRCPC; Psy. Staff, Hawkesbury & District General Hospital; Langs: Bilingual(French/English); (613)632-0139; Fax. (613)632-4791.

ROCHELEAU, Michael G; 402-1245 Esquimalt Rd, Victoria BC V9A 3P2; Cal'80; FRCPC; PhysMed&Rehab (Stroke). Staff Physician, Vancouver Island Health Authority; (250)598-9922; Fax. (250)598-9983.

ROCHETTE, Andre; SAAQ, S21-333 boul Jean-Lesage, Quebec QC G1K 8Z2; Laval'78; (418)528-3899; Fax. (418)644-2041; andre.rochette@saaq.gouv.qc.ca.

ROCHETTE, Anne; CLSC Ste-Therese de Blainville, 55 rue Saint-Joseph, Sainte-Therese QC J7E 4Y5; Sher'81; (450)430-4553 x6011

ROCHETTE, Antoine; Ctr Hosp Affilie-St-Sacrement, 1050 ch Sainte-Foy, Quebec QC G1S 4L8; Laval'03; FRCPC; DiagRad. Staff, Centre Hospitalier Affilié Universitaire de Québec - Hôpital du St-Sacrement; (418)682-7511

ROCHETTE, Denis; CSSS de Chicoutimi, 305 rue Saint-Vallier, Chicoutimi QC G7H 5H6; Laval'70; CSPQ; Psy (Adult Psychiatry). Staff, Complexe hospitalier de la Sagamie; Staff, Institut Roland-Saucier; (418)549-5474; Fax. (418)549-7604.

ROCHETTE, Emilien; 304-3436 boul Sainte-Anne, Quebec QC G1E 6Z2; Laval'59; CSPQ; CommunMed (P.Q.) (Family Medicine). (418)667-3341; Fax. (418)667-3820.

ROCHETTE, Linda; Ctr Dermatologique de Quebec, 105-2880 ch des Quatre-Bourgeo, Quebec QC G1V 4X7; Laval'87; FRCPC; Derm. (418)650-3555; Fax. (418)650-1260.

ROCHETTE, Marie; Min de la Sante et Serv Sociau, 11Flr-1075 ch Sainte-Foy, Quebec QC G1S 2M1; Laval'87; CSPQ; FRCPC; CommunMed; Public Health & Preventive Med. Langs: French; (418)266-6750; Fax. (418)266-4609.

ROCHETTE, Pascal; CHUQ-St-Francois d'Assise, 10 rue de l'Espinay, Quebec QC G1L 3L5; Laval'92; Staff Emerg, Centre Hospitalier Universitaire De Québec - Pavillon De St-françois-d'assise; Physician, EVAQ-Avian Ambulance; Prof, Université Laval; (418)525-4444

ROCHETTE, Pierre; Inst Philippe Pinel de Mtl, 10905 boul Henri-Bourassa E, Montreal QC H1C 1H1; Mon'88; CSPQ; FRCPC; Psy. Staff, Hopital Louis-H Lafontaine; Universite de Montreal; (514)684-8461; pierrerochette@videotron.ca.

ROCHON, Alain; ASSS de l'Estrie, 300-300 rue King E, Sherbrooke QC J1G 1B1; Mon'80; MSc; CSPQ; FRCPC; CommunMed (Health Promotion). Med Consultant, Promotion de la Sante; Clin Prof, Universite de Sherbrooke; Langs: Spanish; Bilingual(French/English); (819)829-3400 x42527; Fax. (819)569-8894; arochon.agence05@ssss.gouv.qc.ca.

ROCHON, Antoine; Institut de Cardiologie de Mtl, 5000 rue Belanger, Montreal QC H1T 1C8; Mon'99; CSPQ; FRCPC; Anes. Staff, Institut de Cardiologie de Montréal; (514)376-3330 x3732

ROCHON, Daniele; Clinique Med du Jardin, 15094 boul Henri-Bourassa, Quebec QC G1G 3Z4; Laval'84; (418)628-9074; Fax. (418)628-0267.

ROCHON, Denise T; McGill Student Hlth Serv Ctre, 5500-3600 rue McTavish, Montreal QC H3A 0G3; Ott'77; CSPQ; FRCPC; Psy (Psychodynamic/Psychotherapy)., McGill University; Langs: English; French; (514)398-6019 x09920; Fax. (514)398-5529.

ROCHON, Francois; Hop du Sacre-Coeur de Mtl, 5400 boul Gouin O, Montreal QC H4J 1C5; Sher'81; CSPQ; FRCPC; Anes. Staff, Hôpital du Sacre-Coeur de Montréal; (514)338-2222 x2680

ROCHON, Jean; Institut Nat'l Sante Publique, 2.03-190 boul Cremazie E, Montreal QC H2P 1E2; Laval'66; CPH; CommunMed (Epidemiology). Langs: English; (514)864-1600 x3631; jean.rochon@inspq.qc.ca.

ROCHON, Jean-Louis; Ville du Nord, 2319 rue Sainte-Marie, Sainte-Sophie QC J5J 1M8; Mon'65; Staff Privil, Centre Hospitalier de LaSalle; (450)436-5627; Fax. (450)436-5637.

ROCHON, Louise M A; SMBD Jewish Gen Hosp, 3755 ch Cote-Sainte-Catherine, Montreal QC H3T 1E2; Sher'73; CSPQ; FRCPC; AnatPath. Sr Staff Path, Sir Mortimer B Davis Jewish General; Assoc Prof Pat & ENT, McGill University; (514)340-8274; Fax. (514)340-8102.

ROCHON, Luc J W; 403-595 Montreal Rd, Ottawa ON K1K 4L2; Ott'78 U of Ottawa; FRCPC; IntMed; Gastroent. Staff, Montfort Hospital; Consultant, The Ottawa Hospital - General Campus; Clinical Asst Prof Med, University of Ottawa; Langs: Bilingual(English/French); (613)745-8633; Fax. (613)745-8715.

ROCHON, Lucie; CLSC Kateri, 90 boul Marie-Victorin, Candiac QC J5R 1C1; Mon'85; (450)659-7661; Fax. (450)444-6276.

ROCHON, Marie-Helene; 535 Family Practice, 535 Montreal Rd, Ottawa ON K1K 0V1; Ott'05; CCFP; (613)746-5350; Fax. (613)746-5340.

ROCHON, Michel; CSSS du Sud de Lanaudière, 911 montee des Pionniers, Terrebonne QC J6V 2H2; Mon'93; CSPQ; DiagRad. Staff, Centre Hospitalier Pierre le Gardeur; (450)654-7525

ROCHON, Micheline; CSSS du Granit, 3569 rue Laval, Lac-Megantic QC G6B 1A5; Sher'74; Staff, Carrefour Sante Granit; (819)583-0330

ROCHON, Michelle; Hop du Sacre-Coeur de Mtl, 5400 boul Gouin O, Montreal QC H4J 1C5; Mon'88; CSPQ; FRCPC; Psy (Geriatric Psychiatry). Staff, Hôpital du Sacre-Coeur de Montréal; Universite de Montreal; Langs: Bilingual(French/English); (514)338-3563; Fax. (514)338-4359.

ROCHON, Paula A; Women's College Hosp, 76 Grenville St, Toronto ON M5S 1B2; McM'83; MPH; FRCPC; IntMed; GeriatricMed. Staff, Women's College Hospital; Assoc Staff, Mount Sinai Hospital; Prof Med, University of Toronto; (416)323-6400; Fax. (416)487-3002; paula.rochon@utoronto.ca.

ROCHOWSKI, Andrzej; Queensway-Carleton Hosp, 3045 Baseline Rd, Ottawa ON K2H 8P4; Jagiellonian Univ (Poland)'05; Staff, Queensway Carleton Hospital; (613)721-2000

ROCHWERG, Bram N; McMaster University, MDCL 3101A-1280 Main St W, Hamilton ON L8S 4K1; Ott'09.

ROCHWERGER, Felisa L; 603-1 St Clair Ave E, Toronto ON M4T 2V7; Buenos Aires (Argentina)'60; FRCPC; Psy (Psychoanalysis). Langs: Spanish; (416)922-2220; Fax. (416)928-9401; felevy@rogers.com.

ROCK, Nathalie; Clinique Ped La Courte Echelle, 86 boul Brien, Repentigny QC J6A 5K7; Laval'92; Peds. Staff Peds, Centre Hospitalier Pierre le Gardeur; (450)657-1705; Fax. (450)657-1800.

ROCK, Rejean; 3087 Capelton Rd GD, North Hatley QC J0B 2C0; Mon'78; Langs: Bilingual(English/French); (819)842-4317; Fax. (819)842-1402; rejean.rock@sympatico.ca.

ROCK, William J; 213-150 Montreal Rd, Vanier ON K1L 8H2; Ott'66; FRCOphth; FRCSC; Ophth (Glaucoma). Assoc Staff, The Ottawa Hospital - General Campus; University of Ottawa; Langs: Bilingual(English/French); (613)238-3850; Fax. (613)235-7972; williamrock@hotmail.com.

ROCKEL, Anthony J; Fort Louis Med Clinic, PO Box 250, Placentia NL A0B 2Y0; Otago (New Zealand)'66; MB ChB; CAFCI; ACLS; ATLS; AddicMed; MD(Neurosci); Staff, Placentia Health Centre; Clin Instructor, Memorial University Of Newfoundland; (709)227-2101; Fax. (709)227-2111; tonyrockel@hotmail.com.

ROCKER, Graeme; Queen Elizabeth II HSC-Halifax, 4456-1796 Summer St, Halifax NS B3H 3A7; Oxford (England)'79; MB BCh; MHSc; FRCP; FRCPC; IntMed (Biomedical Ethics). Staff, Queen Elizabeth II Health Sciences Centre - Halifax Infirmary Site; Prof, Dalhousie University; (902)473-6611; Fax. (902)473-6202; gmrocker@dal.ca.

ROCKERBIE, Neil R; Westwind Med Clinic, 107-755 Goldstream Ave, Victoria BC V9B 2X4; Cal'86; CCFP; (250)478-1764; Fax. (250)478-1300.

ROCKMAN, Gerald L; 202-2560 Gerrard St E, Scarborough ON M1N 1W8; Tor'82; Staff, St Michael's Hospital; (416)690-2285; Fax. (647)436-2792.

ROCKMAN, Patricia F; Clairhurst Med Centre, 306-1466 Bathurst St, Toronto ON M5R 3S3; McM'89; CCFP; FCFP; Teach Staff Family Med, University of Toronto; (416)536-5555; Fax. (416)536-3352.

ROCKMAN-GREENBERG, Cheryl; Health Sciences Centre, CE208-820 Sherbrook St, Winnipeg MB R3A 1R9; McG'74; FCCMG; FRCPC; Peds (Metabolic Genetics); MedGenetics. Clin Scientist Genetics, Health Sciences Centre; Dept Head Peds & Child Health/Prof, University of Manitoba; (204)787-1970; Fax. (204)787-1419.

ROCKWELL, Gloria M; Riverside Prof Centre, 401-1919 Riverside Dr, Ottawa ON K1H 1A2; Dal'97; FRCSC; PlasSurg (Breast Surgery). Consultant (All Sites), The Ottawa Hospital - General Campus; Consultant, Children's Hospital of Eastern Ontario (CHEO); Asst Prof, University of Ottawa; (613)736-6555; Fax. (613)736-1822.

ROCKWELL, Helen A; Rapids Family Health Team, 1150 Pontiac Dr, Sarnia ON N7S 3A7; Dal'08; CCFP; (519)339-8949; Fax. (519)339-9022; hrockwell@rapidsfhteam.ca.

ROCKWOOD, Kenneth J; 1421-5955 Veterans Memorial La, Halifax NS B3H 2E1; Mem'85; FRCP; FRCPC; IntMed; GeriatricMed. Prof, Dalhousie University; (902)473-8687; Fax. (902)473-1050; kenneth.rockwood@dal.ca.

ROCKWOOD, Peter R; 342 Pennywell Rd, St. John's NL A1E 1V9; Mem'83; FRCSC; OrthSurg (Trauma Adult Reconstructive Surgery). Ac Staff, Health Sciences Centre; Ac Staff, St Clare's Mercy Hospital; Clin Assoc Prof OrthSurg, Memorial University Of Newfoundland; (709)754-9870; Fax. (709)753-2671; p.rockwood@rogers.com.

ROCKX, Marie A J; AMA Locum Services, 12230 106 Ave NW, Edmonton AB T5N 3Z1; Wes'04; FRCPC; IntMed; Nephrol.

ROD, Kevin; Toronto Poly Clinic, 204-5460 Yonge St, North York ON M2N 6K7; Ahwaz (Iran)'89; DAAPM; CCFP; FCFP; Member, International Society for the Study of Pain; Member, Canadian Pain Society; Dir Chronic Pain Prog, Toronto Poly Clinic; Lecturer DFCM, University of Toronto; Langs: Persian; (416)250-7171; Fax. (416)250-0323.

RODD, Celia J; MUHC-Montreal Children's Hosp, E 315-2300 rue Tupper, Montreal QC H3H 1P3; Tor'85; FRCPC; Peds; Endocrin (P. Q.); Endocrin&Metab. Staff, McGill University Health Centre - Montreal Children's Hospital; assoc Prof, McGill University; Langs: French; (514)412-4400 x22482; celia.rodd@mcgill.ca.

RODD, Peter M; Forensic Assessment & Comm Ser, 10004 104 Ave NW, Edmonton AB T5J 0K1; Alb'88; FRCPC; Psy (Forensic Psychiatry). Staff, Alberta Hospital Edmonton; (780)342-6400; Fax. (780)426-7272.

RODE, Frauke; Sitka Health Centre, 1284 Fairfield Rd, Victoria BC V8V 4W3; Stellenbosch (South Africa)'97; MB ChB; Langs: Afrikaans; (250)598-5158

RODE, Melvin C; Baker Centre, 709-10025 106 St NW, Edmonton AB T5J 1G4; Alb'69; (780)428-7777; Fax. (780)428-7801.

RODE, Paul B; Cranbrook OB/GYN Med Clinic, 225-1629 Baker St, Cranbrook BC V1C 1B4; Stellenbosch (South Africa)'94; MB ChB; FCOG(SA); FRCSC; ObstGyn. Staff, East Kootenay Regional Hospital; (250)426-1124; Fax. (250)426-1164.

RODEN, W Grant; University Hosp of Northern BC, 1475 Edmonton St, Prince George BC V2M 1S2; Alb'89; AB(AP&CP); BMedSci; MD; FASCP; FRCPC; GenPath (Laboratory Medicine). Staff Path, University Hospital of Northern British Columbia; (250)565-2623; Fax. (250)565-2284; grant.roden@northernhealth.ca.

RODES CABAU, Joseph; Hôpital Laval, 2725 ch Sainte-Foy, Quebec QC G1V 4G5; Barcelona (Spain)'89; Staff, Hôpital Laval; (418)656-8711; Fax. (418)656-4544.

RODGER, Marc A; The Ottawa Hosp-Gen Campus, 201-501 Smyth Rd, Ottawa ON K1H 8L6; Ott'92; FRCPC; IntMed; Hem. Staff, The Ottawa Hospital - General Campus; Langs: English; French; (613)737-8899 x74641

RODGER, N Wilson; 458 Central Ave, London ON N6B 2E5; Man'60; FRCPC; IntMed (Diabetes Mellitus); Endocrin&Metab. Emeritus Staff Endocrin & Metab, St Joseph's Hospital - St Joseph's Health Care; University of Western Ontario; (519)432-1521; Fax. (519)679-9658; wrodger@uwo.ca.

RODGERS, Allen J; Peterborough Reg HC-Hospital, 1 Hospital Dr, Peterborough ON K9J 7C6; Dal'78; Staff, Peterborough Regional Health Centre - Hospital Drive; (705)876-5022

RODGERS, Laurren K; 201-410 Josephine St, Nelson BC V1L 1W3; UBC'06; (778)928-5713

RODGERS, Lynne K; Foothills Med Centre, 1403 29 St NW, Calgary AB T2N 2T9; Man'83; FRCPC; IntMed; GeriatricMed. Staff, Foothills Medical Centre; (403)944-1110

RODGERS, Margaret S; Algonquin College, 1385 Woodroffe Ave, Nepean ON K2G 1V8; Qns'71; (613)727-4723 x7222

RODGERS, Tracy L; Ocean View Women's Clinic, 101-1757 Beaufort Ave, Comox BC V9M 1R8; Mem'97; ObstGyn. (250)339-3114; Fax. (250)339-4186.

RODGERSON, James S; 4 King Street Cres, Weston ON M9N 1K6; Tor'59; BA; Staff, Humber River Regional Hospital - Church Street Site; (416)248-1741; Fax. (416)248-8713.

RODGMAN, Graeme M; CFB Petawawa, PO Box 9999 Stn Main 2 Filed Ambulance, Petawawa ON K8H 2X3; Qns'83; (613)687-5511; Fax. (613)588-4880.

RODGMAN, M Susan; CFB Kingston, PO Box 17000 Stn Forces, Kingston ON K7K 7B4; Qns'84; (613)541-5010

RODIER, Francois; Hop Charles LeMoyne, 3120 boul Taschereau, Greenfield Park QC J4V 2H1; Mon'04; FRCPC; IntMed; Respir. Staff, Hopital Charles LeMoyne; (514)466-5000

RODIER, Irwin J; 614-5858 ch Cote-des-Neiges, Montreal QC H3S 1Z1; McG'72; Staff, St Mary's Hospital Centre; Langs: Hebrew; Spanish; French; (514)739-4037

RODIER, Lucie; Centre Medical de l'Hetriere, 201-3520 rue de l'Hetriere, St-Augustin-D-Desm QC G3A 0B4; Laval'96; (418)651-3933; Fax. (418)651-0256.

RODIER, Mitchell; 310-175 av Stillview, Pointe-Claire QC H9R 4S3; McG'04; FRCPC; Psy. (514)630-2010

RODIN, Gary M; Univ Hlth Network-Princess M, 16 724-610 University Ave, Toronto ON M5G 2M9; Man'70; FRCPC; Psy. Staff, Princess Margaret Hospital - University Health Network; Head/Sr Scientist, Toronto General Hospital - UHN; Prof, University of Toronto; (416)946-4504; gary.rodin@uhn.on.ca.

RODIN, Rachel L; Health Canada, 226B-130 Colonnade Rd, Ottawa ON K1A 0K9; Wes'00; FRCPC; CommunMed;CCFP; (613)946-4470

RODRIGO, Judith A; Div of Hematology, 2775 Laurel St, Vancouver BC V5Z 1M9; Alb'05; FRCPC; IntMed; Hem. (604)875-4863

RODRIGUE, Andre; 11325 2e av, Saint-Georges QC G5Y 1W5; Laval'80; Staff, Centre Hospitalier Beauce-Etchemin; (418)227-9216; Fax. (418)227-0164; arodrig@globetrotter.net.

RODRIGUE, Andree C M; 307-595 Montreal Rd, Ottawa ON K1K 4L2; Ott'93; CCFP; FCFP; (613)746-4390; Fax. (613)746-4840.

RODRIGUE, Annick; PO Box 952, Fernie BC V0B 1M0; Laval'05; CCFP.

RODRIGUE, Bertrand; Centre Med Berger Inc, 22-1000 ch Sainte-Foy, Quebec QC G1S 2L6; Laval'67; MSc; Derm. Staff, Centre Hospitalier Affilié Universitaire de Québec - Hôpital du St-Sacrement; (418)687-3012; Fax. (418)687-3013.

RODRIGUE, Bertrand; Clinique Med St-Zacharie, GD 528 15e av, Saint-Zacharie QC G0M 2C0; Laval'69; (418)593-5511

RODRIGUE, Denis; Clin d'Ophtalmologie Lebourgne, 200-777 boul Lebourgneuf, Quebec QC G2J 1C3; Laval'65; Ophth. ac Staff, Centre Hospitalier Affilié Universitaire de Québec - Hôpital De L'Enfant Jésus; Staff, Hôpital Laval; Consultant, Centre Hospitalier Universitaire De Québec - Pavillon De St-françois-d'assise; (418)628-1417; denis.rodrigue@gch.ulaval.ca.

RODRIGUE, Jean; Min de la Sante et Serv Sociau, 1075 ch Sainte-Foy, Quebec QC G1S 2M1; Sher'72; Dir, Reg. Federation des Med. Omnipracticiens du Quebec; Clin Prof, Universite de Montreal; Langs: English; (418)266-6930; jean.rodrigue@msss.gouv.qc.ca.

RODRIGUE, Jean; Ctr Hosp Affilie-Enfant-Jesus, 1401 18e rue, Quebec QC G1J 1Z4; Laval'89; CSPQ; FRCPC; DiagRad. Staff, Centre Hospitalier Affilié Universitaire de Québec - Hôpital De L'Enfant Jésus; (418)649-5782

RODRIGUE, Jean-Marie; Clinique Med de Famille, 400-1200 rue des Soeurs-du-Bon, Quebec QC G1S 0B1; Laval'66; ac Staff, Centre Hospitalier Affilié Universitaire de Québec - Hôpital du St-Sacrement; (418)688-1385; Fax. (418)688-3249.

RODRIGUE, Jean-Philippe; CSSS de Beauce-Etchemin, 1515 17e rue, Saint-Georges QC G5Y 4T8; Sher'07; FRCSC; OrthSurg. Staff, Centre Hospitalier Beauce-Etchemin; (418)228-2031

RODRIGUE, Julie M; 108-4275 Innes Rd, Orleans ON K1C 1T1; Sher'95; (613)830-2242

RODRIGUE, Lise; Centre médicale Centrale, 4-135 rue Saint-Antoine N, Granby QC J2G 5G7; Laval'80; Médecin, Centre Hospitalier de Granby; (450)372-5401; Fax. (450)372-4174.

RODRIGUE, Luc; CSSS de la Haute-Yamaska, 205 boul Leclerc O, Granby QC J2G 1T7; Sher'82; OrthSurg. Chef chirg ortho, Centre Hospitalier de Granby; (450)372-5491; Fax. (450)372-7197.

RODRIGUE, Lucien; CSSS de Portneuf, 700 rue Saint-Cyrille, Saint-Raymond QC G3L 1W1; Laval'86; ac Staff, Centre Hospitalier Universitaire De Québec - Pavillon De St-françois-d'assise; ac Staff, Centre Hospitalier Portneuf; (418)525-4303

RODRIGUE, Pierre Y; Clinique Med de l'Outaouais, 25 ch de la Savane, Gatineau QC J8T 8A4; Laval'66; Langs: English; (819)561-6611; Fax. (819)561-7997.

RODRIGUE, Vincent; CSSS du Sud de Lanaudière, 911 montee des Pionniers, Terrebonne QC J6V 2H2; Mon'07; CCFP; Staff, Centre Hospitalier Pierre le Gardeur; (450)654-7525

RODRIGUE VERHELST, Ariane; Clinique Medicale du Manoir, 1441 av du Manoir, Alma QC G8B 4X3; Sher'08; (418)662-3944

RODRIGUE-VINET, Ani-Raphaelle; Ctr Hosp du Centre la Mauricie, 50 119e rue, Shawinigan QC G9P 5K1; McG'08; OrthSurg (P.Q.). Staff, Centre Hospitalier du Centre la Mauricie; (819)536-7500

RODRIGUE-VINET, Marie-Lou; Ctr Hosp du Centre la Mauricie, 50 119e rue, Shawinigan-Sud QC G9P 5K1; McG'06; MDCM; FRCSC; OrthSurg. Staff, Centre Hospitalier du Centre la Mauricie; (819)536-7500

RODRIGUES, Americo V F; Canadian Forces Supp Unit HCC, 1745 Alta Vista Dr, Ottawa ON K1A 0K6; Tor'86; Staff, Canadian Forces Health Services Centre; Langs: Portuguese; French; (418)844-5000

RODRIGUES, Arthur F; William Osler HC-Brampton, 2100 Bovaird Dr E, Brampton ON L6R 3J7; Tor'87; Staff, William Osler Health System - Brampton Civic Hospital; Langs: Portuguese; (905)494-2120

RODRIGUES, George B; London Reg Cancer Centre, 790 Commissioners Rd E, London ON N6A 4L6; Qns'96; FRCPC; RadOncol. (519)685-8600; Fax. (519)685-8736.

RODRIGUES, Isabel; CLSC du Marigot, 1351 boul des Laurentides, Vimont QC H7M 2Y2; Mon'83; CCFP; FCFP; (450)668-1506; Fax. (450)668-1507; isabel.rodrigues@umontreal.ca.

RODRIGUES, Jude F N; 160-1720 Howard Ave, Windsor ON N8X 5A6; Bombay (India)'79; DABIM; FRCPC; IntMed (Osteoporosis); Rheum. Staff Cons, Windsor Regional Hospital - Metropolitan Site; Court Staff, Hôtel-Dieu Grace Hospital; (519)254-4833; Fax. (519)254-3692.

RODRIGUES, M Susana B; Markham College Med Clinic, 202-474 College St, Toronto ON M6G 1A4; Lisbon (Portugal)'81; (416)969-8909

RODRIGUES, Paulo R D; 100 Queensway W, Mississauga ON L5B 1B8; Porto Alegre (Brazil)'72; FRCPC; DiagRad. Staff, Trillium Health Centre - Mississauga; (905)848-7527

RODRIGUEZ, Amadeo R; Saint Joseph's Comm Health, 2500-2757 King St E, Hamilton ON L8G 5E4; Cordoba (Argentina)'99; (905)573-7777

RODRIGUEZ, Carl P; Royal University Hosp, 103 Hospital Dr, Saskatoon SK S7N 0W8; Alb'04; FRCPC; DiagRad. Staff, Royal University Hospital; (306)655-2402; Fax. (306)655-2370.

RODRIGUEZ, Carlos H; 203-2238 Dundas St W, Toronto ON M6R 3A9; Buenos Aires (Argentina)'69; ABIM; FRCPC; IntMed (Sleep Medicine); Respir. Langs: Italian; Portuguese; Spanish; (416)531-8760; Fax. (416)531-2843.

RODRIGUEZ, Jean-Pierre; Inst Albert Prevost, 6555 boul Gouin O, Montreal QC H4K 1B3; Mon'69; CSPQ; Psy. Staff, Hôpital du Sacre-Coeur de Montréal; (514)338-4203; Fax. (514)338-4023.

RODRIGUEZ, Jennifer M; Southlake Reg Health Centre, 596 Davis Dr, Newmarket ON L3Y 2P9; Santo Tomas (Philippines)'97; FRCPC; AnatPath. Staff, Southlake Regional Health Centre; (905)895-4521

RODRIGUEZ, Joseph; 210-5450 ch de la Cote-des-Nei, Montreal QC H3T 1Y6; Madrid (Spain)'62; FACS; GenSurg. Chef Surgery, St Mary's Hospital Centre; Asst Prof Surg, McGill University; Langs: Italian; French; Portuguese; (514)735-6337; Fax. (514)735-6339.

RODRIGUEZ, Pacita; CSSS du Sud de Lanaudière, 911 montee des Pionniers, Terrebonne QC J6V 2H2; Mon'01; Staff, Centre Hospitalier Pierre le Gardeur; (450)654-7525

RODRIGUEZ, Richie-Ann; Rodriguez Med Clinic, 6-2755 Lougheed Hwy, New Westminster BC V3B 0A9; (Philippines)'00; CCFP; (604)941-6900

RODRIGUEZ, Sylvia L; Guelph Eye MD Clinic, 214-89 Dawson Rd, Guelph ON N1H 1B1; McM'04; BSc; FRCSC; Ophth. Staff, Guelph General Hospital; Langs: Spanish; (519)265-9022

RODRIGUEZ-ELIZALDE, Sebastian; 810 Wilson Ave, North York ON M3K 1E5; Wes'04; OrthSurg. (416)636-8626; Fax. (416)636-8628.

RODRIGUEZ-MARIN, Emilio; The Credit Valley Hosp, 2200 Eglinton Ave W, Mississauga ON L5M 2N1; McG'90; FRCPC; DiagRad (Angiography & Interventional Radiology). Staff, The Hospital For Sick Children; Staff Radiol, The Credit Valley Hospital; Langs: Spanish; (905)813-4537; Fax. (905)813-3042; erm@cvh.on.ca.

RODRIGUEZ MARRERO, Ildegul; 1-459 Russell St, Brandon MB R7A 5H8.

RODRIGUEZ-MATEO, Jean; Calgary Hlth Refugee Program, 23 McDougall Crt NE, Calgary AB T2E 8R3; (Cuba)'00; CCFP; (403)265-3410; Fax. (403)265-3411.

RODRIGUEZ MOYA, Maria del Rosario; 10-517 av des Pins O, Montreal QC H2W 1S4; Alicante (Spain)'83; assoc Prof, McGill University; Langs: Spanish; Bilingual(English/French); (514)398-7375 x0495; Fax. (514)398-4202; charo.rodriguez@mcgill.ca.

RODRIGUEZ NARANJO, Aristides; 181C 22nd St PO Box 226, Battleford SK S0M 0E0; Havana Medical Scholl (Cuba)'90; Staff, St Joseph's Hospital; Langs: Spanish; Portuguese; (306)445-3226; Fax. (306)445-3131; macklinmed@sasktel.net.

RODRIGUEZ-SARMIENTO, Juan G; Nanaimo Reg Gen Hosp, 1200 Dufferin Cres, Nanaimo BC V9S 2B7; Nueva (Colombia)'91; CCFP; CCFP(E.M.); Staff, Nanaimo Regional General Hospital; (250)754-2141

RODWAN, Khaled S O; Allied Health Centre, 225-3737 Wascana Pky, Regina SK S4S 0A2; Al Arab (Libya)'96; FRCSC; OrthSurg (Spine). Staff, Regina General Hospital; Physician, Allied Health Centre; Lecturer, University of Saskatchewan; (306)337-2643; Fax. (306)337-3192; rodwank@hotmail.com.

RODWAN, Omar M A; 361 Main St N, Moose Jaw SK S6H 0W2; Al Fateh (Libya)'98; FRCPC; IntMed. (306)692-5066; Fax. (306)691-5966.

RODWAY, Megan R; Richmond Road Diag & Trmt Ctre, 1820 Richmond Rd SW, Calgary AB T2T 5C7; Man'86; FRCPC; Psy (Anxiety & Mood Disorders). Staff Psy/Clin Asst Prof, Alberta Children's Hospital; (403)955-8942; mrodway@calgaryhealthregion.ca.

RODWAY-NORMAN, Mark T; Orillia Soldier's Mem Hosp, 170 Colborne St W, Orillia ON L3V 2Z3; Man'85; BSc; FRCPC; Psy (Gender Identity Disorder). Staff, Orillia Soldiers' Memorial Hospital; (705)325-2201

RODYNIUK, Andriy Y; Royal Alexandra Hosp, 10240 Kingsway NW, Edmonton AB T5H 3V9; Alb'85; Anes. Staff, University of Alberta Hospital; Staff, Royal Alexandra Hospital; (780)477-4111

ROE, E Bruce; St Boniface Gen Hosp, 409 Tache Ave, Winnipeg MB R2H 2A6; Sask'88; FRCPC; IntMed; Endocrin&Metab. Exec Dir Clin Prog/Chief Medical Officer, St Boniface General Hospital; (204)235-3108; Fax. (204)235-3108.

ROE, Michael; 201-460 Wellington St, St Thomas ON N5R 6H9; Tor'90; BSc(Hon); FRCSC; ObstGyn (Minimal Invasive Surgery). Ac Staff ObstGyn, St Thomas Elgin General Hospital; Aj Prof, University of Western Ontario; (519)637-3987; Fax. (519)637-3980.

ROE, Richard C; Caledonian Med Clinic, 340 Campbell St, Nanaimo BC V9R 3G7; Cal'83; (250)753-3202; Fax. (250)753-1039.

ROEBOTHAM, Roy W; St Joseph's Health Care, PO Box 5777 Stn B 268 Grosvenor St, London ON N6A 4V2; Mem'89; CCFP; CCFP(E.M.); FCFP; Staff, London Health Sciences Centre - University Hospital; Staff, St Joseph's Hospital - St Joseph's Health Care; (519)646-6000 x64227; rroebotham@bigfoot.com.

ROEBUCK, Marvin J; Scarborough CPM Pain Clinic, 425-1200 Markham Rd, Scarborough ON M1H 3C3; Tor'57; LLB; DAB; FAB; DAAPM; FRCPC; Anes (Chronic Pain Management). Court Staff, The Scarborough Hospital - General Campus; (416)438-7080; Fax. (416)438-7072.

ROECK, Kyra D; St Georges Med Clinic, 1315 St. Georges Ave, North Vancouver BC V7L 3J2; UBC'95; CCFP; (604)984-9213; Fax. (604)986-1390.

ROEDDE, M Gretchen; Haileybury Family Hlth Team, 95 Meridian St, Haileybury ON P0J 1K0; McM'77; Court Staff, Temiskaming Hospital; Consultant, Int'l. Health Planning & Training, Euro Health Group; (705)672-3371; groedde@yahoo.com.

ROEDERER, Ghislaine; Inst de Recherche Clin de Mtl, 110 av des Pins O, Montreal QC H2W 1R7; Mon'80; BSc; PhD; Staff, Centre Hospitalier l'Université de Montréal (CHUM) - Hôtel-Dieu; Prof/Prof, Universite de Montreal; Langs: English; (514)987-5600; Fax. (514)987-5732.

ROEHRL, Michael H A; Univ Hlth Network-Toronto Gen, 200 Elizabeth St, Toronto ON M5G 2C4; (Germany)'98; (416)340-4902

ROELENS, Kurt R E; Mount Royal Family Physicians, 701 Avenue P N, Saskatoon SK S7L 2W1; Cape Town (South Africa)'01; MB ChB; BScAg; Physician, Invermay Health Centre; Langs: Afrikaans; (306)382-5854; Fax. (306)382-7477; kurt.roelens@sasktel.net.

ROELFSEMA, Heather J; Orchardview Med Centre, 100-155 Main St E, Grimsby ON L3M 1P2; McM'01; BSc; MSc; CCFP; (905)945-5476; Fax. (905)945-7707.

ROESCH, Marian T; 1010-625 Vancouver St, Prince George BC V2L 5R6; Sask'90; DABOph; FRCSC; Ophth (Glaucoma). Ad Staff Surg, University Hospital of Northern British Columbia; Clin Instructor, University of British Columbia; (250)563-7373

ROESKE, Amy E; Children's Hosp Eastern Ont, 401 Smyth Rd, Ottawa ON K1H 8L1; Ott'04; FRCPC; Anes. Staff, Children's Hospital of Eastern Ontario (CHEO); (613)737-2431

ROESSEL, Mary; 448 10th St, Courtenay BC V9N 1P6; Minnesota-Minneapolis (USA)'87; Staff, St Joseph's General Hospital; Staff, Campbell River Mental Health & Addiction Services; (250)850-2620

ROETS, Louisa F; Moosomin Family Practice Ctre, PO Box 1528, Moosomin SK S0G 3N0; (South Africa)'85; MB ChB; LMCC; Langs: Afrikaans; (306)435-3838; Fax. (306)435-2176.

ROETS, Pieter G W; Moosomin Family Practice Ctre, PO Box 1528, Moosomin SK S0G 3N0; (306)435-3838; Fax. (306)435-2176.

ROETS, Willem G; Ashern Med Clinic, PO Box 110, Ashern MB R0C 0E0; (204)768-9030

ROFAEEL, Ayman S H; Guelph Gen Hosp, 115 Delhi St, Guelph ON N1E 4J4; Mansura (Egypt)'88; FRCPC; Anes. Staff, Guelph General Hospital; (519)837-6440

ROFAIEL, Basma P; 8-2155 Lawrence Ave E, Scarborough ON M1R 5G9; Cairo (Egypt)'83; MB ChB; CCFP; (416)757-7272

ROFEAL, Michael N H; Brookfield Bonnews HC Centre, GD 57 Main St, Brookfield NL A0G 1J0; Assiut University (Egypt)'03; MB ChB; Staff, Brookfield Bonnews Health Care Centre; (709)536-2405

ROGAKOU, Cleo C; Newmarket Med Place, 211-712 Davis Dr, Newmarket ON L3Y 8C3; Tor'80; BSc; FRCSC; OrthSurg (Arthroplasty). Staff, Southlake Regional Health Centre; Langs: Greek; French; (905)898-4328; Fax. (905)898-3249.

ROGALLA, Patrik; NCSB 1C547, 585 University Ave, Toronto ON M5G 2N2; Berlin (Germany)'91; (416)340-4800

ROGAN, Ernest; Family Med Clinic, 236-2 Hebert Rd, St Albert AB T8N 5T8; Alb'84; Psy. Consultant, Wetaskiwin Hospital & Care Centre; Consultant, Alberta Mental Health Clinics; (780)459-2997; Fax. (780)459-2998.

ROGAN, Heather M; West Lambton Community HC, 100-429 Exmouth St, Sarnia ON N7T 5P1; Man'91; BSc; Staff, Bluewater Health - Norman Site; Staff, Bluewater Health - Mitton Site; Staff, Bluewater Health - Charlotte Eleanor Englehart Hospital; (519)344-3017; Fax. (519)344-7535.

ROGANO, Maria A; 403A-1090 Don Mills Rd, North York ON M3C 3R6; Tor'87; Court Staff Family Med, Sunnybrook Health Sciences Centre; Court Staff Family Med, Women's College Hospital; Ac Staff Family Med, North York General Hospital; Langs: Italian; (416)383-0048; Fax. (416)383-0050.

ROGELSTAD, Michael L; Strathroy Middlesex Gen Hosp, 358-395 Carrie St, Strathroy ON N7G 3C9; Wes'83; FRCSC; Ophth. Staff, Strathroy Middlesex General Hospital - Middlesex Hospital Alliance; (519)246-1610; Fax. (519)246-1611.

ROGER, Judith A; Vancouver Gen Hosp, 855 12th Ave W, Vancouver BC V5Z 1M9; Graz (Austria)'75; FRCSC; GenSurg. Staff, Vancouver General Hospital - Centennial Pavillion; Langs: German; French; (604)875-5292

ROGER, Marie-Eve; Ctr Hosp Affilie-Enfant-Jesus, 1401 18e rue, Quebec QC G1J 1Z4; Laval'03; FRCSC; OrthSurg. Staff, Centre Hospitalier Affilié Universitaire de Québec - Hôpital De L'Enfant Jésus; (418)649-0252

ROGER, Michel; CHUM-Hop Notre-Dame, 1560 rue Sherbrooke E, Montreal QC H2L 4M1; Mon'90; BSc(Biol.); MSc; PhD; FRCPC; MedMicrobiol; Microbio & Infect Dis (P.Q.). Staff, Centre Hospitalier l'Université de Montréal (CHUM) - Hôpital Notre-Dame; (514)890-8000 x25802; michel.roger@ssss.gouv.qc.ca.

ROGER-ACHIM, Diane; CLSC des Faubourgs, 1705 rue de la Visitation, Montreal QC H2L 3C3; Sher'73; CCFP; FCFP; (514)527-2361; Fax. (514)527-3134.

ROGERS, Anna E; Sault Area Hosp, 750 Great Northern Rd, Sault Ste. Marie ON P6B 0A8; Wes'92; FRCPC; Psy. Staff, Sault Area Hospital - Sault Ste Marie; Langs: Polish; (705)759-3434

ROGERS, Carolyn; Medica One, 2019 Caroline St, Burlington ON L7R 1L1; McM'90; CCFP; Staff, Grand Valley Institution for Women; (905)333-0311; Fax. (905)333-0911.

ROGERS, Denis; Sechelt Med Clinic, PO Box 638, Sechelt BC V0N 3A0; Galway (Ireland)'68; MB ChB; BAO; LMCC; Ac Staff, St Mary's Hospital; (604)885-2257; denis_rogers@sunshine.net.

ROGERS, James D; 405-390 Brant St, Burlington ON L7R 4J4; Tor'85; AB(CriticalCareMed.); FRCSC; GenSurg; Critical Care Medicine. Staff, Joseph Brant Memorial Hospital; (905)632-8162; Fax. (905)632-9810.

ROGERS, Jamie B; Hilden Med Clinic, RR 1 1174 Highway 2, Brookfield NS B0N 1C0; Dal'91; FRCSC; Ophth. Ophth, Colchester East Hants Health Centre; (902)895-6525; Fax. (902)895-2389.

ROGERS, Janet L; MacEwan Student Centre, 370-2500 University Dr NW, Calgary AB T2N 1N4; Cal'78; CCFP; FCFP; Ac Staff, Foothills Medical Centre; (403)220-5765

ROGERS, Jenny S; 260 Sherbrooke St, New Westminster BC V3L 3M2; UBC'04; FRCPC; Psy. (604)520-4662

ROGERS, John C; Cape Breton Hlthcare Complex, 1482 George St, Sydney NS B1P 1P3; Dal'88; FRCPC; Psy. Staff, Cape Breton Healthcare Complex; (902)567-8091

ROGERS, John M; London X-Ray Associates, 104-450 Central Ave, London ON N6B 2E8; Dal'72; FRCPC; DiagRad (Neuro Radiology). Staff Neuroradiol, St Joseph's Hospital - St Joseph's Health Care; Asst Prof DiagRad & Nuclear Med, University of Western Ontario; (519)672-7900

ROGERS, Joseph E; 4-315 Avenue Rd, Toronto ON M4V 2H2; Tor'60; DPsy; Psy (Psychotherapy & Psychoanalysis). (416)962-7130; Fax. (416)960-4943.

ROGERS, Kieran A; Bramalea Med Centre, 301-18 Kensington Rd, Brampton ON L6T 4S5; Galway (Ireland)'69; (905)791-5822

ROGERS, Kimberly A; Rocky Med Clinic, PO Box 99 Stn Main, Rocky-Mtn-Hse AB T4T 1A1; Alb'92; CCFP; (403)845-2815; Fax. (403)845-2177.

ROGERS, Kimberly A M; Queensway Obs & Gyn, 406-89 Queensway W, Mississauga ON L5B 2V2; McM'96; BHSc; FRCSC; ObstGyn (Urological Gynecology). Staff, Trillium Health Centre - West Toronto; (905)268-9928; Fax. (905)268-9950.

ROGERS, Kristin D; 95 Manston Cres, Hornell Heights ON P0H 1P0; Qns'92; CCFP; (705)494-2011 x2110; kristin.rogers@forces.gc.ca.

ROGERS, Lori A; Health Sciences Centre, 300 Prince Philip Dr, St. John's NL A1B 3V6; Mem'02; CCFP; CCFP(E.M.); Staff, Health Sciences Centre; (709)777-6300

ROGERS, Louise; Midtown Med Clinic, 35 Campbell Ave, St. John's NL A1E 2Z3; Mem'89.

ROGERS, M Bryson; 104-9920 63 Ave NW, Edmonton AB T6E 0G9; Wes'71; AAD; FRCPC; Derm. Consultant/Staff, Northern Lights Health Region; Consultant/Staff, Lloydminster Hospital; Langs: German; French; (780)461-0573; Fax. (780)461-0725.

ROGERS, Neil J; Elgin Family Med Centre, 270 Elgin St, Ottawa ON K2P 1M2; Queensland (Australia)'76; MB BS; (613)237-2121; Fax. (613)237-2087.

ROGERS, Neil R; Medical Arts Centre, 106-650 Terminal Ave, Nanaimo BC V9R 5E2; Cal'99; CCFP; (250)753-3431; Fax. (250)754-6897.

ROGERS, Paul C J; Children's & Women's HC of BC, A123-4480 Oak St, Vancouver BC V6H 3V4; Pretoria (South Africa)'70; MB ChB; DCH(Lond); MBA; FRCP; FRCPC; Peds (Pediatric Hematology Oncology). Staff, BC Children's Hospital; Head Div of Ped HemOncol/Prof, University of British Columbia; Langs: Afrikaans; (604)875-2406; progers@cw.bc.ca.

ROGERS, Peter J; Health Sciences Centre, 300 Prince Philip Dr, St. John's NL A1B 3V6; Mem'01; CCFP; CCFP(E.M.); Staff, Health Sciences Centre; (709)777-6300

ROGERS, Raymond M; Plaza 44, 120-4402 52 Ave, Lloydminster AB T9V 0Y9; Qns'73; ABIM; FRCPC; IntMed. Staff IntMed, Lloydminster Hospital; (780)875-4930; Fax. (780)875-8361.

ROGERS, Tabitha M C; Royal Ottawa Mental Hlth Ctr, 1145 Carling Ave, Ottawa ON K1Z 7K4; Ott'06; FRCPC; Psy. Staff, Royal Ottawa Mental Health Centre - Royal Ottawa Health Care Group; (613)722-6521

ROGERS, William L; The Peterborough Clinic, 201-26 Hospital Dr, Peterborough ON K9J 7C3; Wes'78; FRCSC; Ophth (Cataract). Assoc Staff, Peterborough Regional Health Centre - Hospital Drive; (705)740-6866; Fax. (705)740-6865.

ROGERSON, Janet; Queen Elizabeth Hosp, PO Box 6600 Stn Central 60 Riverside Dr, Charlottetown PE C1A 8T5; Mem'05; CCFP; Queen Elizabeth Hospital; Staff, Sherwood Family Medical Centre; (902)894-2111

ROGERSON, Jennifer E; Delta Health Sciences Centre, 202-4515 Harvest Dr, Delta BC V4K 4L1; UBC'98; CCFP; Physician, Delta Health Sciences Centre; (604)946-6411; Fax. (604)946-0372.

ROGGENSACK, Anne; Foothills Med Centre, 1403 29 St NW, Calgary AB T2N 2T9; Alb'00; BMedSci; FRCSC; ObstGyn (Maternal Fetal Medicine). Staff, Foothills Medical Centre; (403)944-4415

ROGOVEIN, Ted S; St Joseph's Health Centre, 237-30 The Queensway, Toronto ON M6R 1B5; McG'85; FRCPC; IntMed (Critical Care Medicine). Chief Dept of Med, St Joseph's Health Centre; Lecturer, University of Toronto; (416)530-6103; Fax. (416)530-6073; rogodoc@rogers.com.

ROGOZINSKA, Ludwika; Manitoba Clinic, 790 Sherbrook St, Winnipeg MB R3A 1M3; Cracow (Poland)'74; FACOG; FRCSC; ObstGyn. Staff, Health Sciences Centre; Langs: Polish; (204)774-6541; Fax. (204)786-8092.

ROHACHUK, Kenneth H P; Meadowlark Health Centre, 142 Meadowlark Shopping Ctr NW, Edmonton AB T5R 5W9; Alb'88; CCFP; (780)486-7777; Fax. (780)486-7747.

ROHALD, Pamela; St Boniface Hosp, L2035-409 Tache Ave, Winnipeg MB R2H 2A6; Witwatersrand (South Africa)'97; MB ChB; BSc(Physiotherapy); FRCPC; Anes. Staff, St Boniface General Hospital; (204)237-2580

ROHALD, Sharon; Keele Med Place, 403-2830 Keele St, North York ON M3M 3E5; Witwatersrand (South Africa)'87; MB ChB; CCFP; (416)631-6669; Fax. (416)630-3861.

ROHAN, Ivan; 210-5450 ch de la Cote-des-Nei, Montreal QC H3T 1Y6; Bratislava (Slovakia)'73; CCFP; Asst Prof, Concordia Universtiy; adj Prof/Dir CME, Dept of Family Med, McGill University; (514)731-3249

ROHAN, Peter; MUHC-Montreal Chest Institute, 3650 rue Saint-Urbain, Montreal QC H2X 2P4; Mon'86; DOHS; Staff, McGill University Health Centre - Montreal Chest Institute; Langs: English; French; (514)934-1934 x32502; Fax. (514)737-0590; peter.rohan@muhc.mcgill.ca.

ROHATINSKY, Delee M; Primecare Health, 120-109 Quarry Park Blvd SE, Calgary AB T2C 5E7; UBC'01; (403)930-7111; Fax. (403)930-7114.

ROHE, Philippe; CHUM-Hotel-Dieu, 3840 rue Saint-Urbain, Montreal QC H2W 1T8; Paris (France)'99; CCFP; Staff, Centre Hospitalier l'Université de Montréal (CHUM) - Hôtel-Dieu; (514)890-8000 x14996

ROHEKAR, Gina; St Joseph's Health Care, PO Box 5777 Stn B D2 105-268 Grosvenor St, London ON N6A 4V2; Wes'01; FRCPC; IntMed; Rheum. Staff, St Joseph's Hospital - St Joseph's Health Care; (519)646-6242 x1; Fax. (519)646-6348.

ROHEKAR, Sherry; St Joseph's Health Care, PO Box 5777 Stn B D2 105-268 Grosvenor St, London ON N6A 4V2; Wes'01; FRCPC; IntMed; Rheum. Staff, St Joseph's Hospital - St Joseph's Health Care; (519)646-6242 x1; Fax. (519)646-6221.

ROHER, Luna S; 302-1206 Centre St, Thornhill ON L4J 3M9; McM'88; BScN; FRCPC; Psy (Child Psychiatry). Consultant PsyOncol, Mount Sinai Hospital; Court Staff GenPsy, Centre for Addiction & Mental Health (CAMH) - Queen Site; Consultant, York University Counselling Service; Lecturer, University of Toronto; Langs: Spanish.

ROHLAND, Terry A; Rohland Med Inc, PO Box 34 3010 Highway 3, Pubnico NS B0W 2W0; Mem'78; (902)762-3403; Fax. (902)762-2290.

ROHLICEK, Charles V; MUHC-Montreal Children's Hosp, C. 352-2300 rue Tupper, Montreal QC H3H 1P3; McG'87; MSc; PhD(McG); BSc(Hon); FRCPC; Peds (Pediatric Cardiology); Cardiol. Staff, McGill University Health Centre - Montreal Children's Hospital; assoc Prof, McGill University; Langs: Czech; French; (514)412-4423; Fax. (514)412-4391; charles.rohlicek@muhc.mcgill.ca.

ROHLOFF, Jacqueline M M; University of Alberta Hosp, 8440 112 St NW, Edmonton AB T6G 2B7; Alb'96; CCFP; Staff, University of Alberta Hospital; (780)407-8822; jacquelinerohloff@shaw.ca.

ROHN, Susan E; Elk Valley Hosp, PO Box 670 1501 5th Ave, Fernie BC V0B 1M0; McM'94; BSc(Hon.); CCFP; Staff, Elk Valley Hospital; (250)423-4453; susan.rohn@interiorhealth.ca.

ROIFMAN, Chaim M; The Hosp for Sick Children, 7277-555 University Ave, Toronto ON M5G 1X8; Tel-Aviv (Israel)'79; FRCPC; MedScient(Med) (Allergy & Immunology). Sr Scientist Div of Immunology & Allergy, The Hospital For Sick Children; Prof Peds & Immunology, University of Toronto; Langs: Hebrew; Italian; (416)813-8629; Fax. (416)813-8624; chaim.roifman@sickkids.ca.

ROIFMAN, Idan; Sunnybrook Hlth Sciences Ctr, 2075 Bayview Ave, Toronto ON M4N 3M5; Ott'05; FRCPC; IntMed; Cardiol. Staff, Sunnybrook Health Sciences Centre; (416)480-6100

ROITBERG, Inna; North Med Centre, 305-7131 Bathurst St, Thornhill ON L4J 7Z1; Kishinev (Russia (Federation))'72; CCFP; FCFP; Langs: Hebrew; Russian; (905)882-6798; Fax. (905)882-6448.

ROITMAN, Daryl S; North York Gen Hosp, 373-4001 Leslie St, North York ON M2K 1E1; McG'90; FRCPC; IntMed; Hem; MedOncol. Staff, North York General Hospital; Langs: English; French; (416)756-6000

ROJAS-LIEVANO, Fernando; Dr L Richards Ctre d'Oncologie, 37 rue Providence, Moncton NB E1C 8X3; Bogota (Colombia)'86; FRCPC; RadOncol. Staff, Dr Georges-L-Dumont University Hospital Centre; (506)862-3768; Fax. (506)862-4222.

ROJAS OROZCO, Ledy; CSSS de la Vallée de l'Or, 725 6e rue, Val-d'Or QC J9P 3Y1; Bogota (Colombia)'00; ObstGyn (P.Q.). Staff, Centre Hospitalier de Val d'Or; (819)825-5858 x2280; Fax. (819)825-7909.

ROJAS-VASQUEZ, Marta I; University of Alberta Hosp, 8440 112 St NW, Edmonton AB T6G 2B7; Staff, University of Alberta Hospital; (780)407-8798; Fax. (780)407-8821.

ROJEAB, Farghad B Y; R W Large Mem Hosp, 88 Waglisla St, Bella Bella BC V0T 1Z0; (Jordan)'99; Staff, R W Large Memorial Hospital; (250)957-2314; farghad_rojeab@rwlmh.ca.

ROJNICA, Lillian M; Erinoakkids, 2277 South Millway, Mississauga ON L5L 2M5; Tor'82; FRCPC; Peds (Developmental Pediatrics). Langs: Croatian; (905)855-2690; Fax. (905)820-2756.

ROKNI, Farin; 200-8 Place du Commerce, Verdun QC H3E 1N3; Santo Domingo (Dominican Republic)'96; CCFP; Staff, Barrie Memorial Hospital; (514)798-2228; Fax. (514)787-1929.

ROKOSH, Elizabeth T; Misericordia Community Hosp, 16940 87 Ave NW, Edmonton AB T5R 4H5; Ott'95; BSc; FRCPC; IntMed; Critical Care Medicine. Staff, Covenant Health - Misericordia Community Hospital; Clin Lecturer, University of Alberta; Langs: Polish; (780)735-2858; Fax. (780)735-2953.

ROKOSH, Jacquelyne L; Liberton Med Centre, 205-31 Liberton Dr, St. Albert AB T8N 3X6; Alb'86; Staff, Youville Home St Albert; (780)458-5505; Fax. (780)460-1479.

ROKOSS, Michael J; Hamilton HS-General Site, 513-237 Barton St E, Hamilton ON L8L 2X2; Tor'96; BSc; FRCPC; IntMed (Interventional Cardiology); Cardiol. Staff, Hamilton Health Sciences Centre - Hamilton General Hospital; Asst Prof Med, McMaster University; (905)527-4322

ROLA, Philippe; Hop Santa Cabrini Ospedale, 5655 rue Saint-Zotique E, Montreal QC H1T 1P7; McG'95; FRCPC; IntMed. Staff, Hôpital Santa Cabrini Ospedale; (514)252-6584

ROLA-PLESZCZYNSKI, Marek; CHUS-Hop Fleurimont, 3001 12e av N, Sherbrooke QC J1H 5N4; Sher'70; FRCPC; Peds; ClinImmunol&Allergy. Dir Allergy & Immunol, Centre Hospitalier Universitaire de Sherbrooke-Hopital Fleurimont; Prof, Universite de Sherbrooke; Langs: Polish; English; Italian; (819)346-1110 x14851

ROLAND, Elke H; Children's & Women's HC of BC, K3 177-4480 Oak St, Vancouver BC V6H 3V4; Wes'80; FRCPC; Neur (Pediatric Neurology). Ac Staff, BC Children's Hospital; Assoc Prof Peds, University of British Columbia; Langs: German; (604)875-2121; Fax. (604)875-2285.

ROLAND, Kristine J; Vancouver Gen Hosp, 855 12th Ave W, Vancouver BC V5Z 1M9; Qns'01; FRCPC; HemPath. Staff, Vancouver General Hospital - Centennial Pavillion; (604)875-4381

ROLAND, Pierre B; Clinique Med Le Royer, 301-510 boul Saint-Laurent, Montreal QC H2Y 2Y9; Laval'73; Langs: Bilingual(English/French); (514)931-2021; Fax. (514)844-7204; pierreroland@videotron.ca.

ROLANDI, Joseph R; Tamarack Med Clinic, 191-1500 Cranbrook St N, Cranbrook BC V1C 3S8; UBC'89; BSc(Kinesiol); CCFP; FCFP; Ac Staff, East Kootenay Regional Hospital; (250)426-7724; Fax. (250)426-7718.

ROLBIN, Stephen H; Rothbart Centre for Pain Care, 9-4646 Dufferin St, North York ON M3H 5S4; McG'71; BSc; FRCPC; Anes (Disability Assessment). (416)512-6407; Fax. (416)512-6375.

ROLDAN, Hector A; Huntsville Prof Bldg, 205-348 Muskoka Rd 3 N, Huntsville ON P1H 1H8; San Carlos (Guatemala)'88; FACS; FRCSC; GenSurg (Trauma). Staff Surgeon, Huntsville District Memorial Hospital - Muskoka Algonquin Healthcare; Staff, South Muskoka Memorial Hospital - Muskoka Algonquin Healthcare; Langs: Spanish; (705)789-1874; Fax. (705)789-4734.

ROLDAN LOZANO, Luis O; 43-2300 Finch Ave W, North York ON M9M 2Y3; San Salvador (El Salvador)'74; FRCPC; Psy. Staff, Humber River Regional Hospital - Finch Avenue Site; Langs: Spanish; (416)744-7227; Fax. (416)744-8603.

ROLF, J Douglass; Kelowna Respiratory Clinic, 302-3975 Lakeshore Rd, Kelowna BC V1W 1V3; Alb'84; FCCP; FRCPC; IntMed (Chest Disease & Allergy); Respir. (778)477-5805; Fax. (778)477-5807.

ROLFE, Anthony R; 201-496 Topsail Rd, St. John's NL A1E 2C2; Mem'76; Court Staff, St Clare's Mercy Hospital; (709)368-2115; Fax. (709)368-2444.

ROLFSON, Darryl B; Clinical Sciences Bldg, 1 108-11350 83 Ave NW, Edmonton AB T6G 2P4; Alb'93; BSc; MD; FRCPC; IntMed; GeriatricMed. Staff Clinical Sciences Bldg, University of Alberta Hospital; Assoc Prof Med, University of Alberta; (780)492-6233; Fax. (780)492-2874; darryl.rolfson@ualberta.ca.

ROLLAND, Pascale; Coll Quebecois des Med de Fami, 202-3210 av Jacques-Bureau, Laval QC H7P 0A9; (450)973-2228; Fax. (450)973-4329.

ROLLHEISER, Steven P; Royal Inland Hosp, 311 Columbia St, Kamloops BC V2C 2T1; Sask'79; Ac Staff, Royal Inland Hospital; (250)374-5111; Fax. (250)374-1327.

ROLLIN, Marie-France; Clinique Med Fam Hull, 202-15 boul Montclair, Gatineau QC J8Y 2E2; Ott'05; (819)777-7668

ROLLINS, David F; UBC Eye Care Centre, H-2550 Willow St, Vancouver BC V5Z 3N9; UBC'75; FRCSC; Ophth. Ac Staff, Vancouver General Hospital - Centennial Pavillion; (604)875-1521; Fax. (604)875-5070.

ROLLS, Rodney E; WRHA PACT Program, 4-1050 Leila Ave, Winnipeg MB R2P 1W6; Man'99; FRCPC; Psy.

ROMAGNOLI, Cesare; London HSC-University Hosp, PO Box 5339 Stn B 339 Windermere Rd, London ON N6A 5A5; Bologna (Italy)'84; FRCPC; DiagRad. Staff, London Health Sciences Centre - University Hospital; (519)663-3216

ROMAIN, Sandra; William Osler HC-Brampton, 2100 Bovaird Dr E, Brampton ON L6R 3J7; Ott'03; CCFP; Staff, William Osler Health System - Brampton Civic Hospital; Langs: French; (905)494-2120; Fax. (905)494-6563.

ROMAIN, Yveline; CSSS de Sept-Iles, 45 rue du Pere-Divet, Sept-Iles QC G4R 3N7; Mon'88; Ac Staff, Centre Hospitalier Regional de Sept-Iles; Physician, CLSC de Sept-Iles; (418)962-9761

ROMALIS, Garson; 200-1177 Broadway W, Vancouver BC V6H 1G3; UBC'62; FRCSC; ObstGyn (Abortion). Hon Staff, Vancouver General Hospital - Centennial Pavillion; Ac Staff, BC Women's Hospital & Health Centre; Clin Prof ObstGyn, University of British Columbia; (604)875-2000 x6132; garyromalis@gmail.com.

ROMAN, Bassem A W; 3945 17 Ave SW, Calgary AB T3E 0C3; Ain Shams (Egypt)'93; CCFP; (403)242-8633; Fax. (403)424-8884.

ROMAN, Hassem A W; CSSS de Rimouski-Neigette, CP 3150 Succ A 150 av Rouleau, Rimouski QC G5L 5T1; Ain Shams (Egypt)'99; AnatPath (P.Q.). Staff, Hôpital Regional Rimouski; (418)724-3000; Fax. (418)724-8632.

ROMAN, Jean-Pierre; Clinique Med de Vercheres, 90 montee Calixa-Lavallee, Vercheres QC J0L 2R0; Mon'76; Staff, Hôpital Santa Cabrini Ospedale; (450)468-8129

ROMAN, Manal; Linden Ridge Med Centre, E-123 Scurfield Blvd, Winnipeg MB R3Y 1L6; Tanta (Egypt)'89; CCFP; Staff, McCreary / Alonsa Health Centre; (204)488-9988

ROMAN, Michael A; Rockyview Gen Hosp, 7007 14 St SW, Calgary AB T2V 1P9; Wes'04; FRCPC; IntMed; Respir. Staff, Rockyview General Hospital; (403)943-3283; Fax. (403)252-6471.

ROMAN, Miriam; Hotel-Dieu de Levis, 143 rue Wolfe, Levis QC G6V 3Z1; Staff, Hôtel-Dieu de Lévis; (418)835-7113; miriam_roman@ssss.gouv.qc.ca.

ROMAN, Nader S F S; Linden Ridge Med Centre, E-123 Scurfield Blvd, Winnipeg MB R3Y 1L6; Tanta (Egypt)'89; CCFP; (204)488-9988

ROMAN, Ramon; Inst Polychirurgie de Montreal, 8 Place du Commerce, Verdun QC H3E 1N3; National (Mexico)'64; CSPQ; FRCPC; Anes. Langs: Spanish; English; (514)281-2022; Fax. (514)842-8664; roman2038@yahoo.com.

ROMAN, Raymond M; Portage Prof Bldg, 304-5400 Portage Rd, Niagara Falls ON L2G 5X7; Wes'73; DOHS; Physician, Patheon Pharmaceuticals/Oxy Vinyl Canada/Cytec & Lubrizol; (905)358-3434; Fax. (905)358-3434.

ROMAN, Sandra; PAMQ, 200-1 boul Rene-Levesque E, Montreal QC H2X 3Z5; Mon'90; CCFP; Staff, Hopital de la Cite de la santé; (514)397-0888

ROMAN, Sherwyn; Maidstone Med Clinic, PO Box 399, Maidstone SK S0M 1M0; (306)893-2689; Fax. (306)893-4646.

ROMANCHUK, Kenneth G; Alberta Children's Hosp, 2888 Shaganappi Trail NW, Calgary AB T3B 6A8; Sask'76; DABOph; FRCSC; Ophth (Pediatric Ophthalmology). Staff Vision Clinic, Alberta Children's Hospital; Physician, Vision Clinic; Prof Section of Ophth Dept of Surg, University of Calgary; (403)955-7940

ROMANESCU, Craita A; Goodfellow Prof Bldg, 211-170 McEwan Dr E, Bolton ON L7E 4C8; '93; CCFP; (905)857-8508; Fax. (905)857-8518; arinamdoffice@gmail.com.

ROMANO, Clare C; Foothills Med Centre, 1403 29 St NW, Calgary AB T2N 2T9; Wes'87; FRCPC; DiagRad. Staff, Foothills Medical Centre; (403)944-4530; Fax. (403)944-1120.

ROMANO, Kenneth R S; Callingwood Crossing Med Clini, 6905 172 St NW, Edmonton AB T5T 5Y1; Man'71; Ac Staff, Royal Alexandra Hospital; (780)444-0350; Fax. (780)444-0476.

ROMANO, Marilisa; Mount Sinai Hosp Centre, 5690 boul Cavendish, Cote Saint-Luc QC H4W 1S7; Laval'96; CCFP; Staff, Mount Sinai Hospital Center; (514)369-2222

ROMANO, Walter M; St Joseph's Health Care, PO Box 5777 Stn B 268 Grosvenor St, London ON N6A 4V2; Wes'86; FRCPC; DiagRad (Magnetic Resonance Imaging). Staff, St Joseph's Hospital - St Joseph's Health Care; Asst Prof Radiol/Teach Staff ObstGyn, University of Western Ontario; (519)646-6035

ROMANOVSKY, Adam S; University of Alberta Hosp, 8440 112 St NW, Edmonton AB T6G 2B7; Alb'03; FRCPC; IntMed; Critical Care Medicine; Nephrol. Staff, University of Alberta Hospital; (780)407-8822

ROMANOVSKY, Amanda J; Hys Medical Centre, 604-11010 101 St NW, Edmonton AB T5H 4B9; Alb'03; FRCSC; ObstGyn. (780)421-4728; Fax. (780)426-6698.

ROMANOWSKA, Karinka I; Appletree Med Group, 2948 Baseline Rd, Ottawa ON K2H 8T5; (Poland)'99; (613)288-2059

ROMANOWSKI, Andrew; The Peterborough Clinic, 202-26 Hospital Dr, Peterborough ON K9J 7C3; CCFP; (705)740-6855; Fax. (705)740-6881.

ROMANOWSKI, Barbara; College Plaza, 1000-8215 112 St NW, Edmonton AB T6G 2C8; Alb'73; ABIM; FACP; FRCPC; IntMed (HIV). Consultant, Covenant Health - Misericordia Community Hospital; Consultant, Royal Alexandra Hospital; Consultant, University of Alberta Hospital; Clin Prof Med, University of Alberta; (780)436-4900; Fax. (780)436-4920.

ROMAO, Rodrigo L P; IWK Health Centre, PO Box 9000 Rpo CSC 5850-5980 University Ave, Halifax NS B3K 6R8; Sao Paolo (Brazil)'00; Staff, IWK Health Centre; (902)470-8703; Fax. (902)470-7260.

ROMASHIN, Stanislav; 150-7997 Westminster Hwy, Richmond BC V6X 1A4; (Russia (Federation))'91; CCFP; (778)297-4700

ROMATOWSKI, Walter W; Niagara Health Centre, 308-180 Vine St S, St Catharines ON L2R 7P3; Qns'76; FRCPC; IntMed; Gastroent. Staff, Niagara Health System - Ontario Street Site; Staff, Niagara Health System - St Catharines General Site; Langs: Polish; (905)682-8693; Fax. (905)682-0311.

ROMBAUT, Allan J; Rothesay Med Clinic, 11 Gondola Point Rd, Rothesay NB E2E 5J6; Dal'89; CCFP; FCFP; (506)847-7592; Fax. (506)847-7509.

ROMBAUT, Karen R; Rothesay Med Clinic, 11 Gondola Point Rd, Rothesay NB E2E 5J6; Dal'90; CCFP; FCFP; (506)847-7592; Fax. (506)847-7509.

ROMEO, Philippe; Institut de Cardiologie de Mtl, 5000 rue Belanger, Montreal QC H1T 1C8; Mon'02; FRCPC; AnatPath (Cardiovascular Pathology). Staff, Institut de Cardiologie de Montréal; (514)376-3330 x3870

ROMERO CASTRO, Mario E; CSSS de la Cote-de-Gaspe, 215 boul de York O, Gaspe QC G4X 2W2; (Peru)'86; Staff, Centre Hospitalier de Gaspe; (418)368-3301

ROMERO-SIERRA, Cesar P; Main Street Med Centre, 1251 Stittsville Main St, Stittsville ON K2S 2E5; Qns'93; Staff, Health Support Operational Training Unit; (613)831-7372

ROMEY, Juliyana; Fort St John Med Clinic, 10011 96 St, Fort St. John BC V1J 3P3; Linkoping (Sweden)'01; CCFP; (250)785-6677

ROMNEY, Jacques S; Heritage Med Research Centre, 362-107 University Campus NW, Edmonton AB T6G 2S2; Alb'96; FRCPC; IntMed; Endocrin&Metab. (780)407-3636; Fax. (780)407-6702.

ROMNEY, Marc G; St Paul's Hosp, 1081 Burrard St, Vancouver BC V6Z 1Y6; Wes'96; FRCPC; MedMicrobiol. Staff, Providence Health Care - St Paul's Hospital; (604)806-8188; mromney@providencehealth.bc.ca.

ROMPRE, Anne; CLSC Villeray, 1425 rue Jarry E, Montreal QC H2E 1A7; Mon'85; (514)376-4141; Fax. (514)376-4023.

ROMPRE, Dominique; Ctr Hosp de Lasalle, 8585 Tsse Champlain, LaSalle QC H8P 1C1; Mon'07; CCFP; Staff, Centre Hospitalier de LaSalle; (514)362-8000

ROMSA, G Jonathan; London HSC-University Hosp, PO Box 5339 Stn B 339 Windermere Rd, London ON N6A 5A5; Wes'96; FRCPC; IntMed; NuclearMed. Staff, London Health Sciences Centre - University Hospital; (519)663-3433

ROMSA, Nancy K; St Thomas-Elgin Gen Hosp, PO Box 2007 Stn Main 189 Elm St, St Thomas ON N5P 3W2; Tor'97; CCFP; CCFP(E.M.); Staff, St Thomas Elgin General Hospital; Court Staff, Stratford General Hospital - Huron Perth Healthcare Alliance; Langs: English; French; (519)631-2030 x2051

RONA, Mary J; Westmount Med Bldg, 615-5025 rue Sherbrooke O, Montreal QC H4A 1S9; London (England)'76; CCFP; (514)488-5782; Fax. (514)488-0992.

RONA, Zoltan P; Complementary & Integrative Me, 101-8188 Yonge St, Thornhill ON L4J 1W5; McG'77; MSc(Nutrition); Chief Medical Advisor, NAKA Herbs & Vitamins; (905)764-8700; Fax. (905)764-6641; zoltan78@bellnet.ca.

RONALD, Allan R; St Boniface Gen Hosp, C5124-409 Tache Ave, Winnipeg MB R2H 2A6; Man'61; FACP; FRCPC; IntMed (Infectious Diseases); MedMicrobiol. Staff, St Boniface General Hospital; Langs: English; (204)233-8563; aronald@ms.umanitoba.ca.

RONALD, John A; Medical Centre, 24-1515 Dufferin Cres, Nanaimo BC V9S 2B8; Man'99; FRCPC; IntMed; Critical Care Medicine; Respir. (250)753-2446

RONCO, Juan J; Vancouver Gen Hosp, 855 12th Ave W, Vancouver BC V5Z 1M9; Buenos Aires (Argentina)'80; FRCPC; IntMed (Critical Care Medicine). Assoc Dir ICU, Vancouver General Hospital - Centennial Pavillion; Staff, UBC Hospital - Koerner Pavillion; Asst Prof Med, University of British Columbia; Langs: Spanish; French; (604)875-5949; Fax. (604)875-5957; jronco@vanhosp.bc.ca.

RONDEAU, Chantal; CSSS de Laval, 1755 boul Rene-Laennec, Laval QC H7M 3L9; Ott'89; CCFP; CCFP(E.M.); Staff, Hopital de la Cite de la santé; Langs: English; French; (450)668-1010

RONDEAU, Frederique; Clin de Med Fam de Plessisvill, 1971 rue Bilodeau, Plessisville QC G6L 3J1; Laval'10; (819)362-6337

RONDEAU, Genevieve; CHUM-Hop Saint-Luc, 1058 rue Saint-Denis, Montreal QC H2X 3J4; Mon'04; FRCPC; IntMed; Endocrin&Metab. Staff, Centre Hospitalier l'Université De Montréal (CHUM) - Hôpital Saint-luc; (514)890-8000

RONDEAU, Guy; 188C rue Principale, Huberdeau QC J0T 1G0; Mon'60; (819)687-3233; Fax. (819)687-9562.

RONDEAU, Malcolm R V; 815-777 Hornby St, Vancouver BC V6Z 1S4; UBC'80; Assoc Staff, Providence Health Care - St Paul's Hospital; Clinical Asst Prof, University of British Columbia; (604)681-3857; Fax. (604)681-8876.

RONDEAU, Maryse; CSSS de Vaudreuil-Soulanges, RR 1 11 ch de la Cite-des-Jeunes, Saint-Polycarpe QC J0P 1X0; Mon'89; (450)265-3771; maryse_rondeau@rrsss16.gouv.qc.ca.

RONDEAU, Nancy M; CSSS du Suroît, 150 rue Saint-Thomas, Salaber-de-Valleyf QC J6T 6C1; Sher'96; CCFP; CCFP(E.M.); Staff, Centre Hospitalier Régional du Suroît; (450)371-9920 x2157; nancyjean@videotron.ca.

RONDEAU, Pierre; CLSC St-Michel, 3355 rue Jarry E, Montreal QC H1Z 2E5; Mon'77; (514)722-3000 x5575

RONDEAU, Ronald L; Oxford Med Clinic, PO Box 569 111 Medawell Rd, Oxford NS B0M 1P0; Dal'76; (902)447-3078; Fax. (902)447-4599; ronrondeau@hotmail.com.

RONDI, Kevin; St Paul's Hosp, 1018 Burrard St, Vancouver BC V6Z 1Y6; McM'06; FRCPC; Anes. Staff, Providence Health Care - St Paul's Hospital; (604)682-2344

RONDILLA, F Michael A; Wilfrid Laurier Hlth Services, 75 University Ave W, Waterloo ON N2L 3C5; Wes'96; CCFP; FCFP; (519)884-0710 x3146; Fax. (519)885-4865.

RONEN, Gabriel M; McMaster Univ Med Centre, 3A 58-1280 Main St W, Hamilton ON L8S 4K1; Basel (Switzerland)'72; MSc; FRCPC; Neur (Pediatric Neurology). Staff, Hamilton Health Sciences Centre - McMaster Children's Hospital; Assoc Prof Peds, McMaster University; Langs: German; (905)521-2100 x73392; Fax. (905)521-7914.

RONEY, Peter D; Perth-Smiths Falls Dist Hosp, 60 Cornelia St W, Smiths Falls ON K7A 2H9; Ott'83; FRCSC; Urol. Consultant, Rideau Regional Centre; Staff Consultant/Chief Medical Staff, Perth & Smiths Falls District Hospital - Smiths Falls Site; Clin Associate, Kingston General Hospital; Aj Prof Surg Urology, Queen's University; (613)283-7746; Fax. (613)283-9850.

RONSLEY, John C; Burnaby Hosp, 280-3935 Kincaid St, Burnaby BC V5G 2X6; UBC'86; FRCPC; Psy. Staff Outpatient Records, Burnaby Hospital; (604)453-1939

ROOB, Otokar J; 9368 Southfort Dr, Fort Saskatchewan AB T8L 0C5; Safarika (Slovakia)'75; Staff, Fort Saskatchewan Health Centre; Langs: Slovak; Czech; (780)997-0177; Fax. (780)992-2065; ottoroob@telusplanet.net.

ROOB, Otto V; Health Sciences Centre, 300 Prince Philip Dr, St. John's NL A1B 3V6; Alb'03; FRCPC; Anes (Family Medicine). Staff, Health Sciences Centre; (709)737-6300

ROODE, Lourene A; Rockyview Gen Hosp, 7007 14 St SW, Calgary AB T2V 1P9; Pretoria (South Africa)'87; ACLS; ATLS; CCFP; Staff, Rockyview General Hospital; Langs: Afrikaans; (403)943-3000; lourene@drroode.com.

ROODT, Johann; Broadway Med Clinic, 200-41 Broadway St W, Yorkton SK S3N 0L6; (306)783-2555; Fax. (306)783-2557.

ROOKE, Catherine A; 9731 350 Ave PO Box 763, Oliver BC V0H 1T0; Stellenbosch (South Africa)'97; MB ChB; CCFP; (250)485-0359; Fax. (250)485-0362.

ROOKE, J Louise; Clinique Med Montee Paiement, 205-492 boul de l'Hopital, Gatineau QC J8V 2P4; Ott'89; ac Staff Family Med, Hôpital de Gatineau; (819)561-5511

ROOME, Stephen W; 1864 Oak Bay Ave, Victoria BC V8R 1C5; Tor'84; (250)380-1551; Fax. (250)380-2046.

ROONEY, Hugh; 204-440 Boler Rd, London ON N6K 4L2; Wes'85; Staff, St Joseph's Hospital - St Joseph's Health Care; (519)471-0130; Fax. (519)471-2890.

ROONEY, Michael A; 385 St Paul Ave, Brantford ON N3R 4N6; Wes'98; FRCSC; GenSurg. Staff, The Brant Community Healthcare System - Brantford General Hospital Site; (519)753-1242; Fax. (519)753-4925.

ROONEY, Michael E; Royal University Hosp, 103 Hospital Dr, Saskatoon SK S7N 0W8; Sask'93; FRCPC; Anes. Staff, Royal University Hospital; Clinical Asst Prof, University of Saskatchewan; (306)655-1183; Fax. (306)655-1279.

ROONEY, Michael S; 102-955 Major Mackenzie Dr, Vaughan ON L6A 4P9; Tor'82; FRCPC; DiagRad. (289)553-6336; Fax. (289)553-6339.

ROONEY, Rachel A D; Kingston Gen Hosp, V2-76 Stuart St, Kingston ON K7L 2V7; Qns'97; FRCPC; Anes. Staff, Kingston General Hospital; (613)549-6666 x7827

ROONEY, Rebecca A; Avenue Med Centre, 1-221 Brant Ave, Brantford ON N3T 3J2; Wes'98; FRCSC; ObstGyn. Staff, Kingston General Hospital; (519)753-8666

ROOPANI, Seemi H; 7263 Fraser St, Vancouver BC V5X 3V8; Karachi (Pakistan)'04; FRCPC; Peds. Staff, BC Children's Hospital; (604)322-1440

ROOPCHAND-MOHAMMED, Rupa R; Regional Mental HC-St Thomas, PO Box 2004 Stn Main 467 Sunset Dr, St Thomas ON N5P 3V9; West Indies (Jamaica)'80; FRCPC; Psy (Serious Mentally Ill). Consultant Privil, St Thomas Elgin General Hospital; Staff Psy, Regional Mental Health Care-St Joseph's Health Care; Lecturer, University of Western Ontario; (519)631-8510 x49278

ROOPNARIAN, Indra; 405-531 Davis Dr, Newmarket ON L3Y 6P5; Durban (South Africa)'89; MB ChB; CCFP; (905)898-2240; Fax. (905)898-2253.

ROOPRAM, Devicka J; Dr Charles S Curtis Mem Hosp, 178-200 West St, St Anthony NL A0K 4S0; Kiev (Russia (Federation))'86; Staff, Charles S Curtis Memorial Hospital; (709)454-3333

ROOS, Estelle L; 208-803 Chaparral Dr SE, Calgary AB T2X 0E5; (South Africa)'03; Physician, Lakeland College; Langs: Afrikaans; (403)873-7734; Fax. (403)873-7735.

ROOS, Martin R; Royal Columbian Hosp, 330 Columbia St E, New Westminster BC V3L 3W7; Cal'01; FRCPC; Anes. Staff, Royal Columbian Hospital; (604)520-4253

ROOS, Matthys; Rossburn Health Centre, PO Box 40, Rossburn MB R0J 1V0; Pretoria (South Africa)'78; Staff, Rossburn Health Centre; (204)859-2413

ROOS, Paul J; Norway House Indian Hosp, PO Box 730, Norway House MB R0B 1B0; Stellenbosch (South Africa)'69; MB ChB; Staff, Norway House Indian Hospital; (204)359-6731; Fax. (204)359-4413; roos@mts.net.

ROOSMA, Jennifer E; Richmond Health Services, 7000 Westminster Hwy, Richmond BC V6X 1A2; UBC'84; Staff, Peace Arch Hospital; (604)278-9711

ROOTENBERG, Jonathan H; Addiction & Mental Hlth-Clarke, 250 College St, Toronto ON M5T 1R8; Dublin (Ireland)'90; FRCPC; Psy (Forensic Psychiatry). Staff Psy, Centre for Addiction & Mental Health (CAMH) - College Street Site; Staff Psy, Ontario Shores Centre for Mental Health Sciences; Lecturer Psy, University of Toronto; (416)535-8501 x4389; Fax. (416)979-6965; jonathan_rootenberg@camh.net.

ROOTMAN, David S; Univ Hlth Network-Toronto Western Hosp, 6F-399 Bathurst St, Toronto ON M5T 2S8; Tor'82; FRCSC; Ophth (Cornea). Staff, The Hospital For Sick Children; Staff, Toronto Western Hospital - University Health Network; Staff, Toronto General Hospital - UHN; Assoc Prof Ophth, University of Toronto; Langs: Hebrew; (416)603-5401; Fax. (416)603-1993; d.rootman@utoronto.ca.

ROOTMAN, Jack; UBC Eye Care Centre, 2550 Willow St, Vancouver BC V5Z 3N9; Alb'68; FRCS; CRCP; DABOph; FRCSC; Ophth (Oncology). Staff Ophth, Vancouver General Hospital - Centennial Pavillion; Staff, BC Cancer Agency Vancouver Centre; (604)875-4485; Fax. (604)875-4415.

ROOYAKKERS, Daniel J; Huron Commun Family Hlth Team, PO Box 460 32B-1 Centennial Dr, Seaforth ON N0K 1W0; McM'92; Staff, Seaforth Community Hospital - Huron Perth Healthcare Alliance; (519)600-2273; Fax. (519)600-2501; drooyakkers@rogers.com.

ROPCHAN, Glorianne V; Univ Hlth Network-Toronto Gen, 200 Elizabeth St, Toronto ON M5G 2C4; Tor'80; FRCSC; GenSurg; Cardiovasc&ThorSurg. Staff, Toronto General Hospital - UHN; (416)340-4800

ROPELESKI, Mark J; Hotel-Dieu Hosp, 166 Brock St, Kingston ON K7L 5G2; McG'93; FRCPC; IntMed (Inflammatory Bowel Disease); Gastroent. Asst Prof Med, Hotel-Dieu Hospital; Asst Prof Med, Kingston General Hospital; Langs: English; French; (613)544-3400 x2288; Fax. (613)544-3114.

ROPER, Fiona M; Queen Elizabeth II HSC, 1276 South Park St, Halifax NS B3H 2Y9; Aberdeen (Scotland)'75; Anes. Staff, Queen Elizabeth II Health Sciences Centre - Victoria General Site; (902)473-2331; Fax. (902)423-9454.

ROPER, Mark; Clinique Med Roper, 4500 rue Sherbrooke O, Westmount QC H3Z 1E6; RCS (Ireland)'83; BSc; CCFP; FCFP; Dir Prim Care Fam Med, McGill University Health Centre - Montreal General Campus; Dir, Queen Elizabeth Family Medicine Group; Dir, Department General Medicine Montreal; adj Prof Family Med, McGill University; (514)937-8000; Fax. (514)937-8884.

ROPER, Nicole; Charles Clark Health Clinic, 303 9 Ave SW, High River AB T1V 0H2; Cal'09; CCFP; Staff, High River General Hospital; (403)652-2929; Fax. (403)652-1510.

ROPER, Peter D L; Clinique Med Roper, 4500 rue Sherbrooke O, Westmount QC H3Z 1E6; Glasgow (Scotland)'51; DPM(Lond); MRCPsy; FAPA; CSPQ; FRCPC; Psy (Neuro Psychiatry). Ac Staff Behaviour Therapy Unit, Douglas Mental Health University Institute; adj Prof, McGill University; Langs: English; French; (514)845-3809; Fax. (514)845-1777.

ROQUE, Elmer A; Formation Hlth Services Unit, PO Box 17000 Stn Forces 1200 Colville Rd, Victoria BC V9A 7N2; Alb'98; CCFP; FCFP; Staff, Canadian Forces Health Services - Pacific Centre; (250)363-2394

ROQUEYYA, Rubina; Crescent Town Hlth Centre, 4 The Market Place, East York ON M4C 5M1; Chittagong (Bangladesh)'85; CCFP; (416)690-3412; Fax. (416)691-2543.

RORABECK, Cecil H; 400-700 Richmond St, London ON N6A 5C7; Wes'68; DAB; FRCSC; OrthSurg. Ac Staff Surg, London Health Sciences Centre - University Hospital; Prof, University of Western Ontario; (519)434-5000; Fax. (519)679-5069.

RORKE, Stewart; Dr H Bliss Murphy Cancer Ctr, 300 Prince Philip Dr, St. John's NL A1B 3V6; Mem'96; FRCPC; IntMed; MedOncol. Staff, Dr H Bliss Murphy Cancer Centre; (709)777-7802

RORSTAD, Otto P; Richmond Road Diag & Trmt Ctre, 1820 Richmond Rd SW, Calgary AB T2T 5C7; UBC'72; PhD(Exp Med); ABIM; FRCPC; IntMed (Endocrinology & Metabolism). Staff, Foothills Medical Centre; Prof, University of Calgary; (403)955-8328; Fax. (403)955-8249; rorstad@ucalgary.ca.

ROSA, David A; 207-6453 Morrison St, Niagara Falls ON L2E 7H1; Saba (Netherlands Antilles)'07; CCFP; (289)296-2025; Fax. (289)296-2333.

ROSA NETO, Pedro; 6825 boul Lasalle, LaSalle QC H4H 1R3; (Mexico)'90; Neur (P.Q.). (514)766-1009

ROSARIO, Rosa H; Healthways Med Clinic, 865 Portage Ave, Winnipeg MB R3G 0N8; Santo Domingo (Dominican Republic)'66; LMCC; Langs: Spanish; (204)783-6464

ROSATI, Domenic; 7-1221 Limeridge Rd E, Hamilton ON L8W 1Y1; Tor'86; FRCPC; AnatPath (Family Practice). (905)574-9474; Fax. (905)574-7435.

ROSATI, Mark E; Orillia Soldier's Mem Hosp, 170 Colborne St W, Orillia ON L3V 2Z3; Wes'93; CCFP; Assoc Staff, Orillia Soldiers' Memorial Hospital; (705)325-2201 x3248

ROSBOROUGH, Amy M; Centennial CMH & Brain Injury, PO Box 1000 Stn Main, Ponoka AB T4J 1R8; Cal'10; CCFP; Staff, Centennial Centre for Mental Health & Brain Injury; (403)783-7600

ROSCA STREDIE, Gianina; CSSS du Lac-des-Deux-Montagnes, 520 boul Arthur-Sauve, Saint-Eustache QC J7R 5B1; Iasi (Romania)'97; Psy. Staff, Hôpital de Saint-Eustache; (450)473-6811

ROSCOE, Andrew J; Univ Hlth Network-Toronto Gen, 200 Elizabeth St, Toronto ON M5G 2C4; Liverpool (England)'95; Staff, Toronto General Hospital - UHN; (416)340-3227

ROSCOE, Clare L; Children's Hosp Eastern Ont, 401 Smyth Rd, Ottawa ON K1H 8L1; Dal'98; FRCPC; Psy. Staff, The Hospital For Sick Children; (613)737-7600

ROSCOE, Diane L; Vancouver Gen Hosp, JPPN 1112A-855 12th Ave W, Vancouver BC V5Z 1M9; Jefferson(PA) (USA)'83; FRCPC; MedMicrobiol. Staff Microbiol Lab, Vancouver General Hospital - Centennial Pavillion; (604)875-4547

ROSCOE, Janet M; Medical Centre, C11-3000 Lawrence Ave E, Scarborough ON M1P 2V1; McG'71; BSc; ABIM; AB; FACP; FRCPC; IntMed; Nephrol. Ac Staff, The Scarborough Hospital - General Campus; Ac Staff, Bridgepoint Health Centre; Assoc Prof, University of Toronto; (416)438-9000; Fax. (416)438-9677.

ROSCOE, Martin W A; 309-3101 Bloor St W, Etobicoke ON M8X 2W2; Qns'79; FACS; FRCSC; OrthSurg. Staff OrthSurg, Toronto Rehabilitation Institute - University Centre; Staff OrthSurg, Toronto Rehabilitation Institute - University Centre; Head OrthSurg, St Joseph's Health Centre; Asst Prof, University of Toronto; (416)239-8401; Fax. (416)239-8402.

ROSE, Alwyn L E; Albert Park Family Med Centre, 3992 Albert St, Regina SK S4S 3R1; Aberdeen (Scotland)'68; (306)584-3833; Fax. (306)585-3833.

ROSE, Andrea L; Salmon Arm Med Clinic, PO Box 730 581 Hudson Ave, Salmon Arm BC V1E 4N8; UBC'07; CCFP; Staff, Queen Victoria Hospital; (250)832-2321

ROSE, Barry F; Cardiology Consultants, 101-99 Airport rd, St. John's NL A1A 4Y3; Mem'81; ABIM; FACC; FRCPC; IntMed (Interventional Cardiology); Cardiol. Staff, Health Sciences Centre; Clin Prof, Memorial University Of Newfoundland; (709)726-5311; Fax. (709)726-1028; cardiologyconsultants@nfld.net.

ROSE, Chantal E; 101-9006 Edward St, Chilliwack BC V2P 4E1; Necastle-Upon-Tyne (England)'06; (604)701-6866

ROSE, Colin P; 3778 ch de la Cote-des-Neiges, Montreal QC H3H 1V6; McG'71; FRCPC; Cardiol. Staff, McGill University Health Centre - Montreal General Campus; Langs: English; French; (514)501-9325; colros@mac.com.

ROSE, D Keith; Sunnybrook Hlth Sciences Ctre, C132-2075 Bayview Ave, Toronto ON M4N 3M5; Wes'71; FRCPC; Anes. Exec VP/Chief Med Exec, Sunnybrook Health Sciences Centre; (416)480-6181; Fax. (416)480-5970; keith.rose@sunnybrook.ca.

ROSE, David B; Scarborough North Med Arts, 410-4040 Finch Ave E, Scarborough ON M1S 4V5; Tor'80; BSc; FRCPC; IntMed (Infectious Diseases). Ac Staff Med, The Scarborough Hospital - Birchmount Campus; Dept Chief/Med Staff, The Scarborough Hospital - General Campus; (416)321-3846; Fax. (416)321-3848.

ROSE, David L; Univ of Western Ontario, 11-1151 Richmond St, London ON N6A 3K7; Wes'88; (519)661-3030

ROSE, Edward J; Bayshore Med Bldg, 201-3029 Carling Ave, Ottawa ON K2B 8E8; Ott'72; CCFP; FCFP; Assoc Staff, The Ottawa Hospital - Civic Campus; (613)829-7660

ROSE, Gregory W; The Ottawa Hosp-Civic Campus, 470-1053 Carling Ave, Ottawa ON K1Y 4E9; Man'01; FRCPC; IntMed; InfectDis. Staff, The Ottawa Hospital - Civic Campus; (613)761-4155

ROSE, Heather P; Musquodoboit Harbour Med Clin, RR 1 7907 Highway 7, Musquodbt Hbr NS B0J 2L0; Dal'98; FRCPC; Peds. Staff, IWK Health Centre; (902)889-2650; Fax. (902)889-2844; heather.rose@iwk.nshealth.ca.

ROSE, James C; Gateway Med Bldg, 307-2051 McCallum Rd, Abbotsford BC V2S 3N5; McG'83; FRCSC; OrthSurg. (604)852-2900; Fax. (604)852-3688.

ROSE, James N; Cancer Ctr of Southeastern Ont, 25 King St W, Kingston ON K7L 5P9; Wes'07; FRCPC; RadOncol. Staff, Cancer Centre of Southeastern Ontario; (613)544-2631

ROSE, Matthew D B; Boyle McCauley Health Centre, 10628 96 St NW, Edmonton AB T5H 2J2; Alb'97; CCFP; (780)422-7333; Fax. (780)422-7343; matrose@shaw.ca.

ROSE, Nicholas; Vancouver Gen Hosp, 855 12th Ave W, Vancouver BC V5Z 1M9; Ott'05; FRCPC; EmergMed. Staff, Vancouver General Hospital - Centennial Pavillion; (604)875-4995

ROSE, Norbert J; 345 Kennedy Ave, Toronto ON M6P 3C4; Bratislava (Slovakia)'63; Langs: Italian; Slovak; (416)767-9972; Fax. (416)767-3572.

ROSE, Randi K; North York Med Arts Bldg, 327-1333 Sheppard Ave E, North York ON M2J 1V1; McM'97; FRCPC; IntMed; Cardiol. (416)773-1060; Fax. (416)773-1360.

ROSE, Roger C S; Glenridge Med Bldg, 201-1 Belton Blvd, St Catharines ON L2T 3Y4; Birmingham (England)'64; MB ChB; MRCS; LRCP; Ac Staff Family Phys/Chief Family Practice, Niagara Health System - St Catharines General Site; (905)688-3591; Fax. (905)641-5565.

ROSE, Sean R; Peace Arch Hosp, 15521 Russell Ave, White Rock BC V4B 2R4; Mem'83; LMCC; FRCPC; Anes (Critical Care Medicine). Staff Anaes, Peace Arch Hospital; (604)535-4500 x7910; Fax. (604)535-4540.

ROSE, Spencer G; 302-4420 Chatterton Way, Victoria BC V8X 5J2; Qns'03; FRCPC; Peds. (250)881-7349

ROSE, Stuart C; Foothills Med Centre, C231-1403 29 St NW, Calgary AB T2N 2T9; (South Africa)'93; CCFP; CCFP(E.M.); FCFP; Staff, Foothills Medical Centre; (403)944-1315; Fax. (403)944-2419.

ROSE, Terence J; 302-800 Bathurst St, Toronto ON M5R 3M8; West Indies (Jamaica)'64; Court Staff, St Joseph's Health Centre; (416)535-4392

ROSE, Toby H; Provincial Forensic Path Unit, 200-26 Grenville St, Toronto ON M7A 2G9; Sask'77; DABPath; FRCPC; AnatPath (Forensic Pathology). (416)314-4040; toby.rose@ontario.ca.

ROSE, Velene D; Ontario College of Art & Desig, 100 McCaul St, Toronto ON M5T 1W1; West Indies (Jamaica)'72; (416)977-6000; Fax. (416)977-5465.

ROSE-JANES, Nancy; Upper Grand Family Health Team, 205 Queen St E, Fergus ON N1M 1T2; McM'03; CCFP; (519)787-7418

ROSE SEL, Winsley; The Hosp for Sick Children, 7304-555 University Ave, Toronto ON M5G 1X8; (India)'95; (416)813-6273

ROSEBUSH, David J; Guelph Family Health Team, 305-85 Norfolk St, Guelph ON N1H 4J4; McM'05; BSc; CCFP; Staff, Guelph General Hospital; (519)766-1490

ROSEBUSH, Patricia I; Fontbonne Bldg, F416-301 James St S, Hamilton ON L8P 3B6; McM'80; ABNP; FRCPC; Psy (Psycho Pharmacology). Dir Inpatient Psy, Hamilton Health Sciences Centre - McMaster Children's Hospital; Assoc Prof, McMaster University; (905)522-1155; Fax. (905)521-6133.

ROSEMAN, David; Meadowlark Prof Bldg, 270-8702 Meadowlark Rd NW, Edmonton AB T5R 5W5; London (England)'85; FRCPC; Peds. Ad Staff, Royal Alexandra Hospital; Consultant Privil, Edson Healthcare Centre; Consultant Privil, Bonnyville Healthcare Centre; Clin Assoc Prof, University of Alberta; (780)944-1840; Fax. (780)423-3961.

ROSEN, Barry P; Univ Hlth Network-Princess M, M700-610 University Ave, Toronto ON M5G 2M9; Wes'77; FRCSC; ObstGyn (Ovarian Cancer). Ac Staff, Princess Margaret Hospital - University Health Network; Ac Staff, Toronto General Hospital - UHN; Assoc Staff, Sunnybrook Health Sciences Centre; Asst Prof, University of Toronto; (416)946-2254; Fax. (416)946-2288; barry.rosen@uhn.on.ca.

ROSEN, Charles T; 1364 Simcoe St N, Oshawa ON L1G 4X6; Tor'69; BSc(Hon); Staff, Lakeridge Health - Oshawa Site; (905)576-1693; Fax. (905)434-1884.

ROSEN, Cheryl F; Univ Hlth Network-Toronto Western Hosp, 471-399 Bathurst St, Toronto ON M5T 2S8; Tor'80; BSc; LRCPS; ABD; FRCPC; Derm. Staff Derm, Women's College Hospital; Head Div of Derm, Toronto Western Hospital - University Health Network; Assoc Prof, University of Toronto; (416)603-5952; Fax. (416)603-2782.

ROSEN, Clifford A; Hotel-Dieu Grace Hosp, 1030 Ouellette Ave, Windsor ON N9A 1E1; Witwatersrand (South Africa)'92; MB ChB; Staff, Hôtel-Dieu Grace Hospital; (519)973-4444

ROSEN, David C; Summerville Family Hlth Team, 5F-101 Queensway W, Mississauga ON L5B 2P7; Tor'72; DA; Ac Staff, Trillium Health Centre - Mississauga; Court Staff, The Credit Valley Hospital; Langs: Spanish; French; (905)272-9700 x1; Fax. (905)272-1416.

ROSEN, Fred; Medical Centre, C04-3000 Lawrence Ave E, Scarborough ON M1P 2V1; Tor'62; FRCPC; IntMed (Endocrinology). Staff, The Scarborough Hospital - General Campus; (416)438-6673; Fax. (416)438-5069.

ROSEN, Gili; 303-343 Wilson Ave, North York ON M3H 1T1; Tor'88; CCFP; FCFP; Staff Privil, Baycrest Centre for Geriatric Care; Lecturer, University of Toronto; (416)785-8412; Fax. (416)785-8324.

ROSEN, H David; Children's Hosp Eastern Ont, 401 Smyth Rd, Ottawa ON K1H 8L1; Tor'90; FRCPC; Anes. Staff, Children's Hospital of Eastern Ontario (CHEO); (613)737-7600 x2431

ROSEN, Irving B; 205-123 Edward St, Toronto ON M5G 1E2; Tor'54; MD; FRCSC; GenSurg (P.Q.) (Endocrinology). Att Staff Surg, Mount Sinai Hospital; Court Staff Surg, Toronto General Hospital - UHN; Prof, University of Toronto; Langs: Yiddish; (416)813-4181; Fax. (416)597-3343; irosen@mtsinai.on.ca.

ROSEN, Irving E; Toronto Prof Bldg, 205-123 Edward St, Toronto ON M5G 1E2; Tor'60; FRCPC; DiagRad. Staff Radiol, Sunnybrook Health Sciences Centre; Asst Prof, University of Toronto; (416)597-1016 x2310; Fax. (416)597-6610.

ROSEN, Joel; SMBD Jewish Gen Hosp, 3755 ch Cote-Sainte-Catherine, Montreal QC H3T 1E2; McG'68; Ophth (Cornea). Sr Staff Ophth, McGill University Health Centre - Montreal General Campus; Staff Ophth, Sir Mortimer B Davis Jewish General; Consultant, McGill University Health Centre - Montreal Children's Hospital; assoc Prof, McGill University; Langs: French; Italian; (514)340-8611; Fax. (514)340-8215.

ROSEN, Leonard; 208-5885 ch de la Cote-des-Nei, Montreal QC H3S 2T2; Dal'75; DABOS; FAAOS; FRCSC; OrthSurg (Knee Surgery). Consultant OrthSurg, Institut de Réadaptation Gingras-Lindsay de Montréal; Att Staff OrthSurg, Sir Mortimer B Davis Jewish General; adj Conférencier, McGill University; (514)738-1406; Fax. (514)738-8752; rosenmd@hotmail.com.

ROSEN, Nathan A; Dermetics, 8 & 9-3305 Harvester Rd, Burlington ON L7N 3N2; McG'00; DABD; FRCPC; Derm. Asst Prof Med, McMaster University; Langs: English; (905)336-9624; Fax. (905)336-9625.

ROSEN, Noel A; 210-305 Finch Ave W, North York ON M2R 1N2; Tor'68; CCFP; FCFP; Ac Staff, North York General Hospital - Branson Division; Assoc Staff, North York General Hospital; Assoc Staff, St John's Rehabilitation Hospital; Lecturer Family & Commun Med, University of Toronto; (416)226-3300; Fax. (416)226-2849; noel.rosen@utoronto.ca.

ROSEN, Robin J; Thornhill Med Centre, 18 Centre St, Thornhill ON L4J 1E9; Tor'94; BSc; CCFP; (905)889-3634; Fax. (905)889-3986.

ROSEN, Wayne S; Peter Lougheed Centre, 2230-3500 26 Ave NE, Calgary AB T1Y 6J4; Qns'91; FRCSC; GenSurg. Staff, Peter Lougheed Centre; Langs: German; (403)943-4612; Fax. (403)219-3574; waynerosen@hotmail.com.

ROSEN-ZAIDENER, Dalia S; 403-13291 Yonge St, Richmond Hill ON L4E 4L6; Tor'97; BSc(McG); CCFP; Langs: English; French; (905)773-3884

ROSENAUER, Helen L; 101-1001 Broadway W, Vancouver BC V6H 4E4; UBC'06; FRCPC; Psy.

ROSENBAUM, Debbie A; VGH Internal Med Clinic, 7F-2775 Laurel St, Vancouver BC V5Z 1M9; McG'99; FRCPC; IntMed; Nephrol. (604)875-5181

ROSENBAUM, Peter L; McMaster Univ-IAHS Bldg, 408-1400 Main St W, Hamilton ON L8S 1C7; McG'65; BSc; DrMedCh; FRCPC; Peds (Childhood Disability Research). Ac Staff, Hamilton Health Sciences Centre - McMaster University Medical Centre; Prof Peds, McMaster University; Langs: Bilingual(French/English); (905)525-9140 x27834; rosenbau@mcmaster.ca.

ROSENBER, Jacob J; Columbus Med Arts Bldg, 310-8333 Weston Rd, Woodbridge ON L4L 8E2; Tel Aviv (Israel)'00; (905)850-3250

ROSENBERG, Alan M; Royal University Hosp, 103 Hospital Dr, Saskatoon SK S7N 0W8; Sask'74; FRCPC; Peds (Pediatric Rheumatology); Rheum. Ac Staff Peds, Royal University Hospital; Head Peds/Prof Peds, University of Saskatchewan; (306)966-8112; Fax. (306)966-8640; alan.rosenberg@usask.ca.

ROSENBERG, Arthur; SMBD Jewish Gen Hosp, 3755 ch Cote-Sainte-Catherine, Montreal QC H3T 1E2; Qns'61; FRCPC; Hem (P.Q.); IntMed. Sr Physician, Sir Mortimer B Davis Jewish General; assoc Prof, McGill University; (514)340-8214

ROSENBERG, Bruce N; 7-211 Martindale Rd, St Catharines ON L2S 3V7; Sask'78; Pres, Casandra Medical Centre; Pres, St Catharines Medical Centre; (905)646-3814

ROSENBERG, Edwin M; 1700-1959 Upper Water St, Halifax NS B3J 3N2; Dal'65; MRCPsy; FRCPC; Psy (General Adult Psychiatry). (902)420-9833; Fax. (902)425-4170.

ROSENBERG, Eli; Medpoint Hlth Care Centre, 233-355 Wellington St, London ON N6A 3N7; Tor'04; FRCPC; IntMed; Cardiol. Staff, London Health Sciences Centre - Victoria Campus; (519)432-1919

ROSENBERG, Ellen E; St Mary's Hosp Centre, 3830 av Lacombe, Montreal QC H3T 1M5; McG'73; CCFP; FCFP; Staff, St Mary's Hospital Centre; Assoc Prof Family Med, McGill University; Langs: English; French; (514)734-2624; Fax. (514)734-2602.

ROSENBERG, Erin A; The Ottawa Hosp-Gen Campus, 501 Smyth Rd, Ottawa ON K1H 8L6; Ott'07; FRCPC; IntMed; Critical Care Medicine. Staff, The Ottawa Hospital - General Campus; (613)737-8701

ROSENBERG, Frank W; Queensway Prof Centre, 210-190 Sherway Dr, Etobicoke ON M9C 5N2; Tor'72; DABD; FAAD; FRCPC; Derm (Wound Care). Ac Staff Med Derm, Trillium Health Centre - West Toronto; Langs: Italian; Yiddish; (416)626-1535; Fax. (416)626-2307.

ROSENBERG, Hans; The Ottawa Hosp-Civic Campus, 1053 Carling Ave, Ottawa ON K1Y 4E9; Tor'06; CCFP; CCFP(E.M.); Staff, The Ottawa Hospital - Civic Campus; (613)737-8899

ROSENBERG, Herschel; London HSC-Victoria Hosp, PO Box 5010 Stn B 800 Commissioners Rd E, London ON N6A 5W9; Wes'78; MEd; FRCPC; Peds; Cardiol. Staff, London Health Sciences Centre - Victoria Campus; (519)685-8010; Fax. (519)685-8156.

ROSENBERG, J Joel; 105-688 Coxwell Ave, Toronto ON M4C 3B7; Tor'76; Staff, Toronto East General Hospital Inc; (416)469-1149

ROSENBERG, Jacob J; Columbus Med Arts Bldg, 310-8333 Weston Rd, Woodbridge ON L4L 8E2; Tel Aviv (Israel)'00; FRCPC; Peds. (905)850-3250

ROSENBERG, Jean; Centre Medical de Huntington, RR 3 72A rue Chateauguay, Huntingdon QC J0S 1H0; McM'73; Gen Practice, Huntingdon County Hospital Centre; Conférencier, McGill University; Langs: Bilingual(English/French); (450)264-6101; Fax. (450)264-6124.

ROSENBERG, Jodine L; 104-222 Lawrence Ave W, North York ON M5M 4M1; McM'10; CCFP; (416)847-9999; Fax. (416)847-8999.

ROSENBERG, Joseph I; 406-100 Humber College Blvd, Etobicoke ON M9V 5G4; Man'89; FRCPC; IntMed (Critical Care Medicine); Respir. Staff, William Osler Health System - Etobicoke General Hospital; (416)256-9200; Fax. (416)256-9201.

ROSENBERG, Lara M; 501-1110 Sheppard Ave E, North York ON M2K 2W2; Ott'08; CCFP; (416)223-0555; Fax. (416)223-0540.

ROSENBERG, Lawrence; SMBD Jewish Gen Hosp, 3755 ch Cote-Sainte-Catherine, Montreal QC H3T 1E2; McG'79; MSc; PhD; FRCSC; GenSurg (Pancreatic Surgery). Staff, Sir Mortimer B Davis Jewish General; Sr Staff Surg, McGill University Health Centre - Royal Victoria Hospital; Prof Surg & Med, McGill University; Langs: English; French; (514)340-8222 x5733

ROSENBERG, Marsha H; Baycrest Ctre/Geriatric Care, 3560 Bathurst St, North York ON M6A 2E1; Man'86; DABPN; FRCPC; Psy (Child & Adolescent Psychiatry). Coord Psy Day Hospital, Baycrest Centre for Geriatric Care; Lecturer, University of Toronto; (416)785-2500 x2882; Fax. (416)785-2450.

ROSENBERG, Paul J; William Osler HC-Etobicoke, 101 Humber College Blvd, Etobicoke ON M9V 1R8; McM'78; FRCPC; EmergMed. Staff, William Osler Health System - Etobicoke General Hospital; (416)747-3400

ROSENBERG, Resa; Club Tiny Tots, 3550-6900 boul Decarie, Cote Saint-Luc QC H3X 2T8; McG'09; CCFP; (514)342-9911

ROSENBLAT, Henry; 6-315 Avenue Rd, Toronto ON M4V 2H2; Tor'80; FRCPC; Psy. Ac Staff, Humber River Regional Hospital - Keele Street Site; (416)972-9273; henry@the-wire.com.

ROSENBLATT, Bernard; MUHC-Montreal Children's Hosp, A522-2300 rue Tupper, Montreal QC H3H 1P3; McG'72; AB; FRCPC; Neur (Clinical Neurophysiology); Electroenceph (P.Q.). Dir Dept of Neurophysiol & Div of Child Neurol, McGill University Health Centre - Montreal Children's Hospital; Consultant, Sir Mortimer B Davis Jewish General; assoc Prof, McGill University; (514)412-4453; bernard.rosenblatt@muhc.mcgill.ca.

ROSENBLATT, David S; L3 -319-1650 Cedar Avenue, Montreal QC H3G 1A4; McG'70; FCCMG; CSPQ; MedGenetics (P.Q.); MedScient(Med); Peds (P.Q.). Staff, McGill University Health Centre - Montreal General Campus; Head Human Genetics & Prof, McGill University; Langs: Bilingual(English/French); Hebrew; (514)934-1934 x42978; david.rosenblatt@mcgill.ca.

ROSENBLO, Ehud; 1280 Main St W, Hamilton ON L8S 4K1; Tel Aviv (Israel)'03; (905)521-2100

ROSENBLOOD, Geoffrey S; St Joseph's Healthcare, 50 Charlton Ave E, Hamilton ON L8N 4A6; Wes'99; FRCPC; Anes. Staff, St Joseph's Healthcare - Charlton Campus; (905)522-1155 x33853; roseng@mcmaster.ca.

ROSENBLOOM, Alan M; McConnell Med Centre, 128-820 McConnell Ave, Cornwall ON K6H 4M4; McG'86; CCFP; Staff, Cornwall Community Hospital; (613)936-1564; Fax. (613)936-0174.

ROSENBLOOM, Andrea; SGH Medical Mall, 301-3030 Lawrence Ave E, Scarborough ON M1P 2T7; McG'92; FACC; FRCPC; IntMed (Echocardiography); Cardiol. Staff, The Scarborough Hospital - General Campus; Langs: English; French; (416)431-0041; Fax. (416)431-0042.

ROSENBLOOM, Arlene R; Carling-Broadview Med Bldg, 305-770 Broadview Ave, Ottawa ON K2A 3Z3; Ott'81; CCFP; FCFP; Att Staff, The Ottawa Hospital - Civic Campus; (613)728-7700; Fax. (613)728-5848.

ROSENBLOOM, Ehud; McMaster Health Sciences Ctre, 1280 Main St W, Hamilton ON L8S 4K1; Tel Aviv University (Israel)'03; (905)521-2100

ROSENBLOOM, Lorne; SMBD Jewish Gen Hosp, 3755 ch Cote-Sainte-Catherine, Montreal QC H3T 1E2; McG'00; CSPQ; FRCPC; DiagRad. Staff, Sir Mortimer B Davis Jewish General; (514)340-8233

ROSENBLOOM, Marvin B; SMBD Jewish Gen Hosp, 3755 ch Cote-Sainte-Catherine, Montreal QC H3T 1E2; McG'67; CSPQ; FRCPC; DiagRad. Staff, Sir Mortimer B Davis Jewish General; (514)340-8222

ROSENBLUM, Jerry H; PO Box 22043 Rpo Westmount, Waterloo ON N2L 6J7; Tor'78; FRCPC; Anes. Staff, Grand River Hospital - Kitchener/Waterloo Health Centre; Staff, St Mary's General Hospital; Court Staff, Markham Stouffville Hospital; (519)744-7361; Fax. (519)744-7363.

ROSENBLUM, Norman D; The Hosp for Sick Children, 555 University Ave, Toronto ON M5G 1X8; Dal'80; ABPeds; FRCP; FRCPC; Peds (Pediatric Nephrology). Staff Div of Nephrol, The Hospital For Sick Children; Assoc Prof Peds Lab Med Path & Physiol, University of Toronto; (416)813-5667; Fax. (416)813-5252; norman.rosenblum@sickkids.ca.

ROSENBLUM, Rebeccah M; Royal Alexandra Hosp, 541-10240 Kingsway NW, Edmonton AB T5H 3V9; McM'99; FRCPC; EmergMed. Staff, Royal Alexandra Hospital; Langs: Hebrew; (780)735-4442; Fax. (780)735-4916.

ROSENBLUM, Stan; C-221 Mitton St N, Sarnia ON N7T 6H5; Tor'80; FACS; FCCP; FRCSC; Cardiovasc&ThorSurg. Dir, Sarnia Vein Clinic; (519)332-4665; Fax. (519)332-1855; srosenblum@bluewaterhealth.ca.

ROSENBLUTH, Allan B; Toronto East Gen Hosp Inc, H5-825 Coxwell Ave, Toronto ON M4C 3E7; Man'77; FRCPC; Psy. Chief Psy/Med Dir, Toronto East General Hospital Inc; Consultant, Worker's Safety & Insurance Board; Lecturer Psy, University of Toronto; (416)469-6206; Fax. (416)469-6122; alros@tegh.on.ca.

ROSENBLUTH, Michael B; Toronto East Gen Hosp Inc, 825 Coxwell Ave, Toronto ON M4C 3E7; Man'73; FRCPC; Psy (Pharmacotherapy). Vis Staff, Sunnybrook Health Sciences Centre; Ac Staff Psy, Toronto East General Hospital Inc; Asst Prof Psy, University of Toronto; (416)469-6298; Fax. (416)469-6805.

ROSENCZWEIG, Carolyn C; Langley Mem Hosp, 22051 Fraser Hwy, Langley BC V3A 4H4; UBC'99; FRCPC; CCFP; EmergMed. Staff, Langley Memorial Hospital; (604)514-0688

ROSENFELD, Gregory A; University of British Columbia, 5153-2775 Laurel St, Vancouver BC V5Z 1M9; UBC'92; FRCPC; IntMed. (604)875-4111

ROSENFELD, Iris; Workers Comp Board of MB, 333 Broadway, Winnipeg MB R3C 4W3; New York (USA)'02; FRCSC; PlasSurg. Staff, Workers' Comp Board of MB.

ROSENFELD, Michael W; CarePoint Med Centre, 528A Clarke Rd, Coquitlam BC V3J 3X5; UBC'60; CCFP; Ac Staff, Vancouver General Hospital - Centennial Pavillion; Ac Staff, BC Women's Hospital & Health Centre; Ac Staff, BC Children's Hospital; Clin Instructor Family Pract, University of British Columbia; (604)936-9874

ROSENFELD, S Allan; 43-3075 Ridgeway Dr, Mississauga ON L5L 5M6; Tor'84; DOHS; FCBOM; CCFP; Consultant Occupational Med, City of Mississauga; Consultant occup Med, McMaster University; (905)828-6061; Fax. (905)820-9468.

ROSENFELD, Steven A; Credit Valley Prof Bldg, 404-2300 Eglinton Ave W, Mississauga ON L5M 2V8; Tor'79; FRCSC; OrthSurg (Knee Surgery). Ac Staff, The Credit Valley Hospital; (905)820-0888; Fax. (905)569-8007.

ROSENFIELD, Jay D; The Hosp for Sick Children, 555 University Ave, Toronto ON M5G 1X8; Tor'82; MD; MEd; FRCPC; Peds (Developmental/Behavioural Pediatrics). Ac Staff Dev Paeds, The Hospital For Sick Children; Consultant, Holland Bloorview Kids Rehabilitation Hospital; Vice Dean Undergrad Med Educ/Prof, University of Toronto; (416)813-7037; Fax. (416)813-6334.

ROSENGARTEN, Albert M; Rockyview Gen Hosp, 7007 14 St SW, Calgary AB T2V 1P9; McG'76; FRCSC; ObstGyn (Minimal Invasive Surgery). Staff Ob-Gyn, Rockyview General Hospital; Ac Staff, Foothills Medical Centre; Clin Assoc Prof/Chief Gynecology, University of Calgary; (403)943-8733; Fax. (403)943-8677; amrosengarten@telus.net.

ROSENGARTEN, Mark I; City Square, 500-555 12th Ave W, Vancouver BC V5Z 3X7; Witwatersrand (South Africa)'87; FRCSC; ObstGyn. (604)874-6848; Fax. (604)872-5599.

ROSENGREN, A Orin; 023-3545 ch de la Cote-des-Nei, Montreal QC H3H 1V1; McG'74; CCFP; Staff, McGill University Health Centre - Montreal General Campus; (514)935-1197; Fax. (514)935-1310.

ROSENHEK, I Shoel; Windsor Health Centre, 207-700 Tecumseh Rd E, Windsor ON N8X 4T2; McG'79; BSc; BScPharm; IntMed; Cardiol. Langs: English; French; (519)253-8786

ROSENKRANTZ, Alicia H; West Carleton Family Hlth Team, PO Box 218 119 Langstaff Dr, Carp ON K0A 1L0; McM'79; BSc; CCFP; FCFP; (613)839-3271 x133; Fax. (613)839-3273.

ROSENKRANZ, George J; Centennial CMH & Brain Injury, PO Box 1000 Stn Main, Ponoka AB T4J 1R8; Cal'86; BSc; CCFP; FCFP; Staff Centennial Ctre for Mental Hlth & Brain Injury, Centennial Centre for Mental Health & Brain Injury; Langs: Czech; (403)783-7843; Fax. (403)783-7869.

ROSENSTEIN, David M; Toronto East Gen Hosp Inc, 825 Coxwell Ave, Toronto ON M4C 3E7; Tor'97; CCFP; CCFP(E.M.); Staff, Toronto East General Hospital Inc; Langs: Hebrew; (416)469-6435

ROSENSTEIN, Gerald A; 301B-475 Park St, Kitchener ON N2G 4V5; Ott'81; FRCPC; IntMed; Nephrol. Staff, Grand River Hospital - Kitchener/Waterloo Health Centre; Staff, St Mary's General Hospital; (519)743-9742; Fax. (519)743-0369.

ROSENSTEIN, Karen A; Toronto East Gen Hosp Inc, 825 Coxwell Ave, Toronto ON M4C 3E7; Tor'96; BSc; FRCPC; Peds. Staff, Toronto East General Hospital Inc; Clin Asst, Women's College Hospital; (416)469-6580

ROSENSTOCK, Carl B; 10125 118 St NW, Edmonton AB T5K 1Y3; Man'76; (780)482-7511; Fax. (780)488-0747.

ROSENSTOCK, Ted; 1162 Weston Rd, Toronto ON M6M 4P4; Man'76; LMCC; NBME; ABOph; FRCS; FRCSC; Ophth (Cataract Surgery). Staff, North York General Hospital - Branson Division; Staff, Humber River Regional Hospital - Church Street Site; Staff, Humber River Regional Hospital - Finch Avenue Site; (416)248-1660; Fax. (416)614-0427; tedeye@rogers.com.

ROSENTHAL, Alana J; Danforth Pediatrics, 100-235 Danforth Ave, Toronto ON M4K 1N2; Wes'98; FRCPC; Peds; InfectDis. Staff, North York General Hospital; (416)466-1311; arosenthal@sympatico.ca.

ROSENTHAL, David M; 403-4800 Leslie St, North York ON M2J 2K9; Tor'76; DABOG; FSOGC; FACOG; FRCSC; ObstGyn (Endoscopic Surgery). Ac Staff, North York General Hospital; Consultant, Stevenson Memorial Hospital; Asst Prof, University of Toronto; (416)631-9880; Fax. (416)631-9881.

ROSENTHAL, Donald; St Joseph's Healthcare, 50 Charlton Ave E, Hamilton ON L8N 4A6; Tor'58; FRCPC; Derm., St Joseph's Healthcare - Charlton Campus; Head Div of Derm, Hamilton Health Sciences Centre - McMaster Children's Hospital; Prof Med Derm, McMaster University; Langs: English; French; (905)522-4941

ROSENTHAL, Eva E; York-Med Medical Arts Centre, 202-250 Harding Blvd W, Richmond Hill ON L4C 9M7; Tor'90; CCFP; FCFP; Staff, Mackenzie Richmond Hill Hospital; (905)737-8400; Fax. (905)737-4579.

ROSENTHAL, Gary A; Scarborough North Med Arts, 303-4040 Finch Ave E, Scarborough ON M1S 4V5; Tor'85; FRCSC; GenSurg (Laparoscopic Surgery). Ac Staff, The Scarborough Hospital - Birchmount Campus; Langs: English; French; (416)297-9611; Fax. (416)292-2360.

ROSENTHAL, Gary F; 403-5885 ch de la Cote-des-Nei, Montreal QC H3S 2T2; McG'71; AB; Asst Staff, Sir Mortimer B Davis Jewish General; (514)342-2317; Fax. (514)342-1638.

ROSENTHAL, Gillian A; 203-4450 Chatterton Way, Victoria BC V8X 5J2; Manchester (England)'71; MB ChB; MRCS; LRCP; BSc; Ac Staff, Victoria General Hospital; Ac Staff, Royal Jubilee Hospital; (250)380-7171; Fax. (250)380-1631.

ROSENTHAL, Greta; Rosedale Med Centre, 515-600 Sherbourne St, Toronto ON M4X 1W4; Dublin (Ireland)'69; LRCPSI; DRCOG; FRCPC; Psy (Psychotherapy). Lecturer, University of Toronto; (416)922-7990; Fax. (416)482-0197.

ROSENTHAL, Peter; Victoria Gen Hosp, 6-2340 Pembina Hwy, Winnipeg MB R3T 2E8; McG'85; FRCPC; Psy. Staff, Victoria General Hospital; Langs: Hungarian; (204)269-3570; Fax. (204)269-7619.

ROSENTHAL, Robert M; Sheppard Beecroft Med Clinic, 48 Sheppard Ave W, North York ON M2N 1M2; Tor'89; Assoc Staff Family & Community Med, North York General Hospital; Langs: Hebrew; (416)222-1477; Fax. (416)222-5707; kinbobby@hotmail.com.

ROSENTHAL, Stephen E; SMBD Jewish Gen Hosp, 3755 ch Cote-Sainte-Catherine, Montreal QC H3T 1E2; McG'87; CCFP; CCFP(E.M.); EmergMed (P.Q.). Staff, Sir Mortimer B Davis Jewish General; Langs: English; French; (514)340-8222

ROSENTHALL, Leonard; MUHC-Montreal Gen Hosp, 1650 av Cedar, Montreal QC H3G 1A4; McG'56; CSPQ; FRCPC; DiagRad; NuclearMed; RadOncol. Staff, McGill University Health Centre - Montreal General Campus; Langs: English; French; (514)934-1934 x43855

ROSENTHALL, Wendy; King Street Med Arts Centre, 402-71 King St W, Mississauga ON L5B 4A2; McG'79; FRCPC; IntMed (Diabetology); Endocrin&Metab. Ac Staff, Trillium Health Centre - Mississauga; (905)276-7224; Fax. (905)276-2996.

ROSHDY, Osama; SMBD Jewish Gen Hosp, 3755 ch Cote-Sainte-Catherine, Montreal QC H3T 1E2; Tanta (Egypt)'85; Derm (P.Q.). Staff, Sir Mortimer B Davis Jewish General; (514)340-8272

ROSIE, John S; University of Alberta Hosp, 1E7.08-8440 112 St NW, Edmonton AB T6G 2B7; Aberdeen (Scotland)'71; MB ChB; DPsy; MRCPsy; FRCPC; Psy (Psychotherapy). Clin Coord, University of Alberta Hospital; Clin Prof, University of Alberta; (780)407-8330; Fax. (780)407-6470.

ROSIN, Richard A; West Side Mental Health Team, 200-4088 Cambie St, Vancouver BC V5Z 2X8; Southampton (England)'88; FRCPC; Psy. Staff, Richmond Hospital; (604)873-6733

ROSING, Kim; Neepawa Health Centre, PO Box 1240, Neepawa MB R0J 1H0; Man'09; CCFP; Staff, Neepawa District Memorial Hospital; (204)476-2394

ROSLOSKI, Joseph M; 572 Carlton St, St Catharines ON L2M 4X7; Wes'67; (905)934-7951; Fax. (905)934-7951.

ROSMAN, David E; Maple Med Centre, 203-955 Major Mackenzie Dr, Vaughan ON L6A 4P9; Cape Town (South Africa)'78; MB ChB; FRCSC; ObstGyn. Staff, Mackenzie Richmond Hill Hospital; Langs: Afrikaans.

ROSMAN, Michael A; Clinique Med Viau, 4750 rue Jarry E, Saint-Leonard QC H1R 1X8; Ott'65; OrthSurg. Langs: English; French; (514)326-7203

ROSNER, Jodi L S; 404-564 Belmont Ave W, Kitchener ON N2M 5N6; McM'97; FRCPC; Peds. Clinical Asst Prof, McMaster University; (519)745-5290

ROSNER, Sophie; CSSS d'Antoine-Labelle-Mt Laur, RR 1 2561 ch de la Lievre S, Mont-Laurier QC J9L 3G3; Curie (France)'87; Psy (P.Q.). Staff, CSSS d'Antoine-Labelle; Staff, Centre Hospitalier de Granby; (819)623-1234

ROSOLOWSKY, Elizabeth; 311-3001 Tutt St, Kelowna BC V1Y 2H4; California (USA)'01; FRCPC; Peds. (250)712-9960

ROSOPH, Leslie A; North Bay Dermatology Centre, 500 Cassells St, North Bay ON P1B 3Z7; McG'87; FRCPC; Derm;CCFP; CCFP(E. M.); Staff, North Bay Regional Health Centre - Regional Mental Health; Asst Prof, Northern Ontario School of Medicine; Langs: English; French; (705)476-3376; Fax. (705)476-3967.

ROSS, Alexandra; PO Box 21038 Rpo Quispamsis, Rothesay NB E2E 4Z4; Mem'10; CCFP; (506)849-6750; Fax. (506)849-3373.

ROSS, Alison C; Richmond Med Bldg, 302-2020 Richmond Rd, Victoria BC V8R 6R5; UBC'94; FRCSC; GenSurg. (250)592-4313; Fax. (250)592-5020.

ROSS, Anatoly D; Glengarry Mem Hosp, 20260 County Road 43, Alexandria ON K0C 1A0; (Russia (Federation))'91; Staff, Glengarry Memorial Hospital; (613)525-2222

ROSS, Andrea J; Kateri Mem Hosp Centre, PO Box 10, Kahnawake QC J0L 1B0; Wes'00; CCFP; Staff, Kateri Memorial Hospital Centre; (450)638-3930

ROSS, Andrew A; Queen Elizabeth II HSC, 3009-1276 South Park St, Halifax NS B3H 2Y9; Dal'87; FRCPC; DiagRad; NuclearMed. Staff, Queen Elizabeth II Health Sciences Centre - Victoria General Site; (902)473-2825; Fax. (902)473-2018.

ROSS, Andrew M; Rideau Family Med Centre, RR 2, Kingston ON K7L 5H6; Qns'86; Staff Privil Family Med & Att'd Staff, Kingston General Hospital; (613)546-0151

ROSS, Angela M; 32 Princess St, Hamilton ON L9H 2X7; McM'82; CCFP; (905)628-5000

ROSS, Anthony L; Oakville Family Practice Assoc, 208-1060 Speers Rd, Oakville ON L6L 2X4; Birmingham (England)'50; MB ChB; MRCS; LRCP; CCFP; Court Staff, Halton Healthcare Services Corporation - Oakville Site; Med Examiner, Civil Aviation Canada; (905)842-3735; Fax. (905)842-8001.

ROSS, B Catherine; Alberta Children's Hosp, 2888 Shaganappi Trail NW, Calgary AB T3B 6A8; Cal'88; BSc; FRCPC; Peds (Anesthesia); Critical Care Medicine. Staff Critical Care & PICU, Alberta Children's Hospital; Langs: Bilingual(English/French); (403)955-7211; Fax. (403)955-7081.

ROSS, Barbara J; PO Box 448, Port Williams NS B0P 1T0; Dal'92; BSc; CCFP; (902)542-0779; Fax. (902)542-0530.

ROSS, Barbara M; 8-150 Edmonton Ave, Moncton NB E1C 3B9; Dal'81; BSc; FRCPC; Psy. (506)383-2122; Fax. (506)855-6563.

ROSS, Betty L; Workers' Compensation Board, PO Box 2415 Stn Main 9912 107 St NW, Edmonton AB T5J 2S5; Alb'81; ABIM; FAAFP; CCFP; FCFP; Med Advisor, Workers' Comp Board of AB; (780)498-4239; Fax. (780)498-7807.

ROSS, Cameron C; Crossroads Family Practice, 201-45800 Promontory Rd, Chilliwack BC V2R 5Z5; UBC'90; CCFP; Clin Teacher Family Practice, University of British Columbia; (604)858-3725; Fax. (604)858-8625.

ROSS, Catherine A; Hamilton HS-Henderson Site, 204-711 Concession St, Hamilton ON L8V 1C3; McM'88; FRCPC; AnatPath (Hematology Pathology). Staff, Hamilton Health Sciences Centre-Juravinski Site; Physician, The Juravinski Cancer Centre; (905)527-4322 x42074; Fax. (905)575-2553.

ROSS, Dana I; 201-475 Park St, Kitchener ON N2G 4V5; McM'90; MD; FRCSC; ObstGyn. (519)584-0051; Fax. (519)584-2884; drdross@on.aibn.com.

ROSS, Daniel A; Kiwi Pediatrics, 16662 McKenzie Lake Blvd SE, Calgary AB T2Z 1N4; Cal'94; FRCPC; Peds (Developmental Pediatrics). Clinical Asst Prof Peds, University of Calgary; (403)281-2500; Fax. (403)256-2511.

ROSS, Dave; ASSS Monteregie, 1255 rue Beauregard, Longueuil QC J4K 2M3; Mon'88; Physician, Clinique Medical St-Jacques; (450)928-6777

ROSS, David A; Seven Oaks Gen Hosp, 2300 McPhillips St, Winnipeg MB R2V 3M3; Man'79; BAP; BSc; CCFP; FCFP; Ac Staff, Health Sciences Centre; Ac Staff Fam. Practice Residency Prog., Seven Oaks General Hospital; Assoc Prof Family Med., University of Manitoba; (204)632-3203; Fax. (204)694-5697; dross@cc.umanitoba.ca.

ROSS, David B; University of Alberta Hosp, 4A7.056-8440 112 St NW, Edmonton AB T6G 2B7; Tor'81; ABS; ABTS; FRCSC; GenSurg (Adult Congenital Heart Disease); Cardiovasc&ThorSurg. Staff, University of Alberta Hospital; Langs: English; French; (780)407-8047; Fax. (780)407-8054.

ROSS, David; 8-150 Edmonton Ave, Moncton NB E1C 3B9; Dal'81; BSc; CCFP; FCFP; Staff, The Moncton Hospital; Court Staff, Dr Georges-L-Dumont University Hospital Centre; (506)383-2122; Fax. (506)855-6563.

ROSS, David J; Northeast Comm Health Ctre, 14007 50 St NW, Edmonton AB T5A 5E4; Alb'91; CCFP; FCFP; Assoc Prof Med Faculty of Med & Dentistry, University of Alberta; (780)472-5038; Fax. (780)472-5192.

ROSS, David J; Oshawa Clinic, 117 King St E, Oshawa ON L1H 1B9; Qns'78; Respir; IntMed (Sleep Medicine). Staff, Lakeridge Health - Oshawa Site; (905)723-8551; Fax. (905)721-6651.

ROSS, Dawn L; 313-380 Bedford Hwy, Halifax NS B3M 2L4; Dal'82; FRCPC; Psy. (902)493-3034; Fax. (902)445-9572; dawn.ross@ns.sympatico.ca.

ROSS, Donald A; 204-2825 Clearbrook Rd, Abbotsford BC V2T 6S3; UBC'74; CCFP; FCFP; (604)853-8641

ROSS, Donald C; South Walkerville Med Centre, 160-2224 Walker Rd, Windsor ON N8W 5L7; Tor'45; DPsy; DABPN; DAB; FRCPC; Peds (Adolescent Psychiatry); Psy. Asst Prof Psy & Behavioral Neurosciences, Wayne State University (Detroit,Michigan-USA); (519)254-4252; Fax. (519)637-3162.

ROSS, Douglas C; St Joseph's Health Care, PO Box 5777 Stn B 268 Grosvenor St, London ON N6A 4V2; UBC'83; MEd; PlasSurg (Hand Surgery). Chief Div of Plastic Surg, St Joseph's Hospital - St Joseph's Health Care; Assoc Prof, University of Western Ontario; (519)646-6048; Fax. (519)646-6049.

ROSS, Duncan A; 2087 Granite Ave PO Box 279, Merritt BC V1K 1B8; Ott'92; (250)378-5115

ROSS, Edward C; King Med Clinic, 380 Portland St, Dartmouth NS B2Y 1K8; Dal'69; Court Staff, Queen Elizabeth II Health Sciences Centre - Victoria General Site; Court Staff, IWK Health Centre; (902)463-1525; Fax. (902)463-2945.

ROSS, Elizabeth K; 314-888 8th Ave W, Vancouver BC V5Z 3Y1; (Colombia)'97; (604)731-5353

ROSS, Ella A; 213-150 Montreal Rd, Vanier ON K1L 8H2; Volgograd (Russia (Federation))'91; FRCSC; Ophth. Langs: Russian; (613)238-3850; Fax. (613)235-7972.

ROSS, Frances K; Manitoba Clinic, 790 Sherbrook St, Winnipeg MB R3A 1M3; Qns'81; CCFP; FCFP.

ROSS, Francis; Clinique Med Saint-Vincent, 250 rue King E, Sherbrooke QC J1G 1A9; Sher'85; (819)563-0510

ROSS, Frederick J; Bison Primacy Med Clinic, 1-80 Bison Dr, Winnipeg MB R3T 4Z7; Man'73.

ROSS, Gilles; Polyclinique de l'Anse, 78 rue Lemaire, Sept-Iles QC G4S 1A3; Laval'75; (418)962-1212; Fax. (418)962-6327.

ROSS, Heather J; NCSB 11C-1203, 585 University Ave, Toronto ON M5G 2N2; UBC'88; FRCPC; IntMed (Heart Failure); Cardiol. Dir Cardiac Transplant Prog, Toronto General Hospital - UHN; (416)340-3482; Fax. (416)340-4134.

ROSS, H; Victoria Emerg Phys Mgmt Ltd, 325-1627 Fort St, Victoria BC V8R 1H8; Mem'96; FRCPC; EmergMed. (250)479-6442; Fax. (250)479-1472.

ROSS, Ian G; London HSC-University Hosp, PO Box 5339 Stn B 339 Windermere Rd, London ON N6A 5A5; Qns'99; FRCPC; DiagRad. Staff, London Health Sciences Centre - University Hospital; (519)685-8500

ROSS, J Benjamin; 305-5171 221A St, Langley BC V2Y 0A2; UBC'93; BSc; FRCSC; GenSurg (Endoscopy). Ac Staff, Langley Memorial Hospital; (604)534-9288; Fax. (604)534-9958.

ROSS, James A; Lady Minto Hosp Cochrane, PO Box 4000 241 8th St, Cochrane ON P0L 1C0; Man'82; Staff, Lady Minto Hospital Cochrane; (705)272-4278

ROSS, James F; Portage Clinic Inc, 140 9th St SE, Portage La Prairie MB R1N 3V5; Man'69; FACS; FRCSC; GenSurg. Staff, Portage District General Hospital; Asst Prof, University of Manitoba; (204)857-3445; Fax. (204)239-1278; jross@shaw.ca.

ROSS, James W M; London HSC-Victoria Hosp, PO Box 5010 Stn B 800 Commissioners Rd W, London ON N6A 5W9; Dal'04; FRCPC; Psy. Staff, London Health Sciences Centre - Victoria Campus; (519)685-8500; Fax. (519)667-6564.

ROSS, Jean; Centre Med Sillery, 1270 av William, Quebec QC G1S 4G1; Laval'76; Staff, Centre Hospitalier Universitaire de Quebec-CHUL; Dir méd, SSQ Groupe Financier; (418)688-0664; Fax. (418)688-4601; jeanross@videotron.ca.

ROSS, Jeffrey S; Royal Columbian Hosp, 330 Columbia St E, New Westminster BC V3L 3W7; Man'81; FRCPC; IntMed; NuclearMed. Staff Nuclear Med, Burnaby Hospital; Staff Nuclear Med, Royal Columbian Hospital; (604)520-4434; Fax. (604)520-4444.

ROSS, Jennifer A; 108-284 Helmcken Rd, Victoria BC V9B 1T2; Qns'00; CCFP; (250)480-7333

ROSS, Jessica N; Medical Assoc of Port Perry, 462 Paxton St, Port Perry ON L9L 1L9; (Australia)'07; CCFP; (905)985-2895

ROSS, Joan E; 429 Exmouth St, Sarnia ON N7T 5P1; Qns'86; BSc; FRCSC; GenSurg. Staff GenSurg, Bluewater Health - Mitton Site; Staff GenSurg, Bluewater Health - Norman Site; (519)344-3017; Fax. (519)344-6436.

ROSS, Joel E; 351 Christie St, Toronto ON M6G 3C3; Ott'98; CCFP; CCFP(E.M.); Staff, Markham Stouffville Hospital.

ROSS, John A; Queen Elizabeth II HSC-Halifax, 3021-1796 Summer St, Halifax NS B3H 3A7; Wes'86; MD; FRCPC; EmergMed. Staff, Queen Elizabeth II Health Sciences Centre - Halifax Infirmary Site; Chief Emerg Med, Queen Elizabeth II Health Sciences Centre - Victoria General Site; Chief Dept of Emerg Med, Capital Health Centre; Head Emerg Med/Prof, Dalhousie University; (902)473-2164; Fax. (902)473-3617; johnross@dal.ca.

ROSS, Julie; Clinique Med du Jardin, 15094 boul Henri-Bourassa, Quebec QC G1G 3Z4; Sher'83; CCFP; (418)628-9074; Fax. (418)628-0267.

ROSS, Katherine M; Medical Place Primary Care Ctr, 202-170 Queensway W, Mississauga ON L5B 3A8; Tor'79; CCFP; (905)275-0023; Fax. (905)275-4001.

ROSS, Kathleen M F; Medicalwest, 212-3001 Gordon Ave, Coquitlam BC V3C 2K7; UBC'92; Staff, Royal Columbian Hospital; Staff, Eagle Ridge Hospital & Health Care Centre; (604)944-4077; Fax. (604)944-0677.

ROSS, Laurie M; Rockyview Prof Centre, 258-1011 Glenmore Trail SW, Calgary AB T2V 4R6; Alb'02; CCFP; Staff, Rockyview General Hospital; (403)640-0600; Fax. (403)253-0124; laur1@telus.net.

ROSS, Lonny L; Health Sciences Centre, GC413-820 Sherbrook St, Winnipeg MB R3A 1R9; Man'97; FRCPC; PlasSurg. Staff, Health Sciences Centre; (204)774-6511

ROSS, Marilyn J; 222-425 36 St NE, Calgary AB T2A 6K3; Cal'77; CCFP; FCFP; (403)235-1770; Fax. (403)272-9923.

ROSS, Mark R; Millard Health Centre, 131 Airport Rd NW, Edmonton AB T5G 0W6; Alb'96; BSc; CCFP; (780)498-3285

ROSS, Michael S; Yonge-Eglinton Med Centre, 59A Admiral Rd, Toronto ON M5R 2L4; Tor'74; FRCPC; Psy (P.Q.) (Occupational Psychiatry). (416)567-8141; mross@mindatwork.com.

ROSS, Nagui A M; Queentario Plaza, 2325 Hurontario St, Mississauga ON L5A 4C7; Ain Shams (Egypt)'80; MB ChB; MSc; CCFP; Staff, Shouldice Hospital; Langs: Arabic; rossna2@yahoo.com.

ROSS, Naomi; Pacific Region Occup Health, 657 37th Ave W, Vancouver BC V5Z 1K6; Tor'83; (604)264-2812

ROSS, Peter K; CSSS Ouest-de-l'Ile, 5000-1405 Rte Transcanadienne, Dorval QC H9P 2V9; Sher'92; (514)630-2225 x3120

ROSS, Scott A; Sturgeon Community Hosp, 201 Boudreau Rd, St. Albert AB T8N 6C4; Alb'94; CCFP; CCFP(E.M.); Staff, Sturgeon Community Hospital; (780)418-8229; Fax. (780)460-6376.

ROSS, Shelley N; 7155 Kingsway PO Box 63008 Rpo Highgate, Burnaby BC V5E 4J4; Alb'74; BMedSci; MCFP; CCFP; FCFP; Ac Staff, Burnaby Hospital; Pres, British Columbia Medical Association; (604)439-8993

ROSS, Simon A; 203-2820 Birch St, Vancouver BC V6H 2T6; Cape Town (South Africa)'82; MB ChB; DA(UK); Staff/Chief of Staff, Cormorant Island Health Centre; Physician, Mount Waddington CHC; (604)616-0834

ROSS, Stacey A; Courtice Health Centre, 2F-1450 Highway 2, Courtice ON L1E 3C3; Tor'95; CCFP; (905)721-4946; Fax. (905)721-6170.

ROSS, Stephen G; 210-250 Lawrence Ave W, Toronto ON M5M 1B2; Qns'77; MEd; CCFP; Langs: English; French; (416)789-5012; Fax. (416)789-5072.

ROSS, Stuart A; 102-5940 Macleod Trail SW, Calgary AB T2H 0K2; Otago (New Zealand)'65; MB ChB; FRACP; FRCPC; IntMed (Diabetes). Staff, Foothills Medical Centre; Prof, University of Calgary; (403)288-3224; Fax. (403)288-6409; stuart.ross@lmc.ca.

ROSS, Terrance A; Regina Qu'Appelle HR-Regina, 1440 14th Ave, Regina SK S4P 0W5; Sask'97; CCFP; CCFP(E.M.); Staff, Regina General Hospital; (306)766-4213; Fax. (306)766-4357.

ROSS, Theodore M; Women's College Hosp, E245-76 Grenville St, Toronto ON M5S 1B2; Tor'75; ABS; AB; FACS; FRCSC; GenSurg (Colon & Rectal Surgery). Ac Staff, Women's College Hospital; Ac Staff, Sunnybrook Health Sciences Centre; Assoc Prof Surg, University of Toronto; (416)922-6853; Fax. (416)323-6187; ted.ross@sunnybrook.ca.

ROSS, Theresa A; Chisel Peak Med Centre, PO Box 2769 417 10 Ave, Invermere BC V0A 1K0; Dal'87; CCFP; (250)341-6900; Fax. (250)341-3226.

ROSS, Todd K; Associated Radiologists, 300-140 Wall St, Saskatoon SK S7K 1N4; Sask'99; FRCPC; DiagRad. (306)244-1167; Fax. (306)244-2911.

ROSS, Valerie A; Rockingham Ridge Plaza, 30 Farnham Gate Rd, Halifax NS B3M 3W8; Dal'87; CCFP; CCFP(E.M.); Staff, Hubbards Med. Clinic; (902)443-8388; Fax. (902)443-9887.

ROSS, Wendy J; Penticton Reg Hosp, 550 Carmi Ave, Penticton BC V2A 3G6; Flinders (Australia)'99; Staff, Penticton Regional Hospital; (250)492-9032; Fax. (250)492-9036.

ROSS, William H; Medical Bldg, 400-805 Broadway W, Vancouver BC V5Z 1K1; Wes'67; FRCSC; Ophth (Vitreo Retina). Ac Staff, Providence Health Care - St Paul's Hospital; Ac Staff, Vancouver General Hospital - Centennial Pavillion; Clin Prof Ophth, University of British Columbia; (604)874-0404; Fax. (604)874-0099.

ROSSBACH, Valery M J; Hawkesbury Dist Gen Hosp, 1111 Ghislain St, Hawkesbury ON K6A 3G5; Ott'05; CCFP; Staff, Hawkesbury & District General Hospital; (613)632-1111

ROSSER, Stuart J; Royal Alexandra Hosp, CSC 310-10240 Kingsway NW, Edmonton AB T5H 3V9; Alb'88; FRCPC; IntMed; Critical Care Medicine; InfectDis. Staff, Royal Alexandra Hospital; (780)735-5491; Fax. (780)735-5088.

ROSSER, Timothy D; Regina Qu'Appelle HR-Regina, 1440 14th Ave, Regina SK S4P 0W5; Alb'01; FRCPC; Anes. Staff, Regina General Hospital; (306)766-4252; Fax. (306)766-4443.

ROSSER, Walter W; Family Med Centre, PO Box 8888 Stn Main 220 Bagot St, Kingston ON K7L 5E9; Qns'67; MRCGPract(UK); CCFP; FCFP; Consultant, Toronto General Hospital - UHN; Consultant, Sunnybrook Health Sciences Centre; Teach Staff, Queen's University; Langs: English; French; (613)533-9303; Fax. (613)544-9899.

ROSSET, Jennifer E; Bayview-Finch Med Clinic, 105-3292 Bayview Ave, North York ON M2M 4J5; Wes'01; CCFP; (416)445-4067; Fax. (416)445-0206.

ROSSET, Michael A; Queensway Prof Centre, 417-190 Sherway Dr, Etobicoke ON M9C 5N2; Tor'68; FRCSC; ObstGyn. Staff, Trillium Health Centre - West Toronto; (416)622-6057; Fax. (416)622-8772.

ROSSI, Carlo; CFB Petawawa, PO Box 9999 Stn Main 2 Field Ambulance, Petawawa ON K8H 2X3; McG'08; CCFP; (613)687-5511

ROSSI, Christine M; Algoma District Health Group, 240 McNabb St, Sault Ste. Marie ON P6B 1Y5; Wes'82; CCFP; FCFP; Staff, Sault Area Hospital - Sault Ste Marie; (705)759-5612; Fax. (705)759-5683.

ROSSI, Lilah R N; 116-555 12th Ave W, Vancouver BC V5Z 3X7; UBC'96; BSc; CCFP; Staff, BC Women's Hospital & Health Centre; (604)879-3900

ROSSI, Miriam F.; The Hosp for Sick Children, 555 University Ave, Toronto ON M5G 1X8; New York(NY) (USA)'70; ABPeds; FAAP; FRCPC; Peds (Adolescent Medicine). Med Staff, The Hospital For Sick Children; Prof Peds, University of Toronto; Langs: Italian; (416)813-6146; Fax. (416)813-5392; miriam.rossi@utoronto.ca.

ROSSI, Sikina F; Lansdowne Professional Ctr II, 145-3066 Shelbourne St, Victoria BC V8R 6T9; UBC'88; FRCPC; Derm. (250)370-1250; Fax. (250)370-1269.

ROSSIGNOL, Elsa; Hop Ste-Justine, 3175 ch Cote-Sainte-Catherine, Montreal QC H3T 1C5; McG'00; FRCPC; Peds; Neur. Staff, Hôpital Ste-Justine; (514)345-4931

ROSSIGNOL, Guy; GMF Lafontaine, 242 rue Lafontaine, Riviere-du-Loup QC G5R 3A7; Laval'76; Staff, Centre Hospitalier Regional du Grand-Portage; (418)862-3110; Fax. (418)862-9656.

ROSSIGNOL, Michel; 10 083-2021 av Union, Montreal QC H3A 2S9; Sher'82; CSPQ; FRCPC; CommunMed (Epidemiology); OccupMed. ac Staff, Centre Hospitalier l'Université de Montréal (CHUM) - Hôpital Notre-Dame; Ac Staff, Hopital Maisonneuve-Rosemont; Teach Staff, McGill University; Langs: Bilingual(French/English); (514)864-7968; Fax. (514)873-1369; michel.rossignol@inesss.qc.ca.

ROSSIGNOL, Serge; Universite de Montreal, CP 6128 Succ Centre Ville, Montreal QC H3C 3J7; Mon'66; MSc; PhD; Dir, Equipe de Recherche en Readaptation Sensorimotrice-SMRRT; (514)343-6371; Fax. (514)343-2111.

ROSSITER, Andrew M; Centenial Med Centre, PO Box 674 Rpo Centennial Sq, Mount Pearl NL A1N 2X1; Mem'00; CCFP; (709)368-0033

ROSSITER, John P; Queen's Univ-Richardson Lab, 201-88 Stuart St, Kingston ON K7L 3N6; Cork (Ireland)'84; MB ChB; MRCPath; FRCPC; NeurPath. Att Staff Path, Kingston General Hospital; Att Staff, Hotel-Dieu Hospital; Assoc Prof Path, Queen's University; Langs: English; French; (613)533-6306; Fax. (613)533-2907.

ROSSITER, Lea M; Spadina Health Centre, 404-720 Spadina Ave, Toronto ON M5S 2T9; Tor'81; CCFP; FCFP; Assoc Staff Family Practice Unit, Women's College Hospital; Lecturer Family & Commun Med, University of Toronto; Langs: Spanish; (416)928-0920; Fax. (416)928-7426.

ROSSITER, Liesl C; Mission Hills Med Clinic, 240-32530 Lougheed Hwy, Mission BC V2V 1A5; (South Africa)'98; CCFP; (604)826-7751

ROSSMAN, David W; UBC Eye Care Centre, S1-2550 Willow St, Vancouver BC V5Z 3N9; UBC'99; FRCSC; Ophth. Staff, UBC Eye Care Centre; (604)875-4316

ROSSMAN, Lloyd H; Woodroffe South Med Bldg, 202-1637 Woodroffe Ave, Nepean ON K2G 1W2; Tor'72; DABFP; CCFP; FCFP; Clin Preceptor, University of Ottawa; (613)723-5635; Fax. (613)723-5918.

ROSSMAN, Richard L; Medical Arts Bldg, 311-1 Young St, Hamilton ON L8N 1T8; Ott'70; FRCPC; Gastroent (Internal Medicine). Ac Staff, Hamilton Health Sciences Centre - McMaster University Medical Centre; Court Staff, St Joseph's Healthcare - Charlton Campus; Clin Assoc Prof, McMaster University; (905)525-2779; Fax. (905)525-1723.

ROSSNAGEL, Arthur P; Bramalea City Centre, 389-25 Peel Centre Dr, Brampton ON L6T 3R5; Wes'81; (905)793-7077; Fax. (905)793-7506.

ROSSO, Dominic; Trillium Hlth Ctr-Mississauga, 100 Queensway W, Mississauga ON L5B 1B8; Ott'90; FRCPC; DiagRad (Neuro Radiology). Staff, Trillium Health Centre - Mississauga; (905)848-7100; Fax. (905)848-7349.

ROSSOS, Peter G; Univ Hlth Network-Toronto Gen, 9N 975-200 Elizabeth St, Toronto ON M5G 2C4; Tor'86; FRCPC; IntMed (Therapeutic Endoscopy); Gastroent. Staff Physician, Toronto General Hospital - UHN; Assoc Prof Med, University of Toronto; (416)340-5333; Fax. (416)340-5335.

ROSSOUW, Francois P; Victoria Hosp, PO Box 3000 Stn Main 1200 24th St W, Prince Albert SK S6V 5T4; Pretoria (South Africa)'91; MB ChB; CCFP; CCFP(E.M.); Staff, Victoria Hospital; (306)765-6216; Fax. (306)765-6224.

ROSSOUW, Jacobus P; Regina Qu'Appelle HR-Regina, 1440 14th Ave, Regina SK S4P 0W5; Staff, Regina General Hospital; (306)766-4500; Fax. (306)766-4357.

ROSSOUW, Jacques; East Hill Med Walk-In Clinic, 610-3020 22 St, Red Deer AB T4R 3J5; Stellenbosch (South Africa)'99; MB ChB; (403)343-0115; Fax. (403)343-8551.

ROSSOUW, Linell; Medical Clinic, 147A Albert St N, Regina SK S4R 3B8; Stellenbosch (South Africa)'86; MB BS; MB ChB; Langs: Afrikaans; German; (306)525-6466; Fax. (306)525-6403; medclinic@sasktel.net.

ROSSOUW, Pieter A; 6962 Alberni St, Powell River BC V8A 2C1; Stellenbosch (South Africa)'86; MB ChB; CCFP; FCFP; Langs: Afrikaans; (604)485-4877; Fax. (604)485-9566; pietros@shaw.ca.

ROSSOUW, Vincent E; Beverly Med Centre, 201-2763 Beverly St, Duncan BC V9L 6X2; Stellenbosch (South Africa)'96; MB ChB; Langs: Afrikaans; (250)597-3390

ROSSY, Paul E; 75 boul Saint-Jean-Baptiste, Chateauguay QC J6J 3H6; McG'80; FRCPC; Peds. Staff, McGill University Health Centre - Montreal General Campus; (450)691-0061

ROSTA, Neil I N; Grey Bruce HS-Owen Sound, PO Box 1800 Stn Main 1800 8th St E, Owen Sound ON N4K 6M9; Qns'94; FRCPC; DiagRad;CCFP; Staff, Grey Bruce Health Services - Owen Sound; (519)376-2121; Fax. (519)372-3954.

ROSTAMI, Maryam; Concession Wentworth Med Clini, 503 Concession St, Hamilton ON L9A 1C1; McM'00; CCFP; Langs: Persian; French; (289)396-6605; Fax. (289)396-1025.

ROSTAS, Aaron G; Queensway-Carleton Hosp, 3045 Baseline Rd, Ottawa ON K2H 8P4; Tor'07; Anes. (613)721-2000

ROSTAS, Peter A; Keele Med Place, 301-2830 Keele St, North York ON M3M 3E5; Bologna (Italy)'82; Sr Staff, Humber River Regional Hospital - Church Street Site; Langs: Italian; (416)630-1615; Fax. (416)630-5720.

ROSTOM, Alaa M K A; TRW Bldg, 3280 Hospital Dr NW, Calgary AB T2N 4Z6; Ott'92; FRCPC; IntMed; Gastroent. Physician, Health Research Innovation Centre; (403)592-5089; Fax. (403)592-5090.

ROSTOM, Amr; Univ Hlth Network-Princess M, 15 108-610 University Ave, Toronto ON M5G 2M9; Ain Shams (Egypt)'75; MSc; CCFP; Staff, Princess Margaret Hospital - University Health Network; Langs: Arabic; (416)946-2120; amrostom@hotmail.com.

ROSTON, Christina E B; 2018 Park Royal S, West Vancouver BC V7T 2W4; UBC'78; FRCPC; Anes. (604)922-4498

ROSTVIG, Jeffrey; 101-15850 26th Ave, Surrey BC V3S 2N6; Manchester (England)'78; MB ChB; CCFP; (604)542-7788

ROSU, Liliana; CSSS du Sud de Lanaudière, 911 montee des Pionniers, Terrebonne QC J6V 2H2; Bucharest (Romania)'78; Neur (P.Q.). Staff, Centre Hospitalier Pierre le Gardeur; (450)654-7525; Fax. (450)585-5939.

ROSZELL, Sheri L; Thamesview Family Health Team, 465 Grand Ave W, Chatham ON N7L 1C5; McM'97; CCFP; CCFP(E.M.); FCFP; Ac Staff, Chatham-Kent Health Alliance; Aj Prof Clinical Family Med, University of Western Ontario; Langs: Bilingual(French/English); (519)352-3210; Fax. (519)352-2176.

ROTAPLE, Michael J; Mount Sinai Hosp Centre, 5690 boul Cavendish, Cote Saint-Luc QC H4W 1S7; McG'79; FRCPC; IntMed; Respir. Staff, Mount Sinai Hospital Center; Staff, Centre Hospitalier Laurentien; (514)369-2222; Fax. (514)369-2225.

ROTARI-GHIDIRIM, Nadejda; CSSS de Manicouagan, 635 boul Joliet, Baie-Comeau QC G5C 1P1; (Moldova)'94; CCFP; Staff, Centre Hospitalier Régional Baie-Comeau; (418)589-3701

ROTARU, Carmen; Children's Hosp Eastern Ont, 401 Smyth Rd, Ottawa ON K1H 8L1; (Romania)'96; Staff, Children's Hospital of Eastern Ontario (CHEO); (613)737-7600

ROTBARD, Morris; Victoria Health Centre, 521 Victoria Park Ave, Scarborough ON M4C 5H1; Tor'71; BSc; CCFP; FCFP; Staff, The Scarborough Hospital - General Campus; Ac Staff, Providence Healthcare; Staff, Toronto East General Hospital Inc; (416)694-1400; Fax. (416)694-1985.

ROTECKA, Joanna M; BC Women's Hosp & Health Ctre, 4500 Oak St, Vancouver BC V6H 3N1; Gdansk (Poland)'84; FRCPC; Peds. Staff, BC Women's Hospital & Health Centre; (604)875-2424

ROTENBERG, Brian W; St Joseph's Health Care, PO Box 5777 Stn B E3 104-268 Grosvenor St, London ON N6A 4V2; Tor'00; FRCSC; Otol. Staff, St Joseph's Hospital - St Joseph's Health Care; (519)646-6320

ROTH, Barry A; Tillsonburg Med Centre, 200 Broadway St, Tillsonburg ON N4G 5A7; Tor'87; BSc; (519)842-4231; Fax. (519)842-6955.

ROTH, Daniel E; Central Alberta Med Imaging, 4312 54 Ave, Red Deer AB T4N 4M1; Alb'77; FRCPC; DiagRad. (403)343-6172; Fax. (403)346-5044.

ROTH, Daniel E; The Hosp for Sick Children, BW 10F-555 University Ave, Toronto ON M5G 1X8; UBC'02; FRCPC; Peds. Staff, The Hospital For Sick Children; (416)813-7654

ROTH, Harold G; Rocky Med Clinic, PO Box 99 Stn Main, Rocky-Mtn-Hse AB T4T 1A1; Alb'71; (403)845-2815; Fax. (403)845-2177.

ROTH, Johannes; Children's Hosp Eastern Ont, 401 Smyth Rd, Ottawa ON K1H 8L1; Tubingen (Germany)'96; Staff, Children's Hospital of Eastern Ontario (CHEO); (613)737-7600

ROTH, Kathryn E; St Joseph's Health Care, PO Box 5777 Stn B B2 501-268 Grosvenor St, London ON N6A 4V2; Wes'03; FRCSC; Otol (Head & Neck Surgery). Staff, St Joseph's Hospital - St Joseph's Health Care; (519)646-6124

ROTH, Kirk M; 1844 Coronation Blvd, Cambridge ON N3H 3R9; Qns'07; FRCSC; Urol. (519)650-4510; Fax. (519)650-6045.

ROTH, Leah H; 491 Eglinton Ave W, Toronto ON M5N 1A8; McM'98; BSc; FRCPC; Peds. Staff Peds, North York General Hospital; (416)782-6111; Fax. (416)782-5515.

ROTH, Lee S; SGH Medical Mall, 301-3030 Lawrence Ave E, Scarborough ON M1P 2T7; Wes'05; BSc(Hon); MSc; FRCPC; IntMed; Gastroent. (416)926-0262; Fax. (416)926-0936.

ROTH, Lisa R; Kincardine Family Health Team, 44 Queen St, Kincardine ON N2Z 3C1; Tor'99; CCFP; (519)396-6767; Fax. (519)396-3199; roth@bmts.com.

ROTH, Nathan L; 317-2330 Kennedy Rd, Scarborough ON M1T 0A2; McG'84; FACOG; FSOGC; FRCSC; ObstGyn (Infertility). Ac Staff, The Scarborough Hospital - Birchmount Campus; Langs: English; French; (416)609-8868; Fax. (416)609-8711.

ROTH, Paula; STD & Sexual Health Clinics, 1 Hughson St N, Hamilton ON L8R 3L5; Tor'76; FRCSC; ObstGyn. Staff, Hamilton Health Sciences Centre - McMaster Children's Hospital; Asst Prof, McMaster University; (905)546-2424

ROTH, Sherryn N; 301-3030 Lawrence Ave E, Toronto ON M1P 2T7; Tor'70; FRCP; FACC; FRCPC; Cardiol (Adult Cardiology); IntMed. Ac Staff, The Scarborough Hospital - General Campus; Staff, St Michael's Hospital; Asst Prof, Sunnybrook Health Sciences Centre; (416)431-0041; Fax. (416)431-0042; s.roth@utoronto.ca.

ROTH, Victoria E; Forensic Psychiatric Services, 2840 Nanaimo St, Victoria BC V8T 4W9; UBC'97; FRCPC; Psy. (250)387-1465

ROTH, Virginia R; The Ottawa Hosp-Gen Campus, G12-501 Smyth Rd, Ottawa ON K1H 8L6; Ott'93; FRCPC; IntMed; InfectDis. Staff, The Ottawa Hospital - General Campus; (613)737-8606; vroth@ottawahospital.on.ca.

ROTHBART, Peter; Rothbart Centre for Pain Care, 9-4646 Dufferin St, North York ON M3H 5S4; Edinburgh (Scotland)'62; MB ChB; DABPM; FRCPC; Anes (Pain Management). Dir, Rothbart Pain Management Clinic; Staff, Rothbart Pain Management Clinic; (416)512-8171; Fax. (416)512-6375; reception@rothbart.com.

ROTHBERG, Randy D; Toronto East Gen Hosp Inc, 825 Coxwell Ave, Toronto ON M4C 3E7; Tor'72; FRCPC; DiagRad. Staff, Toronto East General Hospital Inc; (416)461-8272

ROTHENSTEIN, Jeffrey; Lakeridge Hlth Corp-Oshawa, 1 Hospital Crt, Oshawa ON L1G 2B9; Tor'04; FRCPC; IntMed; MedOncol. Staff, Lakeridge Health - Oshawa Site; (905)576-8711 x2802

ROTHER, Mark J; The Credit Valley Hosp, 2200 Eglinton Ave W, Mississauga ON L5M 2N1; Tor'87; FRCPC; IntMed; MedOncol. Staff, Headwaters Health Care Centre - Orangeville Site; Staff, The Credit Valley Hospital; (905)813-1100 x5135

ROTHFELS, Peter L; Worker's Comp Board, 6951 Westminster Hwy, Richmond BC V7C 1C6; Alb'81; BEd; (604)231-8586; Fax. (604)279-7692; peter.rothfels@worksafebc.com.

ROTHMAN, Ann; SMBD Jewish Gen Hosp, 3755 ch de la Cote-Sainte-Cath, Montreal QC H3T 1E2; McG'83; BSc(Hon); MDCM; CCFP; FCFP; Staff Family Med, Sir Mortimer B Davis Jewish General; adj Prof Family Med, McGill University; Langs: Spanish; French; (514)340-8253; Fax. (514)340-8298.

ROTHMAN, Laura G; PG Medical Education Office, 2F-500 University Ave, Toronto ON M5G 1V7; Tor'07; FRCPC; IntMed; Endocrin&Metab.

ROTHMAN, Steven W; Yonge-Eglinton Med Centre, 202-2401 Yonge St, Toronto ON M4P 3H1; McG'93; CCFP; FCFP; Langs: English; French; (416)322-3700; Fax. (416)322-3707.

ROTHOVA, Anna; Family Med Clinic, 1-2536 Main St, Winnipeg MB R2V 4Y1; Prague (Czech Republic)'76; (204)339-1781

ROTHSCHILD, Carl J; Alan Casamore Centre, 420-1669 Broadway E, Vancouver BC V5N 1V9; Washington(DC) (USA)'68; FRCPC; Psy. Instructor, University of British Columbia; (604)675-3996 x21313

ROTHSCHILD, John M; Foothills Med Centre, 1403 29 St NW, Calgary AB T2N 2T9; McG'69; BSc; FRCSC; Cardiovasc&ThorSurg (Pacemaker Surgery). Ac Staff Pacemaker Clinic, Foothills Medical Centre; Consultant, Peter Lougheed Centre; Consultant, Rockyview General Hospital; Clin Assoc Prof, University of Calgary; Langs: English; French; (403)944-1188; Fax. (403)270-0718.

ROTHSTEIN, Jack; Westmount Med Bldg, 555-5025 rue Sherbrooke O, Montreal QC H4A 1S9; McG'79; MSc; FACS; FRCSC; Otol. Staff, McGill University Health Centre - Montreal Children's Hospital; Staff, Sir Mortimer B Davis Jewish General; Lecturer Otol, McGill University; (514)481-0033; Fax. (514)481-9493.

ROTHSTEIN, Sheila; Active Care, 35B-2121 Carling Ave, Ottawa ON K2A 1H2; Alb'63; (613)761-6777

ROTHWELL, Bruce C; Suitor House, 1004 8 Ave SE, Calgary AB T2G 0M4; Cal'82; FRCSC; GenSurg; Critical Care Medicine. Clin Assoc Prof, University of Calgary; (403)264-6720; Fax. (403)237-0167.

ROTHWELL, Robert S; Columbia Med Bldg, 402-301 Columbia St E, New Westminster BC V3L 3W5; McG'71; DABIM; DAB; FACP; FRCPC; IntMed; Rheum. Consultant, Royal Columbian Hospital; Consultant, Eagle Ridge Hospital & Health Care Centre; Langs: French; (604)526-1712; Fax. (604)525-0539.

ROTMAN, Laurie S; Danforth Birchmount Med Centre, 34-462 Birchmount Rd, Scarborough ON M1K 1N8; Tor'83; Court Staff, The Scarborough Hospital - General Campus; Court Staff, Women's College Hospital; (416)698-9988; Fax. (416)698-1055.

ROTONDO, Terrence G; 2-2029 Cassells St, North Bay ON P1B 4E1; Wes'77; Dip SportMed; Ac Staff, North Bay Regional Health Centre - Regional Mental Health; (705)476-5516; Fax. (705)476-1623.

ROTSTEIN, Coleman M F; Univ Hlth Network-Toronto Gen, NCSB 11 12-200 Elizabeth St, Toronto ON M5G 2C4; Cal'76; ABIM(InfectDis); FRCPC; IntMed (Infectious Diseases). Affil Scientist, Toronto General Hospital - UHN; (416)340-4800

ROTSTEIN, Edward A; Community Schizophrenia Serv, 102E-350 King St E, Hamilton ON L8N 3Y3; Man'70; AB; BSc(Med); FRCPC; Psy (Schizophrenia). Staff, Hamilton Health Sciences Centre - McMaster Children's Hospital; Staff, St Joseph's Healthcare - Charlton Campus; Physician, Wellington Psychiatric Outreach Program; Clinical Asst Prof, McMaster University; (905)527-8515; Fax. (905)527-7301.

ROTSTEIN, J R Jennifer N; 7-383 Main St N, Markham ON L3P 1Z3; McM'02; BSc; CCFP; (905)201-8005; jennifer_rotstein@hotmail.com.

ROTSTEIN, Lorne E; Univ Hlth Network-Toronto Gen, EN10 220-200 Elizabeth St, Toronto ON M5G 2C4; Tor'73; FACS; FRCSC; GenSurg (Head & Neck Surgery). Head Div of GenSurg, Toronto General Hospital - UHN; Staff, Princess Margaret Hospital - University Health Network; Prof Surg/Dir, University of Toronto; (416)340-5195; Fax. (416)340-3808; lorne.rotstein@uhn.on.ca.

ROTSTEIN, Ori D; St Michael's Hosp, CCW16 044-30 Bond St, Toronto ON M5B 1W8; Tor'77; FACS; FRCSC; GenSurg. Chief Surgeon, St Michael's Hospital; Prof, University of Toronto; (416)864-5410; Fax. (416)360-0637.

ROTSTEIN, Stephen I; 204-1262 Don Mills Rd, North York ON M3B 2W7; Tor'83; CCFP; (416)444-6221; Fax. (416)444-6116.

ROTTAPEL, Robert K; St Michael's Hosp, 30 Bond St, Toronto ON M5B 1W8; Washington(DC) (USA)'84; IntMed (Medical Research). Staff, St Michael's Hospital; Teach Staff, University of Toronto; (416)864-5420

ROTTEMBOURG, Diane; CHUS-Hop Fleurimont, 3001 12e av N, Sherbrooke QC J1H 5N4; (France)'03; Staff, Centre Hospitalier Universitaire de Sherbrooke-Hopital Fleurimont; (819)346-1110

ROTTENSTEN, Kirsten L; Markham Stouffville Hosp, PO Box 1800 Stn Main 381 Church St, Markham ON L3P 7P3; McM'88; MHSc; FRCPC; CommunMed. Staff, Markham Stouffville Hospital; (905)472-7074

ROTTGER, P John; Associate Med Clinic, PO Box 549, Pincher Creek AB T0K 1W0; Belfast (Ireland)'78; MB ChB; BAO; Clin Lecturer, University of Calgary; (403)627-3321; Fax. (403)627-2280.

ROTUNDO, Mark J; Marlee Med Centre, 249 Marlee Ave, North York ON M6B 4B8; Tor'93; BSc; CCFP; (416)780-8896; Fax. (416)780-1087.

ROTZINGER, Deborah L; Crowfoot Corner Medicentre, 217-150 Crowfoot Cres NW, Calgary AB T3G 3T2; Cal'90; CCFP; (403)241-8900; Fax. (403)241-8109.

ROUCAUT, Francois-Xavier; Ctr Hosp Trois-Riv-St-Joseph, 731 rue Saint-Julie, Trois-Rivieres QC G9A 1Y1; Staff, Centre Hospitalier Regional de Trois-Rivieres; (819)697-3333

ROUETTE, Daniel; 204-352 av Dorval, Dorval QC H9S 3H8; Mon'79; (514)631-8861; Fax. (514)631-6691.

ROUETTE, Justine; CSSS de Laval, 1755 boul Rene-Laennec, Laval QC H7M 3L9; Mon'06; FRCPC; Peds. Staff, Hopital de la Cite de la santé; (450)668-1010

ROUF, Rehana K; Almonte Gen Hosp, SS 1 75 Spring St, Almonte ON K0A 1A0; Ott'76; CCFP; FCFP; Staff, Almonte General Hospital.

ROUGET, Adrien C; Medical Imaging Consultants, 105-11010 101 St NW, Edmonton AB T5H 4B9; Alb'99; FRCPC; DiagRad. Staff, University of Alberta Hospital; (780)426-1121

ROUGET, Julia E; Tawa Professional Centre, 210-3017 66 St NW, Edmonton AB T6K 4B2; Alb'99; BSc; FRCPC; IntMed (Family Medicine). Staff, Covenant Health - Grey Nuns Community Hospital; Clinical Asst Prof IntMed, University of Alberta Hospital; Langs: German; (780)465-7295; Fax. (780)465-2825; jrouget@shaw.ca.

ROUHANA, Elisson; Hilltop Med Clinic, 140-15321 16 Ave, Surrey BC V4A 1R6; (Lebanon)'00; CCFP; (604)531-5575

ROUHANI, Nassim; London Medicentres, 611 Wonderland Rd N, London ON N6H 4V6; (Other Foreign)'07; (519)471-6686

ROUHANI, Shiva; London Medicentres, 611 Wonderland Rd N, London ON N6H 4V6; (Other Foreign)'07; CCFP; (519)471-6686

ROUIFED, Nora; Clin Saint-Louis, 3165 ch Saint-Louis, Quebec QC G1W 4R4; (Algeria)'86; CCFP; (418)653-1970

ROUILLARD, Gervais; Hotel-Dieu d'Arthabaska, 5 rue des Hospitalieres, Victoriaville QC G6P 6N2; Laval'70; ABOtol; FRCSC; Otol (General Surgery). Staff Gen Surg, Hotel-Dieu d'Arthabaska; assoc Staff, Hôpital Sainte-croix; Langs: English; (819)357-1151 x2025; Fax. (819)357-1680; gervais_rouil@videotron.ca.

ROUILLARD, Jean-Francois; Ctr Hosp Affilie-Enfant-Jesus, 1401 18e rue, Quebec QC G1J 1Z4; Laval'86; CSPQ; FRCPC; Anes. Staff, Centre Hospitalier Affilié Universitaire de Québec - Hôpital De L'Enfant Jésus; (418)649-5803

ROUILLARD, Martin; Hotel-Dieu d'Arthabaska, 5 rue des Hospitalieres, Victoriaville QC G6P 6N2; Sher'91; FRCSC; GenSurg. Staff, Hotel-Dieu d'Arthabaska; assoc Prof, Universite de Sherbrooke; (819)357-2030; Fax. (819)357-6006.

ROUILLARD, Pierre; 2601 ch de la Canardiere, Quebec QC G1J 2G3; Laval'77; LMCC; CSPQ; FRCPC; Psy (Addiction Medicine). ac Staff, Institut Universitaire Sante; Clin Prof, Université Laval; Langs: Bilingual(French/English); (418)663-5000 x6451; Fax. (418)661-6891.

ROUILLARD, Roger; Hotel-Dieu de Quebec, 11 Cote du Palais, Quebec QC G1R 2J6; Laval'74; DABOT; Otol. Ac Staff Otol, Centre Hospitalier Universitaire de Québec (CHUQ) - Siege Social; Teach Staff, Université Laval; (418)691-5151

ROUILLARD-LAFOND, Joelle; CSSS de Lac-Saint Jean-Est, CP 1300 Succ Bureau-Chef 300 boul Champlain S, Alma QC G8B 5W3; Sher'04; FRCPC; Peds. Staff, CSSS de Lac-Saint Jean-Est; Langs: Bilingual(French/English); (418)669-2000 x6674; Fax. (418)662-8003; joelle.rouillard-lafond@gmail.com.

ROUILLIER, Jean; Clinique Med St-Etienne, 2-965 Rte Lagueux, St-Etienne-De-Lauz QC G6J 1T5; Laval'78; (418)831-9538; Fax. (418)831-8552.

ROUKEMA, Henry W; London HS-Victoria Hosp, D4 213-800 Commissioners Rd E, London ON N6A 5W9; Wes'87; MSc(ClinEpidem); FRCPC; Peds (Neonatal & Perinatal Medicine). Staff Neonatologist, London Health Sciences Centre - Victoria Campus; Assoc Prof, University of Western Ontario; (519)685-8500; Fax. (519)646-6123.

ROULEAU, Anne; Centre medical de Cowansville, 101-370 rue de la Riviere, Cowansville QC J2K 1N3; Mon'03; Staff, Hôpital Brome-Missisquoi-Perkins; (450)263-0774

ROULEAU, Brigitte; CSSS de Laval, 1755 boul Rene-Laennec, Laval QC H7M 3L9; Mon'97; Staff, Hopital de la Cite de la santé; (450)668-1010

ROULEAU, Charles D; CLSC de Hull, 85 rue Saint-Redempteur, Gatineau QC J8X 4E6; Ott'93; Langs: English; French; (819)770-6908

ROULEAU, Claude A; CHUQ-St-Francois d'Assise, 10 rue de l'Espinay, Quebec QC G1L 3L5; Laval'62; GenSurg. ac Staff, Centre Hospitalier Universitaire De Québec - Pavillon De St-françois-d'assise; Langs: Bilingual(French/English); (418)525-4444 x2411; Fax. (418)525-2264.

ROULEAU, Claude; 45 rue Maribourg CP 367, Maria QC G0C 1Y0; Laval'70; OrthSurg. (418)759-3990; Fax. (418)759-3032; rouberthmaria@globetrotter.net.

ROULEAU, Daniel; CLSC de Normandin, 1205 rue Saint-Cyrille, Normandin QC G8M 4K1; Mon'87; Staff, Centre Maria-Chapdelaine - CH de Dolbeau-Mistassini; (418)274-1234; Fax. (418)276-6970.

ROULEAU, Danielle; CHUM-Hop Notre-Dame, 1560 rue Sherbrooke E, Montreal QC H2L 4M1; Mon'90; FRCPC; MedMicrobiol; Microbio & Infect Dis (P.Q.); InfectDis (P.Q.). Staff, Centre Hospitalier l'Université de Montréal (CHUM) - Hôpital Notre-Dame; (514)345-4931; Fax. (514)412-7545.

ROULEAU, Dominique; Hop du Sacre-Coeur de Mtl, 5400 boul Gouin O, Montreal QC H4J 1C5; Mon'01; FRCSC; OrthSurg (Shoulder). Staff, Hôpital du Sacre-Coeur de Montréal; (514)338-2222

ROULEAU, Guy A; CHUM-Hop Notre-Dame, 1560 rue Sherbrooke E, Montreal QC H2L 4M1; Ott'80; PhD(Genetics); MedGenetics (P.Q.); Neur. Staff, Centre Hospitalier l'Université de Montréal (CHUM) - Hôpital Notre-Dame; (514)890-8000

ROULEAU, Isabelle; Ctr Hosp du Centre la Mauricie, 50 119e rue, Shawinigan-Sud QC G9P 5K1; Laval'05; Staff, Centre Hospitalier du Centre la Mauricie; (819)536-7500

ROULEAU, J J Clement; CSSS de Rimouski-Neigette, CP 3150 Succ A 150 av Rouleau, Rimouski QC G5L 5T1; Laval'98; CSPQ; FRCPC; Anes. Staff, Hôpital Regional Rimouski; (418)724-8147

ROULEAU, Jacinthe; CHUM-Hop Notre-Dame, 1560 rue Sherbrooke E, Montreal QC H2L 4M1; Laval'01; FRCSC; Ophth. Staff, Centre Hospitalier l'Université de Montréal (CHUM) - Hôpital Notre-Dame; (514)890-8000 x27100

ROULEAU, Jacques; Hôpital Laval, 2725 ch Sainte-Foy, Quebec QC G1V 4G5; Laval'69; FACC; LMCC; FRCP; Cardiol (Hemodynamics). Staff Cardiol & Researcher IUCPQ, Hôpital Laval; Prof Med, Université Laval; Langs: Bilingual(English/French); (418)656-8711 x4657; Fax. (418)656-4544; jacques-r.rouleau@med.ulaval.ca.

ROULEAU, Jean-Francois; Imagix, 104-233 rue Turgeon, Sainte-Therese QC J7E 3J8; Ott'99; CSPQ; FRCPC; DiagRad. Staff, Hôtel-Dieu de Saint-Jérôme; (514)866-6622

ROULEAU, Jean-Francois; Polyclinique St-Jerome, 204-200 rue Durand, Saint-Jerome QC J7Z 7E2; Sher'78; Staff, Hôtel-Dieu de Saint-Jérôme; Langs: Bilingual(French/English); (450)438-2647; Fax. (450)438-5544.

ROULEAU, Jean-Lucien; Institut de Cardiologie de Mtl, S 2070-5000 rue Belanger, Montreal QC H1T 1C8; Ott'74; FRCPC; IntMed; Cardiol. Staff, Institut de Cardiologie de Montréal; Dir Scientific de l'Institut de la sante circulatoire et respiratoire, Instituts de Recherche en Sante du Canada; Doyen, Universite de Montreal; Langs: English; French; (514)593-7431; Fax. (514)376-7070; jean-lucien.rouleau@icm-mhi.org.

ROULEAU, Katherine D; SMH-Wellesley Health Centre, 410 Sherbourne St, Toronto ON M4X 1K2; McG'93; BSc; MDCM; MHSc; CCFP; Dir Family Med Residency Prog, St Michael's Hospital; (416)867-3728

ROULEAU, Louise; Clin de Rhumathologie, 1119 rue Sainte-Marguerite, Trois-Rivieres QC G8Z 1Y2; Sher'75; CSPQ; Rheum (P.Q.). Ac Staff, Centre Hospitalier Regional de Trois-Rivieres; Consultant, CSSS de Trois-Rivières; Rheumatology, CHSLD Le Trifluvien; (819)370-8106; Fax. (819)370-8120.

ROULEAU, Lucie; Clinique de Gynecologie, 24 rue Melancon E, Alma QC G8B 6W3; Laval'80; ObstGyn. Staff, CSSS de Lac-Saint Jean-Est; Langs: English; (418)662-6553; Fax. (418)662-3731.

ROULEAU, Michel; CHUQ-Hotel-Dieu de Quebec, 11 Cote du Palais, Quebec QC G1R 2J6; Laval'72; CSPQ; LMCC; Respir. Staff, Centre Hospitalier Universitaire de Québec (CHUQ) - Siege Social; assoc Prof Med, Université Laval; Langs: English; (418)691-5386; Fax. (418)692-5755.

ROULEAU, Michel O; Clin Sante Jacques-Cartier, 200-1815 rue King O, Sherbrooke QC J1J 2E3; Laval'71; Otol. Staff, Centre Hospitalier Universitaire de Sherbrooke-Hopital Fleurimont; Assoc Member, Centre Hospitalier Universitaire de Sherbrooke-Hôpital Hôtel-Dieu; (819)565-7446; Fax. (819)565-7780.

ROULEAU, Pierre; SAAQ, CP 392 Succ Tour D/L Bourse 800 Tour de la Place, Montreal QC H4Z 1L6; Laval'78; Physician, Societe Assurance Automobile du Quebec; (514)954-7678

ROULEAU, Richard; Clinique Med du Phare, 101-822 boul Sainte-Anne, Rimouski QC G5M 1J5; Laval'97; CCFP; Dir, Hôpital Regional Rimouski; (418)723-5135; Fax. (418)724-2251.

ROULEAU, Yves; Ctr Hosp Anna-Laberge, 200 boul Brisebois, Chateauguay QC J6K 4W8; Mon'94; FRCPC; DiagRad. Staff, Hôpital Anna-Laberge; (450)466-5050; rouleaufunaro@videotron.ca.

ROULEAU, Yves; Ctr de Sante Paul-Gilbert, 9330 boul du Centre-Hospitalie, Charny QC G6X 1L6; Mon'85; Staff, Centre Hospitalier Paul-Gilbert; (418)380-8993

ROULIER, Sebastien; CHUS-Hop Fleurimont, 3001 12e av N, Sherbrooke QC J1H 5N4; Sher'98; FRCPC; Peds (Family Medicine); Critical Care Medicine (P.Q.). Staff, Centre Hospitalier Universitaire de Sherbrooke-Hopital Fleurimont; (819)346-1110

ROULIER, Stephan; Hop du Sacre-Coeur de Mtl, 5400 boul Gouin O, Montreal QC H4J 1C5; Mon'95; CCFP; CCFP(E.M.); Staff, Hôpital du Sacre-Coeur de Montréal; (514)338-2222 x2002; s.roulier@videotron.ca.

ROUMAIN, Marie H C; CSSSG-Hop de Gatineau, CP 2000 Succ Bureau-Chef 909 boul de la Verendrye O, Gatineau QC J8P 7H2; McG'06; MDCM; ObstGyn (P.Q.). Staff, Hôpital de Gatineau; (819)966-6100

ROUMELIOTIS, Paul; Eastern Ontario Health Unit, 1000 rue Pitt, Cornwall ON K6J 5T1; McG'83; MDCM; MPH; FRCPC; Peds (Public Health). Aj Prof Peds, McGill University; Langs: Greek; French; Spanish; (613)933-1375; Fax. (613)938-9707.

ROUMY, Gustave; Hop Charles LeMoyne, 3120 boul Taschereau, Greenfield Park QC J4V 2H1; Beirut (Lebanon)'73; CSPQ; DiagRad. Ac Staff Radiol, Hopital Charles LeMoyne; (450)466-5070

ROUMY, Michele B; Medicentre Lasalle, 101-1500 av Dollard, Lasalle QC H8N 1T5; Laval'72; CSPQ; DiagRad (P.Q.). (514)365-7766; Fax. (514)365-8622.

ROURKE, James T B; Health Sciences Centre, 300 Prince Philip Dr, St. John's NL A1B 3V6; Wes'76; MClSc; LLD; CCFP; CCFP(E.M.); FCFP; Staff, Health Sciences Centre; Dean Faculy of Med/Prof, Memorial University Of Newfoundland; (709)777-6602; Fax. (709)777-6746; dean.medicine@mun.ca.

ROURKE, Keith F; Hys Med Centre, 400-11010 101 St NW, Edmonton AB T5H 4B9; Dal'96; FRCSC; Urol. Staff, University of Alberta Hospital; (780)441-2576; Fax. (780)441-2597.

ROURKE, Leslie L; Health Sciences Centre, 300 Prince Philip Dr, St. John's NL A1B 3V6; Wes'77; MClSc; FAAFP; CCFP; FCFP; Staff, Health Sciences Centre; (709)777-6743

ROURKE, Margaret; Le Marchand Mansion, 407-11523 100 Ave NW, Edmonton AB T5K 0J8; Alb'98; BSc; FRCPC; Psy (Psychotherapy). (780)455-5523; Fax. (780)453-1219; maggierourke@yahoo.ca.

ROURKE, Timothy W; 21-5350 Canotek Rd, Gloucester ON K1J 9E2; Dal'87; MBA; BSc; Staff, Royal Victoria Regional Health Centre; Langs: English; French; (613)747-3413; Fax. (613)747-0581.

ROUSE, Danielle; Clin Prev Vasculaire et Lipide, 1950 boul du Cure-Labelle, Saint-Jerome QC J7Y 1S1; Mon'76; Dir, Clin Prevention de la Maladie Vasculaire et Lipides; Langs: Bilingual(French/English); (450)432-5726; Fax. (450)432-5537.

ROUSE, Frank V; Chamber of Commerce Bldg, 502-345 Lakeshore Rd E, Oakville ON L6J 1J5; Qns'57; Ac Staff, Halton Healthcare Services Corporation - Oakville Site; Physician Outpatient, Joseph Brant Memorial Hospital; (905)845-4511

ROUSE, Tyler B; Stratford Gen Hosp, W3 408-46 General Hospital Dr, Stratford ON N5A 2Y6; Tor'02; FRCPC; AnatPath. Staff, Stratford General Hospital - Huron Perth Healthcare Alliance; (519)272-8210 x2873; Fax. (519)272-8198; tyler.rouse@hpha.ca.

ROUSELLE, David A; York Prof Bldg, 301-679 Davis Dr, Newmarket ON L3Y 5G8; Qns'81; FACOG; FRCSC; ObstGyn. Asst Clin Prof ObstGyn, McMaster University; (905)853-2322; Fax. (905)853-7311.

ROUSHDI, Amani E; Mackenzie Richmond Hill Hosp, 10 Trench St, Richmond Hill ON L4C 4Z3; Alexandria (Egypt)'87; FRCPC; Peds; Nephrol. Staff, Mackenzie Richmond Hill Hospital; (905)883-1212

ROUSSEAU, Andre; Hotel-Dieu de Levis, 143 rue Wolf, Levis QC G6V 3Z1; Mon'80; Peds. Staff Peds, Hôtel-Dieu de Lévis; Langs: Bilingual(French/English); (418)835-7322

ROUSSEAU, Anne; CHUQ-Ctr Hosp Univ Laval, 2705 boul Laurier, Quebec QC G1V 4G2; Laval'99; FRCPC; Peds. Staff, Centre Hospitalier Universitaire de Quebec-CHUL; (418)654-2282; anne.rousseau@mail.chuq.qc.ca.

ROUSSEAU, Anne-Marie; Institute Albert-Prevost, 6555 boul Gouin O, Montreal QC H4K 1B3; Mon'02; Psy. (514)338-2222

ROUSSEAU, Annie; Hôpital Laval, 2725 ch Sainte-Foy, Quebec QC G1V 4G5; Laval'00; CSPQ; FRCPC; Anes; Critical Care Medicine (P.Q.). Staff, Hôpital Laval; (418)656-8711

ROUSSEAU, Annie; CSSS de Saint-Jerome, 290 rue de Montigny, Saint-Jerome QC J7Z 5T3; Mon'02; CCFP; Staff, Hôtel-Dieu de Saint-Jérôme; (450)431-8200; Fax. (450)431-8244.

ROUSSEAU, Annie; Ctr Medi Soleil St-Jean-Sur-Ri, 120-383 boul du Seminaire N, St-Jean-sur-Richel QC J3B 8C5; Laval'95; FRCPC; IntMed; Gastroent. (450)347-7557

ROUSSEAU, Bernard; CSSS de Memphremagog, 50 rue Saint-Patrice E, Magog QC J1X 3X3; Mon'64; FRCPC; IntMed; Gastroent (P.Q.). Ac Staff Med, Centre Hospitalier Universitaire De Québec - Pavillon De St-françois-d'assise; Staff, Centre Hospitalier et CLSC de Memphremagog; assoc Prof, Université Laval; (819)943-3381 x2603

ROUSSEAU, Cecile; CLSC Park Extension, 204.2-7085 rue Hutchison, Montreal QC H3N 1Y9; Sher'77; CSPQ; Psy. Staff, McGill University Health Centre - Montreal Children's Hospital; adj Prof, McGill University; (514)273-3800 x6452; Fax. (514)380-8147.

ROUSSEAU, Celine; Hôpital Ste-Justine, 3175 ch Cote-Sainte-Catherine, Montreal QC H3T 1C5; Laval'77; Microbio & Infect Dis (P.Q.); MedMicrobiol; Peds (P.Q.). Staff, Hôpital Ste-Justine; (514)345-4642; Fax. (514)345-4860.

ROUSSEAU, Claude; CSSS de l'Energie-Ste-Therese, 1705 av Georges, Shawinigan QC G9N 2N1; Laval'73; Staff, CH du Centre-de-la-Mauricie (Ste-Thérèse de Shawinigan); (819)536-7500; claude_rousseau@ssss.gouv.qc.ca.

ROUSSEAU, Claudyne; CSSS de Lac-Saint Jean-Est, CP 1300 Succ Bureau-Chef 300 boul Champlain S, Alma QC G8B 5W3; Sher'90; Peds (Developmental Pediatrics). Staff Peds, CSSS de Lac-Saint Jean-Est; (418)669-2000

ROUSSEAU, Come; CSSS de Chicoutimi, 305 rue Saint-Vallier, Chicoutimi QC G7H 5H6; Laval'67; MedOncol (P.Q.); Hem (P.Q.). Staff, Complexe hospitalier de la Sagamie; Langs: English; (418)541-1000 x2092

ROUSSEAU, Daniel; Clinique Radiologie des Recoll, 1900 boul des Recollets, Trois-Rivieres QC G8Z 4K4; Laval'71; DiagRad. Staff, Centre de santé Cloutier-du-Rivage; (819)373-4126

ROUSSEAU, Daniel; Clinique Daniel Rousseau, 2600 rue Victoria, Lachine QC H8S 1Z3; Mon'82; LMCC; (514)637-0707; Fax. (514)637-5405.

ROUSSEAU, Danielle; Centre Med Dorion Vaudreuil, 600 boul Harwood, Vaudreuil-Dorion QC J7V 6A3; Mon'73; (450)455-9301; Fax. (450)455-8964.

ROUSSEAU, Danny; Clinique Med Pierre-Boucher, 1615 boul Jacques-Cartier E, Longueuil QC J4M 2X1; Laval'98; (450)468-6223; dannyrousseau@hotmail.com.

ROUSSEAU, Erella; Village Med Associates, 27-1077 North Service Rd, Mississauga ON L4Y 1A6; Qns'81; CCFP; FCFP; Court Staff, Trillium Health Centre - Mississauga; (905)949-1700; Fax. (905)949-8625.

ROUSSEAU, Francois; Inst U en Sante Mentale de QC, 2601 ch de la Canardiere, Quebec QC G1J 2G3; Mon'90; MSc; CSPQ; FRCPC; Psy (Clinical Research). Staff Geriatric Psy, Institut Universitaire Sante; Staff Geriatric Psy, Centre Hospitalier Universitaire de Quebec-CHUL; assoc Prof, Université Laval; Affil Membre, McGill University; Langs: English; (418)663-5020 x4261; Fax. (418)663-0494; francois_rousseau@crulrg.ulaval.ca.

ROUSSEAU, Francois; CHUQ-St-Francois d'Assise, 10 rue de l'Espinay, Quebec QC G1L 3L5; Laval'83; CSPQ; FRCPC; MedBiochem (Molecular Genetics). Ac Staff, Centre Hospitalier Universitaire De Québec - Pavillon De St-françois-d'assise; Prof Biochem, Université Laval; (418)525-4470; Fax. (418)525-4429.

ROUSSEAU, Frederic; CHSLD du Centre Mauricie, 1650 6e av, Grand-Mere QC G9T 2K4; Sher'94; Staff, Centre Lafleche Grand-Mere; (819)533-2500

ROUSSEAU, Genevieve D; SoundCare Med Centre, 560-1145 Hunt Club Rd, Ottawa ON K1V 0Y3; Ott'90; FRCSC; ObstGyn (Echography). Staff ObstGyn, The Ottawa Hospital - General Campus; Langs: English; (613)738-2378

ROUSSEAU, Helene; GMF Cote-des-Neiges, 500-5700 ch de la cote-des-Nei, Montreal QC H3T 2A8; Mon'91; CCFP; FCFP; Staff, Sir Mortimer B Davis Jewish General; Staff, McGill University; Langs: English; Spanish; (514)731-8531; Fax. (514)731-0563.

ROUSSEAU, Isabelle; CSSS de Chicoutimi, 144-305 rue Saint-Vallier, Chicoutimi QC G7H 5H6; Mon'93; CSPQ; FRCPC; DiagRad. Staff, Complexe hospitalier de la Sagamie; (418)541-1000

ROUSSEAU, Jacinthe; CLSC Saint-Romuald, 200-1205 boul de la Rive-Sud, Saint-Romuald QC G6W 0J6; Laval'78; Médecin, Centre Hospitalier Paul-Gilbert; Médecin, CSSS Alphonse-Desjardins; (418)380-8991; Fax. (418)839-4190; jacinthe.rousseau@ssss.gouv.qc.ca.

ROUSSEAU, Jean; Place du Golf, 401-28 ch du Golf E, St-Charles-Brromee QC J6E 2B4; Sher'87; FRCSC; OrthSurg. (450)756-8073; Fax. (450)756-8075.

ROUSSEAU, Josee; CSSS Kamouraska-Hop Notre-Dame, 1201 6e av, La Pocatiere QC G0R 1Z0; Sher'06; CCFP; Staff, CSSS de Kamouraska; (418)856-7000; Fax. (418)856-4737.

ROUSSEAU, Julie; Hop du Sacre-Coeur de Mtl, 5400 boul Gouin O, Montreal QC H4J 1C5; Mon'96; FRCPC; IntMed; MedOncol; Hem. Staff, Hôpital du Sacre-Coeur de Montréal; Langs: Bilingual(French/English); (514)338-2222

ROUSSEAU, Julie-Anne; Ctre d'Obst et Gynecologie, 4250 1re av, Quebec QC G1H 2S5; Laval'03; FRCSC; ObstGyn. (418)654-0555

ROUSSEAU, Lise; GMF du Chatel, 200-9465 boul de l'Ormiere, Quebec QC G2B 3K7; Laval'75; (418)843-5141; Fax. (418)843-5343.

ROUSSEAU, Louis; Hôpital Laval, 2725 ch Sainte-Foy, Quebec QC G1V 4G5; Laval'68; CSPQ; Psy. Staff, Hôpital Laval; (418)656-4565; Fax. (418)656-4551.

ROUSSEAU, Louise; Hôpital Ste-Justine, 3175 ch Côte-Sainte-Catherine, Montreal QC H3T 1C5; Mon'74; CSPQ; FRCPC; Psy (Child & Adolescent Psychiatry). Staff, Hôpital du Haut-Richelieu; Ac Staff Child & Adolescent OP Psy Clin, Hôpital Ste-Justine; Langs: English; French; (514)345-4931 x5750; Fax. (514)345-4679; louise_rousseau@ssss.gouv.qc.ca.

ROUSSEAU, M Suzanne R; 205-6070 rue Sherbrooke E, Montreal QC H1N 1C1; Mon'65; Electroenceph (P.Q.); Neur (Pediatric Neurology). adj Prof Med, Universite de Montreal; (514)251-4790; Fax. (514)251-4792; srousseau01@videotron.ca.

ROUSSEAU, Mario; SAAQ-Evaluation Medicale, CP 19600 Succ Terminus N4 34-333 boul Jean-Leasge, Quebec QC G1K 8J6; Laval'84; FRCPC; IntMed. Ac Staff, Centre Hospitalier Universitaire de Québec (CHUQ) - Siege Social; Med Consultant, Soc De L'assurance Automobile; mario.rousseau@saaq.gouv.qc.ca.

ROUSSEAU, Melissa; The Ottawa Hosp-Gen Campus, 501 Smyth Rd, Ottawa ON K1H 8L6; McG'07; MDCM; FRCPC; IntMed. Staff, The Ottawa Hospital - General Campus; (613)798-5555

ROUSSEAU, Pierre; CHUM-Hop Notre-Dame, 1560 rue Sherbrooke E, Montreal QC H2L 4M1; Sher'86; FRCP; DACR; CSPQ; RadOncol (Breast Oncology). Staff, Centre Hospitalier Universitaire de Sherbrooke-Hopital Fleurimont; Staff, Centre Hospitalier l'Université de Montréal (CHUM) - Hôpital Notre-Dame; Clin Asst, Universite de Montreal; Langs: Bilingual(English/French); Spanish; (514)890-8254; pierre.rousseau.chum@ssss.gouv.qc.ca.

ROUSSEAU, Pierre; Hop du Sacre-Coeur de Mtl, 5400 boul Gouin O, Montreal QC H4J 1C5; Mon'82; CSPQ; FRCPC; Anes. Chef Anes, Hôpital du Sacre-Coeur de Montréal; Clinical Asst Prof, Universite de Montreal; Langs: English; (514)338-2222 x2680; Fax. (514)338-2009; pierre_rousseau@videotron.ca.

ROUSSEAU, Serge; 1564 av Van Horne, Outremont QC H2V 1L5; Strasbourg (France)'72; ObstGyn. ac Staff, Centre Hospitalier l'Université de Montréal (CHUM) - Hôtel-Dieu; (514)277-5653; Fax. (514)277-9232.

ROUSSEAU, Sophie; CSSS Pierre Boucher, 1333 boul Jacques-Cartier E, Longueuil QC J4M 2A5; Mon'00; Staff, Centre Hospitalier Pierre Boucher; (450)468-8111

ROUSSEAU, Stephane; Clinique du Havre, 79A rue Jacques-Cartier, Gaspe QC G4X 1M5; Laval'94; PhD; Staff, Centre Hospitalier de Gaspe; (418)368-5609; Fax. (418)368-6498.

ROUSSEAU-HARSANY, Elisabeth; Hôpital Ste-Justine, 3175 ch Cote-Sainte-Catherine, Montreal QC H3T 1C5; Strasbourg (France)'72; FRCPC; Peds. Staff, Hôpital Ste-Justine; (514)345-4788; Fax. (514)345-4822.

ROUSSEAU-LORTIE, Andree; Clinique Med de Hauteville, 4435 boul de Hauteville, Terrebonne QC J6X 2Y6; Mon'74; Staff, CSSS de Thérèse de Blainville; (450)492-3153; Fax. (450)492-9380.

ROUSSEL, Claire N; Southside Med Clinic, 5-640 Prospect St, Fredericton NB E3B 9M7; Mon'95; CCFP; FCFP; Langs: Bilingual(French/English); (506)451-8203; Fax. (506)457-9117.

ROUSSEL, Eric; CSSS Pierre Boucher, 1333 boul Jacques-Cartier E, Longueuil QC J4M 2A5; Mon'06; FRCPC; Anes. Staff, Centre Hospitalier Pierre Boucher; (450)468-8111

ROUSSEL, Guy; 617 Rte de la Montagne RR 1, N-Dame-du-Portage QC G0L 1Y0; Laval'80; Otol (P.Q.). Staff, Centre Hospitalier Regional du Grand-Portage; (418)868-1010

ROUSSEL, Marc; CSSS de Manicouagan, 635 boul Jolliet, Baie-Comeau QC G5C 1P1; Laval'00; CCFP; Staff, Centre Hospitalier Régional Baie-Comeau; (418)589-3701

ROUSSEL, Renee; CLSC Reseau Sante Kamouraska, RR 1 595 av Martin, Saint-Pascal QC G0L 3Y0; Laval'82; Staff, Centre Hospitalier Regional du Grand-Portage; Staff, Agence de santé et des services sociaux de la Montérégie; (418)856-7000 x3100

ROUSSEL, Robin; CHUQ-Ctr Hosp Univ Laval, 2705 boul Laurier, Quebec QC G1V 4G2; Sher'00; Staff, Centre Hospitalier Universitaire de Quebec-CHUL; (418)525-4444

ROUSSEL, Stephane; 18 rue Saint-Omer, Levis QC G6V 5C2; Mon'99; Psy. (418)835-7155; Fax. (418)835-7199.

ROUSSEL-CANUEL, Amelie; CSSS de Beauce-Etchemin, 1515 17e rue, Saint-Georges QC G5Y 4T8; Laval'08; Staff, Centre Hospitalier Beauce-Etchemin; (418)228-2031

ROUSSEL-JOBIN, Aude; CHUQ-Hotel-Dieu de Quebec, 11 Cote du Palais, Quebec QC G1R 2J6; Laval'07; FRCPC; AnatPath. Staff, Centre Hospitalier Universitaire de Québec (CHUQ) - Siege Social; (418)525-4444 x23677

ROUSSELLE, Rejeanne; Clinique Med De Tracadie, PO Box 3634 Stn Main, Tracadie-Sheila NB E1X 1G5; Laval'90; CCFP; Staff Emerg, Hôpital de Tracadie-Sheila; (506)395-1143; Fax. (506)395-1150.

ROUSSEV, Ross; 104-40 Wynford Dr, North York ON M3C 1J5; Tor'85; FRCPC; IntMed (Electromyography); Neur. Staff, Toronto East General Hospital Inc; (416)445-2811; Fax. (416)445-2365.

ROUSSIN, Andre; 601-1851 rue Sherbrooke E, Montreal QC H2K 4L5; Mon'76; FRCPC; IntMed (Vascular Medicine). Chef Laboratoire Vasculaire, Institut de Cardiologie de Montréal; Chef Laboratoire Vasculaire, Centre Hospitalier l'Université de Montréal (CHUM) - Hôpital Notre-Dame; assoc Prof, Universite de Montreal; (514)526-5772; Fax. (514)527-0210; andreroussin@earthlink.net.

ROUSSIN, Brent C; First Nations Inuit Health, 300-391 York Ave, Winnipeg MB R2P 2X8; Man'00; FRCPC; Public Health & Preventive Med;CCFP.

ROUSSOS, Marios; Thunder Bay Reg HSC-T-Bay, 980 Oliver Rd, Thunder Bay ON P7B 6V4; Qns'05; FRCPC; IntMed; Critical Care Medicine. Staff, Thunder Bay Regional Health Sciences Centre; (807)684-6366

ROUSSY, Jacques; Centre Pediatrique de Laval, 300-1150 boul de l'Avenir, Laval QC H7N 6L2; Mon'71; Peds. Staff, Hôtel-Dieu de Lévis; (450)686-0822; Fax. (450)686-2388.

ROUSTAIAN, Kaveh; Pontiac Health Centre, 200 rue Argue, Shawville QC J0X 2Y0; Tehran (Iran)'96; Staff, Pontiac Hospital Centre; (819)347-3851

ROUSTAN DELATOUR, Nicolas L D; Montfort Hosp, 713 Montreal Rd, Ottawa ON K1K 0T2; Ott'04; AnatPath. Staff, The Ottawa Hospital - General Campus; (613)746-4621

ROUTH, John M C; Port Hope Med Centre, 204-249 Ontario St, Port Hope ON L1A 3Y9; Bristol (England)'66; MB ChB; DA; (905)885-5511

ROUTHIER, Brigitte; CLSC Laurier-Station, 135 rue de la Station SS 1, Laurier-Station QC G0S 1N0; Laval'92; Prof Unite Med Familiale, Université Laval; (418)728-3435; Fax. (418)728-3477.

ROUTHIER, Gaetane; Universite Laval, 1050 av de la Medicine, Quebec QC G1V 0A6; Sher'75; LMCC; CSPQ; Gastroent. vice Doyen, Université Laval; (418)654-2168; Fax. (418)654-2164; gaetane.routhier@fmulaval.ca.

ROUTHIER, J J Richard; Polyclinique Med Buckingham, 147 rue Joseph, Gatineau QC J8L 1G3; Ott'82; Staff, CH-CHSLD de Papineau - Pavillon du centre hospitalier; Langs: English; French; (819)986-1034; Fax. (819)986-3308.

ROUTHIER, J O Richard; Social Development Canada, 333 North River Rd, Ottawa ON K1A 0L1; Ott'71; (613)952-2170

ROUTHIER, Line; Clinique Med Fam Chandler, CP 788 60-120 boul Rene-Levesque, Chandler QC G0C 1K0; Laval'93; Staff Emerg, Centre Hospitalier de Chandler; Langs: English; (418)689-3344; Fax. (418)689-6085.

ROUTHIER, Marie-Claude; Centre Med Ste-Foy Inc, 802 av du Chanoine-Scott, Quebec QC G1V 3N4; Laval'94; Physician, CLSC Desjardins Levis; Langs: English; French; (418)653-4931; Fax. (418)653-4797.

ROUTHIER, Nathalie; Hop du Sacre-Coeur de Mtl, 5400 boul Gouin O, Montreal QC H4J 1C5; Laval'02; FRCPC; IntMed. Staff, Hôpital du Sacre-Coeur de Montréal; (514)338-2222

ROUTHIER, Shelley Ann A; 688 Emily St, Hanmer ON P3P 1E4; Qns'95; CCFP; Staff, Health Sciences North-St Joseph's Health Centre; Langs: English; French; (705)969-5560; Fax. (705)969-1402.

ROUTHIER, Valerie; CSSS du Lac-des-Deux-Montagnes, 520 boul Arthur-Sauve, Saint-Eustache QC J7R 5B1; Mon'04; Staff, Hôpital de Saint-Eustache; (450)473-6811

ROUTLEDGE, Robin; PO Box 662 Stn Main, Duncan BC V9L 3Y1; Cal'76; FRCPC; Psy. Ac Staff Psy, Cowichan District Hospital; Physician, Duncan Mental Health Centre; (250)748-7420; Fax. (250)748-7420.

ROUTLEDGE, W Michael; Winnipeg Reg Health Authority, 2-490 Hargrave St, Winnipeg MB R3A 0X7; Man'98; FRCPC; CommunMed;CCFP; (204)940-3610; mroutledge@wrha.mb.ca.

ROUTLEY, Ian G; Lillooet Med Clinic, PO Box 850 107 8th St, Lillooet BC V0K 1V0; UBC'87; (250)256-7505; Fax. (250)256-7591.

ROUTY, Jean-Pierre G; MUHC-Royal Victoria Hosp, 687 av des Pins O, Montreal QC H3A 1A1; Marseille (France)'85; Hem (AIDS/HIV). Staff, McGill University Health Centre - Royal Victoria Hospital; Physician SIDA Health Canada, Government du Quebec; McGill University; (514)843-1558; Fax. (514)843-1418; jean-pierre.routy@mcgill.ca.

ROUVINEZ BOUALI, Nicole G; Children's Hosp Eastern Ont, 401 Smyth Rd, Ottawa ON K1H 8L1; Lausanne (Switzerland)'88; Staff, Children's Hospital of Eastern Ontario (CHEO); (613)737-8561; Fax. (613)737-8889.

ROUX, Alain; Hop Charles LeMoyne, 3120 boul Taschereau, Greenfield Park QC J4V 2H1; Mon'78; Neursurg. Staff, Hopital Charles LeMoyne; (450)466-5000 x3034; alain.roux@videotron.ca.

ROUX, Audrey; Hop Maisonneuve-Rosemont, 5415 boul de l'Assomption, Montreal QC H1T 2M4; Mon'05; FRCPC; RadOncol. Staff, Hopital Maisonneuve-Rosemont; (514)252-3400

ROUX, Christian; CSSS Kamouraska-Hop Notre-Dame, CP 460 1201 6e av, La Pocatiere QC G0R 1Z0; Laval'01; CCFP; Staff, CSSS de Kamouraska; (418)856-7000

ROUX, Daniel; Clinique Med Notre-Dame, 138 rue Notre-Dame S, Sainte-Marie QC G6E 4A4; Laval'80; CCFP; (418)387-5200; Fax. (418)387-5283; daniel_roux@ssss.gouv.qc.ca.

ROUX, Emile V W; 3-679 King George Hwy, Miramichi NB E1V 1N9; Pretoria (South Africa)'96; MB ChB; MMed(ORL); Staff, Miramichi Regional Hospital; Langs: Afrikaans; (506)627-7535; Fax. (506)627-7533.

ROUX, Ettienne; Eljen Med Clinic, 1300 111 Ave, Dawson Creek BC V1G 2X5; Orange Free (South Africa)'03; MB ChB; Langs: Afrikaans; (250)782-7525; Fax. (250)782-3318.

ROUX, Jan G; Virden Med Associates, PO Box 730, Virden MB R0M 2C0; Pretoria (South Africa)'86; Langs: Afrikaans; Zulu; German; (204)748-1345; Fax. (204)748-1640.

ROUX, Jean-Francois; CHUS-Hop Fleurimont, 3001 12e av N, Sherbrooke QC J1H 5N4; Sher'99; FRCPC; IntMed; Cardiol. Staff, Centre Hospitalier Universitaire de Sherbrooke-Hopital Fleurimont; (819)346-1110 x14326

ROUX, Josua P; 201-243 Fouth Ave S, Williams Lake BC V2G 1J8; Pretoria (South Africa)'08; MB ChB; (250)398-8102

ROUX, Larissa; Lifemark Sport Medicine, 160-6111 River Rd, Richmond BC V7C 0A2; Alb'96; MPH; PhD; CCFP; Langs: Russian; French; (604)707-2273

ROUX, Louise; Polyclinique Les Sources, 641 4e rue O, Amos QC J9T 2S1; Laval'95; FRCPC; Neur (Parkinson's Disease). Staff Neurol, CH Hôtel-Dieu d'Amos; Langs: Bilingual(French/English); (819)732-1244; Fax. (819)732-4646; lroux@cableamos.com.

ROUX, Michel; CSSS de Saint-Jerome, 290 rue de Montigny, Saint-Jerome QC J7Z 5T3; Mon'94; CSPQ; FRCPC; Anes. Staff, Hôtel-Dieu de Saint-Jérôme; (450)431-8200

ROUX, Pieter G V D; Chetwynd Centre Med Clinic, PO Box 1485, Chetwynd BC V0C 1J0; Stellenbosch (South Africa)'74; BSc; MB ChB; LMCC; AFOM; (250)788-3234; Fax. (250)788-3237; gerhardtroux@yahoo.ca.

ROUX, Rene; 581 rue Heriot, Drummondville QC J2B 1B8; Sher'72; IntMed. Ac Staff, Hôpital Sainte-croix; (819)472-3212

ROUX, Veronique; 169 Botsford St, Moncton NB E1C 4X4; Sher'03; FRCPC; IntMed; Nephrol. (506)857-3020; Fax. (506)855-2847; veronique.roux@vitalite.nb.ca.

ROUZATI, Amir; Medprime Med Centre, 34C-100 Steeles Ave W, Thornhill ON L4J 7Y1; Man'01; (905)762-9996; Fax. (905)762-0038.

ROUZBAHMAN, Marjan; Univ Hlth Network-Toronto Gen, EW11E 215-200 Elizabeth St, Toronto ON M5G 2C4; Tehran (Iran)'97; FRCPC; AnatPath. Staff, Toronto General Hospital - UHN; (416)340-4564

ROVIS, Katarina; Child & Parent Resource Inst, 600 Sanatorium Rd, London ON N6H 3W7; Zagreb (Croatia)'66; FAAP; FRCPC; Peds (Developmental Pediatrics)., University of Western Ontario; Langs: Croatian; (519)858-2774 x2085; Fax. (519)858-1917.

ROWAN, Declan M; Petawawa Centennial Hlth Ctre, 154 Civic Centre Rd, Petawawa ON K8H 3H5; Trinity College Dublin (Ireland)'94; MB; CCFP; (613)687-7641; Fax. (613)687-6808; drrowanpatients@pcfhc.ca.

ROWAN, J Peter; Oakdale Med Bldg, 308-2065 Finch Ave W, North York ON M3N 2V7; Ott'71; CCFP; CCFP(E.M.); Ac Staff, Humber River Regional Hospital - Finch Avenue Site; (416)741-2217; Fax. (416)741-2349.

ROWAN, Kevin R; North Shore Med Imaging, 139 16th St W, North Vancouver BC V7M 1T3; UBC'98; FRCPC; DiagRad. Staff, Lions Gate Hospital; (604)987-9729; Fax. (604)984-8395.

ROWAN, Robert A; Rideau Valley Health Services, 1221 Greenbank Rd, Ottawa ON K2J 5V7; Ott'74; (613)258-8710

ROWAND, Deborah C; Meadowlark Health Centre, 140 Meadowlark Shopping Ctr NW, Edmonton AB T5R 5W9; Cal'77; (780)489-8470; Fax. (780)484-1620.

ROWAT, Bruce M T; Sun Life Financial Tower, 1600-150 King St W, Toronto ON M5H 1J9; McG'71; FACP; CM; CSPQ; FRCPC; IntMed (Insurance Medicine). Staff Physician Med & Emerg Med, Toronto General Hospital - UHN; Med Dir, Sun Life Assurance Co; Chief/Advisor Medical, Bank of Montreal; Adjunct Assoc Prof, University of Toronto; Langs: English; French; (416)350-8142; Fax. (416)915-0885; rowat@ican.net.

ROWE, Andrea; Cambridge Mem Hosp, 700 Coronation Blvd, Cambridge ON N1R 3G2; (Other Foreign)'06; Staff, Cambridge Memorial Hospital; (519)621-2330

ROWE, Brian H; University of Alberta Hosp, 1G1.43-8440 112 St NW, Edmonton AB T6G 2B7; Ott'84; MSc; CCFP; CCFP(E.M.); Staff Emerg, University of Alberta Hospital; Dir Research/Prof/Assoc Dean Clin Reserch, University of Alberta; (780)407-6707; Fax. (780)407-3982.

ROWE, Charles D; Oshawa Clinic, 117 King St E, Oshawa ON L1H 1B9; Wes'75; BSc; FRCSC; ObstGyn. Ac Staff, Lakeridge Health - Oshawa Site; Queen's University; (905)721-3568; Fax. (905)721-3558.

ROWE, Cheryl J; 86 Dearbourne Ave, Toronto ON M4K 1M7; Dal'80; FRCPC; Psy (Women's Issues). Asst Prof, University of Toronto; (416)469-8064

ROWE, Donald G; Physicians Incorporated, 203-316 Willow St, Truro NS B2N 5A4; Dal'90; BSc(Hons.); MSc; Physician, South Cumberland Community Care Centre; (902)895-3535; Fax. (902)895-3444.

ROWE, Ernest N; London HSC-University Hosp, PO Box 5339 Stn B 339 Windermere Rd, London ON N6A 5A5; Mem'07; FRCSC; Urol. Staff, London Health Sciences Centre - University Hospital; (519)663-3352

ROWE, Helen S; Mercantile Centre, 55 Union St, Saint John NB E2L 5B7; Glasgow (Scotland)'79; MB ChB; FRCPC; Psy (Adult Psychiatry). Staff, Saint John Regional Hospital; (506)658-3737; Fax. (506)658-3739.

ROWE, Judy A; Queen Elizabeth II HSC, 3226-1276 South Park St, Halifax NS B3H 2Y9; Mem'97; FRCPC; DiagRad. Staff, Queen Elizabeth II Health Sciences Centre - Victoria General Site; (902)473-2700; Fax. (902)473-2018.

ROWE, Patrick D; Willow Point Med Clinic, 2116D South Island Hwy, Campbell River BC V9W 1C1; Orange Free State (South Africa)'81; CCFP; (778)420-0770; Fax. (778)420-0772.

ROWE, Patrick D; PO Box 2359 Stn B, Prince George BC V2N 2J8; UBC'92; CCFP; CCFP(E.M.); FCFP.

ROWE, Richard C; Health Sciences Centre, GB409-700 William Ave, Winnipeg MB R3E 0Z3; Adelaide (Australia)'70; MB BS; MEd; FRCPC; IntMed (Endocrinology). Prof IntMed, University of Manitoba; (204)787-3601; Fax. (204)787-4826.

ROWE, Timothy C; BC Women's Hosp & Health Ctre, D6-4500 Oak St, Vancouver BC V6H 3N1; Adelaide (Australia)'71; MB BS; FRCOG; FRCSC; ObstGyn (Infertility). Staff, BC Women's Hospital & Health Centre; (604)875-2534

ROWE MAHON, P Elaine; Stratford Gen Hosp, 46 General Hospital Dr, Stratford ON N5A 2Y6; Mem'85; BSc; BMedSci; FRCPC; AnatPath. Staff, Stratford General Hospital - Huron Perth Healthcare Alliance; (519)272-8210

ROWED, David W; 77 Risebrough Ave, Toronto ON M2M 2E2; Wes'66; BA; FRC; FRCSC; Neursurg (Neuro Surgical Consultant). Staff Surg, Sunnybrook Health Sciences Centre; Prof, University of Toronto; (416)733-0233; Fax. (416)480-6085; david.rowed@hotmail.com.

ROWELL-WONG, Joanne L; 203-3825 Sunset St, Burnaby BC V5G 1T4; UBC'91; CCFP; CCFP(E.M.); (604)434-9515; Fax. (604)434-5984.

ROWEN, John P; St Mary's Hosp Centre, 3830 av Lacombe, Montreal QC H3T 1M5; Qns'89; CCFP; CCFP(E.M.); FCFP; Staff, St Mary's Hospital Centre; (514)345-3511

ROWHANI-SEKI, Neda; Orillia Soldiers Mem Hosp, 170 Colborne St W, Orillia ON L3V 2Z3; Ott'93; MD; CCFP; FCFP; Ac Staff Privil, Orillia Soldiers' Memorial Hospital; (705)325-2201 x0; Fax. (705)327-7233.

ROWICKA, Malgorzata D; Spryfield Family Med Clinic, 315 Herring Cove Rd, Halifax NS B3R 1V5; Warsaw (Poland)'83; Court Staff, IWK Health Centre; Langs: Polish; (902)479-0025; Fax. (902)479-2627.

ROWICKA, Monika M; Eastside Health Centre, 688A East River Rd, New Glasgow NS B2H 3S1; Warsaw (Poland)'83; CCFP; (902)752-3632; Fax. (902)755-5532.

ROWLAND, Gerald C; Tillsonburg Med Clinic, PO Box 516 Stn Main, Tillsonburg ON N4G 4J1; Wes'78; BSc(Hons.); Langs: English; French; (519)842-3682; Fax. (519)842-8711.

ROWLAND, Mary J; North Kingston Comm Health Ctr, 400 Elliott Ave, Kingston ON K7K 6M9; McM'01; CCFP; (613)542-2949

ROWLAND, Richard; Queen's Family Health Team, PO Bag 8888 220 Bagot St, Kingston ON K7L 5E9; Tor'71; MCFP(EM); Langs: English; French; (613)533-9303; Fax. (613)544-9899.

ROWLANDS, Donna R; 72 Brant Ave, Brantford ON N3T 5Z8; Mem'91; CCFP; CCFP(E.M.); Staff, The Brant Community Healthcare System - Brantford General Hospital Site; (519)770-0128

ROWLEY, Christopher J; 178 Main St PO Box 400, Mount Forest ON N0G 2L0; Ott'98; CCFP; (519)509-2100; Fax. (519)509-2102; crowley@mac.com.

ROWLEY, Victor A; 899 12th Ave W, Vancouver BC V5Z 1M9; Alb'78; FRCPC; DiagRad. Ac Staff, Vancouver General Hospital - Centennial Pavillion; (604)875-4770; Fax. (604)875-4228.

ROWLINSON, F Anthony; 281 Ontario St, Collingwood ON L9Y 1N2; Tor'73; Chair Medical Ethics, Collingwood General & Marine Hospital; (705)444-1555; Fax. (705)444-1550.

ROWNTREE, Carol I; Greenwood Fam Physicians, PO Box 5, Sundre AB T0M 1X0; Cal'87; CCFP; FCFP; Clinical Asst Prof, University of Calgary; (403)638-2424; Fax. (403)638-3580.

ROWSELL, Corwyn H; Sunnybrook Hlth Sciences Ctre, E428B-2075 Bayview Ave, Toronto ON M4N 3M5; Tor'00; FRCPC; AnatPath. Staff, Sunnybrook Health Sciences Centre; (416)480-6100 x7751

ROWSOM, John T; The Medical Centre, 707 Charlotte St, Peterborough ON K9J 2X5; Wes'78; FRCSC; GenSurg. Staff GenSurg, Peterborough Regional Health Centre - Hospital Drive; (705)876-4515; Fax. (705)876-4546.

ROWTHORN, Leanne M; Lions Gate Hosp, 231 15th St E, North Vancouver BC V7L 2L7; McM'06; CCFP; CCFP(E.M.); Staff, Lions Gate Hospital; (604)985-6406

ROXBOROUGH, Vaughan S; Oromocto Med Clinic, 1285 Onondaga St, Oromocto NB E2V 2P8; Dal'69; Ac Staff, Oromocto Public Hospital; Court Staff, Dr Everett Chalmers Regional Hospital; (506)357-8445; Fax. (506)357-9351; oromed@nb.aibn.com.

ROXBURGH, Brian; Cape Breton Hlthcare Complex, 1482 George St, Sydney NS B1P 1P3; Glasgow (Scotland)'78; MB ChB; MRCPsy; Staff, Glace Bay Healthcare Facility; Staff, Cape Breton Healthcare Complex; (902)567-7703; Fax. (902)567-7493.

ROXIN, Gheorghe S; Calder Health Care Centre, PO Box 190, Burgeo NL A0N 2H0; Tirgu Mures (Romania)'76; Gen Practice, Calder Health Care Centre; (709)886-3350; Fax. (709)886-3382.

ROXIN, Gyorgy; 1811 9 Ave S, Lethbridge AB T1J 1W6; Mem'05; FRCSC; GenSurg (Colorectal Surgery). Staff, Foothills Medical Centre; (403)317-1890

ROXIN, Sara; Calder Health Care Centre, PO Box 190, Burgeo NL A0N 2H0; Tirgu-Mures (Romania)'76; Gen Physician, Calder Health Care Centre; (709)886-3352; Fax. (709)886-3382.

ROY, A Michael; Aberdeen Hosp, 835 East River Rd, New Glasgow NS B2H 3S6; Sask'02; FRCPC; IntMed. Staff, Aberdeen Regional Hospital; (902)752-7600

ROY, Alain; 1814 boul Saint-Joseph E, Montreal QC H2H 1C7; Mon'83; NBME(USA); Ac Staff, Centre Hospitalier l'Université De Montréal (CHUM) - Hôpital Saint-luc; (514)523-3563

ROY, Alain; Hop Maisonneuve-Rosemont, 5415 boul de l'Assomption, Montreal QC H1T 2M4; Mon'79; FRCSC; OrthSurg (Hips Surgery). Dept Head, Hopital Maisonneuve-Rosemont; Dept Head, Hôpital Santa Cabrini Ospedale; Clin Prof, Universite de Montreal; Langs: Bilingual(French/English); (514)257-0619; Fax. (514)257-1966.

ROY, Alain; GMF Montee de la Baie, 3942 ch Oka, St-Joseph-Du-Lac QC J0N 1M0; Mon'87; Langs: Bilingual(French/English); (450)473-7375; Fax. (450)473-2160.

ROY, Alexandra; Findlay Creek Med Center, 4744 Bank St, Greely ON K4P 3W7; Ott'09; CCFP.

ROY, Aline; Clinique Med l'Edifice Central, 204-31 rue King O, Sherbrooke QC J1H 1N5; Sher'88; Langs: English; (819)346-6111; Fax. (819)346-7184.

ROY, Alphonse; Centre Med Berger, 308-1000 ch Sainte-Foy, Quebec QC G1S 2L6; Laval'67; PlasSurg. Staff, Centre Hospitalier Affilié Universitaire de Québec - Hôpital du St-Sacrement; Staff, Centre Hospitalier Universitaire De Québec - Pavillon De St-françois-d'assise; (418)688-0822; Fax. (418)688-0822.

ROY, Amelia; Clinique Sante Jacques-Cartier, 200-1815 rue King O, Sherbrooke QC J1J 2E3; McG'05; CCFP; Staff, Centre Hospitalier Universitaire de Sherbrooke-Hôpital Hôtel-Dieu; Clin Prof Family Med, Universite de Sherbrooke; Langs: Bilingual(French/English); (819)565-7446; Fax. (819)565-7780.

ROY, Andre; 103-850 Grande Allée O, Quebec QC G1S 1C4; Laval'64; Staff, Centre d'hébergement de Beauceville; (418)527-1416

ROY, Andre; Ctr Hosp Affilie-Enfant-Jesus, 1401 18e rue, Quebec QC G1J 1Z4; Laval'75; IntMed. Ac Staff, Centre Hospitalier Affilié Universitaire de Québec - Hôpital du St-Sacrement; Staff, Centre Hospitalier Affilié Universitaire de Québec - Hôpital De L'Enfant Jésus; (418)649-5882

ROY, Andre; Clinique familiale des Hauts-B, 99 boul des Hauts-Bois, Sainte-Julie QC J3E 3J9; Laval'72; Langs: Bilingual(French/English); (450)649-2490; Fax. (450)649-2218.

ROY, Andre; Centre Med Durocher, 140 rue Saint-Vallier O, Quebec QC G1K 1K1; Mon'74; Ac Staff, CSSS de Quebec-Sud; (418)529-0291; Fax. (418)529-7405.

ROY, Andre; Clinique de Physiatrie, 130-100 ch Rockland, Mont-Royal QC H3P 2V9; Mon'93; FRCPC; PhysMed&Rehab. Staff, Institut de Réadaptation Gingras-Lindsay de Montréal; (514)907-0063

ROY, Andre F; CHUM-Hop St-Luc, 1058 rue Saint-Denis, Montreal QC H2X 3J4; Mon'85; FRCSC; GenSurg (Hepatobiliary Transplant Surgery). Staff Surg & HepatoBiliary & Endoscopy, Centre Hospitalier l'Université De Montréal (CHUM) - Hôpital Saint-luc; Physician, Government du Quebec; assoc Prof, Universite de Montreal; (514)890-8000 x36146; Fax. (514)281-6147.

ROY, Andre G; Hotel-Dieu de Levis, 143 rue Wolfe, Levis QC G6V 3Z1; Laval'85; CSPQ; FRCPC; Anes. ac Staff, Hôtel-Dieu de Lévis; (418)835-7121; Fax. (418)835-3969; morphee@ssss.gouv.qc.ca.

ROY, Andre L; 245-919 Centre St NW, Calgary AB T2E 2P6; Sher'79; FRCPC; IntMed (Cardiology).

ROY, Ann-Veronique; Ctr Hosp Laurentien, 234 rue Saint-Vincent, Ste-Agathe-des-Mts QC J8C 2B8; Mon'07; Peds. Staff, Centre Hospitalier Laurentien; (819)324-4000

ROY, Anne; MUHC-Royal Victoria Hosp, 687 av des Pins O, Montreal QC H3A 1A1; Laval'75; CSPQ; FRCPC; DiagRad. Staff, McGill University Health Centre - Royal Victoria Hospital; (514)934-1934

ROY, Annie; CSSS de Laval, 1755 boul Rene-Laennec, Laval QC H7M 3L9; Mon'92; FRCPC; IntMed; Cardiol. Staff Cardiol, Hopital de la Cite de la santé; (450)668-1010

ROY, Anthony; Ctr Hosp de la Rég de L'Amiant, 1717 rue Notre-Dame E, Thetford Mines QC G6G 2V4; Laval'06; FRCSC; GenSurg. Staff, Hopital du CSS de la Region de Thetford.

ROY, Bernadette; Ctr Hosp de Charlevoix, 74 rue Ambroise-Fafard, Baie-Saint-Paul QC G3Z 2J6; Sher'90; Staff, CSSS de Charlevoix; Langs: English; (418)435-5150

ROY, Bruno; 603 9e av, Beauceville QC G5X 1J2; Laval'74; (418)774-3100

ROY, Carmella A; SMBD Jewish Gen Hosp, A530-3755 ch Cote-Sainte-Cathe, Montreal QC H3T 1E2; Dal'93; CSPQ; FRCPC; Psy. Clin Asst, Sir Mortimer B Davis Jewish General; Langs: Spanish; French; (514)340-8222 x5897; carmella@vl.videotron.ca.

ROY, Carolyne D; 100-311 McArthur Ave, Vanier ON K1L 8M3; Ott'85; CCFP; Staff, The Ottawa Hospital - General Campus; Teacher, University of Ottawa; (613)749-1414; Fax. (613)749-2007.

ROY, Christiane; CLSC Kateri, 90 boul Marie-Victorin, Candiac QC J5R 1C1; Mon'89; (450)659-7661; Fax. (450)444-6276.

ROY, Christiane; CHSLD Cartierville, 12235 rue Grenet, Montreal QC H4J 2N9; Mon'88; Staff, Hôpital du Sacre-Coeur de Montréal; (514)337-7300

ROY, Christine; GMF Centre de santé, 3745 rue Georges-Couture, Drummondville QC J2B 7P4; Sher'88; ac Staff, Hôpital Sainte-croix; (819)477-2231; Fax. (819)477-1122.

ROY, Christine; CSSS Becancour Nicolet-Yamaska, 216 rue Principale, Fortierville QC G0S 1J0; Laval'07; CCFP; (819)287-4442

ROY, Claude C; Hôpital Ste-Justine, 3175 ch Cote-Sainte-Catherine, Montreal QC H3T 1C5; Laval'54; Gastroent (P.Q.); Peds. Staff Gastroent Nutrition Serv, Hôpital Ste-Justine; Emeritus Prof, Universite de Montreal; Langs: Bilingual(French/English); (514)345-4931 x6202; Fax. (514)345-4999; claude.roy@recherche-ste-justine.qc.ca.

ROY, Daniel; CHUM-Hop Notre-Dame, 1560 rue Sherbrooke E, Montreal QC H2L 4M1; Mon'84; CSPQ; FRCPC; DiagRad. Staff, Centre Hospitalier l'Université de Montréal (CHUM) - Hôpital Notre-Dame; (514)890-8000 x25856; daniel.roy.chum@ssss.gouv.qc.ca.

ROY, Daniel; 286 rue de Normandie, Sainte-Julie QC J3E 1A7; Mon'76; Staff Perinatal, Centre Hospitalier Pierre Boucher; (450)649-1593; Fax. (450)649-0361.

ROY, Daniel J; 36 rue du Pont, Saint-Leonard NB E7E 1Y1; Mon'93; Langs: English; (506)423-6669; Fax. (506)423-6446.

ROY, Danielle M; Prairie Trail Med Centre, 100-1345 Taylor Ave, Winnipeg MB R3M 3Y9; Man'04; CCFP; (204)475-0088

ROY, Danny; CSSS Cleophas-Claveau, CP 38 succ La Baie 1000 rue du Docteur-Desgagne, La Baie QC G7B 3P9; Laval'10; CCFP; Staff, CHSLD-CLSC Cleophas-Claveau; (418)544-3381

ROY, Deborah; U of Waterloo Health Service, 200 University Ave W, Waterloo ON N2L 3G1; Alb'74; BMedSci; CCFP; Staff, Grand River Hospital - Kitchener/Waterloo Health Centre; Staff, St Mary's General Hospital; Physician Student Health Services, University Of Waterloo; (519)888-4567; Fax. (519)746-5023.

ROY, Denis; Inst Nat'l de Sante Publique d, 945 rue Wolfe, Quebec QC G1V 5B3; Laval'77; CSPQ; FRCPC; CommunMed. Staff, McGill University Health Centre - Montreal General Campus; (514)864-1600 x5320

ROY, Denis; Institut de Cardiologie de Mtl, 5000 rue Belanger, Montreal QC H1T 1C8; Mon'76; FRCPC; Cardiol (Electrophysiology). gén Dir, Institut de Cardiologie de Montréal; Langs: Bilingual(French/English); (514)376-3330; Fax. (514)593-2540; denis.roy@icm-mhi.org.

ROY, Denis; Sudbury Reg Hosp-Laurentian Si, 41 Ramsey Lake Rd, Sudbury ON P3E 5J1; Ott'72; Nephrol (P.Q.); IntMed. Staff, Health Sciences North-Laurentian Site; Langs: Spanish; French; (705)523-7100

ROY, Denis; Hop Charles LeMoyne, 3120 boul Taschereau, Greenfield Park QC J4V 2H1; Sher'87; CSPQ; FRCPC; Anes. Staff Anes, Hopital Charles LeMoyne; (450)466-5000

ROY, Denis-Claude; Hop Maisonneuve-Rosemont, 5415 boul de l'Assomption, Montreal QC H1T 2M4; Mon'82; ABIM; ABIM(Hem); FRCPC; IntMed (Stem Cell Transplantation); Hem. Dir Research Centre, Hopital Maisonneuve-Rosemont; Aj Prof, McGill University; Prof Med, Universite de Montreal; Langs: English; (514)252-3404; Fax. (514)254-5094; denis-claude.roy@umontreal.ca.

ROY, Diane; Clinique Med Ville Emard, 5824 boul Monk, Montreal QC H4E 3H3; Mon'82; Physician, CSSS de Verdun; Langs: English; (514)767-5307; Fax. (514)767-0217.

ROY, Dominique; CLSC Saint-Hubert, 6800 bboul Cousineau, Saint-Hubert QC J3Y 8Z4; Mon'09; CCFP; (450)443-7407

ROY, Elise; Universite de Sherbrooke, 200-150 Place Charles-Le Moyne, Longueuil QC J4K 0A8; Sher'79; MSc; (450)463-1835 x61823

ROY, Elyse; CLSC-CHSLD La Source, 190 76e rue E, Quebec QC G1H 7K4; Laval'02; Staff, Hotel-Dieu d'Arthabaska; (418)628-2572

ROY, Eric; 22 College St, Toronto ON M5G 1K2; Laval'02; CCFP; (416)922-2672; Fax. (416)922-4254.

ROY, Fabienne; Hopital Regional D'Edmundston, 275 boul Hebert, Edmundston NB E3V 4E4; Laval'94; Staff, Hôpital regional d'Edmundston; (506)739-2610; Fax. (506)736-6610.

ROY, Felix-Nicolas; CHUM-Hotel-Dieu, 3840 rue Saint-Urbain, Montreal QC H2W 1T8; Mon'01; FRCPC; NuclearMed. Staff, Centre Hospitalier l'Université de Montréal (CHUM) - Hôtel-Dieu; (514)890-8000

ROY, France; CSSS de la Region de Thetford, 1717 rue Notre-Dame E, Thetford Mines QC G6G 2V4; Laval'74; CSPQ; FRCPC; Anes. Ac Staff Anes, Hopital du CSS de la Region de Thetford; (418)338-7777

ROY, Francis F; Clinique Chirurgivision T R In, 579 rue Laviolette, Trois-Rivieres QC G9A 1V6; Sher'86; FRCSC; Ophth (Cataract). Med Dir, Clinique Chirurgivision T R Inc; (819)693-5757; Fax. (819)373-9482; communication@chirurgivision.com.

ROY, Francois; Clin Med Belvedere, 202-2235 rue Galt O, Sherbrooke QC J1K 1K6; Sher'05; CCFP; (819)563-4244; Fax. (819)563-8924.

ROY, Genevieve; CHUQ-Ctr Hosp Univ Laval, A 1602-2705 boul Laurier, Quebec QC G1V 4G2; Laval'94; FRCPC; Peds. Clin Prof, Centre Hospitalier Universitaire de Quebec-CHUL; Langs: English; French; (418)656-4141; Fax. (418)654-2158; genevieve.roy@mail.chuq.qc.ca.

ROY, Genevieve; Les Gynecologues Associes, 100-235 boul Rene-Levesque E, Montreal QC H2X 1N8; Mon'97; MPH; FRCSC; ObstGyn. Clinical Asst Prof, Centre Hospitalier l'Université De Montréal (CHUM) - Hôpital Saint-luc; Clinical Asst Prof, Universite de Montreal; Langs: Bilingual(French/English).

ROY, Genevieve; Hotel-Dieu de Levis, 143 rue Wolfe, Levis QC G6V 3Z1; Laval'04; FRCPC; Psy. Staff, Hôtel-Dieu de Lévis; (418)835-7121

ROY, Ghyslain; 325 boul Greber, Gatineau QC J8T 8J3; Sher'87; (819)561-4445; Fax. (819)561-3393.

ROY, Gilles; Clinique Med St-Raphael, 101 rue Principale, St-Raphael-Be QC G0R 4C0; Laval'77; Assoc Staff, Hôtel-Dieu de Lévis; (418)243-2115; Fax. (418)243-2054.

ROY, Gilles J; Cambridge Mem Hosp, 700 Coronation Blvd, Cambridge ON N1R 3G2; Ott'08; CCFP; Staff, Cambridge Memorial Hospital; (519)621-2333

ROY, Gregory L; Woodlawn Med Clinic, 92 Main St, Dartmouth NS B2X 1R5; Dal'75; Ac Staff, Dartmouth General Hospital; (902)434-1500; Fax. (902)434-4368.

ROY, Guy; CHUQ-Ctr Hosp Univ Laval, 2705 boul Laurier, Quebec QC G1V 4G2; Laval'78; FRCSC; GenSurg. Ac Staff, Centre Hospitalier Universitaire de Quebec-CHUL; (418)656-4141 x47449

ROY, Guy; Min de la Sante et Serv Sociau, 1075 ch Sainte-Foy, Quebec QC G1S 2M1; Sher'79; CSPQ; FRCPC; CommunMed. Staff, Centre Hospitalier Universitaire de Quebec-CHUL; (418)266-6763; Fax. (418)266-4609.

ROY, Helene; Regie l'Assurance Maladie QC, Q044-1125 Grande Allee O, Quebec QC G1S 1E7; Laval'86; Chief Service de l'Analyse de la Facturation, Regie de l'Assurance Maladie du Quebec; Langs: Spanish; English; (418)682-5144; helene.roy.md@ramq.gouv.qc.ca.

ROY, Helene; CHUQ-Ctr Hosp Univ Laval, 2705 boul Laurier, Quebec QC G1V 4G2; McG'88; FRCPC; Peds. Staff, Centre Hospitalier Universitaire de Quebec-CHUL; (418)654-2282; Fax. (418)654-2137.

ROY, Indrojit; St Mary's Hosp Centre, 3830 av Lacombe, Montreal QC H3T 1M5; McG'80; CSPQ; FRCPC; AnatPath. Staff Path, St Mary's Hospital Centre; assoc Prof, McGill University; Langs: French; Danish; (514)345-3511 x3731; indrojit.roy@ssss.gouv.qc.ca.

ROY, Isabelle; CHUM-Hop Notre-Dame, 1560 rue Sherbrooke E, Montreal QC H2L 4M1; Mon'95; CSPQ; FRCPC; RadOncol. Staff, Centre Hospitalier l'Université de Montréal (CHUM) - Hôpital Notre-Dame; Langs: Bilingual(English/French); (514)890-8254; Fax. (514)412-7537; isabelle.roy.chum@ssss.gouv.qc.ca.

ROY, Isabelle; CHUQ-St-Francois d'Assise, 10 rue de l'Espinay, Quebec QC G1L 3L5; Laval'97; CCFP; Staff, Centre Hospitalier Universitaire De Québec - Pavillon De St-françois-d'assise; (418)525-4444

ROY, Ivan; Clin Externe de Psychiatrie, 765 rue Roland-Forget, Laval QC H7E 4C1; Laval'69; CSPQ; Psy (P.Q.). (450)668-2620; Fax. (450)668-1077.

ROY, Jacinthe; Clinique Med le Plein-Ciel, 475 boul de la Cote-Vertu, Saint-Laurent QC H4L 1X7; Laval'86; (514)337-3171

ROY, Jacques; Clinique Med de l'Ouest, 2200 boul Dionne, Saint-Georges QC G5Y 3X3; Laval'80; (418)228-2024; Fax. (418)228-7715.

ROY, Jean A; Montfort Academic Family Hlth, 101B-745 Montreal Rd, Ottawa ON K1K 0T1; Ott'86; CCFP; FCFP; Assoc Staff, Montfort Hospital; Vice Dean Office Francophone Affairs/Asst Prof, University of Ottawa; Langs: Spanish; (613)749-4429; Fax. (613)749-7942.

ROY, Jean; Hop Maisonneuve-Rosemont, 5415 boul de l'Assomption, Montreal QC H1T 2M4; Laval'84; ABIM(IntMed); ABIM(Hem); FRCPC; IntMed (Bone Marrow Transplant); Hem. Staff, Hopital Maisonneuve-Rosemont; adj Prof, Universite de Montreal; (514)252-3404; jroy.hmr@ssss.gouv.qc.ca.

ROY, Jean; Clinique Med Les Saules, 100-2780 boul Masson, Quebec QC G1P 1J6; Laval'73; Staff, CSSS de Quebec-Sud; (418)871-4492; Fax. (418)877-4478.

ROY, Jean-Denis; CHUM-Hop St-Luc, 1058 rue Saint-Denis, Montreal QC H2X 3J4; Mon'97; FRCA; CSPQ; FRCPC; Anes; GenPath (P.Q.). Staff, Centre Hospitalier l'Université De Montréal (CHUM) - Hôpital Saint-luc; (514)890-8000 x36581; jean-denis.roy@sympatico.ca.

ROY, Jean-Francois; 150-1165 boul Lebourgneuf, Quebec QC G2K 2C9; Laval'83; FRCSC; OrthSurg (Spine Surgery). Ac Staff, Centre Hospitalier Universitaire De Québec - Pavillon De St-françois-d'assise; Langs: Bilingual(English/French); (418)627-3097; Fax. (418)627-5313.

ROY, Jean-Philippe; 158 rue Principale, Saint-Jacques NB E7B 1W4; Sher'07; CCFP; (506)739-7767; Fax. (506)739-8266.

ROY, Jean-Philippe; Clinique Med du Phare, 101-822 boul Sainte-Anne, Rimouski QC G5M 1J5; Laval'03; Staff, Hôpital Regional Rimouski; (418)723-5135; Fax. (418)724-2251.

ROY, Jean-Pierre; MUHC-Montreal Neurology Inst, 3801 rue University, Montreal QC H3A 2B4; Laval'79; FRCPC; Neur. Staff, McGill University Health Centre - Montreal Neurological Hospital; Assoc Staff, McGill University Health Centre - Royal Victoria Hospital; adj Prof, McGill University; (514)398-1911

ROY, Jean-Sebastien; CSSS de Laval, 1755 boul Rene-Laennec, Laval QC H7M 3L9; Mon'96; CSPQ; FRCPC; Anes. Staff, Hopital de la Cite de la santé; (450)668-1010 x2477

ROY, Jean-Yves; CHUQ-Ctr Hosp Univ Laval, 2705 boul Laurier, Quebec QC G1V 4G2; Laval'79; CSPQ; FRCPC; Psy (Consultation Liaison Pediatric Psychiatry). Ac Staff, Centre Hospitalier Universitaire de Quebec-CHUL; (418)654-2256; Fax. (418)654-2756.

ROY, Johanne; Clinique Med St-Vincent, 250 rue King E, Sherbrooke QC J1G 1A9; Sher'90; (819)563-0510; Fax. (819)564-6889.

ROY, Johanne; CSSS de Temiscouata, CP 310 58 rue de l'Eglise, Notre-Dame-du-Lac QC G0L 1X0; Sher'94; CCFP; Staff, Centre Hospitalier Notre-Dame-du-Lac; (418)899-6751

ROY, Josee-Anne; Hop du Sacre-Coeur de Mtl, 5400 boul Gouin O, Montreal QC H4J 1C5; Mon'87; Hem; IntMed. Staff, Hôpital du Sacre-Coeur de Montréal; (514)338-2150; Fax. (514)338-2631.

ROY, Julie; Clinique Med Saint-Louis, 220-3165 ch Saint-Louis, Quebec QC G1W 4R4; Laval'86; LMCC; Staff, CSSS de la Matapedia; (418)653-1970; Fax. (418)653-9956.

ROY, Julie; GMF La Cigogne, 420-3141 boul Taschereau, Greenfield Park QC J4V 2H2; Sher'02; CCFP; Staff, Hopital Charles LeMoyne; (450)466-7892

ROY, Kamalesh C; Weyburn Med Clinic, 110 3rd St, Weyburn SK S4H 0W2; Calcutta (India)'57; FRCS(Ed); MRCS(Lond); LRCP(Eng); FICS; Staff, Weyburn General Hospital; Staff, Weyburn Community Health Services (Mental Health); (306)842-5404

ROY, Katie; 208-600 boul Dieppe, Dieppe NB E1A 9J8; Sher'08; CCFP.

ROY, Leonard W; Valley Med Clinic, 335 Jubilee St, Duncan BC V9L 1W9; Sask'74; CCFP; FCFP; Chair Med Advisor Committee/Chief Staff, Cowichan District Hospital; Clinical Asst Prof, University of British Columbia; (250)748-8151; Fax. (250)748-8157; lwroy@shaw.ca.

ROY, Louis J; 218-2780 av Raymond, Saint-Hyacinthe QC J2S 5W7; Mon'78; OrthSurg. Ac Staff, Centre Hospitalier Honore-Mercier; (450)774-3930; Fax. (450)250-7476.

ROY, Louis; CSSS de Laval, 1755 boul Rene-Laennec, Laval QC H7M 3L9; Mon'03; FRCSC; OrthSurg. Staff, Hopital de la Cite de la santé; (450)668-1010

ROY, Louis; CLSC La Source, 190 76e rue E, Quebec QC G1H 7K4; Sher'86; Staff, Centre Hospitalier Affilié Universitaire de Québec - Hôpital De L'Enfant Jésus; Langs: Bilingual(French/English); (418)628-5630

ROY, Louis; Hôpital Laval, 2725 ch Sainte-Foy, Quebec QC G1V 4G5; Laval'76; Cardiol (P.Q.). Staff, Hôpital Laval; (418)656-4862; Fax. (418)656-4544.

ROY, Louis-Edouard; Complexe Sante Reine-Elizabeth, 444-2100 av de Marlowe, Montreal QC H4A 3L5; Mon'65; CSPQ; FRCPC; Neur; Electroenceph (P.Q.). Staff, Hopital Maisonneuve-Rosemont; adj Prof, Universite de Montreal; Langs: English; (514)489-8582; Fax. (514)489-1683; louise.edouard_roy@yahoo.ca.

ROY, Louise; CSSS de Montmagny-L'Islet, RR 1 350 boul Tache O, Montmagny QC G5V 3R8; Sher'73; Staff, CSSS de Montmagny-L'Islet; (418)248-0630x5563; Fax. (418)248-0820.

ROY, Louise; CHUM-Hop St-Luc, 1058 rue Saint-Denis, Montreal QC H2X 3J4; Mon'87; CSPQ; Anes. Staff, Centre Hospitalier l'Université De Montréal (CHUM) - Hôpital Saint-luc; (514)890-8358

ROY, Louise; CHUM-Hop St-Luc, 1058 rue Saint-Denis, Montreal QC H2X 3J4; Mon'80; FRCPC; IntMed (Pharmacology); Nephrol. Staff Nephrol/Prof adj clin, Centre Hospitalier l'Université De Montréal (CHUM) - Hôpital Saint-luc; Langs: English; (514)890-8000 x32588; Fax. (514)412-7342; louise.roy@umontreal.ca.

ROY, Luc; Clinique Med St-Louis, 504 rue Saint-Louis, Joliette QC J6E 2Z2; Mon'75; (450)759-0581; Fax. (450)759-0584.

ROY, Lucie E; Clin Fam des Basses Laurentide, 2100 boul Cure-Labelle, Saint-Jerome QC J7Y 1S8; Mon'78; Peds. (450)565-1227

ROY, Lucie E; Regie des Rentes du Quebec, CP 5200 Succ Terminus, Quebec QC G1K 7S9; Laval'75; Staff, Hôtel-Dieu de Lévis; (418)657-8709

ROY, Lucie; CSSS de la Haute-Yamaska, 205 boul Leclerc O, Granby QC J2G 1T7; Mon'86; Staff, Centre Hospitalier de Granby; Staff, Foyer de Val d'Or; (450)372-5491

ROY, Madan M; Hamilton HSC-McMaster Site, PO Box 2000 Stn Lcd 1 3N11G-1200 Main St W, Hamilton ON L8N 3Z5; Bangalore (India)'79; MRCP(UK); FRCPC; Peds (Neonatology). Dir Neonatal Nurseries, Hamilton Health Sciences Centre - McMaster Children's Hospital; Prof, McMaster University; Langs: Hindi; (905)521-2100 x75639; Fax. (905)521-4981.

ROY, Madeleine; Inst de Recherche Clin de Mtl, 110 av des Pins O, Montreal QC H2W 1R7; Laval'64; MSc; principale Chercheur, Institut de Recherche Clin de Montreal; (514)987-5742; Fax. (514)987-5732.

ROY, Marc J; West End Family Care Clinic, 80 Michael Cowpland Dr, Kanata ON K2M 1P6; Ott'94; CCFP; FCFP; Court Staff Privil, Carleton Place & District Memorial Hospital; Langs: English; French; Spanish; (613)599-3321

ROY, Marc-Andre; Inst U en Sante Mentale de QC, 2601 ch de la Canardiere, Quebec QC G1J 2G3; Laval'85; CSPQ; MSc; FRCPC; Psy. VP, Institut Universitaire Sante; Prof Centre de Recherche, Université Laval; (418)663-5741; Fax. (418)663-9540; marc-andre.roy@crulrg.ulaval.ca.

ROY, Marcel; 105-185 rue Acadie, Dieppe NB E1A 1G6; Sher'84; CCFP; (506)862-4182; Fax. (506)862-4179; marcel@health.nb.ca.

ROY, Marie L; Don Mills-Eglinton Med Centre, 100-29 Gervais Dr, North York ON M3C 1Z1; Tor'79; PhD; CCBOM; FRCPC; OccupMed (Toxicology). Court Staff, North York General Hospital; Consultant Orthopeds Holland Centre, Sunnybrook Health Sciences Centre; Med Consultant Occupational & Environmental Med, Marie L Roy Professional Corporation; Aj Prof, University of Toronto; Langs: English; French; (416)449-5511; Fax. (416)449-9334.

ROY, Marie; Hôpital Laval, 2725 ch Sainte-Foy, Quebec QC G1V 4G5; Mon'91; CCFP; Staff, Hôpital Laval; (418)656-4550

ROY, Marie-Andree; Hop du Sacre-Coeur de Mtl, 5400 boul Gouin O, Montreal QC H4J 1C5; Sher'99; CCFP; CCFP(E.M.); Staff, Hôpital du Sacre-Coeur de Montréal; (514)338-2222; Fax. (514)338-2384.

ROY, Marie-Christine; 200-594 av Victoria, Saint-Lambert QC J4P 2J6; Laval'74; ABD; FRCPC; Derm (Laser Dermatology). (450)672-2885; Fax. (450)672-1674; drmerey@bellnet.ca.

ROY, Marie-Christine; Ctr d'Obstetrique/Gynecologie, 4250 av 1Re, Quebec QC G1H 2S5; Laval'94; CSPQ; FRCSC; ObstGyn (Colposcopy). Langs: English; (418)654-0555; Fax. (418)654-1898.

ROY, Marie-Christine; Clinique Leger et Associes, 201-1851 rue Sherbrooke E, Montreal QC H2K 4L5; Mon'93; FRCPC; DiagRad. Staff, Hopital Maisonneuve-Rosemont; (514)523-2121

ROY, Marie-Claude; Ctr Hosp Affilie-Enfant-Jesus, 1401 18e rue, Quebec QC G1J 1Z4; Laval'87; Microbio & Infect Dis (P.Q.); MedMicrobiol (P.Q.) (Infectious Diseases). Staff, Centre Hospitalier Affilié Universitaire de Québec - Hôpital De L'Enfant Jésus; Langs: English; (418)649-0252 x3202

ROY, Marie-Claude; CHUS-Hop Fleurimont, 3001 12e av N, Sherbrooke QC J1H 5N4; Sher'02; Peds. Staff, Centre Hospitalier Universitaire de Sherbrooke-Hopital Fleurimont; (819)346-1110

ROY, Marie-Claude; CHUQ-Ctr Hosp Univ Laval, R1742-2705 boul Laurier, Quebec QC G1V 4G2; Sher'95; FRCPC; Peds; Nephrol. Staff, Centre Hospitalier Universitaire de Quebec-CHUL; (418)654-2282; Fax. (418)654-2137; marie-claude.roy@mail.chuq.qc.ca.

ROY, Marie-Hélène; Hotel-Dieu de Levis, 143 rue Wolfe, Levis QC G6V 3Z1; Laval'91; LMCC; Microbio & Infect Dis (P.Q.); MedMicrobiol (Infectiology). Staff, Hôtel-Dieu de Lévis; (418)835-7121; mhelene_roy@ssss.gouv.qc.ca.

ROY, Marie-Josee; CSSS Pierre-Boucher, 1333 boul Jacques Cartier E, Longueuil QC J4M 2A5; Laval'95; FRCPC; Peds. Staff, Centre Hospitalier Pierre Boucher; Langs: Bilingual(French/English); (450)468-8111

ROY, Marie-Lou; Centre Sante des Etchemins, 331 rue du Sanatorium, Lac-Etchemin QC G0R 1S0; Laval'04; CCFP; Staff, CSSS des Etchemins; (418)625-8001

ROY, Marie-Pierre; Hopital Laval, 2725 ch Sainte-Foy, Quebec QC G1V 4G5; Laval'05; Staff, Hôpital Laval; (418)656-8711

ROY, Mario; Hop Louis-H Lafontaine, 7401 rue Hochelaga, Montreal QC H1N 3M5; Mon'94; CSPQ; BSc(Biol.); FRCPC; Psy (Affective Disorders). assoc Membre, Hopital Louis-H Lafontaine; Ac Member, Douglas Mental Health University Institute; Lecturer, McGill University; Clin Teach Staff, Universite de Montreal; (514)251-4000 x2176

ROY, Martine; Ctr Hosp de Verdun, 4000 boul Lasalle, Verdun QC H4G 2A3; Mon'85; (514)362-1000

ROY, Martine; CLSC Carrefour Sante Jonquiere, 3667 boul Harvey, Jonquiere QC G7X 3A9; Sher'96; Staff Phys, Centre Hospitalier Jonquiere; Physician, CLSC Jonquiere; Langs: English; (418)695-2572; Fax. (418)695-8282; martine.roy@ssss.gouv.qc.ca.

ROY, Martine N; 192-17010 90 Ave NW, Edmonton AB T5T 1L6; Alb'90; FRCSC; ObstGyn (Colposcopy). Ac Staff, Covenant Health - Misericordia Community Hospital; Consultant, Cross Cancer Institute; University of Alberta; Langs: French; (780)483-2901; Fax. (780)483-2910.

ROY, Mathieu; CSSS de Rimouski-Neigette, CP 3150 Succ A 150 av Rouleau, Rimouski QC G5L 5T1; Laval'06; Staff, Hôpital Regional Rimouski; (418)723-7851; Fax. (418)724-8615.

ROY, Mathieu; Clinique Med Pierre Boucher, 1615 boul Jacques-Cartier E, Longueuil QC J4M 2X1; Mon'83; FRCSC; GenSurg. (450)468-6223; Fax. (450)468-5041.

ROY, Maurice J B; Seine Med Centre, 125-142 Centrale Ave, Ste Anne MB R5H 1C3; Mon'85; CCFP; FCFP; Langs: English; (204)422-8811; Fax. (204)422-5876.

ROY, Maurice P; 223 ch Madawaska, Grand Falls NB E3Y 1A5; Mem'87; Staff, Hôpital Général de Grand-Falls; Physician, McCain Foods; Langs: English; French; (506)473-6444; Fax. (506)473-6866.

ROY, Maxime; Direction de Sante Publique de, 1301 rue Sherbrooke E, Montreal QC H2L 1M3; Mon'97; FRCPC; CommunMed; Public Health & Preventive Med. (514)528-2400

ROY, Melanie; Ctr d'Ophth Acadie-Bathurst, 2-939 St. Peter Ave, Bathurst NB E2A 2Z3; Sher'00; FRCSC; Ophth. Staff, Hopital Regional Chaleur; Langs: Bilingual(French/English); (506)548-2722; Fax. (506)548-5722.

ROY, Melanie; CSSSG-Hop de Hull, 116 boul Lionel-Emond, Gatineau QC J8Y 1W7; Laval'05; FRCPC; Anes. Staff, Hull Hospital; (819)595-6000

ROY, Melodie; Clin de Sante Jacques-Cartier, 200-1815 rue King O, Sherbrooke QC J1J 2E3; Sher'07; (819)565-7446; Fax. (819)565-7780.

ROY, Michel A; Clin de Chirurgie Plastique, 504-2960 boul Laurier, Quebec QC G1V 4S1; Laval'72; PlasSurg (P.Q.). Ac Staff, Centre Hospitalier Affilié Universitaire de Québec - Hôpital De L'Enfant Jésus; Associate, Centre Hospitalier Universitaire de Quebec-CHUL; Associate, Jeffery Hale Hospital-Saint Brigid's; (418)682-8827; Fax. (418)659-4791; roymd@videotron.ca.

ROY, Michel G; CLSC Laurier-Station, 135 rue de la Station SS 1, Laurier-Station QC G0S 1N0; Laval'78; (418)728-3435; Fax. (418)728-2233.

ROY, Michel; Hôpital Ste-Justine, 3175 ch Cote-Sainte-Catherine, Montreal QC H3T 1C5; Mon'98; FRCPC; Peds; PedEmergMed (P.Q.). Staff, Hôpital Ste-Justine; (514)345-4931 x4788; mikeroy24@hotmail.com.

ROY, Michel; CHUQ-Hotel-Dieu de Quebec, 11 Cote du Palais, Quebec QC G1R 2J6; Laval'67; FRCSC; ObstGyn (Colposcopy); GynOnco (P.Q.). Consultant, Centre Hospitalier Affilié Universitaire de Québec - Hôpital du St-Sacrement; Staff, Centre Hospitalier Universitaire de Québec (CHUQ) - Siege Social; Prof, Université Laval; Langs: English; (418)691-5392; Fax. (418)691-5720; michel.roy@ogy.ulaval.ca.

ROY, Michel R; CLSC Mer Et Montagnes, 600 av William-May GD, Murdochville QC G0E 1W0; Laval'72; Gen Practice, Installation CLSC Gaspe; (418)784-2572; Fax. (418)784-3629.

ROY, Michelle; Ctre Regional de Sante Mentale, RR 1 242 montee Gagnon, Ste-Anne-d-Plaines QC J0N 1H0; Laval'82; CSPQ; FRCPC; Psy. Staff, Institut Philippe-Pinel de Montreal; (450)478-5960; Fax. (450)478-0638.

ROY, Michelle; GMF Cote-des-Neiges, 5700 ch de la Cote-des-Neiges, Montreal QC H3T 2A8; Mon'95; (514)731-8531; Fax. (514)731-9600.

ROY, Mili; Credit Valley Eye Care, 1-3200 Erin Mills Pkwy, Mississauga ON L5L 1W8; Man'91; BSc(Med); FRCSC; Ophth (Uveitis). Staff, Credit Valley Eye Care; (905)820-3937; Fax. (905)820-0111.

ROY, Mononita; The Ottawa Hosp-Civic Campus, 1053 Carling Ave, Ottawa ON K1Y 4E9; Dal'08; IntMed. Fellow, The Ottawa Hospital - Civic Campus; (613)761-4795

ROY, Nadine; 202-185 av Acadie, Dieppe NB E1A 1G6; Sher'98; CCFP; Staff, Dr Georges-L-Dumont University Hospital Centre; (506)860-7203; Fax. (506)862-1265.

ROY, Nancy; CSSSG-Hop de Gatineau, CP 2000 Succ Bureau-Chef 909 boul de la Verendrye, Gatineau QC J8P 7H2; Laval'95; FRCSC; GenSurg. Staff, Hôpital de Gatineau; Langs: Bilingual(English/French); (819)561-8100; drenancyroy@videotron.ca.

ROY, Nathalie A L; 202-1280 Lasalle Blvd, Sudbury ON P3A 1Y8; Ott'99; BSc(BioChem.); CCFP; Langs: English; French; (705)671-3001; Fax. (705)671-3003.

ROY, Nathalie A M; Polyclinique, 314-874 boul de l'Universite E, Chicoutimi QC G7H 6B9; Sher'88; FRCPC; IntMed (Rehabilitation Medicine); Cardiol. Staff, Complexe hospitalier de la Sagamie; Universite de Sherbrooke; (418)545-0539; Fax. (418)545-1032.

ROY, Nathalie; Clin Med Asbestos, 605 boul Simoneau, Asbestos QC J1T 4G7; Mon'98; (819)879-7447; Fax. (819)879-7881.

ROY, Nathalie; Hotel-Dieu de Levis, 143 rue Wolfe, Levis QC G6V 3Z1; Mon'98; CSPQ; FRCPC; IntMed; Rheum. Staff, Hôtel-Dieu de Lévis; Langs: English; (418)835-7121; Fax. (418)835-7134.

ROY, Olivier; CSSS de Trois-Rivières, 1991 boul du Carmel, Trois-Rivieres QC G8Z 3R9; Laval'98; CCFP; CCFP(E.M.); Staff, CSSS de Trois-Rivières; (819)697-3333

ROY, Paul D; 208-1355 Bank St, Ottawa ON K1H 8K7; Man'90; FRCPC; Psy. Staff Psy, The Ottawa Hospital - General Campus; Asst Prof Psy, University of Ottawa; Langs: English; French; paroy@ottawahospital.on.ca.

ROY, Peter D; Medical & Dental Bldg, 400-3939 50A Ave, Red Deer AB T4N 4E6; Dal'74; MSc; FRCSC; GenSurg. (403)347-9037; Fax. (403)348-8470.

ROY, Pierre; B-106 Commerciale Ave RR 1, Tring-Jonction QC G0N 1X0; Laval'92; (418)426-2026; Fax. (418)426-2519.

ROY, Pierre-Michel; Inst U Geriatrie Sherbrooke, 1036 rue Belvedere S, Sherbrooke QC J1H 4C4; Laval'78; CCFP; ac Staff, CSSS Institut universitaire de gériatrie de Sherbrooke; Staff, Centre Hospitalier Universitaire de Sherbrooke-Hôpital Hôtel-Dieu; (819)821-5100

ROY, Pierre-Olivier; CSSS Les Eskers de l'Abitibi, 622 4e rue O, Amos QC J9T 2S2; Sher'03; FRCPC; IntMed. Staff, CH Hôtel-Dieu d'Amos; (819)732-3341

ROY, Pierre-Olivier; CSSS d'Antoine-Labelle-Mt Laur, RR 1 2561 ch de dla Lievre S, Mont-Laurier QC J9L 3G3; Mon'07; Staff, CSSS d'Antoine-Labelle; (819)623-1234

ROY, Regent; 84 Daniel-Johnson CP 630, Danville QC J0A 1A0; Laval'65; (819)839-3191

ROY, Rejean; Centre Med Berger, 416-1000 ch Sainte-Foy, Quebec QC G1S 2L6; Laval'72; CSPQ; FRCSC; Urol. Ac Staff, Hôpital Laval; (418)266-2876; Fax. (418)266-2879.

ROY, Rejean; Clinique Med Sainte-Claire, GD 88 boul Begin, Sainte-Claire QC G0R 2V0; Mon'73; (418)883-3336; Fax. (418)883-2890.

ROY, Renee; Inst Philippe Pinel de Mtl, 10905 boul Henri-Bourassa E, Montreal QC H1C 1H1; Mon'80; CSPQ; CRCP; FRCPC; Psy (Legal Psychiatry). Staff, Institut Philippe-Pinel de Montreal; Vice Dean Postgrad Med Studies, Universite de Montreal; (514)648-8461 x354; Fax. (514)881-3705.

ROY, Richard; CSSS de la Baie-des-Chaleurs, RR 2 419 boul Perron, Maria QC G0C 1Y0; Laval'76; CSPQ; FRCPC; DiagRad. Staff, CSSS de la Baie-des-Chaleurs; (418)759-3443 x2519; Fax. (418)759-3151.

ROY, Robert P A; 318 Gilmore Ave, Burnaby BC V5C 4R1; Man'91; FRCSC; ObstGyn. Langs: Bilingual(French/English); (604)294-8550; Fax. (604)294-8560; robertproy@yahoo.ca.

ROY, Roger; CLSC Haute-Ville-des-Rivieres, 2400 av d'Estimauville, Quebec QC G1E 7G9; Laval'71; Physician Occupational Health, CSSS de la Vielle Capitale; Langs: Bilingual(French/English); (418)623-1010 x227; Fax. (418)623-7513.

ROY, Roland; Hotel-Dieu de Sorel, 400 av de l'Hotel-Dieu, Sorel-Tracy QC J3P 1N5; Laval'73; AB; CSPQ; Anes. Staff, CSSS du Coeur de l'Isle Hôpital Jean-Talon; Staff, Hôtel-Dieu de Sorel; (450)746-6239

ROY, Sebastien; Cite de la Sante de Laval, 1755 boul Rene-Laennec, Laval QC H7M 3L9; Mon'00; CSPQ; FRCPC; Anes (Intensive Care). Staff, Hopital de la Cite de la santé; Langs: English; (450)668-1010

ROY, Sophie; Clin Med Familiale Cowansville, 499 rue du Sud, Cowansville QC J2K 2X9; Sher'04; (450)263-8890; Fax. (450)263-9737.

ROY, Sophie; CSSS de Beauce-Etchemin, 1515 17e rue, Saint-Georges QC G5Y 4T8; Mon'03; CCFP; CCFP(E.M.); Staff, Centre Hospitalier Beauce-Etchemin; (418)228-2031

ROY, Stephane; CSSS Pierre Boucher, 1333 boul Jacques-Cartier E, Longueuil QC J4M 2A5; Mon'88; Electroenceph (P.Q.); Neur (P.Q.). Staff, Centre Hospitalier Pierre Boucher; (450)468-8111

ROY, Stephane; Direction de la Sante Publique, 1255 rue Beauregard, Longueuil QC J4K 2M3; Sher'86; Consultant, Centre Hospitalier Honore-Mercier; (450)928-6777; Fax. (450)928-3023.

ROY, Suzanne; CLSC Vallee des Forts, 978 boul du Seminaire N, St-Jean-Sur-Richel QC J3A 1E5; Sher'87; CCFP; (450)358-2572

ROY, Suzanne; 678 rue Niverville, Trois-Rivieres QC G9A 2A4; Sher'82; Ac Staff Obst, Centre Hospitalier Regional de Trois-Rivieres; Langs: English; Spanish; (819)697-3033; Fax. (819)233-4731; npelletier@infoteck.qc.ca.

ROY, Sylvain; CSSS Drummond-Hop Sainte-Croix, 570 rue Heriot, Drummondville QC J2B 1C1; Sher'99; CSPQ; FRCPC; DiagRad. Staff, Hôpital Sainte-croix; (819)478-6464 x3200; Fax. (819)478-6480; sylvain.roy@ssss.gouv.qc.ca.

ROY, Sylvie; Centre Medical des Generations, 200-465 rue Bibeau, Saint-Eustache QC J7R 0C8; Mon'92; LMCC; Staff, Hôpital de Saint-Eustache; Langs: English; (450)472-1955; Fax. (450)472-1905; sroy@cm25.ca.

ROY, Valerie; Clin Pediatrique des Mille-Ile, 203-233 rue Turgeon, Sainte-Therese QC J7E 3J8; Laval'93; FRCPC; Peds. Staff, Hôpital de Saint-Eustache; (450)434-8006; Fax. (450)434-8007.

ROY, Veronique-Elisabeth; Clinique de Med Familiale, 101-940 boul des Recollets, Trois-Rivieres QC G8Z 3W9; Sher'08; Staff, CSSS de Trois-Rivières; (819)373-0303

ROY, Viateur; 34 boul Montcalm S, Candiac QC J5R 3M5; Mon'69; LMCC; Physician, CHSLD Mgr Coderre; Langs: Bilingual(French/English); (450)672-6651; Fax. (450)672-6653; vroy01@sympatico.ca.

ROY, W M Lawrence; The Hosp for Sick Children, 2211-555 University Ave, Toronto ON M5G 1X8; Dal'72; FRCPC; Anes (Pediatrics). I-VP Medical, The Hospital For Sick Children; Assoc Prof Anes, University of Toronto; (416)813-7445; Fax. (416)813-7543; lawrence.roy@sickkids.ca.

ROY, William A; Brooklin Med Centre, 1A-5959 Anderson St, Brooklin ON L1M 2E9; Tor'70; (905)655-3321; Fax. (905)655-4848.

ROY, Yvan; Clinique Med l'Assomption, 814 boul l'Ange-Gardien N, L'Assomption QC J5W 4M9; Mon'76; Dir Prof Services, CHSLD Cardinal Inc; Ac Staff, Centre Hospitalier Pierre le Gardeur; Ac Staff, Hopital Maisonneuve-Rosemont; (450)589-5778; Fax. (450)589-5779.

ROY, Yves; Coop Sante Ste-Marguerite, 25 rue des Pins, Ste-Marg-Esterel QC J0T 1L0; McG'84; (450)228-3100; Fax. (450)228-1702.

ROY, Yvon; Clinique Med Rochette, 2372 boul Louis-XIV, Quebec QC G1C 5K1; Laval'84.

ROY-BOULOS, Anne-Marie; Univ of Ottawa Hlth Services, 100 Marie Curie St, Ottawa ON K1N 6N5; Sher'76; FRCPC; Derm. Langs: English; French; (613)564-3950

ROY-FLEISING, Celine; MUHC-Montreal Children's Hosp, 2300 rue Tupper, Montreal QC H3H 1P3; Laval'77; ABPeds; FRCPC; Peds. Assoc Staff, McGill University Health Centre - Montreal Children's Hospital; (514)412-4400; cliniqueviau@videotron.ca.

ROY-LACROIX, Marie-Eve; The Ottawa Hosp-Gen Campus, 501 Smyth Rd, Ottawa ON K1H 8L6; Sher'06; FRCSC; ObstGyn. Staff, The Ottawa Hospital - General Campus; (613)325-7915

ROY-MATTON, Naome; CSSS de l'Energie-Ste-Therese, 1705 av Georges, Shawinigan QC G9N 2N1; Sher'05; FRCSC; ObstGyn. Staff, CH du Centre-de-la-Mauricie (Ste-Thérèse de Shawinigan); (819)536-7500; naome_roy-matton@ssss.gouv.qc.ca.

ROY TALBOT, Vincent; CSSS de la Region de Thetford, 1717 rue Notre-Dame E, Thetford Mines QC G6G 2V4; Mon'10; CCFP; Staff, Hopital du CSS de la Region de Thetford; (418)838-7794

ROYAL, Pierre; Hotel-Dieu de Sorel, 400 av de l'Hotel-Dieu, Sorel-Tracy QC J3P 1N5; Sher'81; FRCSC; GenSurg; EmergMed. Staff, Hôtel-Dieu de Sorel; (450)746-6100

ROYAL, Virginie; Hop Maisonneuve-Rosemont, 5415 boul de l'Assomption, Montreal QC H1T 2M4; Mon'02; FRCPC; AnatPath. Staff, Hopital Maisonneuve-Rosemont; (514)252-3498

ROYE, Charmaine A; Avenue Med Clinic, 221 Brant Ave, Brantford ON N3T 3J3; McG'81; FRCSC; ObstGyn. Langs: English; French; (519)753-8666; Fax. (519)753-3109.

ROYEPPEN, Edmund C; Associate Med Clinic, 400-20 14th St W, Prince Albert SK S6V 3K8; Natal (South Africa)'89; FRCSC; GenSurg. (306)953-1653; Fax. (306)764-3091.

ROYER, Christelle; CSSS de la Haute-Yamaska, 205 boul Leclerc O, Granby QC J2G 1T7; Sher'03; Staff, Centre Hospitalier de Granby; Langs: Bilingual(French/English); (450)375-8000

ROYER, Helene; 575 rue Saint-Amable, Quebec QC G1R 2G4; Laval'82; CCFP; (418)644-1075; Fax. (418)644-7719.

ROYER, Nicole; Clinique Med de Cacouna, RR 1 132-535 rue du Patrimoine, Cacouna QC G0L 1G0; Laval'88; (418)862-2170; Fax. (418)862-2506.

ROYER, Paule; CSSS de Memphremagog, 50 rue Saint-Patrice E, Magog QC J1X 3X3; Sher'88; Médecin Family Med, Centre Hospitalier et CLSC de Memphremagog; (819)843-3381

ROYER, Sandrine; CSSS de Chicoutimi, CP 5006 305 rue Saint-Vallier, Chicoutimi QC G7H 5H6; Mon'06; CCFP; CCFP(E.M.); Staff, Complexe hospitalier de la Sagamie; (418)541-1000

ROYER-LAVAL, Joanie; Clinique Med Sainte-Dorothee, 102-1 boul Samson, Laval QC H7X 3S5; Mon'10; (450)689-6334

ROYLE, Mary-Clare H; The Ottawa Hosp-Civic Campus, 1053 Carling Ave, Ottawa ON K1Y 4E9; Mem'03; FRCPC; Psy. Staff, The Ottawa Hospital - Civic Campus; (613)761-4581

ROZARIO, Duncan R; Chamber of Commerce Bldg, 205-345 Lakeshore Rd E, Oakville ON L6J 1J5; Qns'92; FACS; LMCC; DABS; FRCSC; GenSurg. Staff, Halton Healthcare Services Corporation - Oakville Site; (905)845-3614; Fax. (905)845-4310.

ROZE, Gundars E; Mackenzie Richmond Hill Hosp, 10 Trench St, Richmond Hill ON L4C 4Z3; Tor'94; FRCPC; Anes. Court Staff, Mackenzie Richmond Hill Hospital; Langs: Latvian; French; (905)883-1212

ROZE DES ORDONS, Amanda; The Ottawa Hosp-Gen Campus, 501 Smyth Rd, Ottawa ON K1H 8L6; Alb'06; FRCPC; Anes. Staff, The Ottawa Hospital - General Campus; (613)737-8701

ROZEFORT, Willine R; 6875 boul Lasalle, Verdun QC H4H 1R3; (Mexico)'85; LMCC; MSc; CCFP; FCFP; Dir Interimaire des Services Professionnels et Hospitaliers, Douglas Mental Health University Institute; Langs: Creole; Spanish; English; French; (514)761-6131 x2636; Fax. (514)333-3996.

ROZEHNAL, Jan; 799 Bloor St W, Toronto ON M6G 1L8; Mon'82; Langs: German; French; Czech; Slovak; Italian; (416)533-1330; Fax. (416)533-2740.

ROZEN, Dima; Rothbart Centre for Pain Care, 9-4646 Dufferin St, North York ON M3H 5S4; (Netherlands Antilles)'95; (416)512-6407; Fax. (416)512-6375.

ROZEN, Jamie; CLSC Metro, 1801 boul de Maisonneuve O, Montreal QC H3H 1J9; McG'09; CCFP; (514)934-0354

ROZENBERG, Anna; McMaster University, MDCL 3101A-1280 Main St W, Hamilton ON L8S 4K1; McM'06; FRCPC; Anes.

ROZENBERG, Dmitry; 1110-373 Front St W, Toronto ON M5V 3R7; Ott'08; IntMed. (416)206-8615

ROZENCWAIG, Roman R; Westmount Med Bldg, 355-5025 rue Sherbrooke O, Montreal QC H4A 1S9; McG'73; BSc; Langs: Russian; (514)487-0439; Fax. (514)487-0267.

ROZENFARB, Eva; 518 rue Notre-Dame, Repentigny QC J6A 2T8; Sher'82; AB; FRCPC; Derm. Langs: Polish; French; (450)582-1110; Fax. (450)582-0092.

ROZENTAL-KLINGER, Emmanuel; Campbellton Reg Hosp, PO Box 880 Stn Main 189 Lily Lake Rd, Campbellton NB E3N 3H3; Del Rosario (Colombia)'80; FRCSC; GenSurg. Staff, Hôpital Régional Campbellton.

ROZMUS, Jacob; Children's & Women's HC of BC, A119-4480 Oak St, Vancouver BC V6H 3V4; Alb'05; FRCPC; Peds; PedHemaOncol. Staff, BC Children's Hospital; (604)875-2322

ROZON, Jacques; Centre Med Fontainebleau, 102-10 boul des Chateaux, Blainville QC J7B 1Z5; Sher'82; Staff, Hopital de la Cite de la santé; (450)419-8811; Fax. (450)419-7758.

ROZON-RIVEST, Monique; Centre de Sante de Rigaud, 1 rue Hotel de Ville, Rigaud QC J0P 1P0; Mon'76; (450)451-5336; Fax. (450)451-5214.

ROZWADOWSKI, Marek A; West Coast Gen Hosp, 3949 Port Alberni Hwy, Port Alberni BC V9Y 4S1; Cape Town (South Africa)'75; BSc(Med); CAFCI; Staff, West Coast General Hospital; Langs: Polish; Afrikaans; (250)731-1370

RRAFSHI, Lulzim; South Western Med Ctr, 813 Richmond St, London ON N6A 3H6; (Romania)'97; CCFP; (519)433-4330; Fax. (519)433-4332.

RUANE, Bernard J; 402 Borland St, Williams Lake BC V2G 1R7; Dublin (Ireland)'85; MB ChB; BAO; DCH; CCFP; (250)392-7221

RUBAB, Shehla; Saskatoon City Hosp, 701 Queen St, Saskatoon SK S7K 0M7; Nishtar (Pakistan)'92; Staff, Saskatoon City Hospital; (306)655-8045; Fax. (306)655-8119.

RUBABAZA, Jean-Placide; 7-3100 Brock St N, Whitby ON L1R 3J7; Ott'05; FRCSC; ObstGyn. (905)665-3100; Fax. (905)665-3120.

RUBAIYYAT, Tania; St Joseph Fam Med & Dental Ctr, 346 Platts Lane, London ON N6G 1J1; Dhaka (Bangladesh)'98; CCFP; Staff, London Intercommunity Health Centre - Dundas Street; (519)660-0874; Fax. (519)660-6127.

RUBENCHIK, Illana A; North York Gen Hosp, 4001 Leslie St, North York ON M2K 1E1; Witwatersrand (South Africa)'88; FRCPC; AnatPath. Staff, North York General Hospital; (416)756-6254

RUBENFELD, Gordon D; Sunnybrook Hlth Sciences Ctre, D503-2075 Bayview Ave, Toronto ON M4N 3M5; Philadelphia (USA)'87; Staff, Sunnybrook Health Sciences Centre; (416)480-6100 x2440; Fax. (416)480-6953.

RUBENIS, Andris A; Rouge Valley Extendicare, 551 Conlins Ave, Scarborough ON M1B 5S1; Tor'70; Court Staff, The Scarborough Hospital - General Campus; Court Staff, Toronto East General Hospital Inc; Staff, Rouge Valley Extendicare; Langs: Latvian; (416)282-6768; Fax. (416)282-6766.

RUBENS, Fraser D; Univ of Ottawa Heart Institute, H3401A-40 Ruskin St, Ottawa ON K1Y 4W7; Qns'85; MD; MScPath; FRCSC; GenSurg (Adult Cardiac Surgery); CardiothorSurg. Staff Ottawa Heart Inst, The Ottawa Hospital - Civic Campus; Prof Dept of Surg, University of Ottawa; (613)761-4720; Fax. (613)761-4713; frubens@ottawaheart.ca.

RUBENS, Mark J; 59 Sinclair St, Dartmouth NS B2Y 1R7; Alb'84; FRCPC; Psy (General Adult Psychiatry). Consultant Psy, Dartmouth General Hospital; Staff Psy, The Nova Scotia Hospital; Asst Prof, Dalhousie University; (902)466-5211; Fax. (902)461-1869.

RUBENSTEIN, Elizabeth J; St Lawrence College, 100 Portsmouth Ave, Kingston ON K6V 5X3; McM'00; CCFP; CCFP(E.M.); (613)544-5400

RUBENSTEIN, Heather; GMF Cote-des-Neiges, 324-5700 ch de la cote-des-Nei, Montreal QC H3T 2A6; McG'80; CCFP; Langs: English; French; (514)731-8531; Fax. (514)731-0563.

RUBENSTEIN, Joel D; Sunnybrook Hlth Sciences Ctre, 2075 Bayview Ave, Toronto ON M4N 3M5; Louisville(KY) (USA)'71; FRCPC; DiagRad (Musculoskeletal Imaging). Staff, Sunnybrook Health Sciences Centre; Assoc Prof, University of Toronto; (416)480-4356; Fax. (416)480-5855.

RUBENSTEIN, Warren H; Box 25 60 Murray St, Toronto ON M5T 3L9; Tor'75; CCFP; FCFP; Ac Staff, Mount Sinai Hospital; Assoc Prof, University of Toronto; (416)586-4800 x5160; Fax. (416)586-3175; wrubenstein@mtsinai.on.ca.

RUBENZAHL, Steven E; 211-1315 Finch Ave W, North York ON M3J 2G6; Tor'89; Staff Family & Palliative Med, Humber River Regional Hospital - Finch Avenue Site; Staff Family Med, North York General Hospital; Langs: English; French; (416)630-9061; Fax. (416)630-2990.

RUBIN, Alexandra S; Cardiogenix Med Center, 100-8250 boul Decarie, Montreal QC H4P 2P5; McG'05; CCFP; (514)731-7717; Fax. (514)731-2228.

RUBIN, Barry B; Univ Hlth Network-Toronto Gen, 6EN 222-200 Elizabeth St, Toronto ON M5G 2C4; McG'86; PhD; FRCSC; VascSurg. Head Div of Vascular Surg, Toronto General Hospital - UHN; Prof Surg, University of Toronto; Langs: English; French; (416)340-3645; Fax. (416)340-5029.

RUBIN, Daniel J; Delta Hosp, 5800 Mountain View Blvd, Delta BC V4K 3V6; Man'81; DABEM; Staff, Surrey Memorial Hospital; (604)946-1121

RUBIN, David H; Laurel Med Centre Ltd, 106-888 8th Ave W, Vancouver BC V5Z 3Y1; Man'76; FRCPC; DiagRad. (604)879-7726; Fax. (604)879-7725.

RUBIN, Earl E; MUHC-Montreal Children's Hosp, C 1341-2300 rue Tupper, Montreal QC H3H 1P3; McG'87; Microbio & Infect Dis (P.Q.); MedMicrobiol; InfectDis; Peds (Pediatric Infectious Diseases). Staff, McGill University Health Centre - Montreal Children's Hospital; assoc Prof, McGill University; (514)412-4313

RUBIN, Evelyn T; Wellpoint Health Centre, 9F-1240 Bay St, Toronto ON M5R 2A7; Tor'06; CCFP; (416)969-3260; Fax. (416)971-7718.

RUBIN, Gary M; 491 Church St, Toronto ON M4Y 2C6; Dal'85; BSc; LMCC; DR; DipAmerican Academy of HIV Med; Court Staff, Sunnybrook Health Sciences Centre; Co-Chair, Toronto HIV Primary Care Physicians Group; Lecturer Family & Community Med, University of Toronto; (416)463-6929; Fax. (416)463-6577.

RUBIN, Gordon; 202-5885 ch de la Cote-des-Nei, Montreal QC H3S 2T2; McG'83; CCFP; Staff, Kateri Memorial Hospital Centre; Langs: English; French; (514)342-4522; Fax. (514)342-2441.

RUBIN, Mitchell B; Mount Seymour Clinic, 2F-333 Seymour Blvd, North Vancouver BC V7J 2J4; McG'91; CCFP; FCFP; Langs: English; French; (604)904-7712; Fax. (604)904-7714.

RUBIN, Sharon R; Queensway Prof Centre, 308-190 Sherway Dr, Etobicoke ON M9C 5N2; Tor'87; Staff, Trillium Health Centre - West Toronto; (416)695-9475; Fax. (416)695-9538.

RUBIN, Sheldon H; Professional Arts Bldg, 624-100 Arden St, Moncton NB E1C 4B7; Dal'69; FRCPC; IntMed (Oncology); Hem. Court Staff, Dr Georges-L-Dumont University Hospital Centre; Ac Staff Dept of IntMed, The Moncton Hospital; (506)857-2881; Fax. (506)856-8115; dr.sheldon.rubin@horizonnb.ca.

RUBIN, Steven Z; Foothills Med Centre, 1403 29 St NW, Calgary AB T2N 2T9; Cape Town (South Africa)'66; FRCS(E); FRCSC; GenSurg; PedGenSurg. Staff, Foothills Medical Centre; Langs: Afrikaans; Hebrew; (403)944-4695

RUBIN, Yair; Rockyview Gen Hosp, 7007 14 St SW, Calgary AB T2V 1P9; Ott'96; FRCPC; Anes. Staff, Rockyview General Hospital; (403)943-8720; Fax. (403)252-2798.

RUBINGER, Morel; Cancercare Manitoba, 2073-675 McDermot Ave, Winnipeg MB R3E 0V9; Timisoara (Romania)'77; FRCPC; IntMed; Hem; MedOncol. Staff MedOncol, Health Sciences Centre; Chair, Lymphoma Working Group; A-Dir, Blood & Marrow Transplant Program-Manitoba; Assoc Prof IntMed, University of Manitoba; Langs: Romanian; (204)787-2108; morel.rubinger@cancercare.mb.ca.

RUBINO, Mary; Wellpoint Family Practice, 9F-1240 Bay St, Toronto ON M5R 2A7; McM'85; CCFP; FCFP; Assoc Staff Fam Practice, Women's College Hospital; (416)971-7601; Fax. (416)971-7718.

RUBINO, Michael; Polyclinique Cabrini, 213-5700 rue Saint-Zotique E, Montreal QC H1T 3Y7; McG'82; CCFP; Staff, Hôpital Santa Cabrini Ospedale; (514)254-8434

RUBINSTEIN, Ethan; 501 Basic Sciences Bldg, 543-745 Bannatyne Ave, Winnipeg MB R3E 0J9; Basel (Switzerland)'68; LLB; Staff, St Boniface General Hospital; Staff, Health Sciences Centre; Langs: German; Hebrew; Bilingual(French/English); (204)977-5681; Fax. (204)789-3926; rubinste@cc.manitoba.ca.

RUBINSTEIN-SCHIPPER, Rachel; SMBD Jewish Gen Hosp, 3755 ch Cote-Sainte-Catherine, Montreal QC H3T 1E2; New York(NY) (USA)'83; ABD; ABIM; FRCPC; Derm. Staff, Sir Mortimer B Davis Jewish General; adj Prof, McGill University; Langs: Hebrew; Yiddish; (514)340-8222 x5819

RUBIO, Dominador B; Quinte HC Corp-Belleville Gen, 265 Dundas St E, Belleville ON K8N 5A9; Manila (Philippines)'73; BSc(Psychol); Ac Staff, QHC Belleville General; Ac Staff, QHC Trenton Memorial; Langs: Spanish; (613)969-5511; Fax. (613)969-0229.

RUBIO-REYES, Carlos A; 900-158 Robert Angus Dr, Amherst NS B4H 4R7; (El Salvador)'74; CCFP; (902)660-3388; Fax. (902)660-3389; carubioreyes@hotmail.com.

RUBLEE, Catherine H; 425 Lower Bench Rd, Penticton BC V2A 8V4; Qns'75; FRCSC; ObstGyn. Consultant, Penticton Regional Hospital; (250)490-7496; crublee@telus.net.

RUBY, Ralph R F; St Joseph's Health Care, PO Box 5777 Stn B 268 Grosvenor St, London ON N6A 4V2; Wes'63; FRCSC; Otol. Staff, St Joseph's Hospital - St Joseph's Health Care; Prof, University of Western Ontario; (519)646-6143; Fax. (519)646-6146.

RUCKER, Christian J; Leslie Diamond Ctr, 8151-2775 Laurel St, Vancouver BC V5Z 1M9; Wes'91; CCFP; Staff Chemical Dependency Resource Team, Vancouver General Hospital - Centennial Pavillion; Langs: German; (604)875-4788; Fax. (604)875-4749; christian.rucker@vch.ca.

RUCKER, Diana; Clinical Sciences Bldg, B 139-11350 83 Ave NW, Edmonton AB T6G 2P4; Cal'04; FRCPC; IntMed; GeriatricMed. Staff, University of Alberta Hospital; (780)492-6572; Fax. (780)492-2874.

RUCKER, Joshua C S; Mount Sinai Hospital, 1514-600 University Ave, Toronto ON M5G 1X5; Tor'01; FRCPC; Anes. Staff, Mount Sinai Hospital; (416)946-0608

RUDACHYK, Lila M; Saskatoon City Hosp, 701 Queen St, Saskatoon SK S7K 0M7; Sask'75; BSc; FRCPC; PhysMed&Rehab (Stroke Rehabilitation). Dept Head PhysMed & Rehab, Saskatoon City Hospital; Head PhysMed & Rehab, Saskatoon Health Region Saskatoon Public Health; Dept Head PhysMed & Rehab, University of Saskatchewan; (306)655-8659; Fax. (306)655-8813; lila.rudachyk@saskatoonhealthregion.ca.

RUDAN, John F; Kingston Gen Hosp, 76 Stuart St, Kingston ON K7L 2V7; Qns'81; FRCSC; OrthSurg. Staff, Kingston General Hospital; Dept Head Surgery, Queen's University; (613)549-6666 x3667

RUDD, Michael W; 535 Main St, Kentville NS B4N 1L4; Man'98; FRCSC; ObstGyn. (902)678-9679; Fax. (902)678-9569.

RUDD, William Warren H; Rudd Clinic, 825-123 Edward St, Toronto ON M5G 1E2; Tor'59; FACS; FASCRS; FRCSC; GenSurg (Anorectal Surgery). Langs: German; (416)597-0997; Fax. (416)597-2912.

RUDDIMAN, Alan W; Main Street Med Centre, PO Box 489 36005 97 St, Oliver BC V0H 1T0; Witwatersrand (South Africa)'89; MB ChB; LMCC; Chief Medical Staff, South Okanagan General Hospital; Chair Okanagan M A C, Interior Health Authority Corpoate Office; Member Rural Issues Committee, British Columbia Medical Association; (250)498-3411; Fax. (250)498-0233; ruddimana@shaw.ca.

RUDDOCK, David G S; 206-480 Huronia Rd, Barrie ON L4N 6M2; Tor'72; CCFP; FCFP; Asst Prof Family & Commun Med, University of Toronto; (705)734-1150; Fax. (705)734-6266.

RUDDOCK, Deanne L; Manitoba Clinic, 790 Sherbrook St, Winnipeg MB R3A 1M3; Man'93; BSc; FRCSC; ObstGyn., University of Manitoba; (204)788-5504; Fax. (204)775-6373.

RUDDOCK, Nicholas S; 302-85 Norfolk St, Guelph ON N1H 4J4; Tor'69; Assoc Staff, Guelph General Hospital; Langs: English; French; (519)822-1871; Fax. (519)822-1990; nruddock@gbhs.on.ca.

RUDDOCK, William D J; Norfolk Med Centre, 302-85 Norfolk St, Guelph ON N1H 4J4; Ott'03; CCFP; (519)822-1871; Fax. (519)822-1990; wruddock@gbhs.on.ca.

RUDDY, Catherine; Riverside Prof Centre, 405-1919 Riverside Dr, Ottawa ON K1H 1A2; McM'78; BSc(Hon); FRCPC; Derm. Att Staff, The Ottawa Hospital - Civic Campus; Asst Prof, University of Ottawa; (613)237-4690; Fax. (613)237-9637.

RUDDY, James; Valley Prof Centre, 70 Exhibition St, Kentville NS B4N 4K9; Dundee (Scotland)'84; MB ChB; BMedSci(Hons.); LMCC; FRCSC; Otol (Rhinology). Staff, Valley Regional Hospital; (902)678-3850; Fax. (902)678-3851.

RUDDY, Terrence D; Univ of Ottawa Heart Institute, 40 Ruskin St, Ottawa ON K1Y 4W7; Tor'77; FACC; FRCPC; Cardiol; IntMed. Att Physician, The Ottawa Hospital - Civic Campus; Staff Div of Cardiol, University of Ottawa Heart Institute; Assoc Prof, University of Ottawa; (613)761-4085; Fax. (613)761-4596; truddy@ottawaheart.ca.

RUDERMAN, James; Women's College Hosp, 76 Grenville St, Toronto ON M5S 1B2; Tor'75; CCFP; FCFP; Staff, Women's College Hospital; Assoc Prof Family & Commun Med, University of Toronto; (416)323-6060

RUDGE, Sara K; Medica One, 1400 Main St W, Hamilton ON L8S 1C7; McM'98; CCFP; Staff, Mohawk College; (905)540-4247 x26750; sararudge@hotmail.com.

RUDGE, Trevor D; Red Deer Reg Hosp Centre, PO Box 5030 Stn Postal Box Ctr 3942 50A Ave, Red Deer AB T4N 6R2; Man'02; FRCPC; Anes. Staff, Red Deer Regional Hospital Centre; (403)396-6698

RUDINSKAS, Leona C; 2F-27 John St, York ON M9N 1J4; McG'77; ABIM; ABOnc; ABHaem; FRCPC; IntMed (P.Q.) (Hematological Oncology); MedOncol; Hem. Staff, Humber River Regional Hospital - Church Street Site; Coroner, Metro Toronto; Langs: Lithuanian; French; (416)248-6060; Fax. (416)248-5922.

RUDKIN, Teresa; GMF Cote-des-Neiges, 5700 ch de la Cote-des-Neiges, Montreal QC H3T 2A8; Ott'00; CCFP; (514)731-8531

RUDKOWSKI, Jill C; St Joseph's Healthcare, F507-50 Charlton Ave E, Hamilton ON L8N 4A6; Cal'96; FRCPC; IntMed; Respir. Staff, St Joseph's Healthcare - Charlton Campus; (905)522-1155

RUDKY, Rina; Humber River Reg Hosp-Keele, 2175 Keele St, York ON M6M 3Z4; Tor'98; FRCPC; Psy. Staff, Humber River Regional Hospital - Keele Street Site; (416)658-2022; Fax. (416)658-2009.

RUDLAND, Rand B; Kiewit-Kvaerner Contractors, 102-240 Waterford Bridge Rd, St. John's NL A1E 1E2; UBC'78; randrudland@dccnet.com.

RUDMIK, Lucas R; Foothills Med Centre, 602-1403 29 St NW, Calgary AB T2N 2T9; Cal'04; FRCSC; Otol. Staff, Foothills Medical Centre; (403)944-3628; Fax. (403)944-0989.

RUDNER, Howard L; Medical & Dental Bldg, 211-586 Eglinton Ave E, Toronto ON M4P 1P2; Tor'82; CCFP; FCFP; Clin Asst MedOncol, Sunnybrook Health Sciences Centre; Asst Prof, University of Toronto; (416)322-4911; Fax. (416)322-4940.

RUDNER, Rodica; 506-4430 Bathurst St, North York ON M3H 3S3; Bucharest (Romania)'80; Ac Staff Toronto Rehab Ctre, North York General Hospital - Branson Division; Ac Staff, Women's College Hospital; Langs: Romanian; (416)631-7794

RUDNICK, Abraham; 642-2334 Trent St, Victoria BC V8R 4Z4; Hebrew (Israel)'90; PhD; FRCPC; Psy (Schizophrenia). Physician/Leader Psychosis Prog, Regional Mental Health Care-St Joseph's Health Care; Chair Div of Social & Rural Psy, University of Western Ontario; Langs: Hebrew; (250)370-8396

RUDNICK, Alexander; O'Connor Doctor's Office, 20-1450 O'Connor Dr, East York ON M4B 2T8; Dublin (Ireland)'50.

RUDNICK, Martin; 215-4949 Bathurst St, North York ON M2R 1Y1; Tor'76; Ac Staff, North York General Hospital - Branson Division; (416)221-3211; Fax. (416)221-3216.

RUDNIK, James E; 204-1676 Martin Dr, Surrey BC V4A 6E7; McG'97; FRCPC; IntMed. Staff, Delta Hospital; (604)536-2188; Fax. (604)269-3720.

RUDNIKOFF, Jordana S; The Jacob's Pain Centre, 102-8920 Woodbine Ave, Markham ON L3R 9W9; Qns'98; DAAPM; CCFP; (905)305-9484; Fax. (905)305-7381.

RUDNISKY, Christopher J; Royal Alexandra Hosp, 2316-10240 Kingsway NW, Edmonton AB T5H 3V9; Alb'99; MPH; FRCSC; Ophth (Cataract). Assoc Prof, Royal Alexandra Hospital; (780)735-5013; Fax. (780)735-4969; chris@rudnisky.ca.

RUDNISKY, Eugene J; Meadowlark Prof Bldg, 350-8702 Meadowlark Rd NW, Edmonton AB T5R 5W5; Alb'70; FRCSC; Ophth. (780)484-1012; Fax. (780)489-3545.

RUDOLPH, Florian P; Clinical Sciences Bldg, 152 University Campus NW, Edmonton AB T6G 2G3; (Germany)'98; Staff, University of Alberta Hospital; (780)407-7035; Fax. (780)407-8529.

RUDOLPH, Kathrin S; Red Deer Reg Hosp Centre, 3942 50A Ave, Red Deer AB T4N 4E7; Staff, Red Deer Regional Hospital Centre; (403)343-2123; Fax. (403)343-8068.

RUDOVICA, Jelena; University Park Med Clinic, 182 University Park Dr, Regina SK S4V 1A3; (Latvia)'82; Staff, Regina General Hospital; Staff, Pasqua Hospital; (306)789-5997; Fax. (306)789-3443.

RUDOVICS, Aivars; Regina Qu'Appelle HR-Regina, 1440 14th Ave, Regina SK S4P 0W5; Riga (Latvia)'81; Staff, Regina General Hospital; (306)766-0743; Fax. (306)766-3459.

RUDRICK, Brian F J; Grey Bruce HS-Owen Sound, PO Box 1800 Stn Main 1800 8th St E, Owen Sound ON N4K 6M9; Sask'85; FRCPC; AnatPath. Staff Labs, Grey Bruce Health Services - Owen Sound; (519)376-2121 x2140; Fax. (519)376-4413; brudrick@gbhs.on.ca.

RUDSKI, Lawrence G; SMBD Jewish Gen Hosp, 3755 ch Cote-Sainte-Catherine, Montreal QC H3T 1E2; McG'92; FRCPC; IntMed; Cardiol. Staff, Sir Mortimer B Davis Jewish General; McGill University; (514)340-8283 x2992

RUDSTON-BROWN, Blair C D; 104-1629 Townsite Rd, Nanaimo BC V9S 1N3; UBC'88; FRCSC; GenSurg. (250)753-5319; Fax. (250)753-5772.

RUDWAL, Christopher T; Hop Santa Cabrini Ospedale, 5655 rue Saint-Zotique E, Montreal QC H1T 1P7; Warsaw (Poland)'61; FRCPC; IntMed; Nephrol (P.Q.). Staff, Hôpital Santa Cabrini Ospedale; (514)252-6000

RUEFFER, Peter K; Northfield Med Centre, 206-99 Northfield Dr E, Waterloo ON N2K 3P9; Tor'67; Staff, Grand River Hospital - Freeport Site; Staff, Grand River Hospital - Kitchener/Waterloo Health Centre; Staff, St Mary's General Hospital; Asst Prof Family Practice, University of Western Ontario; (519)744-2592; Fax. (519)744-1197.

RUEL, Daniel R; 5881 Malden Rd, Windsor ON N9H 1S5; Wes'97; CCFP; FCFP; (519)966-3411

RUEL, Joannie; CHUS-Hop Hotel-Dieu, 580 rue Bowen S, Sherbrooke QC J1G 2E8; Sher'06; FRCPC; IntMed; Gastroent. Staff, Centre Hospitalier Universitaire de Sherbrooke-Hôpital Hôtel-Dieu; (819)346-1110

RUEL, Marc; H3402-40 Ruskin St, Ottawa ON K1Y 4W7; Ott'94; MPH; FRFPS; FRCSC; CardSurg (AIDS). Dir Lab Research & Cardiac Surg, University of Ottawa Heart Institute; Asst Dean Clinical & Transitional Research, University of Ottawa; Langs: French; (613)761-4893; Fax. (613)761-5367.

RUEL, Monique A; CHUM-Hotel-Dieu, 3480 rue Saint-Urbain, Montreal QC H2W 1T8; Mon'80; Cardiol; IntMed (Hemodynamics). Staff, Centre Hospitalier l'Université de Montréal (CHUM) - Hôtel-Dieu; (514)890-8000

RUEL, Rejean; Clin Med la Perade, 81 rue Ricard, Ste-Anne-Per QC G0X 2J0; Laval'74; LMCC; (418)325-2777; Fax. (418)325-3521.

RUELLAND, Simon; CLSC Lionel-Charest, 340 rue Clement-Lavoie, Baie-Comeau QC G4Z 3B8; Laval'83; Staff, Centre Hospitalier Régional Baie-Comeau; (418)296-2572; Fax. (418)296-7885.

RUEST, Andree; Algorithme Pharma, 1100 av Beaumont, Mont-Royal QC H3P 3H5; Sher'76; (514)341-6077

RUEST, Ann; Hotel-Dieu de Levis, 143 rue Wolfe, Levis QC G6V 3Z1; Laval'85; Staff, Hôtel-Dieu de Lévis; (418)835-7155; Fax. (418)835-7199.

RUEST, Annie; CHUQ-Hotel-Dieu de Quebec, 11 Cote du Palais, Quebec QC G1R 2J6; Sher'96; FRCPC; IntMed; Microbio & Infect Dis (P.Q.); InfectDis; MedMicrobiol. Staff, Centre Hospitalier Universitaire de Québec (CHUQ) - Siege Social; (418)691-5131; annie.ruest@chuq.qc.ca.

RUEST, Louise; Kings Place, 415-440 King St, Fredericton NB E3B 5H8; Laval'91; CCFP; FCFP; Langs: Bilingual(French/English); (506)450-8280; Fax. (506)450-2999.

RUEST, Pierre; Hôpital Ste-Justine, 3175 ch Cote-Sainte-Catherine, Montreal QC H3T 1C5; Mon'84; CSPQ; FRCPC; Anes. Ac Staff, Hôpital Ste-Justine; (514)345-4931

RUEST, Pierre; Clinique Med de l'Est, 203-100 rue King E, Sherbrooke QC J1G 1A4; Sher'75; (819)563-7225; Fax. (819)563-7271.

RUEST, Richard; Clinique Domus Medica, 306-5601 rue Belanger, Montreal QC H1T 1G3; Mon'73.

RUETHER, Joseph D; Tom Baker Cancer Centre, 1331 29 St NW, Calgary AB T2N 4N2; Alb'87; FRCPC; IntMed (Endocrine/Neuroendocrine Cancer); MedOncol. Staff Oncol, Tom Baker Cancer Centre; Staff, Foothills Medical Centre; Staff, Calgary Health Region; Asst Prof, University of Calgary; (403)521-3093; Fax. (403)283-1651.

RUFFET-BOURDON, Sophie; CSSS du Sud de Lanaudière, 911 montee des Pionniers, Terrebonne QC J6V 2H2; Mon'06; Staff, Centre Hospitalier Pierre le Gardeur; (450)654-7525

RUFFO, Connie J; Windsor Square, 240-1959 152 St, Surrey BC V4A 9E3; UBC'85; BSc; V-Chair, Physician Hlth Prog of BC; (604)531-0888; Fax. (604)531-0881.

RUGGIERO, Donato A; 201-1223 St Clair Ave W, Toronto ON M6E 1B5; Tor'70; BSc(Med); Staff, Humber River Regional Hospital - Church Street Site; Langs: Italian; French; (416)653-0895

RUGGLES, David J M; Providence CCC-St Mary's, PO Box 3600 Stn Main 340 Union St, Kingston ON K7L 5A2; Dal'93; FRCPC; PhysMed&Rehab. Staff, Providence Care - St Mary's of the Lake Hospital Site; (613)544-5220

RUGGLES, Janice L; Pickering Med Centre, 219-1885 Glenanna Rd, Pickering ON L1V 6R6; McM'93; BA; FRCSC; ObstGyn. Staff, Rouge Valley Health System - Ajax & Pickering Health Centre Site; Asst Clin Prof Faculty of Hlth Science, Dept of Ob/Gyn, McMaster University; (905)420-2556; Fax. (905)420-3996; jroffice219@gmail.com.

RUGGLES, Lesley A; Antigonish Mall, 133 Church St, Antigonish NS B2G 2E3; Man'86; Staff, St Martha's Regional Hospital; (902)863-2455; Fax. (902)867-6336.

RUGHUBIR, Nirvashni; Pearl Family Practice, 9-1150 Lorne Park Rd, Mississauga ON L5H 3A5; Natal (South Africa)'99; MB ChB; CCFP; (905)271-5717; Fax. (905)271-5484.

RUIJS, Theodora C G; William Osler HC-Brampton, 2100 Bovaird Dr E, Brampton ON L6R 3J7; Utrecht (Netherlands)'87; FRCPC; GenPath. Staff, William Osler Health System - Brampton Civic Hospital; Langs: Dutch; (905)494-2120; theodora_ruijs@oslerhshc.org.

RUITER, P James A; Salus Global Corp, 200-717 Richmond St, London ON N6A 1S2; Alb'87; Asst Clinical Prof, University of Alberta; Langs: Bilingual(English/French); (519)640-7333; Fax. (519)640-5762.

RUMACK, Eric R; 136 Castlewood Rd, Toronto ON M5N 2L6; Tor'84; DOHS; FCBOM; FACOEM; CCFP; Court Staff, The Scarborough Hospital - General Campus; Court Staff, The Scarborough Hospital - Birchmount Campus; Court Staff, Rouge Valley Health System - Centenary Health Centre Site; Physician Occup Health, Multiple Industrial Affiliations; Lecturer, University of Toronto; (647)822-2896; Fax. (416)488-7151; erumack@sympatico.ca.

RUMAN, Tanya A; Synergy Wellness Centre, 225-501 Bethel Dr, Sherwood Park AB T8H 0N2; Ott'02; CCFP; Staff, Hinton Healthcare Centre; (780)467-4343; Fax. (780)449-4951; hinton@hintonmedical.com.

RUMBALL, W James; Kirkland & District Hosp, PO Box 460 Stn Main 313-145 Government Rd E, Kirkland Lake ON P2N 3J1; Tor'59; FRCSC; GenSurg. Pres Med Staff & Cons Surg, Kirkland & District Hospital; Staff Consultant Surg, Englehart & District Hospital Inc; (705)568-2232; Fax. (705)568-2234; wjr@kdhospital.com.

RUMBALL, William G; The Medical Centre, 707 Charlotte St, Peterborough ON K9J 2X5; Tor'58; Otol. (705)743-6222; Fax. (705)741-1264; wrumball88@cogeco.ca.

RUMBLE, Edward J; 377-5 Fairview Mall Dr, North York ON M2J 2Z1; Tor'72; FRCSC; OrthSurg (Knee Surgery). Staff, North York General Hospital; Langs: English; French; (416)492-5633; Fax. (416)495-1590.

RUMBOLT, Brian R; Assiniboine Clinic, 633 Lodge Ave, Winnipeg MB R3J 0S9; Mem'80; Ac Staff, The Salvation Army Grace Hospital.

RUMM, Ellen B H; Addiction & Mental Hlth-Clarke, 250 College St, Toronto ON M5T 1R8; McM'98; FRCPC; Psy. Staff, Centre for Addiction & Mental Health (CAMH) - College Street Site; (416)979-4747

RUMM, Michael J; Kingsway Med Bldg, 5-2917 Bloor St W, Etobicoke ON M8X 1B4; Tor'75; Court Staff, Trillium Health Centre - Mississauga; Court Staff, Trillium Health Centre - West Toronto; (416)236-2575

RUMNEY, Peter G; Holland Bloorview Kids Rehab, 150 Kilgour Rd, Toronto ON M4G 1R8; Tor'81; FRCPC; Peds (Pediatric Rehabilitation). Consultant, The Hospital For Sick Children; Assoc Prof Peds, University of Toronto; (416)753-6068

RUNCIMAN, Kenneth A C; Powassan & Area FHT, PO Box 39 8 King St, Powassan ON P0H 1Z0; Tor'87; CCFP; FCFP; (705)724-3388; Fax. (705)724-5499.

RUNDLE, John D; Professional Bldg, 303-222 King St E, Bowmanville ON L1C 1P6; Tor'67; Court Staff, Lakeridge Health - Bowmanville Site; (905)623-3042; Fax. (905)623-6397.

RUNDLE, Margaret A; Malvern Med Arts Bldg, 100-1333 Neilson Rd, Scarborough ON M1B 4Y9; Tor'89; CCFP; FCFP; (416)291-7719; Fax. (416)287-3775.

RUNGI, Arne A; Niagara HS-St Catharines, 142 Queenston St, St. Catharines ON L2R 7C6; Qns'05; CCFP; Staff, Niagara Health System - St Catharines General Site; (905)684-7271

RUNGI, George; Market Place Med Clinic, 218 Catharine St, Port Colborne ON L3K 4K8; Tor'69; CCFP; FCFP; Langs: Estonian; (905)835-1197; Fax. (905)835-8839.

RUNGTA, Kamal N; UBC Faculty of Med, 2775 Laurel St, Vancouver BC V5Z 1M9; Tor'79; FRCPC; Psy (Sleep Disorders). Consultant Sleep Disorder Prog, UBC Hospital - Koerner Pavillion; Assoc Dean Postgrad Med Educ/Clin Prof, University of British Columbia; (604)875-4111 x67757; kamal.rungta@ubc.ca.

RUNZER, Timothy D; Burnaby Hosp, 3935 Kincaid St, Burnaby BC V5G 2X6; Alb'95; FRCPC; Anes. Staff, Burnaby Hospital; (604)412-6311; Fax. (604)412-6313.

RUO, Leyo; Hamilton HS-Henderson Site, B3159-711 Concession St, Hamilton ON L8V 1C3; Alb'91; FRCSC; GenSurg. Staff, Hamilton Health Sciences Centre-Juravinski Site; (905)521-2100

RUPARELIA, Bhagwanji C; Riverside Prof Centre, 404-1919 Riverside Dr, Ottawa ON K1H 1A2; Bombay (India)'61; MB BS; DRCOG; MRCOG; FRCSC; ObstGyn. Assoc Staff, The Ottawa Hospital - Civic Campus; Assoc Staff, The Ottawa Hospital - Riverside Campus; (613)523-5000; Fax. (613)521-5231.

RUPARELIA, Meera; Upper Canada Family Hlth Team, 203-309 Park St, Brockville ON K6V 6E5; (Ireland)'06; CCFP; Langs: Hindi; French; Gujarati; (613)925-5977; Fax. (613)925-1238.

RUPARELIA, Raj; Warden Family Practice Walk-In, 3502 Danforth Ave, Scarborough ON M1L 1E1; (United Kingdom)'10; CCFP; (647)984-6172

RUPARELIA, Surendra P; Oshawa Medical Arts Bldg, 101-300 King St W, Oshawa ON L1J 2K1; Sheffield (England)'66; MB ChB; LMCC; Court Staff Family Pract, Lakeridge Health - Oshawa Site; Langs: Gujarati; Hindi; (905)576-8447; Fax. (905)576-8535.

RUPARELIA, Vasant C; 4230 Mitch Owen Rd PO Box 580 Stn Main, Manotick ON K4M 1A5; Bombay (India)'69; MB BS; MCPS; Ac Staff, The Ottawa Hospital - Riverside Campus; Langs: Hindi; Gujarati; (613)692-2571; Fax. (613)692-0271.

RUPERT, Raymond H; Rupert Case Mgmt Inc, 1006 Avenue Rd, Toronto ON M5P 2K8; Tor'72; MBA; Court Staff, Women's College Hospital; Court Staff, Sunnybrook Health Sciences Centre; (416)483-2858; Fax. (416)483-5576; rayrup@rogers.com.

RUPKA, Dennis W; Keary Med Centre, 102A-245 Columbia St E, New Westminster BC V3L 3W4; McM'78; FACC; BSc; FRCPC; IntMed (Echocardiography); Cardiol. Staff, Eagle Ridge Hospital & Health Care Centre; Dir Echocardiography, Royal Columbian Hospital; Consultant Echocardiography, College of Physicians & Surgeons of British Columbia; Asst Clin Prof, University of British Columbia; (604)522-8899; Fax. (604)522-4215.

RUS-SERBAN, Lenuta; Lakeshore Gen Hosp, 160 av Stillview, Pointe-Claire QC H9R 2Y2; Tirgu-Mures (Romania)'86; Staff, Lakeshore General Hospital - Pointe Claire; Langs: Romanian; Hungarian; English; (514)630-2225 x4596

RUSAK, Anysia M; Seniors' Outreach Team, 1665 Grant Ave, Nanaimo BC V9S 5K7; Tor'88; FRCPC; Psy (Geriatric Psychiatry). Staff Senoirs' Outreach Team, Nanaimo Regional General Hospital; (250)755-3301

RUSALOVSKA, Svitlana; 224-329 March Rd, Ottawa ON K2K 2E1; (Ukraine)'94; FRCPC; Psy. (613)592-1001

RUSEN, Jack B; Eaton Place Med Centre, 81-333 St Mary Ave, Winnipeg MB R3C 4A5; Man'70; Staff, St Boniface General Hospital; (204)942-0933; Fax. (204)942-2491.

RUSH, Christopher L; SMBD Jewish Gen Hosp, 3755 ch Cote-Sainte-Catherine, Montreal QC H3T 1E2; McG'82; AB; FRCPC; NuclearMed. Clin Assoc Staff, Sir Mortimer B Davis Jewish General; adj Prof, McGill University; (514)340-8222 x5374; Fax. (514)340-7919.

RUSH, David N; Health Sciences Centre, GE421-820 Sherbrook St, Winnipeg MB R3A 1R9; Tucuman (Argentina)'72; FASN; FACP; MD; FRCPC; IntMed (Nephrology). Staff, Health Sciences Centre; Prof Med, University of Manitoba; Langs: Spanish; (204)787-3437; Fax. (204)787-3326; eroloff@hsc.mb.ca.

RUSH, Nene O S; Family Med Centre, 400 Tache Ave, Winnipeg MB R2H 3C3; Tucuman (Argentina)'75; CCFP; FCFP; Ac Staff Fam Pract, St Boniface General Hospital; University of Manitoba; Langs: Spanish.

RUSH, Perry J; Bathurst-Drewry Med Centre, 202-5927 Bathurst St, North York ON M2R 3T5; McG'81; CSPQ; FRCPC; IntMed; Rheum. Staff, St John's Rehabilitation Hospital; Staff, Baycrest Centre for Geriatric Care; Asst Prof, University of Toronto; (416)225-0040; Fax. (416)225-0048.

RUSHENAS, Alexandre; CSSSG-Hop de Hull, 116 boul Lionel-Emond, Gatineau QC J8Y 1W7; Montpellier I (France)'97; Staff, Hull Hospital; (819)966-6200

RUSHTON, Cheryl; 101-435 Regent St, Fredericton NB E3B 3X6; Ott'96; BSc; CCFP; FCFP; Staff, Dr Everett Chalmers Regional Hospital; (506)458-0233; Fax. (506)457-4760.

RUSIMOVIC, Lynn; St-Anne's Med Centre, 500 Old St Patrick St, Ottawa ON K1N 9G4; Mon'02; CCFP; (613)789-1552; Fax. (613)789-0659.

RUSK, Richard; Manitoba Health, 300 Carlton St, Winnipeg MB R3B 3M9; Man'05; CCFP.

RUSKIN, Ronald; 9-315 Avenue Rd, Toronto ON M4V 2H2; Qns'70; DPsy; DABPN; FRCPC; Psy (Psychotherapy). Sr Staff Out-Patient Psy Dept, Mount Sinai Hospital; Sr Associate Research Trinity College, University of Toronto; Langs: English; French; (416)928-0675; Fax. (416)928-0870; ronaldruskinmd@aol.com.

RUSNAK, Barry W; Manitoba X-Ray Clinic, 3263 Portage Ave, Winnipeg MB R3K 0W6; Man'74; FRCPC; DiagRad. Staff, Portage District General Hospital; (204)832-0273; brusnak@shaw.ca.

RUSNAK, Conrad N; Vancouver Gen Hosp, CP5-855 12th Ave W, Vancouver BC V5Z 1M9; Sask'91; CCFP; Staff, Vancouver General Hospital - Centennial Pavillion; (604)875-4754; Fax. (604)875-5593.

RUSNAK, Jane A M; Glenridge Med Bldg, 208-1 Belton Blvd, St Catharines ON L2T 3Y4; Qns'94; BSc(Hons); CCFP; FCFP; (905)938-0633

RUSNOV, Mladen V; Clinique Domus Medica, 5601 rue Belanger, Montreal QC H1T 1G3; Zagreb (Croatia)'65; FRCSC; GenSurg; ThorSurg. Chef chir thorac/Chef chir vascul, Hôpital Santa Cabrini Ospedale; Langs: Croatian; Italian; English; (514)256-5011; Fax. (514)738-9586; m.rusnov@sympatico.ca.

RUSSEK, Richard P; Grandview Med Ctr Fam Hlth Team, 167 Hespeler Rd, Cambridge ON N1R 3H7; Tor'74; CCFP; FCFP; Staff, Cambridge Memorial Hospital; (519)623-4200

RUSSEL, Jennifer M; BC Women's Hosp & Health Ctre, P2 219-4500 Oak St, Vancouver BC V6H 3N1; McM'05; FRCPC; Psy. Staff, BC Women's Hospital & Health Centre; (604)875-2000 x7068

RUSSELL, Alan D; Leamington & Area Fam Hlth Team, 205-197 Talbot St W, Leamington ON N8H 1N8; Mem'89; BMedSci; Staff, Leamington District Memorial Hospital; (519)322-0977; Fax. (519)322-0237.

RUSSELL, Alan L; Main Street Med Centre, 9-10886 Hurontario St, Brampton ON L7A 3R9; London (England)'63; MB BS; MRCS; LRCP; MRCP(Lond); DAAPM; BSc(Hon); (905)846-9911

RUSSELL, Anthony S; Heritage Med Research Centre, 562-107 University Campus NW, Edmonton AB T6G 2S2; London (England)'63; MB ChB; FRCP; ClinImmunol&Allergy (Rheumatology). Ac Staff, University of Alberta Hospital; Prof Med, University of Alberta; (780)407-6296; asr@ualberta.ca.

RUSSELL, Averil E; Ridge Meadows Hosp & Hlth CC, 11666 Laity St, Maple Ridge BC V2X 5A3; UBC'08; CCFP; Staff, Ridge Meadows Hospital & Health Care Centre; (604)463-4111

RUSSELL, Brian F; Alder Med Centre, 277 Evergreen Rd, Campbell River BC V9W 5Y4; Man'70; FRCPC; Peds. (250)287-7454

RUSSELL, David; East Coast Forensic Psy Hosp, 88 Gloria McCluskey Dr, Dartmouth NS B3B 2B8; Dal'92; BSc(Hon.); Staff, The East Coast Forensic Psychiatry Hospital; (902)219-0998; Fax. (902)460-7337; david.russell@cdha.nshealth.ca.

RUSSELL, Edward S; Royal Inland Hosp, 311 Columbia St, Kamloops BC V2C 2T1; Tor'76; Staff, Royal Inland Hospital; (250)374-5111; Fax. (250)314-2327.

RUSSELL, Elizabeth L; Hollidge Med Centre, B6-130 Hollidge Blvd, Aurora ON L4G 8A3; Tor'97; CCFP; (905)841-5554; Fax. (905)841-0088.

RUSSELL, Elizabeth M; Medical Assoc of Port Perry, 462 Paxton St, Port Perry ON L9L 1L9; Tor'88; Ac Staff, Lakeridge Health - Port Perry Site; (905)985-2895; Fax. (905)985-5403.

RUSSELL, G Gordon Q; Meadowlark Health Centre, 232 Meadowlark Shopping Ctr NW, Edmonton AB T5R 5W9; Liverpool (England)'77; FRCS; FRCSC; OrthSurg (Spine Surgery). Staff, Covenant Health - Misericordia Community Hospital; Clin Assoc Prof, University of Alberta; (780)433-4872; Fax. (780)433-4904.

RUSSELL, Grant; SCOHS-Elisabeth Bruyere Hosp, 43 Bruyere St, Ottawa ON K1N 5C8; Perth (Australia)'83; FRACGP; Staff, SCO Health Service - Élisabeth Bruyère Hospital; (613)562-0050

RUSSELL, Iain S; Talisman Centre, 2225 Macleod Trail SE, Calgary AB T2G 5B6; Alb'91; BSc; FRCSC; OrthSurg (Foot & Ankle Surgery). Clinical Asst Prof, University of Calgary; (403)291-0045; Fax. (403)291-0552.

RUSSELL, J David; St Joseph's Healthcare, M318-50 Charlton Ave E, Hamilton ON L8N 4A6; McM'82; FRCPC; IntMed (Transplant Nephrology); Nephrol. Chief Medicine, St Joseph's Healthcare - Charlton Campus; Assoc Prof Med, McMaster University; (905)522-1155 x33679; Fax. (905)521-6088; russellj@mcmaster.ca.

RUSSELL, James A; St Paul's Hosp, 1081 Burrard St, Vancouver BC V6Z 1Y6; Tor'75; ABIM; FCCP; IntMed (Critical Care Medicine). Staff, Providence Health Care - St Paul's Hospital; (604)806-8272; Fax. (604)806-8599; jrussell@providencehealth.bc.ca.

RUSSELL, James A; Tom Baker Cancer Centre, 1331 29 St NW, Calgary AB T2N 4N2; Cambridge (England)'68; MB ChB; FRCP(Edin); Assoc Staff, Foothills Medical Centre; Dir, Alberta Bone Marrow Transplant Program; Clin Prof, University of Calgary; (403)521-3706; Fax. (403)283-1651; jamesrus@cancerboard.ab.ca.

RUSSELL, Jennifer L; The Hosp for Sick Children, 1725-555 University Ave, Toronto ON M5G 1X8; Ott'91; FRCPC; Peds (Pediatric Cardiology); Cardiol. Staff Cardiol, The Hospital For Sick Children; Assoc Prof, University of Toronto; (416)813-7291; Fax. (416)813-7547.

RUSSELL, Jennifer S W; Addiction Services, 65 Brunswick St, Fredericton NB E3B 1G5; Mem'99; CCFP; Langs: English; French; (506)452-5734

RUSSELL, Jocelyn M; Univ of Ottawa Health Services, 300-100 Marie Curie Pvt, Ottawa ON K1N 1A2; Qns'02; CCFP; (613)564-3950

RUSSELL, Joy K; Fairmont Medical Bldg, 510-750 Broadway W, Vancouver BC V5Z 1H4; UBC'82; CCFP; FCFP; Vis Staff, BC Women's Hospital & Health Centre; Ac Staff, Providence Health Care - St Paul's Hospital; Court Staff, BC Children's Hospital; (604)879-5385; Fax. (604)736-0486.

RUSSELL, Kent R; The Ottawa Hosp-Gen Campus, C2433-501 Smyth Rd, Ottawa ON K1H 8L6; Cal'08; IntMed. Staff, The Ottawa Hospital - General Campus; (613)737-7700

RUSSELL, Laura; MUHC-Montreal Children's Hosp, A604-2300 rue Tupper, Montreal QC H3H 1P3; Indianapolis(IN) (USA)'75; ABP; AB; MedGenetics (P.Q.). Staff, McGill University Health Centre - Montreal Children's Hospital; Teach Staff, McGill University; (514)412-4427; Fax. (514)412-4296.

RUSSELL, Laurie J M; Misericordia Community Hosp, 1N 78-16940 87 Ave NW, Edmonton AB T5R 4H5; Alb'84; BSc; FRCPC; AnatPath (Gynecological Pathology). Staff, Covenant Health - Misericordia Community Hospital; (780)735-2076

RUSSELL, Lois E; 5 Spencer St GD, Picton ON K0K 2T0; Qns'80; CCFP; FCFP; Ac Staff, QHC Prince Edward County Memorial; Assoc Teacher Family Med, Queen's University; (613)476-3298; Fax. (613)476-2770.

RUSSELL, Margaret L; Dept Community Hlth Sciences, 3280 Hospital Dr NW, Calgary AB T2N 4Z6; Cal'76; BSc; PhD; FRCPC; CommunMed; Public Health & Preventive Med. Staff, Foothills Medical Centre; (403)220-4279; Fax. (403)270-7307.

RUSSELL, Marianne T; North Road Med Centre, 435S North Rd, Coquitlam BC V3K 3V9; Sask'88; CCFP; Langs: English; French; (604)936-0411

RUSSELL, Paula M; 135 Davie St PO Box 98055 Rpo Yaletown, Vancouver BC V6Z 2Z7; Tor'85; BSc; CCFP; (604)283-4145

RUSSELL, Robert S; James Paton Mem Hosp, 125 Trans Canada Hwy, Gander NL A1V 1P7; Mem'94; FRCSC; OrthSurg. Staff, James Paton Memorial Hospital; Vis Staff, Central West Reg Health Centre; Teacher Pt-Time, Memorial University Of Newfoundland; (709)256-2500; Fax. (709)256-7800.

RUSSELL, Robert S; Mediclinic, 101-3333 8th St E, Saskatoon SK S7H 4K1; Sask'80; MHSc; DTMH; Langs: Spanish; (306)955-1530; Fax. (306)955-8811.

RUSSELL, Ruth C; MUHC-Montreal Children's Hosp, D578-2300 rue Tupper, Montreal QC H3H 1P3; McG'73; CSPQ; FRCPC; Psy. Staff, McGill University Health Centre - Montreal Children's Hospital; assoc Prof, McGill University; (514)412-4400 x23951; Fax. (514)412-4250.

RUSSELL, Sharon A M D; The Juravinski Cancer Centre, 699 Concession St, Hamilton ON L8V 5C2; McM'89; (905)387-9495; Fax. (905)575-6326.

RUSSELL, Steven B; Medical Assoc of Port Perry, 462 Paxton St, Port Perry ON L9L 1L9; Qns'89; Ac Staff, Lakeridge Health - Port Perry Site; (905)985-2895; Fax. (905)985-5403.

RUSSELL, William; 304-1525 Albion Rd, Etobicoke ON M9V 5G5; Dublin (Ireland)'71; MB ChB; BAO; Staff, William Osler Health System - Etobicoke General Hospital; (416)741-1622; Fax. (416)741-2884.

RUSSELL-MAHONEY, Barbara L; Sioux Lookout Zone Fam Phys, PO Box 4000 Stn Main, Sioux Lookout ON P8T 1K2; Alb'93; CCFP; Staff, Sioux Lookout Meno-Ya-Win Health Centre; Langs: Spanish; French; (807)737-5161; Fax. (807)737-4866.

RUSSENES, Rune T; 108-1940 Lonsdale Ave, North Vancouver BC V7M 2K2; Tor'95; CCFP; (604)987-3357

RUSSILLO, Balbina; Dr B Russillo & M Rappaport Cl, 206-5450 ch de la Cote-des-Nei, Montreal QC H3T 1Y6; Laval'86; CCFP; assoc Prof, St Mary's Hospital Centre; Langs: English; French; (514)345-9121; Fax. (514)345-8844.

RUSTAD, Jennifer A; Fairview Community Health, 359-5 Fairview Mall Dr, North York ON M2J 2Z1; Tor'08; CCFP; (416)640-5298; Fax. (416)642-2238.

RUSTHOVEN, James J; Brant Community HC-Brantford, 200 Terrace Hill St, Brantford ON N3R 1G9; Chicago(IL) (USA)'75; FACP; ABIM(InfectDis.); ABIM(MedOncol.); FRCPC; IntMed; MedOncol. Staff, The Brant Community Healthcare System - Brantford General Hospital Site; Prof Med, McMaster University; (519)751-5585

RUSTOM, Nour; Hop Santa Cabrini Ospedale, 5655 rue Saint-Zotique E, Montreal QC H1T 1P7; Mon'08; Staff, Hôpital Santa Cabrini Ospedale; (514)252-6000

RUSU, Gabriela; GMF de Verdun au 55, 55 av de l'Eglise, Verdun QC H4G 3E7; Mon'09; CCFP; (514)737-2496

RUSU, Viorel-George; Hopital Regional D'Edmundston, 275 boul Hebert, Edmundston NB E3V 4E4; Bucharest (Romania)'77; Staff, Hôpital regional d'Edmundston; (506)739-2200

RUSZKOWSKI, Alexandra D; Oshawa Clinic, 117 King St E, Oshawa ON L1H 1B9; McG'94; FRCSC; PlasSurg (Oncology). Staff, Lakeridge Health - Oshawa Site; Staff, Northumberland Hills Hospital; Langs: Polish; English; (905)723-8551; Fax. (905)723-6319.

RUTA, Thomas S; Victoria Gen Hosp, 1 Hospital Way, Victoria BC V8Z 6R5; Man'81; FRCPC; Anes. Staff, Victoria General Hospital; (250)727-4212

RUTH, Chelsea A; Women's Hosp, WS012-735 Notre Dame Ave, Winnipeg MB R3E 0L8; Man'99; FRCPC; Peds. Staff, BC Children's Hospital.

RUTH, Jonathan; Toronto Grace Hosp, 650 Church St, Toronto ON M4Y 2G5; Tor'81; MSc; FRCPC; IntMed; GeriatricMed. Staff, The Salvation Army Toronto Grace Health Centre; (416)925-2251

RUTHE, Keri S; 203-3811 Chatham St, Richmond BC V7E 2Z4; UBC'10; (604)284-5389

RUTHERFORD, Beverly E; Admirals Clinic, 275 Old Island Hwy, Victoria BC V9B 1G4; Man'80; FRCPC; CCFP; CommunMed. (250)380-9070

RUTHERFORD, Colette M; 417-2863 Ellesmere Rd, Scarborough ON M1E 5E9; Tor'99; FRCSC; ObstGyn. Staff, Rouge Valley Health System - Centenary Health Centre Site; (416)282-4242; Fax. (416)282-3812.

RUTHERFORD, Debra L; 202-86 Angeline St S, Lindsay ON K9V 6C5; Wes'78; Court Staff, Ross Memorial Hospital; (705)324-5870; Fax. (705)324-5877.

RUTHERFORD, Kimberly J; 1780 Broadway W PO Box 14064 Rpo Delamont, Vancouver BC V6J 0B9; McM'10; CCFP.

RUTHERFORD, Michael N; Sudbury Reg Hosp-Laurentian, 41 Ramsey Lake Rd, Sudbury ON P3E 5J1; Qns'94; PhD; FRCPC; AnatPath. Staff, Health Sciences North-Laurentian Site; (705)523-7100; Fax. (705)523-7115.

RUTHERFORD, Patricia A; St Joseph's Healthcare, 50 Charlton Ave E, Hamilton ON L8N 4A6; McM'00; FRCPC; Psy. Staff, St Joseph's Healthcare - Charlton Campus; (905)522-1155

RUTHERFORD, Paul; 185 Inkerman St E, Listowel ON N4W 2N1; Qns'64; Ac Staff Complex Continuing Care Committee, Listowel Memorial Hospital - Listowel Wingham Hospitals Alliance; (519)291-4200; Fax. (519)291-5947.

RUTHERFORD, Philip S; PO Box 504, Armstrong BC V0E 1B0; Qns'85; BSc(Hon); MSc; CCFP; Staff, Vernon Jubilee Hospital; Staff, Pleasant Valley Health Centre; Clinical Asst Prof, University of British Columbia.

RUTHERFORD, Susan M; 209-2494 Danforth Ave, East York ON M4C 1K9; Tor'81; FRCSC; Ophth (Low Vision). Staff, Toronto East General Hospital Inc; Lecturer, University of Toronto; (416)699-9035; Fax. (416)699-9063.

RUTHERFORD, Suzanne; Kemptville Dist Hosp, PO Box 2007 2675 Concession Rd, Kemptville ON K0G 1J0; (Australia)'03; CCFP; Staff, Kemptville District Hospital; (613)258-0100

RUTHNUM, L Poovendren; Cedar Hills Med Clinic, 12860 96 Ave, Surrey BC V3V 6A8; Glasgow (Scotland)'79; MB ChB; MRC(UK); DCH; RC; FRCPC; Peds (Pediatric Critical Care). Asst Prof Peds, University of Saskatchewan; Langs: English; French; (604)584-3531

RUTHNUM, Mandy; Washington Park Med Clinic, E-310 8th St, Courtenay BC V9N 1N3; UBC'00; CCFP; Staff Upper Island Geriatric Outreach Program, St Joseph's General Hospital; Langs: Creole; French; (250)334-9241

RUTHNUM, Manorgaren; Lakeland Plaza, 2-515 Harvey Ave, Kelowna BC V1Y 6C7; Glasgow (Scotland)'73; MB ChB; FRCS(Ed); FAAO; FRCSC; Ophth. Ac Staff Surg, Kelowna General Hospital; (250)762-3545; Fax. (250)762-4397.

RUTKA, James T; The Hosp for Sick Children, 1503-555 University Ave, Toronto ON M5G 1X8; Qns'81; PhD; FRCSC; Neursurg (Brain Tumors). Staff, The Hospital For Sick Children; Prof/Dept Chair Surgery, University of Toronto; (416)813-6425; Fax. (416)813-4975; james.rutka@sickkids.ca.

RUTKA, John A; Univ Hlth Network-Toronto Gen, 8N 873-200 Elizabeth St, Toronto ON M5G 2C4; Qns'79; FRCSC; Otol (Neuro Otolaryngology). Staff, Mount Sinai Hospital; Staff, Toronto General Hospital - UHN; Prof Otol, University of Toronto; (416)340-4630; Fax. (416)340-3327.

RUTKOWSKA-ROKOSZ, Anna; CSSS de la Pointe de Ile, 13926 rue Notre-Dame E, Pte-aux-Trembles QC H1A 1T5; Cracow (Poland)'63; Staff, CSSS de la Pointe de Île; Langs: Polish; (514)642-4050; Fax. (514)498-7505; johanrheaume@pdi.ssss.gouv.qc.ca.

RUTKUNAS, Zita M; CR Clinics Vancouver, 507 Broadway W, Vancouver BC V5Z 1E6; Cal'83; BSc; FRCPC; Peds (Pediatric Emergency Medicine). Staff, BC Children's Hospital; Staff, BC Women's Hospital & Health Centre; Clin Assoc Prof, University of British Columbia; (604)568-7115

RUTLEDGE, David F; Chemong Med Centre FHT, PO Box 330 765 Ward St, Bridgenorth ON K0L 1H0; Wes'95; CCFP; (705)292-5590

RUTLEDGE, Gregory J; St Joseph's Healthcare, 50 Charlton Ave E, Hamilton ON L8N 4A6; McM'02; CCFP; CCFP(E.M.); Staff, St Joseph's Healthcare - Charlton Campus; Staff, Hamilton Health Sciences Centre - Hamilton General Hospital; (905)522-1155; Fax. (905)521-6017.

RUTLEDGE, Jennifer M; University of Alberta Hosp, 4C2-8440 112 St NW, Edmonton AB T6G 2B7; Alb'94; FACC; FAAP; FRCPC; Peds (Pediatric Cardiology). Dir Ped Cardiac Catheterization Lab, University of Alberta Hospital; Asst Prof, University of Alberta; (780)407-8361; Fax. (780)407-3954.

RUTLEDGE, Robert D H; Nova Scotia Cancer Centre, 2025-5820 University Ave, Halifax NS B3H 1V7; Tor'90; FRCPC; RadOncol. Langs: English; French; (902)473-6185; Fax. (902)473-7205; rob.rutledge@cdha.nshealth.ca.

RUTLEDGE, Sharon M; 316 George St, Sarnia ON N7T 4P4; Wes'86; FRCSC; ObstGyn. Ac Staff, Bluewater Health - Norman Site; (519)337-4994; Fax. (519)337-4996.

RUTLEDGE, Timothy F; 4001 Leslie St, North York ON M2K 1E1; Tor'84; CCFP; CCFP(E.M.); FCFP; Dir Med Educ/I-VP Med & Academic Affairs, North York General Hospital; Assoc Prof Family & Community Med, University of Toronto; (416)756-6755; Fax. (416)756-6743.

RUTTENBERG, Jacqueline I; CLSC St-Hubert, 50-6800 boul Cousineau, Saint-Hubert QC J3Y 8Z4; Temple(PA) (USA)'00; CCFP; Fam Med, CSSS Champlain; Langs: English; (450)443-7407; Fax. (450)676-3488; jackie@jazzphoto.ca.

RUZ DEL PINO, Ricardo; 60 Chesley Ave, London ON N5Z 2C1; Mon'07; GenSurg.

RUZIC, Svjetlana; Oakridge Pediatrics, 207-650 41st Ave W, Vancouver BC V5Z 2M9; Belgrade (Serbia)'92; FRCPC; Peds. Staff, BC Children's Hospital; (604)266-1874

RUZICKA, Marcel; The Ottawa Hosp-Riverside, 5 21-1967 Riverside Dr, Ottawa ON K1H 7W9; Prague (Czech Republic)'85; PhD; FRCPC; IntMed (Hypertension); Nephrol. Staff Nephrol, The Ottawa Hospital - Riverside Campus; Assoc Prof Nephrol, University of Ottawa; Langs: Czech; (613)738-8400 x82535; Fax. (613)738-8337.

RUZICKOVA, Martina; Abbie J Lane Memorial Bldg, 7101B-5909 Veterans Memorial L, Halifax NS B3H 2E2; Charles University (Czech Republic)'00; FRCPC; Psy. Staff, Colchester East Hants Health Centre; (902)473-2355; Fax. (902)473-8685.

RUZYCKI, William A; Carry Drive Med Centre, 110-116 Carry Dr SE, Medicine Hat AB T1B 3Z8; Cal'86; CCFP; FCFP; (403)528-3568; Fax. (403)528-3535.

RYAN, Andrea C; Surrey Mem Hosp, 13750 96 Ave, Surrey BC V3V 1Z2; UBC'10; CCFP; Staff, Surrey Memorial Hospital; (604)581-2211

RYAN, C Frank P; The Lung Centre, 7209-2775 Laurel St, Vancouver BC V5Z 1M9; National (Ireland)'79; MB ChB; BAO; FRCPC; FRCPC; Respir; IntMed (Academic Medicine). Ac Staff, Vancouver Coastal Health; Prof, University of British Columbia; (604)875-4241; Fax. (604)875-4695; fryan@interchange.ubc.ca.

RYAN, Christopher J; 410-1200 Burrard St, Vancouver BC V6Z 2C7; UBC'77; BSc; Ac Staff, Providence Health Care - St Paul's Hospital; University of British Columbia; (604)681-7561; Fax. (604)681-6995.

RYAN, Clodagh-Mai; Div of Respirology, 9N 967-585 University, Toronto ON M5G 2N2; Cork (Ireland)'93; FRCPC; IntMed. Staff, Toronto General Hospital - UHN; (416)340-4719; Fax. (416)340-4197.

RYAN, Dale T; St Michael's Hosp, 30 Bond St, Toronto ON M5B 1W8; McM'97; FRCPC; EmergMed. Staff, St Michael's Hospital; (416)864-5095

RYAN, Daniel R; All Well Primary Care Centre, 2835 Mill Woods Rd NW, Edmonton AB T6K 4A9; Alb'74; BMedSci; CCFP; Court Staff, University of Alberta Hospital; Clin Lecturer Family Med, University of Alberta; (780)450-4550; Fax. (780)461-1985.

RYAN, Deirdre M A; BC Women's Hosp & Health Ctre, H214E-4500 Oak St, Vancouver BC V6H 3N1; National (Ireland)'84; FRCPC; Psy. Staff, BC Women's Hospital & Health Centre; (604)875-2025; Fax. (604)875-3115.

RYAN, Douglas R; 426-600 University Ave, Toronto ON M5G 1X5; McG'78; FRCPC; IntMed (Hypertension Nephrology). Assoc Staff, Toronto General Hospital - UHN; Assoc Staff, Mount Sinai Hospital; Asst Prof Med, University of Toronto; (416)586-5174; Fax. (416)586-5174.

RYAN, Edmond A; Heritage Med Research Centre, 362-107 University Campus NW, Edmonton AB T6G 2S2; Dublin (Ireland)'75; FRCPI(Ire); DCH; FRCPC; IntMed; Endocrin&Metab. Staff, University of Alberta Hospital; Prof, University of Alberta; (780)407-3636; Fax. (780)407-6702.

RYAN, Edward A J; Toronto West Fertility Center, 100-56 Aberfoyle Cres, Etobicoke ON M8X 2W4; Dublin (Ireland)'71; MB ChB; BAO; FSOGC; FRCSC; ObstGyn (Infertility). Court Staff, Trillium Health Centre - West Toronto; Court Staff, St Joseph's Health Centre; Lecturer Ob/Gyn, University of Toronto; Langs: French; Gaelic; Spanish; (416)231-4100; Fax. (416)231-0845; dr_ed_ryan@torontofertility.com.

RYAN, Gail L; Children's Hosp Eastern Ont, 401 Smyth Rd, Ottawa ON K1H 8L1; Mem'94; FRCPC; Anes. Staff, Children's Hospital of Eastern Ontario (CHEO); (613)737-2431; gryan@cheo.on.ca.

RYAN, Greg; Mount Sinai Hosp, OPG3 2013-600 University Ave, Toronto ON M5G 1X5; Dublin (Ireland)'79; FRCOG; FSOGC; FRCSC; ObstGyn (Perinatal). Dir Fetal Med Unit, Mount Sinai Hospital; Prof ObstGyn, University of Toronto; Langs: German; Irish; Bilingual(French/English); (416)586-4800 x8415; Fax. (416)586-8617; gryan@mtsinai.on.ca.

RYAN, J Wilbay M; 18-6469 Jeanne d'Arc Blvd N, Orleans ON K1C 2R1; Ott'82.

RYAN, Jacqueline O; Kerrisdale Station Med Clinic, 2077 42nd Ave W, Vancouver BC V6M 2B4; UBC'03; (604)261-9494; Fax. (604)261-9405.

RYAN, John C; University Hosp of Northern BC, 1475 Edmonton St, Prince George BC V2M 1S2; UBC'77; CCFP; CCFP(E.M.); FCFP; Staff/Chief EmergMed, University Hospital of Northern British Columbia; (250)565-2201

RYAN, John G; The Ottawa Hosp-Civic Campus, 1053 Carling Ave, Ottawa ON K1Y 4E9; Dal'89; FRCPC; DiagRad. Staff, The Ottawa Hospital - Civic Campus; (613)722-7000

RYAN, John P; Rockyview Gen Hosp, 7007 14 St SW, Calgary AB T2V 1P9; Dublin (Ireland)'80; MB ChB; BAO; LRCPS; FRCPC; Psy (Geriatric Psychiatry). Staff, Rockyview General Hospital; Clin Assoc Prof, University of Calgary; (403)943-3503; Fax. (403)212-1230.

RYAN, John P; 308 23 Ave SW, Calgary AB T2S 0J2; Cal'73; FRCPC; Rheum; IntMed. Ac Staff, Foothills Medical Centre; Ac Staff, Rockyview General Hospital; Clin Assoc Prof, University of Calgary; (403)228-2345; Fax. (403)245-3488.

RYAN, Kenneth F; 910 10th Ave W, Vancouver BC V5Z 4E3; UBC'06; FRCPC; Anes. (604)875-4111

RYAN, Kenneth J; Oakridge Centre South Tower, 203-650 41st Ave W, Vancouver BC V5Z 2M9; UBC'78; CCFP; FCFP; Ac Staff, Providence Health Care - St Paul's Hospital; Court Staff, Providence Health Care - St Vincent's Hospital-Heather Site; Court Staff, BC Women's Hospital & Health Centre; (604)263-5413

RYAN, Michael E; Broadway Family Health Clinic, 3 Herald Ave, Corner Brook NL A2H 6J2; Mem'08; CCFP; Staff, Western Memorial Regional Hospital.

RYAN, Paula P; Kings Lane Med Clinic, 101-164 Kings Lane, Salt Spring Island BC V8K 2P7; Tor'94; CCFP; Med Staff, Lady Minto Gulf Islands Hospital; Langs: Bilingual(English/French); (250)537-0693; Fax. (250)537-1848; paularyan@shaw.ca.

RYAN, Peter W; Roseville Garden Walk-In Clin, 2525 Rose Ville Garden Dr, Windsor ON N8X 3V6; Sheffield (England)'69; MB ChB; (519)944-3393

RYAN, Robert W J; Coronation Plaza, 102-14310 111 Ave NW, Edmonton AB T5M 3Z7; Cal'05; FRCSC; Neursurg. (780)455-2372; Fax. (780)452-7157.

RYAN, Sean; South Huron Med Centre, 23 Huron St W, Exeter ON N0M 1S5; Dal'05; CCFP; CCFP(E.M.); (519)235-3343

RYAN, Siobhan M; Women's College Hosp, 76 Grenville St, Toronto ON M5S 1B2; Mem'83; FRCPC; Derm. Staff, Women's College Hospital; (416)323-6407; Fax. (416)323-6215.

RYAN, Stephen E; The Ottawa Hosp-Civic Campus, 1053 Carling Ave, Ottawa ON K1Y 4E9; Cal'03; FRCPC; DiagRad. Staff, The Ottawa Hospital - Civic Campus; (613)761-4054

RYAN, T Lerato; Queensway-Carleton Hosp, 3045 Baseline Rd, Ottawa ON K2H 8P4; Qns'07; CCFP; Staff, Queensway Carleton Hospital; (613)721-2000

RYAN, Thomas J; 2F-700 Main St E, Hamilton ON L8M 1K7; Dublin (Ireland)'63; MRC(Lond); FRCP(Lond); FRCPC; IntMed (Diabetes). Med Staff, Hamilton Health Sciences Centre - Hamilton General Hospital; Assoc Prof Clin Med, McMaster University; (905)549-4622; Fax. (905)549-7114.

RYAN DROVER, Anne E; Dr Charles A Janeway Child HC, 3J 312-300 Prince Philip Dr, St. John's NL A1B 3V6; Mem'91; FRCPC; Peds. Staff, Janeway Children's Health & Rehabilitation Centre; Clin Associate Faculty of Med, Memorial University Of Newfoundland; (709)777-6300

RYANS, Katharine A; Humber River Reg Hosp-Finch, 2111 Finch Ave W, North York ON M3N 1N1; McM'04; FRCPC; Anes. Staff, Humber River Regional Hospital - Finch Avenue Site; (416)744-2500

RYBAK, Iouri E; Regional Mental HC-London, PO Box 5532 Stn B 850 Highbury Ave, London ON N6A 4H1; Petrozavodsk (Russia (Federation))'84; FRCPC; Psy. Staff, Regional Mental Health Care-St Joseph's Health Care; (519)455-5110

RYCABEL, Anna; CLSC de Paspebiac, CP 7000 273 boul Gerald-D-Levesque, Paspebiac QC G0C 2K0; Laval'02; Staff, CLSC de Paspebiac; (418)752-2572

RYCHEL, Valerie C; 401-1338 Broadway W, Vancouver BC V6H 1H2; McG'93; FRCSC; ObstGyn. (604)736-7131

RYCHTER, Eva J; Beddington Med Clinic, 207-8120 Beddington Blvd NW, Calgary AB T3K 2A8; Warsaw (Poland)'67; Langs: Polish; (403)275-4611; Fax. (403)275-4613.

RYCKMAN, Bruce A; Selkirk Med Centre, 353 Eveline St, Selkirk MB R1A 1N1; Man'73; Ac Staff, Selkirk & District General Hospital; (204)785-2667; Fax. (204)785-8966.

RYDER, Arthur C; MUHC-Royal Victoria Hosp, 687 av des Pins O, Montreal QC H3A 1A1; McG'83; FRCPC; EmergMed. Ac Staff, McGill University Health Centre - Royal Victoria Hospital; adj Prof, McGill University; (514)843-1610; Fax. (514)843-1638.

RYDER, Gerald B; MacDonald Med Centre, 203-2786 16th Ave W, Vancouver BC V6K 4M1; Tor'68; BScPharm; (604)737-7776; Fax. (604)737-7039.

RYDING, S Louise; 205-2039 Robertson Rd, Ottawa ON K2H 8R2; Qns'94; CCFP; Staff, Halton Healthcare Services Corporation - Oakville Site; (613)828-0896

RYDZ, Emilia; St Paul's Hosp, 1081 Burrard St, Vancouver BC V6Z 1Y6; Alb'04; CCFP; CCFP(E.M.); Staff, Providence Health Care - St Paul's Hospital; (604)682-2344

RYDZ, Frederick; London HSC-Victoria Hosp, PO Box 5010 Stn B 800 Commissioners Rd E, London ON N6A 5W9; Jagiellonian U (Poland)'08; IntMed. Staff, London Health Sciences Centre - Victoria Campus; (519)658-8500

RYDZ, Natalia; Tom Baker Cancer Centre, 1331 29 St NW, Calgary AB T2N 4N2; Alb'05; FRCPC; IntMed; Hem. Staff, Tom Baker Cancer Centre; (403)521-3347; Fax. (403)283-1651.

RYDZIK, M Suzanne; 601-333 Preston St, Ottawa ON K1S 5N4; Ott'78; BSc(Biol.); Langs: Bilingual(English/French); (613)235-8079; Fax. (613)235-5421.

RYE, John G; Victoria Hosp, PO Box 3000 Stn Main 1200 24th St W, Prince Albert SK S6V 5T4; Bristol (England)'77; MRCS; LRCP; FRSM; CCFP; Ac Staff, Victoria Hospital; Coord Palliative Care Rural Family Med Residency Training, University of Saskatchewan; (306)764-5793; Fax. (306)763-5855; docrye@shaw.ca.

RYEBURN, Michael; 203-515 3rd Ave W, Prince Rupert BC V8J 1L9; UBC'91; (250)622-2811

RYERSE, Cynthia L; Dundas Med Centre, 206-17 King St E, Dundas ON L9H 1B7; McM'89; FRCPC; Psy. (905)627-8767

RYERSON, Christopher J; St Paul's Hosp, 8B-1081 Burrard St, Vancouver BC V6Z 1Y6; Wes'04; FRCPC; IntMed; Respir. Staff, Providence Health Care - St Paul's Hospital; (604)806-8818

RYERSON, Lindsay M; University of Alberta Hosp, 4C2-8440 112 St NW, Edmonton AB T6G 2B7; Cal'01; FRCPC; Peds (Pediatric Cardiology); Critical Care Medicine; Cardiol. Staff, University of Alberta Hospital; (780)407-3964; Fax. (780)407-3954.

RYGLEWICZ, Kamila J; 201-13278 Tecumseh Rd E, Windsor ON N8N 3T6; Poznan (Poland)'06; CCFP; (519)979-7878; Fax. (519)979-7872.

RYKSZYNSKI, Cathy M; Surrey Mem Hosp, 13750 96 Ave, Surrey BC V3V 1Z2; Man'86; CCFP; Staff, Surrey Memorial Hospital; (604)581-2211

RYLEY, Alan D C; Sims Square, 406-390 Brant St, Burlington ON L7R 4J4; McM'81; FRCSC; GenSurg. Staff, Joseph Brant Memorial Hospital; Staff, Hamilton Health Sciences Centre - McMaster Children's Hospital; (905)333-3690; Fax. (905)333-1450; adc.ryley@sympatico.ca.

RYPENS, Francoise; Hôpital Ste-Justine, 3175 ch Cote-Sainte-Catherine, Montreal QC H3T 1C5; Brussels (Belgium)'88; CSPQ; DiagRad. Staff, Hôpital Ste-Justine; (514)345-4637; Fax. (514)345-4816.

RYSBERGEN, Jacobus; Imperial Med Clinic, PO Box 180, Imperial SK S0G 2J0; MB ChB; (306)963-2140; Fax. (306)963-2518; rysbergen@yahoo.com.

RYTWINSKI, Z Cecil S; Ottawa Valley Family Hlth Team, PO Box 460 95 Spring St, Almonte ON K0A 1A0; Wes'75; CCFP; FCFP; (613)256-9370; Fax. (613)256-0949.

RYZHAK, Oleh M; 106-2130 Lawrence Ave, Scarborough ON M1R 3A6; (Ukraine)'93; FRCPC; IntMed; Cardiol. Staff, Toronto Western Hospital - University Health Network; (416)603-5815

RZADKI, Edward J J; 103-127 Westmore Dr, Etobicoke ON M9V 3Y6; Tor'60; DPsy; FRCPC; Psy (Depression). Ac Staff Psy Mental Health & Addictions Prog/Dir, William Osler Health System - Etobicoke General Hospital; Langs: Polish; (416)749-3933; Fax. (416)749-3936; edward_rzadki@oslerhc.org.

RZEPECKI, Isabela; Lakeshore Gen Hosp, 160 av Stillview, Pointe-Claire QC H9R 2Y2; Gdansk (Poland)'52; CSPQ; Psy. Staff, Lakeshore General Hospital - Pointe Claire; (514)630-2225 x4208; Fax. (514)630-3056.

RZEPKA, Waldemar P; 170A Rebecca St, Oakville ON L6K 1J6; Szczecin (Poland)'75; Assoc Staff, Halton Healthcare Services Corporation - Oakville Site; Langs: Polish; (905)845-9293

SA, Grace A Y; 5-350 Hespeler Rd, Cambridge ON N1R 7N7; Ott'08; CCFP; (519)621-4071

SAAB, George; Grey Bruce HS-Owen Sound, PO Box 1800 Stn Main 1800 8th St E, Owen Sound ON N4K 6M9; Ott'04; FRCPC; DiagRad. Staff, Grey Bruce Health Services - Owen Sound; (519)376-2121; Fax. (519)372-3954.

SAAB, Marc; CSSS de Rimouski-Neigette, CP 3150 Succ A 150 av Rouleau, Rimouski QC G5L 5T1; Ophth (P.Q.). Staff, Hôpital Regional Rimouski; (418)724-3000

SAAD, Ali G; Saskatoon City Hosp, 701 Queen St, Saskatoon SK S7K 0M7; Staff, Saskatoon City Hospital; (306)655-8755; Fax. (306)655-8399.

SAAD, Antoine; 263 rue Denison E, Granby QC J2H 2R4; Beyrut (Lebanon)'69; AB; ObstGyn (P.Q.). Chef Dept of ObstGyn, Centre Hospitalier de Granby; (450)372-0322; Fax. (450)777-2415.

SAAD, Ehab; St Mary's Clinic, PO Box 45 Stn Main 110 Roe Ave, Gander NL A1V 1W5; Ain Shams (Egypt)'92; CCFP; (709)651-0224

SAAD, Emile; St Luke's Med Clinic, 311 Beaver Bank Rd, Beaver Bank NS B4E 1K1; Claude Bernard (France)'97; CCFP; Langs: Bilingual(English/French); (902)865-2627; Fax. (902)865-2628.

SAAD, Fred; CHUM-Hop Notre-Dame, 1560 rue Sherbrooke E, Montreal QC H2L 4M1; Mon'85; CSPQ; FRCSC; Urol (Uro Oncology). Staff, Centre Hospitalier l'Université de Montréal (CHUM) - Hôpital Notre-Dame; Prof, Universite de Montreal; (514)890-8000 x27466; Fax. (514)412-7620; fredsaad@videotron.ca.

SAAD, Genevieve S; 6-500 Manning Rd, Windsor ON N8N 5H3; Ott'01; CCFP; Langs: French; (519)979-7314

SAAD, Maan H A; South Bank Med Centre, 5-2430 Bank St, Ottawa ON K1V 0T7; Alb'90; PhD(Pharm); CCFP; Langs: Arabic; French; (613)736-6946; Fax. (613)736-6948.

SAAD, Nabil K; Doctors Office, 589 3rd Ave S, Stonewall MB R0C 2Z0; Cairo (Egypt)'60; MB BCh; LRCP(Eng); MRCS(Lond); FRCS(Ed); Staff, Stonewall & District Health Centre; Staff, Selkirk & District General Hospital; Physician, Doctors Office; Langs: Arabic; (204)467-5509; Fax. (204)467-5576; nk_saad@hotmail.com.

SAAD, Nathalie; SMBD Jewish Gen Hosp, 3755 ch Cote-Sainte-Catherine, Montreal QC H3T 1E2; Ott'06; Respir (P.Q.); IntMed. Staff, Sir Mortimer B Davis Jewish General; (514)340-8222

SAAD, Reda S M; Hotel-Dieu Grace Hosp, 1030 Ouellette Ave, Windsor ON N9A 1E1; Alexandria (Egypt)'83; FRCPC; AnatPath. Staff, Hôtel-Dieu Grace Hospital; (519)973-4411

SAAD, Salwa; Churchill Med Centre, 16-3105 Winston Churchill Blvd, Mississauga ON L5L 5S3; Mon'82; Langs: Arabic; French; (905)828-9686; Fax. (905)828-8466.

SAAD, Samy M S; Lakeridge HC-Bowmanville, 47 Liberty St S, Bowmanville ON L1C 2N4; Ain Shams (Egypt)'80; FRCPC; Anes. Staff, Lakeridge Health - Bowmanville Site; (905)623-3331

SAAD, Wadih-Pierre; CSSS du Granit, 3569 rue Laval, Lac-Megantic QC G6B 1A5; Beirut (Lebanon)'74; IntMed. Staff, Carrefour Sante Granit; (819)583-0330

SAAD, Wassim; Jackson Park Health Centre, 105-2475 McDougall St, Windsor ON N8X 3N9; Ott'01; FRCPC; IntMed. Staff, Hôtel-Dieu Grace Hospital; (519)252-9861; Fax. (519)252-7787.

SAADALDEEN, Salwa A; East London Med Centre, 1657 Dundas St, London ON N5W 3C6; Baghdad (Iraq)'84; CCFP; Staff, St Joseph's Hospital - St Joseph's Health Care; Staff, London Health Sciences Centre - University Hospital; Langs: Arabic; (519)951-7178; Fax. (519)455-7103.

SAADE, Antoine; PO Box 3007 Stn Main, Tracadie-Sheila NB E1X 1G5; (Russia (Federation))'84; (506)393-7676; Fax. (506)393-7675.

SAADEDDIN, Abdulrahman; 510-1669 Victoria St, Prince George BC V2L 2L5; Istanbul (Turkey)'94; Staff, University Hospital of Northern British Columbia; (250)565-1212

SAADIA, Roger; Health Sciences Centre, 820 Sherbrook St, Winnipeg MB R3A 1R9; (France)'77; FRCS; Staff, Health Sciences Centre; Prof Trauma Surg, University of Manitoba; Langs: Bilingual(French/English); (204)787-1411; Fax. (204)787-4851; rsaadia@hsc.mb.ca.

SAADIA, Vivien; Salvation Army Grace Gen Hosp, 300 Booth Dr, Winnipeg MB R3J 3M7; Witwatersrand (South Africa)'82; FRCPC; Anes. Staff, The Salvation Army Grace Hospital; (204)837-8311

SAANDAR, Namjilmaa; Medical Arts Centre, C11 BC14-3000 Lawrence Ave E, Scarborough ON M1P 2V1; Mongolia (Other Foreign)'98; (416)438-9000

SAAR, John E; 102-476 Holland Ave, Ottawa ON K1Y 0Z5; Qns'89; CCFP; FCFP; Asst Prof, University of Ottawa; (613)722-6216; Fax. (613)722-2177.

SAARI, Carol-Ann; BC Women's Hosp & Health Ctre, D514A-4500 Oak St, Vancouver BC V6H 3N1; UBC'98; BSc(Hon); MB; FRCPC; Psy (Addictions(Dual Diagnosis)). Staff, BC Women's Hospital & Health Centre; Staff, BC Children's Hospital; (604)875-2345 x6007; casaari@cw.bc.ca.

SAARI, Kendra A; Chapleau & Dist Family Hlth Team, 2 Broomhead Rd, Chapleau ON P0M 1K0; NOSM'10; CCFP; (705)864-0210

SAARI, Stephen J; Chapleau & Dist Family Hlth Team, 2 Broomhead Rd, Chapleau ON P0M 1K0; NOSM'10; CCFP; (705)864-0210

SAARY, M Joan; St Michael's Hosp, SW 4F-30 Bond St, Toronto ON M5B 1W8; Tor'97; MSc; DPhil; FRCPC; OccupMed (Aviation & Space Medicine). Fellow, St Michael's Hospital; Med Examiner Civil Aviation, Air Canada Centre; (416)864-5074; Fax. (416)304-1902; joan.saary@utoronto.ca.

SAAYMAN, Marius J I; Royal Inland Hosp, 311 Columbia St, Kamloops BC V2C 2T1; Stellenbosch (South Africa)'86; MB ChB; FRCPC; Anes. Staff, Royal Inland Hospital; Langs: Afrikaans; (250)314-2620; msaayman@telus.net.

SABA, Paul J; 2600 rue Victoria, Lachine QC H8S 1Z5; McG'80; Staff, CSSS de Dorval-Lachine-Lasalle; (514)634-7168; paul.saba@sympatico.ca.

SABA, Samir E; Institute Albert-Prevost, 6555 boul Gouin O, Montreal QC H4K 1B3; Ain Shams (Egypt)'85; Staff, Hôpital du Sacre-Coeur de Montréal; (514)338-2222 x4245

SABADOS, Wade A; Surrey Mem Hosp, 13750 96 Ave, Surrey BC V3V 1Z2; UBC'96; CCFP; CCFP(E.M.); Staff, Surrey Memorial Hospital; (604)671-1923; Fax. (604)542-2291.

SABAN, Shireen S; Northfield Family Hlth Centre, 206-99 Northfield Dr E, Waterloo ON N2K 3P9; Cape Town (South Africa)'89; MB ChB; Staff, The Brant Community Healthcare System - Brantford General Hospital Site; (519)744-2592

SABANATHAN, Sayanthan; Mission Oaks Med Centre, 32136 Lougheed Hwy, Mission BC V2V 1A4; West Indies (Jamaica)'02; MB BS; CCFP; Langs: Tamil; (604)826-7111

SABAPATHI, Karthik; Harry Medovy House, 2F-671 William Ave, Winnipeg MB R3E 0Z2; Bangalore (India)'98; FRCPC; Anes.

SABAPATHY, Christine A; The Hosp for Sick Children, 9401-555 University Ave, Toronto ON M5G 1X8; McG'05; FRCPC; Peds; PedHemaOncol. Fellow, The Hospital For Sick Children; (416)813-7742

SABARATNAM, Rathi M; Victoria Hosp, PO Box 3000 Stn Main 1200 24th St W, Prince Albert SK S6V 5T4; Staff, Victoria Hospital; (306)765-6000

SABATINO, Assunta C; Lincoln Heights Med Centre, 201-1305 Richmond Rd, Ottawa ON K2B 7Y4; UBC'89; CCFP; FCFP; (613)829-3221; Fax. (613)829-6832.

SABBAGH, Charles N J; Smyth Med Centre, 210-1929 Russell Rd, Ottawa ON K1G 4G3; Ott'00; FRCPC; IntMed; Gastroent. Langs: French; (613)736-1137; Fax. (613)739-1337.

SABBAGH, Ramsey; CSSS du Nord de Lanaudière, 1000 boul Sainte-Anne, Joliette QC J6E 6J2; McG'02; FRCPC; IntMed; Nephrol. Staff, Centre Hospitalier Régional de Lanaudière; (450)759-8222

SABBAGH, Robert; CHUS-Hop Fleurimont, 3001 12e av N, Sherbrooke QC J1H 5N4; Mon'98; CSPQ; FRCSC; Urol (Laparoscopy). Staff, Centre Hospitalier Universitaire de Sherbrooke-Hopital Fleurimont; Langs: Bilingual(English/French); (819)346-1110 x14595; Fax. (819)820-6411; robert.sabbagh@usherbrooke.ca.

SABBAGH, Roland; Montfort Hosp, 713 Montreal Rd, Ottawa ON K1K 0T2; McG'99; FRCPC; IntMed; Cardiol. Staff, Montfort Hospital; Langs: French; (613)746-4621

SABBAGH, Zohreh; 502-402 21st St, Saskatoon SK S7K 0C3; (306)956-3444; Fax. (306)956-3577.

SABBAH, Eric; Ctr Cardiovasculaire Rive-Sud, 200-1615 boul Jacques-Cartier, Longueuil QC J4M 2X1; Mon'91; FRCPC; IntMed; Cardiol. Ac Staff Cardiol, Centre Hospitalier Pierre Boucher; Ac Staff Cardiol, Hôpital Anna-Laberge; Langs: Bilingual(French/English); (450)674-2345; Fax. (450)674-1622.

SABBAH, Osama R S; Univ Hlth Network-Toronto Gen, RFE GS480-200 Elizabeth St, Toronto ON M5G 2C4; Riyadh (Saudi Arabia)'02; FRCPC; EmergMed. Staff, Toronto General Hospital - UHN; (416)340-3856; Fax. (416)340-4300.

SABBAH, Robert; Centre Bois de Boulogne, 425-1575 boul Henri-Bourassa O, Montreal QC H3M 3A9; Mon'84; FRCSC; ObstGyn. Staff, Hôpital du Sacre-Coeur de Montréal; (514)956-1618; Fax. (514)336-8814; rsabbah@videotron.ca.

SABBAH, Sandrine; Cite de la Sante de Laval, 1755 boul Rene-Laennec, Laval QC H7M 3L9; Sher'94; Gastroent (P.Q.) (Internal Medicine). Staff, Hopital de la Cite de la santé; (450)668-1010

SABBAH, Sidney; Hop du Sacre-Coeur de Mtl, 5400 boul Gouin O, Montreal QC H4J 1C5; Mon'81; FRCPC; IntMed; Gastroent. Staff, Hôpital du Sacre-Coeur de Montréal; (514)338-2222

SABE-AFFAKI, Georges; Centre Med Notre-Dame, 1515 rue Notre-Dame, Lachine QC H8S 2E4; Beirut (Lebanon)'72; FRCPC; Cardiol. (514)634-7146; Fax. (514)634-7147.

SABELLA, Olivier; Ctr Hosp Reg Chisasibi, CP 250, Chisasibi QC J0M 1E0; McG'03; CCFP; Staff, Cree Board of Health & Social Services James Bay; (819)855-2844

SABERI, Farzad; 209-4885 Kingsway, Burnaby BC V5H 4T2; McG'01; FRCPC; IntMed; Respir. Staff, Burnaby Hospital; Langs: Persian; (604)568-6685; Fax. (604)568-6653.

SABESKI, Lynne M; 47 Marion St, Winnipeg MB R2H 0S8; Man'96; MB ChB; BSc; FRCSC; ObstGyn. Staff, St Boniface General Hospital; Lecturer, University of Manitoba.

SABETTI, Linda M; Mississauga Med Centre, 420-1420 Burnhamthorpe Rd E, Mississauga ON L4X 2Z9; Tor'89; CCFP; FCFP; Staff, Trillium Health Centre - Mississauga; (905)625-1619; Fax. (905)625-9362.

SABGA, Frederick H; Leamington & Area Fam Hlth Team, 197 Talbot St W, Leamington ON N8H 1N8; (Jamaica)'81; MB BS; BSc; Chief Obst, Leamington District Memorial Hospital; (519)322-1100; ricklor@sympatico.ca.

SABIEH, Sadia; Cambridge Mem Hosp, 700 Coronation St, Cambridge ON N1R 3G2; Lahore (Pakistan)'04; Staff, Cambridge Memorial Hospital; (519)621-2333

SABIN, I Morris; 555-5757 av Decelles, Montreal QC H3S 2C3; McG'50; FACOG; FRCSC; ObstGyn. Staff, Sir Mortimer B Davis Jewish General; adj Prof, McGill University; Langs: French; (514)733-6618; Fax. (514)733-6618.

SABIN, Norman; H-2-3755 ch Cote-Sainte-Cather, Montreal QC H3T 1E2; McG'87; CCFP; CCFP(E.M.); Staff, Sir Mortimer B Davis Jewish General; adj Prof, McGill University; Langs: Bilingual(French/English); (514)340-8222 x8253; Fax. (514)340-7551; norman.sabin@mcgill.ca.

SABINE, Margaret; West Lincoln Mem Hosp, 169 Main St E, Grimsby ON L3M 1P3; McG'68; FRCPC; DiagRad. Assoc Staff, West Lincoln Memorial Hospital; (905)945-2253 x323; mjsabine@sympatico.ca.

SABIR, Aaliya P; Alberta Children's Hosp, 2888 Shaganappi Trail NW, Calgary AB T3B 6A8; Alb'02; FRCPC; Peds. Staff, Alberta Children's Hospital; (403)955-2953

SABIR, M Munawar; Evergreen Med Centre, 8960 152 St, Surrey BC V3R 4E4; Punjab (Pakistan)'61; BSc; MB BS; LRCP; MRCS; OrthSurg (Back Pain). (604)588-8181; Fax. (604)588-8421.

SABIR, Mohamed; Professional Med Clinic, 102-9425 94 Ave, Fort Saskatchewan AB T8L 1N6; Bihar (India)'64; MB BS; LRCP; MRCS(Eng); FRCS(Ed); FRCSC; GenSurg (Endoscopy). Ac Staff Surg, Fort Saskatchewan Health Centre; Clin Lecturer Surg, University of Alberta Hospital; Langs: Urdu; (780)992-0666; Fax. (780)992-0673.

SABIR, Sonia; Markham Stouffville Hosp, PO Box 1800 Stn Main 381 Church St, Markham ON L3P 7P3; Tor'93; CCFP; CCFP(E.M.); FCFP; Staff, Markham Stouffville Hospital; Langs: Bengali; (905)472-7111

SABISTON, Colin P; 214-145 15 St SW, North Vancouver BC V7M 1R9; Ott'79; FRCSC; OrthSurg. (604)980-0883

SABLOFF, Mitchell; The Ottawa Hosp-Gen Campus, 501 Smyth Rd Box 704, Ottawa ON K1H 8L6; McG'95; ABIM; BSc; MSc; MCPS; FRCPC; IntMed (Bone Marrow Transplant). Staff Hematology, The Ottawa Hospital - General Campus; Langs: French; (613)737-8899 x71284; Fax. (613)737-8861; msabloff@ottawahospital.on.ca.

SABO, Marlis T; Surrey Mem Hosp, 13750 96 Ave, Surrey BC V3V 1Z2; Wes'05; FRCSC; OrthSurg. Staff, Surrey Memorial Hospital; (604)450-0824

SABOUBA, Mohammad F; Upper James Med Centre, 609 Upper James St, Hamilton ON L9C 2Y9; Mosul (Iraq)'81; MB ChB; CCFP; Langs: Arabic; (905)575-7230; Fax. (905)575-7191.

SABOURET, Pierre J J; CHUM-Hop Notre-Dame, 1560 rue Sherbrooke E, Montreal QC H2L 4M1; Marseille (France)'77; FRCSC; OrthSurg. Staff, Centre Hospitalier l'Université De Montréal (CHUM) - Hôpital Saint-luc; Staff, Centre Hospitalier l'Université de Montréal (CHUM) - Hôpital Notre-Dame; (514)890-8000

SABOURIN, Alain; 300-990 rue Notre-Dame O, Montreal QC H3C 1K1; Mon'90; (514)937-8020; Fax. (514)937-7510; loccoeur@videotron.ca.

SABOURIN, Alexis; 200-2860 boul Laframboise, Saint-Hyacinthe QC J2S 4Z1; Sher'98; FRCPC; IntMed; Endocrin&Metab. Staff, Centre Hospitalier Honore-Mercier; Langs: Bilingual(French/English); (450)778-3238; Fax. (450)778-3308; alexsab@hotmail.com.

SABOURIN, Francois; Ctr Hosp Laurentien, 234 rue Saint-Vincent, Ste-Agathe-des-Mts QC J8C 2B8; Laval'97; FRCSC; GenSurg. Staff, Centre Hospitalier Laurentien; (819)324-4000

SABOURIN, J Georges; Hys Med Centre, 604-11010 101 St NW, Edmonton AB T5H 4B9; Mon'65; FRCSC; ObstGyn. Ac Staff, Royal Alexandra Hospital; Clinical Asst Prof, University of Alberta; Langs: English; French; (780)421-4728; Fax. (780)426-6698.

SABOURIN, Jeanelle N; Tom Baker Cancer Centre, 1331 29 St NW, Calgary AB T2N 4N2; Ott'07; FRCSC; ObstGyn. Staff, Tom Baker Cancer Centre; (403)521-3721; Fax. (403)403-3573.

SABOURIN, Julie; Polyclinique d'Argenteuil, 201-551 rue Berry, Lachute QC J8H 1S4; Sher'92; CCFP; Staff, Centre Hospitalier d'Argenteuil; (450)562-3751; Fax. (450)562-1852.

SABOURIN, Karine; CLSC des Hautes Laurentides, 757 rue de la Madone, Mont-Laurier QC J9L 1T3; Mon'00; CCFP; Langs: English; (819)623-1228; Fax. (819)440-2999.

SABOURIN, Kenneth B; Ottawa Sport Med Centre, 1370 Clyde Ave, Nepean ON K2G 3H8; Ott'91; Dip SportMed; CCFP; Staff, The Ottawa Hospital - Riverside Campus; Langs: Bilingual(English/French); (613)727-2745; Fax. (613)727-2623.

SABOURIN, Marcel J L; 216-350 Sparks St, Ottawa ON K1R 7S8; Ott'75; FRCSC; Ophth. Court Staff, Queensway Carleton Hospital; Langs: French; (613)235-6576; Fax. (613)567-1160.

SABOURIN, Thierry; Hop Charles Lemoyne, 3120 boul Taschereau, Greenfield Park QC J4V 2H1; Laval'07; DiagRad. Staff, Hopital Charles LeMoyne; (450)466-5000

SABOURIN, Thomas; Centre Hosp Honore-Mercier, 2750 boul Laframboise, Saint-Hyacinthe QC J2S 4Y8; Mon'98; Staff, Centre Hospitalier Honore-Mercier; (450)771-3333

SABRA, Sally M M H; Div of Maternal Fetal Med, 3201-700 University Ave, Toronto ON M5G 1Z5; Cairo (Egypt)'99; (416)586-8660

SABRI, Ali; Cypress Reg Health Centre, 2004 Saskatchewan Dr, Swift Current SK S9H 5M8; (Iran)'04; MMed; (306)778-9537; Fax. (306)778-9588; sbri.ali@gmail.com.

SABRI, Kourosh; Hamilton HS-McMaster Site, PO Box 2000 Stn Lcd 1 1200 Main St W, Hamilton ON L8N 3Z5; (United Kingdom)'94; Staff, Hamilton Health Sciences Centre - McMaster University Medical Centre; Langs: Farsi; (905)521-2100

SABRI, Rida A; Great Lakes Med Centre, B-25 Great Lakes Dr, Brampton ON L6R 2S5; Tripoli (Libya)'91; CCFP; FCFP; Langs: Arabic; (905)494-0302; Fax. (905)494-0754; ridasabri@hotmail.com.

SABRY, Boshra I; Orleans Medical-Dental Centre, 106-2555 St. Joseph Blvd, Orleans ON K1C 1S6; Alexandria (Egypt)'76; FAAP; MB ChB; Langs: Arabic; French; (613)837-8579; Fax. (613)837-9750.

SABUR, Natasha F; Sunridge Landing, 3383 26 Ave NE, Calgary AB T1Y 6J4; Tor'06; FRCPC; IntMed; Respir. Staff, Rockyview General Hospital; (403)943-4971; Fax. (403)943-4017.

SABZI MOBARAKEH, Afshin; J A Hildes Northern Med Unit, T162-770 Bannatyne Ave, Winnipeg MB R3E 0W3; (204)794-4575

SACAMANO, James T; 157-1581 Hillside Ave, Victoria BC V8T 2C1; Columbia(MO) (USA)'69; FRCPC; Psy. Staff, Gorge Road Hospital; (250)213-4425

SACCHINI, Clara; Karma Clinic, 400-18 Pine St, Kitchener ON N2H 5Z8; (Italy)'87; (519)570-0090; Fax. (519)570-3202.

SACCOMANNO, Pamela M; William Osler HC-Brampton, 2100 Bovaird Dr E, Brampton ON L6R 3J7; Glasgow (Scotland)'87; MB ChB; FRCPC; Anes. Court Staff, William Osler Health System - Etobicoke General Hospital; Staff, William Osler Health System - Brampton Civic Hospital; (905)494-6576; sacpa@magic.pmh.on.ca.

SACEVICH, Eugene G; The Northwood Park Health Ctre, 504 Edward St N, Thunder Bay ON P7C 4P9; McM'75; BSc(Hon); MA; Asst Prof Faculty of Med, Northern Ontario School of Medicine-Lakehead University; Langs: Russian; French; (807)286-2005; Fax. (807)286-2685.

SACEVICH, Tegan F; Lakehead Psychiatric Hosp, PO Box 2930 Stn P 580 Algoma St N, Thunder Bay ON P7B 5G4; Tor'05; FRCPC; Psy. Staff, Lakehead Psychiatric Hospital - St. Joseph's Care Group.

SACHAR, Seerat; Royal Victoria Hosp, 201 Georgian Dr, Barrie ON L4M 6M2; (India)'01; Staff, Royal Victoria Regional Health Centre; (705)728-9090

SACHDEV, Bhupinder S; 8685 120 St, Delta BC V4C 6R4; Punjab (India)'70; (604)590-3166

SACHDEVA, Ashok; Kingsbridge Med Centre, 20 Kingsbridge Garden Cir, Mississauga ON L5R 3K7; (India)'88; (905)507-1111

SACHDEVA, Ashok K; Sunridge Prof Centre, 414-2675 36 St NE, Calgary AB T1Y 6H6; Punjab (India)'79; CCFP; (403)250-9111; Fax. (403)250-9112.

SACHDEVA, Herveen K; 10F-277 Victoria St, Toronto ON M5B 1W2; Wes'01; FRCPC; CommunMed. (416)338-1607

SACHDEVA, Jasdip S; 101-3 Conestoga Dr, Brampton ON L6Z 4N5; Tor'93; FRCPC; IntMed; Nephrol. Langs: Punjabi; (905)453-0715; Fax. (905)453-0972.

SACHDEVA, Krishan K; 14 Hospital Crt, Oshawa ON L1G 8A1; Punjab (India)'65; FRCS(Eng); FRCSC; Urol (Incontinence). Ac Staff, Lakeridge Health - Oshawa Site; Ac Staff, Lakeridge Health - Whitby Site; Ac Staff, Lakeridge Health - Bowmanville Site; Langs: Hindi; Punjabi; Urdu; (905)728-5133; Fax. (905)436-0193; ksach96857@aol.com.

SACHDEVA, Nandini; Hamilton HS-McMaster Site, PO Box 2000 Stn Lcd 1 1200 Main St W, Hamilton ON L8N 3Z5; Maharshi Dayanand University (India)'95; (905)521-2100

SACHDEVA, Preeti; 718-123 Edward St, Toronto ON M5G 1E2; Man'96; CCFP; FCFP; (416)971-7730; Fax. (416)408-2802.

SACHDEVA, Rajeev; Royal Ottawa Hlth Care Group, 1145 Carling Ave, Ottawa ON K1Z 7K4; Ott'82; FRCPC; Psy. Staff, Royal Ottawa Mental Health Centre - Royal Ottawa Health Care Group; (613)722-6521; Fax. (613)761-3602.

SACHEDINA, Bashirudin; 200-1A Conestoga Dr, Brampton ON L6Z 4N5; Liverpool (England)'79; FRCPC; IntMed; Gastroent. Consultant Gastroent, William Osler Health System - Brampton Civic Hospital; Langs: Gujarati; (905)454-9230; Fax. (905)454-5733.

SACHEDINA, Gulzar P; 4555 Richardson Rd SW, Calgary AB T3E 7E6; Liverpool (England)'80; MB ChB; FRCPC; Anes (Regional Anesthesia). Ac Staff, Foothills Medical Centre; Med Dir, Advanced Cardiac Life Support; Med Dir, Royal View Surgical Center; Clinical Asst Prof, University of Calgary; Langs: Bilingual(English/French); Gujarati; (403)242-2600; Fax. (403)242-3275.

SACHS, Helen K; 8808 92 St NW, Edmonton AB T6C 3R1; Alb'79; (780)469-7147; Fax. (780)469-3871.

SACKIN, H David; Bussiness Bldg, 414-94 Cumberland St, Toronto ON M5R 1A3; Tor'55; (416)513-0025

SACKMAN, Paul G; Horizon Square Med Centre, 401-3508 32 Ave NE, Calgary AB T1Y 6J2; Cal'77; MPH; FRCPC; CommunMed (Family Medicine). (403)291-5588; Fax. (403)250-6783.

SACKS, Diane P G; 106-1300 Don Mills Rd, North York ON M3B 2W6; Pittsburghh(PA) (USA)'69; FAAP; FRCPC; Peds (Adolescent Medicine). Ac Staff, North York General Hospital; Asst Prof, University of Toronto; (416)444-7751; Fax. (416)444-5752; teendoc75@aol.com.

SACKS, Eileen; Bayside Med Centre, 3 Beck Blvd, Penetanguishene ON L9M 1B9; Wes'05; FRCSC; GenSurg. (705)549-3939; Fax. (705)549-0029.

SACKS, Herbert W; PO Box 78185 Rpo Callingwood, Edmonton AB T5T 6A1; Edinburgh (Scotland)'71; DObst; CCFP; FCFP; Langs: Afrikaans; Dutch; Hebrew; (780)487-7156; Fax. (780)481-2449.

SACKS, Jordana B; North York Doctors, 703-240 Duncan Mill Rd, North York ON M3B 3S6; Tor'02; CCFP; Lecturer, University of Toronto; (416)494-7396; Fax. (416)494-0129.

SACKS, Juliette Y; PO Box 62032 Rpo Westmount, Edmonton AB T5M 4B5; Alb'04; FRCSC; ObstGyn;CCFP; CCFP(E.M.).

SACKSEN, Alain J B; Kempenfelt Health Clinic, 21 Essa Rd, Barrie ON L4N 3K4; Wes'01; CCFP; (705)739-8989; Fax. (705)739-8987; kempenfeltclinic@gmail.com.

SACZEK, Krzysztof; Regina Qu'Appelle HR-Regina, 1440 14th Ave, Regina SK S4P 0W5; Staff, Regina General Hospital; (306)766-4602; Fax. (306)766-3461.

SADAF, Arifa; Hôpital régional Chaleur, 1750 Sunset Dr, Bathurst NB E2A 4L7; Punjab University (Pakistan)'95; Staff, Hopital Regional Chaleur; (506)544-2458

SADAK, Yuksel; Bramalea Med Centre, 504-18 Kensington Rd, Brampton ON L6T 4S5; Istanbul (Turkey)'61; ABIM; FRCPC; IntMed (Cardiology). Ac Staff, William Osler Health System - Brampton Civic Hospital; Langs: Turkish; (905)792-2316; Fax. (905)792-7075.

SADANA, Sumeet; Lifesource Health Centre, 130 Robertson Rd, Nepean ON K2H 5Z1; West Indies (Jamaica)'98; FRCPC; Peds. Staff, Children's Hospital of Eastern Ontario (CHEO); Staff, Queensway Carleton Hospital; (613)828-3122; Fax. (613)828-2010.

SADANAND, Venkatraman; Royal University Hosp, 103 Hospital Dr, Saskatoon SK S7N 0W8; Tor'97; FRCSC; Neursurg. Staff, Royal University Hospital; (306)261-7595

SADANI, Gaelle; Hop du Sacre-Coeur de Mtl, 5400 boul Gouin O, Montreal QC H4J 1C5; Staff, Hôpital du Sacre-Coeur de Montréal; (514)338-2222

SADAVOY, Joel; L1 012-60 Murray St, Toronto ON M5T 3L9; Tor'68; DPsy; FRCPC; Psy (Geriatric Medicine). Prof Med, University of Toronto; (416)586-5262; Fax. (416)586-3231; j.sadavoy@utoronto.ca.

SADDI, Ghada-Maria; Ctr Hosp Anna-Laberge, 200 boul Brisebois, Chateauguay QC J6K 4W8; Damascus (Syria)'94; MSc; CCFP; Staff, Hôpital Anna-Laberge; Langs: Arabic; Polish; French; (450)699-2450

SADDIK, Maruf S; Grey Nuns Community Hosp, 1100 Youville Drive West NW, Edmonton AB T6L 5X8; Baghdad (Iraq)'83; MB ChB; FRCPC; GenPath. Staff LabMed & Path, Covenant Health - Grey Nuns Community Hospital; (780)735-7097; Fax. (780)735-9688; maruf@telusplanet.net.

SADE, Shachar; Sunnybrook Hlth Sciences Ctre, 2075 Bayview Ave, Toronto ON M4N 3M5; Wes'04; FRCPC; AnatPath. Staff, Sunnybrook Health Sciences Centre; (416)480-6100 x83869

SADEGHI TEHRANI, Susan; Northmount Med Centre, 203-145 13th St E, North Vancouver BC V7L 2L4; UBC'03; FRCSC; ObstGyn. (604)980-4867

SADEK, Amel H F; 1-6 Clairmont St, Thorold ON L2V 1R1; Cairo (Egypt)'85; CCFP; Langs: Arabic; (905)680-9703; Fax. (905)680-9705; hany_amelhann5@hotmail.com.

SADEK, Irene; DJ Mackenzie Bldg, 204B-5788 University Ave, Halifax NS B3H 1V8; Cairo (Egypt)'89; MB ChB; FRCPC; HemPath. Chief Hematopathology, Queen Elizabeth II Health Sciences Centre - Victoria General Site; Assoc Prof, Dalhousie University; Langs: Arabic; French; (902)473-2177; Fax. (902)473-4113; irene.sadek@cdha.nshealth.ca.

SADEK, Joseph A; The Nova Scotia Hosp, PO Box 1004 Stn Main 142 EC-300 Pleasant St, Dartmouth NS B2Y 3Z9; Ain Shams (Egypt)'90; MB ChB; FRCPC; Psy. Staff, The Nova Scotia Hospital; (902)237-3002; Fax. (902)406-4447.

SADEK, Mouhannad M; Univ of Ottawa Heart Institute, 40 Ruskin St, Ottawa ON K1Y 4W7; Ott'05; FRCPC; IntMed; Cardiol. Staff, University of Ottawa Heart Institute; (613)761-5000

SADEK-BOTROS, Gamal E; 193 Commissioners Rd W, London ON N6J 1X9; Ain Shams (Egypt)'75; MB ChB; FRCPC; Psy (Addiction Medicine). Langs: Arabic; (519)433-6923; Fax. (519)433-6394.

SADER, Benjamin J; Valley Med Clinic, PO Box 2932 Stn Main 231 2 Ave, Strathmore AB T1P 1L5; Alb'97; CCFP; Staff Emerg, Strathmore District Health Services; (403)934-4444; Fax. (403)934-5218.

SADER, John; Clinique medicale GMF-1851, 101-1851 rue Sherbrooke E, Montreal QC H2K 4L5; Mon'89; (514)524-7564; Fax. (514)527-5251.

SADER, Naeem; Willowgrove Med Group, 2-527 Neilson Rd, Saskatoon SK S7S 1P4; Natal (South Africa)'04; BSc; MB ChB; Staff, Rosthern Hospital; Staff, St Paul's Hospital (Grey Nuns) of Saskatoon; (306)653-1543; Fax. (306)653-0422.

SADER, Paul E; Clinique Med Chemin Chambly, 101-3090 ch Chambly, Longueuil QC J4L 4N5; Mon'93; CCFP; Staff, Centre de Sante Isle-Dieu Matagami; (450)670-5700; Fax. (450)670-8830.

SADERA, Abhimanyu J S; 350 Main St E, Milton ON L9T 1P6; Medical University of the Americas (Saint Kitts-Nevis)'08; CCFP; (905)636-0766

SADIK, Aksam; Baygreen Clinic, 10-8 Green Lane, Thornhill ON L3T 7P7; Assiut (Egypt)'70; CCFP; Langs: Arabic; (905)709-9400; Fax. (905)709-9409.

SADIK, Zaki K; Maple Med Centre, 110-955 Major MacKenzie Dr, Vaughan ON L6A 4P9; Assuit (Egypt)'69; CCFP; Staff, Toronto East General Hospital Inc; Langs: Arabic; French; (289)553-3300; Fax. (289)553-2600.

SADIKALI, Fakhruddin; 501-145 Queenston St, St Catharines ON L2R 2Z9; London (England)'63; MRC; ABIM; DCH; FRCPC; IntMed (Gastroenterology). Staff, Niagara Health System - St Catharines General Site; Langs: Kiswahili; Gujarati; Swahili; Hindi; (905)682-2090; Fax. (905)682-4725.

SADIKOT, Abbas F; MUHC-Montreal Neurology Inst, 109A-3801 rue University, Montreal QC H3A 2B4; McG'84; DAB; PhD(NeuroSci); FRCSC; Neursurg (Brain Tumors). Staff, McGill University Health Centre - Montreal Neurological Hospital; Head Functional Neurosurg, McGill University; (514)398-4305; Fax. (514)398-2811.

SADIKOV, Evgeny A; Allan Blair Cancer Centre, 4101 Dewdney Ave, Regina SK S4T 7T1; Moscow (Russia (Federation))'86; Staff, Pasqua Hospital; Clin Assoc Prof Med, University of Saskatchewan; Langs: Russian; Hebrew; (306)766-2813; Fax. (306)766-5688.

SADINSKY, H Leonard; 106-40 Westmore Dr, Etobicoke ON M9V 4C2; Ott'69; Ac Staff Family Pract, William Osler Health System - Etobicoke General Hospital; Staff, Extendicare Brampton & Mississauga; Langs: Bilingual(French/English); (416)742-8222; Fax. (416)742-0184.

SADIQ, Ammara I; Parkland Med Clinic, 205-505 Queen St, Spruce Grove AB T7X 2V2; (South Africa)'04; MB BCh; (780)962-2001; Fax. (780)962-8176.

SADIQ, Najemus; Taunton Health Centre, SS 201 1290 Keith Ross Dr, Oshawa ON L1H 7K4; Bangalore University (India)'91; CCFP; (905)721-6863; Fax. (905)721-6874.

SADIQ, Shahnaz; Royal Oak Center, 192-8888 Country Hills Blvd NW, Calgary AB T3G 5T4; (Pakistan)'78; MB BS; (403)239-3660; Fax. (403)239-4001.

SADIQ, Shehla; Rouge Valley HS-Centenary, 2867 Ellesmere Rd, Scarborough ON M1E 4B9; Karachi (Pakistan)'99; IntMed. Staff, Rouge Valley Health System - Centenary Health Centre Site; (416)284-8131

SADIQ, Syed Z; The Moncton Hosp, 135 MacBeath Ave, Moncton NB E1C 6Z8; Karachi (Pakistan)'91; MB BS; Staff, The Moncton Hospital; Staff, Moncton Mental Health Clinic; Teach Staff, Dalhousie University; (506)857-5780; Fax. (506)857-5751; dr.syed.sadiq@horizonnb.ca.

SADLER, D James; Foothills Med Centre, 1403 29 St NW, Calgary AB T2N 2T9; (Scotland)'87; Staff, Foothills Medical Centre; (403)944-1969; Fax. (403)944-1687.

SADLER, John T S; 246 James St S, Hamilton ON L8P 3B3; Dundee (Scotland)'67; MB ChB; OrthSurg (Joint Replacement). Staff Surg, Hamilton Health Sciences Centre - Hamilton General Hospital; Asst Prof, McMaster University; Langs: French; (905)522-5594; Fax. (905)522-2113.

SADLER, Laura K; Crossroads Family Practice Inc, 201-5110 St Margarets Bay Rd, Upper Tantallon NS B3Z 1E2; Dal'07; CCFP; (902)826-9096; Fax. (902)820-9399.

SADLER, Margot C; 205-220 Main St, Antigonish NS B2G 2C2; Dal'91; CCFP; FCFP; (902)863-2674; Fax. (902)867-5662.

SADLER, R Mark; Queen Elizabeth II HSC-Halifax, 3829-1796 Summer St, Halifax NS B3H 3A7; Dal'77; FRCPC; Neur (Epilepsy). Staff, Queen Elizabeth II Health Sciences Centre - Halifax Infirmary Site; Prof Med, Dalhousie University; (902)473-7451; Fax. (902)473-4438.

SADOUGHI, Mehdi; Medical Office Bldg, 317-89 Humber College Blvd, Etobicoke ON M9V 4B8; Tehran (Iran)'96; FRCSC; OrthSurg. (416)745-1597

SADOUSKI, Maria M; Kings Lane Med Clinic, 101-164 Kings Lane, Salt Spring Island BC V8K 2P7; Qns'89; CCFP; Staff, Lady Minto Gulf Islands Hospital; (250)538-4800

SADOWNIK, Leslie A; Diamond Health Care Centre, 2775 Laurel St, Vancouver BC V5Z 1M9; Alb'91; FRCSC; ObstGyn. Staff, Vancouver General Hospital - Centennial Pavillion; (604)875-4260; Fax. (604)875-4869.

SADOWSKA, Ewa; Saint John Reg Hosp, PO Box 2100 Stn Main 400 University Ave, Saint John NB E2L 4L2; Bialystok (Poland)'80; FRCP; FRCPC; IntMed; Rheum. Staff, Saint John Regional Hospital; (506)648-6659; Fax. (506)648-6687; ewa.sadowska@horizonnb.ca.

SADOWSKI, Daniel C; Royal Alexandra Hosp, 215-10240 Kingsway NW, Edmonton AB T5H 3V9; Sask'84; ABIM; FRCPC; IntMed; Gastroent. Staff Comm Services Centre, Royal Alexandra Hospital; (780)735-6837; Fax. (780)735-5650.

SADOWSKI, Henry A; 201-1024 Ridgeway Ave, Coquitlam BC V3J 1S5; Tor'71; FRCPC; IntMed (Electromyography); Neur. Staff, Royal Columbian Hospital; (604)936-9941; Fax. (604)936-8507.

SADR, Aida; Vancouver Native Hlth Clinic, 449 Hastings St E, Vancouver BC V6A 1P5; Alb'05; CCFP; Staff, Providence Health Care - St Paul's Hospital; (604)255-9766

SADREHASHEMI, Ladan; Vancouver Gen Hosp, 855 12th Ave W, Vancouver BC V5Z 1M9; Cal'99; FRCPC; Psy. Staff Psychiatric Assessment Unit, Vancouver General Hospital - Centennial Pavillion; (604)875-4018

SADRI, Daryoush; Enhanced Care Clinic, 14872 Yonge St, Aurora ON L4G 1N2; Tehran (Iran)'62; CCFP; Langs: Farsi.

SADRY, Dhun S; Crescent Town Health Ctre, 4 The Market Place, Toronto ON M4C 5M1; Bombay (India)'74; CCFP; Langs: Gujarati; Hindi; Marathi; Urdu; (416)690-3412; Fax. (416)691-2543.

SAEED, Akhter; Bluewater Health-Norman Site, 89 Norman St, Sarnia ON N7T 6S3; Punjab (Pakistan)'85; Staff, Bluewater Health - Norman Site; (519)464-4400

SAEED, Arshad; Cdn Forces Health Services Ctr, 101 Colonel By Dr, Ottawa ON K1A 0K2; Karachi (Pakistan)'79; MB BS; CCFP; FCFP; Staff, Canadian Forces Health Services Centre; Langs: Urdu; Hindi; Punjabi; (613)945-1820; Fax. (613)945-1819.

SAEED, Ayesha L; Roslyn Med Bldg, 200-400 5 Ave SW, Calgary AB T2P 0L6; (Pakistan)'97; CCFP; Langs: Urdu; (403)930-1005; Fax. (403)930-1004.

SAEED, Haider A; Garden City Family Health Team, 22 Ontario St, St Catharines ON L2R 7M3; New York (USA)'05; CCFP; (905)984-3335; Fax. (905)984-6008.

SAEED, Khalid; Queens University, 752 King St W, Kingston ON K7L 4X3; Lahore (Pakistan)'82; MB; BSc; MRCPsy(UK); (613)548-5567; ksaeed@casleregina.com.

SAEED, Khawer; 193 Lemarchant Rd, St. John's NL A1C 2H5; Karachi (Pakistan)'87; Staff, St Clare's Mercy Hospital; (709)777-5500

SAEED, Lina; 906 Brant St, Burlington ON L7R 2J5; Baghdad (Iraq)'01; MB BCh; (905)637-5885; Fax. (905)637-0372.

SAEED, Maheen; Univ of Ottawa Health Service, 300-100 Marie Curie Pvt, Ottawa ON K1N 6N5; Dow Medical College (Pakistan)'98; (613)564-3950

SAEED, Muhammad A; 106-704 Mara St, Sarnia ON N7V 1X4; Sind (Pakistan)'89; MB BS; (519)336-1555; Fax. (519)336-2193; iqra97@hotmail.com.

SAEED, Niloufer; Canamera Med Centre, B5-350 Conestoga Blvd, Cambridge ON N1R 7L7; Osmania (India)'62; MB BS; FRCPC; HemPath (AIDS/HIV). Langs: Urdu; Hindi; (519)621-0437; Fax. (519)623-7342.

SAEED, Perie A; Niagara Med Group Fam Hlth Team, 4421 Queen St, Niagara Falls ON L2E 2L2; McG'87; Ac Staff, Niagara Health System - Greater Niagara General Site; Langs: French; (905)356-2236; Fax. (905)356-2568; webmaster@niagaramedicalgroup.com.

SAEED, Tariq M; 104-160 Dundas St E, Mississauga ON L5A 1W4; Tor'75; CCFP; Staff, Trillium Health Centre - West Toronto; Langs: Urdu; Hindi; (905)276-7252; Fax. (905)276-7256.

SAEEDI-TABAR, Soheil; Mississauga Med Centre, 418-1420 Burnhamthorpe Rd E, Mississauga ON L4X 2Z9; Qns'92; CCFP; FCFP; Langs: Farsi; (905)624-6922; Fax. (905)624-6731.

SAETTLER, Elizabeth B; London Reg Cancer Centre, A3 931A-790 Commissioners Rd E, London ON N6A 4L6; Wes'85; FRCSC; GenSurg; General Surgical Oncology. (519)685-8740

SAETTLER, Erik R J; Orillia Soldier's Mem Hosp, 170 Colborne St W, Orillia ON L3V 2Z3; Tor'01; FRCSC; GenSurg; Critical Care Medicine. Staff, Orillia Soldiers' Memorial Hospital; (705)327-6616

SAEY, Anne-Marie; CSSS de Laval, 1755 boul Rene-Laennec, Laval QC H7M 3L9; Mon'05; CCFP; Staff, Hopital de la Cite de la santé; (450)668-1010

SAFA, Behnam; Sunnybrook Hlth Sciences Ctre, M3 200-2075 Bayview Ave, Toronto ON M4N 3M5; Ott'98; MScPharm; FRCPC; Anes (Regional Anesthesia). Staff, Sunnybrook Health Sciences Centre; Asst Prof, University of Toronto; (416)480-4864

SAFA, Nagi; Hop du Sacre-Coeur de Mtl, 5400 boul Gouin O, Montreal QC H4J 1C5; GenSurg (P.Q.). Staff, Hôpital du Sacre-Coeur de Montréal; (514)338-2222; Fax. (514)338-3515.

SAFADI, Gabriel; Hop Louis-H Lafontaine, 7041 rue Hochelaga, Montreal QC H1N 3M5; Mon'87; CSPQ; FRCPC; Psy. Staff, Hôpital Riviere des Prairies; Staff, Hopital Louis-H Lafontaine; Staff, Hôpital Ste-Justine; (514)251-4000; Fax. (514)251-4027.

SAFAKISH KASHANIFARD, Kyarash; Ocean View Family Practice, 306C-60 Vancouver St, Yarmouth NS B5A 2P5; (Other Foreign)'02; (902)742-3542; Fax. (902)742-0369.

SAFAR, Gregory C; Brant Community HC-Brantford, 200 Terrace Hill St, Brantford ON N3R 1G9; Tor'94; CCFP; CCFP(E.M.); FCFP; Staff, The Brant Community Healthcare System - Brantford General Hospital Site; Langs: English; French; (519)752-7871

SAFAR, Modar A; Alliston Family Health Team, PO Box 280 36 Victoria St W, Alliston ON L9R 1S8; Baghdad (Iraq)'95; CCFP; (705)435-8887

SAFAR ZADEH, Elika; North York Gen Hosp, 4001 Leslie St, Toronto ON M2K 1E1; University of Tehran (Iran)'01; Staff, North York General Hospital; (416)756-6000

SAFAVI, Mahsa; York Medical Green Lane, RR 1 Lcd 1 18120 Yonge St, Newmarket ON L3Y 4V8; Teheran (Iran)'03; CCFP; (905)868-9243

SAFFARI, Hamideh; Springfield Med Clinic, 559 Main St, Oakbank MB R0E 1J2.

SAFFER, Linda S; The Promenade Mall, 302-1 Promenade Cir, Thornhill ON L4J 4P8; Witwatersrand (South Africa)'74; MB BS; FRCPC; Psy. Langs: Hebrew; (905)762-0526

SAFFER, Mark D; The Promenade Mall, 302-1 Promenade Cir, Thornhill ON L4J 4P8; Witwatersrand (South Africa)'70; MB BS; FRCPC; Psy. Langs: Hebrew; (905)762-0525

SAFFREY, James A; St Anthony's Med Centre, 306-582 Goldstream Ave, Victoria BC V9B 2W7; Tor'76; CCFP; FCFP; Staff, Victoria General Hospital; (250)474-1221; Fax. (250)474-3917.

SAFFY, Samantha C; Surrey Mem Hosp, 13750 96 Ave, Surrey BC V3V 1Z2; Pretoria (South Africa)'96; MB BCh; FRCPC; Psy. Staff, Surrey Memorial Hospital; (604)581-2211

SAFI, Sohail; Western Memorial Health Clinic, 3 Herald Ave, Corner Brook NL A2H 4B8; Rawalpindi (India)'88; CCFP; Staff, Western Memorial Regional Hospital; (709)632-2152; Fax. (709)632-2103.

SAFIEDDINE, Najib N; Toronto East Gen Hosp Inc, F117-825 Coxwell Ave, Toronto ON M4C 3E7; Wes'02; ThorSurg (Minimal Invasive Surgery); GenSurg. Staff, Toronto East General Hospital Inc; Staff, Sunnybrook Health Sciences Centre; Lecturer, University of Toronto; Langs: Arabic; Spanish; (416)469-2345; Fax. (416)469-9527.

SAFIEH, Patrick; A1-3492 Weston Rd, North York ON M9M 2W1; Tor'90; CCFP; CCFP(E.M.); FCFP; Chief FamilyMed(EM), Humber River Regional Hospital - Finch Avenue Site; Ac Staff, Humber River Regional Hospital - Church Street Site; Langs: Spanish; French; (416)744-8510; Fax. (416)744-7642.

SAFINIA, Layla; Sunnybrook Hlth Sciences Ctre, M1 600-2075 Bayview Ave, Toronto ON M4N 3M5; Shaheed Beheshti (Iran)'98; FRCPC; IntMed; Neur. Staff, Sunnybrook Health Sciences Centre; (416)480-6100

SAFIR, Irina; Uptown Health Centre, 9325 Yonge St, Richmond Hill ON L4C 0A8; Dniepropetrovsk (Ukraine)'85; CCFP; (905)508-8876

SAFIR, Oleg A; Mount Sinai Hosp, 476A-600 University Ave, Toronto ON M5G 1X5; Dniepropetrovsk (Russia (Federation))'90; FRCSC; OrthSurg. Staff, Mount Sinai Hospital; (416)586-4800 x4611

SAFNECK, Janice R; Health Sciences Centre, MS 459A-820 Sherbrook St, Winnipeg MB R3A 1R9; Man'80; FRCPC; AnatPath. Staff Path, Health Sciences Centre; Staff, Misericordia Health Centre; Assoc Prof Med, University of Manitoba; (204)787-2829; Fax. (204)784-4942; safneck@cc.umanitoba.ca.

SAFRAN, Jaclyn E; Southport Family Practice, 110-10333 Southport Rd SW, Calgary AB T2W 3X6; Alb'84; CCFP; FCFP; Staff, Rockyview General Hospital; (403)258-1960; Fax. (403)253-5735.

SAFRANOVICH, Colin E; Ottewell Med Clinic, 6138 90 Ave NW, Edmonton AB T6B 0P2; Alb'94; (780)468-6409; Fax. (780)469-1261.

SAFRANYOS, Richard G A; Pelham Med Centre, 212-245 Pelham Rd, St Catharines ON L2S 1X8; Tor'90; BSc; PhD; FRCPC; IntMed; GeriatricMed. Staff, Niagara Health System - St Catharines General Site; Staff, Niagara Health System - Welland Hospital Site; Staff, Niagara Health System - Port Colborne General Site; Langs: Hungarian; (905)682-9335; Fax. (905)682-9641.

SAGAR, Stephen M; The Juravinski Cancer Centre, 699 Concession St, Hamilton ON L8V 5C2; London (England)'81; MRC; FRCR; DABR; BSc(Hons.); FRCPC; RadOncol. Physician, The Juravinski Cancer Centre; Prof Oncol, McMaster University; (905)387-9495 x64721; Fax. (905)575-6326; stephen.sagar@hrcc.on.ca.

SAGER, Mark J; 303-2797 Bathurst St, North York ON M6B 4B9; Ott'71; CCFP; FCFP; Staff, Mount Sinai Hospital; (416)787-5646 x3; Fax. (416)787-9049.

SAGGAR, Barjinder; Nanak Med Centre, 4-10725 McLaughlin Rd, Brampton ON L7A 3E5; (Pakistan)'98; CCFP; (905)488-1623

SAGI, Eliyhoo A; Lakeridge Hlth Corp-Oshawa, 1 Hospital Crt, Oshawa ON L1G 2B9; Hebrew (Israel)'76; FRCPC; Psy. Staff Psy, Lakeridge Health - Oshawa Site; Langs: Hebrew; (905)576-8711; Fax. (905)721-4780.

SAGINUR, Michael D; Montfort Hosp, 713 Montreal Rd, Ottawa ON K1K 0T2; Qns'07; FRCPC; Peds. Staff, Montfort Hospital; (613)746-4621

SAGINUR, Raphael; The Ottawa Hosp-Civic Campus, CPC 470-1053 Carling Ave, Ottawa ON K1Y 4E9; McG'73; ABIM; FRCPC; IntMed (Infectious Diseases); MedMicrobiol. Staff, The Ottawa Hospital - Civic Campus; Staff, Queensway Carleton Hospital; Assoc Prof, University of Ottawa; Langs: French; (613)761-4155 x1

SAGLE, Margaret A; Royal Alexandra Hosp, 5S133-10240 Kingsway NW, Edmonton AB T5H 3V9; Wes'79; MSc(McM); FRCSC; ObstGyn (Reproductive Endocrinology & Infertility). Staff 5S131 Lois Hole Hosp Robbins Pav Rah, Royal Alexandra Hospital; Prof/Dept Head ObstGyn, University of Alberta; (780)735-4911; Fax. (780)735-4981.

SAGMAN, Doron; Toronto East Gen Hosp Inc, H5-825 Coxwell Ave, Toronto ON M4C 3E7; Cal'87; FRCPC; Psy (Mood Disorders). Ac Staff Psy, Toronto East General Hospital Inc; Lecturer Psy, University of Toronto; (416)469-6580 x6211; Fax. (416)482-6726; sagmand@gmail.com.

SAGMAN, Uri; Humber River Reg Hosp-Church, 200 Church St, Toronto ON M9N 1N8; Cal'81; FRCPC; IntMed. Staff, Humber River Regional Hospital - Church Street Site; Langs: Hebrew; French; (416)243-4103

SAGORIN, Richard A; Blundell Centre Med Clinic, 186-8180 No. 2 Rd, Richmond BC V7C 5K1; Cape Town (South Africa)'83; MB ChB; CCFP; (604)241-8911; Fax. (604)241-8912.

SAGREDO, Sonya; CSSS de Laval, 1755 boul Rene-Laennec, Laval QC H7M 3L9; Mon'98; CSPQ; FRCPC; DiagRad. Staff, Hopital de la Cite de la santé; (450)668-1010

SAHA, Amal K; Public Gardens Med Clinic, 200-5675 Spring Garden Rd, Halifax NS B3J 1H1; Kiev (Ukraine)'91; CCFP; Langs: Bengali; Russian; (902)425-5440; Fax. (902)482-6019; sahaamal@hotmail.com.

SAHA, Sandipan; Streetsville Med Centre, 8-5425 Creditview Rd, Mississauga ON L5V 2P3; Tor'96; (905)826-1164; Fax. (905)826-1214.

SAHA, Sudip K; William Osler HC-Brampton, 2100 Bovaird Dr E, Brampton ON L6R 3J7; University of Pune (India)'97; Staff, William Osler Health System - Brampton Civic Hospital; (905)494-2120

SAHA, Tarit K; Kingston Gen Hosp, 76 Stuart St, Kingston ON K7L 2V7; Rajasthan (Pakistan)'92; FRCPC; Anes. Staff, Kingston General Hospital; (613)549-6666 x3850

SAHAB, Philippe G; Hop Jean-Talon, 1385 rue Jean-Talon E, Montreal QC H2E 1S6; Beirut (Lebanon)'70; CSPQ; FRCPC; Anes (Cardiovascular Anesthesia). Staff, CSSS du Coeur de l'Isle Hôpital Jean-Talon; (514)495-6767

SAHAI, Anand V; CHUM-Hop St-Luc, 1058 rue Saint-Denis, Montreal QC H2X 3J4; Mon'90; Gastroent; IntMed. Staff, Centre Hospitalier l'Université De Montréal (CHUM) - Hôpital Saint-luc; (514)890-8000 x34373; Fax. (514)412-7372.

SAHAJPAL, Riki; Harmony Med Centre, 110-152 Cleopatra Dr, Nepean ON K2G 5X2; Dal'93; BSc; DAB; FRCSC; Urol (Oncology). Staff, Queensway Carleton Hospital; (613)725-1870; Fax. (613)725-1647.

SAHAJPAL, Viki; Dr Charles A Janeway Child HC, 300 Prince Philip Dr, St. John's NL A1B 3V6; Wes'96; FRCSC; OrthSurg. Staff, Health Sciences Centre; (709)777-6300

SAHAY, Bal Makund; B-221 Mitton St N, Sarnia ON N7T 6H5; Lucknow (India)'56; FESC; FCCP; FRCP(Lond); FACC; FACP; FRCPC; IntMed (Cardiology). Staff, Bluewater Health - Mitton Site; Langs: Hindi; (519)339-1031; Fax. (519)339-7591; balsahay@bellnet.ca.

SAHAY, Sidharth; Guelph Gen Hosp, 115 Delhi St, Guelph ON N1E 4J4; Qns'06; CCFP; CCFP(E.M.); Staff, Grey Bruce Health Services - Owen Sound; (519)837-6440

SAHEB, Nabil E; MUHC-Montreal Gen Hosp, L4 122-1650 av Cedar, Montreal QC H3G 1A4; Cairo (Egypt)'64; FRCSC; Ophth. Staff, McGill University Health Centre - Montreal General Campus; assoc Prof, McGill University; (514)935-2053; Fax. (514)934-8223.

SAHEB, Nathalie; CSSS de Laval, 1755 boul Rene-Laennec, Laval QC H7M 3L9; McG'01; FRCPC; IntMed; Gastroent. Staff, Hopital de la Cite de la santé; (450)668-1010

SAHEBJAM, Solmaz; Univ Hlth Network-Princess M, 5 216-610 University Ave, Toronto ON M5G 2M9; (Iran)'00; FRCPC; IntMed; MedOncol. Staff, Princess Margaret Hospital - University Health Network; (416)946-4501

SAHER, Fouad; Hawkesbury Dist Gen Hosp, 1111 Ghislain St, Hawkesbury ON K6A 3G5; Mohammed V University (Morocco)'82; Staff, Hawkesbury & District General Hospital; (613)632-1111

SAHGAL, Arjun; Sunnybrook Hlth Sciences Ctre, TW-2075 Bayview Ave, Toronto ON M4N 3M5; Ott'01; FRCPC; RadOncol. Radiation Oncologist, Princess Margaret Hospital - University Health Network; Staff Odette Cancer Centre, Sunnybrook Health Sciences Centre; (416)946-6513; Fax. (416)946-4586.

SAHHEED, Wade W; City Centre Med Clinic, 202-3420 Hurontario St, Mississauga ON L5B 4A9; McM'89; CCFP; (905)615-8301

SAHI, Kiranjit; 305-145 Queen St E, Brampton ON L6W 3P8; Punjabi (India)'92; FRCSC; ObstGyn. (905)459-1881; Fax. (905)459-8571.

SAHI, Nidhi; MUHC-Royal Victoria Hosp, 687 av des Pins O, Montreal QC H3A 1A1; Man'05; CCFP; Staff, McGill University Health Centre - Royal Victoria Hospital; (514)934-1934

SAHIHOLNASAB, S Vahid; Richmond Hosp, 7000 Westminster Hwy, Richmond BC V6X 1A2; Pecs (Hungary)'97; MD; FRCPC; IntMed (Geriatric Medicine). Staff, Richmond Hospital; Langs: German; Hungarian; Persian; (778)960-7893; vsahiholnasab@palliserhealth.ca.

SAHJPAUL, Ramesh L; Vancouver Coastal Health, 405-125 13th St E, North Vancouver BC V7L 2L3; Tor'87; FRCSC; Neursurg (Spine). Staff, Lions Gate Hospital; Physician, Providence Health Care - St Paul's Hospital; Langs: Hindi; Punjabi; (604)904-7467; Fax. (604)904-7462.

SAHLAS, Demetrios D J; Hamilton HS-General Site, 237 Barton St E, Hamilton ON L8L 2X2; McM'96; LMCC; BSc; MSc; FRCPC; Neur (Stroke). Court Staff, Sunnybrook Health Sciences Centre; Staff, Hamilton Health Sciences Centre - Hamilton General Hospital; Prof MG DeGroote Stroke Mgmt, McMaster University; Aj Prof, University of Toronto; Langs: Greek; French; (905)527-4322 x46373; sahlas@hhsc.ca.

SAHNI, Paramjit P; Temple Med Clinic, 109-5401 Temple Dr NE, Calgary AB T1Y 3R7; CCFP; Staff, Riverdale Health Centre; (403)293-1698; Fax. (403)293-7373.

SAHNI, Puja K; Med Sciences Bldg-U of Toronto, 6263-1 King's College Circle, Toronto ON M5S 1A8; McM'07; FRCPC; IntMed; Respir.

SAHOTA, Gurpreet S; 103-6490 Old Banff Coach Rd SW, Calgary AB T3H 5R8; UBC'09; CCFP; (403)930-5800

SAHOTA, Perminder S; 113-7500 120 St, Surrey BC V3W 3N1; Ranchi (India)'86; MB BS; (604)572-3535; Fax. (604)572-3560.

SAHOTA, Preena S; Surrey Mem Hosp, 13750 96 Ave, Surrey BC V3V 1Z2; UBC'08; CCFP; Staff, Surrey Memorial Hospital; (604)581-2211

SAHOTA, Surjit S; Saddletowne Med Clinic, 974 Saddletowne Cir NE, Calgary AB T3J 0H5; Bombay (India)'64; MB BS; MCPS; LRCP; MRCS(Lond); (403)590-7710; Fax. (403)590-7113.

SAHOTA, Vickram S; Medical One, C4-2501 Third Line, Oakville ON L6M 5A9; Wes'01; CCFP; (905)618-9934; Fax. (905)469-9936.

SAHSI, Rupinder S; St Mary's Gen Hosp, 911 Queens Blvd, Kitchener ON N2M 1B2; Wes'01; Staff, St Mary's General Hospital; (519)749-6410; Fax. (519)749-6411.

SAHYOUN, Hani N I; Scarborough North Med Arts, 405-4040 Finch Ave E, Scarborough ON M1S 4V5; Alexandria (Egypt)'78; MB ChB; FRCPC; Psy (Psycho Geriatrics). Staff, The Scarborough Hospital - Birchmount Campus; Langs: Italian; French; (416)298-8033; Fax. (416)298-8572.

SAI, Obodai; 2713 Kennedy Rd, Scarborough ON M1T 3H8; Accra (Ghana)'73; FRCPC; Psy. Ac Staff, Markham Stouffville Hospital; Court Staff, The Scarborough Hospital - Birchmount Campus; Langs: Akan; Ga; (416)298-3496; Fax. (416)298-3496.

SAIB, Rachid; Ctr Hosp Soins Psychiatriques, CP 800 1141 rue Royale, Malartic QC J0Y 1Z0; Alger (Algeria)'84; Staff, Hôpital psychiatrique de Malartic; (819)757-4342 x8296; Fax. (819)757-4313.

SAIBIL, Fredric G; Sunnybrook Hlth Sciences Ctre, H52-2075 Bayview Ave, Toronto ON M4N 3M5; McG'67; BSc; FRCPC; Gastroent; IntMed (Inflammatory Bowel Disease). Consultant Gastroent, Sunnybrook Health Sciences Centre; Prof Med, University of Toronto; (416)480-4727; Fax. (416)480-5977; fred.saibil@sunnybrook.ca.

SAIBIL, Romy B; 1942 Avenue Rd, North York ON M5M 4A1; Wes'00; CCFP; (416)780-1100; Fax. (416)780-1104.

SAID, Carla; Hotel-Dieu de Sorel, 400 av de l'Hotel-Dieu, Sorel-Tracy QC J3P 1N5; Staff, Hôtel-Dieu de Sorel; (450)746-6000

SAID, Tewfik; Allan Memorial Institute, 1025 av des Pins O, Montreal QC H3A 1A1; Sher'80; FRCP; CSPQ; FRCPC; Psy (Dynamic Psychotherapy). Staff, McGill University Health Centre - Montreal General Campus; Staff, Allan Memorial Institute; (514)934-1934 x34588; Fax. (514)843-2858; tewfik.said@mcgill.ca.

SAIDENBERG, Elianna; The Ottawa Hosp-Gen Campus, 501 Smyth Rd, Ottawa ON K1H 8L6; McM'02; FRCPC; IntMed (Transfusion Medicine); Hem. Fellow, The Ottawa Hospital - General Campus; (613)798-5555

SAIDI, Kaveh; Polyclinique Cabrini, 211-5700 rue Saint-Zotique E, Montreal QC H1T 3Y7; Teheran (Iran)'62; OrthSurg. (514)996-8182

SAIDI, Kevan; South Hlth & Life Managment Ct, 2-2120 Regent St, Sudbury ON P3E 3Z9; McM'03; FRCSC; OrthSurg. Staff, Mount Sinai Hospital; (705)522-9101

SAIEED, Kamila H; Riverbend Atrium One, 116-200 Rivercrest Dr SE, Calgary AB T2C 2X5; (Egypt)'86; MB ChB; CCFP; (403)236-1500; Fax. (403)236-2839.

SAIEED, Nabil H; Dominion Med Centre, 2383 111 St NW, Edmonton AB T6J 5E5; (Egypt)'78; CCFP; Staff, University of Alberta Hospital; (780)436-0020; Fax. (780)436-0603.

SAIGAL, Saroj; McMaster Universiy, HSC 3A-1280 Main St W, Hamilton ON L8S 4K1; Vikram (India)'61; MB BS; DCH; AB; FRCPC; Peds (Neonatology). Dir Growth & Development Clin, Hamilton Health Sciences Centre - McMaster University Medical Centre; Affil Staff, Hamilton Health Sciences Centre-Juravinski Site; Affil Staff, St Joseph's Healthcare - Charlton Campus; Prof, McMaster University; Langs: Punjabi; (905)521-2100 x76959; Fax. (905)521-5007; saigal@mcmaster.ca.

SAIGER, Gail F; Royal Jubilee Hosp, 1952 Bay St, Victoria BC V8R 1J8; Tor'76; CCFP; FCFP; Staff, Royal Jubilee Hospital; (250)370-8715; Fax. (250)370-8625.

SAIKALI, Emilie; CHUQ-Ctr Hosp Univ Laval, 2705 boul Laurier, Quebec QC G1V 4G2; Rennes (France)'06; Peds (P.Q.). Staff, Centre Hospitalier Universitaire de Quebec-CHUL; (418)656-4141; Fax. (418)654-2771.

SAIKALI, Stephan; Ctr Hosp Affilie-Enfant-Jesus, 1401 18e rue, Quebec QC G1J 1Z4; Rennes (France)'02; AnatPath (P.Q.). Staff, Centre Hospitalier Affilié Universitaire de Québec - Hôpital De L'Enfant Jésus; (418)649-5725

SAILLANT, Catherine; Centre Med de Boucherville, 600 boul du Fort-Saint-Louis, Boucherville QC J4B 1S7; Mon'08; (450)655-7321

SAILS, Alison; Beaumont Med Clinic, 5001A 50 Ave, Beaumont AB T4X 1E7; Alb'89; (780)929-6050; Fax. (780)929-5848; amsails@shaw.ca.

SAINBHEE, Parampreet; Gemini Health Centre, 2010-6708 48 Ave, Camrose AB T4V 4S3; (India)'92; MB BS; CCFP; Langs: Hindi; Punjabi; (780)672-9850; Fax. (780)672-9104.

SAINBHEE, Tejinder; Smith Clinic, 1-6601 48 Ave, Camrose AB T4V 3G8; Punjab (India)'89; MB BS; Consultant, Covenant Health - St Mary's Hospital; Langs: Punjabi; Hindi; (780)608-5879; Fax. (780)608-5880.

SAINCHER, Anurag Q; 101-14815 108 Ave, Surrey BC V3R 1W2; Gujarat (India)'88; MB BS; FRCPC; EmergMed. (604)582-2592

SAINCHER, Rajeev; 101-14815 108 Ave, Surrey BC V3R 1W2; Madras (India)'78; MB ChB; Langs: Hindi; Punjabi; (604)582-2592; Fax. (604)582-5125.

SAINDON, Jacinthe; Ctr Hosp Affilie-Enfant-Jesus, 1401 18e rue, Quebec QC G1J 1Z4; Laval'87; CSPQ; FRCPC; Psy. Staff, Centre Hospitalier Affilié Universitaire de Québec - Hôpital De L'Enfant Jésus; (418)649-5769; Fax. (418)649-5934.

SAINDON, Sophie; Hôpital Ste-Justine, 3175 ch Cote-Sainte-Catherine, Montreal QC H3T 1C5; Laval'92; CSPQ; FRCPC; Anes. Staff, Hôpital Ste-Justine; (514)345-4733

SAINE, Marie-Josee; Le Mediclub, 201-6100 av du Boise, Montreal QC H3S 2W1; Mon'71; (514)739-5646; Fax. (514)739-6773.

SAINE, Michel; 1531-1 Place Ville-Marie, Montreal QC H3B 2B5; Ott'80; (514)397-1370; Fax. (514)397-9899.

SAINI, Joginder K; 100-350 Palladium Dr, Kanata ON K2V 1A8; London (England)'80; Staff, Queensway Carleton Hospital; Langs: Hindi; Punjabi; (613)592-1707; Fax. (613)592-9799.

SAINI, Lalit K; Clinical Sciences Bldg, 4 112-11350 83 Ave NW, Edmonton AB T6G 2G2; Tor'04; FRCPC; IntMed; Hem. (780)407-1584

SAINI, Mandeep S; Regional Treatment Centre, 33344 King Rd, Abbotsford BC V2S 4P4; Liverpool (England)'98; FRCPC; Psy. (604)870-7700 x7737

SAINI, Mukesh C; 3-110 Pertosa Dr, Brampton ON L6X 5E9; Punjab (India)'86; MB BS; Langs: Hindi; Punjabi; Urdu; (905)453-8212; Fax. (905)453-9023.

SAINI, Neel; 1-6601 48 Ave, Camrose AB T4V 3G8; Delhi (India)'92; MB BS; DAB; FRCP; FRCPC; Peds (Developmental Pediatrics). Staff, Covenant Health - St Mary's Hospital; Asst Clin Prof, University of Alberta; (780)608-5887; Fax. (780)608-5895.

SAINI, Preeti; Markham Med Centre, 214-6633 Highway 7, Markham ON L3P 7P2; Wes'96; CCFP; Court Staff, Markham Stouffville Hospital; Langs: Hindi; (905)294-2290; Fax. (905)294-0029.

SAINSBURY, Joanna B; Sturgeon Community Hosp, 201 Boudreau Rd, St. Albert AB T8N 6C4; McM'92; CCFP; CCFP(E.M.); Staff, Sturgeon Community Hospital; (780)418-8229

SAINT-AMANT, Gilles; Clinique Med Berger, 2200 ch de chambly, Longueuil QC J4J 3Z3; Mon'72; Staff, Centre Hospitalier Honore-Mercier; (450)651-5752

SAINT-AMANT, Serge; 2-1 av de l'Eglise, Saint-Antoine NB E4V 1L6; Laval'76; FAAFP; CCFP; FCFP; Staff, Dr Georges-L-Dumont University Hospital Centre; Langs: Creole; English; (506)525-2409; Fax. (506)525-2240.

SAINT-AUBIN, Catherine; Inst Albert-Prevost, 6555 boul Gouin O, Montreal QC H4K 1B3; Mon'04; FRCPC; Psy. (514)338-4474

SAINT-CYR, Claire H; Hôpital Ste-Justine, 3175 ch Cote-Sainte-Catherine, Montreal QC H3T 1C5; Laval'75; FRCPC; Peds (Pediatric Rheumatology). Staff Pediatrics, Hôpital Ste-Justine; Consultant Ped Rheum, Centre de Réadaptation Marie Enfant du CHU Sainte-Justine; Prof adj clin, Universite de Montreal; Langs: Bilingual(French/English); (514)345-4713; Fax. (514)345-4897; claire.saint-cyr@hsj.ssss.gouv.qc.ca.

SAINT-CYR, Claire-Marie; Clin Med Landry Frechette, 890 10e rang, Saint-Wenceslas QC G0Z 1J0; Sher'77.

SAINT-CYR, Mathieu; Ctr Hosp Laurentien, 234 rue Saint-Vincent, Ste-Agathe-Des-Mts QC J8C 2B8; Mon'99; Staff, Centre Hospitalier Laurentien; (819)324-4000

SAINT-DIZIER, Chantal; Clinique medicale Notre-Dame, 120-504 rue Notre-Dame, Repentigny QC J6A 2T8; Mon'87; Langs: Bilingual(French/English); (450)585-3232; Fax. (450)582-9763.

SAINT-GEORGES, Guy; Hop du Sacre-Coeur de Mtl, 5400 boul Gouin O, Montreal QC H4J 1C5; Mon'66; CSPQ; FRCPC; DiagRad. Staff, Hôpital du Sacre-Coeur de Montréal; Universite de Montreal; (514)338-2130; Fax. (514)338-3541.

SAINT-GEORGES, Pierre J; Clin Med Antidouleur Outaouais, 201-195 rue de l'Atmosphere, Gatineau QC J9A 3J1; Mon'90; CCFP; Staff, CSSS de la Vallée de la Gatineau; (819)800-0742

SAINT-HILAIRE, Melanie L; St Boniface Gen Hosp, 409 Tache Ave, Winnipeg MB R2H 2A6; Ott'03; CCFP; Staff, St Boniface General Hospital; (204)233-8563

SAINT-JACQUES, Robert R; Polyclinique Saint-Eustache, 75 rue Grignon, Saint-Eustache QC J7P 4J2; Mon'67; FRCPC; Derm. Langs: Italian; English; (450)773-6777; Fax. (450)491-7470; rob.stjacques@live.ca.

SAINT-JEAN, Claude; CSSS de la Haute-Yamaska, 205 boul Leclerc O, Granby QC J2G 1T7; Mon'94; FRCSC; GenSurg (Endoscopy). Staff, Centre Hospitalier de Granby; (450)375-8000; val.jean@sympatico.ca.

SAINT-JEAN, Maude; Hôpital Ste-Justine, 3175 ch Cote-Sainte-Catherine, Montreal QC H3T 1C5; Mon'99; FRCPC; Peds; Microbio & Infect Dis (P.Q.); MedMicrobiol; InfectDis. Staff, Hôpital Ste-Justine; (514)345-4931 x4643

SAINT-JEAN, Pierre; Pavilion Albert Prevost, 6555 boul Gouin O, Montreal QC H4K 1B3; Mon'70; CSPQ; FRCPC; Psy. Staff Ped Psy, Hôpital du Sacre-Coeur de Montréal; (514)338-4356; Fax. (514)338-4357.

SAINT-LAURENT, Daniel; Pavillon Rosemont, C-5689 boul Rosemont, Montreal QC H1T 2H1; Brest (France)'89; CSPQ; Psy. Staff, Hopital Maisonneuve-Rosemont; Langs: English; (514)252-3810; dstlaurent.hmr@ssss.gouv.qc.ca.

SAINT-LAURENT, Guylaine; Hop Brome-Missisquoi-Perkins, 950 rue Principale, Cowansville QC J2K 1K3; Mon'92; CSPQ; FRCPC; Anes (P.Q.). Staff, Hôpital Brome-Missisquoi-Perkins; (450)266-4342 x5546; Fax. (450)263-3138.

SAINT-LAURENT, Marie; Allan Memorial Institute, 1025 av des Pins O, Montreal QC H3A 1A1; Mon'88; CSPQ; FRCPC; Psy (Mood Disorders). Médecin, McGill University Health Centre - Royal Victoria Hospital; Médecin, Allan Memorial Institute; Prof Faculty, McGill University; Langs: Bilingual(French/English); (514)934-1934 x35534; Fax. (514)934-4468.

SAINT-LOUIS, Jean-Francois; Clinique Med des Cantons, 1474 rue King O, Sherbrooke QC J1J 2C2; Sher'96; Staff, Carrefour de Sante et Services Sociaux-Pavillon St-Louis; (819)565-1955

SAINT-LOUIS, Nathalie M M; Centre Sante Rene-Richard, 32 3e av CP 1300, Chapais QC G0W 1H0; Sher'91; (418)745-2591; Fax. (418)745-3684.

SAINT-MARSEILLE, Sophie; Ctr Hosp Rouyn-Noranda, 4 9e rue, Rouyn-Noranda QC J9X 2B2; Mon'91; FRCSC; GenSurg (Gastroenterology). Chef chir gén, Centre Hospitalier Rouyn-Noranda; (819)764-5131; Fax. (819)764-2900; sstm.rn@sympatico.ca.

SAINT-MARTIN, Christine; MUHC-Montreal Children's Hosp, 2300 rue Tupper, Montreal QC H3H 1P3; Louis Pasteur (France)'93; Staff, McGill University Health Centre - Montreal Children's Hospital; (514)412-4450 x22130

SAINT-MARTIN, Marc; Saint Thomas Comm Health Ctre, 9040 84 Ave NW, Edmonton AB T6C 1E4; Ott'06; CCFP; (780)434-2778; Fax. (780)466-8702.

SAINT-MARTIN, Monique; CHUM-Hop St-Luc, 1058 rue Saint-Denis, Montreal QC H2X 3J4; Mon'79; FRCPC; IntMed; GeriatricMed. Staff, Centre Hospitalier l'Université De Montréal (CHUM) - Hôpital Saint-luc; (514)890-8000 x34980

SAINT-MARTIN, Suzanne; 107 av Duchastel, Outremont QC H2V 3E9; Mon'76; assoc Staff, St Mary's Hospital Centre; Médecin, Hydro-Quebec; Langs: English; (514)270-1258

SAINT-MICHEL, Patrick; Centre Med Robinson, 4 rue Robinson N, Granby QC J2G 8Z9; Sher'90; CCFP; CCFP(E.M.); Staff, Centre Hospitalier de Granby; (450)378-8435; Fax. (450)375-8835.

SAINT-PHARD, Lemercier; Clinique Med Viau, 8465 boul Viau, Saint-Leonard QC H1R 2T6; Port-au-Prince (Haiti)'65; Staff, Hopital Louis-H Lafontaine; (514)326-7203; Fax. (514)326-3656.

SAINT-PHARD, Wouter; CHUM-Hotel-Dieu, 3840 rue Saint-Urbain, Montreal QC H2W 1T8; Sher'04; Cardiol; IntMed. Staff, Centre Hospitalier l'Université de Montréal (CHUM) - Hôtel-Dieu; (514)890-8000

SAINT-PIERRE, Andre; Clinique Med Ste-Adele, 1150 rue du Bourg-Joli, Sainte-Adele QC J8B 1W8; Mon'75; (450)229-6633; Fax. (450)229-5765.

SAINT-PIERRE, Jean-Yves; CHUS-Hop Hotel-Dieu, 580 rue Bowen S, Sherbrooke QC J1G 2E8; Sher'90; CSPQ; FRCPC; Psy. Staff, Centre Hospitalier Universitaire de Sherbrooke-Hôpital Hôtel-Dieu; Langs: English; (819)822-6760; Fax. (819)822-6743.

SAINT-VIL, Dickens; Hôpital Ste-Justine, 3175 ch Cote-Sainte-Catherine, Montreal QC H3T 1C5; McG'84; FACS; FRCSC; GenSurg (Pediatrics); PedGenSurg. ac Staff, Hôpital Ste-Justine; Universite de Montreal; Langs: English; (514)345-4879; Fax. (514)345-4964; dickens_saint-vil@ssss.gouv.qc.ca.

SAINTON, Gilles; CHUS-Hop Hotel-Dieu, 580 rue Bowen S, Sherbrooke QC J1G 2E8; Mon'96; CCFP; Staff, Centre Hospitalier Universitaire de Sherbrooke-Hôpital Hôtel-Dieu; Physician, Centre Hospitalier Universitaire de Sherbrooke-Hopital Fleurimont; (819)346-1110; gsainton@videotron.ca.

SAINTONGE, Jacques P A; Hop Maisonneuve-Rosemont, 5415 boul de l'Assomption, Montreal QC H1T 2M4; Mon'72; FRCPC; Peds (Neonatology). Staff, Hopital Maisonneuve-Rosemont; assoc Prof, Universite de Montreal; (514)252-3400; Fax. (514)252-3515; jacques.saintonge@sympatico.ca.

SAINZ, Beatriz M; Oromocto Prof Bldg, 66 Broad Rd, Oromocto NB E2V 1C2; Dal'78; CCFP; Staff, Oromocto Public Hospital; Staff, Dr Everett Chalmers Regional Hospital; Langs: Spanish; French; (506)357-7134; Fax. (506)357-3712.

SAIRAM, Ashwin M; Clinique A M S, 303 av Dorval, Dorval QC H9S 3H6; McG'02; CCFP; (514)300-1031; Fax. (514)300-1041.

SAIRAM, Charith; Ctre Hosp de Lachine, 650 16e av, Lachine QC H8S 3N5; McG'07; MDCM; FRCPC; IntMed. Staff, CSSS de Dorval-Lachine-Lasalle; (514)637-2351

SAITO, Robert K; Oakdale Med Bldg, 212-2065 Finch Ave W, North York ON M3N 2V7; Tor'75; Ac Staff, Humber River Regional Hospital - Finch Avenue Site; (416)741-6966; Fax. (416)741-6974.

SAITO, Simon; Univ of Ottawa Heart Institute, 40 Ruskin Ave, Ottawa ON K1Y 4W7; McG'95; FRCSC; GenSurg; CardSurg. Staff, University of Ottawa Heart Institute; (613)761-4708

SAJED, Sina; Stone's Mill Family Health Ctr, 25 Mill St, Gananoque ON K7G 2L5; Grigore T Popa University (Romania)'04; BSc; CCFP; Asst Prof Family Med, Queen's University; Langs: Farsi; Romanian; (613)382-3974; Fax. (613)382-4417.

SAJID, Saima; Glen Huron Med Centre, 1 Glenn Hawthorne Blvd, Mississauga ON L5R 0C2; Fatima Jinnah Medical College (Pakistan)'03.

SAJJAN, Kuljit K; BC Women's Hosp & Health Ctre, F326-4500 Oak St, Vancouver BC V6H 3N1; UBC'00; CCFP; Staff, BC Women's Hospital & Health Centre; Langs: Punjabi; (604)875-2029; Fax. (604)875-3197.

SAJO, Ildiko M; Woburn Med Dental Centre, 4129 Lawrence Ave E, Scarborough ON M1E 2S2; McG'76; Langs: Hungarian; (416)439-1991; Fax. (416)439-3593.

SAJOUS, Franck J A; CSSS du Nord de Lanaudière, 1000 boul Sainte-Anne, St-Charles-Brromee QC J6E 6J2; Sher'93; CSPQ; Urol. Staff, Centre Hospitalier Régional de Lanaudière; Langs: Bilingual(French/English); (450)759-8222; Fax. (450)759-7969.

SAJWANI, Tasneem; Dominion Med Centres Ltd, 9122 23 Ave NW, Edmonton AB T6N 1H9; (Pakistan)'03; CCFP; (780)801-3360; Fax. (780)801-3366.

SAKAKIBARA, Todd K; Three Birdges Comm Hlth Ctr, 1292 Hornby St, Vancouver BC V6Z 1W2; UBC'00; CCFP; (604)633-4220; Fax. (604)844-2223.

SAKALUK, Timothy J; PO Box 53539 Rpo West Broadway, Vancouver BC V5Z 4M6; Cal'03; CCFP; (604)742-4010

SAKAMOTO, Terence K; 123 Millennium Pky RR 5 Stn Main, Belleville ON K8N 4Z5; Tor'88; FRCSC; Ophth. Staff, QHC Trenton Memorial; (613)961-7440; Fax. (613)961-1798.

SAKANOVIC, Alenko; CFB Petawawa, PO Box 9999 Stn Main, Petawawa ON K8H 2X3; Ott'09; CCFP; (613)687-5511

SAKELLARIDES, Michel; Medical Centre, 2F-171 Montreal Rd, Cornwall ON K6H 1B2; Mon'88; ac Staff, CHSLD de la MRC de Champlain-Centre Saint-Lambert; Langs: English; (613)932-2123; michel.sakellarides@rrsss16.gouv.qc.ca.

SAKIAN, Nima; 38-4567 Lougheed Hwy, Burnaby BC V5C 3Z6; Saba (Netherlands Antilles)'06; CCFP; (604)294-8540

SAKINOFSKY, Isaac; Addiction & Mental Hlth-Clarke, 250 College St, Toronto ON M5T 1R8; Cape Town (South Africa)'55; MB ChB; DPM(Lond); FRCP(UK); FRCPC; Psy (Suicide Risk). Head Suicidology Prog, Centre for Addiction & Mental Health (CAMH) - College Street Site; Emeritus Prof, University of Toronto; (416)979-4674; Fax. (416)979-6815.

SAKIYAMA, Christine M; Rosedale Wellness Centre, 365 Bloor St E, Toronto ON M4W 3L4; Tor'85; CCFP; (416)577-0610

SAKLA, Mary S S; Selkirk Med Centre, 353 Eveline St, Selkirk MB R1A 1K8; (Other Foreign)'93; CCFP; (204)482-8560

SAKOOR, Ahmed; The Raxlen Clinic, B102-340 College St, Toronto ON M5T 3A9; RCS (Ireland)'66; LRCPS; LMCC; (416)966-3641; Fax. (416)944-9947.

SAKOTIC, George; North York Gen Hosp, 4001 Leslie St, North York ON M2K 1E1; Tor'96; FRCPC; Anes. Staff, North York General Hospital; Langs: Serbian; (416)756-6520

SAKR, Lama; SMBD Jewish Gen Hosp, 3755 ch Cote-Sainte-Catherine, Montreal QC H3T 1E2; Mon'03; FRCPC; IntMed; Respir. Staff, Sir Mortimer B Davis Jewish General; (514)340-8222

SAKSENA, Rajni; Clinique St-Gabriel, 2041 rue Wellington, Montreal QC H3K 1W7; New Delhi (India)'72; CCFP; assoc Prof, McGill University Health Centre - Montreal General Campus; assoc Prof, McGill University; Langs: Khmer; French; (514)931-8661

SAKSUN, Jana M B; 1000-1243 Islington Ave, Etobicoke ON M8X 1Y9; Tor'73; BSc(Hon); FRCPC; Derm. Staff, Women's College Hospital; Court Staff, Trillium Health Centre - West Toronto; Court Staff, St Joseph's Health Centre; (416)231-0100

SAKULS, Peter; 205-1466 Bathurst St, Toronto ON M5R 3S3; McM'88; CCFP; Langs: Latvian; (416)483-8111

SALA, Tanya N; Psychealth Centre, PZ430-771 Bannatyne Ave, Winnipeg MB R3E 3N4; Man'01; FRCPC; Psy (Anxiety & Mood Disorders). (204)787-7078

SALACH-MARKIEWICZ, Krystyna; Trillium Hlth Ctre-Mississauga, 100 Queensway W, Mississauga ON L5B 1B8; Warsaw (Poland)'71; Staff, Trillium Health Centre - Mississauga; Staff, St Joseph's Health Centre; Langs: Polish; Russian; (905)848-7100

SALAH, Joan C; 3-131 King St, North Sydney NS B2A 3S1; Dal'01; CCFP; Staff, Northside General Hospital; (902)794-5900; Fax. (902)794-5930.

SALAHUDDIN, Afroze; Oak Park Family Care Centre, 201 Oak Walk Dr, Oakville ON L6H 6M3; Dow Medical College (Pakistan)'77; CCFP; (905)257-3297

SALAHUDEEN, Shafeequr R; Kingston Gen Hosp, 76 Stuart St, Kingston ON K7L 2V7; Madras (India)'93; FRCPC; DiagRad. Staff, Kingston General Hospital; (613)549-6666

SALAM, Abdul; Taunton Health Centre, SS 201 1290 Keith Ross Dr, Oshawa ON L1H 7K4; Nishtar Medical College (Pakistan)'86; CCFP; (905)721-4163

SALAMA, Gamal M S; Humber River Reg Hosp-Keele, 2175 Keele St, North York ON M6M 3Z4; Cairo (Egypt)'80; FRCPC; Psy. Staff, Humber River Regional Hospital - Keele Street Site; (416)249-8111

SALAMA, Magdy G A; Keele & Rogers Med Centre, 605 Rogers Rd, York ON M6M 1B9; Zagazig (Egypt)'79; CCFP; (416)656-1010; Fax. (416)656-6161.

SALAMA, Said S S; 1118-123 Edward St, Toronto ON M5G 1E2; Alexandria (Egypt)'63; MB ChB; DAB; DAA; FRCPC; Anes (Chronic Pain Management). Langs: Arabic; French; (416)593-7700; Fax. (416)593-7702.

SALAMA, Samih S S; St Joseph's Healthcare, 50 Charlton Ave E, Hamilton ON L8N 4A6; Alexandria (Egypt)'65; MB ChB; DABPath(AnatPath); DABPath(DermatoPathology); FRCPC; AnatPath. Ac Staff, Hamilton Health Sciences Centre - McMaster University Medical Centre; Pathologist, St Joseph's Healthcare - Charlton Campus; Prof Path, McMaster University; Langs: Arabic; Fax. (905)521-6192; ssalama@mcmaster.ca.

SALAMAT, Amirreza; York Medical Clinic, 110-1650 Elgin Mills Rd, Richmond Hill ON L4S 0B2; Ghazvin University (Iran)'92; CCFP; (905)770-3858; Fax. (905)770-1964.

SALAME, Charbel; CSSS de la Vallée de l'Or, 725 6e rue, Val-d'Or QC J9P 3Y1; Beirut (Lebanon)'93; Staff, Centre Hospitalier de Val d'Or; (819)825-6711

SALAMEH, Muwaffaq; St Martha's Doctor's Offices, 23 Bay St, Antigonish NS B2G 2G7; (Jordan)'97; MB BS; Staff, St Martha's Regional Hospital; (902)863-1565; Fax. (902)863-0640.

SALAMI, Gorgin; Hop Santa Cabrini Ospedale, 5655 rue Saint-Zotique E, Montreal QC H1T 1P7; Sher'00; Staff, Hôpital Santa Cabrini Ospedale; Langs: English; (514)252-6000

SALAMON, Elizabeth A; Winnipeg Clinic, 425 St Mary Ave, Winnipeg MB R3C 0N2; Man'80; FRCPC; IntMed; Endocrin&Metab. Assoc Staff, St Boniface General Hospital; Att Physician, Victoria General Hospital; Asst Prof, University of Manitoba; (204)957-3202; Fax. (204)943-3516.

SALAMON, Lisa; Gates of Maple Family Practice, 201-955 Major Mackenzie Dr, Maple ON L6A 4P9; Ott'03; BSc(Hon); CCFP; CCFP(E.M.); Staff Emerg, The Scarborough Hospital - General Campus; (905)417-7899; Fax. (905)417-8905.

SALAMON, Miriam; 507-168 Charlotte St, Ottawa ON K1N 8K6; Sher'80; CCFP; Staff, The Ottawa Hospital - General Campus; Asst Prof Family Med, University of Ottawa; Langs: French; (613)789-0907; Fax. (613)789-3396; msalamon@uottawa.ca.

SALAMOUN, Wassim; Summerside Med Centre, 101-475 Granville St, Summerside PE C1N 3N9; Bordeaux (France)'79; ABOtol; Staff Otolaryngology/Med Dir (Admin), Prince County Hospital; Langs: Arabic; Bilingual(French/English); (902)432-8181; Fax. (902)432-8169; wsalamoun@gov.pe.ca.

SALARIEH, Afshin; Dynacare Kasper Med Lab, 200-10150 102 St NW, Edmonton AB T5J 5E2; (Iran)'97; FRCPC; AnatPath. Staff, Queen Elizabeth II Hospital; (780)451-3702; Fax. (780)452-8488.

SALASIDIS, Gary C; St Mary's Gen Hosp, 469-911 Queens Blvd, Kitchener ON N2M 1B2; McG'90; FRCSC; CardiothorSurg. Staff, Grand River Hospital - Kitchener/Waterloo Health Centre; Staff, Grey Bruce Health Services - Owen Sound; Staff Reg Cardiac Care Ctr, St Mary's General Hospital; Langs: Greek; French; (519)749-6937; Fax. (519)749-6492.

SALASIDIS, Robert; MUHC-Montreal Gen Hosp, 1650 av Cedar, Montreal QC H3G 1A4; McG'86; FRCSC; GenSurg; Critical Care Medicine (P.Q.). Staff, McGill University Health Centre - Montreal General Campus; (514)934-1934 x44334

SALAT, Jan M; Appletree Med Centre, 1309 Carling Ave, Ottawa ON K1Z 7L3; Sask'75; Langs: Czech; French; German; (613)715-9419

SALAT, Peter; Valley Reg Hosp, 150 Exhibition St, Kentville NS B4N 5E3; Alb'04; FRCPC; DiagRad. Staff, Valley Regional Hospital; (902)678-7381

SALATHIEL, Ian P; Royal Victoria Hosp, 201 Georgian Dr, Barrie ON L4M 6M2; Cambridge (England)'88; MB ChB; FRCPC; GenPath. Staff, Royal Victoria Regional Health Centre; (705)728-9090 x43221; Fax. (705)739-5685.

SALAZAR, Anastasio; Foothills Med Centre, 1403 29 St NW, Calgary AB T2N 2T9; (Mexico)'84; Staff, Foothills Medical Centre; (403)944-1149; Fax. (403)944-1277.

SALAZAR, Charlene L; 206-331 Sheddon Ave, Oakville ON L6J 1X8; Alb'05; FRCPC; IntMed; Respir. Staff Respirologist, Halton Healthcare Services Corporation - Oakville Site; (905)842-3366

SALAZAR, Sacha R; Mud Creek Med Clinic, 12 Elm Ave, Wolfville NS B4P 1Z9; West Indies (Jamaica)'01; CCFP; (902)542-3633; Fax. (902)542-2709.

SALCEDO, Juan R; Appletree Med Group, 2948 Baseline Rd, Nepean ON K2H 8T5; Bogota (Colombia)'72; FACP; FRCPC; IntMed; Cardiol. Langs: Spanish; French; (613)288-2059; Fax. (613)288-2060.

SALCICCIOLI, Paul; Kingscross Med Group, 408-18 Kensington Rd, Brampton ON L6T 4S5; Tor'77; CCFP; FCFP; Court Staff, William Osler Health System - Brampton Civic Hospital; Aj Clin Lecturer Family & Community Med, University of Toronto; Langs: Italian; (905)792-2280; Fax. (905)792-9832.

SALDANHA, Carla N; Dr H Bliss Murphy Cancer Ctr, 300 Prince Philip Dr, St. John's NL A1B 3V6; Mem'03; CCFP; Staff, Dr H Bliss Murphy Cancer Centre; (709)777-7602

SALEEB, Ashraf H S; Plateau Med Clinic, F8M-1410 Parkway Blvd, Coquitlam BC V3E 3J7; Cairo (Egypt)'81; MB ChB; CCFP; (604)468-1500; Fax. (604)468-1501.

SALEEM, Ashfaq; Red River Family Medical, 724 Ellice Ave, Winnipeg MB R3G 0B4; Peshawar (Pakistan)'88; CCFP; Fam Med, Vita & District Health Centre; (204)786-4673; Fax. (204)772-9656.

SALEEM, Asifa K; Halton Family Health Centre, 2951 Walker's Line, Burlington ON L7M 4Y1; Karachi (Pakistan)'86; CCFP; (905)336-9617; Fax. (905)336-9638.

SALEEM, Azra K; Regional Mental HC-London, PO Box 5532 Stn B 850 Highbury Ave, London ON N6A 4H1; Karachi (Pakistan)'73; FRCPC; Psy. Staff, Regional Mental Health Care-St Joseph's Health Care; University of Western Ontario; Langs: Urdu; (519)455-5110

SALEEM, Hala; The Doctor's Office, 6435 Erin Mills Pky, Mississauga ON L5N 4H4; Baghdad (Iraq)'85; CCFP; Physician, MCI the Doctors Office; Langs: Arabic; (905)821-1406; Fax. (905)821-1409.

SALEEM, Mohammad; Grand River Hosp-KW Hlth Ctre, PO Box 9056 Stn C 835 King St W, Kitchener ON N2G 1G3; Punjab (India)'95; FRCPC; Psy. Staff, Grand River Hospital - Kitchener/Waterloo Health Centre; (519)749-4300

SALEH, Ahmed S M S; Rockyview Gen Hosp, 7007 14 St SW, Calgary AB T2V 1P9; International Islamic University (Malaysia)'02; CCFP; CCFP(E.M.); Staff, Rockyview General Hospital; (403)943-3000; Fax. (403)943-3449.

SALEH, David S; Children's Hosp Eastern Ont, 401 Smyth Rd, Ottawa ON K1H 8L1; Tor'03; FRCPC; Peds; Endocrin&Metab. Staff, Children's Hospital of Eastern Ontario (CHEO); (613)526-3952

SALEH, Dlair; Saskatoon City Hosp, 701 Queen St, Saskatoon SK S7K 0M7; Staff, Saskatoon City Hospital; (306)655-8000

SALEH, Fady; Univ Hlth Network-Toronto Western Hosp, 8 320-399 Bathurst St, Toronto ON M5T 2S8; Tor'05; FRCSC; GenSurg. Staff, Toronto Western Hospital - University Health Network; (416)603-5599; Fax. (416)603-6458.

SALEH, Fatehia; Ctr Hosp Anna-Laberge, 200 boul Brisebois, Chateauguay QC J6K 4W8; Alb'95; CSPQ; FRCPC; Psy. Staff, Hôpital Anna-Laberge; Langs: Arabic; (450)699-2774; Fax. (450)699-2431; fatehiasaleh@yahoo.ca.

SALEH, Naji; Five West, 520-922 5 Ave SW, Calgary AB T2P 5R4; (Belarus)'93; CCFP; (403)663-1714

SALEH, Wasfy S; Bayshore Med Bldg, 203-3029 Carling Ave, Ottawa ON K2B 8E8; Cairo (Egypt)'57; PhD; DABS; DABU; FRCSC; GenSurg; Urol. Court Staff, Queensway Carleton Hospital; Langs: Arabic; French; (613)726-1687; Fax. (613)726-9731.

SALEH, Zainab A; Grey Nuns Community Hosp, 1100 Youville Drive West NW, Edmonton AB T6L 5X8; Bristol (England)'73; MB ChB; FRCPC; Anes. Ac Staff, Covenant Health - Grey Nuns Community Hospital; Ac Staff, Covenant Health - Misericordia Community Hospital; Asst Prof, University of Alberta; (780)735-7020

SALEH-ELGREDLY, Mona; 7-3095 Glen Erin Dr, Mississauga ON L5L 1J3; Cal'96; FRCSC; GenSurg. Staff, Aberdeen Regional Hospital; (905)607-0022; Fax. (905)607-0013.

SALEHEH SHOSHTARI, Peyman; Horwoods Med Clinic, 104-100 Main St, Whitehorse YT Y1A 2A8; (Iran)'92; CCFP; (867)633-2847; Fax. (867)633-2848.

SALEHI, Leila; William Osler HC-Brampton, 2100 Bovaird Dr E, Brampton ON L6R 3J7; McG'07; MDCM; CCFP; CCFP(E.M.); Staff, William Osler Health System - Brampton Civic Hospital; (905)494-2120

SALEHI BAIDOKHTI, Saghi; Newmarket Med Centre, 6-17725 Yonge St, Newmarket ON L3Y 7C1; (Other Foreign)'04; CCFP.

SALEHIAN, Omid; Hamilton HS-General Site, 418-237 Barton St E, Hamilton ON L8L 2X2; Tor'97; MSc; FACC; FAHA; FRCPC; IntMed (Adult Congenital Heart Disease); Cardiol. Staff, Hamilton Health Sciences Centre - Hamilton General Hospital; Assoc Prof, McMaster University; (905)521-2100; Fax. (905)577-8249.

SALEM, Cherien; Whites Med Clinic, 727 Jane St, York ON M6N 4B3; Tor'00; CCFP; Langs: Arabic; French; (416)763-8880; Fax. (416)763-3444.

SALEM, Eman G; Hotel-Dieu Grace Hosp, 1030 Ouellette Ave, Windsor ON N9A 1E1; Cairo (Egypt)'81; MSc; FRCPC; Anes. Staff, Hôtel-Dieu Grace Hospital; Langs: Arabic; (519)973-4444

SALEM, Fayez F S; Vista Med Centre, 1633B St Mary's Rd, Winnipeg MB R2N 1Z3; Cairo (Egypt)'75; (204)257-3661; Fax. (204)257-3827.

SALEM, Jacques; Centre Bois de Boulogne, 130-1575 boul Henri-Bourassa O, Montreal QC H3M 3A9; Beirut (Lebanon)'62; Ophth. (514)337-1139; Fax. (514)731-7435.

SALEM, Nabil; Clinique Med Joliette, 3841 rue Ontario E, Montreal QC H1W 1S5; Toulouse (France)'72; GenSurg. Staff, Centre Hospitalier de LaSalle; (514)524-3731; Fax. (514)524-0675.

SALEM, Reda; CHUM-Hotel-Dieu, 3840 rue Saint-Urbain, Montreal QC H2W 1T8; Mon'01; FRCPC; IntMed; Cardiol. Staff, Centre Hospitalier l'Université de Montréal (CHUM) - Hôtel-Dieu; (514)890-8000

SALEM, Shia; Mount Sinai Hosp, 600 University Ave, Toronto ON M5G 1X5; Qns'64; FRCPC; DiagRad (Diagnostic Ultrasound). Ac Staff Rad-Medical Imaging, Mount Sinai Hospital; Staff, Women's College Hospital; Assoc Prof, University of Toronto; Teach Staff, University Health Network; (416)586-4800 x4405; Fax. (416)586-1569; ssalem@mtsinai.on.ca.

SALEM, Wesam; 159-2515 90 Ave SW, Calgary AB T2L 0L8; Alb'08; CCFP; (403)281-2020; Fax. (403)281-7785; wsalem@ ualberta.ca.

SALENA, Bruno J; Hamilton HS-McMaster Site, PO Box 2000 Stn Lcd 1 2F57-1200 Main St W, Hamilton ON L8N 3Z5; McM'81; FRCPC; IntMed (Gastroenterology). Ac Staff, Hamilton Health Sciences Centre - McMaster Children's Hospital; Affil Staff, St Joseph's Healthcare - Charlton Campus; Affil Staff, Joseph Brant Memorial Hospital; Assoc. Prof., Med., McMaster University; (905)521-2100 x76782; Fax. (905)523-6048.

SALES, Jack L; Springbank Med Centre, 203-460 Springbank Dr, London ON N6J 0A8; Wes'55; FRCSC; GenSurg (Vasectomy); Urol. (519)652-3999; Fax. (519)652-2957; jlms@hay.net.

SALES, Karl H; Kirkland & District Hosp, PO Box 3000 Stn Main 145 Government Rd E, Kirkland Lake ON P2N 3P4; Mon'77; FRCSC; Ophth. Staff, Kirkland & District Hospital; Langs: Spanish; English; (705)567-5251

SALES, Valerie; Markham Stouffville Hosp, PO Box 1800 Stn Main 381 Church St, Markham ON L3P 7P3; McG'92; FRCPC; Peds; InfectDis (HIV). Staff, University Health Network; Staff, North York General Hospital; Staff, Markham Stouffville Hospital; Langs: French; (905)472-7614; Fax. (905)472-7618.

SALEVSKY, Frederick C; MUHC-Montreal Neurology Inst, 548-3801 rue University, Montreal QC H3A 2B4; Alb'83; CSPQ; FRCPC; Anes. Staff, McGill University Health Centre - Montreal Neurological Hospital; (514)398-5387; Fax. (514)398-1352.

SALGADO, David; 24 Dann Dr PO Box 1065, Hampton NB E5N 8H1; Dal'84; (506)832-5068; Fax. (506)832-3804.

SALGADO BENAVIDES, Carlos E; 400-7000 Emerald Dr, Sherwood Park AB T8H 0P5; (Colombia)'84; CCFP; (780)638-5008; Fax. (780)638-5009.

SALGADO DE LEON, Luis A; Cornwall Prof Bldg, 414-2125 11th Ave, Regina SK S4P 3X3; (Mexico)'69; Ac Staff, Regina General Hospital; Ac Staff, Pasqua Hospital; Langs: Spanish; Portuguese; (306)352-2299; Fax. (306)569-5998.

SALH, Baljinder S; Diamond Health Care Centre, 5153-2775 Laurel St, Vancouver BC V5Z 1M9; Leeds (England)'82; MB ChB; FRCPC; IntMed; Gastroent. Staff Gastroent, Vancouver General Hospital - Centennial Pavillion; Asst Prof Med, University of British Columbia; Langs: Punjabi; (604)875-5287; bsalh@interchange. ubc.ca.

SALIB, Ashraf E A; 197-5 Fairview Mall Dr, North York ON M2J 2Z1; Ain Shams (Egypt)'89; MB ChB; CCFP; (416)493-0346; Fax. (416)493-0336.

SALIB, George E; CSSS de Trois-Rivières, 1991 boul du Carmel, Trois-Rivieres QC G8Z 3R9; Mon'05; FRCSC; PlasSurg. Staff, CSSS de Trois-Rivières; (819)697-3333

SALIB, Jeannette L; Albion Med Group, 205-1525 Albion Rd, Etobicoke ON M9V 5G5; Ain Shams (Egypt)'82; CCFP; Langs: Arabic; (416)744-9973; Fax. (416)744-1447.

SALIB, Michel G; Yorkton Reg Health Centre, 270 Bradbrooke Dr, Yorkton SK S3N 2K6; Ain Shams (Egypt)'72; Staff, Yorkton Regional Health Centre; Langs: Arabic; (306)782-2401; drsalib@ hotmail.com.

SALIB, Samir; CSSS-Hop De Hull, 116 boul Lionel-Émond, Gatineau QC J8Y 1W7; Ain Shams (Egypt)'82; GenSurg (P.Q.). Staff, Hull Hospital; (819)595-6000

SALIB, Shadwa S E; Mississauga Med Centre, A2-3980 Grand Park Dr, Mississauga ON L5B 4M6; (Ireland)'00; CCFP; (905)615-0107; Fax. (905)615-1711.

SALIB, Wagdi; 615 Main St PO Box 389, Swan River MB R0L 1Z0.

SALIBA, Cynthia H; Nelson Med Prof Corp, 301 Victoria Ave, Fort Frances ON P9A 2C1; McM'08; CCFP; (807)274-3287; Fax. (807)274-7882.

SALIBA, Issam; CHUM-Hop Notre-Dame, 1560 rue Sherbrooke E, Montreal QC H2L 4M1; Beirut (Lebanon)'96; FRCSC; Otol. Staff, Centre Hospitalier l'Université de Montréal (CHUM) - Hôpital Notre-Dame; (514)890-8000

SALIBA, Nasri; Clin d'Urologie de Gatineau, 3B-520 boul de l'Hopital, Gatineau QC J8V 2P5; Beirut (Lebanon)'78; CSPQ; FRCSC; Urol (Oncology). ac Staff, Hôpital de Gatineau; Langs: English; Arabic; (819)568-3224; Fax. (819)568-8521.

SALIBA, Nouhad; Clinique Med Physimed, 238-6363 Rte Transcanadienne, Saint-Laurent QC H4T 1Z9; Beirut (Lebanon)'73; FRCPC; IntMed; Endocrin (P.Q.). Staff, Centre Hospitalier de Verdun; salnunu@videotron.ca.

SALIH, Bashar; Concordia Hosp, 1095 Concordia Ave, Winnipeg MB R2K 3S8; Istanbul (Turkey)'02; FRCPC; IntMed. Staff, Concordia General Hospital; (204)667-1560

SALIH, Emad A; Medicine Hat Reg Hosp, 666 5 St SW, Medicine Hat AB T1A 4H6; Ain Shams (Egypt)'95; DABPN; MB BS; FRCPC; Neur (Pain Management). Dir Neurol & Pain Med, Medicine Hat Regional Hospital; (403)528-8121; Fax. (403)529-8020; esalih75@yahoo.com.

SALIH, Raafat B; Headwaters Specialist Clinic, 129-150 Rolling Hills Dr, Orangeville ON L9W 4X8; Khartoum (Sudan)'77; MB BS; FRCS(Ire); FRCSC; GenSurg. Staff, Headwaters Health Care Centre - Orangeville Site; Langs: Arabic; (519)941-3488; Fax. (519)941-3441.

SALIH, Rasha; Lacewood Med Centre, 200-366 Lacewood Dr, Halifax NS B3S 1M7; Iraq (Iraq)'99; MB ChB; CCFP; (902)445-9400

SALIKEN, John C; Madrona Imaging, 1804 Bowen Rd, Nanaimo BC V9S 5W4; Cal'80; ABR; BSc; FRCR; FRCPC; DiagRad (Cryosurgery). Staff, Nanaimo Regional General Hospital; (250)753-4351

SALIM, Asim; 379 St Paul Ave, Brantford ON N3R 4N5; Karachi (Pakistan)'92; MB BS; FRCPC; Peds (Gastroenterology). Assoc Prof, Hamilton Health Sciences Centre - McMaster Children's Hospital; Staff, The Brant Community Healthcare System - Brantford General Hospital Site; Langs: Hindi; Punjabi; Urdu; (519)512-0030; Fax. (519)512-0051; asal66@gmail.com.

SALIM, Muhammad; Allan Blair Cancer Centre, 300-4101 Dewdney Ave, Regina SK S4T 7T1; Karachi (Pakistan)'87; MB BS; (306)766-2213; Fax. (306)766-2688.

SALIM, Syeeda S S; Addiction & Mental Hlth-Clarke, 828-250 College St, Toronto ON M5T 1R8; (India)'00; FRCPC; Psy. Staff, Centre for Addiction & Mental Health (CAMH) - College Street Site; (416)979-6911

SALISBURY, David A; Transport Canada Tower C AARG, 330 Sparks St, Ottawa ON K1A 0N5; Qns'78; MHSc; ABPM; FRCP; FRCPC; CommunMed (Aerospace Medicine). Langs: English; French; (613)990-1311; Fax. (613)990-6623; david.salisbury@ tc.gc.ca.

SALIT, Irving E; Univ Hlth Network-Toronto Gen, EN13-215-200 Elizabeth St, Toronto ON M5G 2C4; McG'71; FRCPC; IntMed (AIDS/HIV). Staff, Toronto General Hospital - UHN; Ac Staff Div of InfectDis, Mount Sinai Hospital; Prof, University of Toronto; Langs: French; (416)340-3697; Fax. (416)340-3357; irving. salit@uhn.ca.

SALJA HALILI, Elvira; St Lawrence Med Clinic, PO Box 772 36 Ottawa St, Morrisburg ON K0C 1X0; University of Pristina (Kosovo)'89; CCFP; (613)543-2963

SALKAUSKIS, Stanley J; Oakdale Med Bldg, 308A-2065 Finch Ave W, North York ON M3N 2V7; Tor'69; CCFP; CCFP(E.M.); Ac Staff Family Med, Humber River Regional Hospital - Finch Avenue Site; Langs: Lithuanian; (416)741-7511; Fax. (416)741-7512.

SALL, Gurjinder P; Le Mediclub au Sanctuarie, 201-6100 av du Boise, Montreal QC H3S 2W1; McG'84; BSc(Hon); Clin Associé Surg, Centre Hospitalier l'Université de Montréal (CHUM) - Hôtel-Dieu; Dir Medical Advisory Committee, Quebec Breast Cancer Fdn; Langs: English; French; (514)739-5646; Fax. (514)739-6773.

SALLAM, Sallam A; Saint John Reg Hosp, PO Box 2100 Stn Main 400 University Ave, Saint John NB E2L 4L2; (Jordan)'98; Staff, Saint John Regional Hospital; (506)721-2222

SALLOUM, Alexandre; Clinique Med Saint-Alexandre, 200-2310 rue Saint-Louis, Gatineau QC J8T 5L7; Mon'95; (819)243-4500; Fax. (819)243-1369; asalloum@medecinefamiliale.com.

SALLOUM, Sadek R; The Moncton Hosp, 135 MacBeath Ave, Moncton NB E1C 6Z8; Damascus (Syria)'97; Staff, The Moncton Hospital; (506)857-5532

SALLOUM, Sharon E; UBC Health Clinic, 310-5950 University Blvd, Vancouver BC V6T 1Z3; McM'82; CCFP; FCFP; Staff, Delta Hospital; Clin Assoc Prof/Assoc Dean MD Undergraduate Program Student Affairs, University of British Columbia; (604)822-5431

SALMAN, Aliya; Mount Sinai Hosp, 1514-600 University Ave, Toronto ON M5G 1X5; Punjab (Pakistan)'89; FRCPC; Anes. Staff, Mount Sinai Hospital; (416)586-4800

SALMAN, Bashar M; White Bay Central Health Centr, PO Box 70 63 Cloud Dr, Roddickton NL A0K 4P0; Baghdad (Iraq)'01; Staff, White Bay Central Health Centre; (709)457-2215

SALMAN, Michael S; Children's Hosp, AE 308-840 Sherbrook St, Winnipeg MB R3A 1S1; London (England)'90; Staff, Health Sciences Centre; (204)787-2414

SALMAN, Raed; CSSS de Rivière-de-Loup, 75 rue Saint-Henri, Riviere-du-Loup QC G5R 2A4; (Syria)'00; Staff, Centre Hospitalier Regional du Grand-Portage; (418)868-1010

SALMAN, Sadik; University of Alberta Hosp, 2F1 30-8440 112 St NW, Edmonton AB T6G 2B7; (Iraq)'96; IntMed. Staff, University of Alberta Hospital; (780)407-1570; Fax. (780)407-3132.

SALMAN-GODIN, Ariane; CHUQ-St-Francois d'Assisse, 10 rue de l'Espinay, Quebec QC G1L 3L5; Sher'02; LMCC; Staff, Centre Hospitalier Universitaire De Québec - Pavillon De St-françois-d'assise; (418)525-3404

SALMANIW, Walter R; 3-1153 Esquimalt Rd, Victoria BC V9A 3N7; Tor'81; Langs: Ukrainian; (250)383-6031

SALMASI, Ghazal; Sunnybrook Hlth Sciences Ctre, T2033-2075 Bayview Ave, Toronto ON M4N 3M5; McM'07; IntMed. Staff, Sunnybrook Health Sciences Centre; (416)480-4662

SALMI DE WATMAN, Silvia C; Sunridge Diagnostic Imaging, 2133 36 St NE, Calgary AB T1Y 5S3; (Argentina)'85; (403)568-7676; Fax. (403)568-7677.

SALMON, Andrea K; London HSC-University Hosp, PO Box 5339 Stn B B7 005-339 Windermere Rd, London ON N6A 5A5; Alb'06; FRCPC; Neur. Staff, London Health Sciences Centre - University Hospital; (519)663-3696

SALMON, Ernest A T; 301 Kingston Rd, Pickering ON L1V 1A1; Tor'66; FACS; FRCS(Eng); FRCSC; GenSurg. Ac Staff, Rouge Valley Health System - Ajax & Pickering Health Centre Site; Court Staff, Rouge Valley Health System - Centenary Health Centre Site; (905)509-5867; Fax. (905)509-7929.

SALMON, Gretchen J; 595 Bradley Ave, London ON N6E 3Z8; Tor'06; (519)680-1721; Fax. (519)680-0434.

SALMON, Joanne; Saint John Reg Hosp, PO Box 2100 Stn Main 400 University Ave, Saint John NB E2L 4L2; Alb'04; FRCPC; IntMed; InfectDis. Staff, Saint John Regional Hospital; (506)648-6000

SALO, Paul T; 3280 Hospital Dr NW, Calgary AB T2N 4Z6; Tor'82; FRCSC; OrthSurg (Spine Surgery). Att Staff, Foothills Medical Centre; Consultant, Peter Lougheed Centre; Consultant, Rockyview General Hospital; Assoc Prof, University of Calgary; (403)220-2159; Fax. (403)270-0617.

SALO, Rosaline; 90 John St S, Stratford ON N5A 2Y8; Tor'80; FRCPC; Psy (Child & Adolescent Psychiatry). Staff, Stratford General Hospital - Huron Perth Healthcare Alliance; Langs: French; (519)272-8236; Fax. (519)272-8226.

SALOMON, Paul S; Eastern Health Community Serv, 5 Coish Pl, Clarenville NL A5A 0C3; Leeds (England)'92; MB ChB; CCFP; Staff, The Dr G B Cross Memorial Hospital; (709)466-6400; Fax. (709)466-5718; paul.salomon@easternhealth.ca.

SALONEN, David C; Univ Hlth Network-Toronto Western Hosp, 3MC42-399 Bathurst St, Toronto ON M5T 2S8; Tor'88; FRCPC; DiagRad. Staff Radiol, Toronto Western Hospital - University Health Network; Teach Staff, University of Toronto; (416)603-5800 x5616; Fax. (416)603-5522.

SALOOJEE, Farzana; Allwood Med Clinic, 102-2752 Allwood St, Abbotsford BC V2T 3R7; Witwatersrand (South Africa)'02; MB ChB; (604)850-6893

SALOOJEE, Navaaz A; The Ottawa Hosp-Gen Campus, 501 Smyth Rd, Ottawa ON K1H 8L6; Qns'93; FRCPC; IntMed; Gastroent. Staff, The Ottawa Hospital - General Campus; (613)737-8899 x76420; Fax. (613)737-8599.

SALOPEK, Anthony P; Heritage Village Medicentre, 2041 111 St NW, Edmonton AB T6J 4V9; Alb'89; (780)438-2306; Fax. (780)461-2632.

SALOPEK, Thomas G; Clinical Sciences Bldg, 2 125-152 University Campus NW, Edmonton AB T6G 2G3; Alb'86; FRCPC; Derm (Dermatology Surgery). (780)407-1257; Fax. (780)407-2996.

SALSALI, Mahnaz; Alberta Hosp Edmonton, PO Box 307 Stn Main 17480 Fort Rd, Edmonton AB T5J 2J7; Tehran (Iran)'90; FRCPC; Psy. Staff, Alberta Hospital Edmonton; Staff, Alberta Mental Health Board; (780)342-5555

SALSBERG, Barry B; 115 Balliol St, Toronto ON M4S 1C2; Tor'66; FRCPC; DiagRad.

SALSBERG, Jennifer M; Bay Dermatology Centre, 536-790 Bay St, Toronto ON M5G 1N8; Ott'07; Derm.

SALSBURY, Peter G; 105 Shipley St PO Box 670, Clinton ON N0M 1L0; Wes'80; CCFP; FCFP; Ac Staff, Clinton Public Hospital - Huron Perth Healthcare Alliance; (519)482-3000; Fax. (519)482-7648.

SALSMAN, Kenneth R; Soldier's Mem Hosp, PO Box 730 462 Main St, Middleton NS B0S 1P0; Dal'00; CCFP; Staff, Soldiers Memorial Hospital; (902)825-3411

SALTEL, Marc E J; The Ottawa Hosp-Civic Campus, B3-1053 Carling Ave, Ottawa ON K1Y 4E9; Ott'01; FRCSC; Urol. Staff, The Ottawa Hospital - Civic Campus; Langs: French; (613)798-5555; Fax. (613)761-5305.

SALTER, Allison E; Gaetz Family Practice, 104-45744 Gaetz St, Chilliwack BC V2R 3P1; Cal'07; CCFP; (604)824-1588

SALTER, Elizabeth; 8348 120 St NW, Edmonton AB T6G 1X2; Alb'61; FRCPC; Peds. Staff, Cross Cancer Institute; (780)437-2060

SALTER, Jennifer E; Dept of Physical Med & Rehab, RR184-800 Sherbrook St, Winnipeg MB R3A 1M4; McM'06; FRCPC; PhysMed&Rehab.

SALTER, MIchael; The Hosp for Sick Children, 555 University Ave, Toronto ON M5G 1X8; Wes'82; Head Neurosciences & Mental Health/Sr Scientist Neurosciences & Mental Health, The Hospital For Sick Children; (416)813-5756; Fax. (416)813-7921; michael.salter@sickkids.ca.

SALTER, Margaret J; 692 Euclid Ave, Toronto ON M6G 2T9; McM'83; FRCSC; PlasSurg. Staff, Sunnybrook Health Sciences Centre; (416)901-9020

SALTER, Martin R; Wynyard Community Hlth Ctre, PO Box 1539, Wynyard SK S0A 4T0; Sask'98; LMCC; CCFP; (306)554-3363; Fax. (306)554-2994.

SALTER, Nancy E; 2500-120 Adelaide St W, Toronto ON M5H 1T1; McM'79; DCPsy; DABPN; FRCPC; Psy (Child Psychiatry). Langs: English; French; (416)922-6904; nesalter@sympatico.ca.

SALTER, Timothy J; Halton Family Health Centre, 201-2951 Walker's Line, Burlington ON L7M 4Y1; Tor'77; CCFP; FCFP; (905)336-3437 x2030; Fax. (905)639-0608.

SALTER-OLIVER, Belynda; Prairie Trails Med Centre, 100-1345 Taylor Ave, Winnipeg MB R3M 3Y9; Man'02; CCFP; (204)475-0088

SALTIEL, Philippe; Ctr Hosp de Verdun, 4000 boul Lasalle, Verdun QC H4G 2A3; McG'79; FRCPC; Neur. Staff, Centre Hospitalier de Verdun; (514)362-1000

SALTSTONE, Scot P; Mental Health Clinic, 120 King St W, North Bay ON P1B 5Z7; McM'94; CCFP; (705)494-3050; Fax. (705)494-3092.

SALTZMAN, Abraham J; Markham College Med Clinic, 404-474 College St, Toronto ON M6G 1A4; Tor'72; BSc; FRCPC; IntMed. (416)920-3933; Fax. (416)920-4814; apptforsaltzman@rogers.com.

SALUJA, Inderpal S; Grand River Hosp-KW Hlth Ctre, PO Box 9056 Stn C 835 King St W, Kitchener ON N2G 1G3; Wes'01; CCFP; CCFP(E.M.); Staff, Grand River Hospital - Kitchener/Waterloo Health Centre; (519)749-4242 x4242

SALUJA, Jasjeet; Dr G B Cross Mem Hosp, 67 Manitoba Dr, Clarenville NL A5A 1K3; Meerut University (India)'04; MB BS; Staff, The Dr G B Cross Memorial Hospital; (709)466-3411

SALUJA, Sanjeet S; MUHC-Royal Victoria Hosp, 687 av des Pins O, Montreal QC H3A 1A1; McG'05; CCFP; CCFP(E.M.); Staff, McGill University Health Centre - Royal Victoria Hospital; (514)934-1934

SALVADOR, Shannon C; Diamond Health Care Centre, 6F-2775 Laurel St, Vancouver BC V5Z 1M9; Alb'04; FRCSC; ObstGyn. (604)875-4268

SALVADORI, Marina I; Children's Hosp of Western Ont, 800 Commissioners Rd E, London ON N6A 4G5; Qns'91; FRCPC; Peds; InfectDis. Staff, London Health Sciences Centre - Victoria Campus; (519)685-8500 x58299; marina.salvadori@lhsc.on.ca.

SALVALAGGIO, Ginetta L; East Edmonton Health Centre, 7910 112 Ave NW, Edmonton AB T5B 0C2; Alb'99; CCFP; FCFP; Langs: English; French; (780)342-1470; Fax. (780)342-4742.

SALVARINOVA-ZIVKOVIC, Meni R; Children's & Women's HC of BC, K3 205-4480 Oak St, Vancouver BC V6H 3V4; Skopje (Macedonia)'89; FRCPC; Peds. Staff, BC Children's Hospital; (604)875-2628

SALVENDY, John T; 710-120 Eglinton Ave E, Toronto ON M4P 1E2; Vienna (Austria)'63; DPsy; FRCPC; Psy (Group Psychotherapy). Consultant/Staff Pt-Time, St Michael's Hospital; Prof Psy, University of Toronto; Langs: German; Hebrew; Hungarian; (416)932-9770

SALVETTI, Yvan; Centre de Sante Nord-Cotiers, RR 1 2 7e rue, Forestville QC G0T 1E0; Mon'89; CCFP; Staff, Centre de santé des Côté-Nord; (418)587-2212; Fax. (418)587-6408.

SALVIAN, Anthony J G; Fairmont Med Bldg, 1214-750 Broadway W, Vancouver BC V5Z 1J2; Wes'75; FRCSC; GenSurg; VascSurg. Ac Staff, Vancouver General Hospital - Centennial Pavillion; (604)874-0532; Fax. (604)874-7806; salvian@interchange.ubc.ca.

SALVINO, Luigi A; 2660 Hastings St E, Vancouver BC V5K 1Z6; UBC'87; CCFP; (604)254-1600; Fax. (604)254-2001.

SALY, Anthony J; Spingbank Med Centre, 307-460 Springbank Dr, London ON N6J 0A8; Tor'89; CCFP; FCFP; (519)858-2727; Fax. (519)858-3868.

SALY, Viera; 2054 Sooke Rd, Victoria BC V9B 1W3; Comenius (Slovakia)'82; MSc; FRCPC; Neur (Headache). Neurologist Neurosciences, Vancouver Island Health Authority; Clinical Asst Prof Faculty of Med, University of British Columbia; Langs: Slovak; (250)474-1664; Fax. (250)474-1683.

SALYANI, M Asif; 2563 Major Mackenzie Dr, Vaughan ON L6A 2E8; Tor'02; FRCSC; Ophth. (289)203-1050

SALYANI, Mohamed A; IGA Plaza, 10-2563 Major Mackenzie Dr, Maple ON L6A 2E8; Tor'93; Langs: Kiswahili; Urdu; (905)303-1900; Fax. (905)303-1196; marianne@megafreight.co.za.

SALZMAN, Deborah A; 200-545 Clyde Ave, West Vancouver BC V7T 1C5; McM'85; Staff, Lions Gate Hospital; (604)669-2273

SALZMAN, James R; Vancouver Coastal H Authority, L5-601 Broadway W, Vancouver BC V5Z 4C2; Wes'86; Staff, UBC Hospital - Koerner Pavillion; Physician Student Health Services, Langara College; (604)875-4111 x68790; Fax. (604)736-3917.

SAM, David X; Health Sciences Centre, 1431-3330 Hospital Dr NW, Calgary AB T2N 4N1; Man'99; FRCPC; IntMed. (403)220-6376; Fax. (403)283-6151.

SAM, Diana L; Psych Health Centre, PZ183-771 Bannatyne Ave, Winnipeg MB R3E 3N4; Man'01; FRCPC; Psy (Child & Adolescent Psychiatry).

SAM, Francis B; 201-2221 Keele St, North York ON M6M 3Z5; Alb'67; FACOG; BSc; FRCSC; ObstGyn (Infertility). Ac Staff, Humber River Regional Hospital - Church Street Site; Langs: Fanti; Ga; Akan; (416)967-0761

SAM, Janie L; Norburn Med Clinic, 200-4012 Hastings St, Burnaby BC V5C 2H9; UBC'88; (604)299-2677; Fax. (604)298-6656.

SAM, Jonathan C M; West Oak Med Clinic, 2495 Old Bronte Rd, Oakville ON L6M 4J2; Tor'07; FRCPC; Peds. (905)582-7533; Fax. (905)582-0766.

SAM, Justina J; North York Gen Hosp, 4001 Leslie St, North York ON M2K 1E1; Tor'07; FRCPC; IntMed; Gastroent. Staff, North York General Hospital; (416)756-6000

SAM, Karl; CSSS de Saint-Jerome, 290 rue de Montigny, Saint-Jerome QC J7Z 5T3; Laval'06; FRCPC; DiagRad. Staff, Hôtel-Dieu de Saint-Jérôme; (450)431-8200

SAM, Renida; CLSC Saint-Henri, 3833 rue Notre-Dame O, Montreal QC H4C 1P8; Mon'00; CCFP; (514)933-7541; Fax. (514)933-2411.

SAM, Veronica K L; Tom Baker Cancer Centre, 1331 29 St NW, Calgary AB T2N 4N2; (Antigua & Barbuda)'01; BSP; CCFP; Staff, Tom Baker Cancer Centre; Langs: Chinese; (403)521-3093; Fax. (403)283-1651.

SAMAAN, Magdy K; Clinique Med de Verdun, 29-55 av de l'Eglise, Verdun QC H4G 3E7; Cairo (Egypt)'72; ObstGyn. (514)761-1017

SAMAAN, Muder C; Hamilton HS-McMaster Site, PO Box 2000 Stn Lcd 1 1200 Main St W, Hamilton ON L8N 3Z5; Dublin (Ireland)'98; Staff, Hamilton Health Sciences Centre - McMaster University Medical Centre; (905)521-2100

SAMAAN, Zainab A; St Joseph's Healthcare, PO Box 585 Stn Lcd 1 100 5th St W, Hamilton ON L8N 3K7; Al-Mustansiriyah (Iraq)'93; Staff, St Joseph's Healthcare Hamilton - West 5th Campus; (905)522-1155; Fax. (905)575-6029.

SAMAD, Arif; 302-6389 Coburg Rd, Halifax NS B3H 2A5; Dal'86; BSc; FRCSC; Ophth (Vitreo Retinal Surgery). Assoc Prof Ophth, Dalhousie University; Langs: Urdu; (902)423-2525; Fax. (902)423-1030; arif.samad@ns.aliantzinc.ca.

SAMAD, Imran; 404-4885 Kingsway, Burnaby BC V5H 4T2; Nishtar (Pakistan)'83; ABOtol; FRCSC; Otol (Facial Plastic Surgery). Staff, Burnaby Hospital; Lecturer, University of British Columbia; Langs: Hindi; Hindko; Punjabi; Urdu; (604)433-5610; Fax. (604)433-5716.

SAMAD, Nabeel B; Queen Elizabeth II HSC, 457C-1276 South Park St, Halifax NS B3H 2Y9; Tribhuvan University (Nepal)'08; MB BS; Staff/Clin Associate, Queen Elizabeth II Health Sciences Centre - Victoria General Site; Langs: Urdu; Arabic; Hindi; Nepali; (902)473-4150; Fax. (902)473-6186; nabeel.samad@cdha.nshealth.ca.

SAMAD, Osman; Guildford Town Ctr Med Clinic, 1269-15170 104 Ave, Surrey BC V3R 1N3; Karachi (Pakistan)'86; Langs: Urdu; (604)588-8764; Fax. (604)588-8761.

SAMADI, Nooshin; 311-531 Davis Dr, Newmarket ON L3Y 6P5; Shaheed Beheshti University (Israel)'94; FRCPC; IntMed. Fellow, London Health Sciences Centre - University Hospital; (905)235-5737; Fax. (905)235-5738.

SAMAGH, Manjot K; Scarborough Hosp-Birchmount, 3030 Birchmount Rd, Scarborough ON M1W 3W3; Wes'02; CCFP; CCFP(E.M.); Staff, The Scarborough Hospital - Birchmount Campus; (416)495-2400

SAMAHA, Mark; 120-1240 av Beaumont, Mont-Royal QC H3P 3E5; Qns'96; BSc; MSc; FRCSC; Otol (Rhinology). Att Staff Otol, St Mary's Hospital Centre; adj Prof, McGill University Health Centre - Royal Victoria Hospital; Asst Prof Otol, McGill University; (514)344-1717; mark_samaha@hotmail.com.

SAMAHA, Samar; All Med Health, 16880 Yonge St, Newmarket ON L3Y 0A3; Ott'01; CCFP; (905)895-9777; Fax. (905)895-9720.

SAMAHIN, A Noel; Toronto East Gen Hosp Inc, 825 Coxwell Ave, Toronto ON M4C 3E7; Peradeniya (Sri Lanka)'64; Anes. Staff-Anes, Toronto East General Hospital Inc; Asst Prof, University of Toronto; (416)469-6212; Fax. (416)469-6874.

SAMANI, Amir A; William Osler HC-Brampton, 2100 Bovaird Dr E, Brampton ON L6R 3J7; Tehran (Iran)'92; FRCPC; GenPath. Staff, William Osler Health System - Brampton Civic Hospital; (905)494-2120

SAMANT, Rajiv S; Ottawa Reg Cancer Centre, 501 Smyth Rd, Ottawa ON K1H 8L6; Dal'88; FRCPC; RadOncol (Gynecologic Oncology). Ac Staff Radiation Oncol Cancer Centre, The Ottawa Hospital - General Campus; Assoc Prof, University of Ottawa; (613)737-7700 x70212; Fax. (613)247-3511.

SAMANTA, Tania; St Joseph's Health Centre, 30 The Queensway, Toronto ON M6R 1B5; Tor'04; FRCPC; Peds; Respir. Staff, St Joseph's Health Centre; (416)530-6625

SAMARASENA, L D Asoka; Dr Charles A Janeway Child HC, 300 Prince Philip Dr, St. John's NL A1B 3V6; Colombo (Sri Lanka)'74; MB BS; FFARCSI; FRCPC; Anes. Staff, Janeway Children's Health & Rehabilitation Centre; Assoc Dean Postgraduate Med Studies, Memorial University Of Newfoundland; (709)777-6300

SAMARASENA, Mallika M; Terrace Clinic, 204-35 Major's Path, St. John's NL A1A 4Z9; Colombo (Sri Lanka)'76; MB BS; Langs: Sinhalese; (709)777-3332

SAMARASINGHE, Dewanmina A; Halton Family Health Centre, 2951 Walker's Line, Burlington ON L7M 4Y1; Colombo (Sri Lanka)'94; CCFP; (905)592-3951; Fax. (905)336-9632.

SAMAROO, Leslie L; Burnaby Square Fam Doctors, 105-7885 6th St, Burnaby BC V3N 3N4; UBC'65; (604)526-1303

SAMBASIVAN, Aarathi S; Montfort Hosp, 713 Montreal Rd, Ottawa ON K1K 0T2; Ott'05; FRCPC; Peds. Staff, Montfort Hospital; (613)746-4621

SAMBOR, Krystine E; 306-125 13th St E, North Vancouver BC V7L 2L3; UBC'98; CCFP; FCFP; (604)929-3431; Fax. (604)988-8193.

SAMBORSKI, Rockford W; Lynn Valley Med & Travel Clin, 102-1200 Lynn Valley Rd, North Vancouver BC V7J 2A2; UBC'95; CCFP; FCFP; Dir CME, West Coast General Hospital; Locum Tenens, Lions Gate Hospital; (604)988-0411; Fax. (604)988-5339.

SAMDUP, Dawa Z; Hotel Dieu Hosp, 166 Brock St, Kingston ON K7L 5G2; Madras (India)'91; FRCPC; Peds. Staff Child Developement Centre, Hotel-Dieu Hospital; (613)544-3400

SAMEDY, Natacha; Ctr Med Prive de l'Assomption, 831 boul l'Ange-Gardien N, L'Assomption QC J5W 1P5; Laval'02; Langs: French; (450)589-3232; Fax. (450)589-7352.

SAMENY, Alireza; Hampton Med Clinic, 6274 199 St NW, Edmonton AB T5T 2K4; (Iran)'98; CCFP; (780)486-7370; Fax. (780)486-7335.

SAMER, Kurt K J; 310-2055 Yukon St, Vancouver BC V5Y 4B7; UBC'75; FRCPC; Anes (Chronic Pain Management). Locum Tenens Privileges, Campbell River & District General Hospital; Physician, False Creek Surgical Centre; Physician, Cambie Surgery Centre; (604)319-7294

SAMESHIMA, Takaki; Queensway Prof Centre, 308-190 Sherway Dr, Etobicoke ON M9C 5N2; Tor'71; FRCPC; IntMed (Gastroenterology). Staff Int Med, Trillium Health Centre - West Toronto; Assoc Staff, St Michael's Hospital; (416)621-3714; Fax. (416)621-1247.

SAMETZ, Joan M; 14035 105 Ave NW PO Box 53001, Edmonton AB T5N 0Z1; Ott'83; CCFP; FCFP.

SAMHAN, Omar; Edmundston Reg Hosp, 275 Hebert Bvd, Edmundston NB E3V 4E4; Staff, Hôpital regional d'Edmundston; (506)739-2360; Fax. (506)739-2248.

SAMI, Amer; Saskatoon Cancer Centre, 20 Campus Dr, Saskatoon SK S7N 4H4; Punjab (Pakistan)'89; MB BS; Staff, Saskatoon Cancer Centre; (306)655-2710; Fax. (306)655-2910.

SAMI, Magdi H; MUHC-Royal Victoria Hosp, M462-687 av des Pins O, Montreal QC H3A 1A1; Cairo (Egypt)'69; MB ChB; FACC; FRCPC; IntMed (Clinical Cardiology); Cardiol. principale Médecin, McGill University Health Centre - Royal Victoria Hospital; Prof Med, McGill University; Langs: Arabic; French; Spanish; (514)843-1416; Fax. (514)843-2813.

SAMI, Pensee A; 272 Cedar St, Sudbury ON P3B 1M7; Cairo (Egypt)'77; Staff, Health Sciences North-Laurentian Site; Langs: Arabic; (705)673-4415

SAMI, Sahar; Markham Prof Centre, 203-2265 Pembina Hwy, Winnipeg MB R3T 5J3; Ain Shams (Egypt)'88; CCFP; (204)261-9881

SAMIEE ZAFARGHANDY, Samira; Children's Hosp Eastern Ont, 401 Smyth Rd, Ottawa ON K1H 8L1; Tehran (Iran)'04; FRCPC; Peds. Staff, Children's Hospital of Eastern Ontario (CHEO); (613)737-7600

SAMII, Leyla; 130-1402 8 Ave NW, Calgary AB T2N 1B9; (Other Foreign)'05; CCFP; (403)284-3711

SAMIKIAN, Karoon; Amherstview Med Centre, 18 Manitou Cres W, Amherstview ON K7N 1S3; McG'88; CCFP; Langs: French; (613)384-4888; Fax. (613)384-0889.

SAMIMI, Mehran; Ridge Meadows Hosp & Hlth CC, 11666 Laity St, Maple Ridge BC V2X 5A3; Tehran (Iran)'74; CCFP; Staff, Ridge Meadows Hospital & Health Care Centre; (604)466-6909

SAMIS, Andrew J W; Kingston Gen Hosp, 76 Stuart St, Kingston ON K7L 2V7; Qns'95; BSc(Hon.); MSc; FRCSC; GenSurg; Critical Care Medicine. Gen Surgeon, QHC Belleville General; Att Staff GI Diseases Research Unit, Hotel-Dieu Hospital; Att Staff, Kingston General Hospital; (613)549-6666; Fax. (613)548-2426.

SAMIS, Gregory A; Peter Lougheed Centre, 3604-3500 26 Ave NE, Calgary AB T1Y 6J4; Alb'91; VascSurg; GenSurg. Staff, Peter Lougheed Centre; (403)943-2523; Fax. (403)291-2734; gregory.samis@calgaryhealthregion.ca.

SAMIS, Scott O; Peter Lougheed Centre, 2403-3500 26 Ave NE, Calgary AB T1Y 6J4; Alb'92; Staff, Peter Lougheed Centre; (403)943-5461; Fax. (403)943-5438; scottsamis@hotmail.com.

SAMIS, William D; York-Finch Med Centre, 316-2115 Finch Ave W, North York ON M3N 2V6; Tor'54; FRCSC; Ophth. Court Staff, Humber River Regional Hospital - Finch Avenue Site; (416)745-6969; Fax. (416)745-6724.

SAMJI, Amirali M; West Eglinton Med Centre, 301-2010 Eglinton Ave W, Toronto ON M6E 2K3; Makerere (Uganda)'70; MB ChB; DMRT; DABR; Court Staff, Toronto General Hospital - UHN; Court Staff, Humber River Regional Hospital - Keele Street Site; Lecturer Family & Community Med, University of Toronto; Langs: Gujarati; Hindi; Swahili; (416)782-3736; Fax. (416)782-4951.

SAMJI, Rahim; Royal Alexandra Hosp, 10240 Kingsway NW, Edmonton AB T5H 3V9; Cal'06; FRCPC; DiagRad. Staff, Royal Alexandra Hospital; (780)735-4777; Fax. (416)792-4139.

SAMLER, Shannon R; 214-145 15th St W, North Vancouver BC V7M 1R9; UBC'06; FRCSC; OrthSurg. (604)980-5779

SAMMARELLI, Patricia; Jubilee Centre, 1823 Fort St, Victoria BC V8R 1J6; Rome (Italy)'91; CCFP; Langs: Spanish; Italian; (250)595-6636

SAMOIL, Darryl P; Colebrook Family Practice, 107-15240 56 Ave, Surrey BC V3S 5K7; Alb'88; CCFP; CCFP(E.M.); FCFP; (778)574-1414

SAMOIL, Mary F S; Dr Rose Farag Med Clinic, 1100 Richmond Ave, Brandon MB R7A 1M6.

SAMOILA, John P; 206-13278 Tecumseh Rd E, Windsor ON N8N 3R6; Saba University (Indonesia)'02; (519)735-1490; Fax. (519)735-6236.

SAMOISETTE, Andre; Societe PSM, 215-1600 boul Curé-Labelle, Laval QC H7V 2W2; Mon'71; Staff, Hopital de la Cite de la santé; Universite de Montreal; (450)688-9271; Fax. (450)688-4665.

SAMOKHVALOV, Andriy V; Addiction & Mental Hlth-ARF, 33 Russell St, Toronto ON M5S 2S1; (Ukraine)'02; Staff, Centre for Addiction & Mental Health (CAMH) - Russell Street Site; (416)535-8501; Fax. (416)595-6821.

SAMOLCZYK, Janet L; Grandview Med Ctr Fam Hlth Team, 167 Hespeler Rd, Cambridge ON N1R 3H7; Tor'75; CCFP; FCFP; Teach Staff, McMaster University; Ac Staff, Cambridge Memorial Hospital; (519)623-4200; Fax. (519)623-2546.

SAMOLCZYK, Thomas A; Grandview Med Ctr Fam Hlth Team, 167 Hespeler Rd, Cambridge ON N1R 3H7; Tor'75; Ac Staff, Cambridge Memorial Hospital; (519)623-4200; Fax. (519)623-2546.

SAMOSH, Martin L; Martin Samosh Med Prof Corp, 201-112 Queenston St, St Catharines ON L2R 2Z4; Tor'83; FRCPC; IntMed (Hematological Oncology); Hem. Ac Staff, Niagara Health System - Ontario Street Site; Ac Staff, Niagara Health System - St Catharines General Site; (905)685-8082; Fax. (905)988-5776.

SAMOTIS-TCHERVENKOV, Linda A; MUHC-Montreal Children's Hosp B260-2300 rue Tupper, Montreal QC H3H 1P3; McG'84; FRCPC; Peds. Staff, McGill University Health Centre - Montreal Children's Hospital; Langs: English; French; (514)412-4433

SAMOUELIAN, Vanessa; CHUM-Hop Notre-Dame, 1560 rue Sherbrooke E, Montreal QC H2L 4M1; Lille (France)'05; GynOnco (P.Q.). Staff, Centre Hospitalier l'Université de Montréal (CHUM) - Hôpital Notre-Dame; (514)890-8000 x27244

SAMOUKOVIC, Gordon; MUHC-Royal Victoria Hosp, 687 av des Pins O, Montreal QC H3A 1A1; UBC'05; CardSurg. Staff, McGill University Health Centre - Royal Victoria Hospital; (514)501-6061

SAMOUR, Fathe M A; US Memorial Health Centre, PO Box 398, St Lawrence NL A0E 2V0; Al-Fateh (Libya)'04; Staff, US Memorial Health Centre; (709)873-2330

SAMOYLOFF, Stephan D; Peach City Medical, 3090 Skaha Lake Rd, Penticton BC V2A 7H2; UBC'90; CCFP; CCFP(E.M.); Staff, Penticton Regional Hospital; (250)276-5050; Fax. (250)276-5051.

SAMPAIO, Marcos; The Ottawa Hosp-Gen Campus, 501 Smyth Rd, Ottawa ON K1H 8L6; Sao Paolo (Brazil)'02; Staff, The Ottawa Hospital - General Campus; (613)737-8571; Fax. (613)737-8830.

SAMPATH, Sharadh; 207-6051 Gilbert Rd, Richmond BC V7C 3V3; UBC'03; FRCSC; GenSurg. (604)276-0952

SAMPHIRE, John; Richmond Med Bldg, 309-2020 Richmond Rd, Victoria BC V8R 6R5; UBC'95; FRCSC; GenSurg (Minimal Invasive Surgery); ThorSurg. (250)595-2820; Fax. (250)598-2850.

SAMPLE, Clifford B; Tawa Centre, 205-3017 66 St NW, Edmonton AB T6K 4B2; Alb'98; FRCSC; GenSurg (Gastrointestinal Surgery). Staff, Covenant Health - Grey Nuns Community Hospital; Clin Assoc Prof, University of Alberta; (780)461-6012; Fax. (780)461-5442.

SAMPSEL, Kari L; The Ottawa Hosp-Gen Campus, 501 Smyth Rd, Ottawa ON K1H 8L6; Qns'03; FRCPC; EmergMed. Staff, The Ottawa Hospital - General Campus; (613)737-8136

SAMPSON, Evan E; 10942 124 St NW, Edmonton AB T5M 0H5; Alb'93; FRCPC; PhysMed&Rehab (Electrodiagnosis). (780)447-4924; Fax. (780)452-5111.

SAMPSON, Gweneth L; Stouffville Med Centre, 2F-34 Civic Ave, Stouffville ON L4A 1H2; Tor'87; CCFP; FCFP; (905)640-3100; Fax. (905)640-5346.

SAMPSON, John E; Queen Elizabeth Hosp, PO Box 6600 Stn Central 60 Riverside Dr, Charlottetown PE C1A 8T5; Dal'87; CCFP; CCFP(E.M.); FCFP; Staff, Queen Elizabeth Hospital; (902)894-2111

SAMPSON, Maria T; Halifax Prof Centre, 629-5991 Spring Garden Rd, Halifax NS B3H 1Y6; Dal'96; BSc(Kinesiol); CCFP; Lecturer Family Practice, Dalhousie University; (902)422-8488; Fax. (902)422-8494.

SAMPSON, Mark E; Health Park, 202-45 Weatherbee Rd, Mira Road NS B1M 0A1; Dal'89; CCFP; CCFP(E.M.); FCFP; (902)564-6149; Fax. (902)564-6149.

SAMPSON, Monica; Dr Charles A Janeway Child HC, 300 Prince Philip Dr, St. John's NL A1B 3V6; Mem'89; CCFP; FCFP; Staff, Janeway Children's Health & Rehabilitation Centre; (709)777-3300

SAMPSON, Olivia J; 115-3195 Granville St, Vancouver BC V6H 3K2; McG'93; CCFP; FCFP; Langs: English; (604)732-0525; Fax. (604)732-1064.

SAMPSON, Sonia D; Health Sciences Centre, 300 Prince Philip Dr, St. John's NL A1B 3V6; UBC'03; FRCPC; Anes. Staff, Health Sciences Centre; (709)737-6300

SAMRA, David; Scarborough Prof Centre, 321-1371 Neilson Rd, Scarborough ON M1B 4Z8; Tor'77; FRCSC; ObstGyn (Colposcopy). Staff ObstGyn, Rouge Valley Health System - Centenary Health Centre Site; Langs: Hebrew; French; Arabic; (416)283-6566; Fax. (416)283-3479; samradavid@hotmail.com.

SAMRAI, Gurinder S; AIM Clinic Orleans, 3-1605 Orleans Blvd, Orleans ON K1C 7E2; Mon'08; CCFP; (613)830-6890

SAMSON, Arnaud; Polyclinique Boreal, 668 rue de Parfondeval, Baie-Comeau QC G5C 3R3; Laval'75; LMCC; Langs: Spanish; (418)589-8536; Fax. (418)589-8302.

SAMSON, Benoit; Hop Charles LeMoyne, 3120 boul Taschereau, Greenfield Park QC J4V 2H1; Sher'82; MedOncol; Hem (P.Q.); IntMed. Staff, Hopital Charles LeMoyne; (450)466-5000 x2318; Fax. (450)466-5066.

SAMSON, Carine; CSSS du Nord de Lanaudière, 1000 boul Saint-Anne, St-Charles-Brromee QC J6E 6J2; Laval'09; CCFP; CCFP(E.M.); Staff, Centre Hospitalier Régional de Lanaudière; (450)759-8222

SAMSON, Caroline; Hop du Sacre-Coeur de Mtl, 5400 boul Gouin O, Montreal QC H4J 1C5; Laval'93; CSPQ; FRCPC; DiagRad. Staff, Hôpital du Sacre-Coeur de Montréal; (514)338-2222; Fax. (514)338-2660.

SAMSON, Christine; Regie des Rentes du Qubec, CP 5200 Succ Terminus, Quebec QC G1K 7S9; Laval'82; Staff, Hôtel-Dieu de Lévis; (418)657-8709 x4150

SAMSON, Daniele; ASSS de la Mauricie, 550 rue Bonaventure, Trois-Rivieres QC G9A 2B5; Laval'89; Staff, CLSC Les Bles d'Or; (819)693-3943

SAMSON, Elizabeth A; Courtice Health Centre, 1450 Highway 2, Courtice ON L1E 3C3; Tor'82; BSc(Windsor); CCFP; (905)721-4051; Fax. (905)721-6184.

SAMSON, Esther; Centre de Sante Valcartier, CP 1000 BDP Succ Forces, Courcelette QC G0A 4Z0; Laval'80; CSPQ; FRCPC; Psy. (418)649-5524; Fax. (418)649-5599; dspsamse@cha.quebec.qc.ca.

SAMSON, Gilles; 3774 boul Frontenac O, Thetford Mines QC G6H 2J8; Laval'84; Staff, Hopital du CSS de la Region de Thetford; Langs: English; (418)423-5040; Fax. (418)423-2842.

SAMSON, Isabelle; Dir de la Sante Publique de l', 3113-300 rue King E, Sherbrooke QC J1G 1B1; Qns'95; FRCPC; CommunMed. Langs: English; French; (819)829-3400

SAMSON, Isabelle; Clinique Saint-Vallier, 201-205 rue Montmagny, Quebec QC G1N 4V3; Laval'93; CCFP; Langs: Spanish; English; (418)266-0351

SAMSON, Isabelle; CSSS de L'Hematite, GD 1 rue de l'Aquilon, Fermont QC G0G 1J0; Laval'10; CCFP; Staff, CLSC de l'Hématite; (418)287-3280

SAMSON, Jacques; Clinique Med de Levis, 300-4975 boul de la Rive-Sud, Levis QC G6V 4Z5; Laval'82; FRCSC; Ophth. Staff, Hôtel-Dieu de Lévis; (418)838-8080; Fax. (418)838-5151; colrs@total.net.

SAMSON, Jacques P; Ctr Hosp de Matane, 333 rue Thibault, Matane QC G4W 2W5; Laval'69; CSPQ; Anes. Staff, Centre Hospitalier de Matane; (418)562-3135

SAMSON, Jonah A; First Care Med Centre, 2590 Commercial Dr, Vancouver BC V5N 4C2; Dal'02; CCFP; (604)871-1535

SAMSON, Julie; CSSS de Laval, 1755 boul Rene-Laennec, Laval QC H7M 3L9; Laval'97; CSPQ; FRCPC; Anes. Staff, Hopital de la Cite de la santé; (450)668-1010 x2477; samsonjulie@hotmail.com.

SAMSON, Julie; CSSS de la Mitis, 800 av du Sanatorium, Mont-Joli QC G5H 3L6; Laval'82; Staff, CSSS de la Mitis; (418)775-7261; Fax. (418)775-1989.

SAMSON, Julie; Timmins Family Health Team, 250-123 Third Ave, Timmins ON P4N 1C6; Ott'95; CCFP; CCFP(E.M.); FCFP; Langs: Bilingual(English/French); (705)264-9151; Fax. (705)268-7444.

SAMSON, Karine; CSSS de Memphremagog, 50 rue Saint-Patrice E, Magog QC J1X 3X3; Sher'10; CCFP; Staff, Centre Hospitalier et CLSC de Memphremagog; (819)843-2572

SAMSON, Kevin; A-175 Alma St PO Box 340, Rockwood ON N0B 2K0; McM'86; (519)856-4611; ksamson@ewfht.ca.

SAMSON, Lindy M; Children's Hosp Eastern Ont, 401 Smyth Rd, Ottawa ON K1H 8L1; McM'90; FRCPC; Peds (AIDS/HIV); InfectDis. Chief Div of Infectious Diseases, Children's Hospital of Eastern Ontario (CHEO); (613)737-7600 x2651; Fax. (613)738-4832; samson@cheo.on.ca.

SAMSON, Line M I; Clinique Med Rock Forest, 4870 boul Bourque, Sherbrooke QC J1N 3S5; Mon'94; (819)820-2673 x58; Fax. (819)820-2112.

SAMSON, Louise M; CHUM-Hotel-Dieu, 3840 rue Saint-Urbain, Montreal QC H2W 1T8; Sher'78; DABR; CSPQ; FRCPC; DiagRad. ac Staff, Centre Hospitalier l'Université de Montréal (CHUM) - Hôtel-Dieu; Prof/Head Radio-Oncol & Nuclear Med, Universite de Montreal; (514)890-8150; Fax. (514)412-7193.

SAMSON, Marc; Ctr Hosp Chauveau, 11999 rue de l'Hopital, Quebec QC G2A 2T7; Laval'92; Ac Staff, Centre Hospitalier Chauveau; (418)842-3651; Fax. (418)842-1948.

SAMSON, Marie; Clinique Med d'Alma, 935 av du Pont S, Alma QC G8B 2V5; Laval'88; Staff, CSSS de Lac-Saint Jean-Est; (418)668-8321; Fax. (418)668-5298; marie.samson@ssss.gouv.qc.ca.

SAMSON, Marie-Eve; CHUQ-Ctr Hosp Univ Laval, 2705 boul Laurier, Quebec QC G1V 4G2; Laval'02; FRCPC; Peds; Critical Care Medicine (P.Q.). Staff, Centre Hospitalier Universitaire de Quebec-CHUL; (418)656-4141

SAMSON, Michel; CHUQ-Ctr Hosp Univ Laval, 2705 boul Laurier, Quebec QC G1V 4G2; Laval'80; Cardiol; IntMed (Clinical Cardiology). Ac Staff, Centre Hospitalier Universitaire de Quebec-CHUL; Université Laval; (418)654-2110; Fax. (418)654-2268.

SAMSON, Mimi; CSSS de la Minganie, CP 190 1035 Prom des Anciens, Havre-Saint-Pierre QC G0G 1P0; Mon'97; Staff, CSSS de la Minganie; (418)538-2212; mimi_samson@ssss.gouv.qc.ca.

SAMSON, Nancy L; 8D Shoal Harbour Dr, Clarenville NL A5A 2C4; Mem'97; CCFP; (709)466-1299; Fax. (709)466-2217.

SAMSON, Nelson; Clinique Med St-Joseph, RR 1 841 av Sainte-Therese, St-Joseph-D-Beauce QC G0S 2V0; Laval'72; (418)397-6891; Fax. (418)397-4170.

SAMSON, Sheri-Lee; Fredericton Med Clinic, 304-1015 Regent St, Fredericton NB E3B 6H5; Dal'99; BSc; FRCSC; ObstGyn. Staff, Dr Everett Chalmers Regional Hospital; (506)457-2113; Fax. (506)459-7073.

SAMSON, Stephanie; Centre Med Ste-Foy Inc, 802 av du Chanoine-Scott, Quebec QC G1V 3N4; Laval'88.

SAMSON, Vicky; Clinique de Med Familiale, 1971 rue Bilodeau, Plessisville QC G6L 3J1; Laval'01; Staff, CLSC de l'Erable; (819)362-6337

SAMSON, Yvan; Hôpital Ste-Justine, 3175 ch Cote-Sainte-Catherine, Montreal QC H3T 1C5; Mon'83; FRCPC; Peds (Pediatric Hematology Oncology); MedOncol (P.Q.); Hem. dir Enquêteur/Dir Etudes de Phase 1 & 2 Pediatric Oncol, Hôpital Ste-Justine; Langs: Bilingual(French/English); (514)345-4931; Fax. (514)345-4884; yvan.samson@umontreal.ca.

SAMSON, Yves; 1080 rue Victoria, Edmundston NB E3V 3T2; Laval'82; (506)648-6822; Fax. (506)648-6878.

SAMSOONDAR, Wayne R; 104-10168 Yonge St, Richmond Hill ON L4C 1T6; West Indies (Jamaica)'80; MB BS; FRCSC; Urol. Staff, Mackenzie Richmond Hill Hospital; (905)737-4224; Fax. (905)737-6046.

SAMU, Peter C; Rosedale Radiologists, B1-600 Sherbourne St, Toronto ON M4X 1W4; Tor'61; CRCP; DiagRad. (416)960-0177; Fax. (416)960-8522.

SAMUEL, Charles; Clin Med Metromedic, 100-1538 rue Sherbrooke O, Montreal QC H3G 1L5; McG'86; Langs: French; (514)932-2122; Fax. (514)939-7154.

SAMUEL, Christopher V; Halton HC Serv Corp-Oakville, 327 Reynolds St, Oakville ON L6J 3L7; McM'09; CCFP; CCFP(E.M.); Staff, Halton Healthcare Services Corporation - Oakville Site; (905)338-4618; Fax. (905)338-4146.

SAMUEL, Daniella J; Humber River Reg Hosp-Finch, 2111 Finch Ave W, North York ON M3N 1N1; McM'03; FRCPC; Anes. Staff, Humber River Regional Hospital - Finch Avenue Site; (416)744-2500

SAMUEL, John P; Meadow Lake Assoc Clinic, PO Box 1510, Meadow Lake SK S9X 1Z1; (306)236-5661; Fax. (306)236-4355.

SAMUEL, John P; 945 22 St, Wainwright AB T9W 1T8; (South Africa)'02; (780)842-3324

SAMUEL, Joyce M; A202-11685 Yonge St, Richmond Hill ON L4E 0K7; McM'10; CCFP; (905)884-6500; Fax. (905)884-6100.

SAMUEL, Justin V; Main Med Clinic, 554 Main St E, Hamilton ON L8M 1J3; Kasturba Medical College (India)'00; (905)540-1000; Fax. (905)540-1001.

SAMUEL, Maged Y N; 202-809 Brant St, Burlington ON L7R 2J4; Cairo (Egypt)'87; CCFP; (905)681-1212; Fax. (905)681-1216.

SAMUEL, Oded; Jane & Finch Family Hlth Team, 136A-1 York Gate Blvd, North York ON M3N 3A1; Tor'78; CCFP; CCFP(E.M.); FCFP; Ac Staff EmergMed, Humber River Regional Hospital - Finch Avenue Site; Court Staff, The Scarborough Hospital - Birchmount Campus; Langs: Hebrew; Hungarian; (416)745-4949; Fax. (416)745-0786.

SAMUEL, Steve E S; 405-4430 Bathurst St, North York ON M3H 3S3; Tor'74; FRCSC; PlasSurg (Cosmetic Surgery). Court Staff, North York General Hospital; Ac Staff, Humber River Regional Hospital - Finch Avenue Site; Langs: Hebrew; Hungarian; German; French; (416)630-2715; Fax. (416)630-7630.

SAMUEL, Susan M; Alberta Children's Hosp, 2888 Shaganappi Trail NW, Calgary AB T3B 6A8; UBC'01; FRCPC; Peds; Nephrol. Staff, Alberta Children's Hospital; (403)955-7211; Fax. (403)955-2203.

SAMUEL-THOMASSIN, Véronique; CSSS Les Eskers de l'Abitibi, 622 4e rue O, Amos QC J9T 2S2; Mon'06; Staff, CH Hôtel-Dieu d'Amos; (819)732-3341

SAMUELS, Charles H; 106-51 Sunpark Drive SE, Calgary AB T2X 3V4; Cal'91; DABSM; CCFP; Med Dir, Centre for Sleep & Human Performance; Clinical Asst Prof, University of Calgary; (403)254-6663; Fax. (403)254-6693; admin@centreforsleep.com.

SAMUELS, Lewis; The Brandon Clinic, 620 Dennis St, Brandon MB R7A 5E7; Mem'00; (204)728-4440

SAMUELS, Peter L; Rockyview Gen Hosp, 7007 14 St SW, Calgary AB T2V 1P9; Cal'92; FRCPC; Anes. Staff, Rockyview General Hospital; (403)943-3410

SAMUELS, Peter M; A2-150 Main St E Family Medical Centre, Grimsby ON L3M 1P1; Qns'98; BSc(Hon)(Hons.); CCFP; Staff, West Lincoln Memorial Hospital; Asst Prof Family Med, McMaster University; (905)945-5424; Fax. (905)945-4772; peter.samuels@cogeco.net.

SAMUELS, Sheri L; Canadian Blood Services, 8249 114 St NW, Edmonton AB T6G 2R8; Alb'94; CCFP; Langs: Spanish; samuel.sheri@gmail.com.

SAMUELSON, Samantha L; Whitehorse Gen Hosp, 5 Hospital Rd, Whitehorse YT Y1A 3H7; Cal'03; FRCSC; GenSurg. Staff, Whitehorse General Hospital; (867)393-8700

SAMWAYS, Michelle L; 361 South Service Rd, Grimsby ON L3M 4E8; McM'93; BSc(Hons.); ABPMR; FRCPC; PhysMed&Rehab. Ac Staff, West Lincoln Memorial Hospital; (905)945-0060; Fax. (905)945-9760.

SAMYCIA, Gary M; Baker Clinic, 100-10405 Jasper Ave NW, Edmonton AB T5J 1G5; Alb'77; Ac Staff, Royal Alexandra Hospital; Clin Instructor, University of Alberta; (780)944-9581; Fax. (780)944-9534.

SAN, Vong-Virienne; CSSS de Laval, 280 boul du Roi-du-Nord, Laval QC H7L 4L2; Sher'97; LMCC; (450)622-5110; Fax. (450)622-4150.

SAN AGUSTIN, D Patrick; Grey Nuns Community Hosp, 1100 Youville Drive West NW, Edmonton AB T6L 5X8; Alb'98; CCFP; CCFP(E.M.); Staff, Covenant Health - Grey Nuns Community Hospital; (780)735-7180; Fax. (780)988-5774.

SAN VICENTE, Juan J; Central Alberta Prof Centre, 101-5201 43 St, Red Deer AB T4N 1C7; (Mexico)'69; FRCSC; Urol. (403)342-1034; Fax. (403)340-8833.

SAN VICENTE, Monica K; Royal University Hosp, G525-103 Hospital Dr, Saskatoon SK S7N 0W8; Sask'04; FRCPC; Anes. Staff, Royal University Hospital; (306)655-1182; Fax. (306)655-1279.

SANAN, Anita; Kelowna Gen Hosp, 2268 Pandosy St, Kelowna BC V1Y 1T2; Man'04; FRCPC; Anes. Staff, Kelowna General Hospital; (250)862-4000

SANANDAJI, Khashayar; The Health Centre of Maple, 2810 Major MacKenzie Dr, Vaughan ON L6A 3L2; Lucknow (India)'92; MB BS; CCFP; Langs: Farsi; Hindi; Kurdish; (905)832-3838

SANATANI, Irina; 205-190 Wortley Rd, London ON N6C 4Y7; McM'00; FRCPC; IntMed. Staff, London Health Sciences Centre - University Hospital; (519)204-6727; Fax. (519)649-5055.

SANATANI, Michael S; London Reg Cancer Centre, 790 Commissioners Rd E, London ON N6A 4L6; Wes'00; FRCPC; IntMed; MedOncol. Staff, London Regional Cancer Center; Langs: German; (519)685-8500

SANATANI, Shubhayan; Children's & Women's HC of BC, 1F9-4480 Oak St, Vancouver BC V6H 3V4; UBC'93; FRCPC; Peds (Electrophysiology); Cardiol. Ac Staff, BC Children's Hospital; Assoc Prof Peds, University of British Columbia; Langs: German; (604)875-3619; Fax. (604)875-3463; ssanatani@cw.bc.ca.

SANBORN, Margaret D; South Bruce Grey HC-Chesley, 39 2nd St SE, Chesley ON N0G 1L0; McM'79; CCFP; FCFP; Fam Med, South Bruce Grey Health Services - Chesley Site; Clinical Asst Prof Family Med, McMaster University; (519)363-2340; msanborn@sbghc.on.ca.

SANCHE, Gilbert; CLSC du Marigot, 1351 boul des Laurentides, Vimont QC H7M 2Y2; Mon'84; CCFP; FCFP; adj Prof, Universite de Montreal; (450)668-1803; Fax. (450)668-1507; gilbert.sanche@umontreal.ca.

SANCHE, Stephanie; Polyclinique Med de Terrebonne, 201-901 boul des Seigneurs, Terrebonne QC J6W 1T8; Mon'08; (450)471-1117

SANCHE, Stephen E; Royal University Hosp, 3766-103 Hospital Dr, Saskatoon SK S7N 0W8; Sask'90; CRCP; FRCPC; IntMed; MedMicrobiol; InfectDis. Staff IntMed & LabMed, Royal University Hospital; Asst Prof Med, University of Saskatchewan; (306)655-6658

SANCHEZ, Adolfo; Markham College Med Clinic, 410-474 College St, Toronto ON M6G 1A4; Valladolid (Spain)'58; FRCPC; Psy. Langs: Portuguese; French; Spanish; (416)925-4679; Fax. (416)925-1336.

SANCHEZ, Angelita R; Sudbury Reg Hosp-Kirkwood, 680 Kirkwood Dr, Sudbury ON P3E 1X3; UE Manila (Philippines)'91; DABPN; FRCPC; Psy (Child & Adolescent Psychiatry). Psychiatrist, Health Sciences North-Kirkwood Site; Asst Prof, Northern Ontario School of Medicine; (705)675-5900 x8234; asanchez@hrsrh.on.ca.

SANCHEZ, Arturo; Markham College Med Clinic, 403-474 College St, Toronto ON M6G 1A4; National (Colombia)'58; DABPed; FRCPC; Peds. Court Staff, Women's College Hospital; Court Staff, St Michael's Hospital; Ac Staff, St Joseph's Health Centre; Langs: Italian; Portuguese; Spanish; (416)922-4702; Fax. (416)922-5492.

SANCHEZ, Federico J; 4972 Dundas St W, Etobicoke ON M9A 1B7; Dal'95; BSc; CCFP; FCFP; Langs: Italian; Spanish; French; (416)233-0404

SANCHEZ, Marie-Alice; Inst Philippe Pinel de Mtl, 10905 boul Henri-Bourassa E, Montreal QC H1C 1H1; Mon'86; CSPQ; FRCPC; Psy. ac Staff, Institut Philippe-Pinel de Montreal; (514)648-8461; Fax. (514)881-3706.

SANCHEZ, Marisol; Hôpital Ste-Justine, 3175 ch Cote-Sainte-Catherine, Montreal QC H3T 1C5; Mon'00; FRCPC; Peds; PedEmergMed. Staff, Hôpital Ste-Justine; Langs: Spanish; English; (514)345-4931 x5885; soleil.sanchez@gmail.com.

SANCHEZ, Miguelle; Ctr Hosp Anna-Laberge, 200 boul Brisebois, Chateauguay QC J6K 4W8; Mon'91; FRCPC; MedMicrobiol; Microbio & Infect Dis (P.Q.). Staff, Hôpital Anna-Laberge; (450)699-2425

SANCHEZ, Millaray; Smyth Med Centre, 200-1929 Russell Rd, Ottawa ON K1G 4G3; (Venezuela)'85; CCFP; FCFP; Lecturer Faculty of Med, University of Ottawa; Langs: Spanish; French; (613)249-0666; Fax. (613)249-0804.

SANCHEZ, Zenia A; 110-1300 Central Pky W, Mississauga ON L5C 4G8; Cebu (Philippines)'83; Court Staff, Trillium Health Centre - Mississauga; Langs: Tagalog; (905)279-5505; Fax. (905)279-5557.

SANCHEZ-ARROYO, Emilio; Ctr de Radiologie du West Isla, 175 av Stillview, Pointe-Claire QC H9R 4S3; Salamanca (Spain)'55; CSPQ; DiagRad. Langs: Spanish; French; (514)697-5025

SANCHEZ-BARACALDO, Lilia M; CHUM-Hotel-Dieu, 3840 rue Saint-Urbain, Montreal QC H2W 1T8; Bogota (Colombia)'87; Staff, Centre Hospitalier l'Université de Montréal (CHUM) - Hôtel-Dieu; (514)890-8000 x14464

SANCHEZ-GUERRERO, Francisco G; 2 005-60 Murray St, Toronto ON M5T 3L9; Universidad de Guadalajara (Mexico)'81; (416)586-4800; Fax. (416)586-8766.

SANCHINI, Edouard R G; CLSC-CHSLD Pat Montreal Est, 13926 rue Notre-Dame E, Pte-aux-Trembles QC H1A 1T5; Mon'76; (514)642-4050; Fax. (514)498-7505.

SANCHO, Frederic; Clinique Med du College, GD 1396 rue Notre-Dame, Saint-Cesaire QC J0L 1T0; Mon'07; CCFP; (450)469-0505; Fax. (450)469-4554.

SANDEJAS, Mario F; 2B-1695 Wonderland Rd N, London ON N6G 4W3; Wes'89; (519)474-0614

SANDER, Donald A; Alberni Med Bldg, 10-3855 9th Ave, Port Alberni BC V9Y 4T9; Cardiff (Wales)'80; (250)724-3442; Fax. (250)724-3442.

SANDER, Ryan A; Lakeside Med Clinic, 3919 8th St E, Saskatoon SK S7H 5M7; Sask'05; CCFP; (306)374-6884; Fax. (306)374-2552; ryan.sander@sasktel.net.

SANDERMAN, Blaine S; University of Alberta Hosp, 1E7 22WCM-8440 112 St NW, Edmonton AB T6G 2B7; Alb'73; FRCPC; Psy. Ac Staff, University of Alberta Hospital; (780)407-6543; Fax. (780)407-6672.

SANDERS, Andrew P; Oakmount Med Centre, 220-809 41st Ave W, Vancouver BC V5Z 2N6; Alb'84; FRCPC; Psy. Staff, Vancouver General Hospital - Centennial Pavillion; Asst Prof, University of British Columbia; (604)261-6883

SANDERS, April D; Sanders Med Clinic, 101-3002 32 Ave, Vernon BC V1T 2L7; UBC'84; BSc; CCFP; FCFP; (250)542-3170; Fax. (250)542-0835.

SANDERS, Barry H; Broadway Med Centre, 230-943 Broadway W, Vancouver BC V5Z 4E1; McM'76; FRCSC; ObstGyn (Endoscopic Surgery). Ac Staff, Vancouver General Hospital - Centennial Pavillion; Ac Staff, BC Women's Hospital & Health Centre; Clin Prof, University of British Columbia; (604)734-2712; Fax. (604)734-8572.

SANDERS, Bruce R; 309-1990 Fort St, Victoria BC V8R 6V4; Wes'80; FRCPC; IntMed; Respir. Staff, Vancouver Island Health Authority; (250)383-0250; Fax. (250)381-7820.

SANDERS, David B; Strathroy Middlesex Gen Hosp, 360-395 Carrie St, Strathroy ON N7G 3C9; Wes'80; BSc(Hon); FRCPC; IntMed. Ac Staff, Strathroy Middlesex General Hospital - Middlesex Hospital Alliance; (519)245-4290; Fax. (519)245-4627.

SANDERS, David H; Rapha Med Centre, 8-50 Tacoma Dr, Dartmouth NS B2W 3E6; Dal'66; MD; (902)464-9399; Fax. (902)464-1910.

SANDERS, David W; London HSC-Victoria Hosp, PO Box 5010 Stn B E4 123-800 Commissioners Rd E, London ON N6A 5W9; Tor'93; FRCSC; OrthSurg. Staff, London Health Sciences Centre - Victoria Campus; (519)685-8300 x58086; Fax. (519)685-8016.

SANDERS, Kenneth C; 674 Concession St, Hamilton ON L8V 4T9; McM'77; FRCSC; GenSurg. Asst Prof, McMaster University; (905)387-1367; Fax. (905)387-4500.

SANDERS, Kevin M; North York Med Arts Bldg, 311-1333 Sheppard Ave E, North York ON M2J 1V1; Tor'99; FRCPC; IntMed; Critical Care Medicine; Respir. Staff, Sunnybrook Health Sciences Centre; (416)494-0586; Fax. (416)494-0915.

SANDERS, Lawrence D; Woodstock Gen Hosp, 310 Juliana Dr, Woodstock ON N4V 0A4; Cape Town (South Africa)'80; MB ChB; FACR; FRCPC; DiagRad (Angiography/Interventional). Staff, Woodstock General Hospital; (519)421-4207; Fax. (519)421-4241.

SANDERS, Mark D L; Ingram Family Physicians, 103-149 Ingram St, Duncan BC V9L 1N8; Sask'94; CCFP; FCFP; (250)746-4401; Fax. (250)746-4473; sandersandmclean@shaw.ca.

SANDERS, Robert W; Medical Arts Bldg, 1402-233 Kennedy St, Winnipeg MB R3C 3J5; Man'77; FRCSC; Ophth.

SANDERS, Stuart B; Sheldon Chumir Centre, G061-1213 4 St SW, Calgary AB T2R 0X7; Manchester (England)'81; MB ChB; FRCPC; Psy (Geriatric Medicine). Clin Assoc Prof Psy/Div Chief, University of Calgary; (403)955-6155; Fax. (403)955-6169.

SANDERS, William D; Sanders Med Inc Vein & Aesthet, 101-3002 32 Ave, Vernon BC V1T 2L7; UBC'84; BSc; CCFP; FCFP; (250)542-3170; Fax. (250)542-0835.

SANDERSON, Brian J G; Hammond Bldg, 407-310 Main St N, Moose Jaw SK S6H 3K1; London (England)'72; MB BS; MRCS; LRCP; DObstRCOG; (306)694-0707; Fax. (306)693-1677.

SANDERSON, Francis L; Saint John Reg Hosp, PO Box 2100 Stn Main 400 University Ave, Saint John NB E2L 4L2; McM'81; FRCSC; ObstGyn (Maternal Fetal Medicine). Staff, Saint John Regional Hospital; Asst Prof, Dalhousie University; (506)648-6822; Fax. (506)652-4720; murmi@reg2.health.nb.ca.

SANDERSON, Kirsty J; 278 4th Ave NE, Moose Jaw SK S6H 0C6; (Other Foreign)'94; (306)694-1717; Fax. (306)693-0575.

SANDERSON, Susan R; Saint John Reg Hosp, PO Box 2100 Stn Main 400 University Ave, Saint John NB E2L 4L2; Tor'82; FRCPC; Peds (Pediatric Endocrinology); Endocrin&Metab. Staff, Saint John Regional Hospital; (506)648-6814; Fax. (506)648-6573.

SANDERSON-GUY, Catherine L; Nepean Med Centre, 409-1 Centrepointe Dr, Nepean ON K2G 6E2; McM'83; Staff, Queensway Carleton Hospital; (613)228-8860; Fax. (613)228-9831.

SANDHA, Gurpal S; Zeidler Ledcor Centre, 130 University Campus NW, Edmonton AB T6G 2X8; Punjab (India)'88; MB BS; DABIM; FRCPC; IntMed (Endoscopic Ultrasound); Gastroent. Asst Prof Med, University of Alberta; Langs: Punjabi; Hindi; (780)492-8170; Fax. (780)492-1699; gurpal.sandha@ualberta.ca.

SANDHAM, J Dean; Brodie Centre, 260-727 McDermot Ave, Winnipeg MB R3E 3P5; Alb'67; FRCPC; IntMed (Critical Care Medicine); Respir. Aj Prof, University of Calgary; Dean, University of Manitoba; (204)789-3485; Fax. (204)789-3928.

SANDHAR, Ajit; 120-7404 King George Blvd, Surrey BC V3W 0L4; CCFP; (604)594-7711

SANDHU, Amarpreet S; Daily Care Med & Walk-In Clini, 497 Laurier Ave, Milton ON L9T 3K8; Guru Nanak Dev University (India)'97; CCFP; (905)878-2700; Fax. (905)878-4050.

SANDHU, Amonpreet K; Alberta Children's Hosp, 2888 Shaganappi Trail NW, Calgary AB T3B 6A8; Man'00; FRCPC; Peds. Staff, Alberta Children's Hospital; Langs: Punjabi; (403)955-2953; Fax. (403)955-3055.

SANDHU, Charanjit S; 121-940 Jane St, Vaughan ON L6A 4H7; Tor'04; FRCPC; OccupMed. (905)303-1080

SANDHU, Dalip S; Panorama Med Clinic, 6-6828 128 St, Surrey BC V3W 4C9; Manchester (England)'77; MB ChB; DRCOG; MRCP; MRCGPract; Langs: Punjabi; (604)590-5756; Fax. (604)590-5728.

SANDHU, Gary G; North Delta Med Clinic, 8919 120 St, Delta BC V4C 6R6; UBC'97; BSc; Langs: Punjabi; (604)598-0710; garygsandhu@gmail.com.

SANDHU, Guninder B S; 1723 Kipling Ave, Etobicoke ON M9R 2Y8; (India)'06.

SANDHU, Harmanjit S; 1-1101 Rutherford Rd, Thornhill ON L4J 0E2; Tor'03; CCFP; (905)763-0674; Fax. (905)763-3918.

SANDHU, Harminder B S; Royal Alexandra Hosp, 10240 Kingsway NW, Edmonton AB T5H 3V9; Dal'94; FRCPC; Anes. Staff, Covenant Health - Misericordia Community Hospital; Staff, Royal Alexandra Hospital; Asst Prof, University of Alberta; (780)735-4010

SANDHU, Indermohan; Grey Bruce HS-Owen Sound, PO Box 1800 Stn Main 1800 8th St E, Owen Sound ON N4K 6M9; Dayanand Medical College (India)'98; Staff, Grey Bruce Health Services - Owen Sound; (519)376-2121

SANDHU, Irwindeep; Clinial Sciences Bldg, 4 112-11350 83 Ave NW, Edmonton AB T6G 2G3; Alb'04; FRCPC; IntMed; Hem. Staff, University of Alberta Hospital; (780)407-1993

SANDHU, Janmeet; 3300 Rutherford Rd, Concord ON L4K 5Z2; Sardar Patel Medical College (India)'04.

SANDHU, Jasbir K; Sandalwood Med Centre, 13-2945 Sandalwood Pky E, Brampton ON L6R 3J6; Ravishankar (India)'73; Langs: Hindi; Punjabi; (905)799-7717; Fax. (905)791-2755.

SANDHU, Jatinder S; 201-7110 120 St, Surrey BC V3W 3M8; Punjab (India)'87; MB BS; FRCPC; Psy. Langs: Punjabi; Hindi; (604)572-0195

SANDHU, Karen A P; Orangeville Family Med Centre, M1-32 First St, Orangeville ON L9W 2E1; Qns'06; CCFP; (519)938-8000; Fax. (519)938-8080.

SANDHU, Manbir S; Eagle Ridge Hosp & HCC, 475 Guildford Way, New Westminster BC V3H 3W9; Dominica (Other Foreign)'05; Staff, Eagle Ridge Hospital & Health Care Centre; Langs: Punjabi; (604)461-2022

SANDHU, Manindar K; Lakeridge Hlth Corp-Oshawa, 1 Hospital Crt, Oshawa ON L1G 2B9; UBC'04; FRCPC; IntMed. Staff, Lakeridge Health - Oshawa Site; Clin Associate, St Michael's Hospital; Toronto General Hospital - UHN; (905)576-8711

SANDHU, Manjot S; Peter Lougheed Centre, 3500 26 Ave NE, Calgary AB T1Y 6J4; Man'02; FRCPC; Anes. Staff, Peter Lougheed Centre; (403)291-8555

SANDHU, Naminder; Alberta Children's Hosp, 2888 Shaganappi Trail NW, Calgary AB T3B 6A8; Cal'07; FRCPC; Peds. Staff, Alberta Children's Hospital; (403)944-7551

SANDHU, Naveen S; 200-101 16th St W, North Vancouver BC V7M 1T3; Dal'07; FRCPC; IntMed. (604)904-0810

SANDHU, Navneet K; 203-520 University Ave W, Waterloo ON N2T 2Z6; J J M Medical College (India)'03; (519)743-3641; Fax. (519)743-1042.

SANDHU, Nimani; B9-1235 Trafalgar Rd, Oakville ON L6H 3P1; Tor'03; CCFP; (905)842-7051

SANDHU, Parampal S; 4-110 Pertosa Dr, Brampton ON L6X 5E9; Guru Nanak (India)'84; CCFP; (905)454-8866; Fax. (905)454-6652.

SANDHU, Parminder K; Sunridge Med Clinic, 9-2681 36 St NE, Calgary AB T1Y 5S3; Punjab (India)'81; CCFP; Langs: Punjabi; Hindi; Urdu; (403)250-3010; Fax. (403)250-3065.

SANDHU, Ravinder S; VIVACARE, 120-6345 120 St, Delta BC V4E 2A6; UBC'76; MB BS; (604)599-9445

SANDHU, Ravinder V; The Credit Valley Hosp, 2200 Eglinton Ave W, Mississauga ON L5M 2N1; Tor'05; FRCPC; Psy. Staff, The Credit Valley Hospital; (905)813-2398; Fax. (905)813-4284.

SANDHU, Roop K; 200-300 Main St N, Brampton ON L6V 4H6; Wes'05; CCFP; (905)451-1806

SANDHU, Roopinder K; University of Alberta Hosp, 2C2-8440 112 St NW, Edmonton AB T6G 2B7; (Dominican Republic)'02; Staff, University of Alberta Hospital; (780)407-2176; Fax. (780)407-6452.

SANDHU, Rupinder K; Guelph Family Health Team, 305-85 Norfolk St, Guelph ON N1H 4J4; Punjab (India)'02; CCFP; (519)836-9440; Fax. (519)836-9530; rsandhu@gbhs.on.ca.

SANDHU, Sabrina; Rockyview Gen Hosp, 7007 14 St SW, Calgary AB T2V 1P9; Cal'04; FRCPC; Anes. Staff, Rockyview General Hospital; (403)943-8720

SANDHU, Sangeeta; St Mary's Hosp Centre, 3830 av Lacombe, Montreal QC H3T 1M5; West Bengal (India)'94; MB BS; MD; FCAP; FASCP; Staff, St Mary's Hospital Centre; (514)345-3511; sangeetasandhu@ssss.gouv.qc.ca.

SANDHU, Sharron; Sunnybrook Hlth Sciences Ctre, 2075 Bayview Ave, Toronto ON M4N 3M5; Belfast (Ireland)'94; Staff, Sunnybrook Health Sciences Centre; (416)480-4580

SANDHU, Sukhbir S; Dauphin Reg Health Centre, 625 3rd St SW, Dauphin MB R7N 1R7; Jiwaji (India)'73; FRCPC; Psy. Psychiatrist, Dauphin Regional Health Centre; Lecturer Family Med, University of Manitoba; Langs: Hindi; Punjabi; (204)638-2103; Fax. (204)638-8622.

SANDHURST, Judith; St Mary's Hosp Centre, 3830 av Lacombe, Montreal QC H3T 1M5; McG'99; CCFP; Staff, St Mary's Hospital Centre; (514)345-3511

SANDINO, Ximena A; Medica One, 2079 Lakeshore Rd, Burlington ON L7R 1E2; Universidad De La Sabana (Colombia)'03; CCFP; (905)333-0911

SANDLAND, Helen; Cumberland Health Authority, 34 Prince Arthur St, Amherst NS B4H 1V6; Mem'84; ObstGyn. (902)661-1090; Fax. (902)667-1125.

SANDLER, Alan N; Joseph Brant Mem Hosp, 1230 North Shore Blvd E, Burlington ON L7S 1W7; Birmingham (England)'71; MB ChB; FRCPC; Anes. Staff, Joseph Brant Memorial Hospital; (905)336-4136

SANDLER, Jack T; 117-89 Humber College Blvd, Etobicoke ON M9V 4B8; Cape Town (South Africa)'71; MB ChB; FRCSC; GenSurg (Thoracic Surgery). Ac Staff, William Osler Health System - Etobicoke General Hospital; (416)741-8895; Fax. (416)741-7332.

SANDLER, Samantha D; LMC Diabetes & Endo Centre, 107-1929 Bayview Ave, East York ON M4G 3E8; Tor'93; FRCPC; IntMed (Endocrinology); Endocrin&Metab. Staff, LMC Diabetes & Endocrinology Centres-Bayview; Staff, LMC Diabetes & Endocrinology Centres-Eglinton; (416)654-2929; Fax. (416)645-2930.

SANDOR, Catherine C; 2-210 Lorraine Ave, Kitchener ON N2B 3T4; Tor'85; Court Staff, Grand River Hospital - Kitchener/Waterloo Health Centre; Court Staff, St Mary's General Hospital; (519)570-1223; Fax. (519)570-9367.

SANDOR, George G S; Children's & Women's HC of BC, 1F27-4480 Oak St, Vancouver BC V6H 3V4; Edinburgh (Scotland)'68; FRCP(Ed); FACC; FRCPC; Peds; PedCardiol. Hd Echocardiography Lab, BC Children's Hospital; Consultant, Vancouver General Hospital - Centennial Pavillion; Prof, University of British Columbia; (604)875-2295; Fax. (604)875-3463; gsandor@cw.bc.ca.

SANDOR, George K B; The Hosp for Sick Children, 555 University Ave, Toronto ON M5G 1X8; Tor'86; FRCDC; DDS; PlasSurg (Cranio Facial Surgery). Coord Oral & Maxillofacial Surg, The Hospital For Sick Children; Staff, Holland Bloorview Kids Rehabilitation Hospital; A-Head, Toronto General Hospital - UHN; Assoc Prof, University of Toronto; Langs: Hungarian; (416)813-1500; gsandor@sickkids.on.ca.

SANDOR, Paul; 3W 400-399 Bathurst St, Toronto ON M5T 2S8; Tor'76; BASc; FRCPC; Psy (Neurology & Psychiatry). Dir, Toronto Western Hospital - University Health Network; Prof Psy, University of Toronto; Langs: Hungarian; Czech; Slovak; (416)603-5794; Fax. (416)603-5182; paul.sandor@uhn.on.ca.

SANDOR, Zsuzsanna S; C-1500 Royal York Rd, Etobicoke ON M9P 3B6; Budapest (Hungary)'79; BA; FRCPC; Psy (Fibromyalgia). Langs: Hungarian; (416)249-6677

SANDOUK, Alain J S; Centre Med Pierrefonds, 12774 boul Gouin O, Pierrefonds QC H8Z 1W5; Montpellier (France)'74; CCFP; FCFP; (514)684-8460 x248

SANDOZ, Jacqueline S; The Ottawa Hosp-Gen Campus, 501 Smyth Rd, Ottawa ON K1H 8L6; Tor'06; FRCPC; IntMed; Respir. Staff, The Ottawa Hospital - General Campus; (613)722-7000

SANDRE, Roger M; 41 Ramsey Lake Rd, Sudbury ON P3E 5J1; McM'89; FRCPC; IntMed; InfectDis. Staff, Health Sciences North-Laurentian Site; (705)523-7074

SANDRIK, Hana; Haugen Medical Group, 23C-3300 Smith Dr, Armstrong BC V0E 1B0; (Other Foreign)'09; CCFP; (250)546-8115

SANDRIN, Franco; Access Med Clinic, 200-17001 Rte Trans-Canada, Kirkland QC H9H 5J1; McG'89; MDCM; MSc; FACC; FRCPC; IntMed (Echocardiography); Cardiol. Langs: Italian; French; (514)694-3940; Fax. (514)694-4646.

SANDS, Alex; St Michael's Hosp, 30 Bond St, Toronto ON M5B 1W8; Tor'95; FRCPC; IntMed; Nephrol. Staff, St Michael's Hospital; (416)360-4000

SANDSTROM, Jonas L; Monashee Med Clinic, PO Box 700 2067 Columbia Ave, Rossland BC V0G 1Y0; Wes'95; CCFP; Langs: Swedish; (250)362-9040; Fax. (250)362-9032.

SANDWITH, Sara A M; 333 Hunt Rd PO Box 3064, Courtenay BC V9N 5N3; McM'09; CCFP; (250)339-2242

SANFACON, Cathie; UMF du Grand Littoral, 100-1205 boul de la Rive S, Levis QC G6W 0J4; Mon'05; CCFP; Physician, UMF de Levis; Clin Conférencier, Université Laval; Langs: Bilingual(French/English); (418)380-8597; Fax. (418)380-8596.

SANFACON, Lorraine; CSSS de la Vallée de l'Or, 725 6e rue, Val-d'Or QC J9P 3Y1; Laval'10; CCFP; Staff, Centre Hospitalier de Val d'Or; (819)825-5858

SANFACON, Martin; CSSS Drummond-Hop Sainte-Croix, 570 rue Heriot, Drummondville QC J2B 1C1; Laval'89; IntMed (Cardiology). Staff, Hôpital Sainte-croix; (819)478-6464; Fax. (819)472-3105.

SANFACON, Valerie; CSSS de Sept-Iles, 45 rue du Pere-Divet, Sept-Iles QC G4R 3N7; McG'07; MDCM; FRCPC; Anes. Staff, Centre Hospitalier Regional de Sept-Iles; (418)962-9761

SANFILIPPO, Anthony J; Kingston Gen Hosp, 76 Stuart St, Kingston ON K7L 2V7; Qns'81; FRCPC; IntMed; Cardiol. Staff, Hotel-Dieu Hospital; Staff, Kingston General Hospital; (613)549-6666 x3225; Fax. (613)548-1387.

SANG, Ian T M; Medical Centre, 205-1939 Kennedy Rd, Scarborough ON M1P 2L9; Edinburgh (Scotland)'75; (416)335-8100; Fax. (416)335-6221.

SANG, Richard T M; Shouldice Hosp, 7750 Bayview Ave, Thornhill ON L3T 4A3; Edinburgh (Scotland)'70; BSc; MB ChB; Staff Surg, Shouldice Hospital; (905)889-1125; Fax. (905)889-4216.

SANGANI, Hemalata J B; Clinique Med Victoria, 201-277 boul Churchill, Greenfield Park QC J4V 2M8; Bombay (India)'67; Langs: Hindi; Marathi; Gujarati; French; (450)465-4980

SANGANI, Mahendra B S; Clinique Med Victoria, 201-277 boul Churchill, Greenfield Park QC J4V 2M8; Bombay (India)'68; Staff, Hopital Charles LeMoyne; Langs: Gujarati; Swahili; French; Hindi; (450)465-4980

SANGARALINGHAM, Sinnadurai S; Glazier Med Centre, 11 Gibb St, Oshawa ON L1H 2J9; London (England)'64; LRCPSI(London); MB BS; DABPed; FRCPC; IntMed (Cardiology). Court Staff, Lakeridge Health - Oshawa Site; Court Staff, Lakeridge Health - Whitby Site; Langs: Tamil; (905)579-1212 x206; Fax. (905)579-2021.

SANGERS, Caroline A; U Cosmetic Inc, 1324 Princess St, Kingston ON K7M 3E2; Ott'96; CCFP; Staff, Perth & Smiths Falls District Hospital - Smiths Falls Site; (613)536-5277

SANGHA, Gurinder S; Children's Hosp of Western Ont, E1 105-800 Commissioners Rd E, London ON N6C 2V5; Tor'04; FRCPC; Peds; PedEmergMed. Staff, Children's Hospital of Western Ontario; (519)685-8500

SANGHA, Harpreet S; Toronto Rehab Hillcrest Centre, 47 Austin Terrace, Toronto ON M5R 1Y8; Wes'05; FRCPC; PhysMed&Rehab. Staff, Parkwood Hospital - St Joseph's Health Care; (519)685-4000

SANGHA, Randeep; Cross Cancer Institute, 11560 University Ave NW, Edmonton AB T6G 1Z2; Alb'02; FRCPC; IntMed (Lung Cancer); MedOncol. Staff, Cross Cancer Institute; (780)432-8757; Fax. (780)432-8888.

SANGHA, Romaine; 457-280 Nelson St, Vancouver BC V6B 2E2; Ross University (Dominican Republic)'06; CCFP.

SANGHE, Parminder S; 13719 72 Ave, Surrey BC V3W 2P2; UBC'94; CCFP; Langs: Punjabi; (604)572-5551; Fax. (604)572-9956.

SANGHE, Satinder K; 13719 72 Ave, Surrey BC V3W 2P2; UBC'98; CCFP; Langs: Punjabi; (604)572-5551; Fax. (604)572-9956.

SANGHERA, Baldev S; Primecare Med Centre, 202-7315 Edmonds St, Burnaby BC V3N 1A7; UBC'95; CCFP; Staff, Royal Columbian Hospital; Clin Instructor Family Pract, University of British Columbia; Langs: Punjabi; Hindi; (604)526-2401; Fax. (604)526-1108.

SANGHERA, Gurinder P; 1 001-60 Murray St, Toronto ON M5T 3L9; Alb'02; FRCSC; Ophth. Langs: Punjabi; Hindi; Urdu; (416)586-4800; Fax. (416)586-5915.

SANGOUL, Firooz; Hop Jean-Talon, 1385 rue Jean-Talon E, Montreal QC H2E 1S6; Tehran (Iran)'65; CSPQ; Anes (P.Q.). Staff, CSSS du Coeur de l'Isle Hôpital Jean-Talon; (514)495-6767

SANGSTER, Donald E F; Orillia Soldiers' Mem Hosp, 170 Colborne St W, Orillia ON L3V 2Z3; CCFP; Staff, Orillia Soldiers' Memorial Hospital; (705)325-2201

SANGSTER, Joan E; Surrey Mem Hosp, 13750 96 Ave, Surrey BC V3V 1Z2; Qns'97; CCFP; Staff, Surrey Memorial Hospital; (604)581-2211

SANGSTER, John F; Thames Valley FHT-Byron Fam Me, 1228 Commissioners Rd W, London ON N6K 1C7; Wes'67; MClSc; CCFP; FCFP; Ac Staff Family Med, London Health Sciences Centre - Victoria Campus; Med Dir, Dearness Home LTC; Prof Family Med, University of Western Ontario; (519)472-9670; Fax. (519)657-1766.

SANGSTER, Robert N; Humber River Reg Hosp-Church, 200 Church St, Toronto ON M9N 1N8; Tor'93; FRCPC; DiagRad. Staff Radiol, Humber River Regional Hospital - Church Street Site; (416)243-4158; Fax. (416)243-4162.

SANGSTER-GIBSON, Susan; Maple Key Clinic Family Hlth Team, D2-1036 Princess St, Kingston ON K7L 1H2; Qns'84; (613)546-9721; Fax. (613)546-2799; sangstergibson@maplefht.ca.

SANHUEZA LUCO, Pablo E R F; Developmental Disabilities Ser, 200-1164 Devonshire Ave, North Bay ON P1B 6X7; Santiago (Chile)'67; FRCPC; Psy. Langs: German; Italian; Portuguese; Spanish; (705)494-3180; Fax. (705)494-3189.

SANJAB, Charbel; Ctr Hosp de LaSalle, 8585 Tsse Champlain, LaSalle QC H8P 1C1; Mon'00; CCFP; Fam Med, Centre Hospitalier de LaSalle; (514)362-8000

SANJEEV, Doraiswamy; London HSC-Victoria Campus, PO Box 5010 Stn B 800 Commissioners Rd E, London ON N6A 5W9; Bangalore (India)'79; MB BS; MRCPsy(UK); DPM; FRCPC; Psy. Staff, London Health Sciences Centre - South Street; Staff, London Health Sciences Centre - Victoria Campus; Assoc Prof, University of Western Ontario; (519)667-6863; Fax. (519)667-6564.

SANK, Leslie G; 5500 206 St, Langley BC V3A 8R3; Stellenbosch (South Africa)'83; Staff, Langley Memorial Hospital; (604)534-4214

SANKAR, Tejas; University of Alberta Hosp, 8440 112 St NW, Edmonton AB T6G 2B7; McG'03; FRCSC; Neursurg. Staff, University of Alberta Hospital; (780)407-3567; Fax. (780)407-8203.

SANKARAN, Koravangattu; Royal University Hosp, 103 Hospital Dr, Saskatoon SK S7N 0W8; Kerala (India)'66; MB BS; DABPed; FAAP; FRCPC; Peds (Critical Care Medicine). Dir Neonatal Services & Perinatal Research Lab, Royal University Hospital; Prof, University of Saskatchewan; (306)966-8131; Fax. (306)975-3767; sankaran@duke.usask.ca.

SANKARAN, Rajini; Saskatoon City Hosp, 701 Queen St, Saskatoon SK S7K 0M7; Kerala (India)'66; MB; FRCPC; PhysMed&Rehab (Psychiatry). Staff PhysMed&Rehab, Saskatoon City Hospital; Assoc Prof, University of Saskatchewan; (306)655-8668; Fax. (306)655-8813.

SANKAT, Nadya; West Mississauga Medical, 3050 Argentia Rd, Mississauga ON L5N 8E1; Jamaica (Jamaica)'00; CCFP; (905)785-3627

SANKAT, Olivia M; Cloverdale Walk-In Clinic, 9-225 The East Mall, Etobicoke ON M9B 6J1; Univ of The West Indies (Trinidad & Tobago)'03; (416)231-7743

SANKEY, Christopher L; Satellite Clinic, 21 Strickland Ave, Toronto ON M6K 3E6; McM'90; CCFP; CCFP(E.M.); Staff, Centre for Addiction & Mental Health (CAMH) - College Street Site; Med Dir, First Step Medical Clinic; Lecturer, University of Toronto; (416)537-9346 x5011; Fax. (416)537-2598.

SANMUGASUNDERAM, Suren; 650-1285 Broadway W, Vancouver BC V6H 3X8; Ott'91; BMedSci; FACS; FRCSC; Ophth (Cataract & Refractive). Ac Staff, Providence Health Care - St Paul's Hospital; University of British Columbia; (604)730-8869; Fax. (604)730-0556.

SANNOUFI, Hassan; La Vie Executive Health Centre, 150-525 Legget Dr, Kanata ON K2K 2W2; Kalinin (Russia (Federation))'97; CCFP; CCFP(E.M.); Physician Emergency Room, Queensway Carleton Hospital; Langs: Arabic; Russian; (613)592-0862; Fax. (613)592-4193; info@laviehealth.com.

SANOGO, Karine; CSSS de Saint-Jerome, 290 rue de Montigny, Saint-Jerome QC J7Z 5T3; Mon'03; FRCPC; EmergMed. Staff, Hôtel-Dieu de Saint-Jérôme; (450)431-8200

SANOU, Racine; Hotel-Dieu De Roberval, 450 rue Brassard, Roberval QC G8H 1B9; (Tunisia)'02; DiagRad (P.Q.). Staff, Hotel-Dieu de Roberval; (418)275-0110

SANSFACON, Chantal; Pavillon Albert-Prevost, 6555 boul Gouin O, Montreal QC H4K 1B3; Mon'86; CSPQ; FRCPC; Psy. Staff, Hôpital du Sacre-Coeur de Montréal; (514)338-4246 x4610

SANSOM, Robert M; South Muskoka Mem Hosp, 75 Ann St, Bracebridge ON P1L 2E4; Qns'99; CCFP; Staff, South Muskoka Memorial Hospital - Muskoka Algonquin Healthcare; (705)645-4404; Fax. (705)646-2211.

SANSOME, David E; 1433 Ontario St, Burlington ON L7S 1G5; Dal'70; (905)632-7818; Fax. (905)728-8699.

SANSOUCY, Yanick; CHUS-Hop Fleurimont, 3001 12e av N, Sherbrooke QC J1H 5N4; Sher'02; FRCPC; Anes. Staff, Centre Hospitalier Universitaire de Sherbrooke-Hopital Fleurimont; (819)346-1110

SANSREGRET, Andree; Hôpital Ste-Justine, 3175 ch Cote-Sainte-Catherine, Montreal QC H3T 1C5; McG'98; FRCSC; ObstGyn (Pediatrics). Clinical Asst Prof, Hôpital Ste-Justine; Clinical Asst Prof, Universite de Montreal; Langs: English; (514)345-4706

SANT, Nadia P; The Ottawa Hosp-Gen Campus, 223-501 Smyth Rd, Ottawa ON K1H 8L6; McG'08; IntMed. Fellow, The Ottawa Hospital - General Campus; (613)737-8899

SANT'ANNA, Ana M G D; MUHC-Montreal Children's Hosp, D 562-2300 rue Tupper, Montreal QC H3H 1P3; Rio De Janerio (Brazil)'89; FRCPC; Gastroent. Staff, McGill University Health Centre - Montreal Children's Hospital; (514)412-4400 x24474

SANT'ANNA, Guilherme M; MUHC-Montreal Children's Hosp, C912-2300 rue Tupper, Montreal QC H3H 1P3; Fluminense (Brazil)'88; FRCPC; Peds. Staff, McGill University Health Centre - Montreal Children's Hospital; (514)412-4400

SANTAGATA, Patrizia; CHUM-Hotel-Dieu, 5e-3840 rue Saint-Urbain, Montreal QC H2W 1T8; Mon'96; Cardiol; IntMed. Staff, Centre Hospitalier l'Université de Montréal (CHUM) - Hôtel-Dieu; (514)890-8000

SANTAGATA, Pietro; 12021 15e av, Montreal QC H1E 0A1; Sher'87; Staff, Centre Rouville; (514)881-8814; Fax. (514)881-0907.

SANTANA MENDEZ, Sergio; Southern Alberta Forensic Psy, 11333 85 St NW, Calgary AB T3R 1J3; (Spain)'83; MB ChB; Staff Forensic Psy, Alberta Hospital Edmonton; Clin Lecturer, University of Alberta; (403)944-6815; Fax. (403)944-6852.

SANTDASANI, Sanjay K H; Brandon Clinic, 620 Dennis St, Brandon MB R7A 5E7.

SANTERRE, Carole; College des Med du Quebec, 2170 boul Rene-Levesque O, Montreal QC H3H 2T8; Mon'83; Staff, Centre Hospitalier de Verdun; (514)933-4441

SANTERRE, Denis; 304 av St-Jerome CP 596 Succ Bureau-Chef, Matane QC G4W 3P5; Laval'76; (418)562-3330; Fax. (418)566-6773.

SANTERRE, Marsha J; Seymour Med Clinic, 200-1530 7th Ave W, Vancouver BC V6J 1S3; McM'04; CCFP; (604)739-5611; Fax. (604)738-2102.

SANTERRE, Mylène; Hôpital de CSC de Lamèque, 29 rue de l'Hopital, Lameque NB E8T 1C5; Sher'09; CCFP; Staff, Hôpital de CSC de Lamèque; (506)344-2261

SANTERRE, Regine; Groupe Med de Trois-Rivieres, 225-1900 boul des Recollets, Trois-Rivieres QC G8Z 4K4; Laval'75; (819)375-6666; Fax. (819)375-3423.

SANTHAKUMAR, Vadivelu; Centre City Med Clinic, 5560 McAdam Rd, Mississauga ON L4Z 1P1; Jaffna (Sri Lanka)'83; MB BS; CCFP; Staff, Trillium Health Centre - Mississauga; Staff, The Credit Valley Hospital; Langs: Tamil; (905)273-6895

SANTHER, Kathiraveloo; Niagara H System-G Niagara, PO Box 1018 Stn Main 5546 Portage Rd, Niagara Falls ON L2E 6X2; Ceylon (Sri Lanka)'67; FRCPC; Psy. Ac Staff, Niagara Health System - Greater Niagara General Site; Niagara Child Development Centre; Langs: Tamil; (905)358-0171 x3809; Fax. (905)358-4954.

SANTHIRAMOHAN, Ratha; Mackenzie Richmond Hill Hosp, 10 Trench St, Richmond Hill ON L4C 4Z3; Jaffna (India)'99; FRCPC; Neur. Staff, Mackenzie Richmond Hill Hospital; (905)883-1212

SANTIKYAN, Sarkis; CSSS du Nord de Lanaudière, 1000 boul Sainte-Anne, St-Charles-Brromee QC J6E 6J2; Mon'75; ABIM; MedOncol (P.Q.); Hem. Chief Dept of Specialized Med, Centre Hospitalier Régional de Lanaudière; (450)759-8222; Fax. (450)759-7861.

SANTO, William D P; 100-272 Lawrence Ave W, Toronto ON M5M 4M1; Tor'75; CCFP; FCFP; Ac Staff, St Michael's Hospital; Court Staff, Sunnybrook Health Sciences Centre; Asst Prof, University of Toronto; (416)789-5146; Fax. (416)789-5147.

SANTORO, Dino; 850 King St W, Kitchener ON N2G 1E8; Man'02; FRCPC; Psy. (519)749-4300

SANTOS, Claudia; St Michael's Hosp, 4 008-30 Bond St, Toronto ON M5B 1W8; Tor'97; FRCPC; IntMed; Critical Care Medicine. Staff, Humber River Regional Hospital - Finch Avenue Site; Langs: Italian; Spanish; Portuguese; French; (416)864-6060 x3198

SANTOS, Cynthia Batangan; Health Sciences Centre, 820 Sherbrook St, Winnipeg MB R3A 1R9; Manila (Philippines)'89; FRCPC; AnatPath. Staff, Health Sciences Centre; (204)787-1657

SANTOS, Gilda D; Univ Hlth Network-Toronto Gen, 11F-200 Elizabeth St, Toronto ON M5G 2C4; Sergipe (Brazil)'88; FRCPC; AnatPath. Staff, Toronto General Hospital - UHN; (416)340-4902

SANTOSHAM, Kristi L; Peter Lougheed Centre, 3500 26 Ave NE, Calgary AB T1Y 6J4; UBC'03; FRCPC; Anes. Staff, Peter Lougheed Centre; (403)943-5554; Fax. (403)943-4474.

SANTSCHI, Miriam; CHUS-Hop Fleurimont, 3001 12e av N, Sherbrooke QC J1H 5N4; Sher'00; FRCPC; Peds; Critical Care Medicine (P.Q.). Staff, Centre Hospitalier Universitaire de Sherbrooke-Hopital Fleurimont; (819)346-1110

SANZ, Geoffrey; Kelowna Gen Hosp, 2268 Pandosy St, Kelowna BC V1Y 1T2; Alb'06; FRCPC; EmergMed. Staff, Kelowna General Hospital; (250)862-4000

SAONA, Robert R; St Paul's Hosp, 1081 Burrard St, Vancouver BC V6Z 1Y6; UBC'06; CCFP; CCFP(E.M.); Staff, Providence Health Care - St Paul's Hospital; (604)682-2344

SAOUD, Fahimy; Ctr Hosp de Lachine, 650 16e av, Lachine QC H8S 3N5; (Haiti)'96; CCFP; Staff, CSSS de Dorval-Lachine-Lasalle; (514)934-1934

SAPERSON, Karen; St Joseph's Mountain H Serv, PO Box 585 Stn Lcd 1 E116A-100 West 5th St, Hamilton ON L8N 3K7; Cape Town (South Africa)'83; FRCPC; Psy (Seniors Mental Health). Att Staff, St Joseph's Healthcare Hamilton - West 5th Campus; Att Staff St Joseph's Comm Health Centre, St Joseph's Healthcare - Charlton Campus; Asst Prof Psy/Assoc Chair Education Dept of Psychiatry, McMaster University; Langs: Afrikaans; (905)522-1155 x6782; Fax. (905)575-3778.

SAPIJASZKO, Mariusz J A; First Edmonton Place, 950-10665 Jasper Ave NW, Edmonton AB T5J 3S9; Cal'94; FRCPC; Derm (Cosmetic Surgery). Med Dir, Western Canada Dermatology Institute; Clin Prof Derm, University of Alberta; (780)424-4440; Fax. (780)424-8794.

SAPIR, Daniel; 308-435 Reynolds St, Oakville ON L6J 3M5; Leicester (England)'90; MB ChB; FRCPC; IntMed; Nephrol. (905)815-8910; Fax. (905)815-8911; ardsapr@gmail.com.

SAPIR-PICHHADZE, Ruth; 585 University Ave, Toronto ON M5G 2N2; Hadassah Medical School (Israel)'02; FRCPC; IntMed; Nephrol. (416)340-4800

SAPLYS, Ramunas F J; 406-71 King St W, Mississauga ON L5B 4A2; Tor'82; FRCSC; OrthSurg (Sports Medicine). Staff, Trillium Health Centre - Mississauga; Langs: Lithuanian; (905)275-0020; Fax. (905)275-1094.

SAPOSNIK, Gustavo; 931-55 Queen St E, Toronto ON M5C 1R6; Buenos Aires (Argentina)'90; MSc; FAHA; Neur. Staff Neurol, St Michael's Hospital; Asst Prof, University of Toronto; Langs: Spanish; (416)864-5155; Fax. (416)864-5150.

SAPOZHNIKOV, Marina; 5218 50 St PO Box 86, Tofield AB T0B 4J0; (Russia (Federation))'86; Clin Lecturer, University of Alberta; Langs: Hebrew; Russian; (780)662-3319; Fax. (780)662-3394.

SAPP, George A; 117 Peninsula Rd PO Box 335, Chester NS B0J 1J0; Dal'66; Ophth., Dalhousie University; (902)275-3786; Fax. (902)422-4400.

SAPP, Heidi L C; DJ MacKenzie Bldg, 719-5788 University Ave, Halifax NS B3H 1V8; Dal'94; BSc; FRCPC; AnatPath (Gastrointestinal & Liver Pathology). Assoc Prof, Queen Elizabeth II Health Sciences Centre - Victoria General Site; (902)473-3143; Fax. (902)473-1049; heidi.sapp@cdha.nshealth.ca.

SAPP, John; Queen Elizabeth II HSC-Halifax, 2501F-1796 Summer St, Halifax NS B3H 3A7; Dal'94; FRCPC; IntMed (Cardiac Electrophysiology); Cardiol. Staff, Queen Elizabeth II Health Sciences Centre - Halifax Infirmary Site; (902)473-4272; Fax. (902)473-3158.

SAPP, M Michelle; William Osler HC-Brampton, 2100 Bovaird Dr E, Brampton ON L6R 3J7; Dal'94; BSc(Hons.); FRCPC; AnatPath. Staff, William Osler Health System - Brampton Civic Hospital; Staff, Lakeridge Health - Oshawa Site; (905)494-2120

SAPRA, Sheetal; Inst of Cosmetic & Laser Surg, 100-1344 Cornwall Rd, Oakville ON L6J 7W5; UBC'84; FRCPC; Derm (Cosmetic & Laser Surgery). Staff, Halton Healthcare Services Corporation - Oakville Site; Langs: Punjabi; (905)842-2262; Fax. (905)842-3625; info@icls.ca.

SAPSFORD, Gavin R; Anaesthetic Services, 213-2186 Oak Bay Ave, Victoria BC V8R 1G3; Stellenbosch (South Africa)'81; MB ChB; MMed; FRCPC; Anes. Langs: Afrikaans; (250)595-7211

SAQQUR, Maher; University of Alberta Hosp, 2E3-8440 112 St, Edmonton AB T6G 2B7; Damascus (Syria)'94; FRCPC; Neur. Staff, University of Alberta Hospital; (780)407-7574; Fax. (780)407-1325.

SARA, William B; Crowsnest Med Clinic, PO Box 370, Bellevue AB T0K 0C0; Tor'68; Ac Staff, Crowsnest Pass Health Centre; (403)562-8804; Fax. (403)562-2905; william@crowsnestpass.com.

SARABIA, Alicia; The Credit Valley Hosp, 2200 Eglinton Ave W, Mississauga ON L5M 2N1; McM'91; FRCPC; IntMed; InfectDis; MedMicrobiol. Staff, The Credit Valley Hospital; Langs: Spanish; (905)813-1100; Fax. (905)813-4536.

SARABIA, Vivian E; Bellwood Hlth Services Inc, 1020 McNicoll Ave, Scarborough ON M1W 2J6; Tor'98; CCFP; FCFP; (416)495-0926; Fax. (416)495-7943.

SARAF, Rajni; 116 Mitton St N, Sarnia ON N7T 6G4; Delhi (India)'75; FRCOG; MRCOG; FRCSC; ObstGyn (Colposcopy). Staff, Bluewater Health - Norman Site; Langs: Hindi; Urdu; Arabic; (519)344-3063; Fax. (519)337-6667.

SARAI, Didar S; 10209 Bramalea Rd, Brampton ON L6R 0C4; Guru Nanak (India)'80; CCFP; Langs: Hindi; Punjabi; Urdu; (905)791-9970

SARAN, Kalwinder S; BC Women's Hosp & Health Ctre, P1 309-4500 Oak St, Vancouver BC V6H 3N1; UBC'05; FRCPC; Psy. Staff, BC Women's Hospital & Health Centre; (604)875-2345

SARAN, Kanwal D S; Prairie Trails Med Centre, 100-1345 Taylor Ave, Winnipeg MB R3M 3Y9; Man'02; CCFP; (204)475-0088

SARAN, Neil; MUHC-Montreal Children's Hosp, C521-2300 rue Tupper, Montreal QC H3H 1P3; UBC'03; FRCSC; OrthSurg. Staff, McGill University Health Centre - Montreal Children's Hospital; (514)934-1934; nsaran@cw.bc.ca.

SARANCHUK, Jeffery W; Health Sciences Centre, AD 203-820 Sherbrook St, Winnipeg MB R3A 1R9; Man'97; FRCSC; Urol (Urological Oncology). Staff, Health Sciences Centre; (204)774-6511

SARAVANABAVANANTHAN, Savithri; 2951 Walker's Line, Burlington ON L7M 4Y1; Tamil Nadu (India)'94; CCFP; (905)336-3437; Fax. (905)336-9634.

SARAZA, Milagros F; Bramalea Health Centre, 302-18 Kensington Rd, Brampton ON L6T 4S5; Santo Tomas (Philippines)'68; Staff, William Osler Health System - Brampton Civic Hospital; Langs: Tagalog; (905)791-5246

SARBIT, Jay L; Kelowna Respiratory Clinic, 302-3975 Lakeshore Rd, Kelowna BC V1W 1V3; Man'70; FRCPC; IntMed; Respir. Staff, Central Alberta Cancer Centre; (778)477-5805; Fax. (778)477-5808; sarbit@telusplanet.net.

SARBIT, M Danielle; 314-3001 Tutt St, Kelowna BC V1Y 2H4; Alb'01; CCFP; (250)763-0101; Fax. (250)763-0114.

SARCA, Dana; 101-5927 Bathurst St, North York ON M2R 3T5; Bucharest (Romania)'93; CCFP; (416)222-7982; Fax. (416)222-7880.

SARDANA, Tarek M; 18-6469 Jeanne d'Arc Blvd N, Orleans ON K1C 2R1; Ott'91; Staff, St Francis Memorial Hospital; Med Officer Aerospace, Dept of National Defence; Langs: German; French; (613)841-8500; Fax. (613)841-5310; t.sardana@aviationmedintl.com.

SARDANA, Varun; 333 Lakeshore Rd W, Mississauga ON L5H 1G9; (India)'06.

SARDIWALLA, Ismail; Cape Breton Hlthcare Complex, 1482 George St, Sydney NS B1P 1P3; Natal (Other Foreign)'76; Staff, Cape Breton Healthcare Complex; (902)567-6142; Fax. (902)567-3786.

SAREEN, Jitender; Psychealth Centre, PZ 430-771 Bannatyne Ave, Winnipeg MB R3E 3N4; Man'95; FRCPC; Psy.

SAREEN, Sanjay; Health Sciences Centre, GH 611-820 Sherbrook St, Winnipeg MB R3A 1R9; Man'99; BSc; FRCPC; Anes. Staff, Health Sciences Centre; Staff, St Boniface General Hospital; (204)774-8511

SARETSKY, Lori A; BC Cancer Agency-Vancouver CC, 600 10th Ave W, Vancouver BC V5Z 4E6; Sask'86; Staff, BC Cancer Agency Vancouver Centre; (604)877-6000; Fax. (604)877-6137.

SARFRAZ, Jawaria; Rufus Guinchard Hlth Care Ctr, PO Box 40, Port Saunders NL A0K 4H0; (Pakistan)'07; MB BS; Staff, Rufus Guinchard Health Centre; (709)861-3533

SARFRAZ, Saad; Leamington Dist Mem Hosp, 194 Talbot St W, Leamington ON N8H 1N9; Quaid-E-Azam (Egypt)'00; CCFP; Staff, Leamington District Memorial Hospital; (519)322-3033

SARGEANT, John K; Rockyview Gen Hosp, 7007 14 St SW, Calgary AB T2V 1P9; Cal'83; FRCPC; Psy. Staff, Rockyview General Hospital; Clin Assoc Prof, University of Calgary; (403)943-3614; Fax. (403)943-3624.

SARGEANT, Robert J; St Michael's Hosp, 4 140-30 Bond St, Toronto ON M5B 1W8; Tor'00; MSc; BSc; FRCPC; IntMed (Geriatric Medicine). Staff Cardinal Carter Wing, St Michael's Hospital; (416)864-5361; Fax. (416)864-5714; sargeantr@smh.toronto.on.ca.

SARGENT, Kimberley D; PO Box 132, Bragg Creek AB T0L 0K0; Cal'07; CCFP.

SARGENT, Michael A; Children's & Women's HC of BC, 1L72-4480 Oak St, Vancouver BC V6H 3V4; Manchester (England)'80; MB ChB; MRC; FRCR; FRCPC; DiagRad (Pediatric Radiology). Staff, BC Children's Hospital; Clin Assoc Prof, University of British Columbia; (604)875-2131; Fax. (604)875-2367; msargent@cw.bc.ca.

SARGENT, Randall W; PO Box 40111 Rpo Canmore Cross, Canmore AB T1W 3H9; Cal'88; CCFP.

SARGIOUS, Monica M; Maternal Child Clinic, 182-1402 8 Ave NW, Calgary AB T2N 1B9; Cal'94; BSc; CCFP; FCFP; (403)289-4312; Fax. (403)289-4377.

SARGIOUS, Peter; Peter Lougheed Centre, 5016-3500 26 Ave NE, Calgary AB T1Y 6J4; Cal'91; FRCPC; IntMed (Diabetology). Staff/Med Dir The Calgaray Health Prog, Peter Lougheed Centre; Asst Prof, University of Calgary; (403)943-5526; Fax. (403)943-4908.

SARGOLZAEI, Fatemeh; West London Family Health Clin, 200-785 Wonderland Rd S, London ON N6K 1M6; (Iran)'97; CCFP; (519)641-6712; Fax. (519)641-6189.

SARIC, Amra; Nova Scotia Rehab Centre, 211-1341 Summer St, Halifax NS B3H 4K4; Sarajevo (Bosnia-Herzegovina)'80; FRCPC; PhysMed&Rehab. Staff, Nova Scotia Rehabilitation Centre; (902)473-1238

SARIC, Djemso; Medicine in Motion Med Clinic, 5-121 Ilsley Ave, Dartmouth NS B3B 1S4; (Bosnia-Herzegovina)'77; CCFP; Staff, Medicine in Motion Medical Centre; (902)468-2774; Fax. (902)468-1359.

SARID, Esther; North York Med Arts Bldg, 141-1333 Sheppard Ave E, North York ON M2J 1V1; Tel Aviv (Israel)'74; FRCPC; Psy. Consultant, North York General Hospital; Langs: Hebrew; (416)491-4335; Fax. (416)491-1719.

SARIDES, Constantine A; Fonthill Family Med Centre, PO Box 920 2 Pancake Lane, Fonthill ON L0S 1E0; McM'83; (905)892-6333; Fax. (905)892-0394.

SARILE, Dioscoro D C; Don Valley Med Centre, 302-855 Broadview Ave, Toronto ON M4K 3Z1; UP (Philippines)'66; Court Staff, Toronto East General Hospital Inc; Langs: Spanish; German; Italian; Tagalog; (416)461-6383; Fax. (416)461-5985.

SARIN, Christopher; Elbow River Healing Lodge, 1213 4 St SW, Calgary AB T2R 0X7; Man'99; FRCPC; CommunMed;CCFP; Staff, Foothills Medical Centre; (403)955-6600; Fax. (403)955-6601.

SARIN, Michael K; 347 Rumsey Rd, Toronto ON M4G 1R7; Punjab (India)'59; MB BS; MRCP(Ed); MRCP(Lond); FCCP; FRCPC; IntMed. Prog Physician Diabetes Exercise & Healthy Lifestyle Prog, Toronto Rehabilitation Institute - University Centre; Court Staff, St Michael's Hospital; Court Staff, West Park Healthcare Centre; Assoc Prof Med, University of Toronto; Langs: Hindi; Punjabi; Urdu; (416)597-3422 x5249; Fax. (416)425-0301; mikesarin257@hotmail.com.

SARIN, Nitin; 510-330 Highway 7 E, Richmond Hill ON L4B 3P8; Tor'03; FRCPC; IntMed (Hepatology); Gastroent. Staff, North York General Hospital; (905)707-5007; Fax. (905)707-5008.

SARKAR, Ujjaini; 94 Charing Cross St, Brantford ON N3R 2H6; Delhi (India)'97; MB BS; FRCPC; IntMed. Staff, Hamilton Health Sciences Centre - McMaster University Medical Centre; (519)754-3536

SARKARIA, Gagandeep S; St Mary's Gen Hosp, 911 Queens Blvd, Kitchener ON N2M 1B2; University of Debrecen (Hungary)'03; FRCPC; IntMed; GeriatricMed. Staff, St Mary's General Hospital; (519)749-6929

SARKER, Arun; Thompson Gen Hosp, 871 Thompson Dr S, Thompson MB R8N 0C8; (Bangladesh)'88; CCFP; Staff, Thompson General Hospital; (204)677-2381

SARKHOSH, Kourosh; Royal Alexandra Hosp, 511-10240 Kingsway NW, Edmonton AB T5H 3V9; Cal'06; FRCSC; GenSurg. Staff, Royal Alexandra Hospital; (780)735-6733; Fax. (780)735-5565.

SARKISIAN, Anthony; Saint John Reg Hosp, PO Box 2100 Stn Main 400 University Ave, Saint John NB E2L 4L2; Lake Erie (USA)'04; Staff, Saint John Regional Hospital; (506)648-6000

SARLI, Ricardo; Brandon Reg Health Centre, 150 McTavish Ave E, Brandon MB R7A 2B3; Staff, Brandon Regional Health Centre.

SARLIEVE, Philippe P; University of Alberta Hosp, 2A2-8440 112 St NW, Edmonton AB T6G 2B7; Universite De Besancon (Other Foreign)'00; Staff, University of Alberta Hospital; (780)407-1210; Fax. (780)407-1202.

SARMA, Dipanka; St Michael's Hosp, 30 Bond St, Toronto ON M5B 1W8; Gauhati (India)'83; Staff, St Michael's Hospital; (416)864-6060

SARMAH, Anita; Sunnybrook Hlth Sciences Ctre, M3 200-2075 Bayview Ave, Toronto ON M4N 3M5; Manchester (England)'91; FRCPC; Anes. Staff, Sunnybrook Health Sciences Centre; (416)480-6100; Fax. (416)480-4040.

SARNA, Justyna R; Area 3 Movement Disorders, 3350 Hospital Dr NW, Calgary AB T2N 4Z5; Cal'05; FRCPC; Neur. Staff, Foothills Medical Centre; (403)944-4364; Fax. (403)944-4063.

SARNA, Magdalena A; Foothills Med Centre, 1403 29 St NW, Calgary AB T2N 2T9; Cal'07; Nephrol; IntMed. Staff, Foothills Medical Centre; (403)944-1110

SARNAT, Harvey B; Alberta Children's Hosp, 2888 Shaganappi Trail NW, Calgary AB T3B 6A8; Chicago(IL) (USA)'66; AB; AB; FRCPC; Neur (Pediatric Neurology). Staff, Alberta Children's Hospital; Langs: Spanish; (403)955-7131; Fax. (403)955-2922.

SARNE, Andrew J; Beaches Med Clinic, 116 Glen Manor Dr, Toronto ON M4E 2X2; London (England)'61; CCFP; FCFP; Langs: Polish; (416)698-0999

SAROYA, Satinder K; McLaughlin Village Med Clinic, 85 Steeles Ave W, Brampton ON L6Y 0K3; Punjabi Univ (India)'95; CCFP; (905)455-9374

SARPAL, Amrita; Alberta Children's Hosp, 2888 Shaganappi Trail NW, Calgary AB T3B 6A8; Cal'04; FRCPC; Peds; Critical Care Medicine. Staff, Alberta Children's Hospital; (403)955-7211

SARRAF, Morad K; Keele-Ingram Prof Centre, 202-2221 Keele St, North York ON M6M 3Z5; Tehran (Iran)'61; FRCSC; ObstGyn. Ac Staff, Humber River Regional Hospital - Keele Street Site; Langs: Persian; (416)245-5555; Fax. (416)245-9832; morysarraf@hotmail.com.

SARRASIN, Francois; CSSS de Laval, D0191-1755 boul Rene-Laennec, Laval QC H7M 3L9; Mon'84; CSPQ; Psy. Staff, Hopital de la Cite de la santé; (450)668-1010; Fax. (450)975-5090.

SARRAT-VEZINA, Mijouk-Ariane; CSSS de St-Jerome, 290 rue de Montigny, Saint-Jerome QC J7Z 5T3; Mon'03; FRCPC; Psy. Staff, Hôtel-Dieu de Saint-Jérôme; (450)432-2777

SARRAZIN, Anne-Marie; CSSS du Nord de Lanaudière, 1000 boul Sainte-Anne, St-Charles-Brromee QC J6E 6J2; Mon'90; Electroenceph (P.Q.); Neur. Staff, Centre Hospitalier Régional de Lanaudière; (450)759-8222 x2900; Fax. (450)755-0077.

SARRAZIN, Frederic; Thunder Bay Reg HSC, 980 Oliver Rd, Thunder Bay ON P7B 6V4; Mon'05; CCFP; CCFP(E.M.); Staff, Thunder Bay Regional Health Sciences Centre; (807)684-6100; Fax. (807)684-6828; fred_zarrazin@yahoo.ca.

SARRAZIN, Gerald; CSSS du Sud de Lanaudière, 911 montee des Pionniers, Terrebonne QC J6V 2H2; Mon'72; Ac Staff, Centre Hospitalier Pierre le Gardeur; Langs: English; (450)654-7525

SARRAZIN, Janik G; CSSS de la Vallée de l'Or, 725 6e rue, Val-d'Or QC J9P 3Y1; Ott'95; CCFP; Otol. Staff, Centre Hospitalier de Val d'Or; Staff, CSSS du Témiscamingue; Staff, Kirkland & District Hospital; Langs: English; (819)825-6711; Fax. (819)825-7921; janik_sarrazin@ssss.gouv.qc.ca.

SARRAZIN, Janik G; Polyclinique Pierre Le Gardeur, 370-950 Montee des Pionniers, Terrebonne QC J6V 1S8; Sher'98; FRCSC; Otol. Staff, Centre Hospitalier Pierre le Gardeur; (450)654-7525

SARRAZIN, Jean-Francois; Hôpital Laval, 2725 ch Sainte-Foy, Quebec QC G1V 4G5; McG'99; FRCPC; IntMed; Cardiol. Staff, Hôpital Laval; (418)656-8711; Fax. (418)656-4581.

SARRAZIN, Jolaine; Clinique medicale Notre-Dame, 120-504 rue Notre-Dame, Repentigny QC J6A 2T8; Mon'00; (450)585-3232

SARRAZIN, Josee; Sunnybrook Hlth Sciences Ctre, 2075 Bayview Ave, Toronto ON M4N 3M5; Mon'88; FRCPC; DiagRad (Abdominal Imaging). Staff, Sunnybrook Health Sciences Centre; Langs: English; (416)480-6100 x5732; Fax. (416)480-5855.

SARRAZIN-VINCELETTE, Lucie; 9469 rue Lajeunesse, Montreal QC H2M 1S5; Mon'70; Ac Staff Family Med, Centre Hospitalier l'Université De Montréal (CHUM) - Hôpital Saint-luc; Clinical Asst Prof Family Med, Universite de Montreal; (514)381-7192; Fax. (514)387-4793.

SARRIA, Ricardo; 5706 19A Ave NW, Edmonton AB T6L 1L8; Philippines (Philippines)'79; Clin Associate Hospitalist, Royal Alexandra Hospital; Fam Med, Capital Care - Norwood; (780)450-1919; Fax. (780)450-1927.

SARROUGE, Tania; Ctr Hosp Rouyn-Noranda, 4 9e rue, Rouyn-Noranda QC J9X 2B2; Staff, Centre Hospitalier Rouyn-Noranda; (819)762-0995

SARTEKIN, S Kemal; Prairie Med Centre, 5-1449 Prairie Ave, Port Coquitlam BC V3B 1S9; Istanbul (Turkey)'87; CCFP; Teach Staff Family Med, Royal Columbian Hospital; Staff, Eagle Ridge Hospital & Health Care Centre; University of British Columbia; Langs: Turkish; French; (604)944-8421; Fax. (604)944-8425.

SARTELET, Herve; Hôpital Ste-Justine, 3175 ch Cote-Sainte-Catherine, Montreal QC H3T 1C5; Grenoble (Russia (Federation))'99; CSPQ; AnatPath (P.Q.). Staff, Hôpital Ste-Justine; (514)345-9649

SARTI, Aimee J; The Ottawa Hosp-Gen Campus, 1562A-501 Smyth Rd, Ottawa ON K1H 8L6; Ott'06; IntMed. Staff, The Ottawa Hospital - General Campus; (613)737-8701; Fax. (613)739-6695.

SARTOR, Jason R; Abbotsford Reg Hosp & Cancer C, 32900 Marshall Rd, Abbotsford BC V2S 0C2; Cal'05; CCFP; CCFP(E.M.); Staff, Abbotsford Regional Hospital & Cancer Centre; (604)851-4756; jason.sartor@spchc.hnet.bc.ca.

SARUK, Cynthia M; 220-1560 Yonge St, Toronto ON M4T 2S9; Alb'78; DABPN; FRCPC; Psy. Member, Toronto Psychoanalytic Society; Member, Canadian Psychoanalytic Society; (416)929-9091; Fax. (416)929-9129; cmsaruk@rogers.com.

SARUP, Brij M; 102-1408 Ernest Ave, London ON N6E 3B2; Punjab (India)'61; Langs: Hindi; Punjabi; Urdu; (519)681-6234; Fax. (519)681-9429.

SARY, Gamil; CLSC Hochelaga-Maisonneuve, 4201 rue Ontario E, Montreal QC H1V 1K2; Louvain (Belgium)'74; LMCC; (514)253-2181

SAS, Sandra L; 6 Matheson St S, Kenora ON P9N 1T5; Tor'91; CCFP; FCFP; Staff, Lake of the Woods District Hospital; (807)468-5749; Fax. (807)468-3363; ssas@lwdh.on.ca.

SAS, Silvia E M; 100-350 Palladium Dr, Kanata ON K2V 1A8; Ott'88; Langs: Spanish; (613)592-1707; Fax. (613)592-9799.

SASAKI, Sharon E; PO Box 580, Erin ON N0B 1T0; Tor'87; BSc; MSc(Neurophysiol.); Staff Family Pract, Guelph General Hospital; (519)833-2946; Fax. (519)833-0640.

SASAL, Joanna T; St Joseph's Health Centre, SSW 332-30 The Queensway, Toronto ON M6R 1B5; Warsaw (Poland)'86; FRCPC; IntMed; Nephrol. Staff, St Joseph's Health Centre; Langs: Polish; (416)530-6227; Fax. (416)530-6233.

SASAN, Amritpal S; William Osler HC-Brampton, 2100 Bovaird Dr E, Brampton ON L6R 3J7; Punjabi (Pakistan)'92; Staff, William Osler Health System - Brampton Civic Hospital; (905)494-2120

SASANI, Najat; Health Park, 403B-45 Weatherbee Rd, Sydney NS B1M 0A1; University of Sana'a (Yemen)'96; MB BS; Peds. (902)270-8011; Fax. (902)270-8012.

SASBRINK-HARKEMA, Ashley; Packham Avenue Med Clinic, 104-335 Packham Ave, Saskatoon SK S7N 4S1; Sask'07; CCFP; CCFP(E.M.); (306)651-7091; Fax. (306)651-7092.

SASLOVE, David W; Markham Stouffville Urgent Car, 100-110 Copper Creek Dr, Markham ON L6B 0P9; Tor'75; MCFP(EM); Att Staff Outdoor, St Michael's Hospital; Ac Staff Emerg Med, Mackenzie Richmond Hill Hospital; Court Staff, Toronto Western Hospital - University Health Network; Instructor Surg, University of Toronto; Langs: German; French; (905)472-8911

SASMAL, Pulin B; Heritage Village Medicentre, 2041 111 St NW, Edmonton AB T6J 4V9; Calcutta (India)'64; MB BS; FRCPC; IntMed. (780)438-2306; Fax. (780)461-2632.

SASSE, Sara G; 3050G Portage Ave, Winnipeg MB R3K 0Y1.

SASSEVILLE, Denis; MUHC-Royal Victoria Hosp, A4 17-687 av des Pins O, Montreal QC H3A 1A1; Laval'72; DABD; CSPQ; FRCPC; Derm (Contact Dermatitis). Staff Derm, McGill University Health Centre - Royal Victoria Hospital; assoc Prof, McGill University; Langs: Bilingual(French/English); (514)934-1934 x34648; Fax. (514)843-1570; denis.sasseville@mcgill.ca.

SASSEVILLE, Elise; Clinique Med du Quartier-Latin, 905 boul Rene-Levesque E, Montreal QC H2L 5B1; Mon'97; CCFP; (514)285-5500; Fax. (514)285-2226; sasseville@videotron.ca.

SASSEVILLE, Francine; Clinique Pierre-Boucher, 1615 boul Jacques-Cartier, Longueuil QC J4M 2X1; Mon'88; Langs: English; (450)468-6223

SASSEVILLE, J A Marc; Hop Louis-H Lafontaine, 7401 rue Hochelaga, Montreal QC H1N 3M5; Mon'82; CSPQ; Psy (Emergency Psychiatry). assoc Staff, Centre Hospitalier Regional de Sept-Iles; Chef Emerg Services, Hopital Louis-H Lafontaine; Pres, CMDP; Prof, Universite de Montreal; (514)251-4050; Fax. (514)251-2498; msassevi@ssss.gouv.qc.ca.

SASSEVILLE, Martin; CRSSS Baie-James-Sante Isle-D, CP 790 130 boul Matagami, Matagami QC J0Y 2A0; Mon'92; Staff, Centre de Sante Isle-Dieu Matagami; Langs: Bilingual(French/English); (819)739-2515; Fax. (819)739-6059.

SASSEVILLE, Nicole D; Hotel-Dieu de Levis, 143 rue Wolfe, Levis QC G6V 3Z1; Laval'85; FRCSC; GenSurg. Staff, Hôtel-Dieu de Lévis; (418)835-7121

SASSEVILLE, Rachel; Ctre de Sante Comm de l'Estrie, 280 Industrial Blvd, Alexandria ON K0C 1A0; Mon'95; CCFP; FCFP; (613)525-5544; Fax. (613)525-3991.

SASSEVILLE, Richard; Clinique Med de Mistassini, 148 boul Saint-Michel, Dolbeau-Mistassini QC G8L 5J8; Laval'79; LMCC; (418)276-3161; Fax. (418)276-4581.

SASSI, Roberto B; St Joseph's Healthcare, PO Box 585 Stn Lcd 1 100 West 5th St, Hamilton ON L8N 3K7; Staff, St Joseph's Healthcare - Charlton Campus; Staff, St Joseph's Healthcare Hamilton - West 5th Campus; (905)522-1155

SASSON, Abraham; Bathurst Med Centre, 208-7117 Bathurst St, Thornhill ON L4J 2J6; Tor'76; Langs: Hebrew; Italian; Arabic; (905)709-4259; Fax. (905)709-2898.

SASSON, Zion S; Mount Sinai Hosp, 1602-600 University Ave, Toronto ON M5G 1X5; Tor'79; FRCPC; IntMed; Cardiol. Staff Cardiol, Mount Sinai Hospital; Staff, Toronto General Hospital - UHN; Assoc Prof, University of Toronto; (416)586-8472; Fax. (416)586-4693.

SASTRY, Sunita G; Univ Hlth Network-Toronto Western Hosp, MCL2 405-399 Bathurst St, Toronto ON M5T 2S8; Bombay (India)'91; MB BS; FRCPC; Anes. Staff, Toronto Western Hospital - University Health Network; (416)603-5118; Fax. (416)603-6494.

SATAKE, Ken; 400-2609 Westview Dr, North Vancouver BC V7N 4M2; UBC'98; BSc; CCFP; (604)980-0012; kensatake@yahoo.com.

SATAR, Abdul M A; Two Hills Med Clinic, PO Box 690 4716 50 Ave, Two Hills AB T0B 4K0; (South Africa)'99; Physician, Two Hills Medical Clinic; (780)657-3337; Fax. (780)657-3382.

SATEI, Vali; East York Town Centre, 27E-45 Overlea Blvd, Toronto ON M4H 1C3; St Lucia (Dominican Republic)'95; CCFP; (416)696-9836

SATENSTEIN, Gary H; Wakefield Med Centre, PO Box 400 777 Riverside Dr, Wakefield QC J0X 3G0; McG'82; CCFP; FCFP; Dir Prof Services, Centre Hospitalier Gatineau Mémorial; Physician, Wakefield Medical Centre; Lecturer Family Med, McGill University; Langs: French; (819)459-2363; Fax. (819)459-2997.

SATHI, Nandini; Wellpoint Family Practice, 9F-1240 Bay St, Toronto ON M5R 2A7; McG'92; Dip SportMed; CCFP; FCFP; Court Staff, Sunnybrook Health Sciences Centre; Ac Staff, Women's College Hospital; Lecturer Family & Commun Med, University of Toronto; (416)969-3260; Fax. (416)971-7718.

SATHIAMOORTHY, Marutha; Burntwood Comm Hlth Resource C, 50 Selkirk Ave, Thompson MB R8N 0M7; University of Jaffna (Sri Lanka)'04; MB BS; Staff, Thompson General Hospital; Physician, Lynn Lake Hospital; Langs: Tamil; (204)677-1779; Fax. (204)677-1755.

SATHIANATHAN, Christie; St Boniface Gen Hosp, BG 007-409 Tache Ave, Winnipeg MB R2H 2A6; Qns'04; FRCPC; IntMed; Nephrol. Staff, St Boniface General Hospital; (204)233-8563

SATHIASEELAN, Seyon; Markham Stouffville Hosp, PO Box 1800 Stn Main 1320B-381 Church St, Markham ON L3P 7P3; Ott'06; CCFP; Staff, Markham Stouffville Hospital; (905)472-7111; Fax. (905)472-7617.

SATHYA, Jinka R; Health Sciences Centre, 300 Prince Philip Dr, St. John's NL A1B 3V6; Bangalore (India)'77; FRCPC; RadOncol. Staff Cancer Care Program, Health Sciences Centre; Langs: Hindi; Kanarese; Telugu; (709)777-6300

SATHYA, Pushpa; Dr Charles A Janeway Child HC, 2J736-300 Prince Philip Dr, St. John's NL A1B 3V6; McM'97; FRCPC; Peds. Staff, Janeway Children's Health & Rehabilitation Centre; Langs: Kanarese; (709)737-6300

SATIN, Richard; SMBD Jewish Gen Hosp, G224 8-3755 ch Cote-Sainte-Cat, Montreal QC H3T 1E2; McG'71; ABR; CSPQ; FRCPC; DiagRad (Interventional Radiology). principale Médecin, Sir Mortimer B Davis Jewish General; assoc Prof, McGill University; Langs: Bilingual(English/French); (514)340-8222; Fax. (514)340-7907; satin@jgh.mcgill.ca.

SATKUNAM, Lalith E; Glenrose Rehab Hosp, 1226-10230 111 Ave NW, Edmonton AB T5G 0B7; Peradeniya (Sri Lanka)'84; MB BS; FRCPC; PhysMed&Rehab (Electromyography). Staff, Glenrose Rehabilitation Hospital; Assoc Prof, University of Alberta; (780)735-8870; Fax. (780)735-6018.

SATKUNAM, Niranjala; Royal Alexandra Hosp, 10240 Kingsway NW, Edmonton AB T5H 3V9; Jaffna (Sri Lanka)'84; MB BS; FRCPC; GenPath (Anatomical Pathology). Clin Assoc Prof, University of Alberta; Langs: Tamil; Sinhalese; (780)735-5388; Fax. (780)735-4715; niranjala.satkunam@albertahealthservices.ca.

SATKUNARATNAM, Abheha; St Michael's Hosp, 30 Bond St, Toronto ON M5B 1W8; Ott'97; FRCSC; ObstGyn (Gynecological Surgery). Staff, St Michael's Hospital; Staff, Women's College Hospital; (416)867-7480; Fax. (416)867-7478.

SATO, Kenneth K; Radiology Consultants Assoc, 120-6707 Elbow Dr SW, Calgary AB T2V 0E3; Man'77; FRCPC; DiagRad. Staff, Calgary Regional Health Authority; (403)777-3004; Fax. (403)777-3008.

SATO, Naomi I; Meadowvale Prof Centre, 320-6855 Meadowvale Town Ctre, Mississauga ON L5N 2Y1; Ott'91; (905)569-2282

SATOK, David A; Rogers Communications Inc, 333 Bloor St E, Toronto ON M4W 1G9; Tor'91; BSc; CCFP; FCFP; Ac Staff, Humber River Regional Hospital - Church Street Site; ac Staff, Mount Sinai Hospital Center; Physician Corporate Health Services, Rogers Communications Inc; Lecturer Community & Family Med, University of Toronto; (416)935-6688; Fax. (416)935-4211.

SATOK, Peter M; 718-123 Edward St, Toronto ON M5G 1E2; Tor'91; Staff, Mount Sinai Hospital; (416)971-7730; Fax. (416)408-2802.

SATTARIAN, Javad; 201-3251 Sheppard Ave E, Scarborough ON M1T 3W5; Tehran (Iran)'76; FRCSC; OrthSurg. Staff, The Scarborough Hospital - Birchmount Campus; Langs: Farsi; (416)491-7700; Fax. (416)491-7885.

SATYA, Suma; Saint John Reg Hosp, PO Box 2100 Stn Main 400 University Ave, Saint John NB E2L 4L2; Sydney (Australia)'02; FRCSC; ObstGyn. Staff, Saint John Regional Hospital; (506)648-6271; Fax. (506)648-6878.

SATYANARAYANA, Bellura S; Vanier Med Centre, 12-325 Vanier Blvd, Bathurst NB E2A 3N1; Mysore (India)'64; MB BS; FACP; FRCPC; IntMed. Staff, Hopital Regional Chaleur; Consultant, Hôpital de l'Enfant-Jésus RHSJ; Consultant, Hôpital de Tracadie-Sheila; (506)546-9648; Fax. (506)546-9648.

SATYANARAYANA, Satyendra; Saint John Reg Hosp, PO Box 2100 Stn Main 400 University Ave, Saint John NB E2L 4L2; Dal'01; FRCPC; Psy. Staff, Saint John Regional Hospital; (506)648-6000

SAUCIER, Claude; GMF Concorde, 300 boul de la Concorde E, Laval QC H7G 2E6; Mon'74; (450)667-5310; Fax. (450)667-5248.

SAUCIER, Danie; Centre de Physiatrie de Quebec, 100-700 boul Lebourgneuf, Quebec QC G2J 1E2; Sher'89; FRCPC; PhysMed&Rehab. Staff Physiatrist, CSSS de la Mitis; (418)622-3371; Fax. (418)622-9004.

SAUCIER, Danielle; Unite de Med Familiale, Y211-2690 ch des Quatre-Bourge, Quebec QC G1V 0B7; Laval'83; CCFP; FCFP; Staff, Hôpital Laval; adj Prof, Université Laval; (418)656-4795; Fax. (418)656-4503.

SAUCIER, Jean-Francois; Hôpital Ste-Justine, 3175 ch Cote Sainte-Catherine, Montreal QC H3T 1C5; Laval'58; CSPQ; FRCPC; Psy (Research). Hon Staff, Hôpital Ste-Justine; Chercheur, Universite de Montreal; Langs: Bilingual(French/English); (514)345-4931 x5703; Fax. (514)345-4635; jean.francois.saucier@umontreal.ca.

SAUCIER, Marie-Claude; Clinique Med Gen Alma, 22 rue Melancon E, Alma QC G8B 6W3; Mon'04; (418)668-2370; Fax. (418)668-0873; marie-claude.saucier@ssss.gouv.qc.ca.

SAUCIER, Maude; Clinique de Med d'Alma, 22 rue Melancon E, Alma QC G8B 6W3; Mon'09; (418)668-2370; Fax. (418)668-0873; maude.saucier@ssss.gouv.qc.ca.

SAUCIUC, Nicoleta D; BC Cancer Ctre-Southern Interi, 399 Royal Ave, Kelowna BC V1Y 5L3; Iasi (Romania)'92; FRCPC; IntMed; MedOncol. Staff, BC Cancer Agency Sindi Ahluwalia Hawkins Centre for the Southern Interior; (250)979-3930; Fax. (250)712-3911.

SAUDER, David A; Ridge Meadows Hosp & Hlth CC, 11666 Laity St, Maple Ridge BC V2X 5A3; UBC'83; CCFP; Staff, Ridge Meadows Hospital & Health Care Centre; (604)667-4755

SAUDER, David J; Saskatoon Ortho & Sports Med, 104-311 Ludlow St, Saskatoon SK S7S 1N6; Sask'00; FRCSC; OrthSurg (Upper Extremity Surgery). Clinical Asst Prof, University of Saskatchewan; (306)955-9800; Fax. (306)955-9801; drdavidsauder@yahoo.ca.

SAUERBREI, Eric E; Kingston Gen Hosp, 76 Stuart St, Kingston ON K7L 2V7; McM'75; FRCPC; DiagRad (Breast Imaging). Dir Diagnostic Ultrasound & Research, Kingston General Hospital; Prof, Queen's University; (613)548-2301; Fax. (613)548-2412; sauerbre@post.queensu.ca.

SAUJANI, Virendra S; 4-3151 Dunmore Rd SE, Medicine Hat AB T1B 2H2; London (England)'79; MB BS; DRCOG; Ac Staff, Medicine Hat Regional Hospital; (403)529-6600; Fax. (403)527-7689.

SAUKS, Toomas P; Owen Sound Med Associates, 2000-1415 1st Ave W, Owen Sound ON N4K 4K8; Tor'72; Court Staff, Grey Bruce Health Services - Owen Sound; Asst Prof Family & Commun Med, University of Toronto; Langs: Estonian; (519)371-8166; Fax. (519)370-4042; tsauks@osfht.ca.

SAUL, Daniel I; The Ottawa Hosp-Civic Campus, 1053 Carling Ave, Ottawa ON K1Y 4E9; Tor'07; FRCPC; Psy. Staff, The Ottawa Hospital - Civic Campus; (613)761-4638

SAUL, David G; 8 Abitibi Ave, North York ON M2M 2V1; Tor'75; Court Staff, The Scarborough Hospital - General Campus; (416)221-3633; Fax. (416)221-5599.

SAUL, Mark E; Wakefield Family Practice Ctre, RR 2 777 ch Riverside, Wakefield QC J0X 3G0; McG'00; CCFP; Staff, Centre Hospitalier Gatineau Mémorial; Langs: Hungarian; Spanish; (819)459-2363

SAUL-DUKE, Beverley; Humboldt Med Clinic, PO Box 220, Humboldt SK S0K 2A0; CCFP; (306)682-2618; Fax. (306)682-4499.

SAULNIER, Catherine; Centre Med Fontainebleau, 102-10 boul des Chateaux, Blainville QC J7B 1Z5; Mon'90; LMCC; Staff, Hopital de la Cite de la santé; (450)419-8811; Fax. (450)419-7758.

SAULNIER, Denis; Clin de Cardiologie de Levis, 600-4975 boul de la Rive-Sud, Levis QC G6V 4Z5; Laval'81; FRCPC; IntMed; Cardiol. Staff, Hôtel-Dieu de Lévis; (418)833-5750; Fax. (418)833-5837.

SAULNIER, Nancy; 201-600 boul Dieppe, Dieppe NB E1A 9J8; Sher'00; CCFP; Clin Asst Oncol, Dr Georges-L-Dumont University Hospital Centre; (506)859-4772

SAULS, Robert J; The Credit Valley Hosp, 2200 Eglinton Ave W, Mississauga ON L5M 2N1; Tor'79; CCFP; CCFP(E.M.); FCFP; Ac Staff, The Credit Valley Hospital; Staff, Carlo Fidani Peel Region Cancer Centre; (905)813-1100 x5125; Fax. (905)813-4024.

SAUMART-DUFOUR, Nicolas; Ctr Hosp Fleury, 2180 rue Fleury E, Montreal QC H2B 1K3; Mon'07; IntMed. Staff, Centre Hospitalier Fleury; (514)384-2000

SAUMET CHILITO, Julio; CHUM-Hop St-Luc, 1058 rue Saint-Denis, Montreal QC H2X 3J4; Univ of the North (South Africa)'02; FRCSC; ObstGyn. Staff, Centre Hospitalier l'Université De Montréal (CHUM) - Hôpital Saint-luc; (519)890-8000

SAUND, Gagandeep K; Finchgate Med Centre, 102-40 Finchgate Blvd, Brampton ON L6T 3J1; Qns'06; FRCPC; Peds. (905)791-6444

SAUNDERS, Anne-Corinne; Alberta Children's Hosp, 2888 Shaganappi Trail NW, Calgary AB T3B 6A8; McM'82; FRCPC; Peds (Palliative Care). Staff Peds Palliative Care, Alberta Children's Hospital; Staff, Foothills Medical Centre; Staff, Peter Lougheed Centre; Teach Staff, University of Calgary; (403)955-5464; Fax. (403)955-5501.

SAUNDERS, Christine E; Primrose Family Med Centre, 35 Primrose Ave, Ottawa ON K1R 0A1; McM'08; CCFP; (613)230-7788

SAUNDERS, Darren D; Canada Place Bldg, 206-107 Shirreff Ave, North Bay ON P1B 7K8; Wes'85; FRCPC; IntMed; Nephrol. Consultant, North Bay Regional Health Centre - Regional Mental Health; (705)495-3495; Fax. (705)474-1148.

SAUNDERS, Derek E; 3461 Cook St, Victoria BC V8X 1B3; Mem'81; Staff, Royal Jubilee Hospital; Staff, Victoria General Hospital; (250)386-6161; Fax. (250)382-0613.

SAUNDERS, Fraser W; 95 King St E, Kingston ON K7L 2Z7; Qns'73; FRCSC; Neursurg. Staff, Kingston General Hospital; Asst Prof, Queen's University; (613)544-1284

SAUNDERS, George H; Parkdale Med Centre, 20 St. Peters Rd, Charlottetown PE C1A 5N4; Dal'73; (902)628-6555

SAUNDERS, James J; 5127 49 St, Rocky-Mtn-House AB T4T 1B8; Cal'83; CCFP; Staff, Rocky Mountain House Health Centre; (403)845-2815; Fax. (403)845-2177; fugacious@shaw.ca.

SAUNDERS, Jane N; Duncan Mental Health, 3088 Gibbins Rd, Duncan BC V9L 1E8; Cape Town (South Africa)'89; MB ChB; MMed; DCH; FCP (SA); PhD; FRCPC; Psy (Geriatric Psychiatry). (250)709-3040; Fax. (250)709-3045.

SAUNDERS, Kathleen B; Complete Medical, 573 Torbay Rd, St. John's NL A1A 5G9; Mem'02; CCFP.

SAUNDERS, Kevin K; Rivergrove Med Clinic, 2-2605 Main St, Winnipeg MB R2V 4W3; Man'84; CCFP; (204)632-0024; Fax. (204)697-2047.

SAUNDERS, Kristopher D; Parkdale Med Centre, 22 St. Peters Rd, Charlottetown PE C1A 5N4; Dal'05; CCFP; (902)367-3650; Fax. (902)367-3651.

SAUNDERS, Linda C; North York Family Health Team, 5179 Yonge St, North York ON M2N 5P5; McM'87; (416)733-0555; Fax. (416)733-0830.

SAUNDERS, Megan A; Women's Hlth in Women's Hands, 500-2 Carlton St, Toronto ON M5B 1J3; Man'99; CCFP; (416)593-7655; Fax. (416)593-5867; megan@whiwh.com.

SAUNDERS, Michael G; 723 King St W, Kitchener ON N2G 1E3; McM'92; FRCSC; GenSurg (Endoscopy). (519)745-2366; Fax. (519)745-9035.

SAUNDERS, Natasha R; The Hosp for Sick Children, 555 University Ave, Toronto ON M5G 1X8; Tor'08; Peds. Staff, The Hospital For Sick Children; (416)813-1500

SAUNDERS, Patrick P R; Metrotown Med Centre, 303-6411 Nelson Ave, Burnaby BC V5H 4H3; McG'84; DAB; FRCSC; Ophth (Cornea/External Disease). Ac Staff, Burnaby Hospital; Consultant, Vancouver General Hospital - Centennial Pavillion; Clinical Asst Prof, University of British Columbia; (604)433-1258; Fax. (604)433-6154.

SAUNDERS, Peter T R; PO Box 158, Fort Qu'Appelle SK S0G 1S0; London (England)'71; LRCP; MRCS; DRCOG; (306)332-4533; Fax. (306)332-4822; dr.psaunders@sasktel.net.

SAUNDERS, Rebecca R; 11526 Jasper Ave NW, Edmonton AB T5K 0M8; Alb'92; CCFP; (780)756-4071

SAUNDERS, Robert C; 203-3825 Sunset St, Burnaby BC V5G 1T4; Dal'75; FRCPC; EmergMed. (604)434-9515; Fax. (604)434-5984.

SAUNDERS, Robin D; West Coast Family Med Clinic, 1300-6660 Sooke Rd, Sooke BC V9Z 0A5; London (England)'74; MB BS; MRC; DCH; DRCOG; Delegate District 1, British Columbia Medical Association; Dir Family Pract & Continuing Med Educ, University of British Columbia; (250)642-4233; Fax. (250)642-6032.

SAUNDERS, Stacey C; Burin Family Practice, PO Box 279 43-45 Main St, Burin NL A0E 1E0; Mem'00; CCFP.

SAUNDERS-REUVERS, Cynthia B; 354 Read St PO Box 550, Merrickville ON K0G 1N0; McM'92; (613)269-3400; Fax. (613)269-4958.

SAUNDERSON, Janet L; 407-235 Danforth Ave, Toronto ON M4K 1N2; McM'84; BSc; FRCPC; Peds (Neonatology). Assoc Staff, Toronto East General Hospital Inc; Assoc Staff, The Hospital For Sick Children; Langs: French; (416)465-7421; Fax. (416)465-6588.

SAUNIER, Dennis E; Gain Med Centre, 1199 Austin Ave, Coquitlam BC V3K 3P4; Cal'82; Staff, Eagle Ridge Hospital & Health Care Centre; (604)939-7345; Fax. (604)939-7781.

SAUNIER, Jeremy G; Polyclinique Medicale Vaudreui, 600 boul Harwood, Vaudreuil-Dorion QC J7V 6A3; UBC'09; CCFP; (450)455-9301

SAUREL, Patrick; 909 boul Saint-Joseph, Drummondville QC J2C 2C4; Mon'85; AB; LMCC; FRCS; FRCSC; Ophth (Medical Retina). Ac Staff, Hôpital Sainte-croix; (819)474-8469; clinique. drsaurel@cgocable.ca.

SAURET, Peter; 203-540 College St, Toronto ON M6G 1A6; McG'85; Langs: Italian; French; Spanish; Portuguese; (416)924-4516

SAURIOL, Diane; Hôpital Ste-Justine, 3175 ch Cote-Sainte-Catherine, Montreal QC H3T 1C5; Mon'84; CSPQ; FRCPC; Psy. Staff, Hôpital Ste-Justine; (514)345-4931 x6109; Fax. (514)345-4679.

SAURIOL, Josee; Hop Charles LeMoyne, 3120 boul Taschereau, Greenfield Park QC J4V 2H1; Mon'95; CSPQ; AnatPath (Genito Urinary Pathology). Staff, Hopital Charles LeMoyne; (450)466-5000; josee_sauriol@hotmail.com.

SAURIOL, Nathalie; Blue Mountains Commun Hlth Ctr, 78 King St E, Thornbury ON N0H 2P0; Qns'96; CCFP; FCFP; Staff, Grey Bruce Health Services - Meaford Site; Langs: French; (519)538-1311; Fax. (519)599-5895.

SAURO, Victor S; 101-115 Bell Farm Road, Barrie ON L4M 5G1; Tor'94; BSc(Hons.); PhD; FRCPC; Peds (Diabetology). Locum Tenens, Royal Victoria Regional Health Centre; Locum Tenens, Hanover & District Hospital; Locum Tenens, South Bruce Grey Health Centre - Walkerton Site; Staff Privil, Grey Bruce Health Services - Owen Sound; Prof Peds, University of Western Ontario; (705)503-2591; Fax. (705)503-2592; saurov@rvh.on.ca.

SAUTHIER, Philippe; CHUM-Notre-Dame, 1560 rue Sherbrooke E, Montreal QC H2L 4M1; Lausanne (Switzerland)'86; DGO; GynOnco (P.Q.) (Obstetrics & Gynecology). Staff, Centre Hospitalier l'Université de Montréal (CHUM) - Hôpital Notre-Dame; Clin Prof, Universite de Montreal; Langs: English; (514)890-8000 x24729; Fax. (514)412-7604; philippe.sauthier@umontreal.ca.

SAUVAGEAU, Anny; 7007 116 St NW, Edmonton AB T6H 5R8; Mon'96; MSc(Neurol); CSPQ; AnatPath; GenPath (P.Q.) (Forensic Pathology). Langs: French; (780)427-4987; anny.sauvageau@gov.ab.ca.

SAUVAGEAU, Chantal; Centre de Sante Publique, 2400 av d'Estimauville, Quebec QC G1E 7G9; Laval'99; CSPQ; MSc; FRCPC; CommunMed. Co-Enquêteur, Dir de Sante Publique de la Capitale-Nationale; Langs: English; (418)666-7000 x368; chantal_sauvageau@ssss.gouv.qc.ca.

SAUVAGEAU, Eric; Hotel-Dieu de Sorel, 400 av de l'Hotel-Dieu, Sorel-Tracy QC J3P 1N5; Mon'04; Staff, Hôtel-Dieu de Sorel; (450)746-6000

SAUVAGEAU, Guy J L; Hop Maisonneuve-Rosemont, 5415 boul de l'Assomption, Montreal QC H1T 2M4; Mon'87; FRCPC; IntMed; Hem. Staff, Hopital Maisonneuve-Rosemont; (514)252-3404

SAUVAGEAU, J Johanne; Hop Charles LeMoyne, 3120 boul Taschereau, Greenfield Park QC J4V 2H1; Sher'01; FRCSC; PlasSurg. Staff, Hopital Charles LeMoyne; (450)466-5000

SAUVAGEAU, Jean-Paul; CSSS de Rivière-de-Loup, 75 rue Saint-Henri, Riviere-Du-Loup QC G5R 2A4; Laval'67; Peds (P.Q.). Chief Dept of Ped, Centre Hospitalier Regional du Grand-Portage; Staff, CLSC des Frontieres; Langs: English; (418)868-1000; Fax. (418)868-3338.

SAUVAGEAU, Jocelyne; CLSC Pont-Rouge, 3 rue du Jardin, Pont-Rouge QC G3H 0A8; Laval'79; (418)873-6062; Fax. (418)873-6064.

SAUVAGEAU, Yolaine; Clinique Med le Norois, 201-641 4e rue O, Amos QC J9T 2S1; Laval'82; CCFP; FCFP; Chef Family Med, CH Hôtel-Dieu d'Amos; Prof, Universite de Montreal; (819)732-3368; Fax. (819)732-3442.

SAUVE, Agathe; Centre Med Roy, 281 rue Roy E, Montreal QC H2W 1M7; Mon'73; (514)499-0986; Fax. (514)499-9419.

SAUVE, Claude; Hop du Sacre-Coeur de Mtl, 5400 boul Gouin O, Montreal QC H4J 1C5; Mon'85; Cardiol; IntMed (Echocardiography). Chief Echocardiograph Lab, Hôpital du Sacre-Coeur de Montréal; Langs: Bilingual(English/French); (514)338-2200; Fax. (514)338-2381; csauve007@videotron.ca.

SAUVE, Frederic; CSSS du Suroît, 150 rue Saint-Thomas, Salaber-de-Valleyf QC J6T 6C1; Mon'04; Staff, Centre Hospitalier Régional du Suroît; (450)371-9925; Fax. (450)377-1372.

SAUVE, Jean-Marc; CSSS de Papineau, 155 rue MacLaren E, Gatineau QC J8L 0C2; Ott'81; CSPQ; FRCPC; Anes. Staff, Hôpital de Papineau; Staff, Hull Hospital; (819)986-4115

SAUVE, Jocelyne; Dir Sante Publique Monteregie, 1255 rue Beauregard, Longueuil QC J4K 2M3; Mon'82; CSPQ; FRCPC; CommunMed. (450)928-6777 x3046

SAUVE, Laura J; Children's & Women's HC of BC, 2D5-4480 Oak St, Vancouver BC V6H 3V4; Cal'00; FRCPC; Peds; InfectDis. Staff, BC Children's Hospital; (604)875-3645

SAUVE, Louise; Dir Sante Publique, 2400 av d'Estimauville, Quebec QC G1E 7G9; Mon'82; MSc(Epidemiol); Staff Public Health, Centre Hospitalier Universitaire de Quebec-CHUL; (418)666-7000; Fax. (418)666-2776.

SAUVE, Louise; Clinique Med Cadillac, 3435 rue Bossuet, Montreal QC H1M 2M1; Mon'89; CCFP; (514)253-1211; Fax. (514)253-5091.

SAUVE, Marie; CSSS de Memphremagog, 50 rue Saint-Patrice E, Magog QC J1X 3X3; Mon'86; FRCSC; GenSurg. Staff, Centre Hospitalier de Chandler; Staff, Centre Hospitalier et CLSC de Memphremagog; Staff, Centre Hospitalier Universitaire de Sherbrooke-Hôpital Hôtel-Dieu; (819)843-3381; mariesauve@videotron.ca.

SAUVE, Marie-Josee; Clinique Med Familiale Clermon, 500-106 boul Notre-Dame, Clermont QC G4A 1G3; Laval'83; Staff, Hôpital de la Malbaie; (418)439-3935; Fax. (418)439-4548.

SAUVE, Marie-Lou; 105-100 boul de Montarville, Boucherville QC J4B 5M4; Mon'07; (450)641-6774; Fax. (450)641-7672.

SAUVE, Michel D; Morrison Centre, 10-9914 Morrison St, Fort McMurray AB T9H 4A4; Ott'83; FACP; FCCP; FRCPC; IntMed; Critical Care Medicine; Gastroent. Langs: Spanish; French; (780)790-9455; Fax. (780)790-9430.

SAUVE, Michel; Clinique Med Havre Sante, 521 boul du Havre, Salaber-de-Valleyf QC J6S 4Z5; Mon'73; (450)371-6444; Fax. (450)371-5315.

SAUVE, Nadine; CHUS-Hop Fleurimont, 3001 12e av N, Sherbrooke QC J1H 5N4; Sher'96; FRCPC; IntMed. Staff, Centre Hospitalier Universitaire de Sherbrooke-Hopital Fleurimont; (819)346-1110 x14949; Fax. (819)820-6406.

SAUVE, Nicolas; Inst de Chir Specialisee de Mt, 112-6100 av du Boise, Montreal QC H3S 2W1; Mon'99; Staff, Hopital de la Cite de la santé; (514)737-6100

SAVA, Cristina; Eastside Health Centre, 688 East River Rd, New Glasgow NS B2H 3S1; CCFP; (902)752-6000; Fax. (902)755-5532.

SAVA, Renata; Pavillon Hayes, 3777 rue Jean-Brillant, Montreal QC H3T 1P2; McG'04; CCFP; (514)345-3511

SAVAGE, Bonita H; Salvation Army Grace Gen Hosp, 300 Booth Dr, Winnipeg MB R3J 3M7; Man'85; FRCPC; Psy. Staff, The Salvation Army Grace Hospital; (204)837-0222; Fax. (204)885-3064.

SAVAGE, D Peter; 8 Third St, Collingwood ON L9Y 1K3; Qns'70; Ac Staff, Collingwood General & Marine Hospital; (705)445-4334; Fax. (705)445-4351.

SAVAGE, Erin C; Canadian Forces Health Servic, 1745 Alta Vista Dr, Ottawa ON K1A 0K6; Dal'00; CCFP; CCFP(E.M.); Physician, Canadian Forces Health Services Centre; (613)945-2126

SAVAGE, Julian; CHUS-Hop Hotel-Dieu, 580 rue Bowen S, Sherbrooke QC J1G 2E8; London (England)'96; Otol (P.Q.) (Otology). Staff, Centre Hospitalier Universitaire de Sherbrooke-Hôpital Hôtel-Dieu; (819)346-1110; Fax. (819)564-5449.

SAVAGE, Kerry J; BC Cancer Agency-Vancouver CC, 600 10th Ave W, Vancouver BC V5Z 4E6; UBC'96; BSc; FRCPC; IntMed; MedOncol. Staff, BC Cancer Agency Vancouver Centre; (604)877-6000

SAVAGE, Luke C; Three Hills Med Clinic, PO Box 1149 779 2 St N, Three Hills AB T0M 2A0; Alb'08; CCFP; Clin Lecturer, University of Calgary; (403)443-5522; Fax. (403)443-5524.

SAVAGE, Marie-Claude; CSSS de la Cote-de-Gaspe, 215 boul de York O, Gaspe QC G4X 2W2; Laval'05; FRCSC; Otol. Staff, Centre Hospitalier de Gaspe; (418)368-3301

SAVAGE, Martha H B; 209-85 Norfolk St, Guelph ON N1H 4J4; Alb'92; FRCPC; Psy (Family Medicine). Staff, Homewood Health Centre; (519)836-1277 x53244

SAVAGE, Paul R G; 7808 Elbow Dr SW, Calgary AB T2V 1K4; Cambridge (England)'73; MB BCh; FRCSC; Ophth (Retina Vitreous Surgery). Ac Staff, Rockyview General Hospital; (403)245-4442; Fax. (403)229-1757.

SAVAGE, Rachel; Hop du Sacre-Coeur de Mtl, 5400 boul Gouin O, Montreal QC H4J 1C5; Mon'90; Staff, Hôpital du Sacre-Coeur de Montréal; (514)338-2050 x2572; Fax. (514)338-2222.

SAVARD, Anne; Clinique Med de la Capitale, 14-4225 4e av O, Quebec QC G1H 6P3; Laval'76; Langs: Bilingual(French/English); (418)628-9921; Fax. (418)628-3203.

SAVARD, Catherine; Clinique Med Mellon, 303-2075 boul Mellon, Jonquiere QC G7S 5Z8; Laval'09; (418)548-1121

SAVARD, Chantal; Clinique Med Deux-Montagnes, 201 9e av, Deux-Montagnes QC J7R 3M1; Sher'83; (450)472-7545

SAVARD, Claude; GMF de Verdun au 55, 23-55 av de l'Eglise, Verdun QC H4G 3E7; Mon'77; Staff, Centre Hospitalier de Verdun; (514)766-8700; Fax. (514)766-8511.

SAVARD, Daniel; CSSS Haut-Richelieu-Rouville, 920 boul du Seminaire N, St-Jean-sur-Richel QC J3A 1B7; Mon'76; FRCPC; Cardiol. Staff, Hôpital du Haut-Richelieu; (450)359-5000 x2222

SAVARD, Gabrielle K; Bowmont Med Clinic, 6535 Bowness Rd NW, Calgary AB T3B 0E8; Cal'98; PhD; CCFP; FCFP; Staff Privil, Foothills Medical Centre; Langs: Spanish; French; Danish; (403)247-9797; Fax. (403)247-0014.

SAVARD, Germain; Clinique Med Chaudiere, 102 18e rue, Saint-Georges QC G5Y 4T9; Laval'88; Staff, Centre Hospitalier Beauce-Etchemin; (418)228-6820; Fax. (418)226-0358.

SAVARD, Gilbert; CSSS de Lac-Saint Jean-Est, CP 1300 Succ Bureau-Chef 300 boul Champlain, Alma QC G8B 5W3; Mon'77; Staff, CSSS de Lac-Saint Jean-Est; (418)669-2000

SAVARD, Gilles; Clinique Med St-Ludger, 48 rue Temiscouata, Riviere-du-Loup QC G5R 2X9; Laval'79; Staff, Centre Hospitalier Regional du Grand-Portage; Langs: Bilingual(French/English); (418)867-8262; Fax. (418)867-3368.

SAVARD, Guylene; MD Health Med Centre, 188 Main St S, Brampton ON L6W 2E2; Mon'85; Langs: Bilingual(French/English); (905)456-7774; Fax. (905)456-1158.

SAVARD, Jean-Francois; Ctr Hosp Affilie-Enfant-Jesus, 1401 18e rue, Quebec QC G1J 1Z4; Laval'98; CSPQ; FRCPC; Anes; Critical Care Medicine (P.Q.). Staff, Centre Hospitalier Affilié Universitaire de Québec - Hôpital De L'Enfant Jésus; (418)649-5807; dsilineg@cha.quebec.qc.ca.

SAVARD, Julie; Centre Med Vaudreuil-Dorion, 600 boul Harwood, Vaudreuil-Dorion QC J7V 6A3; Mon'98; (450)455-9301 x224

SAVARD, Lise; Clinique Sante Camille Michaud, CP 420 2870 rue Lafleche, Saint-Paulin QC J0K 3G0; Laval'82; Staff, CH du Centre-de-la-Mauricie (Ste-Thérèse de Shawinigan); (819)268-2013; lise_savard@ssss.gouv.qc.ca.

SAVARD, Marie-Andree; CLSC de Normandin, 1205 rue Saint-Cyrille, Normandin QC G8M 4K1; Sher'00; MCFP; CCFP; Staff Family Med, Centre Maria-Chapdelaine - CH de Dolbeau-Mistassini; (418)274-1234; Fax. (418)274-6970; docsavard@hotmail.com.

SAVARD, Martin; Unite Med Familiale Maizerets, 2480 ch de la Canardiere, Quebec QC G1J 2G1; Laval'97; CCFP; Staff, Centre Hospitalier Régional Baie-Comeau; (418)661-1413

SAVARD, Martin; Ctr Hosp Affilie-Enfant-Jesus, 1401 18e rue, Quebec QC G1J 1Z4; Laval'01; FRCPC; Neur. Staff, Centre Hospitalier Affilié Universitaire de Québec - Hôpital De L'Enfant Jésus; (418)649-0252

SAVARD, Martine M; Ctr Hosp du Centre la Mauricie, 50 119e rue, Shawinigan-Sud QC G9P 5K1; Sher'94; Staff, Centre Hospitalier du Centre la Mauricie; (819)536-7500

SAVARD, Michael M; Westview Hlth Ctr Stony Plain, 4405 South Park Dr, Stony Plain AB T7Z 2M7; Alb'82; Staff, Westview Health Centre; (780)968-3673; Fax. (780)963-0001.

SAVARD, Michel; Dir Sante Publique des Laurent, 210-1000 rue Labelle, Saint-Jerome QC J7Z 5N6; Mon'76; Staff CommunHealth, Centre Hospitalier Régional du Suroît; (450)432-8735; Fax. (450)436-1761; michel_savard@videotron.ca.

SAVARD, Murray L; Kelowna Gen Hosp, 2268 Pandosy St, Kelowna BC V1Y 1T2; Alb'81; BSc; FRCPC; GenPath. Staff, Kelowna General Hospital; (250)862-4300 x7346; dr.murray.savard@interiorhealth.ca.

SAVARD, Normand; Clin Med Fam Obs d'Mistassini, 2-170 av de l'Eglise, Dolbeau-Mistassini QC G8L 4W6; Laval'79; Ac Staff, Centre Maria-Chapdelaine - CH de Dolbeau-Mistassini; Physician Plant, Produits Forestiers-Abitibi-Bowaters; (418)276-5912; Fax. (418)276-6092.

SAVARD, Pascal; 203-2000 rue Cours le Corbusie, Boisbriand QC J7G 3E8; Laval'84; FAAD; FRCPC; Peds (Pediatric Dermatology); Derm. Ac Staff, Hopital de la Cite de la santé; Langs: French; (450)979-1222; Fax. (450)979-6117.

SAVARD, Patrice; CHUM-Hop St-Luc, 1058 rue Saint-Denis, Montreal QC H2X 3J4; Laval'05; FRCPC; MedMicrobiol; Microbio & Infect Dis (P.Q.). Staff, Centre Hospitalier l'Université De Montréal (CHUM) - Hôpital Saint-luc; (514)890-8000

SAVARD, Patrick; CHUQ-Hosp Univ Laval, 2705 boul Laurier, Quebec QC G1V 4G2; Laval'85; FRCSC; Otol. Staff, Centre Hospitalier Universitaire de Quebec-CHUL; Langs: English; (418)656-4141; Fax. (418)691-5717.

SAVARD, Philippe; CSSS du Lac des Deux Montagnes, 520 bou Arthur-Sauve, Saint-Eustache QC J7R 5B1; Sher'05; FRCSC; GenSurg. Staff, Centre Hospitalier Universitaire de Sherbrooke-Hôpital Hôtel-Dieu; Staff, Hôpital de Saint-Eustache; (450)473-6811; Fax. (450)473-6966.

SAVARD, Pierre; Centre Bois de Boulogne, 505-1575 boul Henri-Bourassa O, Montreal QC H3M 3A9; Laval'91; CSPQ; Psy (Anxiety Disorder). Staff, Hôpital du Sacre-Coeur de Montréal; Universite de Montreal; (514)338-4201; Fax. (514)338-4493.

SAVARD, Pierre; CHUQ-Ctr Hosp Univ Laval, 2705 boul Laurier, Quebec QC G1V 4G2; Laval'77; EmergMed. Staff, Centre Hospitalier Universitaire de Quebec-CHUL; (418)656-4444

SAVARD, Pierre-Alexandre; Ctr Hosp du Centre la Mauricie, 50 119e rue, Shawinigan-Sud QC G9P 5K1; Sher'00; GeriatricMed; IntMed. Staff, Centre Hospitalier du Centre la Mauricie; (819)536-7500

SAVARD, Roger; CSSS de Chicoutimi, CP 5006 succ Racine 305 rue Saint-Vallier, Chicoutimi QC G7H 5H6; Laval'77; FRCPC; MedMicrobiol (Infectious Diseases); Microbio & Infect Dis (P.Q.). Staff, Complexe hospitalier de la Sagamie; (418)541-1000 x2684

SAVARD, Sebastien; CHUQ-Hotel-Dieu de Quebec, 11 Cote du Palais, Quebec QC G1R 2J6; Laval'05; FRCPC; IntMed; Nephrol. Staff, Centre Hospitalier Universitaire de Québec (CHUQ) - Siege Social; (418)525-4444 x15882; Fax. (418)691-5757.

SAVARD, Serge; Savard Serge Phlebologie, 200-550 boul de Mortagne, Boucherville QC J4B 5E4; Mon'78; (450)655-1591; Fax. (450)655-8736.

SAVARD, Sylvie; Centre Med Sainte-Foy, 802 av du Chanoine-Scott, Quebec QC G1V 3N4; Laval'88; Physician, CHSLD St-Raymond; (418)653-4931

SAVARD-COTE, Melanie; GMF Montee de la Baie, RR 22 3942 ch d'Oka, St-Joseph-Du-Lac QC J0N 1M0; Mon'01; CCFP; Staff, Hôpital de Saint-Eustache; Langs: Bilingual(French/English); (450)473-3930; Fax. (450)473-2160.

SAVARD-WOODS, Catherine; UMF Gatineau, 100-500 boul de l'Hopital, Gatineau QC J8V 2P5; Laval'05; (819)966-6380; Fax. (819)966-6175.

SAVARIA, Elyse; Owen Sound Med Centre, 2000-1415 1st Ave W, Owen Sound ON N4K 4K8; Mon'89; LMCC; Ac Staff, Grey Bruce Health Services - Owen Sound; Asst Prof, McMaster University; Langs: French; (519)470-3030; Fax. (519)370-4056.

SAVARIA, Frederick G; Ctr Medi Soleil St-Jean-Sur-Ri, 120-383 boul du Seminaire N, St-Jean-sur-Richel QC J3B 8C5; Sher'92; Staff, Hôpital du Haut-Richelieu; (450)347-7557; Fax. (450)347-3099.

SAVARIA, Jean-Pierre; Clin Med Privee, 206-75 boul des Chateaux, Blainville QC J7B 2A4; Mon'78; (450)434-2009; Fax. (450)433-2010.

SAVASI, Ingrid; Grey Bruce HS-Owen Sound, PO Box 1800 Stn Main 1800 8th St E, Owen Sound ON N4K 6M9; Dal'04; FRCSC; ObstGyn. Staff, Grey Bruce Health Services - Owen Sound; (519)371-8381; Fax. (519)371-8399.

SAVATTERI, Michael; 4279 Hixon St GD, Beamsville ON L0R 1B0; Ott'10; CCFP; (905)563-5315

SAVAYA, Savaya; Dr W H Newhook Comm Hlth Ctre, GD, Whitbourne NL A0B 3K0; Mosul (Other Foreign)'03; MB ChB; Staff, Dr William H Newhook Health Centre; (709)759-2300; savaya@mun.ca.

SAVCHUK, Yuriy; East Van Med Bldg, 201-1750 10th Ave E, Vancouver BC V5N 5K4; Ternopol (Ukraine)'92; CCFP; (604)675-9123; Fax. (604)675-9618.

SAVEDIA-CAYABYAB, Sheila M; 21st Medical Clinic, 502-402 21st St E, Saskatoon SK S7K 0C3; Tor'99; FRCPC; Neur. (306)956-3444

SAVELLI, Gordina E; 730 Concession St, Hamilton ON L8V 1C1; McM'75; BScMed; FRCPC; IntMed (Electromyography); Neur. Consultant Neurol, Hamilton Health Sciences Centre-Juravinski Site; Clinical Asst Prof Med, McMaster University; (905)549-7326; Fax. (905)549-9661.

SAVENKOV, Oleg A; Hamilton HS-McMaster Site, PO Box 2000 Stn Lcd 1 1200 Main St, Hamilton ON L8N 3Z5; Novosibirsk (Russia (Federation))'93; MD; FRCPC; Psy (Child & Adolescent Psychiatry). Staff, Hamilton Health Sciences Centre - McMaster University Medical Centre; Langs: Russian; (905)521-2100

SAVEREUX, Michael; CSSS Haut-Richelieu-Rouville, 920 boul du Seminaire N, St-Jean-Sur-Richel QC J3A 1B7; Sher'94; CSPQ; FRCPC; Psy. Staff, Hôpital du Haut-Richelieu; (450)359-5000 x5450

SAVERIANO, Nellina; 203-631 Queenston Rd, Hamilton ON L8K 6R5; McG'85; BSc; MDCM; DAB; FRCPC; Derm. Chief/Court Staff Derm, Hamilton Health Sciences Centre-Juravinski Site; Ac Staff, St Joseph's Healthcare - Charlton Campus; Asst Prof Clinical, McMaster University; Langs: Italian; French; (905)549-1025; Fax. (905)549-9487.

SAVIC, Mile; 5-150 Sidney St, Belleville ON K8P 5E2; (Serbia)'88; CCFP; Langs: Croatian; Serbian; (613)966-7300; Fax. (613)966-7320; mile_savic@hotmail.com.

SAVILLE, Leyana R; 110-210 Centrum Blvd, Orleans ON K1E 3V7; Ott'07; CCFP; (613)424-8977; Fax. (613)424-9075.

SAVIN, Adrian G; Etobicoke Med Centre, 400 The East Mall, Etobicoke ON M9B 3Z9; Bucarest (Romania)'85; CCFP; Staff, Trillium Health Centre - Mississauga; Langs: Romanian; (416)621-2220; Fax. (416)621-2203; adriansavin@hotmail.com.

SAVITSKY, Trisha A; 600 Riverbend Sq NW, Edmonton AB T6R 2E3; Alb'07; CCFP; (780)434-7234; Fax. (780)988-8903.

SAVLOV, Deena J; The Hosp for Sick Children, 555 University Ave, Toronto ON M5G 1X8; Wes'06; Peds. Staff, The Hospital For Sick Children; (416)813-1500

SAVOIA, Katherine M; Market Mall Prof Bldg, 224A-4935 40 Ave NW, Calgary AB T3A 2N1; Cal'91; CCFP; Langs: Italian; (403)247-2345; Fax. (403)247-6217.

SAVOIE, Anik; 202-185 av Acadie, Dieppe NB E1A 1G6; Sher'04; CCFP; Staff, Dr Georges-L-Dumont University Hospital Centre; Langs: Bilingual(French/English); (506)862-1260; Fax. (506)862-1265.

SAVOIE, Anne-Marie; West Champlain Family Health T, 715 Mackay St, Pembroke ON K8A 0C6; Ott'08; CCFP; (613)735-6750

SAVOIE, Anne-Marie; Hotel-Dieu de Levis, 143 rue Wolfe, Levis QC G6V 3Z1; Laval'96; Staff, Hôtel-Dieu de Lévis; Langs: English; (418)835-7121

SAVOIE, Antonin; Dr Georges-L Dumont Reg Hosp, 330 av Universite, Moncton NB E1C 2Z3; Sher'07; CCFP; Staff, Dr Georges-L-Dumont University Hospital Centre; (506)862-4000

SAVOIE, Isabelle; Hôp Reg Dr Georges-L.-Dumont, 330 av Universite, Moncton NB E1C 2Z3; Mon'89; FRCPC; DiagRad; NuclearMed. Staff, Dr Georges-L-Dumont University Hospital Centre; (506)862-4000

SAVOIE, Janie; Dr Georges-L Dumont Reg Hosp, 330 av Universite, Moncton NB E1C 2Z3; Sher'03; FRCPC; Anes. Staff, Dr Georges-L-Dumont University Hospital Centre; (506)862-4000

SAVOIE, Jean-Pierre; Regie des Rentes du Quebec, 348-2600 boul Laurier, Quebec QC G1V 4T3; Laval'85; (418)657-8709 x4454

SAVOIE, Josee; Hop du Sacre-Coeur de Mtl, 5400 boul Gouin O, Montreal QC H4J 1C5; Mon'88; Staff, Hôpital du Sacre-Coeur de Montréal; (514)338-2050

SAVOIE, Liette; CSSS Les Eskers de l'Abitibi, 622 4e rue O, Amos QC J9T 2S2; Sher'90; FRCPC; Peds. Staff, CH Hôtel-Dieu d'Amos; Langs: English; (819)732-3341; Fax. (819)732-6484; liette_savoie@ssss.gouv.qc.ca.

SAVOIE, Line; CLSC Bordeaux-Cartierville, 11822 av de Bois-De-Boulogne, Montreal QC H3M 2X6; Sher'85; Staff, Hôpital du Sacre-Coeur de Montréal; (514)331-2572; Fax. (514)331-0137.

SAVOIE, Lisa; Hop Charles Lemoyne, 3120 boul Taschereau, Greenfield Park QC J4V 2H1; Sher'99; FRCPC; IntMed; Nephrol. Staff, Hopital Charles LeMoyne; (450)466-5000 x2645

SAVOIE, Louis; CLSC Saint-Marc-Les-Carrieres, 1045 boul Bona-Dussault, St-Mar-des-Carr QC G0A 4B0; Laval'92; LMCC; Langs: English; (418)268-3571; Fax. (418)268-8533.

SAVOIE, Louise; Inst U Geriatrie de Montreal, 4565 ch Queen-Mary, Montreal QC H3W 1W5; Mon'86; Staff, Institut Universitaire de Gériatrie de Montréal; Langs: Bilingual(French/English); (514)340-2800

SAVOIE, Luc; 4290 rue Beaubien E, Montreal QC H1T 1S6; Mon'81; (514)374-6711; Fax. (514)374-2051.

SAVOIE, Marc E; Hôpital régional Chaleur, 1750 Sunset Dr, Bathurst NB E2A 4L7; Laval'01; FRCSC; GenSurg (Bariatric Surgery). Staff, Hopital Regional Chaleur; (506)544-3000

SAVOIE, Marc; 202-404 St. George St, Moncton NB E1C 1X6; Sher'96; FRCSC; Urol. (506)857-9900; Fax. (506)852-9212.

SAVOIE, Marie-France; CSSS de Chicoutimi, 305 av Saint-Vallier, Chicoutimi QC G7H 5H6; Sher'04; CCFP; Staff, Complexe hospitalier de la Sagamie; (418)541-1000

SAVOIE, Mary-Lynn; 681-1403 29 St NW, Calgary AB T2N 2T9; Dal'96; FRCPC; IntMed (Stem Cell Transplantation); Hem. Staff, Tom Baker Cancer Centre; Staff, Foothills Medical Centre; Clinical Asst Prof, University of Calgary; Langs: French; (403)944-1564; lynn.savoie@albertahealthservices.ca.

SAVOIE, Pierre; Radiologie Saint-Sauveur, 70 rue Principale, Saint-Sauveur QC J0R 1R6; Mon'64; CSPQ; DiagRad (P.Q.). (450)227-4000

SAVOIE, Rejean; Dr L Richard Ctre d'Oncologie, 37 rue Providence, Moncton NB E1C 8X3; Laval'77; FRCSC; ObstGyn; GynOnco (P.Q.). (506)862-4344; Fax. (506)862-4222.

SAVOIE, Remi; Dr Georges-L-Dumont, 330 av Universite, Moncton NB E1C 2Z3; Sher'06; FRCPC; DiagRad. Staff, Dr Georges-L-Dumont University Hospital Centre; (506)862-4000

SAVOIE, Veronique; CSSSG-Hop de Hull, 116 boul Lionel-Emond, Gatineau QC J8Y 1W7; Ott'93; BSc; CCFP; CCFP(E.M.); FCFP; Staff, Hull Hospital; (819)595-6000

SAVOURY, Loran W; ENT Consultants, 219-1 Paton St, St. John's NL A1B 4S8; Mem'81; FRCSC; Otol.

SAVOY, Cynthia A; Clinique Med du Marais 101, 101-185 av Acadie, Dieppe NB E1A 1G6; Laval'96; CCFP; Staff, Dr Georges-L-Dumont University Hospital Centre; Prof Ctr de Formation Med du NB, Universite de Sherbrooke; Langs: Bilingual(French/English); (506)855-8805; Fax. (506)388-9109.

SAVOY, Effie; North Side Med Clinic, 915 Central Ave N, Swift Current SK S9H 3V3; Manila (Philippines)'98; CCFP; Vis Physician/Clin Assoc Prof Women's Health, Regina General Hospital; Clin Assoc Prof, University of Saskatchewan; (306)773-9100; Fax. (306)773-9668.

SAVVIDOU, Georgoulla; 102A-658 Danforth Ave, East York ON M4J 5B9; Tor'87; BSc; MSc; Staff, Toronto East General Hospital Inc; Langs: Greek; (416)461-3834; Fax. (416)466-0652.

SAVVOPOULOS, Stavros; 265-6960 Mumford Rd, Halifax NS B3L 4P1; Thessaloniki (Greece)'97; CCFP; Staff, Dartmouth General Hospital; (902)487-0213

SAW, Jacqueline W L; L9-2775 Laurel St, Vancouver BC V5Z 1M9; Ott'96; FRCPC; IntMed; Cardiol. Staff Interventional Cardiol, Vancouver General Hospital - Centennial Pavillion; (604)875-5547

SAWA, Gordon M J; 320-89 Queensway W, Mississauga ON L5B 2V2; Wes'74; FRCPC; Neur. Staff, Trillium Health Centre - Mississauga; Court Staff, St Michael's Hospital; Asst Prof Neurol, University of Toronto; (905)279-5958; Fax. (905)279-0486.

SAWA, Michael T; 925-55 Queen St E, Toronto ON M5C 1R6; McM'02; FRCPC; Neur. (416)864-5326; Fax. (416)864-5339.

SAWA, Russell J; Heritage Plaza, 100-8330 MacLeod Trail SE, Calgary AB T2H 2V2; Wes'75; BA; PhD; CCFP; FCFP; (403)258-3000; Fax. (403)258-0300.

SAWADSKY, Bruce V; Sunnybrook Hlth Sciences Ctre, 2075 Bayview Ave, Toronto ON M4N 3M5; McM'92; CCFP; CCFP(E.M.); Staff Emerg, Sunnybrook Health Sciences Centre; (416)480-4037

SAWAN, Bassem; CHUS-Hop Fleurimont, 3001 12e av N, Sherbrooke QC J1H 5N4; Beirut (Lebanon)'92; CSPQ; AnatPath (P.Q.) (Hematology Pathology). Staff, Centre Hospitalier Universitaire de Sherbrooke-Hopital Fleurimont; Langs: English; French; (819)564-5335; Fax. (819)820-6473.

SAWAN, Hasan M S; Queen's University, 70 Barrie St, Kingston ON K7L 3N6; King Abdul Aziz (Saudi Arabia)'01; FRCSC; OrthSurg. (613)533-2543

SAWAQED, Fadi S; Queen Elizabeth II HSC, 293-1276 South Park St, Halifax NS B3H 2Y9; (Jordan)'03; Staff, Queen Elizabeth II Health Sciences Centre - Victoria General Site; (902)473-5853

SAWATSKY, Errin L; 1-25 12th Ave S, Cranbrook BC V1C 2R8; Sask'04; FRCPC; IntMed. (250)426-1995

SAWATSKY, Katrina A; Rockyview Gen Hosp, 7007 14 St SW, Calgary AB T2V 1P9; Cal'05; CCFP; Staff, Rockyview General Hospital; (403)943-3000

SAWATZKY, Cynthia K; Health Action Centre, 640 Main St, Winnipeg MB R3B 0L8; Man'03; CCFP; (204)940-1626

SAWATZKY, K David; DND Canadian Forces, 5674 Cunard St, Halifax NS B3K 1C6; Alb'80; BMedSci; MSc; Advisor Casualty Support, Canadian Forces Health Services Centre (Atlantic); (902)427-3622

SAWATZKY, Mark E C; Penticton Reg Hosp, 101-550 Carmi Ave, Penticton BC V2A 3G6; Man'02; FRCSC; GenSurg. Staff, Penticton Regional Hospital; (250)493-0134

SAWATZKY, Robert J; Gartree Med Clinic, 510-4400 32 St, Vernon BC V1T 9H2; Sask'84; (250)545-9112; Fax. (250)545-7556.

SAWATZKY, Vernon W; PO Box 950, Keewatin ON P0X 1C0; Man'82; Staff, Lake of the Woods District Hospital.

SAWCHUK, Corey W T; Hamilton HS-General Site, 237 Barton St E, Hamilton ON L8L 2X2; Man'87; FRCPC; Anes. Staff, Hamilton Health Sciences Centre - Hamilton General Hospital; (905)528-4472

SAWCHUK, J Paul; River East Health Access Ctre, 975 Henderson Hwy, Winnipeg MB R2K 4L7; Man'92; CCFP; FCFP; (204)938-5000

SAWH, Veejai D; Capt William Jackman Mem Hosp, 410 Booth Ave, Labrador City NL A2V 2K1; (Guyana)'98; MB BS; Staff, Captain William Jackman Memorial Hospital; (709)944-6878; Fax. (709)944-5449.

SAWHNEY, Gulshan; 102-6990 Derry Rd, Milton ON L9T 7H3; Maulana Azad (India)'80; MB BS; FRCPC; IntMed (Gastroenterology). Langs: Hindi; Punjabi; (905)878-8888; Fax. (905)878-9322.

SAWHNEY, Ravinder P S; BC Cancer Agency-Fraser Valley, 13750 96 Ave, Surrey BC V3V 1Z2; Kashmir (India)'81; MB BS; FRCPC; IntMed; MedOncol. Staff, BC Cancer Agency Fraser Valley Centre; Assoc Staff, Surrey Memorial Hospital; Clinical Asst Prof, University of British Columbia; Langs: Punjabi; Hindi; Kashmiri; (604)930-4028; rsawhney@bccancer.bc.ca.

SAWHNEY, Sandeep; 102-13805 104 Ave, Surrey BC V3T 1W7; New York State (USA)'01; CCFP; (604)594-2714

SAWICKI, Zbigniew A; Hys Med Centre, 206B-11010 101 St NW, Edmonton AB T5H 4B9; (Poland)'66; (780)426-1780; Fax. (780)425-7767.

SAWIRES, Hany F S; Toronto East Gen Hosp Inc, G6001S-825 Coxwell Ave, East York ON M4C 3E7; Ain Shams (Egypt)'97; FRCSC; GenSurg (Surgical Oncology). Staff, Toronto East General Hospital Inc; Langs: Arabic; (416)691-1333; Fax. (416)691-1335.

SAWISKY, Grant R; 16940 127 St NW, Edmonton AB T6V 1B1; Alb'08; CCFP; (780)665-1760; Fax. (780)665-2755.

SAWKA, Andrew N; Vancouver Gen Hosp, 855 12th Ave W, Vancouver BC V5Z 1M9; Man'94; FRCPC; Anes. Staff, Vancouver General Hospital - Centennial Pavillion; (604)875-4304

SAWKA, Annie M; Univ Hlth Network-Toronto Gen, 12EN 212-200 Elizabeth St, Toronto ON M5G 2C4; Man'92; FRCPC; IntMed; Endocrin&Metab. Staff, Toronto General Hospital - UHN; (416)340-3678

SAWKA, Barry W; Grand River Hosp-KW Hlth Ctre, PO Box 9056 Stn C 835 King St W, Kitchener ON N2G 1G3; Alb'85; FRCPC; AnatPath; GenPath. Staff, Grand River Hospital - Kitchener/Waterloo Health Centre; (519)749-4300

SAWKA, Carol A; 1615-620 University Ave, Toronto ON M5G 2L7; Alb'78; ABIM; ABMO; FRCPC; Hem (Oncology/Breast Cancer); MedOncol; IntMed. Consultant, St Michael's Hospital; Consultant/Staff, Sunnybrook Health Sciences Centre - Edmond Odette Cancer Centre; VP Clinical Prog, Cancer Care Ontario - Provincial Office; Prof Med & Health Sciences, University of Toronto; (416)217-1253; carol.sawka@cancercare.on.ca.

SAWKA, Sandra E; Manitoba X-Ray Clinic, 3263 Portage Ave, Winnipeg MB R3K 0W6; Man'97; (204)832-0273

SAWKIW, Raymond B; 1935 Paris St, Sudbury ON P3E 3C6; Wes'75; CCFP; Ac Staff, Health Sciences North-St Joseph's Health Centre; Ac Staff, Health Sciences North - Memorial Site; Ac Staff, Health Sciences North-Laurentian Site; Langs: Slovak; Ukrainian; (705)523-2503

SAWLER, Margaret R; Medicine in Motion Med Clinic, 5-121 Ilsley Ave, Dartmouth NS B3B 1S4; McM'97; CCFP; Staff, Medicine in Motion Medical Centre; (902)468-2774; Fax. (902)468-1359.

SAWONIAK, Robert I; Lakeshore Gen Hosp, 160 av Stillview, Pointe-Claire QC H9R 2Y2; UBC'01; CCFP; CCFP(E.M.); Staff, Lakeshore General Hospital - Pointe Claire; (514)630-2225

SAWULA, Donald A; Pelham Group Health Centre, 110-245 Pelham Rd, St Catharines ON L2S 1X8; Tor'84; FRCSC; GenSurg. Court Staff, Niagara Health System - Ontario Street Site; Ac Staff, Niagara Health System - St Catharines General Site; (905)688-1088; Fax. (905)688-4185.

SAWWAN, Ahmad K H; Capt William Jackman Mem Hosp, 410 Booth Ave, Labrador City NL A2V 2K1; Ain Shams (Egypt)'94; MB BCh; Staff, Captain William Jackman Memorial Hospital; (709)944-2632

SAWYER, Douglas M; Royal Juvilee Hosp, 1952 Bay St, Victoria BC V8R 1J8; Alb'73; AB; AB; FRCPC; AnatPath (Dermatological Pathology). Staff, Royal Jubilee Hospital; (250)370-8435; Fax. (250)370-8069.

SAWYER, Elisabeth M; 203-518 Lake St, Nelson BC V1L 4C6; Ott'02; CCFP; (250)354-4414

SAWYER, Jeremy A; 302-915 Grosvenor Ave, Winnipeg MB R3M 0M5; Man'81; FRCPC; Psy.

SAWYER, Marc R; Centre for Family Medicine, 623-1187 Fischer Hallman Rd, Kitchener ON N2E 4H9; McM'06; CCFP; (519)570-3008; Fax. (519)570-0043.

SAWYER, Michael B; Cross Cancer Institute, 11560 University Ave NW, Edmonton AB T6G 1Z2; Tor'94; FRCPC; IntMed (Clinical Pharmacology); MedOncol. Staff, Cross Cancer Institute; Asst Prof Oncol, University of Alberta; (780)432-8248; Fax. (780)432-8888.

SAWYER, Sarah L; Children's Hosp Eastern Ont, 401 Smyth Rd, Ottawa ON K1H 8L1; Cal'07; FRCPC; MedGenetics. Staff, Children's Hospital of Eastern Ontario (CHEO); (613)737-7600

SAWYER, Scott K; Health Sciences Centre, JL143-820 Sherbrook St, Winnipeg MB R3A 1R9; Man'01; FRCPC; Peds; PedEmergMed. Staff, Health Sciences Centre; (204)774-6511

SAWYERS, Elizabeth A; Parkdale Med Tower, 801-1081 Carling Ave, Ottawa ON K1Y 4G2; Ott'98; BSc(Hon); CCFP; Staff Rehab & Family Med, The Ottawa Hospital - Civic Campus; (613)725-2334; Fax. (613)725-3017.

SAX, Lawrence M; Keele-Ingram Prof Centre, 301-2221 Keele St, North York ON M6M 3Z5; Tor'74; BSc; Assoc Staff Fam & CommunMed, Mount Sinai Hospital; Ac Staff Fam & CommunMed, Humber River Regional Hospital - Keele Street Site; (416)249-3180; Fax. (416)249-2410.

SAX, Solly E; Dr Sol E Sax Med Prof Corp, 17 Ridgevalley Cres, Etobicoke ON M9A 3J7; Tor'78; DOHS; CCBOM; FRCPC; OccupMed (Occupational Health/Administration);CCFP; FCFP; Ac Staff, Women's College Hospital; Med Consultant, DuPont Canada; Media Dir, Hamilton Hospitals Assessment Ctre; Lecturer Occup, University of Toronto; (416)234-2060; Fax. (416)850-5687.

SAXENA, Akash D; 809 Brant St, Burlington ON L7R 2J4; McM'98; FRCPC; IntMed.

SAXENA, Anurag; Royal University Hosp, 103 Hospital Dr, Saskatoon SK S7N 0W8; Delhi (India)'82; MB BS; FACA; FRCPC; AnatPath (Hematology Pathology). Staff Path, Royal University Hospital; Assoc Prof/Dean Postgraduate Med Education, University of Saskatchewan; Langs: Hindi; (306)655-2157

SAXENA, Mitra; Mediclinic, 101-3333 8th St E, Saskatoon SK S7H 4K1; Sask'96; CCFP; Staff, Royal University Hospital; Staff, St Paul's Hospital (Grey Nuns) of Saskatoon; (306)955-1530; Fax. (306)955-8811.

SAXENA, Onkar N; PO Box 430, Lanigan SK S0K 2M0; Lucknow (India)'56; LRCP(UK); MRCS(UK); FRCS(Edin); Chief/Medical Staff, Lanigan Hospital; Langs: Hindi; (306)365-2593; Fax. (306)365-3385.

SAXENA, Pradeep; Milton Trails Med Clinic, 8-6521 Derry Rd, Milton ON L9T 7W1; Kanpur University (India)'79; CCFP; (905)876-0002; Fax. (905)876-0003; miltontrailsmedicalclinic@gmail.com.

SAXENA, Rahul; Galaxy 12 Clinic, 2867 Ellesmere Rd, Scarborough ON M1E 4B9; Ott'94; FRCPC; Peds (Adolescent Medicine). Staff Adolescent Med, The Hospital For Sick Children; Staff, Rouge Valley Health System - Centenary Health Centre Site; (416)281-7476; Fax. (416)281-7313.

SAXENA, Saket; Campbellton Reg Hosp, PO Box 880 Stn Main 189 Lily Lake Rd, Campbellton NB E3N 3H3; (India)'02; Staff, Hôpital Régional Campbellton; (506)789-5000

SAXENA, Shiv K; Grand River Hosp-KW Hlth Ctre, PO Box 9056 Stn C 5F-835 King St W, Kitchener ON N2G 1G3; Lucknow (India)'77; FRCPC; IntMed. Staff, Grand River Hospital - Kitchener/Waterloo Health Centre; (519)749-4300

SAXENA, Will; Chatham-Kent Family Health Team, 30 McNaughton Ave, Wallaceburg ON N8A 1R9; University of Delhi (India)'00; (519)627-1497

SAXINGER, Lynora M; University of Alberta Hosp, 2E419WMC-8440 112 St NW, Edmonton AB T6G 2B7; Sask'96; BSc; FRCPC; IntMed (Education); InfectDis. Staff, University of Alberta Hospital; Assoc Prof InfectDis, University of Alberta; (780)407-7920; Fax. (780)407-7137.

SAXON, Daniel J A; Clinique Med Brunswick, 955 boul Saint-Jean, Pointe-Claire QC H9R 5K3; Dal'91; FRCSC; ObstGyn. Staff, Hôpital Anna-Laberge; (514)426-6677

SAXON, Patricia M; Middleton Collaborative Practi, PO Box 1599 Middleton Stn 452 Main St, Middleton NS B0S 1P0; Dal'08; CCFP; (902)825-1095; Fax. (902)825-6973.

SAYAD, George R; 102-1646 McKenzie Ave, Victoria BC V8N 0A3; Tor'83; CCFP; (250)818-0001; Fax. (250)383-0203.

SAYADI, Hassan; Cape Breton Hlthcare Complex, 1482 George St, Sydney NS B1P 1P3; Univ of Aleppo (Syria)'83; Staff, Cape Breton Healthcare Complex; (902)567-8000

SAYAL, Arun K; North York Gen Hosp, 4001 Leslie St, Toronto ON M2K 1E1; Tor'90; CCFP; CCFP(E.M.); Ac Staff Emerg Dept, North York General Hospital; Lecturer Community & Family Med, University of Toronto; (416)756-6000

SAYAL, Manoj K; Oakville Med Centre, 203-331 Sheddon Ave, Oakville ON L6J 1X8; Tor'90; FRCSC; GenSurg; Critical Care Medicine. Langs: Hindi; Punjabi; (905)618-0098; Fax. (905)618-0100.

SAYANI, Ali; 10818 Jasper Ave PO Box 35083 Rpo Midtown, Edmonton AB T5J 0B7; UBC'08; CCFP; (780)422-7333; Fax. (780)422-7343.

SAYANI, Eshratbanu; 1-2060 Ellesmere Rd, Scarborough ON M1H 2V6; Tor'79; CCFP; FCFP; Assoc Staff, Rouge Valley Health System - Centenary Health Centre Site; Assoc Staff, The Scarborough Hospital - Birchmount Campus; Lecturer DCFM, University of Toronto; Langs: Hindi; Gujarati; Urdu; (416)439-2273; Fax. (416)439-2244.

SAYANI, Farzana A; Foothills Med Centre, 681-1403 29 St NW, Calgary AB T2N 2T9; Cal'01; FRCPC; IntMed; Hem. Staff, Foothills Medical Centre; (403)944-1564

SAYAO, Ana Luiza; St Paul's Hosp, 1081 Burrard St, Vancouver BC V6Z 1Y6; UBC'04; FRCPC; Neur. Staff, Providence Health Care - St Paul's Hospital; (604)806-8206

SAYAR, Mirwais A; 302-310 King St E, Kitchener ON N2G 2L3; Stavropol (Russia (Federation))'92; CCFP; (519)743-2142

SAYED, Ahmed; Royal University Hosp, 103 Hospital Dr, Saskatoon SK S7N 0W8; King Khalid University (Saudi Arabia)'02; FRCPC; IntMed; Cardiol. Staff, Royal University Hospital; (306)655-1000

SAYED, Ebrahim; Niagara H System-Welland, 65 Third St, Welland ON L3B 4W5; Dublin (Ireland)'73; Ac Staff, Niagara Health System - Welland Hospital Site; Langs: Gujarati; Urdu; Zulu; (905)738-4647

SAYED, Qasim R; Van Mills Med Center, D115-1930 Fowler Dr, Mississauga ON L5K 0A1; Punjab (India)'92; MB BS; CCFP; (904)403-8200

SAYED AHMED, Raid M S H; 640 Concession St, Hamilton ON L8V 1B5; Abdul Aziz (Saudi Arabia)'98; FRCSC; ObstGyn. (905)387-1032; Fax. (905)387-9954.

SAYED-ALI, Adham A; 13278 Tecumseh Rd E, Windsor ON N8N 3T6; Belgrade (Serbia)'85; CCFP; (519)979-6345; Fax. (519)979-8085.

SAYEED, Asma; Royal Oak Med Clinic, 192-8888 Country Hills Blvd NW, Calgary AB T3G 5T4; (India)'84; CCFP; (403)239-3660; Fax. (403)239-4001.

SAYEED, M A Raffath; Family Med Clinic, PO Box 800 Stn Main 4615 49th Ave, Lloydminster SK S9V 1C1; Madras (India)'72; LRCP; MRCS; Staff, Lloydminster Hospital; Langs: Tamil; Hindi; Urdu; (306)825-8877; Fax. (306)825-5167; familymed.clinic@sasktel.net.

SAYEED, Muhammad R U; William Osler HC-Brampton, 2100 Bovaird Dr E, Brampton ON L6R 3J7; Karachi (Pakistan)'90; MB BS; FRCPC; Psy. Staff, William Osler Health System - Brampton Civic Hospital; (905)494-2120

SAYEGH, Nabil; Clinique Med Pierre-Boucher, 110-1615 boul Jacques-Cartier, Longueuil QC J4M 2X1; Mon'84; Staff, Centre Hospitalier Pierre Boucher; (450)468-6223; Fax. (450)468-5041.

SAYEGH, Renee; CLSC Verdun Cote-St-Paul, 400 rue de l'Eglise, Verdun QC H4G 2M4; Mon'83; Langs: English; (514)766-0546 x2314; Fax. (514)732-5103.

SAYEH, Naser S; 104-33774 Marshall Rd, Abbotsford BC V2S 1L1; Al-Fateh (Libya)'97; Cardiol; IntMed. Staff Echo Cardiography Lab, Providence Health Care - St Paul's Hospital; (604)870-8715

SAYLOR, Kent D; MUHC-Montreal Children's Hosp, F379-2300 rue Tupper, Montreal QC H3H 1P3; Stanford(CA) (USA)'94; FRCPC; Peds. Staff, McGill University Health Centre - Montreal Children's Hospital; (514)412-4400 x23548; Fax. (514)412-4249.

SAYOUD, Fadila; Hop Marie Clarac, 3530 boul Gouin E, Montreal-Nord QC H1H 1B7; (Other Foreign)'08; Staff, Hopital Marie Clarac; (514)321-8800

SAYUCHCHIYADEVAN, Ganeshan; 14-233 Brady St E, Sudbury ON P3B 4H5; (Sri Lanka)'75; MB BS; LRCP(Eng); MRCS(Eng); FRCSC; Ophth. Langs: Tamil; (705)675-1115; Fax. (705)674-9169.

SBEITY, Samer; Hop Reg d'Edmundston, 275 Hebert Blvd, Edmundston NB E3V 4E4; (Lebanon)'01; Staff, Hôpital regional d'Edmundston; (506)739-2200

SBROCCHI, Anne M; MUHC-Montreal Children's Hosp, 2300 rue Tupper, Montreal QC H3H 1P3; Ott'03; FRCPC; Peds; Endocrin&Metab. Staff, McGill University Health Centre - Montreal Children's Hospital; (514)412-4400

SBROCCHI, Stephanie C; 9-2120 Regent St, Sudbury ON P3E 3Z9; Ott'00; CCFP; Lecturer, Northern Ontario School of Medicine; Langs: Italian; French; (705)524-7419; Fax. (705)524-9087.

SCAFFIDI, Carmen P; CSSS du Lac-Temiscamingue, 22 rue Notre-Dame N, Ville-Marie QC J9V 1W8; Laval'93; CCFP; Staff, CSSS du Témiscamingue; Langs: English; French; (819)629-2420; Fax. (819)629-3257; carmen_scaffidi@ssss.gouv.qc.ca.

SCAIFE, Christopher R; Lake of the Woods Dist Hosp, 21 Sylvan St RR 1 Stn Main, Kenora ON P9N 3W7; McM'85; Lake of the Woods District Hospital; (807)468-9861; Fax. (807)468-3638.

SCAIFE, Gerald D; 199 Ontario St, St Catharines ON L2R 5K8; Wes'76; FRCSC; Ophth. Staff, Niagara Health System - Ontario Street Site; Staff, Niagara Health System - St Catharines General Site; (905)684-1822; Fax. (905)684-4766; scaife@on.aibn.com.

SCALA, G Basil; Trillium Hlth Ctre-Mississauga, 100 Queensway W, Mississauga ON L5B 1B8; McM'90; CCFP; Staff, Trillium Health Centre - Mississauga; (905)848-7100

SCALA, Salvatore J; Danforth Med Centre, 1473 Danforth Ave, Toronto ON M4J 1N5; Tor'58; Langs: Italian; American Sign Language; (416)466-3035; Fax. (416)466-4425.

SCALCO, Andreia Z; Women's College Hosp, 76 Grenville St, Toronto ON M5S 1B2; Sao Paulo (Brazil)'95; FRCPC; Psy. Staff, Hamilton Health Sciences Centre - McMaster University Medical Centre; Staff Psychiatry & BehaviouralNeurosciences, St Joseph's Healthcare Hamilton - West 5th Campus; Staff, Women's College Hospital; Langs: Portuguese; (416)323-6400

SCALCO, Monica Z; Univ Hlth Network-Toronto Western Hosp, 461-399 Bathurst st, Toronto ON M5T 2S8; Sao Paolo (Brazil)'89; FRCPC; Psy. Staff Seniours Mental Health Unit, Ontario Shores Centre for Mental Health Sciences; Staff, Toronto Western Hospital - University Health Network; Langs: Portuguese; (416)603-5974; Fax. (416)603-5049.

SCALES, Damon C; Sunnybrook Hlth Sciences Ctre, D108-2075 Bayview Ave, Toronto ON M4N 3M5; Tor'97; BSc; FRCPC; IntMed; Critical Care Medicine. Staff, Sunnybrook Health Sciences Centre; (416)480-6100; damon.scales@utoronto.ca.

SCALI, Jim N; Port Arthur Health Centre Inc, 194 Court St N, Thunder Bay ON P7A 4V7; Tor'82; CCFP; FCFP; Langs: Italian; (807)346-1000 x7760; Fax. (807)346-6206.

SCALI, Vincent C; Northmount Med Centre, 803-145 13th St E, North Vancouver BC V7L 2L4; McG'71; MDCM; FRCSC; ObstGyn. Ac Staff, Lions Gate Hospital; Consultant, BC Cancer Agency Vancouver Centre; Clin Assoc Prof ObstGyn, University of British Columbia; (604)985-4177; Fax. (604)980-3481; vcscali@shaw.ca.

SCALLAN, Francis; Haldimand War Mem Hosp, 101-206 John St, Dunnville ON N1A 2P7; Dublin (Ireland)'78; Acad Staff Family Med, Haldimand War Memorial Hospital; (905)774-7503; Fax. (905)774-6884.

SCAMAN, Donald R; Cannon Clinic, 4-2151 McCallum Rd, Abbotsford BC V2S 3N9; Alb'74; CCFP; Staff, Abbotsford Regional Hospital & Cancer Centre; (604)853-3314; Fax. (604)853-2171.

SCAMPOLI, Nicola; The Credit Valley Hosp, 2200 Eglinton Ave W, Mississauga ON L5M 2N1; Wes'97; CCFP; CCFP(E.M.); Staff, The Credit Valley Hospital; Langs: Italian; (905)813-4530; Fax. (905)813-4444.

SCAMVOUGERAS, Anton; Neuropsychiatry Unit, 0007-2255 Wesbrook Mall, Vancouver BC V6T 2A1; Cape Town (South Africa)'84; MB ChB; FRCPC; Psy (Neurology & Psychiatry). Staff, UBC Hospital - Koerner Pavillion; Clin Assoc Prof, University of British Columbia; Langs: Afrikaans; (604)822-7298; Fax. (604)822-7105; antons@unixg.ubc.ca.

SCANDAR, Jeannette E; Ctre de sante Comm de l'Estrie, 841 Sydney St, Cornwall ON K6H 3J7; Alexandria (Egypt)'81; MB ChB; CCFP; Langs: Arabic; French; (613)937-2683; m.ghobrial@sympatico.ca.

SCANDIFFIO, Ralph J; Medical Expertise HRSDC, 5A-333 North River Rd, Ottawa ON K1A 0L1; Tor'66; Med Advisor, Income Security Program Branch; (613)952-3622; Fax. (613)954-4927; ralph.scandiffio@hrsdc-rhdcc.gc.ca.

SCANGA, Dante G; Blatcford Field Med Clinic, 11541 Kingsway Ave, Edmonton AB T5G 3E8; (Italy)'80; CCFP; Staff Emerg Room, Westlock Healthcare Centre; Langs: Italian; (780)457-1351; Fax. (780)478-7796.

SCANLAN, Daniel T; 309 Midland Ave, Midland ON L4R 3K8; Dal'96; FRCSC; Ophth. (705)527-7744; Fax. (705)527-6731.

SCANLON, Martin N; Chronic Pain Centre, 160-2210 2 St SW, Calgary AB T2S 3C3; Cal'90; BSc; PhD; Anes (Chronic Pain Management). Staff, Rockyview General Hospital; Clin Assoc Prof, University of Calgary; (403)943-9900; Fax. (403)209-2954.

SCANTLEBURY, Morris H; Alberta Children's Hosp, 2888 Shaganappi Trail NW, Calgary AB T3B 6A8; Staff, Alberta Children's Hospital; (403)955-5737; Fax. (403)955-7609.

SCANTLEBURY, William; Dr Billy Scantlebury Med Centr, 15 Brackley Point Rd, Charlottetown PE C1A 6Y1; Wes'99; (902)892-9881; Fax. (902)892-9878.

SCAPPATURA, F Philip; Travel Med Centre, 609-700 Bay St Box 204, Toronto ON M5G 1Z6; Tor'81; (416)340-8222; Fax. (416)340-8190; pscap@idirect.com.

SCARANELO, Anabel M; Univ Hlth Network-Princess M, 3 922-610 University Ave, Toronto ON M5G 2M9; Estadual de Londrina (Brazil)'89; Staff, Princess Margaret Hospital - University Health Network; Langs: Portuguese; (416)946-4501; Fax. (416)946-6564.

SCARBOROUGH, Francois; Hop de Sacre-Coeur de Mtl, 5400 boul Gouin O, Montreal QC H4J 1C5; Laval'93; CCFP; CCFP(E.M.); Staff, Hôpital du Sacre-Coeur de Montréal; (514)338-2222

SCARFE, Andrew G; Cross Cancer Institute, 11560 University Ave NW, Edmonton AB T6G 1Z2; Alb'96; MD; FRCPC; IntMed; MedOncol. Staff Med Oncol, Cross Cancer Institute; Assoc Prof Oncol, University of Alberta; Langs: French; (780)432-8340; Fax. (780)432-8888.

SCARFE, Sarah E; UBC Student Health Service, M334-2211 Wesbrook Mall, Vancouver BC V6T 1Z3; Alb'00; BSc(Psychol); FRCPC; Psy. (604)822-7689; Fax. (604)822-7889.

SCARFF, Michael A; Aberfoyle Clinic, 102-304 The East Mall, Etobicoke ON M9B 6E2; Wes'61; AB; GenPath. (416)231-7968; Fax. (416)231-7982; reception@aberfoyle.com.

SCARFONE, David J; South Walkerville Med Centre, 140-2224 Walker Rd, Windsor ON N8W 5L7; Wes'82; (519)258-8802; Fax. (519)258-8870.

SCARFONE, Dominique; 825 av Dunlop, Outremont QC H2V 2W6; Mon'75; CSPQ; FRCPC; Psy (P.Q.) (Psychoanalysis). Prof Psychologie, Universite de Montreal; Langs: Italian; English; (514)341-7985

SCARFONE, Peter J; Family Practice Clinic, 103-2462 Howard Ave, Windsor ON N8X 3V6; Wes'83; CCFP; (519)972-8910; Fax. (519)972-8991.

SCARIAH, Swapna A C; Rochdale Walk-In Clinic, 4450 Rochdale Blvd, Regina SK S4X 4P7; (Other Foreign)'03; (306)565-0181

SCARINCI, Christine; Ctre de Readaptation Marie-Enf, 5200 rue Belanger E, Montreal QC H1T 1C9; Mon'96; FRCPC; Peds (Physical Medicine & Rehabilitation). Staff, Centre de Réadaptation Marie Enfant du CHU Sainte-Justine; Staff, Centre Hospitalier Universitaire de Sherbrooke-Hopital Fleurimont; Clin Prof, Universite de Sherbrooke; Langs: Spanish; English; (514)374-1710 x8312; Fax. (514)723-7255.

SCARTH, Brian A; Royal Columbian Hosp, 330 Columbia St E, New Westminster BC V3L 3W7; UBC'91; FRCPC; Psy. Staff, Royal Columbian Hospital; (250)520-4662

SCARTH, Hugh M C; Saint John Reg Hosp, PO Box 2100 Stn Main 400 University Ave, Saint John NB E2L 4L2; Tor'82; FRCSC; GenSurg. Ac Staff Surg, Saint John Regional Hospital; Ac Staff Surg, St Joseph's Hospital; Asst Prof, Dalhousie University; (506)648-7921; Fax. (506)648-7925; scahu@reg2.health.nb.ca.

SCARVELIS, Dimitrios; The Ottawa Hosp-Civic Campus, 1053 Carling Ave, Ottawa ON K1Y 4E9; McG'98; FRCPC; IntMed; Hem. Staff, The Ottawa Hospital - Civic Campus; Langs: English; Greek; (613)722-7000

SCATLIFF, John E; St Boniface Gen Hosp, 409 Tache Ave, Winnipeg MB R2H 2A6; Man'70; FRCPC; Anes (Cardiovascular Anesthesia). Ac Staff, St Boniface General Hospital; Asst Prof, University of Manitoba; (204)233-8563

SCATLIFF, Robert M; Paterson Med Centre, 45 Wolsley St, Kenora ON P9N 3W7; Man'08; CCFP; Staff, Lake of the Woods District Hospital; (807)468-3021

SCHAAL, Peter G H; Holly Street Endoscopy Clinic, 301-40 Holly St, Toronto ON M4S 3C3; McG'68; MDCM; FRCSC; GenSurg (Thoracic Surgery). Surgeon, Trillium Health Centre - West Toronto; Langs: German; French; (416)486-8088; Fax. (416)486-7888; peterschaal@hollyendoscopy.ca.

SCHABAS, Patti A; Campbellford Mem Hosp, PO Box 1027 146 Oliver St, Campbellford ON K0L 1L0; Tor'76; FRCPC; Psy (Child & Adolescent Psychiatry). Staff, Campbellford Memorial Hospital; (705)653-1140

SCHABAS, Richard E; Campbellford Mem Hosp, PO Box 1027 146 Oliver St, Campbellford ON K0L 1L0; Tor'76; MHSc; FRCPC; IntMed (Public Health); CommunMed. Staff, Campbellford Memorial Hospital; Assoc Prof Med, University of Toronto; (705)653-1140

SCHABORT, Ingeborg; Stonechurch Family Health Ctre, 1475 Upper Ottawa St, Hamilton ON L8W 3J6; Stellenbosch (South Africa)'81; CCFP; (905)575-1300; Fax. (905)575-1539.

SCHACHAR, Jaime D; Sunridge Prof Centre, 308-2675 36 St NE, Calgary AB T1Y 6H6; Cal'07; ObstGyn. (403)215-4070; Fax. (403)215-4071.

SCHACHAR, Norman S; Heritage Medical Research Bldg, 436-3330 Hospital Dr NW, Calgary AB T2N 4N1; Tor'70; FRCSC; OrthSurg (Surgical Oncology). Ac Staff, Foothills Medical Centre; Consultant, Alberta Children's Hospital; Prof, University of Calgary; (403)220-3880; Fax. (403)210-9717.

SCHACHAR, Russell J; The Hosp for Sick Children, 555 University Ave, Toronto ON M5G 1X8; Tor'71; FRCPC; Psy. Clin Researcher Psy, The Hospital For Sick Children; Assoc Prof, University of Toronto; (416)813-6564; Fax. (416)813-6565; russell.schachar@sickkids.ca.

SCHACHTER, Debbie C; Addiction & Mental Hlth-Queen, 1131-1001 Queen St W, Toronto ON M6J 1H4; McG'80; FRCPC; Psy. Staff, Centre for Addiction & Mental Health (CAMH) - Queen Site; Staff Psy, Centre for Addiction & Mental Health (CAMH) - College Street Site; Langs: French; (416)535-8501

SCHACHTER, G Daniel; Dermatology Centre, 403-208 Bloor St W, Toronto ON M5S 3B4; Tor'71; FRCPC; Derm (Psoriasis). Ac Staff, Women's College Hospital; Ac Staff, Psoriasis Education & Research Centre; Teacher, University of Toronto; (416)922-7546; Fax. (416)922-4358; dermlaser@unlockyourbeauty.com.

SCHACHTER, Joyce; Harmony Med Centre, 101-152 Cleopatra Dr, Nepean ON K2G 5X2; Ott'94; FRCSC; ObstGyn (Urological Gynecology). Langs: French; (613)728-5863; Fax. (613)728-4745.

SCHACHTER, Michael E; 113-13798 94A Ave, Surrey BC V3V 1N1; Cal'04; Nephrol; IntMed. Staff Med, Vancouver General Hospital - Centennial Pavillion; (604)582-6606

SCHACHTER, Murray A; 1007-120 Donald St, Winnipeg MB R3C 4G2; Man'73; Psy. Staff, Health Sciences Centre; Assoc Prof Psy & Family Med, University of Manitoba.

SCHACHTER, Sam S; 9 James St, Milton ON L9T 2P3; Tor'75; Ac Staff, Halton Healthcare Services Corporation - Milton District Hospital; (905)878-1923; Fax. (905)878-4620.

SCHACTER, Brent A; CancerCare Manitoba, 2055A-675 Mcdermot Ave, Winnipeg MB R3E 0V9; Man'65; BSc(Med); FRCPC; IntMed (Bone Marrow Transplant). Physician, CancerCare Manitoba; Ac Staff, Health Sciences Centre; Prof Med, University of Manitoba; (204)787-2128; Fax. (204)786-0196.

SCHACTER, Gordon B; 215-1135 Adelaide St N, London ON N5Y 5K7; Wes'93; CCFP; FCFP; Aj Prof, University of Western Ontario; (519)673-3900; Fax. (519)673-5627.

SCHACTER, Irving B; Medical & Dental Bldg, 400-1849 Yonge St, Toronto ON M4S 1Y2; Tor'49; FRCSC; Neursurg. (416)489-4917; Fax. (416)489-1477; berneyschacter@yahoo.ca.

SCHACTER, Milton W; Bayview-Finch Med Clinic, 200-3292 Bayview Ave, North York ON M2M 4J5; McG'69; Assoc Staff, North York General Hospital; Assoc Staff, North York General Hospital - Branson Division; (416)222-8555; Fax. (416)222-6707.

SCHAEFER, J Paul; Summerside Med Centre, 101-475 Granville St, Summerside PE C1N 4P7; Dal'64; FACS; FRCSC; GenSurg. Staff, Central Newfoundland Regional Health Centre; Consultant Surg, Western Hospital - Health PEI; Staff, Prince County Hospital; (902)432-8113; Fax. (902)436-2269.

SCHAEFER, Jeffrey P; Foothills Med Center, NT 933-1403 29 St NW, Calgary AB T2N 2T9; Sask'91; MSc; BSc; FACP; FRCPC; IntMed (Internal Medicine). Staff, Rockyview General Hospital; Staff, Foothills Medical Centre; Clin Assoc Prof Med, University Of Calgary; (403)944-1525; Fax. (403)407-7771; jpschaef@ucalgary.ca.

SCHAEFER, Rachel I; Schaefer Med Prof Corp, 314-460 Springbank Dr, London ON N6J 0A8; McM'01; BSc; MCFP; CCFP; Physician, Wortley Village Medical Centre; (519)672-8364; Fax. (519)672-0607; schaeferis@rogers.com.

SCHAEFER, Tanya D; Pharmasave Med Complex, 135 Henry St, Miramichi NB E1V 2N5; Dal'90; (506)627-0002

SCHAEFER-ZIELENIAK, Bozena; Clinique Med de la Cite, 150-175 rue de la Visitation, St-Charles-Brromee QC J6E 4N4; Bozena (Poland)'73; Staff, Centre de Sante Isle-Dieu Matagami; Langs: Polish; (450)759-1444; Fax. (450)759-2036.

SCHAEFERS, Hans-Joachim D; Long Pond Med Clinic, PO Box 14097 Stn Manuels 88 Conception Bay Hwy, St. John's NL A1E 3J1; Gesamthochschule Essen (Germany)'82; CCFP; (709)834-4232

SCHAEFFER, David F; Vancouver Gen Hosp, 855 12th Ave W, Vancouver BC V5Z 1M9; Johannes Gutenburg (Germany)'03; FRCPC; AnatPath (General Pathology). Staff, Vancouver General Hospital - Centennial Pavillion; Langs: German; (604)875-4111

SCHAFER-MACDONALD, Helga T; Lynn Valley Med & Travel Clin, 102-1200 Lynn Valley Rd, North Vancouver BC V7J 2A2; Ludwig Maximilian (Germany)'80; CCFP; Langs: German; (604)988-5389; Fax. (604)988-5339.

SCHAFFENBURG, Jocelyn E R; 203-520 University Ave W, Waterloo ON N2T 2Z6; Tor'78; CCFP; FCFP; (519)743-3641; Fax. (519)743-1042.

SCHAFFER, Ayal; Sunnybrook Hlth Sciences Ctre, FG52-2075 Bayview Ave, Toronto ON M4N 3M5; Tor'96; FRCPC; Psy. Head Mood Disorder Prog, Sunnybrook Health Sciences Centre; Assoc Prof Psy, University of Toronto; (416)480-4070; Fax. (416)480-4613.

SCHAFFER, Nathan; Gordon & Leslie Diamond HCC, 8187-2775 Laurel St, Vancouver BC V5Z 1M9; Alb'88; BMedSci; FRCPC; Psy (Community Psychiatry). Staff, Gordon & Leslie Diamond Health Care Centre; Staff, Vancouver General Hospital - Centennial Pavillion; (604)875-4809; Fax. (604)875-5652.

SCHAFFER, Stephen A; St Boniface Gen Hosp, 3015-409 Tache Ave, Winnipeg MB R2H 2A6; Man'03; FRCPC; IntMed; Critical Care Medicine; Cardiol. Staff, St Boniface General Hospital; (204)237-2053

SCHAFFNER, John P; 14 Kentucky Crt, New Minas NS B4N 4N2; Dal'76; FRCSC; Ophth. (902)678-6639; Fax. (902)678-5649.

SCHAFFRIN, Roger M; Westminster Med Bldg, 408-625 Fifth Ave, New Westminster BC V3M 1X4; Sask'63; ABNM; FACP; BA; PhD; FRCPC; IntMed (Allergy). (604)526-9622; Fax. (604)526-4505.

SCHAFFTER, Margaret L; Summit Centre Family Clinic, 209-200 Boudreau Rd, St. Albert AB T8N 6B9; Alb'78; Staff, Sturgeon Community Hospital; (780)458-7000; Fax. (780)458-8484.

SCHALL, W Albrecht; Humber River Reg Hosp-Church, 200 Church St, York ON M9N 1N8; Pretoria (South Africa)'92; FRCPC; AnatPath;CCFP; Staff, Humber River Regional Hospital - Church Street Site; Langs: German; Afrikaans; (416)249-8111 x4601

SCHALLER, Gerald H; Cape Breton Healthcare Complex, 1482 George St, Sydney NS B1P 1P3; Dal'75; FRCPC; DiagRad (Breast Imaging). Staff Radiol, Queen Elizabeth II Health Sciences Centre - Victoria General Site; Staff Diagnostic Imaging, Cape Breton Healthcare Complex; Asst Prof, Dalhousie University; (902)567-8000; gschaller@hfx.eastlink.ca.

SCHAMAN, John P; Ontario Aerobics Centre, RR 2 1010 Hopewell Creek Rd, Breslau ON N0B 1M0; Tor'75; BSc; Assoc Prof, University of Waterloo; (519)648-2252; Fax. (519)648-3686; jschaman@uwaterloo.ca.

SCHAMBERGER-KEREN, Beatrice M; 1701-2200 Yonge St, Toronto ON M4S 2C6; Valle University (Colombia)'83; Psy (General Adult Psychiatry). Langs: Spanish; (416)484-7478

SCHAMP, Adrianna E; The Group Health Centre, 240 McNabb St, Sault Ste. Marie ON P6B 1Y5; Tor'05; BSc; CCFP; (705)759-1234; Fax. (705)541-2226.

SCHAMPAERT, Erick; Hop du Sacre-Coeur de Mtl, A1179-5400 boul Gouin O, Montreal QC H4J 1C5; Mon'89; FRCPC; IntMed (Coronary Angioplasty); Cardiol. Chef Cardiol, Hôpital du Sacre-Coeur de Montréal; Prof, Universite de Montreal; Langs: Spanish; French; (514)338-2340; Fax. (514)338-2905.

SCHANNE, Roswitha E; Hotel-Dieu d'Arthabaska, 5 rue des Hospitalieres, Victoriaville QC G6P 6N2; Sher'79; Derm. Staff, Hotel-Dieu d'Arthabaska; (819)357-2030

SCHANTZ, Daryl I; Children's Hosp, 685 William Ave, Winnipeg MB R3E 0Z2; Man'04; FRCPC; Peds; Cardiol. Staff, Health Sciences Centre; Staff, Variety Children's Heart Centre; (204)774-6511

SCHAPIRA, Theodor H; Dufferin Vaughan Med Clinic, 2-9200 Dufferin St, Concord ON L4K 0C6; McG'75; CCBOM; Langs: Romanian; French; (905)417-3125; Fax. (905)417-3105.

SCHARF, Lorne H; Cornwall Community Hosp, 840 av McConnell, Cornwall ON K6H 5S5; McG'99; CCFP; CCFP(E.M.); FCFP; Staff, Cornwall Community Hospital; Staff, McGill University Health Centre - Royal Victoria Hospital; Langs: French; (613)938-4240

SCHARF, Nathan D; Youthdale Treatment Centre, 227 Victoria St, Toronto ON M5B 1T8; McG'82; MDCM; FRCPC; Psy (Child & Adolescent Psychiatry). Dir Crisis Services, Youthdale Treatment Centres; (416)363-3751; Fax. (416)363-7945; nscharf@youthdale.ca.

SCHARFENBERGER, Angela V; 10150 121 St NW, Edmonton AB T5N 1K4; Alb'97; FRCSC; OrthSurg (Trauma). (780)434-3668; Fax. (780)434-4859.

SCHARFSTEIN, S Briane; PO Box 887, Porcupine Plain SK S0E 1H0; Sask'76; MBA(Qns); CCFP; FCFP.

SCHATTNER, Ariah J; Lakeridge Health Corp-Oshawa, 1 Hospital Crt, Oshawa ON L1G 2B9; Qns'98; FRCPC; IntMed (Oncology); Hem. Staff, Lakeridge Health - Oshawa Site; Staff, Durham Regional Cancer Centre; Langs: Hebrew; French; (905)576-8711; Fax. (905)721-6103.

SCHATZ, Jennifer R; Parkdale Med Tower, 802-1081 Carling Ave, Ottawa ON K1Y 4G2; Qns'87; CCFP; (613)729-9889; Fax. (613)728-2752.

SCHATZDORFER, Julie E; 596 Davis Dr, Newmarket ON L3Y 2P9; Tor'83; BSc; MD; FRCPC; GenPath. Physician Lab, Southlake Regional Health Centre; (905)895-4521 x2536; Fax. (905)952-2824; jschatz@southlakeregional.org.

SCHATZKER, Joseph; Sunnybrook Hlth Sciences Ctre, M350-2075 Bayview Ave, Toronto ON M4N 3M5; Tor'60; BSc(Med); CM; FRCSC; OrthSurg (Trauma). Ac Staff, Sunnybrook Health Sciences Centre; Prof, University of Toronto; Langs: Polish; German; (416)480-6809; Fax. (416)480-5886.

SCHATZMANN, Markus; 206-470 Bronte St S, Milton ON L9T 2J4; Cal'00; BSc; CCFP; Clinical Asst Prof, McMaster University; Langs: Swedish; German; (905)878-6793; Fax. (905)878-6711.

SCHAUB, J Christian; 1113-55 Garry St, Winnipeg MB R3C 4H4; Zurich (Switzerland)'78; FRCPC; Psy. Langs: German; (204)943-2648

SCHAUS, Claus P; Fredericton Med Clinic, 505-1015 Regent St, Fredericton NB E3B 6H5; Ott'89; FRCSC; GenSurg; VascSurg. (506)458-0302; Fax. (506)457-4767.

SCHECHTER, Martin T; Univ of British Columbia, 2206 East Mall, Vancouver BC V6T 1Z3; McM'81; FRCPC; MedScient(Med). Researcher, Providence Health Care - St Paul's Hospital; Dept Head School of Population & Public Hlth, University of British Columbia; (604)822-3910; martin.schechter@ubc.ca.

SCHECHTER-FI, Tal Tova; The Hosp for Sick Children, 555 University Ave, Toronto ON M5G 1X8; Hebrew University (Israel)'99; Staff, The Hospital For Sick Children; (416)813-5886; Fax. (416)813-5327.

SCHECTER, Bayla E; Yarrow Med Bldg, 320-645 Fort St, Victoria BC V8W 1G2; McG'68; AAFP; (250)382-2104; Fax. (250)382-5156.

SCHECTER, Danial M I; CSC Chigamik CHC, 845 King St, Midland ON L4R 0B7; Mon'08; CCFP; Langs: Bilingual(French/English); (705)527-4154; Fax. (705)526-2870.

SCHEELAR, Leslie R; Clinical Sciences Bldg, 8 120-152 University Campus NW, Edmonton AB T6G 2G3; Alb'98; FRCPC; Anes. Staff Anes, University of Alberta Hospital; (780)407-8861

SCHEEPERS, Eugene; 205B St Laurent Ave, Quesnel BC V2J 2C8; Pretoria (South Africa)'04; MB ChB; (250)992-8948

SCHEEPERS, Louis D V; BC Children's Hosp, 1L7-4480 Oak St, Vancouver BC V6H 3V4; Witwatersrand (South Africa)'88; MB ChB; BSc; FRCPC; Anes (Acute & Chronic Pain). Staff Anes, BC Children's Hospital; Langs: Afrikaans; (604)875-2711

SCHEER, Adena S; Univ Hlth Network-Princess M, 3 130-610 University Ave, Toronto ON M5G 2M9; Tor'06; FRCSC; GenSurg. Staff, Princess Margaret Hospital - University Health Network; (416)946-2000

SCHEER, Aedes N; PO Box 1230, Dawson YT Y0B 1G0; UBC'10; CCFP.

SCHEERES, Jan J; 304-5 Quarry Ridge Rd, Barrie ON L4M 7G1; Pretoria (South Africa)'89; FRCSC; ObstGyn (Colposcopy). Staff, Royal Victoria Regional Health Centre; Langs: Dutch; Afrikaans; (705)739-7611; Fax. (705)739-4119.

SCHEFFLER, Erika J; Glenvalley Med Centre, 207-437 Glenmore Rd, Kelowna BC V1V 1Y5; Sask'03; CCFP; (250)860-5811; Fax. (250)860-2811.

SCHEFFLER, Matthias G; Queen Elizabeth II HSC, 1276 South Park St, Halifax NS B3H 2Y9; Ruprecht-Karis-Universitat Heidelberg (Germany)'95; Staff, Queen Elizabeth II Health Sciences Centre - Victoria General Site; (902)473-3866

SCHEFFLER, Rolf F; Quinte HC Corp-Belleville Gen, 265 Dundas St E, Belleville ON K8N 5A9; Mem'76; DABR; BMedSci; FRCPC; DiagRad. Staff, QHC Belleville General; (613)969-7400

SCHEIBENSTOCK, Elisabeth A; Associate Med Clinic, 123 10th Ave S, Cranbrook BC V1C 2N1; Cal'04; CCFP; Staff Emerg Room, East Kootenay Regional Hospital; (250)426-4231

SCHEID, Frederic J; Clinique Externe des Moulins, 101-1355 rue Grande Allee, Terrebonne QC J6W 4K6; Paris (France)'88; Psy (P.Q.) (Consultation). Langs: English; (450)964-6418; courrier@frederic-scheid.com.

SCHEIFELE, David W; Child & Family Research Instit, A5 174-950 28th Ave W, Vancouver BC V5Z 4H4; Wes'69; MD; FRCPC; Peds (Pediatric Infectious Diseases). Staff, BC Children's Hospital; Dir, Vaccine Evaluation Centre; Sr Researcher, Child & Family Research Institute; Prof Peds, University of British Columbia; (604)875-2422; Fax. (604)875-2635.

SCHEIM, Alyssa; Rockland MD, 110-100 rue Rockland, Mont-Royal QC H3P 2V9; McG'05; CCFP; Langs: Bilingual(English/French); (514)667-3383; Fax. (514)667-3384; info@mediservice.ca.

SCHEINEMANN, Katrin; Hamilton HS-McMaster Site, PO Box 2000 Stn Lcd 1 1200 Main St W, Hamilton ON L8N 3Z5; Wurzburg (Germany)'99; Staff, Hamilton Health Sciences Centre - McMaster Children's Hospital; Langs: German; (905)521-2100

SCHEINMAN, Louis J; William Osler HC-Etobicoke, 101 Humber College Blvd, Etobicoke ON M9V 1R8; Boston(MA) (USA)'75; Ac Staff, William Osler Health System - Etobicoke General Hospital; Langs: French; (416)747-3554; Fax. (416)661-0367.

SCHEIRER, Gregg D; Royal Alexandra Hosp, 10240 Kingsway NW, Edmonton AB T5H 3V9; Alb'89; CCFP; CCFP(E.M.); Staff Emerg, Royal Alexandra Hospital; (780)735-5200; Fax. (780)735-4916.

SCHEIRER, Richard N; Royal Alexandra Hosp, B308-10240 Kingsway NW, Edmonton AB T5H 3V9; Alb'93; FRCPC; EmergMed. Staff, Royal Alexandra Hospital; (780)735-4443; Fax. (780)477-4916.

SCHELBERG, Kenneth; North York Med Arts Bldg, 245-1333 Sheppard Ave E, North York ON M2J 1V1; Tor'75; FRCPC; Peds (Adolescent Medicine). Ac Staff Med/Med Dir, North York General Hospital; Ac Staff, The Hospital For Sick Children; Asst Prof Med, University of Toronto; (416)494-7676; Fax. (416)494-7676.

SCHELEW, Benjamin L; Queen Elizabeth II HSC, 1278 South Park St, Halifax NS B3H 2Y9; Dal'89; FRCPC; Anes. Staff, Queen Elizabeth II Health Sciences Centre - Victoria General Site; (902)473-2331

SCHELL, Andrew J; Peter Lougheed Centre, 3500 26 Ave NE, Calgary AB T1Y 6J4; Alb'03; FRCPC; AnatPath (Family Medicine). Staff, Peter Lougheed Centre; (403)943-4036

SCHELLENBERG, Devin D; BC Cancer Agency-Fraser Valley, 13750 96 Ave, Surrey BC V3V 1Z2; UBC'01; FRCPC; RadOncol. Staff, BC Cancer Agency Fraser Valley Centre; (604)930-4085

SCHELLENBERG, Donald W; Health Sciences Centre, 820 Sherbrook St, Winnipeg MB R3A 1R9; Man'85; Staff, Health Sciences Centre; (204)774-6511

SCHELLENBERG, Duncan A; Centre Med Metro Monk, 2376 rue Allard, Montreal QC H4E 2K9; Man'94; Staff, Centre Hospitalier de LaSalle; Langs: German; French; (514)769-9999; duncan.schellenberg@sympatico.ca.

SCHELLENBERG, John D; ALG Prof Centre, PO Box 369 Stn Main 351 Main St, Winkler MB R6W 4A6; Man'82; Ac Staff, Eden Mental Health Centre; (204)325-8115

SCHELLENBERG, Kenneth L; Squamish Med Clinic, PO Box 389 Stn Main, Squamish BC V8B 0A3; Man'67; (604)892-3535; Fax. (604)892-3545.

SCHELLENBERG, Kerri L; University of Alberta Hosp, 2E3-8440 112 St NW, Edmonton AB T6G 2B7; Sask'02; FRCPC; Neur. Staff, University of Alberta Hospital; (780)407-3638; Fax. (780)407-1325.

SCHELLENBERG, R Robert; St Paul's Hosp, 8F-1081 Burrard St, Vancouver BC V6Z 1Y6; Man'71; FRCPC; IntMed (Allergic Disorders); ClinImmunol&Allergy. Ac Staff Pacific Lung Health Centre, Providence Health Care - St Paul's Hospital; Prof Med, University of British Columbia; (604)806-8818

SCHELLENBERG, William C; Westwood Clinic, 3220 Portage Ave, Winnipeg MB R3K 0Y8; Man'85; (204)832-1363; Fax. (204)896-3445.

SCHEMBRI, Paul J; 218 Meadowlark Shopping Ctr NW, Edmonton AB T5R 5W9; Alb'05; FRCSC; PlasSurg. Staff, University of Alberta Hospital; (780)438-0123; Fax. (780)438-0461.

SCHEMENAUER, Chelsea M; Associate Med Clinic, 400-20 14th St W, Prince Albert SK S6V 3K8; Sask'09; BSc; CCFP; (306)953-1684; Fax. (306)764-3091.

SCHEMITSCH, Emil H; St Michael's Orthopaedic Assoc, 800-55 Queen St E, Toronto ON M5C 1R6; Tor'84; FRCSC; OrthSurg (General Surgery). Head Div of OrthSurg, St Michael's Hospital; Staff, St Michael's Orthopaedic Associates; Prof, University of Toronto; (416)864-6003; Fax. (416)359-1601; schemitsche@smh.toronto.on.ca.

SCHEMMER, Drew C; Georgian Radiology Consultants, 115-121 Wellington St W, Barrie ON L4N 1L2; McM'95; FRCPC; DiagRad. Staff, Royal Victoria Regional Health Centre; (705)726-5759

SCHEMMER, Robert J; Wellington Med Arts Bldg, 217-121 Wellington St W, Barrie ON L4N 1L2; Wes'74; FRCPC; Derm (Cosmetic Dermatology). Langs: German; (705)726-1182; Fax. (705)726-1188.

SCHENK, Christian H; Assertive Comm Trmt Team, 711 12 St W, Vancouver BC V5Z 1M9; UBC'84; FRCPC; Psy. Staff, Vancouver General Hospital - Centennial Pavillion; Langs: Spanish; French; German; (604)675-2461

SCHENKER, Marianne; Medical Arts Bldg, 205-180 Metcalfe St, Ottawa ON K2P 1P5; Ott'62; Langs: German; French; Hungarian; (613)236-4703; Fax. (613)237-4704.

SCHEP, Gerald N; Medical Arts Bldg, 204B-581 Davis Dr, Newmarket ON L3Y 2P6; Wes'81; FRCPC; IntMed; Gastroent. Staff, Southlake Regional Health Centre; Langs: French; (905)898-3710; Fax. (905)898-4401.

SCHEPANSKY, Alexandra; Cross Cancer Institute, 11560 University Ave NW, Edmonton AB T6G 1Z2; Tor'81; FRCSC; ObstGyn (Gynecologic Oncology). Dir Dept of Gyn, Cross Cancer Institute; Staff Community Services Centre, Royal Alexandra Hospital; Assoc Prof Gyn, University of Alberta; Langs: Ukrainian; (780)432-8560; Fax. (780)432-8333.

SCHER, Kim E; Douglas Med Centre, 7-238 Bertie St, Fort Erie ON L2A 1Z3; Cape Town (South Africa)'95; MB ChB; CCFP; Assoc Prof Family Med, McMaster University; Assoc Prof Family Med, Queen's University; Langs: Afrikaans; (905)871-1220; Fax. (905)871-1221.

SCHERBARTH, Sandra E; Riveside Prof Centre, 31 Riverside Dr, Sydney NS B1S 3N1; Man'00; CCFP; Staff, Cape Breton Healthcare Complex; (902)270-3514; Fax. (902)562-5848.

SCHERER, Gilles; Clinique Psychiatrie, 190 rue Labonte, Longueuil QC J4H 2P7; Mon'79; FRCPC; Psy. dép Chef, Hopital Charles LeMoyne; Langs: English; (450)466-5453

SCHERER, Jacques; Centre Med Samson, 202-4599 boul Samson, Laval QC H7W 2H2; Mon'84; Staff, Hôpital du Sacre-Coeur de Montréal; Staff, CSSS St-Jerôme; Langs: English; (450)688-7170; Fax. (450)688-3335.

SCHERER, Nita; Kilborn Med Centre, 215-1385 Bank St, Ottawa ON K1H 8N4; Wes'98; ABOtol; FRCSC; Otol. Staff, Montfort Hospital; Staff, Children's Hospital of Eastern Ontario (CHEO); Consultant, The Ottawa Hospital - General Campus; Court Staff, Bruyère Continuing Care - Saint-Vincent Hospital; Langs: French; (613)562-9000; Fax. (613)562-9898.

SCHERRER, Jacques; Hotel-Dieu de Levis, 143 rue Wolfe, Levis QC G6V 3Z1; Laval'73; FRCPC; DiagRad. Staff, Hôtel-Dieu de Lévis; (418)835-7101; Fax. (418)835-7169.

SCHERRER, Louis-Philippe; Inst Univ Cardiol & Pneumol de, 2725 ch Sainte-Foy, Quebec QC G1V 4G5; Laval'07; DiagRad. Staff, Institut Universitaire Cardiologie & Pneumologie de Quebec; (418)656-8711

SCHERTZER, Robert M; West Coast Glaucoma Centre, 1416-750 Broadway W, Vancouver BC V5Z 1J4; Dal'88; FRCSC; Ophth (Anterior Segment Surgery). Assoc Staff UBC Eye Care Centre, Vancouver General Hospital - Centennial Pavillion; Assoc Prof Ophth, University of British Columbia; Langs: French; (604)873-3937; Fax. (604)873-2937; iguy@interchange.ubc.ca.

SCHERTZER, Stephen J; 1100-1200 73rd Ave W, Vancouver BC V6P 6G5; Sher'83; FRCPC; Psy (Mood Disorders). Staff, Vancouver General Hospital - Centennial Pavillion; Teach Staff Psy, University of British Columbia; Langs: French; (604)267-3034

SCHESKE, Glenn A; Vernon Radiological Assoc Inc, 3100 35 Ave, Vernon BC V1T 2T2; Man'70; FRCPC; DiagRad. Ac Staff, Vernon Jubilee Hospital; (250)545-0747

SCHETTINI VAVAL, Florence A M M; UMF de Repentigny, 135 boul Claude-David, Repentigny QC J6A 1N6; (Haiti)'83; (450)654-2911

SCHEUERMEYER, Frank J; St Paul's Hosp, 1081 Burrard St, Vancouver BC V6Z 1Y6; Alb'02; CCFP; CCFP(E.M.); Staff, Providence Health Care - St Paul's Hospital; Langs: German; (604)682-2344

SCHEUFLER, Peter W; 500-165 Dundas St W, Mississauga ON L5B 2N6; Tor'88; FRCSC; ObstGyn. Consultant, Trillium Health Centre - Mississauga; Langs: German; (905)896-1244; Fax. (905)896-1290.

SCHICK, Elizabeth L; Northwest Edmonton Mall Clinic, 2-17303 Stony Plain Rd NW, Edmonton AB T5S 1B5; Alb'98; CCFP; (780)484-0800; Fax. (780)484-0907.

SCHICK, Erik; Hop Maisonneuve-Rosemont, 5415 boul de l'Assomption, Montreal QC H1T 2M4; Louvain (Belgium)'65; FRCSC; Urol (Incontinence). Staff, Hopital Maisonneuve-Rosemont; ac Staff, Hôpital Ste-Justine; (514)252-3400; Fax. (514)252-3561; eschick@videotron.ca.

SCHICK, Judith E; Primrose Med Centre, 8436 182 St NW, Edmonton AB T5T 1Y7; Alb'73; (780)487-7532; Fax. (780)487-8862.

SCHIEBEL, Nicola E E; South Health Campus, 4448 Front St SE, Calgary AB T3M 1M4; Alb'86; FRCPC; EmergMed. Staff, Foothills Medical Centre; Staff, South Health Campus; (403)956-3000

SCHIECK, David O; Dawson Road Family Med Clinic, 83 Dawson Rd, Guelph ON N1H 1B1; Qns'94; CCFP; Staff, Guelph General Hospital; (519)766-1360; Fax. (519)763-4315.

SCHIEDA, Nicola; The Ottawa Hosp-Civic Campus, C1-1053 Carling Ave, Ottawa ON K1Y 4E9; Ott'06; FRCPC; DiagRad. Staff, The Ottawa Hospital - Civic Campus; (613)722-7000

SCHIEDEL, Jonathan J; Happy Valley Family Hlth Team, PO Box 1120 Stn Main 268 Maiden Lane, St Marys ON N4X 1B7; McM'02; CCFP; CCFP(E.M.); (519)284-3450; Fax. (519)284-4471; jschiedel@stmmc.ca.

SCHIELDROP, Peter; CFB Esquimalt-Hlth Serv Ctre, PO Box 17000 Stn Forces 1200 Colville Rd, Victoria BC V9A 7N2; London (England)'62; MB BS; DPM; FRCPC; Psy. Staff Psy, Royal Jubilee Hospital; Staff, Canadian Forces Health Services; (250)363-4411

SCHIELDROP, Philip J; Mitchell Family Doctors, PO Box 790 7 Frances St, Mitchell ON N0K 1N0; UBC'99; CCFP; CCFP(E.M.); (519)348-8402; Fax. (519)348-8400.

SCHIEMAN, Colin; St Joseph's Healthcare, T 2105 H-50 Charlton Ave E, Hamilton ON L8N 4A6; Cal'03; FRCSC; GenSurg; ThorSurg. Staff, St Joseph's Healthcare - Charlton Campus; (905)522-1155

SCHIEMAN, Steven M; 202-117 10th Ave S, Cranbrook BC V1C 2N1; Cal'00; FRCSC; Urol. Staff, University of Alberta Hospital; (250)489-8014; Fax. (250)489-8076.

SCHIFF, Benjamin Z; St Mary's Hosp Centre, 3830 av Lacombe, Montreal QC H3T 1M5; McG'87; CCFP; Staff, St Mary's Hospital Centre; adj Prof, McGill University; Langs: French; (514)734-2629; Fax. (514)734-2605; bschiff@videotron.ca.

SCHIFF, David P E; St Joseph's Healthcare, 50 Charlton Ave E, Hamilton ON L8N 4A6; Tor'73; FACP; BSc; FACR; FRCPC; DiagRad (Interventional Radiology). Ac Staff, St Joseph's Healthcare - Charlton Campus; Assoc Prof, Hamilton Health Sciences Centre - McMaster Children's Hospital; Assoc Prof, McMaster University; (905)521-6009 x3106; Fax. (905)528-1467; dpeschiff@yahoo.ca.

SCHIFF, Jeffrey; N C S B 11C-1262, 585 University Ave, Toronto ON M5G 2N2; McG'98; FRCPC; IntMed; Nephrol. Staff, Toronto General Hospital - UHN; Langs: Bilingual(French/English); (416)340-4800 x3961

SCHIFF, Karen C; St Joseph's Healthcare, 50 Charlton Ave E, Hamilton ON L8N 4A6; Ott'05; FRCPC; EmergMed. Staff, St Joseph's Healthcare - Charlton Campus; (905)522-1155

SCHIFF, Renee L; Medistat Med Familiale, 4965 rue Saint-Pierre, Roxboro QC H9H 5M9; McG'99; FRCPC; IntMed; Cardiol. Staff, Lakeshore General Hospital - Pointe Claire; (514)624-4774; Fax. (514)624-4704.

SCHIFFER, Laura J; Bayview-Finch Med Clinic, 202-3292 Bayview Ave, North York ON M2M 4J5; McM'89; FRCPC; Neur. Staff, North York General Hospital; (416)229-4179; Fax. (416)222-8088.

SCHIFFRIN, Alicia; E104-SMBD Jewish Gen Hosp, 3755 ch Cote-Sainte-Catherine, Montreal QC H3T 1E2; Buenos Aires (Argentina)'71; Endocrin (P.Q.) (Diabetes). Staff, Sir Mortimer B Davis Jewish General; Prof, McGill University; Langs: French; Spanish; Italian; (514)340-7550; Fax. (514)340-7529.

SCHIFFRIN, Ernesto L; SMBD Jewish Gen Hosp, B127-3755 Cote-Ste-Catherine, Montreal QC H3T 1E2; Buenos Aires (Argentina)'69; PhD(McG); FACP; FRCPC; IntMed (Hypertension). Médecin traitant, Sir Mortimer B Davis Jewish General; Chaire Canada Research Hypertension & Vascular Research, Lady Davies Institute; V-prés Research Dept of Med/Prof Med, McGill University; Langs: Spanish; English; (514)340-8222; Fax. (514)340-7539; ernesto.schiffrin@mcgill.ca.

SCHIFIRNET, Diana E; CSSS des Aurores-Boreales, 679 2e rue E, La Sarre QC J9Z 2X7; Mon'09; CCFP; Staff, CSSS des Aurores Boreales; (819)333-2311; diana_schifirnet@ssss.gouv.qc.ca.

SCHIFKE, William G; Elemental Prof Health Centre, 1600 Pembina Hwy, Winnipeg MB R3T 5Z2; Man'10; (204)475-1600; Fax. (204)475-1601.

SCHILLER, Daniel E; Royal Alexandra Hosp, 204-10240 Kingsway NW, Edmonton AB T5H 3V9; Wes'96; FRCSC; GenSurg; General Surgical Oncology. Staff, Royal Alexandra Hospital; (780)413-7766; Fax. (780)944-8652.

SCHILLER, Petra P; 406-1100 Sheppard Ave E, North York ON M2K 2W1; Qns'92; FRCSC; PlasSurg (Breast Surgery). Staff, North York General Hospital; (416)492-3613; Fax. (416)492-0635.

SCHIMMER, Aaron D; Univ Hlth Network-Princess M, 9 516-610 University Ave, Toronto ON M5G 2M9; Tor'93; FRCPC; IntMed (Clinician Investigator Program); Hem. Staff Clin Investigator Prog, Princess Margaret Hospital - University Health Network; (416)946-2000; aaron.schimmer@uhn.on.ca.

SCHIMPF, James; CFB Health Services Centre, PO Box 10500 Stn Forces, Edmonton AB T5J 4J5; Alb'01; CCFP; Staff, Covenant Health - Grey Nuns Community Hospital; Staff, CFB Health Services Centre; (780)973-4011; Fax. (780)973-1651; james.schimpf@canadianforces.gc.ca.

SCHINCARIOL, Holly P; Teen Health Centre, 1585 Ouellette Ave, Windsor ON N8X 1K5; Wes'97; CCFP; FCFP; (519)253-8481

SCHINDLE, Rebecca L; Health Sciences Centre, GF201-820 Sherbrook St, Winnipeg MB R3A 1R9; Ott'03; FRCPC; EmergMed. Staff, Health Sciences Centre; (204)774-6511

SCHINDLER, David L; Cornwall Comm Hosp-McConnell, PO Box 100 Stn Main 840 McConnell Ave, Cornwall ON K6H 5S5; McG'98; Staff, Cornwall Community Hospital; (613)938-4240

SCHINSTINE, Malcolm; Calgary Lab Services, 223 9-3535 Research Rd NW, Calgary AB T2L 2K8; Staff, Calgary Laboratory Services; (403)770-3569

SCHIPPER, Harvey; St Michael's Hosp, 30 Bond St, Toronto ON M5B 1W8; Tor'72; ABIM(MedOncol); FRCPC; IntMed (Medical Oncology). Staff, St Michael's Hospital; Prof Med, University of Toronto; (416)864-5128; Fax. (416)864-5127.

SCHIPPER, Hyman M; SMBD Jewish Gen Hosp, 3755 ch Cote-Sainte-Catherine, Montreal QC H3T 1E2; McG'82; PhD(Neuroendocrin); FRCPC; Neur (Neuro Degenerative Disoder). Staff, Sir Mortimer B Davis Jewish General; Consultant, Donald Berman Maimonides Geriatric Centre; Prof Neurol & NeurSurg, McGill University; Langs: Yiddish; Hebrew; French; (514)340-8260; Fax. (514)340-7502; hyman.schipper@mcgill.ca.

SCHIPPER, Kristine M; Chesley Med Clinic, PO Box 389, Chesley ON N0G 1L0; Alb'95; BSc; CCFP; Staff, South Bruce Grey Health Services - Chesley Site; (519)363-3220; Fax. (519)363-0385.

SCHIPPER, Mitchell J; SMBD Jewish Gen Hosp, 3755 ch Cote-Sainte-Catherine, Montreal QC H3T 1E2; McG'99; CCFP; Staff, Sir Mortimer B Davis Jewish General; Langs: English; French; (514)340-8222

SCHIPPER, Shirley A; Grey Nuns Family Med Clinic, 2927 66 St NW, Edmonton AB T6K 4C1; Alb'99; CCFP; (780)342-1470; Fax. (780)490-0953; sschippe@cha.ab.ca.

SCHIRALLI, Vanna; St Michael's Hosp Heath Ctre, 4F-410 Sherbourne St, Toronto ON M4X 1K2; Tor'82; CCFP; FCFP; Staff, St Michael's Hospital; Asst Prof, University of Toronto; Langs: Italian; (416)867-3728; Fax. (416)867-3726; v.schiralli@utoronto.ca.

SCHIRMER, Nicholas; Hawkesbury & Dist Gen Hosp, 1111 Ghislain St, Hawkesbury ON K6A 3G5; McM'08; CCFP; CCFP(E.M.); Staff, Hawkesbury & District General Hospital; (613)632-1111

SCHLACHTA, Christopher M; London HSC-University Hosp, PO Box 5339 Stn B 339 Windermere Rd, London ON N6A 5A5; McG'90; MDCM; FRCSC; GenSurg (Surgical Oncology). Med Dir Cdn Surgical Technologies & Advanced Robotics, London Health Sciences Centre - University Hospital; Prof Surg & Oncol, Schulich School of Medicine-University of Western Ontario; (519)663-3478; Fax. (519)663-3481.

SCHLAGINTWEIT, Robert; 1451 Kingsway Ave, Port Coquitlam BC V3C 1S2; UBC'85; Langs: German; (604)468-3455; Fax. (604)468-3457.

SCHLANGER, Agnes M; Kingsway Med Centre, 12-2917 Bloor St W, Etobicoke ON M8X 1B4; Semmelweis (Hungary)'79; Langs: Hungarian; (416)234-5524; Fax. (416)234-9037.

SCHLEBUSCH, Gert H G; London Road Diagnostic Clinic, 481 London Rd, Sarnia ON N7T 4X3; Orange Free State (South Africa)'80; MB ChB; CCFP; (519)344-1121; Fax. (519)344-0115.

SCHLECH III, Walter F; Queen Elizabeth II HSC, ACC 5014-1278 Tower Rd, Halifax NS B3H 2Y9; Cornell(NY) (USA)'75; FACP; ABIM; BA; FRCP; IntMed (Infectious Diseases). Ac Staff, Queen Elizabeth II Health Sciences Centre - Victoria General Site; Head Div of InfectDis, Dalhousie University; (902)473-7742; Fax. (902)473-7394; wfsiii@dal.ca.

SCHLEICH, Martin J; Adelaide Med Centre, 7-1080 Adelaide St, London ON N5Y 2N1; McM'06; CCFP; (519)850-6937; Fax. (519)601-0578.

SCHLEIFER, Maria R; 1-4195 Dundas St W, Toronto ON M8X 1Y4; Ott'80; CCFP; FCFP; Staff, St Joseph's Health Centre; (416)236-8788; Fax. (416)236-0158.

SCHLENTHER, Gunther; Associate Med Clinic, 5215 49 Ave, Ponoka AB T4J 1R5; Orange Free State (South Africa)'93; LMCC; MB ChB; Langs: German; Afrikaans; (780)352-7157; Fax. (780)352-2273.

SCHLESINGER, Robert D; SMBD Jewish Gen Hosp, 3755 ch Cote-Sainte-Catherine, Montreal QC H3T 1E2; McG'75; FRCPC; IntMed; Cardiol. Staff, Sir Mortimer B Davis Jewish General; (514)340-8222 x4850; Fax. (514)340-8117.

SCHLOEGL, Susanne C; Dr Susanne C Schloegl Inc, PO Box 159 203-566 Artisan Lane, Bowen Island BC V0N 1G0; Tor'85; (604)947-9986; Fax. (604)947-9804.

SCHLOSS, Eric H; Hys Med Centre, 504-11010 101 St NW, Edmonton AB T5H 4B9; Alb'63; FRCPC; GenPath; Derm. Ac Staff, University of Alberta Hospital; Dir DermPath/Clin Prof, University of Alberta; (780)432-0803; Fax. (780)439-4642; drschlos@telus.net.

SCHLOSS, Melvin D; MUHC-Montreal Children's Hosp, B240-2300 rue Tupper, Montreal QC H3H 1P3; UBC'66; FACS; FRCSC; Otol (Head & Neck Surgery). assoc Staff, Sir Mortimer B Davis Jewish General; assoc Staff, McGill University Health Centre - Montreal General Campus; ac Staff/Chef otol, McGill University Health Centre - Montreal Children's Hospital; Chef Dept of Otol, McGill University; (514)412-4400; Fax. (514)412-4342; melvin.schloss@mcgill.ca.

SCHLOSSER, Alexandra Y; Lakeridge Health-Oshawa, 1 Hospital Crt, Oshawa ON L1G 2B9; McG'08; CCFP; Staff, Mackenzie Richmond Hill Hospital; Staff, Lakeridge Health - Oshawa Site; (905)576-8711

SCHLOSSER, Gisela E; Penhorn Med Clinic, 120-569 Portland St, Dartmouth NS B2W 2H5; Montpellier (France)'82; CCFP; FCFP; Staff, Lillian Fraser Memorial Hospital / Primary Health Care Centre; (902)469-2579; Fax. (902)469-3386.

SCHLOSSER, Holli-Ellen; York-Finch Med Centre, 203B-2115 Finch Ave W, North York ON M3N 2V6; Tor'77; FRCSC; PlasSurg (Plastic & Reconstructive Surgery). Ac Staff, Humber River Regional Hospital - Finch Avenue Site; (416)512-8640; Fax. (416)512-8641.

SCHLOSSER, Robert J; 17-531 Atkinson Ave, Thornhill ON L4J 8L7; Tor'87; FRCPC; IntMed; Endocrin&Metab. Ac Staff, Mackenzie Richmond Hill Hospital; (905)763-8660; robert.schlosser@lmc.ca.

SCHLOSSMACHER, Michael G; Ottawa Hosp Research Institute, 1462-451 Smyth Rd, Ottawa ON K1H 8M5; Vienna (Austria)'87; ABPN; FRCPC; Neur (Movement Disorders). Staff, The Ottawa Hospital - Civic Campus; Scientist Neurosciences, The Ottawa Hospital-Research Institute; Assoc Prof Div of Neurosciences OHRI/Chair Canada Research in Parkinson Disease, University of Ottawa; Langs: German.

SCHMALFUSS, Peter E H; Goodfellow Prof Bldg, 105-170 McEwan Dr E, Bolton ON L7E 4C8; Tor'65; Ac Staff, Humber River Regional Hospital - Keele Street Site; Langs: German; Italian; French; (905)857-3260; Fax. (905)857-6276.

SCHMALTZ, Heidi N; Bridgeland Seniors' Health Cli, 1070 McDougall Rd NE, Calgary AB T2E 7Z2; McG'99; BSc; FRCPC; IntMed; GeriatricMed. Staff Senior's Health, Peter Lougheed Centre; Langs: Bilingual(English/French); (403)955-1506; Fax. (403)955-1504.

SCHMALZ, Ruth I; PO Box 72011 Rpo Sasamat, Vancouver BC V6R 4P2; UBC'89; (604)632-5769

SCHMELING, Heinrike; Alberta Children's Hosp, 2888 Shaganappi Tr NW, Calgary AB T3B 6A8; Berlin (Germany)'98; Staff Peds, Alberta Children's Hospital; (403)955-7771; Fax. (403)955-7649.

SCHMID, Josie; Prince George Surgery Ctre, 2F-500 Victoria St, Prince George BC V2L 2J9; UBC'95; FRCPC; Anes. (250)563-4077

SCHMIDT, Brian J; Health Sciences Centre, 820 Sherbrook St, Winnipeg MB R3A 1R9; Man'80; BSc(Med); FRCPC; Neur (Adult Neurology). Staff Neurol, Health Sciences Centre; Prof, University of Manitoba; (204)787-2609; Fax. (204)787-1486.

SCHMIDT, Daphne M A; Beausejour Primary Hlth Care, PO Box 550 151 1st St S, Beausejour MB R0E 0C0; Man'95; CCFP; (204)268-4966 x522; Fax. (204)268-4399; dschmidt@neha.mb.ca.

SCHMIDT, Jordan P; London HSC-Victoria Hosp, PO Box 5010 Stn B B2 412-800 Commissioners Rd E, London ON N6A 5W9; Wes'98; FRCSC; ObstGyn (Maternal Fetal Medicine). Staff, London Health Sciences Centre - Victoria Campus; Staff, St Joseph's Hospital - St Joseph's Health Care; (519)646-4062; Fax. (519)646-6213; jordan.schmidt@lhsc.on.ca.

SCHMIDT, Lawrence G; St Joseph's Family Med Centre, 346 Platt's Lane, London ON N6G 1J1; Wes'83; CCFP; FCFP; Ad Staff Privil, London Health Sciences Centre - Victoria Campus; Ad Staff Privil, Parkwood Hospital - St Joseph's Health Care; Ad Staff Privil, St Joseph's Hospital - St Joseph's Health Care; Asst Prof Family Med, University of Western Ontario; (519)672-9660; Fax. (519)672-7727.

SCHMIDT, Matthias H; Queen Elizabeth II HSC-Halifax, 3388-1796 Summer St, Halifax NS B3H 3A7; Tor'94; FRCPC; DiagRad (Neuro Radiology). Staff, Queen Elizabeth II Health Sciences Centre - Victoria General Site; (902)473-2700; Fax. (902)473-2018.

SCHMIDT, Michael; Queen Elizabeth II HSC-Infirma, 10W-1796 Summer St, Halifax NS B3H 3A7; Munich (Germany)'90; FRCPC; Anes. Staff, Queen Elizabeth II Health Sciences Centre - Victoria General Site; Staff, Queen Elizabeth II Health Sciences Centre - Halifax Infirmary Site; (902)473-5280; Fax. (902)425-7814.

SCHMIDT, Timothy; Nicola Med Dental Bldg, 201-321 Nicola St, Kamloops BC V2C 6G6; McG'89; FRCPC; IntMed. (250)377-3892

SCHMIT, Isabelle; Hopital Saint-Sacrement, 1050 ch Sainte-Foy, Quebec QC G1S 4L8; Laval'03; FRCSC; Ophth. Staff, CH St-Sacrement Ltee; Staff, Centre Hospitalier Affilié Universitaire de Québec - Hôpital du St-Sacrement; (418)682-7511; isabelle.schmit@orlo.ulaval.ca.

SCHMIT, Pierre J M; IWK Health Centre, PO Box 9700 Rpo CSC 5850-5980 University Ave, Halifax NS B3K 6R8; Paris (France)'81; Staff Diagnostic Imaging, IWK Health Centre; (902)470-8060; Fax. (902)470-7463.

SCHMITZ, Carmen J; Lighthouse Med Centre, 3-2 Main St S, Bayfield ON N0M 1G0; Cal'06; CCFP; (519)565-4141

SCHMOLZER, Georg M; Royal Alexandra Hosp, 10240 Kingsway NW, Edmonton AB T5H 3V9; Staff, Royal Alexandra Hospital; (780)735-4670; Fax. (780)735-4072.

SCHMUTZ, Gerard; CHUS-Hop Fleurimont, 3001 12e av N, Sherbrooke QC J1H 5N4; Strasbourg (France)'78; Staff, Centre Hospitalier Universitaire de Sherbrooke-Hopital Fleurimont; Prof, Universite de Sherbrooke; (819)346-1110; Fax. (819)820-6423; gerard.schmutz@usherbrooke.ca.

SCHNARE, Kevin P K; Aberdeen Hosp, 835 East River Rd, New Glasgow NS B2H 3S6; Dal'85; Staff, Aberdeen Regional Hospital; (902)752-8311; Fax. (902)752-5116.

SCHNARE, Ted D; Royal Ottawa Hlth Care Group, 1145 Carling Ave, Ottawa ON K1Z 7K4; Ott'87; CCFP; Staff Family Med, Royal Ottawa Mental Health Centre - Royal Ottawa Health Care Group; (613)722-6521; Fax. (613)761-3617.

SCHNARR, Jennifer J; Medical Bldg, 207-18 Pine St, Kitchener ON N2H 5Z8; McM'03; FRCSC; ObstGyn. Staff, Grand River Hospital - Kitchener/Waterloo Health Centre; (519)571-0822; Fax. (519)571-1210.

SCHNECK, Christopher R; Mount St Joseph Hosp, 3080 Prince Edward St, Vancouver BC V5T 3N4; Alb'92; CCFP; CCFP(E.M.); Staff, Providence Health Care - Mount Saint Joseph Hospital; (604)874-1141

SCHNEEWEISS, Suzan; The Hosp for Sick Children, 555 University Ave, Toronto ON M5G 1X8; Tor'87; FRCPC; Peds (Pediatric Emergency Medicine). Staff Emerg Ped, The Hospital For Sick Children; Asst Prof, University of Toronto; Langs: Spanish; (416)813-6232; Fax. (416)813-5043; suzan.schneeweiss@sickkids.ca.

SCHNEIDER, Alexia; Sheep River Med Clinic, PO Box 1560 Stn Main 1-74 Elizabeth St, Okotoks AB T1S 1B5; (403)938-4421; Fax. (403)938-5657.

SCHNEIDER, Carol E; WR125-735 Notre Dame Ave, Winnipeg MB R3E 0L8; Man'94; BSc; FRCS; FRCSC; ObstGyn (Maternal Fetal Medicine). Staff, Health Sciences Centre; (204)787-2995; Fax. (204)787-2920.

SCHNEIDER, Elizabeth A; Sudbury Med Centre, 304-65 Larch St, Sudbury ON P3E 1B8; Ott'82; FRCSC; Neursurg. Staff, Health Sciences North-Ramsey Lake Health Center; (705)671-1081; Fax. (705)671-1547; eschneider@hsnsudbury.ca.

SCHNEIDER, Gerd; 204-474 Holland Ave, Ottawa ON K1Y 0Z5; Tor'70; BSc; CCFP; FCFP; Staff, The Ottawa Hospital - Civic Campus; Preceptor Commun & Family Med, University of Ottawa; Langs: German; Italian; French; (613)729-1608; Fax. (613)729-1886.

SCHNEIDER, Howard; Sheppard Associates, 649 Sheppard Ave W, North York ON M3H 2S4; McG'84; CGPP; CCFP; Langs: French; (416)630-0610; Fax. (416)398-5712; h.schneider7@gmail.com.

SCHNEIDER, Johannes S J; McGuire Lake Specialist Centre, 103-571 6 St NE, Salmon Arm BC V1E 1R6; Asuncion (Paraguay)'83; FRCSC; GenSurg. Vis Consultant, Queen Victoria Hospital; Staff GenSurg, Shuswap Lake General Hospital; Langs: German; Spanish; (250)832-2006; Fax. (250)832-6637.

SCHNEIDER, Kalman M; Thistlewood Diagnostic Associa, 110-8077 Islington Ave, Woodbridge ON L4L 7X7; Tor'67; FRCPC; DiagRad. Staff Chief Radiol, William Osler Health System - Etobicoke General Hospital; (905)856-7061

SCHNEIDER, Kathleen C; 606-1 St Clair Ave E, Toronto ON M4T 2V7; Ott'88; FRCPC; Psy. Langs: Hebrew; Hungarian; (416)963-8266

SCHNEIDER, Kenneth M; Windsor Reg Cancer Centre, 2220 Kildare Rd, Windsor ON N8W 2X3; McM'87; FRCPC; RadOncol. Ac Member, Windsor Regional Hospital - Metropolitan Site; (519)253-5253; Fax. (519)971-9922.

SCHNEIDER, Margaret E; Anaesthesia Associates, 439 Park St, Kitchener ON N2G 1N4; Wes'85; FRCPC; Anes. (519)744-7361; Fax. (519)744-7363.

SCHNEIDER, Mark; Seven Oaks Gen Hosp, 2300 McPhillips St, Winnipeg MB R2V 3M3; Sask'07; CCFP; CCFP(E.M.); Staff, Seven Oaks General Hospital; (204)632-7133

SCHNEIDER, Matthias; Medical Centre, PO Box 5000 LCD 1, Medicine Hat AB T1A 8K7; (403)544-4108

SCHNEIDER, Oliver J; Royal Alexandra Hosp, 10240 Kingsway Ave NW, Edmonton AB T5H 3V9; Alb'77; Anes. Staff, Royal Alexandra Hospital; (780)735-4010; Fax. (780)735-4386.

SCHNEIDER, Prism; Foothills Med Centre, 1403 29 St NW, Calgary AB T2N 2T9; Cal'08; Staff, Foothills Medical Centre; (403)944-1110

SCHNEIDER, Rayfel; The Hosp for Sick Children, E 8253-555 University Ave, Toronto ON M5G 1X8; Witwatersrand (South Africa)'80; MB ChB; FRCPC; Peds (Pediatric Rheumatology). Staff, The Hospital For Sick Children; University of Toronto; (416)813-6228; Fax. (416)813-5230.

SCHNEIDER, Wolfgang E; Hillcrest Med Associates, 117 Jasper St, Hinton AB T7V 2A8; Man'76; CCFP; (780)865-2203; Fax. (780)865-7383.

SCHNEIDER-MACRAE, Margaret L N; Westview Med Clinic, 102-550 Carmi Ave, Penticton BC V2A 3G6; Alb'07; FRCPC; IntMed; Respir. (250)493-0887

SCHNEIDEREIT, Nathan P; 1165 Dufferin Cres, Nanaimo BC V9S 2B5; UBC'99; FRCPC; GenSurg (Colon & Rectal Surgery). Staff Colorectal Surg, Nanaimo Regional General Hospital; (250)754-3315; Fax. (250)754-3316.

SCHNEIDERMAN, David A; Smyth Med Centre, 210-1929 Russell Rd, Ottawa ON K1G 4G3; Ott'00; FRCPC; IntMed (Intensive Care); Respir. Langs: Bilingual(English/French); (613)736-1137; Fax. (613)739-1337.

SCHNEIDERMAN, Gerald; 704-60 St Clair Ave E, Toronto ON M4T 1N5; Wes'58; DPsy(McG); FRCPC; Psy. Member Bereavement Research Team, The Hospital For Sick Children; Emeritus Prof Psy & Peds, University of Toronto; Langs: Yiddish; (416)920-2218; Fax. (416)920-2110; gerald.schneiderman@utoronto.ca.

SCHNEIDERMAN, Jacob H; 921-55 Queen St E, Toronto ON M5C 1R6; Tor'74; BSc; FRCPC; Neur (Epilepsy). Assoc Prof, University of Toronto; (416)864-5506; Fax. (416)864-5636.

SCHNELL, Frank N; Maternal Child Clinic, 300-1402 8 Ave NW, Calgary AB T2N 1B8; Cal'80; FAAFP; CCFP; CCFP(E.M.); FCFP; Staff, Foothills Medical Centre; Clin Assoc Prof, University of Calgary; (403)220-0410; Fax. (403)220-0500.

SCHNELL, Gregory B; Calgary Heart Centre, 403-3280 Hospital Dr NW, Calgary AB T2N 4Z6; Wes'94; FRCPC; IntMed; Cardiol. Staff, Foothills Medical Centre; Staff, Health Research Innovation Centre; (403)521-2227; Fax. (403)283-6360.

SCHNEPF, Trevor; 1-5026 50 St, Red Deer County AB T4S 1P3; (Other Foreign)'06; (403)887-2221

SCHNIDER, Denise L; Terrace Hill Med Clinic, 208-217 Terrace Hill St, Brantford ON N3R 1G8; McM'83; FRCSC; GenSurg. Ac Staff, The Brant Community Healthcare System - Brantford General Hospital Site; (519)759-1914; Fax. (519)759-3605.

SCHNORE, Stephen K; Ninth Valley Family Practice, 1-10 Waterloo St, New Hamburg ON N3A 1V5; Wes'81; CCFP; FCFP; (519)662-1551; Fax. (519)662-1402.

SCHNURR, Clare M; Manotick Med Centre, PO Box 580 Stn Main 5492A South River Rd, Manotick ON K4M 1A5; McM'91; MSc; CCFP; (613)692-2571; Fax. (613)692-0271.

SCHNURR, Joseph A; InspireHealth-Southern Interio, 123-565 Bernard Ave, Kelowna BC V1Y 8R4; Sask'83; (250)861-7125

SCHNURR, Lawrence P; 17 Lakeshore Dr PO Box 1360, Morrisburg ON K0C 1X0; Qns'73; FRCPC; IntMed. Staff, Winchester District Memorial Hospital; Staff Chief, Kemptville District Hospital; (613)543-4550; Fax. (613)543-4550.

SCHOALES, Blair R; West Arthur Place, 302-1265 Arthur St E, Thunder Bay ON P7E 6E7; McM'82; FRCSC; Ophth. Staff, Thunder Bay Regional Health Sciences Centre; (807)623-3744; Fax. (807)622-6885.

SCHOEFFNER, Wolfgang V; Hôpital de l'Enfant-Jésus RHSJ, 1 boul St-Pierre O, Caraquet NB E1W 1B6; Heildelberg (Germany)'70; Staff, Hôpital de l'Enfant-Jésus RHSJ; (506)726-2185

SCHOEMAN, Corne S; Bradbrooke Med Clinic, 273 Bradbrooke Dr, Yorkton SK S3N 3L3; (306)782-3627; Fax. (306)782-3628.

SCHOEMAN, Hendrik N; Lakeridge Health Corp-Oshawa, 1 Hospital Crt, Oshawa ON L1G 2B9; Orange Free State (South Africa)'97; MB ChB; CCFP; Staff, Lakeridge Health - Oshawa Site; Staff, Lakeridge Health - Bowmanville Site; Langs: Afrikaans; (905)576-8711

SCHOEMAN, Meyer; Innisfail Med Clinic, 5031 49 St, Innisfail AB T4G 1A4; Pretoria (South Africa)'99; MB ChB; Langs: Afrikaans; (403)227-3356; Fax. (403)227-2702; shoemie@hotmail.com.

SCHOEMAN, Stefan; Comox Valley Med Clinic, 19-1599 Cliffe Ave, Courtenay BC V9N 2K6; Orange Free State (South Africa)'95; MB ChB; CCFP; CCFP(E.M.); Associate Critical Care, Regina General Hospital; Physician Emerg Room, St Joseph's General Hospital; Langs: Afrikaans; Dutch; (250)898-0202; Fax. (250)334-1597.

SCHOENROTH, Leeanne J; Tom Baker Cancer Centre, 1331 29 St NW, Calgary AB T2N 4N2; Sask'90; FRCPC; IntMed; Rheum. Staff, Tom Baker Cancer Centre; (403)521-3093; Fax. (403)283-1651.

SCHOFFER, Kerrie L; Medical Arts Bldg, 401-5880 Spring Garden Rd, Halifax NS B3H 1Y1; Sask'99; FRCPC; Neur (Movement Disorders). Asst Prof, Dalhousie University; (902)407-3100; Fax. (902)407-3101.

SCHOFIELD, Aurel J; Ctr de Formation Medicine, 165 Massey Ave, Moncton NB E1A 3E9; Laval'78; CCFP; FCFP; Staff, Dr Georges-L-Dumont University Hospital Centre; Dir/Sr Associate Ctre de Formation Med du New Brunswick, Universite de Moncton; (506)863-2249; Fax. (506)863-2284; aurel.schofield@umoncton.ca.

SCHOFIELD, Grant M; Golden Opportuniy Med Clinic, PO Box 1320, Wabasca AB T0G 2K0; Staff, Foothills Medical Centre; Staff, Golden Opportuniy Medical Clinic; (780)865-2203; grant.schofield@albertahealthservices.ca.

SCHOFIELD, John E; PO Box 508, Armstrong BC V0E 1B0; Liverpool (England)'64; MB ChB; Staff, Vernon Jubilee Hospital; (250)546-3148; Fax. (250)546-3166.

SCHOFIELD, Lee M; St Lawrence Health Centre, 1F 3-140 The Esplanade, Toronto ON M4X 1K2; Tor'07; CCFP; Staff, Women's College Hospital; Staff, St Michael's Hospital; (416)864-6000

SCHOFIELD, Michel M E; Univ Hlth Network-Toronto Western Hosp, 2E 422-399 Bathurst St, Toronto ON M5T 2S8; McM'84; MSc(Pharmacol.); Staff, Toronto Western Hospital - University Health Network; (416)603-5881; Fax. (416)603-5392.

SCHOFIELD, Sally A; North York Gen Hosp, 4001 Leslie St, North York ON M2K 1E1; Cal'90; FRCPC; Psy. Staff, North York General Hospital; (416)756-6951; Fax. (416)756-6671.

SCHOGT, Barbara; 302-481 University Ave, Toronto ON M5G 2E9; Tor'81; FRCPC; Psy. Langs: Dutch.

SCHOKKING, Ian D; 3-1230 Alward St, Prince George BC V2M 7B1; Tor'85; MSc(Epidemiol.); CCFP; FCFP; Consultant Psychogeriatric, University Hospital of Northern British Columbia; Clin Instructor Family Med, University of British Columbia; Langs: Dutch; French; Urdu; Nepali; (250)562-1231; Fax. (250)562-1207.

SCHOLES, Lawrence C; Brant Community HC-Brantford, 200 Terrace Hill St, Brantford ON N3R 1G9; Tor'95; Anes. Staff, The Brant Community Healthcare System - Brantford General Hospital Site; (519)751-5508; Fax. (519)751-5550.

SCHOLES, Michelle L; 206-1206 Centre St, Thornhill ON L4J 3M9; McM'03; CCFP; (905)907-9998; Fax. (905)907-9098.

SCHOLEY, James W; Univ Hlth Network-Toronto Gen, 8N 859-200 Elizabeth St, Toronto ON M5G 2C4; UBC'80; FRCPC; IntMed; Nephrol. Staff, Toronto General Hospital - UHN; (416)340-5093; Fax. (416)340-4999.

SCHOLEY, Janis K; Lions Gate Hosp, 231 15th St E, North Vancouver BC V7L 2L7; UBC'83; FRCPC; GenPath. Staff, Lions Gate Hospital; (604)984-5761

SCHOLL, Matthew L; Family Health Centre, 200-2462 Howard Ave, Windsor ON N8X 3V6; Wes'92; CCFP; Staff, Hôtel-Dieu Grace Hospital; Court Staff, Windsor Regional Hospital - Metropolitan Site; Physician Plant, Ford Motor Company; (519)258-4293; Fax. (519)258-4456; mscholl1@cogeco.ca.

SCHOLLENBERG, Edmund G A; College Of Phys & Surg Of NB, 300-1 Hampton Rd, Rothesay NB E2E 5K8; Man'76; BSc(Med); DAB; FAAP; LLB; FRCPC; Peds. Registrar, College of Physicians & Surgeons of New Brunswick; (506)849-5050; Fax. (506)849-5069; info@cpsnb.org.

SCHOLTEN, Monique C; Community Mental Health Ctre, 65 Brunswick St, Fredericton NB E3B 1G5; Dal'03; FRCPC; Psy. Physician, Mental Health Centre; (506)453-2132

SCHOLTEN, Vicki; Centre Hosp de LaSalle, 8585 Terr Champlain, LaSalle QC H8P 1C1; Mem'06; FRCPC; Peds. Staff, Centre Hospitalier de LaSalle; (514)362-8000 x32820

SCHOLTENS, Hendrik A; Carlisle Med Centre, PO Box 311 1493 Centre Rd, Carlisle ON L0R 1H0; Wes'69; CCFP; FCFP; Staff, Hamilton Health Sciences Centre - McMaster Children's Hospital; Court Staff, St Joseph's Healthcare - Charlton Campus; Court Staff, Joseph Brant Memorial Hospital; Asst Prof, McMaster University; Langs: Dutch; (905)689-3301; Fax. (905)689-5772.

SCHOLTENS, Martina; Bridge Clinic, 2450 Ontario St, Vancouver BC V5T 4T7; UBC'00; CCFP; (604)709-6540; Fax. (604)879-9173.

SCHOLTZ, Martin M; PO Box 2907, Smithers BC V0J 2N0; Orange Free State (South Africa)'85; MB ChB; Langs: Afrikaans; (250)847-3097; Fax. (250)847-3320; broadwayclinic@telus.net.

SCHOLTZ, Mervin; The Clinic at Walmart, 620-8249 Eagle Landing Pky, Chilliwack BC V2R 0P9; Orange Free State (South Africa)'98; MB ChB; DOHS; CCFP; Langs: Afrikaans; (877)514-8482

SCHOLZ, John F; Bluewater Health-Norman Site, 89 Norman St, Sarnia ON N7T 6S3; Wes'74; FRCPC; Psy (Inpatient Psychiatry). Staff, Bluewater Health - Norman Site; (519)464-4500 x5304; Fax. (519)464-4516.

SCHONBACH, Karen M; 504-1407 Yonge St, Toronto ON M4T 1Y7; McM'83; Psy (AIDS/HIV). (416)968-6222

SCHONBERGER, Lawrence S; Four Corners Med Bldg, 304-2009 Long Lake Rd, Sudbury ON P3E 6C3; Ott'76; DABOphph; FRCSC; Ophth. Ac Staff, Health Sciences North-St Joseph's Health Centre; (705)560-6740; Fax. (705)560-6744.

SCHONDORF, Ronald; SMBD Jewish Gen Hosp, 3755 ch Cote-Sainte-Catherine, Montreal QC H3T 1E2; McG'84; FRCPC; Neur. Staff, Sir Mortimer B Davis Jewish General; (514)340-8222 x2399; Fax. (514)340-7567.

SCHONFELD, Irving B; 406-5885 ch Cote-des-Neiges, Montreal QC H3S 2T2; McG'76; ClinImmunol&Allergy; Peds. Att Staff, Sir Mortimer B Davis Jewish General; Att Staff, McGill University Health Centre - Montreal Children's Hospital; McGill University; Langs: French; (514)731-0772; Fax. (514)731-3026; schon@videotron.ca.

SCHONKEN, Willem P; Stapleford Med Clinic, 372 McCarthy Blvd N, Regina SK S4R 7M2; (South Africa)'77; (306)545-3000; Fax. (306)545-5584.

SCHOOLING, David G; 57 Forsythe St, Oakville ON L6K 3R7; London (England)'63; MB BS; MRCS; LRCP; Staff, Halton Healthcare Services Corporation - Oakville Site; (905)844-4827

SCHOOMBEE, Glenda G D; Lahey Med Center, 2204-120 5th Ave W, Cochrane AB T4C 0A4; (South Africa)'97; (403)981-6000; Fax. (403)981-6001.

SCHOOMBEE, Willem; Cochrane Urgent Care, 60 Grande Boulevard W, Cochrane AB T4C 2B9; (South Africa)'97; (403)851-6000; Fax. (403)851-9056.

SCHOONBAERT, Ian C; CFB Base Medical Clinic, PO Box 9999 Stn Main 2 Field Ambulance, Petawawa ON K8H 2X3; NOSM'09; CCFP; (613)687-5511

SCHOPF, Bernie W; Dr Bernie Schopf Inc, 3-2168 McCallum Rd, Abbotsford BC V2S 6R6; Wes'92; FRCSC; GenSurg (Surgical Oncology). Staff Surg, Abbotsford Regional Hospital & Cancer Centre; Clin Instructor Surg, University of British Columbia; Langs: German; (604)854-5312; Fax. (604)854-5303.

SCHORR, Samuel; 1025-1122 4 St SW, Calgary AB T2R 1M1; McG'75; FRCPC; IntMed (Nephrology). (403)270-7575; Fax. (403)270-2164.

SCHOULS, Jacquelynn J; 103-1221 Lonsdale Ave, North Vancouver BC V7M 2H5; Alb'88; FRCSC; ObstGyn. Ac Staff, Lions Gate Hospital; (604)980-2800; Fax. (604)980-0808; lynnschouls@shaw.ca.

SCHOVANEK, Stefan P J; St Joseph's Gen Hosp, 2137 Comox Ave, Comox BC V9M 1P2; Alb'91; BMedSci; FRCPC; Psy (Geriatric Psychiatry). Staff, St Joseph's General Hospital; Consultant, Campbell River & District General Hospital; Member Geriatric Psy & Commun Psy, University of British Columbia; Langs: Bilingual(English/French); (250)339-1440; Fax. (250)339-1529.

SCHRADER, Dewi V; Children's & Women's HC of BC, 179-4480 Oak St, Vancouver BC V6H 3V4; Melbourne (Australia)'01; FRCPC; Neur (Clinician Investigator Program). Staff, BC Children's Hospital; (604)875-2345

SCHRAG, Christian H; 102-7 Glenbrook Pl SW, Calgary AB T3E 6W4; Qns'99; FRCSC; PlasSurg. Staff, Foothills Medical Centre; (403)215-5155; Fax. (403)240-4254.

SCHRAM, Carrie A; Women's College Hosp, 76 Grenville St, Toronto ON M5S 1B2; Qns'08; CCFP; Staff, Women's College Hospital; (416)323-6060; Fax. (416)323-6332.

SCHRAM, Gernot; Hopital Gen du Lakeshore, 160 av Stillview, Pointe-Claire QC H9R 2Y2; Eberhard Karl University (Other Foreign)'95; FRCPC; IntMed; Cardiol. Staff, Lakeshore General Hospital - Pointe Claire; Staff, Institut de Cardiologie de Montréal; (514)630-2225

SCHRAMM, David R; Civic Parkdale Clinic, 121-737 Parkdale Ave, Ottawa ON K1Y 1J8; Tor'83; FRCSC; Otol (Head & Neck Surgery). Att Staff, The Ottawa Hospital - Civic Campus; Assoc Prof, University of Ottawa; (613)798-5555; Fax. (613)761-4356.

SCHRAMM, William D; Squamish Gen Hosp, 38140 Behrner Dr, Squamish BC V8B 0J3; Sask'61; FRCPC; DiagRad. Staff Diag Imag, Squamish General Hospital / Hilltop House; Staff, Pemberton Health Centre; Physician, Whistler Health Care Centre; (604)892-6033; Fax. (604)892-6072; schramm@pembertonsurgery.co.uk.

SCHREADER, Alicia G; Bluewater Area Family Hlth Tea, PO Box 98 43 Main St W, Zurich ON N0M 2T0; McM'89; CCFP; (519)236-4314; Fax. (519)236-7508; alicia@womenshealthclinic.co.uk.

SCHREIBER, Julie; Clinique Med de l'Hetriere, 201-3520 rue de L'Hêtriére, Quebec QC G3A 0B4; Laval'01; CCFP; Staff, Centre Hospitalier de Gaspe; Staff, Inuulitsivik Health Centre; (418)651-3933; Fax. (819)988-2434; julie_schreiber@hotmail.com.

SCHREIBER, Martin; St Michael's Health Centre, 9F 133-61 Queen St E, Toronto ON M5C 2T2; Tor'87; FRCPC; IntMed; Nephrol. Staff Physician, St Michael's Hospital; Prof Med, University of Toronto; (416)867-7454; Fax. (416)867-3720; m.schreiber@utoronto.ca.

SCHREIBER, Richard A; Children's & Women's HC of BC, K4 200-4480 Oak St, Vancouver BC V6H 3V4; McG'81; FRCPC; Peds (Gastroenterology). Clin Prof, BC Children's Hospital; University of British Columbia; (604)875-2332; Fax. (604)875-3244.

SCHREIBER, William E; Vancouver Gen Hosp, 855 12th Ave W, Vancouver BC V5Z 1M9; Baylor College of Medicine (TX) (USA)'79; ABPath(ClinPath); Consultant Path, Vancouver General Hospital - Centennial Pavillion; Consultant Path, BC Cancer Agency Vancouver Centre; Prof, University of British Columbia; (604)875-4111 x68204; Fax. (604)875-4025; william.schreiber@vch.ca.

SCHREIBER, Yoko S; The Ottawa Hosp-Civic Campus, CPC470-1053 Carling Ave, Ottawa ON K1Y 4E9; Dal'05; FRCPC; InfectDis; IntMed. Staff, The Ottawa Hospital - Civic Campus; (613)737-8899

SCHREIER, Gil J; London HSC-Victoria Hosp, E1406A-800 Commissioners Rd E, London ON N6A 5W9; Tor'96; CCFP; Staff, London Health Sciences Centre - Victoria Campus; Langs: Hebrew; French; (519)685-8500 x57918; Fax. (519)385-8456.

SCHREVE, Siegfried E; Chetwyn Centre Med Clinic, PO Box 1485 5121 47 Ave, Chetwynd BC V0C 1J0; Stellenbosch (South Africa)'78; MB ChB; (250)788-3234; Fax. (250)788-3237.

SCHRICKER, Thomas P S; MUHC-Royal Victoria Hosp, C5 05-687 av des Pins O, Montreal QC H3A 1A1; Erlangen (Germany)'91; Staff, McGill University Health Centre - Royal Victoria Hospital; (514)934-1934 x34883; Fax. (514)843-1698; thomas.schricker@mcgill.ca.

SCHRIEFERS, Harald M; West Oaks Med Centre, 310-32700 South Fraser Way, Abbotsford BC V2T 4M5; Berlin (Germany)'97; (604)557-9938

SCHRIEMER, Ronnald; Spall Med Centre, 150-1940 Harvey Ave, Kelowna BC V1Y 8J8; Stellenbosch (South Africa)'86; MB ChB; Staff, Kelowna General Hospital; (250)860-9909; Fax. (250)860-9906.

SCHRIVER, Christine M; Primary Health Care Centre, 155-346 John St N, Arnprior ON K7S 2P6; Tor'89; CCFP; (613)623-4273; Fax. (613)623-8269.

SCHROEDER, Adele M; Royal Inland Hosp, 311 Columbia St, Kamloops BC V2C 2T1; UBC'00; CCFP; Staff, Royal Inland Hospital; (250)372-1004

SCHROEDER, Alvin N; Assiniboine Clinic, 633 Lodge Ave, Winnipeg MB R3J 0S9; Man'78.

SCHROEDER, Benjamin D; 32-15300 105 Ave, Surrey BC V3R 6A7; Tor'06; FRCPC; IntMed; Endocrin&Metab. (604)584-3669

SCHROEDER, Garry C B; CancerCare Manitoba, 675 McDermot Ave, Winnipeg MB R3E 0V9; Man'85; FRCPC; RadOncol. Staff, CancerCare Manitoba; (204)787-2173; Fax. (204)786-0194; garry.schroeder@cancercare.mb.ca.

SCHROEDER, Maria-Louise; CancerCare Manitoba, 2011-675 McDermot Ave, Winnipeg MB R3E 0V9; Man'66; Peds (Hematology & Bone Marrow Transplant). Dir HLA Lab/Pediatric Bone Marrow Transplant, CancerCare Manitoba; Prof Peds, University of Manitoba; Langs: French; German; (204)787-7095; Fax. (204)787-2226; marlis.schroeder@cancercare.mb.ca.

SCHROTER, Heidemarie; East Calgary Health Centre, 4715 8 Ave SE, Calgary AB T2A 3N4; Berlin (Germany)'75; FRCPC; Peds. Assoc Staff, Alberta Children's Hospital; Asst Prof, University of Calgary; Langs: German; (403)955-1077; Fax. (403)955-1076.

SCHUBERT, Edward P; Royal University Hosp, 103 Hospital Dr, Saskatoon SK S7N 0W8; Cal'04; FRCPC; Anes. Staff, Royal University Hospital; (306)655-1183; Fax. (306)655-1279.

SCHUBERT, Harold E; UBC Hosp, 2211 Wesbrook Mall, Vancouver BC V6T 2B5; UBC'77; Staff Emerg, UBC Hospital - Koerner Pavillion; (604)822-7662; Fax. (604)822-7573.

SCHUBERT, John D; 234-20 Perron St, St Albert AB T8N 1E4; Alb'75; (780)458-8400; Fax. (780)458-8402.

SCHUBERT, Matthew; Wall Street Med Centre, 370-140 Wall St, Saskatoon SK S7K 1N4; Sask'89; FRCSC; ObstGyn (Prenatal Care). Physician, Wall Street Medical Centre; Asst Prof, University of Saskatchewan; (306)652-4331; Fax. (306)242-4855.

SCHUBERT, Peter J; Thunder Bay Reg HSC-Thunder Ba, 980 Oliver Rd, Thunder Bay ON P7B 6V4; UBC'94; FRCPC; Psy. Staff, Thunder Bay Regional Health Sciences Centre; (807)684-6453; Fax. (807)684-5868.

SCHUBERT, Roderick A; Lakeside Med Clinic, 3919 8th St E, Saskatoon SK S7H 5M7; Sask'05; CCFP; Physician, Lakeside Medical Clinic; (306)374-6884; Fax. (306)374-2552.

SCHUCH, Werner; 202-3005 30 St, Vernon BC V1T 9J5; Pretoria (South Africa)'96; MB ChB; BSc(Hons.Pharm.); CCFP; Staff, Vernon Jubilee Hospital; (250)542-1353; Fax. (250)542-2717.

SCHUCK, Matthew J; Foothills Family Med Centre, PO Bag 460 114 1st St SW, Black Diamond AB T0L 0H0; Sask'02; BSc; CCFP; Clin Assoc Prof, University of Calgary; (403)933-4368; Fax. (403)933-2026.

SCHUENEMANN, Holger J; Clinical Epidemiology & Biosta, 2C16-1280 Main St W, Hamilton ON L8N 4K1; Hannover Medical School (Other Foreign)'93; FRCPC; IntMed. Staff Academic Practice, Hamilton Health Sciences Centre - McMaster University Medical Centre; Langs: German; Italian; (905)525-9140

SCHUH, Andre C; Univ Hlth Network-Princess M, 5 205-610 University Ave, Toronto ON M5G 2M9; Tor'83; FRCPC; IntMed; Hem. Sr Scientist, Princess Margaret Hospital - University Health Network; Langs: German; (416)946-6518; Fax. (416)946-6546.

SCHUH, Suzanne; The Hosp for Sick Children, 555 University Ave, Toronto ON M5G 1X8; Tor'77; FAAP; AB(EmergMed.); FRCPC; Peds (Pediatric Emergency Medicine). Staff Emerg Med, The Hospital For Sick Children; Prof Peds, University of Toronto; Langs: Czech; (416)813-6239; Fax. (416)815-5043; suzanne.schuh@sickkids.ca.

SCHULD, Richard L; Professional Corp, 931 19 St S, Lethbridge AB T1J 3H5; Alb'71; FRCPC; IntMed (Cardiology). Staff, Chinook Regional Hospital; Staff Teacher, University of Calgary; (403)328-0693; Fax. (403)328-0619.

SCHULDHAUS, Dianne E; Yellowbird Family Clinic, 3380 Gateway Blvd NW, Edmonton AB T6J 6V1; Alb'93; BSc(Biology); BA; CCFP; (780)434-2893; Fax. (780)435-1057; dschuldhaus@ybfc.com.

SCHULER, Trevor D; Hys Med Centre, 400-11010 101 St NW, Edmonton AB T5H 4B9; Sask'01; FRCSC; Urol. (780)441-2586; Fax. (780)990-7091.

SCHULL, Michael J; Sunnybrook Hlth Sciences Ctre, G147-2075 Bayview Ave, Toronto ON M4N 3M5; Qns'88; FRCPC; EmergMed. Staff Clinical Epidemiology, Sunnybrook Health Sciences Centre; Staff, Women's College Hospital; Langs: French; (416)480-6100 x3793; Fax. (416)480-6048.

SCHULLER, Deborah R; 302-49 St Clair Ave W, Toronto ON M4V 1K6; McM'85; FRCPC; Psy (Industrial Occupational Medicine). Langs: French.

SCHULMAN, Judy L; JBS Medical Centre, 420-1420 Burnhamthorpe Rd, Mississauga ON L4X 2Z9; Wes'85; (905)625-1619; Fax. (905)625-9362.

SCHULMAN, Sam; Hamilton HS-General Site, 611-237 Barton St E, Hamilton ON L8L 2X2; Stockholm (Sweden)'77; PhD; FRCPC; IntMed (Hematology). Staff Thrombosis Service, Hamilton Health Sciences Centre - Hamilton General Hospital; Staff, Thrombosis Service McMaster Clinic; Prof Med, McMaster University; (905)527-4322; Fax. (905)521-1551; schulms@mcmaster.ca.

SCHULSON, Nicholas G; The Family Practice Clinic, 2778A 104th St, Nanaimo BC V9T 2E4; UBC'72; (250)758-1711; Fax. (250)758-2802.

SCHULTE, Conrad; 10-420 King St, Spruce Grove AB T7X 2C7; Alb'88; BSc; Staff, Westview Health Centre; (780)960-1900; Fax. (780)960-1901.

SCHULTE, Paul A; Regina Qu'Appelle Hlth Region, 1440 14th Ave, Regina SK S4P 0W5; Cal'87; DABR; FRCPC; DiagRad. Staff Radiol & Ultrasound, Regina General Hospital; Assoc Prof, University of Saskatchewan; (306)766-4125; Fax. (306)766-4838.

SCHULTZ, John A; Port Health Clinic, 7-600 Ontario St, St Catharines ON L2N 7H8; Tor'82; (905)684-6066; Fax. (905)684-6317.

SCHULTZ, Karen W; Family Med Centre, PO Box 8888 Stn Main 220 Bagot St, Kingston ON K7L 5E9; Qns'83; CCFP; FCFP; Assoc Staff, Kingston General Hospital; Assoc Staff, Hotel-Dieu Hospital; Queen's University; (613)533-9303; Fax. (613)530-9877.

SCHULTZ, Kirk; A119-4480 Oak St, Vancouver BC V6H 3V4; University of Nebraska Medical Center (USA)'82; Staff HemOncol/Bone Marrow Transplant, BC Children's Hospital; Dir, Childhood Cancer & Blood Research; Prof Peds, University of British Columbia; (604)875-2406; Fax. (604)875-2911; kschultz@mail.ubc.ca.

SCHULTZ, Rodney D; Rockyview Gen Hosp, 7007 14 St SW, Calgary AB T2V 1P9; Sask'93; BSc; FRCPC; Anes. Staff, Rockyview General Hospital; Asst Prof, University of Calgary; (403)943-3410

SCHULTZ, Troy D; 201-3301 24 Ave, Vernon BC V1T 9S8; Alb'06; FRCSC; Urol. (250)542-8715

SCHULZ, Gabriella; 620 rue Paul-Limoges, Saint-Jerome QC J7Z 6Y1; Mon'88; Staff, Hôtel-Dieu de Saint-Jérôme; (450)431-6242

SCHULZ, Jan I; St Mary's Hosp Centre, 3830 av Lacombe, Montreal QC H3T 1M5; Wes'70; ABIM; AB; FACP; ClinImmunol&Allergy; IntMed (Rheumatology). Staff, Royal Victoria Regional Health Centre; Chef Div of Immunol, St Mary's Hospital Centre; assoc Prof Med, McGill University; Langs: Czech; German; French; Russian; (514)345-3511; Fax. (514)734-7401.

SCHULZ, Jane A; Royal Alexandra Hosp, 137 CSC-10240 Kingsway NW, Edmonton AB T5H 3V9; Alb'92; BSc; FRCSC; ObstGyn (Urological Gynecology). Staff, Royal Alexandra Hospital; Staff, Urogynecology Clinic; Assoc Prof ObstGyn, University of Alberta; (780)735-5290; Fax. (780)735-5896; schulz@ualberta.ca.

SCHULZ, Jeffrey D; Royal Jubilee Hosp, 1952 Bay St, Victoria BC V8R 1J8; UBC'09; CCFP; Staff, Royal Jubilee Hospital; (250)370-8000

SCHULZ, Monika; Monika Schulz Prof Corp, 2266 Woodpark Ave SW, Calgary AB T2W 2Z8; Cal'86; FRCPC; Psy (Child & Adolescent Psychiatry). Clin Teacher, University of Calgary; (403)264-3111; Fax. (403)264-0544.

SCHULZ, Valerie M N; London HSC-University Hosp, PO Box 5339 Stn B B10 123-339 Windermere Rd, London ON N6A 5A5; Qns'82; FRCPC; Anes (Pain Management). Staff, London Health Sciences Centre - University Hospital; Staff, St Joseph's Hospital - St Joseph's Health Care; Staff, London Regional Cancer Centre; Teach Staff Palliative Med, University of Western Ontario; (519)685-8500; Fax. (519)657-9840.

SCHULZE, Andreas; The Hosp for Sick Children, 555 University Ave, Toronto ON M5G 1X8; Leipzig (Germany)'87; PhD; FRCPC; Peds (Metabolic Genetics). Med Dir Newborn Screening Prog/Assoc Scientist Reserch Institute Genetics & Genomic Biol Prog/Staff Metabolic Geneticist, The Hospital For Sick Children; Assoc Prof Peds Biochem, University of Toronto; (416)813-7654; Fax. (416)813-5345.

SCHULZE, Andreas H; The Hosp for Sick Children, 555 University Ave, Toronto ON M5G 1X8; Karl Marx University of Leipzig (Germany)'75; Staff Div of Clinical & Metabolic Genetics, The Hospital For Sick Children; (416)813-1500

SCHULZE, Costas J; University of Alberta Hosp, 3H2 17-8440 112 St NW, Edmonton AB T6G 2B7; (Germany)'95; FRCSC; CardSurg. Staff Cardiac Surg, University of Alberta Hospital; (780)407-2186; Fax. (780)407-2184.

SCHULZE, Richard H; Barrie Medical Clinics, 505 Yonge St, Barrie ON L4N 4E2; Wes'71; Staff, Royal Victoria Regional Health Centre; (705)728-0037

SCHULZKUMP, Linda; Phoenix Med Centre, 403-2155 10th Ave, Prince George BC V2M 5J6; Arizona (USA)'90; Staff, Northern Health Authority; (250)563-8878

SCHUMACHER, Albert J; 3019 Tecumseh Rd E, Windsor ON N8W 1G8; Wes'82; Pres, Schumacher Research & Leadership Group; Langs: German; (519)974-5952; Fax. (519)974-6377.

SCHUMACHER, Barbara D I; University of Waterloo, 200 University Ave W, Waterloo ON N2L 3G1; Tor'74; Court Staff, Grand River Hospital - Kitchener/Waterloo Health Centre; Court Staff, St Mary's General Hospital; Dir Health Services, University of Waterloo; (519)888-4068; Fax. (519)746-5023; bschumac@uwaterloo.ca.

SCHUMACHER, Gerhard; Aberdeen Med Centre, 1966 Harrison Way, Kamloops BC V1S 1M9; UBC'82; CCFP; FCFP; Ac Staff, Royal Inland Hospital; Med Examiner Aviation Med, Ministry Of Transportation; Clin Instructor Family Med, University of British Columbia; Langs: German; (250)314-5321; Fax. (250)372-8331; gschumacher@shawbiz.ca.

SCHUMACHER, Paul A; Trail Health Centre, 303-1101 Dewdney Ave, Trail BC V1R 4T1; Tor'01; FRCSC; GenSurg. Staff, Kootenay Boundary Regional Hospital; (250)364-1188

SCHUMAN, Leanne E; George Street Family Practice, 1-1400 George St, White Rock BC V4B 4A3; UBC'94; CCFP; FCFP; (604)536-1686

SCHUMILAS, Harry B; Forest Glen Doctors Office, 700 Strasburg Rd, Kitchener ON N2E 2M2; Tor'93; CCFP; (519)578-4450; Fax. (519)579-1142.

SCHUR, Natalie K; Family Med Clinic, 1-2536 Main St, Winnipeg MB R2V 4Y1; Man'89; BSc; FAAP; FRCPC; Peds. Assoc Staff, Health Sciences Centre; Assoc Staff, St Boniface General Hospital; Assoc. Staff, University of Manitoba; (204)339-1781

SCHURCH, Walter; CHUM-Hotel-Dieu, 3840 rue Saint-Urbain, Montreal QC H2W 1T8; Bern (Switzerland)'68; AnatPath (Renal Pathology). Staff, Centre Hospitalier l'Université de Montréal (CHUM) - Hôtel-Dieu; Langs: Italian; German; English; (514)890-8102; walter.schurch.chum@ssss.gouv.qc.ca.

SCHURINGA, Peter C R; 101-751 Victoria St S, Kitchener ON N2M 5N4; Qns'91; FRCSC; OrthSurg (Hand & Upper Extremity Surgery). (519)576-0620; Fax. (519)576-5729; jips@bellnet.ca.

SCHURTER, Matthew J; 26 Church St S, Sunderland ON L0C 1H0; Qns'05; CCFP; (705)357-2336

SCHURTER, Melissa L; Two Rivers Family Health Team, 12-350 Conestoga Blvd, Cambridge ON N1R 7L7; Tor'08; CCFP; (519)629-4615; Fax. (519)629-4630.

SCHUSSLE, Olivier; Univ of Ottawa Heart Institute, 40 Ruskin St, Ottawa ON K1Y 4W7; Universite Pierre et Marie Curie (France)'98; Fellow Cardiac Surg, University of Ottawa Heart Institute; (613)761-4220

SCHUSSLER, Otto; 208 University Park Dr, Regina SK S4V 1A3; Nuevo Leon (Mexico)'71; Physician, South End Medical Clinic; (306)522-2306; Fax. (306)522-2308.

SCHUSTER, Ernst P; Misericordia Community Hosp, 1NW 15-16940 87 Ave NW, Edmonton AB T5R 4H5; Heidelberg (Germany)'81; CCFP; FCFP; Ac Staff, Covenant Health - Misericordia Community Hospital; (780)735-2585; Fax. (780)735-2588.

SCHUSTER, Lidia M; 402-1630 Pandosy St, Kelowna BC V1X 1P7; Porto Alegre (Brazil)'86; FRCPC; Psy. Staff Active Privil, Kelowna General Hospital; Langs: Portuguese; (250)712-9807; Fax. (250)712-9805.

SCHUSTER, Martin; 50 George St N, Cambridge ON N1S 2M8; McM'90; CCFP; FCFP; Langs: German; (519)740-6437; Fax. (519)623-8642.

SCHUTZ, Christian G; Institute of Mental Health, 4214-5980 University Blvd, Vancouver BC V6T 1Z3; (Germany)'91; (604)827-4362

SCHUURMAN, Irma E; Health First Med Centre, 100-15129 100 Ave, Surrey BC V3R 9P4; UBC'83; CCFP; Langs: Dutch; (604)583-3550; Fax. (604)582-2086.

SCHUURMAN, Joy C; Guelph Family Health Team, 83 Dawson Rd, Guelph ON N1H 1B1; McM'02; BSc; CCFP; (519)766-1360; Fax. (519)766-0469.

SCHUURMANS, S Nanette; Tawa Med Centre, 120-3017 66 St NW, Edmonton AB T6K 4B2; Sask'77; FRCSC; ObstGyn (Menopause). Staff Community Services Centre, Royal Alexandra Hospital; Staff, Covenant Health - Grey Nuns Community Hospital; Clin Prof, University of Alberta; (780)461-6220; Fax. (780)461-4197; nan.schuurmans@albertahealthservices.ca.

SCHWAB, Shirley A; 1022-736 Granville St, Vancouver BC V6Z 1G3; Sask'81; BSc; Clin Instructor College of Med, University of British Columbia; (604)687-7951; Fax. (604)687-7057; sschwab@telus.net.

SCHWAB-LANG, Monika E; Cedar Springs Med Centre, E-960 Cumberland Ave, Burlington ON L7N 3J6; Wes'90; CCFP; FCFP; Assoc Staff, Joseph Brant Memorial Hospital; Langs: German; (905)333-9799; Fax. (905)333-4799.

SCHWALFENBERG, Gerry K; West End Prof Bldg, 301-9509 156 St NW, Edmonton AB T5P 4J5; Alb'79; CCFP; FCFP; Staff, Covenant Health - Misericordia Community Hospital; Clin Assoc Instructor Family Practice, University of Alberta; Langs: German; (780)484-1433; Fax. (780)489-1211; gschwalf@telus.net.

SCHWALM, Jon-David R; Hamilton HS-Gen Site, C3 108-237 Barton St, Hamilton ON L8L 2X2; McM'02; FRCPC; IntMed; Cardiol. Staff, Hamilton Health Sciences Centre - Hamilton General Hospital; (905)577-1423

SCHWANDT, Michael; 8F-790 Bay St, Toronto ON M5G 1N8; Man'07; CCFP; (416)378-2588

SCHWANN, Paula G; Herold Road Family Physicians, 1-325 Herold Rd, Saskatoon SK S7V 1J7; Sask'87; CCFP; FCFP; Physician, Cumberland Medical Clinic; Clin Lecturer, University of Saskatchewan; (306)374-2404; Fax. (306)477-0300.

SCHWARCZ, Deborah; Complexe Sante Reine-Elizabeth, 2100 av Marlowe, Montreal QC H4A 3L5; McG'07; MDCM; CCFP; CCFP(E.M.); Staff, Cree Board of Health & Social Services James Bay; (514)485-5013

SCHWARTZ, Blair C; SMBD Jewish Gen Hosp, G050-3755 ch-Côte-Sainte-Cathe, Montreal QC H3T 1E2; McG'06; MDCM; FRCPC; IntMed; Critical Care Medicine. Staff, Sir Mortimer B Davis Jewish General; (514)340-8222 x4974

SCHWARTZ, Brian I; 300-480 University Ave, Toronto ON M5G 1V2; Tor'76; CCFP; CCFP(E.M.); FCFP; Dir Pre-Hospital Care, Sunnybrook Health Sciences Centre; Dir Emergency Management Support, Ontario Agency for Health; Assoc Prof Family Med, University of Toronto; (647)260-7181; bschwartz@socpc.ca.

SCHWARTZ, Caitlin J; Greenbelt Family Health Team, 1C-3500 Fallowfield Rd, Ottawa ON K2J 4A7; UBC'07; BSc(Hon.); CCFP; Staff Cross App't in Family Med & RadOncol, The Ottawa Hospital - General Campus; Lecturer, University of Ottawa; (613)843-1718

SCHWARTZ, Carol E; Sunnybrook Hlth Sciences Ctre, M 1201-2075 Bayview Ave, Toronto ON M4N 3M5; Tor'80; DAB; FRCSC; Ophth (Retina). Staff, Sunnybrook Health Sciences Centre; Staff, The Scarborough Hospital - Birchmount Campus; Asst Prof, University of Toronto; (416)480-5770; Fax. (416)480-4481.

SCHWARTZ, Clive J; Pickering Med Centre, 206-1885 Glenanna Rd, Pickering ON L1V 6R6; Witwatersrand (South Africa)'79; MB BCh; FRCPC; Peds (Developmental Pediatrics). Staff, The Hospital For Sick Children; Consultant, Rouge Valley Health System - Ajax & Pickering Health Centre Site; Asst Prof, University of Toronto; (905)420-2168; Fax. (866)846-6939; clive.schwartz@utoronto.ca.

SCHWARTZ, Daniel; 100-200 Keary St, New Westminster BC V3L 0A6; UBC'01; FRCPC; IntMed (Hypertension); Nephrol. Staff, Fraser East Nephrology Associates; (604)516-7774

SCHWARTZ, Deborah C; Regent Med Bldg, 335-2184 Broadway W, Vancouver BC V6K 2E1; McM'94; CGP; FRCPC; Psy (Group Psychotherapy). Assoc Med Dir, Group Process Research Institute; Langs: Spanish; (604)261-2445; Fax. (604)261-2447; dschwartz@groupprocess.ca.

SCHWARTZ, E Michael; Jane & Shoreham Med Centre, 104-4640 Jane St, North York ON M3N 2K5; Tor'73; CCFP; CCFP(E.M.); FCFP; Assoc Staff, Humber River Regional Hospital - Finch Avenue Site; (416)667-8900

SCHWARTZ, Earl J; 249 St Clair Ave W, Toronto ON M4V 1R3; Tor'72; (416)964-2052; Fax. (416)964-3287.

SCHWARTZ, Gwynne A; Medicine Professional Corp, 305-3024 Hurontario St, Mississauga ON L5B 4M4; Tor'82; CCFP; Staff, Trillium Health Centre - Mississauga; (905)897-1419; Fax. (905)897-1455.

SCHWARTZ, Hannah; St Mary's Hosp Centre, 3830 av Lacombe, Montreal QC H3T 1M5; McG'03; FRCPC; Psy. Staff, St Mary's Hospital Centre; (514)345-3511

SCHWARTZ, Jacqueline R; Futurity Medical, 305-745 Mount Pleasant Rd, Toronto ON M4S 2N4; Wes'08; CCFP; (416)487-2052; Fax. (416)480-2030.

SCHWARTZ, Kenneth M; Baycrest Ctre for Geriatric Ca, 4C91-3560 Bathurst St, North York ON M6A 2E1; Man'78; FRCPC; Psy. Staff, Baycrest Centre for Geriatric Care; (416)785-2500 x2882; Fax. (416)785-2450.

SCHWARTZ, Kevin; The Hosp for Sick Children, 555 University Ave, Toronto ON M5G 1X8; Tor'07; FRCPC; Peds. Staff, The Hospital For Sick Children; (416)813-6273

SCHWARTZ, Leonard D; 304-915 Grosvenor Ave, Winnipeg MB R3M 0M5; Man'98; FRCPC; Psy.

SCHWARTZ, Leonard; Univ Hlth Network-Toronto Gen, 6EN 232-200 Elizabeth St, Toronto ON M5G 2C4; Tor'64; FRCP; FRCPC; IntMed (Cardiology). Staff, Toronto General Hospital - UHN; Teach Staff Med, University of Toronto; (416)340-3933; Fax. (416)595-6441.

SCHWARTZ, Lisa C; Guelph Gen Hosp, 115 Delhi St, Guelph ON N1E 4J4; Mount Sinai School of Medicine (USA)'01; Staff, Guelph General Hospital; (519)822-5350

SCHWARTZ, Mandy S; Summeridge Health Centre, 26-8707 Dufferin St, Thornhill ON L4J 0A2; Wes'02; CCFP; (905)764-0005; Fax. (905)764-0044.

SCHWARTZ, Martin B; 305-745 Mount Pleasant Rd, Toronto ON M4S 2N4; Tor'75; Langs: Hebrew; (416)487-2052; Fax. (416)480-2030.

SCHWARTZ, Michael L; Sunnybrook Hlth Sciences Ctre, A129-2075 Bayview Ave, Toronto ON M4N 3M5; Tor'67; FRCSC; Neursurg (Radio Surgery). Staff Neuro Surg, Sunnybrook Health Sciences Centre; Prof, University of Toronto; Langs: French; (416)480-4738; Fax. (416)480-6085; m.schwartz@utoronto.ca.

SCHWARTZ, Morton L; Central Med Bldg, 103-1105 Carling Ave, Ottawa ON K1Y 4G5; Ott'77; Ac Staff, The Ottawa Hospital - Civic Campus; (613)798-7070; Fax. (613)798-7061.

SCHWARTZ, Owen D; 1205 18 Ave NW, Calgary AB T2M 0W3; Man'70; BSc; (403)457-5077; Fax. (403)457-5019.

SCHWARTZ, Patricia L T; Student Health Service, M334-2211 Wesbrook Mall, Vancouver BC V6T 1Z3; (Chile)'70; FRCPC; Psy. Ac Staff, UBC Hospital - Koerner Pavillion; Asst Prof, University of British Columbia; (604)822-7689

SCHWARTZ, Paul S; 1-1270 Walker Rd, Windsor ON N8Y 4T4; Ott'85; (519)977-9222; Fax. (519)477-9532.

SCHWARTZ, Rochelle S; Genesis Prof Group, 420-1600 Steeles Ave W, Concord ON L4K 4M2; Tor'83; CCFP; FCFP; Staff Privil, North York General Hospital; Staff Privil, Mackenzie Richmond Hill Hospital; Langs: Yiddish; (905)760-1415; Fax. (905)760-2735.

SCHWARTZ, Robert A; Children's Hosp of Eastern ON, 401 Smyth Rd, Ottawa ON K1H 8L1; Tor'03; FRCPC; Anes. Staff, Children's Hospital of Eastern Ontario (CHEO); (613)737-7600

SCHWARTZ, Roslyn T; 171 College St, Kingston ON K7L 4L9; Ott'79; CCFP; Staff, Kingston General Hospital; Staff, Hotel-Dieu Hospital; Teach Staff Med, Queen's University; Langs: French; (613)548-4396; Fax. (613)548-8011.

SCHWARTZ, Sarah B; The Hosp for Sick Children, 6415B-555 University Ave, Toronto ON M5G 1X8; McG'06; MDCM; FRCPC; Peds. Staff, The Hospital For Sick Children; (416)813-1500

SCHWARTZ, Stacey A; Nelson Place, 200-5675 Spring Garden Rd, Halifax NS B3J 1H1; McG'87; FAAP; Peds; MDCM; FRCPC; Peds. Staff, IWK Health Centre; Asst Prof, Dalhousie University; Langs: French; (902)482-3508; Fax. (902)482-6019.

SCHWARTZ, Steven M; The Hosp for Sick Children, 555 University Ave, Toronto ON M5G 1X8; Wayne State Univ (USA)'88; FRCPC; Peds (Critical Care Medicine); Cardiol. Staff Academic Practice Cardiac Critical Care, The Hospital For Sick Children; (416)813-6186; Fax. (416)813-7299; steven.schwartz@sickkids.ca.

SCHWARTZ, Thomas; Kildare Family Med Associates, 8-7005 ch Kildare, Cote Saint-Luc QC H4W 1C1; McG'84; AB; FAAP; FRCPC; Peds; Endocrin&Metab. Consultant, Sir Mortimer B Davis Jewish General; Langs: Hebrew; Hungarian; French; (514)481-7167; Fax. (514)489-5786.

SCHWARTZMAN, Kevin J; MUHC-Montreal Chest Institute, K1 23-3650 rue Saint-Urbain, Montreal QC H2X 2P4; McG'89; MPH(Harvard); FRCPC; Respir; IntMed (Public Health). Staff, McGill University Health Centre - Montreal Chest Institute; Staff, McGill University Health Centre - Royal Victoria Hospital; assoc Prof Med & Epidemiol, McGill University; Langs: Bilingual(English/French); (514)934-1934 x32153; Fax. (514)843-2083.

SCHWARZ, Duncan K; Grand River Hosp-Freeport HC, 3570 King St E, Kitchener ON N2A 2W1; McM'02; CCFP; Staff, Grand River Hospital - Kitchener/Waterloo Health Centre; (519)749-4300

SCHWARZ, Gaston; Centre Chirurgie Plastique, 1506 av Docteur Penfield, Montreal QC H3G 1B9; Ott'66; FACS; FRCSC; PlasSurg (Aesthetic Surgery). Sr Surgeon, McGill University Health Centre - Montreal General Campus; Sr Surgeon, McGill University Health Centre - Royal Victoria Hospital; assoc Prof, McGill University; Langs: Spanish; French; (514)932-8200; Fax. (514)932-6083; drgschwarz@aol.com.

SCHWARZ, Jorge A; 300-245 av Victoria, Westmount QC H3Z 2M6; Philadelphia(PA) (USA)'77; FRCSC; PlasSurg. Langs: Spanish; French; (514)938-4017; Fax. (514)938-4098.

SCHWARZ, Karl A; MUHC-Montreal Gen Hosp, L9 317-1650 av Cedar, Montreal QC H3G 1A4; George Washington Univ (USA)'01; FRCSC; PlasSurg. Staff, McGill University Health Centre - Montreal General Campus; (514)934-1934

SCHWARZ, Niels E; Nanaimo Reg Gen Hosp, 1200 Dufferin Cres, Nanaimo BC V9S 2B7; McM'92; FACP; FRCPC; IntMed. Staff, Nanaimo Regional General Hospital; Langs: Dutch; French; (250)740-6926

SCHWARZ, Peter J; Northmount Med Centre, 304-145 13th St E, North Vancouver BC V7L 2L4; Otago (New Zealand)'72; MB BCh; CCFP; CCFP(E.M.); FCFP; (604)985-1717; Fax. (604)985-1721.

SCHWARZ, Peter R; 225-275 Second Line W, Sault Ste. Marie ON P6C 2J4; Ott'93; CCFP; Langs: German; (705)256-8585

SCHWARZ, Richard J; 207-9181 Main St, Chilliwack BC V2P 4M9; Wes'85; FRCSC; GenSurg. Consultant Surg, Chilliwack General Hospital; (604)792-9338; Fax. (604)792-4413.

SCHWARZ, Robert D; IWK Health Centre, PO Box 9700 Rpo CSC 5850 University Ave, Halifax NS B3K 6R8; Columbia(NY) (USA)'69; FRCSC; Urol. Staff, IWK Health Centre; Staff, Queen Elizabeth II Health Sciences Centre - Victoria General Site; Prof Urol, Dalhousie University; (902)470-8703; Fax. (902)470-8267; robert.schwarz@iwk.nshealth.ca.

SCHWARZ, Rosemarie R; The Credit Valley Hosp, 2200 Eglinton Ave W, Mississauga ON L5M 2N1; Ott'90; FRCPC; IntMed. Staff, The Credit Valley Hospital; Langs: German; (905)813-2200 x7849; Fax. (905)813-4186; rschwarz@cvh.on.ca.

SCHWARZ, Stephan K W; Ctr for Anesthesia/Analgesia, 413A-2176 Health Sciences Mall, Vancouver BC V6T 1Z3; Gottingen (Germany)'95; FRCPC; Anes. (604)827-3680

SCHWARZ-MICHOROWSKI, Bogdan L; Guelph Comm Health Med Ctre, 3 36-125 Delhi St, Guelph ON N1E 4J5; Warsaw (Poland)'74; PhD; FACC; FACP; FRCPC; IntMed (Echocardiography); Cardiol. Staff, Guelph General Hospital; Staff, St Mary's General Hospital; McMaster University; Langs: Polish; Russian; German; (519)829-3861; Fax. (519)829-2301.

SCHWEGMANN, LLewellyn; Valleyview Health Complex, PO Box 1628, Valleyview AB T0H 3N0; Stellenbosch (South Africa)'79; (780)524-4467; Fax. (780)524-2806.

SCHWEIGEL, Robert C; Surrey Med Arts Bldg, 320-13710 94A Ave, Surrey BC V3V 1N1; UBC'92; FRCSC; OrthSurg. (604)585-8469; Fax. (604)585-8479.

SCHWEIGER, Franzjosef; Professional Arts Bldg, 405-100 Arden St, Moncton NB E1C 4B7; Tor'82; FACG; FACP; FRCPC; IntMed (Hepatology); Gastroent. Ac Staff, The Moncton Hospital; Assoc Prof, Dalhousie University; Assoc Prof, Memorial University Of Newfoundland; Langs: German; French; (506)858-8441; Fax. (506)858-0859.

SCHWEIGERT, Michael K; St Michael' Hosp, 30 Bond St, Toronto ON M5B 1W8; Tor'94; BASc; MBA; FRCPC; OccupMed. Staff Occupational & Environment, St Michael's Hospital; (416)864-5074; Fax. (416)867-3673.

SCHWEIHOFER, Eckhart H C; Bloor-Jane Med Bldg, 210-2425 Bloor St W, Toronto ON M6S 4W4; Berlin (Germany)'68; Ac Staff, St Joseph's Health Centre; Langs: German; (416)763-3023; Fax. (416)763-1230.

SCHWEITZER, Bradley H; The Medical Clinic Associates, 4794A Joyce Ave, Powell River BC V8A 3B6; Sask'84; CCFP; (250)485-6261; Fax. (250)485-2820.

SCHWEITZER, Kelly D; Hotel-Dieu Hosp, J2 019-166 Brock St, Kingston ON K7L 5G2; Sask'07; FRCSC; Ophth. Staff, Hotel-Dieu Hospital; (613)544-3310

SCHWEITZER, Mark E; The Ottawa Hosp-General Campus, 501 Smyth Rd, Ottawa ON K1H 8L6; Buffalo (USA)'86; FRCPC; DiagRad. Staff Medical Imaging, The Ottawa Hospital - General Campus; Dept Chair Radiology, University of Ottawa; (613)761-4982

SCHWEITZER, Michael J; Parkway Prof Bldg, 60 Centennial Pky S, Stoney Creek ON L8G 2C5; Tor'95; CCFP; FCFP; CCFP(E.M.); Court Staff Family Med, Hamilton Health Sciences Centre - McMaster University Medical Centre; Ac Staff Family Med, St Joseph's Healthcare - Charlton Campus; Court Staff Emerg, West Lincoln Memorial Hospital; Langs: Hebrew; (905)662-1234; Fax. (905)662-9422.

SCHWEITZER, Morris; SMBD Jewish Gen Hosp, E104-3755 ch Cote-Ste-Catherin, Montreal QC H3T 1E2; Mem'74; PhD; MD; BSc; FRCP; FRCPC; IntMed (Lipidology); Endocrin (P.Q.). Staff, Sir Mortimer B Davis Jewish General; assoc Prof Med, McGill University; Langs: French; (514)340-8090; Fax. (514)340-7529.

SCHWENTER, Frank; CHUM-Hop Notre-Dame, 1560 rue Sherbrooke E, Montreal QC H2L 4M1; Staff, Centre Hospitalier l'Université de Montréal (CHUM) - Hôpital Notre-Dame; (514)890-8000

SCHWERTFEGER, Lynne I; Timmins Family Health Team, 208-38 Pine St N, Timmins ON P4N 6K6; Tor'91; CCFP; FCFP; Staff, Timmins & District Hospital; Staff, White Pines Health Network; Langs: French; (705)264-5111; Fax. (705)267-4212.

SCIARRA, Carmela; 203-1685 Main St W, Hamilton ON L8S 1G5; McM'96; FRCSC; ObstGyn. Ac Staff ObstGyn, Hamilton Health Sciences Centre - McMaster Children's Hospital; Clinical Asst Prof ObstGyn, McMaster University; Langs: Italian; (905)308-7764; Fax. (905)308-7765.

SCIENCE, Michelle E I; The Hosp for Sick Children, 555 University Ave, Toronto ON M5G 1X8; McM'05; FRCPC; Peds; InfectDis. Staff, The Hospital For Sick Children; (416)813-7807

SCILLEY, Christopher G; London HSC-Victoria Hosp, 800 Commissioners Rd E, London ON N6A 5W9; Qns'80; FRCSC; PlasSurg (Breast Reconstruction). Staff, London Health Sciences Centre - Victoria Campus; Asst Prof, University of Western Ontario; (519)667-6755; Fax. (519)667-6643.

SCLATER, Anne L; 2405-1453 Prince Rd, Windsor ON N9C 3Z4; Mem'83; FACP; MSc; FRCP; FRCPC; IntMed; GeriatricMed. Staff Geriatric Assessment Program, Windsor Regional Hospital - Tayfour Site; (519)257-5111 x72227; Fax. (519)257-5242; asclater@cogeco.ca.

SCLATER, Kevin W; Burke Mountain Med Centre, 210-1465 Salisbury Ave, Port Coquitlam BC V3B 6J3; Cal'90; Med Dir, Crossroads Hospice; (604)941-8277; Fax. (604)941-5622.

SCOATES, Peter J; Royal Columbian Hosp, 330 Columbia St E, New Westminster BC V3L 3W7; UBC'76; DAB; FRCPC; Anes. Staff, Royal Columbian Hospital; (604)520-4602; Fax. (604)521-3298.

SCOCCHIA, Tulio G; T G Scocchia Medicine, 406-25 Charlton Ave E, Hamilton ON L8N 1Y2; McM'80; BSc(PhysTher); FRCPC; IntMed; Rheum. Staff, St Joseph's Healthcare - Charlton Campus; (905)525-0255; Fax. (905)525-9764.

SCOLNIK, Dennis; The Hosp for Sick Children, 555 University Ave, Toronto ON M5G 1X8; (Zimbabwe)'79; MSc; MB ChB; DCH; FRCPC; Peds (Pediatric Emergency Medicine). Staff Physician Emerg Services & Clin Pharmacology & Toxicology/Proj Dir Research Institute, The Hospital For Sick Children; Assoc Prof Peds & Graduate Studies, University of Toronto; Langs: Hebrew; (416)813-7500; Fax. (416)813-5043.

SCOTLAND, Catherine M; Foothills Prof Bldg, 240-1620 29 St NW, Calgary AB T2N 4L7; Alb'88; CCFP; (403)284-1844; Fax. (403)284-1847.

SCOTLAND, Newborne; Associated Med Specialists, 1555 Second Ave, Trail BC V1R 1M3; Albert Einstein (USA)'77; DABIM; FRCPC; IntMed (Hematology). (250)368-3301; Fax. (250)368-5053.

SCOTT, Amanda S; Airport Heights Med Clinic, 40 Airport Heights Dr, St. John's NL A1A 4Z7; Mem'06; CCFP; (709)579-2606

SCOTT, Andrea D; 14030 23 Ave NW, Edmonton AB T6R 3L6; (Other Foreign)'09; CCFP; (780)757-4220

SCOTT, Carol L; Unionville Family Physicians, 301-10 Unionville Gate, Markham ON L3R 0W7; Tor'83; FCBOM; DOHS; BSc; Staff Family Practice Unit, Markham Stouffville Hospital; Langs: English; French; (905)475-3121; Fax. (905)475-4270.

SCOTT, Charles F; Kingston Gen Hosp, 76 Stuart St, Kingston ON K7L 2V7; Wes'03; FRCPC; DiagRad. Staff, Hotel-Dieu Hospital; Staff, Kingston General Hospital; (613)548-2301

SCOTT, Daniel G; Grand Bay Med Clinic, PO Box 3004 Stn Main, Grnd-Bay-Wfld NB E5K 4V3; Dal'83; Ac Staff, Saint John Regional Hospital; (506)738-8426; Fax. (506)738-2946; danscott@nbnet.nb.ca.

SCOTT, Darcy J S; Stanton Terr Health Authority, PO Box 10 550 Byrne Rd, Yellowknife NT X1A 2N1; UBC'07; FRCPC; Peds. Staff, Stanton Territorial Health Authority; (867)669-4111

SCOTT, Dion; Beverly Med Clinic, 201-2763 Beverly St, Duncan BC V9L 6X2; Mem'00; BSc; CCFP; Staff, Victoria General Hospital; Staff, Vernon Jubilee Hospital; Staff Urgent Care Phys, Misericordia Health Centre; (250)597-3390; Fax. (250)597-3391; dionscott@hotmail.com.

SCOTT, Douglas F; Nipigon Health Centre, 125 Hogan Rd, Nipigon ON P0T 2J0; Man'05; CCFP; Langs: French; Italian; (807)887-1644; Fax. (807)887-1645.

SCOTT, Douglas V; Radiology Consultants Assoc, 120A-6707 Elbow Dr SW, Calgary AB T2V 0E3; Alb'88; FRCPC; DiagRad; NuclearMed. (403)777-3005; Fax. (403)777-3008.

SCOTT, Duncan A; 128 Ontario St, Kingston ON K7L 2Y4; Tor'82; FRCPC; Psy (Forensic Psychiatry). Clin Dir, Hotel-Dieu Hospital; Assoc Prof, QHC Belleville General; Providence Care - Mental Health Services; Assoc Prof Psy, Queen's University; (613)546-3116; Fax. (613)544-9793; cosmed4@bellnet.ca.

SCOTT, Elizabeth A F; University of Toronto, 554-155 College St, Toronto ON M5T 1P8; McM'80; FRCPC; CCFP; CommunMed. Assoc Med Officer of Hlth, Toronto Public Health Corporate Office; Teach Staff, University of Toronto; (416)392-7463; Fax. (416)392-0713; escott@toronto.ca.

SCOTT, Elizabeth M; Appletree Med Centre, 3001 Carling Ave, Ottawa ON K2B 7Y6; Ott'75; Staff, Queensway Carleton Hospital; Langs: French; (613)596-2323

SCOTT, F G Ellis; 502 Huron St, Stratford ON N5A 5T7; Wes'64; FRCSC; Otol. Staff, Stratford General Hospital - Huron Perth Healthcare Alliance; Staff, St Marys Memorial Hospital - Huron Perth Healthcare Alliance; (519)273-3811; Fax. (519)273-0915; dr.s@sympatico.ca.

SCOTT, Gregory T; Maple Family Health Team, 235 Gore Rd RR 2, Kingston ON K7L 5H6; Qns'86; CCFP; FCFP; Staff, Kingston General Hospital; Langs: French; (613)546-0151; Fax. (613)546-0157.

SCOTT, Heather E; Peter Lougheed Centre, 3500 26 Ave NE, Calgary AB T1Y 6J4; Sask'98; FRCPC; Psy. Staff Psy, Peter Lougheed Centre; (403)944-9750; Fax. (403)944-9787.

SCOTT, Heather M; IWK Health Centre, PO Box 9700 Rpo CSC G2141-5980 University Ave, Halifax NS B3K 6R8; Dal'88; FRCSC; ObstGyn (Maternal Fetal Medicine). Staff, IWK Health Centre; Assoc Prof, Dalhousie University; (902)420-6614; Fax. (902)425-1125; heather.scott@iwk.nshealth.ca.

SCOTT, Hugh A; Ctr Hosp Afillie-Enfant-Jesus, 1401 18e rue, Quebec QC G1J 1Z4; McM'90; CCFP; CCFP(E.M.); Staff, Centre Hospitalier Affilié Universitaire de Québec - Hôpital De L'Enfant Jésus; Langs: English; French; (418)649-5632; Fax. (418)649-5975.

SCOTT, Ian M; David Strangway Bldg, 300-5950 University Blvd, Vancouver BC V6T 1Z3; McM'91; DOHS; MSc; FRCPC; Public Health & Preventive Med;CCFP; FCFP; CommunMed. Assoc Staff, Vancouver General Hospital - Centennial Pavillion; Assoc Prof, University of British Columbia; (604)822-5431; Fax. (604)822-4069; ianscott@interchange.ubc.ca.

SCOTT, Ian M; Internal Med Associates, 215-1610 37 St SW, Calgary AB T3C 3P1; Cal'98; BSc; FRCPC; IntMed; Critical Care Medicine. Staff, Nanaimo Regional General Hospital; (403)685-9499; Fax. (403)685-9422.

SCOTT, Ian R; 100 Kingswood Dr, Fredericton NB E3B 6Z8; McG'83; FRCPC; DiagRad. Ac Staff, Dr Everett Chalmers Regional Hospital; (506)452-5141

SCOTT, J Rowan; Le Marchand Mansion, 407-11523 100 Ave NW, Edmonton AB T5K 0J8; Alb'80; FRCPC; Psy (Psychotherapy). Asst Prof, University of Alberta; (780)488-0929; Fax. (780)453-1219.

SCOTT, Jaime M; Peterborough Reg Health Centre, 1 Hospital Dr, Peterborough ON K9J 7C6; Sask'87; FRCSC; GenSurg. Staff, Peterborough Regional Health Centre - Hospital Drive; (705)743-2121

SCOTT, James L; Victoria General Hosp, 1 Hospital Way, Victoria BC V8Z 6R5; Mem'91; BSc(Hons); MSc; FRCPC; Neur (Neuro Physiology). Staff, Victoria General Hospital; Langs: Bilingual(French/English); Norwegian; (250)727-4212

SCOTT, James N; Foothills Med Centre, 1403 29 St NW, Calgary AB T2N 2T9; Tor'94; FRCPC; DiagRad (Neuro Radiology). Staff Diagnostic Imaging, Foothills Medical Centre; (403)944-1969; Fax. (403)944-2549.

SCOTT, Jason; Dauphin Med Clinic, 622 3rd St SW, Dauphin MB R7N 1R5; Man'00; CCFP; (204)638-6445; Fax. (204)638-5670; tjps@mts.net.

SCOTT, Jeanette M; Queen Elizabeth II HSC-Victori, 10W-1276 South Park St, Halifax NS B3H 2Y9; Otago (New Zealand)'02; MB ChB; Staff, Queen Elizabeth II Health Sciences Centre - Victoria General Site; (902)473-7736

SCOTT, Jeffrey W; IWK Health Centre, PO Box 9700 Rpo CSC 5850 University Ave, Halifax NS B3K 6R8; Edinburgh (Scotland)'77; MHSc; MHSA; FRCPC; Peds (Public Health). Staff Clinical Trials Research Ctr, IWK Health Centre; Physician, Nova Scotia Health Dept; Asst Prof Peds, Dalhousie University; (902)470-2733; Fax. (902)470-7232; scottj@gov.ns.ca.

SCOTT, Jeremy G; Hilltop Med Clinic, 140-15321 16 Ave, Surrey BC V4A 1R6; Sask'68; BSP; CCFP; FCFP; Ac Staff, Peace Arch Hospital; (604)531-5575; Fax. (604)535-0126.

SCOTT, John F; The Ottawa Hosp-Gen Campus, 5235-501 Smyth Rd, Ottawa ON K1H 8L6; Tor'73; MDiv; Staff Palliative Care, The Ottawa Hospital - General Campus; Langs: French; (613)723-8940

SCOTT, Julia D; Southlake Reg Health Centre, 596 Davis Dr, Newmarket ON L3Y 2P9; McM'97; FRCPC; Anes. Staff, Southlake Regional Health Centre; (905)895-4521; Fax. (905)853-2220.

SCOTT, Kane A; Medical Arts Bldg, 106-73 Cumberland St N, Thunder Bay ON P7A 4L8; McM'86; Staff, Thunder Bay Regional Health Sciences Centre Port-Arthur; (807)344-9797; Fax. (807)344-7226.

SCOTT, Karen A; PO Box 1282, Sechelt BC V0N 3A0; Qns'83; CCFP; FCFP; Ac Staff, St Mary's Hospital; Langs: Bilingual(French/English); (604)885-2384; Fax. (604)885-8876.

SCOTT, Kellie D; Elmwood Family Health Centre, 3-204 First Ave, St Thomas ON N5R 4P5; Ott'03; BSc(Hon.MicroImmunology); CCFP; Aj Prof Family Med, Schulich School of Medicine & Dentistry; (519)631-3223; Fax. (519)631-8005.

SCOTT, Kenneth C; Public Health Agency of Canada, 113B-130 Colonnade Rd, Ottawa ON K1A 0K9; Wes'78; FRCPC; IntMed (Infectious Diseases). Sr Advisor Medical/Asst Deputy Minister's Office Infectious Disease Prevention & Control Branch, Public Health Agency of Canada; (613)941-2089; ken.scott@phac.aspc.gc.ca.

SCOTT, Kirk J I; Avenue Med Clinic, 221 Brant Ave, Brantford ON N3T 3J3; McM'76; CCFP; FCFP; Court Staff, The Brant Community Healthcare System - Brantford General Hospital Site; (519)753-8666; Fax. (519)753-6880.

SCOTT, Krista S; East Van Med Bldg, 304-1750 10 Ave E, Vancouver BC V5N 5K4; UBC'98; FRCSC; Ophth (Cataract Surgery). Langs: Bilingual(French/English); (604)876-7433

SCOTT, Leslie A; London HSC-Victoria Hosp, PO Box 5010 Stn B 800 Commissioners Rd E, London ON N6A 5W9; Qns'81; FRCSC; GenSurg (Breast Surgery); PedGenSurg. Staff, London Health Sciences Centre - Children's Hospital; General Surgery, London Health Sciences Centre - Victoria Campus; Asst Prof, London Health Sciences Centre - University Hospital; Staff, St Joseph's Hospital - St Joseph's Health Care; Asst Prof Surg, University of Western Ontario; (519)685-8571; Fax. (519)685-8241; leslie.scott@lhsc.on.ca.

SCOTT, Lisa; Kincardine Commun Med Clinic, 44 Queen St, Kincardine ON N2Z 3C1; Dal'04; BSc(Biol.); CCFP; (519)396-6768; Fax. (519)396-3199.

SCOTT, M J F Lise; 204-2339 Ogilvie Rd, Gloucester ON K1J 8M6; Ott'80; CCFP; FCFP; Langs: English; (613)842-7960; Fax. (613)842-4428.

SCOTT, Malcolm D S; Meadowlark Health Centre, 200 Meadowlark Shopping Ctr NW, Edmonton AB T5R 5W9; Sask'98; FRCPC; DiagRad; NuclearMed. Staff, University of Alberta Hospital; (780)489-5313; Fax. (780)486-5610.

SCOTT, Mark A; Rockyview Gen Hosp, 7007 14 St SW, Calgary AB T2V 1P9; Cal'05; CCFP; CCFP(E.M.); Staff, Foothills Medical Centre; Staff, Rockyview General Hospital; (403)943-3449

SCOTT, Michael A J; Thunder Bay Reg HSC-T-Bay, 980 Oliver Rd, Thunder Bay ON P7B 6V4; Tor'88; FRCPC; Anes. Dir ICU, Thunder Bay Regional Health Sciences Centre; Staff Asst, Queen's University; (807)684-6000; Fax. (807)346-8015.

SCOTT, Michael D; Ladner Med Centre, 5132 Ladner Trunk Rd, Delta BC V4K 1W3; Cape Town (South Africa)'75; MB ChB; CCFP; FCFP; Staff, Chilliwack General Hospital; (604)940-0917; Fax. (604)940-9827.

SCOTT, Peter D M; Orchard Med Centre, 104-1990 Cooper Rd, Kelowna BC V1Y 8K5; Tor'70; Staff, Kelowna General Hospital; (250)861-3235; Fax. (250)861-3448.

SCOTT, R Brent; Alberta Children's Hosp, 2888 Shaganappi Trail NW, Calgary AB T3B 6A8; McG'76; MSc; MDCM; FRCPC; Peds (Pediatric Gastroenterology). Prof Peds, Alberta Children's Hospital; University of Calgary; (403)955-7327

SCOTT, Rachel R; Hôp Ste-Justine, 3175 ch Cote Saint-Catherine, Montreal QC H3T 1C5; Dal'00; FRCPC; Peds; Endocrin&Metab. Staff, Hôpital Ste-Justine; (514)345-4735

SCOTT, Richard T; Medical Associates, 100-155 Main St E, Grimsby ON L3M 1P2; Qns'84; CCFP; FCFP; Ac Staff, West Lincoln Memorial Hospital; (905)945-5476; Fax. (905)945-7707.

SCOTT, Robert C; 14 Kentucky Crt, New Minas NS B4N 4N2; McM'89; FRCSC; Ophth. Staff, Valley Regional Hospital; Staff, Queen Elizabeth II Health Sciences Centre - Victoria General Site; Staff, Soldiers Memorial Hospital; (902)678-6639; Fax. (902)678-5649.

SCOTT, Robert H; The Scott Clinic, 157 Gerrard St E, Toronto ON M5A 2E4; McG'78; Langs: Spanish; French; (416)962-5771; Fax. (416)962-3430.

SCOTT, Robert J; Ocean Walk Med Centre, 1884 Marine Dr, West Vancouver BC V7V 1J6; UBC'76; CCFP; Ac Staff, Lions Gate Hospital; Court Staff, BC Children's Hospital; Court Staff, Vancouver General Hospital - Centennial Pavillion; Staff, Ocean Walk Medical Centre; Asst Clin Prof, University of British Columbia; (604)925-1884; Fax. (604)922-3591.

SCOTT, Roger; Windsor River Walk-In Clinic, 500 Wyandotte St E, Windsor ON N9A 3H9; Cardiff (Wales)'68; (519)254-1594; Fax. (519)254-8355.

SCOTT, Sara A; Dauphin Med Clinic, 622 3rd St SW, Dauphin MB R7N 1R5; Man'07; CCFP; (204)638-6445; Fax. (204)694-5697.

SCOTT, Selma G; Reginal Fertility Program, 400-2000 Veterans Way NW, Calgary AB T3B 4N2; Wes'79; FRCSC; ObstGyn., Foothills Medical Centre; Clinical Asst Prof, University of Calgary; (403)284-9103; Fax. (403)284-9293; selma.scott@albertahealthservices.ca.

SCOTT, Sheila G; 4712 Bowness Rd NW, Calgary AB T3B 0B4; Wes'78; CCFP; (403)247-1616; Fax. (403)247-0310.

SCOTT, Thomas J P; Dauphin Med Clinic, 622 3rd St SW, Dauphin MB R7N 1R5; Man'00; (204)638-6445

SCOTT, Tracy M; St Paul's Hosp, C303-1081 Burrard St, Vancouver BC V6Z 1Y6; Mem'03; FRCSC; GenSurg. Staff, Providence Health Care - St Paul's Hospital; (604)806-9108

SCOTT, Verna D; Regina Qu'Appelle Hlth Region, 1440 14th Ave, Regina SK S4P 0W5; Sask'91; CCFP; Staff Emerg, Regina General Hospital; (306)766-4500; Fax. (306)766-4357.

SCOTT-DOUGLAS, Nairne W; Foothills Med Centre, 1403 29 St NW, Calgary AB T2N 2T9; Cal'91; PhD; FRCPC; IntMed; Nephrol. Staff, Foothills Medical Centre; Med Dir, Southern Alberta Rural Program; Clin Associate Prof, University of Calgary; (403)944-2804; Fax. (403)270-0055.

SCOTT EHLE, Michelle L; Ingram Family Physicians, 103-149 Ingram St, Duncan BC V9L 1N8; McM'97; CCFP; (250)746-4401

SCOTT-FLEURY, Marie-Helene; Douglas Mental Hlth Univ Inst, 6875 boul Lasalle, LaSalle QC H4H 1R3; Belgium (Belgium)'72; Staff, Douglas Mental Health University Institute; (514)761-6131; Fax. (514)769-1745.

SCOTT-THOMAS, Nancy L E; Carling-Broadview Med Bldg, 201-770 Broadview ave, Ottawa ON K2A 3Z3; Wes'92; CCFP; CCFP(E.M.); Staff, Children's Hospital of Eastern Ontario (CHEO); (613)680-1065; Fax. (613)695-1870.

SCOTTON, Paul S; Dufferin-Caledon Hlth Care Ctr, 100 Rolling Hills Dr, Orangeville ON L9W 4X9; UBC'88; Physician Base Hosp, Hamilton Health Sciences Centre; Staff Emerg, Headwaters Health Care Centre - Orangeville Site; Langs: Italian; (519)278-0257; Fax. (519)941-4707.

SCOVIL, Robert J; 1802 St Margarets Bay Rd, Timberlea NS B3T 1B8; Dal'83; (902)876-0415; Fax. (902)876-1723.

SCOVIL, Susan J; Medicine in Motion Med Centre, 5-121 Lisley Ave, Dartmouth NS B3B 1S4; McM'08; CCFP; Staff, Medicine in Motion Medical Centre; (902)468-2774; Fax. (902)468-1359.

SCOZZAFAVA, Giuseppe J; University of Alberta Hosp, 1F216 WMC-8440 112 St NW, Edmonton AB T6G 2B7; Alb'01; FRCPC; Neur; Critical Care Medicine. Staff Critical Care Program, Foothills Medical Centre; Staff, University of Alberta Hospital; (780)407-7363; Fax. (780)407-6020.

SCRAGG, Richard; Port McNeill Med Clinic, PO Box 253 2126 Mcneill Rd, Port McNeill BC V0N 2R0; (Other Foreign)'84; (250)956-3377; Fax. (250)956-3299.

SCRAPNECK, Ronald A; Concordia Gen Hosp, 1095 Concordia Ave, Winnipeg MB R2K 3S8; Man'91; Staff, Concordia General Hospital; (204)667-1560

SCRIBANTE, Lindi; 209-5704 44 St, Lloydminster AB T9V 2A1; (South Africa)'94; Langs: Afrikaans; (780)875-5501; Fax. (780)875-3183.

SCRIMGER, Rufus A; Cross Cancer Institute, 11560 University Ave NW, Edmonton AB T6G 1Z2; Alb'94; FRCPC; RadOncol (Lung Cancer). Staff RadOncol, Cross Cancer Institute; (780)432-8517; Fax. (780)432-8380.

SCRIMSHAW, Catherine L; Associate Med Clinic, PO Box 549, Pincher Creek AB T0K 1W0; Cal'87; CCFP; FCFP; (403)627-3321; Fax. (403)627-2280.

SCRIVEN, Edward A K; Hamilton HS-General Site, 237 Barton St E, Hamilton ON L8L 2X2; McM'07; FRCSC; OrthSurg. Staff, Hamilton Health Sciences Centre - Hamilton General Hospital; (905)527-4322

SCRIVENS, Blair A; Sandbanks Med Centre, 12 Prince Edward Dr, Wellington ON K0K 3L0; Wes'89; CCFP; Staff, QHC Prince Edward County Memorial; Physician, Sandbanks Medical Centre; (613)399-1281

SCROGGIE, David G; 18 Cornish Rd, Toronto ON M4T 2E2; Tor'64; AB; FRCPC; Psy. Asst Prof, University of Toronto; (416)923-6712

SCROOBY, Ivan G; Atwood Med Clinic, 101-143 Fourth Ave S, Williams Lake BC V2G 1J8; Stellenbosch (South Africa)'97; MB ChB; Langs: Afrikaans; (250)398-5162; Fax. (250)398-5673.

SCRUTON, Joan H; Valley Care Med Clinic, E-310 8th St, Courtenay BC V9N 1N3; Sheffield (England)'73; MB ChB; Ac Staff, St Joseph's General Hospital; (250)331-0500; Fax. (250)331-0553; bcmdoc7@telus.net.

SCUCCIMARRI, Rosie; MUHC-Montreal Children's Hosp, C504-2300 rue Tupper, Montreal QC H3H 1P3; McG'94; FRCPC; Peds (Pediatric Rheumatology); Rheum. Staff, McGill University Health Centre - Montreal Children's Hospital; Langs: English; French; (514)412-4268; Fax. (514)412-4365; rosie.scuccimarri@muhc.mcgill.ca.

SCUDAMORE, Charles H; Liver & Pancreatic Surgery Sec, 5173-2775 Laurel St, Vancouver BC V5Z 1M9; UBC'75; MSc(Surg); FACS; FRCS(Ed); FRCS(Eng); FRCSC; GenSurg (Liver & Pancreas Surgery). Assoc Prof Med/Head, Vancouver General Hospital - Centennial Pavillion; Assoc Prof Med/Dir Surg, UBC Hospital - Koerner Pavillion; Assoc Prof, University of British Columbia; (604)875-4416; Fax. (604)875-5869.

SCULLION, Catherine M; Medical Clinic Person-Ctred Ps, 265 Yorkland Blvd, North York ON M2J 1S5; Tor'88; Staff, The Medical Clinic for Person-Centred Psychotherapy; (416)229-2399

SCULLION, P Gabriel; Guelph Gen Hosp, 115 Delhi St, Guelph ON N1E 4J4; Belfast (Ireland)'73; CCFP; FCFP; Staff, Guelph General Hospital; Clinical Asst Prof Family Med, McMaster University; (519)822-5350

SCULLY, Hugh E; 1503-700 Bay St, Toronto ON M5G 1Z6; Qns'65; FACS; FACC; FRCSC; GenSurg; Cardiovasc&ThorSurg. Staff, Toronto General Hospital - UHN; Prof Surg, University of Toronto; Langs: French; (416)340-3693; Fax. (416)340-3397; hugh.scully@uhn.on.ca.

SCULLY, Linda J; The Ottawa Hosp-Civic Campus, 1053 Carling Ave, Ottawa ON K1Y 4E9; Tor'75; BSc; FRCPC; IntMed (Liver Disease); Gastroent. Ac Staff, The Ottawa Hospital - Civic Campus; Assoc Prof, University of Ottawa; (613)761-4830; Fax. (613)761-5415.

SCULLY, Mary-Frances; Health Sciences Centre, 1758E-300 Prince Philip Dr, St. John's NL A1B 3V6; Dublin (Ireland)'79; MB ChB; MRCPI; DCH; FRCPC; Peds (Malignant Hematoma); Hem. Dir Hemophilia Prog, Health Sciences Centre; Dir, Provincial Hemophilia Program for Nfld & Labrador; Editor Web, Thrombosis Interest Group of Canada; Assoc Prof, Memorial University Of Newfoundland; Langs: French; Irish; (709)777-8066

SCULLY, Michael V; Associate Med Clinic, PO Box 1059 1973 Columbia Ave, Rossland BC V0G 1Y0; Burlington (USA)'96; AAFPhys; Staff Phys, Kootenay Boundary Regional Hospital; Langs: Spanish; French; (250)362-7307; Fax. (250)362-9413.

SCURFIELD, Barbara J; Alberta Prof Bldg, 300-320 23 Ave SW, Calgary AB T2S 0J2; Alb'81; CCFP; Staff, Covenant Health - Banff Mineral Springs Hospital; (403)228-0110; Fax. (403)228-9828.

SCURFIELD, Carol M; Women's Health Clinic, 419 Graham Ave, Winnipeg MB R3C 0M3; Man'80; MSc; CCFP; FCFP; (204)947-1517; Fax. (204)944-0223; cscurfield@womenshealthclinic.org.

SEABERG, Raewyn M; Keele-Ingram Prof Centre, 108-2221 Keele St, North York ON M6M 3Z5; Tor'06; FRCPC; Otol. Staff, Mount Sinai Hospital; (416)244-5506

SEAGER, Mary-Jane; Boyd Med Centre, 318-388 Portage Ave, Winnipeg MB R3C 0C8; Man'85; FRCSC; ObstGyn. Chief Medical Officer/Ac Staff, Victoria General Hospital; Staff, St Boniface General Hospital; University of Manitoba; (204)925-3600; Fax. (204)925-3616.

SEAGRIST, W Scott; 185 Glasgow St, Kitchener ON N2M 2M2; Wes'84; Staff Privil, Woodstock General Hospital; (519)570-3330

SEAH, Stanley K K; R16-1111 rue Saint-Urbain, Montreal QC H2Z 1Y6; Man'61; PhD(Lond); MRCP(Edin); DCMT(Lond); MRCP(Lond); IntMed (Infectious Diseases). Att Médecin, McGill University Health Centre - Montreal General Campus; Consultant, Douglas Mental Health University Institute; Consultant, Hôpital Chinois de Montréal; Prof Med, McGill University; Langs: Cantonese; French; (514)393-1071; Fax. (514)393-9709; sea8524@aol.com.

SEAL, Alexander N; 808-1200 Burrard St, Vancouver BC V6Z 2C7; UBC'05; FRCSC; PlasSurg. (604)569-2895

SEAL, Douglas D; Foothills Med Centre, 1403 29 St NW, Calgary AB T2N 2T9; Alb'93; FRCPC; Anes. Staff Anes, Foothills Medical Centre; (403)944-1430; Fax. (403)944-2425.

SEAL, Iain D; Family Practice Unit, 102-402 Hansen St, Whitehorse YT Y1A 1Y8; Alb'92; Physician, Taiga Medical Clinics Inc; Physician, Family Practice Unit; (867)667-6421

SEAL, Melanie D; Health Sciences Centre, 300 Prince Philip Dr, St. John's NL A1B 3V6; Mem'03; FRCPC; IntMed; MedOncol. Staff, Health Sciences Centre; (709)737-6300

SEAL, Paula S; Gulf Canada Square, 300-401 9 Ave SW, Calgary AB T2P 3C5; Alb'93; FRCPC; DiagRad. (403)284-0230

SEAL, Robert F; University of Alberta Hosp, 1C1 04-8440 112 St NW, Edmonton AB T6G 2B7; Alb'83; BSc; FRCPC; Anes (Pediatric Anesthesia). Staff, University of Alberta Hospital; Dir Ped Cardiac Anes/Clin Assoc Prof Anes & Pain Med, University of Alberta; (780)407-7035; Fax. (780)407-8529; rseal@gpu.srv.ualberta.ca.

SEAL, Shane K F; PO Box 23104 Churchill Square, St. John's NL A1B 4J9; UBC'03; FRCSC; PlasSurg. Staff, Health Sciences Centre.

SEALE, Edward R; St Joseph Family Med Clinic, 100-2555 St. Joseph Blvd, Orleans ON K1C 1S6; McG'92; CCFP; CCFP(E.M.); FCFP; Staff Physician, Montfort Hospital; Langs: French; (613)830-1298; Fax. (613)830-2170.

SEALE, Janet E; Bruyere Academic Family Hlth Team, 75 Bruyere St, Ottawa ON K1N 5C7; Wes'81; BSc(Biochem); CCFP; Staff, Bruyère Academic Family Health Team - Bruyèe Family Medicine Centre; Langs: French; (613)683-4363

SEALEY, Brian J; Victoria Med Centre, 304-304 Victoria Ave N, Hamilton ON L8L 5G4; Birmingham (England)'59; MB ChB; MRCS; LRCP; MRCP(London); FRCPC; IntMed (Cardiology). Staff, Hamilton Health Sciences Centre-Juravinski Site; Clin Assoc Prof, McMaster University; (905)546-8538; Fax. (905)546-0638; doc1234@bellnet.ca.

SEALEY, Robert A D; Shelbourne Med Clinic, 150-3200 Shelbourne St, Victoria BC V8P 5G8; Sask'90; Staff, Vancouver Island Health Authority; Staff, Aberdeen Hospital; Physician, Westside Health Centre; (250)592-3183

SEALY, Sasha L; 101-55 Drury Cove Rd, Saint John NB E2H 2Z8; Mem'06; CCFP; Staff, St Joseph's Hospital; (506)652-3900

SEAMAN, Donald M; 150 Park St, Kentville NS B4N 1M6; Dal'57; MDCM; Staff, Valley Regional Hospital; Med Dir, Evergreen Nursing Home; (902)678-2830; Fax. (902)678-6824.

SEAMAN, James G; Valley Prof Centre, 200-70 Exhibition St, Kentville NS B4N 4K9; Dal'71; (902)678-2525; Fax. (902)678-4550; doctorsoffice@accesswave.ca.

SEAMAN, Kenneth L; 400 Bayfield St, Barrie ON L4M 5A1; Tor'87; (705)721-7770

SEAMAN, Leah V; Inuvik Reg Hlth & Social Serv, PO Box 1999, Inuvik NT X0E 0T0; UBC'89; CCFP; FCFP; Staff/Med Officer of Hlth, Inuvik Regional Hospital; Langs: French; (867)777-8000; Fax. (867)777-8036.

SEAMAN, Sarah J; Forest Hill Med Clinic, 4 Forest Hills Pky, Dartmouth NS B2W 5G7; Dal'02; CCFP; (902)435-5530; Fax. (902)473-4760.

SEAMONE, Christopher D; 800-5991 Spring Garden Rd, Halifax NS B3H 1Y6; Dal'81; BSc(Acadia); DABOph; FRCSC; Ophth (Cornea/External Disease). Med Dir Eye & Tissue Bank, Queen Elizabeth II Health Sciences Centre - Victoria General Site; Med Dir Eye & Tissue Bank, New Brunswick Eye Bank; Assoc Prof Ophth, Dalhousie University; (902)429-2760; Fax. (902)425-0666.

SEAR, Andrew I; Fraserview Med Associates, 32-665 Front St, Quesnel BC V2J 5J5; London (England)'69; MB BS; DA; DObst; CCFP; Ac Staff, G R Baker Memorial Hospital; Member Council, College of Physicians & Surgeons of British Columbia; Clinical Asst Prof Family Pract, University of British Columbia; (250)992-3636; Fax. (250)992-7587.

SEARLE, Lisa C; The Moncton Hosp, 135 MacBeath Ave, Moncton NB E1C 6Z8; Dal'05; CCFP; Staff, The Moncton Hospital; (506)857-5900; Fax. (506)857-5133.

SEARLES, Gordon E; 303-2377 111 Street NW, Edmonton AB T6J 5E5; McM'86; MSc; FACP; FRCPC; IntMed; Derm. Consultant, Royal Alexandra Hospital; Consultant, University of Alberta Hospital; Consultant, Misericordia Health Centre; Clin Prof derm, University of Alberta; (780)424-4464 x6620; Fax. (780)424-2534.

SEARLES, Gregory R; Saint John Reg Hosp, PO Box 2100 Stn Main D3D N-400 University Ave, Saint John NB E2L 4L2; Dal'98; FRCPC; IntMed; Cardiol. Staff, Saint John Regional Hospital; (506)648-7974; Fax. (506)648-7976.

SEARLES, Lynne E; PO Box 74084 Strathcona Rpo SW, Calgary AB T3H 3B6; Cal'98; CCFP.

SEARS, Catherine M; Burnside Family Med Clinic, 2-101 Burnside Rd W, Victoria BC V9A 1B7; Wes'83; BSc(Hon); CCFP; FCFP; Staff, Burnside Family Medical Clinic; (250)598-0678; Fax. (250)598-6367.

SEARS, Gerald A; 727 Westmount Hills Dr, London ON N6K 1B3; Wes'52; FACC; FRCPC; IntMed (Cardiology). Emeritus Prof Med, University of Western Ontario; (519)471-4476; Fax. (519)667-6678.

SEARS, Malcolm R; St Joseph's Healthcare, T3219-50 Charlton Ave E, Hamilton ON L8N 4A6; Otago (New Zealand)'65; MB ChB; FRACP; FRCPC; Respir (Public Health). Staff, St Joseph's Healthcare - Charlton Campus; Physician, Firestone Institute for Respiratory Health; Prof, McMaster University; (905)522-1155 x33286; Fax. (905)521-6132; searsm@mcmaster.ca.

SEARS, Ronald S R; Ross Mem Hosp, 10 Angeline St N, Lindsay ON K9V 4M8; Tor'67; BSc; Medical Staff/Staff Hospitalist, Ross Memorial Hospital; (705)324-6111 x4261; Fax. (705)328-6178; rsearsz@cogeco.ca.

SEARS, Steven T; 18 Silver St PO Box 399, Cobalt ON P0J 1C0; Tor'98; CCFP; FCFP; Staff, Temiskaming Hospital; (705)679-5466; Fax. (705)679-5588.

SEATON, Trevor L C; Victoria Med Centre, 303-304 Victoria Ave N, Hamilton ON L8L 5G4; Mona (Jamaica)'69; FRCPC; IntMed (Gastroenterology). Court Staff, St Joseph's Healthcare - Charlton Campus; Ac Staff, Hamilton Health Sciences Centre-Juravinski Site; Clin Assoc Prof, McMaster University; (905)572-7258; Fax. (905)572-6587; seatont@mcmaster.ca.

SEAWARD, P Gareth R; Ontario Power Generation, 3201-700 University Ave, Toronto ON M5G 1Z6; Witwatersrand (South Africa)'79; MB ChB; FRCSC; ObstGyn (Maternal Fetal Medicine). Head Labor & Delivery, Mount Sinai Hospital; Prof ObstGyn, University of Toronto; Langs: Afrikaans; (416)586-8660; Fax. (416)586-8617.

SEBAG, Igal A; E206-SMBD Jewish Gen Hosp, 3755 ch Cote-Sainte-Catherine, Montreal QC H3T 1E2; Mon'94; DABIM; FRCP; FACC; FRCPC; IntMed; Cardiol. Staff, Sir Mortimer B Davis Jewish General; adj Prof Med, McGill University; (514)340-8222 x2992; Fax. (514)340-7534; igal.sebag@mcgill.ca.

SEBAG, Michael; MUHC-Montreal Gen Hosp, A7 117-1650 av Cedar, Montreal QC H3G 1A4; Tor'00; Hem; IntMed. Staff, McGill University Health Centre - Montreal General Campus; (514)934-1934 x42428

SEBAG, Mikael; CHUM-Hop Notre-Dame, 1560 rue Sherbrooke E, Montreal QC H2L 4M1; Mon'82; Ophth (Macular Diseases). ac Staff, Centre Hospitalier l'Université de Montréal (CHUM) - Hôpital Notre-Dame; adj Prof Ophth, Universite de Montreal; (514)890-6000 x27100

SEBAJANG, Herawaty; CHUM-Hop Notre-Dame, 1560 rue Sherbrooke E, Montreal QC H2L 4M1; Mon'97; FRCSC; GenSurg. Staff, Centre Hospitalier l'Université de Montréal (CHUM) - Hôpital Notre-Dame; Langs: Romanian; (514)890-8000 x26607; Fax. (514)412-7821.

SEBALDT, Rolf J; Charlton Med Centre, 608-25 Charlton Ave E, Hamilton ON L8N 1Y2; McG'79; FACP; FRCPC; IntMed (Osteoporosis); Rheum. Staff, St Joseph's Healthcare - Charlton Campus; Assoc Prof Med/Member Faculty, McMaster University; Langs: German; (905)529-6214; Fax. (905)521-0098; sebaldt@mcmaster.ca.

SEBASTIAN, Anthony R; 401-18 Kensington Rd, Brampton ON L6T 4S5; Mem'79; (905)792-2313; Fax. (905)792-7353.

SEBASTIAN, Antonypillai R; Health Park Med Clinic, 402B-45 Weatherbee Rd, Mira Road NS B1M 0A1; St Georges (Grenada)'95; CCFP; (902)567-1400; Fax. (902)567-2722.

SEBASTIAN, Geron C; Rockwood Med Clinic, 4141 Dixie Rd, Mississauga ON L4W 1V5; Dal'70; (905)625-2990

SEBASTIAN, Justin C; First Edmonton Place, 1370-10665 Jasper Ave NW, Edmonton AB T5J 3S9; Mysore (India)'73; FRCPC; IntMed (Respirology). Staff, Royal Alexandra Hospital; (780)702-3866; Fax. (780)702-3880.

SEBASTIAN, Maleakal S; PO Box 603 Stn Main, New Glasgow NS B2H 5E7; Kerala (India)'58; MB BS; FACS; FICS; GenSurg. Head Div of Gen Surg, Aberdeen Regional Hospital; (902)926-2255; Fax. (902)752-3157.

SEBASTIAN, Robert D; Boundary Med Clinic PO Box 400, Grand Forks BC V0H 1H0; Cal'86; CCFP; Boundary Hospital; (250)442-8233; Fax. (250)442-3949.

SEBASTIANELLI, Alexandra; Hotel Dieu de Quebec, 11 ch Cote du Palais, Quebec QC G1R 3J8; Laval'02; FRCSC; ObstGyn. Staff, Centre Hospitalier Universitaire de Québec (CHUQ) - Siege Social; (418)525-4444

SEBASTIANI, Giada; MUHC-Royal Victoria Hosp, 687 av des Pins O, Montreal QC H3A 1A1; Staff, McGill University Health Centre - Royal Victoria Hospital; (514)654-3955

SEBBA, Richard J; Hollyburn Med Centre, 207A-575 16th St, West Vancouver BC V7V 4Y1; Cape Town (South Africa)'79; MB ChB; (604)926-3484; Fax. (604)926-8176.

SEBBAG, Sarah E; Clinique Vendome, 5175 boul de Maisonneuve O, Montreal QC H4A 1Z3; McG'05; CCFP; CCFP(E.M.); (514)484-2355

SEBBI, Esmael M H; James Paton Mem Hosp, 125 Trans Canada Hwy, Gander NL A1V 1P7; Makerere (Uganda)'86; MB ChB; Staff, James Paton Memorial Hospital; (709)256-5658

SEBIRE, Guillaume; CHUS-Hop Fleurimont, 3001 12e av N, Sherbrooke QC J1H 5N4; Paris (France)'91; Neur (P.Q.). Staff, Centre Hospitalier Universitaire de Sherbrooke-Hopital Fleurimont; (819)346-1110; Fax. (819)564-5398; guillaume.sebire@usherbrooke.ca.

SEBULSKY, Tara L G; 230 Robson Rd W, Kelowna BC V1X 3C8; Wes'02; CCFP; Staff, Kelowna General Hospital; (250)765-9777; Fax. (250)765-1350.

SECCARECCIA, Dori-Lynn M; Sunnybrook Hlth Sciences Ctr, 2075 Bayview Ave, Toronto ON M4N 3M5; Wes'87; CCFP; CCFP(E.M.); Staff, Sunnybrook Health Sciences Centre; Staff, Princess Margaret Hospital - University Health Network; (416)480-6100; Fax. (416)480-5146.

SECCOMBE, David W; 307-2083 Alma St, Vancouver BC V6R 4N6; Cal'81; PhD(Physiol); FRCPC; MedBiochem (Diagnosis). Dir, Canadian Reference Laboratory; Man Dir, Canadian External Quality Assessment Laboratory; Assoc Prof Path & Lab Med, University of British Columbia; (604)418-4683; dseccombe@ceqal.com.

SECERBEGOVIC, Said; Parhelion Med Services Inc PO Box 127, Watson Lake YT Y0A 1C0; Dublin (Ireland)'76; BSc(McM); LRCPSI; Examiner Civil Aviation, Parhelion Medical Services Inc; Langs: German; Serbo-Croatian; (867)536-2565; Fax. (867)536-2506; admin@parhelion.ca.

SECERBEGOVIC, Tanis R; Parhelion Med Services Inc, PO Box 127, Watson Lake YT Y0A 1C0; Cork (Ireland)'07; MB BCh; CCFP; Physician, Parhelion Medical Services Inc; (867)536-2565

SECK, Mamadou S; Clinique de Med Familiale, 6e-2120 rue Sherbrooke E, Montreal QC H2K 1C3; (Bulgaria)'97; Staff, Centre Hospitalier l'Université de Montréal (CHUM) - Hôpital Notre-Dame; (514)527-1958; Fax. (514)527-1649.

SECORD, Jonathan B; 470 South Rd PO Box 330, Gabriola BC V0R 1X0; McM'05; CCFP.

SECRETAN, Charles C; 3403 32 Ave, Vernon BC V1T 2M9; Alb'03; OrthSurg (Clinician Investigator Program). (778)475-6070

SECTER, Barbara A; The Breast Centre, 7121 109 St NW, Edmonton AB T6G 1B9; Alb'64; (780)437-2060; Fax. (780)437-2067.

SEDDIKI, Fatiha; CSSS de Laval, 1755 boul Rene-Laennec, Laval QC H7M 3L9; Alger (Algeria)'93; Peds (P.Q.). Staff, Hopital de la Cite de la santé; Langs: Arabic; English; (450)668-1010

SEDERGREEN, Christopher J H; 171 Wyndham Cres, Anmore BC V3H 4X9; London (England)'74; MB BS; LRCP; MRCS; Langs: Bilingual(English/French); (604)461-3899

SEDGE, Paul A; Cdn Forces Health Serv Centre, 101 Colonel By Drive, Ottawa ON K1A 0K2; Ott'98; FRCPC; Psy. Staff, Canadian Forces Health Services Centre; (506)357-6482

SEDIQ, Aimal; Queen West Med Walk In Clinic, 9-400 Queen St W, Brampton ON L6X 1B3; Ott'01; CCFP; (905)796-5777; Fax. (905)796-5725.

SEDLAK, Tara L; Gordon & Leslie Diamond HCC, 9F-2775 Laurel St, Vancouver BC V5Z 1M9; UBC'05; FRCPC; IntMed; Cardiol. Staff, Gordon & Leslie Diamond Health Care Centre; (604)877-2920

SEDRAN, David; 401-960 Lawrence Ave W, North York ON M6A 3B5; Tor'93; CCFP; FCFP; Staff, Humber River Regional Hospital - Finch Avenue Site; Coroner, City of Toronto; Langs: Italian; (416)256-1150; Fax. (416)256-0742.

SEDRAN, Robert J; Children's Hosp, E1 102-800 Commissioners Rd E, London ON N6A 5W9; Tor'96; FRCPC; EmergMed. (519)685-8500; Fax. (519)667-6769.

SEE, Hilario; North York Med Clinic, 303-2175 Sheppard Ave E, North York ON M2J 1W8; Tor'96; CCFP; (416)492-7700; Fax. (416)492-5776.

SEEAR, Michael D; Children's & Women's HC of BC, 1C31-4480 Oak St, Vancouver BC V6H 3V4; (Zimbabwe)'80; MB ChB; FRCPC; Peds (Pediatric Intensive Care & Respiratory Disease). Staff ICU, BC Children's Hospital; Asst Prof Peds, University of British Columbia; (604)875-2119; Fax. (604)875-3293.

SEED, Michael T M; The Hosp for Sick Children, 555 University Ave, Toronto ON M5G 1X8; Newcastle-Upon-Tyne (England)'98; Fellow Ped Cardiol, The Hospital For Sick Children; (416)813-7467; Fax. (416)813-7547.

SEEGOBIN, Ramesh; Highland Med Centre, B2-3300 Rutherford Rd, Vaughan ON L4K 5Z2; Ross Univ (USA)'94; BSc(Hons); CCFP; (905)303-2229; Fax. (905)303-0437.

SEEGOBIN, Ronald D; Kingston Gen Hosp, 76 Stuart St, Kingston ON K7L 2V7; Oxford (England)'74; FRCPC; Anes. Staff Anes, Kingston General Hospital; Langs: French; (613)548-7822; Fax. (613)548-6066.

SEELEY, Richard A M; St Peter's Hosp, 88 Maplewood Ave, Hamilton ON L8M 1W9; Tor'74; Staff, Hamilton Health Sciences Centre - St Peter's Hospital; (905)544-4983; Fax. (905)544-6674; rseeley@stpetes.ca.

SEELY, Andrew J E; The Ottawa Hosp-Gen Campus, 708-501 Smyth Rd, Ottawa ON K1H 8L6; McG'94; FRCSC; GenSurg; Critical Care Medicine; ThorSurg. Scientist, The Ottawa Hospital - General Campus; Langs: English; (613)737-8899 x74032; Fax. (613)737-8668; aseely@uottawa.ca.

SEELY, Jean M; The Ottawa Hosp-Civic Campus, 1053 Carling Ave, Ottawa ON K1Y 4E9; McG'89; FRCPC; DiagRad. Staff, The Ottawa Hospital - General Campus; Staff Radiol, The Ottawa Hospital - Civic Campus; Langs: Spanish; French; (613)798-5555

SEEMAN, Mary V; Addiction & Mental Hlth-Colleg, 250 College St, Toronto ON M5T 1R8; McG'60; DFAPA; FRCPC; Psy (Adult Psychiatry & Psychotherapy). Staff, Centre for Addiction & Mental Health (CAMH) - College Street Site; Langs: French; Polish; (416)535-8501

SEEMANN, Robert P; Circle Square Prof Centre, 216-11808 St Albert Trail, Edmonton AB T5L 4G4; Sask'97; FRCSC; Otol (Head & Neck Surgery). (780)756-7650; Fax. (780)756-7652.

SEEMAYER, Thomas A; 270 Connemara Cres, Ste-Anne-de-Bellev QC H9W 2N7; Chicago(IL) (USA)'63; GenPath. Staff, Centre Hospitalier Pierre le Gardeur; (514)694-4581; thomas.seemayer@ssss.gouv.qc.ca.

SEETHAPATHY, Vijayakumar; Burnaby Ctr for Addiction & Me, 3405 Willingdon Ave, Burnaby BC V5G 3H4; Bangalore (India)'99; (604)875-4111

SEETHARAMDOO, Patrick S; 720 Sackville Dr, Lower Sackville NS B4E 3A4; Glasgow (Scotland)'65; MB ChB; FRCS(Ed); Court Staff, Queen Elizabeth II Health Sciences Centre - Victoria General Site; (902)865-4551; Fax. (902)865-1929.

SEETHRAM, Kenneth; Pacific Ctre for Reproductive, 500-4601 Canaday Way, Burnaby BC V5G 4X7; Alb'92; FRCSC; ObstGyn. (604)422-7276

SEETNER, A Ashley; 504-89 Queensway W, Mississauga ON L5B 2V2; Man'76; FRCSC; Ophth. Att Staff Surg, Trillium Health Centre - Mississauga; (905)279-1110; Fax. (905)279-1105.

SEEVARATNAM, David M; Kozlov Centre, 240-400 Bayfield St, Barrie ON L4M 5A1; Colombo (Sri Lanka)'74; MB BS; MRCPsy(UK); FRCPC; Psy. Consultant, Stevenson Memorial Hospital; (705)725-8105; Fax. (705)739-1700.

SEEVARATNAM, Loretta M; Clinton Family Health Team, PO Box 69 105 Shipley St, Clinton ON N0M 1L0; Wes'06; CCFP; (519)482-3000

SEFAU, Suleiman O A; Polyclinic, 199 Grafton St, Charlottetown PE C1A 1L2; Al-Fateh (Libya)'92; FRCSC; Ophth. (902)629-8810

SEFCIK, T Wayne; 309-1321 Kensington Close, Calgary AB T2N 3J6; Alb'78; MCFP(EM); Staff, Foothills Medical Centre; (403)650-6141

SEFTEL, Matthew D; CancerCare Manitoba, ON 2081-675 McDermot Ave, Winnipeg MB R3E 0V9; Cape Town (South Africa)'93; FRCPC; IntMed (Medical Oncology); Hem. Staff, Health Sciences Centre; CancerCare Manitoba; Asst Prof, University of Manitoba; matthew.seftel@cancercare.mb.ca.

SEGAL, Audrey O; Bayview-Finch Med Clinic, 301-3292 Bayview Ave, North York ON M2M 4J5; Maryland (USA)'07; FRCPC; Peds; ClinImmunol&Allergy. Staff, The Hospital For Sick Children; (416)733-7772; Fax. (416)224-9880.

SEGAL, Barry M; 400-1681 Chestnut St, Vancouver BC V6J 4M6; Witwatersrand (South Africa)'78; FRCPC; Psy. Ac Staff Psy, Vancouver General Hospital - Centennial Pavillion; (604)737-8609; Fax. (604)737-1140.

SEGAL, Basil; Associated Med Dental Bldg, 101-8140 Cook Rd, Richmond BC V6Y 1V1; Cape Town (South Africa)'75; MB ChB; CCFP; Ac Staff, Richmond Hospital; Asst Prof Family Pract, University of British Columbia; (604)279-8833; Fax. (604)279-8883.

SEGAL, David J; Maple Med Clinic, 103-2025 Broadway W, Vancouver BC V6J 1Z6; Alb'79; PhD(CA); Assoc Staff, Vancouver General Hospital - Centennial Pavillion; Langs: Greek; (604)730-9769; Fax. (604)730-0110.

SEGAL, Eli; D027 SMBD Jewish Gen Hosp, 3755 ch Cote-Sainte-Catherine, Montreal QC H3T 1E2; McG'95; FRCPC; EmergMed. Staff, Sir Mortimer B Davis Jewish General; Langs: English; French; (514)340-8222 x5568

SEGAL, Galit R; Family Physicians, 1-390 Steeles Ave W, Thornhill ON L4J 6X2; Dal'97; CCFP; (905)881-3984; Fax. (905)881-3198.

SEGAL, Jean M; Delta Health Sciences Centre, 102-4515 Harvest Dr, Delta BC V4K 4L1; Cal'86; FRCSC; GenSurg (Herniology). Med Dir, Delta Hospital; Physician, Delta Health Sciences Centre; (604)940-2177; jeanmsegal@hotmail.com.

SEGAL, Jeffrey S; Saint-Mary's Hosp Center, 3830 av Lacombe, Montreal QC H3T 1M5; McG'07; MDCM; FRCPC; IntMed. Staff, St Mary's Hospital Centre; Staff, McGill University Health Centre - Montreal General Campus; (514)345-3511

SEGAL, Lauren M; Club Tiny Tots Med Centre, 3550-6900 boul Decarie, Cote Saint-Luc QC H3X 2T8; McG'05; FRCPC; ClinImmunol&Allergy (P.Q.); Peds. (514)342-9911

SEGAL, Marilyn; A536-SMBD Jewish Gen Hosp, 3755 ch Cote-Sainte-Catherine, Montreal QC H3T 1E2; McG'81; DPsy; FRCPC; Psy (Geriatric Psychiatry). Dir Psychogeriatric Services, Sir Mortimer B Davis Jewish General; McGill University; Langs: English; French; (514)340-7902 x5886; Fax. (514)340-8126.

SEGAL, Mikel K; Royal Columbian Hosp, 330 Columbia St E, New Westminster BC V3L 3W7; UBC'98; CCFP; Staff, Royal Columbian Hospital; (604)520-4001

SEGAL, Orit; Davisville Fam Practice, 600-1881 Yonge St, Toronto ON M4S 3C4; Tor'02; CCFP; (416)932-3172; Fax. (416)440-0238.

SEGAL, Perry M; Rene Le Marchand Mansion, 305A-11523 100 Ave NW, Edmonton AB T5K 0J8; McG'59; BSc; MDCM; MRCPsy; FRCPC; Psy (Dynamic Psychotherapy). (780)488-5733; Fax. (780)488-5735; psegal@shaw.ca.

SEGAL, Phillip H B; Univ Hlth Network-Toronto Gen, EN12 216-200 Elizabeth St, Toronto ON M5G 2C4; Alb'04; FRCPC; IntMed; Endocrin&Metab. Staff, Toronto General Hospital - UHN; (416)340-5329; Fax. (416)340-3314.

SEGAL, Roanne J; Ottawa Reg Cancer Centre, 501 Smyth Rd Box 911, Ottawa ON K1H 8L6; McG'87; FRCPC; IntMed (Breasts); MedOncol. Staff Physician Ottawa Reg Cancer Centre, The Ottawa Hospital - General Campus; Physician MedOncol, Ottawa Regional Cancer Centre; Assoc Prof, University of Ottawa; Langs: Bilingual(English/French); (613)737-7700; rsegal@ottawahospital.on.ca.

SEGAL, Russel S; North York Gen Hosp, 4001 Leslie St, North York ON M2K 1E1; Tor'94; CCFP; CCFP(E.M.); Staff Emerd, North York General Hospital; Teacher, University of Toronto; (416)756-6000 x6001; rsegalmd-05@yahoo.ca.

SEGAL, Samantha; 877 Helena St, Trail BC V1R 3X3; Farmington(CT) (USA)'97; (250)368-3334

SEGAL, Samuel; Fairmont Med Bldg, 718-750 Broadway W, Vancouver BC V5Z 1H6; UBC'70; Ac Staff, Vancouver General Hospital - Centennial Pavillion; (604)873-8325; Fax. (604)873-8326.

SEGAL, Shaun M; Toronto Poly Clinic, 204-5460 Yonge St, North York ON M2N 6K7; Qns'06; CCFP; Physician, Rethink Breast Cancer; Lecturer DFCM, University of Toronto; (416)250-7171; Fax. (416)250-0323; shaun@rethinkbreastcancer.com.

SEGAL, Steven H; Southlake Reg Health Centre, 596 Davis Dr, Newmarket ON L3Y 2P9; Ott'97; FRCPC; Anes; Critical Care Medicine. Staff, Southlake Regional Health Centre; (905)895-4521

SEGAL-ARDMAN, Laura; Centre Hosp de Verdun, 4000 boul Lasalle, LaSalle QC H4G 2A3; McG'05; FRCSC; Ophth. Staff, Centre Hospitalier de Verdun; (514)362-1000

SEGALL, Lorne E; 1721 Lakeshore Rd W, Mississauga ON L5J 1J4; McG'99; FRCSC; Otol (Head & Neck Surgery). Staff, Sunnybrook Health Sciences Centre; (905)607-0033; Fax. (905)607-0036.

SEGATO, Peter M; Mud Creek Medical Co-Op, 12E Elm Ave, Wolfville NS B4P 1Z9; UBC'89; CCFP; Langs: Danish; (902)542-3633; Fax. (902)542-2709.

SEGBEFIA, Catherine I; The Hosp for Sick Children, 555 University Ave, Toronto ON M5G 1X8; Kwame Nkrumah University (Other Foreign)'97; Clin Fellow Hem, The Hospital For Sick Children; (416)813-7459

SEGEDI, Ljubinka; Segedi Medicine Prof Corp, 944 King St W, Kitchener ON N2G 1G4; Belgrade (Serbia)'74; CCFP; Langs: Slovak; Serbian; Croatian; (519)585-1981; Fax. (519)585-2356.

SEGEDI, Maja; 10 145 NU-585 University Ave, Toronto ON M5G 2N2; Tor'05; FRCSC; GenSurg. Staff, Toronto General Hospital - UHN; (416)340-4252

SEGEDI, Therese T N; LL-1107 37 St SW, Calgary AB T3C 1S5; (403)246-7788; Fax. (403)242-8850.

SEGEL, George B; The Hosp for Sick Children, 555 University Ave, Toronto ON M5G 1X8; Thomas Jefferson University (USA)'64; Staff Short Duration, The Hospital For Sick Children; (416)813-5401

SEGEL, Lawrence L; Manulife Financial, 3-200 Bloor St E, Toronto ON M4W 1E5; Qns'76; Staff, Manulife Financial; (416)926-6951; Fax. (416)926-6732; larry_segel@manulife.com.

SEGER, Mark R; 306-125 13th St E, North Vancouver BC V7L 2L3; UBC'89; (604)988-8133; Fax. (604)988-8193.

SEGERS, Isidor; Spall Med Clinic, 150-1940 Harvey Ave, Kelowna BC V1Y 8J8; Pretoria (South Africa)'78; MB ChB; LMCC; Langs: Afrikaans; (250)860-9909

SEGSTRO, Ronald J; Health Sciences Ctr Gen Hosp, GA 709-700 William Ave, Winnipeg MB R3E 0Z3; Man'87; FRCPC; Anes. Staff, Health Sciences Centre; (204)787-3796; Fax. (204)787-3656.

SEGU, Michael K B; Regina Centre Med Clinic, 1957 Osler St, Regina SK S4P 1W3; RCS (Ireland)'64; (306)569-1777; Fax. (306)569-0379.

SEGUIN, Aimee M; Meadow Lake Associate Clinic, PO Box 1510, Meadow Lake SK S9X 1Z1; Sask'09; BSc(Hon.); CCFP; Staff, Meadow Lake Hospital; (306)236-5661; Fax. (306)236-4355.

SEGUIN, Andre M; CSSS de Memphremagog, 50 rue Saint-Patrice E, Magog QC J1X 3X3; Mon'85; Staff, Centre Hospitalier et CLSC de Memphremagog; (819)843-3381; Fax. (819)843-8262.

SEGUIN, Anick; Hotel-Dieu d'Arthabaska, 5 rue des Hospitalieres, Victoriaville QC G6P 6N2; Sher'96; FRCPC; Anes (Anesthesia Surgery). Staff, Hotel-Dieu d'Arthabaska; Langs: English; French; (819)357-2030

SEGUIN, Bernard A; 100-2555 St Joseph Blvd, Orleans ON K1C 1S6; Ott'72; CCFP; FCFP; Vis Staff, Montfort Hospital; Langs: English; (613)830-1298

SEGUIN, Bernard; Clin d'Orthopedie Sagamie, 315-874 boul de l'Universite E, Chicoutimi QC G7H 6B9; Laval'68; OrthSurg. Langs: Bilingual(French/English); (418)549-7450; Fax. (418)549-8661.

SEGUIN, Caroline; Hop Charles LeMoyne, 3120 boul Taschereau, Greenfield Park QC J4V 2H1; Mon'94; DiagRad. Staff, Hopital Charles LeMoyne; (450)466-5000; Fax. (450)466-8887.

SEGUIN, Chantal; MUHC-Montreal Gen Hosp, A7 1171-1650 av Cedar, Montreal QC H3G 1A4; Mon'94; FRCPC; IntMed; MedOncol; Hem. Staff, McGill University Health Centre - Montreal General Campus; Langs: Bilingual(French/English); (514)934-1934

SEGUIN, Daniel R; Clarence-Rockland Fam Hlth Team, 2741 rue Chamberland, Rockland ON K4K 0B4; Ott'92; CCFP; Langs: Bilingual(English/French); (613)446-7677; Fax. (613)446-5737.

SEGUIN, Eric; Clnique Med du Sud-Ouest, 103-4475 rue Bannantyne, Verdun QC H4G 1E3; Mon'90; Langs: Bilingual(French/English); (514)765-3600; Fax. (514)765-9625.

SEGUIN, Gerald L; 1 Champlain St, Plantagenet ON K0B 1L0; Ott'62; Langs: French; (613)673-4644

SEGUIN, Guylaine; CHUS-Hop Fleurimont, 3001 12e av N, Sherbrooke QC J1H 5N4; Sher'92; FRCPC; Anes. Staff, Centre Hospitalier Universitaire de Sherbrooke-Hopital Fleurimont; (819)346-1110

SEGUIN, Jean J; Activecare Caremedics FMC, 103-311 McArthur Ave, Vanier ON K1L 8M3; Ott'99; Dip SportMed; CCFP; Asst Surg, The Ottawa Hospital - Civic Campus; Staff Sport Med Clinic, Carleton University; Langs: English; (613)749-1678; Fax. (613)749-9446.

SEGUIN, John P; 506 Astorville Rd RR 1, Astorville ON P0H 1B0; McM'97; CCFP; (705)752-5521; Fax. (705)752-2193.

SEGUIN, Joseph J Y; CSSSG-Hop de Hull, 400-92 Saint-Raymond, Gatineau QC J8Y 1W4; Ott'74; FRCPC; Psy. Staff, Hull Hospital; Langs: English; (819)966-6525

SEGUIN, Marc; CSSS du Nord de Lanaudière, 1000 boul Sainte-Anne, St-Charles-Brromee QC J6E 6J2; Mon'92; FRCSC; ObstGyn. Staff, Centre Hospitalier Régional de Lanaudière; (450)759-8222

SEGUIN, Marie-Claudel; CSSS Pierre Boucher, 1333 boul Jacques-Cartier E, Longueuil QC J4M 2A5; Mon'97; Staff, Centre Hospitalier Pierre Boucher; (450)468-8111

SEGUIN, Marie-France; Clinique Med Plaza Gatineau, 381 boul Maloney E, Gatineau QC J8P 1E3; Laval'93; Staff, CSSS de Gatineau; (819)663-7393; Fax. (819)669-0077.

SEGUIN, Mario; CHUS-Hop Fleurimont, 3001 12e av N, Sherbrooke QC J1H 5N4; Mon'81; FRCSC; Neursurg. Staff, Centre Hospitalier Universitaire de Sherbrooke-Hopital Fleurimont; Aj Prof, Universite de Sherbrooke; (819)346-1110 x13324; Fax. (819)820-6452.

SEGUIN, Nathalie; Ctr Hosp de Verdun, 4000 boul Lasalle, Verdun QC H4G 2A3; Mon'89; DiagRad. Staff, Centre Hospitalier de Verdun; (514)765-8121

SEGUIN, Pierre; Dir de Sante Publique de Mtl, 1301 rue Sherbrooke E, Montreal QC H2L 1M3; Sher'72; MSc; CommunMed (P.Q.) (Occupational Medicine). Staff, Direction de la Sante Publique de Montreal; (514)528-2400

SEGUIN, Robert W; 198 Dell St, Sudbury ON P3C 2Y3; Ott'69; Att Staff, Health Sciences North - Memorial Site; Att Staff, Health Sciences North-St Joseph's Health Centre; Langs: French; (705)674-3461; Fax. (705)674-8901.

SEGURA, Jose A C; Centre Hosp de Chandler, 451 rue Monseigneur Ross E, Chandler QC G0C 1K0; Santiago (Chile)'73; LMCC; FRCPC; Psy (Community Psychiatry). Staff, Centre Hospitalier l'Université de Montréal (CHUM) - Hôpital Notre-Dame; Médecin, Centre Hospitalier de Chandler; Physician Ped Psy, CLSC de Chandler; Langs: Spanish; English; French; (418)689-2261; cabinet.jasegura@sympatico.ca.

SEGURA, Jose; Niagara H System-Welland Site, 65 Third St, Welland ON L3B 4W6; McG'86; FRCPC; GenPath. Staff, Niagara Health System - Welland Hospital Site; (905)732-6111 x3327

SEHDEV, Dashminder; Hamilton HS-General Site, 237 Barton St E, Hamilton ON L8L 2X2; Wes'06; CCFP; CCFP(E.M.); Staff, Hamilton Health Sciences Centre - Hamilton General Hospital; Langs: Punjabi; French; (905)527-4322

SEHDEV, Sandeep R; William Osler HC-Brampton, 5F-2100 Bovaird Dr E, Brampton ON L6R 3J7; Ott'86; FRCPC; IntMed (Hematology); MedOncol. Staff, William Osler Health System - Brampton Civic Hospital; Staff, The Oncology Group; (905)494-6542; Fax. (905)494-6416.

SEHGAL, Jaishree; Belgage Med Arts Bldg, 102-525 Belmont Ave W, Kitchener ON N2M 5E2; Delhi (India)'76; Langs: Hindi; Punjabi; Urdu; (519)745-7550; Fax. (519)745-5665.

SEHGAL, Parmila; Appletree Med Center, 10/11-680 Rexdale Blvd, Etobicoke ON M9W 0B5; Belfast (Ireland)'75; MB ChB; BAO; Langs: Punjabi; (416)213-9577; Fax. (416)213-9588.

SEHGAL, Tarun; University of Alberta Hosp, 8440 112 St NW, Edmonton AB T6G 2B7; Alb'08; IntMed. Staff, University of Alberta Hospital; (780)407-8822

SEHGAL, Yogi; Centre Noreen Richard, 715 Priestman St, Fredericton NB E3B 5W7; Ott'96; CCFP; Staff, Dr Everett Chalmers Regional Hospital; Langs: French; (506)474-4611

SEHL, John J; 495 Park St, Kitchener ON N2G 1N7; Wes'89; BSc; (519)571-7496; Fax. (519)954-3489.

SEHL, Michael J; 340 Hagey Blvd, Waterloo ON N2L 6R6; Tor'83; Staff, St Mary's General Hospital; (519)747-2677

SEHMER, John M; Oakmont Med Centre, 210-809 41st Ave W, Vancouver BC V5Z 2N6; UBC'77; MSc(IndustMed); CCBOM; Assoc Staff, Vancouver General Hospital - Centennial Pavillion; Clin Assoc Prof Family Pract, University of British Columbia; (604)266-2345; Fax. (604)266-2346.

SEHN, Laurie H; BC Cancer Agency-Vancouver CC, 600 10th Ave W, Vancouver BC V5Z 4E6; McG'91; MedOncol; IntMed. Staff, BC Cancer Agency Vancouver Centre; (604)877-6000 x2746; lsehn@bccancer.bc.ca.

SEHON, Anthony A P; Strathcona Mental Health Team, 330 Heatley Ave, Vancouver BC V6A 3G3; Man'79; FRCPC; Psy (Disability Assessment). Dir Psy Education, Vancouver Coastal Health; Clin Prof Psy, University of British Columbia; (604)253-4401; Fax. (604)253-5194.

SEHRAVAT, Narinder S; Albion-Kipling Med Centre, 305-1525 Albion Rd, Etobicoke ON M9V 5G5; Maharshi Dayanand University (India)'84; CCFP; Langs: Hindi; Punjabi; Urdu; (416)740-2274; Fax. (416)740-6178.

SEIB, Deborah L; Emerald Business Centre, 2009-20 Kingsbridge Garden Cir, Mississauga ON L5R 3K7; McM'93; CCFP; (905)712-4094; Fax. (905)712-3298; drseib@laserandveincosmetics.com.

SEIB, Rachael K; Kingston Gen Hosp, V2-76 Stuart St, Kingston ON K7L 2V7; McM'06; FRCPC; Anes. Staff, Toronto Western Hospital - University Health Network; Staff, Kingston General Hospital; (613)549-6666

SEIBEL, Deborah A; 107 Bottomley Ave S, Saskatoon SK S7N 1K5; Cal'73; DTMH(Lond); CCFP; FCFP; Staff Family Med, Regina Qu'Appelle Health Region; Staff, Saskatoon Health Region; Clinical Asst Prof Family Med, University of Saskatchewan; (306)585-7735; Fax. (306)522-8860.

SEIBEL, Donald G; 4420 36 Ave, Edmonton AB T6L 3S1; Alb'75; CAFCI; (780)487-2770; Fax. (780)487-4204; drseibel@telusplanet.net.

SEID, Cherinet; North Renfrew Family Hlth Team, 117 Banting Dr, Deep River ON K0J 1P0; Addis Ababa University (Other Foreign)'99; CCFP; Langs: Amharic; (613)584-1037; cherinets@drdh.org.

SEID, Ying Suey; 2F-607 Gerrard St E, Toronto ON M4M 1Y2; Tor'77; Fam Med, The Salvation Army Toronto Grace Health Centre; Langs: Chinese; (416)461-7547; Fax. (416)461-7548.

SEIDE, Rony; RSSS des Aurores Boreales, CP 6000 Succ Bureau-Chef 679 2e rue E, La Sarre QC J9Z 2X7; Port-au-Prince (Haiti)'91; CCFP; Staff, Centre Hospitalier La Sarre; Staff, CSSS des Aurores Boreales; (819)333-2311; rony_seide@ssss.gouv.qc.ca.

SEIDELIN, Peter H; Univ Hlth Network-Toronto Gen, EN6-234A-200 Elizabeth St, Toronto ON M5G 2C4; Edinburgh (Scotland)'83; MB ChB; FRCPC; IntMed (Cardiology). Staff, Toronto General Hospital - UHN; Assoc Prof Med, University of Toronto; (416)340-4930; Fax. (416)340-3865.

SEIDEN, Howard S; Front-Frederick Health Service, 14F-365 Bloor St E, Toronto ON M4W 3L4; Tor'77; MSc(Pharmacol.); CCFP; FCFP; Staff, St Michael's Hospital; Staff, Toronto General Hospital - UHN; Owner, CML Health Care; Examiner Civil Aviation/Advisor DAC, United States Homeland Security; (416)362-8614; Fax. (416)362-6070; howard.seiden@seidenhealth.com.

SEIDENFELD, Allan M; Sunnybrook Hlth Sciences Ctre, 301-2075 Bayview Ave, Toronto ON M4N 3M5; Tor'73; FRCP; FRCPC; IntMed (Medical Oncology); Hem. Staff HemOncol, Humber River Regional Hospital - Church Street Site; Staff Med & HemOncol, Sunnybrook Health Sciences Centre - Edmond Odette Cancer Centre; Staff, Sunnybrook Health Sciences Centre; Langs: Hebrew; (416)227-1070 x225; Fax. (416)227-1076; drsis@rogers.com.

SEIDL, Maja M; 111-170 Queensway W, Mississauga ON L5B 3A8; Tor'99; BSc; MHSc; CCFP; FCFP; Langs: Croatian; (905)566-0121; Fax. (905)566-8100.

SEIDL, Mladen; Aderwood Med Clinic, 878 Brown's Line, Etobicoke ON M8W 3W2; Zagreb (Croatia)'64; Langs: Croatian; Russian; Slovenian; (416)503-2541; Fax. (416)503-2549.

SEIDLER, Christine; South River Med Centre, PO Box 579 140 Ottawa Ave W, South River ON P0A 1X0; McM'00; CCFP; Asst Prof, Northern Ontario School of Medicine; Langs: French; (705)386-0512; Fax. (705)386-0716.

SEIDMAN, Ernest G; MUHC-Montreal Children's Hosp, C10 145-1650 Cedar Avenue, Montreal QC H3G 1A4; McG'78; FACG; FRCPC; Peds (Gastroenterology). Staff, McGill University Health Centre - Montreal Children's Hospital; Staff Gastroent, McGill University Health Centre - Montreal General Campus; Prof Med & Peds/Chaire B Kaufman Endower IBD, McGill University; Langs: French; Hebrew; Bilingual(English/French); (514)934-8309; Fax. (514)934-8321; digestivelab@hotmail.com.

SEIDMAN, Sheryl G; Univ Hlth Network-Toronto Gen, 200 Elizabeth St, Toronto ON M5G 2C4; Qns'96; CCFP; Staff, Toronto General Hospital - UHN; Langs: Hebrew; French; (416)340-3111

SEIDMANN, Tamara; St John Reg Hosp Facility, PO Box 2100 Stn Main 400 University Ave, Saint John NB E2L 4L2; Bratislava (Slovakia)'79; FRCPC; Anes. Staff, Horizon Health Network Saint John Public Health; Staff, Saint John Regional Hospital; (506)648-6000; Fax. (506)648-6860.

SEIF, Maged G A; Living Arts Med Centre, 2-4100 Living Arts Dr, Mississauga ON L5B 0C3; Assiut (Egypt)'95; CCFP; Langs: Arabic; (905)270-5600; Fax. (905)270-8830.

SEIF, Mona F M; Churchill Med Clinic, 6-3050 Artesian Dr, Mississauga ON L5M 7P5; Ain Shams University (Egypt)'88; CCFP; (905)607-6495; Fax. (905)607-0881.

SEIF-ZADEH, Atih; MEDWELL Clinic, 2-10288 Yonge St, Richmond Hill ON L4C 3B8; Spartan Health Sciences Univ (Saint Lucia)'98; FRCPC; Psy. Staff, Rouge Valley Health System - Centenary Health Centre Site; Langs: Persian; (905)237-9354

SEIFER, Colette; St Boniface Gen Hosp, Y3006-409 Tache Ave, Winnipeg MB R2H 2A6; Staff Cardiol, St Boniface General Hospital; (204)233-8563

SEIFER, Roman; 1205-72 Donald St, Winnipeg MB R3C 1L7; Dublin (Ireland)'57; MB ChB; Psy. Staff, Health Sciences Centre; (204)942-4964

SEIFERT, Oliver; Gateway Med Clinic, 950-3803 Calgary Trail NW, Edmonton AB T6J 5M8; (Germany)'90; Staff, Cold Lake Healthcare Centre; Langs: German; French; (780)436-7240; Fax. (780)436-8142; drseifert@pobox.com.

SEIFRED, Grant P; Niagara HS-Greater Niagara, 5546 Portage Rd, Niagara Falls ON L2E 6X2; Man'82; FACEP; Staff, Niagara Health System - Greater Niagara General Site; (905)522-4941 x3113

SEIGEL, Karen J; Crowfoot West Business Centre, 210-600 Crowfoot Cres NW, Calgary AB T3G 0B4; Qns'02; CCFP; (403)239-9733; Fax. (403)241-8112.

SEIGEL, Sandra A; LL-107 King St W, Dundas ON L9H 1V1; Tor'86; FRCPC; Peds (Pediatric HIV Disease). Staff Pediatric HIV Clinic, Hamilton Health Sciences Centre - McMaster Children's Hospital; Staff, St Joseph's Healthcare - Charlton Campus; Clin Assoc Prof, McMaster University; (905)628-0054; Fax. (905)628-5701.

SEIGEL, Stuart N; Glenmore Clinic, 1605 Gordon Dr, Kelowna BC V1Y 3G8; Qns'83; BSc; FRCPC; IntMed; Rheum. Att Staff, Kelowna General Hospital; (250)762-3808; Fax. (250)762-4477.

SEIGO, Raymond L; 103-9710 Second St, Sidney BC V8L 3C4; Cal'80; BSc; MSc; FRCPC; IntMed. Staff, Vancouver Island Health Authority; (250)656-4161; Fax. (250)655-1219.

SEIKALY, Hadi R; University of Alberta Hosp, 1E4 33 WMC-8440 112 St NW, Edmonton AB T6G 2B7; Tor'88; FRCSC; Otol (Head & Neck Surgery). Staff, University of Alberta Hospital; Assoc Prof/ Research & Otol/Div Dir Otol Head & Neck Surgery, University of Alberta; (780)407-3691; Fax. (780)407-6059.

SEIPP, Timothy T; Veterans Affairs Canada, 60 Nanaimo Ave W, Penticton BC V2A 1N1; UBC'74; (250)770-4406; Fax. (250)770-4411; timothy.seipp@vac-acc.gc.ca.

SEIT, Shawn C W; 1010-32 South Unionville Ave, Markham ON L3R 9S6; Tor'89; Langs: Cantonese.

SEITZ, Andrew R; Western Med Clinic, 144 6th St, Brandon MB R7A 3N2; Alb'87; (204)727-6451; Fax. (866)672-7951.

SEITZ, Dallas P; Providence Care-Mental Health, PO Box 603 Stn Main 752 King St W, Kingston ON K7L 4X3; Sask'03; FRCPC; Psy. Staff, Providence Care - Mental Health Services; (613)546-1101

SEJEAN, Georges; 306-3535 ch Queen-Mary, Montreal QC H3V 1H8; Beirut (Lebanon)'71; FRCSC; Otol. Staff, Hôpital Santa Cabrini Ospedale; Staff, McGill University Health Centre - Montreal General Campus; (514)738-0175

SEKAR, Arni S C; Parkdale Med Tower, 207-1081 Carling Ave, Ottawa ON K1Y 4G2; Mysore (India)'65; LRCP; MRCS; MRC(UK); FRCPC; IntMed; Gastroent. Court Consultant, Queensway Carleton Hospital; Staff Gastrent, The Ottawa Hospital - Civic Campus; (613)729-3179; Fax. (613)729-1026.

SEKELY, Istvan; Advanced Walk-In Med Clinic, 111-21 Queensway W, Mississauga ON L5B 1B6; Semmelweis (Hungary)'84; CCFP; Court Staff Family Practice, Trillium Health Centre - Mississauga; Langs: Hungarian; (905)897-0788

SEKHAVAT, Houfar; 855 Dieppe Blvd, Dieppe NB E1A 7R8; Sher'00; FRCPC; Ophth (Cataract & Glaucoma). Langs: Spanish; English; Persian; (506)386-6747; Fax. (506)386-8158.

SEKHON, Harmanjatinder S; The Ottawa Hosp-Gen Campus, CCW 4220-501 Smyth Rd Box 117, Ottawa ON K1H 8L6; Magadh University (India)'82; Staff, The Ottawa Hospital - General Campus; (613)737-8899 x79036; Fax. (613)737-8853.

SEKHON, Rajinder S; Tecumseh Manning Med Centre, 202-13278 Tecumseh Rd E, Windsor ON N8N 3T6; Tor'88; CCFP; CCFP(E.M.); FCFP; (519)945-7365; Fax. (519)945-9644.

SEKI, John T; 3-4337 Burnside Line, Orillia ON L3V 6H4; Ott'93; FACS; FRCSC; PlasSurg (Hand & Reconstructive Surgery). Ac Staff, Orillia Soldiers' Memorial Hospital; (705)325-6805; Fax. (705)325-9402.

SEKIGUCHI, Debora R; Health Sciences Centre, MS599R-820 Sherbrook St, Winnipeg MB R3A 1R9; Staff, Health Sciences Centre; (204)774-8511

SEKULA, Zygmunt P; Spryfield Family Med Clinic, 315 Hering Cove Rd, Halifax NS B3R 1V5; Silesian (Poland)'63; Langs: Polish; Russian; Arabic; (902)479-0025; Fax. (902)479-2627.

SEKYI-OTU, Ato; BD 48-2140 North Park Dr, Brampton ON L6S 0C9; Tor'90; MSc; FRCSC; OrthSurg (Post Traumatic Arthritis). Staff, William Osler Health System - Brampton Civic Hospital; (905)454-7924

SELAMAN, Mustafa H; The Salvation Army Grace Hosp, 300 Booth Dr, Winnipeg MB R3J 3M7; Baghdad (Iraq)'84; FRCPC; IntMed; Critical Care Medicine. Staff, The Salvation Army Grace Hospital; (204)837-0391

SELAND, Karen L; University Hosp of Northern BC, 1475 Edmonton St, Prince George BC V2M 1S2; Alb'06; FRCPC; DiagRad. Staff, University Hospital of Northern British Columbia; (250)565-2000

SELAND, T Peter; 901 Steele Rd, Kelowna BC V1W 4X1; Alb'64; Neur. Dep Registrar, College of Physicians & Surgeons of British Columbia; (604)787-2174

SELBY, Deborah M; Sunnybrook Hlth Sciences Ctre, H336-2075 Bayview Ave, Toronto ON M4N 3M5; Tor'89; FRCPC; IntMed (Cardiology). Staff, Sunnybrook Health Sciences Centre; (416)480-6100; Fax. (416)480-5146.

SELBY, Kathryn A; Children's & Women's HC Of BC, K3 146-4480 Oak St, Vancouver BC V6H 3V4; Manchester (England)'79; MB BS; FRCPC; Peds; Neur. Staff, BC Children's Hospital; (604)875-2121; Fax. (604)875-2285.

SELBY, Peter L; Bell Gateway Bldg, 3272-100 Stokes St, Toronto ON M6J 1H4; Bombay (India)'89; MHSc; ASAM; CCFP; FCFP; Consultant, St Joseph's Health Centre; Head Nicotine Dependence Clinic, Centre for Addiction & Mental Health (CAMH) - Russell Street Site; Consultant Clin Pharmacol & Toxicology Dept of Peds, The Hospital For Sick Children; Mother Risk; Asst Prof Family & Commun Med, University of Toronto; Langs: Hindi; Marathi; (416)535-8501 x6019; Fax. (416)595-6728; peter.selby@utoronto.ca.

SELBY, Rita; Sunnybrook Hlth Sciences Ctre, A 459-2075 Bayview Ave, Toronto ON M4N 3M5; Nagpur (India)'91; MB BS; FRCPC; IntMed (Thromboembolism); Hem. Staff Med, Sunnybrook Health Sciences Centre; Asst Prof, University of Toronto; Langs: Hindi; Marathi; Sindhi; (416)480-5105

SELCHEN, Daniel H; St Michael's Hosp, SW 001-30 Bond St, Toronto ON M5B 1W8; Man'80; Neur (Multiple Sclerosis). Head Division of Neurol, St Michael's Hospital; Dir, Regional Stroke Centre; Consultant, Multiple Sclerosis Clinic; (416)864-5855; Fax. (416)864-5581.

SELCHEN, Steven K; Mount Sinai Hosp, 941A-600 University Ave, Toronto ON M5G 1X5; Tor'06; FRCPC; Psy. Staff, Mount Sinai Hospital; (416)586-4800

SELDON, Roger C; Campbell River & Dist Gen Hosp, 375 2nd Ave, Campbell River BC V9W 3V1; Cape Town (South Africa)'87; MB ChB; CCFP; Staff, Campbell River & District General Hospital; Langs: Afrikaans; (250)287-2111; Fax. (250)287-2444.

SELEGEAN, Sorin M; Cobequid Comm Health Centre, 7F-5788 University Ave, Halifax NS B3H 1V8; Universitatea de Med si Farmacie Luliu Hatieganu (Other Foreign)'90; Staff Path & Lab Med, Cobequid Community Health Centre; (902)473-7706; Fax. (902)473-7978; sorin.selegean@cdha.nshealth.ca.

SELEMANI, Salumu; Assertive Comm Treatment Team, 36 Queensway, Grnd-Falls-Windsor NL A2B 1J2; University of Kinshasa (Congo (Democratic Republic))'80; Staff, Central Newfoundland Regional Health Centre; Staff, Western Memorial Regional Hospital.

SELF, Dalton D; Red Deer Reg Hosp Centre, 3942 50A Ave, Red Deer AB T4N 4E7; Alb'96; FRCPC; Anes. Staff, Red Deer Regional Hospital Centre; (403)343-4422

SELHI, Brahm D; Selhi Med Prof Corp, 1121 103rd St, North Battleford SK S9A 1K5; Punjab (India)'76; MB BS; CCFP; Med VP, Battlefords Union Hospital; Physician, Battlefords Medical Centre; (306)445-9459; Fax. (306)445-9450.

SELI UZELAC, Antonia; Halton Healthcare Services, 6F-700 Dorval Dr, Oakville ON L6K 3V3; McM'98; BSc(Hons); FRCPC; Psy. Staff Psy, Halton Healthcare Services Corporation - Oakville Site; Asst Prof, McMaster University; (905)338-4432 x4805; Fax. (905)815-5096.

SELICK, Avram Z; Mackenzie Richmond Hill Hosp, 10 Trench St, Richmond Hill ON L4C 4Z3; Tor'74; Staff, Mackenzie Richmond Hill Hospital; (905)883-1212

SELIGMAN, James V; 306-1017 Wilson Ave, North York ON M3K 1Z1; Tor'81; FRCSC; OrthSurg (Hip & Knee Reconstruction). Chief Surg/Dir Surg Program, Humber River Regional Hospital - Church Street Site; (416)240-9995; Fax. (416)240-9415.

SELIM, Adrien; Centre Hosp Chisasibi, PO Box 250, Chisasibi QC J0M 1E0; McG'09; CCFP; Staff, Cree Board of Health & Social Services James Bay; (819)855-9001; Fax. (819)855-2867.

SELINA, Paul G; Valley Med Imaging, 102-32475 Simon Ave, Abbotsford BC V2T 5E3; Alb'94; (604)859-8998

SELINGER, Gregory E; White Clinic Associates, 100-383 Ellis St, Penticton BC V2A 4L9; Sask'98; LMCC; CCFP; Physician, Primary Care Maternity Clinic; (250)492-3024; Fax. (250)492-2761.

SELISKE, Maureen E; 1-3260 Edgemont Blvd, North Vancouver BC V7R 2P2; Tor'90; CCFP; (604)988-2444

SELK, Amanda; Women's College Hosp, 76 Grenville St, Toronto ON M5S 1B2; Wes'04; FRCSC; ObstGyn. Staff Gynaecology Clinic, Mount Sinai Hospital; Staff Gynecology, Women's College Hospital; (416)323-7744

SELK, Bradley A; Selk Physical Med & EMG, 106-311 Ludlow St, Saskatoon SK S7S 1N6; Sask'05; FRCPC; PhysMed&Rehab. Staff, Saskatoon City Hospital; (306)975-3933; Fax. (306)975-3931.

SELKE, Petra A; Fairmont Med Bldg, 1208-750 Broadway W, Vancouver BC V5Z 1J2; UBC'83; FRCSC; ObstGyn. Ac Staff, BC Women's Hospital & Health Centre; Ac Staff, Vancouver General Hospital - Centennial Pavillion; Clin Assoc Prof, University of British Columbia; (604)872-1260; Fax. (604)872-1261; paselkemd@telus.net.

SELL MARUCCO, Erick F; Children's Hosp Eastern Ont, 401 Smyth Rd, Ottawa ON K1H 8L1; Autonoma de Centro America (Other Foreign)'96; Staff, Children's Hospital of Eastern Ontario (CHEO); Langs: Spanish; (613)737-2393

SELLENS, Catherine S; 237 Barton St E, Hamilton ON L8L 2X2; McM'94; FRCPC; EmergMed. Staff, St Joseph's Healthcare - Charlton Campus; Staff, Hamilton Health Sciences Centre - Hamilton General Hospital; Asst Prof Med, McMaster University; (905)527-4322 x46368

SELLERS, A Ruth; Queen Elizabeth Hosp, PO Box 6600 Stn Central 60 Riverside Dr, Charlottetown PE C1A 8T5; McM'80; FRCPC; GenPath; AnatPath. Staff, Queen Elizabeth Hospital; (902)894-2111; msmacdonald@gov.pe.ca.

SELLERS, Elizabeth A C; Children's Hosp, FE307-685 William Ave, Winnipeg MB R3E 0Z2; Wes'92; FRCPC; Peds (Pediatric Endocrinology & Metabolism); Endocrin&Metab. Staff, Variety Children's Heart Centre; Assoc Prof, University of Manitoba; (204)787-7435; Fax. (204)787-1655; esellers@exchange.hsc.mb.ca.

SELLERS, Laura P; Centretown Commun Health Ctre, 420 Cooper St, Ottawa ON K2P 2N6; Ott'07; CCFP; Staff, The Ottawa Hospital - General Campus; Langs: Bilingual(English/French); (613)233-4697

SELLERS, Laurene R; Grand River Hosp-KW HC, PO Box 9056 Stn C 835 King St, Kitchener ON N2G 1G3; McM'88; CCFP; Ac Staff, Grand River Hospital - Kitchener/Waterloo Health Centre; Ac Staff, St Mary's General Hospital; (519)749-4300; Fax. (519)662-2025.

SELLIAH, Prasanna S; Peel Med Arts Bldg, 202-2120 Northpark Dr, Brampton ON L6S 0C9; Tor'92; FRCPC; Peds. (905)799-9815; Fax. (905)799-5950.

SELLMER, Rory C; Foothills Med Centre, 22-1403 29 St NW, Calgary AB T2N 2T9; Cal'03; FRCPC; Psy. Staff, Foothills Medical Centre; (403)944-1322

SELMAN, W Gary; Gulf Canada Square, 320-401 9 Ave SW, Calgary AB T2P 3C5; Alb'74; FRCSC; GenSurg. Ac Staff, Alberta Children's Hospital; Prof, University Of Calgary; (403)221-4489; Fax. (403)221-4420.

SELMANI, Sabrina; CSSS de Rimouski-Neigette, CP 3150 Succ A 150 av Rouleau, Rimouski QC G5L 5T1; Alger (Algeria)'87; Staff RadOncol, Hôpital Regional Rimouski; Université Laval; (418)724-8362; Fax. (418)724-8247.

SELOSSE, Bruno M R J; Clinique Med De Caraquet, CP 5712, Caraquet NB E1W 1B7; Lille (France)'70; Ac Staff, Hôpital de l'Enfant-Jésus RHSJ; (506)727-3332; Fax. (506)727-7365.

SELTENRICH, Michael E; Nanaimo Reg Gen Hosp, 1200 Dufferin Cres, Nanaimo BC V9S 2B7; Cal'97; FRCPC; Anes. Staff, Nanaimo Regional General Hospital; (250)755-7605

SELTZER, Eric C; Whitby MDM Clinic, 80 Thickson Rd S, Whitby ON L1N 7T2; McG'90; Langs: French; (905)668-6448; Fax. (905)668-4023.

SELUCKY, Michal; Markham Stouffville Hlth Ctre, 404-377 Church St, Markham ON L6B 1A1; Tor'83; ABIM; FRCPC; IntMed; Gastroent. Staff, Markham Stouffville Hospital; (905)472-7125; Fax. (905)472-3007.

SELVAKONE, Meera; Pinnacle Health Sciences Ctre, 2-9651 Yonge St, Richmond Hill ON L4C 1V7; UBC'01; CCFP; (905)780-8823; Fax. (905)780-8821.

SELVANANDAN, Vamini K; Alpine Med Clinic, PO Box 4000 Stn Main 201A-211 Bear St, Banff AB T1L 1J8; Tor'99; CCFP; (403)762-3155

SELVANANTHAN, Manivannan; Finch-Warden Med Walk-In Clin, 6A-3430 Finch Ave E, Scarborough ON M1W 2R5; Moscow (Russia (Federation))'89; CCFP; FCFP; Langs: Tamil; Russian; Sinhalese; (416)496-1990; Fax. (416)496-1984.

SELVANAYAGARAJAH, Selliah; York Med Centre, 10660 Yonge St, Richmond Hill ON L4C 3C9; Ceylon (Sri Lanka)'75; MB BS; LMCC; CCFP; Langs: Tamil; (905)770-9096; Fax. (905)770-4703.

SELVARAJ, Madhavan; Surrey Mental Hlth & Addiction, 11F-13401 108 Ave, Surrey BC V3T 5T3; Tamil Nadu University (India)'00; FRCPC; Psy. (604)953-4900

SELVARAJAH, Prrasonna; Oshawa Health Centre, 1F-247 Simcoe St N, Oshawa ON L1G 4T3; (Other Foreign)'06; CCFP; Langs: Tamil; (905)728-7915

SELVARAJAH, Vijeyakumar; Millwoods Town Ctre Prof Bldg, 333-6203 28 Ave NW, Edmonton AB T6L 6K3; Wes'06; FRCPC; IntMed; Gastroent. (780)705-9933; Fax. (780)705-2895.

SELWYN, B Karen; Harvard Square Mall, 210-801 Mohawk Rd W, Hamilton ON L9C 6C2; McM'83; CCFP; FCFP; (905)389-7327; Fax. (905)389-1600.

SELYANINA, Tatyana; CMC Medical Centre, 777 Dundas St W, Mississauga ON L5C 3B6; Karaganda State Medical Academy (Other Foreign)'00; CCFP; Langs: Russian; (905)949-5330

SELZNER, Markus; NCSB 11 C, 1244-585 University Ave, Toronto ON M5G 2N2; Wilhelms Westphalian University (Other Foreign)'93; Staff, Toronto General Hospital - UHN; Staff, The Banting Institute; (416)340-5230

SELZNER-MALEKKIANI, Nazia; Univ Hlth Network-Toronto Gen, 11NCSB 124-200 Elizabeth St, Toronto ON M5G 2C4; Paris (France)'98; PhD; Staff, Toronto General Hospital - UHN; Langs: German; French; (416)340-3451; Fax. (416)340-3126; nazia.selzner@uhn.on.ca.

SEM, Francis W C; Toronto East Gen & Orth Hosp, 825 Coxwell Ave, Toronto ON M4C 3E7; Tor'92; CCFP; FCFP; CCFP(E.M.); Staff, Toronto East General Hospital Inc; Langs: Cantonese; Mandarin; (416)469-6435

SEMAAN, William; CHUS-Hop Hotel-Dieu, 580 rue Bowen S, Sherbrooke QC J1G 2E8; Beirut (Lebanon)'94; Staff, Centre Hospitalier Universitaire de Sherbrooke-Hôpital Hôtel-Dieu; Langs: Bilingual(English/French); (819)822-6733; Fax. (819)822-6790.

SEMAKA, Frank D; PO Box 24073 Rpo Evergreen, Calgary AB T2Y 0J9; Cal'75; CCFP; FCFP.

SEMAKA, Shirley D; Medical Clinic West Tower, 1001-1726 14 Av NW, Calgary AB T2N 4Y8; Cal'80; MSc; PhD; CCFP; FCFP; (403)284-8666

SEMCZYSZYN, Miroslav V; Stoney Creek Med Walk-In Clin, 140 Centennial Pky N, Hamilton ON L8E 1H9; Tor'93; CCFP; Langs: Ukrainian; Polish; (905)561-9255

SEMELHAGO, Gavin R; 207 Main St W PO Box 890, Palmerston ON N0G 2P0; Tor'89; Staff, North Wellington Health Care - Palmerston & District Hospital; (519)343-5000; Fax. (519)343-3544.

SEMELHAGO, Lloyd C; Hamilton HS-General Site, 723-237 Barton St E, Hamilton ON L8L 2X2; Tor'88; BSc; MSc; FRCSC; GenSurg; CardSurg. Staff/Assoc Prof, Hamilton Health Sciences Centre - Hamilton General Hospital; (905)527-7168; Fax. (905)527-0538.

SEMENIUK, Deborah D; Links Clinic, 104-11910 111 Ave NW, Edmonton AB T5G 3G6; Alb'82; CCFP; FCFP; (780)454-0351; Fax. (780)452-6767.

SEMENIUK, Robert M; 118-2436 Skaha Lake Rd, Penticton BC V2A 6E9; UBC'96; FRCSC; Ophth. (250)770-3233; Fax. (250)770-3288.

SEMENIUK, Ross C; Canadian Forces Health Ctre, PO Box 10500 Stn Forces 1 Field Ambulance, Edmonton AB T5J 4J5; Alb'07; CCFP; Staff, CFB Health Services Centre; (780)973-4011; Fax. (780)973-1655; ross.semeniuk@canadianforces.gc.ca.

SEMENIUK, Trent T; Inst of Comm & Family Psy, 4333 ch Cote-Sainte-Catherine, Montreal QC H3T 1E4; Alb'97; FRCPC; Psy. Staff, Sir Mortimer B Davis Jewish General; Staff, Institute of Community & Family Psychiatry; (514)340-8222 x5163; Fax. (514)340-7507; trent.semeniuk@mcgill.ca.

SEMENJUK, Michelle A; Lakeside Clinic, 202-15379 Castle Downs Rd NW, Edmonton AB T5X 3Y7; Man'97; CCFP; (780)472-7575; Fax. (780)472-7404.

SEMENOV, Igor; Amherst Family Associates, 400-158 Robert Angus Dr, Amherst NS B4H 4R7; Tyumen (Other Foreign)'86; (902)660-3131; Fax. (902)660-3132.

SEMERJIAN, Yves; Bathurst Shopping Mall, 212-1300 St Peter Ave, Bathurst NB E2A 3A6; Sher'06; FRCSC; GenSurg. (506)548-2727; Fax. (506)546-3943.

SEMINIANO, Pascualito A; 103-22190 48 Ave, Langley BC V3A 3N5; Manila (Philippines)'72; FRCPC; Psy. Clin Dir Psychiatric Day Prog, Langley Memorial Hospital; Staff, Langley Mental Health Centre; Clinical Asst Prof, University of British Columbia; Langs: Tagalog; (604)534-8151; Fax. (604)534-6192.

SEMIONOV, Alexandre; MUHC-Montreal Gen Hosp, 1650 av Cedar, Montreal QC H3G 1A4; McG'04; FRCPC; DiagRad. Staff, McGill University Health Centre - Montreal General Campus; (514)934-8084; Fax. (514)934-8263.

SEMLACHER, Eric A; Zeidler Ledcor Centre, 130 University Campus NW, Edmonton AB T6G 2X8; UBC'83; FRCPC; IntMed; Gastroent. Staff, University of Alberta Hospital; Langs: German; (780)492-8152; Fax. (780)492-8153.

SEMMLER, Robert T; Alexander Med Bldg, 208-849 Alexander Crt, Peterborough ON K9J 7H8; Wes'87; FRCPC; Neur (Sleep Medicine). Staff, Peterborough Regional Health Centre - Hospital Drive; (705)743-9509; Fax. (705)743-9509.

SEMOFF, Michael; 8B-1400 Bayly St, Pickering ON L1W 3R2; Tor'80; (905)837-2371; Fax. (905)837-9107.

SEMPLE, John L; Women's College Hosp, 76 Grenville St, Toronto ON M5S 1B2; McM'80; BSc(AAM); MSc(Path.); FACS; FRCSC; PlasSurg (Breast Surgery). Staff Ambulatory Surgery, Women's College Hospital; Consultant, Sunnybrook Health Sciences Centre - Edmond Odette Cancer Centre; Chair, Canadian Breast Cancer Foundation; Prof, University of Toronto; (416)323-7555; Fax. (416)323-7710; jsemple@cbcf.org.

SEMPOWSKI, Ian P; Queens Family Health Team, 115 Clarence St, Kingston ON K7L 5N6; Tor'89; CCFP; CCFP(E.M.); (613)533-9303; Fax. (613)533-9308.

SEMRAU, Stanley R; Dr Stanley Semrau Inc, 347 Foul Bay Rd, Victoria BC V8S 4G6; UBC'80; FRCPC; Psy (Forensic Psychiatry). (250)744-9662; Fax. (604)648-9231; drsemrau@direct.ca.

SEMRET, Makeda; St Mary's Hosp Centre, 3830 rue Lacombe, Montreal QC H3T 1M5; Mon'95; FRCPC; IntMed; MedMicrobiol; InfectDis. Staff, St Mary's Hospital Centre; Staff, McGill University Health Centre - Montreal General Campus; Langs: Amharic; French; (514)345-3511 x3716; makeda.semret@mail.mcgill.ca.

SEMSAR, Alireza; All Saints Springhill Hosp, 10 Princess St, Springhill NS B0M 1X0; (Iran)'95; Staff, All Saints Springhill Hospital; Langs: Farsi; (902)597-2841; Fax. (902)597-2454; alireza.semsar@cha.nshealth.ca.

SEMUS, Michael J; Health Sciences Centre, GC 419-820 Sherbrook St, Winnipeg MB R3A 1R9; Man'06; FRCPC; IntMed. Staff, Health Sciences Centre; (204)774-8511

SEN, Indira; Shouldice Hosp, 7750 Bayview Ave, Thornhill ON L3T 4A3; Mithila (India)'74; Staff, Shouldice Hospital; Langs: Bengali; Hindi; (905)889-1125; indirasen@rogers.com.

SEN, Mithu; London HSC-Victoria Hosp, D2 521-800 Commissioners RD E, London ON N6A 5W9; Cal'95; DABSM; FCCP; FCCMG; FRCPC; IntMed (Sleep Medicine); Critical Care Medicine; Respir. Staff Critical Care Trauma Centre, London Health Sciences Centre - Victoria Campus; (519)667-6577; Fax. (519)685-8089.

SEN, Robin; 1850 Main St, Winnipeg MB R2V 3J4; Man'87; (204)942-3128; Fax. (204)942-3172.

SEN, Roger I; Family Health Centre, C10-1410 Major Mackenzie Dr W, Vaughan ON L6A 4H6; Tor'91; Staff Family Med, North York General Hospital; (905)737-1200; Fax. (905)737-6150.

SENARATNE, Manohara P J; Cedars Prof Park, 2939 66 St NW, Edmonton AB T6K 4C1; Colombo (Sri Lanka)'78; MB BS; LRCP; MRCS; PhD; FRCPC; IntMed; Cardiol. Clin Prof, University of Alberta; (780)463-2184; Fax. (780)450-8359.

SENARATNE, Savitri C; Cedars Prof Park, 2939 66 St NW, Edmonton AB T6K 4C1; Colombo (Sri Lanka)'78; MB BS; ABIM; MRCS; LRCP; FRCPC; IntMed (Geriatric Medicine); Rheum. Staff, Glenrose Rehabilitation Hospital; Asst Prof Med, University of Alberta; Langs: Sinhalese; (780)463-2184; Fax. (780)450-8359.

SENAY, Bobby; CSSS de la Region de Thetford, 1717 rue Notre-Dame E, Thetford Mines QC G6G 2V4; Laval'07; FRCPC; IntMed. Staff, Hopital du CSS de la Region de Thetford; (418)338-7777

SENAY, Helene; CHUQ-Ctr Hosp Univ Laval, F00413-2705 boul Laurier, Quebec QC G1V 4G2; Mon'81; FRCPC; IntMed; MedMicrobiol; InfectDis. Staff Microbiol, Centre Hospitalier Universitaire de Quebec-CHUL; (418)656-4141 x47882; Fax. (418)654-2194; helene.senay@chuq.qc.ca.

SENDER, Rachelle R; LL 1-107 King St W, Dundas ON L9H 1V1; Tor'95; PhD; CCFP; FCFP; Staff, Hamilton Health Sciences Centre; (905)628-0840; Fax. (905)628-0843.

SENDEREWICH, Elizabeth C; Northern Med Unit, T162-770 Bannatyne Ave, Winnipeg MB R3E 0W3; Man'82; Staff, Roblin & District Health Centre; Staff, Northern Medical Unit; (204)789-3711

SENDEROVICH, Helena M; Baycrest Centre Geriatric Care, 3560 Bathurst St, North York ON M6A 2E1; Baskirian State Medical University (Russia (Federation))'80; Staff Family & Commun Med, Baycrest Centre for Geriatric Care; (416)685-5563

SENECAL, Ginette; Clinique de Med familiale, 300 rue Paradis, Sorel-Tracy QC J3P 3G6; Mon'83; (450)743-6060

SENECAL, Jean-Luc; CHUM-Hop Notre-Dame, M4243-1560 rue Sherbrooke E, Montreal QC H2L 4M1; Mon'75; FRCPC; IntMed; Rheum. Staff, Centre Hospitalier l'Université de Montréal (CHUM) - Hôpital Notre-Dame; (514)890-8000 x27131; Fax. (514)412-7548.

SENECAL, Lynne; Hop Maisonneuve-Rosemont, 5415 boul de l'Assomption, Montreal QC H1T 2M4; Mon'96; FRCPC; IntMed (Hemodialysis); Nephrol (P.Q.). Associé, Institut de Cardiologie de Montréal; ac Staff, Hopital Maisonneuve-Rosemont; Langs: Bilingual(French/English); (514)252-3400 x3704; Fax. (514)255-3026; lynnesenecal@hotmail.com.

SENECAL-QUEVILLON, Micheline; 4795 Rang St-Andre S RR 1, St-Cuthbert QC J0K 2C0; Mon'70; (450)835-3616; msenecal@xlpornet.com.

SENECHAL, Alain; CSSS Domaine du Roy, 450 rue Brassard, Roberval QC G8H 1B9; Mon'99; FRCPC; Psy. Staff, Hotel-Dieu de Roberval; (418)275-0110; hdr@ssss.gouv.qc.ca.

SENECHAL, Marie-Claude; Clinique Med Lavaltrie, 89C ch Lavaltrie, Lavaltrie QC J5T 2H5; Mon'98; LMCC; Staff, Centre Hospitalier Pierre le Gardeur; Staff, Clinique Medicale de Lavaltrie; (450)586-1033; Fax. (450)586-4498; mcs@bcom.ca.

SENECHAL, Mario; Hôpital Laval, 2725 ch Sainte-Foy, Quebec QC G1V 4G5; Mon'89; FRCPC; IntMed; Cardiol. Staff, Hôpital Laval; (418)656-8711; Fax. (418)656-4581.

SENECHAL, Melanie L; Niagara HS-St Catharines Gen, 142 Queenston St, St. Catharines ON L2R 7C6; Ott'09; CCFP; CCFP(E. M.); Staff, Health Sciences North-Laurentian Site; (905)323-3683; Fax. (905)684-3226.

SENECHAL, Nicole; 501-285 av Laurier E, Montreal QC H2T 3E7; Laval'73; (514)277-4361 x3234; nicolesenechal@sympatico.ca.

SENECHAL, Sylvie; Regie des Rentes du Quebec, CP 5200 Succ Terminus 2600 boul Laurier, Quebec QC G1K 7S9; Laval'78; Médecin, Regie des Rentes du Quebec; (418)657-8709 x3226; sylvie.senechal@rrq.gouv.qc.ca.

SENECHAL, Sylvie; PO Box 7841 Stn Main, Grand Falls NB E3Z 3E8; Sher'04; CCFP; Langs: Bilingual(French/English); (506)473-9051; Fax. (506)473-4468.

SENEKAL, Daniel; Northern Alberta Eye Institute, 10115 99 Ave, Grande Prairie AB T8V 0S1; Orange Free State (South Africa)'91; MMed(Ophth); Staff, Northern Alberta Eye Institute; Chief Ophth, Alberta Health Services-North Zone; (780)538-9997; Fax. (780)538-9788.

SENEKAL, Margaretha A; Associated Med Centre, PO Box 219 4909 50 Ave, St Paul AB T0A 3A0; (South Africa)'82; MB ChB; MMed; Langs: Afrikaans; (780)645-4411; Fax. (780)645-4566.

SENER, Alp; London HSC-University Hosp, PO Box 5339 Stn B 339 Windermere Rd, London ON N6A 5A5; Cal'02; FRCSC; Urol. Staff, London Health Sciences Centre - University Hospital; Langs: French; Turkish; (519)663-3352

SENGAR, Pankaj S; Oshawa Clinic, 7F-117 King St E, Oshawa ON L1H 1B9; Alb'01; FRCSC; GenSurg. Staff, Lakeridge Health - Oshawa Site; (905)721-6153

SENGAR, Sarit K; Provital Health & Wellness, 204-2031 33 Ave SW, Calgary AB T2T 1Z5; Man'99; Staff, Bowglen Medical Clinic; (403)685-4520; Fax. (403)685-4525; sengarsk@hotmail.com.

SENGER, Christof; BC Women's Hosp & Hlth Ctre, 4500 Oak St, Vancouver BC V6H 3N1; Wurzburg (Germany)'86; FCAP; FRCPC; AnatPath (Pediatric Pathology). Staff, BC Women's Hospital & Health Centre; (604)875-2268; Fax. (604)875-3529.

SENGUPTA, Sandip K; Kingston Gen Hosp, 8 211-76 Stuart St, Kingston ON K7L 2V7; Ott'83; FCAP; FRCPC; GenPath (Breast Pathology). Dep Chief Path, Kingston General Hospital; Med Dir, Clinical Laboratories; Prof Path, Queen's University; (613)549-6666 x4169; Fax. (613)548-6076; sengupta@cliff.path.queensu.ca.

SENIKAS, Andre; 425-900 boul du Seminaire N, St-Jean-Sur-Richel QC J3A 1C3; Sher'70; Staff, Hôpital du Haut-Richelieu; Med Dir, Oerlikon Aerospatiale & Medisys Inc; (450)515-1956; Fax. (450)515-1985; andresen@videotron.ca.

SENIKAS, Vyta M; Society of Obst/Gyn of Canada, 780 Echo Dr, Ottawa ON K1S 5R7; McG'74; MDCM; MBA; FRCSC; ObstGyn (Menopause). Assoc Exec VP, The Society of Obstetricians & Gynaecologists of Canada; Langs: Bilingual(English/French); (613)730-4192; Fax. (613)730-6599.

SENIOR, Peter A; College Plaza, 2000-8215 112 St NW, Edmonton AB T6G 2C8; (Scotland)'93; (780)407-3636; Fax. (780)407-6933.

SENIOR, Richard W; Near North Med Clinic, 201-66 Josephine St, North Bay ON P1B 0A7; Tor'89; (705)495-2685; Fax. (705)495-4128.

SENIOR, Steven L; 150 Strickland St, Lakefield ON K0L 2H0; Ott'73; CCFP; FCFP; Staff, Peterborough Regional Health Centre - Hospital Drive; Asst Clin Prof Family Med, McMaster University; Asst Prof Family Med, Queen's University; (705)652-3318; Fax. (705)652-3945; drsenz@yahoo.ca.

SENIOR, Susan E; Hespeler Med Centre, 12-350 Conestoga Blvd, Cambridge ON N1R 7L7; McM'98; FRCPC; Psy. (519)629-4615

SENNETT, Edward S; Clinique familiale des Pins, 1019 Boul des Pins, Val-d'Or QC J9P 4T2; Tor'79; CCFP; CCFP(E.M.); ac Staff, Centre Hospitalier de Val d'Or; Langs: French; (819)825-8464; Fax. (819)825-1335.

SENNEWALD TESKEY, Lisa M; Primary Care Clinic, 1300-13401 108 Ave, Surrey BC V3T 5T3; UBC'94; BSc; Langs: Spanish; French; (604)953-4940; Fax. (604)953-4949; lisa.sennewald@fraserhealth.ca.

SENNIK, Vir Bhushan; King Street Med Arts Centre, 503-71 King St W, Mississauga ON L5B 4A2; Dublin (Ireland)'71; FAAOS; FRCSC; OrthSurg (Knee Surgery). Consultant, Trillium Health Centre - Mississauga; Langs: Hindi; Punjabi; Gujarati; Urdu; (905)848-5744

SENNIKOV, Alexei; Mackenzie Richmond Hill Hosp, 10 Trench St, Richmond Hill ON L4C 4Z3; Belarussian University (Other Foreign)'96; Staff, Mackenzie Richmond Hill Hospital; (905)883-1212

SENO, Hermenegildo-Rommel R; Regina Qu'Appelle HR-Pasqua, 4101 Dewdney Ave, Regina SK S4T 1A5; Santo Tomas (Philippines)'90; FRCPC; AnatPath (Hematology Pathology). Staff, Pasqua Hospital; Staff, Regina General Hospital; University of Saskatchewan; Langs: Tagalog; (306)766-2266; Fax. (306)766-2752; rrseno@pol.net.

SENRA, Poornima; Vancouver Coastal Health, 200-520 6th Ave W, Vancouver BC V5Z 4H5; Bangalore (India)'96; MB BS; CCFP; Staff, Vancouver Coastal Health; (604)708-5235

SENT, Lorna; 110-3540 41st Ave W, Vancouver BC V6N 3E6; Cape Town (South Africa)'71; MB ChB; CCFP; Assoc Staff, UBC Hospital - Koerner Pavillion; Assoc Staff, Vancouver General Hospital - Centennial Pavillion; Clin Instructor Family Practice, University of British Columbia; (604)261-6361; Fax. (604)261-1656.

SENTERMAN, Mary K; The Ottawa Hosp-Gen Campus, 501 Smyth Rd, Ottawa ON K1H 8L6; Albany Medical College (USA)'73; FRCSC; ObstGyn (Colposcopy); AnatPath. Staff Path & ObstGyn, The Ottawa Hospital - General Campus; Prof Path, University of Ottawa; Langs: French; (613)737-8899 x79082; Fax. (613)737-8853.

SENTHELAL, Sashikala; Trillium Hlth Ctre-Mississauga, 100 Queensway W, Mississauga ON L5B 1B8; Jaffna (Sri Lanka)'83; MB BS; FRCPC; Psy (Psycho Geriatrics). Staff, Trillium Health Centre - Mississauga; Langs: Tamil; Sinhalese; (905)848-7586

SENTHELAL, Senthe S; The Credit Valley Hosp, 2200 Eglinton Ave W, Mississauga ON L5M 2N1; Moscow (Russia (Federation))'84; FRCPC; RadOncol. Staff, The Credit Valley Hospital; Langs: Sinhalese; Tamil; Russian; (905)813-1100 x5000; Fax. (905)813-3962.

SENTHILLMOHAN, Sockalingam; Strait Richmond Hosp, RR 1 138 Hospital Rd, Cleveland NS B0E 1J0; Madurai Kamaraj (India)'89; MB BS; Staff, Strait Richmond Hospital; Langs: Tamil; Sinhalese; (902)625-3100

SENTONGO, Colin; Kemptville Dist Hosp, PO Box 2007 2675 Concession Rd, Kemptville ON K0G 1J0; Universidad Iberoamericana(UNIBE) (Dominican Republic)'03; CCFP; Staff, Kemptville District Hospital; (613)258-6133

SENZANI, Farai D; Spiritwood Health Complex, PO Box 69, Spiritwood SK S0J 2M0; (306)883-4400; Fax. (306)883-2140.

SEOW, Cynthia H; TRW Building, 6D18-3280 Hospital Dr NW, Calgary AB T2N 4N1; (Australia)'99; (403)592-5025; Fax. (403)592-5050.

SEPANDJ, Farshad; 2022 33 Ave SW, Calgary AB T2T 1Z4; Dal'89; FRCPC; IntMed (Transplantation); Nephrol. Staff, Foothills Medical Centre; Clin Assoc Prof, University of Calgary; Langs: Persian; (403)521-0201; Fax. (403)521-0550.

SEPANMAA-LUND, Anne M; Heritage Lane Med Centre, 10835 23 Ave NW, Edmonton AB T6J 7B5; Turku (Finland)'82; Langs: Finnish; Swedish; (780)426-6490; Fax. (780)425-4920.

SEPEHR-ARAE, Arash; SMBD Jewish Gen Hosp, 3755 ch Cote-Sainte-Catherine, Montreal QC H3T 1E2; Mon'01; CSPQ(OrthSurg); OrthSurg (P.Q.). Staff, Sir Mortimer B Davis Jewish General; Teach Staff, Queen's University; (514)340-8222; Fax. (514)340-7595.

SEPPALA, Richard E; The Ottawa Hosp-Gen Campus, 501 Smyth Rd, Ottawa ON K1H 8L6; Tor'75; FRCPC; DiagRad. Staff, The Ottawa Hospital - General Campus; Asst Prof, University of Ottawa; Langs: French; (613)737-8093; Fax. (613)737-8501.

SEQUEIRA, Donovan S; Springdale Med Centre, 15-630 Peter Robertson Blvd, Brampton ON L6R 1T4; Tor'91; (905)793-8868; Fax. (905)793-8957.

SEQUEIRA, Errol J; Streetsville Med Centre, 8-5425 Creditview Rd, Mississauga ON L5V 2P3; Tor'91; MBA; CCFP; FCFP; Staff, The Credit Valley Hospital; Court Staff, Trillium Health Centre - West Toronto; Staff, William Osler Health System - Brampton Civic Hospital; Med Dir, Global Health Strategy Inc; (905)826-1164; Fax. (905)826-1214.

SEQUEIRA, Keith A J; St Joseph's HC-Parkwood Hosp, 801 Commissioners Rd E, London ON N6C 5J1; Tor'94; FRCPC; PhysMed&Rehab. Staff, Parkwood Hospital - St Joseph's Health Care; (519)685-4029; Fax. (519)685-4063.

SEQUEIRA, Richard; Peace River Comm Health Ctre, PO Box 400 Stn Main 10101 68th St, Peace River AB T8S 1T6; Mysore (India)'78; DMRD; CCST(U.K); FRCR(UK); MB BS; Staff Diagnostic Imaging, Peace River Community Health Centre; (780)624-7559; Fax. (780)624-7599; sequeirar@gmail.com.

SEQUEIRA, Stanislaus P; Aberdeen Hosp, 835 East River Rd, New Glasgow NS B2H 3S6; Cal'85; FRCSC; OrthSurg. Staff, Aberdeen Regional Hospital; (902)752-8110

SERB, Abdusalam M; Saint John Reg Hosp, PO Box 2100 Stn Main 400 University Ave, Saint John NB E2L 4L2; Al-Fateh (Libya)'94; Staff, Saint John Regional Hospital; (506)648-2537

SERBAN, Alexandrina; Hopital de Saint-Eustache, 520 boul Arthur-Sauve, Saint-Eustache QC J7R 5B1; Iuliu Hatieganu University (Other Foreign)'95; Respir; IntMed. Staff, Hôpital de Saint-Eustache; (450)473-6811

SEREBRIN, Raold G; 309-1100 Sheppard Ave E, North York ON M2K 2W1; Qns'78; FRCPC; Neur. Ac Staff, North York General Hospital; (416)223-5052; Fax. (416)223-7169.

SEREDA, Andrea M; Centre of Hope Family Hlth Tea, 281 Wellington St, London ON N6B 2L4; Wes'07; CCFP; CCFP(E.M.); Staff, St Joseph's Health Centre; (519)645-2348

SEREDA, Andrew W; Crowfoot Corner Medicentre, 217-150 Crowfoot Cres NW, Calgary AB T3G 3T2; Alb'64; Neur. (403)241-8900; Fax. (403)241-8109.

SEREDA, Brian D; 3462 78 Ave NW, Edmonton AB T6B 2X9; Alb'92; CCFP; (780)478-4631; Fax. (780)395-0900; sereda@shaw.ca.

SEREDA, Daniel D; West Edmonton Med/Esthetic, 2039-8882 170 St NW, Edmonton AB T5T 3J7; Alb'70; (780)444-1935; Fax. (780)444-3092.

SEREDA, Danya A; Continuum Med Care Ltd, 202-520 17th St, West Vancouver BC V7V 3S8; UBC'04; FRCPC; Derm. Langs: Bilingual(English/French); (604)913-8183

SEREDYCZ, Larissa I; Islington Med Clinic, 1004-1243 Islington Ave, Etobicoke ON M8X 1Y9; Man'09; BSc; MSc(Pharm); CCFP; (416)767-7725; Fax. (416)767-9959; lseredycz@gmail.com.

SERELO, Larry G; Dahlstrom Med Clinic, 2-32442 George Ferguson Way, Abbotsford BC V2T 4Y4; Sask'87; (604)853-6667; Fax. (604)853-6658.

SERERO, Charles; Centre Med Saint-Henri, 3966 rue Notre-Dame O, Montreal QC H4C 1R1; Sher'81; Langs: Bilingual(French/English); (514)935-4330; Fax. (514)935-4292; doc.serero@hotmail.com.

SERERO, Didier M; SMBD Jewish Gen Hosp, 3755 ch Cote-Sainte-Catherine, Montreal QC H3T 1E2; McG'97; CCFP; CCFP(E.M.); Staff EmergMed, Sir Mortimer B Davis Jewish General; adj Prof, McGill University; Langs: Spanish; French; Hebrew; (514)340-8222 x5568; Fax. (514)340-7917; didier.serero@mcgill.ca.

SEREZO, Paterno C; 932 Dufferin Ave, Wallaceburg ON N8A 2V6; Manila (Philippines)'72; Langs: Tagalog; (519)627-3327

SERFATY, Samuel; Polyclinique Masson, 200-3425 rue Masson, Montreal QC H1X 1R6; Mon'82; (514)376-9961; Fax. (514)376-8100.

SERGEANT, Myles D; St Peter's Hosp, 88 Maplewood Ave, Hamilton ON L8M 1W9; McM'93; CCFP; FCFP; Staff, Hamilton Health Sciences Centre - St Peter's Hospital; (905)777-3837

SERGEEVA, Danielle; Ridge Meadows Hosp & HCC, 11666 Laity St E, Maple Ridge BC V2X 7G5; Kiev (Ukraine)'84; CCFP; Staff, Ridge Meadows Hospital & Health Care Centre; Langs: Russian; (604)463-4111

SERGERIE, Claude; 400 Impasse de Callieres, Boisbriano QC J7G 3A3; Mon'61; Médecin Cons, Hopital Maisonneuve-Rosemont; Médecin Cons, Centre Hospitalier l'Université de Montréal (CHUM) - Hôpital Notre-Dame; Dir Med, CHSLD d'Acceuil Marcelle Ferron; Langs: English; (514)594-2636; Fax. (514)437-3314.

SERGERIE, Franck; Hotel-Dieu de Levis, 143 rue Wolfe, Levis QC G6V 3Z1; Laval'92; DiagRad. Staff, Hôtel-Dieu de Lévis; (418)835-7101; Fax. (418)835-7169.

SERGERIE, Keven; CSSS Cleophas-Claveau, CP 38 succ La Baie 1000 rue du Docteur-Desgagne, La Baie QC G7B 3P9; Laval'10; CCFP; Staff, CHSLD-CLSC Cleophas-Claveau; (418)544-3381

SERGERIE, Mathieu; Hop Maisonneuve-Rosemont, 5415 boul de l'Assomption, Montreal QC H1T 2M4; Mon'06; IntMed. Staff, Hopital Maisonneuve-Rosemont; (514)252-3400

SERGERIE, Mylene; Clinique Med Sainte-Dorothee, 102-1 boul Samson, Laval QC H7X 3S5; Mon'93; Med Staff, CLSC Ruisseau-Papineau; Langs: Bilingual(French/English); (450)689-6334; Fax. (450)689-6339.

SERGERIE, Pascale; CSSSG-Hop de Hull, 116 boul Lionel-Emond, Gatineau QC J8Y 1W7; Mon'92; Staff, Hull Hospital; (819)595-6000

SERGI, Consolato; University of Alberta Hosp, 5B4 09-8440 112 St NW, Edmonton AB T6G 2B7; (Italy)'89; PhD; MPH; Staff, University of Alberta Hospital; Langs: German; French; Italian; (780)407-7951; Fax. (780)407-3009; sergi@ualberta.ca.

SERIES, Frederic; Hôpital Laval, 2725 ch Sainte-Foy, Quebec QC G1V 4G5; Tours (France)'86; Staff, Hôpital Laval; (418)656-4747; Fax. (418)656-4762.

SERMER, Mathew; Ont Power Generation Bldg, 3269-700 University Ave, Toronto ON M5G 1Z5; Tor'80; FRCSC; ObstGyn (Maternal Fetal Medicine). Assoc Chief ObstGyn/Head Maternal-Fetal Med, Mount Sinai Hospital; Staff Lawrence & Frances Bloomberg, Ontario Power Generation Inc; Prof, University of Toronto; Langs: Slovak; (416)586-3195; Fax. (416)586-5223; mathew.sermer@opg.com.

SERNIK, Julian B; Sunnybrook Hlth Sciences Ctre, 317-2075 Bayview Ave, Toronto ON M4N 3M5; UBC'07; FRCSC; OrthSurg. Staff Orth Surg, Sunnybrook Health Sciences Centre; (416)480-4884

SEROPIAN, Lilliane; 5107 boul de Maisonneuve O, Montreal QC H4A 1Z1; McG'81; FRCSC; ObstGyn. (514)369-0010; Fax. (514)369-0008.

SEROWKA, Pawel A; Anaesthetic Services, 213-2186 Oak Bay Ave, Victoria BC V8R 1G3; McM'99; FRCPC; Anes. Staff, Royal Jubilee Hospital; Langs: Polish; (250)595-7211

SERRA, Danielle; Clinique de Med Saint-Jovite, 805 rue de Saint-Jovite, Mont-Tremblant QC J8E 3J8; Mon'74; Langs: Bilingual(French/English); (819)717-3040; Fax. (819)717-3040.

SERRA, Lydia; 5912 av de l'Esplanade, Montreal QC H2T 3A3; Sher'92; (514)274-6584

SERRA, Stefano; Univ Hlth Network-Toronto Gen, 11E 209-200 Elizabeth St, Toronto ON M5G 2C4; Universita Degli Studi Di Cagliari (Other Foreign)'99; Clin Fellow, Toronto General Hospital - UHN; Langs: Italian; (416)340-4800

SERRANO, Manuel; Hop Louis-H Lafontaine, 7401 rue Hochelaga, Montreal QC H1N 3M5; Madrid (Spain)'63; CSPQ; FRCPC; Psy. ac Staff, Hopital Louis-H Lafontaine; adj Prof, Universite de Montreal; Langs: Spanish; English; (514)251-4000 x3448; Fax. (514)251-4047; manuel.serrano@umontreal.ca.

SERRANO ALMEIDA, Cesar A; Alberta Children's Hosp, 2888 Shaganappi Trail NW, Calgary AB T3B 6A8; (Colombia)'90; Neursurg. Staff, Alberta Children's Hospital; (403)944-4496; Fax. (403)283-5559.

SERRAR, Jamal; Clnique Med Marche Central, 300-9250 boul de l'Acadie, Montreal QC H4N 3C5; Laval'95; Staff, Hôpital de Christ-Roi; (514)384-9462

SERRI, Karim; Hop Du Sacre-Coeur De Mtl, 5400 boul Gouin O, Montreal QC H4J 1C5; Mon'98; Cardiol; IntMed. Staff, Hôpital du Sacre-Coeur de Montréal; (514)338-2200; Fax. (514)338-2381; karimserri@hotmail.com.

SERRI, Omar; CHUM-Hop Notre-Dame, 1560 rue Sherbrooke E, Montreal QC H2L 4M1; Clermont-Ferrand (France)'74; PhD; Endocrin (P.Q.). Staff, Centre Hospitalier l'Université de Montréal (CHUM) - Hôpital Notre-Dame; Prof, Universite de Montreal; (514)890-8000 x26619; Fax. (514)412-7603; omar.serri@umontreal.ca.

SERS, Robert N; St Martha's Doctor's Office, G26-23 Bay St, Antigonish NS B2G 2G7; Dal'76; FRCSC; GenSurg. Ac Staff, St Martha's Regional Hospital; Lecturer Surg, Dalhousie University; Langs: English; French; (902)863-4600; Fax. (902)863-1396.

SERTIC, Joseph; Medical Place Primary Care Ctr, 202-170 Queensway W, Mississauga ON L5B 3A8; Tor'82; CCFP; Langs: Croatian; (905)275-0023; Fax. (905)275-4001.

SERUGA, Bostjan; Univ Hlth Network-Princess M, 5 224-610 University Ave, Toronto ON M5G 2M9; University of Ljubljana (Other Foreign)'98; Clin Fellow MedOncol, Princess Margaret Hospital - University Health Network; (416)946-4501

SERUSHAGO, Bazir A; Market Mall Prof Bldg, 327-4935 40 Ave NW, Calgary AB T3A 2N1; (Congo (Democratic Republic))'80; FRCPC; Peds; ClinImmunol&Allergy. (403)265-4163; Fax. (403)265-4173.

SERVANT, Mylene; CSSS Pierre Boucher, 1333 boul Jacques-Cartier E, Longueuil QC J4M 2A5; Sher'03; FRCPC; Anes; Critical Care Medicine. Staff, Centre Hospitalier Pierre Boucher; (450)468-8111

SERVANT, Stephan; CSSS de Trois-Rivières, 1991 boul du Carmel, Trois-Rivieres QC G8Z 3R9; Mon'99; FRCPC; DiagRad. Staff, CSSS de Trois-Rivières; (819)697-3333 x63535

SERWADDA, Rosemary C M; Central Med Clinic, 6-1061 Central Ave N, Swift Current SK S9H 4Y9; (306)773-5855; Fax. (306)778-3799.

SESHADRI, Angela; Ottawa Cardiovascular Centre, 502-1355 Bank St, Ottawa ON K1H 8K7; Qns'99; FRCPC; Cardiol; Peds. Staff, Children's Hospital of Eastern Ontario (CHEO); (613)738-1584; Fax. (613)738-9097.

SESHADRI, Pieter A; Queen Street Surgical Assoc, 202-610 Queen St, Saskatoon SK S7K 0M8; Tor'93; ATLS; BSc(Hons); FRCSC; GenSurg (Minimal Invasive Surgery). Staff, St Paul's Hospital (Grey Nuns) of Saskatoon; Physician, Queen Street Surgical Associates; Clin Asst Prof, University of Saskatchewan; (306)244-6818; Fax. (306)664-3462; seshadri@shaw.ca.

SESHIA, Jyoti B; University Hosp of Northern BC, 1475 Edmonton St, Prince George BC V2M 1S2; Man'10; CCFP; Staff, University Hospital of Northern British Columbia; (250)565-2000

SESHIA, Mary M K; Women's Hosp, WS 012-735 Notre Dame Ave, Winnipeg MB R3E 0L8; Edinburgh (Scotland)'67; MB ChB; DCH; FRCP(Ed); Sec Head Neonatal/Dir, Health Sciences Centre; Prof, University of Manitoba; (204)787-1853; mseshia@cc.umanitoba.ca.

SESKI, Robert D; Hotel Dieu Grace Hosp, 1030 Ouellette Ave, Windsor ON N9A 1E1; University of Mississippi (USA)'86; Staff, Hôtel-Dieu Grace Hospital; (519)973-4411

SESTAK, Philip M; Spectrum Health, 702-1080 Howe St, Vancouver BC V6Z 2T1; Sask'79; CCFP; Ac Staff, Providence Health Care - St Paul's Hospital; Clin Assoc Prof, University of British Columbia; (604)681-1080; Fax. (604)681-0244.

SESTIER, Francois; Clinique Med 1851, 901-1851 rue Sherbrooke E, Montreal QC H2K 4L5; Nancy (France)'72; PhD(Exp Med); FRCPC; Cardiol (P.Q.) (Insurance Medicine). Staff Cardiol, Centre Hospitalier l'Université de Montréal (CHUM) - Hôtel-Dieu; Staff Cardiol, Hôpital Brome-Missisquoi-Perkins; Clin Prof Med/Dir, Universite de Montreal; Langs: English; (514)738-6476; Fax. (514)738-2333; drsestier@hotmail.com.

SETAYESH, Ahmad R; Tacoma Family Med & Walk-In, 101-58 Tacoma Dr, Dartmouth NS B2W 3E5; Tehran (Iran)'94; CCFP; (902)466-1531; Fax. (902)466-1352.

SETH, Aditya; 195A-1151 10th St SW, Salmon Arm BC V1E 1T2; UBC'07; FRCSC; Ophth. Langs: Hindi; Punjabi; (250)832-1131

SETH, Arun K; Bloor-Jane Med Bldg, 412-2425 Bloor St W, Toronto ON M6S 4W4; Lucknow (India)'62; MB BS; Ac Staff, St Joseph's Health Centre; Staff, Trillium Health Centre - West Toronto; Langs: Hindi; Punjabi; Urdu; (416)767-1117; Fax. (416)767-1118.

SETH, Asha L; Bloor-Jane Med Bldg, 412-2425 Bloor St W, Toronto ON M6S 4W4; Lucknow (India)'63; MB BS; Ac Staff, St Joseph's Health Centre; Hon Staff, Trillium Health Centre - West Toronto; Langs: Hindi; Punjabi; Urdu; (416)767-1117; Fax. (416)767-1118.

SETH, Puneet; McMaster Family Practice, A-690 Main St W, Hamilton ON L8S 1A4; McM'09; CCFP; (905)521-5015; Fax. (905)521-5010.

SETH-SHARMA, Anila; 705-1243 Islington Ave, Etobicoke ON M8X 1Y9; St George's (Grenada)'94; BSc(Hon); MD; ABIM; FRCPC; IntMed. (416)233-8885; Fax. (416)233-6556.

SETHI, Asha D; 10-5268 Memorial Dr NE, Calgary AB T2A 2R1; Guru Nanak (India)'76; MB BS; (403)235-6333; Fax. (403)235-6333.

SETHI, Baldev R; Main Street Med Centre, 1251 Main St, Stittsville ON K2S 2E5; Glasgow (Scotland)'64; MB ChB; FRCS; Staff, Western Hospital - Health PEI; Langs: Hindi; Urdu.

SETHI, Berjinder J; Grand River Hosp-Freeport Site, PO Box 9056 3570 King St E, Kitchener ON N2A 2W1; St George's University (Grenada)'07; FRCPC; Psy. Staff, Grand River Hospital - Freeport Site; (519)749-4300; Fax. (519)894-8308.

SETHI, Jagmeet; Cayuga Diabetes Centre, PO Box 448 11B Cayuga St N, Cayuga ON N0A 1E0; New York Medical College (USA)'97; FRCPC; IntMed. Staff, Niagara Health System - Greater Niagara General Site; Staff, Hamilton Health Sciences Centre-Juravinski Site; Langs: Hindi; Punjabi; (289)370-0170; Fax. (289)370-0339.

SETHI, Krishan; 221-35 Main St, Flin Flon MB R8A 1J7; Glasgow (Scotland)'76; MB ChB; CCFP; Ac Staff, Flin Flon General Hospital Inc; Lecturer Medical Education, University of Manitoba; (204)687-4415; Fax. (204)687-4486.

SETHI, Monica; Summerville Family Health Team, 7F-101 Queensway W, Mississauga ON L5B 2P7; Kasturba Medical College (India)'07; CCFP; (905)272-9900; Fax. (905)272-9977.

SETHI, Rajiv; 204-40 Westmore Dr, Etobicoke ON M9V 4C2; Tor'92; FRCPC; IntMed; Gastroent. Langs: Punjabi; Urdu; (416)745-7300; Fax. (416)745-5300.

SETHI, Ritu; GT Dermatology, 14-318 Guelph St, Georgetown ON L7G 4B5; Tor'95; CCFP; (647)799-3096; Fax. (647)799-4011.

SETHI, Shilpa; Musquodoboit Valley Fam Pract, RR 2 492 Archibald Brook Rd, Middle Musquodoboi NS B0N 1X0; Dagestan State Medical Academy (Other Foreign)'01; Langs: Hindi; Urdu; Punjabi; Russian; (902)384-2834; Fax. (902)384-2719.

SETHI, Subash; Victoria Gen Hosp, 2340 Pembina Hwy, Winnipeg MB R3T 2E8; Glasgow (Scotland)'75; MB ChB; FFARCS(Eng); FRCPC; Anes. Staff Anes, Concordia General Hospital; Staff Anes, Victoria General Hospital; Staff, Misericordia Health Centre; University of Manitoba; (204)269-3570

SETHNA, Rustom H; Markham Stouffville Hlth Ctre, 408-377 Church St, Markham ON L6B 1A1; Bombay (India)'81; MB BS; FRCPC; Psy (Geriatric Psychiatry). Consultant Psy, Markham Stouffville Hospital; Consultant Psy, Sunnybrook Health Sciences Centre; Teacher, University of Toronto; (905)472-5733; Fax. (905)472-5215.

SETHURAM, D Tony; Carlingwood Family Med Ctre, 35B-2121 Carling Ave, Ottawa ON K2A 1H2; Dal'92; BSc(Hon.); CCFP; FCFP; (613)761-6777; Fax. (613)761-7744.

SETIAWAN, Melissa; Chinook Reg Hosp, 960 19 St S, Lethbridge AB T1J 1W5; Alb'05; FRCPC; Anes. Staff, Chinook Regional Hospital; (403)388-6131; Fax. (403)388-6708.

SETO, Gordon W J; Nottingham Medical, 310-664 Wye Rd, Sherwood Park AB T8A 6G3; Alb'08; CCFP; (780)416-3220; Fax. (780)416-3224.

SETO, Mei Fun; Westglen Med Clinic, 108-30 Springborough Blvd SW, Calgary AB T3H 0N9; Cal'75; BSc; (403)240-2221; Fax. (403)240-4670.

SETO, Paul H; Meadowlark Plaza, 15823 87 Ave NW, Edmonton AB T5R 4G7; Alb'78; Langs: Cantonese; (780)489-8822; Fax. (780)489-9188.

SETO, Raymond J; 4 Zina St, Orangeville ON L9W 1E1; Qns'97; FRCSC; Ophth. (519)941-4251; Fax. (519)942-2047.

SETRAK, Rafi F; Niagara HS-St Catharines, PO Box 3018 Stn Main 142 Queenston St, St Catharines ON L2R 7C6; Saddam (Iraq)'93; MB ChB; CCFP; CCFP(E.M.); Staff, Niagara Health System - St Catharines General Site; Langs: Arabic; Armenian; (905)378-4647

SETRAKIAN, Jean C; CHUS-Hop Fleurimont, 3001 12e av N, Sherbrooke QC J1H 5N4; McG'84; FRCPC; IntMed. Staff, Centre Hospitalier Universitaire de Sherbrooke-Hopital Fleurimont; Langs: Armenian; English; (819)346-1110 x14949; Fax. (819)820-6406.

SETT, Sikhor N; Clinical Practice Unit, 4F-810 Sherbrook St, Winnipeg MB R3A 1R8; Calcutta (India)'57; DABOG; FSOGC; FRCSC; ObstGyn. Assoc Prof Obst/Gyn & Reproductive Sciences, Health Sciences Centre; Assoc Prof Obst/Gyn & Reproductive Sciences, University of Manitoba; (204)787-4936; Fax. (204)787-2314; ssett@exchange.hsc.mb.ca.

SETTECASE, Fabio; Sunnybrook Hlth Sciences Ctre, 2075 Bayview Ave, Toronto ON M4N 3M5; Boston (USA)'06; FRCPC; DiagRad. Staff Medical Imaging, Sunnybrook Health Sciences Centre; (416)480-4372

SETTERFIELD, Lance B; Admirals Walk Health Centre, 4903 Lochside Dr, Victoria BC V8Y 2E6; Stellenbosch (South Africa)'83; MB BS; Med Dir, Acacia Dermacare; Langs: Afrikaans; (250)381-7546; info@acaciadermacare.com.

SETTON, Deborah M; St Paul's Hosp, 1081 Burrard St, Vancouver BC V6Z 1Y6; UBC'98; BSc; FRCPC; Anes. Staff Anes, Providence Health Care - St Paul's Hospital; (604)806-8337; Fax. (604)806-8487.

SETTON, Nora S; Clinique Med Nova, 3755 boul Saint-Laurent, Montreal QC H2W 1X8; Mon'84; FRCPC; Peds (Neonatology). Staff, Centre Hospitalier l'Université de Montréal (CHUM) - Hôpital Notre-Dame; Staff, Centre Hospitalier l'Université De Montréal (CHUM) - Hôpital Saint-luc; Prof Peds, Universite de Montreal; (514)987-0080; Fax. (514)987-0075.

SETTY, Yatish N; D-1095 1st Ave W, Owen Sound ON N4K 4K7; Mysore (India)'96; Staff, Grey Bruce Health Services - Owen Sound; Langs: Kanarese; Hindi; (519)371-1278; Fax. (519)371-4718.

SEUFERT, Andrea C; Oasis Med Centre, 101-805 Edmonton Trail NE, Calgary AB T2E 3J8; Cal'92; MSc; BSc; CCFP; Langs: German; (403)265-8814; Fax. (403)265-8859; dr.andrea@shaw.ca.

SEVCIK, William E; University of Alberta Hosp, 1G1 50-8440 112 St NW, Edmonton AB T6G 2B7; Alb'93; FRCPC; EmergMed (Pediatric Emergency Medicine). Staff/Asst Prof Clin Emerg Med, University of Alberta Hospital; (780)407-7047; Fax. (780)407-3314.

SEVERIDE, Susan P; 9923 Jubilee Rd W PO Box 1590, Summerland BC V0H 1Z0; UBC'83; BSc; CCFP; FCFP; Ac Staff, Penticton Regional Hospital; (250)494-0521; Fax. (250)494-7144.

SEVERIN, Diane M; Cross Cancer Institute, 11560 University Ave NW, Edmonton AB T6G 1Z2; Alb'88; FRCPC; RadOncol. Staff, Cross Cancer Institute; Assoc Prof, University of Alberta; (780)432-8783; Fax. (780)432-8380; dianesev@cancerboard.ab.ca.

SEVERIN, Naomi E; Guildford Med Dental Centre, 32-15300 105 Ave, Surrey BC V3R 6A7; Cal'03; FRCPC; IntMed; Endocrin&Metab. Staff, Royal Columbian Hospital.

SEVERS, S Robert F; Grey Bruce HS-Owen Sound, PO Box 1800 Stn Main 1800 8th St E, Owen Sound ON N4K 6M9; McM'79; FRCPC; Anes. Chief of Staff, Grey Bruce Health Services - Owen Sound; (519)376-2121

SEVERY, Philip R; Community Psych Service, 1350 St. Andrews Ave, North Vancouver BC V7L 3L4; Bowman-Gray (USA)'66; AB; FRCPC; EmergMed; Psy. Staff, Lions Gate Hospital; (604)983-6020; Fax. (604)983-6022.

SEVICK, Robert J; Foothills Med Centre, 812 NT-1403 29 St NW, Calgary AB T2N 2T9; Alb'84; FRCPC; DiagRad (Neuro Radiology). Reg Dept Head Clinical Diagnostic Imaging/Staff Diagnostic Imaging, Foothills Medical Centre; Dept Head Radiol, University Of Calgary; (403)944-8003; Fax. (403)270-0713; rob.sevick@albertahealthservices.ca.

SEVIGNY, Bernard; Hotel-Dieu de Levis, 143 rue Wolfe, Levis QC G6V 3Z1; Laval'78; LMCC; FRCPC; Otol (P.Q.) (Administration). Staff, Centre Hospitalier Regional de Sept-Iles; Staff Otol, Hôtel-Dieu de Lévis; (418)835-7121

SEVIOUR, Catherine M; Health Sciences Centre, 300 Prince Philip Dr, St. John's NL A1B 3V6; Mem'92; FRCPC; EmergMed. Staff, Health Sciences Centre; (709)777-6300

SEVIOUR, E Peter; Quidi Vidi Family Practice, 2F-120 Lake Ave, St. John's NL A1A 1H4; Mem'92; CCFP; Langs: English; French; (709)579-5711; Fax. (709)579-8227; secking@aol.com.

SEVIOUR, J Paul; Queen Elizabeth Hosp, PO Box 6600 Stn Central 60 Riverside Dr, Charlottetown PE C1A 8T5; Mem'85; FRCPC; IntMed. Staff, Queen Elizabeth Hospital; (902)894-0114

SEVIOUR, Rosann E; Family Med Clinic, 17-141 Torbay Rd, St. John's NL A1A 2H1; Mem'87; MSc(Epidemiol.); FRCPC; CommunMed. Langs: French; (709)579-4400

SEVITT, Brian M; Queensway Prof Centre, 404-190 Sherway Dr, Etobicoke ON M9C 5N2; Edinburgh (Scotland)'70; MB ChB; FRCPC; IntMed (Cardiology). Staff Cardiol, Trillium Health Centre - Mississauga; Staff Cardiol, Trillium Health Centre - West Toronto; (416)622-8620; Fax. (416)622-8624.

SEWARD, E Glenn; 2-6 River Dr, Angus ON L0M 1B2; Mem'92; (705)424-8884; Fax. (705)424-8886.

SEWCHAND, Kenneth; Alexander Prof Centre, 304-849 Alexander Crt, Peterborough ON K9J 7H8; London (England)'65; MB BS; FRCSC; Otol. (705)743-5391; Fax. (705)745-1101; drksewchand@on.aibn.com.

SEWCHAND, Lionel S; 2 King St W, Hamilton ON L8G 1G8; Cal'84; (905)662-5525; Fax. (905)662-1855.

SEWELL, Gary M; 710 Pembina Hwy, Winnipeg MB R3M 2M6; Man'87.

SEWELL, Louise M; Weeneebayko Gen Hosp, PO Box 34 19 Hospital Dr, Moose Factory ON P0L 1W0; Cal'77; Staff, Weeneebayko General Hospital; (705)658-4544

SEXSMITH, George P; St Paul's Hosp, 1081 Burrard St, Vancouver BC V6Z 1Y6; Alb'83; FRCPC; NuclearMed. Staff, Surrey Memorial Hospital; Staff, Providence Health Care - St Paul's Hospital; Dir Nuclear Med Residency Prog/Asst Clin Prof, University of British Columbia; (604)806-8008; Fax. (604)806-8075.

SEXTON, Emilie; CSSS de la Baie-des-Chaleurs, RR 2 419 boul Perron, Maria QC G0C 1Y0; Laval'09; Staff, CSSS de la Baie-des-Chaleurs; (418)759-3443

SEXTON, Frederick G; London Regional Cancer Centre, 790 Commissioners Rd E, London ON N6A 4L6; Wes'74; Staff, London Regional Cancer Centre; (519)685-8650; Fax. (519)685-8627; frederick.sexton@lhsc.on.ca.

SEXTON, K Briar; 4-1854 First Ave W, Vancouver BC V6J 1G5; Wes'00; Ophth. Langs: Bilingual(English/French); (604)282-7900

SEXTON, Patrick H; 2181 Lorraine Dr, Peterborough ON K9L 1X5; Dal'71; Staff Privil, Peterborough Regional Health Centre - Hospital Drive; (705)745-0100

SEXTON, Tracy L; London Reg Cancer Program, A3 805-790 Commissioners Rd E, London ON N6A 4L6; UBC'02; FRCPC; RadOncol. Staff, London Regional Cancer Center; (519)685-8650; Fax. (519)685-8736.

SEY, Michael S L; London HSC-Victoria Hosp, 800 Commissioner Rd E, London ON N6A 5W9; Tor'07; FRCPC; IntMed; Gastroent. Staff, London Health Sciences Centre - University Hospital; Staff, London Health Sciences Centre - Victoria Campus; (519)667-6582; Fax. (519)667-6820.

SEYBOLD, H E; Guelph Family Health Team, 207-55 Wyndham St N, Guelph ON N1H 7T8; McG'79; CCFP; FCFP; (519)836-1455; Fax. (519)836-1321.

SEYBOLD, William D; 5A-389 Main St, Picton ON K0K 2T0; Qns'82; CCFP; FCFP; Staff, QHC Prince Edward County Memorial; (613)476-7870; Fax. (613)476-6482; wds@sympatico.ca.

SEYED AKHAVAN, Pooneh; Joseph & Wolf Lebovic Bldg, 2 029-60 Murray St, Toronto ON M5T 3L9; Tehran (Iran)'99; FRCPC; IntMed; Rheum. Langs: Farsi; Persian; (416)586-4800; Fax. (416)586-8766.

SEYER, Alain; Clinique Med Sainte-Sophie, 2409 boul Sainte-Sophie, Sainte-Sophie QC J5J 2V3; Mon'87; (450)438-3955; Fax. (450)438-5096.

SEYLER, Susan J S; Greenbrook Family Med Centre, 421 Greenbrook Dr, Kitchener ON N2M 4K1; Wes'91; BSc; CCFP; FCFP; Court Staff, St Mary's General Hospital; Court Staff, Grand River Hospital - Kitchener/Waterloo Health Centre; (519)570-1655; Fax. (519)570-3477.

SEYMOUR, Lesley K; Cancer Research Institute, 10 Stuart St, Kingston ON K7L 3N6; Witwatersrand (South Africa)'78; (613)533-6430

SEYMOUR, Patricia F; Coleman Med Clinic, 186 Kenneth St, Duncan BC V9L 1N4; Wes'89; CCFP; FCFP; Langs: French; (250)746-4102

SEYMOUR, Robert G; Fredericton Med Clinic, 504-1015 Regent St, Fredericton NB E3B 6H5; Dal'76; Ophth. (506)458-0210; Fax. (506)457-4769.

SEYONE, Chanthirasekaram; Univ Hlth Network-Toronto Western Hosp, MP7 428-399 Bathurst St, Toronto ON M5T 2S8; Lusaka (Zambia)'84; MB BS; FRCPC; Psy (Acquired Brain Injury). Dir Acquired Brain Injury Clin, Toronto Western Hospital - University Health Network; Asst Prof, University of Toronto; Langs: Tamil; (416)603-5009; Fax. (416)603-5292.

SFEIR, Antoine; CSSS du Granit, 3569 rue Laval, Lac-Megantic QC G6B 1A5; Beirut (Lebanon)'63; GenSurg (P.Q.). (819)583-0330; Fax. (819)583-5364.

SFRISO, Anna; Hotel-Dieu de Levis, 143 rue Wolfe, Levis QC G6V 3Z1; Mon'97; FRCSC; Otol (Clinical Immunology & Allergy). Che oto-rhino-lary, Hôtel-Dieu de Lévis; Langs: Italian; English; (418)835-7121

SGOUROMITIS, Efthimios T; Foothills Med Centre, 257C-1403 29 St NW, Calgary AB T2N 2T9; Alb'89; FRCPC; Psy. Staff Psy, Foothills Medical Centre; (403)944-2144; Fax. (403)283-4671.

SGRO, Michael D; St Michael's Health Centre, 2F-61 Queen St E, Toronto ON M5C 2T2; Wes'89; FRCPC; Peds. Staff, St Michael's Hospital; Staff, Mount Sinai Hospital; Staff, The Hospital For Sick Children; Asst Prof, University of Toronto; (416)867-3655; Fax. (416)867-3736; sgrom@smh.toronto.on.ca.

SHAABAN, Hani; Cape Breton Reg Hosp, 1482 George St, Sydney NS B1P 1P3; Damascus (Syria)'96; FRCPC; IntMed. Staff, Cape Breton Healthcare Complex; (902)567-8000

SHAARBAF, Raid; Aberdeen Regional Hosp, 835 East River Rd, New Glasgow NS B2H 3S6; Baghdad (Iraq)'99; FRCPC; IntMed. Staff, Aberdeen Regional Hospital; (902)752-2413; Fax. (902)752-2590.

SHABAH, Abdo; Hopital Jean-Talon, 1385 rue Jean-Talon E, Montreal QC H2E 1S6; Mon'02; CCFP; Staff, CSSS du Coeur de l'Isle Hôpital Jean-Talon; (514)495-6767; Fax. (866)664-6285.

SHABAN, Joseph A; 1883 Turner Rd, Windsor ON N8W 3K2; Wes'80; ABIM; AB; FACE; FRCPC; IntMed (Diabetology); Endocrin&Metab. Ac Staff, Hôtel-Dieu Grace Hospital; Staff, Windsor Regional Hospital - Tayfour Site; Chief Med, Windsor Regional Hospital - Metropolitan Site; Staff, Regional Bariatric Assessment & Treatment Centre; Aj Prof Med, University of Western Ontario; Langs: Arabic; (519)977-6050; Fax. (519)977-6057.

SHABANA, Wael M; The Ottawa Hosp-Gen Campus, 501 Smyth Rd, Ottawa ON K1H 8L6; Zagazig Faculty of Medicine (Other Foreign)'96; Staff, The Ottawa Hospital - General Campus; Langs: Dutch; Arabic; (613)737-6111

SHABANI, Faryala K; 1A-219 Main St, Bathurst NB E2A 1A9; Louvain (Belgium)'85; LMCC; Staff, Hopital Regional Chaleur; (506)548-2293; Fax. (506)548-0902.

SHABANI-RAD, Meer-Taher; Foothills Med Centre, 1403 29 St NW, Calgary AB T2N 2T9; Tehran (Iran)'93; FRCPC; AnatPath (Hematology Pathology). Staff Hematopath, Foothills Medical Centre; (403)944-4754; Fax. (403)944-1364.

SHABASH, Osama M; Health Choice Centre, 815 College St, Toronto ON M6G 1C9; Al-Fateh (Libya)'00; CCFP; Langs: Arabic; (416)533-1145; Fax. (416)533-3918.

SHABBIR, Hamid; Pacific Med Clinic, 6176 Fraser St, Vancouver BC V5W 3A1; (Other Foreign)'88; (604)301-9955

SHABBITS, Michael S; The Richmond Hosp, 2005-7000 Westminster Hwy, Richmond BC V6X 1A2; UBC'00; FRCPC; Psy. Staff, Richmond Hospital; Staff, Richmond Mental Health Centre; (604)244-5569; Fax. (604)278-4819.

SHABIB, Gihad M H; Kilborn Med Centre, 515-1385 Bank St, Ottawa ON K1H 8N4; Cairo (Egypt)'78; MB ChB; MRCOG; FRCSC; ObstGyn (Colposcopy). Staff, The Ottawa Hospital - General Campus; Staff, Renfrew Victoria Hospital; Langs: Arabic; (613)721-2907; Fax. (613)721-2908.

SHABSOVE, Harold B; Beaches Fam Practice & Walk-In, 116 Glen Manor Dr, Toronto ON M4E 2X2; Wes'63; (416)698-0999

SHACK, Jason A; Fort Frances Clinic, 301 Victoria Ave, Fort Frances ON P9A 2C1; Tor'00; CCFP; (807)274-3287; Fax. (807)274-7882.

SHACK, Martin N; Bathurst-Drewry Med Centre, 104-5927 Bathurst St, North York ON M2R 3T5; Tor'79; CCFP; FCFP; Ac Staff Family Med, North York General Hospital; Teacher, University of Toronto; (416)223-2040; Fax. (416)223-2234; mshack@sympatico.ca.

SHACKLETON, Christopher R; 3265 Archibald Way, Whistler BC V0N 1B3; UBC'78; FRCSC; IntMed; GenSurg; Nephrol. (604)907-1025

SHADBOLT, Nicole S; Riverside Court Med Clinic, 5-3635 Rivergate Way, Ottawa ON K1V 2A4; McM'07; CCFP; (613)739-3700; Fax. (613)739-7043.

SHADD, Joshua D; Ctre for Studies in Family Med, 245-100 Collip Cir, London ON N6G 4X8; Qns'99; CCFP; Staff, Parkwood Hospital - St Joseph's Health Care; Staff, London Health Sciences Centre - University Hospital; Asst Prof, University of Western Ontario; (519)858-5028; Fax. (519)858-5029.

SHADD, Violet W A; Victoria Westmount Med Centre, B106-751 Victoria St S, Kitchener ON N2M 5N4; Tor'72; (519)748-8510; Fax. (519)742-9717.

SHADMANI, Ramak; 1168A The High St, Coquitlam BC V3B 0C6; Teheran (Iran)'93; CCFP; (778)285-1244

SHADOWITZ, Steven B; Sunnybrook Hlth Sciences Ctre, C410-2075 Bayview Ave, Toronto ON M4N 3M5; McG'89; FRCPC; IntMed. Staff IntMed, Sunnybrook Health Sciences Centre; Lecturer, University of Toronto; Langs: French; (416)480-4290; Fax. (416)480-4563; steve.shadowitz@sunnybrook.ca.

SHADRINA, Anna G; PG Medical Education Office, 2044-451 Smyth Rd, Ottawa ON K1H 8M5; National Medical University (Other Foreign)'07; FRCPC; Anes.

SHAFAI-SARSHAR, Roshan S; Southlake Reg Health Centre, 596 Davis Dr, Newmarket ON L3Y 2P9; Tor'94; FRCPC; IntMed. Staff, Southlake Regional Health Centre; Staff, Mackenzie Richmond Hill Hospital; Langs: Farsi; (905)895-4521; Fax. (905)853-2222.

SHAFER, Robyn T; North York Gen Hosp, 4001 Leslie St, North York ON M2K 1E1; Tor'01; CCFP; CCFP(E.M.); Staff, North York General Hospital; Staff, Medcan Health Management Inc; (416)756-6000

SHAFEY, Mona N; Foothills Med Centre, 1403 29 St NW, Calgary AB T2N 2T9; Ott'03; FRCPC; IntMed; Hem. Staff, Foothills Medical Centre; (403)944-8047; Fax. (403)270-7891.

SHAFFELBURG, Michael D; Valley Prof Centre, 70 Exhibition St, Kentville NS B4N 4K9; Dal'94; FRCPC; Derm. (902)678-6452; Fax. (902)678-4550; lls@easlink.ca.

SHAFFER, Eldon A; 6F-3280 Hospital Dr NW, Calgary AB T2N 4N1; Qns'65; DABIM; FACP; FACG; FRCPC; IntMed (Hepatology); Gastroent. Prof, University Of Calgary; (403)592-5033; Fax. (403)592-5040; shaffer@ucalgary.ca.

SHAFFER, Mark R; North York Family Health Team, PO Box 91130 Rpo Bayview Village 2901 Bayview Ave, North York ON M2K 2Y6; Mem'78; CCFP; FCFP; Ac Staff, North York General Hospital; Asst Prof Family & Comm Med, University of Toronto; Langs: French; (416)733-2284; Fax. (416)491-6428.

SHAFFER, Natalie; Clinique Med Urgence St-Hubert, 5645 rue Grande-Allee, Longueuil QC J4Z 3G3; McG'84; FRCPC; Derm (Laser Dermatology). Langs: French; (450)656-0666; ashamp1@aol.com.

SHAFIE, Marzieh; Highgate Med Centre, 103-7188 Kingsway, Burnaby BC V5E 1G3; Tehran (Iran)'96; CCFP; Staff, Copeman Health Centre; Langs: Farsi; (604)777-9101; Fax. (604)517-1006.

SHAFIEE, Mir; Sault Area Hosp, 750 Great Northern Rd, Sault Ste. Marie ON P6B 0A8; Tehran (Iran)'95; FRCPC; IntMed; Nephrol. Staff Renal Clinic, Sault Area Hospital - Sault Ste Marie; (705)759-3862; Fax. (905)759-4999.

SHAFIEE NYESTANAK, Mohammad A; Univ Hlth Network-Toronto Gen, EN 14 208-200 Elizabeth St, Toronto ON M5G 2C4; Tehran (Iran)'91; IntMed. Staff, Toronto General Hospital - UHN; (416)340-4195; Fax. (416)340-5826.

SHAFIQ, Muhammad; Central Alberta Prof Centre, 184-5201 43 St, Red Deer AB T4N 1C7; Karachi (Pakistan)'88; MB BS; ABIM; Langs: Urdu; (403)348-8790; Fax. (403)348-0985; mshafiqmd@yahoo.com.

SHAFIR, Cary; Guelph Gen Hosp, 115 Delhi St, Guelph ON N1E 4J4; McM'93; CCFP; Staff, Guelph General Hospital; (519)822-5350; Fax. (519)822-2170.

SHAFIR, M Sharon; Univ Hlth Network-Toronto Western Hosp, 2W404-399 Bathurst St, Toronto ON M5T 2S8; Tor'66; CCFP; FCFP; Staff Family Health Centre, Toronto Western Hospital - University Health Network; (416)603-5888 x1; Fax. (416)603-5821.

SHAFIR, Mark; Cambridge Mem Hosp, 700 Coronation Blvd, Cambridge ON N1R 3G2; Qns'89; CCFP; FCFP; Staff, Cambridge Memorial Hospital; (519)621-2333; Fax. (519)740-4921.

SHAFIR, Roslyn S; Baywood Med Centre, 507-95 Bayly St W, Ajax ON L1S 7K8; Tor'85; Staff, Rouge Valley Health System - Ajax & Pickering Health Centre Site; (905)426-1146; Fax. (905)426-5220.

SHAFONSKY, Eric W; Richmond Med Bldg, 405-2020 Richmond Rd, Victoria BC V8R 6R5; McG'90; (250)598-7234; Fax. (250)598-0042.

SHAFRAN, Stephen D; University of Alberta Hosp, 2E4 16WCM-8440 112 St NW, Edmonton AB T6G 2B7; Tor'80; ABIM; FRCPC; FRCPC; InfectDis; IntMed (AIDS/HIV). Consultant, Royal Alexandra Hospital; Consultant, Cross Cancer Institute; Ac Staff, University of Alberta Hospital; Prof, University of Alberta; (780)407-8077; Fax. (780)407-7137; sshafran@ualberta.ca.

SHAFRO, Ariel; Trillium Health Centre-Toronto, 4F-150 Sherway Dr, Etobicoke ON M9C 1A5; Wes'05; FRCPC; Psy. Staff Mental Health Services, Trillium Health Centre - West Toronto; (416)259-6671

SHAFTAR, Osama; 205-505 Queen St, Spruce Grove AB T7X 2V2; (780)962-2001; Fax. (780)962-8176.

SHAGLOUF, Hamdi I; 210-282 Linwell Rd, St Catharines ON L2N 6N5; University of Al Fateh (Libya)'98; CCFP; (905)934-4450; Fax. (905)934-4458.

SHAH, Aanand; Dominion Med Centre, 2383 111 St NW, Edmonton AB T6J 5E5; (Ireland)'04; Staff, University of Alberta Hospital; (780)436-0020; Fax. (780)436-0603.

SHAH, Abker; Superior Family Health Team, 44 Great Northern Rd, Sault Ste. Marie ON P6B 4Y7; Sind Medical College (Other Foreign)'91; CCFP.

SHAH, Amil M; Gordon & Leslie Diamond HCC, 11F-2775 Laurel St, Vancouver BC V5Z 1M9; McG'75; FACP; MDCM; FRCPC; IntMed (Medical Oncology). Ac Staff Med Oncol, BC Cancer Agency Vancouver Centre; Ac Staff, Vancouver General Hospital - Centennial Pavillion; Clin Assoc Prof, University of British Columbia; (604)875-4111 x67895; ashah@bccancer.bc.ca.

SHAH, Amit P; St Thomas-Elgin Gen Hosp, PO Box 2007 Stn Main 189 Elm St, St Thomas ON N5P 3W2; Wes'94; CCFP; CCFP(E.M.); FCFP; Staff Emerg, St Thomas Elgin General Hospital; Langs: Gujarati; (519)631-2020

SHAH, Ashvin; St Boniface Gen Hosp, 409 Tache Ave, Winnipeg MB R2H 2A6; Glasgow (Scotland)'74; MB ChB; FACEP; CCFP; Att Physician Emerg, St Boniface General Hospital; Asst Prof, University of Manitoba; (204)235-3006; Fax. (204)237-2071.

SHAH, Baiju R; Sunnybrook Hlth Sciences Ctre, H145-2075 Bayview Ave, Toronto ON M4N 3M5; Tor'97; PhD; FRCPC; IntMed (Clinician Investigator Program); Endocrin&Metab. Staff, Sunnybrook Health Sciences Centre; Scientist, Institute For Clinical Evaluation; Asst Prof, University of Toronto; (416)480-5914; Fax. (416)480-4250.

SHAH, Bharat; Boyd Med Centre, 412-388 Portage Ave, Winnipeg MB R3C 0C8; Glasgow (Scotland)'75; Ac Staff, Misericordia Health Centre; (204)943-2315; Fax. (204)942-5803.

SHAH, Bharatkumar K; Jane Medical Clinic, 206-2780 Jane St, North York ON M3N 2J2; Baroda (India)'78; Staff, Humber River Regional Hospital - Finch Avenue Site; Langs: Gujarati; Hindi; (416)743-3419; Fax. (416)743-6015.

SHAH, Chandrakant P; Anishnawbe Health Toronto, 225 Queen St E, Toronto ON M5A 1S4; Bombay (India)'62; MB BS; FRCPC; Peds. Staff, Anishnawbe Health Toronto; (416)360-0486; Fax. (416)365-1083; cshah@aht.ca.

SHAH, Chirag R; Mayfair Place, 250-6707 Elbow Dr SW, Calgary AB T2V 0E4; Gujarat (India)'00; FRCSC; Ophth (Medical Retina). Physician, Elbow Retina Centre; Langs: Hindi; Gujarati; Punjabi; (403)255-5561; Fax. (403)255-7764.

SHAH, Hemant A; Univ Hlth Network-Toronto Western Hosp, 6B FP172-399 Bathurst St, Toronto ON M5T 2S8; Tor'03; FRCPC; IntMed (Hepatology); Gastroent. Staff, Toronto Western Hospital - University Health Network; Langs: Gujarati; (416)603-5695; Fax. (416)603-6281.

SHAH, Himanshu H; West Park Walk-In Clinic, 1-456 Holland St W, Bradford ON L3Z 0G1; Indore (India)'83; MB BS; CCFP; (905)551-5500; Fax. (905)551-5400.

SHAH, Inayat A; Delta Mental Health Centre, 6345 120 St, Delta BC V4E 2A6; Physician, Mental Health Clinic; (604)948-7010; inayat.shah@rqhealth.ca.

SHAH, Jay K; McMaster University, HSC 2V-1280 Main St W, Hamilton ON L8S 4K1; Bombay (India)'81; MB BS; FRCPC; Peds (Neonatology). Staff Neonatol, Hamilton Health Sciences Centre - McMaster Children's Hospital; Prof, McMaster University; Langs: Hindi; Gujarati; Marathi; (905)521-2100 x75607; Fax. (905)521-5007.

SHAH, Justin A; Yarrow Med Bldg, 305-645 Fort St, Victoria BC V8W 1G2; UBC'03; FRCPC; IntMed; Gastroent. Langs: Bilingual(English/French); (250)361-1565

SHAH, Manish D; 303-4800 Leslie St, North York ON M2J 2K9; Tor'03; MPhil; BSc; FRCSC; Otol (Head & Neck Surgery). Staff, North York General Hospital; Staff, Toronto General Hospital - UHN; (416)499-5558; Fax. (416)499-9392.

SHAH, Meera; Scarborough Hosp-General Div, 3050 Lawrence Ave E, Scarborough ON M1P 2V5; Tor'07; CCFP; CCFP(E.M.); Staff, The Scarborough Hospital - General Campus; Langs: Gujarati; (416)438-2911

SHAH, Misbah A; Rockyview Gen Hosp, 7007 14 St SW, Calgary AB T2V 1P9; Alb'88; FRCPC; Anes. Staff Anes, Rockyview General Hospital; (403)943-8720

SHAH, Mruna M; West Durham Family Health Team, BE 200B-1105 Kingston Rd, Pickering ON L1V 1B5; Tor'96; BSc; PhmB; CCFP; FCFP; Ac Staff, Rouge Valley Health System - Ajax & Pickering Health Centre Site; (905)420-9999

SHAH, Natavarlal H; 436 Second St E, Cornwall ON K6H 1Z3; Calcutta (India)'64; Ac Staff, Cornwall Community Hospital - Second Street Site; Dir Dept of Emerg, Cornwall Community Hospital; Med Dir, Versa Care, Cornwall; Langs: Bengali; Gujarati; Hindi; (613)938-9684; Fax. (613)938-9746.

SHAH, Prakeshkumar S; Mount Sinai Hosp, 775A-600 University Ave, Toronto ON M5G 1X5; Gujarat (India)'88; MRCP; FRCP; Peds; MSc; MB BS; DCH; FRCPC; Peds (Neonatal & Perinatal Medicine). Staff Neonatol, The Hospital For Sick Children; Staff, Mount Sinai Hospital; Langs: Gujarati; Hindi; (416)586-4761; Fax. (416)586-8745; pshah@mtsinai.on.ca.

SHAH, Pravin C; Strathroy Middlesex Gen Hosp, PO Box 5001 395 Carrie St, Strathroy ON N7G 3C9; Gujarat (India)'65; MB BS; FRCPC; AnatPath (Clinical Pathology); GenPath. Dir Labs, Strathroy Middlesex General Hospital - Middlesex Hospital Alliance; Dir Labs, Four Counties Health Services - Middlesex Hospital Alliance; Aj Prof Path, University of Western Ontario; Langs: Gujarati; Hindi; Urdu; (519)245-5295 x5566; Fax. (519)245-5438.

SHAH, Rajiv R; 5F-61 Queen St E, Toronto ON M5C 2T2; Wes'96; FRCSC; ObstGyn. Staff, St Michael's Hospital; Staff, Women's Health Care Centre; Langs: Gujarati; French; (416)867-7480; Fax. (416)867-7478.

SHAH, Rita; Reach Community Health Ctre, 1145 Commercial Dr, Vancouver BC V5L 3X3; UBC'08; CCFP; (604)254-1354

SHAH, Sachin J; London HSC-University Hosp, PO Box 5339 Stn B ALL 139-339 Windermere Rd, London ON N6A 5A5; Sask'08; IntMed. Staff, London Health Sciences Centre - University Hospital.

SHAH, Sachit P; 102-13805 104 Ave, Surrey BC V3T 1W7; Manchester (England)'85; MB ChB; MRC; CCFP; FCFP; Ac Staff, Surrey Memorial Hospital; Langs: Gujarati; (604)594-2714; Fax. (604)507-3514; sachitshah@yahoo.com.

SHAH, Sameer; Castlemore Family Med Centre, 12 Lauderhill Rd, Brampton ON L6P 2Z1; Wes'10; CCFP; (647)268-9031

SHAH, Sheila; Jane Medical Clinic, 206-2780 Jane St, North York ON M3N 2J2; Mysore (India)'79; Staff, Humber River Regional Hospital - Finch Avenue Site; Langs: Hindi; Gujarati; (416)743-3419; Fax. (416)743-6015.

SHAH, Suryakant K; Dr Charles A Janeway Child HC, 3J108-300 Prince Philip Dr, St. John's NL A1B 3V6; Makerere (Uganda)'71; MB ChB; MMed(Peds.); FAAP; FRCPC; Peds (Pediatric Dermatology); PedCardiol. Staff Peds Cardiol, Janeway Children's Health & Rehabilitation Centre; Prof Peds, Memorial University Of Newfoundland; (709)777-4768; Fax. (709)777-4747; sshah@mun.ca.

SHAH, Syed M H; Medical Arts Clinic, 780 Central Ave N, Swift Current SK S9H 0M3; MMed; PhD; (306)773-2811; Fax. (306)778-4081.

SHAH, Vibhuti S; Mount Sinai Hosp, 775A-600 University Ave, Toronto ON M5G 1X5; Seth (India)'85; FRCPC; Peds (Neonatology). Staff, Mount Sinai Hospital; Langs: Gujarati; Hindi; Marathi; (416)586-4816; Fax. (416)586-8745.

SHAH, Vinod H; Rapelje Lodge, 277 Plymouth Rd, Welland ON L3B 6E3; Man'76; Staff, Niagara Health System - Welland Hospital Site; Langs: Hindi; Gujarati; (905)788-6767

SHAH, Zafar A; London HSC-University Hosp, PO Box 5339 Stn B 339 Windermere Rd, London ON N6A 5A5; Punjab (Pakistan)'60; MB BS; FRCSC; GenSurg. Staff, London Health Sciences Centre - University Hospital; Langs: Urdu; Punjabi; (519)663-3081; Fax. (519)663-3182.

SHAHA, Tarun K; Burrard Health Bldg, 201-1160 Burrard St, Vancouver BC V6Z 2E8; Dhaka (Bangladesh)'94; MB BS; CCFP; Langs: Bengali; (604)558-4044; shaha_tk@hotmail.com.

SHAHAB, Saqib; Population Health Branch, 3475 Albert St, Regina SK S4S 6X6; Rawalpindi (Pakistan)'85; MRCP(UK); MPH(USA); FRCPC; CommunMed (Public Health). Chief MHO, Ministry Of Health-Saskatchewan; (306)787-3220; Fax. (306)787-3237.

SHAHANI, Rohan; Gates of Maple Med Center, 103-2200 Rutherford Rd, Vaughan ON L4K 5V2; Tor'04; FRCSC; Urol (Minimal Invasive Surgery). Assoc Staff, Mackenzie Richmond Hill Hospital; (905)832-8428; Fax. (905)832-6651.

SHAHBAZ, Muhammad; Sunridge Family Med Teaching C, 2685 36 St NE, Calgary AB T1Y 5S3; (Other Foreign)'10; CCFP; Staff, Sunridge Family Medicine Teaching Centre; Langs: Urdu; Punjabi; (403)943-5000; Fax. (403)476-8784.

SHAHBAZI, Nasim; 405-984 Oliver Rd, Thunder Bay ON P7B 7C7; (Iran)'98; FRCPC; IntMed; Nephrol. Langs: Persian; (807)345-7170; Fax. (807)345-5888.

SHAHEED, Wagih K A; 1690 Hillside drive, London ON N6G 3T2; Cairo (Egypt)'61; MB ChB; DCH; MRCP(UK); FRCPC; Peds. Langs: Arabic; (226)777-1152; Fax. (519)645-0145; wagih.shaheed@sympatico.ca.

SHAHEEN, Nighat; Chinguacousy & Sandalwood Med, 6-10671 Chinguacousy Rd, Brampton ON L7A 0N5; Karachi (Pakistan)'79; CCFP; (905)840-4343; Fax. (905)840-4303.

SHAHEEN, Uzma; Radiology Assoc of Regina, 6-2727 Parliament Ave, Regina SK S4S 6X5; Rawalpindi (Pakistan)'85; MB BS; FRCPC; DiagRad. Staff, Radiology Associates of Regina; (306)352-7653; Fax. (306)522-4311.

SHAHI, Bahram; Fort Frances Clinic, 301 Victoria Ave, Fort Frances ON P9A 2C1; Tehran (Iran)'88; FRCSC; GenSurg. Langs: Farsi; Persian; (807)274-3287; Fax. (807)274-7882.

SHAHI, Sundeep; Grand River Reg Cancer Centre, PO Box 9056 Stn C 835 King St W, Kitchener ON N2G 1G3; Ott'01; FRCPC; RadOncol. Staff, Grand River Hospital - Kitchener/Waterloo Health Centre; Staff, Grand River Regional Cancer Centre; Langs: Punjabi; (519)749-4380; sundeep.shahi@grhosp.on.ca.

SHAHID, Azmeh; Youthdale Treatment Centre, 227 Victoria St, Toronto ON M5B 1T8; Karachi (Pakistan)'97; Langs: Urdu; (416)363-3751

SHAHID, Raheel A; Dr Everett Chalmers Reg Hosp, PO Box 9000 Stn A, Fredericton NB E3B 5N5; Lahore (Pakistan)'92; Staff, Dr Everett Chalmers Regional Hospital; (506)452-5400

SHAHID, Riad M A; Surrey Med Bldg, 306-9656 King George Blvd, Surrey BC V3T 2V5; Alexandria (Egypt)'61; MB ChB; FRCSC; OrthSurg (Knee Surgery). Consultant Orth, Surrey Memorial Hospital; Langs: German; French; Arabic; (604)588-9232; Fax. (604)588-9242.

SHAHID, Shaneela; Hamilton HS-McMaster Site, PO Box 2000 Stn Lcd 1 1200 Main St W, Hamilton ON L8N 3Z5; Ziauddin Medical University (Other Foreign)'02; FRCPC; Peds. Staff, Hamilton Health Sciences Centre - McMaster Children's Hospital; (905)525-9140

SHAHIDI, Mazda; CHUS-Hotel-Dieu, 580 rue Bowen S, Sherbrooke QC J1G 2E8; (Iran)'95; Staff, Centre Hospitalier Universitaire de Sherbrooke-Hôpital Hôtel-Dieu; (819)346-1110 x25541; Fax. (819)829-6263.

SHAHIN, David R; 402-5800 boul Cavendish, Cote Saint-Luc QC H4W 2T5; McG'76; Langs: French; (514)487-8550; Fax. (514)487-8552.

SHAHIN, Edmond B N; 7-7005 ch Kildare, Cote Saint-Luc QC H4W 1C1; McG'73; FRCPC; Peds; ClinImmunol&Allergy. Staff Allergy, McGill University Health Centre - Montreal General Campus; Prof Faculty, McGill University; Langs: French; (514)487-8565; Fax. (514)487-8549.

SHAHIN, Jack; Medical Centre, 2204-3000 Lawrence Ave E, Scarborough ON M1P 2V1; McG'81; FRCSC; Otol (Facial Plastic Surgery). Staff, Rouge Valley Health System - Centenary Health Centre Site; Staff, The Scarborough Hospital - General Campus; Langs: Bilingual(English/French); (416)289-1225; Fax. (416)289-0970.

SHAHIN, Jason; MUHC-Royal Victoria Hosp, 687 av des Pins O, Montreal QC H3A 1A1; McG'01; FRCPC; IntMed; Critical Care Medicine; Respir. Staff, McGill University Health Centre - Royal Victoria Hospital; (514)934-1934

SHAHIN, Rita M; Toronto Public Health, 10F-277 Victoria St, Toronto ON M5B 1W2; McG'86; FRCPC; CommunMed. Assoc Med Officer of Hlth, Toronto Public Health Corporate Office; University of Toronto; Langs: French; (416)338-7924; Fax. (416)392-0047; rshahin@toronto.ca.

SHAHIN AZAR, Massoud; Queen Elizabeth II HSC-Halifax, 1796 Summer St, Halifax NS B3H 3A7; Mashhad (Other Foreign)'87; Staff, Queen Elizabeth II Health Sciences Centre - Halifax Infirmary Site; (902)473-7105

SHAHMALAK, Shahzad Z; Cambridge Mem Hosp, 700 Coronation Blvd, Cambridge ON N1R 3G2; Karachi (Pakistan)'89; Staff, Cambridge Memorial Hospital; Langs: Hindi; Urdu; (519)740-4900; Fax. (519)740-4936.

SHAHNAVAZ, Shahryar-Ali; 1-1800 Bank St, Ottawa ON K1V 0W3; McM'05; FRCSC; Otol. (506)649-2885; Fax. (506)632-6955.

SHAHNAWAZ, Muhammad; Victoria Med Bldg, 104-1669 Victoria St, Prince George BC V2L 2L5; Nishtar (Pakistan)'89; MB BS; CCFP; Staff, University Hospital of Northern British Columbia; Langs: Punjabi; (250)562-1160; Fax. (250)562-2580.

SHAHOO, Nirmal K; Centennial CMH & Brain Injury, PO Box 1000 Stn Main, Ponoka AB T4J 1R8; Andhra (India)'83; MB BS; DPM(Ire); Staff Centennial Centre for Mental Health & Brain Injury, Centennial Centre for Mental Health & Brain Injury; Staff, Red Deer Regional Hospital Centre; Clin Teacher Family Med, University of Alberta; Langs: Bengali; Hindi; (403)743-7600; Fax. (403)783-7790.

SHAHPARAKI, Aram; 103-4900 Kingsway, Burnaby BC V5H 2E3; Ott'97; FRCPC; IntMed (Endocrinology). Consultant Endocrinologist, Burnaby Hospital; Langs: Farsi; (604)568-6685

SHAHRIAREE, Pegah; Scarborough Hosp-General Div, 3050 Lawrence Ave E, Scarborough ON M1P 2V5; Shaheed Beheshti University (Iran)'00; FRCPC; IntMed;CCFP; Staff, The Scarborough Hospital - General Campus; Langs: Persian; (416)438-2911

SHAHROKHI, Masoud; Park Royal Village Med Centre, J2-925 Main St, West Vancouver BC V7T 2Z3; Teheran (Iran)'91; CCFP; Staff, Coal Harbour Medical Clinic; Physician, Park Royal Village Medical Centre; Langs: Persian; Farsi; (604)922-7372; Fax. (604)922-7336; masoud.shahrokhi@gmail.com.

SHAHROKHI EBRAHIMIPOUR, Shahriar; Sunnybrook Hlth Sciences Ctr, D716-2075 Bayview Ave, Toronto ON M4N 3M5; Ott'01; FRCSC; GenSurg. Staff Ross Tilley Burn Centre, Sunnybrook Health Sciences Centre; (416)480-5554; Fax. (416)480-4891.

SHAHZAD, Karina; Fifth Avenue Walk-In Clinic, 14 Fifth Ave, Orangeville ON L9W 1G2; Punjab (Pakistan)'89; CCFP; Langs: Punjabi; Urdu; (519)942-0040; Fax. (519)942-0048.

SHAHZAD, Seema; Deloraine Med Centre, PO Box 429, Deloraine MB R0M 0M0; Bahuddi Zakaria U (Pakistan)'96; (204)747-2461

SHAIGETZ, Daniel; Clinique Med Rosemont, 1969 boul Rosemont, Montreal QC H2G 1S9; Mon'83; FRCSC; Urol (General Surgery). Staff, CSSS du Coeur de l'Isle Hôpital Jean-Talon; Staff, CSSS Saint-Leonard et Saint-Michel; (514)274-7344; mes@mailhost.tad.jgh.mcgill.ca.

SHAIK, Mehaboob S; Royal Alexandra Hosp, DTC 5027-10240 Kingsway NW, Edmonton AB T5H 3V9; (India)'85; Staff Neonatal Unit, Royal Alexandra Hospital; Staff, Covenant Health - Grey Nuns Community Hospital; (780)735-4647; Fax. (780)735-4072.

SHAIKH, A Allison; St Josephs Health Care, PO Box 5777 Stn B 268 Grosvenor St, London ON N6A 4V2; Ott'02; FRCPC; DiagRad. Staff, St Joseph's Hospital - St Joseph's Health Care; Langs: Bilingual(English/French); (519)646-6000

SHAIKH, Abdul R; Western Mem Health Clinic, 3 Herald Ave, Corner Brook NL A2H 4B8; Sind (India)'86; MB BS; Staff, Charles S Curtis Memorial Hospital; Staff, Western Memorial Regional Hospital; (709)637-3900

SHAIKH, Bashiruddin N; 304-540 College St, Toronto ON M6G 1A6; Poona (India)'61; MB BS; FRCSC; Urol. Ac Staff, Toronto Western Hospital - University Health Network; Langs: Hindi; Gujarati; Marathi; (416)961-6606; Fax. (416)961-0830.

SHAIKH, Bashirunnisa A; William Osler Health Centre, 106B-100 Humber College Blvd, Etobicoke ON M9V 5G4; Bombay (India)'69; Ac Staff, William Osler Health System - Etobicoke General Hospital; Langs: Gujarati; Hindi; Punjabi; Urdu; (416)746-4777

SHAIKH, Furqan K S; The Hosp for Sick Children, 555 University Ave, Toronto ON M5G 1X8; Qns'03; PedHemaOncol; Peds. Staff Haem/Oncol, The Hospital For Sick Children; (416)813-7500

SHAIKH, M Asif; Abbotsford Reg Hosp & Cancer C, 39200 Marshall Rd, Abbotsford BC V2S 0C2; Mumbai (India)'94; Staff, Abbotsford Regional Hospital & Cancer Centre; (604)851-4710

SHAIKH, Maria-Estrella V; Niagara HS-St Catharines Site, PO Box 3018 Stn Main 142 Queenston St, St Catharines ON L2R 7C6; Albany Medical College (USA)'97; CCFP; Staff, Niagara Health System - St Catharines General Site; (905)684-7272; Fax. (905)704-4414.

SHAIKH, Muhammed; Peterborough Reg HC-Hospital, 1 Hospital Dr, Peterborough ON K9J 7C6; Karachi (Pakistan)'89; Staff, Peterborough Regional Health Centre - Hospital Drive; (705)743-2121

SHAIKH, Nasir; St Boniface Gen Hosp, Y3025-409 Tache Ave, Winnipeg MB R2H 2A6; Karachi (Pakistan)'88; MB BS; ABIM; Staff Cardiol, St Boniface General Hospital; Staff, Health Sciences Centre; Asst Prof Med & Cardiac Sciences, University of Manitoba; Langs: Urdu; Hindi; (204)258-1266; Fax. (204)233-2157.

SHAIKH, Omer S; Rainbow Pediatrics, 304-4256 Portage Rd, Niagara Falls ON L2E 6A4; Karachi (Pakistan)'92; Staff, Niagara Health System - St Catharines General Site; Asst Prof Peds, McMaster University; (905)356-5437; Fax. (905)356-4225.

SHAIKH, S Yasmin; 406-5 Fairview Mall Dr, North York ON M2J 2Z1; Punjab (Pakistan)'82; MB BS; CCFP; Langs: Urdu; Hindi; Punjabi; Persian; (416)492-9598; Fax. (416)492-7921.

SHAIKH, Saeed A; 5-2 Lakeshore Rd, St Catharines ON L2N 7E4; RCS (Ireland)'96; FRCPC; IntMed; Rheum. (905)937-2220; Fax. (905)937-4404.

SHAIKH, Sharmeen; Village Park Med Clinic, 110-937 Fir St, Sherwood Park AB T8A 4N6; (Other Foreign)'02; (780)467-8886; Fax. (780)467-6763.

SHAIKH, Vaquas M; William Osler HC-Brampton, 2100 Bovaird Dr E, Brampton ON L6R 3J7; McM'10; CCFP; Staff, William Osler Health System - Brampton Civic Hospital; (905)494-2120

SHAIKH, Wajid A; 200-4125 Lawrence Ave E, Scarborough ON M1E 2S2; Heidelberg (Germany)'69; DABPed; DABACI; FRCP; FAAAI; FRCPC; Peds (Allergy). Staff, The Scarborough Hospital - General Campus; Langs: German; Hindi; Urdu; (416)281-7722; Fax. (416)281-1770.

SHAIKHOLESLAMI, Roya; 663 Coronation Blvd, Cambridge ON N1R 3G4; Tehran (Iran)'78; Staff, Cambridge Memorial Hospital; Langs: Farsi; (519)622-5500; Fax. (519)622-1030.

SHAINHOUSE, J Zevi; Medical Centre Bldg B, 3303-3000 Lawrence Ave E, Scarborough ON M1P 2V1; Tor'74; ABIM(InfectDis); FRCPC; IntMed (Cardiology). Staff, The Scarborough Hospital - General Campus; Langs: Hebrew; (416)438-7556; Fax. (416)438-7896.

SHAIPANICH, Tawimas; St Paul's Hosp, 8B-1081 Burrard St, Vancouver BC V6Z 1Y6; Rangsit (Thailand)'95; FRCPC; IntMed; Respir. Staff Pacific Lung Health Centre, Providence Health Care - St Paul's Hospital; (604)682-2344 x69388

SHAKER, Emil; Ellerslie Medicentre, 102-9404 Ellerslie Rd SW, Edmonton AB T6X 0K6; '89; CCFP; (780)466-8064; Fax. (780)466-8095.

SHAKER, Marian; Ellerslie Medicentre, 102-9404 Ellerslie Rd SW, Edmonton AB T6X 0K6; (Sudan)'03; CCFP; (780)466-8064; Fax. (780)466-8095.

SHAKER, Marian R; Clandeboye Med Clinic, 210B Clandeboye Ave, Selkirk MB R1A 0X1; (Other Foreign)'01; (204)963-2963; Fax. (204)482-4524.

SHAKER, Shameem; 11-7750 Ranchview Dr NW, Calgary AB T3G 1Y9; (403)452-6240; Fax. (403)452-9626.

SHAKER, Vajdiyeh; Tudor Glen Medicentre, 2520 Tudor Glen Market, St. Albert AB T8N 3V3; (780)458-5776; Fax. (780)460-1908.

SHAKERINIA, Tooraj; Dr Tooraj Shakerina Prof Corp, 603-100 Arden St, Moncton NB E1C 4B7; Dal'92; BSc; FACS; FRCSC; GenSurg. (506)382-4552; Fax. (506)382-6072.

SHAKESPEARE, Timothy J; Clinical Sciences Bldg, 8-152 University Campus NW, Edmonton AB T6G 2G3; (780)407-8887; Fax. (780)407-3200.

SHAKHATREH, Hala D S; Pelham Group Health Centre, 212-245 Pelham Rd, St Catharines ON L2S 1X8; (Jordan)'92; FRCPC; Peds. Langs: Arabic; (905)682-2207; Fax. (905)682-1793.

SHAKIB, Alireza; All Saints Springhill Hosp, PO Box 700 10 Princess St, Springhill NS B0M 1X0; National Medical University (Other Foreign)'01; Staff, All Saints Springhill Hospital; (902)597-3773

SHAKIL, Sadia; Horizon Family Practice, 108-15508 87 Ave NW, Edmonton AB T5R 4G5; (Pakistan)'96; Staff, Parkland Medical Centre; Langs: Hindi; Urdu; Punjabi; (780)757-9786; Fax. (780)757-9789; horizonfamilypractice@gmail.com.

SHALABY, Ashraf M K; Terra Losa Grande Med Clinic, 309-17407 99 Ave NW, Edmonton AB T5T 0W7; (Other Foreign)'85; CCFP; (780)340-8480

SHALABY, Karam; 6 rue Canvin, Kirkland QC H9H 4S4; Cairo (Egypt)'72; FRCSC; ObstGyn. Staff, Sir Mortimer B Davis Jewish General; Staff, Lakeshore General Hospital - Pointe Claire; (514)695-1903; Fax. (514)695-1904.

SHALAN AL-GAZI, Mohanad J; Joseph Brant Mem Hosp, 1230 North Shore Blvd E, Burlington ON L7S 1W7; University of Baghdad (Other Foreign)'83; FRCPC; Peds. Staff, Joseph Brant Memorial Hospital; Langs: Arabic; (905)632-3730

SHALAY, Katherine M; Turnbull Diagnostic Imaging, 170 Simcoe St, Peterborough ON K9H 2H7; Qns'83; AB; FRCPC; DiagRad. Staff, Peterborough Regional Health Centre - Hospital Drive; Staff, Peterborough Regional Health Centre - Rogers St Site; (705)742-3639

SHALBY, Moustafa A M M; R Fraser Elliot Bldg, EB3 805-190 Elizabeth St, Toronto ON M5G 2C4; Cairo (Egypt)'02; IntMed. Staff, Toronto General Hospital - UHN; (416)978-2645

SHALISH, Wissam; The Hosp for Sick Children, 555 University Ave, Toronto ON M5G 1X8; McG'08; Peds (Neonatology). Staff, The Hospital For Sick Children; (416)813-1500

SHALOM-PAZ, Einat; MUHC-Royal Victoria Hosp, 687 av des Pins O, Montreal QC H3A 1A1; Staff, McGill University Health Centre - Royal Victoria Hospital; (514)934-1934

SHAMANNA, Dilip K; Kings Med Clinic, 11-3340 17 Ave SE, Calgary AB T2A 0P9; Cal'80; CCFP; (403)273-8500; Fax. (403)569-0706.

SHAMAS, Mary E; Blind River Family Med Clinic, PO Box 1630 527 Causley St, Blind River ON P0R 1B0; Tor'92; MSc(Queen's); CCFP; Ac Staff Privil, Blind River District Health Centre; Med Dir/Pres, Art of Medicine; (705)356-1666; Fax. (705)356-2403; mshamas@brdhc.on.ca.

SHAMCHUK, David A; Meadowlark Health Centre, 200 Meadowlark Shopping Ctr NW, Edmonton AB T5R 5W9; Alb'80; FRCPC; DiagRad. (780)669-2222; Fax. (780)489-5160.

SHAMEKH, Farzaneh; St Mary's Hosp Centre, 3830 av Lacombe, Montreal QC H3T 1M5; McG'94; FRCPC; IntMed. Staff, St Mary's Hospital Centre; (514)345-3511

SHAMES, Sofia; MUHC-Royal Victoria Hosp, 687 av des Pins O, Montreal QC H3A 1A1; McG'04; Cardiol; IntMed. Staff, McGill University Health Centre - Royal Victoria Hospital; (514)934-1934

SHAMESS, Brian A; Algoma Sports Med Phys Injurie, 105-974 Queen St E, Sault Ste. Marie ON P6A 2C5; Wes'80; Dip SportMed; Staff, Sault Area Hospital - Sault Ste Marie; Clinical Asst Prof, Northern Ontario School of Medicine-Lakehead University; Langs: Spanish; (705)759-2393; Fax. (705)759-4835.

SHAMESS, Charles J; Parkdale Med Tower, 602-1081 Carling Ave, Ottawa ON K1Y 4G2; McG'72; FRCPC; IntMed; Rheum. (613)724-6602

SHAMIM, Safia; Halton HSC Corp-Oakville, 327 Reynolds St, Oakville ON L6J 3L7; Punjab (Pakistan)'01; CCFP; CCFP(E.M.); Staff, Halton Healthcare Services Corporation - Oakville Site; Langs: Urdu; (905)845-2571

SHAMISA, Abdalla R M; 205-1106 Ouellette Ave, Windsor ON N9A 1C9; Tripoli (Libya)'89; FRCSC; Neursurg. Langs: Arabic; (519)973-8771; Fax. (519)973-4690.

SHAMJI, Farid M; The Ottawa Hosp-Gen Campus, 6362-501 Smyth Rd, Ottawa ON K1H 8L6; Newcastle (England)'73; MB BS; FACS; FRCSC; GenSurg (Thoracic Surgery); Cardiovasc&ThorSurg. Staff, The Ottawa Hospital - Civic Campus; Staff, The Ottawa Hospital - General Campus; Prof, University of Ottawa; Langs: Gujarati; Kacchi; (613)737-8899 x74030; Fax. (613)737-8668; fshamji@ottawahospital.on.ca.

SHAMJI, Mohammed F; Univ Hlth Network-Toronto Western Hosp, 4 446-399 Bathurst St, Toronto ON M5T 2S8; Qns'03; Neursurg (Spine Surgery). Staff, Toronto Western Hospital - University Health Network; (416)603-5879; Fax. (416)603-5298.

SHAMJI, Salima; Elizabeth Bruyere Hlth Centre, 423Y-75 Bruyere St, Ottawa ON K1N 5C7; McM'94; CCFP; FCFP; Staff, Bruyère Continuing Care - Elisabeth Bruyere Hospital; (613)562-6262; salima@bruyere.org.

SHAMLIAN, Nathalie; Hop de Sacre-Coeur de Montreal, 5400 boul Gouin O, Montreal QC H4J 1C5; Mon'96; FRCPC; Psy. Staff, Hôpital du Sacre-Coeur de Montréal; (514)338-3563; Fax. (514)338-4359.

SHAMMAS, Amer; The Hosp for Sick Children, 555 University Ave, Toronto ON M5G 1X8; Damascus (Syria)'96; FRCPC; NuclearMed (Diagnostic Radiology). Staff, The Hospital For Sick Children; (416)813-6065; Fax. (416)813-7591; amer.shammas@sickkids.ca.

SHAMMAS, Nouri I; SGH Medical Mall, 501-3030 Lawrence Ave E, Scarborough ON M1P 2T7; Baghdad (Iraq)'69; MB ChB; FACS; FRCSC; PlasSurg. Ac Staff, The Scarborough Hospital - General Campus; Langs: Arabic; (416)439-5744; Fax. (416)438-2863.

SHAMMI, Chekkera M; Ontario Shore Ctre Mental Heal, 700 Gordon St, Whitby ON L1N 5S9; Madras (India)'83; MB BS; DPM(Ire); MRCPsy(U.K.); ASAM; FRCPC; Psy (Schizophrenia). Staff Psy, Ontario Shores Centre for Mental Health Sciences; Staff, Centre for Addiction & Mental Health (CAMH) - College Street Site; Asst Prof, University of Toronto; (416)314-2862; shammic@ontarioshores.ca.

SHAMOUT, Zaki; IWK Health Centre, PO Box 9700 Rpo CSC, Halifax NS B3K 6R8; Alexandria (Egypt)'79; MB ChB; Staff, IWK Health Centre; (902)420-6669; Fax. (902)420-6469.

SHAMS, Merajuddin; Unimedico Family Practice, 110-955 Major MacKenzie Dr W, Vaughan ON L6A 4P9; Kabul (Afghanistan)'83; CCFP; Langs: Pashtu; Dari; Farsi; (289)553-3300; Fax. (289)553-2600.

SHAMS, Nagi S A; Dr Shams Walk-In & Fam Practic, 108-178 John St, Brampton ON L6W 2A4; Cairo (Egypt)'75; MB ChB; CCFP; Langs: Arabic; (905)453-0057; Fax. (905)453-0026.

SHAMS, Sherif A A; 418-5450 ch de la Cote-des-Nei, Montreal QC H3T 1Y6; Cairo (Egypt)'63; FRCSC; ObstGyn. Staff, St Mary's Hospital Centre; (514)731-2097; Fax. (514)342-0838.

SHAMS TABRIZI, Shahram; Capilano Med Clinic, 85-935 Marine Dr, North Vancouver BC V7P 1S3; Islamic Azad (Iran)'96; CCFP; (604)988-3443

SHAMSAH, Abdullah A; The Hosp for Sick Children, 555 University Ave, Toronto ON M5G 1X8; Dublin (Ireland)'95; PedEmergMed; Peds. Staff, The Hospital For Sick Children; (416)813-1500

SHAMSEDDIN, Mohammad K; Kingston Gen Hosp, B3 038-76 Stuart St, Kingston ON K7L 2V7; Damascus (Syria)'98; FRCPC; IntMed; Nephrol. Staff, Kingston General Hospital; (613)549-6666

SHAMSI, Mehrnoosh; Eagle Ridge Hosp & HCC, 475 Guildford Way, Port Moody BC V3H 3W9; Yazd Shahid Sadoughi (Iran)'92; CCFP; Staff, Eagle Ridge Hospital & Health Care Centre; Langs: Farsi; (604)461-2022

SHAMSIAN, Elham; Bank Med Centre, 1935 Bank St, Ottawa ON K1V 8A3; Ott'96; CCFP; FCFP; Langs: Farsi; (613)521-2391; Fax. (613)907-1712.

SHAMSIE, Amina J; Findlay Creek Med Centre, 3-4744 Bank St, Ottawa ON K1T 3W7; Tor'91; CCFP; FCFP; Langs: French; (613)317-2584; Fax. (613)822-2775.

SHAMSUDDIN, Syed; Saint John Reg Hosp, PO Box 2100 Stn Main 400 University Ave, Saint John NB E2L 4L2; Bangalore (India)'93; Staff, Saint John Regional Hospital; (506)648-6000

SHAMSUZZAMAN, Mohammed; Broadway Med Clinic, 1319 Broadway Ave, Regina SK S4P 1E5; Chittagong (Bangladesh)'86; MB BS; CCFP; Physician, Broadway Medical Clinic; (306)757-4114; Fax. (306)565-2297.

SHAMY, April A; E724-SMBD Jewish Gen Hosp, 3755 ch Cote-Sainte-Catherine, Montreal QC H3T 1E2; McG'85; FRCPC; IntMed; Hem. Staff, Sir Mortimer B Davis Jewish General; adj Prof Med, McGill University; Langs: English; French; (514)340-8222; Fax. (514)340-8733.

SHAMY, Michel C F; Foothills Med Centre, 1403 29 St NW, Calgary AB T2N 2T9; Qns'06; FRCPC; Neur. Staff, Foothills Medical Centre; (403)944-8671; Fax. (403)944-1602.

SHAN, Xi; 101-3 Conestoga Dr, Brampton ON L6Z 4N5; McM'00; PhD; FRCPC; IntMed; Nephrol. Staff, William Osler Health System - Etobicoke General Hospital; Staff, William Osler Health System - Brampton Civic Hospital; Langs: Chinese; (905)453-0715; Fax. (905)453-0972.

SHAND, J Gregory E; Phoenix Med Centre, 101-2155 10th Ave, Prince George BC V2M 5J6; Alb'88; FRCPC; DiagRad. Staff, University Hospital of Northern British Columbia; (250)563-1608; Fax. (250)563-1288.

SHANDERA, Raymond H; Shandera & Powell Private Clin, PO Box 716 286 Conception Bay Hwy, Bay Roberts NL A0A 1G0; Mem'73; (709)786-3380; Fax. (709)786-6195.

SHANDLING, Maureen R; Joseph & Wolf Lebovic Hlth Com, L2 208-60 Murray St, Toronto ON M5T 3L9; Alb'81; FRCPC; Neur. Staff, Mount Sinai Hospital; Asst Prof, University of Toronto; (416)586-4800 x8597; Fax. (416)586-8623; mshandling@mtsinai.on.ca.

SHANDRO, Gerald L; Misericordia Community Hosp, 16940 87 Ave NW, Edmonton AB T5R 4H5; Alb'69; Neursurg. Staff, Covenant Health - Misericordia Community Hospital; (780)735-2000

SHANDRO, John T A; PO Box 5203 Stn B, Victoria BC V8R 6N4; Alb'75; FRCPC; Anes. (250)598-9777; Fax. (250)598-9788.

SHANDRO, M Tami-Lee; Grey Nuns Community Hosp, 1100 Youville Drive West NW, Edmonton AB T6L 5X8; Alb'82; CCFP; FCFP; Staff Covenant Health, Covenant Health - Grey Nuns Community Hospital; (780)735-7000; Fax. (780)735-7887.

SHANDRO, W G Bud; ENT Associates, 300-1011 Glenmore Trail SW, Calgary AB T2V 4R6; Alb'71; DAB; ABOtol; FRCSC; Otol (Sleep Apnea). Ac Staff, Peter Lougheed Centre; Ac Staff, Alberta Children's Hospital; Clin Lecturer, University of Calgary; (403)571-5210; Fax. (403)571-5211.

SHANE, H Frederick; B200-1460 Main St, North Vancouver BC V7J 1C8; Man'65; FRCPC; Psy. (778)340-1397

SHANE, Marvin D; Seven Oaks Gen Hosp, 2300 McPhillips St, Winnipeg MB R2V 3M3; Man'69; FRCPC; Psy. Staff Psy, Seven Oaks General Hospital; (204)632-7133

SHANFIELD, Isidore; 400-6000 ch de la Cote-des-Nei, Montreal QC H3S 1Z8; McG'64; PhD; FRCSC; GenSurg. principale Staff Surg, Sir Mortimer B Davis Jewish General; assoc Staff, Hôpital Ste-Justine; adj Prof Surg, McGill University; (514)733-2363; Fax. (514)733-1834.

SHANFIELD, Simon E; Ouellette Health Centre, 1083 Ouellette Ave, Windsor ON N9A 4J8; Wes'05; FRCPC; IntMed. Staff, Hôtel-Dieu Grace Hospital; (519)946-0556; Fax. (519)946-0557.

SHANKAR, Jai Jai S; Queen Elizabeth II HSC, 1276 South Park St, Halifax NS B3H 2Y9; Ranchi University (Other Foreign)'99; MB BS; Staff, Queen Elizabeth II Health Sciences Centre - Victoria General Site; (902)473-5453; Fax. (902)473-2018.

SHANKAR, Lalitha; West End Radiological Imaging, 103-2425 Bloor St W, Toronto ON M6S 4W4; Calcutta (India)'75; AB; FRCPC; DiagRad. Associate, Temiskaming Hospital; Prof Rad & Otol, University of Toronto; Langs: Tamil; Hindi; (416)763-4331; Fax. (416)763-2875.

SHANKARDASS, Kanwal; 62 King St W, Dundas ON L9H 1T8; Makerere (Uganda)'72; Ac Staff, Hamilton Health Sciences Centre - McMaster Children's Hospital; Med Dir, Hamilton Health Sciences Centre - St Peter's Hospital; Court Staff, St Joseph's Healthcare - Charlton Campus; Med Dir, St Peter's at Chedoke Residence Long Term Care; Lecturer Family Med, McMaster University; Langs: Hindi; Punjabi; (905)627-3526; Fax. (905)628-9996.

SHANKS, David J; Jim Pattison Pavilion North, 3300-910 10th Ave W, Vancouver BC V5Z 1M9; McG'07; MDCM; FRCPC; IntMed. (604)875-4111 x69119

SHANKS, Gavin L; Providence CCC-St Mary's, PO Box 3600 Stn Main 340 Union St, Kingston ON K7L 5A2; Qns'66; FRCPC; PhysMed&Rehab (Chronic Pain). Staff RehabMed, Providence Care - St Mary's of the Lake Hospital Site; Prof Rehab Med, Queen's University; (613)549-2763; Fax. (613)544-4614; shanksg@providencecare.ca.

SHANKS, Miriam; University of Alberta Hosp, 2C2 WCM-8440 112 St NW, Edmonton AB T6G 2B7; Pavol Jozef (Slovakia)'96; FRCPC; IntMed (Echocardiography); Cardiol. Staff/Asst Prof, University of Alberta Hospital; Langs: Slovak; Czech; (780)407-3551; Fax. (780)407-6452.

SHANMUGAM, Ganesh; Children's Hosp Eastern Ont, 401 Smyth Rd, Ottawa ON K1H 8L1; Dr G R Medical University (India)'93; CardSurg (Cardiology). Staff, Children's Hospital of Eastern Ontario (CHEO); (613)738-3640; Fax. (613)738-4870.

SHANNON, David J; 4492 rue Sherbrooke O, Westmount QC H3Z 1E6; McG'73; FRCPC; IntMed. principale Médecin, McGill University Health Centre - Montreal General Campus; assoc Prof, McGill University; (514)935-7144; Fax. (514)935-1955; drjdshannon@hotmail.ca.

SHANNON, Janet L; Royal University Hosp, 103 Hospital Dr, Saskatoon SK S7N 0W8; Ott'88; FRCPC; Anes. Assoc Staff Anes, Royal University Hospital; Clin Assoc Prof Anes, University of Saskatchewan; Langs: French; (306)655-1183; Fax. (306)655-1279; janshannon@home.com.

SHANNON, Michael A; 453 Park St, Kitchener ON N2G 1N5; Tor'87; FRCSC; ObstGyn. Staff, Grand River Hospital - Kitchener/Waterloo Health Centre; (519)571-1200; Fax. (519)571-8050.

SHANNON, Michael E; Canadian Fdn Global Health, 605-170 Laurier Ave W, Ottawa ON K1P 5V5; Qns'78; Langs: French; (613)231-8555; Fax. (613)231-3970.

SHANNON, Patrick T; Mount Sinai Hosp, 600 University Ave, Toronto ON M5G 1X5; Tor'92; FRCPC; AnatPath; NeurPath. Staff, Mount Sinai Hospital; (416)586-4200

SHANNON, Robert; Medical Arts Bldg, 508-750 Spadina Cres E, Saskatoon SK S7K 3H3; Belfast (Ireland)'72; MB ChB; FRCSC; OrthSurg. (306)244-5561; Fax. (306)934-4877.

SHANNON, Scott E; 38 King St W, Hamilton ON L9H 1T7; Washington University (USA)'96; Langs: Bilingual(English/French); (905)628-5118

SHANNON, William R; Chemong Reg Med Centre, PO Box 330 765 Ward St, Bridgenorth ON K0L 1H0; Tor'94; MSc; CCFP; Staff, Peterborough Regional Health Centre - Hospital Drive; (705)292-0905; Fax. (705)292-8929.

SHAO, Richard H; Toronto East Gen & Orth Hosp, 825 Coxwell Ave, East York ON M4C 3E7; National (Taiwan)'87; FRCPC; IntMed; MedOncol. Staff Hematology Oncology Clinic, Toronto East General Hospital Inc; Langs: Mandarin; Taiwanese; (416)469-3325; Fax. (416)469-8221.

SHAPAN, Mustafa F; Brandon Reg Health Centre, 150 McTavish Ave E, Brandon MB R7A 2B3; Tripoli (Libya)'84; FRCPC; AnatPath. Staff, Brandon Regional Health Centre; (204)578-4000

SHAPERA, Shane M; 9N 971-585 University Ave, Toronto ON M5G 2N2; Tor'03; FRCPC; IntMed; Respir (Interstitial Lung Disease). Staff, Toronto General Hospital - UHN; (416)340-4174; Fax. (416)340-3254; shane.shapera@gmail.com.

SHAPERO, Gary A; 5-7725 Birchmount Rd, Markham ON L3R 9X3; Tor'88; DAA; CCFP; Staff, The Scarborough Hospital - Birchmount Campus; Staff, Markham Stouffville Hospital; Staff, Toronto General Hospital - UHN; Teach Staff Family & Commun Med, University of Toronto; (905)475-9700; Fax. (905)475-5913.

SHAPERO, Harvey G; Shapero Dermatology Clinic, 300-2065 Finch Ave W, Toronto ON M3N 2V7; Tor'67; FRCPC; Derm (Hyperhidrosis). Court Staff, Humber River Regional Hospital - Finch Avenue Site; Vis Staff, Sunnybrook Health Sciences Centre; Asst Prof, University of Toronto; (416)745-3344

SHAPERO, Jonathan; Oakdale Med Bldg, 300-2065 Finch Ave W, North York ON M3N 2V7; Qns'06; FRCPC; Derm. (416)745-3344; Fax. (416)745-3205.

SHAPERO, Stephen E; Bayview Med Centre, 2722 Bayview Ave, North York ON M2L 1B9; Tor'68; CCFP; Ac Staff, North York General Hospital; (416)730-1212; Fax. (416)730-1216.

SHAPERO, Theodore F; SGH Medical Mall, 214-3030 Lawrence Ave E, Scarborough ON M1P 2T7; Tor'69; FRCPC; IntMed; Gastroent. Assoc Staff, The Scarborough Hospital - General Campus; (416)438-5755; Fax. (416)438-3324.

SHAPIR KAHAN, Marcia H; Rosedale Med Centre, 501-600 Sherbourne St, Toronto ON M4X 1W4; Rio de Janeiro (Brazil)'81; FRCPC; Psy (Child & Adolescent Psychiatry). Langs: Hebrew; Portuguese; Spanish; (416)929-7389; Fax. (416)929-7390.

SHAPIRA, Stacey C; The Toronto GI Clinic, 450-5 Fairview Mall Dr, North York ON M2J 2Z1; Tor'00; FRCPC; IntMed; Gastroent. (416)322-7517; Fax. (416)489-8053.

SHAPIRO, A M James; College Plaza, 2000-8215 112 St NW, Edmonton AB T6G 2C8; Newcastle (England)'88; MB BS; PhD(Exp Surg); FRCSC; GenSurg (Hepatobiliary Surgery). Staff, University of Alberta Hospital; Prof Surg/Dir Clin Islet Transplant Prog/Prof Surg/Dir Clin Islet Transplant Prog, University of Alberta; Langs: English; French; (780)407-7971; Fax. (780)407-8259.

SHAPIRO, Adam J; MUHC-Montreal Children's Hosp, 2300 rue Tupper, Montreal QC H3H 1P3; McG'04; Staff, McGill University Health Centre - Montreal Children's Hospital; (514)412-4444

SHAPIRO, Colin M; Univ Hlth Network-Toronto Western Hosp, MP7 421-399 Bathurst St, Toronto ON M5T 2S8; Witwatersrand (South Africa)'77; PhD; MRCPsy; FRCPC; Psy (Neurology & Psychiatry). Ac Staff Sleep & Alertness Clinic, Toronto Western Hospital - University Health Network; Ac Staff, Toronto Rehabilitation Institute - University Centre; Pres, International Neuropsychiatry Association; Prog Dir, Youthdale Child & Adolescent Sleep Centre; Prof Psy/Dir Psy, University of Toronto; Langs: Afrikaans; (416)603-5273; Fax. (416)603-5292.

SHAPIRO, Gary; Health Canada, 10F-180 Queen St W, Toronto ON M5V 3L7; Tor'77; Med Officer of Hlth Occupational Med, Health Canada; (416)973-6193; Fax. (416)973-5885.

SHAPIRO, Heather M; Ctre for Fertility & Reproduct, 250 Dundas St W, Toronto ON M5G 1Z5; McM'83; FRCSC; ObstGyn (Reproductive Endocrinology). Staff, Mount Sinai Hospital; Staff, Toronto General Hospital - UHN; Asst Prof ObstGyn, University of Toronto; (416)586-4994; Fax. (416)586-8398; rbu@mtsinai.on.ca.

SHAPIRO, Howard S; Toronto Public Health, 2340 Dundas St W, Toronto ON M6P 4A9; Qns'95; FRCPC; CommunMed. (416)338-8562; Fax. (416)633-3418.

SHAPIRO, Jennifer S; Temmy Latner Ctre Pallative Ca, 4F-60 Murray St Box 13, Toronto ON M5T 3L9; McM'04; CCFP; Staff, The Scarborough Hospital - General Campus; (416)586-4800; Fax. (416)686-4804.

SHAPIRO, Jerry; Skin Care Centre, 835 10th Ave W, Vancouver BC V5Z 4E8; McG'81; DAB; FRCPC; Derm. Consultant, Ridge Meadows Hospital & Health Care Centre; Consultant, Vancouver General Hospital - Centennial Pavillion; Dir, UBC Hair Clinic Research Treatment & Transplant Centre; Dir Med & Derm/Clin Prof, University of British Columbia; (604)875-5151; Fax. (604)873-9919; jerry.shapiro@vch.ca.

SHAPIRO, Joanna L; Rexdale Med Centre, 2-123 Rexdale Blvd, Etobicoke ON M9W 1P1; Tor'96; CCFP; Langs: Hebrew; French; (416)743-5853; Fax. (416)743-1358.

SHAPIRO, Jodi L; Ontario Power Generation Bldg, 3095-700 University Ave, Toronto ON M5G 1Z5; Tor'95; FRCSC; ObstGyn. Staff, Mount Sinai Hospital; Asst Prof, University of Toronto; (416)586-8817; Fax. (416)586-4746.

SHAPIRO, Joel A; Medical Clinic Person-Ctred Ps, 403-265 Yorkland Blvd, North York ON M2J 1S5; Wes'07; FRCPC; Psy. Staff, London Health Sciences Centre - Victoria Campus; Staff, The Medical Clinic for Person-Centred Psychotherapy; (416)229-2399; Fax. (416)229-9771.

SHAPIRO, Lori E; Thornhill Dermatology Centre, 302-1137 Centre St, Thornhill ON L4J 3M6; Man'88; FRCPC; IntMed (Clinical Pharmacology); Derm. Staff Dermatology Clinic, Sunnybrook Health Sciences Centre; Physician, Sunnybrook Drug Safety Clinic; (905)695-2020; Fax. (905)695-3800; reception@thornhillderm.com.

SHAPIRO, Marla; 105-3292 Bayview Ave, North York ON M2M 4J5; McG'79; MHSc; FRCPC; CommunMed (Women's Health);CCFP; FCFP; Public Health & Preventive Med. Staff, Toronto General Hospital - UHN; Ac Staff, Toronto Western Hospital - University Health Network; Court Staff, Mount Sinai Hospital; Physician Health & Med Contributor/Host Dr Marla & Friends, Canada AM Bell Media CTV; Assoc Prof Family & Commun Med, University of Toronto; Langs: English; French; (416)445-4067; Fax. (416)445-0206.

SHAPIRO, Michelle J; McMaster University, 1280 Main St W, Hamilton ON L8S 4K1; Cal'02; FRCPC; Neur. (905)521-2100

SHAPIRO, R Jean; Gordon & Leslie Diamond HCC, 5F-2775 Laurel St, Vancouver BC V5Z 1M9; McG'77; ABIM; MDCM; FRCPC; IntMed (Nephrology). Ac Staff/Med Dir Renal Transplantation, Vancouver General Hospital - Centennial Pavillion; Clinical Asst Prof, University of British Columbia; Langs: English; French; (604)875-5950; Fax. (604)875-5952; fjshapiro@interchange.ubc.ca.

SHAPIRO, Robert S; 3010-6900 boul Decarie, Cote Saint-Luc QC H3X 2T8; McG'69; AB; FACS; FRCSC; Otol (Head & Neck Surgery). Staff Otol, McGill University Health Centre - Montreal General Campus; assoc Prof, McGill University; Langs: English; French; (514)345-8852

SHAPIRO, Sergey; 606-1 St Clair Ave E, Toronto ON M4T 2V7; Lvov (Ukraine)'72; AB; FRCPC; Psy. Staff, Women's College Hospital; Langs: Russian; Ukrainian; (416)927-0386 x7355; Fax. (416)927-0540.

SHAPIRO, Solomon M; 1038-790 Bay St Box 51, Toronto ON M5G 1N8; Ott'83; FRCPC; Psy (Child & Adolescent Psychiatry). Staff Child, Centre for Addiction & Mental Health (CAMH) - College Street Site; Head Gender & Sexual Orientation Service, The Hincks-Dellcrest Centre - Toronto; Staff, Mount Sinai Hospital; Asst Prof, University of Toronto; Langs: French; (416)323-9849; Fax. (416)979-4685; solomon_shapiro@camh.net.

SHAPIRO, Stanley A; Applegrove Med Clinic, 135 Applegrove St, Sudbury ON P3C 1N2; Tor'81; Langs: Hebrew; French; (705)669-3111; Fax. (705)669-0499.

SHAPIRO, Thomas E; The Westend Family Care Clinic, 80 Michael Cowpland Dr, Kanata ON K2M 1P6; McG'85; Langs: French; (613)596-3321; Fax. (613)599-3366.

SHAPIRO, Yakov; Cedars Prof Park, 2931 66 St NW, Edmonton AB T6K 4C1; Alb'88; BSc(Hon); FRCPC; Psy (Integrated Psychotherapy). Staff, Covenant Health - Grey Nuns Community Hospital; Med Examiner Independent, IMA Inc; Assoc Prof Psy, University of Alberta; Langs: Russian; (780)490-1014; Fax. (780)462-1155.

SHARABYANI, Feryal; Hopital Juif de Readaptation, 3205 Place Alton Goldbloom, Vaudreuil-Dorion QC J7V 1R2; Mon'96; CCFP; Staff, Jewish Rehabilitation Hospital; Langs: Bilingual(French/English); (450)688-9550; Fax. (450)628-0217.

SHARAD, Sunil; Auburn Centre, 901-570 University Ave E, Waterloo ON N2K 4P2; Mem'87; FRCPC; IntMed (Cardiology). Staff, Grand River Hospital - Kitchener/Waterloo Health Centre; Staff, St Mary's General Hospital; Langs: Punjabi; (519)578-4442; Fax. (519)578-5578.

SHARAF EL-DEAN, Mouhammad Z; Dr G B Cross Mem Hosp, 67 Manitoba Dr, Clarenville NL A5A 1K3; Aleppo (Syria)'95; Staff, The Dr G B Cross Memorial Hospital; (709)466-3411

SHARAFADDINZADEH, Naser; Eastwood Med Clinic, 7919 118 Ave NW, Edmonton AB T5B 0R5; (780)756-3666; Fax. (780)756-2598.

SHARAN, Richa; Tri-Cities Mental Health, 1-2232 Elgin Ave, Port Coquitlam BC V3C 2B2; UBC'84; FRCPC; Psy. Staff, Sherbrooke Centre; (604)777-8400; Fax. (604)777-8411.

SHARAN, Sapna; St Joseph's Health Care, PO Box 5777 Stn B 268 Grosvenor St, London ON N6A 4V2; Jawaharlal Institute (India)'92; Staff, London Health Sciences Centre - South Street; Staff Ivey Eye Institute, St Joseph's Hospital - St Joseph's Health Care; Langs: Hindi; (519)685-8795; Fax. (519)646-6094.

SHARAN, Sumit; Sudbury Reg Hosp-Laurentian, 41 Ramsey Lake Rd, Sudbury ON P3E 5J1; Ott'02; FRCPC; Anes. Staff, Health Sciences North-Laurentian Site; Langs: Hindi; (705)523-7100

SHARDA, Priti; Riverwood Med Clinic, 1295 Pembina Hwy, Winnipeg MB R3T 2B3; (Other Foreign)'08; CCFP.

SHARDA, Rajeshvar K; Medical Arts Bldg, 302-1 Young St, Hamilton ON L8N 1T8; Qns'05; FRCSC; Ophth. Langs: Hindi; Punjabi; Urdu; (905)527-5559; Fax. (905)527-3883.

SHAREEF, Mohammad; Cure & Care Med Centre, C-2024 Albert St, Regina SK S4T 2T7; Karachi (Pakistan)'83; MB BS; Physician, Albert Park Family Medical Centres; (306)584-3833; Fax. (306)585-3833.

SHAREEF, Raghad; Postmaster Med Clinic, 2540 Postmaster Dr, Oakville ON L6M 0N2; University of Al-Mustansiriyah (Iraq)'02; CCFP; Langs: Arabic; (905)844-1700; Fax. (905)844-1705.

SHAREK, Christine E; Baker Clinic, 100-10405 Jasper Ave NW, Edmonton AB T5J 3N4; Alb'78; CCFP; (780)944-9582; Fax. (780)944-9534.

SHARGALL, Yaron; St Joseph's Healthcare, T 2105J-50 Charlton Ave E, Hamilton ON L8N 4A6; Hebrew (Israel)'92; FAMCCP; FRCSC; ThorSurg (Thoracic Oncology). Div Head, St Joseph's Healthcare - Charlton Campus; Court Staff, Toronto General Hospital - UHN; Staff, Sunnybrook Health Sciences Centre; Court Staff, Niagara Health System - Greater Niagara General Site; Assoc Prof, University of Toronto; Assoc Prof, McMaster University; Langs: Hebrew; (905)522-1155; Fax. (905)540-6512.

SHARIATI, Majid; Hamiota District Health Centre, 177 Birch Ave, Hamiota MB R0M 0T0; (Other Foreign)'97; Staff, Hamiota District Health Centre; (204)764-2412; Fax. (204)764-2049; mshariati@arha.ca.

SHARIEFF, Saleem; Grand River Hosp-K W Site, PO Box 9056 Stn C 835 King St W, Kitchener ON N2G 1G3; Karachi (Pakistan)'92; FRCPC; IntMed (Cardiology). Staff, Grand River Hospital - Kitchener/Waterloo Health Centre; Clinical Asst Prof, Hamilton Health Sciences Centre - McMaster Children's Hospital; (519)585-2145; Fax. (519)579-2294.

SHARIEFF, Waseem; Hamilton HS-Juravinski Cancer, 699 Concession St, Hamilton ON L8V 5C2; Karachi (Pakistan)'91; FRCPC; RadOncol. Staff, Hamilton Health Sciences Centre - Juravinski Cancer Centre; Staff, McMaster University; (905)387-9495

SHARIF, Anoosh; Markham Stouffville Hosp, PO Box 1800 Stn Main 381 Church St, Markham ON L3P 7P3; Wes'97; FRCPC; DiagRad; NuclearMed. Staff, Markham Stouffville Hospital; (905)472-7373

SHARIF, Ismail A A; Western Mem Reg Hosp, PO Box 2005 Stn Main 1 Brookfield Ave, Corner Brook NL A2H 6J7; (Jordan)'04; IntMed. Staff, Western Memorial Regional Hospital; (709)637-5000

SHARIF, Jibran; South Health Campus, 4448 Front St SE, Calgary AB T3M 1M4; (Other Foreign)'08; CCFP; CCFP(E.M.); Staff, South Health Campus; (403)956-1111

SHARIF, Manoutch N; St Boniface Clinic, 343 Tache Ave, Winnipeg MB R2H 2A5; Teheran (Iran)'60; LRCP; MRCS(Eng); FRCS; FRCSC; OrthSurg. Staff, St Boniface General Hospital; Staff, Victoria General Hospital; Asst Prof Surg, University of Manitoba; (204)925-9572; Fax. (204)233-4568.

SHARIF, Mohammad S; Surrey Med Bdlg, 300-9656 King George Blvd, Surrey BC V3T 2V5; Punjab (Pakistan)'62; MB BS; MSc; DABS; FACS; FRCSC; GenSurg; VascSurg. Ac Staff, Surrey Memorial Hospital; Langs: Punjabi; Urdu; (604)588-1144; Fax. (604)588-1144.

SHARIF, Nadder; London HSC-Victoria Hosp, PO Box 5010 Stn B 800 Commissioners Rd E, London ON N6A 5W9; Tor'09; CCFP; CCFP(E.M.); Staff, London Health Sciences Centre - Victoria Campus; (519)685-8500

SHARIF, Omar; 300-9656 King George Hwy, Surrey BC V3T 2V5; Sint Eustatius (Netherlands)'08; CCFP; (604)588-1144

SHARIFF, Aftab M; Ottawa Childrens Clinic, 402-1105 Carling Ave, Ottawa ON K1Y 4G5; Mysore (India)'96; FRCPC; Peds. Langs: Hindi; Kanarese; (613)728-5437; Fax. (613)728-8611.

SHARIFF, Fahrin B; 35-7700 Bathurst St, Thornhill ON L4J 7Y3; Tor'96; BSc; CCFP; (905)881-6510; Fax. (905)881-6513.

SHARIFF, Fariduddin K; Manitoba Clinic, 790 Sherbrook St, Winnipeg MB R3A 1M3; Dhaka (Bangladesh)'59; FRCSC; OrthSurg. Ac Staff, The Salvation Army Grace Hospital; (204)788-5762; Fax. (204)783-7163.

SHARIFF, Riaz; North Ajax Med Centre, 475 Westney Rd N, Ajax ON L1T 3H4; Tor'81; Langs: Persian; Swahili; Urdu; (905)427-7767; Fax. (905)427-4339.

SHARIFF, Salima N; Surrey Med Arts Bldg, 102-13798 94A Ave, Surrey BC V3V 1N1; Alb'96; FRCPC; IntMed; Cardiol. (604)582-6500; Fax. (604)588-3122.

SHARIFF, Shiraz B K; Dr Shariff Med Prof Centre, 32-147 Clarence St, Brampton ON L6W 1T2; Nottingham (England)'84; Staff, William Osler Health System - Brampton Civic Hospital; Langs: Gujarati; Hindi; Kacchi; (905)454-0000; Fax. (905)454-4941.

SHARIFF, Tahara J T; Medical Clinic, 102-2752 Allwood St, Abbotsford BC V2T 3R7; Trinity (Ireland)'01; (604)850-6893

SHARIFI, Nader; Valley Oak Med Clinic, 102-10663 King George Blvd, Surrey BC V3T 2X8; Dal'93; BSc; CCFP; Staff, Forensic Psychiatric Hospital; Langs: Arabic; (904)581-4181; Fax. (604)582-8741; nsharifi@forensic.bc.ca.

SHARIFI, Shannon E; North Bay Reg Health Centre, 50 College Dr, North Bay ON P1B 8G5; McM'07; FRCPC; Anes.

SHARIR, Sharon; 404-960 Lawrence Ave W, North York ON M6A 3B5; Tor'95; BSc; MPH; MD; FRCSC; Urol (Uro Oncology). Staff, Humber River Regional Hospital - Church Street Site; Asst Prof, University of Toronto; Langs: Hebrew; (416)256-2737; Fax. (416)256-9098.

SHARKAWY, Abdul Q A; Univ Hlth Network-Toronto Western Hosp, 418 8FEW-399 Bathurst St, Toronto ON M5T 2S8; Alb'98; FRCPC; IntMed (AIDS/HIV); InfectDis. Staff Med, Toronto Western Hospital - University Health Network; Asst Prof Med, University of Toronto; Langs: Arabic; French; (416)603-5800; Fax. (416)603-6495; abdu.sharkawy@uhn.on.ca.

SHARKEY, J Brian; Southwood Med Centre, 3F-2385 Pembina Hwy, Winnipeg MB R3T 2H4; Man'76; CCFP; FCFP; Staff, Victoria General Hospital; (204)261-6300; Fax. (204)261-1390.

SHARKEY, Paul J; 304-749 King St W, Kitchener ON N2G 1E4; Wes'79; FACS; FRCSC; GenSurg (Thoracic Surgery). Staff, Grand River Hospital - Kitchener/Waterloo Health Centre; Staff, St Mary's General Hospital; Asst Prof Surg, McMaster University; Aj Prof Surg, University of Western Ontario; (519)742-7424; Fax. (519)742-9920.

SHARKEY, Rowan D; St Boniface Gen Hosp, M4-409 Tache Ave, Winnipeg MB R2H 2A6; Man'06; FRCPC; Psy. Staff, St Boniface General Hospital; (204)233-8563

SHARKEY, Skye; Bowmont Med Clinic, 6535 Bowness Road NW, Calgary AB T3B 0E8; Man'09; CCFP; (403)247-9797; Fax. (403)247-0014.

SHARKIA, Mohamad; IWK Health Centre, 5850-5980 University Ave, Halifax NS B3K 6R8; Hebrew University (Israel)'95; Staff, IWK Health Centre; (902)470-8888

SHARMA, Ajay; Children's Hosp of Western Ont, B1 170-800 Commissioners Rd E, London ON N6A 5W9; Punjabi (India)'90; FRCPC; Peds. Staff, London Health Sciences Centre - Victoria Campus; Langs: Hindi; Punjabi; (519)685-8379

SHARMA, Amar D; Oak Park Med Clinic, 1-2530 Sixth Line, Oakville ON L6H 6W5; Tor'88; Langs: Punjabi; Hindi; (905)257-1006; Fax. (905)257-0661.

SHARMA, Anil B; 2559 Innes Rd, Gloucester ON K1B 3K1; Ott'79; CCFP; Ac Staff, The Ottawa Hospital - Riverside Campus; (613)824-1666

SHARMA, Anil R; Providence HC-St Paul's Hosp, 1081 Burrard St, Vancouver BC V6Z 1Y6; Sask'07; Staff ENT Clinic, Providence Health Care - St Paul's Hospital; (604)682-2344

SHARMA, Anu K; Travel Med & Vaccination Ctre, 314-1030 Georgia St W, Vancouver BC V6E 2Y3; Ott'91; Langs: Punjabi; (604)681-5656

SHARMA, Anuja; Northumberland Hills Hosp, 1000 DePalma Dr, Cobourg ON K9A 5W6; Gandhi (India)'91; Staff, Northumberland Hills Hospital; (905)372-6811

SHARMA, Arunabh B; Oshawa Clinic, 117 King St E, Oshawa ON L1H 1B9; McG'91; FRCPC; IntMed; Respir. Langs: French; (905)721-4908; Fax. (905)721-6657.

SHARMA, Arya M; Royal Alexandra Hosp, 406 CSC-10240 Kingsway Ave NW, Edmonton AB T5H 3V9; Berlin (Germany)'86; FRCP; Staff, Royal Alexandra Hospital; (780)735-5859; Fax. (780)735-5861.

SHARMA, Ashima; Children & Women's Health Ctre, F326-4500 Oak St, Vancouver BC V6H 3N1; Qns'10; CCFP; Staff, BC Women's Hospital & Health Centre; (604)875-2029

SHARMA, Ashok; Grand River Hosp-Kitchener, PO Box 9056 Stn C 835 King St W, Kitchener ON N2G 1G3; Jaipur (India)'73; FACEP; MCFP(EM); Staff, Grand River Hospital - Kitchener/Waterloo Health Centre; Asst Prof Health Sciences, McMaster University; Langs: Hindi; (519)749-4300 x2507; Fax. (519)749-4293; ashok.sharma@grhosp.ca.

SHARMA, Ashu T; Family Hlth Med Centre, 11-10035 Hurontario St, Brampton ON L6Z 0E6; Ott'89; (905)453-2441; Fax. (905)453-4624.

SHARMA, Atul K; CUSM-Montreal Children's Hosp, 2300 rue Tupper, Montreal QC H3H 1P3; Dal'85; FRCPC; Peds; Nephrol. Staff, McGill University Health Centre - Montreal Children's Hospital; (514)412-4400

SHARMA, Bal Krishan; Bluewater Health-Norman Site, 89 Norman St, Sarnia ON N7T 6S3; Guru Nanak Dev University (India)'89; CCFP; Staff, Bluewater Health - Norman Site; Langs: Hindi; Punjabi; (519)464-4400

SHARMA, Kalpana S; PG Medical Education Office, 92 College St, Toronto ON M5G 1L4; Tor'07; ObstGyn. (647)828-2030

SHARMA, Kamal; Univ of Ottawa Heart Institute, 40 Ruskin St, Ottawa ON K1Y 4W7; Dal'03; FRCPC; IntMed; Cardiol. Staff, University of Ottawa Heart Institute; Langs: Hindi; Nepali; French; (613)761-1934; k_sharma@hotmail.com.

SHARMA, Kawal J; 311-200 Gerrard St E, Toronto ON M5A 2E6; Vikram (India)'61; MB BS; MS(ObstGyn); FRCSC; ObstGyn. Staff, St Joseph's Health Centre; Langs: Hindi; Punjabi; Urdu; (416)969-4000

SHARMA, Krishna B; Carling Respiratory Services, 601-1081 Carling Ave, Ottawa ON K1Y 4G2; Qns'98; FRCPC; IntMed; Respir. Staff, The Ottawa Hospital - Civic Campus; (613)729-8262; Fax. (613)729-7870.

SHARMA, Kristina S; Univ Hosp of British Columbia, 1475 Edmonton St, Prince George BC V2M 1S2; Qns'98; FRCPC; DiagRad. Staff, University Hospital of Northern British Columbia; Staff, Vancouver General Hospital - Centennial Pavillion; (250)565-2728

SHARMA, Leneela; Royal Alexandra Hosp, 10240 Kingsway NW, Edmonton AB T5H 3V9; Sask'95; CCFP; CCFP(E.M.); Staff, Royal Alexandra Hospital; (780)964-1568; Fax. (780)735-4916.

SHARMA, Maheshwar D; Alexandra Hosp, 29 Noxon St, Ingersoll ON N5C 1B8; Punjab (India)'65; MB BS; MRCP; MRCS; FRCPC; IntMed. Staff, Alexandra Hospital; Langs: Hindi; Punjabi; Urdu; (519)485-1700; Fax. (519)485-9606.

SHARMA, Malika; Univ Hlth Network-Toronto Gen, 13E 220-200 Elizabeth St, Toronto ON M5G 2C4; McM'07; FRCPC; IntMed. Staff, Toronto General Hospital - UHN; Langs: Hindi; Punjabi; (416)340-3111

SHARMA, Manas; London HSC-University Hosp, PO Box 5339 Stn B 339 Windermere Rd, London ON N6A 5A5; Gauhati University (India)'96; Staff Neuroradiology, London Health Sciences Centre - University Hospital; Langs: Hindi; Punjabi; (519)663-3203; Fax. (519)663-8803.

SHARMA, Manisha; The Credit Valley Hosp, 2200 Eglinton Ave W, Mississauga ON L5M 2N1; Qns'07; CCFP; Staff, The Credit Valley Hospital; (905)813-1100; Fax. (905)813-4024.

SHARMA, Manisha; Oshawa Clinic, 117 King St E, Oshawa ON L1H 1B9; University of Lucknow (Other Foreign)'92; CCFP; (905)721-4974

SHARMA, Meena P; Univ of Ottawa Health Services, N207-801 King Edward Ave, Ottawa ON K1N 6N5; Bombay (India)'84; Langs: Hindi; Marathi; (613)564-3950; Fax. (613)564-0046.

SHARMA, Monika; Strathroy Middlesex Gen Hosp, 395 Carrie St, Strathroy ON N7G 3J4; Punjab (India)'90; CCFP; Staff, Strathroy Middlesex General Hospital - Middlesex Hospital Alliance; Langs: Hindi; (519)245-5295

SHARMA, Mukul; The Ottawa Hosp-Civic Campus, 2182 C2-1053 Carling Ave, Ottawa ON K1Y 4E9; Dal'86; FRCPC; Neur (Headache). Staff Neurosciences Clinic, The Ottawa Hospital - Civic Campus; Teach Staff Neurol, University of Ottawa; (613)737-8798; Fax. (613)761-5380.

SHARMA, Nakul C; Foothills Med Centre, 8F-1403 29 St NW, Calgary AB T2N 2T9; Sask'05; FRCPC; IntMed; Cardiol. Staff Libin Heart Institute, Foothills Medical Centre; Staff, University of Alberta Hospital; (403)918-0601; Fax. (403)775-4456; ncsharma@ualberta.ca.

SHARMA, Nawal K; 207 2nd Ave N, Saskatoon SK S7K 3P2; Rajasthan (India)'71; MB BS; MRC(UK); ABIM; FACP; FRCPC; IntMed. Clin Chief Dept of Med, Saskatoon City Hospital; Staff, St Paul's Hospital (Grey Nuns) of Saskatoon; Physician, Midtown Medical Centre; Clin Prof Med, University of Saskatchewan; (306)664-8833; Fax. (306)653-3166.

SHARMA, Niti; 101-274 Hurst Dr, Barrie ON L4N 0Z3; Indira Gandhi (India)'94; CCFP; Langs: Hindi; (705)726-6059

SHARMA, Om Prakash; The Hosp for Sick Children, 555 University Ave, Toronto ON M5G 1X8; Nagpur University (India)'90; FRCSC; OrthSurg. Staff, The Hospital For Sick Children; Langs: Urdu; Punjabi; (416)586-4800

SHARMA, Pankaj; Fraser Heights Med Clinic, 106-15966 108 Ave, Surrey BC V4N 5V6; Delhi (India)'89; MB BS; CCFP; FCFP; Langs: Hindi; Punjabi; Urdu; (604)582-8820; Fax. (604)582-2103.

SHARMA, Poonam; North Woodlands Med Centre, 202-40 Shellington Place, Brantford ON N3S 0C5; Punjab (India)'81; MB BS; FRCPC; Psy. Langs: Punjabi; Hindi; (519)751-4317; Fax. (519)751-4321.

SHARMA, Pratibhasri A; Create Fertility Centre, 1100-790 Bay St, Toronto ON M5G 1N8; New Jersey (USA)'01; MD; ABOG; Staff, Sunnybrook Health Sciences Centre; Staff, Women's College Hospital; Physician, Create Fertility Centre; Asst Prof ObstGyn, University of Toronto; Langs: Telugu; (416)323-7727; Fax. (416)323-7334.

SHARMA, Rajat; Queen Elizabeth II HSC-Halifax, 2501B-1796 Summer St, Halifax NS B3H 3A7; Sambalpur (Other Foreign)'91; MB BS; Staff, Queen Elizabeth II Health Sciences Centre - Halifax Infirmary Site; (902)473-4474

SHARMA, Rajeev D; Peter Lougheed Centre, 3500 26 Ave NE, Calgary AB T1Y 6J4; (Australia)'00; CCFP; Staff, Peter Lougheed Centre; (403)943-5461; Fax. (403)943-5438.

SHARMA, Rajrishi; Univ of Western Ontario, M106-1151 Richmond St, London ON N6A 5C1; Alb'06; FRCSC; OrthSurg. Langs: Hindi.

SHARMA, Ramesh K; 33 Centre, 101-3401 33 St, Vernon BC V1T 7X7; London (England)'81; MRC; DRCOG; (250)549-1189; Fax. (250)549-4559.

SHARMA, Rameshwar; Grey Nuns Community Hosp, 1100 Youville Drive West NW, Edmonton AB T6L 5X8; Lucknow (India)'66; MB BS; MRCS(Eng); LRCP(Lond); DA(Ire.); Staff Psy, Covenant Health - Grey Nuns Community Hospital; (780)438-0228

SHARMA, Sandeep K; Chase Med Clinic, 826 Thompson Ave Box 410, Chase BC V0E 1M0; '09; CCFP; (250)679-1420; Fax. (250)679-8815.

SHARMA, Sandeep K; Oakville Med Arts Bldg, 10-358 Reynolds St, Oakville ON L6J 3L9; Wes'93; FRCSC; ObstGyn. Staff ObstGyn, Halton Healthcare Services Corporation - Oakville Site; (905)849-8855; Fax. (905)849-6683.

SHARMA, Sandhya K; 6951 Westminster Hwy, Richmond BC V7C 1C6; Suva (Fiji)'78; (604)273-2266

SHARMA, Sangita; Joseph Brant Mem Hosp, 1230 North Shore Blvd E, Burlington ON L7S 1W7; Sask'00; FRCPC; EmergMed. Staff, Joseph Brant Memorial Hospital; Langs: Hindi; (905)632-3730

SHARMA, Sanjay K; 2933 66 St NW, Edmonton AB T6K 4C1; Alb'94; FRCPC; IntMed; Cardiol. Staff, University of Alberta Hospital; Staff, Covenant Health - Grey Nuns Community Hospital; (780)461-6408; Fax. (780)461-6130.

SHARMA, Sanjay; Hotel-Dieu Hosp, 224B-166 Brock St, Kingston ON K7L 5G2; Dal'91; MSc(Epidemiol); MBA; FRCSC; Ophth (Diabetic Retinopathy). Att Staff, Hotel-Dieu Hospital; Att Staff, Kingston General Hospital; Assoc Prof Dept of Ophth & Epidemiol, Queen's University; (613)544-3400 x2227; Fax. (613)544-5707.

SHARMA, Sanjeev K; Red Deer Med Centre, 202-3947 50A Ave, Red Deer AB T4N 6V7; Punjab (India)'98; MB BS; Staff, Red Deer Regional Hospital Centre; (403)341-4303; Fax. (403)341-4322.

SHARMA, Sanjeev P; Carling-Broadview Med Bldg, 202-770 Broadview Ave, Ottawa ON K2A 3Z3; McG'02; FRCSC; OrthSurg. Langs: Bilingual(French/English); (613)728-9872; Fax. (613)728-8465.

SHARMA, Sanjeev; William Osler HC-Brampton, 2100 Bovaird Dr E, Brampton ON L6R 3J7; McM'97; CCFP; Staff, William Osler Health System - Brampton Civic Hospital; (905)494-2120

SHARMA, Saroo; Hamilton HS-Hamilton Gen Hosp, 237 Barton St E, Hamilton ON L8L 2X2; University of Leicester (Other Foreign)'03; FRCPC; Anes. Staff, Hamilton Health Sciences Centre - Hamilton General Hospital; (905)527-4322

SHARMA, Satyendra; St Boniface Gen Hosp, BG034-409 Tache Ave, Winnipeg MB R2H 2A6; Simla (India)'82; MB BS; DABIM; FRCPC; IntMed; Critical Care Medicine; Respir. Coord Resp/Dir, St Boniface General Hospital; Assoc Prof Respiology/Prog Dir, University of Manitoba; (204)233-8563

SHARMA, Satyendra; Kensington Clinic, 325-340 College St, Toronto ON M5T 3A9; Lucknow (India)'67; MS(OrthSurg); DABPMR; FAB(ElectroDiagMed); MB BS; FRCPC; PhysMed&Rehab (Soft Tissue Injuries). Consultant, Sunnybrook Health Sciences Centre; Staff, Toronto Western Hospital - University Health Network; Med Dir Elke Adler Spasticity Mgmt Clinic/Consultant, Baycrest Centre for Geriatric Care; Asst Prof, University of Toronto; Langs: Hindi; (416)603-2725; Fax. (416)603-2730.

SHARMA, Shakti; Dr Sharma Med Prof Corp, 201-7117 Bathurst St, Thornhill ON L4J 2J6; Punjabi (India)'86; FRCPC; Derm (Skin Cancer). Langs: Hindi; Telugu; (905)763-2526; Fax. (905)763-8595.

SHARMA, Shikhi; West End Med Centre, 510 Prince St, Truro NS B2N 1G1; Aligarth Muslim (India)'81; MB BS; CCFP; Staff, Colchester East Hants Health Centre; Langs: Hindi; Urdu; (902)893-7422; Fax. (902)893-1026.

SHARMA, Shiv R; 204-2772 Danforth Ave, Toronto ON M4C 1L7; Agra (India)'62; AB; CCFP; Langs: Hindi; Punjabi; Swahili; Urdu; (416)690-9280; Fax. (416)690-3927.

SHARMA, Shivani; Middlefield Med Centre, 1-8 Shadlock St, Markham ON L3S 3K9; Nagpur (India)'76; Staff, The Scarborough Hospital - Birchmount Campus; Langs: Hindi; Gujarati; Punjabi; (905)471-8980; Fax. (905)471-9352.

SHARMA, Shreekant; North Woodlands Med Centre, 202-40 Shellington Place, Brantford ON N3S 0C5; Punjab (India)'83; MB BS; FRCPC; Psy (Adult General Psychiatry). Langs: Hindi; Punjabi; Urdu; (519)751-4317; Fax. (519)751-4321.

SHARMA, Subhash C; Four Counties Health Services, 1824 Concesssion Rd RR 3, Newbury ON N0L 1Z0; Leicester (England)'82; DRCOG; DCH; CCFP; FCFP; Staff, Four Counties Health Services - Middlesex Hospital Alliance; Aj Prof Family Med, University of Western Ontario; Langs: Hindi; (519)693-7058; Fax. (519)693-7143.

SHARMA, Sudheer; Edmonton Cardiology Consultant, 350-11010 101 St NW, Edmonton AB T5H 4B9; Alb'96; FRCPC; IntMed; Cardiol. (780)428-3246; Fax. (780)425-0487; sudheersharma@telus.net.

SHARMA, Susan M; Queen's Student Health, 146 Stuart St, Kingston ON K7L 3N6; Dal'95; CCFP; FCFP; (613)533-2506

SHARMA, Sushil K; Physicians Incorporated, 201-316 Willow St, Truro NS B2N 5A4; Aligarh Muslim (India)'81; MB BS; BSc; CCFP; Assoc Staff, Colchester East Hants Health Centre; Langs: Hindi; Punjabi; Urdu; (902)893-2255; Fax. (902)893-4869; sushilkumarsharma@hotmail.com.

SHARMA, Verinder; Regional Mental HC-London, PO Box 5532 Stn B 850 Highbury Ave, London ON N6A 4H1; Punjabi (India)'81; FRCPC; Psy (Mood Disorders). Staff, Regional Mental Health Care-St Joseph's Health Care; Langs: Punjabi; Hindi; (519)455-5110; Fax. (519)455-3011.

SHARMA, Vijay K; Miramichi Med Arts Centre, 13-679 King George Hwy, Miramichi NB E1V 1N9; Dal'87; DAB; FRCSC; Ophth. Langs: English; French; (506)627-1919; Fax. (506)627-1798.

SHARMA, Vijay; Rouge Valley HS-Centenary, 2867 Ellesmere Rd, Scarborough ON M1E 4B9; Lucknow (India)'82; FRCPC; Anes. Staff, Mackenzie Richmond Hill Hospital; Langs: Hindi; Punjabi; Urdu; (416)284-8131 x4054; Fax. (416)281-7453.

SHARMA, Vikas; Saskatoon Eye Surgeons, 704-201 1st Ave S, Saskatoon SK S7K 1J5; Rajasthan (India)'99; FRCSC; Ophth. (306)974-4497; Fax. (306)974-4498.

SHARMA, Vinod K; Belmont Med Centre, 203-535 Belmont Ave W, Kitchener ON N2M 5E9; Rajasthan (India)'78; ABIM; FACG; FRCPC; IntMed; Gastroent. Staff, Grand River Hospital - Freeport Site; Staff, St Mary's General Hospital; Langs: Hindi; (519)576-0204; Fax. (519)576-1237.

SHARMA AUCONE, Rachila; Family Care Med Clinic, 190-9040 Blundell Rd, Richmond BC V6Y 1K3; Maharshi Dayanand (India)'98; CCFP; (604)284-5285

SHARMAN, Asheer; The Credit Valley Hosp, 2200 Eglinton Ave W, Mississauga ON L5M 2N1; Ott'04; FRCPC; IntMed; Critical Care Medicine. Staff, The Credit Valley Hospital; (905)813-2200

SHARMAN, Madan G; Northgate Med Centre, 2711 Avonhurst Dr, Regina SK S4R 3J3; Glasgow (Scotland)'58; MB ChB; DTMH; Ac Staff, Pasqua Hospital; Ac Staff, Regina General Hospital; Ac Staff, Wascana Rehabilitation Centre; Northgate Medical Centre; Langs: Punjabi; Hindi; (306)543-4566; Fax. (306)543-4441.

SHARMAN, Peter E; 156 Currie Rd RR 1, Dutton ON N0L 1J0; Cape Town (South Africa)'81; MB ChB; CCFP; (519)762-0943; Fax. (519)762-0946.

SHARMAN, Suneel; Infinity Health Centre, 39 Lower Simcoe St, Toronto ON M5J 3A6; Man'03; CCFP; (416)504-0628; Fax. (416)504-2009.

SHAROBIM, Monica W; Harwood Med Centre, 320 Harwood Ave S, Ajax ON L1S 2J1; Academy Of Medical Sciences & Technology (Sudan)'07; CCFP; (905)231-1122

SHAROBIM, Nazar R; Harwood Med Centre, 2-320 Harwood Ave S, Ajax ON L1S 2J1; Khartoum (Sudan)'94; MB BS; CCFP; CCFP(E.M.); Staff, Halton Healthcare Services Corporation - Georgetown Hospital; Staff, Rouge Valley Health System - Ajax & Pickering Health Centre Site; Langs: Arabic; (905)231-1122; Fax. (905)231-1124.

SHARON, Raphael F; Meadowlark Prof Bldg, 270-8702 Meadowlark Rd NW, Edmonton AB T5R 5W5; (Netherlands)'00; Langs: Dutch; German; Hebrew; (780)944-1840; Fax. (780)423-3961.

SHARP, Daniel C; Daniel C Sharp Prof Corp, 503-123 March St, Sault Ste. Marie ON P6A 2Z5; Qns'80; DABOph; FRCSC; Ophth. Staff, Sault Area Hospital - Sault Ste Marie; (705)759-8744; Fax. (705)759-8821.

SHARP, Lorraine F; Superior Family Health Team, 48-44 Great Northern Rd, Sault Ste. Marie ON P6B 4Y5; McM'09; CCFP; (705)253-6599; Fax. (705)253-8759.

SHARP, Stephen A; Medical Associates, 200-4012 Hastings St, Burnaby BC V5C 2H9; Sask'95; CCFP; (604)299-2677; Fax. (604)298-6656.

SHARPE, James A; Univ Hlth Network-Toronto Western Hosp, W5 440-399 Bathurst St, Toronto ON M5T 2S8; Wes'66; FRCPC; Neur (Ophthalmology). Sr Scientist, Toronto Western Hospital - University Health Network; Prof Neurol, University of Toronto; (416)603-5660; Fax. (416)603-6222.

SHARPE, Jonathan; Summerside Med Centre, 475 Granville St N, Summerside PE C1N 3N9; CCFP; Staff, Prince County Hospital; (902)432-8181

SHARPE, Kimberley A; Lions Gate Hosp, 231 15th St E, North Vancouver BC V7L 2L7; Dal'00; FRCPC; ObstGyn. Staff, Lions Gate Hospital; (604)988-3131; Fax. (604)984-5838.

SHARPE, Michael D; London HSC-University Hosp, PO Box 5339 Stn B 339 Windermere Rd, London ON N6A 5A5; Wes'80; FRCPC; Anes (Critical Care Medicine). Staff Anes & Critical Care, London Health Sciences Centre - University Hospital; Assoc Prof Anes, University of Western Ontario; (519)663-3282; Fax. (519)663-3150; michael.sharpe@lhsc.on.ca.

SHARPE, Robert J; Royal Columbian Hosp, 330 Columbia St E, New Westminster BC V3L 3W7; Ott'00; FRCPC; Anes; Critical Care Medicine. Staff Intensive Care Unit, Royal Columbian Hospital; (604)520-4253

SHARPE, Sally A; The Four Villages Community, 3446 Dundas St W, Toronto ON M6S 2S1; Dal'83; (416)604-3362; Fax. (416)604-3365.

SHASHA, Faiz F A; Health Trush Med Centre, 300-871 Ottawa St, Windsor ON N8X 2C9; Baghdad (Iraq)'76; MB ChB; CCFP; Langs: Arabic; (519)977-7401; Fax. (519)977-6774.

SHASHA, Faris F; Bay d'Espoir Med Clinic, PO Box 369 4 Church St, St Albans NL A0H 2E0; CCFP; (709)538-3244; Fax. (709)538-3228.

SHASHA, Farkad F A; Lakeshore Cawthra Med Centre, 619 Lakeshore Rd E, Mississauga ON L5G 1H9; Baghdad (Iraq)'96; CCFP; (905)891-2424; Fax. (905)891-1501.

SHASTRY, Anil K; St Joseph's Health Care, PO Box 5777 Stn B 268 Grosvenor St, London ON N6A 4V2; Tor'04; FRCPC; NuclearMed; DiagRad. Staff, St Joseph's Hospital - St Joseph's Health Care; (519)685-8500

SHATSHAT, Souad M; Fenwick Med Centre, 207-5595 Fenwick St, Halifax NS B3H 4M2; Al-Arab (Saudi Arabia)'88; MB ChB; FRCPC; IntMed; Rheum. Assoc Prof, Dalhousie University; Langs: Arabic; (902)446-4010; Fax. (902)446-4012.

SHATSKY, Morley A; Radiology Cons of Winnipeg, 202-233 Kennedy St, Winnipeg MB R3C 3J5; Man'75; FRCPC; DiagRad. Ac Staff, Victoria General Hospital; Ac Staff, Ste Anne Hospital; Ac Staff, Bethesda Hospital Steinbach; mshatsky@sehealth.mb.ca.

SHATZ, Richard M; 202-5858 ch Cote-des-Neiges, Montreal QC H3S 1Z1; Sask'63; FACS; FACOG; FRCSC; ObstGyn. principale Médecin, Sir Mortimer B Davis Jewish General; assoc Prof, McGill University; (514)731-3281; Fax. (514)731-2616; richardshatz@sympatico.ca.

SHAUL, C Harvey; 410-340 College St, Toronto ON M5T 3A9; Tor'57; DMRD; FRCPC; DiagRad. (416)962-3202

SHAUL, Randi C; Univ Hlth Network-Princess M, M 700-610 University Ave, Toronto ON M5G 2M9; Tor'79; Clin Associate GynOncol, Princess Margaret Hospital - University Health Network; Langs: Hebrew; (416)946-2254; Fax. (416)946-2288; randi.shaul@uhn.on.ca.

SHAUL, Richard A; 1A-1152 Morningside Ave, Scarborough ON M1B 3A4; Tor'88; (416)284-2853; Fax. (416)284-4951.

SHAVER, Charles S; Appletree Med Group, 4-2150 Robertson Rd, Ottawa ON K2H 9S1; John Hopkins(MD) (USA)'70; FACP; FRCPC; IntMed. Ac Staff, Queensway Carleton Hospital; Langs: German; French; (613)482-0118; Fax. (613)680-6420.

SHAVER, James H; Royal Victoria Hosp, 201 Georgian Dr, Barrie ON L4M 6M2; Wes'83; CCFP; FCFP; Staff, Royal Victoria Regional Health Centre; Prof Family Med, McMaster University; (705)728-9802; Fax. (705)739-5637; shaverj@rvh.on.ca.

SHAVER, Laurie E; Painswick Med Clinic, 505 Yonge St, Barrie ON L4N 4E1; Wes'83; CCFP; Staff, Royal Victoria Regional Health Centre; (705)721-1689; Fax. (705)721-0724; james.h.shaver@sympatico.ca.

SHAVER, Steven W; B-340 11th St, Courtenay BC V9N 8H5; McM'95; FRCSC; Ophth. (250)334-4030; Fax. (250)338-8155.

SHAW, Anne E; 4F-10 George St, Hamilton ON L8P 1C8; Tor'87; Ac Staff, St Joseph's Healthcare - Charlton Campus; Court Staff, Hamilton Health Sciences Centre - McMaster University Medical Centre; (905)521-6919; Fax. (905)521-6918.

SHAW, Brian M; Dr Brian Shaw Med Prof Corp, 404-111 Main St W, North Bay ON P1B 2T6; McM'86; CCFP; FCFP; Lecturer, University of Ottawa; Asst Prof, Northern Ontario School of Medicine-Laurentian University; (705)476-7400; Fax. (705)476-2585.

SHAW, Cinthia F; 2-32904 Ventura Ave, Abbotsford BC V2S 6J3; Ott'90; CCFP; FCFP; (604)859-1211; Fax. (604)852-8466.

SHAW, Clifford A; Elgin Med Centre, 101-2255 Elgin Ave, Port Coquitlam BC V3C 2B4; UBC'83; Staff, Royal Columbian Hospital; (604)942-7292; Fax. (604)942-9698.

SHAW, Danielle R S; Halton HSC Corp-Oakville, 327 Reynolds St, Oakville ON L6J 3L7; Wes'99; FRCPC; AnatPath (General Pathology). Staff, Halton Healthcare Services Corporation - Oakville Site; (905)845-2571; Fax. (905)845-3376.

SHAW, David R; PO Box 489, Oliver BC V0H 1T0; Qns'73; CCFP; Staff, South Okanagan General Hospital; Court Staff, Penticton Regional Hospital; (250)498-3411; Fax. (250)498-0233; shawd@shaw.ca.

SHAW, Diane E; 2703 Lionel Cres SW, Calgary AB T3E 6B1; Alb'79; (403)246-7040; Fax. (403)246-5358.

SHAW, Dorothy; BC Women's Hosp & Health Ctre, B242-4500 Oak St, Vancouver BC V6H 3N1; Edinburgh (Scotland)'72; MB ChB; FRCSC; ObstGyn (Maternal Fetal Medicine). VP Medical Affairs, BC Women's Hospital & Health Centre; Sr Associate Dean Faculty Affairs/Clin Prof, University of British Columbia; (604)875-2809

SHAW, Elizabeth A; McMaster Family Practice, A-690 Main St W, Hamilton ON L8S 1A4; McM'81; CCFP; FCFP; Staff, Hamilton Health Sciences Centre - McMaster University Medical Centre; Teach Staff Med, McMaster University; (905)521-5016; Fax. (905)521-5010.

SHAW, Emily J; Woodlawn Med Clinic, 92 Main St, Dartmouth NS B2X 1R5; Dal'03; FRCPC; IntMed; Rheum. Staff, Queen Elizabeth II Health Sciences Centre - Victoria General Site; Staff, Nova Scotia Rehabilitation Centre; (902)434-1500

SHAW, Erin R; Bedford Basin Women's Hlth Cli, 208A-967 Bedford Hwy, Bedford NS B4A 1A9; Tor'10; CCFP; (902)444-8706; Fax. (902)444-8721.

SHAW, James C; Women's College Hosp, 76 Grenville St, Toronto ON M5S 1B2; Boston(MA) (USA)'78; FRCPC; Derm. Staff Derm, Women's College Hospital; (416)323-6400; Fax. (416)323-6236.

SHAW, James E; UWO Student Health Services, 11UCC-1151 Richmond St, London ON N6A 3K7; Ott'69; Staff, St Joseph's Hospital - St Joseph's Health Care; Staff Student Health Services, University of Western Ontario; (519)661-3030; Fax. (519)661-3380.

SHAW, Jennifer J; 410-125 13th St E, North Vancouver BC V7L 2L3; Sydney (Australia)'78; MB BS; (604)985-0812; Fax. (604)985-2779.

SHAW, Jinny J; Royal Ottawa Hlth Care Group, 1145 Carling Ave, Ottawa ON K1Z 7K4; Ott'00; CCFP; Staff Medical Services, Royal Ottawa Mental Health Centre - Royal Ottawa Health Care Group; Langs: French; (613)722-6521 x6331

SHAW, John F; Dr John F Shaw Med Prof Corp, 215-700 Tecumseh Rd E, Windsor ON N8X 4T2; London (England)'70; DObstRCOG; MRC; CCFP; FCFP; Ac Staff Dept of GP, Hôtel-Dieu Grace Hospital; (519)258-3200; Fax. (519)258-0245.

SHAW, John M; Royal University Hosp, 103 Hospital Dr, Saskatoon SK S7N 0W8; Staff, Royal University Hospital; (306)966-1848; Fax. (306)966-7988.

SHAW, Julia; Unite de Med Familiale, 500 boul de l'Hopital, Gatineau QC J8V 2P5; Sher'10; CCFP; (819)661-6171

SHAW, Karen; College of Phys & Surgs of SK, 500-321A 21st St E, Saskatoon SK S7K 0C1; Sask'83; BSc; Registrar, College of Physicians & Surgeons of Saskatchewan; Staff Family Med, Saskatoon Health Region Corporate Office; Clinical Asst Prof Family Med, University of Saskatchewan; (306)244-7355; Fax. (306)244-2600; shawk@shin.sk.ca.

SHAW, Kenneth S; MUHC-Montreal Children's Hosp, C814-2300 rue Tupper, Montreal QC H3H 1P3; McG'85; FRCSC; GenSurg; PedGenSurg. Staff, McGill University Health Centre - Montreal Children's Hospital; (514)412-4388; Fax. (514)412-4400.

SHAW, Kerrie A; Credit Valley Med Arts Centre, 302-2000 Credit Valley Rd, Mississauga ON L5M 4N4; Ott'09; CCFP; Langs: Bilingual(English/French); (905)813-3850; Fax. (905)813-3853.

SHAW, Kimberly A; Wilson Centre Fam Practice, 1-2185 Wilson Ave, Port Coquitlam BC V3C 6C1; Sask'86; CCFP; Staff, Royal Columbian Hospital; Physician, Primary Care Obstetrical Clinic; (604)942-7227; Fax. (604)942-7058.

SHAW, Laura K; Kelowna Gen Hosp, 2268 Pandosy St, Kelowna BC V1Y 1T2; UBC'04; CCFP; Staff, Kelowna General Hospital; (250)808-1464

SHAW, Lauren M; Whistler Health Care Centre, 201-4380 Lorimer Rd RR 4, Whistler BC V0N 1B4; Qns'79; CCFP; (604)932-3977; Fax. (604)932-3471.

SHAW, Lorne A W; Anaesthetic Services, 213-2186 Oak Bay Ave, Victoria BC V8R 1G3; UBC'75; FRCPC; Anes. Ac Staff, Victoria General Hospital; (250)595-7211; Fax. (250)595-7211.

SHAW, Lynne M; Westside Integrated Hlth Ctre, 130-180 Wilson St, Victoria BC V9A 7N6; Alb'80; (250)592-3122

SHAW, Marcus D; 214 Med Place, 9F-9909 102 St Box 27, Grande Prairie AB T8V 2V4; Ott'95; BSc; BMedSci; FRCSC; GenSurg (Laparoscopic Surgery). Clin Lecturer Surg, University of Alberta; (780)539-4545; Fax. (780)532-6743.

SHAW, Matthew F; Windsor Reg Hosp-Metropolitan, 1995 Lens Ave, Windsor ON N8W 1L9; Wes'06; CCFP; CCFP(E.M.); Staff, Windsor Regional Hospital - Metropolitan Site; Teach Staff, University of Western Ontario; (519)254-1661

SHAW, Nur Deniz; 246-515 Pender St W, Vancouver BC V6B 6H5; UBC'96; FRCPC; Psy (Trauma). (604)685-7722; Fax. (604)685-7752.

SHAW, Patricia A; Univ Hlth Network-Toronto Gen, E11 444-200 Elizabeth St, Toronto ON M5G 2C4; Tor'76; FRCPC; AnatPath. Staff Path, Toronto General Hospital - UHN; Assoc Prof, University of Toronto; (416)340-4673; patricia.shaw@uhn.ca.

SHAW, Paul S; Canmore Gen Hosp, 1100 Hospital Pl, Canmore AB T1W 1N2; Wes'80; FRCPC; DiagRad. Staff, Canmore General Hospital; (403)678-5600; Fax. (403)678-1276.

SHAW, Philip M; Abbotsford Reg Hosp & CC, 32900 Marshall Rd, Abbotsford BC V2S 0C2; Ott'90; CCFP; CCFP(E.M.); Physician, Abbotsford Regional Hospital & Cancer Centre; (604)851-4700

SHAW, Robert Y; Delta Hosp, 5800 Mountain View Blvd, Delta BC V4K 3V6; Albany(NY) (USA)'95; FRCPC; IntMed. Staff, Delta Hospital; (604)946-1121

SHAW, Sandra A; Victoria Gen Hosp, 2340 Pembina Hwy, Winnipeg MB R3T 2E8; Man'82; CCFP; FCFP; CCFP(E.M.); Staff, Victoria General Hospital; (204)269-3570

SHAW, Sarah N; Taddle Creek Family Hlth Team, 522-790 Bay St Box 58, Toronto ON M5G 1N8; McM'05; CCFP; (416)591-1222; Fax. (416)591-1227.

SHAW, Stuart J; Parry Sound Family Health Team, 57 James St, Parry Sound ON P2A 1T6; McG'90; BSc; MDCM; CCFP; FCFP; Staff, West Parry Sound Health Centre; (705)746-2181; Fax. (705)746-4753.

SHAW, Susan A; Royal University Hosp, 103 Hospital Dr, Saskatoon SK S7N 0W8; Sask'95; FRCPC; Anes (Critical Care Medicine). Staff, Royal University Hospital; Physician, Saskatoon Health Region; Asst Prof, University of Saskatchewan; (306)655-1183; Fax. (306)655-1279; susan.shaw@saskatoonhealthregion.ca.

SHAW, Tammy Y; St Joseph's Health Centre, 30 The Queensway, Toronto ON M6R 1B5; Qns'06; CCFP; IntMed. Staff, St Joseph's Health Centre; (416)530-6000

SHAW-STIFFEL, Thomas A W; The Ottawa Hosp-Gen Campus, LM 11-501 Smyth Rd Box 255, Ottawa ON K1H 8L6; McG'81; FACG; FRCPC; IntMed; Gastroent. Staff, The Ottawa Hospital - General Campus; Langs: French; Spanish; (613)737-8899 x79962; Fax. (613)737-8799.

SHAWESH, Malek H E; Baywood Med Centre, 505-95 Bayly St W, Ajax ON L1S 7K8; Al-Fateh (Libya)'00; FRCPC; IntMed; Gastroent. Staff, Rouge Valley Health System - Ajax & Pickering Health Centre Site; (905)683-1277; Fax. (905)683-1273.

SHAWESH, Salim M; Dr Everett Chalmers Reg Hosp, PO Box 9000 Stn A 700 Priestman St, Fredericton NB E3B 5N5; Al-Fateh (Libya)'99; Staff, Saint John Regional Hospital; Staff, The Moncton Hospital; Staff, Dr Everett Chalmers Regional Hospital; (506)452-5400

SHAWN, David H; 312-4002 Sheppard Ave E, Scarborough ON M1S 1S6; Tor'75; FRCPC; Peds (Developmental/Behavioural Pediatrics). Staff Child Development Clinic, North York General Hospital; (416)292-8226; Fax. (416)292-0655; theshawns@rogers.com.

SHAWUSH, Melad F R; The Landmark Med Centre, 1-4150 Albert St, Regina SK S4S 3R8; Tripoli (Libya)'86; MB ChB; LMCC; FRCPC; Neur (Multiple Sclerosis). Physician, The Landmark Medical Centre; Asst Prof, University of Saskatchewan; Langs: Arabic; (306)584-9200; Fax. (306)584-9282; mshawush@sasktel.net.

SHAWUSH, Mohamed F; Landmark Med Centre, 1-4150 Albert St, Regina SK S4S 3R8; Al-Fateh (Libya)'92; FRCSC; OrthSurg (Lower Extremity Reconstruction). (306)584-9200; Fax. (306)584-9282.

SHAWWA, Allam A K; McKenzie Bldg, 206-5788 University Ave, Halifax NS B3H 1V8; (Jordan)'82; MB BS; FRCPC; GenPath. Staff, Queen Elizabeth II Health Sciences Centre - Victoria General Site; Asst Prof, Dalhousie University; Langs: Arabic; (902)473-6663; Fax. (902)473-4113.

SHAWYER, Anna C; McMaster University, 3101A-1280 Main St W, Hamilton ON L8S 4S4; Tor'06; GenSurg.

SHAYAN, Hossein; 2403-1189 Melville St, Vancouver BC V6E 4T8; UBC'01; FRCSC; GenSurg; CardSurg. Staff, Providence Health Care - St Paul's Hospital; Langs: Farsi; (604)893-8801

SHAYEGAN, Bobby; St Joseph's Healthcare, 50 Charlton Ave E, Hamilton ON L8N 4A6; Tor'99; FRCPC; Urol. Staff McMaster Inst of Urol, St Joseph's Healthcare - Charlton Campus; (905)522-1155; Fax. (905)308-7210; shayeb@mcmaster.ca.

SHAYESTEH ALAM, Maryam; Royal Court Med Centre, 105-5 Quarry Ridge Rd, Barrie ON L4M 7G1; Tehran (Iran)'90; FRCPC; Derm (Skin Cancer). Langs: Farsi; (705)503-6333; Fax. (705)503-6330; derm@sincoderm.com.

SHBASH, Iman A M; 12-1300 Garth St, Hamilton ON L9C 4L7; Al Fateh (Libya)'00; FRCPC; Peds. Staff, The Brant Community Healthcare System - Brantford General Hospital Site; Langs: Arabic; (905)575-0611; Fax. (905)575-7737.

SHCHERBATYKH, Ivan Y; North Woodlands Med Centre, 204-40 Shellington Place, Brantford ON N3S 0C5; Voronez State Medical Academy (Russia (Federation))'01; CCFP; (519)759-6116; Fax. (519)759-7727.

SHE, Alex K; 234 Hastings St E, Vancouver BC V6A 1P1; UBC'98; CCFP; FCFP; (604)688-0351; Fax. (604)688-3592.

SHEA, Catherine L; Royal Ottawa Hlth Care Group, 1145 Carling Ave, Ottawa ON K1Z 7K4; Dal'80; FRCPC; Psy. Staff Psy, Royal Ottawa Mental Health Centre - Royal Ottawa Health Care Group; (613)722-6521; Fax. (613)798-2999.

SHEA, Dawn M; Sherwood Family Med Centre, 15 Brackley Point Rd, Charlottetown PE C1A 6Y1; Dal'91.

SHEA, Donald L; Lady Minto Gulf Islands Hosp, 135 Crofton Rd, Salt Spring Island BC V8K 1T1; McG'69; BA; MDCM; FRCPC; DiagRad. Staff, Lady Minto Gulf Islands Hospital; (250)538-4826; Fax. (250)538-4870; donshea@viha.ca.

SHEA, Philip E P; Elizabeth Village Med Clinic, 104-393 Rymal Rd W, Hamilton ON L9B 1V2; McG'67; CCFP; Court Staff, St Joseph's Healthcare - Charlton Campus; (905)388-4028; Fax. (905)388-3302.

SHEA, Sarah E; IWK Health Centre, PO Box 9700 Rpo CSC 5850-5980 University Ave, Halifax NS B3K 6R8; Cal'80; FRCPC; Peds (Developmental Pediatrics). Dir, IWK Health Centre; Staff, Developmental Pediatrics Clinic; Prof Peds, Dalhousie University; (902)470-8483; Fax. (902)470-7284.

SHEA, Theresa M; Dr Theresa Shea Med Clinic, 6-1230 Alward St, Prince George BC V2M 7B1; Cal'05; CCFP; CCFP(E.M.); (250)563-3024

SHEAHAN, Deirdre C; Central Nfld Reg Health Centre, 50 Union St, Grnd-Falls-Windsor NL A2A 2E1; Mem'04; Staff, Central Newfoundland Regional Health Centre; (709)292-2500

SHEAR, Neil H; Sunnybrook Hlth Sciences Ctre, M1 700-2075 Bayview Ave, Toronto ON M4N 3M5; McM'76; ABIM; ABD; FACP; FRCP; BASc; FRCPC; IntMed (Clinical Pharmacology); Derm. Head Derm, Sunnybrook Health Sciences Centre; Head Derm, Women's College Hospital; Chief Derm, University of Toronto; (416)480-4908; Fax. (416)480-6897; neil.shear@sunnybrook.ca.

SHEAR, Roberta M; SMBD Jewish Gen Hosp, A603-3755 ch Cote-Sainte-Cathe, Montreal QC H3T 1E2; McG'93; FRCSC; ObstGyn (Maternal Fetal Medicine). Staff, Sir Mortimer B Davis Jewish General; Langs: English; French; (514)340-8222 x2950; Fax. (514)340-7941; rshear@nurs.jgh.mcgill.ca.

SHEAR, Robin J; Medical Office, 8000 Bathurst St, Thornhill ON L4J 0B8; McM'92; BSc(OccupTheraphy); CCFP; (905)709-9709; Fax. (905)709-9701.

SHEARER, Carl T; New West Sports Med Centre, 202-65 Richmond St, New Westminster BC V3L 5P5; UBC'88; Physician, Ridge Meadows Care Clinic Inc(East); (604)526-7466; Fax. (604)526-4320.

SHEARER, Lauri-Ann; 101-1001 Broadway W PO Box 756, Vancouver BC V6H 4E4; Ott'00; CCFP; (604)531-7749

SHEARER, Robin S; London Reg Cancer Program, 790 Commissioners Rd E, London ON N6A 4L6; Wes'64; CCFP; FCFP; Staff, London Regional Cancer Center; (519)435-8640

SHEARING, Anthony D; South Muskoka Mem Hosp, 75 Ann St, Bracebridge ON P1L 2E4; Tor'99; CCFP; Staff, South Muskoka Memorial Hospital - Muskoka Algonquin Healthcare; (705)645-4400; Fax. (705)645-1221.

SHEARMAN, John K; Bruyere Academic Fam Hlth Team, 75 Bruyere St, Ottawa ON K1N 5C7; London (England)'64; MB BS; LRCP; MRCS; CCFP; FCFP; Physician, SCO Health Service - Élisabeth Bruyère Hospital; Assoc Prof, University of Ottawa; Langs: French; (613)230-3344; Fax. (613)241-1971.

SHEBIB, Pierre Y; CLSC-CHSLD Pat Montreal-Est, 13926 rue Notre-Dame E, Pte-aux-Trembles QC H1A 1T5; Mon'77; (514)642-4050; Fax. (514)498-7505.

SHECHTMAN, Grant L; Bloor Med Clinic, 844 Bathurst St, Toronto ON M5R 3G1; Sask'78; CCFP; FCFP; Staff Family Med, Mount Sinai Hospital; Teacher Family Med, University of Toronto; (416)534-4214; Fax. (416)534-4582.

SHECTER, Adam C; Grand River Hosp-KW Hlth Ctre, PO Box 9056 Stn C 835 King St W, Kitchener ON N2G 1G3; McM'00; CCFP; CCFP(E.M.); Staff, Grand River Hospital - Kitchener/Waterloo Health Centre; (519)749-4242

SHEDID, Daniel; CHUM-Hop Notre-Dame, 1560 rue Sherbrooke E, Montreal QC H2L 4M1; Laval'97; FRCSC; Neursurg (Spine Surgery). Staff, Centre Hospitalier l'Université de Montréal (CHUM) - Hôpital Notre-Dame; Langs: Arabic; English; (514)890-8000; Fax. (514)412-7816.

SHEDLETZKY, Abraham; Vanier Ctre for Women's Health, 655 Martin St, Milton ON L9T 5E6; Tor'75.

SHEDLETZKY, Carolyn S; Yonge-Eglinton Med Centre, 202-2401 Yonge St, Toronto ON M4P 3H1; McM'08; CCFP; (416)322-3700; Fax. (416)322-3707.

SHEEHAN, Ciaran; 169 Talbot St S, Essex ON N8M 1B7; Dublin (Ireland)'72; (519)776-4217; Fax. (519)776-8347.

SHEEHAN, Hilarie L; William Osler HC-Brampton, 2100 Bovaird Dr E, Brampton ON L6R 3J7; Ott'97; FRCPC; DiagRad. Staff, William Osler Health System - Brampton Civic Hospital; (905)494-2120 x51862

SHEEHAN, Mary C; Medical Arts Bldg, 10-626 Main St, Penticton BC V2A 5C8; Cal'84; CCFP; FCFP; Staff, Penticton Regional Hospital; (250)492-0470; Fax. (250)492-5541.

SHEEHAN, Natalie A; Moncton Med Clinic, 403-860 Mountain Rd, Moncton NB E1C 2N7; Laval'96; CCFP; FCFP; (506)853-5171; Fax. (506)853-5172.

SHEEHAN, Stephen D A; Canadian Forces Hlth Serv Ctr, PO Box 99000 Stn Forces, Halifax NS B3K 5X5; McG'89; MDCM; Staff, Canadian Forces Health Services Centre (Atlantic); (902)721-8890

SHEEHAN, Wayne F; St Joseph's Hosp, 130 Bayard Dr, Saint John NB E2L 3L6; Qns'90; CCFP; FCFP; Staff Griatrics, St Joseph's Hospital; (506)632-5556; Fax. (506)632-5512.

SHEEHY, David N; Shubenacadie Health Centre, PO Box 93, Shubenacadie NS B0N 2H0; Dal'83; (902)758-2242; Fax. (902)758-3870.

SHEEHY, Diane; CLSC La Region-Sherbrooke, 1200 rue King E, Sherbrooke QC J1G 1E4; Laval'96; CCFP; Médecin, CLSC La Region-Sherbrooke; (819)563-2572; Fax. (819)563-8502.

SHEFFIELD, Brian; The Doctor's Office, 9625 Yonge St, Richmond Hill ON L4C 5T2; Tor'71; Staff, North York General Hospital - Branson Division; Staff, North York General Hospital; (905)508-4114; Fax. (905)508-4116.

SHEFFIELD, Robert I; Associates Med Clinic, 123 10th Ave S, Cranbrook BC V1C 2N1; Sask'70; (250)426-4231; Fax. (250)426-4357.

SHEFRIN, Allan E; Children's Hosp of Eastern Ont, 401 Smyth Rd, Ottawa ON K1H 8L1; Ott'04; FRCPC; Peds; PedEmergMed. Staff, Children's Hospital of Eastern Ontario (CHEO); (613)737-7600

SHEFTEL, Raisa; Verdun-Lasalle Med Clinic, 5989 rue de Verdun, Verdun QC H4H 1M6; Wroclaw (Poland)'73; assoc Staff, St Mary's Hospital Centre; Langs: Polish; English; Czech; Russian; (514)766-2151; Fax. (514)766-6462.

SHEHATA, Ester N E; 19-499 Ray Lawson Blvd, Brampton ON L6Y 4E6; Alexandria (Egypt)'91; MB ChB; CCFP; (905)460-1100; Fax. (905)460-1175.

SHEHATA, Esther I; 240-1175 Johnson St, Coquitlam BC V3B 7K1; Cairo (Egypt)'67; MB ChB; CCFP; Langs: Arabic; (604)942-1855; Fax. (604)942-1853; shehataesther@hotmail.com.

SHEHATA, Nadia; 204-1931 Mt Newton Cross Rd, Saanichton BC V8M 2A9; Cal'10; CCFP; (250)652-9227

SHEHATA, Nadine; Mount Sinai Hosp, 6 502 5-600 University Ave, Toronto ON M5G 1X5; Mem'94; MSc; BSc; FRCPC; IntMed (Transfusion Medicine); Hem. Staff, St Michael's Hospital; Assoc Med Dir, Canadian Blood Services; Langs: Arabic; (416)586-4800 x2296; Fax. (416)586-8481.

SHEHATA, Ramez S H; Cambridge Mem Hosp, 700 Coronation Blvd, Cambridge ON N1R 3G2; Cairo (Egypt)'89; FRCPC; Anes. Staff, Cambridge Memorial Hospital; Langs: Arabic; French; (519)621-2333 x2100

SHEHATA, Sarwat W M; Sudbury Reg Hosp-Laurentian, 41 Ramsey Lake Rd, Sudbury ON P3E 5J1; Cairo (Egypt)'82; MB ChB; FRCPC; RadOncol. Staff, Health Sciences North-Laurentian Site; Staff, Northeastern Ontario Regional Cancer Centre; Langs: Arabic; (705)522-6237 x2451; Fax. (705)523-7328.

SHEHATA-FOUAD, Seham Z; Credit River Med Clinic, F001B-6045 Creditview Rd, Mississauga ON L5V 2A8; Alexandria (Egypt)'71; MB ChB; CCFP; Physician, Glen Derry Walk-In Clinic; Physician, Britanny Glen Walk-In Clinic; (905)826-6095; Fax. (905)826-9219.

SHEHZAD, Anees A; Dr Shehzad Incorporated, 788 Victoria Rd, Sydney NS B1N 1J7; Punjab (Pakistan)'86; MB BS; CCFP; Staff, Cape Breton Healthcare Complex; Langs: Punjabi; Urdu; (902)564-8361; Fax. (902)567-6161.

SHEIDOW, Thomas G; Ivey Eye Institute, 268 Grosvenor St, London ON N6A 4V2; Wes'95; MMath; BEd; BMath; FRCSC; Ophth (Vitreo Retinal Surgery). Staff, St Joseph's Hospital - St Joseph's Health Care; Staff Ivey Eye Institute, London Health Sciences Centre - Victoria Campus; Physician, Ivey Eye Institute; Assoc Prof Ophth, University of Western Ontario; (519)685-8133; Fax. (519)646-6355; thomas.sheidow@sjhc.london.on.ca.

SHEIK, Nasreen; Edson Med Centre, PO Box 6660 Stn Main 615 50 St, Edson AB T7E 1V1; (780)723-3366

SHEIK, Uzair; PO Box 876, Logan Lake BC V0K 1W0; Cape Town (South Africa)'05; MB ChB; (250)523-9922

SHEIKH, Adnan M; The Ottawa Hosp-Civic Campus, 1053 Carling Ave, Ottawa ON K1Y 4E9; Bangalore University (India)'93; Staff Diag Imaging, The Ottawa Hospital - Civic Campus; Langs: Urdu; (613)761-4982

SHEIKH, Ahmad S; 1821 Rose St, Regina SK S4P 1Z7; (306)525-0716; Fax. (306)359-1068.

SHEIKH, Amber Z; Stamford Med Centre, 305-4256 Portage Rd, Niagara Falls ON L2E 6A4; Mem'05; FRCSC; Ophth. Staff, Niagara Eye Institute; Langs: Urdu; French; Hindi; (905)358-6121; Fax. (905)358-1626.

SHEIKH, Farrukh B; West Durham Family Health Team, BE 200B-1105 Kingston Rd, Pickering ON L1V 1B5; Punjab (Pakistan)'71; MB BS; MD; Langs: Bengali; Punjabi; Urdu; (905)420-9999; Fax. (905)420-0863.

SHEIKH, Gul Nawaz; Rouge Valley-Ajax & Pickering, 580 Harwood Ave S, Ajax ON L1S 2J4; Kashmir University (India)'78; FRCPC; IntMed. Staff, Rouge Valley Health System - Ajax & Pickering Health Centre Site; Langs: Arabic; Hindi; Kashmiri; Urdu; (905)683-2320

SHEIKH, Khalid M; St Joseph's Hosp, 500-1176 Nicholson Rd, Estevan SK S4A 2V6; Lahore (Pakistan)'76; MB BS; FRCS; Staff, St Joseph's Hospital; Langs: Urdu; Punjabi; (306)637-2750; Fax. (306)637-2752.

SHEIKH, Osmaan; Victoria Gen Hosp, 1 Hospital Way, Victoria BC V8Z 6R5; Ott'10; CCFP; Staff, Victoria General Hospital; (250)727-4212

SHEIKH, Shoaib I; Dr G B Cross Mem Hosp, 67 Manitoba Dr, Clarenville NL A5A 1K3; Locum Tenens, The Dr G B Cross Memorial Hospital; (709)466-3411

SHEIKH, Tasnim K; Rouge Valley HS-Centenary, 2867 Ellesmere Rd, Scarborough ON M1E 4B9; (Pakistan)'68; FCAP; DCP; MCPS; FRCPC; AnatPath (Hematology Pathology). Ac Staff Path & Lab Med, Rouge Valley Health System - Centenary Health Centre Site; Langs: Urdu; Punjabi; (416)281-7253

SHEIN, Howard; Hys Med Centre, 202-11010 101 St NW, Edmonton AB T5H 4B9; Johannesburg (South Africa)'81; MB ChB; FFR(D); FRCPC; DiagRad. (780)426-1121; Fax. (780)425-5979.

SHEINBAUM, Deborah; 3825 Cadboro Bay Rd PO Box 50024 Rpo Fairfield Pla, Victoria BC V8N 4G1; Tor'85; Psy. (250)516-1325

SHEINER, Glenn S; North Park Med Centre, 1365 Lawrence Ave W, North York ON M6L 1A4; McG'79; MDCM; CCFP; CCFP(E.M.); Langs: French; (416)244-4377; Fax. (416)244-1004.

SHEINER, Jamie B; Univ Hlth Network-Princess M, 5 205-610 University Ave, Toronto ON M5G 2M9; Tor'88; BSc; MSc; CCFP; FCFP; Staff, Princess Margaret Hospital - University Health Network; (416)946-4534; Fax. (416)946-2983.

SHEINER, Nathan M; SMBD Jewish Gen Hosp, A508-3755 ch Cote-Sainte-Cathe, Montreal QC H3T 1E2; McG'57; MDCM; ThorSurg (P.Q.); Cardiovasc&ThorSurg (General Surgery). Chef Cardiovasc & Thoracic Surg, Sir Mortimer B Davis Jewish General; Prof Surg, McGill University; Langs: Bilingual(English/French); (514)340-8293; Fax. (514)340-7561.

SHEINER, Richard H; 201-4999 rue Sainte-Catherine, Montreal QC H3Z 1T3; McM'82; FRCPC; Psy. (514)939-2225; Fax. (514)939-1685; drsheiner@videotron.ca.

SHELDON, Karyn R; North Toronto Med Bldg, 211-250 Lawrence Ave W, Toronto ON M5M 1B2; Wes'94; BA; CCFP; FCFP; Court Staff, Women's College Hospital; Court Staff, Sunnybrook Health Sciences Centre; Assoc Prof, University of Toronto; (416)787-3771; Fax. (416)782-3030.

SHELDON, Leslie J; Mount St Joseph Hosp, W1 S-3080 Prince Edward St, Vancouver BC V5T 3N4; Alb'84; BSc(Pharm); FRCPC; Psy (Clinical Psychopharmacology). Staff, Providence Health Care - Mount Saint Joseph Hospital; Clin Instructor Psy, University of British Columbia; (604)877-8159; Fax. (604)877-8157.

SHELDON, Robert S; Cardiovascular Research Group, 3280 Hospital Dr NW, Calgary AB T2N 4N1; Tor'81; PhD; FRCPC; IntMed; Cardiol. Staff Cardiol, Foothills Medical Centre; Prof, University Of Calgary; (403)220-8191; Fax. (403)210-9350; sheldon@ucalgary.ca.

SHELDRICK, Peter G; 11 Victoria Ave, Chatham ON N7L 2Z7; Wes'71; Staff, Chatham-Kent Health Alliance; (519)352-5050; Fax. (519)352-8572.

SHELIG, Khaled S; 1-1580 20th St E, Owen Sound ON N4K 5P5; Al Fateh (Libya)'95; FRCPC; IntMed; Cardiol. Staff, Grey Bruce Health Services - Owen Sound; (519)372-9951; Fax. (519)372-1384.

SHELL, Melanie D C; Family Matters Med Centre, X-730 St Anne's Rd, Winnipeg MB R2N 0A2; Man'07; CCFP; (204)253-5320

SHELLEY, A S Douglas; 205-726 Bloor St W, Toronto ON M6G 1L4; West Indies (Jamaica)'67; (416)588-9650

SHELLEY, Eric S; MOHTLC Hlth Services Branch, 370 Select Dr, Kingston ON K7M 8T4; Qns'74; FRCPC; Anes. Prog Dir Dept of Anes, Queen's University; (613)536-3164

SHELTON, Dominick M; Sunnybrook Hlth Sciences Ctre, 2075 Bayview Ave, Toronto ON M4N 3M5; Tor'91; BSc; MD; CCFP; CCFP(E.M.); FCFP; Staff, Sunnybrook Health Sciences Centre; Staff, The Hospital For Sick Children; Staff, Women's College Hospital; Asst Prof Family & Commun Med, University of Toronto; (416)480-6100 x7207

SHELTON, Lynne J; Country Club Plaza, 410-3025 Portage Ave, Winnipeg MB R3K 2E2; Man'84; FRCPC; Psy.

SHELTON, Paul A; Corydon Neurology Associates, 101-698 Corydon Ave, Winnipeg MB R3M 0X9; Man'79; FRCPC; Neur (Behavioural Neurology). Asst Prof Med, University of Manitoba; (204)284-5551; Fax. (204)284-5626.

SHELTON, Rhidian J; Queen Elizabeth II HSC-Halifax, 6896F-1796 Summer St, Halifax NS B3H 3A7; Sheffield (England)'98; MB ChB; Staff, Queen Elizabeth II Health Sciences Centre - Halifax Infirmary Site.

SHEMESH, Tzela; Physimed Med Center, 121-6363 rte Transcanadienne, Saint-Laurent QC H4T 1Z9; Mon'08; CCFP; (514)747-8888

SHEMIE, Sam D; MUHC-Montreal Children's Hosp, C808-2300 rue Tupper, Montreal QC H3H 1P3; McG'85; FRCPC; Peds; Critical Care Medicine. Staff, McGill University Health Centre - Montreal Children's Hospital; Langs: French; (514)412-4400; sam.shemie@muhc.mcgill.ca.

SHEMILT, Ann Marie; Signal Hill Centre, 5986 Signal Hill Center SW, Calgary AB T3H 3P8; Wes'09; CCFP; (403)240-2660

SHEMILT, Roderick J; 49 Johnston Rd, North Bay ON P1B 8G1; McM'74; CCFP; FCFP; (705)472-5466; Fax. (705)472-9859.

SHEMTOV, Oren M; North York Gen Hosp, 4001 Leslie St, North York ON M2K 1E1; Qns'04; CCFP; CCFP(E.M.); Staff, North York General Hospital; (416)756-6000

SHEN, Angela M; Acqua Med Centre, 118-5811 No. 3 Rd, Richmond BC V6X 4L7; UBC'96; CCFP; FCFP; Langs: Cantonese; (604)279-8881; Fax. (604)244-9222.

SHEN, Kay; St Joseph's Health Centre, 30 The Queensway, Toronto ON M6R 1B5; Tor'96; CCFP; Staff Family Med, St Joseph's Health Centre; (416)530-6860; Fax. (416)530-6160.

SHEN, Khaled A; 61 Arthur St, Truro NS B2N 1X7; Al-Fateh (Libya)'94; MB ChB; CCFP; (902)893-7231

SHENASSA, Hassan; Harmony Med Centre, 110-152 Cleopatra Dr, Ottawa ON K2G 5X2; Sask'89; FACOG; FRCSC; ObstGyn (Endometriosis). Head Gynecology/Dir Gyn Minimally Invasive Surg, The Ottawa Hospital - Civic Campus; Asst Prof, University of Ottawa; Langs: Persian; Farsi; (613)725-1870; Fax. (613)725-1647.

SHENAVA, Ravishankar T; Medical Bldg, 345-600 Tecumseh Rd E, Windsor ON N8X 4X9; Mysore (India)'74; MB BS; FRCPC; Psy. Langs: Kanarese; (519)977-9550; Fax. (519)977-9503.

SHENDE, Vasanti N; 4 44-125 Delhi St, Guelph ON N1E 4J5; Pune (India)'90; MB BS; FRCPC; IntMed (Sleep Medicine); Respir. Langs: Hindi; Marathi; (519)823-1730

SHENDEREY, Alexander I; William Osler HC-Brampton, 2100 Bovaird Dr E, Brampton ON L6R 3J7; Leningrad (Russia (Federation))'84; FRCPC; Anes. Staff, William Osler Health System - Brampton Civic Hospital; Langs: German; (905)494-2120

SHENFIELD, Carey B; 25 King St W, Kingston ON K7L 5P9; FRCPC; RadOncol. (613)544-2631

SHENFIELD, Leisa J; Brockville Gen Hosp, 75 Charles St, Brockville ON K6V 1S8; Wes'92; CCFP; CCFP(E.M.); Staff, Brockville General Hospital - Charles Street; Staff, Kingston General Hospital; (613)345-3847

SHENKER, Hannah R; CLSC Cote des Neiges, 5700 ch Cote-des-Neiges, Montreal QC H3T 2A8; McG'05; CCFP; Staff, Inuulitsivik Health Centre; Staff, GMF Côté-des-Neiges; (514)731-8531; hannah.shenker@mail.mcgill.ca.

SHENKER, Robert L; 50 Albert St, Waterloo ON N2L 3S2; Tor'97; FRCSC; PlasSurg (Clinician Investigator Program). Langs: Hebrew; French; (519)746-1132; Fax. (519)746-0316.

SHENKIER, Tamara N; BC Cancer Agency-Vancouver CC, 4F-600 10th Ave W, Vancouver BC V5Z 4E6; McG'84; FRCPC; IntMed; MedOncol. Staff MedOncol, BC Cancer Agency Vancouver Centre; Staff MedOncol, Vancouver General Hospital - Centennial Pavillion; Clin Assoc Prof, University of British Columbia; (604)877-6000; bng@bccancer.bc.ca.

SHENNAN, Andrew T; Sunnybrook Health Sciences Ctr, M4 230-2075 Bayview Ave, Toronto ON M4N 3M5; Aberdeen (Scotland)'67; MB ChB; MRC; Peds (Neonatology). Staff, Sunnybrook Health Sciences Centre; (416)480-6100

SHENNAN, Carmel F W; Victoria Gen Hosp, 1 Hospital Way, Victoria BC V8Z 6R5; (Zimbabwe)'79; MB ChB; FFARCS; FRCPC; Anes (Dental Anesthesia). Staff, Victoria General Hospital; (250)727-4212

SHENODA, Kamal L M; Greencrest Med Clinic, 2750 Pembina Hwy, Winnipeg MB R3P 2H8; (Other Foreign)'81; CCFP; (204)415-0044; Fax. (204)415-2490.

SHENOUDA, Amir Z; Wall Street Med Bldg, 330-140 Wall St, Saskatoon SK S7K 1N4; Ein Shams (Egypt)'65; MB ChB; Ac Staff, Saskatoon City Hospital; Physician, Wall Street Medical Centre; (306)244-8660; Fax. (306)244-9951.

SHENOUDA, George; MUHC-Montreal Gen Hosp, D5 400-1650 av Cedar, Montreal QC H3G 1A4; Ain Shams (Egypt)'77; FRCPC; RadOncol. Staff, McGill University Health Centre - Montreal General Campus; Staff, Sir Mortimer B Davis Jewish General; assoc Prof, McGill University; (514)934-8040; Fax. (514)934-8392.

SHENOUDA, Mark A; Wall Street Med Bldg, 300-140 Wall St, Saskatoon SK S7K 1N4; Sask'95; LMCC; FRCPC; DiagRad (Interventional Radiology). Staff Radiol, Saskatoon City Hospital; Staff Radiol, St Paul's Hospital (Grey Nuns) of Saskatoon; Physician, Wall Street Medical Centre; (306)244-1167; Fax. (306)244-2911.

SHENOUDA, Mervat E F G; Lakewood Med Clinic, 34 Lakewood Blvd, Winnipeg MB R2J 2M6; '89; CCFP; (204)257-4900

SHENOUDA, Nader N S; Kin Place Health Centre, PO Box 28 689 Main St, Oakbank MB R0E 1J0; CCFP; Staff, Selkirk & District General Hospital; (204)444-2227; Fax. (204)444-7851.

SHENOUDA, Nancy M S; West Brampton Med Centre, 5-80 Clementine Dr, Brampton ON L6Y 0L8; Cairo (Egypt)'89; CCFP; Langs: Arabic; (905)451-1107; Fax. (905)451-0933.

SHENOUDA, Nashwa T M; Family Practice Clinic, 84 Memorial Ave, Grnd-Falls-Windsor NL A2A 1R9; CCFP; Staff, Central Newfoundland Regional Health Centre; (709)489-6688

SHENOUDA, Nazih F; Children's Hosp of Eastern Ont, 401 Smyth Rd, Ottawa ON K1H 8L1; Cairo (Egypt)'80; MSc; FRCPC; DiagRad. Staff, Children's Hospital of Eastern Ontario (CHEO); Langs: Arabic; French; (613)737-7600 x2262

SHENOUDA, Phebe F S; Winnipeg Clinic, 425 St Mary Ave, Winnipeg MB R3C 0N2; '93; CCFP; (204)957-1900

SHENOY, Pradeep; Campbellton Reg Hosp, PO Box 880 Stn Main 189 Lily Lake Rd, Campbellton NB E3N 3H3; Mysore (India)'78; FRCS(UK); DLO(London); FACS; Staff Ear Nose & Throat, Hôpital Régional Campbellton; Specialist Ear Nose & Throat, Centre de santé Communitaire - St-Joseph; (506)789-5000; Fax. (506)684-7148; pks_ent@hotmail.com.

SHEOLAL, Ravitha; William Osler HC-Etobicoke, 101 Humber College Blvd, Etobicoke ON M9V 1R8; Natal University (South Africa)'97; FRCPC; Anes. Staff, William Osler Health System - Etobicoke General Hospital; Staff, The Credit Valley Hospital; (905)813-2200

SHEOPERSHAD, Vitesh; Associate Med Clinic, PO Box 510, Slave Lake AB T0G 2A0; (780)849-4155; Fax. (780)849-4574.

SHEOPERSHAD, Yuktesh; High Prairie Med Clinic, PO Box 449, High Prairie AB T0G 1E0; (780)523-4501; Fax. (780)523-4805.

SHEORAN, Rajeev; Mental Health Centre, 740 Carmi Ave, Penticton BC V2A 8P9; Rajasthan (India)'98; MD; Psy. Staff, Penticton Regional Hospital; Staff, Interior Health Authority South Okanagan Penticton Health Unit; Langs: Hindi; (250)770-3434

SHEPARD, Andrea L; Northwood Park Healtrh Centre, 504 N Edward St, Thunder Bay ON P7C 4P9; Dal'96; CCFP; (807)286-2003; Fax. (807)286-2684.

SHEPEL, Michael L; Royal University Hosp, 103 Hospital Dr, Saskatoon SK S7N 0W8; Cal'03; FRCPC; DiagRad. Staff Medical Imaging, Royal University Hospital; (306)655-2402; Fax. (306)655-2370.

SHEPERTYCKY, Martha R; St Boniface Gen Hosp, BG 034-409 Tache Ave, Winnipeg MB R2H 2A6; Man'97; FRCPC; IntMed; Respir. Staff, St Boniface General Hospital; Staff, The Salvation Army Grace Hospital; Staff, Covenant Health - Misericordia Community Hospital; (204)233-8563

SHEPHARD, Suzanne D; Frontenac Med Associates, 201-791 Princess St, Kingston ON K7L 1E9; Tor'89; CCFP; CCFP(E.M.); FCFP; (613)544-2727; Fax. (613)544-7247.

SHEPHERD, Anne L; 442 Markham St, Toronto ON M6G 2L2; Tor'78; FRCPC; Psy. (416)538-3891; Fax. (416)538-0022.

SHEPHERD, Carolin H; Huron Commun Family Hlth Team, PO Box 460 32B-1 Centennial Dr, Seaforth ON N0K 1W0; Tor'89; Site Chief Emerg, Seaforth Community Hospital - Huron Perth Healthcare Alliance; Aj Prof, University of Western Ontario; Langs: German; (519)600-6000; Fax. (519)600-6010; cshepherd@rogers.com.

SHEPHERD, Debra-Jo; Golden Mile Centre, 216-3806 Albert St, Regina SK S4S 3R2; Sask'92; FRCSC; ObstGyn. Physician, Golden Mile Medical Clinic; (306)586-3116; Fax. (306)586-3118.

SHEPHERD, Frances A; Univ Hlth Network-Princess M, 5 104-610 University Ave, Toronto ON M5G 2M9; Tor'70; FRCPC; IntMed (Medical Oncology); Hem. Staff, Princess Margaret Hospital - University Health Network; Chair Lung Cancer Committee, National Cancer Institute of Canada; Prof Med, University of Toronto; Langs: Bilingual(English/French); (416)946-4522; Fax. (416)946-6546.

SHEPHERD, Jessica G; London HSC-University Hosp, PO Box 5339 Stn B A3 132-339 Windermere Rd, London ON N6A 5A5; West Indies (Jamaica)'83; MB BS; FRCPC; AnatPath. Staff, London Health Sciences Centre - University Hospital; (519)685-8500 x36387; Fax. (519)663-2930; jessica.shepherd@lhsc.on.ca.

SHEPHERD, John D; Leukemia/Bmt Program of BC, 10F-2775 Laurel St, Vancouver BC V5Z 1M9; Cal'81; FRCPC; IntMed; Hem. Ac Staff, Vancouver General Hospital - Centennial Pavillion; Ac Staff, BC Cancer Agency Vancouver Centre; VP, Vancouver Coastal Health; Staff, Leukemia/Bone Marrow Transplantation Prog of BC; Clin Assoc Prof Med, University of British Columbia; (604)875-4863; Fax. (604)875-4763; jshepherd@bccancer.bc.ca.

SHEPHERD, Lisa G; London HSC-Victoria Campus, PO Box 5010 Stn B 800 Commissioners Rd E, London ON N6A 5W9; Qns'85; FRCPC; EmergMed. Staff, London Health Sciences Centre - Victoria Campus; (519)685-8500; lisa.shepherd@lhsc.on.ca.

SHEPHERD, Lois E; Kingston Gen Hosp, 76 Stuart St, Kingston ON K7L 2V7; McG'77; FRCPC; HemPath (Clinical Trials). Med Dir Blood Bank & Immunol, Kingston General Hospital; Physician Coord, Clinical Trials, NCIC-CTG; Asst Prof, Queen's University; Langs: French; (613)549-6666; Fax. (613)548-6076.

SHEPHERD, Lynn J; Carling-Broadview Med Bldg, 309-770 Broadview Ave, Ottawa ON K2A 3Z3; Qns'05; FRCSC; ObstGyn. (613)274-7831; Fax. (613)274-3271.

SHEPHERD, Margaret A; Children's & Women's HC of BC, B321-4480 Oak St, Vancouver BC V6H 3V4; McG'77; FRCPC; Peds. Staff, BC Children's Hospital; Langs: Bilingual(English/French); (604)875-2345

SHEPHERD, Michael A; Dr M A Shepherd Inc, 204-3140 Lakeshore Rd, Kelowna BC V1W 3T1; UBC'75; Staff, Kelowna General Hospital; (250)763-1131; Fax. (250)763-3455.

SHEPHERD, Robert W; McKenzie Prof Centre, 220-1595 McKenzie Ave, Victoria BC V8N 1A4; McG'76; CCFP; Affil Clin Instructor Island Med Program Univ of Victoria, University of British Columbia; Langs: Bilingual(English/French); (250)477-9100; Fax. (250)477-9121.

SHEPHERD, S Lance; Mineral Springs Hosp, PO Box 1050 Stn Main, Banff AB T1L 1H7; UBC'89; CCFP; CCFP(E.M.); Staff, Foothills Medical Centre; Staff, Covenant Health - Banff Mineral Springs Hospital; Clin Teacher, University of Calgary; (403)762-2222; Fax. (403)762-4193.

SHEPHERD, Susan E; Medical Assoc of Port Perry, 462 Paxton St, Port Perry ON L9L 1L9; Tor'97; CCFP; Staff, Lakeridge Health - Port Perry Site; (905)985-2895 x5410; Fax. (905)985-8378.

SHEPHERD, Susan M; SMH-Wellesley Health Centre, 410 Sherbourne St, Toronto ON M4X 1K2; Tor'88; CCFP; FCFP; Staff Teacher, University of Toronto; (416)867-3728; Fax. (416)867-3726.

SHEPPARD, David C R; CFB Wainwright, B633-12 CF Health Services Cen, Denwood AB T0B 1B0; Alb'71; Staff, CFB Wainwright; Langs: German; (780)842-1363; Fax. (780)842-1809.

SHEPPARD, Dawn C; The Ottawa Hosp-Gen Campus, 501 Smyth Rd, Ottawa ON K1H 8L6; Mem'05; FRCPC; IntMed; Hem. Staff, The Ottawa Hospital - General Campus; Teach Staff, Queen's University; (613)737-8899

SHEPPARD, Donald; MUHC-Royal Victoria Hosp, L5 07-687 av des Pins O, Montreal QC H3A 1A1; Tor'93; FRCPC; IntMed; InfectDis; MedMicrobiol. Staff, McGill University Health Centre - Royal Victoria Hospital; (514)934-1934 x36104

SHEPPARD, Duane G; Dartmouth Gen Hosp, 325 Pleasant St, Dartmouth NS B2Y 4G8; Mem'96; BSc; FRCPC; IntMed; Gastroent. Staff, Dartmouth General Hospital; (902)461-9733; Fax. (902)461-9687.

SHEPPARD, George F; Nanaimo Reg Gen Hosp, 1200 Dufferin Cres, Nanaimo BC V9S 2B7; Alb'96; CCFP; CCFP(E.M.); FCFP; Staff, Nanaimo Regional General Hospital; (250)754-2141

SHEPPARD, Gillian A; Paradise Health Complex, 206-1386 Topsail Rd, Paradise NL A1L 1P6; Mem'08; CCFP; CCFP(E.M.); Staff, Health Sciences Centre; (709)782-4445

SHEPPARD, James A G; Kelligrews Med Clinic, PO Box 17160 Stn Main, Conception Bay S NL A1X 3H1; Mem'03; CCFP; (709)834-9679

SHEPPARD, Jeffrey B; Northern Lights Health Region, 7 Hospital St, Fort McMurray AB T9H 1P2; Mem'94; CCFP; Staff, Fort McMurray Community Cancer Centre - Alberta Health Services; Staff, Northern Lights Regional Health Centre; (780)791-6161

SHEPPARD, Kerry J; William Jackman Mem Hosp, 410 Booth Ave, Labrador City NL A2V 2K1; Mem'93; FRCSC; ObstGyn. Staff, Captain William Jackman Memorial Hospital; (709)944-2632

SHEPPARD, Matthew G L; North Bay Reg Health Centre, PO Box 2500 50 College Dr, North Bay ON P1B 5A4; Cal'10; CCFP; Staff, North Bay Regional Health Centre - Regional Mental Health; (403)479-7749

SHEPPARD, Matthew J; The Ottawa Hosp-Civic Campus, B 302-1053 Carling Ave, Ottawa ON K1Y 4E9; Mem'11; Staff, The Ottawa Hospital - Civic Campus; (613)722-7000

SHEPPARD, Miranda E; Springbank Med Centre, 304-460 Springbank Dr, London ON N6J 0A8; Ott'07; CCFP; Staff, Wortley Village Medical Centre; Aj Prof, University of Western Ontario; (519)963-3781; Fax. (519)963-3779.

SHEPPARD, Richard J; SMBD Jewish Gen Hosp, 3755 ch Cote-Sainte-Catherine, Montreal QC H3T 1E2; McG'96; FRCPC; IntMed; Cardiol. Staff, Sir Mortimer B Davis Jewish General; Langs: French; (514)340-8222; Fax. (514)340-7531.

SHEPPARD, Ricki M; Creditview Medical, 14B-1240 Eglinton Ave W, Mississauga ON L5V 1N3; Tor'71; Ac Staff, The Credit Valley Hospital; (905)567-4622; Fax. (905)567-7545.

SHEPPARD, Robert R B; Thunder Bay Reg HSC, 980 Oliver Rd, Thunder Bay ON P7B 6V4; Tor'74; FRCPC; Psy (Forensic Psychiatry). Staff Psy, Thunder Bay Regional Health Sciences Centre; Staff Psy, Waypoint Centre for Mental Health Care; (807)684-6467; Fax. (807)684-5868.

SHEPPARD, Shane D; Saskatoon City Hosp, 701 Queen St, Saskatoon SK S7K 0M7; Sask'84; FRCPC; Anes. Staff, Saskatoon City Hospital; (306)655-8000; Fax. (306)374-0281.

SHEPS, David M; 124 Street Med Group, 10839 124 St NW, Edmonton AB T5M 0H4; Man'97; FRCSC; OrthSurg. (780)453-2953; Fax. (780)453-2964; drsheps@shaw.ca.

SHEPS, Franklin W; MCI The Doctors Office, 4-800 Steeles Ave W, Thornhill ON L4J 7L2; Tor'84; CCFP; CCFP(E.M.); FCFP; Langs: Hebrew; (905)738-6699; Fax. (905)738-6073.

SHEPS, Jordana L; Family Practice Health Centre, 3F-77 Grenville St, Toronto ON M5S 1B3; McM'04; CCFP; Staff, Women's College Hospital; (416)323-6060; Fax. (416)323-6350.

SHEPS, Michael D; Dermatology Clinic, 205 Edmonton St, Winnipeg MB R3C 1R4; Man'72; FRCPC; Derm (Hair Loss). Fax. (204)942-4399.

SHEPS, Rachel L; Humber River Reg Hosp-Church, 200 Church St, Toronto ON M9N 1N8; Tor'09; CCFP; CCFP(E.M.); Staff, Humber River Regional Hospital - Church Street Site; (416)249-8111

SHEPS, Samuel B; School of Population & Public, 2206 East Mall, Vancouver BC V6T 1Z3; Cleveland(OH) (USA)'73; FRCPC; Peds. Prof, University of British Columbia; (604)822-3081; Fax. (604)822-4994.

SHER, Andrew K; Westgate Medicentre, 101-9540 163 St NW, Edmonton AB T5P 3M7; Alb'02; CCFP; (780)489-4976; Fax. (780)481-6761.

SHER, Graham D; Canadian Blood Services, 1800 Alta Vista Dr, Ottawa ON K1G 4J5; Witwatersrand (South Africa)'87; MB ChB; PhD; FRCPC; HemPath (Laboratory Hematology). Staff, Canadian Blood Services; (613)739-2001; Fax. (613)739-2099.

SHERAZI, Syed A R; Abbotsford Reg Hosp & Cancer C, 32900 Marshall Rd, Abbotsford BC V2S 0C2; Peshawar (Pakistan)'96; Staff, Abbotsford Regional Hospital & Cancer Centre; Staff, Mission Memorial Hospital; Langs: Pashtu; Punjabi; (604)851-4700

SHERBANIUK, Richard W; Ziedler Ledcor Centre, 2 36-130 University Campus NW, Edmonton AB T6G 2X8; Alb'52; FACP; FRCPC; IntMed (Gastroenterology). Att Staff, University of Alberta Hospital; Clin Prof Gastroent, University of Alberta; (780)492-8157; Fax. (780)492-8295.

SHERBINO, Jonathan D; Hamilton HS-General Site, 237 Barton St E, Hamilton ON L8L 2X2; Ott'01; FRCPC; EmergMed. Staff Emerg Med, Hamilton Health Sciences Centre - Hamilton General Hospital; (905)527-0271

SHERECK, Evan B; Children's & Women's HC of BC, 4480 Oak St, Vancouver BC V6H 3V4; New Jersey-Piscataway (USA)'01; Staff Ped HemOncol, BC Children's Hospital; (604)875-2406

SHERGHIN, Ahmed S O; Windsor Health Centre, 330-600 Tecumseh Rd E, Windsor ON N8X 4X9; Benghazi (Libya)'80; MB ChB; FRCSC; Urol (Transplantation). Langs: Arabic; (519)254-0050; Fax. (519)254-2873.

SHERGILL, Amarpreet S; Peter Lougheed Centre, 3500 26 Ave NE, Calgary AB T1Y 6J4; (India)'00; CCFP; Staff, Peter Lougheed Centre; (403)943-5461; Fax. (403)943-5438.

SHERGILL, Amninder K; Sunridge Prof Centre, 410-2675 36 St NE, Calgary AB T1Y 6H6; (India)'01; CCFP; (403)717-0812; Fax. (403)717-0810.

SHERGILL, Navi; University of Alberta Hosp, 2A2 41-8440 112 St NW, Edmonton AB T6G 2B7; Saba University (Other Foreign)'06; FRCPC; DiagRad. Staff, University of Alberta Hospital; (780)407-6907

SHERGOLD, David J; Humber River Reg Hosp-Church, 200 Church St, York ON M9N 1N8; McM'90; Staff, Humber River Regional Hospital - Church Street Site; Staff, Humber River Regional Hospital - Finch Avenue Site; (416)747-3857

SHERIDAN, Brian L; Univ Hlth Network-Toronto Gen, 11E 415-200 Elizabeth St, Toronto ON M5G 2C4; Newcastle (England)'68; MB BS; FRCP; FRCPath; FRCPC; HemPath (Laboratory Medicine). Dep Head Lab Hem, Toronto General Hospital - UHN; Staff, St Michael's Hospital; Teach Staff Lab Med & PathBiol, University of Toronto; (416)340-4849; Fax. (416)340-5543; brian.sheridan@uhn.on.ca.

SHERIDAN, David P; Royal University Hosp, 103 Hospital Dr, Saskatoon SK S7N 0W8; Sask'77; FRCPC; IntMed; Hem. Prof Med, Royal University Hospital; Prov Leader Malignant Hematol, Saskatchewan Cancer Agency; (306)655-0600; Fax. (306)655-1809.

SHERIDAN, James J; Cartwright Med Clinic, 11 Cartwright St, Grnd Falls-Windsor NL A2A 1L7; Dublin (Ireland)'82; MB ChB; MRC; FRCPC; IntMed. Staff, Ross Family Medical Centre; Langs: Gaelic; Irish; Italian; Latin; Bilingual(French/English); (709)489-5566; Fax. (709)489-1533; jsheridan@nl.rogers.com.

SHERIDAN, Jay T; Canadian Forces Services Ctre, 101 Colonel By Dr, Ottawa ON K1A 0K2; Qns'97; CCFP; FCFP; Staff, Canadian Forces Health Services Centre; (613)838-4756

SHERIDAN, Mark A; Pacific Avenue Med Centre, 300-149 Pacific Ave, Saskatoon SK S7K 1N8; Sask'75; FRCSC; ObstGyn. Physician, Pacific Avenue Medical Centre; (306)653-5970; Fax. (306)653-5383.

SHERIDAN, William J; Queen Elizabeth II HSC-Summer, 2103-1796 Summer St, Halifax NS B3H 3A7; Mem'79; ABIM; FRCP; ABCD; FRCPC; IntMed; Cardiol. Staff, Queen Elizabeth II Health Sciences Centre - Capital Health; Asst Prof, Dalhousie University; (902)473-7400; Fax. (902)473-2434.

SHERIF, Hesham; Grey Bruce HS-Owen Sound, PO Box 1800 Stn Main 7213-1800 8th St E, Owen Sound ON N4K 6M9; Al-Fateh (Libya)'95; FRCSC; Ophth. Staff, Grey Bruce Health Services - Owen Sound; (519)376-2121; Fax. (519)376-7160.

SHERIFF, Maqbool K; Dr Maqbool K Sheriff Inc, 2-1179 Seafield Cres, Nanaimo BC V9S 4S1; Nairobi (Kenya)'77; MB; FRCPC; IntMed; Rheum. Langs: Gujarati; Kiswahili; (250)754-8012; Fax. (250)754-0910.

SHERK, Peter A; Victoria Gen Hosp, 1 Hospital Way, Victoria BC V8Z 6R5; Tor'97; FRCPC; IntMed; Critical Care Medicine; Respir. Staff, Victoria General Hospital; Staff ICU, Royal Jubilee Hospital; (250)818-4824

SHERKIN, Marc D; York-Finch Med Centre, 216E-2115 Finch Ave W, North York ON M3N 2V6; Tor'77; Respir; IntMed. (416)740-1832; Fax. (416)747-3799.

SHERLOCK, Christopher H; St Paul's Hosp, 632-1081 Burrard St, Vancouver BC V6Z 1Y6; London (England)'73; MB BS; FRCPC; MedMicrobiol (Virology). Dir Diag Virology & Ref Lab, Providence Health Care - St Paul's Hospital; Consultant Virol, Vancouver General Hospital - Centennial Pavillion; Consultant, BC Cancer Agency Vancouver Centre; Clin Prof, University of British Columbia; (604)806-8422; csherloc@interchange.ubc.ca.

SHERLOCK, Donald R; Quinte HC Corp-Belleville Gen, WCA 353-265 Dundas St E, Belleville ON K8N 5A9; Qns'70; CCFP; Physician, QHC Belleville General; Physician, Kenna Stellite Inc; Physician, Crane Canada Inc; (613)966-3421; Fax. (613)966-6608; dsherlock@craneplumbing.ca.

SHERLOCK, Jo-Ann I; Grey Nuns Community Hosp, 23-1100 Youville Drive West NW, Edmonton AB T6L 5X8; UBC'89; BSc; BEd; CCFP; Staff Learning & Development Clinic, Covenant Health - Grey Nuns Community Hospital; (780)735-7346; Fax. (780)735-9537.

SHERLOCK, Mary E; Hamilton HS-McMaster Site, PO Box 2000 Stn Lcd 1 1200 Main St W, Hamilton ON L8N 3Z5; National (Ireland)'00; FRCPC; Peds; Gastroent. Staff Gastroent & Hepatology, The Hospital For Sick Children; Staff, Hamilton Health Sciences Centre - McMaster Children's Hospital; (905)521-2100

SHERLOCK, Rebecca L; Children's & Women's HC of BC, 1R46A-4480 Oak St, Vancouver BC V6H 3V4; Mem'98; FAAP; FRCPC; Peds (Neonatal & Perinatal Medicine). Staff, BC Children's Hospital; Clin Asst Prof, University of British Columbia; (604)875-2135; Fax. (604)875-3106; rsherlock@cw.bc.ca.

SHERLOCK, Richard A G; LL-3017 66 St NW, Edmonton AB T6K 4B2; Alb'80; FRCPC; DiagRad. Staff, Covenant Health - Edmonton General Continuing Care Centre; (780)450-9729; Fax. (780)461-7527.

SHERMAN, Christopher G; Sunnybrook Hlth Sciences Ctre, 2075 Bayview Ave, Toronto ON M4N 3M5; Man'83; FRCPC; AnatPath. Staff, Sunnybrook Health Sciences Centre; Asst Prof, University of Toronto; (416)480-6100 x2126; Fax. (416)480-4271.

SHERMAN, Gregory P; Dingwall Med Group, 40 Goodall St, Dryden ON P8N 1V9; McG'86; CCFP; FCFP.

SHERMAN, Maliha A H; 60 Centennial Pky S, Hamilton ON L8G 2C5; Karachi (Pakistan)'99; CCFP; Langs: Swahili; (905)662-2231; Fax. (905)662-2233.

SHERMAN, Mark H; MUHC-Royal Victoria Hosp, M9 05-687 av des Pins O, Montreal QC H3A 1A1; McG'87; FRCPC; IntMed (Clinical Lipid Disorders); Endocrin&Metab. Staff Endocrin & Metab/Dir, McGill University Health Centre - Royal Victoria Hospital; adj Prof Med, McGill University; Langs: Bilingual(French/English); Hebrew; (514)934-1934 x36879; Fax. (514)982-0825; mark.sherman@mcgill.ca.

SHERMAN, Mark; Victoria Health Comm Co-Op, 547 Michigan St, Victoria BC V8V 1S5; McG'98; CCFP; Langs: Bilingual(English/French); (250)388-7844; Fax. (250)380-0244; msherman@jbcp.bc.ca.

SHERMAN, Morris; NCSB 11-1252-585 University Av, Toronto ON M5G 2N2; Witwatersrand (South Africa)'72; MB BS; DPhil; FRCPC; IntMed (Hepatology). Staff, Toronto General Hospital - UHN; Assoc Prof, University of Toronto; Langs: Afrikaans; (416)340-4756; Fax. (416)591-2107; morris.sherman@uhn.on.ca.

SHERMAN, Philip M; The Hosp for Sick Children, 8409-555 University Ave, Toronto ON M5G 1X8; Cal'77; FRCPC; Peds (Pediatric Gastroenterology). Staff Gastroent, The Hospital For Sick Children; Prof, University of Toronto; (416)813-7734; Fax. (416)813-6531; philip.sherman@sickkids.ca.

SHERMAN, Rajnish K; Royal Alexandra Hosp, 10240 Kingsway NW, Edmonton AB T5H 3V9; Alb'90; CCFP; CCFP(E.M.); FCFP; Staff, Royal Alexandra Hospital; (780)735-4442

SHERMAN, Thomas A; Southland Plaza, 870-10201 Southport Rd SW, Calgary AB T2W 4X9; Alb'78; ABIM; FRCPC; IntMed; Gastroent. (403)259-3729; Fax. (403)252-5191.

SHERMAN, Zoia; Provincial Med Clinic, 1400 Provincial Rd, Windsor ON N8W 5W1; Bucharest (Romania)'83; Staff, Windsor Medical Clinic; Langs: Hebrew; Romanian; Russian; (519)250-6990; Fax. (519)250-6946.

SHERRARD, Adam W G; PO Box 661, Dawson YT Y0B 1G0; Ott'10; CCFP.

SHERRET, David; Crown Med Clinic, 1022-123 Edward St, Toronto ON M5G 1E2; Glasgow (Scotland)'50; MB ChB; DPM; FRCPC; Psy (Psychotherapy). (416)979-7866; Fax. (416)979-7387.

SHERWANI, Aamir S; Ross Mem Hosp, 10 Angeline St N, Lindsay ON K9V 4M8; Punjab (India)'86; MB BS; GenSurg. Staff, Ross Memorial Hospital; (705)324-6111

SHERWIN, Elizabeth A; 65 Ellen St, Blenheim ON N0P 1A0; Qns'79; MPH; CCFP; FCFP; Staff, Chatham-Kent Health Alliance; (519)676-5592; Fax. (519)676-2228.

SHERWIN, Elizabeth D; BC Children's Hosp, 2C50-4480 4480 Oak St, Vancouver BC V6H 3V4; Staff, BC Children's Hospital; (604)875-2120

SHERWIN, Gregory D; Bluewater Health-Norman Site, 89 Norman St, Sarnia ON N7T 6S3; Qns'78; FRCPC; Anes. Staff, Bluewater Health - Norman Site; (519)381-0649; Fax. (519)464-4486.

SHERWIN, Richard D; Haugen Med Group, 23C-3300 Smith Dr, Armstrong BC V0E 1B1; Tor'78; CCFP; Att Staff, Vernon Jubilee Hospital; Clinical Asst Prof, University of British Columbia; (250)546-8115; Fax. (250)546-2553.

SHERWOOD, Margaret L; 105-582 Goldstream Ave, Victoria BC V9B 2W7; Wes'79; (250)478-6242

SHERWOOD, Megan E; In-Patient Psychiatry, W1-715 12 Ave W, Vancouver BC V5Z 1M9; UBC'98; FRCSC; Psy. Staff, Providence Health Care - St Paul's Hospital; Staff, Vancouver General Hospital - Centennial Pavillion; Langs: Spanish; (604)875-4139

SHESHGIRI, Jitendra B; 1-1960 Dundas St W, Mississauga ON L5K 2R9; Karnatak (India)'80; MB BS; FRCS(Glas); CCFP; CCFP(E.M.); FCFP; Att Staff Geriatric Fund Enhancement, West Park Healthcare Centre; Preceptor Family & Community Med, University of Toronto; Langs: Marathi; Hindi; Urdu; Kanarese; (905)822-3993; Fax. (905)822-5522; Sheridanmedical@hotmail.com.

SHESHKO, Nykola; 306-595 Montreal Rd, Ottawa ON K1K 4L2; McG'78; CCFP; FCFP; Langs: Ukrainian; French; (613)744-3236; Fax. (613)744-5624.

SHETE, Charudutt D; TLC Medical Bldg, 102-5171 221A St, Langley BC V2Y 0A2; Pune (India)'82; MB BS; CM; FRCSC; GenSurg (Critical Care Medicine). Langs: Hindi; Punjabi; Urdu; Marathi; (604)539-1526; Fax. (604)539-1528.

SHETE, Shilpa C; 22190 48 Ave, Langley BC V3A 3N5; Bombay (India)'88; FRCPC; Psy. (604)530-3213

SHETH, Hinal; The Medical Place, 799 Bloor St W, Toronto ON M6G 1L8; McM'08; CCFP; Langs: Gujarati; (647)349-0053; Fax. (647)349-0063.

SHETH, Nikita T; Kingsridge Med Centre, 2-2015 Kingsridge Dr, Oakville ON L6M 4Y7; Bombay (India),'97; MB BS; CCFP; Langs: Gujarati; Hindi; Marathi; Punjabi; (905)827-3006; Fax. (905)825-9431.

SHETH, Sachiv; St Paul's Hosp, 2F-1081 Burrard St, Vancouver BC V6Z 1Y6; Georgia (USA)'04; Staff, Providence Health Care - St Paul's Hospital; (604)682-2344

SHETH, Tarang N; Trillium Hlth Ctr-Mississauga, 100 Queensway W, Mississauga ON L5B 1B8; Tor'98; FRCPC; DiagRad. Staff, Trillium Health Centre - Mississauga; Langs: Gujarati; (905)848-7100

SHETH, Tej N; Hamilton HS Corp-Gen Site, 509-237 Barton St E, Hamilton ON L8L 2X2; Tor'98; FRCPC; IntMed; Cardiol. Staff, Hamilton Health Sciences Centre - Hamilton General Hospital; Langs: Gujarati; (905)577-1423; Fax. (905)577-1474.

SHETHWALA, Nahid K; 331-125 Delhi St, Guelph ON N1E 4J5; Mumbai (India)'81; MRCP(UK); FRCPC; Peds. Langs: Hindi; Urdu; (519)822-6405; Fax. (519)822-7591.

SHETTAR, Channabasav B; Yarmouth Reg Hosp, 303-60 Vancouver St, Yarmouth NS B5A 2P5; Karnatak (India)'74; MB BS; BSc; Staff, Yarmouth Regional Hospital; (902)742-3541

SHETTY, Banakesari N; Yarmouth Reg Hosp, 319-60 Vancouver St, Yarmouth NS B5A 2P5; Karnatak (India)'83; MB BS; FRCS(Glas); FRCOphthOph(Eng); FRCSC; Ophth. Staff Ophth, Yarmouth Regional Hospital; (902)742-5097; Fax. (902)742-5097.

SHETTY, Geeta R; 101-140 Niagara St, St Catharines ON L2R 4L4; Bombay (India)'81; MB BS; FRC(Lond); FRCPC; Anes (Chronic Pain Management). Staff, Niagara Health System - St Catharines General Site; Langs: Hindi; Marathi; Kanarese; (905)684-9993; Fax. (905)684-7683.

SHETTY, Karunakara N; Queen Elizabeth Hosp, P O Box 6600 Stn Central 60 Riverside Dr, Charlottetown PE C1A 8T5; Mysore (India)'74; MB BS; DABIM; FACP; FRCPI(Ire); FRCPC; IntMed. Ac Staff IntMed, Queen Elizabeth Hospital; Langs: Hindi; Kanarese; (902)894-2111; Fax. (902)894-2918.

SHETTY, Maithili R; St Paul's Hosp, 1081 Burrard St, Vancouver BC V6Z 1Y6; Wes'04; FRCPC; Psy. Staff, Providence Health Care - St Paul's Hospital; (604)682-2344 x62427

SHETTY, Niren; North York Gen Hosp, 4001 Leslie St, North York ON M2K 1E1; Tor'05; CCFP; Staff, North York General Hospital; (416)756-6000; Fax. (416)756-6024.

SHETTY, Panduranga Y; 177 Russell St N, Sarnia ON N7T 6R2; Mysore (India)'74; MB BS; FRCP(Edin); MRCP(UK); FRCPC; IntMed. Staff, Bluewater Health - Charlotte Eleanor Englehart Hospital; Staff, Bluewater Health - Mitton Site; Langs: Kanarese; (519)332-1811; Fax. (519)332-0366.

SHETTY, Rakshay; The Hosp for Sick Children, 555 University Ave, Toronto ON M5G 1X8; Kasturba Medical College (India)'02; Clin Fellow, The Hospital For Sick Children; (416)813-6484; Fax. (416)813-5313.

SHETTY, Rathnakar B; 101-140 Niagara St, St Catharines ON L2R 4L4; Mysore (India)'73; MB BS; FRCOG; FRCSC; ObstGyn (Colposcopy). Staff, Niagara Health System - Ontario Street Site; Staff ObstGyn, Niagara Health System - St Catharines General Site; Langs: Kanarese; Hindi; Marathi; (905)684-9993; Fax. (905)684-7683.

SHEU, K Y Kevin; Station Square Med Clinic, 146-6200 McKay Ave, Burnaby BC V5H 4L7; Alb'00; CCFP; Langs: Taiwanese; Mandarin; (604)438-8288; Fax. (604)438-8289.

SHEVELL, Michael I; MUHC-Montrel Children's Hosp, C414-2300 rue Tupper, Montreal QC H3H 1P3; McG'84; FRCPC; Neur (Neonatal Neurology). Staff, McGill University Health Centre - Montreal Children's Hospital; Chef Pediatrics/assoc Prof Neurology & Peds, McGill University; Langs: English; French; (514)412-4467; Fax. (514)412-4373; michael.shevell@muhc.mcgill.ca.

SHEW, Raphael E; Cornelia Family Health Group, 91 Cornelia St W, Smiths Falls ON K7A 5L3; Ott'87; BSc; CCFP; Chair Dept of Family Med, Perth & Smiths Falls District Hospital - Smiths Falls Site; (613)283-1142; Fax. (613)283-9730; rrkjshew@hotmail.com.

SHEWCHUK, Jason R; Vancouver Gen Hosp, 899 12th Ave W, Vancouver BC V5Z 1M9; Man'98; FRCPC; DiagRad. Staff, Vancouver General Hospital - Centennial Pavillion; Staff, Royal Columbian Hospital; (604)875-4111

SHEWCHUK, John J; Tisdale Med Clinic, PO Box 1510, Tisdale SK S0E 1T0; Sask'76; BSc; CCFP; FCFP; Staff/Chief Family Med, Tisdale Hospital; Clin Instructor Family Med, University of Saskatchewan; (306)873-2619; Fax. (306)873-4489.

SHEWCHUN, James; PO Box 24 Stn Main RR 4, Fergus ON N1M 2W7; Tor'81; DiagRad. Staff Radiol/Dir Radiol Serv, West Parry Sound Health Centre.

SHI, Dawn D; Waterfront Med Centre, 266B Queens Quay W, Toronto ON M5J 1B5; Shanghai (China)'94; CCFP; Langs: Mandarin; (416)595-9699; Fax. (416)595-9698.

SHI, Kevin; Stein Med Clinic, 188-550 Burrard St, Vancouver BC V6C 2B5; Tor'03; CCFP; CCFP(E.M.); (604)688-5924

SHIAU, Carolyn J; Royal Columbian Hosp, 330 Columbia St E, New Westminster BC V3L 3W7; Tor'06; FRCPC; AnatPath. Staff, Royal Columbian Hospital; (604)520-4310

SHIAU, Judy Y; Ottawa Cardiovascular Centre, 502-1355 Bank St, Ottawa ON K1H 8K7; McG'96; FRCPC; IntMed. Staff, The Ottawa Hospital - General Campus; Langs: French; (613)738-1584; Fax. (613)738-9097; judyshiau@hotmail.com.

SHIBANI, Areej A; Univ of Western Ontario, D1000-1151 Richmond St, London ON N6A 5C1; Al Fateh (Libya)'00; AnatPath. (519)685-8500

SHIBANY, Ashraf G S S; Hampton Med Clinic, 6274 199 St NW, Edmonton AB T5T 2K4; (Other Foreign)'01; CCFP; Staff, Flin Flon General Hospital Inc; (780)486-7370

SHIBATA, Henry R; MUHC-Royal Victoria Hosp, A302-687 av des Pins O, Montreal QC H3A 1A1; Hiroshima (Japan)'55; BSc; MSc(ExpSurg.); FACS; GenSurg (Breast Cancer). Staff, McGill University Health Centre - Royal Victoria Hospital; Emeritus Chairman Medical Advisory Committee, Cedars Cancer Institute; Emeritus Prof Surg & Oncol, McGill University; Langs: Japanese; French; (514)843-1526; Fax. (514)843-1462; henry.shibata@muhc.mcgill.ca.

SHIBATA, Marcelo C; Misericordia Community Hosp, 16940 87 Ave NW, Edmonton AB T5R 4H5; (Brazil)'88; Staff Cardiac Sciences, Covenant Health - Misericordia Community Hospital; Clin Assoc Prof, University of Alberta; Langs: Portuguese; Spanish; (780)735-2255; Fax. (780)735-2257; marcelo.shibata@ualberta.ca.

SHIBATA, Mariko A; 1050 91 St SW, Edmonton AB T6X 0P2; Alb'09; CCFP; (780)463-7050

SHIBIL, Majid; 13608 160 Ave NW, Edmonton AB T6V 0B9; (780)998-2256

SHICHOR, T Miriam; Hamilton HS-Chedoke Site, PO Box 2000 Stn Lcd 1 2U1-1200 Main St W, Hamilton ON L8N 3Z5; Hebrew (Israel)'97; Staff, Hamilton Health Sciences Centre - McMaster University Medical Centre; Langs: Hebrew; (905)521-2100 x75166; Fax. (905)523-1224.

SHICK, Roger D; St Paul's Hosp, 4B 435-1081 Burrard St, Vancouver BC V6Z 1Y6; Man'68; FRCPC; Psy. Ac Staff, Providence Health Care - St Paul's Hospital; (604)682-2344 x62946; Fax. (604)806-8782.

SHICKH, Ali M; Professional Bldg, 301-222 King St E, Bowmanville ON L1C 1P6; Benghazi (Libya)'83; MB ChB; FRCPC; IntMed; Rheum. Staff, Lakeridge Health - Bowmanville Site; Langs: Arabic; (905)697-8022; Fax. (905)697-6218.

SHIELDS, Claude; Ctr Hosp Affilie-Enfant-Jesus, 1401 18e rue, Quebec QC G1J 1Z4; Laval'73; LMCC; Hem (P.Q.); IntMed (Hematological Oncology). Staff, Centre Hospitalier Affilié Universitaire de Québec - Hôpital De L'Enfant Jésus; Langs: English; (418)649-5703; Fax. (418)649-5740.

SHIELDS, Jean; Clinique Med Jean Shields, 531 rue Saint-Joseph, Saint-Raymond QC G3L 1K7; Laval'81; (418)337-4293; Fax. (418)337-4295.

SHIELDS, Jean-Francois; Hotel-Dieu de Levis, 143 rue Wolfe, Levis QC G6V 3Z1; Laval'07; EmergMed (Family Medicine). Staff, Hôpital Laval; (418)835-7121

SHIELDS, Stewart D; Summit Centre, PO Box 23002 RPO Citadel, St. Albert AB T8N 6Z9; Alb'90; CCFP; CCFP(E.M.); Staff, Sturgeon Community Hospital; (780)498-7805

SHIELDS, William R; 1923 9 Ave S, Lethbridge AB T1J 1W8; Alb'82; BMedSci; FRCSC; Urol. Staff, Chinook Regional Hospital; (403)329-6653; Fax. (403)380-4024.

SHIELDS, Yehudi P; 203-1223 St Clair Ave W, Toronto ON M6E 1B5; Tor'62; Assoc Staff, Mount Sinai Hospital; Langs: Yiddish; Hebrew; (416)652-3133; Fax. (416)652-6472.

SHIER, Arthur A; Tsawwassen Med Clinic, 201-1077 56 St, Delta BC V4L 2A2; Man'58; Langs: German; (604)943-1131; Fax. (604)943-2617.

SHIER, Donald J; 2971 Kingston Rd, Scarborough ON M1M 1P1; Tor'57; Staff, The Scarborough Hospital - General Campus; Staff, Rouge Valley Health System - Centenary Health Centre Site; (416)261-4025; Fax. (416)261-9398.

SHIER, Edward C; Phoenix Med Centre, 106-2155 10 Ave, Prince George BC V2M 5J6; UBC'09; CCFP; (250)563-5111

SHIER, Luke R; University of Alberta Hosp, 4B2 19 WCM-8440 112 St NW, Edmonton AB T6G 2B7; Tor'98; FRCPC; IntMed; HemPath; Hem. Staff, University of Alberta Hospital; (780)407-2012; Fax. (780)407-8599.

SHIER, R Michael P; Sunnybrook Hlth Sciences Ctre, B610-2075 Bayview Ave, Toronto ON M4N 3M5; Tor'68; BSc; FRCSC; ObstGyn (Colposcopy)., Sunnybrook Health Sciences Centre; Prof, University of Toronto; (416)480-6726; Fax. (416)480-4713.

SHIEVITZ, Alan L; Trillium Hlth Ctr-Mississauga, 100 Queensway W, Mississauga ON L5B 1B8; Wes'94; CCFP; CCFP(E.M.); Staff, Trillium Health Centre - Mississauga; Coroner, City Of Toronto; (905)848-7600; partyal@rogers.com.

SHIFF, Daniel A; William Osler HC-Brampton, S2 749-2100 Bovaird Dr E, Brampton ON L6R 3J7; Tor'04; FRCPC; DiagRad. Staff, William Osler Health System - Brampton Civic Hospital; (905)494-2120

SHIFF, Dori; SMBD Jewish Gen Hosp, 3755 ch Cote-Sainte-Catherine, Montreal QC H3T 1E2; Mon'08; CCFP; Staff, Sir Mortimer B Davis Jewish General; (514)340-8222

SHIFF, Natalie J; Royal University Hosp, 103 Hospital Dr, Saskatoon SK S7N 0W8; Cal'02; FRCPC; Peds (Clinician Investigator Program); Rheum. Staff, Royal University Hospital; (306)966-8112; Fax. (306)966-8640.

SHIFFMAN, Frank H; Victoria Gen Hosp, 2340 Pembina Hwy, Winnipeg MB R3T 2E8; Man'90; Staff, Victoria General Hospital; (204)269-3570

SHIFFMAN, Howard N; Medical Office, 8000 Bathurst St, Thornhill ON L4J 0B8; Sask'83; CCFP; Lecturer Family Med, The Scarborough Hospital - General Campus; (905)709-9709; Fax. (905)709-9701.

SHIFFMAN, Kevin; Ont Shores Ctre For Mental Hlt, 700 Gordon St, Whitby ON L1N 5S9; Stellenbosch (South Africa)'86; MB ChB; FRCPC; Psy. Staff, Ontario Shores Centre for Mental Health Sciences; Langs: Afrikaans; Hebrew; (905)668-5881; Fax. (905)430-4020; drshiffman@rogers.com.

SHIFFMAN, Norman J; 2533 Danforth Ave, Toronto ON M4C 1L1; Ott'74; FRCPC; Derm. Staff, Toronto East General Hospital Inc; Lecturer Med, University of Toronto; (416)698-5521; Fax. (416)698-5721.

SHIGEISHI, Stephen A; Alpine Med Clinic, PO Bag 4000 Stn Main 211 Bear St, Banff AB T1L 1J8; Qns'00; CCFP; (403)762-3155; Fax. (403)762-5797.

SHIH, Aaron C T; Markland Wood Med Clinic, 4335 Bloor St W, Etobicoke ON M9C 2A5; Tor'97; CCFP; Langs: Mandarin; Taiwanese; (416)695-8878; Fax. (416)695-2622.

SHIH, David; 6311 129 St NW, Edmonton AB T6H 3X9; UBC'74; DPH; FRCPC; Psy (Child & Adolescent Psychiatry). (780)436-2567

SHIH, Elizabeth M; Royal Alexandra Hosp, 541 CSC-10240 Kingsway NW, Edmonton AB T5H 3V9; Alb'07; EmergMed. Staff, Royal Alexandra Hospital; (780)735-4442; Fax. (780)735-4916.

SHIH, Michael; 7-895 Brant St, Burlington ON L7R 2J6; Tor'77; Ac Staff, Joseph Brant Memorial Hospital; Langs: Chinese; (905)639-9006

SHIH, Mike C M; 7-110 Ansley Grove Rd, Woodbridge ON L4L 3R1; Tor'82; Ac Staff, William Osler Health System - Etobicoke General Hospital; Langs: Chinese; (905)851-8319; Fax. (905)851-8319.

SHIH, Peter D; 110-3020 Lincoln Ave, Coquitlam BC V3B 6B4; Man'76; Langs: Cantonese; (604)464-8211; Fax. (604)464-6101.

SHIH, Robert H; Markland Wood Med Clinic, 4335 Bloor St W, Etobicoke ON M9C 2A5; Qns'96; CCFP; FCFP; Langs: Taiwanese; Mandarin; Spanish; (416)695-8878; Fax. (416)695-2622; robertshih@doctor.com.

SHIH, Warren W J; Dartmouth Med Centre, 206-46 Portland St, Dartmouth NS B2Y 1H4; Dal'93; FRCSC; GenSurg. (902)461-4549; Fax. (902)461-9967.

SHIHATA, Shadi S A; Foothills Med Centre, 1403 29 St NW, Calgary AB T2N 2T9; Abdul Aziz (Saudi Arabia)'01; FRCSC; OrthSurg. Staff, Foothills Medical Centre; (403)944-1110

SHIK, John W C; Health Sciences Centre, 5326A-300 Prince Philip Dr, St. John's NL A1B 3V6; Tor'00; FRCPC; IntMed; Nephrol. Ac Staff, Waterford Hospital; Ac Staff, Health Sciences Centre; Asst Prof Med, Memorial University Of Newfoundland; (709)777-6300; Fax. (709)777-6656.

SHILASH, Basil M A; Brampton East Health Centre, 200-300 Main St N, Brampton ON L6V 4H6; Al-Fateh (Libya)'98; CCFP; Langs: Arabic; (905)451-1806; Fax. (905)451-8272.

SHILHAN, Caroline B E; F W Green Medical Clinic, 1629 Baker St, Cranbrook BC V1C 1B4; Ott'04; CCFP; Langs: Bilingual(English/French); (250)426-6601

SHILLER, Mitchell B; 100-14770 boul de Pierrefonds, Pierrefonds QC H9H 4Y6; McG'84; FRCPC; Peds. adj Prof, McGill University Health Centre - Montreal Children's Hospital; (514)696-2442; Fax. (514)624-3099.

SHILLETTO, D W Nicholas; Ontario Ctr for Maternal-Fetal, 310-1333 Sheppard Ave E, North York ON M2J 1V1; Dublin (Ireland)'88; BA; MB BCh; FRCSC; ObstGyn (Maternal Fetal Medicine). Staff Perinatol, North York General Hospital; Court Staff, Mackenzie Richmond Hill Hospital; (416)496-0488; Fax. (416)496-9790; nicholas.shilletto@utoronto.ca.

SHILLINGTON, John R; Sheldon M Chumir Urgent Care, 1213 4 St SW, Calgary AB T2R 0X7; UBC'90; CCFP; (403)955-6011; Fax. (403)955-6023.

SHIM, Katharine J; Durham Reg Cancer Centre, 1 Hospital Crt, Oshawa ON L1G 2B9; McM'04; FRCPC; IntMed; MedOncol. Staff, Lakeridge Health - Oshawa Site; (905)576-8711; Fax. (905)721-6103; kshim@lakeridgehealth.on.ca.

SHIM, Paul S; Brockville Gen Hosp, 75 Charles St, Brockville ON K6V 1S8; Ott'02; FRCSC; OrthSurg. Staff, Brockville General Hospital - Charles Street; (613)498-0368; Fax. (613)498-3961.

SHIMANOVSKY, Ludmila A; Maple Med Centre, 204-955 Major Mackenzie Dr, Vaughan ON L6A 4P9; Leningrad (Russia (Federation))'83; CCFP; Langs: Russian; (905)533-5400; Fax. (905)533-5477; drmilashim@hotmail.com.

SHIME, Jerry; Women's College Hosp, E316-76 Grenville St, Toronto ON M5S 1B2; Tor'64; BA; MSc; FRCSC; ObstGyn (Gynecology). Staff, Women's College Hospital; Prof, University of Toronto; (416)323-6126; Fax. (416)323-6148.

SHIMIZU, Jed; Dominion Med Centre, 2383 111 St NW, Edmonton AB T6J 5E5; UBC'10; CCFP; (780)436-0020; Fax. (780)436-0603.

SHIMON, Laith D; Cape Breton Health Care Comple, 1482 George St, Sydney NS B1P 1P3; Mosul (Iraq)'91; MB ChB; FRCPC; Neur;CCFP; Staff, Cape Breton Healthcare Complex; Langs: Arabic; Assyrian; (902)567-6139; Fax. (902)567-3613.

SHIN, Alice J; West End Family Care Clinic, 80 Michael Cowpland Dr, Ottawa ON K2M 1P6; Ott'09; CCFP; (613)599-3321; Fax. (613)599-3366.

SHIN, Amanda L; 113-1077 56th St, Delta BC V4L 2A2; Sask'01; FRCPC; IntMed. (604)948-0277

SHIN, Anne Y; Mackenzie Richmond Hill Hosp, 10 Trench St, Richmond Hill ON L4C 4Z3; Tor'92; BSc; FRCPC; IntMed. Staff, Mackenzie Richmond Hill Hospital; Langs: Korean; (905)883-1212

SHIN, Doo Ho; Surrey Mem Hosp, 13750 96 Ave, Surrey BC V3V 1Z2; Seoul (South Korea)'68; AB; FRCPC; GenPath; AnatPath. Staff Path, Surrey Memorial Hospital; Staff Path, Royal Columbian Hospital; Langs: Korean; (604)585-5613; Fax. (604)585-5562.

SHIN, Frank; Thames Valley FHT-Whitehills M, 1225 Wonderland Rd N, London ON N6G 2V9; Qns'93; CCFP; FCFP; Staff, London Health Sciences Centre - University Hospital; Staff, Chatham-Kent Health Alliance - Sydenham Hospital Campus; Asst Teacher, University of Western Ontario; (519)472-0040; Fax. (519)472-7732; fshin@uwo.ca.

SHIN, John H; 346-1800 Sheppard Ave E PO Box 78, North York ON M2J 5A7; McM'91; DAB(Ophth); FAAO; FRCSC; Ophth. (416)491-0555; Fax. (416)491-0556.

SHIN, Karen H; Scarborough Hosp-Birchmount, 3030 Birchmount Rd, Scarborough ON M1W 3W3; McM'01; FRCPC; Psy. Staff, Sunnybrook Health Sciences Centre; Staff, The Scarborough Hospital - Birchmount Campus; (416)495-2400; Fax. (416)495-2426.

SHIN, Phillip C; North York Gen Hosp, 4001 Leslie St, North York ON M2K 1E1; Tor'01; FRCPC; IntMed; Critical Care Medicine. Staff, North York General Hospital; (416)756-6000

SHIN, Sharon L; St Michael's Hosp, 3CC 141-30 Bond St, Toronto ON M5B 1W8; Tor'04; FRCPC; DiagRad. Staff, St Michael's Hospital; (416)864-5692; Fax. (416)864-5380.

SHIN, T W Thomas; 113-1077 56th St, Delta BC V4L 2A2; UBC'97; LMCC; FRCPC; IntMed. Staff, University Hospital of Northern British Columbia; (604)948-0277

SHIN, Vincent H; Toronto East Gen & Orth Hosp, 825 Coxwell Ave, East York ON M4C 3E7; Ott'98; FRCPC; DiagRad. Staff, Toronto East General Hospital Inc; (416)469-6076

SHIN, Whun Yong; 210-670 Bloor St W, Toronto ON M6G 1L2; Tor'83; Langs: Korean; (416)530-0007; Fax. (416)530-4566.

SHINDER, Janet; 407-5885 ch Cote-des-Neiges, Montreal QC H3S 2T2; McG'75; FRCSC; ObstGyn (P.Q.). Staff, McGill University Health Centre - Montreal Children's Hospital; Langs: French; (514)735-4933; Fax. (514)735-7811.

SHINDER, Michael E; Clinique MDM, 102-6955 boul Taschereau, Brossard QC J4Z 1A7; Tor'80; Langs: French; (450)656-2310; Fax. (450)656-2619.

SHINDER, Rowen; The Moncton Hosp, 135 Macbeath Ave, Moncton NB E1C 6Z8; Tor'88; FRCPC; AnatPath. Head Anath Path Services, The Moncton Hospital; (506)857-5300

SHINDMAN, Judith A; 112 Ava Road, Toronto ON M6C 1W1; Tor'75; Dep Dir Med Affairs, Sanofi Pasteur Ltd; Langs: French; (416)667-2884; Fax. (416)667-2850.

SHINE, Joseph F; 304-5450 ch Cote-des-Neiges, Montreal QC H3T 1Y6; McM'79; FRCSC; ObstGyn. Staff, St Mary's Hospital Centre; Staff, Sir Mortimer B Davis Jewish General; adj Prof, McGill University; Langs: French; (514)737-4393; Fax. (514)737-5639; jfshine@hotmail.com.

SHINE, Kevin S; The Credit Valley Hosp, 2200 Eglinton Ave W, Mississauga ON L5M 2N1; Tor'84; FRCPC; Anes. Staff, The Credit Valley Hospital; (905)813-2200

SHINE, Robert M; Sudbury Reg Hosp-Laurentian, 41 Ramsey Lake Rd, Sudbury ON P3E 5J1; Dublin (Ireland)'69; MB ChB; Health Sciences North-Laurentian Site; Court Staff, North Bay Regional Health Centre - Kirkwood; Asst Prof Anes, University of Ottawa; (705)675-4733; Fax. (705)671-5458.

SHING, Molly; Foothills Med Centre, 1403 29 St NW, Calgary AB T2N 2T9; Man'96; FRCPC; Anes. Staff Anes, Foothills Medical Centre; (403)944-1430; Fax. (403)944-2425.

SHINK, Christine; Clinique Med du Vieux Fort, 7777 boul de la Rive-Sud, Levis QC G6V 6Z1; Laval'85; Staff, Hôtel-Dieu de Lévis; (418)835-5612; Fax. (418)835-3927.

SHINK, Daniel; Clinique Med Vieux Fort, 7777 boul de la Rive-Sud, Levis QC G6V 6Z1; Laval'89; (418)835-5612; Fax. (418)835-3927.

SHINK, Nancy; Clinique Med Ste-Croix, 6350 rue Principale, Sainte-Croix QC G0S 2H0; Laval'86; Staff, Hôtel-Dieu de Lévis; (418)926-3260; Fax. (418)926-2014; nancy.shink@gmf.gouv.qc.ca.

SHINKARUK, Kelly S; Chronic Pain Centre, 67W-2210 2 St SW, Calgary AB T2S 3C3; Alb'04; Anes. (403)943-9900

SHINOFF, Susan; William Osler Health Centre, 205-100 Humber College Blvd, Etobicoke ON M9V 5G4; Cal'92; FRCSC; ObstGyn. Staff, William Osler Health System - Etobicoke General Hospital; Langs: French; (416)749-3620; Fax. (416)749-3640.

SHINTANI, Jessica M; Khatsalano Med Clinic, 3525 4th Ave W, Vancouver BC V6R 1N9; UBC'84; CCFP; Staff, Westcoast Women's Clinic For Midlife Health; (604)738-9601

SHINYANBOLA, Olafimihan O; Prairie North Health Centre, 4806 50th St, Lloydminster SK S9V 0M9; (306)820-5997; Fax. (306)820-5978.

SHIOZAKI, Ian K; Rideau Med Centre, 2 John St, Newboro ON K0G 1P0; Wes'79; (613)272-2500; Fax. (613)272-2838.

SHIPLEY, James H; Lakeridge Hlth Corp-Oshawa, 1 Hospital Crt, Oshawa ON L1G 2B9; Cal'82; CCFP; CCFP(E.M.); FCFP; Staff, Lakeridge Health - Oshawa Site; (905)576-8711

SHIPLEY, William F; 427 Bridge St E, Belleville ON K8N 1P9; Tor'74; CCFP; FCFP; Asst Prof Adjunct Family Practice, Queen's University; (613)962-1260; Fax. (613)962-4039; shipbill@hotmail.com.

SHIPMAN, Richard R; Dr Bernstein Hlth & Diet Clini, 365 Front St N, Belleville ON K8P 5A5; Cambridge (England)'64; MB ChB; DCH; DRCOG; MRACP; Peds (Bariatric Medicine). Physician, Dr Bernstein Health & Diet Clinic; Staff, Dr Bernstein Health & Diet Clinic; (613)967-2228; Fax. (613)967-5847; richard.shipman@shaw.ca.

SHIR, Yoram; MUHC-Montreal Gen Hosp, E19 133-1650 Av Cedar, Montreal QC H3G 1A4; Jerusalem (Israel)'83; Staff, McGill University Health Centre - Montreal General Campus; (514)934-1934 x48222; Fax. (514)934-8096.

SHIRALI, Hemant R; Ashgrove Med Centre, 307-6633 Highway 7, Markham ON L3P 7P2; Pune (India)'82; MB BS; MCh; FRCSC; OrthSurg (Lower Limb Surgery). Staff OrthSurg, Markham Stouffville Hospital; Langs: Hindi; Marathi; (905)471-2221; Fax. (905)471-1070.

SHIRLEY, Donald A; TLC Medical Centre, 305-5171 221A St, Langley BC V2Y 0A2; West Indies (Jamaica)'70; MB BS; FRCSC; GenSurg. Staff, Langley Memorial Hospital; Staff, Peace Arch Hospital; (604)534-9288; Fax. (604)534-9958.

SHIRLEY, Margaret A; Medical Arts Bldg, 302-42 Glen Allan Dr, Bridgewater NS B4V 3N2; Dal'86; DABIM; PhD; FRCPC; IntMed (Infectious Diseases). Staff, South Shore Regional Hospital; (902)543-5108; Fax. (902)543-0894; mshirley@ca.inter.net.

SHIRRIFF, Michael D; Medical Arts Bldg, 103-30 King St, Trenton ON K8V 6B1; Cal'83; Court Staff, QHC Trenton Memorial; (613)394-4868; Fax. (613)392-2608.

SHIRZAD, Shahin; Vancouver Gen Hosp, 855 12th Ave W, Vancouver BC V5Z 1M9; UBC'05; FRCPC; EmergMed. Staff Emerg, Vancouver General Hospital - Centennial Pavillion; (604)875-4111

SHIU, Dominic; Allwood Med Clinic, 102-2752 Allwood St, Abbotsford BC V2T 3R7; Tor'88; BSc; Langs: Cantonese; (604)850-6893; Fax. (604)850-6896.

SHIU, Patrick K Y; Clover Care Med Clinic, 102-17770 56 Ave, Surrey BC V3S 1C7; Tor'79; Langs: Chinese; (604)574-7883

SHIU, Simon S; 130-5890 No. 3 Rd, Richmond BC V6X 3P6; Alb'77; (604)278-6186; Fax. (604)278-0026.

SHIVAKUMAR, Kuppuswami; Northeast Mental Health Centre, 680 Kirkwood Dr, Sudbury ON P3E 1X3; Tver State Medical Academy (Other Foreign)'92; FRCPC; Psy. Staff, North Bay Regional Health Centre - Kirkwood; Prog Dir Psychiatry, Northern Ontario School of Medicine; (705)675-5900; Fax. (705)671-3031.

SHIVAKUMAR, Ranganayaky; 344 Riverside Dr, Sudbury ON P3E 1H7; Madras (India)'93; FRCPC; IntMed (Hematology Pathology). Staff, Health Sciences North-Laurentian Site; Langs: Tamil; (705)586-3101; Fax. (705)586-3103.

SHIVAKUMAR, Sudeep P; Queen Elizabeth II HSC-Victori, 432-1276 South Park St, Halifax NS B3H 2Y9; Qns'03; FRCPC; IntMed; Hem. Staff, Queen Elizabeth II Health Sciences Centre - Victoria General Site; (902)473-3779; Fax. (902)473-4447.

SHIVDASANI, Kumar; Vancouver Gen Hosp, 855 12th Ave W, Vancouver BC V5Z 1M9; McM'89; CCFP; Staff, Vancouver General Hospital - Centennial Pavillion; Staff, Renu Cosmetic; (604)822-7121

SHIVJI, Farzana; Sheldon M Chumir Urgent Care, 1213 4 St SW, Calgary AB T2R 0X7; Cal'00; CCFP; Physician, Sheldon M Chumir Urgent Care Physician Group; (403)955-6011; Fax. (403)955-6023; farzana.shivji@albertahealthservices.ca.

SHIZAS, Athanasios T; North Oshawa Med Centre, 103-1400 Ritson Rd N, Oshawa ON L1G 7W4; Tor'92; Langs: Greek; (905)579-4615; Fax. (905)433-1838.

SHKLANKA, Karen P; PO Box 74540 Kitsilano Rpo, Vancouver BC V6K 4P4; UBC'88; CCFP; Locum Tenens, Vancouver Island Health Authority; Locum Tenens, Lady Minto Gulf Islands Hospital.

SHKLAR, Jaroslav O; 201-3101 Bloor St W, Etobicoke ON M8X 2W2; Tor'67; Staff Teacher Famiy & CommunMed, Toronto Western Hospital - University Health Network; Asst Prof Family & Commun Med, University of Toronto; Langs: Polish; German; Russian; (416)231-1224; Fax. (416)231-1236.

SHKRUM, Michael J; London HSC-University Campus, PO Box 5339 Stn B 339 Windermere Rd, London ON N6A 5A5; Wes'78; DABAP; FRCPC; AnatPath (Forensic Pathology). Staff, London Health Sciences Centre - University Hospital; (519)685-8500 x36357; Fax. (519)663-2930; mike.shkrum@lhsc.on.ca.

SHLIK, Jakov; Royal Ottawa Hlth Care Group, CB1-1145 Carling Ave, Ottawa ON K1Z 7K4; Tartu (Estonia)'85; PhD; Staff, Royal Ottawa Mental Health Centre - Royal Ottawa Health Care Group; Langs: Estonian; Russian; (613)722-6521; Fax. (613)761-3602.

SHLOMOVITZ, Eran; Mount Sinai Hosp, 440-600 University Ave, Toronto ON M5G 1X5; Wes'06; FRCPC; DiagRad. Staff, Mount Sinai Hospital; Langs: Hebrew; (416)586-8359

SHMOORKOFF, Jeffrey F; Westgate Family Med Clinic, 180-17010 90 Ave NW, Edmonton AB T5T 1L6; Alb'92; BSc; CCFP; Staff, Misericordia Community Hospital; (780)487-4260; Fax. (780)481-6776.

SHMORGUN, Doron; Ottawa Fertility Centre, 955 Green Valley Cres, Ottawa ON K2C 3V4; McM'02; FRCSC; ObstGyn. Staff, Cornwall Community Hospital; Langs: Hebrew; Russian; (613)686-3378; Fax. (613)225-9736.

SHMUILOVICH, Olga; London X-ray Associates, 450 Central Ave, London ON N6B 2E8; Patrice Lumumba People's Friendship Univ (Other Foreign)'00; (519)672-7900

SHNIDER, Maurice; Riverwood Med Centre, 1295 Pembina Hwy, Winnipeg MB R3T 2B3; Man'51; Staff, Victoria General Hospital; Semi-Retired.

SHNISHAH, Abdalrhman A; GP Med Clinic, 12225 99 St, Grande Prairie AB T8V 6X9; Al-Arab Medical University (Other Foreign); CCFP; Langs: Arabic; (780)533-4444; Fax. (780)533-4443.

SHOAIB, Muhammad; Malone Med Clinic, 4955 41st Ave, Drayton Valley AB T7A 1V4; (Other Foreign)'91; (780)542-3366; Fax. (780)542-6207.

SHOBOLA, Oladayo D; Hotel-Dieu Grace Hosp, 1030 Ouellette Ave, Windsor ON N9A 1E1; Ibadan (Nigeria)'87; Staff, Hôtel-Dieu Grace Hospital; (519)973-4411

SHOCHAT, Gina; New Inner City Clinic, 69 Queen St E, Toronto ON M5C 1R8; Cape Town (South Africa)'58; CCFP; Langs: Afrikaans; Yiddish.

SHOEBRIDGE, Jeffrey J; Medical Arts Bldg, 3-165 Plymouth Rd, Welland ON L3B 3E1; Wes'07; FRCSC; Urol. Staff, London Health Sciences Centre - Victoria Campus; (905)735-1375; Fax. (905)735-1696.

SHOEMAKER, Christopher A; North Hamilton Comm Hlth Ctre, 438 Hughson St N, Hamilton ON L8L 4N5; Qns'75; (905)523-6611; Fax. (905)523-8735.

SHOEMAKER, Elisabeth A; Orchardview Med Centre, 100-155 Main St E, Grimsby ON L3M 1P2; Tor'81; CCFP; FCFP; Ac Staff, West Lincoln Memorial Hospital; (905)945-5476; Fax. (905)945-7707.

SHOEMAKER, Gerard J; London HSC-University Hosp, PO Box 5339 Stn B C6 131-339 Windermere Rd, London ON N6A 5A5; McM'95; FRCPC; IntMed; Cardiol. Staff, London Health Sciences Centre - University Hospital; (519)663-3485; Fax. (519)663-3484.

SHOESMITH, Christen L; London HSC-Univ Campus Site, PO Box 5339 Stn B C7 119A-339 Windermere Rd, London ON N6A 5A5; Man'00; FRCPC; Neur (Neuromuscular Diseases). Staff, London Health Sciences Centre - University Hospital; (519)663-3597; Fax. (519)663-3609.

SHOESMITH, David R; Fort St John Med Clinic, 10011 96 St, Fort St. John BC V1J 3P3; (Other Foreign)'10; CCFP; (250)785-6677

SHOESMITH, Trevor W; Highland Family Practice, 107C-1966 Guthrie Rd, Comox BC V9M 3X7; Man'02; CCFP; (250)890-0919; Fax. (250)890-0929.

SHOGAN, Ahmad T K; Grey Bruce Health Services, PO Box 1800 Stn M 1800 8 St E, Owen Sound ON N4K 6M9; (Jordan)'87; AnatPath (Clinical Pathology). Staff, Grey Bruce Health Services - Owen Sound; (519)376-2121

SHOGILEV, Howard P; 2682 Eglinton Ave E, Scarborough ON M1K 2S3; Tor'72; Ac Staff, The Scarborough Hospital - General Campus; (416)269-2100; Fax. (416)269-2147.

SHOHAM-HAZON, Nir; Chaleur Reg Hosp, 1750 Sunset Dr, Bathurst NB E2A 4L7; Semmelweis (Hungary)'03; Staff, Hopital Regional Chaleur; (506)544-3000

SHOICHET, Arnold J; Medicinal Cannabis Resource Ct, 450 Nanaimo St, Vancouver BC V5L 4W3; Tor'69; Assoc Staff, Mission Memorial Hospital; Staff, The Fraser Valley Maternity Group; (604)566-9391

SHOICHET, Roy P; Doctors Hosp Phase 1, 585-340 College St, Toronto ON M5T 3A9; Tor'63; AB; FRCPC; Psy. Ac Staff, Toronto Western Hospital - University Health Network; University of Toronto; (416)603-1435; Fax. (416)603-3208.

SHOICHET, William N; Saanich Med Centre, 3491 Saanich Rd, Victoria BC V8X 1W8; Tor'71; Staff, Royal Jubilee Hospital; Staff, Victoria General Hospital; (250)475-2251; Fax. (250)475-3530.

SHOJA, Sheila; Gordon & Leslie Diamond H C, 8181-2775 Laurel St, Vancouver BC V5Z 1M9; UBC'00; FRCPC; Psy. Staff, Vancouver General Hospital - Centennial Pavillion; Staff, Gordon & Leslie Diamond Health Care Centre; (604)875-4809

SHOJANIA, Kamran; Business Bldg, 802-1200 Burrard St, Vancouver BC V6Z 2C7; UBC'89; LMCC; FACRheum; FRCPC; IntMed; Rheum. Staff, Richmond Hospital; Staff, Vancouver General Hospital - Centennial Pavillion; Staff, Peace Arch Hospital; Dir Clinical Trials, Arthritis Research Centre of Canada; Clinical Asst Prof, University of British Columbia; (604)806-9400; Fax. (604)269-3736.

SHOJANIA, Kaveh G; Sunnybrook Hlth Sciences Ctre, H468-2075 Bayview Ave, Toronto ON M4N 3M5; Man'94; Staff, Sunnybrook Health Sciences Centre; (416)480-6100; Fax. (416)480-6777.

SHOJANIA, Nima; Westside Rheumatology, 101-3685 Brown Rd, Westbank BC V4T 1P7; UBC'96; FRCPC; IntMed; Rheum. (778)754-5559

SHOKEIR, M Omar; 202-15388 24 Ave, Surrey BC V4A 2J2; Sask'91; FRCPC; GenPath. Staff, Calgary Laboratory Services.

SHOKER, Ahmed S A H; St Paul's Hosp, B2 13-1702 20th St W, Saskatoon SK S7M 0Z9; Alexandria (Egypt)'75; MB ChB; FRCPC; IntMed (Transplantation); Nephrol. Staff, St Paul's Hospital (Grey Nuns) of Saskatoon; Prof Med, University of Saskatchewan; Langs: Arabic; (306)655-5934; Fax. (306)655-5959.

SHOKRAVI, Mohammad B; Northmount Med Centre, 903-145 13th St E, North Vancouver BC V7L 2L4; Alb'93; FRCPC; Derm. Langs: Farsi; (604)984-1244; Fax. (604)984-1243.

SHOKRI, Sharareh; Englehart & District FHT, PO Box 1110 63 5th St, Englehart ON P0J 1H0; Tehran (Iran)'93; CCFP; (705)544-2321

SHOKRY, Phoebe E; Markham Stouffville Hosp, PO Box 1800 Stn Main 381 Church St, Markham ON L3P 7P3; Alexandria (Egypt)'72; FRCPC; AnatPath. Med Dir/Chief Path & Lab Med, Markham Stouffville Hospital; Langs: Arabic; (905)472-7046; Fax. (905)472-7133.

SHOLTER, Dalton E; 124 Street Med Group, 10839 124 St NW, Edmonton AB T5M 0H4; Sask'92; FRCPC; IntMed; Rheum. Staff, Royal Alexandra Hospital; Staff, University of Alberta Hospital; Staff, Glenrose Rehabilitation Hospital; (780)455-3138; Fax. (780)455-3394.

SHOLZBERG, Michelle; St Michael's Hosp, 2 080-30 Bond St, Toronto ON M5B 1W8; McG'06; MDCM; FRCPC; IntMed; Hem. Staff, St Michael's Hospital; (416)864-5389; Fax. (416)864-5127.

SHOMAIR, Garry Y; 705-55 Eglinton Ave E, Toronto ON M4P 1G8; Tor'74; DCP; FRCPC; Psy (Child & Adolescent Psychiatry). Consultant Telepsych, The Hospital For Sick Children; Lecturer, University of Toronto; (416)488-5189; Fax. (416)486-8468; Garry@Shomair.com.

SHOMAN, Nael M; St Paul's Hosp, B 410-1702 20th St W, Saskatoon SK S7M 0Z9; Sask'04; FRCSC; Otol (Head & Neck Surgery). Staff, St Paul's Hospital (Grey Nuns) of Saskatoon; (306)655-5904; Fax. (306)655-5892.

SHONE, Neal A; 404-2151 McCallum Rd, Abbotsford BC V2S 3N8; Stellenbosch (South Africa)'86; MB ChB; FRCSC; ObstGyn (Obstetrics). Langs: Afrikaans; (604)870-0407; Fax. (604)870-0207.

SHONUBI, Adeyemi O; Airdrie Med Clinic, 10-620 1 Ave NW, Airdrie AB T4B 2R3; (Other Foreign)'94; CCFP; (403)948-3109; Fax. (403)948-6284.

SHOONER, Caroline A; Queen Charlotte Med Clinic, PO Box 9, Queen Charlotte BC V0T 1S0; McG'96; CCFP; Langs: Czech; French; (250)559-4447; Fax. (250)559-8037.

SHOONER, Karl; Coop Solidarite Shooner-Jauvin, 10A rue Georges, Pierreville QC J0G 1J0; Sher'78; Staff, Hôtel-Dieu de Sorel; (450)568-3296; Fax. (450)568-0333.

SHOPE, Kayode O; 1412 17 St S, Cranbrook BC V1C 4S3; Benin (Nigeria)'95; MB BS; Staff, East Kootenay Regional Hospital; (250)426-5281

SHOPPOFF, Lina A; 58A Anson Dr, Iroquois Falls ON P0K 1E0; Ott'09; CCFP; Langs: Bilingual(English/French); (705)258-4156; Fax. (705)258-4159.

SHORE, Donna A; Carling-Broadview Med Bldg, 302-770 Broadview Ave, Ottawa ON K2A 3Z3; Ott'85; CCFP; FCFP; (613)721-6788; Fax. (613)721-6789.

SHORE, Eliane M; 5F-61 Queen St E, East York ON M4C 2T2; Tor'06; FRCSC; ObstGyn. (416)360-4000; Fax. (416)864-5545.

SHORE, Frederica D; 101-40 Westmore Dr, Etobicoke ON M9V 4C2; Tor'79; Staff, William Osler Health System - Etobicoke General Hospital; Med Advisor, Leasureworld Nursing Home; Med Dir, Humber Valley Terrace; (416)745-0100; Fax. (416)745-6604.

SHORE, Resa S; 4132 Main St, Vancouver BC V5V 3P7; McM'78; FRCPC; Psy (Affective Disorders). Staff, Ridge Meadows Hospital & Health Care Centre; Ac Staff In-Patient Psy, Providence Health Care - St Paul's Hospital; Clin Assoc Prof, University of British Columbia; (604)876-8414

SHORE, Stephen M; 106-20103 40 Ave, Langley BC V3A 2W3; Mem'73; BMedSci; BSc; Clin Assoc Prof Family Practice, University of British Columbia; (604)533-6626; Fax. (604)534-1173.

SHOREY, Sanam S; Brampton Med Bldg, 307-164 Queen St E, Brampton ON L6V 1B4; Tor'99; FRCPC; IntMed (Endocrinology); Endocrin&Metab. Assoc Staff, William Osler Health System - Brampton Civic Hospital; Langs: Hindi; (905)595-0559; Fax. (905)595-0579.

SHORSER, S Ronald; Mount Dennis Med Group, 98 Guestville Ave, Toronto ON M6N 4N6; Tor'80; Staff, Humber River Regional Hospital - Church Street Site; Court Staff, Toronto Western Hospital - University Health Network; Langs: French; (416)763-1171; Fax. (416)763-0573.

SHORT, Christine A; Nova Scotia Rehab Centre, 211-1341 Summer St, Halifax NS B3H 4K4; Dal'94; FRCPC; PhysMed&Rehab (Multiple Sclerosis). Div Chief PM & B Capital Health, Nova Scotia Rehabilitation Centre; Div Chief PM & B Capital Health, Queen Elizabeth II Health Sciences Centre - Victoria General Site; Assoc Prof Med/Div Chief Interim PhysMed & Rehab, Dalhousie University; (902)473-1409; Fax. (902)473-3204.

SHORT, Leo F N; Associate Clinic, 4620A 50 Ave, Innisfail AB T4G 1A6; Belfast (Ireland)'74; MB ChB; MRCGPract(Lond); FRCP; CCFP; FCFP; Staff Family Med, Innisfail Health Centre; (403)227-3301; Fax. (403)227-2856; shortl@telusplanet.net.

SHORT, R Keith; Assertive Comm Treatment Team, 36 Queensway, Grnd-Falls-Windsor NL A2B 1J2; Mem'08; CCFP.

SHORT, Thomas W D; Credit Valley Med Arts Centre, 204-2000 Credit Valley Rd, Mississauga ON L5M 4N4; McM'84; BSc(Hons.); FRCSC; Urol (Surgical Oncology). Ac Staff/Med Dir/Gen Surgeon, The Credit Valley Hospital; (905)820-2263; Fax. (905)820-5746.

SHORTER, Anne Marie; Chalmers Gate X-Ray, 309-328 Hwy 7E, Richmond Hill ON L4B 3P7; McM'84; FRCPC; DiagRad (Mammography). (905)731-4001; Fax. (905)731-1458.

SHORTT, Rodger A D; Briarwood Cosmetic Surg Clinic, 1-406 North Service Rd E, Oakville ON L6H 5R2; Qns'04; FRCSC; PlasSurg. (905)849-4282; Fax. (905)849-4630.

SHORTT, Samuel E D; 16 Green St, Nepean ON K2J 3R2; Wes'77; PhD; CCFP; FCFP; Assoc Staff, Hotel-Dieu Hospital; Assoc Staff, Kingston General Hospital; Prof Family Med Comm Health & Epidemiol, Queen's University; (613)825-9799

SHORTT, Stanley G; 212-911 Yates St, Victoria BC V8V 4X3; Cal'76; FRCSC; Ophth (Retina Vitreous Surgery). Ac Staff, Royal Jubilee Hospital; Ac Staff, Victoria General Hospital; (250)598-1252

SHOTT, Craig A; Brant Comm Healthcare System, 200 Terrace Hill St, Brantford ON N3R 1G9; Dal'98; CCFP; Staff, The Brant Community Healthcare System - Brantford General Hospital Site; Langs: Bilingual(English/French); (519)751-5544 x2908

SHOTT, Paula L; 109 King St W, Dundas ON L9H 1V1; Tor'96; CCFP; (905)628-9200; Fax. (905)628-9600.

SHOUGHARY, Ali T; 700 Mackay St, Pembroke ON K8A 1G6; Beirut (Lebanon)'96; FRCSC; Ophth (Pediatric Ophthalmology). Staff, Pembroke Regional Hospital Inc; Langs: Arabic; (613)717-5054; Fax. (613)735-8311.

SHOUKRALLA, Faten S; Richmond Hill Doctors, 416 Elgin Mills Rd W, Richmond Hill ON L4C 4M2; Cairo (Egypt)'81; MB BS; CCFP; FCFP; Langs: Arabic; (905)787-8881; Fax. (905)787-1577; dr.shoukralla@rogers.com.

SHOUKRY, Sahar S; Steinbach Family Med Centre, 10-333 Loewen Blvd, Steinbach MB R5G 0C3; Staff, Thompson General Hospital; (204)326-3401

SHOULDICE, Earle B; Shouldice Hosp, 7750 Bayview Ave, Thornhill ON L3T 4A3; Wes'61; Staff, Shouldice Hospital; (905)889-1125; Fax. (905)889-4216.

SHOULDICE, Elizabeth H; Queensway Carleton Hosp, 3045 Baseline Rd, Nepean ON K2H 8P4; Dal'05; CCFP; CCFP(E.M.); Staff, Queensway Carleton Hospital; (613)721-2000

SHOULDICE, Michelle K; The Hosp for Sick Children, 555 University Ave, Toronto ON M5G 1X8; McM'94; BSc; MSc; FRCPC; Peds (Child Abuse). Dir Suspected Child Abuse & Neglect Prog/Pediatric Consultation Clinic, The Hospital For Sick Children; Med Consultant Peds, Holland Bloorview Kids Rehabilitation Hospital; Asst Prof, University of Toronto; (416)813-5660; Fax. (416)813-5846.

SHOURIDEH-ZIABARI, Sayed M A; Eagle Ridge Family Health Ctre, 203-480 Huronia Rd, Barrie ON L4N 6M4; (Iran)'94; CCFP; Langs: Farsi; (705)727-7688; Fax. (705)734-6284.

SHOUSH, Suzanne; Peninsula Family Health Team, 24 Moore St, Lions Head ON N0H 1W0; Alb'08; CCFP; Staff, Peninsula Family Health Team - Lions Head; (519)793-3445; Fax. (519)793-4604.

SHOVKIVSKA, Iryna; Foothills Med Centre, 1403 29 St NW, Calgary AB T2N 2T9; (Russia (Federation))'83; Staff, Foothills Medical Centre; (403)473-4550

SHOWLER, Adrienne J; Univ Hlth Network-Toronto Gen, 13EN 1319D-200 Elizabeth St, Toronto ON M5G 2C4; Ott'09; Staff InfectDis, Toronto General Hospital - UHN; (416)340-3505; Fax. (416)340-3357.

SHRAFAT, Nadeem; Cape Breton Healthcare Complex, 1482 George St, Sydney NS B1P 1P3; Karachi (Pakistan)'91; MB BS; Staff, Cape Breton Healthcare Complex; (902)567-8000

SHRAGGE, David L; 9012 138 St NW, Edmonton AB T5R 0E6; Alb'74; FRCPC; EmergMed (Administration). Staff, Covenant Health - Misericordia Community Hospital; Assoc Prof, University of Alberta; (780)484-2386; Fax. (780)481-8123; dshragge@shaw.ca.

SHRAYYEF, Muhammad Z; Trafalgar Prof Centre, 412-1235 Trafalgar Rd, Oakville ON L6H 3P1; (Syria)'97; Staff, The Moncton Hospital; Langs: Arabic; (905)337-0040; Fax. (905)337-0044.

SHREEVE, Joanne P; Dixon Med Centre, 302-531 Davis Dr, Newmarket ON L3Y 6P5; Wes'87; (905)830-5551; Fax. (905)830-5597.

SHRESTHA, Prakash T; Wrinch Mem Hosp, PO Box 999, Hazelton BC V0J 1Y0; Montemorelos (Mexico)'89; CCFP; Staff, Wrinch Memorial Hospital; Langs: Spanish; Nepali; (250)842-5211 x153

SHRESTHA, Sherry K; Wrinch Mem Hosp, PO Bag 999 2510 Hwy 62, Hazelton BC V0J 1Y0; Loma Linda (USA)'75; AAFP; ABFPS; CCFP; Staff, Wrinch Memorial Hospital; Staff, Wrinch Memorial Doctors Clinic; (250)842-5234; Fax. (250)842-5065.

SHRIER, Ian; Concordia Sports Med Centre, 6530 rue Sherbrooke O, Montreal QC H4B 1N5; McG'85; PhD; Langs: French; (514)848-3317; Fax. (514)848-3316.

SHRIKHANDE, Satish; Victoria Mental Hlth Centre, 2328 Trent St, Victoria BC V8R 4Z3; Poona (India)'75; DPM(Ire); MRCP(UK); MB BS; FRCPC; Psy (Schizophrenia). Langs: Hindi; Marathi; (250)370-8162

SHRIQUI, Christian L; CHUQ-Ctr Hosp Univ Laval, 4221-2705 boul Laurier, Quebec QC G1V 4G2; Mon'85; MSc; FRCPC; Psy (Psychotic Disorders). Staff, Centre Hospitalier Universitaire de Quebec-CHUL; Langs: Bilingual(English/French); (418)654-2177; Fax. (418)654-2716; christian.shriqui@mail.chuq.qc.ca.

SHRIVES, David M; Professional Bldg, 301B-222 King St E, Bowmanville ON L1C 1P6; Tor'74; FRCPC; IntMed (Gastroenterology). Staff Consultant, Lakeridge Health - Bowmanville Site; (905)623-2570; Fax. (905)623-4646; dr.shrives@bellnet.ca.

SHRIVES, Heloise; 3-2020 Strachan Rd SE, Medicine Hat AB T1B 0M9; (403)580-1882; Fax. (403)504-5799.

SHROFF, Manohar M; The Hosp for Sick Children, 555 University Ave, Toronto ON M5G 1X8; Bombay (India)'81; ABR; FRCPC; DiagRad. Staff, The Hospital For Sick Children; (416)813-7654; Fax. (416)813-7591; manohar.shroff@sickkids.ca.

SHROM, Jerry B; Manitoba Public Insurance, 800-234 Donald St, Winnipeg MB R3C 1M8; Man'82; Physician, Manitoba Public Insurance; (204)985-7000

SHROTT, Barry H; 772 Dovercourt Rd PO Box 323 Stn E, Toronto ON M6H 4E3; Tor'74; Assoc Staff, Mount Sinai Hospital; Physician, Christie Gardens Nursing Home; Physician, Casa Verde Health Centre; (416)537-2527; Fax. (416)537-1280.

SHTYBEL, Wayne W; 7819D East Saanich Rd, Saanichton BC V8M 2B4; Alb'83; FRCPC; Neur. (250)652-4815; Fax. (250)652-4808.

SHU, Abigail C; Gain Med Centre, 1199 Austin Ave, Coquitlam BC V3K 3P4; UBC'01; (604)939-7345

SHU, Daniel S P; Gain Med Centre, 1199 Austin Ave, Coquitlam BC V3K 3P4; Mem'73; Staff, Royal Columbian Hospital; Staff, Eagle Ridge Hospital & Health Care Centre; Langs: Cantonese; (604)939-7345; Fax. (604)939-7781.

SHU, David H P; 311-301 Columbia St E, New Westminster BC V3L 3W5; UBC'01; BSc; FRCPC; IntMed (Endocrinology); Endocrin&Metab. Staff, Royal Columbian Hospital; (604)787-8808; Fax. (604)787-8806; dave.shu@hotmail.com.

SHU, Krishanthy; London HSC-Victoria Campus, PO Box 5010 Stn B 800 Commissioners Rd E, London ON N6A 5W9; Jaffna (Sri Lanka)'98; CCFP; Staff, London Health Sciences Centre - Victoria Campus; Langs: Sinhalese; Tamil; (519)685-8500

SHU, Raymond M; Maxum Professional Centre, 306-385 Silver Star Blvd, Scarborough ON M1V 0E3; Tor'90; FRCPC; Peds (Consultant Pediatrics). Ac Staff, The Scarborough Hospital - Birchmount Campus; Court Staff, Rouge Valley Health System - Centenary Health Centre Site; Lecturer Peds, University of Toronto; Langs: Cantonese; French; (416)291-1284; Fax. (416)291-8696; raymond.shu@utoronto.ca.

SHU, Y W Maggie; Medical Bldg, 207-701 Sheppard Ave E, North York ON M2K 2Z3; (Hong Kong)'92; FRCPC; Peds (Neonatal & Perinatal Medicine). Staff, North York General Hospital; Langs: Cantonese; (416)901-9251; Fax. (416)901-9657.

SHUAIB, Ashfaq; University of Alberta Hosp, 2E3 13WMC-8440 112 St NW, Edmonton AB T6G 2B7; Khyber (Pakistan)'80; FRCPC; Neur (Headache). Staff, University of Alberta Hospital; Dir Div of Neurol/Prof, University of Alberta; (780)407-3254; Fax. (780)407-1325; ashfaq.shuaib@ualberta.ca.

SHUB, Elliot H; North York Family Health Team, 701-240 Duncan Mill Rd, North York ON M3B 3S6; Cape Town (South Africa)'66; Ac Staff Privil, North York General Hospital; Langs: Hebrew; (416)229-6300; Fax. (416)229-6283.

SHUBA, Lesya M; Queen Elizabeth II HSC, 2035-1276 South Park Rd, Halifax NS B3H 2Y9; Dal'00; PhD; FRCSC; Ophth (Glaucoma). Staff Ophth, Queen Elizabeth II Health Sciences Centre - Victoria General Site; Langs: Russian; (902)473-3410; Fax. (902)473-2839; lshuba@dal.ca.

SHUBAT, J Michael; North Huron FHT-Lucknow, PO Box 160 691 Havelock St, Lucknow ON N0G 2H0; Wes'84; Ac Staff, Wingham & District Hospital - Listowel Wingham Hospitals Alliance; Med Dir, Pinecrest Nursing Home; (519)528-2810; Fax. (519)528-3408.

SHUBLAQ, Wael; Waterford Hosp, 306 Waterford Bridge Rd, St. John's NL A1E 4J8; Alexandria (Egypt)'83; MB ChB; PhD; Staff, Waterford Hospital; Locum Tenens, Health Sciences Centre; Locum Tenens, Carbonear General Hospital; Langs: Arabic; Polish; (709)777-3300

SHUCHMAN, Miriam; 7F-790 Bay St, Toronto ON M5G 1N8; Farmington(CT) (USA)'85; Staff, Women's College Hospital; (416)351-3732; Fax. (416)351-3746.

SHUCKETT, Bruce M; Scarborough Hosp-General Div, 3050 Lawrence Ave E, Scarborough ON M1P 2V5; Man'77; FRCPC; DiagRad. Staff Radiol, The Scarborough Hospital - General Campus; (416)438-2911

SHUCKETT, E Paul; Health Sciences Centre, CE 216-820 Sherbrook St, Winnipeg MB R3A 1S1; Man'75; FRCSC; Ophth (Pediatric Ophthalmology). Staff, Misericordia Health Centre; Staff, Health Sciences Centre; (204)787-4377; Fax. (204)787-4965; shucket@umanitoba.ca.

SHUCKETT, Rhonda; Burrard Health Bldg, 406-1160 Burrard St, Vancouver BC V6Z 2E8; Man'78; FRCPC; Rheum; IntMed. Consultant Rheumatol, Providence Health Care - St Paul's Hospital; Asst Prof, University of British Columbia; (604)683-3958; Fax. (604)683-3917.

SHUEN, Paul K; Sheppard Med Bldg, 301-701 Sheppard Ave E, North York ON M2K 2Z3; Melbourne (Australia)'76; MB BS; MRCOG; FRCSC; ObstGyn (Gynecologic Oncology). Ac Staff, North York General Hospital; Lecturer, University of Toronto; Langs: Cantonese; Mandarin; (416)221-0399; Fax. (416)221-2671.

SHUFELT, Kathryn A; Kawartha Cardiology Clinic, 327 Charlotte St, Peterborough ON K9J 0B2; Ott'00; BSc; FRCPC; IntMed; Cardiol. Staff Cardiol, Peterborough Regional Health Centre - Hospital Drive; (705)775-0145; Fax. (705)775-0128.

SHUFFIELD, James W; 285 Catherine St PO Box 188, Wingham ON N0G 2W0; Fort Worth (USA)'92; CCFP; Staff, Wingham & District Hospital - Listowel Wingham Hospitals Alliance; (519)357-3915; Fax. (519)357-1568.

SHUGAR, Gerald; Addiction & Mental Hlth-Clarke, 250 College St, Toronto ON M5T 1R8; Tor'60; DPsy; FRCPC; Psy. Sr Staff Psy & Teach Staff, Centre for Addiction & Mental Health (CAMH) - College Street Site; (416)979-6861; Fax. (416)979-6815.

SHUGARMAN, Laurel G D; Mackenzie Richmond Hill Hosp, 10 Trench St, Richmond Hill ON L4C 4Z3; McM'75; CCFP; Staff, Mackenzie Richmond Hill Hospital; Langs: Bilingual(English/French); (905)883-1212

SHUHAIBAR, Hafez S; Cambridge Mem Hosp, 700 Coronation Blvd, Cambridge ON N1R 3G2; Beirut (Lebanon)'81; DABPath; FRCPC; AnatPath. Staff Pathologist, Cambridge Memorial Hospital; (519)740-4985

SHUKIN, Evelyn K; 101B-2099 152 St, Surrey BC V4A 4N7; Portland (USA)'75; Assoc Staff, Vancouver General Hospital - Centennial Pavillion; Langs: Russian; (604)531-0212; Fax. (604)536-8959.

SHUKLA, Avanish K; Bayvalley Med Arts Bldg, 102-145 Queenston St, St Catharines ON L2R 2Z9; Lucknow (India)'66; BSc; MB BS; DPM(Lond); MRCPsy(UK); DPM(London); FRCPC; Psy. Staff, Niagara Health System - St Catharines General Site; Staff, Niagara Health System - Ontario Street Site; Staff, Niagara Health System - Greater Niagara General Site; Langs: Hindi; (905)687-8004; Fax. (905)687-8984.

SHUKLA, Dinkar K; Four Corners Med Bldg, 205-2009 Long Lake Rd, Sudbury ON P3E 6C3; Sask'00; FRCPC; IntMed (Interventional Cardiology); Cardiol. (705)674-8148; Fax. (705)674-8919.

SHUKLA, Hemen P; Burton Hall, 60 Grosvenor St, Toronto ON M5S 1B6; Dal'04; Dip SportMed; CCFP; Staff, Women's College Hospital; Lecturer, University of Toronto; Langs: Bilingual(English/French); (416)323-6060 x3; Fax. (416)323-6485.

SHUKLA, Hrishikesh; 6720 Hawthorne Dr, Windsor ON N8T 1J9; McM'98; CCFP; Langs: Hindi; (519)944-2295

SHUKLA, Karunakar; Market Mall Med Clinic, 2325 Preston Ave, Saskatoon SK S7J 2G2; Nagpur (India)'68; Physician, Market Mall Medical Clinic; (306)343-1661; Fax. (306)343-1665.

SHUKLA, Rahul; Dermatology Centre, 132 Yonge St, Hamilton ON L8N 1V6; McM'07; FRCPC; Derm. (905)524-2048

SHUKLA, Romesh C; IWK Health Centre, PO Box 9700 Rpo CSC 5980 University Ave, Halifax NS B3K 6R8; Punjab (India)'70; MB BS; FRCPC; Anes. Staff, IWK Health Centre; Head Anesthesia, Dalhousie University; (902)470-6627; Fax. (902)470-6626.

SHUKLA, Shashi P; 5953 Bilton Lane, Halifax NS B3H 4M3; Punjab (India)'70; MB BS.

SHUKLA, Sushama; Spadina Med Clinic, 2-806 Spadina Cres E, Saskatoon SK S7K 3H4; Indore (India)'67; Langs: Hindi; (306)955-3030; Fax. (306)955-4202.

SHUKLA MOHAN, Ruchika; 984 Broadway St W PO Box 53573 Rpo West Broadway, Vancouver BC V5Z 4M6; UBC'08; CCFP; (604)875-5000

SHUKLE, Jacqueline M C; Appletree Med Centre, 2948 Baseline Rd, Nepean ON K2H 8T5; Sask'96; FRCPC; Derm. Langs: Bilingual(English/French); (613)482-0118; Fax. (613)680-6420.

SHUKLE, Pravin J; Appletree Med Group, 2948 Baseline Rd, Nepean ON K2H 8T5; Sask'94; BSc; FRCPC; IntMed (Cardiology). Staff, Queensway Carleton Hospital; Langs: Gujarati; (613)288-2061; Fax. (613)288-0585.

SHUKOOR, Sajid; Hotel-Dieu Grace Hosp, 1030 Ouellette Ave, Windsor ON N9A 1E1; Lahore (Pakistan)'82; MB BS; FRCPC; AnatPath. Staff Path Lab, Hôtel-Dieu Grace Hospital; Langs: Urdu; (519)973-4411; Fax. (519)258-5124.

SHUKRI ALALOUS, Nidaa; Sturgeon Community Hosp, 201 Boudreau Rd, St. Albert AB T8N 6C4; (Iraq)'89; Staff, Sturgeon Community Hospital; (780)418-8200; Fax. (780)460-7082.

SHULAKEWYCH, Markian O; Queensway-Carleton Hosp, 3045 Baseline Rd, Ottawa ON K2H 8P4; Man'94; FRCPC; DiagRad. Staff, Queensway Carleton Hospital; Staff, The Ottawa Hospital - Civic Campus; (613)721-2000; Fax. (613)721-4706.

SHULDINER, Samuel; 3-5435 rue De Terrebonne, Montreal QC H4A 3R7; Ott'76; Staff, Jewish Eldercare Centre - CHSLD JUIF de Montréal; Langs: French; (514)489-5733; Fax. (514)489-2237; samuel.shuldiner@staff.mcgill.ca.

SHULDINER, Sarit L; University City Mall, 45 Four Winds Dr, North York ON M3J 1K7; Tel Aviv (Israel)'96; CCFP; (416)665-7708; Fax. (416)665-4560.

SHULMAN, Barbara; Specialized Women's Health, H214-4500 Oak St, Vancouver BC V6H 3N1; UBC'98; FRCPC; Psy. Staff, Providence Health Care - St Paul's Hospital; Langs: French; (604)875-2025

SHULMAN, David L; Rothbart Centre for Pain Care, 9-4646 Dufferin St, North York ON M3H 5S4; Tor'73; BSc; DAA; CCFP; FCFP; Ac Staff, Markham Stouffville Hospital; Staff, Wilderman Medical Clinic; Langs: Hebrew; (416)512-6407; Fax. (416)512-6375; louisshulman@hotmail.com.

SHULMAN, Desmond; Central Alberta Prof Centre, 182-5201 43 St, Red Deer AB T4N 1C7; Witwatersrand (South Africa)'67; MB ChB; FCP (SA)(Peds.); Consultant, Red Deer Paediatric Consultants; Langs: Afrikaans; (403)343-6404; Fax. (403)343-6215.

SHULMAN, H Mitchell; MUHC-Royal Victoria Hosp, 687 av des Pins O, Montreal QC H3A 1A1; McG'79; FRCPC; EmergMed. Staff, McGill University Health Centre - Royal Victoria Hospital; adj Prof, McGill University; (514)934-1934 x32557; Fax. (514)334-3620.

SHULMAN, Harry S; Sunnybrook Hlth Sciences Ctre, 2075 Bayview Ave, Toronto ON M4N 3M5; Tor'66; FRCPC; DiagRad. Chief Radiology, Sunnybrook Health Sciences Centre; Prof, University of Toronto; (416)480-6100 x2290; Fax. (416)480-5855.

SHULMAN, Kenneth I; Sunnybrook Hlth Sciences Ctre, 2075 Bayview Ave, Toronto ON M4N 3M5; Tor'73; FRCPsy; FRCPC; Psy (Geriatric Psychiatry). Ac Staff, Sunnybrook Health Sciences Centre; Prof Psy, University of Toronto; Langs: Yiddish; (416)480-4079; Fax. (416)480-6022; ken.shulman@sunnybrook.ca.

SHULMAN, Leslie S; Toronto East Gen & Orth Hosp, 825 Coxwell Ave, Toronto ON M4C 3E7; Cal'00; FRCPC; Anes. Staff, Toronto East General Hospital Inc; (416)461-8272

SHULMAN, Rayzel M; The Hosp For Sick Children, 555 University Ave, Toronto ON M5G 1X8; McM'04; FRCPC; Peds; Endocrin&Metab. Staff, The Hospital For Sick Children; (416)813-8088

SHULMAN, Richard W; Trillium Hlth Ctr-West Toronto, 4F-150 Sherway Dr, Toronto ON M9C 1A5; McG'89; FRCPC; Psy (Geriatric Psychiatry). Staff, Trillium Health Centre - West Toronto; Asst Prof, University of Toronto; (416)521-4057; Fax. (416)521-4072.

SHULMAN, Sandy E; Dr Sandy Shulman Med Clinic, 2550A Finch Ave W, North York ON M9M 2G3; Tor'68; CCFP; FCFP; Court Staff, North York General Hospital - Branson Division; Ac Staff Family Pract, Humber River Regional Hospital - Finch Avenue Site; Asst Prof Family & Commun Med, University of Toronto; Langs: Italian; (416)749-5291; Fax. (416)749-6598; sandy.shulman@utoronto.ca.

SHULMAN, Scott M; North Bay Reg Health Clinic, 208-1500 Fisher St, North Bay ON P1B 2H3; Wes'99; BSc; FRCPC; IntMed; Gastroent. Langs: Bilingual(English/French); (705)476-7737; Fax. (705)476-7177; sshulman@cogeco.net.

SHULMAN, Tanya S; Northgate Square, 208-1500 Fisher St, North Bay ON P1B 2H3; Wes'99; FRCPC; IntMed (Cardiology); Nephrol. Staff Nephrol (All Sites), North Bay Regional Health Centre - Regional Mental Health; (705)476-7377; Fax. (705)476-7177.

SHUM, Andrew J H S; Southlake Reg Health Centre, 596 Davis Dr, Newmarket ON L3Y 2P9; UBC'09; CCFP; CCFP(E.M.); Staff, Southlake Regional Health Centre; (905)895-4521

SHUM, Andrew S C; 304-302 Spadina Ave, Toronto ON M5T 2E7; Tor'76; Assoc Staff Urology, Women's College Hospital; Langs: Cantonese; Mandarin; (416)593-5516; Fax. (416)593-5516.

SHUM, David T; Windsor Reg Hosp-Metropolitan, 1995 Lens Ave, Windsor ON N8W 1L9; (Hong Kong)'75; MB BS; DABPath; FRCPC; AnatPath (Dermatological Pathology). Staff, Windsor Regional Hospital - Metropolitan Site; Langs: Cantonese; (519)254-5577 x52360; Fax. (519)254-6861.

SHUM, H T Peter; Glen Erin Med-Dental Centre, 3-2318 Dunwin Dr, Mississauga ON L5L 1C7; McG'76; Ac Staff, The Credit Valley Hospital; Langs: Cantonese; (905)828-2980; Fax. (905)828-6615.

SHUM, Jeffrey B; London HSC-Campus Site, PO Box 5339 Stn B C8 114-339 Windermere Rd, London ON N6A 5A5; Qns'04; FRCSC; GenSurg; Critical Care Medicine. Staff, London Health Sciences Centre - University Hospital; (519)685-8500

SHUM, Kum Cheung; Lakewood Med Centre, 30 Lakewood Blvd, Winnipeg MB R2J 2M6; Otago (New Zealand)'58; (204)257-3395

SHUM, Michael S L; 5320 Victoria Dr, Vancouver BC V5P 3V7; UBC'82; Langs: Cantonese; (604)685-5504

SHUM-TIM, Dominique; MUHC-Royal Victoria Hosp, S8 73B-687 av des Pins O, Montreal QC H3A 1A1; McG'88; MSc; MDCM; FRCSC; GenSurg (Adult Cardiac Surgery); Cardiovasc&ThorSurg (P.Q.); CardiothorSurg. Staff, McGill University Health Centre - Montreal General Campus; Staff, McGill University Health Centre - Montreal Children's Hospital; Staff, McGill University Health Centre - Royal Victoria Hospital; adj Prof Surg, McGill University; Langs: Chinese; French; (514)934-1934

SHUMAK, Rene S; 140-100 Sheppard Ave E, North York ON M2N 6N5; Tor'65; DMRD; FRCPC; DiagRad (Mammography). Staff, North York Ontario Breast Screening Program; Reg Staff Breast Imaging Lead, Ontario Breast Screening Program; Asst Prof, University of Toronto; (416)512-0605; Fax. (416)298-7470.

SHUMAK, Steven L; Sunnybrook Hlth Sciences Ctre, C410-2075 Bayview Ave, Toronto ON M4N 3M5; Tor'80; ABIM; IntMed (Diabetes). Head Div of IntMed/Chief Med Staff, Sunnybrook Health Sciences Centre; Dir Div of IntMed/Prof, University of Toronto; (416)480-4290; Fax. (416)480-4563; steven.shumak@sunnybrook.ca.

SHUMAN, Earl M; 17 Queen St, Cobourg ON K9A 1M8; McM'77; DDS; (905)372-4196

SHUMAN, Mira R; Sunnybrook Hlth Sciences Ctre, AW-2075 Bayview Ave, Toronto ON M4N 3M5; Qns'09; CCFP; Staff, Sunnybrook Health Sciences Centre; (416)480-4942

SHUMBORSKI, Terry G; North East Med Centre, 7210 144 Ave NW, Edmonton AB T5C 2R7; Alb'76; (780)478-2995; Fax. (780)472-0215.

SHUMKA, David J; Southlake Reg Health Centre, 596 Davis Dr, Newmarket ON L3Y 2P9; Tor'81; MSc(Epidem.); Anes. Staff, Southlake Regional Health Centre; Langs: Ukrainian; (905)895-4521

SHUMSKY, Anne G; Foothills Med Centre, 1403 29 St NW, Calgary AB T2N 2T9; Ott'86; FRCSC; ObstGyn. Staff, Foothills Medical Centre; (403)944-1110

SHUNMUGAM, Revendren; The Brandon Clinic, 620 Dennis St, Brandon MB R7A 5E7; (204)728-4440

SHUPAK, Michael; B-145 Marlee Ave, Toronto ON M6B 3H3; Tor'71; Ac Staff, Humber River Regional Hospital - Keele Street Site; Ac Staff, Mount Sinai Hospital; Court Staff, Toronto Western Hospital - University Health Network; Langs: Hebrew; French; Yiddish; (416)787-0661; Fax. (416)787-3458.

SHUPAK, Rachel; St Michael's Hosp, 3 020-30 Bond St, Toronto ON M5B 1W8; Tor'73; FRCP; FRCPC; IntMed; Rheum. Staff, St Michael's Hospital; Assoc Prof, University of Toronto; (416)864-5550; Fax. (416)864-5549; shupakr@smh.toronto.on.ca.

SHURRAW, Sabin C N; 205-9148 23 Ave NW, Edmonton AB T6N 1H9; Man'02; FRCPC; IntMed (Hypertension); Nephrol. Physician, South Edmonton Nephrology; (780)468-3377; Fax. (780)468-9353.

SHUSTACK, Allan; Royal Alexandra Hosp, 4228-10240 Kingsway NW, Edmonton AB T5H 3V9; McG'75; IntMed; Respir (Critical Care Medicine). Assoc Dir ICU, Royal Alexandra Hospital; (780)735-5172; Fax. (780)735-4032; allan.shustack@shaw.ca.

SHUSTER, Joseph; MUHC-Montreal Gen Hosp, 1650 av Cedar, Montreal QC H3G 1A4; Alb'62; PhD; FRCPC; MedBiochem (P.Q.) (Clinical Immunology & Allergy); MedScient(Med). Dir Div of Clin Immunol & Allergy, McGill University Health Centre - Montreal General Campus; McGill University; Langs: English; French; (514)934-1934 x48036

SHUSTER, Michael; PO Box 2409 Stn Main, Banff AB T1L 1C2; Wes'81; DAB; FRCPC; EmergMed. Staff, Covenant Health - Banff Mineral Springs Hospital; Langs: Spanish; French; (403)762-3521; Fax. (403)762-4193; mshuster@telusplanet.net.

SHUSTIK, Chaim; MUHC-Royal Victoria Hosp, C6 80-687 av des Pins O, Montreal QC H3A 1A1; Tor'71; MedOncol (P.Q.); Hem (P.Q.); IntMed. Staff, McGill University Health Centre - Royal Victoria Hospital; (514)843-1558; Fax. (514)843-1418; chaim.shustik@mcgill.ca.

SHUSTIK, Jesse D; BC Cancer Agency-Fraser Valley, 13750 96 Ave, Surrey BC V3V 1Z2; McG'03; MDCM; FRCPC; IntMed; MedOncol; Hem. Staff, BC Cancer Agency Fraser Valley Centre; Staff, Leukemia/Bone Marrow Transplantation Prog of BC; (604)587-4306; jshustik@bccancer.bc.ca.

SHUTE, Ronald D; Grey Nuns Family Med Centre, 2927 66 St NW, Edmonton AB T6K 4C1; Alb'99; CCFP; (780)342-1470; Fax. (780)490-0953.

SHUTT, Harold K R; 503 Twin Brooks Bay NW, Edmonton AB T6J 6W6; Alb'63; Ophth (Neuro Ophthalmology). Staff, Royal Alexandra Hospital; Clin Prof, University of Alberta; (780)434-6255

SHWE, Kyaw; Weyburn Health Centre, 36 4th St, Weyburn SK S4H 0X7; Rangoon (Burma)'85; MB BS; DA; CCFP; Physician, Weyburn Health Centre; (306)842-5444; Fax. (306)842-5449; shwe@sasktel.net.

SHYAM, Vidur; Kingston Gen Hosp, 76 Stuart St, Kingston ON K7L 2V7; Pradesh (India)'78; FRCPC; Anes (Neonatology). Staff, Kingston General Hospital; Staff, Hotel-Dieu Hospital; Langs: German; (613)548-7827; Fax. (613)548-1375.

SHYAMAL, Gayathri P; 333 Sherbourne St, Toronto ON M5A 2S5; Man'05; CCFP; Langs: Malay; Tamil; (416)324-4180; Fax. (416)324-4181.

SHYLEYKO, Elizabeth M; Sunnyhill Pediatric Clinic, 200-1632 14 Ave NW, Calgary AB T2N 1M7; Lublau (Poland)'79; FRCPC; Peds. (403)284-0001; Fax. (403)284-1593.

SHYLEYKO, Romuald J; Sarcee Med Clinic, 32-4604 37 St SW, Calgary AB T3E 3C9; Lublin (Poland)'73; (403)269-9488; Fax. (403)269-9409.

SHYMCHYK, Michael; Country Hills Medicentre, 220-5149 Country Hills Blvd NW, Calgary AB T3A 5K8; Man'90; (403)241-8848; Fax. (403)241-8849.

SHYSH, Alexander J; Peter Lougheed Centre, 3500 26 Ave NE, Calgary AB T1Y 6J4; Alb'86; FRCPC; Anes (Medical Education). Staff, Peter Lougheed Centre; Clinical Asst Prof, University of Calgary; (403)943-5554; Fax. (403)943-4474.

SI-AHMED, Fatma; Clinique 3000, 3000 rue Belanger, Montreal QC H1Y 1A9; Mon'04; Staff, Clinique Medicale 3000; (514)376-7702

SIA, Michael A; Tom Baker Cancer Centre, 1331 29 St NW, Calgary AB T2N 4N2; Tor'01; FRCPC; RadOncol. Staff, Tom Baker Cancer Centre; (403)521-3095; Fax. (403)283-1651.

SIA, Winnie W K; Royal Alexandra Hosp, 332 CSC-10240 Kingsway NW, Edmonton AB T5H 3V9; Alb'96; FRCPC; IntMed. Staff Comm Services Ctre, Royal Alexandra Hospital; Langs: Cantonese; (780)735-6827; Fax. (780)735-5313.

SIA, Yin Shan; Cariboo Mem Hosp, 517 Sixth Ave N, Williams Lake BC V2G 2G8; (Hong Kong)'93; MB BS; Langs: Cantonese; Mandarin; (250)392-4411

SIA, Ying Tung; Glengarry Memorial Hosp, 20260 County Rd 43, Alexandria ON K0C 1A0; Mon'01; FRCPC; IntMed; Critical Care Medicine; Cardiol. Staff, Glengarry Memorial Hospital; Langs: Cantonese; French; (613)525-2222

SIA-VENUGOPAL, Angeline C; 202-45800 Promontory Rd, Chilliwack BC V2R 5Z5; Mangalore (India)'92; MB BS; Langs: Cantonese; Hokkin; Malay; (604)858-2800; Fax. (604)858-2899; angelinesia@hotmail.com.

SIAL, Zia A; Etobicoke Med Centre FHT, 400 The East Mall, Etobicoke ON M9B 3Z9; Jagiellonian Univ (Poland)'03; BSc; CCFP; Langs: Polish; Urdu; Punjabi; Hindi; (416)621-2220; Fax. (416)621-2203; zia.sial@stjoe.on.ca.

SIAUW, Christina L Y; 206-1717 10 St NW, Calgary AB T2M 4S2; Dal'97; BSc; MSc; MCFP; CCFP; (403)282-9865; Fax. (403)282-9893.

SIBALIS, Stephen J; The Doctors Bldg, 905-208 Bloor St W, Toronto ON M5S 3B4; McM'80; BSc; MSc; FRCPC; Psy (Child Psychiatry). Court Staff, Toronto East General Hospital Inc; (416)923-8666; Fax. (416)466-7250.

SIBBALD, Ian I; PO Box 615, Rossland BC V0G 1Y0; Sask'91; CCFP; FCFP; CCFP(E.M.); Staff, Kootenay Boundary Regional Hospital; Langs: Bilingual(English/French); (250)368-5656

SIBBALD, Matthew G; 500-491 Lawrence Ave W, North York ON M5M 1C7; Tor'04; FRCPC; IntMed; Cardiol. (416)781-9500; Fax. (416)781-7985.

SIBBALD, R Gary; Applewood Village Plaza, 23-1077 North Service Rd, Mississauga ON L4Y 1A6; Tor'74; BSc; ABIM; DAA; FRCPC; IntMed; Derm. Ac Staff, Trillium Health Centre - Mississauga; Ac Staff, Women's College Hospital; Staff, Toronto General Hospital - UHN; Assoc Prof Med/Dir, University of Toronto; (905)273-9009; Fax. (905)273-6409.

SIBILLE, Pascale L R; CSSSG-Hop de Gatineau, CP 2000 Succ Bureau-Chef 909 boul Verendrye O, Gatineau QC J8P 7H2; Mon'88; Staff, Hôpital de Gatineau; Langs: Spanish; English; (819)966-6100

SIBLEY, Aaron K; Royal Alexandra Hosp, 541-10240 Kingsway Ave NW, Edmonton AB T5H 3V9; Dal'03; FRCPC; EmergMed. Staff, Royal Alexandra Hospital; (780)735-4442; Fax. (780)735-4916.

SIBLEY, Caroline A; 317 Main St W, Hamilton ON L8P 1K1; McM'90; FRCSC; ObstGyn. Staff, Hamilton Health Sciences Centre - McMaster Children's Hospital; Clinical Asst Prof ObstGyn, McMaster University; (905)540-8100; Fax. (905)540-9094.

SICARD, Eric; Centre Med Laennec, 101-1100 av Beaumont, Mont-Royal QC H3P 3H5; Laval'89; (514)569-3442

SICARD, Fernand; Clinique Med de l'Est Inc, 100-30 boul Saint-Joseph, Montreal QC H2T 1G9; Mon'62; Otol (P.Q.). (514)845-4240

SICARD, Joanne E; Appletree Med Group, 1008-900 Greenbank Rd, Ottawa ON K2J 1S8; McG'82; CCFP; Langs: French; (613)482-0118; Fax. (613)680-6420.

SICARD, Marie-Eve; CSSS de Trois-Rivières, 1991 boul du Carmel, Trois-Rivieres QC G8Z 3R9; Mon'95; LMCC; FRCPC; RadOncol (Gynecologic Oncology). Staff, CSSS de Trois-Rivières; Langs: Bilingual(French/English); (819)371-5002; Fax. (819)378-9712.

SICARD, Nadine; Direction Gen de la sante publ, 2 03-201 boul Cremazie E, Montreal QC H2M 1L2; Sher'00; FRCPC; CommunMed. Staff, Ministry of Health & Social Services-Quebec; (514)873-9975; nadine.sicard@ottawa.ca.

SICHERI, Dolores A; Thunder Bay Reg Cancer Ctre, 980 Oliver Rd, Thunder Bay ON P7B 6V4; New York (NY) (USA)'76; ABIM; AB(Oncol); AB(Hematol); FRCPC; IntMed (Hematology); MedOncol. Staff, Thunder Bay Regional Health Sciences Centre; Langs: Italian; French; (807)684-7200; Fax. (807)684-5808; sicherid@tbh.net.

SICHILIMA, Tangu; Belgage Med Arts Bldg, 101-525 Belmont Ave W, Kitchener ON N2M 5E2; Manchester (England)'00; FRCPC; Peds. Staff, Grand River Hospital - Kitchener/Waterloo Health Centre; (519)880-3695; Fax. (519)749-2452.

SICHLER, Conrad J; 301-672 Brant St, Burlington ON L7R 2H3; McG'98; CCFP; Att Physician, Joseph Brant Memorial Hospital; Instructor, McMaster University; Langs: Bilingual(French/English); (905)333-5001; Fax. (905)333-9829.

SICKERT, Helga G; Meadowood Med Centre, 1555 St Mary's Rd, Winnipeg MB R2M 5L9; Man'83; (204)255-2389; Fax. (204)254-0730.

SICKINGER, Tina M; Davisville Med & Dental Centre, 204-1849 Yonge St, Toronto ON M4S 1Y2; Tor'84; Peds. (416)488-8876; Fax. (416)488-3969.

SICLAIT, Jaime; Clinique Med de Boisbriand, 877 boul de la Grande-Allee, Boisbriand QC J7G 1W6; Sher'87; CCFP; Langs: English; French; (450)437-4600; Fax. (450)437-7038.

SICOTTE, Claude; Ministry of Employment, 575 rue Saint-Amable, Quebec QC G1R 4Z1; Sher'75; LMCC; (418)644-4645

SICOTTE, Jean-Guy; 309 ch Laurendeau SS 23, Magog QC J1X 0M6; Mon'72; Langs: English; French; (819)843-8380; Fax. (819)847-4850; docjgs@videotron.ca.

SIDANI, Karine; Hop Jean-Talon, 1385 rue Jean-Talon E, Montreal QC H2E 1S6; Sher'10; CCFP; Staff, CSSS du Coeur de l'Isle Hôpital Jean-Talon; (514)495-6767

SIDANI, Paul M; Mediclub du Sanctuaire, 6100 av du Boise, Montreal QC H3S 2W1; Beyrouth (Lebanon)'68; FRCSC; ObstGyn. Staff, St Mary's Hospital Centre; (514)739-5646

SIDANI, Zouhair; Centre ORL Jean-Talon, 203-1384 rue Jean-Talon E, Montreal QC H2E 1S3; Beirut (Lebanon)'74; FACS; FICS; FRCSC; Otol (Clinical Immunology & Allergy). Staff, CSSS du Coeur de l'Isle Hôpital Jean-Talon; Langs: English; (514)273-4461; Fax. (514)273-8401; sidani@sympatico.ca.

SIDDALL, Hugh A; 507-294 Main St, Toronto ON M4C 4X5; Dal'71; Ac Staff, The Scarborough Hospital - General Campus; (416)690-7768; Fax. (416)690-7798.

SIDDALL, Laura S; Two Rivers FHT-Hespeler Med Cl, 12-350 Conestoga Blvd, Cambridge ON N1R 7L7; McM'07; CCFP; (519)629-4615; Fax. (519)629-4630.

SIDDALL, Tamara D; Teen Health Centre, 1585 Ouellette Ave, Windsor ON N8X 1K5; Tor'91; Assoc Instructor Reproductive & Sexual Health, Teen Community Health Centre; (519)253-8481; Fax. (519)253-0891; tsiddall@teenhealthcentre.com.

SIDDHA, Sanjay K; Univ Hlth Network-Toronto Western Hosp, 399 Bathurst St, Toronto ON M5T 2S8; Netaji Subhash Chandra Bose University (India)'90; FRCPC; Derm. Staff, Toronto Western Hospital - University Health Network; (416)603-5800; Fax. (416)603-2782.

SIDDHARTHA, Sanjay; Miramichi Reg Hosp, 500 Water St, Miramichi NB E1V 3G5; Raipur (India)'83; Staff, Miramichi Regional Hospital; Langs: Hindi; Urdu; (506)623-3195; Fax. (506)623-6194; sansid@health.nb.ca.

SIDDIQ, Nayeema; 305 Rusholme Rd, Toronto ON M6H 2Y9; Plymouth (Montserrat)'83; Langs: Bengali; Portuguese; (416)588-7864; Fax. (416)588-9498.

SIDDIQI, Fawaz; London HSC-Victoria Campus, PO Box 5010 Stn B E4002-800 Commissioners Rd E, London ON N6A 5W9; Wes'03; FRCSC; Neursurg. Staff, London Health Sciences Centre - Victoria Campus; Staff, London Health Sciences Centre - University Hospital; (519)685-8500

SIDDIQI, Ferhan S; Univ Hlth Network-Toronto Gen, 12N 243-200 Elizabeth St, Toronto ON M5G 2C4; Tor'08; IntMed. Staff, Toronto General Hospital - UHN; (416)340-3111

SIDDIQI, Nargis; Flin Flon Gen Hosp Inc, PO Box 340 50 Church St, Flin Flon MB R8A 1N2; (Other Foreign)'77; Staff, Flin Flon General Hospital Inc; (204)687-7591

SIDDIQI, Nilofar; Grey Bruce Health Services, PO Box 1800 Stn Main 1800 8th St E, Owen Sound ON N4K 6M9; Punjab (Pakistan)'86; CCFP; Staff, Grey Bruce Health Services - Owen Sound; Aj Prof Family Med, Schulich School of Medicine & Dentistry; Langs: Urdu; Punjabi; Hindi; (519)378-5788; Fax. (519)372-4060; nsiddiqi@gbhs.on.ca.

SIDDIQI, Zaeem A; University of Alberta Hosp, 2E3 11WCM-8440 112 St NW, Edmonton AB T6G 2B7; (Pakistan)'87; PhD; Asst Prof, Queen Elizabeth II Hospital; Asst Prof, University of Alberta Hospital; Asst Prof, University of Alberta; Langs: Urdu; Punjabi; (780)407-1778; Fax. (780)407-1325.

SIDDIQUE, Saquib M; Rouge Valley HS-Ajax/Pickering, 580 Harwood Ave S, Ajax ON L1S 2J4; Bangalore University (India)'96; FRCSC; GenSurg. Staff, Rouge Valley Health System - Ajax & Pickering Health Centre Site; (905)683-2320

SIDDIQUE, Yaseen; Wellpoint Midpark Clinic, 103-240 Midpark Way SE, Calgary AB T2X 1N4; (Other Foreign)'91; (403)256-8213; Fax. (403)254-8795.

SIDDIQUI, Adil F; Doctors Plus Med Centre, 310-505 Main St SW, Airdrie AB T4B 3K3; (Pakistan)'86; CCFP; (403)945-0770; Fax. (403)945-8997.

SIDDIQUI, Adnan S; West Vaughan Med Centre, 3900 Rutherford Rd, Woodbridge ON L4H 3G8; University of Sind (Other Foreign)'92; CCFP; (905)417-5461

SIDDIQUI, Anita K; Lakeshore Gen Hosp, 160 av Stillview, Pointe-Claire QC H9R 2Y2; Aga Khan (Pakistan)'95; MB; BSc; FRCPC; IntMed. Staff, Lakeshore General Hospital - Pointe Claire; (514)630-2225

SIDDIQUI, Faisal S; Ann Thomas Bldg, JJ399-700 William Ave, Winnipeg MB R3E 0Z3; Man'01; FRCPC; Anes; Critical Care Medicine. Staff Critical Care, Health Sciences Centre; (204)774-6511

SIDDIQUI, Farhan; Walk in Clinic, 301-170 McEwan Dr E, Bolton ON L7E 4C8; Wes'04; CCFP; CCFP(E.M.); Langs: Urdu; (905)857-2356; Fax. (905)857-6253.

SIDDIQUI, Farhat; Millbourne Road Med Clinic, 131 Millbourne Road East NW, Edmonton AB T6K 1P6; (780)462-4229; Fax. (780)462-3315.

SIDDIQUI, Iqbal M; Langley Mem Hosp, 22051 Fraser Hwy, Langley BC V3A 4H4; Aga Khan University (Pakistan)'98; MB BS; CCFP; Staff, Langley Memorial Hospital; Langs: Urdu; (604)450-2268

SIDDIQUI, Issar; Arborg & Dist Health Centre, PO Box 10 234 Gislason St, Arborg MB R0C 0A0; (Other Foreign)'93; Staff, Arborg & District Health Centre; (204)376-5247; Fax. (204)376-5356; issars@nursinghomeratings.ca.

SIDDIQUI, Jehan Z; Dr H Bliss Murphy Cancer Ctr, 300 Prince Philip Dr, St. John's NL A1B 3V6; Nishar (Pakistan)'87; MB BS; FRCPC; IntMed; MedOncol. Staff, Dr H Bliss Murphy Cancer Centre; (709)777-7802

SIDDIQUI, Mughina A; St Martha's Reg Hosp, 25 Bay St, Antigonish NS B2G 2G5; Punjab (Pakistan)'89; Staff Anes, St Martha's Regional Hospital; Langs: Urdu; Hindi; Punjabi; (902)863-2830; Fax. (902)867-4431; mughina@yahoo.com.

SIDDIQUI, Muzaffar M; Grey Nuns Community Hosp, 5224-1100 Youville Drive West, Edmonton AB T6L 5X8; (Pakistan)'96; MB BS; FRCPC; Neur (Stroke). Staff Med & Neurol, Covenant Health - Grey Nuns Community Hospital; Clinical Asst Prof Neurol, University of Alberta; Langs: Urdu; Hindi; Punjabi; (780)735-9626; Fax. (780)735-9631.

SIDDIQUI, Nausheen F; Univ of Toronto, 602-500 University Ave, Toronto ON M5G 1V7; Ott'07; FRCPC; IntMed; Nephrol. Langs: Urdu; (416)978-2441

SIDDIQUI, Naveed T; Mount Sinai Hosp, 600 University Ave, Toronto ON M5G 1X5; Karachi (Pakistan)'97; Staff, Mount Sinai Hospital; Langs: Hindi; Punjabi; (416)586-5270; Fax. (416)586-8664.

SIDDIQUI, Nishat A; Bank Med Centre Walk-In Clinic, 1935 Bank St, Ottawa ON K1V 8A3; Vikram (India)'66; MB BS; Physician, Hunt Club Medical Centre; Langs: Urdu; Hindi; (613)521-2391; Fax. (613)521-5443.

SIDDIQUI, Sadia; West Vaughan Med Centre, 3900 Rutherford Rd, Woodbridge ON L4H 3G8; (Pakistan)'96; CCFP; (905)417-5461; Fax. (905)417-5463.

SIDDIQUI, Sameerah; Niagara H System-St Catharines, PO Box 3018 Stn Main 142 Queenston St, St Catharines ON L2R 7C6; Karachi (Pakistan)'04; Staff, Niagara Health System - St Catharines General Site; (905)378-4647

SIDDIQUI, Sanam F; Blck Creek Community Hlth Ctre, 202-1 Yorkgate Blvd, North York ON M3N 3A1; Tor'08; CCFP; (416)246-2388; Fax. (416)650-0971.

SIDDIQUI, Tahira; Rothbart Centre For Pain Care, 9-4646 Dufferin St, North York ON M3H 5S4; Dacca (Bangladesh)'70; MB BS; Anes (P.Q.) (Chronic Pain). Staff Anes, Sunnybrook Health Sciences Centre; Langs: Bengali; Hindi; Urdu; (416)512-6407; Fax. (416)512-6375.

SIDDIQUI, Zubaida; Elliott Lake Family Health Team, 31 Nova Scotia Walk, Elliot Lake ON P5A 1Y9; Peshawar (Pakistan)'93; MB BS; CCFP; Langs: Urdu; Hindi; Punjabi; Persian; Arabic; (705)461-8882; Fax. (705)848-3449.

SIDEL, Michael; SMBD Jewish Gen Hosp, E 005-3755 ch Cote-Sainte-Cath, Montreal QC H3T 1E2; McG'04; FRCPC; Neur. Staff, Sir Mortimer B Davis Jewish General; (514)340-8222

SIDEN, Harold B; BC Women's Hosp & Health Ctr, D606-4500 Oak St, Vancouver BC V6H 3N1; Ann Arbor (USA)'87; FRCPC; Peds. Staff, Sunny Hill Health Centre for Children; Staff, BC Women's Hospital & Health Centre; Fellow Developmental Peds, University of British Columbia; (604)875-2776; Fax. (604)875-2502.

SIDENBERG, Lorne H; Pine Seven Med Centre, 180-4600 Highway 7, Woodbridge ON L4L 4Y7; Tor'74; (905)856-3330; Fax. (905)856-3331.

SIDER, Douglas M; Health Protection & Promotion, 306-480 University Ave, Toronto ON M5G 1V2; Tor'77; FRCPC; CommunMed (Public Health). Langs: Portuguese; (647)260-7313; Fax. (647)260-7600.

SIDERIS, Lucas; Hop Maisonneuve-Rosemont, 5415 boul de l'Assomption, Montreal QC H1T 2M4; Laval'97; FRCSC; GenSurg (Medical Oncology); General Surgical Oncology (P.Q.). Staff, Hopital Maisonneuve-Rosemont; Langs: Greek; English; (514)252-0606

SIDERSON, Miriam A; 201-5651 Riverbend Rd NW, Edmonton AB T6H 5K4; Alb'83; CCFP; FCFP; (780)438-8844; Fax. (780)436-9511.

SIDHOM, Cherine R; St Pierre Med Clinic, PO Box 569, St Pierre Jolys MB R0A 1V0; (Other Foreign)'86; CCFP; Staff, Burntwood Regional Health Authority.

SIDHOM, Mary H; The Village @ Bayers Road, 270-7071 Bayers Rd, Halifax NS B3L 2C2; Cairo (Egypt)'72; MB ChB; MSc; CCFP; Langs: Arabic; (902)454-7666; Fax. (902)454-6555.

SIDHU, Fulroop; BC Children's Hosp, 4500 Oak St, Vancouver BC V6H 3N1; UBC'07; Staff, BC Women's Hospital & Health Centre; Langs: Punjabi; (604)875-2345

SIDHU, Gary; Royal Columbian Hosp, 330 Columbia St E, New Westminster BC V3L 3W7; UBC'03; FRCPC; DiagRad. Staff, Royal Columbian Hospital; (604)520-4253

SIDHU, Gurdip S; Victoria Trail Shopp Centre, 132-550 Clareview Rd NW, Edmonton AB T5A 4H2; Kashmir (India)'76; MB BS; CCFP; (780)478-2735; Fax. (780)472-9089.

SIDHU, Gurmeet; Bramalea & Bovaird Walk-In Cli, 107-10095 Bramalea Rd, Brampton ON L6R 0K1; Sardar Patel Medical College (India)'01; CCFP; Langs: Hindi; Punjabi; Urdu; (905)793-3311; Fax. (905)793-3631.

SIDHU, Gurpreet S; Brantford Med Centre, 100-40 Shellington Place, Brantford ON N3S 0C5; Man'92; Staff, The Brant Community Healthcare System - Brantford General Hospital Site; Langs: Hindi; Punjabi; (519)753-9581; Fax. (905)753-9547.

SIDHU, Gurpreet S; Oxford Recovery Clinic, 502 Oxford St E, London ON N5Y 3H7; Jammu-Kashmir (India)'79; MB BS; MRCPsy(U.K.); FRCPC; Psy (Addiction Medicine). Langs: Hindi; Punjabi; (519)645-6000; Fax. (519)433-5404.

SIDHU, Hameil S; Medical Imaging Consultants, MF-11010 101 St NW, Edmonton AB T5H 4B9; Wes'00; FRCPC; DiagRad. (780)426-1121; Fax. (780)425-5979.

SIDHU, Harkirat S; 10404 111 Ave NW, Edmonton AB T5G 3A2; Alb'94; CCFP; FCFP; (780)944-8675; Fax. (780)944-8677.

SIDHU, Jesse A; Gordon & Leslie Diamond HCC, 8189-2775 Laurel St, Vancouver BC V5Z 1M9; UBC'05; FRCPC; Psy. Staff, Providence Health Care - St Paul's Hospital; (604)875-4809

SIDHU, Jiwan S; Kwantlen Med Clinic, 1-12818 72 Ave, Surrey BC V3W 2M9; UBC'89; CCFP; Langs: Punjabi; (604)572-8161; Fax. (604)572-8108.

SIDHU, Kanwarinder S; 105-6935 120 St, Delta BC V4E 2A8; Hope University School Of Medicine (Belize)'07; CCFP; (604)596-4000

SIDHU, Kuldeep S; North York Gen Hosp, 116-4001 Leslie St, North York ON M2K 1E1; Man'95; CCFP; CCFP(E.M.); Staff, North York General Hospital; Langs: Punjabi; (416)756-6165; Fax. (416)756-6151.

SIDHU, Mandeep K; The Clinic @ Walmart, 1000 Guildford Mall, Surrey BC V3R 1N3; Saurashtra University (Other Foreign)'04; CCFP; Staff, The Scarborough Hospital - General Campus; (604)583-8482

SIDHU, Parbaljit S; Halton HSC Corp-Oakville, 327 Reynolds St, Oakville ON L6J 3L7; Tor'07; CCFP; Staff, Halton Healthcare Services Corporation - Oakville Site; (905)845-2571

SIDHU, Parmjit K; F-2309 McCallum Rd, Abbotsford BC V2S 3N7; Punjab (India)'75; FRCPC; Psy. Reg Chief Psy/Clin Dir/Coord, Abbotsford Regional Hospital & Cancer Centre; Coord Psy, Chilliwack General Hospital; Langs: Hindi; Punjabi; Urdu; (604)854-2001; Fax. (604)854-2078.

SIDHU, Rabinder S; 6-6828 128 St, Surrey BC V3W 4C9; Punjab (India)'86; CCFP; Langs: Hindi; Punjabi; (604)590-5756

SIDHU, Raj K; Bristol Med Clinic, 11A-512 Bristol Rd W, Mississauga ON L5R 3Z1; Guru Nanak (India)'84; MB BS; CCFP; FCFP; Langs: Hindi; Punjabi; (905)501-7712; Fax. (905)501-7714.

SIDHU, Rajreet S S; 201-7110 120 St, Surrey BC V3W 3M8; Bombay (India)'89; FRCPC; Psy. (604)596-7911

SIDHU, Ravindar S; St Paul's Hosp, C318-1081 Burrard St, Vancouver BC V6Z 1Y6; Qns'95; FRCSC; GenSurg; VascSurg. Staff, Providence Health Care - St Paul's Hospital; (604)806-8698; Fax. (604)806-8666.

SIDHU, Rupinder; First Care Med Centre, 2590 Commercial Dr, Vancouver BC V5N 4C2; UBC'93; CCFP; (604)871-1535; Fax. (604)871-1541.

SIDHU, Satinderpal; Westgate Medical, 402-20395 Lougheed Hwy, Maple Ridge BC V2X 2P9; (Other Foreign)'09; (604)465-3900

SIDHU, Shani; 8685 120 St, Delta BC V4C 6R4; Punjab (India)'76; MB BS; (604)590-3166

SIDHU, Shivinder S; 105-6935 120 St, Delta BC V4E 2A8; Poona (India)'76; MB BS; (604)596-4000; Fax. (778)593-9909.

SIDHU, Sue P; Vancouver Gen Hosp, 855 12 Ave W, Vancouver BC V5Z 1M9; Sask'07; GenSurg. Staff Trauma Services, Vancouver General Hospital - Centennial Pavillion; (604)875-5292

SIDHU, Surinder S; 220-50 Sunny Meadow Blvd, Brampton ON L6R 0Y7; Amritsar (India)'74; MB BS; Langs: Hindi; Punjabi; Urdu; (905)789-5944; Fax. (905)789-1376.

SIDHU, Surita; Clinical Sciences Bldg, 8 120-152 University Campus NW, Edmonton AB T6G 2G3; Alb'94; FRCPC; Anes. Staff, University of Alberta Hospital; (780)407-8861; Fax. (780)407-3200.

SIDHU, Tejinder K; Lansdowne Professional Ctr II, 255-3066 Shelbourne St, Victoria BC V8R 6T9; UBC'78; Ac Staff, Vancouver Island Health Authority; Langs: Punjabi; (250)595-1135; Fax. (250)595-7377.

SIDIROPOULOS, Michael; Univ Hlth Network-Toronto Gen, 200 Elizabeth St, Toronto ON M5G 2C4; Tor'07; AnatPath. Staff, Toronto General Hospital - UHN; (416)340-3111

SIDKY, Abdallah Y; 212-2475 Bayswater St, Vancouver BC V6K 4N3; Cairo (Egypt)'52; MB ChB; LRCP; MRCS; DPM(Lond & Edin); FRCPC; Psy (Couple Therapy). Langs: Arabic; French; (604)731-6552; Fax. (604)731-6559.

SIDKY, Adam O; 214-145 15th St E, North Vancouver BC V7M 1R9; Tor'02; FRCSC; OrthSurg. Staff, Lions Gate Hospital; (604)980-8600

SIDLOFSKY, Richard N; Doctor's Office, 101-491 Lawrence Ave W, North York ON M5M 1C7; Qns'99; CCFP; (416)787-5693; Fax. (416)787-8094.

SIDOROV, Jana; Phoenix Med Centre, 306-2155 10th Ave, Prince George BC V2M 5J6; Dal'77; Ac Staff, University Hospital of Northern British Columbia; Langs: Croatian; German; Russian; (250)563-8093; Fax. (250)562-5487.

SIDOROWICZ, Ewa; MUHC-Royal Victoria Hosp, 687 av des Pins O, Montreal QC H3A 1A1; McG'81; FRCPC; IntMed. Chef méd interne, Hopital Maisonneuve-Rosemont; Staff, McGill University Health Centre - Royal Victoria Hospital; (514)843-1515; Fax. (514)843-1582.

SIDRA GERGES, Maged; River West Med Centre, 5-6500 Roblin Blvd, Winnipeg MB R3R 3P9; MB BCh; CCFP; Physician, Four Rivers Medical Clinic; Langs: Arabic; (204)897-9666

SIE, Kian Gwan; 943 O'Connor Dr, East York ON M4B 2S7; Airlangga (Indonesia)'67; CCFP; Court Staff, The Scarborough Hospital - General Campus; Langs: Indonesian; Dutch; (416)755-8281; Fax. (416)755-1352.

SIEBERHAGEN, Janine A; Fort St John Med Clinic, 10011 96 St, Fort St. John BC V1J 3P3; Pretoria (South Africa)'08; (250)785-6677

SIEBERT, Lee F; 358 Oxford St E, London ON N6A 1V7; Alb'72; DOphth; FRCSC; Ophth (Retina Vitreous Surgery). Staff, St Joseph's Hospital - St Joseph's Health Care; Consultant, London Health Sciences Centre - University Hospital; Consultant, London Health Sciences Centre - Victoria Campus; Assoc Prof, University of Western Ontario; Langs: French; (519)672-7570; Fax. (519)672-9914.

SIEDLECKI, Jacqueline B C; Georgian Bay Gen Hosp, PO Box 760 Stn Main 1112 St Andrew's Dr, Midland ON L4R 4P4; Cal'06; CCFP; Staff, Lady Minto Hospital Cochrane; Staff, Georgian Bay General Hospital - Midland; Langs: Polish; (705)526-1300; Fax. (705)526-2007.

SIEGEL, Belle M B; 202A-1685 Main St W, Hamilton ON L8S 1G5; McM'77; FRCPC; Psy (Conjoint Therapy). (905)527-7966; Fax. (905)527-7990.

SIEGEL, Irving J; William Osler HC-Brampton, 2100 Bovaird Dr E, Brampton ON L6R 3J7; Wes'83; Staff, William Osler Health System - Brampton Civic Hospital; Langs: English; French; (905)494-2120

SIEGLING, Cecilia; 1668 Tamarack Ave, Prince George BC V2L 2T3; Pretoria (South Africa)'99; MB ChB; CCFP; Staff, University Hospital of Northern British Columbia; Langs: Afrikaans; (250)564-5474; Fax. (250)564-5482.

SIEKIERSKI, Michal M; St Joseph's Health Care, 50 Charlton Ave E, Hamilton ON L8N 4A6; Wes'88; FRCPC; Psy. Staff, St Joseph's Healthcare Hamilton - West 5th Campus; Staff, St Joseph's Healthcare - Charlton Campus; Asst Prof, McMaster University; Langs: Polish; (905)522-1155; Fax. (905)381-5633.

SIELECKA, Daniela; 314 rue Principale CP 399, Mansonville QC J0E 1X0; Poznan (Poland)'70; LMCC; Staff, Centre Hospitalier et CLSC de Memphremagog; Langs: Polish; English; (450)292-3376; Fax. (450)292-4404; accueilmansonville.mm@gsss.gouv.qc.ca.

SIEMENS, D Robert; Kingston Gen Hosp, E4-76 Stuart St, Kingston ON K7L 2V7; Qns'92; FRCSC; Urol (Oncology). Staff, Kingston General Hospital; Queen's University; (613)548-2411; Fax. (613)545-1970.

SIEMENS, Gwendolyn B J; 101-7343 Hurd St, Mission BC V2V 3H7; UBC'88; CCFP; (604)820-9292; Fax. (604)820-9299.

SIEMENS, Randolph W; 101-7343 Hurd St, Mission BC V2V 3H7; UBC'88; (604)820-9292; Fax. (604)820-9299.

SIEMENS, Ronald K; Royal University Hosp, 103 Hospital Dr, Saskatoon SK S7N 0W8; Sask'82; FRCPC; Peds. Staff Emerg Dept, Royal University Hospital; (306)655-2966; Fax. (306)655-2897.

SIEMIATYCKI, Deborah G; North York Gen Hosp-Branson, 555 Finch Ave W, North York ON M2R 1N5; Sher'88; FRCPC; Peds. Staff Child and Adolescent Health Serv, North York General Hospital - Branson Division; Langs: French; (416)632-8709; Fax. (416)632-8704.

SIEMINOWSKI, Tammy E; Sunnyside Med Arts Centre, 14 St Matthews Rd, Toronto ON M4M 2B5; Tor'93; AAFPhys; CCFP; Court Staff, Toronto General Hospital - UHN; Ac Staff, Bridgepoint Health Centre; (416)461-8251 x1969

SIENIAWSKI, Rafal; Windsor Cardiac Centre, 5-130 Ouellette Pl, Windsor ON N8X 1L9; Cracow (Poland)'03; FRCPC; IntMed (Internal Medicine). (519)250-4449

SIENICKI, Marcin; Burnaby Gen Hosp, 3935 Kincaid St, Burnaby BC V5G 2X6; Dal'96; FRCPC; Psy. Staff Central Team, Burnaby Hospital; Staff, Burnaby Mental Health Services; (604)453-1930

SIENKO, Anna E; Peter Lougheed Centre, 3500 26 Ave NE, Calgary AB T1Y 6J4; Cracow (Poland)'83; BSc; AB; FRCPC; AnatPath (Pulmonary Pathology). Staff, Peter Lougheed Centre; (403)943-4783; Fax. (403)291-2931; anna.sienko@cls.ab.ca.

SIERRA, Sony; LIfe Quest Ctre Reproductive M, 18F-655 Bay St, Toronto ON M5G 2K4; Tor'99; FRCSC; ObstGyn (Infertility). Asst Prof, University of Toronto; (416)217-3971; Fax. (416)217-3972.

SIERRA-DUPONT, Sergio; 700-1538 rue Sherbrooke O, Montreal QC H3G 1L5; National (Mexico)'69; FRCSC; Otol. ac Staff, Hopital Charles LeMoyne; Langs: Spanish; Portuguese; English; (514)931-3263; Fax. (514)939-4018.

SIEU, Nida; Hop du Sacre-Coeur De Montreal, 6555 boul Gouin O, Montreal QC H4K 1B3; Mon'04; FRCPC; Psy. Staff, Hôpital du Sacre-Coeur de Montréal; (514)338-2222; Fax. (514)338-4352.

SIFFLEDEEN, J Shaalan; Town Centre Prof Bldg, 333-6203 28 Ave NW, Edmonton AB T6L 6K3; Alb'05; Gastroent; IntMed (Inflammatory Bowel Disease). (780)705-9933; Fax. (780)705-2895.

SIGAL, Cecil; Fairmont Med Bldg, 1212-750 Broadway W, Vancouver BC V5Z 1J2; UBC'59; DAB; FRCPC; Derm. Hon Staff, Vancouver General Hospital - Centennial Pavillion; Emeritus Prof/Clin Associate, University of British Columbia; (604)879-3424; Fax. (604)879-3425.

SIGAL, Ronald J; Richmond Road Diag & Trmt Ctr, 1898-1820 Richmond Rd SW, Calgary AB T2T 5C7; Cal'87; MPH(Harvard); FRCPC; IntMed (Diabetology); Endocrin&Metab. Prof Med, University of Calgary; Langs: French; (403)955-8327; Fax. (403)955-8249; rsigal2@gmail.com.

SIGALAS, John; 308-2863 Ellesmere Rd, Scarborough ON M1E 5E9; Ioannina (Greece)'84; BSc; FRCPC; IntMed (Diabetology); Endocrin&Metab. Staff, Rouge Valley Health System - Centenary Health Centre Site; Langs: Greek; (416)283-8119; Fax. (416)283-8168; docsigalas@gmail.com.

SIGALET, David L; Alberta Children's Hosp, 2888 Shaganappi Trail NW, Calgary AB T3B 6A8; UBC'83; MSc; PhD(Exp Surg); FRCSC; GenSurg (Transplantation); PedGenSurg. Staff Surg, Alberta Children's Hospital; (403)955-2271; Fax. (403)955-7634; sigalet@ucalgary.ca.

SIGALET, J Phillip; 577 5th Ave, Kamloops BC V2C 3R1; UBC'86; FCFP; Staff, Royal Inland Hospital; Coord Continuing Care Med, TSC-HSA; (250)372-8568; Fax. (250)372-8563.

SIGESMUND, Dayle A; One Medical Place, B2-20 Wynford Dr, North York ON M3C 1J4; Tor'87; FRCSC; Ophth (Pediatric Ophthalmology). Ac Staff, Toronto East General Hospital Inc; University of Toronto; (416)446-5955; Fax. (416)446-1147.

SIGISMUND, John G; The Richmond Hosp, 7000 Westminster Hwy, Richmond BC V6X 1A2; UBC'73; Ac Staff, Richmond Hospital; (604)278-9711

SIGMAN, Eric H; MUHC-Montreal Gen Hosp, 1650 av Cedar, Montreal QC H3G 1A4; McG'95; FRCPC; EmergMed;CCFP; CCFP(E.M.); Staff, McGill University Health Centre - Montreal General Campus; Langs: English; French; (514)934-1934; eric.sigman@sympatico.ca.

SIGMAN, Harvey H; SMBD Jewish Gen Hosp, 3755 ch Cote-Sainte-Catherine, Montreal QC H3T 1E2; McG'57; MSc; DAB; FACS; FRCSC; GenSurg. Chef Div of GenSurg, Sir Mortimer B Davis Jewish General; Prof Surg, McGill University; (514)340-8287; Fax. (514)340-7582; harvey.sigman@mcgill.ca.

SIGMAN, Karen G; MUHC-Motreal Children's Hosp, 2300 rue Tupper, Montreal QC H3H 1P3; Wes'90; FRCPC; Peds; ClinImmunol&Allergy. Staff, McGill University Health Centre - Montreal Children's Hospital; Langs: French; (514)214-4470

SIGMAN, Terry E; MUHC-Montreal Children's Hosp, 2300 rue Tupper, Montreal QC H3H 1P3; McG'91; FRCPC; Peds (Gastroenterology). intérim Dir Div of Gastroent, McGill University Health Centre - Montreal Children's Hospital; (514)412-4400 x24474; Fax. (514)412-4392.

SIGMEN, Jacques; 460 rue de Callieres, Trois-Rivieres QC G8W 1M3; Laval'77; (819)374-2225; jacques.sigmen@sympatico.ca.

SIGOUIN, Daniel; CSSS de l'Antoine-Labelle, 1525 rue de l'Annonciation N, Riviere-Rouge QC J0T 1T0; Mon'89; Staff, Centre de L'Annonciation; (819)275-2118

SIGURDSON, Eric S; Psychealth Centre, 771 Bannatyne Ave, Winnipeg MB R3A 1S1; Man'74; MSc; FRCPC; Psy. Clin Dir Liason Serv, Health Sciences Centre; Consultant Liason Service Child & Adolesc Psy, CancerCare Manitoba; Staff, Psychealth Centre; Prof, University of Manitoba; Fax. (204)787-4975; esigurdson@exchange.hsc.mb.ca.

SIGURDSON, Grant T; Royal Alexandra Hosp, 5002-10240 Kingsway NW, Edmonton AB T5H 3V9; Alb'02; FRCPC; GenPath. Staff, Royal Alexandra Hospital; (780)735-6758; Fax. (780)735-4715.

SIGURDSON, Leif J; Health Sciences Centre, GC 401-820 Sherbrook St, Winnipeg MB R3A 1R9; Qns'92; FRCSC; PlasSurg. Staff, Health Sciences Centre; (204)774-6511

SIGURDSON, Wilfred F; Victoria Mental Health Centre, 2328 Trent St, Victoria BC V8R 4Z3; Man'66; FRCPC; Psy. (250)370-8175; Fax. (250)370-8199.

SIHA, Hany H K; Brentwood Medical, 78 Athabascan Ave, Sherwood Park AB T8A 4E3; (Other Foreign)'98; (780)467-0083; Fax. (780)464-6770.

SIHRA, Sona K; Royal Alexandra Hosp, DTC 5002-10240 Kingsway NW, Edmonton AB T5H 3V9; Alb'02; FRCPC; AnatPath. Staff, Royal Alexandra Hospital; (780)735-4111

SIJAN, Dusan; Windsor Reg Hosp-Metropolitan, 1995 Lens Ave, Windsor ON N8W 1L9; Zagreb (Croatia)'65; Staff, Windsor Regional Hospital - Metropolitan Site; Langs: Croatian; Serbian; (519)254-1661

SIKANDER, Shabana; Levi Walk-In Clinic, 4-7235 Bellshire Gate, Mississauga ON L5N 7X1; Aga Khan (Pakistan)'92; CCFP; Preceptor, University of Toronto; Langs: Hindi; Urdu; Punjabi; (905)795-3535; Fax. (905)795-3838.

SIKANETA, Tabo G; Corporate Med Centre, 10-78 Corporate Dr, Scarborough ON M1H 3G4; McM'96; BSc; FRCPC; IntMed; Nephrol. Staff IntMed & Nephrol, The Scarborough Hospital - General Campus; (416)279-0855; Fax. (416)279-0857.

SIKDER, Mohammed Z; Wetaskiwin Hosp & Care Ctre, 4303-6910 47 St, Wetaskiwin AB T9A 3N3; (Bangladesh)'87; Staff, Wetaskiwin Hospital & Care Centre; (780)361-7100; Fax. (780)361-4315; drsikder@hotmail.com.

SIKHAKHANE, Arnold M; Lonsdale Med Dental Bldg, 108-1940 Lonsdale Ave, North Vancouver BC V7M 2K2; Natal (South Africa)'88; MB ChB; CCFP; (604)987-3347

SIKKA, Sujata S; Trillium Health Centre-Mississ, 100 Queensway W, Mississauga ON L5B 1B8; Tor'99; FRCPC; Anes. Staff, Trillium Health Centre - Mississauga; Langs: Hindi; (905)848-7628

SIKORA, Christopher A; Coronation Plaza, 104-14310 111 Ave NW, Edmonton AB T5M 3Z7; Man'04; FRCPC; CommunMed;CCFP; Public Health & Preventive Med. Physician, Alberta Health Services; (780)342-0252; Fax. (780)342-0248.

SIKORA, Felix J; Winnipeg Clinic, 425 St Mary Ave, Winnipeg MB R3C 0N2; Man'85; (204)957-3217; Fax. (204)957-1860.

SIKORSKI, Robert; Thunder Bay Reg HSC-Thunder Ba, 980 Oliver Rd, Thunder Bay ON P7B 6V4; Ott'06; FRCPC; Anes. Staff, Thunder Bay Regional Health Sciences Centre; Langs: Polish; (807)684-6000; Fax. (807)346-8015.

SIKRI, Rajneesh; 120-135 Queen's Plate Dr, Etobicoke ON M9W 6V1; Yerevan State Medical University (Armenia (Republic))'97; CCFP; Langs: Hindi; Punjabi; (416)342-5140; Fax. (416)342-5148.

SILAGY, Stewart J; Westwood Med Clinic, 3320 Portage Ave, Winnipeg MB R3K 0Z1; Man'95; (204)832-1363

SILBERBERG, Phillip J; Radiology Associates of Regina, 6-2727 Parliament Ave, Regina SK S4S 6X5; Witwatersrand (South Africa)'83; DiagRad. (306)352-7653; Fax. (306)522-4311.

SILBURT, Bruce S; Mayflower Med Clinic, 204-998 Parkland Dr, Halifax NS B3M 0A6; Qns'84; BSc; MSc; CCFP; FCFP; (902)835-1628; Fax. (902)835-1151.

SILCOX, Jo Ann T; 302-717 Richmond St, London ON N6A 1S2; Wes'67; LMCC; CRCP; MDiv; MTS; FRCPC; Psy (Cognitive Therapy). Lecturer Theology, Huron University College; Asst Prof Psy, University of Western Ontario; (519)438-1128; Fax. (519)438-8187; jsilcox@bellnet.ca.

SILCOX, Lisa C; Grand River Hosp-KW Hlth Ctr, PO Box 9056 Stn C 835 King St W, Kitchener ON N2G 1G3; McM'00; BScN; FRCPC; Anes. Staff, St Mary's General Hospital; Staff, Guelph General Hospital; Staff, Grand River Hospital - Kitchener/Waterloo Health Centre; (519)742-3611; Fax. (519)749-4216.

SILECKY, Walter B; Oshawa Clinic, 100-117 King St E, Oshawa ON L1H 1B9; Tor'73; DABIM; FRCPC; IntMed; Rheum. Langs: Ukrainian; (905)723-8551; Fax. (905)723-2541.

SILEIKIENE, Danguole; Red Deer Reg Hosp Centre, 3942 50A Ave, Red Deer AB T4N 4E7; Kaunas (Lithuania)'81; FRCPC; AnatPath (Clinical Pathology). Staff, Red Deer Regional Hospital Centre; Physician, David Thompson Reg Health Centre; Langs: Lithuanian; Russian; (403)343-4707; Fax. (403)343-4877.

SILHA, Josef; Manitoba Clinic, 90 Sherbrook St, Winnipeg MB R3A 1M3; Prague (Czech Republic)'98; FRCPC; Endocrin&Metab; IntMed. Staff, Health Sciences Centre.

SILHOVA, Dasa; Charleswood Med Clinic, 3360 Roblin Blvd, Winnipeg MB R3R 0C5; '98; CCFP; (204)889-7200

SILLER, Theodore N; Scarborough North Med Arts, 205-4040 Finch Ave E, Scarborough ON M1S 4V5; Wes'59; DAB; FACS; FRCSC; OrthSurg (Pediatric Orthopedics). Court Staff, The Scarborough Hospital - Birchmount Campus; Hon Staff, The Hospital For Sick Children; Court Staff, Leamington District Memorial Hospital; Consultant, Erinoak; Langs: Hungarian; French; (416)299-0903; Fax. (416)924-6742.

SILLIMAN, M Lee; Northwest Comm Health Ctre, 525 Simpson St, Thunder Bay ON P7C 3J6; Sask'74; (807)622-8235

SILMBERG, Erik O; Southlake Reg Health Ctre, 596 Davis Dr, Newmarket ON L3Y 2P9; Tor'97; FRCPC; DiagRad. Staff, Southlake Regional Health Centre; (905)895-4521; Fax. (905)830-5972.

SILVA, Coeliflor D; Bloor-Jane Med Bldg, 213-2425 Bloor St W, Toronto ON M6S 4W4; UP (Philippines)'67; Ac Staff, St Joseph's Health Centre; Langs: Tagalog; (416)769-3264; Fax. (416)769-7869.

SILVA, Diana; Natawihin/Nakasuwenik Med Clin, GD, Ile-a-la-Crosse SK S0M 1C0; UBC'09; CCFP; (306)833-2044; Fax. (306)833-2401.

SILVA, Enrique; Pembroke Reg Hosp, 705 Mackay St, Pembroke ON K8A 1G8; Montevideo (Uruguay)'69; FCAP; FRCPC; AnatPath. Dir-Lab Serv/Chief AnatPath, Pembroke Regional Hospital Inc; Langs: Spanish; French; (613)732-3675 x6105; Fax. (613)732-6353.

SILVA, Fidelia A; 247 univesity Ave, Moncton NB E1C 5K4; Sher'96; LMCC; FRCPC; IntMed; Gastroent. Langs: Portuguese; English; (506)857-2285; Fax. (506)852-4340.

SILVA, Harini G; Barhaven Mall Med Clinic, 1002-900 Green Bank Rd, Nepean ON K2J 1S8; Peradeniya (Sri Lanka)'86; CCFP; (613)825-0276; Fax. (613)825-7514.

SILVA, Jaime E; Hamilton HS-General Site, 516-237 Barton St E, Hamilton ON L8L 2X2; Barranquilla (Colombia)'84; FRCPC; Neur (Cerebrovascular Disease). Neurology, Hamilton Health Sciences Centre - Hamilton General Hospital; Asst Prof Neurol, McMaster University; Langs: Spanish; (905)528-5981; Fax. (905)577-8013; spehark@hhsc.on.ca.

SILVA, Mariana; Kingston Gen Hosp, 212 005-76 Stuart St, Kingston ON K7L 2V7; Buenos Aires (Argentina)'81; FRCPC; Peds (Pediatric Hematology Oncology). Att Staff, Hotel-Dieu Hospital; Att Staff, Kingston General Hospital; Prof, Queen's University; Langs: Spanish; (613)549-6666 x3833; Fax. (613)548-2364; mps@queensu.ca.

SILVA, Rachel M; Royal Inland Hospital, 311 Columbia St, Kamloops BC V2C 2T1; UBC'97; FRCPC; Anes. Staff, Royal Inland Hospital; (250)374-5111

SILVA, Vincent E; Medical Centre, 24-1515 Dufferin Cres, Nanaimo BC V9S 2B8; Cape Town (South Africa)'81; MB ChB; FRCPC; IntMed. (250)753-2446; Fax. (250)753-9686.

SILVA GOMEZ, Cecilia V; 132-101 Queensway W, Mississauga ON L5B 2P7; Evangelical University (El Salvador)'04; FRCPC; IntMed; Nephrol. (905)272-1104; Fax. (905)272-1105.

SILVA MARTINEZ, Julio C; Palliser Health Authority, 666 5 St SW, Medicine Hat AB T1A 4H6; FRCPC; AnatPath. Staff, Palliser Health Authority; (403)529-8000

SILVAGGIO, Joseph A; Health Sciences Centre, GB137-820 Sherbrook St, Winnipeg MB R3A 1R9; Tor'97; FRCSC; Neursurg (Neuro Vascular). Staff, Health Sciences Centre; Asst Prof Surg & Radiol, University of Manitoba; (204)787-7563; Fax. (204)787-3851.

SILVANO, Mary J; Heritage Village Medicentre, 2041 111 St NW, Edmonton AB T6J 4V9; (780)438-2306; Fax. (780)461-2632.

SILVANO, Sonia; Hop Maisonneuve-Rosemont, 5415 boul de l'Assomption, Montreal QC H1T 2M4; Mon'06; CCFP; Staff, Hopital Maisonneuve-Rosemont; (514)252-3400

SILVEIRA, Benzil M P; Victoria Hospital, PO Box 3000 Stn Main 1200 24th St W, Prince Albert SK S6V 5T4; Staff, Victoria Hospital; (306)953-8974

SILVEIRA, Jose M A D; St Joseph's Health Centre, 4S4 23-30 The Queensway, Toronto ON M6R 1B5; McM'93; FRCPC; Psy. Staff, St Joseph's Health Centre; Asst Prof Psy, University of Toronto; Langs: Portuguese; (416)530-6780; Fax. (416)530-6076.

SILVER, Barry L; 7-950 ch Herron, Dorval QC H9S 1B3; McG'77; FRCSC; Ophth. Staff, McGill University Health Centre - Montreal General Campus; Langs: French; (514)631-2457; Fax. (514)631-9067.

SILVER, Brian; Generations Family Health Ctre, 104-272 Lawrence Ave W, Toronto ON M5M 4M1; Tor'75; Att Staff Senior's Health Centre, North York General Hospital; Lecturer, University of Toronto; (416)847-9999; Fax. (416)847-8999; generationsfhc@gmail.com.

SILVER, Carla D; Family Matters Med Centre, X-730 St Annes' Rd, Winnipeg MB R2M 2X9; Man'09; CCFP.

SILVER, David A; 209-5885 ch Cote-des-Neiges, Montreal QC H3S 2T2; McG'72; FRCSC; Ophth. Att Staff, Sir Mortimer B Davis Jewish General; Consultant, Donald Berman Maimonides Geriatric Centre; (514)737-7213

SILVER, David M; Generations Family Health Ctre, 104-272 Lawrence Ave W, Toronto ON M5M 4M1; Wes'06; CCFP; (416)847-9999; Fax. (416)847-8999.

SILVER, Eric S; Medical & Dental Bldg, 103-1849 Yonge St, Toronto ON M4S 1Y2; Tor'87; CCFP; FCFP; (416)486-8788; Fax. (416)486-4515.

SILVER, Frank L; Univ Hlth Network-Toronto Western Hosp, WW5 447-399 Bathurst St, Toronto ON M5T 2S8; Tor'78; FRCPC; Neur (Cerebrovascular Disease)., Toronto Western Hospital - University Health Network; Assoc Prof, University of Toronto; (416)603-5800; Fax. (416)603-5768; fsilver@uhnres.utoronto.ca.

SILVER, Ian M F; Kingston Gen Hosp, 76 Stuart St, Kingston ON K7L 2V7; Qns'03; FRCPC; DiagRad. Staff, Kingston General Hospital; Langs: Bilingual(English/French); (613)549-6666; Fax. (613)548-2412.

SILVER, Ivan L; Addiction & Mental Hlth-ARF, 33 Russell St, Toronto ON M5S 2S1; Dal'75; DABPN; FRCPC; Psy (Geriatric Psychiatry). Staff, Centre for Addiction & Mental Health (CAMH) - Russell Street Site; Dir Centre for Faculty Development, St Michael's Hospital; Staff Psy, Sunnybrook Health Sciences Centre; Vice Dean Continuing Educ & Professional Dev/Prof, University of Toronto; (416)535-8501

SILVER, Jeffrey S; Generations Family Health Ctre, 104-272 Lawrence Ave W, Toronto ON M5M 4M1; Wes'06; DTM&H; CCFP; Staff, North York General Hospital; (416)847-9999; Fax. (416)847-8999.

SILVER, Karen L; 210-44 Mapleton Rd, Moncton NB E1C 7W8; Dal'89; CCFP; FCFP; Staff, The Moncton Hospital; (506)870-2417; Fax. (506)870-2576.

SILVER, Lesley C A; Children's Hosp of Eastern Ont, 401 Smyth Rd, Ottawa ON K1H 8L1; Malta (Other Foreign)'01; FRCPC; Anes. Fellow, Children's Hospital of Eastern Ontario (CHEO); (613)737-7600

SILVER, M Margaret; St Martha's Med Centre, 23 Bay St, Antigonish NS B2G 2G7; Dal'76; BSc; FRCSC; Ophth (Cataract). Staff, St Martha's Regional Hospital; Lecturer, Dalhousie University; (902)423-9222; Fax. (902)429-1388.

SILVER, Michael E; St Martha's Reg Hosp, 25 Bay St, Antigonish NS B2G 2G5; Dal'91; FRCPC; DiagRad. Dep Chief, St Martha's Regional Hospital; (902)863-2830; Fax. (902)863-8262; msilver@ns.sympatico.ca.

SILVER, Michael; 208-3850 Finch Ave E, Scarborough ON M1T 3T6; Sher'80; BSc; FRCSC; ObstGyn (Colposcopy). Staff, The Scarborough Hospital - Birchmount Campus; Staff, The Scarborough Hospital - General Campus; Langs: French; (416)299-8292; Fax. (416)299-1442.

SILVER, Norman A; Health Sciences Centre, 840 Sherbrook St, Winnipeg MB R3A 1S1; Man'97; BSc; FRCPC; Peds. Asst Prof Ped Emerg, Health Sciences Centre; Asst Prof, University of Manitoba; (204)774-6511

SILVER, Robert D; Univ Hlth Network-Toronto Western Hosp, 1 439-399 Bathurst St, Toronto ON M5T 2S8; Dal'78; ABIM; FACP; FRCPC; IntMed (Diabetology); Endocrin&Metab. Staff Endocrin, Toronto Western Hospital - University Health Network; Staff, Mount Sinai Hospital; Staff, Sunnybrook Health Sciences Centre; (416)603-6453; Fax. (416)603-7378.

SILVER, Samuel A; R Fraser Elliot Bldg, EB3 805-190 Elizabeth St, Toronto ON M5G 2C4; Tor'08; FRCPC; IntMed. Staff, Toronto General Hospital - UHN; (647)345-3855

SILVER, Shane G; Specialist in Skin Diseases, 203 Edmonton St, Winnipeg MB R3C 1R4; Man'98; FRCPC; Derm. (204)942-4399

SILVER, Shawna E; The Hosp for Sick Children, 555 University Ave, Toronto ON M5G 1X8; McM'07; FRCPC; Peds. Staff, The Hospital For Sick Children; (416)813-7500

SILVER, Sheldon; Britannia Med Centre, 9-5925 Grossbeak Dr, Mississauga ON L5N 6S5; Tor'77; Ac Staff, The Credit Valley Hospital; (905)821-2466; Fax. (905)824-2466.

SILVER, Stuart F; Royal Jubilee Hosp, 1952 Bay St, Victoria BC V8R 1J8; Wes'85; FRCPC; DiagRad. Staff Medical Imaging, Royal Jubilee Hospital; Staff Radiol, Victoria General Hospital; (250)370-8272; Fax. (250)370-8947.

SILVER, William A; 301-2153 Smith St., Regina SK S4P 4G2; McG'56; BSc; MSc; FRCSC; OrthSurg (Adult Reconstructive Surgery). Staff Surg, Regina General Hospital; Pres, Medicare Decisions by Concensus; Clin Associate Prof Surg, University of Saskatchewan; (306)584-1953; wsilver@accesscomm.ca.

SILVERA, Dwight A; Atria II, 101-2235 Sheppard Ave E, North York ON M2J 5B5; McM'01; FRCSC; Ophth (Cornea/External Disease). Staff, Credit Valley Eye Care; (416)492-2002

SILVERBERG, Alexis S W; 971 Pinehill Rd, Peterborough ON K9J 6X3; Qns'86; Langs: French; (705)292-8188; Fax. (705)292-8388; drsilverberg@nexicom.net.

SILVERBERG, David C; The Polyclinic, 407-199 Grafton St, Charlottetown PE C1A 1L2; Tor'73; DABPN; FRCPC; Neur (Clinical Neurology). (902)629-8852

SILVERBERG, Jay D H; Sunnybrook Hlth Sciences Ctre, H 149-2075 Bayview Ave, Toronto ON M4N 3M5; Tor'72; FACP; MACP; FRCPC; IntMed (Thyroid Diseases); Endocrin&Metab. Staff, Sunnybrook Health Sciences Centre; (416)480-4761; Fax. (416)480-5258; jay.silverberg@utoronto.ca.

SILVERBERG, Mark S; Mount Sinai Hosp, 441-600 University Ave, Toronto ON M5G 1X5; Tor'92; PhD; FRCPC; IntMed (Inflammatory Bowel Disease); Gastroent. Staff, Mount Sinai Hospital; Staff, Toronto General Hospital - UHN; Assoc Prof Med, University of Toronto; (416)586-4800 x8236; Fax. (416)619-5524.

SILVERBERG, Samuel; Medical Clinic Bldg, 308-89 Humber College Blvd, Etobicoke ON M9V 4B8; Tor'71; FRCPC; IntMed (Rheumatology). Ac Staff, William Osler Health System - Etobicoke General Hospital; (416)745-8894; Fax. (416)745-5976.

SILVERMAN, Earl D; The Hosp for Sick Children, 555 University Ave, Toronto ON M5G 1X8; Tor'78; FRCPC; Peds (Automotive Medicine); Rheum. Staff, The Hospital For Sick Children; Prof Peds & Immunol, University of Toronto; (416)813-6249; Fax. (416)813-4989; earl.silverman@sickkids.ca.

SILVERMAN, Gregory L; Mount Sinai Hosp, 1514-600 University Ave, Toronto ON M5G 1X5; Tor'04; FRCPC; Anes. Staff Anes & Pain Management, Mount Sinai Hospital; (416)586-5270

SILVERMAN, Howard J; Carling Executive Park, 502-1525 Carling Ave, Ottawa ON K1Z 8R9; Tor'91; AB; FRCSC; PlasSurg (Clinical Immunology & Allergy). Ac Staff, Queensway Carleton Hospital; Ac Staff, Almonte General Hospital; Langs: French; (613)792-4137; Fax. (613)792-1522.

SILVERMAN, Jeffrey A; North York Med Arts Bldg, 311-1333 Sheppard Ave E, North York ON M2J 1V1; Tor'98; FRCPC; IntMed; Hem. Staff, North York General Hospital; (416)494-0586; Fax. (416)494-0915; j.silverman@utoronto.ca.

SILVERMAN, Mark J; 43 Wembley Rd, Toronto ON M6C 2G1; Tor'81; CCFP; (416)652-5307; Fax. (416)486-8660.

SILVERMAN, Mark S; Parkdale Med Tower, 404-1081 Carling Ave, Ottawa ON K1Y 4G2; Ott'83; FACP; FACE; BSc; FRCPC; FRCPC; Endocrin&Metab; IntMed (Diabetes). Staff All Campus, The Ottawa Hospital - General Campus; Asst Prof, University of Ottawa; Langs: French; (613)722-1862; Fax. (613)722-1784; msilverman@cyberus.ca.

SILVERMAN, Melvin; 8N 848-585 University Ave, Toronto ON M5G 2N2; McG'64; BSc; MDCM; FRCPC; IntMed (Nephrology). Sr Physician, Mount Sinai Hospital; Sr Staff Nephrol, Toronto General Hospital - UHN; VP-Research, Canadian Institute for Advanced Research; Prof Med, University of Toronto; Langs: French; (416)340-4064; Fax. (416)340-4951; melvin.silverman@utoronto.ca.

SILVERMAN, Michael S; Baywood Med Centre, 200-95 Bayly St W, Ajax ON L1S 7K8; Tor'85; FRCPC; IntMed (AIDS/HIV); InfectDis. Staff, Rouge Valley Health System - Ajax & Pickering Health Centre Site; Staff IntMed, Lakeridge Health - Oshawa Site; University of Toronto; (905)686-3900; Fax. (905)686-9222.

SILVERMAN, Richard E; 204-400 Tache Ave, Winnipeg MB R2H 3C3; Man'77; FRCSC; GenSurg (Colon & Rectal Surgery). Staff, St Boniface General Hospital; Asst Prof, University of Manitoba.

SILVERMAN, Svetlana; Misericordia Community Hosp, 1N 83-16940 87th Ave, Edmonton AB T5R 4H5; Alb'00; FRCPC; AnatPath. Staff, Covenant Health - Misericordia Community Hospital; (780)735-2778; Fax. (780)735-2870.

SILVERSIDES, Candice K; Hydro Place Bldg, 3155-700 Univeristy Ave, Toronto ON M5G 1Z5; Man'94; FRCPC; IntMed; Cardiol. Staff, Toronto General Hospital - UHN; (416)486-4800

SILVERSTEIN, Carol S; 260-5 Fairview Mall Dr, North York ON M2J 2Z1; Tor'92; CCFP; FCFP; Staff, North York General Hospital; Lecturer Family & Commun Med, University of Toronto; Langs: Hebrew; (416)497-6363; Fax. (416)497-7610.

SILVERSTEIN, Ezra A; UC 1-180 Bloor St W, Toronto ON M5S 2V6; Tor'54; BSc; FRCSC; OrthSurg (Consultation). Consultant, Baycrest Centre for Geriatric Care; Asst Prof/Consultant, Mount Sinai Hospital; Court Staff, St Michael's Hospital; Asst Prof, University of Toronto; Langs: Yiddish; French; German; (416)944-3366; Fax. (416)944-0265.

SILVERSTEIN, Jay M; South Lake Reg Health Ctre, 596 Davis Dr, Newmarket ON L3Y 2P9; Tor'87; Staff, Southlake Regional Health Centre; (905)895-4521 x2222

SILVERSTEIN, Paul V; 604-164 Cumberland St, Toronto ON M5R 1A8; McG'73; FRCPC; Psy. Associate Psy, Centre for Addiction & Mental Health (CAMH) - College Street Site; Lecturer, University of Toronto; (416)506-0605; Fax. (416)979-6815.

SILVERSTONE, Peter H; University of Alberta Hosp, 1G7 17-8440 112 St NW, Edmonton AB T6G 2B7; London (England)'82; MB BS; MRCP; FRCPC; Psy. Staff Psy, University of Alberta Hospital; Prof Psy, University of Alberta; (780)407-6576; Fax. (780)407-6672.

SILVERTHORN, Kelly G; Kootenay Lake Hosp, 3 View St, Nelson BC V1L 2V1; Wes'83; FRCPC; DiagRad. Staff Diag Imaging, Kootenay Lake General Hospital; (250)352-3111 x7137; Fax. (250)354-2328.

SILVERTHORNE, Clifford H; PO Box 80292, Burnaby BC V5H 3X6; UBC'73; Ac Staff, Burnaby Hospital.

SILVESTER, Jocelyn A; Children's Hosp, 840 Sherbrook St, Winnipeg MB R3A 1S1; Dal'08; FRCPC; Peds. Staff, Health Sciences Centre.

SILVESTER, Lois E; 246-246 Artists View Way, Calgary AB T3Z 3N1; Alb'73; CCFP; FCFP; (403)540-7781; Fax. (403)242-6169.

SILVESTRI, Alexandre; 2570 av Vanier, Saint-Hyacinthe QC J2S 6L7; Mon'99; FRCSC; Ophth. (450)774-6224

SILVESTRI, Isabelle; Hop Santa Cabrini Ospedale, 5655 rue Saint-Zotique E, Montreal QC H1T 1P7; Laval'02; FRCPC; IntMed; Respir. Staff, Hôpital Santa Cabrini Ospedale; (514)252-6000

SILVIET-CARRICART, Maite; CHUM-Hotel-Dieu, 3840 rue Saint-Urbain, Montreal QC H2W 1T8; Laval'99; FRCPC; IntMed; Respir. Staff, Centre Hospitalier l'Université de Montréal (CHUM) - Hôtel-Dieu; (514)890-8000 x15660; Fax. (514)412-7123.

SILVIU-DAN, Fanny; MUHC-Montreal Gen Hosp, A6 141 5-1650 av Cedar, Montreal QC H3G 1A4; Bucharest (Romania)'80; ABIM; FRCPC; IntMed; ClinImmunol&Allergy. Staff, McGill University Health Centre - Montreal General Campus; Langs: Romanian; French; (514)934-1934 x42456; fanny.silviudan@muhc.mcgill.ca.

SILVIUS, James L; 7007 14 St SW, Calgary AB T2V 1P9; Alb'84; FRCPC; IntMed; GeriatricMed. Staff Seniors Health, Rockyview General Hospital; Clin Assoc Prof, University of Calgary; (403)943-3441; Fax. (403)212-1230; james.silvius@albertahealthservices.ca.

SIM, Adrian B T; Grey Nuns Community Hosp, 1100 Youville Drive West NW, Edmonton AB T6L 5X8; Alb'03; FRCPC; AnatPath. Staff, Covenant Health - Grey Nuns Community Hospital; (780)735-7875; Fax. (780)735-9688.

SIM, Franklin H; Brockville Gen Hosp, 75 Charles St, Brockville ON K6V 1S8; Alb'94; FRCPC; Psy (Child & Adolescent Psychiatry). Staff, Brockville General Hospital - Charles Street; Staff, Brockville Mental Health Centre - Royal Ottawa Health Care Group; (613)345-5645; Fax. (613)345-7431.

SIM, Keng Howe; Trillium Hlth Ctr-Mississauga, 100 Queensway W, Mississauga ON L5B 1B8; Cal'93; FRCPC; IntMed; Gastroent. Staff, Trillium Health Centre - Mississauga; (905)848-7100

SIM, Lois; University of Alberta Hosp, 1D1-8440 112 St NW, Edmonton AB T6G 2B7; Alb'92; FRCPC; Peds. Staff Ped Ambulatory Clinic, University of Alberta Hospital; (780)407-6370; Fax. (780)407-6414.

SIM, Quan-Yong; Univ of Ottawa Health Services, 300-100 Marie Curie Pvt, Ottawa ON K1N 1A2; Mon'98; BSc; CCFP; Langs: French; (613)564-3950; Fax. (613)564-6627; quanyong@hotmail.com.

SIM, Valerie L; Ctr for Prions & Protein Foldi, 204 EEB-89 University Campus N, Edmonton AB T6G 2M8; Cal'99; FRCPC; Neur. Asst Prof, University of Alberta Hospital; (780)248-1873; Fax. (780)492-1335.

SIM, Wee-Lim; Centre Med de la Plaza, 125-6700 ch Cote-des-Neiges, Montreal QC H3S 2B2; Malaya (Singapore)'67; MB BS; FICS; CSPQ; FRCSC; ObstGyn (Family Planning). Staff Gyn, The Ottawa Hospital - General Campus; Langs: Chinese; (514)342-2941; william.169@hotmail.com.

SIMANTIRAKIS, Emmanuel; Montfort Hosp, 713 Montreal Rd, Ottawa ON K1K 0T2; McG'91; FRCPC; DiagRad (Neuro Radiology). Staff, Montfort Hospital; Staff, The Ottawa Hospital - Civic Campus; Langs: Greek; French; (613)719-0553; mannysim@rogers.com.

SIMANTIRAKIS, Pantelis; Lakeridge Hlth Corp-Oshawa, 1 Hospital Crt, Oshawa ON L1G 2B9; McG'88; FRCPC; Anes. Staff, Lakeridge Health - Oshawa Site; Langs: Greek; (905)576-8711 x3237; Fax. (905)721-4773.

SIMARD, Andre; Andre Simard Med Conseil, 217 rue Terroux, Saint-Lambert QC J4R 2W2; Sher'82; (514)913-3296

SIMARD, Andree-Anne; MUHC-Montreal Gen Hosp, L10 221-1650 av Cedar, Montreal QC H3G 1A4; Laval'96; adj Prof Med, McGill University Health Centre - Montreal General Campus; Médecin, CSSS Jeanne-Mance; Universite de Montreal; Langs: Bilingual(English/French); Spanish; Bilingual(French/English); (514)934-1934 x43973; andree-anne.simard@muhc.mcgill.ca.

SIMARD, Caroline; 204-185 av Acadie, Dieppe NB E1A 1G6; Laval'95; Langs: Bilingual(French/English); (506)389-2200; Fax. (506)388-9366.

SIMARD, Catherine; CSSS de Chicoutimi, CP 5006 305 av Saint-Valier, Chicoutimi QC G7H 5H6; Sher'06; FRCSC; ObstGyn. Staff, Complexe hospitalier de la Sagamie; (418)541-1000

SIMARD, Chantal; Clinique Med Baie St-Paul, 101-4 rue du Moulin, Baie-Saint-Paul QC G3Z 2R8; Laval'82; Staff, CSSS de Charlevoix; (418)435-5760; Fax. (418)435-4137.

SIMARD, Christiane; CSSS du Suroît, 150 rue Saint-Thomas, Salaber-de-Valleyf QC J6T 6C1; Mon'88; ac Staff, Centre Hospitalier Régional du Suroît; (450)371-9920

SIMARD, Dominique; 2004 rue Hocquart, Quebec QC G1V 1N8; Laval'65; (418)683-0934

SIMARD, Eric; Clinique Med Touraine, 2B-520 boul de l'Hopital, Gatineau QC J8V 2P5; Mon'00; Staff, Hôpital de Gatineau; (819)568-0212; Fax. (819)568-6310; lord_dramis@hotmail.com.

SIMARD, Fabien; Clinique Med du Fjord, 1469 boul du Saguenay E, Chicoutimi QC G7H 1H2; Laval'76; FRCSC; ObstGyn (Surgical Oncology). Chef obst & gynécol, Complexe hospitalier de la Sagamie; (418)543-4556; Fax. (418)543-4642.

SIMARD, Fernand; Centre de Pediatrie de Laval, 300-1150 boul de l'Avenir, Laval QC H7N 6L2; Laval'71; FRCPC; Peds (Clinical Immunology & Allergy). (418)549-1034; Fax. (418)696-4673; fesimard@videotron.ca.

SIMARD, France; Clinique Med Optimum, 158-1 Place Laval, Laval QC H7N 1A1; Mon'85; Staff, Hopital de la Cite de la santé; Langs: Bilingual(French/English); (450)668-7400; Fax. (450)668-5855.

SIMARD, Frederic; Clinique Frederic Simard, 24 boul Rene-Levesque E, Quebec QC G1R 2V6; Laval'98; CCFP; CCFP(E.M.); Staff, Hôpital du Sacre-Coeur de Montréal; (418)522-5335

SIMARD, Frederic; GMF de Jonquiere, 3835 boul Harvey, Jonquiere QC G7X 2Z5; Sher'06; CCFP; (418)542-7519

SIMARD, Ginette; Carrefour Med Vallee Richelieu, 665 boul Sir-Wilfrid-Laurier, Beloeil QC J3G 4J1; Laval'83; (450)467-0088; Fax. (450)467-6941.

SIMARD, Helene; Ctr Hosp Affilie-Enfant-Jesus, 1401 18e rue, Quebec QC G1J 1Z4; Laval'90; IntMed. Staff, Centre Hospitalier Affilié Universitaire de Québec - Hôpital De L'Enfant Jésus; (418)649-0252; Fax. (418)649-5913.

SIMARD, Herve; CSSS de Chicoutimi, CP 5006 Succ Racine 305 rue Saint-Vallier, Chicoutimi QC G7H 5H6; Laval'65; MedOncol (P.Q.); Hem (P.Q.) (Hematological Oncology). Staff, Complexe hospitalier de la Sagamie; Consultant, CSSS d'Alma; (418)541-1012; Fax. (418)541-1160.

SIMARD, Hugues; Hôpital Ste-Justine, 3175 Cote Sainte-Catherine, Montreal QC H3T 1C5; Laval'69; Psy. ac Staff, Hôpital Ste-Justine; (514)345-4931; Fax. (514)345-4635.

SIMARD, Jacques; Ctr Hosp de Charlevoix, 74 rue Ambroise-Fafard, Baie-Saint-Paul QC G3Z 2J6; Laval'74; Urol. Staff, CSSS de Charlevoix; (418)435-5150

SIMARD, Jacques; Centre Pediatrique de Laval, 300-1150 boul de l'Avenir, Laval QC H7N 6L2; Sher'70; Peds. Médecin, Centre Pediatrique de Laval; Langs: English; (450)686-0822; Fax. (450)686-2388.

SIMARD, Jean; Polyclinique Med Concorde, 300 boul de la Concorde E, Laval QC H7G 2E6; Laval'72; Urol. (450)667-5310; Fax. (450)965-1801.

SIMARD, Jean-Francois; Centre Med Fafard Enr, 201-975 boul Monseigneur-de-la, Baie-Saint-Paul QC G3Z 2W3; Mon'96; Staff, CSSS de Charlevoix; (418)435-6310

SIMARD, Jennifer M; UMF du Nord de Lanaudire, 50 ch du Golf E, St-Charles-Brromee QC J6E 2B4; Mon'94; CCFP; Langs: Bilingual(French/English); (450)889-5577; Fax. (450)889-4239.

SIMARD, Laurie; Gordon & Leslie Diamond HCC, 5F-2775 Laurel St W, Vancouver BC V5Z 1M9; Mon'06; FRCSC; GenSurg. Staff, Vancouver General Hospital - Centennial Pavillion; Staff, Gordon & Leslie Diamond Health Care Centre; (604)875-4111

SIMARD, Laval; Ctr Hosp Affilie-Enfant-Jesus, 1401 18e rue, Quebec QC G1J 1Z4; Laval'79; FRCPC; Cardiol (P.Q.). ac Staff, Centre Hospitalier Affilié Universitaire de Québec - Hôpital De L'Enfant Jésus; (418)649-0252

SIMARD, Louis; Clin Med Riviere du Moulin, 1388 boul du Saguenay E, Chicoutimi QC G7H 1G8; Laval'87; LMCC; AB; NBME; MCFP; CCFP; Staff Gen Med & Psy, Complexe hospitalier de la Sagamie; Langs: English; (418)549-3564; Fax. (418)549-8463; louis.simard@videotron.ca.

SIMARD, Louis-Marie; Centre Hosp de la Lachine, 650 16e av, Montreal QC H4J 1C5; Laval'76; Staff, Centre Hospitalier de Lachine; Staff, Hôpital du Sacre-Coeur de Montréal; (514)637-2351 x77325; louis-marie.simard@mail.mcgill.ca.

SIMARD, Lyne; CSSS du Nord de Lanaudière, 1000 boul Sainte-Anne, St-Charles-Brromee QC J6E 6J2; Laval'89; FRCPC; Psy (Adult Psychiatry). Staff, Centre Hospitalier Régional de Lanaudière; (450)759-8222 x2004; Fax. (450)759-0011.

SIMARD, Marc; Clinique Med Pierre-Boucher, 260-1333 boul Jacques-Cartier, Longueuil QC J4M 2X1; Laval'76; FRCPC; Respir (P.Q.). Staff, Clinique Medicale Pierre-Boucher; (450)468-6223

SIMARD, Marc; Clinique Med de Nutrition, 360-979 av de Bourgogne, Quebec QC G1W 2L4; Laval'73; Médecin, Clinique Medicale de Nutrition de d'Amaigrissement; (418)652-1121; Fax. (418)652-0055.

SIMARD, Marie C; Clinique Med Montfort, 2185 rue de Montfort, Jonquiere QC G7X 4P6; Laval'91; (418)547-4783; msimard.md@videotron.ca.

SIMARD, Marie-Helene; Ctr Hosp Anna-Laberge, 200 boul Brisebois, Chateauguay QC J6K 4W8; Laval'90; Staff, Hôpital Anna-Laberge; (450)699-2425

SIMARD, Martine; CSSS de Sept-Iles, 45 rue du Pere-Divet, Sept-Iles QC G4R 3N7; Sher'87; FRCSC; ObstGyn. Staff, Centre Hospitalier Regional de Sept-Iles; assoc Membre, Centre Hospitalier Régional Baie-Comeau; assoc Membre, CSSS de la Minganie; (418)962-9761; Fax. (418)961-0734; martine.simard@cgocable.ca.

SIMARD, Martine; CMF Berthier, 788 rue Gilles Villeneuve, Berthierville QC J0K 1A0; Mon'81; (450)836-1393; Fax. (450)836-4814.

SIMARD, Melanie; CSSS du Kamouraska, 1201 6e av, La Pocatiere QC G0R 1Z0; Mon'09; CCFP; (418)856-7000; Fax. (418)856-4737.

SIMARD, Michel; CSSS du Sud de Lanaudière, 911 montee des Pionniers, Terrebonne QC J6V 2H2; Mon'82; Staff, Centre Hospitalier Pierre le Gardeur; (450)654-7525

SIMARD, Michel-Xavier; 255 1re av O, Ste-Anne-des-Mts QC G4V 1E3; Mon'79; Staff, Centre Hospitalier des Monts; (418)763-7676

SIMARD, Michele; CHUQ-Ctr Hosp Univ Laval, RC267-2705 boul Laurier, Quebec QC G1V 4G2; Laval'65; AB; FRCPC; Psy. ac Staff, Centre Hospitalier Universitaire de Quebec-CHUL; (418)654-2256; Fax. (418)654-2756.

SIMARD, Mylene; Clinique Med de la Cite, 101-3801 rue de Montcalm, Jonquiere QC G7X 1W1; Laval'00; Staff, Centre Hospitalier Jonquiere; (418)542-1510; Fax. (418)542-1512.

SIMARD, Normand; CSSS de Chicoutimi, 305 rue Saint-Vallier, Chicoutimi QC G7H 5H6; Laval'64; LMCC; Psy (Clinical Psychiatry). Clin Staff Psy, Complexe hospitalier de la Sagamie; Staff, Institut Roland-Saucier; Langs: English; (418)549-5474; Fax. (418)549-7604.

SIMARD, P Line; CSSS du Rocher-Perce, CP 3300 451 rue Mgr Ross O, Chandler QC G0C 1K0; Laval'68; FFR; FRCPC; DiagRad (Echography). Staff Radiol, Centre Hospitalier de Chandler; Langs: Bilingual(French/English); (418)689-2261; Fax. (418)689-2636.

SIMARD, Raymond; 7-180 rue des Gouverneurs, Rimouski QC G5L 8G1; Sher'80; FRCSC; Ophth (Refractive Surgery). Staff, Hôpital Regional Rimouski; Staff Refractive Surg, Centre Laser Pro Vue; Langs: Bilingual(French/English); (418)723-5008; Fax. (418)721-0375.

SIMARD, Raynald; CSSS de Chicoutimi, 305 rue Saint-Vallier, Chicoutimi QC G7H 5H6; Sher'82; FRCPC; IntMed; MedOncol (P.Q.); Hem. ac Staff Hem, Complexe hospitalier de la Sagamie; (418)541-1000 x2092; Fax. (418)541-1160.

SIMARD, Real; Ctre de sante de Mashteuiatsh, 1160 rue Saint-Edmond, Normandin QC G8M 4M7; Laval'58; (418)274-2026

SIMARD, Robert J; 4904 48 St, Leduc AB T9E 6X4; Alb'93; CCFP; Med Examiner, Province of Alberta; (780)986-2712; Fax. (780)986-0356.

SIMARD, Robert; Dir de la Sante Publique-Mtl, 300 rue King E, Sherbrooke QC J1G 1B1; Sher'81; FRCPC; Public Health & Preventive Med;CCFP; CommunMed (P.Q.). Affil Staff, Hopital Maisonneuve-Rosemont; Staff, Direction de la Sante Publique; Universite de Montreal; (514)829-3400; robert_simard@ssss.gouv.qc.ca.

SIMARD, Steeve; 4457 rue Marquette, Montreal QC H2J 3X7; Mon'95; Staff, Hôpital de Saint-Eustache; Fax. (514)522-5419.

SIMARD, Stephanie; CSSS du Suroît, 150 rue Saint-Thomas, Salaber-de-Valleyf QC J6T 6C1; Sher'03; FRCSC; GenSurg. Staff, Centre Hospitalier Régional du Suroît; (450)371-9925

SIMARD, Sylvain; 120-475 boul Talbot, Chicoutimi QC G7H 4A3; Ott'90; CCFP; FCFP; Langs: English; (418)612-1672; Fax. (418)612-1674.

SIMARD, Sylvain; 852-76 rue Dalhousie, Quebec QC G1K 8W6; Laval'64; PhD; Endocrin (P.Q.) (Diabetology). Langs: English.

SIMARD, Valery; CSSS Haut-Richelieu-Rouville, 920 boul du Seminaire N, St-Jean-Sur-Richel QC J3A 1B7; Mon'98; Staff, Hôpital du Haut-Richelieu; (450)359-5000

SIMARD, Vincent; Hop Sainte-Croix, 570 rue Heriot, Drummondville QC J2B 1C1; Laval'08; CCFP; Staff, Hôpital Sainte-croix; (819)478-6464

SIMARD-CHIU, Leslie A; St James Street Med Clinic, 1600 Portage Ave, Winnipeg MB R3J 0C6; Ott'92; CCFP; Dept Head Biochemistry & Med Genetics, University of Manitoba; (204)831-8460

SIMARD-EMOND, Laurence; CHUM-Hop St-Luc, 1058 rue Saint-Denis, Montreal QC H2X 3J4; Mon'06; ObstGyn. Staff 1, Centre Hospitalier l'Université De Montréal (CHUM) - Hôpital Saint-luc; (514)890-8000

SIMARD-LEBRUN, Adele; Clinique Med de la Maison Nesb, 215 rue du Sud, Cowansville QC J2K 2X5; Laval'05; Ophth. (450)263-8551

SIMARD-RACINE, Genevieve; CSSS de la Matapedia, 135 av Gaetan-Archambault, Amqui QC G5J 2K5; Laval'98; Staff, CSSS de la Matapedia; Langs: Spanish; English; (418)629-6611; Fax. (418)629-4484.

SIMATOS, Gary A; 9508 99A St NW, Edmonton AB T6E 3W6; Mem'94; CCFP; Langs: Bilingual(English/French); (780)915-6993

SIMCHISON, Brian L; Kingston Gen Hosp, 76 Stuart St, Kingston ON K7L 2V7; McM'88; FRCPC; Anes. Staff, Kingston General Hospital; (613)548-7827; Fax. (613)548-1375; simchisb@kgh.kari.net.

SIMCOFF, Micah A; Westshore Maternity & Fam Prac, 101-284 Helmcken Rd, Victoria BC V9B 1T2; Man'03; CCFP; (250)474-7715; Fax. (250)474-6659.

SIMENHOFF, Jacques; Parksville Med Clinic, PO Box 250 154 Memorial Ave W, Parksville BC V9P 2G4; Stellenbosch (South Africa)'93; MB ChB; Staff, Logan Lake Primary Health Centre; Langs: Afrikaans; (250)248-5757

SIMEON, Jovan G; Mental Health Outpatient Serv, 200-311 McArthur Ave, Vanier ON K1L 8M3; Zagreb (Croatia)'59; ABPN; FRCPC; Psy (Child & Adolescent Psychiatry). Contact, Children's Hospital of Eastern Ontario (CHEO); Prof, University of Ottawa; Langs: Greek; Croatian; French; Macedonian; Serbian; (613)738-6990; Fax. (613)738-4891; jsimeon@cheo.on.ca.

SIMETIN, Josee; Clinique Med des Erables, 120-578 Route 138, Neuville QC G0A 2R0; Mon'88; Staff, Centre Hospitalier Chauveau; (418)876-2895; Fax. (418)876-2894.

SIMEUNOVIC, Branko; Windsor Sleep Disorders Clinic, 1100 Ouellette Ave, Windsor ON N9A 1C9; Dal'05; FRCPC; IntMed. Staff, London Health Sciences Centre - Victoria Campus; (519)258-0585; Fax. (519)258-6304.

SIMICE, Jaroslav J; 1822E Comox Ave, Comox BC V9M 3M7; Karlova (Czech Republic)'70; FRCPC; IntMed. Langs: Czech; (250)339-6222; Fax. (250)339-6514.

SIMICE, Peter; Central Alberta Med Imaging, 4312 54 Ave, Red Deer AB T4N 4M1; UBC'00; FRCPC; DiagRad. Staff, Red Deer Regional Hospital Centre; (403)343-6172; Fax. (403)343-6172.

SIMICE, Yana; The Brickyard Clinic, 6010 Brickyard Rd, Nanaimo BC V9V 1S5; UBC'99; CCFP; CCFP(E.M.); Staff, Nanaimo Regional General Hospital; Langs: Czech; (250)390-5200

SIMINOSKI, Kerry G; College Plaza, 8F-8215 112 St NW, Edmonton AB T6G 2C8; Alb'82; ABIM; FRCPC; IntMed (Metabolic Bone Disease); Endocrin&Metab. Staff, University of Alberta Hospital; Dir, Endocrine Centre of Edmonton; (780)434-4784; Fax. (780)439-9977.

SIMINOVITCH, Katherine A; Mount Sinai Hosp, 778D-600 University Ave, Toronto ON M5G 1X5; Tor'76; ABIM; FRCPC; IntMed; Rheum. Staff, Mount Sinai Hospital; (416)586-4800 x8723; Fax. (416)586-8731; ksimin@mshri.on.ca.

SIMION, Oana-Maria; CSSS Haut-Richelieu-Rouville, 920 boul du Seminaire N, St-Jean-sur-Richel QC J3A 1B7; McG'02; Cardiol; IntMed. Staff, Hôpital du Haut-Richelieu; (450)359-5000

SIMION, Sonia; CLSC Notre Dame-de-Grace, 2525 boul Cavendish, Montreal QC H4B 2Y4; Bucarest (Romania)'76; Staff, CLSC Notre Dame-de-Grace; Langs: Romanian; English; (514)485-1677; Fax. (514)485-6506; soniasimion@yahoo.ca.

SIMION, Teodor; CSSS du Sud de Lanaudière, 911 montee des Pionniers, Terrebonne QC J6V 2H2; McG'99; FRCSC; OrthSurg. Staff, Centre Hospitalier Pierre le Gardeur; (450)654-7525

SIMKHOVITCH, Peter; Mackenzie Richmond Hill Hosp, 10 Trench St, Richmond Hill ON L4C 4Z3; Wes'06; CCFP; Staff, Mackenzie Richmond Hill Hospital; Staff Family Med, Sunnybrook Health Sciences Centre; (905)883-2153; Fax. (905)883-2156.

SIMKIN, Ruth E; Health Action Centre, 640 Main St, Winnipeg MB R3B 0L8; Man'80; CCFP; FCFP; Staff, Victoria General Hospital; (204)940-1626; Fax. (204)942-7828.

SIMKIN, Sarah R; Pembroke Reg Hosp, 705 Mackay St, Pembroke ON K8A 1G8; Qns'01; CCFP; Staff, Pembroke Regional Hospital Inc; Langs: Bilingual(English/French); (613)732-2811

SIMKUS, Gerald J; Keary Med Centre, 102-245 Columbia St E, New Westminster BC V3L 3W4; McG'80; MDCM; FRCPC; IntMed (Interventional Cardiology); Cardiol. Dir CATH Lab & CCU, Royal Columbian Hospital; Langs: Bilingual(English/French); (604)524-9571; Fax. (604)524-5322; gerald.simkus@fraserhealth.ca.

SIMKUS, Raymond; Brookswood Family Practice, 4041 200B St, Langley BC V3A 1P1; McG'76; Ac Staff, Langley Memorial Hospital; Physician, Brookswood Family Practice; (604)530-1181; Fax. (604)530-5609.

SIMM, James F; Psychealth Centre, PZ 202-771 Bannatyne Ave, Winnipeg MB R3E 3N4; Man'95; FRCPC; Psy. Physician, Psychealth Centre; jsimm@hsc.mb.ca.

SIMMONDS, Mark K; Clinical Sciences Bldg, 8 120-152 University Campus NW, Edmonton AB T6G 2G3; Bristol (England)'84; MB ChB; FRCA; MRC; LMCC; FRCPC; Anes (Pain Management). Clinical Asst Prof Stollery Children's Anes & Pain Mgmt, University of Alberta Hospital; (780)407-8861; Fax. (780)407-3200.

SIMMONDS, Matthew R; University of Alberta Hosp, 3C1 12-8440 112 St NW, Edmonton AB T6G 2B7; Cal'03; FRCPC; Anes; Critical Care Medicine. Staff, University of Alberta Hospital; (780)407-6755; Fax. (780)407-1228.

SIMMONDS, S Douglas; 810-5010 43 St, Red Deer AB T4N 6H2; Alb'79; FRCPC; IntMed; Gastroent. (403)343-6955; Fax. (403)347-9420.

SIMMONDS, Wrensford F; 204-2494 Danforth Ave, Toronto ON M4C 1K9; Tor'85; MSc; Ac Staff, Toronto East General Hospital Inc; (416)690-9700; Fax. (416)690-3805.

SIMMONS, Brian S; Sunnybrook Health Science Ctre, M4224-2075 Bayview Ave, Toronto ON M4N 3M5; Southampton (England)'77; FRCPC; Peds (Neonatal & Perinatal Medicine). Staff Newborn & Developmental Peds, Women's College Hospital; (416)480-6100; Fax. (416)480-5613.

SIMMONS, Christine E; BC Cancer Agency, 6F-600 10 Ave W, Vancouver BC V5Z 1V6; Qns'01; MSc; FRCPC; IntMed; MedOncol. Staff, BC Cancer Agency Vancouver Centre; (604)877-6000

SIMMONS, Collan J T; Stratford Gen Hosp, 46 General Hospital Dr, Stratford ON N5A 2Y6; Tor'04; FRCPC; Anes. Staff, Stratford General Hospital - Huron Perth Healthcare Alliance; (519)271-2120

SIMMONS, Deanna L; 128-2906 Broadway W, Vancouver BC V6K 2G8; UBC'95; CCFP; (604)261-6366 x3956

SIMMONS, Elizabeth L; Lakeridge Health-Oshawa Site, 1 Hospital Crt, Oshawa ON L1G 2B9; Qns'69; PlasSurg. Staff, Lakeridge Health - Oshawa Site; (905)576-8711

SIMMONS, Grace; 203-30 Crystalridge Dr, Okotoks AB T1S 2C3; (Other Foreign)'95; DCH; MB ChB; MRCGPract; (403)995-0010; Fax. (403)995-0051.

SIMMONS, James D; Goodfellow Prof Bldg, 203-170 McEwan Dr E, Bolton ON L7E 4C8; Dal'67; (905)951-1575; Fax. (905)951-1786.

SIMMONS, Kyra E; Carewest Glenmore Park, 1E-6909 14 St SW, Calgary AB T2V 1P8; Cal'92; BSc; Staff, Rockyview General Hospital; Staff, Carewest Glenmore Park; (403)861-6693; Fax. (403)238-2221; ksimmons_12@yahoo.com.

SIMMONS, Malcolm C; Centennary HC-The Court, 418-2863 Ellesmere Rd, Scarborough ON M1E 5E9; Qns'85; (416)924-2482; Fax. (416)924-2484; info@chtc.ca.

SIMMONS, Maureen L; 216 Macdonald Ave, Belleville ON K8N 3Y7; Qns'78; CCFP; FCFP; (613)962-0976; Fax. (613)969-8086.

SIMMONS, Pamela A; Boniface Park Med Centre, 6-700 Markham Rd, Scarborough ON M1H 2A7; Tor'95; BSc; IntMed. (416)431-7100; Fax. (416)431-7191.

SIMMONS, Rachel A; Howard Mutual Med Centre, PO Box 667 20129 Erie St S, Ridgetown ON N0P 2C0; (USA)'08; CCFP; (519)674-2600

SIMMONS, T Britt; Rockyview Gen Hosp, 7007 14 St SW, Calgary AB T2V 1P9; Alb'81; CCFP; Staff, Rockyview General Hospital; (403)943-3597; Fax. (403)943-8411.

SIMMONS, William W; 300 Plains Rd E, Burlington ON L7T 2C6; Tor'87; FRCPC; IntMed; Cardiol. (905)639-6011; Fax. (905)639-0516.

SIMMS, Allyson; Clinique Med de Coaticook, 206-18 rue du Manege, Coaticook QC J1A 3B3; Sher'92; Staff, Centre Hospitalier de Coaticook; Médecin, Clinique Medicale de Manege; Langs: English; (819)849-4808; Fax. (819)849-7400; allysimms@sympatico.ca.

SIMMS, J David; Saint John Reg Hosp, PO Box 2100 Stn Main 400 University Ave, Saint John NB E2L 4L2; Dal'79; FRCPC; DiagRad. Staff, Saint John Regional Hospital; (506)648-6111

SIMMS, Kathryn A; William Osler HS-Etobicoke, 101 Humber College Blvd, Etobicoke ON M9V 1R8; Ott'03; FRCPC; Anes. Staff, Trillium Health Centre - Mississauga; Staff, North York General Hospital; Staff, William Osler Health System - Etobicoke General Hospital; (416)494-2120

SIMMS, Kiri J M; Vancouver Island Health, 5A-2328 Trent St, Victoria BC V8R 4Z3; McM'93; BScN; FRCPC; Psy. Staff, Vancouver Island Health Authority; Staff, Mental Health Centre; Langs: Bilingual(English/French); (250)370-8000; kiri.simms@viha.ca.

SIMMS, Matthew G; Queen Elizabeth II HSC-VG Site, 10F-1276 South Park St, Halifax NS B3H 2Y9; UBC'03; FRCPC; Anes. Staff, Queen Elizabeth II Health Sciences Centre - Victoria General Site; (902)473-2331

SIMMS, R Gregory; Barrie Allergy Clinic, 402-49 High St, Barrie ON L4N 5J4; Dal'74; FRCPC; Peds (Clinical Immunology & Allergy). (705)726-3412

SIMMS, Richard J; Stevenson Mem Hosp, PO Box 4000 Stn Main 200 Fletcher Cres, Alliston ON L9R 1W7; Dal'74; FSOGC; FRCSC; ObstGyn. Staff, Stevenson Memorial Hospital; (705)435-6281

SIMMS, Robin M; Kootenay Lake Gen Hosp, 3 View St, Nelson BC V1L 2V1; Cal'09; CCFP; Staff, Kootenay Lake General Hospital; (250)352-3111

SIMON, Barry J; 1-989 Eglinton Ave, York ON M6C 2C6; Tor'85; FRCPC; Psy (Couple Therapy). Staff, Centre for Addiction & Mental Health (CAMH) - College Street Site; Staff Psy, Mount Sinai Hospital; Asst Prof Psy, University of Toronto; (416)921-6500; Fax. (416)921-6321; drsimon@rogers.com.

SIMON, Christine J; Cobourg Clinic, PO Box 86 Stn Main 44 University Ave E, Cobourg ON K9A 4K4; Tor'80; CCFP; FCFP; Court Staff, Northumberland Hills Hospital; (905)372-3323; Fax. (905)372-3692; christine.simon@cobourgclinic.ca.

SIMON, Daniel; CLSC Mer et Montagnes, 71 boul St-Francois-Xavier E, Grande-Vallee QC G0E 1K0; Mon'81; CCFP; (418)393-2001; Fax. (418)393-2767.

SIMON, David A; Rideau Valley Health Centre, 1221 Greenbank Rd, Ottawa ON K2J 5V7; Ott'05; FRCSC; OrthSurg. (613)258-8716; Fax. (613)440-3238.

SIMON, Gary S; London HSC-Victoria Hosp, PO Box 5010 Stn B C2 166-800 Commissioners Rd E, London ON N6A 5W9; Dal'77; FRCPC; Anes. Ac Staff, London Health Sciences Centre - Victoria Campus; (519)685-8300; Fax. (519)667-6601.

SIMON, James K; Royal Victoria Hosp, 201 Georgian Dr, Barrie ON L4M 6M2; Tor'93; FRCPC; Anes. Court Staff, Stevenson Memorial Hospital; Anesthetist, Royal Victoria Regional Health Centre; (705)728-9090 x4207; Fax. (705)739-5613; simonj@rvh.on.ca.

SIMON, Jeannine G M; 210-269 boul Saint-Jean, Pointe-Claire QC H9R 3J1; McG'76; MDCM; ABOG; FRCSC; ObstGyn (Infertility). Staff, Lakeshore General Hospital - Pointe Claire; Langs: English; French; (514)697-1417; Fax. (514)697-6144; jeannine51@videotron.ca.

SIMON, Jerome B; Hotel-Dieu Hosp, 166 Brock St, Kingston ON K7L 5G2; Qns'62; FACP; ABIM; FACG; FRCP; FRCPC; IntMed (Gastroenterology). Aj Staff Gastroent, Hotel-Dieu Hospital; Aj Staff, Kingston General Hospital; Emeritus Prof Med, Queen's University; (613)544-3310 x2491; Fax. (613)544-3114; simonj@post.queensu.ca.

SIMON, Jessica E; Foothills Med Centre, 710 ST-1403 29 St NW, Calgary AB T2N 2T9; Edinburgh (England)'95; FRCPC; IntMed. Staff Palliative Care, Foothills Medical Centre; (403)944-2304; Fax. (403)270-9652.

SIMON, Jonathan R; 77 MacLaren St, Ottawa ON K2P 0K5; McG'75; FRCPC; Psy. (613)230-3323

SIMON, Karl D A; PO Box 67041 Rpo Northland Vlg, Calgary AB T2L 2L2; Dal'05; FRCPC; Anes. (403)944-1110

SIMON, L Michael; 719 Millidge Ave, Saint John NB E2K 2N7; Dal'88; CCFP; Ac Staff, Saint John Regional Hospital; Ac Staff, St Joseph's Hospital; Dalhousie University; (506)652-6868; Fax. (506)657-3911.

SIMON, Mathieu; Hôpital Laval, 2725 ch Sainte-Foy, Quebec QC G1V 4G5; Laval'94; FRCPC; IntMed (Intensive Care); Critical Care Medicine; Respir. Prof, Hôpital Laval; Langs: English; (418)656-4747; Fax. (418)656-4762; mathieu.simon@crhl.ulaval.ca.

SIMON, Paul B; Mountain Med Clinic, PO Box 820 108-1700 Garcia St, Merritt BC V1K 1B8; UBC'91; (250)315-1455; Fax. (250)315-1427.

SIMON, Renee; Bureau Dre Renee Simon, 204-2499 rue Saint Georges, Longueuil QC J4R 2T4; Mon'84; FRCSC; GenSurg (Endoscopic Surgery). Staff, Hopital Charles LeMoyne; (450)672-8886

SIMON, Sandra S; Meadowlark Health Centre, 180 Meadowlark Shopping Ctr NW, Edmonton AB T5R 5W9; (India)'79; CCFP; Staff, Covenant Health - Misericordia Community Hospital; (780)484-7574; Fax. (780)486-4142.

SIMON, Sonia H; Scarborough Hosp-Birchmount, 3030 Birchmount Rd, Scarborough ON M1W 3W3; University of Al-Mustansiriyah (Other Foreign)'98; FRCPC; Peds. Staff, The Scarborough Hospital - Birchmount Campus; (416)495-2400

SIMONCELLI, Luc; Hopital Marie-Clarac, 3530 boul Gouin E, Montreal-Nord QC H1H 1B7; Mon'87; Staff, Hopital Marie Clarac; Staff, Hôpital du Sacre-Coeur de Montréal; (514)321-8800

SIMONDS, Patricia E; 11503 124 St NW, Edmonton AB T5M 0K5; Alb'57; RC; Psy. (780)487-4754; Fax. (780)444-9307.

SIMONE, Andrew A; 40 King George's Rd, Etobicoke ON M8X 1L3; Qns'63; CM; FRCPC; Derm. Langs: Spanish; Italian; French; (416)231-2817; Fax. (416)231-6205.

SIMONE, Angelo M; Hurontario Med Clinic, 200-2338 Hurontario St, Mississauga ON L5B 1N1; Tor'90; Endocrin&Metab; Peds (Pediatric Endocrinology). Ac Staff, Trillium Health Centre - Mississauga; Langs: Italian; (905)848-8303; Fax. (905)848-5727; asimone@thc.on.ca.

SIMONE, Carmine; Toronto East Gen Hosp, KW 303-825 Coxwell Ave, Toronto ON M4C 3E7; McM'98; BSc; FRCSC; ThorSurg (Critical Care Medicine). Staff Thoracic Surg, Sunnybrook Health Sciences Centre; Thoracic Surg, Royal Victoria Regional Health Centre; Head Div of Critical Care & Thoracic Surg, Toronto East General Hospital Inc; Langs: Italian; (416)465-9133; Fax. (416)465-9584.

SIMONEAU, Esther; CSSS de Laval, 1755 boul Rene-Laennec, Laval QC H7M 3L9; Mon'00; FRCPC; MedMicrobiol. Staff, Hopital de la Cite de la santé; (450)975-5558

SIMONEAU, Jocelyne; CSSS du Suroît, 150 rue Saint-Thomas, Salaber-de-Valleyf QC J6T 6C1; Mon'71; GenPath (P.Q.) (Cytology). Chef Path Services, Centre Hospitalier Régional du Suroît; Langs: Bilingual(French/English); (450)371-9920 x2093; Fax. (450)371-5275; simoneau.jocelyne@sssrr16.gouv.qc.ca.

SIMONEAU, Noella; CSSS de Rivière-de-Loup, 75 rue Saint-Henri, Riviere-du-Loup QC G5R 2A4; Laval'69; Staff, Centre Hospitalier Regional du Grand-Portage; (418)868-1000 x2923; Fax. (418)868-1035.

SIMONEAU, Roger; 201-301 ch du Club-Marin, Verdun QC H3E 1Z2; Mon'60; Psy (P.Q.). Staff, Centre Hospitalier Fleury; (514)769-1781

SIMONEAU-ROY, Judith; CHUS-Hop Fleurimont, 3001 12e av N, Sherbrooke QC J1H 5N4; Sher'96 Sherbrooke; FRCPC; Endocrin&Metab; Peds. Staff, Centre Hospitalier Universitaire de Sherbrooke-Hopital Fleurimont; Langs: Bilingual(English/French); (819)346-1110 x13147; Fax. (819)564-5398; judith.simoneau-roy@usherbrooke.ca.

SIMONETT, Gillian R; Foothills Med Centre, 1403 29 St NW, Calgary AB T2N 2T9; Wes'06; FRCPC; PhysMed&Rehab. Staff, Foothills Medical Centre; (403)944-2061

SIMONIK, Dagmar; Jane & Shoreham Med Ctre, 102-4640 Jane St, North York ON M3N 2K5; Palacky (Czech Republic)'52; Assoc Staff, Humber River Regional Hospital - Finch Avenue Site; Langs: Czech; Slovak; (416)661-6440; Fax. (416)661-2200.

SIMONIK, Martin; Jane & Shoreham Med Ctre, 102-4640 Jane St, North York ON M3N 2K5; Tor'80; Ac Staff, Humber River Regional Hospital - Finch Avenue Site; Langs: Czech; Slovak; French; (416)661-6440

SIMONS, D Irene; Clinique Med Vendome, 200-5175 boul de Maisonneuve O, Montreal QC H4A 1Z3; McG'67; CCFP; FCFP; Affil Staff Family Pract, McGill University Health Centre - Montreal General Campus; Langs: Bilingual(English/French); (514)484-4712; Fax. (514)484-9828; medicat@sprint.ca.

SIMONS, Derek B; 42 Sir Tristram Pl, Markham ON L3P 2X9; Man'87; FRCPC; IntMed; Cardiol. (416)938-2244

SIMONS, Frances E; Children's Hosp, FE125-685 William St, Winnipeg MB R3E 0Z2; Man'99; Staff Allergy & Immunology, Health Sciences Centre.

SIMONS, Frances E R; Children's Hosp, 840 Sherbrook St, Winnipeg MB R3A 1S1; Man'69; FAAAI; FAAP; FRCPC; Peds (Clinical Immunology & Allergy). Consultant Clinica Immunology & Allergy, Health Sciences Centre; Prof Section of Clinical Immunology & Allergy, University of Manitoba; lmcniven@hsc.mb.ca.

SIMONS, Gertjan; 13-1617 Baker St, Cranbrook BC V1C 1B4; Stellenbosch (South Africa)'91; MB ChB; FRCSC; GenSurg. Staff, East Kootenay Regional Hospital; Langs: Afrikaans; (250)417-2024; Fax. (250)417-2026; nimbexsnr@hotmail.com.

SIMONS, Ian W C; Killarney Med Centre, PO Box 1690, Killarney MB R0K 1G0; Pretoria (South Africa)'65; MB ChB; LMCC; BComm; Langs: Afrikaans; (204)523-4609; Fax. (204)523-7340.

SIMONS, Jeffrey A; Prince Rupert Reg Hosp, 1305 Summit Ave, Prince Rupert BC V8J 2A6; London (England)'67; MB BS; MEd; FRCPC; Peds. Staff, Prince Rupert Regional Hospital; (250)622-6506; Fax. (250)622-6277.

SIMONS, Jonathan M; SMBD Jewish Gen Hosp, 3755 ch Cote-Sainte-Catherine, Montreal QC H3T 1E2; McG'00; CCFP; CCFP(E.M.); Staff, Sir Mortimer B Davis Jewish General; (514)340-8222 x5568

SIMONS, Martin E; Univ Hlth Network-Toronto Western Hosp, 3MC 423-399 Bathurst St, Toronto ON M5T 2S8; Tor'80; BSc; FRCPC; DiagRad (Interventional Radiology). Staff, The Hospital For Sick Children; Staff, Toronto Western Hospital - University Health Network; Staff, Mount Sinai Hospital; Asst Prof, University of Toronto; (416)603-6276; martin.simons@uhn.on.ca.

SIMONS, Richard K; Vancouver Gen Hosp, 855 12th Ave W, Vancouver BC V5Z 1M9; Cambridge (England)'77; MB ChB; FRCS; FACS; FRCSC; GenSurg (Trauma). Med Dir Trauma Program, Vancouver General Hospital - Centennial Pavillion; Staff, Vancouver Coastal Health; Prof Surg, University of British Columbia; (604)875-5094; Fax. (604)875-5348.

SIMONSEN, J Neil; National Microbiology Lab, 1015 Arlington St, Winnipeg MB R3E 3R2; Dal'79; FRCPC; IntMed. Staff, National Microbiology Laboratories; (204)789-6071; neil_simonsen@phac-aspc.gc.ca.

SIMONSON, Donald W; Misericordia Health Centre, 99 Cornish Ave, Winnipeg MB R3C 1A2; Man'84; Staff, Stonewall & District Health Centre; Staff, Misericordia Health Centre; (204)788-8364

SIMONYI-GINDELE, Samuel; Gibson Health Clinic, PO Box 9000 Stn A, Fredericton NB E3B 5N5; UBC'02; CCFP; Staff, Dr Everett Chalmers Regional Hospital; (506)447-4444; Fax. (506)447-4221.

SIMONYI-POIRIER, Marianne; Medecine Familiale Montclair, 207-15 boul Montclair, Gatineau QC J8Y 2E2; Mon'04; CCFP; Staff, CH-CHSLD de Papineau - Pavillon du centre hospitalier; (819)772-2003; Fax. (819)772-4880.

SIMOR, Andrew E; Sunnybrook Hlth Sciences Ctre, B103-2075 Bayview Ave, Toronto ON M4N 3M5; Tor'76; FRCPC; IntMed (Infectious Diseases); MedMicrobiol; InfectDis. Staff Microbiol, Sunnybrook Health Sciences Centre; Prof Lab Med, University of Toronto; (416)480-4549; Fax. (416)480-6990; andrew.simor@sunnybrook.ca.

SIMOS, Demetrios; The Ottawa Hosp-General Site, 501 Smyth Rd Box 900, Ottawa ON K1H 8L6; Ott'07; FRCPC; IntMed; MedOncol. Staff, The Ottawa Hospital Pharmacy-General Campus; (613)798-5555

SIMPSON, Alexander I F; Addiction & Mental Hlth-Queen, 3-1001 Queen St W, Toronto ON M6J 1H4; Staff Law & Mental Health Program, Centre for Addiction & Mental Health (CAMH) - Queen Site; (416)535-8501

SIMPSON, C David; Queen Elizabeth II HSC, 404-1276 South Park St, Halifax NS B3H 2Y9; Qns'77; BSc(Hons); FRCPC; IntMed. Staff, Queen Elizabeth II Health Sciences Centre - Victoria General Site; Prof, Dalhousie University; (902)473-2156; Fax. (902)473-8430.

SIMPSON, Charles D A; IWK Health Centre, PO Box 9700 Rpo CSC 5850-5980 Univesity Ave, Halifax NS B3K 6R8; Qns'04; FRCPC; Peds (Neonatal & Perinatal Medicine). Staff Neonatal Perinatal Med, IWK Health Centre; (902)470-8888

SIMPSON, Charles W; Royal University Hosp, 4515-103 Hospital Dr, Saskatoon SK S7N 0W8; Sask'71; ABOG; FRCSC; ObstGyn (Reproductive Endocrinology & Infertility). Consultant ObstGyn, Royal University Hospital; Clin Prof Obst/Gyn/Consultant, University of Saskatchewan; (306)966-2522; Fax. (306)966-8040; charles.simpson@usask.ca.

SIMPSON, Cheryl L; 36-1960 Appleby Line, Burlington ON L7L 0B7; Tor'09; CCFP; (905)315-9929

SIMPSON, Christine L; Grey Nuns Community Hosp, 1100 Youville Drive West NW, Edmonton AB T6L 5X8; Alb'98; FRCPC; IntMed. Staff, Covenant Health - Grey Nuns Community Hospital; (780)735-7000; Fax. (780)416-9309.

SIMPSON, Christopher S; Kingston Gen Hosp, FAPC L3-76 Stuart St, Kingston ON K7L 2V7; Dal'92; FACC; FRCPC; IntMed (Electrophysiology); Cardiol. Staff, Kingston General Hospital; Chief Cardiol/Prof Med, Queen's University; (613)548-3232; Fax. (613)548-1387; simpsonc@kgh.kari.net.

SIMPSON, Craig A; Lennox & Addington County Gen, 8 Richmond Park Dr, Napanee ON K7R 2Z4; Qns'07; CCFP; CCFP(E.M.); Staff, Lennox & Addington County General Hospital; (613)354-3301

SIMPSON, D Lee; Abbie J Lane Mem Bldg, 8F-5909 Veterans Memorial Lane, Halifax NS B3H 2E2; Ott'99; CCFP; Staff, Queen Elizabeth II Health Sciences Centre - Halifax Infirmary Site; (902)473-4887

SIMPSON, Diane L; Diane L Simpson Med Prof Corp, 496 Maple Ave, Hamilton ON L8K 1K5; McM'85; CCFP; CCFP(E.M.); Staff, Hamilton Health Sciences Centre - Hamilton General Hospital; (905)527-4322; Fax. (905)545-6232.

SIMPSON, E Rand; 408-1100 Sheppard Ave E, North York ON M2K 2W1; Tor'63; FRCSC; Ophth (Ocular Oncology). Dir Ocular Oncol, Princess Margaret Hospital - University Health Network; Staff Ophth, North York General Hospital; Dir, Ontario Cancer Institute; Dir, Ocular Tumour Clinic; Assoc Prof, University of Toronto; Langs: French; (416)226-2227; Fax. (416)226-5829; rand.simpson@uhn.on.ca.

SIMPSON, Ewurabena A; Childrens Hosp of Eastern Ont, 401 Smyth Rd, Ottawa ON K1H 8L1; McG'05; Peds (Pediatric Hematology Oncology). Staff, Children's Hospital of Eastern Ontario (CHEO); (613)737-7600

SIMPSON, Ian M; Western Mem Reg Hosp, PO Box 2005 Stn Main 1 Brookfield Ave, Corner Brook NL A2H 6J7; Cambridge (England)'60; DObstRCOG; CCFP; FCFP; Staff Gerontology, Western Memorial Regional Hospital; (709)637-5000

SIMPSON, J David; Tillsonburg Med Clinic, 154 Rolph St, Tillsonburg ON N4G 3Z1; Wes'73; (519)842-3682

SIMPSON, J Thomas; Woolwich Comm Health Centre, PO Box 370 10 Parkside Dr, St Jacobs ON N0B 2N0; Tor'74; BSc(Hon.); MSc; BEd; CCFP; FCFP; Staff, Grand River Hospital - Kitchener/Waterloo Health Centre; Staff, St Mary's General Hospital; (519)664-3794; Fax. (519)664-2182; 74240.342@compuserve.com.

SIMPSON, Janelle D; 23 Gareth Crt, Dieppe NB E1A 8B4; Dal'98; BSc; CCFP.

SIMPSON, John A; Muskoka Algonquin Healthcare, 100 Frank Miller Dr, Huntsville ON P1H 1H7; McM'99; CCFP; Staff, Huntsville District Memorial Hospital - Muskoka Algonquin Healthcare; (705)789-2311; Fax. (705)789-0057.

SIMPSON, John S A; Foothills Med Centre, 1403 29 St NW, Calgary AB T2N 2T9; Cal'89; FRCPC; Psy. Staff Psy, Foothills Medical Centre; (403)944-1272; Fax. (403)944-8340.

SIMPSON, Jory S; The Banting Institute, 209-100 College St, Toronto ON M5G 1L5; UBC'06; FRCSC; GenSurg. Staff, The Banting Institute; (416)978-5575

SIMPSON, Kathleen L; Thunder Bay Reg HSC, 980 Oliver Rd, Thunder Bay ON P7B 6V4; McM'93; CCFP; Staff, Thunder Bay Regional Health Sciences Centre; (807)684-7200

SIMPSON, M Lynn; Cross Roads ObstGyn Clinic, 303-507 Broadway W, Vancouver BC V5Z 1E6; Wes'76; FRCSC; ObstGyn. Ac Staff, Providence Health Care - St Paul's Hospital; (604)872-5484

SIMPSON, Margaret I; West Market Square, 104-1851 Sirocco Dr SW, Calgary AB T3H 4R5; Ott'85; CCFP; FCFP; Langs: Bilingual(English/French); (403)265-9730; Fax. (403)398-0483.

SIMPSON, Matthew T W; Canadian Forces Base, PO Box 17000 Stn Forces 33 Health Services Centre, Kingston ON K7K 7B4; Ott'07; CCFP; (613)541-5010

SIMPSON, Maurice F; 922B 8 Ave S, Lethbridge AB T1J 1P4; Alb'67; CCFP; CCFP(E.M.); (403)380-3711

SIMPSON, Mia B; St Lawrence Campus Hlth Ctre, PO Box 6000 Stn Main, Kingston ON K7L 5A6; Dal'92; CCFP; (613)544-5532 x1136; Fax. (613)545-3931.

SIMPSON, Nancy C; Glovertown Med Clinic PO Box 190, Glovertown NL A0G 2L0; Mem'96; CCFP; (709)533-2372; Fax. (709)533-1021.

SIMPSON, Noemi S; Associate Med Clinic, 203-10030 106 St, Westlock AB T7P 2K4; (780)349-3341; Fax. (780)349-6686.

SIMPSON, Patricia L; Dr Wayne J Daviduck Prof Corp, 206-51 Inglewood Dr, St. Albert AB T8N 4E7; UBC'82; FRCPC; Psy (Anxiety Disorder). Staff Mental Health Program, Sturgeon Community Hospital; (780)569-5419; Fax. (780)419-6027.

SIMPSON, Richard B; Clairhurst Med Centre, 301-1466 Bathurst St, Toronto ON M5R 3S3; Tor'71; BSc(Hon); FRCPC; Psy (Psychoanalysis). Langs: French; (416)532-7207; Fax. (416)413-0519.

SIMPSON, Robert A; Upper Grand Family Health Team, PO Box 100 71 James St, Elora ON N0B 1S0; Belfast (Ireland)'70; MB ChB; BAO; Staff, Groves Memorial Community Hospital; (519)846-5345; Fax. (519)846-8544; rsimpson@cogeco.ca.

SIMPSON, Robert C; Family Medical Village, 101-197 Talbot St W, Leamington ON N8H 1N8; Tor'81; (519)322-1100; Fax. (519)322-2055.

SIMPSON, Robert J; Fort Macleod Med Clinic, PO Box 1239 744 26th St, Fort Macleod AB T0L 0Z0; Tor'04; BSc(Hon); CCFP; Staff Emerg, Fort MacLeod Health Centre; Med Dir, Fort Macleod Extendicare; (403)553-0066; Fax. (403)553-4549.

SIMPSON, William T; 1569 6th Ave, Prince George BC V2L 3N4; Manchester (England)'72; MB ChB; BSc; FACS; GenSurg. Staff, University Hospital of Northern British Columbia; Clin Assoc Prof Surg, University of British Columbia; (250)564-1946; Fax. (250)564-1915.

SIMROSE, Rebecca L; 100-3280 Hospital Dr NW, Calgary AB T2N 4N1; Sask'84; FRCSC; ObstGyn (Maternal Fetal Medicine). Staff, Foothills Medical Centre; (403)289-9269; Fax. (403)210-8381.

SIMS, Christopher H; Rockyview Gen Hosp, 7007 14 St SW, Calgary AB T2V 1P9; Tor'86; FRCPC; Anes. Staff Anes, Rockyview General Hospital; Langs: French; (403)943-8720; Fax. (403)943-8590.

SIMS, Louise E; Cambridge Mem Hosp, 700 Coronation Blvd, Cambridge ON N1R 3G2; Tor'75; CCFP; FCFP; Staff, Cambridge Memorial Hospital; (519)621-2330; Fax. (519)740-7722.

SIMS, Richard H; St Joseph's Health Centre, MWE-30 The Queensway, Toronto ON M6R 1B5; McG'70; FRCSC; ObstGyn (Obstetrics). Ac Staff, St Joseph's Health Centre; Langs: Portuguese; French; (416)232-4410; Fax. (416)907-9557.

SIMSON, Stanley E; 500 Raglan St N PO Box 371 Stn Main, Renfrew ON K7V 4A6; Wes'58; DPsy; FRCPC; Psy. Consultant Psy, Renfrew Victoria Hospital; (613)432-6423

SIMUNOVIC, Marko R I; The Juravinski Cancer Ctre, B3-711 Concession St, Hamilton ON L8V 1C3; Ott'88; MPH; FRCSC; GenSurg (Colon & Rectal Surgery). Staff, St Joseph's Healthcare - Charlton Campus; Staff, Hamilton Health Sciences Centre-Juravinski Site; Staff, The Juravinski Cancer Centre; Asst Prof Surg/Assoc Member, McMaster University; (905)575-6365

SIN, Donald D H; St Paul's Hosp, 8B-1081 Burrard St, Vancouver BC V6Z 1Y6; Alb'91; FRCPC; IntMed; Respir. Staff Pacific Lung Health Center, Providence Health Care - St Paul's Hospital; Staff, James Hogg Capture Research Centre for Cardiovascular & Pulmonary Diseases; Langs: Korean; (604)806-8818; Fax. (604)806-9274; dsin@mrl.ubc.ca.

SIN, Ignatius C F; Grey Nuns Community Hosp, 1100 Youville Drive West NW, Edmonton AB T6L 5X8; (Hong Kong)'73; MB BS; FRCPC; GenPath. Staff Lab Med, Covenant Health - Grey Nuns Community Hospital; (780)735-7038; Fax. (780)735-9688.

SIN, J H Leo; Rouge Valley HS-Ajax-Pickering, 580 Harwood Ave S, Ajax ON L1S 2J4; Qns'07; CCFP; Staff, Rouge Valley Health System - Ajax & Pickering Health Centre Site; (905)683-2320

SIN, Margaret T W; Hys Med Centre, 202-11010 101 St NW, Edmonton AB T5H 4B9; (Hong Kong)'73; MB BS; FRCPC; DiagRad. Staff, Royal Alexandra Hospital; Clin Prof, University of Alberta; (780)426-1121; Fax. (780)425-5979.

SIN, Philip C; Carefirst Family Health Team, 27-420 Highway 7 E, Richmond Hill ON L4B 3K2; Tor'76; Langs: Cantonese; Mandarin; (905)695-1133; Fax. (905)695-0826; philip.sin@carefirstfht.com.

SIN YAN TOO, Natalie M; 3945 17 Ave SW, Calgary AB T3E 0C3; Wes'05; CCFP; (403)242-8633; Fax. (403)242-8884.

SINAI, Joanne; 200B-3060 Cedar Hill Rd, Victoria BC V8T 3J5; Tor'93; MEd; FRCPC; Psy. Physician, USTAT/Group Mental Health Services; (250)889-6413

SINAJON, Romulo M; 224-40 Finchgate Blvd, Brampton ON L6T 3J1; Southwestern (Philippines)'74; Langs: Tagalog; (905)451-6959

SINASAC, Sarah; Univ Hlth Network-Princess M, M700-610 University Ave, Toronto ON M5G 2M9; McM'06; FRCSC; ObstGyn. Staff, Princess Margaret Hospital - University Health Network; (416)946-4043

SINAVE, Christian P; CHUS-Hop Fleurimot, 3001 12e av N, Sherbrooke QC J1H 5N4; Sher'73; FRCPC; IntMed; MedMicrobiol (P.Q.); InfectDis. Staff, Centre Hospitalier Universitaire de Sherbrooke-Hopital Fleurimont; (819)346-1110 x14414

SINAWAN, Riaz A; Prince George Med Bldg, 201-2155 10th Ave, Prince George BC V2M 5J6; (250)563-1502

SINCLAIR, Brian G; 2200 Oak Bay Ave PO Box 42030, Victoria BC V8R 1G3; Cal'86; AB; FRCPC; Peds (Pediatric Cardiology); Cardiol. Staff, Victoria General Hospital; Staff, Vancouver Island Health Authority; Staff, BC Children's Hospital; Clin Assoc Prof Peds, University of British Columbia.

SINCLAIR, Colin M; Langley Mem Hosp, 22051 Fraser Hwy, Langley BC V3A 4H5; Dundee (Scotland)'96; FRCPC; Anes. Staff, Langley Memorial Hospital; (604)534-4121

SINCLAIR, D Barry; Edmonton Clinic Health Academy, 4531-11405 87 Ave, Edmonton AB T6G 1C9; Cal'81; FRCPC; Neur. Staff Aberhart Centre, University of Alberta Hospital; Staff, Edmonton Clinic Health Academy; (780)248-5567

SINCLAIR, David S; MUHC-Montreal Neurology Inst, 109-3801 rue University, Montreal QC H3A 2B4; Dal'86; FRCSC; Neursurg (Cerebrovascular Surgery). Staff, McGill University Health Centre - Montreal Neurological Hospital; adj Prof NeurSurg., McGill University; (514)398-5609; Fax. (514)398-2811; david.sinclair@muhc.mcgill.ca.

SINCLAIR, Douglas E; St Michaels Hosp, BW1 028-30 Bond St, Toronto ON M5B 1W8; Tor'80; CCFP; CCFP(E.M.); EmergMed. Exec VP/Chief Medical Officer, St Michael's Hospital; Fax. (416)867-3715; sinclaird@smh.ca.

SINCLAIR, Duncan W; 4-418 Talbot St W, Aylmer ON N5H 1K9; Wes'63; Staff, St Thomas Elgin General Hospital; (519)773-9234; Fax. (519)773-8775.

SINCLAIR, Jennifer; The Moncton Hosp, 135 MacBeath Ave, Moncton NB E1C 6Z8; Dal'08; CCFP; Staff, The Moncton Hospital; (506)857-5530

SINCLAIR, John; The Ottawa Hosp-Civic Campus, C2-1053 Carling Ave, Ottawa ON K1Y 4E9; Ott'96; FRCSC; Neursurg. Staff, The Ottawa Hospital - Civic Campus; (613)761-5383; Fax. (613)761-4767.

SINCLAIR, Karine; CSSS Drummond-Hop Sainte-Croix, 570 rue Heriot, Drummondville QC J2B 1C1; Laval'02; FRCSC; OrthSurg. Staff, Hôpital Sainte-croix; (819)478-6464

SINCLAIR, Lesley A; Sunnybrook Hlth Sciences Ctre, 2075 Bayview Ave, Toronto ON M4N 3M5; Wes'85; BSc(Hon)(Hon.); FRCPC; Anes (Cardiovascular Anesthesia). Staff, Sunnybrook Health Sciences Centre; Asst Prof Med, University of Toronto; (416)480-4969; Fax. (416)480-6039; lesley.sinclair@sunnybrook.ca.

SINCLAIR, Michael G; Valley Prof Centre, 200-70 Exhibition St, Kentville NS B4N 4K9; Saba (Netherlands Antilles)'04; CCFP; (902)678-8505; Fax. (902)678-4550.

SINCLAIR, Stephen B; Medical Bldg, 315-250 Harding Blvd W, Richmond Hill ON L4C 9M7; Sask'85; BSc(Hons); MSc; FRCPC; IntMed; Gastroent. Ac Staff, Mackenzie Richmond Hill Hospital; (905)770-4560; Fax. (905)770-4501.

SINCLAIR, Thomas M; 205-743 Railway Ave, Canmore AB T1W 1P2; McG'87; FRCSC; PlasSurg (Breast Surgery). Att Physician, Canmore General Hospital; Att Staff Plastic Surg, Covenant Health - Banff Mineral Springs Hospital; Langs: French; (403)678-2020; Fax. (403)678-2175.

SINCLAIR MILLS, Christa; Senior People's Res in North T, 2F-140 Merton St, Toronto ON M4S 1A1; McM'10; CCFP; (416)481-2590

SINDHAR, Tanbir K; Haney Prof Bldg, 207-11743 224 St, Maple Ridge BC V2X 6A4; Manipal University (India)'01; Staff, Ridge Meadows Hospital & Health Care Centre; (604)466-5822

SINDI, Anees A S; PG Medical Education Office, MDCL 3101A-1280 Main St W, Hamilton ON L8S 4K1; King Abdul Aziz University (Saudi Arabia)'04; FRCPC; IntMed; Respir.

SING, George; The Newmark, 412-4885 Kingsway, Burnaby BC V5H 4T2; Edinburgh (Scotland)'70; MB ChB; DRCOG; DCH; ABIM; MRCP; CRCP; IntMed (Gastroenterology). Ac Staff, Burnaby Hospital; (604)438-5509; Fax. (604)438-5569.

SING, Roland I; 110-210 Memorial Ave, Orillia ON L3V 7V1; Cal'93; FRCSC; Urol. Staff, Orillia Soldiers' Memorial Hospital; (705)325-3603; Fax. (705)325-5483.

SINGAL, Mayank; Complete Care Centre, 4821 Calgary Trail NW, Edmonton AB T6H 5W8; McM'09; CCFP; (780)439-1060; Fax. (780)439-1080.

SINGAL, Mona; Children's & Women's HC of BC, 2L5-4480 Oak St, Vancouver BC V6H 3V4; Man'04; FRCPC; Peds; Critical Care Medicine. Staff, BC Children's Hospital; Langs: Punjabi; (604)875-2161

SINGAL, Neera; 340-790 Bay St, Toronto ON M5G 1N8; Tor'97; FRCSC; Ophth (Cornea & Refractive Surgery). Staff, Toronto East General Hospital Inc; Physician, Kensington Eye Institute; Lecturer, University of Toronto; (416)979-9993; Fax. (416)979-9099; neera.singal@uhn.on.ca.

SINGAL, Rajiv K; Medical Office, 218-840 Coxwell Ave, Toronto ON M4C 5T2; Tor'90; FRCSC; Urol. Staff Urol, Toronto East General Hospital Inc; Langs: Hindi; (416)469-3314; Fax. (416)469-2511; rsingh@tegh.on.ca.

SINGAL, Ram K; Shouldice Hosp, 7750 Bayview Ave, Thornhill ON L3T 4A3; Punjab (India)'61; MB BS; FRCSC; GenSurg (Herniology). Staff, Shouldice Hospital; Langs: Hindi; Urdu; Punjabi; (905)889-1125; Fax. (905)889-4216.

SINGAL, Rohit K; St Boniface Gen Hosp, Y3523-409 Tache Ave, Winnipeg MB R2H 2A6; Man'00; FRCSC; CardSurg; Critical Care Medicine. Staff, St Boniface General Hospital; (204)233-8563

SINGAL, Sewa R; York-Finch Med Centre, 200-2115 Finch Ave W, Toronto ON M3N 2V6; Punjab (India)'72; FRCPC; IntMed (Cardiology). Assoc Staff, The Credit Valley Hospital; Staff, Humber River Regional Hospital - Finch Avenue Site; Langs: Hindi; Punjabi; Urdu; (416)741-6111; Fax. (416)741-6121; sewasingal@hotmail.com.

SINGARAM, Dharumaraj; Bram Centre Med Clinic, 16-7910 Hurontario St, Brampton ON L6Y 0P6; Witwatersrand (South Africa)'84; DCH; MB BCh; MCFP(SA); CCFP; Langs: Afrikaans; (289)752-1571; Fax. (289)752-6439.

SINGARAYER, Chandrakumar; Taunton Health Center, SS 201 1290 Keith Ross Dr, Oshawa ON L1H 7K4; London (England)'94; (905)721-4363; Fax. (905)721-6871.

SINGER, Alexander G; Family Med Centre, 5F-400 Tache Ave, Winnipeg MB R2H 2A6; Dublin (Ireland)'07; CCFP; Staff, St Boniface General Hospital; (204)237-2863; Fax. (204)231-2648.

SINGER, Debrah G C; 111 14-398 Steeles Ave W, Thornhill ON L4J 6X3; McG'90; FRCPC; IntMed; Endocrin&Metab. Langs: Hebrew; French; (905)881-0334; Fax. (905)881-1721; steeles@cardiomatters.com.

SINGER, Gabrielle T; Pinecrest-Queensway CHC, 1365 Richmond Rd, Ottawa ON K2B 6R7; Qns'02; CCFP; Physician, Pinecrest-Queensway Community Health Centre; Langs: Bilingual(English/French); (613)820-2001

SINGER, Henry N; Scarborough Prof Centre, 405-1371 Neilson Rd, Scarborough ON M1B 4Z8; Tor'61; FRCSC; Urol. Ac Staff, Rouge Valley Health System - Centenary Health Centre Site; (416)284-4709; Fax. (416)284-4708.

SINGER, Lianne G; 585 University Ave, Toronto ON M5G 2N2; Tor'93; FRCPC; IntMed (Telehealth); Respir. Staff, Toronto General Hospital - UHN; Asst Prof, University of Toronto; (416)340-4996; Fax. (416)340-3609.

SINGER, Lorne; Grand River Hosp-KW Hlth Ctre, PO Box 9056 Stn C 835 King St W, Kitchener ON N2G 1G3; Tor'75; FRCPC; IntMed. Staff, Grand River Hospital - Kitchener/Waterloo Health Centre; (519)742-3611; Fax. (514)749-4334.

SINGER, Marilyn C; Rivergrove Med Clinic, 2-2605 Main St, Winnipeg MB R2V 4W3; Man'83; CCFP; FCFP.

SINGER, Melissa C; North York Doctors, 703-240 Duncan Mill Rd, North York ON M3B 3S6; Tor'04; CCFP; Staff Family, North York General Hospital; Staff, North York Family Health Team-Central Office; (416)494-7396; Fax. (416)494-0129.

SINGER, Michael A; Bagot Street Med Centre, 182 Bagot St, Kingston ON K7L 3G1; Tor'64; IntMed (Nephrology). (613)542-8361; Fax. (613)546-1321.

SINGER, Michael I; Brunswick Med Centre, 201-955 boul Saint-Jean, Pointe-Claire QC H9R 5K3; Tor'91; FRCPC; Derm. Staff, Sir Mortimer B Davis Jewish General; Staff, Dermatologist Inc; adj Prof, McGill University; Langs: French; (514)461-3929; Fax. (514)426-3323.

SINGER, Michael O; Children's Med Clinic, 212-10720 Yonge St, Richmond Hill ON L4C 3C9; McM'96; FRCPC; Peds. (905)884-5678; Fax. (905)884-3791.

SINGER, Peter A; Mars Centre South Tower, 406-101 College St, Toronto ON M5G 1L7; Tor'84; MPH; FRCPC; IntMed. Sr Scientist, Toronto General Hospital - UHN; Co-Dir, Canadian Program on Genomics & Global Health; Sr Scientist, McLaughlin Centre for Molecular Medicine; Prof Med, University of Toronto; (416)673-6567; Fax. (416)978-6826; peter.singer@utoronto.ca.

SINGER, Raymond; Corydon Primary Care, 102-1001 Corydon Ave, Winnipeg MB R3M 0B6; Tor'72; BSc; CCFP; FCFP; Ac Staff, Victoria General Hospital; Staff, Winnipeg Regional Health Authority; Teach Staff, University of Manitoba; Langs: Hebrew; (204)940-2000

SINGER, Robert B; Galeries des Monts, L4-75 av de la Gare RR 6, Saint-Sauveur QC J0R 1R6; McG'69; (450)227-1864; Fax. (450)227-9221.

SINGER, Robert H; 309-720 Guelph Line, Burlington ON L7R 4E2; McM'80; FRCSC; Ophth. Hd Ophth, Joseph Brant Memorial Hospital; (905)681-3315; Fax. (905)681-6327.

SINGER, Shaun; 7E 466-399 Bathurst St, Toronto ON M5T 2S8; Tor'80; BSc; FRCSC; Ophth (Cataract Surgery)., Toronto Western Hospital - University Health Network; Assoc Staff, Mount Sinai Hospital; Med Dir, Kensington Eye Institute; Teach Staff, University of Toronto; (416)603-6470; Fax. (416)603-2923; shaun.singer@uhn.on.ca.

SINGER, Steven B; St Joseph's Health Centre, 30 The Queensway, Toronto ON M6R 1B5; Ott'98; FRCPC; DiagRad. Staff, St Joseph's Health Centre; (416)530-6001

SINGER, Syndie B; 800-55 Queen St E, Toronto ON M5C 1R6; Tor'06; FRCSC; OrthSurg. (416)864-5392

SINGER, Tamara; Clinique Mondiale, 1-5589 ch Cote-des-Neiges, Montreal QC H3T 1Y8; McG'00; CCFP; (514)733-9899

SINGER, William; LMC Endocrinology Centres, 107-1929 Bayview Ave, East York ON M4G 1E8; London (England)'63; MB BS(Hons); FRCP(E); FACP; FRCPC; IntMed (Endocrinology). Hon Consultant Endocrinol, St Michael's Hospital; Staff, LMC Diabetes & Endocrinology Centres-Bayview; Staff, LMC Diabetes & Endocrinology Centres-Eglinton; Assoc Prof Med & Lab Med, University of Toronto; Langs: Italian; French; German; Spanish; (416)645-2929; Fax. (416)645-2930; wilpatsinger@sympatico.ca.

SINGER-JORDAN, Jonathan R; William Osler HC-Etobicoke, 101 Humber College Blvd, Etobicoke ON M9V 1R8; Edinburgh (Scotland)'72; MB ChB; FRCPC; DiagRad. Staff, William Osler Health System - Etobicoke General Hospital; Langs: Hebrew; (416)747-3400

SINGERMAN, Jennifer D; Univ Hlth Network-Toronto Western Hosp, 399 Bathurst St, Toronto ON M5T 2S8; Tor'07; FRCPC; Neur. Staff, Toronto Western Hospital - University Health Network; (416)603-6422

SINGERMAN, Jonathan; Centre Med du College, 1500 av Atwater, Montreal QC H3Z 1X5; McG'91; CCFP; CCFP(E.M.); FCFP; Boursier, McGill University; Langs: French; (514)989-9935; Fax. (514)937-2564; drjsingerman@gmail.com.

SINGH, Abhay K; Regional Mental HC-London, PO Box 5532 Stn B 850 Highbury Ave, London ON N6A 4H1; Magadh (India)'82; MB BS; FRCPC; Psy. Staff, Regional Mental Health Care-St Joseph's Health Care; Langs: Hindi; (519)455-5110; Fax. (519)455-2919.

SINGH, Amandeep; Finchlea Med Centre, 204-490 Bramalea Rd, Brampton ON L6T 0G1; Saba University School of Medicine (Other Foreign)'03; Langs: Hindi; Punjabi; Urdu; (905)792-6500; Fax. (905)792-6853.

SINGH, Amar; Medical & Dental Bldg, 301-3939 50A Ave, Red Deer AB T4N 4E6; Dhambad (India)'87; MB BS; Assoc Staff, Red Deer Regional Hospital Centre; Clin Lecturer, University of Alberta; Langs: Punjabi; Malay; Hindi; (403)314-1373; Fax. (403)343-2172.

SINGH, Amardip; Ramblewood Med Clinic, 101-14 Ramblewood Dr, Wasaga Beach ON L9Z 0C4; Qns'93; CCFP; Staff, Collingwood General & Marine Hospital; (705)429-1595; Fax. (705)429-6730.

SINGH, Amarendra N; Quinte HC Corp-Belleville Gen, 265 Dundas St E, Belleville ON K8N 5A9; Mithila (India)'60; DPM; DTMH; FRSM; FASCH; FIPA; FRCPsy; FICPM; FRCPC; Psy (Psycho Pharmacology). Chief Psy Academic Unit/Dir Psy Academic Unit, QHC Belleville General; Hotel-Dieu Hospital; Kingston General Hospital; Staff Psychiatrist, Providence Care - St Mary's of the Lake Hospital Site; Prof Psychosomatic Med & Psychopharmacol, World Health Organization; Chair Div of Psychopharmacol/Head Div of Psychopharmacol/Prof Psy & Pharmacol, Queen's University; Langs: Hindi; (613)969-7400 x2244; Fax. (613)969-8448; singha@queensu.ca.

SINGH, Amarjit; Goulet Prof Centre, 201-200 Goulet St, Winnipeg MB R2H 0R8; Agra (India)'65; MB BS; (204)233-4675

SINGH, Ameeta E; Edmonton Gen Cont Care Centre, 3B20-11111 Jasper Ave NW, Edmonton AB T5K 0L4; Nottingham (England)'89; MSc; MB BS; FRCPC; IntMed (HIV); InfectDis. Staff, Covenant Health - Edmonton General Continuing Care Centre; Prof, University of Alberta; (780)342-2300; Fax. (780)425-2194.

SINGH, Anil K; Insight Med Imaging, 200 Meadowlark Shopping Ctr NW, Edmonton AB T5R 5W9; Alb'96; FRCPC; DiagRad; NuclearMed. (780)489-5313; Fax. (780)486-5160.

SINGH, Anita D; London Regional Cancer Centre, 790 Commissioners Rd E, London ON N6A 4L6; Dal'93; BSc; CCFP; Staff, London Health Sciences Centre - London Regional Cancer Centre; Langs: Hindi; (519)685-8500; Fax. (519)685-8624.

SINGH, Anurag; 203-45625 Hodgind Ave, Chilliwack BC V2P 1P2; Guru Nanak Dev (India)'97; MB BS; (604)392-4472

SINGH, Anurita; Mental Hlth & Addiction Servic, 15 Chipman Dr, Kentville NS B4N 3V7; Maharani Laxmi Bai Medical College (Other Foreign)'92; MB BS; (902)365-1701; Fax. (902)678-4917.

SINGH, Arjune B; Humber River Reg Hosp-Finch, 2111 Finch Ave W, North York ON M3N 1N1; New Delhi (India)'80; MB BS; FCCP; FRCPC; IntMed; Respir. Ac Staff IntMed & RespMed, Humber River Regional Hospital - Finch Avenue Site; (416)747-3824

SINGH, Artaj; Primary Care Niagara, 104-6150 Valley Way, Niagara Falls ON L2E 1Y3; McM'85; CCFP; (905)371-1881; Fax. (905)371-1888.

SINGH, Arun K; Humber River Reg Hosp-Church, 200 Church St, Toronto ON M9N 1N8; Magadh University (India)'67; MB BS; GenSurg. Staff, Humber River Regional Hospital - Church Street Site; (416)249-8111

SINGH, Arvind G; 65 Roy Boates Rd PO Box 3000 Stn Main, Summerside PE C1N 2A9; Bombay (India)'94; ABPN; FRCPC; Psy (Child Psychiatry). Staff Psychiatrist, Prince County Hospital; Langs: Hindi; Marathi; Punjabi; (902)724-3332; Fax. (902)724-3336.

SINGH, Ashley M; William Osler HC-Brampton, 2100 Bovaird Dr E, Brampton ON L6R 3J7; Natal (South Africa)'83; MB ChB; FRCPC; Anes. Staff, William Osler Health System - Brampton Civic Hospital; (905)494-2120

SINGH, Ashwani K; 11526 Jasper Ave NW, Edmonton AB T5K 0M8; Alb'91; CCFP; FCFP; (780)428-9333

SINGH, Avash J; Children's & Women's HC of BC, 1R11-4480 Oak St, Vancouver BC V6H 3V4; Delhi (India)'86; MB BS; FAAP; FRCPC; Peds (Neonatal & Perinatal Medicine). Assoc Med Dir ECLS Prog/Staff Neonatol, BC Children's Hospital; Clinical Asst Prof Peds, University of British Columbia; Langs: Hindi; Punjabi; (604)875-2135; Fax. (604)875-3106.

SINGH, Baghat S; Dr Kahlon & Associates, 6950 Nicholson Rd, Delta BC V4E 1Z7; London (England)'98; MB BS; CCFP; (604)596-4211

SINGH, Baldev; St Marys Hosp, 4607 53 St, Camrose AB T4V 1Y5; Staff, Covenant Health - St Mary's Hospital; (780)679-6100; Fax. (780)679-6196.

SINGH, Baljit; 65 Thames St, Chatham ON N7L 1S4; Osmania (India)'84; MB BS; FRCSC; ObstGyn (Gynecology). Ac Staff, Chatham-Kent Health Alliance; Aj Prof, University of Western Ontario; Langs: Hindi; Punjabi; Urdu; (519)352-0800 x3350; Fax. (519)352-4527; baljit23@hotmail.com.

SINGH, Barinder; Hotel-Dieu Hosp, 166 Brock St, Kingston ON K7L 5G2; Cork University (Ireland)'08; CCFP; Staff, Hotel-Dieu Hospital; Langs: Hindi; Punjabi; (613)544-3310

SINGH, Birinder; Patient Networks, 157 Yonge St, Toronto ON M5C 1X7; Wes'04; CCFP; (416)362-8822; Fax. (416)362-8877.

SINGH, Christine B; Three Bridges Comm Hlth Ctre, 1292 Hornby St, Vancouver BC V6Z 1W2; UBC'02; CCFP; Staff, BC Women's Hospital & Health Centre; Langs: Spanish; (604)633-4220; Fax. (604)844-2223.

SINGH, Davindra; AvantDerm, 45 Mill St, Toronto ON M5A 3R6; Qns'94; FRCPC; Derm (Geriatric Medicine);CCFP; CCFP(E.M.); (416)869-3376; Fax. (416)365-7546.

SINGH, Davindra; Southlake Reg Health Centre, 596 Davis Dr, Newmarket ON L3Y 2P9; Tor'00; FRCPC; Anes. Staff, Southlake Regional Health Centre; (905)895-4521 x2216

SINGH, Dharm R; St Joseph's Community Hlth Ctr, 1-280 Victoria St, Dalhousie NB E8C 2R6; Banaras (India)'93; Staff, Centre de santé Communitaire - St-Joseph; (506)684-7300; Fax. (506)684-7148.

SINGH, Dilmohan C; The Doctor's Office, 202-3599 Sheppard Ave E, Scarborough ON M1T 3K8; Man'64; (416)321-2643

SINGH, Farid; Homewood Health Centre, 150 Delhi St, Guelph ON N1E 6K9; Ross University (Other Foreign)'01; Staff, Homewood Health Centre; (519)824-1010; Fax. (519)824-8751.

SINGH, Gita; Boxgrove Med Centre, 204-110 Copper Creek Dr, Markham ON L6B 0P9; McM'00; FRCSC; ObstGyn. Staff Centre for Research on Inner, St Michael's Hospital; Staff, Markham Stouffville Hospital; (905)471-8222

SINGH, Gurbalbir; Plastic Surgery Associates, 240-444 St Mary Ave, Winnipeg MB R3C 3T1; Punjab (India)'70; FRCSC; PlasSurg. Staff, Victoria General Hospital; Staff, St Boniface General Hospital; Asst Prof, University of Manitoba; (204)944-9982; Fax. (204)956-0595.

SINGH, Gurdayal; 5973 Fraser St, Vancouver BC V5W 2Z6; Suva (Fiji)'71; ABIM; FRCPC; IntMed (Cardiology). Langs: Hindi; Punjabi; (604)321-3110; Fax. (604)321-7602; drsingh@telus.net.

SINGH, Gurmeet; University of Alberta Hosp, 3A6 074-8440 112 St NW, Edmonton AB T6G 2B7; Alb'92; FRCSC; CardSurg; Critical Care Medicine. Staff, University of Alberta Hospital; (780)407-8822

SINGH, Gurpreet; Alberta Children's Hosp, 2888 Shaganappi Trail NW, Calgary AB T3B 6A8; Amritsar (India)'91; IntMed. Staff, Alberta Children's Hospital; (403)966-3550; Fax. (403)955-2645.

SINGH, Gurpreet; Richmond Med Centre, 307 Bridge St W, Napanee ON K7R 2G3; University of Delhi (India)'05; (613)354-7386

SINGH, Gurwant; Windsor Square Shopp Centre, 235-1959 152 St, Surrey BC V4A 9E3; Kanpur (India)'91; MB; BSc; FRCPC; Neur (Neuromuscular Diseases). Staff, University of Northern British Columbia; Langs: Hindi; Punjabi; (604)541-2860; Fax. (604)541-2890; gurwantg@gmail.com.

SINGH, Harjot K; 206-1717 10 St NW, Calgary AB T2M 4S2; Cal'92; BSc; Langs: Punjabi; (403)282-9865; Fax. (403)282-9893.

SINGH, Harleen; 232-2130 North Park Dr, Brampton ON L6S 0C9; Gandhi (India)'91; CCFP; Langs: Hindi; Punjabi; Urdu; (905)499-2599

SINGH, Harminder; Health Sciences Centre, 820 Sherbrook St, Winnipeg MB R3A 1R9; Delhi (India)'89; FRCPC; IntMed; Gastroent. Staff, Health Sciences Centre; Staff, John Buhler Research Centre; (204)774-8511

SINGH, Harneet; KW Sleep Laboratory, 180 King St S, Waterloo ON N2J 1P8; All-India Institute of Medical Sciences (India)'02; (519)745-2621

SINGH, Harpal; North Burlington Med Centre, 18-1960 Appleby Line, Burlington ON L7L 0B7; McG'93; MDCM; CCFP; Att Physician, Joseph Brant Memorial Hospital; Att Physician, Brant Centre LTC; Att Physician, Brantwood LTC; Langs: French; (905)319-2000; Fax. (905)319-6292.

SINGH, Ichpal; Bonavista Health Centre, PO Box 1641, Bonavista NL A0C 1B0; Calcutta (India)'83; MB BS; Staff, Bonavista Peninsula Health Centre; Physician, Bonavista Health Centre; Langs: Punjabi; (709)468-5227; Fax. (709)468-7385.

SINGH, Inderbir; 206-101 Queensway W, Mississauga ON L5B 2P7; Tor'90; FRCPC; IntMed (Interventional Cardiology); Cardiol. Staff, Trillium Health Centre - Mississauga; (905)615-0012; Fax. (905)615-8537.

SINGH, Inderjit; Medmart Med Centre, 68A Centennial Pky N, Hamilton ON L8E 1H6; Kashmir University (India)'77; CCFP; Langs: Hindi; Kashmiri; Punjabi; Urdu; (905)560-5800

SINGH, Jagdeep; Niagara H System-St Catharines, 142 Queenston St, St Catharines ON L2R 7C6; Guru Nanak University (India)'92; CCFP; CCFP(E.M.); Staff, Niagara Health System - St Catharines General Site; (905)378-4647

SINGH, Jagdeep; William Osler HC-Brampton, 2100 Bovaird Dr E, Brampton ON L6R 3J7; RCSI (Ireland)'05; FRCPC; IntMed. Staff, William Osler Health System - Brampton Civic Hospital; Langs: Punjabi; (905)494-6481; Fax. (905)494-6481.

SINGH, Jagmohan K; Colchester East Hants Hlth Ctr, 600 Abenaki Rd, Truro NS B2N 5A1; Punjab (India)'86; MB BS; FRCPC; IntMed. Staff, Colchester East Hants Health Centre; Langs: Hindi; Punjabi; (902)897-7177; Fax. (902)897-7176.

SINGH, Jaspal; Valley Women & Children's HC, 60 Aberdeen St, Kentville NS B4N 2N3; Dublin (Ireland)'72; LRCPSI; MRCOG(Lond); FRCSC; ObstGyn. Consultant ObstGyn., Valley Regional Hospital; Langs: Hindi; Punjabi; (902)678-4626; Fax. (902)678-6338.

SINGH, Jeffrey M; Trillium Hlth Ctr-Mississauga, 100 Queensway W, Mississauga ON L5B 1B8; Tor'96; CCFP; CCFP(E.M.); FCFP; Staff Family Med, Trillium Health Centre - Mississauga; Staff, Trillium Health Centre - West Toronto; (905)848-7600

SINGH, Jeffrey M; Univ Hlth Network-Toronto Western Hosp, MCL 411K-399 Bathurst St, Toronto ON M5T 2S8; Tor'99; FRCPC; IntMed; Critical Care Medicine. Staff, Toronto Western Hospital - University Health Network; (416)603-2581

SINGH, Jessica; The Juravinski Cancer Centre, 699 Concession St, Hamilton ON L8V 5C2; Wes'08; IntMed (Medical Oncology). Staff, Hamilton Health Sciences Centre - Juravinski Cancer Centre; (905)387-9495

SINGH, Jit J; 8919 120 St, Delta BC V4C 6R6; Leeds (England)'80; MB ChB; DCH; DRCOG; Staff, Surrey Memorial Hospital; Langs: Punjabi; Hindi; Urdu; (604)598-0710

SINGH, Jitendra; Central Alberta Prof Centre, 115-5201 43 St, Red Deer AB T4N 1C7; Alb'85; BMedSci; FRCPC; IntMed. Staff, Red Deer Regional Hospital Centre; Langs: Hindi; (403)340-2724; Fax. (403)340-2724.

SINGH, Jitendra K; Dundas Centre Med Bldg, 205-220 Dundas St W, Whitby ON L1N 8M7; Ranchi (India)'89; MB BS; ABIM; FRCPC; IntMed (Cardiology). Staff Cardiol & IntMed, Lakeridge Health - Oshawa Site; Langs: Hindi; (905)668-9375; Fax. (905)668-1716; drjk@medicalworld.ca.

SINGH, Jogindra; Baywood Med Centre, 204-95 Bayly St W, Ajax ON L1S 7K8; Punjab (India)'61; MB BS; FRCPC; PhysMed&Rehab (Pain Management). Langs: Hindi; Punjabi; (905)683-9039; Fax. (905)683-4438; dr.j.singh@on.aibn.com.

SINGH, Joy R; Bayshore Physicians Group, 1473 Exmouth St, Sarnia ON N7S 3Y1; Spartan Health Sciences U (Saint Lucia)'97; CCFP; (519)336-6661; Fax. (519)336-6644.

SINGH, Judith M; Falls Urgent Care Centre, 104-6150 Valley Way, Niagara Falls ON L2E 1Y3; McM'85; CCFP; FCFP; (905)371-1881; Fax. (905)371-1888.

SINGH, Kanwal K; 304-8425 120 St, Delta BC V4C 6R2; UBC'86; Langs: Punjabi; (604)590-4447; Fax. (604)590-6260.

SINGH, Kanwarjit; 101-8181 120A St, Surrey BC V3W 3P2; Kashmir (India)'80; MB BS; Langs: Hindi; Punjabi; Urdu; (604)599-6909; Fax. (604)599-4192.

SINGH, Kirandeep; Baycrest Ctre/Geriatric Care, 3560 Bathurst St, Toronto ON M6A 2E1; Bonaire (Netherlands Antilles)'07; Staff, Baycrest Centre for Geriatric Care; (416)785-2500

SINGH, Kishore; Appleby Med Centre, 321 Appleby Line, Burlington ON L7L 2X6; Natal (South Africa)'87; MB ChB; CCFP; Assoc Prof Family Med, McMaster University; (905)632-7775; Fax. (905)632-3762; ksingh@applebymedicalcentre.com.

SINGH, Kulbir I; Inpatient Services, E1-715 12th Ave W, Vancouver BC V5Z 1M9; Ranchi (India)'80; MB BS; MRCPsy(UK); FRCPC; Psy. Ac Staff, Vancouver General Hospital - Centennial Pavillion; Staff, Venture -VCMHS; Clinical Asst Prof, University of British Columbia; Langs: Hindi; Punjabi; Urdu; (604)875-4139; Fax. (604)875-5427.

SINGH, Kulrajmohinder; Northgate Med Centre, 2711 Avonhurst Dr, Regina SK S4R 3J3; Aberdeen (Scotland)'68; Staff, Regina General Hospital; Physician, Northgate Medical Centre; (306)543-4566; Fax. (306)543-4441.

SINGH, Kunwar K; Medical Office, 483 East St N, Sarnia ON N7T 6Y7; Osmania (India)'65; MB BS; FAAP; FCCP; FRCPC; Peds (Attention Deficit Hyperactivity Disorder). Staff, Multi Specialty Walk-In Clinic; Langs: Hindi; Punjabi; French; Telugu; Urdu; (519)336-6311; Fax. (519)336-1430.

SINGH, Lakha; Humber River Reg Hosp-Keele, 2175 Keele St, North York ON M6M 3Z4; Tor'05; FRCPC; Psy. Staff, Humber River Regional Hospital - Keele Street Site; (416)249-8111

SINGH, Lakhbir; Pacific Med Clinic, 6176 Fraser St, Vancouver BC V5W 3A1; Tor'93; BSc; CCFP; FCFP; Clin Instructor Family Practice, University of British Columbia; Langs: Punjabi; (604)301-9955; Fax. (604)301-1566.

SINGH, Madhuri; Taylor Street Med Clinic, 3020 Taylor St E, Saskatoon SK S7H 4J2; Patna (India)'64; Physician, Taylor Street Medical Clinic; (306)374-8082; Fax. (306)374-0047.

SINGH, Manbir; 2-940 King St W, Kitchener ON N2G 1G4; New Delhi (India)'73; MB BS; FRCPC; Psy. Staff, Grand River Hospital - Kitchener/Waterloo Health Centre; Staff, St Mary's General Hospital; Langs: Hindi; Punjabi; (519)745-7113; Fax. (519)745-6804.

SINGH, Minesh; 204-1106 Ouellette Ave, Windsor ON N9A 1C9; Natal (South Africa)'94; MB ChB; FRCSC; GenSurg. Langs: Afrikaans; Hindi; (519)977-9839; Fax. (519)977-7979.

SINGH, Mohinder; PO Box 1150, Swan River MB R0L 1Z0; London (England)'63.

SINGH, Munesh C S; Markham Stouffville Hosp, PO Box 1800 Stn Main 381 Church St, Markham ON L3P 7P3; West Indies (Jamaica)'84; MB BS; FRCPC; Peds. Staff, Markham Stouffville Hospital; (905)472-7373 x6174

SINGH, Nandini J; 19 Woodland Green, Calgary AB T3R 1G6; Bombay (India)'74; MB BS; FRCPC; Psy (Mood Disorders). Staff, Peter Lougheed Centre; Member, Alberta Mental Health Board; Teach Staff, University of Calgary; Langs: Hindi; Marathi; Gujarati; (403)944-9700; Fax. (403)241-2800; singh@telusplanet.net.

SINGH, Narendra C; Humber River Reg Hosp-Finch, 2111 Finch Ave W, North York ON M3N 1N1; Bombay (India)'82; FRCPC; Peds. Staff, Humber River Regional Hospital - Finch Avenue Site; (416)747-3824

SINGH, Narendra; Osler Cardiology Associates, 200-3 Conestoga Dr, Brampton ON L6Z 4N5; Dal'87; ABIM; FACC; FRCPC; IntMed; Cardiol. Langs: Hindi; (905)452-9010

SINGH, Navpreet; Dr Langer & Associates, 180 Sandalwood Pky E, Brampton ON L6Z 1Y4; Tor'04; CCFP; (905)846-9255; Fax. (905)846-2525.

SINGH, Neena L; 344-50 Burnhamthorpe Rd W, Mississauga ON L5B 3C2; Sask'85; (905)896-4588

SINGH, Nina R T R; Hamilton HS-McMaster Site, PO Box 2000 Stn Lcd 1 1200 Main St W, Hamilton ON L8N 3Z5; Wes'97; FRCPC; DiagRad (Telehealth). Fellow, Hamilton Health Sciences Centre - McMaster Children's Hospital; (905)521-2100 x75279; Fax. (905)521-5057.

SINGH, Nitin K; Cold Lake Healthcare Centre, 314 25 St, Cold Lake AB T9M 1G6; Goa Medical College (India)'96; Staff, Cold Lake Healthcare Centre; (780)639-3322; Fax. (780)639-2255.

SINGH, Padamjit M; Professional Bldg, 302-222 King St E, Bowmanville ON L1C 1P6; Poona (India)'70; MB BS; FRCSC; ObstGyn. Langs: Hindi; Punjabi; (905)623-2758; Fax. (905)623-7558.

SINGH, Paramjeet; Markham Family Health Team, 101-377 Church St, Markham ON L6B 1A1; Ott'98; BSc; CCFP; FCFP; (905)471-9999; Fax. (905)471-3627.

SINGH, Paramvinder; Harvest Hills Med Clinic Ltd, 715-500 Country Hills Blvd NE, Calgary AB T3K 4Y7; (India)'99; MB BS; CCFP; Langs: Hindi; Urdu; Punjabi; (403)226-8647; Fax. (403)226-8645; hhmcadmin@shaw.ca.

SINGH, Parul; Humber River Reg Hosp-Church, 200 Church St, Toronto ON M9N 1N8; Man'07; CCFP; CCFP(E.M.); Staff, Humber River Regional Hospital - Church Street Site; Langs: Hindi; French; (416)249-8111

SINGH, Parvinder; Castlemore Med Centre, 105-4515 Ebenezer Rd, Brampton ON L6P 2K7; Gauhati (India)'98; MB BS; CCFP; Langs: Hindi; Punjabi; Urdu; (905)794-5900; Fax. (905)794-5559.

SINGH, R Suneet; Gordon & Leslie Diamond HCC, 5293-2775 Laurel St, Vancouver BC V5Z 1M9; McG'93; BSc; FRCPC; IntMed; Nephrol. Clin Instructor, Vancouver General Hospital - Centennial Pavillion; Staff, Gordon & Leslie Diamond Health Care Centre; University of British Columbia; (604)875-5950; Fax. (604)875-5952.

SINGH, Rajiva R; DMI Professional Bldg, 113-704 Mara St, Point Edward ON N7V 1X4; Sask'85; DAB; FACS; FRCSC; Urol. Ac Staff, Bluewater Health - Mitton Site; Langs: Hindi; (519)344-2949; Fax. (519)344-7727.

SINGH, Ram N; London HSC-Victoria Campus, PO Box 5010 Stn B C2 842-800 Commissioners Rd E, London ON N6A 5W9; Rajendra (India)'81; MB BS; FRCPC; Peds (Pediatric Critical Care); Critical Care Medicine. Dir Ped Critical Care Unit, London Health Sciences Centre - Victoria Campus; Dir-Research Ped Critical Care Unit, Children's Hospital of Western Ontario; Asst Prof, University of Ottawa; Langs: Hindi; (519)685-8386; Fax. (519)685-8766.

SINGH, Ram R; Glenmore Landing, D266-1600 90 Ave SW, Calgary AB T2V 5A8; Agra (India)'56; MB BS; MRC(Ed.); FRCPC; IntMed. Staff, Rockyview General Hospital; Assoc Prof, University Of Calgary; Langs: Punjabi; Hindi; Urdu; (403)252-3314; Fax. (403)640-1223; rrsingh@telusplanet.net.

SINGH, Ramandip; Legacy Sport Med Clinic, 14-160 Meadowood Dr, Winnipeg MB R2M 5L6; Punjab (India)'96; FRCPC; IntMed; Rheum. (204)667-1550

SINGH, Ranjit A; Medical Arts Bldg, 430-1105 Pandora Ave, Victoria BC V8V 3P9; UBC'92; FRCPC; IntMed (Endocrinology); Gastroent. Staff, Vancouver Island Health Authority; Staff Endoscopy, Victoria General Hospital; (250)386-7731; Fax. (250)386-7751.

SINGH, Ranjit; Norfolk Med Centre, 304-85 Norfolk St, Guelph ON N1H 4J4; London (England)'67; MB BS; MRCP; FRCPC; Neur (Electrodiagnostic Medicine). Ac Staff, Guelph General Hospital; Consultant, Homewood Health Centre; Associate Research, Human Biology, U. of Guelph; (519)836-5940; Fax. (519)836-3271.

SINGH, Ravi P; Health Sciences North-Laurenti, 41 Ramsey Lake Rd, Sudbury ON P3E 5J1; Ott'09; CCFP; Staff, Health Sciences North-Laurentian Site; (705)522-7100

SINGH, Ravinder; Medical & Dental Bldg, 300-1221 Algonquin Ave, North Bay ON P1B 4Y3; Ott'01; FRCSC; GenSurg (Minimal Invasive Surgery). Langs: Hindi; Punjabi; (705)472-4646; Fax. (705)476-6543.

SINGH, Ravinderpal; Humber River Reg Hosp-Church, 200 Church St, Toronto ON M9N 1N8; Dayanand Med College (India)'02; Staff, Humber River Regional Hospital - Church Street Site; Langs: Punjabi; (416)249-8111

SINGH, Renate G; Life Flight Air Ambulance, HT 5-900 Ferry Rd, Winnipeg MB R3H 0X8; Man'04; FRCPC; Anes. Staff, St Boniface General Hospital; Staff, Health Sciences Centre; Staff, Seven Oaks General Hospital; Staff, Life Flight Air Ambulance.

SINGH, Ricky D; St Boniface Gen Hosp, 409 Tache Ave, Winnipeg MB R2H 2A6; Man'03; FRCPC; Anes;CCFP; Staff, St Boniface General Hospital; (204)233-8563

SINGH, Rondeep; Royal Alexandra Hosp, 541 CSC-10240 Kingsway Ave NW, Edmonton AB T5H 3V9; Wes'02; CCFP; CCFP(E.M.); Staff, Royal Alexandra Hospital; (780)735-4442; Fax. (780)735-4916.

SINGH, Ruby; Brant Community HC-Brantford, 200 Terrace Hill St, Brantford ON N3R 1G9; Man'08; CCFP; Staff, The Brant Community Healthcare System - Brantford General Hospital Site; (519)751-5544

SINGH, S Sony; The Ottawa Hosp-Riverside, 7F-1967 Riverside Dr, Ottawa ON K1H 7W9; Wes'00; BSc; FRCSC; ObstGyn (General Surgery). Staff Shirley Greenberg Women Health Centre, The Ottawa Hospital - Riverside Campus; Staff, Shirley E Greenberg Women's Health Centre; Langs: Punjabi; (613)738-8400 x81740; Fax. (613)738-8505.

SINGH, Sandhya K V; Black Creek Comm Health Ctre, 5-2202 Jane St, Toronto ON M3M 1A4; American University of the Caribbean (St Maarten)'08; (416)249-8000

SINGH, Santokh; St Mary's Hosp Centre, 4F-3830 sv Lacombe, Montreal QC H3T 1M5; Cal'94; BSc(Hons.); FRCPC; Psy. Staff, St Mary's Hospital Centre; Langs: English; French; (514)734-2684; Fax. (514)734-2625.

SINGH, Sarab M; Sturgeon Community Hosp, 201 Boudreau Rd, St. Albert AB T8N 6C4; Meenut (India)'85; Staff, Sturgeon Community Hospital; (780)418-7310; s_m_smgh@hotmail.com.

SINGH, Sarban; The Country Med Practice Ltd, 201-967 Bedford Hwy, Bedford NS B4A 1A9; Kerala (India)'79; MB BS; LRCP; LRCS; LRCPS; (902)832-1983; Fax. (902)443-5699; canada@accesscable.net.

SINGH, Sarbjit; Colcherster Reg Hosp Annex, 600 Abenaki Rd, Truro NS B2N 5A1; Dal'91; Staff, Colchester East Hants Health Centre; (902)897-7177

SINGH, Sheila K; Hamilton HS-McMaster Children', PO Box 2000 Stn Lcd 1 4E5-1200 Main St W, Hamilton ON L8N 3Z5; McM'97; BSc; PhD; FRCSC; Neursurg (Pediatric Neuro Surgery); Public Health & Preventive Med. Staff, Hamilton Health Sciences Centre - McMaster Children's Hospital; Langs: German; French; (905)521-2100; Fax. (905)521-9992.

SINGH, Sheldon M S; Sunnybrook Hlth Sciences Ctre, A222-2075 Bayview Ave, Toronto ON M4N 3M5; Tor'01; FRCPC; IntMed; Cardiol. Staff, Sunnybrook Health Sciences Centre; (416)480-6100

SINGH, Shiv P; 21-1098 Peter Robertson Blvd, Brampton ON L6R 3A5; Punjab (India)'93; MB ChB; CCFP; Langs: Hindi; Punjabi; (905)458-6999; Fax. (905)458-5202.

SINGH, Simron; Toronto Sunnybrook Cancer Ctr, T2 039TW-2075 Bayview Ave, Toronto ON M4N 3M5; Alb'99; MedOncol; IntMed. Staff, Sunnybrook Health Sciences Centre - Edmond Odette Cancer Centre; Langs: Hindi; Punjabi; (416)480-4928; Fax. (416)480-6002.

SINGH, Sonia A; B-20618 Douglas Cres, Langley BC V3A 4B8; Punjab (India)'96; CCFP; (604)534-7878; Fax. (604)534-1684.

SINGH, Sonia; Peace Arch Hosp, 15521 Russell Ave, White Rock BC V4B 2R4; Qns'85; CCFP; Staff, Peace Arch Hospital; (604)541-5830

SINGH, Stephen B; Queen's Family Health Centre, 220 Bagot St, Kingston ON K7L 3G2; Wes'09; CCFP; (613)533-9303

SINGH, Steve K; Hamilton HS-General Campus, 524-237 Barton St E, Hamilton ON L8L 2X2; Tor'03; FRCSC; CardSurg (General Surgery). Staff, Hamilton Health Sciences Centre - Hamilton General Hospital; (905)527-4322

SINGH, Sudha I; St Joseph's Health Care, PO Box 5777 Stn B 268 Grosvenor St, London ON N6A 4V2; Mem'94; FRCPC; Anes (Obstetrics Anesthesia). Staff, St Joseph's Hospital - St Joseph's Health Care; (519)646-6000

SINGH, Sukhwinder; All Care Med Centre, 101-12827 76 Ave, Surrey BC V3W 2V3; (Other Foreign)'89; CCFP; (604)590-0443

SINGH, Sunira; Surrey Med Arts Bldg, 306-13710 94A Ave, Surrey BC V3V 1N1; Kwazulu-Natal (South Africa)'97; MB ChB; FRCPC; Peds. (604)582-6555

SINGH, Sunita K S; PG Medical Education Office, 602-500 University Ave, Toronto ON M5G 1V7; Tor'07; FRCPC; IntMed; Nephrol. Langs: Bilingual(English/French).

SINGH, Tejinder P; Finch-Midland Med Centre, 404-4190 Finch Ave E, Scarborough ON M1S 4T7; Punjabi (India)'75; MB BS; CCFP; FCFP; Staff, The Scarborough Hospital - Birchmount Campus; Langs: Punjabi; Hindi; Urdu; (416)297-9570; Fax. (866)761-6517.

SINGH, Varsha; South Hill Med Centre, 890A Lillooet St W, Moose Jaw SK S6H 8B4; (306)691-0030; Fax. (306)694-5666.

SINGH, Vidyanand B; Bayshore Physicians Group, 1473 Exmouth St, Sarnia ON N7S 3Y1; American University of the Caribbean (Netherlands Antilles)'98; AAFP; ABFPS; CCFP; Langs: Bilingual(English/French); (519)336-6661; Fax. (519)336-6644.

SINGH, Vijay P; Alberta Hosp Edmonton, PO Box 307 Stn Main 17480 Fort Rd, Edmonton AB T5J 2J7; Bihar (India)'73; MRCPsy(UK); FRCPsy(UK); FRCPC; Psy (Criminal Responsibility). Staff, Alberta Hospital Edmonton; Staff, Alberta Mental Health Board; Clin Lecturer, University of Alberta; Langs: Hindi; (780)472-5376; Fax. (780)342-5595; singh@telusplanet.net.

SINGH AUJLA, Kanwerjit; Temple Family Med Clinic, 109-5401 Temple Dr NE, Calgary AB T1Y 3R7; 99 Patiala (India) MB BS; MS(Otol.); CCFP; Staff, Calgary Health Region; Langs: Hindi; Punjabi; (403)293-1698; Fax. (403)293-7373; templemedical@hotmail.com.

SINGHAI, Rashmi; 404-11861 88 Ave, Delta BC V4C 3C6; UBC'87; BSc; Langs: Hindi; (604)599-0077; Fax. (604)599-8531.

SINGHAL, Ashutosh; Children's & Women's HC of BC, K3 159-4480 Oak St, Vancouver BC V6H 3V4; Alb'97; FRCPC; Neursurg. Staff, BC Children's Hospital; (604)875-2094; Fax. (604)875-3109.

SINGHAL, Manoj K; 3100-11666 Steveston Hwy, Richmond BC V7A 1N6; Lucknow (India)'88; CCFP; (604)448-9595

SINGHAL, Manoj; 3100-11666 Steveston Hwy, Richmond BC V7A 1N6; Alb'94; BSc(Pharm); (604)448-9595; Fax. (604)304-9595.

SINGHAL, Nalini; C614-2888 Shaganappi Trail NW, Calgary AB T3B 6A8; Delhi (India)'71; FRCPC; Peds (Neonatology). Ac Staff Peds, Foothills Medical Centre; Ac Staff, Alberta Children's Hospital; Prof, University of Calgary; Langs: Hindi; (403)955-7251; Fax. (403)944-4892; nalini.singhal@albertahealthservices.ca.

SINGHAL, Nishma; Hamilton HS-General Site, 626-237 Barton St E, Hamilton ON L8L 2X2; McM'00; FRCPC; IntMed; InfectDis. Staff McMaster Clinic Med & InfectDis, Hamilton Health Sciences Centre - Hamilton General Hospital; Langs: Hindi; (905)527-4322; Fax. (905)521-1551.

SINGHAL, Rajni; Humber River Reg Hosp-Church, 200 Church St, Toronto ON M9N 1N8; Ott'00; Nephrol; IntMed. Staff, Humber River Regional Hospital - Church Street Site; (416)249-8111

SINGHAL, Rishi K; Queen Elizabeth II Hosp, 10409 98 St, Grande Prairie AB T8V 2E8; (India)'93; CCST; Consultant Psy, Queen Elizabeth II Hospital; (780)538-7618; Fax. (780)538-7600.

SINGHAM, Janakie; Surrey Med Arts Bldg, 305-13798 94A Ave, Surrey BC V3V 1N1; Qns'04; FRCPC; IntMed; Gastroent. (604)585-9889

SINGLETON, Andrea M; Churchill Square Med Clinic, PO Box 23205 Rpo Churchill Sq 209-10 Rowan St, St. John's NL A1B 4J9; Mem'04; CCFP; (709)722-8561; Fax. (709)722-7350.

SINGLETON, Barry C; Bluewater Health-Norman Site, 89 Norman St, Sarnia ON N7T 6S3; Qns'78; BSc(Eng.); FRCPC; Anes. Ac Staff, Bluewater Health - Mitton Site; Ac Staff, Bluewater Health - Norman Site; (519)464-4500; bsingleton@cogeco.ca.

SINGLETON, David B; Singleton Med Clinic, PO Box 219 224 Wallace St, Hope BC V0X 1L0; UBC'78; BSc; (604)869-7118; Fax. (604)869-3260.

SINGLETON, John D; Rainy River Health Ctre, PO Box 278 113 4th St, Rainy River ON P0W 1L0; McM'88; CCFP; Staff, Rainy River Health Centre - Riverside Health Care Facility; (807)852-3222; Fax. (807)852-3990; j.singleton@rhcf.on.ca.

SINGLETON, Kathleen M; Atlantic Med Clinic, PO Box 29119 Hal Shop Ctre, Halifax NS B3L 4T8; Qns'90; CCFP; Staff, IWK Health Centre; Staff, Cobequid Multiservice Centre; Teach Staff Family Practice, Dalhousie University; (902)455-4333; Fax. (902)455-4034; kaysingleton@hfx.eastlink.ca.

SINGLETON, Paul J W; 850 King St W, Kitchener ON N2G 1E8; McM'87; FRCPC; Psy (Pediatric Psychiatry). Staff, Grand River Hospital - Kitchener/Waterloo Health Centre; (519)749-4300 x2320; Fax. (519)749-4271.

SINGNURKAR, Amit; Hamilton HS-Henderson Site, 711 Concession St, Hamilton ON L8V 1C3; McG'03; FRCPC; NuclearMed. Staff, Hamilton Health Sciences Centre-Juravinski Site; (905)521-2100; Fax. (905)389-4990.

SINGWI, Amita; Univ Hlth Network-Toronto Western Hosp, 2 WW-399 Bathurst St, Toronto ON M5T 2S8; Ott'05; BSc; BEd; CCFP; Staff, Toronto Western Hospital - University Health Network; Langs: Hindi; (416)603-5888 x2; Fax. (416)603-5448.

SINGWI, Sanjeev; Headwaters Health Care Ctre, 100 Rolling Hills Dr, Orangeville ON L9W 4X9; Tor'03; Staff, Headwaters Health Care Centre - Orangeville Site; Langs: Hindi; (519)941-2702; Fax. (519)942-0483.

SINHA, Avinash K; MUHC-Montreal Gen Hosp, D10 144-1650 av Cedar, Montreal QC H3G 1A4; Manchester (England)'93; Staff, McGill University Health Centre - Montreal General Campus; (514)934-1934 x43261; Fax. (514)934-8249.

SINHA, Dave R; Oasis Med Clinic, 250-8730 Country Hills Blvd NW, Calgary AB T3G 0E2; Alb'02; CCFP; (403)262-7424; Fax. (403)262-5528.

SINHA, Dinesh P; Dr Sinha Med Incorporated, 877 Tower Rd, Halifax NS B3H 2Y1; Bihar Ranchi (India)'67; MB BS; Med Dir, Melville Lodge Care Centre; Med Dir, Northwood Care Centre; Langs: Hindi; (902)422-1112; Fax. (902)422-1112.

SINHA, Jayaditya J; Steeplehill Med Centre, 205-650 Kingston Rd, Pickering ON L1V 1A6; Tor'92; BSc(Hon); CCFP; (905)831-4547; Fax. (905)831-5109.

SINHA, Meera; 120 Marion St, Winnipeg MB R2H 0T1; Lucknow (India)'68; MB BS; DObst; FRCSC; ObstGyn. Ac Staff, St Boniface General Hospital; Assoc Staff, Victoria General Hospital; Asst Prof ObstGyn, University of Manitoba; (204)237-6482

SINHA, Nachiketa; Mental Health Services, PO Box 5001, Woodstock NB E7M 5C6; Karnatak (India)'00; (506)325-4419; Fax. (506)325-4610.

SINHA, Neel S; Pacific Med Clinic, 6176 Fraser St, Vancouver BC V5W 3A1; Alb'89; (604)301-9955; Fax. (604)301-1566.

SINHA, Prabhat; Campbellton Reg Hosp, PO Box 880 Stn Main 189 Lily Lake Rd, Campbellton NB E3N 3H3; Darbhanga (Other Foreign)'88; Staff, Hôpital Régional Campbellton; (506)789-5000

SINHA, Roona; Royal University Hosp, 3724-103 Hospital Dr, Saskatoon SK S7N 0W8; Ott'04; FRCPC; Peds; PedHemaOncol. Staff, Royal University Hospital; Langs: Bengali; (306)966-7900; Fax. (306)966-8640; roona.sinha@usask.ca.

SINHA, Sachchida N; 120 Marion St, Winnipeg MB R2H 0T1; Patna (India)'63; FRCP(Ed & Glas); DABIM; FRCPC; IntMed (Cardiology). Staff, St Boniface General Hospital; Asst Prof, University of Manitoba; Langs: Hindi; (204)231-0605; Fax. (204)237-6478.

SINHA, Samir K; Mount Sinai Hosp, 4 475-600 University Ave, Toronto ON M5G 1X5; Wes'02; FRCPC; IntMed; GeriatricMed. Staff, Mount Sinai Hospital; (416)586-7859; Fax. (416)586-5113.

SINHA, Siddhartha R; Tom Baker Cancer Centre, 1331 29 St NW, Calgary AB T2N 4N2; Alb'01; RadOncol. Staff, Tom Baker Cancer Centre; (403)521-3077; Fax. (403)283-1651.

SINHA, Smit S; Univ Hlth Network-Toronto Gen, 224-200 Elizabeth St, Toronto ON M5G 2C4; Alb'93; FRCPC; Psy. Staff, Toronto General Hospital - UHN; (416)340-4800

SINKOWSKI, Kerry L; West Street Health Ctre, 205-216 West St, Simcoe ON N3Y 1S8; Tor'90; (519)428-0444; Fax. (519)428-1725; jterdik@sympatico.ca.

SINN, Barbara A; Capilano Med Clinic, 7905 106 Ave NW, Edmonton AB T6A 1H7; Alb'84; (780)465-0951; Fax. (780)465-6928.

SINN, Ralph D; Capilano Med Clinic, 7905 106 Ave NW, Edmonton AB T6A 1H7; Alb'84; (780)465-0951; Fax. (780)465-6928.

SINNADURAI, Sriharan; Family Med Centre, 10-2677 Kennedy Rd, Scarborough ON M1T 3H8; Madras (India)'91; MB BS; CCFP; (416)412-7300; Fax. (416)412-3400.

SINNAEVE, Linda J E; 196 Grand Ave W, Chatham ON N7L 1C1; Wes'84; ABIM; ABEM; FRCPC; IntMed (Endocrinology); Endocrin&Metab. Ac Staff/Med Advisor Diabetes Educ Centre, Chatham-Kent Health Alliance; (519)354-2777; Fax. (519)354-2783.

SINNARAJAH, Aynharan; Foothills Med Centre, 710 ST-1403 29 St NW, Calgary AB T2N 2T9; Tor'01; CCFP; Staff Palliative & End of Life Care, Foothills Medical Centre; Staff Palliative Care Prog, Peter Lougheed Centre; Langs: Tamil; (403)944-2304; Fax. (403)270-9652.

SINNREICH, Michael; MUHC-Montreal Neurology Inst, 365-3801 rue University, Montreal QC H3A 2B4; (Swaziland)'94; Staff, McGill University Health Centre - Montreal Neurological Hospital; adj Prof, McGill University; (514)398-8528; Fax. (514)398-8310; michael.sinnreich@mcgill.ca.

SINSKY, Anna Barbara; Imagerie des Pionniers, 140-950 Montee des Pionniers, Terrebonne QC J6V 1S8; McG'83; MD; FRCPC; DiagRad (Pediatric Radiology). Staff, Centre Hospitalier Universitaire de Sherbrooke-Hopital Fleurimont; Langs: German; French; (450)581-1424; Fax. (450)581-9395; absinsky@msn.com.

SINTON, Geoffrey; Thorold Med Clinic, 60 Albert St W, Thorold ON L2V 2G7; Liverpool (England)'81; DCH; CCFP; (905)680-2722; Fax. (905)227-2070.

SINUFF, Tasnim; Sunnybrook Health Sciences Ctr, D108-2075 Bayview Ave, Toronto ON M4N 3M5; Alb'94; FRCPC; IntMed; Electroenceph; Respir. Staff Critcal Care Med, Sunnybrook Health Sciences Centre; (416)480-6100 x7694; Fax. (416)480-4999.

SINUKOFF, Warren E; 205-738 Sheppard Ave E, North York ON M2K 1C4; Tor'70; Court Staff, North York General Hospital; (416)226-3433; Fax. (416)733-9965.

SINYOR, Mark J; Sunnybrook Hlth Sciences Ctre, FG52-2075 Bayview Ave, Toronto ON M4N 3M5; Tor'07; Psy. Staff, Sunnybrook Health Sciences Centre; (416)480-4070; Fax. (416)480-4613.

SIOMRA, Stephen W; Oshawa Clinic, 117 King St E, Oshawa ON L1H 1B9; Tor'70; FRCSC; Otol (Head & Neck Surgery). Langs: Ukrainian; (905)721-4300; Fax. (905)721-6650.

SION, David M; 210-2425 Tecumseh Rd E, Windsor ON N8W 1E6; Ott'81; FRCSC; GenSurg; PlasSurg. (519)977-8757; Fax. (519)971-9571.

SIOUFI, Georges; Hop Santa Cabrini Ospedale, 5655 rue Saint-Zotique E, Montreal QC H1T 1P7; Mon'86; FRCSC; OrthSurg (Reconstructive Surgery). Staff, Hôpital Santa Cabrini Ospedale; (514)252-6000

SIOUFI, Gilbert K E; Clinique Med Viau, 204-4750 rue Jarry E, Saint-Leonard QC H1R 1X8; Beyrouth (Lebanon)'74; Staff, Centre Hospitalier l'Université De Montréal (CHUM) - Hôpital Saint-luc; (514)326-7203; Fax. (514)326-3656.

SIOUFI, Guy; 1-5184 boul Pie-IX, Montreal QC H1X 2B6; Sher'85; Peds (Dermatology). (514)723-4152; Fax. (514)722-3939.

SIOUFI, Richard; Centre Hosp Anna-Laberge, 200 boul Brisebois, Chateauguay QC J6K 4W8; McG'92; FRCS; FRCSC; Urol. Staff, Hôpital Anna-Laberge; Langs: Arabic; French; (450)699-2425

SIOUI, Christian; 630 rue Chef-Jean-Picard RR 1, Wendake QC G0A 4V0; Laval'82; (418)843-8638; Fax. (418)843-7323.

SIOW, Yin-Hui; Southlake Reg Health Centre, 596 Davis Dr, Newmarket ON L3Y 2P9; Tor'93; FRCPC; DiagRad; NuclearMed. Staff, Southlake Regional Health Centre; (709)637-5000

SIPPY, Rajinder K; McVean Med Centre, 7-1975 Cottrelle Blvd, Brampton ON L6P 2Z8; University of Delhi (India)'80; CCFP; Langs: Punjabi; Hindi; Urdu; (905)794-5300; Fax. (905)794-5350.

SIRA, Surjeet S; Malton Med Arts Bldg, 201-3530 Derry Rd E, Malton ON L4T 4E3; Birmingham (England)'63; MB ChB; LRCP; MRCS; FRCS; FRCSC; GenSurg. Langs: Italian; Punjabi; (905)672-9229

SIRAJ, Naila; Enhanced Care Clinic, 14872 Yonge St, Aurora ON L4G 1N2; Punjab (India)'01; CCFP; Langs: Punjabi; Urdu; (905)505-0950; Fax. (905)841-9404.

SIRARD, Alain; Hôpital Ste-Justine, 3175 ch Cote-Sainte-Catherine, Montreal QC H3T 1C5; Mon'83; ABPeds; NBME; FRCPC; Peds (P.Q.). Staff, Hôpital Ste-Justine; (514)345-4931

SIRAY, Brian L; Foothills Family Med Centre, PO Box 460 114 1 St SW, Black Diamond AB T0L 0H0; Alb'82; CCFP; FCFP; Asst Prof, University of Calgary; (403)933-4368; Fax. (403)933-2026; bsiray@mdh.ab.ca.

SIRBOVAN, Jane E; Scarborough Hosp-General Div, 3050 Lawrence Ave E, Scarborough ON M1P 2V5; Tor'84; FRCPC; AnatPath. Staff, The Scarborough Hospital - General Campus; (416)438-2911 x6379

SIRCA, Florica C; York Central Hosp, 10 Trench St, Richmond Hill ON L4C 4Z3; Timisoara (Romania)'92; FRCPC; IntMed. Staff, Mackenzie Richmond Hill Hospital; Staff IntMed, Toronto Western Hospital - University Health Network; (905)883-1212

SIRDAR, Emmanuel; CHUM-Hotel-Dieu, 3840 rue Saint-Urbain, Montreal QC H2W 1T8; Sher'97; FRCPC; IntMed. Staff, Centre Hospitalier l'Université de Montréal (CHUM) - Hôtel-Dieu; (514)890-8000

SIRDAR, Marie-Eve; CHUM-Hotel-Dieu, 3840 rue Saint-Urbain, Montreal QC H2W 1T8; Mon'05; IntMed. Staff, Centre Hospitalier l'Université de Montréal (CHUM) - Hôtel-Dieu; (514)890-8000 x14444

SIREK, Ann Maria T; Diabetes Care Centre, 83 Dawson Rd, Guelph ON N1H 1B1; Tor'74; MTS; FRCPC; IntMed (Endocrinology). Vis Endocrinologist, Clair Stewart Mount Forest; Langs: Slovak; (519)840-1964

SIREN, Andrew J E; Port Arthur Health Centre Inc, 194 Court St N, Thunder Bay ON P7A 4V7; Ott'96; BSc; ObstGyn (Obstetric Ultrasound). (807)346-1000; Fax. (807)346-6206.

SIREN, Kenneth P J; Sunnybrook Hlth Sciences Ctre, 2075 Bayview Ave, Toronto ON M4N 3M5; Tor'76; CCFP; CCFP(E.M.); Ac Staff, Mount Sinai Hospital; Court Staff Surg, Sunnybrook Health Sciences Centre; (416)480-6100

SIRHAN, Denis; MUHC-Montreal Neurology Inst, 109-3801 rue University, Montreal QC H3A 2B4; Mon'89; FRCSC; Neursurg. adj Prof, McGill University Health Centre - Montreal Neurological Hospital; adj Prof Neuro Surg, McGill University; Langs: Arabic; French; (514)398-1933; Fax. (514)398-2811; evangelia.ozek@muhc.mcgill.ca.

SIRHAN, Shireen M; 950 rue Principale, Cowansville QC J2K 1K3; McG'03; FRCPC; IntMed; MedOncol; Hem. Staff, Hôpital Brome-Missisquoi-Perkins; Staff, CSSS du Coeur de l'Isle Hôpital Jean-Talon; Langs: French; Arabic; (450)629-4342

SIRIANNI, Faye E; South Maternity & Family Pract, 258-1011 Glenmore Trail SW, Calgary AB T2V 4R6; UBC'08; CCFP; (403)640-0600; Fax. (403)253-0124.

SIRIANNI, Giovanna; Sunnybrook Health Sciences Ctr, 2075 Bayview Ave, Toronto ON M4N 3M5; Tor'03; CCFP; Staff Palliative Care Consultation Team, Sunnybrook Health Sciences Centre; Langs: Italian; French; (416)480-6100

SIRIWARDENA, Komudi P; The Hosp for Sick Children, 555 University Ave, Toronto ON M5G 1X8; Otago (New Zealand)'89; Staff, The Hospital For Sick Children; (416)813-7654; Fax. (416)813-5345.

SIRKIN, Wilma L; North York Gen Hosp, 4001 Leslie St, North York ON M2K 1E1; Witwatersrand (South Africa)'88; FRCPC; AnatPath (Perinatal). Staff, North York General Hospital; University of Toronto; Langs: Afrikaans; (416)756-6248; Fax. (416)756-4294.

SIRKO, Peter M; Hamilton HS-General Site, 237 Barton St E, Hamilton ON L8L 2X2; Qns'87; FRCPC; Anes. Staff, Hamilton Health Sciences Centre - Hamilton General Hospital; Langs: Ukrainian; (905)527-4322

SIRMAN, Mehmet R; Humber River Reg Hosp-Keele, 2175 Keele St, York ON M6M 3Z4; Istanbul (Turkey)'80; FRCPC; Psy. Staff, Humber River Regional Hospital - Keele Street Site; Langs: Turkish; French; (416)658-2007; Fax. (416)658-2074.

SIRNA, Salvatore; Danforth Med Centre, 1473 Danforth Ave, Toronto ON M4J 1N5; Tor'85; Staff, Toronto East General Hospital Inc; Langs: Italian; (416)461-0785; Fax. (416)461-0787.

SIROIS, Alain; Clinique Med de Sillery, 1270 av William, Quebec QC G1S 4G1; Laval'85; FRCPC; Psy. Prof, Université Laval; (418)688-5018; Fax. (418)688-4601.

SIROIS, Carolyne; Centre Med de l'Hetriere, 201-3520 boul de l'Hetriere, Quebec QC G3A 0B4; Laval'98; Staff GP, Hôtel-Dieu de Lévis; Conférencier, Université Laval; (418)651-3933; Fax. (418)651-0256; c.sirois@videotron.ca.

SIROIS, Cateline; Hop du Sacre-Coeur de Mtl, 5400 boul Gouin O, Montreal QC H4J 1C5; Laval'96; ThorSurg; GenSurg. Staff, Hôpital du Sacre-Coeur de Montréal; (514)338-2222 x2050

SIROIS, Chantal; CHUS-Hop Fleurimont, 3001 12e av N, Sherbrooke QC J1H 5N4; Laval'93; FRCSC; GenSurg; ThorSurg. Staff, Centre Hospitalier Universitaire de Sherbrooke-Hopital Fleurimont; (819)346-1110 x12371; Fax. (819)820-6871; chantal.sirois@usherbrooke.ca.

SIROIS, Christian; MUHC-Montreal Gen Hosp, L9 513-1650 av Cedar, Montreal QC H3G 1A4; Laval'92; AB(ThoracicSurg); FRCSC; GenSurg (Surgical Oncology); ThorSurg. Staff, Sir Mortimer B Davis Jewish General; Staff, McGill University Health Centre - Montreal General Campus; adj Prof, McGill University; Langs: Bilingual(English/French); (514)934-1934 x44326; Fax. (514)934-8210.

SIROIS, Claude; Cree Board Health & Social Ser, PO Box 250, Chisasibi QC J0M 1E0; Laval'87; Ophth. Staff, Cree Board of Health & Social Services James Bay; Staff, Centre Hospitalier du Centre la Mauricie; (819)855-2844

SIROIS, Dany; Ctr Hosp du Centre la Mauricie, 50 119e rue, Shawinigan-Sud QC G9P 5K1; Laval'03; Staff, Centre Hospitalier du Centre la Mauricie; (819)536-7500

SIROIS, Francois; Hôpital Laval, 2725 ch Sainte-Foy, Quebec QC G1V 4G5; Laval'69; FRCPC; Psy. Consultant, Hôpital Laval; Clin Prof, Université Laval; (418)656-4565; Fax. (418)656-4551.

SIROIS, Genevieve; Institut de Readaptation, 525 boul Wilfrid-Hamel, Quebec QC G1M 2S8; Laval'04; FRCPC; PhysMed&Rehab. Staff, Institut de Readaption & Deficience Physique de Quebec; (418)529-9141 x6920; genevieve.sirois@irdpq.qc.ca.

SIROIS, Isabelle; Hotel-Dieu de Levis, 143 rue Wolfe, Levis QC G6V 3Z1; Laval'96; Respir; IntMed. Staff, Hôtel-Dieu de Lévis; (514)835-7171; Fax. (514)835-7215.

SIROIS, Josee; Clinique Med Richibucto, 9364 rue Main, Richibucto NB E4W 4C9; Sher'05; CCFP; (506)523-4868; Fax. (506)523-1374.

SIROIS, M M Jeanne; CHVO-Hop de Hull, 116 boul Lionel-Emond, Gatineau QC J8Y 1W7; Ott'86; Staff, Hull Hospital; Langs: Polish; French; (819)966-6200; Fax. (819)771-6890.

SIROIS, Marco; CHUS-Hop Fleurimont, 3001 12e av N, Sherbrooke QC J1H 5N4; Laval'96; FRCSC; GenSurg. Staff, Centre Hospitalier Universitaire de Sherbrooke-Hopital Fleurimont; (819)346-1110 x12371

SIROIS, Marco; CLSC des Frontieres, 1922 rue Saint-Vallier RR 2, Pohenegamook QC G0L 1J0; Laval'86; (418)859-2450; Fax. (418)859-3484.

SIROIS, Marie-Claude; CSSS du Lac-des-Deux-Montagnes, 520 boul Arthur-Sauve, Saint-Eustache QC J7R 5B1; Mon'97; Staff, Hôpital de Saint-Eustache; (450)473-6811

SIROIS, Marthe; 1007-12 rue des Jardins Merici, Quebec QC G1S 4Z8; Laval'74; ac Staff, Centre Hospitalier Affilié Universitaire de Québec - Hôpital du St-Sacrement; Staff, Centre Hospitalier Universitaire de Quebec-CHUL; (418)914-7392

SIROIS, Michel; Keystone Place, 4E-270 Douglas Ave, Bathurst NB E2A 1M9; Laval'87; FRCSC; PlasSurg. (506)548-5340

SIROIS, Michel; Centre Med de l'Hetriere, 201-3520 rue de l'Hetriere, St-Augustin-D-Desm QC G3A 0B4; Laval'74; Staff, Hôpital Laval; assoc Staff, Centre Hospitalier Affilié Universitaire de Québec - Hôpital du St-Sacrement; assoc Staff, Centre Hospitalier Universitaire de Quebec-CHUL; (418)651-3933; Fax. (418)651-0256.

SIROIS, Nathalie; CSSS de Sept-Iles, 45 rue du Pere-Divet, Sept-Iles QC G4R 3N7; Sher'92; AB; FRCPC; Peds. Staff, Centre Hospitalier Regional de Sept-Iles; Langs: Bilingual(French/English); (418)962-9761; Fax. (418)968-2111.

SIROIS, Serge; CSSS Pierre Boucher, 1333 boul Jacques-Cartier E, Longueuil QC J4M 2A5; Sher'74; MSc; CCFP; Staff, Centre Hospitalier Pierre Boucher; ac Staff Psy, Hopital Louis-H Lafontaine; Clin Instructeur, Universite de Montreal; (450)468-8111 x82410

SIROIS-BERGERON, Elise; Hôtel-Dieu de Saint-Jérôme, 290 rue de Montigny, Saint-Jerome QC J7Z 5T3; Mon'05; Neur. Staff, Hôtel-Dieu de Saint-Jérôme; (450)431-8200

SIROTA, Marcia; LL-89 Glen Rush Blvd, Toronto ON M5N 2V2; Mem'86; FRCPC; Psy. Langs: Spanish; French.

SIROUNIS, Demetrios A; St Paul's Hosp, 3F-1081 Burrard St, Vancouver BC V6Z 1Y6; Sask'95; FRCPC; Anes; Critical Care Medicine. Staff, Providence Health Care - St Paul's Hospital; (604)806-8337

SIROUNIS, H Heather E; Royal University Hosp, 103 Hospital Dr, Saskatoon SK S7N 0W8; Sask'99; FRCPC; Anes. Staff Anes, Royal University Hospital; (306)655-1183; Fax. (306)655-1279; heathersirounis@hotmail.com.

SIRRS, Sandra M; Gordon & Leslie Diamond HCC, 4F-2775 Laurel St, Vancouver BC V5Z 1M9; UBC'91; FRCPC; IntMed; Endocrin&Metab. Assoc Staff, Vancouver General Hospital - Centennial Pavillion; Clin Instructor, University of British Columbia; (604)875-5965; Fax. (604)875-5967.

SIRZYK, Jeffrey; Hawkesbury & Dist Gen Hosp, 1111 Ghislain St, Hawkesbury ON K6A 3G5; McG'88; CCFP; CCFP(E.M.); FCFP; Staff, Hawkesbury & District General Hospital; Langs: French; Italian; (613)632-1111

SIS, Banu; University of Alberta Hosp, 5B4 24-8440 112 St NW, Edmonton AB T6G 2R7; Ankara (India)'97; FRCPC; AnatPath. Staff, University of Alberta Hospital; (780)407-8132

SISCA, Lyana I; Thistlewood Prof Centre, 207-8077 Islington Ave, Woodbridge ON L4L 7X7; Dal'05; FRCSC; ObstGyn. (905)850-0004

SISCHEK, Stephanie E; Stonechurch Family Hlth Ctre, 1475 Upper Ottawa St, Hamilton ON L8W 3J6; Man'11; (905)575-1300; Fax. (905)575-7831.

SISCHEK, William J; London Health Sciences Centre, PO Box 5010 Stn B 800 Commissioners Rd E, London ON N6A 5W9; Wes'82; FRCPC; Anes (Cardiovascular Anesthesia). Court Staff, St Joseph's Hospital - St Joseph's Health Care; Staff, London Health Sciences Centre - Victoria Campus; Assoc Prof, University of Western Ontario; (519)685-8525; Fax. (519)685-8275; william.sischek@lhsc.on.ca.

SISCHY, Neville L; 210A-305 Finch Ave W, North York ON M2R 1N2; Witwatersrand (South Africa)'72; Ac Staff, North York General Hospital - Branson Division; Court Staff, North York General Hospital; Langs: Yiddish; (416)226-3302; Fax. (416)849-0434.

SISLER, Jeffrey J; CancerCare Manitoba, 2038-675 McDermot Ave, Winnipeg MB R3E 0V9; Man'85; MClSc; CCFP; FCFP; Staff, St Boniface General Hospital; Dir Primary Care Oncology, Cancer Care Manitoba; Assoc Prof Family Med, University of Manitoba; (204)787-3595; Fax. (204)786-0715.

SISLER, W John; Surrey Mem Hosp, 13750 96 Ave, Surrey BC V3V 1Z2; Man'80; FRCPC; DiagRad. Staff, Surrey Memorial Hospital; (604)585-5637; Fax. (604)588-3370.

SISSONS, Joy L; Medicine Hat Reg Hosp, 666 5 St SW, Medicine Hat AB T1A 4H6; (South Africa)'04; Staff, Medicine Hat Regional Hospital; (403)529-8000

SISSONS, Wendy R; Westmount Med Bldg, 440-5025 rue Sherbrooke O, Montreal QC H4A 1S9; Alb'75; AB; FRCPC; Derm (Pediatric Dermatology). Att Staff, McGill University Health Centre - Montreal Children's Hospital; adj Prof, McGill University; Langs: Bilingual(English/French); (514)487-2440; Fax. (514)487-2350.

SISTO, Alfred; Child & Adolescent Clinic, 37 Thorncliff Pl, Nepean ON K2H 6L5; Liege (Belgium)'80; FRCPC; Peds (Gastroenterology). Consultant, Children's Hospital of Eastern Ontario (CHEO); Consultant, The Ottawa Hospital - Civic Campus; Court Staff, Queensway Carleton Hospital; Langs: Bilingual(French/English); (613)596-1568

SIT, Grace K; Olive Med Clinic, 101-117 17 Ave NE, Calgary AB T2E 1L7; Alb'05; CCFP; (403)276-8866; Fax. (403)230-2000.

SIT, Lindsay A; Heartline Med Clinic, 110-2504 Skaha Lake Rd, Penticton BC V2A 6G1; New York University (USA)'07; CCFP; Staff, Weeneebayko General Hospital; (250)492-3511

SIT, Marisa; Univ Hlth Network-Toronto Western Hosp, 472 7EW-399 Bathurst St, Toronto ON M5T 2S8; Tor'01; FRCSC; Ophth. Staff, Toronto Western Hospital - University Health Network; Langs: Cantonese; (416)603-5591; Fax. (416)603-5720.

SIT, Michelle; 202-4235 Sheppard Ave E, Scarborough ON M1S 1T7; Qns'94; CCFP; FCFP; Court Staff, The Scarborough Hospital - Birchmount Campus; Langs: Cantonese; Mandarin; (416)754-3553; Fax. (416)754-3554.

SIT, Shirley M; Rutherford Med Centre, 3-5283 Rutherford Rd, Woodbridge ON L4H 2T2; Tor'93; BASc; MASc; FAAP; FRCPC; Peds. Staff, Humber River Regional Hospital - Finch Avenue Site; (905)264-8311; Fax. (905)264-0801.

SIT, Sze Wan; St Michael's Hosp Family Unit, 3F-61 Queen St E, Toronto ON M5B 1W8; McG'05; CCFP; Staff, St Michael's Hospital; Staff, Toronto East General Hospital Inc; Langs: Cantonese; French; (416)867-7426; Fax. (416)867-7498.

SITARAM, Kadambi P; Centrepointe Med Centre, 305-1 Centrepointe Dr, Nepean ON K2G 6E2; Mysore (India)'73; MB BS; ABPMR; FRCPC; PhysMed&Rehab. Staff, The Ottawa Hospital Rehabilitation Centre; (613)723-5865

SITARU, Doina; Physical Med Group Clinic, 121-6363 rte Transcanadienne, Saint-Laurent QC H4T 1Z9; (Other Foreign)'98; CCFP; (514)581-1857

SITHAMPARANATHAN, Karthika; Platinum Med Clinic FHG, 3170 Eglinton Ave E, Scarborough ON M1J 2H3; St Bartholomew's & Royal London (England)'05; CCFP; Langs: Tamil; (416)265-2255; Fax. (416)265-6737.

SITHAMPARANATHAN, Kasthuri; York Medical Clinic, 110-1650 Elgin Mills Rd, Richmond Hill ON L4S 0B2; Saba University School of Medicine (Other Foreign)'07; CCFP; (905)770-3858

SITLAND, Troy D; Professional Arts Bldg, 412-100 Arden St, Moncton NB E1C 4B7; Dal'98; FRCSC; Urol. (506)857-4780; Fax. (506)857-4786.

SITWELL, Lucian D; Riverside Prof Centre, 304-1919 Riverside Dr, Ottawa ON K1H 1A2; Ott'83; FRCPC; IntMed (Headache); Neur. Staff, The Ottawa Hospital - General Campus; Staff, Montfort Hospital; Staff, Renfrew Victoria Hospital; University of Ottawa; (613)739-7268; Fax. (613)739-7023; lucian.sitwell@on.aibn.com.

SIU, Connie M; Greig Associates, 5732 Victoria Dr, Vancouver BC V5P 3W6; (Hong Kong)'66; MB BS; FRCPC; DiagRad (Bone Densitometry). Physician, Oakridge Centre South Tower; Clin Prof Radiol, University of British Columbia; Langs: Cantonese; (604)321-6774; Fax. (604)321-6626.

SIU, Danny W; 109-3020 Lincoln Ave, Coquitlam BC V3B 6B4; (Hong Kong)'76; MB BS; Ac Staff, BC Mental Health & Addiction Service; Langs: Cantonese; Mandarin; (604)464-4822; Fax. (604)464-4823.

SIU, Henry Y H; Stonechurch Family Health Ctre, 1475 Upper Ottawa St, Hamilton ON L8W 3J6; Tor'08; CCFP; Physician, Stonechurch Family Health Centre; (905)575-1300

SIU, Kevin D; Able-Care Med Clinic, 56-2991 Lougheed Hwy, New Westminster BC V3B 6J6; Tor'06; CCFP; (604)945-7819; Fax. (604)225-2557.

SIU, Kien G J; Scarborough Comm Mental Hlth, 301-2425 Eglinton Ave E, Scarborough ON M1K 5G8; Melbourne (Australia)'66; MB BS; FRCPC; Psy. Staff, The Scarborough Hospital - General Campus; (416)431-8135; Fax. (416)759-5162.

SIU, King Fun; Bay College Med Centre, 216C-777 Bay St, Toronto ON M5G 2C8; (Hong Kong)'76; MB BS; FRCS(Edin); CCFP; Langs: Cantonese; Mandarin; (416)977-8878; Fax. (416)977-0018; ksiu@pmac.ca.

SIU, Lillian L Y; Univ Hlth Network-Princess M, 5 718-610 University Ave, Toronto ON M5G 2M9; Tor'91; FRCPC; IntMed; MedOncol. Staff, Princess Margaret Hospital - University Health Network; Langs: Chinese; (416)946-2911; Fax. (416)946-4467.

SIU, Maurice K; Addiction & Mental Hlth-Queen, 3-1001 Queen St W, Toronto ON M6J 1H4; Ott'98; FRCPC; Psy. Staff, Centre for Addiction & Mental Health (CAMH) - Queen Site; (416)535-8501 x2959

SIU, May P; 2128 Kensington Rd NW, Calgary AB T2N 3R7; UBC'89; CCFP; Langs: Cantonese; (403)270-8939; Fax. (403)270-8937.

SIU, Samuel C B; C6 005-339 Windermere Rd, London ON N6A 5A5; Alb'83; FRCPC; IntMed; Cardiol. Staff, London Health Sciences Centre - University Hospital; Prof Med, University of Western Ontario; (519)663-3581; Fax. (519)663-3218.

SIU, Sidney K; SRS Consultants Inc, 827 Richmond St, London ON N6A 3H7; Tor'82; DABOT; CIH; FRCPC; OccupMed (Occupational & Environmental Health). Staff, London Health Sciences Centre - University Hospital; Asst Prof, University of Western Ontario; Langs: Chinese; (519)858-4694; Fax. (519)858-4692; srscons@on.aibn.com.

SIU, Tung; Canadian Forces Health Service, PO Box 6550 Stn Forces CFB 4 Wing, Cold Lake AB T9M 2C6; UBC'10; CCFP; Staff, Canadian Forces Health Services; (780)840-8000

SIU, Victoria W M; Allin Clinic, 10155 120 St NW, Edmonton AB T5K 2A2; Tor'82; FCCMG; FRCPC; Peds (Medical Genetics). (780)482-7551

SIU, William W Y; Royal Columbian Hosp, 330 Columbia St E, New Westminster BC V3L 3W7; UBC'94; FRCPC; DiagRad. Staff, Eagle Ridge Hospital & Health Care Centre; Staff, Royal Columbian Hospital; Staff, Medray Imaging; (604)520-4640; Fax. (604)520-4801.

SIU, Winnie W; Markham Stouffville Health Cen, 202-379 Church St, Markham ON L6B 0T1; Tor'10; CCFP; (905)472-2200

SIVACIYAN, Vahe; Toronto West Prof Centre, 415-2425 Bloor St W, Toronto ON M6S 4W4; Tor'72; BSc; ABIM; ABC; ABCD; FRCPC; IntMed (Teaching); Cardiol. Staff, St Michael's Hospital; Ac Staff Med, St Joseph's Health Centre; Asst Prof, University of Toronto; Langs: Armenian; French; Turkish; (416)762-0279; Fax. (416)762-0279.

SIVAGANESANATHAN, Arumugam; Scarborough Hosp-Birchmount, 3030 Birchmount Rd, Scarborough ON M1W 3W3; Ceylon (Sri Lanka)'75; MB BS; FRCA(Eng); FRCPC; Anes (Intensive Care). Staff, The Scarborough Hospital - Birchmount Campus; Langs: Tamil; (416)495-2701; Fax. (416)495-2879.

SIVAHARAN, Ajantha; Glazier Med Centre, 11 Gibb St, Oshawa ON L1H 2J9; Saba University (Netherlands Antilles)'05; (905)579-1212

SIVAJI, Nirmala; Scarborough Hosp-Birchmount, 3030 Birchmount Rd, Scarborough ON M1W 3W3; Colombo (Sri Lanka)'78; MB BS; FFARCSI; FRCPC; Anes (Chronic Pain). Staff, The Scarborough Hospital - Birchmount Campus; Langs: Tamil; (416)495-2400; Fax. (416)495-2879.

SIVAJI, Ponnuthurai; 218-385 Silver Star Blvd, Scarborough ON M1V 0E3; (Sri Lanka)'75; MB BS; LRCPS(Ed); LRCPS(Glas); ABIM; FRCPC; IntMed (Cardiology). Ac Staff, The Scarborough Hospital - Birchmount Campus; Langs: Tamil; Sinhalese; (416)298-0644; Fax. (416)298-4533.

SIVAKUMAR, Chandrasekaran; Rockyview Health Centre, 210-1016 68 Ave SW, Calgary AB T2V 4J2; (India)'89; Staff, Foothills Medical Centre; Staff, Cardiometabolic Evaluation & Risk Assessment Centre; (403)541-0033; Fax. (403)541-0032.

SIVAKUMAR, Panchasheila; Kennedy Med Centre, 2405 Eglinton Ave E, Scarborough ON M1K 2M5; Jaffna (Sri Lanka)'85; MB BS; CCFP; Langs: Tamil; Sinhalese; (416)755-3131; Fax. (416)755-3141.

SIVAKUMAR, Saraswati; 167 Townsend St, Sydney NS B1P 5E4; Dr M G R Medical University (India)'95; FRCSC; Ophth. Staff, Cape Breton Healthcare Complex; (902)539-8461; Fax. (902)539-8543.

SIVAKUMAR, Tharsan; LMC Endocrinology Centres, 110 Copper Creek Dr, Markham ON L6B 0P9; Saba University (Other Foreign)'05; FRCPC; IntMed; Endocrin&Metab. (905)294-0800; Fax. (905)294-0814.

SIVAKUMARAN, Sooriyakumaran T; University of Alberta Hosp, 2C2WMC-8440 112 St NW, Edmonton AB T6G 2B7; McM'94; FRCPC; IntMed (Arrhythmias); Cardiol. Staff, University of Alberta Hospital; Teach Staff Cardiol, University of Alberta; (780)407-6182; Fax. (780)407-7942.

SIVAKUMARAN, Thevaki; Cambridge Mem Hosp, 700 Coronation Blvd, Cambridge ON N1R 3G2; Jaffna (Sri Lanka)'83; MB BS; IntMed. Staff, Cambridge Memorial Hospital; Langs: Tamil; (519)621-2330

SIVALINGAM, Kanchana; Devon Gen Hosp, F-101 Erie St S, Devon AB T9G 1A6; (Sri Lanka)'84; MB BS; LRCP(Eng); MRCS(Eng); LMCC; Staff Hospital Med Clinic, Devon General Hospital; Staff, Hospital Medical Clinic; (780)987-4151; Fax. (780)987-4177.

SIVALINGAM, Paramalingam; Montgomery Med Clinic, 9212 95 Ave NW, Edmonton AB T6C 1Z7; Ceylon (Sri Lanka)'81; MB BS; LRCP(Ed); LRCS(Edin); LRCPS(Glas); Staff, Devon General Hospital; Langs: Tamil; (780)465-4954; Fax. (780)466-4675; psiva@telus.net.

SIVANANTH, Ponnampalam; Centennial Prof Centre, 81 Exhibition St, Kentville NS B4N 1C2; Jaffna (Sri Lanka)'92; MB BS; CCFP; (902)678-2755; Fax. (902)678-5546.

SIVANANTHAN, Kamalanayani; Burntwood Reg Health Authority, 50 Selrikirk Ave, Thompson MB R8N 0M7; (Other Foreign)'83; Staff, Burntwood Regional Health Authority; (204)677-1771

SIVANANTHAN, Shankar; Univ Hlth Network-Toronto Gen, JDE 14 217-200 Elizabeth St, Toronto ON M5G 2C4; Ott'09; (416)340-3155

SIVAPALAN, Shivajan; Bowmanville Prof Bldg, 222 King St E, Bowmanville ON L1C 1P6; St George's University of Grenada (Grenada)'09; CCFP; (905)440-3584; Fax. (905)440-3585.

SIVAPALAN, Sivaseelan; Medica One, 1275 Rymal Rd E, Hamilton ON L8W 3N1; University of Manchester (England)'05; CCFP; (905)387-0005; Fax. (905)387-0010.

SIVAPALASINGAM, Nihilarani; Baycrest Centre Geriatric Care, 3560 Bathurst St, Toronto ON M6A 2E1; University of Jaffna (India)'93; Staff, Baycrest Centre for Geriatric Care; (416)785-2500

SIVARAJAH, Kalawathy; Chaleur Reg Hosp, 1750 Sunset Dr, Bathurst NB E2A 4L7; Peradeniya (Sri Lanka)'85; FRCPC; AnatPath. Staff, Hopital Regional Chaleur; Langs: Sinhalese; Tamil; (506)544-2412; Fax. (506)544-2442.

SIVARAJAN, Venkatesan B; The Hosp For Sick Children, 555 University Ave, Toronto ON M5G 1X8; Tor'98; FRCPC; Peds; Critical Care Medicine; Cardiol. Staff, The Hospital For Sick Children; (416)813-7654; Fax. (416)813-7299; earl.silverman@sickkids.ca.

SIVARAMAN, Sujith K; St-Mary's Hosp Centre, 3830 av Lacombe, Montreal QC H3T 1M5; McG'00; FRCPC; EmergMed. Staff, St Mary's Hospital Centre; (514)345-3511 x3263; Fax. (514)734-2688.

SIVASUBRAMANIAM, Tharsika; Bur Oak Med Centre, 5B-20 Bur Oak Ave, Markham ON L6C 0A2; Medical University of the Americas (Other Foreign)'07; CCFP; (905)887-0042; Fax. (905)887-0054.

SIVASUBRAMANIAN, Velan; St Joseph's Health Centre, SSW 419-30 The Queensway, Toronto ON M6R 1B5; Ott'93; FRCPC; Psy. Staff, St Joseph's Health Centre; (416)530-6717; Fax. (416)530-6774.

SIVASUNDARAM, Ramanan; 102-1621 Albert St, Regina SK S4P 2S5; Jaffna (Sri Lanka)'94; FRCSC; OrthSurg;CCFP; Langs: Sinhalese; Tamil; (306)766-0398; Fax. (306)766-7137.

SIVERS, David R; Sudbury Med Centre, 309-65 Larch St, Sudbury ON P3E 1B8; Wes'77; Staff, Health Sciences North-St Joseph's Health Centre; Staff, Health Sciences North - Memorial Site; Staff, Health Sciences North-Laurentian Site; (705)674-3509; Fax. (705)674-3520.

SIVERTSON, Joanne D; Associate Med Clinic, 222-20 14th St W, Prince Albert SK S6V 3K8; Sask'04; FRCSC; ObstGyn. Physician, Associate Medical Clinic; (306)922-3284; Fax. (306)922-3285.

SIVIERO, Giovanni; Hop Santa Cabrini Ospedale, 5655 rue Saint-Zotique E, Montreal QC H1T 1P7; Laval'91; Staff, Hôpital Santa Cabrini Ospedale; (514)252-6000; Fax. (514)252-6501.

SIVILOTTI, Marco L A; Kingston Gen Hosp, 76 Stuart St, Kingston ON K7L 2V7; Qns'88; BSc(Hons); MSc; FRCPC; EmergMed (Toxicology). Att Staff, Kingston General Hospital; Att Staff, Hotel-Dieu Hospital; Assoc Prof Emerg Med, Queen's University; Langs: French; Italian; (613)548-2368; Fax. (613)548-1374.

SIVJEE, Khalil Y; Sunnybrook Hlth Sciences Ctre, A459-2075 Bayview Ave, Toronto ON M4N 3M5; Connecticut (USA)'94; FRCPC; IntMed; Respir. Staff, Sunnybrook Health Sciences Centre; (416)480-4758

SIVUCHA, Walter J; North Road Med Centre, 435S North Rd, Coquitlam BC V3K 3V9; UBC'66; Staff, Royal Columbian Hospital; (604)936-0411; Fax. (604)931-7022.

SIWAK, Christopher D; Central Alberta Med Imaging, 4312 54 Ave, Red Deer AB T4N 4M1; Cal'95; FRCPC; DiagRad. Staff, Foothills Medical Centre; (403)343-6172; Fax. (403)309-0092.

SIYAM, Sheima A M M; Springdale Prof Bldg, 308-2250 Bovaird Dr E, Brampton ON L6R 0W3; Cairo (Egypt)'01; CCFP; Staff, William Osler Health System - Brampton Civic Hospital; (905)595-2870; Fax. (905)595-2869.

SIYIH, Mahysin; Portage Clinic, 140 9th St SE, Portage la Prairie MB R1N 3V5; (Other Foreign)'99; (204)857-3445

SJAUS, Ana; Queen Elizabeth II HSC, 10W-1276 South Park St, Halifax NS B3H 2Y9; UBC'02; FRCPC; Anes. Staff, Queen Elizabeth II Health Sciences Centre - Victoria General Site; (902)473-3866

SJODIN, Astrid D; Towne Centre Medical, 201-3601 Highway 7 E, Markham ON L3R 0M3; McM'93; CCFP; (905)604-3336; Fax. (905)604-7750.

SKABURSKIS, Martin W; Clinique Med Chateauguay, 120 boul Saint-Jean-Baptiste, Chateauguay QC J6K 3A9; McG'80; Respir; IntMed. ac Staff, Hôpital Anna-Laberge; (450)691-8191

SKAKUM, Kurt K; Psychealth Centre, PZ 277-771 Bannatyne Ave, Winnipeg MB R3E 3N4; Man'94; FRCPC; Psy (Consultation-Liaison). Staff, Health Sciences Centre; Assoc Prof Med & Psy, University of Manitoba; (204)787-3482; Fax. (204)787-7480; kskakum@hsc.mb.ca.

SKAKUM, Ruth G H; Skakum Med Corp, 10 Attley Pl, Winnipeg MB R3P 1N7; Man'95; CCFP; Staff, St Boniface General Hospital; (204)233-8563

SKALA, Richard A; Hamilton HS-General Site, 237 Barton St E, Hamilton ON L8L 2X2; Tor'79; BSc; MSc; FRCPC; Anes. Staff, Hamilton Health Sciences Centre - Hamilton General Hospital; (905)527-0271 x46277

SKALA, William N; Southlake Reg Health Centre, 596 Davis Dr, Newmarket ON L3Y 2P9; Tor'71; DAB; FAB; Anes. Consultant, Southlake Regional Health Centre; (905)895-4521

SKALENDA, Patrick J; St Joseph's Health Centre, 30 The Queensway, Toronto ON M6R 1B5; McG'93; BSc; MHSc; MDCM; CCFP; FCFP; Staff Family Med, St Joseph's Health Centre; Lecturer, University of Toronto; Langs: French; (416)530-6860; Fax. (416)530-6160.

SKALLI, Leila; Institute of Mental Health Que, 2601 ch de la Canardiere, Quebec QC G1J 2G3; Mon'05; Psy. Staff, Institut Universitaire Sante; (418)663-5000

SKALSKA, Ursula; 525 Broadway St W PO Box 20004 Rpo Fairview, Vancouver BC V5Z 0C1; Qns'06; FRCPC; IntMed; Hem.

SKAMENE, Alexander; 200-175 av Stillview, Pointe-Claire QC H9R 4S3; Lausanne (Switzerland)'72; Endocrin (P.Q.); IntMed (P. Q.). ac Staff, Lakeshore General Hospital - Pointe Claire; (514)697-6402; Fax. (514)697-6610.

SKAMENE, Emil; MUHC-Montreal Gen Hosp, A6 149-1650 av Cedar, Montreal QC H3G 1A4; Karlova (Czech Republic)'68; FACP; FRCPC; ClinImmunol&Allergy. principale Médecin, McGill University Health Centre - Montreal General Campus; Chef Centre for Host Resistance, McGill University; (514)934-8038; Fax. (514)934-8570.

SKANES, Allan C; London HSC-University Hosp, PO Box 5339 Stn B 339 Windermere Rd, London ON N6A 5A5; Tor'90; FRCP; FRCPC; IntMed (Arrhythmias); Cardiol. Staff Arrhythmia Service, London Health Sciences Centre - University Hospital; (519)663-3746; Fax. (519)663-3782; askanes@uwo.ca.

SKANES, Melissa D; James Paton Mem Hosp, 125 125 Trans Canada Hwy, Gander NL A1V 1P7; Mem'07; DiagRad. Staff, James Paton Memorial Hospital; (709)256-2500

SKANES, Susan E; 135-667 Champlain St, Dieppe NB E1A 1P6; Mem'83; BMedSci; FRCSC; GenSurg (Hand Surgery); PlasSurg. Staff Plastic & ReconstrSurg, Dr Georges-L-Dumont University Hospital Centre; Staff, The Moncton Hospital; Clin Instructor Med, Dalhousie University; Clin Instructeur Med, Universite de Sherbrooke; Langs: Bilingual(French/English); (506)854-2616; Fax. (506)852-4340.

SKANES, Susan M; 205-350 St George St, Moncton NB E1C 1X1; Mem'95; CCFP; (506)388-8181; Fax. (506)388-8188.

SKANTHAN, Sithamparanathan; Abbotsford Reg Hosp & Cancer C, 32900 Marshall Rd, Abbotsford BC V2S 0C2; Colombo (Sri Lanka)'98; Staff, Abbotsford Regional Hospital & Cancer Centre; (604)851-4775

SKARPATHIOTAKIS, Maria; St Michael's Hosp, 30 Bond St, Toronto ON M5B 1W8; Tor'06; FRCPC; DiagRad. Staff, St Michael's Hospital; Langs: Greek; (416)864-5656

SKARRATT, Kevin H; Sunnybrook Hlth Sciences Ctre, 2075 Bayview Ave, Toronto ON M4N 3M5; Cal'02; CCFP; CCFP(E.M.); Staff, Sunnybrook Health Sciences Centre; (416)480-6100

SKARSGARD, David P; Tom Baker Cancer Centre, 1331 29 St NW, Calgary AB T2N 4N2; Sask'87; FRCPC; RadOncol. Staff, Tom Baker Cancer Centre; (403)521-3077; Fax. (403)283-1651.

SKARSGARD, Erik D; Children's & Women's HC Of BC, KO 110 ACB-4480 Oak St, Vancouver BC V6H 3V4; UBC'85; MSc(Surg.); FAAP; FACS; FRCSC; GenSurg; PedGenSurg. Chief Surg, BC Children's Hospital; Staff, UBC Hospital - Koerner Pavillion; Prof Surg, University of British Columbia; (604)875-3744; Fax. (604)875-2721.

SKARSGARD, Peter L; St Paul's Hosp, 490-1081 Burrard St, Vancouver BC V6Z 1Y6; UBC'92; FRCSC; GenSurg; CardSurg. Staff, Vancouver General Hospital - Centennial Pavillion; Staff, Providence Health Care - St Paul's Hospital; Asst Prof, University of British Columbia; (604)806-9320

SKEAD, Lennard; Brandon Reg Health Centre, 150 McTavish Ave E, Brandon MB R7A 2B3; Staff, Brandon Regional Health Centre; (204)578-4107; Fax. (204)726-9779.

SKEATE, Robert C; Canadian Blood Services, 67 College St, Toronto ON M5G 2M1; University of Minnesota (USA)'98; Assoc Med Dir, Canadian Blood Services; (416)313-4560; Fax. (416)974-9757.

SKEETE, Jason R; Kipling Heights Med Centre, 117-2291 Kipling Ave, Etobicoke ON M9W 4L6; (Other Foreign)'05; CCFP; (416)741-4545

SKEHAN, Anthony M; Anthony Skehan Med Prof Corp, 102-2813 Arthur St E, Thunder Bay ON P7E 5P5; Dublin (Ireland)'79; MB ChB; PhD; FRCS; FRCSC; Urol (Incontinence). Assoc Prof Urology, Thunder Bay Regional Health Sciences Centre; (807)623-0004; Fax. (807)623-3334; dleross@tbaytel.net.

SKEIN, Willem; Associate Med Clinic, PO Box 510 213 3 St, Slave Lake AB T0G 2A0; (780)849-4155; Fax. (780)849-4574.

SKEITH, Kenneth J; Allin Clinic, 10155 120 St NW, Edmonton AB T5K 2A2; Alb'78; FRCPC; IntMed; Rheum. (780)482-7551; Fax. (780)414-5669; ken.skeith@ualberta.ca.

SKELDON, Simon C; Queensway Prof Centre, 410-190 Sherway Dr, Etobicoke ON M9C 5N2; UBC'82; FRCSC; Urol. Ac Staff, Trillium Health Centre - West Toronto; (416)620-1685

SKELTON, Geoffrey G; Toronto East Gen Hosp Inc, 825 Coxwell Ave, Toronto ON M4C 3E7; Cal'10; CCFP; Staff, Toronto East General Hospital Inc; (416)469-6580; Fax. (416)469-6874.

SKENDAJ, Evis; Medical One, C2-2501 Third Line, Oakville ON L6M 5A9; Universiteti i Tiranes (Albania)'00; CCFP; (905)618-9934; Fax. (289)271-1132.

SKENE, David S; The Ottawa Hosp-Gen Campus, 501 Smyth Rd, Ottawa ON K1H 8L6; Qns'63; Anes. Ac Staff, The Ottawa Hospital - General Campus; Assoc Prof, University of Ottawa; (613)737-8187; Fax. (613)737-8189.

SKENE, Patsy; Clinique Med Centre-Ville, 5-167 rue de la Reine, Gaspe QC G4X 2W6; Sher'89; Staff, Centre Hospitalier de Gaspe; (418)368-1811; Fax. (418)368-2616.

SKEPASTS, Peter K; 300-2099 152 St, Surrey BC V4A 4N7; Cal'86; FRCSC; Urol. (604)538-0722; Fax. (604)542-0732.

SKIDMORE, David L; IWK Health Centre, PO Box 9700 Rpo CSC 5850 University Ave, Halifax NS B3K 6R8; Wes'00; FRCPC; Peds (Medical Genetics). Staff, IWK Health Centre; Vis Consultant, Saint John Regional Hospital; Staff, Maritime Medical Genetics Services; (902)470-8007; Fax. (902)470-8709.

SKIDMORE, Gary B; The Ottawa Hosp-Gen Campus, 501 Smyth Rd, Ottawa ON K1H 8L6; Wes'76; DAB; FRCPC; Anes. Ac Staff, The Ottawa Hospital - General Campus; Asst Prof, University of Ottawa; (613)737-8187; Fax. (613)737-8189.

SKIDMORE, Martin B; Sunnybrook Hlth Sciences Ctre, M4 228-2075 Bayview Ave, Toronto ON M4N 3M5; London (England)'72; MB BS; DCH; DObstRCOG; MRCP; FRCPC; Peds (Neonatology). Staff Perinatal Unit, Sunnybrook Health Sciences Centre; Ac Staff, Mount Sinai Hospital; Hon Staff, The Hospital For Sick Children; Ac Staff Newborn & Developmental Peds, Women's College Hospital; Dir Peds & ObstGyn/Asst Prof, University of Toronto; (416)480-6100; martin.skidmore@sw.ca.

SKILLINGS, Robert L; Beaupre Varicose Vein Clinic, 600-1335 Carling Ave, Ottawa ON K1Z 8N8; Wes'83; (613)722-0101

SKILLMAN, Jean L; Two Rivers FHT-Hespeler Med Cl, 12B-350 Conestoga Blvd, Cambridge ON N1R 7L7; Wes'71; CCFP; Ac Staff, Cambridge Memorial Hospital; (519)629-4615; Fax. (519)629-4630; jski2@rogers.com.

SKINNARLAND, Ellen M; Gordon Head Treatment Centre, 103-1595 McKenzie Ave, Victoria BC V8N 1A4; Tor'82; Staff Palliative Care, Victoria Hospice Society; (250)477-4777; Fax. (250)477-5471.

SKINNER, Christopher R R; The Ottawa Hosp-Civic Campus, C2184-1053 Carling Ave, Ottawa ON K1Y 4E9; Qns'79; MD; BEng; DABSM; FRCPC; IntMed (Sleep Medicine); Neur. Staff, Montfort Hospital; Staff Neurol, The Ottawa Hospital - Civic Campus; Staff, CSSS d'Antoine-Labelle; Staff Geog, University of Ottawa; Langs: French; Russian; (613)761-5353; Fax. (613)761-5360.

SKINNER, Gregory J; PO Box 68268 Rpo Crowfoot, Calgary AB T3G 3N8; (Netherlands Antilles)'04; CCFP.

SKINNER, James T; Manitoba Adolescent Trmt Ctre, 505-180 King St, Winnipeg MB R3B 3P7; Man'86; FRCPC; Psy.

SKINNER, Natalie; CHUM-Hop Saint-Luc, 1058 rue Saint-Denis, Montreal QC H2X 3J4; Ott'06; CCFP; CCFP(E.M.); Staff, Centre Hospitalier l'Université de Montréal (CHUM) - Hôpital Notre-Dame; Staff, Centre Hospitalier l'Université De Montréal (CHUM) - Hôpital Saint-luc; (514)890-8000

SKINNER, Roger P; Regional Coroner's Office, 440-366 King St E, Kingston ON K7K 6Y3; McM'84; BA; CCFP; CCFP(E.M.); Reg Med Examiner Supervising Office of the Chief Coroner, Regional Coroner's Office-East Region; (613)544-1596; Fax. (613)544-3473.

SKINNER, Sarah J; Kensington Med Clinic, 6548 Hastings St, Burnaby BC V5B 1S2; Dal'77; Staff, Providence Health Care - St Paul's Hospital; (604)299-9769; Fax. (604)299-9772.

SKINNER, Stuart J; Royal University Hosp, 103 Hospital Dr, Saskatoon SK S7N 0W8; Sask'02; BSc; DTM&H; FRCPC; IntMed (AIDS/HIV); InfectDis. Staff, Royal University Hospital; (306)655-1785; Fax. (306)975-0383.

SKINNER, William A; St Paul's Hosp, 1081 Burrard St, Vancouver BC V6Z 1Y6; Dal'04; Staff, Providence Health Care - St Paul's Hospital; (604)806-9262

SKINNIDER, Brian F; Vancouver Gen Hosp, 855 12th Ave W, Vancouver BC V5Z 1M9; Sask'94; FRCPC; AnatPath. Staff Path, BC Cancer Agency Vancouver Centre; Staff, Vancouver General Hospital - Centennial Pavillion; (604)877-6000; brian.skinnider@vch.ca.

SKINNIDER, Douglas J; Foul Bay Prof Centre, 206A-1964 Fort St, Victoria BC V8R 6R3; Sask'87; FRCPC; IntMed. (250)598-3392; Fax. (250)598-3348.

SKINNIDER, Marie T; 3461 Cook St, Victoria BC V8X 1B3; Sask'87; (250)386-6161

SKIPPEN, Peter W; BC Women's Hosp & Health Ctre, 2L10-4480 Oak St, Vancouver BC V6H 3V4; Queensland (Australia)'79; MB BS; FRCPC; Anes (Critical Care Medicine). Staff, BC Children's Hospital; (604)875-2744; Fax. (604)875-2728.

SKIPPER, R James; Credit Valley Med Arts Ctre, 204-2000 Credit Valley Rd, Mississauga ON L5M 4N4; Wes'86; FRCSC; OrthSurg (Hip & Knee Reconstruction). Staff OrthSurg, The Credit Valley Hospital; (905)820-2016; Fax. (905)820-9008.

SKIRVING, Paul D; Elizabeth Avenue Fam Practice, 116-100 Elizabeth Ave, St. John's NL A1B 1S1; Mem'99; (709)579-5005

SKJENNA, Olaf W; 15 Baslaw Dr, Ottawa ON K1G 5J8; Alb'67; DAvMed; Aj Prof, Aerospace Med., U. of Southern California; (613)736-7489; Fax. (613)521-8649.

SKJODT, Neil M; 80 Sioux Rd, Sherwood Park AB T8A 3X5; Cal'91; FCCP; MSc; DABSM; FRCPC; IntMed; Critical Care Medicine; Respir. Staff, University of Alberta Hospital; (780)449-1434; Fax. (780)449-1435.

SKLADMAN, Irina; Joseph Brant Mem Hosp, 1230 North Shore Blvd, Burlington ON L7S 1W7; Azerbaijan N Narimanov University (Other Foreign)'79; FRCPC; Psy. Staff Mental Health Services, Joseph Brant Memorial Hospital; (905)631-1939

SKLAR, Donald; 407-1100 Sheppard Ave E, North York ON M2K 2W1; Tor'62; DPsy; FRCPC; Psy. Consultant, North York General Hospital; (416)226-6988

SKLAR, Lawrence S; Dr L S Sklar Med Office, 203-100 Humber College Blvd, Etobicoke ON M9V 5G4; Tor'84; PhD; FRCPC; IntMed (Cardiology). Att Staff, William Osler Health System - Etobicoke General Hospital; Att Staff, Trillium Health Centre - West Toronto; Att Staff, William Osler Health System - Brampton Civic Hospital; (416)743-4961; Fax. (416)743-4315.

SKLAR, Marsha C; CSST-Direction Reg de Montreal, CP 3 Succ Pl-desjardins TS-1 Complexe desjardins, Montreal QC H5B 1H1; Laval'86; AnatPath. Médecin, CSST-Direction Regionale Montreal; Langs: English; French; (514)906-3122

SKOCHYLAS, Edwin P; Central Alberta Prof Centre, 100-5201 43 St, Red Deer AB T4N 1C7; Sask'79; FRCSC; Ophth (Cosmetics). Ac Staff, Red Deer Regional Hospital Centre; (403)347-6606; Fax. (403)347-6639.

SKOCYLAK, George W; 303-2299 Dundas St W, Toronto ON M6R 1X7; Tor'72; Court Staff Family Practice, St Joseph's Health Centre; Langs: Ukrainian; Polish; (416)766-7610; Fax. (416)766-5398.

SKOLL, M Amanda L; BC Women's & Hosp & Health Ctr, 2H30-4500 Oak St, Vancouver BC V6H 3N1; Sask'82; FRCSC; ObstGyn (Maternal Fetal Medicine). Staff, Vancouver General Hospital - Centennial Pavillion; Staff, BC Women's Hospital & Health Centre; Assoc Prof, University of British Columbia; Langs: Bilingual(English/French); (604)875-3174; Fax. (604)875-3099.

SKOLNICK, Marvin; 105 Brant Ave, Brantford ON N3T 3H4; Tor'59; FRCPC; Derm (Medical Oncology). (519)756-6477; Fax. (519)756-0347.

SKOMRO, Robert; Royal University Hosp, 103 Hospital Dr, Saskatoon SK S7N 0W8; Sask'93; FRCPC; IntMed; Respir. Staff Respiratory Med, Royal University Hospital; Langs: Polish; Russian; (306)966-2475; Fax. (306)966-8694.

SKORENKI, Andrea H; Hys Med Centre, 120-3017 66 St NW, Edmonton AB T6K 4B2; Cal'05; FRCSC; ObstGyn. Staff, University of Alberta Hospital; (780)461-6220

SKORETZ, Terry G; London HSC-Victoria Hosp, PO Box 5010 Stn B E1 102-800 Commissioners Rd E, London ON N6A 5W9; Wes'98; FRCPC; EmergMed. Staff, London Health Sciences Centre - Victoria Campus; (519)667-6538; Fax. (519)667-6769.

SKORY, Gerald M; 18-16945 Leslie St, Newmarket ON L3Y 9A2; Tor'66; (905)868-8689; Fax. (905)868-9479.

SKORY, Leah M; Barrie Comm Health Centre, 490 Huronia Rd, Barrie ON L4N 6M2; Mem'95; CCFP; FCFP; (705)734-9690; Fax. (905)734-0239.

SKORZEWSKA, Anna K; Univ Hlth Network-Toronto Gen, 8 228EN-200 Elizabeth St, Toronto ON M5G 2C4; Tor'97; FRCPC; Psy (Acute Adult Psychiatry). Staff, Toronto General Hospital - UHN; Locum Tenens, Timmins & District Hospital; Asst Prof, University of Toronto; Langs: French; (416)340-4305; Fax. (416)340-4198; anna.skorzewska@uhn.on.ca.

SKOTNICKI-GRANT, Sandra M; Bay Dermatology Centre, 536-790 Bay St, Toronto ON M5G 1N8; Tor'93; FRCPC; Derm (Allergy). Consultant Occup Med & Allergic Contact Dermatitis, St Michael's Hospital; (416)515-8808; Fax. (416)515-8805.

SKOURAS, Nicholas; 1108-20 Eglinton Ave W, Toronto ON M4R 1K8; Tor'92; FRCS; BSc; DABOph; FRCSC; Ophth (Refractive Surgery). Member, American Board of Ophthalmology; Langs: Greek; (416)590-0445; Fax. (416)590-0446; skourasmd@rogers.com.

SKOV, Carolyn M B; 5-506 71 Ave SW, Calgary AB T2V 4V4; Alb'70; BSc; FRCSC; Ophth (Pediatric Ophthalmology). Ac Staff, Rockyview General Hospital; Ac Staff, Alberta Children's Hospital; Clin Lecturer, University of Calgary; (403)253-6700; Fax. (403)253-2102.

SKOVSBO, Vivian; Peter Lougheed Centre, 3500 26 Ave NE, Calgary AB T1Y 6J4; Dal'97; CCFP; Staff Hospital Program Division of Acute CareAcute Care, Peter Lougheed Centre; (403)943-5461

SKOWRONSKI, Danuta M; BC Centre for Disease Control, 655 12th Ave W, Vancouver BC V5Z 4R4; Qns'89; MHSc; FRCPC; CommunMed (Clinical Immunology & Allergy); Public Health & Preventive Med. Clinical Asst Prof, University of British Columbia; (604)660-6067; Fax. (604)660-0197.

SKRABEK, Pamela J; Cancercare Manitoba, ON 2052-675 McDermot Ave, Winnipeg MB R3E 0V9; Man'05; FRCPC; IntMed; Hem. Staff, CancerCare Manitoba.

SKRABEK, Ryan Q; The Rehabilitation Centre, RR133-800 Sherbrook St, Winnipeg MB R3A 1M4; Man'03; FRCPC; PhysMed&Rehab. Physician, The Rehabilitation Centre; Manitoba Public Insurance; rskrabek@cc.umanitoba.ca.

SKRASTINS, Roland; Toronto East Gen & Orth Hosp, 825 Coxwell Ave, Toronto ON M4C 3E7; Qns'79; DABIM; FRCPC; IntMed; Respir. Ac Staff The Respiratory Centre, Toronto East General Hospital Inc; Lecturer Respirol, University of Toronto; Langs: Latvian; (416)469-7777; Fax. (416)469-7717; rskra@tegh.on.ca.

SKRENES, Bryan D; Children's & Women's HC of BC, F326-4500 Oak St, Vancouver BC V6H 3N1; Witwatersrand (South Africa)'86; MB BCh; Staff Family Practice Centre/Staff Family Practice Residency Program, BC Women's Hospital & Health Centre; Leader Faculty for Curriculum, Family Practice Residency Program, University of British Columbia; (604)875-2029; bskrenes@cw.bc.ca.

SKRINSKAS, Alena M; Hamilton HS-General Site, 3F-237 Barton St E, Hamilton ON L8L 2X2; McM'01; FRCPC; Anes. Staff, Hamilton Health Sciences Centre - Hamilton General Hospital; (905)527-0271

SKRINSKAS, Gailius J; Professional Corporation, 204-1110 Sheppard Ave E, North York ON M2K 2W2; Tor'70; BSc; ABIM; FRCPC; IntMed (Gastroenterology). Ac Staff, North York General Hospital; Langs: Lithuanian; (416)223-9821; Fax. (416)223-4034.

SKROBIK, Yoanna K; Hop Maisonneuve-Rosemont, 5415 boul de l'Assomption, Montreal QC H1T 2M4; Mon'83; ABIM(CriticalCare); FRCPC; IntMed (Intensive Care Medicine). Dir méd ICU, Hopital Maisonneuve-Rosemont; Prof, Universite de Montreal; adj Prof, McGill University; Langs: Polish; Spanish; (514)250-3400 x6229; Fax. (514)939-8891; skrobik@sympatico.ca.

SKRUKWA, Monica J; One World Med Centre, 3575 20 Ave NE, Calgary AB T1Y 6R3; Alb'92; CCFP; FCFP; Langs: Greek; French; (403)248-7955; Fax. (403)285-5013.

SKRYPUCH, Orest W I; C-274 Lynden Rd, Brantford ON N3T 5L8; Wes'80; DAB; FRCSC; Ophth. Chief Ophth, The Brant Community Healthcare System - Brantford General Hospital Site; Langs: Ukrainian; (519)752-1133

SKUBIAK, Michael J; Mount IDA Med Centre, PO Box 1870 Stn Main, Salmon Arm BC V1E 4P9; UBC'92; (250)833-1990; Fax. (250)833-1988.

SKUHERSKA, Romana; Clinique familiale des Pins, 1019 boul des Pins, Val-d'Or QC J9P 4T2; Palacky (Czech Republic)'82; Staff, Centre Hospitalier de Val d'Or; (819)825-9060; Fax. (819)825-1335.

SKULSKY, Marina R; MacEwan Student Centre, 370-2500 University Dr NW, Calgary AB T2N 1N4; Cal'78; CCFP; Assoc Prof, University Of Calgary; (403)220-5765; Fax. (403)282-5218.

SKUPSKY, Gerald; Trafalgar Prof Centre, 300-1235 Trafalgar Rd, Oakville ON L6H 3P1; Tor'69; Staff Family Med, Halton Healthcare Services Corporation - Oakville Site; (905)842-0071; Fax. (905)844-3811.

SKURIDINA, Nataliya; Northmount Med Centre, 304-145 13 St E, North Vancouver BC V7L 2L4; (Ukraine)'89; FRCPC; Public Health & Preventive Med. Langs: Russian; Ukrainian; (604)985-1717

SKUY, Beth J; Danforth-Birchmount Med Ctre, 34-462 Birchmount Rd, Scarborough ON M1K 1N8; Tor'86; CCFP; FCFP; Staff, The Scarborough Hospital - General Campus; (416)698-9988; Fax. (416)698-1055.

SKY, Anastasia; 217 Governor's Rd, Hamilton ON L9H 3J7; Tor'87; (905)777-9600

SKY, Kenneth; Medical Clinic Bldg, 331-89 Humber College Blvd, Etobicoke ON M9V 4B8; Tor'63; Otol. Staff, Toronto General Hospital - UHN; Ac Staff/Consultant, William Osler Health System - Etobicoke General Hospital; Hon Treas, Ontario Medical Association; Clin Instructor, University of Toronto; (416)747-1803; Fax. (416)747-9375.

SLABA, Ingrid; Foothills Med Centre, 1403 29 St NW, Calgary AB T2N 2T9; Staff Critical Care Med, Foothills Medical Centre; (403)944-1110

SLABBERT, Jacobus A; Pasqua Hosp, 4101 Dewdney Ave, Regina SK S4T 1A5; Stellenbosch (South Africa)'90; Staff, Pasqua Hospital; (306)766-2222

SLABBERT, Pieter H; Fraserview Med Associates, 32-665 Front St, Quesnel BC V2J 5J5; Pretoria (South Africa)'03; (250)255-7419

SLABBERT, Willem H; Smith Clinic, 1-6601 48 Ave, Camrose AB T4V 3G8; Orange Free State (South Africa)'82; BSc; MB ChB; Langs: Afrikaans; (780)672-2425

SLABU, Dan L; 2430 Rabbit Hill Rd PO Box 88010 Rpo Rabbit Hill, Edmonton AB T6R 0M5; Cal'06; FRCPC; IntMed.

SLACK, Graham W; BC Cancer Agency, 600 10th Ave W, Vancouver BC V5Z 4E6; UBC'02; FRCPC; GenPath. Staff Path, BC Cancer Agency Vancouver Centre; (604)877-6000

SLACK, Irene S; 3 Wilson St E, Ancaster ON L9G 2B3; McM'78; BScN; CCFP; (905)304-8937; Fax. (905)304-7031.

SLACK, Stephen J; Cottage Med Clinic, PO Box 2140, Jasper AB T0E 1E0; London (England)'87; MB BS; LMCC; MRC; (780)852-4885; Fax. (780)853-2199.

SLADDEN, Christopher S; Western Mem Reg Hosp, PO Box 2005 1 Brookfield Ave, Corner Brook NL A2H 6J7; Cardiff (Wales)'92; MB ChB; MRC; FRCPC; Derm. Staff, Western Memorial Regional Hospital; (709)637-5000

SLADE, Cynthia S; Avalon Specialty Clinic, 573 Torbay Rd, St. John's NL A1A 5G9; Mem'02; FRCPC; Psy. (709)754-3787

SLADE, Debra J; Royal Alexandra Hosp, 137 CSC-10240 Kingsway, Edmonton AB T5H 3V9; UBC'84; CCFP; Staff, Royal Alexandra Hospital; Staff, Urogynecology Clinic; (780)735-5290; Fax. (780)735-5896; slade@ualberta.ca.

SLADEK, Robert G; McGill University Hlth Ctre, 6214-740 av Docteur-Penfield, Montreal QC H3A 1A4; Tor'85; FRCPC; IntMed; Endocrin&Metab. Staff, McGill University Health Centre - Montreal General Campus; (514)398-5458; Fax. (514)398-1738.

SLADEN-DEW, Nicholas S; 202-104 Lower Ganges Rd, Salt Spring Island BC V8K 2S7; Dublin (Ireland)'74; MB ChB; BAO; DRCOG; MPH(Harvard); FRCPC; Psy (Administrative Psychiatry). Consultant Psy, Lady Minto Gulf Islands Hospital; Consultant Psy, Salt Spring Island Commun Services; (250)537-0644; sladen-dew@saltspring.com.

SLADIC, Ana-Sabina; King Street Family Physicians, 2-273 King St E, Kingston ON K7L 3B1; Wes'00; CCFP; Assoc Staff, Kingston General Hospital; Langs: Slovenian; (613)549-4515; Fax. (613)546-4059.

SLAGEL, Bradley E; The Group Health Centre, 240 McNabb St, Sault Ste. Marie ON P6B 1Y5; Tor'03; FRCSC; OrthSurg. (705)759-1234

SLAKOV, Holly A; Lady Minto Gulf Islands Hosp, 135 Crofton Rd, Salt Spring Island BC V8K 1T1; UBC'88; CCFP; Staff, Lady Minto Gulf Islands Hospital; (250)538-4800

SLANEY, Nathalie M C; Four Corners Med Bldg, 310-2009 Long Lake Rd, Sudbury ON P3E 6C3; McM'08; Langs: Bilingual(French/English); (705)222-2741; Fax. (705)222-7293.

SLANINA, John; Sanus Med Clinic, PO Box 10 5216 53 St, Lamont AB T0B 2R0; Timisoara (Romania),'82; Staff Family Med, Mundare Hospital; Staff ER Casual Officer, Camrose Community Cancer Centre; Langs: Romanian; (780)895-2272; Fax. (780)895-2771; sanus@shaw.ca.

SLAOUI, Tarik; Hop du Sacre-Coeur De Montreal, 5400 boul Gouin O, Montreal QC H4J 1C5; Toulouse (France)'05; Staff, Hôpital du Sacre-Coeur de Montréal; (514)338-2222

SLAPCOFF, Barry; Hillside Med Centre, 100 av Metcalfe, Westmount QC H3Z 2H4; McG'87; CCFP; Langs: English; French; (514)931-2162; Fax. (514)931-8436; bws@videotron.ca.

SLATAROF, Youssef A; North Bay Reg Health Centre, 50 College Dr, North Bay ON P1B 0A4; Alexandria (Egypt)'82; Staff, North Bay Regional Health Centre - Regional Mental Health; (705)474-7525

SLATAROFF, Youssef A; North Bay Reg Health Centre, PO Box 2500 50 College Dr, North Bay ON P1B 0A4; Alexandria (Egypt)'82; Psy. Staff, North Bay Regional Health Centre - Regional Mental Health.

SLATER, Jay M; Vancouver Gen Hosp, CP5-855 12th Ave W, Vancouver BC V5Z 1M9; Cal'87; CCFP; Ac Staff, Vancouver General Hospital - Centennial Pavillion; Clin Associate, University of British Columbia; (604)875-4754

SLATER, Jonathan D; Acute Services West, 200-1815 Kirschner Rd, Kelowna BC V1Y 4N7; Cal'81; FRCPC; Peds (Pediatric Emergency Medicine). Med Dir Thompson Cariboo Shuswap/Staff, St Joseph's General Hospital; Sr Med Dir, Acute Services West; Langs: French; (250)319-7875; drjonslater@telus.net.

SLATER, Keith S; Shouldice Hosp, 7750 Bayview Ave, Thornhill ON L3T 4A3; Tor'77; Staff, Shouldice Hospital; (905)889-1125; postoffice@shouldice.com.

SLATER, Marie-Eve; St Mary's Hosp Centre, 3830 av Lacombe, Montreal QC H3T 1C5; McG'02; FRCPC; Anes (Pain Management). Staff, Hôpital Ste-Justine; Staff, St Mary's Hospital Centre; (514)345-3511

SLATKOFF, Robert L; Clinique Radiologie Chomedy, 610 boul Curé-Labelle, Laval QC H7V 2T7; McG'64; DiagRad. (450)670-3102; Fax. (450)687-4149.

SLATKOVSKY, Karen E; Guelph Gen Hosp, 115 Delhi St, Guelph ON N1E 4J4; McG'98; CCFP; CCFP(E.M.); Staff, Guelph General Hospital; Langs: Czech; English; Slovak; (519)837-6440

SLATNIK, Irena; Capilano Med Centre, 10143 50 St NW, Edmonton AB T6A 2C1; Krakow (Poland)'77; (780)468-2911; Fax. (780)462-0029.

SLATNIK, Jacek; Royal Alexandra Hosp, 5002 7-10240 Kingsway NW, Edmonton AB T5H 3V9; Krakow (Poland)'77; FRCPC; AnatPath. Chief Lab, Royal Alexandra Hospital; Langs: Polish; (780)735-5935; Fax. (780)735-4715; jslatnik@cha.ab.ca.

SLATTERY, Margaret A S; Apsley Med Centre, PO Box 278, Apsley ON K0L 1A0; Ott'70; (705)656-4281; Fax. (705)656-4079.

SLAUGHTER, David N; 1 Baby Point Cres, York ON M6S 2B7; McG'70; DABIM; Nephrol; IntMed. Staff, The Credit Valley Hospital; Staff, North York General Hospital; University of Toronto; Langs: French; (416)604-1399; Fax. (416)604-9285.

SLAUGHTER, Graham R D; Sunnybrook Hlth Sciences Ctre, D402-2075 Bayview Ave, Toronto ON M4N 3M5; Wes'05; PhD; FRCPC; IntMed. Staff, Sunnybrook Health Sciences Centre; (416)480-6100; Fax. (416)480-4563.

SLAVCHENKO, Paul T; Lakeridge Hlth Corp-Oshawa, 1 Hospital Crt, Oshawa ON L1G 2B9; Qns'84; FRCPC; Anes. Staff, Lakeridge Health - Oshawa Site; Langs: Ukrainian; (705)576-8711 x3237

SLAVEN, Marissa; Juravinski Cancer Centre, 699 Concession St, Hamilton ON L8V 5C2; McG'91; Physician Palliative Care, The Juravinski Cancer Centre; (905)387-9495

SLAVIK, Dalibor E; Saskatoon East Fam Physicians, 21-2105 8th St E, Saskatoon SK S7H 0T8; Pretoria (South Africa)'84; MB ChB; CCFP; FCFP; Physician, Saskatoon East Family Physicians; Langs: Afrikaans; Czech; German; (306)373-5500; Fax. (306)374-9414.

SLAVINA, Anna; Policlinic Family Medicine, 5-4646 Dufferin St, North York ON M3H 5S4; St Peterburg Medical Academy (Russia (Federation))'91; CCFP; Langs: Russian; (416)222-6160; Fax. (416)222-9604.

SLAWNYCH, Michael P; Foothills Med Centre, 1403 29 St NW, Calgary AB T2N 2T9; Cal'03; FRCPC; IntMed (Palliative Care); Cardiol. Staff, Foothills Medical Centre; (403)944-1110

SLAYTER, Ian M; St Martha's Reg Hosp, 25 Bay St, Antigonish NS B2G 2G5; Dal'74; DABPN; FRCPC; Psy. Staff, St Martha's Regional Hospital; (902)867-4500

SLEETH, Sean P; North Huron FHT-Lucknow, 691 Havelock St, Lucknow ON N0G 2H0; Tor'92; CCFP; (519)528-2810

SLEGR, Marie N; Davisville Med & Dental Bldg, 803-1849 Yonge St, Toronto ON M4S 1Y2; Ott'84; FRCPC; IntMed; Neur. Langs: French; (416)281-6364; Fax. (416)281-5170.

SLEIGHTHOLM, Robert L; Brampton Cosmetic & Med Spa, 400-145 Queen St E, Brampton ON L6W 3P8; Wes'79; BSc(Hon)(Hon); FRCSC; PlasSurg (Cosmetic Surgery). Ac Staff, Humber River Regional Hospital - Finch Avenue Site; Ac Staff, Humber River Regional Hospital - Keele Street Site; Langs: Italian; (905)451-5855; Fax. (905)451-9466; claudia@bramptoncosmetic.com.

SLEIMAN, Asad; Centre Hosp de Granby, 205 boul Leclerc O, Granby QC J2G 1T7; Damascus (Syria)'82; Staff, Centre Hospitalier Régional Baie-Comeau; Staff, Centre Hospitalier de Granby; Langs: Bilingual(English/French); (450)375-8000; asadsleiman@gmail.com.

SLEIMAN, Hassan; 1-5900 36e av, Montreal QC H1T 2Z2; Cairo (Egypt)'79; (514)257-9625; Fax. (514)257-8324.

SLEMKO, Scott F; PO Box 89156 Mackenzie Rpo, Calgary AB T2Z 3W3; Alb'07; CCFP.

SLESSAREV, Marat; Univ Hlth Network-Toronto Gen, EB14 217-200 Elizabeth St, Toronto ON M5G 2C4; Tor'10; Staff, Toronto General Hospital - UHN; (416)340-3155

SLEZIC, Ivo; Trillium Hlth Ctr-Mississauga, 100 Queensway W, Mississauga ON L5B 1B8; Zagreb (Croatia)'68; FRCPC; DiagRad (Angiography). Ac Staff Radiol, Trillium Health Centre - Mississauga; Langs: Croatian; (905)848-7522; Fax. (905)848-4498.

SLIGL, Wendy I; University of Alberta Hosp, 3C1 12-8440 112 St NW, Edmonton AB T6G 2B7; UBC'01; FRCPC; IntMed; Critical Care Medicine; InfectDis. Staff, University of Alberta Hospital; (780)407-6755; Fax. (780)407-1228.

SLINGER, Katherine A; 586 Argus Rd, Oakville ON L6J 3J3; Qns'87; Ac Staff, Halton Healthcare Services Corporation - Oakville Site; (905)842-2410; Fax. (905)842-7376.

SLINGER, Peter D; Univ Hlth Network-Toronto Gen, EN3 441-200 Elizabeth St, Toronto ON M5G 2C4; Wes'73; FRCPC; Anes. Staff, Toronto General Hospital - UHN; Prof Anes, University of Toronto; Langs: French; (416)340-4800 x5164; peter.slinger@uhn.on.ca.

SLINGER, Robert W; Children's Hosp Eastern Ont, 401 Smyth Rd, Ottawa ON K1H 8L1; Qns'90; FRCPC; Peds (Pediatric Infectious Diseases); MedMicrobiol; InfectDis. Staff, Children's Hospital of Eastern Ontario (CHEO); Asst Prof, University of Ottawa; (613)737-7600 x2651; slinger@cheo.on.ca.

SLIPACOFF, Daniel; York-Finch Med Centre, 101-2115 Finch Ave W, North York ON M3N 2V6; Wes'71; FRCPC; DiagRad. Staff, Humber River Regional Hospital - Finch Avenue Site; (416)744-2655; Fax. (416)744-0581.

SLIPP, Frank E; 61 Arthur St, Truro NS B2N 1X7; Dal'70; CCFP; FCFP; Assoc Staff, Colchester East Hants Health Centre; (902)893-7231; Fax. (902)893-2406.

SLIPP, Shanda B; Central Teaching Clinic, 8F-1213 4 St SW, Calgary AB T2R 0X7; Mem'07; CCFP; (403)955-9300; Fax. (403)476-8766.

SLIVCHAK, Jane A M; Fort William Family Hlth Clini, 117 McKellar St S, Thunder Bay ON P7E 1H5; McM'03; CCFP; (807)626-1234; Fax. (807)623-5155.

SLIVKO, Tatiana; Mapleview Med Clinic, 1-225 Mapleview Dr E, Barrie ON L4N 0W5; Vladivostok (Russia (Federation))'96; CCFP; Staff, Englehart & District Hospital Inc; (705)503-5300

SLIWIN, Fay R; Sunnybrook Hlth Sciences Ctre, 2075 Bayview Ave, Toronto ON M4N 3M5; Tor'85; CCFP; FCFP; Staff Health Watch Clinic, Women's College Hospital; Staff Odette Cancer Center, Sunnybrook Health Sciences Centre; Court Staff, North York General Hospital; Consultant, The Hospital For Sick Children; University of Toronto; (416)480-6100; Fax. (416)789-3724.

SLIWIN, Sammy J; 1188B Eglinton Ave W, Toronto ON M6C 2E3; Tor'80; FRCSC; PlasSurg (Cosmetic Surgery). Staff, The Scarborough Hospital - Birchmount Campus; Staff, The Scarborough Hospital - General Campus; Dir, Forest Hill Institute of Aesthetic Plastic Surgery; (416)785-7864; Fax. (416)785-7207.

SLIWOWICZ, David A; Baywood Med Centre, 303-95 Bayly St W, Ajax ON L1S 7K8; Tor'70; Staff, Rouge Valley Health System - Ajax & Pickering Health Centre Site; Staff, Rouge Valley Health System - Centenary Health Centre Site; Asst Prof, University of Toronto; Langs: Yiddish; French; (905)683-6422; Fax. (905)683-6548.

SLIWOWICZ, Kevin; Univ Hlth Network-Toronto Gen, 200 Elizabeth St, Toronto ON M5G 2C4; Man'83; BSc; CCFP; CCFP(E. M.); Staff Emerg, Toronto General Hospital - UHN; (416)340-3856

SLIZHEUSKI, Siarhei; Rouge Valley-Centenary HC, 2867 Ellesmere Rd, Scarborough ON M1E 4B9; Minsk State Medical Institute (Belarus)'94; (416)284-8131

SLOAN, Eileen P; Mount Sinai Hosp, 9F-600 University Ave, Toronto ON M5G 1X5; McM'99; FRCPC; Psy (AIDS/HIV). Staff Psy, Mount Sinai Hospital; Asst Prof Psy, University of Toronto; (416)586-4800 x8693; Fax. (416)586-8654.

SLOAN, Gary W; 1-25 Sherbrook St, Winnipeg MB R3C 2B1; Man'79; FRCPC; Psy (General Adult Psychiatry). Ac Staff Psy, Misericordia Health Centre; (204)788-8119; Fax. (204)786-8480.

SLOAN, I A Jeremy; Headache & Pain Relief Centre, 220-251 Consumers Rd, North York ON M2J 4R3; Cape Town (South Africa)'53; MB ChB; FFARCS(Eng); FAAP; FRCPC; Anes (Chronic Pain). Consultant, The Hospital For Sick Children; Consultant, Sunnybrook Health Sciences Centre; Physician, Headache & Pain Relief Centre; Assoc Prof, University of Toronto; Langs: Afrikaans; (416)493-9762; Fax. (416)493-7043.

SLOAN, James M; MUHC-Royal Victoria Hosp, 687 av des Pins O, Montreal QC H3A 1A1; Dal'73; Anes. Staff, McGill University Health Centre - Royal Victoria Hospital; (514)842-1231 x4880

SLOAN, Jeffrey P E; Sudbury Reg Hosp-Laurentian, 41 Ramsey Lake Rd, Sudbury ON P3E 5J1; Ott'91; FRCPC; Anes. Staff, Health Sciences North-Laurentian Site; Langs: English; French; (705)522-2200

SLOAN, Jeffrey R; B C01-310 Bridge St W, Napanee ON K7R 0A4; Tor'80; CCFP; FCFP; Med Staff, Lennox & Addington County General Hospital; Queen's University; (613)354-7640; Fax. (613)354-7435.

SLOAN, Kevin P; Niagara Dermatology Centre, 102-532 Lake St, St Catharines ON L2N 4H4; Qns'92; FRCPC; Derm. Staff, Niagara Health System - St Catharines General Site; Staff, Niagara Health System - Ontario Street Site; (905)646-2255; Fax. (905)646-2033; info@drkevinsloan.com.

SLOAN, Lisa L; Appletree Med Group, 150 Katimavik Rd, Ottawa ON K2L 4A2; Ott'01; CCFP; (613)592-1539; Fax. (613)592-1024.

SLOAN, Michael J; Carmi Clinic, 114-725 Carmi Ave, Penticton BC V2A 3G8; Glasgow (Scotland)'76; MB ChB; BSc; (250)492-4274; Fax. (250)493-1887.

SLOAN, Richard S; 382 Ramsey Lake Rd, Sudbury ON P3E 6H4; Tor'63; FRCPC; DiagRad. (705)675-8086; Fax. (705)675-6097.

SLOAN, Ryan W; 208-210 Dundas St E, Belleville ON K8N 5G8; Alb'82; (613)968-3543

SLOANE, John A; 223 St Clair Ave W, Toronto ON M4V 1R3; Tor'65; FRCPC; Psy (Psychoanalysis). Assoc Staff, Toronto General Hospital - UHN; Assoc Staff, Centre for Addiction & Mental Health (CAMH) - College Street Site; Asst Prof, University of Toronto; (416)925-7791

SLOBODZIAN, Donna M; Broadway Family Physicians, 1801 Broadway Ave, Saskatoon SK S7H 2B6; Sask'89; CCFP; FCFP; (306)652-2632; Fax. (306)652-2637.

SLOBOGEAN, Myron G P; St Michael's Orthopaedic Assoc, 800-55 Queen St E, Toronto ON M5C 1R6; UBC'06; FRCSC; OrthSurg. (416)864-5880; Fax. (416)359-1601.

SLOCOMBE, Linda M; Grace Maternal Child Clinic, 130-1402 8 Ave NW, Calgary AB T2N 1B8; McG'81; (403)289-9051; Fax. (403)284-3129.

SLODKOWSKA, Elzbieta; Sunnybrook Hlth Sciences Ctre, E4 37-2075 Bayview Ave, Toronto ON M4N 3M5; Gdansk Academy of Medicine (Poland)'00; Staff Anath Path, Sunnybrook Health Sciences Centre; (416)480-4600

SLOKA, Jeffery S; Grand River Hosp-KW Hlth Ctre, PO Box 9056 Stn C 554-835 King St W, Kitchener ON N2G 1G3; Mem'03; FRCPC; Neur (Emergency Medicine). Staff, Grand River Hospital - Kitchener/Waterloo Health Centre; (519)749-4222; Fax. (519)749-4230.

SLOMAN, Leon; Intergenerational Wellness Cen, 5225-80 Workman Way, Toronto ON M6J 1H4; London (England)'56; MRCS; LRCP; DPsy(McG.); FRCPC; Psy (Autism Spectrum Disorders). Staff Psy & Child & Youth, Centre for Addiction & Mental Health (CAMH) - College Street Site; Assoc Prof Psy, University of Toronto; (416)535-8501 x6187; Fax. (416)979-4685; slomanl@rogers.com.

SLOMOVIC, Allan R; Univ Hlth Network-Toronto Western Hosp, 6E 401-399 Bathurst St, Toronto ON M5T 2S8; Mem'79; FRCSC; Ophth (Cataract Surgery). Assoc Prof, Toronto Western Hospital - University Health Network; Chairperson Continuing Professional Development, Canadian Ophtalmological Society; Langs: French; (416)603-5389; Fax. (416)603-6420.

SLOMOVIC, Brant M; Univ Hlth Network-Toronto Gen, G480-200 Elizabeth St, Toronto ON M5G 2C4; Technion (Israel)'02; FRCPC; EmergMed. Staff, Toronto General Hospital - UHN; (416)340-3856

SLONIM, Rodney O N; Mount Sinai Hosp, 929-600 University Ave, Toronto ON M5G 1X5; Man'64; FRCPC; Psy (Psychoanalysis). Staff, Centre for Addiction & Mental Health (CAMH) - College Street Site; Head Crisis Intervention Prog/Staff Psy, Mount Sinai Hospital; Asst Prof Psy, University of Toronto; (416)586-4800 x5353; Fax. (416)586-8654; rslonim@mtsinai.on.ca.

SLOPER, Kirsty R; South Maternity & Family Pract, 258-1011 Glenmore Trail SW, Calgary AB T2V 4R6; UBC'00; CCFP; (403)640-0600; Fax. (403)253-0124.

SLORACH, J Ninian; Chatham Med Clinic, 36 Church St, Miramichi NB E1N 1T1; Glasgow (Scotland)'83; MB ChB; MRCGPract; (506)778-8223; Fax. (506)773-4060.

SLOWEY, Alistair; 63 Orchard St, Brockville ON K6V 2J7; Aberdeen (Scotland)'68; MB ChB; Ac Staff, Brockville General Hospital - Charles Street; Ac Staff, Providence Continuing Care Centre (PCCC) - St Vincent de Paul Hospital; Coroner, Province of Ontario; (613)342-8755; Fax. (613)342-6925.

SLOWEY, Patricia I; 321 Woodridge Rd, Brockville ON K6V 7C9; Aberdeen (Scotland)'68; Court Staff, Brockville General Hospital - Charles Street; Court Staff, Providence Continuing Care Centre (PCCC) - St Vincent de Paul Hospital; (613)342-8755; Fax. (613)342-6925.

SLUTCHUK, Marvin; Lakewood Med Centre, 30 Lakewood Blvd, Winnipeg MB R2J 2M6; Man'68; (204)257-3395

SLUTCHUK, Sean C; Victoria Gen Hosp, 2340 Pembina Hwy, Winnipeg MB R3T 2E8; Man'90; Staff, Victoria General Hospital; University of Manitoba; (204)269-3570

SLUTSKY, Arthur S; St Michael's Hosp, QW4 042-30 Bond St, Toronto ON M5B 1W8; McM'76; ABIM; VP Research, St Michael's Hospital; Dir Interdepartmental Div of Critical Care/Prof Med, University of Toronto; (416)864-5637

SLUTSKY, Morley; 720-999 Broadway W, Vancouver BC V5Z 1K5; Man'92.

SLUZAR, Vladimir S; King Street Med Arts Centre, 205-71 King St W, Mississauga ON L5B 4A2; Wes'82; FRCPC; IntMed; Cardiol. Med Dir Cardiac Wellness Rehab Centre & Heart Function Clinic/Staff Cardiol, Trillium Health Centre - Mississauga; Langs: Ukrainian; (905)897-6144; Fax. (905)897-6145.

SLY, Jane E; 361 Waverley St, Ottawa ON K2P 0W4; McG'84; Langs: French; (613)230-2739

SLY, Lloyd E; Children's Hosp Eastern Ont, 401 Smyth Rd, Ottawa ON K1H 8L1; Tor'78; FRCPC; DiagRad. Staff, Children's Hospital of Eastern Ontario (CHEO); Court Staff, The Ottawa Hospital - General Campus; (613)737-7600 x2632; Fax. (613)738-4811; sly@cheo.on.ca.

SLYFIELD, David G M; York Finch Med Centre, 311-2115 Finch Ave W, North York ON M3N 2V6; London (England)'61; MB BS; DPM; MRCPsy(UK); Ac Staff, Humber River Regional Hospital - Finch Avenue Site; (416)746-3035

SLYSZ, Garth W; Sherwood Family Med Centre, 15 Brackley Point Rd, Charlottetown PE C1A 6Y1; Dal'89; CCFP; (902)566-4734; Fax. (902)367-3188.

SLYTHE, Christine; CSSS de Saint-Jerome, 290 rue de Montigny, Saint-Jerome QC J7Z 5T3; Mon'92; Staff, Hôtel-Dieu de Saint-Jérôme; (450)431-8200

SMAGGUS, Andrew C; London HSC-University Hosp, PO Box 5339 Stn B 339 Windermere Rd, London ON N6A 5A5; Tor'06; FRCPC; IntMed. Staff, London Health Sciences Centre - University Hospital; (519)685-8500; Fax. (519)663-3232.

SMAIL, Kahina; CSSS Pierre Boucher, 1333 boul Jacques-Cartier E, Longueuil QC J4M 2A5; Sher'02; CCFP; CCFP(E.M.); Staff, Centre Hospitalier Pierre Boucher; (450)468-8111

SMAILL, Fiona M; McMaster University Med Ctre, PO Box 2000 Stn Lcd 1 2N16-1200 Main St W, Hamilton ON L8N 3Z5; Otago (New Zealand)'78; MB ChB; FRACP; FRCPC; IntMed (AIDS/HIV); MedMicrobiol; InfectDis. Staff InfectDis & MedMicrobiol, Hamilton Health Sciences Centre - McMaster Children's Hospital; Staff, St Joseph's Healthcare - Charlton Campus; Dept Head Path & Molecular Med, McMaster University; (905)521-5075; Fax. (905)521-5099; smaill@mcmaster.ca.

SMAL, Samuel J; Greencrest Pembina Clinic, B-2750 Pembina Hwy, Winnipeg MB R3T 2H8; Staff, Victoria General Hospital; (204)768-3821

SMALL, Allison M; Huntsville Prof Bldg, 203-348 Muskoka Rd 3 N, Huntsville ON P1H 1H8; Ott'01; CCFP; Staff, Huntsville District Memorial Hospital - Muskoka Algonquin Healthcare; Langs: French; (705)789-3005; Fax. (705)789-3001.

SMALL, David I; G203-SMBD Jewish Gen Hosp, 3755 ch Cote-Sainte-Catherine, Montreal QC H3T 1E2; McG'81; FRCPC; IntMed; Respir (Pulmonary Diseases). Staff Respirology, Sir Mortimer B Davis Jewish General; assoc Prof, McGill University; Langs: Bilingual(English/French); (514)340-8203; Fax. (514)340-7555.

SMALL, David R J; Fontbonne Bldg, 4F-301 James St S, Hamilton ON L8P 3B6; McM'81; FRC; FRCSC; ObstGyn. Chief Dept of Obst/Gyn/Ac Staff, St Joseph's Healthcare - Charlton Campus; Assoc Prof, McMaster University; (905)572-1122; Fax. (905)572-7373; drdavesmall@hotmail.com.

SMALL, Debra S; North York Med Group, 704-240 Duncan Mill Rd, North York ON M3B 3S6; McG'00; CCFP; (416)497-0880; Fax. (416)497-2650.

SMALL, Elizabeth A; Fitzgerald Bldg, 112-150 College St, Toronto ON M5S 3E2; The Flinders Univ of South Australia (Australia)'01; (416)978-6801

SMALL, Fern E; 505-1200 Bay St, Toronto ON M5R 2A5; Tor'76; FRCPC; Psy (Psychoanalysis). Staff Pt-Time, Sunnybrook Health Sciences Centre; University of Toronto; (416)920-9850; Fax. (416)485-4581.

SMALL, Lorne N; The Credit Valley Hosp, 2200 Eglinton Ave W, Mississauga ON L5M 2N1; Technion (Israel)'00; FRCPC; IntMed; InfectDis. Staff, The Credit Valley Hospital; Langs: Hebrew; French; (905)813-2200; Fax. (905)813-4536.

SMALL, Lynda A; 2-1400 Lakeshore Rd W, Mississauga ON L5J 1J1; McM'83; Ac Staff, Halton Healthcare Services Corporation - Oakville Site; (905)823-0300; Fax. (905)823-0144.

SMALL, Peter; SMBD Jewish Gen Hosp, 3755 ch Cote-Sainte-Catherine, Montreal QC H3T 1E2; McG'71; FACP; ABIM; AB; FRCPC; ClinImmunol&Allergy. Dir Div of Clin Immunol & Allery, Sir Mortimer B Davis Jewish General; assoc Prof Med, McGill University; Langs: Bilingual(English/French); (514)340-8291; Fax. (514)340-7589.

SMALL, Stephen J; Jane/Major MacKenzie Med Ctre, 9-2943 Major MacKenzie Dr, Vaughan ON L6A 3N9; Tor'93; CCFP; (416)242-2216; Fax. (416)242-9751.

SMALLHORN, Jeffrey F; Stollery Children's Hosp, WMC 4C2 26-8440 112 St NW, Edmonton AB T6G 2B7; Adelaide (Australia)'73; MB BS; FRACP; FRCPC; Cardiol (Echocardiography). Head Section of Echocardiography/Staff, Stollery Children's Hospital; Prof Peds, University of Alberta; (780)407-7684; Fax. (780)407-3954; jeffreysmallhorn@cha.ab.ca.

SMALLMAN, Donald S; Kingston Eye Institute, 725 Arlington Park Pl, Kingston ON K7M 7E4; Dal'98; FRCSC; Ophth (Cataract & Glaucoma). Att Staff, Hotel-Dieu Hospital; Att Staff, Kingston General Hospital; Physician, Kingston Eye Institute; Asst Prof, Queen's University; Langs: English; French; (613)546-1858; Fax. (613)546-4060.

SMALLMAN, Julia L; Provider Services Branch, 370 Select Dr, Kingston ON K7M 8T4; Qns'93; (613)536-3086

SMALLWOOD, Erin J C; Broadway Family Hlth Clinic, 3 Herald Ave, Corner Brook NL A2H 6J2; Mem'05; CCFP; Staff, Western Memorial Regional Hospital; (709)637-5000; Fax. (709)639-5831.

SMALLWOOD, Katharine R; The Moncton Hosp, 135 MacBeath Ave, Moncton NB E1C 6Z8; Mem'07; ObstGyn. Staff, The Moncton Hospital; (613)549-6666

SMALLWOOD, Mark D; Broadway Family Hlth Clinic, 3 Herald Ave, Corner Brook NL A2H 4B8; Mem'03; CCFP; Staff, Western Memorial Regional Hospital; (709)639-5920; Fax. (709)639-5831.

SMAR, Mary C; Cornwall Med Associates, 8-30 Thirteenth St E, Cornwall ON K6H 6V9; McG'83; CCFP; (613)933-9082; Fax. (613)933-2635.

SMARDON, Roy A; Fairfield Med Trmt Centre, 17-1594 Fairfield Rd, Victoria BC V8S 1G1; UBC'80; Assoc Staff, Royal Jubilee Hospital; (250)592-3496

SMART, Ellen F; Castlegar Med Clinic, 1840 8th Ave, Castlegar BC V1N 2Y2; Portland (USA)'02; Physician, Castlegar Medical Clinic; (250)365-7255; Fax. (250)365-0285.

SMART, Gavin W; 201-2903 32 Ave, Vernon BC V1T 2L6; UBC'84; (250)545-2326; Fax. (250)542-4889.

SMART, J R Alexander; Charleswood Med Clinic, 3360 Roblin Blvd, Winnipeg MB R3R 0C5; Dundee (Scotland)'75; Ac Staff, The Salvation Army Grace Hospital; (204)889-7200; Fax. (204)896-5081.

SMART, John E; Alexander Place Long Term Care, 329 Parkside Dr, Waterdown ON L0R 2H0; Wes'60; BA; Med Dir, Alexander Place Long Term Care; (905)689-2662

SMART, Katharine L; Alberta Children's Hosp, 2888 Shaganappi Trail NW, Calgary AB T3B 6A8; UBC'01; FRCPC; Peds; PedEmergMed. Staff, Thompson General Hospital; Staff, Alberta Children's Hospital; (403)955-7211

SMART, Marlene A; 6F-1213 4 St SW, Calgary AB T2R 0X7; Alb'78; FRCPC; Psy. (403)955-6155; Fax. (403)955-6169.

SMART, Sydney E H; Balmoral Med Arts Facility, 410-1366 Yonge St, Toronto ON M4T 3A7; Cambridge (England)'66; MB ChB; BCh; FRCPC; AnatPath. Langs: Bilingual(English/French); (416)964-2220; Fax. (416)964-5649.

SMART, Victoria M S; Univ Hlth Network-Princess M, 5F-610 University Ave, Toronto ON M5G 2M9; National University of Ireland (Ireland)'08; CCFP; Staff, Princess Margaret Hospital - University Health Network; (416)946-4501

SMART, Wallace D; Lethbridge Centre Tower, 907-400 4 Ave S, Lethbridge AB T1J 4E1; Alb'88; DABPN; MSc; FRCPC; Psy (Child & Adolescent Psychiatry). Consultant, Chinook Regional Hospital; Clinical Asst Prof Psy, University of Alberta; (403)394-2292; Fax. (403)394-2296.

SMATANOVA, Dagmar; BC Cancer Agency-Vanc Isl Ctr, 2410 Lee Ave, Victoria BC V8R 6V5; Universita Palackeho (Czech Republic)'07; CCFP; Staff, BC Cancer Agency Vancouver Island Centre; Langs: Russian; Slovak; (250)712-3906

SMECHER, Curtis A; 32562 Murray Ave, Abbotsford BC V2T 4T5; UBC'96; FRCPC; Anes. Staff, West Coast General Hospital; (604)746-3693

SMEIDA, Khaled S M; Daly Grove Shopping Centre, 4217 23 Ave NW, Edmonton AB T6L 5Z8; (Libya)'98; (780)462-0442; Fax. (780)462-0577.

SMEJA, Christina A; Clinique Eastman, CP 149, Eastmain QC J0M 1W0; Mon'83; Langs: French; (819)977-0241; Fax. (819)977-0342.

SMEJA, Helen; 4839 rue Pierre-Lauzon, Pierrefonds QC H8Y 2C4; McG'85; Langs: Spanish; French; (514)685-8784

SMELSKY, Charlene R; Seven Oaks Gen Hosp, 2300 McPhillips St, Winnipeg MB R2V 3M3; Man'90; BA; CCFP; Staff, Seven Oaks General Hospital; Staff, Victoria General Hospital; Lecturer med, University of Manitoba; Langs: French; (204)632-7133

SMELTZER, Wendy L; 217-1111 Olympic Way SE, Calgary AB T2G 0E6; Tor'80; CCFP; FCFP; (403)538-8881; Fax. (403)262-7076; smeltzerw@shaw.ca.

SMERDELY, Marie S; Cross Cancer Institute, 11560 University Ave NW, Edmonton AB T6G 1Z2; Alb'97; FRCPC; DiagRad. Staff, Cross Cancer Institute; (780)432-8771

SMIALOWSKI, Michal A N; 6802 Tatlayoko Lake Rd PO Box 34, Tatlayoko Lake BC V0L 1W0; Ott'78; CCFP; Ac Staff, Bulkley Valley District Hospital; Langs: Bilingual(English/French); (250)476-1119; sml@xplornet.com.

SMIEJA, Marek J; St Joseph's Healthcare, L424-50 Charlton Ave E, Hamilton ON L8N 4A6; Wes'87; FRCPC; IntMed; InfectDis; MedMicrobiol. Staff Lab Med, St Joseph's Healthcare - Charlton Campus; Langs: Polish; (905)521-6143; Fax. (905)521-6083; smiejam@mcmaster.ca.

SMIGAS, Halina; IWK Health Centre, PO Box 9700 Rpo CSC 5850-5980 University Ave, Halifax NS B3K 6R8; Warsaw (Poland)'78; Staff, IWK Health Centre; (902)470-6669; Fax. (902)420-6469.

SMIL, Eva; Southdale Med Centre, 45 Vermillion Rd, Winnipeg MB R2J 4A1; Prague (Czech Republic)'69; (204)257-0604

SMILE, Sharon C; Holland Bloorview Kids Rehab, 150 Kilgour Rd, Toronto ON M4G 1R8; West Indies (Jamaica)'97; Staff, Holland Bloorview Kids Rehabilitation Hospital; (416)425-6220

SMILJANIC, Sasha R; Lion's Gate Hosp, 231 15th St E, North Vancouver BC V7L 2L7; UBC'02; BSc; FRCPC; IntMed; MedOncol. Staff, Lions Gate Hospital; Staff, St Mary's Hospital; (604)988-3131

SMILJIC, Dino; Bear Street Family Physicians, PO Box 1048 Stn Main 302-220 Bear St, Banff AB T1L 1H6; Sask'95; BSc; CCFP; FCFP; Langs: Serbian; (403)762-4846; Fax. (403)762-2445.

SMILLIE, Mark A; 121 4th Ave W PO Box 5695 Stn Main, High River AB T1V 1M7; Alb'96; CCFP; (403)652-7999; Fax. (403)652-7997.

SMILLIE, Tracey C; Brock Med Clinic, 204-1800 Tranquille Rd, Kamloops BC V2B 3L9; UBC'99; CCFP; (250)554-8768; tracey_smillie@hotmail.com.

SMILOVITCH, Mark; MUHC-Royal Victoria Hosp, M476-687 av des Pins O, Montreal QC H3A 1A1; McG'85; FRCPC; IntMed; Cardiol. Att Staff, McGill University Health Centre - Royal Victoria Hospital; Att Staff, McGill University Health Centre - Montreal General Campus; assoc Prof Med, McGill University; Langs: French; (514)843-1505; Fax. (514)843-2813; mark.smilovitch@muhc.mcgill.ca.

SMILTNIEKS, Barbara M A; Medical Clinic Bldg, 303-89 Humber College Blvd, Etobicoke ON M9V 4B8; Tor'73; FRCPC; Peds. Langs: Polish; (416)743-6063; Fax. (416)743-0101; barbara.smiltnieks@rogers.com.

SMIT, Andries A; Optimum Health Med Clinic, PO Box 69 2035 Charters St, Merritt BC V1K 1B8; Stellenbosch (South Africa)'85; MB ChB; Langs: Afrikaans; (250)378-6010; Fax. (250)378-6242; aasmit@shaw.ca.

SMIT, Bernardus H W G M; White Rock Ortho Surg Ctre, 44-1480 Foster St, White Rock BC V4B 3X7; Man'94; FRCSC; OrthSurg. Staff, Peace Arch Hospital; Langs: Dutch; (604)538-0068; Fax. (604)538-0703.

SMIT, Cecile; West Coast Gen Hosp, 3949 Port Alberni Hwy, Port Alberni BC V9Y 4S1; Pretoria (South Africa)'06; MB ChB; Staff, West Coast General Hospital; Langs: Afrikaans; (250)735-1980

SMIT, Deon F; Stevenson Med Clinic, 210A-6640 Vedder Rd, Chilliwack BC V2R 0J2; Stellenbosch (South Africa)'81; MB ChB; Langs: Afrikaans; (604)858-2245

SMIT, Dirk J; 4780 Roger St, Port Alberni BC V9Y 3Z2; Pretoria (South Africa)'02; MB ChB; Langs: Afrikaans; (250)731-1311

SMIT, Ferdie; Victoria Hosp, 1200 24th St W, Prince Albert SK S6V 5T4; (Other Foreign)'06; Staff, Victoria Hospital; (306)765-6200; Fax. (306)765-6224.

SMIT, Gideon; 3310 32 Ave, Vernon BC V1T 2M6; Stellenbosch (South Africa)'00; MB ChB; Langs: Afrikaans; (250)545-5321

SMIT, Jacques-Henri; 2nd Avenue Med Clinic, 330 2nd Ave W, Prince Rupert BC V8J 1G6; Orange Free State (South Africa)'97; MB ChB; Anes (Emergency Medicine). Langs: Afrikaans; (250)624-5500; Fax. (250)624-4797.

SMIT, Johan; Dr Johan Smit Inc, 4425 Gertrude St, Port Alberni BC V9Y 6J7; Stellenbosch (South Africa)'80; MB ChB; LMCC; Physician, Port Alberni Medical Clinic; Langs: Afrikaans; (250)724-1412; Fax. (250)724-1466.

SMIT, Kenneth H; Main Street Med Services, 4929 50 Ave, Lacombe AB T4L 1K3; Orange Free State (South Africa)'87; MB ChB; Dip(Anes); CCFP; Staff, Lacombe Hospital & Care Centre; Langs: Afrikaans; (403)782-6717; Fax. (403)782-4240.

SMIT, Louwrens E; Cedars Prof Park, 2915 66 St NW, Edmonton AB T6K 4C1; Pretoria (South Africa)'72; MB ChB; FRCPC; Psy (General Adult Psychiatry). Langs: Afrikaans; (780)450-9454; Fax. (780)461-6190.

SMIT, Marcel M; GAMA Integrated Med Centre, PO Box 2060, Warman SK S0K 4S0; Staff, GAMA Integrated Medical Centre; (306)382-5554; Fax. (306)382-5567.

SMIT, Maria J; Watrous Med Clinic, PO Box 1059, Watrous SK S0K 4T0; (Other Foreign)'00; Staff, Long Lake Valley Integrated Facility; (306)946-2075

SMIT, Martina; Surrey Mem Hosp, 13750 96 Ave, Surrey BC V3V 1Z2; New York (USA)'03; Staff, Surrey Memorial Hospital; (604)581-2211

SMIT, Morne M; Fraserview Med Associates, 32-665 Front St, Quesnel BC V2J 5J5; Pretoria (South Africa)'03; MB ChB; CCFP; Langs: Afrikaans; (250)992-3636; Fax. (250)992-7587.

SMIT, Mudi; Glenbrook Med Clinic, 111-4306 Richmond Rd SW, Calgary AB T3E 4P6; (South Africa)'84; MB ChB; CCFP; Clin Associate, Tom Baker Cancer Centre; Langs: Afrikaans; (403)685-5480; Fax. (403)685-5482.

SMIT, Nelis; Fraserview Med Clinic, 665 Front St, Quesnel BC V2J 5J5; Stellenbosch (South Africa)'07; MB ChB; Langs: Afrikaans; (250)992-3636

SMIT, Niel F; 1118 Hammond St PO Box 209, Carstairs AB T0M 0N0; (South Africa)'75; (403)337-3121; Fax. (403)337-3714.

SMIT, Shawn; Idylwyld Med Centre, 2-1216A Idylwyld Dr N, Saskatoon SK S7L 0Z9; (306)652-0400; Fax. (306)978-3166.

SMIT, Willem J E; 103-8386 120 St, Surrey BC V3W 3N4; Pretoria (South Africa)'89; MB ChB; (604)594-9990

SMITH, Aaron C; Westville Med Clinic, PO Box 930, Westville NS B0K 2A0; Dal'06; CCFP; (902)396-4142; Fax. (902)396-1707.

SMITH, Aaron G; Guelph Gen Hosp, 115 Delhi St, Guelph ON N1E 4J4; McM'99; CCFP; CCFP(E.M.); Staff, Guelph General Hospital; (519)837-1401

SMITH, Aidan C; Heritage Pointe Family Med Cli, 330-412 Pine Creek Rd, De Winton AB T0L 0X0; (South Africa)'83; MB ChB; (403)279-4944; Fax. (403)720-3321.

SMITH, Alan D; BC Cancer Agency-Vancouver CC, 600 10th Ave W, Vancouver BC V5Z 4E6; Man'07; MedOncol; IntMed. Staff, BC Cancer Agency Vancouver Centre; (604)877-6000

SMITH, Aleka; Tisdale Med Clinic, PO Box 1510, Tisdale SK S0E 1T0; (306)873-4561; Fax. (306)873-4489.

SMITH, Alexander J; Claro Family Practice, 107-4930 55 Ave, Drayton Valley AB T7A 1W2; Pretoria (South Africa)'82; MB ChB; Staff, Drayton Valley Hospital & Care Centre; Langs: Afrikaans; German; (780)621-0202; Fax. (780)621-0213.

SMITH, Andre H D P; 3985 Mutrie Rd, Vernon BC V1T 8W4; Cape Town (South Africa)'78; MB ChB; FRCPC; Anes.

SMITH, Andrew A N; Niagara on the Lake Family Hlt, PO Box 10 1882 Niagara Stone Rd, Niagara-on-the-Lke ON L0S 1T0; McM'09; CCFP; (905)468-3275; Fax. (905)468-7960; asmith@niagara.com.

SMITH, Andrew J; Health Sciences Centre, 300 Prince Philip Dr, St. John's NL A1B 3V6; Mem'05; CCFP; CCFP(E.M.); Staff, Health Sciences Centre; (709)777-8016

SMITH, Andrew J; Sunnybrook Health Sciences Ctr, T2 025-2075 Bayview Ave, Toronto ON M4N 3M5; Tor'90; FACS; MSc; FRCSC; GenSurg (Colorectal Cancer). Div Head Odette Cancer Centre, Sunnybrook Health Sciences Centre; Assoc Prof, University of Toronto; (416)480-4027; Fax. (416)480-6002.

SMITH, Andrew J K; Addiction & Mental Health -ARF, 33 Russell St, Toronto ON M5S 2S1; McG'92; Staff, Centre for Addiction & Mental Health (CAMH) - Russell Street Site; (416)535-8501 x6019; Fax. (416)595-6821.

SMITH, Andrew N; Dartmouth ENT Associates Inc, 100-35 Baker Dr, Dartmouth NS B2W 0H3; Dal'00; BSc; BEd; FRCSC; Otol (Hearing Loss). Staff, Dartmouth General Hospital; (902)435-8585; Fax. (902)435-8695; neilsmithmd@gmail.com.

SMITH, Anna J; Churchill Square Med Clinic, PO Box 23205 Rpo Churchill Sq 209-10 Rowan St, St. John's NL A1B 4J9; Mem'08; CCFP; (709)722-8561

SMITH, Anna J M; Clinton Health Centre, PO Box 69 105 Shipley St, Clinton ON N0M 1L0; McM'93; CCFP; FCFP; (519)482-3000

SMITH, Anne M; Cancer Ctre of Southeastern On, 25 King St W, Kingston ON K7L 5P9; Edinburgh (Scotland)'71; MRCP(UK); FRCPC; Hem (Lymphoma); MedOncol. Staff, Kingston General Hospital; Staff, Cancer Centre of Southeastern Ontario; Assoc Prof Oncol & Med, Queen's University; (613)544-2631 x4505; Fax. (613)546-8209; anne.smith@krcc.on.ca.

SMITH, Anthony A; Medicine Hat Reg Hosp, 666 5 St SW, Medicine Hat AB T1A 4H6; Qns'75; Ac Staff, Medicine Hat Regional Hospital; (403)529-8839

SMITH, Arnold I; 301-3101 Bloor St W, Etobicoke ON M8X 2W2; Man'74; Staff, Toronto General Hospital - UHN; (416)231-9914; Fax. (416)231-5238.

SMITH, Audrey; CLSC du Rocher-Perce, GD 633 rue Daigneault, Chandler QC G0C 1K0; Laval'88; Médecin, Centre Hospitalier de Chandler; (418)689-2572; Fax. (418)689-2840.

SMITH, Barry J; Quinte Healthcare North Hastin, 1H Manor Lane, Bancroft ON K0L 1C0; Man'06; CCFP; Staff, Queensway Carleton Hospital; (613)332-2825

SMITH, Benjamin M; Montreal Chest Institute, 3650 rue Saint-Urbain, Montreal QC H2X 2P4; McG'05; Respir; IntMed. Staff, McGill University Health Centre - Montreal Chest Institute; (514)934-1934

SMITH, Benjamin M; 2250 Fairview St, Burlington ON L7R 4C7; Dal'03; FRCSC; OrthSurg (Upper Extremity Surgery). Staff, Joseph Brant Memorial Hospital; (905)333-5100; Fax. (905)333-5107.

SMITH, Beverley J; Toronto Grace Health Centre, 6F-650 Church St, Toronto ON M4Y 2G5; Tor'82; CCFP; FCFP; Staff, The Salvation Army Toronto Grace Health Centre; Staff, The Scarborough Hospital - Birchmount Campus; Asst Prof, University of Toronto; (416)925-2251 x261; Fax. (416)925-9136.

SMITH, Bryan V; Kanata Prof Centre, 213-99 Kakulu Rd, Kanata ON K2L 3C8; Ott'81; FRCPC; IntMed. Staff/Chief IntMed, Queensway Carleton Hospital; Langs: French; (613)592-2204

SMITH, Bryar E; R J A Medicentres Cnd Inc, 204-10458 Mayfield Rd NW, Edmonton AB T5P 4P4; UBC'97; CCFP; (780)483-7115

SMITH, C Douglas; The Ottawa Hosp-Riverside, 1967 Riverside Dr Box 37, Ottawa ON K1H 7W9; Ott'76; FRCPC; IntMed; Rheum. Assoc Prof, University of Ottawa; Langs: French; (613)738-8400 x81840; Fax. (613)738-8336.

SMITH, Camala A; Rouge Valley-Ajax & Pickering, 580 Harwood Ave S, Ajax ON L1S 2J4; McM'08; CCFP; Staff, Rouge Valley Health System - Ajax & Pickering Health Centre Site; (905)683-2320

SMITH, Cameron D; 201-22242 48 Ave, Langley BC V3A 3N5; UBC'88; (604)530-5052; Fax. (604)530-5091.

SMITH, Carol A; Workplace Safety & Ins Board, 4F-200 Front St W, Toronto ON M5V 3J1; Tor'79; MHSc; FRCPC; OccupMed;CCFP; Physician, Workplace Safety & Insurance Board; (416)344-3088; Fax. (416)344-2380.

SMITH, Cassandra A; Pender Community Health Centre, 59 Pender St W, Vancouver BC V6B 1R3; Alb'00; CCFP; CCFP(E.M.); Staff, Pender Community Health Centre; (604)669-9181; Fax. (604)688-9775.

SMITH, Catherine A; Access Transcona, 845 Regent Ave, Winnipeg MB R3C 3A9; Man'99; FRCPC; IntMed; InfectDis.

SMITH, Cathryn L; 327 Clifton Ave PO Box 2288, Windsor NS B0N 2T0; Dal'81; (902)798-4720; Fax. (902)798-1137.

SMITH, Cheryl D; IWK Health Centre, PO Box 9700 Rpo CSC 5850-5980 University Ave, Halifax NS B3K 6R8; Dal'89; Staff, IWK Health Centre; Staff, Aberdeen Regional Hospital; (902)470-8888

SMITH, Christopher A; Kingston Gen Hosp, 76 Stuart St, Kingston ON K7L 2V7; London (England)'90; FRCPC; IntMed. Staff, Kingston General Hospital; (613)533-2780; Fax. (613)533-6695.

SMITH, Christopher G; St Clare's Mercy Hosp, 154 LeMarchant Rd, St. John's NL A1C 5B8; Mem'05; FRCSC; GenSurg. Staff, St Clare's Mercy Hospital; (709)777-5000

SMITH, Christopher J; Students Union Bldg, 2 200-66 University Campus NW, Edmonton AB T6G 2J7; Alb'00; CCFP; (780)492-2612; Fax. (780)492-0172.

SMITH, Christopher J; McKinney Med Centre, 206-510 Ingersoll Ave, Woodstock ON N4S 4X9; Ott'75; FRCSC; ObstGyn. Consultant, Alexandra Hospital; Consultant Dept of ObstGyn, Woodstock General Hospital; (519)539-9211

SMITH, Christopher N C; Toronto East Gen Hosp Inc, 825 Coxwell Ave, Toronto ON M4C 3E7; Ott'08; FRCPC; IntMed. Staff, Toronto General Hospital - UHN; Staff, Toronto East General Hospital Inc; (416)461-8272

SMITH, Colum J J; Saskatchewan Cancer Agency, 248-111 Research Dr, Saskatoon SK S7N 3R2; Galway (Ireland)'80; Staff, Saskatoon Cancer Centre; VP Clinical Services/Sr Medical Officer, Saskatchewan Cancer Agency; (306)665-0436; Fax. (306)665-0935; columjsmith@gmail.com.

SMITH, Corne S; Nipawin Med Group, PO Box 2135, Nipawin SK S0E 1E0; Stellenbosch (South Africa)'00; MB ChB; Physician, Nipawin Medical Group; (306)862-4626; drcs_smith@hotmail.com.

SMITH, Cornel; Southside Med Clinic, 4821 Calgary Trail NW, Edmonton AB T6H 5W8; Stellenbosch (South Africa)'05; DA(SA); MB ChB; (780)439-1060

SMITH, Cortney M; Colchester East Hants Hlth Ctr, 600 Abenaki Rd, Truro NS B2N 5A1; Wes'06; CCFP; Staff, Colchester East Hants Health Centre; (902)893-5554

SMITH, Craig A; SMBD Jewish Gen Hosp, 3755 ch Cote-Sainte-Catherine, Montreal QC H3T 1E2; Wes'99; CCFP; CCFP(E.M.); Staff, Sir Mortimer B Davis Jewish General; (514)340-8222 x3989

SMITH, Crystal A; 301-6633 Highway 7, Markham ON L3P 7P2; Cal'97; FRCSC; OrthSurg (Upper Extremity Surgery). Staff, Markham Stouffville Hospital; Langs: French; (905)472-3374; Fax. (905)472-3116.

SMITH, Dalene; Brandon Reg Health Centre, 150 McTavish Ave E, Brandon MB R7A 2B3; CCFP; Staff, Brandon Regional Health Centre; (204)726-1122; Fax. (204)726-4429.

SMITH, Dana R; All Well Primary Care Centre, 2835 Mill Woods Rd, Edmonton AB T6K 4A9; Alb'89; (780)450-4550; Fax. (780)461-1985.

SMITH, Daniel N; Smyth Med Centre, 224-1929 Russell Rd, Ottawa ON K1G 4G3; McG'93; CCFP; Ac Staff Privil, The Ottawa Hospital - General Campus; Langs: French; (613)738-3327; Fax. (613)738-9441.

SMITH, David E; North York Med Arts Bldg, 231-1333 Sheppard Ave E, Toronto ON M2J 1V1; Tor'94; MSc; FRCSC; GenSurg (Laparoscopic Surgery). Staff, North York General Hospital; (416)498-8458; Fax. (416)498-9972.

SMITH, David F; BC Women's Hosp & Hlth Ctre, K1 125-4500 Oak St, Vancouver BC V6H 3N1; Qns'65; FRCPC; Peds. Ac Staff Eating Disorder Clinic, BC Women's Hospital & Health Centre; Consultant, Vancouver General Hospital - Centennial Pavillion; Assoc Prof Peds, University of British Columbia; (604)875-2130; Fax. (604)875-2292.

SMITH, David H; Vernon Mental Health Centre, 1440 14 Ave, Vernon BC V1B 2T1; McG'94; FRCPC; Psy (Adolescent Psychiatry). Staff, Vernon Mental Health Centre; (250)549-5737; david.smith@interiorhealth.ca.

SMITH, David H; London HSC-Victoria Hosp, PO Box 5010 Stn B 800 Commissioners Rd E, London ON N6A 5W9; Sask'91; FRCPC; Anes. Staff, London Health Sciences Centre - Victoria Campus; (519)685-8500; Fax. (519)685-8500.

SMITH, David P; 303-749 King St W, Kitchener ON N2G 1E4; McG'70; FRCPC; Peds (Clinical Immunology & Allergy). Ac Staff, Grand River Hospital - Kitchener/Waterloo Health Centre; Court Staff, St Mary's General Hospital; Langs: French; (519)579-0770

SMITH, David R; North Toronto Med Bldg, 107-250 Lawrence Ave W, Toronto ON M5M 1B2; McG'64; FRCSC; Ophth (Pediatric Ophthalmology). Staff Surg., The Hospital For Sick Children; Staff Surg., Humber River Regional Hospital - Finch Avenue Site; Asst Prof, University of Toronto; (416)783-3375; Fax. (416)783-3376.

SMITH, David R; Kingston Orthopaedic Pain Inst, 500-797 Princess St, Kingston ON K7L 1G1; Columbia (Other Foreign)'91; (613)344-1202; Fax. (613)344-1203.

SMITH, David R F; Avenue Bloor Med Group, 405-208 Bloor St W, Toronto ON M5S 3B4; Tor'54; CCFP; FCFP; Court Staff, Toronto General Hospital - UHN; Physician Student Health Serv, University of Toronto; (416)962-1200; Fax. (416)962-1223.

SMITH, David V B; Princeton Med Centre, PO Box 640, Princeton BC V0X 1W0; Cape Town (South Africa)'69; MB ChB; CCFP; FCFP; Staff, Princeton General Hospital; Langs: Afrikaans; (250)295-0091; Fax. (250)295-0651; pmcdsmith@telus.net.

SMITH, David Y; Colchester East Hants Hlth Ctr, 600 Abenaki Rd, Truro NS B2N 5A1; Dal'74; FRCPC; Anes. Chief Anes, Colchester East Hants Health Centre; (902)893-4321

SMITH, Dean A; King Street Med Arts Centre, 207-71 King St W, Mississauga ON L5B 4A2; Tor'85; FRCSC; Ophth (Refractive Surgery). Staff, Trillium Health Centre - Mississauga; Med Dir, TLC Laser Eye Center; (905)897-2020; Fax. (905)270-8669.

SMITH, Dean F; Foothills Med Centre, 1403 29 St NW, Calgary AB T2N 2T9; Alb'83; BMedSci; FRCPC; GenPath; DiagRad; AnatPath. Staff Diagnostic Imaging, Foothills Medical Centre; (403)944-1110; Fax. (403)944-1687.

SMITH, Dean G; The Richmond Hosp, 7000 Westminster Hwy, Richmond BC V6X 1A2; UBC'85; CCFP; CCFP(E.M.); Staff, Richmond Hospital; Staff Emerg, Providence Health Care - St Vincent's Hospital-Heather Site; (604)244-5151

SMITH, Deborah J; Medical Arts Bldg, 407-5880 Spring Garden Rd, Halifax NS B3H 1Y1; Dal'76; FRCPC; Peds. Staff, IWK Health Centre; (902)422-6421; Fax. (902)423-5485.

SMITH, Deborah L; Sudbury Med Centre, 411-65 Larch St, Sudbury ON P3E 1B8; Wes'88; CCFP; FCFP; (705)675-1564

SMITH, Deborah L; Ontario Vein Clinics, 3F-410 North Service Rd E, Oakville ON L6H 5R2; Tor'81; Staff, Humber River Regional Hospital - Finch Avenue Site; Staff, Toronto General Hospital - UHN; (905)849-1835; Fax. (905)849-3712.

SMITH, Dee Ann M; Waterford Hosp, 306 Waterford Bridge Rd, St. John's NL A1E 4J8; Creighton University (USA)'98; CCFP; Staff, Waterford Hospital; (709)777-3084; Fax. (709)778-3678.

SMITH, Deirdre D; Surrey Prenatal Clinic, 9655 137 St, Surrey BC V3T 4G8; UBC'84; CCFP; (778)395-0085

SMITH, Dereck A; St Anthony's Med Centre, 203-582 Goldstream Ave, Victoria BC V9B 2W7; Sask'72; Ac Staff, Vancouver Island Health Authority; (250)478-1796; Fax. (250)478-7912.

SMITH, Derek B; 12051 1 Rd PO Box 30029 Rpo Moncton, Richmond BC V7E 0A6; Dal'00; FRCSC; OrthSurg. (250)374-5844

SMITH, Derrick M; Alberta Children's Hosp, 2888 Shaganappi Trail NW, Calgary AB T3B 6A8; Cal'84; FRCPC; Peds. Ac Staff, Alberta Children's Hospital; (403)955-7070

SMITH, Derryck H; 505-805 Broadway W, Vancouver BC V5Z 1K1; Wes'74; FRCPC; Psy (Brain Injury Psychiatry). Hd Psy, BC Children's Hospital; Clin Prof Psy, University of British Columbia; (604)879-2200; Fax. (604)879-2248; dhsmith@dhsmith.ca.

SMITH, Dianne E; Trinity Rose Med Clinic, PO Box 2467 105-2034 19 Ave, Didsbury AB T0M 0W0; Alb'07; CCFP; (403)518-8762; Fax. (403)518-8746.

SMITH, Donald A; Village Family Health Team, 102-171 East Liberty St, Toronto ON M6K 3P6; McG'76; BSc(Hons Biochem); MDCM; CCFP; FCFP; Staff (Temporary), South Bruce Grey Health Centre - Kincardine Site; Langs: Spanish; French; (416)599-8348; Fax. (416)599-2001; donald.smith@villagefht.ca.

SMITH, Donald G; Grimsby Med Associates, 100-155 Main St E, Grimsby ON L3M 1P2; Wes'73; Ac Staff, West Lincoln Memorial Hospital; Physician, Grimsby Medical Associates; (905)945-5476; Fax. (905)945-7707.

SMITH, Donald H; 6179 Main St PO Box 1089 Stn Main, Stouffville ON L4A 8A1; Tor'52; Court Staff, Markham Stouffville Hospital; Court Staff, Southlake Regional Health Centre; (905)640-2300; Fax. (905)640-5256.

SMITH, Donald H; 200-2903 32 Ave, Vernon BC V1T 2L6; Dal'93; BSc; MD; (250)542-1141; Fax. (250)542-4889.

SMITH, Donna; Burrard Med Bldg, 590-1144 Burrard St, Vancouver BC V6Z 2A5; UBC'96; FRCSC; OrthSurg (Upper Extremity Surgery). Clin Instructor, University of British Columbia; (604)647-0111; Fax. (604)647-0113.

SMITH, Douglas W; Riverside Prof Centre, 204-1919 Riverside Dr, Ottawa ON K1H 1A2; Tor'92; CCFP; (613)260-2684; Fax. (613)260-8863.

SMITH, Edward J; Les Galeries de Vanier, 102-150 Montreal Rd, Vanier ON K1L 8H2; Ott'81; Langs: French; (613)748-1113; Fax. (613)748-1639.

SMITH, Eileen M; York-Med Medical Arts Centre, 404-250 Harding Blvd W, Richmond Hill ON L4C 9M7; McM'83; FRCPC; Peds. (905)737-9898; Fax. (905)737-8583.

SMITH, Eldon R; Univ of Calgary, G225-3330 Hospital Dr NW, Calgary AB T2N 4N1; Dal'67; FRCPC; IntMed (Cardiology). Emeritus Prof IntMed & Physiology & Biophysics, University of Calgary; (403)220-5500; Fax. (403)283-8878; esmith@ucalgary.ca.

SMITH, Erasmus J; Westhill Centre, 203-1808 Bowen Rd, Nanaimo BC V9S 5W4; Orange Free State (South Africa)'82; MB ChB; FRCSC; OrthSurg (Hip & Knee Arthroplasty). Langs: Afrikaans; (250)754-9244; Fax. (250)754-9255.

SMITH, Eric E; Foothills Med Centre, C1212-1403 29 St NW, Calgary AB T2N 2T9; McG'98; FRCPC; Neur. Staff Clin Neurosciences, Foothills Medical Centre; (403)944-1594; Fax. (403)944-1154.

SMITH, Eric W; Loyalist Family Practice, 2A-150 Sidney St, Belleville ON K8P 5E2; Cal'92; BSc; MSc; CCFP; FCFP; (613)771-0008; Fax. (613)771-1861.

SMITH, Erik R; 400 Tache Ave, Winnipeg MB R2H 3C3; Man'00; CCFP; CCFP(E.M.); Staff, St Boniface General Hospital; Staff, The Salvation Army Grace Hospital; (204)233-8563

SMITH, Erin E; Canadian Forces Health Service, PO Box 6550 Stn Forces, Cold Lake AB T9M 2C6; Man'08; CCFP; Staff, Canadian Forces Health Services; (780)840-8000; Fax. (780)840-7326.

SMITH, Erin S; Algonquin Coll Student Hlth Se, 1385 Woodroffe Ave, Nepean ON K2G 1V8; Wes'97; Physician, Algonquin College; (613)727-4723 x7222

SMITH, Faye E; Allin Clinic, 10155 120 St NW, Edmonton AB T5K 2A2; Wes'89; CCFP; FCFP; (780)482-7551; Fax. (780)488-2056.

SMITH, Frank C; 149-3017 St Clair Ave, Burlington ON L7N 3P5; Bristol (England)'69; MB ChB; FRCSC; OrthSurg (Arthroplasty). Court Staff, St Joseph's Healthcare - Charlton Campus; Ac Staff, Hamilton Health Sciences Centre - McMaster University Medical Centre; Physician, Sir William Osler Health Institute; Clin Assoc Prof Surg, McMaster University; (289)337-1920; Fax. (289)337-8323; franksmith@bellnet.ca.

SMITH, Frederick B; Medical Arts Bldg, 206-121 Wellington St W, Barrie ON L4N 1L4; McG'65; Affil Staff, Royal Victoria Regional Health Centre; (705)728-8530; Fax. (705)728-2004.

SMITH, Frederick J R; Royal Jubilee Hosp, 1952 Bay St, Victoria BC V8T 1J8; Wes'90; FRCPC; DiagRad. Staff Diag Imaging, Victoria General Hospital; Staff, Royal Jubilee Hospital; (250)370-8272

SMITH, Gaetan M; 114 ch du Sommet O, Rimouski QC G5N 1V5; Laval'65; Ophth. Consultant, Hôpital Regional Rimouski; (418)723-9142

SMITH, Garth W; Sheldon M Chumir Health Centre, 1213 4th St SW, Calgary AB T2R 0X7; Cal'07; CCFP; CCFP(E.M.); Staff, Foothills Medical Centre; Staff, University of Alberta Hospital; (403)955-6200

SMITH, Genevieve A; Clinique Med Shawville, 269 rue Main, Shawville QC J0X 2Y0; McG'09; CCFP; (819)647-3943

SMITH, George A; 1758 View Dr, Quesnel BC V2J 6G1; Aberdeen (Scotland)'62; MB ChB; Staff, West Fraser Medical; (250)747-3391

SMITH, George E D; 1-928 Broadview Ave, East York ON M4K 2R1; Belfast (Ireland)'73; MRCPsy; FRCPC; Psy (Pharmacotherapy). (416)469-0656; Fax. (416)469-0656.

SMITH, Graeme N; Kingston Gen Hosp, V4-76 Stuart St, Kingston ON K7L 2V7; Wes'92; PhD; FRCSC; ObstGyn (Maternal Fetal Medicine). Staff, Kingston General Hospital; Staff, Hotel-Dieu Hospital; Queen's University; (613)548-2405; Fax. (613)548-1330; gns@post.queensu.ca.

SMITH, Graeme O; Royal Alexandra Hosp, 10240 Kingsway NW, Edmonton AB T5H 3V9; Dal'99; FRCPC; Anes. Staff Anes, Royal Alexandra Hospital; (780)735-4010; Fax. (780)735-4386.

SMITH, Graham H R; Maple Leaf Med Arts, 501-14 College St, Toronto ON M5G 1K2; McG'88; BSc; MDCM; MMedSci; CCFP; FCFP; Physician, Maple Leaf Medical Clinic; Langs: French; (416)465-0756; Fax. (416)465-8344; graham.smith@mapleleafmedical.com.

SMITH, Grant D; 201-3040 Tutt St, Kelowna BC V1Y 2H5; Alb'74; FRCPC; Psy (General Adult Psychiatry). Ac Staff, Kelowna General Hospital; (250)763-7448; Fax. (250)763-7440.

SMITH, Gregory L; Raymond Med Clinic, PO Box 769 20 Church Ave, Raymond AB T0K 2S0; Alb'00; BMedSci; CCFP; Staff, Raymond Health Centre; Langs: English; French; (403)752-3337; Fax. (403)752-4967.

SMITH, H James; 194 Court St N Port Arthur Health Centre, Thunder Bay ON P7A 4V7; Qns'59; FRCP; FRCPC; IntMed (Cardiology). Staff, Thunder Bay Regional Health Sciences Centre Port-Arthur; Staff, St Joseph's Care Group - St Joseph's Hospital; (807)346-1000; Fax. (807)346-6251.

SMITH, Harold M B; Dr Harold MB Smith Med Prof Co, 19 Second Ave N, Yorkton SK S3N 1G1; Sask'89; FRCSC; Ophth (Cataract & Glaucoma). (306)782-4646; Fax. (306)782-4650.

SMITH, Heather; University Hosp of Northern BC, 1475 Edmonton St, Prince George BC V2M 1S2; UBC'08; CCFP; Staff, University Hospital of Northern British Columbia; (250)565-2000

SMITH, Helen L; Fraserview Med Clinic, 32-665 Front St, Quesnel BC V2J 5J5; London (England)'89; (250)992-3636

SMITH, Helene; Avery Health Clinic, 32-665 Front St, Quesnel BC V2J 5J5; Pretoria (South Africa)'03; MB ChB; Langs: Afrikaans; (250)992-3636; Fax. (250)992-7587.

SMITH, Hugh W E; The Salvation Army Grace Hosp, 300 Booth Dr, Winnipeg MB R3J 3M7; Man'70; FRCPC; IntMed (Cardiology). Staff, The Salvation Army Grace Hospital; Staff, Concordia General Hospital; (204)837-0391

SMITH, Ian F; William Osler HC-Brampton, 2100 Bovaird Dr E, Brampton ON L6R 3J7; Tor'75; FACS; FRCSC; GenSurg (Vascular Surgery). Chief of Staff, William Osler Health System - Brampton Civic Hospital; (905)494-2120; Fax. (905)494-6506.

SMITH, Ira A; David L MacIntosh Sport Med Cl, 55 Harbord St, Toronto ON M5S 2W6; Tor'98; CCFP; (416)978-4678; Fax. (416)971-2846.

SMITH, J Michael H; 161 15 St E, North Vancouver BC V7L 2P7; Witwatersrand (South Africa)'73; MB ChB; DCH(Lond); FRCSC; Otol (General ENT). Staff, Lions Gate Hospital; (604)985-6614; Fax. (604)988-1936.

SMITH, Jacques; Ctr Hosp St-Joseph de Malbaie, CP 340 Succ Bureau-chef 303 rue Saint-Etienne, La Malbaie QC G5A 1T8; Laval'72; MS(Minn.); FRCSC; GenSurg. Staff, Hôpital de la Malbaie; (418)665-1711

SMITH, James B; IWK Health Centre, PO Box 9700 Rpo CSC 5850-5980 University Ave, Halifax NS B3K 6R8; McG'69; Anes. Staff, IWK Health Centre; (902)470-8888

SMITH, Jan D W; 301-9200 Mary St, Chilliwack BC V2P 4H6; Pretoria (South Africa)'88; MB ChB; MMed; FCOG(SA); FRCSC; ObstGyn (Pelvic Surgery). Staff/Dept Head ObstGyn, Chilliwack General Hospital; Langs: Afrikaans; (604)702-9600; Fax. (604)702-9601; dewaal2@telus.net.

SMITH, Jason C; The Court Med Clinic, 306-2863 Ellesmere Rd, Scarborough ON M1E 5E9; Cal'01; FRCSC; OrthSurg. Staff, Rouge Valley Health System - Centenary Health Centre Site; (416)284-8131; Fax. (416)284-4510.

SMITH, Jean-Marc C; The Medical Group, 32243 Hurd St, Mission BC V2V 3J9; UBC'86; BSc; CCFP; (604)826-6231; Fax. (604)820-1174.

SMITH, Jeanette E; Forensic Psychiatry, 305-1245 Broadway W, Vancouver BC V6H 1G7; London (England)'83; MB BS; MRCPsy; FRCPC; Psy (Forensic Psychiatry). Clinical Asst Prof, University of British Columbia; (604)733-5722; Fax. (604)739-3734; jsmith@forensic.bc.ca.

SMITH, Jenni; 214-168 13 St E, North Vancouver BC V7L 4W8; UBC'01; FRCSC; GenSurg. Langs: Bilingual(English/French); (604)929-2990; Fax. (604)924-0705.

SMITH, Jennifer L; Malvern Med Clinic, 100-1333 Neilson Rd, Scarborough ON M1B 4Y9; Tor'89; Staff, Toronto East General Hospital Inc; (416)291-7719; Fax. (416)287-3775.

SMITH, Joanna D; Royal University Hosp, 103 Hospital Dr, Saskatoon SK S7N 0W8; Sask'06; CCFP; CCFP(E.M.); Staff, Pasqua Hospital; Staff, Royal University Hospital; (306)655-1363; Fax. (306)655-1011.

SMITH, Johannes L A D; Corinthia Park Med Clinic, 10-4302 50 St, Leduc AB T9E 6J9; Orange Free State (South Africa)'76; LMCC; MB ChB; (780)986-6222; Fax. (780)986-2205.

SMITH, John D; Mineville Med Centre, 4 Peter Crt, Mineville NS B2Z 1K2; Dal'77; BEng; Staff, Queen Elizabeth II Health Sciences Centre - Victoria General Site; Teacher Pt-Time, Dalhousie University; (902)829-3278; Fax. (902)829-2549; john@smith.ns.ca.

SMITH, John R; Credit Valley Med Arts Ctre, 502-2000 Credit Valley Rd, Mississauga ON L5M 4N4; McM'86; FRCSC; ObstGyn (Maternal Fetal Medicine). (905)820-8748; Fax. (905)820-0255.

SMITH, John R M; Four Rivers Med Clinic, 647 Broadway, Winnipeg MB R3C 0X2; London (England)'67; MB BS; LRCP; MRCS; MCFP; FCFP; (204)940-6001; Fax. (204)940-6003.

SMITH, John S; 7154 120 St, Surrey BC V3W 3M8; Oxford (England)'60; BCh; MRC; FRCPC; IntMed. (604)590-5811

SMITH, John T; 103-1811 Victoria St, Prince George BC V2L 2L6; Dublin (Ireland)'73; MB BCh; BAO; FRCPC; IntMed; Respir. Ac Staff/Chief Respir, University Hospital of Northern British Columbia; (250)564-1876; Fax. (250)561-7022.

SMITH, Jonathan G; Collingwood Health Centre, 106-186 Erie St, Collingwood ON L9Y 4T3; McM'04; CCFP; Staff, Collingwood General & Marine Hospital; (705)445-2311; Fax. (705)445-2313.

SMITH, Judith M A; Lakeridge Health Corp-Oshawa, 1 Hospital Crt, Oshawa ON L1G 2B9; McM'94; CCFP; Staff, Lakeridge Health - Oshawa Site; (905)576-8711 x3237

SMITH, Julia A; Windsor Reg Hosp-Metropolitan, 1995 Lens Ave, Windsor ON N8W 1L9; Tor'94; FRCPC; Anes. Staff, Windsor Regional Hospital - Metropolitan Site; Langs: French; (519)254-5577 x52201

SMITH, Julie E; Univ of Lethbridge Hlth Ctre, SU 020-4401 University Dr W, Lethbridge AB T1K 3M4; Qns'86; BSc; CCFP; CCFP(E.M.); FCFP; Staff, Chinook Regional Hospital; Physician Students Health Centre, University of Lethbridge; (403)329-2484; Fax. (403)329-2466; smith@uleth.ca.

SMITH, Karen A; Peterborough Reg HC-Hospital, 1 Hospital Dr, Peterborough ON K9J 7C6; Dal'95; MSc(NeuroSciences); BSc(Pharmacol); FRCPC; Psy (Geriatric Psychiatry). Staff, Peterborough Regional Health Centre - Hospital Drive; (705)876-5076; Fax. (705)876-5160.

SMITH, Karen L; York Med Health Centre, C-17215 Leslie St, Newmarket ON L3Y 8E4; Sask'75; Assoc Staff, Southlake Regional Health Centre; (905)853-0404; Fax. (905)853-3702.

SMITH, Karen M; Providence CCC-St Mary's, PO Box 3600 Stn Main 340 Union St, Kingston ON K7L 5A2; Qns'82; FAB; FAB; FRCPC; PhysMed&Rehab (Spinal Cord Injury). Assoc Prof Rehab Med, Providence Care - St Mary's of the Lake Hospital Site; (613)544-1894; Fax. (613)544-8640; kms1@post.queensu.ca.

SMITH, Karlene I; Findlay Creek Med Centre, 3-4744 Bank St, Ottawa ON K1T 3W7; Ott'09; CCFP; (613)317-2584; Fax. (613)822-2775.

SMITH, Kelley R; 8A Shoal Harbour Dr, Clarenville NL A5A 2C4; Mem'99; CCFP; (709)466-5100; Fax. (709)466-5801.

SMITH, Kenneth A; Cosmetic Surg & Skin Care Clin, 805 Fairfield Rd, Victoria BC V8V 0A7; Sask'82; FRCSC; PlasSurg (Cosmetic Surgery). Staff Privil, Vancouver Island Health Authority; (250)595-3888; Fax. (250)595-8835; info@kasmithplastics.ca.

SMITH, Kenneth D; Victoria Gen Hosp, 1 Hospital Way, Victoria BC V8Z 6R5; UBC'92; CCFP; Staff, Victoria General Hospital; (250)727-4325; Fax. (250)727-4003.

SMITH, Kevin C; Niagara Falls Derm & Skin Care, 201-6453 Morrison St, Niagara Falls ON L2E 7H1; Alb'83; BSc; FRCPC; Derm (Botox & Fillers). (905)356-5335; Fax. (905)356-8362; ksmithderm@gmail.com.

SMITH, Kevin D; Ottawa Carleton Eye Care Centr, 410-2255 Carling Ave, Ottawa ON K2B 7Z5; McG'85; MDCM; FRCSC; Ophth. Langs: English; French; (613)596-0300; Fax. (613)596-0848.

SMITH, Kevin F; Vernon Jubilee Hosp, 2101 32 St, Vernon BC V1T 5L2; Qns'94; FRCPC; Anes. Staff, Vernon Jubilee Hospital; (250)558-1282; Fax. (250)545-5602.

SMITH, Kevin G; Medical Assoc of Port Perry, 462 Paxton St, Port Perry ON L9L 1L9; UBC'85; Ac Staff, Lakeridge Health - Port Perry Site; (905)985-2895; Fax. (905)985-8931.

SMITH, Kevin J; Rouge Valley HS-Ajax-Pickering, 580 Harwood Ave S, Ajax ON L1S 2J4; Cal'98; FRCPC; Anes (Acute & Chronic Pain). Staff, Rouge Valley Health System - Ajax & Pickering Health Centre Site; (905)683-2320 x1288; Fax. (905)427-7090; kevsmith@rogers.com.

SMITH, Kevin R; St Paul's Hosp, 1081 Burrard St, Vancouver BC V6Z 1Y6; Staff, Providence Health Care - St Paul's Hospital; (604)682-2344

SMITH, Kiara K; 4 Villages CHC Dundas Site, 3446 Dundas St W, Toronto ON M6S 2S1; Wes'07; CCFP; Staff, St Joseph's Health Centre; (416)604-3362; Fax. (416)604-3365.

SMITH, Kirsten L; North York Med Arts Bldg, 315-1333 Sheppard Ave E, North York ON M2J 1V1; Wes'99; FRCSC; ObstGyn. Staff, North York General Hospital; (416)494-2400; Fax. (416)494-8758.

SMITH, Larry W; Royal Jubilee Hosp, 1952 Bay St, Victoria BC V8R 1J8; Alb'74; Staff, Royal Jubilee Hospital; (250)319-6238

SMITH, Laurel L; Drumheller Assoc Physicians, PO Box 5600 140 Riverside Dr E, Drumheller AB T0J 0Y0; Alb'93; FRCSC; ObstGyn. (403)823-3345; Fax. (403)823-7823.

SMITH, Lauren; 77 Hunter St E, Hamilton ON L8N 1M4; Qns'07; ObstGyn. (905)521-2788

SMITH, Leonard F G; Stenton Terr Health Authority PO Box 10 Stn Main, Yellowknife NT X1A 2N1; Alb'79; FRCSC; Ophth. Staff Ophth, Stanton Territorial Health Authority; (867)873-3577; dragonsmith@theedge.ca.

SMITH, Lesley J; Univ of Alberta Hosp-SCC/WCM, 1A1 11-8440 112 St NW, Edmonton AB T6G 2B7; Manchester (England)'78; MRC; Peds (Family Medicine) (Pediatric Gastroenterology). Staff, University of Alberta Hospital; Langs: English; French; (780)407-7755; Fax. (780)407-1828.

SMITH, Linda L; Dominion Med Centres Ltd, 9122 23 Ave NW, Edmonton AB T6N 1H9; Ott'00; CCFP; Ad Staff, Covenant Health - Misericordia Community Hospital; Staff, University of Alberta Hospital; Clin Teacher, University of Alberta; (780)801-3360; Fax. (780)801-3366.

SMITH, Linda Y M; F W Green Med Centre, 1629 Baker St, Cranbrook BC V1C 1B4; Sask'77; CCFP; FCFP; (250)426-6601; Fax. (250)426-6470.

SMITH, Lloyd C; St Joseph's Health Centre, SWW 240-30 The Queensway, Toronto ON M6R 1B5; Sask'83; FRCSC; GenSurg. Chief Surgery, St Joseph's Health Centre; Assoc Prof Surg, University of Toronto; (416)530-6033; Fax. (416)530-6044; smithl@stjoe.on.ca.

SMITH, Lorie A; Vancouver Native Hlth Society, 449 Hastings St E, Vancouver BC V6A 1P5; Tor'78; CCFP; Physician, Vancouver Native Health Society; (604)255-9766; Fax. (604)254-5750.

SMITH, Louis F; Dakota Med Centre, 17-845 Dakota St, Winnipeg MB R2M 5M3; Orange Free State (South Africa)'96; MB ChB; BSc; CCFP; Staff, Vita & District Health Centre; Langs: Afrikaans; (204)254-2087

SMITH, Luella M P; The Moncton Hosp, 135 MacBeath Ave, Moncton NB E1C 6Z8; Dal'73; DTM&H; BSc; FCFP; DrMedCh; CCFP; CCFP(E.M.); FCFP; Ac Staff Emerg, The Moncton Hospital; (506)857-5353; Fax. (506)857-5360; samphire2004@yahoo.ca.

SMITH, M Josephine; Haldimand War Mem Hosp, 101-206 John St, Dunnville ON N1A 2P7; Dublin (Ireland)'79; DCH; DObst; MRCGPract(UK); Staff, Haldimand War Memorial Hospital; (905)774-7503; Fax. (905)774-6884; scallan@infinity.net.

SMITH, M Robin; 23-3015 62 St SW, Edmonton AB T6L 5X8; Alb'73; CCFP; FCFP; Staff, Covenant Health - Grey Nuns Community Hospital; Staff, Covenant Health - Misericordia Community Hospital; Asst Prof Family Med, University of Alberta; (780)735-9939; Fax. (780)735-9537; rsmith@cha.ab.ca.

SMITH, M C Patricia; NORD-ASKI Family Health Team, PO Box 727 Stn Main 1403 Edward St, Hearst ON P0L 1N0; McG'83; CCFP; Ac Staff, Hôpital Notre Dame Hospital - Hearst; Langs: French; (705)362-7364; Fax. (705)372-6177; patsmith57@gmail.com.

SMITH, Malcolm W; 905 rue Faudel, Tracadie-Sheila NB E1X 1C1; Manchester (England)'69; MB ChB; DMRD; (506)395-2051; Fax. (506)393-6052.

SMITH, Margaret G; Vancouver Island Cancer Clinic, 2410 Lee Ave, Victoria BC V8R 6V5; Alb'76; Staff, Royal Jubilee Hospital; Staff, BC Cancer Agency Vancouver Island Centre; Clin Teacher Oncol, University of British Columbia; (250)519-5572; Fax. (250)519-2017.

SMITH, Marian H; Foothills Med Centre, 1403 29 St NW, Calgary AB T2N 2T9; Alb'83; FRCPC; Anes. Staff Anes, Foothills Medical Centre; (403)944-1430; Fax. (403)944-2425.

SMITH, Mark A; Carling-Broadview Med Bldg, 308-770 Broadview Ave, Ottawa ON K2A 3Z3; Dal'88; FRCPC; IntMed; Respir. Staff, Queensway Carleton Hospital; (613)725-9374; Fax. (613)725-9195.

SMITH, Marlene W; St Joseph's Health Centre, PO Box 630, Ile-a-la-Crosse SK S0M 1C0; Qns'90; Staff, St Joseph's Hospital; (306)833-2016; Fax. (306)833-3020; msmith@sasktel.net.

SMITH, Marnie L; Centre for Family Medicine, 10B Victoria St S, Kitchener ON N2G 1C5; McM'10; CCFP; Staff, Centre for Family Medicine - Health Sciences Campus Site; (519)783-0024

SMITH, Mary J; Janeway Child Hlth & Rehab Ctr, 300 Prince Philip Dr, St. John's NL A1B 3V6; McM'06; FRCPC; Peds. Staff, Janeway Children's Health & Rehabilitation Centre; (709)777-6300

SMITH, Megan E; Health Sciences Centre, 300 Prince Philip Dr, St. John's NL A1B 3V6; Mem'09; CCFP; CCFP(E.M.); Staff, Health Sciences Centre; (709)737-6300

SMITH, Michael A P; Mississauga Colonoscopy Ctr, 202B-2021 Cliff Rd, Mississauga ON L5A 3N7; Dublin (Ireland)'69; MB ChB; BAO; FRCS(Lond & Ed); FRCSC; GenSurg (Colon & Rectal Surgery). (905)270-4446; Fax. (905)279-3337.

SMITH, Michael J W; Athabasca Prof Bldg, 4903 51 St, Athabasca AB T9S 1E7; Birmingham (England)'71; MB ChB; Ac Staff, Athabasca Healthcare Centre; Member, Pharmaceutical & Therapeutics Committee; (780)675-2498; Fax. (780)675-5924; michaels@telusplanet.net.

SMITH, Michael M; University Hosp of Northern BC, 1475 Edmonton St, Prince George BC V2M 1S2; Dal'02; CCFP; CCFP(E.M.); Staff, University Hospital of Northern British Columbia; (250)565-2000

SMITH, Miles J C; Riverside Med Clinic, 307-1101 Dewdney Ave, Trail BC V1R 4T1; Alb'99; BSc(Hons); CCFP; (250)368-8802; Fax. (250)368-8813.

SMITH, Murdock A; Sydney Family Practice Centre, 196 Kings Rd, Sydney NS B1S 1A1; Dal'69; CCFP; FCFP; Ac Staff, Cape Breton Healthcare Complex; Med Advisor, Worker's Compensation Board of NS; Physician Med Advisor, Harbourstone Enhanced Care & Children's Home; Preceptor Family Med, Dalhousie University; (902)567-0040; Fax. (902)539-9250.

SMITH, Muriel F; Dr Everett Chalmers Reg Hosp, PO Box 9000 Stn A, Fredericton NB E3B 5N5; Dal'70; FACP; FRCPC; GenPath; AnatPath. Staff Path, Dr Everett Chalmers Regional Hospital; (506)452-5479; dr.muriel.smith@horizonnb.ca.

SMITH, Nancy I; Stamford Med Centre, 305-4256 Portage Rd, Niagara Falls ON L2E 6A4; Qns'69; FRCSC; Ophth. (905)358-6121; Fax. (905)358-1626.

SMITH, Norman A; Orleans Urgent Care Clinic, 1220 Prom Place d'Orleans, Orleans ON K1C 2L9; Qns'70; FRCPC; EmergMed. (613)841-5389

SMITH, Oakley D; 206-688 Coxwell Ave, Toronto ON M4C 3B7; Tor'82; FRCSC; Otol (Facial Plastic Surgery). Staff, The Scarborough Hospital - Birchmount Campus; Chief, Toronto East General Hospital Inc; Staff, Sunnybrook Health Sciences Centre; Staff Part-Time, North York General Hospital; Asst Prof Otol, University of Toronto; Langs: French; (416)465-5795; Fax. (416)465-5701; oakleysmith@bellnet.ca.

SMITH, Pamela A T; 200-440 Boler Rd, London ON N6K 4L2; Qns'84; BSc; CCFP; FCFP; Court Staff, London Health Sciences Centre - University Hospital; Court Staff, London Health Sciences Centre - Victoria Campus; Med Staff Assoc, St Joseph's Hospital - St Joseph's Health Care; (519)471-2929; Fax. (519)471-1082.

SMITH, Pamela M; Windsor Reg Hosp-Metropolitan, 1995 Lens Ave, Windsor ON N8W 1L9; Manchester (England)'76; MB ChB; BSc; LMCC; FRCPC; AnatPath (Medical Oncology). Staff Path, Windsor Regional Hospital - Metropolitan Site; (519)254-1661

SMITH, Patricia A; McMaster Univ Medical Centre, PO Box 2000 Stn Lcd 1 4D12-1200 Main St W, Hamilton ON L8N 3Z5; Cape Town (South Africa)'88; FRCOG; MSc; MB BS; FRCSC; ObstGyn (Maternal Fetal Medicine). Staff, Hamilton Health Sciences Centre - McMaster Children's Hospital; Assoc Prof, McMaster University; Langs: Afrikaans; (905)521-2100 x76210; Fax. (905)521-2675; pasmith@mcmaster.ca.

SMITH, Patricia E; Grand River Hosp-KW Hlth Ctre, PO Box 9056 Stn C 835 King St W, Kitchener ON N2G 1G3; McM'82; CCFP; FCFP; Staff, Grand River Hospital - Kitchener/Waterloo Health Centre; (519)749-4300

SMITH, Patricia J; Student Health Clinic, PO Box 4400 Stn A, Fredericton NB E3B 5A3; Dal'87; CCFP; FCFP; Staff Student Health Clinic, University of New Brunswick; (506)453-4837; Fax. (506)452-6087; smithp@whscc.nb.ca.

SMITH, Patricia L; Spadina Health Centre, 404-720 Spadina Ave, Toronto ON M5S 2T9; McM'08; CCFP; Staff, Anne Johnston Health Station; (416)928-0920; Fax. (416)928-7426.

SMITH, Patricia R; Associate Med Clinic, 201-836 1 Ave NW, Airdrie AB T4B 0V2; Cal'87; BSc; LMCC; CCFP; Staff, Dr Patricia Smith Airdrie Urgent Care; Staff, Midway Healthcare Centre; (403)948-6422; Fax. (403)948-4492.

SMITH, Patricia R; Lakeview Med Centre, 13-1945 McKercher Dr, Saskatoon SK S7J 4M4; Sask'06; CCFP; (306)244-5100; Fax. (306)244-5115.

SMITH, Patrick X; 7875 Riverside Dr, Windsor ON N8S 1E1; Tor'83; (519)974-4444; Fax. (519)974-1395.

SMITH, Paula C; Kanata North Med Centre, 832 March Rd, Kanata ON K2W 0C9; Mem'99; BSc(Hon); MCFP; CCFP; (613)599-5599; Fax. (613)599-1005.

SMITH, Peter J; Norburn Med Clinic, 200-4012 Hastings St, Burnaby BC V5C 2H9; Belfast (Ireland)'79; MB ChB; BAO; (604)299-2677; Fax. (604)298-6656.

SMITH, Peter K L; Woodlawn Med Consultants, 92 Main St, Dartmouth NS B2X 1R5; Dal'82; FRCPC; IntMed (Gastroenterology). (902)434-1500; Fax. (902)434-4837.

SMITH, Philip L; Niagara H-System-St Catharines, PO Box 3018 Stn Main 142 Queenston St, St Catharines ON L2R 7C6; Ott'85; FRCPC; Anes. Staff, Niagara Health System - St Catharines General Site; (905)684-7271; Fax. (905)323-7562.

SMITH, Philip M; Cape Breton Hlthcare Complex, 1482 George St, Sydney NS B1P 1P3; Dal'85; FRCSC; GenSurg. Staff, Cape Breton Healthcare Complex; (902)567-8041; Fax. (902)567-8043.

SMITH, Philippe; Hôpital Anna-Laberge, 200 boul Brisebois, Chateauguay QC J6K 4W8; Mon'09; CCFP; Staff, Hôpital Anna-Laberge; (450)699-2525

SMITH, Phillip J; 95 Meridian Ave, Haileybury ON P0J 1K0; Queensland (Australia)'88; MB; BSc; CCFP; (705)672-3371

SMITH, Preston A; C206-5849 University Ave, Halifax NS B3H 4H7; Dal'81; CCFP; FCFP; Senior Assoc Dean, Dalhousie University; (902)494-7830; Fax. (902)474-7119.

SMITH, Quentin A; Crossroads Family Practice, 201-45800 Promontory Rd, Chilliwack BC V2R 5Z5; Cape Town (South Africa)'87; MB ChB; LMCC; CCFP; FCFP; Staff, Chilliwack General Hospital; Clinical Asst Prof, University of British Columbia; Langs: Afrikaans; (604)858-3725; Fax. (604)858-8625.

SMITH, R Garth; Hotel-Dieu Hosp, 166 Brock St, Kingston ON K7L 5G2; West Indies (Jamaica)'81; MB BS; FRCPC; Peds (Acquired Brain Injury). Consultant Peds, Kingston General Hospital; Staff Child Development Clinic, Hotel-Dieu Hospital; Asst Prof Peds, Queen's University; (613)544-3310 x3324; Fax. (613)545-3557; gs3@queensu.ca.

SMITH, R Matthew M; The Langley Business Ctre, 180-8700 200 St, Langley BC V2Y 0G4; UBC'96; FRCSC; GenSurg; VascSurg. (604)888-7505

SMITH, R Stephen; Dr Everett Chalmers Reg Hosp, PO Box 9000 Stn A, Fredericton NB E3B 5N5; Mem'88; CCFP; FCFP; Staff, Dr Everett Chalmers Regional Hospital; (506)458-0233

SMITH, R Vaughn; St Joseph's Hosp, 130 Bayard Dr, Saint John NB E2L 3L6; Dal'80; CCFP; FCFP; Staff, St Joseph's Hospital; (506)632-5740; Fax. (506)632-5657.

SMITH, Randell J; Commonwealth Med Clinic, 77 Commonwealth Ave, Mount Pearl NL A1N 1W7; Mem'76; (709)364-7555; Fax. (709)364-7554.

SMITH, Reilly G; Foothills Med Centre, 1403 29 St NW, Calgary AB T2N 2T9; Alb'04; FRCPC; Psy. Staff, Foothills Medical Centre; (403)944-1321; Fax. (403)944-2400.

SMITH, Riley A L; Dauphin Med Clinic, 622 3rd St SW, Dauphin MB R7N 1R7; Man'08; CCFP; (250)592-3479; Fax. (250)361-3422.

SMITH, Robert A; Sudbury Med Centre, 411-65 Larch St, Sudbury ON P3E 1B8; Wes'88; FRCSC; GenSurg. Staff, Health Sciences North-St Joseph's Health Centre; Staff, Health Sciences North - Memorial Site; (705)675-1564; Fax. (705)675-2572.

SMITH, Robert G; 4-25 Front Ave W, Brockville ON K6V 4J2; Tor'93; FRCPC; Psy (Assertive Commun Treatment). Att Staff Elmgrove Unit & Service Dir, Brockville Mental Health Centre - Royal Ottawa Health Care Group; (613)342-2522; Fax. (613)345-4111.

SMITH, Robert G J; Selkirk Med Centre, 353 Eveline St, Selkirk MB R1A 1N1; Man'69; FRCPC; Peds. Ac Staff, Selkirk & District General Hospital; Ac Staff, Health Sciences Centre; (204)482-5777

SMITH, Robert M; The Langley Business Center, 180-8700 200 St, Langley BC V2Y 0G4; McG'79; (604)888-7505

SMITH, Robert M; Windsor Reg Hosp-Metropolitan, 1995 Lens Ave, Windsor ON N8W 1L9; Glasgow (Scotland)'76; MB ChB; DMRD; FRCPC; DiagRad. Associate Radiol, Windsor Regional Hospital - Metropolitan Site; (519)254-1661; Fax. (519)254-0163; robert_smith@wrh.on.ca.

SMITH, Roger M L; Univ Hlth Network-Toronto Western Hosp, 3M C428-399 Bathurst St, Toronto ON M5T 2S8; Edinburgh (Scotland)'77; Staff, Toronto Western Hospital - University Health Network; Langs: French; (416)603-5800 x2583; Fax. (416)603-4257.

SMITH, Roy W; Meadowood Med Centre, 1555 St Mary's Rd, Winnipeg MB R2M 5L9; Man'79; CCFP; FCFP; Assoc Lecturer, University of Manitoba; (204)255-6973; Fax. (204)254-0730.

SMITH, Ruth E; Advanced Walk-In Med Clinic, 111-21 Queensway W, Mississauga ON L5B 1B6; McM'85; DAA; FRCPC; PhysMed&Rehab (Family Medicine). (905)277-2933

SMITH, Ryan S; London HSC-University Campus, PO Box 5339 Stn B B3 218-339 Winderemere Rd, London ON N6A 5A5; Cal'08; Staff, London Health Sciences Centre - University Hospital.

SMITH, Sally L; BC Cancer Agency-Vanc Island, 2410 Lee Ave, Victoria BC V8R 6V5; UBC'02; FRCPC; RadOncol. Staff, BC Cancer Agency Vancouver Island Centre; (250)519-5577

SMITH, Samuel A; Prince Rupert Reg Hosp, 221-1305 Summit Ave, Prince Rupert BC V8J 2A6; Pretoria (South Africa)'82; MB ChB; MMed; LMCC; Ac Staff, Prince Rupert Regional Hospital; Langs: Afrikaans; (250)622-6501; Fax. (250)622-6502; alf.smith@northernhealth.ca.

SMITH, Sarah C; Nanaimo Mental Hlth & Addictio, 3F-528 Wentworth St, Nanaimo BC V9R 3E4; Dal'95; FRCPC; Psy. Staff, Nanaimo Regional General Hospital; (250)739-5868

SMITH, Sarah J; CLSC Cote-des-Neiges, 5700 ch Cote-des-Neiges, Montreal QC H3T 2A8; Dal'08; CCFP; (514)731-8531; sjsmith4@dal.ca.

SMITH, Sarah; CLSC de la Jacques-Cartier, A-11999 rue de l'Hopital, Quebec QC G2A 2T7; Laval'05; Staff, Centre Hospitalier Regional du Grand-Portage; (418)843-2572

SMITH, Scott A; Kilborn Med Centre, 1385 Bank St, Ottawa ON K1H 8N4; Wes'97; CCFP; (613)523-7440; Fax. (613)523-7440.

SMITH, Scott; Kelowna Gen Hosp, 2268 Pandosy St, Kelowna BC V1Y 1T2; Tor'08; CCFP; Staff, Kelowna General Hospital; (250)862-4000

SMITH, Scott T; Claresholm Med Centre, PO Box 2050, Claresholm AB T0L 0T0; Alb'08; CCFP; (403)625-4484; Fax. (403)625-3969.

SMITH, Shane A; CF Health Services Centre, PO Box 99000 Stn Forces Halifax, Halifax NS B3K 1C8; Dal'09; CCFP; Staff, Canadian Forces Health Services Centre (Atlantic); (902)721-8700

SMITH, Shannon E; Smithville Family Health Ctre, PO Box 218 230 Canboro St, Smithville ON L0R 2A0; Ott'04; CCFP; Staff, Smithville Family Health Centre; (905)957-3328; Fax. (905)957-2475; ssmith@cogeco.ca.

SMITH, Sharyn J; Stratford Gen Hosp, 46 General Hospital Dr, Stratford ON N5A 2Y6; Ott'91; FRCPC; AnatPath. Staff, Stratford General Hospital - Huron Perth Healthcare Alliance; (519)272-8210; sharyn.smith@hpha.ca.

SMITH, Sheena M H; ACT Peterborough, 226 Charlotte St, Peterborough ON K9J 2T8; Dal'86; (705)740-0228; Fax. (705)740-0223.

SMITH, Sheila C; PO Box 102, Smithers BC V0J 2N0; Qns'97; CCFP.

SMITH, Sheila M; Regina Qu'Appelle HR-Regina, 1440 14th Ave, Regina SK S4P 0W5; Sask'95; CCFP; CCFP(E.M.); FCFP; Staff Emerg, Regina General Hospital; (306)766-4213; Fax. (306)766-4357.

SMITH, Shelley D B; Justik Med Clinic, 8225 105 St NW, Edmonton AB T6E 4H2; Alb'97; CCFP; (780)432-0211; Fax. (780)439-9349.

SMITH, Shelley M; JBS Medical Centre, 420-1420 Burnhamthorpe Rd E, Mississauga ON L4X 2Z9; Tor'86; CCFP; Court Staff, Toronto Western Hospital - University Health Network; Court Staff, Trillium Health Centre - Mississauga; Asst Prof, University of Toronto; (905)625-1619; Fax. (905)625-9362.

SMITH, Shona E; South Hlth & Life Managment Ct, 2-2120 Regent St, Sudbury ON P3E 3Z9; McM'03; FRCSC; GenSurg; ThorSurg. (705)522-9101

SMITH, Stanley G; Springbank Med Centre, 209-460 Springbank Dr, London ON N6J 0A8; Dublin (Ireland)'60; MB ChB; CCFP; FCFP; Emeritus Prof, University of Western Ontario; (519)659-2002; Fax. (226)781-0852; sgsmith2@uwo.ca.

SMITH, Stanley S; Professional Corp, 7524 Elbow Dr SW, Calgary AB T2V 1K1; Alb'65; FAAOO; FRCSC; Ophth (Cataract). Staff, Rockyview General Hospital; Asst Prof Ophth, University of Calgary; (403)255-1555; Fax. (403)252-1007; sssmith@shaw.ca.

SMITH, Stephanie W; University of Alberta Hosp, 2E4 16-8440 112 St NW, Edmonton AB T6G 2B7; Dal'01; MSc; FRCPC; IntMed (AIDS/HIV); InfectDis. Dir Residency Training for Infectious Diseases/Staff, University of Alberta Hospital; (780)407-2826; Fax. (780)407-7137.

SMITH, Stephen A; Sault Area Hosp-Sault Ste Mari, 750 Great Northern Rd, Sault Ste. Marie ON P6B 0A8; McM'09; CCFP; Staff, Sault Area Hospital - Sault Ste Marie; (705)759-3434

SMITH, Steven I; Baywood Med Centre, 300-95 Bayly St W, Ajax ON L1S 7K8; Tor'81; FRCSC; Urol. Ac Staff, Lakeridge Health - Oshawa Site; Ac Staff, Rouge Valley Health System - Ajax & Pickering Health Centre Site; Ac Staff, Lakeridge Health - Whitby Site; (905)426-9426; Fax. (905)426-9322.

SMITH, Stuart J; Belmont Prof Centre, 409-564 Belmont Ave W, Kitchener ON N2M 5N6; McM'86; FRCPC; IntMed (Heart Failure); Cardiol. Staff, St Mary's General Hospital; (519)584-1104; Fax. (519)584-0959; westheightscardiology@bellnet.ca.

SMITH, Stuart W; Oakridge Plaza, 385-5780 Cambie St, Vancouver BC V5Z 3A7; UBC'79; FRCSC; Ophth. Ac Staff, Vancouver General Hospital - Centennial Pavillion; Teach Staff Med, University of British Columbia; (604)327-5014; Fax. (604)327-5014.

SMITH, Susan C; 202-436 Gilmour St, Ottawa ON K2P 0R8; Qns'66; FRCPC; Psy. (613)232-9513; Fax. (613)744-8528.

SMITH, Susan E; Nashwaaksis Med Clinic, 475 Brookside Dr, Fredericton NB E3A 8V4; Dal'77; Ac Staff, Dr Everett Chalmers Regional Hospital; (506)458-1331; Fax. (506)458-1326; ses@nbnet.nb.ca.

SMITH, Susan L M; Midhurst Health Centre, 30 Spence Ave SS 33, Midhurst ON L0L 1X1; Qns'82; CCFP; FCFP; Affil Staff, Royal Victoria Regional Health Centre; (705)735-0922; Fax. (705)735-1530.

SMITH, Terrence C; PO BOX 769, Raymond AB T0K 2S0; Alb'74; Staff, Raymond Health Centre; Staff, Magrath Community Health; (403)752-3337; Fax. (403)752-4967; tsmith@mox.chr.ab.ca.

SMITH, Terry A; Ctre Hosp de Verdun, 4000 boul Lasalle, Verdun QC H4G 2A3; UBC'84; FRCPC; IntMed; Respir. Staff, Centre Hospitalier de Verdun; Staff, CSSS de Dorval-Lachine-Lasalle; Staff, Hôpital Anna-Laberge; (514)362-1000

SMITH, Terry S; Sunnybrook Hlth Sciences Ctre, D108-2075 Bayview Ave, Toronto ON M4N 3M5; Tor'85; FRCPC; IntMed; Critical Care Medicine; Anes. Staff, Sunnybrook Health Sciences Centre; (416)480-4522; Fax. (416)480-4999.

SMITH, Thirza E; Pacific Avenue Med Centre, 300-149 Pacific Ave, Saskatoon SK S7K 1N8; Sask'73; FRCSC; ObstGyn. Ac Staff ObstGyn, Saskatoon City Hospital; Consultant, St Paul's Hospital (Grey Nuns) of Saskatoon; Ac Staff, Royal University Hospital; Clin Prof, University of Saskatchewan; (306)653-5970; Fax. (306)653-5383.

SMITH, Thomas J; ENT Consultants, 219-1 Paton St, St. John's NL A1B 4S8; Dal'71; FRCSC; Otol (Head & Neck Surgery). (709)579-1003

SMITH, Trent J; 202-474 Columbia St, Kamloops BC V2C 2T5; Alb'97; BPE; MD; MRCP; FRCPC; Peds (Neonatology). Staff Peds, Royal Inland Hospital; Clin Staff Peds, University of British Columbia; (250)374-3300; Fax. (250)374-8837.

SMITH, Tyler W; Gordon & Leslie Diamond HCC, 10F-2775 Laurel St, Vancouver BC V5Z 1M9; UBC'06; FRCPC; HemPath. Staff, Gordon & Leslie Diamond Health Care Centre; (604)875-4863

SMITH, Valerie F; Gemini Health Centre, 2010-6708 48 Ave, Camrose AB T4V 4S3; Cal'96; BSc; CCFP; FCFP; Staff, Covenant Health - St Mary's Hospital; (780)672-9850; Fax. (780)672-9104.

SMITH, Verne P; Gabriola Med Clinic, PO Box 200, Gabriola BC V0R 1X0; UBC'58; (250)247-9922; Fax. (250)247-9162.

SMITH, W Gary; Medical Arts Bldg, 17 Dunedin St, Orillia ON L3V 5T3; Tor'75; AB; FAAP; FRCPC; Peds (Neonatology). Prog Med Dir, Orillia Soldiers' Memorial Hospital; Assoc Prof Peds, University of Toronto; Langs: English; French; (705)327-9131; Fax. (705)327-9189.

SMITH, Wayne J; CHUS-Hop Hotel-Dieu, 580 rue Bowen S, Sherbrooke QC J1G 2E8; Sher'72; EmergMed. ac Staff, Centre Hospitalier Universitaire de Sherbrooke-Hôpital Hôtel-Dieu; (819)822-6710; Fax. (819)822-6773.

SMITH, Wayne M; Hollyburn Med Centre, 207D-575 16th St, West Vancouver BC V7V 4Y1; Cal'80; BSc(Hons); MSc; Staff/Head Gen Practice, Lions Gate Hospital; (604)922-7234; Fax. (604)926-3541.

SMITH, Wendy L; Northern Med Unit, T162-770 Bannatyne Ave, Winnipeg MB R3E 0W3; Mem'87; CCFP; FCFP; (204)789-3711; Fax. (204)774-8919; wendylab@shaw.ca.

SMITH, Willard A D; West Parry South Health Centre, 6 Albert St, Parry Sound ON P2A 3A4; Dal'02; CCFP; Locum Tenens, Timmins & District Hospital; Staff, Lady Minto Hospital Cochrane; (705)746-4540

SMITH-AUGUSTE, Jacqueline A; 810 Wilson Ave, North York ON M3K 1E5; Cal'96; BSc; MSA; FRCSC; OrthSurg (Trauma). Staff OrthSurg & Medical Staff, Humber River Regional Hospital - Church Street Site; Langs: Spanish; French; (647)347-7218

SMITH-GORVIE, Telisha J; Univ Hlth Network-Toronto Gen, RFE GS480-200 Elizabeth St, Toronto ON M5G 2C4; Man'05; FRCPC; EmergMed. Langs: Bilingual(English/French); (416)340-3111

SMITH-PELLETTIER, I Carolyn; B-21 Devere Dr, Guelph ON N1G 2T2; Qns'69; Court Staff, Guelph General Hospital; Court Staff, Homewood Health Centre; (519)823-5410; Fax. (519)824-5707.

SMITH-WINDSOR, Thomas B; Associate Med Clinic, 400-20 14th St W, Prince Albert SK S6V 3K8; Sask'89; CCFP; FCFP; Physician, Associate Medical Clinic; Clin Assoc Prof Family Med/Coord Rural Division/Assoc Dean Rural & Northern Med Education, University of Saskatchewan; (306)953-1664; Fax. (306)764-3091; dr.tom@sasktel.net.

SMITHERAM, Amanda; Saint John Reg Hosp, PO Box 2100 400 University Ave, Saint John NB E2L 4L2; Dal'06; Staff, Saint John Regional Hospital; (506)648-6000

SMITHERINGALE, Alma J; 11-1110 Sheppard Ave E, North York ON M2K 2W2; London (England)'75; MB BS; FRCSC; Otol (Pediatric Otolaryngology). Staff, North York General Hospital; Assoc Prof, University of Toronto; Langs: French; (416)226-5012; Fax. (416)226-5010.

SMITHERS, Denise L; 202-3607 31 St, Vernon BC V1T 5J4; UBC'00; CCFP; (250)545-5433

SMITS, Cheryl L; 208-190 Wortley Rd, London ON N6C 4Y7; Wes'05; CCFP; (519)438-5101; Fax. (519)438-0369.

SMOLARKIEWICZ, Marek A; Stephenville Comm Med Clinic, 1 Washington Dr, Stephenville NL A2N 2V5; Lublin (Poland)'70; Staff, Janeway Children's Health & Rehabilitation Centre; Langs: Polish; Russian; (709)643-5656

SMOLEY, Lester B; 645-1 av Holiday, Pointe-Claire QC H9R 5N3; McG'78; AB; FRCPC; IntMed (P.Q.); Derm. (514)630-6699; Fax. (514)630-3347.

SMOLINSKI, Walter J; 221 Ellerdale St, Saint John NB E2J 3S4; Dal'84; (506)634-7877; Fax. (506)634-7878.

SMOLKIN, Mark A; 24-2917 Bloor St W, Etobicoke ON M8X 1B4; Qns'91; BA; CCFP; FCFP; Staff, Runnymede Healthcare Centre; (416)944-8431

SMOLKIN, Robert D; Appletree Med Group, 2948 Baseline Rd, Ottawa ON K2H 8T5; Qns'61; Staff, The Ottawa Hospital - Civic Campus; Asst Prof Family Med, University of Ottawa; (613)288-2059; Fax. (613)288-2060.

SMOLLA, Robert; Clinique de Med Familiale, 300 rue Paradis, Sorel-Tracy QC J3P 3G6; Mon'76; (450)908-0508; Fax. (450)908-0508.

SMOSARSKI, David J; Hamilton Family Health, M4-414 Victoria Ave N, Hamilton ON L8L 5G8; McG'88; Langs: French; (905)529-5221

SMRZ, Iva; 701-133 Prince William St, Saint John NB E2L 2B5; Mem'96; FRCSC; Ophth. Ac Staff, Saint John Regional Hospital; Ac Staff, St Joseph's Hospital; Langs: Czech; (506)649-5311; Fax. (506)642-3149.

SMUCZEK, Joseph A; North Appleby Med Centre, 1960 Appleby Line, Burlington ON L7L 6M6; McM'09; CCFP; (905)319-2000

SMULA, Vaclav; Sunnybrook Holland Ortho Arthr, 43 Wellesley St E, Toronto ON M4Y 1H1; Tor'76; MSc; PhD; Staff, Sunnybrook Health Sciences Centre - Holland Orthopaedic & Arthritic Centre; Langs: Czech; (416)967-8504; Fax. (416)967-4214.

SMULLEN, Merril J; Goodfellow Prof Bldg, 206-170 McEwan Dr E, Bolton ON L7E 4C8; Glasgow (Scotland)'76; MB ChB; DRCOG; Ac Staff Family Pract, William Osler Health System - Etobicoke General Hospital; (905)857-3474; Fax. (905)857-3437.

SMUSHKIN, Galina; 130-180 Wilson St, Victoria BC V9A 7N6; Northwestern University (USA)'04; Langs: Russian; French; (250)385-5255

SMUTS, Elvira T; Rockyview Gen Hosp, 5A 253-7007 14 St SW, Calgary AB T2V 1P9; (South Africa)'83; MB ChB; Staff, Foothills Medical Centre; Staff, Rockyview General Hospital; Staff Palliative Care, Chinook Regional Hospital; (403)943-8774

SMYLIE, Janet K; St Michael's Hosp, 30 Bond St, Toronto ON M5B 1W8; Qns'93; CCFP; FCFP; Staff Ctr for Research on Inner City Health, St Michael's Hospital; (416)864-6060

SMYLIE, Michael G B; Cross Cancer Institute, 11560 University Ave NW, Edmonton AB T6G 1Z2; Leicester (England)'87; FRCPC; IntMed; MedOncol. Staff/Clin Researcher, Cross Cancer Institute; Assoc Prof Oncol, University of Alberta; Langs: French; (780)432-8757

SMYLIE, Paul C; Cobblestone Clinic, 1-3414A 28 Ave, Vernon BC V1T 1W9; Leicester (England)'89; MB ChB; FRCPC; IntMed; Cardiol. Staff, Vernon Jubilee Hospital; (250)542-6033; Fax. (250)542-6023; malako@shaw.ca.

SMYTH, Allan J; Jim Pattison Outpatient Care, 9750 140 St, Surrey BC V3T 0G9; Otago (New Zealand)'66; MB ChB; FRCPC; Neur. Staff, Surrey Memorial Hospital; (604)582-4561

SMYTH, Barbara J; Richmond Square, 70-3915 51 St SW, Calgary AB T3E 6N1; Alb'89; CCFP; FCFP; (403)229-2273; Fax. (403)246-9688.

SMYTH, Catherine E; The Ottawa Hosp-Gen Campus, 501 Smyth Rd, Ottawa ON K1H 8L6; McM'96; FRCPC; Anes. Staff, The Ottawa Hospital - General Campus; Langs: French; (613)737-8187; Fax. (613)737-8189.

SMYTH, Daniel J; The Moncton Hosp, 135 MacBeath Ave, Moncton NB E1C 6Z8; Dal'06; FRCPC; IntMed; InfectDis. Staff, The Moncton Hospital; (506)857-5111

SMYTH, David J E; 4904 48 St, Leduc AB T9E 6X4; Alb'93; CCFP; (780)986-2712; Fax. (780)986-0356.

SMYTH, Harley S; Trillium Health Ctre-Missisaug, 100 Queensway W, Mississauga ON L5B 1B8; Qns'63; MA(Oxon); DPhil(Oxon); BA; Neursurg (Neuro Endocrinology). Staff, Trillium Health Centre - Mississauga; Langs: Italian; French; (905)848-7580; Fax. (416)521-4082.

SMYTH, John A; BC Women's Health & HC, 1R47-4500 Oak St, Vancouver BC V6H 3N1; Irish Conjoint Board (Ireland)'72; LRCPSI; FRCPC; Peds (Neonatology). Staff Pediatrics/Neonatology, BC Women's Hospital & Health Centre; Ac Staff, BC Children's Hospital; Clin Assoc Prof, University of British Columbia; (604)875-2135; Fax. (604)875-3106; jsmyth@cw.bc.ca.

SMYTH, Karl R; The Ottawa Hosp-Civic Campus, 1053 Carling Ave, Ottawa ON K1Y 4E9; Mem'98; FRCPC; DiagRad;CCFP; Fellow, The Ottawa Hospital - Civic Campus; (613)761-4054; Fax. (613)761-4476.

SMYTH, Kimberley A; Alberta Children's Hosp, 2888 Shanagappi Trail NW, Calgary AB T3B 6A8; Alb'05; FRCPC; Neur. Staff, Alberta Children's Hospital; (403)955-2296; Fax. (403)955-7609.

SMYTH, Patricia; CLSC Les Aboiteaux, 101-708 4e av, La Pocatiere QC G0R 1Z0; Laval'90; Chef pneumo, CSSS de Kamouraska; Staff, CLSC Les Aboiteaux; Langs: English; (418)856-7000 x6000; Fax. (418)856-5108; patricia.smyth.csssv@ssss.gouv.qc.ca.

SMYTH, Penelope S; University of Alberta Hosp, 2E323 WMC-8440 112 St NW, Edmonton AB T6G 2B7; Alb'97; BSc; FRCPC; Neur (Multiple Sclerosis). Staff, Vancouver General Hospital - Centennial Pavillion; Staff, University of Alberta Hospital; Clin Instructor, University of British Columbia; (780)407-2734; Fax. (780)407-1325.

SMYTH, Richard R J; Sleep Surgery Centre, 303-2963 Glen Dr, Coquitlam BC V3B 2P7; London (England)'74; MB BS; LRCP; FRCS; FRCSC; Otol (Sleep Apnea). Staff, Royal Columbian Hospital; Staff, Eagle Ridge Hospital & Health Care Centre; Founder/Dir, Sleep Surgery Centre; Aj Prof Science, Thompson Rivers University; (604)941-8474; Fax. (604)941-2455.

SMYTH, Robert J; South Lake Reg Health Centre, 596 Davis Dr, Newmarket ON L3Y 2P9; Cal'89; MSc; BPHE; FRCPC; Anes (Critical Care Medicine). Staff Anes, Southlake Regional Health Centre; (905)895-4521; Fax. (905)853-2213; rsmith@southlakeregional.org.

SMYTH, Thomas J; North Muskoka Med Clinic, 202-29 Main St E, Huntsville ON P1H 2C6; Belfast (Ireland)'68; MB ChB; BAO; Court Staff, Huntsville District Memorial Hospital - Muskoka Algonquin Healthcare; (705)789-5581; Fax. (705)788-7888.

SMYTH, William-Lee R; West Parry Sound Health Ctre, 6 Albert St, Parry Sound ON P2A 3A4; Qns'92; FRCSC; OrthSurg. Staff, West Parry Sound Health Centre; (705)746-4540; Fax. (705)773-4634.

SMYTHE, Donna E; Kingsway Med Bldg, 6-2917 Bloor St W, Etobicoke ON M8X 1B4; Wes'84; BSc; FRCSC; Ophth;CCFP; FCFP; Ac Staff, Trillium Health Centre - West Toronto; Court Staff, The Credit Valley Hospital; (416)231-5200; Fax. (416)231-8369.

SMYTHE, John F; Kingston Gen Hosp, W3 304-76 Stuart St, Kingston ON K7L 2V7; Qns'84; FRCPC; Peds; Cardiol. Staff, Kingston General Hospital; Att Staff, Hotel-Dieu Hospital; A-Dept Head Peds, Queen's University; (613)548-3232; Fax. (613)548-1368.

SNADDEN, David; Northern Sport Centre-UNBC, 3333 University Way, Prince George BC V2N 4Z9; Dundee (Scotland)'77; MB ChB; CCFP; Staff, University Hospital of Northern British Columbia; University of British Columbia; (250)960-6172; Fax. (250)960-5512.

SNAIDERMAN, Abraham; Toronto Rehab Inst-Univ Ctr, E5 113 1-550 University Ave, Toronto ON M5G 2A2; National University of Mexico (Mexico)'83; FRCPC; Psy (Brain Injury Psychiatry). Staff Neuro Rehab Prog, Toronto Rehabilitation Institute - University Centre; Dir, NeuroPsychiatry Clinic; Lecturer Psy, University of Toronto; Langs: Hebrew; (416)597-3422

SNAIR, Patti J; Musquodoboit Valley Fam Pract, RR 2 492 Archibald Brook Rd, Midle Musquodoboit NS B0N 1X0; Dal'04; CCFP; Physician, Canadian Forces Health Services Centre (Atlantic); (902)384-2834

SNAJDROVA, Lenka; PO Box 200, Richards Landing ON P0R 1J0; Ott'01; CCFP; CCFP(E.M.); Staff, Sault Area Hospital - Sault Ste Marie; Langs: Slovak; (705)246-2477; Fax. (705)246-0487.

SNAPE, Clive; MD Health Med Centre-Brampton, 186 Main St S, Brampton ON L6W 2E2; Dublin (Ireland)'70; (905)456-7774; Fax. (905)456-1158.

SNARR, M Michelle; 85 Bolton St, Bobcaygeon ON K0M 1A0; Qns'86; CCFP; FCFP; Court Staff, Ross Memorial Hospital; Asst Prof Family Med, Queen's University; (705)738-6136; Fax. (705)738-3771.

SNE, Niv; Hamilton HS-General Site, 6N 604-237 Barton St E, Hamilton ON L8L 2X2; Ott'98; FRCSC; GenSurg. Staff, Hamilton Health Sciences Centre - Hamilton General Hospital; Langs: Hebrew; (905)527-0271

SNEAD III, Orlando C; The Hosp for Sick Children, 555 University Ave, Toronto ON M5G 1X8; Hebrew (Israel)'70; FRCPC; Neur. Staff, The Hospital For Sick Children; (416)813-1500; Fax. (416)813-7839; carter.snead@sickkids.ca.

SNEATH, Jason R; 3F-835 10th Ave W, Vancouver BC V5Z 4E8; Man'08; (604)875-4747

SNEDDON, Kadre A K; Mill Cove Med Centre, 208A-965 Bedford Hwy, Bedford NS B4A 1A9; Mem'02; CCFP; (902)444-8706; Fax. (902)444-8721.

SNELGROVE, Christine; Dr Charles A Janeway Child HC, 300 Prince Philip Dr, St. John's NL A1B 3V6; Mem'96; FRCPC; Psy (Child & Adolescent Psychiatry). Staff, Janeway Children's Health & Rehabilitation Centre; (709)777-4312; Fax. (709)722-0408.

SNELGROVE, W John; Sunnyside Med Arts Centre, 509-27 Roncesvalles Ave, Toronto ON M6R 3B2; UBC'82; FRCPC; Psy (Adult Services & Child Abuse). Consultant Psy, University of Waterloo; (416)534-3212; Fax. (416)534-2298; dr.snelgrove@gmail.com.

SNELL, Laura J; Sunnybrook Hlth Sciences Ctre, M1 519A-2075 Bayview Ave, Toronto ON M4N 3M5; Wes'03; FRCSC; PlasSurg. Staff Breast Surgical Team, Sunnybrook Health Sciences Centre - Edmond Odette Cancer Centre; (416)480-6069; Fax. (416)480-5795.

SNELL, Linda S; MUHC-Royal Victoria Hosp, A4 21-687 av des Pins O, Montreal QC H3A 1A1; Alb'75; ABIM; FACP; FRCPC; IntMed. Dir Div of IntMed & Staff, McGill University Health Centre - Royal Victoria Hospital; Prof/V-prés Dept of Med/Membre Core Faculty Ctre for Med Educ, McGill University; (514)934-1934 x34132; Fax. (514)843-8182.

SNELL, Timothy G; 1265 Onondaga St, Oromocto NB E2V 2P8; Mem'93; CCFP; Ac Staff, Oromocto Public Hospital; Teach Staff, Dalhousie University; (506)357-8459; Fax. (506)357-2238.

SNELLING, Carolyn M H; Stittsville Med Centre, PO Box 1030 Stn Main 1-1339 Main St, Stittsville ON K2S 1C6; Qns'04; CCFP; (613)836-5083; Fax. (613)836-2451.

SNIDER, Bernice E; The Two Hundred, 202-200 St Clair Ave W, Toronto ON M4V 1R1; Tor'62; (416)921-2744; Fax. (416)921-2303.

SNIDER, Carolyn E; St Boniface Gen Hosp, L1019-409 Tache Ave, Winnipeg MB R2H 2A6; McM'03; FRCPC; EmergMed. Staff, St Boniface General Hospital; Staff, Health Sciences Centre; (204)233-8563

SNIDER, D David; 3F-476 Peel St, Woodstock ON N4S 1K1; Wes'83; FRCSC; ObstGyn (Gynecologic Oncology). Staff, Woodstock General Hospital; Staff, Tillsonburg District Memorial Hospital; (519)533-0865; Fax. (519)533-0947.

SNIDER, Douglas D; Royal Alexandra Hosp, L3-10240 Kingsway NW, Edmonton AB T5H 3V9; Alb'99; FRCPC; Anes. Staff, Royal Alexandra Hospital; (780)735-4111

SNIDER, Hannah L; Wellesley Township Hlth Ctre, PO Box 187 1180 Queens Bush Rd, Wellesley ON N0B 2T0; McM'06; CCFP; (519)656-9025

SNIDER, John M; Sudbury Med Centre, 410-65 Larch St, Sudbury ON P3E 1B8; Wes'96; BSc; FRCSC; GenSurg. Staff, Health Sciences North-St Joseph's Health Centre; (705)674-4677; Fax. (705)674-8756; johnsnider2001@hotmail.com.

SNIDER, Matthew G; 115-675 Queen St S, Kitchener ON N2M 1A1; Wes'04; FRCSC; OrthSurg. Staff, St Mary's General Hospital; Staff, Grand River Hospital - Kitchener/Waterloo Health Centre; (519)603-0662

SNIDER, Stacey L; Avon Family Med Center, 511 Huron St, Stratford ON N5A 5T8; McM'00; CCFP; Staff, Stratford General Hospital - Huron Perth Healthcare Alliance; Aj Prof, University of Western Ontario; (519)508-1212; Fax. (519)508-1240.

SNIDER-ADLER, Melissa A; First Step Med Oshawa, 32 Simcoe St S, Oshawa ON L1H 4G2; Wes'97; CCFP; (905)720-0506

SNIDERMAN, Allan D; MUHC-Royal Victoria Hosp, 687 av des Pins O, Montreal QC H3A 1A1; Tor'65; FRCPC; IntMed; Cardiol (P.Q.). principale Médecin, McGill University Health Centre - Royal Victoria Hospital; Prof Experimental Med, McGill University; (514)934-1934; allan.sniderman@muhc.mcgill.ca.

SNIDERMAN, Barry P; 511-360 Bloor St W, Toronto ON M5S 1X1; Tor'65; FRCSC; Ophth. Staff, Mount Sinai Hospital; Staff, Baycrest Centre for Geriatric Care; University of Toronto; (416)961-8244; Fax. (416)961-0489.

SNIDERMAN, Jacob B; 2454 13th Ave W, Vancouver BC V6K 2S8; Qns'64; MCFP; CCFP; FCFP; Staff, Squamish General Hospital / Hilltop House; Staff, Providence Health Care - Mount Saint Joseph Hospital; (604)731-2952; Fax. (604)731-2925; jsnidey@gmail.com.

SNIDERMAN, Kenneth W; Univ Hlth Network-Toronto Gen, 200 Elizabeth St, Toronto ON M5G 2C4; Tor'70; MD(Med.); ABR; MB; DABR; FRCP; LMCC; FRCPC; DiagRad (Interventional Radiology). Staff Diagnostic Imaging, Mount Sinai Hospital; Staff, Toronto General Hospital - UHN; Court Staff, Sunnybrook Health Sciences Centre; Court Staff, The Hospital For Sick Children; Assoc Prof, University of Toronto; (416)340-4800 x3393; Fax. (416)593-0502.

SNIHURA, Robert; RBC Royal Bank-North Tower, 11F-200 Bay St, Toronto ON M5J 2J5; Tor'69; MD; FRCP; FRCPC; IntMed (Administrative Medicine). Vice Pres/Chief/Med Dir, RBC Financial Group; Langs: Ukrainian; (416)955-2351; Fax. (416)974-4383; robert.snihura@rbc.com.

SNODGRASS, Graham P; CML Health Care Imaging, 106-180 Vine St S, St Catharines ON L2R 7P3; Otago (New Zealand)'65; MB ChB; FRCPC; DiagRad. (905)684-6388; Fax. (905)684-6389.

SNODGRASS, James A R; Cook Medical Bldg, 328-1175 Cook St, Victoria BC V8V 4A1; Qns'89; CCFP; FCFP; Langs: Bilingual(English/French); (250)385-3465; Fax. (250)385-4532.

SNOOK, Jody E R; North Okanagan Paediatric Clin, 3-2802 34th St, Vernon BC V1T 5X1; UBC'05; FRCPC; Peds. (250)558-5506

SNOOK, Wayne R; Place Centrum Med Centre, 110-210 Centrum Blvd, Orleans ON K1E 3V7; McM'81; BSc; Officer Health Services, Royal Canadian Mounted Police; Langs: French; (613)991-0968; Fax. (613)834-3227.

SNOVIDA, Lioubov; Leila Med Clinic, 630 Leila Ave, Winnipeg MB R2V 3N7; (204)632-0024

SNOW, D Martyn; Fenwick Med Centre, 311-5595 Fenwick St, Halifax NS B3H 4M2; University of Edinburgh (Scotland)'97.

SNOW, Debbie G; Koffler Student Services Ctre, 214 College St, Toronto ON M5T 2Z9; Tor'90; MSc(OccupMed.); CCFP; FCFP; Court Staff, Women's College Hospital; Court Staff, St Michael's Hospital; (416)978-8030; Fax. (416)971-2089.

SNOW, Pamela A; Health Sciences Centre, 300 Prince Philip Dr, St. John's NL A1B 3V6; Mem'95; CCFP; FCFP; Staff Family Practice Unit, Health Sciences Centre; Asst Prof Family Med, Memorial University Of Newfoundland; (709)777-7795; Fax. (709)777-7916.

SNOW, Stephanie L; Queen Elizabeth II HSC-Victori, 456-1276 South Park St, Halifax NS B3H 2Y9; Dal'05; FRCPC; IntMed; MedOncol. Staff, Queen Elizabeth II Health Sciences Centre - Victoria General Site; (902)473-6019; Fax. (902)473-6286.

SNOW, William M F; 316 St. Peters Rd, Sydney NS B1P 4R1; Dal'71; FRCSC; Ophth. Consultant, Cape Breton Healthcare Complex; (902)539-4497; Fax. (902)539-4700; w.snow@ns.sympatico.ca.

SNOWDON, Bruce A; Windsor Health Unit, 354-1720 Howard Ave, Windsor ON N8X 5A6; Qns'81; FRCSC; PlasSurg. (519)252-4209; Fax. (519)252-0262.

SNOWDON, Jaime F; Dr Georges L Dumont Univ HC, 330 University Ave, Moncton NB E1C 2Z3; Dal'07; FRCPC; AnatPath (General Pathology). Staff, Dr Georges-L-Dumont University Hospital Centre; (506)862-4000

SNOZYK, Patricia T; Cook Street Village Health Cen, 200-1075 Pendergast St, Victoria BC V8X 0A1; Cal'89; CCFP; (250)477-5433

SNYDER, Brian L; Canadian Mental Health Assoc, 710-3601 Hwy 7 E, Markham ON L3R 0M3; Tor'86; FRCPC; Psy. (905)853-8477; Fax. (905)477-5564.

SNYDER, D Bruce; Health Link Family Practice Cl, B10-350 Conestoga Blvd, Cambridge ON N1R 7L7; Tor'71; Affil Staff, Cambridge Memorial Hospital; (519)740-5010; Fax. (519)740-6010.

SNYDER, Donna A; 4025 Elberta Ave, Niagara Falls ON L2E 6G1; Qns'69; DECH; FRCPC; Peds (Behavioural Pediatrics). (905)354-2052

SNYDER, Douglas R; 103-535 Belmont Ave W, Kitchener ON N2M 5E9; Tor'93; CCFP; FCFP; (519)578-8050; Fax. (519)578-9955.

SNYDER, Laurel J; Lake of the Woods Dist Hosp, 21 Sylvan St RR 1 Stn Main, Kenora ON P9N 3W7; Man'96; BSc; CCFP; CCFP(E.M.); FCFP; Staff, Lake of the Woods District Hospital; (807)468-9861 x231; Fax. (807)468-4316; laurels_72@yahoo.com.

SNYDER, Nathan A; 1575 Clarkson Rd, Mississauga ON L5J 2X1; Tor'90; CCFP; Ac Staff, Halton Healthcare Services Corporation - Oakville Site; University of Toronto; (905)822-4800; Fax. (905)822-1358.

SNYMAN, Adam J; Univ Hlth Network-Toronto Gen, EN 3-200 Elizabeth St, Toronto ON M5G 2C4; Orange Free State (South Africa)'97; FRCPC; Anes. Staff, Toronto General Hospital - UHN; Langs: Afrikaans; (416)340-3111; Fax. (416)340-3698.

SNYMAN, Annamarie; Lloydminster Clinic, 5120 46 St, Lloydminster AB T9V 2P7; Stellenbosch (South Africa)'88; MB ChB; Staff, Lloydminster Hospital; Physician, Jubilee Home; Physician, Lloydminster Medical Clinic; Physician, Dr Cooke Extended Care Centre; (780)875-2221; Fax. (780)875-0605.

SNYMAN, Ernst R; Smith Clinic, 1-6601 48 Ave, Camrose AB T4V 3G8; Pretoria (South Africa)'77; BSc; MB ChB; Staff, Covenant Health - St Mary's Hospital; (780)672-2425; Fax. (780)608-5896.

SNYMAN, Gertie P; 316 8 Ave W PO Box 700 Stn Main, Brooks AB T1R 1B6; (403)793-8883; Fax. (403)793-8890.

SNYMAN, Marianna S; 103A-45793 Luckakuck Way, Chilliwack BC V2R 5S3; Stellenbosch (South Africa)'86; MB ChB; LMCC; Langs: Afrikaans; (604)824-9797; drmsnyman@gmail.com.

SNYMAN, Marius R; White Clinic Associates, 100-383 Ellis St, Penticton BC V2A 4L9; Pretoria (South Africa)'94; MB ChB; CCFP; Langs: Afrikaans; (250)492-3024; mariuss@sasktel.net.

SO, Alan I; Gordon & Leslie Diamond HCC, L6-2775 Laurel St, Vancouver BC V5Z 1M9; Alb'97; FRCSC; Urol (Prostate Cancer). Staff, The Prostate Centre; Physician, Gordon & Leslie Diamond Health Care Centre; Assoc Prof, University of British Columbia; (604)875-5003; Fax. (604)875-5604; asomd@hotmail.org.

SO, Boris; Patient Networks, 157 Yonge St, Toronto ON M5C 1X7; Wes'04; CCFP; Assoc Prof, University of Toronto; (416)362-8822; Fax. (416)362-8877.

SO, C Benny; Foothills Med Centre, 1403 29 St NW, Calgary AB T2N 2T9; (Hong Kong)'80; FRCPC; DiagRad. Staff Diagnostic Radiol, Foothills Medical Centre; (403)944-1969; Fax. (403)670-1687.

SO, Cindy H; Southlake Reg Health Centre, 596 Davis Dr, Newmarket ON L3Y 2P9; Tor'07; CCFP; Staff, Southlake Regional Health Centre; (905)895-4521; Fax. (905)952-3050.

SO, Derek Y; Univ of Ottawa Heart Institute, 40 Ruskin Ave, Ottawa ON K1Y 4W7; Tor'97; FRCPC; IntMed; Cardiol. Staff, University of Ottawa Heart Institute; (613)761-4708; Fax. (613)761-4338.

SO, Dominic C Y; The Doctor's Office, 6435 Erin Mills Pky, Mississauga ON L5N 3P3; Tor'92; BSc; CCFP; Lecturer Family & Community Med, University of Toronto; (905)821-1406; Fax. (905)821-1409.

SO, Genhee; St Joseph's Healthcare, 50 Charlton Ave E, Hamilton ON L8N 4A6; McM'01; FRCPC; DiagRad. Staff, St Joseph's Healthcare - Charlton Campus; (905)522-1155

SO, Jeffrey S; Credit Valley Prof Bldg, 509-2300 Eglinton Ave W, Mississauga ON L5M 2V8; Wes'06; FRCPC; IntMed; Gastroent. (905)569-9546; Fax. (905)569-9987.

SO, Joyce; Lakeridge Hlth Corp-Oshawa, 1 Hospital Crt, Oshawa ON L1G 2B9; Tor'01; FRCPC; MedGenetics. Staff, Lakeridge Health - Oshawa Site; Langs: German; (905)433-2733; Fax. (905)721-6122.

SO, Stevenson K F; 8-1170 Burnhamthorpe Rd W, Mississauga ON L5C 4E6; (Hong Kong)'79; MRCP(UK); DCH(Lond); FHKAM(Peds.); LMCC; Langs: Cantonese; Mandarin; (905)272-1099; Fax. (905)272-8546.

SO, Vay Chi; UMF Lanaudiere Sud, 135 boul Claude-David, Repentigny QC J6A 1N6; Mon'98; (450)654-7229

SO, William I; Clearview Med Centre, 4950 137 Ave, Edmonton AB T5Y 2V4; Alb'91; CCFP; FCFP; (780)478-1999; Fax. (780)478-1166.

SO, Yan P; 202-1120 Austin Ave, Coquitlam BC V3K 3P5; UBC'58; Staff, Royal Columbian Hospital; Langs: Cantonese; (604)936-9911; Fax. (604)936-3285.

SOARE, C Alexander; St Joseph's Health Centre, 30 The Queensway, Toronto ON M6R 1B5; Tor'09; CCFP; Staff, St Joseph's Health Centre; (416)530-6000

SOARES, Claudio D N; Women's Health Concerns Clinic, FB 638-301 James St S, Hamilton ON L8P 3B6; Sao Paulo (Brazil)'89; FRCPC; Psy (Women's Mental Health). Staff, St Joseph's Healthcare - Charlton Campus; Dir/Acad Head Mood Disorder Prog, Women's Health Concerns Clinic; Assoc Prof, McMaster University; Langs: Portuguese; (905)522-1155 x32059; Fax. (905)521-6098.

SOARES, Mark A; Trillium Hlth Ctr-Mississauga, 100 Queensway W, Mississauga ON L5B 1B8; Bombay (India)'82; MB BS; DAB; FRCPC; AnatPath (Hematology Pathology). Staff Lab Med, Trillium Health Centre - Mississauga; (905)848-7297

SOBEL, Mara L; McMaster University, 1280 Main St W, Hamilton ON L8S 4K1; Ott'07; FRCSC; ObstGyn. Teacher, McMaster University; (905)521-2100

SOBERMAN, Dov D; Scarborough Hosp-Birchmount, 3030 Birchmount Rd, Scarborough ON M1W 3W3; Wes'92; CCFP; CCFP(E.M.); Ac Staff, The Scarborough Hospital - Birchmount Campus; Ac Staff, The Scarborough Hospital - General Campus; Ac Staff Emerg, Rouge Valley Health System - Centenary Health Centre Site; (416)495-2550

SOBERS, Godfrey; Bathurst Med/Dental Clinic, 301-800 Bathurst St, Toronto ON M5R 3M8; West Indies (Jamaica)'67; (416)535-4134; Fax. (416)535-4035.

SOBEY, Alan V F; University of Alberta Hosp, 3C1 12 WCM-8440 112 St NW, Edmonton AB T6G 2B7; Alb'91; FRCSC; GenSurg; Critical Care Medicine. Staff, University of Alberta Hospital; (780)860-5270; Fax. (780)229-0775.

SOBEY, Paul W H; Keary Med Centre, 107-245 Columbia St E, New Westminster BC V3L 3W4; Alb'86; CCFP; Staff, Royal Columbian Hospital; (604)521-7784; Fax. (604)521-7785; psobey@pol.net.

SOBH, Donia M A K; Queen Elizabeth II HSC, 1278 Tower Rd, Halifax NS B3H 2Y9; Mansoura University (Other Foreign)'03; Staff, Queen Elizabeth II Health Sciences Centre - Victoria General Site; (902)473-5453; Fax. (902)473-2018.

SOBH, Hoda M; Queen Elizabeth II Hosp, 1796 Summer St, Halifax NS B3H 3A7; Mansoura University (Other Foreign)'07; Staff, Queen Elizabeth II Health Sciences Centre - Halifax Infirmary Site; (902)473-2700

SOBIERA, Ruthanne M; Peterborough Reg Health Centre, 1 Hospital Dr, Peterborough ON K9J 7C5; Ott'92; DiagRad. Staff, Peterborough Regional Health Centre - Hospital Drive; (705)743-2121

SOBKIN, Paul R; Royal Jubilee Hosp, 1952 Bay St, Victoria BC V8R 1J8; UBC'92; FRCPC; DiagRad. Staff, Royal Jubilee Hospital; (250)370-8318

SOBKOWSKI, Wojciech W; Professional Arts Bldg, 2B-570 King St, Welland ON L3B 3L2; Gdansk (Poland)'83; FRCPC; IntMed. Langs: Polish; (905)732-7544; Fax. (905)732-2038; sobkowski@primus.ca.

SOBOL, Isaac H; First Nations Inuit Health Cen, 406-1138 Melville St, Vancouver BC V6E 4S3; Qns'85; MD; MCFP; MPH; CCFP; Reg Medical Officer, First Nations Inuit Health Centre; (604)666-9092

SOBOLESKI, Donald A A; Hotel-Dieu Hosp, 166 Brock St, Kingston ON K7L 5G2; Cal'87; FRCPC; DiagRad (Pediatric Radiology). Staff, Hotel-Dieu Hospital; (613)544-3310

SOBOLEV, Igor; Clinical Sciences Bldg, 8 120-152 University Campus NW, Edmonton AB T6G 2G3; (Russia (Federation))'95; FRCPC; Anes (Pain Management). Staff Anes & Pain Med, University of Alberta Hospital; (780)407-8861; Fax. (780)407-3200.

SOBOLOFF, Michael J; 722 Dovercourt Rd PO Box 416, Toronto ON M6H 4E3; Tor'66; CCFP; FCFP; Staff, Trillium Health Centre - Mississauga; Staff, Mount Sinai Hospital; Staff, Toronto General Hospital - UHN; (416)537-2527; Fax. (416)537-1280.

SOBOWALE, Oluyomi A; The Medical Centre, 707 Charlotte St, Peterborough ON K9J 7B3; Ibadan (Nigeria)'81; MB BS; FRCOG; FACOG; FRCSC; ObstGyn (Urogynecology). Staff ObstGyn, Peterborough Regional Health Centre - Hospital Drive; Assoc Staff ObstGyn, Queen's University; Langs: Yoruba; Ibo; (705)876-4529; Fax. (705)743-1449; osobowale@themedicalcentre.net.

SOBOWALE, Opeyemi A; Kildonan Med Centre, 2300 McPhillips St, Winnipeg MB R2V 3M3; (Other Foreign)'01; CCFP.

SOBREIRA, Elizabete M; CSSS du Suroît, 150 rue Saint-Thomas, Salaber-de-Valleyf QC J6T 6C1; Mon'06; CCFP; Staff, Centre Hospitalier Régional du Suroît; (450)371-9920; Fax. (450)377-1372.

SOBRIAN, Jules; 67 King St W PO Box 339, Omemee ON K0L 2W0; Tor'62; (705)799-5230

SOCCAR, Esther A M; Bank Med Centre, 1935 Bank St, Ottawa ON K1V 8A3; Alexandria (Egypt)'84; CCFP; Langs: Arabic; French; (613)521-2391; Fax. (613)521-5443.

SOCHANIWSKYJ, Orest T; 106-210 Memorial Ave, Orillia ON L3V 7V1; Tor'85; CCFP; (705)327-7984; Fax. (705)327-8004.

SOCHETT, Etienne B; The Hosp for Sick Children, 5114-555 University Ave, Toronto ON M5G 1X8; Pretoria (South Africa)'74; MB ChB; DCH; FRCPC; Peds (Bone Densitometry); Endocrin&Metab. Staff, The Hospital For Sick Children; (416)813-7041; Fax. (416)813-6304; etienne.sochett@sickkids.ca.

SOCHOCKA, Elisabeth K; B202-6941 Derry Rd, Milton ON L9T 7H5; Lodz (Poland)'78; Langs: Polish; Russian; Italian; (905)693-9961; Fax. (905)693-0982.

SOCHOCKI, Michael P; Health Sciences Centre, GC 419-820 Sherbrook St, Winnipeg MB R3A 1R9; Man'06; FRCPC; IntMed. Staff, Health Sciences Centre; (204)774-8511

SOCHOWSKI, Randall A; Fort Royal Med Bldg, 335-1900 Richmond Ave, Victoria BC V8R 4R2; UBC'83; FRCPC; IntMed; Cardiol. Staff, Royal Jubilee Hospital; Staff, Victoria General Hospital; (250)595-1551; Fax. (250)595-6793.

SOCKALINGAM, Sanjeev; Univ Hlth Network-Toronto Gen, 8EN 228-200 Elizabeth St, Toronto ON M5G 2C4; Man'03; FRCPC; Psy. Staff, Toronto General Hospital - UHN; (416)340-3762; Fax. (416)340-4198.

SOCRANSKY, Steven J; Sudbury Reg Hosp-Laurentian, 41 Ramsey Lake Rd, Sudbury ON P3E 5J1; McG'91; FRCPC; EmergMed. Staff, Health Sciences North-Laurentian Site; Langs: Spanish; French; (705)675-4700

SODER, Christian M; IWK Health Centre, PO Box 9700 Rpo CSC 5850-5980 University Ave, Halifax NS B3K 6R8; Alb'75; LMCC; NBME; BMedSci; FRCPC; FRCPC; Anes (Critical Care Medicine); Peds. Dir Paediatric Intensive Care, IWK Health Centre; Assoc Prof Peds & Anaes, Dalhousie University; Langs: German; (902)470-8031; Fax. (902)470-7425; chris.soder@iwk.nshealth.ca.

SODERMAN, Robert M; 41953 Sparta Line RR 1, Union ON N0L 2L0; Wes'80; FRCPC; Anes.

SODHI, Parvinder K; Queen Elizabeth II Hosp, 10W-1276 South Park St, Halifax NS B3H 2Y9; Bangalore (India)'00; MB BS; Anes. Staff, Queen Elizabeth II Health Sciences Centre - Victoria General Site; (902)473-2331; Fax. (902)423-9454.

SODHI, Sumeet K; Univ Hlth Network-Toronto Western Hosp, 2W404-399 Bathurst St, Toronto ON M5T 2S8; Tor'97; CCFP; Medical Staff, Toronto Western Hospital - University Health Network; Langs: Bilingual(English/French); (416)603-5888 x2

SODHI, Vijay; 208 Greenway St S PO Box 400, Crystal City MB R0K 0N0; (Other Foreign)'03; Staff, Rock Lake Health District Hospital; (204)873-2424; Fax. (204)873-2206.

SOEDER, Samantha P; Rapids Family Health Team, 1150 Pontiac Dr, Sarnia ON N7S 3A7; McM'08; CCFP; (519)339-8949; Fax. (519)339-9022; ssoeder@rapidsfhteam.ca.

SOEHN, Scott A; Beaumont Family Med Assoc, 4-5102 49 Ave, Beaumont AB T4X 1E4; Cal'97; CCFP; (780)929-5400; Fax. (780)929-2126.

SOENEN, Gary M; West Street Health Centre, 202-216 West St, Simcoe ON N3Y 1S8; Alb'83; FRCSC; GenSurg. (519)426-3366; Fax. (519)426-3267; gmsoenen@amtelecom.net.

SOETAERT, Shayne C J; Shayne Soetaert Prof Corp, PO Box 2380, Fernie BC V0B 1M0; Alb'92; CCFP; (250)423-6404; Fax. (250)423-7227.

SOFRONOVA, Elionora P; Northfield Med Centre, 206-99 Northfield Dr E, Waterloo ON N2K 3P9; N Testemitanu State Medical University (Other Foreign)'79; CCFP; Langs: Romanian; Russian; (519)744-2592; esofronova@ewfht.ca.

SOGBEIN, S Kolawole; Medical & Dental Bldg, 401-1221 Algonquin Ave, North Bay ON P1B 4Y3; Ibadan (Nigeria)'73; MB BS; FICS; FACS; DABU; FRCSC; Urol (Urodynamics). Staff Consultant, North Bay Regional Health Centre - Regional Mental Health; Asst Prof Surg, Northern Ontario School of Medicine; Langs: Yoruba; (705)474-1884; Fax. (705)474-6261; ssogbein@cogeco.ca.

SOGBESAN, Enitan A; St Joseph's Comm Health Centre, 2757 King St E, Hamilton ON L8G 5E4; Lagos (Nigeria)'86; FRCSC; Ophth. Staff, St Joseph's Healthcare Hamilton - King Campus; (905)552-1155; esogbesan@mcmaster.ca.

SOGHRATI, Kamyar; Credit Valley Med Arts Centre, 512-2000 Credit Valley Rd, Mississauga ON L5M 4N4; Tor'01; FRCPC; IntMed; Respir. (905)569-1700; Fax. (905)828-1690.

SOH, Joo-Meng; Trillium Hlth Ctr-Mississauga, 100 Queensway W, Mississauga ON L5B 1B8; Tor'98; FRCPC; IntMed. Staff, Trillium Health Centre - Mississauga; (905)848-7100

SOHAIL, Mohammad K; Creative Psychotherapy Clinic, 213 Byron St S, Whitby ON L1N 4P7; Peshawar (Pakistan)'74; FRCPC; Psy. Langs: Persian; Urdu; (905)666-7253; Fax. (905)666-4397; welcome@drsohail.com.

SOHAL, Avtar S; The Wharton Med Clinic, 14-414 Victoria Ave N, Hamilton ON L8L 5G8; Wes'00; FRCPC; IntMed (Family Medicine); Nephrol. Staff, Halton Healthcare Services Corporation - Oakville Site; Langs: Punjabi; (905)527-7663; Fax. (905)527-7665.

SOHAL, Barjinder S; The Medical Place, 300-799 Bloor St W, Toronto ON M6G 1L8; Man'01; CCFP; Langs: Punjabi; (647)349-0053; Fax. (647)349-0063.

SOHAL, Jasdeep S; Southdale Family Med Centre, 395 Southdale Rd E, London ON N6E 1A2; (Other Foreign)'00; CCFP; (519)691-0100

SOHAL, Parmjit S; 15156 Fraser Hwy, Surrey BC V3R 3P1; Alb'95; BSc; MSc; PhD; CCFP; FCFP; Staff Privil, Surrey Memorial Hospital; Clinical Asst Prof Family Pract, University of British Columbia; Langs: Punjabi; Hindi; (604)585-9696; Fax. (604)585-9688; drsohal@shaw.ca.

SOHI, Davedeep S; Womens College Hosp, 76 Grenville St, Toronto ON M5S 1B2; UBC'08; IntMed. Staff, Women's College Hospital; (416)323-6400

SOHI, Herpreet S; 504-960 Lawrence Ave W, North York ON M6A 3B5; Wes'91; FACS; FRCSC; GenSurg (Endoscopic Surgery). Ac Staff, Humber River Regional Hospital - Finch Avenue Site; Staff, Humber River Regional Hospital - Church Street Site; Lecturer, University of Toronto; Langs: Punjabi; (416)782-2616; Fax. (416)782-5899.

SOHI, Julia; Hopital Jean-Talon, 1385 rue Jean-Talon E, Montreal QC H2E 1S6; Mon'03; CCFP; Staff, Centre Hospitalier Rouyn-Noranda; Staff, CSSS du Coeur de l'Isle Hôpital Jean-Talon; (514)495-6767

SOHI, Kultar S; Hermitage Med Clinic, PO Box 40, Hermitage NL A0H 1S0; Kerala (India)'83; MB BS; (709)883-2222; Fax. (709)883-2292.

SOHI, Paul S; Saint John Reg Hosp Facility, PO Box 2100 Stn Main 400 University Ave, Saint John NB E2L 4L2; McG'88; FRCPC; IntMed (Hypertension); Nephrol. Staff, Saint John Regional Hospital; Asst Prof Med, Dalhousie University; (506)648-6843; Fax. (506)648-7796.

SOHI, Ravinder K; 43-3075 Ridgeway Dr, Mississauga ON L5L 5M6; Alb'93; BMedSci; CCFP; FCFP; Lecturer Family & Community Med, University of Toronto; Langs: Punjabi; (905)828-6061; Fax. (905)820-9468.

SOHLA, Anand; Tillsonburg Family Physicians, 594 Broadway St, Tillsonburg ON N4G 5K9; Wes'86; Staff, Tillsonburg District Memorial Hospital; Langs: Hindi; (519)842-3636; Fax. (519)842-9522.

SOHMER, Benjamin; Univ of Ottawa Heart Institute, H2410-40 Ruskin St, Ottawa ON K1Y 4W7; Dal'00; FRCPC; Anes. Staff, University of Ottawa Heart Institute; (613)761-4379; Fax. (613)761-4925.

SOHMER, Stephen; North Island Orthopaedics, 301-909 Island Hwy, Campbell River BC V9W 2C2; McG'01; MDCM; FRCSC; OrthSurg (Sports Medicine). Langs: Bilingual(English/French); (250)287-2174; Fax. (250)287-2679.

SOHN, Adrian B T; Guelph Family Health Team, 83 Dawson Rd, Guelph ON N1H 1B1; McM'85; CCFP; Staff, Guelph General Hospital; Langs: Hausa; French; (519)837-2242; Fax. (519)763-4315.

SOHN, Brenda; St Joseph's Health Centre, 30 The Queensway, Toronto ON M6R 1B5; Wes'07; ObstGyn. Staff, St Joseph's Health Centre; (416)530-6000

SOHN, Melanie; William Osler HC-Brampton, S1 184-2100 Bovaird Dr E, Brampton ON L6R 3J7; Alb'05; CCFP; CCFP(E.M.); Staff, William Osler Health System - Brampton Civic Hospital; (905)494-2120

SOIBELMAN, Felix; University of Alberta Hosp, 1A7 19-8440 112 St NW, Edmonton AB T6G 2B7; Alb'01; FRCPC; EmergMed. Staff Emerg Med, University of Alberta Hospital; (780)407-8433; Fax. (780)407-3314.

SOICHER, Avrum A; Finchgate Med Centre, 216-40 Finchgate Blvd, Brampton ON L6T 3J1; McG'90; FRCPC; IntMed; Respir. Staff, William Osler Health System - Brampton Civic Hospital; Langs: French; (905)456-2456; Fax. (905)456-8768.

SOIN, Jasminder P; Elbow River Healing Lodge, 1213 4 St SW, Calgary AB T2R 0X7; Qns'03; CCFP; Staff, Elbow River Healing Lodge; (403)955-6600

SOJAT, Alexander J; Community Psych Service, 1350 St. Andrews Ave, North Vancouver BC V7L 3L4; Warwick Medical School (England)'08; MB ChB; Staff, Gordon & Leslie Diamond Health Care Centre; (604)983-6020

SOKAL, John E M; Health Sciences Centre, GF 201-820 Sherbrook St, Winnipeg MB R3A 1R9; Man'89; BSc(Med); CCFP; CCFP(E.M.); Ac Staff, Health Sciences Centre; (204)774-6511

SOKAR-TODD, Hanan B; 107-3305 Harvester Rd, Burlington ON L7N 3N2; McM'08; MSc; PhD(UK); CCFP; Clinical Asst Prof, McMaster University; (905)630-5988; Fax. (905)635-5805.

SOKLOFSKE, Barry A; Medicine Hat Reg Hosp, 666 5 St SW, Medicine Hat AB T1A 4H6; Alb'79; Anes. Staff, Medicine Hat Regional Hospital; (403)529-8000; Fax. (403)528-8101.

SOKO, Phinda D; Albert Park Family Med Centre, 3992 Albert St, Regina SK S4S 3R1; (Other Foreign)'83; (306)584-3833; Fax. (306)585-3833.

SOKOL, Denis S; Lake Country Family Practice, 1-9966 Pollard Rd, Winfield BC V4V 1Z4; Sask'76; BSc; (250)766-3938; Fax. (250)766-5231.

SOKOL, Lorne W; 111-1649 Dufferin St, Toronto ON M6H 4H5; Tor'85; CAFCI; CCFP; FCFP; Langs: Italian; (416)654-9993; Fax. (416)654-3432.

SOKOLENKO, Marina; Canadian Forces Hlth Serv Ctre, PO Box 99000 Stn Forces Operational Trauma, Halifax NS B3K 5X5; Riga (Russia (Federation))'87; FRCPC; Psy. Staff, Canadian Forces Health Services Centre (Atlantic); (902)721-8884; Fax. (902)721-1295.

SOKOLIC, Larry J; Family Health Team, 2 Water Lane, Kirkland Lake ON P2N 3M6; Philadelphia (USA)'87; (705)567-2224; Fax. (705)567-3838.

SOKOLIES, Rex B; Seven Oaks Gen Hosp, 2300 McPhillips St, Winnipeg MB R2V 3M3; Man'93; BSc; CCFP; Staff Emerg, Seven Oaks General Hospital; University of Manitoba; Langs: German; (204)632-7133; Fax. (204)697-1896; rsokolies@sogh.mb.ca.

SOKOLOFF, Dina R; Nepean Med Centre, 101-1 Centrepointe Dr, Ottawa ON K2G 6E2; Ott'91; CCFP; FCFP; Langs: French; Hebrew; (613)224-6339

SOKOLON, Daryl G; The Medical Centre FHT, PO Box 4200 Stn Main 707 Charlotte St, Peterborough ON K9J 7B3; Sask'88; Staff, Peterborough Regional Health Centre - Hospital Drive; (705)743-6222; Fax. (705)743-6288.

SOKOLOV, Stephen T H; Addiction & Mental Hlth-Clarke, 4301-100 Stokes St, Toronto ON M6J 1H4; Man'87; FRCPC; Psy (Mood Disorders). Staff, Centre for Addiction & Mental Health (CAMH) - College Street Site; Asst Prof Psy, University of Toronto; (416)535-8501 x4521; Fax. (416)979-6821.

SOKOLOVA, Elena A; Ontario Reg Stroke Network, 201-984 Oliver Rd, Thunder Bay ON P7B 7C7; Moscow Medical Stomatology Institute (Russia (Federation))'97; Langs: Russian; (807)684-6700; Fax. (807)684-5883.

SOKOLOWSKA, Anna M; Central Med Bldg, 104A-1105 Carling Ave, Ottawa ON K1Y 4G5; Edinburgh (Scotland)'46; FRCPC; Psy. Langs: Polish; (613)729-8713

SOKOLOWSKI, Colleen A; Red Deer Reg Hosp Centre, PO Box 5030 Stn Postal Box Ctr 3F-3942 50A Ave, Red Deer AB T4N 6R2; Qns'96; FRCPC; IntMed; Critical Care Medicine (Respirology). Staff, Red Deer Regional Hospital Centre; (403)343-4446; Fax. (403)358-4342.

SOKOLOWSKI, Danuta; Roblin Med Clinic, 200A Thompson Dr, Winnipeg MB R3J 3E1; (Poland)'71; Langs: Polish.

SOKOLUK, Craig A; Toronto East Gen & Orth Hosp, K407-825 Coxwell Ave, Toronto ON M4C 3E7; Cal'89; ABIM; FRCPC; IntMed; Rheum. Ac Staff Rheumatol, Toronto East General Hospital Inc; (416)778-9692; Fax. (416)778-7669.

SOLAND, Valerie L; CHUM-Hop Notre-Dame, 1560 rue Sherbrooke E, Montreal QC H2L 4M1; Sher'88; FRCPC; Neur (Movement Disorders); Electroenceph (P.Q.). Staff, Centre Hospitalier l'Université de Montréal (CHUM) - Hôpital Notre-Dame; Langs: Bilingual(French/English); (514)890-8123; Fax. (514)412-7711; vsoland@videotron.ca.

SOLANO, Edward B; 203-3040 Tutt St, Kelowna BC V1Y 2H5; Alb'94; MSc; FRCSC; GenSurg (Hepatobiliary & Pancreatic Surgery). Staff General Surgeon, Kelowna General Hospital; (250)763-2226; Fax. (250)861-5937.

SOLANO SALAZAR, Tanya G; The Hosp for Sick Children, 555 University Ave, Toronto ON M5G 1X8; (Costa Rica)'04; Staff, The Hospital For Sick Children; (416)813-7654

SOLARIC, Bojana; Univ Hlth Network-Toronto Gen, 200 Elizabeth St, Toronto ON M5G 2C4; Belgrade (Serbia)'59; DAB; FRCPC; Anes (Cardiovascular Anesthesia). Staff, Toronto General Hospital - UHN; Asst Prof, University of Toronto; Langs: Serbian; (416)340-4800

SOLARICH, Stoyan; North York Med Arts Bldg, 306-1333 Sheppard Ave E, North York ON M2J 1V1; Belgrade (Serbia)'54; Assoc Staff, North York General Hospital; Langs: Croatian; Serbian; (416)494-7452; Fax. (416)494-6180.

SOLARTE THOMAS, Carlos E; University of Alberta Hosp, 2 133 CSB-8440 112 St NW, Edmonton AB T6G 2B7; Universidad del Cauca (Other Foreign)'94; Staff, University of Alberta Hospital; (780)407-6417; Fax. (780)407-6881.

SOLBRIG, Marylou V; Health Sciences Centre, GF543-820 Sherbrook St, Winnipeg MB R3A 1R9; Staff, Health Sciences Centre; (204)774-8511

SOLCOVA, Silvia; Tamarack Med Clinic, 191-1500 Cranbrook St N, Cranbrook BC V1C 3S8; P J Safarik (Slovakia)'98; CCFP; (250)426-7724; Fax. (250)426-0671.

SOLDEVILA, Emmanuel; Clinique Med 3000 Inc, 3000 rue Belanger, Montreal QC H1Y 1A9; Laval'87; Staff, CSSS de la Minganie; ac Staff, CSSS de Quebec-Sud; Staff, Centre Hospitalier Universitaire De Québec - Pavillon De St-françois-d'assise; (514)376-7702

SOLE, Michael J; 4N 488-585 University Ave, Toronto ON M5G 2N2; Tor'66; ABIM; FRCPC; Cardiol (Hypertension). Staff, Toronto General Hospital - UHN; Staff, Toronto Western Hospital - University Health Network; Staff, Mount Sinai Hospital; Prof Med & Physiol, University of Toronto; (416)340-3471; Fax. (416)340-4030; michael.sole@uhn.on.ca.

SOLES, John A; Clearwater Med Centre, 258 Park Dr, Clearwater BC V0E 1N0; UBC'86; (250)674-3319; Fax. (250)674-2470.

SOLEZ, Kim; University of Alberta Hosp, 5B4 02-8440 112 St NW, Edmonton AB T6G 2B7; Rochester(NY) (USA)'72; FRCPC; AnatPath. Staff, University of Alberta Hospital; Teach Staff Path, University of Alberta; (780)407-2607; Fax. (780)407-2608; kim.solez@ualberta.ca.

SOLH, Ziad; Hamilton HS-McMaster Site, PO Box 2000 Stn Lcd 1 1200 Main St W, Hamilton ON L8N 3Z5; Ott'06; FRCPC; Peds. Staff, Hamilton Health Sciences Centre - McMaster University Medical Centre; (905)521-2100

SOLIGNAC, Alain L; Ctr Hosp de Verdun, 4000 boul Lasalle, Verdun QC H4G 2A3; Paris (France)'68; Cardiol (P.Q.). ac Staff, Centre Hospitalier de Verdun; (514)362-1000 x2447

SOLIMAN, Ahmed O M; St Michael's Hosp, 30 Bond St, Toronto ON M5B 1W8; Asyut University (Other Foreign)'98; Anes. (416)864-5071

SOLIMAN, Ehab S; Stellarton Med Centre, PO Box 2600 10 Jubilee Ave, Stellarton NS B0K 1S0; Ain Shams (Egypt)'86; MB ChB; CCFP; FCFP; Staff, Aberdeen Regional Hospital; Langs: Arabic; (902)752-0575; Fax. (902)752-0568; dr.ehabsoliman@gmail.com.

SOLIMAN, Gamal M L; D-210 Martindale Rd, St Catharines ON L2R 6P9; Cairo (Egypt)'78; MB ChB; ABIM; MSc; FRCPC; IntMed; Nephrol. Langs: Arabic; (905)346-0170; Fax. (905)346-0338; gsoliman@primus.ca.

SOLIMAN, Hany; Odette Sunnybrook Cancer Ctre, T2 181-2075 Bayview Ave, Toronto ON M4N 3M5; Tor'05; FRCPC; RadOncol. Staff, The Credit Valley Hospital; Staff, Sunnybrook Health Sciences Centre; Langs: Arabic; (416)480-4951

SOLIMAN, Henry; Radimed West Island, 215 rue Frobisher, Pointe-Claire QC H9R 4R9; Alexandria (Egypt)'69; DiagRad (P.Q.). Staff, Lakeshore General Hospital - Pointe Claire; (514)697-9941; Fax. (514)697-3711.

SOLIMAN, Karim A F; Lakeridge Hlth Corp-Oshawa, 1 Hospital Crt, Oshawa ON L1G 2B9; Ott'05; FRCPC; IntMed; Critical Care Medicine. Staff, Lakeridge Health - Oshawa Site; (905)985-7321

SOLIMAN, Magdi F L; Wheat City Med Clinic, C1-1711C Kirkcaldy Dr, Brandon MB R7A 0B9; (204)727-1711; Fax. (204)727-1707.

SOLIMAN, Samuel R H; Newlife Fertility Centre, 3-263 Queen St E, Brampton ON L6W 4K6; Cairo (Egypt)'85; FRCSC; ObstGyn (Infertility). Staff, William Osler Health System - Brampton Civic Hospital; (905)453-8477; Fax. (905)453-8234; drsoliman@newlifefertility.com.

SOLIMAN, Samy; St Thomas Elgin Gen Hosp, 189 Elm St, St Thomas ON N5R 5C4; Ain Shams (Egypt)'82; FRCPC; IntMed. Staff, St Thomas Elgin General Hospital; Langs: Arabic; (519)631-2020; Fax. (519)631-1825.

SOLIMAN, Sherine S R; 101-586 Argus Rd, Oakville ON L6J 3J3; Ain Shams (Egypt)'93; CCFP; Ac Staff, Halton Healthcare Services Corporation - Oakville Site; (905)842-2410; Fax. (905)842-7376.

SOLIMAN, Wassim G F; William Osler HC-Brampton, 2100 Bovaird Dr E, Brampton ON L6R 3J7; Cairo (Egypt)'81; MB ChB; FRCPC; Psy (Adolescent Psychiatry). Staff, William Osler Health System - Brampton Civic Hospital; Staff, Regional Mental Health Care-St Joseph's Health Care; Langs: Arabic; (905)494-2120

SOLIMANO, Alfonso J; Children's & Women's HC of BC, 1R46-4480 Oak St, Vancouver BC V6H 3V4; Lima (Peru)'78; ABPeds; AB; FRCPC; Peds (Neonatology). Ac Staff, BC Children's Hospital; Ac Staff, BC Women's Hospital & Health Centre; Clin Prof, University of British Columbia; Langs: Spanish; (604)875-2135; Fax. (604)875-3106.

SOLISH, Nowell J; Women's College Hosp, 76 Grenville St, Toronto ON M5S 1B2; Tor'90; FRCPC; Derm. Staff, Women's College Hospital; (416)323-7732; Fax. (416)323-6306.

SOLLARS, Susan J; Main Med Centre, BC-194B Main St, Ottawa ON K1S 1C2; Sask'80; (613)233-7317; drsollars@gmail.com.

SOLLAZZO, David J; St Joseph's Healthcare, 50 Charlton Ave E, Hamilton ON L8N 4A6; McM'08; CCFP; CCFP(E.M.); Staff, St Joseph's Healthcare - Charlton Campus; Langs: Bilingual(English/French); (905)522-1155

SOLLAZZO, John N; Mackenzie Richmond Hill Hosp, 10 Trench St, Richmond Hill ON L4C 4Z3; Tor'07; CCFP; CCFP(E.M.); Staff, Mackenzie Richmond Hill Hospital; Langs: Bilingual(English/French); (905)883-1212

SOLLEREDER, Gordon J; Allin Clinic, 10155 120 St NW, Edmonton AB T5K 2A2; Alb'77; (780)482-7551; Fax. (780)488-2056.

SOLMON, Jordan B; Jane-Finch Family Health Team, 136A-1 Yorkgate Blvd Box 105, North York ON M3N 3A1; Wes'98; CCFP; Langs: Spanish; (416)745-4555; Fax. (416)745-0786; jb_solmon@hotmail.com.

SOLMUNDSON, Kara P; Copeman Healthcare Centre, 400-1128 Hornby St, Vancouver BC V6Z 2L4; Man'06; CCFP; (604)707-2273

SOLNIK, M Charles; City Centre Med Clinic, 101-3420 Hurontario St, Mississauga ON L5B 4A9; Tor'79; Staff, Trillium Health Centre - Mississauga; Langs: Hebrew; (905)273-3176

SOLOMON, Jill K; The Scarborough Hosp-Gen Div, 3050 Lawrence Ave E, Scarborough ON M1P 2V5; McG'98; FRCPC; Peds. Staff, The Scarborough Hospital - General Campus; Langs: Bilingual(French/English); (416)970-7474; Fax. (416)287-3775.

SOLOMON, Leigh; North York Gen Hosp, 4001 Leslie St, North York ON M2K 1E1; McM'83; FRCPC; Psy. Med Staff, North York General Hospital; Lecturer, University of Toronto; (416)756-6655; Fax. (416)756-6671.

SOLOMON, Leon D; 107-5775 ch Cote-des-Neiges, Montreal QC H3S 2S9; Sask'64; DAB; FRCSC; Ophth (Cataract & Refractive). principale Staff Ophth, Sir Mortimer B Davis Jewish General; assoc Prof, McGill University; (514)341-3335; Fax. (514)341-4240.

SOLOMON, Leslie J; Club Tiny Tots, 3550-6900 boul Decarie, Cote Saint-Luc QC H3X 2T8; McG'03; BSc(Physiol); CCFP; Langs: French; (514)342-9911; Fax. (514)342-2911.

SOLOMON, Leslie V; 1483 Main St W, Hamilton ON L8S 1E1; Tor'72; CCFP; FCFP; Assoc Staff, St Joseph's Healthcare - Charlton Campus; Active Teach. Staff, McMaster University; Langs: Hungarian; (905)523-6114; Fax. (905)523-1616.

SOLOMON, M A Andrew; 1867 Lenester Ave, Ottawa ON K2A 3X5; Marseille (France)'76; DPsy; FRCPC; Psy (Cognitive Therapy). Consultant, The Ottawa Hospital - General Campus; Clin Lecturer Psy, University of Ottawa; Langs: Bilingual(English/French); (613)231-4952; Fax. (613)231-4956.

SOLOMON, Martin L; SMBD Jewish Gen Hosp, 3755 ch Cote-Sainte-Catherine, Montreal QC H3T 1E2; Qns'61; DPsy; Psy (Child Psychiatry & Family Therapy). Staff, Sir Mortimer B Davis Jewish General; adj Prof, McGill University; Langs: Bilingual(French/English); (514)340-8222 x5619; Fax. (514)340-7930; mls@magnet.ca.

SOLOMON, Melinda P; The Hosp for Sick Children, 4534-555 University Ave, Toronto ON M5G 1X8; Tor'93; Peds; FRCPC; Peds (Pediatric Respiratory Medicine); Respir. Staff, The Hospital For Sick Children; Assoc Prof Peds, University of Toronto; (416)813-6248; Fax. (416)813-6246; melinda.solomon@sickkids.ca.

SOLOMON, Muriel G; 508 15 Ave SW, Calgary AB T2R 0R2; Alb'75; CCFP; FCFP; Court Staff, Rockyview General Hospital; Langs: Urdu; (403)398-5449; Fax. (403)229-1759.

SOLOMON, Natalia; University of Alberta Hosp, 2B3 12-8440 112 St NW, Edmonton AB T6G 2B7; Vitebsk Medical Institute (Other Foreign)'95; FRCPC; MedMicrobiol (Infectious Diseases). Staff Katz Group Centre, University of Alberta Hospital; Staff Microbiol, Provincial Laboratory for Public Health for Northern Alberta; Clinical Asst Prof, University of Alberta; Langs: Russian; Hebrew; (780)407-7242; Fax. (780)407-3864.

SOLOMON, Peter H; Hull Hosp, 116 boul Lionel-Emond, Gatineau QC J8Y 1W7; McG'88; BSc; FRCPC; Anes. Staff, Hull Hospital; adj Prof Anes, McGill University; Langs: English; French; (819)595-6000; petersolomon@sympatico.ca.

SOLOMON, Philip R; 57 Centre St, Thornhill ON L4J 1G2; Tor'94; FRCSC; Otol (Head & Neck Surgery). Staff, St Michael's Hospital; Staff, Mackenzie Richmond Hill Hospital; Staff, William Osler Health System - Etobicoke General Hospital; Lecturer, University of Toronto; (905)764-0774; Fax. (905)881-2393.

SOLOMON, Robert S; Markham College Med Clinic, 401-474 College St, Toronto ON M6G 1A4; Dal'89; BSc(Anatomy); DAB(Derm.); FRCPC; Derm. Langs: French; (416)921-0880; Fax. (416)921-0088.

SOLOMON, Sukumar D; Brandongate Med Clinic, 6-4025 Brandon Gate Dr, Mississauga ON L4T 3Z9; Ott'78; Langs: Sinhalese; Tamil; (905)978-2831

SOLOMONS, Kevin; 211-2628 Granville St, Vancouver BC V6H 4B4; Cape Town (South Africa)'78; MB ChB; FRCPC; Psy (Geriatric Psychiatry). Staff Psy, UBC Hospital - Koerner Pavillion; (604)733-3557

SOLONYNA, Daniel; Lakeshore Gen Hosp, 310-175 av Stillview, Pointe-Claire QC H9R 4S3; Strasbourg (France)'79; FRCPC; Psy. Staff, Lakeshore General Hospital - Pointe Claire; Langs: French; (514)630-2010 x2015; Fax. (514)630-5184.

SOLORZANO GUTIERREZ, Silma; CSSS de Saint-Jerome, 290 rue de Montigny, Saint-Jerome QC J7Z 5T3; Staff, Hôtel-Dieu de Saint-Jérôme; (450)432-2777

SOLOW, Henry L; Markham Stouffville Hlth Ctre, 407-377 Church St, Markham ON L6B 1A1; McM'84; ABIM; FRCPC; IntMed (Hematology)., Markham Stouffville Hospital; Associate Med, Princess Margaret Hospital - University Health Network; Langs: Polish; (905)472-7072; Fax. (905)472-0529.

SOLTANI-KHORSHIDI, Nazila; 6-2755 Lougheed Hwy, Port Coquitlam BC V3B 5Y9; (Other Foreign)'02; CCFP; (604)552-9140

SOLTY, Heidi L; Sunridge Adult Mental Health, 200-2580 32 St NE, Calgary AB T1Y 7M8; Cal'05; FRCPC; Psy. Staff, Peter Lougheed Centre; (403)944-9749; Fax. (403)944-9787.

SOLTYS, George I M; 406-2984 boul Taschereau, Greenfield Park QC J4V 2G9; Rennes (France)'80; FRCPC; IntMed; Nephrol. Chef Nephrol, Hopital Charles LeMoyne; Langs: French; (450)671-7160; Fax. (450)466-5045; george.soltys@rrsss16.gouv.qc.ca.

SOLTYS, Katherine M; Ottawa Reg Cancer Centre, 503 Smyth Rd, Ottawa ON K1H 1C4; Sask'87; Staff, The Ottawa Hospital - General Campus; Physician, Ottawa Regional Cancer Centre; (613)737-7700; Fax. (613)247-3504.

SOLVEN, Frederick G; Fredericton Med Clinic, 302-1015 Regent St, Fredericton NB E3B 6H5; UBC'76; FRCPC; IntMed. (506)457-4787; Fax. (506)458-0478.

SOLWAY, Eric W; High Park Health Centre, 410-2333 Dundas St W, Toronto ON M6R 3A6; Tor'91; CCFP; Staff, St Joseph's Health Centre; (416)537-7000; Fax. (416)537-0132.

SOLYLO, G Michael A; St Mary's Gen Hosp, 911 Queen's Blvd, Kitchener ON N2M 1B2; Wes'94; FRCPC; Anes. Staff, St Mary's General Hospital; (519)744-3311

SOLYMOSS, Susan; St Mary's Hosp Centre, 3830 av Lacombe, Montreal QC H3T 1M5; McG'81; FRCPC; IntMed; Hem. Staff, McGill University Health Centre - Montreal General Campus; Chef hématol, St Mary's Hospital Centre; Langs: French; (514)345-3511 x3136

SOLYOM, Ildiko E; Oakmont Med Centre, 220-809 41st Ave W, Vancouver BC V5Z 2N6; Budapest (Hungary)'51; FRCPC; Psy. Langs: Hungarian; (604)261-6454; Fax. (604)261-6454; ildi21@shaw.ca.

SOMAIAH, Nayana T; Regent Park Comm Health Centre, 465 Dundas St E, Toronto ON M5A 2B2; Bangalore (India)'91; CCFP; (416)203-4507; Fax. (416)364-0822.

SOMAN, Teesta B; The Hosp For Sick Children, 555 University Ave, Toronto ON M5G 1X8; Delhi (India)'93; Staff, The Hospital For Sick Children; Langs: Bengali; Hindi; (416)813-5668

SOMANI, Arif; McMaster Univ Health Sciences, 1280 Main St W, Hamilton ON L8S 4K1; Tor'93; FRCPC; Peds; Critical Care Medicine. (905)521-2100; Fax. (905)570-8973.

SOMANI, Karim; 224 King St E, Brockville ON K6V 1C6; Alb'02; FRCSC; GenSurg. (613)498-0192; Fax. (613)498-0194.

SOMANI, Mansurali R; Fairmont Centre, 7-32540 Logan Ave, Mission BC V2V 6G3; Sambalpur (India)'72; DObst(Dublin); DRCOG(Lond); CCFP; FCFP; Langs: Gujarati; Hindi; Punjabi; (604)826-4159; Fax. (604)826-4860; a_msomani@shaw.ca.

SOMANI, Parviz N; Parkland Med Associates, 205-505 Queen St, Spruce Grove AB T7X 2V2; Nairobi (Kenya)'73; (780)962-2001; Fax. (780)962-8176.

SOMANI, Rizwan; Glover Med Clinic, 101-5796 Glover Rd, Langley BC V3A 4H9; Leeds (England)'88; MB ChB; DCH; MRC; (604)530-3233; Fax. (604)534-4580.

SOMANI, Rizwan; Alberta Retina Consultants, 400-10924 107 Ave NW, Edmonton AB T5H 0X5; Tor'01; FRCSC; Ophth (Retina). Assoc Prof, Royal Alexandra Hospital; (780)448-1801; Fax. (780)448-1809.

SOMANI, Salim; Parkland Med Associates, 205-505 Queen St, Spruce Grove AB T7X 2V2; Nairobi (Kenya)'73; (780)962-2001; Fax. (780)962-8176.

SOMANI, Shelyn; Northwest Wellness Centre, 10031 100 Ave, Grande Prairie AB T8V 0V2; (Grenada)'06; (780)532-2205; Fax. (780)532-0037; shelyn_s@yahoo.com.

SOMANI, Sohel; 401-7900 Hurontario St, Brampton ON L6Y 0P6; Tor'98; FRCSC; Ophth. Ac Staff Ophth, Humber River Regional Hospital - Finch Avenue Site; Assoc Staff, Princess Margaret Hospital - University Health Network; Asst Prof Ophth & Vision Sciences, University of Toronto; Langs: Gujarati; (905)456-9500; Fax. (905)456-9508; s.somani@utoronto.ca.

SOMASEKARAM, Gnanasekaram; Centennial Prof Centre, 81 Exhibition St, Kentville NS B4N 1C2; Jaffna University (India)'99; MB BS; (902)678-3466

SOMASUNDARAM, Uthayakumaran; Dr Charles A Janeway CHC, 3J 228-300 Prince Philip Dr, St. John's NL A1B 3V6; Jaffna (Sri Lanka)'92; MB BS; CCFP; Staff Surgery Day Care, Janeway Children's Health & Rehabilitation Centre; (709)570-1788

SOMER, Jerry A; 290 Markham Rd, Scarborough ON M1J 3C5; Tor'74; Staff, The Scarborough Hospital - General Campus; (416)266-8000; Fax. (416)266-8007; drsomer@rogers.com.

SOMERA, Saundra-Lisa; Ctr Hosp de Verdun, 4000 boul Lasalle, Verdun QC H4G 2A3; Mon'91; Staff, Centre Hospitalier de Verdun; Langs: English; (514)362-1000

SOMERS, Andrea D; Medcan Health Mgmt Inc, 1500-150 York St, Toronto ON M5H 3S5; McM'03; CCFP; CCFP(E.M.); Staff, Toronto General Hospital - UHN; Staff, Medcan Health Management Inc; (416)350-5688; Fax. (146)350-5981.

SOMERS, Gino R; The Hosp For Sick Children, 555 University Ave, Toronto ON M5G 1X8; Monash (Australia)'91; Staff, The Hospital For Sick Children; (416)813-5430; Fax. (416)813-5974; gino.somers@sickkids.ca.

SOMERS, Patrick A; Spryfield Family Med Clinic, 315 Herring Cove Rd, Halifax NS B3R 1V5; Dublin (Ireland)'87; MB ChB; CCFP; (902)479-0025; Fax. (902)479-2627.

SOMERS, Sangeeta R; James Paton Mem Hosp, 125 Trans Canada Hwy, Gander NL A1V 1P7; Natal (South Africa)'84; FRCPC; AnatPath. Pathologist, James Paton Memorial Hospital; (709)256-5705; Fax. (709)256-5674; ssomers@cehcib.nf.ca.

SOMERS, Sat; McMaster Univ Med Centre, 1200 Main St W, Hamilton ON L8N 3Z5; Sheffield (England)'68; MB ChB; DABR; FRCPC; DiagRad (Gastrointestinal Radiology). Staff, Hamilton Health Sciences Centre - McMaster Children's Hospital; Staff, Guelph General Hospital; Teach Staff, McMaster University; (905)690-3171; somers@mcmaster.ca.

SOMERSALL, Allan C; 100 City Centre Dr, Mississauga ON L5B 2C9; Tor'89; PhD; (416)356-1770; Fax. (905)833-4281.

SOMERSALL, Lee-Anne A; Harborn Med Associates, 510-89 Queens Way W, Mississauga ON L5B 2V2; Washington(DC) (USA)'04; CCFP; (905)273-4380; Fax. (905)273-4335.

SOMERSET, David A; Gulf Canada Square, 300-401 9 Ave SW, Calgary AB T2P 3C5; Southampton (England)'92; FRCSC; ObstGyn. (403)284-0230; Fax. (403)210-8397.

SOMERTON, Stephen C; Terrace Hill Med Centre, 217 Terrace Hill St, Brantford ON N3R 1G8; McM'78; BSc; FRCPC; IntMed (Gastroenterology). Ac Staff, The Brant Community Healthcare System - Brantford General Hospital Site; Court Staff, The Brant Community Healthcare System - Willett Hospital Site; (519)756-3830; Fax. (519)756-6315.

SOMERVILLE, Glasier M; 600-2200 Yonge St, Toronto ON M4S 2C6; Dal'60; Ophth. (416)638-7223; Fax. (416)638-7379.

SOMERVILLE, Jeffrey A; 1165 Dufferin Cres, Nanaimo BC V9S 2B5; Sask'87; FRCSC; ObstGyn. Staff, Nanaimo Regional General Hospital; (250)753-9396

SOMERVILLE, Josephine H; 600-2200 Yonge St, Toronto ON M4S 2C6; Dal'60; FRCPC; PhysMed&Rehab. Staff, Toronto Rehabilitation Institute - University Centre; (416)638-7223; Fax. (416)638-7379.

SOMERVILLE, Peter J; Guelph Renal Clinic, 73 Delhi St, Guelph ON N1E 6L9; Adelaide (Australia)'68; ABIM; FRACP; FRCPC; Nephrol (P.Q.) (Calcium Metabolism); IntMed. Staff, Guelph General Hospital; Staff, Grand River Hospital - Kitchener/Waterloo Health Centre; Consultant, St Joseph's Healthcare - Charlton Campus; Physician, Guelph Renal Clinic; Langs: French; (519)822-7664; Fax. (519)822-0701.

SOMERVILLE, Susan E; 205-272 Lawrence Ave W, Toronto ON M5M 4M1; Tor'86; Court Staff, North York General Hospital; (416)787-7516; Fax. (416)787-7528.

SOMERVILLE, Tara L; 786 Goderich St, Port Elgin ON N0H 2C3; UBC'05; CCFP; (519)832-9600; Fax. (519)832-9602.

SOMMA, Jacques; Hôpital Laval, 2725 ch Sainte-Foy, Quebec QC G1V 4G5; Mon'91; FRCPC; Anes. Staff, Hôpital Laval; (418)656-8711

SOMMA, Maurice; CHUM-Hop Notre-Dame, 1560 rue Sherbrooke E, Montreal QC H2L 4M1; Beirut (Lebanon)'62; MSc; Endocrin (P.Q.); IntMed (P.Q.) (Alternative Medicine). Dir Labs Endocrin, Centre Hospitalier l'Université de Montréal (CHUM) - Hôpital Notre-Dame; Prof, Universite de Montreal; Langs: Arabic; English; (514)890-8200 x27059

SOMMER, Doron D; Hamilton HSC-McMaster Site, PO Box 2000 Stn Lcd 1 3V1-1200 Main St W, Hamilton ON L8N 3Z5; Tor'95; FRCSC; Otol (Head & Neck Surgery). Staff ENT Clinic, Hamilton Health Sciences Centre - McMaster University Medical Centre; Staff, Hamilton Health Sciences Centre - Hamilton General Hospital; Clin Assoc Prof Surg, McMaster University; Langs: Hebrew; (905)521-2100; Fax. (905)521-8552.

SOMMER, Hillel M; Associated Sports & Spine Phys, A-2020 Corydon Ave, Winnipeg MB R3P 0N2; Man'88; FRCPC; PhysMed&Rehab. Staff, Health Sciences Centre; Att'd. Phys., The Rehabilitation Centre; Asst Prof, University of Manitoba; Langs: French; Hebrew; (204)988-5040; Fax. (204)988-5049; hsommer@cc.umanitoba.ca.

SOMMER, Leeor Z; St Joseph's Health Centre, 30 The Queensway, Toronto ON M6R 1B5; Tor'00; CCFP; CCFP(E.M.); Staff, St Joseph's Health Centre; Langs: Hebrew; (416)530-6004

SOMMER, Linda E; Tisdale Med Clinic, PO Box 1510, Tisdale SK S0E 1T0; Man'76; Ac Staff, Tisdale Hospital; (306)873-4561; Fax. (306)873-4489.

SOMMER, Markus; Valley Reg Hosp, 150 Exhibition St, Kentville NS B4N 5E3; Tubingen (Germany)'00; Staff, Valley Regional Hospital; (902)678-7381

SOMMERFELD, Martin R; Hilltop Med Clinic, 140-15321 16th Ave, Surrey BC V4A 1R6; Sask'81; CCFP; Staff, St Michael's Hospital; Staff, Toronto General Hospital - UHN; (604)531-5575

SOMMERFELDT, T Drew; The Campbell Clinic, 160 Columbia Blvd W, Lethbridge AB T1K 4J4; Alb'79; BMedSci; CCFP; FCFP; Ac Staff, Chinook Regional Hospital; Langs: German; (403)381-7000; Fax. (403)381-8250.

SOMMERS, Frank G; 406-360 Bloor St W, Toronto ON M5S 1X1; Tor'70; FRCPC; Psy (Sexual Dysfunction). (416)922-7335; Fax. (416)922-7512.

SOMMERS, Jack G; 2615 Northwood Terr, Halifax NS B3K 3S5; Dal'74; CCFP; FCFP; Ac Staff Family Med, Queen Elizabeth II Health Sciences Centre - Victoria General Site; Court Staff, IWK Health Centre; Dir Health Services, Northwood Manor; Dir Health Services, Northwood Centre; Lecturer, Dalhousie University; (902)423-6141; Fax. (902)453-6857.

SOMMERS, Janet M; Colchester East Hants Hlth Ctr, 600 Abenaki Rd, Truro NS B2N 5A1; Dal'05; CCFP; CCFP(E.M.); Staff, Colchester East Hants Health Centre; (902)893-5556; Fax. (902)893-5552.

SOMMERS, Ryan B; Village Family Physicians, 275 Pictou Rd, Truro NS B2N 2S7; Dal'06; CCFP; (902)895-1232; Fax. (902)897-9749.

SOMMERVILLE, Andrew I; Aberdeen Med Centre, 1966 Harrison Way, Kamloops BC V1S 1M9; Tor'92; (250)314-5342; Fax. (250)372-8331.

SOMMI, Kevin J B; 123-19150 Lougheed Hwy, Pitt Meadows BC V3Y 2H6; London (England)'70; MB BS; Staff, Ridge Meadows Hospital & Health Care Centre; (604)465-0750; Fax. (604)465-0120.

SOMOGYI, Daniel M; 206-2900 Steeles Ave E, Thornhill ON L3T 4X1; McM'94; CSCN(Emerg); CASM; DABPMR; FRCPC; CCFP; PhysMed&Rehab. Langs: Bilingual(English/French); (905)881-6667

SOMSKA, Elena; 307-622 College St, Toronto ON M6G 1B6; Bratislava (Slovakia)'67; Court Staff, Toronto General Hospital - UHN; Langs: Slovak; German; French; Polish; Czech; Russian; (416)588-3182; Fax. (416)516-4999.

SOMYK, Kostiantyn I; Centre Hosp Reg Baie-Comeau, 635 boul Laurier, Baie-Comeau QC G5C 1P1; (Other Foreign)'97; CCFP; Staff, Centre Hospitalier Régional Baie-Comeau; (418)589-3701

SON, Florina; CSSS du Suroît, 150 rue Saint-Thomas, Salaber-de-Valleyf QC J6T 6C1; Cluj-Napoca (Poland)'87; Staff, Centre Hospitalier Régional du Suroît; (450)371-9220; Fax. (450)371-9920.

SON, Wai Kon; Chilliwack Gen Hosp, 45600 Menholm Rd, Chilliwack BC V2P 1P7; Witwatersrand (South Africa)'85; MB ChB; FRCPC; IntMed (Cardiology). Staff, Chilliwack General Hospital; (604)795-4141

SON-HING, Quintin R; Business Bldg, 808-1200 Burrard St, Vancouver BC V6Z 2C7; Cape Town (South Africa)'71; FRCSC; PlasSurg (Cosmetics). Langs: Mandarin; (604)689-1844; Fax. (604)689-9177.

SONBOL, Soliman M; Ontario Shores Ctr Mental HS, PO Box 613 700 Gordon St, Whitby ON L1N 5S9; Cairo (Egypt)'72; MB ChB; FRCPC; Psy. Staff, Ontario Shores Centre for Mental Health Sciences; Langs: Arabic; (905)668-5881; Fax. (905)430-4032.

SONDHI, Asha P; 404 Medical Clinic, 46-1111 Davis Dr, Newmarket ON L3Y 8X2; Patna (India)'76; CCFP; FCFP; Langs: Hindi; Punjabi; (905)868-8330; Fax. (905)868-8332.

SONDHI, Jitin; Alexandra Med Centre, 29 Noxon St, Ingersoll ON N5C 1B8; Tor'07; CCFP; Langs: Hindi; Punjabi; (519)485-9617

SONEA, Michael J; 203-5122 rue Sherbrooke O, Montreal QC H4A 1T1; McG'80; FRCPC; Derm. Langs: Romanian; French; (514)486-3867; Fax. (514)486-8930.

SONEFF, Cynthia M; Westgrove Prof Bldg, 310-10230 142 St NW, Edmonton AB T5N 3Y6; Alb'05; CCFP; Staff, Covenant Health - Misericordia Community Hospital; (780)455-3311; Fax. (780)451-4404.

SONEJI, Neilesh; St Michael's Hosp, MCL2 405-30 Bond St, Toronto ON M5B 1W8; Tor'07; FRCPC; Anes. Staff, Toronto Western Hospital - University Health Network.

SONEJI, Prachi; Patient Networks, 157 Yonge St, Toronto ON M5C 1X7; McM'06; CCFP; Physician, Patient Networks; (416)362-8822; Fax. (416)362-8877.

SONG, Anne; Pinecrest-Queensway CHC, 203-1365 Richmond Rd, Ottawa ON K2B 6R7; Ott'89; CCFP; FCFP; Physician, Pinecrest-Queensway Community Health Centre; Langs: French; (613)820-2001; Fax. (613)820-2006.

SONG, Helen B; Guelph Family Health Team, 21 Yarmouth St, Guelph ON N1H 4G2; Xuzhou Medical College (Other Foreign)'77; CCFP; Langs: Mandarin; (519)822-7831; Fax. (519)822-6234.

SONG, Howard H; EN213 13-585 University Ave, Toronto ON M5G 2N2; Tor'06; FRCPC; IntMed; InfectDis. Staff, Toronto General Hospital - UHN; Langs: Bilingual(English/French); (416)340-3505

SONG, John J; Finchgate Med Centre, 204-40 Finchgate Blvd, Brampton ON L6T 3J1; Tor'87; CCFP; (905)790-2880; Fax. (905)790-1549.

SONG, John Y; Medical Arts Bldg, 8-165 Plymouth Rd, Welland ON L3B 3E1; Qns'93; FRCSC; OrthSurg (Arthroplasty). (905)734-9434; Fax. (905)734-7584.

SONG, Kevin W; Leukemia/BMT Program of BC, 10F-2775 Laurel St, Vancouver BC V5Z 1M9; McG'95; MDCM; FRCPC; IntMed; Hem. Staff, Vancouver General Hospital - Centennial Pavillion; Staff Hematology Administration, Leukemia/Bone Marrow Transplantation Prog of BC; (604)875-4863; ksong@bccancer.bc.ca.

SONG, Sue Chiat; PO Box 74582 Kitsilano Rpo, Vancouver BC V6K 4P4; Tor'97; CCFP; FCFP.

SONG, Tom T Y; Medical Arts Bldg, 5-165 Plymouth Rd, Welland ON L3B 3E1; Wes'89; FRCSC; Urol. Staff, Niagara Health System - Welland Hospital Site; Staff, Niagara Health System - Greater Niagara General Site; Staff, Niagara Health System - St Catharines General Site; Clinical Asst Prof Surg, McMaster University; Aj Prof Surg, University of Western Ontario; (905)735-6013; Fax. (905)735-7880; tsong@niagarahealth.on.ca.

SONG, Wei-Yi; Eric Martin Pavillion, 2334 Trent St, Victoria BC V8R 4Z3; Hunan (China)'89; MB; FRCPC; Psy (Mood Disorders). Staff, Mental Health Centre; Langs: Mandarin; (250)370-8155; Fax. (250)370-8199; wei.song@viha.ca.

SONG, Xinni; The Ottawa Hosp-Gen Campus, 501 Smyth Rd Box 912, Ottawa ON K1H 8L6; Ott'00; FRCPC; IntMed; MedOncol (Family Medicine). Staff, The Ottawa Hospital - General Campus; Physician, Ottawa Regional Cancer Centre; (613)737-8899

SONI, Anil T; Willoughby Med Centre, B1A-20202 66 Ave, Langley BC V2Y 1P3; Mangalore (India)'88; MB BS; CCFP; (604)514-8800; Fax. (604)514-8692.

SONI, Anita; St Boniface Gen Hosp, Y3005-409 Tache Ave, Winnipeg MB R2H 2A6; Man'98; FRCPC; IntMed; Cardiol. Staff Cardiol, St Boniface General Hospital; (204)258-1000; Fax. (204)233-2157.

SONI, Deepa; The Credit Valley Hosp, 2200 Eglinton Ave W, Mississauga ON L5M 2N1; Qns'96; BSc; CCFP; CCFP(E.M.); Staff, The Credit Valley Hospital; Langs: Gujarati; French; (905)813-2200

SONI, Ebrahim; Beach Med Clinic, 350 Beech Ave, Toronto ON M4E 3T8; Witwatersrand (South Africa)'62; MB BCh; CCFP; (416)694-1126; Fax. (416)691-5040.

SONI, Jorge; Addiction & Mental Hlth-Clarke, G60-250 College St, Toronto ON M5T 1R8; National (Mexico)'78; FRCPC; Psy (In-Patient Hospital Psychiatry). Staff, Centre for Addiction & Mental Health (CAMH) - College Street Site; Langs: Spanish; (416)979-4747; Fax. (416)583-4614.

SONI, Nandini R; Variety Children's Heart Ctre, FE 241-685 William Ave, Winnipeg MB R3E 0Z2; Man'91; FRCPC; Peds; PedCardiol. Staff, Health Sciences Centre; Staff, Variety Children's Heart Centre; (204)787-2410; Fax. (204)787-2004; rsoni@exchange.hsc.mb.ca.

SONI, Naveen K; Walkley Med Centre, 1852 Bank St, Ottawa ON K1V 7Z8; Sask'98; CCFP; (613)526-5200; Fax. (613)719-7807.

SONI, Nisha; Walkley Med Centre, 1852 Bank St, Ottawa ON K1V 7Z8; Sask'04; CCFP; (613)526-5200; Fax. (613)719-7807.

SONI, Ramesh K; Burlington Prof Centre, 402-3155 Harvester Rd, Burlington ON L7N 3V2; Manchester (England)'66; MB ChB; Langs: Hindi; Punjabi; (905)632-2977; Fax. (905)632-7960; meshisoni@hotmail.com.

SONI, Rekha; Ermineskin Med Clinic, 301-2377 111 St NW, Edmonton AB T6J 5E5; (India)'90; CCFP; Staff, University of Alberta Hospital; (780)436-8731; Fax. (780)434-8732.

SONI, Sushane; Selkirk & District Gen Hosp, PO Box 5000 Stn Main 100 Easton Dr, Selkirk MB R1A 2M2; Man'91; FRCPC; DiagRad. Staff, Selkirk & District General Hospital; (204)482-5800

SONIER, Paul W; Cheticamp Med Clinic, PO Box 220, Cheticamp NS B0E 1H0; Laval'95; CCFP; (902)224-3110; Fax. (902)224-1905.

SONMOR, Frederick S; 530 25 St SE, Salmon Arm BC V1E 1C8; Sask'75; (250)832-3411; Fax. (250)804-5232.

SONNENBERG, Barend J; Workers' Comp Board, PO Box 1879 Stn Main, Edmonton AB T5J 2P2; S.Africa (South Africa)'89; Physician, Workers' Comp Board of AB; Langs: Afrikaans; (780)498-3839; Fax. (780)498-7808.

SONNENBERG, Brian H; University of Alberta Hosp, 2C2WCM-8440 112 St NW, Edmonton AB T6G 2B7; Tor'92; FRCPC; IntMed; Cardiol. Staff, University of Alberta Hospital; (780)407-7403; Fax. (780)407-6452.

SONNENBERG, Lyn K; Glenrose Rehab Hosp, 198-10230 111 Ave NW, Edmonton AB T5G 0B7; McM'03; BSc(Hons); MSc; FRCPC; Peds (Developmental Pediatrics). Staff, Glenrose Rehabilitation Hospital; Asst Prof, University of Alberta; (780)735-7913; Fax. (780)735-8200.

SONNICHSEN, David G; Kootenay Med Centre, 601 Kootenay St, Nelson BC V1L 1L1; UBC'08; (250)352-2230

SONPAR, Prabhu; Smyth Associate Clinic, 4904 48 St, Leduc AB T9E 6X4; Bombay (India)'83; MB BS; CCFP; Staff, Leduc Community Hospital; Langs: Hindi; (780)986-2712; Fax. (780)986-0356.

SONSHINE, Jodi E; 704-240 Duncan Mill Rd, North York ON M3B 3S6; Tor'99; BSc; CCFP; Ac Staff, North York General Hospital; (416)497-0880; Fax. (416)497-2650.

SOO, B H Norman; Medical Clinic, 406-1110 Sheppard Ave E, North York ON M2K 2W2; Tor'91; Langs: Cantonese; Mandarin; (416)733-4151; Fax. (416)733-9977.

SOO, Isaac; PO Box 52197 RPO Garneau, Edmonton AB T6G 2T5; Alb'07; Gastroent; IntMed. Staff, University of Alberta Hospital.

SOO, Stephanie M; Family Practice Health Centre, 3F-77 Grenville St, Toronto ON M5S 1B3; Wes'08; CCFP; (416)323-6060; Fax. (416)323-6402.

SOO, Tony Y; Primacy Med Clinic, 1792 Trans Canada Way SE, Medicine Hat AB T1B 4C6; (Hong Kong)'71; DABIM; FRCPC; IntMed. Ac Staff, Medicine Hat Regional Hospital; (403)502-8939; Fax. (403)502-8955.

SOO, Victoria; 1-1695 Wonderland Rd N, London ON N6G 4W3; Bowman Gray of Wake Forest University (USA)'06; CCFP; (519)473-6654; Fax. (519)474-9779.

SOOCHAN, Diana C; Postgrad Med Education Office, 602-500 University Ave, Toronto ON M5G 1V7; Alb'06; DiagRad.

SOOD, Alok; Gladwin Med Centre, 106-2955 Gladwin Rd, Abbotsford BC V2T 5T4; Punjab (India)'87; MB BS; CCFP; Staff Family Practice, Gladwin Medical Centre; Langs: Punjabi; Hindi; Urdu; (604)851-5677; Fax. (604)851-5688; aloksood@hotmail.com.

SOOD, Alok Pal; Albany Med Clinic, 807 Broadview Ave, Toronto ON M4K 2P8; McG'92; CCFP; Langs: Spanish; French; (416)461-9471; Fax. (416)461-2710.

SOOD, Balbhadar D; William Osler HC-Etobicoke, 101 Humber College Blvd, Etobicoke ON M9V 1R8; Punjab (India)'62; MB BS; MRC; FRCPC; Psy (Consultation-Liaison). Staff, William Osler Health System - Etobicoke General Hospital; Consultant, William Osler Health System - Brampton Civic Hospital; Langs: Punjabi; Hindi; Urdu; (416)494-2120 x57701; Fax. (416)747-3350.

SOOD, Brijendra; 4712 Bowness Rd NW, Calgary AB T3B 0B4; Birmingham (England)'54; MB ChB; MRCS; LRCP; FRCS(Ed); Med Examiner, Civil Aviation & Federal Government Jobs; Langs: Swahili; Punjabi; Hindi; (403)288-2495; Fax. (403)247-0310; brijsood@shaw.ca.

SOOD, Danesh; Wellness Centre, 305-1366 Yonge St, Toronto ON M4T 3A7; Wes'05; CCFP; Staff, Toronto Western Hospital - University Health Network; (416)962-2964; Fax. (416)962-2526.

SOOD, Manish M; St Boniface Gen Hosp, BG 007-409 Tache Ave, Winnipeg MB R2H 2A6; Tor'02; FRCPC; IntMed; Nephrol. Staff, St Boniface General Hospital; (204)233-8563

SOOD, Narinder; Regina Community Clinic, 1106 Winnipeg St, Regina SK S4R 1J6; Agra (India)'62; MB BS; LRCP(Lond); MRCS(Eng); Physician, Regina Community Clinic; (306)543-7880; Fax. (306)543-6888; sood@reginacommunityclinic.ca.

SOOD, Nidhi; South Health Campus, 4448 Front St SE, Calgary AB T3M 1M4; Ott'05; FRCPC; IntMed. Staff, South Health Campus; (403)956-1111

SOOD, Om Prakash; Transcona Med Clinic, 4936 4th Ave, Regina SK S4T 0J3; Agra (India)'62; LRCP(Lond); MRCS(Eng); FRCS(Eng.Ed); FRCSC; GenSurg. Consultant Surg, Pasqua Hospital; Consultant Surg, Regina General Hospital; Physician, Transcona Medical Clinic; Asst Prof Surg, University of Saskatchewan; (306)775-2688; Fax. (306)543-4633.

SOOD, Priya D; St Josephs Health Sciences Ctr, 30 The Queensway, Toronto ON M6R 1B5; Tor'05; CCFP; (416)530-6860; Fax. (416)530-6160.

SOOD, Rajesh K; Edson Med Centre, PO Box 6660 Stn Main, Edson AB T7E 1V1; (780)723-3366; Fax. (780)723-3437.

SOOD, Rickesh; Headwaters Health Care Centre, 100 Rolling Hills Dr, Orangeville ON L9W 4X9; McM'04; Staff, Headwaters Health Care Centre - Orangeville Site; (519)941-2702; Fax. (519)942-0483.

SOODAN, Baldev S; St Lawrence Med Bldg, 7-614 Second St E, Cornwall ON K6H 1Z8; Jammu-Kashmir (India)'68; MB BS; FRCPC; IntMed (Gastroenterology). Staff Privil, Cornwall Community Hospital; Staff Privil, Cornwall Community Hospital - Second Street Site; Langs: Punjabi; Urdu; (613)938-0620; Fax. (613)938-1239.

SOOKDEO, Sunel; WOHC-Brampton Civic Hosp, 2100 Bovaird Dr E, Brampton ON L6R 3J7; Witwatersrand (South Africa)'95; MB ChB; FACR; FRCPC; DiagRad (Musculoskeletal);CCFP; CCFP(E.M.); Staff Medical Imaging, William Osler Health System - Brampton Civic Hospital; (905)494-2120; Fax. (905)494-6614; sookdeo@hotmail.com.

SOOKHAI, Nicole K; Rexdale Comm Health Centre, 8 Taber Rd, Etobicoke ON M9W 3A4; McM'07; CCFP; Staff, Toronto Western Hospital - University Health Network; (416)744-0066; Fax. (416)744-1881.

SOOKHOO, Siuchan; Manitoba XRay Clinic, 3263 Portage Ave, Winnipeg MB R3K 0W6; (204)832-0273

SOOKNANAN, Avita; 206-815 College St, Toronto ON M6G 1C9; McM'08; CCFP; (416)923-5500; Fax. (416)923-2249.

SOOKRAM, Sunil M; University of Alberta Hosp, 1G1 50WCM-8440 112 St NW, Edmonton AB T6G 2B7; Qns'96; FRCPC; EmergMed (Aviation). Staff/Clin Assoc Prof, University of Alberta Hospital; (780)407-7047; Fax. (866)259-7429; sfookram@telusplanet.net.

SOOLSMA, Serge J; Bowmont Med Clinic, 6535 Bowness Rd NW, Calgary AB T3B 0E8; UBC'02; CCFP; (403)247-9797; Fax. (403)247-0014.

SOON, Gordon S; St Joseph's Health Centre, 30 The Queensway, Toronto ON M6R 1B5; UBC'06; FRCPC; Peds; Rheum. Staff, North York General Hospital; Staff, St Joseph's Health Centre; (416)756-6000

SOON, Shawn J; Dr Shawn J Soon Med Clinic, 2F-4240 Sheppard Ave E, Scarborough ON M1S 1T5; McM'01; FRCSC; Urol (Uro Oncology). Staff, The Scarborough Hospital - General Campus; Staff, The Scarborough Hospital - Birchmount Campus; Langs: French; Mandarin; (416)628-4997; Fax. (416)850-4146.

SOON-SHIONG, Gregory; Pinnacle Health Sciences Ctre, 9651 Yonge St, Richmond Hill ON L4C 1V7; Witwatersrand (South Africa)'81; MB ChB; FRCSC; OrthSurg. Staff, Mackenzie Richmond Hill Hospital; (905)883-6614; Fax. (905)883-6904.

SOONG, Anna S K; Ridgpoint Med Centre, 10815 Yonge St, Richmond Hill ON L4C 3E3; Tor'88; Langs: Cantonese; (905)770-3004; Fax. (905)770-5663.

SOONG, Christine; Mount Sinai Hosp, 428-600 University Ave, Toronto ON M5G 1X5; Wes'01; CCFP; Staff, Mount Sinai Hospital; Langs: Mandarin; (416)586-4800

SOONG, Elaine E; Justik Med Clinic, 8225 105 St NW, Edmonton AB T6E 4H2; Alb'02; CCFP; (780)432-0211

SOONG, John H; Misericordia Community Hosp, 16940 87 Ave NW, Edmonton AB T5R 4H5; Alb'82; FRCPC; Anes. Staff Anes, Covenant Health - Misericordia Community Hospital; (780)735-2863; Fax. (780)735-2967.

SOONG, Patrick Y; Family Health Centre, 200-2462 Howard Ave, Windsor ON N8X 3V6; Wes'93; CCFP; FCFP; Ac Staff, Windsor Regional Hospital - Tayfour Site; (519)258-9484; Fax. (519)258-9774.

SOOR, Gursharan S; Dufferin Area Family Health Te, 140 Rolling Hills Dr, Orangeville ON L9W 4X8; Tor'10; CCFP; (519)941-7575; gursharan.soor@utoronto.ca.

SOORIABALAN, Thuraisamy; Rouge Valley HS-Centenary HC, 2867 Ellesmere Rd, Scarborough ON M1E 4B9; (Sri Lanka)'73; MB BS; MRCPsy(UK); FRCPC; Psy. Consultant, Rouge Valley Health System - Centenary Health Centre Site; Langs: Tamil; (416)281-7318; Fax. (416)281-7320.

SOOS-KAPUSY, Eva D; MUHC-Montreal Gen Hosp, 2300 rue Tupper, Montreal QC H3H 1P3; Tirgu-Mures (Romania)'89; CCFP; Staff, McGill University Health Centre - Montreal Children's Hospital; (514)412-4400

SOOWAMBER, Mohunlall; Clinique Med l'Esperance, 4261 rue Sainte-Catherine E, Montreal QC H1V 1X5; Besancon (France)'81; (514)254-3686; Fax. (514)254-5258.

SOPARKAR, Gautam R; Gautam Soparkar Med Prof Corp, 325 Wellington St, Sarnia ON N7T 1H4; New Delhi (India)'81; MB BS; MRC(UK); DABIM; FRCPC; IntMed (Respirology). Staff, Bluewater Health - Norman Site; Langs: Hindi; (519)344-5011; Fax. (519)344-7875.

SOPER, Juliet; Regina Gen Hosp, 1440 14th Ave, Regina SK S4P 0W5; Auckland (New Zealand)'97; FRCPC; Peds. Staff, Regina General Hospital; (306)766-4444

SOPER, Paul; Glenrose Rehab Hosp, 329-10230 111 Ave NW, Edmonton AB T5G 0B7; Alb'02; FRCPC; Psy. Staff, University of Alberta Hospital; Staff Glenrose ADHD Clinic, Glenrose Rehabilitation Hospital; (780)735-7928; Fax. (780)735-6067.

SORAISHAM, Amuchou S; Foothills Med Centre, C211-1403 29 St NW, Calgary AB T2N 2T9; Pondicherry (India)'95; MB BS; FRCPC; Peds (Neonatal & Perinatal). Staff Peds, Foothills Medical Centre; Asst Prof Peds, University of Calgary; Langs: Hindi; (403)944-1615; Fax. (403)944-4892; amuchou.soraisham@calgaryhealthregion.ca.

SORENI, Noam; St Joseph's Healthcare, F409-50 Charlton Ave E, Hamilton ON L8N 4A6; The Hebrew University (Israel)'97; Staff, St Joseph's Healthcare - Charlton Campus; (905)522-1155; Fax. (905)540-6533.

SORENSEN, Anne K; North Oshawa Med Ctre, 103-1400 Ritson Rd N, Oshawa ON L1G 7W4; Qns'93; CCFP; Court Staff Privil, Lakeridge Health - Oshawa Site; (905)579-8111; Fax. (905)433-1838.

SORENSEN, Donna J; 101-190 Pelican Pl, Sylvan Lake AB T4S 1K2; Alb'93; CCFP; Staff Privil, Brooks Health Centre; (403)887-2224; Fax. (403)887-2261.

SORENSEN, Kyla M; 201-211 Dundas St E, Belleville ON K8N 1E2; McM'07; CCFP; (613)968-6300; Fax. (613)968-6303.

SORENSEN, Paul H B; BC Cancer Research Centre, 4 112-675 10th Ave W, Vancouver BC V5Z 1L3; UBC'84; FRCPC; AnatPath. Staff Path, BC Women's Hospital & Health Centre; Langs: Danish; (604)675-8202; Fax. (604)675-8218; psorensen@cw.bc.ca.

SORENSEN, Ronald B; 3405 Rhodes Dr, Windsor ON N8W 5B3; Wes'77; FRCSC; Urol. Assoc Staff, Hôtel-Dieu Grace Hospital; (519)974-8879; Fax. (519)974-9261.

SORENSON, Katherine J; Hillcrest Med Associates, 117 Jasper St, Hinton AB T7V 2A8; Alb'06; CCFP; (780)865-2203; Fax. (780)865-7383.

SORESTAD, Mark A; Westside Med Associates, 3591 Elliott Rd, Westbank BC V4T 1N9; Sask'88; CCFP; Staff, Kelowna General Hospital; (250)768-6920; Fax. (250)768-6907; wsma@shaw.ca.

SORG, Michael K; Crowfoot Business Centre, 3-400 Crowfoot Cres NW, Calgary AB T3G 5H6; McM'04; FRCPC; Peds; ClinImmunol&Allergy.

SORGE, Cindy R; Avenue Med Centre, 221 Brant Ave, Brantford ON N3T 3J2; Tor'05; FRCSC; ObstGyn. (519)753-8666

SORGE, Raymond; Hôp Brome-Missisquoi-Perkins, 950 rue Principale, Cowansville QC J2K 1K3; McG'88; CCFP; CCFP(E.M.); FCFP; Chef Dept of EmergMed, St Mary's Hospital Centre; Staff, Hôpital Brome-Missisquoi-Perkins; Physician, McGill Hockey Team; adj Prof, McGill University; (450)266-5500

SORGINI, Curtis J; 1351 Martindale Rd, Sudbury ON P3E 4J7; Wes'84; FRCSC; Ophth. Staff, Health Sciences North-St Joseph's Health Centre; Staff, Health Sciences North - Memorial Site; Staff, Health Sciences North-Laurentian Site; Langs: French; (705)523-1226

SORHAINDO, Mark A G; Queen Elizabeth II HSC, 1796 Summer St, Halifax NS B3H 3A7; West Indies (Jamaica)'90; MB BS; BSc; Staff, Queen Elizabeth II Health Sciences Centre - Halifax Infirmary Site; Staff, Worker's Compensation Board of NS; (902)860-3244; Fax. (902)473-5625.

SORIAL, Ashraf M G; Mary Berglund CHC, PO Box 450, Ignace ON P0T 1T0; Alexandria (Egypt)'92; MB ChB; Physician, Mary Berglund CHC; Langs: Arabic; (807)934-2251; Fax. (807)934-6552.

SORIAL, Ihab Z N; Lakeridge Hlth Corp-Oshawa, 1 Hospital Crt, Oshawa ON L1G 2B9; Ain Shams (Egypt)'85; MB ChB; FRCPC; Psy. Staff, Lakeridge Health - Oshawa Site; Langs: Arabic; (905)576-8711 x2206; Fax. (905)721-4742; isorial@lakeridgehealth.on.ca.

SORIAL, Mark Z; 2660 James St, Abbotsford BC V2T 3L5; Cairo (Egypt)'81; MB ChB; FRCPC; Peds (Neonatal & Perinatal Medicine). Head/Staff, Abbotsford Regional Hospital & Cancer Centre; Langs: Arabic; (604)853-8912; Fax. (604)853-8312.

SORIAL, Mary L R; York Med Health Centre, C-17215 Leslie St, Newmarket ON L3Y 8E4; Ain Shams University (Egypt)'97; MB BCh; CCFP; Langs: Arabic; (905)853-0404; Fax. (905)853-3702.

SORIANO, Samuel; 258-2155 Leanne Blvd, Mississauga ON L5K 2K8; Cape Town (South Africa)'62; FAAOS; FRCSC; OrthSurg. (905)823-8482; Fax. (905)823-9848.

SORIANO GRONDIN, Jeannette; Glenmore Landing, D272-1600 90 Ave SW, Calgary AB T2V 5A8; Santo Domingo (Dominican Republic)'78; (403)202-0003; Fax. (403)202-0034.

SORIC, Rajka; West Park Healthcare Ctre, R3 10-82 Buttonwood Ave, Toronto ON M6M 2J5; Zagreb (Croatia)'71; MSc; FRCPC; PhysMed&Rehab (Musculoskeletal). Staff, West Park Healthcare Centre; Asst Prof, University of Toronto; Langs: Croatian; Serbian; (416)243-3705; Fax. (416)243-1177.

SORISKY, Alexander M; The Ottawa Hosp-Riverside, 4F-1967 Riverside Dr, Ottawa ON K1H 7W9; McG'82; BSc; MD; CM; FRCPC; MedBiochem; Endocrin&Metab; IntMed. Staff, The Ottawa Hospital - Riverside Campus; Assoc Prof Med, University of Ottawa; Langs: Bilingual(English/French); (613)738-8400 x81941; Fax. (613)738-8261.

SORNARAJAH, Thangarajah; Peterborough Reg HC-Hospital, 1 Hospital Dr, Peterborough ON K9J 7C6; Jaffna (Sri Lanka)'84; MB BS; FRCPC; AnatPath (Dermatological Pathology). Staff, Peterborough Regional Health Centre - Hospital Drive; Langs: Tamil; (705)743-2121

SOROKA, Dana J; Women's Health Care Clinic, 5F-61 Queen St E, Toronto ON M5C 2T2; McG'94; FRCSC; ObstGyn (Urogynecology). Staff, St Michael's Hospital; (416)867-7480; Fax. (416)867-3693.

SOROKA, Steven D; Dickson Med Bldg, 5088-5820 University Ave, Halifax NS B3H 1V8; Sask'90; MSc; FRCPC; IntMed; Nephrol. Prof Med, Dalhousie University; (902)473-2099; Fax. (902)473-2675; steven.soroka@cdha.nshealth.ca.

SOROKAN, S Todd; Royal City Centre, 261-610 Sixth St, New Westminster BC V3L 3C2; Alb'88; FRCPC; Peds (Neonatal & Perinatal Medicine). (604)522-7979; drsorokan@shaw.ca.

SOROKO, Oleg; Hopital Hotel-Dieu de Sorel, 400 av de l'Hotel-Dieu, Sorel-Tracy QC J3P 1N5; Vitebsk State Medical University (Other Foreign)'87; Staff, Hôtel-Dieu de Sorel; (450)746-6000 x6219; Fax. (450)786-6249.

SORRENTO, Vito A; Pine Seven Med Ctre, 180-4600 Highway 7, Woodbridge ON L4L 4Y7; Tor'96; CCFP; CCFP(E.M.); Court Staff, Mackenzie Richmond Hill Hospital; Langs: Italian; (905)856-3330; Fax. (905)856-3331.

SORSDAHL, A Kent; 589 West Gore St, Stratford ON N5A 1L4; Sask'89; FACS; FRCSC; GenSurg. (519)273-4100; Fax. (519)273-3208.

SOSIAK, Theodore S; 204-3101 Bloor St W, Etobicoke ON M8X 2W2; McM'77; Court Staff Fam Med, St Joseph's Health Centre; Staff, Toronto General Hospital - UHN; Staff, Trillium Health Centre - West Toronto; (416)233-3343; Fax. (416)233-0746.

SOSKA, Marc A; Rockyview Gen Hosp, 7007 14 St SW, Calgary AB T2V 1P9; Ott'99; Anes. Staff Anes, Rockyview General Hospital; Staff Anes, Foothills Medical Centre; (403)943-3000; Fax. (403)252-2798.

SOSNOWSKI, Christopher J; 277 Bridge St W, Napanee ON K7R 2G2; Cal'82; CCFP; FCFP; Langs: Polish; (613)354-4725; Fax. (613)354-1322.

SOSNOWSKI, Mark K; Lynnwood Med Centre, 6622 20A St SE, Calgary AB T2C 0R3; Cal'78; CCFP; FCFP; Att Physician, Carewest Long Term Care; Langs: Polish; (403)279-3311; Fax. (403)279-4214; sosnowski@ucalgary.ca.

SOSTARIC, John V; The Surgeons Office, 236 Elm St, St Thomas ON N5R 1J5; Wes'04; FRCSC; GenSurg (Surgical Oncology). Staff, St Thomas Elgin General Hospital; (519)631-0567; Fax. (519)631-0921; sandypickersg.11@yahoo.com.

SOTH, Mark D; St Joseph's Healthcare, T2116-50 Charlton Ave E, Hamilton ON L8N 4A6; McM'00; FRCPC; IntMed; Critical Care Medicine; Respir. Staff, St Joseph's Healthcare - Charlton Campus; Staff, Hamilton Health Sciences Centre - McMaster Children's Hospital; Asst Prof, McMaster University; (905)522-1155 x4935; Fax. (905)645-8274.

SOTHILINGAM, Subramanian; North Bramelea Med Clinic, 202-9780 Bramalea Rd, Brampton ON L6S 2P1; Peradeniya (Sri Lanka)'76; MB BS; DCH(Ire); DObst(Ire.); CCFP; Ac Staff, Royal University Hospital; Ac Staff, St Paul's Hospital (Grey Nuns) of Saskatoon; Ac Staff, Saskatoon City Hospital; Langs: Sinhalese; Tamil; (905)791-2390

SOTO, Julio C; Institut National Sante Publiq, 190 boul Cremazie E, Montreal QC H2P 1E2; Cayetano Heredia (Peru)'77; MSc(Microbiol.); PhD(PublicHealth); CommunMed (P.Q.) (Infectious Diseases). Staff, Centre Hospitalier l'Université de Montréal (CHUM) - Hôpital Notre-Dame; Médecin, Institut National de Sante Publique du Quebec; Langs: Spanish; English; Portuguese; (514)864-1600 x3215; Fax. (514)864-7646; julio.c.soto.chum@ssss.gouv.qc.ca.

SOTO DE MACHAT, Grace G; Maple Med Centre, 110-955 Major MacKenzie Dr W, Vaughan ON L6A 4P9; Lima (Peru)'96; CCFP; Langs: Spanish; (289)553-3300; Fax. (289)553-2600.

SOTO MOLINA, Juan A; Westgrove Clinic, 102A-505 Queen St, Spruce Grove AB T7X 2V2; San Marcos (Other Foreign)'00; CCFP; (780)960-4102; Fax. (780)962-8176.

SOTO-MORENO, Lourdes; Yarmouth Reg Hosp, 60 Vancouver St, Yarmouth NS B5A 2P5; Puerto Rico (Brazil)'91; Staff, Yarmouth Regional Hospital; (902)742-3541

SOTOMI, Omopelola O; 202-3998 Albert St, Regina SK S4S 3R1; Ibadan (Nigeria)'98; FRCPC; Peds. (306)569-3333; Fax. (306)545-8042.

SOTTO, Alain G; Finchlea Med Centre, 204-490 Bramalea Rd, Brampton ON L6T 0G1; Tor'87; BSc(Hons); FCBOM; Ac Staff, William Osler Health System - Brampton Civic Hospital; Chief Physician, Ontario Power Generation; Med Consultant Occupational, Toronto Transit Commission; Langs: French; (905)792-6500; Fax. (905)792-6853.

SOTTOSANTI, Maria; Children's Hosp of Western Ont, 800 Commissioners Rd E, London ON N6C 2V5; Qns'06; FRCPC; Peds. Staff, Children's Hospital of Western Ontario; (519)685-8500

SOUAID, Jean-Pierre; Carling-Broadview Med Bldg, 310-770 Broadview Ave, Ottawa ON K2A 3Z3; McG'95; BSc; MDCM; ABOtol; FRCS; FRCSC; Otol. Staff, The Ottawa Hospital - Civic Campus; Ac Staff, Queensway Carleton Hospital; Langs: French; (613)729-4991; Fax. (613)729-1701; jpsouaid@hotmail.com.

SOUBBOTINA, Janna; Langley Mem Hosp, 22051 Fraser Hwy, Langley BC V3A 4H4; Tyumen (Russia (Federation))'87; CCFP; Staff, Langley Memorial Hospital; Langs: Russian; (604)534-4121

SOUBIRAN, Eric; Centre Hosp Honore-Mercier, 2750 boul Laframboise, Saint-Hyacinthe QC J2S 4Y8; Sher'75; Staff, Centre Hospitalier Honore-Mercier; Langs: Bilingual(French/English); (450)771-3333 x4214; eric.soubiran@hy.cgocable.ca.

SOUCHON, Frederique; Clin de Migraine de Montreal, 420-1600 boul Henri-Bourassa O, Montreal QC H3M 3E2; Mon'92; FRCPC; Neur (Migraines); Electroenceph (P.Q.). Staff, Centre Hospitalier Pierre Boucher; Staff, Centre Hospitalier l'Université de Montréal (CHUM) - Hôpital Notre-Dame; Langs: Spanish; English; (514)337-0432; Fax. (514)337-0942.

SOUCIE, F Pierre; Centre Med Ruby, 102-361 Main St E, Hawkesbury ON K6A 1A8; Ott'85; Langs: English; (613)632-0605; Fax. (613)632-7073.

SOUCIE, Francois D; Clin Med Fam D'Edmundston, 50 av Bateman, Edmundston NB E3V 4A4; Sher'06; BSc; CCFP; Staff, Hôpital regional d'Edmundston; Langs: Bilingual(French/English); (506)735-4783; Fax. (506)739-1008; fsoucie@hotmail.com.

SOUCIE, Jean-Joseph; Clinique de Med Interne, 20 rue Carrier, Edmundston NB E3V 3Y1; Laval'69; IntMed (P.Q.) (Cardiology). (506)739-9511; Fax. (506)735-8118; cllin.med.int@nb.aibn.com.

SOUCIE, S Pierre; SCOHS-Elizabeth Bruyere Hosp, 43 Bruyere St, Ottawa ON K1N 5C8; Ott'64; CCFP; FCFP; SCO Health Service - Élisabeth Bruyère Hospital; Med Dir Eastern Ontario, Ontario Telemedicine Network; Assoc Prof Family Med, University of Ottawa; Langs: English; (613)562-6322; Fax. (613)562-6013; papadoc@rogers.com.

SOUCY, Cathya; CLSC Rimouski-Neigette, 165 rue des Gouverneurs, Rimouski QC G5L 7R2; Mon'94; Staff, Hôpital Regional Rimouski; Staff Hyperbaric Med, Institute Maritime du Quebec; Langs: Bilingual(French/English); (418)727-5493; csoucy@imq.qc.ca.

SOUCY, Claudette; CSSS de Saint-Jerome, 290 rue de Montigny, Saint-Jerome QC J7Z 5T3; Laval'72; ac Staff, Hôtel-Dieu de Saint-Jérôme; Staff, Hôpital du Sacre-Coeur de Montréal; (450)431-8392

SOUCY, Elaine; Credit Valley Prof Bldg, 209-2300 Eglinton Ave W, Mississauga ON L5M 2V8; Mon'92; FRCPC; IntMed; Rheum. Staff, Halton Healthcare Services Corporation - Oakville Site; Langs: French; (905)607-8334; Fax. (905)607-8184.

SOUCY, Eric; Centre Hosp Fleury, 2180 rue Fleury E, Montreal QC H2B 1K3; Mon'95; Staff, Centre Hospitalier de LaSalle; Staff, Centre Hospitalier Fleury; (514)381-9311

SOUCY, Francois C; 1625 rue Fradet, Drummondville QC J2B 1N7; Laval'65.

SOUCY, Frederic; Hopital Saint-Francois-D'Assis, 10 rue de L'Espinay, Quebec QC G1L 3L5; Laval'01; FRCSC; Urol. Staff, Centre Hospitalier Universitaire De Québec - Pavillon De St-françois-d'assise; Langs: English; (418)525-4444

SOUCY, Genevieve; Ctr Hosp Affilie-Enfant-Jesus, 1401 18e rue, Quebec QC G1J 1Z4; Laval'07; InfectDis (P.Q.); MedMicrobiol. Staff, Centre Hospitalier Affilié Universitaire de Québec - Hôpital De L'Enfant Jésus; (418)649-0252

SOUCY, Genevieve; CSSS de la Cote-de-Gaspe, 215 boul de York O, Gaspe QC G4X 2W2; Mon'05; GenSurg. Staff, Centre Hospitalier de Gaspe; (418)368-3301

SOUCY, Genevieve; CSSS de Rivière-de-Loup, 75 rue Saint-Henri, Riviere-du-Loup QC G5R 2A4; Mon'00; Staff, Centre Hospitalier Regional du Grand-Portage; (418)868-1000; Fax. (418)868-1032.

SOUCY, Genevieve; CHUM-Hop St-Luc, 1058 rue Saint-Denis, Montreal QC H2X 3J4; Mon'03; FRCPC; AnatPath. Staff, Centre Hospitalier l'Université De Montréal (CHUM) - Hôpital Saint-luc; (514)890-8000 x25765

SOUCY, J L Rene; Canadian Med Protective Assoc, PO Box 8225 Stn T 875 Carling Ave, Ottawa ON K1S 5P1; Ott'79; BSc(Hon.Biol.); CCFP; Staff, Canadian Medical Protective Association; Langs: English; French; (613)725-2000

SOUCY, J R L Michel; CLSC Gaston Belanger, CP 590 113-30 rue Ferland, Sorel-Tracy QC J3P 3C7; Ott'77; Staff, Hôpital Richelieu; (450)746-4545 x5154; Fax. (450)746-7489; jrlmsoucy@yahoo.com.

SOUCY, Jacques; Ctr Hosp Affilie-Enfant-Jesus, 1401 18e rue, Quebec QC G1J 1Z4; Laval'66; FRCPC; Derm. ac Staff, Centre Hospitalier Affilié Universitaire de Québec - Hôpital De L'Enfant Jésus; ac Staff, CSSS de Quebec-Sud; (418)649-5520

SOUCY, Jean-Francois; Hôpital Ste-Justine, 3175 ch Cote-Sainte-Catherine, Montreal QC H3T 1C5; Mon'02; FRCPC; MedGenetics. Staff, Hôpital Ste-Justine; Staff, McGill University Health Centre - Montreal Children's Hospital; (514)345-4931

SOUCY, Jean-Paul; CHUM-Hop Notre-Dame, 1560 rue Sherbrooke E, Montreal QC H2L 4M1; Mon'80; ABNM; FRFPS; MSc; FRCPC; NuclearMed. Coord PET Unit, McGill University Health Centre - Montreal Neurological Hospital; Staff, Centre Hospitalier l'Université de Montréal (CHUM) - Hôpital Notre-Dame; Langs: English; (514)890-8280

SOUCY, Louis J; Royal Ottawa Hlth Care Group, 1145 Carling Ave, Ottawa ON K1Z 7K4; UBC'88; FRCPC; Psy. Ac Staff, Royal Ottawa Mental Health Centre - Royal Ottawa Health Care Group; Asst Prof, University of Ottawa; (613)722-6521; Fax. (613)722-7686; lsoucy@ottawahospital.on.ca.

SOUCY, Marc; CHUS-Hop Fleurimont, 3001 12e av N, Sherbrooke QC J1H 5N4; Sher'95; FRCPC; Peds. Staff, Centre Hospitalier Universitaire de Sherbrooke-Hopital Fleurimont; Langs: English; (819)346-1110; Fax. (819)564-5398; marc.soucy@usherbrooke.ca.

SOUCY, Marieke; CSSS de Témiscouta, 103 7e rue E, Degelis QC G5T 1Y6; Ott'02; CCFP; (418)853-2572; Fax. (418)853-3852.

SOUCY, Marina; 54 Av Bateman, Edmundston NB E3V 4A4; Sher'88; CCFP; Staff, Hôpital regional d'Edmundston; (506)739-5949; Fax. (506)739-9066.

SOUCY, Michele; Centre Med Brunswick, 401-955 boul Saint-Jean, Pointe-Claire QC H9R 5K3; Mon'80; MSc; Médecin Occupational Med, CLSC Lac St-Louis; Langs: English; (514)459-3428

SOUCY, Renee; CSSS du Rocher-Perce, CP 3300 451 rue Mgr Ross, Chandler QC G0C 1K0; McG'91; FRCSC; ObstGyn. Staff ObstGyn, Centre Hospitalier de Chandler; Langs: English; French; (418)689-2261; Fax. (418)689-6131.

SOUCY-HIRTLE, Fernande; Maison Michel-Sarrazin, 2101 ch Saint-Louis, Quebec QC G1T 1P5; Laval'60; Médecin, Maison Michel Sarrazin; Langs: English; (418)688-0878; Fax. (418)688-9372; fsoucy-hirtle@sympatico.ca.

SOUDEK JR, Dusan; Dartmouth Med Centre, 310-46 Portland St, Dartmouth NS B2Y 1H4; Qns'84; Langs: Czech; (902)465-4535; Fax. (902)464-4906.

SOUF, Shawki A; 706-2125 11th Ave, Regina SK S4P 3X3; Al-Fateh (Libya)'96; FRCSC; PlasSurg. (306)546-4460; Fax. (306)546-4461.

SOUHAMI, Luis; MUHC-Montreal Gen Hosp, D5400-1650 av Cedar, Montreal QC H3G 1A4; Rio-de-Janeiro (Brazil)'72; ABR; FRCPC; RadOncol (P.Q.) (Medical Oncology). Staff, McGill University Health Centre - Montreal General Campus; Sr Staff, McGill University Health Centre - Royal Victoria Hospital; Sr Staff, Sir Mortimer B Davis Jewish General; Prof RadOncol & Prof, McGill University; Langs: Spanish; Portuguese; French; (514)934-8040; Fax. (514)934-8220; luis.souhami@muhc.mcgill.ca.

SOUISSI, Hassen; Ctr Sante Tulattavik de l'Unga, CP 149, Kuujjuaq QC J0M 1C0; Sher'09; CCFP; Staff, Centre de sante Tulattavik de l'Ungava; (819)964-2905

SOUISSI, Kamel; CSSS de la Vallée de l'Or, 725 6e rue, Val-d'Or QC J9P 3Y1; (Tunisia)'04; Staff, Centre Hospitalier de Val d'Or; Langs: Arabic; English; (819)825-6711; Fax. (819)825-7919.

SOULAMA, Yamatien; CSSS de la Vallée de la Gatine, 309 boul Desjardins, Maniwaki QC J9E 2E7; (Other Foreign)'05; CCFP; Staff, CSSS de la Vallée de la Gatineau; (819)449-4690

SOULARD, Caroline; CSSS d'Argenteuil, 145 av de la Providence, Lachute QC J8H 4C7; Laval'10; CCFP; Staff, Centre Hospitalier d'Argenteuil; (450)562-3761

SOULARD, Isabelle; Hop Charles Lemoyne, 3120 boul Taschereau, Greenfield Park QC J4V 2H1; Sher'96; Psy. Staff, Hopital Charles LeMoyne; (450)466-5020; Fax. (450)466-5420.

SOULARD, Mario; Clinique East Angus, 1A-150 rue Angus S, East Angus QC J0B 1R0; Sher'96; (819)832-2438; Fax. (819)832-2104.

SOULELLIS, Constantine A; MUHC-Montreal Gen Hosp, 1650 av Cedar, Montreal QC H3G 1A4; McG'02; FRCPC; IntMed; Gastroent. Staff, McGill University Health Centre - Montreal General Campus; (514)934-1934; Fax. (514)934-8531.

SOULEZ, Gilles; CHUM-Hop Notre-Dame, 1560 rue Sherbrooke E, Montreal QC H2L 4M1; Paris (France)'88; FRCPC; DiagRad (P.Q.) (Interventional Radiology). ac Staff, Centre Hospitalier l'Université de Montréal (CHUM) - Hôpital Notre-Dame; dép Chef Radio, Radio-Oncology & Nuclear Med, Universite de Montreal; Langs: English; (514)890-8250; Fax. (514)412-7547; gilles.soulez@videotron.ca.

SOULIERE, Danielle; Medi Centre Chomedey, 610 boul Cure-Labelle, Laval QC H7V 2T7; Mon'90; Staff, CSSS de la Minganie; (450)687-6452

SOULIERE, Louise; Dir de la Sante Publique, 300-300 rue King E, Sherbrooke QC J1G 1B1; Mon'82; BSc(BioChem.); Clin Prof, Universite de Sherbrooke; (819)829-3400 x42455; Fax. (819)569-8894.

SOULIERE, Sheila F; BC Cancer Agency-Vanc Isl Ctr, 2410 Lee Ave, Victoria BC V8R 6V5; Tor'94; MD; FRCPC; IntMed (Breast Cancer); MedOncol. Staff, BC Cancer Agency Vancouver Island Centre; (250)519-5571; Fax. (250)519-5590.

SOULIERE, Vicky; Hop du Sacre-Coeur de Mtl, 5400 boul Gouin O, Montreal QC H4J 1C5; Sher'96; FRCPC; IntMed; Cardiol. Staff, Hôpital du Sacre-Coeur de Montréal; (514)338-2222; Fax. (514)338-2381; vickysouliere@yahoo.ca.

SOULIERES, Annie; Clinique Med Plateau Mont-Roya, 103-1374 rue Mont-Royal E, Montreal QC H2J 1Y7; Laval'92; FRCPC; Psy. Staff, Centre Hospitalier Régional de Lanaudière; (514)527-3997; Fax. (514)527-3994.

SOULIERES, Christine; CLSC de Pierrefonds, 13800 boul Gouin O, Pierrefonds QC H8Z 3H6; Mon'87; (514)626-2572; Fax. (514)626-8857.

SOULIERES, Denis; CHUM-Hop Notre-Dame, 1560 rue Sherbrooke E, Montreal QC H2L 4M1; Laval'91; MSc; FRCPC; Peds; MedOncol (P.Q.); Hem. Staff, Centre Hospitalier l'Université de Montréal (CHUM) - Hôpital Notre-Dame; (514)890-8000 x25381; denise.poirier.chum@ssss.gouv.qc.ca.

SOULIGNY, Julie S; 108-4275 Innes Rd, Orleans ON K1C 1T1; Ott'02; Langs: Bilingual(French/English); (613)830-2242; Fax. (613)830-2313.

SOULIGNY, Lyne H; Centre Med Ruby, 101-361 Main St E, Hawkesbury ON K6A 1A8; Mon'96; BSc(Biol.); CCFP; Staff, Hawkesbury & District General Hospital; Langs: Bilingual(French/English); (613)632-0605; Fax. (613)632-7073.

SOULIOS, Christos; 308-658 Danforth Ave, Toronto ON M4J 5B9; Thessaloniki (Greece)'80; FRCPC; Psy. Staff, North York General Hospital; Langs: Greek; (416)778-6534; Fax. (416)778-9990.

SOULTAN, Majed; CSSS du Pontiac, 200 rue Argue, Shawville QC J0X 2Y0; Sher'00; CCFP; Staff, Hull Hospital; (819)647-3851

SOUMBASIS, Elias; Caleo Health Crowfoot West, 340-600 Crowfoot Cres NW, Calgary AB T3G 0B4; Orange Free State (South Africa)'91; MB ChB; CCFP; Langs: Greek; Afrikaans; (403)452-0999; Fax. (403)452-0995.

SOUMIS, Anne; CSSS Pierre-De Sorel, 400 av de l'Hotel-Dieu, Sorel-Tracy QC J3P 1N5; Mon'06; Staff, Hôtel-Dieu de Sorel; (450)746-6000

SOURIAL, Fibi B W; Bramalea City Centre, 25 Peel Centre Dr, Brampton ON L6T 3R5; Cairo (Egypt)'74; CCFP; Langs: Arabic; French; (905)793-7077

SOURISSEAU, Louise A; 310-6411 Buswell St, Richmond BC V6Y 2G5; UBC'85; (604)278-6838; Fax. (604)278-8826.

SOURKES, Myra; Univ Hlth Network-Toronto Western Hosp, 435-399 Bathurst St, Toronto ON M5T 2S8; McG'77; FRCPC; IntMed; Electroenceph (P.Q.); Neur. Staff, Toronto Western Hospital - University Health Network; Staff, Toronto Rehabilitation Institute - University Centre; Langs: French; (416)603-5922; Fax. (416)603-7096.

SOUROVTSEVA, Elena A; Halton HSC Corp-Oakville, 327 Reynolds St, Oakville ON L6J 3L7; Saratov (Russia (Federation))'93; CCFP; Staff, Niagara Health System - Welland Hospital Site; Staff, Halton Healthcare Services Corporation - Oakville Site; Langs: Russian; (905)845-2571

SOUSA-POZA, Joaquin F; 1011 Morgan Rd SS 2 C17, Galiano BC V0N 1P0; Santiago (Spain)'62; DSc(Med); DPsy(McG); FRCPC; Psy (Psychotherapy). Langs: French; Spanish; (250)539-2359; jfsousapoza@gulfislands.com.

SOUSSOU, David; Glace Bay Healthcare Complex, 300 South St, Glace Bay NS B1A 1W5; American University of the Carribean (Other Foreign)'04; Staff, Sterling Medical Centre; (902)849-5511; Fax. (902)849-9005.

SOUSTER, Jenny D; University of Alberta Hosp, 2D WCM-8440 112 St NW, Edmonton AB T6G 2B7; Cal'04; FRCSC; Neursurg. Staff, University of Alberta Hospital; (780)407-8822

SOUSTER, Matthew; University of Alberta Hosp, 8440 112 St NW, Edmonton AB T6G 2B7; Sask'08; Staff, University of Alberta Hospital; (780)407-8822

SOUSTER, Timothy P W; PO Box 1467, Sundre AB T0M 1X0; Cal'06; BSc; CCFP; (403)638-2424; Fax. (403)638-3580.

SOUTAR, W Blake; Pine-Seven Office Park, 301-4610 Highway 7, Woodbridge ON L4L 4Y7; Tor'74; Court Staff, Humber River Regional Hospital - Finch Avenue Site; (905)265-7577; Fax. (905)265-7266.

SOUTER, Anne L; 1-1261 Beaverbrook Ave, London ON N6H 0G6; McM'85; BScN; CCFP; FCFP; Court Staff, St Joseph's Hospital - St Joseph's Health Care; (519)642-2077; Fax. (519)432-6921.

SOUTER, Francis C G; Canadian Forces Supp Unit HCC, 136B-1745 Alta Vista Dr, Ottawa ON K1A 0K6; Qns'69; MHSc; Mgr BWTMCM Project, Canadian Forces Health Services Centre; (613)945-6304; Fax. (613)990-2295.

SOUTHCOTT, John D; X-Ray Associates, 112-11811 Tecumseh Rd E, Tecumseh ON N8N 1L8; Wes'79; FRCPC; DiagRad. (519)979-2255

SOUTHCOTT, W Peter; 176 Essex St, Sarnia ON N7T 4R9; Wes'76; BSc; FRCSC; OrthSurg. Ac Staff, Bluewater Health - Mitton Site; Ac Staff, Bluewater Health - Norman Site; Assoc Staff, Bluewater Health - Charlotte Eleanor Englehart Hospital; (519)336-4100; Fax. (519)336-0570.

SOUTHEY, R George H; Dorval Med Assoc Fam Hlth Team, 104-465 Morden Rd, Oakville ON L6K 3W6; Qns'81; CCFP; FCFP; Ac Staff, Halton Healthcare Services Corporation - Oakville Site; (905)842-7154; Fax. (905)842-3604; gsouthey@cogeco.ca.

SOUTTER, D Ian; 611-581 Davis Dr, Newmarket ON L3Y 2P6; Qns'78; FRCSC; GenSurg (Surgical Oncology). Ac Staff, Southlake Regional Health Centre; (905)853-4448; Fax. (905)853-7411.

SOVIO, Olli M; 2080 McCallum Rd, Abbotsford BC V2S 3N4; UBC'74; FRCSC; OrthSurg. Consultant OrthSurg, Abbotsford Regional Hospital & Cancer Centre; Consultant, 100 Mile House District General Hospital; Consultant, Mission Memorial Hospital; Langs: Finnish; (604)852-1886; Fax. (604)852-3889.

SOVRAN, Steven A; Univ Hlth Network-Toronto Gen, RFE3 805-200 Elizabeth St, Toronto ON M5G 2C4; Wes'06; IntMed. Staff, Toronto General Hospital - UHN; (416)461-8272

SOWA, Bernard; Foothills Med Centre, 1403 29 St NW, Calgary AB T2N 2T9; Accra (Ghana)'76; MB ChB; FRCPC; Psy (General Adult Psychiatry). Staff, Foothills Medical Centre; Med Staff, Alberta Hospital Edmonton; Consultant, Cross Cancer Institute; Clin Prof, University of Alberta; (403)944-8298

SOWA, Bernard; University of Alberta Hosp, 8440 112 St NW, Edmonton AB T6G 2B7; Alb'06; Staff, University of Alberta Hospital; (780)407-8822

SOWERBY, Leigh J; St Josephs Health Care, PO Box 5777 Stn B 268 Grosvenor St, London ON N6A 4V2; Cal'06; FRCSC; Otol (Head & Neck Surgery). Staff, St Joseph's Hospital - St Joseph's Health Care; (519)646-6100

SOWERY, Richard S D; 482 Burlington Ave, Burlington ON L7S 1R5; Qns'00; BScH; MSc; DABU; FRCSC; Urol (Uro Oncology). Staff, Joseph Brant Memorial Hospital; (905)637-3900; Fax. (905)637-5557.

SOYEGE, Adeloye O; Moose Jaw Union Hosp, 455 Fairford St E, Moose Jaw SK S6H 1H3; Staff, Moose Jaw Union Hospital; (306)691-6684; Fax. (306)691-6686.

SOYEGE, Oyebanjo A; Synergy Wellness Centre, 221-501 Bethel Dr, Sherwood Park AB T8H 0N2; (Nigeria)'91; CCFP; (780)464-0123

SOYLU, Hanifi; WS 012-735 Notre Dame Ave, Winnipeg MB R3E 0L8; Erciyes Universitesi (Other Foreign)'89.

SPACEK, Alena M; The Ottawa Hosp-Civic Campus, 1053 Carling Ave, Ottawa ON K1Y 4E9; Ott'01; CCFP; CCFP(E.M.); Staff, The Ottawa Hospital - Civic Campus; Langs: Czech; (613)798-5555

SPACEK, Elena; Inst de Readaptation de Mtl, 6300 av de Darlington, Montreal QC H3S 2J4; Sher'95; FRCPC; PhysMed&Rehab. Staff, Institut de Réadaptation Gingras-Lindsay de Montréal; Langs: Slovak; English; (514)340-2085; Fax. (514)340-2775; espacek@hotmail.com.

SPACEK, Jan; Ctre de Readaptation de l'Estr, 2665 Place des Platanes, Sherbrooke QC J1G 4Z5; Bratislava (Slovakia)'72; DCMT; DGS; Langs: Slovak; Italian; Russian; Czech; (819)820-0460; Fax. (819)820-0211; jspacek@videotron.ca.

SPACEK, Katerina B; West End Family Care Clinic, 80 Michael Cowpland Dr, Ottawa ON K2M 1P6; Dal'08; CCFP; (613)599-3321; Fax. (613)599-3366.

SPACEK, Kimberly L; Maitland Valley Family Hlth Team, 180 Cambria Rd N, Goderich ON N7A 4N8; Ott'00; CCFP; CCFP(E.M.); Staff, Weeneebayko General Hospital; Staff, Westend Family Care Clinic Family Health Team; Langs: Czech; (519)524-6060; Fax. (519)525-5225.

SPACEK, Stan Z; Maitland Valley Family Hlth Team, 180 Cambria Rd N, Goderich ON N7A 4N8; Ott'00; CCFP; CCFP(E.M.); Staff, Weeneebayko General Hospital; Langs: Czech; (519)524-6060; Fax. (519)524-5225.

SPACEY, Sian D; UBC Hospital, S127-2211 Wesbrook Mall, Vancouver BC V6T 2B5; London (England)'92; BSc; MB BS; FRCPC; Neur (Headache). Staff Medical Clinic, UBC Hospital - Koerner Pavillion; Staff, Vancouver General Hospital - Centennial Pavillion; Assoc Prof/Dir Clinical Investigation Prog, University of British Columbia; (604)822-1728; Fax. (604)822-7897.

SPACKMAN, Keith E; PO Box 5550 Stn Main, High River AB T1V 1M6; Cal'79; (403)652-2929; Fax. (403)652-1510.

SPADAFORA, Peter J; 108-21 Surrey St W, Guelph ON N1H 3R3; Tor'95; CCFP; Staff, Guelph General Hospital; Langs: Italian; (519)823-2190; Fax. (519)823-2191.

SPADAFORA, Salvatore M; Mount Sinai Hosp, 5F-600 University Ave, Toronto ON M5G 1X5; Tor'90; FRCPC; Anes (Medical Education). Staff, Mount Sinai Hospital; Vice Dean PG Med Education, University of Toronto; (416)978-6709; Fax. (416)978-7144.

SPADAFORA, Silvana; Sault Area Hosp, 750 Great Northern Rd, Sault Ste. Marie ON P6B 0A8; Ott'88; BSc; FRCPC; IntMed; MedOncol. Staff Algoma Reg Cancer Prog, Sault Area Hospital - Sault Ste Marie; Assoc Consultant, North Eastern Ontario Reg Cancer Centre; Section Leader Internal Med, Northern Ontario School of Medicine; Langs: Italian; French; (705)759-3434 x4450; Fax. (705)759-3815.

SPADY, Michael J; Sheldon M Chumir Urgent Care, 1213 4 St SW, Calgary AB T2R 0X7; Alb'97; CCFP; Physician, Sheldon M Chumir Urgent Care Physician Group; (403)955-6007; Fax. (403)955-6023; michael.spady@albertahealthservices.ca.

SPAFFORD, Peter D; Wall Street Med Clinic, 230-140 Wall St, Saskatoon SK S7K 1N4; Sask'87; FRCS; FRCSC; Otol (Cancer Head & Neck). Ac Staff, St Paul's Hospital (Grey Nuns) of Saskatoon; Ac Staff, Saskatoon City Hospital; Assoc Prof/Ac Staff, Royal University Hospital; Sec Executive Council, Canadian Society of Otolaryngology; Assoc Prof Surg, University of Saskatchewan; (306)242-2346; Fax. (306)244-8864.

SPAIC, Tamara; St Joseph's Health Care, PO Box 5777 Stn B 268 Grosvenor St, London ON N6A 4V2; Mem'04; MSc; BSc; FRCPC; IntMed; Endocrin&Metab. Staff, St Joseph's Hospital - St Joseph's Health Care; Staff, London Health Sciences Centre - London Regional Cancer Centre; Asst Prof, University of Western Ontario; Langs: Yugoslavian; (519)646-6370; Fax. (519)646-6109.

SPAK, Andrew C D; 5966 Mullen Way NW, Edmonton AB T6R 0S9; Alb'00; CCFP; (780)801-1220; Fax. (780)801-1225.

SPANER, David E; Toronto Sunnybrook Reg Cancer, 2075 Bayview Ave, Toronto ON M4N 3M5; Alb'84; PhD(Immunol); FRCPC; IntMed. (416)480-5248; Fax. (416)480-6002.

SPANER, Donna-Mary S; Toronto Grace Hosp, 650 Church St, Toronto ON M4Y 2G5; Alb'84; CCFP; FCFP; Staff Palliative Care, The Salvation Army Toronto Grace Health Centre; (416)925-2251 x201; Fax. (416)925-9136.

SPANER, Douglas L; Groot Dermasurgery Centre, 204-9670 142 St NW, Edmonton AB T5N 4B2; Alb'79; FRCPC; Psy. Staff, Regional Mental Health Services-Edmonton; (780)451-1424; Fax. (780)451-1626; dlspaner@shaw.ca.

SPANER, Shelley J; Radiology Consultants Assoc, 120-6707 Elbow Dr SW, Calgary AB T2V 0E3; Alb'96; FRCPC; DiagRad. (403)777-3003; Fax. (403)777-3008.

SPANGEHL, G Werner; George Street Fam Practice, 1-1400 George St, White Rock BC V4B 4A3; Sask'87; BSc; Staff/Med Dir, Peace Arch Hospital; Langs: German; (604)536-1686; Fax. (604)536-6440; spangehl@shaw.ca.

SPANGENBERG, Benjamin; Associate Med Clinic, 203-10030 106 St, Westlock AB T7P 2K4; Free State University (South Africa) MB ChB; (780)349-3341; Fax. (780)349-6686.

SPANGENBERG, David F; Maidstone Med Clinic, PO Box 399, Maidstone SK S0M 1M0; (306)893-2689; Fax. (306)893-4646.

SPANGLET, Offir; 25 Joseph St, Kitchener ON N2G 4X6; Tor'97; FRCPC; IntMed. (519)578-2100

SPANO, Frank A; Synergy Centre, 1635 Hyde Park Rd, London ON N6H 5L7; Wes'09; CCFP; (519)266-3600

SPANO, Joseph J; 457 London Rd, Sarnia ON N7T 4W9; Wes'77; Staff GP, Bluewater Health - Norman Site; Staff GP, Bluewater Health - Mitton Site; Langs: Italian; French; (519)344-3085

SPANO GRECO, Giuseppe; Avenue Bloor Med Group, 405-208 Bloor St W, Toronto ON M5S 3B4; Tor'92; BSc; Langs: Italian; (416)962-1207; Fax. (416)962-1223.

SPANSWICK, Christopher C; Chronic Pain Centre, 160-2210 2 St SW, Calgary AB T2S 3C3; Manchester (England)'73; FRCA; MB ChB; Med Leader, Calgary Pain Program; Clinical Asst Prof Anes, University of Calgary; (403)943-9900; Fax. (403)209-2954; chris.spanswick@albertahealthservices.ca.

SPARANESE, Amerigo D; Royal Oak Ctre Med Clinic Ltd, 105-4442 West Saanich Rd, Victoria BC V8Z 3E9; Man'76; CCFP; Langs: Italian; (250)479-6721; Fax. (250)727-6751.

SPARAVALO, Nebojsa; Queen Elizabeth II HSC, 257-1276 South Park St, Halifax NS B3H 2Y9; Bosnia-Hercegovina (Bosnia-Herzegovina)'75; Staff, Queen Elizabeth II Health Sciences Centre - Victoria General Site; (902)473-7845; Fax. (902)473-1475.

SPARKES, David M; Foothills Prof Bldg, 170-1620 29 St NW, Calgary AB T2N 4L7; Iowa City(IA) (USA)'70; Ac Staff, Foothills Medical Centre; (403)221-9340; Fax. (403)221-9336.

SPARKES, Rebecca L; Alberta Children's Hosp, 2888 Shaganappi Trail NW, Calgary AB T3B 6A8; Alb'03; FRCPC; MedGenetics. Staff Inherited Metabolic Diseases, Alberta Children's Hospital; (403)955-7587; Fax. (403)955-3091.

SPARKS, George W; Colwood Prof Centre, 202-1910 Sooke Rd, Victoria BC V9B 1V7; Cal'85; CCFP; FCFP; (250)474-0800; Fax. (250)474-5310.

SPARLING, Terence G; BC Cancer Agency-Vanc Isl Ctr, 2410 Lee Ave, Victoria BC V8R 6V5; Qns'72; ABIM; FRCPC; IntMed; Hem. Staff MedOncol, BC Cancer Agency Vancouver Island Centre; (250)519-5500

SPARROW, Andrew K; University Hlth Ntwk-Toronto Western Hosp, WW 2F-399 Bathurst St, Toronto ON M5T 2S8; Qns'08; CCFP; Staff Family Health Team, Toronto Western Hospital - University Health Network; (416)603-5888; Fax. (416)603-5821.

SPARROW, Carl D; Murray Clinic-Valley Mall, 1 Mount Bernard Ave, Corner Brook NL A2H 6Y5; Mem'78; CCFP; FCFP; Staff, Western Memorial Regional Hospital; (709)785-5141; Fax. (709)785-5705.

SPARROW, Nicholas R; Gibsons Med Clinic, RR 8 8-821 Gibsons Way, Gibsons BC V0N 1V8; London (England)'01; MB BS; CCFP; (604)886-2868

SPARROW, Robert K; Stratford Gen Hosp, 46 General Hospital Dr, Stratford ON N5A 2Y6; Mem'75; DiagRad. Staff Radiol, London Health Sciences Centre - Victoria Campus; Staff, Stratford General Hospital - Huron Perth Healthcare Alliance; Assoc Prof Radiol, University of Western Ontario; (519)272-8210; Fax. (519)271-7137.

SPARTACO, Navaro; Miramichi Reg Hosp, 500 Water St, Miramichi NB E1V 3G5; Damascus (Syria)'94; Staff, Miramichi Regional Hospital; (506)623-3000

SPATZ, Alan; SMBD Jewish Gen Hosp, 3755 ch Cote-Sainte-Catherine, Montreal QC H3T 1E2; Paris (France)'92; AnatPath. Staff Path, Sir Mortimer B Davis Jewish General; (514)340-8222

SPAVOR, Maria L; Edmonton Clinic Health Academy, 11405 87 Ave, Edmonton AB T6G 1C9; Alb'97; FRCPC; Peds. Staff Peds, University of Alberta Hospital; Staff, Edmonton Clinic Health Academy; (780)248-5530

SPAXMAN, Thomas L; Brantford Med Centre, 40 Shellington Place, Brantford ON N3S 0C5; McM'97; CCFP; (519)753-9581; Fax. (519)753-9547.

SPAYNE, Jacqueline A; Toronto Sunnybrook Cancer Ctre, 2075 Bayview Ave, Toronto ON M4N 3M5; Tor'99; BSc; PhD; FRCPC; RadOncol. Staff Odette Cancer Centre, Sunnybrook Health Sciences Centre; Staff, Toronto East General Hospital Inc; Staff, Royal Victoria Regional Health Centre; (416)480-4974; Fax. (416)480-6002.

SPAZIANI, Robert; St Joseph's Healthcare, MW H417-50 Charlton Ave E, Hamilton ON L8N 4A6; McM'99; BSc(Hon); FRCPC; IntMed; Gastroent. Staff Gastroent, St Joseph's Healthcare - Charlton Campus; Asst Prof Med, McMaster University; (905)522-1155; Fax. (905)521-6064.

SPEARS, Benjamin; Charlottetown Area Health Ctr, 10-1 Rochford St, Charlottetown PE C1A 9L2; London (England)'65; DPM; MRCS; LRCP; MRCPsy; Ac Staff, Queen Elizabeth Hospital; Clin Instructor Psy, Dalhousie University; (902)628-6258

SPEARS, Danna A; Univ Hlth Network-Toronto Gen, 4NU 492-200 Elizabeth St, Toronto ON M5G 2C4; Qns'00; FRCPC; IntMed; Cardiol. Staff, Toronto General Hospital - UHN; (416)340-3535; Fax. (647)693-7543.

SPEARS, John C; Women's College Hosp, 762-76 Grenville St, Toronto ON M5S 1B2; Wes'57; FRCPC; IntMed (Cardiology). Consultant, Women's College Hospital; Asst Prof Med, University of Toronto; (416)323-7701; Fax. (416)323-6304.

SPEARS, Julian; St Michael's Hosp, 30 Bond St, Toronto ON M5B 1W8; Dal'98; FACS; SM; FRCSC; Neursurg (Vascular Neuro Surgery). Staff NeuroSurg & Endovascular, St Michael's Hospital; (416)864-5667; Fax. (416)864-5644.

SPEER, Margaret L; Eveline Street Clinic, 66 Eveline St, Selkirk MB R1A 1K6; Man'85; CCFP; (204)785-5550; Fax. (204)785-8966.

SPEERT, David P; Child & Family Research Inst, A5 175-950 28th Ave W, Vancouver BC V5Z 4H4; Columbia (USA)'73; FRCPC; Peds (Infectious Diseases). Ac Staff, BC Children's Hospital; Prof Peds, University of British Columbia; (604)875-2438; dspeert@cw.bc.ca.

SPEES, Richard C; 1653 Montreal Rd, Ottawa ON K1J 6N6; McG'76; FRCPC; Psy. Langs: Spanish; French; (613)594-0307; Fax. (613)594-8941.

SPEIRS, John W D; Windsor Radiology Associates, 1568 Ouellette Ave, Windsor ON N8X 1K7; UBC'91; FRCPC; DiagRad.

SPELAY, Jodi L; Medical Arts Bldg, 222-750 Spadina Cres E, Saskatoon SK S7K 3H3; Sask'92; FRCSC; GenSurg; VascSurg. Assoc Prof, St Paul's Hospital (Grey Nuns) of Saskatoon; Chair Med Capital Equipment Comm/Board Member/Rep Assembly, Saskatchewan Medical Association; (306)653-3366; Fax. (306)653-8832.

SPELLISCY, Shawn D; Kelowna Gen Hosp, 2268 Pandosy St, Kelowna BC V1Y 1T2; Alb'77; FRCPC; EmergMed. Staff, Kelowna General Hospital; (250)862-4495

SPENARD, Jean-Raymond; Ctre Med Pierre-Boucher, 370-1615 boul Jacques-Cartier, Longueuil QC J4M 2X1; Mon'83; FRCSC; Otol (Head & Neck Surgery). ac Staff, Centre Hospitalier Pierre Boucher; (450)647-4307

SPENCE, Ann K; 108-450 Central Ave, London ON N6B 2E8; Wes'70; MSc; CCFP; FCFP; Assoc Staff, St Joseph's Hospital - St Joseph's Health Care; Assoc Staff Med, London Health Sciences Centre - Victoria Campus; University of Western Ontario; (519)672-3020; Fax. (519)672-6090.

SPENCE, Brian J; Professional Corp, 67 Scenic Park Cres NW, Calgary AB T3L 1R8; Alb'71; CCFP; (403)239-7881; Fax. (403)241-6856.

SPENCE, Catherine A; Queen West Commun Health Ctre, 168 Bathurst St, Toronto ON M5V 2R4; Tor'87; Court Staff Privil, Women's College Hospital; Court Staff Privil, Toronto General Hospital - UHN; (416)703-8480; Fax. (416)703-8479.

SPENCE, David C; Alberta Hosp Edmonton PO Box 307 Stn Main, Edmonton AB T5J 2J7; Dal'89; FRCPC; Psy. Staff, Alberta Hospital Edmonton; (780)342-5452; Fax. (780)472-5411.

SPENCE, Edwin B; 4744 Bank St, Ottawa ON K1T 3W7; Orange Free State (South Africa)'96; MB BS; Physician Cancer Care, Pinawa Hospital; Langs: Afrikaans; Sotho; (613)317-2584; Fax. (613)822-2775; espence@neha.mb.ca.

SPENCE, Frank P; Bridgeland Med Bldg, 306-803 1 Ave NE, Calgary AB T2E 7C5; Qns'82; FRCPC; IntMed (Interventional Cardiology); Cardiol. Staff, Foothills Medical Centre; Clin Asst Prof, University of Calgary; (403)215-2212; Fax. (403)215-2208; stent@shaw.ca.

SPENCE, J David; 1400 Western Rd, London ON N6G 2V4; Wes'70; BA; MBA; FAHA; FRCP; DrMedCh; FRCPC; IntMed (Stroke Prevention); Neur. Staff, London Health Sciences Centre - University Hospital; Dir, The Robarts Research Institute; Prof Stroke Prevention & Atheroslerosis Centre/Member Stroke Team/Teach Staff Neurol & Clin Pharmacol, University of Western Ontario; Langs: Spanish; (519)931-5731; Fax. (519)931-5737; dspence@robarts.ca.

SPENCE, James W; Royal Jubilee Hosp, 4-1952 Bay St, Victoria BC V8R 1J8; UBC'94; BSc; MSc; FRCPC; IntMed. Staff, Royal Jubilee Hospital; Staff, Cowichan District Hospital; (250)519-1829; Fax. (250)370-8762; jimspence@viha.ca.

SPENCE, Jeffrey D; 309-460 Springbank Dr, London ON N6J 0A8; Wes'95; CCFP; FCFP; (519)858-0013; Fax. (519)858-3713; office.oldsouthfho@gmail.com.

SPENCE, Julia M; St Michael's Hosp, 30 Bond St, Toronto ON M5B 1W8; Qns'87; DAB; FRCPC; EmergMed. Staff, St Michael's Hospital; Staff, Sunnybrook Health Sciences Centre; Asst Prof, University of Toronto; (416)864-5095; Fax. (416)864-5341.

SPENCE, Norma L; Maternal Child Clinic, 130-1402 8 Ave NW, Calgary AB T2N 1B9; Alb'88; CCFP; FCFP; (403)509-3080; Fax. (403)509-3082.

SPENCE, William J E; 407-200 St Clair Ave W, Toronto ON M4V 1R1; Qns'49; FRCSC; GenSurg. Staff, Toronto General Hospital - UHN; Assoc Prof, University of Toronto.

SPENCER, Adam O; Alberta Children's Hosp, 2888 Shaganappi Trail NW, Calgary AB T3B 6A8; McM'05; FRCPC; Anes. Staff, Alberta Children's Hospital; (403)955-7810; Fax. (403)955-7606.

SPENCER, Andrew; Guardian Med Arts Bldg, 206-1950 Algonquin Ave, North Bay ON P1B 4Z2; Wes'89; Staff, North Bay Regional Health Centre - Regional Mental Health; (705)472-1030; Fax. (705)472-4466.

SPENCER, Brian P; Shelbourne Med Clinic, 150-3200 Shelbourne St, Victoria BC V8P 5G8; Alb'75; (250)598-2427; Fax. (250)598-2489.

SPENCER, Frederick A; St Joseph's Healthcare, H319-50 Charlton Ave E, Hamilton ON L8N 4A6; McG'91; FRCPC; Cardiol (Thromboembolism). Staff, St Joseph's Healthcare - Charlton Campus; Prof, McMaster University; (905)522-1155

SPENCER, G Todd; Health Sciences North-Laurenti, 41 Ramsey Lake Rd, Sudbury ON P3E 5J1; NOSM'09; CCFP; Staff, Health Sciences North-Laurentian Site; Staff, St Joseph's General Hospital Elliot Lake; (705)561-3057

SPENCER, George R; Associated Physicians, 2425 Bevan Ave, Sidney BC V8L 4R5; Edinburgh (Scotland)'73; BSc; MB ChB; FRCS(Ed); Ac Staff, Saanich Peninsula Hospital; (250)656-1164; Fax. (250)656-7870.

SPENCER, Gordon J; 646 Main St, Glace Bay NS B1A 4Y1; Dal'92; Physician, Glace Bay Integrated Health Care System; (902)842-1596

SPENCER, J Alan; Fort Frances Clinic, 301 Victoria Ave, Fort Frances ON P9A 2C1; Leeds (England)'61; DRCOG; FRCS; FACS; MB BS; MB ChB; FRCSC; GenSurg. Consultant Surg, La Verendrye Hospital - Riverside Health Care Facility; (807)274-3287; Fax. (807)274-7875.

SPENCER, Joanne; Atikokan Family Health Team, PO Box 1450 123 Marks St, Atikokan ON P0T 1C0; McM'91; (807)597-2721; Fax. (807)597-4632.

SPENCER, John A; 385 The West Mall, Etobicoke ON M9C 1E7; Tor'74; DOphth; FRCSC; Ophth. (416)622-1864; Fax. (416)622-1215.

SPENCER, Jon R L; Canada Place Bldg, 200-107 Shirreff Ave, North Bay ON P1B 7K8; Tor'61; FRCSC; Ophth. Staff, North Bay Regional Health Centre - Regional Mental Health; Consultant, Work Safety & Insurance Board; Langs: French; (705)474-7480; Fax. (705)474-6981.

SPENCER, Kevin D; Winchester Dist Mem Hosp, 566 Louise St, Winchester ON K0C 2K0; Dal'09; CCFP; Staff, Winchester District Memorial Hospital; (613)774-2422

SPENCER, Lesley M; Perth & Smiths Falls Dist Hosp, 60 Cornelia St W, Smiths Falls ON K7A 2H9; Dal'05; CCFP; Staff, SCO Health Service - Élisabeth Bruyère Hospital; Staff, Perth & Smiths Falls District Hospital - Smiths Falls Site; (613)283-2330

SPENCER, Louis R; One Med Place, 302-20 Wynford Dr, North York ON M3C 1J4; Cambridge (England)'49; LRCP; MB ChB; Court Staff, North York General Hospital; (416)441-2118; Fax. (416)441-2119.

SPENCER, Mandy L; Paterson Med Centre, 45 Wolsley St, Kenora ON P9N 3W7; NOSM'09; CCFP; Staff, Lake of the Woods District Hospital; (807)468-3021

SPENCER, Martin H; Seafield Med Bldg, 5-1179 Seafield Cres, Nanaimo BC V9S 4S1; Chicago (USA)'72; FRCSC; Ophth. Staff, Nanaimo Regional General Hospital; Physician, Medical Clinic; Langs: German; Spanish; French; (250)753-3323; Fax. (250)753-1165.

SPENCER, Nigel J; 201-16 Green St, Nepean ON K2J 3R2; Ott'82; (613)825-8397; Fax. (613)825-9687.

SPENCER, Paul S; 1 Klauck St, Fort Erie ON L2A 3P2; Tor'84; Med Dir, Crescent Park Lodge; (905)871-7996

SPENCER, Perry W; 12 Princess St, St Stephen NB E3L 2E8; Dal'75; BSc; ACLS; FCFP; LMCC; CCFP; FCFP; Staff Chief Obst, Charlotte County Hospital; Dep Chief Facility Staff, Saint John Regional Hospital; Asst Prof Family Med, Memorial University Of Newfoundland; Asst Prof Family Med, Dalhousie University; (506)466-5973; Fax. (506)466-5741.

SPENCER, Steven; Kootenay Boundary Reg Hosp, 1200 Hospital Bench, Trail BC V1R 4M1; Wes'88; Staff, Kootenay Boundary Regional Hospital; (250)368-3311

SPENCER NETTO, Fernando A C; Sunnybrook Hlth Sciences Ctre, H115-2075 Bayview Ave, Toronto ON M4N 3M5; Universidade Federal De Pernambuco (Other Foreign)'94; FRCSC; GenSurg (Trauma). Staff, Toronto Western Hospital - University Health Network; Clin Associate, Sunnybrook Health Sciences Centre; Langs: Portuguese; (416)480-6100

SPENLER, Valerie S M S; Anaesthesia Associates, 439 Park St, Kitchener ON N2G 1N4; Sask'85; FRCPC; Anes. (519)744-7361; Fax. (519)744-7363.

SPENSER, Helen R; CHEO Med Clinic, 200-311 McArthur Ave, Vanier ON K1L 8M3; McM'88; MSW; FRCPC; Psy;CCFP; Staff, Children's Hospital of Eastern Ontario (CHEO); Asst Prof Med & Psy, University of Ottawa; Langs: French; (613)738-6990 x251; Fax. (613)738-4891.

SPENSIERI, Donato; Pine Seven Med Centre, 205-4600 Highway 7, Woodbridge ON L4L 4Y7; Tor'75; Ac Staff, William Osler Health System - Etobicoke General Hospital; Ac Staff, Humber River Regional Hospital - Finch Avenue Site; Langs: Italian; (905)850-7788; Fax. (905)850-7790.

SPERANZA, Giovanna; Hopital Charles LeMoyne, 3120 boul Taschereau, Longueuil QC J4V 2H1; McG'04; MedOncol; IntMed. Staff, Hopital Charles LeMoyne; (450)466-5000

SPERBER, Gregory; Edmonton Clinic Health Academy, Edmonton Clinic Health Academy 5383-11405 87 Ave NW, Edmonton AB T6G 1C9; Witwatersrand (South Africa)'56; MSc; PhD; DMD; Staff, Edmonton Clinic Health Academy; Prof, University of Alberta; (780)492-5194; Fax. (780)492-7536; gsperber@ualberta.ca.

SPERDUTO, Michel N; Pontiac Health Centre, 200 rue Argue, Shawville QC J0X 2Y0; (Haiti)'81; Staff, Pontiac Hospital Centre; (819)662-2211

SPERKA, Paul J; Lifemark Health Institute, 230 Meadowlark Shopping Ctr NW, Edmonton AB T5R 5W9; Comenius (Slovakia)'71; FRCPC; OccupMed (Industrial Occupational Medicine). Langs: Slovak; Czech; (780)429-4761; Fax. (780)425-4274; paul.sperka@lifemark.ca.

SPERLICH, Catherine; Hop Charles LeMoyne, 3120 boul Taschereau, Greenfield Park QC J4V 2H1; Mon'99; FRCPC; Hem (Medical Oncology); IntMed. Staff, Hopital Charles LeMoyne; (450)466-5000 x2318; Fax. (450)466-5066; catherine.sperlich@videotron.ca.

SPERLING, Bradley D; 239B 5th Ave N, Saskatoon SK S7K 2P2; Sask'88; CCFP; Physician, Diseases of the Ageing; (306)382-4300; Fax. (306)382-7095.

SPERLING, Zdenka; 204-1865 Marine Dr, West Vancouver BC V7V 1J7; UBC'84; (604)913-1111

SPETTIGUE, Wendy J; Children's Hosp of Eastern Ont, 401 Smyth Rd, Ottawa ON K1H 8L1; Qns'91; FRCPC; Psy. Staff Psy, Children's Hospital of Eastern Ontario (CHEO); (613)737-7600 x3609; wspettigue@cheo.on.ca.

SPEVACK, Leslie M; North York Med Arts Bldg, 222-1333 Sheppard Ave E, North York ON M2J 1V1; Wes'88; FRCSC; Urol. Ac Staff, North York General Hospital; Court Staff, The Scarborough Hospital - Birchmount Campus; Court Staff, Rouge Valley Health System - Centenary Health Centre Site; Staff, North York General Hospital - Branson Division; (416)494-7888; Fax. (416)494-3070.

SPICE, Ronald N; Okotoks Hlth & Wellness Ctre, 11 Cimarron Common, Okotoks AB T1S 2E9; Alb'85; CCFP; FCFP; Med Staff, Claresholm General Hospital; (403)995-2714; Fax. (403)995-2619.

SPICER, Dwight L; Fairview Med Clinic, 222 Fairview Dr, Brantford ON N3R 2W9; McM'82; CCFP; FCFP; Ac Staff, The Brant Community Healthcare System - Brantford General Hospital Site; (519)756-8340; Fax. (519)752-2256.

SPICER, Finlay R; 206-6112 Quinpool Rd, Halifax NS B3L 1A3; Dal'86; (902)420-1635; Fax. (902)420-0025.

SPICER, Jonathan; MUHC-Montreal Gen Hosp, 1650 av Cedar, Montreal QC H3G 1A4; McG'05; FRCSC; GenSurg. Staff, McGill University Health Centre - Montreal General Campus; (514)934-1934

SPICER, Sharron L; Alberta Children's Hosp, 2888 Shaganappi Trail NW, Calgary AB T3B 6A8; Cal'95; FRCPC; Peds. Staff, Alberta Children's Hospital; (403)955-7211; Fax. (403)955-7649.

SPICER, Tara L; Port Arthur Health Centre, 194 Court St N, Thunder Bay ON P7B 2X8; NOSM'09; CCFP; Staff, Thunder Bay Regional Health Sciences Centre Port-Arthur; (807)346-1000; Fax. (807)346-6206.

SPIEGEL, Lynn R; The Hosp for Sick Children, 555 University Ave, Toronto ON M5G 1X8; McG'87; FAAP; MDCM; FRCPC; Peds (Pediatric Rheumatology). Assoc Prof Rheumatol, The Hospital For Sick Children; Staff Ped Rheumatol, Richmond Hill Children's Clinic; Asst Prof, University of Toronto; (416)813-6117; Fax. (416)813-4989.

SPIEGEL, Sanford M; Diagnostic Radiology Sevices L, 408-658 Danforth Ave, East York ON M4J 5B9; Tor'78; FRCPC; DiagRad. Asst Prof, University of Toronto; Langs: Hebrew; (416)465-1726; Fax. (416)465-5695.

SPIEGELMAN, Jamie; Humber River Reg Hosp-Finch, 2111 Finch Ave W, North York ON M3N 1N1; Tor'05; FRCPC; IntMed; Critical Care Medicine. Staff, Toronto General Hospital - UHN; Staff, Humber River Regional Hospital - Finch Avenue Site; (416)340-4485

SPIELMAN, John M; Kenora Med Centre, RR 1 Stn Main 45 Wolsley St, Kenora ON P9N 3W7; Madison(WI) (USA)'79; FRCSC; GenSurg. Staff, Lake of the Woods District Hospital; (807)468-5410; Fax. (807)468-8009.

SPIELMANN, Audrey L; Lions Gate Hosp, 231 15th St E, North Vancouver BC V7L 2L7; UBC'92; BSc; FRCPC; DiagRad. Staff, Lions Gate Hospital; University of British Columbia; (604)988-3131

SPIER, Phyllis; North Med Centre, 306-7131 Bathurst St, Thornhill ON L4J 7Z1; Tor'68; FAAP; Court Staff, North York General Hospital; (905)886-9705; Fax. (905)886-4154.

SPIER, Sheldon; Children's & Women's HC of BC, 4480 Oak St, Vancouver BC V6H 3V4; McG'77; FRCPC; Peds; Respir. Staff, BC Children's Hospital; (604)875-2119

SPIER, Stanley; North Med Centre, 306-7131 Bathurst St, Thornhill ON L4J 7Z1; Tor'68; FRCPC; Derm. Langs: Yiddish; French; (905)886-9705; Fax. (905)886-4154.

SPIERS, Anne-Marie C; Beaumont Med Clinic, 5001A 50 Ave, Beaumont AB T4X 1E7; Alb'07; (780)929-6050; Fax. (780)929-5848.

SPIERS, Caroline; Beaumont Med Clinic, 5001A 50 Ave, Beaumont AB T4X 1E7; Alb'07; CCFP; Langs: Bilingual(English/French); (780)929-6050; Fax. (780)929-5848.

SPIERS, Patrick A; Meadowlark Health Centre, 200 Meadowlark Shopping Ctr NW, Edmonton AB T5R 5W9; Alb'04; FRCPC; DiagRad. (780)489-8430; Fax. (780)481-6630.

SPIERS, S John; Medical Place, 360 Huron St, Stratford ON N5A 5T5; Belfast (Ireland)'73; MB ChB; BAO; Staff, Stratford General Hospital - Huron Perth Healthcare Alliance; Coroner, Milverton County.

SPIERS, Thomas C; Meadowlark Health Centre, 200 Meadowlark Shopping Ctr NW, Edmonton AB T5R 5W9; Alb'72; FRCPC; DiagRad. Ac Staff, Covenant Health - Misericordia Community Hospital; Assoc Prof, University of Alberta; (780)489-5313; Fax. (780)486-5160.

SPIES, Cornelius A; Broadway Med Clinic, 205-41A Broadway St W, Yorkton SK S3N 0L6; Orange Free State (South Africa)'94; MB ChB; MMed; FRCSC; ObstGyn (Endoscopic Gynecology Surgery). Staff, Yorkton Regional Health Centre; Obstetrics & Gynecology, St Peter's Hospital; (306)782-5525; Fax. (306)782-3616; cornelius.spies@shr.sk.ca.

SPIESS, Andre J; Towne Centre Medical, 18-2475 Dobbin Rd, Westbank BC V4T 2E9; Dal'89; (250)768-8315; Fax. (250)768-8326.

SPIESS, Michael P; University of Calgary-HSC, 3330 Hospital Dr NW, Calgary AB T2N 4N1; Cal'07; OrthSurg. Staff, University of Calgary; (403)220-2724; Fax. (403)220-1185.

SPIESS, Steven D; 405 Sackville Dr, Lower Sackville NS B4C 2R9; Dal'92; Hlth Serv Off, Royal Canadian Mounted Police; (902)865-7555; steven.spiess@nshi.ca.

SPIGELBLATT, Linda S; Hop Maisonneuve-Rosemont, 5415 boul de l'Assomption, Montreal QC H1T 2M4; McG'72; BSc; FRCPC; Peds (Alternative Medicine). Consultant, Hôpital Ste-Justine; assoc Prof, Hopital Maisonneuve-Rosemont; assoc Prof, Universite de Montreal; Langs: English; French; (514)252-3807; Fax. (514)252-3545.

SPIKA, John S; Public Health Agency of Canada, 6502A-130 Colonnade Rd, Ottawa ON K1A 0K9; Minneapolis(MN) (USA)'74; Langs: French; (613)948-7929; Fax. (613)946-3135.

SPILLER, Allison E; Kingston Gen Hosp, C7-76 Stuart St, Kingston ON K7L 2V7; McM'97; FRCPC; Neur (Epilepsy). Staff, Kingston General Hospital; (613)549-6666 x6242; Fax. (613)548-1341.

SPILLER, Mark A; Kirkland & District Gen Hosp, 145 Government Rd, Kirkland Lake ON P2N 3P4; Tor'89; Head Emerg & Fam Med/Chief of Staff, Kirkland & District Hospital; (705)567-5251

SPINDLER, Eric E; The Ottawa Hosp-Civic Campus, D6-1053 Carling Ave, Ottawa ON K1Y 4E9; Dal'74; FRCPC; Psy (In-Patient Hospital Psychiatry). Staff, Royal Ottawa Mental Health Centre - Royal Ottawa Health Care Group; Staff, The Ottawa Hospital - Civic Campus; Staff, The Ottawa Hospital - General Campus; (613)761-4588; Fax. (613)761-4177.

SPINK, Amy W A; Royal Jubilee Hosp, 1952 Bay St, Victoria BC V8R 1J8; UBC'07; CCFP; Staff, Royal Jubilee Hospital; (250)370-8000

SPINK JR., Donald R; Brookdale Family Clinic, 304 Bellevue St, Peterborough ON K9H 5G1; Qns'81; BSc; MSc; CCFP; Staff, Peterborough Regional Health Centre - Hospital Drive; Med Advisor, Extendicare-Peterborough; Med Dir, Fairhaven Home for Senior Citizens; (705)743-7101; Fax. (705)743-7104; donspink@hotmail.com.

SPINNER, Miriam R; St Joseph's Healthcare, 50 Charlton Ave E, Hamilton ON L8N 4A6; Baltimore(MD) (USA)'68; AB(Psy.); FRCPC; Psy (Child & Adolescent Psychiatry). Ac Staff McMaster Psychiatric Unit, St Joseph's Healthcare - Charlton Campus; Assoc Prof, McMaster University; (905)522-4941 x33535; Fax. (905)540-6516.

SPIRIDIGLIOZZI, Mary; Rockland MD, 110-100 ch Rockland, Saint-Leonard QC H1R 2T6; McG'87; (514)326-7203; Fax. (514)326-3656.

SPIROU, Christos; 13278 Tecumseh Rd E, Tecumseh ON N8N 1M2; Wes'89; CCFP; Physician, Essex Walk-In Clinic; Physician, Tilburg Walk-In Clinic; Langs: Greek; (519)735-2558; Fax. (519)735-2530.

SPITALE, Naomi S; Carling-Broadview Med Bldg, 303-770 Broadview Ave, Ottawa ON K2A 3Z3; Tor'05; FRCPC; IntMed; Respir. Staff, The Ottawa Hospital - General Campus; (613)722-9900; Fax. (613)722-9100.

SPITHOFF, Daren; Gibson Med Associates, 211-1100 Sunshine Coast Hwy, Gibsons BC V0N 1V7; McM'07; CCFP; Staff, Vancouver General Hospital - Centennial Pavillion; (604)886-2868

SPITHOFF, Sheryl M; St Joseph's Hlth Centre, 30 The Queensway, Toronto ON M6R 1B5; McM'01; CCFP; Staff, St Joseph's Health Centre; (416)530-6000; sheryl.spithoff@pchc.on.ca.

SPITTEL, Devin M; PO Box 278 Stn Del Ctr, Maple Ridge BC V2X 7G2; Alb'68; BSc; DAB; FACS; FRCSC; GenSurg.

SPITZER, Rachel F; Mount Sinai Hosp, 3F-600 University Ave, Toronto ON M5G 1X5; McM'01; BSc; MPH; FRCSC; ObstGyn (Pediatric & Adolescent Gynecology). Staff, The Hospital For Sick Children; Staff, Mount Sinai Hospital; Asst Prof, University of Toronto; Langs: French; Hebrew; (416)586-4822; Fax. (416)586-4657.

SPIVAK, Harold I; St Michael's Hosp, CCW17 002B-30 Bond St, Toronto ON M5B 1W8; Man'86; FRCPC; Psy. Staff Mental Health Serv, St Michael's Hospital; (416)864-3085; Fax. (416)864-5480.

SPIVAK, Mitchel H; Rockyview Gen Hosp, 7007 14 St SW, Calgary AB T2V 1P9; McG'97; FRCPC; Psy. Staff, Rockyview General Hospital; (403)943-8704; Fax. (403)259-6289.

SPLAWINSKI, Jan B; 3407 27 Ave, Vernon BC V1T 1S2; Cal'91; BSc; MSc; FRCSC; OrthSurg (Spine Surgery). Staff, Vernon Jubilee Hospital; Langs: Polish; (250)545-1339; Fax. (250)545-1035; jsvoa@shaw.ca.

SPLINTER, Karen L N; Sudbury Med Centre, 301-65 Larch St, Sudbury ON P3E 1B8; Ott'07; FRCSC; ObstGyn. (705)222-0492; Fax. (705)222-7226.

SPLINTER, William M; Children's Hosp of Eastern Ont, 401 Smyth Rd, Ottawa ON K1H 8L1; Qns'83; FRCPC; Anes (Palliative Care). Staff Anes, Children's Hospital of Eastern Ontario (CHEO); Assoc Staff, The Ottawa Hospital - General Campus; Assoc Staff, The Ottawa Hospital - Civic Campus; Assoc Prof, University of Ottawa; (613)737-2431; Fax. (613)738-4815.

SPODEK, Jeffrey M; Scarborough Prof Centre, 405-1371 Neilson Road, Scarborough ON M1B 4Z8; Wes'98; MD(Hons.); BSc; FRCSC; Urol. Ac Staff, Rouge Valley Health System - Centenary Health Centre Site; Court Staff, The Scarborough Hospital - General Campus; Court Staff, North York General Hospital; (416)284-0233; Fax. (416)284-0974.

SPOONER, Betty A; La Ronge Med Clinic, PO Box 240, La Ronge SK S0J 1L0; Sask'74; CCFP; FCFP; Staff, La Ronge Health Centre; Physician, La Ronge Medical Clinic; (306)425-2174; Fax. (306)425-4199.

SPOONER, Devin A; University Hosp of Northern BC, 1475 Edmonton St, Prince George BC V2M 1S2; UBC'98; CCFP; CCFP(E.M.); Staff, University Hospital of Northern British Columbia; (250)565-2000; Fax. (250)565-2343.

SPOONER, G Richard; Grey Nuns Family Med Centre, 2927 66 St NW, Edmonton AB T6K 4C1; Sask'74; MD; CCFP; FCFP; Staff, Covenant Health - Grey Nuns Community Hospital; Physician, Grey Nuns Family Medicine Centre; Prof/Dept Chair Family Med, University of Alberta; (780)342-1470; Fax. (780)490-0953; rick.spooner@ualberta.ca.

SPOONER, G Robin; Elgin Med Centre, 101-2255 Elgin Ave, Port Coquitlam BC V3C 2B4; Otago (New Zealand)'81; MB ChB; (604)942-7292

SPOONER, Lorinda G; Vancouver Coastal Health, 1141 Melville St, Vancouver BC V6E 4E5; Cal'92; CCFP; FCFP; Physician, Vancouver Drug Court; (604)775-0144

SPOONER, Marcia A; 68 Bridge St, Carleton Place ON K7C 2V3; Ott'07; CCFP; Langs: Bilingual(English/French); (613)257-4793; Fax. (613)257-4794.

SPORINA, Jan; Rockyview Gen Hosp, 7007 14 St SW, Calgary AB T2V 1P9; (Czech Republic)'83; FRCPC; IntMed. Staff, Rockyview General Hospital; (403)943-8693; Fax. (403)943-8535.

SPOTSWOOD, Wayne J; Queen's University, 18 Barrie St, Kingston ON K7L 3J6; Qns'70; FRCPC; EmergMed;CCFP; CCFP(E.M.); Staff Emerg Med, Queen's University; (613)548-2368; Fax. (613)548-1374.

SPOUGE, Alison R I; London HSC-University Hosp, PO Box 5339 Stn B 339 Windermere Rd, London ON N6A 5A5; UBC'83; FRCPC; DiagRad. Staff, London Health Sciences Centre - University Hospital; (519)663-3648; Fax. (519)663-8803.

SPOUGE, David J; North Shore Med Imaging, 139 16th St W, North Vancouver BC V7M 1T3; UBC'86; FRCPC; DiagRad. (604)987-9729; Fax. (604)984-8395.

SPRACKLIN, Ann E; South Shore Reg Hosp, 90 Glen Allan Dr, Bridgewater NS B4V 3S6; Mem'98; FRCPC; DiagRad. Staff, South Shore Regional Hospital; (902)527-5227; Fax. (902)543-9793.

SPRAGUE, John H; Rimrock Med Clinic, 14-5201 50 St, Leduc AB T9E 6T4; Alb'62; BSc; FRCPC; IntMed (Hypertension). Ac Staff, Leduc Community Hospital; (780)986-1714; Fax. (780)986-1824.

SPRAGUE, Nancy L; Rimrock Med Clinic, 14-5201 50 St, Leduc AB T9E 6T4; Alb'76; BSc; (780)986-1714; Fax. (780)986-1824.

SPRATLIN, Jennifer L; Cross Cancer Institute, 11560 University Ave NW, Edmonton AB T6G 1Z2; Alb'01; FRCPC; IntMed (Clinical Trials); MedOncol. Staff, Cross Cancer Institute; (780)432-8513; Fax. (780)432-8888.

SPRATT, Elizabeth E; Hamilton HS-General Site, 237 Barton St E, Hamilton ON L8L 2X2; Mem'80; BMedSci; Asst Cardiac Surg OR, Hamilton Health Sciences Centre - Hamilton General Hospital; (905)527-4322 x46277

SPRATT, Laura L M; 301-3491 Saanich Rd, Victoria BC V8X 1W8; McG'86; MDCM; CCFP; FCFP; (250)475-2251; Fax. (250)475-3530.

SPREAD, Carole-Yvonne; Aberdeen Reg Hosp, 835 East River Rd, New Glasgow NS B2H 3S6; Alb'87; FRCSC; GenSurg. Staff, Aberdeen Regional Hospital; (902)752-1187; Fax. (902)752-2262.

SPRING, Beverly F; Vancouver Home Hospice, 300-999 Broadway W, Vancouver BC V5Z 1K5; McM'80; Assoc Staff, Providence Health Care - St Paul's Hospital; Physician, Vancouver Home Hospice Palliative Care Service; (604)742-4010

SPRING, Elise S; 303-294 Main St, Toronto ON M4C 4X5; McM'83; (416)699-2667; Fax. (416)699-8791.

SPRING, Lawrence R; Pukatawagan Nursing Station, GD, Pukatawagan MB R0B 1G0; Man'99; CCFP; Staff, Pukatawagan Nursing Station; (204)553-2271

SPRING, Melanie J; Trillium Health Ctre-Mississau, 100 Queensway W, Mississauga ON L5B 1B8; Qns'04; FRCPC; IntMed. Staff, Trillium Health Centre - Mississauga; (905)848-7100

SPRING, Paul; 440 Jarvis St, Toronto ON M4Y 2H4; Tor'69; DABPN; FRCPC; Psy (Child & Adolescent Psychiatry). Consultant Child Psy, Lakeridge Health - Oshawa Site; Consultant, The Hincks-Dellcrest Centre - Toronto; Asst Prof, University of Toronto; (416)924-1164 x6075

SPRINGATE, Russell P; Two Rivers FHT-Healthlink, 10-350 Conestoga Blvd, Cambridge ON N1R 7L7; Cal'75; CCFP; FCFP; Staff, Cambridge Memorial Hospital; Clin Assoc Prof Family Med, McMaster University; (519)740-5010; Fax. (519)740-6010.

SPRINGER, Colvin D; Windsor Reg Cancer Centre, 2220 Kildare Rd, Windsor ON N8W 2X3; West Indies (Jamaica)'78; FACR; FRCPC; RadOncol. Staff, Windsor Regional Hospital - Metropolitan Site; Radiation Oncology, Windsor Regional Hospital - Windsor Regional Cancer Centre; (519)253-5253; Fax. (519)255-8679; colvin_springer@wrh.on.ca.

SPRINGER, Jonathon E; Bloor-Jane Med Bldg, 513-2425 Bloor St W, Toronto ON M6S 4W4; Tor'94; FRCPC; IntMed; Gastroent. Staff Gastroent, St Joseph's Health Centre; (416)766-4587; Fax. (416)766-5076.

SPRINGLE, Milan A; Trafalgar Med Clinic, 200-1235 Trafalgar Rd, Oakville ON L6H 3P1; Tor'68; Physician, Maplehurst Correctional Centre; Physician, Syl Apps Youth Centre; (905)844-3281; Fax. (905)849-1076.

SPRINGLE, Stephen W; Georgian Prof Centre, 003-125 Bell Farm Rd, Barrie ON L4M 6L2; Tor'88; Staff, Royal Victoria Regional Health Centre; (705)728-4225; Fax. (705)728-5936.

SPRINGUEL, Andre; Regie l'Assurance Maladie QC, Q004-1125 rue Grand Allee O, Quebec QC G1S 1E7; Sher'80; Staff, Regie de l'Assurance Maladie du Quebec; (418)682-5144 x5255; Fax. (418)643-3858; andre.springuel@saaq.gouv.qc.ca.

SPROAT, Janet E; Cambridge Mem Hosp, 700 Coronation Blvd, Cambridge ON N1R 3G2; McM'80; MSc; PlasSurg (Clinical Oncology). Staff, Hamilton Health Sciences Centre - Hamilton General Hospital; Court Staff Juravinski Cancer Centre, Cambridge Memorial Hospital; Physician, Hamilton Regional Cancer Centre; Clin Assoc Prof, McMaster University; (519)621-2330 x2340

SPROUL, Cathryn D; Medical Assoc Clinic, 305-1101 Dewdney Ave, Trail BC V1R 4T1; Dal'90; BSc(Biology); FRCSC; OrthSurg. (250)364-1799; Fax. (250)368-8886.

SPROUL, M Jane; Medical Bldg, 1703-805 Broadway W, Vancouver BC V5Z 1K1; Qns'76; FRCSC; PlasSurg. (604)872-6717

SPROULE, Donald A; St Mary's Hosp Centre, 3830 av Lacombe, Montreal QC H3T 1M5; McG'86; CCFP; FCFP; ac Staff Family Med, St Mary's Hospital Centre; adj Prof, McGill University; (514)345-3511; Fax. (514)734-2602; dsproule@ssss.gouv.qc.ca.

SPROULE, James; Queen Elizabeth II HSC-Halifax, 4867-1796 Summer St, Halifax NS B3H 3A7; Galway (Ireland)'94; MB BCh; BAO; Staff, Queen Elizabeth II Health Sciences Centre - Halifax Infirmary Site; (902)473-7137; Fax. (902)473-7137.

SPROULE, James R; Canadian Med Protective Assoc, 875 Carling Ave, Ottawa ON K1S 5P1; McG'83; MBA; Dip SportMed; CCFP; CCFP(E.M.); Physician, Canadian Medical Protective Association; (613)725-2000; Fax. (613)725-1300; jsproule@cmpa.org.

SPROULE, Julie S; Maternity Care Clinic, 109-178 96 Ave NE, Calgary AB T3K 6G4; Staff, Maternity Care Clinic; (403)735-4922

SPROULE, Pamela; Tudor Village Clock Tower, 105-1315 Summit Dr, Kamloops BC V2C 5R9; Cal'93; FRCSC; ObstGyn. Ac Medical Staff, Royal Inland Hospital; (250)377-4949; Fax. (250)377-4664.

SPROULE, Timothy R; 605 McCowan Rd, Scarborough ON M1J 1J9; Alb'80; FRCSC; PlasSurg (Burns). Ac Staff, The Scarborough Hospital - General Campus; Court Staff, Sunnybrook Health Sciences Centre; Court Staff, Rouge Valley Health System - Centenary Health Centre Site; Lecturer Plastic Surg, University of Toronto; (416)439-1718; Fax. (416)439-2526; admin@plasticos.ca.

SPRUYT, Marlene E; Temiskaming Health Unit, 43-247 Whitewood Ave Box 1090, New Liskeard ON P0J 1P0; Ott'84; CCFP; FCFP; Ac Staff, Manitoulin Health Centre - Mindemoya Site; (705)647-4305 x2223; Fax. (705)647-5779; marlene.spruyt@ontariomed.ca.

SPRUYT, O Wilhelm; PO Box 359, Spirit River AB T0H 3G0; (South Africa)'72; (780)864-3962; Fax. (780)864-4491.

SPRY, Geoffrey A; Caledonian Med Clinic, 340 Campbell St, Nanaimo BC V9R 3G7; Monash (Australia)'72; BSc(Med.); DObstRCOG; FRACGP; MB BS; (250)753-3202; Fax. (250)753-1039.

SPUDAS, Alexander J; Victoria Terrace Med Centre, 210-1448 Lawrence Ave E, North York ON M4A 2V6; Mainz (Germany)'61; Ac Staff, The Scarborough Hospital - General Campus; Court Staff, Rouge Valley Health System - Centenary Health Centre Site; Staff Pt-Time, Ontario Shores Centre for Mental Health Sciences; Langs: German; Lithuanian; (416)751-0082; Fax. (416)752-4935.

SPUNT, Ronald S; Centre de Med Familiale, 75 av de la Gare, Saint-Sauveur QC J0R 1R6; McG'71; (450)227-1864; Fax. (450)227-9221.

SPUREK, Monika J; Pelham Group Health Centre, 101-245 Pelham Rd, St Catharines ON L2S 1X8; Wroclaw (Poland)'98; FRCPC; IntMed; Cardiol. Staff, Niagara Health System - St Catharines General Site; (905)685-0707; Fax. (905)685-0703.

SPURLL, Gwendoline M; MUHC-Royal Victoria Hosp, C6 82-687 av des Pins O, Montreal QC H3A 1A1; Man'74; FRCPC; Hem (Laboratory Medicine). Staff, McGill University Health Centre - Royal Victoria Hospital; assoc Prof, McGill University; Langs: English; French; (514)843-1558; Fax. (514)843-1418; gwendoline@spurll.mcgill.ca.

SPURRELL, David W; Lakeridge Health Corp-Oshawa, 1 Hospital Crt, Oshawa ON L1G 2B9; Tor'04; FRCPC; Anes. Staff, Lakeridge Health - Oshawa Site; (905)576-8711; Fax. (905)743-5946.

SQUAREY, Kyna J; Health Sciences Centre, 300 Prince Philip Dr, St. John's NL A1B 3V6; Mem'99; BSc; FRCPC; Neur (Movement Disorders). Staff, Health Sciences Centre; Langs: Bilingual(English/French); (709)737-6300

SQUARZOLO, Melanie A M; Sudbury Reg Hosp-Laurentian, 41 Ramsey Lake Rd, Sudbury ON P3E 5J1; Tor'05; CCFP; CCFP(E.M.); Staff, Health Sciences North-Laurentian Site; (705)675-4790

SQUIBB, Stephanie A; Newhook Comm Health Centre, PO Box 449, Whitbourne NL A0B 3K0; Mem'98; CCFP; (709)759-2300; Fax. (709)759-2387.

SQUIRE, Daniel S; 342 Pennywell Rd, St. John's NL A1E 1V9; Mem'83; FRCSC; OrthSurg. Att Staff, St Clare's Mercy Hospital; Att Staff, Health Sciences Centre; (709)579-6339; Fax. (709)753-2671.

SQUIRE, Pamela L; Broadway Med Centre, 930-943 Broadway W, Vancouver BC V5Z 4E1; Sask'88; CCFP; Staff, Lions Gate Hospital; University of British Columbia; (604)737-7122

SQUIRES, Edward M; Dalbrent Med Centre, 200-3604 52 Ave NW, Calgary AB T2L 1V9; Qns'68; Med Staff Assoc, Foothills Medical Centre; Staff Teacher, University of Calgary; (403)284-2261; Fax. (403)284-9434.

SQUIRES, James S; Guelph Med Place, 201B-83 Dawson Rd, Guelph ON N1H 1B1; Tor'80; FRCPC; EmergMed. Physician, Guelph Emergency Medical Services.

SQUIRES, Philip J R; Cambridge Prof Centre, 205-386 Cambria St, Stratford ON N5A 1J4; Cal'73; FAAP; DTMH; FRCPC; Peds. Staff, Stratford General Hospital - Huron Perth Healthcare Alliance; Staff, Wingham & District Hospital - Listowel Wingham Hospitals Alliance; University of Western Ontario; Langs: French; (519)271-2545; Fax. (519)271-6026.

SQUIRES, Suzanne R; Westgrove Clinic, 201-505 Queen St, Spruce Grove AB T7X 2V2; Alb'01; CCFP; (780)962-9888; Fax. (780)960-5298.

SQUIRES, Tina E; Southern Med Centre, 390 Topsail Rd, St. John's NL A1E 2B8; Mem'96; CCFP; (709)364-9556; Fax. (709)364-9408.

SQUIRES, W Gordon D; One Med Place, 215-20 Wynford Dr, North York ON M3C 1J4; Qns'73; DAB; FRCSC; Ophth. Lecturer, University of Toronto; (416)441-1313; Fax. (416)441-6138.

SQUIRES, William E; Timmins & District Gen Hosp, 700 Ross Ave E, Timmins ON P4N 8P2; Ott'01; FRCSC; GenSurg. Staff, Timmins & District Hospital; (705)267-6331

SRADJ, Naila; Clinique Med Le Plein Ciel, 475 boul de la Cote-Vertu, Saint-Laurent QC H4L 1X7; (Algeria)'00; (514)337-3171

SREBRNJAK, Margaret J; The Credit Vally Hosp, 2200 Eglinton Ave W, Mississauga ON L5M 2N1; Tor'92; FRCPC; Anes. Staff, Women's College Hospital; Staff, The Credit Valley Hospital; (905)813-2200

SREEHARSHA, Boraiah; Univ Hlth Network-Princess M, 974-610 University Ave, Toronto ON M5G 2M9; Mysore University (India)'01; DiagRad. Staff, Princess Margaret Hospital - University Health Network; (416)946-4501

SREENIVASAN, Barathi R; St John's Rehab Hosp, 285 Cummer Ave, North York ON M2M 2G1; Dal'98; FRCPC; PhysMed&Rehab. Staff, Sunnybrook Health Sciences Centre; Staff, St John's Rehabilitation Hospital; (416)226-6780

SREENIVASAN, Bobby; Magrath Med Clinic, 308-14127 23 Ave NW, Edmonton AB T6R 0G4; Alb'02; CCFP; (780)430-8788; Fax. (780)435-3134.

SREENIVASAN, Gayatri M; Gordon & Leslie Diamond HCC, 10149-2775 Laurel St, Vancouver BC V5Z 1M9; UBC'96; BSc; FRCPC; IntMed; Hem. Staff, Gordon & Leslie Diamond Health Care Centre; Staff, Vancouver General Hospital - Centennial Pavillion; Clinical Asst Prof Hematology, University of British Columbia; (604)875-4952; Fax. (604)875-4763.

SREENIVASAN, Vidya A; The Rehabilitation Centre, 1200-505 Smyth Rd, Ottawa ON K1H 8M2; Dal'00; FRCPC; PhysMed&Rehab. Assoc Staff Rehab Med, The Ottawa Hospital Rehabilitation Centre; (613)737-7350; Fax. (613)737-9638.

SRICHANDRA, Withaya; Manitoba Clinic, 790 Sherbrook St, Winnipeg MB R3A 1M3; Dublin (Ireland)'61; MB ChB; MRC; FRCSC; ObstGyn (Colposcopy). Assoc Staff, Health Sciences Centre; Assoc Staff, The Salvation Army Grace Hospital; Clin Teacher ObstGyn, University of Manitoba; (204)788-5704; Fax. (204)789-9235.

SRIDHAR, Guruswamy; Regina Qu'Appelle HR-Regina, 1440 14th Ave, Regina SK S4P 0W5; Madras (India)'81; MB; BSc; MRC(UK); FRCP; FRCPC; IntMed (Sleep Medicine); Respir. Staff Sleep Clinic, Regina General Hospital; Asst Prof, University of Saskatchewan; (306)766-4881; Fax. (306)766-4882; g.sridhar@rqhealth.ca.

SRIDHAR, Jami; Campbellton Reg Hosp, PO Box 880 Stn Main 189 Lily Lake Rd, Campbellton NB E3N 3H3; M K C G University (India)'89; Staff, Hôpital Régional Campbellton; Langs: Hindi; Telugu; Oriya; (506)789-5000; Fax. (506)789-5190; jamisridhar@hotmail.com.

SRIDHAR, Kollipara; Western Mem Reg Hosp, PO Box 2005 Stn Main 1 Brookfield Ave, Corner Brook NL A2H 6J7; Sri Venkatesvara University (Sri Lanka)'86; MB BS; FRCPC; Anes. Staff, Western Memorial Regional Hospital; (709)637-5000

SRIDHAR, Krishnakumar; London HSC-University Hosp, PO Box 5339 Stn B 339 Windermere Rd, London ON N6A 5A5; Wes'87; FRCPC; IntMed (Interventional Cardiology); Cardiol. Staff, London Health Sciences Centre - University Hospital; Asst Prof Med, University of Western Ontario; (519)663-3474; Fax. (519)663-2997.

SRIDHAR, Shrikant K; Dawson Creek Med Clinic, 816 103 Ave, Dawson Creek BC V1G 2G1; (Ireland)'07; MB BCh; BAO; (250)782-5271

SRIDHAR, Srikala S; UHN-Princess Margaret Hosp, 5 110-610 University Ave, Toronto ON M5G 2M9; Ott'98; FRCPC; IntMed (Breast Oncology); MedOncol. Staff MedOncol, Princess Margaret Hospital - University Health Network; Langs: English; French; (416)946-4501 x2520; Fax. (416)946-6546; srikala.sridhar@uhn.on.ca.

SRIDHAR, Srilata K; Lakeridge Health-Bowmanville, 47 Liberty St S, Bowmanville ON L1C 2N4; Ott'05; FRCPC; IntMed; Critical Care Medicine. Staff, Mount Sinai Hospital; Staff, Lakeridge Health - Bowmanville Site; (905)623-3331; Fax. (905)697-5115.

SRIGLEY, Jocelyn A; Univ Hlth Network-Toronto Gen, 9 C S B-200 Elizabeth St, Toronto ON M5G 2C4; Tor'06; FRCPC; IntMed; InfectDis; MedMicrobiol. Staff, Toronto General Hospital - UHN; (416)340-4800

SRIGLEY, John R; The Credit Valley Hosp, 2200 Eglinton Ave W, Mississauga ON L5M 2N1; Tor'77; AB(CytoPath); FRCPC; AnatPath (Urology). Consultant Oncol & Urologic Path, The Credit Valley Hospital; Prof, McMaster University; (905)813-2696; jsrigley@cvh.on.ca.

SRIHARAN, Thushiyanthy; Family Med Centre, 10-2677 Kennedy Rd, Scarborough ON M1T 3B5; Madras (India)'89; MB BS; CCFP; Langs: Tamil; (416)412-7300; Fax. (416)412-3400.

SRIHARSHA, Hindupuram V; Orillia Med/Dental Centre, 102-16 O'Brien St, Orillia ON L3V 5S2; Bangalore (India)'67; MB BS; FRCPC; IntMed (Nephrology). Staff, South Muskoka Memorial Hospital - Muskoka Algonquin Healthcare; Staff, Orillia Soldiers' Memorial Hospital; Langs: Kanarese; Tamil; Telugu; (705)326-1242; Fax. (705)327-9818.

SRIKANTHAN, Amirrtha; Univ Hlth Network-Princess M, 5 110-610 University Ave, Toronto ON M5G 2M9; Qns'08; FRCPC; IntMed. (416)946-2000

SRIKISSON, Nirupa; The Malone Med Clinic, 4955 41 Ave, Drayton Valley AB T7A 1V4; (South Africa)'95; (780)542-3366; Fax. (780)542-6207.

SRINATHAN, Sadeesh K; Health Sciences Centre, GE 611-820 Sherbrook St, Winnipeg MB R3A 1R9; McM'91; FRCSC; GenSurg; ThorSurg. Staff, Health Sciences Centre; (204)774-8511

SRINIVAS, Sathish; Herzig Eye Institute, 210-131 Bloor St W, Toronto ON M5S 1R1; Dr M G R Medical University (India)'95; (416)929-2020; Fax. (416)929-0232.

SRINIVASAGAM, Vuthamy M R; Regina Gen Hosp, 1440 14th Ave, Regina SK S4P 0W5; Staff NICU, Regina General Hospital; (306)766-6161; Fax. (306)766-4557.

SRINIVASAN, Anjana; SMBD Jewish Gen Hosp, H231 1-3755 Cote-Sainte-Cather, Montreal QC H3T 1E2; McG'00; CCFP; Staff, Sir Mortimer B Davis Jewish General; adj Prof, McGill University; (514)340-8222 x3269; Fax. (514)340-8634.

SRINIVASAN, Anuradha; Carefirst Family Health Team, 27-420 Hwy 7 E, Richmond Hill ON L4B 3K2; Andhra (India)'74; DCH; Staff, The Scarborough Hospital - General Campus; Staff, The Scarborough Hospital - Birchmount Campus; Langs: Tamil; (905)695-1133; Fax. (905)695-0826; anuradha.srinivasan@carefirstfht.com.

SRINIVASAN, Coimbatore V; Univ Hlth Network-Toronto Gen, 200 Elizabeth St, Toronto ON M5G 2C4; Bangalore University (India)'96; FRCPC; Anes. Staff, Toronto General Hospital - UHN; (416)340-4800 x6960; Fax. (416)340-3698.

SRINIVASAN, Ganesh; Health Sciences Centre, 820 Sherbrook St, Winnipeg MB R3A 1R9; Staff, Health Sciences Centre; Staff, St Boniface General Hospital; (204)774-8511

SRINIVASAN, Ilavajady; The Hosp for Sick Children, 555 University Ave, Toronto ON M5G 1X8; Thanjavur Medical College (India)'94; FRCPC; Anes. Staff, The Hospital For Sick Children; (416)813-7445

SRINIVASAN, Janaki; 518 Eglinton Ave E, Toronto ON M4P 1N6; Bangalore (India)'74; MB BS; FRCPC; Psy (Mood Disorders). Staff, Centre for Addiction & Mental Health (CAMH) - College Street Site; Consultant, North York General Hospital; Lecturer, University of Toronto; Langs: Tamil; (416)489-1984; Fax. (416)489-0278.

SRINIVASAN, Kalyani; Fredericton Med Clinic, 103-435 Regent St, Fredericton NB E3B 3X6; Madras (India)'79; MB BS; DCH; CCFP; Ac Staff, Dr Everett Chalmers Regional Hospital; (506)458-0290; Fax. (506)458-0312; ksrinik@yahoo.com.

SRINIVASAN, Vasundhara; 204-3269 Bloor St W, Etobicoke ON M8X 1E2; Mysore (India)'73; FRCPC; Psy. Staff Teacher, Centre for Addiction & Mental Health (CAMH) - Queen Site; Psychologist Cons, Ontario Correctional Institute; University of Toronto; Langs: Kanarese; Telugu; (416)560-1949

SRIRAM, Konya R V; Victoria Hosp, PO Box 3000 Stn Main 1200 24th St W, Prince Albert SK S6V 5T4; Madras (India)'66; MB BS; FRCPC; Anes. Staff, Victoria Hospital; (306)961-0104

SRIRAM, Priya N; Associate Med Clinic, 400-20 14th St W, Prince Albert SK S6V 3K8; (Other Foreign)'95; CCFP; Staff, Shellbrook Primary Care Clinic; Staff, Family Doctor Walk-In Clinic; (306)764-1513; Fax. (306)764-3091.

SRIRANGARAJAN, Ramani; Strait Richmond Hosp, 138 Hospital Rd RR 1, Cleveland NS B0E 1J0; Jaffna (Sri Lanka)'85; MB BS; CCFP; Staff Emerg, Strait Richmond Hospital; Locum Tenens Emerg, Aberdeen Regional Hospital; Langs: Tamil; (902)625-3100; Fax. (902)625-3770.

SRIVAMADEVAN, Maheswaran; Oak Ridges Med Centre, 303-13291 Yonge St, Richmond Hill ON L4E 4L6; Qns'00; FRCPC; IntMed; Cardiol. Langs: Tamil; (905)751-2941; Fax. (905)751-0107.

SRIVASTAVA, Amresh K; Regional Mental HC-St Thomas, PO Box 2004 Stn Main F160-467 Sunset Dr, St Thomas ON N5P 3V9; Indore University (India)'79; FRCPC; Psy. Staff, Regional Mental Health Care-St Joseph's Health Care; (519)631-8510; Fax. (519)631-2512.

SRIVASTAVA, Anil; Ontario Shores Ctr Mental HS, 700 Gordon St, Whitby ON L1N 5S9; Qns'03; FRCPC; Psy. Staff, Ontario Shores Centre for Mental Health Sciences; (905)668-5881

SRIVASTAVA, Anita; St Joseph's Health Centre, 30 The Queensway, Toronto ON M6R 1B5; Tor'96; CCFP; Staff, St Joseph's Health Centre; (416)530-6860; Fax. (416)530-6160.

SRIVASTAVA, Swati; Campbellton Reg Hosp, PO Box 880 189 Lily Lake Rd, Campbellton NB E3N 3H3; Staff, Hôpital Régional Campbellton; (506)789-5000

SRIVATSA, Kousthub K; Colchester East Hants Hlth Ctr, 600 Abenaki Rd, Truro NS B2N 5A1; Mumbai (India)'99; MB BS; Staff, Colchester East Hants Health Centre; (902)893-4321

SROLOVITZ, Herbert D; G122-SMBD Jewish Gen Hosp, 3755 ch Cote-Sainte-Catherine, Montreal QC H3T 1E2; Basel (Switzerland)'66; DTM; FRCPC; GenPath (Anatomical Pathology). assoc Staff, Sir Mortimer B Davis Jewish General; (514)340-8222 x5473; Fax. (514)340-8102.

SROUR, David; Southlake Reg Health Centre, 596 Davis Dr, Newmarket ON L3Y 2P9; McM'07; CCFP; Staff, Southlake Regional Health Centre; (905)895-4521

SROUR, Leila F; PO Box 19017 Rpo Fourth Ave, Vancouver BC V6K 4R8; Uberlandia (Brazil)'84; FRCPC; CommunMed. Langs: Portuguese.

SROUR, Myriam; MUHC-Montreal Children's Hosp, A508-2300 rue Tupper, Montreal QC H3H 1P3; McG'01; Neur. Staff, McGill University Health Centre - Montreal Children's Hospital; (514)412-4466

SROUR, Nadim; The Ottawa Hosp-Civic Campus, 1053 Carling Ave, Ottawa ON K1Y 4E9; Sher'03; FRCPC; Respir; IntMed (Clinician Investigator Program). Staff, The Ottawa Hospital - Civic Campus; Langs: Bilingual(English/French); (613)798-5555; Fax. (613)761-5333.

SSEGUYA-LWANGA, David; Cape Breton Hlthcare Complex, 1482 George St, Sydney NS B1P 1P3; Makerere (Uganda)'88; MB ChB; Staff Anes, Cape Breton Healthcare Complex; (902)567-7832

ST-AMAND, Hugo; Hôpital de Gatineau, 909 boul de la Verendrye O, Gatineau QC J8P 7H2; Laval'03; FRCSC; PlasSurg (Esthetic Plastic Surgery). div Chef Plastic Surg/Staff, Hôpital de Gatineau; Langs: Bilingual(French/English); (819)966-6100; Fax. (819)966-6297.

ST-AMAND, Marc A; London HSC-University Hosp, PO Box 5339 Stn B 339 Windermere Rd, London ON N6A 5A5; Ott'90; FRCPC; Anes. Asst Prof, London Health Sciences Centre - University Hospital; Langs: French; (519)663-3384

ST AMAND, Ruth A O; 210-1685 Main St W, Hamilton ON L8S 1G5; McM'82; CCFP; FCFP; (905)527-2266

ST AMAND, Timothy A; Niagara Hlth System-Niagara, 142 Queenston St, St Catharines ON L2R 7C6; McM'02; CCFP; CCFP(E.M.); Staff, Niagara Health System - St Catharines General Site; (905)384-7271 x45200

ST AMANT, Krista M; Credit Valley Family Health Te, 101-2300 Eglinton Ave W, Mississauga ON L5M 2V8; NOSM'10; CCFP; (905)813-3850

ST-AMANT, Lincey; Centre Hosp de Val d'Or, 725 6e rue, Val-d'Or QC J9P 3Y1; Sher'10; CCFP; Staff, Centre Hospitalier de Val d'Or; (819)825-5858

ST-AMANT, Manon; CSSS de la Matapedia, 135 av Gaetan-Archambault, Amqui QC G5J 2K5; Laval'00; Staff, CSSS de la Matapedia; (418)629-2211

ST-AMANT-CARDIN, Dolores; 600 boul Harwood, Vaudreuil-Dorion QC J7V 6A3; Mon'07; (450)455-9301

ST-AMOUR, Annie; Barrie Mem Hosp, CP 2000 28 rue Gayle, Ormstown QC J0S 1K0; Mon'97; Staff, Barrie Memorial Hospital; (450)829-2321

ST-AMOUR, Dominic; Centre de Phlebologie, 916 boul Saint-Joseph E, Montreal QC H2J 1K6; Laval'98; Staff, Centre Hospitalier l'Université de Montréal (CHUM) - Hôpital Notre-Dame; (514)526-8888

ST-AMOUR, Eric; Clinique Med Cité des jeunes, 200-214 boul de Cite-des-Jeune, Gatineau QC J8Y 6S8; Ott'94; CCFP; Staff, Hull Hospital; Langs: French; (819)776-6582; Fax. (819)595-0422.

ST-AMOUR, Jeanne; Polyclinique St-Martin, 604-1435 boul Saint-Martin O, Laval QC H7S 2C6; Mon'74; (450)668-3310; Fax. (450)668-9347.

ST-AMOUR, Marie; Dir de la Sante Publique, 1255 rue Beauregard, Longueuil QC J4K 2M3; Sher'96; CSPQ; FRCPC; CommunMed; Public Health & Preventive Med (Infectious Diseases). Staff, Hopital Charles LeMoyne; Langs: English; (450)928-6777 x3126; Fax. (450)928-3023.

ST-AMOUR, Nicole D; 2109 Ottawa St, Windsor ON N8Y 1R8; Ott'01; BSc(Hon); CCFP; (519)945-1171; Fax. (519)945-1173.

ST-AMOUR, Pascale; Ctr Hosp Gatineau Memorial, CP 160 101 ch Burnside, Wakefield QC J0X 3G0; Laval'06; CCFP; Staff, Centre Hospitalier Gatineau Mémorial; (819)459-1112

ST-ANDRE, Carmen; Clinique Med Place Beaumont, 1200 boul Rome, Brossard QC J4W 3H3; Paris (France)'84; Staff, Centre Hospitalier l'Université de Montréal (CHUM) - Hôtel-Dieu; (450)671-6170

ST-ANDRE, Elise; CHUM-Hop Notre-Dame, 1560 rue Sherbrooke E, Montreal QC H2L 4M1; Mon'91; CSPQ; FRCPC; Psy (Depression). Staff, Centre Hospitalier l'Université de Montréal (CHUM) - Hôpital Notre-Dame; (514)890-8000 x25673

ST-ANDRE, Martin; Hôpital Ste-Justine, 3175 ch Cote Sainte-Catherine, Montreal QC H3T 1C5; McG'86; CSPQ; FRCPC; Psy (Adult Psychiatry). Liaison Cons, Hôpital Ste-Justine; adj Prof Psy, Universite de Montreal; (514)345-4931

ST-ANTOINE, Josee; CLSC-d'Hebergement Valcourt, 1150 rue Champlain, Valcourt QC J0E 2L0; Mon'79; (450)532-3191

ST-ANTOINE, Pierre; CHUM-Hop Notre-Dame, 1560 rue Sherbrooke E, Montreal QC H2L 4M1; Mon'73; FRCPC; MedMicrobiol; Microbio & Infect Dis (P.Q.). Staff, Centre Hospitalier l'Université de Montréal (CHUM) - Hôpital Notre-Dame; (514)890-8000 x25801; pierre.st-antoine.chum@ssss.gouv.qc.ca.

ST-ARNAUD, Charles; CHUS-Hopital Hotel-Dieu, 580 rue Bowen S, Sherbrooke QC J1G 2E8; McG'06; MDCM; FRCPC; IntMed; Critical Care Medicine. Staff, Centre Hospitalier Universitaire de Sherbrooke-Hôpital Hôtel-Dieu; (819)346-1110

ST-ARNAUD, Claude; 490 rue Bonaventure, Trois-Rivieres QC G9A 2B4; Mon'89; Ophth (P.Q.). (819)375-4040; Fax. (819)375-3117.

ST-ARNAUD, Daniel; Hotel-Dieu de Levis, 143 rue Wolfe, Levis QC G6V 3Z1; Laval'05; CCFP; CCFP(E.M.); Staff, Hôtel-Dieu de Lévis; (418)835-7121

ST-ARNAUD, Karine; Hop du Sacre-Coeur de Mtl, 5400 boul Gouin O, Montreal QC H4J 1C5; Mon'05; CCFP; CCFP(E.M.); Staff, Hôpital du Sacre-Coeur de Montréal; (514)338-2222

ST-ARNAUD, Nancy; Coop de Solidarite Ste-Gertrud, 6445 rue des Pins, Becancour QC G9H 3K9; Mon'09; CCFP; FCFP; (819)297-2911; Fax. (819)297-2707.

ST-ARNAUD, Philippe; Hop du Sacre-Coeur de Mtl, 5400 boul Gouin O, Montreal QC H4J 1C5; Sher'06; CCFP; CCFP(E.M.); Staff, Hôpital du Sacre-Coeur de Montréal; (514)338-2222

ST-ARNEAULT, Renald; Centre Med Boucherville, 201-600 boul du Fort-St-Louis, Boucherville QC J4B 1S7; Mon'82; Langs: English; (450)655-7321; Fax. (450)655-6311.

ST-AUBIN, Diane; Centre Med de Beauport, 737 av Royale, Quebec QC G1E 1Z1; Sher'86; CCFP; (418)667-7114; Fax. (418)667-5843.

ST-AUBIN, Jean-Jacques; 1702-441 av President-Kennedy, Montreal QC H3A 0A4; Mon'77; LMCC; Staff, Hôpital de l'Archipel; (514)840-5496

ST-CERNY, Jose; DSPPE de Monteregie, 1255 rue Beauregard, Longueuil QC J4K 2M3; Sher'77; (450)920-6777 x5407; Fax. (450)928-6763.

ST-COEUR, Rachelle; Dr Georges-L Dumont Reg Hosp, 330 av Universite, Moncton NB E1C 2Z3; Sher'03; CCFP; CCFP(E.M.); Staff, Dr Georges-L-Dumont University Hospital Centre; (506)862-4113

ST CROIX, Eileen M; James Paton Mem Hosp, 125 Trans Canada Hwy, Gander NL A1V 1P7; Mem'75; FCFP; Staff, James Paton Memorial Hospital; (709)256-5552; Fax. (709)256-5470.

ST-CYR, Dominique; Winchester Dist Mem Hosp, 566 Louise St, Winchester ON K0C 2K0; Mon'87; FRCSC; ObstGyn (Colposcopy). Staff, Winchester District Memorial Hospital; Langs: Bilingual(French/English); (613)774-2420 x6110

ST-CYR, Julie; St Mary's Hosp Centre, 3830 av Lacombe, Montreal QC H3T 1M5; McG'81; ABACPath; CSPQ; FRCPC; MedBiochem; AnatPath. Consultant, Centre Hospitalier Laurentien; Dir Biochem, St Mary's Hospital Centre; assoc Prof, McGill University; Langs: French; (514)345-3511; julie.st-cyr@ssss.gouv.qc.ca.

ST-CYR, Michel; Polyclinique, 220-874 boul de l'Universite E, Chicoutimi QC G7H 6B9; Laval'81; Staff, Complexe hospitalier de la Sagamie; (418)545-1217; Fax. (418)545-4782.

ST-CYR, Yvan; 397-2600 boul Laurier, Quebec QC G1V 4T3; Laval'68; LMCC; OrthSurg (P.Q.) (Pediatric Orthopedics). ac Staff, Centre Hospitalier Universitaire de Quebec-CHUL; Langs: Bilingual(French/English); (418)623-1610; Fax. (418)623-8926.

ST-CYR MONACO, Amélie; Centre Med des Generations, 200-465 rue Bibeau, Saint-Eustache QC J7R 0C8; Mon'09; CCFP; (450)472-1955

ST-DENIS, Pierre; CHUM-Hop Notre-Dame, 1560 rue Sherbrooke E, Montreal QC H2L 4M1; Mon'75; CSPQ; FRCPC; Psy. Staff, Centre Hospitalier l'Université de Montréal (CHUM) - Hôpital Notre-Dame; Clin Teacher, Universite de Montreal; (514)890-8000 x25667

ST-DENIS-DEMERS, Monique; Hop Charles LeMoyne, 3120 boul Taschereau, Greenfield Park QC J4V 2H1; Mon'79; Peds. Staff, Hopital Charles LeMoyne; (450)466-5050

ST-FRANCOIS, Bernard; Clinique Med Hickson, 3805 rue de Verdun, Verdun QC H4G 1K8; Mon'73; ac Staff, Centre Hospitalier de Verdun; (514)769-9671; Fax. (514)769-9676.

ST-GELAIS, Donald; CSSS de Port-Cartier, 3 rue de Shelter Bay, Port-Cartier QC G5B 2W9; Laval'85; Staff, CLSC-CSSS de Port-Cartier; (418)766-2715

ST-GELAIS, Line; CSSS de l'Hématite, GD 1 rue de l'Aquillon, Fermont QC G0G 1J0; Sher'89; Staff, CLSC de l'Hématite; (418)287-5461

ST-GELAIS, Philippe; Clinique Oculus, 10665 1re av, Saint-Georges QC G5Y 6X8; Sher'04; FRCPC; Ophth. Langs: Bilingual(French/English); (418)226-0300; Fax. (418)226-0301.

ST GEORGE-HYSLOP, Peter H; Tanz Neuroscience Bldg, 118-6 Queen's Park Cres, Toronto ON M5S 3H2; Ott'76; FRCPC; IntMed (Inherited Neurological Disorders); Neur. Staff, Toronto Western Hospital - University Health Network; Teach Staff, University of Toronto.

ST-GEORGES, Catherine; CSSS Drummond-Hop Sainte-Croix, 570 rue Heriot, Drummondville QC J2B 1C1; Sher'04; FRCPC; IntMed. Staff, Hôpital Sainte-croix; (819)478-6464

ST-GEORGES, Fernand; Hôpital Laval, 2725 Ch Sainte-Foy, Quebec QC G1V 4G5; Laval'65; Gastroent; IntMed. Staff, Hôpital Laval; (418)656-4511; Fax. (418)656-4587.

ST-GEORGES, Marc J E; CSSS de Laval, 1755 boul Rene-Laennec, Laval QC H7M 3L9; Mon'94; Staff, Hopital de la Cite de la santé; (450)668-1010; Fax. (450)688-2504.

ST-GEORGES, Regent; CSSS de Rimouski-Neigette, CP 3150 Succ A 150 av Rouleau, Rimouski QC G5L 5T1; Laval'88; FRCSC; GenSurg. Staff, Hôpital Regional Rimouski; (418)723-7851

ST-GERMAIN, Antoine; CLSC Longueuil Ouest, 201 boul Cure-Poirier O, Longueuil QC J4J 2G4; Sher'93; CCFP; (450)651-9830

ST-GERMAIN, Isabelle; CSSS de Maskinonge, 10 rue Jonathan RR 1, St-Alexis-D-Monts QC J0K 1V0; Mon'95; (819)265-2572; Fax. (819)268-2505.

ST-GERMAIN, Jean-Francois; Hop Maisonneuve-Rosemont, 5415 boul de l'Assomption, Montreal QC H1T 2M4; Mon'74; CSPQ; Anes. Staff, Hopital Maisonneuve-Rosemont; (514)252-3426; Fax. (514)252-3542.

ST-GERMAIN, Lorraine; Clinique Med St-Redempteur, 266 rue Thibault, Matane QC G4W 2V9; Sher'89; Staff, Centre Hospitalier de Matane; (418)562-6133; Fax. (418)562-6947.

ST-GERMAIN, Marc-Andre; Hop Charles-LeMoyne, 3120 boul Taschereau, Greenfield Park QC J4V 2H1; Mon'00; CSPQ; Psy. Staff, Hopital Charles LeMoyne; (450)466-5000 x2008; Fax. (450)466-5404.

ST-GERMAIN, Myriam; Clinique Med St-Antoine, 609 9e rue, Saint-Jerome QC J7Z 2Z2; Mon'98; CCFP; (450)432-3308; Fax. (450)432-1004.

ST-GERMAIN, Pascal; Ctr Hosp Affilie-Enfant-Jesus, 1401 18e rue, Quebec QC G1J 1Z4; Sher'93; FRCSC; GenSurg. Staff, Centre Hospitalier Affilié Universitaire de Québec - Hôpital De L'Enfant Jésus; Langs: Bilingual(French/English); (418)649-0252

ST-GERMAIN, Paul; Hotel-Dieu de Sorel, 400 av de l'Hotel-Dieu, Sorel-Tracy QC J3P 1N5; Sher'71; MedOncol (P.Q.); Hem (P.Q.). Staff, Hôtel-Dieu de Sorel; (450)746-6000; Fax. (450)746-6028.

ST-GERMAIN, Pierre; CLSC-CHSLD Champagnat, 978 boul du Seminaire N, St-Jean-Sur-Richel QC J3A 1E5; Sher'92; Staff, CLSC-CHLSD Champagnat Vallee des Forts; (450)358-2572

ST GERMAINE, Ronald L; 214 Med Place, 9F-9909 102 St Box 27, Grande Prairie AB T8V 2V4; Alb'97; BSc; FRCSC; GenSurg (Family Medicine). (780)539-4545; Fax. (780)532-6743.

ST GODARD, Edward E; St Boniface Gen Hosp, 409 Tache Ave, Winnipeg MB R2H 2A6; Man'04; CCFP; Staff, St Boniface General Hospital; Staff, Riverview Health Centre; (204)233-8563

ST GODDARD, Jennifer M; Portage Clinic Inc, 140 9th St SE, Portage la Prairie MB R1N 3V5; Man'06; CCFP; (204)857-3445; Fax. (204)239-1278.

ST-HILAIRE, Denis; CSSS de Jonquiere, CP 1200 Stn Pdf Jonquiere 2230 rue de l'Hopital, Jonquiere QC G7X 7X2; Laval'75; CSPQ; Anes. Staff, Centre Hospitalier Jonquiere; (418)695-7700 x2105; Fax. (418)695-7747.

ST-HILAIRE, Eve; Hôpital Georges-L Dumont, 330 av Universite, Moncton NB E1C 2Z3; Sher'02; FRCPC; IntMed (Medical Oncology); Hem. Staff, Dr Georges-L-Dumont University Hospital Centre; Langs: Bilingual(French/English); (506)862-4030; eve_st-hilaire@vitalite.nb.ca.

ST-HILAIRE, Fritz; Clinique Med Perrier, 10-10794 rue Lajeunesse, Montreal QC H3L 2E8; Port-au-Prince (Haiti)'65; ac Staff ObstGyn, Hôpital Ste-Justine; (514)383-0559; Fax. (514)383-3430; sthf@sympatico.ca.

ST-HILAIRE, Gerard; CSSS de Temiscouata, CP 310 58 rue de l'Eglise, Notre-Dame-du-Lac QC G0L 1X0; Laval'63; CSPQ; Anes (P.Q.). Chef anesth, Centre Hospitalier Notre-Dame-du-Lac; (418)899-6751

ST-HILAIRE, Gilles; 215-3031 rue des Chatelets, Quebec QC G1V 3Y8; Laval'65; CSPQ; Psy (P.Q.). Clin Staff Psy, Institut Universitaire Sante; (418)652-8749

ST-HILAIRE, Jason J; Bridges Comm Health Centre, 177 King St, Port Colborne ON L3K 4G5; McG'99; CCFP; Langs: Bilingual(English/French); (289)476-5017; Fax. (289)479-5018.

ST-HILAIRE, Jean; Policlinique St-Martin, 604-1435 boul Saint-Martin O, Laval QC H7S 2C6; Laval'81; (450)668-3310

ST-HILAIRE, Karine; Hotel-Dieu de Quebec, 11 Cote du Palais, Quebec QC G1R 2J6; Laval'06; CCFP; Staff, Centre Hospitalier Universitaire de Québec (CHUQ) - Siege Social; Staff, Centre de santé Cloutier-du-Rivage; (418)525-4444

ST-HILAIRE, Lyette; CSSS de Laval, 280 boul du Roi-Du-Nord, Laval QC H7L 4L2; Mon'88; (450)622-5110

ST-HILAIRE, Michel; Inst of Mental Health Quebec, 2601 ch de la Canardiere, Quebec QC G1J 2G3; Laval'07; FRCPC; Psy. Staff, Institut Universitaire Santé; (418)663-5000

ST-HILAIRE, Richard; CSSS de Beauce-Etchemin, 1515 17e rue, Saint-Georges QC G5Y 4T8; Laval'67; FRCPC; Cardiol (P.Q.). Staff, Centre Hospitalier Beauce-Etchemin; (418)228-2031

ST-HILAIRE, Sophie; Bureau Med IVAC, CP 6056 Succ Centre-Ville 1199 av de Bleury, Montreal QC H3C 4E1; Mon'90; LMCC; CSPQ; FRCPC; Psy (Adult Psychiatry). Staff, Direction des Services Medicaux-CSST; Langs: Bilingual(French/English); (514)906-3019; Fax. (514)906-3029; sophiesthilaire@hotmail.com.

ST-JACQUES, Caroline; CSSS du Sud de Lanaudière, 911 montee des Pionniers, Terrebonne QC J6V 2H2; Mon'06; CCFP; Staff, Centre Hospitalier Pierre le Gardeur; (450)654-7525; Fax. (450)470-2640.

ST-JACQUES, Frederic; CSSS du Nord de Lanaudiere, 1000 boul Sainte-Anne, St-Charles-Brromee QC J6E 6J2; Mon'06; ObstGyn. Staff, Centre Hospitalier Régional de Lanaudière; (450)759-8222

ST-JACQUES, Helene M; 5689 boul Rosemont, Montreal QC H1T 2H1; Mon'77; CSPQ; Psy (Adult Psychiatry). Staff, Centre Hospitalier Universitaire de Québec (CHUQ) - Siege Social; Staff, Hopital Maisonneuve-Rosemont; Asst Prof Psy, Universite de Montreal; (514)252-3400

ST-JACQUES, Lina; Clinique CMI, 240-2040 boul Marie-Laurin, Saint-Laurent QC H4R 1J9; Mon'82; (514)747-9936; Fax. (514)747-9331.

ST-JACQUES, Marie; Westmount Med Bldg, 440-5025 rue Sherbrooke O, Montreal QC H4A 1S9; Mon'78; FRCPC; Derm. Staff, McGill University Health Centre - Royal Victoria Hospital; Chef derma, St Mary's Hospital Centre; Clin Assoc Prof, McGill University; (514)487-2440; Fax. (514)482-2350.

ST JACQUES, Nicole S; Westfort Village Walk-In Clini, 129 Fredrica St W, Thunder Bay ON P7E 3V8; NOSM'09; CCFP; (807)473-5410; Fax. (807)285-0266.

ST JAMES, Sarah A; Sheddon Avenue Med Assoc, 308-331 Sheddon Ave, Oakville ON L6J 1X8; Ott'95; CCFP; (905)845-8771; Fax. (905)845-8379.

ST-JEAN, Benoit; Montfort Hosp, 713 Montreal Rd, Ottawa ON K1K 0T2; Sher'90; FRCSC; GenSurg. Chief Surg/Staff, Montfort Hospital; Langs: Bilingual(French/English); (613)746-4621

ST-JEAN, Bernard; Hôpital de la Malbaie, CP 340 Succ Bureau-Chef 303 rue Saint-Etienne, La Malbaie QC G5A 1T8; Mon'76; CSPQ; Anes., Hôpital de la Malbaie; Staff, Centre Hospitalier de Chandler; Langs: English; (418)665-1700

ST-JEAN, Catherine; CSSS des Aurores Boreales, CP 6000 Succ Bureau-Chef 679 2e rue E, La Sarre QC J9Z 2X7; Mon'05; CCFP; Staff, Centre Hospitalier La Sarre; (819)333-2311

ST-JEAN, Edith; 200-2860 boul Laframboise, Saint-Hyacinthe QC J2S 4Z1; Sher'91; FRCPC; IntMed; Endocrin (P.Q.); Endocrin&Metab. Staff, Centre d hebergement de l Hôtel-Dieu de Saint-Hyacinthe; Langs: Bilingual(French/English); (450)778-3238; Fax. (450)778-3308.

ST-JEAN, Gilles; GMF Concorde, 300 boul de la Concorde E, Laval QC H7G 2E6; Mon'94; (450)667-5310

ST-JEAN, Lise A; CHUM-Hop Notre-Dame, 1560 rue Sherbrooke E, Montreal QC H2L 4M1; Mon'81; FRCPC; MedMicrobiol; Microbio & Infect Dis (P.Q.). Staff, Centre Hospitalier l'Université de Montréal (CHUM) - Hôpital Notre-Dame; (514)890-8000 x25103

ST-JEAN, Mireille C; Ottawa Hosp-Family Med Ctre, 210 Melrose Ave, Ottawa ON K1Y 4K7; Sher'96; CCFP; FCFP; Langs: Bilingual(English/French); (613)761-4334; Fax. (613)761-4453.

ST-JEAN, Pierre; 1055 rue de Bruxelles, Montreal QC H1L 5Z4; Mon'76; (514)353-3110; Fax. (514)353-5808.

ST JOHN, A Brian; 202-29 Toronto St S PO Box 189 Stn Main, Uxbridge ON L9P 1M7; Ott'79; BSc; Ac Staff, Markham Stouffville Hospital - Uxbridge Site; Court Staff, Markham Stouffville Hospital; (905)852-6141; Fax. (905)852-6727.

ST JOHN, Kimberly A; Dr Charles A Janeway Child HC, 4J 129-300 Prince Philip Dr, St. John's NL A1B 3V6; Mem'83; FRCPC; Psy (Child & Adolescent Psychiatry). Staff, Janeway Children's Health & Rehabilitation Centre; Assoc Prof Med, Memorial University Of Newfoundland; (709)777-4197; Fax. (709)722-0408; hcc.stjk@hccsj.nf.ca.

ST JOHN, Philip D; Health Sciences Centre, GE 547-820 Sherbrook St, Winnipeg MB R3A 1R9; Man'90; MPH; FRCPC; IntMed (Neurology); GeriatricMed. Staff, Health Sciences Centre; Langs: English; French; (204)774-6511

ST JOHN, Valerie E; Veterans Affairs, 1039 Princess Ave, Brandon MB R7A 4J5; Man'63; Semi-Retired.

ST-JULIEN, Louis J; 2665 av Sainte-Anne, Saint-Hyacinthe QC J2S 5J4; Mon'69; (450)774-3981; Fax. (450)774-3031.

ST-LAURENT, Carol A; 23 Health Services Centre, PO Box 17000 Stn Forces 17 Wing, Winnipeg MB R3J 3Y5; Man'10; CCFP; Staff, Canadian Forces Base.

ST-LAURENT, Claude-Andre; CSSS Sud Lanaudiere, 135 boul Claude-David, Repentigny QC J6A 1N6; Sher'78; CCFP; Staff, Centre Hospitalier Pierre le Gardeur; (450)654-2911; Fax. (450)654-2762.

ST-LAURENT, Jean-Yves; Clin Sante-Voyage de Montreal, 101-6865 rue Sherbrooke E, Montreal QC H1N 1C7; Laval'77; FRCSC; PlasSurg (Micro Surgery). (514)254-9420

ST-LAURENT, Johanne; Dre Johanne St-Laurent, RR 2 886 boul Perron, Maria QC G0C 1Y0; Laval'78; (418)364-1399; Fax. (418)364-1391.

ST-LAURENT, Judith; Hop Santa Cabrini Ospedale, 5655 rue saint-Zotique E, Montreal QC H1T 1P7; Sher'90; Staff, Hôpital Santa Cabrini Ospedale; (514)252-6000

ST-LAURENT, Maurice; CHUQ-Ctr Hosp Univ Laval, 2705 boul Laurier, Quebec QC G1V 4G2; Laval'74; FRCPC; IntMed; GeriatricMed. ac Staff, Centre Hospitalier Universitaire de Quebec-CHUL; (418)656-4141; Fax. (418)654-2757; geriatrie.pchul@dechuq.ulaval.ca.

ST-LAURENT, Michel; GMF Concorde, 300 boul de la Concorde E, Laval QC H7G 2E6; Mon'76; (450)667-5310; Fax. (450)667-5248.

ST-LAURENT, Renaud; Clinique Musa Mundi Inc, 501-185 rue Dorval, Dorval QC H9S 5J9; Mon'80; Langs: Bilingual(French/English); (514)828-0002

ST-LAURENT-GAGNON, M H L Therese; Ctr Readaptation Marie Enfant, 5200 rue Belanger, Montreal QC H1T 1C9; Mon'74; AB; MSc(Epidemiol.); FRCPC; Peds. Staff, Centre de Réadaptation Marie Enfant du CHU Sainte-Justine; Clin Prof, Universite de Montreal; (514)374-1710

ST-LAURENT LEMERLE, Catherine; CHUQ-Ctr Hosp Univ Laval, 2705 boul Laurier, Quebec QC G1V 4G2; Laval'08; Peds. Staff, Centre Hospitalier Universitaire de Quebec-CHUL; (418)656-4141

ST LOUIS, Eugene L; Burlington Prof Centre, 310-3155 Harvester Rd, Burlington ON L7N 3V2; Qns'68; DMRD; FRCPC; DiagRad. Staff, Joseph Brant Memorial Hospital; (905)637-6608

ST-LOUIS, Gilles; CHUM-Hop Notre-Dame, 1560 rue Sherbrooke E, Montreal QC H2L 4M1; Mon'70; Nephrol (P.Q.); IntMed. Acad Staff, Centre Hospitalier l'Université de Montréal (CHUM) - Hôpital Notre-Dame; (514)890-8000 x26616

ST-LOUIS, Jean; Hop Maisonneuve-Rosemont, 5415 boul de l'Assomption, Montreal QC H1T 2M4; McG'83; FRCPC; IntMed; MedOncol (P.Q.); Hem. Staff, Hopital Maisonneuve-Rosemont; Universite de Montreal; (514)252-3404 x3404; Fax. (514)254-5094.

ST-LOUIS, Jean; Clinique Med Saint-Pierre, 85 rue Saint-Pierre, Saint-Constant QC J5A 2G8; McG'90; IntMed (Respirology). Staff, Hôpital Anna-Laberge; (450)845-4646

ST-LOUIS, Pia; CSSS Kamouraska-Hop Notre-Dame, CP 460 1201 6e av, La Pocatiere QC G0R 1Z0; Mon'00; Staff, CSSS de Kamouraska; (418)856-7000; Fax. (418)856-4737.

ST-MARSEILLE, Melanie; Ctre Hosp de Verdun, 4000 boul Lasalle, Verdun QC H4G 2A3; Mon'03; CCFP; Staff, Centre Hospitalier de Verdun; (514)362-1000

ST-MARTIN, Annie; Clinique Med Lauzon, 213 rue Saint-Joseph, Levis QC G6V 1C8; Sher'91; ac Staff, Hôtel-Dieu de Lévis; (418)833-2473; Fax. (418)833-6954.

ST MARTIN, Blair A; Hys Med Centre, 400-11010 101 St NW, Edmonton AB T5H 4B9; Alb'05; FRCSC; Urol. Staff, University of Alberta Hospital; Langs: Bilingual(English/French); (780)428-6911; Fax. (780)441-2590.

ST-MARTIN, Maurice; NE Specialized Geriatric Servi, E-960 Notre Dame Ave, Sudbury ON P3A 2T4; Qns'80; Staff Geriatric Lead, Health Sciences North-St Joseph's Health Centre; Med Dir Attending MD, Pioneer Manor Long-Term Care Facility; Chief of Staff, St Joseph's Complex Continuing Care Hospital; Langs: French; (705)524-5911; Fax. (705)524-7954.

ST-MAURICE, Francois; 001-2424 boul Lapiniere, Longueuil QC J4Z 2K9; Laval'86; Cardiol (P.Q.); IntMed. (450)676-0808

ST-MICHEL, Pierre; Clinique Procrea, 301-1361 av Beaumont, Mont-Royal QC H3P 2W3; Mon'76; FRCSC; ObstGyn. (514)345-8535

ST-ONGE, Anick; CSSS Drummond-Hop Sainte-Croix, 570 rue Heriot, Drummondville QC J2B 1C1; Laval'96; ObstGyn. Staff, Hôpital Sainte-croix; (819)478-6464

ST-ONGE, Benoit; Clinique Med de Francheville, 111-1220 rue Jean-Nicolet, Trois-Rivieres QC G9A 1B2; Mon'86; (819)373-0947; Fax. (819)373-8512.

ST-ONGE, Chantal; CSSS Drummond-Hop Sainte-Croix, 570 rue Heriot, Drummondville QC J2B 1C1; Sher'01; Staff, Hôpital Sainte-croix; (819)478-6464 x2410

ST-ONGE, Gerard R; 314 Rte de l'Anse-au-Persil, Riviere-du-Loup QC G5R 5Z6; Mon'68; CSPQ; Psy (P.Q.); GenSurg. Staff Psy, Centre Hospitalier Regional du Grand-Portage; (418)894-7621 x294; Fax. (418)868-0530; papa.doc@videotron.ca.

ST-ONGE, Gisele; Urgence Brossard, 7601 boul Taschereau, Brossard QC J4Y 1A2; Mon'65; Peds (P.Q.). (450)462-0863; Fax. (450)462-0174.

ST-ONGE, Joye A; St Joseph's Healthcare, F402-50 Charlton Ave E, Hamilton ON L8N 4A6; Qns'98; FRCPC; IntMed; GeriatricMed. Staff, St Joseph's Healthcare - Charlton Campus; Asst Prof, McMaster University; (905)540-6529; Fax. (905)521-6068.

ST-ONGE, Michel; Carrefour Med Vallee Richelieu, 665 boul Sir-Wilfrid-Laurier, Beloeil QC J3G 4J1; Mon'70; assoc Staff, Centre Hospitalier Honore-Mercier; Langs: English; (450)467-0088; Fax. (450)467-4936.

ST-ONGE, Nathalie; GMF Venta et Marees, 201-391 av Brochu, Sept-Iles QC G4R 4S7; Sher'85; LMCC; Staff, Centre Hospitalier Regional de Sept-Iles; Langs: English; (418)968-1234; Fax. (418)962-4488.

ST-ONGE, Nicole; CHUQ-Hop St-Fancois d'Asisse, 10 rue de l'Espinay, Quebec QC G1L 3L5; Laval'01; Staff, Centre Hospitalier Universitaire De Québec - Pavillon De St-françois-d'assise; (418)525-4444; Fax. (418)525-4006.

ST-ONGE, Odette; CHUQ-Ctr Hosp Univ Laval, 2705 boul Laurier, Quebec QC G1V 4G2; Sher'79; CSPQ; DiagRad. Staff Radiol, Centre Hospitalier Universitaire de Quebec-CHUL; (418)654-2258

ST-ONGE, Robert; Clinique Med de Waterloo, CP 760 100-4900 rue Foster, Waterloo QC J0E 2N0; Sher'84; CCFP; (450)539-1102; Fax. (450)539-2551; roberts@santecourville.com.

ST-ONGE, Sophie; Hopital Laval, 2725 ch Sainte-Foy, Quebec QC G1V 4G5; Laval'91; CSPQ; FRCPC; Anes. Staff, Hôpital Laval; (418)656-4870

ST-ONGE, Sylvain; CLSC-CHSLD-Meilleur, 193 rue Notre-Dame, Repentigny QC J5Z 3C4; Mon'97; Staff, Centre Hospitalier Pierre le Gardeur; (450)654-9012 x322

ST PETERS, Craig B; Parkland Med Clinic, 203-998 Parkland Dr, Halifax NS B3M 0A6; Dal'94; CCFP; (902)404-7737; Fax. (902)404-7066.

ST-PIERRE, Andre; Hôpital Laval, 2725 ch Sainte-Foy, Quebec QC G1V 4G5; Laval'78; CSPQ; FRCPC; Anes. Staff, Hôpital Laval; (418)656-8711; Fax. (418)656-4504.

ST-PIERRE, Andre J; Centre Med Sillery, 1270 av William, Quebec QC G1S 4G1; Laval'75; (418)688-0664; Fax. (418)688-4601.

ST-PIERRE, Anne; Institut de Rhumatologie, 1551 rue Ontario E, Montreal QC H2L 1S6; Mon'80; CSPQ; Rheum (P.Q.); IntMed (P.Q.). Staff, Centre Hospitalier l'Université De Montréal (CHUM) - Hôpital Saint-luc; (514)523-3305; Fax. (514)523-5973.

ST-PIERRE, Antoine; Centre Med St-Redempteur, 210-600 116 Rte, Saint-Nicolas QC G7A 4X8; Laval'99; (418)831-3677

ST-PIERRE, Brigitte; CSSS de Saint-Jerome, 290 rue de Montigny, Saint-Jerome QC J7Z 5T3; Laval'92; Staff, Hôtel-Dieu de Saint-Jérôme; (450)431-8200 x8266

ST-PIERRE, Bruno; 200-620 rue King E CP 21501 Csp Ste-Famille, Sherbrooke QC J1G 5K2; Sher'81; FRCPC; IntMed; Endocrin&Metab. ac Staff, Centre Hospitalier Universitaire de Sherbrooke-Hôpital Hôtel-Dieu; adj Staff, Centre Hospitalier Universitaire de Sherbrooke-Hopital Fleurimont; (819)563-2734; Fax. (819)563-0260.

ST-PIERRE, Caroline; Hopital Laval, 2725 ch Sainte-Foy, Quebec QC G1V 4G5; Laval'06; Staff, Hôpital Laval; (418)656-8711; Fax. (418)657-7558.

ST-PIERRE, Catherine; CHUS-Hop Fleurimont, 3001 12e av N, Sherbrooke QC J1H 5N4; Sher'93; FRCPC; IntMed (Pain Management); Critical Care Medicine (P.Q.). Staff, Centre Hospitalier Universitaire de Sherbrooke-Hopital Fleurimont; (819)346-1110; Fax. (819)820-6406; catherine.st-pierre@usherbrooke.ca.

ST-PIERRE, Claude; Clinique des Med d'Urgence, 632 rue Bowen S, Sherbrooke QC J1G 2E9; Sher'74; ac Staff, Centre Hospitalier Universitaire de Sherbrooke-Hôpital Hôtel-Dieu; Chef, Clinique des Medicale d'Urgence; Clin Prof Pt-Time, Universite de Sherbrooke; (819)822-2700; Fax. (819)822-2027.

ST-PIERRE, Denis; Clin MD Audet Bedard St-Pierre, 110-4850 boul Henri-Bourassa, Quebec QC G1H 3A7; Laval'79; Staff, CSSS de Quebec-Sud; (418)661-6959; Fax. (418)661-1016.

ST-PIERRE, Denys; Centre Med de l'Hetriere, 201-3520 rue de l'Hetriere, St-Augustin-D-Desm QC G3A 0B4; Laval'70; assoc Staff, Hôpital Laval; (418)651-3933; Fax. (418)651-0256.

ST-PIERRE, Florence; CLSC Marigot, 1351 boul des Laurentides, Vimont QC H7M 2Y2; Mon'05; (450)668-1803

ST-PIERRE, France; CLSC-CSSS d'Argenteuil, 145 av de la Providence, Lachute QC J8H 4C7; Mon'85; (450)562-0271

ST-PIERRE, Frederic; Hotel-Dieu de Montmagny, RR 1 350 boul Tache O, Montmagny QC G5V 3R8; Laval'80; CSPQ; Anes (Emergency Medicine). Staff, CSSS de Montmagny-L'Islet; Staff, Centre Hospitalier Regional du Grand-Portage; Langs: Bilingual(French/English); (418)248-0630; frederic.st-pierre@sympatico.ca.

ST-PIERRE, Guy; Clinique Med 3000 Inc, 3000 rue Belanger, Montreal QC H1Y 1A9; Mon'79; (514)376-7702; Fax. (514)376-2639.

ST-PIERRE, Jacques; Ctr Metropolitan Chir Plastiqu, 999 rue de Salaberry, Montreal QC H3L 1L2; Mon'86; CSPQ; FRCPC; Anes. Staff, Centre Hospitalier Fleury; (514)332-7091

ST-PIERRE, Jean-Paul; Clinique 30 Saint-Joseph, 100-30 boul Saint-Joseph E, Montreal QC H2T 1G9; Mon'68; ClinImmunol&Allergy (P.Q.). Staff, Hôpital Ste-Justine; (514)845-4240; Fax. (514)845-5493.

ST-PIERRE, Julie; Clin de Pediatrie du Saguenay, 475 boul Talbot, Chicoutimi QC G7H 4A3; Laval'06; FRCPC; Peds. (418)549-1034; Fax. (418)696-4673.

ST-PIERRE, Katie; CSSS Alphonse Desjardins-UMF, 100-1205 boul de la Rive-Sud, Levis QC G6W 0J4; Laval'08; (418)380-8597; Fax. (418)380-8596.

ST-PIERRE, Louis; Clinique Med de Mont-Joli, 1385 boul Benoit-Gaboury, Mont-Joli QC G5H 4B1; Laval'72; Chef Gen Med, CSSS de la Mitis; (418)775-5353; Fax. (418)775-0025.

ST-PIERRE, Louise; Clinique Familiale la Providen, 16405 av Bourdages S, Saint-Hyacinthe QC J2T 4G9; Mon'76; LMCC; Staff, Centre Hospitalier Honore-Mercier; (450)773-1322; Fax. (450)773-9909.

ST-PIERRE, Luc; Clinique Gynecologique, 102-39 rue Laurier E, Victoriaville QC G6P 6P6; Laval'80; FRCSC; ObstGyn. Ac Staff, Hotel-Dieu d'Arthabaska; Universite de Sherbrooke; Langs: English; (819)357-4073; Fax. (819)357-4075.

ST-PIERRE, Melanie; CHUQ-Hotel-Dieu de Quebec, 11 Cote Du Palais, Quebec QC G1R 2J6; Laval'00; Staff, Centre Hospitalier Universitaire de Québec (CHUQ) - Siege Social; (418)691-5151; Fax. (418)691-5793; melstpierre@hotmail.com.

ST-PIERRE, Michel; CHUS-Hop Fleurimont, 3001 12e av N, Sherbrooke QC J1H 5N4; Sher'72; PhysMed&Rehab; OrthSurg (P.Q.). Staff, Centre Hospitalier Universitaire de Sherbrooke-Hopital Fleurimont; Prof Med, Universite de Sherbrooke; (819)346-1110; Fax. (819)820-6420.

ST-PIERRE, Michel; CSSS du Rocher-Perce, CP 3300 451 rue Mgr Ross E, Chandler QC G0C 1K0; Mon'82; PhysMed&Rehab. Staff, Centre Hospitalier de Chandler; (418)689-2261; Fax. (418)689-5049.

ST-PIERRE, Monique; ASSS de la Capitale-Nationale-, 555 boul Wilfrid-Hamel, Quebec QC G1M 3X7; Laval'87; (418)525-1500

ST-PIERRE, Nancy; Hopital Montfort, 713 Montreal Rd, Ottawa ON K1K 0T2; Laval'06; CCFP; Staff, Montfort Hospital; Langs: Bilingual(French/English); (613)746-4621; Fax. (613)748-4939.

ST-PIERRE, Nicole Y M; 204-185 av Acadie, Dieppe NB E1A 1G6; Laval'83; Staff, Dr Georges-L-Dumont University Hospital Centre; (506)853-7887; Fax. (506)388-9366; stpierren@health.nb.ca.

ST-PIERRE, Raymond; 304-369 boul Fiset, Sorel-Tracy QC J3P 3R3; Mon'62; Otol. Staff, Hôtel-Dieu de Sorel; (450)743-5909

ST-PIERRE, Richard; Clinique Med Monteuil, 200-4650 boul des Laurentides, Laval QC H7K 2J4; Laval'87; Staff, Centre Hospitalier d'Argenteuil; (450)628-8717

ST-PIERRE, Sylvain; 110-2880 ch Quatre-Bourgeois, Quebec QC G1V 4X7; Laval'75; CSPQ; FRCS; FRCSC; Otol (Apnea). assoc Staff, Hôpital Laval; ac Staff Otol Services, Centre Hospitalier Affilié Universitaire de Québec - Hôpital De L'Enfant Jésus; Clin Prof, Université Laval; (418)653-8717; Fax. (418)653-7199; sylvainst-pierre@sympatico.ca.

ST-PIERRE, Taunya A; Sports Med Centre, 1565 Maple Grove Rd, Ottawa ON K2V 1A3; Ott'06; FRCPC; PhysMed&Rehab. (613)591-3939

ST-PIERRE, Yohann; Hôpital Reg Rimouski, 150 av Rouleau, Rimouski QC G5L 5T1; Laval'07; FRCPC; Peds. Staff, Hôpital Regional Rimouski; (418)724-3000

ST-PIERRE, Yves; CLSC-CHSLD du Haut St-Francois, RR 3 460 2E Avenue, Weedon QC J0B 3J0; Laval'62; Staff, CSSS du Haut-Saint-François; Consultant, Centre Hospitalier Universitaire de Sherbrooke-Hôpital Hôtel-Dieu; Physician, Foyer de Weedon Inc; (450)877-3434; Fax. (450)877-5272.

ST ROSE, Auton D F; Northern Health Authority, 1015-299 Victoria St, Prince George BC V2L 5B8; UBC'95; CCFP; FCFP; Staff, Northern Health Authority; (250)563-6334; Fax. (250)563-6308.

ST ROSE, John E M; 804-1189 Talwood Crt, Peterborough ON K9J 7X4; Juarez (Mexico)'79; PhD; Court Staff, QHC North Hastings; Langs: French; (705)876-7045; Fax. (705)876-7734. Semi-Retired.

ST-SAUVEUR, David; Ctr Hosp de Matane, 333 rue Thibault, Matane QC G4W 2W5; Sher'10; CCFP; Staff, Centre Hospitalier de Matane; (418)562-3135

ST VINCENT, Anthony M; River East Med Clinic, 9A-1795 Henderson Hwy, Winnipeg MB R2G 1P3; Man'86; (204)338-7917; Fax. (204)334-0398.

ST-YVES, Chantal; Clinique Med Dagenais, 2065 boul des Laurentides, Laval QC H7M 4M2; Mon'85; (450)975-1557; Fax. (450)975-1557.

ST-YVES, Marie; Clinique Med Shawinigan-Sud, 200-2355 5e av, Shawinigan-Sud QC G9P 1P4; Mon'86; (819)537-6205; Fax. (819)537-5596; marie.st-yves@gmf.gouv.qc.ca.

STAAB, Randolf A; The Credit Valley Hosp, 2411-2200 Eglinton Ave W, Mississauga ON L5M 2N1; Alb'94; FRCPC; Psy. Staff, The Credit Valley Hospital; Langs: German; (905)813-4505; Fax. (905)813-4284.

STABLER, Christopher D; 201-595 Columbia St W, Kamloops BC V2C 1K7; Wes'79; FRCPC; IntMed (Palliative Care); Gastroent. Staff, Royal Inland Hospital; Langs: Spanish; (250)372-9600; Fax. (250)377-8294.

STABLES, Sabrina M; 502-1881 Yonge St, Toronto ON M4S 3C4; Tor'86; Langs: French; (416)539-9598; Fax. (416)539-0802.

STACEY, Brett; Selkirk & District Gen Hosp, PO Box 5000 Stn Main 100 Easton Dr, Selkirk MB R1A 2M2; Man'01; CCFP; Staff, Selkirk & District General Hospital; (204)482-5800; Fax. (204)482-9464.

STACEY, Campbell A; Worker's Comp Board of MB, 333 Broadway, Winnipeg MB R3C 4W3; Man'86; CCFP; Staff, The Salvation Army Grace Hospital; Staff, Victoria General Hospital; Staff, Misericordia Health Centre; Staff, Workers' Comp Board of MB.

STACEY, Cooper B; Dartmouth Med Centre, 203-46 Portland St, Dartmouth NS B2Y 1H4; McG'78; CCFP; FCFP; (902)465-4543; Fax. (902)469-2400.

STACEY, Matthew D G; Kingston Gen Hosp, 76 Stuart St, Kingston ON K7L 2V7; Tor'08; CCFP; CCFP(E.M.); Staff, Kingston General Hospital; (613)549-6666; Fax. (613)548-1374.

STACEY, Shean F; Foothills Med Centre, C229-1403 29 St NW, Calgary AB T2N 2T9; Cal'97; FRCPC; Anes. Staff Anes, Foothills Medical Centre; (403)944-1430; Fax. (403)944-2425.

STACH, Misty J; NW Comm Mental Health Ctr, 280-1620 29 St NW, Calgary AB T2N 4L7; Alb'03; FRCPC; Psy. Staff Psy, RVH Day Treatment Program; Staff Psy, Diagnostic & Treatment Centre; (403)297-7345; Fax. (403)297-4543.

STACHON, Andrea C; Addiction & Mental Hlth-Colleg, 250 College St, Toronto ON M5T 1R8; Parana (Argentina)'01; Staff, Centre for Addiction & Mental Health (CAMH) - College Street Site; (416)535-8501

STACHOWICZ, Tyler; Salvation Army Grace Gen Hosp, 300 Booth Dr, Winnipeg MB R3J 3M7; Man'08; CCFP; CCFP(E.M.); Staff, The Salvation Army Grace Hospital; Staff, Victoria General Hospital; (204)837-0391

STACHULA, Robert B J; 214-2238 Dundas St W, Toronto ON M6R 3A9; Tor'68; Ac Staff, St Joseph's Health Centre; Langs: Polish; (416)535-6657; Fax. (416)535-8938.

STACKHOUSE, Dianne L; Cambridge Med Clinic, 2112 Lakeview Rd, Cambridge-Narrows NB E4C 1N6; Dal'74; BSc; LMCC; Court Staff Privil, The Moncton Hospital; Court Staff Privil, Saint John Regional Hospital; Court Staff Privil, Sussex Health Centre; (506)488-2240; Fax. (506)488-2974.

STACPOOLE, Rebecca A; 4279 Hixon St, Beamsville ON L0R 1B0; Wes'07; MSc; CCFP; (905)563-5315; Fax. (905)563-0933.

STADNICK, Ellamae; University Of Ottawa Heart Ins, H1295-40 Ruskin St, Ottawa ON K1Y 4W7; UBC'04; FRCPC; IntMed; Cardiol. Staff, University of Ottawa Heart Institute; (613)761-4059; Fax. (613)761-4877.

STADNYK, Andrew M; Mindemoya Med Clinic, PO Box 150 2120B Hwy 551, Mindemoya ON P0P 1S0; Sask'77; Ac Staff, Manitoulin Health Centre - Mindemoya Site; (705)377-5371; Fax. (705)377-5372.

STAFFORD, Sara G; 32-15300 105 Ave, Surrey BC V3R 6A7; McG'05; FRCPC; IntMed; Endocrin&Metab. (604)584-3669

STAFFORD, Susan E; Women's College Hosp, W579-76 Grosvenor St, Toronto ON M5S 1B2; Tor'69; FRCPC; IntMed; Gastroent. Ac Staff, Women's College Hospital; (416)968-3425; Fax. (416)323-6518.

STAGER, Andrew C; Lions Gate Hosp, 231 15th St E, North Vancouver BC V7L 2L7; Qns'92; MSc; Dip(SportsMed); CCFP; CCFP(E.M.); Staff, Lions Gate Hospital; Asst Prof, University of British Columbia; (604)230-4315; Fax. (604)681-6682.

STAGG, Andrew P; Royal Alexandra Hosp, 10240 Kingsway Ave NW, Edmonton AB T5H 3V9; Alb'96; CCFP; CCFP(E.M.); Staff, Royal Alexandra Hospital; (780)735-4442; Fax. (780)735-4916.

STAGG, Marie-France; Clin Med Riviere du Moulin, 1388 boul du Saguenay E, Chicoutimi QC G7H 1G8; Sher'06; (418)549-3564; Fax. (418)541-1159.

STAHL, Gordon M; Vancouver Family Health Centre, 100-2732 Hastings St E, Vancouver BC V5K 1Z9; UBC'77; CCFP; FCFP; Vis Staff, Vancouver General Hospital - Centennial Pavillion; Ac Staff, Providence Health Care - St Vincent's Hospital-Heather Site; Clin Assoc Prof Family Med, University of British Columbia; Langs: English; French; (604)253-3166; Fax. (604)253-2048.

STAHLBRAND, Erik A; Avenue Med Centre, 221 Brant Ave, Brantford ON N3T 3J2; Wes'80; BMath; Court Staff, The Brant Community Healthcare System - Brantford General Hospital Site; (519)753-8666; Fax. (519)753-6880.

STAIBANO, Filippo M; 80-360 Hwy 8, Stoney Creek ON L8G 1E8; Tor'78; CCFP; FCFP; Ac Staff, St Joseph's Healthcare - Charlton Campus; Langs: Italian; (905)662-1318; Fax. (905)662-7898.

STAIRS, Heather J; D1-1285 Onondaga St, Oromocto NB E2V 2P8; Dal'90; Ac Staff, Oromocto Public Hospital; Court Staff, Dr Everett Chalmers Regional Hospital; (506)357-3463; Fax. (506)357-6853.

STAIT-GARDNER, Lia Z; Malvern Med Arts Bldg, 100-1333 Neilson Rd, Scarborough ON M1B 4Y9; Ott'91; CCFP; FCFP; Staff, Rouge Valley Health System - Centenary Health Centre Site; (416)291-7719; Fax. (416)287-3775.

STAJKOVIC, Svetlana; Cornerstone Med Centre, 28-1200 37 St SW, Calgary AB T3C 1S2; University of Nis (Other Foreign)'94; FRCPC; IntMed (Rheumatology). Staff, University of Calgary; (403)264-1895; Fax. (403)264-7015.

STAKIW, Julie; Saskatoon Cancer Centre, 20 Campus Dr, Saskatoon SK S7N 4H4; Sask'01; FRCPC; IntMed (Medical Oncology); Hem. Staff, Saskatoon Cancer Centre; (306)655-2980 x5135; Fax. (306)655-2278.

STAKIW, Kenneth J; St Paul's Hosp, 1702 20th St W, Saskatoon SK S7M 0Z9; Sask'72; CCFP; FCFP; Staff, St Paul's Hospital (Grey Nuns) of Saskatoon; (306)655-5869; Fax. (306)655-5918; kstakiw@shaw.ca.

STAL, Jeffrey M; Women's College Hosp, 579-76 Grenville St, Toronto ON M5S 1B2; Wes'92; BSc; FRCPC; IntMed; Gastroent. Ac Staff, Women's College Hospital; Asst Prof, University of Toronto; (416)323-6400; jeffreystal@yahoo.ca.

STALDER, Lisa J; PO Box 323, Radisson SK S0K 3L0; Sask'78; CCFP.

STALINSKA, Teresa M; Sunnyside Med Arts Centre, 505-27 Roncesvalles Ave, Toronto ON M6R 3B2; Gdansk (Poland)'72; Langs: Polish; (416)530-4966; Fax. (416)530-4457.

STALKER, M John B; Kingston Med Arts Bldg, 209-800 Princess St, Kingston ON K7L 5E4; Tor'54; IntMed (General Medicine). (613)547-0311; Fax. (613)547-0312; jstalker@cogeco.ca.

STALKER, Penelope E; Broadway Family Physicians, 1801 Broadway Ave, Saskatoon SK S7H 2B6; Sask'89; CCFP; (306)652-2632; Fax. (306)652-2637; pstalker@sasktel.net.

STALKER, Robert E; 6152 Linden St, Halifax NS B3H 2K8; Dal'77; Dip SportMed; (902)425-9601; Fax. (902)425-9446; robertstalker@eastlink.ca.

STALL, Richard J; St Joseph Health Centre, 30 The Queensway, Toronto ON M6R 1B5; Man'78; DABPN; FRCPC; Psy;CCFP; FCFP; Med Dir Psy Consultation-Liaison Service, St Joseph's Health Centre; (416)975-8864; Fax. (416)530-6076; richard.stall@gmail.com.

STALLWOOD, George R; 2-510 Concession St, Hamilton ON L9A 1C4; Tor'78; FRCPC; Cardiol; IntMed. Coord ICU & Attd Staff Phys, Hamilton Health Sciences Centre-Juravinski Site; Asst Prof, McMaster University; (905)387-3561; Fax. (905)387-0398.

STALLWOOD, Mark I; Thunder Bay Reg Hlth Sciences, 980 Oliver Rd, Thunder Bay ON P7B 6V4; Liverpool (United Kingdom)'93; FRCPC; Anes. Staff, Thunder Bay Regional Health Sciences Centre; (807)684-6000

STALS, Roelof L; Holley Clinic, 348 Front St, Quesnel BC V2J 2K3; Stellenbosch (South Africa)'00; MB ChB; (250)992-2158; Fax. (250)992-9391.

STAMLER, Christopher J; Wawa Family Health Team, 17 Government Rd, Wawa ON P0S 1K0; Tor'10; CCFP; (705)856-1313; Fax. (705)856-9550.

STAMLER, James M; The Spence Clinic, 500-1265 Arthur St E, Thunder Bay ON P7E 5H7; Ott'80; CCFP; FCFP; (807)626-1106; Fax. (807)626-1142.

STAMM, Holly A; Forensic Psychiatric Hosp, 70 Colony Farm Rd, New Westminster BC V3C 5X9; Cal'06; CCFP; Staff, Forensic Psychiatric Hospital; (604)524-7700; hstamm@forensic.bc.ca.

STAMP, Gary W; 204-49 Emma St, Guelph ON N1E 6X1; McM'87; FRCSC; OrthSurg. Staff, Guelph General Hospital; (519)821-3474; Fax. (519)821-8872.

STAMPA, Leonore D; PO Box 3955 Stn Main, Olds AB T4H 1P6; Stellenbosch (South Africa)'85; MB ChB; BSc(Physiol); CCFP; Langs: German; Afrikaans; (403)556-7130; Fax. (403)556-1944.

STANASEL, Cristina-Alexandra; CSSS de Laval, 1755 boul Rene-Laennec, Laval QC H7M 3L9; Ovidius Constanta University (Other Foreign)'00; AnatPath. Staff, Hopital de la Cite de la santé; (450)668-1010

STANBOROUGH, Jack R; Regional Supervising Coroner, 13F-119 King St W, Hamilton ON L8P 4Y7; McM'88; CCFP; CCFP(E.M.); Coroner Reg Supervisor, Regional Coroner's Office; (905)546-8200; Fax. (905)546-8210; jack.stanborough@ontario.ca.

STANBROOK, Matthew J B; Univ Hlth Network-Toronto Western Hosp, 7EW-450-399 Bathurst St, Toronto ON M5T 2S8; Tor'95; BSc; PhD; FRCPC; Respir; IntMed (Asthma). Staff Asthma & Airway Centre, Toronto Western Hospital - University Health Network; Staff, Mount Sinai Hospital; Asst Prof Med, University of Toronto; (416)603-5767; Fax. (416)603-5375; matthew.stanbrook@uhn.on.ca.

STANCER, Karen L; 203-1448 Commercial Dr, Vancouver BC V5L 3X9; Tor'85; CCFP; Langs: Bilingual(English/French); (604)255-6565

STANCHEVA, Blaga A; Dr B Stancheva Med Clinic, 215-888 8th Ave W, Vancouver BC V5Z 3Y1; (Bulgaria)'88; CCFP; Staff Obst, BC Women's Hospital & Health Centre; Staff Obst, Providence Health Care - St Paul's Hospital; Langs: Bulgarian; Russian; (604)872-0305; Fax. (604)639-2689.

STANCIU, Adela E; CLSC de Metro, 300-1801 boul de Maisonneuve O, Montreal QC H3H 1J9; Carol Davila Univ (Other Foreign)'97; CCFP; Médecin, CLSC de Metro; (514)934-0354; Fax. (514)934-6155; astanciu@ssss.gouv.qc.ca.

STANCIU, Constantin; Hôpital Ste-Justine, 6830-3175 Cote-Sainte-Catherin, Montreal QC H3T 1C5; Mon'82; FRCSC; OrthSurg. Ac Staff, Hôpital Ste-Justine; (514)345-4876; constantin_stanciu@ssss.gouv.qc.ca.

STANCU, Diana C; Continuum Med Care, 202-520 17th St, West Vancouver BC V7V 3S8; Bucharest (Romania)'86; CCFP; Staff, Royal Columbian Hospital; Langs: Romanian; (604)913-8183; Fax. (604)913-8804.

STANDER, Isabella C; Stone Cross Clinic, PO Box 357 114 First Ave W, Maidstone SK S0M 1M0; (South Africa)'04; MB ChB; (306)893-1220; Fax. (306)893-1221; isstander@yahoo.com.

STANDER, Joseph M; Cold Lake Health Centre, 206-314 25 St, Cold Lake AB T9M 1G6; Stellenbosch (South Africa)'86; MB ChB; Staff, Cold Lake Healthcare Centre; Physician, Lakeland Medical Clinic; (780)639-3001; Fax. (780)639-3009.

STANDLEY, Jonathan M S; Corrections Canada-Milhaven In, 5775 Bath Rd, Bath ON K0H 1G0; Cambridge (England)'59; Langs: Spanish; French; (613)351-8232

STANFORD, Timothy R; 201-128 Penetang St, Barrie ON L4M 1V6; Dublin (Ireland)'78; CCFP; FCFP; Court Staff, Royal Victoria Regional Health Centre; Lecturer, University of Toronto; Langs: French; (705)726-4681; Fax. (705)739-8404.

STANG, Antonia S; Alberta Children's Hosp, 2888 Shanagappi Trail NW, Calgary AB T3B 6A8; McG'01; FRCPC; Peds; PedEmergMed. Staff Peds, Alberta Children's Hospital; (403)955-7493; Fax. (403)955-3065.

STANGER, Hilda A D; Haney Prof Bldg, 207-11743 224 St, Maple Ridge BC V2X 6A4; London (England)'65; MB BS; LRCP; MRCS; FACC; FRCPC; IntMed (Cardiology). Staff IntMed, Ridge Meadows Hospital & Health Care Centre; (604)463-8712; Fax. (604)466-8703.

STANGER, Michael A; Rebalance MD, 104-3551 Blanshard St, Victoria BC V8Z 0B9; McG'67; AB; MDCM; FRCSC; OrthSurg (Arthroplasty). Staff, Vancouver Island Health Authority; Clin Instructor Family Pract, University of British Columbia; Langs: French; (250)940-4444

STANHOPE, Alan L; Braeside Med Centre, 111-1919 Southland Dr SW, Calgary AB T2W 0K1; London (England)'66; MB BS; MRCS; LRCP; (403)258-2133; Fax. (403)258-2162; stanhope@lycos.com.

STANICH, Warren R; Bowmont Med Clinic, 6535 Bowness Rd NW, Calgary AB T3B 0E8; Alb'94; BSc; Staff, Foothills Medical Centre; (403)247-9797; Fax. (403)247-0014.

STANIFORTH, Sean M; Lions Gate Hosp, 231 15th St E, North Vancouver BC V7L 2L7; Cal'01; CCFP; CCFP(E.M.); Staff, Lions Gate Hospital; (604)988-3131

STANILAND, Terri L; Country Hills Village, PO Box 418 234-5149 Country Hills Blvd NW, Calgary AB T3A 5K8; Alb'87; CCFP; FCFP; (403)247-9797; Fax. (403)247-0014.

STANIMIR, Gerald W; MUHC-Royal Victoria Hosp, F9 26-687 av des Pins O, Montreal QC H3A 1A1; Mon'75; FRCSC; ObstGyn (Gynecologic Oncology). Staff, McGill University Health Centre - Royal Victoria Hospital; Dir GynOncol, McGill University; Langs: Bilingual(English/French); (514)934-1934 x35332; Fax. (514)843-2830; gerald.stanimir@muhc.mcgill.ca.

STANISH, William D; Fenwick Med Centre, 311-5595 Fenwick St, Halifax NS B3H 4M2; Dal'70; FACS; FRCSC; OrthSurg (Sports Medicine). Staff, Queen Elizabeth II Health Sciences Centre - Halifax Infirmary Site; Dir, Ortho & Sport Med Clinic of N.S.; Prof, Dalhousie University; (902)421-7525; Fax. (902)429-7138.

STANKO, Lorraine K; Health Sciences Centre, AE2-820 Sherbrook St, Winnipeg MB R3A 1R9; Man'93; FRCPC; Anes. Staff Harry Medovy House, Health Sciences Centre; (204)774-6511

STANKOVA, Jitka; MUHC-Montreal Children's Hosp, B 300-2300 rue Tupper, Montreal QC H3H 1P3; Karlova (Czech Republic)'93; Staff, McGill University Health Centre - Montreal Children's Hospital; Langs: German; Russian; Czech; (514)412-4400 x24434; Fax. (514)412-4301.

STANLEY, Blair D; Waneta Primary Care Clinic, 242-8100 Rock Island Hwy, Trail BC V1R 4N7; UBC'92; BSc; CCFP; FCFP; Staff Family Pract, Kootenay Boundary Regional Hospital; Clin Instructor Family Pract/Coord REAP Rural Undergrad Med, University of British Columbia; (250)368-0053; Fax. (250)368-0054.

STANLEY, Katherine S; Sunnybrook Hlth Sciences Ctre, D108-2075 Bayview Ave, Toronto ON M4N 3M5; McG'08; IntMed (Critical Care Medicine). Staff, Sunnybrook Health Sciences Centre; (416)480-6100

STANLEY, R Norm; 380-5655 Cambie St, Vancouver BC V5Z 3A4; UBC'66; CCFP; FCFP; Ac Staff, Vancouver General Hospital - Centennial Pavillion; (604)261-8155; Fax. (604)261-8337; drrnstan@telus.net.

STANLEY, Ronald L; Whistler Health Care Centre, 201-4380 Lorimer Rd RR 4, Whistler BC V0N 1B4; Wes'82; (604)932-4911; Fax. (604)932-4992.

STANLEY, Wayne E; Lindsay Prof Bldg, 14-65 Angeline St N, Lindsay ON K9V 5N7; Pretoria (South Africa)'91; MB ChB; LMCC; CCFP; Staff Emerg, Ross Memorial Hospital; Physician, Lindsay Muskies Hockey Club; Physician/Sec-Treas District 6, Ontario Medical Association; Langs: Afrikaans; German; (705)324-3420; Fax. (705)324-1950.

STANNERS, Bruce K; Owen Sound Med Associates, 2000-1415 1st Ave W, Owen Sound ON N4K 4K8; Tor'82; Dip SportMed; CCFP; FCFP; Staff, Grey Bruce Health Services - Owen Sound; (519)470-3030; j.bstanners@sympatico.ca.

STANOJLOVIC, Snezana; 445 rue Saint-Viateur, Joliette QC J6E 3A9; Mon'78; (450)759-4222; Fax. (450)759-8748; docteurstan@hotmail.com.

STANSBERRY, Patricia E; Synergy Wellness Centre, 221-501 Bethel Dr, Sherwood Park AB T8H 0N2; Alb'75; (780)467-4140; Fax. (780)449-5138.

STANTON, Eric B; St Joseph's Healthcare, 50 Charlton Ave E, Hamilton ON L8N 4A6; McM'76; FRCPC; Cardiol (Invasive Cardiology). Staff, St Joseph's Healthcare - Charlton Campus; Assoc Prof, McMaster University; (905)521-6058; Fax. (905)521-6068; stantone@mcmaster.ca.

STANTON, W Thomas H; A-170D Rebecca St, Oakville ON L6K 1J6; Qns'89; CCFP; (905)842-2174; Fax. (905)842-8071.

STANWICK, Richard S; 430-1900 Richmond Ave, Victoria BC V8R 4R2; Man'73; FAAP; MSc; BSc; FRCPC; Peds; Public Health & Preventive Med; CommunMed. Chief Med Officer of Hlth, Vancouver Island Health Authority; Aj Prof, University of Victoria; (250)519-3406; Fax. (250)519-3441; richard.stanwick@viha.ca.

STANWOOD, Murray D; 275 Island Hwy, Victoria BC V9B 1G4; UBC'79; Staff, Vancouver Island Health Authority; (250)380-9070; Fax. (250)727-2899; mstanwood@shaw.ca.

STANZELEIT, Cheri A; Foothills Prof Bldg, 120-1620 29 St NW, Calgary AB T2N 4L7; Cal'91; FRCPC; Peds. Physician, Ladybug Pediatrics; (403)531-9757; Fax. (403)531-9752; grosjean@shaw.ca.

STANZL, Valerie I; PO Box 1924 Stn Main, Lethbridge AB T1J 4K5; UBC'91; FRCSC; ObstGyn. Langs: English; French; (403)329-9147

STAPLES, Catherine A; Kelowna Med Imaging, 101-3330 Richter St, Kelowna BC V1W 4V5; Wes'84; FRCPC; DiagRad (Thoracic). Staff, Kelowna General Hospital; (250)762-4420; Fax. (250)860-8348; cstaples@kelownamedicalimaging.com.

STAPLES, John A; Sunnybrook Hlth Sciences Ctre, GG06-2075 Bayview Ave, Toronto ON M4N 3M5; Alb'04; FRCPC; IntMed. Staff, Sunnybrook Health Sciences Centre; (416)480-4055

STAPLES, Kristy L; Greenbelt Family Health Team, 1C-3500 Fallowfield Rd, Ottawa ON K2J 4A7; Ott'05; (613)843-1718

STAPLES, Robert K; Queen Elizabeth II Hosp, 10409 98 St, Grande Prairie AB T8V 2E8; McM'81; BSc; Staff, Queen Elizabeth II Hospital; (780)538-7460; Fax. (780)532-9303.

STAPLETON, Andrew J; 152 High St PO Box 1108, Sutton West ON L0E 1R0; Qns'74; Ac Staff, Southlake Regional Health Centre; (905)722-9011; Fax. (905)722-9376.

STAPLETON, John K; Cambridge Med Place, 695 Coronation Blvd, Cambridge ON N1R 7J9; Wes'71; FRCSC; OrthSurg. Ac Staff, Cambridge Memorial Hospital; (519)623-7200; Fax. (519)623-7200.

STAPLETON, Melanie P; Peter Lougheed Centre, 3500 26 Ave NE, Calgary AB T1Y 6J4; Cal'99; BSc; FRCPC; IntMed; Gastroent. Staff, Peter Lougheed Centre; (403)943-5708; Fax. (403)943-4471.

STAPLETON, Robert J; Leamington Dist Mem Hosp, 194 Talbot St W, Leamington ON N8H 1N9; Man'97; CCFP; Staff, Leamington District Memorial Hospital; (519)326-2373; Fax. (519)322-5584.

STAPON, Elaine S; 102-7370 Sierra Morena Blvd SW, Calgary AB T3H 4H9; Man'78; (403)217-2222; Fax. (403)240-9272.

STAPPER BUITRAGO, Ingrid S; King Street Med Arts Centre, 404-71 King St W, Mississauga ON L5B 4A2; Pontificia Universidad Javeriana (Other Foreign)'98; CCFP; (905)270-3636

STAR, Janet A; Medical & Dental Bldg, 204-1849 Yonge St, Toronto ON M4S 1Y2; McG'84; FRCPC; Peds. Court Staff, Mount Sinai Hospital; Court Staff, Women's College Hospital; Langs: French; (416)486-0720; Fax. (416)488-7777.

STARE, Liga; Springbank Med Centre, 206-460 Springbank Dr, London ON N6J 0A8; Riga (Latvia)'85; FRCPC; Peds. (519)641-8687

STARK, David G; Minor Emergency Clinic, 180 Vine St, St Catharines ON L2R 7P3; McM'90; BSc; (905)641-7588; Fax. (905)682-5411.

STARK, Donald F; Hycroft Med Bldg, 207-3195 Granville St, Vancouver BC V6H 3K2; Alb'75; FRCPC; IntMed; ClinImmunol&Allergy. Ac Staff, Providence Health Care - St Paul's Hospital; Physician, Medical Clinic; Delta Health Sciences Centre; University of British Columbia; (604)734-4848

STARKE, Bruce T; Golden Med Clinic, PO Box 1170, Golden BC V0A 1H0; Cape Town (South Africa)'79; MB ChB; Langs: Afrikaans; (250)344-2211; Fax. (250)344-7620.

STARKE, Carola G; Mom Care Docs Allin Clinic, 10155 120 St NW, Edmonton AB T5K 2A2; Alb'81; CCFP; FCFP; (780)482-7551; Fax. (780)701-5397.

STARKE, Victor A; Surrey Med Bldg, 200-9656 King George Blvd, Surrey BC V3T 2V5; Stellenbosch (South Africa)'86; MB ChB; (604)581-4611; Fax. (604)581-2652; andrestarke@shaw.ca.

STARKO, Michael J J; Westgrove Medicentre, 10232 142 St NW, Edmonton AB T5N 2N8; Alb'83; (780)452-0281; Fax. (780)452-1381.

STARKO, Robert J; Keary Med Centre, 203-245 Columbia St E, New Westminster BC V3L 3W4; Alb'89; FRCPC; IntMed (Endocrinology); Nephrol. Staff, Abbotsford Regional Hospital & Cancer Centre; (604)525-9666; Fax. (604)525-2173.

STARKS, Stephanie A; Klondyke Med Clinic, 1-3089 3rd Ave, Whitehorse YT Y1A 5B3; Sask'81; CCFP; Physician, Klondyke Medical Clinic; (867)668-4060; Fax. (867)668-2592.

STAROK, Carina N; 202-460 Springbank Dr, London ON N6J 0A8; Wes'87; CCFP; FCFP; Staff, St Joseph's Hospital - St Joseph's Health Care; (519)672-0060; Fax. (519)661-0597.

STAROSELSKY, Arthur; 210-31 Disera Dr, Thornhill ON L4J 0A7; Doneck Medical University (Other Foreign)'89; CCFP; Staff, Royal Victoria Regional Health Centre; Langs: Hebrew; Russian; Ukrainian; (905)771-7755; Fax. (905)771-7752.

STAROSTA, Philippe E; Kanata North Med Centre, 832 March Rd, Kanata ON K2W 0C9; McG'85; CCFP; Langs: French; (613)599-5599; Fax. (613)599-1005.

STARR, David M; 671 Sheppard Ave W, Toronto ON M3H 2S4; Tor'83; FRCSC; GenSurg. Staff, Humber River Regional Hospital - Finch Avenue Site; (416)749-2332; Fax. (416)749-9712.

STARR, Joseph A; North York Med Arts Bldg, 211-1333 Sheppard Ave E, North York ON M2J 1V1; Tor'64; FACS; FRCSC; PlasSurg (Cosmetic Surgery). Ac Staff Plastic Surg, North York General Hospital; (416)494-7422; Fax. (416)494-3197.

STARR, Michael R; 209-269 boul Saint-Jean, Pointe-Claire QC H9R 3J1; Ott'84; FRCPC; IntMed; Rheum. Staff, McGill University Health Centre - Montreal General Campus; Langs: French; (514)697-0134; Fax. (514)697-5937.

STARR, Stephen H; 1520 Fort St, Victoria BC V8S 5J2; Tor'87; (250)598-1621; Fax. (866)623-2560.

STARRA, Ronald F; CSSSG-Hop De Gatineau, CP 2000 Succ Bureau-Chef 909 boul de la Verendrye, Gatineau QC J8P 7H2; Wes'85; FRCPC; IntMed (Respirology). Staff, Hôpital de Gatineau; Langs: French; (819)561-8100

STARREVELD, Elout; Hys Med Centre, 610-11010 101 St NW, Edmonton AB T5H 4B9; Amsterdam (Netherlands)'64; AB; FRCPC; Neur (Epilepsy). Ac Staff, Royal Alexandra Hospital; Ac Staff, Glenrose Rehabilitation Hospital; Clin Assoc Prof Med & Psy, University of Alberta; Langs: Dutch; (780)428-9540; Fax. (780)428-9539.

STARREVELD, Yves P; Foothills Med Centre, 12F-1403 29 St NW, Calgary AB T2N 2T9; Qns'96; PhD(MedBiophysics); FRCSC; Neursurg (Epilepsy). Staff, Foothills Medical Centre; Langs: Dutch; (403)944-1877; Fax. (403)283-2270.

STAS, Romas V; Ajax Med Arts Bldg, 206-601 Harwood Ave S, Ajax ON L1S 2J5; Tor'69; Staff Core Phys Rehab Unit, Rouge Valley Health System - Centenary Health Centre Site; Assoc Chief Staff/Staff Core Phys Rehab Unit, Rouge Valley Health System - Ajax & Pickering Health Centre Site; Langs: Lithuanian; (905)683-3573; Fax. (905)683-3236; rom.stas@sympatico.ca.

STASIAK, Dorota; Centre Hosp de Val-d'Or, 725 6e rue, Val-d'Or QC J9P 3Y1; McG'05; DiagRad. Staff, Centre Hospitalier de Val d'Or; (819)825-5858

STASIAK, Ewa M; Centre Med de la Plaza, 125-6700 ch Cote-des-Neiges, Montreal QC H3S 2B2; Krakow (Poland)'82; Staff, CHSLD Centre-Ville de Montréal; Staff, Jewish Rehabilitation Hospital; Langs: Polish; French; (514)342-2941; Fax. (514)342-3976.

STASIAK, Ferdinand M; 100-120 16th St W, North Vancouver BC V7M 3N6; Cracow (Poland)'80; Langs: Polish; French; (604)985-3330; Fax. (604)986-3316.

STASIAK, Jerome; SMBD Jewish Gen Hosp, 3755 ch Cote-Sainte-Catherine, Montreal QC H3T 1E2; Krakow (Poland)'82; AB; FACEP; EmergMed (P.Q.). Staff Emerg, Sir Mortimer B Davis Jewish General; adj Prof Family Med, McGill University; (514)340-8222 x5568

STASIAK, Lidia M; 250 9-3151 Lakeshore Rd, Kelowna BC V1W 3S9; Cal'09; CCFP; Staff, Victoria General Hospital.

STASIUK, Russell B P; 4057 Mt Seymour Pky, North Vancouver BC V7G 1Z8; Man'65; BSc(Med); FRCPC; Anes. Ac Staff, Vancouver General Hospital - Centennial Pavillion; (604)929-5178

STASSEN, C Frederik; Bagot Street Med Centre, 182 Bagot St, Kingston ON K7L 3G1; Qns'73; (613)542-8783; Fax. (613)546-1321.

STASSEN, Kobus C; South Health Campus, 4448 Front St SE, Calgary AB T3M 1M4; Stellenbosch (South Africa)'90; MB ChB; CCFP; CCFP(E.M.); FCFP; Staff, Peter Lougheed Centre; Staff, South Health Campus; (403)956-1111

STASSEN, Leanda; Wetaskiwin Fam Med Practice, 5107 50 St, Wetaskiwin AB T9A 1K1; (Other Foreign)'05; (780)352-3010; Fax. (780)352-7413.

STATE, Jonathon P; Sandwich Comm Health Centre, PO Box 7391 749 Felix Ave, Windsor ON N9C 4E9; Tor'94; CCFP; (519)258-6002; Fax. (519)258-7896.

STATHER, David R; Health Sciences Centre, 1402-3330 Hospital Dr NW, Calgary AB T2N 4N1; Qns'00; FRCPC; IntMed; Critical Care Medicine; Respir. Staff, Health Sciences Centre; (403)210-3866; Fax. (403)944-1577.

STAUDENMAIER, Christa; Centre Med Haut-Richelieu, 405-900 boul du Seminaire N, St-Jean-Sur-Richel QC J3A 1C3; Sher'76; FRCSC; Ophth (Neuro Ophthalmology). ac Staff, McGill University Health Centre - Montreal Children's Hospital; ac Staff, Hôpital du Haut-Richelieu; Prof Faculty, McGill University; Langs: German; French; (450)348-9229; Fax. (450)348-9220; cstaudenmaier@bellnet.ca.

STAUNTON, Marie; Univ Hlth Network-Princess M, 3 962-610 University Ave, Toronto ON M5G 2M9; National (Ireland)'94; Staff, Princess Margaret Hospital - University Health Network; (416)946-4501; Fax. (416)946-6564.

STAVRAKAKI, Chrissoula S; 201 Winding Way, Nepean ON K2C 3H1; Thessaloniki (Greece)'70; PhD; MRCPsy; FRCPC; Psy (Child Psychiatry & Developmental Disorders). Langs: Greek; (613)825-7092

STAVRINIDIS, Sophie; Physimed, 121-6363 rte Transcanadienne, Saint-Laurent QC H4T 1Z9; Mon'89; FRCPC; IntMed; Cardiol. Staff, CSSS du Coeur de l'Isle Hôpital Jean-Talon; Staff, Hopital Marie Clarac; (514)747-8888

STAVRO SHOLDOFF, Thomas C; Rouge Valley-Centenary HC, 2867 Ellesmere Rd, Scarborough ON M1E 4B9; RCS (Ireland)'84; Staff, Rouge Valley Health System - Centenary Health Centre Site; Langs: Macedonian; (416)284-8131

STE-MARIE, Gaston; Medicentre St-Remi ENR, 901 rue Notre-Dame, Saint-Remi QC J0L 2L0; Mon'75; (450)454-3913; Fax. (450)454-3958.

STE-MARIE, Lise; 101A-621 ch Ozias-Leduc, Beloeil QC J3H 2M7; Mon'78; (450)467-0444; Fax. (450)467-0442.

STE-MARIE, Louis-Georges; Pavillon Edouard-Asselin, 264 boul Rene-Levesque E, Montreal QC H2X 1P1; Mon'76; Endocrin (P.Q.) (Metabolic Bone Disease). Staff, Centre Hospitalier l'Université De Montréal (CHUM) - Hôpital Saint-luc; Langs: English; French; (514)890-8310 x35708

STE-MARIE, Micheline T; F393-2300 rue Tupper, Montreal QC H3H 1P3; Mon'67; MD(Nutrition); FRCPC; Peds (Pediatric Gastroenterology); Gastroent (P.Q.). ac Staff, McGill University Health Centre - Montreal Children's Hospital; assoc Prof Peds, McGill University; Langs: English; French; (514)412-4306; Fax. (514)412-4332.

STE-MARIE, Pierre; 104-177 rue St Joseph, Ste-Martine QC J0S 1V0; Sher'74; (450)427-3742

STE-MARIE, Pierre; Institut ORL Montreal, 201-1361 av Beaumont, Mont-Royal QC H3P 2W3; Sher'71; FRCSC; Otol (Maxillo Facial Surgery). Staff, Hôpital du Sacre-Coeur de Montréal; (514)343-5244

STE-MARIE, Raymond; CHUS-Hop Hotel-Dieu, 580 rue Bowen S, Sherbrooke QC J1G 2E8; Sher'71; CSPQ; FRCPC; DiagRad. ac Staff, Centre Hospitalier Universitaire de Sherbrooke-Hôpital Hôtel-Dieu; (819)346-1110 x22300

STEACIE, Adam D; Upper Canada Family Health Team, 203-309 Park St, Brockville ON K6V 2H8; Qns'85; MSc(Virology); CCFP; FCFP; Staff/Consultant Palliative Care, Brockville General Hospital - Charles Street; (613)345-0918; Fax. (613)345-0865.

STEAD, Lori M; Meadowlark Place Prof Centre, 408-8708 155 St NW, Edmonton AB T5R 1W2; Mem'05; Gastroent; IntMed. (780)930-1915; Fax. (780)930-1916.

STEARN, Donovan; Village Mall Med Clinic, 6320 50 Ave, Red Deer AB T4N 4C6; (403)314-5357; Fax. (403)314-5307.

STEARNS, Eric L; Interlake Surgical Association, 210D Clandeboye Ave, Selkirk MB R1A 0X1; Man'78; FRCSC; ObstGyn. Asst Prof, University of Manitoba.

STEBEN, Marc; Clinique A rue McGill Inc, 900-407 rue McGill, Montreal QC H2Y 2G3; Mon'78; DSc; CCFP; FCFP; ac Staff, Centre Hospitalier l'Université de Montréal (CHUM) - Hôpital Notre-Dame; Staff, Institut National de Sante Publique du Quebec; Prof Social & Preventive Med, Universite de Montreal; Langs: Spanish; English; (514)787-0055; Fax. (514)787-0066; marc.steben@sympatico.ca.

STEBLECKI, Lisa J; Misericordia Community Hosp, 16940 87 Ave NW, Edmonton AB T5R 4H5; Alb'97; BSc; MPH; CCFP; Staff, Covenant Health - Misericordia Community Hospital; Asst Prof Family Med, University of Alberta; (780)735-2800; Fax. (780)735-2857.

STECHER, Robert D; West Carlton Family Hlth Team, PO Box 218 119 Langstaff Dr, Carp ON K0A 1L0; Witwatersrand (South Africa)'93; MB ChB; CCFP; Langs: Afrikaans; (613)839-3271; Fax. (613)839-3273.

STECHO, Terence J; Univ of Waterloo Health Safety, 200 University Ave W, Waterloo ON N2L 3G1; McM'81; (519)885-1211

STECIUK, Paige E; Atrium Prof Bldg, 305-190 Cundles Rd E, Barrie ON L4M 4S5; McM'92; CCFP; FCFP; Assoc Staff, Royal Victoria Regional Health Centre; (705)726-2060; Fax. (705)726-4826.

STECIUK, William P; Clinic 217, 217 Talbot St, St Thomas ON N5P 1B1; Wes'75; Langs: Ukrainian; (519)631-9040

STECKLEY, Jamie L; Grand River Hosp-KW, PO Box 9056 Stn C 5F-835 King St W, Kitchener ON N2G 1G3; Alb'04; FRCPC; Neur. Staff, Grand River Hospital - Kitchener/Waterloo Health Centre; (519)749-4234; Fax. (519)749-4230.

STECUM, Ronald E; CFB Halifax CDU3 CF H Serv, PO Box 99000 Stn Forces, Halifax NS B3K 5X5; McG'06; MDCM; CCFP; Staff, Canadian Forces Health Services Centre (Atlantic); (902)721-8766

STECYK, Robert W; Fort Saskatchewan Med Clinic, 9421 94 Ave, Fort Saskatchewan AB T8L 1N6; Alb'75; Staff, Fort Saskatchewan Health Centre; Staff, Lamont Health Care Centre; (780)998-2231; Fax. (780)998-4399.

STEDMAN JR., Alfred S; Parkdale Med Tower, 403-1081 Carling Ave, Ottawa ON K1Y 4G2; Dublin (Ireland)'69; LRCPSI; FRCS; FACS; FRCSC; GenSurg. (613)725-3721; Fax. (613)725-3053.

STEED, Barrie L; Sunridge Diagnostic Imaging, 2133 36 St NE, Calgary AB T1Y 5S3; Alb'65; DiagRad. (403)568-7676; Fax. (403)568-7677.

STEED, Clayne A; Raymond Med Clinic, PO Box 769 Stn Main 20 Church Ave, Raymond AB T0K 2S0; Alb'75; Assoc Staff, Raymond Health Centre; Board Member, Canadian Medical Association; (403)752-3337; Fax. (403)752-4967.

STEED, Helen L W; Cross Cancer Institute, 11560 University Ave NW, Edmonton AB T6G 1Z2; Alb'97; FRCSC; ObstGyn (Gynecologic Oncology). Staff Gyn Oncol, Cross Cancer Institute; Staff Obst/Gyn, Royal Alexandra Hospital; (780)432-8560; Fax. (780)432-8333.

STEED, Joel D; Calgary Women's Specialty, 201-178 96 Ave NE, Calgary AB T3K 6G4; Cal'97; FRCSC; ObstGyn. Physician, Maternity Care Clinic; (403)806-2496; Fax. (403)806-2497.

STEED, Merrill D; Family Med Center, 2931 20 Ave S, Lethbridge AB T1K 3M5; Alb'85; CCFP; Staff, Covenant Health - St Michael's Health Centre; Staff, Chinook Regional Hospital; (403)328-2326; Fax. (403)327-0123.

STEED, Michael W; Radiology Associates, 1122 Scenic Dr S, Lethbridge AB T1K 7E5; Alb'86; MB ChB; FRCPC; DiagRad. Staff DiagRad, Chinook Regional Hospital; (403)328-1122; Fax. (403)328-1218.

STEED, Regan C; Raymond Med Clinic, PO Box 769 Stn Main 20 Church Ave, Raymond AB T0K 2S0; Cal'09; CCFP; (403)752-3337; Fax. (403)752-4967.

STEED, Wade B; Associate Med Centre, 5016 48 Ave, Taber AB T1G 1R8; Alb'87; (403)223-3525; Fax. (403)223-9020.

STEED, Wesley B; Associate Med Centre, 5016 48 Ave, Taber AB T1G 1R8; Alb'89; Ac Staff, Taber Health Centre; (403)223-3525; Fax. (403)223-9020.

STEEL, Andrew C; 11C 1141-585 University Ave, Toronto ON M5G 2N2; London (England)'96; FRCPC; Anes. Staff, Toronto General Hospital - UHN; (416)340-4746; Fax. (416)340-3698.

STEEL, Graham J; University of Alberta Hosp, 1C1 04-8440 112 St NW, Edmonton AB T6G 2B7; Alb'05; FRCPC; Anes. Staff, University of Alberta Hospital; (780)407-7035; Fax. (780)407-8529.

STEEL, Stefanie; Townsite Med Clinic, 512 Campbell St, Nanaimo BC V9R 3H1; Stellenbosch (South Africa)'05; MB ChB; CCFP; Staff Obst & Privil, Nanaimo Regional General Hospital; Langs: Afrikaans; (250)619-9125; Fax. (250)755-1408.

STEEL, W Dale; The Campbell Clinic, 160 Columbia Blvd W, Lethbridge AB T1K 4J4; Alb'77; CCFP; FCFP; Ac Staff, Covenant Health - St Michael's Health Centre; Ac Staff, Chinook Regional Hospital; (403)381-7000; Fax. (403)381-8250.

STEELE, Alexander A; North Bay Reg Health Centre, 50 College Dr, North Bay ON P1B 0A4; McG'71; BSc; MDCM; FRCPC; AnatPath (Laboratory Medicine). Staff, North Bay Regional Health Centre - Regional Mental Health; (705)474-8600 x2115; Fax. (705)495-7988.

STEELE, Andrew W; Oshawa Clinic, 117 King St E, Oshawa ON L1H 1B9; Tor'91; FRCPC; IntMed (Dialysis); Nephrol. Med Dir/Sec Chief Nephrol, Lakeridge Health - Oshawa Site; Ac Staff, Lakeridge Health - Whitby Site; (905)721-4337; Fax. (905)723-1495.

STEELE, Ann-Leone; Cole Harbour Family Med Ctre, 203-240 Baker St, Dartmouth NS B2W 6L4; Dal'89; CCFP; (902)435-6312; Fax. (902)434-7920.

STEELE, Bart E; 494 Fred St PO Box 30, Winchester ON K0C 2K0; Qns'89; CCFP; FCFP; Staff, Winchester District Memorial Hospital; (613)774-0915; Fax. (613)774-0916.

STEELE, Brian T; LL-107 King St W, Dundas ON L9H 1V1; Belfast (Ireland)'69; MB ChB; MRCP(UK); FRCPC; Peds (Pediatric Nephrology). (905)628-9879; Fax. (905)628-5701.

STEELE, Curtis A; Community Mental Hlth Serv, 109-7071 Bayers Rd, Halifax NS B3L 2C2; Tulane(LA) (USA)'58; AB; Staff Psy, Capital Health District Authority; Teach Staff Psy, Dalhousie University; (902)454-1400; Fax. (902)454-1434.

STEELE, Dale R; City Square East Tower, 500-555 12th Ave W, Vancouver BC V5Z 3X7; Dal'87; FRCSC; ObstGyn. (604)872-1899; Fax. (604)872-5599.

STEELE, Donna M; 202-55 Queen St E, Toronto ON M5C 1R6; Tor'80; FRCSC; ObstGyn (Family Medicine). Ac Staff, St Michael's Hospital; Asst Prof, University of Toronto; (416)864-5240; Fax. (416)864-5144.

STEELE, J MacGregor; Alberta Children's Hosp, C4 438-2888 Shaganappi Trail N, Calgary AB T3B 6A8; Ott'97; FRCPC; Peds; Hem. Staff Peds, Alberta Children's Hospital; (403)955-7155; Fax. (403)955-7393.

STEELE, Leah S; SMH-Wellesley Health Centre, MF-277 Victoria St, Toronto ON M5B 1W2; McM'96; CCFP; Staff Methadone Works, St Michael's Hospital; (416)392-0520; leah.steele@utoronto.ca.

STEELE, Linda G M; South Huron Hosp, 24 Huron St W SS 2 Stn Main, Exeter ON N0M 1S2; Qns'78; PhD(Chem); CCFP; FCFP; Staff, South Huron Hospital Association; (519)238-6346; Fax. (519)235-3405.

STEELE, Liora R; Mitchell Family Doctors, PO Box 790 7 Francis St, Mitchell ON N0K 1N0; Man'94; CCFP; Langs: French; (519)348-8402; Fax. (519)348-8400.

STEELE, Lisa M J; Royal Inland Hosp, 311 Columbia St, Kamloops BC V2C 2T1; New York (USA)'93; ABPath; ABNPath; Staff, Royal Inland Hospital; (250)314-2669

STEELE, Margaret M; London HSC-Children's Hosp, PO Box 5010 Stn B B8 148-800 Commissioners Rd E, London ON N6A 5W9; Wes'87; FRCPC; Psy (Child & Adolescent Psychiatry). Member Child & Adolescent Mental Health Care Program, London Health Sciences Centre - Children's Hospital; Prof Psy/Vice Dean Hospital & Interfaculty Relations, University of Western Ontario; (519)667-6671; Fax. (519)685-8595; margaret.steele@lhsc.on.ca.

STEELE, Stephen S; Kingston Gen Hosp, 76 Stuart St, Kingston ON K7L 2V7; Tor'99; FRCSC; Urol (Pediatric Urology). Staff Urol, Kingston General Hospital; (613)548-6090; Fax. (613)545-1970.

STEEN, Andrea R; 2-1275 Walker Rd, Windsor ON N8Y 4X9; McM'89; CCFP; FCFP; Staff Psy Hospitalist, Hôtel-Dieu Grace Hospital; Staff Hospitalist, Windsor Regional Hospital - Metropolitan Site; (519)253-9116; Fax. (519)253-5404.

STEEN, Rebecca E; 160 Dundurn St S, Hamilton ON L8P 4K3; McM'00; CCFP; Staff, St Joseph's Healthcare - Charlton Campus; Staff, Hamilton Health Sciences Centre - McMaster Children's Hospital; (905)528-5480; Fax. (905)528-2884.

STEENBERG, Lourens J; Northside Med Clinic, 915 Central Ave N, Swift Current SK S9H 3V3; Pretoria (South Africa)'98; Physician, New Hope Clinic; (306)773-9100; Fax. (306)773-9668.

STEENBERG, Melane; Northside Med Clinic, 915 Central Ave N, Swift Current SK S9H 3V3; Pretoria (South Africa)'97; Langs: Afrikaans; (306)773-9100; mel.lou@sasktel.net.

STEENKAMP, Elsabe; Kootenay-Boundary Reg Hosp, 1200 Hospital Bench, Trail BC V1R 4M1; Pretoria (South Africa)'84; MB ChB; FRCPC; DiagRad. Staff, Kootenay Boundary Regional Hospital; (250)368-3311

STEENKAMP, Jakobus W; Cut Knife Med Clinic, PO Box 69, Cut Knife SK S0M 0N0; Stellenbosch (South Africa)'90; DA; MB ChB; Staff, Maidstone Health Complex; Physician, Neilburg Medical Clinic; Langs: Afrikaans; (306)398-2301; Fax. (306)398-2369.

STEER, Robert K; 14B-900 Oxford St E, London ON N5Y 5A1; Wes'79; CCFP; FCFP; Langs: Dutch; (519)451-0720; Fax. (519)451-4370.

STEEVES, Alexander L; 9983 Highway 3 PO Box 209, Mahone Bay NS B0J 2E0; Dal'71; CCFP; FCFP; Staff, Fishermen's Memorial Hospital; (902)624-8373; Fax. (902)624-1524.

STEEVES, Brian R; 26A Market St, Antigonish NS B2G 3B4; Dal'72; Staff, St Martha's Regional Hospital; Media Dir, R K Macdonald Nursing Home; (902)863-1775; Fax. (902)863-0572.

STEEVES, Daniel C; Bigelow Fowler Clinic, 1605 9 Ave S, Lethbridge AB T1J 1W2; Dal'82; BSc(Biol); Staff, Covenant Health - St Michael's Health Centre; Langs: English; French; (403)327-3121; Fax. (403)327-3905.

STEEVES, Emily N; Hillside Med Centre, PO Box 700 Stn Main 541 3rd Ave, Ladysmith BC V9G 1A5; UBC'02; (250)245-2235; Fax. (250)245-3094.

STEEVES, Jeffrey H; 900-157 Hampton Rd, Rothesay NB E2E 2R3; Dal'88; BSc; FRCSC; Ophth. (506)633-8220; Fax. (506)634-3908.

STEEVES, John M; Dalhoulsie Med New Brunwick, PO Box 5050 Stn Main 100 Tucker Park Rd, Saint John NB E2L 4L5; Dal'74; BSc; FRCSC; OrthSurg (Pediatric Orthopedics). Assoc Dean Dalhousie Med New Brunswick, Dalhousie University; (506)648-6000; Fax. (506)648-6833.

STEEVES, Mark A; Montfort Orthopaedic Group, 202-595 Montreal Rd, Ottawa ON K1K 4L2; Mem'05; FRCSC; OrthSurg. Langs: Bilingual(English/French); (613)746-6745; Fax. (613)746-6008.

STEEVES, Thomas D L; 906-55 Queen St E, Toronto ON M5C 1R6; Sask'02; FRCPC; Neur (Movement Disorders). Staff, St Michael's Hospital; Langs: Bilingual(English/French); (416)864-5505; Fax. (416)864-5635.

STEFAN, Mark A; Direction Sante Publique de La, A-800 boul Chomedey, Laval QC H7V 3Y4; Qns'02; BSc; MPH; CommunMed (P.Q.); Public Health & Preventive Med (Infectious Diseases). Staff, Direction Sante Publique de Laval; Med Consultant Prevention & Promotion, Health Canada; Langs: Bilingual(English/French); (450)978-2000 x2098; Fax. (450)978-2100; stefan_reg13@ssss.gouv.qc.ca.

STEFAN, Raluca A; Sunnybrook Hlth Sciences Ctre, C753-2075 Bayview Ave, Toronto ON M4N 3M5; Tor'05; FRCPC; EmergMed. Staff, Sunnybrook Health Sciences Centre; (416)480-6100

STEFANAC, Mile; Halton HCS Corp-Georgetown, 1 Princess Anne Dr, Georgetown ON L7G 2B8; Sydney (Australia)'06; CCFP; CCFP(E.M.); Staff, Halton Healthcare Services Corporation - Georgetown Hospital; Staff, Hamilton Health Sciences Centre - McMaster Children's Hospital; (905)873-0111

STEFANCZYK-SAPIEHA, Lilianna; Hamilton HS-Henderson Site, 711 Concession St, Hamilton ON L8V 1C3; (Poland)'82; CCFP; Hamilton Health Sciences Centre-Juravinski Site; Physician, The Juravinski Cancer Centre; Langs: Polish; (905)527-4322 x42482; Fax. (905)574-9520.

STEFANEK, Wendy L; Crowfoot Village Fam Practice, 210-600 Crowfoot Cres NW, Calgary AB T3G 0B4; Alb'98; CCFP; (403)239-9733; Fax. (403)241-8112.

STEFANELLI, John D; Royal Inland Hosp, 311 Columbia St, Kamloops BC V2C 2T1; Cal'76; FRCPC; GenPath. Staff Path, Royal Inland Hospital; (250)314-2681; Fax. (250)314-2505.

STEFANELLI, Mark G; Health Sciences Centre, 300 Prince Philip Dr, St. John's NL A1B 3V6; UBC'88; FRCPC; IntMed; Neur. Staff Neurol, Health Sciences Centre; Clinical Asst Prof, Memorial University Of Newfoundland; (709)777-6594; Fax. (709)777-6656; mstefane@mun.ca.

STEFANELLI, Michael N; Inpatient Assessment Unit, 7900 Fraser Park Dr, Burnaby BC V5J 5H1; UBC'88; FRCPC; Psy (Adolescent Psychiatry). (778)452-2219; Fax. (778)452-2220.

STEFANIK, Paula L; 206-5359 Dundas St W, Etobicoke ON M9B 1B1; Tor'79; CCFP; CCFP(E.M.); (416)231-1855; Fax. (416)231-0024.

STEFANISON, Henry J; Atrium Prof Bldg, SS 103 301-190 Cundles Rd E, Barrie ON L4M 4S5; Qns'80; FRCSC; GenSurg. Staff, Royal Victoria Regional Health Centre; Langs: Bilingual(English/French); (705)726-0585; Fax. (705)726-2733.

STEFANIU, Rodica; Humber River Reg Hosp-Keele, 2175 Keele St, York ON M6M 3Z4; Bucharest (Romania)'78; FRCPC; Psy (Emergency Psychiatry). Ac Staff, Humber River Regional Hospital - Keele Street Site; Langs: Romanian; French; (416)658-2022 x2146; Fax. (416)658-2009.

STEFANOS, Michael G F; Headwaters Health Care Centre, 100 Rolling Hills Dr, Orangeville ON L9W 4X9; Cairo (Egypt)'95; FRCPC; DiagRad. Staff, Headwaters Health Care Centre - Orangeville Site; Staff, The Credit Valley Hospital; (519)941-2410 x2400; michael.stefanos@utoronto.ca.

STEFANOVIC, Aleksandra; JPPN 1117-899 12th Ave W, Vancouver BC V5Z 1M9; Ott'03; FRCPC; IntMed; MedMicrobiol; InfectDis. Staff, Vancouver General Hospital - Centennial Pavillion; Langs: Spanish; Serbian; (604)875-5634

STEFANOVICH, Chris P; Enhanced Care Clinic, 3857 Lakeshore Blvd W, Etobicoke ON M8W 0A2; Tor'74; CCFP; FCFP; Staff, Women's College Hospital; Staff, Toronto Rehabilitation Institute - University Centre; Lecturer Family & Commun Med, University of Toronto; Langs: Macedonian; Bulgarian; Serbian; Croatian; (416)354-2640; Fax. (416)729-2008; christefano@hotmail.com.

STEFANOVICI, Camelia; Health Sciences Centre, 820 Sherbrook St, Winnipeg MB R3A 1R9; Iasi University (Other Foreign)'84; FRCPC; GenPath. Staff, Health Sciences Centre; Staff, St Boniface General Hospital; Staff, Diagnostic Services of Manitoba; Asst Prof, University of Manitoba; (204)787-8988

STEFANSKI, Katherine E; Toronto East Gen & Orth Hosp, 825 Coxwell Ave, East York ON M4C 3E7; Tor'05; CCFP; CCFP(E.M.); Staff, Toronto East General Hospital Inc; (416)469-6580

STEFANSSON, Donald A; Don Mills-Eglinton Med Centre, 100-29 Gervais Dr, North York ON M3C 1Z1; Man'76; Ac Staff, North York General Hospital; (416)449-3355; Fax. (416)449-9334.

STEFANYK, Harold N; Nicola Med Dental Bldg, 305-321 Nicola St, Kamloops BC V2C 6G6; Alb'87; CCFP; FCFP; (250)374-8813; Fax. (250)374-7946.

STEFANYSHEN, Grant S; Misericordia Health Centre, 99 Cornish Ave, Winnipeg MB R3C 1A2; Man'92; BSc; BA; CCFP; Staff Misericordia Urgent Care, Misericordia Health Centre; (204)788-8186; Fax. (204)774-8919.

STEFFEN, Robert M; Family Physicians Group, PO Box 2170, Melfort SK S0E 1A0; Stellenbosch (South Africa)'98; MB BS; CCFP; Physician, Family Physicians Group; Langs: Afrikaans; (306)752-5222; Fax. (306)752-5233.

STEFFENHAGEN, Nikolai E A; The Ottawa Hosp-Civic Campus, 1053 Carling Ave, Ottawa ON K1Y 4E9; Staff, The Ottawa Hospital - Civic Campus; (613)798-5555

STEFFENS, Gregory M; Wellington Med Arts Bldg, 306-121 Wellington St W, Barrie ON L4N 1L2; McM'89; CCFP; FCFP; (705)728-6952; Fax. (705)728-5393.

STEFIUK, Donald L; City Centre Fam Physicians, 100-514 Queen St, Saskatoon SK S7K 0M5; Sask'77; MCFP; Staff, Saskatoon City Hospital; Physician, City Centre Family Physicians; University of Saskatchewan; (306)244-3016; Fax. (306)244-4737.

STEFOPULOS, Thomas; Ross Memorial Hosp, 10 Angeline St N, Lindsay ON K9V 4M8; Qns'85; Staff, Ross Memorial Hospital; Langs: Hungarian; Macedonian; (705)328-6143; Fax. (705)328-6164.

STEFOU, Vasia; Medical Bldg, 303-1615 Dufferin St, Toronto ON M6H 4H4; Sofia (Bulgaria)'80; Langs: Greek; Macedonian; Russian; Bulgarian; (416)652-3000; Fax. (416)652-3007.

STEFURAK, Taresa L; Toronto East Gen & Orth Hosp, C304-825 Coxwell Ave, East York ON M4C 3E7; Tor'94; BSc; MSc; FRCPC; Neur (Dementia). Ac Staff, Toronto East General Hospital Inc; Ac Staff, Toronto Western Hospital - University Health Network; Asst Prof Neurol, University of Toronto; (416)469-6406; Fax. (416)469-6584.

STEG, Doris; Herzl CRIU Walk-In Clinic, 500-5858 ch Cote-des-Neiges, Montreal QC H3S 1Z1; McG'78; (514)340-8311

STEGARU, Astrid E; Centre Med des Generations, 200-465 rue Bibeau, Saint-Eustache QC J7R 0C8; IASI (Other Foreign)'97; CCFP; Officier scientifique, Centre Hospitalier Regional de Sept-Iles; Langs: Bilingual(English/French); (450)472-1955

STEGER, Katherine A; Douglas Mental Hlth Univ Insti, 6875 boul LaSalle, LaSalle QC H4H 1R3; Dallas (USA)'05; Psy. Staff, Douglas Mental Health University Institute; (514)761-6131

STEGNAJIC, Snezana; 407-658 Danforth Ave, East York ON M4J 5B9; Tor'91; BSc; MSc; CCFP; Langs: Croatian; Serbian; French; (416)462-2700; Fax. (416)462-2702.

STEIGER, Roberta A; Harvest Hills Med Clinic, 715-500 Country Hills Blvd NE, Calgary AB T3K 4Y7; Cal'04; CCFP; (403)226-8647; Fax. (403)226-8645.

STEIGERWALD, Ronald G; St Boniface Gen Hosp, 409 Tache Ave, Winnipeg MB R2H 2A6; Man'79; FRCPC; EmergMed. Ac Staff, St Boniface General Hospital; Asst Prof, University of Manitoba; (204)235-3006; Fax. (204)237-2071; steiger@cc.umanitoba.ca.

STEIMAN, Amanda J; Univ Hlth Network-Toronto Western Hosp, EW-399 Bathurst St, Toronto ON M5T 2S8; Wes'06; FRCPC; IntMed; Rheum. Staff, Toronto Western Hospital - University Health Network; (416)603-5905

STEIN, Adam M; 417-220 Duncan Mill Rd, North York ON M3B 3J5; Witwatersrand (South Africa)'75; FRCPC; Psy. Court Staff, North York General Hospital; (416)222-0136; Fax. (416)222-7398.

STEIN, Barry L; MUHC-Montreal Gen Hosp, D16 128-1650 av Cedar, Montreal QC H3G 1A4; McG'85; DABS; DABCRS; FRCSC; GenSurg (Colon & Rectal Surgery). Dir Centre for Colon & Rectal Surg, McGill University Health Centre - Montreal General Campus; adj Prof, McGill University; Langs: French; (514)934-8486; Fax. (514)934-8487; colorectal@muhc.mcgill.ca.

STEIN, Bernard A; North York Gen Hosp, 805E-4001 Leslie St, North York ON M2K 1E1; Tor'64; FRCPC; Psy. Staff, North York General Hospital; Assoc Prof, University of Toronto; (416)756-5991; Fax. (416)756-6671; bstein@nygh.on.ca.

STEIN, Debra G; The Hincks-Dellcrest Centre, 508-114 Maitland St, Toronto ON M4Y 1E1; Tor'01; FRCPC; Psy. Staff Psy, Mount Sinai Hospital; Langs: Bilingual(English/French); (416)972-1935; Fax. (416)924-9170.

STEIN, Harold A; Bochner Eye Institute, 40 Prince Arthur Ave, Toronto ON M5R 1A9; Tor'53; DOMS; MSc; FRCSC; Ophth. Att Staff, Mount Sinai Hospital; Att Staff, The Scarborough Hospital - General Campus; Dir, Bochner Eye Institute; Prof Ophth, University of Toronto; (416)921-2131; Fax. (416)966-8917; hstein@bochner.com.

STEIN, Jack L; Medical Centre, 2207-3000 Lawrence Ave E, Scarborough ON M1P 2V1; Tor'62; FRCPC; IntMed. Ac Staff, The Scarborough Hospital - General Campus; Assoc Staff, Sunnybrook Health Sciences Centre; (416)438-5900; Fax. (416)438-5182.

STEIN, Jeffrey C; Royal University Hosp, 3670-103 Hospital Dr Box 32, Saskatoon SK S7N 0W8; Man'85; CRCP; FRCPC; IntMed (Cardiology). Staff Cardiol, Royal University Hospital; Langs: French; (306)655-6851; Fax. (306)655-6854.

STEIN, Jeffrey R; Stein Med Clinic, 188-550 Burrard St, Vancouver BC V6C 2B5; UBC'88; (604)688-5924

STEIN, John D; Queen Elizabeth II HSC-Halifax, 4446-1796 Summer St, Halifax NS B3H 3A7; Wes'03; PlasSurg. Staff, Queen Elizabeth II Health Sciences Centre - Halifax Infirmary Site; (902)473-3681; Fax. (902)425-9525.

STEIN, Jonathan D; Bloor-Jane Med Bldg, 215-2425 Bloor St W, Toronto ON M6S 4W4; McM'03; MHSc; FRCPC; Rheum; IntMed. Staff, St Joseph's Health Centre; (416)604-0053

STEIN, Lawrence A; MUHC-Royal Victoria Hosp, 687 av des Pins O, Montreal QC H3A 1A1; McG'68; DiagRad. Chef DiagRad, McGill University Health Centre - Royal Victoria Hospital; assoc Prof, McGill University; (514)934-1934 x34377; Fax. (514)843-1517; lawrence.stein@muhc.mcgill.ca.

STEIN, Marvin D; 203-219 St Clair Ave W, Toronto ON M4V 1R3; Tor'68; FRCPC; Psy. Staff, North York General Hospital; (416)923-4915; Fax. (416)923-4915.

STEIN, Michael A; 400-5300 ch Cote-des-Neiges, Montreal QC H3T 1Y3; McG'92; MDCM; FRCPC; IntMed; Rheum. Staff, St Mary's Hospital Centre; Langs: French; (514)734-7400; Fax. (514)734-7401.

STEIN, Naomi B; 65 av Hillside, Westmount QC H3Z 1W1; McG'69; Peds. Staff OPD, Hôpital Ste-Justine; Langs: English; French; (514)931-2524; Fax. (514)931-2625; naomibstein@hotmail.com.

STEIN, Nina R; Hamilton HS-McMaster Site, PO Box 2000 Stn Lcd 1 1200 Main St W, Hamilton ON L8N 3Z5; University of Rio Grande Sul (Brazil)'04; Staff, Hamilton Health Sciences Centre - McMaster University Medical Centre; Langs: Portuguese; (905)521-2100

STEIN, Nolan-Paul A; 301-1615 Dufferin St, Toronto ON M6H 4H4; Dal'81; Ac Staff, Humber River Regional Hospital - Finch Avenue Site; Court Staff, St Joseph's Health Centre; Langs: Spanish; French; (416)533-1131; Fax. (416)533-4933.

STEIN, Paul B; 310-2902 Broadway W, Vancouver BC V6K 2G8; London (England)'62; MB; BSc; FRCPC; Psy. (604)218-4194; Fax. (604)732-6446.

STEIN, Raymond D; Rosedale Med Centre, 415-600 Sherbourne St, Toronto ON M4X 1W4; Cape Town (South Africa)'68; MB ChB; DABIM; DAB; FRCPC; IntMed; ClinImmunol&Allergy. Assoc Staff, Toronto General Hospital - UHN; Lecturer Med, University of Toronto; Langs: Afrikaans; (416)961-2933; Fax. (416)961-3016.

STEIN, Raymond M; Bochner Eye Institute, 40 Prince Arthur Ave, Toronto ON M5R 1A9; Tor'82; FRCSC; Ophth. Staff, The Scarborough Hospital - General Campus; Staff, Mount Sinai Hospital; Physician, Bochner Eye Institute; Asst Prof, University of Toronto; (416)921-2131; rstein@bochner.com.

STEIN, Richard A M; 406-89 Queensway W, Mississauga ON L5B 2V2; Qns'03; FRCSC; ObstGyn. (905)268-9928; Fax. (905)268-9950.

STEIN, Robert I; Paediatric Endocrinologist, PO Box 5010 Stn B B1 158-800 Commissioners Rd E, London ON N6A 5W9; McG'97; BSc; FRCPC; Peds (Pediatric Endocrinology); Endocrin&Metab. Staff, London Health Sciences Centre - Victoria Campus; Assoc Prof, University of Western Ontario; Langs: Bilingual(French/English); (519)685-8139; Fax. (519)685-8105; robert.stein@lhsc.on.ca.

STEINBART, Murray R; Kinplace Health Complex, PO Box 28, Oakbank MB R0E 1J0; Man'69; BSc(Med.); DPsy; FRCPC; Psy. Physician Community Mental Health Prog, South Eastman Health Unit; Physician Community Mental Health Prog, Interlake-Eastern Regional Health Authority Stonewall; Fax. (204)444-7851.

STEINBERG, Andrew P; Service d'Urologie Rive-Sud, 304-3234 boul Taschereau, Longueuil QC J4V 2H3; McG'96; FRCSC; Urol (Minimal Invasive Urology). (450)671-2945; Fax. (450)671-8045; steinba@me.com.

STEINBERG, Carolyn R; The Richmond Hosp, 7000 Westminster Hwy, Richmond BC V6X 1A2; Tor'76; FRCPC; Psy (Child Psychiatry). Staff Richmond Health Services, Richmond Hospital; Langs: German; (604)278-9711

STEINBERG, Hedy; Yonge-Eglinton Med Centre, 210-2401 Yonge St, Toronto ON M4P 3H1; Tor'88; CCFP; FCFP; Court Staff, Mount Sinai Hospital; (416)485-9044; Fax. (416)485-8525.

STEINBERG, Jeffrey M; 414 Kenneth Ave, North York ON M2N 4W1; Wes'79; Staff, North York General Hospital - Branson Division; Staff, North York General Hospital; (416)222-2331; Fax. (416)222-2394.

STEINBERG, Johannes L; 45420 Hodgins Ave, Chilliwack BC V2P 1P6; Pretoria (South Africa)'78; MB ChB; MMed(Otol); FRCSC; Otol (Head & Neck Surgery). Langs: Afrikaans; (604)792-6921

STEINBERG, Leah J; Mount Sinai Hosp, 1001B-600 University Ave, Toronto ON M5G 1X5; McM'96; CCFP; FCFP; Staff, Mount Sinai Hospital; (416)586-4800 x4253; Fax. (416)586-4804.

STEINBERG, Malcolm H; BC Centre for Disease Control, 655 12th Ave W, Vancouver BC V5Z 4R4; Witwatersrand (South Africa)'84; MB ChB; (604)660-6162; malcolm.steinberg@bccdc.ca.

STEINBERG, Paul I; Psychotherapy Program, 420-5950 University Blvd, Vancouver BC V6T 1Z3; Tor'75; FRCPC; Psy (Psychoanalysis). Consultant Psy, Vancouver Acute Health Services; Clin Prof Psy, University of British Columbia; (604)827-4235; Fax. (604)827-4106.

STEINBERG, Robert J G; Psychealth Centre, PX 119-771 Bannatyne Ave, Winnipeg MB R3E 3N4; Man'77; AB; FRCPC; Psy (Psychotherapy (Adolescent & Adult)). Staff, Psychealth Centre; rsteinberg@exchange.hsc.mb.ca.

STEINBERG, Steven G; 202-133 Main St W, North Bay ON P1B 2T6; Tor'76.

STEINBERG, Wilfred M; Dr W M Steinberg Med Clinic, 503-55 Queen St E, Toronto ON M5C 1R6; Tor'66; FRCSC; ObstGyn (Colposcopy). Ac Staff, St Michael's Hospital; Asst Prof, University of Toronto; (416)864-5738; Fax. (416)864-5795; steinbergw@smh.toronto.on.ca.

STEINBOK, Paul; Children's & Women's HC of BC, K3 159-4480 Oak St, Vancouver BC V6H 3V4; West Indies (Jamaica)'71; MB BS; BSc; DAB; FRCSC; Neursurg (Pediatric Neuro Surgery). Consultant, Vancouver General Hospital - Centennial Pavillion; Hd Neursurg, BC Children's Hospital; Prof, University of British Columbia; (604)875-2094; Fax. (604)875-3109; psteinbok@cw.bc.ca.

STEINBRECHER, Urs P; Div of Gastroenterology, 5153-2775 Laurel St, Vancouver BC V5Z 1M9; Alb'76; DABIM; BMedSci; MD; FRCP; FRCPC; IntMed; Gastroent. Staff Gastroent, Vancouver General Hospital - Centennial Pavillion; Staff, Gordon & Leslie Diamond Health Care Centre; Prof Med, University of British Columbia; (604)875-5039; Fax. (604)875-5447.

STEINEGG, Cathleen M; The Hosp for Sick Children, BW 7442-555 University Ave, Toronto ON M5G 1X8; Nebraska (USA)'98; Staff, The Hospital For Sick Children; (416)813-5169; Fax. (416)813-5392.

STEINEGGER, Cathleen M; The Hosp for Sick Children, 555 University Ave, Toronto ON M5G 1X8; University of Nebraska (USA)'98; Staff Adolescent Med, The Hospital For Sick Children; (416)813-5169; Fax. (416)813-5392.

STEINER, George; Univ Hlth Network-Toronto Gen, 200 Elizabeth St, Toronto ON M5G 2C4; UBC'60; FRCPC; IntMed (Endocrinology & Metabolism). Staff, Toronto General Hospital - UHN; Staff, LMC Diabetes & Endocrinology Centres-Bayview; Staff, LMC Diabetes & Endocrinology Centres-Eglinton; Emeritus Prof Med & Physiol, University of Toronto; Langs: French; (416)340-4133; Fax. (416)340-3314; george.steiner@uhn.on.ca.

STEINER, Meir; Women's Health Concerns Clinic, 301 James St S, Hamilton ON L8P 3B6; Tel Aviv (Israel)'68; PhD; FRCPC; Psy. Ac Staff, St Joseph's Healthcare - Charlton Campus; Court Staff, Hamilton Health Sciences Centre - Hamilton General Hospital; Staff Founding Director, Women's Health Concerns Clinic; Prof Psy, McMaster University; Instructor Medical Sciences, University of Toronto; Langs: German; Hebrew; (905)522-1155 x3605; Fax. (905)521-6098.

STEINER, Theodore S; Heather Pavillon, D452-2733 Heather St, Vancouver BC V5Z 1M9; Durham (England),Virginia (USA)'92; FRCPC; IntMed (Infectious Diseases). Assoc Prof InfectDis, University of British Columbia; (604)875-4588; Fax. (604)875-4013.

STEINER, Warren; MUHC-Montreal Gen Hosp, B6 221-1650 av Cedar, Montreal QC H3G 1A4; McG'83; FRCPC; Psy. Dir Outpatient & Comm Psy, McGill University Health Centre - Montreal General Campus; assoc Prof, McGill University; Langs: French; (514)934-1934 x42052; Fax. (514)934-8237; warren.steiner@mcgill.ca.

STEINGART, Allan B; 260 Queen St W PO Box 60044 Queen Berverly PO, Toronto ON M5V 0C5; McM'81; FRCPC; Psy. Staff, Baycrest Centre for Geriatric Care; (905)709-1470; Fax. (905)780-1470; allan.steingart@gmail.com.

STEINGART, Christopher R; Sanguen Health Centre, 29 Young St E, Waterloo ON N2J 2L4; Cal'93; FRCPC; IntMed (AIDS/HIV). Dir, Sanguen Health Centre; (519)603-0223; csteingart@sanguen.com.

STEINHART, A Hillary; Mount Sinai Hosp, 445-600 University Ave, Toronto ON M5G 1X5; Tor'84; MSc; FRCPC; IntMed (Inflammatory Bowel Disease); Gastroent. Staff, Mount Sinai Hospital; Assoc Prof Med, University of Toronto; (416)586-4800 x5121; Fax. (416)586-3174.

STEINHART, Brian D; 30 Bond St, Toronto ON M5B 1W8; Ott'78; FRCPC; EmergMed. Staff Emerg & Trauma Services, St Michael's Hospital; Assoc Prof Med, University of Toronto; (416)864-5095; steinhartb@smh.toronto.on.ca.

STEINHART, Norman S; 28 Maxwell Ave, Toronto ON M5P 2B5; Tor'81; (416)481-0540; Fax. (416)481-9275.

STEINHAUER, Elizabeth L; 4640 17 Ave NW, Calgary AB T3B 0P3; Cal'80; (403)247-8808; Fax. (403)247-8807.

STEINHOFF, Gary E J; 200-1121 Yates St, Victoria BC V8V 3N1; Ott'75; FRCSC; Urol. Staff, Royal Jubilee Hospital; (250)381-3747; Fax. (250)381-3748.

STEININGER, Jodi L; Gulf Canada Square, 362-401 9 Ave SW, Calgary AB T2P 3C5; Qns'92; BSc(Hons.); CCFP; (403)221-4424; Fax. (403)221-4426.

STEINITZ, Daniel K; Quinte Healthcare-Belleville, WCA3 67-265 Dundas St E, Belleville ON K8N 5A9; Dal'97; FRCSC; OrthSurg (Hand & Wrist Surgery). Chief OrthSurg, QHC Belleville General; Langs: German; French; (613)968-2844; Fax. (613)968-4850; mdortho@hotmail.com.

STEINITZ, Tracy L F; Quinte HC Corp-Belleville Gen, 265 Dundas St E, Belleville ON K8N 5A9; Dal'97; BSc; CCFP; CCFP(E.M.); Staff, QHC Belleville General; Langs: French; (613)969-7400

STEINKE, David E; University of Alberta Hosp, 2D102WC-8440 112 St NW, Edmonton AB T6G 2B7; Sask'83; FRCSC; Neursurg. Ac Staff, University of Alberta Hospital; (780)492-1776; Fax. (780)492-8203.

STEINMAN, Raymond W; Eastwood Med Clinic, 101-1346 Kingston Rd, Scarborough ON M1N 1P9; Tor'69; (416)698-0883; Fax. (416)491-9117.

STEINMAN, Robert J; Clinique de l'Alternative, 2034 rue Saint-Hubert, Montreal QC H2L 3Z5; McG'71; (514)281-9848; Fax. (514)281-8057.

STEINMETZ, Oren K; MUHC-Royal Victoria Hosp, S10 18-687 av des Pins O, Montreal QC H3A 1A1; McG'87; FRCSC; GenSurg; VascSurg. Staff, McGill University Health Centre - Royal Victoria Hospital; (514)842-1231; Fax. (514)843-1730; oren.steinmetz@muhc.mcgill.ca.

STEINMETZ, Peter O; St Mary's Hosp Centre, 3830 av Lacombe, Montreal QC H3T 1M5; McG'91; Staff, St Mary's Hospital Centre; (514)345-3511; Fax. (514)734-2663.

STEINNAGEL, Brenda L; Functional Rehabilitation Inc, 115 King St W, Dundas ON L9H 1V1; McM'93; CCFP; FCFP; Staff, Work Safety & Insurance Board.

STEINRATHS, Michelle R; Victoria Gen Hosp, 1 Hospital Way, Victoria BC V8Z 6R5; UBC'01; FRCPC; MedGenetics. Staff Path & Med Genetics, Victoria General Hospital; (250)727-4461; Fax. (250)727-4295.

STEINRUCK, Martin W; Centuria Medical, 2-1499 Gordon Dr, Kelowna BC V1Y 9R2; UBC'77; CCFP; Staff, Kelowna General Hospital; Langs: German; French; (250)763-5152; Fax. (250)763-6263.

STEINSON, David S; Gain Med Centre, 1199 Austin Ave, Coquitlam BC V3K 3P4; UBC'95; CCFP; (604)939-7345; Fax. (604)939-7781.

STEIRMAN, Michael; Markham Stouffville Hosp, PO Box 1800 Stn Main 381 Church St, Markham ON L3P 7P3; McG'84; FRCPC; DiagRad. Staff Radiol, Markham Stouffville Hospital; Langs: French; (905)472-7093; Fax. (905)472-7078.

STEJAR, Dana C; Sault Area Hosp, 750 Great Northern Rd, Sault Ste. Marie ON P6B 0A8; Bucharest (Romania)'97; FRCPC; Psy. Staff, Sault Area Hospital - Sault Ste Marie; (705)759-3434

STEL, Karen G; Danforth Med Centre, 880 Danforth Rd, Scarborough ON M1K 1H8; Tor'99; CCFP; Physician, International Medical Services; Langs: Dutch; French; (416)264-4848; Fax. (416)264-0547.

STEL, Patrick R; Cool Aid Comm Health Centre, 713 Johnson St, Victoria BC V8W 1M8; UBC'95; Physician, Cool Aid Community Health Centre; Langs: Spanish; (250)385-1466; Fax. (250)383-1327.

STELFOX, Henry T; Calgary Heart Centre, 3E34-3280 Hospital Dr NW, Calgary AB T2N 4Z6; Alb'95; PhD; Critical Care Medicine; IntMed (Trauma). Staff Critical Care, Foothills Medical Centre; Staff Teaching Research & Wellness, Health Research Innovation Centre; Langs: Polish; (403)944-2334; Fax. (403)283-9994.

STELMASCHUK, Myron E; CBI Health Group, 1707-1632 14 Ave NW, Calgary AB T2N 1M7; Cal'95; CCFP; (403)221-0944; Fax. (866)410-8556.

STELZER, Hans J; Alexander Prof Bldg, 201-849 Alexander Crt, Peterborough ON K9J 7H8; McM'75; DABIM; FCCP; FRCPC; Respir (Respirology); IntMed. Staff, Peterborough Regional Health Centre - Hospital Drive; Langs: German; (705)748-5443; Fax. (705)748-5449.

STELZER, Josef; 603-555 River Ave, Winnipeg MB R3L 0E3; Buenos Aires (Argentina)'63; Langs: Spanish; French; Hebrew.

STELZER-CHILTON, Ashleigh D; Seymour Health Centre Ltd, 1530 7th Ave W, Vancouver BC V6J 1S3; McM'03; CCFP; Langs: German; French; (604)739-5614; Fax. (604)738-1487.

STELZL, Glenn E; Squamish Med Clinic, PO Box 389 Stn Main, Squamish BC V8B 0A3; UBC'91; Langs: German; (604)892-3535; Fax. (604)892-3545.

STEMERDINK, Christopher J; Guelph Family Health Team, 207-55 Wyndham St N, Guelph ON N1H 7T8; Tor'01; BSc; MSc; CCFP; Langs: French; (519)836-1443; Fax. (519)836-1321; cstem@sympatico.ca.

STEMPIEN, James E; St Paul's Hosp, 1702 20th St W, Saskatoon SK S7M 0Z9; Tor'84; BSc; CCFP; CCFP(E.M.); FCFP; Staff, St Paul's Hospital (Grey Nuns) of Saskatoon; Langs: French; (306)655-5846; Fax. (306)655-5555.

STEMPIEN, Matthew W; Joseph Brant Mem Hosp, 1230 North Shore Blvd E, Burlington ON L7S 1W7; Wes'77; CCFP; CCFP(E.M.); Staff Emerg, Joseph Brant Memorial Hospital; (905)336-4116; Fax. (905)336-6484.

STENDARDO, Vincenzo R; Appletreee Med Group, 275 Dundas St W, Toronto ON M5T 1G1; Cal'06; CCFP; (647)772-2370; Fax. (416)367-4301.

STENDEL, Mitchell H; SMBD-Jewish Gen Hosp, D010-3755 Cote-Sainte-Catherin, Montreal QC H3T 1E2; McG'94; CCFP; CCFP(E.M.); Staff, Sir Mortimer B Davis Jewish General; Langs: English; (514)340-8222 x5568

STENDER, Jennifer S; Major's Path Family Practice, 301-35 Major's Path, St. John's NL A1A 4Z9; Mem'90; (709)579-2324

STENDER, Mark W; Family Practice Associates, 6155 North St, Halifax NS B3K 5R3; Mem'93; Dip(SportsMed); CCFP; FCFP; Clin Associate, Queen Elizabeth II Health Sciences Centre - Victoria General Site; (902)453-3511; Fax. (902)454-9010.

STENERSON, Paul E; College Plaza Prof Bldg, 406-8215 112 St NW, Edmonton AB T6G 2C8; McM'87; FRCPC; Neur. (780)432-1866; Fax. (780)432-1989.

STENHOUSE, James K; St Boniface Gen Hosp, 409 Tache Ave, Winnipeg MB R2H 2A6; Man'78; Ac Staff, St Boniface General Hospital; (204)233-8563; Fax. (204)231-0640.

STENN, Peter G; Humber River Reg Hosp-Keele, 2175 Keele St, York ON M6M 3Z4; Wes'85; FRCPC; Psy. Staff, Humber River Regional Hospital - Keele Street Site; (416)658-2038; Fax. (416)658-2074.

STENNING, David L; Orangeville Family Med Ctre, M1-32 First St, Orangeville ON L9W 2E1; Wes'98; CCFP; FCFP; (519)938-8000; Fax. (519)938-8080.

STENSTROM, Robert J; St Paul's Hosp, 1081 Burrard St, Vancouver BC V6Z 1Y6; McM'98; DSc; PhD; CCFP; CCFP(E.M.); Dir Research Dept of Emerg Med, Providence Health Care - St Paul's Hospital; Langs: English; French; (604)806-8480; Fax. (604)806-8488.

STENT, Paul A; Fort St James Med Clinic PO Box 1149, Fort St. James BC V0J 1P0; Witwatersrand (South Africa)'85; MB ChB; Clin Instructor Family Practice, University of British Columbia; (250)996-8291; Fax. (250)996-8212.

STEPANKO, Rosemarie; Lendrum Family Clinic, 5526 111 St NW, Edmonton AB T6H 3E9; Alb'77; CCFP; Clin Assoc Prof, University of Alberta; (780)436-3422; Fax. (780)436-3441.

STEPHAN, Ernest F; Parksville Med Clinic, PO Box 250 Stn Main 154 Memorial Ave W, Parksville BC V9P 2G4; Stellenbosch (South Africa)'82; MB ChB; Langs: Afrikaans; (250)248-5757; Fax. (250)248-2128.

STEPHAN, G Paul; 3-2650 Lawrence Ave E, Scarborough ON M1R 2S1; Tor'76; BSc(Hons.Biochem); Court Staff, The Scarborough Hospital - General Campus; Court Staff, Toronto East General Hospital Inc; Med Examiner, Quality Underwriting Services; Med Examiner Insurance, Rapid Med(Toronto/Oshawa); (416)752-3233; Fax. (416)752-3326; paul_stephan@qus.ca.

STEPHAN, Jarad S; AHS Chronic Pain Centre, 160-2210 2 St SW, Calgary AB T2S 3C3; Alb'06; Anes. Staff, University of Alberta Hospital; Staff, Calgary Health Region Chronic Pain Centre; (403)943-9900; Fax. (403)209-2954.

STEPHANY, Harold E; 303-22112 52 Ave, Langley BC V2Y 2M6; UBC'71; Langs: German; (604)530-0056; Fax. (604)530-4718.

STEPHEN, Christopher M; Markham Stouffville Hosp, PO Box 1800 Stn Main 381 Church St, Markham ON L3P 7P3; Tor'84; FRCPC; DiagRad. Staff Diag Imaging, Markham Stouffville Hospital; (905)472-7020; Fax. (905)472-7078.

STEPHEN, David H; Dr Poon's Metabolic Diet Clini, 6-375 Kingston Rd, Pickering ON L1V 1A3; Tor'59; (905)509-6888; Fax. (905)509-0663.

STEPHEN, David J G; Sunnybrook Hlth Sciences Ctre, MG365-2075 Bayview Ave, Toronto ON M4N 3M5; Man'85; BSc; FRCSC; OrthSurg (Lower Extremity Medicine). Staff OrthSurg, Sunnybrook Health Sciences Centre; (416)480-6100 x7105; Fax. (416)480-5886.

STEPHEN, J Daniel; 309-2021 Cliff Rd, Mississauga ON L5A 3N7; Tor'75; CCFP; Staff, Medcan Health Management Inc; Med Consultant, Honeywell - Aerospace Toronto; (905)276-8900; Fax. (905)276-8911; daniel.stephen@honeywell.com.

STEPHEN, James W M; Royal Inland Hosp, 311 Columbia St, Kamloops BC V2C 2T1; Sask'79; DABPath; FRCPC; GenPath; AnatPath. Staff, Royal Inland Hospital; (250)314-2669; Fax. (250)314-2505.

STEPHEN, Lorne J; Oshawa Clinic, 117 King St E, Oshawa ON L1H 1B9; Tor'69; Court Staff, Lakeridge Health - Oshawa Site; (905)723-8551; Fax. (905)721-6664.

STEPHEN, Wesley J; Hamilton HS-Henderson Campus, 711 Concession St, Hamilton ON L8V 1C3; Dal'85; FRCSC; GenSurg (Colon & Rectal Surgery). Ac Staff, Hamilton Health Sciences Centre - McMaster Children's Hospital; Staff, Hamilton Health Sciences Centre-Juravinski Site; Staff, The Juravinski Cancer Centre; (905)521-2100; Fax. (905)528-9388.

STEPHEN GNANARAJ, Leo P; Maidstone Med Clinic, PO Box 399, Maidstone SK S0M 1M0; (Other Foreign)'02; CCFP; (306)893-2689; Fax. (306)893-4646.

STEPHENS, Donald S; Queen Elizabeth Hosp, PO Box 6600 Stn Central 60 Riverside Dr, Charlottetown PE C1A 8T5; Dal'74; Court Staff, Queen Elizabeth Hospital; (902)894-2111

STEPHENS, Janine W; Etobicoke Med Centre, 400 The East Mall, Etobicoke ON M9B 3Z9; Tor'01; CCFP; (416)621-2220; Fax. (416)621-2203.

STEPHENS, John D; Koala Laboratories, 126-15355 24th Ave, Surrey BC V4A 2H9; University of Sydney Medical School (Australia) MRCOG(UK); MB BS; FRCOG(U.K); FACOG(USA); LMCC; Med Dir, Koala Laboratories; (604)805-6253; jdskoala@aol.com.

STEPHENS, Mary H; Clinical Sciences Bldg, 8 110-8440 112 St NW, Edmonton AB T6G 2B7; Wes'86; FACS; FRCSC; GenSurg (Critical Care Medicine). Staff, University of Alberta Hospital; Clin Prof, University of Alberta; Langs: Dutch; (780)433-3107; Fax. (780)433-0289.

STEPHENSEN, Michael C; Assiniboine Clinic, 633 Lodge Ave, Winnipeg MB R3J 0S9; Man'93; CCFP; FCFP; (204)958-6710; Fax. (204)897-7314.

STEPHENSON, Anne L; St Michael's Hosp, 6 040-30 Bond St, Toronto ON M5B 1W8; Tor'95; FRCPC; IntMed; Respir. Staff, St Michael's Hospital; (416)864-5431

STEPHENSON, Catherine A; BC Women's Hosp & Health Ctre, 1L2-4500 Oak St, Vancouver BC V6H 3N1; Newcastle (England)'81; MB BS; FRCPC; Anes. Staff, BC Women's Hospital & Health Centre; Clin Teacher, University of British Columbia; (604)875-2424

STEPHENSON, Christina A; Haliburton Family Med Ctre, PO Box 870 7217 Gelert Rd, Haliburton ON K0M 1S0; Ott'86; Staff, Haliburton Highlands Health Services - Haliburton Site; (705)457-1212; Fax. (705)457-3955.

STEPHENSON, Elizabeth A; The Hosp For Sick Children, 555 University Ave, Toronto ON M5G 1X8; Columbia(NY) (USA)'96; ABPeds; Staff Cardiol, The Hospital For Sick Children; University of Toronto; (416)813-5850; Fax. (416)813-6540; elizabeth.stephenson@sickkids.ca.

STEPHENSON, Jenny P; Toronto Dominion Bank Tower, PO Box 48 Stn Toronto Dom, Toronto ON M5K 1E6; Wes'81; (416)601-7754

STEPHENSON, Linda A; 2-10 King George Crt, Saint John NB E2K 0H5; McG'90; (506)634-8706; Fax. (506)634-6654.

STEPHENSON, Marie-France; Chaleur Reg Hosp, 1750 Sunset Dr, Bathurst NB E2A 4L7; Sher'06; Otol (Head & Neck Surgery). Staff, Hopital Regional Chaleur; (506)544-3000

STEPHENSON, Megan A; Huntsville Prof Bldg, 102-348 Muskoka Rd 3 N, Huntsville ON P1H 1H8; Wes'97; CCFP; FCFP; Staff, Huntsville District Memorial Hospital - Muskoka Algonquin Healthcare; Staff, Fairvern Nursing Home; (705)789-4377; Fax. (705)789-1640.

STEPHENSON, Michael C; 2F-761 Jane St, York ON M6N 4B4; Qns'06; CCFP; (416)760-8677; Fax. (416)693-1330.

STEPHENSON, Michael J; 105-323 Wilson St E, Ancaster ON L9G 4A8; Otago (New Zealand)'72; MSc; DTMH; CCFP; FCFP; Staff, St Joseph's Healthcare - Charlton Campus; Ac Staff, Hamilton Health Sciences Centre - Hamilton General Hospital; Clin Assoc Prof, McMaster University; (905)648-1112; Fax. (905)648-2033.

STEPHENSON, Paul K; 5515 rue St-Jacques, Montreal QC H4A 2E3; Qns'80; FRCSC; OrthSurg (Joint Replacement). Staff, St Mary's Hospital Centre; Langs: French; (514)489-8216; Fax. (514)731-4634.

STEPHENSON, Susan L; Guelph Family Health Team, 21 Yarmouth St, Guelph ON N1H 4G2; Mem'89; (519)822-7831; drsue@bellnet.ca.

STEPHURE, David K; Alberta Children's Hosp, C3 376-2888 Shaganappi Trail N, Calgary AB T3B 6A8; Cal'78; FAAP(Peds); FRCPC; Peds (Pediatric Endocrinology). Staff Ped Endoctrinology, Alberta Children's Hospital; Assoc Prof Peds, University of Calgary; (403)955-7819; Fax. (403)955-5001.

STEPLEWSKI, Jacek D; Mediclinic, 101-3301 8th St E, Saskatoon SK S7H 4K1; Gdansk (Poland)'88; (306)955-1530; Fax. (306)955-8811.

STEPNEY, Sandra K; 110-20103 40 Ave, Langley BC V3A 2W3; UBC'85; BSc; (604)533-1334; Fax. (604)533-4241.

STERESCU, Anca E; Hôpital Ste-Justine, 3175 ch Cote-Sainte-Catherine, Montreal QC H3T 1C5; Mon'99; FRCPC; Peds (Nutrition). Staff, Hôpital Ste-Justine; (514)345-4931; Fax. (514)345-4744; anca.sterescu.hsj@ssss.gouv.qc.ca.

STERGIOPOULOS, Victoria; St Michael's Hosp, CCW 17F-30 Bond St, Toronto ON M5B 1W8; Dal'97; FRCPC; Psy. Staff, St Michael's Hospital; Langs: Greek; (416)864-3085

STERLIN, Carlo; Clinique Externe de Psy, 7345 rue Garnier, Montreal QC H2E 2A1; Port-au-Prince (Haiti)'56; Psy (Transcultural Psychiatry). Langs: Spanish; French; (514)729-3036; Fax. (514)495-6774.

STERLING, George D; Hys Med Centre, 202-11010 101 St NW, Edmonton AB T5H 4B9; Alb'84; FRCPC; DiagRad (Diagnostic Ultrasound). Staff Radiol, Royal Alexandra Hospital; Clin Teacher, University of Alberta; (780)426-1121; Fax. (780)425-5979.

STERN, Alex; Baywood Med Centre, 506-95 Bayly St W, Ajax ON L1S 7K8; Tor'91; BSc; CCFP; Staff, Rouge Valley Health System - Ajax & Pickering Health Centre Site; Langs: Hungarian; (905)428-0210; Fax. (905)428-0449.

STERN, Andrea; Unison Hlth & Commun Services, 12 Flemington Rd, North York ON M6A 2N4; Man'80; BSc; CCFP; CCFP(E.M.); (416)787-1661; Fax. (416)787-3761.

STERN, Dennis J; 48 Oak Ridge Rd S, Parry Sound ON P2A 2W9; London (England)'60; MB BS; MRCS; LRCP; Staff, West Parry Sound Health Centre; Physician, Lakeland Ltc; (705)746-5635; Fax. (705)746-7232; djstern@zeuter.com.

STERN, Donna; St Mary's Hosp Centre, 3830 av Lacombe, Montreal QC H3T 1M5; McG'74; MedOncol (P.Q.); Hem (P.Q.). ac Staff, St Mary's Hospital Centre; adj Médecin Med, McGill University Health Centre - Royal Victoria Hospital; assoc Prof, McGill University; (514)734-2679; Fax. (514)734-2795.

STERN, Eben L; Scarborough Prof Centre, 112-1371 Neilson Rd, Scarborough ON M1B 4Z8; Tor'85; Staff Family Med, Rouge Valley Health System - Centenary Health Centre Site; (416)287-9100; Fax. (416)287-0261.

STERN, Errol; SMBD Jewish Gen Hosp, D 010-3755 Cote-Sainte-Catheri, Montreal QC H3T 1E2; McG'82; FACEP; FRCPC; EmergMed. Staff, Sir Mortimer B Davis Jewish General; Langs: Bilingual(English/French); (514)340-8222 x3446; Fax. (514)340-7917.

STERN, Hartley S; B 119-SMBD Jewish Gen Hosp, 3755 ch Cote-Sainte-Catherine, Montreal QC H3T 1E2; Tor'74; FRCSC; GenSurg (Surgical Oncology). Dir exéc, Sir Mortimer B Davis Jewish General; Langs: French; (514)340-8222 x5111; Fax. (514)340-7530.

STERN, Jerry; SMBD Jewish Gen Hosp, 3755 ch Cote-Sainte-Catherine, Montreal QC H3T 1E2; McG'75; BSc; AB; FRCPC; DiagRad; NuclearMed. Staff, Cornwall Community Hospital - Second Street Site; Staff, Sir Mortimer B Davis Jewish General; Langs: French; (514)340-8222; Fax. (514)340-7919.

STERN, Lara; 4018 rue Sainte-Catherine O, Montreal QC H3Z 1P2; McG'98; FRCPC; Psy. Staff, McGill University Health Centre - Montreal Children's Hospital; (514)412-4449; Fax. (514)412-4346.

STERN, Meira; SMBD-Jewish Gen Hosp, 3755 ch Cote-Sainte-Catherine, Montreal QC H3T 1E2; McG'01; CCFP; Staff, Sir Mortimer B Davis Jewish General; (514)340-8253; Fax. (514)340-8298.

STERN, Richard B; 1437 Belcher St PO Box 300, Port Williams NS B0P 1T0; London (England)'69; MRC; FCCP; FACP; FRCPC; IntMed. Staff, Valley Regional Hospital; Hon Teacher Med, Dalhousie University; (902)542-0584; Fax. (902)542-7218.

STERN, Richard J; Lansdowne Prof Bldg, 140-1641 Hillside Ave, Victoria BC V8T 5G1; Cape Town (South Africa)'72; MB ChB; FRCPC; Psy (Child & Adolescent Psychiatry). Staff, Queen Alexandra Centre for Children's Health; (250)592-4346; Fax. (250)592-5755.

STERN, Robert J; Woodstock Med Family Hlth Org, 204-959 Dundas St E, Woodstock ON N4S 1H2; Tor'89; Staff Med, Woodstock General Hospital; Langs: Hungarian; (519)539-5622

STERN, Sheryl; Health Sciences Centre, GG 345-820 Sherbrook St, Winnipeg MB R3A 1R9; Man'84; MSc(Microbiol.); FRCPC; NuclearMed. Staff Nuclear Med, Health Sciences Centre; Asst Prof, University of Manitoba; (204)787-3375; Fax. (204)787-3090; sstern@hsc.mb.ca.

STERN, Solomon B; Argus Med Centre, 202-581 Argus Rd, Oakville ON L6J 3J4; Tor'82; (905)338-9900; Fax. (905)338-9904; sstern@bellnet.ca.

STERN, Stephen J; Ajax Med Arts Bldg, 103-601 Harwood Ave S, Ajax ON L1S 2J5; Tor'71; Ac Staff, Rouge Valley Health System - Ajax & Pickering Health Centre Site; (905)683-0162; Fax. (905)683-3518.

STERNADEL, Jerzy; 102-477 King St, Welland ON L3B 3K4; Warsaw (Poland)'79; PhD; FRCSC; ObstGyn. Langs: Polish; (905)788-1406; Fax. (905)788-9674.

STERNBERG, Harvey H; Edmonton Clinic, 1A 102-11400 University Ave, Edmonton AB T5G 1Z1; Alb'68; CCFP; FCFP; Staff Family Med Clnic, University of Alberta Hospital; (780)407-7755; Fax. (780)407-1828.

STERNBERG, Leonard; Women's College Hosp, 765-76 Grenville St, Toronto ON M5S 1B2; Tor'71; FRCPC; IntMed (Teaching & Administration); Cardiol. Ac Staff Cardiol, Women's College Hospital; Assoc Staff, Toronto Western Hospital - University Health Network; Assoc Staff, Sunnybrook Health Sciences Centre; Assoc Prof, University of Toronto; (416)323-7556; Fax. (416)323-6304.

STERNS, Laurence D; Western Cardiology Assoc, 335-1900 Richmond Ave, Victoria BC V8R 4R2; Alb'85; FRCPC; IntMed (Electrophysiology); Cardiol. Staff, Vancouver Island Health Authority; (250)595-1551; Fax. (250)595-1000.

STERNTHAL, David S; 1712-808 Nelson St, Vancouver BC V6Z 2H2; Ott'89; BSc; MD; FRCPC; Psy (AIDS/HIV). (604)685-5611; Fax. (604)683-2194.

STETSKO, Samuel D; Royal Alexandra Hosp, 10240 Kingsway NW, Edmonton AB T5H 3V9; Alb'99; FRCPC; Anes. Staff, Royal Alexandra Hospital; (780)735-4010; Fax. (780)735-4386.

STETSKO, Terry P; Royal Alexandra Hosp, 10240 Kingsway NW, Edmonton AB T5H 3V9; Alb'72; Staff, Royal Alexandra Hospital; (780)735-4442

STEVANOVSKI, Peter; Malton Med Arts Bldg, 110-3530 Derry Rd E, Mississauga ON L4T 4E3; Tor'05; CCFP; (905)672-2273; Fax. (905)672-0487.

STEVEN, David A; London HSC-University Hosp, PO Box 5339 Stn B A10 323-339 Windermere Rd, London ON N6A 5A5; Man'96; FRCSC; Neursurg. Staff, London Health Sciences Centre - University Hospital; Langs: French; (519)663-3297; Fax. (519)663-3296.

STEVENS, Annette C; PO Box 29174 Okanagan Mission, Kelowna BC V1W 4A7; McM'90; FRCPC; Psy.

STEVENS, Brett J D; 2104 Old Lakeshore Rd, Burlington ON L7R 1A3; McM'92; FRCPC; IntMed; Cardiol. (905)634-2504; Fax. (905)632-1126.

STEVENS, Christiaan S M; Royal Victoria Hosp, 201 Georgian Dr, Barrie ON L4M 6M2; Tor'03; FRCPC; RadOncol. Staff Regional Cancer Program, Royal Victoria Regional Health Centre; Langs: Bilingual(English/French); (705)728-9802

STEVENS, David C L; 1937 Lee Ave, Victoria BC V8R 4W9; Man'68; Assoc Staff, Royal Jubilee Hospital; Assoc Staff, Victoria General Hospital; (250)598-5107; Fax. (250)598-5722.

STEVENS, David G; 115-675 Queen St S, Waterloo ON N2J 1C4; Tor'91; BSc; FRCSC; OrthSurg. (519)603-0623; Fax. (519)603-0625.

STEVENS, David J; Victoria Square Med Clinic, PO Box 5700 Stn Main 2030-2345 10th Ave W, Prince Albert SK S6V 7V6; London (England)'78; MB BS; LRCP; FRCS; Staff Otol, Victoria Hospital; Physician, Victoria Square Medical Clinic; (306)763-2623; Fax. (306)953-8931.

STEVENS, Gillian T; North Burlington Med Centre, 18-1960 Appleby Line, Burlington ON L7L 0B7; McM'90; (905)319-2000; Fax. (905)319-6292.

STEVENS, Holly E; 101-1301 Main St, Penticton BC V2A 5E9; Tor'78; DAB; BSc; FRCSC; Otol. Staff Consultant, Penticton Regional Hospital; Assoc Prof Clinical, University of British Columbia; (250)492-8440; Fax. (250)492-8441; drholly@shawbiz.ca.

STEVENS, Howard; Etobicoke Med Centre, 400 The East Mall, Etobicoke ON M9B 3Z9; Tor'68; Ac Staff, Trillium Health Centre - West Toronto; (416)621-2220; Fax. (416)621-2203; dr.h.stevens@emcfht.ca.

STEVENS, James D; Battlefords Union Hosp, 1092 107th St, North Battleford SK S9A 1Z1; Cape Town (South Africa)'92; MB ChB; FRCPC; DiagRad. Staff, Battlefords Union Hospital; (306)446-6600

STEVENS, John A; Family Focus Med Clinic, 201-240 Baker Dr, Dartmouth NS B2W 6L4; Dal'82; (902)420-6060

STEVENS, Jonathan P; Royal Alexandra Hosp, NICU-10240 Kingsway Ave NW, Edmonton AB T5H 3V9; Manchester (England)'89; MRCP(UK); BSc; MSc; MB ChB; FRCPC; Peds (Neonatal & Perinatal Medicine). Staff NICU, Royal Alexandra Hospital; (780)735-4670

STEVENS, Katrina G; Kingston Family Health Team, 200-2437 Princess St, Kingston ON K7M 3G1; McG'87; Assoc Staff Family Med, Kingston General Hospital; Langs: French; (613)546-6652; kstevens@kfhn.net.

STEVENS, Kelly A J; University of Alberta Hosp, 1D1 WCM-8440 112 St NW, Edmonton AB T6G 2B7; Alb'04; FRCPC; Peds. Staff Pediatrics Ambulatory Clinic, University of Alberta Hospital; (780)407-8822

STEVENS, Kyle D; 13214 Kelly Ave PO Box 1620, Summerland BC V0H 1Z0; UBC'02; CCFP; (250)494-3432; Fax. (250)494-4392.

STEVENS, Liisa H; Perth & Smith Falls Dist Hosp, 60 Cornelia St W, Smiths Falls ON K7A 2H9; Ott'05; CCFP; Staff, Perth & Smiths Falls District Hospital - Smiths Falls Site; Langs: Bilingual(English/French); (613)283-2330

STEVENS, Louis-Mathieu; CHUM-Hotel-Dieu Hosp, 2 420-3840 rue Saint-Urbain, Montreal QC H2W 1T8; Laval'00; FRCSC; CardSurg (Robotics). Staff Centre Cardiovasculaire de CHUM, Centre Hospitalier l'Université de Montréal (CHUM) - Hôtel-Dieu; Clin Assoc Prof, Centre Recherche du CHUM; Langs: Bilingual(French/English); (514)890-8131; Fax. (514)412-7231; lm.stevens@videotron.ca.

STEVENS, Rob F; Parry Sound Family Health Team, 15 James St, Parry Sound ON P2A 1T4; Ott'05; CCFP; (705)746-9382; Fax. (705)746-7758.

STEVENS, Robert L; Grand River Hosp-KW Hlth Ctre, PO Box 9056 Stn C 835 King St, Kitchener ON N2G 1G3; Qns'88; FRCPC; IntMed;CCFP; Hem. Staff, Grand River Hospital - Kitchener/Waterloo Health Centre; Staff, Grand River Regional Cancer Centre; (519)749-4370; robert.stevens@grhosp.on.ca.

STEVENS, Samuel D; Centrepoint Plaza, 201-68 William St, Brockville ON K6V 4V5; Ott'86; FRCSC; Ophth. Langs: French; (613)342-1254; Fax. (613)342-7728.

STEVENS, Sarah C; IWK Health Centre, PO Box 9700 Rpo CSC 5850-5980 University Ave, Halifax NS B3K 6R8; Dal'86; FRCPC; Anes (Pain Management). Staff, IWK Health Centre; Asst Prof, Dalhousie University; Langs: Bilingual(English/French); (902)470-8251; Fax. (902)470-7911.

STEVENS LEBEL, Miriane; Hop Brome-Missisquoi-Perkins, 950 rue Principale, Cowansville QC J2K 1K3; Sher'06; GenSurg. Staff, Hôpital Brome-Missisquoi-Perkins; Staff, Carrefour Sante Granit; Staff, CSSS du Granit; (450)263-2220

STEVENSON, C Marie; Hawkwood Village Med Clinic, 20-217 Hawksbrow Dr NW, Calgary AB T3G 3K2; Cal'89; (403)777-2757; Fax. (403)777-2755.

STEVENSON, Cameron M; 407-797 Princess St, Kingston ON K7L 1G1; Qns'55; MDCM; FRCPC; Psy. Staff, Kingston General Hospital; Consultant, Hotel-Dieu Hospital; Assoc Staff, Providence Care - Mental Health Services; Member, Consent & Capacity Board of Ontario; Assoc Prof Psy, Queen's University; (613)544-0683; Fax. (613)389-4051.

STEVENSON, Carolynn; Peace Arch Hosp, 15521 Russell Ave, White Rock BC V4B 2R4; UBC'01; CCFP; Staff, Peace Arch Hospital; (604)542-0248

STEVENSON, Colin G; McMaster Family Med Centre, 690 Main St W, Hamilton ON L8S 1A4; Qns'02; CCFP; Langs: French; (905)521-5016; Fax. (905)521-5010.

STEVENSON, Giles W; Prince Rupert Reg Hosp, 1305 Summit Dr, Prince Rupert BC V8J 2A6; Oxford (England)'63; DMRD; FRCP; FFR; FRCR; FRCPC; DiagRad (Gastrointestinal Disorders). Staff Radiol, Prince Rupert Regional Hospital; Staff, CML X-Ray & Ultrasound; (250)624-2171; gilesws@shaw.ca.

STEVENSON, J Milton; Guisachan Family Medicine, 105-2395 Gordon Dr, Kelowna BC V1W 3X7; Cal'78; (250)860-5888; Fax. (250)860-5880.

STEVENSON, Kevin W; Vernon Mental Health Centre, 1440 14 Ave, Vernon BC V1B 2T1; Alb'89; FRCPC; Psy. Staff, Vernon Mental Health Centre; (250)549-5737; kevin.stevenson@interiorhealth.ca.

STEVENSON, Kevin W; Royal University Hosp, 103 Hospital Dr, Saskatoon SK S7N 0W8; Sask'04; FRCSC; GenSurg; Critical Care Medicine. Staff, Royal University Hospital; (306)655-1000

STEVENSON, Lindsay J; University Village Med Clinic, 228-2155 Allison Rd, Vancouver BC V6T 1T5; Qns'09; CCFP; (604)222-2273

STEVENSON, Lisa M; Richmond Square Med Centre, 70-3915 51 St SW, Calgary AB T3E 6N1; Ott'89; CCFP; (403)229-2273; Fax. (403)246-9688.

STEVENSON, Peter; 675 Queen St S, Kitchener ON N2M 1A1; Manchester (England)'75; MB ChB; MRC; FRCS; FRCSC; OrthSurg (Spine Surgery). Staff, Grand River Hospital - Freeport Site; Chief Surg, St Mary's General Hospital; Assoc Prof Kinesiology, University of Waterloo; (519)603-0662

STEVENSON, Robert F; 21 Alworth Pl, Sault Ste. Marie ON P6B 5W5; McG'69; FRCSC; Ophth. Court Staff, St Joseph's General Hospital Elliot Lake; Court Staff Ophth, Sault Area Hospital - Sault Ste Marie; Langs: French; (705)946-5068; Fax. (705)946-2854.

STEVENSON, Robert S; Saint John Med Clinic, 299 Metcalf St, Saint John NB E2K 4P8; Dal'00; FRCPC; IntMed;CCFP; Cardiol. (506)696-4422; Fax. (506)633-1487.

STEVENSON, Ronald W D; UBC Hospital-Purdy Pavillion, M41-2221 Westbrook Mall, Vancouver BC V6T 1Z9; Cal'75; FRCPC; Psy (Sexual Medicine). Ac Staff Psy, Vancouver General Hospital - Centennial Pavillion; Consultant Psychiatrist, Youth Court Services(Burnaby); Staff, UBC Hospital - Purdy Pavillion; Clin Assoc Prof, University of British Columbia; (604)875-8282; Fax. (604)875-8249; rwds@interchange.ubc.ca.

STEVENSON, Sandra J; The Group Health Ctre, 240 McNabb St, Sault Ste. Marie ON P6B 1Y5; Wes'96; FRCPC; Peds. (705)759-1234; Fax. (705)541-2304.

STEVENSON, Skai F J; Diamond Head Med Clinic, PO Box 9200 Stn Main, Squamish BC V8B 0C1; Wes'76; CCFP; FCFP; (604)892-3544; Fax. (604)892-3542.

STEVENSON, Thomas H; 713-1489 Marine Dr, West Vancouver BC V7T 1B8; Dublin (Ireland)'74; MB ChB; BAO; CCFP; FCFP; Vis Staff, Vancouver General Hospital - Centennial Pavillion; (604)253-3166; Fax. (604)253-2048.

STEVENSON, W Rodney; Westville Med Clinic, PO Box 930 1875 Main St, Westville NS B0K 2A0; Dal'68; BSc; Staff, Aberdeen Regional Hospital; Riverton Adult Residential Centre; (902)396-4142; Fax. (902)396-1707.

STEVENSON, William T; Queen Elizabeth II Hosp, 10409 98 St, Grande Prairie AB T8V 2E8; UBC'02; Staff, Queen Elizabeth II Hospital; (780)538-7100

STEVERMAN, Allen I; Jewish Rehabilitation Hosp, 3205 Place Alton-Goldbloom, Laval QC H7V 1R2; Mon'00; CCFP; Médecin, Jewish Rehabilitation Hospital; Médecin, Centre Hospitalier l'Université de Montréal (CHUM) - Hôtel-Dieu; Langs: Bilingual(English/French); (450)688-9550; Fax. (450)688-7229.

STEWARD, Wayne W; The Vernon Family Pract Assoc, 103-3310 32 Ave, Vernon BC V1T 2M6; Alb'66; (778)475-5810; Fax. (778)475-5812.

STEWARDSON, Julie A; Newcastle Village Med Assoc, 87 Mill St N, Newcastle ON L1B 1H8; Qns'07; BSc; CCFP; Staff Med Obst & ER, Lakeridge Health - Bowmanville Site; (905)987-1896; Fax. (905)987-9894.

STEWART, Adam M; Central Hastings Fam Hlth Team, MF-52 St Lawrence St E, Madoc ON K0K 2K0; Wes'07; CCFP; (613)473-4134; Fax. (613)473-4740.

STEWART, Alan R; Interior Health Authority, 220-1815 Kirschner Rd, Kelowna BC V1Y 4N7; McM'85; FRCPC; IntMed (Hospital Administration). Staff, Interior Health Authority; (250)870-4691

STEWART, Andrea K; Montfort Hosp, 713 Montreal Rd, Ottawa ON K1K 0T2; McM'02; FRCPC; Psy. Staff, Royal Ottawa Mental Health Centre - Royal Ottawa Health Care Group; Staff, Montfort Hospital; Langs: Bilingual(English/French); (613)746-4621; Fax. (613)907-8002.

STEWART, Andrew; Halifax Infirmary, 6896-1796 Summer St, Halifax NS B3H 3A7; (Other Foreign)'98; Staff, Queen Elizabeth II Health Sciences Centre - Victoria General Site; (902)473-2184; Fax. (902)473-6293.

STEWART, Andrew E F; L4-30 Dupont St E, Waterloo ON N2J 2G9; McM'04; FRCSC; ObstGyn. (519)746-7878; Fax. (519)746-7877.

STEWART, Ann M; Casey House, 9 Huntley St, Toronto ON M4Y 2K8; Tor'05; CCFP; (416)962-4040; Fax. (416)962-5147.

STEWART, Aviva T; Pembroke Reg Hosp, 705 Mackay St, Pembroke ON K8A 1G8; Qns'95; CCFP; CCFP(E.M.); Staff, Pembroke Regional Hospital Inc; Associate Emerg, Children's Hospital of Eastern Ontario (CHEO); Langs: Bilingual(English/French); (613)732-2811; aj@stewartmail.org.

STEWART, Barbara A; Lethbridge Cancer Centre, 960 19 St S, Lethbridge AB T1J 1W5; Alb'82; FRCPC; Anes. Staff Anes, Royal Alexandra Hospital; Staff, Lethbridge Cancer Centre; (403)388-6131

STEWART, Boyd E M; Weyburn Health Centre, 36 4th St, Weyburn SK S4H 0X7; Sask'74; Staff, Weyburn General Hospital; Staff, Weyburn Health Centre; (306)842-5444; Fax. (306)842-5449; dr.b.stewart@sasktel.net.

STEWART, Bradley E; CFB Halifax CFHSC (A) CDU 3, PO Box 99000 Stn Forces, Halifax NS B3K 5X5; McM'08; Staff, Canadian Forces Health Services Centre (Atlantic); Langs: Bilingual(English/French); (902)721-8764; Fax. (902)721-7535.

STEWART, Bradley J; Hys Med Centre, 600-11010 101 St NW, Edmonton AB T5H 4B9; Sask'93; CRCP; FRCPC; Neur (Migraines). Asst Prof, University of Alberta; (780)413-1710; Fax. (780)421-1786.

STEWART, Brian D; Foothills South Tower, 710-3031 Hospital Dr NW, Calgary AB T2N 2T8; Alb'77; BSc; FRCPC; CCFP; EmergMed (Palliative Care);CCFP(E.M.); Staff, Tom Baker Cancer Centre; Staff Emerg Med, Rockyview General Hospital; (403)944-2304; Fax. (403)270-9652; briand.stewart@calgaryhealthregion.ca.

STEWART, Brian G; Hamilton HS-Henderson Site, 711 Concession St, Hamilton ON L8V 1C3; Tor'06; FRCPC; DiagRad. Staff, Hamilton Health Sciences Centre-Juravinski Site; (905)389-4411

STEWART, Bruce G; Royal Oak Centre, 192-8888 Country Hills Blvd NW, Calgary AB T3G 5T4; Cal'77; CCFP; FCFP; (403)239-3660; Fax. (403)239-4001.

STEWART, Bruce M; Canadian Trauma Consultants, 1125-65 Queen St W, Toronto ON M5H 2M5; Tor'58; FRCPC; Neur. Staff Consultant Neurol, West Park Healthcare Centre; (416)863-1581; Fax. (416)863-1905.

STEWART, Calvin M; Family Med Centre, 2931 20 Ave S, Lethbridge AB T1K 3M5; Alb'69; CCFP; FCFP; Staff, Chinook Regional Hospital; Assoc Staff, Covenant Health - St Michael's Health Centre; (403)328-2326; Fax. (403)327-0123.

STEWART, Christine E; Royal Victoria Reg Health Cent, 201 Georgian Dr, Barrie ON L4M 6M2; Wes'86; CCFP; FCFP; Ac Staff, Royal Victoria Regional Health Centre; (705)792-3333; Fax. (705)728-4120.

STEWART, Christopher C; 201-290 Spring St, Summerside PE C1N 1B8; Dal'87; FRCPC; Psy (Intensive Psychotherapy).

STEWART, Christopher J; 865 3 St NW, Medicine Hat AB T1A 7P7; Cal'74; (403)529-5885; Fax. (403)529-5850.

STEWART, Craig L; Bramalea Med Centre, 401A-18 Kensington St, Brampton ON L6T 4S5; Tor'04; FRCSC; Otol. Staff, Toronto General Hospital - UHN; (905)791-4356; Fax. (905)791-4487.

STEWART, D Greg; Huntsville Prof Bldg, 104-348 Muskoka Rd 3 N, Huntsville ON P1H 1H8; Mem'90; Staff, Huntsville District Memorial Hospital - Muskoka Algonquin Healthcare; Langs: Spanish; (705)789-2355; Fax. (705)789-1051.

STEWART, Darryl F; Sturgeon Community Hosp, 201 Boudreau Rd, St Albert AB T8N 6C4; Qns'77; Staff, Sturgeon Community Hospital; (780)418-8229; Fax. (780)418-8376.

STEWART, Darryl S; Beaumont Med Clinic, 5001A 50 Ave, Beaumont AB T4X 1E7; Alb'79; (780)929-6050; Fax. (780)929-5848.

STEWART, David C; Family Med Centre, 2931 20 Ave S, Lethbridge AB T1K 3M5; Cal'97; CCFP; FCFP; (403)328-2326; Fax. (403)327-0123.

STEWART, David I; Cornwall Med Centre, GD, Cornwall PE C0A 1H0; Dal'76; CCFP; FCFP; Staff, Queen Elizabeth Hospital; (902)566-2117; Fax. (902)569-1201.

STEWART, David J; The Ottawa Hosp-Gen Campus, 501 Smyth Rd, Ottawa ON K1H 8L6; Qns'74; ABIM; FRCPC; IntMed; MedOncol. Staff, The Ottawa Hospital - General Campus; Langs: French; (613)737-7700

STEWART, Donald J; Woolwich Comm Health Centre, PO Box 370 10 Parkside Dr, St Jacobs ON N0B 2N0; Tor'74; MCFP(EM); (519)664-3794; Fax. (519)664-2182.

STEWART, Donald W; Regent Med Bldg, 435-2184 Broadway W, Vancouver BC V6K 2E1; UBC'57; (604)732-1348; Fax. (604)732-1372.

STEWART, Donna E; Univ Hlth Network-Toronto Gen, EN7 229-200 Elizabeth St, Toronto ON M5G 2C4; Qns'67; DPsy; FRCPC; Psy (Women's Mental Health). Dir Women's Health/Sr Scientist Research Institute, Toronto General Hospital - UHN; Pres, International Association of Women's Mental Health; Member Board & Zonal Representative, World Psychiatric Association; Disting Fellow, American Psychiatric Association; Disting Fellow, Canadian Psychiatric Association; Prof, University of Toronto; (416)340-3846; Fax. (416)340-4185; donna.stewart@uhn.on.ca.

STEWART, Douglas A; Tom Baker Cancer Centre, 1331 29 St NW, Calgary AB T2N 4N2; Alb'87; MD; FRCPC; IntMed; MedOncol. Staff, Tom Baker Cancer Centre; Staff, Foothills Medical Centre; Prof, University of Calgary; (403)521-3347; Fax. (403)283-1651.

STEWART, Duncan J; The Ottawa Hosp-Gen Campus, 5206-501 Smyth Rd, Ottawa ON K1H 8L6; McG'77; FRCPC; IntMed; Cardiol. Staff, University of Ottawa Heart Institute; CEO/Dir, Ottawa Hosp Research Institute; Langs: German; French; (613)737-8899; Fax. (613)739-6294; dstewart@ohri.ca.

STEWART, Dwight J; 14 St Andrews St, Cambridge ON N1S 1M3; Cal'93; PhD; FRCPC; Neur (Movement Disorders). Staff, Grand River Hospital - Freeport Site; Staff, St Mary's General Hospital; Staff, Grand River Hospital - Kitchener/Waterloo Health Centre; (519)624-2121; Fax. (519)624-1949.

STEWART, G Ivan; 34 Barrie St, Kingston ON K7L 3J7; Belfast (Ireland)'77; MB ChB; BAO; Dep Head Family Med, Providence Care - St Mary's of the Lake Hospital Site; Assoc Staff, Kingston General Hospital; Assoc Staff, Hotel-Dieu Hospital; Asst Prof Family Med, Queen's University; (613)384-0064; Fax. (613)384-9386.

STEWART, Graeme G R; Queens Road Med Clinic, 64 Queens Rd, Sackville NB E4L 4G9; Dal'83; (506)536-2040; Fax. (506)536-2055.

STEWART, Graham M; Hants North Health Centre, PO Box 46 4539 Highway 215, Noel NS B0N 2C0; Glasgow (Scotland)'71; MB ChB; CIH(Dundee); AFOM(London); Ac Staff Family Med, Colchester East Hants Health Centre; Staff, Hants North Health Centre; (902)369-2080; Fax. (902)369-2220.

STEWART, Gregory E; Star FHT-Tavistock Comm Hlth I, 80 Maria St, Tavistock ON N0B 2R0; Ott'09; CCFP; (519)655-2322

STEWART, Hugh V; Family Med Centre, 2931 20 Ave S, Lethbridge AB T1K 3M5; Alb'70; Staff, Chinook Regional Hospital; (403)328-2326; Fax. (403)327-0123.

STEWART, I Maureen; Riverside Prof Centre, 302-1919 Riverside Dr, Ottawa ON K1H 1A2; Qns'70; (613)523-0923; Fax. (613)523-3828.

STEWART, Jacqueline C; 577 Carmi Ave, Penticton BC V2A 3G7; Tor'82; BSc(Hon); BEd; FRCPC; IntMed (Rheumatoid Arthritis); Rheum. Ac Staff, Penticton Regional Hospital; (250)487-1007; Fax. (250)487-1027.

STEWART, James A; MUHC-Montreal Gen Hosp, 1650 av Cedar, Montreal QC H3G 1A4; Sask'72; FACP; ABIM; FRCPC; IntMed; Cardiol. Staff, McGill University Health Centre - Montreal General Campus; assoc Prof, McGill University; Langs: English; French; (514)934-1934

STEWART, James G; 111 Cameron St, Moncton NB E1C 5Y7; Dal'84; (506)859-4429; Fax. (506)382-5801.

STEWART, James I; Alberta Hip & Knee Clinic, 335-401 9 Ave SW, Calgary AB T2P 3C5; Sask'87; FRCSC; OrthSurg (Shoulder & Knee Reconstruction). Clin Lecturer, University of Calgary; (403)221-4358; Fax. (403)221-4387.

STEWART, James K; Meadowlark Health Centre, 184 Meadowlark Shopping Ctr NW, Edmonton AB T5R 5W9; Alb'02; FRCSC; GenSurg. Staff, University of Alberta Hospital; Langs: Bilingual(English/French); (780)484-1122; Fax. (780)489-4121.

STEWART, James T; Ferris Med Clinic, 5-41 Lakeshore Dr, North Bay ON P1A 2A1; (New Zealand)'88; CCFP; (705)495-4000; Fax. (705)495-4007.

STEWART, James W; Ferris Med Clinic, 5-41 Lakeshore Dr, North Bay ON P1A 2A1; Tor'01; CCFP; Staff, North Bay Regional Health Centre - Regional Mental Health; (705)495-4000; Fax. (705)495-4007.

STEWART, Jeremie R; Sudbury Reg Hosp-Laurentian Si, 41 Ramsey Lake Rd, Sudbury ON P3E 5J1; Ott'06; FRCPC; Anes. Staff, Health Sciences North-Laurentian Site; Langs: Bilingual(English/French); (705)522-7100

STEWART, Jessica N; MUHC-Montreal Children's Hosp, 2300 rue Tupper, Montreal QC H3H 1P3; McG'01; FRCPC; Peds; PedEmergMed; EmergMed. Staff, McGill University Health Centre - Montreal Children's Hospital; (514)412-4400

STEWART, Jodie P; Group Health Centre, 240 McNabb St, Sault Ste. Marie ON P6B 1Y5; McM'98; CCFP; Physician, Group Health Centre; (705)759-3434; Fax. (705)759-5668.

STEWART, John A; King Street Med Arts Ctre, 505-71 King St W, Mississauga ON L5B 4A2; Tor'78; FRCSC; OrthSurg. Staff, Trillium Health Centre - Mississauga; (905)848-4362; Fax. (905)848-4362.

STEWART, John D; Northmount Med Centre, 204-145 13th St E, North Vancouver BC V7L 2L4; Kingston (Jamaica)'69; MB BS; FRCP(UK); FRCPC; Neur (Neuromuscular Diseases). Staff, Lions Gate Hospital; Langs: Bilingual(English/French); (604)924-4009; Fax. (604)924-4006; john.stewart@telus.net.

STEWART, John I; Medical Assoc of Port Perry, 462 Paxton St, Port Perry ON L9L 1L9; Wes'72; Court Staff, Lakeridge Health - Port Perry Site; (905)985-9718; Fax. (905)985-8521.

STEWART, John M; Belgage Med Arts Bldg, 209-525 Belmont Ave W, Kitchener ON N2M 5E2; Wes'79; BSc(Hons.); (519)744-4431; Fax. (519)744-6836.

STEWART, John P; Orleans Urgent Care Clinic, 100-1220 Place D'Orleans Dr, Orleans ON K1C 7K3; McM'86; Staff, The Ottawa Hospital - Civic Campus; Langs: French; (613)841-5389; Fax. (613)841-5393.

STEWART, John S; 12 Prince William St, St Stephen NB E3L 1R5; Dal'75; Ac Staff, Charlotte County Hospital; (506)466-1757

STEWART, John W; Queen Elizabeth II HSC-Halifax, 2148-1796 Summer St, Halifax NS B3H 3A7; Dal'63; FACC; FRCPC; IntMed (Cardiology). Staff, Queen Elizabeth II Health Sciences Centre - Halifax Infirmary Site; Asst Prof Med Cardiol, Dalhousie University; (902)473-2809; Fax. (902)473-2434.

STEWART, Julia R; Burnaby Hosp, 3935 Kincaid St, Burnaby BC V5G 2X6; Mon'99; CCFP; Staff, Burnaby Hospital; Langs: Bilingual(English/French); (604)434-4211

STEWART, Justine N; Reach Community Health Ctre, 1145 Commercial Dr, Vancouver BC V5L 3X3; UBC'96; CCFP; FCFP; Ac Staff, Providence Health Care - St Paul's Hospital; (604)254-1354; Fax. (604)258-9190.

STEWART, Keir M; Queen Elizabeth II HSC-Halifax, 2266-1796 Summer St, Halifax NS B3H 3A7; Dal'80; BSc; FRCSC; GenSurg; Cardiovasc&ThorSurg. Staff, Queen Elizabeth II Health Sciences Centre - Halifax Infirmary Site; (902)473-2717; Fax. (902)473-4448.

STEWART, Kenneth C; Royal Alexandra Hosp, 417 CSC-10240 Kingsway NW, Edmonton AB T5H 3V9; Alb'93; RC; FRCSC; GenSurg (Medical Oncology); ThorSurg. Staff, Royal Alexandra Hospital; Pres Section of Thoracic Surg, Alberta Medical Association; Assoc Prof, University of Alberta; (780)735-4243; Fax. (780)735-4245; kenstewart@cha.ab.ca.

STEWART, Kristofor B; 21st Medical Clinic, 502-402 21st St E, Saskatoon SK S7K 0C3; Sask'04; BScPharm; FRCPC; IntMed (AIDS/HIV). Dir Educational SPH Medicine/Clin Assoc Prof, University of Saskatchewan; (306)956-3444; Fax. (306)956-3577.

STEWART, Laura L; BC Women's Hosp & Health Ctr, K4 208-4500 Oak St, Vancouver BC V6H 3N1; Cal'83; FRCPC; Peds (Pediatric Endocrinology); Endocrin&Metab. Staff, BC Women's Hospital & Health Centre; Clin Assoc Prof Ped Endocrin, University of British Columbia; (604)875-2624

STEWART, Lindsay C; Queensway-Carleton Hosp, 3045 Baseline Rd, Nepean ON K2H 8P4; McG'89; CCFP; CCFP(E.M.); Staff, Queensway Carleton Hospital; Langs: French; (613)721-2000

STEWART, Lois M; Family Physicians, 101-610 Queen St, Saskatoon SK S7K 0M8; Sask'74; Ac Staff Family Pract, Saskatoon City Hospital; Ac Staff, Royal University Hospital; Clin Teacher, University of Saskatchewan; (306)244-0766; Fax. (306)665-8838.

STEWART, Lori K; Hamilton HS-Henderson Site, 711 Concession St, Hamilton ON L8V 1C3; Wes'92; BSc; FRCPC; DiagRad. Staff, Hamilton Health Sciences Centre-Juravinski Site; (905)527-4322 x42261; Fax. (905)575-2660.

STEWART, Marie-Diane; CSSS de Saint-Jérôme, 290 rue Montigny, Saint-Jerome QC J7Z 5T3; Mon'91; FRCPC; IntMed; Gastroent. Staff, Hôtel-Dieu de Saint-Jérôme; (450)431-8201

STEWART, Marilyn J; Seeley's Bay Med Centre, 1-106 Drynan Way, Seeleys Bay ON K0H 2N0; Dal'90; BSc(Chem.); CCFP; FCFP; (613)387-3120; Fax. (613)387-2842.

STEWART, Mark A H; 2201-188 Esplanade St E, North Vancouver BC V7L 4Y1; Man'75; FRCPC; EmergMed. (604)537-3412

STEWART, Martin C; Medical Assoc of Port Perry, 462 Paxton St, Port Perry ON L9L 1L9; Qns'90; FRCSC; CCFP; GenSurg. (905)985-9758; Fax. (905)985-8931.

STEWART, Mary F M; 202-1407 Yonge St, Toronto ON M4T 1Y7; Tor'75; FRCPC; Psy (Psychotherapy & Psychoanalysis). (416)921-4875

STEWART, Megan S; Comox Valley Med Clinic, 19-3199 Cliffe Ave, Courtenay BC V9N 2L9; UBC'95; (250)334-1512

STEWART, Neil A; Piper Creek Clinic, 200-3215 49 Ave, Red Deer AB T4M 0M8; Alb'73; Staff GP, Red Deer Regional Hospital Centre; (403)986-7265; Fax. (403)986-7604.

STEWART, P David; 209 Third Ave, Ottawa ON K1S 2K2; Ann Arbor (USA)'69; CCFP; CCFP(E.M.); FCFP; Ac Staff Med, The Ottawa Hospital - Civic Campus; (613)567-3640; Fax. (613)737-7886.

STEWART, Pamela A; Addiction & Mental Hlth-ARF, 33 Russell St, Toronto ON M5S 2S1; Tor'87; FRCPC; Psy;CCFP; Staff, Centre for Addiction & Mental Health (CAMH) - Russell Street Site; Staff, Mount Sinai Hospital; University of Toronto; (416)535-8501 x6687; Fax. (416)595-6399; pamela_stewart@camh.net.

STEWART, Paula J; District Health Unit, 458 Laurier Blvd, Brockville ON K6V 7A3; Wes'77; FRCPC; CommunMed (Public Health). Dir Chronic Disease Survaillance, Public Health Agency of Canada; Clin Assoc Prof Epidemiol & Comm Med, University of Ottawa; (613)345-5685; Fax. (613)345-2879; paula_stewart@phac.aspc.qc.ca.

STEWART, Philippe J; Avon Family Med Centre, 511 Huron St, Stratford ON N5A 5T8; Alb'11; (519)508-1212

STEWART, R Jay; 126 May St S, Thunder Bay ON P7E 1A9; Qns'96; MSc; BScH; FRCPC; Psy (Suicide Risk). Coroner, City Of Thunder Bay; Asst Prof, Northern Ontario School of Medicine; (807)623-3929; Fax. (807)622-5633; rjsmd@tbaytel.net.

STEWART, Rebekah A L; Vernon Jubilee Hosp, 2101 32 St, Vernon BC V1T 5L2; Cambridge (England)'89; MB ChB; FRCPC; DiagRad. Staff, Vernon Jubilee Hospital; (250)558-1200

STEWART, Robert J; 9111Q-61 Queen St E, Toronto ON M5C 2T2; Qns'88; FRCSC; Urol (Renal Transplant). Ac Staff Urol, St Michael's Hospital; Asst Prof Surg, University of Toronto; (416)867-3686; Fax. (416)867-3675; stewartr@smh.toronto.on.ca.

STEWART, Robert L; Queen Elizabeth II HSC-Halifax, 2146-1796 Summer St, Halifax NS B3H 3A7; Dal'01; FRCPC; IntMed; Cardiol. Staff, Queen Elizabeth II Health Sciences Centre - Halifax Infirmary Site; (902)473-7871; Fax. (902)473-7277.

STEWART, Robin K; Nanaimo Reg Gen Hosp, 1200 Dufferin Cres, Nanaimo BC V9S 2B7; UBC'93; CCFP; CCFP(E.M.); Staff, Nanaimo Regional General Hospital; (250)755-7627

STEWART, Rosemary N; Fairmont Med Bldg, 1116-750 Broadway W, Vancouver BC V5Z 1H3; Alb'74; PhysMed&Rehab (Brain Injury). (604)872-7611; Fax. (604)872-7684.

STEWART, S Evelyn; Child & Family Research Instit, A3 118-938 28th Ave W, Vancouver BC V5Z 4H4; Dal'96; FRCPC; Psy. Staff, Child & Family Research Institute; (604)875-2226

STEWART, Sabrina; Wall Street Med Bldg, 370-140 Wall St, Saskatoon SK S7K 1N4; Sask'97; FRCSC; ObstGyn. Physician, Wall Street Medical Centre; (306)652-4331; Fax. (306)242-4855.

STEWART, Samuel J; Victoria Emerg Phys Mgmt Ltd, 325-1627 Fort St, Victoria BC V8R 1H8; Tor'66; FACEP; FRCPC; EmergMed. (250)479-1442; Fax. (250)479-1472.

STEWART, Susan E; Queen Elizabeth Hosp, PO Box 6600 Stn Central 60 Riverside Dr, Charlottetown PE C1A 8T5; Dal'87; FRCPC; Psy. Staff, Queen Elizabeth Hospital; (902)894-2111 x2121; Fax. (902)894-2973.

STEWART, Tara L; Univ of Alberta Hosp-SCC/WCM, 8440 112 St NW, Edmonton AB T6G 2B7; Alb'08; Staff, University of Alberta Hospital; (780)407-8822

STEWART, Terry J; Alberta Children's Hosp, 2888 Shaganappi Trail NW, Calgary AB T3B 6A8; UBC'79; BSc; DABA; MD; Anes (Pediatric Anesthesia). Ac Staff, Alberta Children's Hospital; Med Dir, Hyperbaric Oxygen Therapy Clinics Inc; (403)955-7810; Fax. (403)955-7606; terry.stewart@calgaryhealthregion.ca.

STEWART, Thomas E; Mount Sinai Hosp, 427-600 University Ave, Toronto ON M5G 1X5; Ott'88; FRCPC; IntMed; Critical Care Medicine. Physician-in-Charge, Mount Sinai Hospital; Prof Med & Anes, University of Toronto; (416)586-8774; Fax. (416)586-5981.

STEWART, Trina L; Summerside Med Centre, 475 Granville St N, Summerside PE C1N 3N9; Mem'98; CCFP; Staff, Prince County Hospital; Assoc Prof Family Med, Dalhousie University; (902)432-8181; info@peibotox.com.

STEWART, Wendy A; Paediatric Neurology Clinic, 54B Marr Rd, Rothesay NB E2E 3K7; Cal'95; MSc; PhD; FRCPC; Peds (Pediatric Neurology); Neur. Staff, Saint John Regional Hospital; Court Staff, The Moncton Hospital; Associate, Dalhousie University; (506)848-4622; Fax. (506)848-4659.

STEWART-HUNTER, George C; Vermilion Health Centre, 5720 50 Ave, Vermilion AB T9X 1K7; London (England)'46; MB ChB; LRCP; MRCS; FRCOG; Staff, Vermilion Health Centre; Staff, Islay Assisted Living; Physician, Alberta East Central Health Region; (780)853-5305; Fax. (780)853-4786; s.hunter@ech.ab.ca.

STEWART-PATTERSON, Christopher; 817-4438 10th Ave W, Vancouver BC V6R 4R8; Cal'88; (604)830-8063; Fax. (604)830-7147.

STEYL, Jolien A; Atwood Med Clinic, 101-143 4th Ave S, Williams Lake BC V2G 1J8; Orange Free State (South Africa)'05; MB ChB; Langs: Afrikaans; (250)398-5162

STEYN, Antony W; Medical Centre, RR 6 1095 9th Concession Rd, Claremont ON L1Y 1A3; Sydney (Australia)'66; MB BS; FRCPC; IntMed (Cardiology). Staff Pt-Time, Toronto East General Hospital Inc; Langs: Dutch; (905)649-2114; Fax. (905)649-2114.

STEYN, Chris; St Joseph's Health Care, PO Box 5777 Stn B D0 213-268 Grosvenor St, London ON N6A 4V2; Pretoria (South Africa)'98; MB ChB; CCFP; Staff, St Joseph's Hospital - St Joseph's Health Care; Langs: Afrikaans; (519)646-6309

STEYN, Daniela; Associate Med Clinic, 203-10030 106 St, Westlock AB T7P 2K4; Pretoria (South Africa)'06; MB ChB(UP); Staff, Westlock Healthcare Centre; (780)349-3341; Fax. (780)349-6686.

STEYN, Frederick W; 2181 Woodthrush St PO Box 114 Stn A, Nanaimo BC V9R 5K4; Pretoria (South Africa)'82; MB ChB; (250)735-8676

STEYN, Frederik M; Associated Med Clinic, PO Box 510 10017 101 Ave, Lac La Biche AB T0A 2C0; (South Africa)'04; (780)623-4421; Fax. (780)623-1920; clinic91@telusplanet.net.

STEYN, Jacobus A; Victoria Hospital, PO Box 3000 Stn Main 1200 24th St W, Prince Albert SK S6V 5T4; Orange Free State (South Africa)'90; MB BS; LMCC; Staff, Victoria Hospital; Langs: Afrikaans; (306)765-6216; Fax. (306)765-6224; kobus.s@sasktel.net.

STEYN, Jacobus H; Royal Inland Hosp, 311 Columbia St, Kamloops BC V2C 2T1; Orange Free State (South Africa)'97; MB ChB; Staff, Royal Inland Hospital; Langs: Afrikaans; (250)314-2577

STEYN, Jacobus J; 102-135 Ormond St, Brockville ON K6V 5Y2; Pretoria (South Africa)'87; MB ChB; FRCPC; IntMed;CCFP; Chief IntMed, Brockville General Hospital - Charles Street; Langs: Afrikaans; (613)342-4454; Fax. (613)342-8065.

STEYN, Janus; North Okanagan Health Unit, 1440 14 Ave, Vernon BC V1B 2T1; Stellenbosch (South Africa)'01; MB ChB; FCP (SA); Staff, Vernon Mental Health Centre; Langs: Afrikaans; (250)549-5737; Fax. (250)549-6358; dr.janus.steyn@interiorhealth.ca.

STEYN, Johan W; Dr Steyn Med Office, PO Box 28, Kipling SK S0G 2S0; Witwatersrand (South Africa)'75; MB ChB; Physician, Kipling Medical Clinic; (306)736-2155; Fax. (306)736-2156; steyn@sasktel.net.

STEYN, Mariette; 135 Ormond St, Brockville ON K6V 5Y2; Pretoria (South Africa)'87; MB ChB; CCFP; Langs: Afrikaans; (613)342-0714; Fax. (613)342-8065.

STEYN, Marius F; PO Box 39, Lantzville BC V0R 2H0; Pretoria (South Africa)'95; MB ChB; BSc(Pharm); CCFP; Langs: Afrikaans; steynm@shaw.ca.

STEYN, Morrison F; Medical Arts Centre, 127-770 6 St SW, Medicine Hat AB T1A 4J6; (South Africa)'82; MB ChB; MMed(Psy); Consultant Psy, Medicine Hat Regional Hospital; Langs: Afrikaans; (403)526-1551; Fax. (403)526-1505.

STEYN, Pierre G; 423 Bronson Ave, Ottawa ON K1R 6J5; Cape Town (South Africa)'70; MSc; MB ChB; Langs: Afrikaans; Dutch; (613)235-9472; Fax. (613)235-4355.

STICH, Beverley R; Oliver PCN at The Allin Clinic, 10155 120 St NW, Edmonton AB T5K 2A2; Man'79; FRCPC; Psy (Administrative Psychiatry). Clin Assoc Prof Psy, University of Alberta; (780)482-7551; Fax. (780)482-3533; bstich@edmontonoliverpcn.com.

STICKNEY, John R; Upper Grand Family Health Team, 753 Tower St S, Fergus ON N1M 2R2; Tor'76; Staff, Groves Memorial Community Hospital; Court Staff, Guelph General Hospital; (519)843-4380; Fax. (519)843-3211.

STIDHAM, Gregory L; Kingston Gen Hosp, W3 316-76 Stuart St, Kingston ON K7L 2V7; Ohio (USA)'76; Peds (Critical Care Medicine). Staff, Kingston General Hospital; (613)549-6666; Fax. (613)548-1369.

STIEB, David M; Air Health Effects Research, 3 029-269 Laurier Ave W, Ottawa ON K1A 0K9; Qns'87; MSc(McM); FRCPC; CommunMed. Physician Air Health Effects, Health Canada; Aj Prof Epidemiol & Commun Med, University of Ottawa; (613)957-3132; Fax. (613)954-7612; dave_stieb@hc-sc.gc.ca.

STIEGELMAR, Robert E; 11202 76 Ave NW, Edmonton AB T6G 0K1; Alb'90; BSc; FRCSC; OrthSurg (Reconstructive Surgery). Staff, University of Alberta Hospital; Staff, Sturgeon Community Hospital; (780)439-4945; Fax. (780)439-0396; stiegelmar@hotmail.com.

STIELL, Andrew P; The Ottawa Hosp-Civic Campus, 1053 Carling Ave, Ottawa ON K1Y 4E9; UBC'08; CCFP; CCFP(E.M.); Staff, The Ottawa Hospital - Civic Campus; Langs: Bilingual(English/French); (613)798-5555

STIELL, Ian G; The Ottawa Hosp-Civic Campus, 1053 Carling Ave, Ottawa ON K1Y 4E9; Wes'75; DAB; FACEP; FRCPC; EmergMed. Ac Staff Emerg Med, The Ottawa Hospital - Civic Campus; Staff, Ottawa Health Research Institute; Dept Chair Emerg Med, University of Ottawa; (613)798-5555 x18683; istiell@ohri.ca.

STIGANT, Caroline E; 201-1990 Fort St, Victoria BC V8R 6V4; UBC'97; FRCPC; IntMed; Nephrol. (250)598-3895; Fax. (250)598-5469.

STIHARU, Simona; Medistat Med Familiale, 4965 rue Saint-Pierre, Pierrefonds QC H9H 5M9; Bucarest (Romania)'81; CCFP; Staff In-Patient, Centre Hospitalier d'Argenteuil; Langs: Romanian; French; (514)624-4774; Fax. (514)624-4704.

STIKAROVSKA, Irena; BC Women's Hosp & Health Ctr, 4500 Oak St, Vancouver BC V6H 3N1; Mon'06; FRCPC; Psy. Staff, BC Women's Hospital & Health Centre; (604)875-2345 x5571

STILL, Douglas K; Jim Pattison Outpatient & Surg, 9750 140 St, Surrey BC V3T 0G9; Alb'70; FRCSC; ObstGyn. Staff Maternal Fetal Med, Surrey Memorial Hospital; (604)582-4558; dkstill@shaw.ca.

STILL, Janet E; Carleton Univ Hlth Services, 2600-1125 Colonel By Dr, Ottawa ON K1S 5B6; Tor'78; Physician, Carleton University; Langs: French; (613)520-6674; Fax. (613)520-4059.

STILL, Susan M; St Mary's Hosp Centre, 3830 av Lacombe, Montreal QC H3T 1M5; Tor'76; BSc; MSc; CCFP; FCFP; Staff, St Mary's Hospital Centre; (514)734-2624; Fax. (514)734-2602; sstill@ssss.gouv.qc.ca.

STILLER, Calvin R; 528 Waterloo St, London ON N6B 2P9; Sask'65; FRCPC; IntMed (Nephrology). Consultant, London Health Sciences Centre - University Hospital; Prof, University of Western Ontario; (519)858-1582; Fax. (519)858-9785.

STILLING, Lee S; Peter Lougheed Centre, 3500 26 Ave NE, Calgary AB T1Y 6J4; Alb'77; FRCPC; Anes. Staff, Peter Lougheed Centre; Asst Prof Anes, University of Calgary; (403)943-5721; Fax. (403)255-1929.

STILLMAN, Karen L; 77 Brae St PO Box 490, Almonte ON K0A 1A0; Mem'95; BSc; FRCSC; ObstGyn (Prenatal Care). Langs: English; French; (613)256-8500; Fax. (613)256-8700.

STILWELL, Moira E; St Paul's Hosp, 1081 Burrard St, Vancouver BC V6Z 1Y6; Cal'77; FRCPC; DiagRad; NuclearMed. Staff Nuclear Med, Providence Health Care - St Paul's Hospital; (604)631-5008; Fax. (604)631-5075.

STIMAC, John M; Dr John Stimac Cardiology, 507-304 Victoria Ave N, Hamilton ON L8L 5G4; Tor'82; Cardiol; IntMed. Langs: French; (905)966-0880

STIMEC, Jennifer; The Hosp for Sick Children, 555 Elizabeth St, Toronto ON M5G 1X8; Tor'00; FRCPC; DiagRad. Staff Med Imaging, The Hospital For Sick Children; (416)813-6888; jennifer@stimec@sickkids.ca.

STIMPSON, Rochelle L M; 370 Broadway E PO Box 95045 Rpo Kingsgate, Vancouver BC V5T 4T8; McM'08; CCFP; (604)875-2029

STIMPSON, Ross E J; Health Sciences Centre, GF 432-820 Sherbrook St, Winnipeg MB R3A 1R9; Man'76; FRCSC; GenSurg (Critical Care Medicine). Staff, Health Sciences Centre; Asst Prof Surg, University of Manitoba; (204)787-2881; Fax. (204)787-4063; rstimpson@hsc.mb.ca.

STINSON, Andrea H; Gibsons Med Clinic, 211-1100 Sunshine Coast Hwy, Gibsons BC V0N 1V7; UBC'00; BSc; MD; CCFP; Staff, St Mary's Hospital; (604)886-2868; Fax. (604)886-9716.

STINSON, Dora A; IWK Health Centre, PO Box 9700 5980 University Ave, Halifax NS B3K 6R8; Wes'63; FRCP; FRCPC; Peds (Neonatal & Perinatal Medicine). Staff Neonatologist, IWK Health Centre; Assoc Prof Neonatologist, Dalhousie University; (902)470-6679; Fax. (902)470-6469; dora.stinson@iwk.nshealth.ca.

STINSON, J Michelle; Grand River Cardiology, 103-7 Grand Ave S, Cambridge ON N1S 2L3; McM'84; FRCPC; IntMed; Cardiol. Staff, Ontario Diagnostic Cardiology; Staff, Ontario Diagnostic Cardiology; (519)623-8611

STINSON, R William; Royal Inland Hosp, 311 Columbia St, Kamloops BC V2C 2T1; Cal'88; Staff, Royal Inland Hospital; (250)374-5111

STINTON, Donald A K; Tower Centre, 422-131 9 Ave SW, Calgary AB T2P 1K1; Cal'74; BSc; CCFP; (403)265-3001; Fax. (403)266-8869.

STINTON, Laura M; Health Research Innovation Ctr, 3280 Hospital Dr NW, Calgary AB T2N 4Z6; Cal'06; FRCPC; IntMed; Gastroent. Staff, Health Research Innovation Centre; (403)592-5025; Fax. (403)592-5050.

STIP, Emmanuel; CHUM-Hopital Notre-Dame, 1560 rue Sherbrooke E, Montreal QC H2L 4M1; Angers (France)'85; FRCPC; Psy (P.Q.). Staff, Centre Hospitalier l'Université de Montréal (CHUM) - Hôpital Notre-Dame; Staff, Hopital Louis-H Lafontaine; Staff, Hotel-Dieu du Sacre-Coeur de Jesus de Quebec; Member, Centre de Recherche Fernand Seguin; Universite de Montreal; (514)890-7658; stip-e@chu-caen.fr.

STIRCU, Cristina E; James Snow Medical, 51 James Snow Pky S, Milton ON L9T 0R3; University of Medicine and Pharmacy (Romania)'96; CCFP; (905)636-1050; Fax. (905)636-1090.

STIRK, Linda J; North York Gen Hosp, 4001 Leslie St, North York ON M2K 1E1; McG'81; FACOG; PhD; MDCM; FRCSC; ObstGyn. Staff, North York General Hospital; University of Toronto; Langs: Bilingual(English/French); (416)756-6002; Fax. (416)487-4147.

STIRLING, Alena M; Royal University Hosp, 103 Hospital Dr, Saskatoon SK S7N 0W8; Sask'05; FRCPC; Anes. Staff, Royal University Hospital; (306)655-1183; Fax. (306)655-1279.

STIRLING, Denise S; Trafalgar Prof Centre, 318-1235 Trafalgar Rd, Oakville ON L6H 3P1; McM'90; BSc; FRCPC; Neur. Consultant Neurol, Halton Healthcare Services Corporation - Oakville Site; (905)849-1322; Fax. (905)849-1323.

STIRLING, Michael J; St Joseph's Gen Hosp, 70 Spine Rd, Elliot Lake ON P5A 1X2; Qns'00; BA(Hon); MBA; FRCSC; GenSurg (Vascular Surgery). Staff, St Joseph's General Hospital Elliot Lake; (705)848-7182; Fax. (705)848-9006.

STIRLING, Robert G; Health Canada, 11F 133-180 Queen St W, Toronto ON M5V 3L7; Tor'94; MHSc; MSc(Physiol.); FRCPC; CommunMed (Infectious Diseases). (416)952-2209; Fax. (416)973-0009.

STIRRETT, Glenna M; 1280 Lasalle Blvd, Sudbury ON P3A 1Y8; Cal'92; CCFP; Staff, Health Sciences North-St Joseph's Health Centre; (705)560-2227

STITT, James C; The Richmond Hosp, 7000 Westminster Hwy, Richmond BC V6X 1A2; Wes'89; CCFP; CCFP(E.M.); Staff Emerg Dept, Richmond Hospital; Clinical Asst Prof, University of British Columbia; (604)244-5151; Fax. (604)244-5194.

STITT, Robert B; Scarborough Hosp-General Div, 3050 Lawrence Ave E, Scarborough ON M1P 2V5; Tor'61; GenSurg (Breast Surgery). Assoc Staff, The Scarborough Hospital - General Campus; (416)431-8120; Fax. (416)431-8221.

STITZ, Marshall Y; Associated Sports & Spine Phys, A-2020 Corydon Ave, Winnipeg MB R3P 0N2; Man'90; FRCPC; PhysMed&Rehab (Occupational Medicine). (204)988-5040; Fax. (204)988-5049; mstitz@mymts.net.

STIVER, H Grant; Div Of Infectious Diseases, D452-2733 Heather St, Vancouver BC V5Z 1M9; Man'68; FRCPC; IntMed (Infectious Diseases). A-Head InfectDis, Vancouver General Hospital - Centennial Pavillion; Prof/A-Head InfectDis, University of British Columbia; (604)875-4588; Fax. (604)875-4013.

STOBART, Kent; Edmonton Clinic Health Academy, 3 529-11405 87 Ave NW, Edmonton AB T6G 1C9; Tor'84; MSc(Qns); FRCPC; Peds (Pediatric Hematology Oncology). Staff, University of Alberta Hospital; Ac Staff, Edmonton Zone Edmonton Public Health Services; Ac Staff, Alberta Cancer Board; Staff, Edmonton Clinic Health Academy; Assoc Prof Peds & Educational/Assoc Dean Undergraduate Med Educational, University of Alberta; Langs: French; (780)248-5524; Fax. (780)407-7476; kent.stobart@gmail.com.

STOBBE, Karl E; Quest CHC, 145 Queenston St, St. Catharines ON L2R 2Z9; Wes'82; CCFP; CCFP(E.M.); FCFP; Staff, West Lincoln Memorial Hospital; Staff Niagara Reg Campus, Niagara Health System - St Catharines General Site; Staff Niagara Reg Campus, Brock University; Langs: German; (905)688-2558; Fax. (905)688-4678.

STOBIE, Shannon B; 20B-385 Frederick St, Kitchener ON N2H 2P2; McM'96; CCFP; FCFP; (519)747-1200; Fax. (519)747-1560.

STOBO, R Benjamin; Athens Dist Family Health Team, PO Box 99 9 Wellington St E, Athens ON K0E 1B0; Ott'87; CCFP; Staff, Brockville General Hospital - Charles Street; (613)924-2623; Fax. (613)924-2276; bstobo@edhospital.on.ca.

STOCEK, Rudolph F; Courtyard Med Clinic, 12-380 Main St, Hartland NB E7P 2N2; Mem'91; Med Dir, The Central Carleton Nursing Home; Med Dir, Carleton York Emergency Medical Services; (506)375-4250; Fax. (506)375-1992.

STOCK, Susan R; 190 boul Crémazie E, Montreal QC H2P 1E2; McM'78; MSc(Epidemiol.); CSPQ; FRCPC; OccupMed (Industrial Occupational Medicine); CommunMed (P.Q.). Staff, Centre Hospitalier l'Université de Montréal (CHUM) - Hôpital Notre-Dame; Aj Prof Epidemiol, McGill University; Clin Prof Public Health, Universite de Montreal; Langs: French; (514)864-1600 x3206; Fax. (514)864-7646; susan.stock@inspq.qc.ca.

STOCK, Suzanne L; 104-145 15th St W, North Vancouver BC V7M 1R9; Qns'97; FRCPC; Peds (Pediatric Endocrinology); Endocrin&Metab. Clin Instructor, University of British Columbia; (604)924-3133; Fax. (604)980-8393; dr_sue@telus.net.

STOCKBURGER, Dena L; Millwoods Family Clinic, 104-2551 Hewes Way NW, Edmonton AB T6L 6W6; Alb'91; CCFP; (780)462-2767; Fax. (780)463-7025.

STOCKBURGER, J Mark; Hinton Med Clinic, 102 Allen Cove, Hinton AB T7V 2A6; Alb'95; CCFP; (780)865-3338; Fax. (780)865-2024.

STOCKDILL, James D; Lansdowne Prof Bldg, 270-1641 Hillside Ave, Victoria BC V8T 5G1; McM'76; CCFP; FCFP; Staff, Royal Jubilee Hospital; (250)595-2452; Fax. (250)592-3897.

STOCKENSTROM, Eric E; 1-2187 4th Ave W, Vancouver BC V6K 1N7; Pretoria (South Africa)'82; MB ChB; Langs: Afrikaans; (604)733-3010; Fax. (604)736-3820.

STOCKLER-IPSIROGLU, Gerda S; Children's & Women's HC of BC, B321-4480 Oak St, Vancouver BC V6H 3V4; Graz(Austria) (Austria)'83; FRCPC; Neur. Staff, BC Children's Hospital; Langs: German; Italian; (604)875-2628

STOCKS, Alison M; Sea Cove Med Clinic, 201-1757 Beaufort Ave, Comox BC V9M 1R8; Colorado (USA)'98; CCFP; (250)339-5335

STOCKS, Christina I; Lethbridge Med Clinic, 300 3 St S, Lethbridge AB T1J 1Y9; Pretoria (South Africa)'02; Langs: Afrikaans; (403)394-2002; Fax. (403)394-2066.

STOCKWELL, Margaret J; Health Canada Tunney's Pasture, 101 Tunney's Pasture Dr, Ottawa ON K1A 0K9; Tor'74; FRCPC; Peds. (613)948-7825; Fax. (613)941-1183.

STODDARD, Douglas W; Toronto SEMI, 601-2 Sheppard Ave E, North York ON M2N 5Y7; Tor'89; Dip SportMed(SportsMed); Physician, Toronto Sports & Exercise Medicine Institute; (416)223-7364; Fax. (416)223-8048.

STODDARD, Peter C; Moncton Med Clinic, 208-860 Mountain Rd, Moncton NB E1C 2N7; Dal'71; CCFP; FCFP; Ac Staff, The Moncton Hospital; (506)853-5160; Fax. (506)383-5743.

STODDART, Karen L; Canadian Forces Hlth Services, 713 Montreal Rd, Ottawa ON K1A 0K2; Cal'01; CCFP; Staff, Canadian Forces Health Services Centre; (613)945-6600

STODDART, Todd A; 204-42 Glen Allan Dr, Bridgewater NS B4V 3N2; Dal'98; FRCSC; GenSurg. Staff Surg, South Shore Regional Hospital; (902)530-3540; Fax. (902)543-4590; stoddart4@hotmail.com.

STOESSER, Michael J P; 481 London Rd, Sarnia ON N7T 4X3; RCS (Ireland)'83; (519)337-3443; Fax. (519)332-8214.

STOESSL, A Jonathan; 2211 Wesbrook Mall, Vancouver BC V6T 2B5; Wes'79; FRCPC; Neur (Movement Disorders). Staff Pacific Parkinson's Res Centre, UBC Hospital - Koerner Pavillion; Staff, Vancouver Coastal Health; Prof Med, University of British Columbia; (604)822-7967; Fax. (604)822-7866; jstoessl@mail.ubc.ca.

STOFFEL, Sandra S; Sheldon M Chumir Urgent Care, 1213 4 St SW, Calgary AB T2R 0X7; Sask'87; FRCPC; CommunMed. (403)955-6011

STOFFMAN, Jayson M; Cancercare Manitoba, ON 2017-675 McDermot Ave, Winnipeg MB R3E 0V9; Qns'98; FRCPC; Peds (Pediatric Hematology Oncology); Hem. Staff, CancerCare Manitoba; Asst Prof Peds & Child Health, University of Manitoba; Langs: French; (204)787-4372; jayson.stoffman@cancercare.mb.ca.

STOFFMAN, John M; 351 Oxford St E, London ON N6A 1V6; Wes'68; FRCPC; Peds. Consultant, London Health Sciences Centre - Victoria Campus; Consultant, St Joseph's Hospital - St Joseph's Health Care; Assoc Prof, University of Western Ontario; (519)672-9803; Fax. (519)672-3355.

STOGRE, Rosemary A; Palisade Gardens, LL-240 Chapel St, Cobourg ON K9A 0E3; Ott'71; Langs: Spanish; (905)372-1174; Fax. (905)372-1182.

STOGRYN, Dale A G; 101-1032 Austin Ave, Coquitlam BC V3K 3P3; Alb'73; CCFP; FCFP; Staff, Royal Columbian Hospital; Clin Prof Family Med, University of British Columbia; (604)939-2441; Fax. (604)939-2420; dstogryn@shaw.ca.

STOGRYN, Joan R; Austin Family Physicians, 102-1015 Austin Ave, Coquitlam BC V3K 3N9; Alb'73; CCFP; FCFP; Court Staff, Royal Columbian Hospital; Court Staff, Eagle Ridge Hospital & Health Care Centre; Member Board of Directors, College of Physicians & Surgeons of British Columbia; Clin Instructor Family Med, University of British Columbia; (604)939-9251; Fax. (604)939-2592.

STOGRYN, Krista M; 220 First St PO Box 189, Tofino BC V0R 2Z0; UBC'05; BSc(Hons); CCFP; (250)725-3282

STOGRYN, Russell D; St Andrew's Plaza, 108-20611 Fraser Hwy, Langley BC V3A 4G4; Man'73; FRCSC; Urol. Staff, Richmond Hospital; Staff, BC Children's Hospital; Staff, Providence Health Care - St Vincent's Hospital-Heather Site; (604)530-2388; Fax. (604)532-9389.

STOIAN, Cristina A; Alberta Children's Hosp, 2888 Shaganappi Trail NW, Calgary AB T3B 6A8; Bucharest (Romania)'90; FRCPC; Peds. Staff, Alberta Children's Hospital; (403)955-2953; Fax. (403)955-3055.

STOJANOVIC, Mileva; Richmond Plaza, 136-3715 51 St SW, Calgary AB T3E 6V2; (Other Foreign)'04; CCFP; (403)686-6967; Fax. (403)686-3736.

STOJANOVIC, Sanja; Ctre Réadaptation Marie Enfant, 5200 rue Belanger, Montreal QC H1T 1C9; Paris (France)'91; CSPQ; Peds (P.Q.). Staff, Hôpital Ste-Justine; (514)374-1710 x8150; sanja.stojanovic.hsi@ssss.gouv.qc.ca.

STOKER, D Brent; Peterborough Family Hlth Team, 26 Hospital Dr, Peterborough ON K9J 7C3; Ott'81; CCFP; (705)740-6864; Fax. (705)740-6858; bstoker@ptboclinic.com.

STOKES, Aidan; IWK Health Centre, PO Box 9700 Rpo CSC 5850-5980 University Ave, Halifax NS B3K 6R8; Dublin (Ireland)'64; MB BS; DCH; DPH; DPM; FRCPC; Psy (Child & Adolescent Psychiatry). Ac Staff, IWK Health Centre; Consultant, Queen Elizabeth II Health Sciences Centre - Victoria General Site; Asst Prof, Dalhousie University; (902)470-8375; Fax. (902)470-8937; astokes@dal.ca.

STOKES, Erika L; The Richmond Hosp, 7000 Westminster Hwy, Richmond BC V6X 1A2; Mem'06; Staff, Richmond Hospital; (604)278-9711

STOKES, Philip M A; Peter Lougheed Centre, 3500 26 Ave NE, Calgary AB T1Y 6J4; Bristol (England)'89; MB BS; MRC; LMCC; FRCPC; Psy. Staff, Peter Lougheed Centre; (403)943-4904; Fax. (403)943-4815.

STOKES, Robert; Cape Breton Reg Hosp, 1482 George St, Sydney NS B1P 1P3; Liverpool (England)'72; MB ChB; CCFP; CCFP(E.M.); Staff, Cape Breton Healthcare Complex; (902)567-8000

STOKES, Shelley M; Glenmore Landing, A301-1600 90 Ave SW, Calgary AB T2V 5A8; Cal'90; CCFP; Med Staff, Rockyview General Hospital; (403)246-0200; Fax. (403)301-0046.

STOKL, Stephen B; Dixon Med Centre, 306-531 Davis Dr, Newmarket ON L3Y 6P5; Tor'77; FRCPC; Psy (Bipolar Disease). Chief Psy, Southlake Regional Health Centre; Lecturer Psy, University of Toronto; (905)898-5415; Fax. (905)898-6371; dr.stokl@rogers.com.

STOKREEF, G John C; Couchiching Family Health Team, 206A-119 Memorial Ave, Orillia ON L3V 5X1; Qns'89; Staff, Orillia Soldiers' Memorial Hospital; (705)326-6763; Fax. (705)326-8117.

STOLAR, Marguerite A; Columbia Med Bldg, 403-301 Columbia St E, New Westminster BC V3L 3W5; McM'83; FRCPC; IntMed; Rheum. Staff, Eagle Ridge Hospital & Health Care Centre; Staff, Royal Columbian Hospital; (604)526-2140; Fax. (604)526-2279.

STOLEE, Karen A; Dr Bernstein Health & Diet Cli, 6465 Millcreek Dr, Mississauga ON L5N 5R3; Ott'83; PhysMed&Rehab. (905)813-4001

STOLEE, Kathrine J; Perth-Smith's Falls Dist Hosp, 33 Drummond St W, Perth ON K7H 2K1; McM'86; FRCPC; PhysMed&Rehab. Staff, Perth & Smiths Falls District Hospital - Perth Site (Great War Memorial Site); (613)267-6777; Fax. (613)267-6559.

STOLL, David L; La Ronge Med Clinic, PO Box 240, La Ronge SK S0J 1L0; Sask'02; CCFP; Physician, La Ronge Medical Clinic; (306)425-2174; Fax. (306)425-4199; davidstoll@hotmail.com.

STOLL, Michael B; Family Physicians Group, PO Box 2170 1121 Main St, Melfort SK S0E 1A0; Sask'07; CCFP; (306)752-4493; Fax. (306)752-4496.

STOLL, Stephen; Lawrence Park X-Ray & Ultras, 250 Lawrence Ave W, Toronto ON M5M 1B2; Tor'79; FRCPC; DiagRad. (416)787-0229; Fax. (416)787-0220.

STOLLER, Jacqueline S; Women's College Hosp, 10F-76 Grenville St, Toronto ON M5S 1B2; McM'10; CCFP; Staff Sport CARE, Women's College Hospital; (416)323-6479

STOLLER, Julius L; Seymour Med Clinic, 200-1530 7th Ave W, Vancouver BC V6J 1S3; St Andrews (Scotland)'58; FRCS; FRCS; FACS; GenSurg. Hon Staff GenSurg, Vancouver General Hospital - Centennial Pavillion; Clin Prof Emeritus, University of British Columbia; (604)739-5612; Fax. (604)738-1587; stoller@interchange.ubc.ca.

STOLLER, Rebecca A; North York Doctors, 703-240 Duncan Mill Rd, North York ON M3B 3S6; McM'02; CCFP; Staff, North York General Hospital; Staff, The Scarborough Hospital - General Campus; Staff, North York Family Health Team-Central Office; (416)494-7396; Fax. (416)494-0129.

STOLLERY, Daniel E; Grey Nuns Community Hosp, 2018-1100 Youville Drive West, Edmonton AB T6L 5X8; Alb'79; FRCPC; IntMed (Critical Care Medicine); Respir. Staff, Covenant Health - Grey Nuns Community Hospital; Staff, University of Alberta Hospital; (780)438-0572; Fax. (780)439-7860.

STOLOVITZ, Cynthia; 3431 rue Stanley, Montreal QC H3A 1S2; Sher'86; CCFP; CCFP(E.M.); FCFP; Staff Emerg, McGill University Health Centre - Royal Victoria Hospital; Staff Family Med, St Mary's Hospital Centre; Langs: French; Hebrew; (514)488-4849; Fax. (514)488-3338.

STOLTZ, Katherine J; 12-277 Welland Ave, St Catharines ON L2R 2P7; McM'86; BA; FRCPC; IntMed; Neur. Vis Consultant, Niagara Health System - Greater Niagara General Site; Vis Consultant, Niagara Health System - St Catharines General Site; Langs: French; (905)688-1037; Fax. (905)688-3988; kstoltz@cogeco.ca.

STOLTZE, David A; Royal Inland Hosp, 311 Columbia St, Kamloops BC V2C 2T1; (Other Foreign)'76; CCFP; Staff, Royal Inland Hospital; (250)374-5111

STONE, Angela M; Sunnybrook Hlth Sciences Ctre, C7 16-2075 Bayview Ave, Toronto ON M4N 3M5; McM'05; FRCPC; EmergMed; Critical Care Medicine. Staff, Sunnybrook Health Sciences Centre; (416)480-6018

STONE, Anthony B; Professional Bldg, 3100-222 King St E, Bowmanville ON L1C 1P6; Tor'90; CCFP; (905)623-2355; Fax. (905)623-9607.

STONE, Catherine M; Medicine in Motion Med Centre, 121 Ilsley Ave, Dartmouth NS B3B 1S4; Newcastle-Upon-tine (England)'01; MB BS; Staff, Medicine in Motion Medical Centre; (902)463-2774; Fax. (902)468-1359.

STONE, Elaine; 202-2238 Dundas St W, Toronto ON M6R 3A9; Tor'76; ABIM; FRCPC; IntMed; Endocrin&Metab. Head Div of Endocrin, St Joseph's Health Centre; University of Toronto; (416)588-5219; Fax. (416)588-5221; e.stonemd@on.aibn.com.

STONE, Eric W; Cardiology Consultants, 101-99 Airport Rd, St. John's NL A1A 4Y3; Mem'77; FRCPC; IntMed (Clinical); Cardiol. Staff Cardiol, Health Sciences Centre; Memorial University Of Newfoundland; (709)726-5311; Fax. (709)726-1028; cardiologyconsultants@nfld.net.

STONE, Erin K; Primrose Family Med Centre, 35 Primrose Ave, Ottawa ON K1R 0A1; McM'06; CCFP; (613)230-7788; Fax. (613)230-7778; erinkeelystone@gmail.com.

STONE, James A; Bridgeland Med Bldg, 306-803 1 Ave NE, Calgary AB T2E 7C5; Qns'84; PhD(CA); FRCPC; IntMed (Cardiac Imaging); Cardiol. Staff, Alberta Health Services; Clin Prof Med, University of Calgary; (403)571-8614; Fax. (403)571-6973.

STONE, James E; Rebalance MD, 104-3551 Blanshard St, Victoria BC V8Z 0B9; Dublin (Ireland)'99; MB BCh; BAO; FRCSC; OrthSurg (Sports Injuries). (250)384-4121; Fax. (250)385-9600.

STONE, James M; 525 Park Rd N, Brantford ON N3R 7K8; Man'87; DDS; MSc; DOMFS; Staff, The Brant Community Healthcare System - Brantford General Hospital Site; (519)754-1204; Fax. (519)754-4750.

STONE, Jasper D; Souris Med Associates, PO Box 400, Souris MB R0K 2C0; (204)483-2147

STONE, Jonathan F; 110-857 Grand Ave W, Chatham ON N7L 4T1; Qns'93; FRCSC; OrthSurg. Staff, Chatham-Kent Health Alliance; (519)436-1100; Fax. (519)436-1106; jstone17@cogeco.ca.

STONE, Karina A; Addiction & Mental Hlth-Clarke, 250 College St, Toronto ON M5T 1R8; Central University (Other Foreign)'03; FRCPC; Psy. Staff, Centre for Addiction & Mental Health (CAMH) - College Street Site; (416)535-8501

STONE, Laura D; Mount Sinai Hosp, 206-600 University Ave, Toronto ON M5G 1X5; Wes'10; CCFP; Staff, Sunnybrook Health Sciences Centre; Staff, Mount Sinai Hospital; (416)586-5058

STONE, Mark C; Ross Memorial Hosp, 10 Angeline St N, Lindsay ON K9V 4M8; Tor'07; CCFP; Staff, Ross Memorial Hospital; (705)324-6111; Fax. (705)328-6144.

STONE, Mervyn A; 202-86 Angeline St S, Lindsay ON K9V 6C5; Tor'77; CCFP; Staff, Ross Memorial Hospital; (705)324-5870; Fax. (705)324-5877.

STONE, Norman C; St Clare's Mercy Hosp, SM 326-154 Lemarchant Rd, St. John's NL A1C 5B8; Mem'93; FRCSC; OrthSurg. Staff, St Clare's Mercy Hospital; (709)777-5843

STONE, O Evans; Coldwater Med Centre, PO Box 489 45 River Rd, Coldwater ON L0K 1E0; Tor'70; (705)686-3335; Fax. (705)686-3837.

STONE, Pamela J; Gulf Canada Square, 340-401 9 Ave SW, Calgary AB T2P 3C5; Qns'84; FRCPC; Peds (Vascular Birthmark). Staff Peds & Vascular Birthmark Clinic, Alberta Children's Hospital; Clinical Asst Prof, University of Calgary; (403)221-4434; Fax. (403)221-4466.

STONE, Peter C A; Belleville Med Arts Bldg, 302-210 Dundas St E, Belleville ON K8N 5G8; Qns'68; FRCSC; Otol. Chief Otol, QHC Belleville General; (613)966-3922; Fax. (613)966-2054.

STONE, Samuel B; Sudbury Reg Hosp-Laurentian, 41 Ramsey Lake Rd, Sudbury ON P3E 5J1; McM'05; CCFP; CCFP(E.M.); Staff, Health Sciences North-Laurentian Site; (705)522-7100

STONE, Sarah J; St Paul's Hosp, 5F-1081 Burrard St, Vancouver BC V6Z 1Y6; UBC'98; CCFP; Staff, Providence Health Care - St Paul's Hospital; (604)806-8060; Fax. (604)806-9311.

STONE, Susan J V; Seaton House, 339 George St, North York ON M5N 2A2; Tor'76; CCFP; FCFP; Staff, St Michael's Hospital; Staff, Toronto General Hospital - UHN; Langs: French; (416)338-3187; Fax. (416)392-6616.

STONE, Trevor B; 403-233 Nelsin's Cres, New Westminster BC V3L 0E4; Mem'99; FRCSC; OrthSurg. (604)526-4606

STONEHAM, Grant W; Royal University Hosp, 103 Hospital Dr Box 204, Saskatoon SK S7N 0W8; Cal'90; FRCPC; DiagRad. Staff Med Imaging, Royal University Hospital; (306)655-2402; Fax. (306)655-2370.

STONEHOCKER, Brian K; University of Alberta Hosp, 1E6 13-8440 112 St NW, Edmonton AB T6G 2B7; Alb'96; FRCPC; Psy. Staff, University of Alberta Hospital; (780)407-6566; Fax. (780)407-6672.

STONEHOCKER, John L; PO Box 2149 Stn Main, Stony Plain AB T7Z 1X6; Alb'80; CCFP; CCFP(E.M.); Staff, Westview Health Centre; (780)968-3673; Fax. (780)963-6919.

STONEMAN, H Richard; North York Gen Hosp, 4001 Leslie St, North York ON M2K 1E1; Wes'79; DABR; FRCPC; DiagRad (Vascular & Interventional Radiology). Ac Staff Diag Imaging, North York General Hospital; (416)756-6005; Fax. (416)756-6370.

STONESTREET, Cong Y; 102-634 Van Horn St, Penticton BC V2A 4L1; Shanghai Medical University (China)'88; Langs: Chinese; (778)588-0875

STONG, Martha M J; Couchiching Family Health Team, 103-119 Memorial Ave, Orillia ON L3V 5X1; McM'92; (705)326-3549; Fax. (705)326-9529.

STOPAINIG, Robert; Misericordia Community Hosp, 1NW 15-16940 87 Ave NW, Edmonton AB T5R 4H5; Vienna (Austria)'96; CCFP; Staff, Covenant Health - Misericordia Community Hospital; Langs: German; (780)735-2585; Fax. (780)735-2588; stopain@telusplanet.net.

STOPFORTH, James G; Stevenson Med Clinic, 210A-6640 Vedder Rd, Chilliwack BC V2R 0J2; Pretoria (South Africa)'85; MB ChB; CCFP; Langs: Afrikaans; (604)858-2246; Fax. (604)858-4498.

STOPFORTH, Jeanne; Stevenson Med Clinic, 210A-6640 Vedder Rd, Chilliwack BC V2R 0J2; Pretoria (South Africa)'89; MB ChB; Langs: Afrikaans; (604)858-2246; Fax. (604)858-4498.

STOPPS, Richard G; 190 Catharine St S, Hamilton ON L8N 2K3; McM'74; BSc; FACOG; FSOGC(C); FRCSC; ObstGyn (Infertility). Ac Staff, St Joseph's Healthcare - Charlton Campus; Associate, Hamilton Health Sciences Centre - McMaster Children's Hospital; Clin Associate, ISIS Regional Fertility Centre; Asst Prof, McMaster University; (905)523-0626; Fax. (905)523-0627.

STORCK, Aric J; Foothills Med Centre, C231-1403 29 St NW, Calgary AB T2N 2T9; Tor'02; FRCPC; EmergMed. Staff Emerg Med, Foothills Medical Centre; (403)944-8430; Fax. (403)944-2419.

STOREK, Jan; University of Calgary, 1869-3330 Hospital Dr NW, Calgary AB T2N 4N1; (Czech Republic)'84; Staff, Tom Baker Cancer Centre; Staff, Foothills Medical Centre; Assoc Prof, University of Calgary; (403)210-8630; Fax. (403)210-8176.

STOREY, Benjamin L; 1016 20 St S, Lethbridge AB T1K 2C9; Cal'05; FRCSC; OrthSurg. Staff, Foothills Medical Centre; (403)394-3720; Fax. (403)327-9571.

STOREY, David G W; PO Box 61530 Rpo Brookswood, Langley BC V3A 8C8; Ott'80; FRCPC; Anes. Staff, Langley Memorial Hospital; Langs: French; (604)534-4121; Fax. (604)534-8283.

STOREY, David L; Whitehorse Gen Hosp, 5 Hospital Rd, Whitehorse YT Y1A 3H7; McM'72; FRCSC; GenSurg. Staff, Whitehorse General Hospital; Staff, Yukon Surgical Clinic; (867)393-8908; Fax. (867)667-6512.

STOREY, Elaine A; Chinook Reg Hosp, 960 19 St S, Lethbridge AB T1J 1W5; Cal'05; Staff, Chinook Regional Hospital; (403)388-6111

STORM, Hendrik W; Thompson Gen Hosp, 871 Thompson Dr, Thompson MB R8N 0C8; (Other Foreign)'79; Staff, Thompson General Hospital; (204)677-2381

STOROSCHUK, Gregory W; Pan Am Sports Med Centre, 75 Poseidon Bay, Winnipeg MB R3M 3E4; Man'91; (204)925-1550; Fax. (204)452-5362.

STOROZ, Linda L; Kelowna Gen Hosp, 2268 Pandosy St, Kelowna BC V1Y 1T2; Alb'80; FAAP; FRCPC; Peds (Neonatology). Staff, Kelowna General Hospital; (250)862-4000

STORR, Martin A; Health Sciences Centre, 3330 Hospital Dr NW, Calgary AB T2N 2T9; (Germany)'97; Assoc Prof, University of Calgary; (403)592-5015; Fax. (403)592-5090.

STORR, Michael; Kingston Gen Hosp, Kidd 10-76 Stuart St, Kingston ON K7L 2V7; Wes'86; BSc; FRCPC; Peds (Neonatology). Staff Child Development Centre, Hotel-Dieu Hospital; Staff Ward Chief Inpatient Ped Serv, Kingston General Hospital; Asst Prof, Queen's University; (613)549-6666 x3103; Fax. (613)548-1369; storrm@kgh.kari.net.

STORRIER, Melville; 33 CF Health Services Kingston, PO Box 17000 Stn Forces, Kingston ON K7K 7B4; Sask'99; CCFP; Staff, Canadian Forces Base Kingston; Langs: Bilingual(English/French); (613)541-5010; melville.storrier@forces.gc.ca.

STORRING, John M; MUHC Montreal Gen Hosp, A7 129-1650 av Cedar, Montreal QC H3G 1A4; McG'00; FRCPC; IntMed; Hem. Staff, McGill University Health Centre - Montreal General Campus; (514)934-1934 x42428; john.storring@mcgill.ca.

STORSLEY, Leroy J; Health Sciences Centre, GE421-820 Sherbrook St, Winnipeg MB R3A 1R9; Man'98; BSc; MD; FRCPC; FRCPC; Nephrol; IntMed. Staff, Health Sciences Centre; Asst Prof, University of Manitoba; (204)787-3583; lstorsley@exchange.hsc.mb.ca.

STORWICK, Gregory S; 3F-1222 11 Ave SW, Calgary AB T3C 0M4; Cal'88; FRCPC; Derm. Staff, Foothills Medical Centre; Clin Asst Prof, University of Calgary; (403)286-0086; Fax. (403)288-7804.

STORY, Betty-Anne; 353 St Paul Ave, Brantford ON N3R 4N3; Dal'99; MD; PhD; CCFP; FCFP; (519)753-2519; Fax. (519)753-8912.

STORY, Carol L; Pacific Spirit Comm Hlth Ctre, 2110 43rd Ave W, Vancouver BC V6M 2E1; UBC'87; CCFP; FCFP; Assoc Staff, Providence Health Care - St Paul's Hospital; (604)267-2697; Fax. (604)261-7253.

STOSKI, Douglas M; Meadowlark Health Centre, 200 Meadowlark Shopping Ctr NW, Edmonton AB T5R 5W9; Man'90; FRCPC; DiagRad. (780)489-5313; Fax. (780)486-5160.

STOSKI, Roxann M; Manitoba X-Ray Clinic, 3263 Portage Ave, Winnipeg MB R3K 0W6; Man'94; BSc(Hon); FRCPC; DiagRad. Lecturer, University of Manitoba; (204)832-0273

STOTHART, Danielle C; Penticton Reg Hosp, 550 Carmi Ave, Penticton BC V2A 3G6; Ott'05; Staff, Penticton Regional Hospital; (250)492-4000

STOTHART, Tonja L; Queensway-Carleton Hosp, 3045 Baseline Rd, Nepean ON K2H 8P4; Ott'98; CCFP; Staff, Queensway Carleton Hospital; Langs: Bilingual(English/French); (613)721-4710

STOTHERS, Keith A; Burrard Med Bldg, 560-1144 Burrard St, Vancouver BC V6Z 2A5; UBC'87; BComm; MB; MHSc; FRCSC; OrthSurg (Sports Medicine). Staff, Providence Health Care - St Paul's Hospital; Clin Instructor, University of British Columbia; (604)629-9252; Fax. (604)629-9282.

STOTHERS, Mary-Ann L; UBC Hospital, 1B F329-2211 Wesbrook Mall, Vancouver BC V6T 2B5; UBC'87; FRCSC; Urol. Staff The Bladder Care Centre, UBC Hospital - Koerner Pavillion; (604)822-7616; Fax. (604)822-7591.

STOTLAND, Brian R; Bayview Business Centre, 216-16700 Bayview Ave, Newmarket ON L3X 1W1; McG'91; FRCPC; IntMed (Inflammatory Bowel Disease); Gastroent. Langs: French; (905)836-4173; Fax. (905)836-9038; bstotland@rogers.com.

STOTLAND, Peter K; North York Med Arts Bldg, 314-1333 Sheppard Ave E, North York ON M2J 1V1; Tor'02; FRCSC; GenSurg (Surgical Oncology). Staff Surg, The Banting Institute; Asst Prof Surg, University of Toronto; (647)258-9960; Fax. (647)258-9965; p.stotland@utoronto.ca.

STOTTS, Grant J; The Ottawa Hospital-Civic Camp, C2184-1053 Carling Ave, Ottawa ON K1Y 4E9; Cal'94; FRCPC; Neur. Staff, The Ottawa Hospital - Civic Campus; (613)761-5353 x3; Fax. (613)761-5360; gstotts@ottawahospital.on.ca.

STOVEL, Duncan C; Univ Of Victoria Health Serv, PO Box 1700 Stn CSC, Victoria BC V8W 2Y2; Man'69; FRCPC; Psy.

STOVEL, Laura E; University of Alberta Hosp, 1E1 01-8440 112 St NW, Edmonton AB T6G 2B7; Alb'97; BA; FRCPC; Psy (Group Psychotherapy). Staff Psy/Prog Dir Psy Residency Program, University of Alberta Hospital; Asst Prof, University of Alberta; (780)407-8725; Fax. (780)407-6470.

STOVER, Laura L; Hamilton HS-General Campus, 237 Barton St E, Hamilton ON L8L 2X2; McM'98; FRCPC; Anes. Staff, Hamilton Health Sciences Centre - Hamilton General Hospital; (905)521-2100

STOWE, Robert M; UBC Neuropsychiatry Program, 2255 Wesbrook Mall, Vancouver BC V6T 2A1; Qns'80; FRCPC; Neur (Behavioural Neurology). Staff, BC Mental Health & Addiction Service; Ac Staff, Vancouver General Hospital - Centennial Pavillion; Clin Assoc Prof Psy & Neurol, University of British Columbia; (604)822-7292; Fax. (604)822-7491.

STOYKO, Larry E; PO Box 396, Didsbury AB T0M 0W0; Alb'77; BSc(Hons.); (403)335-1974; Fax. (403)335-1974.

STRAATHOF, Danny; Royal Columbian Hosp, 330 Columbia St E, New Westminster BC V3L 3W7; Alb'93; FRCPC; AnatPath. Staff Path, Royal Columbian Hospital; Consultant Staff Path, BC Children's Hospital; (604)520-4350; Fax. (604)520-4409.

STRAATMAN, Lynn P; 1690 Matthews Ave, Vancouver BC V6J 2T2; Tor'91; FRCPC; Peds (Cardiology). Staff, BC Women's Hospital & Health Centre; Staff Cardiol, Providence Health Care - St Paul's Hospital; (604)731-4847

STRACHAN, Peter G; King Street Med Arts Centre, 204-71 King St W, Mississauga ON L5B 4A2; Tor'64; FRCPC; Peds. Staff, Trillium Health Centre - Mississauga; Court Staff, The Credit Valley Hospital; Court Staff Peds, The Hospital For Sick Children; Assoc Prof, University of Toronto; (905)279-0212; Fax. (905)279-1447.

STRACHAN, Ritchie J; Victoria Gen Hosp, 2340 Pembina Hwy, Winnipeg MB R3T 2E8; Man'93; Staff, Victoria General Hospital; (204)269-3570

STRADER, Bruce E; 270 Argyle St PO Box 475 Stn Main, Renfrew ON K7V 4A6; McG'71; Ac Staff, Renfrew Victoria Hospital; (613)432-9022; Fax. (613)432-5329.

STRAFELLA, Antonio P; Univ Hlth Network-Toronto Western Hosp, MCL7 417-399 Bathurst St, Toronto ON M5T 2S8; Bologna (Italy)'90; FRCPC; Neur. Sr Scientist, Toronto Western Hospital - University Health Network; Langs: Italian; French; (416)603-5706

STRAHLENDORF, Caron; Children's & Women's HC of BC, A119-4480 Oak St, Vancouver BC V6H 3V4; Witwatersrand (South Africa)'85; MB ChB; Staff, BC Children's Hospital; Langs: Afrikaans; (604)875-3576; Fax. (604)875-2911.

STRAKA, Pavel F; Humber River Reg Hosp-Church, 200 Church St, York ON M9N 1N8; Aberdeen (Scotland)'74; MB ChB; FFARCS(Eng); FRCPC; Anes (Acute & Chronic Pain). Staff, Humber River Regional Hospital - Church Street Site; Langs: Czech; (416)243-4154

STRAKACZ, Marta; Cree Board Hlth & Social Serv, PO Box 250, Chisasibi QC J0M 1E0; McG'01; CCFP; CCFP(E.M.); Staff, Cree Board of Health & Social Services James Bay; (819)855-9001

STRAND, Timothy C O; 63 Airport Rd, St. John's NL A1A 4Y3; Alb'97; FRCSC; ObstGyn (Laparoscopy). Staff, Health Sciences Centre; timothy.strand@easternhealth.ca.

STRANG, Barbara K; The Juravinski Cancer Centre, 699 Concession St, Hamilton ON L8V 5C2; Qns'91; BSc(Hons.); MSc(Epid.); FRCPC; RadOncol. Court Staff, Joseph Brant Memorial Hospital; Staff, The Juravinski Cancer Centre; Assoc Prof, McMaster University; (905)387-9495; Fax. (905)575-6326.

STRANG, David G; Deer Lodge Centre Inc, 2109 Portage Ave, Winnipeg MB R3J 0L3; Man'86; MB BS; BSc(Med.); FRCPC; IntMed; GeriatricMed. Asst Prof IntMed, University of Manitoba; (204)837-1301

STRANG, John D; Halton Family Health Centre, 2951 Walker's Line, Burlington ON L7M 4Y1; Alb'91; (905)592-2272; Fax. (905)336-9627.

STRANG, Lucy J; Oakville Trafalgar Mem Hosp, 327 Reynolds St, Oakville ON L6J 3L7; McM'05; CCFP; Staff, Halton Healthcare Services Corporation - Oakville Site; (905)845-2571

STRANG, Robert A; Nova Scotia Dept of Health, PO BOX 488 Stn Central 1894 Barrington St, Halifax NS B3J 2R8; UBC'90; FRCPC; CommunMed; Public Health & Preventive Med. A-Med Officer of Hlth, Nova Scotia Dept of Health; (902)424-2358; Fax. (902)424-4716; strangra@gov.ns.ca.

STRANGES, Gregory A; Pan Am Sports Med Centre, 75 Poseidon Bay, Winnipeg MB R3M 3E4; Man'01; FRCPC; OrthSurg. (204)925-1550

STRANGWAY, James F; LL3-5 Quarry Ridge Rd, Barrie ON L4M 7G1; Tor'69; Ac Staff, Royal Victoria Regional Health Centre; (705)728-4423; Fax. (705)728-7327; fstrangway@rogers.com.

STRANK, Randall T; Humber River Reg Hosp-Church, 200 Church St, Toronto ON M9N 1N8; Man'97; BSc; CCFP; Staff, Humber River Regional Hospital - Church Street Site; (416)249-8111

STRANK, Robert L; Haig Clinic, 601 6 Ave S, Lethbridge AB T1J 0Z2; Man'89; CCFP; Ac Staff, Chinook Regional Hospital; (403)328-6641; Fax. (403)328-6118.

STRANK, Roydon K; Dakota Med Clinic, 17-845 Regent Ave W, Winnipeg MB R2C 3A9; Man'98; CCFP; (204)938-5700

STRASBERG, Jessica E; Jane-Finch Family Health Team, 136A-1 Yorkgate Blvd Box 105, North York ON M3N 3A1; McM'05; MEd; CCFP; (416)745-4555; Fax. (416)745-0786.

STRASBERG, Suzanne R; Jane-Finch Family Health Team, 136A-1 Yorkgate Blvd Box 105, North York ON M3N 3A1; Tor'92; CCFP; (416)745-4555; Fax. (416)745-0786.

STRASBERG, Zeno; LL-4800 Leslie St, North York ON M2J 2K9; McG'64; DABR; FRCPC; DiagRad (Neuro Radiology). Staff Radiol, Lakeridge Health - Oshawa Site; Locum Tenens, Orillia Soldiers' Memorial Hospital; (416)493-1011; Fax. (416)493-1019; zenoandevy@rogers.com.

STRASFELD, Maurice; 825 East River Rd, New Glasgow NS B2H 3S6; Tor'80; BSc; MSc; Staff Ophthalmology, Aberdeen Regional Hospital; Langs: Yiddish; French; (902)755-1840; Fax. (888)755-1415; drstrasfeld@cpmail.ca.

STRASSER, Roger P; Northern Ontario School of Med, 263-935 Ramsey Lake Rd, Sudbury ON P3E 2C6; Monash (Australia)'77; MB BS; BMedSci; MClSc; Dean/CEO/Prof, Northern Ontario School of Medicine; (705)671-3874 x3363; Fax. (705)675-4858.

STRASZAK, Irena M; Laurel Med Centre, 300-888 8th Ave W, Vancouver BC V5Z 3Y1; McM'86; MHA; FRCPC; Psy. Clinical Asst Prof Psy, University of British Columbia; Langs: Bilingual(English/French); (604)222-9699

STRASZAK-SURI, Marina A; Centrepointe Med Consultants, 106 Centrepointe Dr, Nepean ON K2G 6B1; Ott'86; FRCSC; ObstGyn (Ultrasound). Asst Prof, University of Ottawa; Langs: Polish; French; (613)224-4135; Fax. (613)224-7228.

STRATFORD, Andrew F C; Port Hope Med Centre, 209-249 Ontario St, Port Hope ON L1A 3Y9; Qns'00; FRCSC; GenSurg (Family Medicine). (905)885-2949; Fax. (905)885-0716.

STRATFORD, Philip A T; Cobourg Health Centre, 203-316 King St E, Cobourg ON K9A 5R8; Qns'92; DA; CCFP; Langs: Spanish; French; (905)373-1280; Fax. (905)373-9335.

STRATIS, Anna K; Pender Community Health Centre, 59 Pender St W, Vancouver BC V6B 1R3; Dal'07; CCFP; Staff, Pender Community Health Centre; (604)669-9181

STRATMANN, Hanka H E A; Woodbridge Urgent Care Centre, 2-400 Highway 7, Woodbridge ON L4L 8Z2; Tor'02; CCFP; Langs: Spanish; German; French; (905)851-3777

STRATTON, Faith; Health & Community Services, PO Box 8700 Stn A, St. John's NL A1B 4J6; Mem'74; MHSc; Staff, Health & Community Services; Clinical Asst Prof Commun Med, Memorial University Of Newfoundland; (709)729-3430

STRAUB, Deborah L; Aberdeen Hosp, 835 East River Rd, New Glasgow NS B2H 3S6; Dal'92; CCFP; CCFP(E.M.); Staff, Aberdeen Regional Hospital; (902)752-8311; Fax. (902)752-5116.

STRAUS, Sharon E; St Michael's Hosp, 2 026-30 Bond St, Toronto ON M5B 1W8; Tor'90; FRCPC; IntMed; GeriatricMed. Staff, St Michael's Hospital; (416)864-3068; Fax. (416)864-5805.

STRAUSS, Barry I; Unionville Family Physicians, 301-10 Unionville Gate, Markham ON L3R 0W7; Tor'92; MSc; BSc; CCFP; Ac Staff, Markham Stouffville Hospital; Coroner, York Region; (905)475-3121; Fax. (905)475-4270.

STRAUSS, Bradley H; Sunnybrook Hlth Sciences Ctre, D408-2075 Bayview Ave, Toronto ON M4N 3M5; Tor'82; PhD; FRCPC; IntMed (Interventional Cardiology); Cardiol. Staff, Sunnybrook Health Sciences Centre; Staff, St Michael's Hospital; Prof, University of Toronto; (416)480-6066; Fax. (416)480-6174.

STRAUSS, Frederik J; Properties Med Clinic, 5-5102 Rundlehorn Dr NE, Calgary AB T1Y 1C1; Stellenbosch (South Africa)'81; MB ChB; LMCC; Staff, Properties Medical Clinic; Langs: Afrikaans; (403)280-2700; Fax. (403)285-2641; fjstrauss@telus.net.

STRAUSS, Hans D; 504-2300 Eglinton Ave W, Mississauga ON L5M 2V8; Tor'72; FACC; FCCP; FRCPC; IntMed; Cardiol. Ac Staff, Toronto Rehabilitation Institute - University Centre; Consultant, Centre for Addiction & Mental Health (CAMH) - Russell Street Site; Dir CCU, The Credit Valley Hospital; Asst Prof, University of Toronto; Langs: German; (905)820-5533; Fax. (905)820-6342.

STRAUSS, Jacoba C; 3223 17 Ave SW, Calgary AB T3E 7S1; Stellenbosch (South Africa)'83; MB ChB; DCH(SA); LMCC; Langs: Afrikaans; (403)255-1166; Fax. (403)252-0444.

STRAUSS, John S; Addiction & Mental Hlth-Clarke, 250 College St, Toronto ON M5T 1R8; Tor'92; FRCPC; Psy. Staff, Centre for Addiction & Mental Health (CAMH) - College Street Site; (416)535-8501 x4302

STRAUSS, Martin H; 107-4800 Leslie St, North York ON M2J 2K9; Tor'79; FACC; FRCPC; IntMed; Cardiol. (416)730-0938; Fax. (416)229-6162.

STRAUSS, Matthew S; PG Medical Education Office, M106-1151 Richmond St, London ON N6A 5C1; Wes'08; IntMed.

STRAUSS, Paul L; B1-350 Conestoga Blvd, Cambridge ON N1R 7L7; Tor'91; BSc; FRCSC; ObstGyn. Ac Staff, Cambridge Memorial Hospital; (519)622-5990; Fax. (519)622-5567.

STRAUSS, Pieter; Gladwin Centre, 203-2955 Gladwin Rd, Abbotsford BC V2T 5T4; Orange Free State (South Africa)'84; MB ChB; MMed; FRCPC; Psy. Dept Head, Abbotsford Regional Hospital & Cancer Centre; Langs: Afrikaans; (604)852-8565; Fax. (604)852-0121.

STRAUTS, Zigurts; Windsor Square Shopp Centre, 136-1959 152 St, Surrey BC V4A 9E3; Cal'82; BSc; (604)541-1053; Fax. (604)541-1093.

STRAWBRIDGE, Peter W; Keswick Med Centre, 183 Simcoe Ave, Keswick ON L4P 2H6; Tor'74; Ac Staff, Southlake Regional Health Centre; (905)476-4387; Fax. (905)476-4358.

STRAZA, Lorne D; Pacific Place Mall, 958-999 36 St NE, Calgary AB T2A 7X6; Sask'83; CCFP; (403)387-3300; Fax. (403)387-3305.

STRBAN, Martin; Medical Bldg, 308-18 Pine St, Kitchener ON N2H 5Z8; Qns'87; BSc(Hons.); FRCPC; IntMed; Respir. Ac Staff, Grand River Hospital - Kitchener/Waterloo Health Centre; Ac Staff, St Mary's General Hospital; Langs: Slovak; (519)745-3505; Fax. (519)745-7975.

STRECKER, Harvey D; 212-1676 Martin Dr, Surrey BC V4A 6E7; Cal'87; FRCSC; Otol (Head & Neck Surgery). (604)538-5524; Fax. (604)538-5429.

STREET, Donald G; Village Med Clinic, PO Box 1720 190 Horse Lake Rd, 100 Mile House BC V0K 2E0; UBC'77; Ac Staff, 100 Mile House District General Hospital; (250)395-3000; Fax. (250)395-3055.

STREET, Harry W; 30-2050 Sumas Way, Abbotsford BC V2S 2C7; UBC'94; (604)504-7145; Fax. (604)504-7195.

STREET, John T; Blusson Spinal Cord Centre, 6F-818 10th Ave W, Vancouver BC V5Z 1M9; Cork (Ireland)'93; FRCSI; FRCS; PhD; MB BCh; BAO; Staff, Vancouver General Hospital - Centennial Pavillion; Teach Staff Combined Neurosurgical & Orthopaedic Spine Prog, University of British Columbia; Langs: Gaelic; (604)875-5328; Fax. (604)875-5858.

STREET, Lesley E; Foothills Med Centre, 1403 29 St NW, Calgary AB T2N 2T9; Cal'05; FRCPC; IntMed; Hem. Staff, Foothills Medical Centre; (403)944-1564; Fax. (403)944-2102.

STREET, Robert M; Royal Columbian Hosp, 330 Columbia St E, New Westminster BC V3L 3W7; Mem'83; BMedSci; FRCPC; EmergMed. Staff, Royal Columbian Hospital; Asst Dir Surg/Prof, University of British Columbia; (604)520-4253

STREHLKE, Claudia T; 214 Med Place, 1226-9909 102 St Box 46, Grande Prairie AB T8V 2V4; Alb'65; FRCPC; IntMed. Staff, Queen Elizabeth II Hospital; Langs: German; (780)539-3303; Fax. (780)539-3909; cdnoma@hotmail.com.

STREICH, Robert J; Castlegar Med Associates, 1008 Columbia Ave, Castlegar BC V1N 1H2; UBC'76; MCFP; (250)365-2161; Fax. (250)365-2171; robert.streich@interiorhealth.ca.

STREIFF, Raphael; CSSS des Basques, 550 rue Notre-Dame E, Trois-Pistoles QC G0L 4K0; Universite Nancy (France)'98; Staff, Centre Hospitalier Trois-Pistoles; (418)851-3700

STREILEIN, Karen F; Kinsmen Children's Centre, 1319 Colony St, Saskatoon SK S7N 2Z1; Sask'81; FRCPC; Peds (Developmental Pediatrics). Staff Peds, Royal University Hospital; Physician, Kinsmen Children's Centre; (306)655-1006; Fax. (306)655-1449; kstr100@hotmail.com.

STRELIOFF, George D; Woodbine Med Centre, B 9-76 Arlington Dr, Keswick ON L4P 0A9; Sask'82; DAB; BSc; Staff, Southlake Regional Health Centre; (905)476-0308; Fax. (905)476-1079.

STRENG-COETZEE, Ilana; Downtown Med Clinic, PO Box 1866, Unity SK S0K 4L0; (306)228-4450; Fax. (306)228-4277.

STRESMAN, Elaine J; Hotel Dieu Grace Hosp, 7F-1030 Ouellette Ave, Windsor ON N9A 1E1; McM'00; CCFP; Staff, Hôtel-Dieu Grace Hospital; (519)973-4444; doc_elaine@yahoo.ca.

STRETCH, Neal C; Hanover Med Associates, 118 7th Ave, Hanover ON N4N 2G9; Tor'82; BASc; MASc; CCFP; FCFP; Staff, Hanover & District Hospital; Asst Prof, University of Ottawa; (519)364-2820; Fax. (519)364-3965.

STREUTKER, Catherine J; St Michael's Hosp, 2CC099-30 Bond St, Toronto ON M5B 1W8; Tor'94; FRCPC; AnatPath. Staff, St Michael's Hospital; (416)360-4000 x2363; Fax. (416)864-5648.

STREVEL, Elizabeth L; The Credit Valley Hosp, 2200 Eglinton Ave W, Mississauga ON L5M 2N1; Wes'03; FRCPC; IntMed; MedOncol. Staff Peel Regional Cancer Centre, The Credit Valley Hospital; (905)813-2200; Fax. (905)813-4024.

STRICKLAND, Carol A; Orillia Soldiers' Mem Hosp, 170 Colborne St W, Orillia ON L3V 2Z3; Wes'80; BA(Hons); CCFP; Ac Staff, Orillia Soldiers' Memorial Hospital; Associate Clin Prof, McMaster University; Clin Assoc Prof/Preceptor, University of Toronto; (705)325-2201

STRICKLER, Albert C; Trillium Health Centre-Missisa, 100 Queensway W, Mississauga ON L5B 1B8; Tor'58; DOHS; CCBOM; FACOM; Staff, Trillium Health Centre - West Toronto; Trillium Health Centre - Mississauga; Asst Prof, University of Toronto; (905)848-7100

STRIGLER, Stephen; Downtown Doctors Med Ctre, 418-720 Spadina Ave, Toronto ON M5S 2T9; Tor'84; CCFP; Langs: French; (416)929-1530; Fax. (416)929-7398.

STRIJACK, Bradford J; Surrey Med Arts Bldg, 113-13798 94A Ave, Surrey BC V3V 1N1; (604)581-4441

STRIJAK, Bradford J; Gordon & Leslie Diamond HCC, 5F-2775 Laurel St, Vancouver BC V5Z 1M9; Man'05; FRCPC; IntMed; Nephrol. Physician, Gordon & Leslie Diamond Health Care Centre; (604)875-5950

STRIKE, Jessica S; Lancaster Med Clinic, 2450 Lancaster Rd, Ottawa ON K1B 5N3; Ott'06; CCFP; Langs: Bilingual(English/French); (613)738-9119

STRILCHUK, Douglas A J; Yellowbird Family Clinic, 3380 Gateway Blvd, Edmonton AB T6J 6V1; Alb'84; (780)434-2893; Fax. (780)435-1057; dstrilchuk@ybfc.com.

STRINGER, David G; Centenary Hlth Centre, 2863 Ellesmere Rd, Scarborough ON M1E 5E9; Qns'86; FRCPC; Anes. Staff Anes, Rouge Valley Health System - Centenary Health Centre Site; (416)281-7454; Fax. (416)281-7453.

STRINGER, Elizabeth; IWK Health Centre, PO Box 9700 Rpo CSC 5850 University Ave, Halifax NS B3K 6R8; Dal'01; FRCPC; Peds (Pediatric Rheumatology); Rheum. Staff Ped Rheum, IWK Health Centre; (902)470-8827; Fax. (902)470-7217; elizbeth.stringer@iwk.nshealth.ca.

STRINGER, Katherine C; Ross Family Med Centre, 100 Forest Rd, St. John's NL A1A 3Z9; Cape Town (South Africa)'94; MB ChB; CCFP; Physician, Dr Leonard A Miller Centre; (709)579-5005; Fax. (709)579-5278; katherine.stringer@med.mun.ca.

STRINGER, L Judith; Vancouver Breast Feeding Ctre, 340-943 Broadway W, Vancouver BC V5Z 4E1; London (England)'70; MB BS; DObstRCOG; MRCGPract; (604)738-1912; Fax. (604)738-1231.

STRINGER, Vernon M; Parkdale Med Tower, 802-1081 Carling Ave, Ottawa ON K1Y 4G2; Qns'87; (613)729-9989; Fax. (613)728-2752.

STRITZKE, Amelie I; Surrey Mem Hosp, 13750 96 Ave, Surrey BC V3V 1Z2; Johann Wolfgang Goethe University (Germany)'03; FRCPC; Peds (Neonatal & Perinatal Medicine). Staff, Surrey Memorial Hospital; (604)581-2211

STROBACH, Helene G; Clinique de l'Esprit, 100-5252 boul Maisonneuve O, Montreal QC H4A 3S5; McG'78; MSc; Langs: French; (514)931-1659; Fax. (514)483-6386.

STRODE, Kelly K; Guelph Med Place, 210-83 Dawson Rd, Guelph ON N1H 1B1; McM'05; FRCSC; ObstGyn. Staff, Guelph General Hospital; (519)821-2440

STROESCU, Daniela V; River Park Med Centre, 4-1500 Dakota St, Winnipeg MB R2N 3Y7.

STROKER, Claire; Off Site Adolescent Clinic, 3640 Wells St, Windsor ON N9C 1T9; University of Kansas (USA)'80; (519)258-0484

STROM, Brian S; The West Mall Health Centre, 1-290 The West Mall, Etobicoke ON M9C 1C6; Tor'81; (416)621-4461; Fax. (416)620-7476.

STROMBERG, Lana M; Dominion Med Centres Ltd, 9122 23 Ave NW, Edmonton AB T6N 1H9; Cal'03; CCFP; (780)801-3360; Fax. (780)801-3366.

STROMBERG, Susan J; UBC Hospital, 2211 Wesbrook Mall, Vancouver BC V6T 2B5; UBC'85; CCFP; CCFP(E.M.); Ac Staff, UBC Hospital - Koerner Pavillion; Med Coord Station 262, BC Ambulance Service; Clin Instructor, University of British Columbia; (604)822-7662; Fax. (604)822-7573.

STROME, Janet E; Burlington Prof Centre, 303-3155 Harvester Rd, Burlington ON L7N 3V2; Tor'80; MSc; CCFP; FCFP; Ac Staff, Joseph Brant Memorial Hospital; (905)681-3035; Fax. (905)681-0132.

STRONELL, Roger D; 307-18 Pine St, Kitchener ON N2H 5Z8; McG'71; DABR; FRCPC; DiagRad (Medical Informatics). Langs: Hebrew; French; (519)570-3660; drstronell@on.aibn.com.

STRONG, David G; Calgary Health Region, 10101 Southport Rd SW, Calgary AB T2W 3N2; Alb'84; FRCPC; CommunMed. Staff, Calgary Health Region; (403)943-0272

STRONG, Grant C; Calgary Trail Medicentre, 1-10407 51 Ave NW, Edmonton AB T6H 0K4; Alb'70; Staff, Calgary Trail Medicentres; (780)436-8071; Fax. (780)435-6034.

STRONG, James E; Special Pathogens Program, 1015 Arlington St, Winnipeg MB R3E 3R2; Cal'97; FRCPC; Peds. Staff Children's Hosp, Health Sciences Centre; Head Special Pathogens Prog, Diagnostic & Therapeutics Special Pathogens.

STRONG, Julie K; Lacewood Med Centre, 366 Lacewood Dr, Halifax NS B3S 1M7; Dublin (Ireland)'79; MB ChB; (902)445-9400

STRONG, Michael J; London HSC-University Hosp, PO Box 5339 Stn B C7-120-339 Windermere Rd, London ON N6A 5A5; Qns'82; FRCPC; Neur (Amyotrophic Lateral Sclerosis). Ac Staff, London Health Sciences Centre - University Hospital; Dean/Dept Chair Robarts Research Intstitute, University of Western Ontario; (519)663-3874; Fax. (519)663-3609.

STRONGE, David M; Sows Ear Med Clinic, 7186 Lantzville Rd, Lantzville BC V0R 2H0; London (England)'65; CCFP; (250)390-4542; Fax. (250)390-4561.

STRONGER, Lyle N W; 1217-233 Kennedy St, Winnipeg MB R3C 3J5; Man'02; FRCPC; IntMed; Cardiol.

STRONKS, John E; B-372 Lacroix St, Chatham ON N7M 2W3; Tor'87; CCFP; FCFP; (519)355-1515; Fax. (519)355-1192.

STROTHER, Douglas; Alberta Children's Hosp, 2888 Shaganappi Trail NW, Calgary AB T3B 6A8; Omaha(NE) (USA)'82; BA; MD; ABPeds; ABPeds(HemOncol); Ac Staff, Alberta Children's Hospital; Ac Staff, Foothills Medical Centre; (403)955-7203; Fax. (403)955-2645; doug.strother@albertahealthservices.ca.

STROTHER, Ralph T; 380-1201 5 St SW, Calgary AB T2R 0Y6; Alb'81; CCFP; FCFP; (403)680-2855; Fax. (403)215-7319.

STROUD, Lynfa F; Sunnybrook Hlth Sciences Ctre, D4 70A-2075 Bayview Ave, Toronto ON M4N 3M5; Tor'00; FRCPC; IntMed. Staff, Sunnybrook Health Sciences Centre; (416)480-4244; Fax. (416)480-6191.

STROUD, Richard R; PO Box 274, Fallis AB T0E 0V0; Alb'79; CCFP; Staff, Royal Alexandra Hospital; (780)735-4111

STROVSKAIA, Galina; Panorama Village Med Clinic, 103-15157 56 Ave, Surrey BC V3S 9A5; Sverdlovsk (Russia (Federation))'85; LMCC; CCFP; Langs: Russian; (604)574-0481

STROVSKI, Semion; Panorama Village Med Clinic, 103-15157 56 Ave, Surrey BC V3S 9A5; Sverdlovsk (Russia (Federation))'84; LMCC; CCFP; Langs: Russian; (604)574-0481

STROZ, Edward S; 1122 Islington Ave, Etobicoke ON M8Z 4S2; Tor'60; CCFP; Ac Staff, St Joseph's Health Centre; (416)231-3077; Fax. (416)231-0328.

STROZ, Peter M; Mackenzie Richmond Hill Hosp, 10 Trench St, Richmond Hill ON L4C 4Z3; Tor'88; FRCPC; DiagRad. Staff, Mackenzie Richmond Hill Hospital; (905)883-1212; Fax. (905)883-0772.

STRUBE, Y N Johanna; Hotel-Dieu Hosp, JM6 016-166 Brock St, Kingston ON K7L 5G2; Qns'04; FRCSC; Ophth. Staff, Hotel-Dieu Hospital; (613)544-3310

STRUCK, Wolfgang M; Hys Med Centre, 303-11010 101 St NW, Edmonton AB T5H 4B9; Alb'74; FRCSC; GenSurg. Staff, University of Alberta Hospital; (780)424-0571; Fax. (780)426-6711.

STRUEBY, Brian J D; Mental Health Centre, 2328 Trent St, Victoria BC V8R 4Z3; Sask'91; FRCPC; Psy. Staff, Mental Health Centre; (250)370-8000; brian.strueby@viha.ca.

STRUK, Daniel W; Sudbury Reg Hosp-Laurentian, 41 Ramsey Lake Rd, Sudbury ON P3E 5J1; Wes'94; FRCPC; DiagRad. Staff, Health Sciences North-Laurentian Site; (705)522-2200; Fax. (705)523-7017.

STRUMAS, Nick; Hamilton HS-McMaster Site, PO Box 2000 Stn Lcd 1 4E9-1200 Main St W, Hamilton ON L8N 3Z5; Tor'95; FRCSC; PlasSurg. Staff, Hamilton Health Sciences Centre - McMaster Children's Hospital; Langs: Macedonian; (905)521-2100; Fax. (905)521-9992.

STRUMPFER, Talita; Colwood Med Treatment Ctre, 102-1910 Sooke Rd, Victoria BC V9B 1V7; Stellenbosch (South Africa)'92; CCFP; (250)478-8833

STRUMPHER, Johann W; St Boniface Gen Hosp, 409 Tache Ave, Winnipeg MB R2H 2A6; Stellenbosch (South Africa)'89; MB ChB; FRCPC; Anes; Critical Care Medicine. Staff, St Boniface General Hospital; (204)233-8563

STRUTHERS, Andrew W; 1309 St. Peter Ave, Bathurst NB E2A 3A7; Sheffield (England)'65; MB ChB; FRCS; Sr Staff, Hopital Regional Chaleur; (506)548-3080

STRUTHERS, Graham D N; Worker's Comp Board, PO Box 4700 Stn Terminal, Vancouver BC V6B 1J1; UBC'89; CCFP; Staff, Workers' Compensation Board; (604)232-7036

STRUZIK, Lukasz; South Georgetown Med Clinic, 2-333 Mountainview Rd S, Georgetown ON L7G 6E8; Tor'06; CCFP; Staff, St Joseph's Health Centre; Langs: Polish; (905)417-7771; Fax. (905)417-1377.

STRYDE, Peter C; 207 Gammon Lake Dr, Dartmouth NS B2Z 1T9; Mem'10.

STRYDE, Trevor S; Medical Assoc of Port Perry, 462 Paxton St, Port Perry ON L9L 1L9; Mem'93; FRCSC; GenSurg. (905)985-9758; Fax. (905)985-8931.

STRYDOM, Carin S; Queen Elizabeth II Hosp, 10409 98 St, Grande Prairie AB T8V 2E8; Stellenbosch (South Africa)'94; MB ChB; CCFP; Staff OR, Queen Elizabeth II Hospital; Langs: Afrikaans; (780)538-7588; Fax. (780)538-7364.

STRYDOM, David P J; Vegreville Family Clinic, PO Box 219, Vegreville AB T9C 1R2; Pretoria (South Africa)'00; MB ChB; Physician, Eckville Medical Clinic; (780)632-6414; Fax. (780)632-6404; slmc@shaw.ca.

STRYDOM, Eben A; Family Physicians Group, PO Box 2170, Melfort SK S0E 1A0; Stellenbosch (South Africa)'97; BSc(Hons); MB ChB; Physician, Family Physicians Group; (306)752-3375; Fax. (306)752-5293.

STRYDOM, Gerhardus J; Coast Medical, 1018 Seymour St, Vancouver BC V6B 3M6; Witwatersrand (South Africa)'86; MB ChB; Staff, Abbotsford Regional Hospital & Cancer Centre; Langs: Afrikaans; (604)569-3632

STRYDOM, Heinre; Lakewood Common Med Clinic, 411C Herold Crt, Saskatoon SK S7V 0A7; Stellenbosch (South Africa)'94; MB ChB; Physician, Lakewood Common Medical Clinic; Langs: Afrikaans; (306)933-2868; Fax. (306)933-2865; hsstrydoms@hotmail.com.

STRYDOM, Hendrik G; High Level Med Clinic, 11202 100 Ave, High Level AB T0H 1Z0; (780)926-2286; Fax. (780)926-3550.

STRYDOM, Henriette; The Medical Clinic Associates, 4794 Joyce Ave, Powell River BC V8A 3B6; Orange Free State (South Africa)'04; MB ChB; Langs: Afrikaans; (604)485-6261; Fax. (604)485-2820.

STRYDOM, Jacobus; Park Avenue Med Centre, 4F-4634 Park Ave, Terrace BC V8G 1V7; Stellenbosch (South Africa)'94; MB ChB; Langs: Afrikaans; (250)615-5058; Fax. (250)615-5014.

STRYDOM, Marthinus; Workers' Comp Board, 9912 107 St, Edmonton AB T5K 1G5; Stellenbosch (South Africa)'91; Staff, Queen Elizabeth II Hospital; Staff, Workers' Comp Board; (780)498-4736; Fax. (780)498-7808; strydom@imaginet.co.za.

STRYDOM, Nardia; Laurel Med Centre Ltd, 304-888 8th Ave W, Vancouver BC V5Z 3Y1; Cape Town (South Africa)'86; MB ChB; (604)874-0261; Fax. (604)874-3099.

STRYKER, Rodrick K; Saskatoon Nephrology Group, 434-230 Avenue R South, Saskatoon SK S7M 2Z1; Sask'01; FRCPC; IntMed; Nephrol. Physician, Saskatoon Nephrology Group; (306)934-3300; Fax. (306)934-3355.

STRYKER, Trina D; Regina Gen Hosp, 2C-1440 14 Ave, Regina SK S4P 0W5; Sask'05; FRCSC; ObstGyn (Maternal Fetal Medicine). Staff, Regina General Hospital; (306)766-4368; Fax. (306)766-4453.

STRYTVEEN, Charly A; Grandin Med Clinic, 1 St Ann St, St. Albert AB T8N 2E8; Alb'92; CCFP; (780)459-5581

STRZELCZAK, Dariusz; Miramichi Reg Hosp, 500 Water St, Miramichi NB E1V 3G5; Warsaw (Poland)'85; FRCPC; AnatPath. Staff, Miramichi Regional Hospital; (506)623-3000

STRZELCZYK, Jacek J; St Boniface Gen Hosp, 409-409 Tache Ave, Winnipeg MB R2H 2A6; Tor'02; FRCPC; DiagRad. Staff, St Boniface General Hospital; (204)233-8563

STUART, Andrew J; British Army Training Unit Suf, PO BOX 5000 LCD 1, Medicine Hat AB T1A 8K7; (403)544-4108

STUART, Carmen M; Fredericton Med Clinic, 103-435 Regent St, Fredericton NB E3B 3X6; Mem'93; CCFP; (506)458-0303; Fax. (506)458-0312.

STUART, David S; Kingsway Plaza Phase III, 705-4980 Kingsway, Burnaby BC V5H 4K7; Stanford(CA) (USA)'78; FRCPC; IntMed; MedOncol. (604)261-1021; Fax. (604)434-5053.

STUART, Gary A; 302-132 Parkdale Ave S, Hamilton ON L8K 3P3; Tor'74; (905)547-4207; Fax. (905)547-4207.

STUART, Gavin C E; UBC-Faculty of Medicine, 317-2194 Health Sciences Mall, Vancouver BC V6T 1Z6; Wes'76; DABOG; FACOG; DABG; FRCSC; ObstGyn (Gynecology). Physician, Medical Clinic; Dean Vice-Provost Health, University of British Columbia; (604)822-5767; Fax. (604)822-8017; gstuart@medd.med.ubc.ca.

STUART, Howard R; St Mary's Hosp Centre, 3830 av Lacombe, Montreal QC H3T 1M5; McG'90; CCFP; CCFP(E.M.); Staff, St Mary's Hospital Centre; Staff, Sir Mortimer B Davis Jewish General; adj Prof Family Med, McGill University; Langs: French; (514)345-3511; Fax. (514)458-1596.

STUART, Katherine A; PO Box 42031 Rpo Guildford, Surrey BC V3R 1S5; UBC'01; CCFP.

STUART, Lucille; Whitehorse Med Services Ltd, 406 Lambert St, Whitehorse YT Y1A 1Z7; Dal'89; CCFP; FCFP; Staff, Whitehorse Medical Services Ltd; Langs: German; French; (867)393-6600; Fax. (867)393-6601.

STUART, Philip F; North York Med Arts Bldg, 340-1333 Sheppard Ave, North York ON M2J 1V1; Tor'69; PhD(Microbiol); FRCPC; MedMicrobiol (Tropical & Travel Medicine). Langs: Spanish; French; (416)447-3324; Fax. (416)498-1589.

STUART, Thomas; Vernon Radiological Associates, 3100 35th Ave, Vernon BC V1T 2T1; Dal'74; DABR; FRCR; FRCPC; DiagRad. Staff, Royal Jubilee Hospital; (250)545-0747; tomastuart@shaw.ca.

STUBBINS, Robert I; 3 Simcoe St, Penetanguishene ON L9M 1V2; Qns'78; Ac Staff, Georgian Bay General Hospital - Midland; (705)549-3153; Fax. (705)549-3566.

STUBBS, Barbara E; UHN-Toronto Western Hosp, 2W404-399 Bathurst St, Toronto ON M5T 2S8; Tor'81; CCFP; FCFP; Staff, Toronto Western Hospital - University Health Network; Assoc Prof Family & Commun Med, University of Toronto; (416)603-5888 x1; Fax. (416)603-5821.

STUBBS, Esther R; Campbell River & Dist Gen Hosp, 375 2nd Ave, Campbell River BC V9W 3V1; Qns'05; BSc; CCFP; CCFP(E.M.); Staff, Campbell River & District General Hospital; (250)850-2141

STUBBS, J Mark; 231 46 Ave W PO BOX 1990, Claresholm AB T0L 0T0; Alb'79; (403)468-2141; Fax. (403)468-2141.

STUBBS, Michael D; Alberta Children's Hosp, 2888 Shaganappi Trail NW, Calgary AB T3B 6A8; Cal'06; FRCPC; Psy. Staff, Alberta Children's Hospital; (403)944-7344

STUBBS, Peter J S; The Bluewater Surgical Centre, 106-704 Mara St, Point Edward ON N7V 1X4; (USA)'02.

STUBBS, Robert H; St Michael's Hosp, 30 Bond St, Toronto ON M5B 1W8; Tor'73; DAB; FACS; FRCSC; PlasSurg (Cosmetic Surgery). Staff, St Michael's Hospital; Dir, Cosmetic Surgicentre; (416)864-5110; rhs@psurg.com.

STUBEDA, Iryna; Queen Elizabeth II HSC-Halifax, 6896-1796 Summer St, Halifax NS B3H 3A7; Grodno University (Belarus)'93; Staff, Queen Elizabeth II Health Sciences Centre - Halifax Infirmary Site; (902)473-2700

STUBEDA, Yury V; PO Box 646, Berwick NS B0P 1E0; Dal'10.

STUBINGTON, David; 2005 boul Graham, Mont-Royal QC H3R 1H5; London (England)'49; FRCPC; IntMed (Clinical Cardiology); Cardiol (P.Q.). (514)733-9361

STUCHLY, Joanna Z; Heritage Family Med Centre, 8330 Macleod Trail SE, Calgary AB T2H 2V2; Kracow (Poland)'62; PhD; Langs: Polish; (403)258-3000; Fax. (403)258-0300.

STUCKEY, Emma Flora; 150 Joshua Rd, Orangeville ON L9W 4W5; Ott'79; Fax. (416)510-6870; pstuckey@scottsinfo.com.

STUCKEY, W Mitchell; 80 Valleybrook Dr, North York ON M3B 2S9; Sask'97; (416)442-5600; Fax. (416)510-6870; pstuckey@scottsdirectories.com.

STUCKEY, Valerie A; Centre Med Nazareth, 1771 av Dollard, LaSalle QC H8N 1T9; McG'05; CCFP; Staff, Kateri Memorial Hospital Centre; (514)368-5500; Fax. (514)368-0056.

STUCKLESS, Teri L; Dr H Bliss Murphy Cancer Ctre, 300 Prince Philip Dr, St. John's NL A1B 3V6; Mem'03; FRCPC; RadOncol. Staff, Health Sciences Centre; Staff Cancer Care Program, Dr H Bliss Murphy Cancer Centre; (709)777-6480; Fax. (709)753-0927.

STUDER, Lea H; PO Box 21207 Rpo Terwillegar, Edmonton AB T6R 2V4; Alb'82; FRCPC; Psy. Staff, Alberta Hospital Edmonton; Asst Prof Psy, University of Alberta; (780)342-5555

STUDNIBERG, Allan P; Agincourt Med Centre, 2020 Brimley Rd, Scarborough ON M1S 4R7; Tor'79; Ac Staff, Rouge Valley Health System - Centenary Health Centre Site; Assoc Staff, The Scarborough Hospital - General Campus; (416)293-2404

STUGLIN, Carlo; Saskatoon Cardiol Consultants, 920-606 Spadina Cres E, Saskatoon SK S7K 3H1; Sask'97; FRCPC; IntMed; Cardiol. (306)975-9000

STULBERG, Jennifer R; St Clair Med Clinic, 50 St Clair Ave E, Toronto ON M4T 1M9; Tor'06; CCFP; (416)921-1066; Fax. (416)921-8459.

STULTZ, Timothy; 243 Harbour Dr, Summerside PE C1N 5R1; Dal'92; Staff Geriatric Med, Prince County Hospital; (902)888-3659

STUMPF, Elisabeth M; 3761 Rte Brassard, Shipshaw QC G7P 1C6; Laval'86; Physician, CHSLD Jonquiere; Langs: Bilingual(French/English); (418)695-9998; Fax. (418)695-9998.

STUMPF, Erika; Hop Maisonneuve-Rosemont, 5415 boul de l'Assomption, Montreal QC H1T 2M4; Mon'99; Neur. Staff, Hopital Maisonneuve-Rosemont; Langs: English; (514)252-3400; Fax. (514)252-3529.

STUMPF, Michael; 610 boul Cure-Labelle, Laval QC H7V 2T7; Mon'88; ac Membre, Hopital de la Cite de la santé; Langs: English; (450)687-6452; Fax. (450)687-3243; micstumpf@videotron.ca.

STUPARYK, Robert M; Lakeridge Health Corp-Oshawa, 1 Hospital Crt, Oshawa ON L1G 2B9; Wes'93; CCFP; CCFP(E.M.); FCFP; Staff, Rouge Valley Health System - Centenary Health Centre Site; Staff, The Scarborough Hospital - General Campus; Staff, Lakeridge Health - Oshawa Site; (905)576-8711; Fax. (905)721-4749.

STURGE, Cecil C; Western Bay Med Clinic, PO Box 10, Western Bay NL A0A 4J0; Dal'72.

STURGEON, Jeremy F G; MUHC-Royal Victoria Hosp, 687 av des Pins O, Montreal QC H3A 1A1; London (England)'68; MB BS; FRCPC; FRCPC; MedOncol (P.Q.); IntMed (Gynecological Cancer). Dir MedOncol, McGill University Health Centre - Royal Victoria Hospital; Dir Med Oncol, McGill University Health Centre - Montreal General Campus; Langs: Bilingual(English/French); (514)934-8492; Fax. (514)934-8363; jeremy.sturgeon@muhc.mcgill.ca.

STURGEON, Mary-Ellen; Oak Bay Med Centre, 159-2515 90 Ave SW, Calgary AB T2V 0L8; Cal'88; (403)281-2020; Fax. (403)281-7785.

STURGEON, Simon; 2197 Hunt Cres, Burlington ON L7M 3E2; Alb'91; Fax. (416)510-6870.

STURM, Esther R W; Bayview-Finch Med Clinic, 301-3292 Bayview Ave, North York ON M2M 4J5; Tor'84; MScN; CCFP; Staff, North York General Hospital; Langs: Hebrew; (416)222-2200; Fax. (416)224-9880.

STURM, Heshy; 202-441 Clark Ave W, Thornhill ON L4J 6W8; Tor'78; Peds. Langs: Hebrew; (905)764-5114

STURMAN, Dubravka; Markham Stouffville Hosp, PO Box 1800 Stn Main 381 Church St, Markham ON L3P 7P3; Zagreb (Croatia)'64; GenPath. Staff, Markham Stouffville Hospital; Langs: Croatian; (905)472-7044

STURMER, Marcio L; Hop du Sacre-Coeur de Mtl, 5400 boul Gouin O, Montreal QC H4J 1C5; Rio Grande (Brazil)'94; Staff, Hôpital du Sacre-Coeur de Montréal; (514)338-2222; Fax. (514)338-3410.

STURMWIND, Jakob; Shelbourne Med Clinic, 150-3200 Shelbourne St, Victoria BC V8P 5G8; Alb'75; CCFP; Ac Staff, Royal Jubilee Hospital; Assoc Staff, Victoria General Hospital; (250)592-8485; Fax. (250)598-2489.

STURMY, S Paul; 205-220 Main St, Antigonish NS B2G 2C2; Dal'75; CCFP; (902)863-3201; Fax. (902)867-5662.

STURWOLD, Nichole M; Marathon Family Health Team, PO Box 399 22 Peninsula Rd, Marathon ON P0T 2E0; Dublin (Ireland)'10; MB BCh; BAO; CCFP; (807)229-3243

STUSHNOFF, James J; South Hill Med Clinic, 890A Lillooet St W, Moose Jaw SK S6H 8B4; Sask'06; Staff, South Hill Medical Centre; Physician, Saskatchewan Medical Association; (306)691-0030; Fax. (306)694-5666.

STUTZ, Eric M; North York Family Health Team, 702-240 Duncan Mill Rd, North York ON M3B 3S6; Tor'07; CCFP; Staff, North York General Hospital; Staff, North York Family Health Team-Central Office; (416)494-7435; Fax. (416)494-4819.

STYFFE, Philip T; Care Point Med Centre, 711 Pender St W, Vancouver BC V6C 3T2; UBC'83; Vis Staff, Vancouver General Hospital - Centennial Pavillion; (604)687-4858

STYLES, Janet K; Queen Elizabeth II HSC, 2105-1796 Summer St, Halifax NS B3H 4S3; Mem'05; FRCPC; IntMed; Cardiol. Staff, Queen Elizabeth II Health Sciences Centre - Halifax Infirmary Site; (902)473-4941; Fax. (902)473-2434.

STYLES, Scott G; 728 Anderson St, Whitby ON L1N 3V6; McM'00; FRCPC; Peds. (905)666-0039; Fax. (905)666-0618.

STYRA, Rima G; Univ Hlth Network-The Toronto, EN8 219-200 Elizabeth St, Toronto ON M5G 2C4; Tor'81; FRCPC; Psy. Assoc Prof, Toronto General Hospital - UHN; Asst Prof, University of Toronto; Langs: Lithuanian; (416)340-4825; Fax. (416)340-4198; rima.styra@uhn.on.ca.

STYRSKY, Eva M; Humber River Reg Hosp-Keele, 2175 Keele St, York ON M6M 3Z4; Tor'80; FRCPC; Psy. Staff, Humber River Regional Hospital - Keele Street Site; (416)658-2062; Fax. (416)658-2009.

STYS, Anna M; Aspen Med Clinic, 221-339 Aspen Glen Landing SW, Calgary AB T3H 0N6; Ott'84; CCFP; (403)263-7997; Fax. (403)263-7996.

STYS, Peter K; Foothills Med Centre, 12F-1403 29 St NW, Calgary AB T2N 2T9; Ott'84; FRCPC; Neur. Staff, Foothills Medical Centre; Staff, Hotchkiss Brain Institute; Staff, University of Calgary; (403)944-1447; Fax. (403)944-1154.

SU, Antonio J; CSSS de Laval, 1755 boul Rene-Laennec, Laval QC H7M 3L9; Laval'04; Anes. Staff, Hopital de la Cite de la santé; (450)975-5342

SU, Charles H; Winchester District Mem Hosp, 566 Louise St, Winchester ON K0C 2K0; Wes'98; CCFP; CCFP(E.M.); Staff/Chief EmergMed, Winchester District Memorial Hospital; Dir Distributed Med Education, University of Ottawa; (613)774-2420

SU, Didacus; Villa Marconi Nursing Home, 1026 Baseline Rd, Ottawa ON K2C 0A6; Ott'67; CCFP; FCFP; Staff, Queensway Carleton Hospital; Staff, Villa Marconi Nursing Home; Langs: Chinese; (613)224-0194; Fax. (613)224-0573.

SU, Jason W S; Durham Sports Centre, 1883 Kingston Rd, Pickering ON L1V 1C9; Tor'96; BScPharm; Dip(SportsMed); CCFP; Staff, Rouge Valley Health System - Centenary Health Centre Site; Physician, Athletics Commissioner; Staff, SPC Sports Performance Center; Clin Researcher, University of Toronto; Langs: Mandarin; (905)428-9370; Fax. (905)428-2396.

SU, Jean; MUHC-Royal Victoria Hosp, 687 av des Pins O, Montreal QC H3A 1A1; Cal'96; CCFP; CCFP(E.M.); Staff, McGill University Health Centre - Royal Victoria Hospital; (514)934-1934 x34277; Fax. (514)843-2852.

SU, Jenny C; Lions Gate Hosp, 231 15th St E, North Vancouver BC V7L 2L7; UBC'03; FRCPC; DiagRad. Staff, Lions Gate Hospital; (604)988-3131

SU, Michael C T; Foothills Med Centre, 1403 29 St NW, Calgary AB T2N 2T9; Ott'96; CCFP; CCFP(E.M.); Staff, Foothills Medical Centre; (403)944-1315

SU, Shih-Hann; CHUM-Hop Notre-Dame, 1560 rue Sherbrooke E, Montreal QC H2L 4M1; Mon'03; FRCPC; MedMicrobiol; InfectDis (P.Q.). Staff, Centre Hospitalier l'Université de Montréal (CHUM) - Hôpital Notre-Dame; (514)890-8000

SU, Winnie; Regent Med Bldg, 250-2184 Broadway W, Vancouver BC V6K 2E1; UBC'00; CCFP; (604)733-5181; Fax. (604)733-5184.

SU, Xiao Y; Source Unique Clinic, 219 Main St E, Hawkesbury ON K6A 1A1; Mon'10; CCFP; (613)632-4185

SUAZO HIDALGO, Lina M; Salveo Family Med Clinic, B8-6455 MacLeod Trail SW, Calgary AB T2H 0K8; (Other Foreign)'96; CCFP; Langs: Spanish; (403)444-0428; Fax. (403)537-0029.

SUBAI, Ziad; Centre Med Urgence d'Anjou, 103-7811 boul Louis-H.-Lafonta, Anjou QC H1K 4E4; Beirut (Lebanon)'69; (514)353-7892; Fax. (514)355-1935.

SUBBARAO, Padmaja; The Hosp for Sick Children, 4534-555 University Ave, Toronto ON M5G 1X8; Tor'94; MSc(Epidem.); FRCPC; Peds (Pediatric Respirology); Respir. Staff, The Hospital For Sick Children; Asst Prof, University of Toronto; (416)813-6167; Fax. (416)813-6246.

SUBERU, Ganiyu B; Weyburn Mental Health Centre, PO Box 2003 Stn Main, Weyburn SK S4H 2Z9; Lagos University (Other Foreign)'96; FRCPC; Psy. Chief Psy, Weyburn Community Health Services (Mental Health); (306)842-2665; Fax. (306)842-8690.

SUBHANI, Khaja N; Gladstone Prof Centre, 6155 North St, Halifax NS B3K 5R3; Osmania (India)'62; (902)453-3511; Fax. (902)454-9010.

SUBLETT, Stirling F; Cambridge Mem Hosp, 700 Coronation Blvd, Cambridge ON N1R 3G2; Tor'73; Staff, Cambridge Memorial Hospital; (519)621-2330

SUBRAMAN, Priya; Regional Mental Health Care, PO Box 5532 Stn B 850 Highbury Ave, London ON N6A 4H1; Rajah Muthiah Medical College (India)'91; Staff, Regional Mental Health Care-St Joseph's Health Care; (519)455-5110

SUBRAMANIAM, Suresh; South Health Campus, 4448 Front St SE, Calgary AB T3M 1M4; Dr M G R Medical University (India)'00; FRCPC; Neur. Staff, Foothills Medical Centre; Staff, South Health Campus; (403)956-2461; Fax. (403)956-2992.

SUBRAMANIAM, Tharani; Bowmanville Prof Bldg, 2101-222 King St E, Bowmanville ON L1C 1P6; Kursk State Medical University (Other Foreign)'04; CCFP; (905)697-3607

SUBRAMANIAN, Anantasivan; Niagara Falls Med Centre, 304-6453 Morrison St, Niagara Falls ON L2E 7H1; Bombay (India)'88; MS; FRCSC; GenSurg. Langs: Hindi; Marathi; Tamil; (289)296-0499; anants65@yahoo.com.

SUBRAMANIAN, Aravind; The Doctor's Office, 4701B 130th Ave SE, Calgary AB T2Z 4J2; Joao Pessoa (Brazil)'96; Physician, The Doctors Office; Langs: Portuguese; Spanish; Tamil; (403)232-1000; Fax. (403)257-6353.

SUBRAMANIAN, Ganesh K; The Sleep Disorders Clinic, 7-55 Frid St, Hamilton ON L8P 4M3; Wes'06; FRCPC; IntMed; Respir. (905)529-3068

SUBRAMANIAN, Thangamani; Shakti Med Clinic, 1309 Main St W, Hamilton ON L8S 1C5; Madras (India)'70; DObstRCOG; CCFP; FCFP; Ac Staff Family Pract, Hamilton Health Sciences Centre - McMaster University Medical Centre; Court Staff, St Joseph's Healthcare - Charlton Campus; Court Staff, Hamilton Health Sciences Centre-Juravinski Site; Asst Prof Family Med, McMaster University; Langs: Hindi; Malayalam; Tamil; (905)529-6560; Fax. (905)529-6573.

SUBZWARI, Sayed; PO Box 541, Nakusp BC V0G 1R0; (Other Foreign)'96; CCFP.

SUCHAK, Amar A; Londown Towne Square, 120-6707 Elbow Drive SW, Calgary AB T2V 0E3; Man'02; FRCPC; DiagRad. Staff, University of Alberta Hospital.

SUCHAK, Nayana A; Towne Centre Medical, 201-3601 Highway 7 E, Markham ON L3R 0M3; Man'96; CCFP; (905)604-3336; Fax. (905)604-7750.

SUCHAROV, Maxwell S; 208-2760 Broadway W, Vancouver BC V6K 2G4; McG'70; MDCM; FRCPC; Psy. (604)732-0011; Fax. (604)266-6849.

SUCHET, Ian B; Radiology Associates of Regina, 6-2727 Parliament Ave, Regina SK S4S 6X5; Witwatersrand (South Africa)'82; MB ChB; FRCPC; DiagRad. Ac Staff Radiol, Regina General Hospital; Physician, Radiology Associates of Regina; (306)352-7653; Fax. (306)522-4311; is@accesscomm.ca.

SUCHOWERSKY, Oksana; University of Alberta Hosp, 23E.32 WMC-8440 112 St, Edmonton AB T6G 2B7; Cal'78; FCCMG; FRCPC; Neur (Medical Genetics). Ac Staff Neurological Sciences, Foothills Medical Centre; Consultant, Alberta Children's Hospital; Dept Head Med Genetics/Prof, University of Calgary; Langs: Ukrainian; (780)407-7497; Fax. (780)407-1325; oksana.suchowersky@albertahealthservices.ca.

SUCIU, Cristina-Delia; Brant Community HC-Brantford, 200 Terrace Hill St, Brantford ON N3R 1G9; Cluj (Romania)'81; FRCPC; Anes. Staff, The Brant Community Healthcare System - Brantford General Hospital Site; Langs: Romanian; (519)751-5508

SUCIU, Valentin S; 207-285 Aurora Cres, Kelowna BC V1X 7N6; Cluj (Romania)'81; CCFP; (250)765-8220; Fax. (250)765-9015.

SUD, Abhimanyu; 200-236 Avenue Rd, Toronto ON M5R 2J4; Tor'09; CCFP; Lecturer Family Med/Clin Assoc Prof Pain Management, University of Toronto; (416)922-2000; Fax. (416)922-2005.

SUD, Anil K; Four Rivers Med Clinic, 878 Main St, Winnipeg MB R2W 3P1; Man'92; Staff, Seven Oaks General Hospital.

SUD, Sachin; Trillium Hlth Ctre-Mississauga, 100 Queensway W, Mississauga ON L5B 1B8; Wes'03; FRCPC; IntMed (Critical Care Medicine). Staff, Trillium Health Centre - Mississauga; (905)848-7663; Fax. (905)804-7744.

SUD, Shelly; The Ottawa Hosp-Gen Campus, 501 Smyth Rd, Ottawa ON K1H 8L6; McG'03; CCFP; IntMed. Staff Medical Oncology Training Program, The Ottawa Hospital - General Campus; Langs: Hindi; French; (613)722-7000

SUDAI, Tamar; Don Valley Med Associates, 216-1333 Sheppard Ave E, North York ON M2J 1V1; McG'83; CCFP; FCFP; Assoc Staff, North York General Hospital; Lecturer Family & Commun Med, University of Toronto; Langs: Hebrew; French; (416)498-4445; Fax. (416)498-3114; tsudai@baycrest.org.

SUDBURY, Ian D; 2001 107 St, Blairmore AB T0K 0E0; Cal'10; CCFP; (403)562-8804

SUDBURY, M Susan F; Peterborough Reg Health Ctre, 1 Hospital Dr, Peterborough ON K9J 7C6; Qns'84; FRCPC; IntMed; Rheum. Staff, Peterborough Regional Health Centre - Hospital Drive; (705)743-2121

SUDDABY, Kenneth W G; 900-275 Slater St, Ottawa ON K1P 5H9; Man'89; FRCPC; Psy (Couples & Family Therapy). (613)230-1916; Fax. (613)822-5182.

SUDHARSHAN, Namratha; 6-1109 Summerside Dr SW, Edmonton AB T6X 0H5; Bangalore University (India)'00; FRCPC; Neur. (780)469-3434; Fax. (780)469-5979.

SUDOL, Malgorzata M; Alder Med Clinic, 1211 8th Ave W, Vancouver BC V6H 1C7; Alb'04; FRCPC; PhysMed&Rehab. Staff, G F Strong Rehabilitation Centre; (604)734-2553

SUE, Donna; 203-3825 Sunset St, Burnaby BC V5G 1T4; UBC'89; Langs: Cantonese; (604)434-9515; Fax. (604)434-5984.

SUE, Michelle T; West Mississauga Medical, 3050 Argentia Rd, Mississauga ON L5N 8E1; Tor'99; BSc; CCFP; (905)785-3627; Fax. (905)785-3628.

SUE, Sammy C W; Markham Stouffville Hosp, PO Box 1800 Stn Main 381 Church St, Markham ON L3P 7P3; Tor'06; CCFP; CCFP(E.M.); Staff, Markham Stouffville Hospital; (905)472-7000

SUE-A-QUAN, Andrew I; St Joseph's Health Centre, 30 The Queensway, Toronto ON M6R 1B5; Tor'94; CCFP; CCFP(E.M.); Staff, Rouge Valley Health System - Centenary Health Centre Site; Staff, St Joseph's Health Centre; (416)530-6000

SUE-A-QUAN, Errol A; Medical Centre, 206-1939 Kennedy Rd, Scarborough ON M1P 2L9; Edinburgh (Scotland)'63; FRCS; DABOS; OrthSurg (Feet Seating & Mobility). Ac Staff, Rouge Valley Health System - Centenary Health Centre Site; (416)282-9200; Fax. (416)282-0906.

SUE-A-QUAN, Gregory T; St Joseph's Health Centre, 30 The Queensway, Toronto ON M6R 1B5; Wes'94; FRCPC; IntMed. Staff, St Joseph's Health Centre; (416)530-6000 x3722; Fax. (416)530-6107.

SUE-A-QUAN, Penelope A; Medical Centre, 206-1939 Kennedy Rd, Scarborough ON M1P 2L9; Edinburgh (Scotland)'64; (416)282-9200; Fax. (416)282-0906.

SUE-CHUE-LAM, Andrew K; Mackenzie Richmond Hill Hosp, 10 Trench St, Richmond Hill ON L4C 4Z3; Tor'78; FRCPC; AnatPath. Staff, The Credit Valley Hospital; Staff, Mackenzie Richmond Hill Hospital; (905)883-1212

SUE-CHUE-LAM, Jerry; Campbellford Mem Hosp, PO Box 1027 146 Oliver Rd, Carrying Place ON K0K 1L0; Aberdeen (Scotland)'71; MB ChB; DAB; FRCSC; GenSurg. Staff, Campbellford Memorial Hospital; (705)653-1140

SUEN, Kenneth C H; 1103-1483 Homer St, Vancouver BC V6Z 3C7; (Hong Kong)'65; DAB; FRCPC; AnatPath; GenPath. Consultant Path, Vancouver General Hospital - Centennial Pavillion; Clin Prof, University of British Columbia; (604)899-0240; Fax. (604)899-0240.

SUEN, Wai Yeung W; 9052 208 St NW, Edmonton AB T5T 1X6; Alb'70.

SUES-MCKAY, Heather A; Brampton Nuclear Services, 28-470 Chrysler Dr, Brampton ON L6S 0C1; Qns'97; CCFP; CCFP(E.M.); Staff, Mount Sinai Hospital; (905)791-3458

SUESS, Andrew M; The Hosp for Sick Children, 555 University Ave, Toronto ON M5G 1X8; Wes'06; FRCPC; Anes. Staff Anesthesia & Pain Med, The Hospital For Sick Children; (416)813-7500

SUESS, Christine J; 10 Montreal Rd, Cornwall ON K6H 1B1; Chicago (USA)'96; BA; FRCSC; Ophth. Chief Ophthalmology Service/Staff, Cornwall Community Hospital; (613)936-9130; Fax. (613)936-9727.

SUGA RAK, Michelle S; 204-2425 Tecumseh Rd E, Windsor ON N8W 1E6; Wes'00; FRCSC; ObstGyn. (519)254-6461

SUGAI, Michael K; 102-27 Major Mackenzie Dr E, Richmond Hill ON L4C 1G6; McM'78; FRCPC; IntMed; Rheum. Ac Staff Int Med, Mackenzie Richmond Hill Hospital; Court Consultant, Southlake Regional Health Centre; Court Consultant, Markham Stouffville Hospital; (905)883-0500; Fax. (905)883-0501.

SUGAMORI, Mark E; Riverview Med Group, 205 Queen St E, Fergus ON N1M 1T2; Tor'89; BASc; MASc; CCFP; FCFP; Staff, Groves Memorial Community Hospital; (519)787-7418; Fax. (519)787-7421; mark.sugamori2@sympatico.ca.

SUGAR, Linda M; Sunnybrook Hlth Sciences Ctre, 2075 Bayview Ave, Toronto ON M4N 3M5; McM'75; FRCPC; IntMed; AnatPath. Staff, Sunnybrook Health Sciences Centre; Asst Prof, University of Toronto; (416)480-4120

SUGAR, Paul S; 6412 Bay St, West Vancouver BC V7W 2H1; Tor'73; Ac Staff, Lions Gate Hospital; (604)984-5738; Fax. (604)984-3798.

SUGARS, Benjamin J A; Misericordia Community Hosp, 16940 87 Ave NW, Edmonton AB T5R 4H5; Cal'07; FRCPC; IntMed. Staff, Covenant Health - Misericordia Community Hospital; (780)735-2000; Fax. (780)735-9091.

SUGARS, John G; Lethbridge Mental Hlth Clinic, 200 5 Ave S, Lethbridge AB T1J 4C7; Queensland (Australia)'63; MB; BSc; FRCPC; Psy. Staff, Lethbridge Mental Health Clinic; (403)381-5260

SUGARS, William P; Hys Med Centre, 202-11010 101 St NW, Edmonton AB T5H 4B9; Alb'93; FRCPC; DiagRad. (780)426-1121; Fax. (780)425-5979.

SUGDEN, Stuart R; Elkford Healthcare Centre, PO Box 250 212 Alpine Way, Elkford BC V0B 1H0; New South Wales (Australia)'91; MB BS; (250)865-2215; Fax. (250)865-7289.

SUGGITT, Terry E; North Perth Family Health Team, 185 Inkerman St E, Listowel ON N4W 2N1; Ott'00; CCFP; (519)291-4200; Fax. (519)291-5947.

SUGIMOTO, Akira K; London HSC-Victoria Hosp, PO Box 5010 Stn B 800 Commissioners Rd E, London ON N6A 5W9; Wes'90; FRCSC; ObstGyn (Surgical Oncology). Staff, London Health Sciences Centre - Victoria Campus; (519)685-8088; Fax. (519)685-8176.

SUGIYAMA, I F H James; Taddle Creek Connection, B102-726 Bloor St W, Toronto ON M6G 4A1; Tor'86; Ac Staff, St Joseph's Health Centre; Langs: Spanish; (416)964-0800; Fax. (416)964-2935.

SUH, Daniel; Uxbridge Family Health Clinic, B-2 Elgin Park Dr, Uxbridge ON L9P 0B1; Nottingham (England)'08; CCFP; (905)852-1009; Fax. (905)852-3531.

SUH, Huhn Soo; East Kootenay Reg Hosp, 13 24th Ave N, Cranbrook BC V1C 3H9; Kyungpook (South Korea)'63; DAB; FASCP; Dir Labs/Head Path, East Kootenay Regional Hospital; (250)426-5281; Fax. (250)426-8052.

SUH, Kathryn N; The Ottawa Hosp-Civic Campus, 1053 Carling Ave, Ottawa ON K1Y 4E9; Ott'89; FRCPC; IntMed; InfectDis. Staff, The Ottawa Hospital - Civic Campus; Assoc Prof Med & Peds, University of Ottawa; (613)761-4155; Fax. (613)761-5260.

SUH, Matthew C K; 201-436 Gilmour St, Ottawa ON K2P 0R8; Seoul (Korea)'57; DPsy(McG.); FRCPC; Psy (Psychoanalysis). Consultant, The Ottawa Hospital - General Campus; Consultant, Royal Ottawa Mental Health Centre - Royal Ottawa Health Care Group; Member, Canadian Institute of Psychoanalysis; Clin Assoc Prof Psy, University of Ottawa; (613)234-7573; Fax. (613)744-8528; matthew.suh@mcgill.ca.

SUH, Sung-Hee; Guildford Med Clinic, 14650 104 Ave, Surrey BC V3R 1M3; (Other Foreign)'03; CCFP; (604)582-8985

SUH, Young S; St Luke Family Practice, 5-5761 Glover Rd, Langley BC V3A 8M8; Alb'86; CCFP; FCFP; Langs: Korean; (604)530-5825; Fax. (604)530-5828.

SUHADOLC, Thomas G; Smithville Family Health Ctre, PO Box 218 230 Canboro St, Smithville ON L0R 2A0; Tor'81; CCFP; FCFP; Ac Staff, West Lincoln Memorial Hospital; Teach Staff Family Med, McMaster University; (905)957-3328; Fax. (905)957-2475.

SUHAIL, Tariq; Belgage Med Arts Bldg, 104-525 Belmont Ave W, Kitchener ON N2M 5E2; Karachi (Pakistan)'91; FRCPC; IntMed (Rheumatology). (519)743-5858

SUHANI, N Gabriel; 111 rue Saint-Laurent, Saint-Eustache QC J7P 3Z5; Iuliu Hatieganu University of Medicine & Pharmacy (Romania)'94; FRCPC; Psy (Adult & Individual Psychotherapy). Staff Psy, Hôpital de Saint-Eustache; Langs: Romanian; English; (450)473-1720; Fax. (450)473-6369; gsuhani2@yahoo.fr.

SUJANA KUMAR, Shoba; Women's College Hosp, 4F-76 Grenville St, Toronto ON M5S 1B2; Wes'03; FRCPC; IntMed; Endocrin&Metab. Staff Endocrin Program, Women's College Hospital; (416)323-6013; Fax. (416)323-6534.

SUK, Allison L; Montebello Med Centre, 8-118 Lake St, St. Catharines ON L2R 5Y4; Wes'03; CCFP; (905)685-6555; Fax. (905)685-6558.

SUK, Andy G; 401A-101 Queensway W, Mississauga ON L5B 2P7; McG'97; FRCPC; IntMed (Diabetology); Endocrin&Metab. Staff, Trillium Health Centre - Mississauga; Langs: Mandarin; (905)272-9232; Fax. (905)272-8984.

SUK, Jean C; Riverside Prof Centre, 205-1919 Riverside Dr, Ottawa ON K1H 1A2; McG'87; FRCPC; Peds. Langs: French; (613)737-3121; Fax. (613)737-6048.

SUKE, Ralph; Saugeen Shores Med Bldg, 36 Grey St N, Southampton ON N0H 2L0; McM'79; CCFP; FCFP; Staff, South Bruce Grey Health Centre - Kincardine Site; (519)797-3805; Fax. (519)797-2674; rmsuke@hotmail.com.

SUKERMAN, Darren J; Summerville Family Health Team, 211-190 Sherway Dr, Etobicoke ON M9C 5N2; Columbia Medicine & Health Sciences with Ben Gurion University (Israel)'02; BSc(Physiology); BEd; Staff/Member Medical Education Committee/Leader Family Practice, Trillium Health Centre - West Toronto; Prof part-Time Dept of Med/Site Coord Trillium-ASCM 1 Mississauga Academy of Med, University of Toronto; (416)621-9700; Fax. (416)621-4438; dsukerman@thc.on.ca.

SUKERMAN, Sydney; 202-717 Richmond St, London ON N6A 1S2; Tor'72; FRCSC; Otol (Head & Neck Surgery). Ac Staff, London Health Sciences Centre - Victoria Campus; Ac Staff, St Joseph's Hospital - St Joseph's Health Care; Consultant, Woodstock General Hospital; Assoc Prof, University of Western Ontario; (519)672-4700; Fax. (519)672-7323; drssukerman@on.aibn.com.

SUKHAI, Natasha P; William Osler HC-Etobicoke, 101 Humber College Blvd, Etobicoke ON M9V 1R8; Ott'06; CCFP; Staff, William Osler Health System - Etobicoke General Hospital; (416)494-2120

SUKHERA, Javeed I; London HSC-Victoria Hosp, PO Box 5010 Snt B 800 Commissioners Rd E, London ON N6A 5W9; Ben Gurion (Israel)'07; Staff, London Health Sciences Centre - Victoria Campus; (519)685-8500; Fax. (519)685-8595.

SUKHRANI, Geeta; Tawa Centre, 219-3017 66 St NW, Edmonton AB T6K 4B2; Delhi (India)'76; FRCPC; Peds. (780)463-2863; Fax. (780)450-0360.

SUKKAR, Ghassan A A; The Hosp for Sick Children, 555 University Ave, Toronto ON M5G 1X8; King Abdul Aziz U (Saudi Arabia)'03; Staff, The Hospital For Sick Children; (416)813-5711; Fax. (416)813-1500.

SUKKHU, Visham; Prince Albert Med Clinic, 681 15th St W, Prince Albert SK S6V 7H9; Natal (South Africa)'94; MB ChB; Physician, Prince Albert Medical Clinic; (306)764-1505; Fax. (306)764-7775; visham_s@yahoo.com.

SUKOSD, Eva; Saint Joseph's Hosp, 130 Bayard Dr, Saint John NB E2L 3L6; (Romania)'81; Staff, Saint John Regional Hospital; Staff, St Joseph's Hospital; (506)632-5508; Fax. (506)632-5598.

SULA, Sharon L; 1479 Indian Grove, Mississauga ON L5H 2S5; Tor'79; CCFP; FCFP; Ac Staff, Trillium Health Centre - Mississauga; (905)274-7225; Fax. (905)271-4322.

SULAIMAN, Ibrahim H H; Thompson Gen Hosp, 871 Thompson Dr S, Thompson MB R8N 0C8; Al-Fateh (Libya)'98; FRCPC; Anes. Staff, Thompson General Hospital; Staff, Northern Health Thompson Regional Office; (204)778-1576

SULAIMAN, Mahabat H A; Minnedosa Med Group, PO Box 810 120 Second Ave SW, Minnedosa MB R0J 1E0; '86; (204)868-5062; Fax. (204)867-2986.

SULEIMAN, Ali M; Plaza II Mall, 613A-8600 Franklin Ave, Fort McMurray AB T9H 4G8; (780)748-2974; Fax. (780)748-2978.

SULEIMAN, Thomas; 102-8585 160 St, Surrey BC V4N 1G4; Wurzburg (Germany)'73; CCFP; Staff Emerg & Man Power Committee, Surrey Memorial Hospital; Clin Assoc Prof, University of British Columbia; (604)593-5085

SULEMAN, Mohamed R; True North Imaging, 200-751 Victoria St S, Kitchener ON N2M 5N4; Makerere (Uganda)'72; FRCPC; DiagRad. Staff, Guelph General Hospital; Langs: Kacchi; (519)570-2198; Fax. (519)570-3405.

SULEMAN, Shiraz; Bramalea Med Centre, 207-18 Kensington Rd, Brampton ON L6T 4S5; Natal (South Africa)'87; MB ChB; FACOG; FRCSC; ObstGyn. Langs: Hindi; (905)792-5027; Fax. (905)792-0631.

SULIKOWSKI, Angelina; Niagara H System-Welland Site, 65 Third St, Welland ON L3B 4W6; Academy of Medicine (USA)'00; CCFP; Staff, Niagara Health System - Welland Hospital Site; (905)738-4647

SULIMAN, Asem S M; St Mary's Health Centre, PO Box 353, St Marys NL A0B 3B0; Locum Tenens, Dr Walter Templeman Health Centre; Physician, St Mary's Health Centre; (709)525-2980; asem.suliman@easternhealth.ca.

SULL, Thomas J; Mackenzie Richmond Hill Hosp, 10 Trench St, Richmond Hill ON L4C 4Z3; Tor'07; CCFP; CCFP(E.M.); Staff, Mackenzie Richmond Hill Hospital; (905)883-1212; Fax. (905)883-2138.

SULLIVAN, Arthur K; 508-465 Richmond Rd, Ottawa ON K2A 1Z1; Vermont (USA)'71; FRCPC; Hem (Psychiatric Oncology); Psy. Court Staff Psy, Queensway Carleton Hospital; Consultant staff, The Ottawa Hospital - General Campus; (613)422-3843; Fax. (613)422-4998.

SULLIVAN, Barry J; 203-3040 Tutt St, Kelowna BC V1Y 2H5; Tor'91; FRCSC; GenSurg. Staff, Kelowna General Hospital; Langs: Bilingual(English/French); (250)763-2226; Fax. (250)861-5937.

SULLIVAN, Brian J M; 70 Ferguson Ave N, Hamilton ON L8R 1L4; Tor'79; ABIM; FRCPC; Cardiol (Clinical Cardiology); IntMed. Court Staff, Hamilton Health Sciences Centre - McMaster Children's Hospital; Ac Staff Cardiol, St Joseph's Healthcare - Charlton Campus; Asst Prof Med, McMaster University; (905)529-8926; Fax. (905)529-2280.

SULLIVAN, David B; Thamesview Family Health Team, 103-20 Emma St, Chatham ON N7L 5K5; RCS (Ireland)'84; MB ChB; CCFP; Staff, Chatham-Kent Health Alliance; (519)352-2476; Fax. (519)354-9011.

SULLIVAN, Glendon E; Saint John Reg Hosp, PO Box 2100 Stn Main 400 University Ave, Saint John NB E2L 4L2; Lexington(KY) (USA)'83; FACP; FCCP; ABIM; FRCPC; IntMed (Respirology). Staff, Saint John Regional Hospital; (506)648-6000

SULLIVAN, Hugh P C; Sullivan Cardiology, 70 Ferguson Ave N, Hamilton ON L8R 1L4; McM'83; BSc(Tor); FRCPC; IntMed; Cardiol. Ac Staff, St Joseph's Healthcare - Charlton Campus; Staff, Sullivan Cardiology Associates; Asst Prof Med, McMaster University; (905)529-8926; Fax. (905)529-2280.

SULLIVAN, James D; Clinique Med St-Jacques, 101-5515 rue Saint-Jacques, Montreal QC H4A 2E3; McG'62; MSc; FRCSC; OrthSurg (Sports Medicine). assoc Staff, St Mary's Hospital Centre; Conférencier Orth, McGill University; Langs: Bilingual(English/French); (514)489-8216; Fax. (514)489-8061.

SULLIVAN, John A P; Queen Elizabeth II HSC-Halifax, 2268-1796 Summer St, Halifax NS B3H 3A7; Dal'74; FRCSC; Cardiovasc&ThorSurg. Staff, Queen Elizabeth II Health Sciences Centre - Halifax Infirmary Site; (902)473-7933; Fax. (902)473-4448; john.sullivan@dal.ca.

SULLIVAN, John H; Canso Med Clinic, PO Box 162 1760 Union St, Canso NS B0H 1H0; Dal'71; GenSurg. Staff, South Shore Regional Hospital; (902)366-2171; Fax. (902)366-2556.

SULLIVAN, John M; Bridgewater Family Practice, 450 Lahave St, Bridgewater NS B4V 4A3; Dal'81; (902)543-9923; Fax. (902)543-6260.

SULLIVAN, Kathleen M C; Burrard Health Bldg, 407-1160 Burrard St, Vancouver BC V6Z 2E8; Tor'88; FRCSC; Ophth (AIDS/HIV). Staff, Providence Health Care - St Paul's Hospital; University of British Columbia; (604)685-6348; Fax. (604)638-6135.

SULLIVAN, Liezl; Alder Med Centre, 277 Evergreen RD, Campbell River BC V9W 5Y4; Pretoria (South Africa)'94; CCFP; (250)287-7454

SULLIVAN, Michael E; Southlake Reg Health Centre, 596 Davis Dr, Newmarket ON L3Y 2P9; Ott'86; FRCPC; Anes. Staff Anes & Critical Care, Southlake Regional Health Centre; University of Toronto; (905)895-4521

SULLIVAN, Michael J J; Sullivan Cardiology, 70 Ferguson Ave N, Hamilton ON L8R 1L4; McM'76; ABIM; FRCPC; IntMed; Cardiol. Staff Cardiol, St Joseph's Healthcare - Charlton Campus; Assoc Prof Med, McMaster University; (905)529-8926; Fax. (905)529-2280.

SULLIVAN, Patrick D; Kennedy Services Complex, 7B-20 Kennedy Dr, Sussex NB E4E 2P1; Dal'74; Staff, Sussex Health Centre; (506)432-4300; Fax. (506)432-4306.

SULLIVAN, Patrick J; The Ottawa Hosp-Civic Campus, PO Box 249C B310-1053 Carling Ave, Ottawa ON K1Y 4E9; Tor'83; FRCPC; Anes. Staff, The Ottawa Hospital - Civic Campus; University of Ottawa; (613)761-4169; Fax. (613)761-5209.

SULLIVAN, Patrick J; Patient Networks, 157 Yonge St, Toronto ON M5C 1X7; Wes'04; CCFP; Staff, The Ottawa Hospital - Civic Campus; Langs: Bilingual(English/French); (416)362-8822; Fax. (416)362-8877.

SULLIVAN, Paul A; St Joseph's Health Centre, 220-30 The Queensway, Toronto ON M6R 1B5; Tor'96; FRCSC; GenSurg (Laparoscopic Surgery). Staff, St Joseph's Health Centre; Court Staff, Toronto East General Hospital Inc; (416)530-6030; Fax. (416)530-6520.

SULLIVAN, Peter J; Three Sisters Obst & Fam Med C, 106-75 Dyrgas Gate, Canmore AB T1W 0A6; Dal'08; CCFP; (403)609-9095; Fax. (403)609-7232; peterjohnsullivan@hotmail.com.

SULLIVAN, Shelley E; Killick Health Services Inc, 54 Union St, Grnd-Falls-Windsor NL A2A 2E2; Mem'98; CCFP; Staff, Central Newfoundland Regional Health Centre; (709)292-8400; Fax. (709)292-8443.

SULLIVAN, Thomas J; Trinity Conception Med Assoc, PO Box 903 Stn Main 16 Goff Ave, Carbonear NL A1Y 1C4; Mem'75; Ac Staff, Carbonear General Hospital; (709)596-5135; Fax. (709)596-0212.

SULLIVAN, Tracy; Carling-Broadview Med Bldg, B7-770 Broadview Ave, Ottawa ON K2A 3Z3; UBC'85; (613)761-1919; Fax. (613)761-1357.

SULLIVAN, William F; Family Practice Unit, 3F-61 Queen St E, Toronto ON M5C 2T2; Tor'86; BSc; PhD(Philosophy); CCFP; Staff Family & Commun Med, St Michael's Hospital; Staff Family Med, Surrey Place Centre; Assoc Prof Family & Commun Med, University of Toronto; (416)867-7426; Fax. (416)867-7498; bill.sullivan@utoronto.ca.

SULLOVEY, Amanda J; Sunnybrook Hlth Sciences Ctre, FG 29-2075 Bayview Ave, Toronto ON M4N 3M5; Ott'04; FRCPC; Psy. Staff, Sunnybrook Health Sciences Centre; (416)480-5677; Fax. (416)480-6878.

SULLOVEY, Carl A; Medical & Dental Bldg, 702-586 Eglinton Ave E, Toronto ON M4P 1P2; McG'77; CCFP; Court Staff, The Scarborough Hospital - General Campus; Court Staff, Rouge Valley Health System - Centenary Health Centre Site; Court Staff Family Pract, Sunnybrook Health Sciences Centre; (416)483-8796; Fax. (416)322-5286.

SULLY, Irma-Nancy; AMSPM, 330 Sparks St, Ottawa ON K1A 0N8; Ott'98; CCFP; Staff, Health Canada; Langs: Creole; French; (613)993-9436

SULLY LETAL, Jillian C; 1207 18A St NW, Calgary AB T2N 2H5; Sask'03; FRCPC; Anes. Staff, Foothills Medical Centre; (403)992-8862

SULOWSKI, Christopher A; McMaster Univ-Children's Hosp, HSC 3A-1280 Main St W, Hamilton ON L8S 4K1; Tor'06; FRCPC; Peds; PedEmergMed. Staff, McMaster University; (905)521-2100

SULPHER, Jeffrey A; Univ of Ottawa, 2044-451 Smyth Rd, Ottawa ON K1H 8M5; Qns'08; FRCPC; IntMed.

SULTAN, Daria A; CSSS Bordeaux-Cartierville, 555 boul Gouin O, Montreal QC H3L 1K5; Iasi (Romania)'89; Staff, CSSS des Sources d'Asbestos; Staff, Pavillon Notre-Dame de la Merci; Langs: English; Romanian; (514)331-3025; Fax. (514)331-2053; lastdaria@hotmail.com.

SULTAN, Ghazala; Chatham-Kent Family Health Team, 207-20 Emma St, Chatham ON N7L 5K5; Punjab (Pakistan)'85; CCFP; Staff Family Health Team, Chatham-Kent Health Alliance; Aj Prof Family Med, University of Western Ontario; Langs: Urdu; Hindi; Punjabi; (519)354-2172; Fax. (519)354-0886.

SULTAN, Khaleel H S H; London HSC-University Campus, PO Box 5339 Stn B 339 Windermere Rd, London ON N6A 5A5; RCS (Ireland)'01; Gastroent; IntMed. Staff Gastroent, London Health Sciences Centre - University Hospital; (519)685-8500

SULTAN, Mahmud M T; Grantham Plaza, B2-400 Scott St, St Catharines ON L2M 3W4; Al-Arab Medical University (Libya)'90; MB BCh; CCFP; Langs: Arabic; (905)937-0000; Fax. (905)937-0030.

SULTAN, Mazen; Ctr Hosp du Centre la Mauricie, 50 119e rue, Shawinigan-Sud QC G9P 5K1; Alger (Algeria)'86; Ophth (P.Q.). Staff, Centre Hospitalier du Centre la Mauricie; Langs: Bilingual(French/English); (819)536-7500; mazen.sultan@cgocable.ca.

SULTAN, Nabil M; London HSC-Victoria Hosp, PO Box 5010 Stn B A2 337-800 Commissioners Rd E, London ON N6A 5W9; Wes'04; FRCPC; IntMed; Nephrol. Staff, London Health Sciences Centre - Victoria Campus; Staff, London Health Sciences Centre - University Hospital; Langs: Arabic; (519)685-8385

SULTAN, Omar; Regina Arrhythmia Centre, 2500A 11th Ave, Regina SK S4P 0K5; St Kitts & Nevis University (Other Foreign)'02; FRCPC; IntMed (Cardiac Electrophysiology); Cardiol. Med Dir, Electrophysiology & Pacemaker Clinic; Med Dir, Regina Qu'Appelle Health Region; Langs: Hindi; French; Spanish; Urdu; (306)522-0831; Fax. (306)522-0834; sultanoffice@sasktel.net.

SULTAN, Soraya G S; McGill University Hlth Centre, P3 066-1025 av des Pins O, Montreal QC H3A 1A1; McG'86; BSc(Hon); CSPQ; DrMedCh; FRCPC; Psy (Sleep Disorders). Consultant, McGill University Health Centre - Royal Victoria Hospital; Staff, Allan Memorial Institute; adj Prof Psy, McGill University; Langs: French; (514)934-1934 x35503; Fax. (514)843-2858; sgs.etc@gmail.com.

SULTANA, Roksana; Riverview Health Centre, 1 Morley Ave, Winnipeg MB R3L 2P4; Dacca (Bangladesh)'75; Staff, Riverview Health Centre; (204)452-3411

SULTANA, Samar; Landsdowne Shopp Centre, 5124 122 St NW, Edmonton AB T6H 3S3; (Other Foreign)'99; CCFP; (780)437-8818; Fax. (780)439-5557.

SULTANA, Shahida; Markham Stouffville Hosp, PO Box 1800 Stn Main 381 Church St, Markham ON L3P 7P3; Chittagong (Pakistan)'94; FRCPC; IntMed. Staff, Markham Stouffville Hospital; Langs: Bengali; (905)472-7000

SULTANEM, Ibrahim A; Ctr Hosp du Centre la Mauricie, 50 119e rue, Shawinigan-Sud QC G9P 5K1; Damascus (Syria)'89; IntMed. Staff, Centre Hospitalier Universitaire de Sherbrooke-Hopital Fleurimont; (819)536-7500; Fax. (819)536-7649; ibrahim.sultanem@tr.cgocable.ca.

SULTANEM, Khalil; SMBD Jewish Gen Hosp, G002-3755 ch Cote-Sainte-Cathe, Montreal QC H3T 1E2; Sher'90; FRCPC; RadOncol (Therapeutic Radiology). Staff, Sir Mortimer B Davis Jewish General; Langs: Arabic; English; (514)340-8288; Fax. (514)340-7548; ksultane@roc.jgh.mcgill.ca.

SULTANIAN, Richard A; Zeidler Ledcor Centre, 2 20A-130 University Campus NW, Edmonton AB T6G 2X8; Alb'05; Gastroent; IntMed. Staff, University of Alberta Hospital; (780)492-1458; Fax. (780)492-8148.

SULYMA, Lelia Y L; Broadview Med Centre, 202-741 Broadview Ave, Toronto ON M4K 3Y3; Cal'79; (416)778-7355; Fax. (416)778-1518.

SULYMAN, Mutiat O; East Coast Forensic Hosp, 88 Gloria McCluskey Dr, Dartmouth NS B3B 2B8; Usman Danfodyo University College (Other Foreign)'99; MB BS; Staff, The East Coast Forensic Psychiatry Hospital; (902)460-7300; mutiat.sulyman@cdha.nshealth.ca.

SULZ, Carey J; Parksville Med Clinic, PO Box 250 Stn Main 154 Memorial Ave W, Parksville BC V9P 2G4; Cal'92; (250)248-5757; Fax. (250)248-2128.

SUM, Edric C H; 301-3024 Hurontario St, Mississauga ON L5B 4M4; (Hong Kong)'70; Ac Staff, Trillium Health Centre - Mississauga; Langs: Cantonese; Mandarin; (905)273-7171; Fax. (905)273-9990.

SUMANAC, Katica; 203-60 Hatt St, Dundas ON L9H 7T6; Belgrade (Serbia)'82; CCFP; Langs: Croatian; Serbian; (905)627-1800; Fax. (905)627-1700; kates@sumanac.com.

SUMAR, Shahirose; Eagle Ridge Hosp & Hlth CC, 475 Guildford Way, Port Moody BC V3H 3W9; UBC'91; Staff, Eagle Ridge Hospital & Health Care Centre; (604)461-2022

SUMMERS, Leslie B; Ross Mem Hosp, 10 Angeline St N, Lindsay ON K9V 4M8; Glasgow (Scotland)'68; MB ChB; Staff, Ross Memorial Hospital; (705)324-6111; Fax. (705)328-2817; lesliebcan@netscape.net.

SUMNER, Glen L; Foothills Med Centre, C822B-1403 29th St NW, Calgary AB T2N 2T9; Qns'90; BSc(Hons); FRCPC; IntMed (Cardiac Pacing); Cardiol. Staff, Foothills Medical Centre; Physician, Libin Cardiovascular Institute; Asst Prof Med, University of Calgary; Langs: Bilingual(English/French); (403)944-3258; Fax. (403)944-3262.

SUMNER, Michael G; Erin Mills Med Centre, PO Box 80 E229A-5100 Erin Mills Pky, Mississauga ON L5M 4Z5; Hahnemann(PA) (USA)'66; DABPN(P); FRCPC; Psy (General Psychiatry & Neurological Psychiatry & Mino). (905)593-9269

SUN, Alexander Y; 5-815-610 University Ave, Toronto ON M5G 2M9; Tor'89; AB; FRCPC; RadOncol. Staff, Princess Margaret Hospital - University Health Network; (416)946-2126; Fax. (416)946-6561.

SUN, Anna K; 101-4695 Hastings St, Burnaby BC V5C 2K6; UBC'97; CCFP; Staff, Metrotown Centre; (604)298-7201; Fax. (604)291-6176.

SUN, Charles Y; Victoria Emerg Phys Mgmt Ltd, 325-1627 Fort St, Victoria BC V8R 1H8; Wes'71; FRCPC; EmergMed. (250)479-1442

SUN, Christina H Y; Glazier Med Centre, 11 Gibb St, Oshawa ON L1H 2J9; Ceylon (Sri Lanka)'90; MB BS; FRCSC; ObstGyn. Staff, Lakeridge Health - Oshawa Site; (905)579-1212; Fax. (905)579-2021.

SUN, Christopher K; Queensway Prof Centre, 102-190 Sherway Dr, Etobicoke ON M9C 5N2; Qns'08; CCFP; (416)622-4762; Fax. (416)622-4763.

SUN, Clement K; Addiction Centre of Toronto, 1288 Danforth Ave, Toronto ON M4J 1M6; Tor'74; Physician, Addiction Centre of Toronto; (416)462-0228; Fax. (416)461-7690; clement.sun@albertahealthservices.ca.

SUN, Dongmei; London HSC-Victoria Hosp, 800 Commissioners Rd E, London ON N6A 5W9; Shanghai Medical University (China)'93; FRCPC; IntMed. Staff, London Health Sciences Centre - University Hospital; Staff, London Health Sciences Centre - Victoria Campus; (519)685-8500

SUN, Gavin R; Vulcan Med Clinic, PO Box 419 610 Elizabeth St, Vulcan AB T0L 2B0; Johannesburg (South Africa)'06; MB BCh; CCFP; (403)485-2216; Fax. (403)485-2218.

SUN, Hao; Mapleton Health Centre, 11 Andrews Dr W, Drayton ON N0G 1P0; Ott'10.

SUN, I-Chia W; Crossroads Clinics, 350-507 Broadway W, Vancouver BC V5Z 1E6; Sask'99; CCFP; (604)568-1337

SUN, J Jianhang; Westlock Healthcare Centre, 10220 93 St, Westlock AB T7P 2G4; Shanghai (China)'86; Staff, Westlock Healthcare Centre; (780)349-3301

SUN, Jenet H F; Richmond Public Market, 2270-8260 Westminster Hwy, Richmond BC V6X 3Y2; UBC'89; Staff, Richmond Hospital; Langs: Chinese; (604)821-1112; Fax. (604)821-1274.

SUN, John C L; CBI Health Centre, 202-940 Goldstream Ave, Victoria BC V9B 2Y4; Cal'95; BSc(Hons.); FRCSC; Neursurg (Spine). Clinical Faculty, University of British Columbia; Langs: Mandarin; (250)391-7850; Fax. (250)391-6668; landrade@cbi.ca.

SUN, Joyce; 620-943 Broadway W, Vancouver BC V5Z 1K3; UBC'88; CCFP; FCFP; Staff, Surrey Memorial Hospital; Langs: Cantonese; Mandarin; (604)738-8030; Fax. (604)738-8021.

SUN, Kathryn A; McGill Sport Med Clinic, 475 av des Pins O, Montreal QC H2W 1S4; McG'02; CCFP; (514)398-4035; Fax. (514)398-4035; ksu13@hotmail.com.

SUN, Keith L; Royal Columbian Hosp, 330 Columbia St E, New Westminster BC V3L 3W7; Sask'03; FRCPC; Anes. Staff Anes, Royal Columbian Hospital; Langs: Cantonese; (604)520-4253

SUN, Louise Y P; The Ottawa Hosp-Civic Campus, 1053 Carling Ave, Ottawa ON K1Y 4E9; McM'08; Staff Anes, The Ottawa Hospital - Civic Campus; (613)722-7000

SUN, Ning-Zi; Hopital Chinois de Montreal, 189 av Viger E, Montreal QC H2X 3Y9; McG'07; MDCM; IntMed. Staff, Hôpital Chinois de Montréal; (514)871-0961

SUN, Ping; Health Sciences Centre, MS5595-820 Sherbrook St, Winnipeg MB R3A 1R9; Shandong Medical University (China)'95; FRCPC; HemPath. Staff, Health Sciences Centre; (204)787-8513

SUN, Rosemarie H L; Care Point Med Centre, 140-555 Sixth St, New Westminster BC V3L 5H1; Colombo (Sri Lanka)'82; MB BS; CCFP; (604)523-1166; Fax. (604)523-1722.

SUN, Siwen; CLSC-CHSLD PAT Montreal Est, 13926 rue Notre-Dame E, Montreal QC H1A 1T5; McG'10; MDCM; CCFP; (514)494-4924

SUN, Sophie; BC Cancer Agency-Vancouver CC, 4567-600 10th Ave W, Vancouver BC V5Z 4E6; Tor'00; FRCPC; IntMed; MedOncol. Staff, BC Cancer Agency Vancouver Centre; (604)877-6000 x2730; Fax. (604)877-0585.

SUN, W David; Hampton Med Clinic, 6274 199 St NW, Edmonton AB T5T 2K4; McG'09; CCFP; (780)486-7370; Fax. (780)486-7335.

SUN, Xiaoli; The Ottawa Hosp-Gen Campus, 501 Smyth Rd, Ottawa ON K1H 8L6; Nanjing Medical College (China)'98; Staff, The Ottawa Hospital - General Campus; (613)737-8561

SUN, Yi-Hui; Hawkwood Village Med Clinic, 20-217 Hawksbrow Dr NW, Calgary AB T3G 3K2; Capital University of Medical Sciences (Other Foreign)'85; PhD; CCFP; Staff, Foothills Medical Centre; Langs: Chinese; (403)777-2757; Fax. (403)777-2755.

SUNDAR, Ishaan P; Regina Qu'Appelle HC-Regina, 1440 14th Ave, Regina SK S4P 0W5; Lucknow (India)'94; MB BS; CCFP; Staff, Regina General Hospital; (306)766-4444

SUNDARALINGAM, Nirmala; Ontario Shores Ctr Mental HS, PO Box 613 700 Gordon St, Whitby ON L1N 5S9; Ceylon (Sri Lanka)'76; MB BS; MRCPsy(UK); FRCPC; Psy (Child & Adolescent Psychiatry). Staff Psy/Med Dir Adolescent Young Adults/Dual Diagnosis, Ontario Shores Centre for Mental Health Sciences; Langs: Tamil; (905)668-5881

SUNDARALINGAM, Theepa; Rouge Valley-Centenary HC, 2867 Ellesmere Rd, Scarborough ON M1E 4B9; Tor'07; FRCPC; IntMed; MedOncol. Staff, Rouge Valley Health System - Centenary Health Centre Site; (416)281-7483

SUNDARAM, Arun N E; Univ Hlth Network-Toronto Western Hosp, 5F-399 Bathurst St, Toronto ON M5T 2S8; Rajiv Gandhi (India)'97; FRCPC; Neur (Neuro Ophthalmology). Staff, Toronto Western Hospital - University Health Network; Langs: Kanarese; (416)603-5660; Fax. (416)603-6222.

SUNDARAM, Manickavasagam; Lakeridge Health Corp-Oshawa, 1 Hospital Crt, Oshawa ON L1G 2B9; Alb'02; CCFP; Staff, Lakeridge Health - Oshawa Site; Langs: French; (905)576-8711; Fax. (905)721-7763.

SUNDARAM, Sujatha; Medical & Dental Bldg, 216-1849 Yonge St, Toronto ON M4S 1Y2; Mem'90; CCFP; (416)487-9309; Fax. (416)487-9790.

SUNDARARAJAN, Kanchanamala; Dr Kanchana Sundar Inc, 6637 Hwy 1, Kentville NS B4R 1B7; Stanley Medical College (Other Foreign)'89; MB BS; (902)679-6650; Fax. (902)679-1739.

SUNDARESAN, R Sudhir; The Ottawa Hosp-Gen Campus, 6361-501 Smyth Rd, Ottawa ON K1H 8L6; Ott'83; FRCSC; GenSurg (Surgical Oncology); ThorSurg. Chief Thoracic Surg, The Ottawa Hospital - General Campus; Dept Chair Surgery(interim), University of Ottawa; Langs: Bilingual(English/French); (613)737-8899; Fax. (613)737-8668; ssundaresan@ottawahospital.on.ca.

SUNDARESWARAN, Shanthini; 204-160 Dundas St E, Mississauga ON L5A 1W4; (Cuba)'87; CCFP; Langs: Spanish; Tamil; Sinhalese; (905)270-9111; Fax. (905)270-9114; shanthy88@hotmail.com.

SUNDBY, Kirk A; 1729B Comox Ave, Comox BC V9M 3M2; UBC'79; FRCSC; OrthSurg. Staff, Royal Inland Hospital; (250)941-0080

SUNDER, Ravi K B; Royal Inland Hosp, 311 Columbia St, Kamloops BC V2C 2T1; Tor'08; CCFP; CCFP(E.M.); Staff, Royal Inland Hospital; (250)374-5111

SUNDERJI, Nadiya A; St Josephs Health Centre, SWW 445-30 The Queensway, Toronto ON M6R 1B5; Wes'03; FRCPC; Psy. Staff Women's Mental Health, Women's College Hospital; Staff, St Joseph's Health Centre; (416)530-6486; Fax. (416)530-6076.

SUNDERJI, Salim H J; 2320 Main St, London ON N6P 1A9; Nairobi (Kenya)'73; MB ChB; CCFP; FCFP; Aj Prof Med, University of Western Ontario; (519)652-5996; Fax. (519)652-1694.

SUNDERLAND, Dorothy J; 27 Third St, Collingwood ON L9Y 1K4; McM'87; CCFP; Ac Staff, Collingwood General & Marine Hospital; Langs: French; (705)445-4111; Fax. (705)445-8250; cmc@cois.on.ca.

SUNDERLAND, Ian R P; 602-750 Spadina Cres E, Saskatoon SK S7K 3H1; Washington University (USA)'05; FRCSC; PlasSurg. (306)653-7766; Fax. (306)653-7768.

SUNDERLAND, Mark P; 694 Seymour St, Kamloops BC V2C 2H2; Qns'73; ABPS; FACS; FRCSC; PlasSurg. Ac Staff, Royal Inland Hospital; (250)374-9722; Fax. (250)374-9758.

SUNDVICK, Sharon M; 101-1032 Austin Ave, Coquitlam BC V3K 3P3; UBC'89; (604)939-2441; Fax. (604)939-2420.

SUNEJA, Sumeet K; Regional Kidney Wellness Cntre, 3 Conestoga Blvd, Brampton ON L6Z 4N5; McM'01; Nephrol; IntMed. Staff, William Osler Health System - Brampton Civic Hospital; Langs: Punjabi; Urdu; Hindi; (905)497-0114; Fax. (905)497-7114.

SUNENBLICK, Robert E; 370-4060 rue Sainte-Catherine, Westmount QC H3Z 2Z3; Philadelphia (USA)'74; (514)488-5553; Fax. (514)807-5380.

SUNERH, Pal S; 303-1525 Albion Rd, Etobicoke ON M9V 5G5; Punjab (India)'78; Staff, William Osler Health System - Etobicoke General Hospital; Langs: Hindi; Punjabi; Urdu; (416)748-9600; Fax. (416)748-3092.

SUNG, Deborah H; Fairmount Med Clinic, 7811 Fairmount Dr SE, Calgary AB T2H 0X8; Cal'03; CCFP; (403)242-7300; Fax. (403)242-7302.

SUNG, Emily E K C; E-1001 Austin Ave, New Westminster BC V3K 3N9; UBC'09; CCFP; (604)937-2520

SUNG, Henry M H; Vancouver Gen Hosp, 855 12th Ave W, Vancouver BC V5Z 1M9; UBC'77; FRCPC; Anes. Ac Staff, Vancouver General Hospital - Centennial Pavillion; Clin Assoc Prof, University of British Columbia; (604)875-4304; Fax. (604)875-5209.

SUNG, Hyun J; Glenrose Rehab Hosp, 10230 111 Ave NW, Edmonton AB T5G 0B7; (Other Foreign)'98; CCFP; Staff, Glenrose Rehabilitation Hospital; (780)735-7999

SUNG, Lillian; The Hosp for Sick Children, 555 University Ave, Toronto ON M5G 1X8; Ott'93; FRCPC; Peds; Hem; InfectDis. Staff Peds, The Hospital For Sick Children; (416)813-5287; Fax. (416)813-5979.

SUNG, Patrick P W; PO Box 741 Stn Main, Vegreville AB T9C 1R8; Alb'83; Staff, Covenant Health - St Joseph's General Hospital; Langs: Cantonese; Mandarin; Spanish; (780)632-2811; Fax. (780)632-6182.

SUNG, Yong Kyung; Univ Hlth Network-The Toronto, 200 Elizabeth St, Toronto ON M5G 2C4; Wes'91; Staff, Toronto General Hospital - UHN; (416)715-5317

SUNKARA, Madhava R; Forest Lawn Medicentre, 1814 33 St SE, Calgary AB T2B 0T4; (403)235-5651; Fax. (403)248-1741.

SUNNER, Parveen K; University of Alberta Hosp, 8440 112 St NW, Edmonton AB T6G 2B7; Alb'07; DiagRad. Staff, University of Alberta Hospital; (780)407-6810; Fax. (780)407-6176.

SUNNER, Sohail; 16-2120 North Park Dr, Brampton ON L6S 0C9; Saba (Netherlands Antilles)'06; CCFP; Langs: Punjabi; (905)792-0100; Fax. (905)792-0190.

SUNSHINE, Stanley L; Medical Bldg, 1101-805 Broadway W, Vancouver BC V5Z 1K1; UBC'60; CCFP; FCFP; Att Staff, Vancouver General Hospital - Centennial Pavillion; Chairman Medical Review Panel, Work Safety & Insurance Board of BC; Instructor, University of British Columbia; (604)879-5271; Fax. (604)879-8712; stanley.sunshine@worksafebc.com.

SUPALA-BERGER, Agnes Z; St Joseph's Health Centre, 30 The Queensway, Toronto ON M6R 1B5; Munich (Germany)'93; FRCPC; Neur. Staff, St Joseph's Health Centre; Langs: German; Hungarian; (416)530-6000

SUPERINA-BELL, Diann J; St Michael's Hosp, 30 Bond St, Toronto ON M5B 1W8; McG'75; MDCM; FRCPC; Peds (Developmental Pediatrics). Staff, St Michael's Hospital; University of Toronto; Langs: Spanish; Portuguese; French; Italian; (416)489-7690

SUPERSTEIN, Rosanne; Hôpital Ste-Justine, 3175 ch Cote Saiinte-Catherine, Montreal QC H3T 1C5; McG'94; FRCSC; Ophth. assoc Membre, Centre Hospitalier l'Université de Montréal (CHUM) - Hôpital Notre-Dame; assoc Membre, Hôpital Ste-Justine; Staff, McGill University Health Centre - Montreal Children's Hospital; assoc Membre, Universite de Montreal; (514)345-2347 x2; Fax. (514)345-4880; rosanne.superstein@mcgill.ca.

SUPPAL, Priya; Shoppers World Med Centre, 106-499 Main St S, Brampton ON L6Y 1N7; McM'92; CCFP; FCFP; Staff, William Osler Health System - Brampton Civic Hospital; Langs: Hindi; Punjabi; (905)796-6570; Fax. (905)796-3977.

SUPPES, Robert J; Sault Area Hosp, 750 Great Northern Rd, Sault Ste. Marie ON P6B 0A8; Man'08; CCFP; Staff, Sault Area Hospital - Sault Ste Marie; (705)297-9722

SUPPIAH, Nagappan; Health Sciences Centre, 300 Prince Philip Dr, St. John's NL A1B 3V6; Madras (India)'74; MB BS; FRCPC; Anes (Obstetrics Anesthesia). Staff Anes, Health Sciences Centre; Langs: Tamil; (709)777-6540; Fax. (709)777-6506.

SUR, Monalisa; Hamilton HS-Henderson Site, 100-711 Concession St, Hamilton ON L8V 1C3; Punjab (India)'89; MRCPath(UK); FRCPC; AnatPath (Surgical Pathology). Staff/Assoc Prof, Hamilton Health Sciences Centre-Juravinski Site; Langs: Hindi; Bengali; Punjabi; (905)527-4322 x42033; Fax. (905)389-1698.

SUR, Ranjan K; The Juravinski Cancer Centre, 699 Concession St, Hamilton ON L8V 5C2; Osmania (India)'84; PhD; FRCPC; RadOncol. Staff, Hamilton Health Sciences Centre-Juravinski Site; Staff, Hamilton Health Sciences Centre - McMaster Children's Hospital; Prof, McMaster University; Langs: Hindi; Bengali; (905)387-9711; Fax. (905)575-6326.

SUR, Smeeksha S; Medical Office, 21-1098 Peter Robertson Blvd, Brampton ON L6R 3A5; Punjab (India)'97; MB BS; FRCPC; Peds (Allergy). Langs: Hindi; Punjabi; Urdu; (905)458-6999; Fax. (905)458-5202.

SURAJBALLI, Hemchand; The Pas Health Complex, PO Box 240, The Pas MB R9A 1K4; Natal (South Africa)'80; MB ChB; CCFP; Staff/Anesthetist, St. Anthony General Hospital; Langs: Hindi; (204)623-6431

SURANGIWALA, Sabiha M; Meadowvale Prof Centre, 102-6855 Meadowvale Town Ctre, Mississauga ON L5N 2Y1; Pune (India)'93; DOMS; MB BS; CCFP; Langs: Hindi; Urdu; Marathi; (905)567-9900; Fax. (905)567-9011.

SURANI, Karim S; 417-751 3 St SW, Calgary AB T2P 4K8; Alb'81; CCFP; (403)234-0066; Fax. (403)233-8679.

SURANYI, Leslie; St Lawrence Med Bldg, 5-614 Second St E, Cornwall ON K6H 1Z8; Budapest (Hungary)'67; FRCPC; Neur (Neuro Physiology). Langs: Hungarian; (613)936-1366; Fax. (613)347-1068.

SURANYI-CADOTTE, Barbara E; Douglas Mental Hlth Univ Inst, 6875 boul Lasalle, Verdun QC H4H 1R3; Montpellier (France)'75; MSc; FRCPC; Psy (Psycho Geriatrics). ac Staff, Douglas Mental Health University Institute; assoc Prof, McGill University; Langs: Hungarian; (514)761-6131

SURAPANENI, Ramakrishna R; 487 Park St, Kitchener ON N2G 1N7; Karnatack (India)'72; MB BS; FRCPC; Psy. Langs: Hindi; Telugu; (519)744-5656; Fax. (519)744-6751.

SURBEY, Glenn D; Abbey Family Medicine, 2307 Khalsa Gate, Oakville ON L6M 4J2; Qns'86; CASM; CCFP; Staff, Halton Healthcare Services Corporation - Oakville Site; (905)847-1133; Fax. (905)847-9782.

SURBEY, Manindar; Scottsdale Med Centre, 100-101 Nicholson Rd, Delta BC V4E 1Z7; Sask'81; Langs: Spanish; Punjabi; (604)596-4211

SURESH, Hemalatha; Thorncliffe Family Med Clinic, 14-5440 4 St NW, Calgary AB T2K 1A8; Rangaraya (India)'74; MB BS; LRCP(Ed); LRCS(Scot.); CCFP; FCFP; (403)730-0224; Fax. (403)274-2136.

SURESH, Mulluvila R K; 14-5440 4 St NW, Calgary AB T2K 1A8; Kerala (India)'76; MB BS; LRCP(Ed); LRCS(Ed); LRCPS(Glas); (403)730-0224; Fax. (403)274-2136.

SURETTE, Joel Y; Yarmouth Reg Hosp, 60 Vancouver St, Yarmouth NS B5A 2P5; Dal'03; FRCPC; DiagRad. Staff Imaging Dept, Yarmouth Regional Hospital; (902)742-3542; Fax. (902)742-1238.

SURGENOR, Colum J; Associate Clinic, 5215 49 Ave, Wetaskiwin AB T9A 0R1; Dublin (Ireland)'79; MB ChB; BAO; (780)352-7157; Fax. (780)352-2273.

SURGENOR, Hannah; 4313 Gallant Ave, North Vancouver BC V7G 2C1; Manchester (England)'01; MB ChB; (604)929-5222

SURI, Michelle D; Isis Women's Health Clinic, 144-1402 8 Ave NW, Calgary AB T2N 1B9; Man'04; FRCSC; ObstGyn. Staff, Foothills Medical Centre; (403)289-8996; Fax. (403)289-8956.

SURI, Permjit S; Centrepointe Med Consultants, 106 Centrepointe Dr, Nepean ON K2G 6B1; Jiwaji (India)'78; FRCPC; IntMed (Infectious Diseases). Langs: Swahili; Punjabi; Gujarati; Hindi; Urdu; (613)224-6151 x22; Fax. (613)224-7228; travelmedclinic@rogers.com.

SURI, Pravesh K; Cornwall Prof Bldg, 415-2125 11th Ave, Regina SK S4P 3X3; Punjab (India)'65; (306)525-8355; Fax. (306)352-2213.

SURI, Rakesh M R; Pasqua Hosp, 4F-4101 Dewdney Ave, Regina SK S4T 1A5; Tor'95; FRCSC; GenSurg; CardSurg. Staff, Pasqua Hospital; (306)766-2222

SURI, Reena; Royal Oak Med Clinic, 192-8888 Country Hills Blvd, Calgary AB T3G 5T4; Cal'05; CCFP; (403)239-3660; rsuri.braich@gmail.com.

SURI, Rita; Hopital Saint-Luc, 1058 rue Saint-Denis, Montreal QC H2X 3J4; Sask'97; MSc; FRCPC; IntMed; Nephrol. Staff, Centre Hospitalier l'Université De Montréal (CHUM) - Hôpital Saint-luc; Langs: French; (514)890-8000

SURI, Shashi; Regina Qu'Appelle HR-Pasqua, 100-4101 Dewdney Ave, Regina SK S4T 1A5; Delhi (India)'69; FRCPC; Anes. Staff OR/Head Anes, Regina General Hospital; Clin Asst Prof, University of Saskatchewan; (306)766-2222

SURKA, Milosh S; Terra Nova Health Services, 160-3675 Westminster Hwy, Richmond BC V7C 5V2; Bratislava (Slovakia)'74; Physician, Tao Rehabilitation Clinic; Langs: Slovak; Czech; Polish; (604)278-9525 x9527

SURKAN, David L; 102-383 Ellis St, Penticton BC V2A 4K9; Sask'77; Ac Staff, Penticton Regional Hospital; (250)492-2022; Fax. (250)492-1022.

SURKAN, Donald G; Associate Med Clinic, 400-20 14th St W, Prince Albert SK S6V 3K8; Sask'80; LMCC; (306)953-1657; Fax. (306)764-3091.

SURKAN, John M; Dr J M Surkan Med Clinic, 620 Winnipeg St, Penticton BC V2A 5M9; Sask'83; Staff, Penticton Regional Hospital; (250)492-8802; Fax. (250)492-0610.

SURKAN, Michael W; White Clinic Associates, 100-383 Ellis St, Penticton BC V2A 4L9; Sask'75; CCFP; FCFP; Ac Staff, Penticton Regional Hospital; (250)492-3024; Fax. (250)492-2761.

SURKES, Jan; 112-20644 Eastleigh Cres, Langley BC V3A 4C4; Wes'86; FRCPC; IntMed; Cardiol (Echocardiography). Staff, Langley Memorial Hospital; (604)533-8803; Fax. (604)533-8581.

SURMA, Beata; 2F-333 Lakeshore Rd W, Mississauga ON L5H 1G9; Poznan University of Medical Sciences (Other Foreign)'04; (905)274-7055

SURMAWALA, Shahida; Westgate Medicentre, 101-9540 163rd St, Edmonton AB T5P 3M7; (Pakistan)'84; MB BS; CCFP; Clin Associate, Grey Nuns Community Hospital; Clin Associate, University of Alberta Hospital; Langs: Urdu; Kacchi; Punjabi; (780)489-4976; Fax. (780)481-6761.

SUROWANIEC, Tadeusz; Hopital du Suroit, 150 rue Saint-Thomas, Salaber-de-Valleyf QC J6T 6C1; McG'94; FRCSC; GenSurg. Staff, Hôpital Brome-Missisquoi-Perkins; Staff, Centre Hospitalier Régional du Suroît; (450)371-9920

SURPRENANT, Anne; CSSS Memphremagog, 435 rue Dufferin, Stanstead QC J0B 3E2; Mon'97; Staff, Centre Hospitalier Regional de Sept-Iles; Langs: English; (819)876-7521

SURRY, Susan A M; Simcoe Muskoka Dist Hlth Unit, 15 Sperling Dr, Barrie ON L4M 6K9; Wes'97; FRCPC; Peds (Public Health). (705)721-7520 x7398; Fax. (705)721-1495.

SURTI, Bhadreshchandra V; Regional Mental HC-Lodon, PO Box 5532 Stn B 850 Highbury Ave, London ON N6A 4H1; Gujarat (India)'75; MB BS; DPsy; FRCPC; Psy (Psycho Pharmacology & Psychotherapy). Staff, Regional Mental Health Care-St Joseph's Health Care; Consultant, London Health Sciences Centre - South Street; Consultant, Thunder Bay Regional Health Sciences Centre Port-Arthur; Assoc Prof, University of Western Ontario; Langs: Gujarati; Hindi; Urdu; (519)455-5110; Fax. (519)455-2677.

SURTIE, Elmo A; Royal University Hosp, 103 Hospital Dr, Saskatoon SK S7N 0W8; Stellenbosch (South Africa)'85; MB ChB; FRCPC; Anes. Staff, Royal University Hospital; (306)655-1183; Fax. (306)655-1279.

SURTIE, Faizel R; Rochdale Crossing Med Clinic, 7-5875 Rochdale Blvd, Regina SK S4X 2P9; Accra (Ghana)'81; MB ChB; (306)205-8020; Fax. (306)205-8023.

SURYANARAYAN, Deepa; Hamilton HS-McMaster Site, PO Box 2000 Stn Lcd 1 3W11-1200 Main St W, Hamilton ON L8N 3Z5; Mysore (India)'00; IntMed (Hematology).

SURYAVANSHI, Rajeev K; A-568 Christina St N, Sarnia ON N7T 5W6; Gorakhpur University (India)'89; MS; FRCSI; FRCSC; GenSurg (Laparoscopy). Aj Prof GenSurg, University of Western Ontario; Langs: Hindi; Punjabi; Urdu; (519)336-1800; Fax. (519)336-1801.

SURYAVANSHI, Shveta; Suryavanshi Med Clinic, A-568 Christina St N, Sarnia ON N7T 5W6; Gorakhpur University (India)'93; CCFP; Langs: Hindi; Punjabi; (519)336-1800; Fax. (519)336-1801.

SURYAVANSHI, Sudhir K; Warm & Cozy Personal Care Home, 502 Paton Cres, Saskatoon SK S7W 0B8; (Other Foreign)'89; (306)653-2273; Fax. (306)653-2279.

SUSANTO, Aida T; After Hours Med Clinic, 775 Strand Blvd, Kingston ON K7P 2S7; Tor'76; (613)546-5506

SUSIL, Monica; 25 Black Lake Rd, Lively ON P3Y 1J3; Saba Medical University (Other Foreign)'08; CCFP; Langs: Czech; French; (705)692-1018

SUSINI, Vincenzo R; Geraldston Dist Hosp, 500 Hogarth Ave W, Geraldton ON P0T 1M0; Saba (Netherlands Antilles)'07; Staff, Geraldton District Hospital; Langs: Italian; (807)854-1862; vsusini@geraldtondh.com.

SUSKIN, Neville G; London HSC-University Hosp, PO Box 5339 Stn B C6 124G-339 Windermere Rd, London ON N6A 5A5; Cape Town (South Africa)'84; MB ChB; MSc; FACC; FRCPC; Cardiol (Internal Medicine). Med Dir Cardiac Rehab & Secondary Prevention Prog, London Health Sciences Centre - University Hospital; (519)663-3488; Fax. (519)663-3583.

SUSMAN, Edison; 7-5550 Lawrence Ave E, Scarborough ON M1C 3B2; Tor'84; ATLS; ACLS; Staff, The Scarborough Hospital - General Campus; Staff, Rouge Valley Health System - Centenary Health Centre Site; Langs: Hebrew; Yiddish; (416)283-3700; Fax. (416)283-1453.

SUSS, Roger G; Victoria Gen Hosp, 2340 Pembina Hwy, Winnipeg MB R3T 2E8; Man'88; CCFP; CCFP(E.M.); FCFP; Staff, Victoria General Hospital; (204)269-3570

SUSSER, M Marc; Business Bldg, 401-400 Tache Ave, Winnipeg MB R2H 3C3; Man'83; (204)231-5500; Fax. (204)231-3319.

SUSSET, Veronique; Centre de Read Lucie-Bruneau, 2275 Av Laurier E, Montreal QC H2H 2N8; Paris (France)'53; FRCPC; PhysMed&Rehab (Alternative Medicine). Consultant, Centre de Readaptation Lucie-Bruneau; Langs: Bilingual(French/English); (514)527-4521 x2271; Fax. (514)527-6637.

SUSSEX, Bruce A; Health Sciences Centre, 1291-300 Prince Philip Dr, St. John's NL A1B 3V6; Melbourne (Australia)'74; MSc(ExpMed.); FRCPC; IntMed (Heart Failure); Cardiol. Ac Staff Med & Cardiol, Health Sciences Centre; Prof, Memorial University Of Newfoundland; (709)777-7337; Fax. (709)777-8069.

SUSSMAN, Gordon L; Medical Research, 202 St Clair Ave W, Toronto ON M4V 1R2; Wes'77; FACP; ABIM; FAAAAI; FRCPC; IntMed; ClinImmunol&Allergy. Prof Med, University of Toronto; (416)944-8333

SUSSMAN, Jack W; Keele Med Place, 2830 Keele St, North York ON M3M 3E5; Tor'74; Ac Staff, Humber River Regional Hospital - Finch Avenue Site; (416)633-6812; Fax. (416)633-6187.

SUSSMAN, Jillian; North York Gen Hosp-Branson, 555 Finch Ave W, North York ON M2R 1N5; Cal'03; FRCPC; Psy (Child & Adolescent Psychiatry). Staff, North York General Hospital - Branson Division; (416)632-8709; Fax. (416)632-8704.

SUSSMAN, Jonathan; The Juravinski Cancer Centre, 4 204-699 Concession St, Hamilton ON L8V 5C2; Tor'90; FRCPC; RadOncol;CCFP; Staff, The Juravinski Cancer Centre; Assoc Prof, McMaster University; Langs: German; French; (905)387-9495; Fax. (905)575-6326.

SUSSMAN, Sidney; Medical Imaging, NCSB1C 556-585 University Ave, Toronto ON M5G 2N2; Wes'76; FRCPC; DiagRad. Staff, Toronto General Hospital - UHN; Staff, Princess Margaret Hospital - University Health Network; Staff, Baycrest Centre for Geriatric Care; (416)340-4800 x3372; Fax. (416)593-0502.

SUSTRIK, Ryan A; St Boniface Gen Hosp, 409 Tache Ave, Winnipeg MB R2H 2A6; Alb'07; FRCPC; EmergMed. Staff, St Boniface General Hospital; (204)233-8563

SUSZEK, J Jeffrey G; Brant Community HC-Brantford, 200 Terrace Hill St, Brantford ON N3R 1G9; Tor'94; BSc; CCFP; CCFP(E.M.); FCFP; Staff Emerg Room, The Brant Community Healthcare System - Brantford General Hospital Site; (519)752-7871

SUTANDAR, Kalam; Univ Hlth Network-Toronto Gen, 8EN 220-200 Elizabeth St, Toronto ON M5G 2C4; Qns'05; FRCPC; Psy. Staff, Toronto General Hospital - UHN; (416)340-3111; Fax. (416)340-4198.

SUTANDAR, Marilyn; A-110 Queens Plate Dr, Etobicoke ON M9W 0B4; Ott'06; FRCSC; ObstGyn. Staff, William Osler Health System - Etobicoke General Hospital; (416)745-0770; Fax. (416)745-1377.

SUTANTO, Ian H; PO Box 88064 Rpo Rabbit Hill, Edmonton AB T6R 0M5; Alb'10; CCFP.

SUTCLIFFE, Graham V; Dr G V Sutcliffe Inc, 4425 Gertrude St, Port Alberni BC V9Y 6J7; Cardiff (Wales)'74; MB ChB; MRCGPract; DRCOG; Staff, West Coast General Hospital; (250)723-5822; Fax. (250)723-7304.

SUTCLIFFE, Ian T; Hôpital de Gatineau, 909 boul de la Verendrye, Gatineau QC J8P 7H2; Ott'05; FRCPC; IntMed; Gastroent. Staff, Hôpital de Gatineau; (819)966-6100

SUTCLIFFE, Penelope A; Sudbury & Dist & Health Unit, 1300 Paris St, Sudbury ON P3E 3A3; Tor'92; MHSc; FRCPC; CommunMed; Public Health & Preventive Med. Staff, Sudbury & District Health Unit Corporate Office; Langs: Bilingual(English/French); (705)522-9200 x291; Fax. (705)677-9606.

SUTCLIFFE, Steven D I; UBC Hospital, 2211 Wesbsrook Mall, Vancouver BC V6T 2B5; Sask'89; ABIM; FRCPC; IntMed (AIDS/HIV). Staff, UBC Hospital - Koerner Pavillion; Langs: German; (604)822-7121; Fax. (604)822-1796.

SUTHERLAND, Christy I; 1060 Howe St, Vancouver BC V6Z 1P5; Dal'08; CCFP; (604)682-0505

SUTHERLAND, David J; Central Health Consultants, 129 Lincoln Rd, Grnd-Falls-Windsor NL A2A 1P3; Dal'84; FRCSC; Urol. Ac Staff, Central Newfoundland Regional Health Centre.

SUTHERLAND, Donald F; St Joseph's Hosp, 130 Bayard Dr, Saint John NB E2L 3L6; Dal'89; CCFP; Staff, St Joseph's Hospital; Staff, Saint John Regional Hospital; Teach Staff, Dalhousie University; (506)632-5625; Fax. (506)632-5512.

SUTHERLAND, Donna E; Health Sciences Centre, GB 421-820 Sherbrook St, Winnipeg MB R3A 1R9; Man'92; FRCSC; Otol (Head & Neck Surgery). Staff, Health Sciences Centre; Asst Prof, University of Manitoba; (204)787-3349; Fax. (204)787-1727.

SUTHERLAND, Eleanor W; 204-474 Holland Ave, Ottawa ON K1Y 0Z5; Alb'53; Member, College Of Family Physicians Of Canada-Ontario; (613)729-1608; Fax. (613)729-1886.

SUTHERLAND, Eric N; Pan Am Pain Clinic, 75 Poseidon Bay, Winnipeg MB R3M 3E4; Man'92; FRCPC; Anes. Staff, Health Sciences Centre; Staff, Pain Management Centre.

SUTHERLAND, Francis R; Foothills Med Centre, 10F-1403 29 St NW, Calgary AB T2N 2T9; Cal'82; FRCSC; GenSurg (Hepatobiliary & Pancreatic Surgery). Staff Oncol, Tom Baker Cancer Centre; Staff, Foothills Medical Centre; Staff Teacher, University of Calgary; (403)944-1233; Fax. (403)944-3502; francis.sutherland@calgaryhealthregion.ca.

SUTHERLAND, Garnette R; Foothills Med Centre, 1403 29 St NW, Calgary AB T2N 2T9; Man'78; FRCSC; Neursurg. Ac Staff NeuroSurg, Foothills Medical Centre; (403)210-8557; Fax. (403)283-2270.

SUTHERLAND, George R; St Martha's Reg Hosp, 25 Bay St, Antigonish NS B2G 2G5; Dal'82; Staff, St Martha's Regional Hospital; (902)863-2830; Fax. (902)867-4432.

SUTHERLAND, Heather; Leukemia/BMT Program of BC, 10149-2775 Laurel St, Vancouver BC V5Z 1M9; Sask'80; PhD; FRCPC; IntMed (Bone Marrow Transplant); Hem. Ac Staff, Vancouver General Hospital - Centennial Pavillion; Staff Leukemia/Bone Marrow Transplantation Prog of BC, BC Cancer Agency Vancouver Centre; (604)875-4863

SUTHERLAND, I Scott; Medical Arts Bldg, 202-233 Kennedy St, Winnipeg MB R3C 3J5; Man'80; FRCPC; DiagRad (Neuro Radiology).

SUTHERLAND, James G; Boyd Med Centre, 412-388 Portage Ave, Winnipeg MB R3C 0C8; Man'82; Staff, Misericordia Health Centre; (204)943-6437

SUTHERLAND, Jeffrey; Halton Hills FHT-Guelph Street, UL-171 Guelph St, Georgetown ON L7G 4A1; Dal'91; CCFP; FCFP; Med Staff Family Med, Halton Healthcare Services Corporation - Georgetown Hospital; (905)877-4123; Fax. (905)873-8882.

SUTHERLAND, John D; University of Alberta Hosp, 2D2 14-8440 112 St, Edmonton AB T6G 2B7; Alb'00; FRCSC; GenSurg. Staff, University of Alberta Hospital; (780)407-8822; Fax. (780)407-7394.

SUTHERLAND, Judith A; BC Cancer Ctre-South Interior, 399 Royal Ave, Kelowna BC V1Y 5L3; Cal'87; BSc; MSc; FRCPC; IntMed; MedOncol; Hem. Staff, BC Cancer Agency Sindi Ahluwalia Hawkins Centre for the Southern Interior; Ac Staff, Kelowna General Hospital; Staff, BC Cancer Agency Vancouver Centre; (250)712-3996; Fax. (250)712-3911; jsutherl@bccancer.bc.ca.

SUTHERLAND, Karen E; Manitoba Adolescent Trmt Ctre, 120 Tecumseh St, Winnipeg MB R3E 2A9; Man'85; FRCPC; Psy (Child & Adolescent Psychiatry). Staff, Manitoba Adolescent Treatment Centre; (204)477-6391; ksutherland@matc.ca.

SUTHERLAND, Kathleen M; River City Med Clinic, PO Box 369 Stn A, Campbell River BC V9W 5B6; Cape Town (South Africa)'92; MB ChB; (250)287-2111; Fax. (250)287-2444.

SUTHERLAND, Katrine C; 4313 Gallant Ave, North Vancouver BC V7G 2C1; Glasgow (Scotland)'72; MB ChB; (604)929-5222; Fax. (604)929-3256.

SUTHERLAND, Kenneth B; Quinte Healthcare Corp-Bellevi, 265 Dundas St E, Belleville ON K8N 5A9; Dal'82; FRCPC; DiagRad., QHC Belleville General; Head Dept of Diagnostic Radiol, Queen's University; (613)969-7400 x2025; Fax. (613)969-5561.

SUTHERLAND, Kenneth S; Bay Street Walk-In Med Ctre, 960 3rd Ave E, Owen Sound ON N4K 2K9; Sask'70; Ac Staff, Grey Bruce Health Services - Owen Sound; Dir, Bay Street Walk-In Medical Centre; (519)376-4865; Fax. (519)376-4409.

SUTHERLAND, Kristiina A; North Bay Reg Health Centre, 680 Kirkwood Dr, Sudbury ON P3E 1X3; McM'06; FRCPC; Psy. Staff, North Bay Regional Health Centre - Kirkwood; (705)675-5900

SUTHERLAND, Lisa J C; PO Box 4791, Rothesay NB E2E 5X5; Dal'90; CCFP; FCFP; (506)849-8509; Fax. (506)849-8777.

SUTHERLAND, Lloyd R; 3330 Hospital Dr NW, Calgary AB T2N 4N1; McG'73; ABIM; AB; FACP; Gastroent; IntMed. Ac Staff, Foothills Medical Centre; (403)220-4696; Fax. (403)266-3618.

SUTHERLAND, Michelle; Morgan Creek Site Clinic, 106-15252 32 Ave, Surrey BC V3S 0R7; Poznan (Poland)'05; (604)542-4885

SUTHERLAND, Robert L; Alder Med Centre, 277 Evergreen Rd, Campbell River BC V9W 5Y4; Cape Town (South Africa)'87; MB ChB; CCFP; Staff ER, Campbell River & District General Hospital; Langs: Afrikaans; (250)287-7441; Fax. (250)287-4384.

SUTHERLAND, William E; Waycobah Med Centre, PO Box 351 93 Reservation Rd, Whycocomagh NS B0E 3M0; McM'08; (902)756-2156

SUTTER, F Michelle; Victoria Med Bldg, 315-1669 Victoria St, Prince George BC V2L 2L5; UBC'87; FRCS; FRCSC; GenSurg (Surgical Oncology). Staff GenSurg, University Hospital of Northern British Columbia; Assoc Prof, University of British Columbia; (250)562-2634; Fax. (250)562-2631.

SUTTER, Joan A; The Brandon Clinic, 620 Dennis St, Brandon MB R7A 5E7; Man'76; FRCSC; ObstGyn. Ac Staff, Brandon Regional Health Centre; (204)571-7135; Fax. (204)726-1765.

SUTTON, Ann; CHUQ-Ctr Hosp Univ Laval, 2705 boul Laurier, Quebec QC G1V 4G2; Laval'78; FRCPC; Gastroent (P.Q.). Clin Prof, Centre Hospitalier Universitaire de Quebec-CHUL; Langs: English; (418)654-2168; Fax. (418)654-2164; ann.sutton@chuq.qc.ca.

SUTTON, Bruce M; Park Towers, 106-400 Walmer Rd, Toronto ON M5P 2X7; Tor'83; FRCPC; Psy. Ac Staff, St Michael's Hospital; University of Toronto; (416)975-9554

SUTTON, Evelyn D; Nova Scotia Rehab Centre, 245-1341 Summer St, Halifax NS B3H 4K4; Dal'84; FRCPC; IntMed (Scleroderma); Rheum. Staff, Queen Elizabeth II Health Sciences Centre - Halifax Infirmary Site; Head Div of Rheumatology, Nova Scotia Rehabilitation Centre; Asst Dean Admissions/Prof Med, Dalhousie University; (902)473-7040; Fax. (902)473-7019; evelyn.sutton@cdha.nshealth.ca.

SUTTON, Frank R; Rockyview Prof Centre, 24-1011 Glenmore Trail SW, Calgary AB T2V 4R6; Alb'72; BSc; FRCSC; PlasSurg. (403)228-4211; Fax. (403)228-3362.

SUTTON, Gregory; Kelligrews Med Clinic, PO Box 17160, Conception-Bay-S NL A1X 3H1; Mem'05; CCFP; (709)834-2171

SUTTON, Hugh F S; Alta Vision Plus, 200-9401 Franklin Ave, Fort McMurray AB T9H 3Z7; London (England)'70; MB BS; DABOph; FAAO; FRCSC; Ophth (Laser Surgery). Staff, Seymour Medical Clinic; Staff, Central Eye Clinic; (780)790-2020; Fax. (780)743-8869.

SUTTON, Ian R; Health Sciences Centre, GG 5MS 261-820 Sherbrook St, Winnipeg MB R3A 1R9; Man'86; FRCPC; Anes. Staff, Health Sciences Centre; (204)774-6511

SUTTON, John R; Concordia Physio Sport, 262-7005 boul Taschereau, Longueuil QC J4Z 1A7; McG'73; FRCSC; OrthSurg. ac Staff, St Mary's Hospital Centre; (450)445-1556; Fax. (450)445-2998.

SUTTON, Neal S; 189 Acton Ave, Toronto ON M3H 4H6; Tor'82; (416)633-4843

SUTTON, Robert E; 312/314-688 Coxwell Ave, Toronto ON M4C 3B7; London (England)'63; MB BS; FRCPC; Peds. Att Staff, The Hospital For Sick Children; (416)465-2485; Fax. (416)465-7488.

SUTTON, Roger A L; BC Women's Hosp & Health Ctre, 4500 Oak St, Vancouver BC V6H 3N1; Oxford (England)'60; MB BCh; FRCP; FACP; FRCPC; IntMed (Nephrology). Med Dir Osteoporosis Clinic, BC Women's Hospital & Health Centre; Consultant, BC Children's Hospital; Emeritus Staff Limited, Vancouver General Hospital - Centennial Pavillion; Physician, Urology Stone Clinic; Emeritus Prof Med, University of British Columbia; (604)875-2018

SUTTON, Susan K; 100-20 Heritage Meadows Rd SE, Calgary AB T2H 3C1; Alb'90; CCFP; FCFP; (403)252-8851; Fax. (403)252-1765.

SUTTON-BROWN, Martin A; Jim Pattison Outpatient Care, 9750 140 St, Surrey BC V3T 0G9; Cal'02; FRCPC; Neur. Staff, Foothills Medical Centre; (604)582-4561

SUTTORP, Vivien V; 801 1 Ave S, Lethbridge AB T1J 4L5; UBC'94; BSc; MPH; CCFP; FCFP; Langs: Dutch; German; (403)388-6014; Fax. (403)320-0145.

SUZUKI, Aya; 257-346 John St N, Arnprior ON K7S 2P6; Tor'04; CCFP; (613)623-2048; Fax. (613)623-6719.

SVARC, Emile D; Complexe Sante Reine-Elizabeth, 412-2100 Av De Marlowe, Montreal QC H4A 3L5; Zagreb (Croatia)'62; DAB; FRCSC; Ophth. ac Staff, Sir Mortimer B Davis Jewish General; ac Staff, St Mary's Hospital Centre; ac Staff, Mount Sinai Hospital Center; Conférencier, McGill University; Langs: Croatian; French; Hebrew; Italian; Russian; Serbian; (514)485-5096; Fax. (514)485-5002.

SVARTBERG, Martin; Mount Sinai Hosp, 936-600 University Ave, Toronto ON M5G 1X5; Oslo (Norway)'78; PhD; MD; Psy. Staff, Mount Sinai Hospital; Langs: Danish; Norwegian; Swedish; (416)596-4200

SVED, Michael H; Minto Plaza, 1007-655 Bay St, Toronto ON M5G 2K4; Ott'88; FRCSC; ObstGyn. Staff, St Michael's Hospital; (416)408-4248; Fax. (416)408-0407.

SVEINBJORNSON, Timothy P; Anesthesia & Perioperative Med, 330 Columbia St E, New Westminster BC V3L 3W7; Ott'88; FRCPC; Anes. Staff Anes, Providence Health Care - St Paul's Staff, Royal Columbian Hospital; (604)528-5002

SVENTEK, Pavol; CSSS de la Vallée de l'Or, 725 6e rue, Val-d'Or QC J9P 3Y1; Bratislava (Slovakia),'80; CCFP; Staff, Centre Hospitalier de Val d'Or; Langs: Slovak; Czech; French; (819)825-6711; Fax. (819)825-7919.

SVIHOVEC, William J; Clinique CAMU, 100-1144 rue Saint-Laurent O, Longueuil QC J4K 1E5; McG'75; Langs: French; (450)651-5700; Fax. (450)651-9700.

SVIHRA, Martin W; Univ Hlth Network-Toronto Western Hosp, 9E 409-399 Bathurst St, Toronto ON M5T 2S8; Ott'03; FRCPC; Psy. Staff Community Mental Health, Toronto Western Hospital - University Health Network; (416)603-5605; Fax. (416)603-5490.

SVITEK, Jessica C; Centre Med & Prof de Dorval, 667 ch Bord-du-Lac Lakeshore, Dorval QC H9S 2B7; Laval'03; CCFP; Médecin, Hôpital Santa Cabrini Ospedale; Staff, CSSS de la Pointe de l'Île; Langs: English; (514)633-1510

SVOBODA, Tomislav; Seaton House Family Hlth Team, 339 George St, Toronto ON M5A 2N2; Tor'95; BSc; MSc; FRCPC; CCFP; CommunMed (Public Health). Court Staff, St Michael's Hospital; Langs: Croatian; (416)397-5598; Fax. (416)392-5587; tomislav.svoboda@utoronto.ca.

SVORKDAL, Nelson J; Royal Jubilee Hosp, 1952 Bay St, Victoria BC V8R 1J8; Sask'90; FRCPC; Anes. Staff, Royal Jubilee Hospital; (250)519-1836; Fax. (250)519-1837.

SVYSTONYUK, Oleksandr I; 306-581 Davis Dr, Newmarket ON L3Y 2P6; Chernovzy (Russia (Federation))'93; FRCSC; ObstGyn. Langs: Russian; Ukrainian; (905)952-2885; Fax. (905)952-2886.

SWADI, Omar Q M; Toronto Rubb Clinic, 825-123 Edward St, Toronto ON M5G 1E2; Baghdad (Iraq)'92; FRCPC; Anes. Staff, Timmins & District Hospital; Langs: Arabic; (416)888-1950

SWAIH, Omar M O; 15345 97 St NW, Edmonton AB T5X 5V3; Al Fateh (Libya)'04; CCFP; Gen Physician, Fogo Island Health Centre; (780)457-6060; Fax. (780)457-6111.

SWAIN, Ann E; Valley Prof Centre, 210-70 Exhibition St, Kentville NS B4N 4K9; Dal'96; CCFP; Staff, Western Kings Memorial Health Centre; Teach Staff, Acadia University; (902)679-0536

SWAIN, Gordon J; Peterborough Reg HC-Hospital, CCW 4968-1 Hospital Dr, Peterborough ON K9J 7C6; Qns'97; FRCPC; IntMed; Hem. Staff, Peterborough Regional Health Centre - Hospital Drive; (705)740-9326

SWAIN, Mark G; Calgary Heart Centre, 4AA20-3280 Hospital Dr NW, Calgary AB T2N 4Z6; Qns'85; FRCPC; IntMed (Hepatology); Gastroent. Staff, Foothills Medical Centre; Physician, Health Research Innovation Centre; Assoc Prof Med/Chair, University of Calgary; (403)592-5010; Fax. (403)592-5080; swain@ucalgary.ca.

SWAIN, Valerie J; St James Street Med Clinic, 1600 Portage Ave, Winnipeg MB R3J 0C6; Man'83; (204)774-1868; Fax. (204)774-7303.

SWAINE, Frederick B; WOHC-Brampton Civic Hosp, S3 443-2100 Bovaird Dr E, Brampton ON L6R 3J7; Qns'80; MBA; FRCPC; GenPath. Staff, William Osler Health System - Brampton Civic Hospital; (905)494-2120

SWAINSON, Jennifer N; Misericordia Community Hosp, 3F-16940 87 Ave NW, Edmonton AB T5R 4H5; Alb'04; FRCPC; Psy. Staff Cabrini Center, Covenant Health - Misericordia Community Hospital; (780)735-2594; Fax. (780)735-2595.

SWAINSON, Stephen J; 101-190 Pelican Place, Red Deer County AB T4S 1K2; Alb'09; CCFP; Staff Alberta Rural Family, University of Alberta Hospital; (403)887-2224; Fax. (403)887-2261.

SWALES, David W; Pineridge X-Ray, 555 George St N, Peterborough ON K9H 3S1; McG'61; BSc; CSPQ; DiagRad (Nuclear Medicine). Staff, Deep River & District Hospital; Staff, St Francis Memorial Hospital; Staff, Renfrew Victoria Hospital; (705)745-1058

SWALES, William C; Peterborough Reg HC-Hospital, 1 Hospital Dr, Peterborough ON K9J 7C6; McG'88; Staff, Peterborough Regional Health Centre - Hospital Drive; (705)876-5060

SWALLOW, Carol J; Mount Sinai Hosp, 1225-600 University Ave, Toronto ON M5G 1X5; Tor'84; PhD; FACS; FRCSC; GenSurg (Surgical Oncology). Professor - Dept of Surgery, Mount Sinai Hospital; Staff Surg, Princess Margaret Hospital - University Health Network; Assoc Prof Surg, University of Toronto; (416)586-4800 x1558; Fax. (416)586-8392; cswallow@mtsinai.on.ca.

SWAMI, Kamla A; 320-1861 Robertson Rd, Ottawa ON K2H 1B9; Tor'89; Staff, Queensway Carleton Hospital; (613)801-0035 x106; Fax. (613)801-0036.

SWAMINATH, Anand; Juravinski Cancer Centre, 699 Concession St, Hamilton ON L8V 5C2; Ott'04; RadOncol. Staff, Princess Margaret Hospital - University Health Network; (905)387-9711

SWAMINATH, Sam; Chatham Jail, 17 Seventh St, Chatham ON N7M 4J9; Osmania (India)'72; MB BS; DPM; MRCPsy; FRCPC; Psy (Forensic Psychiatry). Staff Psy & Forensic Prog, Regional Mental Health Care-St Joseph's Health Care; Asst Prof, University of Western Ontario; Langs: Hindi; Urdu; Tamil; Telugu; Kanarese.

SWAMINATHAN, Aparna; St Joseph's Hlth - Fam Med Ctr, 30 The Queensway, Toronto ON M6R 1B5; Dublin (Ireland)'06; CCFP; Staff Family Med Centre, St Joseph's Health Centre; Langs: Bilingual(English/French); (416)530-6860; Fax. (416)530-6160.

SWAMINATHAN, Sunita; Univ Hlth Network-Toronto Gen, 200 Elizabeth St, Toronto ON M5G 2C4; Cal'08; CCFP; CCFP(E.M.); Staff, Toronto General Hospital - UHN; (416)340-3111

SWAMY, Gandhaparimala N A; Dr Swamy Med Prof Corp, 102-1316 Central Ave, Prince Albert SK S6V 6P5; Bangalore (India)'69; LRCP(Lond); MRCS(Eng); (306)763-7525; Fax. (306)763-7525.

SWAMY, Ganesh; Foothills Med Centre, 1018-1403 29 St NW, Calgary AB T2N 2T9; Ott'97; FRCSC; OrthSurg. Staff, Foothills Medical Centre; Langs: Tamil; French; (403)944-4487; Fax. (403)451-1545.

SWAMY, Guruswamy N; 309 Commissioners Rd W, London ON N6J 1Y4; Karnatak (India)'71; MB BS; MRCPsy(UK); FRCPC; Psy. Staff, Regional Mental Health Care-St Joseph's Health Care; Staff, Strathroy Middlesex General Hospital - Middlesex Hospital Alliance; Asst Prof, University of Western Ontario; Langs: Kanarese; (519)474-4191; Fax. (519)473-7284.

SWAMY, Pramod; Hillside Med Clinic, PO Box 700 541 3rd Ave, Ladysmith BC V9G 1A5; Sask'03; CCFP; (250)245-2235; Fax. (250)245-3094.

SWAN, Amber C; Dr Everett Chalmers Hosp, PO Box 9000 Stn A 700 rue Priestman, Fredericton NB E3B 5N5; Dal'03; BSc; CCFP; Staff, Dr Everett Chalmers Regional Hospital; (506)452-5199; Fax. (506)452-5233.

SWAN, Andrew C; Richmond Med Bldg, 101-2020 Richmond Ave, Victoria BC V8R 6R5; Man'73; CCFP; FCFP; Langs: English; French; (250)477-7284

SWAN, David M A; 208-3930 Shelbourne St, Victoria BC V8P 5P6; Alb'72; FRCPC; Psy (General Adult Psychiatry). Ac Staff, Royal Jubilee Hospital; Staff, Victoria General Hospital; Consultant, BC Cancer Agency Vancouver Island Centre; (250)721-1117; Fax. (250)721-5678.

SWAN, Donald W; 225 Fairview Dr PO Box 28017 Rpo N Park Plaza, Brantford ON N3R 7X5; Dal'74; Court Staff, The Brant Community Healthcare System - Brantford General Hospital Site; (519)759-4060; Fax. (519)759-8807.

SWAN, James H; Scarborough Prof Centre, 406-1371 Neilson Rd, Scarborough ON M1B 4Z8; Qns'71; FACC; FRCPC; IntMed. Ac Staff, St Michael's Hospital; Ac Staff, Rouge Valley Health System - Centenary Health Centre Site; Lecturer Med, University of Toronto; (416)281-9499; Fax. (416)283-5705.

SWAN, John; Saint John Reg Hosp, PO Box 2100, Saint John NB E2L 4L2; Mem'05; FRCPC; DiagRad. Staff, Saint John Regional Hospital; (506)648-6000

SWAN, Kathryn M; Fairview Med Arts Centre, 208-2200 Fairview St, Burlington ON L7R 4H9; University College (Ireland)'07; CCFP; (905)632-2542

SWAN, Nadine T; Linden Med Clinic, PO Box 303 Stn Del Centre 7-385 Broadway St, Yorkton SK S3N 2W1; Pretoria (South Africa)'00; MB ChB; (306)783-7926; Fax. (306)783-7932.

SWANEPOEL, Abraham C J; Cottage Med Clinic, PO Box 2140 300 Miette Ave, Jasper AB T0E 1E0; (South Africa)'83; MB ChB; Physician, Cottage Medical Clinic; Langs: Afrikaans; (780)852-4885; Fax. (780)852-2199.

SWANEPOEL, Richard D; Village Mall Med Clinic, 6320 50 Ave, Red Deer AB T4N 4C6; (South Africa)'94; MB ChB; (403)314-5357; Fax. (403)314-5307.

SWANEPOEL, Walter E; Glenboro Health Dist Hosp, PO Box 310 219 Murray St, Glenboro MB R0K 0X0; Orange Free State (South Africa)'76; Staff, Glenboro Health District Hospital; (204)827-2438; Fax. (204)827-2741.

SWANEPOEL, Wilhelm A; 105-22838 Lougheed Hwy, Maple Ridge BC V2X 2V6; Pretoria (South Africa)'74; MB ChB; (604)467-4166; Fax. (604)467-5240.

SWANN, David R; 626 3 Ave NW, Calgary AB T2N 0J1; Alb'73; FRCPC; CommunMed (Infectious Diseases). Clin Assoc Prof Commun Med, University of Alberta; (403)270-2145; Fax. (403)670-0827.

SWANN, Frederick W; Ingram Family Physicians, 103-149 Ingram St, Duncan BC V9L 1N8; UBC'78; (250)746-4401; Fax. (250)746-4473.

SWANN, Lauren; Crossroads Family Practice, 201-45800 Promontory Rd, Chilliwack BC V2R 5Z5; UBC'08; CCFP; Staff, Chilliwack General Hospital; (604)858-3725

SWANSON, J Graham; Caroline Family Hlth Team-BFMG, 208-3155 Harvester Rd, Burlington ON L7N 3V2; Wes'71; CCFP; FCFP; Ac Staff Family Med, Joseph Brant Memorial Hospital; Court Staff, Hamilton Health Sciences Centre - Hamilton General Hospital; Clinical Asst Prof Family Med, McMaster University; (905)333-8222; Fax. (905)333-9343.

SWANSON, Kevin J; Courtenay Med Clinic, 788 Grant Ave, Courtenay BC V9N 2T3; Alb'96; CCFP; FCFP; (250)334-2445; Fax. (250)334-2642.

SWANSON, Mark A; Orillia Soldier's Mem Hosp, 170 Colborne St W, Orillia ON L3V 2Z3; Wes'76; FRCPC; DiagRad., Orillia Soldiers' Memorial Hospital; (705)325-2201 x3270

SWANSON, Murray C J; Cabrini Centre, F4-16811 88 Ave NW, Edmonton AB T5R 5Y6; Alb'84; FRCPC; Psy. Med Staff, Covenant Health - Misericordia Community Hospital; Clin Assoc Prof, University of Alberta; (780)735-2934; Fax. (780)735-2973.

SWARBRECK, Brian S; 40-180 Parsons Rd, Alliston ON L9R 1E8; Tor'81; Ac Staff, Stevenson Memorial Hospital; (705)435-5633; Fax. (705)435-2860.

SWART, Henry C; Summerside Med Centre, 1-475 Granville St, Summerside PE C1N 3N9; Stellenbosch (South Africa)'82; MB ChB; FCOG(SA)(SA); Staff ObstGyn, Prince County Hospital; Langs: German; Afrikaans; Dutch; (902)432-8121; Fax. (902)436-9660; hncs@islandtelecom.com.

SWART, Ignatius; Valleyview Health Complex, PO Box 1628, Valleyview AB T0H 3N0; (South Africa)'05; (780)524-3323; Fax. (780)524-2806.

SWART, Johan J; Oasis Med Centre, 201-175 Chestermere Station Wa, Chestermere AB T1X 1V2; Pretoria (South Africa)'75; MB ChB; Staff Privil, Victoria Hospital; Staff, Properties Medical Clinic; Physician, South Hill Medical Practice; (403)266-1192; Fax. (403)266-1194.

SWART, Maritza; Woodstock Gen Hosp, 310 Juliana Dr, Woodstock ON N4V 0A4; Pretoria (South Africa)'99; MB ChB; Staff, Woodstock General Hospital; (519)421-4211

SWART, Matthys L; High Prairie Assoc Clinic, PO Box 1350, High Prairie AB T0G 1E0; (South Africa)'04.

SWART, Petrus A; Dept of Anes, 2449-910 10th Ave W, Vancouver BC V5Z 1M9; Stellenbosch (South Africa)'83; MB ChB; DA; FRCPC; Anes. Staff, Vancouver General Hospital - Centennial Pavillion; (604)875-4304

SWART, Petrus J; Regina Qu'Appelle HR-Pasqua, 4101 Dewdney Ave, Regina SK S4T 1A5; Staff, Pasqua Hospital; (306)766-2222

SWART, Pieter D; Mid-Island Med Clinic, PO Box 310 744 Memorial Hwy, Qualicum Beach BC V9K 1S8; Witwatersrand (South Africa)'75; MB BCh; Physician, Parksville Walk-In Clinic; (250)752-3284; Fax. (250)752-3519; drpdswart@gmail.com.

SWART, Rosalie D; Group One Med Associates, 1111 Springfield Rd, Kelowna BC V1Y 8R7; Wes'92; CCFP; Staff, Kelowna General Hospital; (250)762-4246; Fax. (250)762-4041.

SWART, Servaas D K; 101-595 Columbia St W, Kamloops BC V2C 1K7; Orange Free State (South Africa)'99; MB ChB; (250)372-3223

SWART, Vandeurs; Coventry Hills Family Care Ctr, 105-100 Country Village Rd NE, Calgary AB T3K 5Z2; Stellenbosch (South Africa)'84; Langs: Afrikaans; (403)226-6715; Fax. (403)226-6748.

SWART, Wayne; Lloydminster Med Clinic, 5120 46 St, Lloydminster AB T9V 2P7; Alb'81; (780)875-2221; Fax. (780)875-0605.

SWART, Werner; Lloydminster Med Clinic, 5120 46 St, Lloydminster AB T9V 2P7; Pretoria (South Africa)'04; MB ChB; Physician, Lloydminster Medical Clinic; (780)875-2221; Fax. (780)875-0605.

SWARTS, Petrus J E; Easthill Med Walk-In Clinic, 610-3020 22 St, Red Deer AB T4R 3J5; Stellenbosch (South Africa)'88; (403)343-0115; Fax. (403)343-8551; ehwalkin@telus.net.

SWARTZ, Carin; Associate Clinic, 5215A 49 Ave, Wetaskiwin AB T9A 0R1; (South Africa)'93; MB ChB; LMCC; Langs: Afrikaans; German; (780)352-7157; Fax. (780)352-2273.

SWARTZ, David A; Toronto Grace Hosp, 650 Church St, Toronto ON M4Y 2G5; Tor'76; Staff Palliative Care Prog, The Salvation Army Toronto Grace Health Centre; (416)925-2251 x201; Fax. (416)925-9136; dswartz@torontograce.org.

SWARTZ, David S; Mackenzie Richmond Hill Hosp, 10 Trench St, Richmond Hill ON L4C 4Z3; Qns'90; CCFP; CCFP(E.M.); Staff, Mackenzie Richmond Hill Hospital; (905)883-2241

SWARTZ, Erik N; 7000 Westminster Hwy, Richmond BC V6X 1A2; UBC'99; BSc; MSc; LMCC; LRCP; MRCP; AddicMed; ABPeds; DABPed; FAAP; FRCP; FRCPC; Peds (Medical Informatics). Att Physician, BC Children's Hospital; Staff Child Health Centre, Richmond Hospital; Clin Assoc Prof, University of British Columbia; (604)233-3222; Fax. (604)233-5620.

SWARTZ, Jo S; Children's Hosp, AE403-840 Sherbrook St, Winnipeg MB R3A 1S1; Man'78; FRCPC; Anes. Asst Prof/Ac Staff Children's Hosp, Health Sciences Centre; (204)787-2560; Fax. (204)787-1560.

SWARTZ, Richard H; Sunnybrook Hlth Sciences Ctre, A442-2075 Bayview Ave, Toronto ON M4N 3M5; Tor'04; FRCPC; Neur. Staff, Sunnybrook Health Sciences Centre; (416)480-4866

SWATI, Ismatun; Chaleur Reg Hosp, 1750 Sunset Dr, Bathurst NB E2A 4L7; Dhaka (Other Foreign)'96; Staff, Hopital Regional Chaleur; (506)544-3000

SWAYZE, Allan G; 305W-200 St Clair Ave W, Toronto ON M4V 1R1; Tor'63; DPsy; FRCPC; Psy (Genetic Psychiatry). Sr Consultant Staff, North York General Hospital; Asst Prof Psy, University of Toronto; (416)789-3458; Fax. (416)789-5168.

SWAYZE, Ian G; Addiction & Mental Hlth-Queen, 1001 Queen St W, Toronto ON M6J 1H4; Wes'92; FRCPC; Psy. Staff, Centre for Addiction & Mental Health (CAMH) - Queen Site; (416)535-8501; Fax. (416)583-1324.

SWAYZE, Kathleen A; Garden City Family Health Team, 22 Ontario St, St Catharines ON L2R 7M3; McM'87; CCFP; FCFP; Asst Prof Clinical/ Students Affairs Niagara Campus/Dir Michael G DeGroote School of Med, McMaster University; Med Dir, Ridley College; (905)984-3335; Fax. (905)984-6008.

SWEDAN, Ahmed M; Leamington District Mem Hosp, 194 Talbot St W, Leamington ON N8H 1N9; Al Fateh (Libya)'03; CCFP; CCFP(E.M.); Staff, Leamington District Memorial Hospital; (519)322-2501; Fax. (519)322-0702.

SWEDLO, Dean C; Foothills Med Centre, C222-1403 29 ST NW, Calgary AB T2N 2T9; Man'05; Critical Care Medicine; Anes. Staff, Foothills Medical Centre; Staff, Peter Lougheed Centre; (403)944-1110

SWEENEY, Clodagh M; Hamilton HS-Chedoke Site, PO Box 2000 Stn Lcd 1 3A 511-1200 Maint St W, Hamilton ON L8N 3Z5; Belfast (Ireland)'93; Staff, Hamilton Health Sciences Centre - McMaster University Medical Centre; (905)521-2100; Fax. (905)308-7548.

SWEENEY, Desmond H M; Royal Jubilee Hosp, 1952 Bay St, Victoria BC V8R 1J8; UBC'04; Anes. Staff, Royal Jubilee Hospital; (250)370-8000

SWEENEY, George D; Hollidge Med Centre, B6-130 Hollidge Blvd, Aurora ON L4G 8A3; Cape Town (South Africa)'58; MB ChB; PhD; MedScient(Med) (Geriatric Medicine)., Southlake Regional Health Centre; (905)841-5554; Fax. (905)841-0088.

SWEENEY, Maureen F; Live Young Med Centre, 103-9845 Resthaven Dr, Sidney BC V8L 3E7; UBC'87; (250)654-0383; Fax. (250)412-4448.

SWEENEY, Mila Silva; 80 Valleybrook Dr, North York ON M3B 2S9; Manila (Philippines)'86; (416)442-5600; Fax. (416)510-5128.

SWEENEY, Trevor A; St Clare's Mercy Hosp, 154 Lemarchant Rd, St. John's NL A1C 5B8; Mem'01; FRCPC; Anes. Staff Anes, St Clare's Mercy Hospital; (709)777-5000

SWEENY, Margo J; Westcoast Family Practice Ctre, 2775 Laurel St, Vancouver BC V5Z 1M9; UBC'84; CCFP; FCFP; Staff, BC Women's Hospital & Health Centre; Staff, Vancouver General Hospital - Centennial Pavillion; (604)875-5691; Fax. (604)875-5694.

SWEET, Blythe A; Rockyview Gen Hosp, 7007 14 St SW, Calgary AB T2V 1P9; UBC'00; FRCPC; Anes. Staff, Rockyview General Hospital; (403)943-8720

SWEET, Daniel C; Rideau Valley Health Centre, 1221 Greenbank Rd, Ottawa ON K2J 5V7; Ott'82; ASAM; Anes (Addiction Medicine). (613)258-8710; Fax. (613)440-3238.

SWEET, David D; Vancouver Gen Hosp, 855 12th Ave W, Vancouver BC V5Z 1M9; Alb'02; FRCPC; EmergMed; Critical Care Medicine. Staff, Vancouver General Hospital - Centennial Pavillion; (604)875-4995

SWEET, H Bruce; Thunder Bay Med Centre, 110-63 Algoma St N, Thunder Bay ON P7A 4Z6; Wes'76; (807)345-7555; Fax. (807)345-1891; sweetb@tbaytel.net.

SWEET, Joan M; Univ Hlth Network-Toronto Gen, 11 444E-200 Elizabeth St, Toronto ON M5G 2C4; Tor'77; FACP; FRCPC; AnatPath. Staff, Toronto General Hospital - UHN; Asst Prof Path, University of Toronto; (416)340-4563; Fax. (416)340-5517.

SWEET, Lamont E; Office of Chief Med of Health, PO Box 2000 Stn Central 2F-11 Kent St, Charlottetown PE C1A 7N8; McG'67; Peds (Epidemiology). Chief Med of Health, PEI Health & Social Services; (902)368-4996; Fax. (902)368-4969; lesweet@gov.pe.ca.

SWEET, Margaret E; 201-984 Oliver Rd, Thunder Bay ON P7B 7C7; McM'86; BSc(Hons); FAB; FAB; FRCPC; Neur. Langs: French; (807)684-6707

SWEET, Susan M; 100-2109 Ottawa St, Windsor ON N8Y 1R8; Ott'02; PhD; CCFP; Assoc Prof, University of Western Ontario; (519)252-9990; Fax. (519)252-2602.

SWEET JR, Robert C G; MUHC-Montreal Gen Hosp, A2 141-1650 av Cedar, Montreal QC H3G 1A4; McG'79; FRCSC; Otol (Neuro Otolaryngology). assoc Staff, McGill University Health Centre - Montreal General Campus; Adj Otol, McGill University Health Centre - Royal Victoria Hospital; Adj Otol, Sir Mortimer B Davis Jewish General; adj Prof, McGill University; Langs: French; (514)934-8018; Fax. (514)934-8422; robert.sweet@mcgill.ca.

SWEETLAND, Robert J; Health Sciences Centre, 820 Sherbrook St, Winnipeg MB R3A 1R9; Man'86; Staff, Health Sciences Centre; (204)774-6511

SWEEZEY, Neil B; The Hosp for Sick Children, 555 University Ave, Toronto ON M5G 1X8; Qns'80; BSc; MD; LMCC; FRCPC; Peds (Pediatric Respiratory Medicine); Respir. Staff Respiratory Med, The Hospital For Sick Children; Assoc Prof Peds & Physiol, University of Toronto; Langs: Bilingual(French/English); (416)813-5128; Fax. (416)813-5771; neil.sweezey@sickkids.ca.

SWEKLA, Michaela; Cambridge Mem Hosp, 700 Coronation Blvd, Cambridge ON N1R 3G2; Bratislava (Slovakia)'94; Staff, Cambridge Memorial Hospital; Langs: Czech; German; Slovak; (519)621-2333

SWENERTON, Jean E; BC Women's Hosp & Health Ctre, 1Q72-4500 Oak St, Vancouver BC V6H 3N1; UBC'69; FRCPC; Anes (Obstetrics Anesthesia). Clin Assoc Prof, BC Women's Hospital & Health Centre; Clin Assoc Prof, University of British Columbia; Langs: Bilingual(English/French); (604)875-2158

SWENIA, Mohamed M M; 604-8600 Franklin ave, Fort McMurray AB T9H 4G8; Tripoli (Libya)'81; MB ChB; FRCSC; GenSurg (Gastrointestinal Endoscopy). Langs: Arabic; (780)743-3444; Fax. (780)743-3278; mswenia@telusplanet.net.

SWENOR, Rachel; Ctr Hosp du Centre la Mauricie, 50 119e rue, Shawinigan QC G9P 5K7; Laval'06; Psy. Staff, Centre Hospitalier du Centre la Mauricie; (819)536-7500

SWENSON, Brigit A; New Heights Comm Hlth Centre, 12 Flemington Rd, North York ON M6A 2N4; Dal'00; CCFP; Langs: Spanish; (416)787-1661; Fax. (416)787-3761.

SWENSON, J Robert; The Ottawa Hosp-Gen Campus, 501 Smyth Rd Box 400, Ottawa ON K1H 8L6; Ott'80; FRCPC; Psy (Consultant Liaison Psychiatry). Ac Staff, The Ottawa Hospital Rehabilitation Centre; Dep Head Gen Campus/Dir, The Ottawa Hospital - General Campus; Assoc Prof, University of Ottawa; Langs: French; (613)737-8083; Fax. (613)739-9980; jrswenson@ottawahospital.on.ca.

SWERSKY, Joanne F; Meadowlark Health Centre, 200 Meadowlark Shopping Ctr NW, Edmonton AB T5R 5W9; Witwatersrand (South Africa)'76; MB ChB; FRCPC; DiagRad (General Radiology Ultrasound & Mammography). Ac Staff, Covenant Health - Misericordia Community Hospital; Asst Prof, University of Alberta; (780)489-7851; Fax. (780)486-5160.

SWICA, Leszek J; Cypress Reg Hosp, 2004 Saskatchewan Dr, Swift Current SK S9H 5M8; Wroclaw (Poland)'78; FRCPC; Anes. Staff, Cypress Regional Hospital; Langs: Polish; (306)778-9529; Fax. (306)778-9419; leszek@ns.sympatico.ca.

SWIDINSKY, Teddi L D; Timmins & Dist Hosp, 700 Ross Ave E, Timmins ON P4N 8P2; Man'03; GenSurg. Staff, Timmins & District Hospital; (705)267-2131

SWIECA, Richard O; CSSS du Suroît, 150 rue Saint-Thomas, Salaber-de-Valleyf QC J6T 6C1; McG'84; DAB; FRCSC; Ophth. Staff, Centre Hospitalier Régional du Suroît; Langs: French; (450)371-9920; Fax. (450)371-7454; doctorswieca@bellnet.ca.

SWIEGERS, Roxanne L; Health Matters Med Clinic, 102-3215 Dunmore Rd SE, Medicine Hat AB T1B 2H2; Stellenbosch (South Africa)'84; MB ChB; CCFP; Staff, Medicine Hat Regional Hospital; Langs: Afrikaans; (403)504-0450; Fax. (403)529-4601.

SWIERCZEK, Janusz S; 102-304 The East Mall, Etobicoke ON M9B 6E2; Krakow (Poland)'66; PhD; FRCPC; Psy (Mood Disorders). Consultant, Workmens' Comp Board; Langs: Polish; (416)231-7968; Fax. (416)231-7982.

SWIFT, Alexander B; Saint Mary's Health Clinic, 923 Robie St, Halifax NS B3H 3C3; McM'96; CCFP; CCFP(E.M.); FCFP; (902)496-8727; Fax. (902)496-8222.

SWIFT, Arthur; 4131 rue Sherbrooke O, Westmount QC H3Z 1B7; McG'81; FRCSC; PlasSurg (Aesthetic Surgery). Staff, Mount Sinai Hospital Center; (514)933-2353; Fax. (514)933-7087; drarthurswift@qc.aibn.com.

SWIFT, Elena R; Bedford Family Care Associates, 204-967 Bedford Hwy, Bedford NS B4A 1A9; McM'97; CCFP; (902)835-6200; Fax. (902)832-7100; erswift@hfx.eastlink.ca.

SWIFT, John E; 611 Wonderland Rd N, London ON N6H 4V6; London (England)'64; MRCS; LRCP; MB BS; CCFP; FCFP; Staff, Medicentres Canada; (519)471-6686; Fax. (519)471-2801; gardenpall@live.ca.

SWIFT, Margaret E; Ridge Meadows Hosp & Hlth CC, 11666 Laity St, Maple Ridge BC V2X 5A3; Mem'80; CCFP; Staff, Ridge Meadows Hospital & Health Care Centre; (604)463-4111

SWIFT, Valerie A; Courtice Health Centre, 1450 Highway 2, Courtice ON L1E 3C3; Qns'83; CCFP; FCFP; Court Staff, Lakeridge Health - Oshawa Site; (905)721-3539; Fax. (905)721-6189.

SWIGGUM, Elizabeth A; Royal Jubilee Hosp, 1952 Bay St, Victoria BC V8R 1J8; Dal'98; FRCPC; IntMed; Cardiol. Staff, Royal Jubilee Hospital; (250)519-1601; Fax. (250)370-8267.

SWIGGUM, Susan M M; Canadian Med Protective Assoc, PO Box 8225 Stn T 875 Carling Ave, Ottawa ON K1S 5P1; Ott'76; DAB; FRCPC; Derm. Staff, Canadian Medical Protective Association; Fax. (613)725-1300.

SWINAMER, Deanna L; Family Practice Associates, 6155 North St, Halifax NS B3K 5R3; Alb'92; BSc(Nutrition); MSc(ExperMed); CCFP; FCFP; (902)453-3511; Fax. (902)454-9010.

SWINAMER, Stuart A; London HSC-University Hosp, PO Box 5339 Stn B B6 120-339 Windermere Rd, London ON N6A 5A5; Wes'92; Staff, London Health Sciences Centre - University Hospital; (519)685-8500 x33098; Fax. (519)679-6414.

SWINKELS, Helena M; Central City Tower, 400-13450 102 Ave, Surrey BC V3T 4M5; UBC'93; FRCPC; CommunMed;CCFP; FCFP; Public Health & Preventive Med. Staff, Office of the Medical Health Officer; (604)587-7892; Fax. (604)930-5414.

SWINSON, Richard P; Fontbonne Bldg, F611-301 James St S, Hamilton ON L8P 3B6; Liverpool (England)'63; MB ChB; DPM; FRCPsy; FCPA; FRCPC; Psy. Assoc Staff, Toronto General Hospital - UHN; Med Dir Anxiety Treatment & Research Centre, St Joseph's Healthcare - Charlton Campus; Emeritus Prof, McMaster University; (905)522-1155 x34964; Fax. (905)521-6120; swinsonr@mcmaster.ca.

SWINTON, Andrew A; Core Family Med Clinic, 222-80 Chippewa Rd, Sherwood Park AB T8A 4W6; Alb'89; CCFP; FCFP; (780)464-9661; Fax. (780)417-0656.

SWIRSKY, Jacqueline E; Roslyn Med Bldg, 200-400 5th Ave SW, Calgary AB T2P 0L6; Cal'09; CCFP; (403)930-1005; Fax. (403)930-1004.

SWIRSKY, Karen N; St Michael's Hosp, 30 Bond St, Toronto ON M5B 1W8; McM'07; CCFP; Staff Family Practice Unit, St Michael's Hospital; (416)867-7426; Fax. (416)867-7498.

SWIRSKY, S Neil; Seven Oaks Gen Hosp, 2300 McPhillips St, Winnipeg MB R2V 3M3; Man'75; FRCPC; EmergMed (Hospital Administration). Staff, Seven Oaks General Hospital; Med Advisor Driver & Vehicle Licensing, Ministry of Transportation; Assoc Prof Emerg Med, University of Manitoba; (204)632-3113

SWISTON, John R; Gordon & Leslie Diamond HCC, 7243-2775 Laurel St, Vancouver BC V5Z 1M9; Alb'00; FRCPC; IntMed (Clinician Investigator Program); Respir. Staff, Gordon & Leslie Diamond Health Care Centre; (604)875-4122; Fax. (604)875-4695.

SWITAKOWSKI, Peter K; Univ Hlth Network-Toronto Gen, 200 Elizabeth St, Toronto ON M5G 2C4; Wes'01; CCFP; CCFP(E.M.); Staff, Toronto General Hospital - UHN; Langs: Polish; (416)340-3946

SWITCHUK, Marianna; Monarch Laser & Wellness Ctre, 15 Empress Ave, Hamilton ON L9A 1M1; Tor'92; (905)388-2400; Fax. (905)388-2405.

SWITZER, Connie M; Tawa Centre, 217-3017 66 St NW, Edmonton AB T6K 4B2; Alb'74; FRCPC; IntMed (Therapeutic Endoscopy); Gastroent. Ac Staff, Covenant Health - Grey Nuns Community Hospital; Clin Prof Med, University of Alberta; (780)450-1807; Fax. (780)461-9876.

SWITZER, Neil T; Radiology Consultants Assoc, 120-6707 Elbow Dr SW, Calgary AB T2V 0E3; Man'96; FRCPC; DiagRad. (403)777-3003

SWITZER, Philip J; Greig Associates, 5732 Victoria Dr, Vancouver BC V5P 3W6; McG'68; FRCPC; DiagRad. Staff, Oakridge Centre South Tower; Seymour Medical Clinic; Clin Prof Radiol, University of British Columbia; (604)321-6774; Fax. (604)321-6626.

SWITZER, Rosanna M; Murakami Med Clinic, PO Box 1000, Hope BC V0X 1L0; UBC'07; CCFP; (604)869-5648

SWOBODA, Ewa; Sunnyside Med Arts Centre, 410-27 Roncesvalles Ave, Toronto ON M6R 3B2; Wroclaw (Poland)'87; FRCPC; Psy (Child & Adolescent Psychiatry). Langs: Polish; Russian; (647)438-7177; Fax. (647)430-7855.

SWOPE, Sheila A; PO Box 389, Squamish BC V8B 0A3; UBC'87; (604)892-3535; Fax. (604)892-3545.

SY, Candice; Eagle Ridge Hosp & HCC, 475 Guilford Way, New Westminster BC V3H 3W9; UBC'07; CCFP; Staff, Eagle Ridge Hospital & Health Care Centre; (250)370-8000

SY, John C; 730 Bradley Ave, London ON N6E 1J8; Manila (Philippines)'70; Langs: Chinese; Tagalog; (519)681-6990; Fax. (519)681-6316.

SY, Keiyan; The Banting Institute, 110-100 College St, Toronto ON M5G 1L5; Tor'07; AnatPath. Staff, The Banting Institute; (416)978-7535

SY, Magdalena G; Stadium Med Centre, 21-1941 Uxbridge Dr NW, Calgary AB T2N 2V2; (403)248-8807; Fax. (403)403-2488.

SY, Peter Y; Tomken Shopp Ctre, 925 Rathburn Rd E, Mississauga ON L4W 4C3; Far Eastern University (Philippines)'77; Assoc Staff, Trillium Health Centre - Mississauga; Langs: Chinese; Tagalog; (905)848-6633; Fax. (905)848-6635.

SY, Richmond G; Riverside Prof Centre, 206-1919 Riverside Dr, Ottawa ON K1H 1A2; UBC'96; FRCPC; IntMed; Gastroent. Staff, The Ottawa Hospital - General Campus; (613)738-8400; Fax. (613)738-8391.

SY, William Y; Finch-Midland Med Centre, 203-4190 Finch Ave E, Scarborough ON M1S 4T7; Far Eastern (Philippines)'75; FRCPC; Psy. Langs: Mandarin; Tagalog; (416)299-8060; Fax. (416)299-9046.

SYAL, Abeer; Murrayville Health Care Centre, 202-22112 52 Ave, Langley BC V2Y 2M6; Wes'03; FRCSC; OrthSurg. (604)534-3235

SYAL, Suresh; 2A-80 Glen Shields Ave, Concord ON L4K 1T7; Tor'88; Assoc Staff Family Pract, Toronto General Hospital - UHN; Langs: Hindi; Punjabi; (905)738-9141; Fax. (905)695-2700.

SYAN, Gurcharan S; Gurcharan S Syan Med Prof Corp, 102-430 Notre Dame Ave, Sudbury ON P3C 5K7; Punjab (India)'77; MB BS; MRC(UK); Cardiol; IntMed. Staff, Health Sciences North - Memorial Site; Langs: Punjabi; Arabic; Hindi; (705)671-3650; Fax. (705)671-9130.

SYAN, Rajinder S; 206 MacKenzie St N, Sarnia ON N7T 6K9; Punjab (Pakistan)'85; MB BS; FRCPC; IntMed (Family Medicine). (519)337-0444; Fax. (519)337-5444.

SYAN, Swaran K; Medi Aesthethics Solutions, 200-430 Notre Dame Ave, Sudbury ON P3C 5K7; Punjabi (India)'77; MB BS; CCFP; Staff, Health Sciences North-St Joseph's Health Centre; Staff, Health Sciences North - Memorial Site; Staff, Health Sciences North-Laurentian Site; Langs: Hindi; Punjabi; (705)523-1036; Fax. (705)523-4589.

SYDOR, Devin T; Kingston Gen Hosp, V2-76 Stuart St, Kingston ON K7L 2V7; UBC'05; FRCPC; Anes. Staff, Kingston General Hospital; (613)548-7827

SYED, A Shaista; Jane & Shoreham Med Ctre, 103-4640 Jane St, North York ON M3N 2K5; Punjab (Pakistan)'67; CCFP; Court Staff Family Practice Unit, St Michael's Hospital; Ac Staff, Humber River Regional Hospital - Finch Avenue Site; Coord Medical Written Exam, College Of Family Physicians Of Canada-Ontario; Langs: Urdu; Hindi; Punjabi; (416)665-1641; Fax. (416)661-8297.

SYED, Abdul R; Royal Victoria Hospital, 2432-201 Georgian Dr, Barrie ON L4M 6M2; Osmania (India)'80; AB; Staff, Royal Victoria Regional Health Centre; Langs: Urdu; Hindi; (705)728-9090; Fax. (705)739-5685.

SYED, Abu A; Medical Bldg, 200-86 Angeline St S, Lindsay ON K9V 6C5; Osmania (India)'80; FRCPC; IntMed (Respirology). Court Consultant, Ross Memorial Hospital; Langs: Hindi; Urdu; (705)328-2019; Fax. (705)328-1842; abuasyed@bellnet.ca.

SYED, Ali A; William Osler HC-Etobicoke, 101 Humber College Blvd, Etobicoke ON M9V 1R8; Aurangabad (India)'69; MB BS; FRCPC; Anes. Staff, William Osler Health System - Etobicoke General Hospital; Langs: Hindi; Urdu; (416)747-3554

SYED, Arif M; 6-1010 Dream Crest Rd, Mississauga ON L5V 3A4; Alb'97; FRCPC; Psy. Langs: Urdu; (905)813-9674; Fax. (905)813-9459.

SYED, Atyab A N; Ziedler Ledcor Centre, 130 University Campus NW, Edmonton AB T6G 2X8; Punjab (India)'01; FRCPC; IntMed; Gastroent. (780)248-1033; Fax. (780)444-8339.

SYED, Badruddin; Westend Walk-In Med Clinic, 411 Confederation Dr, Saskatoon SK S7L 5C3; Bangalore (India)'73; LMCC; Staff, St Paul's Hospital (Grey Nuns) of Saskatoon; Staff, Saskatoon City Hospital; Staff, Royal University Hospital; Physician, Westend Walk-In Medical Clinic; (306)382-6333; Fax. (306)382-6381.

SYED, Husnain; Nanaimo Reg Gen Hosp, 1200 Dufferin Cres, Nanaimo BC V9S 2B7; Staff, Nanaimo Regional General Hospital; (250)755-7691

SYED, Ikramuddin; Etobicoke Urgent Care Centre, 10-25 Woodbine Downs Blvd, Etobicoke ON M9W 6N5; Universidad Iberoamericana(UNIBE) (Other Foreign)'05; CCFP; Langs: Spanish; Urdu; (416)741-2273

SYED, Jaffer A; London HSC-University Hosp, PO Box 5339 Stn B C6 117B-339 Windermere Rd, London ON N6A 5A5; Tor'98; FRCPC; IntMed; Cardiol. Staff, London Health Sciences Centre - University Hospital; Langs: Urdu; (519)663-3536; Fax. (519)434-3278.

SYED, Khalid A; Univ Hlth Network-Toronto Western Hosp, 446 EW1-399 Bathurst St, Toronto ON M5T 2S8; Tor'99; FRCSC; OrthSurg. Staff, Toronto Western Hospital - University Health Network; Langs: Hindi; Urdu; Fax. (416)603-5281.

SYED, Naseeruddin; Landsdowne Place Walk In Clini, 769 Borden Ave, Peterborough ON K9J 0B6; Andhra (India)'81; (705)775-0444; Fax. (705)775-0437.

SYED, Nazia; Mackenzie Richmond Hill Hosp, 10 Trench St, Richmond Hill ON L4C 4Z3; Maharashtra University (India)'05; FRCPC; IntMed. Staff, Mackenzie Richmond Hill Hospital; Langs: Hindi; (905)883-1212

SYED, Saadat A S; Jane & Shoreham Med Ctre, 103-4640 Jane St, North York ON M3N 2K5; Dublin (Ireland)'61; MRCS(Eng); FRCOG; LRCPSI; CCFP; Ac Staff, Humber River Regional Hospital - Finch Avenue Site; Humber River Regional Hospital - Church Street Site; Langs: Urdu; Punjabi; Swahili; Italian; Hindi; (416)665-1641; Fax. (416)661-8297; saada29@hotmail.com.

SYED, Shahid; River Valley Med Clinic, 106 Lambert St, Whitehorse YT Y1A 1Z2; (Pakistan)'85; Physician, River Valley Medical Clinic; (867)667-6491

SYED, Sumairah A; Health For All Family Health T, 202-379 Church St, Markham ON L6B 0T1; Southampton (England)'03; CCFP; Staff, Sunnybrook Health Sciences Centre; Langs: Urdu; (905)472-2200; Fax. (905)472-5662.

SYED, Summer; Hamilton HS-General Site, 3F-237 Barton St E, Hamilton ON L8L 2X2; Tor'00; FRCPC; Anes. Staff, Hamilton Health Sciences Centre - Hamilton General Hospital; (905)527-0271; Fax. (905)577-8223.

SYED, Tahniat S; Markham Pediatric Hlth Centre, 207-5293 Hwy 7, Markham ON L3P 1B8; The Medical College of Pennsylvania (USA)'96; (905)471-7787

SYED, Uzma; Rouge Valley HC-Centenary, 2867 Ellesmere Rd, Scarborough ON M1E 4B9; Karachi (Pakistan)'99; FRCPC; IntMed. Staff, Rouge Valley Health System - Centenary Health Centre Site; Langs: Urdu; Hindi; (416)284-3118; Fax. (416)281-7384.

SYED, Yasmeen; Markham Plaza, 2-1221 Markham Rd, Scarborough ON M1H 3E2; Punjab (Pakistan)'80; Staff, Rouge Valley Health System - Centenary Health Centre Site; Langs: Punjabi; Hindi; Urdu; (416)439-1377; Fax. (416)913-1434.

SYED, Zareen; Rouge Valley HS-Centenary, 2867 Ellesmere Rd, Scarborough ON M1E 4B9; Karachi (Pakistan)'99; MB BS; MD; FRCPC; IntMed (Geriatric Medicine). Staff, Rouge Valley Health System - Centenary Health Centre Site; Langs: Urdu; (416)284-3118; Fax. (416)281-7384.

SYED, Zohair H; 100-101 Queensway W, Mississauga ON L5B 2P7; Wes'10; CCFP; (905)949-0801; Fax. (905)949-0803.

SYEDA, Naheed G; Foothills Med Centre, U37-1403 29 St NW, Calgary AB T2N 2T9; (Pakistan)'83; Staff Renal, Foothills Medical Centre; (403)944-1137; Fax. (403)944-2810.

SYGAL, Vitaly; St Mary's Hosp Centre, 3830 av Lacombe, Montreal QC H3T 1M5; McG'03; DiagRad. Staff, St Mary's Hospital Centre; (514)345-3511

SYKES, Glen C; Drumheller Assoc Physicians, PO Box 5600, Drumheller AB T0J 0Y0; (403)823-3345; Fax. (403)823-7823.

SYKES, Lucinda J; Meditation for Health, 509-720 Spadina Ave, Toronto ON M5S 2T9; Tor'77; (416)413-9158; info@meditationforhealth.com.

SYKINIOTIS, John; Inst Univ de Geriatrie de Mtl, 4565 ch Queen-Mary, Montreal QC H3W 1W5; Sher'88; CCFP; FCFP; Staff, Institut Universitaire de Gériatrie de Montréal; (514)340-2800

SYLVAIN, Jacques P E; Harmony Med Center, 106-152 Cleopatra Dr, Ottawa ON K2G 5X2; McG'74; FACOG; FRCSC; ObstGyn (High Risk Pregnancy). Staff, The Ottawa Hospital - Civic Campus; Asst Prof, University of Ottawa; Langs: French; (613)729-7352; Fax. (613)729-4633.

SYLVAIN, Michel; CHUQ-Ctr Hosp Univ Laval, 1235-2705 boul Laurier, Quebec QC G1V 4G2; Laval'89; Electroenceph (P.Q.); Neur. Staff, Centre Hospitalier Universitaire de Quebec-CHUL; (418)654-2708; Fax. (418)654-2710.

SYLVAIN, Pierre-Luc; Ctr Hosp de Matane, 333 rue Thibault, Matane QC G4W 2W5; Laval'02; Staff, Centre Hospitalier de Matane; Langs: Spanish; English; (418)562-3135; Fax. (418)562-9374.

SYLVAIN, Sonia; UMF Laurier, 2875 boul Laurier, Quebec QC G1V 4G2; Laval'96; CCFP; Staff, Centre Hospitalier Universitaire de Quebec-CHUL; (418)654-2701; Fax. (418)654-2138.

SYLVAIN-LUCIEN, Joseph; GMG de Grand-Mere, 200-1050 8e rue, Grand-Mere QC G9T 4K4; Michoacana (Mexico)'83; Staff, Centre Lafleche Grand-Mere; (819)538-8888; Fax. (819)538-1812.

SYLVESTER, Heather A; Special Services Unit, 90 John St S, Stratford ON N5A 2Y8; Wes'86; BSc(Hons.); CCFP; Assoc Staff Mental Health, Stratford General Hospital - Huron Perth Healthcare Alliance; (519)272-8210 x2563; Fax. (519)272-8226.

SYLVESTER, Michael J; Queens Family Health Team, 106B-115 Clarence St, Kingston ON K7L 5N6; Ott'93; CCFP; FCFP; Langs: French; (613)533-9303

SYLVESTRE, Alma D; Hop Maisonneuve-Rosemont, 5415 boul de l'Assomption, Montreal QC H1T 2M4; Mon'02; FRCPC; RadOncol (Lung). Chef du dépt, Hopital Maisonneuve-Rosemont; (514)252-3425; Fax. (514)252-3556.

SYLVESTRE, Amélie; CSSS BC-UMF Maria, 419 rue Perron, Maria QC G0C 1Y0; Mon'06; Staff, CSSS de la Baie-des-Chaleurs; (418)759-1336; Fax. (418)759-1344.

SYLVESTRE, Andre; CSSSG-Hop De Gatineau, CP 2000 Succ Bureau-Chef 909 boul de la Verendrye O, Gatineau QC J8P 7H2; McG'78; Staff, Hôpital de Gatineau; (819)561-8100

SYLVESTRE, Camille V; Hôpital Ste-Justine, 3175 ch Cote-Sainte-Catherine, Montreal QC H3T 1C5; McG'95; FRCSC; ObstGyn (Gynecological Reproductive Endocrinology). Staff, Hôpital Ste-Justine; (514)345-4931

SYLVESTRE, Chantal; CSSS de l'Ouest de l'Ile, 13800 boul Gouin O, Pierrefonds QC H8Z 3H6; Mon'88; Médecin, CSSS de l'Ouest de l'Ile; (514)626-2572; Fax. (514)624-7486.

SYLVESTRE, Guy; 260-2040 boul Marcel-Laurin, Saint-Laurent QC H4R 1J9; Mon'71; Derm (Esthetic Dermatology). ac Staff, Hôpital du Sacre-Coeur de Montréal; (514)387-6433; Fax. (514)387-6041; dermato@qc.aira.com.

SYLVESTRE, Jacques; Clinique Med de Rawdon, 201-3240 1e av, Rawdon QC J0K 1S0; Mon'79; (450)834-2304; Fax. (450)834-3345.

SYLVESTRE, Marie-Claude; CSSG-Hop de Gatineau, CP 2000 Succ Bureau-Chef 909 boul de la Verendrye O, Gatineau QC J8P 7H2; Sher'84; Anes. ac Staff, Hôpital de Gatineau; (819)561-8299

SYLVESTRE, Nicolas; GMF Des Seigneurs, 201-901 boul des Seigneurs, Terrebonne QC J6W 1T8; Sher'08; CCFP; Staff, Centre Hospitalier Pierre le Gardeur; (450)471-1117

SYLVESTRE, Pierre A; 6250 av Newman, Montreal QC H4E 4K4; Mon'72; (514)765-8000

SYLVESTRE, Pierre-Alexandre; CSSS de Laval, 1755 boul Rene-Laennec, Laval QC H7M 3L9; Laval'07; Staff, Hopital de la Cite de la santé; (450)668-1010; Fax. (450)975-5545.

SYLWESTROWICZ, Anna M; Victoria Gen Hosp, 1 Hospital Way, Victoria BC V8Z 6R5; Man'91; FRCPC; Anes. Staff Anes, Victoria General Hospital; Staff, Anaesthetic Services; Langs: Polish; (250)727-4152

SYLWESTROWICZ, Thomas A; Dr T A Sylwestrowicz Med Inc, 182 Wall St, Saskatoon SK S7K 1N4; Gdansk (Poland)'67; PhD; FRCPC; IntMed (Gastroenterology). Physician, Quance East Medical Clinic; Ac Staff, Saskatoon Health Region; Clin Prof Med, University of Saskatchewan; Langs: Polish; (306)477-2800; Fax. (306)477-2821.

SYME, Colin W; 201-174 Harwood Ave S, Ajax ON L1S 2H6; Edinburgh (Scotland)'68; Langs: French; (905)686-4424; Fax. (905)686-4761.

SYME, Roderick G; Bayshore Med Bldg, 302-3029 Carling Ave, Ottawa ON K2B 8E8; McM'80; DAB; FACS; FRCSC; GenSurg; VascSurg. Staff Surg, Queensway Carleton Hospital; (613)820-9403; Fax. (613)820-3738.

SYMINGTON, David J; Health Services Complex, 2-20 Kennedy Dr, Sussex NB E4E 2P1; Alb'82; Staff, Sussex Health Centre; (506)432-6866; Fax. (506)433-8329.

SYMINGTON, Ian R; City of Lakes Fam Hlth Team, C-960 Notre Dame Ave, Sudbury ON P3A 2T4; Ott'01; CCFP; Staff, Health Sciences North-St Joseph's Health Centre; (705)222-8326; Fax. (705)566-7617.

SYMMES, John C; York Prof Bldg, 100-679 Davis Dr, Newmarket ON L3Y 5G8; Tor'73; FRCPC; IntMed; Cardiol. (905)898-4073; Fax. (905)898-3437.

SYMON, Andrea L; Herold Road Family Physicians, 1-325 Herold Rd, Saskatoon SK S7V 1J7; Sask'09; CCFP; (306)374-2404; Fax. (306)477-0300.

SYMON, Keith; 6548 Hastings St, Burnaby BC V5B 1S2; Cape Town (South Africa)'82; MB ChB; Langs: Hebrew; (604)299-9769; Fax. (604)299-9772; ksymon@axionet.com.

SYMONDS, Christopher J; Richmond Road Diagnostic Ctre, 1820 Richmond Rd SW, Calgary AB T2T 5C7; UBC'88; ABIM; FRCPC; IntMed (Endocrinology); Endocrin&Metab. Staff Endocrin, Foothills Medical Centre; Staff, Calgary Regional Health Authority; Clinical Asst Prof Med, University Of Calgary; (403)955-8328; Fax. (403)955-8249; cjsymond@ucalgary.ca.

SYMONDS, J Christopher; 136-1 Market Square, Saint John NB E2L 4Z6; Mem'96; BSc(Biol.); FRCSC; Ophth (Cataract). Assoc Staff Ophth, Saint John Regional Hospital; (506)633-8282; Fax. (506)634-3908.

SYMONS, Sean P; Sunnybrook Hlth Sciences Ctre, 2075 Bayview Ave, Toronto ON M4N 3M5; Tor'95; FRCPC; DiagRad. Staff, Sunnybrook Health Sciences Centre; (416)480-5729

SYMS, Jonathan B; Addiction & Mental Hlth-Queen, 1113-1001 Queen St W, Toronto ON M6J 1H4; Qns'04; CCFP; CCFP; Staff, Centre for Addiction & Mental Health (CAMH) - Queen Site; (416)535-8501 x2971; Fax. (416)583-1284.

SYNNES, Anne R; Children's & Women's HC of BC, 1R13-4480 Oak St, Vancouver BC V6H 3V4; McG'81; MDCM; MHSc; FRCPC; Peds (Neonatal & Perinatal Medicine). Staff, BC Children's Hospital; Clin Associate Prof, University of British Columbia; Langs: Norwegian; French; (604)875-2135; Fax. (604)875-3106.

SYNNOTT, Dominique; Centre Méd Rockland, S100-100 ch Rockland, Mont-Royal QC H3P 2V9; Mon'87; LMCC; FRCSC; GenSurg (Oncology/Breast Cancer). Staff, Hôpital du Sacre-Coeur de Montréal; Prof, Universite de Montreal; Clin Prof, Université Laval; Langs: Bilingual(French/English); (514)331-4322; Fax. (514)331-8683.

SYNNOTT, Jocelyne; Clinique de Peds de Rimouski, 301-161 av Rouleau, Rimouski QC G5L 5T3; Sher'88; FRCPC; Peds. Staff, Hôpital Regional Rimouski; (418)724-4221; Fax. (418)725-3025.

SYPOSZ, Benedykt S; Parkdale Med Tower, 802-1081 Carling Ave, Ottawa ON K1Y 4G2; Tor'78; CCFP; FCFP; Staff, The Ottawa Hospital - Civic Campus; Clin Teacher Family Med, University of Ottawa; (613)725-2335; Fax. (613)728-2752.

SYRNYK, Jeffrey A; McKenzie Family Practice, 71 High St SE, Calgary AB T2Z 3T9; Alb'92; CCFP; (403)257-0500; Fax. (403)257-3186.

SYSAK, Daniel G; Red Deer Reg Hosp Centre, PO Box 5030 Stn Postal Box Ctr 3942 50A Ave, Red Deer AB T4N 4E7; Cal'93; Anes. Staff, Red Deer Regional Hospital Centre; (403)343-4768

SYSLAK, Paul H; William Osler HC-Brampton, 2100 Bovaird Dr E, Brampton ON L6R 3J7; Man'94; FRCPC; CCFP; Anes. Staff, William Osler Health System - Brampton Civic Hospital; (905)494-2120

SYTY-GOLDA, Marie B; Hamilton Downtown Med Ctre, 101-432 Main St E, Hamilton ON L8N 1J9; Wroclaw (Poland)'80; Ac Staff, Hamilton Health Sciences Centre - Juravinski Cancer Centre; Ac Staff, Hamilton Health Sciences Centre - McMaster Children's Hospital; Court Staff, St Joseph's Healthcare - Charlton Campus; Ac Staff, Hamilton Health Sciences Centre - Hamilton General Hospital; Clinical Asst Prof Family Med, McMaster University; Langs: Polish; (905)529-2423; Fax. (905)522-2600.

SZABO, Angelika F; The Coleman Clinic, 186 Kenneth St, Duncan BC V9L 1N4; Wes'87; Staff, Cowichan District Hospital; (250)746-4102; Fax. (250)746-5960.

SZABO, Eileen M; 101-315 5th Ave N, Saskatoon SK S7K 5Z8; Szeged (Hungary)'91; BSc; ABIM; FRCPC; IntMed (Dermatology). Staff, Saskatoon City Hospital; Clinical Asst Prof, Royal University Hospital; Clinical Asst Prof, University of Saskatchewan; Langs: Hungarian; French; (306)651-3900; Fax. (306)978-5276.

SZABO, Elod Z; The Hosp for Sick Children, 555 University Ave, Toronto ON M5G 1X8; Szeged (Other Foreign)'95; FRCPC; Anes. Staff, The Hospital For Sick Children; Langs: Hungarian; (416)813-7445

SZABO, Gabriel; CSSS du Suroît, 150 rue Saint-Thomas, Salaber-de-Valleyf QC J6T 6C1; Univ of Med & Pharm Targu Mures (Romania)'94; Staff, Centre Hospitalier Régional du Suroît; Langs: Romanian; English; (450)371-9920 x2228; Fax. (450)377-5604.

SZABO, Jason T; MUHC-Montreal Gen Hosp, A5 123-1650 av Cedar, Montreal QC H3G 1A4; Alb'89; CCFP; Staff, McGill University Health Centre - Montreal General Campus; Staff, St Mary's Hospital Centre; (514)934-8070; Fax. (514)937-1424.

SZABO, Michael S; University Health Network, 190 Elizabeth St, Toronto ON M5G 2C4; McM'94; BSc(Hons.); CCFP; CCFP(E.M.); Staff, Toronto General Hospital - UHN; Langs: French; (416)340-3946

SZABO, S C Mary; Copeman Health Care Center, 400-628 12 Ave SW, Calgary AB T2R 0H6; Cal'82; CCFP; CCFP(E.M.); FCFP; (403)270-2273; Fax. (403)521-2250.

SZABO, Thomas F; Coperman Health Care Centre, 400-628 12 Ave SW, Calgary AB T2R 0H6; Cal'79; CCFP; CCFP(E.M.); FCFP; (403)270-2273; Fax. (403)251-2250.

SZACHNOWSKA, Violetta I; Parksville After Hours Clinic, PO Box 250 Stn Main 154 Memorial Ave W, Parksville BC V9P 2G4; Szczecin (Poland)'88; CCFP; Langs: Polish; (250)248-7200; Fax. (250)248-2128.

SZAJKOWSKI, Stanley; Parkview Prof Centre, 205-2110 Main St, Winnipeg MB R2V 2C2; Man'72; BSc(Med); Langs: Polish; (204)339-1744; Fax. (204)334-2309.

SZAJKOWSKI, Terrence P; Prairie Trails Med Centre, 1345 Taylor Ave, Winnipeg MB R3M 3Y9; Man'07; CCFP; (204)475-0088

SZAKACS, Thomas A; Brant Community HC-Brantford, 200 Terrace Hill St, Brantford ON N3R 1G9; McM'02; DTM&H; FRCPC; IntMed (Family Medicine); InfectDis. Staff, The Brant Community Healthcare System - Brantford General Hospital Site; (519)751-5544; Fax. (519)752-7809.

SZAKY, Esther A; York Med Bldg, 205-250 Harding Blvd, Richmond Hill ON L4C 9M7; Semmelweis (Hungary)'79; FRCPC; IntMed; Nephrol. Langs: Hungarian; (905)508-5911; Fax. (905)508-2972.

SZALAY, David A; Hamilton HSC-Hamilton Gen, 237 Barton St E, Hamilton ON L8L 2X2; Tor'91; FRCSC; GenSurg; VascSurg. Staff, Hamilton Health Sciences Centre - Hamilton General Hospital; Staff, St Joseph's Healthcare - Charlton Campus; Assoc Prof, McMaster University; (905)527-4322; Fax. (905)521-0440.

SZARKA, Istvan L; 672 Upper James St, Hamilton ON L9C 2Z3; McM'83; CCFP; Staff Privil, Hamilton Health Sciences Centre - McMaster Children's Hospital; Court Staff Privil, St Joseph's Healthcare - Charlton Campus; McMaster University; Langs: Polish; Hungarian; (905)389-2253; Fax. (905)575-4669.

SZARVAS, Szilvia; Western Mem Reg Hosp, PO Box 2005 Stn Main 1 Brookfield Ave, Corner Brook NL A2H 6J7; Szeged (Hungary)'95; Staff, Western Memorial Regional Hospital; (709)637-5000

SZASZ, John; 2-695 Canterbury St, Woodstock ON N4S 8W7; Wes'54; Ophth. Staff, Woodstock General Hospital; Staff, Alexandra Hospital; Langs: Hungarian; (519)537-3871; Fax. (519)537-2917.

SZATMARI, Peter; McMaster University, 207-1280 Main St W, Hamilton ON L8S 4K1; McM'76; FRCPC; Psy. Staff, Hamilton Health Sciences Centre - McMaster University Medical Centre; Prof, McMaster University; (905)521-2100 x77364; Fax. (905)574-6665; szatmar@mcmaster.ca.

SZCZEPANIK, Dorota M; Carlington Comm Hlth Services, 900 Merivale Rd, Ottawa ON K1Z 5Z8; Academy of Medicine (Poland)'98; CCFP; (613)722-2161

SZCZESNY, Krystian M; 43 Prince Arthur St PO Box 698 Stn Main, Amherst NS B4H 4B8; Wroclaw (Poland)'81; FRCPC; IntMed (Gastroenterology). Staff IntMed, Cumberland Regional Health Care Center; Staff, North Cumberland Memorial Hospital; Staff, All Saints Springhill Hospital; (902)667-1017; Fax. (902)667-0664.

SZCZYGIELSKI, Blazej I; Ctre de Tulattavik de l'Ungava, PO Box 149, Kuujjuaq QC J0M 1C0; UBC'06; CCFP; CCFP(E.M.); Staff, Centre de sante Tulattavik de l'Ungava; Langs: Polish; French; (819)964-2905; Fax. (819)964-6353.

SZE, Augustine Y S; The Credit Valley Hosp, 2200 Eglinton Ave W, Mississauga ON L5M 2N1; Wes'99; FRCPC; Anes. Staff, The Credit Valley Hospital; (905)813-2200; augsze@aol.com.

SZE, Jacqueline Y M; Scarborough Comm Mental Hlth, 301-2425 Eglinton Ave E, Scarborough ON M1K 5G8; Tor'06; FRCPC; Psy. Staff, Hotel-Dieu Hospital; (416)431-8200; Fax. (416)759-5162.

SZE, Mabel C; Downtown Commun Hlth Clinic, 569 Powell St, Vancouver BC V6A 1F8; Tor'07; CCFP; Staff, Downtown Community Health Clinic; Langs: Cantonese; Mandarin; (604)255-3151

SZE, Michael M K; 201-236 Georgia St E, Vancouver BC V6A 1Z7; Tor'77; DAB; CCFP; CCFP(E.M.); FCFP; (604)689-8969; Fax. (604)689-8930; mksze@hotmail.com.

SZE, Shirley W M; Royal Inland Hosp, 5F AT-311 Columbia St, Kamloops BC V2C 2T1; Alb'76; CCFP; FCFP; Assoc Staff Vascular Improvement Clinic, Royal Inland Hospital; Staff, VIP Clinic; (250)314-2727; Fax. (250)374-0122.

SZEGO, Peter L; MUHC-Royal Victoria Hosp, R2 27-687 av des Pins O, Montreal QC H3A 1A1; McG'65; BSc; CSPQ; FRCPC; IntMed (Therapeutic Endoscopy); Gastroent. Consultant, St Mary's Hospital Centre; Staff Gastroent, McGill University Health Centre - Royal Victoria Hospital; assoc Prof, McGill University; Langs: Hungarian; French; (514)843-1616; Fax. (514)843-1421.

SZELAG, Marek A; Atrium Prof Bldg, 203-190 Cundles Rd E, Barrie ON L4M 4S5; Gdansk (Poland)'86; CCFP; Associate Family Med, Royal Victoria Regional Health Centre; Langs: Polish; (705)726-1198; Fax. (705)726-6229.

SZELAZEK, Joanna T; Manitoba Adolescent Trmt Ctre, 228 Maryland St, Winnipeg MB R3G 1L6; Man'95; BSc; FRCPC; Psy (Child & Adolescent Psychiatry). Langs: Polish.

SZENDREY, James J; Whitby Med Clinic, 200 Brock St N, Whitby ON L1N 4H5; Qns'88; CCFP; (905)668-3378; Fax. (905)668-3807.

SZENTGYORGYI, Eva M; Univ Hlth Network-Toronto Gen, EW 11E-200 Elizabeth St, Toronto ON M5G 2C4; Semmelweis (Hungary)'74; FRCPC; AnatPath. Staff, Toronto General Hospital - UHN; Langs: Hungarian; (416)340-5203

SZERB, Jennifer J; Queen Elizabeth II HSC-Halifax, 5F-1796 Summer St, Halifax NS B3H 3A7; Dal'84; FRCPC; Anes. Staff, Queen Elizabeth II Health Sciences Centre - Halifax Infirmary Site; (902)473-4326

SZERESZEWSKI, Abraham; Queenston Med & Dental Ctre, 204-631 Queenston Rd, Hamilton ON L8K 6R5; Qns'74; CCFP; FCFP; (905)561-2932; Fax. (905)561-4882.

SZETO, Christopher C; Sudbury Reg Hosp-Laurentian, 41 Ramsey Lake Rd, Sudbury ON P3E 5J1; Mem'02; FRCSC; Otol. Staff, Health Sciences North-Laurentian Site; Staff, Health Sciences North-Ramsey Lake Health Center; (705)673-6836; cszeto@hsnsudbury.ca.

SZETO, Isabella W; Headwaters Health Care Centre, 100 Rolling Hills Dr, Orangeville ON L9W 4X9; Wes'01; CCFP; Staff, Headwaters Health Care Centre - Orangeville Site; Langs: Cantonese; (519)941-2410

SZETO, Kenneth P C; Szeto Choy & Partners, 203A-3636 Steeles Ave E, Markham ON L3R 1K9; Tor'82; BSc; Langs: Cantonese; Mandarin; (905)477-5679; Fax. (905)477-5632.

SZETO, Michael; The Ottawa Hosp-Gen Campus, CCW 1401-501 Smyth Rd, Ottawa ON K1H 8L6; Tor'01; FRCPC; Anes. Staff, The Ottawa Hospital - General Campus; (613)737-8187

SZEZEPANIAK, Theresa M S; 203-9123 Mary St, Chilliwack BC V2P 4H7; Leicester (England)'97; MB ChB; DRCOG; (604)795-9161

SZIKLAS, Tibor J; Medical Arts Bldg, 218-1538 rue Sherbrooke O, Montreal QC H3G 1L5; Budapest (Hungary)'53; Staff, Catherine Booth Hospital; assoc Staff, St Mary's Hospital Centre; Langs: Hungarian; French; (514)935-7149

SZILAGYI, Alison J; Front-Frederick Health Service, 14F-365 Bloor St E, Toronto ON M4W 3L4; McG'04; CCFP; (416)362-8777; Fax. (416)362-7879.

SZILAGYI, Andrew; SMBD Jewish Gen Hosp, E110-3755 Cote-Ste-Catherine, Montreal QC H3T 1E2; McG'74; FRCPC; IntMed (P.Q.); Gastroent. Staff, Sir Mortimer B Davis Jewish General; Staff Teacher, McGill University; Langs: Hungarian; French; (514)340-8144; Fax. (514)340-8282.

SZILVASSY, Imre Z; 264 Concession St, Hamilton ON L9A 1B2; Debrecen (Hungary)'84; Langs: German; Hungarian; (905)383-1921; Fax. (905)383-6562.

SZIRMAY-KALOS, Tibor Z; 201-386 Cambria St, Stratford ON N5A 1J4; Budapest (Hungary)'87; FRCSC; ObstGyn. Staff, Listowel Memorial Hospital - Listowel Wingham Hospitals Alliance; Langs: Hungarian; (519)272-1999; Fax. (519)272-9888.

SZKOTAK, Artur J; University of Alberta Hosp, 4B1 34-8440 112 St NW, Edmonton AB T6G 2B7; Alb'05; FRCPC; HemPath. Staff, University of Alberta Hospital; (780)407-1407; Fax. (780)407-8599.

SZKRUMELAK, Nadia; Allan Memorial Inst, 1025 av des Pins O, Montreal QC H3A 1A1; McG'80; FRCPC; Psy. Staff, McGill University Health Centre - Royal Victoria Hospital; Médecin, Allan Memorial Institute; Langs: French; (514)934-1934 x35683; Fax. (514)843-2858.

SZKUP, Beata E; Royal University Hosp, 103 Hospital Dr, Saskatoon SK S7N 0W8; Warsaw (Poland)'88; FRCPC; Anes. Staff, Royal University Hospital; (306)655-1000

SZKUP, Leszek P; Royal University Hosp, 103 Hospital Dr, Saskatoon SK S7N 0W8; Warsaw (Poland)'85; FRCPC; DiagRad. Asst Prof Med Imaging, Royal University Hospital; Langs: Polish; (306)655-2402; Fax. (306)665-0830.

SZLANTA, Agata; Providence CCC-St Mary's, PO Box 3600 Stn Main 340 Union St, Kingston ON K7L 5A2; Mon'07; CCFP; Staff, Providence Care - St Mary's of the Lake Hospital Site; Langs: Bilingual(English/French); (613)544-5220; Fax. (613)544-4017.

SZMITKO, Paul E; PG Medical Education Office, 2F-500 University Ave, Toronto ON M5G 1V7; Tor'05; FRCPC; IntMed; Cardiol. (416)978-6976

SZMUILOWICZ, Julio; Dr Julio Szmuilowicz Med Corp, 46 Edgecombe Ave, Toronto ON M5N 2X3; (Mexico)'73; DABPN; FRCPC; Psy (Psychoanalysis). Asst Prof, University of Toronto; Langs: Spanish; Hebrew; Portuguese; Yiddish; (416)783-3330; Fax. (416)783-3330.

SZMUILOWICZ, Sharon; Mount Sinai Hosp, 937-600 University Ave, Toronto ON M5G 1X5; Tor'04; FRCPC; Psy. Staff, Mount Sinai Hospital; Langs: Spanish; (416)586-4800; Fax. (416)586-8654.

SZOMBATHY, Stanley P; 1812 Marshall St, Kelowna BC V1Y 2B7; Sask'83; BSc; FRCPC; Peds (Allergy). Staff Peds, Kelowna General Hospital; (250)868-2442; Fax. (250)868-3422; sszombathy@telus.net.

SZOZDA, Timothy J P; Belmont Prof Centre, 200-564 Belmont Ave W, Kitchener ON N2M 5N6; Wes'86; CCFP; FCFP; Staff, Grand River Hospital - Kitchener/Waterloo Health Centre; Staff, St Mary's General Hospital; (519)742-2046; Fax. (519)742-3607.

SZPAKOWICZ, Mikolaj D; Surrey Mem Hosp, 13750 96 Ave, Surrey BC V3V 1Z2; Ott'00; CCFP; CCFP(E.M.); Staff, Surrey Memorial Hospital; Langs: Polish; (604)581-2211

SZPAKOWSKI, Pawel P; Hamilton HSC-Henderson Site, 711 Concession St, Hamilton ON L8V 1C3; Gdansk (Poland)'02; CCFP; Staff, Hamilton Health Sciences Centre-Juravinski Site; (905)521-2100

SZPEJDA, Monika A; Niagara Health Centre, 206-180 Vine St S, St Catharines ON L2R 7P3; Cracow (Poland)'80; FRCPC; Peds. Staff, Niagara Health System - St Catharines General Site; Langs: Polish; (905)682-0122; Fax. (905)682-1429.

SZPEJDA, Witold J; Niagara H System-St Catharine, PO Box 3018 Stn Main 142 Queenston St, St Catharines ON L2R 7C6; Cracow (Poland)'80; FRCPC; Anes. Staff, Niagara Health System - St Catharines General Site; Staff, Niagara Health System - Ontario Street Site; Langs: Polish; (905)684-7271 x45561; Fax. (905)684-1468.

SZPILBERG, Michael; Plaza Cote-des-Neiges, 125-6700 ch Cote-des-Neiges, Montreal QC H3S 2B2; Cracow (Poland)'75; Langs: Polish; Russian; (514)342-2941; Fax. (514)342-3976; szpil@videotron.ca.

SZPINDEL, Isaac I E; 32 Park Rd, Toronto ON M4W 2N4; McM'92; Langs: Hebrew; Yiddish; French; (416)598-9344; Fax. (416)598-8198.

SZTRAMKO, Richard W K; St Paul's Hosp, 9F-1081 Burrard St, Vancouver BC V6Z 1Y6; Tor'07; GeriatricMed; IntMed. Staff SPH Elder Care, Providence Health Care - St Paul's Hospital; (604)682-2344

SZTUCZKA, Waldemar J; Southland Court Med Clinic, 333-10601 Southport Rd SW, Calgary AB T2W 3M6; Gdansk (Poland)'78; (403)271-1000

SZTUKOWSKI, Izabela; Alberta Children's Hosp, 2888 Shaganappi Trail NW, Calgary AB T3B 6A8; Alb'02; FRCPC; Peds; PedEmergMed; EmergMed. Staff Pediatric Emerg, Alberta Children's Hospital; (403)955-7070; Fax. (403)955-7398.

SZTUKOWSKI, Teresa M; Scenic Acres Med Centre, 8555 Scurfield Dr NW, Calgary AB T3L 1Z6; Silesian (Poland)'75; CCFP; FCFP; Langs: Polish; (403)547-2255; Fax. (403)547-2254.

SZUDEK, Ewa A; Medical Arts Bldg, 407-5880 Spring Garden Rd, Halifax NS B3H 1Y1; Warsaw (Poland)'73; FRCPC; Peds (Neonatology)., Dalhousie University; Langs: Polish; (902)422-6421; Fax. (902)423-5485; eszudek@dal.ca.

SZUDEK, Jacek; PO Box 21189 Terwillegar PO, Edmonton AB T6R 2V4; Dal'06; Otol (Head & Neck Surgery); IntMed. Staff, University of Alberta Hospital; (780)407-6640

SZUL, J Michael; College of Phys & Surg of Ont, 80 College St, Toronto ON M5G 2E2; Man'74; CCFP; FCFP; Physician, Ukrainian Canadian Care Centre; Member, College of Physicians & Surgeons of Ontario; (416)967-2600; Fax. (416)967-2616.

SZULC, Elizabeth K; Vodden Med Arts Centre, 100-36 Vodden St E, Brampton ON L6V 4H4; Szczecin (Poland)'80; Langs: Polish; (905)450-5278

SZUMACHER, Ewa F; Sunnybrook Hlth Sciences Ctre, 2075 Bayview Ave, Toronto ON M4N 3M5; Lodz (Poland)'82; FRCPC; RadOncol. Staff, Sunnybrook Health Sciences Centre; Staff, Sunnybrook Health Sciences Centre - Edmond Odette Cancer Centre; Asst Prof, University of Toronto; Langs: Polish; French; Russian; (416)480-6000 x2802; Fax. (416)480-6002.

SZUMSKI, Roman G; National Research Council, 1015-100 Sussex Dr, Ottawa ON K1A 0R6; Qns'84; FRCPC; GenPath. VP Life Sciences, National Research Council; Langs: Bilingual(English/French); (613)993-9244; roman.szumski@nrc-cnrc.gc.ca.

SZWAJCER, David; Cancer Care Manitoba, ON 2064-675 McDermot Ave, Winnipeg MB R3B 0V9; Wes'00; FRCPC; IntMed (Medical Oncology); Hem. Staff, Health Sciences Centre; Physician, CancerCare Manitoba; (204)787-2197

SZYMANSKA, Aleksandra; Central Square Med Clinic, 1209 Main St, Smithers BC V0J 2N0; McM'08; CCFP; Langs: Polish; (250)428-8873

SZYMANSKI, Jan F; Saint John Reg Hosp, PO Box 2100 Stn Main 400 University Ave, Saint John NB E2L 4L2; Poznan (Poland)'79; Staff, Saint John Regional Hospital; (506)648-6000

SZYMANSKI, Waldemar A; Allin Clinic, 10155 120 St NW, Edmonton AB T5K 2A2; Poznan (Poland)'74; PhD; FRCPC; Peds (Pediatric Gastroenterology). Med Staff, Royal Alexandra Hospital; Staff Privil, University of Alberta Hospital; Staff, University of Alberta; Langs: Polish; Russian; (780)482-7551; Fax. (780)488-2056.

SZYMCZAK, Peter S; PG Medical Education Office, 70 Barrie St, Kingston ON K7L 3N6; Poznan University (Poland)'07; Psy.

SZYMONOWICZ, Wanda M; Credit Valley Hosp, 2200 Eglinton Ave W, Mississauga ON L5M 2N1; McM'77; FRCPC; Peds. Dir Level II Nursery, The Credit Valley Hospital; Staff, Pediatric Medical Clinic; Langs: Italian; French; Polish; Spanish; Portuguese; Romanian; (905)813-4120; Fax. (905)813-4128.

T'IEN, Wallace; Datmouth Med Centre, 206-46 Portland St, Dartmouth NS B2Y 1H4; Dal'80; FRCSC; Urol. (902)407-3668; Fax. (902)407-4053.

T'IEN, Willis L; D-2002 Comox Ave, Comox BC V9M 3M6; Dal'77; FRCSC; GenSurg. (250)339-7115; Fax. (250)339-7115.

TA, Diana; CSSS de la Vallée de l'Or, 725 6e rue, Val-d'Or QC J9P 3Y1; Mon'07; CCFP; Staff, Centre Hospitalier de Val d'Or; (819)825-6711

TA, Hien Minh; Mackenzie Richmond Hill Hosp, 10 Trench St, Richmond Hill ON L4C 4Z3; Dal'91; FRCPC; Anes;CCFP; FCFP; Staff, Mackenzie Richmond Hill Hospital; Langs: Vietnamese; (905)883-1212

TA, Thuan C; Gaetz Family Practice, 101-45744 Gaetz St, Chilliwack BC V2R 3P1; London (England)'92; MB BS; CCFP; (604)847-3782; Fax. (604)847-3789.

TA, To-Quyen; 202-535 boul Sir-Wilfrid-Lauri, Beloeil QC J3G 5E9; Laval'89; Ophth (P.Q.) (Glaucoma). (450)464-0821; Fax. (450)464-8799.

TA, Tuyet Phi; Polyclinique Rosemont, 3377 boul Rosemont, Montreal QC H1X 1K4; Sher'97; Staff, Hôpital Chinois de Montréal; Langs: Chinese; Vietnamese; English; (514)798-8688; Fax. (514)798-8680.

TAABAZUI, Mary-Margaret; London HSC-South Street Site, 583-375 South St, London ON N6A 4G5; Havana (Cuba)'95; FRCPC; IntMed. Staff, London Health Sciences Centre - South Street; Staff, London Health Sciences Centre - Victoria Campus; (519)667-6843

TAABAZUING, Mary-Margaret; London HSC-Victoria Hosp, PO Box 5010 800 Commissioners Rd E, London ON N6A 4G5; Havana Higher Institute of Medical Sciences (Cuba)'95; FRCPC; IntMed. Staff, London Health Sciences Centre - Children's Hospital; Langs: Spanish; (519)685-8500

TAAM, Jason E W D; Clinical Sciences Bldg, CSB 8120-152 University Campus, Edmonton AB T6G 2G3; Man'03; FRCPC; Anes. Staff, University of Alberta Hospital; Langs: Bilingual(English/French); (780)407-8822

TABACK, Shayne P; Children's Hosp, 840 Sherbrook St, Winnipeg MB R3A 1R9; Man'89; FRCPC; Peds (Pediatric Endocrinology); Endocrin&Metab. Prov Staff Med, Health Sciences Centre; Staff, John Buhler Research Centre; Asst Prof Med, University of Manitoba; tabacksp@cc.umanitoba.ca.

TABAH, Meryl A; Lakeshore Gen Hosp, 160 av Stillview, Pointe-Claire QC H9R 2Y2; Laval'07; CCFP; CCFP(E.M.); Staff, Lakeshore General Hospital - Pointe Claire; (514)630-2225

TABAH, Nicolas; CSSS de Manicouagan, 635 boul Jolliet, Baie-Comeau QC G5C 1P1; Sher'01; FRCPC; DiagRad. Staff, Centre Hospitalier Régional Baie-Comeau; (418)589-3701

TABAH, Roger J; MUHC-Montreal Gen Hosp, L9 413-1650 av Cedar, Montreal QC H3G 1A4; McG'80; FRCSC; GenSurg (Endocrinology Surgery). Staff, McGill University Health Centre - Royal Victoria Hospital; Staff, McGill University Health Centre - Montreal General Campus; assoc Prof Surg, McGill University; Langs: French; (514)934-1934 x44333; Fax. (514)934-8210.

TABAKIAN, Ohan; CSSS Bordeaux-Cartierville, 555 boul Gouin O, Montreal QC H3L 1K5; Beirut (Lebanon)'64; Staff, Pavillon Notre-Dame de la Merci; (514)331-3020

TABARI, Mohammad; 208-1585 Markham Rd, Scarborough ON M1B 2W1; Tehran (Iran)'94; FRCSC; GenSurg (Critical Care Medicine). Staff/Gen Surgeon, The Scarborough Hospital - General Campus; Langs: Farsi; Persian; (416)439-9253; Fax. (416)439-2552.

TABARMANAF, Tofigh; Burnaby Hosp, 3935 Kincaid St, Burnaby BC V5G 2X6; Santiago Technological (Dominican Republic)'98; CCFP; Staff Hospitalist Program, Burnaby Hospital; (604)434-4211

TABARSI, Aref; Campbell River & Dist Gen Hosp, 375 2nd Ave, Campbell River BC V9W 3V1; UBC'95; FRCPC; GenPath (Cytology). Staff, Campbell River & District General Hospital; Langs: Persian; (250)850-2141

TABASSUM, Farah J; Four Villages Comm Health Ctr, 1700 Bloor St W, Toronto ON M6P 4C3; McG'99; CCFP; FCFP; (416)604-3361; Fax. (416)604-3367.

TABBANE, Karim; Douglas Mental Hlth Univ Inst, 6875 boul Lasalle, LaSalle QC H4H 1R3; Staff, Douglas Mental Health University Institute; (514)761-6131

TABET, Jean-Claude; CHUM-Hop Notre-Dame, 1560 rue Sherbrooke E, Montreal QC H2L 4M1; Mon'82; FRCSC; Otol (Head & Neck Surgery). Chef Serv, Centre Hospitalier l'Université de Montréal (CHUM) - Hôpital Notre-Dame; adj Prof, Universite de Montreal; (514)890-8000 x27201

TABIB, Mohamed A; Windsor Reg Hosp-Metropolitan, 1995 Lens Ave, Windsor ON N8W 1L9; Al-Fateh (Libya)'99; MB ChB; FRCPC; DiagRad. Staff, Windsor Regional Hospital - Metropolitan Site; Langs: Arabic; Spanish; (519)254-3150

TABLOIE, Farshid; Scarborough Hosp-Birchmount, 3030 Birchmount Rd, Scarborough ON M1W 3W3; Tehran (Iran)'98; FRCSC; OrthSurg. Staff, The Scarborough Hospital - Birchmount Campus; Langs: Farsi; Persian; (416)495-2600

TABOR, Thomas K; 701-440 Central Ave, London ON N6B 2E5; Qns'08; CCFP; Langs: Bilingual(English/French); (519)601-7577; Fax. (519)601-7737.

TABORI, Uri Y; The Hosp For Sick Children, 555 University Ave, Toronto ON M5G 1X8; Hadassah (Israel)'96; Staff, The Hospital For Sick Children; (416)813-7654 x1503; Fax. (416)813-8024; uri.tabori@sickkids.ca.

TACKABERRY, Kelly M J; PO Box 80044 Rpo Beacon Hill, Calgary AB T3R 0B2; Alb'10; CCFP.

TADDEO, Danielle; Hôpital Ste-Justine, 3175 ch Cote-Sainte-Catherine, Montreal QC H3T 1C5; Mon'89; FRCPC; Peds (Adolescent Medicine). Staff, Hôpital Ste-Justine; Clin Prof, Universite de Montreal; (514)345-4722; Fax. (514)345-4778.

TADDEUCCI, Sean; 1122-736 Granville St, Vancouver BC V6Z 1G3; UBC'90; (604)687-5328; Fax. (604)687-5328.

TADEPALLI, Srinivasa R; Whitehorse Med Services Ltd, 406 Lambert St, Whitehorse YT Y1A 1Z7; Mysore (India)'93; MB BS; FRCSI; Pres, Whitehorse General Hospital; Pres, College of Physicians & Surgeons of Yukon; Physician, Whitehorse Medical Services Ltd; (867)393-6600; Fax. (867)393-6601.

TADIBOYINA, Venu T; Scarborough Hosp-General Div, 3050 Lawrence Ave E, Scarborough ON M1P 2V5; Wes'06; FRCPC; IntMed. Staff, The Scarborough Hospital - General Campus; (416)431-8200

TADROS, Ayman E; Bonaventure Med Clinic, 101-12427 Bonaventure Dr SE, Calgary AB T2J 3N8; Assiut (Egypt)'98; MB ChB; CCFP; Physician, River Valley Medical Clinic; (403)225-9499

TADROS, Cherif; Western Med Assessment, 17204 106A Ave NW, Edmonton AB T5S 1E6; Mon'85; FRCSC; OrthSurg. Staff, Western Medical Assessments; Langs: English; French; (780)433-1191; ctadros@sympatico.ca.

TADROS, Ibtissam F H; 301-1065 Canadian Pl, Mississauga ON L4W 3C2; Ain Shams University (Egypt)'96; CCFP; Langs: Arabic; (905)624-5230; Fax. (905)624-6787.

TADROS, Mina; Maple Med Clinic, 2-1079 Maple Ave, Milton ON L9T 0A5; Medical Univ of Americas (USA)'04; MS; BSc; CCFP; (905)636-7600; Fax. (905)636-7601.

TADROS, Monir L; Markham College Med Clinic, 409-474 College St, Toronto ON M6G 1A4; Cairo (Egypt)'62; FRCSC; Ophth (Cataract). Langs: Arabic; (416)922-7198; Fax. (416)922-4081.

TADROS, Peter; 404 Old Tecumseh Rd, Windsor ON N8N 3S8; Sask'65; CRCP; FRCPC; DiagRad (Angiography). Hon Staff Radiol, Hôtel-Dieu Grace Hospital; Aj Prof, University of Western Ontario; (519)479-8551; Fax. (519)979-8128.

TADROS, Shaheer; The Ottawa Hosp-Gen Campus, 501 Smyth Rd Box 202, Ottawa ON K1H 8L6; Mem'80; FRCSC; GenSurg. Staff, The Ottawa Hospital - General Campus; Assoc Staff, The Ottawa Hospital - Riverside Campus; Langs: Arabic; French; (613)737-8899

TADROS, Sharif W; Burlington Med Centre, 2400 Guelph Line, Burlington ON L7P 4M7; Mem'84; Staff, Trillium Health Centre - Mississauga; Langs: Arabic; Lithuanian; French; (905)336-1221

TADROS, William I; 10153 King George Hwy PO Box 3110, Surrey BC V3T 2W1; Cairo (Egypt)'79; MB ChB; (604)951-0885

TADROSS, Alphonse; Upper River Valley Hosp, 11300 130 Rte, Watervil-Carleton NB E7P 0A4; Assiut (Egypt)'73; Staff, Upper River Valley Hospital - Waterville; (506)375-2943

TADROSS, Emmanuel H; Grand River Hosp-KW Hlth Ctre, PO Box 9056 Stn C 835 King St W, Kitchener ON N2G 1G3; Cairo (Egypt)'63; MRCPsy(Eng); DAB; MB ChB; FRCPC; Psy (Child Psychiatry). Staff, Grand River Hospital - Kitchener/Waterloo Health Centre; Staff, St Mary's General Hospital; Staff, Grand River Hospital - Freeport Site; Med Dir, Sunlife Canada; Langs: Arabic; French; (519)745-0511

TADROSS, Latif A A S; Guelph Gen Hosp, 115 Delhi St, Guelph ON N1E 4J4; Ain Shams (Egypt)'74; MB ChB; FRCPC; AnatPath; GenPath. Staff, Guelph General Hospital; Langs: Arabic; (519)837-6440 x2880; ltadross@gghorg.ca.

TADROUS, Zakaria L T; Tadrous Eye Centre, 102-34143 Marshall Rd, Abbotsford BC V2S 1L8; Ain Shams (Egypt)'82; FRCS(Glas. Ed); MB ChB; FRCSC; Ophth (Cataract). Staff, Chilliwack General Hospital; Staff, Abbotsford Regional Hospital & Cancer Centre; Staff, Mission Memorial Hospital; Langs: Arabic; Punjabi; (604)852-2040; Fax. (604)852-2045; ztadrous@telus.net.

TAEEB, Hussein A A; Access Med Centre, 13718 113A St, Edmonton AB T5X 4H7; Al Fateh (Libya)'02; CCFP; (780)456-3067; Fax. (780)478-6384.

TAERK, Gary S; 102-300 St Clair Ave W, Toronto ON M4V 1S4; Tor'73; FRCPC; Psy (Psychoanalysis). Associate Psy, Toronto General Hospital - UHN; Asst Prof, University of Toronto; (416)969-9795; Fax. (416)484-9227.

TAFLER, Gitta E; 289 Inglewood Dr, Toronto ON M4T 1J2; Tor'71; FRCPC; Psy. (416)483-1959; Fax. (416)483-8042.

TAGALAKIS, Vasiliki V; SMBD Jewish Gen Hosp, 3755 ch Cote-Sainte-Catherine, Montreal QC H3T 1E2; McG'96; FRCPC; IntMed. Staff, Sir Mortimer B Davis Jewish General; (514)340-8222 x4974; Fax. (514)340-7905.

TAGBOTO, Senyo K; Central Med Clinic, 6-1061 Central Ave N, Swift Current SK S9H 4Y9; (England)'87; CCST(UK); MSc; MRCP(UK); FRCP(Ed); FRCPC; IntMed; Nephrol. Consultant IntMed & Nephrol, Cypress Regional Hospital; (306)773-5855; Fax. (306)778-3799.

TAGEMOUATI, Mohammed; 160 av Stillview, Pointe claire QC H9R 2Y2; Mohammed V (Morocco)'95; Staff, Centre Hospitalier de Val d'Or; Langs: English; Arabic; French; (819)630-2225 x2699; tagahmed@yahoo.fr.

TAGGART, Jason J; Alberta Children's Hosp, 2888 Shaganappi Trail NW, Calgary AB T3B 6A8; Dal'05; FRCPC; Psy. Staff, Alberta Children's Hospital; (403)955-3077

TAGGART, Linda R; Univ Hlth Network-Toronto Gen, 13N 213-200 Elizabeth St, Toronto ON M5G 2C4; Tor'07; InfectDis; IntMed. Staff, Toronto General Hospital - UHN; (416)340-3505; Fax. (416)340-3357.

TAGGESELL, Richard J; Misericordia Comm Hosp & HC, 16940 87 Ave NW, Edmonton AB T5R 4H5; Oxford (England)'81; MB ChB; FRCPC; Anes. Staff, Covenant Health - Misericordia Community Hospital; Staff, Saanich Peninsula Hospital; (780)735-2863

TAGLIABUE, Giovanni; Foothills Med Centre, 1403 29 St NW, Calgary AB T2N 2T9; Staff, Foothills Medical Centre; (403)944-1570; Fax. (403)283-4994.

TAGUCHI, Yoshinori; MUHC-Royal Victoria Hosp, S6 86-687 av des Pins O, Montreal QC H3A 1A1; McG'59; PhD(Exp Med); FRCSC; Urol. Staff, McGill University Health Centre - Royal Victoria Hospital; (514)843-1525

TAHA, Hussam A A; Jeffrey's Med Clinic, GD, Jeffrey's NL A0N 1P0; Al-Nahrain University (Other Foreign)'02; CCFP; (709)660-2607

TAHA, Monir; Halton Region Health, 1151 Bronte Rd, Oakville ON L6M 3L1; Tor'87; MHSc; FRCPC; CommunMed (Public Health);CCFP; FCFP; Assoc Med Officer of Hlth, Halton Region Health; (905)825-6000 x7806; Fax. (905)825-1444.

TAHAINEH, Sakher M H; Health Sciences Centre, 300 Prince Philip Dr, St. John's NL A1B 3V6; (Jordan)'03; MB BS; Staff, Health Sciences Centre; (709)737-6300

TAHAN, Majd; CSSS du Suroît, 150 rue Saint-Thomas, Salaber-de-Valleyf QC J6T 6C1; Aleppo (Syria)'86; FRCPC; IntMed. Staff, Centre Hospitalier Régional du Suroît; Langs: English; French; (450)371-9925; Fax. (450)371-7454.

TAHER, Altaf; Health Sciences Centre, 1539C-300 Prince Philip Dr, St. John's NL A1B 3V6; Karnatak University Dharwar (India)'88; FRCPC; AnatPath. Staff, Health Sciences Centre; (709)737-6300

TAHER, Fakhruddin; Trillium Hlth Ctr-West Toronto, 150 Sherway Dr, Etobicoke ON M9C 1A5; Karachi (Pakistan)'79; FRCPC; IntMed. Staff, Trillium Health Centre - West Toronto; Langs: Urdu; (416)521-4196

TAHER, Ismail T A; Lewisporte Med Clinic, PO Box 1195, Lewisporte NL A0G 3A0; U of Garyounis (Libya)'02; MB ChB; Staff, Western Memorial Regional Hospital.

TAHER, Karim; Orillia Soldier's Mem Hosp, 170 Colborne St W, Orillia ON L3V 2Z3; Tor'94; BScChemEng; CCFP; Staff Anes, Orillia Soldiers' Memorial Hospital; (705)325-2201 x3248; Fax. (705)325-3181; kstaher@osmh.on.ca.

TAHER, Muba S; Keystone Dermatology Institute, 303-2377 111 St NW, Edmonton AB T6J 5E5; Alb'99; FRCPC; Derm (Dermatology Surgery). Clinical Asst Prof Derm, University of Alberta; (780)439-7546; Fax. (780)988-6647.

TAHER, Taha H; 2933 66 St NW, Edmonton AB T6K 4C1; Alb'98; FRCPC; IntMed; Cardiol. Staff, University of Alberta Hospital; (780)485-6669; Fax. (780)485-6835.

TAHER, Zaki A; Keystone Dermatology Institute, 303-2377 111 St NW, Edmonton AB T6J 5E5; Alb'06; (780)439-7546; Fax. (780)988-6647.

TAHERI, Sepideh; Springbank Paediatric Serv Inc, 206-460 Springbank Dr, London ON N6J 0A8; University of Edinburgh (Scotland)'89; (519)641-8687

TAHERI-ANARAKI, Atousa; Richmond Hill After Hours Clin, 301 High Tech Rd, Richmond Hill ON L4B 4R2; Islami Azad University (Saudi Arabia)'96; CCFP; (905)709-4274

TAHILIANI, Manoj; 104A-300 King St W, Oshawa ON L1J 2K1; Ott'00; FRCPC; IntMed; Cardiol. Staff Invasive Cardiol, Lakeridge Health - Oshawa Site; (905)245-0616; Fax. (905)245-0618.

TAHILIANI, Ravi; 104A-300 King St W, Oshawa ON L1J 2K1; Mem'98; FRCPC; IntMed; Cardiol. Staff Cardiol, Lakeridge Health - Port Perry Site; Chief Cardiol, Lakeridge Health - Oshawa Site; (905)245-0616; Fax. (905)245-0618.

TAHIR, Ferhana; Family Care Med Centre, 104-3050 Garden St, Whitby ON L1R 2G7; Nishtar Medical College (Pakistan)'03; CCFP; CCFP(E.M.); (905)430-5305; Fax. (905)430-6416.

TAHIR, Ismail T A; Family Med Clinic, 484-490 Main St, Lewisporte NL A0G 3A0; (Other Foreign)'02; CCFP; (709)360-7511; Fax. (709)535-0172.

TAHIR, Laeeq A; Moncton Med Clinic, 404-860 Mountain Rd, Moncton NB E1C 2N7; Islamia (Pakistan)'85; MB BS; MD; FRCP; FRCPC; Psy (Anxiety & Mood Disorders). Consultant Psy, The Moncton Hospital; Asst Prof, Dalhousie University; Langs: Urdu; Hindi; Punjabi; (506)857-5893; Fax. (506)857-5894; latahir@serha.ca.

TAHIRA, Shamim; Burntwood Comm Hlth Resource, 50 Selkirk Ave, Thompson MB R8N 0M7; (Other Foreign)'91; CCFP; Physician, Burntwood Regional Health Authority; (204)677-1777; Fax. (204)677-1755.

TAHIRKHELI, Surriya J; The Ottawa Hosp-Gen Campus, 501 Smyth Rd, Ottawa ON K1H 8L6; Punjab (Pakistan)'73; FRCPC; Psy. Staff, The Ottawa Hospital - General Campus; Langs: Punjabi; Urdu; (613)737-8010; Fax. (613)739-8115.

TAHLAN, Pramil; 7 Jack Poole Dr, Woodstock ON N4S 8V9; Rajasthan (India)'71; MB BS; FRCPC; Psy. Consultant, Woodstock General Hospital; Langs: Hindi; (519)421-1235; Fax. (519)290-2280.

TAI, Chao; Hys Med Centre, 610-11010 101 St NW, Edmonton AB T5H 4B9; (Singapore)'69; MB BS; FRCPC; Neur (Neuromuscular Diseases). Ac Staff, University of Alberta Hospital; Consultant, Royal Alexandra Hospital; Consultant, Glenrose Rehabilitation Hospital; Clin Assoc Prof, University of Alberta; Langs: Chinese; (780)428-9538; Fax. (780)428-9539.

TAI, Charles C F; 204-5678 Granville St, Vancouver BC V6M 3C5; Alb'95; FRCPC; IntMed; Neur. Langs: Cantonese; (604)269-3729; Fax. (604)269-3723.

TAI, Christine J Y; McNeely Med Clinic, 455 McNeely Ave, Carleton Place ON K7C 4S6; The Flinders University (Australia)'07; CCFP; (613)253-2233

TAI, Davina J; Saskatoon Nephrology Group, 434-230 Avenue R S, Saskatoon SK S7M 2Z1; Sask'04; MSc; FRCPC; IntMed; Nephrol. Clinical Asst Prof, University of Saskatchewan; (306)934-3300; Fax. (306)934-3355.

TAI, Derek Y H; 813 Richmond St, London ON N6A 3H6; McM'07; CCFP; Langs: Cantonese; (519)433-4330

TAI, Emelda M; 207-294 Main St, Toronto ON M4C 4X5; Malaya (Singapore)'59; MB BS; Langs: Mandarin; Cantonese; Thai; (416)698-2226; Fax. (416)698-6346.

TAI, Evelyn K; 226 Meadowvale Prof Centre, 6855 Meadowvale Town Ctre Cir, Mississauga ON L5N 2Y1; Tor'81; CCFP; FCFP; Langs: Cantonese; Mandarin; (905)821-2114; Fax. (905)821-1360.

TAI, Isabella T W; Div of Gastroenterology, 5153-2775 Laurel St, Vancouver BC V5Z 1M9; Tor'95; FRCPC; IntMed; Gastroent. Staff, Vancouver General Hospital - Centennial Pavillion; Langs: Mandarin; Portuguese; (604)875-5640; Fax. (604)875-5447.

TAI, Linda C L; 4186 Dunbar St, Vancouver BC V6S 2E7; UBC'92; (604)739-9881; Fax. (604)739-9803.

TAI, Lucas; 201-1011 Dufferin St, Toronto ON M6H 4B5; Tor'80; Langs: Mandarin; Taiwanese; (416)531-9925; Fax. (416)531-6599.

TAI, Peter C; Univ Health Network-Toronto Western Hosp, 446 5 WW-399 Bathurst St, Toronto ON M5T 2S8; Alb'00; ABPN; FRCPC; Neur (Epilepsy). Staff, Toronto Western Hospital - University Health Network; (416)603-5685; Fax. (416)603-5768.

TAI, R W Melissa; 505-18 Wynford Dr, North York ON M3C 3S2; Tor'93; FRCSC; ObstGyn (Urological Gynecology). Staff, Toronto East General Hospital Inc; Lecturer ObstGyn, University of Toronto; Langs: Mandarin; (416)385-3431; Fax. (416)385-1945.

TAI, T H Patricia; Allan Blair Cancer Centre, 300-4101 Dewdney Ave, Regina SK S4T 7T1; (Hong Kong)'84; MB BS; FRCR(Eng); DMRT; FRCPC; RadOncol. Staff, Allan Blair Cancer Centre; Prof, University of Saskatchewan; Langs: Chinese; (306)766-2288; Fax. (306)766-2688.

TAI-POW, J Malcolm; Scarborough Hosp-Birchmount, 3030 Birchmount Rd, Scarborough ON M1W 3W3; Tor'84; FRCPC; Anes. Staff, The Scarborough Hospital - Birchmount Campus; (416)495-2561

TAIANI, Edward J; 14 Kentucky Crt, New Minas NS B4N 4N2; Dal'77; FRCSC; Ophth. (902)678-6639; Fax. (902)678-5649.

TAILFEATHERS, Esther E; PO Box 842, Stand Off AB T0L 1Y0; (USA)'98; Physician, Blood Tribe Department of Health Inc; etail08@hotmail.com.

TAILLEFER, Catherine; Hôpital Ste-Justine, 3175 ch Cote Sainte-Catherine, Montreal QC H3T 1C5; Mon'03; FRCSC; ObstGyn (Maternal Fetal Medicine). Staff, Hopital Maisonneuve-Rosemont; Staff, Hôpital Ste-Justine; (514)345-4931

TAILLEFER, Jean; Institut de Cardiologie de Mtl, 5000 rue Belanger, Montreal QC H1T 1C8; Mon'69; FRCPC; Anes (Cardiovascular Anesthesia). Staff, Institut de Cardiologie de Montréal; Clin Assoc Prof, Universite de Montreal; (514)376-3330; Fax. (514)376-8784; jean.taillefer@icm-mhi.org.

TAILLEFER, Michel; 107 ch du Lac Millette CP 189, Saint-Sauveur QC J0R 1R0; Mon'82; Langs: English; French; (450)227-9933; Fax. (450)227-4900.

TAILLEFER, Normand; Medicale Sportive de Laval, 3095 Autoroute Laval O, Laval QC H7P 4W5; Mon'81; (450)682-2324; Fax. (450)682-9759.

TAILLEFER, Raymond; CSSS Haut-Richelieu-Rouville, 920 boul du Seminaire N, St-Jean-Richelieu QC J3A 1B7; Mon'79; AB; FRCPC; NuclearMed (Nuclear Cardiology). Staff, Hôpital du Haut-Richelieu; Prof Nuclear Med, Universite de Montreal; Langs: Bilingual(French/English); (450)359-5000 x5100; Fax. (450)359-5198; rtaillefer@hotmail.com.

TAILLEFER, Simon; CLSC & Centre Petite Nation, 14 rue St-Andre, St-Andre-Avellin QC J0V 1W0; Mon'06; Médecin, CLSC & Centre d'Hebergement Petite Nation; (819)983-7341; Fax. (819)983-3495.

TAILLEUR, Luc; CHUQ-St-Francois d'Assise, 10 rue de l'Espinay, Quebec QC G1L 3L5; Laval'97; Staff, Centre Hospitalier Universitaire De Québec - Pavillon De St-françois-d'assise; (418)525-4444; luc.tailleur@chuq.qc.ca.

TAILLON, A Monique; Stan Cassidy Centre for Rehab, 800 Priestman St, Fredericton NB E3B 0C7; Ott'88; BSc; FRCPC; PhysMed&Rehab. Hd PhysMed&Rehab, Stan Cassidy Centre for Rehabilitation; Ac Staff, Dr Everett Chalmers Regional Hospital; Langs: Bilingual(French/English); (506)452-5183; Fax. (506)447-4749.

TAILLON, David; Hopital Charles Lemoyne, 3120 boul Taschereau, Longueuil QC J4V 2H1; Mon'03; Staff, Hopital Charles LeMoyne; Staff, Centre Hospitalier Régional de Lanaudière; (450)466-5000

TAILLON, Jean-Paul; 775 Route 263, Disraeli QC G0N 1E0; Mon'68; (418)449-4915

TAILLON, Joseph E A C; CSSS de la Region de Theford, 1717 rue Notre-Dame E, Thetford Mines QC G6G 2V4; Mon'78; FRCPC; IntMed (Geriatric Medicine). ac Staff, Centre Hospitalier Universitaire de Quebec-CHUL; assoc Staff, Centre Hospitalier Chauveau; Staff, Hopital du CSS de la Region de Thetford; Prof, Institut Universitaire Cardiologie & Pneumologie de Quebec; pers Prof, Université Laval; Langs: English; (418)338-7729; Fax. (418)338-7734; carl.taillon@chuq.qc.ca.

TAILLON, Mario R; Saskatoon Ortho & Sports Med C, 104-311 Ludlow St, Saskatoon SK S7S 1N6; Sask'87; FRCSC; OrthSurg. (306)651-0800; Fax. (306)651-0801.

TAILLON, Paul A; 3-1945 McKercher Dr, Saskatoon SK S7J 4M4; Sask'82; Dip SportMed(SportMed); CCFP; Langs: English; French; (306)653-0112; Fax. (306)653-5995.

TAILLON, Pierre; Comm des Lesions Professionell, 211-2800 boul Saint-Martin O, Laval QC H7T 2S9; Mon'72; (450)680-6255

TAILOR, Adarsh; Royal Victoria Hosp, 201 Georgian Dr, Barrie ON L4M 6M2; Man'02; FRCPC; IntMed; Respir. Staff, Royal Victoria Regional Health Centre; Langs: Gujarati; (705)728-9802

TAILOR, Chetna; 402-267 O'Connor St, Ottawa ON K2P 1V3; Wes'04; FRCPC; IntMed; Endocrin&Metab. (613)234-2594

TAINSH, Susan M M; Scott Clinic, 775 Monaghan Rd s, Peterborough ON K9J 5K2; McM'82; FRCPC; IntMed (Chronic Pain); GeriatricMed. Staff, Peterborough Regional Health Centre - Hospital Drive; (705)743-4255; Fax. (705)743-4250.

TAIT, Glendon R; Abbie J Lane Mem Bldg, 7101B-5909 Veterans Memorial L, Halifax NS B3H 2E2; Cal'04; FRCPC; Psy. Staff, Queen Elizabeth II Health Sciences Centre - Victoria General Site; (902)473-2492; Fax. (902)473-1422.

TAIT, Heather M; 604-100 Arden St, Moncton NB E1C 4B7; Wes'97; FRCSC; GenSurg. (506)857-5144; Fax. (506)857-5062.

TAIT, John H; Doctors Bldg, 305-955 Queen St E, Sault Ste. Marie ON P6A 2C3; Qns'70; FRCSC; OrthSurg. Ac Staff, Sault Area Hospital - Sault Ste Marie; (705)759-5650

TAIT, Margaret V; The Group Health Centre, 240 McNabb St, Sault Ste. Marie ON P6B 1Y5; Qns'70; FRCPC; DiagRad. (705)759-1234

TAIWO, Olumide A; Plaza 2 Shopping Ctr, 616-8600 Franklin Ave, Fort McMurray AB T9H 4G8; Ilorin (Nigeria)'91; MB BS; CCFP; (780)714-6665; Fax. (780)714-5021.

TAIWO, Tolulola O; Red Deer Reg Hosp Centre, 3942 50A Ave, Red Deer AB T4N 6R2; Ilorin (Nigeria)'95; MB BS; MSc; MPH; CCFP; Staff, Red Deer Regional Hospital Centre; Staff Palliative Care, Northern Lights Regional Health Centre; Assoc Lecturer, University of Alberta; (403)348-8815; Fax. (403)309-2802; ttaiwo@nlhr.ca.

TAJ, Amer J; Jame Paton Mem Hosp, 125 Trans Canada Hwy, Gander NL A1V 1P7; Punjab (India)'86; MB BS; Staff, James Paton Memorial Hospital; (709)256-5632

TAJ, Anita A; Mental Health Centre, PO Box 3003 Stn Main, Prince Albert SK S6V 6G1; King Edward Medical University (Other Foreign)'96; MB BS; MRCPsy; Consultant Psy, Prince Albert Parkland Health Region; Langs: Urdu; (306)765-6055; Fax. (306)765-6349.

TAJIRIAN, Tania; Village Family Health Team, 102-171 Liberty St E, Toronto ON M6K 3P6; Ott'03; CCFP; Staff, Centre for Addiction & Mental Health (CAMH) - College Street Site; Langs: Arabic; Armenian; (416)599-8348; Fax. (416)599-2001; tania.tajirian@villagefht.ca.

TAK, Farzana Y; Windsor Reg Children's Centre, 3901 Connaught Ave, Windsor ON N9C 4H4; Lahore (Pakistan)'84; DABPN; Staff, Windsor Regional Hospital - Metropolitan Site; (519)257-5215; Fax. (519)257-5212.

TAKACH LAPNER, Sarah L D; Postgrad Med Education Office, MDCL 3101A-1280 Main St W, Hamilton ON L8S 4K1; Tor'06; Hem; IntMed. (604)278-9116

TAKACS, Ernest S; 931 Heacock Rd NW, Edmonton AB T6R 2L9; Alb'65; (780)988-6659; Fax. (780)437-9491.

TAKACS, Jennifer M L; Univ of Waterloo Health Servic, 200 University Ave W, Waterloo ON N2L 3G1; Ott'05; CCFP; Physician, University of Waterloo; (519)888-4096; Fax. (519)746-5023.

TAKAHASHI, Jennifer L; Nicola Neurology Clinic, 203-321 Nicola St, Kamloops BC V2C 6G6; Qns'98; BSc; FRCPC; Neur (Movement Disorders). Staff Neurol, Royal Inland Hospital; Staff Neurol, Hillside Tertiary Psychiatric Centre; (250)314-9912; Fax. (250)372-1381.

TAKAHASHI MONROY, Takeshi; Windsor Health Centre, 119-700 Tecumseh Rd E, Windsor ON N8X 4T2; Guadalajara (Mexico)'90; FRCSC; GenSurg. Staff, Windsor Health Centre; Langs: Spanish; (519)419-0972; Fax. (519)419-0793.

TAKANO, Tomoko; MUHC-Royal Victoria Hosp, R228-687 av des Pins O, Montreal QC H3A 1A1; Tokyo (Japan)'86; PhD; Staff Nephrol, McGill University Health Centre - Royal Victoria Hospital; adj Prof, McGill University; Langs: Japanese; (514)842-1231 x35208; Fax. (514)843-2815.

TAKARO, Timothy K; Simon Fraser University, BH 11300-8888 University Dr, Burnaby BC V5A 1S6; North Carolina (USA)'85; Physician, Simon Fraser University; (778)782-7186

TAKATS, Laszlo N; Allin Clinic, 10155 120 St NW, Edmonton AB T5K 2A2; Alb'63; IntMed (Geriatric Medicine). Asst Prof, University of Alberta; Langs: Hungarian; (780)482-7551; Fax. (780)414-5669.

TAKAYA, Sachiko; 21st Medical Clinic, 502-402 21st St E, Saskatoon SK S7K 0C3; Sask'94; CRCP; FRCPC; IntMed (AIDS/HIV); InfectDis. Langs: Japanese; (306)956-3444; Fax. (306)956-3577.

TAKEUCHI, Lawrence; Royal Inland Hosp, 311 Columbia St, Kamloops BC V2C 2T1; McM'89; MSc; FRCPC; Anes (Critical Care Medicine). Staff, Royal Inland Hospital; (250)374-5111 x2620

TAKHAR, Amandeep; Haynes Hall-Family Med, 101-115 Clarence St, Kingston ON K7L 3N6; Tor'10; CCFP.

TAKHAR, Amitoj K; 15 Allan Dr, Bolton ON L7E 2B5; University of Lucknow (Other Foreign)'03; CCFP; (905)951-1234

TAKHAR, Baldeep; B6A-350 Conestoga Blvd, Cambridge ON N1R 7L7; Manchester (England)'90; MB ChB; DCH; DRCOG; (519)620-7044; Fax. (519)623-7342.

TAKHAR, Jatinder; Regional Mental HC-London, PO Box 5532 Stn B 850 Highbury Ave, London ON N6A 4H1; Jammu-Kashmir (India)'78; MB BS; FRCPC; Psy. Consultant Collaborative Care Prog & Transition Into Primary Care Psychiatry, Regional Mental Health Care-St Joseph's Health Care; Assoc Dean Cont Professional Development/Prof, University of Western Ontario; Langs: Hindi; Punjabi; (519)455-5110 x47185; Fax. (519)455-2262; jatinder.takhar@sjhc.london.on.ca.

TAKHAR, Sneeta K; 4474 Joyce Ave, Powell River BC V8A 3A6; Tor'94; FRCPC; IntMed. (604)485-5340; Fax. (604)485-5341; sneeta_t@yahoo.com.

TAKLA, Nagwa A; Niagara Health Centre, 201-180 Vine St S, St Catharines ON L2R 7P3; Ain Shams (Egypt)'78; MB ChB; CCFP; Langs: Arabic; French; (905)682-5196; Fax. (905)682-9317.

TAKROURI, Heba S R; Hamilton HS-McMaste Site, PO Box 2000 Stn Lcd 1 1200 Main St W, Hamilton ON L8N 3Z5; (Jordan)'03; Staff, Hamilton Health Sciences Centre - McMaster Children's Hospital; (905)521-2100

TAKTAK, Assaad; Centre Hosp Rouyn-Noranda, 4 9e rue, Rouyn-Noranda QC J9X 2B2; (Lebanon)'98; Staff, Centre Hospitalier Rouyn-Noranda; (819)764-5131; Fax. (819)764-2900.

TAL, David T; St Joseph's Health Centre, 30 The Queensway, Toronto ON M6R 1B5; Albert Einstein College of Medicine (USA)'85; FRCPC; IntMed (Driving Medicine); GeriatricMed. Staff, St Joseph's Health Centre; Langs: Hebrew; (416)530-6532; Fax. (416)530-6472; a.g.e.matters@rogers.com.

TALAAT, Mohamed S; B54-3940 ch Cote-des-Neiges, Montreal QC H3H 1W2; Tor'79; (514)383-1515

TALAJIC, Mario; Institut de Cardiologie de Mtl, 5000 rue Belanger, Montreal QC H1T 1C8; Ott'80; Cardiol; IntMed (Electrophysiology). Staff Cardiol & electrophysiol, Institut de Cardiologie de Montréal; dép Chef Med/Chef, Universite de Montreal; Langs: Bilingual(English/French); (514)376-3330; Fax. (514)376-1355.

TALARICO, Brian N; Crisis Program-NBRHC, 304-120 King St W, North Bay ON P1B 5Z7; Wes'94; FRCPC; Psy. Staff, North Bay Regional Health Centre - Regional Mental Health; (705)494-3050; Fax. (705)476-2730.

TALARICO, Susanna; The Hosp for Sick Children, 555 University Ave, Toronto ON M5G 1X8; Ott'07; FRCPC; Peds. Staff, The Hospital For Sick Children; (416)813-1500

TALATI, Hetal H; Peterborough Reg HC-Hospital, 1 Hospital Dr, Peterborough ON K9J 7C6; Gujarat (India)'95; FRCPC; GenPath. Staff, Peterborough Regional Health Centre - Hospital Drive; (705)743-2121

TALBALLA, Hala A H; Ravines Med Centre, 2-535 Larry Uteck Blvd, Halifax NS B3M 0E3; Ahfad University for Women (Sudan)'00; (902)407-4382; Fax. (902)407-4381.

TALBOT, Claire F; Langara Coll Student Hlth Serv, 100 49th Ave W, Vancouver BC V5Y 2Z6; UBC'79; BSc; Staff Palliative Care, Providence Health Care - St Paul's Hospital; Physician, Langara College; (604)323-5256; Fax. (604)323-5487.

TALBOT, Danielle; Cite de la sante de Laval, 1755 boul Rene-Laennec, Laval QC H7M 3L9; Mon'91; FRCPC; IntMed; MedOncol; Hem. Chef hématol, Hopital de la Cite de la santé; Fax. (450)975-5044.

TALBOT, Genevieve; Ctr Hosp de Verdun, 4000 boul Lasalle, Verdun QC H4G 2A3; Sher'94; Staff, Centre Hospitalier de Verdun; (514)362-1000; Fax. (514)362-2823.

TALBOT, J H Bernard; Ctr de Readaptation Lucie-Brun, 2275 Av Laurier E, Montreal QC H2H 2N8; Laval'58; FRCPC; PhysMed&Rehab (Geriatric Medicine). Staff, Centre de Readaptation Lucie-Bruneau; Staff, Centre Hospitalier Jacques Viger; Consultant, Centre de Readaptation La Maison(Rouyn-Noranda); (514)527-4527 x217; Fax. (514)527-0979; bernard.talbot@ssss.gouv.qc.ca.

TALBOT, Jacques; Inst Philippe Pinel de Mtl, 10905 rue Henri-Bourassa E, Montreal QC H1C 1H1; Laval'65; Psy (Legal Psychiatry). Staff, Institut Philippe-Pinel de Montreal; Langs: English; (514)648-8461; Fax. (514)881-3783.

TALBOT, Jacques R; 1404-5115 boul de l'Assomption, Montreal QC H1T 4B2; Mon'69; Membre, Canadian Society of Phlebology; (514)256-8195; Fax. (514)585-2472; jac.talbot@sympatico.ca.

TALBOT, James A; 9758 86 Ave NW, Edmonton AB T6E 2L4; Tor'85; FRCPC; MedMicrobiol (Public Health). Assoc Prof Clinical Lab Med & path/Assoc Prof Adjunct Public Health Sciences, University of Alberta; (780)707-2711; Fax. (780)413-7603.

TALBOT, Jean; 7 rue du Pere-Jogues, Quebec QC G2A 2Y8; Laval'66; MedBiochem (P.Q.). Chef Med Biol, Centre Hospitalier Universitaire de Québec (CHUQ) - Siege Social; Consultant, Jeffery Hale Hospital-Saint Brigid's; Sec, Université Laval; (418)842-2228; Fax. (418)691-5709.

TALBOT, Jeanne D; Ottawa Inst of Cognitive Thera, 200-411 Roosevelt Ave, Ottawa ON K2A 3X9; Mon'93; FRCPC; Psy. (613)820-9931; Fax. (613)820-9996.

TALBOT, Jeannine; Clin de la Migraine de Montrea, 420-1600 boul Henri-Bourassa O, Montreal QC H3M 3E2; Laval'72; Electroenceph (P.Q.); Neur (P.Q.). ac Staff, Hôpital du Sacre-Coeur de Montréal; (514)337-0433

TALBOT, Jessica; Polyclinique d'Argenteuil, 201-551 rue Berry, Lachute QC J8H 1S4; Mon'07; CCFP; (450)562-3751; Fax. (450)562-1852.

TALBOT, Jo-Ann; Saint John Reg Hosp, PO Box 2100 Stn Main 400 University Ave, Saint John NB E2L 4L2; Man'96; FRCPC; EmergMed. Staff, Saint John Regional Hospital; Langs: English; French; (506)648-6000

TALBOT, Karine; Clinique Med de Pontiac-du-Lac, CP 4099 Succ A 10300 ch Sainte-Marguerite, Trois-Rivieres QC G9B 7Y6; Laval'98; Médecin, CSSS Cloutier-Durivage; Langs: English; (819)377-5015; Fax. (819)377-5550.

TALBOT, Linda A; CLSC Arthur-Buies, 430 rue Labelle, Saint-Jerome QC J7Z 5L3; Mon'74; (450)431-2221; Fax. (450)565-0133.

TALBOT, Marie-Claude; CLSC Camirand, 95 rue Camirand, Sherbrooke QC J1H 4J6; Sher'09; (819)780-2222

TALBOT, Marie-Pier; Cite de la sante de Laval, 1755 boul Rene-Laennec, Laval QC H7M 3L9; Mon'10; Staff, Hopital de la Cite de la santé; (450)668-1010

TALBOT, Martin; CHUM-Hop Saint-Luc, 1058 rue Saint-Denis, Montreal QC H2X 3J4; Mon'96; FRCPC; Anes. Staff, Centre Hospitalier l'Université De Montréal (CHUM) - Hôpital Saint-luc; (514)345-3511 x3344

TALBOT, Maxime; Quartier General Forces, CP 4000 Succ K 20-6363 rue Notre-Dame E, Montreal QC H1N 3R9; Laval'99; FRCSC; OrthSurg. Staff, McGill University Health Centre - Montreal General Campus; Médecin, Quartier General Forces Canadiennes; (514)252-2777

TALBOT, Michel N; CSSS du Suroît, 150 rue Saint-Thomas, Salaber-de-Valleyf QC J6T 6C1; Mon'69; FRCSC; GenSurg. Staff, Centre Hospitalier Régional du Suroît; (450)371-9925

TALBOT, Nathalie; 501A rte Principale CP 520, Daveluyville QC G0Z 1C0; Sher'89; assoc Staff, Hôpital Sainte-croix; (819)367-2714

TALBOT, Yves R; 4F-60 Murray St Box 25, Toronto ON M5T 3L9; Sher'71; FRCPC; Peds (Family Medicine). Acad Staff Family & Comm Med, Mount Sinai Hospital; Teach Staff Family Med/Hlth Admin, University of Toronto; (416)586-4800 x5160; Fax. (416)586-8885.

TALBOT-BOLDUC, Anne-France; Centre Hosp Reg Chisasibi, CP 250, Chisasibi QC J0M 1E0; Laval'07; CCFP; Staff, Cree Board of Health & Social Services James Bay; (819)855-2844

TALBOT-JONES, Robert; T J Medical Associates, 152-15277 Castle Downs Rd NW, Edmonton AB T5X 3N5; St Andrews (Scotland)'71; MB ChB; (780)472-2273; Fax. (780)473-2276.

TALBOT JR., Paul; Recherches Clinical Inc, 300-1750 av de Vitre, Quebec QC G1J 1Z6; Laval'67; FACC; Cardiol (P.Q.) (Clinical Research). ac Staff Cardiol, Centre Hospitalier Affilié Universitaire de Québec - Hôpital De L'Enfant Jésus; Clin Prof, Université Laval; Langs: English; (418)663-9371; Fax. (418)663-8639; recherches.clinicar@bellnet.ca.

TALEB, Samir; Restigouche Hosp Centre, 63 Gallant Dr, Campbellton NB E3N 2T5; University: Rijeka (Other Foreign)'90; Staff, Restigouche Hospital Centre; Langs: Arabic; Croatian; (506)789-6721; Fax. (506)789-6726; samirtaleb99@gmail.com.

TALENTO, Riccoh R; Kennedy Heights Med Clinic, 11944 88 Ave, Delta BC V4C 3C8; UBC'89; (604)543-5531; Fax. (604)648-9445.

TALIANO, John P; Niagara Health Centre, 208-180 Vine St S, St Catharines ON L2R 7P3; Dublin (Ireland)'88; FAAFP; Langs: English; French; (905)641-9582; Fax. (905)641-9420.

TALIB, Ashnoor S; Gates of Maple Family Practice, 201-955 Major MacKenzie Dr W, Vaughan ON L6A 4P9; McM'05; CCFP; Staff, Royal Health Care Centre; Langs: Gujarati; Kacchi; (905)417-7899; Fax. (905)417-8905.

TALIBI, Tal Talip; 11231 151 St NW, Edmonton AB T5M 4B8; Istanbul (Turkey)'57; Staff, University of Alberta Hospital; Staff Med, Royal Alexandra Hospital; (780)471-5454; Fax. (780)454-7210.

TALKO, Peter; Clinique Med de Shawville, PO Box 700 269 Main St, Shawville QC J0X 2Y0; McG'81; Langs: English; French; (819)647-2924; Fax. (819)647-2845.

TALLEVI, Christie L; London Medicentre, 611 Wonderland Rd N, London ON N6H 4V6; McM'06; CCFP; (519)471-6686; Fax. (519)471-2801.

TALLMADGE, Caroline; The Ottawa Hosp-Civic Campus, 1053 Carling Ave, Ottawa ON K1Y 4E9; McM'86; Anes. Staff, The Ottawa Hospital - Civic Campus; (613)798-5555; Fax. (613)798-5554.

TALLMEISTER, Alan H; Scarborough Hosp-Birchmount, 3030 Birchmount Rd, Scarborough ON M1W 3W3; Tor'81; FRCPC; Anes (Administration). Court Staff, Rouge Valley Health System - Centenary Health Centre Site; Ac Staff Anes, The Scarborough Hospital - Birchmount Campus; Court Staff Anes, Markham Stouffville Hospital; Langs: Estonian; German; (416)495-2561; Fax. (416)495-2562.

TALLON, John M; Emergency & Health Services, 302-2955 Virtual Way, Vancouver BC V5M 4X6; Tor'84; MSc; FRCPC; EmergMed (Trauma). (604)660-6910

TALLON, Stephen G; London East Med Centre, 295 Saskatoon St, London ON N5W 6A2; Wes'86; CCFP; FCFP; Staff Family Med, St Joseph's Hospital - St Joseph's Health Care; (519)659-3006; Fax. (519)659-8575.

TALLOS, Peter B; BC Cancer Agency-Fraser Valley, 13750 96 Ave, Surrey BC V3V 1Z2; Sydney (Australia)'69; MB BS; Staff, BC Cancer Agency Fraser Valley Centre; (604)930-4028

TALMAN, Marianne R; Hamilton HS-General Site, 423-237 Barton St E, Hamilton ON L8L 2X2; McM'92; FRCPC; IntMed. Staff, Hamilton Health Sciences Centre - Hamilton General Hospital; (905)521-2100

TALON, Charles E; Clinique Med Berger, 2200 ch de Chambly, Longueuil QC J4J 3Z3; Laval'67; Langs: Spanish; English; (450)651-7331; Fax. (450)646-9130.

TALPUR, Jehanara; Western Mem Reg Hosp, PO Box 2005 Stn Main 1 Brookfield Ave, Corner Brook NL A2H 6J7; Sind (Pakistan)'76; MB BS; Chief Psy, Western Memorial Regional Hospital; (709)637-5601

TALSKY, Mark A; Walter MacKenzie HSC, 1E1-132 University Campus NW, Edmonton AB T6G 2R7; Tor'07; Psy. Teach Staff, University of Alberta; (780)407-6938

TALUKDAR, Chiranjib; Golden Mile Centre, 208-3806 Albert St, Regina SK S4S 3R2; Dhaka (Bangladesh)'67; MB BS; DCH(Glas); DAB; FAAP; FRCPC; Peds (Pediatric Dermatology). Att Staff Peds, Pasqua Hospital; Dir Peds Asthma Clinic/Chair Peds, Regina General Hospital; Clin Prof Peds & College of Med, University of Saskatchewan; Langs: Bengali; Urdu; Hindi; Burmese; Chakma; French; (306)569-1565; Fax. (306)569-3353; chiranjib_talukdar@hotmail.com.

TALUKDAR, Momtaz H; 281 Stone Rd E, Guelph ON N1G 5J5; University of Chittagong (Bangladesh)'80; CCFP; Langs: Bengali; (519)823-5133

TALUKDAR, Sneha P; Broadway Med Clinic, 1319 Broadway Ave, Regina SK S4P 1E5; DhaKa (Bangladesh)'72; Staff Privil, Pasqua Hospital; Physician, Broadway Medical Clinic; (306)757-4114; Fax. (306)565-2297.

TALWALKAR, P Aravind; King Street Med Arts Centre, 201-71 King St W, Mississauga ON L5B 4A2; Bombay (India)'66; MB BS; MCPS; LMCC; Court Staff, Trillium Health Centre - West Toronto; Court Staff, Trillium Health Centre - Mississauga; Langs: Hindi; Marathi; (905)273-4700; Fax. (905)273-4978.

TALWAR, K K Joan; University of Alberta Hosp, 8440 112 St NW, Edmonton AB T6G 2B7; Tor'07; Peds. Staff, University of Alberta Hospital; (780)407-8822

TALWAR, Manoj K; 5-900 King St W, Kitchener ON N2G 1G5; Sask'87; FRCSC; GenSurg (Cardiovascular & Thoracic Surgery); ThorSurg; CardiothorSurg. Staff, Grand River Hospital - Kitchener/Waterloo Health Centre; Staff, St Mary's General Hospital; Consultant Privil Thoracic Surg, Guelph General Hospital; (519)579-1522; Fax. (519)579-5598.

TALWAR, Shalin R; Allin Med Clinic, 10155 120 St NW, Edmonton AB T5K 2A2; (Other Foreign)'07; CCFP; (780)482-7551

TAM, Alvin H; 202-3000 Highway 7, Markham ON L3R 6E1; Man'03; CCFP; (905)480-1050; Fax. (905)480-0898.

TAM, Amy S; Grand River Reg Cancer Ctre, PO Box 9056 Stn C 835 King St W, Kitchener ON N2G 1G3; Tor'02; FRCPC; IntMed; Hem. Staff, Grand River Hospital - Kitchener/Waterloo Health Centre; Staff, Grand River Regional Cancer Centre; (519)749-4370 x3512; Fax. (519)749-4378; amy.tam@grhosp.on.ca.

TAM, Christina; Burlington After Hours Clinic, 183-2025 Guelph Line, Burlington ON L7P 4M8; Wes'83; (905)681-7755; Fax. (905)333-1960.

TAM, Christopher H; Ontario Shores Ctr Mental HS, PO Box 613 700 Gordon St, Whitby ON L1N 5S9; Tor'02; FRCPC; Psy. Staff, Ontario Shores Centre for Mental Health Sciences; (905)430-4055

TAM, Christopher K H; 1857 Lawrence Ave E, Scarborough ON M1R 2Y3; (Hong Kong)'84; MB BS; MRC(UK); DCH; DTM; Court Staff, The Scarborough Hospital - General Campus; Langs: Cantonese; Mandarin; (416)759-6723; Fax. (416)759-6723.

TAM, Christopher W M; Southcentre Med Clinic, 159-100 Anderson Rd SE, Calgary AB T2J 3V1; Alb'93; CCFP; (403)271-8288; Fax. (403)225-8298.

TAM, Daphne C; Oakridge Centre South Tower, 226-650 41st Ave W, Vancouver BC V5Z 2M9; UBC'97; CCFP; FCFP; Langs: Cantonese; Mandarin; (604)263-5666; Fax. (604)267-3360.

TAM, David W; Oakville Med Centre, 204-331 Sheddon Ave, Oakville ON L6J 1X8; Tor'91; FRCSC; ObstGyn. Staff, Halton Healthcare Services Corporation - Oakville Site; Langs: Cantonese; (905)337-2191; Fax. (905)337-2300.

TAM, Denise H; 10-78 Corporate Dr, Scarborough ON M1H 3G4; Northwestern (USA)'02; FRCPC; IntMed; Nephrol. Langs: Bilingual(English/French); (416)279-0855; Fax. (416)279-0857.

TAM, Diamond Y F; Credit Valley Eye Care, 1-3200 Erin Mills Pky, Mississauga ON L5L 1W8; (Ireland)'03; Staff, Credit Valley Eye Care; Langs: Cantonese; (905)820-3937

TAM, Dorothy; William Osler HC-Etobicoke, 101 Humber College Blvd, Etobicoke ON M9V 1R8; Qns'06; FRCPC; Anes. Staff, William Osler Health System - Etobicoke General Hospital; (416)747-3554

TAM, Edward; Fairmount Med Bldg, 305-750 Broadway W, Vancouver BC V5Z 1H2; Dal'05; FRCPC; IntMed. (604)876-5122

TAM, Edwin M; UBC-Dept of Psychiatry, 0007-2255 Wesbrook Mall, Vancouver BC V6T 2A1; McG'89; FRCPC; Psy. Clin Researcher, Vancouver General Hospital - Centennial Pavillion; Clin Researcher, UBC Hospital - Koerner Pavillion; Clin Assoc Prof, University of British Columbia; Langs: Cantonese; French; (604)822-7325; Fax. (604)822-7922.

TAM, Emily J S; 7-291 Davis Dr, Newmarket ON L3Y 2N6; McM'06; FRCPC; PhysMed&Rehab. (905)898-5777

TAM, Emily W Y; The Hosp for Sick Children, 555 University Ave, Toronto ON M5G 1X8; McG'03; FRCPC; Neur. Staff, The Hospital For Sick Children; (416)813-1500

TAM, Eric S L; Eye MD Institute, 401-7900 Hurontario St, Brampton ON L6Y 0P6; Tor'98; FRCSC; Ophth. Staff, Mount Sinai Hospital; Staff, William Osler Health System - Brampton Civic Hospital; Physician, Eye MD Institute; University of Toronto; (905)456-9500; Fax. (905)456-9508.

TAM, Florence M S; Summit Centre, 206-200 Boudreau Rd, St. Albert AB T8N 6B9; Alb'97; FRCSC; ObstGyn. Clinical Asst Prof, University of Alberta; (780)459-1121; Fax. (780)459-0128.

TAM, Hon-Yin A; Daily Care Med & Walk in Clini, 4-497 Laurier Ave, Milton ON L9T 3K8; Wes'74; Ac Staff, Halton Healthcare Services Corporation - Milton District Hospital; Langs: Cantonese; (905)878-8700; Fax. (905)878-2220.

TAM, James W L; St Boniface Gen Hosp, Y3015-409 Tache Ave, Winnipeg MB R2H 2A6; Tor'89; FRCPC; IntMed (Echocardiography); Cardiol. Sec Chief Cardiol, St Boniface General Hospital; (204)233-8563; Fax. (204)233-9162; jtam@exchange.hsc.mb.ca.

TAM, John K W; Tower Prof Centre, 5520 50 Ave, Wetaskiwin AB T9A 0T3; Alb'77; Staff, Wetaskiwin Hospital & Care Centre; (780)352-9700; Fax. (780)352-9739.

TAM, Jonny H S; Dr Jonny Tam Med Prof Corp, 203-959 Dundas St E, Woodstock ON N4S 1H2; Mem'91; Langs: Chinese; (519)537-6229; Fax. (519)537-2402.

TAM, K Felix; 465 Main St, Vancouver BC V6A 2T7; Dundee (Scotland)'82; MB ChB; DCH; Court Staff, BC Women's Hospital & Health Centre; Court Staff, Providence Health Care - Mount Saint Joseph Hospital; Langs: Cantonese; Mandarin; (604)683-2727; Fax. (604)688-6323.

TAM, Kin-Hung; Quinte HC Corp-Belleville Gen, 265 Dundas St E, Belleville ON K8N 5A9; Tor'76; Physician, QHC Belleville General; Langs: Chinese; (613)969-7400 x2434

TAM, Larissa E; Scarborough North Med Arts, 305-4040 Finch Ave E, Scarborough ON M1S 4V5; Tor'96; FRCSC; ObstGyn. Ac Staff, The Scarborough Hospital - General Campus; (416)299-4750; Fax. (416)299-7595.

TAM, Mae Yit M; 15450 Vine Ave, White Rock BC V4B 2T4; Sask'89; FRCSC; Ophth (Glaucoma). Assoc Consultant, Peace Arch Hospital; Langs: Cantonese; (604)531-3212; Fax. (604)531-4012.

TAM, Martina Y T; 10 Clark St W, Leamington ON N8H 1E4; Wes'76; Langs: Chinese; (519)326-6621

TAM, Michael C C; CML Health Care, 100-5 Fairview Mall Dr, North York ON M2J 2Z1; Alb'63; DAB; FRCPC; DiagRad. Langs: Chinese; (416)508-7659

TAM, Paul Y W; Corporate Med Centre, 10-78 Corporate Dr, Scarborough ON M1H 3G4; (Hong Kong)'73; MB BS; FACP; FRCPC; IntMed (Nephrology). Med Dir Nephrol/Dialysis Prog, The Scarborough Hospital - General Campus; Langs: Cantonese; (416)279-0855 x238; Fax. (416)279-0857.

TAM, Penny K; Gordon & Leslie Diamond HCC, 7F-2775 Laurel St, Vancouver BC V5Z 1M9; Qns'06; FRCPC; IntMed. Staff, Providence Health Care - St Paul's Hospital; Staff, Gordon & Leslie Diamond Health Care Centre; Staff, Vancouver General Hospital - Centennial Pavillion; (604)875-5181

TAM, Peter; Northbrook Med Centre, 12357 Hwy 41 RR 1, Northbrook ON K0H 2G0; McM'88; (613)336-8888; Fax. (613)336-2819.

TAM, Robert C; 606 Caledonia Rd, Toronto ON M6E 4V5; McG'67; Langs: Cantonese; (416)787-7627; Fax. (416)787-2375.

TAM, Ronald K H; Children's Hosp Eastern Ont, 401 Smyth Rd, Ottawa ON K1H 8L1; Man'91; FRCPC; Peds. Staff, Children's Hospital of Eastern Ontario (CHEO); Langs: Chinese; French; (613)737-2328; Fax. (613)738-4852; rtam@cheo.on.ca.

TAM, Sandy W; Westgate Family Med Clinic, 180-17010 90 Ave NW, Edmonton AB T5T 1L6; Alb'02; CCFP; (780)487-4260; Fax. (780)481-6776.

TAM, Stephanie; Toronto East Gen Hosp Inc, 825 Coxwell Ave, Toronto ON M4C 3E7; Tor'07; FRCSC; Urol. Staff, Toronto East General Hospital Inc; (416)461-8272; Fax. (416)469-6106.

TAM, Sydney P; 333 Sherbourne St, Toronto ON M5A 2S5; Ott'91; CCFP; Staff, Markham Stouffville Hospital; Langs: Chinese; French; (416)324-4180; Fax. (416)324-4181.

TAM, Terence K Y; Saanich Peninsula Hosp, 2166 Mount Newton Cross Rd, Saanichton BC V8M 2B2; Tor'97; CCFP; CCFP(E.M.); Staff, Saanich Peninsula Hospital; (250)652-3911

TAM, Thomas C; 201-2772 Danforth Ave, Toronto ON M4C 1L7; Tor'72; Staff, Toronto East General Hospital Inc; Langs: Mandarin; (416)691-2600

TAM, Thomas T M; Strathcona Family Med Centre, 246-30 Springborough Blvd SW, Calgary AB T3H 0N9; Cal'96; CCFP; (403)777-9935

TAM, Thomas W H; London East Med Centre, 295 Saskatoon St, London ON N5W 6A2; Tor'93; CCFP; FCFP; Staff Pt-Time, St Joseph's Hospital - St Joseph's Health Care; Staff Pt-Time, London Health Sciences Centre - Victoria Campus; Langs: Chinese; (519)659-1900; Fax. (519)659-8575.

TAM, Vincent C; Tom Baker Cancer Centre, 1331 29 St NW, Calgary AB T2N 4N2; Ott'05; FRCPC; IntMed; MedOncol. Staff, Tom Baker Cancer Centre; (403)680-1578

TAM, Vincent S; William Osler HC-Etobicoke, 101 Humber College Blvd, Etobicoke ON M9V 1R8; National (Taiwan)'68; FRCPC; Anes. Staff, William Osler Health System - Etobicoke General Hospital; (416)747-3554

TAM, W S Theresa; Public Health Agency of Cda, AL 6201A-100 Colonnade Rd, Ottawa ON K1A 0K9; Nottingham (England)'89; BMedSci; FRCPC; Peds (International Health); InfectDis. Physician, Public Health Agency of Canada; Langs: Cantonese; (613)957-0316; Fax. (613)948-7783; theresa.tam@phac-aspc.gc.ca.

TAM, William Y; St Joseph's Healthcare, 50 Charlton Ave E, Hamilton ON L8N 4A6; (Hong Kong)'72; PhD; MRCPsy; FRCPC; Psy. Ac Staff, St Joseph's Healthcare - Charlton Campus; Pt-Time Assoc. Clin. Prof., McMaster University; Langs: Chinese; (905)522-4941

TAM, Wilson W; 5873 Victoria Dr, Vancouver BC V5P 3W5; UBC'75; Court Staff, Providence Health Care - Mount Saint Joseph Hospital; Court Staff, Providence Health Care - St Vincent's Hospital-Heather Site; Court Staff, BC Women's Hospital & Health Centre; Langs: Cantonese; Mandarin; (604)321-1911

TAM, Wing-Hei; Windsor Reg Hosp-Metropolitan, 1995 Lens Ave, Windsor ON N8W 1L9; (Taiwan)'70; FRCPC; DiagRad. Ac Staff, Windsor Regional Hospital - Metropolitan Site; Langs: Cantonese; Mandarin; (519)254-1661

TAM, Winston T L; Guildford Med Dental Centre, 31-15300 105 Ave, Surrey BC V3R 6A7; Tor'96; BSc; CSPQ; FRCSC; ObstGyn (Prenatal Care). Staff, Surrey Memorial Hospital; Langs: Cantonese; Mandarin; (604)953-0335; Fax. (604)953-0338.

TAM-QUYEN, Marie-Therese; Ctr Hosp de Lachine, 650 16e av, Lachine QC H8S 3N5; Laval'07; CCFP; Staff, CSSS de Dorval-Lachine-Lasalle; (514)637-2351

TAMAKLOE, Barnaby E A; Toronto East Gen & Orth Hosp, 825 Coxwell Ave, East York ON M4C 3E7; Accra (Ghana)'76; MB ChB; FRCPC; Psy (Mood Disorders). Consultant Psy, Toronto East General Hospital Inc; Sr Staff Psy/Pres Medical Staff, Ontario Shores Centre for Mental Health Sciences; Langs: Akan; Ga; (416)469-6198; Fax. (416)469-6805.

TAMALE, John R; Brant Community HS-Willet Site, 238 Grand River St N, Paris ON N3L 2N7; Makerere (Uganda)'90; MB BS; CCFP; CCFP(E.M.); Staff, West Haldimand General Hospital; Staff, The Brant Community Healthcare System - Willett Hospital Site; (519)442-7400; j.tamale@rogers.com.

TAMAN, Sara M; The Albany Clinic, 807 Broadview Ave, Toronto ON M4K 2P8; Tor'72; CCFP; FCFP; Staff, Toronto General Hospital - UHN; Staff, Women's College Hospital; (416)461-9471; Fax. (416)461-2710; sara.taman@utoronto.ca.

TAMANAHA, Loree M L; Forcemedic, 1021 rue Jean-Talon E, Montreal QC H2R 1V6; McG'09; CCFP; (514)787-1818

TAMARI, Erez; Credit Valley Prof Bldg, 410-2300 Eglinton Ave W, Mississauga ON L5M 2V8; Tor'83; Ac Staff Family Med, The Credit Valley Hospital; (905)820-2646; Fax. (905)820-7828.

TAMARI, Itamar E; Stonegate Comm Health Centre, 150 Berry Rd, Etobicoke ON M8Y 1W3; Tor'92; CCFP; FCFP; Court Staff, St Joseph's Health Centre; Langs: Hebrew; (416)231-7070; Fax. (416)231-6903.

TAMAYO ESTRADA, Catalina M; The Hosp for Sick Children, 555 University Ave, Toronto ON M5G 1X8; Universidad Pontificia Bolivariana (Other Foreign)'00; Peds (Pediatric Cardiology). Staff, The Hospital For Sick Children; (416)813-7467; Fax. (416)813-7547.

TAMAYO MENDOZA, Jesus; Brandon Reg Health Centre, 150 McTavish Ave E, Brandon MB R7A 2B3; Lasalle (Mexico)'88; Staff, Brandon Regional Health Centre; (204)726-1122

TAMAZ, Raja; CHUM-Hotel-Dieu, 3840 rue Saint-Urbain, Montreal QC H2W 1T8; Laval'02; FRCPC; IntMed; Gastroent. Staff, Centre Hospitalier l'Université de Montréal (CHUM) - Hôtel-Dieu; (514)890-8000 x14980; raja.tamaz@umontreal.ca.

TAMBAKIS, Maria L; London HSC-Victoria Hosp, PO Box 5010 Stn B 800 Commissioners Rd E, London ON N6A 5W9; Ott'10; CCFP; Staff, London Health Sciences Centre - Victoria Campus; (519)685-8500

TAMBASCO, Domenica; King West Village Med Centre, 201-626 King St W, Toronto ON M5V 1M7; Napoli (Italy)'01; CCFP; Langs: Italian; French; Spanish; (416)703-1313; Fax. (416)703-1310; domenicatambasco@yahoo.ca.

TAMBAY, Robert; 207-1081 Carling Ave, Ottawa ON K1Y 4G2; McG'95; FRCPC; IntMed; Gastroent. Langs: Italian; French; Spanish; (613)729-3179; Fax. (613)729-1026.

TAMBLYN, C David; 236 Ontario St, Stratford ON N5A 3H5; Wes'67; FACP; FRCPC; IntMed. Ac Staff, Stratford General Hospital - Huron Perth Healthcare Alliance; (519)273-2681; Fax. (519)273-4533; tamblyns@sympatico.ca.

TAMBLYN, Susan E; 85 Neal Ave, Stratford ON N5A 5A7; Wes'67; DPH; FRCPC; CommunMed (Public Health). (519)273-0827; Fax. (519)273-1431.

TAMBOLI, Mharukh Y; 207-421 Richmond Rd, Ottawa ON K2A 4H1; UBC'76; Staff, The Ottawa Hospital - General Campus; Langs: Gujarati; (613)729-1773; Fax. (613)729-8612.

TAMBOLINE, Colin R; 1-2379 Bevan Ave, Sidney BC V8L 4M9; UBC'91; PhD; (250)656-4143; Fax. (250)656-9285.

TAMILIA, Michael; E104-SMBD Jewish Gen Hosp, 3755 ch Cote-Sainte-Catherine, Montreal QC H3T 1E2; Milano (Italy)'84; FRCPC; IntMed; Endocrin&Metab. Staff, Sir Mortimer B Davis Jewish General; (514)340-8250; Fax. (514)340-7510.

TAMIR, Diana; Mount Sinai Hosp, EN3 462-600 University Ave, Toronto ON M5G 1X5; Tor'02; FRCPC; Anes. Staff, Toronto General Hospital - UHN; Staff, Mount Sinai Hospital; (416)340-5164; Fax. (416)340-3698.

TAMPIERI, Donatella; MUHC-Montreal Neurological Ins, 540A-3801 rue University, Montreal QC H3A 2B4; Bologna (Italy)'82; FRCPC; DiagRad. Consultant NeuroRad, McGill University Health Centre - Royal Victoria Hospital; Consultant, Sir Mortimer B Davis Jewish General; ac Staff Radiol, McGill University Health Centre - Montreal Neurological Hospital; Consultant, McGill University Health Centre - Montreal Children's Hospital; Prof DiagRad, McGill University; Langs: Italian; (514)398-1908; Fax. (514)398-7213.

TAMPLIN, Richard E I; Town Plaza Med Clinic, 40-4314 Main St RR 4, Whistler BC V0N 1B4; Galway (Ireland)'73; MB BCh; (604)905-7089; Fax. (604)905-7039.

TAN, A Lawrence; Health Sciences Centre, GE611-820 Sherbrook St, Winnipeg MB R3A 1R9; McG'88; FRCSC; GenSurg; ThorSurg. Staff, Health Sciences Centre; Assoc Prof, University of Manitoba; (204)787-3791; Fax. (204)787-7143; ltan@exchange.hsc.mb.ca.

TAN, Adrienne O; Univ Hlth Network-Toronto Gen, 8EN 229-200 Elizabeth St, Toronto ON M5G 2C4; UBC'02; FRCPC; Psy. Staff, Toronto General Hospital - UHN; (416)340-4800; Fax. (416)340-4198.

TAN, Alexander Y; 353-7105 Chebucto Rd, Halifax NS B3L 4W8; Dal'01; FRCSC; Ophth. (902)453-3937; Fax. (902)453-3959.

TAN, Allan; Queen Spadina Med Centre, 455 Queen St W, Toronto ON M5V 2A9; McM'03; CCFP; Langs: Mandarin; (416)869-3627; Fax. (416)703-3962.

TAN, Amy Y Y; Grey Nuns Family Med Centre, 2927 66 St NW, Edmonton AB T6K 4C1; Cal'02; CCFP; (780)342-1470; Fax. (780)490-0953.

TAN, Ann; Abbotsford Reg Hosp & Cancer C, 32900 Marshall Rd, Abbotsford BC V2S 0C2; Wes'04; Staff, Abbotsford Regional Hospital & Cancer Centre; Staff, BC Cancer Agency Abbotsford Centre; (604)851-4710

TAN, B J Nicholas; Golden Med Clinic, PO Box 1170 826 9 Ave S, Golden BC V0A 1H0; Tor'04; Langs: Cantonese; Mandarin; (604)897-9092; Fax. (250)344-7620.

TAN, Ben J K; Royal University Hosp, 3729-103 Hospital Dr, Saskatoon SK S7N 0W8; Tor'84; FRCPC; Peds; InfectDis. Staff, Royal University Hospital; (306)655-1777

TAN, Brenda P; Affinity Med Clinic, 2186-3779 Sexsmith Rd, Richmond BC V6X 3Z9; Tor'97; BSc; CCFP; Langs: Cantonese; (778)297-7992; Fax. (778)297-7995.

TAN, Charles C; Bayview Woods Med Centre, 610 Major Mackenzie Dr E, Richmond Hill ON L4C 1J9; Laval'92; PhD; Court Staff, Mackenzie Richmond Hill Hospital; Physician, Bayview Woods Medical Centre; Langs: French; Taiwanese; Fukinese; (905)770-7500; Fax. (905)737-2383.

TAN, Chin Chai; Empire Med Centre, 204 Freshwater Rd, St. John's NL A1C 2P5; Dublin (Ireland)'68; LMCC; Ac Staff, St Clare's Mercy Hospital; Staff, Health Care Corporation Of St John's; Langs: Chinese; Malay; (709)579-7391

TAN, Chin Kien; Rosedale Med Centre, 504-600 Sherbourne St, Toronto ON M4X 1W4; Tor'74; Staff, Toronto Western Hospital - University Health Network; Langs: Cantonese; Mandarin; (416)928-1883; Fax. (416)447-5917; ck.tan@sympatico.ca.

TAN, Chong-Jet; Humber River Reg Hosp-Finch, 2111 Finch Ave W, Toronto ON M3N 1N1; Dal'95; MD; FRCPC; Anes. Staff, Humber River Regional Hospital - Finch Avenue Site; (416)744-2500; Fax. (416)747-3773.

TAN, Christopher Y K; 207-7130 Warden Ave, Markham ON L3R 1S2; Ott'07; CCFP; Langs: Chinese; (905)470-1117; Fax. (905)470-1115.

TAN, Darrell H S; St Michael's Hosp, 4CC R4 179-30 Bond St, Toronto ON M5B 1W8; Tor'02; InfectDis; IntMed (AIDS/HIV). Staff, Toronto General Hospital - UHN; Clin Associate, St Michael's Hospital; Langs: Spanish; Cantonese; French; (416)864-5696; Fax. (416)864-5310.

TAN, Edward; Portage Med Clinic, 140 9 St SE, Portage la Prairie MB R1N 3V5; Man'10; CCFP.

TAN, James; The Credit Valley Hosp, 2200 Eglinton Ave W, Mississauga ON L5M 2N1; McM'07; CCFP; CCFP(E.M.); Staff, The Credit Valley Hospital; (905)813-4530

TAN, Jensen C C; 504-960 Lawrence Ave W, North York ON M6A 3B5; Tor'04; FRCSC; GenSurg (Clinician Investigator Program). Langs: Cantonese; (416)782-2616

TAN, Jerry K L; South Walkerville Med Centre, 300-2224 Walker Rd, Windsor ON N8W 5L7; Qns'84; FRCPC; IntMed; Derm. Staff, Windsor Regional Hospital - Metropolitan Site; (519)971-8874; Fax. (519)971-8672.

TAN, K W Andre; 3-307A Bridge St W, Napanee ON K7R 3V3; McG'89; MDCM; FRCSC; Otol. Consultant, Lennox & Addington County General Hospital; Assoc Prof, Queen's University; Langs: Chinese; (613)409-8888; Fax. (613)409-8889.

TAN, Kennard E K; Royal Jubilee Hosp, 1952 Bay St, Victoria BC V8R 1J8; Alb'06; MedMicrobiol. Staff, Vancouver General Hospital - Centennial Pavillion; Staff, Royal Jubilee Hospital; (250)370-8325

TAN, Kiat T; Royal University Hosp, 103 Hospital Dr, Saskatoon SK S7N 0W8; Leicester (England)'99; FRCPC; DiagRad. Staff Med Imaging, Royal University Hospital; (306)655-2402; Fax. (360)655-2370.

TAN, Kim-Weng; Orleans Medical-Dental Ctre, 210-2555 St. Joseph Blvd, Orleans ON K1C 1S6; Dublin (Ireland)'65; MB ChB; FACC; FCCP; FRCPC; IntMed (Cardiology). (613)824-7798; Fax. (613)824-4391.

TAN, Kong Teng; Dept of Medical Imaging, 1C 572-585 University Ave, Toronto ON M5G 2N2; Queen's (Ireland)'94; FRCPC; DiagRad. Staff, Toronto General Hospital - UHN; (416)823-0929; Fax. (416)593-0502.

TAN, Lana S; K W Hospice Palliative Care, 298 Lawrence Ave, Kitchener ON N2M 1Y4; Tor'02; CCFP; Staff, Grand River Hospital - Kitchener/Waterloo Health Centre; Staff, New Vision Family Health Team - Greenbrook; Physician, K W Hospice Palliative Care; (519)578-9757

TAN, Lee Puan; Windsor Allergy & Asthma, 1407 Ottawa St, Windsor ON N8X 2G1; Santo Tomas (Philippines)'63; FRCPC; IntMed (Asthma). Langs: Chinese; Tagalog; (519)258-4356; Fax. (519)258-9918.

TAN, Lisa L Y; Station Square Med Clinic, 146-6200 Mckay Ave, Burnaby BC V5H 4L7; UBC'00; CCFP; (604)438-8288

TAN, Melissa C Y; Peace Arch Hosp, 15521 Russell Ave, White Rock BC V4B 2R4; Tor'08; CCFP; CCFP(E.M.); Staff, Peace Arch Hospital; (604)531-5512

TAN, Michelle W; Heatlh Care Services, 6951 Westminster Hwy, Richmond BC V7C 1C6; Tor'90; CCFP; Langs: Cantonese; Mandarin; Fookien; Hokkin; Malay; Teochew; (604)231-8888

TAN, Patrick B; Brampton Gastroenterology, 12-470 Chrysler Dr, Brampton ON L6S 0C1; Mem'02; FRCPC; IntMed; Gastroent. Langs: Bilingual(English/French); (905)790-6362; Fax. (905)790-6612.

TAN, Peter K H; Surrey Med Arts Bldg, 117-13798 94A Ave, Surrey BC V3V 1N1; UBC'86; FRCPC; FRCPC; Cardiol; IntMed (Lipid Disorders). Ac Staff, Surrey Memorial Hospital; (604)581-4300; Fax. (604)588-3122; pkhtan@aol.com.

TAN, Richard Y; Windsor Health Centre, 155-1720 Howard Ave, Windsor ON N8X 5A6; Ott'99; BSc; FRCPC; IntMed; Critical Care Medicine; Respir. Staff, Hôtel-Dieu Grace Hospital; Staff, Windsor Regional Hospital - Metropolitan Site; (519)255-7964; Fax. (519)255-9320.

TAN, Rita; Hop Du Sacre-Coeur De Montreal, 5400 boul Gouin O, Montreal QC H4J 1C5; Mon'06; Staff, Hôpital du Sacre-Coeur de Montréal; (514)338-2383; Fax. (514)338-3155.

TAN, Romeo B; 4119 Bathurst St, North York ON M3H 3P4; Manila (Philippines)'87; CCFP; Langs: Tagalog; (647)352-6188; Fax. (647)352-9288.

TAN, Rusung; Child & Family Research Instit, A4 148-950 28 Ave W, Vancouver BC V5Z 4H4; UBC'86; FRCPC; MedMicrobiol. Staff, BC Children's Hospital; (604)875-3605

TAN, Seang Lin; MUHC-Royal Victoria Hosp, F6 10-687 av des Pins O, Montreal QC H3A 1A1; National (Singapore)'77; MB BS; FRCOG; FRCSC; ObstGyn (Reproductive Medicine). Médecin, McGill University Health Centre - Royal Victoria Hospital; Dir méd Montreal Reproductive Centre/Prof, McGill University; Langs: Mandarin; Cantonese; French; (514)369-0688; Fax. (514)934-2518; seanglin.tan@muhc.mcgill.ca.

TAN, Siew-Wan; Westglen Med Clinic, 108-30 Springborough Blvd SW, Calgary AB T3H 0N9; Cal'02; CCFP; (403)240-2221; Fax. (403)240-4670.

TAN, Teng Hin; Briarhill Med Centre, 58A-2700 Dufferin St, Toronto ON M6B 4J3; Tor'80; (416)256-2650; Fax. (416)256-5831.

TAN, Thuang Kim; 405-855 Broadview Ave, Toronto ON M4K 3Z1; Alb'71; BSc; Court Staff, St Michael's Hospital; Langs: Chinese; (416)967-9220; Fax. (416)967-9276.

TAN, Tjien-King; Shouldice Hosp, 7750 Bayview Ave, Thornhill ON L3T 4A3; Erlangen (Germany)'66; Staff, Shouldice Hospital; Langs: German; Indonesian; Dutch; (905)889-1125; Fax. (905)889-4216.

TAN, Weiping; 1136-2929 Barnet Hwy PO Box 52513 Rpo Coquitlam Ctr, New Westminster BC V3B 7J4; Beijing (China),'97; PhD; CCFP; (604)496-5183

TAN-DY, Cherrie R; Surrey Mem Hosp, 13750 96 Ave, Surrey BC V3V 1Z2; Boston(MA) (USA)'96; ABPeds; CRCP; DABPed; FAAP; PhC; FRCPC; Peds (Neonatal & Perinatal Medicine). Staff Neonatal Intensive Care Unit, Surrey Memorial Hospital; Site Leader Island Med Prog, University of British Columbia; (604)581-2211; cherrie.tan-dy@viha.ca.

TAN-HOGG, Wan-Cheng; St Paul's Hosp, 166-1081 Burrard St, Vancouver BC V6Z 1Y6; Aberdeen (Scotland)'73; Staff, Providence Health Care - St Paul's Hospital; Staff, Capture Centre for Cardiopulmonary Research; (604)806-8346

TAN-JARVIS, Vilma S; Vellore Village Med Centre, 16A-9750 Weston Rd, Woodbridge ON L4H 2Z7; Manila (Philippines)'87; AB(Philosophy); CCFP; Langs: Tagalog; (905)652-2000; Fax. (905)652-1835.

TAN-TAM, Clara C H; Surrey Mem Hosp, 13750 96 Ave, Surrey BC V3V 1Z2; UBC'06; Staff, Surrey Memorial Hospital; (604)581-2211

TANAKA, Asae; Medical Bldg, 120-6180 Blundell Rd, Richmond BC V7C 4W7; UBC'93; CCFP; FCFP; Langs: Japanese; (604)271-1314; Fax. (604)241-8615.

TANAKA, Karen R; 302-372 Hollandview Trail, Aurora ON L4G 0A5; McM'84; CCFP; FCFP; Staff, Southlake Regional Health Centre; (905)750-0080; Fax. (905)750-0085.

TANAKA, Peter M; St Joseph's Health Care, PO Box 5777 Stn B 268 Grosvenor St, London ON N6A 4V2; Wes'95; CCFP; CCFP(E.M.); FCFP; Staff Teacher, St Joseph's Hospital - St Joseph's Health Care; (519)646-6000 x4227; Fax. (519)646-6038.

TANAKA, Roderick T; Doctor's on Bayview, 15900 Bayview Ave, Aurora ON L4G 7Y3; Tor'82; CCFP; Ac Staff, Southlake Regional Health Centre; (905)726-9755; Fax. (905)726-9631.

TANAKA, Steven H; St Joseph's Health Centre, 30 The Queensway, Toronto ON M6R 1B5; UBC'00; FRCPC; Anes. Staff, St Joseph's Health Centre; (416)530-6090

TANCIU, Nicolae; 510-600 rue de la Montagne, Montreal QC H3C 4S4; Bucharest (Romania)'54; PhD; LMCC; (514)934-9924

TANCON, Gino; Valley Care Med Clinic, E-310 8th St, Courtenay BC V9N 1N3; UBC'73; BSc; Langs: Italian; (250)331-0500; Fax. (250)331-0553.

TANCON, Scott M A; Peter Lougheed Centre, 3500 26 Ave NE, Calgary AB T1Y 6J4; UBC'08; CCFP; CCFP(E.M.); Staff, Peter Lougheed Centre; (403)943-4999; Fax. (403)943-4018.

TANDAN, Tara C A; Murrayville Health Care Centre, 104-22112 52 Ave, Langley BC V2Y 2M6; McM'97; FRCPC; Peds (Adolescent Medicine). Staff Eating Disorders, BC Children's Hospital; (604)514-7777; Fax. (604)534-8016.

TANDAN, Ved R; Hamilton HS-Henderson Site, 711 Concession St, Hamilton ON L8V 1C3; Tor'89; FRCSC; GenSurg (Hepatobiliary & Pancreatic Surgery). Staff, St Joseph's Healthcare - Charlton Campus; Staff, Hamilton Health Sciences Centre-Juravinski Site; Staff, Hamilton Regional Cancer Centre; Assoc Prof Surg & Clin Epidemiol Biotatistics, McMaster University; (905)521-2100

TANDAREANU, Luminita; Hop Santa Cabrini Ospedale, 5655 rue Saint-Zotique E, Montreal QC H1T 1P7; (Romania)'90; CCFP; Staff, Hôpital Santa Cabrini Ospedale; Langs: Romanian; Bilingual(French/English); (514)252-6000; Fax. (514)252-6636; l_tandareanu@yahoo.ca.

TANDON, Anu; Sunnybrook Hlth Sciences Ctre, A459-2075 Bayview Ave, Toronto ON M4N 3M5; Tor'01; Respir (Sleep Medicine); IntMed. Staff, Sunnybrook Health Sciences Centre; Staff, Women's College Hospital; Langs: Hindi; (416)480-4758; Fax. (416)480-5153.

TANDON, Naveen; Two Rivers FHT-Hespeler Med Cl, B5-350 Conestoga Blvd, Cambridge ON N1R 7L7; Sask'03; (519)621-0437

TANDON, Puneeta; Zeidler Ledcor Centre, 1-28A-130 University Campus, Edmonton AB T6G 2X8; Sask'00; FRCPC; IntMed; Gastroent. Langs: Hindi; (780)492-9844; Fax. (780)492-9873; ptandon@ualberta.ca.

TANDON, Ramesh K; Westend Walk-In Med Clinic, 411 Confederation Dr, Saskatoon SK S7L 5C3; Agra (India)'66; MB BS; LRCP; MRCS(Eng); Physician, Westend Walk-In Medical Clinic; (306)382-6333; Fax. (306)382-6381.

TANDON, Vikas; St Joseph's Healthcare, F543-50 Charlton Ave E, Hamilton ON L8N 4A6; McM'03; FRCPC; IntMed; Cardiol. Staff, University of Ottawa Heart Institute; Staff, St Joseph's Healthcare - Charlton Campus; Langs: Hindi; Punjabi; (905)521-6058

TANEDA, Barbara L; 302-22112 52 Ave, Langley BC V2Y 2M6; Tor'90; ObstGyn. (604)533-0551

TANEJA, Ravi; London HSC-University Hosp, PO Box 5339 Stn B 339 Windermere Rd, London ON N6A 5A5; Armed Forces Medical College (India)'87; FRCPC; Anes. Staff, London Health Sciences Centre - University Hospital; Langs: Punjabi; Hindi; (519)663-3270; Fax. (519)663-2957.

TANFERNA, Rosaria; Polyclinique Med Pierre Gardeu, 300-1000 Montee des Pioniers, Terrebonne QC J6V 1S8; Mon'88; CCFP; Staff, Hopital Maisonneuve-Rosemont; (450)657-5799; Fax. (450)657-1809.

TANG, Alan C; Professional Arts Bldg, 2D-570 King St, Welland ON L3B 3L2; Wes'89; FRCSC; Otol (Head & Neck Surgery). Staff, Niagara Health System - Welland Hospital Site; (905)788-1711; Fax. (905)788-2332.

TANG, Alexander W L; North York Gen Hosp, 4001 Leslie St, North York ON M2K 1E1; Tor'76; FRCPC; Anes. Staff, North York General Hospital; Langs: English; French; (416)756-6002; Fax. (416)756-6520.

TANG, Allan S; Hys Med Centre, 202-11010 101 St NW, Edmonton AB T5H 4B9; Ott'76; BSc; DABR; FRCPC; DiagRad. Staff, Covenant Health - Edmonton General Continuing Care Centre; Clin Instructor, University of Alberta; (780)426-1121; Fax. (780)425-5979.

TANG, Anthony S L; Western Cardiology Assoc, 335-1900 Richmond Ave, Victoria BC V8R 4R2; Tor'77; BSc; FRCPC; IntMed (Electrophysiology); Cardiol. Langs: Cantonese; (250)595-1551

TANG, Bao Quy; General Surgery Associates, 230-1555 McKenzie Ave, Victoria BC V8N 1A4; Wes'97; DABS; FRCSC; GenSurg (Laparoscopic Surgery). Staff, Royal Jubilee Hospital; Staff, Victoria General Hospital; Langs: Cantonese; (250)220-8932; Fax. (250)220-8926.

TANG, Betty W; Child & Youth Mental Hlth Serv, 2F-152 15th St E, North Vancouver BC V7L 2R1; Ott'97; FRCPC; Psy (Child & Adolescent Psychiatry). Staff, Chilliwack General Hospital; Consultant Development Disabilities Mental Health Serv, Child & Youth Mental Health Services; (604)984-3795; betty.tang@rghealth.ca.

TANG, Cathy; University of Alberta Hosp, 1C1 04-8440 112 St NW, Edmonton AB T6G 2B7; Sask'83; FRCPC; Anes. Staff Anes, University of Alberta Hospital; (780)407-7035; Fax. (780)407-3200.

TANG, Christine E; The Credit Valley Hosp, 2200 Eglinton Ave W, Mississauga ON L5M 2N1; McG'82; CCFP; CCFP(E.M.); Staff, The Credit Valley Hospital; Staff, Nipigon District Memorial Hospital; Langs: English; French; (905)813-4466; Fax. (905)813-4477; ctang@ndmh.ca.

TANG, Christine L; 340-135 Queen's Plate Dr, Etobicoke ON M9W 6V1; UBC'93; BSc(Hons.); MSc; FRCSC; PlasSurg (Breasts). Ac Staff Cosmetic Reconstruction Surg, William Osler Health System - Etobicoke General Hospital; (416)740-0428; Fax. (416)740-3490.

TANG, Clementine; City Square Pediatrics, 495-555 12th Ave W, Vancouver BC V5Z 3X7; McG'99; FRCPC; Peds. Langs: Mandarin; Fookien; Tagalog; (604)730-5622 x5

TANG, David T T; Queen Elizabeth II HSC, 4714-1796 Summer St, Halifax NS B3H 3A7; UBC'06; FRCSC; PlasSurg. Staff, Queen Elizabeth II Health Sciences Centre - Halifax Infirmary Site; Staff, Halifax Infirmary Plastic Surgery; (902)473-1740; Fax. (902)425-2592.

TANG, Dominic M H; Group Health Centre, 240 McNabb St, Sault Ste. Marie ON P6B 1Y5; Man'68; Staff Psy, Sault Area Hospital - Sault Ste Marie; Langs: Cantonese; (705)759-1234; Fax. (705)759-5528.

TANG, Godwin P Y; Chalmers Med Office, 8-360 Highway 7 E, Richmond Hill ON L4B 3Y7; Tor'95; CCFP; FCFP; Langs: Chinese; (905)881-0900; Fax. (905)881-0906.

TANG, Gordon L S; Greystone Med Walk-In Clinic, C1D-8 Greystone Walk Dr, Scarborough ON M1K 5J2; (Hong Kong)'84; CCFP; FCFP; Court Staff, The Scarborough Hospital - General Campus; Langs: Cantonese; (416)266-1818; Fax. (416)266-0800; gordontang@rogers.com.

TANG, Howard H L; 406-15940 Fraser Hwy, Surrey BC V4N 0X8; Tor'77; (604)502-7228; Fax. (604)502-7229.

TANG, Hung-Yip; Hillcrest Mall Doctor's Office, 9350 Yonge St, Richmond Hill ON L4C 5G2; Tor'81; Staff, Mackenzie Richmond Hill Hospital; Langs: Cantonese; Mandarin; (905)883-1599; Fax. (905)883-0416.

TANG, Ian; BC College of Family Physician, 350-1665 Broadway Ave W, Vancouver BC V6J 1X1; Physician, BC College of Family Physicians; (604)736-1877; Fax. (604)736-4675.

TANG, Jianqing; Hop Charles LeMoyne, 3120 boul Taschereau, Greenfield Park QC J4V 2H1; Shanghai (China)'83; FRCPC; MedBiochem. Staff, Hopital Charles LeMoyne; (450)466-5000

TANG, Joanna W; 5F-101 Queensway W, Mississauga ON L5B 2P7; Tor'09; CCFP; (905)272-9700

TANG, Jonathan D; Mount Saint Joseph Hosp, CC 3A-3080 Prince Edward St, Vancouver BC V5T 3N4; UBC'04; FRCPC; Cardiol; IntMed. Staff, Providence Health Care - Mount Saint Joseph Hospital; Staff, Providence Health Care - St Paul's Hospital; (604)877-8192

TANG, Judy M; 1199 Lynn Valley Rd PO Box 16035, North Vancouver BC V7J 3S9; UBC'10; CCFP; (604)734-7125

TANG, Julian W; Alberta Provincial Laboratory, 2B1 03WCM-8440 112 St NW, Edmonton AB T6G 2J2; Staff, University of Alberta Hospital; Staff, Alberta Provincial Laboratory; (780)407-3068; Fax. (780)407-8984; julian.tang@albertahealthservices.ca.

TANG, Karen; Foothills Med Centre, 1403 29 St NW, Calgary AB T2N 2T9; Alb'08; FRCPC; IntMed. Staff, Foothills Medical Centre; (403)944-1110

TANG, Keith Y K; Delta Med Centre, 140-4977 Trennant St, Delta BC V4K 2K5; Tor'07; CCFP; (604)946-7661

TANG, Kenneth; Markham Stouffville Hosp, PO Box 1800 Stn Main 381 Church St, Markham ON L3P 7P3; Stellenbosch (South Africa)'92; MB ChB; LMCC; FRCPC; Anes. Staff Anes, Markham Stouffville Hospital; (905)472-7074

TANG, Lan; Unimedico Family Practice, 110-955 Major MacKenzie Dr, Vaughan ON L6A 4P9; (Other Foreign)'84; Langs: Mandarin; (289)553-3300; Fax. (289)553-2600.

TANG, Lawrence L; 1097 Nelson St, Nanaimo BC V9S 2K1; LRCPS (Ireland)'76; FRCSI; FRCSC; PlasSurg (Cosmetic Surgery). Staff, Nanaimo Regional General Hospital; (250)753-6441; Fax. (250)753-6012.

TANG, Patricia A; Tom Baker Cancer Centre, 1331 29 St NW, Calgary AB T2N 4N2; Alb'00; BSc; FRCPC; IntMed; MedOncol. Staff MedOncol, Tom Baker Cancer Centre; (403)521-3093; Fax. (403)283-1651.

TANG, Patrick H; 103-73 Delhi St, Guelph ON N1E 6L9; McM'07; EmergMed. (519)837-1401

TANG, Patrick K C; BC Centre for Disease Control, 655 12th Ave W, Vancouver BC V5Z 4R4; UBC'99; FRCPC; MedMicrobiol. Staff, BCCDC Public Health; (604)660-3231; Fax. (604)660-1360.

TANG, Q T An; CHUM-Hopital Saint-Luc, 2117-1058 rue Saint-Denis, Montreal QC H2X 3J4; Sher'00; FRCPC; DiagRad. Staff, Centre Hospitalier l'Université De Montréal (CHUM) - Hôpital Saint-luc; (514)944-4213

TANG, Quoc Kiet; CSSS St-Leonard & St-Michel, 7400 boul Saint-Michel, Montreal QC H2A 2Z8; Saigon (Vietnam)'77; Staff, Centre Hospitalier Jacques Viger; (514)270-9271

TANG, Raymond K; Vancouver Gen Hosp, 2449-899 12th Ave W, Vancouver BC V5Z 1M9; Tor'01; FRCPC; Anes. Staff, Vancouver General Hospital - Centennial Pavillion; (604)875-4304

TANG, S C Albert; Appletree Med Group, 1582 Bank St, Ottawa ON K1H 7Z5; Ott'74; CCFP; Ac Staff, Queensway Carleton Hospital; Ac Staff, The Ottawa Hospital - Civic Campus; Clin Lecturer Family Med, University of Ottawa; Langs: Chinese; (613)482-0118; Fax. (613)680-6420.

TANG, S P Allan; Westminster Med Bldg, 404-625 Fifth Ave, New Westminster BC V3M 1X4; McG'70; Med Staff, Royal Columbian Hospital; (604)521-2515; Fax. (604)521-2515.

TANG, Samuel L T; The Richmond Hosp, 7000 Westminster Hwy, Richmond BC V6X 1A2; Tor'03; FRCPC; Anes. Staff, Richmond Hospital; (604)278-9711

TANG, Shangguo; Hamilton HS-McMaster Site, PO Box 2000 Stn Lcd 1 2N27-1200 Main St, Hamilton ON L8N 3Z5; Luzhou (China)'83; FRCPC; AnatPath. Staff Path & Molecular Med, Hamilton Health Sciences Centre - McMaster Children's Hospital; Staff, Hamilton Health Sciences Centre - McMaster University Medical Centre; Staff, Hamilton Health Sciences Centre-Juravinski Site; Langs: Mandarin; (905)521-2100

TANG, Thanh Q; CLSC Saint-Michel, 3355 rue Jarry E, Montreal QC H1Z 2E5; McG'06; MDCM; CCFP; (514)374-8223

TANG, Timothy K K; Foothills Med Centre, C229-1403 29 St NW, Calgary AB T2N 2T9; UBC'74; FRCPC; Anes (Cardiovascular Anesthesia). Staff Anes, Foothills Medical Centre; (403)944-1430; Fax. (403)944-2425.

TANG, Tin-Yan; Com El Med Bldg, 103-2620 Commercial Dr, Vancouver BC V5N 4C4; (Hong Kong)'71; MB BS; Langs: Cantonese; Mandarin; (604)872-2565; Fax. (604)872-2566.

TANG, Vincent W; Family Med Practice, 240-5655 Cambie St, Vancouver BC V5Z 3A4; Man'84; Langs: Cantonese; Mandarin; (604)321-7679; Fax. (604)321-0707.

TANG-WAI, David F; Univ Hlth Network-Toronto Western Hosp, 5WW 441-399 Bathurst St, Toronto ON M5T 2S8; McG'96; FRCPC; Neur. Staff, Toronto Western Hospital - University Health Network; Langs: Bilingual(French/English); (416)603-2581; Fax. (416)603-5768.

TANG-WAI, Raymond M; Rockyview Gen Hosp, 4A 147-7007 14 St SW, Calgary AB T2V 1P9; Man'99; FRCPC; Psy. Staff Urgent Assessment, Rockyview General Hospital; (403)943-3808; Fax. (403)259-6289.

TANG-WAI, Richard F; Edmonton Clinic Health Academy, 4 588-11405 87 Ave NW, Edmonton AB T6G 1C9; McG'99; FRCPC; Neur. Staff, Edmonton Clinic Health Academy; (780)407-2064; Fax. (888)353-1163.

TANG-WAI, Robert; 429 Princess Ave, Brandon MB R7A 0N8; Galway (Ireland)'69; MB ChB; BAO; FRCPC; Neur (Clinical Neurology). Dir Clin Neurophysiol/Ac Staff/Consultant, Brandon Regional Health Centre; Consultant, Assiniboine Centre; (204)727-1894; Fax. (204)728-6171.

TANGHE-LAPOINTE, Karina; CSSS du Suroît, 150 rue Saint-Thomas, Salaber-de-Valleyf QC J6T 6C1; Mon'97; Staff, Centre Hospitalier Régional du Suroît; (450)321-2477

TANGJERD, Norvin E; Moose Jaw Ultrasound Clinic, 1021 9th Ave NW, Moose Jaw SK S6H 8C6; Sask'78; FRCPC; DiagRad (Ultrasound). Physician, Moose Jaw Ultrasound Clinic; (306)693-1925; Fax. (306)693-1924.

TANGRI, Navdeep; Seven Oaks Gen Hosp, 2PD 13-2300 McPhillips St, Winnipeg MB R2V 3M3; Man'04; FRCPC; IntMed; Nephrol. Staff, Seven Oaks General Hospital; (204)632-7133

TANGRI, Vikram; London HSC-University Campus, PO Box 5339 Stn B 339 Windermere Rd, London ON N6A 5A5; Wes'08; IntMed. Staff, London Health Sciences Centre - University Hospital; (519)685-8500

TANGUAY, Agnes M J; Caremedics Med Centre, 18-1910 St Laurent Blvd, Ottawa ON K1G 1A4; Mon'86; Langs: Bilingual(French/English); (613)523-5550; Fax. (613)523-5580.

TANGUAY, Alain; Hotel-Dieu de Levis, 143 rue Wolfe, Levis QC G6V 3Z1; Laval'80; ac Staff, Hôtel-Dieu de Lévis; (418)835-7122; Fax. (418)835-7191.

TANGUAY, Alain G; CSSSG-Hop de Hull, 116 boul Lionel-Emond, Gatineau QC J8Y 1W7; Ott'89; CCFP; CCFP(E.M.); FCFP; Staff, Hull Hospital; Langs: English; (819)595-6000

TANGUAY, Andre; Clinique Medicale, 101-254 boul Cure-Labelle, Sainte-Rose QC H7L 3A2; Mon'71; (450)622-3603; Fax. (450)622-3605; tanand20_siril@ssss.gouv.qc.ca.

TANGUAY, Caroline; GMF Centre Med du Parc, 101-84 rue du Court, Granby QC J2G 4Y5; Mon'94; CCFP; Staff, Centre Hospitalier de Granby; Langs: English; (450)375-1161; Fax. (450)375-7740.

TANGUAY, Caroline; Clinique Med de Montmagny, 100-83 Av de la Fabrique, Montmagny QC G5V 2J3; Laval'99; LMCC; Staff, CSSS de Montmagny-L'Islet; Langs: Bilingual(French/English); (418)248-4933; caroline.tanguay@gmf.gouv.qc.ca.

TANGUAY, Caroline; Lab Sciences Judiciairies, 12E-1701 rue Parthenais, Montreal QC H2K 3S7; Mon'99; FRCPC; AnatPath (Forensic Pathology). Staff, Laboratory Sciences Judiciairies & Medico Legal; (514)873-3300; caroline.tanguay@msp.gouv.qc.ca.

TANGUAY, Daniel; Institut de Cardiologie de Mtl, 5000 rue Belanger, Montreal QC H1T 1C8; Mon'87; Staff, Institut de Cardiologie de Montréal; (514)593-2511; Fax. (514)593-2540.

TANGUAY, Elisabeth; Centre Med Centrale, 4-135 rue Saint-Antoine N, Granby QC J2G 5G7; Sher'05; (450)372-5401

TANGUAY, Frederic; Centre Hosp le Gardeur, 911 montée des Pionniers, Terrebonne QC J6V 2H2; Mon'06; FRCSC; OrthSurg. Staff, Centre Hospitalier Pierre le Gardeur; (450)654-7525; Fax. (450)470-2640.

TANGUAY, Jacques; 45 rue Principale, Granby QC J2G 2T7; Mon'72; DAB; FAAD; Derm. (450)372-4233; Fax. (450)372-8182.

TANGUAY, Jean-Francois; Institut de Cardiologie de Mtl, E 5530-5000 rue Belanger, Montreal QC H1T 1C8; Mon'87; FACC; FESC; FAHA; FRCPC; IntMed (Interventional Cardiology); Cardiol. Staff Interventional Cardiol, Institut de Cardiologie de Montréal; Prof, McGill University; Prof, Universite de Montreal; Langs: Bilingual(French/English); (514)376-3330 x3375; Fax. (514)593-2596.

TANGUAY, Jeffrey J; Univ Hlth Network-Toronto Gen, 200 Elizabeth Sr, Toronto ON M5G 2C4; Wes'03; FRCPC; AnatPath (Forensic Pathology). Staff, Toronto General Hospital - UHN; Physician, Forensic Pathology Unit; (416)340-3325

TANGUAY, Karen E; 52 Elbow River Rd, Calgary AB T3Z 2V2; Cal'94; BSc(Hons.); MSc; FRCPC; Psy. (403)686-6200; Fax. (403)686-6200.

TANGUAY, Marie-Claude; CSSS Pierre Boucher, 1333 boul Jacqes-Cartier E, Longueuil QC J4M 2A5; Mon'96; FRCSC; ObstGyn. Staff, Centre Hospitalier Pierre Boucher; Langs: Bilingual(French/English); (450)468-8111; Fax. (450)468-3309.

TANGUAY, Nicole; Hop Louis-H Lafontaine, 7401 rue Hochelaga, Montreal QC H1N 3M5; Mon'62; LMCC; Staff Psy, Hopital Louis-H Lafontaine; (514)251-4000 x3000; Fax. (514)257-2498.

TANGUAY, Simon; MUHC-Montreal Gen Hosp, L8 318-1650 av Cedar, Montreal QC H3G 1A4; Sher'87; FRCSC; Urol. Staff, McGill University Health Centre - Montreal General Campus; (514)934-8535; Fax. (514)934-8297.

TANGUAY, Stephane; Hôtel-Dieu de Lévis, 143 rue Wolfe, Levis QC G6V 3Z1; Laval'88; FRCPC; Psy. Staff, Institut Universitaire Sante; Staff, Hôtel-Dieu de Lévis; (418)835-7121

TANGUAY-BERNARD, Marie-Michèle; CSSS- IUGS, 1200 rue King E, Sherbrooke QC J1G 1E4; Sher'09; CCFP; Staff, CLSC La Region-Sherbrooke; (819)780-2222

TANHA, Farzad; 102-2216 McCallum Rd, Abbotsford BC V2S 3P3; Sask'93; FRCPC; Neur. (604)870-8736; Fax. (604)870-8746.

TANHUANCO-KHO, Grace Y; Royal Jubilee Hosp, 5F-1952 Bay St, Victoria BC V8R 1J8; UP (Philippines)'81; AB(AP&CP); FRCPC; GenPath; AnatPath. Staff, Royal Jubilee Hospital; Langs: Fukinese; Tagalog; (250)370-8837

TANIGUCHI, Alan; McMaster Innovation Park, 201A-175 Longwood Rd S, Hamilton ON L8P 0A1; Alb'88; Staff, Hamilton Health Sciences Centre - McMaster Children's Hospital; (905)525-9140

TANIOUS, Lawrence F; West Durham Family Health Team, 200B-1105 Kingston Rd, Pickering ON L1V 1B5; Assiut (Egypt)'74; MB ChB; Staff, Rouge Valley Health System - Ajax & Pickering Health Centre Site; Member/Med Dir Community Nursing Home, Hospice Durham Board - Palliative Care Committee Durham West; Langs: Arabic; (905)420-9999

TANIS, Emile J; CSSS du Lac-Témiscamingue, 22 rue Notre-Dame N, Ville-Marie QC J9V 1W8; Port-au-Prince (Haiti)'80; Staff, CSSS du Témiscamingue; (819)629-2420; Fax. (819)629-3257; emile_tanis@ssss.gouv.qc.ca.

TANJOUR, Mazen; Alberta Children's Hosp, 2888 Shaganappi Trail NW, Calgary AB T3B 6A8; Damascus (Syria)'98; Staff, Alberta Children's Hospital; (403)955-7894; Fax. (403)955-2646.

TANKEL, Jonathan; Hys Med Centre, 510-11010 101 St NW, Edmonton AB T5H 4B9; Witwatersrand (South Africa)'86; MB BCh; FRCSC; ObstGyn. Ac Staff, Royal Alexandra Hospital; Asst Prof ObstGyn, University of Alberta; Langs: Afrikaans; (780)414-0782; Fax. (780)414-0784; jtankel@shaw.ca.

TANKEL, Keith; Cross Cancer Institute, 11560 University Ave NW, Edmonton AB T6G 1Z2; Witwatersrand (South Africa)'93; MB ChB; FRCPC; RadOncol. Staff, Cross Cancer Institute; (780)432-8771; Fax. (780)432-8771.

TANNA, Gemini V; Sunnybrook Hlth Sciences Ctre, A239-2075 Bayview Ave, Toronto ON M4N 3M5; Tor'98; FRCPC; IntMed; Nephrol. Staff, Sunnybrook Health Sciences Centre; Langs: Gujarati; (416)480-6100

TANNENBAUM, Cara B; Inst Univ Geriatrie de Mtl, 4565 ch Queen-Mary, Montreal QC H3W 1W5; McG'94; GeriatricMed; IntMed. Staff, Institut Universitaire de Gériatrie de Montréal; (514)340-3540 x2526; Fax. (514)340-3530.

TANNENBAUM, David W; Ray D Wolfe Family Med, 4F-60 Murray St Box 25, Toronto ON M5T 3L9; McG'77; CCFP; FCFP; Pres, Ontario College of Family Physicians; Assoc Prof, University of Toronto; Langs: English; French; (416)586-4800 x3190; Fax. (416)586-3175; david.tannenbaum@utoronto.ca.

TANNENBAUM, Hyman; 740-4060 rue Sainte-Catherine, Westmount QC H3Z 2Z3; McG'69; FACP; FRCPC; IntMed (Osteo Arthritis); ClinImmunol&Allergy; Rheum. principale Médecin, McGill University Health Centre - Montreal General Campus; Dir, Rheumatic Disease Centre of Montreal; assoc Prof, McGill University; (514)932-7438; Fax. (514)932-1469.

TANNENBAUM, Joanne A; Meadowlands Fam Health Centre, 888 Meadowlands Dr, Ottawa ON K2C 3R2; McG'00; CCFP; Physician, Meadowlands Family Health Centre; Langs: Hebrew; French; (613)228-2882; Fax. (613)228-2856.

TANNENBAUM, Terry-Nan; Montreal Reg Hlth & Social Ser, 1301 rue Sherbrooke E, Montreal QC H2L 1M3; Cal'78; MPH; FRCPC; CommunMed (Infectious Diseases);CCFP; FCFP; Public Health & Preventive Med. Staff, McGill University Health Centre - Montreal General Campus; Staff, Sir Mortimer B Davis Jewish General; Médecin Public Health Dept, Montreal Regional Health & Social Services; assoc Prof Family Med/adj Prof, McGill University; Langs: English; French; (514)528-2400 x3375; Fax. (514)528-2461; ttannenb@santepub-mtl-qc.ca.

TANNER, Erika L; 309-1580 Merivale Rd, Ottawa ON K2G 4B5; Dal'04; CCFP; (613)226-4030; Fax. (613)225-3891.

TANNER, Keith L; Sunnybrook Hlth Sciences Ctre, M3 200-2075 Bayview Ave, Toronto ON M4N 3M5; Tor'93; FRCPC; Anes. Staff, Sunnybrook Health Sciences Centre; (416)480-4864; Fax. (416)480-6039.

TANNER, Wayne R; St Michael's Hosp, 7 080-30 Bond St, Toronto ON M5B 1W8; Tor'72; FRCSC; GenSurg; VascSurg. Ac Staff Vascular Surg, St Michael's Hospital; Lecturer VascSurg, University of Toronto; (416)864-5154; Fax. (416)864-6012.

TANNIR, Hassan; 102-794 rue Frechette, Longueuil QC J4J 5C9; Beirut (Lebanon)'73; (450)674-0714; Fax. (450)674-8641.

TANNIS, Anita D; 119-2419 Bellevue Ave, West Vancouver BC V7V 4T4; McM'90; CCFP; Langs: Latvian; French; (604)922-6181; Fax. (604)922-6360.

TANNOCK, Ian F; Univ Hlth Network-Princess M, 5 208-610 University Ave, Toronto ON M5G 2M9; Philadelphia(PA) (USA)'74; PhD; FRCPC; IntMed (Medical Oncology). Sr Scientist, Princess Margaret Hospital - University Health Network; Researcher, Ontario Cancer Institute; Prof Med & Medical Biophysics, University of Toronto; Langs: Bilingual(English/French); (416)946-2245; Fax. (416)946-4563; ian.tannock@uhn.on.ca.

TANNOUS, Rosemonde E; Stamford Med Centre, 306-4256 Portage Rd, Niagara Falls ON L2E 6A4; Ain Shams (Egypt)'77; MB ChB; ABIM; FRCPC; IntMed (Hypertension); Cardiol. Staff Consultant IntMed & Cardiol, Niagara Health System - Greater Niagara General Site; Langs: Arabic; French; (905)354-1895; Fax. (905)354-5097.

TANNOUS, Waguih N; Clin Med Gen Bois de Boulogne, 310-1575 boul Henri-Bourassa O, Montreal QC H3M 3A9; Ain Shams (Egypt)'80; CCFP; Langs: Arabic; French; (514)336-1117; Fax. (514)336-3378.

TANO, David S; Foothills Med Centre, AW 260A-1403 29 St NW, Calgary AB T2N 2T9; Alb'96; FRCPC; Psy (Forensic Psychiatry). Staff, Foothills Medical Centre; Staff, Peter Lougheed Centre; (403)944-6800; Fax. (403)944-6852.

TANOUBI, Issam; Hop Maisonneuve-Rosemont, 5415 boul de l'Assomption, Montreal QC H1T 2M4; (Tunisia)'03; Staff, Hopital Maisonneuve-Rosemont; (514)252-3426; Fax. (514)252-3542.

TANSEY, Patrick A H; York-Finch Med Centre, 305-2115 Finch Ave W, North York ON M3N 2V6; RCS (Ireland)'90; FRCSC; OrthSurg. Staff, Humber River Regional Hospital - Finch Avenue Site; (416)746-1818; Fax. (416)746-1815.

TANSKI, Jennifer A; Market Mall Med Clinic, 2325 Preston Ave, Saskatoon SK S7J 2G2; Witwatersrand (South Africa)'83; MB ChB; Staff, Royal University Hospital; Staff, Saskatoon City Hospital; Staff, St Paul's Hospital (Grey Nuns) of Saskatoon; (306)374-2777; Fax. (306)374-2778.

TANSWELL, A Keith; The Hosp for Sick Children, 555 University Ave, Toronto ON M5G 1X8; London (England)'69; MRCS; MB BS; DObstRCOG; MRCP; FRCPC; Peds (Neonatal Intensive Care). Staff Neonatol, The Hospital For Sick Children; Prof Peds, University of Toronto; (416)813-6344; Fax. (416)813-8724; keith.tanswell@sickkids.ca.

TANTON, Elizabeth L; 100-5791 No. 3 Rd, Richmond BC V6X 2C9; Wes'83; AB; FRCPC; DiagRad (Neuro Radiology). Staff, Burnaby Hospital; Staff, Richmond Hospital; (604)278-9152; Fax. (604)278-9291; btanton@telus.net.

TANTON, Robert L; High Sreet Family Med Centre, 101-49 High St, Barrie ON L4N 5J4; Dal'90; CCFP; FCFP; Staff, Royal Victoria Regional Health Centre; (705)728-5780; Fax. (705)728-8371.

TANUSEPUTRO, Peter; Appletree Med Group, 2-1582 Bank St, Ottawa ON K1H 7Z5; Tor'08; FRCPC; Public Health & Preventive Med;CCFP; (613)731-6620; Fax. (613)731-6622.

TANYOUS, Manal S R; Burnaby Centre for Mental Heal, 3405 Willingdon Ave, Burnaby BC V5G 3H3; (Other Foreign)'95; CCFP; (604)675-3950

TANZER, Herbert; North York Med Arts Bldg, 202-1333 Sheppard Ave E, North York ON M2J 1V1; Tor'64; FRCSC; Ophth (Medical Retina). Ac Staff, North York General Hospital; Consultant, Princess Margaret Hospital - University Health Network; Langs: Bilingual(English/French); (416)494-7455; Fax. (416)494-4833.

TANZER, Michael; MUHC-Montreal Gen Hosp, B5 159 3-1650 av Cedar, Montreal QC H3G 1A4; McG'84; FRCSC; OrthSurg. Staff, McGill University Health Centre - Montreal General Campus; (514)934-8240; tanzerm@gmail.com.

TANZER, Russell S; North York Gen Hosp, 4001 Leslie St, North York ON M2K 1E1; Tor'72; Staff, North York General Hospital; (416)756-6001

TANZOLA, Robert C; Kingston Gen Hosp, V2-76 Stuart St, Kingston ON K7L 2V7; Qns'01; FRCPC; Anes. Staff, Kingston General Hospital; (613)548-7827; Fax. (613)548-1375.

TAO, Sha; Dominion Health Centres, 2383 111 St NW, Edmonton AB T6J 5E5; Sichuan (China)'82; Staff, University of Alberta Hospital; Staff, Royal Alexandra Hospital; Langs: Mandarin; (780)436-0020; Fax. (780)436-0603.

TAO, Tina Maria M L; Kingsway Med Bldg, 24-2917 Bloor St W, Toronto ON M8X 1B4; Wes'93; FRCPC; Psy (Child Psychiatry). (416)922-6897; Fax. (416)944-8432.

TAPARDEL, Anca F; Univ of Alberta Hosp SCC/WCM, 2F1 12-8440 112 St NW, Edmonton AB T6G 2B7; Bucharest (Romania)'98; FRCPC; IntMed. Staff Privil, Royal Alexandra Hospital; Staff, University of Alberta Hospital; Langs: Romanian; (780)407-1570; ancatapardel@med.ualberta.ca.

TAPARIA, Minakshi S; 1 112H-11350 83 Ave, Edmonton AB T6G 2B7; (India)'94; MB; BSc; MRCPath; Staff, University of Alberta Hospital; Teach Staff, University of Alberta; Langs: Hindi; (780)407-6232; Fax. (780)407-2680.

TAPARIA, Sanjay; Dr Wayne J Daviduck Prof Corp, 201-51 Inglewood Dr, St. Albert AB T8N 4E7; (India)'93; MB BS; Staff, Covenant Health - Grey Nuns Community Hospital; (780)569-5470; Fax. (780)569-5472.

TAPIERO, Bruce; Hôpital Ste-Justine, 3175 ch Cote-Sainte-Catherine, Montreal QC H3T 1C5; Mon'88; FRCPC; Peds. Staff, Hôpital Ste-Justine; (514)345-4931; Fax. (514)345-4822; bruce_tapiero@ssss.gouv.qc.ca.

TAPP, Carly A; Rexdale Community Htlh Ctr, 8 Taber Rd, Etobicoke ON M9W 3A4; Man'02; CCFP; (416)744-6312; Fax. (416)744-1881.

TAPPAY, Joel K; University of Calgary, 2500 University Ave NW, Calgary AB T2N 1N4; Cal'09; CCFP; (403)210-9355; Fax. (403)282-5218.

TAPPER, C Mark; St Joseph's Gen Hosp, 2137 Comox Ave, Comox BC V9M 1P2; Oxford (England)'75; MB ChB; FRCPC; Psy. Consultant, St Joseph's General Hospital; (250)339-1493; Fax. (250)339-1578.

TAPPER, Jason; Manitoba Clinic, 790 Sherbrook St, Winnipeg MB R3A 1M3; Man'06; Peds. (204)774-6541

TAQI, Esmaeel; Alberta Children's Hosp, 2888 Shaganappi Trail NW, Calgary AB T3B 6A8; King Abdul Aziz (Saudi Arabia)'00; PedGenSurg; GenSurg. Staff, Alberta Children's Hospital; (403)955-2848; Fax. (403)955-7634.

TARABAIN, Osman A; Jackson Park Health Centre, 150-2475 McDougall Ave, Windsor ON N8X 3N9; Kuala Lumpur (Malaysia) BSc; FRCPC; IntMed (Cardiology). Staff, Windsor Regional Hospital - Metropolitan Site; Staff, Hôtel-Dieu Grace Hospital; Asst Prof, University of Western Ontario; Langs: Arabic; (519)252-9861

TARADASH, Jay B; The Two Hundred, 218-200 St Clair Ave W, Toronto ON M4V 1R1; Tor'68; DABD; FRCPC; Derm. Court Staff, Women's College Hospital; Asst Prof, University of Toronto; (416)961-7731; Fax. (416)961-7673.

TARAKDJIAN, Megerditch; 301-1600 boul Cure Labelle, Laval QC H7V 2W2; Aleppo (Syria)'78; (450)978-9173; Fax. (450)978-0782.

TARAKDJIAN, Noushig; Hop Santa Cabrini Ospedale, 5655 rue Saint-Zotique E, Montreal QC H1T 1P7; Mon'07; DiagRad. Staff, Hôpital Santa Cabrini Ospedale; (514)252-6000

TARAKJI, Ahmad R; Yarmouth Reg Hosp, 405-60 Vancouver St, Yarmouth NS B5A 2P5; Aleppo (Syria)'97; DABIM; FRCPC; IntMed (Geriatric Medicine); Nephrol. Med Dir Renal Dialysis Unit, Yarmouth Regional Hospital; Pres Nephrol, Hypertension Maritime Clinic Inc; Langs: Arabic; (902)749-0553; Fax. (902)742-3976; dartca@eastlink.ca.

TARANGER, Lawrence A; Medical Arts Bldg, 537-750 Spadina Cres E, Saskatoon SK S7K 3H3; Alb'62; FRCSC; Urol (Medical Oncology). Ac Staff, Royal University Hospital; Ac Staff, Saskatoon City Hospital; Ac Staff, St Paul's Hospital (Grey Nuns) of Saskatoon; Clin Prof, University of Saskatchewan; (306)653-3255; Fax. (306)653-4386; dr.l.taranger@sasktel.net.

TARANTINO, Leopold; Polyclinique Cabrini, 204-5700 rue Saint-Zotique E, Montreal QC H1T 3Y7; Naples (Italy)'56; Otol. Staff, Centre Hospitalier l'Université de Montréal (CHUM) - Hôtel-Dieu; Staff, Polyclinique Cabrini; (514)259-6741

TARANU, Corina; Clinique Med Mondiale, 1-5589 ch Cote-des-Neiges, Montreal QC H3T 2T2; Bucharest (Romania)'81; Staff, CLSC-CHSLD De Rosemont; (514)733-9899

TARAS, Fernand J; 110-100 ch Rockland, Mont-Royal QC H3P 2V9; Mon'81; Staff, St Mary's Hospital Centre; Staff, Metro Medic Clinic; (514)667-3383; ftaras@rockland,d.com.

TARAS, Lisa H; Occupational Health Clinic, 1218-171 Slater St, Ottawa ON K1A 0K9; McG'91; CCFP; Medical Officer Specialized Health Services Directorate, Health Canada; Langs: Spanish; French; (613)946-6583; Fax. (613)990-9397.

TARASIEWICZ, Iwona R; 987 King St E, Hamilton ON L8M 1C6; Kracow (Poland)'81; CCFP; Staff, St Joseph's Healthcare - Charlton Campus; Langs: Polish; (905)545-0049; Fax. (905)545-9797.

TARASKA, Victoria K; The Derm Centre, 1385 Grant Ave, Winnipeg MB R3N 1Z2; Man'92; FRCPC; Derm (Cosmetic Dermatology). Physician, First Glance Aesthetic Clinic; (204)474-1221; Fax. (204)897-1221.

TARASKA, Vincent A; Winnipeg Clinic, 425 St Mary Ave, Winnipeg MB R3C 0N2; Man'69; FACP; FCCP; FRCPC; IntMed (Respiratory Disease). Ac Staff, Victoria General Hospital; Staff, Health Sciences Centre; Asst Prof, University of Manitoba; (204)957-3220; Fax. (204)957-7410.

TARATIBU, Mozwa B; Pinehouse Med Clinic, 147-211 Pinehouse Dr, Saskatoon SK S7K 0G5; (Other Foreign)'80; (306)668-6333; Fax. (306)249-2499.

TARAZI, Fadi; Dr Fadi Tarazi Inc, 202-3825 Sunset St, Burnaby BC V5G 1T4; McG'91; FRCSC; OrthSurg (Shoulder). Staff OrthSurg, Burnaby Hospital; Staff, False Creek Surgical Centre; Langs: Arabic; French; (604)294-8209; Fax. (604)294-8614.

TARAZONA RAMIREZ, Angela M; Avenida Bonavista Shopp Ctre, 438-12445 Lake Fraser Dr SE, Calgary AB T2J 7A4; (Colombia)'97; CCFP; Staff, Foothills Medical Centre; (403)452-7167; Fax. (403)452-7170.

TARCAK, Norbert; CLSC Lac Saint-Louis, 180 av Cartier, Pointe-Claire QC H9S 4S1; Komensky (Slovakia)'84; Staff, CLSC Lac St-Louis; (514)697-4110

TARDIF, Alain; Clinique Med Neufchatel, 101-2425 boul Bastien, Quebec QC G2B 1B3; Laval'82; (418)843-3771; Fax. (418)843-3865; atardif@sympatico.ca.

TARDIF, Caroline; Centre Hosp Fleury, 2180 rue Fleury E, Montreal QC H2B 1K3; Mon'04; FRCSC; GenSurg. Staff, Centre Hospitalier Fleury; (514)381-9311

TARDIF, Chantal; Clinique Med Grand-Boulevard, 200-353 boul des Bois-Francs S, Victoriaville QC G6P 4T2; Mon'93; Staff, Hotel-Dieu d'Arthabaska; Langs: Bilingual(French/English); (819)818-0266

TARDIF, Daniel; Primum Experts-Conseils, 143 ch Fleming, Cantley QC J8V 3B4; Mon'86; MBA; Langs: English; French; (819)962-6160; Fax. (819)607-0891.

TARDIF, Denis; Polyclinique de Montreal, 209-12245 rue Grenet, Montreal QC H4J 2J6; Laval'78; FRCSC; Ophth. ac Staff, Hôpital du Sacre-Coeur de Montréal; Staff, Polyclinique de Montreal; (514)332-4009; Fax. (514)331-2428.

TARDIF, Dominique; CSSS Becancour-Nicolet-Yamaska, 675 rue Saint-Jean-Baptiste, Nicolet QC J3T 1S4; Laval'96; MSc; Staff, Hôpital de Christ-Roi; (819)293-2071; Fax. (819)293-2024.

TARDIF, Eric; CSSS De Saint-Jerome, 290 rue de Montigny, Saint-Jerome QC J7Z 5T3; Mon'03; FRCSC; GenSurg. Staff, Hôtel-Dieu de Saint-Jérôme; (450)431-8200

TARDIF, Eric; CSSS de Beauce-Etchemin, 1515 17e rue, Saint-Georges QC G5Y 4T8; Laval'94; Staff, Centre Hospitalier Beauce-Etchemin; (418)228-2031

TARDIF, Frederic; CSSS de Chicoutimi, 305 rue Saint-Vallier, Chicoutimi QC G7H 5H6; Laval'97; Staff, Complexe hospitalier de la Sagamie; (418)541-1000

TARDIF, Gaetan; Toronto Rehab Institute, 550 University Ave, Toronto ON M5G 2A2; Laval'81; Dip(ElectroDiagMed); Dip SportMed(SportsMed); FRCPC; PhysMed&Rehab (Sports Medicine). Med Prog Dir Rehab & Post Acute Care/Chief Psy, Toronto Rehabilitation Institute - University Centre; Med Prog Dir Rehab & Post Acute Care, University Health Network; Dir Div of Physiatry, University of Toronto; Langs: French; (416)597-3422 x3730; Fax. (416)597-7114.

TARDIF, Isabelle; CSSS Pierre Boucher, 1333 boul Jacques-Cartier E, Longueuil QC J4M 2A5; Mon'98; CCFP; Staff, Centre Hospitalier Pierre Boucher; (450)468-8111

TARDIF, Isabelle; CLSC Bordeaux-Cartierville, 11822 av de Bois-De-Boulogne, Montreal QC H3M 2X6; Mon'97; CCFP; Staff, Hôpital de Saint-Eustache; Staff, CLSC Bordeaux-Cartierville; adj Dir program Family Med Unit, Universite de Montreal; Langs: Bilingual(French/English); (514)331-2572; Fax. (514)331-5130.

TARDIF, Jacques; Clinique ORL, 305-200 rue Durand, Saint-Jerome QC J7Z 7E2; Mon'65; Otol. Consultant, Hôtel-Dieu de Saint-Jérôme; Staff, Clinique Otolaryngology; (450)229-5795; Fax. (450)229-4850.

TARDIF, Jean-Claude; Institut de Cardiologie de Mtl, 5000 rue Belanger, Montreal QC H1T 1C8; Mon'87; FRCPC; IntMed; Cardiol. Dir Research Ctr & Intravascular Ultrasound Core Lab/Chaire CIHR Research, Institut de Cardiologie de Montréal; assoc Prof Med, Universite de Montreal; Langs: Bilingual(English/French); (514)376-3330; Fax. (514)593-2500; jean-claude.tardif@icm-mhi.org.

TARDIF, Johanne; CHAQ-Hop du Saint-Sacrement, 1050 ch Sainte-Foy, Quebec QC G1S 4L8; Laval'97; MSc; Staff, Centre Hospitalier Affilié Universitaire de Québec - Hôpital du St-Sacrement; Staff, Centre Hospitalier Portneuf; Staff, Institut Prive de Chirurgie Laser & Esthetique; (418)682-7878

TARDIF, Louise; CLSC Olivier-Guimond, 5810 rue Sherbrooke E, Montreal QC H1N 1B2; Montpellier (France)'72; Langs: Bilingual(French/English); (514)255-2365; Fax. (514)255-3353.

TARDIF, Marc; Centre Med de Riviere-du-Loup, 242 rue Lafontaine, Riviere-du-Loup QC G5R 3A7; Laval'88; Staff, Centre Hospitalier Regional du Grand-Portage; (418)862-3110; Fax. (418)862-9656.

TARDIF, Michel; Carrefour Med Centre, 200-3030 boul Le Carrefour, Laval QC H7T 2P5; McG'74; Staff, McGill University Health Centre - Montreal General Campus; (450)686-8899; Fax. (450)686-7466.

TARDIF, Michele; 3060-5199 rue Sherbrooke E, Montreal QC H1T 3X2; Laval'01; FRCSC; PlasSurg (Reconstructive Surgery). Staff, Hopital Maisonneuve-Rosemont; Langs: Spanish; English; (514)252-3400; Fax. (514)253-3331.

TARDIF, Patrick; CSSS de Laval, 1755 boul Rene-Laennec, Laval QC H7M 3L9; Mon'05; Staff, Hopital de la Cite de la santé; (450)668-1010

TARDIF, Pierre; 110-9 av Lanning, Saint-Sauveur QC J0R 1R6; Mon'82; (450)227-8799; Fax. (450)227-9976.

TARDIF, Sylvie; CHUS-Hopital Fleurimont, 3001 12e av N, Sherbrooke QC J1H 5N4; Sher'85; FRCSC; Otol (Head & Neck Surgery). ac Staff, Centre Hospitalier de Granby; assoc Staff, Centre Hospitalier Universitaire de Sherbrooke-Hopital Fleurimont; (819)346-1110

TARDIF, Yves; Ctr Hosp Affilie-Enfant-Jesus, 1401 18e rue, Quebec QC G1J 1Z4; Laval'75; MCFP(EM); EmergMed (P.Q.) (Emergency Family Medicine). Staff Emerg, Centre Hospitalier Affilié Universitaire de Québec - Hôpital De L'Enfant Jésus; (418)649-5632; Fax. (418)649-5775.

TARDIF, Yvon-Maurice; Centre oculaire de Quebec, 50-2480 ch Sainte-Foy, Quebec QC G1V 1T6; Laval'70; Ophth. Consultant, Centre Hospitalier Universitaire De Québec - Pavillon De St-françois-d'assise; ac Staff, Centre Hospitalier Universitaire de Quebec-CHUL; assoc Staff, Centre Hospitalier Affilié Universitaire de Québec - Hôpital du St-Sacrement; adj Prof, Université Laval; (418)780-6345

TARDY, Solange; 500 boul Rene-Levesque O, Montreal QC H2Z 1W7; Mon'80; ACLS; Membre, Tribunal Administratif du Quebec; Langs: English; (514)873-8030; Fax. (514)873-8288.

TAREK, Shaul Y; The Credit Valley Hosp, 2200 Eglinton Ave W, Mississauga ON L5M 2N1; McM'07; CCFP; CCFP(E.M.); Staff, The Credit Valley Hospital; (905)813-2200

TAREMI, Mojgan; Southlake Reg Health Centre, 596 Davis Dr, Newmarket ON L3Y 2P9; Tehran (Iran)'97; FRCPC; RadOncol. Staff, Southlake Regional Health Centre; Staff, Princess Margaret Hospital - University Health Network; Langs: Farsi; (905)595-4521

TARGETT, Matthew M; Valley Prof Centre, 200-70 ExhibitionSt, Kentville NS B4N 4K9; Saba (Netherlands Antilles)'07; CCFP; (902)678-8505

TARGONSKY, Elisha D; The Credit Valley Hosp, 2200 Eglinton Ave W, Mississauga ON L5M 2N1; Qns'09; CCFP; CCFP(E.M.); Staff, The Credit Valley Hospital; (905)813-4171

TARGOWNIK, Laura E; John Buhler Research Centre, 805G-715 McDermot Ave, Winnipeg MB R3E 3P4; Man'97; FRCPC; IntMed; Gastroent. Staff John Buhler Research Centre, Health Sciences Centre; Assoc Prof Med, University of Manitoba; (204)480-1311; Fax. (204)789-3972.

TARHONI, Mohamed M; Dr Leonard A Miller Centre, 100 Forest Rd, St. John's NL A1A 3Z9; Staff, Dr Leonard A Miller Centre; (709)777-8119; mohamed.tarhoni@med.mun.ca.

TARHUNI, Wadea M; Moose Jaw Cardiac Centre, 361 Main St N, Moose Jaw SK S6H 0W2; Al-Fateh (Libya)'91; MB BCh(Hon.); FACC; FACP; FRCPC; IntMed; Cardiol. Staff, Windsor Cardiac Centre; Assoc Prof, University of Saskatchewan; Langs: Arabic.

TARI, Stephane; Hop Maisonneuve-Rosemont, 5415 boul de l'Assomption, Montreal QC H1T 2M4; Sher'87; Staff, Hopital Maisonneuve-Rosemont; (514)252-3400

TARIQ, Hanzla; Brameast Family Health Network, 38-2130 North Park Dr, Brampton ON L6S 0C9; McM'10; CCFP; (905)792-2211

TARIQ, Khalida P; Dominion Med Centres Ltd, 9122 23 Ave NW, Edmonton AB T6N 1H9; (Pakistan)'80; CCFP; Physician, Dr Bernstein Health & Diet Clinic; Langs: Urdu; Punjabi; Hindi; (780)801-3360; Fax. (780)801-3366.

TARIQ, Marium; Howard Mutual Med Centre, PO Box 667 20129 Erie St S, Ridgetown ON N0P 2C0; (Other Foreign)'08; CCFP; (519)397-5455

TARIQ, Muhammad; Beautiful Plains Comm Med Clin, PO Box 70 499 Mountain Ave, Neepawa MB R0J 1H0.

TARLO, Susan M; Univ Hlth Network-Toronto Western Hosp, EW7 449-399 Bathurst St, Toronto ON M5T 2S8; London (England)'69; MB BS; MRCP; MRCS; LRCP; FRCPC; IntMed (Clinical Immunology & Allergy); Respir. Staff Respiratory Phys, Toronto Western Hospital - University Health Network; Staff Gage Occup & Environmental Hlth Unit, St Michael's Hospital; Prof Med & Public Health Services, University of Toronto; (416)603-5177; Fax. (416)603-6763.

TARMAN, Vera I; Vera Ingrid Tarman Med Prof, 24 Monteith St, Toronto ON M4Y 1K7; McM'92; MSc; CCFP; FCFP; Instructor, St Michael's Hospital; Instructor, University of Toronto; (416)323-3660; Fax. (416)323-4778.

TARNOPOLSKY, Mark A; McMaster Children's Hosp, 2H26-1200 Main St W, Hamilton ON L8N 3Z5; McM'88; PhD; FRCPC; PhysMed&Rehab (Neuro Metabolism). Prof Peds & Med, Hamilton Health Sciences Centre - McMaster Children's Hospital; Dir, Neurometabolic & Neuromuscular Clinic; Prof Peds & Med, McMaster University; (905)521-7933 x76593; Fax. (905)521-2638.

TAROMI, Bejzad; King Street Med Arts Centre, 504-71 King St W, Mississauga ON L5B 4A2; Tehran (Iran)'97; FRCSC; OrthSurg. (905)306-1449

TARR, Garnett M; Desert Doctors' Clinic, PO Box 860, Osoyoos BC V0H 1V0; Stellenbosch (South Africa)'89; MB ChB; BSc(Hons.); Staff, South Okanagan General Hospital; Langs: Afrikaans; Dutch; (250)495-6565; Fax. (250)495-6051; tarrg@shaw.ca.

TARRANT, Gary M; Ross Family Med Centre, 6F-100 Forest Rd, St. John's NL A1A 3Z9; Mem'80; CGP; CCFP; FCFP; Ross Family Medical Centre; (709)777-6301; Fax. (709)777-8323; gary.tarrant@med.mun.ca.

TARSHIS, Jordan C; Sunnybrook Hlth Sciences Ctre, M3 200-2075 Bayview Ave, Toronto ON M4N 3M5; McM'91; FRCPC; Anes. Staff, Sunnybrook Health Sciences Centre; Asst Prof, University of Toronto; (416)480-4864; Fax. (416)480-6039.

TARSHIS, Lorne M; Institute of Cosmetic Surgery, 31 Alvin Ave, Toronto ON M4T 2A7; Tor'71; DAB; FACS; FRCSC; Otol (Cosmetic Surgery). Consultant, Sunnybrook Health Sciences Centre; Court Staff, St Michael's Hospital; Asst Prof, University of Toronto; (416)926-8122; Fax. (416)926-8841; info@cosmeticscanada.com.

TARSHIS, Tanya J; 23 Lonsdale Rd, Toronto ON M4V 1W4; Tor'85; Langs: Italian; (416)515-9595; Fax. (416)515-9779.

TARSHIS, W Lisa; North York Doctors, 703-240 Duncan Mill Rd, North York ON M3B 3S6; McM'89; BSc; CCFP; FCFP; Ac Staff, North York General Hospital; Staff, North York Family Health Team-Central Office; Lecturer, University of Toronto; (416)494-7396; Fax. (416)494-0129.

TARTARO, Piero; Sunnybrook Hlth Sciences Ctre, HG 64-2075 Bayview Ave, Toronto ON M4N 3M5; Tor'03; FRCPC; IntMed; Gastroent. Ac Staff, Royal Victoria Regional Health Centre; Court Staff, Stevenson Memorial Hospital; Staff, Sunnybrook Health Sciences Centre; (416)480-6799; Fax. (416)480-5977.

TARUKANDIRWA, Callisto; Central Alberta Prof Centre, 220-5201 43 St, Red Deer AB T4N 1C7; (Zimbabwe)'88; MB ChB; FRCPC; IntMed (Medical Oncology). Staff Internist, Red Deer Regional Hospital Centre; Staff Internist & Med Oncol, Alberta Cancer Board; (403)347-8755; Fax. (403)986-8068.

TARULLI, Giuseppe P; Humber River Reg Hosp-Church, 200 Church St, Toronto ON M9N 1N8; Padova (Italy)'79; DABR; RVT; FRCPC; DiagRad (Interventional Cardiology). Staff, Humber River Regional Hospital - Church Street Site; Pres, Ontario Association of Radiologist; Asst Prof Radiol, McMaster University; Langs: Italian; (416)243-4660; Fax. (416)243-4377.

TARUMI, Yoko; Royal Alexandra Hosp, 3228-10240 Kingsway NW, Edmonton AB T5H 3V9; Sapporo (Japan)'91; Staff Palliative Care Prog, Royal Alexandra Hospital; Langs: Japanese; (780)735-4038; Fax. (780)735-5880; ytarumi@cha.ab.ca.

TARUN, A S M Noorullah; St Claude Clinic, PO Box 269 149 Cypress Ave, St Claude MB R0G 1Z0; (Other Foreign)'93; CCFP; (204)379-2281

TARZWELL, Robert R; Lions Gate Hosp, 231 15 St E, North Vancouver BC V7L 2L7; Man'01; FRCPC; Psy; NuclearMed. Staff, Providence Health Care - St Paul's Hospital; Staff, Lions Gate Hospital; (604)988-3131

TASCHEREAU, Charles; Polyclinique Med des Ponts, SS 90 120-1100 boul de la Rive-Sud, Saint-Romuald QC G6W 5M6; Laval'85; (418)834-1177; Fax. (418)834-9275; cm.taschereau.md@videotron.ca.

TASCONA, Daniel J; Orillia Soldiers' Mem Hosp, 170 Colborne St W, Orillia ON L3V 2Z3; Tor'04; FRCPC; IntMed; Nephrol. Staff, Orillia Soldiers' Memorial Hospital; Langs: Bilingual(English/French); (705)325-2201

TASHAROFI KIA, Mina; Appletree Med Centre, 9625 Yonge St, Richmond Hill ON L4C 5T2; McM'07; CCFP; (647)722-2370; Fax. (416)367-4301.

TASKER, Ronald R; Univ Hlth Network-Toronto Western Hosp, 4W 437-399 Bathurst St, Toronto ON M5T 2S8; Tor'52; BA; MA; FRCSC; Neursurg (Neurology). Med Dir Neurology Clinic, Toronto Rehabilitation Institute - University Centre; Hon Staff NeuroSurg, Toronto Western Hospital - University Health Network; Emeritus Prof, University of Toronto; (416)603-5771; Fax. (416)603-5298.

TASNEEM, Muhammad; Family Med Clinic, 1-790 Burnhamthorpe Rd W, Mississauga ON L5C 4G3; Punjab (Pakistan)'88; MB BS; LMCC; CCFP; Staff, Glenashton Medical Centre; Physician, Peel Family Medical & Walk-In Clinic; Staff, New Best Care Medical Centre; Langs: Hindi; Punjabi; Urdu; (905)897-9000

TASOVAC-BABIC, Radmila; Hôp Reg d'Edmundston, 275 boul Hebert, Edmundston NB E3V 4E4; Sarajevo (Bosnia-Herzegovina),Sarajevo (Bosnia-Herzegovina)'78; CCFP; Staff, Hôpital regional d'Edmundston; (506)739-2200

TASSE, Eliane; CSSS de la Haute-Gaspésie, 50 rue de Belvedere, Ste-Anne-des-Monts QC G4V 1X4; Mon'10; Staff, Centre Hospitalier des Monts; (418)763-2261

TASSE, Jacynthe; CSSS de Portneuf, 700 rue Saint-Cyrille, Saint-Raymond QC G3L 1W1; Sher'01; CCFP; Staff, Centre Hospitalier Portneuf; (418)337-4611; jacynthe_tasse@hotmail.com.

TASSE, Michel; CSSS de Saint-Jerome, 290 rue de Montigny, Saint-Jerome QC J7Z 5T3; Mon'80; FRCSC; OrthSurg. Staff, Hôtel-Dieu de Saint-Jérôme; (450)431-8200; Fax. (450)565-1099.

TASSE, Pierre; Hôtel-Dieu Sainte-Jérôme, 290 rue de Montigny, Saint-Jerome QC J7Z 5T3; McG'84; OrthSurg. Staff, Hôtel-Dieu de Saint-Jérôme; (450)431-8200

TASSI, Hisham H; Thompson Gen Hosp, 871 Thompson Dr, Thompson MB R8N 0C8; Kursk (Russia (Federation)),'99; BSc; FACP; Staff, Thompson General Hospital; (204)677-2381; Fax. (204)778-1462; info@drtassi.com.

TASSIS, Andreas; Digestive Health Clinic, 510-330 Hwy 7 E, Richmond Hill ON L4B 3P8; Institute of Medicine (Other Foreign)'90; FRCSC; GenSurg. Langs: Greek; (905)707-5007

TASSOT, Pierre-Marie; 509 rue Adoncour, Longueuil QC J4G 2M6; Beirut (Lebanon)'81; FRCSC; Ophth. (450)646-7788

TATARYN, Brian L; Hamilton HS-General Site, 237 Barton St E, Hamilton ON L8L 2X2; Man'95; CCFP; CCFP(E.M.); Staff, Hamilton Health Sciences Centre - McMaster Children's Hospital; Staff, Hamilton Health Sciences Centre-Juravinski Site; Staff, Hamilton Health Sciences Centre - Hamilton General Hospital; (905)521-2100

TATARYN, Donna N; Westmount Med Bldg, 605-5025 rue Sherbrooke O, Montreal QC H4A 1S9; Alb'74; FRCSC; GenSurg. ac Staff, St Mary's Hospital Centre; Ac Staff, McGill University Health Centre - Montreal Children's Hospital; (514)488-4582; Fax. (514)488-5268.

TATARYN, Ivanna V; Hys Med Centre, 207-11010 101 St NW, Edmonton AB T5H 4B9; Alb'72; DAB; FACOG; FRCSC; ObstGyn (Reproductive Endocrinology & Infertility). Staff Infertility Clinic, Royal Alexandra Hospital; Staff, University of Alberta Hospital; Clin Prof, University of Alberta; Langs: Ukrainian; (780)420-1771; Fax. (780)425-9299; itataryn@gpu.srv.ualberta.ca.

TATE, Laura J; Medical Office, 304-840 Coxwell Ave, Toronto ON M4C 5T2; Tor'83; FRCSC; PlasSurg. Chief Surg, Toronto East General Hospital Inc; Asst Prof Surg, University of Toronto; (416)696-6581; Fax. (416)696-6056.

TATEBE, Rodney Y; 579 Martin St, Penticton BC V2A 5L5; Alb'75; FRCSC; OrthSurg. Staff, Penticton Regional Hospital; (250)493-7195; Fax. (250)493-0422.

TATEMICHI, Sue R; 440 Highland Ave, Fredericton NB E3A 5X1; Tor'85; CCFP; FCFP; Dir Family Med Teaching Unit, Dr Everett Chalmers Regional Hospital; Assoc Prof, Dalhousie University; Langs: English; French; (506)452-2760; Fax. (506)459-2998.

TATHAM, Richard H B; Medical Arts Bldg, 10-626 Main St, Penticton BC V2A 5C8; London (England)'87; BSc(Hons.); MB BS; LMCC; CCFP; Physician, White Clinic Associates; Langs: English; French; (250)492-0470; Fax. (250)492-5541.

TATHAM, Robert B; Medical Centre, 3304-3000 Lawrence Ave E, Scarborough ON M1P 2V1; Tor'80; DABOT; FRCSC; Otol (Head & Neck Surgery). Staff, The Scarborough Hospital - General Campus; Staff, Rouge Valley Health System - Centenary Health Centre Site; (416)438-6292; Fax. (416)438-6405.

TATLAY, Kiran D K; Venture Place, 100-2525 Rose Ville Garden Dr, Windsor ON N8T 3J8; Qns'95; BSc(Hon.); CCFP; Langs: Punjabi; (519)945-4474; Fax. (519)944-1703.

TATLIDIL, Cuneyt; Vallley Reg Hosp, 150 Exhibition St, Kentville NS B4N 5E3; Dal'02; FRCPC; AnatPath. Staff, Valley Regional Hospital; (902)678-7381

TATOR, Charles H; Univ Hlth Network-Toronto Western Hosp, 4W 433-399 Bathurst St, Toronto ON M5T 2S8; Tor'61; PhD; FACS; FRCSC; Neursurg (Spinal Cord Injury). Staff, Toronto Western Hospital - University Health Network; Prof, University of Toronto; (416)603-5889; Fax. (416)603-5298; charles.tator@uhn.on.ca.

TATTERSALL, Philippa J; 210-1685 Main St W, Hamilton ON L8S 1G5; McM'88; Staff, St Joseph's Healthcare Hamilton - West 5th Campus; Physician Mental Health Program, Hamilton Family Health Team; Langs: Portuguese; French.

TATTUM, Leah E; SGH Medical Mall, 407-3030 Lawrence Ave E, Scarborough ON M1P 2T7; Northwestern(IL) (USA)'99; FRCPC; Peds. Staff, The Scarborough Hospital - General Campus; (416)431-5292; Fax. (416)431-4011.

TATU, Dan-Marius; CSSSG-Hop de Hull, 116 Boul Lionel-Emond, Gatineau QC J8Y 1W7; Bucharest (Romania)'85; FRCPC; IntMed. Staff, Hull Hospital; (819)595-6104; Fax. (819)595-6039.

TATUCH, Yuriy M; Don Mills Family Health Team, 200-20 Wynford Dr, North York ON M3C 1J4; Tor'98; CCFP; Langs: Ukrainian; (416)444-6161; Fax. (416)444-5849.

TATZEL, Timothy R; Thorold Med Clinic, 60 Albert St W, Thorold ON L2V 2G7; Tor'81; BSc; CCFP; FCFP; Court Staff, Niagara Health System - St Catharines General Site; Langs: German; (905)227-5255; Fax. (905)227-2070.

TAU, Mahlodi E; Blackmarsh Family Care Centre, 260 Blackmarsh Rd, St. John's NL A1E 1T2; Natal (South Africa)'99; MB ChB; Staff, Carbonear General Hospital.

TAUB, Dina S; 110-10333 Southport Rd SW, Calgary AB T2W 3X6; Tor'99; CCFP; (403)258-1960; Fax. (403)253-5735.

TAUB, Kenneth J; Foothills Med Centre, 1403 29 St NW, Calgary AB T2N 2T9; Ott'69; ABIM; FRCPC; IntMed; Nephrol (P.Q.). Ac Staff, Foothills Medical Centre; Assoc Prof, University of Calgary; (403)944-2510; Fax. (403)944-3199.

TAUB, Nadine S; 10085 Whalley Blvd, Surrey BC V3T 4G1; Man'07; CCFP; (604)582-5826

TAUB, Sherry J; 309-9555 Yonge St, Richmond Hill ON L4C 9M5; Man'82; DABPN; (905)508-3422; Fax. (905)508-7025.

TAUBNER, Eric P; PO Box 37094 Rpo Lynwood, Edmonton AB T5R 5Y2; Alb'73; DABPN; FRCPC; Psy. Ac Staff, Covenant Health - Misericordia Community Hospital; (780)425-1787

TAUCER, Fabiano A S; Montfort Hosp, 713 Montreal Rd, Ottawa ON K1K 0T2; Tor'79; FRCPC; NuclearMed; DiagRad. Staff Diag Imag, Montfort Hospital; Asst Prof, University of Ottawa; Langs: Italian; French; (613)746-4621 x2276; Fax. (613)748-4951.

TAUH, Mangi N; Capital City Women's Centre, 196-17010 90 Ave NW, Edmonton AB T5T 1L6; Sask'96; BSc; BEd; FRCSC; ObstGyn (Menopause). Staff/Coord Education, Covenant Health - Misericordia Community Hospital; Langs: Hindi; (780)439-2007; Fax. (780)439-3080.

TAUNTON, Jack E; Allan McGavin Sports Med Ctr, 3055 Wesbrook Mall, Vancouver BC V6T 1Z3; UBC'76; Vis Staff Acute Care Unit, UBC Hospital - Koerner Pavillion; Prof Family Pract, University of British Columbia; (604)822-3614; Fax. (604)822-9058; jtaunton@interchange.ubc.ca.

TAUQIR NAQVI, Syeda N; Woodstock Gen Hosp, 505-310 Juliana Dr, Woodstock ON N4V 0A4; Punjab (Pakistan)'95; FRCPC; AnatPath. Staff Path Lab, Woodstock General Hospital; Langs: Urdu; Hindi; Punjabi; (519)421-4211; stauqir@wgh.on.ca.

TAUSEEF, Nazia; Courtice Health Centre, 1450 Hwy 2, Courtice ON L1E 3C3; Peshawar (India)'89; FRCSC; ObstGyn. Staff, Lakeridge Health - Oshawa Site; Langs: Hindi; Punjabi; (905)721-4992

TAUSSKY, Daniel M; CHUM-Hop Notre-Dame, 1560 rue Sherbrooke E, Montreal QC H2L 4M1; Basel (Switzerland)'95; Staff, Centre Hospitalier l'Université de Montréal (CHUM) - Hôpital Notre-Dame; (514)890-8254; dantaussky@hotmail.com.

TAUTKUS, Robert F; Heart Lake Med Centre, 204-10425 Kennedy Rd, Brampton ON L6Z 0A4; Tor'81; CCFP; FCFP; Langs: English; French; (905)846-3777; Fax. (905)846-4498.

TAVARES, Alexandre G; Child & Adolescent Trmt Ctre, 1240 10th St, Brandon MB R7A 7L6; Sao Paolo (Brazil)'98; FRCPC; Psy.

TAVARES, Grace E E; Squamish Med Clinic, PO Box 389 Stn Main 37979 Cleaveland Ave, Squamish BC V8B 0A3; Tor'01; CCFP; (604)892-3535; Fax. (604)892-3545.

TAVARIA, Ashdin; Peace Arch Hosp, 15521 Russell Ave, White Rock BC V4B 2R4; St George's (Grenada)'05; Staff Elder Health, Peace Arch Hospital; (604)535-4577

TAVASSOLI, Massoud; CSSS-Hopital De Hull, 116 boul Lionel-Emond, Gatineau QC J8Y 1W7; Mon'01; GenSurg. Staff, Hull Hospital; (819)966-6200; masstavass@hotmail.com.

TAVASSOLI, Mohammed; Clinique Med 3600, 3600 rue Ontario E, Montreal QC H1W 1R7; Paris (France)'71; GenSurg. (514)526-2556; Fax. (514)526-9212.

TAVAZZANI, Franco G; Brameast Family Health Org, 48-2140 North Park Dr, Brampton ON L6S 0C9; Wes'96; FRCSC; OrthSurg (Sports Injuries). Staff, Mackenzie Richmond Hill Hospital; Langs: English; French; (905)790-9595; Fax. (905)790-9590.

TAVENOR, Anthony J; Medical Consultants of Nfld, 304-2 Herald Ave, Corner Brook NL A2H 4B5; Mem'85; FRCPC; IntMed; Gastroent. Staff, Western Memorial Regional Hospital; (709)639-9181; Fax. (709)639-1210.

TAVERNIER, Joseph; Huronia Med Centre, PO Box 790 Stn Main, Midland ON L4R 4P4; Dartmouth(NH) (USA)'74; FRCSC; GenSurg (Endoscopy). Chief Surg, Georgian Bay General Hospital - Midland; (705)526-3338; Fax. (705)526-4240; jotav@csolve.net.

TAVES, Abram; 3107 35 Ave, Vernon BC V1T 2T2; Man'74; FRCSC; GenSurg. Staff, Vernon Jubilee Hospital; (250)545-6443; Fax. (250)545-8212.

TAVES, Donald H; London X-Ray Associates, 104-450 Central Ave, London ON N6B 2E8; Wes'81; FRCPC; DiagRad (Administration). Staff, St Joseph's Hospital - St Joseph's Health Care; Prof Med, University of Western Ontario; (519)672-5270; Fax. (519)672-2724.

TAWADROS, Mamdouh B E; Dr Rose Farag Med Clinic, 1100 Richmond Ave, Brandon MB R7A 1M6; Cairo (Egypt) MB BCh; Physician Family Med, Wheat City Medical Clinic.

TAWADROS, Patrick; Credit Valley Surgical Assoc, 2207 Dunwin Dr, Mississauga ON L5L 1X1; Tor'02; FRCSC; GenSurg (Clinician Investigator Program). (905)820-3633; Fax. (905)820-3352.

TAWADROSS, Sherif M S; Milton Family Care Centre, 820 Main St E, Milton ON L9T 0J4; (Egypt)'91; CCFP; (905)864-9898; Fax. (905)864-9393.

TAWAGI, F Georges; Harmony Med Centre, 101-152 Cleopatra Dr, Nepean ON K2G 5X2; Mon'82; ObstGyn. Staff, The Ottawa Hospital - Civic Campus; Asst Prof, University of Ottawa; Langs: English; French; (613)728-6212; Fax. (613)728-3866.

TAWAR, Vinod C; Kwantlen Med Clinic, 1-12818 72 Ave, Surrey BC V3W 2M9; Cebu (Philippines)'85; MSc(Pharm); CCFP; (604)572-8161; Fax. (604)572-8108.

TAWFIK, Abdeldaim M; Barrhead Clinic Holdings Ltd, PO Box 4540 Stn Main, Barrhead AB T7N 1A4; Craiova (Romania)'82; MB BS; (780)674-2231; Fax. (780)674-2447.

TAWFIK, Viola L; Whitemouth Dist Health Centre, PO Box 219 75 Hospital St, Whitemouth MB R0E 2G0; (Other Foreign)'85; Staff, Whitemouth District Health Centre; (204)348-7191; tawfikv@neha.mb.ca.

TAWFIK HELMY, Safaa; Roblin District Health Centre, PO Box 940 15 Hospital St, Roblin MB R0L 1P0; CCFP; Staff, Roblin & District Health Centre; (204)937-8740

TAWILE, Carolyne; Centre Med Brunswick, 203-955 rue Saint-Jean, Pointe-Claire QC H9R 5K3; Laval'92; FRCSC; PlasSurg. Staff, Lakeshore General Hospital - Pointe Claire; Staff, Hopital Charles LeMoyne; (514)459-3045; Fax. (514)426-9059.

TAY, Jason; The Ottawa Hosp-Gen Campus, L2279-501 Smyth Rd, Ottawa ON K1H 8L6; Dublin (Ireland)'98; FRCPC; IntMed; Hem. Staff, The Ottawa Hospital - General Campus; (613)722-7000

TAY, Keng Y; London HSC-Victoria Hosp, 800 Commissioners Rd W, London ON N6A 5W4; New South Wales (Australia)'97; FRCPC; DiagRad. Staff, London Health Sciences Centre - Victoria Campus; Langs: Cantonese; Mandarin; (519)685-8500; Fax. (519)685-8592.

TAYAB, Syed M A; Niagara HS-Douglas Mem Site, 230 Bertie St, Fort Erie ON L2A 1Z2; Dacca (Bangladesh)'62; MB BS; FRCPC; IntMed (Cardiology). Staff, Niagara Health System - Douglas Memorial Hospital Site; Langs: Bengali; (905)871-7342; Fax. (905)871-7395.

TAYAG, Christel M; 113-2462 Howard Ave, Windsor ON N8X 3V6; Angeles University Foundation (Other Foreign)'01; BSc; CCFP; Langs: Tagalog; (519)946-0246; Fax. (519)258-2169.

TAYFOUR, Fouad; South Walkerville Med Centre, 198-2224 Walker Rd, Windsor ON N8W 5L7; Damascus (Syria)'79; FRCSC; Ophth (Retina Vitreous Surgery). Staff, Hôtel-Dieu Grace Hospital; Staff, Windsor Regional Hospital - Metropolitan Site; Langs: Arabic; (519)255-7922; Fax. (519)252-7223.

TAYLOR, Allan J; National Defence Headquarters, 101 Colonel By Dr, Ottawa ON K1A 0K2; Qns'08; CCFP; Staff, Canadian Forces Health Services Centre; Langs: Bilingual(English/French); (613)218-5594

TAYLOR, Amanda B; McMaster Univ Campus Hlth Ctr, 1280 Main St W, Hamilton ON L8S 4K1; McM'05; CCFP; Staff, McMaster University; (905)525-9140 x27717

TAYLOR, Andrea C; Streetsville Med Centre, 8-5425 Creditview Rd, Mississauga ON L5V 2P3; McM'04; CCFP; (905)826-1164

TAYLOR, Andrew W; Peninsula Eye Associates, 504-5400 Portage Rd, Niagara Falls ON L2G 5X7; Tor'91; BSc; DABOph; FRCSC; Ophth (Refractive Surgery). Chief Ophth, Niagara Health System - Greater Niagara General Site; (905)356-3311; Fax. (905)356-3595; ataylor@lasikprovision.com.

TAYLOR, Anthony S; Royal Columbian Hosp, 330 Columbia St E, New Westminster BC V3L 3W7; Alb'85; MBA; FRCPC; EmergMed (Quality of Care). Staff Emerg Room, Royal Columbian Hospital; Consultant, Convergent Health Care; (604)520-4000; astaylor@shaw.ca.

TAYLOR, Ardythe E; Breast Cancer Support Care, 414-301 14th St NW, Calgary AB T2N 2A1; Cal'86; CCFP; FCFP; Clin Associate, Tom Baker Cancer Centre; Med Dir, Breast Cancer Supportive Care; (403)270-2242; Fax. (403)270-2251.

TAYLOR, Brett W; IWK Health Centre, PO Box 9700 Rpo CSC 5850-5980 University Ave, Halifax NS B3K 6R8; Sask'84; FRCPC; Peds (Pediatric Asthma). Staff, IWK Health Centre; (902)428-8823; Fax. (902)470-3248.

TAYLOR, Brian G; Royal University Hosp, 103 Hospital Dr, Saskatoon SK S7N 0W8; Alb'07; FRCPC; Anes. Staff, Royal University Hospital; (306)655-1183; Fax. (306)655-1279.

TAYLOR, Brian M; London HSC-University Hosp, PO Box 5339 Stn B 80F12-339 Windermere Rd, London ON N6A 5A5; Wes'75; DAB; FACS; FRCSC; GenSurg (Colon & Rectal Surgery). Chief GenSurg, London Health Sciences Centre - University Hospital; Chair Div of GenSurg & Assoc Prof, University of Western Ontario; (519)663-3209; Fax. (519)663-3052.

TAYLOR, Brian V; Health Centre of Bradford, 2-456 Holland St W, Bradford ON L3Z 0G1; Tor'99; (905)775-4999; Fax. (905)775-4909.

TAYLOR, Bryan S; Keele Med Place, 403-2830 Keele St, North York ON M3M 3E5; Witwatersrand (South Africa)'87; MB ChB; CCFP; Langs: Hebrew; (416)631-6669; Fax. (416)630-3861.

TAYLOR, Bryce R; Univ Hlth Network-Toronto Gen, EN10 213-200 Elizabeth St, Toronto ON M5G 2C4; Tor'68; FACS; FRCSC; GenSurg (Endoscopic Surgery). Staff, Toronto General Hospital - UHN; Langs: English; French; (416)340-3558; Fax. (416)340-4211.

TAYLOR, Cameron R; Carmi Clinic, 124-725 Carmi Ave, Penticton BC V2A 3G8; Cal'86; BSc; FRCSC; OrthSurg (Sports Medicine). Staff OrthSurg, Penticton Regional Hospital; (250)492-8030; Fax. (250)492-8032.

TAYLOR, Carolyn M; St Paul's Hosp, B476A-1081 Burrard St, Vancouver BC V6Z 1Y6; UBC'01; FRCPC; Cardiol; IntMed (Clinician Investigator Program). Staff, Providence Health Care - St Paul's Hospital; (604)806-8785

TAYLOR, Carolyn V; Clairhurst Med Centre, 201-1466 Bathurst St, Toronto ON M5R 3S3; Tor'99; BSc(Hon.); MSc; FRCPC; Peds. Staff, The Hospital For Sick Children; (416)531-3331; Fax. (416)531-1639.

TAYLOR, Catherine Y; Trillium Hlth Ctr-Mississauga, 100 Queensway W, Mississauga ON L5B 1B8; Tor'96; FRCPC; Peds (Neonatal & Perinatal Medicine). Staff, Trillium Health Centre - Mississauga; (905)848-7100; cy.taylor@utoronto.ca.

TAYLOR, Charlene; Comm Addiction & Mental Hlth, PO Box 5166 101 Nanticoke Creek Pky, Townsend ON N0A 1S0; McM'84; FRCPC; Psy. Psychiatrist, Community Addiction & Mental Health Services; (519)587-4658; Fax. (519)587-4118.

TAYLOR, Christine G; Brief Intervention Unit Hlth C, 715 12 Ave W, Vancouver BC V5Z 1M9; Alb'94; FRCPC; Psy. Staff, Vancouver General Hospital - Centennial Pavillion; Staff, Providence Health Care - St Paul's Hospital; Staff, Brief Intervention Unit Health Centre; Staff, Whistler Health Care Centre; (604)875-4111 x21412

TAYLOR, Christine M; 1105-20 Eglinton Ave W PO Box 2066, Toronto ON M4R 1K8; Tor'88; FRCPC; Psy. Staff Psy, Sunnybrook Health Sciences Centre; Lecturer Med, University of Toronto; (416)485-4802; Fax. (416)485-4802.

TAYLOR, Christopher D; 301-1625 Oak Bay Ave, Victoria BC V8R 1B1; UBC'93; FRCSC; PlasSurg (Hand Microsurgery). Div Head Plastic Surg, VIHA-South; Clin Instructor, University of British Columbia; (250)595-6009; Fax. (250)595-4077.

TAYLOR, Colin L; Central Alberta Med Imaging, 4312 54 Ave, Red Deer AB T4N 4M1; Wes'98; FRCPC; DiagRad. (403)343-6172; Fax. (403)343-6159.

TAYLOR, Dale B; Hazelwood Med Clinic, 302-16088 84 Ave, Surrey BC V4N 0V9; UBC'81; Staff, Surrey Memorial Hospital; (604)507-0623; Fax. (604)507-0624.

TAYLOR, David C; Gordon & Leslie Diamond HCC, 4213-2775 Laurel St, Vancouver BC V5Z 1M9; UBC'78; FRCSC; GenSurg; VascSurg. Head VascSurg, Vancouver General Hospital - Centennial Pavillion; Staff, Gordon & Leslie Diamond Health Care Centre; Assoc. Prof. & Hd., University of British Columbia; (604)875-5540; Fax. (604)875-5542; dctaylor@interchange.ubc.ca.

TAYLOR, David C; London HSC-Victoria Hosp, PO Box 5010 Stn B 4F ZE-800 Commissioners Rd E, London ON N6A 5W9; Wes'70; FRCS; FRCPC; OrthSurg; EmergMed. Staff, London Health Sciences Centre - University Hospital; Staff, London Health Sciences Centre - Victoria Campus; Clin Assoc Prof Med, University of Western Ontario; (519)685-8055 x55365; Fax. (519)685-8059.

TAYLOR, David R; Queen's Univ Etherington Hall, 3039-94 Stuart St, Kingston ON K7L 3N6; Columbia University (Colombia)'03; (613)533-6796

TAYLOR, Donna K; Kincardine Physicians Group, 44 Queen St, Kincardine ON N2Z 3C1; Wes'77; Ac Staff, South Bruce Grey Health Centre - Kincardine Site; Aj Prof, University of Western Ontario; (519)396-2600; Fax. (519)396-6177.

TAYLOR, Douglas S; 215 Lemarchant Rd, St. John's NL A1C 2H5; Edinburgh (Scotland)'62; MB ChB; FRCPC; IntMed. Ac Staff, St Clare's Mercy Hospital; Consultant, Health Sciences Centre; Clinical Asst Prof Discipline of Med, Memorial University Of Newfoundland; (709)579-3251

TAYLOR, Dylan A; University of Alberta Hosp, 2C2 WCM-8440 112 St NW, Edmonton AB T6G 2B7; Alb'81; FRCPC; IntMed (Clinical Cardiology); Cardiol. Clin Dir Stollery Chidren's Adult Echocardiography Lab, University of Alberta Hospital; Head Diagnostic Cardiac Sciences Prog, Alberta Health Services; Clin Prof Med, University of Alberta; (780)407-1575; Fax. (780)407-6452; dtaylor@cha.ab.ca.

TAYLOR, E Kent; 445 Inglehart St N, Oakville ON L6J 3J5; Tor'81; LMCC; BSc(Hon); DABD; MD; MSc; FRCP; FRCPC; Derm (Hair Transplantation). (905)844-8800; Fax. (905)844-8200; ktay@cogeco.ca.

TAYLOR, Elaine M; AL0701A-Health Canada, 200 Tunney's Pasture Driveway, Ottawa ON K1A 0K9; Tor'82; CCFP; FCFP; Att Staff, The Ottawa Hospital - Civic Campus; Teacher, University of Ottawa; Langs: English; French; (613)941-8306; Fax. (613)954-2354.

TAYLOR, Elizabeth L; Genesis Fertility Centre, 300-1367 Broadway W, Vancouver BC V6H 4A7; Dal'98; FRCSC; ObstGyn (Gynecology). Clin Instructor, University of British Columbia; (604)879-3032; Fax. (604)875-1432.

TAYLOR, Geoffrey D; University of Alberta Hosp, 2E4 16-8440 112 St NW, Edmonton AB T6G 2B7; Sask'77; FRCPC; IntMed; InfectDis. Dir Stollery Children's Infection Control Unit, University of Alberta Hospital; Prof Med, University of Alberta; (780)407-7786; Fax. (780)407-7137; geoff.taylor@ualberta.ca.

TAYLOR, Gerald M J; 1263 Canford Cres, Mississauga ON L5J 3M9; Tor'73; AAFP; CCFP; Staff, Halton Healthcare Services Corporation - Oakville Site; (905)823-3615; Fax. (905)823-9995.

TAYLOR, Glenn P; The Hosp for Sick Children, 555 University Ave, Toronto ON M5G 1X8; UBC'76; FRCPC; AnatPath. Staff, The Hospital For Sick Children; (416)813-5971; Fax. (416)813-2156; glenn.taylor@sickkids.ca.

TAYLOR, Gordon; 301-1111 Lonsdale Ave, North Vancouver BC V7M 2H4; UBC'90; BA; (604)990-0008; Fax. (604)986-8492.

TAYLOR, Gregory W; Public Health Agency of Canada, AL 6701B-120 Colonnade Rd, Ottawa ON K1A 0K9; Dal'83; FRCPC; CommunMed (Public Health). (613)946-5072; Fax. (613)952-3196; gregory_taylor@phac.-aspc.gc.ca.

TAYLOR, Gretta; Abbie J Lane Mem Bldg, 6L-5909 Veteran's Memorial Lan, Halifax NS B3H 2E2; Mon'00; CCFP; Langs: Spanish; Polish; French; gretta.taylor@cdha.nshealth.ca.

TAYLOR, Hallie A; Sunnybrook Hlth Sciences Ctre, 2075 Bayview Ave, Toronto ON M4N 3M5; Man'05; FRCPC; DiagRad. Staff, Sunnybrook Health Sciences Centre; (416)480-6100

TAYLOR, Heather L; Preventous Collaborative Healt, 1635 17 Ave SW, Calgary AB T2T 0E5; UBC'03; CCFP; (403)229-0129; Fax. (403)398-0193.

TAYLOR, Hilary J C; South Shore Reg Hosp, 90 Glen Allan Dr, Bridgewater NS B4V 3S6; London (England)'67; MB BS; LRCP; MRCS; FFARCS; FRCPC; Anes. Ac Staff, South Shore Regional Hospital; (902)543-4603; Fax. (902)543-8618.

TAYLOR, Hugh R; 703-400 Tache Ave, Winnipeg MB R2H 3C3; Man'87; FRCSC; GenSurg (Minimal Access Surgery). Staff, St Boniface General Hospital; Staff, Concordia General Hospital; University of Manitoba; (204)237-7195; Fax. (204)233-3344; hrtaylor@shaw.ca.

TAYLOR, Ieleen S; 101-190 Pelican Pl, Sylvan Lake AB T4S 1K2; Alb'95; CCFP; Staff, Red Deer Regional Hospital Centre; (403)887-2224; Fax. (403)887-2261.

TAYLOR, J Robert D; Riverside Prof Centre, 203-1919 Riverside Dr, Ottawa ON K1H 1A2; Dal'78; Staff, The Ottawa Hospital - Riverside Campus; (613)731-3015; Fax. (613)731-3021.

TAYLOR, J Grant; 605 James St N, Hamilton ON L8L 1J9; Universidad Del Noreste (Mexico)'81; (905)529-8558; Fax. (905)577-6306.

TAYLOR, J Robert M; 256-39 Robertson Rd, Ottawa ON K2H 8R2; Tor'71; FRCPC; IntMed (Hematology Pathology); Hem. Consultant Ottawa Reg Cancer Centre, The Ottawa Hospital - General Campus; Dir-Lab Serv/Chief LabMed, Queensway Carleton Hospital; Langs: English; French; (613)725-9852; Fax. (613)695-9852.

TAYLOR, J E Scott; PO Box 99000 Stn Forces CF Health Services Centre, Halifax NS B3K 5X5; Dal'84; FRCSC; OrthSurg. Chief Surg, Canadian Forces Health Services Centre (Atlantic); Court Staff Orth, Queen Elizabeth II Health Sciences Centre - Victoria General Site; Locum Tenens, Valley Regional Hospital; (902)721-8801; Fax. (902)721-0356; scott.taylor@forces.gc.ca.

TAYLOR, James D N; Foul Bay Prof Centre, 312-1964 Fort St, Victoria BC V8R 6R3; McG'83; AB; Ophth (Cataract Surgery). Ac Staff, Vancouver Island Health Authority; Langs: English; French; (250)595-1223; Fax. (250)595-5422.

TAYLOR, James; Central Toronto Comm Hlth Ctr, 168 Bathurst St, Toronto ON M5V 2R4; McG'07; MDCM; CCFP; (416)703-8480; Fax. (416)703-8479.

TAYLOR, James M; Peterborough Reg HC-Hosp Dr, 1 Hospital Dr, Peterborough ON K9J 7C6; Ross University (USA)'02; FRCPC; Anes. Staff, Peterborough Regional Health Centre - Hospital Drive; (705)876-5038; Fax. (705)876-5105.

TAYLOR, Jana L; MUHC-Montreal Gen Hosp, 1650 av Cedar, Montreal QC H3G 1A4; McG'99; FRCPC; DiagRad (Thoracic Radiology). Staff, McGill University Health Centre - Montreal General Campus; (514)934-1934; jana.taylor@muhc.mcgill.ca.

TAYLOR, John A; Upper Appleby Med Associates, 36-1960 Appleby Line N, Burlington ON L7L 0B7; Tor'89; (905)315-9929; Fax. (905)315-9314.

TAYLOR, John C; Millard Health Centre, 131 Airport Rd NW, Edmonton AB T5G 0W6; (Other Foreign)'69; (780)498-3284; Fax. (780)498-3806.

TAYLOR, John C; Millard Health Centre, 131 Airport Rd, Edmonton AB T6G 0W6; Wes'72; DTMH; EmergMed. (780)498-3284; Fax. (780)498-3806.

TAYLOR, John D; 93 Monk St PO Box 820, Chapleau ON P0M 1K0; Tor'61; Court Staff, Lady Dunn Health Centre; Langs: English; French; (705)864-1393; Fax. (705)864-2722; jdtaylor@lseri.com.

TAYLOR, John P T F; 140 Cameron St, Sarnia ON N7V 4A8; Pretoria (South Africa)'80; FRCS(Ed); FRCSC; GenSurg (Endoscopy). Langs: Dutch; French.

TAYLOR, John R; 100 Rolling Hills Dr, Orangeville ON L9W 4X9; Qns'63; FACS; FRCSC; PlasSurg (Cosmetic Surgery). Staff, Headwaters Health Care Centre - Orangeville Site; (905)925-6029; Fax. (905)925-6425.

TAYLOR, Jonathan; 200-82 Tacoma Dr, Dartmouth NS B2W 3E5; Dal'82; (902)435-8202; Fax. (902)435-4294.

TAYLOR, Jonathan S; 100-1410 Mayor Magrath Dr S, Lethbridge AB T1K 2R3; Qns'99; FRCSC; Urol. (403)524-1401; Fax. (403)524-1403.

TAYLOR, Katherine L; The Hosp For Sick Children, 555 University Ave, Toronto ON M5G 1X8; Newcastle (Australia)'94; Staff, The Hospital For Sick Children; (416)813-7445; Fax. (416)813-7543.

TAYLOR, Kenneth N; Dr Kenneth & Taylor Medicine, 216-245 Pelham Rd, St Catharines ON L2S 1X8; Ott'72; Staff, Niagara Health System - St Catharines General Site; Staff, Niagara Health System - Ontario Street Site; (905)988-9277; Fax. (905)688-2652.

TAYLOR, Kerri-Ann S; The Group Health Centre, 240 McNabb St, Sault Ste. Marie ON P6B 1Y5; McM'00; BSc(Hon); FRCSC; GenSurg. Staff Surg, Sault Area Hospital - Sault Ste Marie; (705)759-7234 x5651; Fax. (705)759-5659.

TAYLOR, Kimball J; Cardston Med Clinic, PO Box 550, Cardston AB T0K 0K0; Alb'79; AAFP; Pres/Staff, Cardston Hospital; (403)653-3311; Fax. (403)653-1098.

TAYLOR, Lindsay E; Lockview Med Clinic, 203-667 Sackville Dr, Lower Sackville NS B4C 2S4; UBC'09; (902)252-3011; Fax. (902)252-3012.

TAYLOR, Lorraine; Mood Disorders Clinic, 400-723 Rymal Rd W, Hamilton ON L9B 2W2; McM'86; FRCPC; Psy. (905)522-1384; Fax. (905)522-2738.

TAYLOR, Marian R; PO Box 3433 Stn Main, Leduc AB T9E 6M2; Alb'70.

TAYLOR, Marianne J; 399 Royal Ave, Kelowna BC V1Y 5L3; Wes'85; FRCPC; IntMed; MedOncol. Staff, BC Cancer Agency Sindi Ahluwalia Hawkins Centre for the Southern Interior; Staff, Kelowna General Hospital; Clinical Asst Prof, University of British Columbia; (250)979-6620; Fax. (250)712-3911.

TAYLOR, Mark C; Bluewater Health-Norman Site, 89 Norman St, Sarnia ON N7T 6S3; Tor'80; MSc; FRCSC; GenSurg (Hepatobiliary Surgery). VP Medial Affairs, Bluewater Health - Norman Site; Staff, Lakeridge Health - Bowmanville Site; Staff, Lakeridge Health - Oshawa Site; (519)464-4529

TAYLOR, Martha L; Greenbrook Family Med Ctre, 421 Greenbrook Dr, Kitchener ON N2M 4K1; Qns'86; CCFP; FCFP; Staff, St Mary's General Hospital; Staff, Grand River Hospital - Kitchener/Waterloo Health Centre; Staff, New Vision Family Health Team - Greenbrook; (519)570-1655; Fax. (519)570-3477.

TAYLOR, Martin; 425-100 Richmond St W, Toronto ON M5H 3K6; Wes'59; (416)360-8208; Fax. (416)360-0692.

TAYLOR, Mary M; Riverside Prof Centre, 303-1919 Riverside Dr, Ottawa ON K1H 1A2; Ott'86; (613)731-2781; Fax. (613)731-0085; drtaylor@bellnet.ca.

TAYLOR, Megan M; Castlegar Med Associates, 1008 Columbia Ave, Castlegar BC V1N 1H2; Alb'97; CCFP; Staff Admitting Privileges, Kootenay Boundary Regional Hospital; (250)365-2161; Fax. (250)365-2171; casmedassociates@hotmail.com.

TAYLOR, Michael D; The Hosp for Sick Children, 1504-555 University Ave, Toronto ON M5G 1X8; Wes'94; FRCSC; Neursurg (Clinician Investigator Program). Clin Investigator Program, The Hospital For Sick Children; (416)813-6125; Fax. (416)813-4975; mdtaylor@sickkids.ca.

TAYLOR, Michael J; Markham-Stouffville Hosp, PO Box 1800 Stn Main 381 Church St, Markham ON L3P 7P3; Ott'99; CCFP; CCFP(E.M.); Staff, Markham Stouffville Hospital; (905)472-7111

TAYLOR, Michael R; Children's Hosp of Eastern Ont, 401 Smyth Rd, Ottawa ON K1H 8L1; Cal'90; CCFP; CCFP(E.M.); FCFP; Staff, Children's Hospital of Eastern Ontario (CHEO); Langs: Spanish; French; American Sign Language; (613)737-7600

TAYLOR, Murray F; Kingston Gen Hosp, 76 Stuart St, Kingston ON K7L 2V7; Qns'70; EmergMed. Staff, Kingston General Hospital; Att Staff, Niagara Health System - Ontario Street Site; Lecturer Surg, Queen's University; (613)548-2368

TAYLOR, Pamela L; Whitby Med Arts Bldg, 204-1615 Dundas St E, Whitby ON L1N 2L1; University of Southampton (England)'99; CCFP; (289)240-7962; Fax. (289)240-7964.

TAYLOR, Paul A; Burrard Health Bldg, 602-1160 Burrard St, Vancouver BC V6Z 2E8; London (England)'74; MB BS; FRCPC; IntMed; Nephrol. Ac Staff, Providence Health Care - St Paul's Hospital; Vis Staff, Lions Gate Hospital; Clin Assoc Prof, University of British Columbia; (604)681-7191; Fax. (604)681-4482; ptaylor@providencehealth.bc.ca.

TAYLOR, R Dale; Canadian Med Protective Assoc, 875 Carling Ave, Ottawa ON K1S 5P1; Tor'81; FRCSC; GenSurg. Staff, Canadian Medical Protective Association; (613)725-2000; Fax. (613)725-1300.

TAYLOR, Rhonda V; The Credit Valley Hosp, 2200 Eglinton Ave W, Mississauga ON L5M 2N1; McM'98; CCFP; CCFP(E.M.); Staff, The Credit Valley Hospital; (905)813-4141

TAYLOR, Richard S; Victoria Gen Hosp, 1 Hospital Way, Victoria BC V8Z 6R5; London (England)'80; MB BS; FRCPC; Peds (Consultant Pediatrics). Staff Neonatology, Victoria General Hospital; Assoc Prof, University of British Columbia; (250)727-4151; Fax. (250)727-4042.

TAYLOR, Richard W; Care Point Med Centre, 711 Pender St W, Vancouver BC V6C 3T2; McG'73; CCFP; Assoc Staff Family Med, Providence Health Care - St Paul's Hospital; (604)689-1103; Fax. (604)687-4860.

TAYLOR, Robert A; Kootenay Lake Med Clinic, 1140 Lakeside Dr, Nelson BC V1L 5Z3; UBC'94; (250)352-4666; Fax. (250)352-4696.

TAYLOR, Robert H; 3100-910 10th Ave W, Vancouver BC V5Z 1M9; McG'70; FRCSC; GenSurg (Breasts). Consultant Surg, BC Cancer Agency Vancouver Island Centre; Ac Staff, Providence Health Care - Mount Saint Joseph Hospital; Clin Assoc Prof, University of British Columbia; Langs: Bilingual(English/French); (604)875-5372; rhtaylor@interchange.ubc.ca.

TAYLOR, Robin S L; Colchester East Hants Health, 600-600 Abenaki Rd, Truro NS B2N 5A1; Cal'05; FRCPC; PH (Community Medicine); Public Health & Preventive Med. Staff, Colchester East Hants Health Authority Truro Public Health Office; (902)893-5820; Fax. (902)893-5839.

TAYLOR, Roger M; Brant Community HC-Brantford, 200 Terrace Hill St, Brantford ON N3R 1G9; Tor'94; Anes. Staff, The Brant Community Healthcare System - Brantford General Hospital Site; (905)751-5508; Fax. (519)751-5550; rtrtaylor@excite.com.

TAYLOR, Ronald P; Regina Qu'Appelle HR-Regina, 1440 14th Ave, Regina SK S4P 0W5; Sask'00; LMCC; CCFP; CCFP(E.M.); Staff, Regina General Hospital; (306)766-4500; Fax. (306)766-4357; fadreus@hotmail.com.

TAYLOR, Ronald W; 19 Alvin Ave, Toronto ON M4T 2A7; Tor'77; Staff Family Pract/Dir S C Cooper Sports Med Clinic, Mount Sinai Hospital; Physician, Toronto Blue Jays Baseball Club; Lecturer, University of Toronto; (416)921-2172; Fax. (416)921-2360.

TAYLOR, Rosemarie A; Lockview Med Clinic, 207-159 Cobequid Rd, Lower Sackville NS B4C 2N1; Dal'74; BSc(Hon); (902)832-2311; Fax. (902)832-2312.

TAYLOR, Ross; The Moncton Hosp, 135 MacBeath Ave, Moncton NB E1C 6Z8; UBC'10; CCFP; Staff Family Medicine Medical Education Office, The Moncton Hospital; (506)857-5111

TAYLOR, Ruth L; Royal Ottawa Hlth Care Group, 1145 Carling Ave, Ottawa ON K1Z 7K4; Ott'02; BScChemEng; MSc; FRCPC; Psy (Concurrent Disorders). Staff Disorders Program, Royal Ottawa Mental Health Centre - Royal Ottawa Health Care Group; Consultant Admitting Privileges, The Ottawa Hospital - General Campus; (613)722-6521

TAYLOR, S Mark; Dickson Med Bldg, 3052-5820 University Ave, Halifax NS B3H 1V7; Wes'95; FRCSC; Otol (Facial Plastic Surgery). Staff, Queen Elizabeth II Health Sciences Centre - Victoria General Site; (902)473-5752; Fax. (902)473-4016; smtaylorwashu@yahoo.com.

TAYLOR, Sandra L; 301-1625 Oak Bay Ave, Victoria BC V8R 1B1; Cal'81; (250)595-6009; Fax. (250)595-4077.

TAYLOR, Sara B; PO Box 22070 Rpo Westpark, Red Deer AB T4N 6X4; Wes'98; CCFP.

TAYLOR, Sara K; BC Cancer Ctre-Southern Interi, 399 Royal Ave, Kelowna BC V1Y 5L3; McG'03; FRCPC; IntMed; MedOncol. Staff, BC Cancer Agency Sindi Ahluwalia Hawkins Centre for the Southern Interior; (250)712-3900

TAYLOR, Sean W; Kingston Gen Hosp, C7-76 Stuart St, Kingston ON K7L 2V7; Dal'04; FRCPC; Neur. Staff, Kingston General Hospital; (613)549-6666; Fax. (613)548-1341.

TAYLOR, Shira G; Taddle Creek Connection, B102-726 Bloor St W, Toronto ON M6G 4A1; Tor'07; CCFP; (416)964-0800; Fax. (416)964-2935.

TAYLOR, Stephen A; Beamsville Med Centre FHT, PO Box 430 4279 Hixon St, Beamsville ON L0R 1B0; McG'81; CCFP; FCFP; Staff, West Lincoln Memorial Hospital; (905)563-5315; Fax. (905)563-0933.

TAYLOR, Steven J; 1187 Fischer Hallman Rd, Kitchener ON N2E 4H9; Qns'87; BSc; Staff, Grand River Hospital - Kitchener/Waterloo Health Centre; Staff, St Mary's General Hospital; (519)570-1200; Fax. (519)570-1214.

TAYLOR, Susan A; West Coast Gen Hosp, 3949 Port Alberni Hwy, Port Alberni BC V9Y 4S1; McM'80; FRCPC; IntMed (Menopause). Staff, West Coast General Hospital; (250)731-1370

TAYLOR, Susan M; Your Total Health Centre, 302-2330 Kennedy Rd, Scarborough ON M1T 0A2; Tor'86; Ac Staff, The Scarborough Hospital - Birchmount Campus; (416)298-1303; Fax. (416)298-4872.

TAYLOR, Susan N; Boyd Med Centre, 318-388 Portage Ave, Winnipeg MB R3C 0C8; Man'87; FRCSC; ObstGyn. Staff, St Boniface General Hospital; Lecturer, University of Manitoba; (204)925-3600; Fax. (204)925-3616.

TAYLOR, Taryn-Lise; Carleton Sports Med Clinic, 1125 Colonel By Dr, Ottawa ON K1S 5B6; Ott'04; MSc; Dip SportMed; CCFP; Surg Asst Orth, Montfort Hospital; Physician, Carleton Sports Med Clinic; Physician, Med Team Clinic; (613)520-3510; Fax. (613)520-3974.

TAYLOR, Thomas G; 18-1710 Ellis St, Kelowna BC V1Y 2B5; UBC'74; CCFP; FCFP; (250)763-5427

TAYLOR, Tracy L; Foothills Prof Bldg, 120-1620 29 St NW, Calgary AB T2N 4L7; Cal'03; FRCPC; Peds. Staff, Alberta Children's Hospital; (403)531-9757; Fax. (403)531-9752.

TAYLOR, Trudy A; Nova Scotia Rehab Centre, 245-1341 Summer St, Halifax NS B3H 4K4; Dal'01; FRCPC; IntMed; Rheum. Staff Rehab, Queen Elizabeth II Health Sciences Centre - Victoria General Site; (902)473-7040; Fax. (902)473-7019.

TAYLOR, Valerie H; Women's College Hosp, 9F-76 Grenville St, Toronto ON M5S 1B2; Mem'99; BMedSci; FRCPC; Psy (Mood Disorders). Staff Centre for Mountain Health Services, St Joseph's Healthcare Hamilton - West 5th Campus; Staff Psy (All Sites), Hamilton Health Sciences Centre - McMaster Children's Hospital; Staff, Women's College Hospital; (416)323-6400; Fax. (416)323-7718.

TAYLOR, Vicki L; Professional Arts Bldg, 625-100 Arden St, Moncton NB E1C 4B7; Mem'83; DAB; FRCSC; Ophth (Retina). Court Staff, Dr Georges-L-Dumont University Hospital Centre; Ac Staff, The Moncton Hospital; Dir, TLC Excimer Laser Centre; (506)383-2992; Fax. (506)854-4869.

TAYLOR, William H; 205-1370 Don Mills Rd, North York ON M3B 3N7; Tor'61; FRCSC; GenSurg (Psychotherapy); PedGenSurg. (416)449-3700; Fax. (416)449-2862; gnpn@msn.com.

TAYLOR, William H; Royal Victoria Hosp, 201 Georgian Dr, Barrie ON L4M 6M2; Tor'92; Anes. Staff, Royal Victoria Regional Health Centre; Langs: Bilingual(English/French); (705)728-9802

TAYLOR, William J; Hotel-Dieu Grace Hosp, 1030 Ouellette Ave, Windsor ON N9A 1E1; Ott'83; FRCPC; Anes. Staff Anes, Hôtel-Dieu Grace Hospital; Langs: English; French; (519)973-4421; Fax. (519)255-2130.

TAYLOR, William J; Moncton Med Clinic, 202-860 Mountain Rd, Moncton NB E1C 2N7; Dal'72; CCFP; FCFP; Staff, The Moncton Hospital; Assoc Prof, Dalhousie University; (506)853-5165; Fax. (506)853-5134.

TAYLOR, William J B; Hys Med Centre, 202-11010 101 St NW, Edmonton AB T5H 4B9; Alb'81; FRCPC; DiagRad. (780)426-1121; Fax. (780)425-5979.

TAYLOR, William L; Medical Arts Bldg, 206-121 Wellington St W, Barrie ON L4N 1L2; Tor'70; Staff, Royal Victoria Regional Health Centre; (705)737-4944

TAYLOR, William N; Richmond Health Science Ctre, 650-555 WBroadway, Vancouver BC V5Z 1C6; Witwatersrand (South Africa)'71; MB ChB; FRCS(Ed); FACS; FRCSC; Urol. Clin Assoc Prof, Vancouver General Hospital - Centennial Pavillion; Staff, Richmond Hospital; Consultant Urol, False Creek Surgical Centre; Physician, Metrovan Urology; Clin Assoc Prof Surg, University of British Columbia; (604)739-9695; Fax. (604)709-9676; williamntaylor@gmail.com.

TAYLOR, William P; Dermatology Office, 728 6 St SW, Medicine Hat AB T1A 4J5; Alb'79; BMedSci; FRCPC; Derm (Skin Cancer). Consultant, Medicine Hat Regional Hospital; (403)529-0010; Fax. (403)529-0033; taylor@shaw.ca.

TAYLOR CLARKE, Rebecca J; PO Box 448, Port Williams NS B0P 1T0; Dal'97; CCFP; (902)542-0779; Fax. (902)542-0530.

TAYLOR-FUREY, Allison N; Dr Charles A Janeway Child HC, 300 Prince Philip Dr, St. John's NL A1B 3V6; Mem'01; CCFP; Staff Dr Charles A Janeway Child Health Centre, Health Sciences Centre; (709)777-4575

TAYLOR GJEVRE, Regina M; Royal University Hosp, 103 Hospital Dr, Saskatoon SK S7N 0W8; Mem'87; FRCPC; IntMed; Rheum. Staff, Royal University Hospital; (306)966-8262; Fax. (306)966-8381; r.gjevre@usask.ca.

TAYLOR-WALL, Suzanne E M; 1-1261 Beaverbrook Ave, London ON N6H 0G6; Wes'08; CCFP; (519)642-2077; Fax. (519)642-1725.

TAYNEN, Howard D; 407-390 Brant St, Burlington ON L7R 4J4; Qns'73; FRCPC; Psy (Psychotherapy). (905)632-2112

TAYYEB, Tahir; Queen Elizabeth II Hosp, 10409 98 St, Grande Prairie AB T8V 2E8; Nishtar (Pakistan)'88; Staff ObstGyn, Queen Elizabeth II Hospital; (780)538-2190; Fax. (780)538-7621.

TAZKARJI, M Bachir; Trillium Summerville Teaching, 7F-101 Queensway W, Mississauga ON L5B 2P7; Aleppo Medical School (Syria)'97; CCFP; Att Physician, Geriatric Rehabilitation Institute; Teach Staff Family Med, University of Toronto; (905)272-9900; Fax. (905)272-9977.

TAZZEO, James I; Couchiching Family Health Team, 104A-119 Memorial Ave, Orillia ON L3V 5X1; McM'94; CCFP; Staff, Orillia Soldiers' Memorial Hospital; (705)329-0310; Fax. (705)329-0352.

TBAKHI, Abdelghani I A; Hotel Dieu Grace Hosp, 1030 Ouellette Ave, Windsor ON N9A 1E1; (Jordan)'86; Staff, Hôtel-Dieu Grace Hospital; (519)973-4411

TCHERENKOVA, Inaa A; La Loche Health Centre, PO Box 1, La Loche SK S0M 1G0; Leningrad (Russia (Federation))'93; CCFP; Staff, La Loche Health Centre and Hospital; Langs: Russian; (306)822-3201; Fax. (306)822-2798.

TCHERNI, Marly B L; Regina Qu'Appelle HR-Regina, 6-4101 Dewdney Ave, Regina SK S4T 1A5; Man'98; FRCSC; GenSurg (Family Medicine). Gen Surgeon, Pasqua Hospital; (306)566-6181; Fax. (306)566-6188.

TCHERNOV, Andrei G; North Med Centre, 103-7131 Bathurst St, Thornhill ON L4J 7Z1; Moscow (Russia (Federation))'86; AB; CCFP; Langs: Russian; (905)763-6682; Fax. (905)763-1705.

TCHERVENKOV, Christo I; MUHC-Montreal Children's Hosp, C829-2300 rue Tupper, Montreal QC H3H 1P3; McG'78; FRCSC; GenSurg; Cardiovasc&ThorSurg. ac Staff, McGill University Health Centre - Montreal General Campus; ac Staff, McGill University Health Centre - Royal Victoria Hospital; Prof Surg, McGill University; Langs: Bulgarian; French; (514)412-4400 x22394; Fax. (514)412-4330; christo.tchervenkov@muhc.mcgill.ca.

TCHERVENKOV, Jean I; MUHC-Royal Victoria Hosp, S10 26-687 av des Pins O, Montreal QC H3A 1A1; McG'80; FRCSC; GenSurg. Staff, McGill University Health Centre - Royal Victoria Hospital; Langs: English; French; (514)842-1231 x34042; tchervenkov@hotmail.com.

TCHERVENKOV, Sophia B; 500-5450 ch de la Cote-des-Nei, Montreal QC H3T 1Y6; McG'84; FRCSC; ObstGyn (AIDS/HIV). Staff, St Mary's Hospital Centre; Langs: Polish; French; (514)344-5188

TCHERVENKOVA, Milka A; 7385 Place Malraux, Brossard QC J4Y 1S5; Sofia (Bulgaria)'56; Staff, Hopital Charles LeMoyne; Langs: Bulgarian; French; Russian; (450)678-9400; Fax. (450)678-1500.

TE, Luis D; 107-31 Fairview Blvd, St Albert AB T8N 3M5; Manila (Philippines)'56; FRCPC; IntMed (Clinical Immunology & Allergy). Att Staff, Royal Alexandra Hospital; Med Staff, University of Alberta; (780)458-8999; Fax. (780)458-3121.

TE-JUATCO, Lillien; Lougheed Plaza, 240-9600 Cameron St, Burnaby BC V3J 7N3; UBC'84; (604)421-1027

TEAGUE, Kevin R; Anaesthesia Assoc of London, 100 Piccadilly St, London ON N6A 1R8; Cal'02; FRCPC; Anes. (519)685-8500

TEAGUE, Paul E R; Minor-Emerg Clinic, 180 Vine St S, St Catharines ON L2R 7P3; Tor'65; CCFP; (905)682-5411

TEAKLES, Joseph; 3-1116A Mountain Rd, Moncton NB E1C 2T3; Mon'01; CCFP; (506)383-4339; Fax. (506)854-6574.

TEAL, Barbara A; Harvard Square Mall, 202-801 Mohawk Rd W, Hamilton ON L9C 6C2; McM'83; CCFP; FCFP; (905)388-2447; Fax. (905)387-3965.

TEAL, Patricia K; Douglas Med Centre, 238 Bertie St, Fort Erie ON L2A 1Z3; Wes'69; FRCSC; Ophth (Cataract). Chief Ophth, Niagara Health System - Douglas Memorial Hospital Site; (905)871-6737; Fax. (905)871-9893; info@tealcosmeticlaser.com.

TEAL, Philip A; Gordon & Leslie Diamond HCC, 8289-2775 Laurel St, Vancouver BC V5Z 1M9; Alb'74; FRCPC; EmergMed (Headache); Neur. Ac Staff, Vancouver General Hospital - Centennial Pavillion; Chair, Canadian Stroke Consortium; Staff, Gordon & Leslie Diamond Health Care Centre; Staff Teacher, University of British Columbia; (604)875-5515; Fax. (604)875-5514; teal@interchange.ubc.ca.

TEAPE-HUMPHREY, Lorna T; Westbram Family Physicians, 104-100 Pertosa Dr, Brampton ON L6X 0H9; West Indies (Jamaica)'90; CCFP; (905)451-1244; Fax. (905)451-6955.

TEASDALE, Francois; 6A-5955 av Wilderton, Montreal QC H3S 2V1; Mon'66; FRCPC; Peds (Neonatology). ac Staff/Prof Peds & Section of Perinatol, Hôpital Ste-Justine; Prof Peds, Universite de Montreal; Langs: Bilingual(French/English); (514)737-5791

TEASELL, Lynne D; Foothills Family Practice, 102-30 Crystalridge Dr, Okotoks AB T1S 2C3; McM'93; BSc; Staff, High River General Hospital; Langs: English; French; (403)938-5455; Fax. (403)938-4749.

TEASELL, Robert W; St Joseph's HC-Parkwood Hosp, 801 Commissioners Rd E, London ON N6C 5J1; Wes'81; FRCPC; PhysMed&Rehab (Pain & Disability Evaluation). Staff, Parkwood Hospital - St Joseph's Health Care; Prof, University of Western Ontario; (519)685-4559; Fax. (519)685-4023.

TEBBENHAM, Troy E; Thunder Bay Reg HSC-T-Bay, 980 Oliver Rd, Thunder Bay ON P7B 6V4; Qns'96; FRCPC; EmergMed. Staff, Thunder Bay Regional Health Sciences Centre; (807)684-6100

TEBBUTT, L Christopher; Georgian Prof Centre, 300-125 Bell Farm Rd, Barrie ON L4M 6L2; Wes'88; FRCPC; IntMed (Respirology). (705)725-9699; Fax. (705)733-8350; allen.tebbutt@sympatico.ca.

TEBBUTT-SPEIRS, Susan M R; Penticton Reg Hosp, 550 Carmi Ave, Penticton BC V2A 3G6; UBC'93; FRCPC; GenPath. Staff, Penticton Regional Hospital; (250)492-4000 x2340

TEBOUL, Barbara K; CSSS du Suroît, 150 rue Saint-Thomas, Salaber-de-Valleyf QC J6T 6C1; McG'91; Ophth. ac Staff, Centre Hospitalier Régional du Suroît; ac Staff, St Mary's Hospital Centre; Langs: English; French; (450)371-9920; Fax. (450)371-7454.

TEBOUL, Eric A; 290 rue de Montigny, Saint-Jerome QC J7Z 5T3; McG'87; CRCP; Psy (Emergency Psychiatry). Staff, Hôtel-Dieu de Saint-Jérôme; Langs: English; French; (450)432-2777; Fax. (450)431-8207; ericteboul@videotron.ca.

TEBOUL, Nathalie; Clinique Med Riel, 455 boul Riel, Gatineau QC J8Z 2J8; McG'91; MDCM; FRCSC; Ophth (Cataract Surgery). Staff, Montfort Hospital; Staff, CSSS de Gatineau; Staff, Downtown Ophthalmologists; Langs: English; French; (819)777-7416; Fax. (819)777-5061.

TECIMER, Sandy N; Rowntree Health Centre, 11-2687 Kipling Ave, Etobicoke ON M9V 5G6; McM'04; CCFP; (416)744-1680

TECTOR, Susan E; Hopital Montfort, 713 Montreal Rd, Ottawa ON K1K 0T2; McG'98; CCFP; CCFP(E.M.); Staff, Montfort Hospital; Langs: French; (613)746-4621

TEE, James B; Alberta Children's Hosp, 2888 Shaganappi Trail NW, Calgary AB T3B 6A8; Tor'99; FRCPC; Peds; Nephrol. Staff, Alberta Children's Hospital; (403)955-7913; Fax. (619)566-5812.

TEE, Rodney K; Nepean Med Centre, 409-1 Centrepointe Dr, Nepean ON K2G 6E2; Newcastle (England)'72; MRCGPract; DRCOG; Ac Staff, Queensway Carleton Hospital; (613)228-8860; Fax. (613)228-9831.

TEED, D Lionel; Dr Everett Chalmers Reg Hosp, PO Box 9000 Stn A, Fredericton NB E3B 5N5; Dal'68; AB; FRCPC; DiagRad (Nuclear Medicine). Staff, Dr Everett Chalmers Regional Hospital; (506)452-5136; Fax. (506)452-5646.

TEEFY, Patrick J; London HSC-University Hosp, PO Box 5339 Stn B 339 Windermere Rd, London ON N6A 5A5; Ott'86; FRCPC; IntMed (Interventional Cardiology); Cardiol. Staff, London Health Sciences Centre - University Hospital; (519)663-3075; Fax. (519)663-3516; teefyp@lhsc.on.ca.

TEEHAN, Michael D; Abbie J Lane Memorial Bldg, 3041-5909 Veterans Memorial La, Halifax NS B3H 2E2; Dublin (Ireland)'77; DCH; MRC; MRCPsy; LRCPS; FRCPC; Psy. Psychiatrist, Queen Elizabeth II Health Sciences Centre - Victoria General Site; Asst Dean Student Affairs/Assoc Prof, Dalhousie University; Langs: Gaelic; (902)473-7134; Fax. (902)429-2028.

TEEL, Warren D; Occupational Health Clinic, 171 Kendall St, Sarnia ON N7V 4G6; Wes'90; (519)337-4627; Fax. (519)337-9442.

TEELUCKSINGH, George D; Agincourt Prof Centre, 324-2330 Kennedy Rd, Scarborough ON M1T 0A2; London (England)'58; MB BS; Staff, North York General Hospital; Staff, The Scarborough Hospital - Birchmount Campus; Staff Family Med, The Scarborough Hospital - General Campus; (416)497-6484; Fax. (416)497-6815.

TEEPLE, Lori E; Bluewater Area Family Hlth Tea, 43 Main St, Zurich ON N0M 2T0; Ott'86; CCFP; CCFP(E.M.); FCFP; VP Med Aff/Chief Staff, St Thomas Elgin General Hospital; Langs: English; French; (519)236-4314; lori@womenshealthclinic.co.uk.

TEES, David A; Saint John Med Clinic, 295-299 Metcalf St, Saint John NB E2K 4P8; Mem'86; FRCSC; Otol (Head & Neck Surgery). Staff, Saint John Regional Hospital; Dept Head Otol/Med Dir Surgical Services, Regional Health Authority Region 5; Clin Instructor, Dalhousie University; (506)634-1115; Fax. (506)636-9002; dtees@nbnet.nb.ca.

TEETAERT, Matthew A; Hawkesbury Dist Gen Hosp, 1111 Ghislain St, Hawkesbury ON K6A 3G5; Man'09; CCFP; Staff, Hawkesbury & District General Hospital; (613)632-1111

TEFERI, Amde M; Homewood Health Centre, 150 Delhi St, Guelph ON N1E 6K9; Addis Ababa (Ethiopia)'76; MD; BSc; MPH; FRCPC; Psy. Staff, Homewood Health Centre; Langs: Tigrigna; Amharic; (519)824-1010 x145; Fax. (519)767-3577; tefeamde@homewood.org.

TEH, M C Matthew; C12-8380 Kennedy Rd, Markham ON L3R 0W4; Alb'86; Langs: Mandarin; Cantonese; (905)946-0882; Fax. (905)946-0436.

TEHFE, Moustapha; CHUM-Hop Notre-Dame, 1560 rue Sherbrooke E, Montreal QC H2L 4M1; (Lebanon)'98; Staff, Centre Hospitalier l'Université de Montréal (CHUM) - Hôpital Notre-Dame; (514)890-8000 x25381; Fax. (514)412-7803.

TEHRANIFAR, Mitra; Kateri Mem Hosp Centre, 10 River Rd, Kahnawake QC J0L 1B0; Staff, Kateri Memorial Hospital Centre; (450)638-3930; Fax. (450)638-4634.

TEHRANIPOUR, Neda; CSSS du Lac-des-Deux-Montagnes, 520 boul Arthur-Sauve, Saint-Eustache QC J7R 5B1; Shahid Beheshti Univ of Medical Sciences (Other Foreign)'04; FRCPC; DiagRad. Staff, Hôpital de Saint-Eustache; (450)473-6811

TEICHMAN, Joel M H; St Paul's Hosp, C307-1081 Burrard St, Vancouver BC V6Z 1Y6; McG'87; FRCSC; Urol (General Surgery). Staff Urol, Providence Health Care - St Paul's Hospital; Langs: Bilingual(English/French); (604)806-8266; Fax. (604)806-8666.

TEICHROB, Deanna M; Nicola Med Dental Bldg, 400-321 Nicola St, Kamloops BC V2C 6G6; UBC'03; FRCPC; IntMed. (250)314-3601

TEIJEIRA, F Javier; CHUS-Hop Fleurimont, 3001 12e av N, Sherbrooke QC J1H 5N4; Navarra (Spain)'67; PhD(Spain); FRCSC; Cardiovasc&ThorSurg (P.Q.); CardSurg. Staff, Centre Hospitalier Universitaire de Sherbrooke-Hopital Fleurimont; (819)346-1110 x14356

TEILLET, Marc E; Selkirk Mental Health Centre, PO Box 9600 Stn Main, Selkirk MB R1A 2B5; Man'86; FRCPC; Psy (Chronic Care). Staff Psy, Selkirk Mental Health Centre; (204)482-3810; Fax. (204)482-6390.

TEIN, Ingrid; The Hosp for Sick Children, 555 University Ave, Toronto ON M5G 1X8; Tor'79; BSc; FRCPC; Peds (Pediatric Neurology). Staff, The Hospital For Sick Children; Langs: Estonian; French; (416)813-5668; Fax. (416)813-6334; ingrid.tein@sickkids.ca.

TEIRA, Pierre; Hôpital Ste-Justine, 3175 ch Cote-Sainte-Catherine, Montreal QC H3T 1C5; Toulouse (France)'05; Staff, Hôpital Ste-Justine; (514)345-4931 x6912; Fax. (514)345-4884; pierre.teira.hsj@ssss.gouv.qc.ca.

TEITEL, Jerome M; St Michael's Hosp, 2 080Q-30 Bond St, Toronto ON M5B 1W8; Tor'73; FRCPC; Hem; IntMed. Head Hem, St Michael's Hospital; Prof, University of Toronto; (416)864-5128

TEITEL, Jesse D; 311-4800 Leslie St, North York ON M2J 2K9; Tor'82; CCFP; Staff, North York General Hospital; Staff, Rouge Valley Health System - Centenary Health Centre Site; Langs: Hebrew; (416)229-2380; Fax. (416)229-2513.

TEITELBAUM, Earl J; 180-5 Fairview Mall Dr, North York ON M2J 2Z1; McG'84; FRCPC; IntMed; Cardiol. Staff, North York General Hospital; (416)633-1780; Fax. (416)633-6530.

TEITELBAUM, Ivor; Yorkview Med Centre, 104-3695 Keele St, North York ON M3J 1N2; Witwatersrand (South Africa)'80; Langs: Afrikaans; Hebrew; (416)633-3711; Fax. (416)633-0521.

TEITELBAUM, Jeanne S; MUHC-Montreal Neurology Inst, 3801 rue University, Montreal QC H3A 2B4; Mon'80; FRCPC; Neur. Dir program, McGill University Health Centre - Montreal Neurological Hospital; assoc Prof, Universite de Montreal; assoc Prof, McGill University; (514)398-6644 x00400; Fax. (514)398-1352; jeanne.teitelbaum@muhc.mcgill.ca.

TEITELBAUM, Louise E; Providence Care-Mental Health, PO Box 603 Stn Main 752 King St W, Kingston ON K7L 4X3; Mon'85; BSc; FRCPC; Psy (Geriatric Psychiatry). Staff, Providence Care - Mental Health Services; Asst Prof Psy, Queen's University; (613)546-1101; Fax. (613)548-5569.

TEITELBAUM, Peter S; Riverside Prof Centre, 411-1919 Riverside Dr, Ottawa ON K1H 1A2; Ott'70; Langs: Italian; French; Norwegian; (613)733-5553; Fax. (613)733-2689.

TEITELBAUM, Stanley; 260-5 Fairview Mall Dr, North York ON M2J 2Z1; Tor'72; CCFP; FCFP; Ac Staff, North York General Hospital; Asst Prof Family & Commun Med, University of Toronto; (416)497-6363; Fax. (416)497-7610.

TEIXEIRA, Fernando J; St Michael's Hosp, 30 Bond St, Toronto ON M5B 1W8; Tor'97; FRCPC; EmergMed. Staff Emerg, St Michael's Hospital; (416)864-5095

TEIXEIRA, Frederick A; Don Mills-Eglinton Med Centre, 100-29 Gervais Dr, North York ON M3C 1Z1; Tor'70; (416)449-6525; Fax. (416)449-9334.

TEIXEIRA, Marc A; Nanaimo Reg Gen Hosp, 1200 Dufferin Cres, Nanaimo BC V9S 2B7; Qns'94; CCFP; CCFP(E.M.); Staff, Nanaimo Regional General Hospital; (250)755-7627; Fax. (250)755-7660.

TEJPAR, Ismet; 3300-950 10 Ave, Vancouver BC V5Z 1M9; Wes'86; Staff, Vancouver General Hospital - Centennial Pavillion; (604)875-4073

TEJPAR, Shamim J; 282 Erie St, Stratford ON N5A 2N2; Shiraz (Iran)'78; FAAP; FRCPC; Peds. Staff Peds, Stratford General Hospital - Huron Perth Healthcare Alliance; Consultant Privil Peds, Seaforth Community Hospital - Huron Perth Healthcare Alliance; Staff, Listowel Memorial Hospital - Listowel Wingham Hospitals Alliance; Assoc Dean Rural & Regional Med, University of Western Ontario; Langs: Gujarati; Kacchi; (519)273-4252; Fax. (519)273-7830; stejpar@rogers.com.

TEKANO, Kenneth J; Lonsdale Med & Dental Bldg, 108-1940 Lonsdale Ave, North Vancouver BC V7M 2K2; UBC'84; (604)987-3357

TEKLE, Abedom; 302-5171 221A St, Langley BC V2Y 0A2; Sask'94; BSc(Biochem); Staff, Langley Memorial Hospital; Langs: Tigrigna; (604)539-7733; Fax. (604)539-7713.

TEKU, Edo; St Joseph's Hlth Ctr Urban FHT, 511-27 Roncesvalles Ave, Toronto ON M6R 3B2; Palacky (Czech Republic)'85; CCFP; FCFP; Langs: Amharic; Czech; (416)539-8181; Fax. (416)539-8797.

TELANG, Harshad; 303-984 Oliver Rd, Thunder Bay ON P7B 7C7; Ott'92; FRCS; FRCSC; GenSurg. Staff, Thunder Bay Regional Health Sciences Centre; Assoc Prof, Northern Ontario School of Medicine-Lakehead University; Langs: Bilingual(English/French); (807)345-4500; Fax. (807)345-4501.

TELCH, Joseph; 209-548 Carlton Rd, Markham ON L3R 0C6; National (Mexico)'69; MSc; FRCPC; Peds (Clinical Nutrition). Consultant Peds, North York General Hospital; Consultant Clin Nutrition, Holland Bloorview Kids Rehabilitation Hospital; Consultant, Erin Oak Treatment Centre for Children; Lecturer Peds, University of Toronto; Langs: Spanish; Hebrew; Portuguese; (905)477-7560; Fax. (905)477-7857; joseph.telch@utoronto.ca.

TELFER, Charles D; Surrey Med Arts Bldg, 320-13710 94A Ave, Surrey BC V3V 1N1; Alb'81; FRCSC; OrthSurg. (604)585-8469; Fax. (604)585-8479.

TELFER, Christine J; 203-350 St George St, Moncton NB E1C 1X1; Alb'80; CCFP; FCFP; Staff, The Moncton Hospital; Staff, Dr Georges-L-Dumont University Hospital Centre; (506)857-8045

TELFORD, Edward; 1-188 Sunset Dr, St Thomas ON N5R 3B9; Wes'80; CCFP; FCFP; Court Staff, St Thomas Elgin General Hospital; (519)633-1100; Fax. (519)633-1122.

TELFORD, Gordon O; Richmond Med Bldg, 103-2020 Richmond Rd, Victoria BC V8R 6R5; Alb'73; FAAD; Derm; IntMed (Infectious Diseases). Dir Psoriasis Unit, Royal Jubilee Hospital; Staff, Victoria General Hospital; Clin Instructor Med, University of British Columbia; (250)595-3424; Fax. (250)598-5766.

TELFORD, Jennifer J; Pacific Gastroenterology Assoc, 770-1190 Hornby St, Vancouver BC V6Z 2K5; UBC'96; BSc(Hon); MPH; ABIM; FRCPC; IntMed; Gastroent. Prof Gastroent, Providence Health Care - St Paul's Hospital; Clinical Asst Prof, University of British Columbia; (604)688-6332; Fax. (604)689-2004.

TELIKICHARLA KANDALA, Narsimhachary; Park Avenue Med Centre, 203-4634 Park Ave, Terrace BC V8G 1V7; Poona (India)'71; MB BS; Langs: Hindi; Marathi; Telugu; (250)638-4082

TELIO, David; Kingsway Plaza Phase III, 705-4980 Kingsway, Burnaby BC V5H 4K7; Tor'06; FRCPC; IntMed; MedOncol; Hem. Staff, Gordon & Leslie Diamond Health Care Centre; Staff, BC Cancer Agency Vancouver Centre; (604)434-5001

TELIO, Summer L; Outpatient Psy Program Hlth Ct, 715 12th Ave, Vancouver BC V5Z 1M9; Tor'06; FRCPC; Psy. Staff, Vancouver General Hospital - Centennial Pavillion; Staff, Outpatient Psychiatry Program Health Centre; (604)875-4794

TELLEZ-ZENTENO, Jose F; Royal University Hosp, 1622-103 Hospital Dr Box 26, Saskatoon SK S7N 0W8; Mexico (Mexico)'96; MSc; PhD; Staff Neurol, Royal University Hospital; Assoc Prof, University of Saskatchewan; Langs: Spanish; (306)655-1000; Fax. (306)966-8008.

TELLIER, Claudia; MUHC-Royal Victoria Hosp, 687 av des Pins O, Montreal QC H3A 1A1; Laval'07; IntMed. Staff, McGill University Health Centre - Royal Victoria Hospital; (514)934-1934

TELLIER, Genevieve; Hôpital Ste-Justine, 3175 ch Cote-Sainte-Catherine, Montreal QC H3T 1C5; Mon'81; FRCPC; Psy. Prof, Universite de Montreal; (514)345-4931 x2882; Fax. (514)345-2187; genevieve.tellier.hsj@ssss.gouv.qc.ca.

TELLIER, Guy; Clinique Med de Mirabel, CP 1059 13714 boul du Cure-Labelle, Mirabel QC J7J 1A1; Mon'82; Staff, Hôtel-Dieu de Saint-Jérôme; (450)435-7666; Fax. (450)435-1716; gtellier@omnispec.ca.

TELLIER, Lyne; Clin de Gynecologique de Levis, 400-4975 boul de la Rive-Sud, Levis QC G6V 4Z5; Laval'91; FRCSC; ObstGyn (Colposcopy). Staff, Hôtel-Dieu de Lévis; Langs: English; (418)833-1522; Fax. (418)833-1526.

TELLIER, Pierre-Paul; McGill Univ Student Hlth Serv, 3600 rue McTavish, Montreal QC H3A 0G3; Ott'76; CCFP; FCFP; Médecin Student Health Services, McGill University; (514)398-6017; Fax. (514)398-2559.

TELLIER, Raymond J M; Provincial Laboratory, 3030 Hospital Dr NW, Calgary AB T2N 4W4; Sher'86; MSc(Microbiol.); CSPQ; BSc(Physics); FRCPC; MedMicrobiol. Assoc Prof, University of Calgary; Langs: English; French; (403)944-2724; Fax. (403)283-0142; raymond.tellier@albertahealthservices.ca.

TELNER, Adam H; LMC Endocrinology Centres, 107-1929 Bayview Ave, East York ON M4G 3E8; McG'72; MSc; FACP; FRCPC; IntMed (Endocrinology); Endocrin&Metab., LMC Diabetes & Endocrinology Centres-Barrie; Staff, LMC Diabetes & Endocrinology Centres-Bayview; Langs: French; (416)645-2929; Fax. (416)645-2930; adam.telner@lmc.ca.

TELNER, Deanna E; Family Health Centre, 105-840 Coxwell Ave, Toronto ON M4C 5T2; Ott'99; CCFP; Staff, Toronto East General Hospital Inc; (416)469-6464; Fax. (416)469-6164.

TELTSCHER, Marty S; Centre Hosp de Lachine, 650 16e av, Lachine QC H8S 3N5; McG'04; FRCPC; IntMed; MedMicrobiol; InfectDis. Staff, CSSS de Dorval-Lachine-Lasalle; (514)637-2351 x77125

TEMAN, Carolin J; Foothills Med Center, C1136-1403 29 St NW, Calgary AB T2N 2T9; Staff, Foothills Medical Centre; Staff, Calgary Laboratory Services; (403)944-8041; Fax. (403)944-8998.

TEMAN, Paul T; Business Bldg, 300-295 Midpark Way SE, Calgary AB T2X 2A8; (403)254-6400; Fax. (403)254-6403.

TEMINS, Carol A; 220 Meadowvale Prof Centre, 6855 Meadowvale Town Ctre Cir, Mississauga ON L5N 2Y1; Tor'86; CCFP; Court Staff Family Med, The Credit Valley Hospital; (905)826-6013; Fax. (905)826-0980.

TEMKIT, Abdelkader; CSSSG-Hop de Hull, 116 boul Lionel-Emond, Gatineau QC J8Y 1W7; Alger (Algeria)'77; IntMed; Staff, Hull Hospital; Langs: French; (819)595-6000 x6035; Fax. (819)595-6325; abdtemk@yahoo.com.

TEMMAR, Rabia; CHUS-Hop Fleurimont, 3001 12e av N, Sherbrooke QC J1H 5N4; Alger (Algeria)'96; Staff, Centre Hospitalier Universitaire de Sherbrooke-Hopital Fleurimont; (819)346-1110

TEMPIER, Raymond P L; Montfort Hosp, 713 Montreal Rd, Ottawa ON K1K 0T2; Marseille (France)'78; MSc; FRCPC; Psy (Public Health). Staff, Montfort Hospital; Langs: English; German; (613)746-4621; Fax. (613)748-4838.

TEMPLE, Becky A; Fort St John Med Clinic, 10011 96 St, Fort St. John BC V1J 3P3; UBC'81; CCFP; Med Dir NE, Fort St John Hospital & Health Centre; (250)785-6677; Fax. (250)787-0109.

TEMPLE, Bryan K; 110-89 Queensway W, Mississauga ON L5B 2V2; Tor'81; FRCPC; IntMed; Neur. Staff, Trillium Health Centre - Mississauga; (905)566-9330; Fax. (905)566-5683.

TEMPLE, Michael J; The Hosp for Sick Children, 555 University Ave, Toronto ON M5G 1X8; Wes'92; FRCPC; DiagRad (Pediatric Interventional Radiology). Staff, The Hospital For Sick Children; (416)813-6039; Fax. (416)813-2139; michael.temple@sickkids.ca.

TEMPLE, Michelle T; Children's Hosp of Eastern Ont, 401 Smyth Rd, Ottawa ON K1H 8L1; Mem'03; FRCPC; Psy. Staff, Children's Hospital of Eastern Ontario (CHEO); (613)737-2260

TEMPLE, Walley J; Tom Baker Cancer Centre, 1331 29 St NW, Calgary AB T2N 4N2; Qns'70; FACS; FRCSC; GenSurg (Surgical Oncology). Dir Surgical Oncol, Foothills Medical Centre; Staff/Chief Div Sugrical Oncology, Tom Baker Cancer Centre; Prof, University of Calgary; (403)521-3914; Fax. (403)521-3744.

TEMPLE-OBERLE, Claire F; Tom Baker Cance Centre, 1331 29 St NW, Calgary AB T2N 4N2; Qns'96; FRCSC; PlasSurg. Staff, Tom Baker Cancer Centre; (403)521-3275; Fax. (403)944-3926.

TEMPLEMAN, F David; 151 Pine Valley Dr, London ON N6J 4M2; Alb'02; DipChild&AdolescPsy; FRCPC; Psy (Child & Adolescent Psychiatry). (519)435-6499; Fax. (866)504-3115.

TEMPLETON, Christina G; Dr Charles A Janeway Child Hc, 300 Prince Philip Dr, St. John's NL A1B 3V6; Mem'95; FRCPC; Peds (Pediatric Cardiology); Cardiol. Staff, Janeway Children's Health & Rehabilitation Centre; (709)777-4462

TEMPLETON, W Robert; 1900 Fort St, Victoria BC V8R 1J8; Belfast (Ireland)'64; Consultant Genetics, Vancouver Island Health Authority; Asst Prof, University of British Columbia; (250)370-8509; Fax. (250)370-8285.

TEN HOVE, Martin W; Hotel-Dieu Hosp, 166 Brock St, Kingston ON K7L 5G2; Qns'89; FRCSC; Ophth (Neuro Ophthalmology). Staff, Hotel-Dieu Hospital; (613)544-3400 x3388; Fax. (613)544-3041; tenhove@post.queensu.ca.

TENASCHUK, Danny S; Montfort Hosp, 713 Montreal Rd, Ottawa ON K1K 0T2; Tor'83; DiagRad. Staff, Montfort Hospital; Langs: English; French; (613)746-4621 x2508; Fax. (613)748-4921.

TENBY, Lionel; Dr Lionel Tenby Fam Med Clinic, 160-3920 Francis Rd, Richmond BC V7C 1J7; London (England)'55; MB BS; MRCS; LRCP(Eng); LMCC; Ac Staff, Richmond Hospital; Langs: German; Yiddish; French; Spanish; (604)277-7171; Fax. (604)277-1966.

TENENBAUM, Jerry; 202-2179 Yonge St, Toronto ON M4S 2A9; Tor'73; FRCPC; IntMed; Rheum. (416)546-4316; Fax. (416)551-0386.

TENENBEIN, Marshall S; Harry Medovy House, 2F-671 William Ave, Winnipeg MB R3E 0Z2; Man'05; FRCPC; Anes.

TENENBEIN, Milton; Children's Hosp, JL 143-840 Sherbrook St, Winnipeg MB R3A 1S1; Man'73; AB; FRCPC; Peds. Dir Emerg Serv, Health Sciences Centre; Dir, Manitoba Poison Control Centre; Prof, University of Manitoba; (204)787-2445; Fax. (204)787-4807.

TENENBEIN, Paul K; Univ Hlth Network-Toronto Western Hosp, 399 Bathurst St, Toronto ON M5T 2S8; Man'00; FRCPC; Anes. Staff, Toronto Western Hospital - University Health Network; (416)603-5118

TENG, Billy B; The Richmond Gen Hosp, 7000 Westminster Hwy, Richmond BC V6X 1A2; UBC'02; FRCPC; GenPath. Staff, Richmond Hospital; (604)278-5160

TENG, Carolyn J; 100-30 Prospect St, Newmarket ON L3Y 3S9; Tor'01; FRCSC; CardSurg. Staff, St Michael's Hospital; (905)895-4521; Fax. (905)868-8371.

TENG, Sophia C; Hayyan Healthcare Clinic, 8-9301 Bathurst St, Richmond Hill ON L4C 9S2; Saba University School of Medicine (Other Foreign)'09; (905)237-7472

TENHUNEN, Linda M; Sudbury Reg Hosp-Laurentian, 41 Ramsey Lake Rd, Sudbury ON P3E 5J1; Ott'83; Staff Northeastern Ont Reg Cancer Ctre, Health Sciences North-Laurentian Site; (705)522-6237 x2451; Fax. (705)523-7329.

TENKI, Michael C; Rodney Med Clinic, PO Box 249 226 Furnival Rd, Rodney ON N0L 2C0; Dal'99; (519)785-0456; Fax. (519)785-2064.

TENN-LYN, Nicole A; Trillium Hlth Ctr-Mississauga, 100 Queensway W, Mississauga ON L5B 1B8; McM'00; FRCPC; EmergMed. Staff EmergMed, Trillium Health Centre - Mississauga; (905)848-7600

TENNANKORE, Karthik K; Univ Hlth Network-Toronto Gen, 200 Elizabeth St, Toronto ON M5G 2C4; Wes'06; FRCPC; IntMed; Nephrol. Staff, Toronto General Hospital - UHN; (416)340-3111

TENNANT, Matthew T S; Alberta Retina Consultants, 400-10924 107 Ave NW, Edmonton AB T5H 0X5; UBC'96; FRCSC; Ophth. Staff, Royal Alexandra Hospital; (780)448-1801; Fax. (780)448-1809.

TENNANT, Sarah C; South Shore Regional Hosp, 90 Glen Allan Dr, Bridgewater NS B4V 3S6; UBC'09; CCFP; Staff, South Shore Regional Hospital; (902)543-4603

TENNEN, Gayla B; Sunnybrook Hlth Sciences Ctre, FG 29-2075 Bayview Ave, Toronto ON M4N 3M5; McM'01; FRCPC; Psy. Staff, Sunnybrook Health Sciences Centre; (416)480-6100

TENNENHOUSE, Ronald S; Woodbridge Urgent Care Centre, 2-4000 Highway 7, Woodbridge ON L4L 8Z2; Man'76; CCFP; Staff, William Osler Health System - Etobicoke General Hospital; (905)851-3777; Fax. (905)851-0682.

TENNENT, Alison C; Cooperative Health Centre, 110 8th St E, Prince Albert SK S6V 0V7; Mem'95; BSc; FRCSC; ObstGyn. (306)922-3284; Fax. (306)922-3285; alison_tennent@hotmail.com.

TENOVE, R John; Nanton Med Clinic, PO Box 940 2214 20th St, Nanton AB T0L 1R0; Alb'76; Gen Practice, High River General Hospital; (403)646-2218; Fax. (403)646-3046.

TEO, Astra L; 204-2401 Yonge St, Toronto ON M4P 3H1; Tor'09; CCFP; (416)485-2222; Fax. (416)485-2276.

TEO, Iris Y H; The Ottawa Hosp-Gen Campus, 4F-501 Smyth Rd, Ottawa ON K1H 8L6; Qns'05; FRCPC; AnatPath. Staff, The Ottawa Hospital - General Campus; (613)798-5555

TEO, Koon Kang; Hamilton HS-General Site, C2 106-237 Barton St E, Hamilton ON L8L 2X2; Dublin (Ireland)'78; MB ChB; PhD; FRCPI(Ire); LRCPSI; FRCPC; Cardiol. Staff, Hamilton Health Sciences Centre - Hamilton General Hospital; Prof, McMaster University; (905)521-2100 x76222; Fax. (905)527-9642.

TEO, Michele M; Heritage Med Research Centre, 562-107 University Campus NW, Edmonton AB T6G 2S2; Alb'05; Rheum; IntMed. Staff, Heritage Medical Research Centre; (780)407-2121; Fax. (780)407-6055; mteo@cha.ab.ca.

TEO, Su-Ting; Ryerson Health Centre, 350 Victoria Ave, Toronto ON M5B 2K3; Mem'96; BSc; BMedSci; MCFP; CCFP; (416)979-5070; Fax. (416)979-5073.

TEO, Swee L; Pan Am Clinic, 75 Poseidon Bay, Winnipeg MB R3M 3E4; (Other Foreign)'04; CCFP; (204)927-2772

TEODORESCU, Cristina; Centre Med Nazareth, 1771 av Dollard, LaSalle QC H8N 1T9; Lucian Blaga (Other Foreign)'99; CCFP; (514)368-5500; Fax. (514)368-0056.

TEODORESCU, I Valentina; Whitby Clinic, 200 Brock St N, Whitby ON L1N 4H5; Timisoara (Romania)'86; CCFP; (905)668-3378; Fax. (905)668-3807.

TEODORESCU, Otilia; Atlantic Med Clinic, PO Box 29119 Rpo Hal Shop Ctre, Halifax NS B3L 4T8; (Romania)'98; CCFP; (902)482-0301; Fax. (902)455-4034.

TEODORINI, Irving K; 276 Linwell Rd, St Catharines ON L2N 1S7; Dublin (Ireland)'65; MB ChB; BAO; (905)934-9492; Fax. (905)934-9499.

TEOFILOV, Ivan K; Dr Nayar & Associates, 125-750 Spadina Cres E, Saskatoon SK S7K 3H3; Varna (Bulgaria)'93; LMCC; Staff, Saskatchewan Medical Association; (306)652-5414; Fax. (306)652-5554.

TEOH, Desiree A; Foothills Med Centre, 1403 29 St NW, Calgary AB T2N 2T9; Qns'03; FRCPC; Anes. Staff, Foothills Medical Centre; (403)944-1430; Fax. (403)944-2425.

TEOH, Johnny C; The Pediclinic, 505-11010 101 St NW, Edmonton AB T5H 4B9; Man'90; BSc; FRCPC; Peds. Att Staff, Royal Alexandra Hospital; Consultant Staff, Glenrose Rehabilitation Hospital; Att Staff, Stollery Children's Hospital; Asst Prof, University of Alberta; Langs: Mandarin; (780)414-6812; Fax. (780)428-0852.

TEOH, Kevin H T; 100-30 Prospect St, Newmarket ON L3Y 3S9; Tor'82; FRCSC; GenSurg; Cardiovasc&ThorSurg. Ac Staff, Hamilton Health Sciences Centre - Hamilton General Hospital; Asst Prof, McMaster University; (905)836-4600; Fax. (905)868-8371.

TEOLIS, Jean-Pierre; Clinique Domus Medica, 409-5601 rue Belanger, Montreal QC H1T 1G3; Mon'65; Langs: Italian; English; (514)256-5011; Fax. (514)325-5687.

TEOLIS, Stefan; GMF Concorde, 300 boul de la Concorde E, Laval QC H7G 2E6; Mon'92; CCFP; Staff ObstGyn, Hopital de la Cite de la santé; Langs: Italian; English; (450)667-5310; Fax. (450)667-5248; teoste20_siril@gouv.qc.ca.

TEPER, Shane H; Queen Square Doctors FHT, 201-366 Main St N, Brampton ON L6V 1P8; Ott'92; CCFP; CCFP(E.M.); Ac Staff, The Scarborough Hospital - General Campus; Ac Staff, Rouge Valley Health System - Centenary Health Centre Site; Ac Staff, William Osler Health System - Brampton Civic Hospital; (905)455-1455; Fax. (905)455-5498.

TEPLINSKY, Avery L; Malvern Med Arts Bldg, 100-1333 Neilson Rd, Scarborough ON M1B 4Y9; Tor'75; CCFP; Ac Staff, Rouge Valley Health System - Centenary Health Centre Site; Court Staff, The Scarborough Hospital - General Campus; Court Staff, The Scarborough Hospital - Birchmount Campus; (416)291-7719; Fax. (416)287-3775.

TEPLITSKY, Mark; 700-55 Eglinton Ave E, Toronto ON M4P 1G8; McG'72; FRCPC; Psy. Ac Staff, Toronto East General Hospital Inc; (416)922-4285; Fax. (416)483-1911.

TEPLITSKY, Yoella; Anishnawbe Health Toronto, 225 Queen St E, Toronto ON M5A 1S4; Mem'08; CCFP; (416)360-0486; Fax. (416)365-1083.

TEPPER, Jamie L; Oshawa Clinic, 117 King St E, Oshawa ON L1H 1B9; McG'93; FRCPC; IntMed; ClinImmunol&Allergy. Langs: English; French; (905)721-3597; Fax. (905)721-6658.

TEPPER, Joshua D; Sanctuary Health Clinic, 25 Charles St E, Toronto ON M4Y 1R9; McM'98; CCFP; (416)922-0628; Fax. (416)922-4961.

TEPPER, Martin L; Canadian Forces Supp Unit HCC, 1745 Alta Vista Dr, Ottawa ON K1A 0K6; Tor'72; FRCPC; CommunMed. Staff, Canadian Forces Health Services Centre; (613)945-6600

TEPPER, Stephen J; Bridgepoint Hosp, 14 Saint Matthews Rd, Toronto ON M4M 2B5; McG'93; CCFP; Staff, Bridgepoint Health Centre; Staff, Sunnybrook Health Sciences Centre; (416)461-8251

TEPPERMAN, Arnold D; The Court, 317-2863 Ellesmere Rd, Scarborough ON M1E 5E9; Tor'68; FRCPC; IntMed (Medical Oncology). Staff, Rouge Valley Health System - Centenary Health Centre Site; (416)282-9333; Fax. (416)282-7078.

TEPPERMAN, Perry S; The Physical Med Clinic, 207-390 Steeles Ave W, Thornhill ON L4J 6X2; Tor'73; BSc; FRCPC; PhysMed&Rehab (Chronic Pain). Court Staff, North York General Hospital - Branson Division; Court Staff, Sunnybrook Health Sciences Centre; Asst Prof Med, University of Toronto; (905)764-8558; Fax. (905)764-0175; teppe@rogers.com.

TER BRUGGE, Karel G; Univ Hlth Network-Toronto Western Hosp, 399 Bathurst St, Toronto ON M5T 2S8; Utrecht (Netherlands)'68; FRCPC; DiagRad (Cerebrovascular Surgery). Head NeuroRadiol, Toronto Western Hospital - University Health Network; Head Interventional NeuroRadiol, The Hospital For Sick Children; Prof Radiol, University of Toronto; Langs: Dutch; (416)603-5266; Fax. (416)603-4257; karel.terbrugge@uhn.on.ca.

TER KEURS, Hendrik; Health Research Innovation Ctr, 68-3280 Hospital Dr NW, Calgary AB T2N 4Z6; Leiden (Netherlands)'72; PhD; FRCPC; IntMed (Cardiology). Staff Cardiol, Foothills Medical Centre; Prof, Health Research Innovation Centre; Prof Med & Physiol, University of Calgary; Langs: French; Dutch; German; (403)220-4525; Fax. (403)210-9739; terkeurs@ucalgary.ca.

TER KUILE, Sonia A; Village Family Health Team, 102-171 East Liberty St, Toronto ON M6K 3P6; McG'09; CCFP; (416)599-8348; Fax. (416)599-2001.

TERADA, Sharon L; 108-359 Riverside Dr, Sudbury ON P3E 1H5; Tor'94; BSc; CCFP; (705)688-1359; Fax. (705)688-1422.

TERBLANCHE, L Marthinus W T; PO Box 1462 Stn A, Prince George BC V2L 4V4; Stellenbosch (South Africa)'93; MB ChB; FRCPC; Anes. (250)301-0327

TERBLANCHE, Ockert C; Royal Alexandra Hosp, 10240 Kingsway NW, Edmonton AB T5H 3V9; Stellenbosch (South Africa)'85; FRCPC; Anes. Staff, Royal Alexandra Hospital; Langs: Afrikaans; (780)735-4010

TERCIER, John A; Kelowna Gen Hosp, 2268 Pandosy St, Kelowna BC V1Y 1T2; Alb'77; FRCPC; EmergMed. Staff, Kelowna General Hospital; (250)862-4495

TERENZI, Kristin A; Thistlewood Prof Centre, 307-8077 Islington Ave, Woodbridge ON L4L 7X7; Wes'91; BSc(Hon.); CCFP; FCFP; Langs: Italian; (905)856-8086; Fax. (905)856-2756.

TEREPA, Mary I; Lenore Centre Med Clinic, 4-123 Lenore Dr, Saskatoon SK S7K 7H9; Man'96; CCFP; Physician, Lenore Drive Medical Clinic; Langs: Ukrainian; (306)242-6700; Fax. (306)242-1168.

TEREPOSKY, Lynne M; 314-3001 Tutt St, Kelowna BC V1Y 2H4; UBC'90; CCFP; Clin Assoc Prof, University of British Columbia; (250)763-0101; Fax. (250)763-0114.

TERESI, James E; Mount Sinai Hosp, 1514-600 University Ave, Toronto ON M5G 1X5; Tor'95; FRCPC; Anes (Acute Pain Management). Staff, Mount Sinai Hospital; Clin Associate, Toronto General Hospital - UHN; Asst Prof, University of Toronto; (416)586-5270; Fax. (416)586-8664.

TERESPOLSKY, Deborah; The Credit Valley Hosp, 2200 Eglinton Ave W, Mississauga ON L5M 2N1; Witwatersrand (South Africa)'84; MB ChB; FCCMG; FRCPC; Peds (Clinical Genetics). Staff Genetics Clinic, The Credit Valley Hospital; (905)813-4104; Fax. (905)813-4347; dterespolsky@cvh.on.ca.

TERLIEN, Paul C; Ingram Family Physicians, 103-149 Ingram St, Duncan BC V9L 1N8; Witwatersrand (South Africa)'79; MB ChB; CCFP; FCFP; Langs: Afrikaans; (250)746-4401; Fax. (250)746-4473.

TERLINGEN, Melissa M; Great Slave Med Clinic, 5005 53 St, Yellowknife NT X1A 1V5; UBC'97; CCFP; (867)920-4211; Fax. (867)873-5912.

TERMANSEN, Paul E; 1350 St. Andrews Ave, North Vancouver BC V7L 3L4; UBC'61; DPsy; FRCPC; Psy. Ac Staff, Lions Gate Hospital; Dir, Lions Gate Institute of Psychotherapy; Med Dir, North Shore Mental Health Centre; Clin Assoc Prof, University of British Columbia; (604)924-3111; Fax. (604)924-3103.

TERNAMIAN, Artin M; Bloor-Jane Med Bldg, 402-2425 Bloor St W, Toronto ON M6S 4W4; Alexandria (Egypt)'72; MB ChB; ObstGyn (Colposcopy). Ac Staff, St Joseph's Health Centre; Ac Staff, Trillium Health Centre - West Toronto; Ac Staff, Toronto Rehabilitation Institute - University Centre; Asst Prof ObstGyn, University of Toronto; Langs: Armenian; Arabic; French; (416)766-1144

TERPSTRA, Collin R; 204B-375 University Ave E, Waterloo ON N2K 3M7; Wes'07; FRCPC; IntMed; ClinImmunol&Allergy. (509)578-1500; Fax. (519)800-3732.

TERRAS, Jean-Claude; Clinique Medicale, 5884 Route 17, Saint-Quentin NB E8A 2J1; Lyon (France)'69; Staff, Hôtel-Dieu St-Joseph de Saint-Quentin; Langs: English; (506)235-2467; Fax. (506)235-3522.

TERRAULT, Daniel; Clin Med La Cite Place du Parc, 900-300 rue Léo-Pariseau, Montreal QC H2X 4B3; Mon'73; Staff, Centre Hospitalier l'Université de Montréal (CHUM) - Hôtel-Dieu; (514)281-1722; Fax. (514)281-6697.

TERRAULT, Stephane; CSSS Les Eskers de l'Abitibi, 622 4e rue O, Amos QC J9T 2S2; Mon'97; Staff, CH Hôtel-Dieu d'Amos; (819)732-3341

TERRETT, Luke A; The Ottawa Hosp-Civic Campus, 1053 Carling Ave, Ottawa ON K1Y 4E9; UBC'06; FRCPC; EmergMed. Staff, The Ottawa Hospital - Civic Campus; (613)789-5555

TERRIAULT, Paul; Hop du Sacre-Coeur de Mtl, 5400 boul Gouin O, Montreal QC H4J 1C5; Sher'82; Cardiol; IntMed. Staff, Hôpital du Sacre-Coeur de Montréal; (514)338-2200

TERRIFF, Blake A; 2460 Naramata Rd RR 1, Naramata BC V0H 1N0; Alb'78; FRCPC; DiagRad. Med Dir, Penticton Regional Hospital; (250)496-5263

TERRY, Jefferson; Hamilton HS-McMaster Site, PO Box 2000 Stn Lcd 1 2N17-1200 Main St W, Hamilton ON L8N 3Z5; Cal'03; PhD; FRCPC; AnatPath (General Pathology). Staff, Hamilton Health Sciences Centre - McMaster Children's Hospital; (905)521-2100

TERRY, Timothy J; Cross Cancer Institute, 11560 University Ave NW, Edmonton AB T6G 1Z2; Dublin (Ireland)'72; MB BS; BAO; FRCR(UK); FRCPC; DiagRad. Staff Radiol, Cross Cancer Institute; Physician, Alberta Health Services; Clin Assoc Prof, University of Alberta; (780)432-8741; Fax. (780)432-8552.

TESCH, Marvin R; Queen Elizabeth Hosp, PO Box 6600 Stn Central 60 Riverside Dr, Charlottetown PE C1A 8T5; UBC'82; FRCPC; GenPath. Staff, Queen Elizabeth Hospital; (902)894-2302

TESCHKE, M Jill; Valley Ridge Family Physicians, 321-11245 Valley Ridge Dr NW, Calgary AB T3B 5V4; Cal'92; (403)282-3806; Fax. (403)284-5601.

TESFAYE, Yoseph; Hop Riviere-des-Prairies, 7070 boul Perras, Montreal QC H1E 1A4; Brussels (Belgium)'79; PhD(Biochem); Staff, Hôpital Riviere des Prairies; Staff, Providence Notre-Dame-de-Lourdes Inc; Langs: Tigrigna; Amharic; French; (514)323-7260 x2484; Fax. (514)328-3539.

TESHIMA, Christopher W; Zeidler Ledcor Centre, 2 28-130 University Campus NW, Edmonton AB T6G 2X8; Tor'03; MSc(ClinEpi); FRCPC; IntMed (Therapeutic Endoscopy); Gastroent. Asst Prof, University of Alberta; (780)248-1673; Fax. (780)492-9416; teshima@ualberta.ca.

TESHIMA, John S; Sunnybrook Hlth Sciences Ctre, FW-2075 Bayview Ave, Toronto ON M4N 3M5; Tor'94; BSc(Hon); MEd; FRCPC; Psy (Adolescent Psychiatry). Staff Psy, Sunnybrook Health Sciences Centre; Staff, The Hospital For Sick Children; Asst Prof, University of Toronto; (416)480-6100 x3077; Fax. (416)480-6818.

TESIOROWSKI, Alicja; 205-125 13th St E, North Vancouver BC V7L 2L3; Wroclaw (Poland)'81; CCFP; Langs: Polish; (604)985-9551; Fax. (604)985-1037.

TESKEY, Jennifer F; Children's Hosp, 840 Sherbrook St, Winnipeg MB R3A 1S1; Cal'00; FRCPC; Peds. Staff, Health Sciences Centre; (204)774-6511

TESKEY, Lindsay S; The Credit Valley Hosp, 2200 Eglinton Ave W, Mississauga ON L5M 2N1; Tor'02; FRCPC; Peds; Nephrol. Staff, The Credit Valley Hospital; (416)813-4120; Fax. (416)813-4128.

TESKEY, Luke M; Walk-In-Clinic, 103-8386 Scott Rd, Surrey BC V3W 3N4; McG'86; Langs: English; French; (604)594-9990

TESKEY, Robert J; Saint John Reg Hosp, PO Box 2100 Stn Main 400 University Ave, Saint John NB E2L 4L2; Ott'84; FRCPC; FRCPC; Cardiol; IntMed (Critical Care Medicine). Staff Interventional Cardiol, Saint John Regional Hospital; Physician, New Brunswick Heart Centre; Langs: Bilingual(French/English); (506)648-6101; Fax. (506)648-6110; rteskey@dal.ca.

TESLER, Janet; The Doctor's Office, 13-205 Marycroft Ave, Woodbridge ON L4L 5X8; Tor'04; CCFP; (905)856-2100; Fax. (905)856-2101; jtesler@mcimed.com.

TESLER-MABE, Carlos; GF-715 12th Ave W, Vancouver BC V5Z 1N1; UBC'95; FRCPC; Psy. Staff, Vancouver General Hospital - Centennial Pavillion; Langs: Spanish; (604)875-4794; Fax. (604)875-5368; ctesler-mabe@forensic.bc.ca.

TESLUK, Raymond P; 1-50 Cavan St PO Box 360 Stn Main, Port Hope ON L1A 3W4; Tor'67; CCFP; FCFP; Coroner, Port Hope Area; Langs: Ukrainian; (905)885-8221; Fax. (905)885-6995; atease@eagle.ca.

TESLUK, W Anne; 1-50 Cavan St PO Box 360 Stn Main, Port Hope ON L1A 3W4; Tor'67; CCFP; FCFP; Ac Staff, Northumberland Hills Hospital; (905)885-8221; Fax. (905)885-6995; atease@eagle.ca.

TESOLIN-LAVOIE, Maude; CHUQ-Hotel-Dieu de Quebec, 11 Cote du Palais, Quebec QC G1R 2J6; Laval'98; FRCPC; DiagRad (Family Medicine). Staff, Centre Hospitalier Universitaire de Québec (CHUQ) - Siege Social; (418)691-5151

TESSARO, Mark J; Victoria General Hosp, 1 Hospital Way, Victoria BC V8Z 6R5; UBC'10; CCFP; Staff, Victoria General Hospital; (250)727-4212

TESSIER, Barbara; Dir de la Sante Publique, 363 rte Cameron, Sainte-Marie QC G6E 3E2; Laval'76; (418)389-1551; Fax. (418)389-1540; barbara_tessier@ssss.gouv.qc.ca.

TESSIER, Claude; CHUQ-Hotel-Dieu de Quebec, 11 Cote Du Palais, Quebec QC G1R 2J6; Laval'67; MedOncol (P.Q.); Hem (P. Q.) (Ovarian Disorders). Staff, Centre Hospitalier Universitaire de Québec (CHUQ) - Siege Social; ac Staff, Hôtel-Dieu de Lévis; assoc Staff, CSSS de Quebec-Sud; (418)691-5280

TESSIER, Daniel; Inst U Geriatrie Sherbrooke, 375 rue Argyll, Sherbrooke QC J1J 3H5; Sher'78; FRCPC; IntMed; GeriatricMed. Staff, Institut Universitaire de Geriatrie de Sherbrooke-Pavillon Argyll; Staff, Centre Hospitalier Universitaire de Sherbrooke-Hopital Fleurimont; Langs: Spanish; English; (819)780-2220 x46254; Fax. (819)829-7145; csssiugs@ssss.gouv.qc.ca.

TESSIER, Dominique; Clinique du Quartier Latin, 905 boul Rene-Levesque E, Montreal QC H2L 5B1; Mon'81; CCFP; FCFP; Staff, Centre Hospitalier l'Université de Montréal (CHUM) - Hôpital Notre-Dame; Langs: Portuguese; Bilingual(English/French); (514)285-5500; Fax. (514)285-2226; dr.dominique.tessier@medisys.ca.

TESSIER, Elisabeth; Clinique Med Pierre-Bertrand, 212-303 boul Pierre-Bertrand, Quebec QC G1M 3L7; Laval'87; ac Staff, CSSS de Quebec-Sud; (418)683-2724; Fax. (418)683-8861.

TESSIER, Francine; BC Women's Hosp & Health Ctre, 1U2-4500 Oak St, Vancouver BC V6H 3N1; Mon'89; FRCSC; ObstGyn (Maternal Fetal Medicine). Staff Maternal Fetal Med, BC Women's Hospital & Health Centre; Clinical Asst Prof, University of British Columbia; Langs: Bilingual(French/English); (604)875-3075; Fax. (604)875-3864.

TESSIER, Genevieve; Cite de la sante de Laval, 1755 boul Rene-Laennec, Laval QC H7M 3L9; Sher'08; Staff, Hopital de la Cite de la santé; (450)668-1010

TESSIER, Genevieve; Hop Maisonneuve-Rosemont, 5415 boul de l'Assomption, Montreal QC H1T 2M4; Mon'98; FRCPC; IntMed; Gastroent. Staff, Hopital Maisonneuve-Rosemont; (514)252-3400

TESSIER, Gilbert; Clinique Radio des Recolletes, 185-1900 boul des Recollets, Trois-Rivieres QC G8Z 4K4; Mon'80; FRCPC; DiagRad. Staff, Centre de santé Cloutier-du-Rivage; (819)373-1603; Fax. (819)373-1604.

TESSIER, Guylaine; Clinique Med Saint-Alexandre, 200-2310 rue Saint-Louis, Gatineau QC J8T 5L7; Sher'88; CCFP; Staff Emerg/Med Prof, Hôpital de Gatineau; Affil Prof, McGill University; Langs: English; French; (819)243-4500; Fax. (819)243-1369; gtessier@medecinefamiliale.com.

TESSIER, J L Pierre F; Royal Ottawa Hlth Care Group, 1145 Carling Ave, Ottawa ON K1Z 7K4; Sher'76; FRCPC; Psy. Staff Psy, Royal Ottawa Mental Health Centre - Royal Ottawa Health Care Group; (613)722-6521 x6366

TESSIER, Jean-Francois; Clinique Med du Boise Langevin, 130-288 rue Pierre-Saindon, Rimouski QC G5L 9A8; Mon'81; (418)724-4672

TESSIER, Jocelyne; Canadian Med Protective Assoc, 875 Carling Ave, Ottawa ON K1S 5P1; Mon'82; FRCSC; Urol. Staff, Canadian Medical Protective Association; (613)725-2000

TESSIER, Jocelyne; Ch Saint-Joseph De La Tuque, 885 boul Ducharme, La Tuque QC G9X 3C1; Laval'83; FRCPC; Psy. Staff, Centre Hospitalier Saint-Joseph de la Turque; (819)523-4581

TESSIER, Johanne; CSSS de Beauce-Etchemin, 1515 17e rue, Saint-Georges QC G5Y 4T8; Laval'93; FRCPC; Anes. Staff, Centre Hospitalier Beauce-Etchemin; (418)228-2031 x5000; Fax. (418)227-9452; johannetessier@cgocable.ca.

TESSIER, Julie L; Kingston Gen Hosp, 76 Stuart St, Kingston ON K7L 2V7; Qns'95; FRCSC; ObstGyn. Staff, Kingston General Hospital; Langs: English; French; (613)548-1327; Fax. (613)548-1330.

TESSIER, Levis; Clinique Med St-Stanislas, 1380 rue Principale, St-Stanislas-D-Cha QC G0X 3E0; Laval'76; (418)328-8417; Fax. (418)328-8446.

TESSIER, Lorraine; Centre Med Jean-Talon, 302-1392 rue Jean-Talon E, Montreal QC H2E 1S4; Mon'73; Staff, Hôpital du Sacre-Coeur de Montréal; Med Consultant, Sigma Assistel; Langs: English; (514)658-4726; Fax. (514)658-5090; tessierdoc@hotmail.com.

TESSIER, Louis; Hopital Jean-Talon, 1385 rue Jean-Talon E, Montreal QC H2E 1S6; Mon'99; FRCPC; Psy. Staff, CSSS du Coeur de l'Isle Hôpital Jean-Talon; (514)495-6767

TESSIER, Michel; Hôpital Laval, 2725 ch Sainte-Foy, Quebec QC G1V 4G5; Laval'90; LMCC; FRCP; BSc(Hon); CSPQ; MSc; FRCPC; NuclearMed. Staff, Hôpital Laval; Langs: Bilingual(French/English); (418)656-4580; Fax. (418)656-4857; michel.tessier@rad.ulaval.ca.

TESSIER, Paule; Centre Med Ste-Foy Inc, 802 av du Chanoine-Scott, Quebec QC G1V 3N4; Laval'86; (418)653-4931; Fax. (418)653-4797.

TESSIER, Pierre C; Hopital Montfort, 713 Montreal Rd, Ottawa ON K1K 0T2; Sher'78; MBA; CCFP; FCFP; Staff, Montfort Hospital; Physician, Equipe de sante Familiale de l'Est d'Ottawa; Langs: Spanish; English; French; (613)746-4621

TESSIER, Pierre; Hop Sacre-Coeur de Montreal, 5400 boul Gouin O, Montreal QC H4J 1C5; Mon'88; Cardiol; IntMed. Staff, Hôpital du Sacre-Coeur de Montréal; (514)338-2340

TESSIER, Sylvie; UMF Nord Lanaudiere, 50 ch du Golf E, St-Charles-Brromee QC J6E 2B4; Mon'87; CCFP; (450)759-3060

TESSIER, Yves; CHUQ-Hop Saint-Sacrement, 1050 ch Sainte-Foy, Quebec QC G1S 4L8; Laval'65; FRCPC; Cardiol. ac Staff Cardiol, Centre Hospitalier Affilié Universitaire de Québec - Hôpital du St-Sacrement; (418)682-7500; Fax. (418)688-9567.

TESSLER, Bernard B; Keary Med Centre, 207-245 Columbia St E, New Westminster BC V3L 3W4; Man'63; DAB; FRCPC; Neur. (604)526-1848; Fax. (604)526-1847.

TESSLER, Karen M; 804-55 Queen St E, Toronto ON M5C 1R6; Man'77; FRCSC; ObstGyn. Ac Staff, St Michael's Hospital; Asst Prof, University of Toronto; (416)860-0160; Fax. (416)860-0811.

TESSLER, Lisa S; Sparling East Med Centre, PO Box 820 402 2 Ave, Fernie BC V0B 1M0; Man'93; BSc; CCFP; (250)423-4442; Fax. (250)423-3424.

TESSLER, Michael J; 5975 av Notre-Dame de Grace, Montreal QC H4A 1M9; Man'81; Anes. Staff, Sir Mortimer B Davis Jewish General; assoc Prof, McGill University; Langs: English; French; (514)488-1519

TETELBAUM, Maria; Family Dental & Healthcare Ctr, 1635 Hyde Park Rd, London ON N6H 5L7; Bucarest (Romania)'95; CCFP; (519)266-3600

TETLEY, Christopher D; Saanich Peninsula Hosp, 2166 Mount Newton Cross Rd, Saanichton BC V8M 2B2; UBC'03; CCFP; CCFP(E.M.); Staff, Saanich Peninsula Hospital; (250)652-3911

TETRAULT, Claire; 301-300 boul Churchill, Greenfield Park QC J4V 2N2; Mon'67; FAAD; Derm. (450)465-1801

TETRAULT, Isabelle; Ctr Hosp Affilie-Enfant-Jesus, 1401 18e rue, Quebec QC G1J 1Z4; Laval'95; FRCPC; MedMicrobiol. Staff, Centre Hospitalier Affilié Universitaire de Québec - Hôpital De L'Enfant Jésus; (418)649-0252 x3202

TETRAULT, Louise-Marie; U of Ottawa Health Services, 300-100 Marie Curie Pvt, Ottawa ON K1N 1A2; Ott'77; Langs: English; French; (613)564-3950; Fax. (613)564-6627.

TETREAULT, Guy; GMF Centre de santé, 3745 rue Georges-Couture, Drummondville QC J2B 7P4; Mon'90; CCFP; ac Staff, Hôpital Sainte-croix; Langs: English; (819)477-2231; Fax. (819)477-1122.

TÉTREAULT, Laurie; Hop Santa Cabrini Ospedale, 5655 reu Sainte-Zotique E, Montreal QC H1T 1P7; Mon'09; CCFP; Staff, Hôpital Santa Cabrini Ospedale; (514)252-6000

TETREAULT, Martine; Service Med Prive, 105-100 boul de Montarville, Boucherville QC J4B 5M4; Mon'95; (450)641-6774; Fax. (450)641-7672.

TETREAULT, Michel F; St Boniface Gen Hosp, 409 Tache Ave, Winnipeg MB R2H 2A6; Mon'76; FRCPC; EmergMed;CCFP; CCFP(E.M.); Exec Dir Clinical Prog & C M O, St Boniface General Hospital; (204)237-2317; Fax. (204)237-0891.

TETREAULT, Patrice; CHUM-Hop Notre-Dame, 1560 rue Sherbrooke E, Montreal QC H2L 4M1; McG'95; FRCSC; OrthSurg. Staff, Centre Hospitalier l'Université de Montréal (CHUM) - Hôpital Notre-Dame; (514)890-8000 x25900

TETREAULT, Pierre L J; CSSS Pierre Boucher, 1333 boul Jacques-Cartier E, Longueuil QC J4M 2A5; Sher'74; AB; Psy. Chef Dept of Psy, Centre Hospitalier Pierre Boucher; (450)468-8401

TETREAULT, Stephane; Hop Charles Lemoyne, 3120 boul Taschereau, Greenfield Park QC J4V 2H1; Mon'88; CCFP; CCFP(E.M.); Staff Emerg, Hopital Charles LeMoyne; (450)466-5050; Fax. (450)671-0884.

TETREAULT, Sylvie; Centre Med Saint-Francois, 200-2125 boul Lemire, Drummondville QC J2B 8N8; Sher'82; ac Staff, Hôpital Sainte-croix; (819)477-6793; Fax. (819)477-6962.

TETREAULT-DESLANDES, Marieve; Clinique de Med Familiale, 6e-2120 rue Sherbrooke E, Montreal QC H2K 1C3; Mon'08; CCFP; (514)527-1958; Fax. (514)527-1649.

TETU, Bernard; CHA-Hopital Saint-Sacrement, 1050 ch Sainte-Foy, Quebec QC G1S 4L8; Laval'79; FRCPC; AnatPath. Staff Path, Centre Hospitalier Universitaire de Québec (CHUQ) - Siege Social; Staff, Centre Hospitalier Affilié Universitaire de Québec - Hôpital du St-Sacrement; Prof, Université Laval; (418)682-7511; bernard.tetu@chuq.qc.ca.

TETU, Christian; 1364 rue Saint-Jacques, L'Ancienne-Lorette QC G2E 2X1; Laval'77; Staff, Centre Hospitalier Universitaire de Quebec-CHUL; (418)872-4904; Fax. (418)877-2981.

TETU, Felix-Andre; 298-2600 boul Laurier, Quebec QC G1V 4T3; Laval'75; PlasSurg (Reconstructive Surgery). ac Staff, Centre Hospitalier Affilié Universitaire de Québec - Hôpital du St-Sacrement; (418)681-1000; Fax. (418)681-0032; docteurtetu@videotron.ca.

TETU, Marie A; Centre Med de l'Hetriere, 201-3520 rue de l'Hetriere, St-Augustin-D-Desm QC G3A 0B4; Laval'77; Consultant, Hôpital Laval; Staff Psy, Centre Hospitalier Universitaire de Québec (CHUQ) - Siege Social; (418)651-3933; Fax. (418)651-0256.

TETZ, Doreen J; 3646D Denman Rd PO Box 80, Denman Island BC V0R 1T0; UBC'83; CCFP; (250)335-2260

TETZ, Rhonda L M; 10-69 Dunlop St, Red Deer AB T4R 2H6; (USA)'96; (403)347-8611

TEVAARWERK, Gerald J M; Jubilee Centre, 1823 Fort St, Victoria BC V8R 1J6; Wes'65; FRCPC; IntMed (Endocrinology); Endocrin&Metab. Langs: German; (250)370-1828; Fax. (250)592-2248; tevaar@telus.net.

TEVENDALE, Suzi; Royal Inland Hosp, 311 Columbia St, Kamloops BC V2C 2T1; UBC'87; Staff, Royal Inland Hospital; (250)314-2734

TEW, William L; London Medical-Dental Bldg, 102-450 Central Ave, London ON N6B 2E8; Wes'53; FACS; FACOG; FRCSC; ObstGyn (Obstetrics). Consultant, South Huron Hospital Association; Aj Prof ObstGyn, University of Western Ontario; (519)672-1421; Fax. (519)672-1426.

TEWFIK, Marc A; MUHC-Royal Victoria Hosp, E4 41-687 av des Pins O, Montreal QC H3A 1A1; McG'03; FRCSC; Otol. Staff, McGill University Health Centre - Royal Victoria Hospital; (514)582-0908; Fax. (514)843-1403.

TEWFIK, Sherif; Fairview Mall, Box 239 334-1800 Sheppard Ave E, North York ON M2J 5A7; Cairo (Egypt)'72; MB ChB; FRCPC; Psy (Developmental Disability). Consultant Psy, North York General Hospital; Langs: Arabic; (416)499-7337; Fax. (416)499-7339.

TEWFIK, Tewfik L; MUHC-Montreal Children's Hosp, B240-2300 rue Tupper, Montreal QC H3H 1P3; Alexandria (Egypt)'69; DS; AB; Otol (Pediatric Otolaryngology). Staff, McGill University Health Centre - Montreal Children's Hospital; Prof, McGill University Health Centre - Montreal General Campus; Staff, McGill University Health Centre - Royal Victoria Hospital; Langs: Arabic; French; (514)412-4304; Fax. (514)412-4342; ted.tewfik@mcgill.ca.

TEWFIK, Yvette-Nelly; CLSC Metro, 1801 boul de Maisonneuve O, Montreal QC H3H 1J9; Mon'04; CCFP; (514)934-0354; Fax. (514)934-3776.

TEWFIK MOUSSA, Laila; Princess Avenue Med Clinic, 45657 Princess Ave, Chilliwack BC V2P 2B7; Alexandria (Egypt)'79; ASAM; MB ChB; FRCPC; CCFP; FCFP; Psy (Addiction Medicine). Langs: Arabic; (604)792-4909; Fax. (604)792-4909.

TEXTOR, Catherine; Northern Health Authority, 908-299 Victoria St, Prince George BC V2L 5B8; UBC'01; CCFP; CCFP(E.M.); Staff, Northern Health Authority; University of British Columbia; (250)563-4706; Fax. (250)563-4549.

THA, Susan P L; Dept of Path, JPN1-910 10th Ave W, Vancouver BC V5Z 1M9; UBC'76; PhD; FRCPC; AnatPath. Staff, Vancouver General Hospital - Centennial Pavillion; Clinical Asst Prof Path, University of British Columbia; Langs: English; French; (604)875-4111 x61179; Fax. (604)264-1979.

THACKER, Kenneth E J; Port Arthur Health Centre Inc, 194 Court St, Thunder Bay ON P7A 4V7; Qns'94; CCFP; Staff, Thunder Bay Regional Health Sciences Centre; (807)345-2332

THACKERAY, Sharron J; Veteran's Affairs Canada, 320-1321 Blanshard St, Victoria BC V8W 3B3; Sask'78; CCFP; FCFP; Staff, Veterans Affairs Canada; (250)363-0134

THACKERAY, Victor T; Worker's Comp Board, 200-1881 Scarth St, Regina SK S4P 4L1; Sask'76; CCFP; FCFP; Physician, Worker's Comp Board of SK; (306)787-4996; vthackeray@ucbsnsk.com.

THAELL, John F; South Health Campus, 4448 Front St SE, Calgary AB T3M 1M4; Alb'71; FACP; FRCPC; Hem (Oncology); IntMed. Ac Staff, Tom Baker Cancer Centre; Staff, South Health Campus; Clin Assoc Prof, University of Calgary; (403)956-2489; Fax. (403)956-2994; jthaell@ucalgary.ca.

THAI, Dine C K; Clinique Med Hochelaga, 9080 rue Hochelaga, Montreal QC H1L 2N9; Mon'10; (514)353-8742

THAI, H M Vincent; University of Alberta Hosp, 8440 112 St NW, Edmonton AB T6G 2B7; (Singapore)'94; MB BS; MRC(UK); CCFP; Dir Palliative Care Prog, University of Alberta Hospital; Asst Prof, University of Alberta; Langs: Mandarin; Cantonese; Hokkin; (780)407-2840; Fax. (780)407-1394.

THAI, Hoang Lan; 103-601 rue Adoncour, Longueuil QC J4G 2M6; Mon'87; FRCPC; IntMed; Gastroent. (450)647-2422

THAI, Minh-Thu; CSSS du Temiscamingue, 22 Notre-Dame N, Longueuil QC J3V 1W8; McG'10; MDCM; CCFP; (819)629-2420

THAI, Nga; Clinique Med Notre-Dame, 504 rue Notre-Dame, Repentigny QC J6A 2T8; Mon'93; CCFP; ac Staff, Centre Hospitalier Pierre le Gardeur; (450)585-1620; Fax. (450)841-3322.

THAI, Quynh-Nhu; Hop Santa Cabrini Ospedale, 5655 rue Saint-Zotique E, Montreal QC H1T 1P7; Mon'93; CCFP; Staff, Hôpital Santa Cabrini Ospedale; (514)252-6546

THAI, Wayne; North Kipling Health Centre, 3-2700 Kipling Ave, Etobicoke ON M9V 4P2; Alb'98; CCFP; FCFP; (416)747-8501

THAIN, Lisa M F; Maple Med Centre, 216-955 Major Mackenzie Dr W, Vaughan ON L6A 4P9; Tor'88; DABR; FRCPC; DiagRad (Body Imaging). Ac Staff, Southlake Regional Health Centre; Court Staff, Mackenzie Richmond Hill Hospital; (905)508-5040; Fax. (289)553-5042.

THAIN, Mary E; Five Counties Children's Ctre, 872 Dutton Rd, Peterborough ON K9H 7G1; Qns'69; FRCPC; Peds. Ac Staff Ped, Peterborough Regional Health Centre - Hospital Drive; Med Dir, Five Counties Children's Centre; (705)748-2221; Fax. (705)748-3526; mthain@fivecounties.on.ca.

THAIN, Michael J; Red Deer Reg Hosp Centre, PO Box 5030 Stn Postal Box Ctr 3942 50 Ave, Red Deer AB T4N 4E7; Alb'70; Ac Staff, Red Deer Regional Hospital Centre; (403)343-4422; Fax. (403)341-5148; mthain@parsonsclinic.ca.

THAIN, Sou K; Kingston Reg Cancer Centre, 25 King St W, Kingston ON K7L 5P9; Rangoon (Burma)'79; MB BS; FRCPC; RadOncol. Physician, Kingston Regional Cancer Centre; Langs: Burmese; Hindi; Tamil; Telugu; (613)544-2630 x4139; sou.thain@krcc.on.ca.

THAKERSEE, Bhavna K; 250 Dundas St E, Waterdown ON L0R 2H4; Natal (South Africa)'97; MB ChB; LMCC; CCFP; Langs: Hindi; Afrikaans; Gujarati; Zulu; (905)690-0962; Fax. (905)690-0963.

THAKKAR, Elizabeth; Shawville Med Clinic, 138-70 Shawville Blvd SE, Calgary AB T2Y 2Z3; Calcutta (India)'60; DCH; LRCP; MRCS; LMCC; MB BS; Langs: Hindi; Malayalam; (403)254-8703; Fax. (403)254-8609.

THAKKAR, Kirit V; Malton Med Group, 22-7330 Goreway Dr, Mississauga ON L4T 4J2; Bombay (India)'75; Langs: Gujarati; Hindi; Punjabi; (905)677-4200; Fax. (905)677-0541.

THAKORE, Siddharth; Alberta Children's Hosp, 2888 Shaganappi Trail NW, Calgary AB T3B 6A8; Cal'06; FRCPC; Peds. Staff, Alberta Children's Hospital; (403)955-7211

THAKORLAL, Harilal; Main & Marine Med Clinic, 235 Marine Dr SE, Vancouver BC V5X 2S4; Otago (New Zealand)'67; Langs: Hindi; Gujarati; (604)322-3011; Fax. (604)322-2827.

THAKRAR, Amar; Hotel Dieu Hosp, B2-166 Brock St, Kingston ON K7L 5G2; Sask'05; FRCPC; IntMed; Cardiol. Staff, Kingston General Hospital; Staff, Hotel-Dieu Hospital; (613)544-3400; Fax. (613)544-7250.

THAKRAR, Mansukhlal L; 216-8338 18 St SE PO Box 10089 Rpo Riverbend, Calgary AB T2C 5E2; Makerere (Uganda)'67; MRCS(Eng); LRCP(Lond); Langs: Gujarati; (403)236-2344; Fax. (403)236-2383.

THAKRAR, Mitesh V; Peter Lougheed Centre, 3500 26 Ave NE, Calgary AB T1Y 6J4; Cal'05; FRCPC; IntMed; Respir. Staff, Foothills Medical Centre; Staff, Peter Lougheed Centre; (403)943-4833; Fax. (403)943-4017.

THAKRAR, Sheena; 5-2120 Regent St, Sudbury ON P3E 3Z9; Sask'99; MCFP; CCFP; FCFP; (705)222-3737; Fax. (705)222-4259.

THAKUR, Aruna K; Health & Counselling Services, MBC 0154-8888 University Dr, Burnaby BC V5A 1S6; Gujarat (India)'64; MB BS; LRCP; MRCS; FRCPC; Psy (Acute & Chronic Pain). Staff, Simon Fraser University; (778)782-3692

THAKUR, Nathan; Midpark Family Med Centre, 100-290 Midpark Way SE, Calgary AB T2X 1P1; Sask'09; CCFP; (403)254-8405

THAKUR, Varsha; The Hosp for Sick Children, 555 University Ave, Toronto ON M5G 1X8; Wes'03; FRCPC; Peds. Staff The Labatt Familiy Health Centre, The Hospital For Sick Children; (416)582-9648

THALABOT, Marie-Claude; CSSS de Manicouagan, 635 boul Jolliet, Baie-Comeau QC G5C 1P1; Laval'05; FRCSC; ObstGyn. Staff, Centre Hospitalier Régional Baie-Comeau; (418)589-3701

THAM, C W Joseph; Dept of Neuropsychiatry, 2-2255 Wesbrook Mall, Vancouver BC V6T 2A1; Alb'96; FRCPC; Psy (Neurology & Psychiatry). Consultant, BC Mental Health & Addiction Service; Clin Researcher, UBC Hospital - Koerner Pavillion; Consultant, George Pearson Centre; University of British Columbia; (604)822-7549

THAM, Edythe B; Stollery Children's Hosp, 4C2-8440 112 St NW, Edmonton AB T6G 2B7; (Australia)'94; Staff, Stollery Children's Hospital; Staff, University of Alberta Hospital; (780)407-3355; Fax. (780)407-3854; etham@ualberta.ca.

THAM, Elizabeth; Etobicoke Urgent Care Clinic, 25 Woodbine Downs Blvd, Etobicoke ON M9W 6N5; Tor'92; BSc; CCFP; FCFP; Staff, William Osler Health System - Etobicoke General Hospital; Langs: Cantonese; (416)741-2273; Fax. (416)741-3542.

THAM, Pooi-Lin; 499 Oxford St E, London ON N5Y 3H8; Tor'74; CCFP; FCFP; Ac Staff, London Health Sciences Centre - Victoria Campus; Ac Staff, Parkwood Hospital - St Joseph's Health Care; Court Staff, St Joseph's Hospital - St Joseph's Health Care; Langs: Cantonese; Mandarin; (519)672-8618

THAMBIRAJ, Joshua R; Westgrove Medicentre, 10232 142 St NW, Edmonton AB T5N 2N8; (780)452-0281; Fax. (780)452-1381.

THAMILVAANAN, Paramanathan; Windsor Reg Hosp-Metropolitan, 1995 Lens Ave, Windsor ON N8W 1L9; Medical Academy of Lativa (Other Foreign)'02; CCFP; CCFP(E.M.); Staff, Windsor Regional Hospital - Metropolitan Site; (519)254-5577

THAMILVAANAN, Shanthi; 1190 Tecumseh Rd E, Windsor ON N8W 1B4; Jaffna (Sri Lanka)'93; MB BS; CCFP; (519)977-8899; Fax. (519)977-8866.

THAMOTHARAM, Niththialuxmy; Finch-Warden Med Walk-In Clin, 6A-3430 Finch Ave E, Scarborough ON M1W 2R5; Colombo (Sri Lanka)'85; MB BS; CCFP; Langs: Sinhalese; Tamil; (416)496-1990; Fax. (416)496-1984.

THAMPI, Nisha; The Hosp for Sick Children, 1447-555 University Ave, Toronto ON M5G 1X8; Tor'06; FRCPC; Peds; InfectDis. Staff, The Hospital For Sick Children; (416)813-7807

THAN, Thi Ngoc T; 201-3025 Hurontario St, Mississauga ON L5A 2H1; Ho Chiminh (Vietnam)'88; CCFP; Langs: Vietnamese; (905)270-8878; Fax. (905)270-2188.

THAN TRONG, An; Hop Santa Cabrini Ospedale, 5655 rue Saint-Zotique E, Montreal QC H1T 1P7; Saigon (Vietnam)'73; FRCSC; GenSurg. Staff, Hôpital Santa Cabrini Ospedale; Staff, Hopital Louis-H Lafontaine; Langs: Vietnamese; English; (514)252-6000

THANAMAYOORAN, Siva; Cape Breton Healhcare Complex, 1482 George St, Sydney NS B1P 1P3; Nsukka (Nigeria)'91; MB BS; FRCPC; IntMed; Nephrol. Staff, Cape Breton Healthcare Complex; (902)567-7276; Fax. (902)567-7277; thanas@cbdha.nshealth.ca.

THANASSOULIS, George; MUHC-Royal Victoria Hosp, 687 av des Pins O, Montreal QC H3A 1A1; Tor'01; FRCPC; IntMed; Cardiol. Staff, McGill University Health Centre - Royal Victoria Hospital; (514)934-1934

THANGAROOPAN, Arulanantham; Rouge Valley-Ajax & Pickering, 580 Harwood Ave S, Ajax ON L1S 2J4; (Sri Lanka)'70; MB BS; MRCPsy(UK); FRCPC; Psy (Anxiety & Mood Disorders). Staff Psy, Rouge Valley Health System - Ajax & Pickering Health Centre Site; Langs: Tamil; (905)683-2320 x3275; Fax. (905)683-8527.

THANGAROOPAN, Arulnmozhy; 105-712 Davis Dr, Newmarket ON L3Y 8C3; Dal'98; FRCPC; IntMed; Cardiol. Staff Cardiologist, Toronto General Hospital - UHN; Langs: Tamil; (905)953-7917; Fax. (905)953-0046.

THANGASAMY, Rajasekaran; Fenton Med Centre, 4-2 Fenton Rd, Markham ON L3R 7B4; Annamalai (India)'94; MB BS; (905)948-9455; Fax. (905)948-0570.

THANGAVELU, Dheshnie; Victoria Hosp, 1200 24th St W, Prince Albert SK S6V 5T4; Staff, Victoria Hospital; (306)765-6000

THANH, Christine; Ctr Hosp Anna-Laberge, 200 boul Brisebois, Chateauguay QC J6K 4W8; Mon'10; Staff, Hôpital Anna-Laberge; (450)699-2425

THANH, Lan Quang; Clinique de Gastroenterologie, 202-895 boul du Seminaire N, St-Jean-Sur-Richel QC J3A 1J2; Saigon (Vietnam)'69; FRCPC; Gastroent (P.Q.). Staff, Hôpital du Haut-Richelieu; Langs: Vietnamese; English; (450)359-7575; Fax. (450)359-7577; thanhqlan@yahoo.com.

THAPAR, Natasha; Univ Hlth Network-Toronto Gen, 3 805-190 Elizabeth St, Toronto ON M5G 2C4; Alb'07; FRCPC; IntMed. Staff, Toronto General Hospital - UHN; (416)978-2645; Fax. (416)340-3179.

THAPAR, Tania; Doctors Plus Med Centre, 310-505 Main St SW, Airdrie AB T4B 3K3; (Other Foreign)'08; CCFP; (403)906-9865

THAPAR, Vijay K; Millboourne Road Med Clinic, 131 Millbourne Road East NW, Edmonton AB T6K 1P6; Delhi (India)'66; MB BS; MRCS; LRCP; CCFP; Court Staff, University of Alberta Hospital; Langs: Urdu; Punjabi; (780)462-4229; Fax. (780)462-3315; vktprofco@aol.com.

THARANI, Yasmin; Fraser Highway Med Clinic, 27109 Fraser Hwy, Aldergrove BC V4W 3R2; Alb'99; (604)856-1717

THARMARATNAM, Thadsha; Mackenzie Richmond Hill Hosp, 10 Trench St, Richmond Hill ON L4C 4Z3; Qns'06; CCFP; CCFP(E.M.); Staff, Mackenzie Richmond Hill Hospital; (905)883-1212

THARMARATNAM, Uma M; Mount Sinai Hosp, 600 University Ave, Toronto ON M5G 1X5; Colombo (Sri Lanka)'76; MB BS; FFARCSI; FRCPC; Anes (Obstetrics Anesthesia). Staff Anes & Pain Med, Mount Sinai Hospital; Langs: Tamil; (416)586-4800 x5270; Fax. (416)586-8664; utharma@hotmail.com.

THARMARATNAM, Yasho; 3-2466 Eglinton Ave E, Scarborough ON M1K 5J8; Colombo (Sri Lanka)'81; MB BS; CCFP; Langs: Tamil; (416)266-7786; Fax. (416)266-2256.

THARSON, Carolyn C; 502-1355 Bank St, Ottawa ON K1H 8K7; Albany (USA)'00; FRCPC; IntMed. (613)738-1584; Fax. (613)738-9097.

THASSANAPAFF, Vatinee; Oshawa Clinic, 117 King St E, Oshawa ON L1H 1B9; Ross University (Dominica)'07; (905)721-6166; Fax. (905)721-6604.

THATTE, Smita V; Royal Ottawa Hlth Care Group, 1145 Carling Ave, Ottawa ON K1Z 7K4; Nagpur (India)'81; FRCPC; Psy (Child & Adolescent Psychiatry). Staff, Royal Ottawa Mental Health Centre - Royal Ottawa Health Care Group; Asst Prof, University of Ottawa; Langs: Marathi; Hindi; (613)722-6521 x6511; Fax. (613)761-3603; sthatte@rogers.com.

THAULI, Gulraj; Norburn Med Associates, 200-4012 Hastings St, Burnaby BC V5C 2H9; UBC'89; Assoc Staff, Burnaby Hospital; (604)299-2677; Fax. (604)298-6656.

THAUVETTE, Daniel; Ctr Hosp Affilie-Enfant-Jesus, 1401 18e rue, Quebec QC G1J 1Z4; Laval'96; FRCSC; GenSurg; Critical Care Medicine. Staff, Centre Hospitalier Affilié Universitaire de Québec - Hôpital De L'Enfant Jésus; (418)649-0252

THAVANATHAN, Mylvaganam J M; Paton Med Centre, 218A-1 Paton St, St. John's NL A1B 4S8; Ceylon (Sri Lanka)'73; MB BS; LRCP; MRCS(Eng); FRCS(Ed); FRCSC; GenSurg. (709)722-9526

THAVENDIRANATHAN, Paaladinesh; Osler Cardiology Associates, 200-3 Conestoga Dr, Brampton ON L6Z 4N5; Tor'03; FRCPC; IntMed; Cardiol. (905)453-6938; Fax. (905)452-1052.

THAVUNDAYIL, Joseph X; Douglas Mental Hlth Univ Inst, 6875 boul Lasalle, Verdun QC H4H 1R3; Kerala (India)'73; MB BS; Staff, Douglas Mental Health University Institute; Asst Prof Psy, McGill University; Langs: Malayalam; Bilingual(French/English); (514)761-6131 x3400; Fax. (514)762-3040; thajos@douglas.mcgill.ca.

THAYAPARAN, Jeyasakthy J; Mackenzie Richmond Hill Hosp, 10 Trench St, Richmond Hill ON L4C 4Z3; Jaffna (Sri Lanka)'94; MD; ABIM; FRCPC; IntMed (Geriatric Medicine). Staff, Mackenzie Richmond Hill Hospital; Langs: Sinhalese; Tamil; (905)883-1212 x3889; Fax. (905)883-2181; jthayaparan@yorkcentral.on.ca.

THAYAPAREN, Yasotha; North Ajax Med Clinic, 475 Westney Rd N, Ajax ON L1T 3H4; (Sri Lanka)'01; CCFP; (905)427-7767; Fax. (905)427-4339.

THE, B L Linda; 502-1110 Finch Ave W, North York ON M3J 2T2; Freiberg (Germany)'70; FRCSC; ObstGyn. Staff, North York General Hospital - Branson Division; Langs: German; Indonesian; (416)630-3614; Fax. (416)630-0377.

THEAKSTON, Karl D; London HSC-University Hosp, PO Box 5339 Stn B 339 Windermere Rd, London ON N6A 5A5; Qns'85; Staff, London Health Sciences Centre - University Hospital; (519)663-3200; Fax. (519)663-3013.

THEAL, Jeremy J T; North York Gen Hosp, 4001 Leslie St, North York ON M2K 1E1; Tor'99; FRCPC; IntMed (Therapeutic Endoscopy); Gastroent. Staff, North York General Hospital; (416)756-6000; Fax. (416)352-1729.

THEAL, Michael D; Regional Cardiology Services, 208-564 Belmont Ave W, Kitchener ON N2M 5N6; Dal'96; FRCPC; IntMed (Interventional Cardiology); Cardiol. Staff, St Mary's General Hospital; Staff, Grand River Hospital - Kitchener/Waterloo Health Centre; (519)576-3099; Fax. (519)576-3112.

THEBAUD, Bernard C F; University of Alberta Hosp, 3A3 13-8440 112 St NW, Edmonton AB T6G 2B7; Louis Pasteur Universite (France)'95; PhD; FRCPC; Peds (Neonatal & Perinatal Medicine). Prof Peds/Staff Med, University of Alberta Hospital; Prof Peds, University of Alberta; Langs: German; French; (780)407-1305; Fax. (780)407-3030.

THEBAULT, Marguerite; CLSC Jean Olivier-Chenier, 29 ch d'Oka, St-Eustache QC J7R 1K6; Sher'79; (450)491-1233; Fax. (450)791-3424.

THEBERGE, Helene; Clinique Med St-Joseph, 841 av Sainte-Therese RR 1, St-Joseph-D-Beauce QC G0S 2V0; Laval'77; (418)397-6891

THEBERGE, Jacques; CSSS de Maskinonge, 2841 rue Lafleche, Saint-Paulin QC J0K 3G0; Laval'88; CCFP; FCFP; Staff, CSSS de Maskinongé; (819)268-2572

THEBERGE, Josee; CSSS de la Vallée de l'Or, 725 6e rue, Val-d'Or QC J9P 3Y1; Sher'84; Psy (Depression). Staff, Centre Hospitalier de Val d'Or; Langs: English; (819)825-5858; Fax. (819)825-7937.

THEBERGE, Lise; 270-65 rue Belvedere N, Sherbrooke QC J1H 4A7; Sher'80; (819)822-4991

THEBERGE, Valerie; CHUQ-Hotel-dieu de Quebec, 11 ch Cote du Palais, Quebec QC G1R 2J6; Sher'04; FRCPC; RadOncol. Staff, Centre Hospitalier Universitaire de Québec (CHUQ) - Siege Social; (418)691-5264; Fax. (418)691-5268.

THEILLIEZ, Boris; CSSS de Gatineau, 116 boul Lionel-Emond, Gatineau QC J8Y 1W7; Jean Monnet Saint-Etienne (Other Foreign)'00; Staff, Hull Hospital; (819)966-6104; Fax. (819)966-6077.

THELLEN, Jean; 701 rue Bourgogne, Mont-Saint-Hilaire QC J3H 3Y4; Laval'70; Langs: Bilingual(French/English); (450)467-0075

THEMAN, Kirsten D; Bloor Med Clinic, 844 Bathurst St, Toronto ON M5R 3G1; Qns'08; CCFP; (416)534-4214; Fax. (416)534-4582.

THEMAN, M Allison; Grandview Heights Med Clinic, 12313 63 Ave NW, Edmonton AB T6H 1R4; Alb'78; CCFP; FCFP; (780)437-1968; Fax. (780)438-4395.

THEMAN, Trevor W; College of Phys & Surgs of AB, 2700-10020 100 St NW, Edmonton AB T5J 0N3; Alb'74; FRCSC; GenSurg. Registrar, College of Physicians & Surgeons of Alberta; Aj Prof Clinical, University of Alberta; (780)969-4970; Fax. (780)420-0651; trevor.theman@cpsa.ab.ca.

THENG, Pei Shih; Family Med Centre, 387 Cedar St, Simcoe ON N3Y 2J2; Mem'02; (519)426-4821

THENGANATT, John; 9N 965-585 University Ave, Toronto ON M5G 2N2; Qns'01; FRCPC; IntMed; Respir. Staff, Toronto General Hospital - UHN; (416)340-4591; Fax. (416)340-3109.

THENGANATT, Lilly; Thorncliffe Med Centre, A6-45 Overlea Blvd, East York ON M4H 1C3; Munich (Germany)'70; CCFP; FCFP; Langs: German; French; Malayalam; (416)696-9836 x333; Fax. (416)696-8080.

THEOBALD, Geoffrey M; The Doctor's Office, 387-25 Peel Centre Dr, Brampton ON L6T 3R5; London (England)'61; MB BS; LRCP; MRCS; (905)793-7077

THEODORE, Gene M; 700 Main St PO Box 1180, Swan River MB R0L 1Z0; Man'64; Staff GP, Swan Valley Health Facilities; (204)734-4504; Fax. (204)734-4504; genetheo@mts.net.

THEODORE, Sylvie; 215-874 boul de l'Universite E, Chicoutimi QC G7H 6B9; Laval'03; FRCPC; Neur. Staff, Complexe hospitalier de la Sagamie; (418)549-9571; Fax. (418)549-8631.

THEODORESCU, Paul; Base Militaire de Valcartier, CP 1000 Bdp Succ Forces, Courcelette QC G0A 4Z0; Sher'09; CCFP; Staff, Centre de Sante Valcartier; (418)844-5000

THEODOROPOULOS, John S; Mount Sinai Hosp, 476C-600 University Ave, Toronto ON M5G 1X5; Qns'99; FRCSC; OrthSurg. Staff, The Hospital For Sick Children; Langs: Greek; French; (416)586-4800; Fax. (416)586-8501.

THEODOROU, Maria E; Quinte Health CC- Belleville, 265 Dundas st E, Belleville ON K8N 5A9; Tor'99; FRCPC; IntMed. Chief IntMed, QHC Belleville General; (613)544-5479; Fax. (613)544-5479.

THEODULE, Jean-Claude; Ctr de Readaptation Lucie-Brun, 2275 av Laurier E, Montreal QC H2H 2N8; Port-au-Prince (Haiti)'71; Staff, Centre de Readaptation Lucie-Bruneau; (514)527-4527; Fax. (514)527-6637.

THEOHAR, Carl; 1016-790 Bay St, Toronto ON M5G 1N8; Tor'62; FICPM; FRCPC; Psy (Psychosomatic Medicine). (416)923-1786

THEORET, Chantal; CHUS-Hop Fleurimont, 3001 12e av N, Sherbrooke QC J1H 5N4; Sher'93; FRCSC; OrthSurg (Pediatric Orthopedics). Staff, Centre Hospitalier Universitaire de Sherbrooke-Hopital Fleurimont; (819)346-1110 x14233; Fax. (819)820-6410.

THEORET, Christina M; Royal University Hosp, 103 Hospital Dr, Saskatoon SK S7N 0W8; Sask'05; FRCPC; DiagRad. Staff, Royal University Hospital; (306)655-2371; Fax. (306)655-2370.

THEORET, Francois A J; 207-1062 Ghislain St, Hawkesbury ON K6A 3B2; Ott'77; CCFP; FCFP; Langs: English; French; (613)632-8547; Fax. (613)632-8549.

THEORET, Gilles; CSSS de Laval, 1755 boul Rene-Laennec, Laval QC H7M 3L9; Mon'77; AnatPath. Staff, Hopital de la Cite de la santé; (450)975-5302; Fax. (450)975-5061.

THEORET, Johanne; CLSC Pt Services Haute-Ville, 55 ch Sainte-Foy, Quebec QC G1R 1S9; Mon'83; CCFP; FCFP; ac Staff, Centre Hospitalier Affilié Universitaire de Québec - Hôpital du St-Sacrement; (418)641-2572; Fax. (418)641-0078.

THEORET, Jonathan; St Paul's Hosp, 1081 Burrard St, Vancouver BC V6Z 1Y6; McG'06; MDCM; EmergMed. Staff, Royal Columbian Hospital; Staff, Providence Health Care - St Paul's Hospital; (604)682-2344

THEORET, Mylene; CHUS-Hop Fleurimont, 3001 12e av N, Sherbrooke QC J1H 5N4; Sher'00; FRCPC; Anes. Staff, Centre Hospitalier Universitaire de Sherbrooke-Hopital Fleurimont; (819)346-1110

THERAPONDOS, Georgios P; Univ Hlth Network-Toronto Gen, NCSB 11 12-200 Elizabeth St, Toronto ON M5G 2C4; Edinburgh (Scotland)'92; Dir Clinical Trials Multiorgan Transplant Prog/Staff, Toronto General Hospital - UHN; (416)340-4248; Fax. (416)340-4041.

THERASSE, Eric; CHUM-Hotel-Dieu, 3840 rue Saint-Urbain, Montreal QC H2W 1T8; Laval'86; FRCPC; DiagRad (Angioradiology). Staff, Centre Hospitalier l'Université de Montréal (CHUM) - Hôtel-Dieu; (514)890-8150; Fax. (514)412-7193; eric.therasse.chum@ssss.gouv.qc.ca.

THERIAULT, A Nathanaelle; Agence de la Capitale National, 2400 av d'Estimauville, Quebec QC G1E 7G9; Laval'02; MSc; FRCPC; CommunMed (Infectious Diseases); Public Health & Preventive Med. Langs: Bilingual(French/English); (418)666-7000 x393; Fax. (418)666-2776.

THERIAULT, Anne; Ctre Univ de Sante McGill, 304-2155 rue Guy, Montreal QC H3H 2R9; Mon'86; Staff Employee Health Office, McGill University Health Centre - Montreal General Campus; Médecin, Centre Universitaire de Sante McGill; (514)934-1934 x42385; anne.theriault@muhc.mcgill.ca.

THERIAULT, Benoit; Centre Hosp Hotel-Dieu d'Amos, 622 4e rue, Amos QC J9T 2S2; Laval'05; FRCPC; IntMed. Staff, CH Hôtel-Dieu d'Amos; (819)732-3341

THERIAULT, Catherine; CHUQ-Hotel-Dieu de Quebec, 11 ch Cote Du Palais, Quebec QC G1R 2J6; Laval'92; FRCPC; AnatPath (Hematology Pathology). Staff, Centre Hospitalier Universitaire de Québec (CHUQ) - Siege Social; (418)691-5233; Fax. (418)691-5226.

THERIAULT, Claude; Clinique St-Barnabe, 202-176 av Rouleau, Rimouski QC G5L 8W1; Sher'76; FRCSC; PlasSurg. (418)722-4433; Fax. (418)722-4995.

THERIAULT, Claudine; CHUQ-St-Francois d'Assise, 10 rue de l'Espinay, Quebec QC G1L 3L5; Sher'94; FRCPC; IntMed (Echocardiography); Cardiol. Staff, Centre Hospitalier Universitaire De Québec - Pavillon De St-françois-d'assise; (418)525-4319; Fax. (418)525-4444.

THERIAULT, Cynthia H; Dr Everett Chalmers Hosp, PO Box 9000 Stn A 700 Priestman St, Fredericton NB E3B 5N5; Dal'02; FRCPC; DiagRad. Staff, The Moncton Hospital; Staff River Valley Health, Dr Everett Chalmers Regional Hospital; (506)452-5136

THERIAULT, Denise; CSST Chaudiere-Appalaches, 835 rue de la Concorde, Levis QC G6W 7P7; Laval'76; ac Staff, Hôtel-Dieu de Lévis; Staff, CSST-Chaudiere-Appalaches; (418)839-2500

THERIAULT, Dominique; Les Assoc de Gynecologues, 1299 boul Concorde E, Laval QC H7N 5T4; Mon'89; ObstGyn (Echography). Staff ObstGyn, Hopital de la Cite de la santé; (450)668-3250; Fax. (450)668-7595.

THERIAULT, Eric; 4037 ch St-Paul, Laterriere QC G7N 1C3; Sher'97; CCFP.

THERIAULT, Gilles; MUHC-Montreal Chest Institute, 3650 rue Saint-Urbain, Montreal QC H2X 2P4; Laval'66; CommunMed (P.Q.) (Industrial Occupational Medicine). Staff Commun Health, McGill University Health Centre - Montreal General Campus; Staff, Hopital Maisonneuve-Rosemont; Staff, McGill University Health Centre - Montreal Chest Institute; Prof Occup Health, McGill University; Langs: English; (514)934-1934 x32622; Fax. (514)843-2070.

THERIAULT, Guy; Clinique Fam d'Arthabaska, 2-39 rue Laurier E, Victoriaville QC G6P 6P6; Sher'81; (819)357-9322

THERIAULT, Guylene; Clinique Med Saint-Alexandre, 2310 rue Saint-Louis, Gatineau QC J8T 5L7; Mon'94; CCFP; Staff, Hôpital de Gatineau; Médecin, Unite de Medicine Familiale; (819)966-6171

THERIAULT, J Francois A; South Richter Prof Bldg, 207-3330 Richter St, Kelowna BC V1W 4V5; Alb'87; BSc; FRCSC; Ophth (Lacrimal). Staff Ophth, Kelowna General Hospital; Clinical Asst Prof Visual Science & Ophth, University of British Columbia; Langs: Bilingual(English/French); (250)868-3866; Fax. (250)868-3858.

THERIAULT, J Germain-Michel; Clinique Med Saint-Louis, 220-3165 ch Saint-Louis, Quebec QC G1W 4R4; Laval'72; Médecin, Groupe Sante Medisys; adj Prof Physical Educ, Université Laval; Langs: English; (418)653-1970; Fax. (418)653-9956.

THERIAULT, Josee; Sudbury Reg Hosp-Laurentian, 41 Ramsey Lake Rd, Sudbury ON P3E 5J1; Mon'97; FRCPC; IntMed; Critical Care Medicine. Staff, Health Sciences North-Laurentian Site; Langs: Bilingual(French/English); (705)523-7100; josee.theriault@sympatico.ca.

THERIAULT, Julie F; Ctr Hosp de l'Universite Laval, 2705 boul Laurier, Quebec QC G1V 4G2; Laval'98; CCFP; Staff, Centre Hospitalier Universitaire de Quebec-CHUL; (418)654-2255; Fax. (418)654-2757.

THERIAULT, Julie J; Clin Med Pierre-Bertrand, 212-303 boul Pierre-Bertrand, Quebec QC G1M 3L7; Laval'98; CCFP; Staff, Centre Hospitalier Universitaire de Quebec-CHUL; (418)683-2724; Fax. (418)683-8861.

THERIAULT, Lise; CLSC Haute-Ville, 55 ch Sainte-Foy, Quebec QC G1R 1S9; Laval'03; Staff, CSSS de Kamouraska; Staff, CSSS Haute-Ville; (418)641-2572; lise.theriault@irdpq.qc.ca.

THERIAULT, Louis F J; 203-140 Champlain St, Dieppe NB E1A 1N8; Laval'88; FRCPC; Psy (Mood Disorders). Dir Psychiatric Prog, Dr Georges-L-Dumont University Hospital Centre; Langs: Bilingual(French/English); (506)856-5926; Fax. (506)855-2324; louist@rrsb.nb.ca.

THERIAULT, Luce; 56 av Bateman, Edmundston NB E3V 4A4; Sher'06; CCFP; Staff, Hôpital regional d'Edmundston; (506)735-4437; Fax. (506)739-7265.

THERIAULT, Lyne; Clinique Med des Bois-Francs, 101 rue Demers E, Princeville QC G6L 4E8; Sher'84; LMCC; ac Staff, Hotel-Dieu d'Arthabaska; Langs: English; (819)364-2150; Fax. (819)364-6057.

THERIAULT, M Y Diane; Dartmouth Med Centre, 206-44 Portland St, Dartmouth NS B2Y 1H3; Dal'83; FRCPC; IntMed (Osteoporosis); Rheum. Langs: English; French; (902)407-4053; Fax. (902)407-4575.

THERIAULT, Marie-Claude; CSSS de la Baie-des-Chaleurs, RR 2 419 boul Perron, Maria QC G0C 1Y0; Sher'94; FRCPC; DiagRad. (418)759-3443 x2159; Fax. (418)759-3151.

THERIAULT, Marie-Noel; CSSS du Lac-Temiscamingue, 22 rue Notre-Dame N, Ville-Marie QC J9V 1W8; Sher'00; Staff, CSSS du Témiscamingue; (819)629-2420; marie-noel_theriault@ssss.gouv.qc.ca.

THERIAULT, Martine; Clinique Med Nepisiguit, 950 Picot Ave, Bathurst NB E2A 4Z9; Sher'10; CCFP; (506)546-6696

THERIAULT, Maryse; Clinique Med Nepisiguit, 950 ave Picot, Bathurst NB E2A 4Z9; Sher'08; CCFP; (506)546-6696; Fax. (506)545-7723.

THERIAULT, Melanie; MUHC-Montreal Gen Hosp, 1650 av Cedar, Montreal QC H3G 1A4; Mon'03; FRCPC; DiagRad. Staff, Hôpital du Sacre-Coeur de Montréal; Staff, McGill University Health Centre - Montreal General Campus; (514)934-1934

THERIAULT, Mimi; Hotel-Dieu de Levis, 143 rue Wolfe, Levis QC G6V 3Z1; Laval'07; FRCPC; Derm. Staff, Hôtel-Dieu de Lévis; (418)835-7121

THERIAULT, Nancy; Clinique Gyn de Trois-Rivieres, 2237 7e av, Trois-Rivieres QC G8Z 3E2; Laval'94; FRCSC; ObstGyn. (819)379-5350

THERIAULT, Nicole; 8228 rue Sainte-Claire, Montreal QC H1L 1W7; Sher'79; (514)354-2949

THERIAULT, Normand; Centre Med St-Redempteur, 210-600 Rte 116, Saint-Nicolas QC G7A 4X8; Laval'83; (418)831-4455; Fax. (418)831-7967; normand.theriault@gmf.gouv.qc.ca.

THERIAULT, P Scott; East Coast Forensic Psy Hosp, 88 Gloria McCluskey Ave, Dartmouth NS B3B 2B8; Dal'86; FRCPC; Psy (Forensic Psychiatry). Staff, The East Coast Forensic Psychiatry Hospital; Assoc Prof, Dalhousie University; (902)460-7300 x7334; Fax. (902)460-7337.

THERIAULT, Patrick; Citizenship & Immigration Cana, 219 av Laurier O, Ottawa ON K1A 1L1; Laval'90; CCFP; Staff, Citizenship & Immigration Canada; Langs: Spanish; (613)941-8336; Fax. (613)941-2179; Patrick.theriault@cicoge.ca.

THERIAULT, Pierre; CLSC Malauze, GD 107 132 Rte O, Saint-Omer QC G0C 2Z0; Laval'79; Médecin, CLSC de Malauze; (418)364-7064

THERIAULT, Serge; CMF Berthier, CP 1230 788 rue Gilles-Villeneuve, Berthierville QC J0K 1A0; Mon'79; (450)836-4212; Fax. (450)836-4814.

THERIAULT, Stephane; CSSS de Rivière-du-Loup, 75 rue Saint-Henri, Riviere-du-Loup QC G5R 2A4; Sher'92; FRCPC; Anes (Cardiology). Staff, Centre Hospitalier Regional de Sept-Iles; Staff, Centre Hospitalier Regional du Grand-Portage; (418)868-1010 x2923

THERIAULT, Stephane; Ctr Hosp Laurentien, 234 rue Saint-Vincent, Ste-Agathe-Des-Mts QC J8C 2B8; Mon'94; Staff, Centre Hospitalier Laurentien; (819)324-4000; Fax. (819)324-4010.

THERIAULT-VIGER, Nicolas; 200-2924 boul Taschereau, Greenfield Park QC J4V 2G8; Mon'92; Psy. (450)466-8486

THERIEN, Genevieve; CHAQ-Hop de l'Enfant-Jesus, 1401 18e rue, Quebec QC G1J 1Z4; Laval'02; FRCPC; Derm (Esthetic Dermatology). Staff, Centre Hospitalier Affilié Universitaire de Québec - Hôpital De L'Enfant Jésus; Staff, Clinique de Vinci; Langs: Bilingual(French/English); (418)649-5520; Fax. (418)649-5527.

THERIEN, Manon; CSSS de la Haute-Yamaska, 205 boul Leclerc O, Granby QC J2G 1T7; Sher'89; FRCPC; Psy. Staff, Centre Hospitalier de Granby; (450)375-8001; Fax. (450)372-2235.

THERIEN, Serge; Clinique sante Jacques-Cartier, 200-1815 rue King O, Sherbrooke QC J1J 2E3; Sher'71; FRCPC; Peds (Public Health). Langs: English; (819)565-7774; Fax. (819)565-7780.

THERMANN, Angela G; BC Cancer Agency, 4481-600 10 Ave W, Vancouver BC V5Z 4E6; Witwatersrand (South Africa)'88; MB ChB; Staff GPO RadOncol, BC Cancer Agency Vancouver Centre; Staff, Richmond Hospital; Staff, Stein Medical Clinic; Langs: German; Afrikaans; (604)877-6000 x3241

THERON, Jan J H; 2A-1743 Comox Ave, Comox BC V9M 3M2; Orange Free State (South Africa)'85; MB ChB; MMed; FRCPC; Peds. Langs: Afrikaans; (250)941-0042

THERON, Karina; The Maple Tree Clinic, 1181 6th Ave NE, Salmon Arm BC V1E 2S5; Pretoria (South Africa)'93; MB ChB; Staff, Shuswap Lake General Hospital; Langs: Afrikaans; (250)832-9361; Fax. (250)833-4781.

THERON, Paul S; Mission Hills Med Clinic, 240-32530 Lougheed Hwy, Mission BC V2V 1A5; (604)820-7751

THERON, Ronelle; University of Alberta Hosp, 8440 112 St NW, Edmonton AB T6G 2B7; (South Africa)'02; MB ChB; Staff, University of Alberta Hospital; (780)407-8822

THEROUX, Julie; Ctre Hosp de Lachine, 650 16e av, Lachine QC H8S 3N5; Mon'03; Staff, CSSS de Dorval-Lachine-Lasalle; (514)637-2351; therouxj@aol.com.

THEROUX, Marie-Claude; Clinique Med l'Envolee, 5025 rue de Salaberry, Montreal QC H4J 1J1; Mon'89; ac Staff, Hôpital du Sacre-Coeur de Montréal; (514)331-2323; Fax. (514)333-8534.

THEROUX, Pierre; Institut de Cardiologie de Mtl, 5000 rue Belanger, Montreal QC H1T 1C8; Mon'67; FACC; Cardiol. ac Staff, Institut de Cardiologie de Montréal; Prof Med, Universite de Montreal; Langs: English; (514)376-3330 x3616; Fax. (514)376-1076.

THERRIAULT, Natalie; Hull Hospital, 116 boul Lionel-Emond, Gatineau QC J8Y 1W7; Mon'90; BSc; FRCSC; OrthSurg (Osteoporosis). Staff, CSSS de Gatineau; Staff, Hull Hospital; Langs: Bilingual(French/English); (819)595-6000

THERRIEN, Andre; Ctr de Sante Vallee-Gatineau, 309 boul desjardins, Maniwaki QC J9E 2E7; McG'79; Staff, CSSS de la Vallée de la Gatineau; (819)449-2300; Fax. (819)449-6137.

THERRIEN, Anne-Marie; CSSSG-Hop De Gatineau, 101-500 boul de l'Hopital, Gatineau QC J8V 2P5; Ott'04; Staff, Hôpital de Gatineau; Langs: English; (819)561-8171; amtherrien@hotmail.com.

THERRIEN, Arawn A A; Stone's Mill Family Hlth Ctre, 25 Mill St, Gananoque ON K7G 2L5; Dal'01; CCFP; Physician, Stone's Mill Family Health Centre; Langs: Portuguese; (613)382-3974; Fax. (613)382-4417.

THERRIEN, Elyse; CSSS de Laval, 1755 boul Rene-Laennec, Laval QC H7M 3L9; Mon'03; Peds. Staff, Hopital de la Cite de la santé; (450)668-1010

THERRIEN, Gaston J E; 96 rue du Mont-Marie, Levis QC G6V 1W8; Mon'76; (418)838-9804; Fax. (418)838-3996.

THERRIEN, Ghislaine; Clinique Med Ste-Adele, 1150 rue du Bourg-Joli, Sainte-Adele QC J8B 1W8; Mon'77; (450)229-6633; Fax. (450)229-5765.

THERRIEN, Guenievre; Burnaby Centre for Mental Heal, 3405 Willingdon Ave, Burnaby BC V5G 3H3; Mon'08; CCFP; (604)675-3950

THERRIEN, Guy; Centre Hosp St-Eustache, 520 boul Arthur-Sauve, Saint-Eustache QC J7R 5B1; Mon'99; CCFP; Staff, Hôpital de réadaptation Villa Medica; Staff, Hôpital de Saint-Eustache; (514)288-8201; Fax. (514)288-9355.

THERRIEN, J Jean A G; 305-1062 Ghislain St, Hawkesbury ON K6A 3B2; Mon'82; Staff, Hawkesbury & District General Hospital; Langs: Bilingual(French/English); (613)632-2779; Fax. (613)632-4011; therrien.jean@gmail.com.

THERRIEN, Jocelyne; Clinique Medi-Val, 100-408 rue Jeanne-Mance, Salaber-de-Valleyf QC J6T 4G1; Mon'82; Staff, Centre Hospitalier Régional du Suroît; (450)370-3507; Fax. (450)370-3395.

THERRIEN, Joelle; CSSS de Trois-Rivières, 1991 boul du Carmel, Trois-Rivieres QC G8Z 3R9; Mon'08; Staff, CSSS de Trois-Rivières; (819)697-3333

THERRIEN, Judith; SMBD Jewish Gen Hosp, 3755 ch Cote-Sainte-Catherine, Montreal QC H3T 1E2; McG'91; Cardiol; IntMed. Staff, Sir Mortimer B Davis Jewish General; (514)340-8222; Fax. (514)340-7534.

THERRIEN, Marc; CSSSG-Hop de Hull, 116 Boul Lionel-Emond, Gatineau QC J8Y 1W7; Sher'94; Electroenceph (P.Q.); Neur. Staff, Hull Hospital; (819)595-6212; Fax. (819)595-6213.

THERRIEN, Michel; Clinique Med Lemoyne, 203-2499 rue Saint-Georges, Lemoyne QC J4R 2T4; Mon'69; Staff, Hopital Charles LeMoyne; (450)672-6652; Fax. (450)672-6653.

THERRIEN, Michel; Clinique MD-Plus, 60 ch du Golf E, Joliette QC J6E 2B4; Mon'87; Staff, Centre Hospitalier Régional de Lanaudière; (450)759-9995

THERRIEN, Mylene; CSSS de la Cote-de-Gaspe, 215 boul de York O, Gaspe QC G4X 2W2; Laval'10; CCFP; Staff, Centre Hospitalier de Gaspe; (418)368-3301

THERRIEN, Rene; Clinique Med St-Louis, 220-3165 ch Saint-Louis, Quebec QC G1W 4R4; Laval'77; Staff, Centre Hospitalier Universitaire de Québec (CHUQ) - Siege Social; (418)653-1970

THERRIEN, Sylvie; Commission Sante Securite Trav, 2-2710 rue Bachand, Saint-Hyacinthe QC J2S 8B6; Laval'75; Consultant, Commission Sante Securite Travail; Langs: Bilingual(French/English); (450)771-3900 x3768; Fax. (450)771-3520; sylvie.therrien@csst.qc.ca.

THESS, Bernard A J; Portage Clinic Satellite Offic, 59 Royal Rd N, Portage la Prairie MB R1N 1T9.

THEVATHASAN, Kayalvili; Guelph Gen Hosp, 115 Delhi St, Guelph ON N1E 4J4; Jaffna (Sri Lanka)'93; Staff, Guelph General Hospital; Langs: Tamil; (519)822-5350

THIAB, Ali S; Portage Med Clinic, 402-5400 Portage Rd, Niagara Falls ON L2G 5X7; Baghad (Iraq)'96; MB ChB; CCFP; Langs: Arabic.

THIAGARAJAH, Arjuna; 815-4438 10 Ave W, Vancouver BC V6R 4R8; Alb'01; Staff, Calgary Trail Medicentres.

THIARA, Parminder K; 282-220 4 Ave SE, Calgary AB T2G 4X3; Alb'01; FRCPC; CommunMed;CCFP; Staff, Foothills Medical Centre; Staff, Health Canada; (403)861-8447; parminder_thiara@hc-sc.gc.ca.

THIARA, Rajpal S; Glenrose Rehab Hosp, 1226-10230 111 Ave NW, Edmonton AB T5G 0B7; Qns'01; FRCPC; PhysMed&Rehab (Neurology). Staff, Glenrose Rehabilitation Hospital; (780)735-8208; Fax. (780)735-6018.

THIBAUDEAU, Johanne; Polyclin Med Pierre LeGardeur, 300-1000 montee des Pionniers, Terrebonne QC J6V 1S8; Mon'82; Staff, Hopital de la Cite de la santé; Staff, Polyclinique Medicale Pierre-Le-Gardeur; Langs: English; (450)657-1313

THIBAUDEAU, Pascale; Queen Elizabeth II HSC, 1796 Summer St, Halifax NS B3H 3A7; McG'07; MDCM; OrthSurg. Staff, Queen Elizabeth II Health Sciences Centre - Halifax Infirmary Site; (902)473-7337; Fax. (902)473-7370.

THIBAUDEAU, Sylvain; CLSC de la Haute-Yamaska, 294 rue Deragon, Granby QC J2G 5J5; Sher'90; Staff, Centre Hospitalier de Granby; (450)375-8000 x6517; Fax. (450)375-1304.

THIBAUDEAU, Sylvie; CLSC de Paspebiac, CP 7000 273 boul Gerard-D-Levesque, Paspebiac QC G0C 2K0; Mon'83; Médecin, CLSC de Paspebiac; Langs: English; (418)752-2572 x238

THIBAULT, A Alfred; Hop Louis-H Lafontaine, 7401 rue Hochelaga, Montreal QC H1N 3M5; Mon'64; FRCPC; Psy. Staff, Hopital Louis-H Lafontaine; Staff, Hôpital du Sacre-Coeur de Montréal; (514)251-4000

THIBAULT, Anne; CLSC Lamater, 1317 boul des Seigneurs, Terrebonne QC J6W 5B1; Mon'92; Médecin, CLSC Lamater; (450)471-2881 x4056; Fax. (450)471-6763.

THIBAULT, Annie; Clinique Med du Sud-Ouest, 4475 rue Bannantyne, Verdun QC H4G 1E2; Mon'09; CCFP; (514)765-3600

THIBAULT, Audrey; Clinique Med Familiale Chandle, CP 788 60B boul Rene-Levesque E, Chandler QC G0C 1K0; Sher'08; (418)689-3344

THIBAULT, Bernard; Institut de Cardiologie de Mtl, 5000 rue Belanger, Montreal QC H1T 1C8; Mon'87; Cardiol; IntMed. Staff, Institut de Cardiologie de Montréal; (514)376-3330; Fax. (514)593-2161.

THIBAULT, Caroline; Ctr Hosp de LaSalle, 8585 Tsse Champlain, LaSalle QC H8P 1C1; Sher'99; CCFP; Staff Emerg, Centre Hospitalier de LaSalle; Langs: English; French; (514)362-8000; carolinethibault80@hotmail.com.

THIBAULT, Claude; CHUQ-St-Francoise d'Assise, B1 520-10 rue de l'Espinay, Quebec QC G1L 3L5; Mon'89; FRCSC; GenSurg (Colon & Rectal Surgery). Staff, Centre Hospitalier Universitaire De Québec - Pavillon De St-françois-d'assise; adj Prof/Dir Surgery Program, Université Laval; Langs: Bilingual(French/English); (418)525-4444 x52619; Fax. (418)525-4162.

THIBAULT, Elise; CSSS de Laval, 111-1755 boul Rene-Laennec, Laval QC H7M 3L9; Mon'00; FRCPC; GenSurg (Varicose Veins); VascSurg. Staff, Hopital de la Cite de la santé; Staff, Poly Clinique Medicale Concorde; Langs: Bilingual(French/English); (450)668-1010; elisethibault@hotmail.com.

THIBAULT, Emilie; CLSC de Windsor, 23 rue Ambroise-Dearden, Windsor QC J1S 1G8; Sher'08; Staff, Carrefour de Sante et Services Sociaux-Pavillon St-Louis; (819)845-2751

THIBAULT, Ginette; CSSS d'Argenteuil, 145 av de la Providence, Lachute QC J8H 4C7; Mon'72; Staff, Centre Hospitalier d'Argenteuil; Langs: English; (450)562-3761; Fax. (450)566-3311.

THIBAULT, Isabelle; Sunnybrook Hlth Sciences Ctre, 2075 Bayview Ave, Toronto ON M4N 3M5; Laval'07; RadOncol. Staff, Sunnybrook Health Sciences Centre; (416)480-6100

THIBAULT, Jean; Comm Sante Securite Travail, 901 boul Talbot, Chicoutimi QC G7H 6N7; Laval'58; Médecin, Commission Sante Securite Travail; (418)696-5200

THIBAULT, Julie; CSSS Drummond-Hop Sainte-Croix, 570 rue Heriot, Drummondville QC J2B 1C1; Sher'03; Staff, Hôpital Sainte-croix; (819)478-6464

THIBAULT, Julie; Centre Hosp Honore-Mercier, 2750 boul Laframboise, Saint-Hyacinthe QC J2S 4Y8; McG'99; CCFP; CCFP(E.M.); Staff, Centre Hospitalier Honore-Mercier; (450)771-3333

THIBAULT, Julie; 103-1691 boul Louis-Frechette, Nicolet QC J3T 1Z6; Laval'92; Staff, Hôpital de Christ-Roi; (819)293-2022; Fax. (819)293-2024.

THIBAULT, Louis; CSSS Pierre Boucher, 1333 boul Jacques-Cartier E, Longueuil QC J4M 2A5; Sher'87; Electroenceph (P.Q.); Neur. Staff, Centre Hospitalier Pierre Boucher; (450)468-8111

THIBAULT, Louise; Dr Georges-L Dumont Reg Hosp, 330 av Universite, Moncton NB E1C 2Z3; Sher'80; FRCPC; MedMicrobiol. Ac Staff Med Microbiol, Dr Georges-L-Dumont University Hospital Centre; (506)862-4140; Fax. (506)862-4827.

THIBAULT, Louise; Clin Med de la Rose des Ventes, 3498 boul Sainte-Rose, Laval QC H7P 4K7; Mon'88; Médecin, Clinique Med la Rose des Vents; (450)624-1844; Fax. (450)624-1866.

THIBAULT, Manon; Ctr Hosp Affilie-Enfant-Jesus, 1401 18e rue, Quebec QC G1J 1Z4; Laval'77; FRCPC; Neur (Epilepsy); Electroenceph (P.Q.). Staff, Centre Hospitalier Affilié Universitaire de Québec - Hôpital De L'Enfant Jésus; Clin Prof, Université Laval; Langs: Bilingual(French/English); (418)649-5882; Fax. (418)649-5915.

THIBAULT, Marc; CSSS de la Baie-des-Chaleurs, RR 2 419 boul Perron, Maria QC G0C 1Y0; Laval'92; Staff, CSSS de la Baie-des-Chaleurs; (418)759-3443

THIBAULT, Marcel; Centre Medical Fusey, 101-200 rue Fusey, Trois-Rivieres QC G8T 2V8; Laval'73; Staff GP, Hôpital de la Malbaie; (819)378-7811

THIBAULT, Marie-Eve; Clin du Perinatalite Trois-Riv, 100-4900 boul des Forges, Trois-Rivieres QC G8Y 1X1; Sher'05; CCFP; Staff, CSSS de Trois-Rivières; (819)697-3333; Fax. (819)373-0765.

THIBAULT, Marie-Frederique; CHUM-Hop Notre-Dame, 1560 rue Sherbrooke E, Montreal QC H2L 4M1; Mon'98; Staff, Centre Hospitalier l'Université de Montréal (CHUM) - Hôpital Notre-Dame; Médecin, CLSC Montcalm; (514)890-8000 x26727; marie-frederique.thibault@ssss.gouv.qc.ca.

THIBAULT, Marie-Josee; CSSS de Sept-Iles, 45 rue Pere-Divet, Sept-Iles QC G4R 3N7; Mon'88; FRCPC; Derm. Staff, Centre Hospitalier Regional de Sept-Iles; (418)962-9761; Fax. (418)962-1858.

THIBAULT, Maurice; Hop Maisonneuve-Rosemont, 5415 boul de l'Assomption, Montreal QC H1T 2M4; Mon'66; Chief Geriatric Servs, Hopital Maisonneuve-Rosemont; Clin Teacher Family Med, Universite de Montreal; (514)252-3869; Fax. (514)252-3573; maurice.thibault@umontreal.ca.

THIBAULT, Nicolas; CFB Edmonton-1 FD Ambulance, CP 10500 succ Forces 162 Churchill Blvd, Edmonton AB T5J 4J5; Mon'98; CCFP; Staff, CFB Health Services Centre; Langs: Spanish; English; (780)973-4011

THIBAULT, Nicole; Jardins du Haut-Saint-Laurent, 4770 rue Saint-Felix, St-Augustin-D-Desm QC G3A 0K1; Laval'84; (418)872-4936; Fax. (418)872-4245.

THIBAULT, Nicole; Clinique Med Solumed, 1-8230 Boul Taschereau, Brossard QC J4X 1C2; Mon'85; LMCC; Langs: English; (450)466-0003; Fax. (450)466-0022.

THIBAULT, Pierre-Marc; Hosp du Centre la Mauricie, 50 119e rue, Shawinigan QC G9P 5K1; Laval'09; Staff, Centre Hospitalier du Centre la Mauricie; (819)536-7500

THIBAULT, Roger; Clinique Med Mirabel, CP 1059 13714 boul Cure Labelle, Mirabel QC J7J 1A1; Laval'67; (450)435-7666; Fax. (450)435-1716.

THIBAULT, Sebastien; CSSS de Trois-Rivières, 1991 boul du Carmel, Trois-Rivieres QC G8Z 3R9; Mon'01; Staff, CSSS de Trois-Rivières; Langs: English; (819)697-3333; Fax. (819)372-3535; seb_tibo@hotmail.com.

THIBAULT, Sonia; CLSC Ahuntsic, 1165 boul Henri-Bourassa E, Montreal QC H2C 3K2; Mon'91; (514)384-2000 x8404; Fax. (514)381-1486.

THIBAULT, Suzanne; Centre Med Varennes, 201-2082 Rte Marie-Victorin, Varennes QC J3X 2C7; McG'80; Langs: Bilingual(French/English); (450)652-2959; Fax. (450)652-3792.

THIBAULT, Suzanne; Centre Med Racine, 2490 1re av, Quebec QC G1L 5A8; Laval'79; (418)640-2565; Fax. (418)640-2578.

THIBAULT, Veronic; Centre Hosp le Gardeur, 911 Montee des Pionniers, Terrebonne QC J6V 2H2; Mon'07; CCFP; Staff, Centre Hospitalier Pierre le Gardeur; Staff, CLSC de Richelieu; (450)654-7525

THIBAULT-CHABOT, Isabelle; Hop Charles Lemoyne, 3120 boul Taschereau, Greenfield Park QC J4V 2H1; Sher'00; Psy. Staff, Hopital Charles LeMoyne; (450)466-5020

THIBEAULT, Amy B; South Hills Tertiary Psy Rehab, 100-945 Southill St, Kamloops BC V2B 7Z9; McM'01; FRCPC; Psy. (250)554-5590

THIBEAULT, Claude; 502-8500 rue Saint-Charles, Brossard QC J4X 2Z8; Sher'72; LMCC; BA; Vis Prof Clinical Med Branch, University of Texas; Langs: Bilingual(French/English); (450)923-6826; ctebo@videotron.ca.

THIBEAULT, Danny; Chaleur Reg Hosp, 1750 Sunset Dr, Bathurst NB E2A 4L7; Laval'05; ACLS; ATLS; CCFP; Staff Emerg, Hopital Regional Chaleur; Langs: Bilingual(French/English); (506)544-2000

THIBEAULT, Laurent; CSSS de Manicouagan, 635 boul Jolliet, Baie-Comeau QC G5C 1P1; Laval'96; Psy. Staff, Centre Hospitalier Régional Baie-Comeau; (418)589-3701

THIBEAULT, Lynda; Dir de la Sante de Montreal, TA-1301 rue Sherbrooke E, Montreal QC H2L 1M3; Laval'90; FRCPC; CommunMed. Médecin, Agence de Sante Services Sociaux; (514)342-0902 x3963; lthibeault_reg13@ssss.gouv.qc.ca.

THIBEAULT, Marie-Helene; Clinique Med de Pintendre, 5-792 rte du President-Kennedy, Pintendre QC G6C 1C8; Sher'07; (418)837-6943; Fax. (418)837-0487.

THIBEAULT, Marie-Marthe; Hopital l'Hotel-Dieu de Quebec, 11 Cote du Palais, Quebec QC G1R 2J6; Laval'87; FRCPC; Derm. ac Membre, Centre Hospitalier Universitaire de Québec (CHUQ) - Siege Social; (418)691-5200

THIBEAULT, Roseline; CHUQ-Ctre Hop Univ Laval, R 1742-2705 boul Laurier, Quebec QC G1V 4G2; Laval'01; FRCPC; Peds; InfectDis. Staff, Centre Hospitalier Universitaire de Quebec-CHUL; Langs: Bilingual(French/English); (418)525-4444; Fax. (418)654-2137; roseline.thibeault@mail.chuq.qc.ca.

THIBEAULT, Yves; 169 Botsford St, Moncton NB E1C 4X4; Mon'92; FRCPC; IntMed; Nephrol. (506)857-3020; Fax. (506)855-2847.

THIBEAULT-CARON, Helene; 75 rue de la Montagne GD, St-Boniface-D-Shaw QC G0X 2L0; Laval'78; (819)535-2108

THIBEAULT-EYBALIN, Marie-Pierre; CHUQ-Ctr Hosp Univ Laval, A 1842-2705 boul Laurier, Quebec QC G1V 4G2; McG'05; FRCPC; Neur. Staff, Centre Hospitalier Universitaire de Quebec-CHUL; (418)654-2787

THIBERT, Alain; Clinique Medi-Val, 100-408 rue Jeanne Mance, Salaber-de-Valleyf QC J6T 4G1; Mon'82; Staff, Centre Hospitalier Régional du Suroît; (450)370-3387; Fax. (450)370-3395.

THIBERT, Gilberte; Lakeshore Gen Hosp, 160 av Stillview, Pointe-Claire QC H9R 2Y2; Mon'78; FRCPC; IntMed (P.Q.) (Gastroenterology). Staff, Lakeshore General Hospital - Pointe Claire; (514)630-2225; Fax. (514)695-6369.

THIBERT, Jean-Francois; Centre Hosp de Verdun, 4000 boul Lasalle, LaSalle QC H4G 2A3; Mon'01; CCFP; CCFP(E.M.); Staff, Montfort Hospital; Staff, Centre Hospitalier de Verdun; (514)362-1000

THIBERT, Mark R; Harbourview Med Clinic, 43 Court St N, Thunder Bay ON P7A 4T5; Wes'83; BSc(Biology); FRCSC; GenSurg; PlasSurg. Pres Medical Staff, St Joseph's Care Group - St Joseph's Hospital; Ac Staff, Thunder Bay Regional Health Sciences Centre; Prof Med, McMaster University; (807)346-5939; Fax. (807)346-5497.

THIBERT, Robert F; 304-450 Central Ave, London ON N6B 2E8; Wes'85; FRCPC; IntMed (Cardiology). (519)439-9851; Fax. (519)439-4806.

THIBODEAU, Alain; Clinique Med Legardeurois, 130-155 reu Notre-Dame, Repentigny QC J5Z 3C4; Mon'88; Staff Emerg, Hopital Maisonneuve-Rosemont; Staff Teacher, Universite de Montreal; (450)582-5551; Fax. (450)582-2718.

THIBODEAU, Alfred E; 7-767 Maple Ave, Burlington ON L7S 2K1; Wes'56; Staff, Joseph Brant Memorial Hospital; (905)639-5162; Fax. (905)639-3034; athibodeau@rogers.ca.

THIBODEAU, Daniel; CHUS-Hop Fleurimont, 3001 12e av N, Sherbrooke QC J1H 5N4; Sher'80; FRCSC; ObstGyn. Staff, Centre Hospitalier Universitaire de Sherbrooke-Hopital Fleurimont; Staff Teacher, Universite de Sherbrooke; Langs: English; (819)346-1110; daniel.thibodeau@usherbrooke.ca.

THIBODEAU, Daniele; 103-185 av Acadie, Dieppe NB E1A 1G6; Mon'97; CCFP; Langs: English; (506)388-0808; Fax. (506)388-0801.

THIBODEAU, Denis L; Kaslo Primary Health Centre, PO Box 670 673 A Ave, Kaslo BC V0G 1M0; Mem'95; (250)353-2291

THIBODEAU, Emilie; Polyclinique St-Eustache, 75 rue Grignon, Saint-Eustache QC J7P 4J2; Mon'07; CCFP; (450)473-6882

THIBODEAU, Jacinthe; Institut de Cardiologie de Mtl, 5000 rue Belanger, Montreal QC H1T 1C8; Mon'79; ac Staff, Institut de Cardiologie de Montréal; (514)376-3330; Fax. (514)376-4766.

THIBODEAU, Jacques; 126 ch du Lac Chaud RR 1, La Macaza QC J0T 1R0; Laval'72; CCFP; FCFP.

THIBODEAU, James A; CFB Edmonton Garrison, PO Box 10500 Stn Forces 1 Field Ambulance, Edmonton AB T5J 4J5; Mem'05; CCFP; Staff, Edmonton Garrison Health Services Centre; james.thibodeau@forces.gc.ca.

THIBODEAU, Jean-Louis; 41 rue Anna, Saint-Jacques NB E7B 1B2; Sher'75; Consultant Health Care Hosp Serv Branch, New Brunswick Power Group of Companies; Langs: English; French; jthibodeau@nbpower.com.

THIBODEAU, Marie-Pierre; CHUM-Hop Notre-Dame, 1560 rue Sherbrooke E, Montreal QC H2L 4M1; Mon'04; FRCPC; GeriatricMed; IntMed. Staff, Centre Hospitalier l'Université de Montréal (CHUM) - Hôpital Notre-Dame; (514)890-8000

THIBODEAU, Martin; Clin Med Specialisee-Psyche, 400-400 av Laurier O, Montreal QC H2V 2K7; Mon'93; FRCPC; Psy. (514)279-4141; Fax. (514)279-4101.

THIBODEAU, Melina J M; Tuscany Med Clinic, 102-1646 McKenzie AVe, Victoria BC V8N 0A3; Dal'97; Dip SportMed; CCFP; (250)818-0001; Fax. (250)383-0203.

THIBODEAU, Michel E; Hawkesbury Dist Gen Hosp, 1111 Ghislain St, Hawkesbury ON K6A 3G5; Mon'98; FRCPC; IntMed. Staff, Hawkesbury & District General Hospital; Langs: Bilingual(French/English); (613)632-1111; Fax. (613)636-6175.

THIBODEAU, Micheline; CHUM-Hop Notre-Dame, 1560 rue Sherbrooke E, Montreal QC H2L 4M1; Mon'81; FRCPC; DiagRad. Staff, Centre Hospitalier l'Université de Montréal (CHUM) - Hôpital Notre-Dame; Clin Adj, Universite de Montreal; (514)890-8250

THIBODEAU, Nicole; Hop du Saint-Sacrement, 1050 ch Sainte-Foy, Quebec QC G1S 4L8; Laval'84; Psy. Staff, Centre Hospitalier Affilié Universitaire de Québec - Hôpital du St-Sacrement; (418)682-7898; Fax. (418)682-7959.

THIBODEAU, Pierre G; CHUM-Hop St-Luc, 1058 rue Saint-Denis, Montreal QC H2X 3J4; Mon'84; Staff, Centre Hospitalier l'Université De Montréal (CHUM) - Hôpital Saint-luc; (514)890-8000 x36441; Fax. (514)412-7432.

THIBODEAU, Pierre; CSSS d'Argenteuil, 145 av de la Providence, Lachute QC J8H 4C7; Sher'76; Staff, Douglas Mental Health University Institute; Staff, Centre Hospitalier d'Argenteuil; Langs: Bilingual(French/English); (514)562-3761 x8433; pierre.thibodeau@douglas.mcgill.ca.

THIBODEAU, Raymond; CSSS du Nord de Lanaudière, 1000 boul Sainte-Anne, St-Charles-Brromee QC J6E 6J2; Sher'87; CCFP; FCFP; ac Staff, Centre Hospitalier Régional de Lanaudière; (450)759-8222; Fax. (450)759-5213.

THIBODEAU, Renee; 401-955 boul Saint-Jean, Pointe-Claire QC H9R 5K3; Sher'80; (514)459-3428; Fax. (514)426-3323.

THIBOUTOT, Francois; CHUQ-Hotel-Dieu de Quebec, 11 Cote du Palais, Quebec QC G1R 2J6; Laval'02; FRCPC; Anes; Critical Care Medicine. Staff, Centre Hospitalier Universitaire de Québec (CHUQ) - Siege Social; (418)525-4444

THICKE, Brian C; Peel Village Med Centre, 28 Rambler Dr, Brampton ON L6W 1E2; Wes'56; BA; Ac Staff, William Osler Health System - Brampton Civic Hospital; Med Dir, Tullamore Nursing Home; Med Examiner Civil Aviation, Ministry of Transportation; (905)451-5586; Fax. (905)451-1233.

THICKE, Steven C; Saanich Peninsula Hosp, 2166 Mount Newton Cross Rd, Saanichton BC V8M 2B2; UBC'81; Staff, Saanich Peninsula Hospital; (250)652-3911

THIDA, Ma Khin; 201-1160 Burrard St, Vancouver BC V6Z 2E8; Dhakka (India)'94; MB BS; CCFP; Langs: Hindi; Urdu; Burmese; Bengali; (604)558-4044; mkthida@hotmail.com.

THIEL, Alexander; SMBD Jewish Gen Hosp, 3755 ch Cote-Sainte-Catherine, Montreal QC H3T 1E2; Bonn (Germany)'94; Staff, Sir Mortimer B Davis Jewish General; (514)340-8222 x5844; Fax. (514)340-7510; alexander.thiel@mcgill.ca.

THIEL, John A; Parliament Place, 100-2631 28th Ave, Regina SK S4S 6X3; Sask'91; BSc; MSc; FRCSC; ObstGyn (Operative Laparoscopy). Staff, Regina General Hospital; Staff, St Joseph's Hospital; Asst Prof, University of Saskatchewan; (306)586-1800; Fax. (306)586-3511.

THIELE-KUNTZ, Amy M; Royal Victoria Hosp, 201 Georgian Dr, Barrie ON L4M 6M2; Dal'96; FRCPC; Anes. Anesthetist, Royal Victoria Regional Health Centre; (705)728-9090

THIEM, Sasha C; Fairview Comm Health Centre, 359-5 Fairview Mall Dr, North York ON M2J 2Z1; Man'09; CCFP; (416)640-5298; Fax. (416)642-2238.

THIEN, Vincent V S; Scarborough North Med Arts, 406-4040 Finch Ave E, Scarborough ON M1S 4V5; UBC'99; FRCPC; IntMed; Gastroent. Staff, The Scarborough Hospital - Birchmount Campus; Langs: Hakka; (416)335-4669; Fax. (416)335-4672.

THIESEN, Aducio L; University of Alberta Hosp, 5B4 57-8440 112 St NW, Edmonton AB T6G 2B7; (Brazil)'94; FRCPC; AnatPath. Staff, University of Alberta Hospital; (780)407-2861; Fax. (780)407-3009.

THIESSEN, Barton P; Health Sciences Centre, 300 Prince Philip Dr, St. John's NL A1B 3V6; UBC'04; FRCPC; Anes. Staff, Health Sciences Centre; (709)777-6300

THIESSEN, Brian A; Gordon & Leslie Diamond HCC, 8275A-2775 Laurel St, Vancouver BC V5Z 1M9; Sask'90; FRCPC; Neur (Neuro Oncology). Ac Staff, Vancouver General Hospital - Centennial Pavillion; Ac Staff, BC Cancer Agency Vancouver Centre; Staff, Gordon & Leslie Diamond Health Care Centre; Clinical Asst Prof Med, University of British Columbia; (604)875-5352; Fax. (604)875-5351.

THIESSEN, Mark D; Saanich Plaza Med Clinic, 3544 Blanshard St, Victoria BC V8X 1W3; UBC'89; (250)475-3331; Fax. (250)475-1157.

THIESSEN, Myron N; South Eastman Health Clinic, PO Box 470, La Broquerie MB R0A 0W0; Man'88; CCFP; VP Medical Services, Southern Health/Santé Sud Corporate Office La Broquerie.

THIESSEN, Paul N; Fairmont Med Bldg, 1314-750 Broadway W, Vancouver BC V5Z 1J3; Alb'74; FRCPC; Peds (Neonatology). Ac Staff, BC Women's Hospital & Health Centre; Ac Staff, BC Children's Hospital; Med Dir Spinal Cord Clinic, BC Cancer Agency Vancouver Centre; Clin Prof Peds, University of British Columbia; (604)879-4564; Fax. (604)879-5191.

THIESSEN, Trent E; 203-610 Queen St, Saskatoon SK S7K 0M8; Sask'98; FRCSC; OrthSurg (Lower Extremity Reconstruction). Clin Asst Prof, University of Saskatchewan; (306)244-5533; Fax. (306)244-4545; aussiedocnurse@yahoo.ca.

THIFFAULT, Gilbert; Medigestal Inc, 101-2655 boul Daniel-Johnson, Laval QC H7P 5Y2; Laval'65; BSc; MB BS; FRCSC; OrthSurg (P.Q.). Médecin, Medigestal Inc; Langs: English; (450)688-4451; Fax. (450)688-5018.

THIFFAULT, Jocelyne; Clinique Med St-Francois, 201-8495 rue Adrien, Laval QC H7A 1J9; Mon'75; Staff, Hopital de la Cite de la santé; Langs: Spanish; English; (450)665-1622; Fax. (450)665-0240.

THIFFEAULT, Line; Clin d'Expertise Med du Quebec, 440-979 boul de Bourgogne, Quebec QC G1W 2L4; Laval'88; FRCPC; Psy. Staff, Centre Hospitalier Universitaire de Quebec-CHUL; (418)654-3268

THILLAINADARAJAH, Pandaram; Dr Thillai Inc, 1-13665 96 Ave, Surrey BC V3V 1Z1; Ceylon (Sri Lanka)'70; MB BS; MRCPsy; DPM; FRCPC; Psy (Affective Disorders). Consultant Psy, Surrey Memorial Hospital; Langs: Tamil; (604)582-0156; Fax. (604)581-0110.

THILLE, Suzanne M L; St Boniface Gen Hosp, E4003-409 Tache Ave, Winnipeg MB R2H 2A6; Ott'91; FRCPC; IntMed; GeriatricMed. Staff, St Boniface General Hospital; (204)233-8563

THIMM, Andreas J; Woodbridge Med Centre, A13-9600 Islingston Ave, Woodbridge ON L4H 2T1; Ross University (USA)'08; (905)893-8085

THIND, Charanjit K; Connaigre Peninsula Comm HC, PO Box 70 1 Alexander Ave, Harbour Breton NL A0H 1P0; Punjab University (India)'87; MB BS; Staff, Connaigre Peninsula Community Health Centre; (709)885-2359; charanjit.thind@easternhealth.ca.

THIPPHAVONG, Seng; Women's College Hosp, W267-76 Grenville St, Toronto ON M5S 1B2; Wes'04; FRCPC; DiagRad. Staff, Women's College Hospital; (416)323-6113

THIRLWELL, Celeste J; Sleep Disorders Clinic, 580-340 College St, Toronto ON M5T 3A9; McM'00; FRCPC; Psy. Langs: Spanish; French; (416)603-9531

THIRLWELL, Michael P; MUHC-Montreal Gen Hosp, A7 130-1650 av Cedar, Montreal QC H3G 1A4; McG'66; ABIM; FACP; MDCM; FRCPC; IntMed (Palliative Care); MedOncol. Dir MedOncol, McGill University Health Centre - Montreal General Campus; Staff, McGill University Health Centre - Royal Victoria Hospital; Staff, St Mary's Hospital Centre; Prof MedOncol, McGill University; Langs: Cantonese; French; (514)934-8075

THIRSK, Robert B; Canadian Space Agency, 6767 Route De L'aeroport, Longueuil QC J3Y 8Y9; McG'82; BSc; SM; MBA; Staff, Canadian Institute of Health Research; Langs: English; French; (450)926-4702; rthirsk@cihr-irsc.gc.ca.

THIRSK, Warren S; North Edmonton Health Centre, 14007 50 St NW, Edmonton AB T5A 5E4; McM'97; FRCPC; EmergMed (Sports Medicine). Staff, Royal Alexandra Hospital; (780)342-4123; Fax. (780)342-4186.

THIRUGNANAM, Subarna; Markham Stouffville Hosp, PO Box 1800 Stn Main 381 Church St, Markham ON L3P 7P3; Tor'05; FRCPC; IntMed; Critical Care Medicine. Staff, Markham Stouffville Hospital; Langs: Tamil; (905)472-7000

THIRUGNANASAMPANTHAPILLAI, Vakeesan; Fogal Medical Centre, 7-8920 Highway 50, Brampton ON L6P 3A3; (New Zealand)'87; FRNZCGP; CCFP; Langs: Tamil; Sinhalese; (905)915-8778; Fax. (905)915-8780.

THISDALE, Jean; Polyclinique St-Eustache, 75 rue Grignon, St-Eustache QC J7P 4J2; Mon'79; Langs: Portuguese; English; (450)472-0447; Fax. (450)473-1916.

THISTLE, Brent E; Western Mem Reg Hosp, PO Box 2005 Stn Main 1 Brookfield Ave, Corner Brook NL A2H 6J7; (Ireland)'05; CCFP; Staff, Western Memorial Regional Hospital; (709)637-5000

THIVIERGE, Benoit E; Hop du Sacre-Coeur de Mtl, 5400 Boul Gouin O, Montreal QC H4J 1C5; Mon'78; FRCPC; MedMicrobiol. Med Consultant, Pavillon Notre-Dame de la Merci; ac Staff, Hôpital du Sacre-Coeur de Montréal; (514)338-2222 x2157; Fax. (514)338-2909.

THIVIERGE, Caroll; Clinique Med Pasteur, 770 1re av, Quebec QC G1L 3K2; Laval'65; Ac Staff, CSSS de Quebec-Sud; Langs: English; (418)529-0042 x4; Fax. (418)529-4924; thiviergeca@hotmail.com.

THIVIERGE, Claude-Yves; Dir de la Sante Publique Mtl, 1301 rue Sherbrooke E, Montreal QC H2L 1M3; Sher'83; Staff, Direction de Sante Publique de Montreal; (514)528-2400; Fax. (514)528-2425.

THIVIERGE, Isabelle; Hotel-Dieu de Levis, 143 rue Wolfe, Levis QC G6V 3Z1; Laval'96; GeriatricMed; Gastroent (P.Q.); IntMed. Staff, Hôtel-Dieu de Lévis; (418)835-7121

THIVIERGE, Jean-Claude; Clinique Med Racine, 201-900 boul Raymond, Quebec QC G1B 3G3; Laval'66; adj Staff Geriatric, Centre d'hebergement Saint-Augustin; Médecin, Clinique Medical Montmorency; (418)667-8068; Fax. (418)667-8131.

THIVIERGE, Marie-France; CSSS du Nord de Lanaudière, 1000 boul Sainte-Anne, Joliette QC J6E 6J2; Mon'06; IntMed. Staff, Centre Hospitalier Régional de Lanaudière; (450)759-8222

THIVIERGE, Maryse; CHUQ-St-Francoise d'Assise, C2639-10 rue de l'Espinay, Quebec QC G1L 3L5; Laval'97; CCFP; Staff, Centre Hospitalier Universitaire De Québec - Pavillon De St-françois-d'assise; (418)525-4425; Fax. (418)525-4322.

THIVIERGE, Robert L; Hôpital Ste-Justine, 3175 ch Cote-Sainte-Catherine, Montreal QC H3T 1C5; Laval'68; FAAP; FRCPC; Peds. Clin Assoc Prof/Staff, Hôpital Ste-Justine; vice Doyen Ass't, Universite de Montreal; (514)345-4675; Fax. (514)345-4822; robert.thivierge@umontreal.ca.

THIVIERGE, Robert; 86 rue Sainte-Anne, Ste-Anne-De-Bellev QC H9X 1L8; Mon'78; (514)457-7186; Fax. (514)457-7186.

THIYAGARAJAN, Senthil K; Niagara H System-Welland Site, 65 Third St, Welland ON L3B 4W6; Dr M G R Medical University (India)'96; FRCPC; Anes. Staff, Niagara Health System - Welland Hospital Site; Langs: Tamil; (905)732-6111

THIYAGARATNAM, Pathmini; The Richmond Hosp, 7000 Westminster Hwy, Richmond BC V6X 1A2; (Sri Lanka)'72; MB BS; MRCP(UK); FRCPC; GenPath. Ac Staff Path, Richmond Hospital; (604)278-9711; Fax. (604)244-5162.

THOBANI, Shafik U F; Lions Gate Hosp, 231 15th Ave E, North Vancouver BC V7L 2L7; London (England)'81; MB BS; FRCPC; Anes (Acute Pain Management). Staff, Lions Gate Hospital; (604)984-5709; Fax. (604)984-5729.

THOBANI, Yasmin; B-796 Burnhamthorpe Rd W, Mississauga ON L5C 2R9; UBC'75; Court Staff, Trillium Health Centre - Mississauga; Langs: Gujarati; Hindi; (905)272-4770; Fax. (905)272-4733; drthobani@rogers.com.

THOBIE, Gisele; Hopital Louis-H Lafontaine, 7401 rue Hochelaga, Montreal QC H1N 3M5; Dijon (France)'72; Anes (P.Q.). ac Staff, CSSS de Dorval-Lachine-Lasalle; Staff, Douglas Mental Health University Institute; Staff, Hopital Louis-H Lafontaine; (514)251-4000 x2730

THOM, Cheryl M; Calgary Women's Imaging Centre, 20 Richard Way SW, Calgary AB T3E 7M9; Alb'80; FRCPC; DiagRad (Mammography). (403)685-3123; Fax. (403)685-3235; cthom@womensimaging.ca.

THOMA, Achilleas; Dr A Thoma Med Prof Corp, 101-206 James St S, Hamilton ON L8P 3A9; McM'76; FACS; FRCSC; PlasSurg (Cosmetic Surgery). Court Staff, Joseph Brant Memorial Hospital; Court Staff, Hamilton Health Sciences Centre; Ac Staff PlasSurg, St Joseph's Healthcare Hamilton - King Campus; Clin Prof Surg, McMaster University; Langs: Greek; (905)523-0019; Fax. (905)523-0229.

THOMAS, Andrew J; CPHC Comm Family Hlth Team, 6-555 California Ave Box 338, Brockville ON K6V 5V5; University of Cape Town (South Africa)'86; MB ChB; CCFP; FCFP; Ac Staff, Brockville General Hospital - Charles Street; Coroner, Province of Ontario; Aj Prof, Queen's University; Clin Prof, University of Ottawa; (613)342-4076; Fax. (613)342-6578; athomas@cphcare.ca.

THOMAS, Anthony D; Wawa Family Health Team, PO Box 1218 17 Government Rd, Wawa ON P0S 1K0; London (England)'70; MB BS; Ac Staff, QHC Trenton Memorial; (705)856-1313; Fax. (705)856-9550.

THOMAS, Biju K; Rochdale Walk-In Clinic, 4450 Rochdale Blvd, Regina SK S4X 4P7; (Other Foreign)'03; (306)565-0181

THOMAS, Bruce; Women's College Hosp, 76 Grenville St, Toronto ON M5S 1B2; Tor'62; FRCSC; ObstGyn. Staff, Women's College Hospital; (416)323-7744; Fax. (416)323-6237.

THOMAS, C Kuncheria; Espanola Reg Hosp & Hlth Ctre, 825 McKinnon Dr, Espanola ON P5E 1R4; Kerala (India)'81; MB BS; CCFP; CCFP(E.M.); Staff, Espanola Regional Hospital and Health Centre; Staff Emerg Room, Pembroke Regional Hospital Inc; Court Staff Emerg Room, Southlake Regional Health Centre; Court Staff Emerg Room, The Scarborough Hospital - General Campus; Staff, Kemptville District Hospital; Langs: Malayalam; (705)869-1420; Fax. (705)869-3081.

THOMAS, Chandra M; Foothills Med Centre, 1403 29 St NW, Calgary AB T2N 2T9; Cal'01; FRCPC; IntMed (Palliative Care); Nephrol. Staff, Peter Lougheed Centre; Staff, Foothills Medical Centre; Staff Nephrol, Alberta Health Services-Calgary Zone; Clinical Asst Prof, University of Calgary; (403)944-3962; Fax. (403)944-3199.

THOMAS, Charlene H; Towers Med Clinic, 120-100 Elizabeth Ave, St. John's NL A1B 1S1; Mem'01; CCFP; (709)753-9900; Fax. (709)753-6716.

THOMAS, Christin; Toronto East Gen Hosp Inc, B112-825 Coxwell Ave, Toronto ON M4C 3E7; Man'10; CCFP; Staff, Toronto East General Hospital Inc; (416)461-8272

THOMAS, D Richard R; Laurel Med Centre Ltd, 314-888 8th Ave W, Vancouver BC V5Z 3Y1; London (England)'78; MB BS; LRCP; MRCS; FRCPC; Derm. Staff, Vancouver General Hospital - Centennial Pavillion; Asst Prof, University of British Columbia; Langs: Welsh; (604)731-5353; Fax. (604)731-6166.

THOMAS, Daina; University of Alberta Hosp, 8440 112 St NW, Edmonton AB T6G 2B7; Cal'07; PedEmergMed; Peds. Staff, University of Alberta Hospital; Teach Staff, University of Calgary; (780)407-8822

THOMAS, Danielle A; 214 College St, Toronto ON M5T 2Z9; McG'83; FRCPC; Psy., University of Toronto; (416)978-8070

THOMAS, David; Centre Hosp le Gardeur, 911 Montee des Pionniers, Terrebonne QC J6V 2H2; Cardiff (Wales)'72; Anes (P.Q.). Staff, Centre Hospitalier Pierre le Gardeur; Staff, Hôpital Santa Cabrini Ospedale; (450)654-7525

THOMAS, David M; Family Practice Med Clinic, PO Box 1230, Port-aux-Basques NL A0M 1C0; Mem'06; CCFP; Chief of Staff, Dr Charles L Legrow Health Centre; (709)695-6295; Fax. (709)695-6296.

THOMAS, Eddie; Clinique Med du Carrefour, 1005 Rte Lagueux, St-Etienne-De-Lauz QC G6J 1J8; Laval'93; Staff, Centre Hospitalier Chauveau; (418)836-2002; Fax. (418)836-2070; eddie.thomas@videotron.ca.

THOMAS, Elizabeth; Vancouver Gen Hosp, 855 12th Ave W, Vancouver BC V5Z 1M9; Madras (India)'72; MB BS; FRCPath; FRCPC; MedMicrobiol. Staff, Vancouver General Hospital - Centennial Pavillion; (604)875-4111

THOMAS, Eric K; Stratford Family Health Team, 102-342 Erie St, Stratford ON N5A 2N4; Qns'84; Staff, Stratford General Hospital - Huron Perth Healthcare Alliance; (519)271-5831; Fax. (519)271-5930.

THOMAS, Eva E; BC Women's Hosp & Hlth Ctre, K4 222-4500 Oak St, Vancouver BC V6H 3N1; Uppsala (Sweden)'76; PhD; FRCPC; MedMicrobiol. Staff, BC Women's Hospital & Health Centre; Asst Prof, University of British Columbia; Langs: Swedish; (604)875-2622; Fax. (604)875-2950.

THOMAS, G Ross; Tantramar Commun Health Centre, 1-2 Main St, Sackville NB E4L 4A3; Dal'85; CCFP; Staff, Sackville Memorial Hospital; (506)536-0210; Fax. (506)536-0761.

THOMAS, Gene F; Iron Ore Company of Canada, PO Box 1000, Labrador City NL A2V 2L8; Mem'01; Staff, Iron Ore Company of Canada; (709)944-8353; Fax. (709)944-8079.

THOMAS, Gillian M; Sunnybrook Odette Cancer Ctr, T2 161-2075 Bayview Ave, Toronto ON M4N 3M5; Tor'70; FRCPC; RadOncol (Gynecological Cancer) (Gynecologic Oncology). Staff RadOncol Research Centre, Sunnybrook Health Sciences Centre; Staff, Sunnybrook Health Sciences Centre - Edmond Odette Cancer Centre; Prof RadOncol & ObstGyn, University of Toronto; (416)480-6165; Fax. (416)480-6002; gillian.thomas@sunnybrook.ca.

THOMAS, Gordon R; Royal Ottawa Mental Hlth Ctre, 1145 Carling Ave, Ottawa ON K1Z 7K4; Cal'03; FRCPC; Psy. Staff, Royal Ottawa Mental Health Centre - Royal Ottawa Health Care Group; (613)722-6521; Fax. (613)798-2999.

THOMAS, Jacqueline A; Hydro Place Bldg, OPG 3093-700 University Ave, Toronto ON M5G 1Z5; McM'96; FRCSC; ObstGyn. (416)586-4632; Fax. (416)586-5216.

THOMAS, Jennifer E; 715 McKay St, Pembroke ON K8A 2J8; McM'08; CCFP; (613)735-1089

THOMAS, Jennifer L; Sharing Care Med Clinic, 204-1800 Tranquille Rd, Kamloops BC V2B 3L9; Cal'85; (250)554-8768

THOMAS, Jill M; Dr J M Thomas Med Prof Corp, 2500-1 Dundas St W, Toronto ON M5G 1Z3; Wes'97; CCFP; (416)642-2350

THOMAS, John A; Rockyview Gen Hosp, 7007 14 St SW, Calgary AB T2V 1P9; Galway (Ireland)'71; FRCPC; Anes. Staff Anes, Rockyview General Hospital; (403)943-3410; Fax. (403)287-1456.

THOMAS, Jonathan B; Peninsula FHT-Lions Head, 24 Moore St, Lions Head ON N0H 1W0; Qns'06; CCFP; (519)793-3445

THOMAS, Karen E; The Hosp for Sick Children, 555 University Ave, Toronto ON M5G 1X8; Oxford (England)'90; FRCPC; DiagRad. Staff, The Hospital For Sick Children; (416)813-1500; Fax. (416)813-7591; karen.thomas@sickkids.ca.

THOMAS, Kenneth C; Foothills Med Centre, MT 0440-1403 29 St NW, Calgary AB T2N 2T9; Qns'97; FRCSC; OrthSurg. Staff Surg, Foothills Medical Centre; (403)944-3070; Fax. (403)270-8004.

THOMAS, Lyle S; Red Deer Reg Hosp Centre, PO Box 5030 Stn Postal Box Ctr 3942 50A Ave, Red Deer AB T4N 6R2; Alb'98; CCFP; CCFP(E.M.); Staff Emerg, Red Deer Regional Hospital Centre; (403)343-4444

THOMAS, Mary C; Glenridge Med Bldg, 204-1 Belton Blvd, St Catharines ON L2T 3Y4; Tor'79; CCFP; FCFP; Staff, Niagara Health System - St Catharines General Site; Staff, Niagara Health System - Ontario Street Site; (905)688-2229

THOMAS, Mary; South East Toronto Family Heal, 105-840 Coxwell Ave, Toronto ON M4C 5T2; Melbourne (Australia)'91; MB BS; CCFP; Staff, Toronto East General Hospital Inc; Langs: Greek; (416)469-6464; Fax. (416)469-6164.

THOMAS, Mary Ann; Alberta Children's Hosp, C3 438-2888 Shaganappi Trail, Calgary AB T3B 6A8; McG'99; CCMG; FRCPC; MedGenetics (Cytogenetics). Staff Medical Genetics, Alberta Children's Hospital; Asst Prof, University of Calgary; Langs: French; (403)955-7460; Fax. (403)955-2701.

THOMAS, Mary-Janet; Gamma Daycare Laboratory, 750 Peter Morand Cres, Ottawa ON K1G 6S4; Tor'67; AnatPath. Staff, The Ottawa Hospital - Civic Campus; (613)729-0200

THOMAS, Michelle L; Patterson Med Clinic, 45 Wolsley St RR 1 Stn Main, Kenora ON P9N 3W7; Man'96; CCFP; FCFP; (807)468-3021; Fax. (807)468-6964; nfathomas@hotmail.com.

THOMAS, Nancy; CHUQ-Ctr Hosp Univ Laval, 2705 boul Laurier, Quebec QC G1V 4G2; Laval'92; FABOG; FRCSC; ObstGyn (Obstetrics) (Maternal Fetal Medicine). Staff CME Perinatol, Centre Hospitalier Universitaire de Quebec-CHUL; Aj Prof Perinatol, Université Laval; Langs: Bilingual(French/English); (418)525-4444; Fax. (418)577-2058; nancy.thomas@ogy.ulaval.ca.

THOMAS, Nell; East Wellington Family Hlth Team, 1-6 Thompson Cres, Erin ON N0B 1T0; NOSM'09; BA; MClSc; CCFP; (519)833-9396; Fax. (519)833-9838.

THOMAS, Paul; 650 rue Saint-Charles O, Longueuil QC J4H 1G9; Sher'76; Langs: Bilingual(French/English); (450)442-3326; Fax. (450)442-9399.

THOMAS, Peter; Medical & Dental Bldg, 308-586 Eglinton Ave E, Toronto ON M4P 1P2; London (England)'68; MB BS; FRCP; FCCP; FACP; FRCPC; IntMed (Respiratory Sleep Disorders). Staff, St Michael's Hospital; Staff, Lakeridge Health - Whitby Site; Assoc Prof Med, University of Toronto; (647)427-5091

THOMAS, Rejean; Clinique Med l'Actuel, 1130-1001 de Maisonneuve E, Montreal QC H2L 4P9; Laval'79; (514)524-3642 x230; Fax. (514)524-3831; rthomas@lactuel.ca.

THOMAS, Richard D; Huronia Med Centre, PO Box 790 Stn Main 103-1070 Hugel Ave, Midland ON L4R 4P4; Qns'78; CASM(SportMed); BA(Hons.); CCFP; Ac Staff Anes, Georgian Bay General Hospital - Midland; (705)526-8482; Fax. (705)526-8789; rthomas1121@rogers.com.

THOMAS, Richard P; Kingston Gen Hosp, V4-76 Stuart St, Kingston ON K7L 2V7; Ott'82; FRCSC; ObstGyn. Staff, Kingston General Hospital; Asst Prof, Queen's University; Langs: English; French; Bilingual(English/French); (613)548-6067; Fax. (613)548-1330; thomasr@queensu.ca.

THOMAS, Robert G; Central Alberta Prof Centre, 155-5201 43 St, Red Deer AB T4N 1C7; UBC'76; FRCSC; Urol. (403)358-7654; Fax. (403)348-2940.

THOMAS, Robert S; Thames Valley FHT-Windermere S, 301-460 Wellington St, St Thomas ON N5R 6H9; Wes'68; Staff, St Thomas Elgin General Hospital; (519)631-5670; Fax. (519)631-8570.

THOMAS, Roger E; Sheldon Shumir Centre, 1213 4 St SW, Calgary AB T2R 0X7; McM'77; PhD; MRC; AB; CCFP; Prof Family Med, University of Calgary; Langs: German; French; (403)955-9300; Fax. (403)476-8766.

THOMAS, Roger H; Richmond Health Science Ctre, 550-6091 Gilbert Rd, Richmond BC V7C 5L9; Birmingham (England)'77; MB ChB; FRCS; FRCSC; Ophth. Ac Staff, Richmond Hospital; Court Staff, Delta Hospital; Langs: German; French; (604)273-1128; Fax. (604)278-3316; thomasr@shaw.ca.

THOMAS, Sajni S; 66 Waterloo St, Saint John NB E2L 3P4; Dal'80; Staff, St Joseph's Hospital; Staff, Saint John Regional Hospital; (506)634-1110; Fax. (506)634-0571.

THOMAS, Shawn T; Concordia Health Associates, 102-1155 Concordia Ave, Winnipeg MB R2K 2M9; Man'02; CCFP; (204)415-0322

THOMAS, Shira; Arbour Med Clinic, 281 Stone Rd E, Guelph ON N1G 5J5; McM'95; BSc; CCFP; Staff, Guelph General Hospital; (519)823-5133; Fax. (519)827-0255.

THOMAS, Sophia; Hotel-Dieu Grace Hosp, 1030 Ouellette Ave, Windsor ON N9A 1E1; Wes'96; CCFP; Staff, Hôtel-Dieu Grace Hospital; Langs: Bilingual(English/French); (519)973-4444

THOMAS, Sumesh P; McMaster University, HSC 4F-1280 Main St W, Hamilton ON L8S 4K1; Benin (Nigeria)'90; FRCPC; Peds (Neonatology). Teach Staff, McMaster University; (905)521-2100; Fax. (905)521-5007.

THOMAS, Sunu S; Univ Hlth Network-Toronto Western Hosp, EW5 559-399 Bathurst St, Toronto ON M5T 2S8; Tor'05; Cardiol; IntMed. Staff, St Michael's Hospital; (416)603-5815

THOMAS, Tara J; Hamilton HS-General Site, 3F-237 Barton St E, Hamilton ON L8L 2X2; McM'06; FRCPC; Anes. Staff, Hamilton Health Sciences Centre - Hamilton General Hospital; (905)527-4322

THOMAS, Tina E; Hop de l'Enfant Jesus, 1401 18E rue, Quebec QC G1J 1Z4; Mon'97; FRCSC; Neursurg (Neuro Oncology). Staff, Centre Hospitalier Affilié Universitaire de Québec - Hôpital De L'Enfant Jésus; (418)649-0252; Fax. (418)649-5988.

THOMAS, Trace S; 203-1819 Beaufort Ave, Comox BC V9M 1R9; UBC'94; FRCPC; IntMed. Staff, St Joseph's General Hospital; (250)339-9500; Fax. (250)339-9535.

THOMAS, Valsa; 500 Oxford St E, London ON N5Y 3H7; Kerala (India)'72; Ac Staff, St Joseph's Hospital - St Joseph's Health Care; Court Staff, London Health Sciences Centre - Victoria Campus; Langs: Malayalam; (519)434-5841; Fax. (519)434-5841.

THOMAS, Wendy M; Univ of Western Ontario, 11-1151 Richmond St, London ON N6A 3K7; Tor'06; CCFP; (519)661-3030

THOMAS, Yves; GMF Shawinigan Sud, 200-2355 5e av, Shawinigan-Sud QC G9P 1P4; Louvain (France)'88; (819)537-6205

THOMAS FILS-AIME, Claudette; CLSC Parc Extension, 7085 rue Hutchison, Montreal QC H3N 1Y9; Toluca (Mexico)'81; Langs: Spanish; English; Creole; (514)273-9591

THOMAS-GUY, Catherine; CP 83542 Csp Garnier, Montreal QC H2J 4E9; Sher'94; (514)362-8387; Fax. (450)466-4219.

THOMASSE, Michele D; Mountain View Med Clinic, 201-1789 KLO Rd, Kelowna BC V1W 3P3; Sask'89; CCFP; Langs: English; French; (250)860-6799; Fax. (250)860-6798.

THOMASSE, Robert L; Aspen Med Centre, 21-429 Tranquille Rd, Kamloops BC V2B 3G9; Sask'96; (250)376-7242; Fax. (250)376-2282.

THOMASSIN, Bruce G; 7316 rue Sherbrooke O, Montreal QC H4B 1R7; McG'79; assoc Médecin, St Mary's Hospital Centre; (514)486-7318; Fax. (514)486-7639.

THOMASSIN, David; Hôtel-Dieu de Lévis, 143 rue Wolfe, Levis QC G6V 3Z1; Laval'09; CCFP; CCFP(E.M.); Staff, Hôtel-Dieu de Lévis; (418)835-7105

THOMASSIN, Josyane; Medi-Centre Kirkland, 2971 boul Saint-Charles, Kirkland QC H9H 3B5; McG'86; CCFP; FCFP; Staff, Centre Hospitalier de LaSalle; Médecin, Medi-Centre Kirkland; Langs: Bilingual(English/French); (514)426-2311; Fax. (514)697-3929.

THOMASSIN, Michael G; 7316 rue Sherbrooke O, Montreal QC H4B 1R7; McG'75; BSc; MDCM; CCFP; FCFP; Ac Staff, St Mary's Hospital Centre; Langs: English; French; (514)486-7318; Fax. (514)486-7639.

THOMASSIN-GIRARD, Caroline; Clinique Externe de Pedopsy, 200-2924 Boul Taschereau, Greenfield Park QC J4V 2G8; Sher'95; Psy (Pediatric Psychiatry). Staff Ped Psy, Hopital Charles LeMoyne; Staff Ped Psy, Centre Hospitalier de Granby; (450)466-8486; Fax. (450)466-8789.

THOMERE, Serge H J; CMR Saint-Bruno URFI, 265 boul Seigneurial O, Longueuil QC J3V 2H4; Pierre & Marie Curie Universite (France)'78; (450)441-5503 x8424

THOMMASEN, Harvey V; PO Box 18, Hagensborg BC V0T 1H0; UBC'87; CCFP; FCFP; Physician, Haida Gwaii North Hosp & Health Centre; Clin Prof, University of British Columbia; (250)982-3208; Fax. (250)982-3208.

THOMPSON, A Ian; Chesley Med Clinic, PO Box 160 Stn Main 33 2nd Ave SE, Chesley ON N0G 1L0; Qns'79; CCFP; FCFP; Pres, South Bruce Grey Health Services - Chesley Site; (519)363-3220; Fax. (519)363-0385; ithompson@sbghc.on.ca.

THOMPSON, Aaron M S; St Michael's Hosp, 30 Bond St, Toronto ON M5B 1W8; Ott'03; FRCPC; OccupMed. Staff, St Michael's Hospital; Staff, Occupational Health Clinic; (416)867-7470; Fax. (416)864-5870.

THOMPSON, Adam M; Courtenay Med Associates, 201-1350 England Ave, Courtenay BC V9N 8X6; (Other Foreign)'94; CCFP; (250)334-4411; Fax. (250)338-1245.

THOMPSON, Agnes J; Bowmont Med Clinic, 6535 Bowness Rd NW, Calgary AB T3B 0E8; (403)247-9797; Fax. (403)247-0014.

THOMPSON, Alan A; Alexander Prof Bldg, 301-849 Alexander Crt, Peterborough ON K9J 7H8; Qns'82; FRCSC; GenSurg; VascSurg. (705)743-6760; Fax. (705)743-9912.

THOMPSON, Andrew C; London HSC-Victoria Hosp, PO Box 5010 Stn B E1 102-800 Commissioners Rd E, London ON N6A 5W9; Wes'97; FRCPC; EmergMed. Staff, London Health Sciences Centre - Victoria Campus; (519)667-6530; Fax. (519)667-6538.

THOMPSON, Andrew E; St Joseph's Health Care, PO Box 5777 Stn B D2 162-268 Grosvenor St, London ON N6A 4V2; Wes'98; FRCPC; IntMed; Rheum. Staff, St Joseph's Hospital - St Joseph's Health Care; (519)646-6337; Fax. (519)646-6338.

THOMPSON, Andrew L; Lion's Gate Hosp, 231 15th St E, North Vancouver BC V7L 2L7; Mem'02; FRCPC; DiagRad. Staff, Lions Gate Hospital; Staff, North Shore Medical Imaging; (604)988-3131

THOMPSON, Angela D; Red Deer Reg Hosp Centre, PO Box 5030 Stn Postal Box Ctr 3942 50A Ave, Red Deer AB T4N 6R2; Sask'87; FRCPC; AnatPath. Staff, Red Deer Regional Hospital Centre; (403)343-4735; Fax. (403)343-4877.

THOMPSON, Ann E; Coleman Clinic, 186 Kenneth St, Duncan BC V9L 1N4; UBC'87; (250)746-4102; Fax. (250)746-5960.

THOMPSON, Anne M; Hycroft Med Bldg, 115-3195 Granville St, Vancouver BC V6H 3K2; Cal'78; CCFP; FCFP; Ac Staff, BC Women's Hospital & Health Centre; Ac Staff, BC Children's Hospital; (604)732-0525; Fax. (604)732-1064.

THOMPSON, Bridget E; 253-99 Fifth Ave, Ottawa ON K1S 5P5; Qns'07; CCFP; (613)224-8505

THOMPSON, Calvin P; The Ottawa Hosp-Gen Campus, 501 Smyth Rd, Ottawa ON K1H 8L6; Ott'95; FRCPC; Anes. Staff, The Ottawa Hospital - General Campus; Langs: English; French; (613)737-8187; Fax. (613)737-8189.

THOMPSON, Carly A; Royal Victoria Hosp, 201 Georgian Dr, Barrie ON L4M 6M2; McM'06; CCFP; CCFP(E.M.); Staff, Royal Victoria Regional Health Centre; (705)728-9802

THOMPSON, Caroline J; Scarborough Hosp-Gen Div, 3050 Lawrence Ave E, Scarborough ON M1P 2V5; Wes'01; CCFP; CCFP(E.M.); Staff, The Scarborough Hospital - General Campus; (416)438-2911

THOMPSON, Charles V; 1128-1550 Kingston Rd, Pickering ON L1V 6W9; Tor'02; FRCSC; OrthSurg. Staff, Toronto East General Hospital Inc; Staff, Mount Sinai Hospital.

THOMPSON, Christopher R; St Paul's Hosp, 2350-1081 Burrard St, Vancouver BC V6Z 1Y6; McG'77; FACC; FRFPS; FRCPC; Cardiol (Clinical Cardiology). Dir Cardiac Echo Lab, Providence Health Care - St Paul's Hospital; Clin Assoc Prof Med, University of British Columbia; (604)806-8018; Fax. (604)806-8410; cthompson@providencehealth.bc.ca.

THOMPSON, Darren J; Provincial Assessment Centre, 28-3405 Willingdon Ave, Burnaby BC V5G 3H4; Alb'93; DABPN; BMedSci; FRCPC; Psy (Geriatric Psychiatry). Staff, The Provincial Assessment Centre; Clinical Asst Prof, University of British Columbia; (604)660-0228

THOMPSON, David C; 640 North St PO Box 508, Dresden ON N0P 1M0; Qns'82; CCFP; FCFP; (519)683-2082; Fax. (519)683-6085.

THOMPSON, David K; Avenue Med Clinic, 221 Brant Ave, Brantford ON N3T 3J3; Qns'82; CCFP; FCFP; Ac Staff, The Brant Community Healthcare System - Brantford General Hospital Site; Langs: English; French; (519)753-8666; Fax. (519)753-6880.

THOMPSON, David M; Gordon & Leslie Diamond HCC, 4107-2775 Laurel St, Vancouver BC V5Z 1M9; UBC'78; FRCPC; IntMed (Endocrinology). Staff, UBC Hospital - Koerner Pavillion; Staff, Vancouver General Hospital - Centennial Pavillion; Staff, Gordon & Leslie Diamond Health Care Centre; (604)875-5996; Fax. (604)875-5925.

THOMPSON, Deborah L; IWK Health Centre, PO Box 9700 Rpo CSC 5850 University Ave, Halifax NS B3K 6R8; Dal'76; FRCPC; DiagRad. Staff, IWK Health Centre; (902)470-8060; Fax. (902)470-7463.

THOMPSON, Diana P G; New Best Care Med Centre, 4-790 Burnhamthorpe Rd W, Mississauga ON L5C 4G3; (Jamaica)'99; CCFP; Staff, New Best Care Medical Centre; (905)848-8686; Fax. (905)848-8796.

THOMPSON, Donald S; Peterborough Clinic FHT, 202-26 Hospital Dr, Peterborough ON K9J 7C3; Birmingham (England)'71; MB ChB; DA; Staff, Peterborough Regional Health Centre - Hospital Drive; Coroner, Peterborough Area; Pres/Coroner, Ontario Coroners Association; (705)740-6860; Fax. (705)740-6881.

THOMPSON, Douglas J; The Jenny Trout Centre, 204-342 Erie St, Stratford ON N5A 2N4; Tor'73; BSc(Hon); CCFP; Ac Staff, Stratford General Hospital - Huron Perth Healthcare Alliance; (519)271-2061; Fax. (519)271-8255.

THOMPSON, Elisabeth J; Westgrove Clinic, 201-505 Queen St, Spruce Grove AB T7X 2V2; Cal'94; CCFP; FCFP; (780)962-9888; Fax. (780)960-5298.

THOMPSON, Elizabeth B; Brant Community HC-Brantford, 200 Terrace Hill St, Brantford ON N3R 1G9; Mem'85; Staff, The Brant Community Healthcare System - Brantford General Hospital Site; (519)752-7871; Fax. (519)751-5507.

THOMPSON, Elizabeth; Victoria Gen Hosp, 1 Hospital Way, Victoria BC V8Z 6R5; McM'07; CCFP; Staff, Victoria General Hospital; (250)727-4212

THOMPSON, Ellen N; B22-550 Terminal Ave, Ottawa ON K1G 0Z3; Newcastle (England)'70; MB BS; FRCPC; Anes (Chronic Pain Management). Staff, The Ottawa Hospital - Civic Campus; Clinical Asst Prof, University of Ottawa; Langs: Danish; Norwegian; Swedish; (613)731-4770; Fax. (613)731-6201.

THOMPSON, Elu M; Springborough Prof Centre, 108-30 Springborough Blvd, Calgary AB T3H 0N9; McG'75; BSc; MDCM; ObstGyn. Staff, Rockyview General Hospital; (403)240-2221; Fax. (403)240-4670.

THOMPSON, Erin E; Piper Creek Med Clinic, 200-3215 49 Ave, Red Deer AB T4N 0M8; Alb'10; CCFP; (403)986-7265; Fax. (403)986-7604.

THOMPSON, Franklin C; Lions Gate Hosp, 231 15th St E, North Vancouver BC V7L 2L7; UBC'71; MCFP(EM); Staff Emerg, Lions Gate Hospital; (604)984-5799; Fax. (604)984-5828.

THOMPSON, Geoffrey B; 84 Chartwell Crt, Fredericton NB E3B 7A1; Mem'87; FRCPC; Anes.

THOMPSON, Graham C; Alberta Chidren's Hosp, 2888 Shaganappi Trail NW, Calgary AB T3B 6A8; Wes'00; FRCPC; Peds (Pediatric Emergency Medicine). Staff Emerg Med, Alberta Children's Hospital; (403)955-7295; Fax. (403)955-7552.

THOMPSON, Gregory; River Valley ENT Associates, 340 Brunswick St, Fredericton NB E3B 1H1; Dal'03; BSc; PhD; FRCSC; Otol (Head & Neck Surgery). Staff, Oromocto Public Hospital; Staff, Dr Everett Chalmers Regional Hospital; (506)457-3100; Fax. (506)457-3101; thompson@rivervalleyent.ca.

THOMPSON, Gregory K; Univ Hlth Network-Princess M, 610 University Ave, Toronto ON M5G 2M9; Dal'76; Staff, Princess Margaret Hospital - University Health Network; (416)946-2000

THOMPSON, Guy W S; London HSC-University Hosp, PO Boc 5339 Stn B ALL 113-339 Windermere Ave, London ON N6A 5A5; Wes'85; FRCP; FRCPC; IntMed (AIDS/HIV); InfectDis. Staff InfectDis, London Health Sciences Centre - University Hospital; (519)663-3849; Fax. (519)663-3232.

THOMPSON, Ian B; North Shore Family Health Team, PO Box 760 415 Scotia St, Schreiber ON P0T 2S0; Qns'91; CCFP; FCFP; Staff, The McCausland Hospital; Langs: Spanish; (807)824-2934; Fax. (807)824-2758.

THOMPSON, J Paul; Orthopaedic & Spinal Surgery, 214-145 13th St E, North Vancouver BC V7L 2L4; Wes'81; FRCSC; OrthSurg. Ac Staff, Providence Health Care - Mount Saint Joseph Hospital; Clin Instructor Orthopeds, University of British Columbia; (604)980-0883; Fax. (604)980-4759.

THOMPSON, James; Royal Jubilee Hosp, 1952 Bay St, Victoria BC V8R 1J8; UBC'98; FRCPC; EmergMed. Staff, Victoria General Hospital; Staff, Royal Jubilee Hospital; (250)370-8000

THOMPSON, James M; Dept of Veteran's Affairs, PO Box 7700 Stn Central, Charlottetown PE C1A 8M9; Cal'84; CCFP; CCFP(E.M.); FCFP; Staff, Queen Elizabeth Hospital; Physician, Veterans Affairs Canada; (902)566-8888; james.thompson@vac-acc.gc.ca.

THOMPSON, Jannette J; 270-5 Fairview Mall Dr, North York ON M2J 2Z1; West Indies (Jamaica)'94; CCFP; Langs: Spanish; (416)493-5244; Fax. (416)493-6225.

THOMPSON, Jean-Pierre; 286 rue de Normandie, Sainte-Julie QC J3E 1A7; Mon'76; Staff, Centre Hospitalier Honore-Mercier; Langs: Bilingual(French/English); (450)649-1593; Fax. (450)649-0361.

THOMPSON, Jeannine M; PO Box 31012, Langley BC V1M 0A9; Qns'05; CCFP.

THOMPSON, John L; 708-1155 Robson St, Vancouver BC V6E 1B5; Alb'81; (604)696-5244

THOMPSON, Judith A; St Joseph's Health Centre, 30 The Queensway, Toronto ON M6R 1B5; Tor'92; BSc; CCFP; FCFP; Staff Family Med Centre, St Joseph's Health Centre; Asst Prof ENR Physician Lead, University of Toronto; (416)530-6860; Fax. (416)530-6160; thompj@stjoe.on.ca.

THOMPSON, Karen M; Annapolis Valley Hlth Adult Me, 15 Chipman Dr, Kentville NS B4N 3V7; Mem'04; FRCPC; Psy. Staff, Annapolis Valley Health Adult Mental Health Program; (902)364-1701; Fax. (902)678-4917.

THOMPSON, Katherine M E; Mediclinic, 101-3333 8th St E, Saskatoon SK S7H 4K1; Tor'09; BSc; MSc; CCFP; (306)955-1530; Fax. (306)955-8811.

THOMPSON, Keith A; 213-1135 Adelaide St N, London ON N5Y 5K7; Wes'87; CCFP; FCFP; (519)660-1220; Fax. (519)660-8739.

THOMPSON, Kerry; Trillium Hlth Ctre-Mississauga, 100 Queensway W, Mississauga ON L5B 1B8; Ott'07; FRCPC; IntMed. Staff, Trillium Health Centre - Mississauga; (905)848-7557

THOMPSON, Krista L; Tantallon Family Practice, 202-5110 St Margarets Bay Rd, Upper Tantallon NS B3Z 1E2; Mem'88; BMedSci; CCFP; (902)826-2744; Fax. (902)826-2887; kltsmbmc@eastlink.ca.

THOMPSON, Margaret A; The Hosp for Sick Children, 2426-555 University Ave, Toronto ON M5G 1X8; Tor'82; FACMT; FRCPC; EmergMed (Toxicology). Staff, The Hospital For Sick Children; Staff Emerg, St Michael's Hospital; Med Dir, Ontario Poison Centre; (416)813-8870; Fax. (416)813-7489; margaret.thompson@sickkids.ca.

THOMPSON, Marian P; 220 Victoria Rd S, Guelph ON N1E 5R1; Tor'81; MSc; FRCSC; Ophth. Staff, Guelph General Hospital; (519)824-0733; Fax. (519)824-1348.

THOMPSON, Maureen E; Parry Sound Family Health Team, 15 James St, Parry Sound ON P2A 1T4; Wes'74; BSc; Ac Staff Family Med, West Parry Sound Health Centre; (705)746-9382; Fax. (705)746-7758.

THOMPSON, Melanie L; A2701-1600 90 Ave SW PO Box 72089 Rpo Glenmore Land, Calgary AB T2V 5H9; Cal'03; CCFP; (403)700-6329; Fax. (403)238-1517.

THOMPSON, Michael A; PO Box 430, Coronation AB T0C 1C0; (403)578-3232; Fax. (403)578-3235.

THOMPSON, Michael R; Pender Island Med Centre, 5715 Canal Rd, Pender Island BC V0N 2M1; Mangalore (India)'88; MB BS; (250)629-3233; Fax. (250)629-3234.

THOMPSON, Pamela A; Stonechurch Family Health Ctre, 1475 Upper Ottawa St, Hamilton ON L8W 3J6; McM'80; CCFP; FCFP; (905)574-1444; Fax. (905)575-9892.

THOMPSON, Pamela J; Business Bldg, 105-150 Crowfoot Cres NW, Calgary AB T3G 3T2; Alb'02; CCFP.

THOMPSON, Paul; 1503-625 av Président-Kennedy, Montreal QC H3A 1K2; Mon'74; FRCSC; Ophth. Staff, Centre Hospitalier l'Université de Montréal (CHUM) - Hôpital Notre-Dame; Langs: English; (514)849-9215; Fax. (514)849-5115.

THOMPSON, Penelope J; Hamilton HS-McMaster Site, PO Box 2000 Stn Lcd 1 MDCL 2202-1200 Main St W, Hamilton ON L8N 3Z5; McM'86; FRCPC; Peds (Neonatal & Perinatal Medicine). Staff, Hamilton Health Sciences Centre - McMaster University Medical Centre; (905)525-9140

THOMPSON, Robert G; Southland Plaza, 870-10201 Southport Rd SW, Calgary AB T2W 4X9; McG'75; FRCPC; IntMed; Gastroent. Ac Staff, Rockyview General Hospital; (403)259-3729; Fax. (403)252-5191.

THOMPSON, Robert J; Foothills Med Centre, 1403 29 St NW, Calgary AB T2N 2T9; Man'04; FRCPC; Anes. Staff, Foothills Medical Centre; (403)944-1430; Fax. (403)270-2268.

THOMPSON, Robert J; Ingram Family Physicians, 103-149 Ingram St, Duncan BC V9L 1N8; UBC'80; (250)746-4401

THOMPSON, Robert P; 808-1200 Burrard St, Vancouver BC V6Z 2C7; Sask'66; FRCSC; PlasSurg (Cosmetic Surgery). (604)681-5158

THOMPSON, Ryan M; Transcona Access, 845 Regent Ave W, Winnipeg MB R2C 3A9; Man'04; CCFP; rthompson@slmhc.on.ca.

THOMPSON, Sarah J; Mental Health Services, 3F-55 Union St, Saint John NB E2L 5B7; Dal'00; FRCPC; Psy (Geriatric Psychiatry). (506)658-3737

THOMPSON, Stephanie E; Research Transition Facility, 3064-8308 114 St NW, Edmonton AB T6G 2V2; Dal'06; FRCPC; IntMed; Nephrol. (780)407-8822; Fax. (780)407-3270.

THOMPSON, Stephen R; A34-481 North Service Rd W, Oakville ON L6M 2V6; Sydney (Australia)'05; FRCSC; OrthSurg. (905)844-7706; Fax. (905)844-7808.

THOMPSON, Susan E; Cumberland Reg Hlth Care Ctre, 19428 Highway 2, Amherst NS B4H 1N6; Mem'88; FRCPC; DiagRad. Staff, The Moncton Hospital; (902)667-3361

THOMPSON, Thomas R; A-194 Provencher Blvd, Winnipeg MB R2H 0G3; Man'83; MSc; BSc; FRCPC; Psy (Forensic Psychiatry - Adult). Member Manitoba Justice Review Board (Criminal Code), Province of Manitoba; Langs: French; Spanish; (204)237-8738; Fax. (204)237-8738; tomthomp@mts.net.

THOMPSON, Tracey A; Gatineau Cosmetic Surg Clinic, 3A-520 boul de l'Hopital, Gatineau QC J8V 2P5; Qns'91; FRCSC; PlasSurg (Breast Reconstruction). Staff, Hôpital de Gatineau; Staff, Queensway Carleton Hospital; Langs: English; French; (819)561-8739; Fax. (819)561-6929; info@cliniquegatineau.com.

THOMPSON, W Kevin; Southlake Reg Health Ctre, 596 Davis Dr, Newmarket ON L3Y 2P9; Tor'72; FRCPC; Anes. Staff Anes, Southlake Regional Health Centre; (905)853-2216 x2668; Fax. (905)853-2213.

THOMPSON, William M; St Joseph's Gen Hosp, 2137 Comox Ave, Comox BC V9M 1P2; Newcastle (England)'63; MB BS; DMRD(Ed); FRCPC; DiagRad; NuclearMed. Staff X-Ray Dept, St Joseph's General Hospital; (250)339-1420

THOMS, John W; Dr H Bliss Murphy Cancer Ctre, 300 Prince Philip Dr, St. John's NL A1B 3V6; Mem'04; FRCPC; RadOncol. Staff, Dr H Bliss Murphy Cancer Centre; (709)777-7602

THOMSEN, Anne Marie; 201-520 17th St, West Vancouver BC V7V 3S8; Alb'90; (604)913-8183; Fax. (604)913-8804.

THOMSEN, J Eric; B-274 Lynden Rd, Brantford ON N3T 5L8; Wes'89; FRCSC; Ophth. (519)758-8626; Fax. (519)758-9848.

THOMSON, Alan B R; University of Alberta Hosp, 2F1-8440 112 St NW, Edmonton AB T6G 2B7; Qns'67; MSc; PhD; FRCPC; Gastroent; IntMed. Staff, University of Alberta Hospital; Prof Med, University of Alberta; (780)492-8154; Fax. (780)492-7964; alan.thomson@ualberta.ca.

THOMSON, Alexandra E; Kingsfoil Med Clinic, 764 Bernard Ave, Kelowna BC V1Y 6P5; Wes'96; BSc; CCFP; Staff, Kelowna General Hospital; (250)979-0003; Fax. (250)979-0004.

THOMSON, Andrea L; Hamilton HS-Henderson Site, 711 Concession St, Hamilton ON L8V 1C3; McM'04; FRCPC; DiagRad. Staff, Hamilton Health Sciences Centre-Juravinski Site; (905)521-2100

THOMSON, Benjamin K A; London HSC-University Hosp, PO Box 5339 Stn B 339 Windermere Rd, London ON N6A 5A5; Cork (Ireland)'07; FRCPC; IntMed; Nephrol. Staff, London Health Sciences Centre - University Hospital; (519)685-8300

THOMSON, Brent R J; 1835 Corydon Ave, Winnipeg MB R3N 0K6; Man'82; CCBOM; CCFP; FCFP; (204)983-6330; Fax. (204)983-8534.

THOMSON, Bruce W; 100-302 The East Mall, Etobicoke ON M9B 6C7; Tor'63; GenPath. (416)231-7968; Fax. (416)231-7982; reception@aberfoyle.com.

THOMSON, Carol A; Old Quebec Street Mall, 208-55 Wyndham St N, Guelph ON N1H 7T8; McM'90; CCFP; FCFP; Court Staff, Homewood Health Centre; Court Staff, St Joseph's Health Centre; Court Staff, Guelph General Hospital; (519)837-1270; Fax. (519)767-2262.

THOMSON, Carolyn J; Dalhousie Family Medicine, 6960 Mumford Rd, Halifax NS B3L 4P1; Dal'89; BSc; CCFP; FCFP; Court Staff, IWK Health Centre; Teach Staff, Dalhousie Family Medicine; (902)473-4700; Fax. (902)473-8548; c.thomson@ns.sympatico.ca.

THOMSON, Christopher J; Medical Arts Bldg, 602-750 Spadina Cres E, Saskatoon SK S7K 3H3; Sask'02; FRCSC; PlasSurg (Hand & Wrist Surgery). (306)653-7766; Fax. (306)653-7768.

THOMSON, David B; East Van Med Bldg, 406-1750 10th Ave E, Vancouver BC V5N 5K4; UBC'86; CCFP; Ac Staff, Vancouver General Hospital - Centennial Pavillion; (604)872-1672; Fax. (604)872-7032.

THOMSON, David M; Peninsula FHT-Lions Head, 24 Moore St, Lions Head ON N0H 1W0; Dal'90; BSc(Hon); CCFP; FCFP; Site Chief/Preceptor ROMP, Grey Bruce Health Services - Lion's Head; Med Examiner, Transport Canada; Med Dir, Golden Dawn Nursing Home; Lecturer, University of Toronto; Aj Prof Med, University of Western Ontario; (519)793-3445; Fax. (519)793-4604; thomsond@tc.gc.ca.

THOMSON, David M P; MUHC-Mnotreal Gen Hosp, A6 149-1650 av Cedar, Montreal QC H3G 1A4; Wes'64; PhD(Lond); CSPQ; FRCP; FRCPC; IntMed (Allergy); ClinImmunol&Allergy. principale Médecin Clin Immunol & Allergy, McGill University Health Centre - Montreal General Campus; Prof Med, McGill University; Langs: Bilingual(English/French); (514)934-8038; Fax. (514)934-8570; david.thomson@muhc.mcgill.ca.

THOMSON, Diane R L; Ingram Family Physicians, 103-149 Ingram St, Duncan BC V9L 1N8; UBC'84; CCFP; FCFP; (250)746-4401

THOMSON, Dorothy J; Royal University Hosp, 103 Hospital Dr, Saskatoon SK S7N 0W8; Qns'79; FRCSC; Cardiovasc&ThorSurg. Ac Staff Surg, Royal University Hospital; (306)966-8170; Fax. (306)966-6932.

THOMSON, Glen T D; Thomson House, 1835 Corydon Ave, Winnipeg MB R3N 0K6; Man'81; FRCPC; IntMed (Ankylosing Spondylitis); Rheum. Dir, Center for Inflamatory & Arthritis Disease Studies; Assoc Prof, University of Manitoba; (204)947-1766

THOMSON, Gregory W; Argus Med Centre, 300-581 Argus Rd, Oakville ON L6J 3J4; Qns'76; Med Dir Rehab & Geriatrics Prog, Halton Healthcare Services Corporation - Oakville Site; Med Dir, Villages of Halton Region; (905)338-9900; Fax. (905)338-9904; gthomson@haltonhealthcare.on.ca.

THOMSON, Ian R; St Boniface Gen Hosp, 409 Tache Ave, Winnipeg MB R2H 2A6; Man'71; MB ChB; FRCPC; Anes. Staff, St Boniface General Hospital; (204)233-8563

THOMSON, James G; Hamilton HS-Henderson Site, 711 Concession St, Hamilton ON L8V 1C3; Edinburgh (Scotland)'69; MB ChB; DMRD; FRCR; FRCPC; DiagRad (Diagnostic Imaging). Ac Staff Radiol, Hamilton Health Sciences Centre-Juravinski Site; Clin Assoc Prof, McMaster University; (905)389-4411; Fax. (905)575-2660.

THOMSON, John G; B2-194 Main St, Ottawa ON K1S 1C2; Ott'78; FRCPC; IntMed; Rheum. Staff (All Sites), The Ottawa Hospital - General Campus; Asst Prof, University of Ottawa; Langs: English; French; (613)232-2604; Fax. (613)232-2779; thomper@sympatico.ca.

THOMSON, Julie J; Maternal Child Clinic, 130-1402 8 Ave NW, Calgary AB T2N 1B9; Cal'03; CCFP; (403)284-8711

THOMSON, June A K; King Street Med Arts Centre, 407-71 King St W, Mississauga ON L5B 4A2; Tor'63; Ac Staff, Trillium Health Centre - Mississauga; (905)279-1340; Fax. (905)279-0382.

THOMSON, Katherine A; Fairview Med Arts Centre, 208-2200 Fairview St, Burlington ON L7R 4H9; McM'01; CCFP; (905)333-5245; Fax. (905)632-2617.

THOMSON, Leanne M; Kincardine Community Med Clini, 44 Queen St, Kincardine ON N2Z 3C1; McM'92; CCFP; FCFP; Staff, South Bruce Grey Health Centre - Kincardine Site; Langs: English; French; (519)396-6769; Fax. (519)396-6707.

THOMSON, Margaret B; Alberta Children's Hosp, 2888 Shaganappi Trail NW, Calgary AB T3B 6A8; McG'89; FRCPC; Peds (Diabetes). Staff, Alberta Children's Hospital; (403)955-7070; Fax. (403)955-7869.

THOMSON, Mari-Lynn; Newell Associates Clinic, PO Box 280 Stn Main 220 4th St W, Brooks AB T1R 1B3; Belfast (Ireland)'90; Staff, Brooks Health Centre; (403)362-5501; Fax. (403)362-8426.

THOMSON, Mark F; Abc Medical Clinic, 9842 101 Ave, Fort St. John BC V1J 2B2; Cape Town (South Africa)'88; MB ChB; (250)785-1220; Fax. (250)785-9750.

THOMSON, Merrin M; Grey Bruce HS-Owen Sound, PO Box 1800 Stn Main 1800 8th St E, Owen Sound ON N4K 6M9; McM'76; FCFP; Staff, Grey Bruce Health Services - Owen Sound; (519)376-2121 x2345

THOMSON, Robert J; Min of Hlth & Long-Term Care, PO Box 168 Stn Main 370 Select Dr, Kingston ON K7L 5V1; Ott'73; Med Consultant, Provider Services Branch-OHIP; (613)536-3054

THOMSON, Scott M; Grey Bruce HS-Owen Sound, PO Box 1400 Stn Main 1800 8th St E, Owen Sound ON N4K 6M9; Tor'85; FRCPC; DiagRad. Staff, Grey Bruce Health Services - Owen Sound; (519)376-2121; Fax. (519)372-3954.

THOMSON, Sydney L; Gordon & Leslie Diamond HCC, 6F-2775 Laurel St, Vancouver BC V5Z 1M9; UBC'85; FRCSC; ObstGyn (Sexual Medicine). Assoc Staff Gyn, Vancouver General Hospital - Centennial Pavillion; Staff, Gordon & Leslie Diamond Health Care Centre; Clinical Asst Prof, University of British Columbia; (604)875-4260 x4268; Fax. (604)875-4869.

THOMSON, Thomas A; BC Cancer Agency-Vancouver CC, 600 10th Ave W, Vancouver BC V5Z 4E6; UBC'72; BSc; FRCPC; GenPath (Surgical Oncology). Staff, BC Cancer Agency Vancouver Centre; Clin Assoc Prof, University of British Columbia; (604)877-6000; Fax. (604)873-5384; tthomson@bccancer.bc.ca.

THOMSON, Tracy C; Gaia Collaborative Medicine, 101-75 Dyrgas Gate, Canmore AB T1W 0A6; Wes'91; HBSc; CCFP; (403)675-4242; Fax. (403)675-4243; info@gaiaclinic.ca.

THOMSON, Valerie R; 26 Forbes St, Cambridge ON N3C 2E2; Tor'84; BScN; Affil Staff Outpatient Mental Health, Cambridge Memorial Hospital; (519)658-4615; Fax. (519)658-4630.

THOMSON, Veronica M; 6217-2850 Shaughnessy St, Port Coquitlam BC V3C 6K5; Dublin (Ireland)'74.

THONG, Chee Nyok; Medical Bldg, 809-805 Broadway W, Vancouver BC V5Z 1K1; Dublin (Ireland)'72; LRCPSI; FRCSI; FRCSC; Otol. Ac Staff, BC Children's Hospital; Vis Staff, Providence Health Care - St Paul's Hospital; Staff, Boundary Park Medical Centre; Dir, British Columbia Ear Bank; Clin Assoc Prof, University of British Columbia; Langs: Cantonese; Hakka; Indonesian; Malay; (604)872-4566

THONGTHAI, Kanyabhorn; Postgrad Med Education Office, 602-500 University Ave, Toronto ON M5G 1V7; Chulalongkorn University (Thailand)'04; FRCPC; IntMed.

THONI, Andrea J; Dartmouth Gen Hosp, 2309A-325 Pleasant St, Dartmouth NS B2Y 4G8; McM'97; FRCPC; GenPath;CCFP; Staff, Dartmouth General Hospital; (902)465-8306; Fax. (902)465-8558.

THORBURN, James P; Janeway Children's Hlth & Reha, 300 Prince Philip Dr, St. John's NL A1B 3V6; Mem'10; CCFP; Staff, Janeway Children's Health & Rehabilitation Centre; (709)777-6300

THORDARSON, Ian T; Royal Columbian Hosp, 330 Columbia St E, New Westminster BC V3L 3W7; UBC'91; FRCPC; EmergMed;CCFP; CCFP(E.M.); FCFP; Staff, Royal Columbian Hospital; (604)520-4640

THORLAKSON, Derek P; Salvation Army Grace Hosp, 300 Booth Dr, Winnipeg MB R3J 3M7; Man'85; Staff, Misericordia Health Centre; Staff, The Salvation Army Grace Hospital; (204)837-0391

THORLAKSON, Ian J; Victoria Gen Hosp, 2340 Pembina Hwy, Winnipeg MB R3T 2E8; Man'93; Staff, Victoria General Hospital; (204)269-3570

THORLAKSON, Robert H; Winnipeg Clinic, 425 St Mary Ave, Winnipeg MB R3C 0N2; Man'49; FRCS; FACS; FRCSC; GenSurg. Ac Staff, Health Sciences Centre; Ac Staff, Seven Oaks General Hospital; Prof, University of Manitoba; (204)957-1900; Fax. (204)943-2164.

THORNE, J Carter; 43 Lundys Lane, Newmarket ON L3Y 3R7; Tor'76; ABIM; FACP; FACRheum; FRCPC; IntMed (Adult Rheumatology); Rheum. Consultant/Ac Staff, Southlake Regional Health Centre; Court Staff Cons Staff, Royal Victoria Regional Health Centre; VP, Canadian Rheumatology Association; Prin Investigator, The Arthritis Program Research Group Inc; Teacher, University of Toronto; (905)895-0525; Fax. (905)895-6536.

THORNE, James D; Canadian Sport Medicine, 2424 University Dr NW, Calgary AB T2N 3Y9; Alb'82; BSc; CCFP; (403)289-8959; Fax. (403)284-9139.

THORNE, Mary J; East Kootenay Reg Hosp, 13 24th Ave N, Cranbrook BC V1C 3H9; Tor'87; BSc; MSc; CCFP(E.M.); CCFP(E.M.); Staff, East Kootenay Regional Hospital; (250)426-5281

THORNE, Susan F; 333 Main St PO Box 190, Liverpool NS B0T 1K0; Dal'91; BSc; CCFP; FCFP; Ac Staff, Queens General Hospital; (902)354-4855; Fax. (902)354-7301.

THORNE, Tracey E; Gabriola Med Clinic, PO Box 200 377 Berry Point Rd, Gabriola BC V0R 1X0; Dal'07; CCFP; (250)247-9922

THORNELOE, W David; Dixie Road Med Associates, 2200 Dixie Rd, Mississauga ON L4Y 1Z4; Tor'76; CCFP; FCFP; Staff, Trillium Health Centre - Mississauga; (905)279-1700; Fax. (905)897-9167.

THORNER, Paul S; The Hosp for Sick Children, 555 University Ave, Toronto ON M5G 1X8; Tor'78; PhD; FCAP; FRCPC; AnatPath. Assoc Head Div of Path, The Hospital For Sick Children; Prof Path, University of Toronto; (416)813-5108; Fax. (416)813-5974.

THORNER, Richard S; Dixie Road Med Associates, 2200 Dixie Rd, Mississauga ON L4Y 1Z4; Tor'64; CCFP; FCFP; Ac Staff Family Med, Trillium Health Centre - Mississauga; (905)279-1700; Fax. (905)897-9167.

THORNHILL, George M; 1283 Manawagonish Rd, Saint John NB E2M 3X8; Dal'69; (506)635-8889; Fax. (506)674-1166; maxwel@nb.aibn.com.

THORNLEY, Glenn D; Georgian Prof Centre, 203-125 Bell Farm Rd, Barrie ON L4M 6L2; Qns'75; FRCSC; Otol (General Surgery). Otolaryngology, Huronia Regional Centre; Staff, Royal Victoria Regional Health Centre; Otolaryngology, Collingwood General & Marine Hospital; (705)737-3422; Fax. (705)725-7330.

THORNTON, John F R; 205-1246 Yonge St, Toronto ON M4T 1W5; Dublin (Ireland)'72; MB ChB; BAO; FRCPC; Psy (Chronic Pain). (416)926-8944; Fax. (416)926-8944.

THORNTON, Mary D; Peterborough Reg HC-Hospital, 1 Hospital Dr, Peterborough ON K9J 7C6; Laval'90; FRCPC; Psy (Psycho Pharmacology). Staff, Peterborough Regional Health Centre - Hospital Drive; (705)876-5028; Fax. (705)876-5013.

THORNTON, Pamela J; Peace Arch Hosp, 15521 Russell Ave, White Rock BC V4B 2R4; UBC'97; FRCPC; IntMed; GeriatricMed. Staff Elder Health, Peace Arch Hospital; (604)535-4577; Fax. (604)535-4587.

THORNTON, Peter N; Strathcona Family Med Centre, 246-30 Springborough Blvd SW, Calgary AB T3H 0N9; Tor'91; CCFP; (403)777-9935; Fax. (403)777-9938.

THORNTON, Tanya H; Happy Valley Family Hlth Team, PO Box 1120 268 Maiden Lane, St Marys ON N4X 1B7; Tor'02; CCFP; (519)284-3450; Fax. (519)284-4471; tthornton@stmmc.ca.

THOROGOOD, Mark D; The Avenues Clinic, 2801C 13th Ave, Medicine Hat AB T1A 3R1; (Zimbabwe)'82; MB ChB; LMCC; DCH(SA); CCFP; FCFP; Physician, Medicine Hat Regional Hospital; Physician, Primary Care Network; (403)526-1950; Fax. (403)526-1930.

THOROGOOD, William D; Delhi Family Health Team, 105 Main Street of Delhi, Delhi ON N4B 2L8; McM'94; CCFP; Staff, Norfolk General Hospital; Staff, West Haldimand General Hospital; (519)582-2323 x222; Fax. (519)582-1513.

THORPE, B Patricia; Fredericton Med Clinic, 203-1015 Regent St, Fredericton NB E3B 6H5; Dal'74; Staff, Dr Everett Chalmers Regional Hospital; (506)458-0237; Fax. (506)459-3302.

THORPE, Dominic J; Royal Jubilee Hosp, 1952 Bay St, Victoria BC V8R 1J8; UBC'88; Staff, Royal Jubilee Hospital; (250)370-8000 x2085

THORPE, John B; West Street Health Centre, 302-216 West St, Simcoe ON N3Y 1S8; Qns'76; FRCSC; Ophth. (519)426-9851; Fax. (519)426-6154.

THORPE, Lilian U; Saskatoon City Hosp, 7027-701 Queen St, Saskatoon SK S7K 0M7; Tor'82; FRCPC; Psy (Geriatric Psychiatry). Staff Geriatric Special Prog, Saskatoon City Hospital; Chair Section of Geriatric Psy, Canadian Psychiatric Association; Clin Prof Psy, University of Saskatchewan; Langs: German; (306)655-7997; Fax. (306)655-7995; thorpel@sdh.sk.ca.

THORPE, Marilyn B; London Medical-Dental Bldg, 204-450 Central Ave, London ON N6B 2E8; McM'86; FRCPC; Psy (Adolescent Psychiatry). Asst Prof, University of Western Ontario; (519)433-1123

THORPE, R Brandon; South Hill Med Clinic, 890A Lillooet St W, Moose Jaw SK S6H 8B4; Witwatersrand (South Africa)'89; MB ChB; Prov Med Dir Acute & Emerg Med Services, Ministry Of Health-Saskatchewan; Chief Family Pract/Reg Med Acute & Emerg Med Services/Dir Teen Wellness Clinic, Five Hills Health Region; Physician, South Hill Medical Centre; (306)691-0030; Fax. (306)694-5666.

THORPE, William R; North Middlesex Comm Clinic, PO Box 490 268 Parkhill Main St, Parkhill ON N0M 2K0; Qns'75; MSc(Pharm.); Court Staff, Strathroy Middlesex General Hospital - Middlesex Hospital Alliance; Consultant Med, Workplace Safety & Insurance Board; (519)294-6881; Fax. (519)294-6982; admin@nmcmc.ca.

THORSON, J Douglas; Kingsland Med Clinic, 7712 Elbow Dr SW, Calgary AB T2V 1K2; Cal'74; Ac Staff Geriatric Rehab, Rockyview General Hospital; Ac Staff, Bethany Care Centre; Member, Southern Alberta Regional Geriatric Program; Physician, Chinook Nursing Homes; Physician, Mayfair Nursing Homes; Beverly Nursing Homes; (403)252-6681; Fax. (403)252-9741.

THORSTEINSON, Larry S; 675 Ripple Rd, Sudbury ON P3E 3P5; Qns'72; FACEP; CCFP; CCFP(E.M.); Staff, Health Sciences North - Memorial Site; University of Ottawa; Langs: English; French; (705)671-3008

THORSTEINSON, V James; Three Bridges Comm Health Ctre, 1292 Hornby St, Vancouver BC V6Z 1W2; Man'73; CCFP; FCFP; Staff, Three Bridges Community Health Centre; Exec Dir, BC College of Family Physicians; Staff Providence Hlthcare & Vancouver Commun, Vancouver Coastal Health; Assoc Prof Family Pract, University of British Columbia; (604)633-4220

THOTTINGAL, Antony P; Boyd Med Centre, 803-388 Portage Ave, Winnipeg MB R3C 0C8; Kasturba (India)'64.

THOTTINGAL, Paul A; Boyd Bldg, 803-388 Portage Ave, Winnipeg MB R3C 0C8; Man'95; FRCPC; IntMed; InfectDis.

THOUIN, Dominique; CSSS de la Cote-de-Gaspe, 215 boul de York O, Gaspe QC G4X 2W2; Mon'93; FRCPC; Psy. Staff, Centre Hospitalier de Gaspe; (418)368-3301 x4220; Fax. (418)368-3481.

THOUIN, Susan K; Scarborough Hosp-Gen Div, 3050 Lawrence Ave E, Scarborough ON M1P 2V5; Tor'06; CCFP; CCFP(E.M.); Staff, The Scarborough Hospital - General Campus; Staff, Lakeridge Health - Port Perry Site; (416)438-2911; Fax. (416)431-8204.

THOW, David P; Oshawa Clinic, 117 King St E, Oshawa ON L1H 1B9; Man'87; CCFP; FCFP; (905)721-6969; Fax. (905)721-6605.

THRASHER, Sarah M; Kerrisdale Travel & Immunizati, 2077 42nd Ave W, Vancouver BC V6M 2B4; UBC'70; (604)261-9494

THRENDYLE, Kenneth L; 1494 St Clair Pky PO Box 220, Courtright ON N0N 1H0; Wes'55; (519)867-2644; Fax. (519)867-3573.

THUAT, Nam; St Michael's Family Health Ctr, 13930 74 St NW, Edmonton AB T5C 3H7; Alb'01; CCFP; Langs: Vietnamese; (780)457-1600; Fax. (780)472-4799.

THUAUDET, Danielle; 611-4022 av de Kent, Montreal QC H3S 1N6; Mon'73; Staff, McGill University Health Centre - Royal Victoria Hospital; Fax. (514)731-4563.

THULL-FREEDMAN, Jennifer D; Alberta Children's Hosp, 2888 Shaganappi Trail NW, Calgary AB T3B 6A8; Thomas Jefferson University (USA)'97; Staff, Alberta Children's Hospital; (403)955-7093; Fax. (403)955-7552; jdthull@yahoo.com.

THUOT, Amelie; CSSS Haut-Richelieu-Rouville, 920 boul du Seminaire N, St-Jean-Sur-Richel QC J3A 1B7; Sher'99; FRCPC; MedMicrobiol (Infectious Diseases). Staff InfectDis, Hôpital du Haut-Richelieu; Langs: English; (450)359-5000 x5200

THUOT, Evelyne; Clinique Externe de Psychiatri, 10345 rue Papineau, Montreal QC H1A 0A1; Sher'04; FRCPC; Psy. Staff, Centre Hospitalier Fleury; (514)383-5080

THUOT, Francois J L; CHUQ-Hotel-Dieu de Quebec, 11 Cote Du Palais, Quebec QC G1R 2J6; Sher'95; FRCSC; Otol. Staff, Centre Hospitalier Universitaire de Québec (CHUQ) - Siege Social; (418)525-4444

THUOT, Pierre; 105-1055 12e av N, Fleurimont QC J1E 2X4; Mon'69; (819)821-2142; Fax. (819)821-0248.

THURAIRAJAH, Indranee; Addiction & Mental Hlth-Queen, 1001 Queen St W, Toronto ON M6J 1H4; Peradeniya (Sri Lanka)'67; MB BS; FRCPC; Psy (General Adult Psychiatry). Staff, Centre for Addiction & Mental Health (CAMH) - Queen Site; Langs: Tamil; (416)535-8501

THURAIRAJAH, Rajeswary; Trillium Hlth Ctre-Mississauga, 100 Queensway W, Mississauga ON L5B 1B8; (Sri Lanka)'70; MRC(Eng); FRCSC; ObstGyn (Prenatal Care). Staff, Trillium Health Centre - Mississauga; Langs: Tamil; (905)848-7100

THURBER, Lynette A; 100-5791 No 3 Rd, Richmond BC V6X 2C9; UBC'75; FRCPC; DiagRad. Staff Radiol, Burnaby Hospital; Staff Radiol, Richmond Hospital; (604)278-9152; Fax. (604)278-9291.

THURGOOD, Ann M; Dalhousie Health Services, 1459 Oxford St, Halifax NS B3H 2R4; Dal'93; FRCPC; Psy. Staff, Canadian Forces Health Services Centre (Atlantic); (902)494-2171

THURGOOD, Elaine N; Oxford Med Centre, 312 Oxford St W, London ON N6H 4N7; UBC'81; (519)432-6786; Fax. (519)432-3292.

THURGUR, Claire H; Vernon Jubilee Hosp, 2101 32 St, Vernon BC V1T 5L2; Tor'02; FRCPC; DiagRad. Staff, Vernon Jubilee Hospital; (250)558-1200

THURGUR, Lisa D; Sunnybrook Hlth Sciences Ctre, C753-2075 Bayview Ave, Toronto ON M4N 3M5; Cal'02; EmergMed (Clinical Pharmacology). Staff, Sunnybrook Health Sciences Centre; Langs: Bilingual(English/French); (416)480-4037

THURLEY, Jane; Psychiatric Associates, 202-10 Alcorn Ave, Toronto ON M4V 3A9; Tor'86; FRCPC; Psy. (416)944-1279; Fax. (416)975-0129.

THURLING, M Lynne; Groves Mem Community Hosp, 140-235 Union St E, Fergus ON N1M 1W3; McM'78; PhD; FRCPC; Psy (Adult Psychiatry). Staff, Groves Memorial Community Hospital; Asst Prof, University of Toronto; Langs: English; French; (519)787-3791; Fax. (519)843-7420.

THURSTON, Peter R; Riverside Prof Centre, 312-1919 Riverside Dr, Ottawa ON K1H 1A2; Ott'74; BSc; FRCSC; OrthSurg (Arthroplasty). Staff, The Ottawa Hospital - General Campus; Consultant, Renfrew Victoria Hospital; Langs: English; French; (613)736-7615; Fax. (613)733-3651.

THURSTON, Wendy A; St Joseph's Health Centre, 30 The Queensway, Toronto ON M6R 1B5; Tor'83; BSc; FRCPC; DiagRad (Abdominal Imaging). Dept Chief Diagnostic Imaging, St Joseph's Health Centre; Asst Prof, University of Toronto; (416)530-6027; Fax. (416)530-6025; thursw@stjoe.on.ca.

THWALA, Andrea B; Flin Flon Gen Hosp Inc, PO Box 340 500 Church St, Flin Flon MB R8A 1N2; BSc; MB ChB; Staff, Flin Flon General Hospital Inc; (204)687-7591

THWIN, Noreen; Parry Sound Family Health Team, 15 James St, Parry Sound ON P2A 1T4; Rangoon (Burma)'78; MB BS; (705)746-9382; Fax. (705)746-7758.

THYAGU, Santhosh; Univ Hlth Network-Princess M, 5F-610 University Ave, Toronto ON M5G 2M9; Kerala (India)'92; Staff, Princess Margaret Hospital - University Health Network; (416)946-4501; Fax. (416)946-2105.

THYER, Linda N; UBC Student Health Services, M334-2211 Wesbrook Mall, Vancouver BC V6T 1Z3; McG'94; CCFP; Staff, University of British Columbia Student Health Services; Langs: Bilingual(French/English); (604)822-7011

TIAB, George A; Beautiful Plains Comm Med Clin, PO Box 70 499 Mountain Ave, Neepawa MB R0J 1H0.

TIAH, Ai Lin; Fairmont Med Bldg, 1314-750 Broadway W, Vancouver BC V5Z 1J3; RCS (Ireland)'00; FRCPC; Peds. Staff, Providence Health Care - St Paul's Hospital; (604)879-4564

TIBBET, Juliana S; Toronto East Gen & Orth Hosp, J6100-825 Coxwell Ave, East York ON M4C 3E7; Tor'01; FRCPC; Anes. Staff, Toronto East General Hospital Inc; (416)461-8272

TIBBLES, Lee Anne; HSC-Faculty of Med, 4A12-3280 Hospital Dr NW, Calgary AB T2N 4Z6; Ott'89; BSc(Hon); FRCPC; IntMed (Transplantation); Nephrol. Asst Prof, University of Calgary; (403)220-2064; Fax. (403)283-1267; tibbles@ucalgary.ca.

TIBBO, Jamie J; ENT Consultants, 219-1 Paton St, St. John's NL A1B 4S8; Mem'04; Otol (Head & Neck Surgery). (709)579-1003

TIBBO, Perry M; 207-725 Coronation Blvd, Cambridge ON N1R 7S9; Mem'84; (519)620-2775; Fax. (519)620-2540.

TIBBO, Philip G; Abbey J Lane Memorial Bldg, 3030-5909 Veteran's Memorial L, Halifax NS B3H 2E2; Mem'91; FRCPC; Psy. (902)473-1678

TIBONI, Maria-Elena; St Joseph's Healthcare, 50 Charlton Ave E, Hamilton ON L8N 4A6; Buenos Aires (Argentina)'91; FRCPC; IntMed. Staff, St Joseph's Healthcare - Charlton Campus; Langs: Italian; Spanish; French; (905)522-1155; Fax. (905)521-6068.

TICEA, Marilena C; Old Orchard Med Clinic, 11-4429 Kingsway, Burnaby BC V5H 2A1; Bucharest (Romania)'94; CCFP; (604)431-6585

TICHY, Danusa; Park Royal Med Clinic, 560-580 Park Royal N, West Vancouver BC V7T 1H9; Safarika (Slovakia)'69; Vis Staff, Providence Health Care - St Vincent's Hospital-Heather Site; Consultant, Surrey Memorial Hospital; Staff, Park Royal Medical Clinic; (604)922-7390

TICK, Heather S; Cdn Mem Chiropractic College, 6100 Leslie St, North York ON M2H 3J1; Tor'82; CAFCI; CCFP; Staff, Canadian Memorial Chiropractic College; (416)482-2340; Fax. (416)646-1115.

TICKTIN, Stephen J; Sunnyside Med Arts Centre, 404-27 Roncesvalles Ave, Toronto ON M6R 3B2; Tor'73; BA; MRCPsy; MA; (905)709-9279

TICOLL, Brian; Markham Stouffville Health Ctr, 408-377 Church St, Markham ON L6B 1A1; Sher'80; FRCPC; Psy. Ac Staff, Markham Stouffville Hospital; Langs: Spanish; Italian; French; (905)472-5733; Fax. (905)472-5215.

TIDD, Christopher M; London HSC-Victoria Hosp, PO Box 5010 Stn B A2 550-800 Commissioners Rd E, London ON N6A 5W9; New York (USA)'97; Psy. Staff, London Health Sciences Centre - Victoria Campus; Staff, Regional Mental Health Care-St Joseph's Health Care; (519)685-8500

TIDMARSH, Mary E L; Fairmont Med Bldg, 1314-750 Broadway W, Vancouver BC V5Z 1J3; McG'77; BSc; MDCM; FRCPC; Psy (Autism). Staff Psy, Dr Thiessen & Associates Paediatric Clinic; Staff Psy/Consultant Interior Reg Health Authority, Fraser Health Authority Corporate Office; Langs: Bilingual(English/French); (604)374-4255; lee.tidmarsh@fraserhealth.ca.

TIEDE, Roger H; East Kootenay Reg Hosp, 13 24 Ave N, Cranbrook BC V1C 3H9; Man'90; G R Baker Memorial Hospital; Staff, East Kootenay Regional Hospital; Langs: German; (250)489-6432; rtiede@goldcity.net.

TIEDEMANN, Rodger E; Univ Hlth Network-Princess M, 9 721-610 University Ave, Toronto ON M5G 2M9; Auckland (New Zealand)'98; Staff, Princess Margaret Hospital - University Health Network; (416)946-2359; Fax. (416)946-6546.

TIEDJE, I E Henry; Killaloe Med Centre, RR 2 45 Mill St PO Box 5, Killaloe ON K0J 2A0; Tor'73; CCFP; Chief Medical Staff, St Francis Memorial Hospital; Court Staff, Pembroke Regional Hospital Inc; Province of Ontario; (613)757-2095; Fax. (613)757-3680.

TIEGS, Richard G; 944 Queen's Blvd, Kitchener ON N2M 1B4; Wes'71; (519)579-3020; Fax. (519)579-3893.

TIEN, Homer C; Sunnybrook Hlth Sciences Ctre, H186-2075 Bayview Ave, Toronto ON M4N 3M5; McM'92; FRCSC; GenSurg (Trauma). Staff, Sunnybrook Health Sciences Centre; Langs: Chinese; (416)480-5850; Fax. (416)480-5851.

TIEN, Teri C Y; Kingsway Med Clinic, 4645 Kingsway, Burnaby BC V5H 2B3; Alb'06; CCFP; (604)558-2611

TIERNEY, Anne J; Foothills Med Centre, 1403-1403 29 St, Calgary AB T2N 2T9; National (Ireland)'76; DCH; DObst; MRC; FRCP; FRCPC; Peds (Neonatology). Staff NICU, Foothills Medical Centre; (403)944-1939; Fax. (403)944-4892; anne.tierney@calgaryhealthregion.ca.

TIERNEY, James J; Western Mem Reg Hosp, PO Box 2005 Stn Main 1 Brookfield Ave, Corner Brook NL A2H 6J7; Galway (Ireland)'70; MB ChB; BAO; Locum Tenens, Sir Thomas Roddick Hospital; Staff, Western Memorial Regional Hospital; (709)637-5000

TIERNEY, Shauna L; Health Point Care Centre, 1454 Hillside Ave, Victoria BC V8T 2B7; UBC'06; CCFP; (250)370-5637; Fax. (604)225-2557.

TIESSEN, Alan C; Peter Lougheed Centre, 3500 26 Ave NE, Calgary AB T1Y 6J4; Cal'93; FRCPC; Anes. Staff Anes, Peter Lougheed Centre; (403)943-5554; Fax. (403)943-4474.

TIETZE, Linda; Medicine Professional Corp, 110-2425 Tecumseh Rd E, Windsor ON N8W 1E6; Tor'96; FRCSC; Otol (Head & Neck Surgery). Ac Staff, Windsor Regional Hospital - Metropolitan Site; Ac Staff, Hôtel-Dieu Grace Hospital; (519)252-9196; Fax. (519)256-8926.

TIGCHELAAR, Sandra R; Couchiching Family Health Team, 201C-119 Memorial Ave, Orillia ON L3V 5X1; Qns'96; CCFP; FCFP; (705)326-2208; Fax. (705)325-9498.

TIGCHELAAR, Timothy C; Orillia Soldier's Mem Hosp, 170 Colborne St W, Orillia ON L3V 2Z3; Qns'97; CCFP; CCFP(E.M.); FCFP; Staff, Orillia Soldiers' Memorial Hospital; (705)325-2201

TIGERT, Scott S; 502-2000 Credit Valley Rd, Mississauga ON L5M 4N4; Tor'89; FRCSC; ObstGyn. (905)820-8748; Fax. (905)820-0255.

TIGHE, Bryan F; Penticton Reg Hosp, 101-550 Carmi Ave, Penticton BC V2A 3G6; Dublin (Ireland)'74; MB ChB; BAO; FRCS(I); FRCSC; GenSurg. Staff, Penticton Regional Hospital; (250)493-7750

TIGHE, Spencer A; Pinecrest Queensway Act Team, 215B-1365 Richmond Rd, Ottawa ON K2B 6R7; Tor'86; FRCPC; Psy (Clinical Research). Physician, Pinecrest-Queensway Community Health Centre; (613)820-4922 x465; Fax. (613)820-3995.

TIGUERT, Rabi; Centre Med Berger Inc, 416-1000 ch Sainte-Foy, Quebec QC G1S 2L6; Alger (Algeria)'86; assoc Prof, Université Laval; Langs: Arabic; (418)266-2879; Fax. (418)266-2879.

TIHAL, Hirawan; 200-180 James St S, Hamilton ON L8P 4V1; McM'74; FRCPC; IntMed; Cardiol. Asst Prof Med, McMaster University; (905)523-0244; Fax. (905)523-0284; htihal@hotmail.com.

TIISLAR, Milvi K; Royal Jubilee Hosp, 1952 Bay St, Victoria BC V8R 1J8; Tor'08; CCFP; Staff, Royal Jubilee Hospital; Langs: Bilingual(English/French); (250)370-8000

TIJSSEN, Janice A; The Hosp For Sick Children, 555 University Ave, Toronto ON M5G 1X8; McG'06; MDCM; FRCPC; Peds (Critical Care Medicine). Staff, The Hospital For Sick Children; Langs: Bilingual(English/French); (416)813-1500

TIKHONOVA, Elina; 205-125 13th St E, North Vancouver BC V7L 2L3; Minsk (Belarus)'91; CCFP; (604)985-9551

TIKKANEN, Kaarina V; 404 Medical Clinic, 39-1111 Davis Dr, Newmarket ON L3Y 8X2; Tor'83; CCFP; (905)895-1992; Fax. (905)898-2553.

TIKKISETTY, Bhanu P; The Landmark Med Centre, 7-4150 Albert St, Regina SK S4S 3R8; Rangaraya (Other Foreign)'95; FRCPC; IntMed; Nephrol. Physician, The Landmark Medical Centre; (306)352-3018; Fax. (306)352-1476; btikkisetty@sasktel.net.

TILBE, Kim S; 402-65 Larch St., Sudbury ON P3E 1B8; McM'83; MSc; FRCPC; IntMed (Gastroenterology). Ac Staff, Health Sciences North - Memorial Site; Court Staff, Stevenson Memorial Hospital; Reg Dir Internal Med, Northern Ontario School of Medicine-Lakehead University; (705)670-8911; Fax. (705)670-8592; gi.tilbe@bellnet.ca.

TILBROOK, Devon S J; Sioux Lookout Zone Fam Phys, PO Box 4000, Sioux Lookout ON P8T 1K2; Qns'06; CCFP; (807)737-5160; Fax. (807)737-4364.

TILDESLEY, Hugh D; 410-1033 Davie St, Vancouver BC V6E 1M7; McG'75; ABIM; FRCPC; IntMed (Diabetes). Ac Staff, Providence Health Care - St Paul's Hospital; Consultant, Kelowna General Hospital; Consultant, Vancouver General Hospital - Centennial Pavillion; Prof Med, University of British Columbia; (604)689-1055; Fax. (604)689-2955.

TILE, Lianne E; Univ Hlth Network-Toronto Gen, EN7 222-200 Elizabeth St, Toronto ON M5G 2C4; Qns'92; ABIM; BSc; MEd; FRCPC; IntMed. Staff, Mount Sinai Hospital; Staff, Toronto General Hospital - UHN; (416)340-4842; Fax. (416)340-3750; lianne_tile@hotmail.com.

TILE, Marvin; Sunnybrook Hlth Sciences Ctre, MG 301-2075 Bayview Ave, Toronto ON M4N 3M5; Tor'57; LMCC(Med); LRCP; FRCSC; OrthSurg (General Orthopedics). Staff OrthSurg, Sunnybrook Health Sciences Centre; Member, Order of Canada; Emeritus Prof Surg, University of Toronto; (416)480-4941; Fax. (416)480-5886.

TILLER, Barbara A; 1296 Pacific Blvd, Vancouver BC V6Z 2V1; Dal'86; CCFP; (604)633-2474

TILLER, Shawn R; James Paton Mem Hosp, 125 Trans Canada Hwy, Gander NL A1V 1P7; Mem'95; CCFP; Staff, James Paton Memorial Hospital; (709)256-2500

TILLEY, Alison E; Brockville Gen Hosp, 75 Charles St, Brockville ON K6V 1S8; Wes'06; FRCSC; GenSurg. Staff, Kingston General Hospital; Staff, Brockville General Hospital - Charles Street; (613)945-5645

TILLEY, David A; Maple Leaf Medical, GF-70 Carlton St, Toronto ON M5B 1L6; Dal'82; (416)960-0145; Fax. (416)960-0489.

TILLEY, David L; Family Practice Associates, 200-6155 North St, Halifax NS B3K 5R3; Dal'87; (902)453-3511; Fax. (902)454-9010.

TILLEY, Joy; Churchill Square Med Clinic, PO Box 23205 Rpo Churchill Sq 209-8 Rowan St, St. John's NL A1B 4J9; Mem'05; CCFP; (709)722-8561; Fax. (709)722-7350.

TILLEY, Peter A G; BC Women's Hosp & Hlth Ctre, 2G11-4500 Oak St, Vancouver BC V6H 3N1; UBC'86; FRCPC; MedMicrobiol. Staff, BC Women's Hospital & Health Centre; (604)875-2345 x6694

TILLEY, Stephen E; Foothills Med Centre, 1403 29 St NW, Calgary AB T2N 2T9; Mem'08; FRCPC; IntMed (Cardiology). Staff, Foothills Medical Centre; (403)944-8119; Fax. (403)944-2757.

TILLIM, Jeremy D; HSC-Faculty of Med, 3330-3330 Hospital Dr NW, Calgary AB T2N 4N1; University of Nevada (USA)'85; CCFP; CCFP(E.M.); Teach Staff, University of Calgary; (403)220-8737; Fax. (403)210-8165.

TILLMANN, Mary P; 404-49 St Clair Ave W, Toronto ON M4V 1K6; McM'85; CCFP; FCFP; Staff, Sun Life Assurance Co; Asst Prof, University of Toronto; (416)920-6965

TILLMANN, William D; First Med Group, 125-210 Memorial Ave, Orillia ON L3V 7V1; Wes'86; CCFP; FCFP; Staff, Orillia Soldiers' Memorial Hospital; (705)329-1223; Fax. (705)329-3255.

TILLOTSON, Edward C; Bridlewood Mall, 153A-2900 Warden Ave, Scarborough ON M1W 2S8; Tor'71; Court Staff, North York General Hospital; (416)498-1771; Fax. (416)498-7548.

TILSWORTH, Richard H; Strathroy Middlesex Gen Hosp, 395 Carrie St, Strathroy ON N7G 3J4; Wes'73; BSc; FRCPC; Anes (Acute Pain Management). Dir Acute Pain Management, London Health Sciences Centre - Victoria Campus; Staff, Strathroy Middlesex General Hospital - Middlesex Hospital Alliance; (519)245-1550

TIMAR-BANU, Olimpia M; Clinique Med Pelletier, 300-8330 boul Taschereau, Longueuil QC J4X 1C2; Bruxelles (Belgium)'94; CCFP; Médecin, Clinique Medicale Pelletier; Langs: Romanian; English; (450)465-5379; Fax. (514)412-7584.

TIMARAC, Ratka; 301-132 Parkdale Ave S, Hamilton ON L8K 3P3; Belgrade (Serbia)'72; Staff, Hamilton Health Sciences Centre-Juravinski Site; Langs: Yugoslavian; Serbian; (905)549-6616; Fax. (905)549-5015.

TIMKO, Julie B; Family Med Centre, A2-150 Main St E, Grimsby ON L3M 1P1; Dal'08; CCFP; (905)945-5424

TIMKO, Livius; Guildford Health Centre, LL3-15300 105 Ave, Surrey BC V3R 6A7; Prague (Czech Republic)'58; FRCPC; DiagRad. (604)581-1101

TIMMERMANN, Scott A; Life Mark Health Centre, 2225 Macleod Trail SE, Calgary AB T2G 5B6; McM'95; BSc; BEd; FRCSC; OrthSurg (Knee Reconstructive Surgery). (403)291-0045; Fax. (403)291-0552.

TIMMONS, Amelie; CLSC d'Hebergement Valcourt, 1150 rue Champlain, Valcourt QC J0E 2L0; Sher'99; (450)532-3191

TIMMONS, Pauline M; 20B-385 Frederick St, Kitchener ON N2H 2P2; McM'01; CCFP; (519)747-1200; Fax. (519)747-1560.

TIMOL, Farzana; Prince of Wales Med Clinic, 2055 Prince of Wales Dr, Regina SK S4V 3A3; Pretoria (South Africa)'03; LMCC; MB ChB; Physician, North Battleford Medical Clinic; (306)546-2005; Fax. (306)546-4055.

TIMOL, Shehnaz; CMC Med Centre, 7720 Markham Rd, Markham ON L3S 3K1; Howard University (USA)'07; CCFP; (905)471-5330

TIMONERA, Elizabeth R; Humber River Reg Hosp-Church, 200 Church St, York ON M9N 1N8; University of the East (Philippines)'89; FRCPC; AnatPath. Staff, Humber River Regional Hospital - Church Street Site; (416)249-8111 x8017

TIMOTHEE, Jean-Robert; 103-2944 boul Taschereau, Greenfield Park QC J4V 2G8; Lille (France)'71; CSPQ; Cardiol (P.Q.). assoc Staff, Hopital Charles LeMoyne; Langs: English; (450)465-8679; Fax. (450)465-5095.

TIMOTHY, Toma J; 1545 Johnston Ave, White Rock BC V4B 3Z6; UBC'09; CCFP; (604)560-6161

TIMPSON, Deborah J; Pembroke Reg Hosp, 705 Mackay St, Pembroke ON K8A 1G8; McM'94; FRCPC; PhysMed&Rehab. Chief Rehab, Pembroke Regional Hospital Inc; (613)732-3675; Fax. (613)732-2224; timpson@nrtco.net.

TIN, Lancelot K; Credit Valley Prof Bldg, 307-2300 Eglinton Ave W, Mississauga ON L5M 2V8; Philadelphia(PA) (USA)'83; FRCSC; GenSurg. Langs: Cantonese; Mandarin; (905)569-7976; Fax. (905)569-8296.

TIN, Wendy W T; Dr Wendy Tin Med Prof Corp, 502-2125 11th Ave, Regina SK S4P 3X3; Alb'97; FRCSC; GenSurg. Staff, Pasqua Hospital; (306)352-9280; Fax. (306)352-9281.

TINAWI, Paul; Hop Santa Cabrini Ospedale, 5655 rue Saint-Zotique E, Montreal QC H1T 1P7; Mon'99; CCFP; Staff, Hôpital Santa Cabrini Ospedale; (514)252-6000

TINAWI, Simon; MUHC-Montreal Gen Hosp, L7 510-1650 av Cedar, Montreal QC H3G 1A4; Sher'80; FRCPC; PhysMed&Rehab (Musculoskeletal Medicine). Staff, McGill University Health Centre - Montreal General Campus; Consultant, Centre Readaptation Constance-Lethbridge; Langs: English; Arabic; (514)934-1934 x44185; Fax. (514)934-8265; simon.tinawi@muhc.mcgill.ca.

TINCKAM, Kathryn J; UHN Reg HLA Laboratory, 307-67 College St, Toronto ON M5G 2M1; Man'97; BSc; MMedSci; FRCPC; IntMed (Renal Transplant); Nephrol.. Staff, Toronto Western Hospital - University Health Network; (416)340-4995

TINCOCA, Lorenzo P; Hotel-Dieu de Sorel, 400 Av de l'Hotel-Dieu, Sorel-Tracy QC J3P 1N5; Bucarest (Romania)'85; FRCPC; IntMed. Staff, Hôtel-Dieu de Sorel; Langs: French; (450)746-6000

TING, Andrew Y C; University of Alberta Hosp, 8440 112 St NW, Edmonton AB T6G 2B7; Alb'07; Ophth. Staff, University of Alberta Hospital; (780)407-8822

TING, Helen C I; Laurel Med Centre, 215-888 8th Ave W, Vancouver BC V5Z 3Y1; UBC'00; CCFP; Langs: Mandarin; (604)872-0345; Fax. (604)639-2689.

TING, John U L; 10751 King George Blvd, Surrey BC V3T 2X6; Singapore (Singapore)'72; MB BS; Langs: Mandarin; (604)581-2611

TING, Justin W; 3055 Wesbrook Mall, Vancouver BC V6T 1Z3; Man'09; CCFP; Staff, University of British Columbia; (604)822-3614

TING, K H George; Joseph Brant Mem Hosp, 1230 North Shore Blvd E, Burlington ON L7S 1W7; McG'90; FRCPC; DiagRad. Staff, Joseph Brant Memorial Hospital; Langs: Chinese; (905)632-3737

TING, Lucy P; PO Box 39011 Point Grey, Vancouver BC V6R 4P1.

TING, Patricia; Gulf Canada Square, 315-401 9 Ave SW, Calgary AB T2P 3C5; Cal'05; FRCPC; Derm. (403)263-0661

TING, Peter L; 7255 Fraser St, Vancouver BC V5X 3V8; Ott'65; Langs: Malay; Hokkin; Foochow; Mandarin; (604)325-4907

TING, Robert H; Corporate Med Centre, 10-78 Corporate Dr, Scarborough ON M1H 3G4; Wes'88; FRCPC; IntMed; Nephrol. Staff, The Scarborough Hospital - General Campus; Langs: Mandarin; Chinese; (416)279-0855 x238; Fax. (416)279-0857.

TING, Sherwin C; Cross Roads Clinic, 350-507 Broadway St W, Vancouver BC V5Z 1E6; UBC'04; CCFP; (604)568-7229

TING, Y Z Heather; University of Alberta Hosp, 1C1 04-8440 112 St NW, Edmonton AB T6G 2B7; Dal'07; FRCPC; Anes. Staff, University of Alberta Hospital; (780)445-7542; Fax. (780)407-8529.

MALONE, Christina Ting; Manotick Med Centre, 5230 Mitch Owens Rd, Manotick ON K4M 1B2; Ott'89; CCFP; FCFP; (613)692-2571; Fax. (613)692-0271.

TINGEY, David P; St Joseph's Health Care, PO Box 5777 Stn B 268 Grosvenor St, London ON N6A 4V2; Wes'85; FRCSC; Ophth (Glaucoma). Staff Ivey Eye Institute, St Joseph's Hospital - St Joseph's Health Care; Staff, London Health Sciences Centre - University Hospital; Staff, London Health Sciences Centre - Victoria Campus; Assoc Prof, University of Western Ontario; (519)685-8351; Fax. (519)646-6248.

TINGLEY, Brenda M; Brookside Mall Walk-In Clinic, 2-435 Brookside Dr, Fredericton NB E3A 8V4; Dal'79; Staff, Dr Everett Chalmers Regional Hospital; (506)455-7551

TINGLEY, David R; 208 Edgett Ave, Moncton NB E1C 7B7; Dal'77; FRCPC; DiagRad. Staff, The Moncton Hospital; (506)859-7516; Fax. (506)855-9855.

TINGLEY, Erin M; Gibson Health Clinic, PO Box 9000 Stn A, Fredericton NB E3B 5N5; Alb'99; CCFP; Staff, Dr Everett Chalmers Regional Hospital; (506)447-4444; Fax. (506)447-4221; emrtingley@hotmail.com.

TINGURIA, Mukund B; Brant Community HC-Brantford, 200 Terrace Hill St, Brantford ON N3R 1G9; Nagpur (India)'80; FRCPC; AnatPath. Staff, The Brant Community Healthcare System - Brantford General Hospital Site; Langs: Hindi; (519)751-5544

TINH-PHU, Audrey; CSSS de Vallée de la Gatineau, 309 boul Desjardins, Maniwaki QC J9E 2E7; Strasbourg (France)'06; Staff, CSSS de la Vallée de la Gatineau; (819)449-4690

TINITS, Peter; Stratford Gen Hosp, 46 General Hospital Dr, Stratford ON N5A 2Y6; Tor'76; FRCPC; Anes. Ac Staff, Stratford General Hospital - Huron Perth Healthcare Alliance; Langs: Estonian; (519)271-2120; Fax. (519)272-8221.

TINK, Wendy L H; Sheldon Shumuik Centre, 8F-1213 4 St SW, Calgary AB T2R 0X7; Cal'82; BSc; CCFP; FCFP; Clinical Asst Prof Regional Clinical Dept of Family Med, Calgary Health Region; (403)955-9300; Fax. (403)476-8765; wendy.tink@calgaryhealthregion.ca.

TINKER, Anna; BC Cancer Agency-Vancouver CC, 600 10th Ave W, Vancouver BC V5Z 4E6; Cal'99; FRCPC; IntMed; MedOncol. Staff, BC Cancer Agency Vancouver Centre; (604)877-6000; Fax. (604)872-4596.

TINMOUTH, Alan T; The Ottawa Hosp-Gen Campus, 501 Smyth Rd Box 201, Ottawa ON K1H 8L6; Cal'94; ABIM; FRCPC; IntMed; Hem. Staff/Staff, The Ottawa Hospital - General Campus; Asst Prof Med, University of Ottawa; Langs: English; French; (613)737-8899; Fax. (613)739-6266; atinmouth@ottawahospital.on.ca.

TINMOUTH, Jill M; Sunnybrook Hlth Sciences Ctre, HG 40-2075 Bayview Ave, Toronto ON M4N 3M5; New York(NY) (USA)'95; PhD; FRCPC; IntMed (Gastrointestinal Disorders); Gastroent. Staff, Sunnybrook Health Sciences Centre; Langs: Bilingual(English/French); (416)480-5910; Fax. (416)480-4845.

TINMOUTH, William W; 202-1532 Cliffe Ave, Courtenay BC V9N 2K4; Wes'97; FRCSC; Urol (Endocrinology). Consultant Surgs, St Joseph's General Hospital; Consultant Surgs, Campbell River & District General Hospital; Langs: Bilingual(English/French); (250)338-7763; Fax. (250)703-2225.

TINNEY, Ward T; Westgate Med Clinic, 402-20395 Lougheed Hwy, Maple Ridge BC V2X 2P9; UBC'81; BSc; (604)465-3900

TINTSCHEFF, Mary M; Halton HCS Corp-Oakville, 327 Reynolds St, Oakville ON L6J 3L7; Tor'78; FRCPC; Anes. Staff, Halton Healthcare Services Corporation - Oakville Site; (905)338-4647

TIONG, Irving Y H; Humber River Reg Hosp-Church, 200 Church St, York ON M9N 1N8; McG'98; FRCPC; IntMed; Cardiol. Staff, Humber River Regional Hospital - Church Street Site; (416)236-2783; Fax. (416)236-2783.

TIPPLE, Marion A; Children's & Women's HC of BC, 1F3-4480 Oak St, Vancouver BC V6H 3V4; London (England)'68; MB BS; FRCP(E); FRCPC; Peds (Electrophysiology); PedCardiol. Ac Staff, BC Children's Hospital; Ac Staff, Royal Columbian Hospital; Clin Prof, University of British Columbia; Langs: Japanese; French; (604)875-3233; Fax. (604)875-2774; pedcard@interchange.ubc.ca.

TIRADO, Rossana M; 206-210 Centrum Blvd, Orleans ON K1E 3V7; Sher'88; FRCPC; Peds. Ac Staff Special Care Nursery, The Ottawa Hospital - Civic Campus; Langs: Spanish; French; (613)794-9901; rtirado@rogers.com.

TIRET, Bertrand-Philippe; Ctr Hosp Pierre-Janet, 20 rue Pharand, Gatineau QC J9A 1K7; Nancy (France)'88; Prés Med Evaluation Serv & Pharm, Centre Hospitalier Pierre-Janet; (819)776-8086; Fax. (819)771-4727.

TIRKOS, S Sam; South East Toronto Family Hlth, 1871 Danforth Ave, Toronto ON M4C 1J3; Tor'07; CCFP; (416)699-7775

TIRMIZI, Lubna T; Pickering Holistic Health Ctre, 220-1101 Kingston Rd, Pickering ON L1V 1B5; Wes'00; CCFP; Langs: Hindi; Punjabi; Urdu; (905)831-9797; Fax. (905)839-9984.

TIROVOLAS, Konstantinos; 324 Lakeshore Rd E, Mississauga ON L5G 1H4; Athens (Greece)'73; FRCPC; Psy (Child & Adolescent Psychiatry). Langs: Greek; (905)274-8914; Fax. (905)274-1654.

TIRSCHMANN, Gunnar; Klondyke Med Clinic, 1-3089 3rd Ave, Whitehorse YT Y1A 5B3; (Germany)'98; CCFP; Physician, Klondyke Medical Clinic; (867)668-4060; Fax. (867)668-4067.

TISCHENKO, Alexander; St Boniface Gen Hosp, Y3539-409 Tache Ave, Winnipeg MB R2H 2A6; Odessa (Ukraine)'89; PhD; FRCPC; IntMed (Cardiac Electrophysiology); Cardiol. Staff Cardiol, St Boniface General Hospital; Asst Prof, University of Manitoba; Langs: Russian; Ukrainian; (204)237-2977; Fax. (204)233-8755.

TISCHLER, Aron M; North Shore Eye Associates, 102-1111 Lonsdale Ave, North Vancouver BC V7M 2H4; UBC'80; FRCSC; Ophth. (604)988-1166; Fax. (604)988-0166.

TISDALE, Britton E; William Osler HC-Brampton, 2100 Bovaird Dr E, Brampton ON L6R 3J7; Qns'03; Urol. Staff, William Osler Health System - Brampton Civic Hospital; (905)494-2120

TISDALL, Gordon W; 1104-50 Prince Arthur Ave, Toronto ON M5R 1B5; Tor'64; DPsy; FRCPC; Psy. Consultant, Centre for Addiction & Mental Health (CAMH) - College Street Site; Asst Prof, University of Toronto; (416)923-2979

TISHER, Carolyn R; Health Source Med Clinic, 473 Dupont St, Toronto ON M6G 1Y6; UBC'03; CCFP; (416)588-1888; Fax. (416)588-0388.

TISHLER, Steven J; 600-101 Queensway W, Mississauga ON L5B 2P7; Tor'90; FRCPC; IntMed; Cardiol. Staff Cardiol, Trillium Health Centre - Mississauga; Assoc Staff, Toronto General Hospital - UHN; (905)306-8404; Fax. (905)277-0136.

TISSERA, Ponsuge A D; Brandon Clinic, 620 Dennis St, Brandon MB R7A 5E7; (Other Foreign)'83; (204)728-4440

TISSOT, Brian D; Sudbury Reg Hosp-Laurentian Si, 41 Ramsey Lake Rd, Sudbury ON P3E 5J1; Tor'86; CCFP; CCFP(E.M.); Staff, Health Sciences North-St Joseph's Health Centre; Staff, Health Sciences North-Laurentian Site; (705)675-4700

TISSOT, Jean-Marie; CLSC de la Jacques-Cartier, 041-11999A rue de l'Hopital, Quebec QC G2A 2T7; Mon'70; Prés CME, Centre Hospitalier Chauveau; Langs: English; (418)843-2572; Fax. (418)843-3880.

TITA, Ioana; Family Practice Clinic, 103-15955 Airport Rd, Caledon East ON L7C 1H9; University of Medicine & Pharmacy (Other Foreign)'01; CCFP; Langs: Romanian; (905)584-9377

TITHECOTT, Gary A; 202 King St W, Chatham ON N7M 1E5; Wes'79; FRCPC; Peds. Consultant, Chatham-Kent Health Alliance; Consultant, Chatham-Kent Health Alliance - Sydenham Hospital Campus; Assoc Dean Undergraduate Med Education/Aj Prof, University of Western Ontario; (519)351-9322; Fax. (519)351-9323.

TITIS, Apostolus; Taunton Health Centre, SS 201 1290 Keith Ross Dr, Oshawa ON L1H 7K4; (Ireland)'05; CCFP; Langs: Greek; (905)721-4160

TITLE, Lawrence M; Halifax Infirmary, 6896J-1796 Summer St, Halifax NS B3H 3A7; Tor'84; FRCPC; IntMed (Interventional Cardiology); Cardiol. Att Staff Cardiol, Queen Elizabeth II Health Sciences Centre - Victoria General Site; Asst Prof, Dalhousie University; (902)473-8470; Fax. (902)473-6293; ltitle@dal.ca.

TITRI ZAIBAK, Nabyla; CSSS de Gatineau, 104 rue Lois, Gatineau QC J8Y 3R7; (Algeria)'86; (819)776-7660 x7442; Fax. (819)770-5490.

TITTLEY, Camille M L; PRG Medical Inc, 836 Upper James St, Hamilton ON L9C 3A4; Ott'85; Langs: Bilingual(French/English); (905)385-6777

TITTLEY, Jacques G; Hamilton HS-General Site, 5N 508-237 Barton St E, Hamilton ON L8L 2X2; Ott'83; FRCSC; GenSurg; VascSurg. Staff, Hamilton Health Sciences Centre - Hamilton General Hospital; Langs: French; (905)527-4322; Fax. (905)521-1284.

TITTLEY, Matthieu; CHUS Hop Hotel-Dieu, 580 rue Bowen S, Sherbrooke QC J1G 2E8; Laval'03; FRCPC; Psy (Psychotic Disorders). Aj Prof, Centre Hospitalier Universitaire de Sherbrooke-Hôpital Hôtel-Dieu; (819)346-1110; Fax. (819)829-6263; matthieu.tittley@usherbrooke.ca.

TITUS, Jolene J; Meadow Lake Associate Clinic, PO Box 1510, Meadow Lake SK S9X 1Z1; (306)236-5661; Fax. (306)236-4355.

TITUS, Roselin T; The Salvation Army Grace Hosp, 300 Booth Dr, Winnipeg MB R3J 3M7; Man'06; CCFP; Staff, The Salvation Army Grace Hospital; (204)837-0391

TIU, Stephen S; Trillium Health Ctre-Mississau, 100 Queensway W, Mississauga ON L5B 1B8; UBC'93; BSc; CCFP; CCFP(E.M.); Staff, Trillium Health Centre - Mississauga; (905)848-7100

TJADEN, Janice M; 195A-1151 10 Ave SW, Salmon Arm BC V1E 1T3; UBC'91; FRCSC; Ophth. (250)832-1131; Fax. (250)832-1106.

TJAHJADI, Anindita; Children's Hosp Eastern Ont, 401 Smyth Rd, Ottawa ON K1H 8L1; UBC'07; FRCPC; Peds. Staff, Children's Hospital of Eastern Ontario (CHEO); Langs: Indonesian; (613)737-7600

TJAN, Eng-Tjie; ENT Consultants, 219-1 Paton St, St. John's NL A1B 4S8; National (Taiwan)'64; FRCSC; Otol. Staff, Janeway Children's Health & Rehabilitation Centre; Langs: Chinese; (709)579-1003; Fax. (709)579-1708.

TJAN, Eugenie U; Sheridan Health, 44B-2225 Erin Mills Parkway, Mississauga ON L5K 1T9; Tor'91; Staff Family Med, The Credit Valley Hospital; Langs: Indonesian; (905)403-9595

TJANDRAWIDJAJA, Michael C; William Osler Hosp-Brampton, 2100 Bovaird Dr E, Brampton ON L6R 3J7; Alb'04; FRCPC; IntMed; Cardiol. Staff, William Osler Health System - Brampton Civic Hospital; (905)494-6221; Fax. (905)494-6717.

TJIA, Sabine P Y; LaSalle Medicale, 200-8190 boul Newman, LaSalle QC H8N 1X9; Mon'93; Langs: English; (514)368-8666; Fax. (514)368-9477.

TJON, Peter E; 208-9889 Highway 48, Markham ON L6E 0B7; Tor'95; CCFP; (905)294-4467; Fax. (905)294-8925.

TJONG, Joshua K; 969 Queen St, Sault Ste. Marie ON P6A 2C4; Cal'94; MSc; PhD; FRCPC; DiagRad., Sault Area Hospital - Sault Ste Marie; Langs: Indonesian; Mandarin; Chinese; (705)759-3434; jf.tjong@rogers.com.

TKACHUK, Douglas C; Life Labs, 100 International Blvd, Etobicoke ON M9W 6J6; Man'82; FRCPC; AnatPath. Staff, Princess Margaret Hospital - University Health Network; (416)675-4530; Fax. (416)213-4206.

TKALYCH, Paul J; Mayfair Place Med Centre, 313-6707 Elbow Dr SW, Calgary AB T2V 0E5; Sask'83; Staff, Rockyview General Hospital; Langs: Ukrainian; Russian; (403)252-6022; Fax. (403)253-1923.

TKATCH, Shelin; 300-2626 Croydon Dr, Surrey BC V3S 0S8; UBC'95; FRCSC; ObstGyn. Staff ObstGyn, Peace Arch Hospital; (604)531-3915; Fax. (604)531-3724.

TLHAPE, Daniel R; Drumheller Assoc Physicians, PO Box 5600 140 Riverside Dr E, Drumheller AB T0J 0Y0; (Other Foreign)'99; (403)823-3345; Fax. (403)823-7823.

TLILI, Messaoud; Hop Marie Clarac, 3530 boul Gouin E, Montreal-Nord QC H1H 1B7; (Algeria)'77; CCFP; Staff, Hopital Marie Clarac; (514)321-8800

TLUSTY, Eva; Oakville Diagnostic Imaging, B4-1235 Trafalgar Rd, Oakville ON L6H 3P1; Prague (Czech Republic)'66; FRCPC; DiagRad (Ultrasound). Langs: Czech; (905)845-0014; Fax. (905)845-0018.

TNANI, Amel K; CSSS de Chicoutimi, CP 5006 305 rue Saint-Vallier, Chicoutimi QC G7H 5H6; (Tunisia)'98; Staff, Complexe hospitalier de la Sagamie; (418)541-1000

TO, Agnes S; 2005-7000 Westminster Highway, Richmond BC V6X 1A2; UBC'02; MCPS; FRCPC; Psy. Staff, Richmond Hospital; Langs: Chinese; Cantonese; Mandarin; (604)244-5144; Fax. (604)278-4819.

TO, Dinh Vu; Community Link Med Clinic, 114 Woodlawn Rd, Dartmouth NS B2W 2S7; Ho Chi Minh (Vietnam)'92; LMCC; CCFP; Staff, The Nova Scotia Hospital; Langs: Vietnamese; (902)462-7138; Fax. (902)462-3028; vudinhto@yahoo.com.

TO, Howard K H; Black Creek GHC, 5-2202 Jane St, Toronto ON M3M 1A4; Tor'94; CCFP; (416)249-8000; Fax. (416)249-4594; howard.to@bcchc.com.

TO, K H Kent; St Michael's Hosp, 30 Bond St, Toronto ON M5B 1W8; McG'08; CCFP; Staff Family Practice Unit, St Michael's Hospital; (416)867-7426; Fax. (416)867-7498.

TO, Karen C; St Joseph's Healthcare, M304-50 Charlton Ave E, Hamilton ON L8N 4A6; McM'06; FRCPC; IntMed; Nephrol. Staff, St Joseph's Healthcare - Charlton Campus; (905)522-1155; Fax. (905)521-6153.

TO, My Lan; Centre Med Fam de Gatineau, 201-908 boul Maloney E, Gatineau QC J8P 1H5; McG'01; (819)663-9676; Fax. (819)663-9326.

TO, Toan Bao; Medical Clinic Bldg, 218-89 Humber College Blvd, Etobicoke ON M9V 4B8; Saigon (Vietnam)'81; FRCPC; IntMed (Adult Cardiology); Cardiol. Dir CCU, William Osler Health System - Etobicoke General Hospital; Assoc Staff Cardiol, Toronto Western Hospital - University Health Network; Clin Instructor, University of Toronto; Langs: Vietnamese; (416)743-3636; Fax. (416)743-5961; totoa@magic.pmh.on.ca.

TO, Tuyet Anh; Clinique Med Mira, 1560 boul de Rome, Brossard QC J4W 3A1; Mon'86; Staff, Centre Hospitalier de Verdun; (450)466-1880

TOAL, Kevin F; St Michael's Family Health Ctr, 13930 74 St NW, Edmonton AB T5C 3H7; Belfast (Ireland)'66; MB ChB; BAO; (780)406-4883; Fax. (780)406-4882.

TOAL, Satish C; Saint John Reg Hosp, PO Box 2100 Stn Main 400 University Ave, Saint John NB E2L 4L2; Nagpur (India)'94; Staff, Saint John Regional Hospital; (506)649-2713; Fax. (506)648-6110.

TOAL, Stephen; Allin Clinic, 10155 120 St NW, Edmonton AB T5K 2A2; Alb'95; CCFP; (780)482-7551; Fax. (780)488-2056.

TOANE, E Benjamin; 6304 129 Ave NW, Edmonton AB T5A 0G1; Alb'73; (780)478-1031; Fax. (780)478-1205.

TOBE, Lauren E; Scarborough Prof Centre, 406-1371 Neilson Rd, Scarborough ON M1B 4Z8; McM'99; FRCPC; IntMed. (416)281-9499; Fax. (416)283-5705.

TOBE, Sheldon W; Sunnybrook Hlth Sciences Ctre, A240-2075 Bayview Ave, Toronto ON M4N 3M5; Cal'85; FRCPC; IntMed; Nephrol. Staff, Sunnybrook Health Sciences Centre; Assoc Prof Med, University of Toronto; (416)480-6901; Fax. (416)480-6940.

TOBER, Alfred E; St Paul's Hosp, 1081 Burrard St, Vancouver BC V6Z 1Y6; Man'91; FRCPC; EmergMed. Staff, Health Sciences Centre; Staff, Providence Health Care - St Paul's Hospital; Seven Oaks General Hospital; St Boniface General Hospital; Langs: German; (604)682-2344

TOBER, Gerald P; Smith Clinic, 1-6601 48 Ave, Camrose AB T4V 3G8; Alb'76; Ac Staff, Covenant Health - St Mary's Hospital; (780)672-2424; Fax. (780)608-5897.

TOBERT, Gregory J; 6668 Fraser St, Vancouver BC V5X 3T5; UBC'79; CCFP; FCFP; Ac Staff, Providence Health Care - Mount Saint Joseph Hospital; Assoc Staff, Vancouver General Hospital - Centennial Pavillion; Ac Staff, BC Children's Hospital; Clin Asst Prof Family Med, University of British Columbia; (604)321-6651; Fax. (604)325-3915.

TOBIA, Bernard; Northbrook Med Centre, 12357 Hwy 41 RR 1, Northbrook ON K0H 2G0; Dublin (Ireland)'81; (613)336-8888

TOBIAS, Guy; Mackenzie Richmond Hill Hosp, 10 Trench St, Richmond Hill ON L4C 4Z3; Wes'06; CCFP; Staff, Mackenzie Richmond Hill Hospital; (905)883-1212

TOBIN, Cathryn E; 210-5293 Highway 7, Markham ON L3P 7M7; McM'86; FRCPC; Peds (Pediatric & Adolescent Medicine). Court Staff, Markham Stouffville Hospital; (905)201-9633; Fax. (905)201-9382.

TOBIN, Cheryl L; Cape Breton Reg Hosp, 1482 George St, Sydney NS B1P 1P3; Mem'06; CCFP; Staff Palliative Care, Cape Breton Healthcare Complex; (902)567-7804; Fax. (902)567-8062.

TOBIN, D Jonathan; Greenboro Family Med Center, 25 Tapiola Cres, Ottawa ON K1T 2J7; Tor'83; CCFP; Langs: Hebrew; (613)738-0303; Fax. (613)738-8950.

TOBIN, John A; 60 Av Bateman, Edmundston NB E3V 4X6; Laval'89; (506)735-8891; Fax. (506)739-9050; jtobin@health.nb.ca.

TOBIN, Thomas E; Guelph Family Health Team, 101-83 Dawson Rd, Guelph ON N1H 1B1; Wes'88; CCFP; (519)766-1360; Fax. (519)766-0469.

TOBLER, Kathleen R; Alberta Children's Hosp, 2888 Shaganappi Trail NW, Calgary AB T3B 6A8; Cal'91; FRCPC; Peds (Pediatric Critical Care). Staff Pediatric Intensivist, Alberta Children's Hospital; Dir Pediatric Residency Training Prog, University of Calgary; (403)955-7769; Fax. (403)955-7081.

TODARY FAHMY, Yvette P; River West Med Centre, 6500 Roblin Blvd, Winnipeg MB R3R 3P9; (Other Foreign)'88; CCFP; (204)897-9666

TODD, Andrea M; Royal University Hosp, 103 Hospital Dr, Saskatoon SK S7N 0W8; Tor'03; FRCPC; Anes. Staff, Royal University Hospital; (306)655-1183; Fax. (306)655-1279.

TODD, Bruce L S; Whitehorse Med Services Ltd, 406 Lambert St, Whitehorse YT Y1A 1Z7; McG'76; Staff, Whitehorse General Hospital; Physician, Whitehorse Medical Services Ltd; (867)393-6633; Fax. (867)393-6601.

TODD, Crystal F; Birchwood Prof Centre, 24 Kentucky Crt, New Minas NS B4N 4N2; Dal'03; BSc; CCFP; (902)681-1080; Fax. (902)681-1600.

TODD, David C; Joseph Brant Mem Hosp, 1230 North Shore Blvd, Burlington ON L7S 1W7; McM'99; FRCPC; IntMed; Respir. Staff, Joseph Brant Memorial Hospital; Staff, St Joseph's Healthcare - Charlton Campus; (905)632-3730

TODD, David M; Market Mall Prof Centre, 312-4935 40 Ave NW, Calgary AB T3A 2N1; Alb'70; CCFP; (403)247-2345; Fax. (403)247-6217.

TODD, Gerald T; 400-11010 101 St NW, Edmonton AB T5H 4B9; Alb'84; BSc; FRCSC; Urol (Oncology). Staff, Cross Cancer Institute; Staff, University of Alberta Hospital; Assoc Prof, University of Alberta; (780)441-2577; Fax. (780)441-2587.

TODD, John D; Windsor Square Shopp Centre, 201-1959 152 St, Surrey BC V4A 9E3; Cal'74; GenSurg (Surgical Oncology). Surg Asst, Surrey Memorial Hospital; Locum Tenens, Fraser Health Authority; (604)535-0525; Fax. (604)535-0698; dr_todd@shaw.ca.

TODD, Jonathan K; 899 12 Ave W, Vancouver BC V5Z 1M9; Qns'06; FRCPC; IntMed (Echocardiography); Cardiol. Staff Echo Dept, Gordon & Leslie Diamond Health Care Centre; (604)875-4111

TODD, Judith M; Codsell Medical, 1 Codsell Ave, North York ON M3H 3V6; Cal'92; CCFP; FCFP; (416)398-7355; Fax. (416)398-7353.

TODD, Leslie A; Business Bldg, 217-150 Crowfoot Cres NW, Calgary AB T3G 3T2; UBC'92; CCFP; FCFP; (403)241-8900; Fax. (403)241-8109.

TODD, Robert J; Eskasoni Primary Care Clinic, PO Box 7745 44 Spencer's Lane, Eskasoni NS B1W 1B3; Dal'01; CCFP; Staff, Cape Breton Healthcare Complex; (902)379-2500; Fax. (902)379-2271.

TODD, Stanley D L; Brant Community HC-Brantford, 200 Terrace Hill St, Brantford ON N3R 1G9; Tor'95; AnatPath. Staff, The Brant Community Healthcare System - Brantford General Hospital Site; (519)752-7871

TODD, Susan E; 4733 49 St, Red Deer AB T4N 1T6; Alb'85; FRCPC; Psy. Staff, Red Deer Regional Hospital Centre; (403)340-7046; Fax. (403)340-5217; susan.todd@albertahealthservices.ca.

TODD, Thomas R J; Canadian Med Protective Assn, PO Box 8225 Stn T CSC 875 Carling Ave, Ottawa ON K1G 3H7; Qns'69; FRCSC; GenSurg (Critical Care Medicine); ThorSurg. (613)725-9965

TODEROVICH, Eugene; R J A Medicentres Cnd Inc, 204-10458 Mayfield Rd, Edmonton AB T5P 4P4; Alb'72; (780)483-7115; Fax. (780)484-6531.

TODOROV, Christo; Hop Louis-H Lafontaine, 7401 rue Hochelaga, Montreal QC H1N 3M5; Leningrad (Russia (Federation))'72; MSc; Psy (P.Q.) (Anxiety Disorder). Staff, Hopital Louis-H Lafontaine; Langs: Russian; French; Bulgarian; (514)251-4000; Fax. (514)251-7527.

TODOROV, Krasimir G; 480-3033 Immel St, Abbotsford BC V2S 6S2; Varna (Bulgaria)'94; Langs: Bulgarian; (604)852-6781; Fax. (604)852-0869.

TODOROVIC, Cedomirka; Rocky Point Med Clinic, 2523 St John's St, Port Moody BC V3H 2B3; Belgrade (Serbia)'82; CCFP; Physician, Rocky Point Medical Clinic; Langs: Croatian; Serbian; (604)936-7277; Fax. (604)936-7112.

TODORUK, Dennis N; Rene Lemarchand Mansion, 401-11523 100 Ave NW, Edmonton AB T5K 0J8; Alb'71; FRCPC; IntMed; Gastroent. Asst Prof, University of Alberta; (780)488-6867; Fax. (780)488-3654.

TOEG, Abraham; Sturgeon Community Hosp, 201 Boudreau Rd, St Albert AB T8N 6C4; (Israel)'86; Staff, Medicine Hat Regional Hospital; Staff, Sturgeon Community Hospital; Physician, Okotoks Health & Wellness Centre; (780)418-2000

TOEWS, Bernhard J; 204-1118 Austin Ave, Coquitlam BC V3K 3P5; Man'72; Chief Gen Pract, Royal Columbian Hospital; Physician Occup Med, New Wesminster Police; Langs: Dutch; German; (604)936-1315; Fax. (604)936-9010.

TOEWS, Gertrude J; Selkirk Family Medicine, 307-1101 Dewdney Ave, Trail BC V1R 4T1; Alb'72; Staff, Kootenay Boundary Regional Hospital; (250)368-8802; Fax. (250)368-8813.

TOEWS, John A; 2020 18 St NW, Calgary AB T2M 3T1; Man'69; FRCPC; Psy. Ac Staff Psy, Foothills Medical Centre; (403)220-0022; Fax. (403)210-2080.

TOEWS, Karen A; Steinbach Family Med Centre, 10-333 Loewen Blvd, Steinbach MB R5G 0C3; Man'94; CCFP; FCFP; (204)326-3401

TOEWS, Ronald P; 5-100 Highland Rd W, Kitchener ON N2M 3B5; Tor'83; BSc; CCFP; FCFP; Court Staff, St Mary's General Hospital; Court Staff, Grand River Hospital - Kitchener/Waterloo Health Centre; Langs: German; (519)742-3600; Fax. (519)742-3386.

TOFFELMIRE, Edwin B; Kingston Gen Hosp, 76 Stuart St, Kingston ON K7L 2V7; McG'81; FRCPC; IntMed. Staff, Hotel-Dieu Hospital; Consultant, Providence Care - St Mary's of the Lake Hospital Site; Med Dir Renal Unit, Kingston General Hospital; Staff Teacher, Queen's University; (613)548-1366

TOFFOLI, Daniela; MUHC-Montreal Children's Hosp, D168 2-2300 rue Tupper, Montreal QC H3H 1P3; McG'04; Ophth. Staff, McGill University Health Centre - Montreal Children's Hospital; (514)412-4400 x22891

TOFFOLI-ZADRA, Nadia D; Maple Med Centre, 210-955 Major MacKenzie Dr, Vaughan ON L6A 4P9; Tor'94; CCFP; FCFP; Staff, Mackenzie Richmond Hill Hospital; Langs: Italian; (905)832-2201; Fax. (905)832-2246.

TOFFOLO, Denny; Victoria Med Centre, 306-304 Victoria Ave N, Hamilton ON L8L 5G4; McM'84; Langs: Italian; (905)572-9180; Fax. (905)572-9022.

TOFT, Ian P; St Thomas-Elgin Gen Hosp, PO Box 2007 Stn Main 189 Elm St, St Thomas ON N5P 3W2; Tor'96; CCFP; FCFP; Staff, St Thomas Elgin General Hospital; Langs: English; French; (519)631-2020

TOGNOTTI, Darin M T; PO Box 18130 Rpo Heritage Mtn, Port Moody BC V3H 0A2; UBC'95; CCFP; CCFP(E.M.); (604)822-7121

TOGURI, Allan G; SGH Medical Mall, 510-3030 Lawrenve Ave E, Scarborough ON M1P 2T7; Tor'69; AB(Urol.); FACS; BSc(Hon.); FRCSC; Urol (Surgical Oncology). Exec Dir, Society of Urologic Surgeons of Ontario; Aj Prof Surg, University of Toronto; Langs: Japanese; German; (416)439-8913; Fax. (416)439-0784.

TOHME, Juliette; Markham Walk-In Clinic, 3607 Hwy 7, Markham ON L3R 8W6; (Other Foreign)'93; CCFP; (905)474-5764; Fax. (905)604-9401.

TOHME, Serge; Ctr Hosp de Verdun, 4000 boul Lasalle, Verdun QC H4G 2A3; Beirut (Lebanon)'81; FRCSC; OrthSurg. Staff, Centre Hospitalier de Verdun; (514)362-1000

TOI, Ants; Univ Hlth Network-Princess M, 4 833-610 University Ave, Toronto ON M5G 2M9; Tor'66; DMRD; FRCPC; DiagRad (Ultrasound). Staff, Princess Margaret Hospital - University Health Network; Staff, Toronto General Hospital - UHN; Staff, Mount Sinai Hospital; Assoc Prof Radiol, University of Toronto; Langs: Estonian; (416)946-4501; Fax. (416)946-2805; atoi@mtsinai.on.ca.

TOKAR, Judith L; 280 Welland Ave, St Catharines ON L2R 2P9; McM'81; BSc; FRCPC; Neur (Neuromuscular Diseases). Staff, Niagara Health System - St Catharines General Site; Staff, Niagara Health System - Greater Niagara General Site; Staff, Niagara Health System - Niagara-on-the-Lake Hospital Site; (905)687-3615; Fax. (905)687-6550.

TOKAREWICZ, Alexander C; St Joseph's Health Centre, PO Box 5777 Stn B 268 Grosvenor St, London ON N6A 4V2; Wes'71; DAB; FRCOphth; FRCSC; Ophth (Cornea). Staff, St Joseph's Hospital - St Joseph's Health Care; Ac Staff, London Health Sciences Centre - Victoria Campus; Consultant, London Health Sciences Centre - University Hospital; Assoc Prof Ophth, University of Western Ontario; Langs: Ukrainian; (519)646-6233; Fax. (519)646-6129.

TOKAREWICZ, John P M; 201 Talbot St, Leamington ON N8H 3X5; Wes'82; BSc; CCFP; FCFP; (519)322-2826; Fax. (519)322-0874.

TOKARYK, Robert A M; Medical Arts Bldg, 427-750 Spadina Cres E, Saskatoon SK S7K 3H3; Sask'71; BA; FRCSC; PlasSurg. (306)665-8886; Fax. (306)934-0775; dr.tokaryk@sasktel.net.

TOKIC, Vesna; Seymour Med Clinic, 1530 7th Ave W, Vancouver BC V6J 1S3; Prague (Czech Republic)'97; CCFP; Langs: Serbo-Croatian; Czech; (604)739-5611; Fax. (604)738-2102.

TOLBA, Marwan; St Joseph's Health Centre, 1-280 Victoria St, Dalhousie NB E8C 2R6; Damascus (Syria)'95; CCFP; Staff, Hôpital Régional Campbellton; Staff, Centre de santé Communitaire - St-Joseph; (506)684-7727; Fax. (506)684-7747.

TOLEDANO, Baruch J; Hôpital Ste-Justine, 3403-3175 ch Cote-Sainte-Cathe, Montreal QC H3T 1C5; McG'89; FRCPC; Peds (Critical Care Medicine). Staff, Hôpital Ste-Justine; (514)345-4675; Fax. (514)345-7731; baruch_toledano@umontreal.ca.

TOLEDANO, Daniel R; 301-1263 St Clair Ave W, Toronto ON M6E 1B8; Tor'86; Ac Staff, St Joseph's Health Centre; Langs: English; French; (416)656-9219; Fax. (416)656-4981.

TOLEDANO, Karine; Institut de Cardiologie de Mtl, 5000 rue Belanger, Montreal QC H1T 1C8; McG'00; FRCPC; Anes. Staff, Institut de Cardiologie de Montréal; (514)376-3330; Fax. (514)376-8784; ktole@hotmail.com.

TOLEDANO, Thierry E; Centre Hosp de Lachine, 650 16e av, Lachine QC H8S 3N5; McG'05; IntMed. Staff, Centre Hospitalier de Lachine; (514)637-2351; thierry.toledano@mail.mcgill.ca.

TOLEVA, Olga I; University of Alberta Hosp, 2C2WCM-8440 112 St NW, Edmonton AB T6G 2B7; Sofia University (Bulgaria)'98; FRCPC; IntMed;CCFP; Cardiol. Staff, University of Alberta Hospital; (780)969-9786

TOLHURST, Elizabeth A; North York Gen Hosp, 4001 Leslie St, North York ON M2K 1E1; Qns'03; CCFP; CCFP(E.M.); Staff Emerg Med, North York General Hospital; (416)756-6000

TOLKIN, Jonathan B; 212-4800 Leslie St, North York ON M2J 2K9; Dublin (Ireland)'79; MB ChB; FRCPC; Peds. Staff, North York General Hospital; (416)497-1987; Fax. (416)497-0712.

TOLLESTRUP, Jonathon B; Dahl Clinic, PO Box 310, Magrath AB T0K 1J0; Cal'92; CCFP; FCFP; (403)758-3363; Fax. (403)758-6845.

TOLLESTRUP, Wallace R; Raymond Med Clinic, PO Box 769 Stn Main 20 Church Ave, Raymond AB T0K 2S0; Alb'77; (403)752-3337; Fax. (403)752-4967.

TOLMIE, Johan; Coronation Med Clinic, PO Box 430, Coronation AB T0C 1C0; (South Africa)'85; MB ChB; CCFP; (403)578-3232; Fax. (403)578-3235.

TOLMIE, Wendy I; 8023 Highway 7 RR 2, Guelph ON N1H 6H8; Ott'87; BPE; (519)822-1717; Fax. (519)822-0093.

TOLSZCZUK, Michelle; La Cite Med Tour Belle-Cour, 221-2590 boul Laurier, Quebec QC G1V 4M6; Laval'88; Staff, Centre Hospitalier Universitaire de Sherbrooke-Hôpital Hôtel-Dieu; (418)659-3336; michtols@gmail.com.

TOLTON, Alexander D; Churchill Health Centre, PO Box 2500, Churchill MB R0B 0E0; Man'87; CCFP; FCFP; Staff, Churchill Health Centre; (204)675-8318

TOLTON, Rani G; 4-7758 Kent Blvd, Brockville ON K6V 7J9; Man'95; CCFP; FCFP; Staff, Canadian Forces Base Kingston; (613)341-8954; Fax. (613)341-8954; rani.tolton@forces.gc.ca.

TOM, Roger W J; Central City Med Clinic, 3110-10153 King George Blvd, Surrey BC V3T 2W1; Ott'88; (604)951-0885; Fax. (604)951-0689.

TOM, Tony P T; 103-3325 Kingsway, Vancouver BC V5R 5K6; Cal'84; CCFP; Langs: Chinese; (604)431-5008; Fax. (604)431-5007.

TOM-PACK, Maurice; Mount Sinai Hosp, 600 University Ave, Toronto ON M5G 1X5; West Indies (Other Foreign)'03; FRCSC; OrthSurg. Staff, Mount Sinai Hospital; (416)596-4200

TOMA, Alina; St Michael's Hosp, 30 Bond St, Toronto ON M5B 1W8; Qns'05; FRCPC; EmergMed; Critical Care Medicine; IntMed. Staff, St Michael's Hospital; Langs: Romanian; (416)360-4000

TOMA, Antoun A M; Derry Med Clinic, 16B-3221 Derry Rd W, Mississauga ON L5N 7L7; Ain Shams (Egypt)'80; MB ChB; CCFP; FCFP; Langs: Arabic; (905)824-0005; Fax. (905)824-7440.

TOMA, Azhar M; Kipling Heights Med Centre, 117B-2291 Kipling Ave, Etobicoke ON M9W 4L6; Baghdad (Iraq)'02; MB ChB; CCFP; Staff, Bramalea Community Health Centre; Langs: Arabic; (416)740-2895

TOMA, Cristian; Welcome Med Clinic, 105-7885 6th St, Burnaby BC V3N 3N4; Iasi (Romania)'87; CCFP; (604)526-8905

TOMA, Emil; CHUM-Hotel-Dieu, 3840 rue Saint-Urbain, Montreal QC H2W 1T8; Bucharest (Romania)'66; FRCPC; MedMicrobiol (AIDS). Staff, Centre Hospitalier l'Université de Montréal (CHUM) - Hôtel-Dieu; (514)890-8000 x14063; Fax. (514)412-7234.

TOMA, Lily; Royal Oak Oasis Med Clinic, 250-8730 Country Hills Blvd NW, Calgary AB T3G 0E2; Timisoara (Romania)'87; LMCC; CCFP; Staff Privil, Rockyview General Hospital; Langs: Romanian; (403)262-7787; Fax. (403)262-7786.

TOMA, Mustafa; St Paul's Hosp, 475A-1081 Burrard St, Vancouver BC V6Z 1Y6; UBC'03; FRCPC; IntMed; Cardiol. Staff, Providence Health Care - St Paul's Hospital; (604)806-7356

TOMA, Nicola; St Mary's Hosp Centre, 3830 Lacombe, Montreal QC H3T 1M5; Mon'02; MSc; MCFP; FCFP; Staff, St Mary's Hospital Centre; Staff, McGill University Health Centre - Montreal General Campus; Staff, McGill University Health Centre - Royal Victoria Hospital; Fellow, Sir Mortimer B Davis Jewish General; Fellow, McGill University; Langs: Romanian; (514)345-3511 x3453; ntoma@videotron.ca.

TOMA, Sarah G; Mediclinic, 9116 82 Ave NW, Edmonton AB T6C 0Z5; Baghdad (Iraq)'68; Langs: Arabic; Assyrian; (780)465-0522; Fax. (780)465-0436.

TOMA, Tamer S; Family Focus Med Clinic, 201-240 Baker Dr, Dartmouth NS B2W 6L4; Ain shams (Egypt)'98; MB BCh; CCFP; Langs: Arabic; (902)462-0893; Fax. (902)462-2015.

TOMA, Warda S; Lions Gate Hosp, 231 15th St E, North Vancouver BC V7L 2L7; McG'08; Peds. Staff, Lions Gate Hospital; (604)988-3131

TOMAN, John D; 507-18 Kensington Rd, Brampton ON L6T 4S5; Tor'74; BSc; (905)792-2228; Fax. (905)792-2275.

TOMANEK, Anna I; Cochrane Primary Care Centre, 103-100 Grande Blvd W, Cochrane AB T4C 0S4; Knalubu (Poland)'89; CCFP; Langs: Polish; (403)932-2089; Fax. (403)932-1820.

TOMASHPOLSKAYA, Janny; Humber Valley Ultrasound Inc, 2630 Kipling Ave, Etobicoke ON M9V 4B9; Odessa (Ukraine)'61; FRCPC; DiagRad. Ac Staff, Women's College Hospital; Langs: Russian; (416)748-8434; Fax. (416)748-6158.

TOMASZEWSKI, Christopher; Dr C Tomaszewski MD Inc, 103-1015 Austin Ave, Coquitlam BC V3K 3N9; Lodz (Poland)'79; Staff, Eagle Ridge Hospital & Health Care Centre; Staff, Royal Columbian Hospital; (604)931-4885; Fax. (604)931-4847; ctomaszewski_mdinc@shawlink.ca.

TOMBLER, Richard D; 1500 Power Dam Dr RR 2 Lcd 1, Cornwall ON K6H 5R6; Ott'77; FRCSC; OrthSurg (Sports Medicine). Staff, Cornwall Community Hospital; Langs: English; French; (613)938-2990; Fax. (613)938-5082.

TOMBLIN, Joan L; Royal Columbian Hosp, 330 Columbia St E, New Westminster BC V3L 3W7; McG'72; FRCPC; MedMicrobiol. Staff Lab, Royal Columbian Hospital; (604)520-4347

TOMC, John E; 204-2425 Tecumseh Rd E, Windsor ON N8W 1E6; Ott'87; FRCSC; ObstGyn (Infertility). Clin Teacher, University of Western Ontario; (519)254-6461; Fax. (519)254-1349.

TOMCZAK-BOJARSKI, Anna B; Sudbury Reg Hosp-Laurentian, 41 Ramsey Lake Rd, Sudbury ON P3E 5J1; Warsaw (Poland)'81; FRCPC; AnatPath. Staff, Health Sciences North-St Joseph's Health Centre; Staff, Health Sciences North-Laurentian Site; Langs: Polish; (705)674-3181

TOMEN, Mark E; Dr Mark Tomen Prof Centre, 208-240 Grand Ave W, Chatham ON N7L 1C1; Wes'86; Staff, Chatham-Kent Health Alliance; (519)352-1251; Fax. (519)354-2721.

TOMES, Ladislav; Toronto East Gen Hosp Inc, 825 Coxwell Ave, Toronto ON M4C 3E7; Purkyne University (Czech Republic)'96; FRCPC; AnatPath. Staff, Toronto East General Hospital Inc; Langs: Czech; (416)461-8272

TOMI, Salem S; Lessard Med Clinic, 6633 177 St, Edmonton AB T5T 4K3; Al-Fateh (Libya)'98; (780)757-7999; Fax. (780)757-7991.

TOMI, Zohair S; Alpha Dermatology Centre, 111-1 Paton St, St. John's NL A1B 4S8; Tripoli (Libya)'89; MB ChB; FRCPC; Derm. (709)753-5525

TOMIAK, Anna T; Kingston Reg Cancer Centre, 25 King St W, Kingston ON K7L 5P9; Qns'87; FRCPC; IntMed; MedOncol. Staff, Kingston Regional Cancer Centre; (613)544-2631 x4503; Fax. (613)548-8201; anna.tomiak@krcc.on.ca.

TOMIAK, Eva M; Children's Hosp of Eastern Ont, 401 Smyth Rd, Ottawa ON K1H 8L1; Qns'84; FRCPC; IntMed (Medical Genetics); MedOncol. Staff, Children's Hospital of Eastern Ontario (CHEO); Langs: English; French; (613)737-7600; Fax. (613)738-4822.

TOMINI, Stephen R; 200 Fletcher Cres PO Box 4000 Stn Main, Alliston ON L9R 1W7; Ott'03; BMus; BSc; Staff, Stevenson Memorial Hospital; (705)435-6281

TOMITA, Todd M; Broadway Forensic Group, 305-1245 Broadway W, Vancouver BC V6H 1G7; Tor'95; FRCPC; Psy (Forensic Psychiatry). Staff, Regional Treatment Centre & Pacific Institution; (604)733-5722; ttomita@forensic.bc.ca.

TOMKIEWICZ, Robert P; Grey Nuns Community Hosp, 41-1100 Youville Drive West NW, Edmonton AB T6L 5X8; (Poland)'86; Staff, Covenant Health - Grey Nuns Community Hospital; (780)735-7042; Fax. (780)735-7285.

TOMLIN, Heather A; 1221-3266 Yonge St, Toronto ON M4N 3P6; Ott'92; FRCPC; DiagRad (Acupuncture). Langs: German; French.

TOMLIN PROCYK, Jennifer L T; North York Gen Hosp, 4001 Leslie St, North York ON M2K 1E1; Tor'03; CCFP; CCFP(E.M.); Staff, North York General Hospital; (416)756-6000; Fax. (416)756-6822.

TOMLINSON, Charles W; Hamilton HS-Hamilton Gen, 237 Barton St E, Hamilton ON L8L 2X2; Man'76; PhD; FACC; FRCPC; IntMed (Cardiology). Staff Cardiol, Hamilton Health Sciences Centre-Juravinski Site; Staff, Hamilton Health Sciences Centre - Hamilton General Hospital; Assoc Prof Cardiol, McMaster University; (905)521-9533; Fax. (905)527-1467; tomlins@hhsc.ca.

TOMLINSON, Corey L; Richmond Med Bldg, 302-2020 Richmond Ave, Victoria BC V8R 6R5; Alb'07; FRCSC; GenSurg. Staff, University of Alberta Hospital; (250)592-4313

TOMLINSON, Donna A; Avon Family Med Centre, 511 Huron St, Stratford ON N5A 5T8; Wes'88; (519)508-1212; Fax. (519)508-1240.

TOMLINSON, H Mary M; The Nova Scotia Hosp, PO Box 1004 Stn Main, Dartmouth NS B2Y 3Z9; London (England)'71; MRCS; LRCP; Psy. Ac Staff, The Nova Scotia Hospital; Lecturer Psy, Dalhousie University; (902)464-3043; Fax. (902)464-3044.

TOMLINSON, R Bruce; St Marys Mem Hosp, PO Box 940 Stn Main 267 Queen St, St Marys ON N4X 1B6; Wes'85; Staff, St Marys Memorial Hospital - Huron Perth Healthcare Alliance; (519)284-1330

TOMLINSON, Robert C K; The Hosp For Sick Children, 555 University Ave, Toronto ON M5G 1X8; Glasgow (Scotland)'94; Staff Neonatal Intensive Care Unit, The Hospital For Sick Children; (416)813-6925; Fax. (416)813-5245.

TOMM, Bill G; 3410 28 Ave, Vernon BC V1T 1W9; Cal'78; FRCPC; Psy (Psychotherapy). (250)549-0483; Fax. (250)542-0954.

TOMM, Karl M; Henry Huang Bldg, 300-2204 2 St NW, Calgary AB T2S 3C2; Alb'63; FRCPC; Psy (Family Therapy). (403)802-1680; Fax. (403)270-7446.

TOMMASINI, Robert; Yonge-Eglinton Med Centre, 207-2401 Yonge St, Toronto ON M4P 3H1; Dublin (Ireland)'86; MB ChB; BAO; LRCP; LRCS; CCFP; Langs: Italian; (416)483-8382; Fax. (416)483-6690.

TOMNEY, Patricia A; Chatham-Kent Health Alliance, PO Box 2030 Stn Main 80 Grand Ave W, Chatham ON N7M 5L9; Dal'85; BSc; MSc; DiagRad. Staff, Chatham-Kent Health Alliance; (519)352-6400 x6530; Fax. (519)437-6040.

TOMPALSKI, Sherry L; CFB Petawawa, PO Box 9999 Stn Main S 111-101 Menin Rd, Petawawa ON K8H 2X3; UBC'86; FRCPC; Psy. (613)601-3470

TOMPKINS, Beverly A; The Burke Institute, 210-1333 8 St SW, Calgary AB T2R 1M6; Cal'91; (403)802-1772; Fax. (403)802-1762.

TOMPKINS, Brent W; Dr H Bliss Murphy Cancer Ctre, 300 Prince Philip Dr, St. John's NL A1B 3V6; Mem'96; FRCPC; RadOncol. Staff Dr Bliss Murphy Cancer Center, Health Sciences Centre; (709)777-7805

TOMPKINS, Brock J F; Northwood Med Centre, 35 Springbank Ave N, Woodstock ON N4S 7P6; Tor'96; BSc(Hons.); CCFP; (519)539-1112; Fax. (519)537-2944.

TOMPKINS, Kirsty A; Health Sciences Centre, 300 Prince Philip Dr, St. John's NL A1B 3V6; Mem'92; FRCPC; IntMed (Clinician Investigator Program); Hem. Staff Clinician Investigator Program, Health Sciences Centre; (709)777-8062

TOMSON, William G; Worker's Compensation Board, 6951 Westminster Hwy, Richmond BC V7C 1C6; Tor'70; FACSM; FAAFP; FAASM; Sr Advisor Med, WorkSafe BC; (604)276-5130; Fax. (604)279-7408; wtomson@cheo.on.ca.

TOMY, Kerry L; 200C-392 Academy Rd, Winnipeg MB R3N 0B8.

TOMY, Nadia N; University of Alberta Hosp, 1E1-8440 112 St NW, Edmonton AB T6G 2B7; Ott'02; FRCPC; Psy. Staff, University of Alberta Hospital; (780)407-8330; Fax. (780)407-6470.

TOMY, R Halim; Concordia Gen Hosp, 1095 Concordia Ave, Winnipeg MB R2K 3S8; Man'95; CCFP; FCFP; CCFP(E.M.); Staff, Concordia General Hospital; (204)667-1560

TON, Sau Nu Thi; Centre Med 325, 425 boul Cure-Poirier O, Longueuil QC J4J 2H3; Hue (Vietnam)'76; (450)679-6666; Fax. (450)679-6446; sntton@videotron.ca.

TON-NU, Thanh-Thao; CSSS du Nord de Lanaudière, 1000 boul Sainte-Anne, St-Charles-Brromee QC J6E 6J2; Mon'97; FRCPC; IntMed (Cardiac Radiology & Echocardiogram); Cardiol. Staff, Lakeshore General Hospital - Pointe Claire; Staff, Centre Hospitalier de Verdun; Langs: French; Vietnamese; (450)759-8222

TON-THAT, Quoc-Huy; 4469 av Christophe-Colomb, Montreal QC H2J 3G4; McG'05; CCFP; CCFP(E.M.); Langs: Vietnamese; French; (514)971-5711

TON-THAT, Quoc-Tuan; CSSS du Suroît, 150 rue Saint-Thomas, Salaber-de-Valleyf QC J6T 6C1; Mon'87; FRCPC; NuclearMed. Staff, Centre Hospitalier Régional du Suroît; (450)371-9920; Fax. (450)694-0495.

TON-THAT, Trac; Centre Lucie-Bruneau, 2275 av Laurier E, Montreal QC H2H 2N8; Saigon (Vietnam)'75; Staff, Centre de Readaptation Lucie-Bruneau; (514)527-4527 x2225; Fax. (514)527-6637.

TONDREAU, Genevieve; Hop Maisonneuve-Rosemont, 5415 boul de l'Assomption, Montreal QC H1T 2M4; Mon'90; CCFP; FCFP; Prof/Chef méd fam, Hopital Maisonneuve-Rosemont; Clin Prof, Universite de Montreal; (514)252-3400 x4513; Fax. (514)252-3854.

TONEFF, Christopher J; 120-1636 Main St, Penticton BC V2A 5G8; McM'92; (250)492-3336; Fax. (250)492-3338.

TONELLI, Marcello A; Clinical Sciences Bldg, 7 129-152 University Campus NW, Edmonton AB T6G 2G3; Wes'95; FRCPC; IntMed; Nephrol. Staff, University of Alberta Hospital; (780)407-8520; Fax. (780)407-7878; mtonelli-admin@med.alberta.ca.

TONER, Lee V; Health Sciences North, 41 Ramsey Lake Rd, Sudbury ON P3E 5J1; Dal'98; CCFP; CCFP(E.M.); Staff, Health Sciences North-St Joseph's Health Centre; Section Leader Emergency Med, Northern Ontario School of Medicine-Laurentian University; Langs: Bilingual(English/French); (705)675-4700; Fax. (705)675-4794.

TONG, Amy Y M; Health Sciences Centre, 300 Prince Philip Dr, St. John's NL A1B 3V6; (Hong Kong)'76; MB BS; FRCPC; IntMed. Staff, Health Sciences Centre; (709)777-8662

TONG, Christina; Clinique Med Roper, 4500 rue Sherbrooke O, Westmount QC H3Z 1E6; McG'94; BSc(Hon.); CCFP; FCFP; Langs: English; French; (514)937-8000; Fax. (514)937-8884.

TONG, Daniel Y; 2105 Commercial Dr, Vancouver BC V5N 4B3; Alb'71; BSc; MSc; Ac Staff, Providence Health Care - Mount Saint Joseph Hospital; Court Staff, BC Women's Hospital & Health Centre; Langs: Cantonese; Mandarin; French; (604)254-7262; Fax. (604)254-7263.

TONG, Jennifer N; Red Lake Med Associates, PO Box 311 51G Hwy 105, Red Lake ON P0V 2M0; Wes'08; CCFP; (807)727-2617; Fax. (807)727-3122.

TONG, Jennifer Y; Collingwood Med Clinic, 350-3150 54 Ave E, Vancouver BC V5S 1Z1; UBC'03; CCFP; (604)435-3388

TONG, Kevin L F; East Van Med Bldg, 506-1750 10th Ave E, Vancouver BC V5N 5K4; Rio de Janeiro (Brazil)'85; Vis Staff, Vancouver General Hospital - Centennial Pavillion; Clinical Asst Prof, University of British Columbia; Langs: Mandarin; Taiwanese; Portuguese; Chinese; Fukinese; Spanish; (604)873-2022; Fax. (604)873-0292; kevin-tong@shaw.ca.

TONG, Lawrence; York Institute of Plastic Surg, 199 Avenue Rd, Toronto ON M5R 2J3; Tor'95; FRCSC; PlasSurg. Staff, York Institute of Plastic Surgery; (416)972-0999

TONG, Maorong; Port Arthur Health Centre Inc, 194 Court St N, Thunder Bay ON P7A 4V7; Bengbu Medical College (China)'84; CCFP; Langs: Mandarin; Japanese; (807)346-1000

TONG, Melissa G Y; Surrey Eye Associates, 13490 104 Ave, Surrey BC V3T 1V8; Thomas Jefferson University (USA)'07; FRCSC; Ophth. (604)588-6001

TONG, Nhan Thien; Family Med Clinic, 59-4801 Keele St, North York ON M3J 3A4; Wes'89; Ac Staff Family Med, Humber River Regional Hospital - Finch Avenue Site; Langs: Vietnamese; (416)398-7523; Fax. (416)398-7524.

TONG, Norman T; PO Box 26077 Rpo Ctrl Richmond, Richmond BC V6Y 3V3; Witwatersrand (South Africa)'76; MB ChB; (604)818-6821

TONG, Raymond Q L; 102-12005 238B St, Maple Ridge BC V4R 1W1; Dal'66; Ac Staff, Ridge Meadows Hospital & Health Care Centre; (604)476-9705; Fax. (604)467-5240.

TONG, Shu Kow; Carefirst Family Health Team, 27-420 Highway 7 E, Richmond Hill ON L4B 3K2; Manchester (England)'79; FRSM; Court Staff, The Scarborough Hospital - Birchmount Campus; Ac Staff, The Scarborough Hospital - General Campus; Langs: Cantonese; (905)695-1133; Fax. (905)695-0826.

TONG, Vicki M; University Village Med Clinic, 228-2155 Allison Rd, Vancouver BC V6T 1T5; UBC'01; CCFP; (604)222-2273; Fax. (604)222-3403.

TONG, Vince; Aquarius Med Clinic, 202-179 Davie St, Vancouver BC V6Z 2Y1; Wes'00; CCFP; (604)669-7772; Fax. (604)669-7772.

TONG, Xiaoxing C; Grand River Hosp K W HC, PO Box 9056 Stn C 835 King St W, Kitchener ON N2G 1G3; Tor'05; CCFP; CCFP(E.M.); Staff, St Mary's General Hospital; Staff Emerg, Grand River Hospital - Kitchener/Waterloo Health Centre; (519)749-4242

TONGUE, Antonio G; CSSS- Hop de Hull, 116 boul Lionel-Emond, Gatineau QC J8Y 1W7; Laval'03; FRCPC; DiagRad. Staff, Hull Hospital; (819)966-6200 x6028; 001.agt@gmail.com.

TONKIN, Katia S; Cross Cancer Institute, 11560 University Ave NW, Edmonton AB T6G 1Z2; London (England)'78; MB BS; LMCC; MRC; FRCPC; IntMed (Breast Cancer); MedOncol. Staff, Cross Cancer Institute; Assoc Prof, University of Alberta; (780)432-8514; Fax. (780)432-8888; katia.tonkin@albertahealthservices.ca.

TONN, Debra J; La Ronge Med Clinic, PO Box 240, La Ronge SK S0J 1L0; Sask'05; CCFP; Physician, La Ronge Medical Clinic; (306)425-2174; Fax. (306)425-4199.

TONNU, Lienchi; Clinique Plateau Mont-Royal, 1374 av du Mont-Royal E, Montreal QC H2J 1Y7; Saigon (Vietnam)'75; (514)527-3997

TONOGAI, Wayne T; Kelowna Gen Hosp, 2268 Pandosy St, Kelowna BC V1Y 1T2; Wes'88; FRCPC; DiagRad. Staff, Kelowna General Hospital; (250)862-4454

TONON, Kristen A; West Carleton Family Hlth Team, PO Box 218 119 Langstaff Dr, Carp ON K0A 1L0; McM'99; CCFP; (613)839-3271; Fax. (613)839-3273.

TONSETH, Rolf P; BC Cancer Agency, 600 10 Ave W, Vancouver BC V5Z 4E6; UBC'88; FRCPC; DiagRad; NuclearMed. Staff, BC Cancer Agency Vancouver Centre; (604)707-5979

TOOFANI, Roya; MCI Medical Clinics INC, 200-160 Eglinton Ave E, Toronto ON M4P 3B5; Man'97; Physician, North Hamilton Community Health Centre; (905)529-4040; toofani@nhchc.ca.

TOOGOOD, Jillian A; East Elgin Family Health Team, 2-418 Talbot St W, Aylmer ON N5H 1K9; The Flinders Univ of South Australia (Australia)'10; (519)765-1280

TOOLE, Douglas R; The Medical Clinic Associates, 4794A Joyce Ave, Powell River BC V8A 3B6; UBC'72; (604)485-6261; Fax. (604)485-2820.

TOOLE, John W P; Specialist in Skin Diseases, 205 Edmonton St, Winnipeg MB R3C 1R4; Man'72; BSc; ABD; FRCPC; Derm. Chief Derm, Winnipeg Regional Health Authority; Head Section of Derm/Prof Med, University of Manitoba; (204)943-8245; Fax. (204)942-4399.

TOOLEY, Camilla M; Florenceville Med Clinic, 2-23 McCain St, Florenceville NB E7L 3J5; Dal'82; (506)392-6268; Fax. (506)392-5501.

TOOMING, Vello E T; Halton HCS Corp-Milton, 7030 Derry Rd, Milton ON L9T 7H6; Wes'79; Ac Staff, Halton Healthcare Services Corporation - Milton District Hospital; Physician, Maplehurst Detention Centre; (905)878-2383

TOONG, Ying Lai H; 701-123 Edward St, Toronto ON M5G 1E2; Shantung Medical College (China)'62; Assoc Staff, Toronto Western Hospital - University Health Network; Langs: Cantonese; Mandarin; Shanghai; (416)977-2833; Fax. (416)977-1335.

TOOP, Jo-Ann D; Jo-Ann Toop Med Prof Corp, RR 1 18840 Beaverbrook Rd, Martintown ON K0C 1S0; McG'87; (613)528-4402; Fax. (613)528-4623.

TOOR, Dalvinder S; 6425 Main St, Vancouver BC V5W 2V5; Punjab (India)'77; MB BS; CCFP; Langs: Hindi; Punjabi; Urdu; (604)568-5667; Fax. (604)568-6697.

TOOR, Gurdev S; West Winds Med Clinic, 2130-4818 Westwinds Dr NE, Calgary AB T3J 3Z5; (403)293-5454; Fax. (403)293-1511.

TOOR, Jaspreet K; St Joseph's Healthcare, 50 Charlton Ave E, Hamilton ON L8N 4A6; Punjab (India)'99; MB BS; FRCPC; AnatPath. Staff, St Joseph's Healthcare - Charlton Campus; (905)522-4941; jaspreet.toor@cdha.nshealth.ca.

TOOTH, Kerry J; Toronto East Gen & Orth Hosp, 825 Coxwell Ave, East York ON M4C 3E7; Tor'93; FRCPC; DiagRad. Staff, Toronto East General Hospital Inc; (416)461-8272

TOOTOOSIS, Janet J; North Battleford Med Clinic, 102-11427 Railway Ave E, North Battleford SK S9A 3G8; Sask'99; CCFP; Physician, North Battleford Medical Clinic; (306)445-4415; Fax. (306)445-5145.

TOP, Karina A M; IWK Health Centre, PO Box 9700 Rpo CSC 5850-5980 University Ave, Halifax NS B3K 6R8; Dal'05; FRCPC; Peds; InfectDis. Staff, IWK Health Centre; (902)470-6343; Fax. (902)470-7232.

TOPAKIAN, Arman; 2100-504 rue Notre-Dame, Repentigny QC J6A 2T8; Istanbul (Turkey)'66; CSPQ; FRCSC; ObstGyn (P.Q.). Langs: Bilingual(English/French); (450)654-6973; Fax. (450)582-1573.

TOPHAM, Darren J; Synthesis Proactive Med Inc, 817A 49 Ave SW, Calgary AB T2S 1G8; Cal'91; CCFP; Staff Operating Room, Rockyview General Hospital; Physician, Synthesis Proactive Medicine Inc; Med Dir Dermedics Advanced Med Aesthetics/Physician Orthopedics Assist, Britannia Dermedics; Physician, Health Resource Centre; (403)984-4313; Fax. (403)984-4314; dctopham@shaw.ca.

TOPIC, Delilah L; BC Cancer Agency Southern Int, 399 Royal Ave, Kelowna BC V1Y 5L3; Tor'06; FRCPC; IntMed; MedOncol. Staff, BC Cancer Agency Sindi Ahluwalia Hawkins Centre for the Southern Interior; (250)712-3930

TOPLACK, Christina M; 201-5663 Cornwallis St, Halifax NS B3K 1B6; McM'91; CCFP; (902)425-4157; Fax. (902)542-0875.

TOPP, Bruce R; 205-272 Lawrence Ave W, Toronto ON M5M 4M1; Tor'85; BSc; Dip SportMed; CCFP; Staff, North York General Hospital; Staff, Sunnybrook Health Sciences Centre; (416)787-7516; Fax. (416)787-7528.

TOPP, Trevor J; Queen Elizabeth II HSC, 8 813-1276 South Park St, Halifax NS B3H 2Y9; Alb'88; ATLS; BSc; MD; FACS; FRCS; FRCSC; GenSurg; Critical Care Medicine. Staff, Queen Elizabeth II Health Sciences Centre - Victoria General Site; Asst Prof Med & Surg, Dalhousie University; (902)473-5131; Fax. (902)473-2299; tjtopp@dal.ca.

TOPPIN, Dennis I; Royal City Med Bldg, 203-250 Keary St, New Westminster BC V3L 5E7; West Indies (Jamaica)'67; MB BS; FRCSC; GenSurg; Cardiovasc&ThorSurg. Ac Staff, Royal Columbian Hospital; (604)525-6232; Fax. (604)525-0483.

TOPPIN, James L; West Arthur Place, 304-1265 Arthur St E, Thunder Bay ON P7E 6E7; Tor'81; Staff, Thunder Bay Regional Health Sciences Centre; (807)625-0055; Fax. (807)625-6504.

TOPPING, Claude; Ctr Hosp Affilie-Enfant-Jesus, 1401 18e rue, Quebec QC G1J 1Z4; Laval'81; CCFP; CCFP(E.M.); FCFP; EmergMed. Staff Emerg, Centre Hospitalier Affilié Universitaire de Québec - Hôpital De L'Enfant Jésus; Dir Prog de Formation Complementaire & Emerg Med, Université Laval; (418)649-5632; Fax. (418)656-5252.

TOPPS, David A; Sheldon Shumuik Centre, 8F-1213 4 St SW, Calgary AB T2R 0X7; Aberdeen (Scotland)'80; MB ChB; MRCGPract; CCFP; FCFP; (403)955-9500; Fax. (403)476-8766.

TOPPS, Maureen H; Sheldon M Chumir Health Centre, 1213 4 St SW, Calgary AB T2R 0X7; Aberdeen (Scotland)'82; MB ChB; CCFP; FCFP; Staff, Sheldon M Chumir Urgent Care Physician Group; (403)955-9300; maureen.topps@albertahealthservices.ca.

TOPSTAD, Dawnelle R; PO Box 67158 Rpo Northland Vil, Calgary AB T2L 2L2; Alb'89; FRCSC; GenSurg. Staff, Red Deer Regional Hospital Centre.

TOPTCHIEVA, Anna A; Toronto East Gen & Orth Hosp, 825 Coxwell Ave, East York ON M4C 3E7; Dal'02; FRCPC; Anes. Staff, Toronto East General Hospital Inc; Langs: Russian; Ukrainian; (416)461-8272; Fax. (416)469-6874.

TORAN, Victor A; 2301 Weston Rd, York ON M9N 1Z7; Tor'76; FRCSC; Otol (Head & Neck Surgery). Sr Staff, Humber River Regional Hospital - Church Street Site; Langs: German; Slovak; (416)241-6701; Fax. (416)249-2008.

TORBEY, Camille; 104-9840 97 Ave, Grande Prairie AB T8V 7K2; Beyrouth (Lebanon)'82; FRCSC; Urol. Staff, Queen Elizabeth II Hospital; (780)538-4315; Fax. (780)538-1596.

TORBIAK, Carl W; Meadowlark Health Centre, 200 Meadowlark Shopping Ctr NW, Edmonton AB T5R 5W9; Man'90; FRCPC; DiagRad. Staff, Covenant Health - Misericordia Community Hospital; Clin Instructor DiagRad, University of Alberta; (780)489-7851; Fax. (780)489-5160.

TORBIAK, Raymond P; Joseph Brant Mem Hosp, 1230 North Shore Blvd E, Burlington ON L7S 1W7; Man'83; FRCPC; DiagRad (Angiography). Vis Staff, Hamilton Health Sciences Centre - McMaster Children's Hospital; Staff, Hamilton Health Sciences Centre-Juravinski Site; Staff, Joseph Brant Memorial Hospital; Asst Prof Radiol, McMaster University; (905)632-3730; Fax. (905)336-6480.

TORBICKI, Edward A; Anaesthesie Associates, 2F-439 Park St, Kitchener ON N2G 1N4; Ott'82; FRCPC; Anes. Staff, St Mary's General Hospital; Staff, Grand River Hospital - Kitchener/Waterloo Health Centre; Langs: Polish; (519)744-7361; Fax. (519)744-7363.

TORBIN, Lauren B; Davisville Fam Practice, 612-1881 Yonge St, Toronto ON M4S 3C4; Tor'78; (416)488-0123; Fax. (416)488-9804.

TORDJMAN, Philippe; Clin Med Maisonneuve Rosemont, RC60-5345 boul l'Assomption, Montreal QC H1T 4B3; Mon'95; CCFP; CCFP(E.M.); Staff, Centre Hospitalier Fleury; (514)257-7000; Fax. (514)257-7003; ptordjman@videotron.ca.

TOREN, Andrew J; CHAQ-Hop Saint-Sacrement, 1050 ch Sainte-Foy, Quebec QC G1S 4L8; Tor'06; FRCSC; Ophth. Staff, Centre Hospitalier Affilié Universitaire de Québec - Hôpital du St-Sacrement; (418)682-7904

TOREN, Paul J; The Prostate Centre, 2660 Oak St, Vancouver BC V6H 3Z6; Qns'06; FRCSC; Urol. Staff, The Prostate Centre; (604)875-7111 x21762

TORESON, Jeffrey A; 303-321 Nicola St, Kamloops BC V2C 6G6; Alb'05; FRCSC; OrthSurg. (250)434-6400

TORFASON, Lois A; Student Wellness Centre, MEH 370-2500 University Dr NW, Calgary AB T2N 1N4; Cal'88; BA(Psych); BN; (403)210-9355; Fax. (403)282-5218.

TORGERSON, Cory S; 31-70 Yorkville Ave, Toronto ON M5R 1B9; Tor'02; FRCSC; Otol (Head & Neck Surgery). Staff, Sunnybrook Health Sciences Centre; (647)343-0207; Fax. (647)343-0277; info@drtorgerson.com.

TORIGIAN, Michael A; 4421 Queen St, Niagara Falls ON L2E 2L2; (Antigua & Barbuda)'03; CCFP; (905)356-2236; Fax. (905)356-2568.

TORIZ, Luis; Hôtel-Dieu de Saint-Jérôme, 290 rue Montigny, Saint-Jerome QC J7Z 5T3; (Mexico)'70; OrthSurg (P.Q.). ac Staff, Hôtel-Dieu de Saint-Jérôme; assoc Staff, CSSS d'Antoine-Labelle; Langs: Spanish; English; (450)431-8200

TORKIAN-VALASHANI, Bahman; Harmony Med Clinic, 1385 Harmony Rd N, Oshawa ON L1H 7K5; Shaheed Beheshti University (Iran)'94; CCFP; Langs: Farsi; (905)436-9646; Fax. (905)436-9666.

TORLAKOVIC, Emina; Univ Hlth Network-Toronto Gen, 411-200 Elizabeth St, Toronto ON M5G 2C4; Zagreb (Croatia)'86; Staff, Toronto General Hospital - UHN; (416)340-4800; Fax. (416)340-5543.

TORLAKOVIC, Goran; William Osler HC-Etobicoke, 101 Humber College Blvd, Etobicoke ON M9V 1R8; Zagreb (Croatia)'87; FRCPC; AnatPath. Staff, William Osler Health System - Etobicoke General Hospital; (416)494-2120; goran.torlakovic@saskatoonhealthregion.com.

TORNE-PEREZ, Montserrat; Windsor Reg Hosp-Tayfour Site, 1453 Prince Rd, Windsor ON N9C 3Z4; Universidad del Cauca (Colombia)'97; Staff, Windsor Regional Hospital - Tayfour Site; (519)254-5577

TORNG, Shirley; Simon Fraser Health Authority, 309-301 Columbia St E, New Westminster BC V3L 3W5; Mem'96; FRCPC; IntMed; Nephrol. Staff, Royal Columbian Hospital; Staff, Surrey Memorial Hospital; (604)515-1175; Fax. (604)777-5615; nephoffice@gmail.com.

TOROK, Kim M; Port Hope Comm Health Centre, 99 Toronto Rd, Port Hope ON L1A 3S4; Qns'96; CCFP; FCFP; Asst Prof, Northern Ontario School of Medicine; (905)885-2626; Fax. (905)885-2646.

TOROK, Maria T; Dartmouth Med Centre, 301-46 Portland St, Dartmouth NS B2Y 1H4; Debrecen (Hungary)'63; FRCPC; Peds. Langs: Hungarian; Polish; (902)465-8720; Fax. (902)465-8712.

TOROK-BOTH, Clinton J; Misericordia Comm Hosp & HC, 16940 87 Ave NW, Edmonton AB T5R 4H5; Alb'00; FRCPC; Anes; Critical Care Medicine. Staff Critical Care Clinic, Covenant Health - Misericordia Community Hospital; (780)735-2858; Fax. (780)735-2953.

TOROK-BOTH, George A; Smith Clinic, 1-6601 48 Ave, Camrose AB T4V 3G8; Alb'96; CCFP; Staff, Covenant Health - St Mary's Hospital; (780)672-2425; Fax. (780)608-5897.

TOROSSI, Gregory A; Concordia Gen Hosp, 1095 Concordia Ave, Winnipeg MB R2K 3S8; Man'91; Staff/Site Mgr Emerg, Concordia General Hospital; Assoc Staff Emerg, Victoria General Hospital; University of Manitoba; (204)667-1560

TORRANCE, Shona M; Faculty of Health Sciences, 4D 14B-1280 Main St W, Hamilton ON L8S 4K1; McM'03; FRCSC; ObstGyn (Maternal Fetal Medicine). Staff, Hamilton Health Sciences Centre - McMaster Children's Hospital; (905)521-2100; Fax. (905)527-2675.

TORRAVILLE, Douglas A; James Paton Mem Hosp, 125 Trans Canada Hwy, Gander NL A1V 1P7; Mem'81; ObstGyn (Urogynecology). Staff, James Paton Memorial Hospital; Staff, Central Newfoundland Regional Health Centre; Staff, Captain William Jackman Memorial Hospital; (709)256-2500; dlmtorraville@msn.com.

TORRES, Carlos H; The Ottawa Hosp-Civic Campus, 1053 Carling Ave, Ottawa ON K1Y 4E9; Pontificia Universidad Javeriana (Other Foreign)'96; Staff, The Ottawa Hospital - Civic Campus; Langs: Bilingual(English/French); (613)798-5555

TORRES, Frank X; Health Sciences Centre, 300 Prince Philip Dr, St. John's NL A1B 3V6; University of Guadalajara (Mexico)'83; Staff, Health Sciences Centre; (709)737-6300

TORRES, Monica M; London HSC-Victoria Campus, 800 Commissioners Rd E, London ON N6A 5W9; Javier Pontifical University (Dominican Republic)'01; FRCSC; GenSurg. Staff, Alexandra Marine & General Hospital; Staff, London Health Sciences Centre - Victoria Campus; (519)685-8500

TORRES-BALLEN, Myriam; Ctre Hosp Rouyn-Noranda, 4 9e rue, Rouyn-Noranda QC J9X 2B2; (Colombia)'88; Staff, Centre Hospitalier Rouyn-Noranda; Staff, CSSS de Rouyn-Noranda; (819)762-5599; Fax. (819)762-0230.

TORRES JIMENEZ, Monica; Alexandra Marine & Gen Hosp, 120 Napier St, Goderich ON N7A 1W5; Pontificia Universidad Javeriana (Other Foreign)'98; Staff, Alexandra Marine & General Hospital; Langs: Spanish; (519)524-8323

TORRES MARTINEZ, Nestor E; 70 Charles St, Brockville ON K6V 1T3; McG'94; CCFP; Langs: Spanish; French; (613)345-1549; Fax. (613)345-5296.

TORRES-PARDO, Carlos I; MUHC-Royal Victoria Hosp, 687 av des Pins O, Montreal QC H3A 1A1; Bogota (Colombia)'93; Staff, McGill University Health Centre - Royal Victoria Hospital; (514)842-1231; Fax. (514)843-1517.

TORRES ROJAS, Gisset D L C; CSSS de Laval, 280 boul Roi du Nord, Laval QC H7L 4L2; Havana (Cuba)'91; CCFP; Staff, CSSS de la Vallée de la Gatineau; (450)622-5110

TORRES-TREJO, Alejandro; Juravinski Cancer Centre, 699 Concession St, Hamilton ON L8V 5C2; (Mexico)'89; Staff, Hamilton Health Sciences Centre - Juravinski Cancer Centre; (905)387-9495; Fax. (905)575-6326.

TORRI, Vamsee; Allan Blair Cancer Centre, 4101 Dewdney Ave, Regina SK S4T 7T1; Staff, Allan Blair Cancer Centre; (306)766-2213; Fax. (306)766-2777.

TORRIBLE, Susan J; Geriatric Assessment, 453 Prince Rd, Windsor ON N9C 3Z4; Cal'96; FRCPC; IntMed; GeriatricMed. (519)257-5112; Fax. (519)257-5242.

TORRIE, Ian D; Canadian Forces Supp Unit HCC, 1745 Alta Vista Dr, Ottawa ON K1A 0K6; Mem'94; Staff OpMed 1, Canadian Forces Health Services Centre; (613)945-6600 x3627; Fax. (613)945-6668.

TORRIE, Julie C; Lahey Med Centre, 2204-120 5 Ave, Cochrane AB T4C 0A4; (Other Foreign)'07; CCFP; (403)981-6000; Fax. (403)981-6001.

TORRIE, Kathleen A; Sows Ear Med Clinic, PO Box 190 7186 Lantzville Rd, Lantzville BC V0R 2H0; UBC'90; Ac Staff, Nanaimo Regional General Hospital; (250)390-4542; Fax. (250)390-4561.

TORRIE, Ryan D; Associate Med Centre, 5016 48 Ave, Taber AB T1G 1R8; (USA)'03; CCFP; (403)223-3525; Fax. (403)229-9020.

TORRIERO, Melissa J; Maternity Care Clinic, 109-178 96 Ave NE, Calgary AB T3K 6G4; Cal'06; CCFP; Staff, Maternity Care Clinic; Langs: Bilingual(English/French); (403)735-4922

TORS, Adrienne; 206-4040 Finch Ave E, Scarborough ON M1S 4V5; Tor'89; Staff Family Pract, The Scarborough Hospital - Birchmount Campus; Langs: Cantonese; (416)495-7972; Fax. (416)495-1418.

TORSHER, Kevin J; Rockyview Gen Hosp, 7007 14 St SW, Calgary AB T2V 1P9; Alb'91; FRCPC; Anes. Staff, Rockyview General Hospital; (403)943-8720; Fax. (403)943-8242.

TORSTENSEN, Eric T; Rebalance MD, 104-3551 Blanshard St, Victoria BC V8Z 0B9; Cal'93; FRCSC; OrthSurg (Foot & Ankle Surgery). (250)940-4444

TOSCANO, Marie; Clinique de Dermatologie, 110-500 boul Greber, Gatineau QC J8T 7W3; Sher'87; FRCPC; Derm. Staff, Hull Hospital; Staff, CH-CHSLD de Papineau - Pavillon du centre hospitalier; Langs: Italian; English; (819)561-5553; Fax. (819)561-5554.

TOSEFSKY, Merrick; Able-Care Med Clinic, 56-2991 Lougheed Hwy, Coquitlam BC V3B 6J6; Witwatersrand (South Africa)'84; MB ChB; Assoc Staff, Royal Columbian Hospital; Assoc Staff/Med Dir, Eagle Ridge Hospital & Health Care Centre; (604)945-7819; Fax. (604)945-2884.

TOSIKYAN, Axel; Hop du Sacre-Coeur de Mtl, 5400 boul Gouin O, Montreal QC H4J 1C5; McG'99; MedOncol; IntMed; Hem. Staff, Hôpital du Sacre-Coeur de Montréal; Langs: Armenian; Turkish; (514)338-2150; Fax. (514)338-2631; tosik99@yahoo.com.

TOSONI, Caroline M A; 1-1180 Place D'Orleans Dr, Orleans ON K1C 7K3; McM'95; BPs; CCFP; Langs: English; French; (613)830-7615; Fax. (613)824-6807.

TOSTI, Roberto; Pavillon Antoine Gauvreau, 18 rue Saint-Omer, Levis QC G6V 5C2; Mon'92; FRCPC; Psy. Staff, Hôtel-Dieu de Lévis; (418)835-7155

TOSTOWARYK, Karen J; Carling-Broadview Med Bldg, 304-770 Broadview Ave, Ottawa ON K2A 3Z3; McM'84; Surg Asst, The Ottawa Hospital - General Campus; Surg Asst, Queensway Carleton Hospital; (613)728-0161; Fax. (613)728-0122.

TOTH, Adam A; Queensway Prof Centre, 403-190 Sherway Dr, Etobicoke ON M9C 5N2; Wes'91; FRCSC; Otol (Head & Neck Surgery). Staff Otol, Trillium Health Centre - Mississauga; Langs: French; (416)695-2772; Fax. (416)695-2199.

TOTH, Agnes; Perth & Smiths Falls Dist Hosp, 60 Cornelia St W, Smiths Falls ON K7A 2H9; Wes'07; CCFP; Staff, Perth & Smiths Falls District Hospital - Smiths Falls Site; (613)283-2330

TOTH, Cory C; Heritage Med Research Bldg, 155-3330 Hospital Dr NW, Calgary AB T2N 4N1; Sask'97; BSc(Physics); FAAN; FRCPC; Neur (P.Q.) (Neuromuscular Diseases). (403)220-8831; Fax. (403)283-8731; corytoth@shaw.ca.

TOTH, Darryl P; 210-2425 Tecumseh Rd E, Windsor ON N8W 1E6; Wes'90; FRCPC; Derm. (519)971-7546; Fax. (519)971-9571.

TOTH, Ellen L; Heritage Med Research Centre, 107-362 University Campus NW, Edmonton AB T6G 2S2; Buenos Aires (Argentina)'78; ABIM; FRCPC; IntMed (Diabetes); Endocrin&Metab. Staff, University of Alberta Hospital; Prof, University of Alberta; (780)407-3636; Fax. (780)407-6702; ellen.toth@ualberta.ca.

TOTH, Gary A; Cowichan District Hosp, 3045 Gibbins Rd, Duncan BC V9L 1E5; UBC'87; BSc; CCFP; CCFP(E.M.); Med Staff Assoc, Cowichan District Hospital; (250)746-4141

TOTH, Joseph; MUHC-Royal Victoria Hosp, 48070-687 av des Pins O, Montreal QC H3A 1A1; Budapest (Hungary)'56; DiagRad. Staff, McGill University Health Centre - Royal Victoria Hospital; Langs: Hungarian; French; (514)934-1934

TOTH, Julius L R; York Thoracic Surgery Assoc, 56 Prospect St, Newmarket ON L3Y 3S9; Tor'85; MSc; DAB; FACS; FCCP; FRCSC; GenSurg; Critical Care Medicine; ThorSurg. Staff, Headwaters Health Care Centre - Orangeville Site; Consultant Thoracic Surg, Orillia Soldiers' Memorial Hospital; Staff, Southlake Regional Health Centre; Langs: Hungarian; (905)853-5864; Fax. (905)853-5865; jtoth@bellnet.ca.

TOTH, Michael L; 6-418 Talbot St W, Aylmer ON N5H 1K9; Wes'84; CCFP; FCFP; Staff, St Thomas Elgin General Hospital; (519)773-5336; Fax. (519)773-5337.

TOTH, Peter; The Credit Valley Hosp, 2200 Eglinton Ave W, Mississauga ON L5M 2N1; McM'92; CCFP; CCFP(E.M.); FCFP; Pres/Medical Staff, The Credit Valley Hospital; Langs: Slovak; (905)813-2200

TOTHILL, Andrea E; Seymour Med Clinic, 1530 7 Ave W, Vancouver BC V6J 1S3; UBC'98; FRCPC; IntMed; Critical Care Medicine; Respir. (604)738-2151

TOTOUNCHIAN, Fatemeh; Careview Med Centre, 214-3001 Gordon Ave, New Westminster BC V3C 2K7; Teheran (Iran)'96; (604)941-7700

TOUBASSI, Diana; Toronto Western FHT, 2W 428-399 Bathurst St, Toronto ON M5T 2S8; Tor'06; CCFP; Staff, Toronto Western Hospital - University Health Network; (416)603-5888; Fax. (416)603-5448.

TOUCHBURN, Andre P; Hopital George-L Dumont, 330 University Ave, Moncton NB E1C 2Z3; McG'91; CCFP; CCFP(E.M.); Staff, Dr Georges-L-Dumont University Hospital Centre; Langs: German; French; (506)312-3533; Fax. (506)869-2039.

TOUCHETTE, Catherine; CHUQ-Hôp de L'Enfant Jésus, 1401 18e rue, Quebec QC G1J 1Z4; Laval'05; FRCPC; Psy. Staff, Centre Hospitalier Affilié Universitaire de Québec - Hôpital De L'Enfant Jésus; (418)349-0252

TOUCHETTE, Jean-Sebastien; Ctr Hosp Laurentien, 234 rue Saint-Vincent, Ste-Agathe-des-Mts QC J8C 2B8; Laval'07; Staff, Centre Hospitalier Laurentien; (819)324-4000; jstouchette@hotmail.com.

TOUCHETTE, Matthieu; CHUS-Hop Hotel-Dieu, 580 rue Bowen S, Sherbrooke QC J1G 2E8; Sher'99; FRCPC; IntMed. Staff, Centre Hospitalier Universitaire de Sherbrooke-Hôpital Hôtel-Dieu; Staff, Centre Hospitalier Universitaire de Sherbrooke-Hopital Fleurimont; Langs: English; (819)346-1110; matthieu.touchette@usherbrooke.ca.

TOUCHETTE, Michel; Polyclinique Med Fabreville, 380 boul Cure-Labelle, Laval QC H7P 5L3; Mon'67; Vis Staff, Hôpital de Saint-Eustache; Vis Staff, Hopital de la Cite de la santé; (450)628-5800; Fax. (450)628-0217.

TOUCHIE, Claire E; The Ottawa Hosp-Gen Campus, CPCR L2135-501 Smyth Rd Box 20, Ottawa ON K1H 8L6; McG'90; FRCPC; IntMed (AIDS/HIV); InfectDis; MedMicrobiol. Staff, The Ottawa Hospital - General Campus; Assoc Prof, University of Ottawa; Langs: French; (613)739-6747

TOUCHIE, Harold W; Fredericton Med Clinic, 407-1015 Regent St, Fredericton NB E3B 6H5; Dal'67; OrthSurg. (506)458-0275; Fax. (506)457-4712.

TOUCHIE, Jane E; Dr Everett Chalmers Reg Hosp, PO Box 9000 Stn A 700 Priestman St, Fredericton NB E3B 5N5; Dal'89; Staff, Dr Everett Chalmers Regional Hospital; (506)452-5400

TOUCHIE, Michael J; Ottawa Reg Cancer Centre, 503 Smyth Rd, Ottawa ON K1H 1C4; Mem'87; Physician, Ottawa Regional Cancer Centre; Langs: English; French; (613)737-7700

TOUEG, Jacques; Polyclinique Concorde, 225-300 boul de la Concode E, Laval QC H7G 2E6; Mon'95; FRCSC; OrthSurg (Arthroscopy). Langs: Italian; English; (450)668-3840

TOUGAS, Manon; Hamilton HS-Henderson Site, 711 Concession St, Hamilton ON L8V 1C3; Mon'89; FRCPC; IntMed; Critical Care Medicine. Staff, Hamilton Health Sciences Centre-Juravinski Site; Langs: Bilingual(English/French); (905)527-4322 x42111

TOULANY, Alene A; The Hosp for Sick Children, 555 University Ave, Toronto ON M5G 1X8; Dal'06; FRCPC; Peds (Adolescent Medicine). Staff, The Hospital For Sick Children; (416)813-7500; Fax. (416)813-5392.

TOULOUSE, Krystel; CHUS-Hop Fleurimont, 3001 12e av N, Sherbrooke QC J1H 5N4; Sher'07; FRCPC; Peds. Staff, Centre Hospitalier Universitaire de Sherbrooke-Hopital Fleurimont; (819)346-1110

TOUMA, Georges; CSSS de la Baie-des-Chaleurs, RR 2 419 boul Perron, Maria QC G0C 1Y0; Aleppo (Syria)'74; Staff, CSSS de la Baie-des-Chaleurs; (418)759-3443

TOUMA, Nadine J; Asclepios Med Clinic, 2-750 Taylor Creek Dr, Orleans ON K1C 1T1; Mon'05; CCFP; Langs: Bilingual(French/English); (613)830-8388

TOUMA, Naji J; Kingston Gen Hosp, E4-76 Stuart St, Kingston ON K7L 2V7; Wes'03; BASc; FRCSC; Urol (Minimal Invasive Urology). Staff, Kingston General Hospital; Langs: Bilingual(English/French); (613)549-6666; Fax. (613)545-1970.

TOUMA, Zahi N; Univ Hlth Network-Toronto Western Hosp, 1 415EW-399 Bathurst St, Toronto ON M5T 2S8; Kursk State Medical University (Other Foreign)'99; Staff, Toronto Western Hospital - University Health Network; (416)603-5800

TOUNTAS, Apostolos A; Business Bldg, 404-1017 Wilson Ave, North York ON M3K 1Z1; Athens (Greece)'71; FRCSC; OrthSurg (Foot & Ankle Surgery). Staff, Humber River Regional Hospital - Church Street Site; Langs: Greek; (416)398-9624; Fax. (416)398-9626; aatountas@rogers.com.

TOUPIN, Genevieve; Hotel-Dieu de Levis, 143 rue Wolfe, Levis QC G6V 3Z1; Sher'97; FRCPC; Psy. Staff, Hôtel-Dieu de Lévis; Langs: English; (418)835-7121

TOUPIN, Jacques R; 400 Rang Point-Du-Jour S, L'Assomption QC J5W 1H7; Mon'71; (450)589-7416

TOUPIN, Line; CLSC St-Leonard, 5540 rue Jarry E, Saint-Leonard QC H1P 1T9; Mon'79; (514)328-3460; Fax. (514)328-1468.

TOUPIN, M A M Carole; A-8371 boul Newman, LaSalle QC H8N 1Y4; Mon'76; (514)363-3231

TOUPIN, Manon; Direction de la Sante Publique, 550 rue Bonaventure, Trois-Rivieres QC G9A 2B5; Sher'88; MB; CSPQ; MPH; MSc; CommunMed (P.Q.) (Mental Illness). (819)693-3636; Fax. (819)373-1627.

TOUPIN, Melissa; The Ottawa Hosp-Gen Campus, 501 Smyth Rd, Ottawa ON K1H 8L6; Tor'07; Hem; IntMed. Staff Ottawa Blood Disease Centre, The Ottawa Hospital - General Campus; (613)719-2518

TOUPIN, Michael E; 39 rue Andrea, Dieppe NB E1A 8L2; Sher'96; FRCPC; DiagRad (Interventional Radiology).

TOUPIN, Yves; Clinique Chirurgie Plastique, 101-111 boul de l'Hopital, Gatineau QC J8T 7V1; Laval'82; FRCSC; PlasSurg. Staff PlasticSurg, Hôpital de Gatineau; (819)561-1123; Fax. (819)561-6100; yvestoupin@bellnet.ca.

TOURANGEAU, Francine; CSSS de Rimouski-Neigette, CP 3150 Succ A 150 av Rouleau, Rimouski QC G5L 5T1; Mon'81; FRCPC; MedMicrobiol. Staff Med Microbiol & InfectDis, Hôpital Regional Rimouski; (418)724-8336; Fax. (418)724-8619.

TOURANGEAU, June A D; Forest Hill Inst of Aesthetic, 1188B Eglinton Ave W, Toronto ON M6C 2E3; Ott'64; Anes. Langs: English; French; (416)785-7864; Fax. (416)785-7207.

TOURANGEAU-LARIVIERE, Marie-Eve; CSSS de Rivière-du-Loup, 75 rue Saint-Henri, Riviere-du-Loup QC G5R 2A4; Laval'08; CCFP; Staff, Centre Hospitalier Regional du Grand-Portage; (418)868-1000

TOURE, Lossany E; Hotel-Dieu d'Arthabaska, 5 rue des Hospitaliers, Victoriaville QC G6P 6N2; Sher'07; GenSurg. Staff, Hotel-Dieu d'Arthabaska; (819)357-2030

TOURIAN, Leon; Ctr de Sante de l'Universite M, 1025 av des Pins O, Montreal QC H3A 1A1; Laval'08; (514)934-1934 x35575

TOURIGNY, Andre; Ctr Hosp Affilie-St-Sacrement, L2-1050 ch Sainte-Foy, Quebec QC G1S 4L8; Laval'80; FRCPC; CommunMed (P.Q.); Public Health & Preventive Med. Staff, Centre Hospitalier Affilié Universitaire de Québec - Hôpital du St-Sacrement; (418)682-7511 x4830; Fax. (418)682-7998.

TOURIGNY, Daniel; Medi-Centre Chomedey, 610 Boul Cure-Labelle, Laval QC H7V 2T7; Mon'70; FRCPC; Peds. Staff Peds, Hopital de la Cite de la santé; Staff, Centre Hosp Ambulatoire Reg de Laval; (450)687-6452; Fax. (450)781-4487.

TOURIGNY, Marc E; Ctr Hosp Anna-Laberge, 200 boul Brisebois, Chateauguay QC J6K 4W8; Laval'78; FRCPC; Gastroent. Staff, Hôpital Anna-Laberge; (450)699-2425

TOURIGNY, Paul D; Foothills Med Centre, 1403 29 St NW, Calgary AB T2N 2T9; Qns'01; FRCPC; EmergMed. Staff Emerg Med, Foothills Medical Centre; (403)944-1635; Fax. (403)670-2400.

TOURIGNY, Richard; Clinique Med Pierre-Bertrand, 103-303 boul Pierre-Bertrand, Quebec QC G1M 3L7; Laval'87; FRCSC; Ophth. Langs: English; (418)683-3348; Fax. (418)683-4448.

TOURIGNY-RIVARD, Marie F; Royal Ottawa Hlth Care Group, 1145 Carling Ave, Ottawa ON K1Z 7K4; Mon'74; DAB; FRCPC; Psy (Geriatric Psychiatry). Clin Dir Geriatric Psy Prog, Royal Ottawa Mental Health Centre - Royal Ottawa Health Care Group; Assoc Prof Royal Ottawa Mental Health Center, University of Ottawa; (613)722-6521 x6506; Fax. (613)798-2999.

TOURIN, Olga; Peak Pulmonary Consulting Inc, 3-400 Crowfoot Cres NW, Calgary AB T3G 5H7; Minsk Medical Institute (Belarus)'93; FRCPC; IntMed; Respir. (855)738-7325; Fax. (855)738-7325.

TOURJMAN, Smadar V; Hopital Louis-H. Lafontaine, 7401 rue Hochelaga, Montreal QC H1N 3M5; McG'84; FRCPC; Psy. Staff, Centre Hospitalier l'Université de Montréal (CHUM) - Hôpital Notre-Dame; Hopital Louis-H Lafontaine; (514)251-4000; stourjman@hotmail.com.

TOURNOUX, Francis B M; Centre Cardio-Vasculaire, 3847 rue Saint-Urbain, Montreal QC H2W 1T8; Staff, Centre Hospitalier l'Université de Montréal (CHUM) - Hôtel-Dieu; (514)890-8000 x5438

TOURVILLE, Eric; CHAQ-Hop Saint-Sacrement, 1050 ch Sainte-Foy, Quebec QC G1S 4L8; Laval'99; FRCSC; Ophth. Staff, Centre Hospitalier Universitaire de Quebec-CHUL; (418)682-7511; Fax. (418)682-7534.

TOURVILLE, Yves V; 149 sent de l'Equerre, Baie-Saint-Paul QC G3Z 2Y2; Laval'66; GenSurg. Staff, CSSS de Charlevoix; (418)435-6604

TOUSIGNANT, Benoit; Hotel-Dieu De Levis, 143 rue Wolfe, Levis QC G6V 3Z1; Laval'00; FRCPC; Anes. Staff, Hôtel-Dieu de Lévis; (418)835-7121 x3218; bentous@hotmail.com.

TOUSIGNANT, Claude P J; St Michael's Hosp, 30 Bond St, Toronto ON M5B 1W8; Ott'87; FRCPC; Anes; Critical Care Medicine. Staff, St Michael's Hospital; Langs: English; French; (416)360-4000; Fax. (416)864-6014.

TOUSIGNANT, Eric; Hotel-Dieu d'Arthabaska, 5 rue des Hopitalieres, Victoriaville QC G6P 6N2; Laval'06; FRCPC; IntMed. Staff, Hotel-Dieu d'Arthabaska; (819)357-2030 x2300

TOUSIGNANT, Jacqueline; 201-2115 boul Casavant O, Saint-Hyacinthe QC J2S 7E5; Mon'80; FRCPC; Derm. (450)774-7621; Fax. (450)250-6000.

TOUSIGNANT, Jean; CSSS de Trois-Rivières, 1991 boul du Carmel, Trois-Rivieres QC G8Z 3R9; Laval'72; FRCPC; Anes. ac Staff (All Sites), CSSS de Trois-Rivières; Langs: Spanish; English; French; (819)697-3333

TOUSIGNANT, Julie; Centre Hospitalier Sagamie, 305 rue Saint-Vallier, Chicoutimi QC G7H 5H6; Laval'97; FRCSC; GenSurg. gén Chirurgien, Complexe hospitalier de la Sagamie; (418)541-1000

TOUSIGNANT, Karine; Polyclinique des Recollets, 1900 boul des Recollets, Trois-Rivieres QC G8Z 4K4; Sher'00; Nephrol; IntMed. Staff, CSSS de Trois-Rivières; (819)373-1202

TOUSIGNANT, Maryse; Ctr Hosp Laurentien, 234 rue Saint-Vincent, Ste-Agathe-Des-Mts QC J8C 2B8; Laval'98; Staff, Centre Hospitalier Laurentien; (819)324-4000 x4779; Fax. (819)324-4092.

TOUSIGNANT, Maude; Centre Hosp Honore-Mercier, 2750 boul Laframboise, Saint-Hyacinthe QC J2S 4Y8; Staff, Centre Hospitalier Honore-Mercier; Staff, Centre de santé des Côté-Nord; (450)771-3333

TOUSIGNANT, Michel P; Clinique Drs Lefevbre et Tousi, 513 5e av, Grand-Mere QC G9T 2M5; Laval'71; Langs: English; French; (819)533-5721; Fax. (819)533-5337.

TOUSIGNANT, Michelle M; Royal Alexandra Hosp, 10240 Kingsway NW, Edmonton AB T5H 3V9; UBC'08; CCFP; CCFP(E.M.); Staff, Royal Alexandra Hospital; (780)735-4111

TOUSIGNANT, Pierre; Dir de la Sante Publique-Mtl, 1301 rue Sherbrooke E, Montreal QC H2L 1M3; Laval'73; FRCPC; IntMed; CommunMed. Med Consultant Clin Epidemiol, Hopital Maisonneuve-Rosemont; Staff Comm Health Dept, McGill University Health Centre - Royal Victoria Hospital; assoc Prof Med, McGill University; (514)528-2400 x3569; Fax. (514)528-2512; ptousi@santepub-mtl.qc.ca.

TOUSIGNANT, Sebastien; Hotel-Dieu de Levis, 143 rue Wolfe, Levis QC G6V 3Z1; Laval'03; FRCPC; Anes. Staff, Hôtel-Dieu de Lévis; (418)835-7121

TOUSIGNANT, Sylvie; CSSS Memphremagog, RR 4 435 rue Dufferin, Stanstead QC J0B 3E0; Sher'82; (819)876-7521; syltousignant@videotron.ca.

TOUSSAINT, M Junie B; Don Valley Med Centre, 207-855 Broadview Ave, Toronto ON M4K 3Z1; Cal'83; Court Staff, St Michael's Hospital; Langs: English; French; (416)463-1323; Fax. (416)463-1718.

TOUSSAINT, Martin; CSSS de Montmagny l'Islet, RR 2 2-4 rue de la Madone, Saint-Eugene QC G0R 1X0; Mon'74; MSc; Médecin, CSSS St Eugene; Médecin, CSSS de Montmagny l'Islet; Langs: English; (418)247-3927; Fax. (418)247-7613; mtoussaint@videotron.ca.

TOUSSAINT, Sebastien; CSSS Haut-Richelieu-Rouville, 978 boul du Seminaire N, St-Jean-sur-Richel QC J3A 1E5; Laval'95; Staff, CSSS de la Baie-des-Chaleurs; Staff, CLSC-CHLSD Champagnat Vallee des Forts; (450)358-2572

TOUSSAINT, Simon; Clinique Med Dr Simon Toussain, 1475 Place Lamontagne, Becancour QC G9H 0A6; Mon'04; (819)233-9600; Fax. (819)233-9601.

TOUSSI, Tahmouresse; 1392 rue Sherbrooke E, Montreal QC H2L 1M4; Lausanne (Switzerland)'60; Peds (Palliative Care). ac Staff, Centre Hospitalier l'Université de Montréal (CHUM) - Hôpital Notre-Dame; Ac Staff, Hôpital Ste-Justine; Clin Teacher, Universite de Montreal; Langs: Persian; (514)525-1112; Fax. (514)525-7691.

TOUTANT, Robert; 102-810 av Joffre, Quebec QC G1S 3L7; Mon'68; DiagRad (P.Q.). ac Staff, Hotel-Dieu de Roberval; (418)524-4109; toutant_robert@sympatico.ca.

TOUW, Andrew J; Timmins & District Hosp, 700 Ross Ave E, Timmins ON P4N 8P2; Wes'04; CCFP; Staff, Timmins & District Hospital; (705)267-2131; Fax. (705)267-6325.

TOUYZ, Rhian M; Family Medicine Clinic, 2100 av Marlowe, Montreal QC H4A 3L5; Witwatersrand (South Africa)'84; MB ChB; MSc(Med.); PhD; Médecin Family Med, McGill University; (514)934-8080; Fax. (514)934-8385.

TOUZEL, Christine; CSSS de Rimouski-Neigette, CP 3150 Succ A 150 av Rouleau, Rimouski QC G5L 5T1; Sher'07; IntMed. Staff, Hôpital Regional Rimouski; (418)724-3000

TOUZEL, Elizabeth L; C 01-310 Bridge St W, Napanee ON K7R 0A4; Qns'85; CCFP; FCFP; Staff, Lennox & Addington County General Hospital; (613)354-2858; Fax. (613)354-6495.

TOUZEL, Thomas A; 310 Bridge St W, Napanee ON K7R 2G4; Qns'85; Staff/Pres Med Staff, Lennox & Addington County General Hospital; (613)354-2858; Fax. (613)354-6495; ttouzel@lacgh.napanee.on.ca.

TOUZIN, Eric S; Sioux Lookout Meno-Ya-Win HC, PO Box 909 Stn Main 11 Fifth Ave, Sioux Lookout ON P8T 1B4; Ott'02; FRCSC; GenSurg. Staff, Sioux Lookout Meno-Ya-Win Health Centre; Langs: Bilingual(English/French); (807)737-3030; Fax. (807)737-6282; etouzin@slmhc.on.ca.

TOWHEED, Tanveer E; Queen's Univ Etherington Hall, 2066-94 Stuart St, Kingston ON K7L 3N6; Qns'89; MSc(Epidem.); DABIM(Rheum.); FACP; FRCPC; IntMed; Rheum. Staff, Kingston General Hospital; Staff, Hotel-Dieu Hospital; Staff, Providence Care - St Mary's of the Lake Hospital Site; Assoc Prof Med, Queen's University; Langs: Urdu; (613)533-6896; Fax. (613)533-2189; tt5@queensu.ca.

TOWILL, Garry A; Capeda Med Clinic Inc, 103-8386 12 St, Surrey BC V3W 3N4; Sask'76; CCFP; FCFP; (604)594-9990; Fax. (604)594-4362.

TOWNLEY, John B; 315-89 Humber College Blvd, Etobicoke ON M9V 4B8; Cambridge (England)'98; FRCSC; OrthSurg. (416)741-9271; Fax. (416)745-9146.

TOWNLEY, Richard; Cardiology Associates, 2606 Pandosy St, Kelowna BC V1Y 1V6; UBC'97; FRCPC; IntMed; Cardiol. Staff, St Boniface General Hospital; (250)762-9211

TOWNS, Dale K K; Canadian Blood Services, F4-737 13 Ave SW, Calgary AB T2R 1J1; Sask'82; FRCPC; Anes (Transfusion Medicine). Staff Anes, Foothills Medical Centre; Med Dir, Canadian Blood Services; Clinical Asst Prof, University of Calgary; (403)410-2676; Fax. (403)410-2799; dale.towns@blood.ca.

TOWNS, Kathryn A; Southlake Reg Health Centre, 596 Davis Dr, Newmarket ON L3Y 2P9; Tor'06; FRCPC; IntMed; MedOncol. Staff Stronach Reg Cancer Centre, Southlake Regional Health Centre; (905)895-4521; Fax. (905)952-2818.

TOWNSEND, Anthony L; Westminster Med Bldg, 204-625 Fifth Ave, New Westminster BC V3M 1X4; Cape Town (South Africa)'63; DAB; FRCSC; Ophth (Anterior Segment Surgery). Consultant, Royal Columbian Hospital; Consultant, Ridge Meadows Hospital & Health Care Centre; (604)521-3232; Fax. (604)521-3824.

TOWNSEND, Judy A; 10942 124 St NW, Edmonton AB T5M 0H5; Cal'94; FRCPC; PhysMed&Rehab. (780)447-4924; Fax. (780)452-5111.

TOWNSEND, Marria M; Three Bridges Health Care Ctre, 1292 Hornby St, Vancouver BC V6Z 1W2; UBC'05; CCFP; (604)736-9844; Fax. (604)844-2223.

TOWNSEND, Philip A; 605-267 O'Connor St, Ottawa ON K2P 1V3; Qns'86; (613)567-4199

TOWNSEND, Tiffany N; Gordon & Leslie Diamond HCC, 8271-2775 Laurel St, Vancouver BC V5Z 1M9; McG'99; FRCPC; Neur. Staff, Vancouver General Hospital - Centennial Pavillion; Staff Epilepsy Clinic, Gordon & Leslie Diamond Health Care Centre; Langs: Bilingual(English/French); (604)875-4402

TOWNSLEY, Carol A; Women's College Hosp, 6E-76 Grenville St, Toronto ON M5S 1B2; McG'99; CCFP; Staff ACTT Clinic, Women's College Hospital; Staff, Princess Margaret Hospital - University Health Network; Langs: English; French; (416)323-6400; Fax. (416)323-6001.

TOWNSON, Andrea F; G F Strong Rehabilitation Ctre, 4255 Laurel St, Vancouver BC V5Z 2G9; Qns'91; FRCPC; PhysMed&Rehab. Staff, G F Strong Rehabilitation Centre; Langs: Bilingual(English/French); (604)714-4112; Fax. (604)737-6251.

TOY, Jonathan W M; 303-14310 111 Ave NW, Edmonton AB T5M 2P4; Man'04; FRCSC; PlasSurg. (780)758-3377; Fax. (780)758-3232; office.drtoy@gmail.com.

TOY, William; Ctr Hosp de LaSalle, 8585 Tsse Champlain, LaSalle QC H8P 1C1; Tor'94; Staff, Centre Hospitalier de LaSalle; Langs: English; French; (514)362-8000 x1429

TOYE, Baldwin W; The Ottawa Hosp-Gen Campus, 3955A-501 Smyth Rd Box 115, Ottawa ON K1H 8L6; Tor'82; FRCPC; IntMed; MedMicrobiol; InfectDis. Staff Microbiologist & InfectiousDis, The Ottawa Hospital - General Campus; Assoc Prof, University of Ottawa; Fax. (613)737-8323.

TOYE, Jennifer M; University of Alberta Hosp, 3A3 13 WMC-8440 112 St NW, Edmonton AB T6G 2B7; Sask'05; FRCPC; Peds (Neonatal & Perinatal Medicine). Staff, University of Alberta Hospital; (780)407-8822

TOYE, John W; 170 Colborne St W, Orillia ON L3V 2Z3; Qns'78; DAB(HandSurg); FRCSC; PlasSurg (Melanoma). Ac Staff, Orillia Soldiers' Memorial Hospital; Langs: Spanish; French; (705)327-1436; Fax. (705)327-1872; johntoye@rogers.com.

TOYE, Julie; CLSC Loungueuil Ouest, 201 boul Cure-Poirier O, Longueuil QC J4J 2G4; Mon'04; Médecin, CLSC Longueuil Ouest; (450)651-9830; julie.toye@cssspb.qc.ca.

TOYE, Paul L; Foothills Prof Bldg, 350-1620 29 St NW, Calgary AB T2N 4L7; Tor'80; (403)282-1245; Fax. (403)282-9545.

TOYONAGA, Vernon M; Courtice Health Centre, 300-1450 Highway 2, Courtice ON L1E 3C3; Tor'90; (905)721-3526; Fax. (905)721-4369.

TOYOTA, Brian D; Gordon & Leslie Diamond HCC, 8117-2775 Laurel St, Vancouver BC V5Z 1M9; McG'84; FRCSC; Neursurg. Staff, Vancouver General Hospital - Centennial Pavillion; Staff, BC Cancer Agency Vancouver Centre; Staff, Gordon & Leslie Diamond Health Care Centre; (604)875-5233; btoyota@telus.net.

TOYOTA, Jane C; West Park Healthcare Centre, 82 Buttonwood Ave, York ON M6M 2J5; Tor'77; Court Staff, West Park Healthcare Centre; Staff, Momiji Wellness Centre; (416)243-3600; j.toyota@utoronto.ca.

TOZE, Cynthia L; Leukemia/BMT Program of BC, 10149-2775 Laurel St, Vancouver BC V5Z 1M9; Qns'86; ABIM; FRCP; MHSc; MCPS; MD; LMCC; FRCPC; IntMed (Hematology & Bone Marrow Transplant); Hem. Ac Staff Hem, BC Cancer Agency Vancouver Centre; Ac Staff, Vancouver General Hospital - Centennial Pavillion; Asst Prof, University of British Columbia; (604)875-4863 x63168; ctoze@bccancer.bc.ca.

TOZER, Nancy M; 401-955 boul Saint-Jean, Pointe-Claire QC H9R 5K3; Tor'78; CCFP; FCFP; ac Staff, Lakeshore General Hospital - Pointe Claire; Langs: English; French; (514)695-0165; Fax. (514)695-0991.

TOZER, Richard G; The Juravinski Cancer Centre, 699 Concession St, Hamilton ON L8V 5C2; McM'90; BSc(Hon.); PhD; FRCPC; IntMed (Breasts); MedOncol. Head Systemic Therapy/Head Supportive Care/Staff MedOncol, The Juravinski Cancer Centre; Assoc Prof, McMaster University; (905)387-9495 x64604; Fax. (905)575-6326.

TOZLOVANU-PASKAL, Viorika; CSSS de Papineau, 500 rue Belanger, Gatineau QC J8L 2M4; Kichinev (Moldova)'79; CCFP; Staff, CH-CHSLD de Papineau - Pavillon du centre hospitalier; (819)986-4115; tozlovanu@hotmail.com.

TOZMAN, Seymour; The Colonnade, 416-131 Bloor St W, Toronto ON M5S 1R1; Tor'63; CSPQ(Psy); DABPN(Psy); Psy (P. Q.) (Work Injuries). (416)921-0315; Fax. (416)921-9437.

TOZZI, Daniel P; Medical Arts Bldg, 1000-1538 rue Sherbrooke O, Montreal QC H3G 1L5; McG'73; Langs: Italian; English; (514)933-2778; Fax. (514)871-9863; info@villemariemed.com.

TRABELSI, Asma; Montfort Hosp, 713 Montreal Rd, Ottawa ON K1K 0T2; Faculte de Medecine de Sfax (Tunisia)'02; CCFP; Staff, Montfort Hospital; (613)746-4621

TRABOULSEE, Anthony L; UBC Hospital, S199-2211 Wesbrook Mall, Vancouver BC V6T 2B5; Dal'94; BSc(Biol/Med); FRCPC; Neur (Multiple Sclerosis). Staff MS Clinic, UBC Hospital - Koerner Pavillion; Asst Prof, University of British Columbia; (604)822-0788; Fax. (604)822-7703.

TRABOULSI, Mouhieddin; Calgary Heart Centre, 403-3280 Hospital Dr NW, Calgary AB T2N 4Z6; Damascus (Syria)'79; FRCPC; IntMed; Cardiol. Staff Cardiol, Foothills Medical Centre; Staff, Health Research Innovation Centre; Clin Assoc Prof, University of Calgary; Langs: Arabic; (403)521-2227; Fax. (403)283-6360.

TRACEY, John P; Dr John P Tracey Med Prof Corp, 210-157 Queen St E, Brampton ON L6W 3X4; Dublin (Ireland)'71; CCFP; FCFP; (905)457-7566; Fax. (905)457-7611.

TRACEY, Joshua; Saint John Reg Hosp, PO Box 2100 400 University Ave, Saint John NB E2L 4L2; Mem'09; CCFP; Staff, Saint John Regional Hospital; (506)648-6000

TRACEY, Kevin P; Hotel-Dieu Grace Hosp, 4F-1030 Ouellette Ave, Windsor ON N9A 1E1; Mem'81; AB; FRCPC; NuclearMed. Dir Dept of NuclearMed, Hôtel-Dieu Grace Hospital; (519)973-4417; Fax. (519)973-4667.

TRACEY, Scott J; Greenbelt Family Health Team, 3500 Fallowfield Rd, Ottawa ON K2J 4A7; Wes'07; CCFP; (613)843-1718; Fax. (613)843-0201.

TRACHTENBERG, John; 3-208-620 University Ave, Toronto ON M5G 2M9; McG'73; FRCSC; Urol (Urological Oncology). Staff, Princess Margaret Hospital - University Health Network; Prof, University of Toronto; Langs: English; French; (416)946-2100 x1; Fax. (416)598-9997; john.trachtenberg@uhn.on.ca.

TRACY, Gary E; Niagara H System-Welland Site, 65 Third St, Welland ON L3B 4W6; Qns'75; FRCPC; DiagRad. Staff, Niagara Health System - Welland Hospital Site; (905)732-6111 x3289

TRACY, Susanne; Leamington District Mem Hosp, 194 Talbot St W, Leamington ON N8H 1N9; St Matthew's Unviersity (Other Foreign)'03; Staff, Leamington District Memorial Hospital; (519)322-4933; Fax. (519)322-1952.

TRADOUNSKY, Golda E; Mount Sinai Hosp Centre, 5690 boul Cavendish, Cote Saint-Luc QC H4W 1S7; Mon'95; CCFP; Staff, Mount Sinai Hospital Center; Langs: English; (514)369-2222 x3200; Fax. (514)369-0873; dr_golda@yahoo.ca.

TRAFALGAR, Barbara; 3170 Longmeadow Rd, Burlington ON L7M 2X6; McM'97.

TRAGER, Chaim J; A-20 Torbay Rd, Markham ON L3R 1G6; Dal'73; Langs: English; French; (905)415-1940; Fax. (416)449-1633.

TRAGER, Morris E; Family Practice Associates, 200-6155 North St, Halifax NS B3K 5R3; Dal'74; Staff, Queen Elizabeth II Health Sciences Centre - Victoria General Site; Staff, IWK Health Centre; Physician Occupational Health, Nova Scotia Liqour Commission; (902)453-3511; Fax. (902)454-9010.

TRAHAN, Andre G; 1381 rue Notre-Dame CP 130, St-Maurice QC G0X 2X0; Laval'65; Staff, Centre de santé Cloutier-du-Rivage; Staff, CSSS de Trois-Rivières; (819)379-7272; Fax. (819)379-2702; drtrahan@drtrahan.com.

TRAHAN, Gilles; 1100 boul Saint-Sacrement, Shawinigan QC G9N 6W4; Laval'75; (819)539-0765 x702; Fax. (819)539-0849; gilles.trahan@alcan.com.

TRAHAN, J Simon-Pierre; Russell Med Centre, PO Box 70 Stn Main 110 Craig St, Russell ON K4R 1C7; Ott'83; Assoc Staff Emerg, Winchester District Memorial Hospital; Langs: English; French; (613)445-3220; Fax. (613)445-3659.

TRAHAN, Linda; CSSS Pierre Boucher, 1333 boul Jacques-Cartier E, Longueuil QC J4M 2A5; Mon'89; FRCPC; Psy. Staff, Centre Hospitalier Pierre Boucher; (450)468-8401

TRAHAN, Sabine; Hop Maisonneuve-Rosemont, 5415 boul de l'Assomption, Montreal QC H1T 2M4; Mon'99; Staff, Hopital Maisonneuve-Rosemont; (514)252-3400

TRAHAN, Sylvain; Hôpital Laval, 2725 ch Sainte-Foy, Quebec QC G1V 4G5; Laval'01; FRCPC; AnatPath. Staff, Hôpital Laval; (418)656-8711 x5323; Fax. (418)656-4571.

TRAHEY, Julia C; Health Sciences Centre, 1273-300 Prince Philip Dr, St. John's NL A1B 3V6; Mem'86; FRCPC; IntMed. Staff, Health Sciences Centre; Staff, Newfoundland & Labrador Cancer Treatment Centre; Clinical Asst Prof, Memorial University Of Newfoundland; (709)777-8652

TRAIFOROS, Eirene R; Foothills Med Centre, C231-1403 112 St NW, Calgary AB T2N 2T9; Sask'03; CCFP; CCFP(E.M.); Staff, Strathmore District Health Services; Staff, Foothills Medical Centre; (403)944-1635; Fax. (403)944-2419.

TRAIL, Carla N; CPHC Brockville Fam Hlth Team, PO Box 338 6-555 California Ave, Brockville ON K6V 5V5; McM'06; CCFP; Langs: Bilingual(English/French); (613)342-4076; Fax. (613)342-6578; ctrail@cphcare.ca.

TRAILL, Larisa M; Windsor Reg Hosp-Metropolitan, 1995 Lens Ave, Windsor ON N8W 1L9; (Grenada)'05; Staff, Windsor Regional Hospital - Metropolitan Site; (519)254-5577

TRAIN, Anthony D; Life Medical Clinic, PO Box 1406 Stn Main 4740 50th Ave, Whitecourt AB T7S 1P3; (780)706-7080; Fax. (780)706-7064.

TRAIN, Harriet P; Overbrook Med Centre, 110-120 Overbrook Place, North York ON M3H 4P8; Tor'75; (416)633-4984; Fax. (416)633-4446.

TRAINOR, Shannon E; Lakeridge Hlth Corp-Oshawa, C2 160C-1 Hospital Crt, Oshawa ON L1G 2B9; Tor'97; FRCSC; GenSurg; ThorSurg. Staff, Lakeridge Health - Oshawa Site; (905)576-8711; Fax. (905)433-4577.

TRAINOR, W Brian; Guelph Family Health Team, 103-21 Surrey St W, Guelph ON N1H 3R3; Wes'79; BSc; CCFP; FCFP; Staff, Guelph General Hospital; Staff, St Joseph's Hospital - St Joseph's Health Care; Staff, Homewood Health Centre; (519)837-1170; Fax. (519)837-1240.

TRAJAN, Marc; Medical Centre, 24-1515 Dufferin Cres, Nanaimo BC V9S 2B8; UBC'68; FRCPC; IntMed; Respir. (250)753-2446; Fax. (250)753-9686.

TRAJANO, Janet D; Winnipeg Clinic, 425 St Mary Ave, Winnipeg MB R3C 0N2; Cebu (Philippines)'99.

TRAM, B V Jenny; Bristol Family Physicians, 102-2315 Bristol Cir, Oakville ON L6H 6P8; Qns'03; CCFP; (905)287-2035; Fax. (905)287-2036.

TRAM, Carolyn Q N; Sunnybrook Hlth Sciences Ctre, 2075 Bayview Ave, Toronto ON M4N 3M5; Tor'08; FRCPC; IntMed (Critical Care Medicine). Staff, Sunnybrook Health Sciences Centre; (416)480-6100

TRAM, Khai Minh; 103-302 Spadina Ave, Toronto ON M5T 2E7; (Vietnam)'78; FRCPC; IntMed. Staff, St Michael's Hospital; Clin Instructor, University of Toronto; Langs: Vietnamese; (416)203-6866; Fax. (416)203-9580.

TRAMBAKOULOS, Dimitra; 402-235 Danforth Ave, Toronto ON M4K 1N2; Ott'03; CCFP; (416)466-4290; Fax. (416)466-4393.

TRAMBITAS, Camelia A; Taunton Health Centre, SS 201 3F-1290 Keith Ross Dr, Oshawa ON L1H 7K4; Univ of Medicine and Pharmacy (Other Foreign)'88; CCFP; Langs: Romanian; (905)721-4300 x5266

TRAN, Anh T N; F 26-3175 Rutherford Rd, Concord ON L4K 5Y6; Ott'08; CCFP; Langs: Vietnamese; (905)761-5482; Fax. (905)761-0523.

TRAN, Anthony L; Dominion Med Centres Ltd, 9122 23 Ave NW, Edmonton AB T6N 1H9; Alb'08; CCFP; (780)801-3360; Fax. (780)801-3366.

TRAN, Bernie B C; Norfinch Med Centre, 105-2100 Finch Ave W, North York ON M3N 2Z9; Tor'91; Langs: Vietnamese; French; (416)667-8796; Fax. (416)667-8796.

TRAN, Boi Anh; Clinique Med Chambly, 2200 Ch De Chambly, Longueuil QC J4J 3Z3; Mon'84; Staff, CHSLD Lucille-Teasdale; Langs: Vietnamese; English; (450)651-7331

TRAN, Cao Phanh; Clinique Familiale Pasteur, 5415 rue Grande Allee, Longueuil QC J4Z 3G9; Saigon (Vietnam)'75; (450)445-3600

TRAN, Cao Thang; Clinique Med 3600, 3600 rue Ontario E, Montreal QC H1W 1R2; Saigon (Vietnam)'69; (514)526-2556; Fax. (514)526-9212.

TRAN, D Jeffrey; The Hosp for Sick Children, 555 University Ave, Toronto ON M5G 1X8; Tor'93; FRCPC; Peds; InfectDis. Staff, The Hospital For Sick Children; Langs: Vietnamese; (416)813-6268

TRAN, David V B; Griffiths Med Clinic, 28-5201 50 St, Leduc AB T9E 6T4; Dal'97; CCFP; (780)986-6200; Fax. (780)986-5200.

TRAN, Diane; 202-2125 rue Jean-Talon E, Montreal QC H2E 1V4; Mon'05; FRCPC; Derm. (514)728-9203

TRAN, Diem Thu T; Univ of Ottawa Heart Institute, 40 Ruskin St, Ottawa ON K1Y 4W7; Qns'04; FRCPC; Anes. Staff, University of Ottawa Heart Institute; Langs: Vietnamese; (613)798-5555; Fax. (613)761-4925.

TRAN, Duy; Hop Maisonneuve-Rosemont, 5415 boul de l'Assomption, Montreal QC H1T 2M4; Mon'05; FRCPC; IntMed; Nephrol. Staff, Hopital Maisonneuve-Rosemont; (514)252-3400; Fax. (514)252-3506.

TRAN, Emmanuelle; Clin Med de Metabetchouan, 20 rue Saint-Basile, Metab-L-A-La-Croix QC G8G 1S9; Mon'91; (418)349-8933; Fax. (418)349-8082.

TRAN, Franklin T V; 104-200 Consilium Place PO Box 63, Scarborough ON M1H 3E4; McG'97; FRCSC; OrthSurg (Arthroscopy). Dir Orth/Staff, The Scarborough Hospital - General Campus; (416)479-8686; Fax. (416)296-8816.

TRAN, Hanh-Khiem; Hop Charles Lemoyne, 3120 boul Taschereau, Greenfield Park QC J4V 2H1; Mon'95; Gastroent (P. Q.); IntMed (P.Q.). Staff, Hopital Charles LeMoyne; (450)466-5000; Fax. (450)466-5036.

TRAN, Hieu Duc; CSSS de la Mitis, 800 av du Sanatorium, Mont-Joli QC G5H 3L6; Saigon (Vietnam)'78; Staff, CSSS de la Mitis; (418)775-7261

TRAN, Jean-Cao P; GMF Centre de santé, 3745 rue Georges-Couture, Drummondville QC J2B 7P4; Sher'03; CCFP; Staff, Hôpital Sainte-croix; (819)477-2231; Fax. (819)477-1122.

TRAN, Kham Quang; Toronto East Gen & Orth Hosp, 825 Coxwell Ave, East York ON M4C 3E7; Tor'91; FRCPC; IntMed; Critical Care Medicine; Respir. Staff, Toronto East General Hospital Inc; Langs: Vietnamese; (416)469-6333

TRAN, Kim A T; Postgrad Med Education Office, 602-500 University Ave, Toronto ON M5G 1V7; McM'08; Peds.

TRAN, M A Marie; Service externe de psychiatrie, 230-383 boul du Seminaire N, St-Jean-sur-Richel QC J3B 8C5; Mon'06; FRCPC; Psy. Staff, Hôpital du Haut-Richelieu; (450)346-2222

TRAN, Mai Tuyet; Copeman Health Care Centre, 400-628 12 Ave SW, Calgary AB T2R 0H6; Cal'03; CCFP; (403)270-2273

TRAN, Maithy N; Univ Hlth Network-Toronto Gen, 3 805-190 Elizabeth St, Toronto ON M5G 2C4; Wes'07; FRCPC; IntMed. Staff, Toronto General Hospital - UHN; (416)380-5428; Fax. (416)978-7230.

TRAN, Margaret H M; Oakridge Centre South Tower, 203-650 41st Ave W, Vancouver BC V5Z 2M9; Cal'90; BSc; CCFP; FCFP; Staff, BC Women's Hospital & Health Centre; Staff, Providence Health Care - Mount Saint Joseph Hospital; Langs: Cantonese; Mandarin; (604)263-6222; Fax. (604)263-9297.

TRAN, Mong Lam; Clin Med Beaubien-des-Erables, 2175 rue Beaubien E, Montreal QC H2G 1M5; Saigon (Vietnam)'68; LMCC; (514)722-0083; Fax. (514)721-7219; lammongtran@yahoo.com.

TRAN, Nguu Tu; Centre Med 425, 425 boul Cure-Poirier O, Longueuil QC J4J 2H3; Laval'84; (450)679-6666; Fax. (450)679-6446.

TRAN, Nguyen X D; CHSLD Ruisseau-Papineau, 350 boul Samson, Laval QC H7X 1J4; Sher'93; (450)689-0933

TRAN, Ninh Ngoc; Public Health Services, 4F-1 Hughson St N, Hamilton ON L8R 3L5; Qns'04; FRCPC; CommunMed;CCFP; Langs: Bilingual(English/French); (905)546-2424

TRAN, P P Peter; 925-123 Edward St, Toronto ON M5G 1E2; Tor'93; FRCPC; Psy (Psycho Geriatrics). Staff Commun Mental Health OP Prog, The Scarborough Hospital - General Campus; Langs: Vietnamese; (416)597-1616; Fax. (416)597-2073.

TRAN, Paul C D; Hopital Pierre-Boucher, 1333 boul Jacques-Cartier E, Longueuil QC J4M 2A5; Sher'07; Respir; IntMed. Staff, Centre Hospitalier Pierre Boucher; (450)468-8111

TRAN, Peter; Chipman Health Centre, 9 Civic Crt, Chipman NB E4A 2H8; Dal'96; CCFP; Chief Staff/Med Dir, Queens North Community Health Centre; (506)339-7650; Fax. (506)339-7652.

TRAN, Phu Manh; Langley Mem Hosp, 22051 Fraser Hwy, Langley BC V3A 4H4; Cal'91; CCFP; CCFP(E.M.); Staff, Langley Memorial Hospital; Staff, Shuswap Lake General Hospital; Langs: Vietnamese; (604)261-3053; phusly99@yahoo.com.

TRAN, Preston T P; Woodbridge Urgent Care Centre, 2-4000 Highway 7, Woodbridge ON L4L 8Z2; McG'91; CCFP; FCFP; (905)851-3777; Fax. (905)851-0682.

TRAN, Quang Hieu D; MUHC-Montreal Gen Hosp, 1650 av Cedar, Montreal QC H3G 1A4; Mon'98; FRCPC; Anes. Staff, McGill University Health Centre - Montreal General Campus; (514)934-1934 x43261

TRAN, Quang Hieu; CLSC Riviere-des-Prairies, 8655 boul Perras, Montreal QC H1E 4M7; Saigon (Vietnam)'74; (514)494-4924; Fax. (514)494-0135.

TRAN, Quoc Hung; 55 Centre St, Chatham ON N7M 4W1; Qns'95; FRCPC; IntMed. Staff, Chatham-Kent Health Alliance; Langs: Vietnamese; (519)351-6647; Fax. (519)351-6827.

TRAN, Quoc Tan; Broadway & Burrard Med Clinic, 1816 Broadway W, Vancouver BC V6J 1Y9; Mem'92; (604)736-1888

TRAN, Quynh Mong; Bridgeland Prof Centre, 305-1010 1 Ave NE, Calgary AB T2E 7W7; Alb'00; FRCSC; ObstGyn. Staff, Peter Lougheed Centre; (403)266-3030; Fax. (403)266-3050.

TRAN, S Stanley; Scarborough Gastroent Assoc, 208-1585 Markham Rd, Scarborough ON M1B 2W1; McG'95; FRCPC; IntMed (Hepatology); Gastroent. Staff, The Scarborough Hospital - General Campus; Langs: English; Vietnamese; (416)439-9253; Fax. (416)439-3875.

TRAN, Simone M P; PO Box 1575 Stn A, Fredericton NB E3B 5G2; Dal'93; BSc(Hon); BA; FRCPC; Psy. Staff, Psy, Saint John Regional Hospital; Psychiatrist, Centracare; simone.tran@gnb.ca.

TRAN, T G Joe; South Common Med Centre, 3-2110 Burnhamthorpe Rd W, Mississauga ON L5L 5Z5; Qns'91; Langs: Vietnamese; French; (905)820-3209; Fax. (905)820-2576.

TRAN, T S Paul; CSSS du Suroît, 150 rue Saint-Thomas, Salaber-de-Valleyf QC J6T 6C1; Mon'87; FRCPC; IntMed. Staff, Centre Hospitalier Régional du Suroît; (450)371-9920; Fax. (450)371-7454.

TRAN, Tanya; PO Box 62007 Rpo Westmount, Edmonton AB T5M 4B5; Cal'02; CCFP.

TRAN, Teresa B C; Vaughan CHC Bldg A, 206-9401 Jane St, Vaughan ON L6A 4H7; Tor'92; CCFP; FCFP; Langs: Vietnamese; French; (905)303-8490; Fax. (905)832-0093.

TRAN, Thai Hoa; The Hosp for Sick Children, BW 9401-555 University Ave, Toronto ON M5G 1X8; McG'08; FRCPC; Peds (Hematological Oncology). (416)235-8215; Fax. (416)813-5327.

TRAN, Thi Bich T; 1209 rue Belanger, Montreal QC H2S 1H7; Hue (Vietnam)'74; (514)279-3802

TRAN, Thi Cuc P; Mandalay Med Clinic, 70 Mandalay Dr, Winnipeg MB R2P 1V8; Saigon (Vietnam)'78; Staff, Seven Oaks General Hospital; (204)633-6840; Fax. (204)633-6840.

TRAN, Thi-My-Linh; Centre Med Metro Monk, 2376 rue Allard, Montreal QC H4E 2K9; Sher'94; Langs: Bilingual(French/English); (514)769-9999; Fax. (514)769-9008.

TRAN, Thien-Chuong; Centre Hosp Honore-Mercier, 2750 boul Laframboise, Saint-Hyacinthe QC J2S 4Y8; Mon'02; CCFP; Staff, Centre Hospitalier Regional de Sept-Iles; Staff, Centre Hospitalier Honore-Mercier; (450)771-3333

TRAN, Thu-Hang; SMBD Jewish Gen Hosp, 3755 ch Cote-Sainte-Catherine, Montreal QC H3T 1E2; McG'93; CCFP; CCFP(E.M.); Staff, Sir Mortimer B Davis Jewish General; Langs: Vietnamese; English; (514)340-8222

TRAN, Tri Minh; Reseau SSSS Aurores Boreales, CP 6000 Succ Bureau-Chef 679 2e rue E, La Sarre QC J9Z 2X7; Mon'98; CCFP; Staff, Centre Hospitalier La Sarre; (819)333-2311; Fax. (819)339-2729.

TRAN, Trong Quang; Hop Maisonneuve-Rosemont, 5689 boul Rosemont, Montreal QC H1T 2M4; Sher'05; Psy. Staff, Hopital Maisonneuve-Rosemont; (514)252-3914

TRAN, Van Cuong; Centre de Read Lucie-Bruneau, 2275 av Laurier E, Montreal QC H2H 2N8; Saigon (Vietnam)'82; Médecin, Centre de Readaptation Lucie-Bruneau; (514)527-4521; Fax. (514)527-7968.

TRAN, Van Nham; 2565A Hurontario St, Mississauga ON L5A 2G4; Saigon (Vietnam)'70; Langs: Vietnamese; French; (905)896-4270

TRAN, Van-Chung; 202-302 Spadina Ave, Toronto ON M5T 2E7; Saigon (Vietnam)'81; CCFP; Langs: Vietnamese; (416)977-2864; Fax. (416)977-2864; vctran2007@gmail.com.

TRAN, Van-Dung; Clin Med Beaubien-des-Erables, 2175 rue Beaubien E, Montreal QC H2G 1M5; Saigon (Vietnam)'75; Langs: Vietnamese; French; (514)722-0083

TRAN, Van-Kim; Clinique Med d'Urgence Leger, 101-5900 boul Leger, Montreal-Nord QC H1G 1K9; Saigon (Vietnam)'63; (514)327-4200; Fax. (514)327-4201.

TRAN, Viet Tan; 406-595 Montreal Rd, Ottawa ON K1K 4L2; McG'96; FRCSC; Urol. Langs: Vietnamese; French; (613)741-8634; Fax. (613)741-6229.

TRAN, Vu-Kiet; 113-385 Silver Star Blvd, Scarborough ON M1V 0E3; Sher'97; CCFP; CCFP(E.M.); FCFP; Staff, Toronto Western Hospital - University Health Network; Langs: Cantonese; French; (416)551-2888

TRAN, Xia Tiang; Clinique Med Carron's, 999 boul Saint-Laurent, Montreal QC H2Z 1J4; Mon'01; CCFP; Staff, Clinique Medicale Carron; (514)861-9154; Fax. (514)861-8447.

TRAN, Xia-Hoe; Clinique Med Carron, 995 boul Saint-Laurent, Montreal QC H2Z 1J4; Sher'97; Staff, Centre Hospitalier l'Université De Montréal (CHUM) - Hôpital Saint-luc; Médecin, Clinique Medicale Carron; Langs: Chinese; English; (514)861-9154; Fax. (514)861-8447.

TRAN, Yasuo; CSSS Les Eskers de l'Abitibi, 622 4e rue O, Amos QC J9T 2S2; Mon'07; Staff, CH Hôtel-Dieu d'Amos; (819)732-3341

TRAN-DAVIES, Nhung; Calmar Med Clinic, PO Box 1079 4741 50 Ave, Calmar AB T0C 0V0; Alb'02; CCFP; Staff, Devon General Hospital; Langs: Vietnamese; (780)985-3344; Fax. (780)985-3877.

TRAN HUU, Yen; Medical Clinic, PO Box 1539 118 rue Principale, Saint-Jacques NB E7B 1A2; Iberoamericana (Mexico)'97; Staff, Hôpital regional d'Edmundston; (506)739-6992; Fax. (506)739-9546.

TRAN-LE, Hong Phuc; Clinique familiale des Pins, 1019 boul des Pins, Val-d'Or QC J9P 4T2; Sher'92; CCFP; FCFP; Staff, Centre Hospitalier de Val d'Or; (819)825-9060; Fax. (819)825-1335.

TRAN NGOC, Cuong; The Credit Valley Hosp, 2200 Eglinton Ave W, Mississauga ON L5M 2N1; McG'89; FRCPC; DiagRad. Staff, The Credit Valley Hospital; Langs: Vietnamese; English; (905)813-3978; Fax. (905)813-3042.

TRAN NGUYEN, Quoc Viet; Hop Jean-Talon, 1385 rue Jean-Talon E, Montreal QC H2E 1S6; Sher'97; Staff, CSSS du Coeur de l'Isle Hôpital Jean-Talon; (514)495-6767

TRAN NGUYEN, Thi Thu; Inst de Readaptation de Mtl, 6300 av de Darlington, Montreal QC H3S 2J4; Saigon (Vietnam)'79; Staff, Institut de Réadaptation Gingras-Lindsay de Montréal; (514)340-2085; Fax. (514)340-2149; jnolet@ssss.gouv.qc.ca.

TRAN-THANH, Danh; CHUM-Hotel-Dieu, 3840 rue Saint-Urbain, Montreal QC H2W 1T8; Mon'02; FRCSC; AnatPath. Staff, Centre Hospitalier l'Université de Montréal (CHUM) - Hôtel-Dieu; (514)890-8000

TRAN-VAN, Bernard; Clinique Ortho Laurentienne, 18-500 Boul des Laurentides, Saint-Jerome QC J7Z 4M2; Paris (France)'72; OrthSurg. (450)436-8482; Fax. (450)436-7427.

TRANG, Amy J; Humber River Reg Hosp-Church, 200 Church St, Toronto ON M9N 1N8; Tor'06; FRCPC; Anes. Staff Anes, St Michael's Hospital; Staff, Humber River Regional Hospital - Church Street Site; (416)249-8111

TRANG, Nguyen; 157-346 John St N, Arnprior ON K7S 2P6; Sher'99; CCFP; Staff, Arnprior & District Memorial Hospital; Langs: Vietnamese; English; (613)623-7964; Fax. (613)623-7965.

TRANG, The Vinh; CSSS de la Haute-Yamaska, 205 boul Leclerc O, Granby QC J2G 1T7; Sher'95; Anes. Staff, Centre Hospitalier de Granby; (450)375-8000 x2219

TRANMER, Jennifer E; Lansdowne Professional Ctr II, 235-3066 Shelbourne St, Victoria BC V8R 6T9; Qns'07; CCFP; Staff, Royal Jubilee Hospital; (250)592-6988

TRANQUI, John; 203-7125 Goreway Dr, Mississauga ON L4T 4H3; Tor'90; Langs: English; French; (905)677-8554; Fax. (905)677-8150.

TRANSUE, Sarah; Hôpital Reg d'Edmundston, 275 Hebert Blvd, Edmundston NB E3V 4E4; Michigan (USA); Staff, Hôpital regional d'Edmundston; (506)739-2200

TRANT, Alison M S; 100-11 Rosemount Ave, Ottawa ON K1Y 4R8; Ott'87; (613)724-5852; Fax. (613)724-9965.

TRANT, Donald F; Georgetown Med Associates, 199 Princess Anne Dr, Georgetown ON L7G 2B8; Tor'74; CCFP; FCFP; Pres Patient Prog/Court Staff, Halton Healthcare Services Corporation - Georgetown Hospital; (905)873-3000; Fax. (905)873-0800.

TRANULIS, Constantin; Hopital Louis-H Lafontaine, 7401 rue Hochelaga, Montreal QC H1N 3M5; Mon'01; FRCPC; Psy. Staff, Hopital Louis-H Lafontaine; Staff, Institute of Community & Family Psychiatry; (514)282-6060

TRAPLIN, Steven J; Guelph Family Health Team, 311-85 Norfolk St, Guelph ON N1H 4J4; McM'83; (519)836-7861; Fax. (519)836-8842; s.traplin@ontariomd.ca.

TRAPMAN, Johan L; Jane-Clair Med Centre, 2F-2698 Jane St, North York ON M3L 1S5; Leiden (Netherlands)'58; Staff, Humber River Regional Hospital - Keele Street Site; Staff, Humber River Regional Hospital - Finch Avenue Site; Langs: Dutch; German; (416)743-2041; Fax. (416)743-2045.

TRATCH, Alexandre; CHUM-Hopital Hotel-Dieu, 3840 rue Saint-Urbain, Montreal QC H2W 1T8; Laval'05; FRCPC; EmergMed. Staff, Centre Hospitalier l'Université de Montréal (CHUM) - Hôtel-Dieu; (514)890-8000

TRATTNER, Raquel; Centre Med Brunswick, 955 boul Saint-Jean, Pointe-Claire QC H9R 4Z7; McG'08; CCFP; (514)426-6677; Fax. (514)426-3323.

TRAUB-WERNER, Daniel Z; 43 Oriole Gardens, Toronto ON M4V 1V9; Buenos Aires (Argentina)'69; FRCPC; Psy (Psychoanalysis). Member, Canadian Psychoanalytic Society; Langs: Spanish; (416)920-3585

TRAUBICI, Jeffrey; The Hosp for Sick Children, 555 University Ave, Toronto ON M5G 1X8; Chicago(IL) (USA)'94; FRCPC; DiagRad. Staff, The Hospital For Sick Children; (416)813-6276; Fax. (416)813-7591; jeffrey.traubici@sickkids.ca.

TRAUTMAN, Allen F; 1921 10 Ave S, Lethbridge AB T1K 0B8; Alb'76; FRCSC; GenSurg. (403)380-4777; Fax. (403)380-3416.

TRAVERS, Andrew H; Emergency Health Services, 160-237 Brownlow Ave, Dartmouth NS B3B 2C5; Dal'94; FRCPC; EmergMed. Staff, Queen Elizabeth II Health Sciences Centre - Victoria General Site; (902)424-1729; Fax. (902)424-1781; traverah@gov.ns.ca.

TRAVERS, Sean A; North Bay Reg Health Centre, PO Box 2500 50 College Dr, North Bay ON P1B 0A4; Ott'95; FRCPC; Anes. Staff, North Bay Regional Health Centre - Regional Mental Health; Langs: English; French; (705)474-8600

TRAVERSE, Lionel D B; PO Box 112 Stn Mount Lehman, Abbotsford BC V4X 2P7; Paris (France)'80; DAB; FAAP; FRCPC; Peds (Neonatology). Langs: Spanish; English.

TRAVLOS, Andrew; Pacific Rehab Medicine, 140-943 Broadway W, Vancouver BC V5Z 4E1; Witwatersrand (South Africa)'84; MB ChB; FRCPC; PhysMed&Rehab (Neuromuscular Diseases). Staff Med/Med Mgr, Vancouver General Hospital - Centennial Pavillion; Clin Assoc Prof, University of British Columbia; Langs: Greek; Afrikaans; (604)733-2222; Fax. (604)733-2202; rehabmd@pacificrehab.net.

TRAYNOR, Michael D; BC Children's Hosp, 4480 Oak St, Vancouver BC V6H 3V4; UBC'95; FRCPC; Anes. Staff, BC Children's Hospital; Langs: Bilingual(English/French); (604)875-2345

TRAYNOR, Shirley M M; Braeside Med Centre Ltd, 111-1919 Southland Dr SW, Calgary AB T2W 0K1; Dublin (Ireland)'84; MB ChB; MRC(Eng); DCH; DObst; (403)258-2133; Fax. (403)258-2162.

TREASURER, Haren M; Business Bldg, 104-1017 Wilson Ave, North York ON M3K 1Z1; Wes'03; CCFP; (416)630-9329

TREASURER, Sushila M; Business Bldg, 104-1017 Wilson Ave, North York ON M3K 1Z1; Bombay (India)'68; Langs: Gujarati; Hindi; (416)630-9329; Fax. (416)630-3700.

TREBELL, Joanne R; 202-135 15th St E, North Vancouver BC V7L 2P7; UBC'86; (604)980-0919; Fax. (604)980-0244.

TRECARTEN, Mark A; Queensway-Carleton Hosp, 3045 Baseline Rd, Nepean ON K2H 8P4; Ott'85; CCFP; CCFP(E.M.); Staff, Queensway Carleton Hospital; (613)721-4710

TREDGET, Edward E; University of Alberta Hosp, 2D2 31-8440 112 St NW, Edmonton AB T6G 2B7; Alb'76; FRCSC; PlasSurg (Burns). Staff, University of Alberta Hospital; Prof Med/Dir, University of Alberta; (780)407-6979; Fax. (780)407-7394; etredget@ualberta.ca.

TREEHUBA, Kathryn E; PO Box 5037 Lcd Merivale, Nepean ON K2C 3H3; Wes'78; FRCSC; ObstGyn. Fax. (613)722-4103.

TREGOBOV, L Earl; Surrey Mem Hosp, 13750 96 Ave, Surrey BC V3V 1Z2; Man'89; FRCPC; DiagRad. Staff, Surrey Memorial Hospital; (604)588-3365; Fax. (604)588-3370.

TREGONING, Shaun K; D-2309 McCallum Rd, Abbotsford BC V2S 3N7; Witwatersrand (South Africa)'89; MB ChB; FCOG(SA); FRCSC; ObstGyn (Pelvic Floor Surgery). Staff, Abbotsford Regional Hospital & Cancer Centre; Clinical Asst Prof, University of British Columbia; Langs: Dutch; Afrikaans; Tagalog; Chinese; (604)557-1111; Fax. (604)557-1188; drshauntregoning@telus.net.

TREHERNE, Kerri A D; Alexandra Comm Health Centre, 101-1318 Centre St NE, Calgary AB T2E 2R7; Alb'94; BSc; CCFP; FCFP; (403)266-2622; Fax. (403)266-2692.

TREHERNE, Stephen E; 4500 rue Sherbrooke O, Westmount QC H3Z 1E6; McG'83; FRCPC; Peds. ac Staff, McGill University Health Centre - Montreal Children's Hospital; (514)932-4975; Fax. (514)932-9984.

TREIGYS, Darius; CSSS des Aurores Boreales, 679 2e rue E, La Sarre QC J9Z 2X7; Kaunas University (Other Foreign)'91; Staff, Centre Hospitalier La Sarre; (819)333-2311; Fax. (819)333-4227.

TREILHARD, John B; Whitby Clinic, 200 Brock St N, Whitby ON L1N 4H5; McM'83; BSc(Hons); MA; PhD; Ac Staff Emerg Med & Family Pract, Humber River Regional Hospital - Church Street Site; Langs: Bilingual(English/French); (905)427-0183; Fax. (905)668-3807.

TREISSMAN, Mark J B Y E; 240-546 St Paul St, Kamloops BC V2C 5T1; Wes'91; FRCSC; ObstGyn. (250)374-7722; Fax. (250)374-0446.

TREISSMAN, Simon P I D; 1723 High Ricardo Way, Kamloops BC V2E 1L3; Tor'90; FRCSC; Urol. (250)851-1364

TREKI, Ibrahim M; 1190 Tecumseh Rd E, Windsor ON N8W 1B4; Al-Fateh (Libya)'98; FRCPC; IntMed (Endocrinology & Metabolism). Staff, Hôtel-Dieu Grace Hospital; Staff, Windsor Regional Hospital - Tayfour Site; Staff, Windsor Regional Hospital - Metropolitan Site; Staff, Regional Bariatric Assessment & Treatment Centre; Aj Associate Prof, University of Western Ontario; Langs: Arabic; (519)253-6777; Fax. (519)253-2594.

TRELEAVEN, Darin J; St Joseph's Healthcare, 50 Charlton Ave E, Hamilton ON L8N 4A6; McM'95; FRCPC; IntMed; Nephrol. Staff, St Joseph's Healthcare - Charlton Campus; Langs: English; French; (905)522-4941

TRELLES, Francisco; Centre Hosp Univ du Quebec, 2705 boul Laurier, Quebec QC G1V 4G2; Mon'00; Gastroent; IntMed. Staff, Hôpital Regional Rimouski; Staff, Centre Hospitalier Universitaire de Quebec-CHUL; Langs: English; (418)654-2168; Fax. (418)654-2164.

TRELOAR, Murray E; Gamma-Dynacare Med Labs, 1100 Bennett Road, Bowmanville ON L1C 3K5; Tor'75; FCAP; FRCPC; GenPath., Lakeridge Health - Oshawa Site; Med Consultant, Gamma Dynacare Labs; Lecturer Path, University of Toronto; (905)576-8711 x3405; mtreloar@lakeridgehealth.on.ca.

TREMAINE, Robert D L; Atlantic Derm Consultants, 401-6155 North St, Halifax NS B3K 5R3; Dal'82; FRCPC; Derm (Phototherapy). Staff, IWK Health Centre; Staff Derm, Queen Elizabeth II Health Sciences Centre - Victoria General Site; Lecturer Med, Dalhousie University; (902)455-7273; rob.tremaine@ns.sympatico.ca.

TREMBLAY, Alain; 94 rue Joseph-W-Fleury, Alma QC G8E 2K2; Sher'75; Staff, CSSS de Lac-Saint Jean-Est; (418)347-4696; Fax. (418)347-4697; altrem29@hotmail.com.

TREMBLAY, Alain; Polyclinique Med Buckingham, 147 rue Joseph, Gatineau QC J8L 1G3; Mon'76; FRCPC; Psy. (819)986-1034

TREMBLAY, Alain; HSC-Faculty of Med, 3330 Hospital Dr NW, Calgary AB T2N 4N1; McG'95; FRCPC; IntMed (Interventional Pulmonary Medicine); Respir. Staff, Foothills Medical Centre; Staff, Tom Baker Cancer Centre; Clinical Asst Prof, University of Calgary; Langs: English; French; (403)210-3866; Fax. (403)944-1577; atrembla@ucalgary.ca.

TREMBLAY, Anik; CSSS de Beauce-Etchemin, 1515 17e rue, Saint-Georges QC G5Y 4T8; Laval'98; Staff, Centre Hospitalier Beauce-Etchemin; (418)228-2031; Fax. (418)226-0358.

TREMBLAY, Annie; CHUQ-Hotel-Dieu de Quebec, 11 Cote Du Palais, Quebec QC G1R 2J6; Laval'95; FRCPC; Psy (Psychiatric Oncology). Staff, Centre Hospitalier Universitaire de Québec (CHUQ) - Siege Social; (418)525-4444 x15808; Fax. (418)691-5019; tremblaya@hotmail.com.

TREMBLAY, Annie; Clinique Med de Montmagny, 100-83 av de la Fabrique, Montmagny QC G5V 2J3; Laval'92; (418)248-4933; Fax. (418)248-2778; annietremblay@gmf.gouv.qc.ca.

TREMBLAY, Annie; Hop Maisonneuve-Rosemot, 5415 boul de l'Assomption, Montreal QC H1T 2M4; Mon'02; FRCPC; IntMed; Cardiol. Staff, Hopital Maisonneuve-Rosemont; (514)252-3812

TREMBLAY, Anouk; CSSS de Trois-Rivières, 1991 boul du Carmel, Trois-Rivieres QC G8Z 3R9; Laval'99; MedOncol; Hem; IntMed. Staff, CSSS de Trois-Rivières; Langs: Bilingual(French/English); (819)697-3333 x63474; Fax. (819)372-3529.

TREMBLAY, Benoit P; CHUQ-Hotel-Dieu de Quebec, 11 Cote Du Palais, Quebec QC G1R 2J6; Laval'81; Cardiol; IntMed (Hemodynamics). ac Staff, Centre Hospitalier Universitaire de Québec (CHUQ) - Siege Social; (418)691-5151; Fax. (418)691-5415.

TREMBLAY, Bianca; CSSS Maria-Chapdelaine, 2000 av du Sacre-Coeur, Dolbeau-Mistassini QC G8L 2R5; Sher'08; Staff, Centre Maria-Chapdelaine - CH de Dolbeau-Mistassini; (418)276-1234; Fax. (418)276-4355.

TREMBLAY, Bruno; Clinique Med de Courville, 1049 av Larue, Quebec QC G1C 1J5; Laval'78; Langs: English; (418)661-0097; Fax. (418)661-0307.

TREMBLAY, Candide; CSSS du Sud de Lanaudière, 911 montee des Pionniers, Terrebonne QC J6V 2H2; Laval'79; Respir. Staff, Centre Hospitalier Pierre le Gardeur; (450)654-7525; Fax. (450)654-4296.

TREMBLAY, Carole; CSSS de Trois-Rivières, 1991 boul du Carmel, Trois-Rivieres QC G8Z 3R9; Mon'94; MedMicrobiol. Staff, Centre Hospitalier Regional de Trois-Rivieres; Staff, CSSS de Trois-Rivières; Staff, Hôtel-Dieu de Saint-Jérôme; (819)697-3333; cmarietremblay@hotmail.com.

TREMBLAY, Caroline; Clinique Med Pierre-Bertrand, 203-303 boul Pierre-Bertrand, Quebec QC G1M 3L7; Laval'00; (418)688-0872; Fax. (418)688-4951.

TREMBLAY, Catherine; St Michael's Hosp, 30 Bond St, Toronto ON M5B 1W8; Mon'05; ObstGyn. Staff ObstGyn, St Michael's Hospital; Langs: Bilingual(English/French); (416)360-4000

TREMBLAY, Cecile; CHUM-Hotel-Dieu, E7 355-3840 rue Saint-Urbain, Montreal QC H2W 1T8; Mon'92; FRCPC; MedMicrobiol (Infectious Diseases). Staff, Centre Hospitalier l'Université de Montréal (CHUM) - Hôtel-Dieu; (514)890-8000

TREMBLAY, Chantal; Clinique Med St-Louis, 504 rue St-Louis, Joliette QC J6E 2Z2; Mon'77; LMCC; Médecin, Clinique Med St-Louis; (450)759-0581; Fax. (450)759-0584; mariadechantal@hotmail.com.

TREMBLAY, Chantal; CSSS de la Vallee-de-l'Or, 2311-725 6e rue, Val-d'Or QC J9P 3Y1; Mon'89; Clin Staff, Hôpital psychiatrique de Malartic; Staff, Centre Hospitalier de Val d'Or; Staff, Maison de la Source Gabriel; Langs: Bilingual(French/English); (819)825-5858; Fax. (819)757-6034; chantal_tremblay@ssss.gouv.qc.ca.

TREMBLAY, Chantal; 200-731 rue Galt O, Sherbrooke QC J1H 1Z1; Sher'75; FRCSC; Otol (Head & Neck Surgery). ac Staff, Centre Hospitalier Universitaire de Sherbrooke-Hôpital Hôtel-Dieu; Consultant, Centre Hospitalier Universitaire de Sherbrooke-Hopital Fleurimont; pers Prof, Universite de Sherbrooke; (819)564-8662; Fax. (819)564-1294.

TREMBLAY, Chantale; CSSS de Chicoutimi, 305 rue Saint-Vallier, Chicoutimi QC G7H 5H6; Laval'77; Staff, Complexe hospitalier de la Sagamie; (418)541-1000; Fax. (418)541-1160.

TREMBLAY, Charles; CSSS de la Vallée de l'Or, 725 6e rue, Val-d'Or QC J9P 3Y1; Laval'73; FRCPC; IntMed; Respir (P.Q.). Staff, Centre Hospitalier de Val d'Or; (819)825-6711

TREMBLAY, Christine; Clinique Med Adoncour, 200-505 rue Adoncour, Longueuil QC J4G 2M6; Mon'83; Médecin, Clinique Medicale Adoncour; (450)646-4445; Fax. (450)646-5526.

TREMBLAY, Christine; CSSS de Laval, SS62-1755 boul Rene-Laennec, Laval QC H7M 3L9; Sher'96; FRCPC; IntMed; MedOncol; Hem. Staff, Hopital de la Cite de la santé; (450)668-1010; Fax. (450)975-5044.

TREMBLAY, Claude A; CHUQ-Hotel-Dieu de Quebec, 11 Cote Du Palais, Quebec QC G1R 2J6; Laval'77; FRCPC; MedMicrobiol (Infectious Diseases). Staff Microbiol & InfectDis, Centre Hospitalier Universitaire de Québec (CHUQ) - Siege Social; Clin Assoc Prof, Université Laval; (418)691-5131; claude.tremblay@chuq.qc.ca.

TREMBLAY, Claude; 75 2e rue Sartigan RR 2, Saint-Georges QC G5Y 5B8; Laval'65; (418)228-5752; Fax. (418)228-5752.

TREMBLAY, Claude; Polyclinique Med des Ponts, SS 90 120-1100 boul de la Rive-Sud, Saint-Romuald QC G6W 5M6; Laval'88; (418)834-1177

TREMBLAY, Claude; Hotel-Dieu de Levis, 143 rue Wolfe, Levis QC G6V 3Z1; Laval'84; DiagRad. Staff, Diag Radiol, Hôtel-Dieu de Lévis; (418)691-5131; Fax. (418)691-5457.

TREMBLAY, Denis; CHUQ-Hotel-Dieu de Quebec, 11 Cote Du Palais, Quebec QC G1R 2J6; Laval'91; Anes. Staff, Centre Hospitalier Universitaire de Québec (CHUQ) - Siege Social; (418)691-5151; denisj1962@hotmail.com.

TREMBLAY, Diane; Ctr Hosp du Centre la Mauricie, 50 119e rue, Shawinigan-Sud QC G9P 5K1; Laval'82; Staff, Centre Hospitalier du Centre la Mauricie; (819)536-7500 x3141

TREMBLAY, Dominic; CSSS de Trois-Rivières, 1991 boul du Carmel, Trois-Rivieres QC G8Z 3R9; Sher'06; FRCPC; NuclearMed. Staff, CSSS de Trois-Rivières; (819)697-3333

TREMBLAY, Dominique; Les Gynecologues Laval, 1299 boul de la Concorde O, Laval QC H7N 5T4; Mon'94; ObstGyn. Médecin, Les Gynecologues Associates Laval; (450)668-3250; Fax. (450)668-7595; bobi2@videotron.ca.

TREMBLAY, Dominique; Clinique Med du Centre, 2020 boul Rene Gauthier, Varennes QC J3X 1N9; Laval'88; (450)652-2222; Fax. (450)652-3970.

TREMBLAY, Dominique M; Hop Maisonneuve-Rosemont, 5415 boul de l'Assomption, Montreal QC H1T 2M4; Mon'05; FRCSC; PlasSurg. Staff, Hopital Maisonneuve-Rosemont; (514)252-3400

TREMBLAY, Emilie; Centre Hosp Reg de Lanaudiere, 1000 boul Sainte-Anne, St-Charles-Brromee QC J6E 6J2; Staff, Centre Hospitalier Régional de Lanaudière; (450)759-8222

TREMBLAY, Emilie; CLSC Pasbebiac, RR 2 273 boul Gerard-D.-Levesque O, Paspebiac QC G0C 2K0; Mon'10; CCFP; Staff, CLSC de Paspebiac; (418)752-2572

TREMBLAY, Eric; St Mary's Hosp Centre, 3830 av Lacombe, Montreal QC H3T 1M5; McG'91; Staff, St Mary's Hospital Centre; (514)345-3511 x3412

TREMBLAY, Florence; St Marys Family Med Centre, 3777 rue Jean-Brillant, Montreal QC H3T 1M5; Laval'04; CCFP; Staff, St Mary's Hospital Centre; Langs: Bilingual(French/English); (514)345-3511

TREMBLAY, Florence; GMF la Cigogne, 420-3141 boul Taschereau, Longueuil QC J4V 2H2; Sher'08; (450)466-7892

TREMBLAY, Francine; MUHC-Royal Victoria Hosp, S9 30-687 av des Pins O, Montreal QC H3A 1A1; Mon'84; FRCSC; GenSurg; General Surgical Oncology (P.Q.). Staff, McGill University Health Centre - Royal Victoria Hospital; (514)934-1934 x36313; Fax. (514)843-1434; francine.tremblay@muhc.mcgill.ca.

TREMBLAY, Francois; Hop Maisonneuve-Rosemont, 5415 boul de l'Assomption, Montreal QC H1T 2M4; Mon'99; Staff Emerg, Hopital Maisonneuve-Rosemont; (514)252-3400

TREMBLAY, Francois; CHUM-Hotel-Dieu, 3840 rue Saint-Urbain, Montreal QC H2W 1T8; Mon'07; FRCSC; IntMed; Respir. Staff, Centre Hospitalier l'Université de Montréal (CHUM) - Hôtel-Dieu; (514)890-8000

TREMBLAY, Frederic; Hop Santa Cabrini Ospedale, 5655 rue Saint-Zotique E, Montreal QC H1T 1P7; Laval'02; CCFP; CCFP(E.M.); Staff, Hôpital Santa Cabrini Ospedale; (514)252-6000

TREMBLAY, Genevieve; Dir de Sante Publique, 2400 av d'Estimauville, Quebec QC G1E 7G9; Laval'74; MPH; FRCPC; CommunMed; Public Health & Preventive Med. Med Consultant, Dir de Sante Publique de la Capitale-Nationale; Langs: English; (418)666-7000 x402; Fax. (418)666-2776; genevieve_tremblay@ssss.gouv.qc.ca.

TREMBLAY, Genevieve; Ctr Jeunesse de l'Estrie Val d, 8475 ch Blanchette, Sherbrooke QC J1N 3A3; Mon'02; CCFP; Staff, St Mary's Hospital Centre; (819)864-4221; Fax. (819)864-0671.

TREMBLAY, Gerald; Polyclinique du Saguenay, 314-874 Boul de l'Universite E, Chicoutimi QC G7H 6B9; Laval'70; Cardiol (P.Q.) (Echocardiography). (418)545-0539; Fax. (418)545-1032; g.tremblay@sympatico.ca.

TREMBLAY, Gilles R; Centre Med St-Urbain, 611-3875 rue Saint-Urbain, Montreal QC H2W 1V1; McG'71; MSc; FACS; FAAOS; FRCSC; OrthSurg (Accident Evaluation). Consultant, Hôpital Ste-Justine; principale Staff OrthSurg, Centre Hospitalier l'Université de Montréal (CHUM) - Hôtel-Dieu; assoc Prof Surg & Graduate Studies, Universite de Montreal; Langs: English; French; (514)844-8272; Fax. (514)844-8843; surort@qc.aibn.com.

TREMBLAY, Guy; Hotel-Dieu du Sacre-Coeur, 1 av du Sacre-Coeur, Quebec QC G1N 2W1; Laval'67; Psy (P.Q.). Staff, Hotel-Dieu du Sacre-Coeur de Jesus de Quebec; (418)529-6851 x452

TREMBLAY, Guy-Luc; 990 St Peter Ave, Bathurst NB E2A 2Z4; Laval'84; Otol (P.Q.). Ac Staff, Hopital Regional Chaleur; (506)546-8999; Fax. (506)546-1457.

TREMBLAY, Helene; Clinique Med du Quartier, 1191 av Cartier, Quebec QC G1R 2S9; Laval'87; Langs: Bilingual(French/English); (418)522-1911; Fax. (418)522-1789.

TREMBLAY, Helene; Clinique Medi-Plus, 4100 3e av O, Quebec QC G1H 6E1; Laval'79; LMCC; Langs: English; (418)622-6969; Fax. (418)622-2037; tremblay.h@videotron.ca.

TREMBLAY, Hugues; Clinique Med St-Redempteur, 266 rue Thibault, Matane QC G4W 2V9; Laval'77; (418)562-6133; Fax. (418)562-6947.

TREMBLAY, Isabelle; Hop du Sacre-Coeur de Mtl, 5400 boul Gouin O, Montreal QC H4J 1C5; Sher'97; FRCPC; Anes. Staff, Hôpital du Sacre-Coeur de Montréal; (514)338-2222 x2140; Fax. (514)338-2009.

TREMBLAY, Guy; CHAQ-Hopital du Sacrement, 1050 ch Sainte-Foy, Quebec QC G1S 4L8; Laval'70; CSPQ; FRCPC; Cardiol (Industrial Occupational Medicine). ac Staff, Centre Hospitalier Affilié Universitaire de Québec - Hôpital du St-Sacrement; Affil Staff, Université Laval; (418)682-7511; tremblay.cmb@videotron.ca.

TREMBLAY, Jacques; Douglas Mental Hlth Univ Inst, 6875 boul Lasalle, Verdun QC H4H 1R3; Mon'70; MSc; Prés, Douglas Mental Health University Institute; Langs: Spanish; English; French; (514)761-6131; trejac@douglas.mcgill.ca.

TREMBLAY, Jacques; Hop Maisonneuve-Rosemont, 5415 boul de l'Assomption, Montreal QC H1T 2M4; Mon'74; Respir (P.Q.) (Internal Medicine). Staff, Hopital Maisonneuve-Rosemont; (514)252-3400; Fax. (514)252-3434.

TREMBLAY, Jean; 9 ch des Lacs, Lac-Beauport QC G3B 1C1; Laval'71; (418)849-8091; Fax. (418)849-1663; jean.tremblay@travail.gouv.qc.ca.

TREMBLAY, Jean-Denis; Clinique Med Familiale Dolbeau, 1521 rue des Erables, Dolbeau-Mistassini QC G8L 1C4; Laval'76; Médecin Family Med, Centre Maria-Chapdelaine - CH de Dolbeau-Mistassini; Langs: Bilingual(French/English); (418)276-0041; Fax. (418)276-7170.

TREMBLAY, Jean-Francois; CHUM-Hotel-Dieu, 3840 rue Saint-Urbain, Montreal QC H2W 1T8; McG'98; Derm. Staff, Centre Hospitalier l'Université de Montréal (CHUM) - Hôtel-Dieu; (514)890-8000

TREMBLAY, Jean-Francois; Hop Maisonneuve-Rosemont, 5415 boul de l'Assomption, Montreal QC H1T 2M4; Mon'92; Cardiol; IntMed. Staff, Hopital Maisonneuve-Rosemont; (514)252-3400; Fax. (514)282-3529.

TREMBLAY, Jean-Guy; Ctr Hosp Univ de Quebec-CHUL, 2705 boul Laurier, Quebec QC G1V 4G2; Laval'70; ac Staff, Centre Hospitalier Universitaire de Quebec-CHUL; (418)654-2167

TREMBLAY, Jean-Luc; Clinique de Rhumatologie, 1119 rue Sainte-Marguerite, Trois-Rivieres QC G8Z 1Y2; Mon'94; FRCPC; IntMed; Rheum. (819)370-8106; Fax. (819)370-8120.

TREMBLAY, Jean-Philippe; Hôp Sainte Anne de Beaupré, 11000 rue des Montagnards, Beaupre QC G0A 1E0; Laval'92; Staff, Centre Hospitalier Universitaire De Québec - Pavillon De St-françois-d'assise; Staff, Hôpital Sainte Anne de Beaupré; (418)827-3726

TREMBLAY, Jocelyn; Clinique Med du Phare, 101-822 boul Sainte-Anne, Rimouski QC G5M 1J5; Mon'98; (418)723-5135

TREMBLAY, Joey E J; Lady Minto Hosp Cochrane, PO Box 4000 241 8th St, Cochrane ON P0L 1C0; Ott'09; CCFP; Staff, Lady Minto Hospital Cochrane; (705)272-7200

TREMBLAY, Johanne; Service de l'Evaluation Med SE, CP 7777 Succ Terminus 207-2600 boul Laurier, Quebec QC G1K 7T4; Laval'85; Médecin, CSST-Chaudiere-Appalaches; (418)657-8709

TREMBLAY, Julie; CSSS de Saint-Jerome, 290 rue de Montigny, Saint-Jerome QC J7Z 5T3; Sher'06; MedMicrobiol. Staff, CSSS St-Jerôme; (450)432-2777

TREMBLAY, Julie; Inst U en Sante Mentale de QC, 2601 ch de la Canardiere, Quebec QC G1J 2G3; Laval'91; FRCPC; Psy. Staff, Institut Universitaire Sante; (418)663-5721; Fax. (418)663-5758.

TREMBLAY, Lambert; Clinique Med Saint-Louis, 220-3165 ch Saint-Louis, Quebec QC G1W 4R4; Laval'64; Psy. Staff, Centre Hospitalier Universitaire de Québec (CHUQ) - Siege Social; (418)653-1970; Fax. (418)691-5019.

TREMBLAY, Lise; Hôpital Laval, 2725 ch Sainte-Foy, Quebec QC G1V 4G5; Laval'99; FRCPC; IntMed (Family Medicine); Respir. Staff Pneumologie, Hôpital Laval; (418)656-8711; Fax. (418)656-5252; tli12@hotmail.com.

TREMBLAY, Lorraine N; Sunnybrook Hlth Sciences Ctre, H171-2075 Bayview Ave, Toronto ON M4N 3M5; Wes'91; FRCSC; GenSurg (Clinician Investigator Program). Staff, Sunnybrook Health Sciences Centre; Langs: English; French; (416)480-5255; Fax. (416)480-5499.

TREMBLAY, Louise J; Clinique Statcare, 104-175 av Stillview, Pointe-Claire QC H9R 4S3; Ott'81; CCFP; (514)694-9282

TREMBLAY, Louise; Centre Med Boucherville, 201-600 boul du Fort-Saint-Lou, Boucherville QC J4B 1S7; Laval'82; (450)655-7321; Fax. (450)655-6311.

TREMBLAY, Luc; CLSC Samuel de Champlain, 100-5811 boul Taschereau, Brossard QC J4Z 1A5; Mon'83; (450)445-4452; Fax. (450)445-5535.

TREMBLAY, Madeleine D; Vancouver Gen Hosp, 855 12th Ave W, Vancouver BC V5Z 1M9; Sher'78; FRCPC; Psy (Adult Psychiatry). Ac Staff, Vancouver General Hospital - Centennial Pavillion; Asst Prof, University of British Columbia; Langs: Bilingual(English/French); (604)875-4111 x54018; Fax. (604)875-4226.

TREMBLAY, Madeleine; Clinique Med de la Cite, 101-3801 rue De Montcalm, Jonquiere QC G7X 1W1; Laval'85; (418)542-1510; Fax. (418)542-1512.

TREMBLAY, Marc-Andre; CSSS de Lac-Saint Jean-Est, CP 1300 Succ Bureau-chef 300 boul Champlain S, Alma QC G8B 5W3; Sher'04; MSc; FRCSC; OrthSurg. Staff, CSSS de Lac-Saint Jean-Est; Langs: Bilingual(French/English); (418)669-2000; Fax. (418)668-9685.

TREMBLAY, Marie-Claude; Institut de l'Oeil des Laurent, 1400 boul de la Grande-Allée, Sainte-Therese QC J7G 2Z8; Mon'88; FRCSC; Ophth. assoc Staff, Complexe hospitalier de la Sagamie; Staff, Hôpital du Sacre-Coeur de Montréal; Staff, Centre Hospitalier Fleury; Médecin, Institut de l'Oeil des Laurentides; Prof adj clin, Universite de Montreal; Langs: English; French; (450)419-7819

TREMBLAY, Marie-Claude S; Clinique Varices, 333 rue Montee Sanche, Boisbriand QC J7G 2E6; Laval'97; Langs: English; (450)434-7706

TREMBLAY, Marie-Eve; Ctr Hosp Laurentien, 234 rue Saint-Vincent, Ste-Agathe-des-Mts QC J8C 2B8; Mon'06; CCFP; Staff, Centre Hospitalier Laurentien; Staff, Centre Hospitalier Régional du Suroît; (819)324-4000

TREMBLAY, Marie-France; Clinique Med Blainville, 205-519 boul Cure-Labelle, Blainville QC J7C 2H6; Mon'81; Langs: Bilingual(French/English); (450)433-1112; Fax. (450)430-1274.

TREMBLAY, Marie-Helene; Clinique Saint-Redempteur, 210-600 Rte 116, Saint-Nicolas QC G7A 4X8; Mon'93; Staff, Hôtel-Dieu de Lévis; (418)831-4455; marie-helene.tremblay@gmf.gouv.qc.ca.

TREMBLAY, Marie-Helene; CHUQ-Hop de l'Enfant-Jesus, 1401 18e rue, Quebec QC G1J 1Z4; Mon'03; FRCPC; Anes. Staff, Centre Hospitalier Affilié Universitaire de Québec - Hôpital De L'Enfant Jésus; (418)649-0252

TREMBLAY, Marino; Clinique Med de Rawdon, 201-3240 1ere av, Rawdon QC J0K 1S0; Laval'74; (450)834-2304; Fax. (450)834-3345.

TREMBLAY, Marjolaine; CHUQ-Hotel-Dieu de Quebec, 11 Cote Du Palais, Quebec QC G1R 2J6; Laval'87; Staff, Centre Hospitalier Universitaire de Québec (CHUQ) - Siege Social; (418)691-5151

TREMBLAY, Marjorie; Hop du Sacre-Coeur de Mtl, 5400 boul Gouin O, Montreal QC H4J 1C5; Sher'01; Staff, Hôpital du Sacre-Coeur de Montréal; (514)338-2050

TREMBLAY, Martin; Expertise Neurosciences, 101 av Laurier O, Montreal QC H2T 2N6; Mon'91; FRCPC; Psy. Staff, Centre Hospitalier l'Université de Montréal (CHUM) - Hôpital Notre-Dame; (514)526-1648; Fax. (514)526-2016.

TREMBLAY, Maryse; CSSS de Manicouagan, 635 boul Jolliet, Baie-Comeau QC G5C 1P1; Laval'02; FRCPC; Anes. Staff, Centre Hospitalier Régional Baie-Comeau; (418)589-3701 x2786

TREMBLAY, Maxime; CSSS Pierre Boucher, 1333 boul Jacques-Cartier E, Longueuil QC J4M 2A5; Sher'97; FRCPC; DiagRad. Staff, Centre Hospitalier Pierre Boucher; (450)468-8157

TREMBLAY, Melissa; CSSS de la Sagamie, 305 rue Saint-Vallier, Chicoutimi QC G7H 5H6; Laval'01; CCFP; CCFP(E.M.); Staff, Complexe hospitalier de la Sagamie; (418)541-1234; Fax. (418)541-1000.

TREMBLAY, Michel; GMF Polyclinique des Ponts, 120-1100 boul de la Rive-Sud, Saint-Romuald QC G6W 5M6; Laval'84; Prés, Svc Technologiques Ac Inc; Langs: Bilingual(French/English); (418)835-5612; Fax. (418)834-9275; pcpsecretariat@hotmail.com.

TREMBLAY, Michele M; 1145 Carling Ave, Ottawa ON K1Z 7K4; Ott'83; FRCPC; Psy (Geriatric Psychiatry). Staff, Royal Ottawa Mental Health Centre - Royal Ottawa Health Care Group; Asst Prof, University of Ottawa; Langs: French; English; (613)722-6521 x6905; Fax. (613)798-2999.

TREMBLAY, Michele; Inst National Sante Publique, 190 boul Crémazie E, Montreal QC H2P 1E2; Laval'79; Med Consultant, Institut National de Sante Publique du Quebec; Langs: Bilingual(English/French); (514)864-1600 x3509; Fax. (514)864-1616; michele.tremblay@inspq.qc.ca.

TREMBLAY, Michele; Dir de la Sante Publique-Mtl, 1301 rue Sherbrooke E, Montreal QC H2L 1M3; Mon'79; FRCPC; CommunMed. (514)528-2400; Fax. (514)528-2452.

TREMBLAY, Micheline; Hop Jeffery Hale, 1250 ch Sainte-Foy, Quebec QC G1S 2M6; Laval'81; CCFP; FCFP; Staff, Jeffery Hale Hospital-Saint Brigid's; Clin Prof Med, Université Laval; Langs: Bilingual(French/English); (418)683-4471; Fax. (418)864-2266.

TREMBLAY, Monique; Clin Med Garnison St-Jean, CP 100 Succ Bureau-Chef, Richelain QC J0J 1R0; Laval'91; FRCPC; Psy. Staff, Centre Hospitalier Pierre Boucher; (450)358-7099 x7656

TREMBLAY, Myriam; CHUQ-St-Francois d'Assise, 10 rue de l'Espinay, Quebec QC G1L 3L5; Laval'88; ac Staff Family Med, Centre Hospitalier Universitaire De Québec - Pavillon De St-françois-d'assise; (418)525-4351; Fax. (418)525-4322.

TREMBLAY, Nancy; Clinique Med Belanger, 300-3871 reu Belanger, Montreal QC H1X 3M7; Laval'92; FRCPC; Psy. Staff, Centre Hospitalier Régional Baie-Comeau; (514)722-1166

TREMBLAY, Nathalie; Clinique Med Plateau Marquette, 200-731 rue Galt O, Sherbrooke QC J1H 1Z1; Sher'97; Staff, Centre Hospitalier Universitaire de Sherbrooke-Hopital Fleurimont; (819)564-8662; Fax. (819)564-1294.

TREMBLAY, Nathalie; CSSS Nicolet-Yamaska, 675 rue Saint-Jean-Baptiste, Nicolet QC J3T 1S4; Laval'90; Staff, Hôpital de Christ-Roi; (819)293-2071

TREMBLAY, Nicolas; Hopital Laval, 2725 ch Sainte-Foy, Quebec QC G1V 4G5; Laval'06; CCFP; Staff, Centre Hospitalier de Gaspe; Staff, Hôpital Laval; Staff, Hôpital de l'Archipel; (418)656-8711

TREMBLAY, Normand A G; CSSS Pierre Boucher, 1333 boul Jacques-Cartier E, Longueuil QC J4M 2A5; Ott'65; FRCPC; Anes. Staff, Centre Hospitalier Pierre Boucher; (450)468-8111; mrnt@videotron.ca.

TREMBLAY, Pamela M; Glazier Med Centre, 11 Gibb St, Oshawa ON L1H 2J9; Tor'81; FRCSC; ObstGyn. Staff, Lakeridge Health - Oshawa Site; (905)579-1212; Fax. (905)579-2021.

TREMBLAY, Pascale; Clinique Med Mellon, 303-2075 boul Mellon, Jonquiere QC G7S 5Z8; Mon'98; Physician, CSSS Carrefour Sante Jonquiere; Langs: English; (418)548-1121; Fax. (418)548-5345.

TREMBLAY, Patrice; Ctr Hosp de Matane, 333 rue Thibault, Matane QC G4W 2W5; Mon'93; LMCC; Staff, Centre Hospitalier de Matane; (418)562-3135

TREMBLAY, Paul-Benoit; Agence de Sante & Services, 930 rue Jacques-Cartier E, Chicoutimi QC G7H 7K9; Laval'69; Médecin, Hydro-Quebec; Med Consultant, Agence de sante & Services Sociaux; (418)545-4980 x341; Fax. (418)545-4718.

TREMBLAY, Philippe; CHUQ-Ctr Hosp Univ Laval, RC 157-2705 boul Laurier, Quebec QC G1V 4G2; Laval'99; FRCPC; Psy. Staff, Centre Hospitalier Universitaire de Quebec-CHUL; (418)654-2121; Fax. (418)654-2132.

TREMBLAY, Pierre G; CHUQ-Ctr Hosp Univ Laval, RC 267-2705 boul Laurier, Quebec QC G1V 4G2; Laval'83; FRCPC; Psy (Pediatric Psychiatry). ac Staff, Centre Hospitalier Universitaire de Quebec-CHUL; (418)654-2256; Fax. (418)654-2756; pierreg.tremblay@mail.chuq.qc.ca.

TREMBLAY, Pierre H; Hop Riviere-des-Prairies, 7070 boul Perras, Montreal QC H1E 1A4; Laval'73; FRCPC; Psy (Community Psychiatry). Physician-in-Charge, Hôpital Riviere des Prairies; Consultant, Hopital Maisonneuve-Rosemont; Prof Psy, Universite de Montreal; (514)328-3503; Fax. (514)323-4163; pierreh.tremblay.hrdp@ssss.gouv.qc.ca.

TREMBLAY, Pierre; Hôpital régional Chaleur, 1750 Sunset Dr, Bathurst NB E2A 4L7; Sher'00; Staff, Hopital Regional Chaleur; (506)544-3000

TREMBLAY, Pierre; Clinique Pediatrique Sainte-Fo, 295-2600 boul Laurier, Quebec QC G1V 4T3; Sher'79; FRCPC; Peds. Staff, Complexe hospitalier de la Sagamie; (418)658-0906; Fax. (418)652-7094; ptremblayear@videotron.ca.

TREMBLAY, Pierre; Clinique Med Bromont, C101-82 boul de Bromont, Bromont QC J2L 2K3; Laval'68; Langs: English; (450)534-5474; Fax. (450)534-1725.

TREMBLAY, Pierre; CHUQ-Ctr Hosp Univ Laval, 2705 boul Laurier, Quebec QC G1V 4G2; Mon'81; FRCPC; Anes. Staff, Centre Hospitalier Universitaire de Quebec-CHUL; (418)656-4141; Fax. (418)654-2774.

TREMBLAY, Pierre-Michel; Dr George L Dumont Reg HC, 330 Univesity Ave, Moncton NB E1C 2Z3; Laval'84; Ac Staff Emerg, Dr Georges-L-Dumont University Hospital Centre; Langs: English; French; (506)862-4230

TREMBLAY, Pierre-Paul; Centre de sante Haute-Gaspesie, 50 rue Belvedere, Ste-Anne-des-Monts QC G4V 1X4; Laval'72; Med Staff, Centre Hospitalier de Matane; Staff, Centre Hospitalier des Monts; (418)763-2261

TREMBLAY, Pierre-Paul; Clinique Med St-Liboire, 104-54 rue Saint Patrice, Saint-Liboire QC J0H 1R0; Mon'90; Staff, Centre Hospitalier Honore-Mercier; (450)793-4414; Fax. (450)793-2615.

TREMBLAY, Rene M; Ctr Hosp Affilie-St-Sacrement, 1050 ch Sainte-Foy, Quebec QC G1S 4L8; Sher'70; FRCPC; Gastroent (P.Q.). Staff, Centre Hospitalier Affilié Universitaire de Québec - Hôpital du St-Sacrement; Clin Prof, Université Laval; Langs: English; (418)682-7646; Fax. (418)682-7588.

TREMBLAY, Richard; CSSS de Laval, 1755 boul Rene-Laennec, Laval QC H7M 3L9; McG'95; Nephrol; IntMed. Staff, Hopital de la Cite de la santé; Langs: English; (450)668-1010; Fax. (450)975-5072.

TREMBLAY, Robert; Clinique Fam des Prairies, 310 boul Antonio-Barrette, N-D-Des-Prairies QC J6E 1G2; Sher'85; Staff, Centre Hospitalier Régional de Lanaudière; Langs: English; (450)752-1050; Fax. (450)752-2965.

TREMBLAY, Roger J P R; Edifice Bldg, CP 100 Succ Bureau-Chef 41 C SVC S FC, Richelain QC J0J 1R0; Ott'91; FCFP; CCFP; FCFP; Médecin, National Defence Montreal Detachment Services Group; (450)358-7099 x7113; tremblay.jpr@forces.gc.ca.

TREMBLAY, Roger; 2965 1re av, Quebec QC G1L 3P2; Laval'77; CCFP; Associate, Centre Hospitalier Universitaire De Québec - Pavillon De St-françois-d'assise; (418)627-4000; Fax. (418)628-0293.

TREMBLAY, Roger T; McConnell Med Centre, 216-820 Mcconnell Ave, Cornwall ON K6H 4M4; Laval'93; CCFP; (613)933-4790; Fax. (613)933-3511.

TREMBLAY, Roland R; CHUQ-Ctr Hosp Univ Laval, G-00250-2705 boul Laurier, Quebec QC G1V 4G2; Laval'64; DSc; BPhil; FACP; PhD; FRCPC; MedScient(Med) (Endocrinology & Andrology); Endocrin (P.Q.). ac Staff, Centre Hospitalier Universitaire de Quebec-CHUL; Consultant, Hôpital de la Malbaie; Langs: English; (418)654-2733; Fax. (418)654-2215; roland.r.tremblay@crchul.ulaval.ca.

TREMBLAY, Ronald; St Lawrence College, 2 Belmont St, Cornwall ON K6H 4Z1; McG'82; Physician, St Lawrence College; Langs: Bilingual(English/French); (613)932-9895; rtremblay@sl.on.ca.

TREMBLAY, Samuel L; Hôpital De L'Enfant Jésus, 1401 18e rue, Quebec QC G1J 1Z4; Laval'07; FRCPC; IntMed. Staff, Centre Hospitalier Affilié Universitaire de Québec - Hôpital De L'Enfant Jésus; (418)649-0252

TREMBLAY, Sandra; Hotel-Dieu de Levis, 143 rue Wolfe, Levis QC G6V 3Z1; Laval'90; FRCSC; Neur; Electroenceph (P.Q.). Staff, Hôtel-Dieu de Lévis; Staff, Hopital du CSS de la Region de Thetford; Staff, Centre Hospitalier Paul-Gilbert; (418)835-7121; Fax. (418)835-7212.

TREMBLAY, Serge; 5 2e ave CP 128, Forestville QC G0T 1E0; Laval'78; (418)587-2229; Fax. (418)584-2420.

TREMBLAY, Serge Y; 3995 montee Saint-Hubert, Longueuil QC J3Y 4K2; Laval'78; (450)676-6911; Fax. (450)676-4097.

TREMBLAY, Sonia; CLSC Rene-Cassin, 600-5800 boul Cavendish, Cote Saint-Luc QC H4W 2T5; Mon'05; CCFP; (514)488-9163; Fax. (514)485-2978.

TREMBLAY, Sophie; BC Children's Hosp, 4480 Oak St, Vancouver BC V6H 3N1; Mon'95; FRCPC; Peds (Neonatal & Perinatal Medicine). Staff, BC Women's Hospital & Health Centre; (604)875-2135

TREMBLAY, Stephane D; Centre De Sante Paul-Gilbert, 9330 boul du Centre-Hospitalie, Levis QC G6X 1L6; Laval'94; FRCPC; EmergMed (P.Q.). Staff, Hôtel-Dieu de Lévis; Staff, Centre Hospitalier Paul-Gilbert; (418)380-8993

TREMBLAY, Stephane; CHUS-Hop Fleurimont, 3001 12e av N, Sherbrooke QC J1H 5N4; Sher'91; FRCPC; Peds. Staff, Centre Hospitalier Universitaire de Sherbrooke-Hopital Fleurimont; (819)346-1110; Fax. (819)820-6420.

TREMBLAY, Suzanne; Clinique Med d'Alma, 935 av Du Pont S, Alma QC G8B 2V5; Laval'85; Staff, CSSS de Lac-Saint Jean-Est; (418)668-6121; Fax. (418)668-5298.

TREMBLAY, Sylvie S; Ctr Hosp du Centre la Mauricie, 50 119e rue, Shawinigan-Sud QC G9P 5K1; Mon'92; FRCSC; Otol (Head & Neck Surgery). Staff, Centre Hospitalier du Centre la Mauricie; (819)536-7609; Fax. (819)536-7619; pierre.gauthier@tr.cgocable.ca.

TREMBLAY, Sylvie; Societe Assurance Automobile, S2 1-260 rue de l'Estuaire, Quebec QC G1K 8Z3; Laval'78; Langs: Bilingual(French/English); (418)528-5356; Fax. (418)528-1223.

TREMBLAY, Sylvie; Centre Med Drummond, 60 rue Loring, Drummondville QC J2C 7Y9; McG'89; Langs: Bilingual(French/English); (819)477-2500; Fax. (819)477-6249.

TREMBLAY, Thierry; CSSS de la Vallée de l'Or, 725 6e rue, Val-d'Or QC J9P 3Y1; Sher'94; FRCSC; Urol. Staff, Centre Hospitalier de Val d'Or; (819)825-6711; Fax. (819)825-7927; ttremblay@cablevision.qc.ca.

TREMBLAY, Valerie M C; Medical & Dental Bldg, 300-1221 Algonquin Ave, North Bay ON P1B 4Y3; Sher'04; FRCSC; Otol (Head & Neck Surgery). Langs: Bilingual(French/English); (705)472-2646; Fax. (705)476-6543.

TREMBLAY, Vanessa; Hopital de Saint-Eustache, 520 boul Arthur-Sauve, Saint-Eustache QC J7R 5B1; Sher'03; FRCPC; IntMed. Staff, Hotel-Dieu d'Arthabaska; Staff, Hôpital de Saint-Eustache; (450)473-6811

TREMBLAY, Yves; Hop Santa Cabrini Ospedale, 5655 rue Saint-Zotique E, Montreal QC H1T 1P7; Sher'93; FRCSC; GenSurg (P.Q.) (Intensive Care). Staff, Hôpital Santa Cabrini Ospedale; Universite de Montreal; (514)252-6000; tremblayy@hotmail.com.

TREMBLAY-ALLAN, Fannie; CSSS Maria-Chapdelaine, 2000 boul Sacre-Coeur, Dolbeau-Mistassini QC G8L 2R5; Laval'00; FRCSC; GenSurg (Laparoscopy). Staff, Centre Maria-Chapdelaine - CH de Dolbeau-Mistassini; Staff, Lakeshore General Hospital - Pointe Claire; Langs: English; (418)276-1234; Fax. (418)276-4355.

TREMBLAY-BOUCHARD, Emilie; CSSSG-Hop de Gatineau, CP 2000 Succ Bureau-Chef 909 boul le Verendry O, Gatineau QC J8P 7H2; Sher'06; CCFP; Staff, Hôpital de Gatineau; (819)966-6100

TREMBLAY-COUTU, Eleonore; Hopital Charles LeMoyne, 3120 boul Taschereau, Longueuil QC J4V 2H1; Mon'05; Anes. Staff, Centre Hospitalier l'Université de Montréal (CHUM) - Hôpital Notre-Dame; Staff, Hopital Charles LeMoyne; (450)466-5000

TREMBLAY-GONTHIER, Elise; CSSS de la Baie-des-Chaleurs, 419 boul Perron, Maria QC G0C 1Y0; Laval'07; CCFP; Staff, CSSS de la Baie-des-Chaleurs; (418)759-3443

TREMBLAY-JOLICOEUR, Claudine; Pavillon Albert-Prevost, 6555 boul Gouin O, Montreal QC H4K 1B3; Sher'76; FRCPC; Psy (Pediatric Psychiatry). Staff, Hôpital du Sacre-Coeur de Montréal; Clin Prof, Universite de Montreal; (514)338-4356; Fax. (514)338-4357.

TREMBLAY LAROCHE, Dave; Ctr Hosp Affilie-Enfant-Jesus, 1401 18e rue, Quebec QC G1J 1Z4; Laval'08; FRCPC; IntMed. Staff, Centre Hospitalier Affilié Universitaire de Québec - Hôpital De L'Enfant Jésus; (418)649-0252

TREMBLAY-REINHARDT, Nicolas-Olivier; Hotel-Dieu de Roberval, 450 rue Brassard, Roberval QC G8H 1B9; Mon'04; Staff, Hôpital de l'Archipel; Staff, Hotel-Dieu de Roberval; Langs: Spanish; English; (418)275-0110

TREMBLAY-TANGUAY, Charles; CSSS du Rocher Percé, CP 3300 451 rue Mgr Ross, Chandler QC G0C 1K0; Laval'07; CCFP; Staff, Centre Hospitalier de Chandler; (418)689-2261

TREMBLAY TREMPE, Renee; CRSSS de la Baie-James, 51 3e rue, Chibougamau QC G8P 1N1; Sher'06; CCFP; Staff, CRSSS de la Baie-James; (418)748-2676

TREMBLAY-WURTELE, Diane; CLSC des Maskoutains, 1015 rue Gauthier, Saint-Hyacinthe QC J2S 8T2; Mon'74; Médecin, CLSC-CHSLD des Maskoutains; (450)778-2572 x6065; Fax. (450)778-1899; diane.tremblay@rrsss16.gouv.qc.ca.

TREMEER, Cory B; Associated Radiologists, 300-140 Wall St, Saskatoon SK S7K 1N4; Sask'05; FRCPC; DiagRad. (306)244-1167; Fax. (306)244-2911.

TREMPE, Dominique; Hop Maisonneuve-Rosemont, 5415 boul de l'Assomption, Montreal QC H1T 2M4; Mon'84; Staff, Hopital Maisonneuve-Rosemont; (514)252-3400

TREMPE, Germain L; Hop du Sacre-Coeur de Mtl, 5400 boul Gouin O, Montreal QC H4J 1C5; Mon'66; MedOncol (P.Q.); HemPath; Hem (P.Q.) (Hematological Oncology). ac Staff, Hôpital du Sacre-Coeur de Montréal; Langs: Bilingual(English/French); (514)338-2150; Fax. (514)338-2631.

TREMPE, Jocelyne; 10890 rue Waverly, Montreal QC H3L 2W8; Mon'66; DPH; (514)332-1112

TREMPE, Laurent; 3921 rue Saint-Denis, Montreal QC H2W 2M4; Mon'72; (514)287-9294

TREMPE-GOURDEAU, Suzanne; Groupe Sante Medisys, 410-3165 ch Saint-Louis, Quebec QC G1W 4R4; Laval'74; Member Medical Evaluator, Regis des Rentes du Quebec; Staff, Groupe Sante Medisys; Langs: Bilingual(French/English); (418)681-0167; Fax. (418)681-4564; suzanne.trempe@medisys.ca.

TREMPE-MASSON, Catherine; Clinique Med des Sommets, 1070 rue Principale E, Ste-Agathe-des-Mts QC J8C 1L6; Mon'01; Staff, Hôpital de l'Archipel; (819)321-1212

TRENHOLM, Arthur D; Public Gardens Med Clinic, 200-5675 Spring Garden Rd, Halifax NS B3J 1H1; Dal'71; (902)425-5440; Fax. (902)482-6019.

TRENHOLM, E Jo-Anne; Orleans Family Health Clinic, 101-210 Centrum Blvd, Orleans ON K1E 3V7; Dal'77; CCFP; FCFP; (613)837-5454; Fax. (613)837-3781.

TRENHOLM, J Andrew; Queen Elizabeth II HSC, 4510A-1796 Summer St, Halifax NS B3H 3A7; Dal'96; FRCSC; OrthSurg (Trauma Surgery). Staff, Queen Elizabeth II Health Sciences Centre - Halifax Infirmary Site; Langs: Bilingual(English/French); (902)473-5311; Fax. (902)425-7382; trean@reg2.health.nb.ca.

TRENHOLM, Richard L; Huntsville Prof Bldg, 202-348 Muskoka Rd 3 N, Huntsville ON P1H 1H8; McM'00; BSc; MSc; CCFP; Langs: Bilingual(English/French); (705)788-3623; Fax. (705)788-3624; rich.trenholm@mahc.ca.

TRENHOLME, Brenda J; Riverside Family Medicine, PO Box 1955, Rossland BC V0G 1Y0; UBC'83; (250)368-7022

TRENKER, David C; Southdale Med Clinic, 395 Southdale Rd E, London ON N6E 1A2; Wes'90; Staff, Regional Mental Health Care-St Joseph's Health Care; (519)691-0100; Fax. (519)691-1172.

TRENKER, Richard S; 402-111 Main St W, North Bay ON P1B 2T6; Qns'88; Staff, North Bay Regional Health Centre - Regional Mental Health; (705)494-8877; Fax. (705)494-9915.

TREPANIER, Claude; Ctr Hosp Affilie-Enfant-Jesus, 1401 18e rue, Quebec QC G1J 1Z4; Laval'77; Anes. ac Staff, Centre Hospitalier Affilié Universitaire de Québec - Hôpital De L'Enfant Jésus; pers Prof, Université Laval; (418)649-5803; Fax. (418)649-5936.

TRÉPANIER, David; Centre Serv Sociaux Manicouaga, 835 boul Jolliet, Baie-Comeau QC G5C 1P1; Laval'09; CCFP; Staff, Centre Hospitalier Régional Baie-Comeau; (418)589-3701

TREPANIER, Gerald P; Medical Imaging Consultants, 202-11010 101 St NW, Edmonton AB T5H 4B9; Alb'77; FRCPC; DiagRad. (780)426-1121; Fax. (780)425-5979.

TREPANIER, Jean R; Place Vanier, TA 5F-333 North River Rd, Ottawa ON K1A 0L1; Ott'77; Langs: English; French; (613)954-5692

TREPANIER, Jean-Pierre; Agence de santé de Lanaudiere, 245 rue du Cure-Majeau, Joliette QC J6E 8S8; Sher'00; FRCPC; CommunMed (Public Health). Langs: Bilingual(French/English); (450)759-1157 x4497; Fax. (450)759-5149; jean-pierre_trepanier@ssss.gouv.qc.ca.

TREPANIER, Josee; Centre Med Iberville, 101-235 2e Av, St-Jean-Sur-Richel QC J2X 2B2; Mon'87; (450)347-5548; Fax. (450)347-4091.

TREPANIER, Line; Clinique sante de Thetford, 2000-926 rue Labbe, Thetford Mines QC G6G 2A8; Laval'84; Staff, Hopital du CSS de la Region de Thetford; Langs: English; (418)338-4581; Fax. (418)338-4584.

TREPANIER, Louise; CLSC Riviere des Prairies, 8655 boul Perras, Montreal QC H1E 4M7; Mon'82; CCFP; Médecin, Hopital Maisonneuve-Rosemont; Clin Supvr Family Med, Universite de Montreal; Langs: Bilingual(French/English); (514)494-4924; Fax. (514)494-4235.

TREPANIER, Madeleine; Clinique Med des Sommets, 1070 rue Principale, Ste-Agathe-des-Mts QC J8C 1L6; Mon'04; CCFP; CCFP(E.M.); Staff, Centre Hospitalier Rouyn-Noranda; (819)321-1212; Fax. (819)321-3232.

TREPANIER, Marie C; 125-100 boul de Montarville, Boucherville QC J4B 5M4; Ott'71; (450)449-0022; Fax. (450)449-0227.

TREPANIER, Paul J; Madrona Imaging Westhill Ctre, A-1804 Bowen Rd, Nanaimo BC V9S 5W4; Alb'87; FRCPC; DiagRad. Staff, UBC Hospital - Koerner Pavillion; (250)753-4351; Fax. (250)753-0856.

TREPANIER, Stephane; Agence Serv Sociaux Cote-Nord, 691 rue Jalbert, Baie-Comeau QC G5C 2A1; Sher'06; FRCPC; Public Health & Preventive Med. Staff, Agence de développement de réseaux locaux des services de santé et des services sociaux de la Côte-Nord; (418)589-9845; Fax. (418)589-8574.

TREPEL, Simon P; Manitoba Adolescent Trmt Ctre, 120 Tecumseh St, Winnipeg MB R3E 2A9; Man'01; FRCPC; Psy.

TRERICE, Deborah A; Royal Oak Centre Med Clinic, 105-4442 West Saanich Rd, Victoria BC V8Z 3E9; Qns'90; CCFP; (250)479-6721; Fax. (250)727-6751.

TRESOOR, Tracy L; Roblin Med Centre, PO Box 1030, Roblin MB R0L 1P0; Man'85; CCFP; (204)937-8312

TRETIAK, Wendy D; Youville Centre, 6-845 Dakota St, Winnipeg MB R2M 5M3; Man'95; CCFP; FCFP; (204)255-4840; Fax. (204)255-4903.

TRETIAKOV, Michael; Country Hills Village, 220-5149 Country Hills Village, Calgary AB T3A 5K8; (403)241-8848; Fax. (403)241-8849.

TREVENEN, Cynthia L; Alberta Children's Hosp, 2888 Shaganappi Trail NW, Calgary AB T3B 6A8; Man'67; BSc; FRCPC; AnatPath (Pediatric Pathology). Ac Staff, Alberta Children's Hospital; Clin Prof, University of Calgary; (403)955-7386; Fax. (403)955-2321; cynthia.trevenen@cls.ab.ca.

TREVOR, Andrew W; St Joseph's Life Care Centre, 15-99 Wayne Gretzky Pky, Brantford ON N3S 6T6; Assam (India)'72; Staff, The Brant Community Healthcare System - Brantford General Hospital Site; Langs: Hindi; (519)759-7372; Fax. (519)759-4343.

TREW, Michael E; Foothills Med Centre, 1403 29 St NW, Calgary AB T2N 2T9; Sask'77; BSc(Med.); FRCPC; Psy (Consultant Liaison Psychiatry). Staff, Foothills Medical Centre; Sr Med Dir Addiction & Mental Health, Alberta Health Services; Teach Staff, University of Calgary; (403)943-0427; Fax. (403)943-6830; michael.trew@calgaryhealthregion.ca.

TREYVAUD, Stephane N; Dr S Treyvaud Med Prof Corp, 408-345 Lakeshore Rd E, Oakville ON L6J 1J5; Basel (Switzerland)'79; FRCPC; Psy (Psychoanalysis). Langs: German; French; Italian; (905)338-1386; Fax. (905)338-2717; halltrey@sympatico.ca.

TRIANTAFILLOU, Mark; McGill Centre, PO Box 2000 Stn Central 55 McGill Ave, Charlottetown PE C1A 7N8; Athens (Greece)'60; DPM; MRCPsy; Staff, Hillsborough Hospital & Special Care Centre; Dir Mental Health, Prince Edward Island Health Department; Consultant Psy, Community Mental Health; Langs: Greek; (902)368-4911; mltriantafillou@ihis.org.

TRIASSI ASPER, Maria; Thistlewood Prof Centre, 306-8077 Islington Ave, Woodbridge ON L4L 7X7; Tor'98; FRCP; FRCPC; Peds; ClinImmunol&Allergy. Clin Staff, The Hospital For Sick Children; Lecturer, University of Toronto; Langs: Italian; (905)856-8714

TRICKEY, Brian H; Urgent Care Centre, 945 Gardiners Rd, Kingston ON K7M 7H4; Ott'76; (613)389-3348

TRIFFAULT, Olivier; Ctr Hosp Pierre-Janet, 20 rue Pharand, Gatineau QC J9A 1K7; Rennes (France)'90; FRCPC; Psy. Dir, Centre Hospitalier Pierre-Janet; (819)771-7761; Fax. (819)771-2908; olivier_triffault@ssss.gouv.qc.ca.

TRIFIRO, Mark A; E104-SMBD Jewish Gen Hosp, 3755 ch Cote-Sainte-Catherine, Montreal QC H3T 1E2; McG'79; FRCPC; IntMed. Staff Endocrin, Sir Mortimer B Davis Jewish General; assoc Prof Med, McGill University; Langs: English; French; (514)340-8222 x5445; Fax. (514)340-7529.

TRIFIRO, Silvana G; Hop Santa Cabrini Ospedale, 5655 rue Saint-Zotique E, Montreal QC H1T 1P7; McG'83; FRCPC; IntMed; MedMicrobiol; InfectDis. Staff, Hôpital Santa Cabrini Ospedale; (514)252-6000 x7130; Fax. (514)252-6592; trifiro_silvana@ssss.gouv.qc.ca.

TRIFIS, Mokhtar H M; Eastwood Med Clinic, 7919 118 Ave NW, Edmonton AB T5B 0R5; (780)756-3666; Fax. (780)756-2534.

TRIGAZIS, Leonidas; Goodfellow Prof Bldg, 105-170 McEwan Dr E, Bolton ON L7E 4C8; Tor'02; PhD; BSc; CCFP; Langs: Greek; (905)857-3260; Fax. (905)857-6276.

TRIKI, Msod A M; Bay St George Med Clinic, 129 Montana Dr, Stephenville NL A2N 2T4; (Other Foreign)'00; CCFP; Staff, Rufus Guinchard Health Centre; Staff, Bay St George Medical Clinic; (709)643-6635

TRIMBLE, Nancy E; 200-128 Penetang St, Barrie ON L4M 1V6; Tor'87; CCFP; Ac Staff, Royal Victoria Regional Health Centre; (705)726-9790; Fax. (705)726-0827.

TRINDER, Tammy C; Surrey Mem Hosp, 13750 96 Ave, Surrey BC V3V 1Z2; McM'01; CCFP; Staff, Surrey Memorial Hospital; (604)581-2211

TRINH, Ba-Chinh; Clinique de radiologie Viau, 203-4750 rue Jarry E, Saint-Leonard QC H1R 1X9; Mon'94; FRCPC; DiagRad. (514)326-9850; Fax. (514)326-9851.

TRINH, Ba-Truc; Hop Cite de la Sante de Laval, 1755 boul Rene-Laennec, Laval QC H7M 3L9; Mon'96; FRCSC; Otol (Endocrinology Surgery). Staff, Hopital de la Cite de la santé; Chief Otol Division, Hôpital du Sacre-Coeur de Montréal; Langs: Vietnamese; English; (450)668-1010

TRINH, Bich Hang; Centre de Sante Hymus, 1700 boul Hymus, Kirkland QC H9J 2W2; Saigon (Vietnam)'75; (514)426-7161; Fax. (514)426-0325.

TRINH, Emilie B K; Polyclinique, 103-12905 rue Sherbrooke E, Pte-aux-Trembles QC H1A 1B9; Mon'10; CCFP; (514)498-4050

TRINH, Grace H; Pacific Med Clinic, F33-4300 Steeles Ave E, Markham ON L3R 0Y5; (Other Foreign)'87; CCFP; (905)604-7889; Fax. (905)604-7890.

TRINH, Hang Kim T; Steinbach Family Med Centre, 10-333 Loewen Blvd, Steinbach MB R5G 0C3; Man'04; CCFP; (204)326-3401; Fax. (204)326-3899.

TRINH, Hue Co; Pacific Med Centre, FF33-4300 Steeles Ave E, Markham ON L3R 0Y5; Saigon (Vietnam)'87; (905)604-7889; Fax. (905)604-7890.

TRINH, K Y Denny; 303-2189 Yonge St, Toronto ON M4S 2B2; McM'91; FRCPC; IntMed. Staff, Toronto General Hospital - UHN; Langs: Chinese; Vietnamese; (416)481-7720; Fax. (416)481-9903.

TRINH, Kien V; Ancaster Sport Med Centre, 1015 Golf Links Rd, Ancaster ON L9K 1L6; Wes'92; CAFCI; Dip SportMed; FCAMA; MSc; CCFP; FCFP; Ac Staff, Hamilton Health Sciences Centre - Hamilton General Hospital; Court Staff, St Joseph's Healthcare - Charlton Campus; Langs: Chinese; (905)648-4425; Fax. (905)648-4426.

TRINH, L Hang Bich; Dr H Trinh Med Office, 3-3033 Palstan Rd, Mississauga ON L4Y 4E7; Medical & Pharmaceutical University (Vietnam)'93; CCFP; Langs: Vietnamese; (905)270-4567

TRINH, Nathalie; Centre ORL Jean-Talon, 203-1384 rue Jean-Talon E, Montreal QC H2E 1S3; McG'95; FRCSC; Otol. Staff, CSSS du Coeur de l'Isle Hôpital Jean-Talon; Staff, CSSS de Dorval-Lachine-Lasalle; Langs: Vietnamese; French; (514)273-4461; Fax. (514)273-8401.

TRINH, Ngoc Chau; Clinique Med de l'Ile, 182 rue Montcalm, Gatineau QC J8Y 3B5; Saigon (Vietnam)'75; Ac Staff, Hull Hospital; Langs: Vietnamese; French; (819)777-3771; Fax. (819)777-1106; ngoc.trinh@sympatico.ca.

TRINH, Quoc-Dien; CHUM-Hopital Saint-Luc, 1058 rue Saint-Denis, Montreal QC H2X 3J4; Mon'05; FRCSC; Urol. Staff, Centre Hospitalier l'Université De Montréal (CHUM) - Hôpital Saint-luc; (514)890-8000

TRINH, Thao Trang; Unite de Med Familiale, 135 boul Claude-David, Repentigny QC J6A 1N6; Mon'97; CCFP; Médecin, CLSC-CHSLD Meilleur; (450)654-2911; Fax. (450)654-0359.

TRINH, Thomas Q N; Langley Mem Hosp, 22051 Fraser Hwy, Langley BC V3A 4H4; Sher'96; LMCC; CCFP; Ac Staff, Langley Memorial Hospital; Langs: Vietnamese; French; (604)587-5555

TRINH, Tony; Foothills Med Centre, 1403 29 St W, Calgary AB T2N 2T9; Cal'06; Staff, Foothills Medical Centre; (403)944-1110; Fax. (403)210-9205.

TRINH, Tram K; Chatham-Kent Health Alliance, PO Box 2030 Stn Main 80 Grand Ave W, Chatham ON N7L 1B5; Sher'02; FRCSC; GenSurg. Staff, Chatham-Kent Health Alliance; (519)355-1888; Fax. (519)355-0086.

TRINH, Trevor; Sports Med Centre, 2500 University Dr NW, Calgary AB T2N 1N4; Alb'09; CCFP; (403)220-8518; Fax. (403)282-6170.

TRINH TAN, Frederick; Ctr Hosp Fleury, 2180 rue Fleury E, Montreal QC H2B 1K3; Mon'10; CFP; FamilyMed. Staff, Centre Hospitalier Fleury; (514)384-2000

TRINKAUS, Martina A; St Michael's Hosp, 2 0842W-30 Bond St, Toronto ON M5B 1W8; Tor'04; FRCPC; IntMed; Hem. Staff, St Michael's Hospital; Lecturer, University of Toronto; (416)864-5632; Fax. (416)864-3055.

TRINKAUS, Mateya E; Markham Stouffville Health Ctr, 407-377 Church St, Markham ON L6B 1A1; Tor'04; FRCPC; IntMed; MedOncol. Staff, Markham Stouffville Health Centre; (905)472-7072; Fax. (905)472-0529.

TRINOS, Baieruss M; Toronto Rehab Inst-Univ Ctr, 550 University Ave, Toronto ON M5G 2A2; Medical University of the Americas (Other Foreign)'09; CCFP; Staff, Toronto Rehabilitation Institute - University Centre; (416)597-3422; Fax. (416)351-8120.

TRIOLET, William O; St Mary's Hospital Centre, 3830 Lacombe Ave, Montreal QC H3T 1M5; Tor'81; Anes (AIDS/HIV). Staff, St Mary's Hospital Centre; adj Prof, McGill University; (514)345-3511 x3344; Fax. (514)734-2683; w.o.triolet.inc@Gmail.com.

TRIPATHI, Davender K; Medical Arts Bldg, 208-581 Davis Dr, Newmarket ON L3Y 2P6; Patiala (India)'83; MB BS; FRCPC; IntMed; Gastroent. Consultant, Southlake Regional Health Centre; Langs: Hindi; Punjabi; (905)952-2210; Fax. (905)952-2218.

TRIPODI, Anthony L J; Royal View X-Ray, 103-1436 Royal York Rd, Etobicoke ON M9P 3A9; Tor'68; DMRD; FRCPC; DiagRad. Langs: Italian; (416)247-5486; Fax. (416)241-9138.

TRIPODI, Deanna; Whistler Health Care Centre, RR 4 4380 Lorimer Rd, Whistler BC V0N 1B4; Cal'04; CCFP; CCFP(E.M.); (604)932-3977; Fax. (604)932-0660.

TRIPP, Julie A; Family Med Centre, 611 Wonderland Rd N, London ON N6H 4V6; McM'05; CCFP; (519)471-6686; Fax. (519)471-2801.

TRISCOTT, Jean A C; Glenrose Rehab Hosp, 1259-10230 111 Ave NW, Edmonton AB T5G 0B7; Alb'81; BSc; BEd; FAAFP; CCFP; FCFP; Dir Div of Care of Elderly, University of Alberta Hospital; Staff, Glenrose Rehabilitation Hospital; Prof, University of Alberta; (780)735-8882; Fax. (780)735-8846; jeantriscott@capitalhealth.ca.

TRISTER, Neil L; 305-5858 ch Cote-des-Neiges, Montreal QC H3S 1Z1; McG'70; Clin Adj Family Pract, Sir Mortimer B Davis Jewish General; (514)735-1604; Fax. (514)735-1605.

TRITES, Jonathan R B; Dickson Bldg, 3045-5820 University Ave, Halifax NS B3H 1V7; Dal'94; FRCSC; Otol (Head & Neck Surgery). Att Staff, Queen Elizabeth II Health Sciences Centre - Victoria General Site; Asst Prof Surg, Dalhousie University; (902)473-3784; Fax. (902)473-3816; jonathan.trites@cdha.nshealth.ca.

TRITES, Kimberly L; Saint John Regional Hosp, PO Box 2100 Stn Main 400 University Ave, Saint John NB E2L 3L6; Dal'03; FRCSC; ObstGyn. Staff, Saint John Regional Hospital; Lecturer, Dalhousie University; Asst Prof, Memorial University Of Newfoundland; (902)895-4478; Fax. (506)648-6875.

TRIVEDI, Vijay K; Regina Qu'Appelle HR-Regina, 1440 14th Ave, Regina SK S4P 0W5; Bombay (India)'80; MB BS; DABN; CDD; FRCPC; NuclearMed (Nuclear Cardiology). Staff Nuclear Med, Regina General Hospital; Staff Nuclear Med, Pasqua Hospital; (306)766-4156; Fax. (306)766-4134.

TRIVIERI, Maria G; R Fraser Elliott Bldg, 3 805-190 Elizabeth St, Toronto ON M5G 2C4; Pisa (Italy)'97; FRCPC; IntMed. Staff, Toronto General Hospital - UHN; Langs: Italian; French; (416)978-2645

TRNKA, Peter; Children's & Women's HC of BC, K4 152-4480 Oak St, Vancouver BC V6H 3V4; Comenius (Slovakia)'90; Staff, BC Children's Hospital; (604)875-2272; Fax. (604)875-3649; ptrnka@cw.bc.ca.

TROCHIMCHUK, Teegan M; Thunder Bay Med Centre, 470-63 Algoma St N, Thunder Bay ON P7A 4Z6; Ott'07; CCFP; (807)344-8475

TROFIMUK, J Timothy; Griffiths Med Clinic, 28-5201 50 St, Leduc AB T9E 6T4; Alb'82; CCFP; Ac Staff, Leduc Community Hospital; (780)986-6200; Fax. (780)986-5200.

TROJAN, Daria A; MUHC-Montreal Neurology Inst, 3801 rue University, Montreal QC H3A 2B4; Farmington(CT) (USA)'84; MSc; FRCPC; PhysMed&Rehab (Neurologic Rehab). Staff, McGill University Health Centre - Montreal Neurological Hospital; Staff, Jewish Rehabilitation Hospital; assoc Prof Neurol, McGill University; Affil Prof Med, Universite de Montreal; Langs: Ukrainian; French; (514)398-8911; Fax. (514)398-2745.

TROJANOWSKI, Elizabeth M; Unionville Family Physicians, 201-10 Unionville Gate, Markham ON L3R 0W7; Wroclaw (Poland)'75; Staff, Lakeridge Health - Whitby Site; Langs: Polish; (905)305-7642; Fax. (905)305-7495.

TROJANOWSKI, Jan A; Vancouver Gen Hosp, 855 12 Ave W, Vancouver BC V5Z 1N1; Dal'05; FRCPC; EmergMed; Critical Care Medicine. Staff, Vancouver General Hospital - Centennial Pavillion; (604)581-2211

TROLLIP, Jean J; Canadian Forces Services Ctre, 101 Colonel By Drive, Ottawa ON K1A 0K2; Pretoria (South Africa)'00; CCFP; Physician, Canadian Forces Health Services Centre; Langs: Afrikaans; (613)838-8790

TROLLOPE, A Karen; McMaster Family Practice, A-690 Main St W, Hamilton ON L8S 1A4; Dal'82; CCFP; Staff, Hamilton Health Sciences Centre - McMaster University Medical Centre; Langs: Hindi; French; (905)521-5015; Fax. (905)521-5010; pkumar38@cogeco.ca.

TROMP, Margaret M; Picton Clinic, RR 2 5C-389 Main St, Picton ON K0K 2T0; Tor'85; CCFP; FCFP; (613)476-7870; Fax. (613)476-6482.

TRON, Victor A; Quenn's Univ-Richardson Lab, 88 Stuart St, Kingston ON K7L 3N6; Alb'82; FRCPC; AnatPath. Dept Head Pathol & Molecular Med, Queen's University; (613)533-2850

TROP, Isabelle; CHUM-Hotel-Dieu, 301-3840 rue Saint-Urbain, Montreal QC H2W 1T8; McG'94; FRCPC; DiagRad (Breasts). Staff, Centre Hospitalier l'Université de Montréal (CHUM) - Hôtel-Dieu; Langs: Spanish; English; (514)890-8059; Fax. (514)412-7237.

TROP, Sebastien; St Michael's Hosp, 30 Bond St, Toronto ON M5B 1W8; McG'02; FRCSC; CardSurg; Critical Care Medicine. Staff Cardiovasc & Thoracic Surg, St Michael's Hospital; Langs: Bilingual(French/English); (416)864-5303

TROPE, Graham E; Univ Hlth Network-Toronto Western Hosp, 6 411EW-399 Bathurst St, Toronto ON M5T 2S8; Witwatersrand (South Africa)'73; MB ChB; FRCS(Ed); PhD; FRCSC; Ophth (Glaucoma). Sr Scientist, Toronto Western Hospital - University Health Network; Prof Ophth, University of Toronto; (416)603-5800 x5317

TROPPER, J R Guy; Avant Garde Medical, 260-550 boul De Mortagne, Longueuil QC J4B 5E4; Sher'83; FACS; AB; FRCSC; Otol (Head & Neck Surgery). Staff, Allergy Medical Clinic; Langs: Bilingual(French/English); (450)641-0155; gtroppermd@cogeco.net.

TROPPER, Martin; Clinique Radiologie Granby, 66 rue Court, Granby QC J2G 4Y5; Laval'87; DiagRad. Staff, Centre Hospitalier de Granby; (450)378-0167

TROPPMANN, Leticia A; Univ of Ottawa Heart Institute, 40 Ruskin St, Ottawa ON K1Y 4W7; Ott'05; FRCPC; IntMed. Staff, University of Ottawa Heart Institute; (613)761-5000

TROQUET, Jean-Marc; MUHC-Montreal Gen Hosp, 1650 av Cedar, Montreal QC H3G 1A4; McG'95; EmergMed. Staff, McGill University Health Centre - Montreal General Campus; (514)934-1934

TROSSMAN, Bernard; Davisville Med & Dental Centre, 412-1849 Yonge St, Toronto ON M4S 1Y2; McG'57; FRCPC; Psy (Psychotherapy). (416)962-2980; Fax. (416)962-3123.

TROSTER, Myron; Stratford Gen Hosp, 46 General Hospital Dr, Stratford ON N5A 2Y6; Tor'65; AnatPath; GenPath. Staff, Stratford General Hospital - Huron Perth Healthcare Alliance; Langs: French; Yiddish; (519)272-8210 x2881; Fax. (519)272-8198; michael.troster@hpha.ca.

TROTT, Barbara E; Seymour Health Centre, 1530 7th Ave W, Vancouver BC V6J 1S3; California (USA)'91; Staff, Campbell River & District General Hospital; Langs: Spanish; (604)738-2151

TROTT, Jeffrey N; 9-2275 Westoak Trails Blvd, Oakville ON L6M 3W6; Cal'83; FRCPC; Neur. Ac Staff, Halton Healthcare Services Corporation - Georgetown Hospital; Instructor Med, University of Toronto; (905)338-8550

TROTTER, Judy E; PM & R, 257 King St W, Dundas ON L9H 1V8; McM'74; FRCPC; PhysMed&Rehab. Staff, Hamilton Health Sciences Centre - McMaster University Medical Centre; McMaster University; (905)628-3966; Fax. (905)628-3968; judytrotter@execulink.com.

TROTTER, Martin J; Calgary Lab Services, 9-3535 Research Rd NW, Calgary AB T2L 2K8; UBC'85; BSc; PhD; FRCPC; AnatPath (Dermatological Pathology). Head Derm Path, Calgary Laboratory Services; Assoc Prof, University of Calgary; (403)770-3202; Fax. (403)770-3741; martin.trotter@cls.ab.ca.

TROTTER, Theresa; Tom Baker Cancer Centre, 1331 29 St NW, Calgary AB T2N 4N2; UBC'85; BSc; FRCPC; RadOncol. Staff RadOncol, Tom Baker Cancer Centre; Staff, Foothills Medical Centre; Staff Teacher, University of Calgary; (403)521-3708; Fax. (403)283-1651; theresat@cancerboard.ab.ca.

TROTTERSHAW, Terralene L; 7105 West Saanich Rd, Brentwood Bay BC V8M 1P7; Man'87; Ad Staff Privil, Saanich Peninsula Hospital; (250)652-3637; Fax. (250)652-4898.

TROTTIER, Anne-Marie; Clinique Rockland MD, 100 ch Rockland, Mont-Royal QC H3P 2V9; Mon'98; Anes. Staff, Centre Hospitalier Pierre le Gardeur; (514)667-3383

TROTTIER, Antonio G; Neuro Rive-Sud, 250-4896 boul Taschereau, Greenfield Park QC J4V 2J2; Ott'71; Electroenceph (P.Q.); Neur (P.Q.). ac Staff, Hopital Charles LeMoyne; Langs: English; (450)672-1931; Fax. (450)672-3308; nrs@videotron.ca.

TROTTIER, Benoit; Clinique Med l'Actuel, 1130-1001 boul Maisonneuve E, Montreal QC H2L 4P9; Mon'85; Staff, Centre Hospitalier l'Université De Montréal (CHUM) - Hôpital Saint-luc; (514)524-1001; Fax. (514)524-3831.

TROTTIER, Cloe; CSSS du Sud de Lanaudière, 911 montee des Pionniers, Terrebonne QC J6V 2H2; Mon'04; CCFP; Staff, Centre Hospitalier Pierre le Gardeur; (450)654-7525

TROTTIER, Daniel C J; Montfort Hosp, 713 Montreal Rd, Ottawa ON K1K 0T2; Ott'03; FRCSC; GenSurg. Staff, The Ottawa Hospital - General Campus; Staff, Montfort Hospital; Langs: Bilingual(English/French); (613)746-4621; Fax. (613)748-4914.

TROTTIER, Daniel; 2385 boul Masson, Quebec QC G1P 1J3; Laval'88; (418)871-0970

TROTTIER, Francois; Clin Radiologie Saint-Pascal, 1900 av Mailloux, Quebec QC G1J 5B9; Laval'89; FRCPC; DiagRad. Staff, Centre Hospitalier de Matane; (418)667-6041

TROTTIER, Gregory T; Scarborough Prof Centre, 207-1371 Nelson Rd, Scarborough ON M1B 4Z8; Cal'04; FRCSC; Urol. (647)360-1155; Fax. (647)350-1055.

TROTTIER, Julie; 15-2020 boul Rene-Gaultier, Varennes QC J3X 1N9; Mon'89; Staff, Centre Hospitalier Pierre Boucher; (450)652-2222; Fax. (450)652-3970.

TROTTIER, Marc; 944 6e av, Grand-Mere QC G9T 2J1; Laval'84; (819)533-5783; Fax. (819)533-5759.

TROTTIER, Marielle; Clinique Med de la Marine, 101-303 Boul de la Marine, Varennes QC J3X 2G6; Mon'89; Langs: Bilingual(French/English); (450)652-9616; Fax. (450)652-4345.

TROTTIER, Mikael; Hopital Laval, 2725 ch Sainte-Foy, Quebec QC G1V 4G5; Sher'04; FRCPC; NuclearMed. Staff Institut Universitaire Cardiologie & Pneumologie de Quebec, Hôpital Laval; (418)656-8711

TROTTIER, Mylene; Inst Nat'l de Sante Publique, 190 boul Cremazie E, Montreal QC H2P 1E2; Mon'83; Langs: English; (514)864-1600 x3230; Fax. (514)864-1616; mylene.trottier@inspq.qc.ca.

TROTTIER, Patrice; Centre Med de la Montagne, 457 boul Laurier, Mont-Saint-Hilaire QC J3H 3P2; Mon'84; (450)464-1777; Fax. (450)464-1779; ptrottier@cmmontagne.com.

TROTTIER, Pierre; Clin d'Ophtalmologie Saguenay, 150 boul Barrette, Chicoutimi QC G7H 7W8; Sher'04; FRCSC; Ophth. Staff, CSSS de Lac-Saint Jean-Est; (418)545-2571; pierre.trottier@ssss.gouv.qc.ca.

TROTTIER, Richard; 191 Prom Saint-Louis SS 54, N-D-D-L'ILe-Perrot QC J7V 7P2; Mon'82; (514)365-3775; Fax. (514)365-3775.

TROTTIER, Sylvie; Hôpital Laval, 2725 ch Sainte-Foy, Quebec QC G1V 4G5; McG'82; MSc; FRCPC; MedMicrobiol (AIDS/HIV). Chef Med Biology, Hôpital Laval; Chef Microbiology InfectDis & Immunol, Université Laval; Langs: English; Bilingual(French/English); (418)656-8711 x5579; sylvie.trottier@crchul.ulaval.ca.

TROTTIER, Vincent; Ctr Hosp Affilie-Hop l'Enfant, 1401 18e rue, Quebec QC G1J 1Z4; Mon'99; FRCSC; GenSurg; Critical Care Medicine. Staff, Centre Hospitalier Affilié Universitaire de Québec - Hôpital De L'Enfant Jésus; (418)649-0252 x6317; Fax. (418)649-5579.

TROTTIER, Yolaine; Marketed Health Product, 200 Tunney's Pasture, Ottawa ON K1A 0K9; Laval'81; Staff, Hôpital de Gatineau; (613)954-4518

TROTTIER-HEBERT, Valerie; Inst of Mental Health Quebec, 2601 ch de la Canardiere, Quebec QC G1J 2G3; Sher'06; FRCPC; Psy. Staff, Institut Universitaire Sante; Staff, Centre Hospitalier Affilié Universitaire de Québec - Hôpital De L'Enfant Jésus; (418)663-5000

TROUGHTON, K Mark; Peterborough Reg HC-Hospital, 1 Hospital Dr, Peterborough ON K9J 7C6; Qns'87; CCFP; CCFP(E.M.); FCFP; Staff, Peterborough Regional Health Centre - Hospital Drive; (705)743-2121

TROUGHTON, Timothy; Family Practice Associates, PO Box 2010 223 16th Ave, Creston BC V0B 1G0; Belfast (Ireland)'92; MRCGPract; DCH; MB BCh; DRCOG; BCh; Pres, Creston Valley Medical Society; Clin Instructor, University of British Columbia; (250)428-9371; Fax. (250)428-9350.

TROUTON, Konia J; Vancouver Island Women's Clini, 104-284 Helmcken Rd, Victoria BC V9B 1T2; Qns'90; MPH; CCFP; FCFP; Langs: Bilingual(English/French); (250)480-7338; Fax. (250)480-7339.

TROW, Rory M; Medical Clinic, PO Box 730 Stn Main, Salmon Arm BC V1E 4N8; Cape Town (South Africa)'94; MB ChB; MMed(PainManagement); (250)832-6094; Fax. (250)832-5235.

TROYANOV, Stephan; Hop du Sacre-Coeur de Mtl, 5400 boul Gouin O, Montreal QC H4J 1C5; Mon'97; FRCPC; IntMed; Nephrol. Staff, Hôpital du Sacre-Coeur de Montréal; (514)338-2883

TROYANOV, Yves; Polyclinique de Montreal, 410-12245 rue Grenet, Montreal QC H4J 2J6; Laval'94; ABIM; FRCPC; IntMed; Rheum. Staff, Hôpital du Sacre-Coeur de Montréal; (514)334-9112; Fax. (514)334-2945.

TRPKOV, Kiril; Rockyview Gen Hosp, 7007 14 St SW, Calgary AB T2V 1P9; Skopje (Macedonia)'87; FRCPC; AnatPath (Surgical Pathology). Staff Path, Rockyview General Hospital; Asst Prof Path & Lab Med, University of Calgary; Langs: Macedonian; French; (403)943-3443; Fax. (403)943-3333; kiril.trpkov@cls.ab.ca.

TRUANT, Gregory S; 101-186 Albert St, London ON N6A 1M1; Wes'78; FRCPC; Psy (Adult Psychiatry). Assoc Prof Psy, University of Western Ontario; (519)645-7154; Fax. (519)645-7594.

TRUCHAN, Margaret B; 202-514 Queen St, Saskatoon SK S7K 0M5; Liege (Belgium)'83; FRCPC; IntMed (Rheumatology). Assoc Prof Med, Royal University Hospital; Langs: Polish; Italian; French; (306)242-4041; Fax. (306)664-9921.

TRUCHON, Josee; SMBD-Jewish Gen Hosp, 3755 ch Côte-Sainte-Catherine, Montreal QC H3T 1E2; Laval'97; ObstGyn (Echography Obstetrics & Gynecology). Staff, Sir Mortimer B Davis Jewish General; (514)340-8222

TRUCHON, Michel L; Bonfield Med Centre, PO Box 304 105 Landon St, Bonfield ON P0H 1E0; Ott'80; BSc; Langs: English; French; (705)776-3655; Fax. (705)776-1940.

TRUCHON, Rene; CHUQ-Ctr Hosp Univ Laval, 2206-2705 boul Laurier, Quebec QC G1V 4G2; Laval'78; FRCPC; Anes. ac Staff, Centre Hospitalier Universitaire de Quebec-CHUL; Université Laval; (418)656-4141; Fax. (418)654-2774.

TRUCHON, Sophie; CHUQ-Ctr Hosp Univ Laval, 2100-2705 boul Laurier, Quebec QC G1V 4G2; Laval'00; FRCPC; DiagRad. Staff, Centre Hospitalier Universitaire de Quebec-CHUL; (418)654-2258

TRUCHON, Valery; Clinique Medicale GMF-1851, 101-1851 rue Sherbrooke E, Montreal QC H2K 4L5; Mon'07; CCFP; (514)524-7564

TRUDEAU, Alain; Hotel-Dieu de Roberval, 450 rue Brassard, Roberval QC G8H 1B9; Sher'83; GenSurg. Staff, Hotel-Dieu de Roberval; (418)275-0110

TRUDEAU, Chantal D; Professional Arts Bldg, 402-100 Arden St, Moncton NB E1C 4B7; Dijon (France)'84; FRCPC; IntMed; Cardiol. Staff, The Moncton Hospital; Langs: French; (506)855-2588; Fax. (506)856-5194.

TRUDEAU, Dorothee; CLSC des Faubourgs, 1250 rue Sanguinet, Montreal QC H2X 3E7; Mon'71; (514)527-2361

TRUDEAU, Gisele; Agence de Sante Serv Sociaux, 2400 av d'Estimauville, Quebec QC G1E 7G9; Mon'81; Staff, Complexe hospitalier de la Sagamie; Médecin, Agence de la santé et des services sociaux de la Capitale-Nationale; (418)666-7000; Fax. (418)666-2776.

TRUDEAU, Jacqueline D; Vancouver Gen Hosp, 855 12th Ave W, Vancouver BC V5Z 1M9; UBC'08; Staff, Vancouver General Hospital - Centennial Pavillion; (604)875-4111

TRUDEAU, Jean-Bernard; College des Med Du Quebec, 2170 boul Rene-Levesque O, Montreal QC H3H 2T8; Sher'82; Douglas Mental Health University Institute; Staff, College des Medecins du Quebec; (514)933-4441 x5350; Fax. (514)933-5374.

TRUDEAU, Judith; Hotel-Dieu de Levis, 143 rue Wolfe, Levis QC G6V 3Z1; Laval'02; FRCPC; IntMed; Rheum. Staff, Hôtel-Dieu de Lévis; (418)835-7121

TRUDEAU, Luc; Clin Prevention Cardiovasculai, H 132-5790 ch Cote-des Neiges, Montreal QC H3S 1Y9; Mon'84; FRCPC; IntMed (P.Q.) (Hypertension). Staff Clinique de Prevention Cardiovasculaire, Sir Mortimer B Davis Jewish General; adj Prof Med, McGill University; Langs: English; (514)340-8222 x4030; Fax. (514)340-8732.

TRUDEAU, Marc; Medicine Hat Reg Hosp, 666 5 St SW, Medicine Hat AB T1A 4H6; Mon'82; CSPQ; MedOncol; IntMed. Staff The Margery E Yuill Cancer Centre, Medicine Hat Regional Hospital; Langs: English; French; (403)529-8817; Fax. (403)529-8007.

TRUDEAU, Marie-Helene; Clinique Externe de Psychiatri, 279 rue de la Providence, Granby QC J2G 4S7; Mon'95; FRCPC; Psy (Adult Psychiatry). Staff, Centre Hospitalier de Granby; (450)375-8001; Fax. (450)372-2235.

TRUDEAU, Maureen E; Sunnybrook Odette Cancer Ctr, T2 023-2075 Bayview Ave, Toronto ON M4N 3M5; Tor'81; ABIM; FRCPC; IntMed (Breast Cancer); MedOncol. Head Med Oncol & Hematol, Sunnybrook Health Sciences Centre; Head Systemic Therapy Prog, Sunnybrook Health Sciences Centre - Edmond Odette Cancer Centre; Prof, University of Toronto; (416)480-5145; Fax. (416)480-6002.

TRUDEAU, Michel; Clinique med Deux-Montagnes, 201 9e av, Deux-Montagnes QC J7R 3M1; Mon'77; (450)472-7520; mictrudeau@videotron.ca.

TRUDEAU, Nadine; Hotel-Dieu du Sacre-Coeur, 1 av du Sacre-Coeur, Quebec QC G1N 2W1; Mon'93; FRCPC; Psy. Psychiatre, Hotel-Dieu du Sacre-Coeur de Jesus de Quebec; (418)529-6851 x451; Fax. (819)691-0750.

TRUDEAU, Nicolas; CLSC de Saint-Jerome, 1000 rue Labelle, Saint-Jerome QC J7Z 5N6; Laval'05; (450)432-2777

TRUDEAU, Patrick; Clin de Chirurgie du Saguenay, 200-874 boul de l'Universite E, Chicoutimi QC G7H 6B9; Mon'93; FRCSC; GenSurg (Telehealth). ac Staff, Complexe hospitalier de la Sagamie; Langs: Bilingual(French/English).

TRUDEAU, Pierre; Clinique Med de sante R Cliche, 291 rte 108, Beauceville QC G5X 2Z4; Laval'79; (418)774-9878; Fax. (418)774-9891.

TRUDEAU, Pierre; CLSC des Mille-Iles, 4731 boul Levesque E, Laval QC H7C 1M9; Mon'83; Staff, CLSC des Milles-Iles; Langs: Bilingual(French/English); (450)661-2572; Fax. (450)661-5322.

TRUDEAU, Robert; 30 boul Kane CP 306 Succ Bureau-Chef, La Malbaie QC G5A 1T8; Mon'77; (418)665-4193

TRUDEAU, Sonia; Hop Louis-H Lafontaine, 4144-7401 rue Hochelaga, Montreal QC H1N 3M5; Laval'84; FRCPC; Psy. Staff, Hopital Louis-H Lafontaine; Langs: Bilingual(French/English); (514)251-4000; Fax. (514)251-4059; trudeau.sonia@videotron.ca.

TRUDEAU, Sylvie; CLSC Jardin du Quebec, 2 rue Ste-Famille CP 1110, Saint-Remi QC J0L 2L0; Sher'79; (450)454-4671; Fax. (450)454-4538.

TRUDEAU, Terrence R; Public Health Services, CP 5001 Stn Lcd 1 81 rue Albert, Moncton NB E1C 8R3; Ott'75; Psy. (506)856-2546; Fax. (506)869-6252.

TRUDEAU, Vincent; STM-Service de Sante, 8840-800 rue de la Gauchetiere, Montreal QC H5A 1J6; Mon'79; ac Staff, Hôpital du Sacre-Coeur de Montréal; (514)280-4783; Fax. (514)280-6150; vincent.trudeau@stm.info.

TRUDEAU-MARTEL, Adele; Centre Med Haut-Richelieu, 415-900 boul du Seminaire N, St-Jean-Sur-Richel QC J3A 1C3; Mon'66; FRCPC; Derm. (450)348-1778; Fax. (450)348-0982.

TRUDEL, Andre-Jean; Clinique Med Centrale, 2e-2050 rue Regent, Saint-Hubert QC J4T 3R5; Mon'88; (450)678-9194; Fax. (450)678-0915.

TRUDEL, Claude; Clinique Med Concorde, 303-300 boul de la Concorde E, Laval QC H7G 2E6; Mon'78; FRCSC; Urol. dép Chef, Hopital de la Cite de la santé; (450)667-5310; Fax. (450)667-2163.

TRUDEL, Claudine; Ctr Hosp du Centre la Mauricie, 50 119e rue, Shawinigan-Sud QC G9P 5K1; Laval'10; CCFP; Staff, Centre Hospitalier du Centre la Mauricie; (819)536-7500

TRUDEL, Eric; CSSS des-Deux-Montagnes, 520 boul Arthur-Sauve, Saint-Eustache QC J7R 5B1; Sher'02; FRCPC; Anes. Staff, Hôpital de Saint-Eustache; (450)473-6811; Fax. (450)473-6966.

TRUDEL, Francois; Polyclinique d'Argenteuil, 201-551 rue Berry, Lachute QC J8H 1S4; Mon'85; Staff, Centre Hospitalier Fleury; (450)562-3751; Fax. (450)562-1852.

TRUDEL, Guillaume; CLSC Kateri, 90 boul Marie-Victorin, Candiac QC J5R 1C1; Laval'85; (450)659-7661; Fax. (450)444-6276.

TRUDEL, Guy; The Rehabilitation Centre, 505 Smyth Rd, Ottawa ON K1H 8M2; Laval'88; MSc; FRCPC; PhysMed&Rehab. Staff, The Ottawa Hospital Rehabilitation Centre; Consultant, SCO Health Service - Élisabeth Bruyère Hospital; Consultant, The Ottawa Hospital - General Campus; Prof PhysMed&Rehab, University of Ottawa; Langs: Bilingual(French/English); (613)737-8899 x75591; Fax. (613)739-6864.

TRUDEL, Jacques; Clinique Med Memphre, 200-323 rue Sherbrooke, Magog QC J1X 2R9; Mon'76; Consultant, Centre Hospitalier Universitaire de Sherbrooke-Hopital Fleurimont; (819)847-1313; Fax. (819)847-3529.

TRUDEL, Jean-Francois; Inst U Geriatrie Sherbrooke, 375 rue Argyll, Sherbrooke QC J1J 3H5; Sher'78; MMedSci; FRCPC; Psy (Geriatric Psychiatry). Staff, Institut Universitaire de Geriatrie de Sherbrooke-Pavillon Argyll; adj Prof, Universite de Sherbrooke; Langs: English; (819)821-5103; Fax. (819)829-7137.

TRUDEL, Jean-René; 706-2197 Riverside Dr, Ottawa ON K1H 7X3; Mon'80; DABPN; CSPQ; FRCPC; Psy (Psycho Pharmacology). Langs: Bilingual(French/English); (613)800-5402; Fax. (613)523-1243.

TRUDEL, Jean-Sebastien; Hopital du Haut Richelieu, 920 boul du Seminaire N, St-Jean-sur-Richel QC J3A 1B7; Sher'99; FRCPC; DiagRad. Staff, Hôpital du Haut-Richelieu; Staff, Hopital Charles LeMoyne; (450)359-5000

TRUDEL, Jocelyn; GMF de Grand-Mere, 200-1050 8e rue, Grand-Mere QC G9T 4L4; Laval'83; (819)538-1099; Fax. (819)538-3686.

TRUDEL, Judith; CSSS de l'Energie, 50 119e rue, Shawinigan QC G9N 2N1; Sher'01; FRCPC; Peds. (819)536-7526; Fax. (819)536-7572; judith_trudel@ssss.gouv.qc.ca.

TRUDEL, Karen; City Square Paediatrics, 495-555 12th Ave W, Vancouver BC V5Z 3X7; McG'06; MDCM; FRCPC; Peds. (604)730-5622

TRUDEL, Louise; Centre Hosp Honore-Mercier, 2750 boul Laframboise, Saint-Hyacinthe QC J2S 4Y8; Mon'86; Staff, Centre Hospitalier Honore-Mercier; (450)771-3333

TRUDEL, Manon; Clinique Med Riviere du Moulin, 1388 boul du Saguenay E, Chicoutimi QC G7H 1G8; Sher'96; Langs: English; (418)549-3564; Fax. (418)549-8463.

TRUDEL, Melissa; Clinique Med Shawinigan-Sud, 200-2355 5e av, Shawinigan-Sud QC G9P 1P4; Sher'05; CCFP; (819)537-6205; melissa.trudel@gmf.gouv.qc.ca.

TRUDEL, Odile; Clinique Med l'Avenir, 200-1150 boul de l'Avenir, Laval QC H7N 6L2; Mon'81; (450)680-1150; Fax. (450)680-1151.

TRUDEL, Philippe J H; Grandview Med Ctr Fam Hlth Team, 167 Hespeler Rd, Cambridge ON N1R 3H7; Tor'74; BSc; Affil Staff, Cambridge Memorial Hospital; (519)623-4200; Fax. (519)623-2546.

TRUDEL, Robert; CSSS de Laval, 1755 boul Rene-Laennec, Laval QC H7M 3L9; Mon'83; FRCPC; DiagRad. Staff, Hopital de la Cite de la santé; (450)668-1010 x2551; Fax. (514)428-3864; roberttrudel@mac.com.

TRUDEL, Suzanne M; Univ Hlth Network-Princess M, DMOH5 110-610 University Ave, Toronto ON M5G 2M9; Tor'94; FRCPC; IntMed (Medical Oncology); Hem. Scientist, Princess Margaret Hospital - University Health Network; Langs: English; French; (416)946-4566; Fax. (416)946-2087; strudel@uhnres.utoronto.ca.

TRUDEL, Sylvain; CSSS du Rocher-Perce, CP 3300 451 rue Mgr Ross, Chandler QC G0C 1K0; Laval'97; CCFP; CCFP(E.M.); FCFP; Staff, Centre Hospitalier de Chandler; (418)689-2261; Fax. (418)689-5551.

TRUDEL-BRUN, Amelie; Ctr Hosp de Verdun, 4000 Boul Lasalle, Verdun QC H4G 2A3; Laval'01; Staff, Centre Hospitalier de Verdun; (514)362-1000 x2141; Fax. (514)765-7306.

TRUDELLE, Louis; Medi-Centre Chomedey, 610 boul Cure-Labelle, Laval QC H7V 2T7; Mon'82; Staff, Hopital de la Cite de la santé; (450)687-6452; Fax. (450)687-3243.

TRUEMAN, Gillian M; 26 Canadian Forces Health Serv, PO Box 5000 Stn Main 14 Wing Greenwood, Greenwood NS B0P 1N0; Tor'79; BSc; BEd; Physician, Canadian Forces Health Services Centre; (902)765-1494 x5046; Fax. (902)765-1278.

TRUFFER, Eric; CSSS de Trois-Rivières, 1991 boul du Carmel, Trois-Rivieres QC G8Z 3R9; Sher'95; FRCSC; Neursurg. Staff, CSSS de Trois-Rivières; (819)697-3333; Fax. (819)370-6681; etruffer@hotmail.com.

TRUFFY, Gilles; CLSC-CHSLD d'Autray, 30 rue St-Gabriel CP 870, St-Gabriel-D-Brand QC J0K 2N0; Mon'77; (450)835-4705; Fax. (450)835-7217.

TRUMAN, Tony L; 135 Dundas St E, Belleville ON K8N 1C3; Qns'77; CCFP; (613)966-9169; Fax. (613)966-0854.

TRUONG, Barney T H; Saigon Med & Dental Bldg, 202-1817 48 St SE, Calgary AB T2B 1L9; Alb'05; CCFP; Langs: Vietnamese; (403)235-5151; Fax. (403)235-5114; truongclinic86@yahoo.ca.

TRUONG, Catherine; Halton HCS Corp-Milton, 7030 Derry Rd, Milton ON L9T 7H6; UBC'03; CCFP; CCFP(E.M.); Staff, Halton Healthcare Services Corporation - Milton District Hospital; (905)878-2383

TRUONG, Cong Phuc; Ctr de Sante MRC Maskinonge, 450 2e rue, Louiseville QC J5V 1V3; Saigon (Vietnam)'74; Staff, CSSS de Maskinongé; Langs: Vietnamese; Chinese; French; (819)228-9486; Fax. (819)228-2973.

TRUONG, Dang-Toan; Queensway-Carleton Hosp, 3045 Baseline Rd, Nepean ON K2H 8P4; McG'88; FRCPC; DiagRad. Staff, Queensway Carleton Hospital; Langs: Vietnamese; French; (613)721-4700 x2701

TRUONG, Do Huu; Saigon Med & Dental Bldg, 202-1817 48 St SE, Calgary AB T2B 1L9; Saigon (Vietnam)'73; Staff, Peter Lougheed Centre; Langs: Vietnamese; (403)235-5151; Fax. (403)235-5114.

TRUONG, Francoise; Trillium Hlth Ctre-Mississauga, 100 Queensway W, Mississauga ON L5B 1B8; Mon'02; FRCPC; AnatPath. Staff, William Osler Health System - Brampton Civic Hospital; Staff, William Osler Health System - Etobicoke General Hospital; Langs: Bilingual(French/English); (905)848-7580

TRUONG, Hau Van; Rosedale Med Centre, 507-600 Sherbourne St, Toronto ON M4X 1W4; McM'02; FRCPC; Psy.

TRUONG, James; Callander Lakeside Med Clinic, PO Box 520 299 Main St N, Callander ON P0H 1H0; Qns'98; Staff, North Bay Regional Health Centre - Regional Mental Health; Langs: Bilingual(English/French); (705)752-1004

TRUONG, Kim L L; Saigon Med & Dental Bldg, 202-1817 48 St SE, Calgary AB T2B 1L9; Saigon (Vietnam)'75; Staff, Peter Lougheed Centre; Langs: Vietnamese; Cantonese; (403)272-9666; Fax. (403)235-5114.

TRUONG, Long P T; Canadian Field Hosp, PO Box 999 Stn Main, Petawawa ON K8H 2X3; Ott'10; CCFP; Staff, Base Hospital-CFB Petawawa; (613)687-5511

TRUONG, Minh-Dung; 5428 av Victoria, Montreal QC H3W 2P4; McG'90; Staff, Centre Hospitalier de LaSalle; (514)731-9899

TRUONG, Ngoc-Uyen T T; Hop Maisonneuve-Rosemont, 5415 boul de l'Assomption, Montreal QC H1T 2M4; Laval'93; FRCPC; IntMed; Endocrin&Metab. Staff, Hopital Maisonneuve-Rosemont; (514)252-3400

TRUONG, Patrick D C; Niagara H S-Greater Niagara Ge, 5546 Portage Rd, Niagara Falls ON L2E 6X2; Laval'97; FRCPC; Anes. Staff, Niagara Health System - Greater Niagara General Site; Langs: Bilingual(French/English); (905)358-0171

TRUONG, Pauline T; BC Cancer Agency-Vanc Isl Ctr, 2410 Lee Ave, Victoria BC V8R 6V5; McG'90; MDCM; FRCPC; RadOncol. Staff, BC Cancer Agency Vancouver Island Centre; Langs: Vietnamese; French; (250)519-5500; Fax. (250)519-2018.

TRUONG, Quyen; 5415 boul Grande-Allee, Brossard QC J4Z 3G9; Kiel (Germany)'80; (450)445-3600; Fax. (450)445-7140.

TRUONG, Theresa; Alexandra Comm Health Centre, 101-1318 Centre St NE, Calgary AB T2E 2R7; Cal'07; CCFP; (403)266-2622; Fax. (403)266-2692.

TRUONG, Thi Kim N; 2-12315 boul Rolland, Montreal-Nord QC H1G 6A6; Saigon (Vietnam)'75; (514)326-1919; Fax. (514)748-6323.

TRUONG, Thuy-Tien; Centre Med Boucherville, 201-600 boul du Fort-Saint-Lou, Boucherville QC J4B 1S7; McG'87; Derm. (450)665-7321; Fax. (450)665-6311.

TRUONG, Tinh Dinh; 498 Kingsway St, Vancouver BC V5T 3J9; Saigon (Vietnam)'79; Langs: Vietnamese; (604)876-9907; Fax. (604)876-9927.

TRUONG, Tony H; Alberta Children's Hosp, 2888 Shaganappi Trail NW, Calgary AB T3B 6A8; Cal'02; FRCPC; Peds (Pediatric Hematology Oncology). Staff, Alberta Children's Hospital; (403)955-7203; Fax. (403)955-2645.

TRUONG, Tuyet Lan; 208A-269 boul Saint-Jean, Pointe-Claire QC H9R 3J1; Laval'83; Langs: Vietnamese; English; (514)694-2524; Fax. (514)694-2820.

TRUONG, Vu Ngoc; Metrotown Med Centre, 306-6411 Nelson Ave, Burnaby BC V5H 4H3; UBC'00; FRCSC; Urol (Laparoscopy). Urology, Burnaby Hospital; Staff Urol, Royal Columbian Hospital; Staff Urol, Eagle Ridge Hospital & Health Care Centre; Clin Instructor Urologic Sciences, University of British Columbia; (604)433-2305; Fax. (604)433-2306.

TRUONG, Walter; The Hosp for Sick Children, S107-555 University Ave, Toronto ON M5G 1X8; Ohio State University (USA)'05; FRCSC; OrthSurg. Staff, The Hospital For Sick Children; (416)813-1500

TRUONG HONG, Bao Son; CLSC-CHSLD Saint-Laurent, 1055 av Sainte-Croix, Saint-Laurent QC H4L 3Z2; Sher'98; (514)748-6381; Fax. (514)748-6323.

TRUS, Michola R; Hamilton HS-Henderson Site, 203-711 Concession St, Hamilton ON L8V 1C3; Dal'90; FRCPC; IntMed; Hem. Staff Hematol, Hamilton Health Sciences Centre - Juravinski Cancer Centre; Hematology, Hamilton Health Sciences Centre-Juravinski Site; (905)527-4322 x42035; Fax. (905)575-2553.

TRUSCOTT, Bruce O; Albany Med Clinic, 807 Broadview Ave, Toronto ON M4K 2P8; Tor'69; Staff, Toronto East General Hospital Inc; (416)461-9471; Fax. (416)462-2027.

TRUSCOTT, David H R; 6919 Lamont Crt SW, Calgary AB T3E 6G6; Alb'55; FAAP; FRCPC; Peds. Staff, Rockyview General Hospital; Staff, Alberta Children's Hospital; Assoc Prof Peds, University of Calgary; rtruscot@telus.net.

TRUSDALE, Paisley W; Sault Area Hosp, 750 Great Northern Rd, Sault Ste. Marie ON P6B 0A8; Man'07; CCFP; CCFP(E.M.); Staff, Thunder Bay Regional Health Sciences Centre; Staff, Sault Area Hospital - Sault Ste Marie; (705)759-3434

TRUSDALE, Terry N W; St Joseph's Hosp, PO Box 3251 Stn P 35 Algoma St N, Thunder Bay ON P7B 5G7; Glasgow (Scotland)'73; MB ChB; DObstRCOG; CCFP; FCFP; Staff, St Joseph's Care Group - St Joseph's Hospital; Staff, Thunder Bay Regional Health Sciences Centre; Physician Student Health Services, Canadian Federation College; (807)343-2431

TRUTEAU, Michel; Clinique Domus Medica, 301-5601 rue Belanger, Montreal QC H1T 1G3; Mon'71; assoc Staff, Lakeshore General Hospital - Pointe Claire; ac Staff, Hôpital Santa Cabrini Ospedale; (514)256-5011; Fax. (514)259-7903.

TRUTER, Andre; 101-9717 Third St, Sidney BC V8L 3A3; Orange Free State (South Africa)'96; FRCSC; GenSurg. (250)656-8121

TRUTER, Rene; Moose Jaw Union Hosp, 455 Fairford St E, Moose Jaw SK S6H 1H3; Staff, Moose Jaw Union Hospital; (306)694-0200

TRUTSOV, Zdravko B; Vancouver Gen Hosp, 855 12 Ave W, Vancouver BC V5Z 1M9; I P Pavlov Higher Medical Institute (Other Foreign)'93; FRCPC; IntMed. Staff, Vancouver General Hospital - Centennial Pavillion; (604)875-4111

TRZCIENIECKA, Anna A; Delhi Commun Health Centre, 105 Main Street of Delhi, Delhi ON N4B 2L8; Wroclaw (Poland)'93; AAFPhys; DABFP; CCFP; Staff, Norfolk General Hospital; Langs: Polish; Russian; (519)582-2323; Fax. (519)582-3770; drtrzcina@hotmail.com.

TSAFNAT, Tamar; Mitchell Family Doctors, PO Box 790 7 Frances St, Mitchell ON N0K 1N0; McM'99; CCFP; (519)348-8402; Fax. (519)348-8400.

TSAI, Ellen; Canadian Med Protective Assoc, 875 Carling Ave, Ottawa ON K1S 5P1; Qns'91; MHSc; FRCPC; Peds (Pediatric Critical Care). Med Dir Ped Intensive Care Services, Kingston General Hospital; Staff, Canadian Medical Protective Association; Asst Prof, Queen's University; Langs: Mandarin; Chinese; French; (613)725-9965; tsaie@kgh.kari.net.

TSAI, Ellie L; Kingston Med Arts Centre, 206-800 Princess St, Kingston ON K7L 5E4; Wes'97; BSc; FRCPC; IntMed; ClinImmunol&Allergy. (613)546-6673; Fax. (613)544-3288.

TSAI, Eve C; The Ottawa Hosp-Civic Campus, C2-1053 Carling Ave, Ottawa ON K1Y 4E9; Tor'95; PhD; FRCSC; Neursurg (Spine). Assoc Scientist, The Ottawa Hospital - Civic Campus; Asst Prof, University of Ottawa; (613)761-5383 x3; Fax. (613)761-4967; etsai@ohri.ca.

TSAI, Gina Y; St Josephs Hosp Allergy Clinic, B3 110-268 Grosvenor St, London ON N6A 4V2; UBC'08; IntMed. Staff, London Health Sciences Centre - South Street; Staff, St Joseph's Hospital - St Joseph's Health Care; Staff, St Josephs Hospital Allergy Clinic; (519)685-8167; Fax. (519)685-8274.

TSAI, Hua-Lin; 2015 Centre St NW, Calgary AB T2E 2S9; Tor'81; FRCPC; Anes. Staff, Rockyview General Hospital; (403)247-8777

TSAI, Jason Y S; 202-3555 Don Mills Rd, North York ON M2H 3N3; National (Taiwan)'76; Court Staff, North York General Hospital; Court Staff, The Scarborough Hospital - Birchmount Campus; Langs: Fukinese; Mandarin; Taiwanese; (416)493-9511; Fax. (416)493-1797.

TSAI, Olivia C; Rouge Valley HS-Centenary, 2867 Ellesmere Rd, Scarborough ON M1E 4B9; Tor'98; FRCPC; Anes. Staff, Rouge Valley Health System - Centenary Health Centre Site; (416)284-8131

TSAI, Scott S W; Hamilton HS-Henderson Campus, 711 Concession St, Hamilton ON L8V 1C3; Tor'96; FRCPC; DiagRad. Staff, Hamilton Health Sciences Centre-Juravinski Site; (905)527-4322

TSAI, Shian-Yih; Wilson Med Centre, 130 Wilson St, Hamilton ON L8R 1E2; National (Taiwan)'57; AB; FRCSC; Urol (Dialysis). Ac Staff, St Joseph's Healthcare - Charlton Campus; Asst Prof Surg, McMaster University; Langs: Chinese; Japanese; (905)526-6250; Fax. (905)526-9754.

TSAI, Vance C; Gateway Hlth & Wellness Ctre, 208-2051 McCallum Rd, Abbotsford BC V2S 3N5; Tor'01; BSc; MSc; FRCSC; Otol (Head & Neck Surgery). Clin Instructor Surg, University of British Columbia; Langs: Mandarin; (604)864-0747; Fax. (604)864-0706.

TSAI, Willis H; Rockyview Gen Hosp, 7007 14 St SW, Calgary AB T2V 1P9; Tor'91; AB; FRCPC; IntMed; Respir. Staff, Rockyview General Hospital; Staff, Foothills Medical Centre; University of Calgary; Langs: English; French; (403)943-3283; Fax. (403)252-6471.

TSAKALAKI, Anna; Clinique Med Santé-Equilibre, 77 rue Vanier, Gatineau QC J9H 1X4; Laval'88; CCFP; FCFP; Langs: Greek; English; (819)684-7171; Fax. (819)685-0406.

TSAKIRIDIS, Theodoros; Juravinski Cancer Centre, 699 Concession St, Hamilton ON L8V 5C2; Tor'01; PhD; FRCPC; RadOncol (Lung Cancer). Staff, Niagara Health System - Ontario Street Site; Physician, Hamilton Health Sciences Centre - Juravinski Cancer Centre; Teach Staff, McMaster University; Langs: Greek; (905)387-9711 x64704; Fax. (905)575-6326.

TSAMPALIEROS, Anne K; Chidlren's Hosp Eastern Ont, 401 Smyth Rd, Ottawa ON K1H 8L1; Ott'06; FRCPC; Peds; Nephrol. Staff, Children's Hospital of Eastern Ontario (CHEO); (613)737-7600

TSANACLIS, Alexandre; CHUS-Hop Fleurimont, 3001 12e av N, Sherbrooke QC J1H 5N4; Sao Paolo (Brazil)'71; Staff, Centre Hospitalier Universitaire de Sherbrooke-Hopital Fleurimont; (819)346-1110 x15960; Fax. (819)564-5377.

TSANACLIS, Ana-Maria C; CHUS-Hop Fleurimont, 3001 12e av N, Sherbrooke QC J1H 5N4; Sao Paolo (Brazil)'71; Staff, Centre Hospitalier Universitaire de Sherbrooke-Hopital Fleurimont; assoc Prof, Universite de Sherbrooke; Langs: Portuguese; English; Spanish; (819)346-1110 x15939; Fax. (819)820-6473.

TSANDELIS, Nickoli; Belgage Med Arts Centre, 208-525 Belmont Ave W, Kitchener ON N2M 5E2; Wes'78; FRCSC; ObstGyn. Staff, Grand River Hospital - Kitchener/Waterloo Health Centre; Langs: Greek; (519)742-1090; Fax. (519)741-8929.

TSANG, Albert H; St Michal's Hosp Academic-FHT, 938-790 Bay St, Toronto ON M5G 1N8; Tor'95; CCFP; Langs: Chinese; (416)928-2220; Fax. (416)928-2219.

TSANG, Allan Y; 2270-3700 No. 3 Rd, Richmond BC V6X 3X2; UBC'95; (604)273-0990; Fax. (604)273-0716.

TSANG, Andy H K; 6-52 Holland St E PO Box 1209 Stn Main, Bradford ON L3Z 2B6; Tor'88; Assoc Staff, Southlake Regional Health Centre; (905)775-0081; Fax. (905)775-9290.

TSANG, Ann S Y; 218-4002 Sheppard Ave E, Scarborough ON M1S 4R5; Sydney (Australia)'82; CCFP; Staff, The Scarborough Hospital - General Campus; Staff, North York General Hospital; Langs: Chinese; (416)497-9999; Fax. (416)497-1990.

TSANG, Bernice; Southlake Reg Health Centre, 596 Davis Dr, Newmarket ON L3Y 2P9; UBC'99; FRCPC; IntMed; Cardiol. Staff, Southlake Regional Health Centre; Langs: Cantonese; (905)895-4521 x2946; Fax. (905)952-2823.

TSANG, Bonnie; University of Alberta Hosp, 8440 112 St NW, Edmonton AB T6G 2B7; Wes'08; Staff, University of Alberta Hospital; (780)407-8822

TSANG, David T S; Parker Place Med Clinic, 1550-4380 No 3 Rd, Richmond BC V6X 3V7; (Hong Kong)'57; DPH; MB BS; FRCPC; Derm. (604)273-9899; Fax. (604)273-9977.

TSANG, Henry H K; University Hosp of Northern BC, 1475 Edmonton St, Prince George BC V2M 1S2; UBC'83; FRCSC; ObstGyn (Maternal Fetal Medicine). Staff, University Hospital of Northern British Columbia; Langs: Chinese; (250)960-2288; Fax. (250)562-8838.

TSANG, Ian K; 1417-750 Broadway W, Vancouver BC V5Z 1J4; (Taiwan)'63; MB; FRCPC; IntMed; Rheum. Clin Prof Emeritus, Vancouver General Hospital - Centennial Pavillion; Emeritus Prof, University of British Columbia; Langs: Cantonese; Mandarin; (604)708-8225; Fax. (604)708-8291.

TSANG, Janius; CSSS Coeur de Hop Jean-Talon, 1385 rue Jean-Talon E, Montreal QC H2E 1S6; Cal'04; FRCPC; Anes. Staff, St Mary's Hospital Centre; Staff, CSSS du Coeur de l'Isle Hôpital Jean-Talon; (514)495-6767 x6365

TSANG, Jennifer L; Sunnybrook Hlth Sciences Ctre, D108-2075 Bayview Ave, Toronto ON M4N 3M5; Ott'03; FRCPC; IntMed; Critical Care Medicine. Staff, Sunnybrook Health Sciences Centre - Edmond Odette Cancer Centre; Staff, Toronto General Hospital - UHN; Staff, The Scarborough Hospital - General Campus; Langs: Cantonese; (416)480-6100

TSANG, Jim H C; Jim H C Tsang Med Prof Corp, 417-1420 Burnhamthorpe Rd E, Mississauga ON L4X 2Z9; Tor'92; Langs: Chinese; (905)206-1883; Fax. (905)206-9634.

TSANG, John C; Regina Qu'Appelle HR-Regina, 1440 14th Ave, Regina SK S4P 0W5; McG'92; FRCSC; CardSurg. Staff CVT Associates, Regina General Hospital; (306)766-6900; Fax. (306)766-6920.

TSANG, John Y C; Vancouver Gen Hosp, 855 12th Ave W, Vancouver BC V5Z 1M9; Tor'74; ABIM; DABA; FACP; FAMCCP; FRCPC; Anes (Critical Care Medicine). Staff, Vancouver General Hospital - Centennial Pavillion; Staff, Providence Health Care - St Paul's Hospital; Staff, James Hogg Capture Research Centre for Cardiovascular & Pulmonary Diseases; Langs: Cantonese; (604)875-5949; jtsang@interchange.ubc.ca.

TSANG, Joseph W T; 138-3150 3150 54 Ave E, Vancouver BC V5S 1Z1; McG'68; Vis Staff, Vancouver General Hospital - Centennial Pavillion; Langs: Chinese; (604)875-5949

TSANG, Kam-Yuen; 167A Woodbridge Ave, Woodbridge ON L4L 2S6; Tor'75; Langs: Chinese; (905)851-1121; Fax. (905)851-1937.

TSANG, Katherine; University Hosp of Northern BC, 1475 Edmonton St, Prince George BC V2M 1S2; Cal'88; BSc(Hons.); FRCPC; AnatPath (Surgical Pathology). Staff, University Hospital of Northern British Columbia; (250)565-2421; Fax. (250)565-2664.

TSANG, Mae T; St Boniface Gen Hosp, 409 Tache Ave, Winnipeg MB R2H 2A6; Man'03; FRCPC; Anes. Staff, St Boniface General Hospital; (204)233-8563

TSANG, Michael B; Hamilton HS-General Site, 237 Barton St E, Hamilton ON L8L 2X2; UBC'07; FRCPC; IntMed. Staff, Hamilton Health Sciences Centre - Hamilton General Hospital; Langs: Cantonese; (905)527-4322

TSANG, Michael S M; Jubilee Square, 33-280 West Beaver Creek Rd, Richmond Hill ON L4B 3Z1; (Hong Kong)'71; CCFP; FCFP; Langs: Cantonese; Mandarin; (905)762-1111; Fax. (905)762-1112.

TSANG, Monica C W; Collingwood Med Clinic, 138-3150 54th Ave E, Vancouver BC V5S 1Z1; Alb'06; CCFP; Langs: Chinese; (604)437-1888

TSANG, Nicole; South Vancouver Mental Health, 220-1200 73rd Ave W, Vancouver BC V6P 6G5; Wes'06; FRCPC; Psy. Staff, South Vancouver Mental Health Team; Staff, Early Psychosis Intervention; (604)266-6124; ntsang@telus.net.

TSANG, Peter W K; Gordon & Leslie Diamond HCC, 10F-2775 Laurel St, Vancouver BC V5Z 1M9; Wes'86; FRCPC; IntMed (Cardiology); Hem. Staff, Vancouver General Hospital - Centennial Pavillion; Staff, BC Women's Hospital & Health Centre; Staff Cardiol, Gordon & Leslie Diamond Health Care Centre; Med Consultant, Canadian Blood Services; Clin Instructor, University of British Columbia; Langs: Cantonese; (604)875-4952; Fax. (604)875-4763.

TSANG, Philip; Civic Family Med Centre, 210 Melrose Ave, Ottawa ON K1Y 4K7; Tor'10; CCFP; (613)761-4334

TSANG, Raymond W M; Sheppard Med Bldg, 201-701 Sheppard Ave E, North York ON M2K 2Z3; Tor'99; Langs: Cantonese; (416)913-6130; Fax. (647)435-6730; raymond.tsang@utoronto.ca.

TSANG, Richard W C; Univ Hlth Network-Princess M, 610 University Ave, Toronto ON M5G 2M9; Ott'81; FRCPC; IntMed; RadOncol. Staff, Princess Margaret Hospital - University Health Network; Prof, University of Toronto; (416)946-2123; Fax. (416)946-4586.

TSANG, Roger; Tom Baker Cancer Centre, 1331 29 St NW, Calgary AB T2N 4N2; Alb'04; FRCPC; IntMed; MedOncol. Staff, Tom Baker Cancer Centre; Staff, University of Alberta Hospital; Staff, Cross Cancer Institute; (403)521-3688; Fax. (403)283-1651.

TSANG, Teresa S M; Gordon & Leslie Diamond HCC, 9F-2775 Laurel St, Vancouver BC V5Z 1M9; Alb'89; FRCPC; IntMed (Adult Cardiology); Cardiol. Staff, Vancouver General Hospital - Centennial Pavillion; Langs: Cantonese; (604)875-5067

TSANG, Victor T L; Oakmont Med Centre, 250-809 41st Ave W, Vancouver BC V5Z 2N6; Tor'95; FRCSC; GenSurg. Staff, Providence Health Care - Mount Saint Joseph Hospital; Staff, Providence Health Care - St Vincent's Hospital-Heather Site; Langs: Cantonese; French; (604)261-5434; Fax. (604)261-2064.

TSANG, W Y Eliza; Cachet Family Physicians, 2-9255 Woodbine Ave, Markham ON L6C 1Y9; Mon'00; CCFP; Langs: Mandarin; Cantonese; French; (905)887-2222; Fax. (905)887-3655.

TSANG, Wendy W C; 31 Centre St S, Brampton ON L6W 2X7; Qns'03; FRCPC; IntMed; Cardiol.

TSANG CHENG, Joyce S S; Student Health Services, M334-2211 Wesbrook Mall, Vancouver BC V6T 2B5; Alb'95; CCFP; (604)822-7011

TSAO, Jonathan R; The Credit Valley Hosp, 2200 Eglinton Ave W, Mississauga ON L5M 2N1; Tor'85; FRCPC; RadOncol. Consultant Staff, Trillium Health Centre - West Toronto; Staff, The Credit Valley Hospital; Consultant Staff, William Osler Health System - Brampton Civic Hospital; Langs: French; (905)813-1100 x5000; Fax. (905)813-3962; jtsao@cvh.on.ca.

TSAO, May N; Toronto Sunnybrook Reg Cancer, 2075 Bayview Ave, Toronto ON M4N 3M5; Tor'93; FRCPC; RadOncol. Staff, Sunnybrook Health Sciences Centre; (416)480-4806; Fax. (416)480-6002; may.tsao@sw.ca.

TSAO, Ming-Sound; Univ Hlth Network-Toronto Gen, 11EA24-200 Elizabeth St, Toronto ON M5G 2C4; UBC'76; FRCPC; AnatPath. Sr Scientist, Princess Margaret Hospital - University Health Network; Staff, Toronto General Hospital - UHN; Prof Path, University of Toronto; Langs: Chinese; Indonesian; (416)340-4737; Fax. (416)340-5517.

TSAO, Smiley G S; 102-10 Unionville Gate, Unionville ON L3R 0W7; Tor'88; CCFP; FCFP; Med Staff, The Scarborough Hospital - Birchmount Campus; Med Examiner, Clarica; Langs: Mandarin; Cantonese; Taiwanese; Fookien; Shanghai; (905)305-8687; Fax. (905)305-8685; dr_s_tsao@yahoo.ca.

TSAPARAS, Panagiotis F; 222-601 Sixth St, New Westminster BC V3L 3C1; Cal'00; FRCSC; Otol (Head & Neck Surgery). (604)521-5301; Fax. (604)521-5311; yotistsaparas@yahoo.com.

TSATOUMAS, Maria; MUHC-Montreal Gen Hosp, 1650 av Cedar, Montreal QC H3G 1A4; McG'98; FRCPC; DiagRad. Staff, McGill University Health Centre - Montreal General Campus; (514)934-1934 x43851

TSATSARONIS, Eleftheria; 208-2238 Dundas St W, Toronto ON M6R 3A9; Cologne (Germany)'68; Court Staff, Toronto Western Hospital - University Health Network; Langs: Greek; (416)533-3314; Fax. (416)533-5853.

TSCHEN, H H Steve; 1291 Ouellette Ave, Windsor ON N8X 1J3; Zurich (Switzerland)'73; Langs: Chinese; German; Japanese; (519)258-3429; Fax. (519)258-7252.

TSCHIRHART, Jeffrey D; 7-140 Queensway Dr E, Simcoe ON N3Y 4Y7; Wes'90; Ac Staff, Norfolk General Hospital; (519)426-0011; Fax. (519)426-1671.

TSE, Anna; Agincourt Med Centre, 2020 Brimley Rd, Scarborough ON M1S 4R7; McM'09; CCFP; (416)293-2404; Fax. (416)321-1359.

TSE, Anthony C H; 705-5799 Yonge St, North York ON M2M 3V3; Canton (China)'56; Langs: Cantonese; Mandarin; (416)221-8612; Fax. (416)221-8784.

TSE, Brian L; Medical Assoc of Port Perry, 462 Paxton St, Port Perry ON L9L 1L9; Wes'09; CCFP; (905)985-2895; Fax. (905)985-5403.

TSE, Chingying; Burnhamthorpe Mall, 202-666 Burnhamthorpe Rd, Etobicoke ON M9C 2Z4; Tor'80; Langs: Chinese; (416)622-9220

TSE, Chun Wing; CLSC Notre Dame-de-Grace, 2525 boul Cavendish, Montreal QC H4B 2Y4; McG'09; CCFP; Staff, CLSC Notre Dame-de-Grace; (514)484-7878

TSE, Edward T W; Cornwall Prof Bldg, 400-2125 11th Ave, Regina SK S4P 3X3; McG'76; FRCSC; Urol. (306)757-0658; Fax. (306)757-6440.

TSE, Frances W M; McMaster University, 1280 Main St W, Hamilton ON L8S 4K1; Cal'98; FRCPC; IntMed; Gastroent. Staff, Hamilton Health Sciences Centre - McMaster Children's Hospital; Teach Staff, McMaster University; Langs: Cantonese; Mandarin; (905)521-2100

TSE, Geoffrey N W; Surrey Mem Hosp, 13750 96 Ave, Surrey BC V3V 1Z2; (Hong Kong)'64; MB BS; FRCS(Ed); DABS; FRCSC; GenSurg (Colon & Rectal Surgery). Att Staff Surg, Surrey Memorial Hospital; Langs: Cantonese; Mandarin; Chinese; (604)763-5412; Fax. (604)588-3320; gntse18@yahoo.com.

TSE, Helen S; Market Mall Prof Bldg, 301-4935 40 Ave NW, Calgary AB T3A 2N1; Cal'81; CCFP; FCFP; (403)286-4924; Fax. (403)247-2644.

TSE, Janet L; PO Box 86093 Rpo Marda Loop, Calgary AB T2T 6B7; Alb'08; CCFP.

TSE, Jennifer E; 10818 Jasper Ave PO Box 35086 Rpo Midtown, Edmonton AB T5J 0B7; Alb'05; CCFP; Staff, Calgary Foothills Primary Care Network; Locum Tenens, Alberta Medical Association; Locum Tenens, Calgary Health Region.

TSE, Jennifer E; 852 119 St SW, Edmonton AB T6W 0J1; Alb'01; BSc; CCFP; (780)988-2615; Fax. (780)988-2609.

TSE, Joanne S; Westbrook Prof Bldg, 205-1610 37 St SW, Calgary AB T3C 3P1; Cal'87; BSc; Langs: Chinese; (403)242-7788; Fax. (403)242-3279.

TSE, Kenneth K Y; St Joseph's Healthcare, 50 Charlton Ave E, Hamilton ON L8N 4A6; Monash (Australia)'67; MB BS; FRCPC; Anes. Ac Staff, St Joseph's Healthcare - Charlton Campus; Clin Assoc Prof, McMaster University; Langs: Cantonese; (905)522-4941 x3853

TSE, Leonard W H; Univ Hlth Network-Toronto Gen, EN6 220-200 Elizabeth St, Toronto ON M5G 2C4; Tor'97; MASc; FRCSC; GenSurg (Vascular & Endovascular Surgery); VascSurg. Staff, Toronto General Hospital - UHN; Asst Prof, University of Toronto; Langs: French; Chinese; (416)340-4805; Fax. (416)340-5029.

TSE, Luke B S; 501 McBride St, Prince Rupert BC V8J 3G5; (Hong Kong)'80; MB BS; CCFP; Langs: Cantonese; Hakka; Mandarin; (250)622-6340; Fax. (250)624-3526.

TSE, Man Buen; Medical Dental Centre, 303-2780 Jane St, North York ON M3N 2J2; Tor'76; FRCSC; ObstGyn. Ac Staff, Humber River Regional Hospital - Church Street Site; Ac Staff, Humber River Regional Hospital - Finch Avenue Site; Langs: Chinese; (416)748-3030; Fax. (416)748-3031.

TSE, Olivia Q; 4484 rue Sherbrooke O, Westmount QC H3Z 1E6; McG'86; Peds. adj Prof Peds, McGill University; (514)933-4490

TSE, Sandra T; Children's Hosp Eastern Ont, 401 Smyth Rd, Ottawa ON K1H 8L1; Alb'90; FRCPC; Peds. Staff, Children's Hospital of Eastern Ontario (CHEO); (613)737-2318; Fax. (613)738-4852.

TSE, Shirley M L; The Hosp for Sick Children, 8253-555 University Ave, Toronto ON M5G 1X8; Tor'95; FRCPC; Peds (Pediatric Rheumatology); Rheum. Prog Dir/Assoc Prof, The Hospital For Sick Children; Langs: Cantonese; (416)813-6117; Fax. (416)813-4989.

TSE, Wai Ching; St James Street Med Clinic, 1600 Portage Ave, Winnipeg MB R3J 0C6; Man'94; CCFP; FCFP; Med Officer of Hlth, National Microbiology Laboratories; Staff, Health Canada; (204)783-0349

TSE, Wing Kin; 210-4235 Sheppard AVe E, Scarborough ON M1S 1T7; Wes'74; Ac Staff, The Scarborough Hospital - General Campus; Court Staff, Toronto East General Hospital Inc; Court Staff, The Scarborough Hospital - Birchmount Campus; Langs: Chinese; (416)298-9715; Fax. (416)298-9715.

TSE, Yvonne Y W; Univ Hlth Network-Toronto Gen, 200 Elizabeth St, Toronto ON M5G 2C4; McM'08; FRCPC; IntMed. Staff Gastroent, Toronto General Hospital - UHN; (416)340-4800

TSE-CHANG, Alena W; 2430 Rabbit Hill Rd NW PO Box 88033 Rpo Rabbit Hill, Edmonton AB T6R 0M5; Alb'05; FRCPC; Peds; InfectDis. Staff, University of Alberta Hospital; Teach Staff, University of Alberta; (780)994-3373; Fax. (780)758-3373.

TSE HING YUEN, Stephanie; London HSC-University Hosp, PO Box 5339 Stn B 339 Windermere Rd, London ON N6A 5A5; RCS (Ireland)'10; CCFP; Staff, London Health Sciences Centre - University Hospital; (519)685-8300

TSEGA, Edemariam; Hamilton HS-McMaster Site, 3X-1200 Main St W, Hamilton ON L8N 3Z5; McG'65; MDCM; DCMT(Lond); PhD; FRCPC; IntMed (Gastroenterology). Acad Staff, Hamilton Health Sciences Centre-Juravinski Site; Staff, Hamilton Health Sciences Centre - McMaster University Medical Centre; Langs: Amharic; (905)521-2100; Fax. (905)521-2629.

TSEKREKOS, Stephen N; Canadian Forces Supp Unit HCC, 1745 Alta Vista Dr, Ottawa ON K1A 0K6; Cal'99; FRCPC; OccupMed. Staff Directorate of Force Health Protection, Canadian Forces Health Services Centre; (613)945-6782; Fax. (613)945-6823.

TSENG, George W; Broadway Station Med Clinic, 2516 Commercial Dr, Vancouver BC V5N 4C2; UBC'98; CCFP; CCFP(E.M.); FCFP; Staff, Aberdeen Health Centre; Langs: Mandarin; (604)872-5377

TSENG, Jui-Teng; 1504-10160 115 St NW, Edmonton AB T5K 1T6; (Taiwan)'63.

TSENG, Leo; Lakeridge Hlth Corp-Oshawa, 1 Hospital Crt, Oshawa ON L1G 2B9; Qns'06; FRCPC; PhysMed&Rehab. Staff, Lakeridge Health - Oshawa Site; (905)576-8711; Fax. (905)721-4735.

TSENG, Michael; Addiction & Mental Hlth-Clarke, 11F-250 College St, Toronto ON M5T 1R8; Cal'02; FRCPC; Psy. Staff, Centre for Addiction & Mental Health (CAMH) - College Street Site; (416)535-8501

TSENG, Nora C; 3-7398 Edmonds St, Burnaby BC V3N 1A8; Qns'82; (604)524-8541; Fax. (604)524-8526.

TSHABALALA, Augustine K; Leader Med Clinic, PO Box 638, Leader SK S0N 1H0; Physician, Leader Medical Clinic; (306)628-4584; Fax. (306)628-3998.

TSHATSHELA, Mzikayise; Riveside Health Complex, PO Box 628, Turtleford SK S0M 2Y0; Staff, Riverside Health Complex; (306)845-2277; Fax. (306)845-4434.

TSHIBUMBU, Josiane M; CHSLD Foyer du Bonheur, 125 rue Lionel Emond, Gatineau QC J8Y 5S8; Lubumbashi (Other Foreign)'96; CCFP; (819)966-6410 x215

TSHIYOMBO, Tshala; Confederation Family Med Clini, 8B-300 Confederation Dr, Saskatoon SK S7L 4T6; (Ivory Coast)'85; Staff, Bengough Health Centre; Physician, Confederation Family Medical Clinic; (306)956-7775; Fax. (306)956-7779.

TSIAPRAILIS, Alexandros; Erin Mills Med Centre, E229A-5100 Erin Mills Pky, Mississauga ON L5M 4Z5; Tor'99; BSc(Hon.); MSc(Neurosciences); FRCPC; Neur. Ac Staff, The Credit Valley Hospital; (905)607-2600; Fax. (905)607-9292.

TSIEN, Cynthia; Univ Hlth Network-Toronto Gen, 10EN 224-200 Elizabeth St, Toronto ON M5G 2C4; McG'04; Gastroent; IntMed. Staff, Toronto General Hospital - UHN; (416)340-3111

TSIHLIAS, John; Etobicoke Urology Associates, 207-100 Humber College Blvd, Etobicoke ON M9V 5G4; Tor'91; MSc; FRCSC; Urol (Urological Oncology). Staff, William Osler Health System - Etobicoke General Hospital; Langs: Greek; (416)746-4805; Fax. (416)742-2139; j.tsihlias@utoronto.ca.

TSIKATA, Setorme A; Parkland Med Associates, 205-505 Queen St, Spruce Grove AB T7X 2V2; (Ghana)'98; BSc; MSc; MB ChB; CCFP; Staff, Covenant Health - Misericordia Community Hospital; Langs: Twi; Ga; Fanti; Ewe; (780)962-2001; Fax. (780)962-8176.

TSIMIKLIS, Catherine; Hop Sacre-Coeur de Montreal, 5400 boul Gouin O, Montreal QC H4J 1C5; Mon'03; FRCPC; MedMicrobiol. Staff, Hôpital du Sacre-Coeur de Montréal; Dir Gender Equity Issues, University of Ottawa; (514)338-2222 x7275

TSIMIKLIS, Georgios; Merivale Cardiovascular Cons, 201-1370 Clyde Ave, Ottawa ON K2H 3H8; McG'04; FRCPC; IntMed; Cardiol. Staff, Kingston General Hospital; (613)722-8086; Fax. (613)761-1944.

TSIN, Karen W; Scarborough North Med Arts, 207-4040 Finch Ave E, Scarborough ON M1S 4V5; Tor'95; CCFP; Langs: Cantonese; (416)754-2727; Fax. (416)754-2728.

TSIN, Thomas T Y; Thistlewood Diagnostic Assoc, 110-8077 Islington Ave, Woodbridge ON L4L 7X7; (Hong Kong)'68; FRCPC; DiagRad; NuclearMed. Staff, William Osler Health System - Etobicoke General Hospital; Langs: Chinese; (905)856-7061

TSIODRAS, Athanasios; Hop Santa Cabrini Ospedale, 5655 rue Saint-Zotique E, Montreal QC H1T 1P7; McG'07; MDCM; CCFP; Staff, Hôpital Santa Cabrini Ospedale; Staff, Centre Hospitalier de Lachine; Staff, CSSS de Dorval-Lachine-Lasalle; (514)252-1535; athanasios.tsiodras@mail.mcgill.ca.

TSIPURAS, Dennis J; Ctr de Radiologie Ouest Island, 350-175 av Stillview, Pointe-Claire QC H9R 4S3; McG'68; BSc; MDCM; FRCPC; DiagRad. (514)697-9940; Fax. (514)697-3711.

TSOI, Edward Y K; The Medical Centre, 2-137 King St, Estevan SK S4A 2T5; Belfast (Ireland)'81; MB ChB; BAO; MRC(UK); CCFP; FCFP; Staff, St Joseph's Hospital; (306)634-6444; Fax. (306)634-9187.

TSOI, Keith S K; St Joseph's Healthcare, H421 MW-50 Charlton Ave E, Hamilton ON L8N 4A6; Tor'02; FRCPC; IntMed; Gastroent. Staff, St Joseph's Healthcare - Charlton Campus; Langs: Cantonese; (905)522-1155; Fax. (905)308-7201.

TSOI, Michael T; Peter Lougheed Centre, 3500 26 Ave NE, Calgary AB T1Y 6J4; Alb'01; CCFP; Staff, Peter Lougheed Centre; (403)943-5461; Fax. (403)943-5438.

TSOUKAS, Alexander; Montreal Sleep Clinic, 4427 Sherbrooke O, Montreal QC H3Z 1E5; McG'08; IntMed. (514)938-0995

TSOUKAS, Christos M; 804 rue Jean-Talon O, Montreal QC H3N 1S4; Athens (Greece)'77; ABIM; FACP; FRCPC; IntMed (AIDS). Staff, McGill University Health Centre - Montreal General Campus; Langs: French; Greek; (514)272-0707; Fax. (514)272-2278; chris.tsoukas@muhc.mcgill.ca.

TSOUKAS, Georges; MUHC-Montreal Gen Hosp, C6 260-1650 av Cedar, Montreal QC H3G 1A4; McG'68; BSc; FRCPC; Endocrin (P.Q.) (Diabetology); IntMed. Staff, McGill University Health Centre - Montreal General Campus; assoc Prof Med, McGill University; Langs: Spanish; Greek; French; (514)934-8000

TSOUKAS, Michael; 804 rue Jean-Talon O, Montreal QC H3N 1S4; Dublin (Ireland)'08; IntMed. (514)270-4384

TSOULIS, Christopher J; Guelph Medical Place 2, 107-89 Dawson Rd, Guelph ON N1H 1B1; McM'84; PhD; FRCPC; Derm. Consultant, Grand River Hospital - Freeport Site; Consultant, Guelph General Hospital; (519)836-7326; Fax. (519)763-5440.

TSOULOS, Panagiotis; CLSC du Plateau Mont-Royal, 4625 av de Lorimier, Montreal QC H2H 2B4; McG'10; MDCM; CCFP; (514)521-7663

TSUCHIDA, William S; 525 Park Rd N, Brantford ON N3R 7K8; McM'76; (519)756-3530; Fax. (519)756-0454.

TSUCHIYA, Shauna C; Royal Inland Hosp, 311 Columbia St, Kamloops BC V2C 2T1; Tor'09; CCFP; Staff, Royal Inland Hospital; (250)374-5111

TSUI, Alice S Y; Windsor Reg Hosp-Metropolitan, 1995 Lens Ave, Windsor ON N8W 1L9; Wes'99; CCFP; CCFP(E.M.); Staff, Leamington District Memorial Hospital; Staff, Windsor Regional Hospital - Metropolitan Site; Staff, Hôtel-Dieu Grace Hospital; (519)254-5577

TSUI, Andrew K W; 137 Roncesvalles Ave, Toronto ON M6R 2L2; Wes'00; CCFP; (416)534-6699; Fax. (416)534-0172.

TSUI, Ban C; Clinical Sciences Bldg, 8 120-152 University Campus NW, Edmonton AB T6G 2G3; Dal'95; FRCPC; Anes. Staff, University of Alberta Hospital; (780)407-8861; Fax. (780)407-3200.

TSUI, Connie C W; 5570 Joyce St, Vancouver BC V5R 4H6; UBC'92; CCFP; Langs: Cantonese; (604)430-2311; Fax. (604)430-2350.

TSUI, Elaine Y L; Yee Hong Med Centre, 60 Scottfield Dr, Scarborough ON M1S 5T7; (Hong Kong)'85; MB BS; FRCPC; IntMed; Endocrin&Metab. Assoc Staff, Mount Sinai Hospital; University of Toronto; Langs: Cantonese; Mandarin; (416)940-4818; Fax. (416)321-5705; elaine_tsui@yahoo.com.

TSUI, Floria P L; Northeast Comm Health Ctre, 14007 50 St NW, Edmonton AB T5A 5E4; UBC'85; FRCSC; ObstGyn. Ac Staff, Royal Alexandra Hospital; University of Alberta; (780)342-4050

TSUI, I L Helen; A6-4261 Highway 7, Unionville ON L3R 9W6; (Hong Kong)'83; MB BS; FRCP; FAAP(Peds); FRCPC; Peds (Pediatric Emergency Medicine). Clin Teacher, The Hospital For Sick Children; Staff Community Peds, Markham Stouffville Hospital; Langs: Cantonese; Mandarin; (905)477-2211; Fax. (905)477-5615.

TSUI, Joseph K; Pacific Parkinson Research Ctr, M36-2221 Wesbrook Mall, Vancouver BC V6T 2B5; (Hong Kong)'74; MB BS; MRCP(UK); FRCPC; Neur (Botox Injection)., Vancouver General Hospital - Centennial Pavillion; Staff, UBC Hospital - Koerner Pavillion; Physician, Pacific Parkinson Research Centre; Langs: Cantonese; Mandarin; (604)822-7682; Fax. (604)822-7866.

TSUI, Kwan-Cheung; York-Finch Med Centre, 101-2115 Finch Ave W, North York ON M3N 2V6; (Hong Kong)'76; MB BS; FRCPC; DiagRad (Ultrasound). Staff, Humber River Regional Hospital - Finch Avenue Site; Langs: Chinese; (416)744-2655; Fax. (416)744-0581.

TSUI, On Shun; Crystal Square Mall, 1612-4500 Kingsway, Burnaby BC V5H 2A9; Adelaide (Australia)'06; MB BS; (604)436-1231

TSUI, Simon Y T; Corporate Med Centre, 10-78 Corporate Dr, Scarborough ON M1H 3G4; (Hong Kong)'94; FRCPC; IntMed; Nephrol. Staff, Mackenzie Richmond Hill Hospital; Langs: Cantonese; (416)279-0855; Fax. (416)279-0857.

TSUI, Vincent T; St Joseph's Health Centre, 30 The Queensway, Toronto ON M6R 1B5; Wes'06; FRCPC; IntMed; GeriatricMed. Staff, St Joseph's Health Centre; Langs: Cantonese; (416)530-6532; Fax. (416)530-6585.

TSUI, Winston W H; 610-22470 Dewdney Trunk Rd, Maple Ridge BC V2X 5Z6; Qns'00; FRCPC; Cardiol; IntMed. (604)467-8482

TSUJIKAWA, Ronald K; MCI The Doctor's Office, 32-4604 37 St SW, Calgary AB T3E 3C9; UBC'72; (403)269-9488; Fax. (403)269-9409.

TSUNEYOS, Hiroshi; Univ Hlth Network-Toronto Gen, 200 Elizabeth St, Toronto ON M5G 2C4; Tottori Daigaku Igakubu (Japan)'94; Staff, Toronto General Hospital - UHN; (416)340-4789

TSUNG, David; PO Box 60624 Grandville Park P, Vancouver BC V6H 4B9; Dal'99.

TSUYUKI, Kurt T; The Surrey Eye Care Centre, 13490 104 Ave, Surrey BC V3T 1V8; UBC'89; FACS; FRCSC; Ophth. Consultant, Cariboo Memorial Hospital and Health Centre; Chair Div of Ophth, Surrey Memorial Hospital; Consultant, Royal Columbian Hospital; Consultant, Eagle Ridge Hospital & Health Care Centre; (604)951-0076; Fax. (604)951-9588; kurt_tsuyuki@telus.net.

TSUYUKI, Sean H; Manitoba X-Ray Clinic, 3263 Portage Ave, Winnipeg MB R3K 0W6; Man'88; FRCPC; DiagRad.

TSVETKOV, Elena V; The Ottawa Hosp-Gen Campus, 501 Smyth Rd, Ottawa ON K1H 8L6; Riga Stradins University (Other Foreign)'83; FRCPC; IntMed (Medical Oncology). Staff, The Ottawa Hospital - General Campus; (613)792-0432

TSZE, Kwok-Khin; BC Women's Hosp & Health Ctre, 4500 Oak St, Vancouver BC V6H 3N1; National (Taiwan)'74; Staff, BC Women's Hospital & Health Centre; (604)875-2136

TU, David T; Vancouver Native Health Clinic, 449 Hastings St E, Vancouver BC V6A 1P5; McM'98; CCFP; Langs: Mandarin; (604)255-9766; Fax. (604)254-5763.

TU, Geming S; 825 Oxford St E, London ON N5Y 3J8; Tor'88; Staff, London Health Sciences Centre - University Hospital; Staff, St Joseph's Hospital - St Joseph's Health Care; Langs: Mandarin; (519)673-0159; Fax. (519)673-5384.

TU, Jack V; Sunnybrook Hlth Sciences Ctre, G106-2075 Bayview Ave, Toronto ON M4N 3M5; Wes'88; PhD; MSc; FRCPC; IntMed (Cardiology). Staff, Sunnybrook Health Sciences Centre; Prof, University of Toronto; (416)480-4700; Fax. (416)480-6048.

TU, Karen; Univ Hlth Network-Toronto Western Hosp, 2W404-399 Bathurst St, Toronto ON M5T 2S8; Tor'92; MD; MSc; CCFP; FCFP; Physician, Toronto Western Hospital - University Health Network; Scientist, Institute for Clinical Evaluative Sciences; Assoc Prof Family & Commun Med, University of Toronto; (416)603-5888 x2; Fax. (416)603-5821; k.tu@utoronto.ca.

TU, Khue; Centre Medical 425, 425 boul Cure-Poirier O, Longueuil QC J4J 2H3; Mon'89; Staff, Centre Hospitalier Pierre Boucher; (450)679-6666; Fax. (450)679-6446.

TU, Kimphry M; Surrey Mem Hosp, 13750 96 Ave, Surrey BC V3V 1Z2; Alb'99; CCFP; CCFP(E.M.); Staff, Surrey Memorial Hospital; (604)581-2211; Fax. (604)588-3377.

TU, Le Mai; CHUS-Hop Fleurimont, 4109-3001 12e av N, Sherbrooke QC J1H 5N4; Sher'87; FRCSC; Urol (Female Urology). Staff Urology Services, Centre Hospitalier Universitaire de Sherbrooke-Hopital Fleurimont; (819)346-1110; Fax. (819)820-6411; le.mai.tu@usherbrooke.ca.

TU, My-Linh; 202-5450 ch Cote-des-Neiges, Montreal QC H3T 1Y6; Saigon (Vietnam)'72; Staff, St Mary's Hospital Centre; Staff, Sir Mortimer B Davis Jewish General; Staff Teacher, McGill University; (514)733-8883; Fax. (514)733-4896.

TUBETTI-GOODINE, Roseanne; 870 Main St PO Box 9093, Woodstock NB E7M 0B2; Dal'81; CCFP; FCFP; Assoc Instructor Family Med, Dalhousie University; (506)328-3115; Fax. (506)328-2247.

TUBIN, Stanislaw; Southside Hlth & Life Mgmt Ctr, 2-2120 Regent St, Sudbury ON P3E 3Z9; Ott'89; FRCSC; OrthSurg (Adult Reconstructive Surgery). Staff, Health Sciences North - Memorial Site; (705)522-9101; Fax. (705)522-5744.

TUCCI, Marisa A; Hôpital Ste-Justine, 3175 ch Cote-Sainte-Catherine, Montreal QC H3T 1C5; Mon'87; FRCPC; Peds (Critical Care Medicine). Staff, Hôpital Ste-Justine; adj Prof, Universite de Montreal; Langs: Italian; English; (514)345-4931 x3261; Fax. (514)345-7731; marisa.tucci@recherche-ste-justine.qc.ca.

TUCHAK, Carmen C; Glenrose Rehab Hosp, 1228-10230 111 Ave NW, Edmonton AB T5G 0B7; Cal'94; BSc(Hon); FRCPC; PhysMed&Rehab. Staff, Glenrose Rehabilitation Hospital; Asst Prof, University of Alberta; (780)735-8218; Fax. (780)735-6018.

TUCK, Alan B; London HSC-University Hosp, PO Box 5339 Stn B 339 Windermere Rd, London ON N6A 5A5; Wes'85; PhD(Microbiol & Immunol; FRCPC; AnatPath (Breast Pathology). Staff, London Health Sciences Centre - University Hospital; Prof Path & Oncol, University of Western Ontario; (519)685-8500 x36361; Fax. (519)663-2930; atuck@uwo.ca.

TUCK, James A; Medical Assoc of Port Perry, 462 Paxton St, Port Perry ON L9L 1L9; Mem'90; Staff, Lakeridge Health - Port Perry Site; (905)985-2895 x5420; Fax. (905)985-3464.

TUCK, Sarah E; Powassan & Area FHT, 8 King St, Powassan ON P0H 1Z0; McG'10; MDCM; CCFP; (705)724-1020

TUCKER, A George; Air Canada Med Clinic, PO Box 6002 Stn Toronto Amf, Mississauga ON L5P 1B4; Tor'57; BA; BSc; FRCPC; IntMed. Med Consultant, Air Canada Medical Clinic; (905)676-2400; Fax. (905)676-2402.

TUCKER, Devin; City Centre Health, 100-8160 Cook Rd, Richmond BC V6Y 1T8; Tor'98; CCFP; (604)233-5699

TUCKER, Elrie C; 101-1832 rue Sherbrooke O, Montreal QC H3H 1E4; McG'61; BSc; MDCM; CSPQ; FRCSC; ObstGyn. Staff, McGill University Health Centre - Royal Victoria Hospital; Langs: English; French; (514)937-8432; Fax. (514)933-5929.

TUCKER, Joan M; North York Gen Hosp-Branson, 129-555 Finch Ave W, North York ON M2R 1N5; McG'89; FRCPC; Psy (Adolescent Psychiatry). Staff, North York General Hospital - Branson Division; University of Toronto; Langs: English; French; (416)635-2410; Fax. (416)635-2428; jtucker@nygh.on.ca.

TUCKER, John H; Valley Regional Hosp, 150 Exhibition St, Kentville NS B4N 5E3; Wes'87; FRCPC; Anes; Critical Care Medicine. Staff, Valley Regional Hospital; (902)300-0233

TUCKER, Lori V; BC Women's Hosp & Health Ctre, K4 120-4500 Oak St, Vancouver BC V6H 3N1; Boston (USA)'83; Staff Resident Education, BC Women's Hospital & Health Centre; (604)875-2437; Fax. (604)875-3141.

TUCKER, Nancy A; The Joseph & Wolf Lebovic Bldg, 1 001-60 Murray St, Toronto ON M5T 3L9; Wes'87; Ophth (Oculo Plastic Surgery). Langs: French; (416)586-4800; Fax. (416)586-5915.

TUCKER, S Walter; Wabana Med Clinic, PO Box 699, Bell Island NL A0A 4H0; Dublin (Ireland)'73.

TUCKER, Sarah A; Riverside Med Clinic, 304-1101 Dewdney Ave, Trail BC V1R 4T1; UBC'08; CCFP; (250)368-5656

TUCKER, Tara L; BCC-Elisabeth Bruyere Hosp, 284 J-43 Bruyere St, Ottawa ON K1N 5C8; Mem'90; BMedSci; FRCPC; Peds (Palliative Care). Staff, SCO Health Service - Élisabeth Bruyère Hospital; Dir Faculty Wellness Program, University of Ottawa; (613)562-0050

TUCKER, William S; 47 Glenview Ave, Toronto ON M4R 1P5; Tor'68; FRCSC; Neursurg.

TUDOR, Manuela G; Arbour Med Centre, 281 Stone Rd E, Guelph ON N1G 5J5; Timisoara (Romania)'97; CCFP; (519)823-5133

TUDORESCU, Aurel; CSSS Haut-Richelieu-Rouville, 920 boul du Seminaire N, St-Jean-sur-Richel QC J3A 1B7; Bucharest (Romania)'77; Neur. Staff, Hôpital du Haut-Richelieu; (450)359-5000

TUFESCU, Tudor V; Section of Orthopaedics, AD4-720 McDermot Ave, Winnipeg MB R3E 0T3; Qns'00; FRCSC; OrthSurg. Staff, Health Sciences Centre.

TUFFNELL, Clayton E E; 202-2190 West Railway St, Abbotsford BC V2S 2E2; UBC'02; FRCSC; ObstGyn. (604)859-7725

TUGALEV, Oleg; Woodstock Gen Hosp, 310 Juliana Dr, Woodstock ON N4V 0A4; Donesk Medical Institute (Russia (Federation))'91; FRCPC; PhysMed&Rehab (Physiology). Staff, Woodstock General Hospital; Langs: Russian; Ukrainian; (519)421-4224; Fax. (519)421-4079.

TUGALEVA, Elena; London HS-University Campus, PO Box 5339 Stn B 339 Windermere Rd, London ON N6A 5A5; Donetsk (Russia (Federation))'91; FRCPC; AnatPath (Forensic Pathology). Staff, London Health Sciences Centre - University Hospital; Physician Forensic Path, Province of Ontario; Langs: Russian; Ukrainian; (519)685-8500; Fax. (519)663-2930.

TUGAULT, Julie; Clinique Med 2 Tours, A-1001 rue University, Montreal QC H3B 4L4; Mon'95; (514)954-4444; Fax. (514)954-4446.

TUGG, Lorne A; St Michael's Hosp, 30 Bond St, Toronto ON M5B 1W8; McM'89; FRCPC; Psy. Staff Psy, St Michael's Hospital; Teacher, University of Toronto; (416)864-3084; Fax. (416)864-5480.

TUGWELL, Barna D; Queen Elizabeth II HSC, 7F-1276 South Park St, Halifax NS B3H 2Y9; Harvard (USA)'98; FRCPC; IntMed; Endocrin&Metab (Diabetology). Staff, Queen Elizabeth II Health Sciences Centre - Victoria General Site; (902)473-3723; Fax. (902)473-5912.

TUGWELL, Peter S L; Center For Global Health, 202-1 Stewart St, Ottawa ON K1N 6N5; London (England)'69; MSc(Clin.Epidem); FRCP; FACP; FRCPC; IntMed (Rheumatology). (613)562-5800 x1945

TUHAN MIRZA BARANOWSKI, Izolda L; Timmins & District Hosp, 700 Ross Ave E, Timmins ON P4N 8P2; Ott'97; FRCPC; Psy. Staff, Timmins & District Hospital; Langs: Polish; French; (705)360-6036; Fax. (705)264-6525.

TUJIK, Karla L; Sudbury Reg Hosp-Laurentian, 41 Ramsey Lake Rd, Sudbury ON P3E 5J1; UBC'99; CCFP; CCFP(E.M.); Staff, Health Sciences North-Laurentian Site; Staff, Health Sciences North-St Joseph's Health Centre; (705)523-7100

TUKA, Andrea; Canadian Forces Health Service, PO Box 17000 Stn Forces, Victoria BC V9A 7N2; Budapest (Hungary)'93; FRCPC; Psy. Staff Mental Health Services, Canadian Forces Health Services; Langs: Hungarian; (250)363-4411

TUKARAM, Khoday T; 416-5450 ch Cote-des-Neiges, Montreal QC H3T 1Y6; Mysore (India)'58; MB BS; FRCSC; Urol. Staff, St Mary's Hospital Centre; (514)739-8078; Fax. (514)737-0336.

TUKKER, Roderick P; Vancouver Gen Hosp, 855 12th Ave W, Vancouver BC V5Z 1M9; Qns'93; CCFP; Staff, Vancouver General Hospital - Centennial Pavillion; (604)822-7121

TULAI, Cristina; 211-75 Albert St, Ottawa ON K1P 5E7; Bucharest (Romania)'79; Langs: Romanian; (613)238-2626; Fax. (613)238-2626.

TULANDI, Tati; Centre de sante Queen Elizabet, 2100 av de Marlowe, Montreal QC H4A 3L5; (Indonesia)'72; Staff, McGill University Health Centre - Royal Victoria Hospital; (514)934-1934; Fax. (514)934-8385.

TULANDI, Thomas; Clinique Med le Norois, 201-641 4e rue O, Amos QC J9T 2S1; Mon'05; (819)732-3368

TULANDI, Togas; MUHC-Royal Victoria Hosp, WP F6-687 av des Pins O, Montreal QC H3A 1A1; (Indonesia),Harvard (USA)'71; ABOG; FACOG; MSCHC; FRCSC; ObstGyn (Minimal Invasive Surgery). Chaire Milton Leong in Reproductive Med/Prof Obst/Gyn, McGill University; Langs: Bilingual(English/French); (514)934-1934 x31391; Fax. (514)843-1448.

TULI, Raman; 500-1565 Carling Ave, Ottawa ON K1Z 8R1; McG'90; FRCSC; Ophth (Vitreo Retinal Surgery). Langs: English; French; (613)226-5455; Fax. (613)226-9478.

TULI, Vikas; York Med Health Centre, J-17215 Leslie St, Newmarket ON L3Y 8E4; Tor'96; BSc(Hons); FRCSC; OrthSurg (Hand Wrist & Elbow Surgery). Staff, Southlake Regional Health Centre; (905)953-0864; Fax. (905)953-8405.

TULIN, Caroline; Hop Maisonneuve-Rosemont, 5415 boul de l'Assomption, Montreal QC H1T 2M4; Mon'01; Staff, Hopital Maisonneuve-Rosemont; (514)252-3400

TULIN, Michel; Cenre Med de Chambly, 205-1101 boul Brassard, Chambly QC J3L 5R4; Montpellier (France)'65; Gastroent (P.Q.). Langs: Bilingual(English/French); (450)658-6601; Fax. (450)658-7849.

TULIPAN, Tanya M; Reproductive Mental Health Ser, 5850 University Ave, Halifax NS B3K 6R8; Wes'02; FRCPC; Psy. Staff, IWK Health Centre; Staff, The Nova Scotia Hospital; (902)499-5335

TULK, Stephen E; SCHC The Hub, 2660 Eglinton Ave E, Scarborough ON M1K 2S3; Tor'77; BSc(AAM); CMI; CCFP; FCFP; Court Staff Privil, Toronto East General Hospital Inc; Teacher Medical Illustration, Ontario College of Art & Design; Teacher Anatomy, Art Gallery Of Ontario; (416)642-9445; Fax. (416)284-1964; stephen_tulk@ago.net.

TULL, Russell G; Group Health Centre, 240 McNabb St, Sault Ste. Marie ON P6B 1Y5; UBC'04; CCFP; (705)759-1234; Fax. (705)541-2287.

TULLIO, Gerald C; Peel Med Arts Bldg, 500-145 Queen St E, Brampton ON L6W 3P8; Ott'96; FRCPC; Neur (Neuro Physiology). Staff, William Osler Health System - Brampton Civic Hospital; (905)456-8010; Fax. (905)456-3885.

TULLIS, D Elizabeth; St Michael's Hosp, 6 049-30 Bond St, Toronto ON M5B 1W8; Tor'85; FRCPC; IntMed (Cystic Fibrosis); Respir. Head Respirol, St Michael's Hospital; Assoc Prof Med/Prog Dir, University of Toronto; (416)864-5406; Fax. (416)864-5922; tullise@smh.toronto.on.ca.

TULLIS, Gary D; Metrotown Med Centre, 204-6411 Nelson Ave, Burnaby BC V5H 4H3; Sask'79; FRCPC; Derm. (604)433-4721; Fax. (604)433-4883; drtullis@shaw.ca.

TULLOCH, Heather V; Health Sciences Centre, AE 203-820 Sherbrook St, Winnipeg MB R3A 1R9; Man'87; FRCPC; Anes. Staff, Health Sciences Centre; (204)774-6511

TULLY, Shawn A; 201-301 Columbia St E, New Westminster BC V3L 3W5; Man'04; CCFP; (604)526-4655; Fax. (604)526-7656.

TULSIANI, Suresh R K; Dr S R Tulsiani Inc, 365-3066 Shelbourne St, Victoria BC V8R 6T9; Jammu-Kashmir (India)'76; DCH(Ire); FAAP; FRCPC; Peds (Neonatal & Perinatal Medicine). Consultant Ped, Victoria General Hospital; Clinical Asst Prof Peds, University of British Columbia; Clinical Asst Prof Ped, University Of Victoria; (250)595-0595; Fax. (250)595-5321.

TULVING, Linda; Student Wellness Centre, 1280 Main St W, Hamilton ON L8S 4S4; Cal'85; BSc; MA; CCFP; FCFP; Dir Campus Health, McMaster University; (905)525-9140 x27700

TUMBACH, Janna L; Associate Famiy Phys Clinic, 262 2nd Ave NE, Swift Current SK S9H 2C8; Sask'04; CCFP; Commun Teach Staff Academic Family Med, University of Saskatchewan; (306)773-1555; Fax. (306)773-6817.

TUMBER, Hardeep S; Surlang Med Clinic, 106-19475 Fraser Hwy, Surrey BC V3S 6K7; Sask'85; LMCC; Staff, BC Mental Health & Addiction Service; Langs: Punjabi; (604)533-5051; Fax. (604)533-8353.

TUMBER, P Paul S; Univ Hlth Network-Toronto Western Hosp, 2 405 MCL-399 Bathurst St, Toronto ON M5T 2S8; Sask'91; FRCPC; Anes. Staff, Toronto Western Hospital - University Health Network; Langs: Punjabi; (416)603-5118; Fax. (416)603-6494.

TUMI, Kamaleddin H; Barrie Plastic & Cosmetic Surg, 102-34 Quarry Ridge Rd, Barrie ON L4M 7G1; Al-Fateh (Libya),'86; MB BS; FRCSC; PlasSurg (Hand Surgery). Hd PlasSurg, Royal Victoria Regional Health Centre; Langs: Arabic; (705)737-9235; Fax. (705)737-9469; info@barrieplasticsurgery.com.

TUMILTY, Joseph A; James Paton Mem Hosp, 125 Trans Canada Hwy, Gander NL A1V 1P7; Dal'91; BSc; FRCSC; OrthSurg. Staff, James Paton Memorial Hospital; Clin Instructor, Memorial University Of Newfoundland; (709)256-5701; jtumilty@nl.rogers.com.

TUNDE-BYASS, Modupe O J; 440-5 Fairview Mall Dr, North York ON M2J 2Z1; Ibadan (Nigeria)'87; MB BS; MRCOG; FRCSC; ObstGyn. Staff, North York General Hospital; Langs: Yoruba; (416)497-4999; Fax. (416)497-0011.

TUNG, Amrik S; 12811 96 Ave, Surrey BC V3V 6V9; Karnatak (India)'78; (604)588-7976

TUNG, Amy S L; Doctors on Bayview, 15900 Bayview Ave, Aurora ON L4G 7Y3; Tor'08; CCFP; (905)726-9755

TUNG, Andrew S; 301-2151 McCallum Rd, Abbotsford BC V2S 3N8; UBC'06; FRCSC; PlasSurg. (604)850-0750

TUNG, Dean J; University of Alberta Hosp, 5B4 13-8440 112 St NW, Edmonton AB T6G 2B7; UBC'04; FRCPC; GenPath. Staff, University of Alberta Hospital; (780)407-2124

TUNG, Frances Y; East Liberty Med Clinic, 105-901 King St W, Toronto ON M5V 3H5; Tor'75; BSc; CCFP; FCFP; Lecturer, St Michael's Hospital; Lecturer, University of Toronto; Langs: Cantonese; (416)599-6000; Fax. (855)498-5062.

TUNG, Guat Khim; UBC Hospital, 2211 Wesbrook Mall, Vancouver BC V6T 2B5; Sheffield (England)'87; MB ChB; CCFP; Staff, UBC Hospital - Koerner Pavillion; (604)822-7520

TUNG, Julie; PO Box 18117 RPO Heritage Mtn, New Westminster BC V3H 0A2; McM'98; CCFP; Staff, Eagle Ridge Hospital & Health Care Centre; (604)420-9252

TUNG, K K Stanley; 211-1033 Davie St, Vancouver BC V6E 1M7; Man'89; BSc; IntMed (Cardiology). Clinical Asst Prof, Providence Health Care - St Paul's Hospital; Langs: Cantonese; Mandarin; (604)806-8174; Fax. (604)806-8344.

TUNG, Kenneth S H; Sacrborough North Med Arts, 308-4040 Finch Ave E, Scarborough ON M1S 4V5; Tor'83; Staff, The Scarborough Hospital - Birchmount Campus; Staff, William Osler Health System - Etobicoke General Hospital; Langs: Mandarin; Taiwanese; (416)754-2801; Fax. (647)258-0422.

TUNG, Parampal P; McKenzie Towne Medical, 102-620 McKenzie Towne Dr SE, Calgary AB T2Z 0Y6; (Other Foreign)'04; BSc; BMedSci; CCFP; (403)262-6311; Fax. (403)262-5911.

TUNG, Taranjit S; Health Sciences Centre, AD420-820 Sherbrook St, Winnipeg MB R3A 1R9; Sask'07; FRCSC; OrthSurg. Staff, Health Sciences Centre; (204)787-1219

TUNG, Tommy H T; Woodbine Med Centre, B 9-76 Arlington Dr, Keswick ON L4P 0A9; Tor'79; Assoc Staff, Southlake Regional Health Centre; Langs: Chinese; (905)476-0308; Fax. (905)476-1079.

TUNKS, Eldon R; Regional Rehab Centre, 237 Barton St E, Hamilton ON L8L 2X2; Tor'69; FRCPC; Psy (Chronic Pain Management). Ac Staff Regional Rehab Centre, Hamilton Health Sciences Centre - Hamilton General Hospital; Emeritus Prof Psy, McMaster University; Langs: Italian; (905)521-2100 x77038; Fax. (905)521-7954.

TUNKS, Marcel G; St Josephs Healthcare, T2127-50 Charlton Ave E, Hamilton ON L8N 4A6; Tor'04; FRCPC; IntMed; Respir. Staff, St Joseph's Healthcare - Charlton Campus; (905)522-1155

TUNNICLIFFE, Brian W; CPHC Gananoque Community FHT, 338 Herbert St, Gananoque ON K7G 1R1; Tor'68; (613)382-7383; Fax. (613)382-7323.

TUNZI, Christina R; Spadina Health Centre, 404-720 Spadina Ave, Toronto ON M5S 2T9; Tor'04; CCFP; (416)928-0920; Fax. (416)928-7426.

TUORI, Christopher T; M C I The Doctors Office, 255 Morningside Ave, Scarborough ON M1E 3E6; Tor'75; Ac Staff, Rouge Valley Health System - Centenary Health Centre Site; (416)284-1020

TUPCHONG, Michele A; Ashgrove Med Centre, 302-6633 Highway 7, Markham ON L3P 7P2; Tor'94; FRCPC; IntMed; Rheum. (905)471-4402; Fax. (905)471-1903.

TUPPAL, Raj K; Oshawa Clinic, 117 King St E, Oshawa ON L1H 1B9; Mem'85; FRCPC; IntMed; Derm. Assoc Staff, Lakeridge Health - Oshawa Site; (905)721-3563 x3563; Fax. (905)721-3557.

TUPPER, Astrid E; Rockyview Gen Hosp, 7007 14 St SW, Calgary AB T2V 1P9; Cal'00; CCFP; Staff, Rockyview General Hospital; Langs: German; French; (403)943-3000; astrid.tupper@calgaryhealthregion.ca.

TUPPER, Janet K; Haig Clinic, 601 6 Ave S, Lethbridge AB T1J 0Z2; UBC'00; CCFP; Staff, Chinook Regional Hospital; Staff, Sexual Health Clinic-Alberta; Clin Preceptor, University of Alberta; Clin Preceptor, University of Calgary; (403)328-6641; Fax. (403)328-6118.

TUPPER, Jennifer I L; Mineral Spring Hosp, PO Box 1050 305 Lynx St, Banff AB T1L 1H7; UBC'99; CCFP; CCFP(E.M.); Staff, Covenant Health - Banff Mineral Springs Hospital; Langs: English; French; (403)762-2222

TUPPER, Vashti E; Real Canadian Super Store, 1205 Oxford St W, London ON N6H 1V9; Wes'84; BA; CCFP; FCFP; Ad Staff Privil, St Joseph's Hospital - St Joseph's Health Care; (519)672-8460; Fax. (519)672-4947; jtupper@sympatico.ca.

TURA, Alfredo; 2-1836 Comox Ave, Comox BC V9M 3M7; Pisa (Italy)'99; CCFP; Langs: Italian; (250)702-3242

TURABIAN, B Michael; The Brandon Clinic, 620 Dennis St, Brandon MB R7A 5E7; Man'72; FRCPC; IntMed (Cardiology). Dir Echocardiography & Pacemaker Serv, Brandon Regional Health Centre; (204)728-4440; Fax. (204)726-1765; turabian@westman.wave.ca.

TURBIDE, Christian; 120-500 Mapleton Rd, Moncton NB E1G 0N3; Sher'98; FRCPC; IntMed (Family Medicine); Gastroent.

TURBIDE, Manon; CSSS de la Vallée de l'Or, 725 6e rue, Val-d'Or QC J9P 3Y1; Sher'90; FRCSC; ObstGyn. Staff, Centre Hospitalier de Val d'Or; Langs: Bilingual(French/English); (819)825-6711; Fax. (819)825-7948.

TURBIDE, Pascale; CSSS de Sept-Iles, 45 rue du Pere-Divet, Sept-Iles QC G4R 3N7; Laval'90; FRCSC; Ophth. Staff, Centre Hospitalier Regional de Sept-Iles; Langs: Bilingual(French/English); (418)962-9761 x2696; Fax. (418)962-8699; dauphin@globetrotter.net.

TURBIDE, Pierre; CSSS de la Matapedia, 135 av Gaetan Archambeault, Amqui QC G5J 2K5; Mon'93; CCFP; Staff, CSSS de la Matapedia; (418)629-2211; Fax. (418)629-4484.

TURBIN, Dmitry; St Paul's Hosp, 1081 Burrard St, Vancouver BC V6Z 1T6; Moscow Medical-Stomatology Institute (Russia (Federation))'90; FRCPC; AnatPath. Staff, Providence Health Care - St Paul's Hospital; (604)682-2344

TURBIS, Carole; CSSS de Sept-Iles, 405 av Brochu, Sept-Iles QC G4R 2W9; Laval'77; LMCC; Staff Services Communautaire, Centre Hospitalier Regional de Sept-Iles; (418)962-2572 x4114; Fax. (418)962-1858.

TURCHEN, Barry J; 480-3033 Immel St, Abbotsford BC V2S 6S2; Man'79; Ac Staff, Abbotsford Regional Hospital & Cancer Centre; (604)852-6781; Fax. (604)852-0869.

TURCHIN, Diana C; Trillium Health Ctre-Mississau, 100 Queensway W, Mississauga ON L5B 1B8; Tor'89; FRCSC; OrthSurg (Knee Surgery). Staff Orth, Trillium Health Centre - Mississauga; (905)848-7100

TURCHIN, Irina; Fredericton Med Clinic, 501B-1015 Regent St, Fredericton NB E3B 6H5; Cal'04; FRCPC; Derm. Staff, Hopital Regional Chaleur.

TURCHIN, Kathrin M; Harbourfront Medical, 4-8 York St, Toronto ON M5J 2Y2; Tor'09; CCFP; Langs: Bilingual(English/French); (416)366-2273; Fax. (416)366-5665.

TURCOT, Alice; ASSS-Chaudiere Appalaches, 363 rue Cameron, Sainte-Marie QC G6E 3E2; Laval'76; FRCPC; OccupMed. ac Staff, Hôtel-Dieu de Lévis; Staff, Agence de la santé et des services sociaux de Chaudière-Appalaches; (418)389-1523; Fax. (418)389-1525.

TURCOT, Catherine; Clinique Med Familiale de Verd, 4000 boul Lasalle, LaSalle QC H4G 2A3; Mon'05; CCFP; Staff, Barrie Memorial Hospital; (514)765-7325; Fax. (514)362-2823.

TURCOT, France; Pavillon Rosemont, 5689 boul Rosemont, Montreal QC H1T 2H1; Mon'77; FRCPC; Psy. Staff, Hopital Maisonneuve-Rosemont; (514)252-3910 x4873; Fax. (514)252-3810.

TURCOT, Francis; CSSS du Suroît, 150 rue Saint-Thomas, Salaber-de-Valleyf QC J6T 6C1; Mon'06; Staff, Centre Hospitalier Régional du Suroît; (450)371-9920

TURCOT, Josee; UMF Maisonneuve-Rosemont, 5689-boul Rosemont, Montreal QC H1T 2H1; Mon'08; Staff, Hopital Maisonneuve-Rosemont; (514)252-3400 x4513; Fax. (514)252-3754.

TURCOT, Olivier; Hôtel-Dieu de Lévis, 143 rue Wolfe, Levis QC G6V 3Z1; Laval'01; CCFP; CCFP(E.M.); Staff, Hôtel-Dieu de Lévis; (819)697-3333

TURCOT, Richard; Polyclinique de Trois-Rivieres, 365-1900 boul des Recollets, Trois-Rivieres QC G8Z 4K4; Laval'71; IntMed (P.Q.); Nephrol (P.Q.). ac Staff, Centre Hospitalier Regional de Trois-Rivieres; (819)373-1202; Fax. (819)693-1845; richardturcot@cgocable.ca.

TURCOT, Roger; Clinique Medi-Plus, 4100 3e av O, Quebec QC G1H 6E1; Laval'73; (418)622-6969; Fax. (418)622-2037.

TURCOTTE, Alain; CSSS de Laval, 1755 boul Rene-Laennec, Laval QC H7M 3L9; Mon'88; Staff, Hopital de la Cite de la santé; (450)975-5444; Fax. (450)975-5497; aturcotte@videotron.ca.

TURCOTTE, Alain F; Societe Ass Automobile du QC, S2 36-333 boul Jean-Lesage, Quebec QC G1K 8J6; Laval'86; Médecin, Societe Assurance Automobile du Quebec; (418)528-3923

TURCOTTE, Angele; Centre De L'Osteoporose, 100-1200 av de Germain-des-Prè, Quebec QC G1V 3M7; Laval'77; FRCPC; IntMed (P.Q.); Rheum. (418)650-2671; Fax. (418)650-3916.

TURCOTTE, Anna-Marie; GMF de Trois-Rivieres, 1900 boul des Recollets, Trois-Rivieres QC G8Z 4K4; Sher'10; (819)375-6666

TURCOTTE, Annick; UMF Charles Lemoyne, 201-299 boul Sir-Wilfrid-Lauri, Saint-Lambert QC J4R 2L1; Sher'94; CCFP; (450)466-5630; Fax. (450)466-5631.

TURCOTTE, Antoine; CSSS De Saint-Jerome, 290 rue de Montigny, Saint-Jerome QC J7Z 5T3; Sher'03; FRCSC; OrthSurg. Staff, Hôtel-Dieu de Saint-Jérôme; (450)431-8200

TURCOTTE, Bernard; CMF Berthier, GD 788 av Gilles-Villeneuve, Berthierville QC J0K 1A0; Mon'83; Staff, Centre Hospitalier Régional de Lanaudière; (514)836-4212; Fax. (450)836-4814.

TURCOTTE, Carole; Centre Hosp Honore-Mercier, 2750 boul Laframboise, Saint-Hyacinthe QC J2S 4Y8; Laval'88; Anes (P.Q.). Staff, Centre Hospitalier Honore-Mercier; (450)771-3353; Fax. (450)771-3282.

TURCOTTE, Chantal; Clinique Plexo Mediclub, 201-6100 av du Boise, Montreal QC H3S 2W1; Laval'84; LMCC; admin Associé, Clinique Plexo Mediclub; Langs: English; (514)739-5646; Fax. (514)739-6773.

TURCOTTE, Claudine; Hôtel-Dieu de Lévis, 143 rue Wolfe, Levis QC G6V 3Z1; Mon'99; FRCPC; Psy. Staff, Hôtel-Dieu de Lévis; (418)835-7155; Fax. (418)835-7199.

TURCOTTE, Elisabeth; CLSC Salaberry-de-Valleyfield, 71 rue Maden, Salaber-de-Valleyf QC J6S 3V4; Sher'09; (450)371-0143

TURCOTTE, Eric; CHUS-Hop Fleurimont, 3001 12e av N, Sherbrooke QC J1H 5N4; Sher'97; MRCP; FRCP; RC; FRCPC; NuclearMed (Nuclear Cardiology). Staff, Centre Hospitalier Universitaire de Sherbrooke-Hopital Fleurimont; Langs: Bilingual(French/English); (819)820-6490; e.turcotte@usherbrooke.ca.

TURCOTTE, Francois; Clinique des Med d'Urgence, 632 rue Bowen S, Sherbrooke QC J1G 2E9; Sher'84; (819)822-2700

TURCOTTE, Genevieve; CLSC de Sherbrooke, 1200 rue King E, Sherbrooke QC J1G 1E4; Mon'99; CCFP; Médecin, CLSC La Region-Sherbrooke; (819)780-2222

TURCOTTE, Gilles; Ctr Hosp Affilie-Enfant-Jesus, 1401 18e rue, Quebec QC G1J 1Z4; Laval'66; MedBiochem (P.Q.). Sec Med Biochem Service, Centre Hospitalier Affilié Universitaire de Québec - Hôpital De L'Enfant Jésus; ac Staff Med Biochem, CSSS de Montmagny-L'Islet; ac Staff Med Biochem, CSSS de Kamouraska; Clin Prof, Université Laval; Langs: English; Bilingual(French/English); (418)649-0252 x3305; Fax. (418)649-5796; gilles.turcotte.cha@ssss.gouv.qc.ca.

TURCOTTE, Jacques; Clin d'Expertises Med Quebec, 440-979 av de Bourgogne, Quebec QC G1W 2L4; Laval'78; Médecin, Clinique d'Expertises Med du Quebec Inc; (418)654-3268

TURCOTTE, Jean; Clinique Med Jean-Turcotte, 655 boul des Erables, Valcourt QC J0E 2L0; Sher'77; CCFP; (450)532-3464; Fax. (450)532-3989; jturc@cooptel.qc.ca.

TURCOTTE, Jean; Centre Med le Mesnil, 300-1300 boul Lebourgneuf, Quebec QC G2K 2N1; Laval'72; FRCPC; Cardiol. (418)624-1800; Fax. (418)624-1820; jaturc2000@yahoo.com.

TURCOTTE, Jean; Clinique Med Hickson, 3805 rue de Verdun, Verdun QC H4G 1K8; Mon'67; Staff, Centre Hospitalier de Verdun; Langs: English; (514)769-9671; Fax. (514)769-9676.

TURCOTTE, Jean T; CHUS-Hop Fleurimont, 3001 12e av N, Sherbrooke QC J1H 5N4; Laval'72; Staff, Centre Hospitalier Universitaire de Sherbrooke-Hopital Fleurimont; (819)346-1110

TURCOTTE, Jean-Francois; 1401 18e rue, Quebec QC G1J 1Z4; Laval'74 Laval; DAB; FRCS; FRCSC; Neursurg (Neuro Vascular). Chef Services/ac Staff Neurosurgs, Centre Hospitalier Affilié Universitaire de Québec - Hôpital De L'Enfant Jésus; Clin Prof Surg, Université Laval; Langs: Bilingual(French/English); French; (418)649-5734; Fax. (418)649-5988.

TURCOTTE, Jean-Jacques; Centre Hosp Honore-Mercier, 2750 boul Laframboise, Saint-Hyacinthe QC J2S 4Y8; Laval'66; Peds. Staff, Centre Hospitalier Honore-Mercier; (450)771-3333; Fax. (450)771-3552.

TURCOTTE, Jean-Marc; Ctr Hosp Affilie-Enfant-Jesus, 1401 18e rue, Quebec QC G1J 1Z4; Laval'65; FRCPC; DiagRad. Staff Radiol, Centre Hospitalier Affilié Universitaire de Québec - Hôpital De L'Enfant Jésus; (418)649-5782; Fax. (418)649-5972.

TURCOTTE, Jean-Robert; Hop du Sacre-Coeur de Mtl, 5400 boul Gouin O, Montreal QC H4J 1C5; Sher'74; MPH(Harvard); FRCPC; Psy. ac Staff, Hôpital du Sacre-Coeur de Montréal; (514)338-2070; Fax. (514)338-3187.

TURCOTTE, Jessie; Hôtel dieu St-Joseph, 21 rue Canada, Saint-Quentin NB E8A 2P6; Sher'05; CCFP; Staff, Hôtel-Dieu St-Joseph de Saint-Quentin; (506)235-2300; jturcotte@nbnet.nb.ca.

TURCOTTE, Julie; Clinique des Troubles Anxieux, 505-1575 rue Henri-Bourassa O, Montreal QC H3M 3A9; Laval'92; FRCPC; Psy. Staff, Hôpital du Sacre-Coeur de Montréal; adj Prof, Universite de Montreal; (514)338-2070

TURCOTTE, Karen E; Ottawa Valley Family Health Te, 95 Spring St, Almonte ON K0A 1A0; Tor'09; CCFP; (613)256-9370; Fax. (613)256-0949.

TURCOTTE, Karine; Hôpital de Saint-Eustache, 520 boul Arthur-Sauve, Saint-Eustache QC J7R 5B1; Sher'07; Staff, Centre Hospitalier de Chandler; Staff, Hôpital de Saint-Eustache; (450)473-6811

TURCOTTE, Marie L; Dryden Reg Health Centre, PO Box 3003 Stn Main 58 Goodall St, Dryden ON P8N 2Z6; Cal'04; Staff, Dryden Regional Health Centre; (807)223-8200

TURCOTTE, Martine; CSSS de Laval, 1755 boul Rene-Laennec, Laval QC H7M 3L9; Mon'98; Staff, Hopital de la Cite de la santé; (450)668-1010

TURCOTTE, Maryse; Hotel-Dieu de Levis, 143 rue Wolfe, Levis QC G6V 3Z1; Laval'82; Dir-svcs prof, Hôtel-Dieu de Lévis; (418)835-7111; Fax. (418)835-7196.

TURCOTTE, Michel; Clinique Med de la Capitale, 14-4225 4e av O, Quebec QC G1H 6P3; Laval'69; ac Staff, Centre Hospitalier Universitaire De Québec - Pavillon De St-françois-d'assise; (418)628-9921; Fax. (418)628-3203.

TURCOTTE, Pierre; Clin d'Opthalmologie de la Cit, 10-2600 boul Laurier, Quebec QC G1V 4T3; Laval'82; FRCSC; Ophth (Retina). Médecin, Clinique d'Opthalmologie de la Cite; (418)650-2395; Fax. (418)654-1580; ptem@sympatico.ca.

TURCOTTE, Renee; U M F Dieppe, 105-185 av Acadie-Piece, Dieppe NB E1A 1G6; Laval'77; Staff, Elsipogtog Health Centre; Clin Prof, Universite de Sherbrooke; Clin Prof, University of Moncton; Langs: Bilingual(French/English); (506)862-4182; Fax. (506)862-4179.

TURCOTTE, Robert; MUHC-Montreal Gen Hosp, B5 159 6-1650 av Cedar, Montreal QC H3G 1A4; Mon'82; FRCSC; OrthSurg (Musculo Skeletal Oncology). Chef OrthSurg, McGill University Health Centre - Montreal General Campus; assoc Prof, McGill University; Langs: Bilingual(French/English); (514)934-1394 x42266; Fax. (514)934-8453; robert.turcotte@muhc.mcgill.ca.

TURCOTTE, Robin; Institute Albert Prevost, 6555 boul Gouin O, Montreal QC H4K 1B3; Mon'83; Staff, Centre Hospitalier Pierre Boucher; (514)338-4246; Fax. (514)338-4391.

TURCOTTE, Roc; Hôpital Laval, 2725 ch Sainte-Foy, Quebec QC G1V 4G5; Laval'89; DiagRad. Staff, Hôpital Laval; (418)656-4512; Fax. (418)878-2738; rocturcotte@videotron.ca.

TURCOTTE, Suzanne; CLSC de Sherbrooke, 50 rue Camirand, Sherbrooke QC J1H 4J5; Laval'87; (819)563-2572; Fax. (819)823-0415.

TURCOTTE-LAGACE, Mathieu; Hop Charles Lemoyne, 3120 boul Taschereau, Greenfield Park QC J4V 2H1; Laval'01; CCFP; CCFP(E.M.); Staff, Hopital Charles LeMoyne; Langs: English; (450)466-5000

TURECKI, Gustavo X; Douglas Mental Hlth Univ Inst, 6875 boul Lasalle, Verdun QC H4H 1R3; Sao Paolo (Brazil)'89; MSc; PhD; Staff, Douglas Mental Health University Institute; adj Prof Psy, McGill University; (514)761-6131; Fax. (514)886-4466.

TUREK, Caroline A; Brooklin Med Centre, A1-5959 Anderson St, Brooklin ON L1M 2E9; Tor'90; (905)655-3321; Fax. (905)655-4848.

TUREK, Michele A; The Ottawa Hosp-Gen Campus, 501 Smyth Rd, Ottawa ON K1H 8L6; McG'77; FRCPC; IntMed; Cardiol. Ac Staff Med, The Ottawa Hospital - General Campus; Dept Head Med/Assoc Prof, University of Ottawa; Langs: Bilingual(English/French); (613)737-8810; Fax. (613)739-6727; mturek@ottawahospital.on.ca.

TURENNE, Annette Y M; 61009 Range Rd 454 PO Box 7006 Stn Main, Bonnyville AB T9N 2H4; Alb'88; (780)826-2215; Fax. (780)826-2914.

TURENNE, Francois; Clinique Med de Lavaltrie, 1400 rue Notre-Dame, Lavaltrie QC J5T 1M6; Mon'96; Staff, Centre Hospitalier Pierre le Gardeur; (450)586-1033; Fax. (450)586-4498.

TURENNE, Hubert; CSSS du Sud de Lanaudière, 911 montee des Pionniers, Terrebonne QC J6V 2H2; Port-au-Prince (Haiti)'84; Staff, Centre Hospitalier Pierre le Gardeur; (450)654-7525 x31184; Fax. (450)470-2645; hubertturenne@videotron.ca.

TURENNE, Yves; CLSC Champagnat Vallee Forts, 978 boul du Seminaire N, St-Jean-sur-Richel QC J3A 1E5; Mon'87; Staff, CLSC-CHLSD Champagnat Vallee des Forts; (450)358-2578

TURGEON, Eugene W T; East Street Med Arts Centre, 304-170 East St, Sault Ste. Marie ON P6A 3C6; Tor'70; CCFP; FCFP; Ac Staff, Sault Area Hospital - Sault Ste Marie; (705)759-3355; Fax. (705)759-6299.

TURGEON, Francoise; CSSS Jonquiere, 2230 rue de l'Hopital, Jonquiere QC G7X 7X2; Sher'98; Staff, Centre Hospitalier Jonquiere; Langs: Spanish; English; (418)695-7700; francoise.turgeon@ssss.gouv.qc.ca.

TURGEON, Frederic; Clinique Med Soleil, 64 1re av O, Amos QC J9T 1T8; Mon'91; CCFP; FCFP; Staff, CH Hôtel-Dieu d'Amos; (819)732-8341; Fax. (819)732-1642.

TURGEON, Genevieve; Hop Charles LeMoyne, 3120 boul Taschereau, Greenfield Park QC J4V 2H1; Sher'02; Staff, Hopital Charles LeMoyne; (450)466-5000

TURGEON, Jean; Hôpital Ste-Justine, 3175 ch Cote-Sainte-Catherine, Montreal QC H3T 1C5; Mon'84; FRCPC; Peds (Hospitalist). ac Staff, Hôpital Ste-Justine; Clin Assoc Prof, Universite de Montreal; Langs: Bilingual(French/English); (514)345-4675; Fax. (514)345-4822; jean.turgeon@umontreal.ca.

TURGEON, Jean-Martin; CSSS Drummond-Hop Sainte-Croix, 570 rue Heriot, Drummondville QC J2B 1C1; Laval'94; OrthSurg. Staff, Hôpital Sainte-croix; (819)478-6464

TURGEON, Josee-Anne; Centre de Sante Valcartier, CP 1000 Succ Forces, Courcelette QC G0A 4Z0; Laval'96; FRCPC; Psy. Staff, Hôtel-Dieu de Lévis; Médecin, Centre de Sante Valcartier; (418)844-5000 x5802; Fax. (418)844-7606.

TURGEON, Manon; Clinique Med le Gardeurois, 130-155 rue Notre-Dame, Repentigny QC J5Z 3C4; Mon'76; Langs: English; (450)582-5551; Fax. (450)582-2718.

TURGEON, Marie-Eve; Clin Familiale de St-Lambert, 209 rue de Woodstock, Saint-Lambert QC J4P 1W7; Mon'00; (450)466-8583; Fax. (450)466-4072.

TURGEON, Marie-Helene; Clinique Med de Levis, 100-4975 boul de la Rive-Sud, Levis QC G6V 4Z5; Laval'90; FRCPC; Psy. Staff, CSSS de Montmagny-L'Islet; (418)833-5810

TURGEON, Michel; Centre Med Ste-Foy Inc, 802 av du Chanoine-Scott, Quebec QC G1V 3N4; Laval'83; (418)653-4931; Fax. (418)653-4797.

TURGEON, Michel; Clinique Med du Cuivre, 12 rue Gamble E, Rouyn-Noranda QC J9X 3B7; Laval'85; (819)764-9441; Fax. (819)764-5792.

TURGEON, Mireille; CSSS Therese de Blainville, 125 rue Duquet, Sainte-Therese QC J7E 0A5; Laval'95; Staff, Hôpital de Saint-Eustache; (450)430-4553 x6604; Fax. (450)430-3859.

TURGEON, Nathalie; CHUQ-Hotel-Dieu de Quebec, 11 Cote du Palais, Quebec QC G1R 2J6; Laval'92; FRCPC; MedMicrobiol (Infectious Diseases). Staff, Centre Hospitalier Universitaire de Québec (CHUQ) - Siege Social; adj Prof, Universite de Montreal; Langs: English; French; (418)691-5131

TURGEON, Pierre L; Hotel-Dieu de Sorel, 400 av de l'Hotel-Dieu, Sorel-Tracy QC J3P 1N5; Mon'67; MedMicrobiol. Staff, Hôtel-Dieu de Sorel; (450)746-6000 x7221; Fax. (450)746-6018.

TURGEON, Pierre-Paul; CSSS Haut-Richelieu-Rouville, 920 bou du Seminaire N, St-Jean-sur-Richel QC J3A 1B7; Mon'74; AB; FRCPC; AnatPath. Staff, Hôpital du Haut-Richelieu; (450)359-5000 x2202; Fax. (450)359-5237.

TURGEON, Pierre-Victor; 500-235 boul René-Lévesque E, Montreal QC H2X 1N8; Mon'77; (514)395-9090; Fax. (514)395-8877.

TURGEON, Renee; CHUQ-Ctr Hosp Univ Laval, 2705 boul Laurier, Quebec QC G1V 4G2; Laval'96; Staff, Centre Hospitalier Universitaire de Quebec-CHUL; (418)656-4141

TURGEON, Sebastien; UMF Nord de Lanaudiere, 50 ch du Golf E, St-Charles-Brromee QC J6E 2B4; Sher'00; CCFP; Staff, Centre Hospitalier Régional de Lanaudière; (450)759-3060; Fax. (450)759-7799.

TURGEON, Susie A; 3998 Main St, Vancouver BC V5V 3P2; McM'82; CCFP; Clin Instructor, University of British Columbia; (604)873-3666; Fax. (604)875-8790.

TURGEON, Thomas R; Concordia Hip & Knee Institute, 310-1155 Concordia Ave, Winnipeg MB R2K 2M9; Wes'98; FRCSC; OrthSurg (Adult Reconstructive Surgery). Staff, Concordia General Hospital; Asst Prof Surg, University of Manitoba.

TURGEON-FOURNIER, Alexis; CHAQ-Hop De l'Enfant-Jesus, 1401 18e rue, Quebec QC G1J 1Z4; Laval'99; LMCC; FRCPC; Anes (Critical Care Medicine). Staff, Centre Hospitalier Affilié Universitaire de Québec - Hôpital De L'Enfant Jésus; Langs: English; (418)649-0252; alexisturgeon@yahoo.ca.

TURINECK, David T; Smooth Rock Falls Hosp, PO Box 219 107 Kelly Rd, Smooth Rock Falls ON P0L 2B0; Dublin (Ireland)'84; Staff, Smooth Rock Falls Hospital; Langs: English; French; (705)338-2781; Fax. (705)338-2933.

TURK, Allison H; Mount Pleasant Fam Practice, 245 Eglinton Ave E, Toronto ON M4P 3B7; Tor'88; BSc; CCFP; FCFP; (416)485-7663; Fax. (416)485-2671.

TURKISTANI, Yosra A A; London HSC-University Hosp, PO Box 5339 Stn B 339 Windermere Rd, London ON N6A 5A5; Umm Al Qura University (Other Foreign)'06; IntMed. Staff, London Health Sciences Centre - University Hospital; (519)663-3511

TURKSTRA, Ian; Thames Valley Family Hlth Team, RR 5 22262 Mill Rd, Mount Brydges ON N0L 1W0; Wes'09; CCFP; (519)264-2800; iant@smhc.net.

TURKSTRA, Timothy P; London HSC-University Hosp, PO Box 5339 Stn B C3104-339 Windermere Rd, London ON N6A 5A5; McM'00; FRCPC; Anes (Neuro Anesthesia). Staff Anes, London Health Sciences Centre - University Hospital; (519)663-3283

TURLAPATI, Padmini N; Ashgrove Med Centre, 306-6633 Highway 7, Markham ON L3P 7P2; Delhi (India)'63; MD; DCH; FRCPC; Peds (Developmental/Behavioural Pediatrics). Staff Peds, Markham Stouffville Hospital; Langs: Tamil; Hindi; Telugu; (905)471-8074; Fax. (905)471-8043; pturlapati@yahoo.ca.

TURLEY, Conor B; Credit Valley Med Arts Bldg, 511-2000 Credit Valley Rd, Mississauga ON L5M 4N4; Dublin (Ireland)'80; MB ChB; BAO; FRCS; FRCSC; PlasSurg (Plastic & Reconstructive Surgery). Staff, The Credit Valley Hospital; Staff, Peel Cancer Centre; Teach Staff, University of Toronto; (905)820-2453; Fax. (905)820-0812; info@drcturley.ca.

TURLEY, Jolanda C; Primrose Family Med Unit, 35 Primrose Ave, Ottawa ON K1R 0A1; McG'97; CCFP; Langs: Dutch; French; Spanish; (613)230-7788; Fax. (613)230-7778.

TURLEY, Judith J E; St Michael's Hosp, 3Q-30 Bond St, Toronto ON M5B 1W8; Tor'66; FRCPC; Neur. Staff Neurophysiology Lab, St Michael's Hospital; (416)864-5193; Fax. (416)864-6095.

TURLIUK, Robert C; 4052 New St, Burlington ON L7L 1S9; Wes'88; DOHS; (905)637-2323; Fax. (905)637-7875.

TURMEL, Andre; Ctr Hosp Affilie-Enfant-Jesus, 1401 18e rue, Quebec QC G1J 1Z4; Mon'86; Neursurg (P.Q.). Staff, Centre Hospitalier Affilié Universitaire de Québec - Hôpital De L'Enfant Jésus; (418)649-5734; Fax. (418)649-5915.

TURMEL, Bruno; Direction de la Sante Publique, 2.03-201 boul Cremazie E, Montreal QC H2M 1L2; Mon'83; Med Consultant, Ministre Sante & Services Social du Quebec; Langs: Bilingual(English/French); (514)873-1592; Fax. (514)864-2778; bruno.turmel@msss.gouv.qc.ca.

TURMEL, France; Le "388" Saint-Vallier, 388 rue Saint-Vallier O, Quebec QC G1K 1K6; Laval'72; Psy (P.Q.). (418)522-1555; Fax. (418)683-1935.

TURMEL, Linda; Clinique Med Sainte-Claire, GD 88 boul Begin, Sainte-Claire QC G0R 2V0; Laval'09; CCFP; (418)883-3336

TURMEL, Roger; Agence Santé et Serv Sociaux, 288 rue Pierre-Saindon, Rimouski QC G5L 9A8; Laval'92; FRCPC; Psy (Consultation-Liaison). Staff Psy, Hôpital Regional Rimouski; (418)724-5231

TURMEL, Serge; 19-930 ch du Fleuve, Les Cedres QC J7T 0C9; Laval'77; chef Coroner, City Of Quebec; (450)264-4661; serge.turmel@ville.quebec.qc.ca.

TURMEL, Yvan; Centre Med Ste-Anne, 100-10459 Boul Sainte Anne, St-Anne-Beaup QC G0A 3C0; Laval'74; Coroner Capitale Nationale Quebec, Edifice Wilfirid-Derome; Langs: Bilingual(French/English); (418)827-3444; yvan.turmel@msp.gouv.qc.ca.

TURMEL, Yves; Clin Med Plateau Marquette, 200-731 rue Galt O, Sherbrooke QC J1H 1Z1; Mon'79; Physician, CHSLD La Maison Blanche de North Hatley; Langs: English; (819)564-8662; Fax. (819)564-1294.

TURNBULL, D Ian; 5F-20 Dundas St W, Toronto ON M5G 2C2; McG'62; DABPath; MDCM; GenPath. (416)314-4260

TURNBULL, Geoffrey K; Wren Turnbull Medical Inc, 6123 Jubilee Rd, Halifax NS B3H 2E8; Qns'78; FRCPC; IntMed; Gastroent. Ac Staff, Queen Elizabeth II Health Sciences Centre - Victoria General Site; Prof Med, Dalhousie University; (902)473-4140; Fax. (902)473-4406; turnbull@dal.ca.

TURNBULL, Ian M; Laurel Med Centre Ltd, 202-888 8th Ave W, Vancouver BC V5Z 3Y1; UBC'57; FRCSC; Neursurg. (604)879-1925; Fax. (604)872-7394.

TURNBULL, Jeffrey M; The Ottawa Hosp-Gen Campus, LM12-501 Smyth Rd Box 100, Ottawa ON K1H 8L6; Qns'78; FRCPC; IntMed. Staff Chief, The Ottawa Hospital - General Campus; Prof Med, University of Ottawa; (613)737-8459

TURNBULL, Jennifer E S; Hop de Montreal pour Enfants, 2300 rue Tupper, Montreal QC H3H 1P3; Qns'05; FRCPC; Peds; PedEmergMed. Staff, McGill University Health Centre - Montreal Children's Hospital; (514)412-4400

TURNBULL, John D; Hamilton HS-McMaster Site, PO Box 2000 Stn Lcd 1 4U7-1200 Main St W, Hamilton ON L8N 3Z5; Wes'80; FRCPC; IntMed; Neur. Staff, Hamilton Health Sciences Centre - McMaster Children's Hospital; Langs: English; French; (905)521-2100 x76365; Fax. (905)521-2656; turnbull@mcmaster.ca.

TURNBULL, John R; 202-857 Grand Ave W, Chatham ON N7L 4T1; Wes'90; FRCSC; OrthSurg. (519)351-8200; Fax. (519)351-8118.

TURNBULL, Robert G; Tawa Centre, 205-3017 66 St NW, Edmonton AB T6K 4B2; Alb'89; FRCSC; GenSurg; VascSurg. Ad Staff, University of Alberta Hospital; Ad Staff, Covenant Health - Grey Nuns Community Hospital; Clinical Asst Prof, University of Alberta; (780)461-6012; Fax. (780)461-5442.

TURNBULL, Ruth L; Ladner Centre Medical, 513 Ladner Trunk Rd, Delta BC V4K 1W3; Sask'85; BSc(Chem.); (604)940-0321

TURNELL, Roger W; Royal Alexandra Hosp, 5S 131-10240 Kingsway NW, Edmonton AB T5H 3V9; McG'78; DAB; FACOG; FSOGC; FRCSC; ObstGyn (Maternal Fetal Medicine). Staff Perinatol, Royal Alexandra Hospital; Caritas Health Group-Edmonton; Prof ObstGyn, University of Alberta; (780)735-4812; Fax. (780)735-4981.

TURNER, A Robert; Cross Cancer Institute, 11560 University Ave NW, Edmonton AB T6G 1Z2; McG'72; DrMedCh; ABIM; CSPQ; MDCM; FRCPC; IntMed (P.Q.) (Hematological Oncology); Hem; MedOncol. Staff Clin Hem, University of Alberta Hospital; Sr Specialist, Cross Cancer Institute; Staff MedOncol, Alberta Health Services; (780)432-8514; Fax. (780)432-8888.

TURNER, Andrew J; 305-984 Oliver Rd, Thunder Bay ON P7B 7C7; Mem'81; FRCSC; Otol (Head & Neck Surgery). Staff Otol (All Sites), Thunder Bay Regional Health Sciences Centre; Asst Prof/Chief Surg, Northern Ontario School of Medicine-Lakehead University; (807)344-4334; Fax. (807)344-4111; turner@tbaytel.com.

TURNER, Bradley J; 5017 47A Ave, Delta BC V4K 1T9; Alb'83; Staff, Delta Hospital; (604)946-1168; Fax. (604)946-4251.

TURNER, Caroline A; Sheldon M Chumir Health Centre, 1213 4 St SW, Calgary AB T2R 0X7; Cal'09; CCFP; Staff Urgent Care Centre, Sheldon M Chumir Urgent Care Physician Group; (403)955-6200; caroline.turner@albertahealthservices.ca.

TURNER, Charles G W; Hants Community Hosp, 89 Payzant Dr, Windsor NS B0N 2T0; Dal'77; FRCPC; DiagRad. Staff, Hants Community Hospital; (902)792-2079; Fax. (902)792-2094.

TURNER, Christopher B; Banff Mineral Springs Hosp, PO Box 1050 Stn Main, Banff AB T1L 1H7; Alb'88; CCFP; CCFP(E.M.); FCFP; Staff, Covenant Health - Banff Mineral Springs Hospital; (403)762-2222; Fax. (403)762-4193.

TURNER, Cory C; Oshawa Clinic, 117 King St E, Oshawa ON L1H 1B9; Tor'88; FRCPC; Derm (Cosmetics). (905)723-8551; Fax. (905)721-3513.

TURNER, D Christopher; AL0701-BHPB7 Health Canada, 200 Tunney's Pasture Driveway, Ottawa ON K1A 0K9; Dal'77; BSc(Acadia); FAAP; FRCPC; Peds (Pediatric Hematology Oncology). Medical Officer Marketed Health Product directorate, Health Canada; Langs: English; French; (613)954-6522; Fax. (613)952-7738.

TURNER, David R; Brandon Reg Health Centre, 150 McTavish Ave E, Brandon MB R7A 2B3; London (England)'79; MB BS; FFARCS; BSc; FRCPC; Anes (Chronic Pain Management). Staff Anes, Brandon Regional Health Centre; (204)726-1122; Fax. (204)728-0528.

TURNER, Diana L; Carewest-Sarcee, 3504 Sarcee Rd SW, Calgary AB T3E 4T4; Cal'93; MSc; CCFP; FCFP; (403)686-8140; Fax. (403)686-8127.

TURNER, Frances N; Greenbrook Family Med Centre, 421 Greenbrook Dr, Kitchener ON N2M 4K1; Tor'85; CCFP; FCFP; (519)570-1655; Fax. (519)570-3477.

TURNER, Francois; Hotel-Dieu d'Arthabaska, 5 rue des Hospitalieres, Victoriaville QC G6P 6N2; Laval'07; Staff, Hotel-Dieu d'Arthabaska; (819)357-2030

TURNER, Genevieve; CLSC du Richelieu-Point, 1394 rue Notre-Dame, Saint-Cesaire QC J0L 1T0; Mon'98; Staff, Hôpital du Haut-Richelieu; (450)469-0269

TURNER, Holtby M; 38 King St W, Dundas ON L9H 1T7; McM'87; CCFP; FCFP; Assoc Staff FamMed, Hamilton Health Sciences Centre - McMaster Children's Hospital; (905)628-5118; Fax. (905)628-1739.

TURNER, Howard M; MUHC-Montreal Gen Hosp, A5 123-1650 av Cedar, Montreal QC H3G 1A4; Washington(DC) (USA)'91; FRCPC; IntMed (P.Q.). Staff, Douglas Mental Health University Institute; Att Staff, McGill University Health Centre - Montreal General Campus; Langs: English; French; (514)934-8070; Fax. (514)937-1424.

TURNER, J Garth E; Hys Med Centre, 202-11010 101 St NW, Edmonton AB T5H 4B9; Sask'70; FRCPC; DiagRad. Staff Radiol, Royal Alexandra Hospital; Clinical Asst Prof, University of Alberta Hospital.

TURNER, J Patricia; 109 King St W, Dundas ON L9H 1V1; McM'87; BSc(PT); CCFP; FCFP; (905)628-9200; Fax. (905)628-9600.

TURNER, Jodie R; East Kootenay Reg Hosp, 13 24th Ave N, Cranbrook BC V1C 3H9; McG'08; CCFP; CCFP(E.M.); Staff, East Kootenay Regional Hospital; (250)426-5281

TURNER, Joel P; D010-SMBD Jewish Gen Hosp, 3755 ch Cote-Sainte-Catherine, Montreal QC H3T 1E2; McG'97; FRCPC; EmergMed. Staff, Sir Mortimer B Davis Jewish General; Langs: English; French; (514)340-8222 x3898

TURNER, John J; York Prof Bldg, 220-679 Davis Dr, Newmarket ON L3Y 5G8; Tor'62; FRCPC; Derm. Staff, Toronto Western Hospital - University Health Network; Ac Staff, Southlake Regional Health Centre; Hon Staff, North York General Hospital - Branson Division; Asst Prof, University of Toronto; (905)895-6661; Fax. (905)895-7148.

TURNER, Julia A; Child & Youth Mental Health, 300-3003 St Johns St, Port Moody BC V3H 2C4; Witwatersrand (South Africa)'85; MB ChB; FFPsy; FRCPC; Psy. Staff, Ridge Meadows Hospital & Health Care Centre; (604)469-7600

TURNER, Justine M; Edmonton Clinic Health Academy, 11405 87 Ave NW, Edmonton AB T6G 1C9; Perth (Australia)'91; Staff, University of Alberta Hospital; Staff, Stollery Children's Hospital; Staff, Edmonton Clinic Health Academy; (780)248-5570; Fax. (780)248-5627.

TURNER, Katherine A; Natawihin/Nakasuwenik Med Clin, GD, Ile-a-la-Crosse SK S0M 1C0; McM'09; CCFP; (306)833-2044; Fax. (306)833-2401.

TURNER, Kim E; Kingston Gen Hosp, 76 Stuart St, Kingston ON K7L 2V7; McM'85; MSc; BSc; FRCPC; Anes. Staff, Kingston General Hospital; Assoc Prof, Queen's University; (613)548-7827; Fax. (613)548-1375.

TURNER, Lary J; Appletree Med Centre, 207-267 O'Connor St, Ottawa ON K2P 1V3; Tor'60; FRCPC; IntMed (Gastroenterology). Asst Prof Med, University of Ottawa; (613)567-8000; Fax. (613)567-8022; larryjturner@rogers.com.

TURNER, Laurence J; Royal City Med Bldg, 208-250 Keary St, New Westminster BC V3L 5E7; London (England)'69; MB BS; LRCP; MRCS; FACS; MA; FRCSC; GenSurg (Abdominal Surgery). Staff Consultant Surg, Royal Columbian Hospital; Staff Consultant, Eagle Ridge Hospital & Health Care Centre; Clin Assoc Prof Surg, University of British Columbia; (604)526-3721; Fax. (604)526-3811.

TURNER, Lesley A; Dr Charles H Janeway Child HC, 300 Prince Philip Dr, St. John's NL A1B 3V6; Mem'97; FRCPC; Peds (Medical Genetics). Staff, Janeway Children's Health & Rehabilitation Centre; (709)777-4390

TURNER, Lisa A; 84 Dufferin Ave, Saint John NB E2K 2T8; Dal'02; CCFP.

TURNER, M Dawn; Mitchell Family Doctors, PO Box 790 7 Frances St, Mitchell ON N0K 1N0; Mem'03; CCFP; Staff Family Med, Stratford General Hospital - Huron Perth Healthcare Alliance; (519)348-8402; Fax. (519)348-8400.

TURNER, Marci R; Malvern Med Centre, 100-1333 Neilson Rd, Scarborough ON M1B 4Y9; Wes'07; FRCPC; IntMed; Endocrin&Metab; ObstGyn. Staff, The Scarborough Hospital - Birchmount Campus; (416)291-7719; Fax. (416)287-3775.

TURNER, Maria D; Mitchell Family Doctors, PO Box 790 7 Francis St, Mitchell ON N0K 1N0; Mem'03; CCFP; (519)348-8402; Fax. (519)348-8400.

TURNER, Mark O; Windsor Square Shopp Centre, 241-1959 152 St, Surrey BC V4A 9E3; McG'85; FRCPC; IntMed; Respir. Staff, Peace Arch Hospital; Clinical Asst Prof Med, University of British Columbia; Langs: English; French; (604)531-5781; Fax. (604)531-5791.

TURNER, Mary Ann S; Fort Med Clinic, 101-6603 132 Ave NW, Edmonton AB T5C 2A4; Baltimore(MD) (USA)'76; (780)476-1388; Fax. (780)473-3530.

TURNER, Michel; 210-900 boul du Seminaire N, St-Jean-Sur-Richel QC J3A 1C3; Mon'70; (450)348-1118; Fax. (450)348-9998.

TURNER, Paul V; Perth Med Clinic, 14 Isabella St, Perth ON K7H 2W6; Wes'76; CCFP; FCFP; (613)267-2574; Fax. (613)267-3723.

TURNER, Penny A; Mackenzie Richmond Hill Hosp, 10 Trench St, Richmond Hill ON L4C 4Z3; Alb'98; FRCPC; IntMed; Nephrol. Staff, Mackenzie Richmond Hill Hospital; (905)883-2065; Fax. (905)883-2065.

TURNER, Peter G; 301-720 Guelph Line, Burlington ON L7R 4E2; Otago (New Zealand)'71; MB ChB; FRCPC; Psy (Mood Disorders). Consultant Staff Continuing Care Clinic, Joseph Brant Memorial Hospital; Consultant Psy, Halton Healthcare Services Corporation - Oakville Site; Member, St Joseph's Healthcare Hamilton - West 5th Campus; Staff, Schizophrenia Mood & Anxiety Disorders Clinic; Asst Clin Prof Psy & Behavioural Sciences, McMaster University; Langs: German; (905)631-9650; Fax. (905)631-9549.

TURNER, R Douglas; Burnham Med Clinic, 103-380 Burnham St, Peterborough ON K9H 1T6; Qns'72; (705)748-4041; Fax. (705)748-3907.

TURNER, Richard H; Manning Med Clinic, GD, Manning AB T0H 2M0; Leeds (England)'75; MB ChB; MRCS; LRCP; CCFP; (780)836-2811

TURNER, Richard J; Medical Imaging Cons Hys Ctre, 105-11010 101 St NW, Edmonton AB T5H 4B9; Alb'96; FRCPC; DiagRad. (780)426-1121; Fax. (780)425-5979.

TURNER, Robert B; Aesthetic Solutions, 10-1250 Waverley St, Winnipeg MB R3T 6C6; Man'89; FRCSC; PlasSurg. (204)927-3500

TURNER, Robert L; Westgrove Med Clinic, 200-10230 142 St NW, Edmonton AB T5N 3Y6; Alb'94; CCFP; (780)454-4242; Fax. (780)454-4224.

TURNER, Roy; Rockyview Gen Hosp, 7007 14 St SW, Calgary AB T2V 1P9; Cal'98; BSc(Physiology); FRCPC; Psy. Staff, Rockyview General Hospital; (403)943-3808; Fax. (403)259-6289.

TURNER, S Patrick D; University Hosp of Northern BC, 1475 Edmonton St, Prince George BC V2M 1S2; UBC'97; CCFP; CCFP(E.M.); Staff, University Hospital of Northern British Columbia; (250)565-2000; Fax. (250)565-2466.

TURNER, Sheldon A; Weston Med Centre, 1953 Weston Rd, York ON M9N 1W8; McM'80; CCFP; Assoc Staff, Humber River Regional Hospital - Church Street Site; Instructor, Sunnybrook Health Sciences Centre; Instructor, University of Toronto; (416)248-5539; Fax. (416)248-0520.

TURNER, Shelley A M; Anishnawbe Mushkiki, 29 Royston Crt, Thunder Bay ON P7B 2L2; McM'06; CCFP; Associate Family & ER, Grey Bruce Health Services - Lion's Head; Associate, Collingwood General & Marine Hospital; (807)343-4843; Fax. (807)343-4728; turners@tc.gc.ca.

TURNER, Simon R; University of Alberta Hosp, 8440 112 St NW, Edmonton AB T6G 2B7; Alb'07; Staff, University of Alberta Hospital; (780)407-8822

TURNER, Stephen A; Centre Hosp Fleury, 2180 rue Fleury E, Montreal QC H2B 1K3; Qns'98; FRCPC; IntMed; MedMicrobiol; InfectDis. Staff, Centre Hospitalier Fleury; (514)381-9311 x5063

TURNER, Steven L; 4607 50 Ave PO Box 3955 Stn Main, Olds AB T4H 1P6; Cal'87; CCFP; FCFP; Chief FamilyMed, Olds Hospital & Care Centre; (403)556-7130; Fax. (403)556-1944.

TURNER, Stuart G; Rockyview Gen Hosp, 7007 14 St SW, Calgary AB T2V 1P9; UBC'76; FRCPC; EmergMed. Staff Emerg, Rockyview General Hospital; (403)943-3449; Fax. (403)943-3220.

TURNER, Suzanne D; St Michael's Hosp, 30 Bond St, Toronto ON M5B 1W8; Tor'10; CCFP; Staff, St Michael's Hospital; (416)360-4000

TURNER, Timothy J; 302-717 Richmond St, London ON N6A 1S2; Wes'72; FRCPC; Psy. Aj Prof Psy, University of Western Ontario; (519)438-1128; Fax. (519)438-8187.

TURNER, Troy W S; Edmonton Clinic Health Academy, 11405 87 Ave, Edmonton AB T6G 1C9; Sask'96; LMCC; FRCPC; Peds (Pediatric Emergency Medicine). Att Staff Ped, University of Alberta Hospital; Staff, Edmonton Clinic Health Academy; Clin Teacher Med, University of Alberta; (780)248-5575; Fax. (780)248-5625; twstmd@hotmail.com.

TURNER, Tyrone S; St Joseph's Health Centre, 4SSW-423-30 The Queensway, Toronto ON M6R 1B5; Qns'71; FRCPC; Psy (Hospitalist);CCFP; Staff Psy, St Joseph's Health Centre; Staff Psy, Sault Area Hospital - Sault Ste Marie; Lecturer, University of Toronto; (416)530-6788; Fax. (416)530-6076.

TURNER-GOMES, Sophronia O; Finchgate Med Centre, 312-40 Finchgate Blvd, Brampton ON L6T 3J1; Edinburgh (Scotland)'75; FRCPC; Peds (Pediatric Cardiology); Cardiol. (905)792-2314; Fax. (905)792-3901.

TURNHAM, Lucy M; Children's & Women's HC Of BC, 1A41-4480 Oak St, Vancouver BC V6H 3V4; UBC'89; BA; MB; Clin Associate HemOncol, BC Children's Hospital; Langs: Spanish; French; (604)875-3575; Fax. (604)875-3414; lturnham@cw.bc.ca.

TURPIE, Alexander G G; Hamilton HS-General Site, 237 Barton St E, Hamilton ON L8L 2X2; Glasgow (Scotland)'62; FRCP(Lond); FRCP; FACP; FACC; FRCPC; IntMed (Thrombosis). Emeritus Staff, Hamilton Health Sciences Centre - Hamilton General Hospital; Prof, McMaster University; (905)527-1710; turpiea@mcmaster.ca.

TURPIE, Fiona H I; Hamilton HS-McMaster Site, PO Box 2000 Stn Lcd 1 1200 Main St W, Hamilton ON L8N 3Z5; McM'94; Anes; IntMed. Staff, Hamilton Health Sciences Centre - McMaster Children's Hospital; (905)521-2100; Fax. (905)521-5090.

TURPIE, Irene D; East Region Mental Hlth Serv, 2757 King St E, Hamilton ON L8G 5E4; Glasgow (Scotland)'64; MB ChB; MSc; FACP; FRCPC; IntMed; GeriatricMed. Med Dir Health for Older Adults Prog, St Joseph's Centre for Ambulatory Health Services; Physician, East Region Mental Health Services; Dir Div of Geriatric Med, McMaster University; (905)573-4804; turpiei@mcmaster.ca.

TURPIN, Galina; Silverfern Walk-In Clinic, 160 Jubilee St, Duncan BC V9L 1W7; (Other Foreign)'87; CCFP; (250)709-9600

TURPIN, Sophie M B; Hôpital Ste-Justine, 3175 ch Cote-Sainte-Catherine, Montreal QC H3T 1C5; Mon'88; FRCPC; NuclearMed. Staff, Centre Hospitalier l'Université de Montréal (CHUM) - Hôtel-Dieu; Staff, Hôpital Ste-Justine; (514)345-4684

TURQUI, Farida; Centre Hosp de LaSalle, 8585 tsse Champlain, LaSalle QC H8P 1C1; (Other Foreign)'02; CCFP; Staff, Centre Hospitalier de LaSalle; (514)363-3985

TURSKI, Edgar R; 1-1230 Alward St, Prince George BC V2M 7B1; UBC'79; CCFP; FCFP; Ac Staff, University Hospital of Northern British Columbia; (250)563-8151; Fax. (250)563-9211; edturski@shaw.ca.

TURVEY, Erin A; Guelph Family Health Team, 83 Dawson Rd, Guelph ON N1H 1B1; McM'03; CCFP; (519)766-1360

TURVEY, Stuart E; Children's & Women's HC of BC, B321-4480 Oak St, Vancouver BC V6H 3V4; Sydney (Australia)'96; FRCPC; Peds; ClinImmunol&Allergy. Staff, BC Children's Hospital; (604)875-2345

TUSHINSKI, Morris; Family Physicians, 1-390 Steeles Ave W, Thornhill ON L4J 6X2; Tor'75; CCFP; FCFP; Staff, Sunnybrook Health Sciences Centre; Staff, Mackenzie Richmond Hill Hospital; Staff, St John's Rehabilitation Hospital; University of Toronto; (905)881-3984; Fax. (905)881-3198.

TUSZYNSKA, Hanna M; Hamilton HS-General Site, 237 Barton St E, Hamilton ON L8L 2X2; Gdansk (Poland)'85; FRCPC; Anes. Fellow, Hamilton Health Sciences Centre - Hamilton General Hospital; Langs: Spanish; Polish; (905)527-4322 x6698

TUTERS, Kaspars B; 9-315 Avenue Rd, Toronto ON M4V 2H2; Tor'63; FRCPC; Psy. Asst Prof, University of Toronto; Langs: Latvian; German; (416)964-6777; Fax. (416)964-8647; k.tuters@utoronto.ca.

TUTSCHKA, Bridget K; Thames Valley FHT-W London, 2F-785 Wonderland Rd S, London ON N6K 1M6; Dal'06; CCFP; Langs: Bilingual(English/French); (519)641-6712; Fax. (519)641-6189; btutschka@uwo.ca.

TUTTLE, Irene M; 10D-67 Caroline St S, Hamilton ON L8P 3K6; Aberdeen (Scotland)'70; MB ChB; DObst; RC.

TUTTLE, John R; Rockyview Gen Hosp, 7007 14 St SW, Calgary AB T2V 1P9; Cal'82; FRCPC; Psy. Staff Addictions & Mental Health, Rockyview General Hospital; (403)943-8704; Fax. (403)259-6289.

TUTTLE, Peggy F; Carbonear Gen Hosp, 86 Highroad S, Carbonear NL A1Y 1A4; Mem'07; GenSurg. Staff, Carbonear General Hospital; (709)945-5111

TUTUNCUOGLU, Suleyman O; Northern Lights Health Region, 7 Hospital St., Fort McMurray AB T9H 1P2; (Turkey)'87; Staff, Northern Lights Regional Health Centre; (780)791-6151; Fax. (780)791-6057.

TUVEL, Brandon R; Kootenay Lake Gen Hosp, 426-3 View St, Nelson BC V1L 2V1; Qns'08; FRCPC; IntMed. Staff, Kootenay Lake General Hospital; (250)352-3111

TUVIVOVICH, Victoria E; CSSS du Suroit, 201-181 rue Victoria, Salaber-de-Valleyf QC J6T 1A7; Kazkov (Ukraine)'85; Staff, Centre Hospitalier Régional du Suroît; Langs: Russian; French; Ukrainian; Hebrew; (450)373-6252; Fax. (450)371-4910.

TUWOR, George; PO Box 158, Fort Qu'Appelle SK S0G 1S0; (England)'92; CCFP; (306)332-4460; Fax. (306)332-4822.

TUYP, Evert J; 218-3030 Lincoln Ave, Coquitlam BC V3B 6B4; Wes'79; DABD; FRCPC; Derm. Consultant, Royal Columbian Hospital; Clinical Asst Prof, University of British Columbia; (604)941-3342

TWEED, W Arnold; The Salvation Army Grace Hosp, 300 Booth Dr, Winnipeg MB R3J 3M7; Man'64; MD; FRCPC; Anes. Staff, The Salvation Army Grace Hospital; (204)837-0391; arnold.tweed@uhn.on.ca.

TWEEDDALE, Mary E; Mackenzie Richmond Hill Hosp, 10 Trench St, Richmond Hill ON L4C 4Z3; Tor'78; MSc; FRCPC; IntMed (Oncology); Hem. Staff, Mackenzie Richmond Hill Hospital; Lecturer, University of Toronto; (905)883-1212 x3590; Fax. (905)883-2156.

TWEEDIE, Edward J; London HSC-University Hosp, PO Box 5339 Stn B 339 Windermere Rd, London ON N6A 5A5; Wes'90; FRCPC; AnatPath (Forensic Pathology). Staff, London Health Sciences Centre - University Hospital; Assoc Prof Path, University of Western Ontario; (519)685-8500 x36351; Fax. (519)663-2930.

TWEEDIE, James W; Perth Med Clinic, 14 Isabella St, Perth ON K7H 2W6; Qns'55; Ac Staff, Perth & Smiths Falls District Hospital - Perth Site (Great War Memorial Site); (613)267-5687; Fax. (613)267-3745.

TWEEDIE, T Cameron; Owen Sound Med Centre, 2000-1415 1st Ave W, Owen Sound ON N4K 4K8; Wes'88; CCFP; CCFP(E.M.); FCFP; Ac Staff, Grey Bruce Health Services - Owen Sound; (519)376-9561; Fax. (519)370-4041.

TWEEDLE, Shelley D; Royal Columbian Hosp, 330 Columbia St E, New Westminster BC V3L 3W7; UBC'06; Anes. Staff, Vancouver General Hospital - Centennial Pavillion; Staff, Royal Columbian Hospital; (604)520-4605

TWEEL, Douglas K H; Polyclinic Prof Centre Inc, 201-199 Grafton St, Charlottetown PE C1A 1L2; Dal'80; BSc; (902)629-8843; Fax. (902)628-6024.

TWELKER, Sunny S; Thunder Bay Reg HSC, 980 Oliver Rd, Thunder Bay ON P7B 6V4; Cal'02; CCFP; CCFP(E.M.); Staff, Thunder Bay Regional Health Sciences Centre; (807)684-6000

TWEMLOW, Diane W; Central Med Bldg, 401-1105 Carling Ave, Ottawa ON K1Y 4G5; Ott'78; CCFP; FCFP; Staff, The Ottawa Hospital - Civic Campus; Asst Prof Family Med, University of Ottawa; (613)729-5812; Fax. (613)729-2867.

TWEMLOW, Gregory D; Quinte HC Corp-Belleville Gen, 265 Dundas St E, Belleville ON K8N 5A9; Ott'83; FRCPC; GenPath. Associate/Chief Path, QHC Belleville General; (613)969-5511; Fax. (613)968-9912.

TWIDDY, Ronald R; 104 Main St PO Box 1540, Brighton ON K0K 1H0; Qns'80; Ac Staff, QHC Trenton Memorial; (613)475-1285; Fax. (613)475-1287.

TWISS, Jennifer E; Hamilton HS-McMaster Site, PO Box 2000 Stn Lcd 1 1200 Main St W, Hamilton ON L8N 3Z5; Cal'05; FRCPC; Peds. Staff, Hamilton Health Sciences Centre - McMaster Children's Hospital; (905)521-2100

TWIST, David L; Pain Management Clinic, 9750 140 St, Surrey BC V3T 0G9; Sask'86; FRCPC; Anes (Pain Management). Staff, BC Cancer Agency Fraser Valley Centre; Staff, Surrey Memorial Hospital; (604)582-4587

TWOMEY, Ciaran F; Clinical Sciences Bldg, 8152-152 University Campus NW, Edmonton AB T6G 2G3; (Ireland)'94; Staff, University of Alberta Hospital; (780)407-8861

TWUM-BARIMA, David Y; Trafalgar Prof Centre, 412-1235 Trafalgar Rd, Oakville ON L6H 3P1; Accra (Ghana)'74; MSc; MB ChB; FRCPC; IntMed (Endocrinology). Langs: Akan; (905)337-0040; Fax. (905)337-0044; yaw.twum-barima@lmc.ca.

TY, Patricia L; McKenzie Prof Centre, 200-1595 McKenzie Ave, Victoria BC V8N 1A4; UBC'91; (250)721-4105

TYBERG, Jeffrey P; Sunnybrook Health Sciences Ctr, C753-2075 Bayview Ave, Toronto ON M4N 3M5; McG'85; FRCPC; EmergMed. Med Dir/Chief Emerg Serv, Toronto East General Hospital Inc; Staff, Sunnybrook Health Sciences Centre; Asst Prof Med, University of Toronto; (416)480-6100; Fax. (416)480-4704.

TYEBKHAN, Juzer M; Royal Alexandra Hosp, 10240 Kingsway NW, Edmonton AB T5H 3V9; London (England)'85; MB BS; MRCP(UK); FRCPC; Peds (Neonatal & Perinatal Medicine). Staff Neonatol, Royal Alexandra Hospital; Asst Prof Peds, University of Alberta; Langs: Gujarati; (780)735-4670; Fax. (780)735-4072; Juzer.Tyebkhan@capitalhealth.ca.

TYLDESLEY, Scott K; BC Cancer Agency-Vancouver CC, 600 10th Ave W, Vancouver BC V5Z 4E6; UBC'93; FRCPC; RadOncol. Staff, BC Cancer Agency Vancouver Centre; (604)877-6000; Fax. (604)708-2000.

TYLER, Ingrid V L; OAHPP, 300-480 University Ave, Toronto ON M5G 1V2; UBC'02; CCFP; Public Health & Preventive Med; CommunMed. Staff Family Hlth Centre, Toronto Western Hospital - University Health Network; (647)260-7302; Fax. (647)260-7600.

TYLER, James B; 200-128 Penetang St, Barrie ON L4M 1V6; Ross University (Dominica)'02.

TYLER, Joan C; Lorraine Wing Tower C, 201 Deacon St, Pembroke ON K8A 2J6; Ott'83; CCFP; FCFP; Staff, Pembroke Regional Hospital Inc; Langs: Bilingual(French/English); (613)732-5777; Fax. (613)732-5774; jctyler@sympatico.ca.

TYLER, Melissa J; Family Med Centre, 220 Bagot St, Kingston ON K7L 3G2; UBC'08; CCFP; (613)533-9303

TYMCHAK, Wayne J; University of Alberta Hosp, 2C2 WCM-8440 112 St NW, Edmonton AB T6G 2B7; Alb'79; FRCPC; IntMed (Intensive Care); Cardiol. Dir Stollery Children's Cardiac Cath Lab & Reg Anticoagulation Clinic/CCU, University of Alberta Hospital; Prof Med, University of Alberta; Langs: Ukrainian; (780)407-1574; Fax. (780)407-6452.

TYMCHAK, Zane A; Wall Street Med Bldg, 220-140 Wall St, Saskatoon SK S7K 1N4; Sask'83; (306)653-5522; Fax. (306)653-1723.

TYMIANSKI, Michael; Univ Hlth Network-Toronto Western Hosp, WW4 435-399 Bathurst St, Toronto ON M5T 2S8; Tor'87; PhD; FRCSC; Neursurg. Sr Scientist, Toronto Western Hospital - University Health Network; (416)603-5896; Fax. (416)603-5298.

TYNAN, Iain E T; Nicola Med Dental Bldg, 400-321 Nicola St, Kamloops BC V2C 6G6; UBC'90; FRCPC; IntMed. (250)314-3601

TYNAN, Jennifer R; Royal University Hosp, 103 Hospital Dr, Saskatoon SK S7N 0W8; Sask'05; FRCPC; DiagRad. Staff, Royal University Hospital; Langs: Bilingual(English/French); (306)655-2371; Fax. (306)655-2370.

TYNAN, Maebh E; Dr E Medical & Travel Clinic, 5-4550 Ebenezer Rd, Brampton ON L6P 2R2; Dublin (Ireland)'84; CCFP; (905)794-4277; Fax. (905)794-7211.

TYNDALL, Mark W; The Ottawa Hosp-Gen Campus, G8-501 Smyth Rd, Ottawa ON K1H 8L6; McM'85; DSc; FRCPC; IntMed (Infectious Diseases-HIV/AIDS). Staff, The Ottawa Hospital - General Campus; (613)737-8899; mtyndall@cfenet.ubc.ca.

TYNDEL, Felix J; Bridlewood Prof Centre, 208-3443 Finch Ave E, Scarborough ON M1W 2S1; Tor'79; BSc; FRCPC; IntMed (Neuro Ophthalmology); Neur. Staff, The Scarborough Hospital - Birchmount Campus; Assoc Staff, Toronto Western Hospital - University Health Network; Asst Prof Neurol, University of Toronto; Langs: German; (416)773-0418; Fax. (416)773-0109.

TYNSKI, Gregory F; 535 Main St, Kentville NS B4N 1L4; Dal'87; FRCSC; ObstGyn. Staff ObsGyn, Valley Regional Hospital; (902)678-9679; Fax. (902)678-9569.

TYRELL, Benjamin D; Hilltop Med Clinic, 140-15321 16 Ave, Surrey BC V4A 1R6; London (England)'88; (604)531-5575

TYRRELL, Allison O; 107-3885 Duke of York Blvd, Mississauga ON L5B 0E4; Ross University (USA)'00; (905)366-4441; Fax. (905)366-4443.

TYRRELL, Benjamin; Edmonton Cardiology Cons, 350-11010 101 St NW, Edmonton AB T5H 4B9; Wes'00; FRCPC; IntMed (Interventional Cardiology); Cardiol. Staff, Royal Alexandra Hospital; Staff, University of Alberta Hospital; (780)428-3246; Fax. (780)425-0487.

TYRRELL, D Lorne J; Katz-Rexall Centre, 6010-1A University Campus NW, Edmonton AB T6G 2E1; Alb'68; PhD(Pharm); FRCPC; IntMed (Infectious Diseases). Ac Staff, Cross Cancer Institute; Consultant, Royal Alexandra Hospital; Ac Staff, University of Alberta Hospital; Prof Med Microbiol & Immunol, University of Alberta; (780)492-8415; Fax. (780)492-5304.

TYRRELL, Derek J; Pert Med Clinic, 14 Isabella St, Perth ON K7H 2W6; Dublin (Ireland)'73; MB ChB; DObstRCOG; DCH; (613)267-3742; Fax. (613)267-3745.

TYSDAL, Margaret A; Professional Med Associates, 550 Main St N, Moose Jaw SK S6H 3K3; Sask'76; Staff, Moose Jaw Union Hospital; Staff, Professional Medical Associates; (306)694-1061; Fax. (306)692-2080.

TYSDALE, Kim G; 4-246 Dundas St S, Cambridge ON N1R 8A8; McM'87; CCFP; FCFP; (519)623-4131; Fax. (519)623-4119.

TYSON, Caroline B; Royal Cloumbian Hosp, 330 Columbia St E, New Westminster BC V3L 3W7; UBC'03; FRCPC; EmergMed. Staff, Royal Columbian Hospital; (604)520-4253

TYSON, John E A; RR 3, Clifford ON N0G 1M0; Wes'60; FACS; AB; FACOG; FRCSC; ObstGyn (Reproductive Endocrinology). Dir-Dev, Society of Gynecologic Investigations; Med Dir, CARE Health Resources; (519)338-3499; Fax. (519)338-3888; jtcare@aol.com.

TYSON, Nerissa A; 300-149 Pacifice Ave N, Saskatoon SK S7K 1N8; Cal'07; ObstGyn. (306)653-5970; Fax. (306)653-5383.

TYSON, Thom V; Appletree Med Centre, 2948 Baseline Rd, Ottawa ON K2H 8T5; Qns'89; Langs: English; French; (613)288-0417; Fax. (613)288-2060.

TYTUS, Richard H; 700 Main St E, Hamilton ON L8M 1K7; McM'80; CCFP; FCFP; (905)545-1376; ricktytus@aol.com.

TZAKAS, Peter; 1871 Danforth Ave, Toronto ON M4C 1J4; Birmingham (England)'06; CCFP; (416)699-7775; Fax. (416)699-7776.

TZANETOS, Katina; Univ Hlth Network-Toronto Gen, 14EN 224-200 Elizabeth St, Toronto ON M5G 2C4; McM'97; FRCPC; IntMed (Clinician Investigator Program). Staff, Toronto General Hospital - UHN; Langs: Greek; (416)340-5189; Fax. (416)595-5826.

TZENEFF, Simeon G; Medical Expertise Division, 178-333 North River Rd, Ottawa ON K1A 0L1; Ott'69; Langs: English; French; (613)941-6943; Fax. (613)952-8466.

TZEROVSKA, Rayka I; Lakeridge Health Corp-Oshawa, 1 Hospital Crt, Oshawa ON L1G 2B9; Sofia (Bulgaria)'82; FRCPC; Anes (Cardiovascular Anesthesia). Staff, Lakeridge Health - Oshawa Site; (905)576-8711

TZIOUGRAS, Petra; D-170 Rebecca St, Oakville ON L6K 1J6; Wes'87; Staff, Halton Healthcare Services Corporation - Oakville Site; (905)842-2174; Fax. (905)842-8071; drptziougras@live.ca.

TZOUANNIS, Nicholas; Inst Geriatrie de Sherbrooke, 375 rue Argyll, Sherbrooke QC J1J 3H5; Sher'06; CCFP; Staff, Institut Universitaire de Geriatrie de Sherbrooke-Pavillon Argyll; (819)780-2222

UBAIDAT, Manaf; Hopital Regional Chaleur, 1750 Sunset Dr, Bathurst NB E2A 4L7; (Jordan)'94; AnatPath (Clinical Pathology). Staff, Hopital Regional Chaleur; (506)544-2330

UBANI, Nelson C; 305-5950 ch Cote-des-Neiges, Montreal QC H3S 1Z6; McG'67; BSc(Hons.); GenSurg.

UBEDA, Ivan; CSSS de la Haute-Gaspésie, 50 rue du Belvedere, Ste-Anne-des-Monts QC G4V 1X4; Laval'10; CCFP; Staff, Centre Hospitalier des Monts; (418)763-2261

UBHI, Jagdeep S; 401-223 Nelson's Cres, New Westminster BC V3L 0E4; Sask'94; FRCSC; ObstGyn. Staff, Royal Columbian Hospital; Staff, Eagle Ridge Hospital & Health Care Centre; Langs: Punjabi; Hindi; (604)777-1703; Fax. (604)777-1761.

UBHI, Mandeep S; 21st Medical Clinic, 502-402 21st St E, Saskatoon SK S7K 0C3; Sask'96; CRCP; FRCPC; IntMed; Respir. Langs: Punjabi; (306)956-3444; Fax. (306)956-3577.

UBHI, Perminder S; 2137 4 Ave NW, Calgary AB T2N 0N6; London (England)'80; FRCPC; PhysMed&Rehab. Staff Psy, Foothills Medical Centre; Asst Prof Clin Neurosciences, University of Calgary; Langs: Punjabi; (403)670-7020; Fax. (403)670-7022.

UBHI, Ram S; West Winds Med Clinic, 2130-4818 Westwinds Dr NE, Calgary AB T3J 3Z5; Cardiff (Wales)'67; MB ChB; Langs: Punjabi; Hindi; Urdu; (403)293-5454; Fax. (403)293-1511.

UBHI, Surinder K; Medi Plus II, 1146-4818 Westwinds Dr NE, Calgary AB T3J 3Z5; Punjab (India)'68; MB BS; MRCS(Eng); LRCP(Lond); CCFP; Langs: Punjabi; Hindi; Urdu; (403)293-5454; Fax. (403)293-1511.

UBHI, Verjinderpal S; 5B-1474 Pickwick Dr, Mississauga ON L5V 2G2; London (England)'80; DCH; DRCOG; MRCGPract; CCFP; Staff, The Credit Valley Hospital; Langs: Swahili; Punjabi; Hindi; (905)812-0700; Fax. (905)812-7501.

UCAR, Colin D; Timmins & District Hosp, 700 Ross Ave E, Timmins ON P4N 8P2; Wes'99; MA; CCFP; Locum Tenens, Timmins & District Hospital; (519)614-2112

UCHMAN, Dubravka; Medical Arts Centre, 103-650 Terminal Ave S, Nanaimo BC V9R 5E2; UBC'09; CCFP; (250)753-3431

UDAYA SHANKAR, Sachidanandam; Oshawa Clinic, 117 King St E, Oshawa ON L1H 1B9; Madras (India)'76; FRCPC; Psy. (905)721-3529; Fax. (905)721-3516.

UDAYASANKAR, Vijayalakshmi; Victoria Square Med Clinic, 218-2345 10th Ave W, Prince Albert SK S6V 7V6; Dr M G R Medical University (India)'95; MRCOG(UK); FRCSC; ObstGyn. (306)764-9266; Fax. (306)764-9267.

UDDIN, A H M Jamal; Markham College Med Clinic, 402-474 College St, Toronto ON M6G 1A4; Dacca (Bangladesh)'58; ABIM; FRCPC; IntMed (Rheumatology). Ac Staff, North York General Hospital - Branson Division; Langs: Bengali; Hindi; Urdu; (416)922-4335; Fax. (416)922-7905; ju511@rogers.com.

UDDIN, Fatima; 225 Queen St E, Toronto ON M5A 1S4; Tor'08; CCFP; Langs: Bengali; (416)360-0486; Fax. (416)365-1083.

UDDIN, Iftikhar; Lloydminster Hosp, 3820 43 Ave, Lloydminster SK S9V 1Y5; Staff, Lloydminster Hospital; (306)820-6000

UDDIN, Sameena; The Credit Valley Hosp, 2200 Eglinton Ave W, Mississauga ON L5M 2N1; Wes'03; FRCSC; ThorSurg (Thoracic Oncology); GenSurg. Staff, The Credit Valley Hospital; Langs: Urdu; French; Hindi; (905)813-1100 x1841; Fax. (905)813-4024.

UDECHUKWU, Maurice U; St Clare's Mercy Hosp, 154 LeMarchant Rd, St. John's NL A1C 5B8; Ibadan (Nigeria)'87; ABIM; Staff, St Clare's Mercy Hospital; (709)777-5000

UDELL, Jacob A; Women's College Hosp, 76 Grenville St, Toronto ON M5S 1B2; Tor'03; FRCPC; IntMed; Cardiol. Staff, Women's College Hospital; (416)323-7723; Fax. (416)323-6304.

UDJUS TEITELBAUM, Kristin; Children's Hosp Eastern Ont, 401 Smyth Rd, Ottawa ON K1H 8L1; Bergen (Norway)'74; FRCPC; DiagRad. Staff, Children's Hospital of Eastern Ontario (CHEO); Asst Prof, University of Ottawa; Langs: Norwegian; (613)737-2305; Fax. (613)737-2306.

UDOEYOP, Emmanuel U J; 117 First St E, Cornwall ON K6H 1K8; Ibadan (Nigeria)'83; MRCOG(UK); FWACS; FRCSC; ObstGyn (Urogynecology). Clinical Asst Prof, University of Ottawa; Langs: Ibibio; Yoruba; (613)932-2800; Fax. (613)936-2700.

UDOEYOP, Victoria I; 671 River Rd, Gloucester ON K1V 2G2; Univesity of Jos (Nigeria)'92; MB BS; CCFP; (613)822-0487; Fax. (613)822-0073.

UDOLU, Owhoede J; Cape Breton Reg Hosp, 1482 George St, Sydney NS B1P 1P3; University of Port Harcourt (Other Foreign)'98; FRCPC; Psy. Staff, Cape Breton Healthcare Complex; (902)567-7730

UDUPA, Sharmila; Children's Hosp of Eastern Ont, 401 Smyth Rd, Ottawa ON K1H 8L1; McG'07; MDCM; Peds (Cardiology). Staff, Children's Hospital of Eastern Ontario (CHEO); (613)737-7600

UDWADIA, Rushad T; Westminster Med Bldg, 701-625 Fifth Ave, New Westminster BC V3M 1X4; Bombay (India)'84; FICS; MB BS; FACS; MS; FRCSC; GenSurg (Trauma). Langs: Punjabi; Hindi; Farsi; (604)524-3133; Fax. (604)524-6716.

UETRECHT, Jack P; University of Toronto, 144 College St, Toronto ON M5S 3M2; Ohio State University (USA)'75; PhD; FACP; Staff, Sunnybrook Health Sciences Centre; Prof Faculty of Pharmacy, University of Toronto; (416)978-8939

UFFEN, Kenneth F; Grey Bruce Health Services, 369 Mary St, Wiarton ON N0H 2T0; Tor'76; CCFP; FCFP; Prog Dir Post Grads/Chair, North York General Hospital; Staff, Grey Bruce Health Services - Wiarton Site; Staff E W Bickle Centre, Toronto Rehabilitation Institute - Queen Elizabeth Centre; Asst Prof Med, University of Toronto; (519)534-2411; Fax. (519)534-2413.

UGABI, Solomon; 721 Millidge Ave, Saint John NB E2K 2N7; Zaporozhye (Other Foreign)'86.

UGARTE TORRES, Alejandra; Rockyview Gen Hosp, 7007 14 St SW, Calgary AB T2V 1P9; Staff, Rockyview General Hospital.

UGOLINI, Patricia; Hop Maisonneuve-Rosemont, 5415 boul de l'Assomption, Montreal QC H1T 2M4; Mon'92; FRCPC; DiagRad (Cardiovascular Imaging). Staff, Hopital Maisonneuve-Rosemont; Staff, Institut de Cardiologie de Montréal; assoc Staff, Centre Hospitalier l'Université De Montréal (CHUM) - Hôpital Saint-luc; pers Prof, Universite de Montreal; Langs: English; (514)252-3535; Fax. (514)252-3537; pugolini.hmr@ssss.gouv.qc.ca.

UGWOKE, Ethelbert T C; James Paton Mem Hosp, 125 Trans Canada Hwy, Gander NL A1V 1P7; (Nigeria)'87; MB BS; Staff, James Paton Memorial Hospital; (709)256-2500

UGWUMBA, Rukevwe; Downtown Physician's Clinic, 3125E Woodhams Dr, Regina SK S4V 2R5; Benin (Nigeria)'93; LRCS; MRCGPract; DTMH; LRCP; LMCC; LMSSA; MB BS; MSc; PhD; MCFP; CCFP; (306)522-3043; Fax. (306)525-0154.

UH, Mitchell; Business Bldg, 800-1200 Burrard St, Vancouver BC V6Z 2C7; UBC'08; IntMed. (604)806-9400

UHLIG, Eric L P; Downtown Doctors Med Centre, 418-720 Spadina Ave, Toronto ON M5S 2T9; Tor'84; MASc; DIH; Staff, Salvation Army Harbour Light Centre; (416)929-1530; Fax. (416)929-7398.

UHLIR, Anne Marie; Clinique Med Ste-Croix, 6350 rue Principale, Sainte-Croix QC G0S 2H0; McG'91; Langs: Bilingual(English/French); (418)926-3260; Fax. (418)926-2014; amuhlir@hotmail.com.

UHLMAN, Dorothy L; BC Cancer Agency-Abbotsford, 32900 Marshall Rd, Abbotsford BC V2S 0C2; Michigan (USA)'83; FRCPC; IntMed. Staff, Abbotsford Regional Hospital & Cancer Centre; (604)851-4710 x64532

UHOEGBU, Chimdi U; Cape Breton Reg Hosp, 1482 George St, Sydney NS B1P 1P3; (Nigeria)'94; MB BS; Staff, Cape Breton Healthcare Complex; (902)567-8000

UHTHOFF, Peter A F; Children's Hosp Eastern Ont, 401 Smyth Rd, Ottawa ON K1H 8L1; Ott'91; Staff, Children's Hospital of Eastern Ontario (CHEO); Langs: English; French; (613)737-2420

UHTHOFF MUNRO, Sylvia; Centre Med Ste-Anne, 500 Old St. Patrick St, Ottawa ON K1N 9G4; Ott'86; Staff, The Ottawa Hospital - General Campus; Langs: German; French; (613)789-1552; Fax. (613)789-0659.

UJJAINWALLA, Mark H; Smyth Med Centre, 122-1929 Russell Rd, Ottawa ON K1G 4G3; Ott'81; Staff, The Ottawa Hospital - Riverside Campus; Staff, Children's Hospital of Eastern Ontario (CHEO); (613)731-7535; Fax. (613)731-7536.

UKABAM, Sylvester O; Regina Internal Med Specialist, 1821 Rose St, Regina SK S4P 1Z7; Ibadan (Nigeria)'74; MB BS; FRCP; Consultant Gastroent, Pasqua Hospital; Consultant Gastroent, Regina General Hospital; Consultant Gastroent, Wascana Rehabilitation Centre; Regina Internal Medicine Specialists; Clin Assoc Prof, University of Saskatchewan; Langs: Ibo; (306)565-2093; Fax. (306)359-1068; sukabam@sasktel.net.

UKANI, Hanif; 201-2502 St John's St, Port Moody BC V3H 2B4; Cal'98; FRCSC; PlasSurg (Hand Surgery). Clin Instructor Div of PlasSurg, University of British Columbia; (604)931-1893; Fax. (604)931-1894; info@plasticsurgerybc.ca.

UKPEH, Henry A; 410-1200 Hospital Bench, Trail BC V1R 4M1; Ilorin (Nigeria)'83; MB BS; FAAP; FRCPC; Peds (Consultant Pediatrics). Staff, Kootenay Boundary Regional Hospital; Clin Assoc Prof Peds/Consultant, University of British Columbia; (250)364-2556; Fax. (250)368-3196; doctorukpeh@gmail.com.

UKRAINETZ, Owen M; Bigelow Fowler Clinic, 1605 9 Ave S, Lethbridge AB T1J 1W2; Sask'95; CCFP; (403)327-3121; Fax. (403)327-5593.

UKRAINETZ, Philip J; Alberta Children's Hosp, 2888 Shaganappi Trail NW, Calgary AB T3B 6A8; Cal'98; FRCPC; EmergMed. Staff, Alberta Children's Hospital; (403)955-7211

UL HAQ, Huma Z; Mel Lloyd Family Health Team, 167 Centre St, Shelburne ON L0N 1S4; Fatima Jinnah Medical College (Pakistan)'89; CCFP; Staff, Mel Lloyd Family Health Team; Langs: Hindi; Punjabi; Urdu; (519)925-0017; Fax. (519)925-6717.

ULAN, Susan R; Telus Plaza South, 2700-10020 100 St NW, Edmonton AB T5J 0N3; Wes'88; CCFP; Admin Senior Med Advisor, College of Physicians & Surgeons of Alberta; (780)969-4930; Fax. (780)420-0651.

ULECKAS, Gintaras T; North York Gen Hosp, 4001 Leslie St, North York ON M2K 1E1; Qns'93; CCFP; Staff, North York General Hospital - Branson Division; Staff, North York General Hospital; Langs: Lithuanian; French; (416)756-6000

ULECKAS, Jurate K; Polyclinique Concorde, 300 boul de la Concorde E, Laval QC H7G 2E6; Tor'87; FRCSC; Ophth (Pediatric Ophthalmology). Langs: Lithuanian; French; Spanish; (450)667-5310; Fax. (450)667-8329; jurate@videotron.ca.

ULIC, Bogdan-Christian I; Mount Sinai Hosp, 913-600 University Ave, Toronto ON M5G 1X5; Bucarest (Romania)'82; FRCPC; Psy. Staff, Mount Sinai Hospital; Langs: Romanian; (416)596-4200; Fax. (416)596-3149.

ULIC, Liliana; Southlake Reg Health Centre, W3-596 Davis Dr, Newmarket ON L3Y 2P9; Bucharest (Romania)'82; FRCPC; Psy. Staff, Southlake Regional Health Centre; Langs: Romanian; (905)895-4529; Fax. (416)447-8608.

ULJANITSKI, Sofia; Vaughan Comm Health Centre, 206A-9401 Jane St, Vaughan ON L6A 4H7; Russian State Medical University (Russia (Federation))'98; CCFP; (905)303-8490; Fax. (905)832-0093.

ULLAH, Farid; 115-1856 Ambrosi Rd, Kelowna BC V1Y 4R9; (Pakistan)'87; MB BS; MRCPsy; DPM; Staff, Interior Health Authority Central Okanagan Kelowna Health Unit; Langs: Urdu; Hindi; Punjabi; (778)478-0624

ULLAH, Hidayat; Scenic Acres Med Clinic, 8555 Scurfield Dr NW, Calgary AB T3L 1Z6; Karachi (Pakistan)'65; MB; BSc; LRCP; MRCS; FRCS(Eng & Ed); Langs: Urdu; (403)547-2255; Fax. (403)547-2254.

ULLAH, Ismat; Lenore Centre Med Clinic, 4-123 Lenore Dr, Saskatoon SK S7K 7H9; (Other Foreign)'89; (306)242-6700; Fax. (306)242-1168.

ULLAH, Saif; University of Alberta Hosp, 2E4 21W-8440 112 St NW, Edmonton AB T6G 2B7; Punjab University (Pakistan)'02; Respir; IntMed. Staff Pumonary Med, University of Alberta Hospital; (780)407-8822

ULLMAN, Doris B; North Woodlands Med Centre, 204-40 Shellington Place, Brantford ON N3S 0C5; McM'82; BMath; CCFP; Langs: German; (519)759-6116; Fax. (519)759-7727.

ULLMARK, Nicole P; Montfort Hosp, 713 Montreal Rd, Ottawa ON K1K 0T2; Wes'02; CCFP; Staff, Montfort Hospital; Staff, Canadian Forces Health Services Centre; (613)945-1367; Fax. (613)945-1348; nicole@smith.ns.ca.

ULLYATT, Kim J; Western Mem Reg Hosp, PO Box 2005 Stn Main 1 Brookfield Ave, Corner Brook NL A2H 6J7; Orange Free State (South Africa)'95; MB ChB; Staff, Western Memorial Regional Hospital; (709)637-5000

ULLYOT, Suzanne C; Misericordia Health Centre, 302-99 Cornish Ave, Winnipeg MB R3C 1A2; Man'71; FRCPC; Anes (Pediatric Anesthesia). Staff Pediatric Dental Program, Misericordia Health Centre; Assoc Prof, University of Manitoba; (204)788-6581

ULMER, Brian G; Medical Arts Bldg, 222-750 Spadina Cres E, Saskatoon SK S7K 3H3; Sask'83; BSc(Adv); FRCSC; GenSurg; VascSurg. (306)653-3366; Fax. (306)653-8832; ulmervasc@sasktel.net.

ULMER, Marcie J; 606-625 Fifth Ave, New Westminster BC V3M 1X4; Sask'02; FRCPC; Derm. (204)528-3961

ULYSSE, Marc-Andre; Clinique Med de Vimont, 1768C boul des Laurentides, Laval QC H7M 2P6; Port-au-Prince (Haiti)'58; (450)663-8300; Fax. (450)663-8301.

UM, Gregory T H; Main Street Square, 1-381 Main St N, Markham ON L3P 1Z3; Tor'92; Langs: Korean; (905)471-4795; Fax. (905)471-4796.

UMAMAHESWARAN-MAHARAJ, Meera; Rouge Valley-Ajax & Pickering, 580 Harwood Ave S, Ajax ON L1S 2J4; West Indies (Other Foreign)'03; FRCPC; Peds. Staff, Rouge Valley Health System - Ajax & Pickering Health Centre Site; (905)683-2320

UMAPATHY, Dhiviya; Hôpital du Haut-Richelieu, 920 boul du Seminaire N, St-Jean-sur-Richel QC J3A 1B7; Mon'05; FRCPC; Respir; IntMed. Staff, Hôpital du Haut-Richelieu; (450)359-5000

UMAR, Amir; Cumberland Med Hlth Services, 33 Havelock St, Amherst NS B4H 4W1; Karachi (Pakistan)'90; MB; BSc; Staff, The Moncton Hospital; (902)667-3879; Fax. (902)667-5959.

UMAR, Imran; Saint John Reg Hosp, PO Box 2100 Stn Main 400 University Ave, Saint John NB E2L 4L2; Punjab (India)'87; Staff, Saint John Regional Hospital; (506)648-6501

UMAR-KHITAB, Asher A; Ajax Med Arts Bldg, 106-601 Harwood Ave S, Ajax ON L1S 2J5; Wes'97; FRCSC; GenSurg. Staff, Rouge Valley Health System - Ajax & Pickering Health Centre Site; (905)427-6399; Fax. (905)427-9174.

UMEDALY, Hamed S; UBC Dept of Anes, JPP2N 2449-910 10th Ave W, Vancouver BC V5Z 1M9; UBC'86; FRC; ACLS; FRCPC; Anes. Staff, Vancouver General Hospital - Centennial Pavillion; Clin Assoc Prof Med Div of Cardiac & Thoracic Anaesthesia, University of British Columbia; (604)875-4304; Fax. (604)875-5209; humedaly@vanhosp.bc.ca.

UMEH, Jude I; Highlands Health Network, 150 Rolling Hills Dr, Orangeville ON L9W 4X8; Enugu (Nigeria)'86; MB BS; LMCC; MRCOG; FRCOG; FRCSC; ObstGyn. Langs: Ibo; (519)940-8775; Fax. (519)940-0355; jiumeh@yahoo.ca.

UMEMOTO, Lorne N; Clin d'Allergie Pediatrie de Q, 102-2880 ch des Quatre-Bourgeo, Quebec QC G1V 4X7; Tor'70; FRCPC; Peds (Allergy & Respirology); ClinImmunol&Allergy (P.Q.). ac Staff, Centre Hospitalier Affilié Universitaire de Québec - Hôpital du St-Sacrement; Langs: English; French; (418)682-2300; Fax. (418)657-6898.

UMER, Hafiz M; Halton HCS Corp-Milton, 7030 Derry Rd, Milton ON L9T 7H6; Jimma University (Other Foreign)'00; CCFP; CCFP(E.M.); Staff, Halton Healthcare Services Corporation - Milton District Hospital; (905)876-7038; Fax. (905)876-7000.

UMMAT, Samira; 930-943 Broadway W, Vancouver BC V5Z 4E1; Delhi (India)'88; MB; BSc; FRCPC; PhysMed&Rehab. Langs: Punjabi; Hindi; (604)737-7375; Fax. (604)737-7325.

UMMAT, Sunil K; Broadway Med Centre, 930-943 Broadway W, Vancouver BC V5Z 4E1; Dal'86; FRCSC; Otol. Langs: Hindi; (604)737-7375; Fax. (604)737-7325.

UMOQUIT, Andres B; Boniface Park Med Centre, 7-700 Markham Rd, Scarborough ON M1H 2A7; Southwestern (Philippines)'72; Staff, North York General Hospital - Branson Division; Langs: Tagalog; Spanish; (416)289-0779; Fax. (416)289-7900.

UMRAN, Tamim; Business Bldg, 1000-1200 Burrard St, Vancouver BC V6Z 2C7; UBC'04; FRCSC; OrthSurg. Staff, Vancouver General Hospital - Centennial Pavillion; Staff, Gordon & Leslie Diamond Health Care Centre; (604)629-9259

UN, C C Victor; North York Gen Hosp, 4001 Leslie St, Toronto ON M2K 1E1; Edinburgh (Scotland)'86; MB ChB; FRCA; FRCPC; Anes. Staff, North York General Hospital; (416)756-6265

UNARKET, Bhikubhai D; Family Care Med Centre, 112-55 Castleridge Blvd NE, Calgary AB T3J 3J8; London (England)'69; MB BS; LRCP; MRCS; Langs: Gujarati; Hindi; (403)280-5500; Fax. (403)293-2207.

UNARKET, Milan; Bridgepoint Hosp, 205B-14 St Matthews Rd, Toronto ON M4M 2B5; Sask'00; FRCPC; PhysMed&Rehab. Staff, Bridgepoint Health Centre; (416)461-8251; Fax. (416)470-6714.

UNDERELL, J Roderick; Abbotsford Reg Hosp & CC, 32900 Marshall Rd, Abbotsford BC V2S 0C2; Tor'76; FRCPC; Anes. Reg Chief of Staff, Abbotsford Regional Hospital & Cancer Centre; (604)851-4709

UNDERWOOD, Heather; G F Strong Rehabilitation Ctre, 4255 Laurel St, Vancouver BC V5Z 2G9; McM'96; FRCPC; PhysMed&Rehab. Staff, G F Strong Rehabilitation Centre; Staff, Alder Medical Clinic; (604)714-4113

UNDSETH, Audrey L; Glenmore Landing Vein Clinic, D267-1600 90 Ave SW, Calgary AB T2V 5A8; Cal'98; CCFP; FCFP; (403)253-2555; Fax. (403)640-4247.

UNG, Berton Y K; 1256 Danforth Rd, Scarborough ON M1J 1E5; Tor'93; CCFP; Staff, The Scarborough Hospital - Birchmount Campus; Staff FamMed, The Scarborough Hospital - General Campus; Staff, Yae Hong Centre for Geriatric Care; Langs: Cantonese; French; Mandarin; (416)261-3500; Fax. (416)266-9400.

UNG, Chantelle Y W; Victoria Terrace Med Centre, 302-1448 Lawrence Ave E, North York ON M4A 2V6; Dal'94; FRCPC; Derm. Langs: Cantonese; French; (416)750-8400; Fax. (416)750-1091.

UNG, Karen; The Richmond Hosp, 2510-7000 Westminster Hwy, Richmond BC V6X 1A2; UBC'05; FRCPC; GenPath. Staff, Richmond Hospital; (604)278-9711 x4234

UNG, Muoy; CLSC Bordeaux-Cartierville, 11822 av du Bois-De-Boulogne, Montreal QC H3M 2X6; Mon'99; Staff, Hôpital de Saint-Eustache; Universite de Montreal; Langs: Chinese; (514)331-2288 x2500; Fax. (514)331-0137.

UNG, Yee C; Odette Cancer Centre, 2075 Bayview Ave, Toronto ON M4N 3M5; Alb'85; FRCPC; RadOncol. Staff, Sunnybrook Health Sciences Centre; Assoc Prof, University of Toronto; (416)480-4951; Fax. (416)480-6002.

UNG-DATTA, Sheila M L; 100-20 Heritage Meadows Dr SE, Calgary AB T2H 3C1; Cal'05; CCFP; (403)252-8851; Fax. (403)252-1765.

UNGAR, Clifford N; 2523 St Johns St, Port Moody BC V3H 2B3; McG'81; (604)936-7277; Fax. (604)936-7112.

UNGAR, Thomas E; North York Gen Hosp, 4001 Leslie St, North York ON M2K 1E1; Tor'87; ACLS; ATLS; AB; FRCPC; Psy;CCFP; FCFP; Ac Staff Psy, North York General Hospital; Asst Prof Psy, University of Toronto; (416)756-6080; Fax. (416)756-6319.

UNGARIAN, Jillian L R; Dauphin Med Clinic, 622 3rd St SW, Dauphin MB R7N 1R5; (Other Foreign)'07; CCFP; (204)638-6445; Fax. (204)638-5670.

UNGER, Andrea G; Brant Community HC-Brantford, 200 Terrace Hill St, Brantford ON N3R 1G9; McM'97; CCFP; CCFP(E.M.); FCFP; Staff, The Brant Community Healthcare System - Brantford General Hospital Site; (519)752-7871; aunger99@yahoo.com.

UNGER, Barbara E; Rockyview Gen Hosp, 7007 14 St SW, Calgary AB T2V 1P9; Sask'63; Staff, Rockyview General Hospital; (403)943-3410

UNGER, Bernard; SMBD Jewish Gen Hosp, D010-3755 ch Cote-Ste-Catherin, Montreal QC H3T 1E2; Mon'82; CSPQ; CCFP; CCFP(E.M.); FCFP; EmergMed (P.Q.). Staff, Sir Mortimer B Davis Jewish General; adj Prof, McGill University; Langs: English; French; (514)340-8222 x3898; Fax. (514)340-7917; bernard.unger@mcgill.ca.

UNGER, Bertram J; Health Sciences Centre, 820 Sherbrook St, Winnipeg MB R3A 1R9; Man'90; Staff, Health Sciences Centre; Staff, St Boniface General Hospital; (204)774-8511

UNGER, Byron P; Alberta Surgical Centre, 202-14310 111 Ave NW, Edmonton AB T5M 3Z7; Sask'93; FRCPC; Anes. Staff, University of Alberta Hospital; (780)488-2724; Fax. (780)488-2774.

UNGER, D Terrance; D Terry Unger Prof Corp, 206-200 Boudreau Rd, St. Albert AB T8N 6B9; Alb'73; BMedSci; FRCOG; FRCSC; ObstGyn (Minimal Invasive Pelvic Surgery). Ac Staff, Sturgeon Community Hospital; Asst Clin Prof, University of Alberta; (780)459-1104; Fax. (780)459-0128.

UNGER, David A; Care Point Med Centre, 1123 Davie St, Vancouver BC V6E 1N2; Sask'92; CCFP; FCFP; Staff, Providence Health Care - St Paul's Hospital; Staff, Aquarium Medical Clinic; (604)915-9517; dave@theedge.ca.

UNGER, Jason B A; Associate Med Clinic, PO Box 7590 Stn Main 10011 101 St, Peace River AB T8S 1T2; Man'03; CCFP; (780)459-1104; Fax. (780)459-0128.

UNGER, Jeffrey J; Saanich Peninsula Hosp, 2166 Mount Newton Cross Rd, Saanichton BC V8M 2B2; Ott'96; CCFP; CCFP(E.M.); FCFP; Staff, Saanich Peninsula Hospital; (250)652-7550; Fax. (250)544-5014.

UNGER, Kathy D; Family Med Associates, 5021 51 St, Lacombe AB T4L 2A3; Cal'05; CCFP; (403)782-3351; Fax. (403)782-5879.

UNGER, Mark A; The Credit Valley Hosp, 2200 Eglinton Ave W, Mississauga ON L5M 2N1; Tor'06; CCFP; Staff, The Credit Valley Hospital; Langs: Bilingual(English/French); (905)813-2200

UNGER, Matthew R; Family Med Associates, 5021 51 St, Lacombe AB T4L 2A3; Man'07; CCFP; (403)782-3351; Fax. (403)782-5879.

UNGER, Sharon L; Mount Sinai Hosp, 775A-600 University Ave, Toronto ON M5G 1X5; Dal'91; BSc; FRCPC; Peds (Neonatal & Perinatal Medicine). Staff, Mount Sinai Hospital; Asst Prof, University of Toronto; Langs: English; French; (416)586-4800 x8593; Fax. (416)586-8745; sunger@mtsinai.on.ca.

UNGER, Waldemar G; Broadway Med Centre, 230-943 Broadway W, Vancouver BC V5Z 4E1; UBC'69; FRCSC; ObstGyn. Sr Consultant, Vancouver General Hospital - Centennial Pavillion; Staff, BC Women's Hospital & Health Centre; Clin Associate Prof, University Of British Columbia; Langs: German; (604)734-2712; Fax. (604)734-8572.

UNGER, Walter P; Hair Transplantation Men/Women, 214-99 Yorkville Ave, Toronto ON M5R 3K5; Tor'63; FACP; FRCPC; Derm (Hair Transplantation). Assoc Prof Med, University of Toronto; Clin Prof Derm, Mount Sinai School of Medicine (New York,USA); (416)944-9393; Fax. (416)944-9774.

UNGERER, Danel; Associate Med Clinic, 25 St Michael St, St. Albert AB T8N 1C7; Pretoria (South Africa) MB ChB; Langs: Afrikaans; (780)458-1234; Fax. (780)460-7941.

UNIAT, Linda M; Retina Imaging Centre Ltd, 402-11010 101 St NW, Edmonton AB T5H 4B9; Alb'77; FRCS; FRCSC; Ophth (Retina Vitreous Surgery). Ac Staff, Royal Alexandra Hospital; Clin Assoc Prof, University of Alberta; Langs: French; Ukrainian; (780)421-0460; Fax. (780)425-5062.

UNIKOWSKY, Bernie; MUHC-Montreal Gen Hosp, L4 525-1650 av Cedar, Montreal QC H3G 1A4; McG'75; ABIM; FRCPC; IntMed; Nephrol. Staff, McGill University Health Centre - Montreal General Campus; assoc Prof Med, McGill University; (514)934-1934 x44035; Fax. (514)934-8248.

UNOH, Emma S; 115 Maclean Place, Welland ON L3B 5X9; Ibadan (Nigeria)'00; MB BS; MRCPsy(UK); MPH; FRCPC; Psy. (905)650-3403; Fax. (289)273-2810.

UNRUH, Helmut W; Health Sciences Centre, GE 611-820 Sherbrook St, Winnipeg MB R3A 1R9; Man'76; FRCSC; GenSurg; ThorSurg. Staff, Health Sciences Centre; Prof, University of Manitoba; (204)787-3791; Fax. (204)787-7143; hunruh@hsc.mb.ca.

UNSWORTH, Declan P; PO Box 1373, Jasper AB T0E 1E0; Sask'08; CCFP.

UNSWORTH, Roderick J; Prince Albert Comm Clinic, 110 8th St E, Prince Albert SK S6V 0V7; Dublin (Ireland)'70; DCH; DObst; DRCOG(Eng); Physician, Prince Albert Community Clinic; (306)763-6464; Fax. (306)763-2101.

UNWALA, Fatima E; CSC St-Thomas Comm Hlth Ctr, 9040 84 Ave NW, Edmonton AB T6C 1E4; Alb'04; Staff, Royal Alexandra Hospital; (780)434-2778; Fax. (780)466-8702.

UNWALA, Hussein A; Alberta Children's Hosp, 2888 Shaganappi Tr NW, Calgary AB T3B 6A8; Alb'05; PedEmergMed; Peds. Staff, Alberta Children's Hospital; (403)955-7211

UONG DINH, Bich Thao; CSSS de Laval, 1755 boul Rene-Laennec, Laval QC H7M 3L9; Mon'01; CCFP; Staff, Hopital de la Cite de la santé; (450)668-1010

UPADHYAY, Amitkumar S; Aurora Med Centre, 201-15017 Yonge St, Aurora ON L4G 1M5; Gujarat (India)'99; ABEM; CCFP; Staff, Stevenson Memorial Hospital; Staff, Southlake Regional Health Centre; Langs: Hindi; Gujarati; (905)727-4241; Fax. (905)727-4288; zau296@yahoo.com.

UPADHYAY, Rajat; Foothills Med Centre, C231-1403 29 St NW, Calgary AB T2N 2T9; Man'02; CCFP; CCFP(E.M.); Staff, Foothills Medical Centre; Langs: Hindi; Nepali; (403)944-2726

UPADHYE, Suneel; St Joseph's Healthcare, 50 Charlton Ave E, Hamilton ON L8N 4A6; Qns'96; FRCPC; EmergMed. Staff, Hamilton Health Sciences Centre - Hamilton General Hospital; Staff, St Joseph's Healthcare - Charlton Campus; Staff, Hamilton Health Sciences Centre - McMaster Children's Hospital; (905)522-1155; suneel_upadhye@hotmail.com.

UPAL, Faiza; Halton Hills Family Health Team, 199 Princess Anne Dr, Georgetown ON L7G 0E3; McM'09; CCFP; Langs: Urdu; (905)873-3000

UPENIEKS, John A; 278 The West Mall, Etobicoke ON M9C 1C5; Tor'85; Staff, Trillium Health Centre - Mississauga; (416)621-3253; Fax. (416)622-2699.

UPENIEKS, Maria; 278 The West Mall, Etobicoke ON M9C 1C5; Tor'85; CCFP; (416)621-3253; Fax. (416)622-2699.

UPENIEKS, Richard L; St Mary's Gen Hosp, 911 Queens Blvd, Kitchener ON N2M 1B2; Tor'87; CCFP; Staff, St Mary's General Hospital; Langs: Latvian; (519)744-3311

UPFOLD, Jane A; 99 Horton St W, London ON N6J 4Y6; Wes'81; CCFP; CCFP(E.M.); Staff, London Health Sciences Centre - Victoria Campus; Physician, Wortley Village Medical Centre; (519)434-9768

UPITIS, Jennifer A; Oak Ridges Aesthetics Centre, 401-13291 Yonge St, Richmond Hill ON L4E 4L6; Alb'00; DDerm(Derm,Harvard); (905)773-1599; Fax. (905)773-3515; info@ordc.ca.

UPNEJA, Harpreet K; Windsor Reg Hosp-Western, 1453 Prince Rd, Windsor ON N9C 3Z4; Kanpur University (India)'88; FRCPC; IntMed. Staff, Windsor Regional Hospital - Tayfour Site; Langs: Hindi; Punjabi; (519)257-5166; Fax. (519)257-5161.

UPPAL, Gayatri; Pearly Rideau Veterans Hlth Ct, 1750 Russel Rd, Ottawa ON K1G 5Z6; Punjab (India)'90; CCFP; Langs: Hindi; Punjabi; (613)526-7170

UPPAL, Jaishree; Primary Care Physician, 239 George St, Sarnia ON N7T 4P1; Baroda (India)'77; Staff, Bluewater Health - Norman Site; Staff, Bluewater Health - Mitton Site; Langs: Hindi; (519)332-4699; Fax. (519)332-3236.

UPPAL, Loveleen; 715 12 Ave W, Vancouver BC V5Z 1M9; Caribbean (Other Foreign)'03; Psy. Staff, Vancouver General Hospital - Centennial Pavillion; (604)875-4111

UPPAL, Rakesh; 5-900 Ray Lawson Blvd, Brampton ON L6Y 5H7; Punjab (India)'80; MB BS; Langs: Hindi; Punjabi; Urdu; (905)452-0026; Fax. (905)452-1974.

UPPAL, Sonia; Abbotsford Mental Health Ctre, 11-32700 George Ferguson Way, Abbotsford BC V2T 4V6; Guru Nanak (India)'82; MB BS; FRCPC; Psy. Ac Staff, Abbotsford Regional Hospital & Cancer Centre; Langs: Punjabi; Hindi; Urdu; (604)870-7800; Fax. (604)870-7801.

UPSHUR, Ross E G; Sunnybrook Hlth Sciences Ctre, A100-2075 Bayview Ave, Toronto ON M4N 3M5; McM'86; MSc; FRCPC; CommunMed (Family Medicine). Staff, Sunnybrook Health Sciences Centre; Teach Staff Family & Commun Med, University of Toronto; Teach Staff Family & Commun Med, McMaster University; (416)480-4931; Fax. (416)480-6038; rupshur@idirect.com.

UPTON, Adrian R M; Hamilton HS-McMaster Site, PO Box 2000 Stn Lcd 1 R4U8-1200 Main St W, Hamilton ON L8N 3Z5; Cambridge (England)'65; MB ChB; LRCP; MRCS; FRCPC; Neur. Prof/Head Div of Neur, Hamilton Health Sciences Centre - McMaster Children's Hospital; Dir Neurological & Epilepsy Clinics & Diag Neurophysiology, St Joseph's Healthcare - Charlton Campus; Langs: English; French; (905)521-2100 x76372; Fax. (905)521-2656; uptona@hhsc.ca.

UPTON, Julia E M; The Hosp for Sick Children, 7272-555 University Ave, Toronto ON M5G 1X8; Wes'02; FRCPC; IntMed; ClinImmunol&Allergy. Staff Clinical Immunol & Allergy, The Hospital For Sick Children; (416)813-8626; julia.upton@sickkids.ca.

UPTON, Kenneth J; Women's Health Care, 3206 35 St, Vernon BC V1T 6B7; Cape Town (South Africa)'81; MB ChB; FRCSC; ObstGyn. Langs: Afrikaans; (250)503-1552; Fax. (250)275-3171; womenshealth@shawbiz.ca.

UR, Ehud; Gordon & Leslie Diamond HCC, 4116-2775 Laurel St, Vancouver BC V5Z 1M9; London (England)'82; MB BS; MRC; IntMed (Diabetology). Staff, Gordon & Leslie Diamond Health Care Centre; Staff Endocrinology, Providence Health Care - St Paul's Hospital; (604)875-5929

UR RAHMAN, Asad; Regina Gen Hosp, 1440 14th Ave, Regina SK S4P 0W5; Staff, Regina General Hospital; (306)766-4444

URBACH, David R; Univ Hlth Network-Toronto Gen, 10NU 214-200 Elizabeth St, Toronto ON M5G 2C4; Tor'93; MSc; FRCSC; GenSurg (Endocrinology Surgery). Staff, Toronto General Hospital - UHN; Assoc Prof Surg, University of Toronto; (416)340-4284; Fax. (416)340-4211; david.urbach@uhn.on.ca.

URBACH, Stacey L; The Hosp for Sick Children, 555 University Ave, Toronto ON M5G 1X8; Tor'95; MPH; FRCPC; Peds (Pediatric Endocrinology); Endocrin&Metab. Staff, The Hospital For Sick Children; (416)813-7763; Fax. (416)813-6304.

URBACK, Percy G; Raxlen Associates, B102-340 College St, Toronto ON M5T 3A9; Tor'53; FRCPC; IntMed (Gastroenterology). Chief, Raxlen Associates Clinic; Langs: Portuguese; (416)925-8011; Fax. (416)944-9947.

URBACK, Robert K; 401-960 Lawrence Ave W, North York ON M6A 3B5; Tor'84; CCFP; FCFP; Staff, Humber River Regional Hospital - Keele Street Site; (416)256-1150; Fax. (416)256-0742.

URBAIN, Jean-Luc C P; Brantford Gen Hosp, 200 Terrace Hill St, Brantford ON N3R 1G9; Louvain (Belgium)'80; PhD; FRCPC; NuclearMed (Medical Oncology). Staff, The Brant Community Healthcare System - Brantford General Hospital Site; Langs: French; (519)751-5544

URBAIN, Melanie; Dr Georges L-Dumont Reg Hosp, 330 av Universite, Moncton NB E1C 2Z3; Sher'99; CCFP; Staff, Dr Georges-L-Dumont University Hospital Centre; (506)862-4000

URBAN, George S; St Anthony's Med Centre, 206-582 Goldstream Ave, Victoria BC V9B 2W7; Wes'80; BSc; Assoc Staff, Royal Jubilee Hospital; Ac Staff, Victoria General Hospital; (250)478-2133; Fax. (250)474-2783; gsurban@telus.net.

URBAN, Thomas M; Brady Clinic, 101-359 Riverside Dr, Sudbury ON P3E 1H5; Tor'91; CCFP; FCFP; (705)688-8833; Fax. (705)688-8646.

URBANKIEWICZ, Lester R; Toronto East Gen & Orth Hosp, 825 Coxwell Ave, Toronto ON M4C 3E7; Tor'81; FRCPC; Anes. Staff, Toronto East General Hospital Inc; (416)461-8272

URBANSKI, R Pierre; Centre Med Pour Enfants, 1791 av Dollard, Lasalle QC H8N 1T9; McG'77; AB; ABP; Peds (Neonatology). Staff Neonatal Unit, Centre Hospitalier de LaSalle; Staff, Lakeshore General Hospital - Pointe Claire; Staff EmergMed, McGill University Health Centre - Montreal Children's Hospital; Langs: Polish; French; (514)368-0441; Fax. (514)368-0445.

URBANSKI, Stefan J; Foothills Med Centre, 1403 29 St NW, Calgary AB T2N 2T9; Warsaw (Poland)'75; FRCPC; AnatPath. Staff AnatPath, Foothills Medical Centre; Staff, Calgary Laboratory Services; Prof, University of Calgary; (403)944-4751; Fax. (403)944-4748; stefan.urbanski@cls.ab.ca.

URBANTKE, Elizabeth A; Woodstock Gen Hosp, 310 Juliana Dr, Woodstock ON N4V 0A4; Tor'95; BSc; CCFP; CCFP(E.M.); FCFP; Staff, Woodstock General Hospital; (519)421-4222; Fax. (519)421-4256.

UREN, Kelly J; Valley Reg Hosp, 150 Exhibition St, Kentville NS B4N 5E3; UBC'86; ATLS; DAB(Path.); DMJ; FRCPC; AnatPath (Forensic Pathology). Ac Staff, Valley Regional Hospital; Ac Staff, Yarmouth Regional Hospital; (902)698-1894; Fax. (902)679-3811.

URETSKY, Aubrey D; Capital City Women's Centre, 196-17010 90 Ave NW, Edmonton AB T5T 1L6; Alb'04; BSc; MSc; FRCSC; ObstGyn. (780)439-2007; Fax. (780)439-3080.

URETSKY, H Richard; Capital City Women's Centre, 196-17010 90 Ave NW, Edmonton AB T5T 1L6; Alb'70; FACOG; BSc; FRCOG; FRCSC; ObstGyn. Langs: German; French; Hebrew; (780)439-2007; Fax. (780)439-3080; ccwc@telus.net.

URFER, Francois N; 400-1 Main St, Hawkesbury ON K6A 1A1; Lausanne (Switzerland)'80; Staff, Hawkesbury & District General Hospital; Langs: German; English; (613)632-0173; Fax. (613)632-2417; francois.urfer@sympatico.ca.

URMSON, Andrew T; Saskatoon Ortho & Sports Med C, 104-311 Ludlow St, Saskatoon SK S7S 1N6; Sask'03; FRCSC; OrthSurg. (306)242-5543; Fax. (306)242-5592.

URMSON, Kristine I; Royal University Hosp, 103 Hospital Dr, Saskatoon SK S7N 0W8; Sask'00; FRCPC; Anes. Staff, Royal University Hospital; (306)655-1183; Fax. (306)655-1279.

URNESS, Douglas; Centennial CMH & Brain Injury, PO Box 1000 Stn Main, Ponoka AB T4J 1R8; Alb'83; FRCPC; Psy (General Adult Psychiatry). Ac Staff, Centennial Centre for Mental Health & Brain Injury; Clin Dept Head, Central Zone Mental Health; Staff, Alberta Community Mental Health Clinic; Asst Prof Commun Health, University of Calgary; (403)783-7643; Fax. (403)783-7790.

UROWITZ, Edwin P; Rouge Valley HS-Centenary, 202-2863 Ellesmere Rd, Scarborough ON M1E 5E9; Tor'73; FACS; FRCSC; OrthSurg. Ac Staff, Rouge Valley Health System - Centenary Health Centre Site; (416)281-8878; Fax. (416)281-8959.

UROWITZ, Murray B; Univ Hlth Network-Toronto Western Hosp, 1E409-399 Bathurst St, Toronto ON M5T 2S8; Tor'63; FACP; FRCP; FRCPC; IntMed (Rheumatology). Sr Scientist, Toronto Western Hospital - University Health Network; Staff, Princess Margaret Hospital - University Health Network; Staff, Mount Sinai Hospital; Prof, University of Toronto; Langs: Hebrew; (416)603-5828; Fax. (416)603-9387.

URQUHART, Robert J; Peter Lougheed Centre, 3500 26 St NE, Calgary AB T1Y 6J4; Man'03; FRCPC; Psy. Staff, Peter Lougheed Centre; (403)943-5737

URSANI, Nafisa Ali A; Halton Healthcare Serv Corp, 327 Reynolds St, Oakville ON L6J 3L7; University of Sind (Other Foreign)'89; MB BS; FRCPC; AnatPath. Staff, Halton Healthcare Services Corporation - Oakville Site; (905)338-4690; Fax. (905)845-3376.

URSCHEL, Simon; University of Alberta Hosp, 4C2 32-8440 112 St NW, Edmonton AB T6G 2B7; Staff, University of Alberta Hospital; (780)492-3253; Fax. (780)407-3310.

URSEL, Peter G; Lindsay Prof Bldg, 3-65 Angeline St N, Lindsay ON K9V 5N7; Ott'85; (705)328-1747; Fax. (705)328-1650; afursel@cogeco.ca.

URSELL, Melanie R M; South Muskoka Med Centre, 230 Manitoba St, Bracebridge ON P1L 2E1; Tor'97; BSc; MSc; Neur (Multiple Sclerosis). Lecturer, University of Toronto; (705)646-2800; Fax. (705)646-2803.

URSON, Shoshana; Mackenzie Richmond Hill Hosp, 10 Trench St, Richmond Hill ON L4C 4Z3; Jerusalem (Israel)'77; AB; FRCPC; Psy (Adult General Psychiatry). Staff, Mackenzie Richmond Hill Hospital; Langs: Russian; Hebrew; (905)832-1406 x2204; Fax. (905)832-1952.

URSULIAK, Zenovia B J; NS Early Psychosis Program, 3F-5909 Veterans Memorial Lane, Halifax NS B3H 2E2; Cal'01; FRCPC; Psy (Early Psychosis). (902)473-3812; Fax. (902)473-3456; zenovia.ursuliak@cdha.nshealth.ca.

URTASUN, Raul C; Cross Cancer Institute, 11560 University Ave NW, Edmonton AB T6G 1Z2; Buenos Aires (Argentina)'59; DABR; FRCPC; RadOncol (Tumor). Staff, Cross Cancer Institute; Consultant, University of Alberta Hospital; Langs: Spanish; (780)432-8516; Fax. (780)432-8380; raulurtas@cancerboard.ab.com.

URTON, Jack I M; Athabasca Health Authority, PO Box 124, Black Lake SK S0J 0H0; Sask'77; Staff, La Loche Health Centre and Hospital; (306)439-2200; Fax. (306)439-2210; j.urton@sasktel.net.

URTON, Todd E; 401-190 Wellington St, Kingston ON K7L 3E4; Qns'02; FRCSC; Ophth. Staff, Hotel-Dieu Hospital; (613)546-1858; Fax. (613)546-4060.

USHA, Sama P; The Specialist's Clinic, 301-220 Dundas St W, Whitby ON L1N 8M7; Madras (India)'65; FRCPC; Psy. Langs: Tamil; (905)430-3058; Fax. (905)668-3156.

USHER, Ann K; Consort Med Centre, PO Box 58, Consort AB T0C 1B0; Wes'72; BSc; FACOG; FRCSC; ObstGyn (Infertility). (403)577-3737; Fax. (403)577-3739.

USHER, Darren J; The Royal Victoria Hosp, 201 Georgian Dr, Barrie ON L4M 6M2; McM'04; FRCPC; EmergMed. Staff, Royal Victoria Regional Health Centre; (705)728-9090

USHER, Olive E; Consort Med Centre, PO Box 58, Consort AB T0C 1B0; (403)577-3737; Fax. (403)577-3739.

USHKO, Allan W; University of Alberta Hosp, 8440 112 St NW, Edmonton AB T6G 2B7; Alb'92; CCFP; CCFP(E.M.); Staff Emerg, University of Alberta Hospital; (780)407-8433

USMAN, Abida; 305-300 John St, Thornhill ON L3T 5W4; Peshawar (Pakistan)'77; Staff, North York General Hospital - Branson Division; Langs: Urdu; Punjabi; (905)764-5253; Fax. (905)764-6979.

USMAN, Muhammad U; Cape Breton Reg Hosp, 1482 George St, Sydney NS B1P 1P3; Punjab (Pakistan)'97; MB BS; Staff, Cape Breton Healthcare Complex; (902)578-5056

USMANI, Nawaid H; Cross Cancer Institute, 11560 University Ave NW, Edmonton AB T6G 1Z2; McM'01; FRCPC; RadOncol (Surgical Oncology). Staff RadOncol, Cross Cancer Institute; Asst Prof, University of Alberta; (780)432-8518; Fax. (780)432-8380.

USTINA, Judith K; Garneau Prof Centre, 407-11044 51 Ave NW, Edmonton AB T6H 5B4; Alb'82; FRCPC; Psy (Child Psychiatry). Staff, Glenrose Rehabilitation Hospital; Staff, Royal Alexandra Hospital; University of Alberta; (780)438-6181; Fax. (780)437-3499.

UTHMAN, Elmonttasir M; St Clare's Mercy Hosp, 154 LeMarchant Rd, St. John's NL A1C 5B8; University of Khartoum (Sudan)'95; MB BS; Staff, St Clare's Mercy Hospital; Staff, Carbonear General Hospital; (709)777-5000

UTIGARD, Dale K; Crowfoot Village Prof Centre, 201-60 Crowfoot Cres NW, Calgary AB T3G 3J9; Alb'08; CCFP; (403)374-0244; Fax. (403)374-0354.

UTTLEY, Steven R; Family Medical Centre, 101 Joseph St, Pembroke ON K8A 8C9; Ott'05; CCFP; Langs: Bilingual(English/French); (613)732-6662; Fax. (613)732-6666.

UWABOR, Wisdom O; Health District #10, PO Box 400, Virden MB R0M 2C0; (Other Foreign)'95; (204)748-1345

UWAIFO, Victor O; Waypoint Mental Health Care, 500 Church St, Penetanguishene ON L9M 1G3; University of Benin (Other Foreign)'03; Staff, Waypoint Centre for Mental Health Care; (705)549-3181

UWALAKA, Anne N; Fort Macleod Med Clinic, PO Box 820, Fort MacLeod AB T0L 0Z0; (403)553-3351; Fax. (403)553-4774.

UWIERA, Trina C; University of Alberta Hosp, 2C3 82-8440 112 St NW, Edmonton AB T6G 2B7; Sask'00; FRCSC; Otol (Pediatric Otolaryngology). Staff, Stollery Children's Hospital; Staff, University of Alberta Hospital; Assoc Prof Surg, University of Alberta; Langs: Bilingual(English/French); (780)407-3866; Fax. (780)407-2004.

UXA, Amar K; Univ Hlth Network-Toronto Gen, 4NU 508-200 Elizabeth St, Toronto ON M5G 2C4; Bundelkhand (India)'94; Staff, Toronto General Hospital - UHN; Asst Prof, University of Toronto; (416)340-4598; Fax. (416)340-4418.

UY, Antonio F; Peterborough Clinic, 26 Hospital Dr, Peterborough ON K9J 7C3; Cebu (Philippines)'88; CCFP; Langs: Cebuano; Tagalog; (705)740-6884; Fax. (705)740-6863; aaanthoniouy@gmail.com.

UYEDA, Linda E; 16033 108 Ave PO Box 74055, Surrey BC V4N 5H9; UBC'99; Staff, Forensic Psychiatric Hospital; (604)614-7688; luyeda@forensic.bc.ca.

UYIRWOTH, Gabriel; Golden Opportunity Med Clinic, PO Box 1320 881A Mistassiniy Rd S, Wabasca AB T0G 2K0; (Uganda)'81; Staff, Golden Opportuniy Medical Clinic; (780)891-2847; Fax. (780)628-3148; gabriel.uyirwoth@albertahealthservices.ca.

UYS, Tharina; The Brandon Clinic, 620 Dennis St, Brandon MB R7A 5E7; Orange Free State (South Africa)'85; MB ChB; Langs: Afrikaans; (204)728-4440

UZARAGA, Isabella M; BC Cancer Agency-Vanc Isl Ctr, 2410 Lee Ave, Victoria BC V8R 6V5; Cape Town (South Africa),'88; Staff Pain & Symptom Management, BC Cancer Agency Vancouver Island Centre; (250)519-5656

UZOHO, Festus O; Blairmore Med Clinic, 225 Betts Ave, Saskatoon SK S7M 1L2; (Other Foreign)'89; CCFP; (306)652-6400; Fax. (306)652-6403.

VACCANI, Jean-Philippe; Children's Hosp Eastern Ont, 401 Smyth Rd, Ottawa ON K1H 8L1; Ott'97; FRCSC; Otol (Head & Neck Surgery). Staff, Children's Hospital of Eastern Ontario (CHEO); Langs: French; Italian; (613)737-7600 x2706; Fax. (613)738-4122; vaccani@cheo.on.ca.

VACHET, Mylene J; Clarence-Rockland Fam Hlth Team, 2741 rue Chamberland, Rockland ON K4K 0B4; Ott'87; CCFP; Langs: English; French; (613)446-7677; Fax. (613)446-5737.

VACHHANI, Luv; Pine Valley Med Centre, 7700 Pine Valley Dr, Woodbridge ON L4L 2X4; Saba University (Netherlands Antilles)'06; CCFP; Staff, Pine Valley Medical Centre; (905)851-1234; Fax. (905)851-4548.

VACHHRAJANI, Hareshkumar V; Saskatoon Cancer Centre, 20 Campus Dr, Saskatoon SK S7N 4H4; Saurashtra (India)'72; MB BS; FRCR; Staff RadOncol, Royal University Hospital; Staff, Saskatoon Cancer Centre; Clin Asst Med, University of Saskatchewan; (306)655-2739; Fax. (306)655-2639.

VACHON, Andre; Clinique Med Familiale, 422 15e rue O, La Guadeloupe QC G0M 1G0; Laval'69; Langs: Bilingual(French/English); (418)459-6090; Fax. (418)459-6030; cliniquefamiliale@hb.sympatico.ca.

VACHON, Andree; Clinique Med St-Louis, 220-3165 ch Saint-Louis, Quebec QC G1W 4R4; Laval'77; (418)653-1970; Fax. (418)653-9956.

VACHON, Caroline; Clinique Med Saint-Luc, 264 boul Saint-Luc, St-Jean-Sur-Richel QC J2W 1C3; Laval'89; (450)348-6124

VACHON, Francine; Clinique Med Saint-Marc, 1295 boul Saint-Sacrement, Shawinigan QC G9N 3M8; Sher'77; Staff, CH du Centre-de-la-Mauricie (Ste-Thérèse de Shawinigan); (819)539-2999; francine_vachon@ssss.gouv.qc.ca.

VACHON, Francois; Médi Centre Chomedey, 610 boul Cure-Labelle, Laval QC H7V 2T7; Mon'10; (450)687-6452

VACHON, Guylaine; CSSS de Laval, 1755 boul Rene-Laennec, Laval QC H7M 3L9; Laval'83; EmergMed (P.Q.). Staff, Hopital de la Cite de la santé; (450)668-1010

VACHON, Jean-Francois; Clinique Med de Verdun, 5-4074 boul Lasalle, LaSalle QC H4G 2A2; Laval'85; FRCPC; Psy. (514)439-4119

VACHON, Louis; 225-214 boul Cite-des-Jeunes, Gatineau QC J8Y 6S8; Ott'77; FRCPC; Cardiol. Staff, CSSS de la Baie-des-Chaleurs; (819)775-3344; Fax. (819)775-3345.

VACHON, Louise; Clinique Med Plaza Gatineau, 381 Boul Maloney E, Gatineau QC J8P 1E3; Laval'82; (819)669-7393; Fax. (819)669-0077.

VACHON, Marie-France; Clinique Med de Levis, 100-4975 boul de la Rive-Sud, Levis QC G6V 4Z5; Laval'75; ac Staff, Hôtel-Dieu de Lévis; Langs: English; (418)833-5810; Fax. (418)833-2720.

VACHON, Marie-Louise C; CHUQ-Hopital Laval, S 796-2705 boul Laurier, Quebec QC G1V 4G2; Sher'02; FRCPC; MedMicrobiol. Staff, Centre Hospitalier Universitaire de Quebec-CHUL; (418)525-4444

VACHON, Mario; Clinique Med Chateauguay, 120 boul Saint-Jean-Baptiste, Chateauguay QC J6K 3A9; Mon'80; (450)691-8191; Fax. (450)691-8568.

VACHON, Michel; Clinique Med 3000 Inc, 3000 rue Belanger, Montreal QC H1Y 1A9; Mon'82; (514)376-7702; Fax. (514)376-2639.

VACHON, Natalie; CRSSS Hop de Chibougamau, 51 3e rue, Chibougamau QC G8P 1N1; Laval'96; FRCPC; Psy (Forensic Psychiatry). dép Chef, CRSSS de la Baie-James; Langs: Bilingual(French/English); (418)748-2676

VACHON, Pierre; 10445 1re av, Saint-Georges QC G5Y 6X8; Laval'84; FRCSC; OrthSurg. assoc Staff, Carrefour Sante Granit; ac Staff, Centre Hospitalier Beauce-Etchemin; (418)228-2899; Fax. (418)228-2875.

VACRI, Chantal; Clinique Med Blainville, 519 boul du Cure-Labelle, Sainte-Therese QC J7C 2H6; Mon'88; Staff Obst & GenMed, Hôpital de Saint-Eustache; (450)430-2222; Fax. (450)433-1274.

VACY-LYLE, Mark J; Southland Court Med Clinic, 228-10601 Southport Rd SW, Calgary AB T2W 3M6; Cape Town (South Africa)'80; MB ChB; (403)225-8013; Fax. (403)225-8892.

VADAS, Peter; St Michael's Hosp, CW 8 161-30 Bond St, Toronto ON M5B 1W8; Tor'83; BSc; PhD; FACP; FRCPC; IntMed (Anaphylaxis); ClinImmunol&Allergy. Head Div of Allergy & Clin Immunol, St Michael's Hospital; Med Dir, Regional Anaphylaxis Clinic; Assoc Prof, University of Toronto; Langs: Hungarian; (416)864-5777; Fax. (416)864-3033.

VADASZ, Gabriel A; Bloor Park Med Centre, 307-726 Bloor St W, Toronto ON M6G 4A1; Tor'77; CCFP; FCFP; Langs: Italian; French; Spanish; (416)535-2255; Fax. (416)535-5041.

VADEBONCOEUR, Alain-Michel; Institut de Cardiologie de Mtl, 5000 rue Belanger, Montreal QC H1T 1C8; Mon'88; EmergMed (P.Q.). Staff, Institut de Cardiologie de Montréal; (514)376-3330 x2092; Fax. (514)221-3229.

VADEBONCOEUR, Bonita A; Burnside Family Med Clinic, 2-101 Burnside Rd W, Victoria BC V9A 1B7; UBC'91; Staff, Canadian Forces Health Services - Pacific Centre; Staff, Colwood Medical Treatment Centre; (250)381-4353

VADEBONCOEUR, Christina M; 401 Smyth Rd, Ottawa ON K1H 8L1; UBC'90; BSc; DrMedCh; FRCPC; Peds (Palliative Care). Staff, Children's Hospital of Eastern Ontario (CHEO); Consultant Perinatal Med Palliative Care, The Ottawa Hospital - General Campus; (613)737-7600 x2679; Fax. (613)523-3617; vadeboncoeur@cheo.on.ca.

VADEBONCOEUR, Marielle; Imagix-Radiologie Brossard, 2340 boul Lapiniere, Brossard QC J4Z 2K7; Mon'71; LMCC; LRCPS; DiagRad. (450)656-1220; Fax. (450)656-3513; mariellevad@hotmail.com.

VADEBONCOEUR, Roger; Inst Readaptation Gingras-Lind, 6300 av de Darlington, Montreal QC H3S 2J4; Laval'69; PhysMed&Rehab (Palliative Care). Staff, Institut de Réadaptation Gingras-Lindsay de Montréal; Langs: Bilingual(French/English); (514)340-2770; Fax. (514)340-2775; roger.vadeboncoeur@ssss.gouv.qc.ca.

VADERA, Rajiv; St Joseph's Healthcare, 50 Charlton Ave E, Hamilton ON L8N 4A6; Qns'89; CCFP; CCFP(E.M.); FCFP; Staff, St Joseph's Healthcare - Charlton Campus; (905)522-1150 x8510

VADNAIS, Marjorie; Hôpital Ste-Justine, 3175 ch Cote-Sainte-Catherine, Montreal QC H3T 1C5; Mon'04; FRCPC; Psy. Staff, Hôpital Ste-Justine; (514)345-4931

VADOR, Gunjan M; Scarborough Hosp-Birchmount, 3030 Birchmount Rd, Scarborough ON M1W 3W3; Bombay (India)'89; MB BS; FRCPC; IntMed. Staff, The Scarborough Hospital - Birchmount Campus; Langs: Hindi; Gujarati; Marathi; (416)495-2576; Fax. (416)495-2579.

VADYSINGHE, Amal; Office of Chief Med Examiner, 210-1 Wesley Ave, Winnipeg MB R3C 4C6.

VAEZI, Aref; Bloor-Dufferin Med Centre, 204-1011 Dufferin St, Toronto ON M6H 4B5; McM'87; CCFP; Ac Staff, Humber River Regional Hospital - Keele Street Site; Physician, Canadian Centre for Victims of Torture; Clin Preceptor, University of Toronto; Langs: Farsi; Persian; (416)531-3535; Fax. (416)486-7996.

VAFIADIS, Petros; CSSS de Saint-Jerome, 290 rue de Montigny, Saint-Jerome QC J7Z 5T3; McG'02; FRCSC; GenSurg. Staff, Hôtel-Dieu de Saint-Jérôme; (450)431-8201

VAGA, Kristin H; Postgrad Med Education Office, 70 Barrie St, Kingston ON K7L 3N6; Tor'09; CCFP; CCFP(E.M.).

VAGHADIA, Himat; Vancouver Gen Hosp, JPP 2449-855 12th Ave W, Vancouver BC V5Z 1M9; London (England)'79; BSc(Hon.); MHSc; FFARCS; MB BS; FRCS; FRCPC; Anes (Ambulatory Anesthesia). Ac Staff, Vancouver General Hospital - Centennial Pavillion; Clin Assoc Prof Anes Health Care & Epidemiol, University of British Columbia; Langs: Gujarati; Hindi; Swahili; Punjabi; (604)875-4575; Fax. (604)875-5209; Himat.Vaghadia@vch.ca.

VAGO, Agnes; Toronto East Gen & Orth Hosp, 825 Coxwell Ave, Toronto ON M4C 3E7; Debrecen (Hungary)'74; FRCPC; AnatPath. Staff, Toronto East General Hospital Inc; Langs: Hungarian; (416)469-6580; Fax. (416)469-6359.

VAHDAT, Jamie H; Medical Arts Bldg, 7-165 Plymouth Rd, Welland ON L3B 3E1; Sask'92; BSc(Hons.); FRCSC; Ophth (Cataract & Refractive). Ac Staff, Niagara Health System - Welland Hospital Site; (905)734-6716; Fax. (905)734-7647.

VAHIDY, Seemin A; 5706 19A Ave NW, Edmonton AB T6L 1L8; Karachi (Pakistan)'82; MB BS; Langs: Urdu; Hindi; Punjabi; (780)450-1919; Fax. (780)450-1927.

VAIDESWARAN, Sangeeta; Colborne Family Med Centre, 612 Colborne St, London ON N6B 2V2; Ranchi (India)'87; MB BS; CCFP; FCFP; Langs: Tamil; Hindi; (519)673-1962; Fax. (519)673-3758.

VAIDYA, Ann R; PO Box 89140 Mackenzie Rpo, Calgary AB T2Z 3W3; Cal'05; CCFP; (403)984-4877; Fax. (403)984-4877.

VAIDYA, Shailla; Carleton & Church Walk In Clin, 60 Carleton St, Toronto ON M5B 1J2; Dal'99; CCFP; CCFP(E.M.); Langs: English; French; (416)646-1890; Fax. (416)646-1892; svaidya@mtsinai.on.ca.

VAIDYANATH, Chantal G; Toronto Rehab Inst-Univ Ctre, 10 1073-550 University Ave, Toronto ON M5G 2A2; Wes'01; FRCPC; PhysMed&Rehab (Brain Injury Rehabilitation). Staff, Toronto Rehabilitation Institute - University Centre; (416)597-3422; Fax. (416)597-7107.

VAIDYANATHAN, Chandraprabha; Children Hosp of Eastern Ont, 401 Smyth Rd, Ottawa ON K1H 8L1; Madras (India)'71; MB BS; FRCPC; Peds (Emergency & General Pediatrics). Physician Emerg, Children's Hospital of Eastern Ontario (CHEO); Asst Prof, University of Ottawa; Langs: Tamil; (613)737-7600

VAIDYANATHAN, Prema; 110 Queen's Plate Dr, Etobicoke ON M9W 0B4; Calcutta (India)'85; MB BS; FACOG; DObst(Ire.); FRCOG; FRCSC; ObstGyn. Staff, William Osler Health System - Etobicoke General Hospital; Langs: Hindi; Tamil; Bengali; (416)741-2079

VAIDYANATHAN, Sammy; 200-65 Queen St W, Toronto ON M5H 2M5; (Other Foreign)'06; CCFP; CCFP(E.M.); Staff, Humber River Regional Hospital - Finch Avenue Site.

VAIDYANATHAN, Sankar; Finchlea Med Centre, 204-490 Bramalea Rd, Brampton ON L6T 0G1; Calcutta (India)'81; MRC; CCFP; ObstGyn. Staff, William Osler Health System - Etobicoke General Hospital; Staff, William Osler Health System - Brampton Civic Hospital; Langs: Bengali; Hindi; Punjabi; Tamil; (905)792-6500; Fax. (905)792-6853.

VAIL, Gordon R; Hotel-Dieu Grace Hosp, 1030 Ouellette Ave, Windsor ON N9A 1E1; Tor'00; CCFP; CCFP(E.M.); Staff, Hôtel-Dieu Grace Hospital; (519)973-4401; Fax. (519)252-3632.

VAILLANCOURT, Catherine; Clinique Med St-Louis, 220-3165 ch St-Louis, Quebec QC G1W 4R4; Sher'03; (418)653-1970

VAILLANCOURT, Christian; The Ottawa Hosp-Civic Campus, 1053 Carling Ave, Ottawa ON K1Y 4E9; Mon'94; LMCC; AB; FRCPC; EmergMed. Staff, The Ottawa Hospital - Civic Campus; Langs: Bilingual(French/English); (613)798-5555; Fax. (613)761-4936.

VAILLANCOURT, Christopher A; Millidge Place, 707 Millidge Ave, Saint John NB E2K 2N7; Ott'90; CCFP; CCFP(E.M.); (506)696-6544; Fax. (506)696-0787.

VAILLANCOURT, Claude; Sun Life Canada, 1155 rue Metcalfe, Montreal QC H3B 2V9; Mon'68; Consultant Med, Sun Life Canada; Langs: Bilingual(English/French); (514)866-6411 x5608; vaillancourtc@sympatico.ca.

VAILLANCOURT, Francois; Clinique Med du Cuivre, 12 rue Gamble E, Rouyn-Noranda QC J9X 3B7; Ott'79; (819)764-4569

VAILLANCOURT, Guy; CSSS du Sud de Lanaudière, 911 montee des Pionniers, Terrebonne QC J6V 2H2; Mon'82; FRCPC; Anes. Staff, Centre Hospitalier Pierre le Gardeur; Universite de Montreal; (450)654-7525; Fax. (450)470-2602.

VAILLANCOURT, Isabelle; CLSC de Sherbrooke, 50 rue Camirand, Sherbrooke QC J1H 4J5; Sher'78; Prof Family Med, Universite de Sherbrooke; (819)565-2572; Fax. (819)565-2509; ivaillancourt@gaby-travel.com.

VAILLANCOURT, Jean-Philippe; Hôpital Sainte-Croix, 570 rue Heriot, Drummondville QC J2B 1C1; Sher'06; Psy. Staff, Hôpital Sainte-croix; (819)478-6464 x3402

VAILLANCOURT, Luc; CHUQ Hotel-Dieu de Quebec, 11 Cote-du-Palais, Quebec QC G1R 2J6; Laval'85; FRCSC; Ophth; AnatPath. Staff, Centre Hospitalier Universitaire de Québec (CHUQ) - Siege Social; Pathologiste, Hôtel-Dieu de Lévis; (418)525-4444

VAILLANCOURT, Lucie; CHUQ-St-Fracois d'Assise, 10 rue de l'Espinay, Quebec QC G1L 3L5; Laval'85; ac Staff, Centre Hospitalier Universitaire De Québec - Pavillon De St-françois-d'assise; (418)525-4397; Fax. (418)525-4424.

VAILLANCOURT, Martin; CSSS de Chicoutimi, 305 rue Saint-Vallier, Chicoutimi QC G7H 5H6; Mon'01; FRCPC; Anes. Staff, Complexe hospitalier de la Sagamie; (418)541-1000 x2217

VAILLANCOURT, Raymonde; Clinique Sante Jacques-Cartier, 200-1815 rue King O, Sherbrooke QC J1J 2E3; Mon'74; CCFP; FCFP; Staff, Centre Hospitalier Universitaire de Sherbrooke-Hopital Fleurimont; Chef Dept of Reg Gen Med Esrie, Universite de Sherbrooke; Langs: Bilingual(French/English); (819)565-7446; Fax. (819)565-7780.

VAILLANCOURT, Rosaire; Hôpital Laval, 2725 ch Sainte-Foy, Quebec QC G1V 4G5; Mon'81; FRCSC; GenSurg (Surgical Oncology); Cardiovasc&ThorSurg. Staff, Hôpital Laval; adj Prof, Université Laval; Langs: Bilingual(French/English); (418)656-8711; Fax. (418)656-4762.

VAILLANCOURT, Suzanne M; MUHC-Montreal Children's Hosp, 2300 rue Tupper, Montreal QC H3H 1P3; Cal'00; Peds (Pediatric Emergency Medicine). Staff, McGill University Health Centre - Montreal Children's Hospital; (514)412-4400

VAILLANCOURT, Yvon; GMF Concorde, 300 boul de la Concorde E, Laval QC H7G 2E6; McG'72; (450)667-5310; Fax. (450)667-5248.

VAILLANT, Nathalie; CLSC des Mille-Iles, 4731 boul Levesque E, Laval QC H7C 1M9; Mon'90; (450)661-5370; Fax. (450)661-9147.

VAIR, Donald B; Queen Elizabeth II HSC, 8 806-1276 South Park St, Halifax NS B3H 2Y9; Dal'76; FRCSC; GenSurg (P.Q.) (Biliary Surgery). Court Staff, IWK Health Centre; Ac Staff, Queen Elizabeth II Health Sciences Centre - Victoria General Site; Assoc Prof, Dalhousie University; (902)473-3242; Fax. (902)473-5939; brock.vair@dal.ca.

VAIRAVANATHAN, Rajani; Toronto East Gen & Orth Hosp, 825 Coxwell Ave, East York ON M4C 3E7; Tor'02; CCFP; CCFP(E.M.); Staff, Toronto East General Hospital Inc; Langs: Tamil; (416)469-6580 x7734

VAISH, Saurabh; Allwood Med Clinic, 102-2752 Allwood St, Abbotsford BC V2T 3R7; Lucknow (India)'98; MB BS; DABEM; CCFP; Staff, Abbotsford Regional Hospital & Cancer Centre; Teach Staff, University of British Columbia; (604)850-6893; Fax. (604)850-6896.

VAISHNAV, Vandana; Prince County Hosp, PO Box 3000 65 Roy Boates Ave, Summerside PE C1N 3G6; Rajasthan University (Other Foreign)'95; FRCPC; Anes. Staff, Prince County Hospital; (902)438-4200

VAISLER, Barry J; Northmount Med Centre, 604-145 13th St E, North Vancouver BC V7L 2L4; Wes'72; FRCSC; OrthSurg (Hand Surgery). Ac Staff, Lions Gate Hospital; (604)987-1711; Fax. (604)987-9171; bvaisler@hotmail.com.

VAITEKUNAS, Susan; SMBD Jewish Gen Hosp, 3755 ch Cote-Sainte-Catherine, Montreal QC H3T 1E2; McG'86; Staff, Sir Mortimer B Davis Jewish General; (514)340-8222 x3829; Fax. (514)340-7547.

VAITHIANATHAN, Kandiah; Medical Centre, 109-2100 Ellesmere Rd, Scarborough ON M1H 3B7; Colombo (Sri Lanka)'79; LRCP(Ed); LRCS(Ed); CCFP; FCFP; Langs: Tamil; (416)438-2496; Fax. (416)438-8290.

VAITHILINGAM, Dushandhan S; 400 The West Mall, Etobicoke ON M9C 5S1; Tor'89; (416)626-6383; Fax. (416)626-6326.

VAITHILINGAM, Sudhama S; 4309 Harold Ave, South Porcupine ON P0N 1H0; Dublin (Ireland)'72; DCH; LRCPSI; FRCS; Member Infect Control, Timmins & District Hospital; Med Advisor, Extendicare Nursing Home; Assoc Prof Clinical Science, Northern Ontario School of Medicine; (705)235-3123; Fax. (705)235-3920.

VAJCNER, Glen A; Suitor House, 1004 8 Ave SE, Calgary AB T2G 0M4; Man'06; FRCSC; GenSurg. (403)264-6720; Fax. (403)351-1679.

VAJID, Muhammad A; Peterborough Reg Health Centre, 1 Hospital Dr, Peterborough ON K9J 7C6; Sind Medical College (Other Foreign)'86; Staff, Peterborough Regional Health Centre - Hospital Drive; (705)743-2121

VAJPEYI, Rajkumar; Univ Hlth Network-Toronto Gen, E11 209-200 Elizabeth St, Toronto ON M5G 2C4; Calcutta (India)'81; FRCPC; AnatPath (General Pathology). Staff, Toronto General Hospital - UHN; Langs: Bengali; Hindi; Punjabi; (416)340-4827

VAJRAVELU, Pavithra; View Med Family Practice, 1449 View Cres, Delta BC V4L 2K2; (Other Foreign)'02; (604)943-6999

VAJSAR, Jiri; The Hosp for Sick Children, 555 University Ave, Toronto ON M5G 1X8; Prague (Czech Republic)'76; FRCPC; Neur. Staff, The Hospital For Sick Children; Assoc Prof, University of Toronto; (416)813-7500; Fax. (416)813-6334; jiri.vajsar@sickkids.ca.

VAKANI, M Tariq; Dixie Medical Group, 113-1055 Canadian Place, Mississauga ON L4W 0C2; Karachi (Pakistan)'79; MRCP(UK); FACC; FRCPC; IntMed (Hypertension); Cardiol. Locum Tenens Cardiol, Joseph Brant Memorial Hospital; Langs: Hindi; Gujarati; Urdu; (905)212-9600; tariqvakani@gmail.com.

VAKEESAN, Sivaraji; Fogal Medical Centre, 7-8920 Highway 50, Brampton ON L6P 3A3; (Other Foreign)'87; CCFP; Langs: Tamil; (905)915-8778; Fax. (905)915-8780.

VAKHARIA, Narendra R; Queen Elizabeth II HSC, 1276 South Park St, Halifax NS B3H 2Y9; Dal'93; FRCPC; Anes. Staff, IWK Health Centre; Staff, Queen Elizabeth II Health Sciences Centre - Victoria General Site; Asst Prof, Dalhousie University; (902)473-2331

VAKIL, Ankitkumar P; Doctors Plus Med Centre, 310-505 Main St SW, Airdrie AB T4B 3K3; (403)945-0770; Fax. (403)945-8997.

VAKIL, Catherine R; Family Med Centre, 220 Bagot St, Kingston ON K7L 5E9; Ott'85; CCFP; FCFP; Staff, Kingston General Hospital; Langs: Bilingual(French/English); (613)533-9303; Fax. (613)549-0426; cv4@post.queensu.ca.

VAKILHA, Mehrdad; 1 Somerset Pl PO Box 209, Somerset MB R0G 2L0; Shaheed Beheshti University (Other Foreign)'97; (204)744-2265; Fax. (204)744-2511.

VAKILITAHAMI, Habib; Northern Medical Unit, T162-770 Bannatyne Ave, Winnipeg MB R3E 0W3; (Other Foreign)'90; (204)789-3711

VAKTOR, Peter; 480-550 rue Sherbrooke O, Montreal QC H3A 1B9; Montpellier (France)'77; BSc; adj Médecin, McGill University Health Centre - Royal Victoria Hospital; Langs: Hungarian; French; (514)284-1006; Fax. (514)284-1021; pvak@cam.org.

VALA, Francis H; 230-150 Esplanade St W, North Vancouver BC V7M 1A3; Shiraz (Iran)'94; CCFP; Langs: Farsi; (604)980-2128

VALADE, Andre; Clinique Med 3000 Inc, 3000 rue Belanger, Montreal QC H1Y 1A9; Mon'85; Staff, Hôpital Santa Cabrini Ospedale; (514)376-7702; Fax. (514)376-2639.

VALADKA, Mikas A; 303-2150 Bloor St W, Toronto ON M6S 1M8; Julius Maximilian University (Germany)'80; Ac Staff, St Joseph's Health Centre; Langs: German; Lithuanian; (416)769-2415; Fax. (416)767-5337.

VALADKA, Saulius M; Halton Healthcare Serv-Oakvill, 327 Reynolds St, Oakville ON L6J 3L7; Qns'01; FRCPC; DiagRad. Staff, Halton Healthcare Services Corporation - Oakville Site; Langs: Lithuanian; (905)845-2571; svaladka@haltonhealthcare.on.ca.

VALANI, Rahim A; Hamilton HS-General Site, 237 Barton St E, Hamilton ON L8L 2X2; Qns'99; FRCPC; EmergMed;CCFP; CCFP(E.M.); Staff, Hamilton Health Sciences Centre - Hamilton General Hospital; (905)521-2100

VALCOURT, Dieudonné; CSSS de Gatineau, 949 rue de la Verendrye, Gatineau QC J8T 7H2; Port-au-Prince (Haiti)'01; IntMed. (819)966-6100

VALCOURT, Edith E; Montfort Med Centre, 5-1968 Portobello Blvd, Orleans ON K4A 4E7; Ott'02; FRCSC; ObstGyn. Ac Staff, Montfort Hospital; Langs: Bilingual(English/French); (613)837-7033 x6; Fax. (613)837-5781.

VALDECANAS, Georgina G; Rockyview Gen Hosp, 4580-7007 14 St SW, Calgary AB T2V 1P9; (Other Foreign)'92; CCFP; Staff, Rockyview General Hospital; (403)943-3597; Fax. (403)943-8411.

VALDIVIA, Olga E; Centre d'Urgence Salaberry, 2758 rue de Salaberry, Montreal QC H3M 1L3; Mon'01; CCFP; Staff, Hôpital de Saint-Eustache; (514)337-4772

VALE, John W; 14-85 Church St, Mississauga ON L5M 1M6; Tor'71; FRCSC; GenSurg. Ac Staff, Trillium Health Centre - West Toronto; (905)812-8003

VALE, Noah A; 4G Spadina Ave, Toronto ON M5V 3Z9; McM'08; CCFP; Fax. (416)367-4301.

VALENTE, Maria; Harbourview Clinic, 43 Court St N, Thunder Bay ON P7A 4T5; Tor'92; Langs: Italian; (807)344-7877; Fax. (807)346-8687.

VALENTI, David A; MUHC-Royal Victoria Hosp, A451-687 av des Pins O, Montreal QC H3A 1A1; McG'92; FRCPC; DiagRad. Staff, McGill University Health Centre - Royal Victoria Hospital; Langs: English; French; (514)843-1545; Fax. (514)843-1517; david.valenti@muhc.mcgill.ca.

VALENTINE, Karen A; Foothills Med Centre, C210-1403 29 St NW, Calgary AB T2N 2T9; Cal'90; FRCPC; IntMed; Hem. Staff Hematol, Foothills Medical Centre; (403)944-4451; Fax. (403)944-1647.

VALENTINIS, Alissia R; Taddle Creek Family Health Team, 522-790 Bay St E Box 58, Toronto ON M5G 1N8; Ott'03; BSc; CCFP; Staff, St Michael's Hospital; Staff, Women's College Hospital; Langs: Italian; (416)591-1222; Fax. (416)591-1227.

VALENTINO, Pamela; The Hosp for Sick Children, 555 University Ave, Toronto ON M5G 1X8; McG'07; MDCM; FRCPC; Peds; Gastroent. Staff, The Hospital For Sick Children; Langs: Italian; French; (416)813-1500

VALERIOTE, Josee; Clinique Chirurgie Orthopediqu, 126 rue St-Louis, Longueuil QC J4R 2L5; Sher'05; FRCSC; OrthSurg. (450)672-1212

VALETTAS, Nicholas; Hamilton HS-General Site, 509-237 Barton St E, Hamilton ON L8L 2X2; Tor'93; ABCD; FRCPC; FRCPC; Cardiol; IntMed (Interventional Cardiology). Staff, Hamilton Health Sciences Centre-Juravinski Site; Staff McMaster Clinic, Hamilton Health Sciences Centre - Hamilton General Hospital; Assoc Prof, McMaster University; Langs: French; Greek; (905)574-0953; Fax. (905)574-8417; valettn@mcmaster.ca.

VALIA, Bhavna; 306-267 O'Connor St, Ottawa ON K2P 1V3; Wes'81; CCFP; Langs: Gujarati; French; (613)233-6652; Fax. (613)233-0981.

VALIANTE, Taufik A; Univ Hlth Network-Toronto Western Hosp, WW4W 436-399 Bathurst St, Toronto ON M5T 2S8; Tor'97; FRCSC; Neursurg (Epilepsy). Staff, Toronto Western Hospital - University Health Network; (416)603-5460; Fax. (416)603-5298.

VALIKANGAS, Eija M; CML Health Centre, 520-790 Bay St, Toronto ON M5G 1N8; Helsinki (Finland)'73; FRCPC; DiagRad. Langs: Finnish; (416)260-1974; Fax. (416)260-1687.

VALIMOHAMED, Farah; Royal Columbian Hosp, 330 Columbia St E, New Westminster BC V3L 3W7; UBC'95; FRCPC; Anes. Staff, Royal Columbian Hospital; (604)520-4602

VALIN, Sharonie S; North York Gen Hosp, 4S-4001 Leslie St, North York ON M2K 1E1; Tor'00; CCFP; Staff Family Med, North York General Hospital; Langs: Hebrew; (416)756-6980; Fax. (416)756-6979.

VALIQUET, Stacey K; Thames Valley FHT-Victoria Fam, 60 Chesley Ave, London ON N5Z 2C1; Wes'00; CCFP; CCFP(E.M.); Staff, London Health Sciences Centre - Victoria Campus; (519)433-8424; Fax. (519)433-2244; stacey.valiquet@lhsc.on.ca.

VALIQUETTE, Alain; Clinique Med Deux-Montagnes, 201 9e av, Deux-Montagnes QC J7R 3M1; Mon'79; Staff, Hôpital de Saint-Eustache; (450)472-7520 x4; Fax. (450)472-0886.

VALIQUETTE, Celine; CLSC des Maskoutains, 1015 rue Gauthier, Saint-Hyacinthe QC J2S 8T2; Mon'85; (450)778-2572; Fax. (450)771-3701.

VALIQUETTE, Louis; CHUS-Hop Fleurimont, 3001 12e av N, Sherbrooke QC J1H 5N4; Sher'95; MSc; FRCP; LMCC; FRCPC; IntMed (Epidemiology & Clinical Epidemiology); InfectDis; MedMicrobiol. Staff, Centre Hospitalier Universitaire de Sherbrooke-Hopital Fleurimont; (819)346-1110; Fax. (819)829-3286; louis.valiquette@usherbrooke.ca.

VALIQUETTE, Louise; Dir de protection Sante publiq, 2 03-201 boul Cremazie E, Montreal QC H2M 1L2; Mon'86; FRCPC; CommunMed. Staff, Hopital Maisonneuve-Rosemont; Staff, Ministry of Health & Social Services-Quebec; (514)873-1289; lvalique@santepub-mtl.qc.ca.

VALIQUETTE, Luc; Les Urologues Assoc de Mtl, 301-235 boul Rene-Levesque E, Montreal QC H2X 1N8; Mon'78; FACS; FRCSC; Urol (Erectile Dysfunction). Staff Urol, Centre Hospitalier l'Université De Montréal (CHUM) - Hôpital Saint-luc; Médecin, Les Urologues Ass du CHUM; dép Chef Surgery, Universite de Montreal; Langs: English; (514)861-0213; Fax. (514)861-3021.

VALIQUETTE, Noemie; Clinique Med Memphre, 200-323 rue Sherbrooke, Magog QC J1X 2R9; Sher'87; Langs: Bilingual(French/English); (819)847-1313; Fax. (819)847-3529.

VALIQUETTE-LAVIGNE, Mylene; Centre Hosp Honore-Mercier, 2750 boul Laframboise, Saint-Hyacinthe QC J2S 4Y8; Mon'04; FRCPC; Psy. Staff, Centre Hospitalier Honore-Mercier; (450)771-3222

VALIULIS, Algis P J; Taunton Surgical Centre, 1290 Keith Ross Dr, Oakville ON L6H 7K4; Tor'78; BSc; FACS; FRCSC; GenSurg (Laparoscopy). Staff, Lakeridge Health - Oshawa Site; Langs: Lithuanian; (905)723-8551; Fax. (905)721-6642.

VALJI, Azim M; Royal Alexandra Hosp, 415-10240 Kingsway NW, Edmonton AB T5H 3V9; Alb'89; FRCSC; GenSurg; ThorSurg. Staff, Royal Alexandra Hospital; (780)735-4583; Fax. (780)735-4245.

VALJI, Shairose; Royal Alexandra Hosp, 415-10240 Kingsway NW, Edmonton AB T5H 3V9; Alb'92; CCFP; Staff Commun Services Ctre, Royal Alexandra Hospital; (780)735-4488; Fax. (780)735-4245.

VALKOVA, Vanelia V; Carbonear Gen Hosp, 86 Highroad S, Carbonear NL A1Y 1A4; Pleven Medical University of Bulgaria (Bulgaria)'91; Staff, Carbonear General Hospital; (709)945-5111

VALLABH, Pravesh K; University of Alberta Hosp, 1E7 21WMC-8440 112 St NW, Edmonton AB T6G 2B7; Natal (South Africa)'97; MB ChB; FRCPC; Psy;CCFP; Staff Multidisciplinary Pain Centre, University of Alberta Hospital; Langs: Gujarati; Hindi; Zulu; (780)407-8638

VALLABHANENI, M Rao; 692 Euclid Ave, Toronto ON M6G 2T9; Andhra (India)'73; MB BS; FRCPC; Psy. Staff, Mount Sinai Hospital; Langs: Telugu; (416)901-9020; Fax. (416)901-7217.

VALLANCE, Hilary D; Children's & Women's HC Of BC, 2F22-4480 Oak St, Vancouver BC V6H 3V4; UBC'87; FRCPC; MedBiochem (Biochemical Genetics). Staff, BC Children's Hospital; Clin Assoc Prof, University of British Columbia; (604)875-2551; Fax. (604)875-3434; hvallance@cw.bc.ca.

VALLANCE, Maelor; St Paul's Hosp, 1081 Burrard St, Vancouver BC V6Z 1Y6; Glasgow (Scotland)'58; MB ChB; DPM; FRCPsy; FRCPC; Psy (Medico Legal Psychiatry). Hon Staff Outpatient Psy, Providence Health Care - St Paul's Hospital; Hon Staff, Vancouver General Hospital - Centennial Pavillion; Clin Prof Emeritus, University of British Columbia; (604)682-2344 x62415; Fax. (604)806-8941; maelor@hotmail.com.

VALLEE, Chantal; Hop Charles Lemoyne, 3120 boul Taschereau, Greenfield Park QC J4V 2H1; Sher'98; FRCPC; IntMed (Cardiology). Staff, Hopital Charles LeMoyne; Prof, Universite de Sherbrooke; Langs: Bilingual(English/French); (450)466-5000 x2880; Fax. (450)466-5768; chantal.vallee@usherbrooke.ca.

VALLEE, Helene; Clinique Med Chaudiere, 102 18e rue, Saint-Georges QC G5Y 4T9; Laval'88; LMCC; adj Staff HemOncol, Centre Hospitalier Beauce-Etchemin; Langs: Bilingual(French/English); (418)228-6820; Fax. (418)226-0358.

VALLEE, Isabelle; 14 Wing Greenwood, PO Box 5000 Stn Main Greenwood 26 CF Health Services, Greenwood NS B0P 1N0; Sher'10; CCFP; Staff, Canadian Forces Base-Greenwood; (902)765-1494

VALLEE, Jacynthe; Centre Med de la Vallee, 1-22 av du Pont, Amqui QC G5J 3T5; Laval'82; (418)629-6611; Fax. (418)629-4484.

VALLEE, Michel; Hop Maisonneuve-Rosemont, 5415 boul de l'Assomption, Montreal QC H1T 2M4; Laval'00; CSPQ; FRCPC; IntMed (Hypertension); Nephrol. Staff, Hopital Maisonneuve-Rosemont; (514)252-3400

VALLEE, Michele; Regie des Rentes du Quebec, 2600 boul Laurier, Quebec QC G1V 4T3; Laval'85; Staff, Centre Hospitalier Portneuf; Médecin, Regie des Rentes du Quebec; (418)657-8709 x3670; Fax. (418)528-0404; michele.vallee@rrq.gouv.qc.ca.

VALLEE, Nicole; Regie l'Assurance Maladie QC, Q 044-1125 Grande Allee O, Quebec QC G1S 1E7; Laval'84; GenSurg. Staff, Centre Hospitalier Affilié Universitaire de Québec - Hôpital du St-Sacrement; Médecin, Regie de l'Assurance Maladie du Quebec; (418)682-5144

VALLEE, Pierre; Clinique Med du Sud-Ouest, 3-4475 rue Bannatyne, Verdun QC H4G 1E2; Laval'70; Médecin, Clinique Med du Sud-Ouest; Médecin, Clinique Medicale de l'Ouest; Langs: Bilingual(French/English); (514)765-3600; Fax. (514)765-9625; pierre.vallee@gms.gouv.qc.ca.

VALLEE, Rene; Centre Med Ste-Anne, 100-10974 boul Sainte-Anne, Beaupre QC G0A 1E0; Laval'73; (418)827-4022; Fax. (418)827-4964.

VALLEE, Sophie; Polyclinique Med de Terrebonne, 201-901 boul des Seigneurs, Terrebonne QC J6W 1T8; Laval'97; Staff, Centre Hospitalier Pierre le Gardeur; (450)471-1117; Fax. (450)471-8043; drsop@videotron.ca.

VALLEE, Sophie-Lisa; Clinique Med 201, 104 rue Sainte-Agathe, Ste-Agathe-Des-Mts QC J8C 2K3; Sher'81; (819)326-3464; Fax. (819)326-8801; s.l.vallee@sympatico.ca.

VALLENTYNE, Stephen W; 210-347 Leon Ave, Kelowna BC V1Y 8C7; Man'83; FRCPC; PhysMed&Rehab. Med Dir Work Capacity Evaluation Prog, Kelowna General Hospital; (250)762-2330

VALLETTE, Sophie; CHUM-Hop Notre-Dame, 1560 rue Sherbrooke E, Montreal QC H2L 4M1; Marseille (France)'99; PhD(Neurosciences); FRCPC; Endocrin&Metab (Neuro Endocrinology). Prof, Centre Hospitalier l'Université de Montréal (CHUM) - Hôpital Notre-Dame; Langs: English; (514)890-8000 x25223; Fax. (514)412-7692; sophie.vallette@ircm.qc.ca.

VALLIANT, Lew H; 256 Wellington St, Kingston ON K7K 2Z1; Qns'76; AB; FAAFP; CCFP; FCFP; Assoc Staff, Hotel-Dieu Hospital; Assoc Staff, Kingston General Hospital; (613)542-1988

VALLIERES, Andree; Ctr de Med Familiale Gatineau, 908 boul Maloney E, Gatineau QC J8P 1H5; Sher'06; CCFP; (819)663-7711; Fax. (819)663-9326.

VALLIERES, Bertrand J; CSSS de Trois-Rivières, 1991 boul du Carmel, Trois-Rivieres QC G8Z 3R9; Sher'71; AB; NuclearMed. Staff, CSSS de Trois-Rivières; (819)378-9854; Fax. (819)378-9814.

VALLIERES, Camil; Clinique Med du Cartier, 1191 av Cartier, Quebec QC G1R 2S9; Laval'78; LMCC; Staff, Jeffery Hale Hospital-Saint Brigid's; Médecin, Clinique Medicale du Cartier; (418)522-1911; Fax. (418)522-1789.

VALLIERES, Francois; CSSSRT, 1717 rue Notre-Dame N, Thetford Mines QC G6G 2V4; Laval'93; Staff, Hopital du CSS de la Region de Thetford; (418)338-7777

VALLIERES, Gerald; Anapharm Inc, 2500 rue Einstein, Quebec QC G1P 0A2; Laval'82; Médecin, Pharmanet Canada Inc; (418)527-3067; Fax. (418)527-3456.

VALLIERES, Isabelle; CHUQ-Hotel-Dieu de Quebec, 11 Cote du Palais, Quebec QC G1R 2J6; Laval'98; FRCPC; RadOncol (Lymphoma & Myeloma). Staff, Centre Hospitalier Universitaire de Québec (CHUQ) - Siege Social; Langs: Bilingual(French/English); (418)691-5264; Fax. (418)691-5268; isabelle.vallieres@mail.chuq.qc.ca.

VALLIERES, M Beth; Dunbar Family Practice, 5-350 Hespeler Rd, Cambridge ON N1R 7N7; Qns'88; CCFP; CCFP(E.M.); FCFP; Staff, Cambridge Memorial Hospital; Staff, Stirling Heights Long Term Care Facility; Langs: English; French; (519)624-8934; Fax. (519)624-1576.

VALLIERES, Marcel; Clinique Med Ste-Marthe, 1770 rue Notre-Dame Est, Trois-Rivieres QC G8T 4J3; Laval'79; ac Staff, CSSS de Trois-Rivières; Médecin, Centre Medicale Ste-Marthe; (819)373-9887; Fax. (819)371-9894.

VALLIERES, Martin; CSSS de Beauce-Etchemin, 1515 17e rue, Saint-Georges QC G5Y 4T8; Laval'95; Staff, Centre Hospitalier Beauce-Etchemin; (418)228-2031

VALLIERES, Michel; CHUQ-Hotel-Dieu de Quebec, 11 Cote du Palais, Quebec QC G1R 2J6; Laval'70; FRCPC; IntMed. Staff, Centre Hospitalier Universitaire de Québec (CHUQ) - Siege Social; adj Prof, Université Laval; (418)691-5087; Fax. (418)691-5266.

VALLIERES, Nathalie; Clinique Med Carre St-Lambert, 100A-299 Boul Sir-Wilfrid-Laur, Saint-Lambert QC J4R 2L1; Sher'00; Staff, Hopital Charles LeMoyne; Langs: Bilingual(French/English); (450)465-6551; Fax. (450)465-9810.

VALLIERES-PILON, Julia; SMBD Jewish Gen Hosp, 3755 ch Cote-Sainte-Catherine, Montreal QC H3T 1E2; Mon'10; CCFP; Staff, Sir Mortimer B Davis Jewish General; (514)340-8222

VALLY, Tomas; West Coast Family Med Clinic, PO Box 880 1300-6660 Sooke Rd, Sooke BC V9Z 1H8; UBC'90; CCFP; (250)642-3913; Fax. (250)642-6620.

VALMANA, Anton; 4733 49 St, Red Deer AB T4N 1T6; (403)340-7046; Fax. (403)340-5217.

VALNICEK, Stanislav; Kelowna Gen Hosp, 2268 Pandosy St, Kelowna BC V1Y 1T2; Prague (Czech Republic)'57; FACOG; FRCSC; ObstGyn. Staff, Kelowna General Hospital; Langs: Czech; (250)862-4000; stanv@shaw.ca.

VALNICEK, Stanley M; Okanagan Plastic Surgery Centr, 401-3320 Richter St, Kelowna BC V1W 4V5; Sask'86; FRCSC; PlasSurg (Cosmetics). Staff Surgical Floor, Okanagan Plastic Surgery Centre; Dir Skin Care floor, Okanagan Skin Care Centre; Clinical Asst Prof, University of British Columbia; (250)868-9290; Fax. (250)868-9704.

VALOIS, Carol; UMF Charles Lemoyne, 201-299 boul Sir-Wilfrid-Lauri, Saint-Lambert QC J4R 2L1; Mon'82; CCFP; FCFP; Prof Family Med, Universite de Sherbrooke; Langs: Bilingual(French/English); (450)466-5630; Fax. (450)466-5631.

VALOIS, Chantal; Cooperative de Sante, 206-1937 Ch Du Village, St-Adolphe-D'Howrd QC J0T 2B0; Mon'94; Physician, CLSC des Pays d'Enhaut; Langs: Bilingual(French/English); (819)327-3534; Fax. (819)327-3332.

VALOIS, Joyce; Centre Med Blouin Valois, 100B-299 boul Sir-Wilfrid-Laur, Saint-Lambert QC J4R 2L1; Mon'83; CCFP; FCFP; Langs: English; (450)465-5541; Fax. (450)465-7358.

VALOIS, Lucie; Clinique Méd Mascouche, 100-1025 Montee Masson, Mascouche QC J7K 2L9; Mon'81; CCFP; (450)474-6000; Fax. (450)474-6666.

VALOIS, M S Nadine; CSSS de Trois-Rivières, 1991 boul du Carmel, Trois-Rivieres QC G8Z 3R9; Laval'02; FRCPC; Peds. Staff, CSSS de Trois-Rivières; (819)697-3333

VALOIS, Maria; Toronto East Gen Hosp Inc, 825 Coxwell Ave, Toronto ON M4C 3E7; Mon'95; PhD; FRCPC; IntMed (Adverse Drug Reactions). Staff, The Scarborough Hospital - Birchmount Campus; Staff, Toronto East General Hospital Inc; Langs: American Sign Language; French; (416)461-8272; mvalois@tsh.to.

VALOIS, Marie-Michelle; Hôpital de Christ-Roi, 675 rue Saint-Jean-Baptiste, Nicolet QC J3T 1S4; Mon'08; Staff, Hôpital de Christ-Roi; (819)293-2071

VALOIS, Maxime; Ctr Hosp de Verdun, 4000 boul Lasalle, Verdun QC H4G 2A3; Sher'02; CCFP; CCFP(E.M.); Staff, Centre Hospitalier de Verdun; (514)362-1000; maxvalois@hotmail.com.

VALOIS GOMEZ, Teresa A; MUHC-Montreal Children's Hosp, C 118-2300 rue Tupper, Montreal QC H3H 1P3; Caracas (Venezuela)'96; Anes (P.Q.) (Pediatric Anesthesia). Staff, McGill University Health Centre - Montreal Children's Hospital; (514)412-4400 x22463; Fax. (514)412-4341; teresa.valois@muhc.mcgill.ca.

VALTCHANOVA, Zdravka P; North Side Med Clinic, 915 Central Ave N, Swift Current SK S9H 3V3; Varna (Bulgaria)'91; CCFP; Physician, Southwest Medi-Centre; (306)773-9100; Fax. (306)773-9668.

VALTUILLE, Lucas S; University of Alberta Hosp, 8440 112 St NW, Edmonton AB T6G 2B7; Staff, University of Alberta Hospital; (780)407-8822; Fax. (780)407-6452.

VALYI, Lajos; Ajax Family Care Centre, 30 Kingston Rd W, Ajax ON L1T 4K8; Budapest (Hungary)'77; CCFP; CCFP(E.M.); FCFP; Physician, Canadian Forces Base; Langs: Hungarian; (905)721-6884; Fax. (905)721-6873.

VAN, Ngoc Binh; Clinton Public Hosp, 98 Shipley St, Clinton ON N0M 1L0; Medical University of the Americas (Other Foreign)'09; Staff, Clinton Public Hospital - Huron Perth Healthcare Alliance; (519)482-3447

VAN, Quang; CHSLD Emilie-Gamelin, 1440 rue Dufresne, Montreal QC H2K 3J3; Laval'93; (514)527-8921

VAN, Thomas T C; One-Stop Med Centre, 1A-3585 Lawrence Ave E, Scarborough ON M1G 1P4; Tor'94; CCFP; Langs: Cantonese; Vietnamese; (416)431-0736; Fax. (416)431-0648.

VAN, Victor B C; Georgetown Med Associates, 199 Princess Anne Dr, Georgetown ON L7G 0E3; Alb'06; CCFP; Langs: Cantonese; (905)873-3000; Fax. (905)873-0800.

VAN AARDT, Jan A N; 204-18730 Fraser Hwy, Surrey BC V3S 7Y4; Pretoria (South Africa)'06; (604)575-0501

VAN AARDT, Renier G; Eagles Landing, 510 Prince St, Truro NS B2N 1G1; Stellenbosch (South Africa)'91; MB ChB; CCFP; Consultant, Allergan; Preceptor, Coherent Amt Inc; Med Dir, Vitality Medi Spa; Langs: Afrikaans; Flemish; (902)893-7613; Fax. (902)893-8070; drvanaardt@nslaser.com.

VAN ADEL, Brian A; London HSC-University Hosp, PO Box 5339 Stn B C7 128-339 Windermere Rd, London ON N6A 5A5; McM'05; FRCPC; Neur. Staff, London Health Sciences Centre - University Hospital; (519)685-8500

VAN AERDE, Arne; Foothills Family Med Centre, PO Bag 460 114 1 St SW, Black Diamond AB T0L 0H0; Alb'09; CCFP; (403)933-4368

VAN AERDE, John E E; Central City Tower, 400-13450 102 Ave, Surrey BC V3T 0H1; Leuven (Belgium)'78; PhD(MedSci); FRCPC; Peds (Neonatology). Staff Collaborative Practice & Quality Improvement, Stollery Children's Hospital; Reg Dir New Born Med Stollery Children's, University of Alberta Hospital; Associate School of Leadership Studies, Royal Roads University; Clin Prof Peds & Neonatology, University of Alberta; Langs: German; Dutch; French; Flemish; (604)587-4600; jvanaerd@cha.ab.ca.

VAN AERDE, Lisa; 6681 Mary Ellen Dr PO Box 41010, Nanaimo BC V9T 6M7; UBC'10; CCFP; (250)668-8575

VAN AERDE, Tim; 6681 Mary Ellen Dr PO Box 41010 Rpo Woodgrove, Nanaimo BC V9T 6M7; Alb'05; CCFP; CCFP(E.M.); (250)668-8575

VAN AGGELEN, Debra J; 201-1555 Marine Dr, West Vancouver BC V7V 1H9; UBC'85; Staff, Lions Gate Hospital; (604)926-1515; Fax. (604)926-1545.

VAN ALLEN, Margot I; BC Women's Hosp & Health Ctre, C234-4500 Oak St, Vancouver BC V6H 3N1; Chicago (USA)'77; FRCPC; MedGenetics. Staff Med Genetics, BC Women's Hospital & Health Centre; (604)875-2157

VAN ALPHEN, Katarina M; Owen Sound Med Centre, 2000-1415 1st Ave W, Owen Sound ON N4K 4K8; Tor'84; CCFP; Court Staff Privil, Grey Bruce Health Services - Owen Sound; (519)470-3030; Fax. (519)370-4058.

VAN ALSTYNE, Murray A; Dauphin Med Clinic, 622 3rd St SW, Dauphin MB R7N 1R5; Man'83; CCFP; Ac Staff, Dauphin Regional Health Centre; (204)638-6445; Fax. (204)638-5670.

VAN AMERINGEN, Michael A; Fontbonne Bldg, 4F 439-301 James St S, Hamilton ON L8P 3B6; McM'80; FRCPC; Psy (Anxiety Disorder);CCFP; Court Staff Psy, Hamilton Health Sciences Centre - McMaster University Medical Centre; Ac Staff Psy, St Joseph's Healthcare - Charlton Campus; Assoc Prof Psy & Behavioural Neurosciences, McMaster University; Langs: Cantonese; (905)522-1155; Fax. (905)540-6533.

VAN AMEYDE, Kenneth J L; Health Sciences Centre, GC 419-820 Sherbrook St, Winnipeg MB R3A 1R9; Alb'79; FRCPC; IntMed. Ac Staff, Health Sciences Centre; (204)787-3735; Fax. (204)787-4826; kvanameyde@exchange.hsc.mb.ca.

VAN AMSTEL, Leanne L; Health Sciences Centre, 820 Sherbrook St, Winnipeg MB R3A 1R9; Dal'02; FRCPC; DiagRad. Staff, Health Sciences Centre; (204)774-8511

VAN ANDEL, Morris; College of Phys & Surgs of BC, 300-669 Howe St, Vancouver BC V6C 0B4; UBC'68; CCFP; Staff, College of Physicians & Surgeons of British Columbia; Langs: Dutch; (604)733-7758

VAN ARKEL, Elsbeth C; Lynnwood Med Centre, 6622 20A St SE, Calgary AB T2C 0R3; Holland (Netherlands)'93; Langs: Dutch; (403)279-3311; Fax. (403)279-4214.

VAN ARSDELL, Glen S; The Hosp for Sick Children, 555 University Ave, Toronto ON M5G 1X8; Loma Linda(CA) (USA)'86; FRCSC; CardSurg (Cardiovascular & Thoracic Surgery). Staff, The Hospital For Sick Children; (416)813-6420; Fax. (416)813-7984; glen.vanarsdell@sickkids.ca.

VAN AS, Nicolaas; Bluewater Health-Norman Site, 89 Norman St, Sarnia ON N7T 6S3; Stellenbosch (South Africa)'95; MB ChB; CCFP; CCFP(E.M.); Staff, Bluewater Health - Norman Site; Langs: Dutch; (519)464-4400; Fax. (519)541-1143.

VAN ASSCHE, Gert A A; Mount Sinai Hosp, 437-600 University Ave, Toronto ON M5G 1X5; Louvain (Belgium)'92; Staff, Mount Sinai Hospital; (416)596-4200; Fax. (416)586-8899.

VAN BAARDWIJK, S Charles; Burlington Med Arts Bldg, 761 Brant St, Burlington ON L7R 2H7; Wes'86; Staff, Joseph Brant Memorial Hospital; (905)681-3191; Fax. (905)681-6613.

VAN BAARDWIJK, Susan L; Harvard Square Mall, 205-801 Mohawk Rd W, Hamilton ON L9C 6C2; Wes'87; (905)389-0349; Fax. (905)389-1707.

VAN BENDEGEM, Jack P; 204-99 Sinclair Ave, Georgetown ON L7G 5G1; Tor'85; BSc; Staff, Halton Healthcare Services Corporation - Georgetown Hospital; (905)873-3344; Fax. (905)873-8094.

VAN BOEKEL, Patricia E; Stratford Gen Hosp, 46 General Hospital Dr, Stratford ON N5A 2Y6; Mem'98; CCFP; CCFP(E.M.); Staff, Stratford General Hospital - Huron Perth Healthcare Alliance; (519)272-8210

VAN BOXEL, Paul J; Cumberland Reg Hlth Care Ctr, 19428 Hwy 2 RR 6, Amherst NS B4H 1N6; Cape Town (South Africa)'62; MB ChB; FRCSC; GenSurg (Surgical Oncology). Staff, Cumberland Regional Health Care Center; Langs: Dutch; (902)667-3361; Fax. (902)667-1920.

VAN BREDA, Alta; Southwest Medi-Centre, 500-1 Springs Dr, Swift Current SK S9H 3X6; (306)773-4681; Fax. (306)778-3449.

VAN BRENK, Bert; The Medical Centre, PO Box 4200 Stn Main 707 Charlotte St, Peterborough ON K9J 7B3; Tor'93; BSc; FRCSC; PlasSurg. Ac Staff, Peterborough Regional Health Centre - Hospital Drive; (705)876-4521; Fax. (705)743-7874.

VAN BUSSEL, Elisabeth M; Regional Mental HC-London, PO Box 5532 Stn B K172-850 Highbury Ave, London ON N6A 4H1; Tor'92; FRCPC; Psy (Geriatric Psychiatry). Staff Regional Psychogeriatric Program, Regional Mental Health Care-St Joseph's Health Care; Staff Psychogeriatric Program, Parkwood Hospital - St Joseph's Health Care; (519)455-5110

VAN BUSSEL, Jared J; The Associate Clinic, PO Box 549 1222 Bev MacLachlin Dr, Pincher Creek AB T0K 1W0; Alb'05; CCFP; Staff, Foothills Medical Centre; (403)627-3321; Fax. (403)627-1782.

VAN BUUREN, John C; Gain Med Centre, 1199 Austin Ave, Coquitlam BC V3K 3P4; Dal'84; Staff, Royal Columbian Hospital; (604)939-7345; Fax. (604)939-7781.

VAN BUYNDER, Paul; Fraser Health, 400-13450 102nd Ave, Surrey BC V3T 0H1; Melbourne (Australia)'80; (604)587-7890

VAN CAESEELE, Paul G; 750 William Ave PO Box 8450 Stn Main, Winnipeg MB R3E 3J7; Man'95; FRCPC; MedMicrobiol. Staff, Cadham Provincial Laboratories; (204)945-6123; Fax. (204)780-4770; paul.vancaeseele@gov.mb.ca.

VAN CAMPENHOUT, Isabelle; Hop Charles Lemoyne, 3120 boul Taschereau, Greenfield Park QC J4V 2H1; Mon'89; FRCPC; DiagRad. Staff, Hopital Charles LeMoyne; (450)466-5000 x2030

VAN DAALEN, Erica; St Thomas-Elgin Gen Hosp, PO Box 2007 Stn Main 189 Elm St, St Thomas ON N5P 3W2; Tor'06; CCFP; CCFP(E.M.); Staff, St Thomas Elgin General Hospital; (519)631-2030

VAN DAM, Darren J; Ilderton Med Clinic, 36 Heritage Dr, Ilderton ON N0M 2A0; Qns'08; CCFP; (519)666-1610

VAN DE KAMP, Schaana M; Royal University Hosp, 103 Hospital Dr, Saskatoon SK S7N 0W8; Sask'07; CCFP; CCFP(E.M.); Staff, Royal University Hospital; (306)655-1383; Fax. (306)655-1258.

VAN DE MOSSELAER, Gregory J; Misericordia Health Centre, 99 Cornish Ave, Winnipeg MB R3C 1A2; Man'91; CCFP; Staff, Misericordia Health Centre; (204)774-6581

VAN DE VELDE, Rochelle S; Winnipeg Clinic, 425 St Mary Ave, Winnipeg MB R3C 0N2; Man'98; FRCPC; Derm.

VAN DE VENTER, Gavin E; Meadow Lake Assoc Clinic, PO Box 1510, Meadow Lake SK S9X 1Z1; Pretoria (South Africa)'93; MB ChB; BSc(Hons); LMCC; Meadow Lake Hospital; Staff, Meadow Lake Associate Clinic; (306)236-5661; Fax. (306)236-4355.

VAN DEN AKKER, Machiel T; The Hosp for Sick Children, 555 University Ave, Toronto ON M5G 1X8; Amsterdam (Netherlands)'91; Fellow, The Hospital For Sick Children; (416)813-1500

VAN DEN BERG, Daniel J H; Associate Clinic, 5215 49 Ave, Wetaskiwin AB T9A 0R1; (South Africa)'82; (780)352-7157; Fax. (780)352-2273.

VAN DEN BERG, Lucretia; 202-2179 Yonge St, Toronto ON M4S 2A9; Pretoria (South Africa)'75; MB ChB; ABIM; FACP; FRCPC; IntMed (Endocrinology). Langs: Afrikaans; (416)546-4316

VAN DEN BERG, Marietta; Surrey Mem Hosp, 13750 96 Ave, Surrey BC V3V 1Z2; Pretoria (South Africa)'88; MB ChB; FRCPC; Psy. Staff, Surrey Memorial Hospital; (604)581-2211

VAN DEN BIGGELAAR, Jane C; 12-1917 4th Ave W Box 12, Vancouver BC V6J 1M7; Tor'91; CCFP; CCFP(E.M.); (778)847-8838; Fax. (604)737-4907.

VAN DEN BREKEL, Antoinette M; Seymour Med Clinic, S3-1530 7 Ave W, Vancouver BC V6J 1S3; McG'91; MDCM; FRCPC; Peds (Newborn Medicine). Staff, Providence Health Care - St Paul's Hospital; Langs: Bilingual(French/English); (604)738-2151; avandenbrekel@telus.net.

VAN DEN ELZEN, Marketa; Burnaby Hosp, 3935 Kincaid St, Burnaby BC V5G 2X6; Loma Linda University (USA)'01; FRCPC; Neur. Staff Neurology Clinic, Burnaby Hospital; (604)434-4211

VAN DEN ELZEN, Peter; Children's & Women's HC of BC, 2K29-4480 Oak St, Vancouver BC V6H 3V4; Cal'99; Staff, BC Children's Hospital; (604)875-2345 x7343; Fax. (604)875-3479.

VAN DEN EYNDE, Frederique; Douglas Mental Hlth Univ Inst, 6875 boul Lasalle, Montreal QC H4H 1R3; Staff, Douglas Mental Health University Institute; (514)761-6131

VAN DEN HEEVER, Jesaja W; St Boniface Gen Hosp, L2035-409 Tache Ave, Winnipeg MB R2H 2A6; Orange Free State (South Africa)'93; MB BS; FRCPC; Anes. Staff, St Boniface General Hospital; (204)233-8563

VAN DEN HEEVER, Zacharias A N; Clinical Sciences Bldg, 8 120-152 University Campus NW, Edmonton AB T6G 2G3; (South Africa)'03; Staff, Northern Lights Regional Health Centre; Staff, University of Alberta Hospital; (780)407-1877

VAN DEN HOF, Michiel C; IWK Health Centre, PO Box 9700 Rpo CSC, Halifax NS B3K 6R8; Dal'80; FRCSC; ObstGyn (High Risk Obstetrics). Staff, IWK Health Centre; Prof, Dalhousie University; (902)470-6605; Fax. (902)425-1125; michiel_vandenhof@iwk.nshealth.ca.

VAN DER BERG, Jan D; Red Deer Med Centre, 106-3947 50A Ave, Red Deer AB T4N 6V7; Stellenbosch (South Africa)'78; MB ChB; MMed(Int); Head Div of Gen IntMed, Red Deer Regional Hospital Centre; Langs: Afrikaans; German; (403)314-4174; Fax. (403)314-4177.

VAN DER BERG, Nicolaas M; Medical Arts Clinic, 780 Central Ave N, Swift Current SK S9H 0M3; (Other Foreign)'01; (306)773-2811; Fax. (306)778-4081.

VAN DER BYL, Gwynneth L; Steinbach Med Clinic, 10-333 Loewen Blvd, Steinbach MB R5G 0C3; (Other Foreign)'98; (204)326-8867; Fax. (204)326-4818.

VAN DER GOES, Theresa A; Dr Theresa A van der Goes Inc, 1624 Woobank Rd, Nanaimo BC V9X 1M8; Cal'94; CCFP; Clin Instructor, University of British Columbia; (250)754-3218; Fax. (250)754-3852.

VAN DER HOUT, David M; Yorkview Med Centre, 3695 Keele St, North York ON M3J 1N2; McM'79; CCFP; Med Dir, The Salvation Army Toronto Grace Health Centre; Ac Staff, Humber River Regional Hospital - Finch Avenue Site; (416)633-3711; Fax. (416)633-0521.

VAN DER JAGT, Richard H C; The Ottawa Hosp-Gen Campus, 7208-501 Smyth Rd, Ottawa ON K1H 8L6; McM'83; FRCPC; IntMed; Hem (Lymphoma & Myeloma). Ac Staff Hem, The Ottawa Hospital - General Campus; Affil Investigator Clin Epidemiol, Ottawa Health Research Institute; Assoc Prof Med & Hematol, University of Ottawa; Langs: Dutch; (613)737-8804; rvanderjagt@toh.on.ca.

VAN DER KAMP, Nicholas H; Burnham Med Services, 105-380 Burnham St, Peterborough ON K9H 1T6; McM'91; CCFP; FCFP; (705)741-3489; Fax. (705)741-3715.

VAN DER KWAST, Theodorus H; Univ Hlth Network-Toronto Gen, 200 Elizabeth St, Toronto ON M5G 2C4; Erasmus (Netherlands)'80; FRCPC; GenPath (Urology). Staff, Toronto General Hospital - UHN; (416)340-4597; Fax. (416)340-5517.

VAN DER LINDE, Erich P; Newell Associate Clinic, PO Box 280 Stn main 220 4th St W, Brooks AB T1R 1B3; CCFP; (403)362-5501; Fax. (403)362-8426.

VAN DER LINDE, Etienne; Dr G B Cross Mem Hosp, 67 Manitoba Dr, Clarenville NL A5A 1K3; Stellenbosch (South Africa)'84; MB ChB; LMCC; MCFP; Chief Emerg Med, The Dr G B Cross Memorial Hospital; Langs: Dutch; Afrikaans; Flemish; (709)466-3411; Fax. (709)466-5553; evdlinde@nf.sympatico.ca.

VAN DER LINDEN, Marjorie A; 3491 Saanich Rd, Victoria BC V8X 1W8; UBC'93; CCFP; FCFP; (250)475-2251; Fax. (250)475-3530.

VAN DER LOO, Sara E; Atikokan Family Health Team, PO Box 1450 123 Marks St, Atikokan ON P0T 1C0; Ott'02; CCFP; (807)597-2721; Fax. (807)597-4632.

VAN DER LUGT, Hubertus; East Kootenay Reg Hosp, 13 24th Ave N, Cranbrook BC V1C 3H9; Orange Free State (South Africa)'92; MB ChB; MMed(Psy); FRCPC; Psy. Staff Psy, East Kootenay Regional Hospital; Langs: Afrikaans; (250)426-5281 x6499; Fax. (250)417-6180.

VAN DER MEER, Isabelle R; Work Safe of BC, 6951 Westminster Hwy, Vancouver BC V6B 5L5; Stellenbosch (South Africa)'84; MB ChB; (604)232-7169

VAN DER MERWE, Abraham J; The Malone Med Clinic, 4955 41 Ave, Drayton Valley AB T7A 1V4; (South Africa)'88; MB ChB; (780)542-3366; Fax. (780)542-6207.

VAN DER MERWE, Adam B; 211 Lakeshore Pl, Saskatoon SK S7J 3T7; Pretoria (South Africa)'99; MB ChB; Langs: Afrikaans.

VAN DER MERWE, Christina J; Abbotsford Reg Hosp & Cancer C, 32900 Marshall Rd, Abbotsford BC V2S 0C2; Orange Free State (South Africa)'88; MB ChB; Staff, Abbotsford Regional Hospital & Cancer Centre; (604)615-2552

VAN DER MERWE, Cornelis M; Alberta/Saskatchewan Wellness, 3-5202 12th St, Lloydminster AB T9V 0W1; (South Africa)'03; MB ChB; Dip(MentalHealth); Langs: Afrikaans; (780)875-5200; Fax. (780)875-9258.

VAN DER MERWE, Daniel F; 101-3949 Maple Way, Port Alberni BC V9Y 0B2; Pretoria (South Africa)'91; MB ChB; Staff, East Kootenay Regional Hospital; Langs: Afrikaans; (250)723-3211

VAN DER MERWE, Daniel T H; West Coast Gen Hosp, 101-3949 Maple Way, Port Alberni BC V9Y 4S1; Stellenbosch (South Africa)'81; MB ChB; MMed; Staff, West Coast General Hospital; Langs: Afrikaans; German; (250)723-3211 x1

VAN DER MERWE, Dirk J; Gulf Canada Square, 300-401 9 Ave SW, Calgary AB T2P 3C5; Stellenbosch (South Africa)'99; MB ChB; (403)284-0230

VAN DER MERWE, Errol J; The Medical Clinic, PO Box 998 2025 Granite Ave, Merritt BC V1K 1B8; Pretoria (South Africa)'77; MB ChB; Langs: Afrikaans; (250)378-6222; Fax. (250)378-6227.

VAN DER MERWE, Estie; Edson Med Centre, PO Box 6660 Stn Main 616 50 St, Edson AB T7E 1V1; (South Africa)'05; LMCC; Langs: Afrikaans; (780)723-3366; Fax. (780)723-3437.

VAN DER MERWE, Francina J; Cameron Med Clinic, 302 Cameron St, Williams Lake BC V2G 1S9; Stellenbosch (South Africa)'00; MB ChB; Langs: Afrikaans; (250)305-1102; Fax. (250)305-1138.

VAN DER MERWE, Gerrit F; Hys Med Centre, 202-11010 101 St NW, Edmonton AB T5H 4B9; (South Africa)'85; MB ChB; (780)426-1121; Fax. (780)425-5979.

VAN DER MERWE, Henrik; Regina Qu'Appelle HR-Regina Ge, 1440 14th Ave, Regina SK S4P 0W5; Orange Free State (South Africa) MB ChB; Staff, Regina General Hospital; (306)766-4444

VAN DER MERWE, Herman S; Elkhorn Med Clinic, GD, Elkhorn MB R0M 0N0; Stellenbosch (South Africa)'95; MB ChB; CCFP; FCFP; Staff, Southeast Integrated Care Centre - Moosomin; Coord EMS, Pipestone Health District; Physician, Elkhorn Medical Clinic; Moosomin Family Practice Centre; Coord COPS, Saskatchewan Cares-Moosomin Centre; Langs: Afrikaans.

VAN DER MERWE, Ignatius; Kitimat Gen Hosp & Health Ctr, 920 Lahakas Blvd S, Kitimat BC V8C 2S3; Pretoria (South Africa)'90; MB ChB; LMCC; FRCSC; OrthSurg. Staff, Kitimat Hospital & Health Centre; (250)632-8669; Fax. (250)632-8668.

VAN DER MERWE, Jacobus J J; West Hill Med Clinic, 1A-2995 2nd Ave W, Prince Albert SK S6V 5V5; (306)865-8500; Fax. (306)765-8501.

VAN DER MERWE, Jan G; Regina Qu'Appelle HC-Pasqua, 4101 Dewdney Ave, Regina SK S4T 1A5; Pretoria (South Africa)'90; MB ChB; MMedAnes; Staff, Pasqua Hospital; (306)766-2295; Fax. (306)766-2842.

VAN DER MERWE, Johann V; Mayfair Place, 236-6707 Elbow Dr SW, Calgary AB T2V 0E4; Pretoria (South Africa)'84; MB ChB; LMCC; Langs: Afrikaans; (403)259-3300; Fax. (403)259-3355.

VAN DER MERWE, Johannes M; 3114-910 10th Ave W, Vancouver BC V5Z 4E3; Pretoria (South Africa)'00; MB ChB; FRCSC; OrthSurg. Langs: Afrikaans; (604)875-4111

VAN DER MERWE, John S; Border City Clinic, 2707 50th Ave, Lloydminster SK S9V 2A8; (306)825-4427; Fax. (306)825-2028.

VAN DER MERWE, Marius; Ramblewood Med Clinic, 101-14 Ramblewood Dr, Wasaga Beach ON L9Z 0C4; University of Stellenbosch (South Africa)'88; (705)429-8270

VAN DER MERWE, Neville D; Nipawin Med Group, PO Box 2135, Nipawin SK S0E 1E0; (Other Foreign)'04; (306)862-4626; Fax. (306)862-3522.

VAN DER MERWE, Phillip W; Vasectomy Clinic, 201-2303 4 St SW, Calgary AB T2S 2S7; Stellenbosch (South Africa)'88; MB ChB; CCFP; Langs: Afrikaans; (403)640-4320; Fax. (403)640-4397.

VAN DER MERWE, Schalk W; Moose Jaw Union Hosp, 455 Fairford St E, Moose Jaw SK S6H 1H3; Staff, Moose Jaw Union Hospital; (306)694-0250

VAN DER MERWE, Shirley G; Aberdeen Med Clinic, 1966 Harrison Way, Vernon BC V1B 1M9; Cape Town (South Africa)'98; MB ChB; Staff, Aberdeen Medical Clinic; Langs: Afrikaans; Zulu; (250)672-9795; Fax. (250)672-9726.

VAN DER MERWE, Vanessa; Saskatoon City Hosp, 701 Queen St, Saskatoon SK S7K 0M7; Pretoria (South Africa)'00; MB ChB; Staff Rehab Services, Saskatoon City Hospital; (306)655-8000

VAN DER MERWE, Wynand A; Battlefords Union Hosp, 1092 107th St, North Battleford SK S9A 1Z1; Staff, Battlefords Union Hospital; (306)446-6948

VAN DER POLL, Annerien M; Campbell Clinic, 430 Mayor Magrath Dr S, Lethbridge AB T1J 3M1; Pretoria (South Africa)'90; MB ChB; (403)328-8101; Fax. (403)328-8150.

VAN DER POLL, Corneil X; Campbell Clinic, 430 Mayor Magrath Dr S, Lethbridge AB T1J 3M1; Stellenbosch (South Africa)'89; MB ChB; LMCC; (403)328-8101; Fax. (403)328-8150.

VAN DER ROSS, Richard R; Family Physicians Group, PO Box 2170, Melfort SK S0E 1A0; Stellenbosch (South Africa)'98; MB ChB; BSc; Physician, Family Physicians Group; (306)752-5757; Fax. (306)752-7252; richardvdr@gmail.com.

VAN DER VYVER, Izak A; 13214 Kelly Ave PO Box 1620, Summerland BC V0H 1Z0; Pretoria (South Africa)'06; MB ChB; Staff, Port Hardy Hospital; Langs: Afrikaans; (250)494-3432

VAN DER VYVER, Johannes D; 4607 50 Ave PO Box 3955 Stn Main, Olds AB T4H 1P6; (South Africa)'84; MB ChB; CCFP; (403)556-7130

VAN DER VYVER, Marthinus J; Sunnybrook Hlth Sciences Ctr, 2075 Bayview Ave, Toronto ON M4N 3M5; Stellenbosch (South Africa)'88; MMed; FRCPC; Anes (Obstetrics Anesthesia). Staff, Sunnybrook Health Sciences Centre; Asst Prof, University of Toronto; Langs: Afrikaans; (416)480-6100; Fax. (416)480-6039.

VAN DER VYVER, Susanna M; Ancron Med Centre, 108-402 Baker St, Nelson BC V1L 4H8; Orange Free State (South Africa)'05; MB ChB; Langs: Afrikaans; (250)352-9144; Fax. (250)352-9141.

VAN DER WAL, Michael; Anaesthetic Services, 213-2186 Oak Bay Ave, Victoria BC V8R 1G3; Cape Town (South Africa)'81; MB ChB; FRCPC; Anes. Staff, Royal Jubilee Hospital; (250)595-7211; Fax. (250)595-7211.

VAN DER WALT, Johannes C; Wetaskiwin Family Med Practice, 5107 50 St, Wetaskiwin AB T9A 1K1; Stellenbosch (South Africa)'07; MB ChB; Langs: Afrikaans; (780)352-3010; Fax. (780)352-7413.

VAN DER WALT, Louiza; Supermed Family Pract Clinic, 1D-595 Ontario St, Welland ON L3B 0B3; Pretoria (South Africa)'89; MB ChB; CCFP; FCFP; Staff, Niagara Health System - Welland Hospital Site; Langs: Afrikaans; (905)734-8777; Fax. (905)734-4358.

VAN DER WALT, Marthinus; Redwater Capital Health Clinic, PO Box 393 4808 49th Ave, Redwater AB T0A 2W0; Bethlehem (Israel)'90; MB ChB; (780)942-4780; Fax. (780)942-4787.

VAN DER WALT, Petrus J; Bonnyville Med Clinic, PO Box 1007 Stn Main, Bonnyville AB T9N 2J7; (780)826-3346; Fax. (780)826-6362.

VAN DER WALT, Petrus J; Lakeland Med Clinic, 206-314 25 St, Cold Lake AB T9M 1G6; Stellenbosch (South Africa)'86; MB ChB; Langs: Afrikaans; (780)639-3001; Fax. (780)639-3009.

VAN DER WART, Adriaan D F; Second Avenue Med Clinic, 330 2nd Ave, Prince Rupert BC V8J 1G6; Pretoria (South Africa)'97; BSc(Hons Pharm); MB ChB; CCFP; Staff, Second Avenue Medical Clinic; Langs: Afrikaans; (250)624-5500; Fax. (250)624-4797.

VAN DER WATT, Gabriel J E; Coventry Hill Family Care Ctre, 105-100 Country Village Rd NE, Calgary AB T3K 5Z2; Stellenbosch (South Africa)'81; MB ChB; Physician, Calgary Foothills Primary Care Network; Langs: Afrikaans; (403)226-6475; Fax. (403)226-6748.

VAN DER WATT, Hendrik H; Bonnyville Med Clinic, PO Box 1007 Stn Main 4610 50 Ave, Bonnyville AB T9N 2J7; (780)826-3346

VAN DER WATT, Leon; Regina Gen Hosp, L2-1440 14th Ave, Regina SK S4P 0W5; Pretoria (South Africa)'05; MB ChB; Staff, Regina General Hospital; Langs: Afrikaans; (306)766-4444

VAN DER WATT, Morne J; Chilliwack Gen Hosp, 45606 Menholm Rd, Chilliwack BC V2P 1P7; Pretoria (South Africa)'99; MB ChB; CCFP; CCFP(E.M.); Staff, Chilliwack General Hospital; (604)702-4756; Fax. (604)791-3125.

VAN DER WATT, Sharne; Bonnyville Med Clinic, PO Box 1007 Stn Main 4610 50 Ave, Bonnyville AB T9N 2J7; (South Africa)'07; MB ChB; (780)826-3346; Fax. (780)826-6362.

VAN DER WESTHUIZEN, Christiaan L; Family Health Clinic, PO Box 4127 Stn Main, Ponoka AB T4J 1R5; Stellenbosch (South Africa)'94; MB ChB; CCFP; Langs: Afrikaans; (403)783-5305

VAN DER WESTHUIZEN, Frans W; High Prairie Assoc Clinic, PO Box 1350, High Prairie AB T0G 1E0; Free State (South Africa)'05; MB ChB; (780)523-2868; Fax. (780)523-2875.

VAN DER WESTHUIZEN, Gerhard; Southland Court Med Clinic, 228-10601 Southport Rd SW, Calgary AB T2W 3M6; Pretoria (South Africa)'79; MB ChB; Langs: English; French; (403)225-8803; Fax. (403)225-8892; gerhard55@shaw.ca.

VAN DER WESTHUIZEN, Izak J; Family Health Clinic, PO Box 4127 Stn Main Bay 10-5011 48 Ave, Ponoka AB T4J 1R5; Stellenbosch (South Africa)'94; MB ChB; CCFP; FCFP; (403)783-5305; Fax. (403)783-8722.

VAN DER WESTHUIZEN, Lucas C; Elgin Med Centre, 101-2255 Elgin Ave, Port Coquitlam BC V3C 2B4; (604)942-7292

VAN DER WESTHUIZEN, Marinus; Rockyview Gen Hosp, 7007 14 St SW, Calgary AB T2V 1P9; Staff, Dr Cooke Extended Care Centre; Staff, Rockyview General Hospital; Staff, Border City Medical Clinic; (403)943-3000

VAN DER WESTHUIZEN, Nick G; Royal Jubilee Hosp, 1952 Bay St, Victoria BC V8R 1J8; Rhodesia (Zimbabwe)'79; LRCS; LRCPS(Glas); MMed(Path); MB ChB; FRCPC; AnatPath. Staff Path, Royal Jubilee Hospital; (250)370-8465; Fax. (250)370-8069.

VAN DER WESTHUIZEN, Solomon H; 3-2020 Strachan Rd SE, Medicine Hat AB T1B 0M9; (Other Foreign)'91; CCFP; (403)580-1882; Fax. (403)504-5799.

VAN DER WESTHUYZEN, Willem J; 568 Mountainview Sq, Kitimat BC V8C 2N2; Stellenbosch (South Africa)'84; MB ChB; Staff, Kitimat Hospital & Health Centre; (250)632-3135

VAN DER WEYDE, Marlene P; Elderwood Med Clinic, PO Box 17 102-664 Beach Rd, Qualicum Beach BC V9K 1S7; Tor'95; BSc; MSc; CCFP; (250)738-1166; Fax. (250)738-1167.

VAN DER ZWEEP, John B; Lasik MD Inc, 400-123 2nd Ave S, Saskatoon SK S7K 7E6; Man'01; FRCSC; Ophth. (306)651-7243; Fax. (306)651-7246.

VAN DEVENTER, Tharine; Bonnyville Med Clinic, PO Bag 1007 Stn Main 4610 50 St, Bonnyville AB T9N 2J7; Free State (South Africa)'00; MB ChB; (780)826-3346; Fax. (780)826-6362.

VAN DIEPEN, Sean F P; University of Alberta Hosp, 2C2 WMC-8440 112 St NW, Edmonton AB T6G 2B7; Tor'04; FRCPC; IntMed; Cardiol. Staff, University of Alberta Hospital; (780)407-6507; Fax. (780)407-7485.

VAN DOESBURG, Nicolaas H; Hôpital Ste-Justine, 3175 ch Cote-Sainte-Catherine, Montreal QC H3T 1C5; Mon'74; FRCPC; Peds; Cardiol (P.Q.); PedCardiol. Staff, Hôpital Ste-Justine; adj Prof, Universite de Montreal; (514)345-4654; Fax. (514)345-4896; nicolaas_van_doesburg@ssss.gouv.qc.ca.

VAN DONKERSGOED, Lubbertus; Windsor Square Family Practice, 240-1959 152 St, Surrey BC V4A 9E3; Pretoria (South Africa)'91; MB ChB; LMCC; CCFP; (604)531-0888; Fax. (604)582-2086.

VAN DORP, Johannes; Wiarton Med Centre, PO Box 749 202-369 Mary St, Wiarton ON N0H 2T0; Wes'76; Staff, Grey Bruce Health Services - Wiarton Site; Langs: Dutch; French; (519)534-0310; Fax. (519)534-5252.

VAN DORP, Nelvia M D; Grey Bruce Health Services, 369 Mary St, Wiarton ON N0H 2T0; Wes'06; CCFP; Staff, Grey Bruce Health Services - Wiarton Site; (519)534-1700; Fax. (519)534-1744.

VAN DORSSER, John G; Scott Clinic, 775 Monaghan Rd S, Peterborough ON K9J 5K2; Qns'70; Court Staff, Peterborough Regional Health Centre - Hospital Drive; (705)748-4710; Fax. (705)742-7661.

VAN DUSEN, Diane S; Cobourg Med Clinic, PO Box 86 Stn Main 44 University Ave E, Cobourg ON K9A 4K4; Tor'71; CCFP; FCFP; Court Staff Privil, Northumberland Hills Hospital; (905)372-3323; Fax. (905)372-3692.

VAN DUYSE, Stan G; Westmount Med Center, 550-1 Car Westmount, Montreal QC H3Z 2P9; McG'71; Langs: Dutch; French; (514)934-2334 x296; Fax. (514)931-2929.

VAN DYK, Aletta H; Foothills Med Centre, 928-1403 29 St NW, Calgary AB T2N 2T9; Orange Free State (South Africa)'81; MB ChB; LMCC; Staff, Foothills Medical Centre; Langs: Afrikaans; (403)944-2800; Fax. (403)283-7365.

VAN DYK, Frederick P; Avery Health Clinic, 31-665 Front St, Quesnel BC V2J 5J5; Stellenbosch (South Africa)'90; MB ChB; Langs: Afrikaans; (250)992-8322

VAN DYK, Jessie; The Hosp for Sick Children, 602-555 University Ave, Toronto ON M5G 1X8; Pretoria (South Africa)'01; Staff, The Hospital For Sick Children; (416)813-6927

VAN DYK, Johannes B; 202-474 Columbia St, Kamloops BC V2C 2T5; Stellenbosch (South Africa)'98; MB ChB; (250)374-3300

VAN DYK, Werner W A; Seven Oaks Gen Hosp, 2300 McPhillips St, Winnipeg MB R2V 3M3; Pretoria (South Africa)'97; ATLS; LMCC; CCFP; CCFP(E.M.); Staff, Seven Oaks General Hospital; Staff, Selkirk & District General Hospital; Langs: Afrikaans; (204)632-7133

VAN DYKE, Christiane; CHUM-Hotel-Dieu, 3840 rue Saint-Urbain, Montreal QC H2W 1T8; Mon'89; Staff, Centre Hospitalier l'Université de Montréal (CHUM) - Hôtel-Dieu; (514)281-1722

VAN EEDEN, Donavan C; Langenburg Health Centre, PO Box 370, Langenburg SK S0A 2A0; Pretoria (South Africa)'99; MB ChB; Staff, St Anthony's Hospital; Staff, Yorkton Regional Health Centre; (306)743-2446; Fax. (306)743-2448.

VAN EEDEN, Jean L; Fort St John Med Clinic, 10011 96 St, Fort St. John BC V1J 3P3; Stellenbosch (South Africa)'00; (250)785-6677

VAN EEDEN, Johannes H; Bayswater Med Clinic, 207-2475 Bayswater St, Vancouver BC V6K 4N3; Pretoria (South Africa)'87; MB ChB; LMCC; Asst Prof, University of British Columbia; Langs: Afrikaans; (604)734-2614; Fax. (604)736-8585.

VAN EEDEN, Stephanus F; St Paul's Hosp, 1081 Burrard St, Vancouver BC V6Z 1Y6; Stellenbosch (South Africa)'75; MB ChB; PhD; FRCPC; IntMed (Respirology). Staff Pacific Lung Health Centre, Providence Health Care - St Paul's Hospital; Staff, Capture Centre for Cardiopulmonary Research; Asst Prof, University of British Columbia; Langs: Afrikaans; (604)682-2344 x68818

VAN ES, Caroline M; 106-3960 Quadra St, Victoria BC V8X 4A3; Ott'84; (250)727-3737

VAN ESSEN, Krista M; 100-20 Heritage Meadows Dr SE, Calgary AB T2H 3C1; Cal'03; CCFP; (403)252-8851; Fax. (403)252-1765.

VAN ESSEN, Susanne N; Niagara H System-St Catharines, PO Box 3018 Stn Main 142 Queenston St, St. Catharines ON L2R 7C6; Ott'07; Staff, Niagara Health System - St Catharines General Site; (905)378-4647

VAN ESSEN, Suzanne N; Niagara HS-St Catharines, 142 Queenston St, St. Catharines ON L2R 7C6; Ott'07; CCFP; CCFP(E.M.); Staff, Niagara Health System - St Catharines General Site; (905)378-4647

VAN EYK, Nancy A; IWK Health Centre, PO Box 9700 Rpo CSC G2141-5850 University Ave, Halifax NS B3K 6R8; Ott'95; FRCSC; ObstGyn (Pediatric & Adolescent Gynecology). Staff, IWK Health Centre; (902)470-7491; Fax. (902)425-1125.

VAN GELDER, Jacob R; Western Memorial Health Clinic, 3 Herald Ave, Corner Brook NL A2H 4B8; Amsterdam (Netherlands)'80; Staff, Western Memorial Regional Hospital; Clin Lecturer Peds, Memorial University Of Newfoundland; (709)637-3900

VAN GEND, Richard F; Mageta Med Centre, 110-20528 Lougheed Hwy, Maple Ridge BC V2X 2P8; Staff, Pinawa Hospital; Staff, Lac du Bonnet District Health Centre; (604)465-1100

VAN GENTEVOORT, Marlene A; Pembroke Reg Hosp, 705 Mackay St, Pembroke ON K8A 1G8; Wes'87; FRCPC; DiagRad. Med Dir Diag Imaging, Pembroke Regional Hospital Inc; (613)732-3675 x6308; Fax. (613)732-6342; mvangentevoort@pemgenhos.org.

VAN GOOR, John H; Southland Court Med Clinic, 233-10601 Southport Rd SW, Calgary AB T2W 3M6; Alb'65; (403)221-4373; Fax. (403)221-4390.

VAN GULIK, Michael G F; William Osler HC-Etobicoke, 101 Humber College Blvd, Etobicoke ON M9V 1R8; Otago (New Zealand)'94; FRCPC; Anes. Staff, William Osler Health System - Etobicoke General Hospital; (416)494-2120

VAN HEERDE, Johannes C; Signal Road Med Clinic, 108 Wolverine Dr, Fort McMurray AB T9H 4Y7; Cape Town (South Africa)'92; MB BS; Langs: Afrikaans; (780)790-9342; Fax. (780)791-0221; jvanheerde@shaw.ca.

VAN HEERDEN, Aletta J; Professional Med Associates, 550 Main St N, Moose Jaw SK S6H 3K3; Orange Free State (South Africa)'85; MB ChB; LMCC; Physician, Professional Medical Associates; Langs: Afrikaans; (306)694-2082; Fax. (306)692-2080.

VAN HEERDEN, Alida; City Centre Mall, 28-5201 50 St, Leduc AB T9E 6T4; Pretoria (South Africa)'99; MB ChB; Staff, Leduc Community Hospital; Langs: Afrikaans; (780)986-6200; Fax. (780)986-5200.

VAN HEERDEN, Andre; Westside Med Associates, 3591 Elliott Rd, Kelowna BC V4T 1N9; Pretoria (South Africa)'82; MB ChB; CCFP; FCFP; Langs: Afrikaans; (250)768-7656; Fax. (250)768-6907; avanheerden@shaw.ca.

VAN HEERDEN, Andries C; Broadway Med Clinic, 75-41 Broadway St W, Yorkton SK S3N 0L6; Pretoria (South Africa)'94; MB ChB; (306)783-2555; Fax. (306)783-2557.

VAN HEERDEN, Auret H; Spall Medical Clinic, 150-1940 Harvey Ave, Kelowna BC V1Y 8J8; (South Africa)'79; MB ChB; (250)860-9909; Fax. (250)860-9906.

VAN HEERDEN, Gert B; Professional Med Associates, 550 Main St N, Moose Jaw SK S6H 3K3; Orange Free State (South Africa)'84; MB ChB; Staff, Moose Jaw Union Hospital; Staff, Professional Medical Associates; Langs: Afrikaans; (306)694-2082; Fax. (306)692-2080.

VAN HEERDEN, Hendrik G; Nipawin Med Group, PO Box 2135 63-211 7th Av E, Nipawin SK S0E 1E0; Cape Town (South Africa)'71; LMCC; MB ChB; Physician, Nipawin Medical Group; Langs: German; Afrikaans; (360)862-4626; Fax. (306)862-3522.

VAN HEERDEN, Jacobus J; Stapleford Med Clinic, 372 McCarthy Blvd N, Regina SK S4R 7M2; Stellenbosch (South Africa)'79; MB ChB; Physician, Stapleford Medical Clinic; (306)545-3000; Fax. (306)545-5584; kobiev@accesscomm.ca.

VAN HEERDEN, Johannes A W; Aberdeen Med Centre, 1966 Harrison Way, Kamloops BC V1S 1M9; Orange Free State (South Africa)'04; MB ChB; (250)314-5311

VAN HEERDEN, Lizaan; Fraserview Med Associates, 32-665 Front St, Quesnel BC V2J 5J5; Orange Free State (South Africa)'04; MB ChB; Langs: Afrikaans; (250)992-3636

VAN HEERDEN, Martha M; Nipawin Med Group, PO Box 2135, Nipawin SK S0E 1E0; MB ChB; Staff, Nipawin Hospital; Physician, Nipawin Medical Group; (306)862-4626; martha@nipawin.com.

VAN HEERDEN, Pieter W; Fort Vermillion Med Clinic, PO Box 306, Fort Vermilion AB T0H 1N0; Stellenbosch (South Africa)'87; MB ChB; (780)927-3213; Fax. (780)927-4664; pwvanheerden@hotmail.com.

VAN HEES, Jacqueline M; The Cornwall Comm Hosp, PO Box 100 Stn Main 840 McConnell Ave, Cornwall ON K6H 5S5; Tor'87; CCFP; CCFP(E.M.); FCFP; Cornwall Community Hospital; Staff, Cornwall Community Hospital - Second Street Site; Staff, Winchester District Memorial Hospital; Staff, Perth & Smiths Falls District Hospital - Smiths Falls Site; Langs: Dutch; French; (613)938-4240 x2227; Fax. (613)938-5552.

VAN HEEST, Rardi D; 210-245 Columbia St E, New Westminster BC V3L 3W4; UBC'98; BSc; MA; FRCSC; GenSurg (Trauma). Clin Instructor, University of British Columbia; (604)522-7737; Fax. (604)522-1571.

VAN HEININGEN, Willem P J; Wellesley Township Commun HC, PO Box 187 1180 Queen's Bush Rd, Wellesley ON N0B 2T0; McM'10; CCFP; Staff, Woolwich Community Health Centre - Wellesley Site; (519)656-9025

VAN HELDER, Tomas; Hamilton HS-McMaster Site, PO Box 2000 Stn Lcd 1 1B7B-1200 Main St W, Hamilton ON L8N 3Z5; McM'94; FRCPC; Anes. Staff, Hamilton Health Sciences Centre - McMaster University Medical Centre; (905)525-9140; Fax. (905)524-2911.

VAN HOOGENHUIZE, William; PO Box 176, Shelburne ON L0N 1S0; Wes'57; FACAAI; FAAEM; ABAI; Member, American Academy of Environmental Medicine; Member, American College of Allergy Asthma & Immunology; Member, Canadian Society of Allergy & Clinical Immunology; (877)348-4782; Fax. (519)925-0901; mvanhoogenhuize@aol.com.

VAN HOOREN, Tamara A; London HSC-Victoria Hosp, PO Box 5010 Stn B B1 137-800 Commissioners Rd E, London ON N6A 5W9; Ott'05; FRCPC; Peds. Staff, London Health Sciences Centre - Victoria Campus; (519)685-8500; Fax. (519)685-8156.

VAN HOOYDONK, Vincent L; The BidWell Clinic, 93 Bidwell St, Tillsonburg ON N4G 3V1; Wes'73; Staff Anes, Alexandra Hospital; Staff Anes, Tillsonburg District Memorial Hospital; Staff, Woodstock General Hospital; Langs: Flemish; Dutch; (519)842-3105; Fax. (519)688-3800; vincent.vanhooydonk@sympatico.ca.

VAN HORNE, Wayne A; Assiniboine Clinic, 633 Lodge Ave, Winnipeg MB R3J 0S9; Man'66; CCFP; Ac Staff, The Salvation Army Grace Hospital; Lecturer Family Med, University of Manitoba; (204)988-9600; Fax. (204)888-1750.

VAN HOUWELINGEN, Andrew P; St Thomas-Elgin Gen Hosp, PO Box 2007 Stn Main 189 Elm St, St Thomas ON N5R 5C4; Tor'05; FRCSC; OrthSurg. Staff, St Thomas Elgin General Hospital; (519)637-8308; Fax. (519)637-7727.

VAN IDERSTINE, Edward V; University Hosp of Northern BC, 1475 Edmonton St, Prince George BC V2M 1S2; UBC'87; FRCPC; GenPath (Hematology Pathology). Staff Lab/Chief InfectDis, University Hospital of Northern British Columbia; (250)565-2421; Fax. (250)565-2284.

VAN IERSEL, Rebecca I; 200-100 Colborne St W, Orillia ON L3V 2Y9; Qns'05; CCFP; Staff, Orillia Soldiers' Memorial Hospital; (705)327-3330; Fax. (705)327-7675.

VAN IMPE, Jeffrey J H; Waypoint Centre for Mental HC, 500 Church St, Penetanguishene ON L9M 1G3; Wes'05; FRCPC; Psy. Staff, Waypoint Centre for Mental Health Care; (705)549-3181

VAN INEVELD, Cornelia H M; St Boniface Gen Hosp, E4003-409 Tache Ave, Winnipeg MB R2H 2A6; Man'89; MSc; FRCPC; IntMed; GeriatricMed. Staff, St Boniface General Hospital; Langs: Dutch; (204)237-2410; cineveld@cc.umanitoba.ca.

VAN JAARSVELD, Anshia; Cold Lake Health Centre, 205-314 25 St, Cold Lake AB T9M 1G6; (South Africa)'03; MB ChB; Staff, Cold Lake Healthcare Centre; (780)639-3180; Fax. (780)639-3181.

VAN JAARSVELD, Barend P; Chelsea Court Health Centre, 779 Chelsea St, Brockville ON K6V 6J8; Pretoria (South Africa)'89; CCFP; (613)342-1199; Fax. (613)342-2900.

VAN JAARSVELD, Iris M; Moosomin Family Practice Ctre, PO Box 1528, Moosomin SK S0G 3N0; Physician, Moosomin Family Practice Centre; (306)435-3838; Fax. (306)435-2178.

VAN JAARSVELD, Juliana B; Tisdale Med Clinic, PO Box 1510, Tisdale SK S0E 1T0; (306)873-4561; Fax. (306)873-4489.

VAN JAARSVELDT, Hendrik S M; Associate Med Clinic, 203-10030 106 St, Westlock AB T7P 2K4; Stellenbosch (South Africa)'96; MB ChB; (780)349-3341; Fax. (780)349-6686.

VAN JAARSVELDT, Werner D; Pembina Med Clinic, 2251 Pembina Hwy, Winnipeg MB R3T 2H1; Stellenbosch (South Africa)'96; MB ChB; CCFP; Langs: Afrikaans; (204)415-9022

VAN KAMPEN, Janice Y; Niagara H System-St Catharines, 142 Queenston St, St Catharines ON L2R 7C6; McM'97; MA; BA; FRCPC; Psy (Adult Psychiatry). Staff, Niagara Health System - St Catharines General Site; (905)378-4647

VAN KARNEBEEK, Clara D; BC Children's Hosp, K3 201-4480 Oak St, Vancouver BC V6H 3V4; Amsterdam (Netherlands)'03; Staff Peds & Biochemical Diseases, BC Children's Hospital; Langs: Dutch; (604)875-2628

VAN LAEKEN, Nancy Y; 1788-1111 Georgia St W, Vancouver BC V6E 4M3; Ott'81; FRCSC; PlasSurg (Breast Surgery). Staff, Vancouver General Hospital - Centennial Pavillion; Ac Staff, Providence Health Care - St Paul's Hospital; Staff, BC Children's Hospital; Staff, Providence Health Care - Mount Saint Joseph Hospital; University of British Columbia; (604)669-1633; Fax. (604)669-4516.

VAN LEEUWEN, Jennifer F; Peterborough Reg HC-Hosp, 1 Hospital Dr, Peterborough ON K9J 7C6; Tor'93; CCFP; Staff, Peterborough Regional Health Centre - Hospital Drive; (705)743-2121

VAN LEEVE, Karenza; 280-546 St Paul St, Kamloops BC V2C 5T1; Cape Town (South Africa)'93; MMed(Peds); MB ChB; FRCPC; Peds (Neonatology). Staff Peds, Interior Health Authority-Royal Inland.

VAN LIEROP, Muriel J; 205-200 Finch Ave W, North York ON M2R 3W4; London (England)'68; MB BS; (416)229-1993; Fax. (416)229-0527.

VAN LIESHOUT, Ryan J; Fontbonne Bldg, 301 James St S, Hamilton ON L8P 3B6; Ott'04; FRCPC; Psy. Staff, Hamilton Health Sciences Centre - McMaster Children's Hospital; Staff, St Joseph's Healthcare Hamilton - West 5th Campus; (905)522-1155; Fax. (905)521-6098.

VAN LOON, J David; Millbrook Med Centre, PO Box 290, Millbrook ON L0A 1G0; Tor'68; CCFP; (705)932-2772; Fax. (705)932-4089.

VAN MANEN, Michael A; University of Alberta Hosp, 3A3 13-8440 112 St NW, Edmonton AB T6G 2B7; Alb'05; Peds (Neonatal & Perinatal Medicine). Staff, University of Alberta Hospital; (780)407-8822

VAN MIDDLESWORTH, Karen E; Southside Med Clinic, 208-640 Prospect St, Fredericton NB E3B 9M7; Man'07; CCFP; (506)455-2657; Fax. (506)455-2658.

VAN NIEKERK, Adria R; Virden Med Associates, PO Box 730, Virden MB R0M 2C0; Stellenbosch (South Africa)'80; MB ChB.

VAN NIEKERK, Christopher; Crestview Med Clinic, 102-204 O'Connell Dr, Corner Brook NL A2H 5N4; Cape Town (South Africa)'78; MB ChB; Staff, Western Memorial Regional Hospital.

VAN NIEKERK, Dirk J T; BC Cancer Agency-Vancouver CC, 600 10th Ave W, Vancouver BC V5Z 4E6; Pretoria (South Africa)'82; MB ChB; MMed; FRCPC; AnatPath. Staff, BC Cancer Agency Vancouver Centre; Langs: Afrikaans; Fax. (604)877-2061.

VAN NIEKERK, Etienne; Dr CW Wiebe Med Centre, 385 Main St, Winkler MB R6W 1J2; MB ChB; (204)325-4312; Fax. (204)325-4594.

VAN NIEKERK, Izak J M; Family Med Associates, 5021 51 St, Lacombe AB T4L 2A3; Stellenbosch (South Africa)'92; MB ChB; MBA; Langs: Afrikaans; (403)782-3351; Fax. (403)782-5879.

VAN NIEKERK, Jozef W; 439 6 Ave SW, Medicine Hat AB T1A 5A9; Pretoria (South Africa)'98; MB ChB; MMed; (403)487-5152; Fax. (403)487-5153.

VAN NIEKERK, Petrus J; Park Avenue Med Centre, 3F-4634 Park Ave, Terrace BC V8G 1V7; (Other Foreign)'08; Langs: Afrikaans; (250)615-5005

VAN NOPPEN, Beth-Anne; Perth Med Clinic, 14 Isabella St, Perth ON K7H 2W6; Ott'92; CCFP; Staff Teacher/Dir, QHC North Hastings; (613)267-1660; Fax. (613)267-5706.

VAN NOPPEN, Boudewyn J; Perth Med Clinic, 14 Isabella St, Perth ON K7H 2W6; Ott'93; CCFP; Assoc Staff, QHC North Hastings; (613)267-1660; Fax. (613)267-5706.

VAN OLM, John M J; 22-1815 Varsity Estates Dr NW, Calgary AB T3B 3Y7; Man'77; (403)286-4903; Fax. (403)288-0310.

VAN OLM, T M Matthew J; Glenmore Landing, D272-1600 90 Ave SW, Calgary AB T2V 5A8; Amsterdam (Netherlands)'73; ABIM; FRCPC; IntMed (Environmental Medicine); Respir. Staff, Rockyview General Hospital; Clinical Asst Prof, University of Calgary; Langs: Dutch; German; French; (403)288-7965; Fax. (403)202-0034.

VAN ONSELEN, Eugene; PO Box 232, Saulnierville NS B0W 2Z0; Pretoria (South Africa)'90; MB ChB; CCFP; (902)769-2911; Fax. (902)769-2507.

VAN OOSTROM, Trevor M; Nanaimo Reg Gen Hosp, 1200 Dufferin Cres, Nanaimo BC V9S 2B7; Ott'99; FRCPC; Anes. Staff, Nanaimo Regional General Hospital; (250)755-7691

VAN PRAET, Oliver M; Univ Hlth Network-Toronto Gen, 200 Elizabeth St, Toronto ON M5G 2C4; McG'06; MDCM; CCFP; CCFP(E.M.); Staff, Toronto General Hospital - UHN; (416)340-3856

VAN RAALTE, Vanessa A; Royal Jubilee Hosp, 1952 Bay St, Victoria BC V8R 1J8; UBC'94; FRCPC; DiagRad. Staff, Royal Jubilee Hospital; (250)370-8000

VAN RAAY, Michelle S; 508 15 Ave SW, Calgary AB T2R 0R2; Alb'99; CCFP; (403)398-5449; Fax. (403)229-1759.

VAN REEKUM, Robert; Hamilton HS-McMaster Site, PO Box 2000 Stn Lcd 1, Hamilton ON L8N 3Z5; McM'85; FRCPC; Psy (Neurology & Psychiatry). Staff Acquired Brain Injury Program, Hamilton Health Sciences Centre - McMaster University Medical Centre; (416)487-4414

VAN RENSBURG, Adriaan E; Univ Hlth Network-Toronto Gen, EN3 464-200 Elizabeth St, Toronto ON M5G 2C4; Stellenbosch (South Africa)'93; FRCPC; Anes. Staff, Toronto General Hospital - UHN; (416)715-7595

VAN RENSBURG, Benjamin W; ABC Medical Clinic, 9842 101 Ave, Fort St John BC V1J 2B2; Pretoria (South Africa)'79; MB ChB; (250)785-1220; Fax. (250)785-9750; bendosa@hotmail.com.

VAN RENSBURG, Corne J; Dakota Med Centre, 17-845 Dakota St, Winnipeg MB R2M 5M3; Pretoria (South Africa)'00; CCFP; (204)232-7056

VAN RENSBURG, Deon R; Green Med Clinic, 1629 Baker St, Cranbrook BC V1C 1B4; Pretoria (South Africa)'02; MB ChB; BSc; (250)417-4777; Fax. (250)426-6470.

VAN RENSBURG, Esias R; Sunnyhill Health Centre, 3644 Slocan St, Vancouver BC V5M 3E8; Pretoria (South Africa)'87; MB ChB; MMed; FRCPC; Peds (Pediatric Emergency Medicine). Langs: Afrikaans; (604)453-8300

VAN RENSBURG, Pieter D J; The Brandon Clinic, 620 Dennis St, Brandon MB R7A 5E7; (204)728-4440

VAN RHIJN, Peter R; Streetsville Med Centre, 8-5425 Creditview Rd, Mississauga ON L5V 2P3; Leiden (Netherlands)'70; Ac Staff, The Credit Valley Hospital; Langs: Dutch; German; (905)826-1164; Fax. (905)826-1214.

VAN RIETSCHOTEN, Walter A; Associates Med Clinic, 123 10th Ave S, Cranbrook BC V1C 2N1; UBC'76; BSc; CCFP; FCFP; (250)426-4231; Fax. (250)426-4357.

VAN RIJN, Theo A; 4372 10th Ave W, Vancouver BC V6R 2H7; Tor'71; FRCPC; PhysMed&Rehab. Assoc Staff, G F Strong Rehabilitation Centre; Consultant, Vancouver General Hospital - Centennial Pavillion; Asst Prof, University of British Columbia; (604)222-8383

VAN ROOI, Henrietta M; Carewest Glenmore Park, 6909 14 St SW, Calgary AB T2V 1P8; Cape Town (South Africa)'87; MB ChB; CCFP; Staff, Carewest Glenmore Park; Staff, Rockyview General Hospital; Staff Day Hosp, Carewest Sarcee Hospice; Langs: Afrikaans; (403)640-6480; Fax. (403)258-7681.

VAN ROOIJEN, Tersia; Cariboo Mem Hosp & Hlth Ctre, 517 6 Ave N, Williams Lake BC V2G 2G8; Stellenbosch (South Africa)'04; MB ChB; Staff, Cariboo Memorial Hospital and Health Centre; Langs: Afrikaans; (250)392-4411

VAN ROOY, Charles H; 102-909 Island Hwy, Campbell River BC V9W 2C2; Pretoria (South Africa)'87; MB ChB; MMed; FRCSC; Otol (Head & Neck Surgery). (250)830-0707; Fax. (250)830-0701.

VAN ROOYEN, Calin L; Viking Med Clinic, 5301 51 St, Viking AB T0B 4N0; (South Africa)'02; Langs: Afrikaans; (403)336-4780; Fax. (403)336-2020; calin_vanrooyen@yahoo.ca.

VAN ROOYEN, Elizabeth E M; Oasis Med Clinic, 504-3 Stonegate Dr NW, Airdrie AB T4B 0N2; (Other Foreign)'06; (403)945-8216; Fax. (403)945-8276.

VAN ROOYEN, Frederick C; 12 West Med Clinic, 130-227 11 Ave SW, Calgary AB T2R 1R9; Stellenbosch (South Africa)'85; MB ChB; PhD; (403)210-0121; Fax. (403)210-0320.

VAN ROOYEN, Gert I; Tiffin Med Clinic, 3-230 Aberdeen Blvd, Midland ON L4R 5N4; Pretoria (South Africa)'89; CCFP; (705)526-4992; Fax. (705)527-6338.

VAN ROOYEN, Hendrik M; Fort Vermilion Med Clinic, PO Box 306 4506 47th St, Fort Vermilion AB T0H 1N0; Stellenbosch (South Africa)'81; MB ChB; Staff, St Theresa General Hospital; (780)927-3213; Fax. (780)927-4664; docthys@gmail.com.

VAN ROOYEN, Hugo M; Regina Qu'Appelle HR -Regina, 1440 14th Ave, Regina SK S4P 0W5; (Other Foreign)'04; CCFP; Staff, Regina General Hospital; (306)766-4215; Fax. (306)766-4357.

VAN ROOYEN, Marthinus B; Bonnyville Med Clinic, PO Box 1007 Stn Main 4610 50 St, Bonnyville AB T9N 2J7; (South Africa)'05; MB ChB; (780)826-3346; Fax. (780)826-6362.

VAN ROOYEN, Marthinus L; South Sherbrook Hlth Centre, 88 Sherbrook St, Winnipeg MB R3C 2B3.

VAN ROOYEN, Peter J; Golden Mile Centre, 27-3806 Albert St, Regina SK S4S 3R2; Pretoria (South Africa)'86; MB ChB; (306)789-3200; Fax. (306)789-3154.

VAN ROOYEN, Renske; The Clinic at Walmart, 620-8249 Eagle Landing Pky, Chilliwack BC V2R 0P9; (Other Foreign)'06; MB ChB; (604)792-8482

VAN ROSSUM, Nicole; CHUS-Hop Fleurimont, 3001 12e av N, Sherbrooke QC J1H 5N4; Sher'95; FRCPC; IntMed; Endocrin&Metab. Staff, Centre Hospitalier Universitaire de Sherbrooke-Hopital Fleurimont; Langs: Bilingual(English/French); (819)346-1110; nvanrossum@hotmail.com.

VAN SCHAGEN, Carolyn M; 201-22242 48 Ave, Langley BC V3A 3N5; UBC'93; CCFP; FCFP; (604)530-5052; Fax. (604)530-5091.

VAN SCHAIK, Charmaine S; Southlake Reg Health Centre, 596 Davis Dr, Newmarket ON L3Y 2P9; McM'95; FRCPC; Peds. Staff, Southlake Regional Health Centre; (905)895-4521

VAN SCHALKWYK, Andries S; Kitimat Gen Hosp & Health Ctr, 920 Lahakas Blvd S, Kitimat BC V8C 2S3; Stellenbosch (South Africa)'97; MB ChB; CCFP; Staff, Kitimat Hospital & Health Centre; (250)632-8679; Fax. (250)632-8631.

VAN SCHALKWYK, Daniel J; Life Medical Clinic, PO Box 1406 Stn Main 4740 50 Ave, Whitecourt AB T7S 1P3; (South Africa)'97; Langs: Afrikaans; (780)706-7080; Fax. (780)706-7064.

VAN SCHALKWYK, Johanna M; 3-271 Ingram St, Duncan BC V9L 1P3; Stellenbosch (South Africa)'97; MB ChB; (250)597-0366; Fax. (250)597-0480.

VAN SCHALKWYK, Julianne E; Cross Roads ObstGyn, 330-507 Broadway W, Vancouver BC V5Z 1E6; Dal'99; MSc; FRCSC; ObstGyn (Infectious Diseases). Staff ObstGyn, BC Women's Hospital & Health Centre; Clinical Asst Prof, University of British Columbia; (604)872-5484; Fax. (604)708-0748.

VAN SCHALKWYK, Matthys C; Sylvan Med Centre, 5007 46 St, Sylvan Lake AB T4S 1C2; (Other Foreign)'06; (403)887-2221; Fax. (403)887-3777.

VAN SCHOOR, J Tinie; 115-579 Kingston Rd, Toronto ON M4E 1R3; Witwatersrand (South Africa)'66; MB BCh; CCFP; FCFP; (416)691-0238; Fax. (416)691-6038.

VAN SITTERT, Jacobus J; 401-1757 Beaufort Ave, Comox BC V9M 1R8; Pretoria (South Africa)'83; MB ChB; MMed; FRCSC; OrthSurg. Langs: Afrikaans; (250)890-3661

VAN SITTERT, Lambert W; Niagara H System-Welland Site, 65 Third St, Welland ON L3B 4W6; Pretoria (South Africa)'89; MB ChB; CCFP; CCFP(E.M.); Staff, Niagara Health System - Welland Hospital Site; Langs: Afrikaans; (905)732-6111 x3250

VAN SLYKE, Tiffany; Westgrove Clinic, 201-505 Queen St, Spruce Grove AB T7X 2V2; Qns'09; CCFP; (780)960-5297

VAN SPALL, Harriette G C; Hamilton HS-General Site, C3 117-237 Barton St, Hamilton ON L8L 2X2; Tor'02; FRCPC; IntMed; Cardiol. Staff, Hamilton Health Sciences Centre - Hamilton General Hospital; Staff, Mount Sinai Hospital; (905)527-4322

VAN STADEN, Johannes J; 2010 Braun Bay, Regina SK S4V 0L5; Pretoria (South Africa)'84; MB ChB; (306)585-3487; Fax. (306)248-8219; vanstadenj@dlcwest.com.

VAN STERTHEM, Marie-Josee; Medicentre Pincourt, 88 5e av, Pincourt QC J7V 5K7; Mon'79; Langs: Bilingual(French/English); (514)425-1000; Fax. (514)425-1288.

VAN STRAALEN, Rosemary T; Trafalgar Med Centre, 200-1235 Trafalgar Rd, Oakville ON L6H 3P1; McM'91; (905)844-3281; Fax. (905)849-1076.

VAN STRAATEN, Jacobus P L; Bigelow-Fowler Med Clinic, 1605 9 Ave S, Lethbridge AB T1J 1W2; Orange Free State (South Africa)'98; MB ChB; Langs: Afrikaans; (403)328-3121; Fax. (403)327-3905.

VAN STRALEN, Judy P M; 206-1637 Woodroffe Ave, Nepean ON K2G 1W2; McM'99; FRCPC; Peds. Consultant Staff, Children's Hospital of Eastern Ontario (CHEO); (613)726-7355; Fax. (613)726-7567.

VAN TONDER, Cornelius P; Midpark Family Med Centre, 150-290 Midpark Way SE, Calgary AB T2X 1P1; Orange Free State (South Africa)'90; MB ChB; LMCC; Physician, Northern Family Practice; (403)201-2726; Fax. (403)201-2710.

VAN TONDER, Janna; Mokala Medical, 161A-31 Southridge Dr, Okotoks AB T1S 2N3; Pretoria (South Africa)'94; MB ChB; LMCC; (403)995-5740; Fax. (403)995-5743.

VAN TONDER, Petrus J; Abbotsford Reg Hosp & Cancer C, 32900 Marshall Rd, Abbotsford BC V2S 0C2; (South Africa)'88; CCFP; CCFP(E.M.); Staff, Abbotsford Regional Hospital & Cancer Centre; (604)851-4700

VAN TONGEL, Alexander G C; Pan Am Clinic, 75 Poseidon Bay, Winnipeg MB R3M 3E4; (204)927-2772

VAN UUM, Stanislaus H M; St Joseph's Health Care, PO Box 5777 Stn B B5 120-268 Grosvenor St, London ON N6A 4V2; Nijmegen (Netherlands)'89; PhD; FRCPC; IntMed; Endocrin&Metab. Staff, St Joseph's Hospital - St Joseph's Health Care; Assoc Prof, University of Western Ontario; Langs: Dutch; German; (519)646-6000 x64070; Fax. (519)646-6058; stan.vanuum@sjhc.london.on.ca.

VAN VEENHUYZEN, Eleanor J; Daysland Med Centre, PO Box 160, Daysland AB T0B 1A0; (Other Foreign)'80; (780)374-3944; Fax. (780)374-2433.

VAN VLIET, Aaron J; Medical & Dental Bldg, 208-1221 Algonquin Ave, North Bay ON P1B 4Y3; Tor'05; FRCSC; OrthSurg. (705)472-0221; Fax. (705)472-9686.

VAN VLIET, Deborah; Newmarket Med Place, 101A-712 Davis Dr, Newmarket ON L3Y 8C3; Tor'94; FRCSC; PlasSurg (Breast Surgery). (905)898-1814; Fax. (905)898-7698.

VAN VLIET, Guy; Hôpital Ste-Justine, 3175 ch Cote-Sainte-Catherine, Montreal QC H3T 1C5; Brussels (Belgium)'76; Endocrin (P.Q.) (Pediatric Endocrinology). Staff, Hôpital Ste-Justine; Prof Peds, Universite de Montreal; Langs: Dutch; English; (514)345-4735

VAN VLIET, Michael; Northern Medical Unit, T162-770 Bannatyne Ave, Winnipeg MB R3E 0W3; Ross University (Dominica)'06; CCFP; Staff, Northern Medical Unit; (204)789-3711

VAN VLYMEN, Janet M; Kingston Gen Hosp, 76 Stuart St, Kingston ON K7L 2V7; Qns'90; FRCPC; Anes. Staff, Kingston General Hospital; (613)549-7827; Fax. (613)548-1375.

VAN VO, Thi Hai; Ctr Hosp de Verdun, 4000 boul Lasalle, LaSalle QC H4G 2A3; Sher'98; FRCPC; IntMed; Nephrol. Staff, Centre Hospitalier de Verdun; (514)362-1000 x1000; Fax. (514)362-2958.

VAN VOLKINGBURGH, David R; Wellington Med Arts Bldg, 303-121 Wellington St W, Barrie ON L4N 1L2; Qns'62; Staff, Royal Victoria Regional Health Centre; (705)728-5536; Fax. (705)728-4885.

VAN VUUREN, Hermanus; Battlefords Union Hosp, 1092 107th St, North Battleford SK S9A 1Z1; Staff, Battlefords Union Hospital; (306)446-6600

VAN VUUREN, Marius J; Trans Canada Med Centre, 152-1440 52 St NE, Calgary AB T2A 4T8; Orange Free State (South Africa)'95; MB ChB; CCFP; (403)272-3627; Fax. (403)272-3647; marlandiu@shaw.ca.

VAN WALRAVEN, Adrianus A; Grand River Hosp K-W HC, PO Box 9056 Stn C 835 King St W, Kitchener ON N2G 1G3; Tor'78; FRCPC; IntMed. Staff, Grand River Hospital - Kitchener/Waterloo Health Centre; Ac Staff, Stratford General Hospital - Huron Perth Healthcare Alliance; (519)749-4300

VAN WALRAVEN, Carl G; The Ottawa Hosp-Civic Campus, A S B1-003-1053 Carling Ave, Ottawa ON K1Y 4E9; Tor'91; FRCPC; IntMed. Staff, The Ottawa Hospital - Civic Campus; Staff, Ottawa Health Research Institute; (613)761-4903; Fax. (613)761-5492; cvanwalraven@ohri.ca.

VAN WERT, Ryan J F; Markham Stouffville Hosp, PO Box 1800 Stn Main 381 Church St, Markham ON L3P 7P3; Tor'06; FRCPC; IntMed. Staff, Markham Stouffville Hospital; (905)472-7000

VAN WEST, Cornel P; Dr G B Cross Mem Hosp, 67 Manitoba Dr, Clarenville NL A5A 1K3; Staff, The Dr G B Cross Memorial Hospital; Staff, Burin Peninsula Health Care Centre; (709)466-3411

VAN WESTENBRUGGE, John A; Gimbel Eye Centre, 450-4935 40 Ave NW, Calgary AB T3A 2N1; Alb'78; DAB; FRCSC; Ophth. Staff, Rockyview General Hospital; (403)286-3022; Fax. (403)286-2943; jvanwestj@telus.com.

VAN WIJK, Jan E; Medical Cons of West Nfld, 304-2 Herald Ave, Corner Brook NL A2H 4B5; Stellenbosch (South Africa)'75; MB ChB; Staff, Western Memorial Regional Hospital; (709)639-9181

VAN WILTENBURG, Robert T; 100-3001 Gordon Ave, New Westminster BC V3C 2K7; Alb'87; FRCPC; DiagRad. (604)941-7611; Fax. (604)942-4612.

VAN WYCK, Lloyd G; The Best You Clinic, 202-1545 Carling Ave, Ottawa ON K1Z 8P9; Wes'80; FRCSC; PlasSurg. Asst Prof, The Ottawa Hospital - Civic Campus; Staff, Children's Hospital of Eastern Ontario (CHEO); University of Ottawa; (613)722-7912; Fax. (613)722-2291; Plasticsurgery@videotron.ca.

VAN WYK, Andre R; Fort Langley Med Clinic, PO Box 99 Stn Fort Langley 23148 96 Ave, Langley BC V1M 2R4; Stellenbosch (South Africa)'88; MB ChB; MBA; CCFP; FCFP; Ac Staff, Langley Memorial Hospital; Preceptor, University of British Columbia; Langs: Afrikaans; German; Dutch; (604)888-2433; dr.a.vanwyk@shaw.ca.

VAN WYK, Bernize; City Centre Med Clinic, 284 City Centre Dr, Kitimat BC V8C 1T6; Orange Free State (South Africa)'04; MB ChB; (250)632-6131

VAN WYK, Elmo; Stevenson Med Clinic, 210A-6640 Vedder Rd, Chilliwack BC V2R 0J2; Stellenbosch (South Africa)'95; (604)703-2030; Fax. (604)796-0221.

VAN WYK, Gerritt C B; Professional Med Associates, 550 Main St N, Moose Jaw SK S6H 3K3; Orange Free State (South Africa)'78; MMed(Urol.); Staff, Professional Medical Associates; (306)694-2082; Fax. (306)692-2080.

VAN WYK, Gregory D; Infinity Med Centre, 300-5440 45 St, Red Deer AB T4N 1L1; Pretoria (South Africa)'88; MB ChB; (403)348-2991; Fax. (403)348-2993; glccg@telusplanet.net.

VAN WYK, Hadriaan S; Cariboo Mem Hosp, 517 Sixth Ave N, Williams Lake BC V2G 2G8; Stellenbosch (South Africa)'04; MB ChB; Staff, Cariboo Memorial Hospital and Health Centre; Langs: Afrikaans; (250)267-5543

VAN WYK, Karen; Pacific Med Clinic, 2032 Kingsway, Vancouver BC V5N 2T3; University of Cape Town (South Africa)'06; MB ChB; (604)874-5555

VAN WYK, Louis; Two Hills Med Clinic, PO Box 690, Two Hills AB T0B 4K0; (South Africa)'82; MB ChB; Physician, Two Hills Medical Clinic; (780)657-3337; Fax. (780)657-3382; twohill1@telusplanet.net.

VAN WYK, Mariette; Foothills Med Centre, G28-1403 29 St NW, Calgary AB T2N 2T9; Pretoria (South Africa)'87; MB ChB; LMCC; Staff, Foothills Medical Centre; (403)944-2900

VAN WYK, Schalk S; Garrison Medical, 2-45555 Market Way W, Chilliwack BC V2R 0M5; Stellenbosch (South Africa)'95; CCFP; (604)846-8812

VAN WYK, Stephanie; James Paton Mem Hosp, 125 Trans Canada Hwy, Gander NL A1V 1P7; Orange Free State (South Africa)'78; MB ChB; James Paton Memorial Hospital; (709)256-5423

VAN WYLICK, Richard C; Hotel-Dieu Hosp, 382C-166 Brock St, Kingston ON K7L 5G2; Qns'94; FRCPC; Peds (Child Abuse). Att Staff, Hotel-Dieu Hospital; Staff, Kingston General Hospital; Asst Prof, Queen's University; Langs: Bilingual(English/French); (613)544-3400 x3359; Fax. (613)544-3559; richard.vanwylick@queensu.ca.

VAN WYNGAARDEN, Case B; Northern Lights Reg Health Ctr, 7 Hospital St, Fort McMurray AB T9H 1P2; Cal'04; FRCPC; DiagRad. Staff, Northern Lights Regional Health Centre; (780)791-6024

VAN ZANTEN, Audrey; Dr Nayar & Associates, 125-750 Spadina Cres, Saskatoon SK S7K 3H3; Pretoria (South Africa)'95; MB ChB; DRCOG; Physician, Kelvington Medical Clinic; Langs: Afrikaans; (306)652-5414; Fax. (306)652-5554.

VAN ZANTEN, Sander J; Zeidler Ledcor Centre, 2 14A-130 University Campus NW, Edmonton AB T6G 2X8; Amsterdam (Netherlands)'79; MPH(Harvard); FRCPC; IntMed; Gastroent. Staff Zeidler Ledcor Centre/Div Dir GI, University of Alberta Hospital; Sec Head Regional GI, Edmonton Zone Edmonton Public Health Services; Langs: Dutch; Spanish; (780)492-9840; Fax. (780)492-9865.

VAN ZUIDEN, Lowell J; Alberta Hip & Knee Clinic, 335-401 9 Ave SW, Calgary AB T2P 3C5; McM'76; BASc; MBA; FRCSC; OrthSurg (Adult Reconstructive Surgery). Ac Staff, Rockyview General Hospital; Assoc Prof Surg, University of Calgary; (403)221-4321; Fax. (403)221-4387; lvz@orthosurgeons.ca.

VAN ZYL, Andre; Dr O Brown & Dr A Van Zyl Inc, 4556 Gertrude St, Port Alberni BC V9Y 6K1; Stellenbosch (South Africa)'74; CCFP; Staff, West Coast General Hospital; Langs: Afrikaans; (250)723-5514; Fax. (250)724-2465.

VAN ZYL, Andre T; James Paton Mem Hosp, PO Box 250 125 Trans Canada Hwy, Gander NL A1V 1P7; Pretoria (South Africa)'84; MB ChB; Staff, James Paton Memorial Hospital; Staff, Janeway Children's Health & Rehabilitation Centre; Physician, Dr Hugh Twomey Health Care Centre; Langs: Afrikaans; (709)256-2500

VAN ZYL, Anneleen; Dr O Brown & Dr A Van Zyl Inc, 4556 Gertrude St, Port Alberni BC V9Y 6K1; Stellenbosch (South Africa)'98; MB ChB; Langs: Afrikaans; (250)724-0166; Fax. (250)724-2465; brownvanzyl@shaw.ca.

VAN ZYL, Cornelius J; Grey Bruce H S-Owen Sound, PO Box 1800 Stn Main 1800 8th St E, Owen Sound ON N4K 6M9; Stellenbosch (South Africa)'85; MB ChB; LMCC; DCH; CCFP; CCFP(E.M.); Staff, Grey Bruce Health Services - Owen Sound; Langs: Afrikaans; (519)372-5920 x2030

VAN ZYL, Hendrik P; Royal Inland Hosp, 311 Columbia St, Kamloops BC V2C 2T1; Stellenbosch (South Africa)'93; MB ChB; CCFP; CCFP(E.M.); Staff, Royal Inland Hospital; (250)314-2100

VAN ZYL, Johan L; Melville Med Associates, PO Box 209, Melville SK S0A 2P0; Pretoria (South Africa)'73; MB ChB; BSc(Hon); PhmB; Staff Family Med, St Peter's Hospital; (306)728-4466; Fax. (306)728-3093.

VAN ZYL, Johannes P; Victoria Med Bldg, 302-1669 Victoria St, Prince George BC V2L 2L5; Stellenbosch (South Africa)'94; MB ChB; FRCSC; OrthSurg (Sports Medicine). Staff, University Hospital of Northern British Columbia; Langs: Afrikaans; (250)563-2272; Fax. (250)563-2962.

VAN ZYL, Leendert P C; Georgian Prof Centre, 003-125 Bell Farm Rd, Barrie ON L4M 6L2; Pretoria (South Africa)'97; MB ChB; Langs: Afrikaans; (705)721-5991; Fax. (705)728-5936.

VAN ZYL, Lizette; Owen Sound Family Health Team, 1415 1st Ave W, Owen Sound ON N4K 4K8; Stellenbosch (South Africa)'85; MB ChB; DCH; LMCC; CCFP; Langs: Afrikaans; (519)470-3030; Fax. (519)470-3035.

VAN ZYL, Louis T; Sleep & Alertness Clinic, 2 263-750 Dundas St W, Toronto ON M6J 1E9; Pretoria (South Africa)'74; MB ChB; MMed; FRCPC; Psy (Consultant Liaison Psychiatry). Consultant Sleep Med & Medical Psychiatry, Sleep Ontario Clinics; Emeritus Prof Psy, Queen's University; Langs: Afrikaans; (416)603-5723; Fax. (416)603-5258.

VAN ZYL, Maria-Louise; 403B-3210 25 Ave, Vernon BC V1T 1P1; Pretoria (South Africa)'76; CCFP; Langs: Afrikaans; (250)549-2722; Fax. (250)549-2715.

VAN ZYL, Matheus C; 9805 103 St PO Box 130, Sexsmith AB T0H 3C0; (South Africa)'84; (780)568-2277; Fax. (780)568-2299; chrisvanzyl@hotmail.com.

VAN ZYL, Shaun; PO Box 160, Kimberley BC V1A 2Y6; Stellenbosch (South Africa)'97; Staff ER, East Kootenay Regional Hospital; (250)427-4861; Fax. (250)427-2082.

VAN ZYL, Stephanus A; Rocky Med Clinic, PO Box 99 Stn Main, Rocky-Mtn-Hse AB T4T 1A1; (South Africa)'94; MB ChB; (403)845-2815; Fax. (403)845-2177.

VAN ZYL, Stephanus D; University of Alberta Hosp, 10-8440 112 St NW, Edmonton AB T6G 2B7; Stellenbosch (South Africa)'02; MB ChB; Staff, University of Alberta Hospital; (780)407-6154; stefvanzyl@hotmail.com.

VAN ZYL, Stephanus F; Mediclinic, 101-3333 8th St E, Saskatoon SK S7H 4K1; Pretoria (South Africa)'05; MB ChB; CCFP; Staff, St Paul's Hospital (Grey Nuns) of Saskatoon; Staff, Saskatoon City Hospital; (306)955-1530; Fax. (306)955-8811.

VAN ZYL, William P; Eastwood Med Centre, 201-1346 Kingston Rd, Scarborough ON M1N 1P9; Dundee (Scotland)'73; MB ChB; Staff, Toronto East General Hospital Inc; Langs: Afrikaans; (416)690-8112; Fax. (416)690-8113.

VANASELJA, Reet; Rosedale Med Centre, 510-600 Sherbourne St, Toronto ON M4X 1W4; Tor'74; CCFP; Langs: Estonian; (416)323-1414; Fax. (416)323-1411.

VANASSE, Alain; CHUS-Hop Fleurimont, 3001 12e av N, Sherbrooke QC J1H 5N4; Sher'77; CCFP; FCFP; Staff, Centre Hospitalier Universitaire de Sherbrooke-Hopital Fleurimont; (819)564-5329; Fax. (819)564-5424; alain.vanasse@usherbrooke.ca.

VANASSE, Catherine; Inst Geriatrie de Sherbrooke, 375 av Argyll, Sherbrooke QC J1J 3H5; Sher'82; Staff, Institut Universitaire de Geriatrie de Sherbrooke-Pavillon Argyll; Langs: English; (819)780-2220 x46223; Fax. (819)829-7146.

VANASSE, Francois; Clinique Med Saint-Louis, 3165 ch Saint-Louis, Quebec QC G1W 4R4; Mon'84; Staff, Jeffery Hale Hospital-Saint Brigid's; assoc Staff, Centre Hospitalier Universitaire De Québec - Pavillon De St-françois-d'assise; (418)653-1970; francois.vanasse@ssss.gouv.qc.ca.

VANASSE, Madeleine; Institut de Cardiologie de Mtl, 5000 rue Belanger, Montreal QC H1T 1C8; Sher'83; IntMed. Staff, Institut de Cardiologie de Montréal; (514)376-3330; Fax. (514)593-2540.

VANASSE, Louise; U of Ottawa Health Services, 300-100 Marie Curie Pvt, Ottawa ON K1N 1A2; Mon'80; MPH; CCFP; FCFP; Langs: English; (613)564-3950; Fax. (613)564-6627.

VANASSE, Michel; Hôpital Ste-Justine, 3175 ch Cote-Ste-Catherine, Montreal QC H3T 1C5; Mon'69; FRCPC; Neur; Electroenceph (P.Q.). ac Staff, Centre de Réadaptation Marie Enfant du CHU Sainte-Justine; ac Staff, Hôpital Ste-Justine; (514)345-4653; Fax. (514)345-4787; mmvanasse@videotron.ca.

VANAST, Walter J; Kateri Mem Hosp Centre, CP 10, Kahnawake QC J0L 1B0; Tor'66; FRCPC; Neur. Staff, Kateri Memorial Hospital Centre; Langs: Dutch; French; (450)638-3930

VANDAL, Claude; Clinique Med St-David, 4497 boul de la Rive-Sud, Levis QC G6W 6M9; Laval'78; CCFP; CCFP; Langs: Bilingual(English/French); (418)833-4791; Fax. (418)837-0254; claude.vandal@videotron.ca.

VANDAL, Johanne; 10800 rue Berri, Montreal QC H3L 2H4; Mon'76; ac Staff, Hôpital du Sacre-Coeur de Montréal; Staff, Centre Hospitalier Fleury; (514)388-8002

VANDAL, Lyne; Clinique Med des Saules, 100-2780 boul Masson, Quebec QC G1P 1J6; Laval'88; Staff, CSSS de Quebec-Sud; (418)871-4492

VANDAL, Marie-Claude; Centre Med Laennec, 200-1750 av de Vitre, Quebec QC G1J 1Z6; Laval'90; Cardiol (P.Q.); IntMed. (418)663-2858; Fax. (418)663-2352.

VANDANA, Neeraj; Yarmouth Reg Hosp, 80 Vancouver St, Yarmouth NS B5A 2P5; Dr S N Medical College (Other Foreign)'88; Staff, Yarmouth Regional Hospital; (902)742-3541

VANDEGRIEND, Richarad A; Gordon & Leslie Diamond HCC, 604-8775 Laurel St, Vancouver BC V5Z 1M9; Alb'08; IntMed. Staff, Gordon & Leslie Diamond Health Care Centre; (604)875-4111 x69821

VANDELLI, Stefania; CLSC Bordeau Cartierville, 11822 av Bois-de-Boulogne, Montreal QC H3M 2X6; Laval'06; CCFP; (514)331-2572

VANDEMOORTELE, Sylvere; CLSC Saint-Hubert, 6800 boul Cousineau, Saint-Hubert QC J3Y 8Z4; Mon'73; Clin Prof, Universite de Montreal; (450)443-7400; Fax. (450)676-3488; sylverevan@hotmail.com.

VANDEMOORTELE, Thomas; CHUM-Hop Notre-Dame, 1560 rue Sherbrooke E, Montreal QC H2L 4M1; Mon'04; FRCPC; IntMed; Critical Care Medicine; Respir. Staff, Centre Hospitalier l'Université de Montréal (CHUM) - Hôpital Notre-Dame; Staff, Centre Hospitalier l'Université de Montréal (CHUM) - Hôtel-Dieu; (514)890-8000

VANDENBERG, Alison P; Markham Med Centre, 214-6633 Highway 7, Markham ON L3P 7P2; Dal'77; BSc; Staff, Markham Stouffville Hospital; (905)294-2290; Fax. (905)294-0029; alison.vandenberg@9mail.com.

VANDENBERG, Ingrid L; Lakehead Psychiatric Hosp, PO Box 2930 Stn P 540 Algoma St N, Thunder Bay ON P7B 5G4; McM'82; FRCPC; Psy. Staff, Lakehead Psychiatric Hospital - St. Joseph's Care Group; (807)343-4300

VANDENBERG, Theodore A; London Reg Cancer Centre, A3 944-790 Commissioners Rd E, London ON N6A 4L6; Ott'79; FRCPC; IntMed; MedOncol. Staff, London Health Sciences Centre - Victoria Campus; Staff Oncol, London Regional Cancer Program; Prof Oncol, University of Western Ontario; Langs: English; French; (519)685-8640; Fax. (519)685-8624.

VANDENBROUCKE-MENU, Franck; CHUM-Hop St-Luc, 1058 rue Saint-Denis, Montreal QC H2X 3J4; Breslau (Other Foreign)'99; Staff, Centre Hospitalier l'Université De Montréal (CHUM) - Hôpital Saint-luc; (514)890-8000 x36146; Fax. (514)412-7380; frank.vandenbroucke.chum@ssss.gouv.qc.ca.

VANDER BEEK, Laura E; Hamilton HS-Juravinski Site, 711 Concession St, Hamilton ON L8V 1C3; McM'07; FRCSC; GenSurg. Staff, Hamilton Health Sciences Centre-Juravinski Site; (905)521-2100

VANDER KLIPPE, Stephen W; Wingham Med Centre, 285 Catherine St, Wingham ON N0G 2W0; Ott'09; CCFP; (519)357-3915; Fax. (519)357-1568.

VANDER LEEK, Timothy K; College Plaza, 903-8215 112 St NW, Edmonton AB T6G 2C8; Alb'94; FRCPC; Peds; ClinImmunol&Allergy. (780)413-6689; Fax. (780)413-7254.

VANDER MEER, Rachel L; Juravinski Cancer Centre, 699 Concession St, Hamilton ON L8V 5C2; Wes'07; MedOncol; IntMed. Staff, Hamilton Health Sciences Centre - Juravinski Cancer Centre; (905)387-9495

VANDER STELT, Ruth E; CLSC Quyon, 164 rue Clarendon CP 278, Quyon QC J0X 2V0; Laval'92; CCFP; FCFP; Staff, Pontiac Hospital Centre; Langs: English; (819)458-2848; Fax. (819)458-2470.

VANDERBECK, R Lindsay; 2F-117 Cedar St, Sudbury ON P3E 1A9; Qns'81; CCFP; FCFP; (705)673-8353; Fax. (705)673-7245.

VANDERBURGH, J David H; Thunder Bay Reg HSC-T-Bay, 980 Oliver Rd, Thunder Bay ON P7B 6V4; McM'08; CCFP; CCFP(E.M.); Staff, Thunder Bay Regional Health Sciences Centre; (807)684-6000; Fax. (807)346-8113.

VANDERBURGH, Leslie C; William Osler HC-Brampton, 2100 Bovaird Dr E, Brampton ON L6R 3J7; Wes'89; FRCPC; DiagRad. Staff, William Osler Health System - Brampton Civic Hospital; Asst Prof, University of Toronto; (905)494-2120 x58149; Fax. (905)494-6614.

VANDERFLUIT, Rhonda L; Bayswater Family Practice, 200-2475 Bayswater St, Vancouver BC V6K 4N3; UBC'07; CCFP; (604)731-0091

VANDERKOOI, Otto G; Alberta Children's Hosp, 2888 Shaganappi Trail NW, Calgary AB T3B 6A8; Alb'98; FRCPC; Peds (Pediatric Infectious Diseases); MedMicrobiol; InfectDis. Staff InfectDis, Alberta Children's Hospital; (403)955-7813

VANDERKOOY, John D; Grand River Hosp-KW HC, PO Box 9056 835 King St W, Kitchener ON N2G 1G3; Qns'02; BScHons; FRCPC; Psy (Child & Adolescent Psychiatry). Staff, Grand River Hospital - Kitchener/Waterloo Health Centre; (519)749-4300; Fax. (519)749-4301.

VANDERKOOY, John; PO Box 569, Harriston ON N0G 1Z0; Wes'71; Assoc Staff, North Wellington Health Care - Palmerston & District Hospital; Langs: Dutch; (519)338-2922; Fax. (519)338-5435.

VANDERMEULEN, John A; Hamilton HS-McMaster Site, PO Box 2000 Stn Lcd 1 1200 Main St W, Hamilton ON L8N 3Z5; Tor'84; PhD; FRCPC; Peds (Pediatric Endocrinology); Endocrin&Metab. Staff Sect of Ped Endocrin&Metabolism, Hamilton Health Sciences Centre - McMaster Children's Hospital; Affil Staff, St Joseph's Healthcare - Charlton Campus; Assoc Prof, McMaster University; (905)521-2100 x73716; Fax. (905)308-7548; vmeulen@mcmaster.ca.

VANDERPUTTEN, Marilyn R; 2-3855 9 Ave, Port Alberni BC V9Y 4T9; Cal'05; FRCSC; GenSurg. Staff, Peace Arch Hospital; (250)724-6596

VANDERSCHUREN, Abel; Ctr Hosp Affilie-Enfant-Jesus, 1401 18e rue, Quebec QC G1J 1Z4; Staff, Centre Hospitalier Affilié Universitaire de Québec - Hôpital De L'Enfant Jésus; (418)649-0252

VANDERSLUIS, Ronald; Scarborough North Med Arts, LL2-4040 Finch Ave E, Scarborough ON M1S 4V5; Tor'89; FRCSC; OrthSurg (Knee & Shoulder). Staff, The Scarborough Hospital - Birchmount Campus; Staff, One Medical Place Hosp; Langs: Dutch; (416)335-5055; Fax. (416)335-6183; ronvandersluis@bellnet.ca.

VANDERSLUIS, Rudolf; Lakeridge Hlth Corp-Oshawa, 1 Hospital Crt, Oshawa ON L1G 2B9; Tor'81; FRCPC; EmergMed;CCFP; CCFP(E.M.); FCFP; Ac Staff, Lakeridge Health - Oshawa Site; Staff, Sunnybrook Health Sciences Centre; Staff, Mount Sinai Hospital; University of Toronto; Langs: Dutch; (905)576-8711

VANDERSPEK, Susan C; 101-650 Sheppard Ave E, North York ON M2K 3E4; McM'08; CCFP; (416)222-7775; Fax. (416)222-7785.

VANDERWATER, Charles L; Tollendale Christian Ret Villa, 101-274 Hurst Dr, Barrie ON L4N 0Z3; Qns'80; MCFP; Ac Staff, Royal Victoria Regional Health Centre; (705)726-1191; Fax. (705)726-8015.

VANDERWERT, Ruwani T; Seven Oaks Gen Hosp, 5F-2300 McPhillips St, Winnipeg MB R2V 3M3; Man'99; FRCPC; Psy. Staff, Seven Oaks General Hospital; (204)632-7133

VANDERZWAN, Jonas B; Strathroy Med Clinic, 74 Front St E, Strathroy ON N7G 1Y7; Tor'02; CCFP; (519)245-0430; Fax. (519)245-5870.

VANDEWAETERE, Anik R M; Caremedics Hunt Club Clinic, 201-2446 Bank St, Ottawa ON K1V 1A4; Ott'89; CCFP; FCFP; Langs: English; French; (613)739-0998; Fax. (613)739-1485; travelmedicineottawa@rogers.com.

VANDEWALLE, Philip L; 31 Caradoc St N, Strathroy ON N7G 2M5; Wes'90; CCFP; FCFP; Staff, London Health Sciences Centre - Victoria Campus; Staff, Strathroy Middlesex General Hospital - Middlesex Hospital Alliance; Teach Staff Family Med, University of Western Ontario; (519)245-3590; Fax. (519)245-6032; vandewal@uwo.ca.

VANDEYAR, Thivian; St Thomas-Elgin Gen Hosp, PO Box 2007 Stn Main 189 Elm St, St Thomas ON N5P 3W2; Wes'07; CCFP; CCFP(E.M.); Staff, St Thomas Elgin General Hospital; (519)631-2030; Fax. (519)631-4106.

VANDOR, Thomas A; Centre Med Ormstown, RR 4 24 rue Gale, Ormstown QC J0S 1K0; McG'73; Staff, Barrie Memorial Hospital; (450)829-2331; Fax. (450)829-3636.

VANDORPE, Robert A; Queen Elizabeth II HSC-Halifax, 1796 Summer St, Halifax NS B3H 3A7; Dal'82; FRCPC; DiagRad (Neuro Radiology). Staff, Queen Elizabeth II Health Sciences Centre - Halifax Infirmary Site; Teach Staff, Dalhousie University; (902)473-4910; Fax. (902)473-5323.

VANDYCKE, Laurent; Clinique Med Pierre-Boucher, 1615 boul Jacques-Cartier E, Longueuil QC J4M 2X1; Mon'94; (450)468-6223; Fax. (450)468-5041.

VANEK, Arthur W; Dr Arthur Vanek Med Prof Corp, 211-2238 Dundas St W, Toronto ON M6R 3A9; Tor'80; ABIM; FRCPC; IntMed; Respir (Sleep Apnea). Head Respirology/Allergy, St Joseph's Health Centre; (416)538-2872; Fax. (416)538-2873.

VANEK, Irene J; St Michael's Hosp, 4025-30 Bond St, Toronto ON M5B 1W8; Purkyne (Czech Republic)'68; DAB; FRCSC; Ophth (Medical Ophthalmology). Staff AFT Position, St Michael's Hospital; Langs: Czech; German; (416)864-5945

VANEK, J Nicholas; Medical Clinic Person-Ctred Ps, 403-265 Yorkland Blvd, North York ON M2J 1S5; Purkyne (Czech Republic)'68; Staff, The Medical Clinic for Person-Centred Psychotherapy; Langs: Czech; (416)229-2399; Fax. (416)229-9771.

VANEY, Dagny L; 6681 Mary Ellen Dr PO Box 41045 Rpo Woodgrove, Nanaimo BC V9T 6M7; Alb'90; CCFP; FCFP; (250)754-5545

VANGURP, J Gerald; Clinique Medicale GMF-1851, 101-1851 Sherbrooke St E, Montreal QC H2K 4L5; Dal'76; Langs: English; French; (514)524-7564; Fax. (514)527-5251.

VANHOOF, Ronald A; 203-170 Simcoe St, Peterborough ON K9H 2H7; Tor'81; Staff, Peterborough Regional Health Centre - Hospital Drive; (705)748-4011; Fax. (705)741-6340; rvanhoof@prhc.on.ca.

VANHOUTTE, Paul-Robert V; Saint John Reg Hosp, PO Box 2100 Stn Main 400 University Ave, Saint John NB E2L 4L2; RCS (Ireland)'02; CCFP; Staff, Saint John Regional Hospital; Langs: Flemish; French; (506)648-6000

VANHUYSEN, Marie; MUHC-Montreal Gen Campus, L8 512-1650 av Cedar, Montreal QC H3G 1A4; Lille II (France)'05; Staff, McGill University Health Centre - Montreal General Campus; (514)934-1934

VANIA, Mariam; High Tech Pain Mgmt Office, 109-1575 Steeles Ave E, North York ON M2M 3Y7; Witwatersrand (South Africa)'61; MB ChB; FRCPC; Psy (Child & Adolescent Psychiatry). Langs: Afrikaans; Gujarati; (416)225-4442; Fax. (416)733-9032.

VANIA, Shera; Scarborough Prof Centre, 308-1371 Neilson Rd, Scarborough ON M1B 4Z8; Tor'89; Ac Staff, Rouge Valley Health System - Centenary Health Centre Site; (416)283-7701; Fax. (416)283-7108.

VANIER, Claude; Hop Louis-H Lafontaine, 7401 rue Hochelaga, Montreal QC H1N 3M5; Mon'80; FRCPC; Psy (Electroconvulsive Therapy). Staff, Hopital Louis-H Lafontaine; Prof adj clin, Universite de Montreal; (514)251-4000; Fax. (514)251-4054; claude.vanier@videotron.ca.

VANIER, Kelly L; 107-121 Dundas St E, Belleville ON K8N 1C3; McM'03; FRCPC; Peds. (613)968-8288; Fax. (613)968-6433.

VANIER, Laurent; Hop Charles-LeMoyne, 3120 boul Taschereau, Greenfield Park QC J4V 2H1; Mon'97; CCFP; CCFP(E.M.); Staff, Hopital Charles LeMoyne; (450)466-5000 x2780; Fax. (450)466-5051.

VANIER, Lyne; Centre de Sante Valcartier, CP 1000 Bdp Succ Forces, Courcelette QC G0A 4Z0; Laval'84; FRCPC; Psy (Clinical Psychiatry). Staff, Institut Universitaire Sante; Médecin, Centre de Sante Valcartier; Supvr Psy, Université Laval; (418)844-5000 x5802; Fax. (418)844-6987.

VANIER, Mylene; Hop du Sacre-Coeur de Mtl, 5400 boul Gouin O, Montreal QC H4J 1C5; Laval'05; Staff, Hôpital du Sacre-Coeur de Montréal; (514)338-2222

VANIER, Rejean; Clinique Med de l'Avenir, 200-1150 boul de l'Avenir, Laval QC H7N 6L2; Laval'78; (450)680-1150; Fax. (450)680-1151.

VANIER, Stephane; Hop du Sacre-Coeur de Mtl, 5400 boul Gouin O, Montreal QC H4J 1C5; Mon'89; CCFP; FCFP; ac Staff, Hôpital du Sacre-Coeur de Montréal; Langs: English; (514)338-2383; Fax. (514)338-3155.

VANKA, Thomas; Drummond Med Bldg, 810-1414 rue Drummond, Montreal QC H3G 1W1; Montpellier (France)'74; (514)843-5577; Fax. (514)843-5817.

VANLERBERGHE, Kenneth R; Kings Cross Doctors Office, 17 Kings Cross Rd, Brampton ON L6T 3V5; Tor'92; CCFP; (905)799-9144; Fax. (905)799-1250.

VANN, Patricia M; Northwestern Health Unit, 75D Van Horne Ave, Dryden ON P8N 2B2; McM'85; CCFP; FCFP; (807)223-8777; Fax. (807)737-5754.

VANNELLI, Anthony M; London HSC-University Hosp, PO Box 5339 Stn B 339 Windermere Rd, London ON N6A 5A5; Wes'85; FRCPC; Anes (Cardiovascular Anesthesia). Staff, London Health Sciences Centre - University Hospital; Langs: Italian; (519)685-8500 x3338

VANNER, Stephen J; Hotel-Dieu Hosp, 166 Brock St, Kingston ON K7L 5G2; Qns'83; MSc; FRCPC; IntMed; Gastroent. Staff, Hotel-Dieu Hospital; Att Staff, Kingston General Hospital; Consultant, Providence Care - St Mary's of the Lake Hospital Site; Prof, Queen's University; (613)544-3400 x2332; Fax. (613)544-3114; vanners@hdh.kari.net.

VANOUNOU, Tsafrir; SMBD Jewish Gen Hosp, 3755 ch Cote-Sainte-Catherine, Montreal QC H3T 1E2; McG'99; FRCSC; GenSurg. Staff, Sir Mortimer B Davis Jewish General; (514)340-8222

VANSPALL, Gordon D; Quinte HC-Belleville Gen Hosp, 265 Dundas St E, Belleville ON K8N 5A9; Bangalore (India)'70; MB BS; FRCPC; Anes (Critical Care Medicine). Staff, QHC Belleville General; (613)939-7400

VANT, Thomas E; Dalbrent Med Centre, 110-3604 52 Ave NW, Calgary AB T2L 1V9; Alb'88; CCFP; Med Dir, Accident Rehabilitation Centre; Med Dir, Intermed Safety; (403)282-9445; Fax. (403)284-0093.

VANT VOORT, M Joan; Aurora Med Centre, 200-15017 Yonge St, Aurora ON L4G 1M5; Tor'88; BSc; CCFP; FCFP; (905)727-9481; Fax. (905)727-6280.

VANTANAJAL, Jimmy S; Sheldon M Chumir Health Centre, 1213 4 St SW, Calgary AB T2R 0X7; (Other Foreign)'08; CCFP; (403)955-9300; jimmy.vantanajal@albertahealthservices.ca.

VANTELON, Jean-Marie; Dr L Richard Ctre D'Oncologie, 37 rue Providence, Moncton NB E1C 8X3; Paris (France)'97; Staff, Dr Georges-L-Dumont University Hospital Centre; Langs: French; (506)862-4030; Fax. (506)862-4222; jmvantelon@hotmail.com.

VANTOMME, Sylvia B; Hillsdale Med Clinic, 1380G 23rd Ave., Regina SK S4S 3S5; Sask'86; CCFP; FCFP; (306)584-1533; Fax. (306)584-1767.

VANUKURU, Venkata R; Hilltop Med Clinic, 140-15321 16 Ave, Surrey BC V4A 1R6; Vijayawada (India)'89; MB BS; CCFP; (604)531-5575

VANVAT, Jarnail S; Sandalwood Med Centre, 5-2945 Sandalwood Pky E, Brampton ON L6R 3J6; Sask'05; CCFP; Langs: Punjabi; (905)463-1337; Fax. (905)463-1338.

VARADARASA, Arulanandam; William Osler HC-Brampton, 2100 Bovaird Dr E, Brampton ON L6R 3J7; Jaffna (Sri Lanka)'87; MB BS; FRCPC; IntMed. Staff, William Osler Health System - Brampton Civic Hospital; Langs: Sinhalese; Tamil; (905)494-2120; Fax. (905)494-6206.

VARADI, Robert G; West Park Healthcare Centre, 82 Buttonwood Ave, York ON M6M 2J5; McG'02; FRCPC; IntMed; Respir. Staff, West Park Healthcare Centre; Langs: Bilingual(English/French); (416)243-8947; Fax. (416)243-8947.

VARANO, Kristopher; Centre for Family Medicine, 10B Victoria St S, Kitchener ON N2G 1C5; Wes'10; CCFP; (519)783-0023

VARAPRAVAN, Sreelatha P; Regional Mental Health Care, PO Box 5532 Stn B 850 Highbury Ave, London ON N6A 4H1; Mysore (India)'95; MB BS; FRCPC; Psy. Assoc Prof Mood & Anxiety Unit, Regional Mental Health Care-St Joseph's Health Care; Langs: Hindi; (519)455-5110; Fax. (519)455-2919.

VARDAR, Gonul; Albany Med Clinic, 807 Broadview Ave, Toronto ON M4K 2P8; Izmir (Turkey)'65; Langs: Turkish; (416)461-9471; Fax. (416)461-2710.

VARDY, Cathy L; Janeway Children's Hlth & Reha, 2711-300 Prince Philip Dr, St. John's NL A1B 3V6; Mem'83; FRCPC; Peds. Staff, Health Sciences Centre; Staff, Janeway Children's Health & Rehabilitation Centre; Chair Clinical Disciplines Peds/Asst Prof, Memorial University Of Newfoundland; (709)777-4606

VARDY, Pamela Y; 4-1116 Mountain Rd, Moncton NB E1C 2T3; Mem'98; CCFP; (506)854-2300; Fax. (506)857-5013.

VARDY, Rhonda M; Mackenzie Richmond Hill Hosp, 10 Trench St, Richmond Hill ON L4C 4Z3; Mem'89; FRCPC; Psy (Child & Adolescent Psychiatry). Staff Shaw Clinic, Mackenzie Richmond Hill Hospital; (905)883-1212; Fax. (905)883-2144.

VARELAS, Michael A N; The Richmond Hosp, 7000 Westminster Hwy, Richmond BC V6X 1A2; UBC'83; FRCPC; Neur (Adult Neurology). Consultant, Vancouver General Hospital - Centennial Pavillion; Ac Staff, Richmond Hospital; Asst Prof, University of British Columbia; (604)937-0331; Fax. (604)269-3763.

VARENBUT, Michael; Oak Ridges Med Centre, 403-13291 Yonge St, Richmond Hill ON L4E 4L6; Tor'91; DAB; CCFP; FCFP; Staff, Mackenzie Richmond Hill Hospital; Staff, Southlake Regional Health Centre; Staff, Sunnybrook Health Sciences Centre; Teach Staff Med, University of Toronto; Langs: Hebrew; Russian; (905)773-7759; Fax. (905)773-1325; laura@prototype.ca.

VAREY, Peter A; 63 Park Ave, Brantford ON N3S 5H4; McM'88; FRCPC; PhysMed&Rehab (Electrodiagnosis). (519)756-1865; Fax. (519)756-7092.

VARGA, Caroline; CSSS du Sud de Lanaudière, 911 montee des Pionniers, Terrebonne QC J6V 2H2; Laval'04; FRCPC; Neur. Staff Neur, Centre Hospitalier Pierre le Gardeur; Langs: Bilingual(French/English); (450)654-7525; Fax. (450)470-4296.

VARGA, Marica; St Joseph's Health Centre, 30 The Queensway, Toronto ON M6R 1B5; Bucharest (Romania)'75; ABIM; FRCPC; IntMed (Geriatric Medicine); GeriatricMed. Consultant, Runnymede Healthcare Centre; Consultant, West Park Healthcare Centre; Langs: Greek; French; Italian; Romanian; (416)530-6532; Fax. (416)530-6585.

VARGA-SOLYMOSS, Susan M; Westmount Square Med Clinic, T1 550-1 car Westmount, Westmount QC H3Z 2P9; Budapest (Hungary)'53; FRCPC; IntMed (Diabetology); Endocrin (P.Q.). Staff, McGill University Health Centre - Montreal General Campus; (514)934-2334 x297; Fax. (514)931-2929.

VARGAS, Danilo R; 206-9808 King George Hwy, Surrey BC V3T 2V6; UP (Philippines)'71; BSc; FRCSC; Otol (Hearing Loss). Ac Staff, Surrey Memorial Hospital; Consultant, Peace Arch Hospital; Clin Instructor Surg, University of British Columbia; Langs: Tagalog; (604)582-0208; Fax. (604)588-7551.

VARGAS DREYER, Maria G; CHUM-Hotel-Dieu, 3840 rue Saint-Urbain, Montreal QC H2W 1T8; Venezia (Italy)'86; Staff, Centre Hospitalier l'Université de Montréal (CHUM) - Hôtel-Dieu; (514)890-8000

VARGHESE, Boji; Four Corners Med Bldg, 410-2009 Long Lake Rd, Sudbury ON P3E 6C3; Bangalore (India)'89; FRCPC; IntMed; Endocrin&Metab. Langs: Malayalam; (705)523-5663

VARGHESE, Sunil A; The Ottawa Hosp-Gen Campus, 501 Smyth Rd, Ottawa ON K1H 8L6; Qns'07; InfectDis; IntMed. Staff, The Ottawa Hospital - General Campus; (613)737-7777

VARI, Barbara J; St Lawrence Health Centre, 3-140 The Esplanade, Toronto ON M5A 4P5; McM'89; CCFP; FCFP; Staff, St Michael's Hospital; University of Toronto; (416)864-6000; Fax. (416)360-4902.

VARIEUR, Stephen P; Huntsville Prof Bldg, 201-348 Muskoka Rd 3 N, Huntsville ON P1H 1H8; McM'94; CCFP; CCFP(E.M.); (705)789-6137; Fax. (705)789-6175.

VARIN, Ginette; Centre de Sante Integrale, RR 5 1-160 rue Pope, Cookshire QC J0B 1M0; Mon'78; (819)875-5535; Fax. (819)875-3631.

VARIN, Jean R; Dr Jean Varin Orthopediste, 455 boul de l'Hopital, Gatineau QC J8T 7X7; Laval'82; MRCS; FRCS; BMedSci; CSPQ; DMJ; FRCSC; OrthSurg (Assessment-Clinical Impairment & Disability). Staff, Montfort Hospital; Langs: Bilingual(French/English); (819)243-8782 x3; Fax. (819)243-7081.

VARIN, Sylvain; Clinique Med l'Assomption, 5345 boul de l'Assomption, Montreal QC H1T 4B3; Mon'82; (514)257-7000

VARKUL, Mark D; William Osler Health Centre, 202-100 Humber College Blvd, Etobicoke ON M9V 5G4; Tor'95; FRCPC; IntMed (Critical Care Medicine); Respir. Staff IntMed, William Osler Health System - Etobicoke General Hospital; (416)746-1011; Fax. (416)746-1411.

VARLESE, Fabio; Baycrest Ctre/Geriatric Care, 1C16-3560 Bathurst St, North York ON M6A 2E1; Rome (Italy)'91; FRCPC; IntMed; GeriatricMed. Staff, Baycrest Centre for Geriatric Care; Consultant, Mount Sinai Hospital; Langs: Italian; (416)785-2500; Fax. (416)785-2863; fvarlese@baycrest.org.

VARLEY, Kevin R; Brandon Reg Health Centre, 150 McTavish Ave E, Brandon MB R7A 2B3; Qns'05; FRCPC; Psy. Staff, Brandon Regional Health Centre; (204)578-4000

VARMA, Amrit B; Winnipeg Clinic, 425 St Mary Ave, Winnipeg MB R3C 0N2; Glasgow (Scotland)'71; MB ChB; FRCSC; Otol (Rhinology). Ac Staff, Victoria General Hospital; Winnipeg Clinic; University of Manitoba; Langs: Punjabi; (204)957-3228; Fax. (204)943-1900; avarma@winnipegclinic.com.

VARMA, Devesh K; Credit Valley Eye Care, 1-3200 Erin Mills Pky, Mississauga ON L5L 1W8; Dal'04; FRCSC; Ophth. Staff, Credit Valley Eye Care; Langs: Hindi; French; (905)820-3937

VARMA, Divya J; Dartmouth Med Centre, 210-46 Portland St, Dartmouth NS B2Y 1H4; Dal'97; CCFP; Staff, Dartmouth General Hospital; Staff, IWK Health Centre; Langs: Hindi; (902)465-8714; Fax. (902)464-4903; divyainhalifax@hotmail.com.

VARMA, Gokuldas R; MD Medical Centre, 1801 Eglinton Ave W, Toronto ON M6E 2H8; Rome (Italy)'77; MASc; Court Staff Family Practice, Humber River Regional Hospital - Finch Avenue Site; Assoc Staff, Toronto General Hospital - UHN; Lecturer Med, University of Toronto; Langs: Italian; Malayalam; Hindi; (416)657-1321; Fax. (416)657-8482.

VARMA, Neel B; Winnipeg Med Clinic, 130-2855 Pembina Hwy, Winnipeg MB R3T 2H5; Man'03.

VARMA, P Victor; Chatham-Kent Health Alliance, PO Box 2030 Stn Main 80 Grand Ave W, Chatham ON N7M 5L9; Alb'96; FRCPC; DiagRad. Staff, Chatham-Kent Health Alliance; (519)352-6400

VARMA, Prem K; Southbank Med Centre, 5-2430 Bank St, Ottawa ON K1V 0T7; Assam Medical College (India)'68; Langs: Hindi; (613)737-7400; Fax. (613)736-6948.

VARMA, Renatta; 4000 Dewdney Ave, Regina SK S4T 1A2; Sask'98; FRCSC; Ophth (Vitreo Retinal Surgery). Board Member, Horizon Laser Vision Centre; (306)522-1092; Fax. (306)522-0507.

VARMA, Shanta; Hamilton Comm Health Centre, M1B-414 Victoria Ave N, Hamilton ON L8L 5G8; Tor'07; CCFP; Physician, Mohawk College; (905)540-4247; Fax. (905)528-0517.

VARMA, Sonal; Kingston Gen Hosp, 76 Stuart St, Kingston ON K7L 2V7; Mahatma Gandhi Memorial Medical College (India)'01; AnatPath. Staff, Kingston General Hospital; (613)548-6035

VARMA, Sonya; NW Calgary Diabetes Centre, 150-1620 29 St NW, Calgary AB T2N 4L7; Sask'97; ABIM; FRCP; FRCPC; IntMed (Diabetology). Staff Med, Covenant Health - Misericordia Community Hospital; Dir, North West Calgary Diabetes Centre; (403)282-3200; Fax. (403)282-3223; varma@me.com.

VARNER, Catherine E; Mount Sinai Hosp, 206-600 University Ave, Toronto ON M5G 1X5; North Carolina (USA)'08; CCFP; CCFP(E.M.); Staff, Mount Sinai Hospital; (416)586-5058; Fax. (416)586-4719.

VARNEY, Ian G; 902-1849 Yonge St, Toronto ON M4T 3A7; Tor'81; CCFP; FCFP; (416)487-1060; Fax. (416)487-0137.

VARRIN, Angela E; 322 Dominion St, Renfrew ON K7V 1H4; Ott'10; CCFP.

VARSAVA, Michael E; Hotel-Dieu Grace Hosp, 1030 Ouellette Ave, Windsor ON N9A 1E1; Tor'77; Staff, Hôtel-Dieu Grace Hospital; (519)973-4401

VARSHNEY, Nishi K; Sunnybrook Hlth Sciences Ctre, H479-2075 Bayview Ave, Toronto ON M4N 3M5; Cal'07; FRCPC; IntMed (Geriatric Medicine). Staff, Sunnybrook Health Sciences Centre; (416)480-6100

VARTANIAN, Astghik; Clinique Med Alpha Medic, 1253 rue Guy, Montreal QC H3H 2K5; Yerevan (Russia (Federation))'67; Langs: Russian; Armenian; English; (514)933-8383

VARTAZARMIAN, Garabed; Clinique Med Fleury, 2157 rue Fleury E, Montreal QC H2B 1K1; Sofia (Bulgaria)'58; (514)388-2600

VARTAZARMIAN, Raphael; CSSS de Laval, 1755 boul Rene-Laennec, Laval QC H7M 3L9; McG'05; Staff, Hopital de la Cite de la santé; (450)668-1010

VARTIAN, Michele; Clinique Med l'Envolee, 5025 rue de Salaberry, Montreal QC H4J 1J1; Mon'91; FRCPC; Peds (Ambulatory Pediatrics). Staff, Hopital de la Cite de la santé; Langs: Spanish; English; (514)331-2323; Fax. (514)333-8534.

VARTIC-IFTENE, Felicia; Hotel Dieu Hosp, 166 Brock St, Kingston ON K7L 5G2; Cluj (Other Foreign)'84; Staff, Hotel-Dieu Hospital; (613)544-3400

VARTY, Barbara F; Haliburton Highlands Family Cl, PO Box 870 7217 Gelert Rd, Haliburton ON K0M 1S0; Tor'75; (705)457-1212; Fax. (705)457-3955.

VARTY, Christopher B; Rouge Valley-Centenary HC, 2867 Ellesmere Rd, Scarborough ON M1E 4B9; Tor'67; FRCPC; Anes. Staff, Rouge Valley Health System - Centenary Health Centre Site; Langs: English; French; (416)284-8131

VARTY, Kimberly M; Atikokan Family Health Team, PO Box 1450 123 Marks St, Atikokan ON P0T 1C0; NOSM'09; CCFP; (807)597-2721

VARTY, T Douglas; Fredericton Med Clinic, 206-1015 Regent St, Fredericton NB E3B 6H5; Dal'95; CCFP; Assoc Staff, Dr Everett Chalmers Regional Hospital.

VARUGHESE, Elizabeth A; White Rock Med Clinic, 101-15451 Russell Ave, White Rock BC V4B 2R5; Sask'87; Staff Maternity Clinic, Peace Arch Hospital; Staff, Peace Arch Community Medical Centre; (604)531-5595; Fax. (604)531-9818.

VARUGHESE, Jobin; Queen Square Doctors FHT, 201-366 Main St N, Brampton ON L6V 1P8; (Other Foreign)'05; (905)455-1331

VARVARIKOS, Mariette; CHUM-Hop Notre-Dame, 1560 rue Sherbrooke E, Montreal QC H2L 4M1; Mon'95; LMCC; CCFP; CCFP(E.M.); FCFP; Staff, Centre Hospitalier l'Université de Montréal (CHUM) - Hôpital Notre-Dame; Langs: Greek; Spanish; English; (514)890-8000

VARY, Ana R; Clinique Med Luso, 1 av Mont-Royal E, Montreal QC H2T 1N4; Bogota (Colombia)'75; (514)849-2391; Fax. (514)849-2394.

VARY, Christiane; CLSC Riviere-des-Prairies, 8655 boul Perras, Montreal QC H1E 4M7; Mon'09; CCFP; (514)494-4924

VARY, John R; Clinique d'Urologie, 307-176 av Rouleau, Rimouski QC G5L 8W1; Mon'76; FRCSC; Urol. Langs: English; French; (418)724-6262; Fax. (418)722-6265; varyriki@gocable.ca.

VAS, Antonio B L; Upper Ottawa Med Clinic, 2-1447 Upper Ottawa St, Hamilton ON L8W 3J6; Dublin (Ireland)'71; Ac Staff, St Joseph's Healthcare - Charlton Campus; (905)389-4976; Fax. (905)389-2326.

VAS, David W; Lakeshore Gen Hosp, 160 av Stillview, Pointe-Claire QC H9R 2Y2; Mon'97; CCFP; CCFP(E.M.); Staff, Lakeshore General Hospital - Pointe Claire; Langs: German; Hebrew; Hungarian; (514)630-2225

VASA, Priya P; St James Town Health Centre, 410 Sherbourne St, Toronto ON M4X 1K2; Tor'09; CCFP; (416)864-3096

VASANJI, Adil N; Rabbit Hill Med Clinic, 14030 23 Ave NW, Edmonton AB T6R 3L6; Alb'09; CCFP; (780)757-4220

VASANTHAN, Veeragathy; Peninsula Health Care Corp, 67A Manitoba Dr, Clarenville NL A5A 1K3; Colombo (Sri Lanka)'82; MB BS; Staff, Peninsula Health Care Corporation; Clinical Asst Prof, Memorial University Of Newfoundland; Langs: Sinhalese; Tamil; (709)466-3411; Fax. (709)466-5372.

VASARHELYI, Edward M; London HSC-University Campus, PO Box 5339 339 Windermere Rd, London ON N6A 5A5; Qns'05; FRCSC; OrthSurg. Staff, London Health Sciences Centre - University Hospital; (519)663-3413; Fax. (519)663-3417.

VASCONCELOS, Jose A; The Brandon Clinic, 620 Dennis St, Brandon MB R7A 5E7; Recife (Brazil)'56; FRCPsy; FRCPC; Psy (Adult General Psychiatry). Consultant, Brandon Regional Health Centre; Langs: Spanish; Portuguese; (204)571-7135 x156; Fax. (204)726-1765.

VASDEV, Shawn; Addiction & Mental Health-Coll, 250 College St, Toronto ON M5T 1R8; Ott'07; FRCPC; Psy. Staff, Centre for Addiction & Mental Health (CAMH) - College Street Site; (416)535-8501

VASELENAK, Sharon A; Yellowbird Family Clinic, 3380 Gateway Blvd NW, Edmonton AB T6J 6V1; Alb'81; CCFP; FCFP; (780)434-2893; Fax. (780)435-1057.

VASEY, Kirsten N; Workplace Safety & Ins Board, 2485 Ouellette Ave, Windsor ON N8X 1L5; Qns'02; CCFP; Staff, Workplace Safety & Insurance Board; (519)966-0660

VASHISHT, Shashi; Ackroyd Med Clinic, 105-8056 King George Blvd, Vancouver BC V5W 5B5; Jabalpur (India)'67; MB BS; Langs: Hindi; Punjabi; (604)593-5499

VASIL, Dany; Hotel-Dieu d'Arthabaska, 5 rue des Hospitalieres, Victoriaville QC G6P 6N2; Sher'88; FRCPC; Anes (P.Q.). Staff, Hotel-Dieu d'Arthabaska; (819)357-2030

VASIL, Lisa; Castlegar Med Clinic, 1101 3rd St, Castlegar BC V1N 2A1; McG'98; CCFP; (250)365-7717; Fax. (250)365-0347.

VASIL, Nancy; Pavillon Rosemont, 5e-5689 boul Rosemont, Montreal QC H1T 2H1; Sher'91; LMCC; FRCPC; Psy (Consultation-Liaison). Staff, Hopital Maisonneuve-Rosemont; Clin Prof, Universite de Montreal; (514)252-3914; Fax. (514)252-3810.

VASILE, Gabriela; Eagle Ridge Hosp & Health CC, 475 Guildford Way, Port Moody BC V3H 3W9; Iasi (Romania)'91; CCFP; Staff, Eagle Ridge Hospital & Health Care Centre; Langs: Romanian; French; (604)313-2921

VASILESCU, Ovidiu; 232-5 Fairview Mall Dr, North York ON M2J 2Z1; Faculte De Medicina Generala Din CraiovaCraiova (Romania)'85; CCFP; Langs: Romanian; (416)492-2960; Fax. (416)492-4025.

VASILEVSKY, Carol-Ann; SMBD Jewish Gen Hosp, 3755 ch Cote-Sainte-Catherine, Montreal QC H3T 1E2; McG'80; AB; FACS; FRCSC; GenSurg (Colon & Rectal Surgery). Dir 2nd Year Surgery Course, Sir Mortimer B Davis Jewish General; adj Prof, McGill University; (514)731-2479; Fax. (514)340-7560; carol-ann.vasilevsky@mcgill.ca.

VASILEVSKY, Murray L; MUHC-Montreal Gen Hosp, 1650 av Cedar, Montreal QC H3G 1A4; McG'75; FRCPC; IntMed (Hypertension); Nephrol (P.Q.). Dir Nephrol, McGill University Health Centre - Montreal General Campus; assoc Prof, McGill University; (514)934-1934 x44034; Fax. (514)934-8248; murray.vasilevsky@muhc.mcgill.ca.

VASILIE, Yvonne B; Lakeshore Gen Hosp, 160 Stillview Ave, Pointe-Claire QC H9R 2Y2; Bucarest (Romania)'92; FRCSC; ObstGyn. Staff, Lakeshore General Hospital - Pointe Claire; Langs: Romanian; English; (514)630-2225

VASILIKAKI-BAKER, Helen; McGill Univ Student Hlth Serv, 3600 rue McTavish, Montreal QC H3A 1Y2; Dal'87; CCFP; adj Prof Family Med, McGill University; (514)398-6017; Fax. (514)398-2559.

VASILIOU, Denise M; Toronto East Gen & Orth Hosp, 825 Coxwell Ave, East York ON M4C 3E7; Tor'01; FRCPC; IntMed. Staff, Toronto East General Hospital Inc; Langs: Greek; French; (416)461-8272

VASILIU, Irene M; St Joseph's Care Group, 35 Algoma St N, Thunder Bay ON P7B 5G7; Bucharest (Romania)'93; (807)344-4600; Fax. (807)344-2419.

VASKA, Solomon R; Riversdale Med Walk-In Clinic, 341 20th St W, Saskatoon SK S7M 0X1; Andhra (India)'70; MB BS; (306)651-1699; Fax. (306)651-1698.

VASOVICH, Inge; 4-65 Mall Rd, Hamilton ON L8V 5B8; Wes'70; Staff, St Joseph's Healthcare - Charlton Campus; Staff, Hamilton Health Sciences Centre - McMaster University Medical Centre; Langs: Yugoslavian; German; Serbian; (905)574-4033; Fax. (905)574-8479.

VASQUEZ, Arthur R; Central Park Med Clinic, 104-3965 Kingsway, Burnaby BC V5H 1Y8; Sask'91; (604)434-8781

VASQUEZ, Manuel O; 300-2045 Dufferin St, York ON M6E 3R4; Lima (Peru)'58; Staff, Humber River Regional Hospital - Church Street Site; Langs: Italian; Spanish; (416)651-2340; Fax. (416)651-7472.

VASQUEZ, Raul A; Bayview Mall Med Office, 50-470 Dundas St E, Belleville ON K8N 1G1; Universidad Central De Venezuela (Venezuela)'97; CCFP; Langs: Spanish; (613)966-4045; Fax. (613)966-0072.

VASQUEZ, Virgilio B; Associate Family Physicians Cl, 262 2nd Ave NE, Swift Current SK S9H 2C8; Santo Tomas (Philippines)'61; DAB; FACS; FRCSC; GenSurg. (306)773-1555; Fax. (306)773-6817.

VASS, Sylvie; CSSS de Chicoutimi, CP 5006 succ bureau-chef 305 rue Saint-Vallier, Chicoutimi QC G7H 5H6; Sher'85; FRCPC; RadOncol. Staff, Complexe hospitalier de la Sagamie; (418)549-2195

VASSAR, Elizabeth V; Vancouve Gen Hosp, 5D-855 12 Ave W, Vancouver BC V5Z 1M9; Poznan University (Other Foreign)'06; FRCPC; Psy. Staff, Vancouver General Hospital - Centennial Pavillion.

VASSEL, Jennifer L; 370 Broadway Ave E PO Box 95045 Rpo Kingsgate, Vancouver BC V5T 4T8; UBC'10; CCFP; (604)873-3558

VASSILIOU, Demetra; Parkdale Med Bldg, 301-1081 Carling Ave, Ottawa ON K1Y 4G2; McG'87; FRCSC; ObstGyn. Staff, The Ottawa Hospital - Civic Campus; University of Ottawa; Langs: Greek; French; (613)729-6113; Fax. (613)691-1276; demetraoffice@rogers.com.

VASSILIOU, Melina; MUHC-Montreal Gen Hosp, L9 313-1650 av Cedar, Montreal QC H3G 1A4; McG'01; FRCSC; GenSurg (Laparoscopic Surgery). Staff, McGill University Health Centre - Montreal General Campus; adj Prof, McGill University; Langs: Bilingual(French/English); (514)934-1934 x44330; Fax. (514)934-8210; melina.vassiliou@mcgill.ca.

VASSILYADI, Michael; Children's Hosp Eastern Ont, 401 Smyth Rd, Ottawa ON K1H 8L1 Neurosurgery; McG'90; MSc; FACS; FAAP; BSc(Hon); CM; LMCC; FRCSC; Neursurg (Pediatric Neuro Surgery). Ac Staff Ped Neuro Surg/Investigator Research Institute, Children's Hospital of Eastern Ontario (CHEO); Dir Chapter, Think First; Assoc Prof Surg & Peds, University of Ottawa; Langs: French; Greek; (613)738-3985; Fax. (613)738-4293.

VASSOS, Laurie J; Acadia Med Centre, 3310 8th St E, Saskatoon SK S7H 5M3; Sask'80; Physician, Acadia Medical Centre; (306)373-6000; Fax. (306)477-5000.

VASTARDIS, Alexander D; Vancouver Gen Hosp, JPN 3500-855 12th Ave W, Vancouver BC V5Z 1M9; UBC'00; CCFP; Staff, Vancouver General Hospital - Centennial Pavillion; (604)875-5027

VASUDEV, Akshya; London HSC-Victoria Campus, PO Box 5010 Stn B ZA 4-800 Commissioners Rd E, London ON N6A 5W9; University of Delhi (India)'96; Staff, London Health Sciences Centre - Victoria Campus; Langs: Hindi; Punjabi; (519)685-8500

VASUDEV, Kamini; London HSC-Victoria Campus, PO Box 5010 Stn B 800 Commissioners Rd E, London ON N6A 5W9; University of Delhi (India)'96; Staff, London Health Sciences Centre - Victoria Campus; (519)685-8500

VASUDEV, Pooja; Cambridge Mem Hosp, 700 Coronation Blvd, Cambridge ON N1R 3G2; Delhi (India)'01; FRCPC; AnatPath. Staff, Cambridge Memorial Hospital; (519)621-2330

VASUDEVA, Pratibha R; 150 Rolling Hills Dr Box 110, Orangeville ON L9W 4X8; Sardar Patel (India)'77; MB BS; MS; Staff, Headwaters Health Care Centre - Orangeville Site; (519)943-1094; Fax. (519)943-1095.

VASUDEVAN, Mudalodu V; Forest Glade Med Centre, 3145 Forest Glade Dr, Windsor ON N8R 1W6; Bangalore (India)'71; MB BS; Langs: Kanarese; Telugu; Hindi; (519)739-2888; Fax. (519)739-2848.

VASYLEVYCH, Nataliya V; The Doctor's Office, 1011 Upper Middle Rd E, Oakville ON L6H 4L1; Zaporozskij Medicinskij Institut (Other Foreign)'98; CCFP; Langs: Russian; (905)849-7007; Fax. (905)849-7883.

VAT, Sopharat; CHUM-Hopital Hotel-Dieu, 3840 Saint-Urbain, Montreal QC H2W 1T8; Mon'07; Respir; IntMed. Staff, Centre Hospitalier l'Université de Montréal (CHUM) - Hôtel-Dieu; Staff, Centre Hospitalier Régional de Lanaudière; (514)890-8444

VATS, Arun R; Greenwood Mall Med Centre, PO Box 1022 963 Central Ave, Greenwood NS B0P 1N0; Dal'91; Ac Staff/Pres Med Staff, Western Kings Memorial Health Centre; Ac Staff, Valley Regional Hospital; (902)765-4688; Fax. (902)765-4688.

VATTHEUER, Annabel G; Southwood Med Centre, 3F-2385 Pembina Hwy, Winnipeg MB R3T 2H4; Man'87; (204)988-1590; Fax. (204)988-1595.

VATTHEUER, Frank B; Psychealth Centre, PX362-771 Bannatyne Ave, Winnipeg MB R3E 3N4; Man'85; FRCPC; Psy. Staff, Psychealth Centre; (204)787-3887; Fax. (204)787-3380; fvattheuer@exchange.hsc.mb.ca.

VATTURI, Ravi S; Dr Charles S Curtis Mem Hosp, 178-200 West St, St Anthony NL A0K 4S0; Andhara (India)'84; MB BS; Charles S Curtis Memorial Hospital; (709)454-3333

VAUCHER, Michel P; Hop Louis-H Lafontaine, 7401 rue Hochelaga, Montreal QC H1N 3M5; Staff, Hopital Louis-H Lafontaine; (514)251-4000

VAUCHER, Robert-Yves; Clinique Med du Lac, 33 rue Saint-Patrice E, Magog QC J1X 5B7; Mon'90; FRCPC; Neur (P.Q.). Staff, Hopital Louis-H Lafontaine; (819)843-2944

VAUDRY, John S; Paterson Med Centre, 45 Wolsley St RR 1 Stn Main, Kenora ON P9N 3W7; Cal'82; (807)468-4433; Fax. (807)468-5565.

VAUDRY, Wendy L A; Edmonton Clinic Health Academy, 3 588D-11405 87 Ave, Edmonton AB T6G 1C9; McG'82; FRCPC; Peds; InfectDis. Staff, Stollery Children's Hospital; Staff, Edmonton Clinic Health Academy; Prof, University of Alberta; (780)248-5540

VAUGEOIS, Alain; Polyclinique du Cap, 110-700 boul Thibeau, Trois-Rivieres QC G8T 7A1; Mon'94; CCFP; Physician, Centre Investigation Cliniques Mauricie; Langs: Bilingual(French/English); (819)373-6516; Fax. (819)373-6516.

VAUGHAN, Brendan G; 110-10333 Southport Rd SW, Calgary AB T2W 3X6; Cal'01; CCFP; (403)258-1960; Fax. (403)253-5735.

VAUGHAN, Derek J; 50-1063 Talbot St PO Box 20033 Rpo Centre, St Thomas ON N5P 4H4; Qns'88; CCFP; CCFP(E.M.); FCFP; Staff Privil, St Thomas Elgin General Hospital; Aj Prof Family Med, University of Western Ontario; (519)637-2424; Fax. (519)637-2537.

VAUGHAN, Edward D; E D Vaughan Med Prof Corp, 505-1221 Algonquin Ave, North Bay ON P1B 4Y3; Manchester (England)'66; (705)476-1530; Fax. (705)476-1840.

VAUGHAN, George E R; Chatham-Kent Family Health Team, 9-30 McNaughton Ave, Wallaceburg ON N8A 1R9; Cambridge (England)'61; MB ChB; FRCS(Eng); FRCSC; GenSurg (Endoscopy). Staff Surg, Chatham-Kent Health Alliance - Sydenham Hospital Campus; Staff, Chatham-Kent Family Health Teams Inc. - Wallaceburg Site; (519)627-1497

VAUGHAN, Gerrard A; Wellington Med Clinic, 84C-3200 North Island Hwy, Nanaimo BC V9T 1W1; UBC'73; Ac Staff, Nanaimo Regional General Hospital; (250)740-2100; Fax. (250)740-2114.

VAUGHAN, Joanne; 100-235 Danforth Ave, Toronto ON M4K 1N2; McG'90; FRCPC; Peds; Critical Care Medicine. (416)466-1311; Fax. (416)466-9629.

VAUGHAN, Matthew M; Northumberland Hills Hosp, 1000 DePalma Dr, Cobourg ON K9A 5W6; Sheffield (England)'91; MSc; DABR; FRCR(London); Dir Diagnostic Imaging, Northumberland Hills Hospital; (905)372-6811; Fax. (905)372-4243.

VAUGHAN, Michael W; 135-5325 Cordova Bay Rd, Victoria BC V8Y 2L3; Mem'76; BA; BSc; BMedSci; Staff, Victoria General Hospital; Staff, Royal Jubilee Hospital; Staff Fam Med, University of Victoria; Clin Instructor, University of British Columbia; (250)385-6115; Fax. (250)385-8153.

VAUGHAN, Michele L; Courtice Health Centre, 1450 Highway 2, Courtice ON L1E 3C3; Wes'89; CCFP; FCFP; Assoc Staff, Lakeridge Health - Oshawa Site; (905)721-3539; Fax. (905)721-3526.

VAUGHAN, Peter W; South Shore Reg Hosp, 90 Glen Allan Dr, Bridgewater NS B4V 3S6; McM'82; MPH(John Hopkins); Med Dir/VP/CEO, South Shore Regional Hospital; Assoc Prof, Dalhousie University; Langs: English; French; (902)527-5271; Fax. (902)527-5269; pvaughn@ssdha.nshealth.ca.

VAUGHAN, R L Robert; 1442 County Rd RR 1, Carrying Place ON K0K 1L0; Qns'63; CCFP; Hon Staff, QHC Belleville General; Staff, Belmont Long Term Care; Staff, Crown Ridge Nursing Home; Queen's University; (613)967-1661

VAUGHAN, Stephen D; South Health Campus, 4448 Front St SE, Calgary AB T3M 1M4; Mem'07; FRCPC; IntMed; InfectDis. Staff, Rockyview General Hospital; Staff, South Health Campus; (403)956-1111

VAUGHAN-JACKSON, Julian D; East End Health Centre, 2-4 Mount Cashel Rd, St. John's NL A1A 1X7; London (England)'67; MB BS; LRCP; MRCS; (709)753-1450

VAUGHAN-NEIL, Edward F; Scarborough Hosp-General Div, 3050 Lawrence Ave E, Scarborough ON M1P 2V5; Oxford (England)'66; MB ChB; FACC; ABNM; MRCS; FRCPC; IntMed; NuclearMed; Cardiol. Staff NuclearMed, The Scarborough Hospital - General Campus; (416)431-8106; Fax. (416)431-8103.

VAUSE, Tannys D R; Ottawa Fertility Centre, 200-955 Green Valley Cres, Ottawa ON K2C 3V4; Man'03; FRCSC; ObstGyn (Reproductive Endocrinology). Staff, Ottawa Fertility Centre; Asst Prof, University of Ottawa; (613)686-3378; Fax. (613)225-9736.

VAUTOUR, Line M; MUHC-Royal Victoria Hosp, M9 05-687 av des Pins O, Montreal QC H3A 1A1; Tor'92; BSc; MSc; FRCP; FRCPC; IntMed (Endocrinology); Endocrin&Metab. Asst Physician, McGill University Health Centre - Royal Victoria Hospital; Asst Physician, McGill University Health Centre - Montreal General Campus; adj Prof, McGill University; Langs: English; French; (514)934-1934 x3510; Fax. (514)982-0825; line.vautour@mcgill.ca.

VAUTOUR, Marc; Dr Georges L-Dumont Reg Hosp, 330 av Universite, Moncton NB E1C 2Z3; Mon'99; FRCPC; Psy. Staff, Dr Georges-L-Dumont University Hospital Centre; (506)862-4000

VAVASSIS, Peter; Hop Maisonneuve-Rosemont, 5415 boul de l'Assomption, Montreal QC H1T 2M4; Mon'01; FRCPC; RadOncol. Staff, Hopital Maisonneuve-Rosemont; (514)252-3425; Fax. (514)252-3556.

VAVOUGIOS, George; Doctors on Bayview, 15900 Bayview Ave, Aurora ON L4G 7Y3; Wes'96; CCFP; FCFP; Langs: Greek; (905)726-9755; Fax. (905)726-9631.

VAVOUGIOS, James; 202-245 Danforth Ave, Toronto ON M4K 1N2; Tor'82; CCFP; FCFP; Langs: Greek; (416)461-1171; Fax. (416)461-1172.

VAYALUMKAL, Antony J; Medical Arts Bldg, 520-1 Young St, Hamilton ON L8N 1T8; Kerala (India)'73; DAB; FRCSC; Ophth. Langs: Malayalam; (905)527-4323; Fax. (905)527-1301.

VAYALUMKAL, Joseph; Alberta Children's Hosp, C4 619-2888 Shaganappi Trail N, Calgary AB T3B 6A8; McM'00; FRCPC; Peds; InfectDis. Staff, Alberta Children's Hospital; (403)955-7813; Fax. (403)955-3045.

VAYALUMKAL, Philip X; William Osler HS-Brampton, 2100 Bovaird Dr E, Brampton ON L6R 3J7; Tor'06; CCFP; CCFP(E.M.); Staff, William Osler Health System - Brampton Civic Hospital; Langs: Bilingual(English/French); (905)494-2120

VAYANI, Haji A; Dr Everett Chalmers Hosp, PO Box 9000 Stn A, Fredericton NB E3B 5N5; Karachi (Pakistan)'83; Staff, Dr Everett Chalmers Regional Hospital; (506)452-5231

VAZ, Camila M; 408-3101 Bloor St W, Etobicoke ON M8X 2W2; Bombay (India)'86; MB BS; FRCPC; Peds; Endocrin&Metab. Staff, The Hospital For Sick Children; (416)236-1654

VAZ, Gerald A; Gershaw Med Centre, 1-809 Bullivant Cres SW, Medicine Hat AB T1A 5G6; Mysore (India)'69; MB BS; DCH; DABPed; FRCPC; Peds. Staff Peds, Medicine Hat Regional Hospital; Asst Clin Prof, University of Calgary; (403)527-4448; Fax. (403)528-4988.

VAZ, Glenn F; North Okanagan Women's Health, 303-3210 25 Ave, Vernon BC V1T 1P1; UBC'93; FRCPC; IntMed. (250)503-0818; Fax. (250)503-0820.

VAZ, Reena F; Oakpark Med Clinic, 1-2530 Sixth Line, Oakville ON L6H 6W5; Alb'96; (905)257-1006; Fax. (905)257-0661.

VAZ, Simone S; William Osler HC-Brampton, 2100 Bovaird Dr E, Brampton ON L6R 3J7; McM'99; FRCPC; Peds (Neonatal & Perinatal Medicine). Staff, William Osler Health System - Brampton Civic Hospital; (905)494-2120; Fax. (905)494-6594.

VAZE, Medini; Dr Medini Vaze Med Clinic, PO Box 74101 Rpo Strathcona, Calgary AB T3H 3B6; UBC'03; CCFP; Staff, Peter Lougheed Centre; (403)943-5735

VAZIRI, Mojgan; Lions Gate Hosp, 231 15th St E, North Vancouver BC V7L 2L7; Tehran (Iran)'88; FRCPC; AnatPath. Staff, Lions Gate Hospital; Langs: Farsi; (604)984-5758; mojgan.vaziri@vch.ca.

VEALE, A Christine; Polyclinic Prof Centre Inc, 199 Grafton St, Charlottetown PE C1A 1L2; Dal'79; BSc; Staff, Queen Elizabeth Hospital; (902)629-8818; Fax. (902)566-9251.

VEALE, John L; 33 Church St S, Ajax ON L1S 6A6; Dublin (Ireland)'68; MB ChB; FRCPC; Peds. Langs: Gaelic; (905)683-0200

VEALE, Kimberly D; Phoenix Med Centre, 406-2155 10th Ave, Prince George BC V2M 5J6; Cal'04; CCFP; (250)564-7360; Fax. (250)564-1977.

VEALE, Pamela M; Alberta Children's Hosp, 2888 Shaganappi Trail NW, Calgary AB T3B 6A8; Cal'93; FRCPC; Peds (Developmental Pediatrics). Staff Child Development Centre, Alberta Children's Hospital; Asst Prof Peds, University of Calgary; (403)955-5912; Fax. (403)955-5896.

VEALL, John W; Lions Gate Hosp, 231 15 St E, North Vancouver BC V7L 2L7; Qns'01; FRCPC; Anes. Staff, Royal Columbian Hospital; Staff, Lions Gate Hospital; (604)988-3131

VEALL, Martin B; 9292 Highway 93 PO Box 1 RR 2 Stn Main, Midland ON L4R 4K4; Tor'86; CCFP; Langs: German; (705)527-7959; Fax. (705)527-1773.

VEARNCOMBE, Mary E; Sunnybrook Hlth Sciences Ctre, B103-2075 Bayview Ave, Toronto ON M4N 3M5; Tor'73; FRCPC; MedMicrobiol. Staff, Sunnybrook Health Sciences Centre; Assoc Prof, University of Toronto; (416)480-4243; Fax. (416)480-6990.

VEASEY, Duncan A; Annapolis Valley Health, 15 Chipman Dr, Kentville NS B4N 3V7; London (England)'77; MB BS; Staff, Annapolis Valley Health Adult Mental Health Program; (902)679-2870

VEASEY, Jack B; Hants Community Hosp, 89 Payzant Dr, Windsor NS B0N 2T0; Dal'02; CCFP; Staff, Hants Community Hospital; Medical Officer, Canadian Forces Health Services Centre (Atlantic); Physician Emerg, Capital Health District Authority; (902)792-2059; veasey.jb@forces.gc.ca.

VECCHIARELLI, John A; Norfinch Med Centre, 103-2100 Finch Ave W, North York ON M3N 2Z9; Tor'79; Langs: Italian; Spanish; (416)739-7878; Fax. (416)739-7818.

VECCHIO, Michael J; 212-1315 Finch Ave W, North York ON M3J 2G6; Tor'76; Ac Staff, Humber River Regional Hospital - Finch Avenue Site; Langs: Italian; French; Spanish; (416)630-7426; Fax. (416)630-2741.

VECCHIO, Silvano R; St Michael's Family Health Ctr, 13930 74 St NW, Edmonton AB T5C 3H7; Alb'69; BSc; Langs: Italian; French; (780)457-1600; Fax. (780)472-4799.

VEDD, Vipal; Royal Inland Hosp, 311 Columbia St, Kamloops BC V2C 2T1; UBC'05; FRCPC; DiagRad. Staff, Royal Inland Hospital; (250)374-5111

VEDEL, Isabelle; SMBD-Jewish Gen Hosp, 3755 ch Cote-Sainte-Catherine, Montreal QC H3T 1E2; Universite Rene Descartes (France)'03; Staff, Centre de Medecine Familiale Herzl; (514)340-8222 x1990

VEDELAGO, Harry R; Homewood Health Centre, 150 Delhi St, Guelph ON N1E 6K9; McM'94; CCFP; FCFP; Staff, Homewood Health Centre; Langs: Greek; (519)824-1010 x398; Fax. (519)767-3536.

VEENEMA, Christopher T; Queen Square Doctors FHT, 201-366 Main St N, Brampton ON L6V 1P8; Qns'09; CCFP; (905)455-1331; Fax. (905)455-5498.

VEENHUYZEN, George D; Foothills Med Centre, C836-1403 29 St NW, Calgary AB T2N 2T9; Man'94; FRCPC; IntMed (Electroencephalography); Cardiol. Staff, Foothills Medical Centre; Staff Cardiol, University of Calgary; Langs: Greek; (403)944-3282; Fax. (403)944-2906.

VEENMAN, Gerrit; Homewood Health Centre, 150 Delhi St, Guelph ON N1E 6K9; Wes'69; Staff Addiction Med, Homewood Health Centre; Langs: Dutch; (519)824-1010; Fax. (519)767-3536; veengary@homework.org.

VEENSTRA, Fedde; Owen Sound Family Health Team, 2000-1415 1st Ave W, Owen Sound ON N4K 4K8; Wes'76; CCFP; CCFP(E.M.); Langs: Dutch; (519)376-5700; Fax. (519)370-4044; eastview@bellnet.ca.

VEENSTRA, Jacob; Springdale Med Centre, 15-630 Peter Robertson Blvd, Brampton ON L6R 1T4; Wes'71; Langs: Dutch; (905)793-8868; Fax. (905)793-8957.

VEER, A Adriana; Boardwalk Prof Centre, 220 Water St, Charlottetown PE C1A 9M5; Wes'98; CCFP; Staff, Queen Elizabeth Hospital; Dalhousie University; Langs: English; French; (902)620-2037

VEERAPEN, Valmiki; Quinsam Med Clinic, 280-1400 Dogwood St, Campbell River BC V9W 3A6; Cape Town (South Africa)'01; MB ChB; CCFP; Langs: French; (250)286-3053; Fax. (250)286-0504.

VEGAS, Annette L; Univ Hlth Network-Toronto Gen, 200 Elizabeth St, Toronto ON M5G 2C4; McG'84; FRCPC; Anes (Cardiovascular Anesthesia). Staff, Toronto General Hospital - UHN; University of Toronto; (416)340-3242; Fax. (416)340-3698.

VEGIARD, Chantal; Centre d'Accueil de Lachine, 650 Place d'Accueil, Lachine QC H8S 3Z5; Mon'90; (514)634-7161 x2222

VEGSUND, Bjorn C; Lions Gate Hosp, 231 15th St E, North Vancouver BC V7L 2L7; UBC'08; CCFP; CCFP(E.M.); Staff, Lions Gate Hospital; (604)988-3131

VEIDLINGER, Otto F; 320-790 Bay St, Toronto ON M5G 1N8; Tor'60; BSc(Med); FRCPC; Neur. Langs: German; Hungarian; (416)921-2121; Fax. (416)929-7316; otto.veidlinger@utoronto.ca.

VEIKLE, Conrad J; Lakeside Med Clinic, 3919 8th St E, Saskatoon SK S7H 5M7; Sask'08; CCFP; (306)374-6884; Fax. (306)374-2552.

VEILLETTE, Andre; Inst de Recherche Clin de Mtl, 1105-110 av des Pins O, Montreal QC H2W 1R7; Laval'81; FRCPC; IntMed; MedOncol. Staff, McGill University Health Centre - Montreal General Campus; (514)987-5561; Fax. (514)987-5562.

VEILLETTE, Bruno; Clinique Med Gen d'Alma, 22 rue Melancon E, Alma QC G8B 6W3; Sher'82; Staff, CSSS de Lac-Saint Jean-Est; (418)668-2370; Fax. (418)668-0873; bruno.veillette@ssss.gouv.qc.ca.

VEILLETTE, Christian J H; Univ Hllth Network-Toronto Western Hosp, W1 440-399 Bathurst St, Toronto ON M5T 2S8; Cal'98; MSc; FRCSC; OrthSurg (Upper Extremity & Arthroscopic Surgery). Staff Shoulder & Elbow Surg, Toronto Western Hospital - University Health Network; Asst Prof OrthSurg, University of Toronto; (416)603-5929; Fax. (416)223-6624.

VEILLETTE, Helene; Ctr Hosp Affilie-Enfant-Jesus, 1401 18e rue, Quebec QC G1J 1Z4; Laval'05; Derm. Staff, Centre Hospitalier Affilié Universitaire de Québec - Hôpital De L'Enfant Jésus; (418)649-5520

VEILLETTE, Julie; CLSC Rimouski-Neigette, 165 rue des Gouverneurs, Rimouski QC G5L 7R2; Sher'99; CCFP; ac Staff, CSSS de la Mitis; assoc Staff, Hôpital Regional Rimouski; (418)723-1222; Fax. (418)723-7668.

VEILLETTE, Rejean; Commission Scolaire de Mtl, 3737 rue Sherbrooke E, Montreal QC H1X 3B3; Laval'62; Med Consultant, School Commission of Montreal; Langs: Bilingual(French/English); (514)596-6043; Fax. (514)596-7454.

VEILLETTE, Rene; Direction de la Sante Publique, 222-363 route Cameron, Sainte-Marie QC G6E 3E2; Laval'93; CommunMed (P.Q.). Staff, Hôtel-Dieu de Lévis; (418)389-1557; Fax. (418)389-1525; rene_veillette@ssss.gouv.qc.ca.

VEILLETTE, Yves; Hop Maisonneuve-Rosemont, 5415 boul de l'Assomption, Montreal QC H1T 2M4; Laval'77; LMCC; FRCPC; Anes (Pain Management). Staff/Aj Prof, Hopital Maisonneuve-Rosemont; adj Prof, Universite de Montreal; Langs: Bilingual(French/English); (514)252-3400; Fax. (514)252-3532.

VEILLEUX, Alain; 201-3550 rue de Cherbourg, Trois-Rivieres QC G8Y 6S6; Laval'83; Staff, Centre Hospitalier Regional de Trois-Rivieres; (819)379-7756; Fax. (819)374-9156.

VEILLEUX, Annie; Hôpital Ste-Justine, 3175 ch Cote-Sainte-Catherine, Montreal QC H3T 1C5; Laval'76; FRCPC; Peds (Developmental Pediatrics). Ac Staff, Hôpital Ste-Justine; adj Prof, Universite de Montreal; (514)345-4789; Fax. (514)345-2321; annie.veilleux.hsj@ssss.gouv.qc.ca.

VEILLEUX, Bertrand; Clinique Med MD Plus, 301-1100 av Beaumont, Mont-Royal QC H3P 3H5; Mon'83; FRCPC; Derm. Staff, Centre Hospitalier l'Université De Montréal (CHUM) - Hôpital Saint-luc; (514)738-4445; Fax. (514)738-8284; bertrandveilleux@hotmail.com.

VEILLEUX, Blandine; 540 Rte Taylor, Saint-Georges QC G5Y 5C2; Laval'73; Staff, Centre Hospitalier Beauce-Etchemin; (418)228-7381; Fax. (418)228-7606; blandine.veilleux@globetrotter.net.

VEILLEUX, Brigitte; Clinique Med Mont-Ste-Anne, 100-10974 boul Ste-Anne, Beaupre QC G0A 1E0; Laval'85; LMCC; Physician, CHSLD Foyer L'Accueil St George; Médecin, Clinique Medicale St-Martin; Langs: Bilingual(French/English); (418)827-4022; Fax. (418)827-4964.

VEILLEUX, Caroline; GMF le Gardeurois, 130-155 rue Notre-Dame, Repentigny QC J5Z 3C4; Sher'07; CCFP; (450)582-5551; Fax. (450)582-2718.

VEILLEUX, Chantal; CHUQ-Hotel-Dieu de Quebec, 11 Cote du Palais, Quebec QC G1R 2J6; Laval'88; FRCPC; GenPath (P.Q.); AnatPath. Staff, Centre Hospitalier Universitaire de Québec (CHUQ) - Siege Social; (418)691-5233; Fax. (418)691-5225.

VEILLEUX, Francine; 101-1800 boul le Corbusier, Laval QC H7S 2K1; Sher'79; MSc(Epidemiology & Biostatistic); FRCPC; Electroenceph (P.Q.); Neur (P.Q.). (450)686-0100; Fax. (450)686-0252.

VEILLEUX, Johanne; CSSS de Trois-Rivières, 1991 boul du Carmel, Trois-Rivieres QC G8Z 3R9; Laval'89; FRCPC; Psy. Staff, CSSS de Trois-Rivières; Staff, Institut Universitaire Sante; (819)697-3333

VEILLEUX, John; 219 Chilcott Cres, Newmarket ON L3X 3G6; Laval'05; Tel. (416)510-6843; Email: jvlabatt@gmail.com

VEILLEUX, Julien R; Min Emploie Solidarite Sociale, 575 rue Saint-Amable, Quebec QC G1R 4Z1; Sher'72; CommunMed (Administration). Médecin, Ministry De La Solidarite Sociale; (418)644-4646; julien.veilleux@mess.gouv.qc.ca.

VEILLEUX, Leon-Jean; CHUS-Hop Hotel-Dieu, 580 rue Bowen S, Sherbrooke QC J1G 2E8; Sher'77; Anes. Staff, Centre Hospitalier Universitaire de Sherbrooke-Hôpital Hôtel-Dieu; Dir Professional Services & Anes, Canadian Armed Forces; (819)346-1110; Fax. (819)564-5300.

VEILLEUX, Marie-Christine; Clinique Med de Touraine, 2B-520 boul de l'Hopital, Gatineau QC J8V 2P5; Sher'91; Staff, Hôpital de Gatineau; Langs: Bilingual(French/English); (819)568-0212; Fax. (819)568-6310.

VEILLEUX, Marie-Christine; Clinique Med Val-Belair, 202-1147 boul Pie-XI N, Quebec QC G3K 2P8; Laval'05; Médecin, CSSS de Becancour-Nicolet-Yamaska; (418)843-2473; Fax. (418)843-0224.

VEILLEUX, Martin J P L; Hop du Sacre-Coeur de Mtl, 5400 boul Gouin O, Montreal QC H4J 1C5; Laval'85; FRCPC; NuclearMed. Staff, Hôpital du Sacre-Coeur de Montréal; (514)338-2244; Fax. (514)338-3686; martveil@videotron.ca.

VEILLEUX, Martin; Montreal Neurological Hosp, 138-3801 rue University, Montreal QC H3A 2B4; Sher'79 Université de Sherbrooke; FRCPC; Neur (Epilepsy); Electroenceph (P.Q.). Staff, McGill University Health Centre - Montreal Neurological Hospital; Langs: Bilingual(French/English); (514)398-8553; Fax. (514)398-2745; martin.veilleux@mcgill.ca.

VEILLEUX, Martine; Centre Med Saint-Vallier, 201-205 rue Montmagny, Quebec QC G1N 4V3; Mon'92; Staff, Jeffery Hale Hospital-Saint Brigid's; (418)688-0872; Fax. (418)688-4951.

VEILLEUX, Raymond; CHUQ-St-Francois D'Assise, 10 rue de l'Espinay, Quebec QC G1L 3L5; Laval'04; FRCPC; Anes. Staff, Centre Hospitalier Universitaire De Québec - Pavillon De St-françois-d'assise; (418)525-4444

VEILLEUX, Richard; Clinique Med du Carrefour, 805 boul Frontenac E, Thetford Mines QC G6G 6L5; Mon'94; (418)335-3553; Fax. (418)335-9309.

VEILLEUX, Sarto; Centre Med de Beauport, 737 av Royale, Quebec QC G1E 1Z1; Laval'77; LMCC; Langs: English; (418)667-7114; Fax. (418)667-5843.

VEILLEUX-LECLERC, Sylvie; 1004 rue du Haut-Bois, Quebec QC G1Y 2Y3; Laval'79; Staff, Hôpital Laval; Assoc Staff, Centre Hospitalier Universitaire De Québec - Pavillon De St-françois-d'assise; (418)658-7671

VEILLEUX-LEMIEUX, Maude; Centre Hosp Universite Laval, 1742-2705 boul Laurier, Quebec QC G1V 4G2; Laval'05; FRCPC; Peds (Adolescent Medicine). Staff, Centre Hospitalier Universitaire de Quebec-CHUL; (418)525-4444; Fax. (418)654-2137.

VEINISH, Shelley L; Baycrest Ctre/Geriatric Care, 1C11-3560 Bathurst St, North York ON M6A 2E1; McM'85; FRCPC; IntMed; GeriatricMed. Consultant Geriatrics, Markham Stouffville Hospital; Consultant Geriatrics, Mount Sinai Hospital; Asst Prof, University of Toronto; Langs: Bilingual(English/French); (416)785-2500 x2621; Fax. (416)785-2863; sveinish@utoronto.ca.

VEINOT, John P; The Ottawa Hosp-Gen Campus, CCW 4121-501 Smyth Rd Box 117, Ottawa ON K1H 8L6; Dal'88; ABPath; FRCP; FRCPC; AnatPath (Laboratory Medicine). Staff LabMed/Clin Investigator, The Ottawa Hospital - Civic Campus; Staff, University of Ottawa Heart Institute; Staff, The Ottawa Hospital - General Campus; Dept Chair Pathology & Lab Med/Assoc Prof, University of Ottawa; (613)737-8294; Fax. (613)737-8712; jpveinot@ottawahospital.on.ca.

VEINOT-NASH, Janet L; Dalhousie Family Medicine, 265-6960 Mumford Rd, Halifax NS B3L 4P1; Dal'79; CCFP; FCFP; Staff, Queen Elizabeth II Health Sciences Centre - Victoria General Site; Staff, IWK Health Centre; (902)473-4700

VEISMAN, Aneta; Medical & Dental Bldg, 500-1849 Yonge St, Toronto ON M4S 1Y2; Jassy (Romania)'66; FRCPC; Psy. Langs: Romanian; (416)481-3030

VEITH, Martin; Victoria Hosp, PO Box 3000 Stn Main 1200 4th St W, Prince Albert SK S6V 5T4; (Other Foreign)'00; MB ChB; Staff Emerg, Victoria Hospital; Langs: Afrikaans; (306)765-6000

VEITH, Sylvia H; Prince Albert Commun Clinic, 110 8th St E, Prince Albert SK S6V 0V7; Physician, Prince Albert Community Clinic; (306)763-6464; veith@shaw.ca.

VEKEMANS, Gaelle; Plexo Mediclub du Sanctuaire, 6100 av du Boise, Montreal QC H3S 2W1; Sher'93; FRCPC; Peds. Staff, Hopital de la Cite de la santé; (514)739-5646

VEKSLER, Anna L; Westmount Square Med Imaging, C210-1 Car Westmount, Montreal QC H3Z 2P9; McG'88; FRCPC; DiagRad. Staff, McGill University Health Centre - Royal Victoria Hospital; Langs: English; French; (514)939-9764; Fax. (514)939-9363.

VELA, Kanna J; West Durham Family Health Team, 200B-1105 Kingston Rd, Pickering ON L1V 1B5; Tor'08; (905)420-3370; Fax. (905)420-6458.

VELAMOOR, Varadaraj R; Trellis Mental Hlth & Dev Serv, 147 Delhi St, Guelph ON N1E 4J3; Osmania (India)'70; MB; BSc; DPM; MRC(UK); FRCPC; Psy. Langs: Tamil; Hindi; (519)821-2060

VELASQUEZ MALVEHY, Juan M; Niagara H System-St Catharines, PO Box 3018 Stn Main 142 Queenston St, St Catharines ON L2R 7C6; Valle (Mexico)'80; FRCPC; IntMed. Staff, Niagara Health System - St Catharines General Site; Langs: Spanish; (905)684-7271; Fax. (905)323-7559.

VELAZQUEZ, Ricardo J; Cowichan Med Centre, 3106 Gibbins Rd, Duncan BC V9L 1E8; Valle (Colombia)'82; FRCSC; OrthSurg (Arthroplasty). Staff, Cowichan District Hospital; Langs: Spanish; (250)715-1565; Fax. (250)715-1569.

VELDHUIS, Keimpe; London HSC-Victoria Hosp, PO Box 5010 Stn B 800 Commissioners Rd E, London ON N6A 5W9; Qns'65; FRCPC; IntMed. Consultant, London Health Sciences Centre - Victoria Campus; Consultant, St Joseph's Hospital - St Joseph's Health Care; Clin Asst, London Regional Cancer Centre; Aj Prof Clin, University of Western Ontario; Langs: Dutch; German; French; (519)685-8650; Fax. (519)685-8627.

VELDHUIS, Kim A; George Street Family Practice, 1-1400 George St, White Rock BC V4B 4A3; Amsterdam (Netherlands)'05; CCFP; (604)536-1686; Fax. (604)536-6440.

VELDHUYZEN VAN ZANTEN, Sander J O; Queen Elizabeth II HSC, 928-1276 South Park St, Halifax NS B3H 2Y9; Amsterdam (Netherlands)'82; Staff, Queen Elizabeth II Health Sciences Centre - Victoria General Site; (902)473-4647; Fax. (902)473-5548.

VELEHORSCHI, Corina M; Windsor Reg Hosp-Western Camp, 2616-1453 Prince Rd, Windsor ON N9C 3Z4; Iasi (Italy)'96; FRCPC; Psy (Geriatric Psychiatry). Staff, Windsor Regional Hospital - Tayfour Site; Staff, Hôtel-Dieu Grace Hospital; Langs: Romanian; (519)257-5111

VELEZ, Gloria C; MCI The Doctor's Office, 4099 Erin Mills Pky, Mississauga ON L5L 3P9; University of Antioquia (Colombia)'95; CCFP; Langs: Spanish; (905)820-3310; Fax. (905)820-3312.

VELIANOU, James L; Hamilton HS-General Site, 508-237 Barton St E, Hamilton ON L8L 2X2; McM'92; FRCPC; IntMed (Interventional Cardiology); Cardiol. Dir CCU, Hamilton Health Sciences Centre - Hamilton General Hospital; Langs: Greek; (905)526-7616; Fax. (905)527-4463.

VELICARIA, Laing P; White River Med Clinic, PO Box 278 102 Winnipeg St, White River ON P0M 3G0; Far Eastern (Philippines)'72; Court Staff, Lady Dunn Health Centre; Court Staff, Wilson Memorial General Hospital; Langs: Tagalog; (807)822-2320; Fax. (807)822-2686; laing.velicaria@gmial.com.

VELJANOVA PEEVA, Elizabeth; Clin Externe Sante Mentale, 200-237 boul Saint-Jean-Baptis, Chateauguay QC J6K 3C3; Skopje (Macedonia)'78; Psy. (450)692-0002

VELJI, Azim M; 201-4383 Portage Rd, Niagara Falls ON L2E 6A6; Ott'77; DOHS; FAAFP; CCFP; Staff, Niagara Health System - Greater Niagara General Site; Physician, Casino Niagara; Langs: Gujarati; Hindi; (905)356-9076; Fax. (905)354-6535.

VELJI, Iman; Barrhead Clinic, PO Box 4540 Stn Main, Barrhead AB T7N 1A4; (780)674-2231

VELJKOVIC, Andrea N; 108-10 Webster St, Kentville NS B4N 1H7; Alb'04; FRCSC; OrthSurg. (902)679-3399; Fax. (902)679-3350.

VELLANI, Azizadin S; 302-1525 Robson St, Vancouver BC V6G 1C3; Dublin (Ireland)'78; Ac Staff, Providence Health Care - St Paul's Hospital; Langs: Gujarati; (604)684-6055; Fax. (604)684-6055.

VELLANI, Zahir S; Crestwood Med & Dental Bldg, 208-6051 Gilbert Rd, Richmond BC V7C 3V3; Manchester (England)'77; CCFP; FCFP; Ac Staff, Richmond Hospital; (604)278-0090; Fax. (604)278-0061.

VELLATHOTTAM, Andrew G; 6F-520 Ellesmere Rd, Scarborough ON M1R 0B1; Wes'09; CCFP; Staff, Toronto Western Hospital - University Health Network; (416)751-5600; Fax. (416)751-3600.

VELLEND, Hillar; Mount Sinai Hosp, R415-600 University Ave, Toronto ON M5G 1X5; Tor'68; ABIM; FRCP; FRCPC; IntMed (Infectious Diseases-HIV/AIDS); InfectDis. Staff, Toronto General Hospital - UHN; Staff, Mount Sinai Hospital; Langs: Estonian; (416)586-8474; Fax. (416)586-8350; hvellend@mtsinai.on.ca.

VELMURUGIAH, Rhenugadevi; All Well Primary Care Centre, 4217 23 Ave NW, Edmonton AB T6L 5Z8; Jaffna (Sri Lanka)'83; MB BS; CCFP; Langs: Tamil; (780)462-0442; Fax. (780)462-0577.

VELMURUGIAH, Velupillai; Barrhead Health Care Centre, 4815 51 Ave, Barrhead AB T7N 1M1; Colombo (Sri Lanka)'82; MB BS; FRCS(Eng); DLO(Eng); Staff, Barrhead Healthcare Centre; (780)674-9436; Fax. (780)674-9432.

VELOS, Pamela; 205-2801 Keele St, North York ON M3M 2G6; Tor'79; DAB; FACS; FRCSC; Ophth (Cataract Surgery). Langs: Greek; French; (416)633-5226; Fax. (416)633-5135.

VELOSO, Felix M; The Medical Centre, 7-4101 Dewdney Ave, Regina SK S4T 1A5; Manila (Philippines)'61; FRCPC; Neur. Staff, Pasqua Hospital; Staff, Regina General Hospital; Clin Prof Neurol, University of Saskatchewan; (306)525-3586; Fax. (306)522-7566.

VELSHER, Lea S; North York Gen Hosp, 4001 Leslie St, North York ON M2K 1E1; McG'80; FCCMG; FRCPC; Peds (Prenatal Care) (Clinical Genetics). Court Staff, Rouge Valley Health System - Centenary Health Centre Site; Ac Staff Genetics, North York General Hospital; University of Toronto; Langs: Hebrew; French; (416)756-6345 x4390; Fax. (416)756-6727.

VELTHUYSEN, Elsa; Brandon Reg Health Centre, 150 McTavish Ave E, Brandon MB R7A 2B3; CCFP; Staff, Brandon Regional Health Centre; (204)726-1122

VELTHUYSEN, Gerrit C; Holley Clinic, 348 Front St, Quesnel BC V2J 2K3; Pretoria (South Africa)'91; MB ChB; Langs: Afrikaans; (250)992-2159

VELTHUYSEN, Johann; Brandon Reg Health Centre, 150 McTavish Ave E, Brandon MB R7A 2B3; Staff, Brandon Regional Health Centre; (204)726-1122

VELTMAN, Albina; Hamilton Assertive Comm Team, 204-52 Cannon St W, Hamilton ON L8R 2B5; Wes'03; FRCPC; Psy. Staff, Hamilton Assertive Community Team; Langs: Russian; (905)525-4273; Fax. (905)525-4926.

VELURI, Ramamohan; Northeast Mental Hlth Centre, 680 Kirkwood Dr, Sudbury ON P3E 1X3; Andhra (India)'76; MB BS; MRCPsy(UK); FRCPC; Psy (Medico Legal Issues)., North Bay Regional Health Centre - Kirkwood; Asst Prof, Northern Ontario School of Medicine; Asst Prof Psy, University of Western Ontario; Langs: Persian; Telugu; (705)670-8989; Fax. (705)670-8898.

VENANCE, Shannon L; London HSC-University Hosp, PO Box 5339 Stn B 339 Windermere Rd, London ON N6A 5A5; Ott'97; FRCPC; Neur (Neuromuscular Diseases). Staff Clinical Neurological Services, London Health Sciences Centre - University Hospital; (519)663-3337; Fax. (519)663-3328.

VENCHIARUTTI, Nadia; Maple Med Centre, 210-955 Major Mckenzie Dr, Vaughan ON L6A 4P9; Tor'96; CCFP; FCFP; Staff, Mackenzie Richmond Hill Hospital; Langs: Italian; (905)832-2201; Fax. (905)832-2246.

VENDER, Ronald B; Dermatology Centre, 132 Young St, Hamilton ON L8N 1V6; Mem'86; BMedSci; FRCPC; Derm. Ac Staff, St Joseph's Healthcare - Charlton Campus; Court Staff (All Sites), Hamilton Health Sciences Centre - McMaster Children's Hospital; Assoc Prof Derm, McMaster University; Langs: English; French; (905)524-2049; Fax. (905)524-1152.

VENDITTI, Marcello W; Boyd Med Centre, 388 Portage Ave, Winnipeg MB R3C 0C8; Man'05; CCFP; (204)925-3600

VENDITTOLI, Pascal-Andre; Hop Maisonneuve-Rosemont, 5415 boul de l'Assomption, Montreal QC H1T 2M4; Laval'96; FRCSC; OrthSurg. Staff, Hopital Maisonneuve-Rosemont; (514)252-3400; Fax. (514)252-0115.

VENIER, Elisa A; Davisville Med & Dental Centre, 216-1849 Yonge St, Toronto ON M4S 1Y2; Tor'87; Langs: Italian; (416)487-9309; Fax. (416)487-9790.

VENKAT RAGHAVAN, Lakshmi; Univ Hlth Network-Toronto Western Hosp, 399 Bathurst St, Toronto ON M5T 2S8; Madras (India)'93; FRCPC; Anes. Staff, Toronto Western Hospital - University Health Network; Langs: Tamil; (416)603-5118; Fax. (416)603-6494.

VENKATACHALAM, Viswanathan C; Queen Elizabeth II HSC, 6896F-1796 Summer St, Halifax NS B3K 6A3; Bombay (India)'94; MB BS; Staff, Queen Elizabeth II Health Sciences Centre - Halifax Infirmary Site; (902)473-2700

VENKATARAMAN, Murali; 13214 Kelly Ave PO Box 1620, Summerland BC V0H 1Z0; UBC'91; BSc; Ac Staff, Penticton Regional Hospital; (250)494-3432; Fax. (250)494-4392.

VENKATARANGAM, George J M; 325 Model Farm Rd, Quispamsis NB E2G 1M3; Madras (India)'63; MB BS; LMCC; Anes (Pain Management). Ac Staff, Saint John Regional Hospital; (506)847-3535; Fax. (506)847-3536.

VENKATARANGAM, Nina E N; 523-1200 Markham Rd, Scarborough ON M1H 3C3; Mem'91; BSc; BMedSci; AB; FRCSC; ObstGyn. Staff, The Scarborough Hospital - General Campus; Langs: English; French; (416)439-2335; Fax. (416)439-3078.

VENKATESAN, Bogeswari; 678 Colborne St, London ON N6A 3Z3; Madras (India)'72; MB BS; FRCPC; Psy. Langs: Tamil; (519)642-7699

VENKATESAN, Nithya; Victoria Gen Hosp, 2340 Pembina Hwy, Winnipeg MB R3T 2E8; Dr MGR Medical University (India)'97; ABIM; FRCPC; IntMed. Staff Medical Office, Victoria General Hospital; Lecturer, University of Manitoba; (204)269-3570

VENKATESAN, Varagur M; London Reg Cancer Centre, A3 907-790 Commissioners Rd E, London ON N6A 4L6; Bangalore (India)'72; MB BS; FRCS(E); FRCPC; RadOncol. Staff, London Regional Cancer Center; Assoc Prof Oncol, University of Western Ontario; Langs: Tamil; (519)685-8650; Fax. (519)685-8627.

VENKATESH, Thiruganasam; The Ottawa Hosp-Civic Campus, F6-1053 Carling Ave, Ottawa ON K1Y 4E9; TamilNadu Dr. MGR Medical University (India)'93; MB BS; CCFP; CCFP(E.M.); Staff Clinical Epidemiology Program, The Ottawa Hospital - Civic Campus; Langs: Tamil; (613)798-5555; Fax. (613)761-5351; pondyvenki@yahoo.com.

VENKATESH, Vikram; Grand River Hosp K-W HC, PO Box 9056 Stn C 835 King St W, Kitchener ON N2G 1G3; Tor'05; DiagRad. Staff, Grand River Hospital - Kitchener/Waterloo Health Centre; (519)749-4300

VENKATESH, Vugranam C; Surrey Med Arts Bldg, 306-13710 94A Ave, Surrey BC V3V 1N1; Madras (India)'80; MB BS; FRCPC; Peds. Staff, BC Children's Hospital; (604)582-6555; Fax. (604)582-6578.

VENKATESWARAN, Sunita; Children Hosp of Eastern Ont, 401 Smyth Rd, Ottawa ON K1H 8L1; Wes'01; Neur; Peds. Staff, Children's Hospital of Eastern Ontario (CHEO); Langs: Tamil; French; (613)737-7600

VENNAM, Ramesh B; Regina Med Centre, 100-2550 12th Ave, Regina SK S4P 3X1; (306)566-4120; Fax. (306)566-4150.

VENNE, Anne-Marie; CLSC Olivier-Guimond, 5810 rue Sherbrooke E, Montreal QC H1N 1B2; Mon'86; (514)255-2365; Fax. (514)255-3353.

VENNE, Danielle; CLSC Kateri, 90 boul Marie-Victorin, Candiac QC J5R 1C1; Mon'79; (450)659-7661; Fax. (450)444-6276.

VENNE, Sophie; 109-1400 boul Edouard, Longueuil QC J4T 3T2; Sher'89; FRCSC; ObstGyn (Colposcopy). Staff ObstGyn, Hopital Charles LeMoyne; Staff Commun Med, CLSC Kateri; Langs: Bilingual(French/English); (450)923-2870; Fax. (450)923-4025.

VENNE, Suzanne; Clin Med la Cite Place du Parc, 900-300 rue Léo-Pariseau, Montreal QC H2X 4B3; Mon'74; ac Staff, Centre Hospitalier l'Université de Montréal (CHUM) - Hôtel-Dieu; (514)281-1722; Fax. (514)281-6697.

VENNE, Sylvie; Ministre Sante Service Socieux, RC 03-201 boul Cremazie E, Montreal QC H2M 1L5; Mon'79; Staff, Ministry of Health & Social Services-Quebec; (450)436-8622 x2279; sylvie_venne@ssss.gouv.qc.ca.

VENNER, Christopher P; Cross Cancer Institute, 11560 University Ave NW, Edmonton AB T6G 1Z2; Cal'05; Hem; IntMed. Staff, Cross Cancer Institute; (780)432-8757

VENNER, Peter M; Cross Cancer Institute, 11560 University Ave NW, Edmonton AB T6G 1Z2; Alb'73; FRCP; FRCPC; IntMed (Hospital Based); MedOncol. Att Staff, University of Alberta Hospital; Att Staff Med Oncology, Cross Cancer Institute; Prof Oncol, University of Alberta; (780)432-8756; Fax. (780)432-8888; peterven@cancerboard.ab.ca.

VENNETTILLI, Marco C; Royal Court Med Centre, LL2-1 Quarry Ridge Rd, Barrie ON L4M 7G1; McM'05; FRCSC; OrthSurg (Upper Extremity Surgery). Staff, Royal Victoria Hospital of Barrie's Community Care Centre for Substance Abuse; (705)797-8801

VENTER, Anton; Chetwynd Centre Med Clinic, PO Box 1485, Chetwynd BC V0C 1J0; Pretoria (South Africa)'86; MB ChB; Langs: Afrikaans; (250)788-3234; Fax. (250)788-3237.

VENTER, Dirk J; Stonewall & Dist Health Ctr, 589 3rd Ave S, Stonewall MB R0C 2Z0; Pretoria (South Africa)'74; MB ChB; Staff, Stonewall & District Health Centre; (204)467-5514; Fax. (204)467-5576.

VENTER, Hendrik J; 526 Mary St PO Box 564, Shoal Lake MB R0J 1Z0; Pretoria (South Africa)'84; Chief/Medical Staff, Shoal Lake/Strathclair Health Centre; (204)759-2755; Fax. (204)754-2264.

VENTER, Hendrik L; Welland McMaster Family Hlth Team, PO Box 920 2 Pancake Lane, Fonthill ON L0S 1E0; Pretoria (South Africa)'85; MB ChB; CCFP; Langs: Afrikaans; (905)892-4859; Fax. (905)892-0394.

VENTER, Herman C A; Mount IDA Med Centre, PO Box 1870 Stn Main 200 Trans Canada Hwy W, Salmon Arm BC V1E 4P9; Orange Free State (South Africa)'99; MB ChB; Staff, Shuswap Lake General Hospital; Langs: Afrikaans; (250)833-1990; Fax. (250)833-1988.

VENTER, J Christiaan; Wetaskiwin Fam Med Practice, 5107 50 St, Wetaskiwin AB T9A 1K1; (South Africa)'93; MB ChB; CCFP; Langs: Afrikaans; (780)352-3010; Fax. (780)352-7413.

VENTER, Jan F; Shaughnessy Health, 500-916 Broadway St W, Vancouver BC V5Z 1K7; Orange Free State (South Africa)'95; MB ChB; CCFP; Langs: Afrikaans; (604)283-2350

VENTER, Lizanne; Whitecourt Healthcare Centre, 20 Sunset Blvd, Whitecourt AB T7S 1M8; (South Africa)'04; Staff, Whitecourt Healthcare Centre; (780)778-2285; Fax. (780)778-3350; lizannemd@yahoo.ca.

VENTER, Ruan F; Wainwright Clinic, 501 10 St, Wainwright AB T9W 1R5; (780)842-3341; Fax. (780)842-5858.

VENTER, Wikus; South Calgary Health Centre, 31 Sunpark Plaza SE, Calgary AB T2X 3W5; Pretoria (South Africa)'89; MB ChB; CCFP; (403)943-9476

VENTRESCA, Mario R; Portal Village Market, 248 Killaly St W, Port Colborne ON L3K 6A6; Wes'82; FRCSC; Ophth (Vitreo Retina). Chief Surg, Niagara Health System - Port Colborne General Site; Langs: Italian; French; (905)834-5611; Fax. (905)834-5612.

VENTURA, Karyna; Hôpital régional Chaleur, 1750 Sunset Dr, Bathurst NB E2A 4L7; Manila (Philippines)'95; Staff, Hopital Regional Chaleur; (506)544-3000

VENTUREYRA, Enrique C G; Children's Hosp Eastern Ont, 401 Smyth Rd, Ottawa ON K1H 8L1; La Plata (Argentina)'70; FACS; FRCSC; Neursurg (Pediatric Neuro Surgery). Chief Div of NeuroSurg, Children's Hospital of Eastern Ontario (CHEO); Consultant NeuroSurg, The Ottawa Hospital - General Campus; Assoc Staff NeuroSurg, The Ottawa Hospital - Civic Campus; Prof, University of Ottawa; Langs: Spanish; (613)737-2316; Fax. (613)738-4840.

VENTURI, David B; Sheridan Med Associates, 1-1960 Dundas St W, Mississauga ON L5K 2R9; Tor'84; (905)822-3993; Fax. (905)822-5522.

VENUGOPAL, Raghu; R Fraser Elliott Bldg, 190 Elizabeth St, Toronto ON M5G 2C4; Dal'01; FRCPC; EmergMed. Staff, Toronto General Hospital - UHN; (416)340-3947

VENUGOPAL, Vikram; Queens Square, 1802-45 Alderney Dr, Dartmouth NS B2Y 2N6; Bangalore (India)'72; MB BS; FRCS(Ed); MCh(Liverpool); FRCSC; OrthSurg (Joint Replacement). Consultant/Physician, Dartmouth General Hospital; Lecturer Ortho Surg, Dalhousie University; (902)469-9667; Fax. (902)469-4753.

VENUMBAKA, Abaya; Insight Med Centre, 502 4 Ave SW, Medicine Hat AB T1A 5A1; Madras (India)'78; MRCPsy(UK); Ad Staff Child & Adolescent Psy, Medicine Hat Regional Hospital; (403)527-2999; Fax. (403)527-7720.

VENUMBAKA, S Anand; Insight Med Centre, 502 4 Ave SW, Medicine Hat AB T1A 5A1; (India)'74; LMCC; MRCPsy; (403)527-2999; Fax. (403)527-7720.

VERA MAC, Vanessa I; Credit Valley Eye Care, 1-3200 Erin Mills Pky, Mississauga ON L5L 1W8; Universidad Del Zulia (Other Foreign)'02; Clin Fellow, Credit Valley Eye Care; (905)820-3937

VERA SILVA, V Antonio; First Care Med Clinic, 104-500 Sheppard Ave E, North York ON M2N 6H7; 80Trujillo (Peru)'83; CCFP; Langs: Spanish; (416)644-5561; Fax. (416)644-5564.

VERA SUAREZ, Caridad; Clinique de Dermatologie, 133 rue Bernard, Joliette QC J6E 2C4; Mon'05; FRCPC; Derm. (450)759-3505; Fax. (450)756-8879.

VERBEEK, Johannes H; Paediatric Associates, 651 Ross Ave E, Timmins ON P4N 8T4; Qns'63; MPH; FRCPC; GenPath (Dermatology); Peds. Staff Ped, Timmins & District Hospital; Langs: Dutch; (705)264-3599; Fax. (705)264-7130.

VERBEEK, P Richard; Sunnybrook Hlth Sciences Ctre, BG 15-2075 Bayview Ave, Toronto ON M4N 3M5; McG'83; FRCPC; EmergMed. Staff Emergency Services, Sunnybrook Health Sciences Centre; Asst Prof, University of Toronto; (416)480-4037; Fax. (416)480-4704.

VERBEEK, Willem C; 651 Ross Ave E, Timmins ON P4N 8T4; National University of Ireland (Ireland)'96; MB ChB; Dip SportMed; FRCPC; Peds (Sports Medicine). Staff, Timmins & District Hospital; (705)264-3599; Fax. (705)264-7130.

VERBEETEN, Bernard C; Medical Centre, 2374 Eglinton Ave E, Scarborough ON M1K 2P4; Tor'73; FRCPC; DiagRad. (416)757-4254; Fax. (416)751-2421.

VERBEETEN, Karen M; Fitzgerald Bldg, 112-150 College St, Toronto ON M5S 3E2; Tor'06; FRCPC; DiagRad; NuclearMed. Langs: Bilingual(English/French); (416)807-8018

VERBEETEN, Yvonne D; Balmoral Health Group, 405-1366 Yonge St, Toronto ON M4T 3A7; Tor'76; CCFP; Ac Staff, Women's College Hospital; Lecturer Med, University of Toronto; Langs: German; (416)923-5767; Fax. (416)923-5125.

VERBONAC, Garth S J; Saunte Med Clinic, 101-15850 28th Ave, Maple Ridge BC V3Z 2N6; UBC'95; CCFP; (604)531-4131; Fax. (604)531-0126; garthsj@shaw.ca.

VERBURG, Adrian J E; 102-20 Emma St, Chatham ON N7L 5K5; Wes'81; Staff, Chatham-Kent Health Alliance; Langs: Dutch; (519)354-3515; Fax. (519)354-6458.

VERBURG, Lucas; WD Stevenson Med Complex, PO Box 1628, Valleyview AB T0H 3N0; Pretoria (South Africa)'90; CCFP; FCFP; (780)524-4469; Fax. (780)524-2806.

VERCAUTEREN, Suzanne M; BC Children's Hosp, 4480 Oak St, Vancouver BC V6H 3N1; Utrecht (Netherlands)'99; FRCPC; HemPath. Staff, BC Children's Hospital; (604)875-2939

VERCHERE, Cynthia G; Children's & Women's HC Of BC, A242-4480 Oak St Box 150, Vancouver BC V6H 3V4; UBC'88; FRCSC; PlasSurg. Ac Staff Plastic Surg Clinic, BC Children's Hospital; Staff, Plastic Surgery Clinic; Clin Instructor, University of British Columbia; (604)875-3758; Fax. (604)875-2749.

VERDANT, Alain G; Hop du Sacre-Coeur de Mtl, C5060-5400 boul Gouin O, Montreal QC H4J 1C5; Mon'67; FRCSC; GenSurg; Cardiovasc&ThorSurg. ac Staff, Hôpital du Sacre-Coeur de Montréal; (514)338-2170; Fax. (514)338-3313.

VERDEJO-AGUILAR, N Alfonso; Burrard Health Bldg, 705-1160 Burrard St, Vancouver BC V6Z 2E8; Autonomus National (Mexico)'71; FRCPC; IntMed; Rheum. Langs: Spanish; (604)688-6143; Fax. (604)688-6714.

VERDEJO ARANCIBIA, Adriana A; St Joseph's Health Centre, 7-280 Victoria St, Dalhousie NB E8C 2X2; (Chile)'99.

VERDIZAD, P Ariana; 101-12165 Harris Rd, Pitt Meadows BC V3Y 2E9; Stanbul-Capa (Turkey)'87; CCFP; Langs: Farsi; Turkish; (604)465-0556

VERDON, Josee; MUHC-Royal Victoria Hosp, M8 12-687 av des Pins O, Montreal QC H3A 1A1; Mon'81; FRCPC; IntMed; GeriatricMed. Staff, McGill University Health Centre - Royal Victoria Hospital; Langs: English; French; (514)934-1934 x34499; josee.verdon@muhc.mcgill.ca.

VERDONCK, Olivier; Hop Maisonneuve-Rosemont, 5415 boul de l'Assomption, Montreal QC H1T 2M4; Universite de Bordeaux (France)'06; Staff, Hopital Maisonneuve-Rosemont; (514)252-3400

VERDONK, Robert D; CMC Medical Clinic, 1471 Harmony Rd, Oshawa ON L1H 7K5; Alb'90; CCFP; (905)576-5330; Fax. (905)576-5354.

VERDOORN, Marius; Fort Vermilion Med Clinic, PO Box 306, Fort Vermilion AB T0H 1N0; Stellenbosch (South Africa)'83; MB BCh; Med Staff, St Theresa General Hospital; (780)927-3213; Fax. (780)927-4664; verdoom@iafrcia.com.

VERDURMEN, Maria T; Guisachan Family Medicine, 105-2395 Gordon Dr, Kelowna BC V1W 3S7; UBC'94; CCFP; (250)860-5888

VERDUYN, Ashley M; Patient Networks, 157 Yonge St, Toronto ON M5C 1X7; McM'05; CCFP; (416)362-8822; Fax. (416)362-8877.

VERDUYN, Robin F; Toronto Rehab Inst-Lyndhurst, 520 Sutherland Dr, Toronto ON M4G 3V9; McM'08; CCFP; Staff, Toronto Rehabilitation Institute - Lyndhurst Centre; (416)597-3422

VERDY, Isabelle; Mediclub du Sanctuaire, 6100 av du Boise, Montreal QC H3S 2W1; Mon'85; Peds. (514)739-7521; Fax. (514)739-6773.

VERES, Agnes I; Women's Health Clinic, 419 Graham Ave, Winnipeg MB R3C 0M3; Man'72; (204)947-1517

VERES, Lisa; Dr Lisa Veres Prof Centre, 130-1641 Hillside Ave, Victoria BC V8T 5G1; UBC'91; BSc; Staff Privil, Vancouver Island Health Authority; (250)595-4151; Fax. (250)598-7125.

VERESEZAN, Alexa P; 105-262 Oxford St E, London ON N6A 1T8; Cluj (Romania)'89; FRCPC; Psy. Langs: Romanian; Fax. (519)473-1489.

VERGE, Jacqueline L; Summerhill Med Clinic, 207-130 Conception Bay Hwy, Conception Bay S NL A1W 3A6; Mem'86; (709)834-2039; Fax. (709)834-9649.

VERGEL DE DIOS, Oscar M; Windsor Reg Hosp-Metropolitan, 1995 Lens Ave, Windsor ON N8W 1L9; Manila (Philippines)'72; Anes (Pain Control). Staff, Windsor Regional Hospital - Metropolitan Site; (519)254-1661

VERGER, Pierre; 203 av Universite, Moncton NB E1C 5K4; Toulouse (Other Foreign)'93; (506)388-4549; Fax. (506)388-2145.

VERGIDIS, Dimitrios; Thunder Bay Reg HSC-T-Bay, 980 Oliver Rd, Thunder Bay ON P7B 6V4; Alb'83; FRCPC; IntMed (Hematological Oncology); Hem. Staff, Northwestern Ontario Regional Cancer Centre - Cancer Care Ontario; Staff, Thunder Bay Regional Health Sciences Centre; Staff, Cancer Care Ontario - Provincial Office; Asst Prof, McMaster University; Langs: Greek; (807)684-7200

VERGIS, Ashley S; St Boniface Gen Hosp, Z3039-409 Tache Ave, Winnipeg MB R2H 2A6; Man'02; FRCSC; GenSurg. Staff, St Boniface General Hospital; (204)233-8563

VERHEUL, Glenn R; Saint John Reg Hosp, PO Box 2100 Stn Main 400 University Ave, Saint John NB E2L 4L2; UBC'92; CCFP; CCFP(E.M.); FCFP; Staff, Saint John Regional Hospital; (506)648-6000

VERHOEFF, Nicolaas P L G; Baycrest Ctre/Geriatric Care, PB 762-3560 Bathurst St, North York ON M6A 2E1; Rotterdam (Netherlands)'88; PhD; FRCPC; Psy (Geriatric Psychiatry). Staff Psychiatrist Kunin-Lunenfeld Applied Research Unit, Baycrest Centre for Geriatric Care; Assoc Prof Geriatric Psy, University of Toronto; Langs: Spanish; Dutch; German; French; (416)785-2500 x2167; Fax. (416)785-4230.

VERHOVSEK, Madeleine M; St Joseph's Healthcare, L208-50 Charlton Ave E, Hamilton ON L8N 4A6; McM'04; FRCPC; IntMed; Hem. Staff, St Joseph's Healthcare - Charlton Campus; (905)521-6024

VERHULST, Lorne A; Shelbourne Med Clinic, 150-3200 Shelbourne St, Victoria BC V8P 1G8; Alb'78; MPA(Harvard); Med Consultant, Ministry of Health Planning; (250)590-8275

VERI, John-Paul; Alexander Prof Bldg, 204A-849 Alexander Crt, Peterborough ON K9J 7H8; McG'96; FRCSC; OrthSurg. Langs: English; French; (705)874-5005; Fax. (705)874-5007.

VERITY, Robert A; Dynacare Kasper Med Labs, 200-10150 102 St NW, Edmonton AB T5J 5E2; Sask'95; FRCPC; MedMicrobiol. Staff, Alberta Provincial Laboratory of Public Health; Asst Prof Med Microbiol & Immunol, University of Alberta; (780)451-3702; Fax. (780)454-2845; rverity@cha.ab.ca.

VERITY, Shawn D; Pan Am Sports Med Clinic, 75 Poseidon Bay, Winnipeg MB R3M 3E4; Man'06; CCFP; (204)925-1550

VERKLEY, Elspeth C; Midpark Family Med Centre, 100-290 Midpark Way SE, Calgary AB T2X 1P1; Cal'99; CCFP; (403)254-8405; Fax. (403)254-6585.

VERMA, A Tony; 146-6200 McKay Ave, Burnaby BC V5H 4L7; UBC'04; CCFP; (604)438-8288

VERMA, Aikta; Sunnybrook Hlth Sciences Ctre, C753-2075 Bayview Ave, Toronto ON M4N 3M5; Ott'07; FRCPC; EmergMed. Staff, Sunnybrook Health Sciences Centre; (416)480-6018; Fax. (416)480-6797.

VERMA, Ashok K; Radiology Associates of Regina, 6-2727 Parliament Ave, Regina SK S4S 6X5; Poona (India)'67; DCH; DMRD; FRCR; FRCPC; DiagRad. Staff, Regina General Hospital; Physician, Radiology Associates of Regina; Langs: Hindi; Punjabi; (306)352-7653; Fax. (306)522-4311; verma_4321@hotmail.com.

VERMA, Atul; MUHC-Royal Victoria Hosp, M4 76-687 av des Pins O, Montreal QC H3A 1A1; Tor'97; FRCPC; IntMed; Cardiol. Staff, McGill University Health Centre - Royal Victoria Hospital; (514)843-5837

VERMA, Bharti; Duffus Health Centre, 208-7071 Bayers Rd, Halifax NS B3L 2C2; Dal'84; CCFP; Ac Staff, Queen Elizabeth II Health Sciences Centre - Victoria General Site; Dalhousie University; (902)453-4585; Fax. (902)453-5657.

VERMA, Geetika E; Aberhart Centre One, 8329-11402 University Ave NW, Edmonton AB T6G 2J3; Tor'01; FRCPC; IntMed (Tuberculosis); Respir. (780)407-1348; Fax. (780)407-1429.

VERMA, Kamla R; Albert Park Family Med Centre, 3992 Albert St, Regina SK S4S 3R1; Punjab (India)'70; MB BS; FRCPC; Psy. Staff, Regina General Hospital; Physician, Albert Park Family Medical Centres; Langs: Hindi; Punjabi; (306)584-3833; Fax. (306)585-3833.

VERMA, Kumud; 206-8425 120 St, Delta BC V4C 5R2; Man'93; BSc; CCFP; Langs: Hindi; Punjabi.

VERMA, Manhar L B N; 82 Wentworth Terr SW, Calgary AB T3H 0C9; Glasgow (Scotland)'72; MB ChB; FRCPC; Anes. Ac Staff, Rockyview General Hospital; Ac Staff, Peter Lougheed Centre; Ac Staff, Foothills Medical Centre; Asst Prof, University of Calgary; Langs: Hindi; Punjabi; (403)278-7425; Fax. (403)278-4484.

VERMA, Manisha; Univ Hlth Network-Toronto Western Hosp, WW2F-399 Bathurst St, Toronto ON M5T 2S8; Tor'10; CCFP; Staff, Toronto Western Hospital - University Health Network; (416)603-5888; Fax. (416)603-5821.

VERMA, Mradula R; Parkview Prof Centre, 202-2110 Main St, Winnipeg MB R2V 2C2; Lucknow (India)'68; MB BS; DABPed; FRCPC; Peds. (204)338-7707

VERMA, Mukesh K; Health Sciences Centre, 300 Prince Philip Dr, St. John's NL A1B 3V6; Delhi (India)'83; MB BS; RadOncol. Staff H Bliss Murphy Cancer Centre, Health Sciences Centre; (709)777-6300

VERMA, Narpendra; 50 Cindy Lane RR 1, Lisle ON L0M 1M0; Guru Nanak (India)'74; Staff, Stevenson Memorial Hospital; Langs: Punjabi; Hindi; (705)435-8878; vermanick@hotmail.com.

VERMA, Neil; Mackenzie Richmond Hill Hosp, 10 Trench St, Richmond Hill ON L4C 4Z3; Tor'04; CCFP; CCFP(E.M.); Staff, Mackenzie Richmond Hill Hospital; Langs: Spanish; Punjabi; French; (905)883-1212

VERMA, Pramod K; Cedars Prof Park, 2911 66 St NW, Edmonton AB T6K 4C1; Delhi (India)'82; FRCSC; ObstGyn. Staff, Covenant Health - Grey Nuns Community Hospital; Langs: Urdu; Gujarati; Hindi; Punjabi; (780)450-2400; Fax. (780)450-6471.

VERMA, Prem A; Dept of Veteran's Affairs, PO Box 7700 Stn Central, Charlottetown PE C1A 8M9; Indore (India)'61; Court Staff Privil, Western Hospital - Health PEI; Court Staff Privil, Community Hospital Inc; Med Advisor, Veterans Affairs Canada; Langs: Hindi; Punjabi; (902)566-8972; prem.verma@vac-acc.gc.ca.

VERMA, Rishi; Carepoint Clinic, 711 Pender St W, Vancouver BC V6C 1K6; Sask'01; CCFP; Staff, Carepoint Clinic; (604)687-4858

VERMA, Sarita; Univ Hlth Network-Toronto Western Hosp, 3W442-399 Bathurst St, Toronto ON M5T 2S8; McM'91; CCFP; FCFP; Staff, Toronto Western Hospital - University Health Network; Dep Dean Faculty of Med, University of Toronto; (416)603-2581; Fax. (416)603-5233.

VERMA, Serena; UBC Health Clinic, 310-5950 University Blvd, Vancouver BC V6T 1Z3; Tor'06; CCFP; (604)822-5431

VERMA, Shailendra; The Ottawa Hosp-Gen Campus, 501 Smyth Rd, Ottawa ON K1H 8L6; Qns'79; FRCPC; IntMed (Breast Cancer); MedOncol. Ac Staff, The Ottawa Hospital - General Campus; Asst Prof Med, University of Ottawa; Langs: Hindi; French; (613)737-7700 x6747

VERMA, Subhash C; Stephenville Crossing Med Clin, PO Box 370 Stn Main, Stephenville-Cross NL A0N 2C0; Punjab (India)'89; MB BS; Langs: Punjabi; (709)646-2233

VERMA, Subodh; St Michael's Hosp, 8 003-30 Bond St, Toronto ON M5B 1W8; Cal'00; FRCSC; CardSurg (Cardiology). Staff Terrence Donnelly Heart Centre Cardiovasc & Thoracic Surg/Assoc Prof, St Michael's Hospital; (416)864-5303; Fax. (416)864-5881; vermasu@smh.toronto.on.ca.

VERMA, Sunil; Sunnybrook Hlth Sciences Ctre, TW-2075 Bayview Ave, Toronto ON M4N 3M5; Alb'98; FRCPC; IntMed (Breast Cancer); MedOncol. Staff, Sunnybrook Health Sciences Centre; (416)480-5248; Fax. (416)480-6002; vermamd@hotmail.com.

VERMA, Vinod K; Guild Family Clinic, 82 Dearham Wood, Scarborough ON M1E 1S4; Delhi (India)'81; MB BS; Langs: Hindi; (416)208-5833; Fax. (416)208-5844.

VERMAAK, Anita; Riverdale Health Services Ctre, PO Box 428 512 Quebec St, Rivers MB R0K 1X0; (Other Foreign)'95; MB ChB; Staff, Riverdale Health Centre; (204)328-5321

VERMAAK, Christoffel J; Lynn Lake Hosp, PO Box 2030, Lynn Lake MB R0B 0W0; Staff, Lynn Lake Hospital; (204)356-2474; cvermaak@brha.mb.ca.

VERMAAK, David M; 103-300 Merganser Dr W, Chestermere AB T1X 1L6; Cape Town (South Africa)'88; MB ChB; (403)235-3343; Fax. (403)235-3359.

VERMAAK, Jan A; Professional Med Associates, 550 Main St N, Moose Jaw SK S6H 3K3; (306)694-2082; Fax. (306)692-2080.

VERMAAT, Jentien H; Scarborough Hosp-Birchmount, 3030 Birchmount Rd, Scarborough ON M1W 3W3; Cape Town (South Africa)'79; MB ChB; FRCPC; Peds. Staff Pediatrics Clinic, The Scarborough Hospital - Birchmount Campus; Langs: Dutch; (416)495-2886; Fax. (416)495-2538.

VERMETTE, Audrey; CSSS Les Eskers de l'Abitibi, 622 4e rue O, Amos QC J9T 2S2; Sher'03; FRCPC; Anes. Staff, CH Hôtel-Dieu d'Amos; (819)732-3341 x2356

VERMETTE, Johanne; 61 rue de l'Anse, St-Jean-des-Piles QC G0X 2V0; Laval'86; (819)538-6105

VERMETTE, M Gabrielle; Service de Pedopsychiatrie, 6550 rue Saint-Georges, Levis QC G6V 6X2; Laval'81; (418)835-7121 x4114; Fax. (418)838-8873.

VERMETTE, Suzie; CSSS de Saint-Jerome, 290 rue de Montigny, Saint-Jerome QC J7Z 5T3; Mon'98; Staff, Hôtel-Dieu de Saint-Jérôme; (450)431-8200

VERMEULEN, Abraham P M; Gardiner Park Mall, 358 University Park Dr, Regina SK S4V 2Z6; Stellenbosch (South Africa)'81; MB ChB; CCFP; (306)719-1500

VERMOOTEN, Carel A; Western Mem Reg Hosp, PO Box 2005 Stn Main 1 Brookfield Ave, Corner Brook NL A2H 6J7; Orange Free State (South Africa)'80; MB ChB; DA; MMed; Chief/Staff, Western Memorial Regional Hospital; (709)637-5000; Fax. (709)634-8107; cavermooten@nf.sympatico.ca.

VERNACCHIA, Carlo; Polyclinique Cabrini, 210-5700 rue Saint-Zotique E, Montreal QC H1T 3Y7; Mon'74; Langs: Italian; English; (514)256-1362; Fax. (514)256-2599.

VERNEC, Alan R; Kinatex Sports Physio, 600-1538 rue Sherbrooke O, Montreal QC H3G 1L5; McG'85; Clin Conférencier, Centre Hospitalier l'Université de Montréal (CHUM) - Hôpital Notre-Dame; Clin Prof, Sir Mortimer B Davis Jewish General; Physician, Athletics Canada; Langs: Bilingual(English/French); (514)939-1416; Fax. (514)939-6185.

VERNIQUET, Andrew J W; James Paton Mem Hosp, 125 Trans Canada Hwy, Gander NL A1V 1P7; Bristol (England)'74; MB ChB; FRCPC; Anes. Staff, James Paton Memorial Hospital; Staff, The Dr G B Cross Memorial Hospital; (709)256-2500

VERNON, Errol E; Health Canada, 835-9700 Jasper Ave NW, Edmonton AB T5J 4C3; West Indies (Jamaica)'78; Staff, Public Service Occupational Health Program; errol.vernon@hc.sc.qc.ca.

VERNON, James D; 227 King St S PO Box 1601, Waterloo ON N2J 4C5; Wes'75; FRCPC; EmergMed. (519)888-3900

VERNOOY, Catherine M; Active Care Med Group, 1108 Klondike Rd, Ottawa ON K2K 0G1; Qns'97; CCFP; (613)254-9777; Fax. (613)254-9778.

VERNY, Thomas R; 48 Albert St, Stratford ON N5A 3K3; Tor'61; DPsy; FRCPC; Psy (Couple Therapy). Langs: German; (519)271-5174; Fax. (519)271-5174.

VERONES, Patricia M; Justik Med Clinic, 8225 105 St NW, Edmonton AB T6E 4H2; Alb'97; CCFP; FCFP; (780)432-0211; Fax. (780)439-9349.

VERONNEAU, Andre; Clin Saint-Laurent-du-Fleuve, 9010 Rte Marie-Victorin RR 2, Contrecoeur QC J0L 1C0; Mon'78; Langs: English; (450)746-3841; Fax. (450)746-3840; ave.md@videotron.ca.

VEROUKIS, Stasa; Children's Hosp, JL379-840 Sherbrook St, Winnipeg MB R3A 1R9; Man'02; FRCPC; Peds; Critical Care Medicine. Staff, Health Sciences Centre; (204)774-8511

VERRALL, John R; Associated Radiologists of SK, 300-140 Wall St, Saskatoon SK S7K 1N4; Sask'97; FRCPC; DiagRad. Physician, Associated Radiologists of Saskatoon; (306)244-1167; Fax. (306)244-2911.

VERREAULT, Denis; 8720 av Royale RR 3, Chateau-Richer QC G0A 1N0; Laval'64; ac Staff, Centre Hospitalier Affilié Universitaire de Québec - Hôpital De L'Enfant Jésus; (418)824-4220; Fax. (418)824-5220.

VERREAULT, France; Clinique Med Elysee, 451 rue des Champs-Elysees, Chicoutimi QC G7H 2W3; Laval'96; Médecin, CLSC Mission; (418)545-2323; Fax. (418)545-2756.

VERREAULT, Guy; Clinique Med d'Alma, 935 av du Pont S, Alma QC G8B 2V5; Laval'83; Staff, CSSS de Lac-Saint Jean-Est; Médecin, Clinique Medicale de Alma; (418)668-6121; Fax. (418)668-5298.

VERREAULT, Jean; CHUS-Hop Fleurimont, 3001 12e av N, Sherbrooke QC J1H 5N4; Sher'83; LMCC; FRCPC; NuclearMed. Staff, Centre Hospitalier Universitaire de Sherbrooke-Hopital Fleurimont; Clin Prof, Universite de Sherbrooke; Langs: English; (819)346-1110 x13659; Fax. (819)820-6490; jean.verreault@usherbrooke.ca.

VERREAULT, Jean-Pierre; Ctr d'Obstetrique/Gynecologie, 4250 1re av, Quebec QC G1H 2S5; Laval'74; FRCSC; ObstGyn (Ultrasound). Staff, Centre Hospitalier Universitaire De Québec - Pavillon De St-françois-d'assise; (418)654-0555; Fax. (418)654-1898.

VERREAULT, Nina; CHUQ-Hop Laval, H1340-2705 bou Laurier, Quebec QC G1V 4G2; Laval'00; FRCPC; Peds; ClinImmunol&Allergy. Staff, Centre Hospitalier Universitaire de Quebec-CHUL; Langs: English; (418)654-2240

VERREAULT, Rene; UMF Laval, 2690 ch des Quatre-Bourgeois, Quebec QC G1V 0B7; Laval'89; MSc(Epidemiol.); PhD(Epidemiol); CCFP; Staff, Hôpital Laval; Staff, Centre Hospitalier Affilié Universitaire de Québec - Hôpital du St-Sacrement; Staff, Centre Hospitalier Affilié Universitaire de Québec - Hôpital De L'Enfant Jésus; assoc Prof, Université Laval; (418)656-8711; Fax. (418)656-4503; rene.verreault@msp.ulaval.ca.

VERREAULT, Steve; Ctr Hosp Affilie-Enfant-Jesus, 1401 18e rue, Quebec QC G1J 1Z4; Laval'97; FRCPC; Neur (Cerebrovascular Disease). Staff, Centre Hospitalier Affilié Universitaire de Québec - Hôpital De L'Enfant Jésus; (418)649-5892; Fax. (418)649-5896.

VERRELLI, Mauro; St Boniface Gen Hosp, 409 Tache Ave, Winnipeg MB R2H 2A6; Padova (Italy)'90; FACP; FRCPC; IntMed; Nephrol. Ac Staff Sect of Nephrol, St Boniface General Hospital; Asst Prof, University of Manitoba; Langs: Italian; (204)237-2121; Fax. (204)233-2770; verrelli@cc.umanitoba.ca.

VERRET, Benoit; CSSS de Rivière-de-Loup, 75 rue Saint-Henri, Riviere-Du-Loup QC G5R 2A4; Laval'93; FRCPC; IntMed (Cardiology). Staff, Centre Hospitalier Regional du Grand-Portage; Langs: Bilingual(French/English); (418)868-1000 x2560; Fax. (418)868-1059; verretb@videotron.ca.

VERRET, Gaston; Clinique Gaston Verret, 554 Cote Joyeuse, Saint-Raymond QC G3L 4B1; Laval'72; assoc Staff, Centre Hospitalier Portneuf; (418)337-2236 x2241; Fax. (418)337-4019.

VERRET, Gilles W; 29788 Route 134, Dalhousie Junction NB E3N 6A6; Laval'81; LMCC; FRCSC; OrthSurg. Med Dir Orth Serv, Hôpital Régional Campbellton; (506)684-5390; Fax. (506)684-5390.

VERRET, Louis; Ctr Hosp Affilie-Enfant-Jesus, D2000-1401 18e rue, Quebec QC G1J 1Z4; Laval'95; CSPQ; MFOM; LMCC; MRCP; FRC; FRCPC; Neur (Alzheimer's Disease). Staff, Centre Hospitalier Affilié Universitaire de Québec - Hôpital De L'Enfant Jésus; Langs: English; (418)649-5980; Fax. (418)649-5981; verretl@videotron.ca.

VERRET, Nadine; Hotel-Dieu de Levis, 143 rue Wolfe, Levis QC G6V 3Z1; Laval'99; ObstGyn. Staff, Hôtel-Dieu de Lévis; (418)835-7121

VERRET, Simon; Ctr Hosp Affilie-Enfant-Jesus, D2622-1401 18e rue, Quebec QC G1J 1Z4; Laval'65; FRCPC; Peds; Electroenceph (P.Q.); Neur (Pediatric Neurology). ac Staff, Centre Hospitalier Affilié Universitaire de Québec - Hôpital De L'Enfant Jésus; Consultant, Centre Hospitalier Universitaire de Quebec-CHUL; Consultant, Centre Hospitalier Universitaire De Québec - Pavillon De St-françois-d'assise; (418)649-5980; Fax. (418)649-5981; simon.verret@fmed.ulaval.ca.

VERRET-DAIGNEAULT, Genevieve; Clinique Med de l'Alternative, 2034 rue Saint-Hubert, Montreal QC H2L 3Z5; Mon'05; CCFP; (514)281-9848

VERRETTE, Pierre; Centre Med Jeffery Hale, 305-1248 ch Sainte-Foy, Quebec QC G1S 2M5; Laval'73; (418)681-7854; Fax. (418)681-6173.

VERRETTE, Sylvie; CSST-Dir des Services Medicaux, 6e-1199 rue de Bleury, Montreal QC H3B 3J1; Laval'87; BACC(Psych); Langs: Bilingual(French/English); (514)906-3003; Fax. (514)906-3001; sylvie.verrette@csst.qc.ca.

VERRICO, Howard J; 20800 Lougheed Hwy PO Box 326 Stn Del Ctr, Maple Ridge BC V2X 7G2; Tor'85; (604)463-4111

VERRIER, Pierre; Hop Sacre-Coeur de Montreal, 5400 boul Gouin O, Montreal QC H4J 1C5; Sher'74; CSPQ; Psy (Consultation-Liaison). Staff Psychosomatic Services, Hôpital du Sacre-Coeur de Montréal; Staff Family Med & Psy Program, Universite de Montreal; Langs: English; (514)338-2070; Fax. (514)338-3187; p.verrier@umontreal.ca.

VERRIER-FRECHETTE, Veronique; CHUS-Hop Fleurimont, 3001 12e av N, Sherbrooke QC J1H 5N4; Sher'96; CCFP; CCFP(E.M.); Staff, Centre Hospitalier Universitaire de Sherbrooke-Hopital Fleurimont; (819)346-1110; Fax. (819)820-6420.

VERRILLI, David V; Village Family Health Team, 102-171 East Liberty St, Toronto ON M6K 3P6; Mem'09; CCFP; (416)599-8348; Fax. (416)599-2001; david.verrilli@villagefht.ca.

VERRYN-STUART, Ian T; Valley Prof Centre, 200-70 Exhibition St, Kentville NS B4N 4K9; Dal'76; Staff, Valley Regional Hospital; (902)678-2525; Fax. (902)678-4550.

VERSCHELDEN, Paul; CSSS de Laval, 1755 boul Rene-Laennec, Laval QC H7M 3L9; Mon'88; Respir; IntMed. Staff, Hopital de la Cite de la santé; (450)668-1010; Fax. (450)975-5545.

VERSCHUREN, Rex E; Lapsley Family Doctors, 13 Lapsley Rd, Scarborough ON M1B 1K1; Tor'87; CCFP; FCFP; Pres Med Staff Society/Ac Staff, Rouge Valley Health System - Centenary Health Centre Site; Langs: Dutch; French; (416)754-9595; Fax. (416)754-3946.

VERSNICK, Eric J A; Colchester East Hants Hlth Ctr, 600 Abenaki Rd, Truro NS B2N 5A1; Tor'96; FRCPC; DiagRad. Staff, Colchester East Hants Health Centre; Staff, Queen Elizabeth II Health Sciences Centre - Victoria General Site; (902)893-4321; Fax. (902)893-5534.

VERSTER, Gerhardus H J; Oasis Med Clinic, 2145 Louie Dr, Westbank BC V4T 3E6; Stellenbosch (South Africa)'83; MB ChB; CCFP; (250)768-7656

VERSTER, Ryno J; Dr G B Cross Mem Hosp, 67 Manitoba Dr, Clarenville NL A5A 1K3; Cape Town (South Africa)'97; MB ChB; Staff, The Dr G B Cross Memorial Hospital; (709)466-3411

VERSTER, Servaas W D; Willows Med Clinic, 1300 111 Ave, Dawson Creek BC V1G 2X5; Stellenbosch (South Africa)'76; MB ChB; (250)782-7525

VERSTRATEN, Karin L; Highstreet House, 311-933 17 Ave SW, Calgary AB T2T 5R6; Cal'88; FRCSC; Ophth (Cataract & Glaucoma). Staff, Rockyview General Hospital; Asst Prof, University of Calgary; (403)245-3304; Fax. (403)245-9675; verstratenoffice@telus.net.

VERTES, George E; SGH Medical Mall, 302-3030 Lawrence Ave E, Scarborough ON M1P 2T7; McG'79; FRCPC; Cardiol; IntMed. Staff, The Scarborough Hospital - General Campus; Langs: Hungarian; French; (416)265-3676; Fax. (416)265-2645; georgevertes@rogers.com.

VERTESI, Leslie; Royal Columbian Hosp, 330 Columbia St E, New Westminster BC V3L 3W7; Tor'70; MHSc; FRCPC; EmergMed (Public Health). Med Dir, Royal Columbian Hospital; Med Dir, Eagle Ridge Hospital & Health Care Centre; Asst Prof, University of British Columbia; (604)520-4253; Fax. (604)648-8023.

VERTINSKY, Alexandra T; Vancouver Gen Hosp, 855 12th Ave W, Vancouver BC V5Z 1M9; UBC'00; FRCPC; DiagRad. Staff, Vancouver General Hospital - Centennial Pavillion; (604)875-4111

VERTUE, Peter J; South Hill Med Centre, 890A Lillooet St W, Moose Jaw SK S6H 8B4; (Other Foreign)'04; (306)684-0833; Fax. (306)694-5666.

VERVAECK, Colette Y T B; PO Box 1449, Didsbury AB T0M 0W0; Louvain (Belgium)'87; Staff, Didsbury District Health Services; Langs: English; French; (403)335-3669; Fax. (403)335-3679.

VERVAEKE, Robert J; 304-1335 Carling Ave, Ottawa ON K1Z 8N8; Ott'84; FRCPC; Psy. (613)728-5672; Fax. (613)728-5672.

VERVILLE, Marcel; 400-671 2e rue E, La Sarre QC J9Z 3J7; Mon'79; ac Staff, Centre Hospitalier La Sarre; Noranda-Rondorie Horne; (819)339-5661; Fax. (819)339-3015.

VERWEY, Drikus; Oasis Med Clinic, 2145 Louie Dr, Westbank BC V4T 3E6; Stellenbosch (South Africa)'98; MB ChB; (250)768-7656

VESCAN, Allan D; Mount Sinai Hosp, 401-600 University Ave, Toronto ON M5G 1X5; Wes'01; BSc; FRCSC; Otol (Rhinology). Staff, Mount Sinai Hospital; Lecturer, University of Toronto; (416)586-4439; Fax. (416)586-8600.

VESELINOVIC, Aleksandra; Phoenix Med Centre, 203-2155 10th Ave, Prince George BC V2M 5J6; Rijeka (Croatia)'77; FRCSC; Ophth. Staff, University Hospital of Northern British Columbia; (250)563-2363; Fax. (250)563-5058.

VESPRINI, Daniel J; Sunnybrook Hlth Sciences Ctre, T2 11-2075 Bayview Ave, Toronto ON M4N 3M5; Tor'02; FRCPC; RadOncol. Staff, Sunnybrook Health Sciences Centre; (416)480-4806; Fax. (416)480-6002.

VESTVIK, Sandra; Steel Head Med Centre, PO Box 1238 3202 14th St, Houston BC V0J 1Z0; UBC'90; Staff, Houston Health Centre; Staff, Bulkley Valley District Hospital; (250)845-4039

VETERE, Phyllis-Marie; MUHC-Montreal Gen Hosp, 1650 av Cedar, Montreal QC H3G 1A4; Mem'90; Staff, McGill University Health Centre - Montreal General Campus; Langs: Italian; Norwegian; French; (514)934-8090

VETHAMUTHU, Jennifer M; Children's Hosp of Eastern Ont, 401 Smyth Rd, Ottawa ON K1H 8L1; Ott'01; FRCPC; Peds; Nephrol. Staff Peds Nephrol, Children's Hospital of Eastern Ontario (CHEO); Langs: Bilingual(English/French); (613)737-7600; Fax. (613)738-3254.

VETHANAYAGAM, Dilini P; University of Alberta Hosp, 2E4 29 WMC-8440 112 St NW, Edmonton AB T6G 2B7; Alb'92; BSc; FRCPC; IntMed (Asthma); Respir. Staff Adult Pulmonary, University of Alberta Hospital; Asst Prof, University of Alberta; Langs: Tamil; (780)407-1479; Fax. (780)407-6384; dilini@ualberta.ca.

VETISKA, Frantisek; Oakville Peds Urgent Care Clin, 2540 Postmaster Dr, Oakville ON L6M 5A8; Praque (Czech Republic)'62; Langs: Czech; Polish; Russian; (905)847-5437

VETSCH, Elizabeth A; Grandview Heights Med Clinic, 12313 63 Ave NW, Edmonton AB T6H 1R4; Alb'75; CCFP; (780)437-1968; Fax. (780)438-4395.

VETTERGREEN, Frances M; Gulf Canada Square, 370-401 9 Ave SW, Calgary AB T2P 3C5; Cal'93; CCFP; FCFP; (403)221-4467; Fax. (403)221-4442.

VETTERS, John M; Stratford Gen Hosp, 46 General Hospital Dr, Stratford ON N5A 2Y6; Glasgow (Scotland)'62; MB ChB; FRCPath; FRCPC; AnatPath. Associate Path, Stratford General Hospital - Huron Perth Healthcare Alliance; (519)271-2120; Fax. (519)272-8198; john.vetters@hpha.ca.

VETTESE, Antonio; Credit Valley Prof Bldg, 407-2300 Eglinton Ave W, Mississauga ON L5M 2V8; Tor'80; FRCSC; Ophth. Ac Staff, The Credit Valley Hospital; Court Staff, Trillium Health Centre - Mississauga; Court Staff, William Osler Health System - Brampton Civic Hospital; Langs: Italian; French; (905)820-0097; Fax. (905)820-6944.

VEZINA, Andre; PAMQ-Prog Aide Med Quebec, 200-1 boul Rene-Levesque E, Montreal QC H2X 3Z5; Laval'76; Staff, College des Medecins du Quebec; (514)397-0888; Fax. (514)397-0654.

VEZINA, Andree; CHUQ-Ctr Hosp Univ Laval, 2705 boul Laurier, Quebec QC G1V 4G2; Laval'84; Staff, Centre Hospitalier Universitaire de Quebec-CHUL; Prof Emerg Med, Université Laval; (418)656-4141; Fax. (418)691-5717.

VEZINA, Catherine; MUHC-Montreal Children's Hosp, 2300 rue Tupper, Montreal QC H3H 1P3; Laval'04; PedHemaOncol (P.Q.); Peds. Staff, McGill University Health Centre - Montreal Children's Hospital; (514)412-4400 x24445; Fax. (514)412-4301.

VEZINA, Claude T J; Timmins & Dist Hosp, 700 Ross Ave E, Timmins ON P4N 8P2; Ott'77; FRCPC; DiagRad. Staff/Med Dir Diag Imag, Timmins & District Hospital; Langs: English; French; (705)360-6069; Fax. (705)267-6395.

VEZINA, Daniel; Cite de la Sante de Laval, 1755 boul Rene-Laennec, Laval QC H7M 3L9; Laval'95; FRCPC; Anes. Staff, Hopital de la Cite de la santé; (450)668-1010

VEZINA, Danielle; CSSS de Laval, 1755 boul Rene-Laennec, Laval QC H7M 3L9; Mon'79; FRCPC; IntMed (Hospitalist); Nephrol. Staff, Hopital de la Cite de la santé; Langs: English; (450)668-1010

VEZINA, Diane; Centre Med Racine, 201-900 boul Raymond, Quebec QC G1B 3G3; Mon'86; (418)667-8066; Fax. (418)667-8131.

VEZINA, Francine; CHUQ-Ctr Hosp Univ Laval, 2705 boul Laurier, Quebec QC G1V 4G2; Laval'84; Staff, Centre Hospitalier Universitaire de Quebec-CHUL; (418)654-2255; Fax. (418)654-2173.

VEZINA, Francine; CHUQ-St-Francois d'Assise, 10 rue de l'Espinay, Quebec QC G1L 3L5; Laval'83; Staff, Centre Hospitalier Universitaire De Québec - Pavillon De St-françois-d'assise; (418)525-4397

VEZINA, Francois; CHUS-Hotel-Dieu, 580 Bowen Sud, Sherbrooke QC J1G 2E8; Sher'01; FRCSC; OrthSurg (Sports Medicine). Chef cabinet, Centre Hospitalier Universitaire de Sherbrooke-Hopital Fleurimont; Chef cabinet, Centre Hospitalier Universitaire de Sherbrooke-Hôpital Hôtel-Dieu; Staff, Centre Hospitalier et CLSC de Memphremagog; Aj Prof, Universite de Sherbrooke; Langs: Bilingual(French/English); (819)346-1110 x28304; Fax. (819)822-6725; orthopedie-med@usherbrooke.ca.

VEZINA, Gilles; Centre de Sante Integrale, RR 5 1-160 rue Pope, Cookshire QC J0B 1M0; Laval'65; Langs: Bilingual(English/French); (819)875-5535; Fax. (819)875-3631; gvezina@omni-med.com.

VEZINA, Jacques W; CHUM-Hop St-Luc, 1058 rue Saint-Denis, Montreal QC H2X 3J4; Laval'81; Staff, Centre Hospitalier l'Université De Montréal (CHUM) - Hôpital Saint-luc; (514)890-8000

VEZINA, Jean-Philippe; Ctr Hosp Affilie-Hop-Enfant Je, 1401 18e rue, Quebec QC G1J 1Z4; Laval'04; FRCSC; Otol (Head & Neck Surgery). Staff, Centre Hospitalier Affilié Universitaire de Québec - Hôpital De L'Enfant Jésus; (418)649-0252

VEZINA, Julie; CSST Chaudiere-Appalaches, 835 rue de la Concorde, Levis QC G6W 7P7; Laval'88; Staff, CSST-Chaudiere-Appalaches; Médecin, Societe Assurance Automobile du Quebec; (418)839-2500; julie.vezina@csst.qc.ca.

VEZINA, Lise; Ctre d'Hebergement Limoilou, 1401 ch de la Canardiere, Quebec QC G1J 0A6; Laval'91; Staff, Institut Universitaire Sante; (418)529-6571 x7034; Fax. (418)524-6807.

VEZINA, Louise; Polyclinique St-Jerome, 206-200 rue Durand, Saint-Jerome QC J7Z 7E2; Laval'80; FRCSC; ObstGyn. (450)565-6332; Fax. (450)436-5488.

VEZINA, Marie-Claude; Hôpital Laval, IUCPQ-2725 ch Sainte-Foy, Quebec QC G1V 4G5; Laval'01; FRCPC; Anes; Critical Care Medicine. Staff, Hôpital Laval; (418)656-8711

VEZINA, Martin; Clinique de Psychiatrie, 2012 boul Rene-Laennec, Laval QC H7M 4J8; Mon'86; FRCPC; Psy (Adult & Child Psychiatry). Staff, Hopital de la Cite de la santé; Staff, Centre Hospitalier Ambulatoire Regional de Laval; (450)662-3665; Fax. (450)662-9124.

VEZINA, Michel; Ctr de Sante Sociaux Vieille, 3e-880 rue Pere-Marquette, Quebec QC G1S 2A4; Laval'70; MPH; FRCPC; CommunMed (Industrial Occupational Medicine). ac Staff, Centre Hospitalier Universitaire de Quebec-CHUL; Consultant, Institut National de Sante Publique; assoc Prof, Université Laval; Langs: English; (418)681-8787 x3800; Fax. (418)687-9694.

VEZINA, Pascale; CSSS du Lac-des-Deux-Montagnes, 520 boul Arthur-Sauve, Saint-Eustache QC J7R 5B1; Mon'90; FRCSC; OrthSurg. Staff, Hôpital de Saint-Eustache; Langs: English; (450)473-7222; Fax. (450)661-2833.

VEZINA, Paul; Clinique Med Haut-Anjou, 45-7500 boul les Galeries d'An, Anjou QC H1M 3M4; Mon'76; (514)493-1999; Fax. (514)493-4428.

VEZINA, Sylvie; Clinique Med l'Actuel, 1130-1001 boul Maisonneuve E, Montreal QC H2L 4P9; Mon'86; (514)524-1001; Fax. (514)524-3831.

VEZINA, William C; London HSC-Victoria Campus, 800 Commissioners Rd E, London ON N6A 5W9; Wes'73; AB; AB; FRCPC; DiagRad; NuclearMed. Staff, London Health Sciences Centre - Victoria Campus; (519)663-3424; Fax. (519)685-8290; william.vezina@lhsc.on.ca.

VEZINA, Yannik; Horizon Feminin, 206-200 rue Durand, Saint-Jerome QC J7Z 7E2; Mon'97; FRCSC; ObstGyn. Staff, Hôtel-Dieu de Saint-Jérôme; (450)436-4228; Fax. (450)436-5488.

VEZINA, Yves; CHUS-Hop Fleurimont, 2616-3001 12e av N, Sherbrooke QC J1H 5N4; Laval'77; FRCPC; IntMed; Respir. ac Staff, Centre Hospitalier Universitaire de Sherbrooke-Hopital Fleurimont; assoc Staff, Hôpital Sainte-croix; (819)822-6735; Fax. (819)822-6763.

VIALLET, Norbert R J; Health Sciences Centre, GB421-820 Sherbrook St, Winnipeg MB R3A 1R9; Man'00; FRCSC; Otol. Staff, Health Sciences Centre; (204)774-6511

VIANZON, Clarita S; Norlyn Med Clinic, 100-309 Hargrave St, Winnipeg MB R3B 2J8; Manila (Philippines)'64; LMCC; Langs: Tagalog; (204)956-0988; Fax. (204)943-9954.

VIANZON EDORA, Daisy M; Formation Health Services Unit, PO Box 17000 Stn Forces, Victoria BC V9A 7N2; UBC'96; BSc; CCFP; Staff, Canadian Forces Health Services - Pacific Centre; Langs: Tagalog; (250)363-4120; Fax. (250)363-4436.

VIAU, Alexandre; Ctr Hosp Rouyn-Noranda, 4 9e Rue, Rouyn-Noranda QC J9X 2B2; Mon'08; Staff, Centre Hospitalier Rouyn-Noranda; (819)764-5131

VIAU, Lucie; Clinique Ext Psychiatrie, 765 rue Roland-Forget, Laval QC H7E 4C1; Mon'89; FRCPC; Psy. Staff, Hopital de la Cite de la santé; (450)668-2620 x2; Fax. (450)668-1077.

VIAU, Melanie; Clinique Familiale Pas-A-Pas, 3650 boul Henri-Bourassa E, Montreal-Nord QC H1H 1J6; Sher'04; (514)328-9797; Fax. (514)328-2672.

VIBIEN, Anne; Centre Hosp Honore-Mercier, 2750 boul Laframboise, Saint-Hyacinthe QC J2S 4Y8; Mon'86; MedMicrobiol. Staff, Centre Hospitalier Honore-Mercier; (450)771-3333 x3535; Fax. (450)771-3510.

VICARUDDIN, Omair; Glenwood Med Clinic, 16114 100A Ave, Edmonton AB T5P 4A1; Alb'06; CCFP; (780)405-7520; Fax. (587)521-1801.

VICARUDDIN, Zehra; Glenwood Med Clinic, 11614 100A Ave, Edmonton AB T5P 4A1; (Pakistan)'04; CCFP; (780)405-7520; Fax. (587)521-1801.

VICAS, Ingrid M O; Foothills Med Centre, C231-1403 29 St NW, Calgary AB T2N 2T9; McG'76; AB; AB; FRCPC; EmergMed (Alternative Medicine). Staff, Foothills Medical Centre; (403)944-7635

VICE, Frances B; Royal Columbian Hosp, 330 Columbia St E, New Westminster BC V3L 3W7; McM'98; FRCPC; AnatPath (General Pathology). Staff, Royal Columbian Hospital; (604)520-4814

VICIAN, Michael; Queen Elizabeth II HSC, 1276 South Park St, Halifax NS B3H 2Y9; Justus-Liebig (Other Foreign)'97; Staff Surg, Queen Elizabeth II Health Sciences Centre - Victoria General Site; (902)473-7015; Fax. (902)473-4442.

VICKAR, Darby K; Trillium Hlth Ctr-Mississauga, 100 Queensway W, Mississauga ON L5B 1B8; Man'81; DiagRad. Staff, Trillium Health Centre - Mississauga; (905)848-7524; Fax. (905)848-7349.

VICKAR, David B; Associated Radiologists, 202-11010 101 St NW, Edmonton AB T5H 4B9; Man'79; FRCPC; DiagRad. (780)426-1121; Fax. (780)988-6069.

VICKAR, Eric L; Psychealth Centre, 771 Bannatyne Ave, Winnipeg MB R3E 3N4; Man'83; DABPN; FRCPC; Psy;CCFP; Dir Child & Adolescent Inpatient Unit, Health Sciences Centre; Staff, Psychealth Centre; Assoc Prof, University of Manitoba; (204)787-3148; Fax. (204)787-4975; evickar@exchange.hsc.mb.ca.

VICKERS, Janet A; Credit Valley Fam Pract Assoc, 205-2300 Eglinton Ave W, Mississauga ON L5M 2V8; Wes'87; BA(Phys.Ed.); CCFP; CCFP(E.M.); FCFP; Staff, The Credit Valley Hospital; (905)820-8144; Fax. (905)820-1631.

VICKERS, Michael M; Tom Baker Cancer Centre, CC110-1331 29 St NW, Calgary AB T2N 4N2; Mem'04; FRCPC; IntMed; MedOncol. Staff, Tom Baker Cancer Centre; (403)521-3707; Fax. (403)283-1651.

VICKERSON, Donald G; Summerside Med Centre, 1-475 Granville St, Summerside PE C1N 3N9; Dal'76; (902)432-8170

VICTOR, Gary H; Dr Walter Anderson Bldg, 2251 Pandosy St, Kelowna BC V1Y 1T1; Dublin (Ireland)'82; FRC; FRCPC; IntMed (Infectious Diseases). Staff, Kelowna General Hospital; (250)862-4398

VICTORY, Rahi; 100-3555 North Service Rd E, Windsor ON N8W 5R7; Qns'98; FRCSC; ObstGyn. (519)544-6400; Fax. (519)944-6406.

VICUS, Danielle L; Sunnybrook Hlth Sciences Ctre, 2075 Bayview Ave, Toronto ON M4N 3M5; Ben Gurion University of the Negev (Other Foreign)'02; Staff, Sunnybrook Health Sciences Centre; Langs: Hebrew; (416)480-4378; Fax. (416)480-6002.

VIDA, Stephen; MUHC-Montreal Gen Hosp, 1650 av Cedar, Montreal QC H3G 1A4; McG'81; FRCPC; Psy (Geriatric Psychiatry). Adj, McGill University Health Centre - Montreal General Campus; Staff, Allan Memorial Institute; adj Prof, McGill University; Langs: Hungarian; French; (514)934-1934

VIDAL, Louise; GMF Plateau Marquette, 200-731 rue Galt O, Sherbrooke QC J1H 1Z1; Sher'88; CCFP; Langs: Bilingual(French/English); (819)564-8662; Fax. (819)564-1294.

VIDAL PERALTA, Bertha C R B; TS Med Center, 692 Euclid Ave, Toronto ON M6G 2T9; Universidad Autonoma De Honduras (Honduras)'91; FRCPC; Psy. Staff, Women's College Hospital; Staff, Centre for Addiction & Mental Health (CAMH) - College Street Site; Langs: Spanish; (416)901-9020; Fax. (416)901-7217.

VIDEN, Lonny H; Lenore Centre Med Clinic, 4-123 Lenore Dr, Saskatoon SK S7K 7H9; Sask'01; BSc; CCFP; (306)242-6700; Fax. (306)242-1168.

VIDYASANKAR, Gokul; The Ottawa Hosp-Gen Campus, 501 Smyth Rd, Ottawa ON K1H 8L6; Mem'09; Staff, The Ottawa Hospital - General Campus; (613)722-7000

VIEGAS, Aiza E; The Doctor's Office, 1011 Upper Middle Rd E, Oakville ON L6H 4L1; Wes'05; CCFP; (905)849-7007; Fax. (905)849-7883.

VIEGAS, Desmond S I; PO Box 36528 Rpo Seafair, Richmond BC V7C 5M4; UBC'92.

VIEIRA, Lucy M; 203A-263 boul Saint-Jean, Pointe-Claire QC H9R 3J1; Ott'90; FRCPC; Neur (Migraines). adj Prof, McGill University Health Centre - Montreal General Campus; Langs: Portuguese; French; (514)695-8886; Fax. (514)695-9860.

VIEIRA, Rose-Anne P; Lakeridge Hlth Corp-Oshawa, 1 Hospital Crt, Oshawa ON L1G 2B9; Tor'93; CCFP; Staff, Lakeridge Health - Oshawa Site; (905)576-8711; Fax. (905)721-7763.

VIEIRA NETO, Leonardo; CSSS de Chicoutimi, CP 162 305 av Saint-Vallier, Chicoutimi QC G7H 5H6; Juiz de Fora (Other Foreign)'97; Staff, Complexe hospitalier de la Sagamie; Langs: Portuguese; English; (418)541-1000; Fax. (418)541-1109; vieiraneto2@hotmail.com.

VIEN, Daniel; CSSS du Lac Temiscamingue, 22 rue Notre-Dame N, Ville-Marie QC J9V 1W8; Sher'89; FRCSC; GenSurg. Staff, CSSS du Témiscamingue; assoc Staff, CH Hôtel-Dieu d'Amos; Médecin, CSST Direction Reg de Quebec; (819)629-2420; daniel_vien@ssss.gouv.qc.ca.

VIEN, Helene; Medvaris, 29-2600 boul Laurier, Quebec QC G1V 4T3; Laval'94; (418)781-0579

VIEN, Jeanne; Clinique Med de Carrefour, 1221 boul Marcotte Roberval, Roberval QC G8H 3B8; Mon'91; Staff, CSSS Domaine-Du-Roy; (418)275-1122; Fax. (418)275-1107; jeanne@leblond.com.

VIEN, Marcel; Clinique Med Familiale Dolbeau, 1521 rue des Erables, Dolbeau-Mistassini QC G8L 1C4; Laval'76; Langs: English; (418)276-0041; Fax. (418)276-7170.

VIENNEAU, Theresa L; Aberdeen Hosp, 835 East River Rd, New Glasgow NS B2H 3S6; Dal'99; FRCPC; Psy. Staff Mental Health Serv, Aberdeen Regional Hospital; Staff, Pictou County Health Authority Public Health Services New Glasgow; (902)755-1137

VIENS, Christian; CHUS-Hop Hotel-Dieu, 580 rue Bowen S, Sherbrooke QC J1G 2E8; Sher'91; Staff, Centre Hospitalier Universitaire de Sherbrooke-Hôpital Hôtel-Dieu; (819)346-1110

VIENS, Claudette; Clinique Med Claudette Viens, RR 1 190 Route 138, Les Bergeronnes QC G0T 1G0; Mon'86; Physician, Direction de la sante Publique(Baie-Comeau); Langs: Spanish; English; (418)232-1118; Fax. (418)232-1118; claudette_viens@ssss.gouv.qc.ca.

VIENS, Daniel L; CSSS Drummond-Hop Sainte-Croix, 570 rue Heriot, Drummondville QC J2B 1C1; Sher'04; FRCPC; IntMed. Staff, Hôpital Sainte-croix; (819)478-6464

VIENS, Gilles; Centre Med Saint-Francois, 200-2125 boul Lemire, Drummondville QC J2B 8N8; Laval'84; ac Staff, Hôpital Sainte-croix; (819)477-6793; Fax. (819)477-6962; gilles_viens@gmf.gouv.qc.ca.

VIENS, Gisele; St Claude Clinic, PO Box 269 149 Cypress Ave, St Claude MB R0G 1Z0; Sher'85; CCFP; FCFP; (204)379-2281; Fax. (204)379-2769.

VIENS, Hugo; Clin Orthopedie Haut-Richelieu, 320-900 boul du Seminaire N, St-Jean-Sur-Richel QC J3A 1C3; Mon'98; FRCSC; OrthSurg. (514)348-6966; Fax. (514)348-0664.

VIENS, Mario; Clinique Sante Jacques-Cartier, 200-1815 rue King O, Sherbrooke QC J1J 2E3; Sher'88; FRCSC; GenSurg (Surgical Oncology). Staff, Centre Hospitalier Universitaire de Sherbrooke-Hôpital Hôtel-Dieu; Clin Prof, Universite de Sherbrooke; Langs: Bilingual(French/English); (819)569-2715; Fax. (819)565-7780.

VIENS, Pierre; 963 rue Vauquelin RR 1, Neuville QC G0A 2R0; Mon'63; MSc; PhD; (418)876-3970; pviens@videotron.ca.

VIERO, Sandra; North York Gen Hosp, 4001 Leslie St, North York ON M2K 1E1; Tor'94; FRCPC; AnatPath. Staff Lab & Path, North York General Hospital; Staff, The Hospital For Sick Children; (416)756-6928; Fax. (416)756-4294.

VIG, Kartar S; Oxford Med Walk-In Clinic, 102-140 Oxford St E, London ON N6A 5R9; Dublin (Ireland)'61; LRCP; LRCS; FRCSC; GenSurg. Langs: Hindi; Punjabi; (519)433-4999; Fax. (519)433-4151.

VIG, Rattanjeet S; South Health Campus, 4448 Front St SE, Calgary AB T3M 1M4; Cal'10; CCFP; Staff, Peter Lougheed Centre; Staff Hospitalist Admin, South Health Campus; (403)956-1111

VIGANO, Antonio A L; MUHC-Montreal Gen Hosp, L10 210-1650 av Cedar, Montreal QC H3G 1A4; Milan (Italy)'88; MSc(Epidemiol.); assoc Staff, Sir Mortimer B Davis Jewish General; Att Staff, McGill University Health Centre - Montreal General Campus; Att Staff, McGill University Health Centre - Royal Victoria Hospital; adj Prof Palliative Care, McGill University; Langs: Italian; French; Spanish; (514)934-1934 x43916; Fax. (514)934-8034.

VIGARS, James S; Baywest Medical, 103-400 Main St W, North Bay ON P1B 2V2; Tor'89; Ac Staff, North Bay Regional Health Centre - Regional Mental Health; Asst Prof, Northern Ontario School of Medicine-Lakehead University; (705)476-1293; Fax. (705)476-1625.

VIGEANT, Alain; Clinique Med de l'Arcadie, 1B rue Marion, Saint-Jacques QC J0K 2R0; Mon'98; CCFP; Staff, Centre Hospitalier Régional de Lanaudière; (450)839-7851; Fax. (450)839-7396.

VIGEANT, Huguette; 1275 av James-Lemoine, Quebec QC G1S 1A1; Laval'71; Med Evaluateur, Regie de l'Assurance Maladie du Quebec; Langs: English; (418)527-7074

VIGEANT, Julie; Clinique Med Saint-Vincent, 250 rue King E, Sherbrooke QC J1G 1A9; Sher'86; LMCC; Langs: Bilingual(French/English); (819)563-0510; Fax. (819)564-6889.

VIGEANT, Patrice; CSSS du Suroît, 150 rue Saint-Thomas, Salaber-de-Valleyf QC J6T 6C1; Sher'89; FRCPC; IntMed; MedMicrobiol; InfectDis. Staff, Centre Hospitalier Régional du Suroît; (450)371-9920 x2109; patrice.vigeant@rrsss16.gouv.qc.ca.

VIGER, Marc D; Medwest Med Clinic, 10A-110 Wedge Rd, Saskatoon SK S7L 6Y4; Sask'05; CCFP; (306)979-6185; Fax. (306)979-6186.

VIGER, Pierre; CSSS du Sud de Lanaudière, 911 montee des Pionniers, Terrebonne QC J6V 2H2; Mon'66; CSPQ; FACS; FRCSC; GenSurg (P.Q.) (Gastroenterology). ac Staff Surg, Centre Hospitalier Pierre le Gardeur; (450)654-7525 x32214; Fax. (450)585-5939.

VIGNA, Victor; 1-646 Huron St, London ON N5Y 4J8; Wes'65; (519)672-1040; Fax. (519)672-1430.

VIGNAULT, Francois; IRM Quebec, 225-1900 av Mailloux, Quebec QC G1J 5B9; Mon'86; FRCPC; DiagRad. Staff, Hôtel-Dieu de Lévis; (418)667-0060; Fax. (418)227-3825.

VIGNEAULT, Annie; Hop Maisonneuve-Rosemont, 5415 boul de l'Assomption, Montreal QC H1T 2M4; Mon'06; CCFP; CCFP(E.M.); Staff, Hopital Maisonneuve-Rosemont; (514)252-3400

VIGNEAULT, Diane; CLSC du Richelieu, 300 ch de Marieville, Richelieu QC J3L 3V8; Sher'89; (450)658-7561; Fax. (450)658-4390.

VIGNEAULT, Eric; CHUQ-Hotel-Dieu de Quebec, 11 Cote Du Palais, Quebec QC G1R 2J6; Mon'92; FRCPC; RadOncol (Therapeutic Radiology). Consultant, Hôtel-Dieu de Lévis; Staff, Centre Hospitalier Universitaire de Québec (CHUQ) - Siege Social; Prof, Université Laval; Langs: Bilingual(French/English); (418)691-5264; Fax. (418)691-5268.

VIGNEAULT, Louise; Hôpital Laval, 2725 ch Sainte-Foy, Quebec QC G1V 4G5; Laval'06; FRCPC; Anes. Staff, Hôpital Laval; (418)656-8711

VIGNEAULT, Marc; GMF Centre de santé, 3745 rue Georges-Couture, Drummondville QC J2B 7P4; Sher'86; ac Staff, Hôpital Sainte-croix; Clin Prof, Universite de Sherbrooke; (819)477-2231; Fax. (819)477-1122.

VIGNERON, Eugene A; West Carleton Family Hlth Team, PO Box 218 119 Langstaff Dr, Carp ON K0A 1L0; Tor'92; CCFP; FCFP; (613)839-3271

VIGNJEVIC, Peter M; Dr P M Vignjevic Med Prof Corp, 203-631 Queenston Rd, Hamilton ON L8K 6R5; Tor'93; ABD; RC; FRC; FRCPC; Derm (Laser Surgery). Staff, St Joseph's Healthcare - Charlton Campus; Staff, Hamilton Health Sciences Centre - Hamilton General Hospital; McMaster University; Langs: Serbo-Croatian; Croatian; Ukrainian; Serbian; Yugoslavian; (905)549-1025; Fax. (905)549-9487; appointments@doctorv.ca.

VIGNOLA, Elise C; Ctr Hosp Rouyn-Noranda, 4 9e rue, Rouyn-Noranda QC J9X 2B2; Mon'10; Staff, Centre Hospitalier Rouyn-Noranda; (819)764-5131

VIGNOLA PIGEON, Laurie; Clinique Med Mascouche, 1025 montee Masson, Mascouche QC J7K 2L9; Laval'06; (450)474-6000; Fax. (450)474-6666.

VIGNUDO, Silvia; Healthway Med Centre, 865 Portage Ave, Winnipeg MB R3G 0N8; (Other Foreign)'89; CCFP; Staff, Vita & District Health Centre; (204)783-6464

VIGOD, Simone N; Women's College Hosp, 956-76 Grenville St, Toronto ON M5S 1B2; Tor'03; MSc; FRCPC; Psy. Staff, Women's College Hospital; (416)323-6230; Fax. (416)323-6356.

VIGUERA SALAZAR, Milagro C; Lucan Med Centre, PO Box 880 280 Main St, Lucan ON N0M 2J0; (Cuba)'93; CCFP; Langs: Spanish; (519)227-4015

VIHERJOKI, Stephen; Dingwall Med Group, PO Box 3011 Stn Main 40 Goodall St, Dryden ON P8N 2Z6; Qns'05; CCFP; Chief Emergency Services, Dryden Regional Health Centre; (807)223-6683; Fax. (807)223-4733.

VIJAY, Nishka R; Pembroke Gen Hosp, 705 MacKay St, Pembroke ON K8A 1G8; Tor'01; FRCPC; Psy. Staff, Pembroke Regional Hospital Inc; (613)732-2811

VIJAY, Raj; Derry Village Clinic, 2-7070 Saint Barbara Blvd, Mississauga ON L5W 0E6; Man'85; CCFP; Physician, Fairview Ten Medical Clinic; Langs: Tamil; Hindi; (905)565-9100; Fax. (905)565-8973.

VIJAY, Sheela M; University of Alberta Hosp, 2F1 28Z-8440 112 St NW, Edmonton AB T6G 2B7; Cal'04; FRCPC; IntMed. Staff, University of Alberta Hospital; (780)407-8822

VIJAYAKANTHAN, Kandiah; Sudbury Med Centre, 306-65 Larch St, Sudbury ON P3E 1B8; Colombo (Sri Lanka)'75; MB BS; MRC; FRCSC; ObstGyn. Staff, Health Sciences North-St Joseph's Health Centre; Langs: Tamil; (705)674-0040; Fax. (705)674-8938.

VIJAYARAGHAVAN, Ram; Rouge Valley Cardiology, 406-1371 Neilson Ave, Scarborough ON M1B 4Z8; Tor'99; BSc; FRCPC; IntMed (Interventional Cardiology); Cardiol. Staff, Rouge Valley Health System - Centenary Health Centre Site; (416)281-9499; Fax. (416)283-5705.

VIJAYARATNAM, Visvalingam; Rosedale Med Centre, 711-600 Sherbourne St, Toronto ON M4X 1W4; Ceylon (Sri Lanka)'74; MB BS; FRCPC; Peds; Gastroent. Langs: Sinhalese; Tamil; (416)929-0929; Fax. (416)929-8084; vvijayaratnam@rogers.com.

VIJH, Meeta; McLaughlin Village Med Clinic, 2F-85 Steeles Ave W, Brampton ON L6Y 0K3; 80Gulbarga (India)'90; MB BS; CCFP; Langs: Punjabi; Hindi; (905)455-9374; Fax. (905)455-9505.

VIK, Astrid L; UBC Hosp, 2211 Wesbrook Mall, Vancouver BC V6T 2B5; UBC'97; FRCPC; Psy. Staff, UBC Hospital - Koerner Pavillion; (604)822-7121; Fax. (604)822-7253.

VIKIS, Elena A T; 401-233 Nelson's Cres, New Westminster BC V3L 0E4; Man'02; FRCSC; GenSurg. Staff, Vancouver General Hospital - Centennial Pavillion; (604)524-2454

VILA, J Michael; Alberta Children's Hosp, 2888 Shaganappi Trail NW, Calgary AB T3B 6A8; Qns'06; FRCPC; Peds. Staff, Alberta Children's Hospital; Staff, Foothills Medical Centre; (403)955-2953

VILA-RODRIGUEZ, Fidel; Neurostimulation Service, 6F-805 12 Ave W, Vancouver BC V5Z 1M9; Barcelona (Spain)'00; FRCPC; Psy. Staff, Vancouver General Hospital - Centennial Pavillion; Staff Neurostimulation Services, University of British Columbia; Langs: Spanish; Catalan; (604)675-2449; fvila-rodriguez@psych.ubc.ca.

VILADEVALL, Hugo; St Mary's Hosp Centre, 3830 av Lacombe, Montreal QC H3T 1M5; McG'04; CCFP; CCFP(E.M.); Staff, McGill University Health Centre - Royal Victoria Hospital; Staff, St Mary's Hospital Centre; (514)345-3511 x2690; jugo.viladevall@mail.mcgill.ca.

VILAGHY, Miklos I; 508-600 Sherbourne St, Toronto ON M4X 1W4; Pecs (Hungary)'65; Langs: Hungarian; (416)922-7726; Fax. (416)922-9447.

VILAIN, Luc S; 801-320 ch de la Rive-Boisee, Pierrefonds QC H8Z 3M2; Santo Domingo (Dominican Republic)'63; ObstGyn (P.Q.). (514)626-8562

VILCINI, Michelle M; The Medical Centre FHT, PO Box 4200 Stn Main 707 Charlotte St, Peterborough ON K9J 7B3; McM'91; CCFP; FCFP; Staff Privil, Peterborough Regional Health Centre - Hospital Drive; (705)876-4520; Fax. (705)743-2997.

VILIS, Donna M; PO Box 160, Pakenham ON K0A 2X0; Ott'74; Ac Staff, Arnprior & District Memorial Hospital; Court Staff, Almonte General Hospital; (613)624-5480; Fax. (613)624-5223.

VILJOEN, Annette; Meadow Lake Assoc Clinic, PO Box 1510, Meadow Lake SK S9X 1Z1; Pretoria (South Africa)'94; MB ChB; Physician, Meadow Lake Associate Clinic; (306)236-5661; Fax. (306)236-4355.

VILJOEN, Jean-Pierre; Haugen Med Group, 23C-3300 Smith Dr, Armstrong BC V0E 1B1; Stellenbosch (South Africa)'98; MB ChB; (250)546-8115; Fax. (250)546-2553.

VILJOEN, Johan A; Dr Viljoen & Durand Vamiliy Me, PO Box 10, Medicine Hat AB T1A 7E6; Orange Free State (South Africa)'76; CCFP; FCFP; (403)487-5450; Fax. (403)487-5451; johanviljoen@mac.com.

VILJOEN, Johan; Bayvalley Med Arts Bldg, 201A-145 Queenston St, St Catharines ON L2R 2Z9; Stellenbosch (South Africa)'81; MB ChB; MMed; FRCSC; ObstGyn (Menopause). Consultant, Niagara Health System - St Catharines General Site; Langs: Afrikaans; (905)684-8395; Fax. (905)684-4717.

VILJOEN, Johann H; Medicross Clinic, 10-69 Dunlop St, Red Deer AB T4R 2H6; Orange Free State (South Africa)'95; BMedSci; MB ChB; LMCC; CCFP; Langs: Afrikaans; (403)347-6811; Fax. (403)347-6899.

VILJOEN, Lourens J; Crossroads Family Practice, 201-45800 Promontory Rd, Chilliwack BC V2R 5Z5; (South Africa)'08; MB ChB; (604)858-3725

VILJOEN, Mark I; Grandview Woodland Addict Serv, 310-1669 Broadway Ave E, Vancouver BC V5N 1V9; Witwatersrand (South Africa)'89; MB ChB; Staff, Maples Adolescent Treatment Centre; Staff, Grandview Woodland Addiction Services; (604)675-3950

VILJOEN, Mighael I; Esterhazy Dist Med Clinic, PO Box 940, Esterhazy SK S0A 0X0; (306)745-6682; Fax. (306)745-2995.

VILJOEN, Rene; Medicross Clinic, 10-69 Dunlop St, Red Deer AB T4R 2H6; (South Africa)'94; MB ChB; CCFP; Langs: Afrikaans; (403)347-6811; Fax. (403)347-6899.

VILJOEN, Willem A; Signature Park Plaza, 100-1919 Sirocco Dr SW, Calgary AB T3H 2Y3; Pretoria (South Africa)'88; MB ChB; Langs: Afrikaans; (403)278-1003; Fax. (403)398-9420; viljoen@nucleus.com.

VILK, Jeffery K; Niagara H System-St Catharines, PO Box 3018 Stn Main 142 Queenston St, St Catharines ON L2R 7C6; Man'93; FRCPC; DiagRad. Staff, Niagara Health System - St Catharines General Site; (905)684-7271 x6538; Fax. (905)684-6990.

VILLA RESTREPO, Diego; BC Cancer Agency, 600 10th Ave W, Vancouver BC V5Z 4E6; Javier Pontifical University (Colombia)'02; FRCPC; IntMed; MedOncol. Staff, BC Cancer Agency Vancouver Centre; Langs: Spanish; (604)877-6000

VILLAGE, Ronald S; Northmount Med Centre, 704-145 13th St E, North Vancouver BC V7L 2L4; UBC'91; (604)988-8588; Fax. (604)988-1344.

VILLALOBOS NARVAEZ, Ethel H; CSSS de Trois-Rivières, 1991 boul du Carmel, Trois-Rivieres QC G9A 1Y1; (Other Foreign)'01; CCFP; (819)697-3333

VILLALON, Reynaldo D M; 111-10090 152 St, Surrey BC V3R 8X8; St Louis (Philippines)'84; (604)581-3550

VILLALPANDO BERUMEN, Juan M; Institute Univ Geriatrie Mtl, 4565 ch Queen-Mary, Montreal QC H3W 1W5; Lasalle (France)'93; Staff, Institut Universitaire de Gériatrie de Montréal; (514)340-1424

VILLANI, Anita; The Hosp for Sick Children, 555 University Ave, Toronto ON M5G 1X8; Ott'07; FRCPC; Peds. Staff, The Hospital For Sick Children; (416)813-7742

VILLANUEVA, Alvin P; Medical Arts Bldg, 202-770 6th St SW, Medicine Hat AB T1A 8M7; (Philippines)'96; Staff, Medicine Hat Regional Hospital; Physician, Palliser Health Authority; (403)487-5313; Fax. (403)487-5305; alvin.villanueva@cls.ab.ca.

VILLANUEVA ARQUINT, Monique; Markham Stouffville Hosp, PO Box 1800 Stn Main 381 Church St, Markham ON L3P 7P3; Tor'92; MSc; PhD; FRCPC; GenPath (Cytology). Staff, Markham Stouffville Hospital; Langs: Spanish; German; French; (905)472-7044; Fax. (905)472-7133.

VILLANYI, Diane; Gordon & Leslie Diamond HCC, 7F-2775 Laurel St, Vancouver BC V5Z 1M9; UBC'05; GeriatricMed; IntMed. Physician, Gordon & Leslie Diamond Health Care Centre; Langs: Bilingual(English/French); (604)875-5706

VILLAR, Erwin; Professional Corp, 931 19 St S, Lethbridge AB T1J 3H5; St Louis University (Other Foreign)'92; FRCPC; IntMed. (403)328-0693; Fax. (403)328-0619.

VILLAR, Giselle C P; BC Women's Hosp & HC, 4500 Oak St, Vancouver BC V6H 3N1; Sao Paolo (Brazil)'92; FRCPC; Anes. Staff, BC Women's Hospital & Health Centre; Langs: Portuguese; (604)875-2158

VILLASENOR, Fernando M; Mageta Med Clinic, 110-20528 Lougheed Hwy, Maple Ridge BC V2X 2P8; Monterrey (Mexico)'84; CCFP; Teach Staff Family Med, University of British Columbia; (604)465-1100

VILLELLA, Giovanni; 104-860 Tecumseh Rd E, Windsor ON N8X 2S5; Tor'01; FRCPC; Psy. Staff, Windsor Regional Hospital - Metropolitan Site; Staff, Hôtel-Dieu Grace Hospital; Aj Prof Med & Dentistry, University of Western Ontario; Langs: Italian; (519)977-8604

VILLEMAIRE, Jean-Marc; CHUQ-Hotel de l'Enfant-Jesus, 1401 18e rue, Quebec QC G1J 1Z4; Mon'86; FRCPC; NuclearMed. Staff, Centre Hospitalier Affilié Universitaire de Québec - Hôpital De L'Enfant Jésus; (418)649-0252

VILLEMAIRE, Pierre A; Clinique Med Masson-Angers, 101-1100 ch Montreal O, Gatineau QC J8M 2A9; Dal'87; Staff, CH-CHSLD de Papineau - Pavillon du Centre d'Accueil; (819)281-1509; Fax. (819)281-1741.

VILLEMURE, Jacques; Clinique Med Frontenac, 24 rue Frontenac, Riviere-du-Loup QC G5R 1S5; Laval'79; ac Staff, Centre Hospitalier Regional du Grand-Portage; (418)862-0333; Fax. (418)868-0505.

VILLEMURE, Louise; 68 4e av, Plaisance QC J0V 1S0; Mon'82; (819)427-5333; Fax. (819)427-8280.

VILLEMURE, Marie-Pier; Inst U Geriatrie Sherbrooke, 1036 rue Belvedere, Sherbrooke QC J1H 4C4; Mon'09; CCFP; Staff, CSSS Institut universitaire de gériatrie de Sherbrooke; (819)780-2222

VILLEMURE, Philippe; CSSS de Lac-Saint Jean-Est, CP 1300 succ Bureau-Chef 300 boul Champlain S, Alma QC G8B 5W3; Sher'06; CCFP; Staff, CSSS de Lac-Saint Jean-Est; (418)669-2000

VILLEMURE, Real; Clinique de Med Familiale, 101 rue Lavoie, Rimouski QC G5L 5Y2; Laval'77; Staff, Hôpital Regional Rimouski; (418)723-5272; Fax. (418)725-2030.

VILLENEUVE, Alain-Fernand; Clinique Med Pasteur, 770 1re av, Quebec QC G1L 3K2; Laval'75; (418)529-9976; Fax. (418)529-4924; monaco@videotron.ca.

VILLENEUVE, Andre; Hotel-Dieu de Levis, 143 rue Wolfe, Levis QC G6V 3Z1; Laval'94; CCFP; CCFP(E.M.); Staff, Hôtel-Dieu de Lévis; (418)835-7122

VILLENEUVE, Andreanne; Hôpital Ste-Justine, 3175 ch Cote-Sainte-Catherine, Montreal QC H3T 1C5; Mon'08; Peds. Staff, Hôpital Ste-Justine; (514)345-4931

VILLENEUVE, Audrey; CSSS de Lac-Saint Jean-Est, CP 1300 Succ Bureau-chef 300 boul Champlain S, Alma QC G8B 5W3; Mon'05; Staff, CSSS de Lac-Saint Jean-Est; (418)669-2000

VILLENEUVE, Audrey; Hôpital de Saint-Eustache, 520 boul Arthur-Sauve, Saint-Eustache QC J7R 5B1; Laval'06; FRCPC; Anes;CCFP; Staff, Hôpital de Saint-Eustache; (450)473-6811

VILLENEUVE, Bertrand; Min de l'Emploi & Solidarite S, 425 rue Saint-Amable, Quebec QC G1R 4Z1; Laval'62; Hem (P.Q.) (Hematological Oncology). ac Staff, Hôpital Laval; assoc Staff, Centre Hospitalier Affilié Universitaire de Québec - Hôpital du St-Sacrement; Consultant, Centre Hospitalier Universitaire De Québec - Pavillon De St-françois-d'assise; Staff, Ministry De La Solidarite Sociale; (418)643-3104; bertrand.villeneuve@mess.gouv.qc.ca.

VILLENEUVE, Carol; Inst U en Sante Mentale de QC, 2601 ch de la Canardiere, Quebec QC G1J 2G3; Laval'72; (418)663-5321; Fax. (418)661-6891.

VILLENEUVE, Carolyne; Clinique Familiale des Prairie, 310 boul Antonio-Barrette, Joliette QC J6E 1G2; Laval'07; CCFP; (450)752-1050

VILLENEUVE, Claude; Hôpital Ste-Justine, 3175 ch Cote-Sainte-Catherine, Montreal QC H3T 1C5; Laval'66; LMCC; Psy (Adolescent Psychiatry). ac Staff, Hôpital Ste-Justine; adj Prof Psy, Universite de Montreal; (514)345-4695; Fax. (514)345-4679.

VILLENEUVE, Diane; Dir de la Sante Publique-Mtl, 1301 rue Sherbrooke E, Montreal QC H2L 1M3; Mon'76; Staff, Hopital Maisonneuve-Rosemont; Clin Instructeur, Universite de Montreal; Langs: Bilingual(French/English); (514)528-2400 x3562; Fax. (514)528-2463; dvillene@santepub-mtl.qc.ca.

VILLENEUVE, Edith; CHUM-Hôpital Notre-Dame, 4E-1560 rue Sherbrooke E, Montreal QC H2L 4M1; Mon'01; FRCPC; IntMed; Rheum. Staff, Centre Hospitalier l'Université de Montréal (CHUM) - Hôpital Notre-Dame; (514)890-8000 x28800; Fax. (514)412-7230.

VILLENEUVE, Edith M B; Hôpital Ste-Justine, B9-3175 ch Cote-Sainte-Catheri, Montreal QC H3T 1C5; Mon'85; Anes (Internal Medicine). ac Staff, Hôpital Ste-Justine; (514)345-4733; Fax. (514)345-4601.

VILLENEUVE, Etienne; UMF Nord de Lanaudière, 50 ch du Golf O, St-Charles-Brromee QC J6E 2B4; Mon'08; CCFP; (450)759-3060; Fax. (450)759-7799.

VILLENEUVE, Evens; Inst of Mental Health Quebec, 2601 ch de la Canardiere, Quebec QC G1J 2G3; Laval'76; FRCPC; Psy (Personality Disorders). rég Psychiatre, Institut Universitaire Sante; dép Chef Services, Clnique Faubourg St-Jean Services; Dir Admissions, Université Laval; (418)663-5321

VILLENEUVE, Francois; CLSC Montcalm, 110 rue Saint-Isidore RR 1, Saint-Esprit QC J0K 2L0; Mon'83; (450)839-3676

VILLENEUVE, Georges-Henri; Clinique Med Gen d'Alma, 22 rue Melancon E, Alma QC G8B 6W3; Laval'73; Staff, CSSS de Lac-Saint Jean-Est; (418)668-2377; Fax. (418)668-0873; georges-henri.villeneuve@ssss.gouv.qc.ca.

VILLENEUVE, Helene; CSSS de Chicoutimi, CP 5006 305 rue Saint-Vallier, Chicoutimi QC G7H 5H6; Mon'93; FRCPC; IntMed (P.Q.); Endocrin&Metab. Staff, Complexe hospitalier de la Sagamie; (418)549-5987; Fax. (418)549-9948.

VILLENEUVE, Hugo; Complexe Hosp de la Sagamie, CP 5006 305 rue St-Vallier, Chicoutimi QC G7H 5H6; Mon'07; FRCPC; RadOncol. Staff, Complexe hospitalier de la Sagamie; (418)549-5987

VILLENEUVE, Isabelle; CHUQ-Hotel-Dieu de Quebec, 11 Cote du Palais, Quebec QC G1R 2J6; Laval'95; Staff, Centre Hospitalier Universitaire de Québec (CHUQ) - Siege Social; (418)691-5042; Fax. (418)691-5024.

VILLENEUVE, Jacques; Hôpital Laval, 2725 ch Sainte-Foy, Quebec QC G1V 4G5; Laval'80; FRCPC; Anes. Staff, Hôpital Laval; Prof, Université Laval; (418)656-8711

VILLENEUVE, Jasmin; DRSP de la Capitale-Nationale, 2400 av d'Estimauville, Quebec QC G1E 7G9; Laval'96; (418)666-7000 x364

VILLENEUVE, Jean; Ctr Hosp Affilie-Enfant-Jesus, 1401 18e rue, Quebec QC G1J 1Z4; Mon'90; CCFP; CCFP(E.M.); EmergMed (P. Q.). Staff, Centre Hospitalier Affilié Universitaire de Québec - Hôpital De L'Enfant Jésus; (418)649-5632

VILLENEUVE, Jean; Clinique Med St-Constant, 102-113 rue Saint-Pierre, Repentigny QC J6A 2G8; Laval'87; (450)632-1630; Fax. (450)632-5242.

VILLENEUVE, Jean-Benoit; Hydro-Quebec, 101-75 boul René-Lévesque O, Montreal QC H2Z 1A4; Laval'73; Médecin, Hydro-Quebec; (514)289-2211 x2981; Fax. (514)289-4158.

VILLENEUVE, Jean-Pierre; Ctr Hosp de Verdun, 4000 boul Lasalle, Verdun QC H4G 2A3; Mon'82; Staff, Centre Hospitalier de Verdun; Clin Adj, Universite de Montreal; (514)362-1000 x4326; Fax. (514)765-7306; mpjpv@sympatico.ca.

VILLENEUVE, Jean-Pierre; CHUM-Hop St-Luc, 1058 rue Saint-Denis, Montreal QC H2X 3J4; Mon'71; Gastroent (P.Q.) (Hepatology). Prof/Clin Prof Research Centre, Centre Hospitalier l'Université De Montréal (CHUM) - Hôpital Saint-luc; Prof, Universite de Montreal; (514)890-8000 x35722; Fax. (514)412-7314.

VILLENEUVE, Josee; Centre De L'Osteoporose, 100-1200 av Germain-des-Pres, Quebec QC G1V 3M7; Laval'86; FRCPC; IntMed. Staff, Centre Hospitalier Universitaire de Quebec-CHUL; Médecin, Centre De L'Osteoporose et De Rhumathologie de Quebec; (418)650-4531; Fax. (418)650-3916.

VILLENEUVE, Lucien; Clinique Med de Saint-Sauveu, RR 6 70 rue Principale, Saint-Sauveur QC J0R 1R6; Mon'81; (450)227-8436

VILLENEUVE, Marc; 401-5600 boul des Galeries, Quebec QC G2K 2H6; Laval'85; FRCSC; ObstGyn. ac Staff, Centre Hospitalier Universitaire De Québec - Pavillon De St-françois-d'assise; (418)260-9555; Fax. (418)260-9556; procrea@videotron.ca.

VILLENEUVE, Marie; Hop Louis H-Lafontaine, 304-7401 rue Hochelaga, Montreal QC H1N 3M5; Laval'00; FRCPC; Psy. Staff, Hopital Louis-H Lafontaine; Langs: English; (514)251-4000

VILLENEUVE, Marie; Centre Med Quatre-Bourgeois, 300-979 av de Bourgogne, Quebec QC G1W 2L4; Laval'85; (418)653-4050; Fax. (418)653-4475.

VILLENEUVE, Michel; Centre Med Drummond, 60 rue Loring, Drummondville QC J2C 7Y9; Mon'85; ac Staff, Hôpital Sainte-croix; (819)477-2500; Fax. (819)477-6249.

VILLENEUVE, Nadia; Clinique Pediatrique Longueuil, 105-2160 ch du Tremblay, Longueuil QC J4N 1A8; Laval'95; FRCPC; Peds. Staff, McGill University Health Centre - Montreal Children's Hospital; (450)448-4621; Fax. (450)448-5403.

VILLENEUVE, Nicole; Clinique Sante de Thetford, 2000-926 rue Labbe, Thetford Mines QC G6G 2A8; Laval'75; (418)338-4581; Fax. (418)338-4584; nicole@centresantethetford.ca.

VILLENEUVE, Patrick J; The Ottawa Hosp-Gen Campus, 6359-501 Smyth Rd Box 902, Ottawa ON K1H 8L6; McG'02; FRCSC; GenSurg (Clinician Investigator Program); ThorSurg. Staff, The Ottawa Hospital - General Campus; Langs: Bilingual(English/French); (613)737-8899; Fax. (613)737-8668.

VILLENEUVE, Pierre; Stronach Reg Cancer Centre, 596 Davis Dr, Newmarket ON L3Y 2P9; McG'04; PhD; FRCPC; IntMed; Hem. Fellow, Princess Margaret Hospital - University Health Network; Langs: Bilingual(English/French); (905)895-4521

VILLENEUVE, Pierre; CSSS du Haut Saint-Maurice, 885 rue Ducharme, La Tuque QC G9X 3C1; Laval'90; Staff EmergMed, Centre Hospitalier Saint-Joseph de la Turque; (819)523-4581

VILLENEUVE, Pierre-Marc; Clinical Sciences Bldg, 11 107-11350 83 Ave, Edmonton AB T6G 2P4; McG'08; IntMed. (780)407-7717

VILLENEUVE, Regis; Clinique Dr Claude Malenfant, 100-1731 3e av, Val-d'Or QC J9P 1W3; Laval'81; cadre Sec Medical, Centre Hospitalier de Val d'Or; (819)824-1802

VILLENEUVE, Simon; Centre Hosp Chauveau, 11999 rue de l'Hopital, Quebec QC G2A 2T7; Laval'05; Staff, Centre Hospitalier Chauveau; (418)842-3651

VILLENEUVE, Suzanne; Clinique Med Pelletier, 300-8330 boul Taschereau, Brossard QC J4X 1C2; Mon'83; (450)465-5379; Fax. (450)465-5615; suzanne.villeneuve@videotron.ca.

VILLENEUVE, Valerie; MUHC-Royal Victoria Hosp, 687 av des Pins O, Montreal QC H3A 1A1; Laval'97; FRCPC; Anes. Staff, McGill University Health Centre - Royal Victoria Hospital; (514)934-1934 x34880

VILLIARD, Jean-Sebastien; CSSS Maria-Chapdelaine, 2000 boul du Sacré-Coeur, Dolbeau-Mistassini QC G8L 2R5; Laval'02; Staff, Centre Maria-Chapdelaine - CH de Dolbeau-Mistassini; (418)276-1234; Fax. (418)276-4355.

VILLIARD, Marie-France; CLSC de la Jacques Cartier, 042-11999A rue de l'Hopital, Quebec QC G2A 2T7; Laval'90; (418)843-2572 x7615; Fax. (418)843-3880.

VILLIARD, Paule; Clinique Med Mercier, 101-464 boul Saint-Jean-Baptis, Mercier QC J6R 2B1; Sher'95; CCFP; Staff, Hôpital Anna-Laberge; (450)699-0539

VILLIARD, Roselyne; Centre Chirurgical de Joliette, 202-222 rue de la Visitation, Joliette QC J6E 4N5; Mon'04; FRCSC; GenSurg. (450)753-7588

VILLOTA, Maurilio; Clinique Med 6930 Papineau Inc, 6930 av Papineau, Montreal QC H2G 2X7; Madrid (Spain)'66; FRCPC; Electroenceph (P.Q.); Neur (P.Q.). Staff, CSSS du Coeur de l'Isle Hôpital Jean-Talon; Staff, Hopital de la Cite de la santé; (514)722-0000; Fax. (514)722-2431; mvillota@videotron.ca.

VILONEL, Etienne E; North Vancouver Med Clinic, 115 16th St W, North Vancouver BC V7M 1T3; Pretoria (South Africa)'05; MB ChB; Langs: Afrikaans; (604)904-8804; evilonel@sasktel.net.

VILORIA, Juan B; Lakeshore Gen Hosp, 160 av Stillview, Pointe-Claire QC H9R 2Y2; Manila (Philippines)'59; FRCPC; AnatPath. Staff, Lakeshore General Hospital - Pointe Claire; Staff, McGill University Health Centre - Montreal General Campus; (514)630-2225 x5530; Fax. (514)630-2053.

VILOS, Angelos G C; PG Medical Education Office, M106-1151 Richmond St, London ON N6A 5C1; Meharry Medical College (Other Foreign)'07; FRCPC; ObstGyn.

VILOS, George A; St Joseph's Health Care, PO Box 5777 Stn B 268 Grosvenor St, London ON N6A 4V2; Wes'74; FACOG; FSOGC; FRCSC; ObstGyn. Ac Staff, St Joseph's Hospital - St Joseph's Health Care; Prof ObstGyn, University of Western Ontario; Langs: Greek; (519)646-6104; Fax. (519)646-6345; george.vilos@sjhc. london.on.ca.

VIMALENDRAN, Suthaharan; The Ottawa Hosp-Gen Campus, 501 Smyth Rd Box 210, Ottawa ON K1H 8L6; Tor'03; FRCPC; IntMed;CCFP; Nephrol. Staff, The Ottawa Hospital - General Campus; (613)737-8726; Fax. (613)737-8250.

VINAY, Patrick; CHUM-Hop Notre-Dame, 1560 rue Sherbrooke E, Montreal QC H2L 4M1; Mon'68; PhD; Nephrol (P.Q.) (Palliative Care). Staff, Centre Hospitalier l'Université de Montréal (CHUM) - Hôpital Notre-Dame; Langs: English; (514)890-8000; Fax. (514)412-7589.

VINCELETTE, Jean; CHUM-Hop St-Luc, 1058 rue Saint-Denis, Montreal QC H2X 3J4; Mon'70; FRCPC; MedMicrobiol. Staff, Centre Hospitalier l'Université De Montréal (CHUM) - Hôpital Saint-luc; Clin Prof, Universite de Montreal; (514)890-8000 x36210; Fax. (514)412-7412.

VINCELETTE, Pierre; Ctr Hosp Rouyn-Noranda, 4 9e rue, Rouyn-Noranda QC J9X 2B2; Mon'72; Peds (Medical Oncology). Chef Neonatology, Centre Hospitalier Rouyn-Noranda; Staff Peds, Centre de Readaptation La Maison(Rouyn-Noranda); (819)764-5131; Fax. (819)797-6887; pierre.vincelette@ssss. gouv.qc.ca.

VINCENT, Andre; Hotel-Dieu de Levis, 143 rue Wolfe, Levis QC G6V 3Z1; Laval'81; MedMicrobiol; IntMed. ac Staff, Hôtel-Dieu de Lévis; assoc Staff, Centre Hospitalier Universitaire de Québec (CHUQ) - Siege Social; (418)835-7121 x3302

VINCENT, Anjali L S; 101-3607 31 St, Vernon BC V1T 5J4; Bangalore (India)'98; MB BS; CCFP; (250)275-6585; Fax. (250)549-1247.

VINCENT, Anne-Marie; Hop Maisonneuve-Rosemont, 5415 boul de l'Assomption, Montreal QC H1T 2M4; Laval'03; PedHemaOncol; Hem; Peds. Staff, Hopital Maisonneuve-Rosemont; (514)252-3400 x4558

VINCENT, Annick; Centre Med de l'Hetriere, 201-3520 rue de l'Hetriere, St-Augustin-D-Desm QC G3A 0B4; Laval'89; FRCPC; Psy. Staff, Institut Universitaire Sante; Langs: English; French; (418)651-3933; Fax. (418)651-0256.

VINCENT, Catherine; CHUM-Hop St-Luc, 1058 rue Saint-Denis, Montreal QC H2X 3J4; Mon'97; FRCPC; IntMed; Gastroent. Staff, Centre Hospitalier l'Université De Montréal (CHUM) - Hôpital Saint-luc; (514)890-8000; Fax. (514)412-7314.

VINCENT, David C; North Woodlands Med Centre, 204-40 Shellington Place, Brantford ON N3S 0C5; McM'81; CCFP; Clin Teach Staff Family Med, McMaster University; (519)759-6116; Fax. (519)759-7727.

VINCENT, Denis R J; Cite Francophone, 138-8627 91 St NW, Edmonton AB T6C 3N1; Alb'87; CCFP; FCFP; Staff, Covenant Health - Grey Nuns Community Hospital; Langs: Spanish; English; (780)450-8635; Fax. (780)401-3104.

VINCENT, Francois; CSSS de Trois-Rivières, 1991 boul du Carmel, Trois-Rivieres QC G8Z 3R9; Mon'94; FRCPC; RadOncol (Medical Oncology). Staff, Hotel-Dieu d'Arthabaska; Staff, Centre Hospitalier Régional de Lanaudière; Staff, CSSS de Trois-Rivières; Consultant, Ministry of Health-Quebec; (819)371-5002; Fax. (819)378-9712; francois_vincent_chrtr@ssss.gouv.qc.ca.

VINCENT, Franklyn A; Northwest Med Group, 30 Farnham Gate Rd, Halifax NS B3M 3W8; Jaffna (Sri Lanka)'93; MB BS; CCFP; Langs: Tamil; Sinhalese; (902)443-8388; Fax. (902)443-9887.

VINCENT, Franklynne K; St Joseph's Health Centre, SWW 232-30 The Queensway, Toronto ON M6R 1B5; Tor'83; MB BS; BSc; FRCPC; Derm. Head Derm, St Joseph's Health Centre; (416)530-6095; Fax. (416)530-6184.

VINCENT, George M F; St Joseph's Health Centre, SWW 234-30 The Queensway, Toronto ON M6R 1B5; Tor'83; FRCSC; OrthSurg (Lower Extremity Reconstruction). Staff, Toronto Western Hospital - University Health Network; Staff, St Joseph's Health Centre; University of Toronto; (416)530-6773; Fax. (416)530-6184; vinceg@stjoe.on.ca.

VINCENT, Gilles; Clinique Fam de St-Hyacinthe, 2955 boul Laframboise, Saint-Hyacinthe QC J2S 4Z3; Mon'72; (450)774-4611; Fax. (450)773-9913.

VINCENT, Gilles; Clinique Med de Francheville, 111-1220 rue Jean-Nicolet, Trois-Rivieres QC G9A 1B2; Laval'81; Staff, CSSS de Trois-Rivières; (819)373-2117; Fax. (819)373-8512.

VINCENT, Guy; Centre Med Saint-Charles, 104-1740 ch Saint Charles, Lachenaie QC J6W 3R3; Mon'87; (450)492-2277; Fax. (450)492-1030.

VINCENT, Hubert; Clinique Med Avenir MD, 220-1575 boul de l'Avenir, Laval QC H7S 2N5; Mon'01; Staff, Centre Hospitalier Affilié Universitaire de Québec - Hôpital du St-Sacrement; (450)696-1025; Fax. (450)696-1019.

VINCENT, Linda S; CSSS de Trois-Rivières, 1991 boul du Carmel, Trois-Rivieres QC G8Z 3R9; Laval'86; FRCPC; RadOncol (P.Q.) (Medical Oncology). Chef, CSSS de Trois-Rivières; (819)371-5002; Fax. (819)378-9712; vinlin@videotron.ca.

VINCENT, Lisa G; Oak Park Family Care Centre, 201 Oak Walk Dr, Oakville ON L6H 6M3; Tor'90; BSc; CCFP; FCFP; Court Staff Family Pract, The Credit Valley Hospital; (905)257-3297; Fax. (905)257-8621.

VINCENT, Mark D; London Reg Cancer Centre, 790 Commissioners Rd E, London ON N6A 4L6; Cape Town (South Africa)'76; MB ChB; MRC; FRCPC; IntMed (Gastrointestinal Disorders); MedOncol. Staff MedOncol, London Health Sciences Centre - Victoria Campus; Assoc Prof, University of Western Ontario; Langs: Afrikaans; (519)685-8640; Fax. (519)685-8624.

VINCENT, Martin; Hop du Sacre-Coeur de Montreal, 5400 boul Gouin O, Montreal QC H4J 1C5; Mon'03; CCFP; CCFP(E.M.); Staff, Hôpital du Sacre-Coeur de Montréal; (514)338-2222

VINCENT, Matthieu; Clinique Med Pierre-Boucher, 1615 boul Jacques-Cartier E, Longueuil QC J4G 1K3; Sher'01; EmergMed. Staff, Clinique Medicale Pierre-Boucher; Langs: English; French; (450)468-6223; matthieu_vincent@hotmail.com.

VINCENT, Matthieu; Centre Hosp Rég du Suroît, 150 150 rue Saint-Thomas, Salaber-de-Valleyf QC J6T 6C1; Mon'09; CCFP; Staff, Centre Hospitalier Régional du Suroît; Staff, Barrie Memorial Hospital; (450)371-9920

VINCENT, Melanie A; Hôpital Ste-Justine, 7950-3175 Cote-Sainte-Catherin, Montreal QC H3T 1C5; McG'98; FRCPC; Peds. Staff, Hôpital Ste-Justine; (514)345-4931; Fax. (514)354-4822.

VINCENT, Merville A; Edgewood Psychiatric Services, 2121 Boxwood Rd, Nanaimo BC V9S 4L2; McM'84; FRCPC; Psy (Addiction Psychiatry). Dir, Edgewood Psychiatric Services; Clin Instructor Psy, University of British Columbia; (250)751-0111; Fax. (250)751-2758.

VINCENT, Nancy E; Chinook Reg Hosp, 960 19 St S, Lethbridge AB T1J 1W5; Dal'82; FRCSC; OrthSurg (Orthopedics). Staff, Covenant Health - St Michael's Health Centre; Chinook Regional Hospital; (403)388-6709; Fax. (403)320-1866.

VINCENT, Natacha; CLSC Richmond, 110 rue Barlow, Richmond QC J0B 2H0; Sher'92; Langs: Bilingual(French/English); (819)542-2777 x55400; Fax. (819)826-3867.

VINCENT, Pierre M; Institute of Mental Health Que, 2601 rue de la Canardière, Quebec QC G1J 2G3; Laval'65; DPsy; Psy. Staff, Centre Hospitalier Affilié Universitaire de Québec - Hôpital De L'Enfant Jésus; Staff, Institut Universitaire Sante; Clin Assoc Prof, Université Laval; Langs: English; (418)663-5781; Fax. (418)663-5758; pierre_vincent@ssss.gouv.qc.ca.

VINCENT, Pierre R; 17 rue Fusey, Trois-Rivieres QC G8T 2T4; Laval'64; (819)375-6282; Fax. (819)691-4048.

VINCENT, Serge; Clinique Med Pointe-Levy, 215 rue Saint-Omer, Levis QC G6V 8N3; Laval'78; (418)835-1767; Fax. (418)835-1787.

VINCENT-GAUDREAULT, Daphne; Centre Andre Boudreau, 910 rue Labelle, Saint-Jerome QC J7Z 5M5; Mon'09; CCFP; (450)432-1395

VINCENT O'KEEFE, Karine; Clinique Medicale, 13555 boul Lacroix, Saint-Georges QC G5Y 1P1; Laval'06; (418)228-8001

VINCER, Michael J; IWK Health Centre, PO Box 9700 Rpo CSC 5850 University Ave, Halifax NS B3K 6R8; Mem'77; FRCPC; Peds (Neonatology). Staff, IWK Health Centre; Assoc Prof Me/Med Dir, Dalhousie University; (902)470-6641; Fax. (902)470-6469.

VINCIC, Lydia M; St Joseph's Healthcare, 50 Charlton Ave E, Hamilton ON L8N 4A6; Ott'84; FRCPC; AnatPath. Staff, St Joseph's Healthcare - Charlton Campus; Assoc Prof, McMaster University; (905)522-1155; Fax. (905)521-6192; vincicl@ mcmaster.ca.

VINDEN, Christopher M; London HSC-Victoria Hosp, E2 218-800 Commissioners Rd E, London ON N6A 5W9; Qns'85; FRCSC; GenSurg. Staff, London Health Sciences Centre - Victoria Campus; Staff, St Joseph's Hospital - St Joseph's Health Care; Assoc Prof, University of Western Ontario; (519)685-8407; Fax. (519)685-8408.

VINDEN, G Dickson; 6 Matheson Beach RR 3, Beaverton ON L0K 1A0; London (England)'53; MB BS; DTMH; Assoc Staff, Ross Memorial Hospital; (705)426-2494; Fax. (705)426-2520; vindens@candlelight.ca.

VINER, Gary S; Ottawa Hosp-Family Med Ctre, 210 Melrose Ave, Ottawa ON K1Y 4K7; Tor'77; CCFP; FCFP; Staff, The Ottawa Hospital - General Campus; Assoc Prof Family Med, University of Ottawa; (613)761-4334; Fax. (613)761-4453.

VINER, Norman M; 533 Golden Ave, Ottawa ON K2A 2E6; Ott'81; (613)728-0399

VINER, Sidney M; Peter Lougheed Centre, ICU-3500 26 Ave NE, Calgary AB T1Y 6J4; Alb'83; ABIM; FRCPC; IntMed (Critical Care Medicine); Respir. Dep Head Critical Care, Peter Lougheed Centre; Staff, Alberta Health Services Calgary; Clin Assoc Prof, University of Calgary; (403)943-4310; Fax. (403)291-1491.

VINET, Elise; Hopital de la Enfant-Jesus, 1401 18e rue, Quebec QC G1J 1Z4; Laval'03; FRCPC; IntMed; Cardiol. Staff, Centre Hospitalier Affilié Universitaire de Québec - Hôpital De L'Enfant Jésus; (418)649-0252

VINET, Evelyne; MIUC-Royal Victoria Hosp, 687 av des Pins O, Montreal QC H3A 1A1; Mon'01; Rheum; IntMed. Staff, McGill University Health Centre - Montreal General Campus; Staff, McGill University Health Centre - Royal Victoria Hospital; (514)934-1934

VINET, Jean-Charles; CSSS Haut-Richelieu-Rouville, 920 boul du Seminaire N, St-Jean-sur-Richel QC J3A 1B7; Mon'05; DiagRad. Staff, Hôpital du Haut-Richelieu; (450)359-5000; Fax. (450)359-5251.

VINET, Pierre; 66 boul de la Concorde E, Laval QC H7G 4S4; Mon'67; (450)663-4014; vinet2@videotron.ca.

VINETTE, Christian; 501A rue Principale CP 520, Daveluyville QC G0Z 1C0; Sher'89; CCFP; FCFP; assoc Staff, Hôpital Sainte-croix; (819)367-2714; Fax. (819)367-2715.

VINETTE, Gaetan; Clinique Med Rock Forest, 1-4870 boul Bourque, Sherbrooke QC J1N 3S5; Sher'79; CCFP; Consultant, Centre Hospitalier Universitaire de Sherbrooke-Hôpital Hôtel-Dieu; (819)820-2673; Fax. (819)820-2112.

VINETTE, Stephane; Polyclinique Saint-Jerome, 102-200 rue Durand, Saint-Jerome QC J7Z 7E2; Mon'90; Staff, Hôtel-Dieu de Saint-Jérôme; (450)431-7666; Fax. (450)431-1275.

VINETTE-AZZI, Julie F; 21-5350 Canotek Rd, Gloucester ON K1J 9E2; Ott'00; CCFP; Staff, Montfort Hospital; Langs: Spanish; French; (613)747-1814; Fax. (613)747-0851.

VINH, Chuong; Ctr Hosp de LaSalle, 8585 Tsse Champlain, LaSalle QC H8P 1C1; Saigon (Vietnam)'84; Staff, Centre Hospitalier de LaSalle; (514)362-8000 x1661

VINH, Donald C; MUHC-Montreal Gen Hosp, A5 156-1650 av Cedar, Montreal QC H3G 1A4; McG'01; FRCPC; IntMed; MedMicrobiol; InfectDis. Staff, McGill University Health Centre - Montreal General Campus; (514)934-1934 x42419

VINNITSKY, Leonid; Central City Med Clinic, 3110-10153 King George Blvd, Surrey BC V3T 2W1; Sverlousk (Russia (Federation))'82; (604)951-0885; Fax. (604)951-0689.

VINSON, Robert S; Woodstock Gen Hosp, 310 Juliana Dr, Woodstock ON N4V 0A4; Sask'76; FRCPC; DiagRad. Staff, Woodstock General Hospital; (519)421-4204 x2362; Fax. (519)421-4241.

VIOLA, Raymond A; Queen's Univ-Palliative Care, 34 Barrie St, Kingston ON K7L 3J7; Tor'80; MSc(Epidem); CCFP; FCFP; Ac Staff, Kingston General Hospital; Ac Staff, Hotel-Dieu Hospital; Staff Cons, Providence Care - St Mary's of the Lake Hospital Site; Assoc Prof Health Sciences, Queen's University; (613)549-6666 x3223; Fax. (613)548-2436; rav@queensu.ca.

VIOLAGO, Francisco C; Winnipeg Clinic, 425 St Mary Ave, Winnipeg MB R3C 0N2; Santo Tomas (Philippines)'55; DABS; FACS; FRCSC; GenSurg; VascSurg. Ac Staff, St Boniface General Hospital; Asst Prof, University of Manitoba; (204)957-1900; Fax. (204)943-2164.

VIOLETTE, Chantal L; Clinique de Med Interne, 20 rue Carrier, Edmundston NB E3V 3Y1; Mon'98; ABIM; FRCPC; IntMed (Endocrinology). Staff IntMed, Hôpital regional d'Edmundston; Langs: Bilingual(French/English); (506)739-9511; Fax. (506)735-8118; clin.med.int@nb.aibn.com.

VIOLETTE, Claude P; Hôpital régional Chaleur, 1750 Sunset Dr, Bathurst NB E2A 4L7; Laval'93; FRCPC; IntMed (Cardiology). Staff IntMed, Hopital Regional Chaleur; Langs: Bilingual(French/English); (506)544-3000; Fax. (506)544-2460; claude.violette@vitalitenb.ca.

VIPLER, Christopher J; 140-4977 Trennant St, Delta BC V4K 2K5; UBC'07; CCFP; (604)946-7661

VIPLER, Sharon K; Panorama Village Med Clinic, 103-15157 Hwy 10, Surrey BC V3S 9A5; UBC'06; CCFP; (604)574-0481

VIPOND, Joseph C F; Foothills Med Centre, C231-1403 29 St NW, Calgary AB T2N 2T9; Alb'96; CCFP; CCFP(E.M.); FCFP; Staff, Foothills Medical Centre; (403)944-1596; Fax. (403)944-2419.

VIPULANANTHAN, Manohary; Brandon Reg Health Centre, AP1-150 McTavish Ave E, Brandon MB R7A 2B3; Colombo (Sri Lanka)'73; MB BS; FRCPC; Psy. Staff, Brandon Regional Health Centre; Langs: Tamil; (204)578-4000

VIPULANANTHAN, Velluppillai; Medical Arts Bldg, 339 Princess Ave, Brandon MB R7A 0N7; Ceylon (Sri Lanka)'73; MB BS; FRCPC; Psy.

VIRA, Farzana; Univ Hlth Network-Toronto Gen, E14 217-200 Elizabeth St, Toronto ON M5G 2C4; Tor'10; Staff, Toronto General Hospital - UHN; (416)340-3155

VIRANI, Hakique N; 10419 102 Ave NW, Edmonton AB T5J 0B4; Cal'01; FRCPC; CommunMed. (780)429-3991; Fax. (780)429-3988.

VIRANI, Mirza R; 112-7155 Woodbine Ave, Markham ON L3R 1A3; Shiraz (Iran)'78; Langs: Urdu; Hindi; Persian; Swahili; (905)470-7999; Fax. (905)470-6333.

VIRANI, Noordin; Creekside Med Clinic, 4-12192 Symons Valley Rd NW, Calgary AB T3P 0A3; (Norway)'90; MSc; DHA; (403)275-6606; Fax. (403)730-0941.

VIRANI, Noorshina S; Foothills Med Centre, 1403 29 St NW, Calgary AB T2N 2T9; Qns'96; FRCP; FRCPC; PhysMed&Rehab (Pain Management). Staff, Foothills Medical Centre; Clinical Asst Prof Neurosciences, University of Calgary; (403)944-4475; Fax. (403)283-2526.

VIRANI, Shaheena; Burnaby Ctr for Mental Hlth &, 3405 Willingdon Ave, Burnaby BC V5G 3H4; (Saint Kitts-Nevis)'99; (604)875-4111

VIRANI, Shahnawaz A; Gordon & Leslie Diamond HCC, 9F-2775 Laurel St, Vancouver BC V5Z 1M9; UBC'99; MSc; ABIM; MPH; FRCPC; IntMed (Heart Failure); Cardiol (Heart Failure). Staff, Vancouver General Hospital - Centennial Pavillion; Assoc Dean, Gordon & Leslie Diamond Health Care Centre; (604)875-5092; Fax. (604)875-5761.

VIRDEE, Manjit S; McLaughlin Village Med Clinic, 85 Steeles Ave W, Brampton ON L6Y 0K3; Poona (India)'86; CCFP; FCFP; Ac Staff Family Med, The Credit Valley Hospital; Langs: Hindi; Punjabi; Urdu; (905)455-9374; Fax. (905)455-9505.

VIRDY, Kiran; MCI The Doctors Office, 4099 Erin Mills Pky, Mississauga ON L5L 3P9; Tor'96; BSc(Hons.); CCFP; (905)820-3310; Fax. (905)820-3312; woodlandmedical@gmail.com.

VIREY, Maselle G; King Street Med Arts Centre, 300-71 King St W, Mississauga ON L5B 4A2; University of the Philippines (Philippines)'78; BSc; DPsy; DABPN; DPsy; FRCPC; Psy. Court Consultant, Trillium Health Centre - Mississauga; Staff, Trillium Health Partners-Mississauga; Lecturer, University of Toronto; Langs: Tagalog; (905)896-1302; Fax. (905)896-8223.

VIRGILI, Philippe C; Hop Reg d'Edmundston, 275 Hebert Blvd, Edmundston NB E3V 4E4; Nice (France)'78; Staff, Hôpital regional d'Edmundston; (506)739-2211; Fax. (506)739-2231.

VIRICK, Mohan S; 316 Rear Kings Rd, Sydney NS B1S 1A8; Christian Medical College (India)'61; MB BS; MPH(Johns Hopkins); Langs: Punjabi; Hindi; Urdu; Burmese; (902)539-6049; Fax. (902)539-4681.

VIRJI, Mumtaz A; BC Children's Hosp, 2D 17-4480 Oak St, Vancouver BC V6H 3V4; Karachi (Pakistan)'89; MB BS; FRCPC; Peds (Nephrology). Staff Peds, BC Children's Hospital; Langs: Kacchi; Urdu; Gujarati; Hindi; (604)875-2130; Fax. (604)875-3021.

VIRK, Roohina; Beaufort Delta Health Social S, PO Bag Service 2, Inuvik NT X0E 0T0; UBC'07; CCFP; Staff Medical Doctors Office, Beaufort-Delta Health & Social Services Authority Inuvik Public Health Unit; (867)777-7246

VIRMANI, Achla R; Douglas Mental Hlth Univ Inst, 6875 boul Lasalle, Verdun QC H4H 1R3; Delhi (India)'80; Staff, Douglas Mental Health University Institute; Langs: Bilingual(French/English); Hindi; Punjabi; Urdu; (514)761-6131; achla.virmani@douglas.mcgill.ca.

VIRMANI, Vivek; The Ottawa Hosp-Gen Campus, 501 Smyth Rd, Ottawa ON K1H 8L6; Aligarh Muslim University (Other Foreign)'02; Staff, The Ottawa Hospital - General Campus; (613)737-8571

VIRRO, Michael R; Markham Fertility Centre, 5F-379 Church St, Markham ON L6B 0T1; Tor'83; FRCSC; ObstGyn (Fertility). Staff, Markham Stouffville Hospital; (905)472-7128; Fax. (905)472-4994; mvirro@interhop.net.

VISBAL AMADOR, Fernando A; 390 Lincoln St, Welland ON L3B 4N4; Bogota (Colombia)'79; FRCPC; Peds. Aj Asst Prof, McMaster University; Langs: Spanish; (905)788-1777; Fax. (905)788-1779.

VISBAL MORENO, A Luis; Kirkland & District Hosp, 313-145 Government Rd E, Kirkland Lake ON P2N 3P4; Cartagena (Colombia)'90; FRCSC; GenSurg. Staff, Kirkland & District Hospital; (705)568-2232; Fax. (705)568-2234.

VISCH, Shawn H R; Plessis Med Centre, 12-801 Regent Ave W, Winnipeg MB R2C 3A7; Man'90; CCFP; FCFP; Staff, Concordia General Hospital; (204)222-4200; Fax. (204)222-8181.

VISCHER, Gisela H; Lions Gate Hosp, 231 15th St E, North Vancouver BC V7L 2L7; Freiburg (Germany)'74; FRCPC; GenPath; AnatPath. Staff Lab Services, Lions Gate Hospital; Langs: German; (604)984-5765; Fax. (604)984-5805.

VISCHOFF, Daniel; Hôpital Ste-Justine, 3175 ch Cote-Sainte-Catherine, Montreal QC H3T 1C5; Lausanne (Switzerland)'80; FRCPC; Anes (P.Q.). Staff, Hôpital Ste-Justine; (514)345-4733; Fax. (514)345-4601.

VISCONTI, Vincenzo; Brentwood Medical, 78 Athabascan Ave, Sherwood Park AB T8A 4E3; Alb'81; Staff, University of Alberta Hospital; (780)467-0083; Fax. (780)464-6770.

VISENTIN, Diana E; D-566 Bryne Dr, Barrie ON L4N 9P6; McM'95; BScN; FRCP; FRCPC; IntMed (Cardiology). Staff, Royal Victoria Regional Health Centre; Langs: Italian; (705)735-4682; Fax. (705)735-4684; de.visentin@sympatico.ca.

VISENTIN, Laura M; Findlay Creek Med Centre, 4744 Bank St, Ottawa ON K1T 0K8; McM'09; CCFP; (613)317-2584; Fax. (613)822-2775.

VISKARI, Danny A; 6435 Dixon Dam Rd, Vernon BC V1B 3J9; UBC'93; FRCPC; Anes. Staff, Vernon Jubilee Hospital; (250)558-3316

VISKONTAS, Darius G; 403-233 Nelson's Cres, New Westminster BC V3L 0E4; Ott'00; FRCSC; OrthSurg (Lower Extremity Reconstruction). (604)777-5577; Fax. (604)777-5644.

VISRAM, Farzin M; Hamilton HS-Henderson Site, 711 Concession St, Hamilton ON L8V 1C3; Tor'95; FRCPC; IntMed; Critical Care Medicine; Respir. Staff, Hamilton Health Sciences Centre-Juravinski Site; (905)389-4411

VISRAM, Hasina; The Ottawa Hosp-Riverside, 1967 Riverside Dr, Ottawa ON K1H 7W9; Qns'08; FRCPC; IntMed. Staff, The Ottawa Hospital - Riverside Campus; (613)722-7000

VISSER, Francois C; Centennial Ctr for Mental Heal, PO Box 1000 Stn Main, Ponoka AB T4J 1R8; Kansas (USA)'94; CCFP; Staff, Centennial Centre for Mental Health & Brain Injury; (403)783-7643; Fax. (403)783-7790.

VISSER, Gerhardt; The Brandon Clinic, 620 Dennis St, Brandon MB R7A 5E7; Pretoria (South Africa)'95; MB ChB; LMCC; (204)728-4440; Fax. (204)726-1765.

VISSER, Hendrik A; Wholeness Family Clinic, PO Box 90, Crapaud PE C0A 1J0; Dal'78; (902)658-2000

VISSER, Hermann B; Medical Arts Clinic, 103-650 Terminal Ave S, Nanaimo BC V9R 5E2; CCFP; Staff, Cross Lake Nursing Station; (250)753-3431

VISSER, Karen A L; Harmony Med Centre, 110-152 Cleopatra Dr, Ottawa ON K2G 5X2; Wes'04; FRCSC; ObstGyn. (613)725-1870; Fax. (613)725-1647.

VISSER, Pieter J; Medical Midtown Clinic, 902 3 Ave, Wainwright AB T9W 1C5; Stellenbosch (South Africa)'86; MB ChB; Langs: Afrikaans; (780)842-6750; Fax. (780)842-6730.

VISSER, Shaun L; Montfort Hosp, 713 Montreal Rd, Ottawa ON K1K 0T2; McG'95; CCFP; CCFP(E.M.); Staff, Montfort Hospital; Langs: English; French; (613)746-4621

VISVANATHA, Lakshmi V; 104-6404 Bowness Rd NW, Calgary AB T3B 0E7; Alb'87; (403)288-3733; Fax. (403)288-8081.

VISVANATHA, Susmita A; Bramalea Med Group, 500-18 Kensington Rd, Brampton ON L6T 4S5; Tor'98; CCFP; FCFP; (905)791-7575; Fax. (905)791-7532.

VISVANATHAN, Kishore; Medical Arts Bldg, 537-750 Spadina Cres E, Saskatoon SK S7K 3H3; Sask'85; Dip; FRCSC; Urol. Div Head Urol, Saskatoon Health Region; Clin Assoc Prof Surg, University of Saskatchewan; (306)653-3255; Fax. (306)653-4386.

VITALE, George D; Foothills Med Centre, 210-1403 29 St NW, Calgary AB T2N 2T9; Ott'99; Nephrol; IntMed. Staff, Foothills Medical Centre; (403)944-2510; Fax. (403)944-3199.

VITALE, William R; 2962 Oxford St, Halifax NS B3L 2W4; McG'76; BS(Summa Cum Laude); MA; PhD; MDCM; FRCPC; Peds (Adolescent Medicine). Assoc Staff, IWK Health Centre; (902)425-3919; Fax. (902)425-3919.

VITALI, Aleksander M; Royal University Hosp, 103 Hospital Dr, Saskatoon SK S7N 0W8; FRCSC; Neursurg. Staff Neurosurg, Royal University Hospital; (306)655-1364; Fax. (306)655-1258.

VITARO, Maryann; Salus Med Centre, 6-3603 Langstaff Rd, Woodbridge ON L4L 9G7; Ott'98; CCFP; Langs: Croatian; (905)856-0771; Fax. (905)856-1619; mvitaro@rogers.com.

VITHALAL, Neetha; Exeter Med Clinic, PO Box 879, 100 Mile House BC V0K 2E0; Witwatersrand (South Africa)'91; MB ChB; CCFP; (250)395-2271; Fax. (250)395-2599.

VITOU, Constantine K; 2101 boul Graham O, Mont-Royal QC H3R 1H6; McG'50; CCFP; FCFP; (514)342-9971; Fax. (514)735-0241.

VITOU, Louise Y; 302A-475 Park St, Kitchener ON N2G 4V5; McG'88; FRCPC; IntMed; Critical Care Medicine; Nephrol. Staff Nephrol, Grand River Hospital - Kitchener/Waterloo Health Centre; Langs: English; French; (519)743-9309; Fax. (519)743-9726.

VITUG, Gene A S; Foothills Prof Bldg, 150-1620 29 St NW, Calgary AB T2N 4L7; Alb'95; CCFP; (403)282-3200; Fax. (403)398-1322.

VITULLO, Bennedetto B; Queen Elizabeth Hosp, PO Box 6600 Stn Central, Charlottetown PE C1A 8T5; McG'75; FAAP; FRCPC; Peds (Neonatology). Staff, Queen Elizabeth Hospital; Langs: Spanish; Italian; French; (902)894-2111

VIVIAN, Anthony C H; Hodgins Prof Bldg, 205-45625 Hodgins Ave, Chilliwack BC V2P 1P2; London (England)'71; ABIM; MRC; MB BS; FRCPC; IntMed. Langs: English; French; (604)792-5540; Fax. (604)792-9284.

VIVIAN, Laura D; Dr Charles A Janeway Child HC, 300 Prince Philip Dr, St. John's NL A1B 3V6; Mem'04; FRCPC; Peds. Staff, Janeway Children's Health & Rehabilitation Centre; Staff, Health Sciences Centre; (709)777-4349

VIVIAN, Mark A; Health Sciences Centre, GA216-820 Sherbrook St, Winnipeg MB R3A 1R9; Man'06; FRCPC; DiagRad. Staff, Health Sciences Centre; (204)774-8511

VIVIER, Hester C; Fort Langley Med Clinic, PO Box 99 Stb Fort Langley 23148 96 Ave, Langley BC V1M 2R4; Stellenbosch (South Africa)'87; MB ChB; CCFP; (604)888-2433

VIVIERS, George F; Niagara Med Prof Centre, PO Box 10 1882 Niagara Stone Rd, Niagara-on-the-Lke ON L0S 1T0; (South Africa)'96; MB ChB; CCFP; (905)468-3275; Fax. (905)468-7960; gviviers@niagara.com.

VIVIERS, Willem F; Battlefords Union Hosp, 1092 107th St, North Battleford SK S9A 1Z1; Staff, Battlefords Union Hospital; (306)446-6600

VIVODA, Edward E; Family Practice & Sports Med, 34A Sydenham St E, Aylmer ON N5H 1L2; Tor'77; ABCFP; CCFP; Court Staff Privil, Tillsonburg District Memorial Hospital; Court Staff Privil, St Thomas Elgin General Hospital; Aj Prof Family Practice, University of Western Ontario; (519)765-1960; Fax. (519)765-2971.

VIVONA, Angelo A; Markham Stouffville Health Ctr, 402-377 Church St, Markham ON L6B 1A1; Tor'94; FRCSC; GenSurg. Staff, Markham Stouffville Hospital; Langs: Italian; (905)472-7122; Fax. (905)472-2290; angelo.vivona@utoronto.ca.

VIZEL, Michael J; 12-250 Wincott Dr, Etobicoke ON M9R 2R5; McG'90; ABIM; FACP; Langs: Bilingual(English/French); (416)249-0002; Fax. (416)249-0842.

VIZEL, Saul; Medical Arts Bldg, 1-715 Coronation Blvd, Cambridge ON N1R 7R1; McG'81; ABIM; FACC; FRCPC; IntMed; Cardiol. Ac Staff, Cambridge Memorial Hospital; Langs: English; French; (519)622-0067; Fax. (519)623-6355.

VIZHUL, Andrey I; Univ Hlth Network-Toronto Gen, EN1 420-200 Elizabeth St, Toronto ON M5G 2C4; Dniepropetrovsk State Medical Academy (Ukraine)'89; Staff, Toronto General Hospital - UHN; (416)340-4363

VIZSOLYI, Peter T; 3461 Cook St, Victoria BC V8X 1B3; UBC'81; CCFP; FCFP; (250)386-6161; Fax. (250)382-0613.

VLAAR, Henry J; 207-45 Stanley St, Ayr ON N0B 1E0; Wes'83; Staff, The Brant Community Healthcare System - Brantford General Hospital Site; Staff, The Brant Community Healthcare System - Willett Hospital Site; Langs: Dutch; (519)632-9153; Fax. (519)632-9578.

VLACHAKI, Maria T; BC Cancer Agency-Vancouver, 2410 Lee Ave, Victoria BC V8R 6V5; Athens (Greece)'87; Staff, BC Cancer Agency Vancouver Island Centre; (250)519-5594

VLACHOS, Helen; CHUS-Hop Fleurimont, 3001 12e av N, Sherbrooke QC J1H 5N4; McG'91; FRCPC; Peds (Neonatology); Respir. Staff, Centre Hospitalier Universitaire de Sherbrooke-Hopital Fleurimont; Langs: Greek; French; (819)346-1110 x14851; Fax. (819)564-5215.

VLADARS, Josef M A; 205-1135 Adelaide St N, London ON N5Y 5K7; Wes'80; CCFP; FCFP; (519)672-5910; Fax. (519)672-3991.

VLAHOS, Donna S; SGH Medical Mall, 205-3030 Lawrence Ave E, Scarborough ON M1P 2T7; Tor'90; CCFP; FCFP; Ac Staff Family Pract, The Scarborough Hospital - General Campus; Langs: Greek; (416)439-7968; Fax. (416)439-3088.

VLAHOS, Susan D; North Shore Treatment Centre, 20A-700 Tranquille Rd, Kamloops BC V2B 3H9; Dal'86; BSc; Ac Staff, Royal Inland Hospital; (250)554-4265

VLAHOVICH, Alexandra R; Halton Healthcare-Georgetown, 1 Princess Anne Dr, Georgetown ON L7G 2B8; Qns'05; CCFP; Ac Staff, Halton Healthcare Services Corporation - Georgetown Hospital; (905)873-0111; Fax. (905)873-2953.

VLAHOVICH, Josip; Dufferin Med Clinic, 2045 Dufferin St, Toronto ON M6E 3R4; Zagreb (Croatia)'65; Assoc Staff, Centre for Addiction & Mental Health (CAMH) - Queen Site; Langs: Croatian; Serbian; (416)656-6500

VLAHOVICH, Slavica; Canadian Forces Hlth Serv Grou, 118-1745 Alta Vista Dr, Ottawa ON K1A 0K6; Ott'79; BSc; Staff, Canadian Forces Health Services Centre; Langs: Bilingual(English/French); (613)945-6896; Fax. (613)945-6668.

VLAOVIC, Branislav; O'Connor Doctor Office, 20-1450 O'Connor Dr, East York ON M4B 2T8; Belgrade (Serbia)'66; Staff, Toronto East General Hospital Inc; Langs: Croatian; Serbian; (416)285-4075

VLAOVIC, Peter D; 305KW-650 Sammon Ave, East York ON M4C 5M5; Tor'99; BSc; FRCSC; Urol (Endoscopy). Staff, Toronto East General Hospital Inc; Lecturer, University of Toronto; Langs: Serbian; (416)465-6008; Fax. (416)465-3901; pvlao@tegh.on.ca.

VLASSCHAERT, John J; Alexander Prof Bldg, 201-849 Alexander Crt, Peterborough ON K9J 7H8; Qns'79; FRCPC; IntMed (Critical Care Medicine); Respir. Staff, Peterborough Regional Health Centre - Hospital Drive; (705)749-2727; Fax. (705)749-2788.

VLATTEN, Arnim; Queen Elizabeth II HSC, 1276 South Park St, Halifax NS B3H 2Y9; Ulm (Germany)'97; Staff, Queen Elizabeth II Health Sciences Centre - Victoria General Site; (902)473-3866

VLCKOVA, Ludmila; Cannon Clinic, 4-2151 McCallum Rd, Abbotsford BC V2S 3N9; Purkyne (Czech Republic)'83; Staff, Abbotsford Regional Hospital & Cancer Centre; Langs: Czech; (604)853-3314; Fax. (604)853-2171.

VLIAGOFTIS, Harissios; Heritage Med Research Centre, 550A-107 University Campus NW, Edmonton AB T6G 2S2; (Greece)'87; Staff, University of Alberta Hospital; Asst Prof Med, University of Alberta; (780)407-7225; Fax. (780)492-5329; hari@ualberta.ca.

VLOK, Nicolaas C; Brandon Clinic, 620 Dennis St, Brandon MB R7A 5E7; Orange Free State (South Africa)'97; MB ChB; LMCC; CCFP; Langs: Afrikaans; (204)728-4440

VO, H D David; CMH Med Centre, 111-1315 Finch Ave W, North York ON M3J 2G6; Hue (Vietnam)'89; CCFP; Langs: Vietnamese; (416)631-6888; Fax. (416)631-6887.

VO, Khanh Hong; Family Med Clinic, 108-2065 Finch Ave W, North York ON M3N 2V7; Hue (Vietnam)'89; CCFP; Staff, Humber River Regional Hospital - Finch Avenue Site; Langs: Vietnamese; (416)746-7506; Fax. (416)746-7553.

VO, Kim; Centre Hosp Fleury, 2180 rue Fleury E, Montreal QC H2B 1K3; Mon'98; FRCSC; GenSurg. Staff, Centre Hospitalier Fleury; (514)381-9311

VO, Minh Ha; Medicentre Lasalle, 207-1500 av Dollard, LaSalle QC H8N 1T5; Sher'91; Langs: Vietnamese; English; (514)366-5732; Fax. (514)366-2474.

VO, Minh Nhat; St. Boniface Gen Hosp, Y3543-409 Tache Ave, Winnipeg MB R2H 2A6; Staff, St Boniface General Hospital; mvo@sbgh.mb.ca.

VO, Tai Thuan; Hop Louis-H Lafontaine, 7401 rue Hochelaga, Montreal QC H1N 3M5; Saigon (Vietnam)'77; Staff, Hopital Louis-H Lafontaine; (514)251-4000; Fax. (514)251-8474.

VO, Tan Tai; 725 6e rue, Val-d'Or QC J9P 3Y1; '74; FRCPC; AnatPath. Staff Med Biol & Path, Centre Hospitalier de Val d'Or; Langs: French; Vietnamese; (819)825-6711; Fax. (819)825-7942; vo_tan_tai@hotmail.com.

VO, Thanh Truc; Hopital Charles-Lemoyne, 3120 boul Taschereau, Longueuil QC J4V 2H1; Mon'02; FRCSC; GenSurg; VascSurg. Staff, Hopital Charles LeMoyne; Staff, Centre Hospitalier Universitaire de Sherbrooke-Hopital Fleurimont; (450)466-5000

VO, Thi Minh D; Medicentre Lasalle, 207-1500 av Dollard, LaSalle QC H8N 1T5; Mon'97; CCFP; Staff Centre Ambulatoire Geriatrie, Hopital de la Cite de la santé; Médecin, Medicentre Lasalle; Langs: Vietnamese; English; (514)766-0546; Fax. (514)765-3265.

VO, Thi Minh T; Ctre d'Hebergement Champlain, 1325 rue Crawford, Verdun QC H4H 2N6; Sher'93; (514)766-8513

VO, Thi Nhu Y; Centre de Med Fam de Gatineau, 201-908 boul Maloney E, Gatineau QC J8P 1H5; Mon'86; Staff, Centre Hospitalier Gatineau Mémorial; Clin Instructor, University of Ottawa; Langs: Vietnamese; English; (819)663-7711; Fax. (819)663-9326.

VO, Thoi Hen; 1380 Queen St W, Toronto ON M6K 1L7; Saigon (Vietnam)'67; Langs: Vietnamese; French; (416)603-1300; Fax. (416)603-1301.

VO, Thuy Tien; Plexo du Sanctuaire, 106-6100 av du Boise, Montreal QC H3S 2W1; Mon'01; FRCPC; Peds; PedEmergMed. Médecin, Medi-Club Au Sanctuaire; (514)739-5646

VO, Thuy-Quynh; CSSS de Manicouagan, 635 rue Joliet, Baie-Comeau QC G5C 1P1; Mon'08; Staff, Centre Hospitalier Régional Baie-Comeau; (418)589-3701

VO, Tuyet Bach; 2-2721 Jane St, North York ON M3L 1S3; Saigon (Vietnam)'78; GenPath (General Practice). Langs: Vietnamese; (416)748-0803; Fax. (416)748-0677.

VO-DOAN, Kim-Loan; Centre ORL Jean-Talon, 203-1384 rue Jean-Talon E, Montreal QC H2E 1S3; Sher'88; DABOph; FRCSC; Otol (Head & Neck Surgery). Staff, CSSS du Coeur de l'Isle Hôpital Jean-Talon; Staff, Hopital Charles LeMoyne; Langs: Vietnamese; English; (514)273-4461; Fax. (514)273-8401.

VO NGUYEN, Lan; Fraser Health Authority, 260 Sherbrooke St, New Westminster BC V3L 3M2; Wes'98; FRCPC; Anes. Staff, Royal Columbian Hospital; Langs: Vietnamese; (604)520-4602

VO-TIGLEY, Emilie T; Royal Oak Centre, 192-8888 Country Hills Blvd NW, Calgary AB T3G 5T4; Cal'98; CCFP; (403)239-3660; Fax. (403)239-4001.

VO VAN, Tuyen; 766 rue Rachel E, Montreal QC H2J 2H5; Mon'84; (514)521-6253

VOADEN, M E Carol; Lawrence Park Med Centre, G8-250 Lawrence Ave W, Toronto ON M5M 1B2; Tor'60; Ac Staff Family Med, North York General Hospital; (416)789-7691; Fax. (416)789-7692.

VOBECKY, J Suzanne; Hôpital Ste-Justine, 3175 Ch Cote-Sainte-Catherine, Montreal QC H3T 1C5; Sher'80; FRCSC; GenSurg; Cardiovasc&ThorSurg (Pediatric Cardiac Surgery). ac Staff, Hôpital Ste-Justine; Langs: Czech; English; (514)345-4676; Fax. (514)345-4917; suzanne_vobecky@ssss.gouv.qc.ca.

VOCELLE, Josee; CSSS de Beauce-Etchemin, 1515 17e rue, Saint-Georges QC G5Y 4T8; Laval'94; Staff, Centre Hospitalier Beauce-Etchemin; (418)228-2031

VOCKENTANZ, Birgit M; Bradley Med Centre, 595 Bradley Ave, London ON N6E 3Z8; Tor'90; (519)680-1721; Fax. (519)680-0434.

VODUC, Kim D; BC Cancer Agency-Vancouver CC, 600 10th Ave W, Vancouver BC V5Z 4E6; Tor'00; FRCPC; RadOncol. Staff, BC Cancer Agency Vancouver Centre; (604)877-6000; Fax. (604)930-4065.

VODUC, Nha; The Ottawa Hosp-Gen Campus, 211-501 Smyth Rd, Ottawa ON K1H 8L6; McG'97; FRCPC; IntMed; Respir. Staff Respirol, The Ottawa Hospital - General Campus; Asst Prof, University of Ottawa; (613)737-8198; Fax. (613)737-8537.

VOEGELIN, Richard E; 102-527 Admiral St, Woodstock ON N4S 5B2; Wes'76; FRCSC; Urol. Consultant, Tillsonburg District Memorial Hospital; Ac Staff, Woodstock General Hospital; Consultant, Alexandra Hospital; (519)539-8575; Fax. (519)539-2994; voegelinr@execulink.com.

VOETMANN, Susanne; Family Practice Clinic, 2778 104 St, Nanaimo BC V9R 2N2; UBC'85; (250)758-1711

VOEUK, Anna; PO Box 52177 Rpo Garneau, Edmonton AB T6G 2T5; Cal'06; CCFP.

VOGEL, Christine P; Guelph Family Health Team, 101-83 Dawson Rd, Guelph ON N1H 1B1; McM'98; CCFP; (519)766-1360

VOGEL, Judith A; Institute of Comm & Family Psy, 150-4333 ch Cote-Sainte-Cather, Montreal QC H3T 1E4; Man'73; FRCPC; Psy (P.Q.) (Family Psychiatry). (514)340-8226

VOGEL, Martin V; McArthur Family Medical, 311 McArthur Ave, Ottawa ON K1L 8M3; Cape Town (South Africa)'85; MB ChB; Member, Canadian Medical Association; Langs: Afrikaans; martin@sma.sk.ca.

VOGEL, Philip L; 4825 50th St PO Box 939, Stettler AB T0C 2L0; (South Africa)'95; MB ChB; LMCC; (403)742-4011; Fax. (403)742-4013.

VOGES-MARTINEZ, Armando; Campbellton Med Clinic, 10 Village Ave, Campbellton NB E3N 3S8; (Mexico)'73; (506)789-0119; Fax. (506)675-2156.

VOGLER, Rachel A; Pacific Med Clinic, 3185 Grandview Hwy, Vancouver BC V5M 2E9; Qns'08; CCFP; (604)434-2222

VOGLIMACCI-STEPHANOPOLI, P; Ctr Hosp Rouyn-Noranda, 4 9e rue, Rouyn-Noranda QC J9X 2B2; Mon'82; FRCPC; IntMed. Staff, Centre Hospitalier Rouyn-Noranda; (819)764-5131

VOGRINCIC, Gerard S; Lions Gate Hosp, 231 15th St E, North Vancouver BC V7L 2L7; Alb'87; FRCPC; GenPath. Staff Path, Lions Gate Hospital; (604)984-5760

VOGT, Kelly; London HSC-University Hosp, PO Box 5339 Stn Main 339 Windermere Rd, London ON N6A 5C1; Wes'07; GenSurg. Staff, London Health Sciences Centre - University Hospital; (519)663-3269

VOGT, Lori A; Mental Health Bldg, 4500 Oak Bay St Box 156, Vancouver BC V6H 3N1; Man'82; BSc; CCST; MD; FRCP; FRCPC; Psy (Child & Adolescent Psychiatry). Consultant Ped Psy, Victoria General Hospital; Staff, Eating Disorder Program in the Capital Region; (604)875-2783

VOGT, Victoria L; Meadow Lake Assoc Clinic, PO Box 1510, Meadow Lake SK S9X 1Z1; Sask'04; CCFP; Staff Internet Consultent, Northern Medical Services; (306)236-5661; Fax. (306)236-4355.

VOHRA, Angeli; Upper Appleby Prof Centre, 26-1960 Appleby Line, Burlington ON L7L 0B7; Ott'05; CCFP; (905)335-6142; Fax. (905)335-5929.

VOHRA, Anita; Taddle Creek Family Health Team, 304-790 Bay St, Toronto ON M5G 1N8; Dal'98; FRCPC; Psy. Staff, Centre for Addiction & Mental Health (CAMH) - Russell Street Site; (416)801-1004; Fax. (416)977-0974.

VOHRA, Asha D; Upper Appleby Prof Centre, 26-1960 Appleby Line, Burlington ON L7L 0B7; Punjab (India)'72; Langs: Punjabi; Hindi; (905)335-9266; Fax. (905)335-5929.

VOHRA, Geeta B; Huntingwood Med Clinic, 2361 Warden Ave, Scarborough ON M1T 1V7; Tor'97; CCFP; (416)299-4999; Fax. (416)299-1422.

VOHRA, Manoj; Colchester East Hants HC, 600 Abenaki Rd, Truro NS B2N 5A1; Dal'88; CCFP; Staff, Colchester East Hants Health Centre; (902)893-5554; Fax. (902)893-2443.

VOHRA, Rajat; 162 Huston St PO Box 419, Burks Falls ON P0A 1C0; Wes'93; BSc; CCFP; Staff Physician, Algonquin Health Centre; Asst Prof Med, Northern Ontario School of Medicine-Laurentian University; (705)382-0002; Fax. (705)382-2220; rajsterv@hotmail.com.

VOHRA, Sanjeev; Surrey Specialized Seniors Cli, 3B-9750 140 St, Surrey BC V3T 0G0; Punjab (Pakistan)'92; MB BS; BSc; FRCPC; IntMed; GeriatricMed. Staff, Surrey Memorial Hospital; Staff, Jim Pattison Outpatient Care and Surgery Centre; (604)582-4550 x76413

VOHRA, Sukh C; Upper Appleby Prof Centre, 26-1960 Appleby Line, Burlington ON L7L 0B7; Punjab (India)'80; Langs: Hindi; Punjabi; (905)335-9266; Fax. (905)335-5929.

VOHRA, Sunita; Edmonton Gen Continuing Care, 8B19-11111 Jasper Ave NW, Edmonton AB T5K 0L4; Dal'94; FRCPC; Peds (Clinical Pharmacology). Staff Stollery Children's Hosp, University of Alberta; (780)342-8592

VOICE, Sandra D; SGH Medical Mall, 512-3030 Lawrence Ave E, Scarborough ON M1P 2T7; Alb'79; FRCSC; PlasSurg. Staff, The Scarborough Hospital - General Campus; Hd PlasSurg, Cosmetic Surgery Hospital; Staff, William Osler Health System - Etobicoke General Hospital; (905)851-7701; Fax. (905)856-4406; voice@sympatico.ca.

VOIGT, Robert F; Spectrum Health, 702-1080 Howe St, Vancouver BC V6Z 2T1; UBC'84; Assoc Staff, Providence Health Care - St Paul's Hospital; Clin Instructor Med, University of British Columbia; (604)681-1080; Fax. (604)681-0244.

VOIGTLANDER-BOLZ, Julia I M; St Michael's Hosp, 30 Bond St, Toronto ON M5B 1W8; Ludwig Maximilian University at Munich (Other Foreign)'98; Staff, St Michael's Hospital; (416)864-5071

VOINESKOS, Aristotle N; Addiction & Mental Hlth-Clarke, 250 College St, Toronto ON M5T 1R8; Tor'03; FRCPC; Psy. Staff, Centre for Addiction & Mental Health (CAMH) - College Street Site; (416)535-8501

VOINESKOS, George; Addiction & Mental Hlth-Clarke, 250 College St, Toronto ON M5T 1R8; Athens (Greece)'62; DPM(Eng); MRC; FRCPC; Psy (Couples & Family Therapy). Sr Psychiatrist/Teacher, Centre for Addiction & Mental Health (CAMH) - College Street Site; Prof Psy, University of Toronto; Langs: Greek; (416)979-6804; Fax. (416)979-6815.

VOINOV, Valentin; Lakeridge Health Oshawa, 1 Hospital Crt, Oshawa ON L1G 2B9; Medical University of Debrecen (Hungary)'06; Staff, Lakeridge Health - Oshawa Site; (905)576-8711

VOISINE, Claude; Polyclinique, 208-874 boul de l'Universite E, Chicoutimi QC G7H 6B9; Laval'65; FRCPC; Psy (P.Q.). (418)545-4488; Fax. (418)545-4782; claudevoisine@videotron.ca.

VOISINE, Jean-Francois; CSSS de Chicoutimi, CP 264 305 rue Saint-Vallier, Chicoutimi QC G7H 5H6; Laval'97; Psy. Staff, Complexe hospitalier de la Sagamie; Staff, Institut Roland-Saucier; (418)549-5477

VOISINE, Pierre; Hôpital Laval, 2725 ch Sainte-Foy, Quebec QC G1V 4G5; Mon'96; FRCSC; CardSurg. Staff, Hôpital Laval; Langs: Bilingual(English/French); (418)656-4717; Fax. (418)656-4707; pierre.voisine@chg.ulaval.ca.

VOJDANI, Merle A; Grand River Hosp-K-W HC, PO Box 9056 Stn C 835 King St W, Kitchener ON N2G 1G3; Manila (Philippines)'81; Staff, Grand River Hospital - Kitchener/Waterloo Health Centre; (519)749-4300

VOJDANI, O Kyle A; Toronto East Gen & Orth Hosp, 825 Coxwell Ave, East York ON M4C 3E7; Mem'05; CCFP; CCFP(E.M.); Staff, Toronto East General Hospital Inc; (416)469-6580

VOJVODICH, Sandra M; Credit Valley Prof Bldg, 207-2300 Eglinton Ave W, Mississauga ON L5M 2V8; Alb'90; FRCSC; Otol (Head & Neck Surgery). Staff, Trillium Health Centre - Mississauga; Staff, The Credit Valley Hospital; (905)820-8952; Fax. (905)820-8306.

VOKAC, Ludmila; Don Mills Family Health Team, 200-20 Wynford Dr, North York ON M3C 1J4; Karlova (Czech Republic)'75; Court Staff, Sunnybrook Health Sciences Centre; Langs: Czech; (416)444-6161; Fax. (416)444-5792.

VOKEY, Keith A; Carbonear Gen Hosp, 86 Highroad South, Carbonear NL A1Y 1A4; Mem'99; FRCPC; Psy. Staff, Carbonear General Hospital; (709)945-5022

VOKEY, Susan E; Southside Hlth & Life Mgmt Ctr, 2-2120 Regent St, Sudbury ON P3E 3Z9; Mem'87; FRCSC; OrthSurg (Hand & Upper Extremity Surgery). Staff (All Sites), Health Sciences North-St Joseph's Health Centre; (705)522-9101; Fax. (705)522-5744.

VOLDENG, Jason S; Grey Nuns Community Hosp, 5027-1100 Youville Drive West, Edmonton AB T6L 5X8; Man'05; CCFP; Staff, Covenant Health - Grey Nuns Community Hospital; (780)735-7000

VOLESKY, Monika; SMBD Jewish Gen Hosp, E003-3755 ch Cote-Sainte-Cathe, Montreal QC H3T 1E2; McG'98; CASM; FRCSC; OrthSurg (Sports Medicine). Chirurgien Orthopaedic, Sir Mortimer B Davis Jewish General; adj Prof, McGill University; Langs: Bilingual(English/French); (514)340-7532; Fax. (514)340-7595.

VOLKOVINSKAIA, Tamara; Grey Nuns Community Hosp, 1100 Youville Drive West NW, Edmonton AB T6L 5X8; (Ukraine)'83; CCFP; Staff, Alberta Hospital Edmonton; Staff, Covenant Health - Grey Nuns Community Hospital.

VOLL, Christopher L; Dr C L Voll Prof Med Corp, 408-333 25th St E, Saskatoon SK S7K 0L4; Witwatersrand (South Africa)'76; MB ChB; MMed; PhD; FRCPC; Neur (Electromyography). Ac Staff, Saskatoon City Hospital; Ac Staff/Dir Stroke Prevention Clinic, Royal University Hospital; Ac Staff, St Paul's Hospital (Grey Nuns) of Saskatoon; Prof, University of Saskatchewan; (306)652-1312; Fax. (306)665-1220.

VOLLANT, Stanley; Pavillon Roger-Gaudry, U23 1-2900 rue Edouard Montpet, Montreal QC H3T 1J4; Mon'89; GenSurg (Gastroenterology). (514)343-6111 x42522; Fax. (514)906-3034.

VOLLINOTI, Carlos A; Clinique Privee d'Echographie, 444-4 rue Taschereau, Gatineau QC J8Y 2V5; Buenos Aires (Argentina)'71; FACOG; CSPQ; FRCSC; ObstGyn (P.Q.). Staff ObstGyn & Echography, Hôpital de Gatineau; Langs: Spanish; English; (819)771-1884; Fax. (819)771-0662.

VOLLRATH, Thilo E; 305-130 Slater St, Ottawa ON K1P 6E2; McG'60; DPsy; FRCPC; Psy. Langs: German; (613)567-7514; Fax. (613)225-4747.

VOLPE, Michael S A; St Boniface Gen Hosp, A8024-409 Tache Ave, Winnipeg MB R2H 2A6; (Other Foreign)'07; CCFP; Staff Palliatiave Care Prog, St Boniface General Hospital; (204)233-8563

VOLPINI, Brie V; St Joseph's Health Centre, 30 The Queensway, Toronto ON M6R 1B5; Qns'06; FRCPC; IntMed. Staff, St Joseph's Health Centre; (416)530-6000

VOLTIC, Laura; 5881 Malden Rd, Windsor ON N9H 1S5; Ott'03; CCFP; Langs: Croatian; (519)966-2473

VOLTZ, Jean-Marc; Ctr Hosp du Centre la Mauricie, 50 119e rue, Shawinigan-Sud QC G9P 5K1; Nancy (France)'90; Staff, Centre Hospitalier du Centre la Mauricie; (819)536-7575; jean-marc.voltz@wanadoo.fr.

VOLZ, Bernhard A; Beamsville Med Ctr Fam Hlth Team, PO Box 430 4279 Hixon St, Beamsville ON L0R 1B0; Tor'93; CCFP; Staff, West Lincoln Memorial Hospital; Langs: German; (905)563-5315; Fax. (905)563-0933.

VOMIERO, Gemma F; Alberta Children's Hosp, 2888 Shaganappi Trail NW, Calgary AB T3B 6A8; McM'98; BSc(Hon); FRCPC; Peds. Staff, Alberta Children's Hospital; (403)955-2953; Fax. (403)955-3055.

VON DADELSZEN, Peter; BC Women's Hosp & Health Ctre, 2H30-4500 Oak St, Vancouver BC V6H 3N1; Otago (New Zealand)'84; MB ChB; BMedSci; MRC; FRANZCOG; FRCSC; ObstGyn (Maternal Fetal Medicine). Staff, BC Women's Hospital & Health Centre; Staff, Vancouver General Hospital - Centennial Pavillion; Staff, Providence Health Care - St Paul's Hospital; Asst Prof, University of British Columbia; Langs: English; French; (604)875-3054; Fax. (604)875-2725.

VON DEHN, Stephanie K; Selkirk Family Med Centre, 307-1101 Dewdney Ave, Trail BC V1R 4T1; McM'04; CCFP; (250)368-8802

VON DER PORTEN, Fern W; Whistler Health Care Center, 4380 Lorimer Rd, Whistler BC V0N 1B4; UBC'01; CCFP; CCFP(E.M.); (604)932-4911; Fax. (604)932-4922.

VON ENGELBRECHTEN, Heidi D; Low Risk Maternity Clinic, 130-1402 8 Ave NW, Calgary AB T2N 1B9; Cal'07; CCFP; (403)509-3080; Fax. (403)509-3082.

VON HANNA, Silvia G; 303-636 Upper James St, Hamilton ON L9C 2Z2; McM'72; (905)383-7364; Fax. (905)538-5495.

VON KUSTER, Kenneth R B; Victoria Gen Hosp, 2340 Pembina Hwy, Winnipeg MB R3T 2E8; Alb'95; FRCPC; GenPath. Staff, Victoria General Hospital; (204)269-3570

VON SCHLEGELL, Ahmad S; William Osler HC-Etobicoke, 101 Humber College Blvd, Etobicoke ON M9V 1R8; Rush Medical College (USA)'05; Staff, William Osler Health System - Etobicoke General Hospital; (416)747-3388

VON SCHROEDER, Herbert P; Univ Hlth Network-Toronto Western Hosp, E2 421-399 Bathurst St, Toronto ON M5T 2S8; UBC'86; MSc; BSc; DABOS; FRCSC; OrthSurg (Hand Surgery). Staff, Toronto Western Hospital - University Health Network; Assoc Prof Hand Program, University of Toronto; Langs: German; (416)603-5641; Fax. (416)603-5813.

VON WESTARP, Christian H A; Royal Jubilee Hosp, 1952 Bay St, Victoria BC V8R 1J8; Dal'70; FRCPC; IntMed (Endocrinology & Metabolism). Ac Staff, Royal Jubilee Hospital; Ac Staff, Victoria General Hospital; (250)370-1110

VONA, Frank G; PO Box 352, Campbellville ON L0P 1B0; McG'86; (905)699-4626; Fax. (905)854-6264.

VONDER MUHLL, Isabelle F; University of Alberta Hosp, 2C2 WCM-8440 112 St NW, Edmonton AB T6G 2B7; UBC'96; BSc; FRCPC; IntMed (Adult Congenital Heart Disease); Cardiol. Asst Prof Cardiol, University of Alberta Hospital; (780)407-3107; Fax. (780)407-6452.

VONDETTE, Michael J; Kerrisdale Prof Centre, 256-2025 42nd Ave W, Vancouver BC V6M 2B5; Dal'75; FRCPC; PhysMed&Rehab. Consultant, Vancouver General Hospital - Centennial Pavillion; Consultant, Providence Health Care - Holy Family Hospital; Consultant, G F Strong Rehabilitation Centre; Asst Prof Med, University of British Columbia; (604)228-1922; mvondette@providencehealth.bc.ca.

VONKEMAN, Hermen; Miramichi Reg Hosp, 500 Water St, Miramichi NB E1V 3G5; Orange Free State (South Africa)'84; MB ChB; MMed; Staff, Miramichi Regional Hospital; (506)627-7007; Fax. (506)627-7009.

VONNIESSEN, Michael; Lakeshore Gen Hosp, 160 av Stillview, Pointe-Claire QC H9R 2Y2; McG'89; CCFP; CCFP(E.M.); Staff, Lakeshore General Hospital - Pointe Claire; Langs: English; French; (514)630-2225 x2044

VOOGHT, Mark T R; Five Hills Health Region, 107-110 Ominica St W, Moose Jaw SK S6H 6V2; Stellenbosch (South Africa)'95; MB ChB; MMed(CommunHealth); Langs: Afrikaans; (306)691-1537; Fax. (306)691-1523.

VOOGJARV, Harry M; Timmins & Dist Hosp, 1583-700 Ross Ave E, Timmins ON P4N 8P2; McM'88; FRCSC; GenSurg; Critical Care Medicine. Chief of Staff, Timmins & District Hospital; Asst Prof, Northern Ontario School of Medicine-Laurentian University; Langs: French; Finnish; (705)267-3566; Fax. (705)267-3566.

VOON, Frederick H S; Royal Jubilee Hosp, 1952 Bay St, Victoria BC V8R 1J8; Alb'01; CCFP; CCFP(E.M.); Staff, Royal Jubilee Hospital; (250)637-8000

VOON, Kevin K S; Brant Business Bldg, 402-672 Brant St, Burlington ON L7R 2H3; Alb'86; CCFP; FCFP; Langs: Chinese; (905)637-1177; Fax. (905)637-5120.

VOON, Victor B H; 528A Clarke Rd, New Westminster BC V3J 3X5; Ott'67; Ac Staff, Royal Columbian Hospital; Ac Staff, Eagle Ridge Hospital & Health Care Centre; (604)936-9874; Fax. (604)936-9741.

VOORE, Peter M; Ctre for Addiction & Mental Hl, 5215E-100 Stokes St, Toronto ON M6J 1H4; Tor'82; FRCPC; Psy. Dir Gen Psy & Women's, Centre for Addiction & Mental Health (CAMH) - College Street Site; Staff, Centre for Addiction & Mental Health; Med Dir, Centre for Addiction & Mental Health Ambulatory Care & Structured Treatments; Assoc Prof, University of Toronto; (416)979-4277; Fax. (416)979-6810.

VOORHEIS, Paul M; Georgian Radiology Consultants, 115-121 Wellington St W, Barrie ON L4N 1L2; Wes'82; FRCPC; DiagRad. Chief DiagRad, Royal Victoria Regional Health Centre; (705)726-4531

VOORNEVELD, Colin R; 304-2299 Dundas St W, Toronto ON M6R 1X7; Ott'82; ABIM; FRCPC; IntMed (Family Medicine); Rheum. Staff, St Joseph's Health Centre; Consultant, Medcom Development; (416)516-4751; Fax. (416)516-8580.

VOORPOSTEL, Margaret W M; Southlake Reg Health Centre, 596 Davis Dr, Newmarket ON L3Y 2P9; Wes'80; Staff, Southlake Regional Health Centre; Langs: Dutch; (905)895-4521

VOPICKA, Avaleen A; Fowler Kennedy Sports Med Clin, PO Box 7005 SC1001-1460 Oxford St E, London ON N5V 1W2; Wes'85; CCFP; CCFP(E.M.); FCFP; Ac Staff, London Health Sciences Centre - University Hospital; (519)452-4230; Fax. (519)452-4415.

VORA, Harshala P; Stonechurch Family Hlth Centre, 1475 Upper Ottawa St, Hamilton ON L8W 3J6; Bombay (India)'94; CCFP; Langs: Gujarati; Hindi; Marathi; (905)575-1300

VORA, Parag K; Hamilton HS-McMaster Site, PO Box 2000 Stn Lcd 1 1200 Main St W, Hamilton ON L8N 3Z5; Bombay (India)'92; FRCPC; DiagRad. Staff, Hamilton Health Sciences Centre - McMaster Children's Hospital; (905)521-2100

VORNBERGER, William J; London Road Diagnostic Clinic, 481 London Rd, Sarnia ON N7T 4X3; St George's University of Grenada (Grenada)'99; (519)336-0339

VOROBEYCHIK, Galina; Burnaby Hosp, 3935 Kincaid St, Burnaby BC V5G 2X6; Moscow (Russia (Federation))'89; FRCPC; Neur (Multiple Sclerosis). Staff Fraser Health Multiple Sclerosis Clinic, Burnaby Hospital; (604)412-6405; Fax. (604)412-6407.

VOROBEYCHIK, Helena; Burnaby Med Centre, M37-4277 Kingsway, Burnaby BC V5H 3Z2; Moskovskjj (Russia (Federation))'83; CCFP; (604)438-9991; Fax. (604)438-9960.

VORONEY, Jon-Paul J; Tom Baker Cancer Centre, 1331 29 St NW, Calgary AB T2N 4N2; Tor'02; FRCPC; RadOncol (Radiosurgery). Staff, Tom Baker Cancer Centre; (403)521-3164; Fax. (403)283-1651.

VOROS, Gabor D; Cambridge Mem Hosp, 700 Coronation Blvd, Cambridge ON N1R 3G2; (Other Foreign)'06; CCFP; Staff, Cambridge Memorial Hospital; (519)621-2330

VOROS, Gyula; Postmaster Med Clinic, 2540 Postmaster Dr, Oakville ON L6M 0N2; Tor'06; BSc; CCFP; Langs: Bilingual(English/French); (905)844-1700; Fax. (905)844-1705.

VOROS, Mario; Peterborough Reg Hlth Centre, 1 Hospital Dr, Peterborough ON K9J 7C6; Qns'99; FRCPC; DiagRad. Staff, Peterborough Regional Health Centre - Hospital Drive; Langs: Slovak; (705)743-2121

VOROS, Sandor; Airdrie Med Centre, 10-620 1 Ave NW, Airdrie AB T4B 2R3; (Slovakia)'96; (403)948-3109; Fax. (403)948-6284.

VOROSOVA, Gertruda; Airdrie Med Clinic, 10-620 1 Ave NW, Airdrie AB T4B 2R3; Comenius University (Slovakia)'96; Staff, Pembina-Manitou Health Centre; (403)948-3109; Fax. (403)948-6284.

VORPS, Harry M; SGH Medical Mall, 204-3030 Lawrence Ave E, Scarborough ON M1P 2T7; Tor'81; BSc; MSc; Ac Staff, The Scarborough Hospital - General Campus; (416)431-1242; Fax. (416)431-0836.

VORSTER, Alewyn P; Tiger Hills Health District, PO Box 191, Treherne MB R0G 2V0; Pretoria (South Africa)'88; Chief/Medical Staff, Tiger Hills Health District; Langs: Afrikaans; (204)723-2133; alewyn_vorster@hc-sc.gc.ca.

VORSTER, Beukes J; Regina Qu'Appelle HR-Regina, 1440 14th Ave, Regina SK S4P 0W5; Stellenbosch (South Africa)'98; MB ChB; Staff, Regina General Hospital; (306)766-4444

VORSTER, Deon J; Wild Rose Med Centre, PO Box 3955 Stn Main 4607 50 Ave, Olds AB T4H 1P6; Pretoria (South Africa)'00; MB ChB; CCFP; (403)556-7130; Fax. (403)556-1944.

VORSTER, Johannes J; Broadway Med Clinic, 200-41 Broadway St W, Yorkton SK S3N 0L6; '03; Langs: Afrikaans; (306)783-2555; Fax. (306)783-2557.

VORSTER, Rene; Broadway Med Clinic, 205-41 Broadway W, Yorkton SK S3N 0L6; (Other Foreign)'05; (306)782-5525; Fax. (306)782-3616.

VORSTER, Sarel; Lindsay Prof Centre, 14-65 Angeline St N, Lindsay ON K9V 5N7; Pretoria (South Africa)'82; MB ChB; LMCC; CCFP; Staff, Ross Memorial Hospital; Langs: Afrikaans; (705)324-6061; Fax. (705)324-2155.

VORTEL, Jerry J; Dr Jerry Vortel Inc, 304-7031 Westminster Hwy, Richmond BC V6X 1A3; Karlova (Czech Republic)'79; FRCPC; IntMed (AIDS/HIV); InfectDis. Consultant, Burnaby Hospital; Consultant, Richmond Hospital; (604)231-9697

VORUGANTI, Lakshmi N P; Halton HSC Corp-Oakville, 327 Reynolds St, Oakville ON L6J 3L7; Andhra (India)'78; MB BS; MRC; MSc; FRCPC; Psy (Academic & Research Practice). Staff, Halton Healthcare Services Corporation - Oakville Site; Langs: Hindi; Telugu; (905)338-4660; Fax. (905)338-4481.

VORUGANTI, Sachi M; The Juravinski Cancer Centre, 699 Concession St, Hamilton ON L8V 5C2; Andhra (India)'80; MB BS; FRCPC; RadOncol. Staff, The Juravinski Cancer Centre; Langs: Hindi; Telugu; (905)387-9495; Fax. (905)575-6326.

VOS, Andre J; Mediclinic, 101-3333 8th St E, Saskatoon SK S7H 4K1; (Other Foreign)'05; CCFP; Staff ICU, St Paul's Hospital (Grey Nuns) of Saskatoon; (306)955-1530; Fax. (306)955-8811.

VOS, Eugene P; 11050 103 Ave, Grande Prairie AB T8V 7H1; Pretoria (South Africa)'86; BSc(Hons); MB ChB; (780)532-2332; Fax. (780)513-2828.

VOS, Patrick M; St Paul's Hosp, 1081 Burrard St, Vancouver BC V6Z 1Y6; Amsterdam (Netherlands)'92; FRCPC; DiagRad. Staff, Providence Health Care - St Paul's Hospital; Langs: Dutch; (604)806-8006

VOSLOO, Dianne L; Health & Counselling Centre, 8888 University Dr, Burnaby BC V5A 1S6; Pretoria (South Africa)'88; MB ChB; CCFP; Physician Student Health Services, Simon Fraser University; Langs: Afrikaans; (778)782-4615; Fax. (778)782-5781.

VOSOUGHI, Reza; Health Sciences Centre, GF543-820 Sherbrook St, Winnipeg MB R3A 1R9; Mashhad University of Medical Science (Other Foreign)'92; FRCPC; Neur. Staff, Health Sciences Centre; (204)774-8511

VOSS, Maurice D; St Joseph's Healthcare, 50 Charlton Ave E, Hamilton ON L8N 4A6; Auckland (New Zealand)'92; MB ChB; FRCPC; DiagRad (Interventional Radiology). Staff, St Joseph's Healthcare - Charlton Campus; Asst Prof, McMaster University; (905)522-1155 x36009

VOSS, Nicholas J S; BC Cancer Agency-Vancouver CC, 600 10th Ave W, Vancouver BC V5Z 4E6; London (England)'69; DMRT; FRCR; FRCPC; RadOncol. Ac Staff RadOncol, BC Cancer Agency Vancouver Centre; Ac Staff, Vancouver General Hospital - Centennial Pavillion; Clin Assoc Prof, University of British Columbia; (604)877-6000; Fax. (604)877-0505.

VOSTRETSOV, Stepan; Parhelion Med Services Inc, PO Box 127, Watson Lake YT Y0A 1C0; Physician, Parhelion Medical Services Inc; (867)536-2316; Fax. (867)536-2506.

VOSTRETSOVA, Nataliya V; Richmond Central Med Clinic, 150-7997 Westminster Hwy, Richmond BC V6X 1A4; Kharkov (Ukraine)'88; FCFP; CCFP; Staff, Surrey Memorial Hospital; Langs: Russian; Ukrainian; (778)297-4700; Fax. (778)297-4800; parus552003@yahoo.ca.

VOSU, Helen A; North York Gen Hosp, 4001 Leslie St, North York ON M2K 1E1; Tor'79; FRCPC; Anes (Cardiovascular Anesthesia). Staff, North York General Hospital; (416)756-6000

VOTH, Arnold J; Hys Med Centre, 608-11010 101 St NW, Edmonton AB T5H 4B9; Sask'66; FACP; LMCC; FRCPC; IntMed (Hematology). Ac Staff, Royal Alexandra Hospital; Consultant, Glenrose Rehabilitation Hospital; Consultant, Cross Cancer Institute; University of Alberta; Langs: German; French; (780)474-8071; Fax. (780)479-2524.

VOTH, Bevan R; Crossroads Family Practice, 201-45800 Promontory Rd, Chilliwack BC V2R 5Z5; UBC'98; MSc; BSc; CCFP; FCFP; Clin Instructor, University of British Columbia; (604)858-3725; Fax. (604)858-8625; bevanvoth@shaw.ca.

VOUDOURIS, Nicholas C; Thornhill Med Centre, 18 Centre St, Thornhill ON L4J 1E9; Cal'84; Ac Staff Family Practice, Mackenzie Richmond Hill Hospital; Langs: Greek; (905)889-3634; Fax. (905)889-3986.

VOURIOT, Daniel D; Bluewater Health - Norman Site, 89 Norman St, Sarnia ON N7T 6S3; Man'95; CCFP; CCFP(E.M.); Staff, Bluewater Health - Norman Site; (519)464-4400

VOURLAS, Anastasios; Insight Diagnostic Imaging Cor, 408-658 Danforth Ave, East York ON M4J 5B9; Tor'85; FRCPC; DiagRad. Langs: Greek; (416)465-1726; Fax. (416)465-5695.

VOUTSILAKOS, Emorphea; Kitsilano Fairview Mental Hlth, 400-1212 Broadway W, Vancouver BC V6H 3V2; UBC'97; FRCPC; Psy. Langs: Greek; (604)736-2881; evoutsilakos@forensic.bc.ca.

VOWINCKEL, Erika A M; Front-Frederick Health Service, 14F-365 Bloor St E, Toronto ON M4W 3L4; Qns'01; BSc; CCFP; (416)362-8777; Fax. (416)362-7879.

VOYER, Danielle; 202-4707 boul des Laurentides, Laval QC H7K 3G4; Mon'75; (450)662-7780; Fax. (450)662-1983.

VOYER, Gilles; CHUS-Hop Fleurimont, 3001 12e av N, Sherbrooke QC J1H 5N4; Sher'74; Dir Centre for Continuing Educ, Centre Hospitalier Universitaire de Sherbrooke-Hopital Fleurimont; Dir Centre for Continuing Education, Universite de Sherbrooke.

VOYER, Isabelle; CSSS de Chicoutimi, 305 rue Saint-Vallier, Chicoutimi QC G7H 5H6; Mon'10; CCFP; Staff, Complexe hospitalier de la Sagamie; (418)541-1000

VOYER, Jean; Clinique Med St-Etienne, 2-965 Rte Lagueux, St-Etienne-De-Lauz QC G6J 1T5; Laval'78; (418)831-9538; Fax. (418)831-8552.

VOYER, Nathalie; CHUS-Hop Hotel-Dieu, 580 rue Bowen S, Sherbrooke QC J1G 2E8; Laval'88; FRCPC; DiagRad (P.Q.). Staff, Centre Hospitalier Universitaire de Sherbrooke-Hôpital Hôtel-Dieu; (819)346-1110

VOYER, Patricia; Clinique Med la Cite, 101-3801 rue de Montcalm, Jonquiere QC G7X 1W1; Laval'85; ac Staff, Centre Hospitalier Jonquiere; (418)542-1510; Fax. (418)542-1512.

VOYER, Stephane M; St Paul's Hosp, 5900-1081 Burrard St, Vancouver BC V6Z 1Y6; McG'05; MDCM; FRCPC; IntMed. Staff, Vancouver General Hospital - Centennial Pavillion; Staff, Gordon & Leslie Diamond Health Care Centre; Staff, Providence Health Care - St Paul's Hospital; Langs: Bilingual(English/French); (604)806-8735

VOYSEY, Mark A; 321 Seaton St, Toronto ON M5A 2T6; Monash (Australia)'78; MB BS; BMedSci; FRCPC; Psy (Child & Adolescent Psychiatry). Consultant, Residential Youth Treatment Centre; (416)925-7749; Fax. (416)925-7749.

VOYVODIC, Blair J; B-49 Mill St, Killaloe ON K0J 2A0; Ott'85; Langs: Bilingual(French/English); (613)757-0847; Fax. (613)757-0847.

VOZAR, Jiri G; 229 Synergy Wellness Centre, 501 Behtel Dr, Sherwood Park AB T8H 0N2; Prague (Czech Republic)'73; FRCPC; Psy. (780)416-8747; Fax. (780)449-5461.

VOZIS, Constantin G; 374 Danforth Ave, Toronto ON M4K 1N8; Sofia (Bulgaria)'55; Staff, North York General Hospital - Branson Division; Langs: Greek; Macedonian; (416)461-1455

VOZIS, Eva E; Medical & Dental Bldg, 710-1849 Yonge St, Toronto ON M4S 1Y2; Tor'74; AnatPath. Langs: Bulgarian; (416)489-6615

VOZORIS, Nicholas T; St Michael's Hosp, 30 Bond St, Toronto ON M5B 1W8; Tor'04; BSc; MHSc; FRCPC; IntMed (Sleep Medicine); Respir. Staff, St Michael's Hospital; (416)864-6026; Fax. (416)864-5649.

VOZORIS, Socrates A; Humber River Reg Hosp-Church, 200 Church St, York ON M9N 1N8; Philadelphia(PA) (USA)'00; FRCPC; IntMed; Cardiol. Staff, Humber River Regional Hospital - Church Street Site; Langs: Greek; (416)236-2783; Fax. (416)236-2783.

VRABEC, George; Royal City Med Bldg, 302-250 Keary St, New Westminster BC V3L 5E7; Prague (Czech Republic)'63; FRCSC; GenSurg; Cardiovasc&ThorSurg. Chief Vasc & ThorSurg, Royal Columbian Hospital; (604)525-6411; Fax. (604)525-6189.

VRABEC, George J; 105-2051 McCallum Rd, Abbotsford BC V2S 3N5; UBC'96; FRCSC; Urol (Minimal Invasive Urology). (604)851-5668; Fax. (604)851-5670.

VRABLIK, Stefan; Ridgeway Clinic, 1001 Ridgeway St E, Thunder Bay ON P7E 5H8; Palacky (Czech Republic)'60; Langs: Slovak; (807)622-0601; Fax. (807)623-0470.

VRAETS, Adrienne C; Hamilton HS-McMaster Site, PO Box 2000 Stn Lcd 1 2U1-1200 Main St W, Hamilton ON L8N 3Z5; Tor'02; FRCPC; Anes. Staff, Hamilton Health Sciences Centre - McMaster University Medical Centre; (905)521-2100

VRAHAS, Voula; MUHC-Royal Victoria Hosp, S7W-687 av des Pins O, Montreal QC H3A 1A1; CCFP; Staff, McGill University Health Centre - Royal Victoria Hospital; (514)934-1934 x35172

VRANA, Andrea P; Lions Gate Hosp, 231 15th St E, North Vancouver BC V7L 2L7; UBC'04; FRCPC; Anes. Staff Anes, Lions Gate Hospital; (604)988-3131

VRETENAR, Doris F; Business Bldg, 514-1200 Burrard St, Vancouver BC V6Z 2C7; Alb'93; FRCPC; Anes. Staff, Vancouver General Hospital - Centennial Pavillion; Langs: Croatian; (604)806-6365; Fax. (604)974-0067.

VREUGDENHIL, Michael J; 4 Anishnaabeg Dr, Muncey ON N0L 1Y0; McM'98; CCFP; FCFP; (519)289-0352

VROOM, W Robbert; College of Phys & Surgs of BC, 300-669 Howe St, Vancouver BC V6C 0B4; McG'75; CCFP; CCFP(E.M.); Staff, Surrey Memorial Hospital; Dep Registrar, College of Physicians & Surgeons of British Columbia; Clin Preceptor, University of British Columbia; Langs: Spanish; Dutch; (604)733-7758; Fax. (604)669-8954.

VU, Binh Thien; 3-695 Canterbury St, Woodstock ON N4S 8W7; Wes'88; Staff, Woodstock General Hospital; Langs: Vietnamese; (519)421-3350

VU, Caroline T N; CLSC Saint-Hubert, 6800 boul Cousineau, Saint-Hubert QC J3Y 8Z4; Sher'03; CCFP; (450)443-7400; Fax. (450)676-4645.

VU, David D V; 302-302 Spadina Ave, Toronto ON M5T 2E7; Saigon (Vietnam)'71; Langs: Vietnamese; French; (416)591-7096; Fax. (416)591-7549.

VU, Dung; Inst Readapt Gingras-Lindsay, 6300 av de Darlington, Montreal QC H3S 2J4; Saigon (Vietnam)'74; LMCC; Staff, Institut de Réadaptation Gingras-Lindsay de Montréal; Langs: Vietnamese; English; (514)340-2085 x2306; Fax. (514)340-2775.

VU, Erik N; Emergency & Critical Care Med, JPPN-910 10th Ave W, Vancouver BC V5Z 1M9; UBC'03; FRCPC; EmergMed; Critical Care Medicine. Staff, Vancouver General Hospital - Centennial Pavillion; Langs: Bilingual(English/French); (604)875-4700; Fax. (604)875-4872.

VU, Lan Huu; Royal Alexandra Hosp, 502-10240 Kingsway NW, Edmonton AB T5H 3V9; Wes'06; FRCSC; GenSurg. Staff, University Hospital of Northern British Columbia; Staff Community Services Ctr, Royal Alexandra Hospital; (780)735-6726; Fax. (780)735-5565.

VU, Manh Huu; Hamilton HS-Hamilton Gen Hosp, 237 Barton St E, Hamilton ON L8L 2X2; McM'83; FRCPC; DiagRad. Staff Diagnostic Imaging, Hamilton Health Sciences Centre - McMaster Children's Hospital; Staff, Hamilton Health Sciences Centre - Hamilton General Hospital; Langs: Vietnamese; (905)521-2100

VU, Mark P; Vanvouver Gen Hosp, 2449-899 12th Ave W, Vancouver BC V5Z 1M9; UBC'01; FRCPC; Anes. Staff, Vancouver General Hospital - Centennial Pavillion; Langs: Bilingual(English/French); (604)875-4304; Fax. (604)875-5209.

VU, Minh Thuy; CLSC St-Leonard, 5540 rue Jarry E, Saint-Leonard QC H1P 1T9; Saigon (Vietnam)'77; (514)328-3460; Fax. (514)328-1468.

VU, N Q Wayne; 2-1329 Fuller St, London ON N5Y 4R1; Wes'99; CCFP; Langs: Vietnamese; (519)455-2200

VU, Ngoc Dien; Centre Med Fleury, 211-2157 rue Fleury E, Montreal QC H2B 1K1; Saigon (Vietnam)'69; ac Staff, Centre Hospitalier Fleury; Langs: English; French; (514)384-8556; Fax. (514)381-9872.

VU, Suzanne; CLSC St-Laurent, 1055 av Sainte-Croix, Saint-Laurent QC H4L 3Z2; Sher'98; (514)748-6381; Fax. (514)748-6323.

VU, T A John; Courtice Health Centre, 1450 Highway 2, Courtice ON L1E 3C3; Ott'91; Langs: French; (905)723-8551 x4808; Fax. (905)721-6186; johnvumd@gmail.com.

VU, The-Hung; Clinique Med Colombus, 312-1140 rue Jean-Talon E, Montreal QC H2R 1V9; Saigon (Vietnam)'69; Langs: Italian; French; Vietnamese; (514)270-2141

VU, Thi Khanh H; CHSLD J H Charbonneau, 3095 rue Sherbrooke E, Montreal QC H1W 1B2; Saigon (Vietnam)'72; Staff, CHSLD Lucille-Teasdale; (514)523-1173

VU, Thi Thuong T; Centre Med Fleury Wilson, 2157 rue Fleury E, Montreal QC H2B 1K1; Mon'86; Langs: Bilingual(French/English); (514)858-6110; Fax. (514)381-9872.

VU, Thi-Trinh T; CHUM-Hop Notre-Dame, 1560 rue Sherbrooke E, Montreal QC H2L 4M1; Laval'99; FRCPC; RadOncol. Staff, Centre Hospitalier l'Université de Montréal (CHUM) - Hôpital Notre-Dame; (514)890-8000

VU, Thien Tai T; CLSC Parc Extension, 7085 rue Hutchison, Montreal QC H3N 1Y9; Sher'98; LMCC; CCFP; Staff, Hôpital du Sacre-Coeur de Montréal; Médecin, CLSC Parc Extension; (514)273-9591; Fax. (514)273-8363.

VU, Thien Tuong V; Hopital Jean-Talon, 1385 rue Jean-Talon E, Montreal QC H2E 1S6; Mon'05; FRCSC; Otol. Staff, CSSS du Coeur de l'Isle Hôpital Jean-Talon; (514)495-6767

VU, Thien-Tuong M; CHUM-Hop St-Luc, 1058 rue Saint-Denis, Montreal QC H2X 3J4; Laval'00; FRCPC; IntMed; GeriatricMed. Staff, Centre Hospitalier l'Université De Montréal (CHUM) - Hôpital Saint-luc; (514)890-8000; Fax. (514)412-7376.

VU, Trevor T C; Abbottsfield Shoppers Mall, 226-3210 118 Ave NW, Edmonton AB T5W 4W1; Alb'88; Langs: Vietnamese; (780)471-2626; Fax. (780)474-0151.

VU, Trung K; Brentwood Family Med Centre, 810-3630 Brentwood Rd NW, Calgary AB T2L 1K8; Alb'96; CCFP; Langs: Vietnamese; (403)289-6631; Fax. (403)289-6575; hpmed@telusplanet.net.

VU-KHANH, Anh-Thu; Centre Med Aylmer-Lucerne, 67 rue du Couvent, Gatineau QC J9H 6A2; Sher'06; CCFP; (819)684-1234; Fax. (819)684-1240.

VU NGOC, Quynh-Phuong; CSSS Pierre Boucher, 1333 rue Jacques-Cartier E, Longueuil QC J4M 2A5; Mon'90; FRCPC; DiagRad. Staff, Centre Hospitalier Pierre Boucher; Langs: Vietnamese; (450)468-8157; Fax. (450)468-8165.

VU-NGUYEN, Caroline X L; CLSC Rene Cassin, 5800 boul Cavendish, Montreal QC H4W 2T5; Mon'90; Médecin, CSSS de Gatineau; Langs: Vietnamese; English; (514)484-7878

VUCEMILO, Ivica; 520-89 Queensway W, Mississauga ON L5B 2V2; Zagreb (Croatia)'94; FRCSC; GenSurg; VascSurg. Staff, Trillium Health Centre - Mississauga; Langs: Croatian; (905)848-7777; Fax. (905)848-6360; ivucemilo@thc.on.ca.

VUILLERMET, Denise; Clinique Med Blainville, 519 boul du Cure-Labelle, Blainville QC J7C 2H6; Sher'84; (450)430-2222; Fax. (450)430-1274.

VUJICIC, Neda; Black Creek Comm Hlth Centre, 5-2202 Jane St, North York ON M3M 1A4; Tor'09; CCFP; Langs: Croatian; Serbian; (416)249-8000

VUJNOVIC, Predrag; Bloor-Jane Med Bldg, 512-2425 Bloor St W, Toronto ON M6S 4W4; Belgrade (Serbia)'60; Ac Staff, St Joseph's Health Centre; Langs: Yugoslavian; Serbian; (416)763-3816

VUJOSEVIC, Darija; Garden City Family Health Team, 7-145 Carlton St, St Catharines ON L2R 1R5; Djuro Pucar Stari Univ (Bosnia-Herzegovina)'89; CCFP; Langs: Serbo-Croatian; (905)988-5600; Fax. (905)988-5622.

VUJOVIC, Olga; London Reg Cancer Centre, 790 Commissioners Rd E, London ON N6A 4L6; Tor'81; FRCPC; RadOncol;CCFP; Staff, London Health Sciences Centre - London Regional Cancer Centre; (519)685-8600; Fax. (519)685-8627.

VUKMIROVIC-POPOVIC, Snezana; Hamilton HS-MUMC, PO Box 2000 Stn Lcd 1 2V 17B-1200 Main St W, Hamilton ON L8N 3Z5; Belgrade (Serbia)'86; FRCPC; AnatPath. Staff, Hamilton Health Sciences Centre - McMaster University Medical Centre; Langs: Serbian; (905)521-2100; Fax. (905)577-0198; popovics@hhsc.ca.

VUKOJEVIC, Duska; Bayview Mall Med Office, 50-470 Dundas St E, Belleville ON K8N 1G1; (Serbia)'92; Assoc Member, QHC Belleville General; Langs: Serbo-Croatian; Croatian; Serbian; (613)966-4045 x2222; Fax. (613)966-0072.

VUKOVIC, Ljubomir; Min of Hlth Long Term Care, 370 Select Dr, Kingston ON K7M 8T4; Sheffield (England)'65; MB ChB; FRCS; Otol (Head & Neck Surgery). Langs: Serbian.

VUKOVIC, Milorad; The Shoniker Clinic, 2877A Ellesmere Rd, Scarborough ON M1E 4C1; Sarajevo (Bosnia-Herzegovina)'86; FRCPC; Psy. Staff, Rouge Valley Health System - Centenary Health Centre Site; Langs: Croatian; Serbian; (416)281-7301; Fax. (416)281-7465.

VUKSANOVIC, Milos; Dauphin Med Clinic, 622 3rd St SW, Dauphin MB R7N 1R5.

VUKSIC, Stanko; Royal Jubilee Hosp, 1952 Bay St, Victoria BC V8R 1J8; UBC'83; FRCPC; Anes. Staff, Royal Jubilee Hospital; (250)370-8000; vuksics@sasktel.net.

VUKUSIC, Alan V; Royal Inland Hosp, 311 Columbia St, Kamloops BC V2C 2T1; UBC'99; CCFP; CCFP(E.M.); Staff, Royal Inland Hospital; (250)314-2425; Fax. (250)314-2327.

VUONG, Te; SMBD Jewish Gen Hosp, G002-3755 ch Cote-Ste-Catherin, Montreal QC H3T 1E2; Mon'81; ABIM; FRCPC; IntMed (Digestive Tumors); RadOncol; MedOncol. Staff, Centre Hospitalier Pierre Boucher; Chef RadioOncology, Sir Mortimer B Davis Jewish General; assoc Prof, McGill University; (514)340-8222 x2073; Fax. (514)340-7548; tvuong@jgh.mcgill.ca.

VUPPUTURI, Sujana K; Malvern Med Centre, 100-1333 Neilson Rd, Scarborough ON M1B 4Y9; Tor'88; (416)291-7719; Fax. (416)287-3775.

VUURMANS, Johannes L T; 102-245 Columbia St E, New Westminster BC V3L 3W4; Amsterdam (Netherlands)'97; Staff, Victoria Heart Institute Foundation; Langs: Dutch; (604)524-9571

VVEDENSKYY, Oleksandr; Vernon Jubilee Hosp, 2101 32 St, Vernon BC V1T 5L2; National Medical University (Other Foreign)'97; FRCPC; Anes. Staff, Vernon Jubilee Hospital; (250)545-2211

VYAS, Mukul N; Main & Marine Med Clinic, 235 Marine Dr SE, Vancouver BC V5X 2S4; Bombay (India)'53; MB BS; MRCP(Lond); FRCPC; IntMed (Cardiology). Langs: Gujarati; Hindi; (604)322-3011

VYSE, Adam D; 121 4th Ave W PO Box 5695 Stn Main, High River AB T1V 1M7; Cal'93; CCFP; FCFP; (403)652-7999; Fax. (403)652-7997.

VYSE, Nancy A; 121 4th Ave SW PO Box 5695 Stn Main, High River AB T1V 1M7; Cal'94; CCFP; (403)652-7999; Fax. (403)652-7997.

VYSELAAR, John R; 100-123 15th St E, North Vancouver BC V7L 2P7; UBC'03; FRCPC; IntMed; Cardiol. (604)980-1031; cardiology@johnvyselaar.com.

VYVER, Ellie E; Alberta Children's Hosp, 2888 Shaganappi Trail NW, Calgary AB T3B 6A8; McM'03; FRCPC; Peds (Adolescent Medicine). Staff, Alberta Children's Hospital; (403)955-2978; Fax. (403)955-7649.

VYVEY, Melissa L; Somerset West CHC, 55 Eccles St, Ottawa ON K1R 6S3; Tor'09; CCFP; (613)238-1220

WACHOWICH, Donna M; Foothills Prof Bldg, 350-1620 29 St NW, Calgary AB T2N 4L7; Alb'82; CCFP; FCFP; Staff Privil Emerg, Rockyview General Hospital; (403)282-1245; Fax. (403)282-9545.

WACHOWSKI, Ireneusz; Misericordia Comm Hosp & H C, 16940 87 Ave NW, Edmonton AB T5R 4H5; Pomeranian (Poland)'86; FRCPC; Anes. Staff, Covenant Health - Misericordia Community Hospital; Langs: Polish; (780)735-2863; Fax. (780)735-2967.

WACHSMUTH, J Rodney; 912-123 Edward St, Toronto ON M5G 1E2; Mem'75; DCPsy; FRCPC; Psy. Staff, The Hospital For Sick Children; Asst Prof Psy, University of Toronto; (416)598-4782; Fax. (416)598-4782.

WACHTEL, Sean L; Kootenay Lake Gen Hosp, 3 View St, Nelson BC V1L 2V1; Leicester (England)'94; MB ChB; CCFP; Staff, Kootenay Lake General Hospital; (250)352-3111 x2345

WACHTLER, Oswald F; Properties MDM Clinic, 5102 Rundlehorn Dr NE, Calgary AB T1Y 1C1; Vienna (Austria)'68; Langs: French; German; (403)280-2700; Fax. (403)285-2641.

WACKER, Kevin P; East Street Med Arts Centre, 104-170 East St, Sault Ste. Marie ON P6A 3C6; Sask'91; (705)256-8351; Fax. (705)759-6865.

WACKETT, Charles J L; Hawkesbury & Dist Gen Hosp, 1111 Ghislain St, Hawkesbury ON K6A 3G5; Ott'06; FRCSC; GenSurg. Staff, Hawkesbury & District General Hospital; (613)632-1111

WACLAWSKI, Eugene; 5-30 University Terrace, 8303 112 St NW, Edmonton AB T6G 1K4; (780)492-1366

WADA, Juhn A; UBC Hospital, 2255 Wesbrook Mall, Vancouver BC V6T 2B5; Hokkaido (Japan)'45; MD(Hon); FRCPC; Neur (Electroencephalography). Hon Consultant Neurol, UBC Hospital - Koerner Pavillion; Emeritus Prof Neurol & Neurosciences, University of British Columbia; Langs: Japanese; (604)822-7358; Fax. (604)822-7268; jwada@interchange.ubc.ca.

WADA, Ryan; 120-6707 Elbow Dr SW, Calgary AB T2Y 0E3; McG'00; FRCPC; DiagRad (Neuro Radiology). (403)777-3007

WADDELL, Andrea E; Univ Hlth Network-Toronto Gen, 8EN 231-200 Elizabeth St, Toronto ON M5G 2C4; Tor'03; FRCPC; Psy. Staff, Toronto General Hospital - UHN; (416)340-4463

WADDELL, Charlotte A; Children's Health Policy Ctre, 2434-515 Hastings St W, Vancouver BC V6B 5K3; McM'91; BSc; MSc; FRCPC; Psy (Child Abuse);CCFP; Consultant, Provincial Child Psychiatry; Assoc Prof Health Sciences/Dir Children's Health Policy Centre, Simon Fraser University; (778)782-7775; Fax. (778)782-7777.

WADDELL, Guy; CHUS-Hop Fleurimont, 3001 12e av N, Sherbrooke QC J1H 5N4; Sher'83; FRCSC; ObstGyn (Endoscopy). Staff, Centre Hospitalier Universitaire de Sherbrooke-Hopital Fleurimont; Chef ObstGyn, Universite de Sherbrooke; Langs: Bilingual(English/French); (819)346-1110; Fax. (819)820-6434; guy.waddell@usherbrooke.ca.

WADDELL, Ian C; Royal University Hosp, 103 Hospital Dr, Saskatoon SK S7N 0W8; Auckland (New Zealand)'87; MB ChB; FRCPC; DiagRad. Staff, Royal University Hospital; (306)655-2372; Fax. (306)655-2387.

WADDELL, James P; 207-55 Queen St E, Toronto ON M5C 1R6; Alb'67; DAB; FRCSC; OrthSurg (Joint Arthroplasty). Staff, St Michael's Hospital; Prof, University of Toronto; (416)864-6001; Fax. (416)864-6010; waddellj@smh.ca.

WADDELL, John M; Weeneebayko Gen Hosp, PO Box 34 19 Hospital Dr, Moose Factory ON P0L 1W0; Tor'89; Staff, Weeneebayko General Hospital; (705)658-4544

WADDELL, Thomas K; Univ Hlth Network-Toronto Gen, NU9 949-200 Elizabeth St, Toronto ON M5G 2C4; Ott'87; FRCSC; GenSurg (Telehealth); ThorSurg. Staff, Toronto General Hospital - UHN; (416)340-3432; Fax. (416)340-4556; tom.waddell@uhn.on.ca.

WADDEN, Ann M; 105-375 Pleasant St, Dartmouth NS B2Y 4N4; Dal'84; Staff, Dartmouth General Hospital; Staff, IWK Health Centre; (902)469-2447; Fax. (902)469-2449.

WADDEN, Michael R; 100 Station Lane, Kentville NS B4N 0A3; Dal'95; CCFP; (902)681-9126; Fax. (902)681-1058; docwadden@kindle.com.

WADDEN, Nancy A T; St Clare's Mercy Hosp, 154 Lemarchant Rd, St. John's NL A1C 5B8; Mem'84; AB; FRCPC; DiagRad (Breast Imaging). Staff, Health Sciences Centre; Staff Radiol, St Clare's Mercy Hospital; Assoc Prof, Memorial University Of Newfoundland; (709)777-5657

WADDEN, Patricia M; Health Sciences Centre, 300 Prince Philip Dr, St. John's NL A1B 3V6; Mem'83; FRCPC; AnatPath; GenPath. Staff Path, Health Sciences Centre; (709)777-6401

WADDEN, Paul C; Victoria Prof Centre, 301-111 Waterloo St, London ON N6B 2M4; Mem'79; FRCPC; Psy. Staff, Bluewater Health - Mitton Site; Ac Staff, Regional Mental Health Care-St Joseph's Health Care; (519)266-6944

WADDEN, Robert A; Renaissance Hair Clinic, 302 Hamilton Ave, St. John's NL A1E 1J9; Dal'91; ABHRS; Staff, Renaissance Hair Replacement Clinic.

WADDINGTON, Ashley; Kingston Gen Hosp, 76 Stuart St, Kingston ON K7L 2V7; McM'06; FRCSC; ObstGyn. Fellow, Kingston General Hospital; (613)542-9473; Fax. (613)533-6779.

WADE, Andrew; 2888 Shaganappi Trail NW, Calgary AB T3B 6A8; Leeds (England),'71; BSc(Hon.); PhD; Staff, Alberta Children's Hospital; (403)955-2980; Fax. (403)955-7798; pedneph@me.com.

WADE, Andrew W; Alberta Children's Hosp, 2888 Shaganappi Trail NW, Calgary AB T3B 6A8; Cal'91; PhD; BSc; FRCPC; Peds (Nephrology). Dir Dialysis/Staff, Alberta Children's Hospital; Assoc Prof Peds, University of Calgary; (403)955-2980; Fax. (403)955-7798.

WADE, Carol L; Credit Valley Obst/Gyn Assoc, 502-2000 Credit Valley Rd, Mississauga ON L5M 4N4; Tor'87; FRCSC; ObstGyn (Urogynecology). Ac Staff ObstGyn, The Credit Valley Hospital; (905)820-8748; Fax. (905)820-0255; cwade@cvh.on.ca.

WADE, David A; Dr D A Wade Prof Corp, 515 Youghall Dr, Bathurst NB E2A 4X7; Dal'73; (506)548-8077; Fax. (506)546-5834.

WADE, Jessica L; Élisabeth Bruyère Hosp, 3JB-43 Bruyere St, Ottawa ON K1N 5C8; Mem'10; CCFP; Staff, SCO Health Service - Élisabeth Bruyère Hospital; (613)532-6335

WADE, John P D; Laurel Med Centre Ltd, 208-888 8th Ave W, Vancouver BC V5Z 3Y1; UBC'80; FRCPC; IntMed; Rheum. Ac Staff, Vancouver General Hospital - Centennial Pavillion; (604)875-1570; Fax. (604)875-1569.

WADE, Leonard R; Vulcan Med Clinic, PO Box 419, Vulcan AB T0L 2B0; Cal'85; CCFP; (403)485-2216; Fax. (403)485-2218.

WADE, N Kevin; Kerrisdale Prof Centre, 345-2025 42nd Ave W, Vancouver BC V6M 2B5; McG'88; FRCPC; IntMed (Cataract Surgery); Ophth. Clin Assoc Prof, University of British Columbia; (604)263-3335

WADE, Phillip S; Canadian Hearing Society, 271 Spadina Rd, Toronto ON M5R 2V3; Tor'70; DDS; FRCSC; Otol (Head & Neck Surgery). Staff Pt-Time, Toronto General Hospital - UHN; Staff, Markham Stouffville Hospital; Physician, The Canadian Hearing Society; Asst Prof, University of Toronto; (416)920-1717; Fax. (416)920-4211; pwade@chs.ca.

WADEHRA, Davinder B S; LMC Brampton, 2130 North Park Dr, Brampton ON L6S 0C9; University of Delhi (India)'02.

WADEY, Veronica M R; Sunnybrook Holland Ortho Arthr, 327-43 Wellesley St E, Toronto ON M4Y 1H1; Cal'96; FRCSC; OrthSurg. Staff, Sunnybrook Health Sciences Centre - Holland Orthopaedic & Arthritic Centre; (416)967-8615; Fax. (416)967-8622.

WADGE, Richard; Fleetwood Place Care Home, 16011 83 Ave, Surrey BC V4N 0N2; UBC'70; Ac Staff, Surrey Memorial Hospital; Med Dir, Fleetwood Paint & Decorating C; Clin Instructor Med, University of British Columbia; (604)590-6860; rwadge@hotmail.com.

WADGE, Sara M; 103-5631 Inlet Ave PO Box 799, Sechelt BC V0N 3A0; UBC'97; FRCPC; IntMed. Staff, St Mary's Hospital; (604)885-7103; Fax. (604)885-7104.

WADGYMAR, J Arturo; 501-2300 Eglinton Ave W, Mississauga ON L5M 2V8; National (Mexico)'75; ABIM; MSc; FACP; FRCPC; IntMed; Nephrol. Staff, The Credit Valley Hospital; Langs: Spanish; (905)820-8770; Fax. (905)820-3703; awadgymar@cvh.on.ca.

WADHERA, Sanjay K; 17-6219 Centre St NW, Calgary AB T2K 0V2; Ott'89; CCFP; (403)274-4428; Fax. (403)274-4824.

WADHWA, Anupma; The Hosp for Sick Children, 7304-555 University Ave, Toronto ON M5G 1X8; Tor'96; FRCPC; Peds; InfectDis. Staff, The Hospital For Sick Children; (416)813-6273; Fax. (416)813-5032.

WADHWA, Atma S; B1-172 Ethel St, Sturgeon Falls ON P2B 1V9; Punjab (India)'58; MB BS; MRCP(Lond); FCCP; FRCPC; IntMed (Cardiology). Chief ICU Dept/Ac Staff, West Nipissing General Hospital; Langs: Hindi; French; Punjabi; (705)753-0540; Fax. (705)753-0689.

WADHWA, Birender P S; Medical Clinic, PO Box 888 Stn Main, Corner Brook NL A2H 6H6; Baba Farid University (Other Foreign)'05; CCFP; Locum Tenens, Western Memorial Regional Hospital; (709)634-1900

WADHWA, Gagan D D; Univ Hlth Network-Princess M, 16 119-610 University Ave, Toronto ON M5G 2M9; Dal'06; FRCPC; IntMed; MedOncol. Staff, Princess Margaret Hospital - University Health Network; (416)946-2000

WADHWA, Kanwar J S; Killick Health Services, 129 Lincoln Rd, Grnd-Falls-Windsor NL A2A 1P3; Baba Farid University (India)'05; MB BS; IntMed. Staff, Central Newfoundland Regional Health Centre.

WADHWA, Mandeep; Uptown Health, 8-9325 Yonge St, Richmond Hill ON L4C 0A8; Delhi (India)'98; CCFP; (905)508-8876

WADHWA, Pradeep; Family Care Med Centre, 112-55 Castleridge Blvd NE, Calgary AB T3J 3J8; London (England)'79; MB BS; DCH; DRCOG; MRC; Langs: Punjabi; (403)280-5500; Fax. (403)293-2207.

WADHWA, Uttam J K; Trillium Hlth Ctr-Mississauga, 1023-100 Queensway W, Mississauga ON L5B 1B8; New Delhi (India)'71; MB BS; FRCPC; Psy (Acute Adult Psychiatry). Staff, Trillium Health Centre - Mississauga; Langs: Hindi; Punjabi; Urdu; Arabic; (905)848-7580; Fax. (905)804-7969.

WADHWA, Vikram S; Health Sciences Centre, GA 216-820 Sherbrook St, Winnipeg MB R3A 1R9; Dal'01; FRCPC; DiagRad. Staff, Health Sciences Centre; (204)787-1328; Fax. (204)787-3118.

WADIA, Yasmin J; Peace Arch Commun Med Clinic, 1545 Johnston Ave, White Rock BC V4B 3Z6; Ranchi (India)'71; Langs: Hindi; Gujarati; (604)535-8496

WADIWALLA, Shamim; Queen Elizabeth II HSC, 431-1276 South Park St, Halifax NS B3H 2Y9; (India)'98; Staff Hematology, Queen Elizabeth II Health Sciences Centre - Victoria General Site; (902)473-7006; Fax. (902)473-4420.

WADSWORTH, Louis D; Children's & Women's HC Of BC, 2K51-4480 Oak St, Vancouver BC V6H 3V4; Manchester (England)'66; MB ChB; FRCP; FRCPC; HemPath. Div Head HemPath, BC Children's Hospital; Consultant, Vancouver General Hospital - Centennial Pavillion; Clin Prof Path, University of British Columbia; (604)875-2306; Fax. (604)875-2815.

WAECHTER, Jason E; Foothills Med Centre, 1403 29 St NW, Calgary AB T2N 2T9; UBC'97; FRCPC; Anes; Critical Care Medicine. Staff, Foothills Medical Centre; (403)944-4636

WAERN, Bryn F; 23 Biggar Ave, Toronto ON M6H 2N5; Tor'67; DPsy; (416)654-1333; Fax. (416)654-1333; brynw@sympatico.ca.

WAESE, Adam S; Hope Team-CMHA, 2F-15150 Yonge St, Aurora ON L4G 1M2; Qns'99; BSc(Hon); FRCPC; Psy (Couple Therapy). Locum Tenens, Temiskaming Hospital; Staff, Canadian Mental Health Agency-Hope Team; Lecturer, University of Toronto; (905)853-8477 x4260; Fax. (905)841-3007.

WAGAR, Donald B; PO Box 12117 Murrayville RPO, Langley BC V3A 9J5; UBC'70.

WAGENAAR, Johannes M B; 173 Fern Rd W, Qualicum Beach BC V9K 1S4; Stellenbosch (South Africa)'79; Staff, Nanaimo Regional General Hospital; Langs: Afrikaans; (250)752-0557; Fax. (250)752-6918.

WAGG, Adrian S; Clinical Sciences Bldg, 1 116-11350 83 Ave, Edmonton AB T6G 2P4; (780)492-5338

WAGG, Brian D; 70 Charles St, Brockville ON K6V 1T3; Ott'76; CCFP; FCFP; Ac Staff, Brockville General Hospital - Charles Street; Ac Staff, Providence Continuing Care Centre (PCCC) - St Vincent de Paul Hospital; (613)345-1458; Fax. (613)345-5296.

WAGG, Ian D; Georgian Bay Gen Hosp, PO Box 760 Stn Main 1112 St Andrew's Dr, Midland ON L4R 4P4; Tor'09; CCFP; Staff, Georgian Bay General Hospital - Midland; (705)526-1300; Fax. (705)526-2007.

WAGG, James P; Saint John Reg Hosp, PO Box 2100 Stn Main 400 University Ave, Saint John NB E2L 4L2; Dal'93; FRCSC; OrthSurg (Trauma). Staff, Saint John Regional Hospital; (506)648-7902; Fax. (506)648-7012; j_wagg@hotmail.com.

WAGG, L Allison; Waypoint Centre for Mental HC, 500 Church St, Penetanguishene ON L9M 1G3; Ott'07; FRCPC; Psy. Staff, Sault Area Hospital - Sault Ste Marie; Staff, Waypoint Centre for Mental Health Care; (705)549-3181

WAGHMARE, Raj; Enhanced Care Clinic, 14872 Yonge St, Aurora ON L4G 1N2; Wes'00; CCFP; Staff, Grey Bruce Health Services - Markdale; Langs: English; French; (905)505-0950

WAGHRAY, Ranjit K; Calgary Lab Services, 9-3535 Research Rd NW, Calgary AB T2L 2K8; Osmania (India)'77; MB BS; FCAP; FRCPC; AnatPath (Cytopath). Staff Calgary Lab Services, Peter Lougheed Centre; Dir Cytopath, Calgary Laboratory Services; Clin Assoc Prof Path, University of Calgary; (403)770-3204; Fax. (403)770-3295; ranjit.waghray@cls.ab.ca.

WAGLER, Amanda M; Upper Grand Family Health Team, LL-205 Queen St E, Fergus ON N1M 1T2; McM'04; CCFP; (519)787-1200; Fax. (519)787-1803.

WAGMAN, David M; Goodfellow Prof Bldg, 202-170 McEwan Dr E, Bolton ON L7E 4C8; McG'89; Staff, William Osler Health System - Etobicoke General Hospital; Langs: English; French; (905)951-7740; Fax. (905)951-7742.

WAGMAN, Robert D; Davisville Med & Dental Centre, 712-1849 Yonge St, Toronto ON M4S 1Y2; Columbia(NY) (USA)'81; DABOph; AB; FRCSC; Ophth (Pediatric Ophthalmology). Staff, Toronto Western Hospital - University Health Network; (416)925-8893; Fax. (416)925-1335.

WAGNER, Brenda L M; 307-7031 Westminster Hwy, Richmond BC V6X 1A3; Ann Arbor (USA)'91; FRCSC; ObstGyn. Dep Head ObstGyn & Co-Clin Prog Manager, BC Women's Hospital & Health Centre; Langs: English; French; (604)270-1434; Fax. (604)270-3431.

WAGNER, Brent G; 103-8585 160 St, Surrey BC V4N 1G4; Alb'90; BMedSci; (604)543-9719

WAGNER, Cheryl A; St Michal's Hosp Academic-FHT, PO Box 36 940-790 Bay St, Toronto ON M5G 1N8; McM'82; CCFP; FCFP; Staff, Toronto General Hospital - UHN; University of Toronto; (416)926-0101; Fax. (416)926-1910.

WAGNER, Christine M; Surrey Prenatal, 2-9655 137 St, Surrey BC V3T 4G8; McM'82; CCFP; FCFP; Staff, Surrey Memorial Hospital; (778)395-0085; Fax. (778)395-0085.

WAGNER, Daniel; Clin Reseau Le Trait D'Union, 38 boul Marie-Victorin, Delson QC J5B 1A9; Mon'70; Prés, Clinique Reseau le Trait d'Union; Langs: Bilingual(French/English); (450)633-0123; Fax. (450)633-1140; wagc@bellnet.ca.

WAGNER, Elisabeth M; Sunridge Prof Centre, 501-2675 36 St NE, Calgary AB T1Y 6H6; Sask'94; BSc; FRCSC; ObstGyn (Laparoscopy). Langs: English; French; (403)219-8333; Fax. (403)250-1496.

WAGNER, Garth A L; 67 Wing Bldg, 102-2210 2 St SW, Calgary AB T2S 3C3; Sask'64; FACS; FRCSC; Otol (Sinusitis). Staff, Alberta Children's Hospital; (403)292-9555; Fax. (403)292-9557; gwagner@ucalgary.ca.

WAGNER, Marie-Helene; Serv Externe de Psychiatrie, 230-383 boul du Seminaire N, St-Jean-sur-Richel QC J3B 8C5; Mon'04; FRCPC; Psy. (450)346-2222

WAGNER, Marie-Soleil; Hôpital Ste-Justine, 3175 ch Cote-Sainte-Catherine, Montreal QC H3T 1C5; Mon'98; FRCSC; ObstGyn. Staff, Hôpital Ste-Justine; (514)345-4706; Fax. (514)345-4648.

WAGNER, Michael B; Edmonton Clinic, L2-11400 University Ave. , Edmonton AB T6G 1Z1; Alb'06; Dip SportMed; CCFP; Physician Glen Sather Sports Med Clinic, University of Alberta; (780)407-5160; Fax. (780)407-5667.

WAGNER, Sheldon I; 403-265 Yorkland Blvd, North York ON M2J 5C7; Tor'68; (416)229-2399; Fax. (416)229-9771.

WAGNER, Susan G; Broadway Family Physicians, 1801 Broadway Ave, Saskatoon SK S7H 2B6; Sask'08; CCFP; (306)652-2632; Fax. (306)652-2637.

WAGONER, Michelle L; Nova Med Centre, 204-496 Topsail Rd, St. John's NL A1E 2C2; Mem'99; (709)745-6682

WAHAB, Nazneem N; Hys Med Centre, 350-11010 101 St NW, Edmonton AB T5H 4B9; Sask'97; FRCPC; IntMed (Echocardiography); Cardiol. Staff, Royal Alexandra Hospital; (780)428-3246; Fax. (780)425-0487.

WAHALAWATTA, Punsara D; Primacy Family First Health Ct, PO Box 51031 375 des Epinettes Ave, Orleans ON K1E 3E6; Saba University (Other Foreign)'06; (613)841-7009; Fax. (613)841-0106.

WAHAY, Leigh R; North Lanark Comm Hlth Centre, 207 Robertson Rd, Lanark ON K0G 1K0; Ott'99; CCFP; Ac Staff, Perth & Smiths Falls District Hospital - Perth Site (Great War Memorial Site); (613)259-2182; Fax. (613)259-5235.

WAHBA, Inas A A; 10125 157 St NW, Edmonton AB T5P 2T9; (Egypt)'87; (780)486-6664; Fax. (780)486-6654.

WAHBA, Mark Y; Royal University Hosp, 103 Hospital Dr, Saskatoon SK S7N 0W8; Sask'00; CCFP; CCFP(E.M.); Staff Emerg, Royal University Hospital; (306)655-1364; Fax. (306)655-1258; drmarkwahba@mac.com.

WAHBA, Odette Z; Kennedy Med Centre, 6-510 Driftcurrent Dr, Mississauga ON L4Z 4B4; Cairo (Egypt)'79; CCFP; Langs: Arabic; (905)568-1173; Fax. (905)568-2621.

WAHBA, Raouf S; Foothills Med Centre, 1403 29 St NW, Calgary AB T2N 2T9; Ain Shams (Egypt)'77; FRCPC; Anes. Staff Anes, Foothills Medical Centre; (403)944-1430

WAHBA, Rasha G S; Credit Landing Med Clinic, 7-224 Lakeshore Rd W, Mississauga ON L5H 1G6; Ain Shams (Egypt)'98; CCFP; Langs: Arabic; (905)271-6455; Fax. (905)271-6492; mmfwahba@hotmail.com.

WAHBA HANNA, Talaat W S; Wheat City Med Clinic, C1-1711 Kirkcaldy Dr, Brandon MB R7A 0B9; (Other Foreign)'84; (204)727-1711

WAHBY, Allen J; 103-860 Tecumseh Rd E, Windsor ON N8X 2S5; Wes'74; Staff, Windsor Regional Hospital - Metropolitan Site; Staff Gen Pract, Hôtel-Dieu Grace Hospital; Langs: Hungarian; (519)254-3552; Fax. (519)254-2077.

WAHEED, Shahzad B; Janeway Children's Hlth & Reha, 300 Prince Philip Dr, St. John's NL A1B 3V6; Karachi University (Pakistan)'97; FRCPC; Peds (Pediatric Critical Care). Staff, Janeway Children's Health & Rehabilitation Centre; (709)777-6300

WAHEED, Waqar; Alberta Children's Hosp, A0 208-2888 Shanagappi Trail, Calgary AB T3B 6A8; Rawalpindi (Pakistan)'97; MB BS; FRCPC; Psy (Child & Adolesc Forensic Psy). Staff Forensic Adolescent Prog, Alberta Children's Hospital; Clin Instructor, University of Alberta; Langs: Urdu; Punjabi; Hindi; (403)955-2214; Fax. (403)955-3108; waqar.waheed@calgaryhealthregion.ca.

WAHHAB, Ramzy; CHUM-Hop Notre-Dame, 1560 rue Sherbrooke E, Montreal QC H2L 4M1; Mon'08; FRCPC; IntMed. Staff, Centre Hospitalier l'Université de Montréal (CHUM) - Hôpital Notre-Dame; (514)890-8000

WAHI, Gita; McMaster Univ-Children's Hosp, 1280 Main St W, Hamilton ON L8S 4K1; Wes'04; FRCPC; Peds. Staff, The Hospital For Sick Children; Staff, McMaster University; (905)521-2100; Fax. (905)308-7548.

WAHI, Shobha; Charlton Med Centre, 302-25 Charlton Ave E, Hamilton ON L8N 1Y2; Punjab (India)'70; FAAP; FRCPC; Peds. Staff Clinical Teaching Unit, St Joseph's Healthcare - Charlton Campus; Clin Assoc Prof, McMaster University; Instructor, University of Toronto; Langs: Hindi; Urdu; (905)523-7920; Fax. (905)523-5121.

WAHID, Salman; Cambridge Mem Hosp, 700 Coronation Blvd, Cambridge ON N1R 3G2; (Pakistan)'94; (519)740-4900; Fax. (519)740-4900.

WAHL, Adalbert E; Rebalance MD, 104-3551 Blanshard St, Victoria BC V8Z 0B9; Alb'71; BSc; FRCSC; OrthSurg (Spinal Injury). Staff, Victoria General Hospital; Staff, Royal Jubilee Hospital; Staff, Gorge Road Hospital; (250)940-4444

WAHL, Marius C; 568 Mountainview Sq, Kitimat BC V8C 2N2; Stellenbosch (South Africa)'85; MB ChB; Langs: Afrikaans; (250)632-4993

WAHL, Patrick D; Health Services Centre, PO Box 17000 Stn Forces B 62-23 Canadian Forces Base, Winnipeg MB R3J 3Y5; Cal'91; CCFP; Staff, Canadian Forces Base.

WAI, Amy C K; Patient Networks, 157 Yonge St, Toronto ON M5C 1X7; Tor'92; CCFP; FCFP; Physician, Patient Networks; (416)362-8822; Fax. (416)362-8877.

WAI, Elaine S S; BC Cancer Agency-Vanc Isl Ctr, 2410 Lee Ave, Victoria BC V8R 6V5; UBC'95; FRCPC; RadOncol. Staff, BC Cancer Agency Vancouver Island Centre; (250)519-5575; Fax. (250)519-2018.

WAI, Eugene K; The Ottawa Hosp-Civic Campus, J 141-1053 Carling Ave, Ottawa ON K1Y 4E9; Tor'94; FRCSC; OrthSurg (Spinal Injury). Staff, The Ottawa Hospital - Civic Campus; (613)761-5555 x19138; Fax. (613)761-4944; ewai@ottawahospital.on.ca.

WAI, Yvonne; Meadowbrook Lane Med Centre, 103E-4581 Highway 7, Unionville ON L3R 1M6; Wes'96; BSc; FRCPC; IntMed; ClinImmunol&Allergy. (905)479-9693

WAIDA, Eiko; North Okanagan Paediatric Clin, 3-2802 34 St, Vernon BC V1T 5X1; Alb'90; FAAP; FRCPC; Peds. Staff, Vernon Jubilee Hospital; Langs: Japanese; (250)558-5506; Fax. (250)558-5108; nopc@shawcable.com.

WAINBERG, Daniel; 101B-1771 Comox Ave, Comox BC V9M 3L9; McM'08; CCFP; (250)339-5780

WAINBERG, Sara J; Toronto Memory Prog, 400-1 Valleybrook Dr, North York ON M3B 2S7; McM'07; CCFP; (416)386-9761

WAIND, Peter B; 105-131 Union St E, Waterloo ON N2J 1C4; McM'80; LMCC; FRCSC; Ophth. Staff, St Mary's General Hospital; Staff, Grand River Hospital - Kitchener/Waterloo Health Centre; Langs: Bilingual(English/French); (519)746-1040; Fax. (519)746-4413; peter.waind@sympatico.ca.

WAINER, Stephen; East Calgary Health Centre, 4715 8 Ave SE, Calgary AB T2A 3N4; Witwatersrand (South Africa)'79; MB ChB; FRCPC; Peds. Staff, Peter Lougheed Centre; Staff, Alberta Children's Hospital; (403)955-1077; Fax. (403)955-1076; wainer@ucalgary.ca.

WAINWRIGHT, Ruth E H; A I M Health Group, 1051 Wonderland Rd S, London ON N6K 3X4; London (England)'58; MB BS; DRCOG; (519)472-2060; Fax. (519)471-7299.

WAISBERG, Jon W; North Toronto Eye Care, 407-2115 Finch Ave W, North York ON M3N 2V6; Wes'67; FRCSC; Ophth. Ac Staff, Humber River Regional Hospital - Finch Avenue Site; Ac Staff, Humber River Regional Hospital - Church Street Site; (416)748-2020; Fax. (416)748-8582; jww43@rogers.com.

WAISGLASS, Barry R; Niagara Falls Comm Health Ctre, PO Box 123 4481 Queen St, Niagara Falls ON L2E 6S8; Ott'73; (905)356-4222; Fax. (905)356-5676.

WAISMAN, Zohar; North York Gen Hosp, U7S 120-4001 Leslie St, North York ON M2K 1E1; McM'95; FRCPC; Psy (Acute & Chronic Pain). Consultant Psy Wasser Pain Clinic, Mount Sinai Hospital; Staff Law & Mental Health Prog, Centre for Addiction & Mental Health (CAMH) - Queen Site; North York General Hospital - Branson Division; Head Inpatient Psy, North York General Hospital; Asst Prof, University of Toronto; Langs: Hebrew; Russian; (416)756-6000 x4246

WAITE, Patricia L; Pine Seven Med Centre, 150-4600 Highway 7, Woodbridge ON L4L 4Y7; Tor'84; CCFP; FCFP; Staff, William Osler Health System - Etobicoke General Hospital; (905)856-1000; Fax. (905)851-9927.

WAITE, Robert P; Weld Street Clinic, PO Box 1060 Stn Main 168 Weld St, Parksville BC V9P 2H1; UBC'92; Staff, Nanaimo Regional General Hospital; (250)248-5677; Fax. (250)248-4287.

WAITSCHIES, Elfriede G; 100-300 Main St N, Brampton ON L6V 4H6; Tor'76; Staff, William Osler Health System - Brampton Civic Hospital; (905)450-0151; Fax. (905)450-7152.

WAITZER, Sloane M; Baywood Med Centre, 200-95 Bayly St W, Ajax ON L1S 7K8; Tor'80; FRCPC; Derm (Cosmetic Dermatology). (905)686-3900

WAIZ, Richard L; 103-20644 Fraser Hwy, Langley BC V3A 4G5; UBC'86; (604)530-4979; Fax. (604)530-2975.

WAJA, Lukmaan; 30 Larocque Rd, North Bay ON P1B 8G3; Witwatersrand (South Africa)'88; MB ChB; FRCSC; ObstGyn. Staff, North Bay Regional Health Centre - Regional Mental Health; Assoc Prof Family Med Prog, Northern Ontario School of Medicine; Langs: Afrikaans; (705)495-3101; Fax. (705)495-8460.

WAJEEH, Mohammed; Yarmouth Reg Hosp, 306-60 Vancouver St, Yarmouth NS B5A 2P5; Baghdad (Iraq)'71; MB ChB; Staff Dr Wajeeh Eye Clinic Ltd, Yarmouth Regional Hospital; (902)742-7678; Fax. (902)742-0928.

WAJSTAUB, Sandra; Cape Breton Reg Hosp, 1482 George St, Sydney NS B1P 1P3; Wes'99; BA; BSc; MBA; FRCPC; RadOncol (Medical Oncology). Staff, Cape Breton Healthcare Complex; Staff RadOncol, Cape Breton Cancer Centre; (902)567-7771; Fax. (902)567-3182.

WAJSZILBER, Marcelo A; CSSS de la Vallée de l'Or, 725 6e rue, Val-d'Or QC J9P 3Y1; Buenos Aires (Argentina)'82; Staff, Centre Hospitalier de Val d'Or; (819)825-6711

WAKEFIELD, J Scott; Peter Lougheed Centre, 3500 26 Ave NE, Calgary AB T1Y 6J4; Cal'93; CCFP; FCFP; Staff, Peter Lougheed Centre; Langs: English; French; (403)943-5461; Fax. (403)943-5438; scottwakefield@shaw.ca.

WAKEFIELD, Jacqueline S G; Foundation for Med Pract Educ, DTC-1280 Main St W, Hamilton ON L8S 4L8; Ann Arbor(MI) (USA)'69; CCFP; FCFP; Staff, Foundation for Medical Practice Education; (905)525-9140; Fax. (905)540-4988.

WAKEFIELD, Robert G; Gordon & Leslie Diamond HCC, 7F-2775 Laurel St, Vancouver BC V5Z 1M9; Stanford(CA) (USA)'73; BSc; MD; FRCP; FACP; FRCPC; IntMed (Geriatric Medicine). Staff, Gordon & Leslie Diamond Health Care Centre; Clin Asst Prof IntMed, University of British Columbia; (604)875-5907; Fax. (604)875-5906.

WAKEFIELD, Tara S; North Side Clinic, 915 Central Ave N, Swift Current SK S9H 3V3; Indiana(IN) (USA)'99; CCFP; (306)773-9100; Fax. (306)773-9668; tarawakefield@hotmail.com.

WAKEGIJIG, Annelind D V; Baawaating Family Health Team, 210 Gran St, Sault Ste. Marie ON P6A 5K9; Alb'97; CCFP; Staff, Sault Area Hospital - Thessalon Division; Staff, Baawaating Family Health Team; Asst Prof, Northern Ontario School of Medicine-Lakehead University; (705)575-7191; Fax. (705)575-7193.

WAKEHAM, Julia C; 1-273 King St E, Kingston ON K7L 3B1; Cal'02; CCFP; (613)766-0110; Fax. (613)766-6017.

WAKELIN, David L; 203-300 Brae Rd, Duncan BC V9L 3T8; UBC'69; FRCSC; Ophth. Ac Staff, Cowichan District Hospital; Consultant, Royal Jubilee Hospital; (250)748-2922; Fax. (250)748-9647; dwakelind@shaw.ca.

WAKELY, Kathryn A; 348 Lyndock St, Corunna ON N0N 1G0; Wes'78; BSc(Hon); Court Staff, Bluewater Health - Mitton Site; Physician, C F Industrial Inc; (519)862-1461; Fax. (519)862-5835.

WAKELY, Laura J; Victoria Gen Hosp, 1 Hospital Way, Victoria BC V8Z 6R5; UBC'07; FRCPC; Anes. Staff, Victoria General Hospital; Staff, Lions Gate Hospital; (250)727-4212

WAKELY, Peter A; 348 Lyndock St PO Box 818, Corunna ON N0N 1G0; Wes'78; Staff, Bluewater Health - Mitton Site; Staff, Bluewater Health - Norman Site; (519)862-1461; Fax. (519)862-5835.

WAKEMAN, M Stewart A; 1-25 Sherbrook St, Winnipeg MB R3C 2B1; Man'81; BSc; FRCPC; Psy (Community Psychiatry). Assoc Staff, Misericordia Health Centre; Registrar Psy, Winnipeg Commun. & Long Term Care Authority.

WAKIL, Georges; Hopital Charles LeMoyne, 3120 boul Taschereau, Longueuil QC J4V 2H1; McG'04; RadOncol. Staff, Hopital Charles LeMoyne; (450)466-5000

WAKIM, Emma G; Medical Bldg, 400-18 Pine St, Kitchener ON N2H 5Z8; McM'97; FRCSC; ObstGyn. (519)570-0090; Fax. (519)570-3202.

WAKS, Joshua A; 305-745 Mount Pleasant Rd, Toronto ON M4S 2N4; Wes'06; CCFP; (416)487-2052; Fax. (416)480-2030.

WAKULICH, Joanne A; Woodbine Med Centre, B9-76 Arlington Dr, Keswick ON L4P 0A9; Alb'90; CCFP; Staff, Southlake Regional Health Centre; (905)476-0308; Fax. (905)476-1079.

WALC, Leslie C; Bayside Med Centre, 3 Beck Blvd, Penetanguishene ON L9M 1B9; Ott'96; BSc; FRCSC; GenSurg. (705)549-3939; Fax. (705)549-0029.

WALD, Rachel M; 5N 517-585 University Ave, Toronto ON M5G 2N2; Tor'98; FRCPC; Peds (Congenital Heart Disease); Cardiol. Assoc Staff, The Hospital For Sick Children; Staff, Toronto General Hospital - UHN; Asst Prof, University of Toronto; (416)340-5502; Fax. (416)340-5014.

WALD, Robert W; Mount Sinai Hosp, 600 University Ave, Toronto ON M5G 1X5; Tor'72; FACC; FACP; ABC; ABIM; BSc(Hon); FRCPC; Cardiol (Cardiac Pacing). Staff Cardiol, Mount Sinai Hospital; Staff Cardiol, Toronto General Hospital - UHN; Assoc Prof Med, University of Toronto; Langs: Hungarian; French; (416)586-5285; Fax. (416)586-8585; rwald@mtsinai.on.ca.

WALD, Ron; St Michael's Hosp, 30 Bond St, Toronto ON M5B 1W8; McG'99; FRCPC; IntMed; Nephrol. Staff, St Michael's Hospital; Langs: Hebrew; French; (416)867-3703; Fax. (416)867-3709.

WALDBILLIG, David K; St Mary's Gen Hosp, 911 Queens Blvd, Kitchener ON N2M 1B2; McM'91; BSc; MSc; CCFP; CCFP(E.M.); Staff Emerg Room, St Mary's General Hospital; Med Dir/Staff, Canadian Forces Base Borden; Supvr Elective, Rural Ontario Medical Program; (519)749-6410; Fax. (519)749-6411; dwaldbillig@gbhs.on.ca.

WALDE, Paul L D; Group Health Centre, 240 McNabb St, Sault Ste. Marie ON P6B 1Y5; London (England)'68; LRCP; MRCS; MRC; ABIM; FRCPC; IntMed; MedOncol. Staff Consultant Algoma Reg Cancer Prog, Sault Area Hospital - Sault Ste Marie; (705)759-5631; Fax. (705)946-5241.

WALDEN, Paul D; Whistler Med Clinic, 4380 Lorimer Rd RR 4, Whistler BC V0N 1B4; Tor'84; BSc; CCFP; Staff, Pine Medical Clinic; (604)932-4911; Fax. (604)932-4992; pwalden@shaw.ca.

WALDENBERG, Samuel S; 395 Queen St S, Hamilton ON L8P 3T8; London (England)'63; DPM; MPhil; MRCPsy; FRCPC; Psy (Pain Management). (905)529-1829; Fax. (905)529-3635.

WALDMAN, Deborah J; 4186 Dunbar St, Vancouver BC V6S 2E7; Qns'93; BSc; CCFP; (604)739-9881; Fax. (604)739-9803; dwaldman@shaw.ca.

WALDMAN, Jeffrey C; Psychealth Centre, PX3-771 Bannatyne Ave, Winnipeg MB R3E 3N4; Qns'98; FRCPC; Psy. Physician, Psychealth Centre; jwaldman@exchange.hsc.mb.ca.

WALDMAN, Lyle H; Westmount Square Med Centre, 1 car Westmount, Montreal QC H3Z 2P9; Louvain (Belgium)'73; Médecin, O-I Canada; Médecin, CLSC Waswanipi; Langs: Spanish; French; (514)934-2334; lylandre@yahoo.com.

WALDMAN, Murray L; St John's Rehab Hosp, 285 Cummer Ave, North York ON M2M 2G1; Man'72; CCFP; CCFP(E.M.); Staff, St John's Rehabilitation Hospital; Teacher, University of Toronto; (416)226-6780; Fax. (416)226-6265; murray.waldman@gmail.com.

WALDOLF, Richard E; Pembroke Reg Hosp, 705 Mackay St, Pembroke ON K8A 1G8; Ott'08; CCFP; Staff, Pembroke Regional Hospital; Langs: Bilingual(English/French); (613)732-2811; richard.waldolf@pemreghos.org.

WALDRON, James B; Gladstone Med Centre, 4095 rue Tupper, Westmount QC H3Z 3E5; Otago (New Zealand)'64; AB; FRCSC; Ophth (Comprehensive Ophthalmology). assoc Staff Ophth, McGill University Health Centre - Montreal General Campus; adj Prof, McGill University; Langs: French; (514)935-0866; Fax. (514)989-7204.

WALDRON, John N; Univ Hlth Network-Princess M, 610 University Ave, Toronto ON M5G 2M9; Qns'88; FRCPC; RadOncol. , Princess Margaret Hospital - University Health Network; Lecturer, University of Toronto; (416)946-2000 x6522; john.waldron@uhn.on.ca.

WALDRON, Leslie A; Urgent Care Centre, 945 Gardiners Rd, Kingston ON K7M 7H4; Cal'94; CCFP; FCFP; Att Staff, QHC North Hastings; Att Staff, Stevenson Memorial Hospital; Langs: English; French; (613)544-0200; Fax. (613)544-4264.

WALDRON, Mark A; Lennox & Addington Gen Hosp, 8 Richmond Park Dr, Napanee ON K7R 2Z4; Tor'94; CCFP; CCFP(E.M.); Staff, Lennox & Addington County General Hospital; (613)354-3301

WALDRON, Ross R; 3591 31 St, Vernon BC V1T 5J4; UBC'86; CCFP; (250)542-1215; Fax. (250)542-0160.

WALE, Jason T; St Joseph's Gen Hosp, 2137 Comox Ave, Comox BC V9M 1P2; UBC'96; CCFP; CCFP(E.M.); Staff Emerg Med & Family Med, St Joseph's General Hospital; Langs: English; French; (250)339-2242; Fax. (250)339-0985.

WALE, Martin C J; Royal Jubilee Hosp, WW 312-1952 Bay St, Victoria BC V8R 1J8; Nottingham (England)'80; Staff, Royal Jubilee Hospital; (250)370-8531

WALELE, Abdul A; 100-3 Connestoga Dr, Brampton ON L6Z 4N5; South Africa (Zimbabwe)'86; MMed; FRCPC; IntMed; Nephrol. Staff, St Joseph's Healthcare - Charlton Campus; (905)216-0238; Fax. (905)497-7114.

WALENTYNOWICZ, Magdalena A; Capital District Mental Health, 500-33 Alderney Dr, Dartmouth NS B2Y 2N4; Krakow (Poland)'77; FRCPC; Psy. Staff Psy, The Nova Scotia Hospital; Staff/Asst Prof, Capital District Mental Health Program; Asst Prof, Dalhousie University; (902)466-1830; Fax. (902)466-1851.

WALER, Oleh R; Pelham Group Health Centre, 216-245 Pelham Rd, St Catharines ON L2S 1X8; Mem'73; Ac Staff, Niagara Health System - St Catharines General Site; Langs: Ukrainian; (905)988-1363; Fax. (905)688-2652.

WALES, Paul W; The Hosp for Sick Children, 1526-555 University Ave, Toronto ON M5G 1X8; UBC'93; BSc; MSc; FRCSC; GenSurg; PedGenSurg. Staff, The Hospital For Sick Children; (416)813-7654 x1490; Fax. (416)813-7477; paul.wales@sickkids.ca.

WALFISH, Paul G; Mount Sinai Hosp, 413 7-600 University Ave, Toronto ON M5G 1X5; Tor'58; FACP; FRCPC; IntMed (Endocrinology). Att Physician Sr, Mount Sinai Hospital; (416)586-4437; Fax. (416)586-8861.

WALGAMA, B G Shiromi D; Howard Ave Walk in Clinic, 124-2462 Howard Ave, Windsor ON N8X 3V6; Colombo (Sri Lanka)'97; CCFP; (519)946-0171; Fax. (519)971-9120.

WALI, Dilip; William Osler HC-Brampton, 2100 Bovaird Dr E, Brampton ON L6R 3J7; Calcutta (India)'83; Staff, William Osler Health System - Brampton Civic Hospital; (905)494-2120

WALIA, Jagdeep S; C4-74 Stuart St, Kingston ON K7L 2V4; Guru Nanek Dev University (India)'98; MedGenetics. (613)548-2467

WALIA, Manjit S; Belgage Med Arts Centre, 203-525 Belmont Ave W, Kitchener ON N2M 5E2; Sheffield (England)'80; MB ChB; FAAP; FRCPC; Peds (Neonatology). Staff, Grand River Hospital - Kitchener/Waterloo Health Centre; Langs: Punjabi; Swahili; (519)744-3301; Fax. (519)744-3637.

WALIA, Tamana; BC Cancer Agency-Abbotsford, 32900 Marshall Rd, Abbotsford BC V2S 0C2; Bangalore (India)'02; Staff, Abbotsford Regional Hospital & Cancer Centre; Langs: Hindi; Punjabi; (604)851-4710

WALJI, Moez B; 408-658 Danforth Ave, Toronto ON M4J 5B9; Tor'81; FRFPS; FRCPC; DiagRad. (416)465-1726; Fax. (416)465-5695.

WALJI, Mohammediqbal F H; Selkirk Mental Health Centre, PO Box 9600 Stn Main 825 Manitoba Ave, Selkirk MB R1A 2B5; Shiraz (Iran)'81; DABPN; FRCPC; Psy (Geriatric Psychiatry). Staff Extended Treatment Unit, Selkirk Mental Health Centre; (204)482-3810; Fax. (204)785-1507; walji.m@shaw.ca.

WALJI, Shahebina; Bridgeland Prof Centre, 206A-1010 1 Ave NE, Calgary AB T2E 7W7; McM'00; BSc; CCFP; (403)272-2962; Fax. (403)457-2960.

WALJI, Shiraz A; 215-11625 Elbow Dr SW, Calgary AB T2W 1G8; Makerere (Uganda)'70; Langs: Gujarati; Kacchi; Hindi; Swahili; (403)281-6518; Fax. (403)251-7068.

WALK, Brian P; Mississauga Med Centre, 410-1420 Burnhamthorpe Rd E, Mississauga ON L4X 2Z9; Tor'91; (905)624-1597; Fax. (905)624-6853.

WALKER, Alfredo E; The Ottawa Hosp-Gen Campus, 4F-501 Smyth Rd Box 117, Ottawa ON K1H 8L6; West Indies (Trinidad & Tobago)'96; (613)737-8899

WALKER, Allan F; Royal Alexandra Hosp, 10240 Kingsway NW, Edmonton AB T5H 3V9; Alb'77; Staff, Royal Alexandra Hospital; (780)735-4442; Fax. (780)735-4916.

WALKER, Angela J; Cabinet Med Prive Rive-Sud, 1 rue d'Aragon, St-Basile-le-Grand QC J3N 1L5; UBC'99; CCFP; Staff Emerg, Sir Mortimer B Davis Jewish General; Langs: English; French; (450)482-3441; Fax. (450)482-3421.

WALKER, Arlene A; Misericordia Health Centre, 99 Cornish Ave, Winnipeg MB R3C 1A2; Man'83; Staff, Misericordia Health Centre; (204)788-8186

WALKER, Blair A M; St Paul's Hosp, 1081 Burrard St, Vancouver BC V6Z 1Y6; UBC'84; FRCPC; AnatPath. Staff, Providence Health Care - St Paul's Hospital; Teach Staff Pulmonary Research Lab, University of British Columbia; (604)806-8581; Fax. (604)806-8158.

WALKER, Brandie L; Foothills Med Centre, 1403 29 St NW, Calgary AB T2N 2T9; Cal'05; FRCPC; IntMed; Respir. Staff, Foothills Medical Centre; (403)944-1110

WALKER, C Robin; St Joseph's Health Care, PO Box 5777 Stn B 268 Grosvenor St, London ON N6A 4V2; Manchester (England)'71; MB ChB; FRCPC; Peds (Neonatology). Staff, London Health Sciences Centre - Victoria Campus; VP Integrated Med, St Joseph's Hospital - St Joseph's Health Care; Langs: English; French; (519)646-6000; Fax. (519)646-6014; robin.walker@sjhc.london.on.ca.

WALKER, Candace M; Villa Caritas, 16515 88 Ave NW, Edmonton AB T5R 0A4; Alb'05; Psy. Staff, University of Alberta Hospital; Staff, Alberta Hospital Edmonton; (780)342-6552; Fax. (780)342-6579.

WALKER, Caroline; CSSS du Rocher-Perce, CP 3300 451 rue Mgr Ross, Chandler QC G0C 1K0; Sher'04; FRCPC; IntMed. Staff, Centre Hospitalier de Chandler; (418)689-2261

WALKER, Carolyn E; 24-301 Metcalfe St, Ottawa ON K2P 1R9; Ott'89; BSc(Hons.); (613)762-2285; calijonah@yahoo.ca.

WALKER, Colin M; The Family Practice Clinic, 2778A 104th St, Nanaimo BC V9T 2E4; Sask'77; Ac Staff, Nanaimo Regional General Hospital; (250)758-1711; Fax. (250)758-2802.

WALKER, David M C; Robert Sutherland Hall, 323-138 Union St, Kingston ON K7L 3N6; Qns'71; FRCPC; IntMed (Emergency Medicine). Att Staff, Kingston General Hospital; Att Staff, Hotel-Dieu Hospital; Dean Health Sciences/Prof, Queen's University; (613)533-6000 x75592; Fax. (613)530-6983; deanfhs@post.queensu.ca.

WALKER, Diane; Medical Bldg, 401-805 Broadway W, Vancouver BC V5Z 1K1; Wes'83; AB; FRCSC; Ophth. (604)874-7533; Fax. (604)874-7534.

WALKER, Douglas R; Kingston Gen Hosp, 76 Stuart St, Kingston ON K7L 2V7; Tor'81; FRCPC; DiagRad (Angiography & Interventional Radiology). Staff, Kingston General Hospital; (613)548-2301; Fax. (613)548-2412.

WALKER, G Ross; Kingston Gen Hosp, 76 Stuart St, Kingston ON K7L 2V7; Wes'82; FRCSC; GenSurg (Breasts). Staff, Kingston General Hospital; Staff, Hotel-Dieu Hospital; Assoc Dean Postgraduate Med Education, Queen's University; (613)549-6666 x4743; Fax. (613)548-2456.

WALKER, George W; Rockyview Gen Hosp, ICU/CCU-7007 14 St SW, Calgary AB T2V 1P9; UBC'83; Staff Coronary Care Unit, Rockyview General Hospital; (403)943-3000

WALKER, Grace V; St Paul's Hosp, 1702 20th St W, Saskatoon SK S7M 0Z9; Sask'83; CCFP; FCFP; Staff, St Paul's Hospital (Grey Nuns) of Saskatoon; Staff, Saskatoon Cancer Centre; (306)655-5530; Fax. (306)655-5518.

WALKER, Harmannus C G; Glace Bay Healthcare Complex, 300 South St, Glace Bay NS B1A 1W5; Tor'64; FRCPC; DiagRad. Staff, Glace Bay Healthcare Facility; (902)842-2832; Fax. (902)849-0287.

WALKER, Ian W; G740-3330 Hospital Dr NW, Calgary AB T2N 4N1; Cal'98; CCFP; CCFP(E.M.); Staff Emerg Med, Foothills Medical Centre; (403)944-1635; Fax. (403)210-8148.

WALKER, Irwin R; Hamilton HS-Juravinski Site, A3 65-711 Concession St, Hamilton ON L8V 1C3; Melbourne (Australia)'65; FRACP; FRCPC; FRCPC; Hem; IntMed. Staff, Hamilton Health Sciences Centre-Juravinski Site; Prof, McMaster University; (905)521-2100 x76384; Fax. (905)575-7320; walkeri@mcmaster.ca.

WALKER, J Roberts; 471 Hibernia St, Stratford ON N5A 5W2; Wes'82; DABOphth; FRCSC; Ophth (Cataract). Staff, Stratford General Hospital - Huron Perth Healthcare Alliance; (519)273-2370; Fax. (519)273-0150.

WALKER, James D; Civic Parkdale Clinic, GE 10-737 Parkdale Ave, Ottawa ON K1Y 1J8; Wes'74; FRCPC; Derm (Pediatric Dermatology). Ac Staff (All Sites), The Ottawa Hospital - General Campus; Consultant, Carleton Place & District Memorial Hospital; Consultant, Children's Hospital of Eastern Ontario (CHEO); Staff, The Ottawa Hospital - Civic Campus; Assoc Prof, University of Ottawa; (613)761-4774

WALKER, James D; 100-2010 Eglinton Ave W, York ON M6E 2K3; Cambridge (England)'84; MB ChB; BSc(Hon.); DABR; FRCPC; DiagRad. Ac Staff, William Osler Health System - Brampton Civic Hospital; (416)781-2050

WALKER, Jamie M; Lions Gate Hosp, 231 15th St E, North Vancouver BC V7L 2L7; Alb'83; FRCPC; Anes. Staff, Lions Gate Hospital; (604)984-5709; Fax. (604)984-5729.

WALKER, Janet A; Keystone Place, 101-270 Douglas Ave, Bathurst NB E2A 1M9; Ott'94; FRCSC; GenSurg (Breast Oncology). Staff, Prince County Hospital; Staff, Aberdeen Regional Hospital; Langs: English; French; (506)548-1711; Fax. (506)548-2711.

WALKER, Jennifer D; 205-125 13th St E, North Vancouver BC V7L 2L3; Ott'90; CCFP; Langs: English; French; (604)985-9551; Fax. (604)985-1037.

WALKER, Jennifer L; University Health Centre, 2 200-66 University Campus NW, Edmonton AB T6G 2J7; Alb'96; CCFP; FCFP; (780)492-2612; Fax. (780)492-0172.

WALKER, Jonathan S D M; Quinsam Med Clinic, 280-1400 Dogwood St, Campbell River BC V9W 3A6; Stellenbosch (South Africa)'85; MB ChB; (250)286-0601; Fax. (250)286-0504.

WALKER, Joseph; Nanaimo Reg Gen Hosp, 1200 Dufferin Cres, Nanaimo BC V9S 2B7; London (England)'70; MB BS; FRCPC; Psy (Geriatric Psychiatry). Staff, Nanaimo Regional General Hospital; Langs: Irish; Gaelic; Spanish; (250)716-7791; Fax. (250)740-2670; joseph.walker@viha.ca.

WALKER, Kathleen J; Stonechurch Family Health Ctre, 1475 Upper Ottawa St, Hamilton ON L8W 3J6; McM'86; CCFP; FCFP; Assoc Staff, Hamilton Health Sciences Centre-Juravinski Site; (905)574-1444; Fax. (905)575-9892.

WALKER, Kenneth J; Forest Med Centre, 15 Main St E, Forest ON N0N 1J0; Tor'83; CCFP; (519)786-2136; Fax. (519)786-4187.

WALKER, Lori L; Alberta Children's Hosp, 2888 Shaganappi Trail NW, Calgary AB T3B 6A8; Man'98; FRCPC; Peds. Staff Cleft Palate Clinic, Alberta Children's Hospital; Staff Asthma Clinic, South Calgary Health Centre; (403)955-2953; Fax. (403)955-3055.

WALKER, M Louise; Ottawa Sport Med Centre, 1370 Clyde Ave, Nepean ON K2G 3H8; Tor'77; BSc; Dip SportMed(SportMed); CCFP; FCFP; Court Staff, The Ottawa Hospital - Civic Campus; Court Staff, SCO Health Service - Élisabeth Bruyère Hospital; Asst Prof Med, University of Ottawa; (613)727-2745; Fax. (613)727-2623; ottawasportmedicinecentre@yahoo.com.

WALKER, Malcolm G; Northern Lights Reg Health Ctr, 7 Hospital St, Fort McMurray AB T9H 1P2; (South Africa)'87; MB ChB; CCFP; Staff, Northern Lights Regional Health Centre; Langs: Afrikaans; Dutch; German; (780)791-6128; Fax. (780)791-6184.

WALKER, Margaret A; Family Practice Clinic, 84 Memorial Ave, Grnd-Falls-Wi NL A2A 1R9; Mem'79; CCFP; (709)489-6687

WALKER, Mark B; Avery Health Clinic, 31-665 Front St, Quesnel BC V2J 5J5; Witwatersrand (South Africa)'73; MB ChB; Exec Member, G R Baker Memorial Hospital; Langs: Afrikaans; (250)992-8322; Fax. (250)992-1563.

WALKER, Mark C; The Ottawa Hosp-Gen Campus, 8420-501 Smyth Rd, Ottawa ON K1H 8L6; Qns'93; FRCSC; ObstGyn (Maternal Fetal Medicine). Scientist, The Ottawa Hospital - General Campus; Prof, University of Ottawa; (613)739-6655; Fax. (613)737-8402; mwalker@ottawahospital.on.ca.

WALKER, Mathieu A D; St Mary's Hosp Centre, 2335-3830 av Lacombe, Montreal QC H3T 1M5; McG'99; FRCP; FRCPC; IntMed (Echocardiography); Cardiol. Staff, St Mary's Hospital Centre; Dir Cardiology Residency Training Program, McGill University; Langs: Bilingual(English/French); (514)734-2614; Fax. (514)734-2766; mathieu.walker@mcgill.ca.

WALKER, Michelle L; Hamilton HS-Henderson Site, 711 Concession St, Hamilton ON L8V 1C3; McM'06; DiagRad. Staff, Hamilton Health Sciences Centre-Juravinski Site; (905)521-2100

WALKER, Paul M; Spectral Diagnostics Inc, 2-135 The West Mall, Toronto ON M9C 1C2; Wes'73; PhD; FRCSC; GenSurg (Critical Care Medicine); VascSurg. Staff Surg, Toronto General Hospital - UHN; Pres/CEO, Spectral Diagnostic Inc; Aj Prof, University of Toronto; (416)626-3233 x2100; Fax. (416)626-2739; pwalker@spectraldx.com.

WALKER, Peter; The Ottawa Hosp-Riverside, 4 08-1967 Riverside Dr, Ottawa ON K1H 7W9; Ott'72; FRCPC; IntMed; Endocrin (P.Q.). Staff, The Ottawa Hospital - Riverside Campus; Prof, University of Ottawa; Langs: French; (613)738-8400; Fax. (613)738-8261; pwalker@uottawa.ca.

WALKER, Randy A; 33477A Mayfair Ave, Abbotsford BC V2S 1P6; Sask'06; FRCSC; Ophth. (604)853-6321

WALKER, Richard E A; Radiology Consultants Assoc, 120-6707 Elbow Dr SW, Calgary AB T2V 0E3; Sask'92; FRCPC; DiagRad. (403)777-3007; Fax. (403)777-3008.

WALKER, Robert M C; Queensway-Carleton Hosp, 3045 Baseline Rd, Ottawa ON K2H 8P4; Dal'77; CCFP; FCFP; Clin Assoc Prof, Queensway Carleton Hospital; (613)520-6674

WALKER, Robin M C; 1-376 Eagle St, Newmarket ON L3Y 8Z4; McM'94; FRCSC; Ophth. Staff, Southlake Regional Health Centre; (905)868-8725; Fax. (905)868-8727.

WALKER, Roxanne E; 100A-3305 Harvester Rd, Burlington ON L7N 3N2; McM'95; FRCPC; Peds (Pediatric Cardiology). Affil Staff, The Hospital For Sick Children; Affil Staff, Joseph Brant Memorial Hospital; (289)337-2716; Fax. (289)337-8396.

WALKER, Shannon L; 152-1848 Main St, Penticton BC V2A 5H3; UBC'87; FRCPC; IntMed (Critical Care Medicine); Respir. Med Dir ICU, Penticton Regional Hospital; Clinical Asst Prof, University of British Columbia; (250)493-4773

WALKER, Shawn T K; 319 15 Ave N PO Box 969, Creston BC V0B 1G0; Sask'91; (250)428-8873

WALKER, Stephen A J; Atlantic Offshore Med Services, PO Box 2442 Stn C 4 Henry St, St. John's NL A1C 6E7; Edinburgh (Scotland)'72; MB ChB; DCH; MRC; (709)722-4074

WALKER, Stephen W; 69 Lake Ave W, Carleton Place ON K7C 1L5; UBC'88; (613)257-1818; Fax. (613)257-5890.

WALKER, Tara L; Wolseley Family Med Clinic, 825 Oxford St E, London ON N5Y 3J8; UBC'96; Staff Family Med, London Health Sciences Centre - South Street; Assoc Staff, Alexandra Hospital; Staff Family Med, St Joseph's Hospital - St Joseph's Health Care; (519)673-0159; Fax. (519)673-5384.

WALKER, William L; Summerside Med Centre, 101-475 Granville St, Summerside PE C1N 4P7; Dal'80; FRCSC; GenSurg. Staff, Prince County Hospital; (902)432-8115; Fax. (902)436-3769; wl.walker@pei.sympatico.ca.

WALKOVICH, Peter; Rouge Valley-Centenary HC, 2867 Ellesmere Rd, Scarborough ON M1E 4B9; McG'59; DAB; FACS; MDCM; FRCSC; GenSurg. Court Staff Surg, Rouge Valley Health System - Centenary Health Centre Site; Langs: Ukrainian; (416)284-8131

WALKTY, Andrew J; Health Sciences Centre, MS673B-820 Sherbrook St, Winnipeg MB R3A 1R9; Man'03; FRCPC; IntMed; MedMicrobiol; InfectDis. Staff, Health Sciences Centre; (204)774-8511

WALL, Alastair R; 21st Medical Clinic, 502-402 21st St E, Saskatoon SK S7K 0C3; Sask'06; FRCPC; IntMed; Critical Care Medicine. (306)956-3444; Fax. (306)956-3577.

WALL, Andrea E; Tantramar Comm Hlth Ctre, 1-2 Main St, Sackville NB E4L 4A3; Dal'03; BSc; CCFP; (506)536-0210; Fax. (506)536-9810.

WALL, Cara L E; Kelowna Gen Hosp, 2268 Pandosy St, Kelowna BC V1Y 1T2; Sask'01; CCFP; Staff, Kelowna General Hospital; (250)864-8360

WALL, Christopher J; Wall Street Med Bldg, 300-140 Wall St, Saskatoon SK S7K 1N4; Sask'03; FRCPC; DiagRad. (306)244-1167; Fax. (306)244-2911.

WALL, David T; Kelowna Gen Hosp, 2268 Pandosy St, Kelowna BC V1Y 1T2; Tor'85; FRCPC; DiagRad. Staff, Kelowna General Hospital; Staff, Kelowna Medical Imaging; (250)862-4454; Fax. (250)862-4458.

WALL, Donna A; CancerCare Manitoba, 675 McDermot Ave, Winnipeg MB R3E 0V9; Man'81; Staff, CancerCare Manitoba; (204)787-2197

WALL, Jane M; Sunnybrook Hlth Sciences Ctre, 2075 Bayview Ave, Toronto ON M4N 3M5; Ott'86; FRCPC; DiagRad. Staff, Sunnybrook Health Sciences Centre; Langs: English; French; (416)480-6100 x7071; Fax. (416)480-5855.

WALL, Leah K; Lincoln Med Centre, 4413 Ontario St, Beamsville ON L0R 1B5; McM'08; CCFP; (905)563-1212

WALL, Mary T; BC Cancer of Southern Interior, 399 Royal Ave, Kelowna BC V1Y 5L3; Mem'90; Staff Kelowna Cancer Clinic, BC Cancer Agency Sindi Ahluwalia Hawkins Centre for the Southern Interior; (250)449-2218; Fax. (250)712-3911.

WALL, Ronald B; Spiritwood Primary Health Care, PO Box 69, Spiritwood SK S0J 2M0; Sask'80; CAS; Court Staff, Royal University Hospital; Asst Dir Family Med/Clin Instructor, University of Saskatchewan; (306)883-4400; Fax. (306)883-2140.

WALL, William J; London HSC-University Hosp, PO Box 5339 Stn B C8 002A-339 Windermere Rd, London ON N6A 5A5; Wes'70; CM; FRCSC; GenSurg (Liver Transplant). Staff, London Health Sciences Centre - University Hospital; Member, Order of Canada; Prof Surg, University of Western Ontario; (519)663-2940; Fax. (519)663-3067; wj.wall@lhsc.on.ca.

WALLACE, Anne A E; W C S Enterprises Inc, 142 Cassandra Blvd, Toronto ON M3A 1S9; Tor'66; CCFP; (416)449-6791; Fax. (416)449-1732; dr.a.wallace@rogers.com.

WALLACE, Carla J; Foothills Med Centre, 1403 29 St NW, Calgary AB T2N 2T9; Alb'81; FRCPC; DiagRad (Neuro Radiology). Staff Diagnostic Imaging, Foothills Medical Centre; Assoc Prof, University of Calgary; (403)944-1969; Fax. (403)944-1120.

WALLACE, Charles J; 16 The Square PO Box 209, Bayfield ON N0M 1G0; London (England)'55; MB BS; LMCC; Court Staff Privil, South Huron Hospital Association; (519)565-2922; Fax. (519)565-5922.

WALLACE, Clarissa; Columbia Med Bldg, 202-301 Columbia St E, New Westminster BC V3L 3W5; Qns'83; FRCPC; IntMed (Diabetology); Endocrin&Metab. Staff IntMed, Royal Columbian Hospital; Clinical Asst Prof Div of Endocrinol, University of British Columbia; (604)522-8399; Fax. (604)522-2635.

WALLACE, Elizabeth M; Outpatient Mental Health, 6F-1213 4 St SW, Calgary AB T2R 0X7; Cal'84; FRCPC; Psy (Psychotherapy & Psychoanalysis). Clin Asst Prof Dept of Psy, University of Calgary; (403)955-6678; Fax. (403)955-6688.

WALLACE, Garry E; Guelph Family Health Team, 83 Dawson Rd, Guelph ON N1H 1B1; Ott'95; CCFP; (519)766-1360; Fax. (519)766-0469.

WALLACE, Gordon J; Canadian Med Protective Assn, PO Box 8225 Stn T CSC 875 Carling Ave, Ottawa ON K1G 3H7; Ott'79; FRCPC; EmergMed. Dir-Educ Risk Management Serv, Canadian Medical Protective Association; Assoc Prof, University of Ottawa; (613)725-9965 x381

WALLACE, M Christopher; Kingston Gen Hosp, V3 363-76 Stuart St, Kingston ON K7L 2V7; Qns'80; FACS; FRCSC; Neursurg (Cerebrovascular Disease). Staff, Kingston General Hospital; Staff, Humber River Regional Hospital - Church Street Site; Prog Dir Div of NeuroSurg, University of Toronto; (613)549-6666; Fax. (613)548-1346.

WALLACE, Sarah G; 400-65 Larch St, Sudbury ON P3E 1B8; Tor'04; FRCSC; ObstGyn. (705)670-9048; Fax. (705)670-9208.

WALLACE, Sharon E; Specialist in Skin Diseases, 205 Edmonton St, Winnipeg MB R3C 1R4; Man'86; (204)943-4922; Fax. (204)942-4399.

WALLACE, Susan M A; Westminster Med Bldg, 706-625 Fifth Ave, New Westminster BC V3M 1X4; Tor'80; FACS; FRCSC; Ophth. Staff, Ridge Meadows Hospital & Health Care Centre; Clinical Asst Prof, University of British Columbia; (604)522-8638; Fax. (604)522-3711.

WALLACE, Thomas H; 102-400 Main St W, North Bay ON P1B 2V2; Wes'82; FRCSC; OrthSurg (Knee Surgery). Ac Staff, North Bay Regional Health Centre - Regional Mental Health; (705)476-9895; Fax. (705)494-1025.

WALLACE, Thomas M; Nicola Med Dental Bldg, 400-321 Nicola St, Kamloops BC V2C 6G6; Dal'02; FRCSC; GenSurg. Staff, Royal Inland Hospital; (250)828-2848; Fax. (250)828-2948.

WALLACE, Timothy D J; Cumberland Reg Hlth Care Ctre, 19428 Hwy 2 RR 6, Amherst NS B4H 1N6; Dal'99; FRCSC; Otol (Facial Plastic Surgery). Consultant, Colchester East Hants Health Centre; Staff, Cumberland Regional Health Care Center; Staff, Bayview Memorial Health Centre; Asst Prof Surg, Dalhousie University; (902)667-5044; Fax. (902)667-5045; tim.wallace@cha.nshealth.ca.

WALLACE, Wendy C; 170 East St, Sault Ste. Marie ON P6A 3C6; McM'10; CCFP; (705)759-1234

WALLACE-CHAU, Dhea; Rockyview Gen Hosp, 7007 14 St SW, Calgary AB T2V 1P9; Sask'98; FRCSC; ObstGyn. Staff, Foothills Medical Centre; Staff, St Joseph's General Hospital; Staff, Rockyview General Hospital; (403)943-8733; Fax. (403)943-8677.

WALLACE-KIMMEL, Eda J; Grand River Hosp-KW Hlth Ctre, PO Box 9056 Stn C 835 King St W, Kitchener ON N2G 1G3; West Indies (Jamaica)'89; FFARCSI; ABR; MB BS; FRCPC; DiagRad. Staff, Grand River Hospital - Kitchener/Waterloo Health Centre; (519)749-4300; Fax. (519)749-4309.

WALLACH, Jean-Philippe; Simon Fraser Health Region, 600-22470 Dewdney Trunk Rd, Maple Ridge BC V2X 5Z6; Wes'07; IntMed. (604)467-5333

WALLANI, Zulfikarali A; Markham Stouffville Health Ctr, 408-377 Church St, Markham ON L6B 1A1; (Tanzania)'72; FRCPC; Psy (Adult Psychiatry). Staff, Markham Stouffville Hospital; Langs: Gujarati; (905)472-5733; Fax. (905)472-5215.

WALLENIUS, Samantha C; Sault Area Hosp, 750 Great Northern Rd, Sault Ste. Marie ON P6B 0A8; Tor'03; FRCPC; Psy. Staff, Sault Area Hospital - Sault Ste Marie; (705)759-3434

WALLER, Julian R L; Brock Med Clinic, 16-1800 Tranquille Rd, Kamloops BC V2B 3L9; Birmingham (England)'88; MRCGPract; MRCS; MB ChB; Physician Diabetes Clinic, Royal Inland Hospital; (250)554-8768; Fax. (250)554-7873.

WALLERSTEIN, Avi; Lasik MD, 1250 boul Rene-Levesque O, Montreal QC H3B 4W8; Qns'91; FRCSC; Ophth (Refractive Surgery). Dir méd, Lasik MD Inc; Langs: Hebrew; Romanian; Yiddish; Hungarian; French; (514)933-0133; Fax. (514)845-0600; stapp@lasikmd.com.

WALLEY, Barbara A; Tom Baker Cancer Centre, 1331 29 St NW, Calgary AB T2N 4N2; Cal'90; BSc; FRCPC; IntMed (Breast Cancer); MedOncol. Staff MedOncol, Tom Baker Cancer Centre; Med Dir Calgary Breast Health Prog, Alberta Health Services Edmonton; Asst Prof Med, University of Calgary; (403)521-3688; Fax. (403)283-1651.

WALLEY, David T; 368 College St PO Box 631, Durham ON N0G 1R0; Sheffield (England)'78; MB ChB; Ac Staff, South Bruce Grey Health Centre - Durham Site; Assoc Staff, Hanover & District Hospital; Med Dir, Rockwood Terrace; (519)369-2510; Fax. (519)369-3831.

WALLEY, Keith R; St Paul's Hosp, 1081 Burrard St, Vancouver BC V6Z 1Y6; Man'81; FRCPC; IntMed (Critical Care Medicine). Assoc Dir ICU, Providence Health Care - St Paul's Hospital; Prof Med, University of British Columbia; (604)806-8136; Fax. (604)806-8351.

WALLEY, Virginia M; Life Labs, 100 International Blvd, Toronto ON M9W 6J6; Wes'78; FRCPC; AnatPath. ON Medical Director, Peterborough Regional Health Centre - Hospital Drive; Med Dir Ontario, Life Labs; (416)675-4530; Fax. (416)213-4206; virginia.walley@lifelabs.com.

WALLI, J Eric; Winnipeg Clinic, 425 St Mary Ave, Winnipeg MB R3C 0N2; Qns'71; FRCPC; IntMed; Gastroent. Asst Prof, University of Manitoba; (204)957-3213; Fax. (204)942-2671.

WALLIK, David W; Caroline Family Hlth Team-CMG, 15-3305 Harvester Rd, Burlington ON L7N 3N2; Tor'84; CCFP; FCFP; Staff, Joseph Brant Memorial Hospital; University of Toronto; Langs: Estonian; (905)632-8007; Fax. (905)681-6341.

WALLING, Ann D; SMBD Jewish Gen Hosp, E206-3755 ch Cote-Sainte-Cathe, Montreal QC H3T 1E2; Laval'84; FRCPC; IntMed (Echocardiography); Cardiol. Staff, Sir Mortimer B Davis Jewish General; assoc Prof Med, McGill University; Langs: Bilingual(French/English); (514)340-8222 x7540; Fax. (514)340-7534.

WALLING, Keith E; 201-667 Sackville Dr, Lower Sackville NS B4C 2S4; St Andrews (Scotland)'56; MB ChB; DPH(St.Andrews); DLO(London); FRCSC; Otol. Emeritus Staff, IWK Health Centre; Emeritus Staff, Queen Elizabeth II Health Sciences Centre - Victoria General Site; Consultant, Dartmouth General Hospital; Emeritus Prof Otol Assist, Dalhousie University; Langs: English; French; (902)865-9951; Fax. (902)865-6440.

WALLING, Marvlyn A; Creditview Medical, B14-1240 Eglinton Ave W, Mississauga ON L5V 1N3; Dal'01; BSc; MSc; CCFP; (905)567-4622; Fax. (905)567-7545.

WALLING, Simon A; IWK Health Centre, PO Box 9700 Rpo CSC 5850 University Ave, Halifax NS B3K 6R8; Dundee (Scotland)'88; MB ChB; FRCSC; Neursurg (Neuro Oncology). Att Staff, IWK Health Centre; Att Staff Neuro Surg, Queen Elizabeth II Health Sciences Centre - Victoria General Site; Staff, Queen Elizabeth II Health Sciences Centre - Halifax Infirmary Site; Asst Prof, Dalhousie University; (902)473-5453; Fax. (902)473-8458.

WALLINGTON, Marion C; 906 Brant St, Burlington ON L7R 2J5; McM'82; (905)637-5885; Fax. (905)637-0372.

WALLINGTON, Tamara A; WOHC-Brampton Civic Hosp, 2100 Bovaird St E, Brampton ON L6R 3J7; McM'97; FRCPC; CommunMed. Staff, William Osler Health System - Brampton Civic Hospital; (905)494-2120

WALLMAN, Daniel A; Whistler Health Care Centre, 4380 Lorimer Rd RR 4, Whistler BC V0N 1B4; McM'87; (604)932-4911; Fax. (604)932-4992.

WALLMAN, Ronald A; Boxgrove Med Arts Centre, 300-110 Copper Creek Dr, Markham ON L6B 0P9; Wes'86; FRCSC; PlasSurg. Staff, Markham Stouffville Hospital; Court Staff, Mackenzie Richmond Hill Hospital; (905)472-7121; Fax. (905)472-6586; ronwallman42@hotmail.com.

WALLOT, Hubert A; Inst U en Sante Mentale de QC, 2601 ch de la Canardiere, Quebec QC G1J 2G3; Sher'72; MPH; PhD; FRCPC; Psy; Public Health & Preventive Med; CommunMed. ac Staff Psy, Institut Universitaire Sante; ac Staff, Centre Hospitalier Universitaire de Quebec-CHUL; Prof, Tele-Universite de l'Ugam; (418)529-2445; Fax. (418)628-6068; wallotha@hotmail.com.

WALLS, Jessica; Mount St Joseph Hosp, 3080 Prince Edward St, Vancouver BC V5T 3N4; UBC'03; FRCPC; DiagRad. Staff, Providence Health Care - Mount Saint Joseph Hospital; (604)874-1141

WALLS, Lori A; Peter Lougheed Centre, 3500 26 Ave NE, Calgary AB T1Y 6J4; Alb'98; CCFP; Staff, Peter Lougheed Centre; (403)943-5461; Fax. (403)266-4366.

WALMAN, Noah; Forest Hill Family Health Cent, 2F-491 Eglinton Ave W, Toronto ON M5N 1A8; (Other Foreign)'07; CCFP; (416)782-6111; Fax. (416)782-5515.

WALMSLEY, Michael J; West G T A Endoscopy, B18 183-2225 Erin Mills Pky, Mississauga ON L5K 1T9; London (England)'63; MB BS; MRCS; LRCP; FRCS(Ed); FRCSC; GenSurg (Gastroenterology). Langs: Croatian; German; (905)823-0223; Fax. (905)823-9780.

WALMSLEY, Roger M; PO Box 250, Cassidy BC V0R 1H0; McM'88; CCFP; CCFP(E.M.); (250)246-8447

WALMSLEY, Sharon L; Univ Hlth Network-Toronto Gen, 13EN 214-200 Elizabeth St, Toronto ON M5G 2C4; Wes'83; FRCPC; IntMed (AIDS/HIV); InfectDis; MedMicrobiol. Ac Staff InfectDis & Microbiol, Toronto General Hospital - UHN; Prof Med, University of Toronto; (416)340-3871; Fax. (416)340-3357; sharon.walmsley@uhn.ca.

WALPOLA, Piyal L; Pickering Med Centre, 205-1885 Glenanna Rd, Pickering ON L1V 6R6; Colombo (Sri Lanka)'93; CCFP; FCFP; Langs: Sinhalese; (905)839-2214; Fax. (905)839-7357.

WALSER-JEBB, Dianne M; 653 Bunting Rd, St Catharines ON L2M 2Z9; McM'80; RN; BScN; CCFP; FCFP; (905)935-4114; Fax. (905)934-4700.

WALSH, Allyn E; Stonechurch Family Health Ctre, 1475 Upper Ottawa St, Hamilton ON L8W 3J6; Wes'76; CCFP; FCFP; Ac Staff, Hamilton Health Sciences Centre; Prof, McMaster University; (905)575-1300; Fax. (905)575-1539.

WALSH, Anne J; Newmarket Med Place, 303-712 Davis Dr, Newmarket ON L3Y 8C3; Glasgow (Scotland)'88; MB ChB; FRCSC; ObstGyn. Staff, Southlake Regional Health Centre; (905)898-6575; Fax. (905)898-6676.

WALSH, Anthony D; Hart Bldg, 202-15 Rowan St, St. John's NL A1B 2X2; Mem'91; FRCPC; Psy. Staff, Health Sciences Centre; (709)579-1583

WALSH, Catharine M; The Hosp For Sick Children, 8417 BW-555 University Ave Box, Toronto ON M5G 1X8; Tor'03; FRCPC; Peds (Clinician Investigator Program); Gastroent. Staff, The Hospital For Sick Children; (416)813-7500; Fax. (416)813-6531.

WALSH, Catherine M; 1-1261 Beaverbrook Ave, London ON N6H 0G6; Wes'83; BSc(Hon); CCFP; FCFP; Staff, Parkwood Hospital - St Joseph's Health Care; Assoc Prof, University of Western Ontario; (519)432-4107; Fax. (519)432-6921.

WALSH, Christopher J; Univ Hlth Network-Toronto Gen, 11C 1194-200 Elizabeth St, Toronto ON M5G 2C4; UBC'08; IntMed. Staff, Toronto General Hospital - UHN; (416)340-4996

WALSH, Claire M; 103-747 Hyde Park Rd, London ON N6H 3S3; Dublin (Ireland)'80; (519)471-6686; Fax. (519)471-2801.

WALSH, Coleen P; Health Sciences Centre, 300 Prince Philip Dr, St. John's NL A1B 3V6; Mem'98; FRCPC; Psy. Staff Psy, Health Sciences Centre; (709)777-7297

WALSH, Colin K; Haig Clinic, 601 6 Ave S, Lethbridge AB T1J 0Z2; Alb'07; CCFP; Staff Admitting Privil, Chinook Regional Hospital; (403)328-6641; Fax. (403)328-6118.

WALSH, Cynthia B; The Ottawa Hosp-Civic Campus, 1053 Carling Ave, Ottawa ON K1Y 4E9; Wes'00; FRCPC; DiagRad. Staff, The Ottawa Hospital - Civic Campus; (613)761-4831

WALSH, Dionne M; Haig Clinic, 601 6 Ave S, Lethbridge AB T1J 0Z2; Alb'07; CCFP; (403)328-6641; Fax. (403)328-6118.

WALSH, Elizabeth A; Dr Charles A Janeway Child HC, 300 Prince Philip Dr, St. John's NL A1B 3V6; Galway (Ireland)'81; MRC; FRCPC; DiagRad. Staff, Janeway Children's Health & Rehabilitation Centre; Clinical Asst Prof, Memorial University Of Newfoundland; (709)777-4169

WALSH, Gilbert D; Labrador Health Centre, PO Box 7000 Stn C 227 Hamilton River Rd, Happy-Valley-Goose NL A0P 1C0; Mem'04; FRCPC; Psy. Staff, Labrador Health Centre; (709)897-2000

WALSH, Gregory J; North Lanark Comm Hlth Centre, 207 Robertson Dr, Lanark ON K0G 1K0; McM'82; CCFP; CCFP(E.M.); FCFP; Ac Staff, Perth & Smiths Falls District Hospital - Perth Site (Great War Memorial Site); Teach Staff Comm & Family Med, University of Ottawa; (613)259-2182; Fax. (613)259-5235.

WALSH, Jennifer D; Saint John Reg Hosp, PO Box 2100 Stn Main 400 University Ave, Saint John NB E2L 4L2; Dal'05; FRCSC; ObstGyn. Staff, Saint John Regional Hospital; (506)648-6000

WALSH, Jennifer; Halton HCS Corp-Oakville, 327 Reynolds St, Oakville ON L6J 3L7; Qns'94; FRCPC; GenPath. Ac Staff Path, Halton Healthcare Services Corporation - Oakville Site; Asst Prof Path & Molecular Med, McMaster University; (905)338-4675; jwalsh@haltonhealthcare.on.ca.

WALSH, Joanna C; London HSC-University Hosp, PO Box 5339 Stn B 339 Windermere Rd, London ON N6A 5A5; (Wales)'99; FRCPC; AnatPath. Staff, London Health Sciences Centre - University Hospital; (519)685-8300

WALSH, John A; Okotoks Hlth & Wellness Ctre, 11 Cimarron Common, Okotoks AB T1S 2E9; Cape Town (South Africa)'74; MB ChB; CCFP; Staff, Saskatoon City Hospital; Ac Staff, St Paul's Hospital (Grey Nuns) of Saskatoon; Clin Instructor Obst & Emerg Med, University of Saskatchewan; (403)995-2600; Fax. (403)995-2656.

WALSH, John M; Westbrook Prof Bldg, 215-1610 37 St SW, Calgary AB T3C 3P1; Alb'86; FRCPC; IntMed. Consultant, Peter Lougheed Centre; Consultant, Brooks Health Centre; Clin Assoc Prof, University of Calgary; (403)284-0777; Fax. (403)685-9422.

WALSH, Julie; Centre Med Donnacona, 420 rte 138, Donnacona QC G3M 1C2; Laval'94; CCFP; Langs: French; (418)285-1122; Fax. (418)285-0006.

WALSH, Kevin J; 560 9 Ave SW, High River AB T1V 1B3; Cal'94; CCFP; (403)652-2200

WALSH, Kilian B; 10-243 Eglinton Ave W, Toronto ON M4R 1B1; Dublin (Ireland)'66; DPM; FRCPC; Psy. (416)545-1827; Fax. (416)545-1827; kbwalsh@bellnet.ca.

WALSH, Kimberley A; Caroline Med Group, 15-3305 Harvester Rd, Burlington ON L7N 3N2; Tor'09; CCFP; (905)632-8007; Fax. (905)632-6341.

WALSH, Marie-Jeanne L; Salveo Family Med Clinic, B8-6455 MacLeod Trail SW, Calgary AB T2H 0K8; Alb'86; CCFP; FCFP; Assoc Prof Med, University of Alberta; (403)444-0428; Fax. (403)537-0029.

WALSH, Mark J; Queen Elizabeth II HSC, 6 202-1276 South Park St, Halifax NS B3H 2Y9; Tor'97; BSc; MSc; FRCSC; GenSurg (Hepatobiliary Surgery). Staff Gen Surg & Multiorgan Transplantation, Queen Elizabeth II Health Sciences Centre - Victoria General Site; Staff, IWK Health Centre; Asst Prof, Dalhousie University; (902)473-5296; Fax. (902)473-5297; mark.walsh@cdma.nshealth.ca.

WALSH, Mary G A; Richmond Street Clinic, 862 Richmond St W, Toronto ON M6J 1C9; Dublin (Ireland)'69; MB ChB; BAO; FRCPC; Psy. Staff, Centre for Addiction & Mental Health (CAMH) - Queen Site; Lecturer Psy, University of Toronto; Langs: Gaelic; (416)535-8501 x2456; Fax. (416)586-1279.

WALSH, Michael J; Chisel Peak Med Clinic, PO Box 2769 417 10 Ave, Invermere BC V0A 1K0; Alb'91; (250)341-6900; Fax. (250)341-3226.

WALSH, Michael W; St Joseph's Healthcare, M303-50 Charlton Ave E, Hamilton ON L8N 4A6; Cal'01; FRCPC; IntMed; Nephrol. Staff, St Joseph's Healthcare - Charlton Campus; (905)522-1155; Fax. (905)521-6153.

WALSH, Noreen M G; DJ Mackenzie Bldg, 721-5788 University Ave, Halifax NS B3H 1V8; Cork (Ireland)'78; FRCPath; MRCP; MB BCh; BAO; FRCPC; AnatPath. Prof, Dalhousie University; (902)473-6897; Fax. (902)473-7978; noreen.walsh@cdha.nshealth.ca.

WALSH, Pamela J; The Moncton Hosp, 135 MacBeath Ave, Moncton NB E1C 6Z8; Dal'79; MCFP(EM); Staff, The Moncton Hospital; (506)857-5353

WALSH, Patric B; 2425 Bevan Ave, Sidney BC V8L 4R5; Manchester (England)'59; MB ChB; Fax. (250)656-7870.

WALSH, Paul E; Holy Rood Med Clinic, PO Box 337, Holyrood NL A0A 2R0; Mem'79; (709)229-7385; Fax. (709)229-3216.

WALSH, Paul F; High Level Med Clinic, 11202 100 Ave SS 1, High Level AB T0H 1Z0; Mem'92; CCFP; (780)926-2286; Fax. (780)926-3550.

WALSH, Paula M; Cabot Square Med Clinic, ML-55 Stavanger Dr, St. John's NL A1A 5E8; Mem'04; CCFP; (709)576-7075

WALSH, Penelope E; 202-275 Ontario St, Kingston ON K7K 2X5; Qns'63; (613)542-9274

WALSH, Philip; Coalition of Family Physicians, 900-45 Sheppard Ave E, North York ON M2N 5W9; McG'67; Staff, Coalition of Family Physicians (COFP); (416)495-8071; Fax. (416)733-2491; philwalsh308@gmail.com.

WALSH, Philippe; Hopital du Haut-Richelieu, 920 boul du Seminaire N, St-Jean-sur-Richel QC J3A 1B7; Mon'97; Urol (Oncology). Staff, Hôpital du Haut-Richelieu; Langs: Bilingual(French/English); (450)359-5000

WALSH, Ronald J; Walsh & Assoc Occupational Hea, 202-289 Pinnacle St, Belleville ON K8N 3B3; Qns'72; DOHS; CCBOM; (613)966-4114; Fax. (613)966-4130; admin@walshandassociates.ca.

WALSH, Scott R A; Sunnybrook Hlth Sciences Ctre, MI 700-2075 Bayview Ave, Toronto ON M4N 3M5; Tor'00; PhD; FRCPC; Derm (AIDS/HIV). Staff, Women's College Hospital; Staff, Sunnybrook Health Sciences Centre; (416)480-6100 x7243; Fax. (416)480-6897.

WALSH, Suzanne L; Calgary Urban Project Society, 1001 10 Ave NW, Calgary AB T2R 0B7; Cal'92; CCFP; (403)221-8780

WALSH-BERGIN, Paula; Assertive Community Treatment, 205-1355 Bank St, Ottawa ON K1H 8K7; McM'93; FRCPC; Psy (Developmental Disability). Staff, Royal Ottawa Mental Health Centre - Royal Ottawa Health Care Group; (613)722-6521; Fax. (613)739-8400.

WALSHE, Kevin J; La Loche Health Centre, Bag Service 1, La Loche SK S0M 1G0; Dublin (Ireland)'68; MB ChB; BAO; Staff, La Loche Health Centre and Hospital; (306)822-3201; Fax. (306)822-2798; k.walshe@sasktel.net.

WALTER, Anthony J; Royal Bank Plaza Med Centre, PO Box 134 Stn Royal Bank LR8-200 Bay St, Toronto ON M5J 2J3; Tor'83; FRCPC; MedMicrobiol; Derm. Staff, Sunnybrook Health Sciences Centre; (416)368-6787 x3; Fax. (416)368-7632.

WALTER, Jens-Erik; MUHC-Royal Victoria Hosp, F8 59-687 av des Pins O, Montreal QC H3A 1A1; UBC'00; FRCSC; ObstGyn (Urological Gynecology). Staff, St Mary's Hospital Centre; Staff, McGill University Health Centre - Royal Victoria Hospital; Dir Div of UroGyn/Staff, McGill University Health Centre - Montreal General Campus; Langs: Bilingual(English/French); (514)934-1934 x44289; Fax. (514)843-1708; jensew8@hotmail.com.

WALTER, Phillip C; Evergreen Med Centre, 8960 152 St, Surrey BC V3R 4E4; UBC'88; (604)588-8181

WALTER, Robert E; Royal Inland Hosp, 311 Columbia St, Kamloops BC V2C 2T1; Qns'85; FRCPC; DiagRad (Diagnostic Imaging). Staff Med Imaging, Royal Inland Hospital; (250)314-2400; Fax. (250)314-2326.

WALTERS, Anupama A; Compass Med Centre, 450-200 Wellington St W, Toronto ON M5V 3C7; Dal'08; CCFP; (416)593-5000; Fax. (416)593-5004.

WALTERS, Brennan M A; Meadowlark Place Prof Centre, 408-8708 155 St NW, Edmonton AB T5R 1W2; Alb'99; FRCPC; IntMed; Gastroent. (780)930-1915; Fax. (780)930-1916.

WALTERS, Dana M; Lake of the Woods Dist Hosp, RR 1 Stn Main 21 Sylvan St, Kenora ON P9N 3W7; St George's University (Grenada)'00; BSc; MD; Staff, Lake of the Woods District Hospital; (807)468-9861; Fax. (807)468-7247.

WALTERS, Daniel J; Lake of the Woods Dist Hosp, RR 1 Stn Main 21 Sylvan St, Kenora ON P9N 3W7; St George's University (Grenada)'00; Staff, Lake of the Woods District Hospital; (807)468-9861

WALTERS, Justin J; St Boniface Gen Hosp, BG 007-409 Tache Ave, Winnipeg MB R2H 2A6; Sask'00; BSc(Hon); FRCPC; IntMed; Nephrol. Staff, St Boniface General Hospital; (204)237-2613; Fax. (204)233-2770.

WALTERS, Lawrence T; Front-Frederick Health Service, 145 Front St E, Toronto ON M5A 1E3; McG'62; CCFP; FCFP; (416)362-8777; Fax. (416)627-7879.

WALTERS, Lawrence T; Front-Frederick Health Service, 1400-365 Bloor St E, Toronto ON M4W 3L4; Tor'88; CCFP; FCFP; Staff Family & CommunMed, Humber River Regional Hospital - Keele Street Site; Staff Family & Commun Med, Toronto General Hospital - UHN; Lecturer Family & CommunMed, University of Toronto; (416)362-8777; Fax. (416)362-7879.

WALTERS, Nicolaas J; Hanna Med Clinic, PO Box 700, Hanna AB T0J 1P0; Staff, Coronation Hospital & Care Centre; Locum Tenens, Carewest Glenmore Park; (403)854-3351; Fax. (403)854-4116; hannamc8@telus.net.

WALTERS, Thomas D; The Hospital for Sick Children, 555 University Avae, Toronto ON M5G 1X8; Perth (Australia)'93; Staff Hepatology & Nutrition, The Hospital For Sick Children; (416)813-5143

WALTI, Herve; CHUS-Hop Fleurimont, 3001 12e av N, Sherbrooke QC J1H 5N4; Paris (France)'82; Chief Peds, Centre Hospitalier Universitaire de Sherbrooke-Hopital Fleurimont; Chef Peds, Universite de Sherbrooke; Langs: English; (819)346-1110 x14634; Fax. (819)564-5398; herve.walti@usherbrooke.ca.

WALTON, Christina R; Grande Cache Med Clinic, PO Box 540 1600A Acorn Plaza, Grande Cache AB T0E 0Y0; UBC'08; CCFP; (780)827-2540; Fax. (780)827-5698.

WALTON, Christine C; Postgrad Med Education Office, 602-500 University Ave, Toronto ON M5G 1V7; McM'05; OrthSurg. Langs: Bilingual(English/French); (416)978-6976

WALTON, J Mark; Hamilton HS-McMaster Site, PO Box 2000 Stn Lcd 1 4E3-1200 Main St W, Hamilton ON L8N 3Z5; Alb'85; AB; MRC; FRCSC; GenSurg (Neonatal); PedGenSurg. Staff, St Joseph's Healthcare - Charlton Campus; Staff, The Credit Valley Hospital; Dir, Hamilton Health Sciences Centre - McMaster Children's Hospital; Asst Dean Postgrad Med Educ, McMaster University; Langs: Bilingual(English/French); (905)521-2100 x75244; Fax. (905)521-9992; waltonj@mcmaster.ca.

WALTON, Jennifer M; Edmonton Clinic Health Academy, 3 577-11405 87th Ave NW, Edmonton AB T6G 1C9; Qns'00; FRCPC; Peds. Staff, University of Alberta Hospital; Staff, Edmonton Clinic Health Academy; (780)428-5510; Fax. (888)790-1081.

WALTON, John C; Stratford Gen Hosp, 46 General Hospital Dr, Stratford ON N5A 2Y6; Wes'72; FRCPC; AnatPath. Staff Lab & Path, Stratford General Hospital - Huron Perth Healthcare Alliance; (519)272-8210 x2891

WALTON, Kimberly J; Queensway-Carleton Hosp, 3045 Baseline Rd, Ottawa ON K2H 8P4; McM'05; FRCPC; Anes. Staff, Queensway Carleton Hospital; Langs: Bilingual(English/French); (613)721-2100

WALTON, Lloyd T; Saskatchewan Worker's Comp, 115 24th St E, Saskatoon SK S7K 1L5; Sask'83; Med Consultant, Saskatchewan Workers Compensation Board; (306)933-6312; Fax. (306)933-8495; lloydwalton@wcbsask.com.

WALTON, Lorne A; Ridge Meadows Hosp & Hlth CC, 11666 Laity St, Maple Ridge BC V2X 5A3; UBC'74; BSc; Staff, Ridge Meadows Hospital & Health Care Centre; (604)463-4111; walton@telus.net.

WALTON, Mark; Bonne Bay Health Centre, PO Box 70 131-13 Main St, Norris Point NL A0K 3V0; London (England)'99; MB ChB; CCFP; Staff, Bonne Bay Health Centre; (709)458-2201

WALTON, Nigel G; Hollyburn Med Centre, 307-575 16th St, West Vancouver BC V7V 4Y1; Liverpool (England)'78; MB ChB; MRCGPract(UK); CCFP; (604)922-0211; Fax. (604)922-8898.

WALTON-KNIGHT, Nicola A; Mount Seymour Clinic, 333 Seymour Blvd, North Vancouver BC V7J 2J4; Leeds (England)'96; CCFP; (604)904-7712

WALZ, Barbara A E; Credit Valley Prof Bldg, 208-2300 Eglinton Ave W, Mississauga ON L5M 2V8; McM'85; DABIM; FRCPC; IntMed (Adult Rheumatology); Rheum. (905)820-9229; Fax. (905)820-3370.

WALZ, Norman C H; Central Alberta Prof Centre, 165-5201 43 St, Red Deer AB T4N 1C7; Tor'82; FRCSC; Urol. Staff, Red Deer Regional Hospital Centre; (403)341-4400; Fax. (403)341-4401.

WAMBERA, Katherine M; 5-7816 Saanich Rd E, Saanichton BC V8M 2B3; Ott'95; MSc(Psy); FRCPC; Peds; Neur (Pediatric Neurology). Staff On-Call Ped Neurol, Victoria General Hospital; Staff Outreach Ped Neurol, Nanaimo Regional General Hospital; (250)652-2009; Fax. (250)652-2085.

WAMBULWA, Charles R; Roseway Hosp, PO Box 610, Shelburne NS B0T 1W0; Howard University (USA)'06; Staff, Roseway Hospital; (902)875-3011

WAN, Andrea W; The Hosp for Sick Children, 555 University Ave, Toronto ON M5G 1X8; Tor'05; Cardiol; Peds. Staff, The Hospital For Sick Children; (416)813-5310

WAN, Andrew W C; 28-7010 Warden Ave, Markham ON L3R 5Y3; (Hong Kong)'83; CCFP; FCFP; Staff, The Scarborough Hospital - General Campus; Langs: Mandarin; Cantonese; (905)415-3773; Fax. (905)415-2313; wanwai@ipoline.com.

WAN, Calvin K N; Dr Walter Anderson Bldg, 1H-2251 Pandosy St, Kelowna BC V1Y 1T1; McM'98; FRCSC; CardSurg. Staff, Vancouver General Hospital - Centennial Pavillion; Staff, Providence Health Care - St Paul's Hospital; Staff, Kelowna General Hospital; Langs: Cantonese; Mandarin; (250)862-4336

WAN, David A; Montebello Med Clinic, 118 Lake St, St Catharines ON L2R 5Y1; Tor'07; CCFP; (905)685-6555; Fax. (905)685-6558.

WAN, John C; 108-8789 Woodbine Ave, Markham ON L3R 9T6; Brussels (Belgium)'83; FRCPC; IntMed (Rheumatology). Langs: Cantonese; (905)604-0815; Fax. (905)604-0816.

WAN, Jonathan F H; MUHC-Montreal Gen Hosp, D5400-1650 av Cedar, Montreal QC H3G 1A4; UBC'02; FRCPC; RadOncol. Staff, McGill University Health Centre - Montreal General Campus; (514)934-8040; Fax. (514)934-8392.

WAN, Peter S K; Boniface Park Med Centre Inc, 6-700 Markham Rd, Scarborough ON M1H 2A7; Tor'88; FRCPC; IntMed (Pain Management). Physician, Toronto Poly Clinic; (416)431-7100; Fax. (416)431-7191; pwan@tpclinic.com.

WAN, Vera A; Montabelo Med Clinic, 118 Lake St, St Catharines ON L2R 5Y1; Tor'07; CCFP; (905)685-6555; Fax. (905)685-6558.

WAN CHOW WAH, Doreen Y L; MUHC-Royal Victoria Hosp, M8 12-687 av des Pins O, Montreal QC H3A 1A1; McG'01; FRCPC; IntMed; GeriatricMed. Staff, McGill University Health Centre - Royal Victoria Hospital; Staff, Sir Mortimer B Davis Jewish General; (514)934-1934 x34677; Fax. (514)843-1738.

WAND, Reginald R; Fraser Health Child & Youth, 9634 King George Blvd, Surrey BC V3T 0G7; Man'72; FRCPC; Psy (Child & Adolescent Psychiatry). Consultant Adolescent Day Treatment Prog, Surrey Memorial Hospital; Staff, Newton/Cloverdale Child & Youth Mental Health Team; Staff, South Surrey/White Rock Child & Youth Mental Health Team; Staff, Fraser Health Child & Youth Neuropsychiatry Clinic; (604)587-3814; rrwand@shaw.ca.

WANDZURA, Michael J; Lakeland Vision Institute, 7-210 15th St E, Prince Albert SK S6V 1G2; Sask'95; FRCSC; Ophth. Physician, South Hill Medical Practice; (306)764-2020; Fax. (306)764-2036; wandz@shaw.ca.

WANES HANA, Maha R; 215 Van Buren St, Kemptville ON K0G 1J0; Cairo (Egypt)'94; CCFP; (613)258-2486

WANG, Alex C; St Mary's Gen Hosp, 911 Queens Blvd, Kitchener ON N2M 1B2; Wes'09; CCFP; Staff, St Mary's General Hospital; (519)744-3311

WANG, Amy R Y; 120-8120 Cook Rd, Richmond BC V6Y 1T9; UBC'09; CCFP; (604)278-5191

WANG, Angela J; Bluewater Health-CEE Site, 2F-450 Blanche St, Petrolia ON N0N 1R0; McM'05; BSc(Hon); MSc; CCFP; Staff, Bluewater Health - Charlotte Eleanor Englehart Hospital; Langs: Mandarin; Taiwanese; (519)882-1300; Fax. (519)882-1312.

WANG, Ay-Ling; Beechwood Forest Med Centre, 2-890 Glasgow St, Kitchener ON N2N 3G6; Tor'85; CCFP; FCFP; Langs: Chinese; (519)744-4293; Fax. (519)744-6424.

WANG, Beatrice; Carey Wang Ctre for Derm Surg, 100-4 Car Westmount, Montreal QC H3Z 2S6; McG'90; BSc; FAAD; CSPQ; MDCM; FRCPC; Derm (Dermatology Surgery). adj Prof, McGill University Health Centre - Royal Victoria Hospital; adj Prof, McGill University; Langs: English; French; (514)788-3300; Fax. (514)788-3202.

WANG, Bing; Kelowna General Hosp, 2268 Pandosy St, Kelowna BC V1Y 1T2; Sichuan Medical College (China)'85; FRCPC; MedMicrobiol. Staff, Kelowna General Hospital; (250)862-4300 x2578

WANG, Bing; Foothills Med Centre, C229-1403 29 St NW, Calgary AB T2N 2T9; Beijing (China)'82; MB; FRCPC; Anes (Neuro Anesthesia). Ac Staff Anes, Foothills Medical Centre; Clinical Asst Prof, University of Calgary; Langs: Chinese; (403)944-1430; Fax. (403)944-2425; bwan@ucalgary.ca.

WANG, Caroline Y M; 125-8120 Cook Rd, Richmond BC V6Y 1T9; UBC'84; Langs: Mandarin; (604)278-5195; Fax. (604)278-2023; wangc@interchange.ubc.ca.

WANG, Chang Shu; CHUS-Hop Fleurimont, 3001 12e av N, Sherbrooke QC J1H 5N4; Nanjing (China)'82; PhD; Staff, Centre Hospitalier Universitaire de Sherbrooke-Hopital Fleurimont; assoc Prof, Université Laval; Langs: English; (819)346-1110 x14652; Fax. (819)820-6445.

WANG, Charlie S K; 2F-353 St Paul Ave, Brantford ON N3R 4N3; Tor'03; FRCPC; IntMed (Clinician Investigator Program); Gastroent. Staff, Toronto General Hospital - UHN; (519)759-8899; Fax. (519)759-1799.

WANG, Chen; Mount Sinai Hosp, 600 University Ave, Toronto ON M5G 1X5; Jiamusi/Harbin (China)'81; FRCPC; HemPath (Laboratory Hematology). Staff, Mount Sinai Hospital; Asst Prof Med, University of Toronto; Langs: Chinese; (416)586-4469; cwang@mtsinai.on.ca.

WANG, Cheng; Cobequid Comm Health Centre, 726-5788 University Ave, Halifax NS B3H 1V8; Tianjin University (China)'95; Staff, Cobequid Community Health Centre; (902)869-6130; cheng.wang@cdha.nshealth.ca.

WANG, Cheng T; St Michael's Hosp, 30 Bond St, Toronto ON M5B 1W8; Tor'92; FRCPC; GenPath;CCFP; Staff Family Med Unit, St Michael's Hospital; Assoc Med Dir Cardiac Wellness & Rehab, Trillium Health Centre - West Toronto; Langs: Mandarin; (416)867-7428; Fax. (416)867-7498; wangt@smh.toronto.on.ca.

WANG, Clayton J; Medical Bldg, 1101-805 Broadway Ave W, Vancouver BC V5Z 1K1; Wes'97; MBA; CCFP; Staff, BC Women's Hospital & Health Centre; Clinical Asst Prof Med, University of British Columbia; Langs: Mandarin; (604)879-5271; Fax. (604)879-8712.

WANG, Dan-Bing; DJ International Health Inc, 2F-3633 Westwinds Dr NE, Calgary AB T3J 5K3; Alb'00; CCFP; (403)266-8050; Fax. (403)663-8821.

WANG, Don; The Ottawa Hosp-Gen Campus, 501 Smyth Rd, Ottawa ON K1H 8L6; Bethune (China)'86; MSc; FCAP; FRCPC; AnatPath (Cytopath). Staff, The Ottawa Hospital - General Campus; Asst Prof, University of Ottawa; Langs: Chinese; (613)737-8292; Fax. (613)737-8853; dwang@ottawahospital.on.ca.

WANG, Emily J; Clinique Med Blainville, 519 boul du Cure-Labelle, Sainte-Therese QC J7C 2H6; McG'99; FRCPC; Derm. (450)430-2221

WANG, Eugene; Forensic Psychiatry Hosp, 70 Colony Farm Rd, New Westminster BC V3C 5X9; Baylor(TX) (USA)'99; FRCPC; Psy. Staff Adult Forensic Psychiatric Community Services, Forensic Psychiatric Hospital; Staff, Vancouver Regional Forensic Clinic; Staff, Surrey Fraser Valley Clinic; (604)524-7700; Fax. (604)660-1206; ewang@forensic.bc.ca.

WANG, Grace T; Fifth Avenue Med Centre, 300-14 Fifth Ave, Orangeville ON L9W 1G2; McM'02; FRCSC; GenSurg. (519)942-1515; Fax. (519)942-5112.

WANG, Haili; University of Alberta Hosp, 2D2 13-8440 112 St NW, Edmonton AB T6G 2B7; Alb'03; FRCSC; GenSurg (Colorectal Surgery). Staff, University of Alberta Hospital; Langs: Mandarin; (780)407-2906; Fax. (780)407-3492.

WANG, Henry; York Med Health Centre, G-17215 Leslie St, Newmarket ON L3Y 8E4; Tor'79; ABIM; FRCPC; IntMed (Endocrinology); Endocrin&Metab. Chief Div of Gastroent, Southlake Regional Health Centre; Langs: Chinese; (905)853-4253

WANG, Hsiu-Li; Region Of Waterloo Public Hlth, 99 Regina St S, Waterloo ON N2J 4V3; Laval'95; FRCPC; CommunMed. Langs: Bilingual(English/French); (519)883-2278

WANG, James C Y; 505-95 Bayly St W, Ajax ON L1S 7K8; Tor'94; FRCPC; IntMed; Gastroent. Staff, Rouge Valley Health System - Ajax & Pickering Health Centre Site; (905)683-0881; Fax. (905)683-1273.

WANG, Jean C Y; Univ Hlth Network-Princess M, 610 University Ave, Toronto ON M5G 2M9; Tor'89; FRCPC; IntMed; Hem. Staff, Princess Margaret Hospital - University Health Network; Staff, Toronto Medical Discovery Team; (416)340-5233

WANG, Jeffry B; Markham Heritage Health Clinic, 130-5970 16th Ave, Markham ON L3P 7R1; Wes'00; CCFP; (905)471-2967; Fax. (905)471-0476.

WANG, Jen-Te; 5-10330 152nd St, Surrey BC V3R 4G8; Yonsei (Korea)'65; Assoc Staff, Surrey Memorial Hospital; Langs: Chinese; (604)588-8811

WANG, Jingwei; Hys Med Centre, 207-11010 101 St NW, Edmonton AB T5H 4B9; Shen Yang (China)'90; FRCSC; ObstGyn. (780)420-1771; Fax. (780)425-9299.

WANG, Jodie L M C; 1150 Franklin Blvd, Cambridge ON N1R 7J2; Sask'89; (519)620-7044

WANG, Kai-Yun; Royal Health Care Centre, 130 Adelaide St W, Toronto ON M5H 3P5; Tor'79; Langs: German; (416)361-6142; Fax. (416)361-1200.

WANG, Li; The Alex Senior Comm Hlth Ctr, 630 9 Ave SE, Calgary AB T2G 4V9; Harbin (China)'80; PhD; CCFP; Physician, The Alex Seniors Health Centre; Langs: Chinese; (403)920-0011; Fax. (403)920-0014.

WANG, Louie T S; Kingston Gen Hosp, 76 Stuart St, Kingston ON K7L 2V7; Wes'88; FRCPC; Anes. Staff, Kingston General Hospital; Staff, Hotel-Dieu Hospital; Asst Prof, Queen's University; (613)548-7827; Fax. (613)548-1375.

WANG, Noreen B; MF-510 Raglan St N, Renfrew ON K7V 1P5; Ott'03; CCFP; CCFP(E.M.); (613)432-4815; Fax. (613)433-9154.

WANG, Paul P Y; Kipling Heights Med Centre, 2291 Kipling Ave, Etobicoke ON M9W 4L6; Tor'89; Staff, William Osler Health System - Etobicoke General Hospital; (416)741-4545; Fax. (416)744-1484.

WANG, Robert Y; Pinnacle Health Sciences Ctr, 9651 Yonge St, Richmond Hill ON L4C 1V7; McM'02; FRCSC; OrthSurg. Langs: Mandarin; (905)918-2212

WANG, Shao-Hua; University of Alberta Hosp, 2H2 34-8440 112 St NW, Edmonton AB T6G 2B7; Harbin (China)'82; MSc; FRCSC; CardSurg (Thoracic Surgery). Staff Stollery Children's Cardio Thoracic Surg, University of Alberta Hospital; Clin Prof, University of Alberta; Langs: Mandarin; (780)407-3630; Fax. (780)407-3631; shaohua.wang@albertahealthservices.ca.

WANG, Shaoli; 256-4255 Arbutus St, Vancouver BC V6J 4R1; Beijing (China)'82; CCFP; Langs: Mandarin; (604)738-5887; Fax. (604)738-5817.

WANG, Sherry X; Saskatoon City Hosp, 7F-701 Queen St, Saskatoon SK S7K 0M7; Tongji Medical College of Huazhong (China)'92; FRCPC; PhysMed&Rehab. Staff, Saskatoon City Hospital; (306)655-8657; Fax. (306)655-8813.

WANG, Thur; 408-12310 102 St, Grande Prairie AB T8V 0N4; Alb'95; MSc; Staff, Queen Elizabeth II Hospital; Langs: Chinese; (780)665-1942

WANG, Ting-Yu; Lakeshore Gen Hosp, 160 av Stillview, Pointe-Claire QC H9R 2Y2; McG'07; MDCM; Endocrin&Metab; IntMed. Staff, Lakeshore General Hospital - Pointe Claire; (514)630-2225

WANG, Wei; Campbellton Reg Hosp, PO Box 880 Stn Main 189 Lily Lake Rd, Campbellton NB E3N 3H3; Shandong (China)'82; Pathologist, Hôpital Régional Campbellton.

WANG, Wen-Shan; 993 Hamilton Rd, London ON N5W 1A4; Dublin (Ireland)'66; MB ChB; BAO; Langs: Mandarin; (519)451-4963; Fax. (519)451-4960.

WANG, Wenjie; Foothills Med Centre, 1403 29 St NW, Calgary AB T2N 2T9; Harbin (China)'95; FRCPC; IntMed (Transplantation); Nephrol. Staff Med, Foothills Medical Centre; Langs: Mandarin; (403)944-5164; Fax. (403)944-5803.

WANG, Xi; Hamilton HS-Henderson Site, 711 Concession St, Hamilton ON L8V 1C3; Man'07; DiagRad. Staff, Hamilton Health Sciences Centre-Juravinski Site; (905)527-4322

WANG, Xiangyu; Foothills Med Centre, 918NT-1403 29 St NW, Calgary AB T2N 2T9; Fujian Medical University (China)'83; FRCPC; IntMed; Nephrol. Staff, Foothills Medical Centre; (403)944-3962; Fax. (403)944-3199.

WANG, Xiaoping; Misericordia Comm Hosp & HC, 16940 87 Ave NW, Edmonton AB T5R 4H5; Georgia (USA)'83; Staff, Covenant Health - Misericordia Community Hospital; Langs: Chinese; (780)735-2611; Fax. (780)439-3837; wang170@hotmail.com.

WANG, Xin-Yong; City Square Med Centre, 126-555 12th Ave W, Burnaby BC V5Z 3X7; McG'96; CCFP; Langs: Chinese; French; (604)568-8377; Fax. (604)568-8370.

WANG, Yan; Perth-Smiths Falls Dist Hosp, 60 Cornelia St W, Smiths Falls ON K7A 2H9; Mon'05; FRCSC; ObstGyn (Urogynecology). Staff, Perth & Smiths Falls District Hospital - Smiths Falls Site; Langs: Chinese; English; (613)283-2330; Fax. (613)283-0048.

WANG, Yinong; Diagnostic & Scientific Centre, C421-3535 Research Rd NW, Calgary AB T2L 2K8; Staff, Calgary Laboratory Services; (403)770-3844; Fax. (403)770-3292.

WANG, Yongdong; Hamilton HS-McMaster Site, PO Box 2000 Stn Lcd 1 1200 Main St W, Hamilton ON L8N 3Z5; Taishan Medical College (Other Foreign)'86; Staff, Hamilton Health Sciences Centre - McMaster Children's Hospital; (905)521-2100

WANG, Yongjin; The Credit Valley Hosp, 2200 Eglinton Ave W, Mississauga ON L5M 2N1; Beijing (China)'87; FRCPC; RadOncol. Staff, The Credit Valley Hospital; Langs: Mandarin; (905)813-1100 x5000; Fax. (905)813-3962.

WANG, Yue; Guildford Family Health, 201-10190 152A St, Surrey BC V3R 1J7; Beijing (China)'89; CCFP; Staff Privil, Surrey Memorial Hospital; Clin Instructor Family Practice Prog, University of British Columbia; Langs: Mandarin; Cantonese; Shanghai; (604)588-1822; Fax. (604)588-1825.

WANG, Yun-Lin; Rosedale Med Centre, 706-600 Sherbourne St, Toronto ON M4X 1W4; Seoul (Korea)'71; Langs: Korean; Mandarin; (416)968-1543; Fax. (416)968-9699; yunwang732@yahoo.ca.

WANG, Zhi; 102-256 rue de Montigny, Saint-Jerome QC J7Z 5P9; Mon'03; FRCSC; OrthSurg. Langs: Chinese; French; (450)565-6793

WANGER, Karen; B C Ambulance Service, 302-2955 Virtual Way, Vancouver BC V5M 4X6; McG'85; MDCM; FRCPC; EmergMed. Assoc Staff Emerg, Providence Health Care - St Paul's Hospital; Med Consultant, British Columbia Ambulance Services; Langs: Bilingual(English/French); (604)660-1381; karen.wanger@gov.bc.ca.

WANIA, Hormuzshaw J; Halton Family Health Centre, 2951 Walker's Line, Burlington ON L7M 4Y1; Karachi (Pakistan)'88; CCFP; (905)336-3437 x2061; Fax. (905)336-9626.

WANIGARATNE, Mihiri M; Students Union Bldg, 2 200-66 University Campus NW, Edmonton AB T6G 2J7; Alb'91; (780)492-2612; Fax. (780)492-0172.

WANIS, Nashat S; Broadway Med Clinic, 215-41 Broadway St W, Yorkton SK S3N 0L6; Cairo (Egypt)'81; FRCSC; GenSurg.

WANIS, Wahan; Medical Bldg, 1702-805 Broadway W, Vancouver BC V5Z 1K1; Rostovski (Russia (Federation))'81; FRCPC; Psy (Cross-Culture Psychiatry). Staff Psy, West End Mental Health Team; Clin Assoc Prof, University of British Columbia; Langs: Arabic; Armenian; Russian; Spanish; (604)875-9066; Fax. (604)875-9056.

WANKLING, Gilbert J; 1624 7th Ave, Prince George BC V2L 3P6; Man'87; GenSurg. (250)561-2700; Fax. (250)561-2794.

WANKLYN, Beverly Jill; Kelowna Gen Hosp, 2268 Pandosy St, Kelowna BC V1Y 1T2; Man'85; FRCPC; GenPath (Cytopath). Staff, Kelowna General Hospital; (250)862-4433

WANLESS, Ian R; DJ MacKenzie Bldg, 740-5788 University Ave, Halifax NS B3H 1V8; McG'71; BSc; DABPath; FRCPC; GenPath (Liver Disease). (902)473-5236; Fax. (902)473-1049; iwanless@eastlink.ca.

WANNAN, Barry W; Elliot Lake Family Health Team, 229-31 Nova Scotia Walk, Elliot Lake ON P5A 1Y9; Wes'67; Ac Staff Diag Imaging, St Joseph's General Hospital Elliot Lake; (705)461-8882; Fax. (705)848-3449.

WANNENBURG, Johan; 3F-65 Henry St, Miramichi NB E1V 2N4; Pretoria (South Africa)'89; (506)623-3353; Fax. (506)623-3356.

WANNER, Nicoelle R E; Health Matters Med Clinic, 102-3215 Dunmore Rd SE, Medicine Hat AB T1B 2H2; Alb'03; CCFP; (403)504-0450; Fax. (403)529-4601.

WANONO, Oshrit; CAMH Pace Clinic, 80 Workman Way, Toronto ON M6J 1H4; McM'07; FRCPC; Psy. Staff, Centre for Addiction & Mental Health (CAMH) - College Street Site; (416)535-8501

WANONO, Revital; Seven Oaks Gen Hosp, 2300 McPhillips St, Winnipeg MB R2V 3M3; Tor'06; FRCPC; IntMed; Respir. Staff, Seven Oaks General Hospital; (204)632-7133

WANSBROUGH, Michael C T; Mount Sinai Hosp, 206-600 University Ave, Toronto ON M5G 1X5; McM'92; CCFP; CCFP(E.M.); Staff, Mount Sinai Hospital; Langs: English; French; (416)586-5058; Fax. (416)586-4719.

WANSON, Annabelle S; Royal University Hosp, 8 145EH-103 Hospital Dr, Saskatoon SK S7N 0W8; University of Sint Eustatius (Other Foreign)'02; FRCPC; Psy. Staff Psy, Royal University Hospital; Staff, Saskatoon City Hospital; (306)655-0879; Fax. (306)966-8237.

WANSON, Laurent P; Royal University Hosp, 120-103 Hospital Dr, Saskatoon SK S7N 0W8; Staff, Royal University Hospital; (306)655-1000; Fax. (306)966-8237.

WANT, David A; Sudbury Reg Hosp-Laurentian, 41 Ramsey Lake Rd, Sudbury ON P3E 5J1; Wes'93; FRCPC; RadOncol. Staff, Health Sciences North-Laurentian Site; Asst Prof Med, University of Ottawa; (705)522-6237 x2451; Fax. (705)523-7329.

WANZEL, Kyle R; Clinician Investigator Program, 600-1243 Islington Ave, Etobicoke ON M8X 1Y9; Tor'98; FRCSC; PlasSurg (Clinician Investigator Program). Asst Prof, University of Toronto; (416)236-2571; Fax. (416)236-4591.

WAPLER, Michel F; Service de Pedopsychiatrie, 6550 rue Saint-Georges, Levis QC G6V 6X2; McG'85; FRCPC; Psy. Staff, Hôtel-Dieu de Lévis; (418)835-7155; Fax. (418)838-8873.

WAQAR, Mohsin; Victoria Med Bldg, 102-1669 Victoria St, Prince George BC V2L 2L5; UBC'10; (250)564-3133

WAR, Leonora B; Cabrini Centre, 411-16811 88 Av NW, Edmonton AB T5R 5Y6; (India)'95; Staff, Covenant Health - Misericordia Community Hospital; (780)735-9377; Fax. (780)735-9397.

WARAICH, Ihsan U; Kennedy Med Clinic, 9-7990 Kennedy Rd S, Brampton ON L6W 0B3; King Edward Medical College (Other Foreign)'02; CCFP; Langs: Hindi; Punjabi; Urdu; (905)455-5445; Fax. (905)455-5665; iwaraich@ahealingplace.ca.

WARAICH, Paul S; Burnaby Hosp, 3935 Kincaid St, Burnaby BC V5G 2X6; McM'96; BSc; MHSc; FRCPC; Psy. Staff, Maples Adolescent Treatment Centre; Staff Burnaby Mental Health Services, Burnaby Hospital; Staff, Providence Health Care - St Paul's Hospital; Assoc Researcher, University of British Columbia; (604)453-1930; Fax. (604)453-1929.

WARBECK, Paul J; Jackson-Hughes Health Centre, PO Box 357 125 Hogan Rd, Nipigon ON P0T 2J0; Qns'84; BSc; CCFP; Staff, Thunder Bay Regional Health Sciences Centre; (807)887-1644; Fax. (807)887-1645.

WARBURTON, Malcolm A; PO Box 370, Paradise Hill SK S0M 2G0; Edinburgh (Scotland)'71; MB ChB; Staff, Paradise Hill Health Centre; (306)344-2330; Fax. (306)344-4982.

WARBURTON, Rebecca; Medical & Dental Bldg, 400-3939 50A Ave, Red Deer AB T4N 4E6; Sask'05; FRCSC; GenSurg. Staff, Red Deer Regional Hospital Centre; (403)347-9037; Fax. (403)347-9038.

WARD, Alan E; Tottenham Med Centre, PO Box 2000 119 Queen St N, Tottenham ON L0G 1W0; Tor'72; Ac Staff, Stevenson Memorial Hospital; (905)936-4211; Fax. (905)936-3493.

WARD, B Megan; 7120 Hurontario St PO Box 667 Rpo Streetsville, Mississauga ON L5M 2C2; McM'85; FRCPC; CommunMed;CCFP; Public Health & Preventive Med. (905)791-7800

WARD, Barbara J; Medical Imaging Consultants, 200-3017 66 St NW, Edmonton AB T6K 4B2; Alb'80; FRCPC; DiagRad. Staff, Covenant Health - Grey Nuns Community Hospital; (780)450-9729; Fax. (780)438-1205.

WARD, Brian J; MUHC-Montreal Gen Hosp, L10 509-1650 av Cedar, Montreal QC H3G 1A4; McG'80; ABIM(InfectDis.); FRCPC; IntMed (P.Q.); MedMicrobiol (P.Q.). Staff, McGill University Health Centre - Montreal General Campus; (514)934-1934 x42810; Fax. (514)934-8347; brian.ward@mcgill.ca.

WARD, Bryan D; Telus Plaza South, 2700-10020 100 St NW, Edmonton AB T5J 0N3; Cal'76; CCFP; FCFP; Member, College of Physicians & Surgeons of Alberta; Clin Teacher Family Med, University of Alberta; (780)969-5004; Fax. (780)428-2712.

WARD, Carol L; Royal Inland Hosp, 311 Columbia St, Kamloops BC V2C 2T1; Qns'87; ABPN; FRCPC; Psy (Geriatric Psychiatry). Staff, Royal Inland Hospital; Physician, Hillside Psychiatric Centre; (250)314-2598; Fax. (250)314-2410; carol.ward@interiorhealth.ca.

WARD, Christopher R; 22-88 Duncan Ave W, Penticton BC V2A 7J7; Queensland (Australia)'01; MB BS; (250)492-2944

WARD, Colin J; Royal Court Med Centre, LL2-1 Quarry Ridge Rd, Barrie ON L4M 7G1; McM'02; FRCSC; GenSurg. Staff, Hamilton Health Sciences Centre - McMaster Children's Hospital; (705)737-0363; Fax. (705)737-2842.

WARD, David G H; Mount St Joseph Hosp, 3080 Prince Edward St, Vancouver BC V5T 3N4; Man'94; FRCPC; Psy (Acute Adult Psychiatry). Staff, Providence Health Care - Mount Saint Joseph Hospital; (604)874-1141 x78391

WARD, David K; 202-14439 104 Ave, Surrey BC V3R 1M1; Tor'80; FRCSC; PlasSurg (Breast Reconstruction). Ac Staff, Surrey Memorial Hospital; Consultant, Royal Columbian Hospital; Med Dir, Valley Surgery Centre; (604)582-2762; Fax. (604)582-2764.

WARD, Donna M; 298 Lawrence Ave, Kitchener ON N2M 1Y4; Tor'75; CCFP; FCFP; Ac Staff, Grand River Hospital - Kitchener/Waterloo Health Centre; Ac Staff Palliative Care, St Mary's General Hospital; A-Med Dir Supportive Care, Grand River Regional Cancer Centre; (519)578-9757; Fax. (519)578-9750.

WARD, Glen K; 305-22112 52 Ave, Langley BC V2Y 2M6; McG'86; PhD; FRCPC; Peds. Staff Ped, Langley Memorial Hospital; Staff Ped, Peace Arch Hospital; Langs: Bilingual(English/French); (604)534-9177

WARD, Gregory J; Central Alberta Prof Centre, 169-5201 43 St, Red Deer AB T4N 1C7; Man'03; FRCPC; IntMed; Gastroent. (403)755-9270; Fax. (403)755-9272.

WARD, Heather A; Royal University Hosp, 100-103 Hospital Dr, Saskatoon SK S7N 0W8; Sask'91; MSc; FRCPC; IntMed; Respir. Staff Med, Royal University Hospital; (306)933-6167; Fax. (306)933-8312.

WARD, Helen C; Royal Ottawa Health Care Group, 1145 Carling Ave, Ottawa ON K1Z 7K4; Cal'96; FRCPC; Psy (Forensic Psychiatry). Staff, Royal Ottawa Mental Health Centre - Royal Ottawa Health Care Group; Asst Prof, University of Ottawa; (613)722-6521 x6936

WARD, Joel W; Pembroke Reg Hosp, 705 Mackay St, Pembroke ON K8A 1G8; Qns'93; CCFP; Staff, Pembroke Regional Hospital Inc; (613)639-9020

WARD, John H; St Paul's Hosp, 1081 Burrard St, Vancouver BC V6Z 1Y6; Tor'83; FRCPC; IntMed; Hem. Ac Staff, Providence Health Care - St Paul's Hospital; (604)806-8480; Fax. (604)806-8488.

WARD, Kenneth M; Cambridge Med Place, 3-695 Coronation Blvd, Cambridge ON N1R 7J9; Qns'74; AB; FACS; FRCSC; Otol. Consultant, St Mary's General Hospital; Consultant, Grand River Hospital - Kitchener/Waterloo Health Centre; Staff, Cambridge Memorial Hospital; (519)622-1250; Fax. (519)622-8932.

WARD, Leanne M; Children's Hosp Eastern Ont, 250H-401 Smyth Rd, Ottawa ON K1H 8L1; McM'93; BSc; FRCPC; Peds (Metabolic Bone Disease); Endocrin&Metab. Staff PedEndocrinol, Children's Hospital of Eastern Ontario (CHEO); Asst Prof, University of Ottawa; Langs: English; French; (613)737-7600; Fax. (613)738-4236.

WARD, Michael A; Professional Bldg, 2101-222 King St E, Bowmanville ON L1C 1P6; Tor'95; BSc; MSc; CCFP; Staff, Lakeridge Health - Bowmanville Site; (905)697-3607; Fax. (905)697-3645.

WARD, Michelle G K; Children's Hosp Eastern Ont, 401 Smyth Rd, Ottawa ON K1H 8L1; McM'99; FRCPC; Peds (Child Abuse). Staff, Children's Hospital of Eastern Ontario (CHEO); Asst Prof, University of Ottawa; Langs: English; French; (613)737-7600 x2571; Fax. (613)738-4834.

WARD, Mylene; Clinician Investigator Program, 105-21 Surrey St W, Guelph ON N1H 3R3; Wes'98; MEd; BSc; FRCSC; GenSurg (Clinician Investigator Program). Ac Staff, Guelph General Hospital; Langs: Bilingual(English/French); (519)836-4830; Fax. (519)836-1341.

WARD, Natalie H; 110-10333 Southport Rd SW, Calgary AB T2W 3X6; Cal'04; CCFP; Staff, Rockyview General Hospital; (403)258-1960; Fax. (403)253-5735.

WARD, Randy R; Clinique Med Jean Coutu, 3-1116A rue Mountain, Moncton NB E1C 2T3; Ott'08; CCFP; (506)857-1106; Fax. (506)855-7537.

WARD, Richard A; Crowfoot Village Fam Practice, 210-600 Crowfoot Cres NW, Calgary AB T3G 0B4; Cal'85; CCFP; FCFP; Physician CDM Lead Calgary Primary Care Network, Foothills Medical Centre; Clin Teacher Family Med/Coord Continuing Med Ed, University of Calgary; (403)239-9733; Fax. (403)241-8112.

WARD, Richard; Univ Hlth Netowork-Toronto Gen, EN887-200 Elizabeth St, Toronto ON M5G 2C4; London (England)'00; Staff, Toronto General Hospital - UHN; (416)340-5233; Fax. (416)340-3799.

WARD, Robert A; Queensway-Carleton Hosp, 3045 Baseline Rd, Ottawa ON K2H 8P4; Qns'80; Staff, University of Ottawa Heart Institute; Staff, Queensway Carleton Hospital; (613)721-2000

WARD, Simon D; Shuswap Lake Gen Hosp, PO Box 520 Stn Main 601 10th St NE, Salmon Arm BC V1E 4N6; Leeds (England)'03; MB ChB; Staff, Shuswap Lake General Hospital; (250)833-3600

WARD, Simon P; Tower Prof Centre, 5520 50 Ave, Wetaskiwin AB T9A 0T3; (South Africa)'05; (780)352-9700; Fax. (780)352-9739.

WARD, Susan E; The Credit Valley Hosp, 2200 Eglinton Ave W, Mississauga ON L5M 2N1; Wes'95; FRCPC; DiagRad. Staff, The Credit Valley Hospital; (905)813-4491; Fax. (905)813-3042.

WARD, Susan J; Carberry Health Centre, PO Box 2000, Carberry MB R0K 0H0; Stellenbosch (South Africa)'87; CCFP; Staff, Carberry Plains Health Centre; (204)834-2126; Fax. (204)834-3808.

WARD, William J; Greenwood Fam Physicians, PO Box 5, Sundre AB T0M 1X0; (403)638-2424; Fax. (403)638-3580.

WARD-SMITH, Rosalind A; North Burlington Med Centre, 18-1960 Appleby Line, Burlington ON L7L 0B7; McM'98; CCFP; Langs: Bilingual(English/French); (905)319-2000; Fax. (905)319-6292.

WARDA, Lynne J; Children's Hosp Emergency, NA335-700 McDermot Ave, Winnipeg MB R3E 0T2; McM'92; FRCPC; Peds. Fellow, Health Sciences Centre.

WARDE, Padraig R D; Univ Hlth Network-Princess M, 610 University Ave, Toronto ON M5G 2M9; Dublin (Ireland)'77; MB ChB; BAO; MRC; FRCPC; RadOncol., Princess Margaret Hospital - University Health Network; Assoc Prof, University of Toronto; (416)946-2122; Fax. (416)946-4586; padraig.warde@rmp.uhn.on.ca.

WARDELL, Florence E B; City Centre Fam Physicians, 100-514 Queen St, Saskatoon SK S7K 0M5; Sask'78; (306)244-3016; Fax. (306)244-4737.

WARDELL, Gaylord C; 107-1424 Southview Dr SE, Medicine Hat AB T1B 4E7; Sask'78; CRCP; FRCPC; Anes (Pain Management). Staff, Medicine Hat Regional Hospital; (403)580-3545; Fax. (403)580-3546.

WARDEN, David H; Stapleford Med Clinic, 372 McCarthy Blvd N, Regina SK S4R 7M2; Sask'77; CCFP; FCFP; Staff, Pasqua Hospital; Staff, Regina General Hospital; Physician, Stapleford Medical Clinic; (306)545-3000; Fax. (306)545-5584.

WARDEN, Sarah J; U of Toronto Health Services, 2F-214 College St, Toronto ON M5T 2Z9; Cal'07; CCFP; Staff, Women's College Hospital; (416)978-8030; Fax. (416)971-2089.

WARDILL, Karen J; Kensington Med Clinic, 6548 Hastings St, Burnaby BC V5B 1S2; Otago (New Zealand)'82; MB BS; DObst; (604)299-9769; Fax. (604)299-9772; karenwardill@hotmail.com.

WARDLE, Andrew P B D; The Credit Valley Hosp, 2200 Eglinton Ave W, Mississauga ON L5M 2N1; Sheffield (England)'71; MB ChB; Anes. Court Staff, The Credit Valley Hospital; (905)820-4466; Fax. (905)338-3199.

WARDLE, Nancy E; 2572 Arbutus Rd, Victoria BC V8N 1W2; McM'79.

WARDMAN, A E Dennis; 2303 41 Ave W PO Box 18143, Vancouver BC V6M 4L3; Alb'95; FRCPC; CommunMed (Aboriginal Health). (604)812-1424

WARE, Mark A; MUHC-Montreal Gen Hosp, E19 145-1650 av Cedar, Montreal QC H3G 1A4; West Indies (Jamaica)'92; MB BS; MSc; Staff, McGill University Health Centre - Montreal General Campus; adj Prof Family Med & Anes, McGill University; Langs: English; French; (514)934-1934; Fax. (514)934-8096; mark.ware@muhc.mcgill.ca.

WARF, Curren W; Youth Health Program, CSB V2 223-950 28 Ave W, Vancouver BC V5Z 4H4; California (USA)'88; MScEd; FSAM; FAAP; Staff Youth Health Program, BC Women's Hospital & Health Centre; (604)875-0000 x4635; cwarf@cw.bc.ca.

WARKENTIN, James P B; Gateway Health & Wellness Ctre, 203-2051 McCallum Rd, Abbotsford BC V2S 3N5; Cal'10; CCFP; (604)855-0677

WARKENTIN, Joel D; Thunder Bay Pediatrics, 588 Arthur St, Thunder Bay ON P7E 5R7; McG'03; MDCM; FAAP; MBA; FRCPC; Peds. Staff, La Verendrye Hospital - Riverside Health Care Facility; Staff, Thunder Bay Regional Health Sciences Centre; Staff, Dryden Regional Health Centre; Lecturer, Northern Ontario School of Medicine-Lakehead University; (807)766-3370; Fax. (807)766-3374.

WARKENTIN, Ray E; Bethesda Reg Health Centre, PO Box 939 Stn Main 316 Henry St, Steinbach MB R5G 1A2; Man'05; CCFP; Staff, Bethesda Hospital Steinbach; (204)326-6411; rwarkentin@sehealth.mb.ca.

WARKENTIN, Theodore E; Hamilton HS-General Site, 1 270B-237 Barton St E, Hamilton ON L8L 2X2; Man'83; FRCPC; IntMed (Platelet Disorders); Hem. Staff Hematologist/Reg Dir Transfusion Med Hamilton Reg Lab Med Program, Hamilton Health Sciences Centre - Hamilton General Hospital; Prof Med Path & Molecular Med, McMaster University; Langs: German; (905)527-0271 x46139; Fax. (905)577-1421.

WARKUS, Thomas; CHUM-Hopital Notre-Dame, 1560 rue Sherbrooke E, Montreal QC H2L 4M1; Lausanne (Other Foreign)'95; Prof adj clin, Centre Hospitalier l'Université de Montréal (CHUM) - Hôpital Notre-Dame; Langs: German; Dutch; (514)890-8000 x23871; Fax. (514)412-7604.

WARMAN CHARDON, Jodi P; Childrens Hosp of Eastern ON, C2-401 Smyth Rd, Ottawa ON K1H 8L1; Ott'06; Neur. Staff, The Ottawa Hospital - Civic Campus; Staff, Children's Hospital of Eastern Ontario (CHEO); (613)737-7600

WARME, Gordon; Addiction & Mental Hlth-Clarke, 250 College St, Toronto ON M5T 1R8; Tor'57; Psy. Staff, Centre for Addiction & Mental Health (CAMH) - College Street Site; Langs: German; (416)535-8501

WARMENHOVEN, Wilhelm H; Lougheed Health Centre, 106-22838 Lougheed Hwy, Maple Ridge BC V2X 2V6; Pretoria (South Africa)'85; MB ChB; Langs: Afrikaans; (604)463-4165; Fax. (604)463-9987; gclinic@telus.net.

WARMINGTON, Lise M; North Edmonton Health Centre, 14007 50 St NW, Edmonton AB T5E 5E4; Alb'01; Peds. Staff, University of Alberta Hospital; Physician, North Edmonton Childen's Centre; (780)342-4168; Fax. (780)342-4196; lmw1@ualberta.ca.

WARNAKULASOORIYA, Riviraj; Lakeshore Health Centre, PO Box 110 1 Steenson Dr, Ashern MB R0C 0E0; CCFP; Staff, Lakeshore Health Centre; (204)768-2461

WARNEBOLDT, Jean A; Eagle Ridge Hosp & Health CC, 475 Guildford Way, Port Moody BC V3H 3W9; UBC'04; CCFP; Staff, Eagle Ridge Hospital & Health Care Centre; (604)461-2022

WARNEKE, Lorne B; Cedars Prof Park, 2915 66 St NW, Edmonton AB T6K 4C1; Alb'67; FRCPC; Psy (Anxiety Disorder). Staff Psy, Covenant Health - Grey Nuns Community Hospital; Clin Prof Psy., University of Alberta; (780)450-9450; Fax. (780)461-6190.

WARNER, Anne-Marie; 1902 Richmond Rd, Victoria BC V8R 4R2; (250)592-3441

WARNER, David W; 142-3000 Lougheed Hwy, Coquitlam BC V3B 1C5; Alb'88; CCFP; (604)945-0100; Fax. (604)945-0171.

WARNER, Ellen; Sunnybrook Hlth Sciences Ctre, 2075 Bayview Ave, Toronto ON M4N 3M5; Tor'80; MSc; FACP; FRCPC; IntMed (Breast Cancer); MedOncol. Consultant, North York General Hospital; Staff, Sunnybrook Health Sciences Centre - Edmond Odette Cancer Centre; Prof Med, University of Toronto; Langs: Hebrew; Yiddish; (416)480-4617; Fax. (416)480-6002; ellen.warner@sunnybrook.ca.

WARNER, John A; 208-3825 Sunset St, Burnaby BC V5G 1T4; UBC'83; FRCSC; Urol (Urological Oncology). Staff, Royal Columbian Hospital; Staff, Burnaby Hospital; (604)439-1272; Fax. (604)430-1213.

WARNER, Leonard C; Bathurst Med Centre, 207-7117 Bathurst St, Thornhill ON L4J 2J6; Tor'84; FRCPC; IntMed; Nephrol. Staff, North York General Hospital; Court Staff, Sunnybrook Health Sciences Centre; Langs: Hebrew; (905)764-0333; Fax. (905)764-7712; lwrenraw@aol.com.

WARNER, Margaret N; MUHC-Royal Victoria Hosp, M7 22-687 av des Pins O, Montreal QC H3A 1A1; Dal'90; FRCPC; IntMed; Hem. Staff, McGill University Health Centre - Royal Victoria Hospital; Langs: English; French; (514)843-1558

WARNER, Michael B; Toronto East Gen Hosp, 825 Coxwell Ave, Toronto ON M4C 3E7; Qns'04; FRCPC; IntMed; Critical Care Medicine. Staff, Toronto East General Hospital Inc; Staff, Toronto General Hospital - UHN; (416)461-8272; mwarner@tegh.on.ca.

WARNER, Simon J; Simon J Warner Medical Inc, 401-805 Broadway W, Vancouver BC V5Z 1K1; Cal'84; FRCSC; Ophth. Ac Staff Eye Care Centre, Vancouver General Hospital - Centennial Pavillion; Clin Instructor, University of British Columbia; (604)874-7533; Fax. (604)874-7534.

WARNER, Tyson S; South Calgary Health Centre, 31 Sunpark Plaza SE, Calgary AB T2X 3W5; UBC'01; CCFP; (403)978-7414

WARNESS, Richard S S; 3-2308 24 St SW, Calgary AB T2T 5H8; Alb'74; (403)242-3064; Fax. (403)249-2275.

WARNICA, J Wayne; Foothills Med Centre, C 849-1403 29 St NW, Calgary AB T2N 2T9; Man'66; FACC; FACP; FRCP; FRCPC; IntMed (Congestive Heart Failure); Cardiol. Staff cardiol, Foothills Medical Centre; Emeritus Prof Cardiac Surg & Med, University of Calgary; (403)944-1020; Fax. (403)944-1592; wwarnica@ucalgary.ca.

WARNICK, Brady M; Royal Columbian Hosp, 330 Columbia St E, New Westminster BC V3L 3W7; UBC'07; Anes. Staff, Royal Columbian Hospital; (604)528-5002

WARNOCK, David L; 314A Cook St, Victoria BC V8V 3X6; UBC'91; BSc; (250)383-0215

WARNOCK, Garth L; Gordon & Leslie Diamond HCC, 5153-2775 Laurel St, Vancouver BC V5Z 1M9; Alb'76; MSc; FRCSC; GenSurg (Transplantation). Staff, Gordon & Leslie Diamond Health Care Centre; Dept Head/Staff, Vancouver General Hospital - Centennial Pavillion; Co-Ed in Chief, Canadian Journal of Surgery; (604)875-5371; Fax. (604)875-5447.

WARNOCK, Thomas F; Stratford Gen Hosp, 46 General Hospital Dr, Stratford ON N5A 2Y6; Edinburgh (Scotland)'74; MB ChB; BSc(MedSci); Staff, Stratford General Hospital - Huron Perth Healthcare Alliance; Langs: English; French; (519)272-8210 x2510; Fax. (519)271-7137.

WARR, David G; Univ Hlth Network-Princess M, 5 204-610 University Ave, Toronto ON M5G 2M9; Qns'78; FRCPC; IntMed; MedOncol. Staff, Princess Margaret Hospital - University Health Network; Assoc Prof Med, University of Toronto; (416)946-2260; Fax. (416)946-6546; david.warr@uhn.on.ca.

WARRACK, Ian M; 43 Aylmer Ave, Ottawa ON K1S 5R4; Aberdeen (Scotland)'66; MB ChB; CCFP; FCFP; Langs: English; French; (613)226-4937; Fax. (613)215-0534.

WARRAICH, Gunwant; The Ottawa Fertility Centre, 955 Green Valley Cres, Ottawa ON K2C 3V4; Man'07; ObstGyn (Infertility Endocrinology). (613)686-3378

WARRAICH, Kanwarjit; Carmedics McArthur, 103-311 McArthur Ave, Ottawa ON K1L 8M3; Medical University of the Americas (Other Foreign)'06; CCFP; (613)749-1678; Fax. (613)749-9446.

WARRAICH, Naseer A; Northwest Co-op Comm Hlth Ctre, 103-61 Tyndall Ave, Winnipeg MB R2X 2T4; Punjab (India)'87; MB BS; CCFP; Staff, Seven Oaks General Hospital.

WARREN, Andrew E; IWK Health Centre, PO Box 9700 Rpo CSC 5850-5980 University Ave, Halifax NS B3K 6R8; Mem'92; FRCPC; Peds (Pediatric Cardiology); Cardiol. Staff Ped Cardiol, IWK Health Centre; Assoc Dean Postgraduate Med Educ/Assoc Prof, Dalhousie University; (902)470-8407; Fax. (902)470-6616; andrew.warren@iwk.nshealth.ca.

WARREN, Bethel F; Univ of Toronto Health Service, 214 College St W, Toronto ON M5S 1A1; Tor'82; CCFP; (416)978-8030

WARREN, Daniel T; CBI Health Centre, 2F-605 Discovery St, Victoria BC V8T 5G4; Cal'04; FRCSC; Neursurg. (250)383-4430

WARREN, David W; London HSC-Victoria Hosp, PO Box 5010 Stn B 800 Commissioners Rd E, London ON N6A 5W9; Wes'82; FAAP; FRCPC; Peds (Child Abuse);CCFP; CCFP(E.M.); FCFP; Staff, London Health Sciences Centre - Victoria Campus; Staff EmergMed, St Joseph's Hospital - St Joseph's Health Care; Assoc Prof, University of Western Ontario; (519)685-8331; Fax. (519)685-8156; david.warren@lhsc.on.ca.

WARREN, E Janet; Conestoga College Student Heal, 299 Doon Valley Dr, Kitchener ON N2G 4M4; Tor'89; CCFP; FCFP; Physician, Conestoga College; (519)763-3344; Fax. (519)748-3509.

WARREN, Heather M; University of Toronto, 602-500 University Ave, Toronto ON M5G 1V7; Mem'05; Cardiol; IntMed. (416)946-0059; Fax. (416)978-7144.

WARREN, James M; Fairmont Med Bldg, 1413-750 Broadway W, Vancouver BC V5Z 1J4; Cambridge (England)'78; MB ChB; CCFP; Ac Staff, Vancouver General Hospital - Centennial Pavillion; (604)876-5405; Fax. (604)876-4440.

WARREN, Jeffrey; The Ottawa Hosp-Gen Campus, 501 Smyth Rd Box 222, Ottawa ON K1H 8L6; Ott'02; FRCSC; Urol. Staff, The Ottawa Hospital - General Campus; (613)798-5555

WARREN, Jessi K; Weyburn Health Centre, 36 4th St, Weyburn SK S4H 0X7; Sask'07; CCFP; Physician, Weyburn Health Centre; (306)842-5444; Fax. (306)842-5449.

WARREN, Jo-Ann L; Village Family Physicians, 275 Pictou Rd, Truro NS B2N 2S7; Mem'92; FRCPC; Psy. Staff, Colchester East Hants Health Centre; (902)895-1232; Fax. (902)897-9749.

WARREN, Katherine J; PO Box 1088, Windsor NS B0N 2T0; Dal'96; FRCPC; Psy (Psychotherapy). Lecturer, Dalhousie University.

WARREN, Kenneth G; Clinical Sciences Bldg, 9 101-152 University Campus NW, Edmonton AB T6G 2G3; Wes'72; FRCPC; Neur (Multiple Sclerosis). Staff, University of Alberta Hospital; Prof Med, University of Alberta; (780)407-3620; Fax. (780)492-1365; kwarren@ualberta.ca.

WARREN, Linda J; Vancouver Breast Centre, 505-750 Broadway W, Vancouver BC V5Z 1H4; UBC'68; FRCPC; DiagRad (Breast Imaging). Ac Staff, BC Women's Hospital & Health Centre; Ac Staff, Vancouver General Hospital - Centennial Pavillion; Consultant, BC Cancer Agency Vancouver Centre; Prov Chief Radiol, Vancouver Screening Mammography Program of BC; Clin Prof Rad, University of British Columbia; (604)879-4177; Fax. (604)879-4147.

WARREN, Louis; CLSC de la Jacques Cartier, 47-11999A de l'Hopital, Quebec QC G2A 2T7; Laval'86; CCFP; FCFP; Prof, Université Laval; (418)843-2572 x7516; Fax. (418)843-3880.

WARREN, Melina D; Royal Jubilee Hosp, 1952 Bay St, Victoria BC V8R 1J8; Cal'05; FRCPC; DiagRad. Staff Imaging Services, Royal Jubilee Hospital; (250)370-8272

WARREN, Paule; CSSS Les Eskers de l'Abitibi, 622 4e rue O, Amos QC J9T 2S2; Laval'92; FRCPC; IntMed. Staff, CH Hôtel-Dieu d'Amos; (819)732-3341; Fax. (819)732-6465.

WARREN, Peter W; West Kelowna Walk-In Fam Pract, 105-2231 Louie Dr, Bank Kelowna BC V4T 3K3; Cal'99; BSc; CCFP; (250)768-6985; Fax. (250)768-5490.

WARREN, Rex C; North Perth Family Health Team, 185 Inkerman St E, Listowel ON N4W 2N1; Qns'83; (519)291-4200; Fax. (519)291-5947.

WARREN, Richard C; Cole Harbour Family Med Ctre, 203-240 Baker St, Dartmouth NS B2W 6L4; Dal'01; CCFP; Staff, Dr Everett Chalmers Regional Hospital; (902)435-6312; Fax. (902)434-7920.

WARREN, Richard J; Vancouver Plastic Surg Centre, 1000-777 Broadway W, Vancouver BC V5Z 4J7; UBC'74; FRCSC; PlasSurg (Cosmetic Surgery). Staff PlasticSurg, Vancouver General Hospital - Centennial Pavillion; Med Dir, Vancouver Plastic Surgery Center; Clin Assoc Prof Surg, University of British Columbia; (604)876-1774; Fax. (604)876-8456; richardwarren@telus.net.

WARREN, Robert G; Greenwood Fam Physicians, PO Box 5 709 1 St NE, Sundre AB T0M 1X0; Cal'09; CCFP; (403)638-2424; Fax. (403)638-3580.

WARREN, Thomas A; 208-331 Sheddon Ave, Oakville ON L6J 1X8; Wes'05; FRCPC; IntMed; MedMicrobiol; InfectDis. Staff, Mount Sinai Hospital; (905)844-5346; Fax. (905)849-6551.

WARREN, Vesta M; Greenwood Fam Physicians, PO Bag 5 709 1 St NE, Sundre AB T0M 1X0; Alb'97; CCFP; FCFP; Staff, Sundre Hospital & Care Centre; Clin Lecturer, University of Alberta; Clin Lecturer, University of Calgary; (403)638-2424; Fax. (403)638-3580.

WARREN, William P; Etobicoke Med Centre, 400 The East Mall, Etobicoke ON M9B 3Z9; Dal'61; FAAAI; FACA; IntMed (Allergy). (416)621-2220; Fax. (416)621-2357; drwpwarren@hotmail.com.

WARRENDER, A Brian; Guisachan Family Medicine, 105-2395 Gordon Dr, Kelowna BC V1W 3X7; Qns'73; Ac Staff, Kelowna General Hospital; (250)860-5888; Fax. (250)860-5880; gfm@shawcable.ca.

WARRIAN, Kevin J; 5340 1 St SW, Calgary AB T2H 0C8; Man'07; FRCSC; Ophth. (403)252-3937; Fax. (403)286-6819.

WARRIAN, R Keith; ST Boniface Gen Hosp, Y3525-409 Tache Ave, Winnipeg MB R2H 2A6; Man'69; FRCSC; GenSurg; Cardiovasc&ThorSurg. Staff, St Boniface General Hospital; (204)233-8563

WARRIAN, W Garnet; PO Box 91550 Stn West Vancouve, West Vancouver BC V7V 3P2; Man'91; FRCPC; Psy.

WARRIAN, William G; Dauphin Med Clinic, 622 3rd Ave St SW, Dauphin MB R7N 1R5; Man'65; CCFP; (204)638-6445; Fax. (204)638-5670.

WARRINER, C Brian; UBC Anesth & Pharmacology, 3300-910 10th Ave W, Vancouver BC V5Z 1M9; UBC'71; FRCPC; Anes (Cardiac Anesthesia). Staff, Vancouver General Hospital - Centennial Pavillion; Staff Anes, Vancouver Coastal Health; Head Anes Pharmacol & Therapeutics/Prof/Dept Head & School Dir Anes, University of British Columbia; (604)875-5855; Fax. (604)875-5344; bwarriner@vanhosp.bc.ca.

WARRINGTON, Cara L E; Surrey Mem Hosp, 13750 96 Ave, Surrey BC V3V 1Z2; UBC'00; Staff, Surrey Memorial Hospital; Staff, Langley Memorial Hospital; (604)581-2211

WARRINGTON, James C; London HSC-Victoria Hosp, PO Box 5010 Stn B B2 369-800 Commissioners Rd E, London ON N6A 5W9; Tor'03; PhD; FRCPC; NuclearMed. Staff, London Health Sciences Centre - Victoria Campus; (519)685-8500; Fax. (519)685-8290.

WARRINGTON, Richard J; Health Sciences Centre, GC 319-820 Sherbrook St, Winnipeg MB R3A 1R9; London (England)'67; MB BS; PhD; BSc(Hons.); FRCPC; IntMed; ClinImmunol&Allergy. Staff, Health Sciences Centre; Prof Med & Immunol, University of Manitoba; (204)787-3186; Fax. (204)787-3216; rwarrington@hsc.mb.ca.

WARSH, Franklin H; Central Community Health Ctre, 359 Talbot St, St Thomas ON N5P 1B7; McM'00; CCFP; (519)633-7989; Fax. (519)633-8467.

WARSH, Jerry J; Addiction & Mental Hlth-Clarke, R20-250 College St, Toronto ON M5T 1R8; Tor'69; PhD; FRCPC; Psy. Head Sect of Biochemical Psy, Centre for Addiction & Mental Health (CAMH) - College Street Site; Prof Psy, University of Toronto; (416)979-4279; Fax. (416)979-4730.

WARSHAWSKI, Frank J; Rockyview Gen Hosp, 7007 14 St SW, Calgary AB T2V 1P9; Alb'76; ABIM; FCCP; FRCPC; IntMed (Cardiovascular Disease); Respir. Staff, Rockyview General Hospital; Staff, Foothills Medical Centre; Staff ICU, Peter Lougheed Centre; Staff, Calgary Health Region; Asst Prof, University of Calgary; (403)943-3788; Fax. (403)212-1241; frank.warshawski@calgaryhealthregion.ca.

WARSHAWSKI, Laurence M; Skin Care Centre, 835 10th Ave W, Vancouver BC V5Z 4E8; UBC'75; FRCPC; Derm (Moles Surgery). Consultant, BC Cancer Agency Sindi Ahluwalia Hawkins Centre for the Southern Interior; Ac Staff, Vancouver General Hospital - Centennial Pavillion; Clin Prof, University of British Columbia; (604)875-4888; Fax. (604)875-4777.

WARSHAWSKI, Patricia A; 8630 120 St, Surrey BC V3W 3N6; UBC'78; Staff, Surrey Memorial Hospital; (604)591-2322; Fax. (604)591-9053.

WARSHAWSKI, Robert S; Hys Med Centre, 202-11010 101 St NW, Edmonton AB T5H 4B9; Alb'75; DABR; DAB; FRCPC; DiagRad (Bone Densitometry); NuclearMed. Staff, Royal Alexandra Hospital; Asst Prof, University of Alberta; (780)426-1121; Fax. (780)425-5979; rwarshawski@shaw.ca.

WARSHAWSKI, S Joseph; 300-1011 Glenmore Trail SW, Calgary AB T2V 4R6; Alb'79; FRCSC; Otol (Head & Neck Surgery). Staff, Calgary Regional Health Authority; (403)571-5215; Fax. (403)571-5204; reception@bsczone.com.

WARSHAWSKI, Thomas J; 208-3330 Richter St, Kelowna BC V1W 4V5; Cal'86; FRCPC; Peds. Staff, Kelowna General Hospital; Chair, Childhood Obesity Foundation; (250)762-0466; Fax. (250)762-0477.

WARSHAWSKY, Bryna F; Middlesex London Health Unit, 101-50 King St, London ON N6A 5L7; McG'86; MHSc; FRCPC; CommunMed. Assoc Med Officer of Hlth, City of London Health Dept; Teach Staff Epidemiol, University of Western Ontario; (519)663-5317; Fax. (519)663-8241; bwarshawsky@london.ca.

WARSHAWSKY, Paul J; B300-SMBD Jewish Gen Hosp, 3755 ch Cote-Sainte-Catherine, Montreal QC H3T 1E2; McG'93; FRCPC; IntMed (Critical Care Medicine); Respir. Staff, Sir Mortimer B Davis Jewish General; (514)340-7500; Fax. (514)340-8133.

WARSI, Mohammed A; Imaging Research Centre, F127-301 James St S, Hamilton ON L8P 3B6; Tor'03; FRCPC; Psy. Langs: Urdu.

WARSI, Mohammed M; Upper River Valley Hosp, 11300 Route 130, Waterville NB E7P 0A4; Karachi (Pakistan)'6; MB BS; Staff, Upper River Valley Hospital - Waterville; Langs: Arabic; Urdu; (506)375-3740

WARSI, Mustafa K; 203-2525 Roseville Gardens Dr, Windsor ON N8T 3J8; Karachi (Pakistan)'98; FRCPC; Psy. Staff, Windsor Regional Hospital - Tayfour Site; (519)944-0283; Fax. (519)944-5383.

WARSI, Shabaz M; Coboconk Comm Med Centre, PO Box 147, Coboconk ON K0M 1K0; Ott'90; (705)454-3375; Fax. (705)454-1534.

WARTELLE-BLADOU, Claire F S; CHUM-Hopital St-Luc, 1058 rue Saint-Denis, Montreal QC H2X 3J4; Universite de la Mediterranee (France)'91; Staff, Centre Hospitalier l'Université De Montréal (CHUM) - Hôpital Saint-luc; (514)890-8000; Fax. (514)412-7314.

WARWARUK, Joslyn A; Teen Health Centre, 1585 Ouellette Ave, Windsor ON N8X 1K5; Wes'90; Staff, Windsor Regional Hospital - Metropolitan Site; (519)253-5481; Fax. (519)253-0891.

WARWICK, Kimberly A; Parry Sound Family Health Team, 75 Bowes St, Parry Sound ON P2A 2L6; Qns'89; CCFP; FCFP; Staff, West Parry Sound Health Centre; (705)746-5595; Fax. (705)746-6576.

WARWICK, Simon P; Greenwood Fam Physicians, PO Box 5, Sundre AB T0M 1X0; (United Kingdom)'04; MB ChB; (403)638-2424

WASAN, Tina; Centre for Womens Health, 404-13291 Yonge St, Richmond Hill ON L4E 4L6; Qns'93; CCFP; FCFP; Staff Health Watch, Women's College Hospital; Physician, Sexual Health Clinic; (905)773-4444; Fax. (905)773-1777.

WASCHKE, Kevin A; MUHC-Montreal Gen Hosp, D7 102-1650 av Cedar, Montreal QC H3G 1A4; McG'98; FRCPC; IntMed (Pancreatobiliary Endoscopy); Gastroent. Langs: French; (514)934-1934 x48899; Fax. (514)934-8531; kevin.waschke@muhc.mcgill.ca.

WASEEM, Zeeshan; Bronte Medical, 78 Jones St, Oakville ON L6L 6C5; Tor'05; FRCPC; PhysMed&Rehab. Staff, Toronto Rehabilitation Institute - University Centre.

WASEF, Mervat S R; Greencrest Clinic, B-2750 Pembina Hwy, Winnipeg MB R3P 2H8; (Other Foreign)'90; CCFP.

WASEF, Mourkus; Hampden Med Clinic, PO Box 10, Hampden NL A0K 2Y0; Alexandria (Egypt)'84; MB ChB; CCFP; (709)455-3111; Fax. (709)455-2232.

WASEF, Nagy S R; Souris Med Associates, PO Box 400, Souris MB R0K 2C0; (Other Foreign)'92; CCFP; (204)483-2147

WASEL, Norman R; Stratica Med Clinic, 200-10140 117 St NW, Edmonton AB T5K 1X3; Man'95; BSc; FRCPC; Derm. Asst Clin Prof, University of Alberta; (780)428-5554; Fax. (780)428-5556; nwasel@look.ca.

WASERMAN, Jack; Humber River Reg Hosp-Keele, 2175 Keele St, Toronto ON M6M 3Z4; McG'75; DAB; DPsy; FRCPC; Psy (Psycho Pharmacology). Physician/Leader Ambulatory Serv, Humber River Regional Hospital - Keele Street Site; (416)658-2022; Fax. (416)658-2074.

WASERMAN, Susan; McMaster Univ Med Centre, HSC 3V49-1280 Main St W, Hamilton ON L8S 4K1; McG'81; BSc; MSc; FRCPC; IntMed; ClinImmunol&Allergy. Att Physician, Hamilton Health Sciences Centre - McMaster Children's Hospital; Staff, St Joseph's Healthcare - Charlton Campus; Prof Med, McMaster University; Langs: English; French; (905)521-2100 x76374; Fax. (905)521-4971.

WASEY, Naureen; St Thomas Surgical Clinic, 4 St Joseph St, St. Albert AB T8N 0B5; Mem'99; FRCSC; GenSurg. (780)459-6633; Fax. (780)459-6609.

WASFI, Atef M; Clinique Med Cadillac, 3435 rue Bossuet, Montreal QC H1M 2M1; Alexandria (Egypt)'94; MB ChB; ac Staff, Centre Hospitalier Rouyn-Noranda; Langs: Arabic; French; (514)253-1211; Fax. (514)253-5091.

WASFY, Samia W; The Doctors Office, 4099 Erin Mills Pkwy, Mississauga ON L5L 3P9; Alexandria (Egypt)'69; MB BCh; DCH; DPH; CCFP; Physician, Queentario Medical Centre; Langs: French; Arabic; (905)820-3310; Fax. (905)820-3312; samiawasty@hotmail.com.

WASH, Walter F; Ermineskin Med Clinic, 301-2377 111 St, Edmonton AB T6J 5E5; Stellenbosh (South Africa)'82; MB ChB; (780)436-8731; Fax. (780)434-8732.

WASHBURN, Robert M; Dr R M Washburn Med Clinic, 5-418 Talbot St W, Aylmer ON N5H 1K9; Dal'73; CCFP; FCFP; Staff Family Med, St Thomas Elgin General Hospital; Court Staff Family Med, Tillsonburg District Memorial Hospital; Aj Prof Clinical, University of Western Ontario; (519)773-8456; Fax. (519)765-1408.

WASI, Parveen; Hamilton HSC-Juravinski Site, 711 Concession St, Hamilton ON L8V 1C3; Mem'87; FRCPC; IntMed; Hem. Staff Juravinski Hosp Site, Hamilton Health Sciences Centre-Juravinski Site; Prof Med, McMaster University; (905)521-2100 x73390; Fax. (905)575-7320.

WASIELEWSKI, Joseph F; Thunder Bay Reg HSC-T-Bay, 980 Oliver Rd, Thunder Bay ON P7B 6V4; Wayne State University (USA)'76; FCAP; FACPath; Chief Pathologist, Thunder Bay Regional Health Sciences Centre; Consultant Path., Life Labs; (807)684-6584 x6590; Fax. (807)684-5878; wasielej@tbh.net.

WASIF, Evet A; Associated Radiologists, 300-140 Wall St, Saskatoon SK S7K 1N4; Cairo (Egypt)'64; FRCPC; DiagRad (Mammography). Dir Diag Rad, Saskatoon City Hospital; Clin Assoc Prof Diag Rad, University of Saskatchewan; Langs: Arabic; French; (306)244-1167; Fax. (306)244-2911; ewasif@shaw.ca.

WASIL, Bushra I; Windsor River Walk-In Clinic, 500 Wyandotte St E, Windsor ON N9A 3H9; Nishtar Medical College (India)'87; CCFP; (519)254-2226

WASILENKO, Lotje; Grey Nuns Community Hosp, 1100 Youville Drive W NW, Edmonton AB T6L 5X8; (Netherlands Antilles)'02; CCFP; Staff, Covenant Health - Grey Nuns Community Hospital; (780)735-7000; Fax. (780)735-7680.

WASLEN, Gregory D; Plastic Surgery Centre, 1030 10 Ave SW, Calgary AB T2R 1M4; Sask'74; FRCSC; PlasSurg (Esthetic Plastic Surgery). Staff Med & Health Resource Centre, Calgary Regional Health Authority; Asst Prof, University of Calgary; Langs: French; Spanish; German; (403)228-1313; Fax. (403)228-1314; plasticsurgerycentre@telus.net.

WASLEN, Thomas A; Associated Radiolgists, 300-140 Wall St, Saskatoon SK S7K 1N4; Sask'91; FRCPC; DiagRad. (306)244-1167; Fax. (306)244-2911.

WASMEIER, Torsten E; Western Mem Reg Hosp, PO Box 2005 Stn Main 1 Brookfield Ave, Corner Brook NL A2H 6J7; Mem'78; Staff, Western Memorial Regional Hospital; (709)637-5000; Fax. (709)637-5327.

WASOWICZ, Marcin; Univ Hlth Network-Toronto Gen, EN3 424-200 Elizabeth St, Toronto ON M5G 2C4; Poznan (Poland)'93; Staff, Toronto General Hospital - UHN; Langs: Polish; (416)340-4800 x3350; Fax. (416)340-3698.

WASS, Hilary; 300-3939 Quadra St, Victoria BC V8X 1J5; Mem'74; FRCPC; Hem (AIDS/HIV); IntMed. (250)480-0400; Fax. (250)480-0458.

WASSEF, Georgina; E-876 Montreal Rd, Ottawa ON K1K 4L3; Ott'96; CCFP; Langs: Arabic; French; (613)742-8182

WASSEF, Hanaa S N; Mulock-Bayview Med Clinic, 30-16700 Bayview Ave, Newmarket ON L3X 1W1; El Minia (Egypt)'92; CCFP; Langs: Arabic; (905)830-0016; Fax. (905)830-0016.

WASSEF, Kawsar K; McConnell Med Centre, 215-820 Mcconnell Ave, Cornwall ON K6H 4M4; Cairo (Egypt)'71; MB ChB; FRCPC; Psy (General Adult Psychiatry). Staff, Cornwall Community Hospital - Second Street Site; Consultant Psy., Tricounty Mental Health (Psychogeriatric Services); Langs: Arabic; (613)938-2328; Fax. (613)938-0537.

WASSEF, Lamia F F; Greenbank Med Centre, 107-139 Greenbank Rd, Nepean ON K2H 9A5; Cairo (Egypt)'93; MB ChB; MSc; CCFP; Langs: Arabic; (613)680-7602; Fax. (613)680-7811.

WASSEF, Magdy W; Clinique Med Pierrefonds, 24-12774 boul Gouin O, Pierrefonds QC H8Z 1W5; Ain Shams (Egypt)'61; AB; FACOG; ac Staff, Lakeshore General Hospital - Pointe Claire; (514)684-8460; Fax. (514)426-8983.

WASSEF, Ramses; CHUM-Hop St-Luc, 1058 rue Saint-Denis, Montreal QC H2X 3J4; Mon'78; ABS; FRCSC; GenSurg (Colon & Rectal Surgery). Staff, Centre Hospitalier l'Université De Montréal (CHUM) - Hôpital Saint-luc; Adj Vice Dean Student Life, Universite de Montreal; Langs: French; (514)890-8000 x34953; Fax. (514)412-7259.

WASSEF, Shadia; St George Med Clinic, 925 Rathburn Rd E, Mississauga ON L4W 4C3; Zagazig (Egypt)'78; MB ChB; CCFP; Staff, Conestoga Medical Centre; (905)949-0123; Fax. (905)949-0124.

WASSENAAR, Willem; Central Clinic, 302-311 Sherbourne St, Toronto ON M5A 3Y1; Wes'70; MSc; MBA; (416)925-1266 x241; Fax. (416)920-6319; wassena@attglobal.net.

WASSER, Edward M I; The Jacobs Pain Centre, 102-8920 Woodbine Ave, Markham ON L3R 9W9; McM'89; DAAPM; CCFP; Staff, Toronto East General Hospital Inc; Staff, St John's Rehabilitation Hospital; Langs: Bilingual(English/French); (905)305-9484; Fax. (905)305-7381.

WASSER, Pnina C; Westmount Med Bldg, 415-5025 rue Sherbrooke O, Montreal QC H4A 1S9; McG'88; CCFP; FCFP; Staff, St Mary's Hospital Centre; McGill University; Langs: English; French; (514)489-4014; Fax. (514)489-1955.

WASSERFALL, Marthinus; Spectrum Health, 702-1080 Howe St, Vancouver BC V6Z 2T1; Stellenbosch (South Africa)'97; MB ChB; CCFP; Langs: Afrikaans; (604)681-1080; Fax. (604)681-0244.

WASSERMAN, Avi; Hotel-Dieu Grace Hosp, 1030 Ouellette Ave, Windsor ON N9A 1E1; Tor'94; FRCPC; IntMed (Cardiology). Staff, Hôtel-Dieu Grace Hospital; Langs: Hebrew; (519)973-4411; Fax. (519)255-2170.

WASSERMAN, David W; Cancer Ctre of Southeastern On, 25 King St W, Kingston ON K7L 5P9; Qns'08; IntMed. (613)544-2630

WASSERMAN, Gary A; 202-1525 Albion Rd, Etobicoke ON M9V 5G5; Tor'72; FRCPC; Derm. (416)743-4267; Fax. (416)743-8737.

WASSERMAN, Jeffrey J; St Michael's Hosp, 30 Bond St, Toronto ON M5B 1W8; Man'86; FRCPC; EmergMed; Anes., St Michael's Hospital; (416)864-5825; Fax. (416)864-6014.

WASSERMAN, Jonathan D; The Hosp for Sick Children, 555 University Ave, Toronto ON M5G 1X8; Harvard (USA)'03; Staff, The Hospital For Sick Children; (416)813-7116; Fax. (416)813-8604.

WASSERMAN, Lori B; Toronto East Gen Hosp Inc, 835 Coxwell Ave, Toronto ON M4C 3E7; Qns'07; FRCPC; Psy. Staff, Toronto East General Hospital Inc; (416)469-6580

WASSERMAN, Lukas J; St Joseph's Healthcare, 50 Charlton Ave E, Hamilton ON L8N 4A6; Stellenbosch (South Africa)'97; FRCSC; GenSurg (Gastroenterology). Staff, St Joseph's Healthcare - Charlton Campus; (905)525-1155

WASSERMAN, Paula R; Rockyview Gen Hosp, 7007 14 St SW, Calgary AB T2V 1P9; Sask'99; FRCPC; Anes. Staff Anes, Rockyview General Hospital; (403)943-3410

WASSERMANN, Delene; 368 Westridge Dr, Williams Lake BC V2G 5J1; Pretoria (South Africa)'07; MB ChB; Langs: Afrikaans; German; (250)267-3962

WASSERSTEIN, David N; Postgrad Med Education Office, 602-500 University Ave, Toronto ON M5G 1V7; Tor'07; OrthSurg.

WASSIF, Ehab B A E; Niagara Med Group Fam Hlth Team, 4421 Queen St, Niagara Falls ON L2E 2L2; Alexandria (Egypt)'95; CCFP; (905)374-2160; Fax. (905)374-0812; ewassif@uwo.ca.

WASSILL, Diane B; Peter Lougheed Centre, 3500 26 Ave NE, Calgary AB T1Y 6J4; Sask'84; FRCPC; Anes. Ac Staff, Peter Lougheed Centre; (403)943-5721; Fax. (403)219-3574.

WASSMANN, Sven; SMBD Jewish Gen Hosp, 3755 ch Cote Ste-Catherine, Montreal QC H3T 1E2; Goettingen (Germany)'98; Staff, Sir Mortimer B Davis Jewish General; (514)340-8222 x8283; Fax. (514)340-7534.

WASSWA-KINTU, Jemima J; 6-2755 Lougheed Hwy, Port Coquitlam BC V3B 5Y9; Makerere (Uganda)'79; MB ChB; (604)944-1773

WASTI, Qasim H; 201-12005 238B St, Maple Ridge BC V4R 1W1; Bahawalpur (Pakistan)'84; MB BS; CCFP; Langs: Punjabi; Hindi; Urdu; (604)463-9200; Fax. (604)463-9203; qasimw@msn.com.

WASTI, Tehmina Q; 201-12005 238B St, Maple Ridge BC V4R 1W1; Aga Khan University (Pakistan)'92; MB BS; CCFP; Langs: Hindi; Urdu; Punjabi; (604)463-9200; Fax. (604)463-9203.

WASTI, Zahid; Kelowna Gen Hosp, 2268 Pandosy St, Kelowna BC V1Y 1T2; Poznan University (Other Foreign)'01; Psy. Staff, Kelowna General Hospital; Langs: Urdu; (250)862-4000

WASTY, S Fasahat H; St Thomas-Elgin Gen Hosp, 189 Elm St, St Thomas ON N5R 5C4; Karachi (Pakistan)'86; MB BS; CRCP; FRCPC; GenPath (Anatomical Pathology). Staff, St Thomas Elgin General Hospital; Langs: Urdu; (519)631-2030 x2080; Fax. (519)637-3222; fwasty@stegh.on.ca.

WASYLENKI, Donald A; St Michael's Hosp, 17F-30 Bond St, Toronto ON M5B 1W8; Sask'71; MSc; FRCPC; Psy. Chief Psychiatrist, St Michael's Hospital; Staff, Centre for Addiction & Mental Health (CAMH) - College Street Site; Chair Psy/Prof, University of Toronto; (416)864-3080; Fax. (416)864-3091.

WASYLENKO, Eric A; Regional Clinical Ethics, 120-10301 Southport Lane SW, Calgary AB T2W 1S7; Cal'82; (403)943-1267; Fax. (403)943-2875.

WASYLYK, Roman Y; Trillium Hlth Ctr-Mississauga, 100 Queensway W, Mississauga ON L5B 1B8; Tor'93; CCFP; CCFP(E.M.); Staff, Trillium Health Centre - Mississauga; Langs: Ukrainian; (905)848-7600

WASZCZUK, Madeleine; 1452 ch du Fleuve, Les Cedres QC J7T 1C8; Ott'65; Psy (P.Q.). (514)731-4080

WAT, Patrick C W; 6179 Main St PO Box 1089 Stn Main, Stouffville ON L4A 8A1; Tor'79; Langs: Cantonese; (905)640-2300; Fax. (905)640-5256.

WAT, S Y Josephine; Hamilton HSC-Henderson Campus, 711 Concession St, Hamilton ON L8V 1C3; London (England)'97; FRCPC; DiagRad. Staff, Hamilton Health Sciences Centre-Juravinski Site; (905)527-4322

WAT, Stephen W; North Edmonton Health Centre, 7910 112 Ave NW, Edmonton AB T5B 0C2; Alb'10; CCFP; (780)342-4740; Fax. (780)342-4742.

WATADA, Brian H; Commercial Street Med Centre, 202-311 Commercial St, Milton ON L9T 3Z9; Tor'96; BSc; MCFP; CCFP; Ac Staff, Halton Healthcare Services Corporation - Milton District Hospital; (905)876-2021; Fax. (905)876-2507; watdab@hotmail.com.

WATANABE, Hiroko; 204-13798 94A Ave, Surrey BC V3V 1N1; McG'64; FACP; MDCM; FRCPC; IntMed; Endocrin&Metab. (604)930-0100; Fax. (604)930-0600.

WATANABE, Mamoru; HSC-Faculty of Med, 3330 Hospital Dr NW, Calgary AB T2N 4N1; McG'57; MD; FRCPC; IntMed (Endocrinology & Metabolism). Staff, Foothills Medical Centre; Emeritus Prof, University of Calgary; (403)220-8725; Fax. (403)270-8025; watanabe@ucalgary.ca.

WATANABE, Sharon M; Cross Cancer Institute, 2001A-11560 University Ave NW, Edmonton AB T6G 1Z2; McG'88; FRCPC; IntMed (Palliative Care); MedOncol. Dir Symptom Control & Palliative, Cross Cancer Institute; Prof Palliative Care Med, University of Alberta; (780)432-8318; Fax. (780)432-8419; sharonwa@cancerboard.ab.ca.

WATANABE, Wei; Coast Med Clinic, 1018 Seymour St, Vancouver BC V6B 3M6; UBC'09; CCFP; (604)569-3632

WATANABE DUFFY, Karen N; Children's Hosp of Eastern Ont, 401 Smyth Rd, Ottawa ON K1H 8L1; Wes'86; CSPQ; FRCPC; IntMed (Rheumatology). Staff, McGill University Health Centre - Montreal Children's Hospital; Staff, Children's Hospital of Eastern Ontario (CHEO); adj Prof/Dir Training Program, McGill University; Langs: Bilingual(English/French); (613)737-7600; Fax. (613)738-4297.

WATCHORN, Adam T S; Banff Mineral Springs Hosp, PO Box 1050 Stn Main, Banff AB T1L 1H7; UBC'09; CCFP; CCFP(E.M.); Staff, Covenant Health - Banff Mineral Springs Hospital; (403)762-2222

WATELLE, Hubert; 102 rue Karine, Duhamel-Ouest QC J9V 1S8; Laval'60; Staff, CSSS du Témiscamingue; (819)629-3536; hubert_watelle@ssss.gouv.qc.ca.

WATELLE, Sylvie; Clinique Med de L'Or, 228 2e rue E, La Sarre QC J9Z 2G9; Laval'86; Médecin, Centre Hospitalier La Sarre; Médecin, Centre Hospitalier St-Jean; Prof, Universite de Montreal; Langs: Bilingual(French/English); (819)339-5617; Fax. (819)339-2729.

WATERHOUSE, Christopher C M; Alberta Children's Hosp, 2888 Shaganappi Trail NW, Calgary AB T3B 6A8; Dal'02; FRCPC; Peds (Pediatric Gastroenterology); Gastroent. Staff, Alberta Children's Hospital; (403)955-7211

WATERMAN, Douglas H; Columbia Med Bldg, 306-301 Columbia St E, New Westminster BC V3L 3W5; Alb'82; BSc; DAB; FACOG; FRCSC; ObstGyn (Laparoscopic Surgery). Ac Staff, Eagle Ridge Hospital & Health Care Centre; Ac Staff, Royal Columbian Hospital; Clin Assoc Prof, University of British Columbia; (604)528-9042; Fax. (604)528-9032.

WATERMAN, Elizabeth J; Pacific Ctre for Reproductive, 500-4601 Canada Way, Burnaby BC V5G 4X7; UBC'02; FRCSC; ObstGyn (Maternal Fetal Medicine). Staff, BC Women's Hospital & Health Centre; Staff, Genesis Fertility Centre; (604)422-7276

WATERMAN, Heather L; Royal Victoria Hosp, 201 Georgian Dr, Barrie ON L4M 6M2; Tor'00; CCFP; CCFP(E.M.); Staff, Royal Victoria Regional Health Centre; (705)728-9090

WATERMAN, Kimberley R; Seafield Med Bldg, 1-1179 Seafield Cres, Nanaimo BC V9S 4S1; UBC'79; FRCPC; Neur (Epilepsy). (250)591-2490

WATERMAN, Nadia J; CSSS Baie-James, CP 1-1650, Chisasibi QC J0M 1E0; Mon'06; CCFP; CCFP(E.M.); Staff, Cree Board of Health & Social Services James Bay; (819)855-9001

WATERS, C Ian; 208-1990 Fort St, Victoria BC V8R 6V4; UBC'77; BSc; FRCPC; IntMed; Respir. Staff, Vancouver Island Health Authority; (250)592-1354; Fax. (250)592-9291.

WATERS, Deborah A; 69 Main St E PO Box 1269, Grand Bend ON N0M 1T0; McM'78; CCFP; FCFP; (519)238-2362; Fax. (519)238-6478.

WATERS, Eugenie F; SCOHS-Elisabeth Bruyere Hosp, 352JB-43 Bruyere St, Ottawa ON K1N 5C8; Wes'10; CCFP; Staff, SCO Health Service - Élisabeth Bruyère Hospital; (613)562-6335

WATERS, Heather M; Stonechurch Family Health Ctre, 1475 Upper Ottawa St, Hamilton ON L8W 3J6; McM'97; CCFP; Ac Staff, St Joseph's Healthcare - Charlton Campus; Court Staff, Hamilton Health Sciences Centre - McMaster Children's Hospital; Asst Prof Family Med, McMaster University; (905)575-7757; Fax. (905)575-7831; watersh@mcmaster.ca.

WATERS, Kellie L; University of Alberta Hosp, 1D1 WMC-8440 112 St NW, Edmonton AB T6G 2B7; Alb'01; FRCPC; Peds. Staff, University of Alberta Hospital; (780)407-6370; Fax. (780)407-6414; kelliewaters@cha.ab.ca.

WATERS, Marnie M; Health Action Centre, 640 Main St, Winnipeg MB R3B 0L8; Man'99; CCFP; (204)940-1626

WATERS, Philip D; MUHC-Royal Victoria Hosp, 687 av des Pins O, Montreal QC H3A 1A1; McG'02; Anes. Staff, McGill University Health Centre - Royal Victoria Hospital; (514)842-1231

WATERS, Shannon; First Nations & Inuit Hlth Reg, 540-757 Hastings St W, Vancouver BC V6C 3E6; UBC'02; BSc; MHSc; MB; FRCP; FRCPC; CommunMed. (604)666-6155; watersshannon@hotmail.com.

WATERS, Terrence S; Vancouver Gen Hosp, 855 12th Ave W, Vancouver BC V5Z 1M9; UBC'76; FRCPC; Anes. Ac Staff Anes, Vancouver General Hospital - Centennial Pavillion; Asst Prof, University of British Columbia; Langs: Spanish; (604)875-4304; Fax. (604)875-5209; terry.waters@vch.ca.

WATERS, Valerie J; The Hosp for Sick Children, 555 University Ave, Toronto ON M5G 1X8; McG'98; FRCPC; Peds; InfectDis. Staff, The Hospital For Sick Children; Langs: Bilingual(English/French); (416)813-1500; Fax. (416)813-8404; valerie.waters@sickkids.ca.

WATERSON, Lydia; Lower Lonsdale Med Centre, 230-150 Esplanade St W, North Vancouver BC V7M 1A3; Orange Free State (South Africa)'84; MB ChB; (604)980-2128

WATERSTON, Sarah E; Hopital de Gatineau, 909 boul la Verendrye O, Gatineau QC J8P 7H2; Ott'07; Peds. Staff, Hôpital de Gatineau; (819)966-6165

WATIER, Alain; CHUS-Hop Hotel-Dieu, 580 rue Bowen S, Sherbrooke QC J1G 2E8; Sher'75; FRCPC; Gastroent. ac Staff, Centre Hospitalier Universitaire de Sherbrooke-Hôpital Hôtel-Dieu; Consultant, Centre Hospitalier Universitaire de Sherbrooke-Hopital Fleurimont; (819)569-2551; Fax. (819)822-6797.

WATKE, Christine A; Maternity Associate, 1510 9 Ave S, Lethbridge AB T1J 1V8; UBC'86; Staff, Chinook Regional Hospital; (403)942-0555; Fax. (403)942-3373.

WATKIN, Daniel; Ramblewood Med Clinic, 101-14 Ramblewood Dr, Wasaga Beach ON L9Z 0C4; Toulouse (France)'82; Staff, Collingwood General & Marine Hospital; Langs: English; French; (705)429-8270; Fax. (705)429-7611.

WATKINS, Drew B; Student Health Services-UCC, 11UCC-1151 Richmond St, London ON N6A 3K7; Tor'89; (519)661-2111; Fax. (519)661-3380; dwatkins@uwo.ca.

WATKINS, J Frederick; Hotel-Dieu Hosp, 385-166 Brock St, Kingston ON K7L 5G2; Dal'83; FRCSC; PlasSurg (Hand Surgery). Staff, Hotel-Dieu Hospital; Staff, Kingston General Hospital; Asst Prof Surg, Queen's University; (613)544-3400 x2300; Fax. (613)544-1658; watkinsf@hdh.kari.net.

WATKINS, Nicola J; Sunpark Prof Centre, 118-40 Sunpark Plaza SE, Calgary AB T2X 3X7; Cal'07; CCFP; (403)254-4000; Fax. (403)254-1282.

WATKINS, William T; Canadian Med Protective Assn, 875 Carling Ave, Ottawa ON K1S 5P1; Wes'95; MCFP; BSc(Hon); CCFP; Dir Professional Services, Canadian Medical Association; Staff, Canadian Medical Protective Association; (613)725-2000; todd.watkins@cma.ca.

WATLER, Crosbie L; Cowichan Med Centre, 3088 Gibbins Rd, Duncan BC V9L 1E8; McM'91; FRCPC; Psy. (250)709-3040; Fax. (250)709-3045.

WATLING, Christopher J; Postgrad Med Education Office, MSB 103-1151 Richmond St, London ON N6A 5C1; Dal'90; MMed; FRCPC; Neur (Neuro Oncology). Ac Staff, London Health Sciences Centre - Victoria Campus; Clin Assoc Prof Clin Neurological Sciences & Oncol/Assoc Dean Postgraduate Med Education, University of Western Ontario; (519)661-2019; Fax. (519)850-2492; chris.watling@lhsc.on.ca.

WATLING, Mark A; Anxiety Trmt & Research Centre, 6F-301 James St S, Hamilton ON L8P 3B6; Dal'94; BSc; FRCPC; Psy (Anxiety Disorder). Staff, St Joseph's Healthcare - Charlton Campus; (905)521-6041

WATMAN, Silvia C; Sunridge Prof Centre, 3-2675 36 St NE, Calgary AB T1Y 6H6; (403)291-3315; Fax. (403)291-9308.

WATRICH, Deanne G; Misericordia Comm Hosp & HC, 16940 87 Ave NW, Edmonton AB T5R 4H5; Sask'93; CCFP; CCFP(E.M.); Staff Emerg, Covenant Health - Misericordia Community Hospital; Staff Emerg, Sturgeon Community Hospital; (780)735-2252; Fax. (780)735-2966.

WATSON, A Elizabeth W; Seven Oaks Gen Hosp, 2300 McPhillips St, Winnipeg MB R2V 3M3; Dublin (Ireland)'79; FRCPC; IntMed; GeriatricMed. Head Dept of Geriatric Med, Seven Oaks General Hospital; Asst Prof, University of Manitoba; (204)632-3117; Fax. (204)697-2065; ewatson@sogh.mb.ca.

WATSON, Adrienne N; Mayflower Med Clinic, 204-998 Parkland Dr, Halifax NS B3M 0A6; Dal'98; CCFP; FCFP; (902)835-1628; Fax. (902)835-1151.

WATSON, Alan F; Victoria Westmount Med Ctre, 202-751 Victoria St S, Kitchener ON N2M 5N4; Dublin (Ireland)'57; BAO; LM(Rotunda); DRCOG; DDS(Hons); (519)744-4000; Fax. (519)744-8265.

WATSON, Andrew; M S I, 230 Brownlow Ave, Dartmouth NS B3B 0G5; London (England)'64; Staff, McGill Centre; (902)468-9700; Fax. (902)490-2275.

WATSON, Andrew C; Cornwall Comm Hosp-McConnell, PO Box 100 Stn Main 840 McConnell Ave, Cornwall ON K6H 5S5; Belfast (Ireland)'82; MB ChB; BAO; Staff, Cornwall Community Hospital - Second Street Site; Staff, Cornwall Community Hospital; Staff, Renfrew Victoria Hospital; (613)938-4080

WATSON, Andrew F; 101-519 Highway 33 W, Kelowna BC V1X 1Y2; Pretoria (South Africa)'87; MB ChB; CCFP; (250)765-7729; Fax. (250)491-1034.

WATSON, Ann E; Jim Pattison Outpatient Care &, 9750 140th St, Surrey BC V3T 0G9; (Other Foreign)'79; (604)582-4582; Fax. (604)582-4591.

WATSON, Bryn A; Chinook Reg Hosp, 960 19 St S, Lethbridge AB T1J 1W5; Cal'99; FRCPC; Anes. Staff, Chinook Regional Hospital; (403)388-6111

WATSON, Christoper P N; 104-89 Humber College Blvd, Etobicoke ON M9V 4B8; Tor'66; FRCPC; Neur (Chronic Pain). Staff, William Osler Health System - Etobicoke General Hospital; Staff, West Park Healthcare Centre; Asst Prof, University of Toronto; (416)239-3494; Fax. (416)239-6365; peter.watson@utoronto.ca.

WATSON, Christopher H C; 202-22 Richmond St, Richmond Hill ON L4C 3Y1; Qns'74; FRCSC; OrthSurg. Att Staff, Mackenzie Richmond Hill Hospital; (905)883-1497; Fax. (905)883-9141; christopher.watson@rogers.com.

WATSON, Diane B; St Lawrence Valley Trmt Ctre, PO Box 5000 1804 Hwy 2, Brockville ON K6V 7N2; UBC'70; FRCPC; Psy (Gender Identity Disorder). (613)341-2870; Fax. (613)341-2884; diane.watson@rohcg.on.ca.

WATSON, G Douglas; Bow River Prof Bldg, 312-4411 16 Ave NW, Calgary AB T3B 0M3; Alb'71; DAB; FRCPC; Psy. (403)571-5166; Fax. (403)571-5167; watsong@telusplanet.net.

WATSON, George K; 17C-815 1st Ave W, Prince Rupert BC V8J 1B3; UBC'80; Att Staff, Prince Rupert Regional Hospital; Med Dir, Acropolis Manor Intermediate Care Home; Clin Instructor, University of British Columbia; (250)624-3331; Fax. (250)624-9464.

WATSON, Hilary A; Maitland Valley Family Hlth Team, 180 Cambria Rd N, Goderich ON N7A 4N8; McM'03; CCFP; Staff, Alexandra Marine & General Hospital; (519)524-6060; Fax. (519)524-5225.

WATSON, Iain S; Main Street Family Health Ctr, 1251 Stittsville Main St, Stittsville ON K2S 2E5; Ott'93; (613)831-7372; Fax. (613)831-6381.

WATSON, Ian J; 103-174 Harwood Ave S, Ajax ON L1S 2H6; Tor'01; CCFP; (905)683-0690; Fax. (905)683-1431.

WATSON, J David; Kingsway Plaza Phase III, 608-4980 Kingsway, Burnaby BC V5H 4K7; Man'83; FRCPC; PhysMed&Rehab. (604)880-2253

WATSON, James T; St Joseph's Health Care, PO Box 5777 Stn B 268 Grosvenor St, London ON N6A 4V2; Wes'81; FRCPC; Anes. Staff, London Health Sciences Centre - University Hospital; Staff, St Joseph's Hospital - St Joseph's Health Care; (519)646-6000 x6421; Fax. (519)646-6116.

WATSON, John B; The Ottawa Hosp-Gen Campus, 1401-501 Smyth Rd, Ottawa ON K1H 8L6; Ott'85; AB; FRCPC; Anes (Pain Management). Staff, The Ottawa Hospital - General Campus; Consultant, SCO Health Service - Élisabeth Bruyère Hospital; Asst Prof, University of Ottawa; Langs: Bilingual(French/English); (613)737-8187; Fax. (613)737-8189; jwatson@ottawahospital.on.ca.

WATSON, Jonathan M; St Joseph's Gen Hosp, 2137 Comox Ave, Comox BC V9M 1P2; Newcastle (England)'92; FRCPC; Anes. Staff Medical Staff Office, St Joseph's General Hospital; (250)339-2242

WATSON, K Randal; 206-101 Queensway W, Mississauga ON L5B 2P7; Tor'83; FRCPC; IntMed (Interventional Cardiology); Cardiol. Staff, Trillium Health Centre - Mississauga; Asst Prof Med, University of Toronto; (905)615-9285; Fax. (905)615-8537.

WATSON, Keith E; Dixon Med Centre, 208-531 Davis Dr, Newmarket ON L3Y 6P5; Wes'73; Ac Staff, Southlake Regional Health Centre; (905)895-6551; Fax. (905)895-9874.

WATSON, Krista P; PO Box 680, Mahone Bay NS B0J 2E0; Dal'99; CCFP; CCFP(E.M.); Staff, Fishermen's Memorial Hospital; (902)527-7040; Fax. (902)634-7328.

WATSON, Leah D; Univ Hlth Network-Toronto Gen, RFE GS480-200 Elizabeth St, Toronto ON M5G 2C4; Man'03; FRCPC; EmergMed. Staff, Toronto General Hospital - UHN; (416)340-3856; Fax. (416)340-4300.

WATSON, Mary E D; Midtown Med Clinic, 35 Campbell Ave, St. John's NL A1E 2Z3; Mem'80; CCFP; FCFP; (709)579-0703; Fax. (709)579-1477.

WATSON, Mary-Lynn; Queen Elizabeth II HSC-Halifax, 355-1796 Summer St, Halifax NS B3H 3A7; Dal'89; CCFP; CCFP(E.M.); Staff, Queen Elizabeth II Health Sciences Centre - Halifax Infirmary Site; (902)473-8457; Fax. (902)473-3617.

WATSON, Matthew T; Cole Harbour Family Med Centre, 203A-240 Baker Dr, Dartmouth NS B2W 6L4; Alb'99; CCFP; FCFP; (902)435-6312; Fax. (902)434-7920.

WATSON, Michael W B; West End Prof Bldg, 211-9509 156 St NW, Edmonton AB T5P 4J5; London (England)'51; MRCS; LRCP; DRCOG; Langs: French; German; (780)483-3253; Fax. (780)483-3212.

WATSON, Misty A E; Heritage Pointe Family Med, 330-412 Pine Creek Rd, De Winton AB T0L 0X0; (403)279-4944; Fax. (403)720-3321.

WATSON, Neil C; Foothills Med Centre, 1403 29 St NW, Calgary AB T2N 2T9; London (England)'79; FRCPC; Anes. Staff Anes, Foothills Medical Centre; (403)944-1430; Fax. (403)944-2425.

WATSON, Norman; Valley Med Clinic, 335 Jubilee St, Duncan BC V9L 1W9; UBC'80; Staff, Canadian Academy of Sports & Exercise Medicine; Clin Assoc Prof Family Med, University of British Columbia; (250)748-8151; Fax. (250)748-8157.

WATSON, Paul A; West Arthur Place, 308-1265 Arthur St E, Thunder Bay ON P7E 6E7; Cal'92; FRCPC; IntMed; Nephrol. Staff, Thunder Bay Regional Health Sciences Centre; (807)622-5452; Fax. (807)622-5710; pvwatson@shawbiz.ca.

WATSON, Peter H; BC Cancer Agency-Vanc Island, 2410 Lee Ave, Victoria BC V8R 6V5; Cambridge (England)'83; MB ChB; FRCPC; AnatPath (Breast Cancer). Staff, BC Cancer Agency Vancouver Island Centre; (250)519-5710; Fax. (250)519-2009.

WATSON, Priya N; 80 Workman Way, Toronto ON M5T 1R8; McM'00; MSc; Psy (Child & Adolescent Psychiatry). Staff, Centre for Addiction & Mental Health (CAMH) - College Street Site; Staff, Centre for Addiction & Mental Health (CAMH) - Queen Site; Langs: Bilingual(English/French); (416)535-8501; Fax. (416)979-4996.

WATSON, Sally J; The Medical Clinic Associates, 4794 Joyce Ave, Powell River BC V8A 3B6; Manchester (England)'97; MB ChB; Langs: Welsh; (604)485-6261; Fax. (604)485-2820.

WATSON, Shayna L; Cancer Ctre Southeastern Ont, 25 King St W, Kingston ON K7L 5P9; McM'92; CCFP; FCFP; Staff, Cancer Centre of Southeastern Ontario; Staff, The Ottawa Hospital - Civic Campus; (613)650-5571

WATSON, Sheila D; Rockyview Gen Hosp, 7007 14 St SW, Calgary AB T2V 1P9; McM'87; BSc; FRCSC; ObstGyn. Ac Staff ObstGyn, Rockyview General Hospital; Langs: English; French; (403)943-8733; Fax. (403)943-8677.

WATSON, Stephen B; Foothills Med Centre, G28-1403 29 Street NW, Calgary AB T2N 2T9; Alb'80; BMedSci; CCFP; FCFP; Assoc Staff Family Med, Foothills Medical Centre; (403)944-2800

WATSON, Timothy W J; Foothills Med Centre, 1079-1403 29 St NW, Calgary AB T2N 2T9; Cal'79; FRCPC; Neur (Stroke). Staff Clin Neurosciences, Foothills Medical Centre; Asst Prof Med, University of Calgary; (403)944-2097; Fax. (403)944-2611; watsont@ucalgary.ca.

WATSON, Wade T A; IWK Health Centre, PO Box 9700 Rpo CSC 5850 University Ave, Halifax NS B3K 6R8; Dal'82; FRCPC; Peds (Pediatric Allergy); ClinImmunol&Allergy. Staff, IWK Health Centre; (902)470-6554

WATSON, William J; St Michael's Hosp, 30 Bond St, Toronto ON M5B 1W8; McG'77; CCFP; FCFP; Staff Family & Med, St Michael's Hospital; Langs: English; French; (416)867-7426; Fax. (416)867-7498; watsonw@smh.toronto.on.ca.

WATSON-CREED, Gaynor B; Public Health Services, 5-7 Mellor Ave, Dartmouth NS B3B 0E8; Dal'99; FRCPC; CommunMed;CCFP; Med Officer of Hlth, Capital Health IWK Health Centre Public Health Dartmouth; (902)481-5883; Fax. (902)481-5803; watsong@cdha.nshealth.ca.

WATT, Anne M; Lions Gate Hosp, 231 15th St E, North Vancouver BC V7L 2L7; Tor'88; CCFP; CCFP(E.M.); FCFP; Staff, Lions Gate Hospital; (604)988-3131; Fax. (604)984-5828.

WATT, Beth C; 103-20644 Fraser Hwy, Langley BC V3A 4G5; UBC'83; (604)530-4979; Fax. (604)530-2975; beth_watt@telus.net.

WATT, Christopher J; Cook Street Village Med Clinic, 101A-230 Cook St, Victoria BC V8V 3X3; Tor'88; (250)222-9999; watti@telus.net.

WATT, Denise A; Foothills Med Centre, C231-1403 29 St NW, Calgary AB T2N 2T9; Qns'99; BSc; CCFP; CCFP(E.M.); Staff, Foothills Medical Centre; (403)944-1635; Fax. (403)944-2419.

WATT, Donald W C; Glenmore Landing Vein Clinic, D267-1600 90 Ave SW, Calgary AB T2V 5A8; Aberdeen (Scotland)'62; DMRD(Lond); FRCPC; DiagRad (Interventional Radiology). Staff, Glenmore Landing Vein Clinic; (403)253-2555; Fax. (403)640-4247.

WATT, Douglas A; 22 Richard St, Sydney Mines NS B1V 2H7; Dal'84; FRCPC; PhysMed&Rehab. Staff, Northside General Hospital; Staff, Cape Breton Healthcare Complex; (902)736-4404; Fax. (902)736-6035; dwatt@ns.sympatico.ca.

WATT, Douglas G D; McGill University, 3655 Prom Sir-William-Osler, Montreal QC H3G 1Y6; McG'69; MSc; PhD; Prof, McGill University; (514)398-6025; Fax. (514)398-8241.

WATT, Elizabeth J; 34333 Renton St., Abbotsford BC V2S 5B7; UBC'85; BSc; CCFP; FCFP; Staff, Abbotsford Regional Hospital & Cancer Centre; Physician Health Services, Fraser Valley Institute; Staff Lead Physician, Abbotsford Youth Health Centre; Staff Botox & Filler, Face Beautiful Cosmedic Spa; Physician, Peardonville House; (604)851-6107; watt_elizabeth@hotmail.com.

WATT, Garth B; 205-6389 Coburg Rd, Halifax NS B3H 2A5; McG'86; MDCM; FRCPC; Psy. Langs: English; French; (902)423-7954; Fax. (902)423-7964.

WATT, Gordon L D; Orleans Urgent Care Centre, 100-1220 Prom Place d'Orleans, Orleans ON K1C 7K3; Qns'66; Court Staff Emerg, The Ottawa Hospital - Civic Campus; Physician Occupational Med, Queensway Carleton Hospital; Physician, Orleans Urgent Care Centre; (613)729-8063; Fax. (613)729-8063.

WATT, James H; 45 St Thomas St, St. Albert AB T8N 6Z1; Wes'83; FRCPC; DiagRad (Musculoskeletal Imaging). Langs: English; French; (780)729-0348

WATT, Janet A; 201-190 Wellington St, Kingston ON K7L 3E4; Qns'91; CCFP; FCFP; (613)542-4181; Fax. (613)547-0004.

WATT, John A; Formation Health Serv Unit, PO Box 17000 Stn Forces 1200 Colville Rd, Victoria BC V9A 7N2; Aberdeen (Scotland)'62; MB ChB; DPM; MRCPsy; FAPA; FRCPC; Psy (Adult Psychiatry). Staff, Canadian Forces Health Services - Pacific Centre; (250)363-4411; Fax. (250)363-4405; sndywtt@yahoo.ca.

WATT, Maggie J; Festubert Family Practice, 350 Festubert St, Duncan BC V9L 3S9; UBC'97; CCFP; FCFP; Staff, Cowichan District Hospital; (250)746-7720; Fax. (250)748-4839.

WATT, Man-Joe; Glenrose Rehab Hosp, 119 GE-10230 111 Ave NW, Edmonton AB T5G 0B7; (Hong Kong)'72; MB BS; AB; FRCPC; Peds (Cerebral Palsy); PhysMed&Rehab. Med Dir Neuromotor Prog & Syncrude Center for Motion & Balance, Glenrose Rehabilitation Hospital; Prof, University of Alberta; Langs: Chinese; (780)735-7918; Fax. (780)735-7907.

WATT, Natalie A M; Glenmore Landing D267-1600 90 Ave SW, Calgary AB T2V 5A8; Cal'91; CCFP; FCFP; (403)253-2555; Fax. (403)640-4247; veins@telusplanet.net.

WATT, Peter D; 404 Medical Clinic, 39-1111 Davis Dr, Newmarket ON L3Y 8X2; Tor'86; BSc; FRCSC; ObstGyn. Asst Prof ObstGyn, McMaster University; Lecturer, University of Toronto; Langs: Bilingual(English/French); (905)836-7100; Fax. (905)836-7062; drwatt@rogers.com.

WATT, William G; The Medical Clinic, 10011 96 St, Fort St. John BC V1J 3P3; Wes'76; (250)785-6677; Fax. (250)787-0109; wwatt@awink.com.

WATTAM, David P; Etherington Hall, 1004-70 Barrie St, Kingston ON K7L 3N6; Qns'79; FRCPC; IntMed. Staff, Hotel-Dieu Hospital; Ac Staff, QHC Belleville General; Consultant, QHC Prince Edward County Memorial; Consultant, Weeneebayko General Hospital; Teach Staff, Queen's University; (613)533-3061

WATTERS, A Kevin; MUHC-Montreal Gen Hosp, 1650 av Cedar, Montreal QC H3G 1A4; McG'75; FRCPC; AnatPath (Dermatological Pathology). Staff, McGill University Health Centre - Montreal General Campus; Assoc Prof Path, McGill University; (514)937-6011 x43840; Fax. (514)934-8296; kevin.watters@muhc.mcgill.ca.

WATTERS, Conrad W L; Hotel-Dieu Hosp, 166 Brock St, Kingston ON K7L 5G2; Wes'74; FRCSC; PlasSurg. Staff, Hotel-Dieu Hospital; (613)544-3400

WATTERS, Elizabeth C; 101-1516 Fairview Rd, Penticton BC V2A 6A3; McM'86; BSc; Staff, Penticton Regional Hospital; (250)493-7141; Fax. (250)493-8366.

WATTERS, James M; The Ottawa Hosp-Civic Campus, 208-1053 Carling Ave, Ottawa ON K1Y 4E9; Tor'77; FACS; FRCSC; GenSurg. Ac Staff Surg, The Ottawa Hospital - Civic Campus; Prof, University of Ottawa; (613)761-4780; Fax. (613)761-4698; jwatters@ohri.ca.

WATTERS, Suzanne E; PO Box 1205 Stn A, Comox BC V9M 7Z8; McM'05; CCFP; Langs: Bilingual(English/French).

WATTERS, William B; Ancaster Prof Arts Bldg, 202-323 Wilson St E, Ancaster ON L9G 4A8; Wes'76; BSc; MSc; DOHS; Ac Staff, St Joseph's Healthcare - Charlton Campus; Court Staff, Hamilton Health Sciences Centre - McMaster University Medical Centre; (905)648-1431; Fax. (905)648-9887.

WATTERSON, James D; The Ottawa Hosp-Gen Campus, 501 Smyth Rd Box 222, Ottawa ON K1H 8L6; Qns'95; FRCSC; Urol. Staff, The Ottawa Hospital - General Campus; (613)737-8373; Fax. (613)737-8982; jwatterson@ottawahospital.on.ca.

WATTERSON, James G; 160 Edelweiss Dr NW, Calgary AB T3A 3R1; Cal'77; FRCPC; Anes.

WATTERSON, John R; Pacific Arthritis Centre, 208-888 8th Ave W, Vancouver BC V5Z 3Y1; UBC'95; BSc; FRCPC; IntMed (Adult Rheumatology); Rheum. Clinical Asst Prof, University of British Columbia; (604)875-8020; Fax. (604)875-8058; jwatterson@shaw.ca.

WATTERSON, Timothy J; Strathcona Mental Health Team, 201-330 Heatley Ave, Vancouver BC V6A 3G3; UBC'71; CCFP; Vis Staff, Vancouver General Hospital - Centennial Pavillion; Staff, Strathcona Mental Health Team; (604)253-4401; Fax. (604)253-5194.

WATTERUD, Donna L; Thamesview Family Health Team, 465 Grand Ave W, Chatham ON N7L 1C5; Qns'80; FCFP; CCFP; Ac Staff, Chatham-Kent Health Alliance; (519)351-6464; Fax. (519)351-4890.

WATTS, Barbara E L; Headwaters Health Care Ctre, 100 Rolling Hills Dr, Orangeville ON L9W 4X9; Tor'82; CCFP; Ac Staff, Headwaters Health Care Centre - Orangeville Site; (519)940-2410; Fax. (519)941-4707.

WATTS, Craig S; Clinique Medic Elle, 500-1980 rue Sherbrooke O, Montreal QC H3H 1E8; McG'74; ABIM; CSPQ; Rheum; ClinImmunol&Allergy; IntMed (Adult Rheumatology). Consultant Rheum, Hopital Ste-Anne; assoc Médecin Rheum, McGill University Health Centre - Montreal General Campus; Staff Rheumatology, Catherine Booth Hospital; adj Prof IntMed & Rheum, McGill University; (514)933-9325; Fax. (514)933-2706; drcraigwatts@qc.aibn.com.

WATTS, Eric D J; Executive Bldg, 310-6411 Buswell St, Richmond BC V6Y 2G5; UBC'80; (604)278-6838; Fax. (604)278-8826.

WATTS, Harold R; Cow Head Med Clinic, PO Box 70, Cow Head NL A0K 2A0; Wes'68; (709)243-2407

WATTS, Helene; CLSC des Mille-Iles, 4731 boul Levesque E, Laval QC H7C 1M9; Laval'86; Médecin, CLSC des Milles-Iles; Langs: Bilingual(French/English); (450)661-2572; Fax. (450)661-9147.

WATTS, Jacqueline; Linden Ridge Med Centre, E-123 Scurfield Blvd, Winnipeg MB R3Y 1L6; Pretoria (South Africa)'89; (204)488-9988

WATTS, Jill A; Chatham Med Clinic, 36 Church St, Miramichi NB E1N 1T1; Mem'86; Staff, Miramichi Regional Hospital; (506)778-8223; Fax. (506)773-4060.

WATTS, Joel C; Institut Philippe Pinel de Mon, 10905 boul Henri-Bourassa E, Montreal QC H1C 1H1; Wes'03; FRCPC; Psy. Staff, Institut Philippe-Pinel de Montreal; (514)648-8461

WATTS, Kingsley F; Runnymede Health Centre, 625 Runnymede Rd, Toronto ON M6S 3A3; Tor'87; BA; CCFP; FCFP; Ac Staff, St Joseph's Health Centre; Staff, Toronto Rehabilitation Institute - Queen Elizabeth Centre; Asst Prof Family Med, University of Toronto; (416)762-7316; wattsk@stjoe.on.ca.

WATTS, Nancy; Clinique Méd familale Jonquièr, 3835 boul Harvey, Jonquiere QC G7X 2Z5; Laval'92; CCFP; Staff, Centre Hospitalier Jonquiere; Langs: Bilingual(French/English); (418)542-7519; Fax. (418)542-6541.

WATTS, Peter W S; Valley Women & Children's HC, 60 Aberdeen St, Kentville NS B4N 2N3; Belfast (Ireland)'66; MB ChB; BAO; DRCOG; FRCOG; ObstGyn. (902)678-4626; Fax. (902)678-6338.

WATTS, Robyn J; Dr Robyn Watts Inc, 201-6051 Gilbert Rd, Richmond BC V7C 3V3; UBC'00; FRCSC; PlasSurg (Breast Surgery). Staff, Coastal Plastic Surgery; Langs: Bilingual(English/French); (604)273-1034; Fax. (604)273-1037; info@coastalplasticsurgery.com.

WATTS, Sylvie; CLSC Saint-Michel, 3355 rue Jarry E, Montreal QC H1Z 2E5; Mon'87; (514)374-8223; Fax. (514)374-5931.

WATTY, Margaret R; Marly Med Clinic, 182-1402 8 Ave NW, Calgary AB T2N 1B8; Alb'85; CCFP; Clin Prof, Foothills Medical Centre; (403)289-4312; Fax. (403)289-4377.

WAUQUAIRE, Catherine; Hotel-Dieu de Sorel, 400 av de l'Hotel-Dieu, Sorel-Tracy QC J3P 1N5; Staff, Hôtel-Dieu de Sorel; (450)746-6000

WAVRANT, Sandrine; Hopital Sainte-Justine, 3175 ch Cote-Sainte-Catherine, Montreal QC H3T 1C5; Lyon (France)'05; Staff, Hôpital Ste-Justine; (514)345-4788

WAWER, Andrew R; Northside Harbor View Hosp, PO Box 399 Stn Main, North Sydney NS B2A 3M4; Dal'83; Chief Emerg Services, Northside General Hospital; (902)794-1515; Fax. (902)794-1184.

WAWER, Ursula B; Sun Tower Bldg, 416-1550 Bedford Hwy, Bedford NS B4A 1E6; Mem'88; FRCPC; Psy. Staff, The East Coast Forensic Psychiatry Hospital; (902)422-5849; Fax. (902)835-6860; ursula.wawer@cdha.nshealth.ca.

WAWRYKO, Paul M; St Boniface Gen Hosp, 409 Tache Ave, Winnipeg MB R2H 2A6; Man'06; FRCPC; AnatPath. Staff, St Boniface General Hospital; (204)233-8563

WAWRYKOW, Teresa M J; Concordia Gen Hosp, 1095 Concordia Ave, Winnipeg MB R2K 3S8; Man'05; CCFP; CCFP(E.M.); Staff, Concordia General Hospital; (204)667-1560

WAWRZYSZYN, Benigna B; IWK Health Centre, PO Box 9700 Rpo CSC 5850-5980 University Ave, Halifax NS B3K 6R8; Wroclaw (Poland)'73; FRCPC; Anes (Pediatrics). Staff, IWK Health Centre; Dalhousie University; (902)470-8305; Fax. (902)470-2911.

WAWRZYSZYN, Janusz; Pier Med Clinic, 788 Victoria Rd, Sydney NS B1N 1J7; Wroclaw (Poland)'70; Staff, Cape Breton Healthcare Complex; Langs: Polish; (902)564-8361; Fax. (902)567-6161.

WAX, Randy S; Lakeridge Hlth Corp-Oshawa, 20213-1 Hospital Crt, Oshawa ON L1G 2B9; Tor'94; DABIM; MD; MEd; FRCP; FRCPC; IntMed (Critical Care Medicine). Med Dir Prog for Resuscitation Educ & Patient Safety, Mount Sinai Hospital; Staff, Lakeridge Health - Oshawa Site; Asst Prof Critical Care, University of Toronto; (905)576-8711; randy.wax@utoronto.ca.

WAXMAN, David H; 100-14770 boul de Pierrefonds, Pierrefonds QC H9H 4Y6; McG'92; FRCPC; Peds. (514)696-2442

WAXMAN, Mark L; East York Med Health Centre, 27E-45 Overlea Blvd, East York ON M4H 1C3; Tor'76; (416)696-9836; Fax. (416)696-8080.

WAXMAN, Marvin; Village Health Centre, 108 Scollard St, Toronto ON M5R 1G2; Tor'69; CCFP; FCFP; Assoc Staff, Mount Sinai Hospital; (416)925-3843; Fax. (416)968-7952.

WAXMAN, Menashe B; Univ Hlth Network-The Toronto, 3GW 558-200 Elizabeth St, Toronto ON M5G 2C4; McG'63; FRCPC; IntMed (Cardiac Electrophysiology). Staff, Toronto General Hospital - UHN; Prof Med, University of Toronto; Langs: English; French; (416)340-3929; Fax. (416)595-1811; menashe.waxman@uhn.on.ca.

WAXMAN, Robyn E; Ont Shores Ctre for Mental Hea, 700 Gordon St, Whitby ON L1M 5S9; Ott'05; FRCPC; Psy. (905)430-4055; Fax. (905)430-4465.

WAY, Daniel O; Carleton Univ Health Services, 2600-1125 Colonel By Dr, Ottawa ON K1S 5B6; Wes'85; CCFP; FCFP; Staff, The Ottawa Hospital - Civic Campus; Physician, Carleton University Health Services; Assoc Prof Family Med, University of Ottawa; (613)520-6674; Fax. (613)520-4059; dway@scohs.on.ca.

WAY, Jeffrey C E; Acadia Med Centre, 202-8330 Fairmount Dr SE, Calgary AB T2H 0Y8; Mem'80; FACS; FRCSC; GenSurg (Trauma). Staff Surg, Calgary Health Region; Clin Lecturer, University of Calgary; (403)252-5674; Fax. (403)252-3938.

WAYDA, Charlene E; Mapleview Med Clinic, 340 Elgin St, Port Colborne ON L3K 6G9; McM'86; Physician, Mapleview Medical Clinic; (905)835-9817; Fax. (905)835-1647.

WAYMOUTH, Heather E; Etherington Hall, 3038-94 Stuart St, Kingston ON K7L 3N6; Cal'08; IntMed (Rheumatology). (613)533-2623; Fax. (613)533-6695.

WAYMOUTH, Patricia L; Lynnwood Med Centre, 6622 20A St SE, Calgary AB T2C 0R3; Qns'73; CCFP; (403)279-3311; Fax. (403)279-4214.

WAYMOUTH, William E W; Algoma District Cancer Program, 750 Great Northern Rd, Sault Ste. Marie ON P6B 0A6; Mem'78; Staff, Sault Area Hospital - Sault Ste Marie; (705)759-3434; Fax. (705)759-3815.

WAZANA, Ashley D; Child Development & Mental Hea, 4335 ch Cote-Sainte-Catherine, Montreal QC H3T 1E4; McM'96; FRCPC; Psy (Pediatric Psychiatry). Staff, Sir Mortimer B Davis Jewish General; Staff, McGill University Health Centre - Montreal Children's Hospital; Staff, Institute of Community & Family Psychiatry; Langs: Spanish; French; (514)340-8210; Fax. (514)340-7903.

WEAGLE, Everett D E; 204-26 North St, Bridgewater NS B4V 2V6; Dal'88; (902)543-2242; Fax. (902)530-3146.

WEATHERALL, Paul I; Loyalist Family Practice, 2A-150 Sidney St, Belleville ON K8P 5E2; Tor'91; (613)771-0008; Fax. (613)771-1861.

WEATHERDON, Derek S; Medical Associates, 100-155 Main St E, Grimsby ON L3M 1P2; Wes'95; CCFP; (905)945-5476

WEATHERHEAD, Debra J; Queensway Carleton Hosp, 3045 Baseline Rd, Ottawa ON K2H 8P4; Dal'90; BSc; CCFP; CCFP(E.M.); FCFP; Staff, Queensway Carleton Hospital; (613)721-2000

WEATHERHEAD, Louis E P; Louis Weatherhead Med Prof Cor, 208-1919 Riverside Dr, Ottawa ON K1H 1A2; The University of West Indies (Jamaica)'78; BSc(Hons.); MB BS; DABD; FRCPC; Derm (Cutaneous Oncology). Ac Staff, The Ottawa Hospital - Civic Campus; Consultant, Ontario Cancer Foundation; Assoc Prof Derm, University of Ottawa; Langs: French; (613)230-8191; Fax. (613)230-4402; lweatherhead@ottawahospital.on.ca.

WEATHERHEAD, Michael F; 203-2494 Danforth Ave, Toronto ON M4C 1K9; Tor'67; (416)698-3898; Fax. (416)698-0272.

WEATHERSTON, Evelyn J; 141 Lake St PO Box 1025 Stn Main, Pembroke ON K8A 6Y6; Wes'77; BA(Hon.); (613)732-3635; Fax. (613)732-9854; drweatherston@bellnet.ca.

WEATHERSTON, Philip M; Sardis Family Practice, 202-45425 Luckakuck Way, Chilliwack BC V2R 2T7; Edinburgh (Scotland)'71; MB ChB; (604)858-9461; Fax. (604)858-9921.

WEAVER, Andrew R; Family Practice Associates, PO Box 2010 223 16 Ave N, Creston BC V0B 1G0; Cal'06; CCFP; (250)428-9371; Fax. (250)428-9350.

WEAVER, Donald F; Queen Elizabeth II HSC-Halifax, 3822-1796 Summer St, Halifax NS B3H 3A7; Qns'81; PhD; FRCPC; Neur (Epilepsy). Staff, Queen Elizabeth II Health Sciences Centre - Halifax Infirmary Site; (902)473-2268; Fax. (902)473-4438.

WEAVER, Gerald B; Providence Care DDCOT, 301-234 Concession St, Kingston ON K7K 6W6; McM'80; FRCPC; Psy.

WEAVER, Joel G R; Nepean Med Centre, 311-1 Centrepointe Dr, Ottawa ON K2G 6E2; Ott'01; FRCSC; GenSurg. (613)225-8433; Fax. (613)274-7535.

WEAVER, Joel H; Chinook Reg Hosp, 960 19 St S, Lethbridge AB T1J 1W5; Alb'94; BMedSci; CASM; CCFP; Staff Geriatrician, Chinook Regional Hospital; Med Dir, Covenant Health - St Michael's Health Centre; Clin Lecturer, University of Alberta; (403)388-6600; Fax. (403)388-6340.

WEAVER, Lana M; Erinoakkids, 2277 South Millway, Mississauga ON L5L 2M5; Tor'96; FRCPC; Peds (Developmental Pediatrics). (905)855-2690 x2469; Fax. (905)820-2756.

WEAVER, Robert G; 4440 Stark St, Richmond BC V7B 1A1; Mem'77; (604)270-1370

WEAVER, William G; South Muskoka Med Centre, 230 Manitoba St, Bracebridge ON P1L 2E1; McM'82; (705)646-7634; Fax. (705)646-0476.

WEBB, Charles D; 102-8584 Granville St, Vancouver BC V6P 4Z7; Cape Town (South Africa)'82; Dir Board Member/Div of Family Practice/V-Chair Div of Family Practice, British Columbia Medical Association; Langs: Afrikaans; (604)266-1496; Fax. (604)266-9011.

WEBB, David A; Easthill Med Walk-In Clinic, 610-3020 22 St, Red Deer AB T4R 3J5; London (England)'72; MB BS; LRCP; MRCS; DA(UK); (403)343-0115; Fax. (403)343-8551; david.webb@impacthealth.ca.

WEBB, G Robert; PO Box 3004 Stn Main, Grnd-Bay-Wfld NB E5K 4V3; Dal'78; BSc; MSc; Ac Staff, Saint John Regional Hospital; Ac Staff, St Joseph's Hospital; GP Assoc Staff, Centracare; Member, College of Family Physicians of Canada-New Brunswick; (506)738-8462; Fax. (506)738-3385; webbr@nbnet.nb.ca.

WEBB, Irma A S; 2 1-555 Concession St, Hamilton ON L8V 1A8; McM'87; CCFP; FCFP; (905)387-0831

WEBB, Janet L; Central Hastings Fam Hlth Team, 52 St Lawrence St E, Madoc ON K0K 2K0; Tor'86; CCFP; FCFP; Med Dir, Caressant Care Marmora; (613)473-4134; Fax. (613)473-4740.

WEBB, Katie A D; Quee's Univ Family Med Centre, 115 Clarence St, Kingston ON K7L 5N6; Ott'06; CCFP; (613)533-9303

WEBB, Margot A; Clayton Heights Med Clinic, 204-18730 Fraser Hwy, Surrey BC V3S 7Y4; (Other Foreign)'06; (604)575-0501

WEBB, Robert J; PO Box 3004 Stn Main, Grnd-Bay-Wfld NB E5K 4V3; Sask'74; DObstRCOG; (506)738-8462; Fax. (506)738-3385.

WEBB, Ronald B; Two Rivers FHT-Hespeler Med Cl, B12-350 Conestoga Blvd, Cambridge ON N1R 7L7; Qns'73; CCFP; FCFP; Staff, Two Rivers Family Health Team - Hespeler Medical Clinic; (519)629-4615; Fax. (519)629-4630.

WEBB, Stephen P; East Reg Mental Health Service, 2757 King St E, Hamilton ON L8G 5E4; McM'84; FRCPC; Psy. Ac Staff, St Joseph's Healthcare - Charlton Campus; (905)573-4801; Fax. (905)573-4802.

WEBB, Susan M; Children's Hosp, 840 Sherbrook St, Winnipeg MB R3A 1S1; Man'78; FRCPC; Peds (Child Abuse). Staff Peds, Health Sciences Centre; Dir Undergraduate Med Educ/Assoc Prof Med, University of Manitoba; (204)787-2401; Fax. (204)787-1468.

WEBB, Timothy R; 33 Health Services Centre, PO Box 17000 Stn Forces, Kingston ON K7K 7B4; Qns'91; (613)541-5010

WEBBER, Douglas L; Vancouver Gen Hosp, JPN1-855 12th Ave W, Vancouver BC V5Z 1M9; UBC'81; BSc; FRCPC; GenPath; AnatPath. Staff Path & Labs, Vancouver General Hospital - Centennial Pavillion; (604)875-4111 x61079; Fax. (604)875-4797.

WEBBER, Eric M; Children's & Women's HC Of BC, KO 123-4480 Oak St, Vancouver BC V6H 3V4; Tor'87; FRCSC; GenSurg; PedGenSurg. Ac Staff, BC Children's Hospital; Assoc Prof, University of British Columbia; (604)875-3744; Fax. (604)875-2721; emwebber@interchange.ubc.ca.

WEBBER, Gail C; Rideau FHT - Lancaster Site, 11-2450 Lancaster Rd, Ottawa ON K1B 5N3; Qns'91; CCFP; FCFP; Staff Family Med, The Ottawa Hospital - General Campus; Teach Staff Family Med, University of Ottawa; (613)738-9119; Fax. (613)738-2736.

WEBBER, Patina D; Royal Jubilee Hosp, 1952 Bay St, Victoria BC V8R 1J8; UBC'97; CCFP; CCFP(E.M.); Staff, Royal Jubilee Hospital; (250)370-8000

WEBBER, Paul F; Royal Victoria Hosp, 201 Georgian Dr, Barrie ON L4M 6M2; Mem'94; FRCPC; Anes. Staff, Royal Victoria Regional Health Centre; (705)728-9090; Fax. (705)739-5613.

WEBER, Amy E; 200-545 Clyde Ave, West Vancouver BC V7T 1C5; UBC'06; CCFP; (604)669-2274

WEBER, Bryce A; Alberta Children's Hosp, 2888 Shaganappi Trail NW, Calgary AB T3B 6A8; Alb'04; FRCSC; Urol (Pediatric Urology). Staff, Alberta Children's Hospital; (403)955-2776; Fax. (403)955-7634.

WEBER, Catherine L C; Lakeshore Gen Hosp, 160 av Stillview, Pointe-Claire QC H9R 2Y2; Man'00; FRCPC; IntMed (Clinician Investigator Program); Nephrol. Staff, Lakeshore General Hospital - Pointe Claire; (514)630-2225

WEBER, Christopher C; Riverside Prof Centre, 301-1919 Riverside Dr, Ottawa ON K1H 1A2; Ott'87; Dip SportMed; BSc; Dip SportMed; Asst Surg & Gen Pract, The Ottawa Hospital - Riverside Campus; Med Examiner Civil Aviation, Transport Canada; Langs: English; French; (613)523-3245; Fax. (613)733-3651.

WEBER, Donald W; 11202 76 Ave NW, Edmonton AB T6G 0K1; Alb'91; FRCSC; OrthSurg. (780)439-4945; Fax. (780)439-0396.

WEBER, Elizabeth A; 411-4430 Bathurst St, North York ON M3H 3S3; McM'80; BScN; FRCPC; IntMed (Asthma); ClinImmunol&Allergy. Court Staff Drug Testing at Drug Safety Clinic, Sunnybrook Health Sciences Centre; Staff IntMed, Humber River Regional Hospital - Finch Avenue Site; Staff Drug Testing, Drug Safety Clinic; Lecturer, University of Toronto; (416)635-5004

WEBER, Florence A; CHUM-Hop St-Luc, 1058 rue Saint-Denis, Montreal QC H2X 3J4; Mon'99; IntMed. Staff, Centre Hospitalier l'Université De Montréal (CHUM) - Hôpital Saint-luc; (514)890-8300

WEBER, Gary G; Simcoe Mall Med Centre, 7-140 Queensway E, Simcoe ON N3Y 4Y7; Wes'79; (519)426-0011; Fax. (519)426-1671.

WEBER, Keith; CFP Gagetown, PO Box 17000 Stn Forces, Oromocto NB E2V 4J5; Sask'03; CCFP; Medical Officer Basic Diving, National Defense-New Brunswick; (506)440-2397

WEBER, Linda J; Parkdale Comm Health Centre, 1229 Queen St W, Toronto ON M6K 1L2; Tor'98; CCFP; Staff, St Joseph's Health Centre; Staff, Parkdale Community Health Centre; (416)537-2455; Fax. (416)537-5133; linda.weber@pchc.on.ca.

WEBER, Marie E; MUHC-Royal Victoria Hosp, S7W-687 av des Pins O, Montreal QC H3A 1A1; McG'97; CCFP; Staff, McGill University Health Centre - Royal Victoria Hospital; Langs: English; French; (514)934-1934 x35172

WEBER, Michael H; MUHC-Montreal Gen Hosp, 1650 av Cedar, Montreal QC H3G 1A4; Man'05; FRCSC; OrthSurg. Staff, McGill University Health Centre - Montreal General Campus; (514)934-1934 x42219

WEBER, Stacie D; 102-5 Quarry Ridge Rd, Barrie ON L4M 7G1; McG'99; CCFP; Langs: English; French; (705)735-4100; Fax. (705)735-4162.

WEBER, Therese T H; Foothills Med Centre, 1403 29 St NW, Calgary AB T2N 2T9; Cal'88; CCFP; Staff, Foothills Medical Centre; (403)944-1110

WEBER-BAYAR, Audrey; CHUM-Hop Notre-Dame, 1560 rue Sherbrooke E, Montreal QC H2L 4M1; Staff, Centre Hospitalier l'Université de Montréal (CHUM) - Hôpital Notre-Dame; (514)890-8000

WEBERPALS, Johanne I; The Ottawa Hosp-Gen Campus, 8168-501 Smyth Rd, Ottawa ON K1H 8L6; Wes'97; MSc; FRCSC; ObstGyn (Gynecologic Oncology). Asst Prof GynOncol, The Ottawa Hospital - General Campus; Clin Instructor Centre for Cancer Therapeutics, The Ottawa Hospital-Research Institute; Langs: Bilingual(English/French); (613)737-8899; Fax. (613)737-8828.

WEBERT, Kathryn E; Canadian Blood Serv Med Office, 35 Stone Church Rd, Ancaster ON L9K 1S5; Wes'96; FRCPC; IntMed (Transfusion Medicine); Hem. Staff, Hamilton Health Sciences Centre - McMaster Children's Hospital; (905)645-6391; Fax. (905)540-5801.

WEBSTER, Christine E; Credit Valley Prof Bldg, 203-2300 Eglinton Ave W, Mississauga ON L5M 2V8; Wes'81; FRCPC; Derm. Ac Staff, The Credit Valley Hospital; Court Staff, Women's College Hospital; Court Staff, The Hospital For Sick Children; (905)820-1748; Fax. (905)820-7445.

WEBSTER, Colleen A; Kingston Family Health Team, 200-2437 Princess St, Kingston ON K7M 3G1; UBC'94; BSc; CCFP; FCFP; (613)546-6652; Fax. (613)546-5292; cwebster@kfhn.net.

WEBSTER, David L; Sudbury Reg Hosp-Laurentian, 41 Ransey Lake Rd, Sudbury ON P3E 5J1; Wes'77; FRCPC; NuclearMed. Ac Staff, Health Sciences North - Memorial Site; Ac Staff, Health Sciences North-St Joseph's Health Centre; Staff, Thunder Bay Regional Health Sciences Centre; Staff, Health Sciences North-Laurentian Site; (705)675-4714; dwebster@hrsrh.on.ca.

WEBSTER, David M; Dr David M Webster Med Clinic, 12 Parade St, Yarmouth NS B5A 3A4; Dal'90; (902)749-1655; Fax. (902)749-0222.

WEBSTER, Duncan V; Saint John Reg Hosp, PO Box 2100 Stn Main 400 University Ave, Saint John NB E2L 4L2; Dal'01; MA; FRCPC; IntMed (Infectious Diseases); MedMicrobiol. Staff, Saint John Regional Hospital; (506)648-6000

WEBSTER, Edwin G; Port Arthur Health Centre Inc, 194 Court St N, Thunder Bay ON P7A 4V7; Wes'82; (807)346-1000; Fax. (807)346-6209.

WEBSTER, J Anne; Anaesthetic Services, 213-2186 Oak Bay Ave, Victoria BC V8R 1G3; Qns'82; FRCPC; Anes. Staff, Victoria General Hospital; (250)595-7211; Fax. (250)595-7211.

WEBSTER, James; Alexander Med Bldg, 210-849 Alexander Crt, Peterborough ON K9J 7H8; Ott'90; CCFP; FCFP; (705)876-1066; Fax. (705)876-8763.

WEBSTER, Jennifer D; Belleville Queen's Univ-FMC, 201-145 Station St, Belleville ON K8N 2S9; Man'05; CCFP; (613)771-1910; Fax. (613)771-1016.

WEBSTER, Marc A; Tom Baker Cancer Centre, 1331 29 St NW, Calgary AB T2N 4N2; Ott'00; FRCPC; IntMed; MedOncol. Staff Med Oncol, Tom Baker Cancer Centre; (403)521-3093; Fax. (403)283-1651.

WEBSTER, Michael C; Medical Care Clinic, 1385 Bank St, Ottawa ON K1H 8N4; University of Newcastle-Upon-Tyne (England)'71; MB BS; DRCOG; CCFP; (613)523-7440

WEBSTER, Peter M; Sunnybrook Hlth Sciences Ctre, A459-2075 Bayview Ave, Toronto ON M4N 3M5; Tor'68; MD; FRCPC; IntMed (Respirology). Staff, Sunnybrook Health Sciences Centre; Asst Prof Med, University of Toronto; Langs: Bilingual(French/English); (416)480-4758; Fax. (416)480-5153; peter.webster@utoronto.ca.

WEBSTER, R Shawn; Vulcan Med Clinic PO Box 419, Vulcan AB T0L 2B0; Alb'82; CCFP; FCFP; Staff, Vulcan Community Health Centre; (403)485-2216; Fax. (403)485-2218; shawn.webster@calgaryhealthregion.ca.

WEBSTER, Randall J W; Bayshore Med Bldg, 104-3029 Carling Ave, Ottawa ON K2B 8E8; Wes'72; FRCPC; IntMed; Gastroent. Consultant Staff, Queensway Carleton Hospital; (613)820-7613; Fax. (613)820-0293.

WEBSTER, Sheila B; Royal City Med Bldg, 103-250 Keary St, New Westminster BC V3L 5E7; UBC'91; FRCPC; IntMed; Respir. (604)525-8822; Fax. (604)525-9470.

WEBSTER, Susan D; Dr Susan Webster Peds Inc, 206-82 Tacoma Dr, Dartmouth NS B2W 3E5; Dal'86; Peds. (902)433-0829; Fax. (902)433-1430.

WEBSTER, Todd M; 209-1101 2nd Ave E, Owen Sound ON N4K 2J1; Qns'98; FRCSC; Urol. Staff, Grey Bruce Health Services - Owen Sound; (519)370-2266; Fax. (519)372-0731.

WEBSTER, W Robert W; Belleville Queen's Univ-FMC, 201-145 Station St, Belleville ON K8N 2S9; Man'01; ATLS; ACLS; BSc; AAFPhys; MD; LMCC; MCFP; AddicMed; CCFP; Ac Staff/Chief Urban Family Med, QHC Belleville General; (613)771-1910; Fax. (613)771-1016; robertwebster2001@hotmail.com.

WEBSTER, Wanda J; 106-316 King St E, Cobourg ON K9A 5R8; Tor'70; Ac Staff, Northumberland Hills Hospital; (905)377-9925; Fax. (905)377-9926.

WECKWORTH, Mary F; 1283 Nanaimo St, Vancouver BC V5L 4T5; Sask'78; Ac Staff, Vancouver General Hospital - Centennial Pavillion; (604)251-6313; Fax. (604)251-1311.

WECKWORTH, Paul F; Medical Arts Bldg, 537-750 Spadina Cres E, Saskatoon SK S7K 3H3; Sask'79; FRCSC; Urol (Pediatric Urology). Staff, St Paul's Hospital (Grey Nuns) of Saskatoon; (306)653-3255; Fax. (306)653-4386.

WECOWSKI, Eveline; Centre Med Laurier, 5661 boul Laurier, Terrebonne QC J7M 1T7; Mon'99; Langs: Bilingual(French/English); (450)477-5364; Fax. (450)477-5634.

WEDEL, Robert J; Associate Med Centre, 5016 48 Ave, Taber AB T1G 1R8; Cal'74; CCFP; FCFP; Ac Staff, Taber Health Centre; Exec Member, College of Family Physicians of Canada-Alberta; Asst Prof Family Med, University of Calgary; Clinical Asst Prof Family Med, University of Alberta; (403)223-3525; Fax. (403)223-9020; wedel@ucalgary.ca.

WEDGE, Charlotte I; One Medical Place, 308-20 Wynford Dr, Toronto ON M3C 1J4; Sask'87; BSc; MD; FRCSC; Ophth (Cataract). Chief Ophth, Toronto East General Hospital Inc; Court Staff, St Michael's Hospital; Staff Surgical Unit, One Medical Place Hosp; Asst Prof, University of Toronto; (416)922-2052; Fax. (416)922-3013.

WEDGE, John H; The Hosp for Sick Children, 555 University Ave, Toronto ON M5G 1X8; Sask'69; DAB; FACS; FRCSC; OrthSurg (Pediatric Orthopedics). Staff Surg, The Hospital For Sick Children; Prof Surg, University of Toronto; (416)813-6944; Fax. (416)813-6692.

WEDGE, Richard; McGill Centre, PO Box 2000 Stn Central 55 McGill Ave, Charlottetown PE C1A 7N8; Dal'86; Med Dir, Prince County Hospital; Staff, McGill Centre; (902)368-4430

WEE, Christine M; Hopital Jean-Talon, 1385 rue Jean-Talon E, Montreal QC H2E 1S6; McG'05; FRCPC; DiagRad. Staff, CSSS du Coeur de l'Isle Hôpital Jean-Talon; (514)495-6767; Fax. (514)495-6734.

WEE, Edgardo Y; 3133 Main St, Vancouver BC V5T 3G8; Manila (Philippines)'77; Vis Staff, Vancouver General Hospital - Centennial Pavillion; Langs: Fookien; Tagalog; (604)873-1107

WEE, Joy Y M; Providence CCC-St Mary's, PO Box 3600 Stn Main 340 Union St, Kingston ON K7L 5A2; UBC'93; BSc; FRCPC; PhysMed&Rehab. Staff, Providence Care - St Mary's of the Lake Hospital Site; Queen's University; Langs: French; (613)544-2143

WEEBEDDA, Upali S K; Stonewall Med Group, 589 3rd Ave S, Stonewall MB R0C 2Z0; Peradeniya (Sri Lanka)'87; CCFP; Staff, Stonewall & District Health Centre; Staff, Selkirk & District General Hospital; (204)467-5514; Fax. (204)467-5576.

WEEKES, Andrew N; 311-1 Centrepointe Dr, Ottawa ON K2G 6E2; Tor'05; FRCSC; GenSurg. (613)225-2525

WEEKES, Darlene A; The Hosp for Sick Children, 555 University Ave, Toronto ON M5G 1X8; Maryland (USA)'06; FRCPC; Anes. Staff, The Hospital For Sick Children; (416)813-7445

WEEKS, Andrew S; 303-216 West St, Simcoe ON N3Y 1S8; Qns'76; FRCPC; IntMed; Cardiol. Staff, Norfolk General Hospital; Langs: English; French; (519)426-7370; Fax. (519)426-9877.

WEEKS, Claire Ann O; G F Strong Rehab Centre, 4255 Laurel St, Vancouver BC V5Z 2G9; Dal'85; PhD(Biochem); PhysMed&Rehab (Spinal Cord Injury). Staff, G F Strong Rehabilitation Centre; Consultant, Vancouver General Hospital - Centennial Pavillion; Clinical Asst Prof, University of British Columbia; (604)734-1313

WEEKS, Sally K; MUHC-Royal Victoria Hosp, 687 av des Pins O, Montreal QC H3A 1A1; London (England)'61; MB BS; Anes (P.Q.). Staff, McGill University Health Centre - Royal Victoria Hospital; (514)934-1934 x34880; Fax. (514)843-1698.

WEEKS, Sarah G; Foothills Med Centre, C849-1403 29 St NW, Calgary AB T2N 2T9; Cal'99; FRCPC; IntMed; Cardiol. Staff, Foothills Medical Centre; (403)944-2480; Fax. (403)944-1592.

WEENING, Bradley S; A34-481 North Service Rd W, Oakville ON L6M 2V6; McM'00; BSc(Hon); BPHE; FRCSC; OrthSurg (Hip & Knee Arthroplasty). Staff, Halton Healthcare Services Corporation - Oakville Site; (905)844-7706; Fax. (905)844-7808.

WEERASEKERA, Priyanthy; Fontbonne Bldg, F442-301 James St S, Hamilton ON L8P 3B6; McM'85; FRCPC; Psy. Ac Staff Anxiety Disorders, St Joseph's Healthcare - Charlton Campus; Assoc Prof Psy/Coord Postgrad & Psychotherapy, McMaster University; (905)522-1155 x3499; Fax. (905)540-6533.

WEERASINGHE, Chandana P; VGH Internal Med Clinic, 7F-2775 Laurel St, Vancouver BC V5Z 1M9; Alb'05; IntMed. Staff Outpatient Clinic, Providence Health Care - St Paul's Hospital; (604)875-5181

WEERASINGHE, Nandanie; Calgary Trail Medicentre, 1-10407 51 Ave NW, Edmonton AB T6H 0K4; Prague (Czech Republic)'72; FAAP; Physician, Calgary Trail Medicentres; Langs: Sinhalese; Czech; (780)436-8071; Fax. (780)435-6034; nandanie@shaw.ca.

WEETMAN, Sara B; St Pau's Hosp, 1702 20th St W, Saskatoon SK S7M 0Z9; Sask'05; CCFP; CCFP(E.M.); Staff, St Paul's Hospital (Grey Nuns) of Saskatoon; (306)655-5000

WEGNER, Sandra L; Kenderdine Med Clinic, 2-50 Kenderdine Rd, Saskatoon SK S7N 3A1; Dal'91; Physician, Kenderdine Medical Clinic; (306)934-6601; Fax. (306)934-6615.

WEGRZYCKI, Wieslaw; Ctr de Sante Vallee-Gatineau, 309 boul desjardins, Maniwaki QC J9E 2E7; Wroclaw (Poland)'79; CCFP; Staff, CSSS de la Vallée de la Gatineau; Langs: Bilingual(French/English); (819)449-4690; Fax. (819)449-6137; bjjw@lino.com.

WEHBI, Elias; The Hosp for Sick Children, 555 University Ave, Toronto ON M5G 1X8; Tor'06; Urol. Staff, The Hospital For Sick Children; (416)813-1500

WEHNER, Timothy M; Keewatin Med Clinic, PO Box 847 904 Ottawa St, Keewatin ON P0X 1C0; Man'90; CCFP; FCFP; (807)547-2818; Fax. (807)547-3285.

WEHRLI, Bret M; London HSC-University Hosp, PO Box 5339 Stn B 339 Windermere Rd, London ON N6A 5A5; Tor'95; FRCPC; AnatPath (General Pathology). Staff, London Health Sciences Centre - University Hospital; (519)685-8500 x36371; Fax. (519)663-2930.

WEHRSPANN, William H; Toronto West Prof Centre, 419-2425 Bloor St W, Toronto ON M6S 4W4; University of Iowa (USA)'71; FRCPC; Psy. (416)769-9619; Fax. (416)769-3517; whwehrspann@rogers.com.

WEI, Alice C C; Univ Hlth Network-The Toronto, 10EN 215-200 Elizabeth St, Toronto ON M5G 2C4; McG'95; MDCM; FACS; MSc; FRCSC; GenSurg (Surgical Oncology). Affil Scientist, Toronto General Hospital - UHN; Staff, Princess Margaret Cancer Centre; Asst Prof Surg, University of Toronto; (416)340-4232; Fax. (416)340-3808.

WEI, Charles C Y; Baywood Med Centre, 401-95 Bayly St W, Ajax ON L1S 7K8; Tor'96; BSc; FRCPC; IntMed (Dialysis); Nephrol. Staff Nephrol, Lakeridge Health - Oshawa Site; Staff Nephrol, Rouge Valley Health System - Ajax & Pickering Health Centre Site; (905)686-3351; Fax. (905)427-2679.

WEI, Ho-Yin; Chalmers Gate Med Bldg, 305-328 Highway 7 E, Richmond Hill ON L4B 3P7; (Hong Kong)'85; MB BS; MRC(UK); CCFP; FCFP; Assoc Staff Fam Med, Mackenzie Richmond Hill Hospital; Langs: Cantonese; (905)763-9622; Fax. (905)763-9621.

WEI, Peter Y; The Lung Health Clinic, 8737 156 St NW, Edmonton AB T5R 1Y5; Alb'05; FRCPC; Respir; IntMed. (780)498-1800; Fax. (780)483-7774.

WEI, Xingchang; Alberta Children's Hosp, 2888 Shaganappi Trail NW, Calgary AB T3B 6A8; West China Medical University (China)'87; Staff Diagnostic Imaging, Alberta Children's Hospital; (403)955-7985; Fax. (403)955-7656.

WEI WEI, Corie; St Michael's Hosp, 30 Bond St, Toronto ON M5B 1W8; Wes'07; FRCPC; DiagRad. Staff, St Michael's Hospital; (416)360-4000

WEICHERT, Gabriele E; The Brickyard Clinic, 6010 Brickyard Rd, Nanaimo BC V9V 1S5; McM'98; FRCPC; Derm. (250)390-5200; Fax. (250)390-5252.

WEICKER, Christopher R; PO Box 730 Stn Main, Salmon Arm BC V1E 4N8; UBC'00; CCFP; (250)832-2321; Fax. (250)832-6095; cweicker@samedicalclinic.com.

WEICKER, Constance M; Goodfellow Prof Bldg, 208-170 McEwan Dr E, Bolton ON L7E 4C8; Tor'86; CCFP; FCFP; Staff, William Osler Health System - Etobicoke General Hospital; (905)951-3696; Fax. (905)951-3698.

WEIDEMAN, Tanya; Cochrane Comm Hlth Centre, 60 Grande Blvd, Cochrane AB T4C 0S4; Pretoria (South Africa)'87; MB ChB; Staff, Cochrane Urgent Care; Langs: Afrikaans; (403)851-6261; Fax. (403)851-6279.

WEIDEMAN, Theodor; 3823 12th Ave W, Vancouver BC V6R 2N9; Cape Town (South Africa)'78; FRCPC; Anes. (604)228-9091

WEIDNER, Marie-France; Centre Hosp Honore-Mercier, 2750 Boul Laframboise, Saint-Hyacinthe QC J2S 4Y8; Mon'99; DiagRad. Staff, Centre Hospitalier Honore-Mercier; (450)771-3333

WEIGEL, Michael A; 104-266 4 St SW, Medicine Hat AB T1A 4E5; Alb'90; FRCPC; IntMed. (403)580-8288; Fax. (403)580-8233.

WEIGENS, David; Hillside Med Centre, 100 av Metcalfe, Westmount QC H3Z 2H4; McG'79; CCFP; Langs: Bilingual(English/French); (514)990-1477; Fax. (514)931-8436.

WEIGENSBERG, Corey N; Scarborough Hosp-General Div, 3050 Lawrence Ave E, Scarborough ON M1P 2V5; McG'86; FRCPC; AnatPath. Assoc Staff Path, The Scarborough Hospital - General Campus; Langs: English; French; (416)438-2911 x6035; Fax. (416)431-8245.

WEIGHMAN, Maurice A T; 5203 49 Ave, Killam AB T0B 2L0; (780)385-3294; Fax. (780)385-3295.

WEIGLEIN, Otto; Centre for Personal Surgery, 520 Locust St, Burlington ON L7S 1V2; Cal'75; FRCSC; PlasSurg (Cosmetic Surgery). Ac Staff Surg, Joseph Brant Memorial Hospital; Court Staff, Halton Healthcare Services Corporation - Oakville Site; Dir, Centre for Personal Surgery; Langs: German; (905)634-5573; Fax. (905)634-5406; otto.weiglein@cosmedicacanada.com.

WEIJER, Charles E; University of Western Ont, 307A-1151 Richmond St, London ON N6A 3K7; Alb'88; FRCPC; Psy.

WEILER, Gabrielle S; Children's Hosp Eastern Ont, 401 Smyth Rd, Ottawa ON K1H 8L1; Ott'97; FRCPC; Peds; Nephrol. Staff, Children's Hospital of Eastern Ontario (CHEO); Langs: Bilingual(English/French); (613)737-7600; Fax. (613)737-2441.

WEILER, Kathleen A; 10-2448 160 St PO Box 38034 Rpo Morgan Height, Surrey BC V3S 6R3; Qns'09; CCFP; (604)616-4302

WEILER, Peter J; One Med Place, 304-840 Coxwell Avenue, Toronto ON M4C 5T2; McM'86; BASc; MASc; FRCSC; OrthSurg (Arthroscopic Surgery). Consultant OrthSurg, Toronto East General Hospital Inc; Consultant OrthSurg, Bridgepoint Health Centre; Asst Prof Surg, University of Toronto; (416)441-2245; Fax. (416)441-2246; pjweiler@pathcom.com.

WEILER, Robert L; St Paul's Hosp, 1702 20th St W, Saskatoon SK S7M 0Z9; Sask'79; FRCPC; Anes. Staff, St Paul's Hospital (Grey Nuns) of Saskatoon; (306)655-5240; Fax. (306)978-8281.

WEILL, Alain F; CHUM-Hop Notre-Dame, 1560 rue Sherbrooke E, Montreal QC H2L 4M1; Paris (France)'93; FRCPC; DiagRad. Staff, Centre Hospitalier l'Université de Montréal (CHUM) - Hôpital Notre-Dame; (514)890-8000 x23780; Fax. (514)612-7567; alain.weill.chum@ssss.gouv.qc.ca.

WEIMAR, Sophie-Anne; Burris Clinic, 300-275 Lansdowne St, Kamloops BC V2C 6J3; Stellenbosch (South Africa)'91; MB ChB; CCFP; Langs: Afrikaans; (250)372-3303; Fax. (250)377-7300.

WEIN, Cheryl R; The Health Centre of Maple, 2810 Major MacKenzie Dr, Vaughan ON L6A 3L2; Tor'00; CCFP; Staff Emerg Room, Humber River Regional Hospital - Keele Street Site; (905)832-3838; Fax. (905)832-9097.

WEIN, Francine B; MUHC-Royal Victoria Hosp, E4 60-687 av des Pins O, Montreal QC H3A 1A1; McG'93; ABOph; FRCSC; Ophth (Neuro Ophthalmology). Staff, McGill University Health Centre - Royal Victoria Hospital; Staff, Sir Mortimer B Davis Jewish General; Langs: Bilingual(English/French); (514)934-1934 x36337; Fax. (514)843-1618.

WEIN, Howard P; Polyclinique Cabrini, 215-5700 rue Saint-Zotique E, Montreal QC H1T 3Y7; Man'58; CSPQ; Electroenceph (P.Q.); Neur (P.Q.) (Clinical Neurology). Associé, Hôpital Santa Cabrini Ospedale; Associate, Louis Hyppolyte Lafontaine Hospital; Langs: Italian; French; (514)737-5243; Fax. (514)733-3922.

WEIN, Theodore H; MUHC-Montreal Gen Hosp, L7305-1650 av Cedar, Montreal QC H3G 1A4; Burlington(VT) (USA)'93; FRCPC; Neur (Stroke). Staff, McGill University Health Centre - Montreal General Campus; (514)934-8058; Fax. (514)934-8265; twein@videotron.ca.

WEINBERG, Anthony L; The Ottawa Hosp-Riverside, 6 52-1967 Riverside Dr, Ottawa ON K1H 7W9; Durham (England)'65; FRCP; FRCPC; IntMed. Staff, The Ottawa Hospital - Riverside Campus; Med Counsellor, WSIAT; Prof Med, University of Ottawa; (613)738-8255; Fax. (613)738-8256.

WEINBERG, Eitan; Scarborough Hosp-Birchmount, 3030 Birchmount Rd, Scarborough ON M1W 3W3; Tor'04; FRCPC; Peds. Staff, The Scarborough Hospital - Birchmount Campus; (416)495-2886

WEINBERG, Elissa J; Shops on Steele Med Centre, 206-2900 Steeles Ave E, Thornhill ON L3T 4X1; Ott'98; CCFP; (905)881-6667

WEINBERG, Erica L; Rouge Valley HS-Centenary, 2867 Ellesmere Rd, Scarborough ON M1E 4B9; Tor'87; BSc; MSc; MPhil; Ac Staff, Rouge Valley Health System - Centenary Health Centre Site; (416)284-8131; Fax. (416)286-8413.

WEINBERG, Eytan N; Concordia Gen Hosp, 1095 Concordia Ave, Winnipeg MB R2K 3S8; Staff, Concordia General Hospital; (204)667-1560

WEINBERG, Garry B; 207-4 Montreal Rd, Cornwall ON K6H 1B1; Man'00; FRCSC; Urol. (613)938-9200; Fax. (613)937-4154.

WEINBERG, Jeffrey N; The Jacobs Pain Centre, 102-8920 Woodbine Ave, Markham ON L3R 9W9; McG'96; Langs: Bilingual(French/English); (905)305-9484; Fax. (905)305-7381.

WEINBERG, Michael J; 247 Queensway Ave W, Mississauga ON L5B 1B9; Tor'90; FRCSC; PlasSurg (Cosmetic Surgery). Staff, Trillium Health Centre - Mississauga; Staff, The Credit Valley Hospital; Langs: Dutch; French; (905)273-3045; Fax. (905)273-3699; michaelweinberg@rogers.com.

WEINBERG, Mitchell L; Medical Examiner's Bldg, 7007 116 St NW, Edmonton AB T6H 5R8; (780)422-4987; Fax. (780)422-1265.

WEINBERG, Robert B; Etobicoke Med Centre, 400 The East Mall, Toronto ON M9B 3Z9; McG'98; CCFP; Langs: English; French; (416)621-2220; Fax. (416)621-2203.

WEINBERG, Terri E; St Gabriel Med Centre, 101-650 Sheppard Ave E, North York ON M2K 3E4; Tor'80; CCFP; FCFP; Ac Staff, North York General Hospital; Langs: English; French; (416)225-5400; Fax. (416)225-7710.

WEINBERGER, Allen N; Pine Seven Med Centre, 180-4600 Highway 7, Woodbridge ON L4L 4Y7; Tor'83; Ac Staff, William Osler Health System - Etobicoke General Hospital; (905)856-3330; Fax. (905)856-3331.

WEINBERGER, Thomas; 2682 Eglinton Ave E, Scarborough ON M1K 2S3; Tor'73; Langs: Hungarian; (416)269-6800

WEINER, Lorne S; 211-75 Albert St, Ottawa ON K1P 5E7; Qns'74; CCFP; (613)238-5963; Fax. (613)238-2626.

WEINER, Marta A; Waterford Hosp, 306 Waterford Bridge Rd, St. John's NL A1E 4J8; Lublin (Poland)'84; FRCPC; Psy. Staff, Waterford Hospital; Staff Start Clinic, St Clare's Mercy Hospital; (709)777-3333

WEINER-BARON, David L; 401-4800 Leslie St, North York ON M2J 2K9; McG'83; FRCPC; IntMed (Therapeutic Endoscopy); Gastroent. Chief Med, North York General Hospital; Staff, Mount Sinai Hospital; Staff, Baycrest Centre for Geriatric Care; Asst Prof Med, University of Toronto; (647)345-2120; Fax. (647)345-2124; dbaron@nygh.on.ca.

WEINERMAN, Brian H; Victoria Gen Hosp, 1 Hospital Way, Victoria BC V8Z 6R5; Man'67; FRC; FRCPC; IntMed (Medical Oncology). Staff, Royal Jubilee Hospital; Staff, Victoria General Hospital; (250)370-8000; brian.weinerman@viha.ca.

WEINGARTEN, David; Shouldice Hosp, PO Box 370 7750 Bayview Ave, Thornhill ON L3T 4A3; Tor'71; Staff, Shouldice Hospital; (905)889-1125

WEINGARTEN, Kevin A; The Hosp for Sick Children, 555 University Ave, Toronto ON M5G 1X8; Tor'05; PedHemaOncol; Peds. Staff, The Hospital For Sick Children; (416)813-1500

WEINGARTEN, Murray D; 303-615 Davis Dr, Newmarket ON L3Y 2R2; Tor'79; FRCPC; IntMed. Staff, Southlake Regional Health Centre; (905)895-3183

WEINGERT, Michael E; Wortley Village Med Centre, 103-190 Wortley Rd, London ON N6C 4Y7; Tor'75; FRCPC; IntMed; Cardiol. Staff, London Health Sciences Centre - Victoria Campus; Staff, St Thomas Elgin General Hospital; Prof Med, University of Western Ontario; (519)642-1101

WEINKAUF, Justin G; University of Alberta Hosp, 2E439 WCM-8440 112 St NW, Edmonton AB T6G 2B7; Sask'97; FRCPC; IntMed; Respir. Staff, University of Alberta Hospital; (780)407-1632; Fax. (780)407-6384.

WEINMAN, Robert D; Statcare, 104-175 av Stillview, Pointe-Claire QC H9R 4S3; Case Western Reserve University (USA)'77; CCFP; Langs: English; French; (514)694-9282

WEINREB, Ilan; Univ Hlth Network-Toronto Gen, 11E 403-200 Elizabeth St, Toronto ON M5G 2C4; Tor'01; FRCPC; AnatPath. Staff, Toronto General Hospital - UHN; (416)340-5146; Fax. (416)340-5517.

WEINROTH, H Judith; Medical Clinic Person-Ctred Ps, 403-265 Yorkland Blvd, North York ON M2J 1S5; Tor'83; MD; MSc; GP Psych. Staff, The Medical Clinic for Person-Centred Psychotherapy; (416)229-2399; Fax. (416)229-9771; weinroth@sympatico.ca.

WEINROTH, Ian S; North York Gen Hosp-Branson, 1S-555 Finch Ave W, North York ON M2R 1N5; Wes'05; FRCPC; Psy. Staff, North York General Hospital - Branson Division; Staff, Mount Sinai Hospital; (416)633-9420

WEINSTEIN, Gary S; Yonge-Eglinton Med Centre, 210-2401 Yonge St, Toronto ON M4P 3H1; Tor'89; (416)486-9600; Fax. (416)486-9227.

WEINSTEIN, Jordan J; St Michael's Health Centre, 9F-61 Queen St E, Toronto ON M5C 2T2; Tor'99; FRCPC; IntMed; Nephrol. Staff Nephrol/Dir ukidney.com/Prof Med, St Michael's Hospital; Langs: Hebrew; (416)867-3703; Fax. (416)593-6275; j.weinstein@utoronto.ca.

WEINSTEIN, Julie L; Wawa Family Health Team, 17 Goverment Rd, Wawa ON P0S 1K0; Tor'08; CCFP; (705)856-1313

WEINSTEIN, Michael J; The Hosp for Sick Children, 7729-555 University Ave, Toronto ON M5G 1X8; Tor'94; FRCPC; Peds. Staff, The Hospital For Sick Children; Asst Prof, University of Toronto; (416)813-1500; Fax. (416)813-8345; michael.weinstein@sickkids.ca.

WEINSTEIN, Miriam G; The Hosp for Sick Children, 10215-555 University Ave, Toronto ON M5G 1X8; Qns'96; FRCPC; Peds; Derm. Staff Ped Derm/Dir Fellowships Derm, The Hospital For Sick Children; Assoc Prof Peds & Med, University of Toronto; (416)813-8186; Fax. (416)813-7909.

WEINSTEIN, Richard D; 201-715 Fischer Hallman Rd, Kitchener ON N2E 4E9; Ott'94; FRCSC; Ophth. Ac Staff, St Mary's General Hospital; (519)745-3690; Fax. (519)745-4856.

WEINSTEIN, Robert P; North York Gen Hosp, 8F-4001 Leslie St, North York ON M2K 1E1; Ott'85; FRCPC; Psy (Psycho Pharmacology). Ac Staff, North York General Hospital; Langs: Bilingual(English/French); (416)756-6655; Fax. (416)756-6671.

WEINSTOCK, David J; 206 Sheppard Ave W, Toronto ON M2N 1N1; Tor'96; FRCSC; Ophth (Cataract Surgery). (416)221-2442; Fax. (416)512-2022.

WEINSTOCK, Michael S; 39 Pleasant Blvd, Toronto ON M4T 1K2; Tor'69; BSc; Langs: Hebrew; (416)967-4446; Fax. (416)967-9406; michael.weinstock79@gmail.com.

WEINSTOCK, S Joseph; 206 Sheppard Ave W, Toronto ON M2N 1N1; Tor'71; DOphth(Sci); FRCSC; Ophth (Vision & Eye Problems) (Laser Refractive Surgery). Staff, Toronto Western Hospital - University Health Network; Assoc Prof, University of Toronto; (416)221-2442; Fax. (416)512-2022.

WEINSTOCK, V Moss; 5-106 Cornell Park Ave, Markham ON L6B 1B6; Tor'98; FRCSC; Ophth. (905)209-0016; Fax. (905)209-0017.

WEINSTOCK-GOLDBERG, Sara; 403-1017 Wilson Ave, North York ON M3K 1Z1; Tor'84; CCFP; FCFP; Court Staff Privileges, Humber River Regional Hospital - Keele Street Site; Langs: Spanish; (416)636-5500; Fax. (416)636-5501.

WEIR, Bryce K A; PO Box 1879 Stn Main, Edmonton AB T5J 2P2; McG'60; BSc; MSc; FACS; DAB; FRCSC; Neursurg. Staff Medical Services, Workers' Comp Board; bryce.weir@wcb.ab.ca.

WEIR, Douglas C; 1704-2200 Yonge St, Toronto ON M4S 2C6; Cal'77; DCH; FRCPC; Psy (Child Psychiatry). (416)488-8628; Fax. (416)488-1082; dcweir@on.aibn.com.

WEIR, E Ruth; Nosehill Med Clinic, 137-1829 Ranchlands Blvd NW, Calgary AB T3G 2A7; UBC'84; CCFP; FCFP; (403)239-8888; Fax. (403)241-1506.

WEIR, Erica; Public Health Branch, 17250 Yonge St, Newmarket ON L3Y 6Z1; Qns'97; FRCPC; CommunMed;CCFP; Public Health & Preventive Med. Physician, Regional Municipality of York; (905)830-4444; Fax. (905)895-3166; erica.weir@york.ca.

WEIR, Heather N; 301-845 St Clair Ave W, Toronto ON M6C 1C3; Dublin (Ireland)'76; MB ChB; BAO; MRCPsy; FRCPC; Psy. Staff Psy, The Hospital For Sick Children; Teacher, University of Toronto; (416)656-8359; Fax. (416)656-8760.

WEIR, Ian H; Royal Jubilee Hosp, 1952 Bay St, Victoria BC V8R 1J8; Alb'86; FRCPC; DiagRad. Staff, Royal Jubilee Hospital; Staff, Victoria General Hospital; (250)370-8272; Fax. (250)370-8594.

WEIR, Jean E; Peterborough Day Clinic, 26 Hospital Dr, Peterborough ON K9J 7C3; Tor'76; CCFP; Langs: Creole; (705)743-2040

WEIR, Lorna M; BC Cancer Agency, 600 10th Ave W, Vancouver BC V5Z 4E6; Qns'85; FRCPC; RadOncol (Breast Cancer). Staff, BC Cancer Agency Vancouver Centre; Assoc Staff, Vancouver General Hospital - Centennial Pavillion; Clin Assoc Prof, University of British Columbia; (604)877-6000

WEIR, Martina J E; Lakeridge Health Corp-Oshawa, 1 Hospital Crt, Oshawa ON L1G 2B9; Tor'90; CCFP; Staff, Lakeridge Health - Oshawa Site; (905)576-8711; Fax. (905)721-7763.

WEIR, Matthew A; London HSC-University Campus, PO Box 5339 Stn B ALL 139A-339 Windermere Rd, London ON N6A 5A5; Qns'03; FRCPC; IntMed; Nephrol. Staff, London Health Sciences Centre - Victoria Campus; Staff, London Health Sciences Centre - University Hospital; (519)663-2998

WEIR, Michael J; Kawartha Urology Assoc, 101-380 Burnham St, Peterborough ON K9H 1T6; Tor'93; FRCSC; Urol. Staff, Peterborough Regional Health Centre - Hospital Drive; (705)743-6480; Fax. (705)585-4885.

WEIR, Michele M; London HSC-University Hosp, PO Box 5339 Stn B 339 Windermere Rd, London ON N6A 5A5; Qns'90; FRCPC; AnatPath (Cytopath). Staff Dept of Path, London Health Sciences Centre - University Hospital; Staff, London Laboratory Services Group; (519)685-8500 x36359

WEIR, Paul T; 287 Huron St, Stratford ON N5A 5T3; McM'81; CASM; Staff, Stratford General Hospital - Huron Perth Healthcare Alliance; (519)271-5320; Fax. (519)271-5324.

WEIR, Rene V; Medical Bldg, 205-1990 Fort St, Victoria BC V8R 6V4; UBC'71; FRCPC; IntMed (Nephrology). (250)595-8811; Fax. (250)595-8503; weir.vna@shaw.ca.

WEIR, Tara G; 403-265 Yorkland Blvd, North York ON M2J 5C7; Tor'00; CCFP; (416)229-2399; Fax. (416)229-9771.

WEIRICH, Martin K; Penticton Reg Hosp, 550 Carmi St, Penticton BC V2A 3G6; Man'85; FRCPC; Anes. Staff, Penticton Regional Hospital; (250)492-4000

WEIS, Ezekiel; Royal Alexandra Hosp, 2319-10240 Kingsway Ave NW, Edmonton AB T5H 3V9; Cal'00; MPH; FRCSC; Ophth (Orbital & Oculoplastics). Staff, Royal Alexandra Hospital; (780)735-4932; Fax. (780)735-4969.

WEISBAUM, Harry; 77 Balsam Ave, Toronto ON M4E 3B8; Tor'70; (416)617-6625; Fax. (416)698-3274.

WEISBERG, Fay G; First Steps Fertility, 215-4025 Yonge St, North York ON M2P 2E3; Man'85; FRCSC; ObstGyn (Infertility). Ac Staff, Women's College Hospital; Asst Prof, University of Toronto; (416)924-4666; Fax. (416)924-7099.

WEISBERG, Lori M; St Joseph's Health Centre, 30 The Queensway, Toronto ON M6R 1B5; Tor'04; FRCPC; Psy. Staff, St Joseph's Health Centre; (416)530-6000

WEISBLOOM, Joy M; Nepean Med Centre, 402-1 Centrepointe Dr, Nepean ON K2G 6E2; McG'81; CCFP; FCFP; Ac Staff General & Family Practice, Queensway Carleton Hospital; Langs: English; French; (613)226-2266; Fax. (613)226-3386.

WEISBORD, Tim; CLSC de Saint-Jerome, 1000 rue Labelle, Saint-Jerome QC J7Z 5N6; McG'69; (450)431-8001 x6212

WEISBROD, Daniel J; 221-2180 Steeles Ave W, Vaughan ON L4K 2Z5; Tor'00; FRCSC; Ophth (Medical Retina). Staff, Sunnybrook Health Sciences Centre - Edmond Odette Cancer Centre; Staff, St Joseph's Health Centre; (905)761-7002; Fax. (905)761-7003.

WEISBROD, Gerald I; North Park Med Centre, D2-1365 Lawrence Ave W, North York ON M6L 1A4; Tor'51; LMCC; Langs: Italian; (416)244-4377; Fax. (416)244-1004.

WEISBROD, Gordon L; 585 University Ave, Toronto ON M5G 2N2; Tor'67; FRCPC; DiagRad. Sr Staff Rad/Chief Div of Chest Imaging/Sr Staff Rad/Chief Div of Chest Imaging, Toronto General Hospital - UHN; Prof Radiol, University of Toronto; (416)340-4800

WEISBROD, Lawrence H; 106-2221 Keele St, North York ON M6M 3Z5; Tor'78; FRCPC; DiagRad. Affil Staff Radiol, Humber River Regional Hospital - Keele Street Site; (416)658-2153; Fax. (416)235-1563.

WEISBROD, Lawrence; One Medical Place, 310-20 Wynford Dr, North York ON M3C 1J4; Tor'93; FRCSC; Ophth (Cataract Surgery). Staff, Sunnybrook Health Sciences Centre; Staff, Toronto East General Hospital Inc; Staff, Baycrest Centre for Geriatric Care; Instructor, University of Toronto; (416)640-0661; Fax. (416)640-0664.

WEISBROD, Matthew J; 2-460 Hume St, Collingwood ON L9Y 1W6; Wes'92; (705)444-7200; Fax. (705)444-7203.

WEISBROD, Mitchell J; Toronto East Gen & Orth Hosp, 825 Coxwell Ave, East York ON M4C 3E7; Tor'95; FRCPC; Anes. Staff, Toronto East General Hospital Inc; (416)469-6212

WEISBROT, Jeffrey J; York-Med Medical Arts Centre, 404-250 Harding Blvd W, Richmond Hill ON L4C 9M7; Tor'85; FRCPC; Peds. Assoc Staff, Mackenzie Richmond Hill Hospital; Assoc Staff, The Hospital For Sick Children; (905)737-9898; Fax. (905)737-8583; jfweisbrot@rogers.com.

WEISDORF, Thea M; SMH-Wellesley Health Centre, 410-410 Sherbourne St, Toronto ON M4X 1K2; Mem'91; CCFP; FCFP; Staff, Centre for Addiction & Mental Health (CAMH) - Russell Street Site; University of Toronto; (416)867-3728; Fax. (416)867-3726.

WEISEL, Richard D; Univ Hlth Network-Toronto Gen, 4N 466-200 Elizabeth St, Toronto ON M5G 2C4; Milwaukee(WI) (USA)'69; MD; FRCSC; Cardiovasc&ThorSurg. Staff Surg, Toronto General Hospital - UHN; Prof Surg, University of Toronto; (416)581-7662; Fax. (416)340-3475; richard.weisel@uhn.on.ca.

WEISENBACHER, Arthur; Central Mall Medical Clinic, 3621 Tecumseh Rd E, Windsor ON N8W 1H8; Tor'98; Physician, Central Mall Medical Centre; (519)948-0011; windsorriver@hotmail.com.

WEISENBURGER, Earle F; Caledonian Clinic Ltd, 340 Campbell St, Nanaimo BC V9R 3G7; Alb'67; Ac Staff, Nanaimo Regional General Hospital; (250)753-3202; Fax. (250)753-1039.

WEISER, Brent A; Keele Ingram Prof Centre, 209-2221 Keele St, Toronto ON M6M 3Z5; Dublin (Ireland)'85; FRCSC; Ophth (Glaucoma). Ac Staff, Humber River Regional Hospital - Church Street Site; Ac Staff, North York General Hospital - Branson Division; Consultant Staff, West Park Healthcare Centre; Ac Staff, Humber River Regional Hospital - Finch Avenue Site; Langs: English; French; (416)249-4255; Fax. (416)249-4791.

WEISER, William J; St Michael's Hosp, 30 Bond St, Toronto ON M5B 1W8; Tor'64; FRCPC; DiagRad. Ac Staff, St Michael's Hospital; (416)864-5672

WEISGERBER, Christopher A; Base Medical Clinic, PO Box 9999 Stn Main, Petawawa ON K8H 2X3; Sask'91; CCFP; Staff, QHC Trenton Memorial; Staff, Base Hospital-CFB Petawawa; Fax. (613)687-5511; weisgerber.ca@forces.gc.ca.

WEISGERBER, Kim J; Victoria Med Bldg, 407-1669 Victoria St, Prince George BC V2L 2L5; Sask'88; Staff, University Hospital of Northern British Columbia; (250)564-6899; Fax. (250)564-7408.

WEISLEDER, Louis M; 404-2300 Eglinton Ave W, Mississauga ON L5M 2V8; Tor'87; FRCSC; OrthSurg (Sports Medicine). Staff Surg, The Credit Valley Hospital; (905)828-1587; Fax. (905)569-8007.

WEISLER, Marvin N; Meadowlark Prof Bldg, 340-8702 Meadowlark Rd NW, Edmonton AB T5R 5W5; Wes'66; FRCSC; Urol. (780)484-0600; Fax. (780)484-0122.

WEISNAGEL, John; Polyclinique Med Concorde, 300 boul de la Concorde E, Laval QC H7G 2E6; Mon'58; ClinImmunol&Allergy (P.Q.); Peds (P.Q.). (450)667-5310; Fax. (450)667-5248.

WEISNAGEL, S John; CHUQ-Ctr Hosp Univ Laval, B0027-2705 boul Laurier, Quebec QC G1V 4G2; Mon'92; ABIM; CSPQ; FRCPC; IntMed (Diabetology); Endocrin (P.Q.); Endocrin&Metab. Staff, Centre Hospitalier Affilié Universitaire de Québec - Hôpital De L'Enfant Jésus; Staff, Centre Hospitalier Universitaire de Quebec-CHUL; assoc Prof, Université Laval; Langs: Bilingual(English/French); (418)654-2169; Fax. (418)654-2792; john.weisnagel@chul.ulaval.ca.

WEISS, Alan A; Gordon & Leslie Diamond HCC, 5F-2775 Laurel St, Vancouver BC V5Z 1M9; UBC'71; ABIM; FRCPC; IntMed (Emergency Medicine); Gastroent. Staff Gastroent, BC Cancer Agency Vancouver Centre; Ac Staff, Vancouver General Hospital - Centennial Pavillion; Staff, Gordon & Leslie Diamond Health Care Centre; Clin Prof Gastroent, University of British Columbia; Langs: Czech; French; (604)875-5474; Fax. (604)875-5373.

WEISS, Andrea M; St Joseph's Health Centre, 30 The Queensway, Toronto ON M6R 1B5; UBC'09; CCFP; Staff, St Joseph's Health Centre; (416)530-6860; Fax. (416)530-6180.

WEISS, Elise C; Western Reg Health Authority, 192 1st Ave W, Souris MB R0K 2C0; Man'82; MSc; CCFP; FCFP; Staff, Brandon Regional Health Centre; VP Medical Services, Prairie Mountain Health Corporate Office Souris; (204)483-5000

WEISS, Elliott P; St Paul's Hosp, 433-1081 Burrard St, Vancouver BC V6Z 1Y6; Tor'82; DABPM; MBA; FRCPC; PhysMed&Rehab (Personal Injury Management Assessment). Consultant, Vancouver General Hospital - Centennial Pavillion; Consultant, Richmond Hospital; Consultant, Burnaby Hospital; Staff, Providence Health Care - St Paul's Hospital; (604)806-8973; Fax. (604)806-9254; eweiss@providencehealth.bc.ca.

WEISS, Helen M; Vancouver Native Hlth Society, 449 Hastings St E, Vancouver BC V6A 1P5; UBC'88; Physician, Vancouver Native Health Society; Langs: French; (604)255-9766; Fax. (604)254-5750.

WEISS, Israel D; North York Gen Hosp, 4001 Leslie St, North York ON M2K 1E1; McG'03; Anes. Staff, North York General Hospital; (416)756-6000

WEISS, Jacqueline R; Weiss ADHD Clinic, 101-585 16 St W, West Vancouver BC V7V 3R8; McG'82; FRCPC; Psy. Staff, BC Women's Hospital & Health Centre; Staff, Providence Health Care - St Paul's Hospital; Med Mgr, Child & Youth Mental Health Services; (604)281-1219

WEISS, Janice M; Malvern Med Centre, 100-1333 Neilson Rd, Scarborough ON M1B 4Y9; Tor'84; CCFP; Staff, Medcan Health Management Inc; (416)291-7719; Fax. (416)287-3775.

WEISS, Karl A; Hop Maisonneuve-Rosemont, 5415 boul de l'Assomption, Montreal QC H1T 2M4; Mon'89; FRCPC; MedMicrobiol (Infectious Diseases). Staff, Hopital Maisonneuve-Rosemont; Prof, McGill University; Prof, Universite de Montreal; Langs: English; (514)252-3400 x2693; Fax. (514)252-3898; weisscan@aol.com.

WEISS, Margaret D; 1488 Gordon Ave, Vancouver BC V6N 3N1; McG'83; FRCPsy; MPhil; FRCPC; Psy (Child Psychiatry). Clin Prof Psy, University of British Columbia; Langs: Bilingual(English/French); (604)875-2738; Fax. (604)875-2099; mweiss@cw.bc.ca.

WEISS, Mark; Bellwood Health Services, 1020 McNicoll Ave, Scarborough ON M1W 2J6; Tor'87; (416)495-0926; Fax. (416)495-7943.

WEISS, Matthew J; CHUQ-Hopital Laval, 2705 boul Laurier, Quebec QC G1V 4G2; Kansas (USA)'03; Peds (Pediatric Critical Care). Staff, Centre Hospitalier Universitaire de Quebec-CHUL; (418)656-7900

WEISS, Ronald S; 29 Clemow Ave, Ottawa ON K1S 2B1; Ott'87; CCFP; FCFP; Staff, Children's Hospital of Eastern Ontario (CHEO); Staff, The Ottawa Hospital - General Campus; Pres., No-Scalpel Vasectomy Inc.; Asst Prof, University of Ottawa; (613)235-3535; Fax. (613)237-8193.

WEISS, Shelly K; The Hosp for Sick Children, 6526-555 University Ave, Toronto ON M5G 1X8; McM'85; FRCPC; Peds; Neur (Pediatric Neurology). Staff Peds, The Hospital For Sick Children; Asst Prof Peds, University of Toronto; (416)813-6332; Fax. (416)813-7096; shelly.weiss@sickkids.ca.

WEISS, William V; 22 Nelson St W, Meaford ON N4L 1R1; Tor'68; Court Staff, Toronto Western Hospital - University Health Network; Med Ed in Chief, NC Press Health Books; Pres Biologistics Med, Computing Consulting Company; (519)538-2821; Fax. (519)538-2383.

WEISSBERGER, Jeffrey M; Markham Family Health Team, 101-377 Church St, Markham ON L6B 1A1; Tor'98; CCFP; FCFP; Staff, Markham Stouffville Hospital; Langs: Hebrew; Hungarian; (905)471-9999; Fax. (905)471-3627.

WEISSGLAS, Issie S; 3755 ch Cote-Sainte-Catherine, Montreal QC H3T 1E2; McG'78; MSc; FACS; FRCS; BSc(Hon); DS; LMCC; MD; FRCSC; GenSurg (P.Q.) (Breast Surgery). Staff, Sir Mortimer B Davis Jewish General; Langs: French; (514)340-8222 x2115; Fax. (514)340-8298; issiew@sympatico.ca.

WEISSGLAS, Juma J M; Sunnybrook Hlth Sciences Ctre, 2075 Bayview Ave, Toronto ON M4N 3M5; McM'06; FRCPC; Psy. Staff, Sunnybrook Health Sciences Centre; (416)480-6100

WEISZ, Dany; The Hosp for Sick Children, 555 University Ave, Toronto ON M5G 1X8; Wes'06; FRCPC; Peds (Neonatal & Perinatal Medicine). Staff, The Hospital For Sick Children; (416)813-8592; Fax. (416)813-5245.

WEISZ, Janet I; 1433 Ontario St, Burlington ON L7S 1G5; McM'82; FAAP; FRCPC; Peds. Chief Peds, Joseph Brant Memorial Hospital; Staff, Hamilton Health Sciences Centre - McMaster Children's Hospital; Clinical Asst Prof, McMaster University; Langs: Hungarian; (905)637-0352; Fax. (905)637-2966.

WEISZ, Samuel I; Meadowlark Health Centre, 224 Meadowlark Shopping Ctr NW, Edmonton AB T5R 5W9; Alb'56; BSc; MS(Med.); FACP; FRCPC; IntMed (Thyroid Diseases). Ac Staff, Covenant Health - Misericordia Community Hospital; (780)484-8474; Fax. (780)489-3836.

WEITEMEYER, Rudolf A; A-145 Columbia St E, New Westminster BC V3L 3W2; Tor'70; BSc; FACS; GenSurg (Gastroenterology). Ac Staff, Eagle Ridge Hospital & Health Care Centre; Ac Staff, Royal Columbian Hospital; Langs: German; (604)521-5986; Fax. (604)521-9122.

WEITZ, Jeffrey I; Hamilton HS-Henderson Site, 237 Barton St E, Hamilton ON L8L 2X2; Ott'76; ABIM(Hem/MedOncol); FACP; FRCPC; Hem (Research). Exec Dir Thrombosis & Atherosclerosis Research Institute, Hamilton Health Sciences Centre-Juravinski Site; Chair Thorombosis, Canada Research in Thrombosis; Prof, McMaster University; (905)574-8550; Fax. (905)575-2646; weitzj@taari.ca.

WEITZMAN, Brian N; The Ottawa Hosp-Gen Campus, 501 Smyth Rd, Ottawa ON K1H 8L6; McG'79; FRCPC; EmergMed;CCFP; CCFP(E.M.); FCFP; Staff, The Ottawa Hospital - General Campus; Langs: Bilingual(English/French); (613)737-8000; Fax. (613)737-8967.

WEITZMAN, Sheila S; The Hosp for Sick Children, 9402-555 University Ave, Toronto ON M5G 1X8; Witwatersrand (South Africa)'68; FRCPC; Peds (Pediatric Oncology). Staff Div of Haem Oncol, The Hospital For Sick Children; Prof, University of Toronto; (416)813-5872; Fax. (416)813-5327; sheila.weitzman@sickkids.ca.

WEIZEL, Harold A E; 601-123 Edward St, Toronto ON M5G 1E2; Tor'47; DAB; FACS; FRCSC; GenSurg (Breast Oncology). Consultant Surg, Toronto General Hospital - UHN; Assoc Prof Surg, University of Toronto; Langs: Yiddish; (416)392-9297; Fax. (416)813-4179; hweizel@on.aibn.com.

WEIZMAN, Adam; Mount Sinai Hosp, 445-600 University Ave, Toronto ON M5G 1X5; Man'06; FRCPC; IntMed; Gastroent. Staff, Mount Sinai Hospital; (416)586-5121; Fax. (416)586-3174.

WEIZMAN, David A; Gates of Maple Med Center, 104-2200 Rutherford Rd, Vaughan ON L4K 5V2; Tor'00; FRCSC; GenSurg. (905)417-7850; Fax. (905)417-4866.

WEIZMAN, Samuel I; North York Med Bldg, 105-1017 Wilson Ave, North York ON M3K 1Z1; Man'72; FRCPC; Peds. (416)633-2000; Fax. (416)633-2000.

WEKA-LUNGUNGA, Charles; Clinique Méd Vanier, 8-325 boul Vanier, Bathurst NB E2A 3N1; Kinshasa (Nigeria)'82; CCFP; Staff, Hopital Regional Chaleur; (506)350-0950; Fax. (506)350-1450.

WEKSBERG, Alfred; North York Med Arts Bldg, 324-1333 Sheppard Ave E, North York ON M2J 1V1; Alb'81; FACP; FRCPC; Derm (Botox Injection). Staff, St Joseph's Care Group - St Joseph's Hospital; Staff, North York General Hospital; Lecturer Med, University of Toronto; Langs: English; French; (416)499-8242; Fax. (416)499-3945; info@drweksberg.com.

WEKSBERG, Rosanna; The Hosp for Sick Children, 555 University Ave, Toronto ON M5G 1X8; Tor'78; FCCMG; FRCPC; Peds (Medical Genetics). Staff Clinical & Metabolic Genetics, The Hospital For Sick Children; Teach Staff Peds, University of Toronto; (416)813-6386; Fax. (416)813-5345; rweksb@sickkids.ca.

WELBOURNE, David R; Thunder Bay Reg HSC-T-Bay, 980 Oliver Rd, Thunder Bay ON P7B 6V4; Ott'89; FRCPC; GenPath. Staff, Thunder Bay Regional Health Sciences Centre; (807)684-6584; Fax. (807)684-5878.

WELCH, Barbara K; 688 Brant St PO Box 1625 Stn Lcd 1, Burlington ON L7R 5A1; Dal'98; BSc; (905)333-1343; Fax. (905)333-6467.

WELCH, David S; Associate Med Clinic, PO Box 7590 Stn Main 10011 101 St, Peace River AB T8S 1T2; Alb'86; CCFP; Staff, Associate Medical Clinic; (780)624-2581; Fax. (780)624-4015.

WELCH, Gilbert J C; Rossmere Med Centre, C-1046 Henderson Hwy, Winnipeg MB R2K 2M5; Man'64.

WELCH, James C; MUHC-Royal Victoria Hosp, 687 av des Pins O, Montreal QC H3A 1A1; Tor'82; FRCPC; EmergMed. Staff, McGill University Health Centre - Royal Victoria Hospital; (514)934-1934; jamescwelch@hotmail.com.

WELCH, John P; Medical Arts Bldg, 307-5880 Spring Garden Rd, Halifax NS B3H 1Y1; Edinburgh (Scotland)'58; MB ChB; PhD; FCCMG.

WELCH, Robert J; The Medical Centre FHT, PO Box 4200 Stn Main 707 Charlotte St, Peterborough ON K9J 7B3; Qns'93; (705)743-6222; Fax. (705)741-1264.

WELCH, Stephen A; London Reg Cancer Centre, A3 917-790 Commissioners Rd E, London ON N6A 4L6; Man'00; FRCPC; IntMed; MedOncol. Staff, London Regional Cancer Center; (519)685-8640; Fax. (519)685-8624; stephen.welch@lhsc.on.ca.

WELCHNER, E Jonathan; 69 Wellington St E, Aurora ON L4G 1H7; Tor'86; (905)503-8000; Fax. (905)503-8100.

WELDER, Clayton A; Medical Clinic, PO Box 730 Stn Main, Salmon Arm BC V1E 4N8; UBC'98; CCFP; FCFP; Member Secretary Treasurer, Shuswap Lake General Hospital; (250)832-6092; Fax. (250)832-5235.

WELDON, Charles J; Clinique Med Maison Nesbitt, 215 rue Du Sud, Cowansville QC J2K 2X5; Sher'78; FRCSC; Ophth. Staff, Hôpital Brome-Missisquoi-Perkins; Langs: English; French; (450)263-8551; Fax. (450)263-8937.

WELDON, Erin R; Health Sciences Centre, 820 Sherbrook St, Winnipeg MB R3A 1R9; Man'00; FRCPC; EmergMed. Staff, Health Sciences Centre; (204)774-6511

WELDON, Mimi B; Nordel Crossing Med Clinic, PO Box 84539 115-12080 Nordel Way, Surrey BC V3W 1P6; Pretoria (South Africa)'96; MB ChB; PhmB; CCFP; Langs: Afrikaans; (604)543-0888

WELIK, Leonard J; Hudson Medicentre, 200-465 rue Main, Hudson QC J0P 1H0; Montpellier (France)'76; (450)458-5393

WELIKOVITCH, Lisa; Foothills Med Centre, C849-1403 29 St NW, Calgary AB T2N 2T9; McM'85; FRCPC; IntMed (Echocardiography); Cardiol. Staff Cardiol, Foothills Medical Centre; Assoc Prof, University of Calgary; (403)944-4243; Fax. (403)944-1592; lisa.welikovitch@calgaryhealthregion.ca.

WELISCH, Eva; London HSC-University Hosp, PO Box 5010 Stn B 800 Commissioners Rd E, London ON N6A 5W9; Berlin (Germany)'87; Staff, London Health Sciences Centre - Victoria Campus; (519)685-8010; Fax. (519)685-8584; eva.welisch@lhsc.on.ca.

WELK, Blayne K; St Joseph's Health Care, PO Box 5777 Stn B B4 667-268 Grosvenor St, London ON N6A 4V2; Wes'04; FRCSC; Urol. Staff, St Joseph's Hospital - St Joseph's Health Care; (519)646-6367; Fax. (519)646-6037.

WELKE, Timothy M; Toronto East Gen Hosp Inc, 6100-825 Coxwell Ave, Toronto ON M4C 3E7; Tor'02; FRCPC; Anes. Staff, Toronto East General Hospital Inc; Staff, Toronto General Hospital - UHN; (416)461-8272

WELLAND, Francis A; 2137 Autumn Breeze Dr N, Mississauga ON L5B 1R3; Sheffield (England)'69; MB ChB; DObstRCOG; Staff, Trillium Health Centre - Mississauga; (416)377-5504

WELLINGTON, Nancy E F; Children's Hosp Western Ont, 800 Commissioners Rd E, London ON N6C 6B5; Tor'80; FRCP; FRCPC; Peds (Emergency Medicine). Staff, Children's Hospital of Western Ontario; Aj Prof Peds, University of Western Ontario; (519)685-8500; vaughn1@brktel.on.ca.

WELLINGTON, Stephen R; Sunny Hill Hlth Ctr For Childr, 3644 Slocan St, Vancouver BC V5M 3E8; Cal'96; FRCPC; Peds. Staff, Sunny Hill Health Centre for Children; (604)453-8300; Fax. (604)453-8390.

WELLMAN, Eleanor; Clinique Med Neufchatel, 101-2425 boul Bastien, Quebec QC G2B 1B3; Ott'75; LMCC; CCFP; Staff Family Med & Geriatrics, Centre Hospitalier Chauveau; Langs: English; French; (418)843-3771; Fax. (418)843-3865.

WELLMAN, Mark B; Old Quebec Street Mall, T28-55 Wyndham St N, Guelph ON N1H 7T8; McM'02; FRCSC; Otol (Head & Neck Surgery). Staff Otol, Guelph General Hospital; (519)822-8833; Fax. (866)318-6851.

WELLS, Anthony R; 937 Mount Pleasant Rd, Toronto ON M4P 2L7; Tor'71; Corp Med Dir, Owens-Corning Canada; (416)484-6760; Fax. (416)484-6761.

WELLS, Calvin R; Royal University Hosp, G807-103 Hospital Dr, Saskatoon SK S7N 0W8; Sask'90; FRCPC; IntMed; Cardiol. Staff, Royal University Hospital; (306)655-6890; Fax. (306)655-6413; calvin.wells@saskatoonhealthregion.ca.

WELLS, Holly D; Pan Imaging, 681 15th St W, Prince Albert SK S6V 7H9; Sask'87; FRCPC; DiagRad (General Radiology & Ultrasound). Physician, Pan Imaging; (306)764-1986; Fax. (306)764-1978; hwells@sasktel.net.

WELLS, Jennie L; St Joseph's HC-Parkwood Hosp, 801 Commissioners Rd E, London ON N6C 5J1; Farmington (USA)'91; MSc; BSc(Hon); FACP; MSc; FRCPC; IntMed; GeriatricMed. Coord Geriatric Rehab Services, Parkwood Hospital - St Joseph's Health Care; Consultant Privil, St Joseph's Hospital - St Joseph's Health Care; Assoc Prof Med/Chair Div of Geriatric Med, University of Western Ontario; Langs: Spanish; (519)685-4021; Fax. (519)685-4093; jennie.wells@sjhc.london.on.ca.

WELLS, John D; Hamilton HS-General Site, 730-237 Barton St E, Hamilton ON L8L 2X2; Tulane University School of Medicine (USA)'73; FRCSC; Neursurg. Att Staff Surg, Hamilton Health Sciences Centre - Hamilton General Hospital; Langs: English; French; (905)522-7432; Fax. (905)527-8998; wellsjoh@hhsc.ca.

WELLS, Laurie L; Waypoint Centre for Mental HC, 500 Church St, Penetanguishene ON L9M 1G3; McM'87; CCFP; Ac Staff, Waypoint Centre for Mental Health Care; (705)549-3181 x2284; Fax. (705)549-2146; lwells@mhcp.on.ca.

WELLS, Mark C; 312-460 Springbank Dr, London ON N6J 0A8; Man'90; Physician, Wortley Village Medical Centre; (519)963-3780; Fax. (519)963-3778.

WELLS, Mary K; 202-35 Major's Path, St. John's NL A1A 4Z9; Mem'86; FRCSC; GenSurg. Langs: English; French; (709)777-5151

WELLS, Neil J; Business Bldg, 808-1200 Burrard St, Vancouver BC V6Z 2C7; UBC'90; FRCSC; PlasSurg (Hand & Wrist Surgery). Asst Prof, University of British Columbia; (604)688-8568; Fax. (604)689-9177.

WELLS, Peter B; Central Med Clinic, 102-150 St Paul St, Collingwood ON L9Y 3P2; McM'80; CCFP; FCFP; Staff, Collingwood General & Marine Hospital; Dir, Rural Ontario Medical Program; Asst Prof, McMaster University; University of Toronto; (705)445-2827; Fax. (705)445-1671; pwells@gbhs.on.ca.

WELLS, Philip J; Dr Philip J Wells Inc, PO Box 190 49A Riverside Ave, Stewiacke NS B0N 2J0; Cape Town (South Africa)'83; Staff, Colchester East Hants Health Centre; (902)639-2484; Fax. (902)639-2380.

WELLS, Philip S; The Ottawa Hosp-Gen Campus, M1857-501 Smyth Rd Box 206, Ottawa ON K1H 8L6; Ott'84; MSc; FRCPC; IntMed (Thrombosis); Hem. Staff, The Ottawa Hospital - General Campus; Dept Chair Med/Prof Med & Clinical Epidemiol, University of Ottawa; (613)737-8755; Fax. (613)737-8851; pwells@oh.on.ca.

WELLS, Richard A; Toronto Sunnybrook Reg Cancer, TW 72058-2075 Bayview Ave, Toronto ON M4N 3M5; Mem'85; PhD(Oxon); FRCP; FRCPC; IntMed (Hematological Oncology); Hem. Staff, Sunnybrook Health Sciences Centre; Asst Prof, University of Toronto; (416)480-5248; Fax. (416)480-6002; richard.wells@sw.ca.

WELLS, Stephen C; Brantford Med Centre, 40 Shellington Place, Brantford ON N3S 0C5; Tor'76; (519)753-9581; Fax. (519)753-9547.

WELLS, Tiffany H; Royal Alexandra Hosp, 55131 RP-10240 Kingsway NW, Edmonton AB T5H 3V9; Wes'03; FRCSC; ObstGyn. Staff, Royal Alexandra Hospital; (780)735-4927; Fax. (780)735-4981.

WELLS, Woodrow A; Univ Hlth Network-Princess M, 5 964-610 University Ave, Toronto ON M5G 2M9; Sask'77; FRCPC; IntMed; RadOncol., Princess Margaret Hospital - University Health Network; (416)946-6513; Fax. (416)946-4442.

WELLWOOD, Alison M; Wolfville Prof Centre, 3-4 Little Rd, Wolfville NS B4P 1P4; Dal'07; CCFP; (902)542-3880; Fax. (902)542-4611.

WELLWOOD, Heather M; Wolfville Prof Centre, 3-4 Little Rd, Wolfville NS B4P 1P4; Dal'74; Ac Staff, Valley Regional Hospital; (902)542-3880; Fax. (902)542-4611; h.wellwood@ns.sympatico.ca.

WELMAN, Johannes; Viking Med Clinic, PO Box 868 5419 50 St, Viking AB T0B 4N0; (780)336-4780; Fax. (780)336-2020.

WELSFORD, Michelle; Hamilton Health Sciences CPER, 201-430 McNeilly Rd, Hamilton ON L8E 5E3; UBC'95; FRCPC; EmergMed. Med Dir Paramedic Base Hosp Prog, Hamilton Health Sciences Centre-Juravinski Site; Staff, Hamilton Health Sciences Centre - Hamilton General Hospital; (905)643-1103; Fax. (905)643-1104.

WELSH, Edward V; 312-3001 Tutt St, Kelowna BC V1Y 2H4; UBC'83; FRCPC; IntMed; Nephrol. Staff, Kelowna General Hospital; (250)861-4847; Fax. (250)861-4831.

WELSH, Lawrence; The Medical Group, 32243 Hurd St, Mission BC V2V 3J9; London (England)'84; MB BS; CCFP; (604)826-6231; Fax. (604)820-1174.

WELSH, Melissa E; Canadian Forces Base Trenton, PO Box 1000 PO Stn Forces, Astra ON K0K 3W0; McM'10; CCFP; Staff, Canadian Forces Base; (613)392-2811

WELSH, Michael M; Radiology Consultants Assoc, 120A-6707 Elbow Dr SW, Calgary AB T2V 0E3; Alb'85; FRCPC; DiagRad. (403)777-3003; Fax. (403)777-3008.

WELSH, Richard M; Gateway Health & Wellness Ctre, 203-2051 McCallum Rd, Abbotsford BC V2S 3N5; UBC'87; CCFP; FCFP; Staff, Abbotsford Regional Hospital & Cancer Centre; (604)855-0677; Fax. (604)855-0722.

WELSH, Robert C; University of Alberta Hosp, 2C200 WCM-8440 112 St NW, Edmonton AB T6G 2B7; Sask'93; ABIM; FRCPC; IntMed; Cardiol. Staff, University of Alberta Hospital; (780)407-3613; Fax. (780)407-6452; rwelsh@cha.ab.ca.

WELT, Michel; Clinique Med le Plein-Ciel, 475 boul de la Cote-Vertu, Saint-Laurent QC H4L 1X7; Mon'78; FRCSC; ObstGyn. Staff, Hôpital du Sacre-Coeur de Montréal; Prof ObstGyn, Universite de Montreal; (514)334-9449; Fax. (514)337-6023; michelwelt@sympatico.ca.

WELTERS, Tania L; Halton HSC Corp-Oakville, 327 Reynolds St, Oakville ON L6J 3L7; McM'02; CCFP; CCFP(E.M.); Staff Emerg, Halton Healthcare Services Corporation - Oakville Site; Langs: Bilingual(English/French); (905)338-4690 x4605; twelter@hotmail.com.

WELTMAN, Glen L; Mount Sinai Hosp, 4F-600 University Ave, Toronto ON M5G 1X5; Tor'90; CCFP; Staff, Mount Sinai Hospital; (416)586-4800 x8824; Fax. (416)586-3230.

WEN, Chuck K; North York Family After Hours, PO Box 91105 Rpo Bayview Village 2901 Bayview Ave, North York ON M2K 2Y6; Tor'07; CCFP; (905)973-3821

WEN, Joseph Y M; Queensway Prof Centre, 412-190 Sherway Dr, Etobicoke ON M9C 5N2; Tor'98; FRCSC; GenSurg (Surgical Oncology). (416)621-3551; Fax. (416)621-3335.

WENDEL, Thomas; East Kootenay Reg Hosp, 13 24th Ave N, Cranbrook BC V1C 3H9; Oregon (USA)'84; Staff, East Kootenay Regional Hospital; Langs: German; (250)426-5281

WENDELBOE, Michael W; Chinook Regional Hosp, 960 19 St S, Lethbridge AB T1J 1W5; Alb'90; FRCPC; GenPath (Anatomical Pathology). Staff, Chinook Regional Hospital; (403)388-6111

WENDLAND, Wilfred; Village Med Clinic, PO Box 1720, 100 Mile House BC V0K 2E0; Sask'67; Physician, Westridge Medical Group; Physician, Medi-Kel F P & Walk-In-Clinic; Langs: German; (250)395-3000; Fax. (250)395-3055.

WENDLING, Lisa C; Russell M Hall Family Hlth Cen, PO Box 550 32 South Court St, Norwich ON N0J 1P0; Wes'95; (519)863-2338; Fax. (519)863-2073; wendlingl@sympatico.ca.

WENG, Andrew P; BC Cancer Agency, 600 10th Ave W, Vancouver BC V5Z 4E6; Chicago (USA)'97; Staff, BC Cancer Agency Vancouver Centre; (604)675-8136; Fax. (604)877-0712.

WENGLE, Larry M; 204-347 College St, Toronto ON M5T 2V8; Tor'72; Staff, Toronto Western Hospital - University Health Network; Langs: Portuguese; Spanish; German; (416)967-6868; Fax. (416)967-9533.

WENNBERG, Richard A; Univ Hlth Network-Toronto Western Hosp, SW 444-399 Bathurst St, Toronto ON M5T 2S8; UBC'90; FRCPC; Neur; Electroenceph (P.Q.). Staff, Toronto Western Hospital - University Health Network; Staff, Toronto General Hospital - UHN; Staff, Mount Sinai Hospital; Asst Prof, University of Toronto; Langs: English; French; (416)603-5402; Fax. (416)603-5768.

WENNER, Gail R; 730-943 Broadway W, Vancouver BC V5Z 4E1; UBC'81; Ac Staff, BC Children's Hospital; Vis Staff, Vancouver General Hospital - Centennial Pavillion; Vis Staff, Providence Health Care - St Paul's Hospital; Corp Physician, Canada Mortgage & Housing Corp.; Clin Instructor, University of British Columbia; (604)734-4454; Fax. (604)734-9791.

WENNING, Joan B; IWK Health Centre, PO Box 9700 Rpo CSC 5850-5980 University Ave, Halifax NS B3K 6R8; Dal'79; FRCSC; ObstGyn. Staff, IWK Health Centre; Assoc Prof, Dalhousie University; (902)470-8365; Fax. (902)425-1125.

WENSKE, Thomas R; London HSC-University Hosp, PO Box 5339 Stn B 339 Windermere Rd, London ON N6A 5A5; Wes'91; Staff, London Health Sciences Centre - University Hospital; Langs: German; (519)685-8500

WENSLEY, David F; Children's & Women's HC of BC, 1C31A-4480 Oak St, Vancouver BC V6H 3V4; London (England)'77; MRC; FRCPC; Peds (Critical Care Medicine); Respir. Staff Ped Critical Care, BC Children's Hospital; Clin Prof Peds, University of British Columbia; (604)875-2119; Fax. (604)875-3293.

WENSVEEN, Quentin J; Misericordia Comm Hosp & HC, 16940 87 Ave NW, Edmonton AB T5R 4H5; Alb'89; FRCPC; Anes. Staff Anes, Covenant Health - Misericordia Community Hospital; (780)735-2863

WENT, John H; Brockville Gen Hosp, 75 Charles St, Brockville ON K7V 1S8; Qns'66; DABR; FRCPC; DiagRad. Staff, Brockville General Hospital - Charles Street; (613)345-5645; Fax. (613)345-8324.

WENTLANDT, Kirsten; Univ Hlth Network-Toronto Gen, 200 Elizabeth St, Toronto ON M5G 2C4; Qns'06; CCFP; Staff, Toronto General Hospital - UHN; (416)340-4800

WENTWORTH, Kathryn; F W Green Med Centre, 1629 Baker St, Cranbrook BC V1C 1B4; Cape Town (South Africa)'99; Langs: Afrikaans; (250)426-6601

WENTWORTH, Paul; Brant Community HC-Brantford, 200 Terrace Hill St, Brantford ON N3R 1G9; Cardiff (Wales)'60; MRCS(Eng); LRCP(Lond); DObstRCOG; FRCPath; FRCPC; GenPath. Staff, The Brant Community Healthcare System - Brantford General Hospital Site; (519)752-7871 x2446; Fax. (519)752-7809.

WENTZEL, Johann D; PO Box 590, Kerrobert SK S0L 1R0; Pretoria (South Africa)'81; Staff, Kerrobert Health Centre; Langs: Afrikaans; (306)834-2289; Fax. (306)834-2389; johann.wentzel@hrha.sk.ca.

WENTZELL, Scott A; Workplace Safety & Ins Board, 200-1113 Jade Crt, Thunder Bay ON P7B 6V3; Dal'91; (807)343-1975

WENTZELL, Tracey M; The Goodhouse Bldg, 93 West St, Corner Brook NL A2H 2Y6; McG'04; FRCSC; OrthSurg. Staff, Western Memorial Regional Hospital.

WENZEL, Dwayne M; Kelowna Gen Hosp, 2268 Pandosy St, Kelowna BC V1Y 1T2; Alb'93; FRCPC; GenPath. Staff, Kelowna General Hospital; (250)862-4300

WEPENER, Frederik J; Barrhead Clinic Holdings, PO Box 4540 Stn Main, Barrhead AB T7N 1A1; (South Africa)'96; (780)674-2231; Fax. (780)674-2447.

WEPENER, Liezl; Barrhead Clinic Holdings, PO Box 4540 Stn Main 5040 49A St, Barrhead AB T7N 1A4; (South Africa)'97; (780)674-2231; Fax. (780)674-2447.

WERB, Marsha R; Medical Dental Centre, 708-586 Eglinton Ave E, Toronto ON M4P 1P2; Tor'73; FRCPC; IntMed (Diabetology); Endocrin&Metab. Court Staff, Women's College Hospital; Court Staff, Sunnybrook Health Sciences Centre; Asst Prof, University of Toronto; (416)322-3198; Fax. (416)322-3725.

WERB, Ronald; 308-1033 Davie St, Vancouver BC V6E 1M7; Cape Town (South Africa)'71; MB ChB; MRCP(UK); FRCPC; IntMed (Nephrology). Ac Staff IntMed & Nephrol, Providence Health Care - St Paul's Hospital; Clin Prof Med, University of British Columbia; Langs: Afrikaans; (604)566-9982

WERB, Solomon M; Dr Sol M Werb & Associates, 206-2797 Bathurst St, Toronto ON M6B 4B9; Alb'72; BSc; Ac Staff, Mount Sinai Hospital; Langs: Yiddish; (416)783-1890; Fax. (416)780-9348.

WERBICKI, James E; Saskatooon City Hosp, 701 Queen St, Saskatoon SK S7K 0M7; Sask'84; CCFP; CCFP(E.M.); FCFP; Staff Emerg Med, Saskatoon City Hospital; Staff, Royal University Hospital; Clin Teacher Family Med, University of Saskatchewan; (306)655-8309; Fax. (306)655-8759.

WERGER, Jeffrey P; Boxgrove Med Arts Centre, 105-110 Copper Creek Dr, Markham ON L6B 0P9; Tor'91; FACS; FRCSC; Otol (Rhinology). Staff, Markham Stouffville Hospital; Instructor Otol, University of Toronto; (905)472-6511; Fax. (905)472-5436.

WERHUN, Robert S; 5803 Main St, Niagara Falls ON L2G 5Z6; McM'96; ABIM; FCCP; FRCPC; IntMed (Cardiology); Respir. Staff, Niagara Health System - Greater Niagara General Site; Langs: Ukrainian; (905)371-1117; Fax. (905)371-9986.

WERIER, Joel M; The Ottawa Hosp-Gen Campus, CCW 1661-501 Smyth Rd, Ottawa ON K1H 8L6; Man'91; FRCSC; OrthSurg (Orthopedic Oncology). Staff, The Ottawa Hospital - General Campus; University of Ottawa; (613)737-8213; Fax. (613)737-8150; jwerier@ottawahospital.on.ca.

WERIER, Jonathon G; Markham Prof Centre, 205-2265 Pembina Hwy, Winnipeg MB R3T 5J3; Man'78; (204)261-9761; Fax. (204)261-9468.

WERKER, Denise H; Public Health Agency of Canada, 6701B-120 Colonnade Rd, Ottawa ON K1A 0K9; Ott'80; MHSc; FRCPC; CommunMed; Public Health & Preventive Med. Langs: English; French; (613)946-3552; Fax. (613)952-4670.

WERKMAN, Isabella M; 4713 48 Ave SS 3, St Paul AB T0A 3A3; (South Africa)'73; MB ChB; MMed(Psych); Staff Psy, Lakeland Health Care; Langs: Afrikaans; Dutch; German; (780)645-3331; Fax. (780)645-1712; neels@telusplanet.net.

WERLE, Jason R; Gulf Canada Square, 335-401 9 Ave SW, Calgary AB T2P 3C5; Sask'94; MD; FRCSC; OrthSurg (Adult Hip & Knee Reconstruction). Ac Staff, Peter Lougheed Centre; Ac Staff, Foothills Medical Centre; Ac Staff, Rockyview General Hospital; Teach Staff Orth Surg, University of Calgary; (403)221-4309; Fax. (403)221-4387.

WERNECK, Christiane C F; 500-89 Queensway W, Mississauga ON L5B 2V2; Universidade Federal de Minas Gerais (Other Foreign)'97; Langs: Portuguese; (905)848-7777; Fax. (905)848-6360.

WERNER, Dietrich; Cobequid Comm Health Centre, 204-5788 University Ave, Halifax NS B3H 1V8; National Autonomous (Honduras)'95; FRCPC; AnatPath. Staff, Queen Elizabeth II Health Sciences Centre - Halifax Infirmary Site; Staff, Cobequid Community Health Centre; (902)527-5068; dietrich.werner@cdha.nshealth.ca.

WERNER, Monica J; Westmount Med Clinic, 11035 Groat Rd NW, Edmonton AB T5M 3J9; UBC'98; Physician, Hobbema Indian Health Services; Langs: German; (780)705-4090; Fax. (780)705-4394.

WERNICKE, Frank; St Joseph's Gen Hosp, 2137 Comox Ave, Comox BC V9M 1P2; Luebeck University (Germany)'90; Staff, St Joseph's General Hospital; Langs: German; (250)890-3712

WERRY, Barbara K; Drs D & B Werry Inc, 500-1144 Burrard St, Vancouver BC V6Z 2A5; Qns'76; FRCPC; Anes. Staff, Ambulatory Surgical Centre Vancouver; (604)629-9258

WERRY, Donald G; Vancouver Bone & Joint Clinic, 500-1144 Burrard St, Vancouver BC V6Z 2A5; Qns'76; FRCSC; OrthSurg (Joint Replacement). Ac Staff Orth, Providence Health Care - St Paul's Hospital; Chairman Board/Board Member, Ambulatory Surgical Centre Vancouver; (604)683-3585; Fax. (604)683-3531; dwerry@vbjc.ca.

WERRY, Elizabeth A; Humber River Reg Hosp-Keele, 2175 Keele St, Toronto ON M6M 3Z4; McM'93; FRCPC; Psy (Adult Psychiatry). Staff, Humber River Regional Hospital - Keele Street Site; (416)658-2022; Fax. (416)658-2074; drelizabethw@hotmail.com.

WERTLEN, Winston G; 307-615 Main St, Yarmouth NS B5A 1K1; Stellenbosch (South Africa)'96; MB ChB; CCFP; (902)742-4528; Fax. (902)742-7216.

WERTMAN, Antoinette; North York Gen Hosp, 4001 Leslie St, North York ON M2K 1E1; Tor'76; BSc; CAFCI; CCFP; CCFP(E.M.); Ac Staff, North York General Hospital; Lecturer, University of Toronto; Langs: Hebrew.

WERTZLER, William F; Foothills Med Centre, C231-1403 29 St NW, Calgary AB T2N 2T9; Cal'83; CCFP; CCFP(E.M.); FCFP; Staff Emerg Med, Foothills Medical Centre; (403)944-1635; Fax. (403)944-2419.

WESA, Mina; BC Women's Hosp & Hlth Ctre, 4500 Oak St, Vancouver BC V6H 3N1; UBC'08; Staff, BC Women's Hospital & Health Centre; (604)875-2000; mwesa@cw.bc.ca.

WESCOTT, Don D; St Martha's Doctor's Office, 23 Bay St, Antigonish NS B2G 2G7; Alb'75; FACOG; FRCSC; ObstGyn. Staff, St Martha's Regional Hospital; (902)863-1558; Fax. (902)863-4200; ddwescott@ns.sympatico.ca.

WESLEY, Shannon J; Nipigon Family Health Team, 125 Hogan Rd, Caramat ON P0T 1J0; Minnesota (USA)'04; CCFP; (807)887-1644; Fax. (807)887-1645.

WESLEY, Steven J; St Joseph's Mountain H Service, PO Box 585 Stn Lcd 1 100 5th St W, Hamilton ON L8N 3K7; Qns'95; LMCC; RC; FRCPC; Psy (Adult Psychiatry & Psychotherapy). Staff, St Joseph's Healthcare Hamilton - West 5th Campus; Staff Psy, Ontario Shores Centre for Mental Health Sciences; Langs: French; (905)522-1155; steven_wesley@hotmail.com.

WESLEY-JAMES, Timothy; Guelph Urology Associates, 205-77 Westmount Rd, Guelph ON N1H 5J1; Qns'83; FRCSC; Urol. Ac Staff, Guelph General Hospital; (519)824-7272; Fax. (519)824-0833.

WESNER, Marni-Lyn; Glen Sather Sport Med Clinic, 11400 University Campus NW, Edmonton AB T6G 1Z1; Sask'94; CCFP; FCFP; (780)407-5160; Fax. (780)407-5667.

WESOLKOWSKA, Anna; Cape Breton Hlthcare Complex, 1482 George St, Sydney NS B1P 1P3; Warsaw (Poland)'66; Staff Family Med. & Psy., Cape Breton Healthcare Complex; Langs: Polish; French; (902)567-8092; Fax. (902)567-7905.

WESOLOWSKA, Ewa B; CHUM-Hotel-Dieu, 3840 rue Saint-Urbain, Montreal QC H2W 1T8; Lodz (Poland)'83; FRCPC; MedBiochem (P.Q.) (Laboratory Medicine). Chef biochimie, Centre Hospitalier l'Université de Montréal (CHUM) - Hôtel-Dieu; Langs: Polish; Russian; French; Slovak; (514)890-8000 x14503; Fax. (514)412-7154; ewa.wesolowska.chum@ssss.gouv.qc.ca.

WESOLOWSKI, Carl A; Royal University Hosp, 103 Hospital Dr, Saskatoon SK S7N 0W8; Wroclaw (Poland)'80; MD; FRCPC; NuclearMed (Family Medicine). Staff, Royal University Hospital; (306)655-1000

WESOLOWSKI, Marta A; Peterborough Family Health Team, LL 02-26 Hospital Dr, Peterborough ON K9J 7C3; (Other Foreign)'08; Langs: Polish; (705)740-6846; Fax. (705)740-6847; mwesolowski@ptboclinic.com.

WESSELS, Johann B; Victoria Hosp, PO Box 3000 Stn Main 1200 24th St W, Prince Albert SK S6V 5T4; Pretoria (South Africa)'86; MB ChB; Staff Emerg Med, Victoria Hospital; (306)765-6000; Fax. (306)763-2871.

WESSELS, Marie-Louise; Victoria General Hosp, 1 Hospital Way, Victoria BC V8Z 5R5; Pretoria (South Africa)'94; MB ChB; CCFP; FCFP; Staff, Victoria General Hospital; Langs: Afrikaans; (250)727-4212

WESSELS, Philip H; 209-5704 44 St, Lloydminster AB T9V 2A1; Pretoria (South Africa)'85; MB ChB; MMed; Langs: Afrikaans; (780)875-2584; Fax. (780)875-3183; pwessels@telusplanet.net.

WESSELS, Wynand; 101-9815 97 St, Grande Prairie AB T8V 8B9; Pretoria (South Africa)'93; MMed(Orth); MB ChB; Staff OrthSurg, Queen Elizabeth II Hospital; (780)402-7181; Fax. (780)402-9829.

WESSLER, Andreas N; Nanaimo Reg Hosp, 1200 Dufferin Cres, Nanaimo BC V9S 2B7; Alb'96; FRCPC; GenPath. Staff, Nanaimo Regional General Hospital; (250)755-7691

WESSON, Trevor; Millenia Clinic, 150 rue Sainte-Catherine O, Montreal QC H5B 1B2; Dal'92; Langs: German; (514)287-2683

WESSON, Virginia A; Mount Sinai Hosp, L1 012 7-60 Murray St, Toronto ON M5T 3L9; Tor'88; MSc; FRCPC; Psy (Geriatric Psychiatry). Staff, Mount Sinai Hospital; (416)586-4800 x6159; Fax. (416)586-3231.

WEST, Amanda L; Health For All Family Health T, 202-379 Church St, Markham ON L6B 0T1; Wes'09; CCFP; (905)472-2200; Fax. (905)472-5662.

WEST, Dixy Lee; Orleans Family Health Clinic, 218-210 Centrum Blvd, Orleans ON K1E 3V7; Alb'80; FRCPC; Psy. Asst Prof Psy, University of Ottawa; (613)841-1615; Fax. (613)841-3818.

WEST, Jacques; Dr Jacques West Inc, 2479 McCallum Rd, Abbotsford BC V2S 3P8; Pretoria (South Africa)'88; MB ChB; Staff, Abbotsford Regional Hospital & Cancer Centre; Langs: Afrikaans; Dutch; (604)852-2279; Fax. (604)852-2863.

WEST, John R; Royal Alexandra Hosp, 10240 Kingsway NW, Edmonton AB T5H 3V9; Wes'87; DAB; FRCPC; AnatPath; GenPath. Staff, Royal Alexandra Hospital; (780)735-5301; Fax. (780)735-4715.

WEST, Kenneth A; Queen Elizabeth II HSC-VG Site, 5087-1276 South Park St, Halifax NS B3H 1V8; Wes'85; FRCPC; IntMed (Transplantation); Nephrol. Staff Physician, Queen Elizabeth II Health Sciences Centre - Victoria General Site; Prof, Dalhousie University; (902)473-5543; Fax. (902)473-2675; kawest@dal.ca.

WEST, L Michael; Dickson Bldg, 5090-5820 University Ave, Halifax NS B3H 1V8; Qns'79; FACP; FRCPC; IntMed; Nephrol. Staff Cons Nephrol, IWK Health Centre; Staff, Queen Elizabeth II Health Sciences Centre - Victoria General Site; Assoc Prof, Dalhousie University; (902)473-4023; Fax. (902)473-2675; michael.west@cdha.nshealth.ca.

WEST, Lori J; Li Ka Shing Research Centre, 6002-1A University Campus NW, Edmonton AB T6G 2E1; New Orleans(LA) (USA)'83; FRCPC; Peds (Pediatric Cardiology). Staff Stollery Children's Cardiol, University of Alberta Hospital; Prof, University of Alberta; Langs: Spanish; (780)492-3200; Fax. (780)492-8239; ljwest@ualberta.ca.

WEST, Michael J; 33 Dundas St, Dundas ON L9H 1A1; Qns'91; CCFP; FCFP; (905)628-6150; Fax. (905)628-1609.

WEST, Michael; Leslie Med Centre, 214-4800 Leslie St, North York ON M2J 2K9; Tor'74; FRCSC; OrthSurg (Hip & Knee Replacement). (416)491-5454; Fax. (416)491-5464.

WEST, Michael; GB 136-820 Sherbrook St, Winnipeg MB R3A 1R9; Man'73; FRCS; FRCSC; Neursurg (Oncology). Co-Dir, Winnipeg Centre for Gamma Knife Surgery; Prof Surg, University of Manitoba; (204)787-7960; Fax. (204)787-3851; mwest@hsc.mb.ca.

WEST, Peter H F; Saint John Reg Hosp, PO Box 2100 Stn Main 400 University Ave, Saint John NB E2L 4L2; Dal'93; FRCPC; IntMed; Critical Care Medicine. Staff, Saint John Regional Hospital; (506)648-6000

WEST, Robert D; Bagot Street Med Centre, 182 Bagot St, Kingston ON K7L 3G1; Cal'76; Assoc Staff, Hotel-Dieu Hospital; Assoc Staff, Kingston General Hospital; Lecturer Family Med, Queen's University; (613)542-8783; Fax. (613)546-1321; admin@bagot.com.

WEST, Susan M; Pitt Meadows Med Clinic, 125-19150 Lougheed Hwy, Surrey BC V3T 2H6; McG'69; Staff, Ridge Meadows Hospital & Health Care Centre; Staff, Pitt Meadows Medical Clinic; (604)465-4911

WEST, William J H; Mapleview Med Clinic, 340 Elgin St, Port Colborne ON L3K 6G9; McM'81; Ac Staff, Niagara Health System - Port Colborne General Site; (905)835-9817; Fax. (905)835-1647.

WEST, William; The Richmond Hosp, 7000 Westminster Hwy, Richmond BC V6X 1A2; McM'97; CCFP; CCFP(E.M.); Staff, Richmond Hospital; (604)244-5585

WESTACOTT, Paul C; Cambridge Mem Hosp, 700 Coronation Blvd, Cambridge ON N1R 3G2; Queensland (Australia)'78; FRCPC; Anes. Staff, Cambridge Memorial Hospital; (519)621-2330 x2100; Fax. (519)740-4906; wesp@golden.net.

WESTBERG, Kirsten I; Plastic & Reconstruction Surg, 120-2950 22 St, Red Deer AB T4R 0H9; Man'96; FRCSC; PlasSurg (Hand Microsurgery). Staff, Red Deer Regional Hospital Centre; (403)350-3323; Fax. (403)350-3324.

WESTBROOK, Christopher J; Lakeridge Health-Port Perry Si, 451 Paxton St, Port Perry ON L9L 1A8; Wes'08; CCFP; Staff, Lakeridge Health - Port Perry Site; (905)985-7321

WESTBY, Donald M; Weymouth Med Clinic, PO Box 220, Weymouth NS B0W 3T0; Dublin (Ireland)'77; MB ChB; BAO; DCH; Assoc Staff, Digby General Hospital; (902)837-5640; Fax. (902)837-5450.

WESTBY, John C; Western Mem Reg Hosp, 1 Brookfield Ave, Corner Brook NL A2H 6J7; Dublin (Ireland)'65; Staff, Western Memorial Regional Hospital; (709)637-5000

WESTBY, Lloyd; 120-1636 Main St, Penticton BC V2A 5G8; UBC'90; CCFP; FCFP; Langs: Norwegian; (250)490-9378; Fax. (250)492-3338.

WESTEN, Evelyn C; 185 Inkerman St E, Listowel ON N4W 2N1; Ott'82; DObst(N.Zealand); Staff/Member Maternal & Newborn Committee, Listowel Memorial Hospital - Listowel Wingham Hospitals Alliance; (519)291-4200; Fax. (519)291-5947.

WESTENBERG, Hendrik H; Maple Family Health Team, 115 Lower Union St, Kingston ON K7L 2N3; Amsterdam (Netherlands)'60; Coroner, City Of Kingston; Coroner, County Of Frontenac; Assessor NEL, Workplace Safety & Insurance Board; Physician Designated Physician, Citizenship & Immigration Canada; Langs: Dutch; German; French; (613)542-7095; Fax. (613)542-2224.

WESTENDORP, Matthew W; Upper Grand Family Health Team, 753 Tower St S, Fergus ON N1M 2R2; Qns'01; BSc(Hons.); CCFP; Staff ER, Groves Memorial Community Hospital; (519)843-4380; Fax. (519)843-3211.

WESTERBERG, Brian D; St Paul's Hosp, P2-1081 Burrard St, Vancouver BC V6Z 1Y6; Qns'89; ABOtol; MHSc; BA; FRCSC; Otol (Head & Neck Surgery). Staff, Providence Health Care - St Paul's Hospital; Staff, Rotary Hearing Clinic-Providence 2; (604)806-8540; Fax. (604)806-8777.

WESTERLUND, John A R; CSSS du Nord de Lanaudiere, 1000 boul Sainte-Anne, St-Charles-Brromee QC J6E 6J2; UBC'84; FRCPC; MedBiochem. Staff, Centre Hospitalier Régional de Lanaudière; Langs: French; (450)759-8222 x2617; Fax. (450)759-3075; john_westerlund@ssss.gouv.qc.ca.

WESTHEUSER, Susan L; Legacy Med Centre, 378 4 Ave S, Lethbridge AB T1J 5E9; Alb'90; CCFP; FCFP; (403)320-1504; Fax. (403)329-3778.

WESTIB, Andreas; Cardiology Consultants, 306-803 1 Ave NE, Calgary AB T2E 7C5; (Germany)'95; Consultant Cardiol, Peter Lougheed Centre; Consultant Cardiol, Rockyview General Hospital; Consultant Cardiol, Foothills Medical Centre; (403)571-8600; Fax. (403)571-8659.

WESTKIRK, Russell C; 904-1 St Clair Ave E, Toronto ON M4T 2V7; Tor'83; FRCPC; Psy. (416)961-0182; Fax. (416)961-7872; russellwestkirk@sympatico.ca.

WESTLAKE, Alice G; The Medical Assoc of Sechelt, PO Box 638 5531 Inlet Ave, Sechelt BC V0N 3A0; Cal'79; BSc; CCFP; (604)885-2257

WESTLAKE, Susan J; Balmoral Med Arts Facility, 405-1366 Yonge St, Toronto ON M4T 3A7; McM'81; CCFP; FCFP; Court Staff Family & Commun Med, Women's College Hospital; Assoc Staff Family & Commun Med, Mount Sinai Hospital; Teacher Family & Commun Med, University of Toronto; (416)923-5767; Fax. (416)923-5125.

WESTLEY, Elizabeth A; Bells Corners Med Group, 103-1956 Robertson Rd, Nepean ON K2H 5B9; Ott'92; BSc; CCFP; (613)596-6427; Fax. (613)596-3162.

WESTLIND, Paul E; Mount Sinai Hosp, 965-600 University Ave, Toronto ON M5G 1X5; McM'96; FRCPC; Psy. Staff, Mount Sinai Hospital; University of Toronto; (416)586-4800 x8540; Fax. (416)586-5970; paul_westlind@camh.net.

WESTMACOTT, Clare W M; 202-56 Lincoln Park, Canmore AB T1W 3E9; Wes'73; CCFP; (403)678-2737; Fax. (403)609-9324; idealhealth@shaw.ca.

WESTON, Bonnie C; 10-838 Somerset St W, Ottawa ON K1R 6R7; Tor'87; ABOph; FRCSC; Ophth (Cornea). (613)237-5533; Fax. (613)237-5534.

WESTON, Lyle E; Professional Arts Bldg, 224-100 Arden St, Moncton NB E1C 4B7; Dal'85; FRCPC; Neur. Ac Staff, The Moncton Hospital; Consultant, Dr Georges-L-Dumont University Hospital Centre; (506)858-8887; Fax. (506)858-8408; westonle@nbnet.nb.ca.

WESTON, W Fenton D; Kingston Family Health Team, 403-800 Princess St, Kingston ON K7L 5E4; Tor'69; DCMT; Staff, Kingston General Hospital; Staff, Ongwanada Resource Centre; Court Staff, Hotel-Dieu Hospital; Staff, Kingston Family Health Team - Princess Street Site; Queen's University; (613)549-2522; Fax. (613)549-0490.

WESTON, William M; 224-1063 King St W, Hamilton ON L8S 4S3; McM'86; BEng; ATLS; FRSM; Clinical Asst Prof Surg, Hamilton Health Sciences Centre - McMaster University Medical Centre; Clinical Asst Prof Surg, McMaster University; (905)516-4900; Fax. (905)304-4900; westonw@globalserve.net.

WESTRA, Yolande N; Queen Elizabeth II Hosp, 10409 98 St, Grande Prairie AB T8V 2E8; Cal'92; FRCPC; IntMed. Staff, Queen Elizabeth II Hospital; (780)830-2844; Fax. (780)830-2843.

WESTREICH, Neal M; Sunnybrook Hlth Sciences Ctre, 2075 Bayview Ave, Toronto ON M4N 3M5; McM'95; FRCPC; Psy. Staff, Sunnybrook Health Sciences Centre; (416)480-4208; Fax. (416)480-6818.

WESTWOOD, David M; Sow's Ear Med Clinic, PO Box 190 7186 Lantzville Rd, Lantzville BC V0R 2H0; Cambridge (England)'65; MB ChB; DObstRCOG; CCFP; (250)390-4542; Fax. (250)390-4561.

WESTWOOD, Michael; Plaza Baie D'Urfe, 14-90 rue Morgan, Baie-D'Urfe QC H9X 3A8; Cape Town (South Africa)'66; MRCP; DCH; FRCPC; Peds (Adolescent Medicine). Att Staff, McGill University Health Centre - Montreal Children's Hospital; Att Staff, Lakeshore General Hospital - Pointe Claire; Assoc Prof Peds, McGill University; Langs: English; French; (514)695-6345; Fax. (514)695-7336; mwestwood@videotron.ca.

WETMORE, Stephen J; Thames Valley FHT-Victoria Fam, 60 Chesley Ave, London ON N5Z 2C1; Tor'75; CCFP; FCFP; Ac Staff, London Health Sciences Centre - Victoria Campus; Ac Staff, Parkwood Hospital - St Joseph's Health Care; Coroner, Province of Ontario; Dept Chair Family Med/Prof Family Med, University of Western Ontario; (519)433-8424; Fax. (519)433-2244; swetmore@uwo.ca.

WETZER, Wolfgang H; 101-7784 East Saanich Rd, Saanichton BC V8M 2B3; McG'78; Staff, Saanich Peninsula Hospital; Staff, Civil Aviation Canada; Langs: German; French; (250)652-9121; Fax. (250)652-0306; w.wetzer@shaw.ca.

WEXLER, Denise M M A; Wellington Dermatology Assoc, 272 Oxford St W, London ON N6H 1S9; Wes'69; FRCPC; Derm. (519)434-2193; Fax. (519)434-9676.

WEXLER, Howard R; St Joseph's Health Care, PO Box 5777 Stn B 268 Grosvenor St, London ON N6A 4V2; Wes'70; FRCPC; Anes (Critical Care Medicine). Staff, St Joseph's Hospital - St Joseph's Health Care; Member Board of Dir, Ontario Medical Association; Asst Prof Anes, University of Western Ontario; (519)646-6000 x64218; Fax. (519)668-8257.

WEXLER, Marvin J; MUHC-Royal Victoria Hosp, S7 30-687 av des Pins O, Montreal QC H3A 1A1; McG'65; MSc; FACS; MDCM; FRCSC; GenSurg (Breast Cancer). principale Chirurgien, McGill University Health Centre - Royal Victoria Hospital; Prof, McGill University; Langs: English; French; (514)934-1934 x35178; Fax. (514)843-1503; marvin.wexler@muhc.mcgill.ca.

WEYERS, Hendrik; Miramichi Reg Hosp, 500 Water St, Miramichi NB E1V 3G5; Pretoria (South Africa)'74; MMed(Orthop); Staff, Miramichi Regional Hospital; (506)623-3970; Fax. (506)623-3971.

WEYMAN, Karen R; St Michael's Hosp, 30 Bond St, Toronto ON M5B 1W8; Tor'89; CCFP; FCFP; Staff, St Michael's Hospital; Asst Prof, University of Toronto; (416)867-7426; Fax. (416)867-7498; weymank@smh.ca.

WEZELMAN, John; 5118 48 St, Castor AB T0C 0X0; London (England)'67; MB BS; DA; Staff, Covenant Health - Our Lady of the Rosary Hospital; (403)882-0004; Fax. (403)882-3525.

WHALEN, Brien A; Main Street Med Centre, 1251 Main St, Stittsville ON K2S 2E5; Mem'92; (613)831-6381; Fax. (613)831-6381.

WHALEN, Julie H; Clinique Med Elmwood, 205-565 Elmwood Dr, Dieppe NB E1A 2X4; Sher'93; CCFP; FCFP; Langs: Bilingual(French/English); (506)857-0035; Fax. (506)384-9099.

WHALEN, Mark G; 10 Village Ave PO Box 66 Stn Main, Campbellton NB E3N 3G1; Sher'81; ABIM; CSPQ; FACP; FRCPC; IntMed. Head IntMed/Med Dir ICU, Hôpital Régional Campbellton; Langs: French; (506)789-1406; Fax. (506)789-1999; mwhalen_md@nb.aibn.com.

WHALEN, Ronald V; Queen Elizabeth Hosp, PO Box 6600 Stn Central 60 Riverside Dr, Charlottetown PE C1A 8T5; Alb'99; CCFP; CCFP(E.M.); Staff, Queen Elizabeth Hospital; (902)894-2111

WHALEN, Sylvia A M; Orleans Family Health Clinic, 101-210 Centrum Blvd, Orleans ON K1E 3V7; Dal'90; CCFP; Langs: English; French; (613)837-5454; Fax. (613)837-3781.

WHALEN-BROWNE, Karen A; Kingston Family Health Team, 202-275 Bagot St, Kingston ON K7L 3G4; Tor'85; BSc(Hons.); CCFP; FCFP; Langs: English; French; (613)549-7477; Fax. (613)549-4920.

WHALEY, Robert S; 131 Howland Dr, Huntsville ON P1H 2P7; Qns'84; (705)789-6455; Fax. (705)789-1403.

WHAN, Deborah E; Two Rivers FHT-Hespeler Med Cl, B12-350 Conestoga Blvd, Cambridge ON N1R 7L7; McM'98; CCFP; Ac Staff, Cambridge Memorial Hospital; (519)629-4615; Fax. (519)629-4630.

WHANG, Paul; Humber River Reg Hosp-Church, 200 Church St, Toronto ON M9N 1N8; Wes'84; FRCPC; Anes. Staff, Humber River Regional Hospital - Church Street Site; (416)243-4154

WHARTON, Sean N; The Wharton Med Clinic, M14-414 Victoria Ave N, Hamilton ON L8L 5G8; Tor'01; FRCPC; IntMed (Cardiology). Staff, Hamilton Health Sciences Centre; (905)527-7663; Fax. (905)527-7665; wharton@whartonmedicalclinic.com.

WHATELY, Christopher G; Brant Community HC-Brantford, 200 Terrace Hill St, Brantford ON N3R 1G9; Qns'78; BSc; DAB; FRCSC; OrthSurg. Staff, The Brant Community Healthcare System - Brantford General Hospital Site; (519)771-6649

WHATLEY, Darren; CPHC Gananoque Community FHT, 338 Herbert St, Gananoque ON K7G 1R1; Saba (Other Foreign)'08; CCFP; (613)382-7383; Fax. (613)382-7323.

WHATLEY, Gordon S; Queen Elizabeth II HSC-Halifax, 1796 Summer St, Halifax NS B3H 3A7; Tor'80; FRCPC; Anes. Staff, Queen Elizabeth II Health Sciences Centre - Halifax Infirmary Site; (902)473-4326; Fax. (902)473-3820.

WHATLEY, Philip L; Emo Community Health Service, PO Box 569, Emo ON P0W 1E0; Man'77; BSc; DTMH; Chief/Medical Staff, Emo Health Centre-Riverside Health Care Facility; (807)482-2323; Fax. (807)482-3089; p.whatley@rhcf.on.ca.

WHATLEY, Richard J; The Peterborough Clinic FHT, 303-26 Hospital Dr, Peterborough ON K9J 7C3; Tor'79; CCFP; FCFP; (705)740-6853; Fax. (705)740-6863; rwhatley@ptboclinic.com.

WHATLEY, Shawn D; Southlake Reg Health Centre, 596 Davis Dr, Newmarket ON L3Y 2P9; Ott'96; CCFP; FCFP; CCFP(E.M.); Staff, Southlake Regional Health Centre; (905)895-4521 x2222

WHEATCROFT, Mark D; St Michael's Hosp, 30 Bond St, Toronto ON M5B 1W8; Staff Vascular Surg, St Michael's Hospital; (416)864-5212; Fax. (416)864-6012.

WHEATLEY, B Matthew; University of Alberta Hosp, 2D102 WCM-8440 112 St NW, Edmonton AB T6G 2B7; Alb'95; BSc; PhD; FRCSC; Neursurg (Epilepsy). Staff, University of Alberta Hospital; (780)407-3567; Fax. (780)407-8203.

WHEATLEY, Brian; 32 Windfield Cres, Kanata ON K2M 2B7; Durham (England)'62; FRCS(Ed); Dir, ECO-ANTH Consulting; (613)592-3934; Fax. (613)592-3934; wheatley@travel-net.com.

WHEATLEY-PRINCE, Paul F; The Ottawa Hosp-Gen Campus, 501 Smyth Rd, Ottawa ON K1H 8L6; Manchester (England)'97; Staff, The Ottawa Hospital - General Campus; (613)737-7700; Fax. (613)247-3511.

WHEELDON, P John; 2135 Norris Avenue PO Box 670, Lumby BC V0E 2G0; Birmingham (England)'60; (250)547-8810; Fax. (250)547-8830; jrwheel2@telus.net.

WHEELER, Bruce H; Extendicare Hillcrest Calgary, 1512 8 Ave NW, Calgary AB T2N 1C1; Cal'74; CCFP; Fax. (403)500-9420.

WHEELER, Devon S; Misericordia Comm Hosp, 16940 87 Ave NW, Edmonton AB T5R 4H5; Sask'08; CCFP; CCFP(E.M.); Staff, Covenant Health - Misericordia Community Hospital; (780)735-2000

WHEELER, James K; 65 Ellen St, Blenheim ON N0P 1A0; Tor'99; CCFP; Staff, Chatham-Kent Health Alliance; Aj Prof Family Med, University of Western Ontario; (519)676-5592; Fax. (519)676-2228.

WHEELER, Jesse J F; The Medical Centre, 707 Charlotte St, Peterborough ON K9J 7B3; Qns'10; CCFP; Med Staff, Peterborough Regional Health Centre - Hospital Drive; (705)876-4554; Fax. (705)431-1449.

WHEELER, Leslie; Dr Charles A Janeway Child HC, 300 Prince Philip Dr, St. John's NL A1B 3V6; Mem'03; FRCPC; Psy. Staff, Janeway Children's Health & Rehabilitation Centre; (709)777-6300

WHEELER, Martin M; Doctors Med Clinic, 215-306 Shelbourne St, Victoria BC V8R 6T9; London (England)'75; MRCS; MB BS; LRCP; CCFP; FCFP; (250)388-4211; mwheeler@edhospital.on.ca.

WHEELER, Maxwell; Bayvalley Med Arts Bldg, 304-145 Queenston St, St Catharines ON L2R 2Z9; Mem'74; BSc; AB; FRCPC; Psy. Consultant, Niagara Health System - Ontario Street Site; (905)685-1515; Fax. (905)685-1152.

WHEELER, Stephen J; Victoria Emerg Phys Mgmt Ltd, 325-1627 Fort St, Victoria BC V8R 1H8; UBC'86; ABEM; BSc; Staff Emerg. Dept., Royal Jubilee Hospital; Med Dir BC Air Ambulance, BC Ambulance Service; (250)479-1442; Fax. (250)479-1472; drwheeler@me.com.

WHEELOCK, W Brian; Saint John Reg Hosp, PO Box 2100 Stn Main 400 University Ave, Saint John NB E2L 4L2; Dal'73; FRCSC; Neursurg. Ac Staff, Saint John Regional Hospital; Asst Prof Surg, Dalhousie University; (506)648-6650; Fax. (506)648-6649.

WHELAN, Barbara L; 102-186 Albert St, London ON N6A 1M1; Dal'84; (519)432-8402; Fax. (519)601-1840.

WHELAN, Chantal I; Carlington Comm Hlth Services, 900 Merivale Rd, Ottawa ON K1Z 5Z8; Tor'85; FRCPC; Psy (Communicative & Learning Disability). Staff, The Ottawa Hospital - General Campus; University of Ottawa; Langs: Bilingual(French/English); (613)722-9731; Fax. (613)722-8244; cwhelan@carlington.ochc.org.

WHELAN, Ciara M; Temmy Latner Centre, 2-60 Murray St, Toronto ON M5T 3L9; Qns'08; CCFP; (416)586-4800

WHELAN, Daniel B; St Michael's Orthopaedic Assoc, 800-55 Queen St E, Toronto ON M5C 1R6; Mem'96; MSc; Dip SportMed; FRCSC; OrthSurg (Sports Medicine). Staff, St Michael's Hospital; Asst Prof, University of Toronto; (416)864-6002; Fax. (416)359-1601; wheland@smh.toronto.on.ca.

WHELAN, Edward P; CML Healthcare Inc, 102-150 Katimavik Rd, Kanata ON K2L 2N2; Qns'80; FRCPC; DiagRad.

WHELAN, James H A; Terrace On The Square, 8-10 Rowan St, St. John's NL A1B 2X1; Mem'89; FRCSC; Ophth (Glaucoma). Ac Staff, Health Sciences Centre; Ac Staff, Janeway Children's Health & Rehabilitation Centre; Asst Prof Surg, Memorial University Of Newfoundland; (709)726-2075; Fax. (709)726-2027.

WHELAN, Jennifer; Belleville Queen's Univ-FMC, 200-145 Station St, Belleville ON K8N 2S9; Dublin (Ireland)'03; CCFP; (613)771-1910; Fax. (613)771-3396.

WHELAN, John M; 1233 7th Ave W, Vancouver BC V6H 1B7; Dublin (Ireland)'67; MB ChB; BAO; FRCPC; Psy. Staff, Powell River General Hospital; (604)731-6177; Fax. (604)875-5652.

WHELAN, John P J; St Joseph's Healthcare, 50 Charlton Ave E, Hamilton ON L8N 4A6; McM'81; FRCSC; Urol. Ac Staff The McMaster Institute of Urology, St Joseph's Healthcare - Charlton Campus; Court Staff, Hamilton Health Sciences Centre - McMaster Children's Hospital; Court Staff, McMaster Institute of Urology; Assoc Prof Surg, McMaster University; (905)521-6014; Fax. (905)528-3043; whelanp@mcmaster.ca.

WHELAN, Patrick J; Markham Stouffville Health Ctr, 402-377 Church St, Markham ON L6B 1A1; Dal'81; FRCSC; GenSurg. Ac Staff, Markham Stouffville Hospital; (905)472-7122; Fax. (905)472-2290.

WHELAN, Thomas F; Saint John Reg Hosp, PO Box 2100 Stn Main 400 University Ave, Saint John NB E2L 4L2; Dal'89; FRCSC; Urol. Staff, Saint John Regional Hospital; (506)648-7801; Fax. (506)648-6894.

WHELAN, Timothy J; The Juravinski Cancer Centre, 4 204-699 Concession St, Hamilton ON L8V 5C2; Oxford (England)'80; FRCPC; IntMed; RadOncol. Staff, Hamilton Health Sciences Centre-Juravinski Site; Assoc Prof Med/Assoc Member, McMaster University; (905)387-9711 x64501; Fax. (905)575-6308; tim.whelan@jcc.hhsc.ca.

WHELAN, Wendy E; Southern Med Clinic, 390 Topsail Rd, St. John's NL A1E 2B8; Mem'77; (709)364-9556

WHELER, David S; 307-2130 Lawrence Ave E, Scarborough ON M1R 3A6; Tor'85; BSc; CCFP; FCFP; Assoc Staff, The Scarborough Hospital - General Campus; (416)751-6141; Fax. (416)751-5270.

WHELER, R James; The Doctor's Office, 1011 Upper Middle Rd E, Oakville ON L6H 4L1; Tor'57; (905)849-7007; Fax. (905)849-7883.

WHELTON, Charles L M; PO Box 396 Stn Main, Parksville BC V9P 2G5; Tor'83; FRCPC; Psy. Staff Psy, Parksville Mental Health & Addiction Services; Staff, Edgewood Treatment Centre.

WHERRETT, Brian A; Hotel-Dieu Hosp, 166 Brock St, Kingston ON K7L 5G2; Qns'58; FRCPC; Peds (Developmental Pediatrics). Consultant Child Development Centre, Hotel-Dieu Hospital; Consultant Peds, Kingston General Hospital; Emeritus Prof Peds, Queen's University; (613)544-3400 x3325; Fax. (613)545-3557.

WHERRETT, Christopher G; The Ottawa Hosp-Gen Campus, 501 Smyth Rd, Ottawa ON K1H 8L6; Wes'88; FRCPC; Anes (Hyperbaric Medicine); Critical Care Medicine. Staff, The Ottawa Hospital - General Campus; Asst Prof, University of Ottawa; (613)737-8187; cwherrett@ottawahospital.on.ca.

WHERRETT, Diane K; The Hosp For Sick Children, 5110-555 University Ave, Toronto ON M5G 1X8; Qns'87; FRCPC; Peds (Pediatric Endocrinology); Endocrin&Metab. Staff Endocrinol, The Hospital For Sick Children; (416)813-8159; Fax. (416)813-6304.

WHERRETT, John R; 501-2727 Yonge St, Toronto ON M4N 3R6; Qns'55; PhD(Lond); FRCPC; Neur. Staff, Toronto Western Hospital - University Health Network; Emeritus Prof, University of Toronto; (416)932-0145; j.wherrett@utoronto.ca.

WHERRETT, Laurie J; 2A-194 King St W, Oshawa ON L1J 2J2; Qns'89; FRCSC; GenSurg; Critical Care Medicine. Ac Staff, Lakeridge Health - Oshawa Site; (905)436-5870; Fax. (905)436-2010.

WHETTER, Christine R; Queensway-Carleton Hosp, 3045 Baseline Rd, Nepean ON K2H 8P4; UBC'99; FRCPC; IntMed. Staff, Queensway Carleton Hospital; (613)721-4842; Fax. (613)721-4785.

WHETTER, Ian C; Northern Connection Med Ctre, LL-425 Elgin Ave, Winnipeg MB R3A 1P2; Man'05; CCFP; (204)940-8777; Fax. (204)940-4387.

WHETTER, Kevin M; St Joseph's Gen Hosp, 2137 Comox Ave, Comox BC V9M 1P2; Man'96; FRCPC; Psy. Staff, St Joseph's General Hospital; (250)890-3712

WHIDDEN, Paul G R; MacLeod Trail Plastic Surgery, 7425 Macleod Trail SW, Calgary AB T2H 0L8; Alb'95; BSc; FRCSC; PlasSurg (Cosmetic Surgery). Clin Teach Staff Plastic Surg, Rockyview General Hospital; Staff, Macleod Trail Plastic Surgery; Staff Teacher, University of Calgary; (403)228-2684; Fax. (403)242-5090; drwhidden@whidden.ca.

WHIDDEN, Peter G; Scarboro Village, 300-1608 17 Ave SW, Calgary AB T2T 0E3; Alb'66; FACS; BA; FRCSC; PlasSurg (Cosmetics). Ac Staff Surgeon, Peter Lougheed Centre; (403)228-2558; Fax. (403)229-3441; whiddenp@telusplanet.net.

WHITAKER, Katherine J; 1863 Oak Bay Ave, Victoria BC V8R 1C6; Dal'86; FRCPC; Psy. (250)595-3127

WHITBY, Peter L; Centre for Family Medicine, 10B Victoria St S, Kitchener ON N2G 1C5; Birmingham (England)'77; MB ChB; CCFP; FCFP; Ac Staff, Grand River Hospital - Kitchener/Waterloo Health Centre; Clinical Asst Prof, McMaster University; (519)783-0021; Fax. (519)783-0031.

WHITE, Adam S; 416-1033 Davie St, Vancouver BC V6E 1M7; UBC'03; FRCPC; IntMed; Endocrin&Metab. Staff, Providence Health Care - St Paul's Hospital; (604)689-1055

WHITE, Alan V M; Lindsay Park Sports Med Ctre, 2225 MacLeod Trail SE Box 50, Calgary AB T2G 5B6; Qns'67; ABIM; FRCPC; IntMed (Cardiac Rehabilitation); Cardiol. (403)571-6950

WHITE, Amie M; PO Box 4427 Stn South CRO, Edmonton AB T6E 4T5; Alb'05; CCFP.

WHITE, Andrea A; London HSC-Victoria Hosp, PO Boc 5010 Stn B B2 441-800 Commissioners Rd E, London ON N6A 5W9; Wes'99; FRCSC; ObstGyn. Staff, London Health Sciences Centre - Victoria Campus; (519)685-8289

WHITE, Andrea A; Lethbridge Centre Mall, 239-200 4 Ave S, Lethbridge AB T1J 4C9; NOSM'10; CCFP; (403)942-0800

WHITE, Bonnie L; Grimsby Med Associates, 100-155 Main St E, Grimsby ON L3M 1P2; Wes'10; CCFP; (905)945-5476; Fax. (905)945-7707.

WHITE, Brian A; The Family Practice Clinic, 2778 104th St, Nanaimo BC V9T 2E4; UBC'71; (250)758-1711; Fax. (250)758-2802.

WHITE, Carol A; Kingston Family Health Team, 500A Gardiners Rd, Kingston ON K7M 7W9; Mem'81; CCFP; FCFP; Assoc Staff, Kingston General Hospital; Asst Prof, Queen's University; (613)389-5974; Fax. (613)389-0804.

WHITE, Carole B T; 203-2825 Clearbrook Rd, Abbotsford BC V2T 6S3; UBC'77; CCFP; Staff, Abbotsford Regional Hospital & Cancer Centre; (604)852-1567; Fax. (604)852-8949; carolwhite@fastmail.fm.

WHITE, Celina D; Cumberland Health Authority, 34 Prince Arthur st, Amherst NS B4H 1V6; Dal'81; Staff, Cumberland Health Authority; Dist Med Continuing Care/Pres Med Staff/Board Member Directors of Doctors NS, District Health Authority 5; (902)661-1090; Fax. (902)667-1125; cdwhite@ns.aliantzinc.ca.

WHITE, Christine A; Etherington Hall, 3032-94 Stuart St, Kingston ON K7L 2V6; Qns'99; FRCPC; IntMed; Nephrol. (613)533-3134; Fax. (613)533-3292.

WHITE, Christine L; 307-595 Montreal Rd, Ottawa ON K1K 4L2; McG'75; CCFP; FCFP; Langs: English; French; (613)746-4390; Fax. (613)746-4840.

WHITE, Christopher M; South Health Campus, 4448 Front St SE, Calgary AB T3M 1M4; McM'92; BSc(Hon.); FRCPC; Neur (Neuromuscular Diseases). Staff Clinical Neurosciences, South Health Campus; (403)943-8500; Fax. (403)640-7615.

WHITE, Christopher W; Associated Radiologists, 300-140 Wall St, Saskatoon SK S7K 1N4; Sask'93; BSc; FRCR; ABR; FRCPC; DiagRad. Physician, Associated Radiologists of Saskatoon; (306)244-1167; Fax. (306)244-2911; cwhite99@shaw.ca.

WHITE, Colin P; The Ottawa Hosp-Gen Campus, 501 Smyth Rd, Ottawa ON K1H 8L6; Mem'07; FRCSC; PlasSurg (Reconstructive Micro Surgery). Staff, The Ottawa Hospital - General Campus; (613)722-7000

WHITE, Colin T; Children's & Women's HC of BC, K4 151-4480 Oak St, Vancouver BC V6H 3V4; Ott'92; BSc; FAAP; FRCPC; Peds; Nephrol. Asst Prof, BC Children's Hospital; (604)875-2272; Fax. (604)875-3649.

WHITE, Craig P; Notre Dame Mem Health Centre, Hospital Lane, Twillingate NL A0G 4M0; Saba University (Netherlands Antilles)'08; CCFP; Staff, Notre Dame Bay Memorial Health Centre; (709)884-2131

WHITE, Damian F A; 105-3949 Maple Way, Port Alberni BC V9Y 0B2; Witwatersrand (South Africa)'91; MB ChB; CCFP; (250)723-3581

WHITE, Darrell J; Queen Elizabeth II HSC, 433-1276 South Park St, Halifax NS B3H 2Y9; Dal'91; FRCPC; IntMed; Hem. Staff, Queen Elizabeth II Health Sciences Centre - Victoria General Site; (902)473-7922; Fax. (902)473-4447.

WHITE, David G; 501-1110 Sheppard Ave E, North York ON M2K 2W2; Tor'75; CCFP; CCFP(E.M.); FCFP; Chief Family Med, North York General Hospital; Assoc Prof Family & Commun Med, University of Toronto; (416)223-0555; Fax. (416)223-0540; david.white@utoronto.ca.

WHITE, Debrah L; Westmount Square Hlth Group, HC 180-1 car Westmount, Westmount QC H3Z 2P9; McG'80; MSc; Associé, Sir Mortimer B Davis Jewish General; Langs: French; (514)934-2334 x221; Fax. (514)934-2929.

WHITE, Ernest J; 3 Shadow Dr RR 6, Guelph ON N1H 6J3; Dal'59; FRCSC; OrthSurg. Staff Surg, Guelph General Hospital; (519)822-4911; Fax. (519)822-1970.

WHITE, Frederick A; 481 Park St, Kitchener ON N2G 1N7; Wes'89; FRCPC; IntMed; ClinImmunol&Allergy. Asst Prof IntMed, McMaster University; (519)578-9999; Fax. (519)578-6109.

WHITE, Gail M C; 603-320 March Rd, Kanata ON K2K 2E3; Qns'83; CCFP; FCFP; Staff/Chief Family Med, Queensway Carleton Hospital; (613)591-1780; Fax. (613)591-9219.

WHITE, Gavin J; Western Mem Reg Hosp, PO Box 2005 Stn Main 1 Brookfield Ave, Corner Brook NL A2H 6J7; Dublin (Ireland)'92; BA; FRCS(Eng); FRCR(Eng); MB; BAO; BCh; Staff, Western Memorial Regional Hospital; (709)637-5000

WHITE, Gerald A; Halton HCS Corp-Oakville, 327 Reynolds St, Oakville ON L6J 3L7; Tor'94; FRCPC; Anes. Staff, Halton Healthcare Services Corporation - Oakville Site; (905)845-2571

WHITE, Gill N; Regina Qu'Appelle HR-Regina, 1440 14th Ave, Regina SK S4P 0W5; Sask'75; CCFP; FCFP; Staff College of Medicine, Regina General Hospital; Staff Teacher, University of Saskatchewan; (306)766-3872; Fax. (306)766-4833.

WHITE, Graham D; Glenboro Health Dist Hosp, PO Box 310, Glenboro MB R0K 0X0; (Other Foreign)'70; MB ChB; LMCC; CCFP; Staff, Glenboro Health District Hospital; (204)827-2438; Fax. (204)827-2741.

WHITE, Graham E; Parksville Med Centre, PO Box 250 154 Memorial Ave W, Parksville BC V9P 2G4; Alb'71; BSc; MSc; CCFP; (250)248-5757; Fax. (250)248-2128.

WHITE, Hubert P; Janeway Children's Hlth & Reha, 300 Prince Philip Dr, St. John's NL A1B 3V6; Mem'77; FRCPC; Psy. Staff, Health Sciences Centre; Staff, Janeway Children's Health & Rehabilitation Centre; (709)777-4483

WHITE, Ian S; 1026 5th Ave PO Box 2469, Invermere BC V0A 1K0; Alb'79; CCFP; Langs: German; French.

WHITE, J Patrick; 4291 Gordon Head Rd, Victoria BC V8N 3Y4; Glasgow (Scotland)'67; Dip SportMed(SportMed); (250)592-6640

WHITE, James A; London HSC-University Hosp, PO Box 5339 Stn B C6 124G-339 Windermere Rd, London ON N6A 5A5; Wes'99; FRCPC; IntMed; Cardiol. Staff, London Health Sciences Centre - University Hospital; (519)663-3511; Fax. (519)663-3743.

WHITE, James P; 4291 Gordon Head Rd, Victoria BC V8N 3Y4; Dal'83; FRCSC; OrthSurg. (250)592-6640

WHITE, Jane; Hop Jeffrey Hale, 1250 ch Sainte-Foy, Quebec QC G1S 2M6; Laval'82; FRCPC; DiagRad. Staff, Jeffery Hale Hospital-Saint Brigid's; Staff, Centre Hospitalier Universitaire de Quebec-CHUL; (418)683-4471

WHITE, Jeffrey A; CFB Gagetown, PO Box 17000 Stn Forces, Oromocto NB E2V 4J5; Dal'84; (506)440-2397

WHITE, Jeffrey V; Paradise Wellness, 204-1386 Topsail Rd, Paradise NL A1L 1P6; Mem'90; BMedSci; CCFP; FCFP; (709)782-4123; Fax. (709)782-4120.

WHITE, Jeremy H; Brooke Radiology, 5791 No. 3 Rd, Richmond BC V6X 2C9; UBC'03; FRCPC; DiagRad. (604)278-9151

WHITE, Joanne E; Terrace on The Square, 8-10 Rowan St, St. John's NL A1B 2X3; Mem'03; FRCSC; ObstGyn. Locum Tenens, Labrador Health Centre; (709)739-6004

WHITE, Jonathan S; Royal Alexandra Hosp, 409 CSC-10240 Kingsway, Edmonton AB T5H 3V9; (United Kingdom)'93; FRCSC; GenSurg. Staff, Royal Alexandra Hospital; (780)735-5147; Fax. (780)735-5459.

WHITE, Juliet; 2 Lyall Ave, Toronto ON M4E 1V8; Tor'72; CCFP; FCFP; (416)699-9823; Fax. (416)699-0459.

WHITE, K Bruce; Brandon Reg Health Centre, 150 McTavish Ave E, Brandon MB R7A 2B3; Dal'86; FRCPC; Anes. Staff Pre-Anaesthetic Clinic, Brandon Regional Health Centre; (204)726-1122; Fax. (204)728-0528.

WHITE, Keith J; Medi-Kel Med Clinic, PO Box 2100 Rpo Banks Centre, Kelowna BC V1X 4K5; Glasgow (Scotland)'77; MB ChB; (250)862-4996

WHITE, Kimberley D; Community Mental Health, 109-7071 Bayers Rd, Halifax NS B3L 2C2; Mem'91; FRCPC; Psy. Staff Psy, Community Mental Health Program; (902)454-1400; Fax. (902)454-1434.

WHITE, Laurie J; Medical & Dental Bldg, 108-1849 Yonge St, Toronto ON M4S 1Y2; Qns'79; (416)481-6103; Fax. (416)481-6104.

WHITE, Lawrence M; Mount Sinai Hosp, 562-600 University Ave, Toronto ON M5G 1X5; Tor'89; FRCPC; DiagRad (Musculoskeletal Imaging). Staff, Toronto General Hospital - UHN; Staff, Mount Sinai Hospital; University of Toronto; (416)586-4800 x5231; Fax. (416)586-8695; lwhite@mtsinai.on.ca.

WHITE, Lisa A; U of Ottawa Health Services, PO Box 450 Stn A 300-100 Marie Curie Pvt, Ottawa ON K1N 1A2; McG'91; CCFP; FCFP; Langs: English; French; (613)564-3950; Fax. (613)564-6627.

WHITE, M Edward; Sherwood Family Med Centre, 15 Brackley Point Rd, Charlottetown PE C1A 6Y1; Wes'92; CCFP; FCFP; Physician, Sherwood Family Medical Centre; Langs: English; French; (902)367-3747; Fax. (902)367-3748.

WHITE, Margaret A; Carleton Univ Health Services, 2600-1125 Colonel By Dr, Ottawa ON K1S 5B6; McM'90; Dip SportMed(SportMed); CCFP; FCFP; (613)520-6674; Fax. (613)520-3851.

WHITE, Martin N; 68 Bridge St, Carleton Place ON K7C 2V3; Ott'72; Staff, Almonte General Hospital; Staff, Carleton Place & District Memorial Hospital; (613)257-4793; Fax. (613)257-4794.

WHITE, Mary E; Queen Elizabeth Hosp, PO Box 6600 Stn Central 60 Riverside Dr, Charlottetown PE C1A 8T5; Alb'03; FRCPC; DiagRad. Staff, Queen Elizabeth Hospital; (902)894-2111

WHITE, Maureen E; Halifax Prof Centre, 420-5991 Spring Garden Rd, Halifax NS B3H 1Y6; Mem'86; CCFP; FCFP; (902)429-6958; Fax. (902)422-4996; mewhite@ns.sympatico.ca.

WHITE, Michael L; Colchester East Hants Hlth Ctr, 600 Abenaki Rd, Truro NS B2N 5A1; London (England)'70; MB BS; DCH; FRCP; FRCPC; Peds (Psychiatry). Clin Associate Child & Adolesc Psy, Colchester East Hants Health Centre; (902)893-5554; Fax. (902)835-2127.

WHITE, Michel B; Hop Ste-Anne, 305 boul Anciens-Combattants, Ste-Anne-de-Bellev QC H9X 1Y9; Mon'93; FRCPC; Psy (Geriatric Psychiatry). Staff, Hopital Ste-Anne; (514)457-3440 x3200

WHITE, Michel; Institut de Cardiologie de Mtl, 5000 rue Belanger, Montreal QC H1T 1C8; Laval'83; FACC; FRCPC; IntMed (Hypertension); Cardiol. Staff, Institut de Cardiologie de Montréal; assoc Prof Med, Universite de Montreal; (514)376-3330 x3935; Fax. (514)593-2575.

WHITE, Nancy A; Peterborough Reg HC-Hospital, 1 Hospital Dr, Peterborough ON K9J 7C6; McM'89; Dip SportMed(SportMed); CCFP; CCFP(E.M.); FCFP; Staff, Peterborough Regional Health Centre - Hospital Drive; Med Dir, Centre for Sports Medicine; (705)876-5022

WHITE, Naomi; Dr Everett Chalmers Reg Hosp, PO Box 9000 Stn A 700 Priestman St, Fredericton NB E3B 5N5; Dal'02; CCFP; Staff, Dr Everett Chalmers Regional Hospital; (506)447-4444

WHITE, Neil G; 201-836 1 Ave NW, Airdrie AB T4B 0V2; Cal'85; CCFP; Clin Lecturer, University of Calgary; (403)948-6422; Fax. (403)948-4492.

WHITE, Neil J; Foothills Med Centre, G33K-1403 29 St NW, Calgary AB T2N 2T9; UBC'04; FRCSC; OrthSurg. Staff, Foothills Medical Centre; Staff, University of Calgary; (403)220-3366; Fax. (403)220-1185.

WHITE, Nicholas; 4539 Marine Ave, Powell River BC V8A 2K5; UBC'91; (604)485-9200; Fax. (604)485-2633.

WHITE, Norman F; Coast Specialists Office, 103-5631 Inlet Ave, Sechelt BC V0N 3A0; McG'62; DPsy; MDCM; Psy (Behavioural Medicine). Emeritus Prof, McMaster University; (604)885-4826; Fax. (604)885-4856.

WHITE, Owen J; Mountain Med Clinic, PO Box 1660, Neepawa MB R0J 1H0; London (England)'72; Staff, Neepawa District Memorial Hospital; (204)476-3381; Fax. (204)476-2156; owhite@arha.ca.

WHITE, Patrick J; Alberta Hospital Edmonton, PO Box 307, Edmonton AB T5J 2J7; National (Ireland)'76; MB ChB; BAO; MRCPsy(UK); Staff, University of Alberta Hospital; Staff, Alberta Hospital Edmonton; Reg Prog Dir Mental Health, Capital Mental Health Authority; Staff Psy, Alberta Mental Health Services; Dept Chair Psy, University of Alberta; (780)342-5456; Fax. (780)342-5368; patrickwhite@cha.ab.ca.

WHITE, Paula M; Centre Hosp Baie-des-Chaleurs, RR 2 419 boul Perron, Maria QC G0C 1Y0; Ott'85; Staff, CSSS de la Baie-des-Chaleurs; Médecin, Clinique des Medecins New-Richmond; Langs: Bilingual(French/English); (418)759-3443

WHITE, Philip; Philip A White Ltd, 203-285 Aurora Cres, Kelowna BC V1X 7N6; London (England)'69; MB BS; CCFP; Staff, Kelowna General Hospital; Med Dir Family Med, BC Cancer Agency Sindi Ahluwalia Hawkins Centre for the Southern Interior; Med Dir/Chair, Family Practice Oncology Network; (250)765-3139; Fax. (250)765-9015.

WHITE, Randall F; Detwiller Pavilion, 2255 Wesbrook Mall, Vancouver BC V6T 2A1; Emoy(GA) (USA)'86; FRCPC; Psy. Staff, Providence Health Care - St Paul's Hospital; Clin Instructor, University of British Columbia; (604)822-7546

WHITE, Richard A; The Peterborough Clinic, 26 Hospital Dr, Peterborough ON K9J 7C3; McG'73; FRCPC; Peds. Ac Staff, Peterborough Regional Health Centre - Hospital Drive; Langs: English; French; (705)740-6845; Fax. (705)740-6897.

WHITE, Robert J; Edson Med Centre, PO Box 6660 Stn Main, Edson AB T7E 1V1; Birmingham (England)'78; (780)723-3366; Fax. (780)723-3437.

WHITE, Robert J; Vanier Med Centre, 9-325 Vanier Blvd, Bathurst NB E2A 3N1; Ott'72; Staff, Hopital Regional Chaleur; (506)546-9263

WHITE, Robert W; Surrey Pediatric Associates, 103-13710 94A Ave, Surrey BC V3V 1N1; Cal'81; FRCPC; Peds. Clin Instructor, University of British Columbia; (604)583-7070; Fax. (604)582-5536.

WHITE, Roger T; Lethbridge Centre Mall, 239-200 4 Ave S, Lethbridge AB T1J 4C9; Alb'08; CCFP; (403)942-0800; Fax. (403)942-0799.

WHITE, Rosemary A; 120-2751 Gladstone St, Halifax NS B3K 4W6; Dal'74; (902)423-8950; Fax. (902)423-6009.

WHITE, Samuel A; Associated Anaes Services, M2A-601 Broadway W, Vancouver BC V5Z 4C2; Belfast (Ireland)'73; FRCPC; Anes. Ac Staff Anes, Vancouver General Hospital - Centennial Pavillion; (604)874-5291

WHITE, Sandra L; Western Med Clinic, 144 6th St, Brandon MB R7A 3N2; Witwatersrand (South Africa)'80; MB ChB; (204)727-6451; Fax. (204)727-4150.

WHITE, Stephen F; Lennox & Addington Gen Hosp, 8 Richmond Park Dr, Napanee ON K7R 2Z4; Qns'93; CCFP; CCFP(E.M.); Staff, Lennox & Addington County General Hospital; (613)354-3301

WHITE, Valerie A; Vancouver Gen Hosp, 855 12th Ave W, Vancouver BC V5Z 1M9; Mem'79; FRCPC; GenPath; AnatPath. Staff Path, Vancouver General Hospital - Centennial Pavillion; Teach Staff, University of British Columbia; (604)875-4111

WHITE, Wendy L; Edmonton Garrison Hlth Serv Ct, PO Box 10500 Stn Forces, Edmonton AB T5J 4J5; UBC'87; FRCPC; Psy (Trauma). Staff Psy Outpatient Dept, Sturgeon Community Hospital; Physician, Edmonton Garrison Health Services Centre; (780)973-4011; Fax. (780)973-1496.

WHITE, William D; Foothills Med Centre, C203-1403 29 St NW, Calgary AB T2N 2T9; Cal'99; FRCPC; Psy (Addiction Psychiatry). Consultant Psy, Foothills Medical Centre; Asst Prof Med, University of Calgary; (403)944-1322; Fax. (403)944-2165; william.white@albertahealthservices.ca.

WHITE-GUAY, Brian; Clinique de Med Familiale, 6e-2120 rue Sherbrooke E, Montreal QC H2K 1C3; Laval'76; FRCPC; CommunMed (Family Medicine); Public Health & Preventive Med. Prof, Universite de Montreal; (514)527-1958; Fax. (514)527-1649.

WHITEACRE, Laura L; York-Finch Med Centre, 411-2115 Finch Ave W, North York ON M3N 2V6; McM'81; BSc; FRCSC; GenSurg. Ac Staff, Humber River Regional Hospital - Finch Avenue Site; Langs: Italian; (416)740-3949; Fax. (416)740-6734.

WHITEHALL, Jeffrey D; Market Place Medical, 47-218 Catharine St, Port Colborne ON L3K 4K8; Qns'90; CCFP; FCFP; (905)834-5855; Fax. (905)835-5833.

WHITEHEAD, Cheryl L; Mount Royal Univ Hlth Services, 4825 Mount Royal Gate SW, Calgary AB T3E 6K6; Sask'74; CCFP; FCFP; Physician Health Services, Mount Royal University; (403)440-6326; Fax. (403)440-6759.

WHITEHEAD, Cynthia R; Women's College Hosp, 76 Grenville St, Toronto ON M5S 1B1; McM'87; CCFP; FCFP; Staff, Toronto Rehabilitation Institute - University Centre; Staff, Women's College Hospital; University of Toronto; (416)323-6060

WHITEHEAD, Jeffrey J; Cdn Forces Health Protection, 1745 Alta Vista Dr, Ottawa ON K1A 0K6; Ott'81; FRCPC; CommunMed (Public Health). Dir DGHS-DND, Canadian Forces Health Services Centre; Aj Prof Epidemiol & Commun Med, University of Ottawa; (613)945-8062 x3984; Fax. (613)945-6823.

WHITEHEAD, Katherine E A; Toronto East Gen Hosp Inc, 825 Coxwell Ave, Toronto ON M4C 3E7; Qns'02; CCFP; CCFP(E.M.); Staff Complex Continuing Care, Toronto East General Hospital Inc; (416)461-8272

WHITEHEAD, Kristine M; Somerset West Comm Hlth Ctre, 55 Eccles St, Ottawa ON K1R 6S3; Tor'92; BSc; CCFP; FCFP; Physician, Somerset West Community Health Centre; Asst Prof, University of Ottawa; (613)238-1220; Fax. (613)235-2982; kwhitehead@swchc.on.ca.

WHITEHEAD, Lori N; St Joseph's Healthcare, T2124-50 Charlton Ave E, Hamilton ON L8N 4A6; Tor'85; FCCP; FRCPC; IntMed (Tuberculosis); Respir. Med Staff Firestone Institute of Respiratory Health, St Joseph's Healthcare - Charlton Campus; Clin Assoc Prof Med, McMaster University; (905)521-6000; Fax. (905)521-6183; lwhitehe@stjosham.on.ca.

WHITEHEAD, Michael J; Royal Inland Hosp, 311 Columbia St, Kamloops BC V2C 2T1; Cape Town (South Africa)'76; MB ChB; FRCPC; Anes. Staff, Royal Inland Hospital; Langs: Afrikaans; (250)314-2620

WHITEHEAD, Stephen M; Public Health Services, 101-310 Idylwyld Dr N, Saskatoon SK S7L 0Z2; Leeds (England)'75; MB ChB; Dep Med Officer of Hlth, Public Health Services; (306)655-4765; Fax. (306)655-4414; steve.whitehead@saskatoon.healthregion.ca.

WHITEHILL, Kellie J; 330-507 Broadway W, Vancouver BC V5Z 1E6; Man'04; FRCSC; ObstGyn. Staff ObstGyn, BC Women's Hospital & Health Centre; (604)872-5484; kwhitehill@cw.bc.ca.

WHITEHOUSE, Sandra R; Children's & Women's HC of BC, A248-4480 Oak St, Vancouver BC V6H 3V4; Sydney (Australia)'79; FRCPC; Peds (Adolescent Health Care). Staff, BC Children's Hospital; (604)875-2970

WHITELEGG, Geraldine M; Vancouver Coastal Hlth Travel, L5-601 Broadway W, Vancouver BC V5Z 4C2; UBC'82; Staff, Vancouver Coastal Health; (604)736-9244

WHITEMAN, Avram D; Clinique Roper, 4500 rue Sherbrooke O, Montreal QC H3Z 1E6; Laval'87; MPH; FCBOM; FACOEM; CCFP; FCFP; Staff, St Mary's Hospital Centre; Att Staff, Donald Berman Maimonides Geriatric Centre; Dir Occup Health Services, Merck Frosst Canada Ltd; Staff, McGill University Health Centre; Staff, Clinique Roper; adj Prof, McGill University; Langs: Bilingual(English/French); (514)937-8000

WHITEMAN, Donald W; 67 Ontario St, Trenton ON K8V 2G8; Alb'69; BSc; DABOph; FRCSC; Ophth. Ac Staff Ophth., QHC Trenton Memorial; (613)394-4545; Fax. (613)394-5048.

WHITESIDE, Catharine I; Univ Hlth Network-Toronto Gen, 8N 845-200 Elizabeth St, Toronto ON M5G 2C4; Tor'75; PhD; FRCPC; IntMed; Nephrol. Staff, Toronto General Hospital - UHN; Dean Faculty of Med/Vice Provost Relations w/ Health Care Inst, University of Toronto; (416)340-4140; Fax. (416)586-9827; catharine.whiteside@utoronto.ca.

WHITFIELD, Bobbi-Jo; Medicine Hat Reg Hosp, 666 5 St SW, Medicine Hat AB T1A 4H6; Cal'00; CCFP; Staff Maternity Clinic, Medicine Hat Regional Hospital; Physician, Palliser Health Authority; (403)502-8644; Fax. (403)528-8123; bobbi-jo.whitfield@cls.ab.ca.

WHITFIELD, Margaret D; 60 Lascelles Blvd, Toronto ON M5P 2E2; Qns'66; DPsy; FRCPC; Psy (Child & Adolescent Psychiatry). (416)481-7510; Fax. (416)481-7510.

WHITFIELD, Michael F; Children's & Women's HC of BC, 1R47-4480 Oak St, Vancouver BC V6H 3V4; Edinburgh (Scotland)'70; MB BS; FRCPC; Peds (Neonatology). Staff Neonatol, BC Children's Hospital; University of British Columbia; (604)875-2135; Fax. (604)875-3106; mwhitfield@cw.bc.ca.

WHITFORD, Amber L L; Central Alberta Prof Centre, 279-5201 43 St, Red Deer AB T4N 1C7; Alb'06; ObstGyn. (403)347-1114; Fax. (403)347-1116.

WHITING, David A; 103-3040 Tutt St, Kelowna BC V1Y 2H5; Cape Town (South Africa)'84; MB ChB; DCH; CCFP; FCFP; (250)860-1622; Fax. (250)762-9051.

WHITING, Natalie M; Royal Jubilee Hospl, 1952 Bay St, Victoria BC V8R 1J8; Qns'96; CCFP; Staff, Royal Jubilee Hospital; Langs: French; (250)370-8715

WHITING, Sharon E; Children's Hosp Eastern Ont, 401 Smyth Rd, Ottawa ON K1H 8L1; West Indies (Jamaica)'77; MB BS; FRCPC; Peds (Pediatric Neurology); Neur. Staff, Children's Hospital of Eastern Ontario (CHEO); Vice Dean Health/Hospital Services, University of Ottawa; Langs: English; French; (613)737-2605; Fax. (613)738-4879.

WHITING, Wilma G; Lakeridge Hlth Corp-Oshawa, 1 Hospital Crt, Oshawa ON L1G 2B9; Tor'83; FRCPC; Anes. Staff, Lakeridge Health - Oshawa Site; Langs: Bilingual(English/French); (905)576-8711 x3237; Fax. (905)721-4848.

WHITLEY, Carol L; 29136 Townshipline Rd, Abbotsford BC V4X 1S1; Wes'77.

WHITLEY, Susan A; Rideau Valley Health Services, 1221 Greenbank Rd, Ottawa ON K2J 5V7; Qns'95; CCFP; FCFP; Court Staff Privil, The Ottawa Hospital - Civic Campus; Langs: English; French; (613)258-8710; Fax. (613)440-3238.

WHITLOCK, James A; The Hosp for Sick Children, 555 University Ave, Toronto ON M5G 1X8; Dal'81; Div Head Haematology/Oncology/Chair Women's Auxiliary Millennium, The Hospital For Sick Children; (416)813-8885; Fax. (416)813-5327; jim.whitlock@sickkids.ca.

WHITLOCK, Pierre; Dr L Richard Centre d'Oncologi, 37 rue Providence, Moncton NB E1C 8X3; Mon'92; FRCPC; IntMed; MedOncol; Hem. Staff HemOncol, Dr Leon Richard Oncology Centre; Prof, Universite de Sherbrooke; Langs: Bilingual(French/English); (506)862-4030; Fax. (506)862-4222.

WHITLOCK, Richard P; Hamilton HS-General Site, C1 114-237 Barton St E, Hamilton ON L8L 2X2; Tor'01; BSc; MSc; FRCSC; CardSurg; Critical Care Medicine. Asst Prof Surg Cardiac Surg & Critical Care, Hamilton Health Sciences Centre - Hamilton General Hospital; Asst Prof Surg, McMaster University; (905)527-4322; Fax. (905)577-8017.

WHITMAN, Lucinda A; Health Sciences Centre, 1518B-300 Prince Philip Dr, St. John's NL A1B 3V6; Mem'80; FRCPC; Hem. Staff, Health Sciences Centre; Assoc Prof Path & Med, Memorial University Of Newfoundland; (709)777-6550

WHITMAN, Richard J; Atwood Med Clinic, 101-143 Fourth Ave S, Williams Lake BC V2G 1J8; Birmingham (England)'69; MB ChB; (250)398-5162; Fax. (250)398-5673.

WHITMORE, Christine A; King Street Med Arts Centre, 401-71 King St W, Mississauga ON L5B 4A2; Qns'85; CCFP; FCFP; Staff, Trillium Health Centre - Mississauga; (905)273-9793; Fax. (905)273-7054.

WHITMORE, Nancy A; Hasegawa Clinic, 156 Waterloo St S, Stratford ON N5A 4B4; Man'87; FAB; MBA; FRCSC; ObstGyn (Administration). (519)271-2822; Fax. (519)271-8533.

WHITNEY, Brenda J; Promenade Village Shoppes, 35-7700 Bathurst St, Thornhill ON L4J 7Y3; Ott'79; CCFP; FCFP; Court Staff, Mackenzie Richmond Hill Hospital; (905)881-6510; Fax. (905)881-6513.

WHITNEY, Diane K; Ridgeway Clinic, 1001 Ridgeway St E, Thunder Bay ON P7E 5H8; Wes'88; FRCPC; Psy (Women's Issues). Staff, Thunder Bay Regional Health Sciences Centre; Asst Prof, University of Western Ontario; Asst Prof, University of Toronto; (807)622-0601; Fax. (807)623-0470.

WHITNEY, J David; Brameast Family Health Org, 38-2130 North Park Dr, Brampton ON L6S 0C9; Tor'74; Ac Staff, William Osler Health System - Brampton Civic Hospital; (905)792-2211; Fax. (905)792-2901.

WHITNEY, Nermin A; King Street Med Arts Centre, 401-71 King St W, Mississauga ON L5B 4A2; Tor'05; CCFP; (905)273-9793; Fax. (905)273-7054.

WHITSITT, Paul F; Durham College Campus Hlth Ctr, SS 201 2000 Simcoe St N, Oshawa ON L1H 7K4; Wes'84; Staff, Lakeridge Health - Oshawa Site; Physician, Provax Travel & Immunization Clinic; Staff Campus Health Centre, Durham College; (905)721-3037

WHITTAKER, Brianne J; Rockyview Maternity & Family P, 258-1011 Glenmore Trail SW, Calgary AB T2V 4R6; Alb'09; CCFP; Staff Low Risk Obst, Rockyview General Hospital; (403)640-0600; Fax. (403)253-0124.

WHITTAKER, David; Port McNeill Med Centre, 2161 McNeill Rd Box 14, Port Mcneill BC V0N 2R0; (Other Foreign)'08; (250)956-3377

WHITTAKER, Elizabeth I; Markham Prof Centre, 307-2265 Pembina Hwy, Winnipeg MB R3T 5J3; Qns'83; (204)275-3769; Fax. (204)269-6574.

WHITTAKER, J Scott; Pacific Gastroenterology Assoc, 770-1190 Hornby St, Vancouver BC V6Z 2K5; UBC'76; FRCPC; Gastroent (Nutrition); IntMed. Staff, Providence Health Care - St Paul's Hospital; Clinical Asst Prof, University of British Columbia; Langs: Bilingual(English/French); (604)688-6332; Fax. (604)689-2004.

WHITTAKER, John S; Pacific Gastroenterology Assoc, 770-1190 Hornby St, Vancouver BC V6Z 2K5; Edinburgh (England)'50; (604)688-6332

WHITTAKER, Mark E; Dingwall Med Group, PO Box 3011 Stn Main, Dryden ON P8N 2Z6; Man'89; BSc(Med); MSc; CCFP; FCFP; Staff, Dryden Regional Health Centre; Asst Prof, Northern Ontario School of Medicine-Laurentian University; (807)223-2258; Fax. (807)223-4733.

WHITTAKER, R Bryn; Auxillary Nursing Home, 14225 94 St NW, Edmonton AB T5E 6C6; Dundee (Scotland)'74; MB ChB; CCFP; FCFP; Staff, Capital Care - Dickinsfield; Physician, Auxillary Nursing Home; Asst Prof Clinical, University of Alberta; (780)496-7581; Fax. (780)496-7584.

WHITTAKER, Stephen; Spratt Med Centre, 1-4188 Spratt Rd, Gloucester ON K1V 0Z6; Tor'85; CCFP; Asst Prof Family Med, University of Ottawa; (613)822-2363; Fax. (613)822-1838.

WHITTAKER, Stuart J; Canadian Forces Base Health Se, PO Box 17000 Stn Forces, Victoria BC V9B 1T2; Dal'09; CCFP; Staff, Canadian Forces Health Services; (250)363-5616

WHITTEMORE, N Blair; MUHC-Montreal Children's Hosp, B336-2300 rue Tupper, Montreal QC H3H 1P3; McG'60; FRCPC; IntMed; Hem (P.Q.). Dir Hem Labs, McGill University Health Centre - Montreal General Campus; Langs: English; French; (514)412-4322; Fax. (514)412-4338; blair.whittemore@muhc.mcgill.ca.

WHITTEN-STOVALL, Richard F; Albany Med Clinic, 807 Broadview Ave, Toronto ON M4K 2P8; Emory University (USA)'77; (416)461-9471

WHITTICK, John D R; Victoria East Med Clinic, 2068 Prince of Wales Dr, Regina SK S4V 3A6; Aberdeen (Scotland)'71; CCFP; FCFP; Staff, Regina General Hospital; Staff, Pasqua Hospital; Physician, Victoria East Medical Clinic; (306)789-4677; Fax. (306)789-3422.

WHITTIER, Michael J; 72 Governors Rd E RR 1, Paris ON N3L 3E1; Tor'81; FRCPC; Anes. (519)448-1005

WHITTINGHAM, Heather A; Hamilton HS-General Site, 415-237 Barton St E, Hamilton ON L8L 2X2; Qns'02; FRCPC; IntMed; Critical Care Medicine. Staff McMaster Clinic, Hamilton Health Sciences Centre - Hamilton General Hospital; (905)527-0271

WHITTINGHAM, Jennifer M; Thunder Bay Reg HSC, 980 Oliver Rd, Thunder Bay ON P7B 6V4; McM'05; FRCPC; Anes. Staff, Thunder Bay Regional Health Sciences Centre; (807)684-6000

WHITTINGTON, Christine A; 100-33774 Marshall Rd, Abbotsford BC V2S 1L1; Queensland (Australia)'79; FABFACRRM; CCFP; FCFP; Staff, Abbotsford Regional Hospital & Cancer Centre; Clin Assoc Prof Family Pract, University of British Columbia; (604)853-2611; Fax. (604)853-2659.

WHITTLE, Daniel J; 2000-1415 1st Ave E, Owen Sound ON N4K 4K8; Tor'86; Staff, Grey Bruce Health Services - Owen Sound; (519)470-3030; Fax. (519)470-3035.

WHITTOM, Renaud; Hop du Sacre-Coeur de Mtl, 5400 boul Gouin O, Montreal QC H4J 1C5; Laval'85; FRCPC; IntMed; MedOncol; Hem. Staff, Hôpital du Sacre-Coeur de Montréal; Prof adj clin, Universite de Montreal; (514)338-2050; Fax. (514)338-2631; renaudw@globetrotter.qc.ca.

WHITTOM, Serge; CHUQ-Hotel-Dieu de Quebec, 11 Cote du Palais, Quebec QC G1R 2J6; Laval'83; Endocrin (P.Q.); IntMed. Staff, Centre Hospitalier Universitaire de Québec (CHUQ) - Siege Social; (418)691-5016

WHITTOM, Steve; Hotel-Dieu de Levis, 143 rue Wolfe, Levis QC G6V 3Z1; Laval'91; Gastroent; IntMed. Staff, Hôtel-Dieu de Lévis; (418)835-7121

WHITTON, Anthony C; The Juravinski Cancer Centre, 699 Concession St, Hamilton ON L8V 5C2; London (England)'78; FRCR; BSc(Hon); MB; BS; FRCPC; RadOncol (Neuro Oncology). Ac Staff, Hamilton Health Sciences Centre-Juravinski Site; Prof Oncology & Peds, McMaster University; (905)387-9711 x64706; Fax. (905)575-6326; anthony.whitton@jcc.hhsc.ca.

WHITTON, Joel L; Medical Arts Bldg, 602-1200 Bay St, Toronto ON M5R 2A5; Tor'72; PhD(MedSci); FRCPC; Psy (Endocrinology). Member United Nations, World Health Organization; Lecturer Medicina Alternativa, Open International University; (416)963-9238; joelwhitton@ctp.net.

WHITTY, C Dennis; 249 Carlton St, St Catharines ON L2N 1B6; Tor'76; MSc; PhD; Staff, Niagara Health System - St Catharines General Site; Staff, Niagara Health System - Ontario Street Site; (905)934-3730; Fax. (905)934-2737; dwhitty@cogeco.net.

WHITTY, Tina M; Royal Victoria Hosp, 201 Georgian Dr, Barrie ON L4M 6M2; Mem'97; FRCPC; Anes. Ac Staff, Royal Victoria Regional Health Centre; (705)728-9802; Fax. (705)726-0822.

WHITTY, Wanda S; Heritage Med Clinic, PO Box 235, Holyrood NL A0A 2R0; Mem'93; CCFP; FCFP; (709)229-7779; Fax. (709)229-7772.

WHYLIE, Barbara; Canadian Cancer Society, 200-10 Alcorn Ave, Toronto ON M4V 3B1; Belfast (Ireland)'65; MB ChB; BAO; Dir Cancer Control Policy, National Cancer Institute of Canada; Dir, Canadian Cancer Society; (416)961-7223; Fax. (416)961-4189; barbara.whylie@uhn.on.ca.

WHYNE, Mitchell S; Royal Victoria Hosp, 201 Georgian Dr, Barrie ON L4M 6M2; Tor'83; CASM(SportsMed); Chief EmergMed, Royal Victoria Regional Health Centre; (705)728-9802 x4121

WHYNOT, Andrew S; 428 St George St, London ON N6A 3B3; Tor'88; CCFP; CCFP(E.M.); FCFP; Staff, Strathroy Middlesex General Hospital - Middlesex Hospital Alliance; (519)702-6271; Fax. (519)439-8718.

WHYNOT, Elizabeth M; 14-6417 Fraser St, Vancouver BC V5W 4B5; Qns'72; CCFP; Pres, BC Women's Hospital & Health Centre; Court Staff, UBC Hospital - Koerner Pavillion; Sr Physician Prog. Support, Children & Women's Health Centre; Clin Instructor Family Pract/Teach Staff, University of British Columbia; (604)805-2068; ewhynot@cw.bc.ca.

WHYTE, Hilary E A; The Hosp for Sick Children, 3898-555 University Ave, Toronto ON M5G 1X8; Dublin (Ireland)'76; MB BCh; BAO; DCH; MSc; FRCPC; Peds (Neonatology). Staff, The Hospital For Sick Children; Med Dir Paediatric, O R N G E (Air Ambulance); (416)813-8829; Fax. (416)813-5245; hilary.whyte@sickkids.ca.

WHYTE, James F H; Medical Clinic Renson Physco, 403-265 Yorkland Blvd, North York ON M2J 5C7; McM'07; CCFP; Assoc Prof, Northern Ontario School of Medicine-Laurentian University; Assoc Prof, Tyndale University College & Seminary; (416)229-2399; Fax. (416)229-9771.

WHYTE, Jennifer A; Family Med Centre, 103-7143 West Saanich Rd, Saanichton BC V8M 1P7; UBC'91; CCFP; (250)652-9191; Fax. (250)652-5576.

WHYTE, Laura M; Cape Breton Reg Hosp, 1482 George St, Sydney NS B1P 1P3; Dal'09; CCFP; Staff, Cape Breton Healthcare Complex; (902)565-8953

WHYTE, Robert A; Faculty of Health Sciences, MDCL 3106-1280 Main St W, Hamilton ON L8S 4K1; McM'97; FRCPC; Anes. Staff, Hamilton Health Sciences Centre - McMaster Children's Hospital; Chair Undergraduate MD Program, McMaster University; (905)525-9140; Fax. (905)546-0349.

WHYTE, Robin K; 5850-5980 University Ave PO Box 9700 Rpo CSC, Halifax NS B3K 6R8; London (England)'70; BSc; MB BS; MRCP(UK); FAAP; FRCP; FRCPC; Peds (Neonatology). Staff Neonatal Ped, IWK Health Centre; Prof, Dalhousie University; (902)470-6466; Fax. (902)470-6938; robin.whyte@dal.ca.

WHYTE, Simon D; Children's & Women's HC of BC, 1L7-4480 Oak St, Vancouver BC V6H 3V4; Newcastle-Upon-Tyne (England)'94; Staff, BC Children's Hospital; (604)875-2711; Fax. (604)875-3221.

WHYTE, Stanley L; Seven Oaks Gen Hosp, 2300 McPhillips St, Winnipeg MB R2V 3M3; Man'92; Staff Emerg, Seven Oaks General Hospital; Staff Emerg, The Salvation Army Grace Hospital; Lecturer Emerg Med, University of Manitoba; (204)632-7133; Fax. (204)694-8276.

WHYTE, Tanya R; Canadian Forces Hlth Services, PO Box 99000 Stn Forces, Halifax NS B3K 5X5; Alb'06; (902)721-8700; Fax. (902)721-8866.

WIATROWSKA, Beata A; Royal Ottawa Mental Hlth Ctr, 1145 Carling Ave, Ottawa ON K1Z 7K4; Wroclaw (Poland)'89; FRCPC; AnatPath (Cytopath); Psy. Staff, Royal Ottawa Mental Health Centre - Royal Ottawa Health Care Group; Langs: Polish; (613)722-6521 x6501

WIATROWSKI, Joe F K; Salvation Army Grace Gen Hosp, 300 Booth Dr, Winnipeg MB R3J 3M7; Man'85; CCFP; CCFP(E.M.); FCFP; Dir Emerg, The Salvation Army Grace Hospital; University of Manitoba; (204)837-8311; jwiatrow@ggh.mb.ca.

WICENTOVICH, Lana M; Haig Clinic, 601 6 Ave S, Lethbridge AB T1J 0Z2; Man'01; CCFP; (403)328-6641; Fax. (403)328-6118.

WICHOLAS, Bertrand L; Children's & Women's HC of BC, 4500 Oak St, Vancouver BC V6H 3N1; Yale (USA)'03; FRCPC; Psy. Staff, BC Women's Hospital & Health Centre; (604)875-2345; bwicholas@cw.bc.ca.

WICHOLAS, Leslie; Children's & Women's HC of BC, B321-4480 Oak St, Vancouver BC V6H 3V4; Cal'98; FRCPC; Psy. Staff, BC Children's Hospital; Staff, BC Women's Hospital & Health Centre; (604)875-2345 x7415

WICKENS, Courtney M; West London Family Hlth Clinic, 200-785 Wonderland Rd S, London ON N6K 1M6; McM'09; CCFP; Staff, University of Western Ontario; (519)641-6712

WICKENS, Jennifer K; McKenzie Prof Centre, 201-1595 McKenzie Ave, Victoria BC V8N 1A4; UBC'91; CCFP; Physician, Royal Oak Centre Medical Clinic Ltd; (250)721-1188; Fax. (250)727-2292.

WICKERT, John C; Shuswap Lake Gen Hosp, PO Box 520 Stn Main 601 10 St NE, Salmon Arm BC V1E 4N6; Alb'80; FRCPC; DiagRad. Staff, Shuswap Lake General Hospital; Staff, Queen Victoria Hospital; (250)833-3600; Fax. (250)833-3628; dr.john.wickert@interiorhealth.ca.

WICKERT, Wayne A; Yorkton Reg Health Centre, 270 Bradbrooke Dr, Yorkton SK S3N 2K6; Alb'76; FRCPC; IntMed; Critical Care Medicine. Staff IntMed, Yorkton Regional Health Centre; (306)782-2401

WICKETT, Claire F; Glenmore Landing, PO Box 72066 1600 90 Ave SW, Calgary AB T2V 5A8; Cal'04; CCFP.

WICKETT, Jamie A E; Thames Valley FHT-Victoria Fam, 60 Chesley Ave, London ON N5Z 2C1; UBC'04; CCFP; (519)433-8424; Fax. (519)433-5796.

WICKETT, Robert G; Grand River Hosp KW Hlth Ctr, PO Box 9056 Stn C 835 King St W, Kitchener ON N2G 1G3; Wes'99; CCFP; CCFP(E.M.); Staff, Grand River Hospital - Kitchener/Waterloo Health Centre; (519)749-4300

WICKHAM, David; RCSC Inc, 2-2168 McCallum Rd, Abbotsford BC V2S 6R6; UBC'82; FRCSC; OrthSurg. Staff, Chilliwack General Hospital; Staff, Abbotsford Regional Hospital & Cancer Centre; (604)853-3381; Fax. (604)853-8096.

WICKHAM, Michael R; Canmore Gen Hosp, 1100 Hospital Place, Canmore AB T1W 1N2; Cal'94; CCFP; CCFP(E.M.); Staff, Canmore General Hospital; (403)678-5536; Fax. (403)678-5069.

WICKLAND-WELLER, Monica L; Rimbey Med Clinic, PO Box 650, Rimbey AB T0C 2J0; Alb'85; (403)843-2256; Fax. (403)843-2255.

WICKLOW, Brandy A; Diabetes Education Resource, FE307-685 William Ave, Winnipeg MB R3E 0Z2; Man'03; FRCPC; Peds; Endocrin&Metab.

WICKLUM, Sonja C; Pure North S'Energy Foundation, 800-326 11 Ave SW, Calgary AB T2R 0C5; Cal'92; CCFP; FCFP; Langs: English; French; (403)457-5077

WICKMAN, Marlene S; Cross Roads Clinics, 350-507 Broadway W, Vancouver BC V5Z 1E6; Man'95; BSc(Hons.); BSc(Med.); CCFP; Staff, Cross Roads Clinics; (604)568-7229

WICKRAMA, Thamara; The Moncton Hosp, 135 MacBeath Ave, Moncton NB E1C 6Z8; Colombo (Sri Lanka)'79; Staff, The Moncton Hospital; (506)857-5111

WICKRAMASINGHE, Senani D; McConnell Med Centre, 209-820 Mcconnell Ave, Cornwall ON K6H 4M4; Colombo (Sri Lanka)'68; MB BS; FRCPC; Peds. Langs: Sinhalese; (613)933-8160

WICKREMASINGHE, Lalya S; Reach Comm Health Centre, 1145 Commercial Dr, Vancouver BC V5L 3X3; Sask'85; Ac Staff, Providence Health Care - St Paul's Hospital; Court Staff, BC Children's Hospital; Clinical Asst Prof Med, University of British Columbia; (604)254-1354; Fax. (604)258-9190.

WICKSTROM, Wendy L; Group One Med Associates, 1111 Springfield Rd, Kelowna BC V1Y 8R7; Wes'87; CCFP; (250)762-4246; Fax. (250)762-4041.

WIDAJEWICZ, Witold J; Forensic Psychiatric Hosp, 70 Colony Farm Rd, Coquitlam BC V3C 5X9; Wroclaw (Poland)'84; MSc; DABPN; FRCPC; Psy. Staff, Forensic Psychiatric Hospital; Physician, Mental Health Addiction Services - Williams Lake; Clin Instructor, University of British Columbia; Langs: Polish; (604)524-7763; Fax. (604)660-1206; wwidajewicz@forensic.bc.ca.

WIDDER, Sandy L; University of Alberta Hosp, 2D4 27-8440 112 St NW, Edmonton AB T6G 2B7; Wes'01; FRCSC; GenSurg; Critical Care Medicine. Staff, University of Alberta Hospital; (780)407-2005; Fax. (780)407-2144.

WIDDIFIELD, Hillary E; Steinbach Family Med Centre, 10-333 Loewen Blvd, Steinbach MB R5G 0C3; (Other Foreign)'09; (204)326-3401

WIDE, Jennifer K; St Paul's Hosp, 1081 Burrard St, Vancouver BC V6Z 1Y6; UBC'06; FRCPC; Psy. Staff, Vancouver General Hospital - Centennial Pavillion; Staff Outpatient Dept, Providence Health Care - St Paul's Hospital; (604)682-2344

WIDEMAN, Anne; Sunnybrook Hlth Sciences Ctre, A112-2075 Bayview Ave, Toronto ON M4N 3M5; McM'95; CCFP; Staff, Sunnybrook Health Sciences Centre; Assoc Staff, North York General Hospital; University of Toronto; (416)480-4942; Fax. (416)480-5774.

WIDJAJA, Elysa; The Hosp for Sick Children, 555 University Ave, Toronto ON M5G 1X8; Melbourne (Australia)'95; Staff, The Hospital For Sick Children; (416)813-7654; Fax. (416)813-7591; elysa.widjaja@sickkids.ca.

WIDJANARKO, Djoen; Sudbury Reg Hosp-Laurentian, 41 Ramsey Lake Rd, Sudbury ON P3E 5J1; Gadjah Mada (Indonesia)'71; Staff, Health Sciences North-Laurentian Site; Staff, Health Sciences North - Memorial Site; Langs: Dutch; Indonesian; (705)671-1000; Fax. (705)675-4780; lwidjanarko@hrsrh.on.ca.

WIDJANARKO, Lianti; Sudbury Reg Hosp-Laurentian, 41 Ramsey Lake Rd, Sudbury ON P3E 5J1; Gadjah Mada (Indonesia)'74; AB; FRCPC; AnatPath. Ac Staff, Health Sciences North - Memorial Site; Staff, Health Sciences North-Laurentian Site; Staff, Health Sciences North-St Joseph's Health Centre; Langs: Indonesian; (705)671-1000; lwidjanarko@hrsrh.on.ca.

WIDMAN, David S; Trillium Hlth Ctr-Mississauga, 100 Queensway W, Mississauga ON L5B 1B8; Wes'92; FRCPC; DiagRad. Staff, Trillium Health Centre - Mississauga; (905)848-7100

WIDMAN, Jody K; Fairlawn Med Centre, 209-2401 Yonge St, Toronto ON M4P 3H1; Tor'93; CCFP; Staff, Bridgepoint Health Centre; (416)322-9933; Fax. (416)322-7097.

WIDMER, Hugues; CHUM- Hopital Saint-Luc, 1058 rue Saint-Denis, Montreal QC H2X 3J4; Mon'97; FRCSC; Urol. Staff, Centre Hospitalier l'Université De Montréal (CHUM) - Hôpital Saint-luc; (514)890-8000

WIDRICH, Guy V; Health Care Med Centre, 301P-1 Promenade Cir, Thornhill ON L4J 4P8; Witwatersrand (South Africa)'89; MB ChB; FRCPC; Peds (Neonatal & Perinatal Medicine). Ac Staff Peds, Humber River Regional Hospital - Finch Avenue Site; Lecturer, University of Toronto; (905)889-1761; Fax. (905)889-0295.

WIEBE, Alison W; Dartmouth Med Centre, 210-46 Portland St, Dartmouth NS B2Y 1H4; UBC'97; CCFP; FCFP; (902)465-4539; Fax. (902)464-4908.

WIEBE, Amanda J; Bradley Med Centre, 2F-595 Bradley Ave, London ON N6E 3Z8; McM'00; CCFP; (519)936-0704; Fax. (519)668-1942; wiebe@bmts.com.

WIEBE, Arthur G; Kincardine Commun Med Clinic, 44 Queen St, Kincardine ON N2Z 3C1; Ott'75; Dip SportMed(SportMed); CCFP; FCFP; Staff, South Bruce Grey Health Centre - Kincardine Site; Aj Prof Family Med, University of Western Ontario; Lecturer, University of Toronto; (519)396-6773; Fax. (519)396-6177.

WIEBE, Bradley K; The Clinic at Walmart, 620-8249 Eagle Landing Pky, Chilliwack BC V2R 0P9; Alb'00; BSc; Staff, The Clinic @ Walmart; (604)792-8482

WIEBE, Carl H B; Vancouver Psychotherapy Ctre, 400-601 Broadway Ave W, Vancouver BC V5Z 4C2; Man'88; FRCPC; Psy. Langs: German; (604)871-4177

WIEBE, Carmen E; BPD CLinic, 33 Russell St, Toronto ON M5S 2S1; Dal'97; FRCPC; Psy. Staff, Centre for Addiction & Mental Health (CAMH) - Queen Site; University of Toronto; (416)535-8501 x2368; Fax. (416)595-6399; carmen_wiebe@camh.net.

WIEBE, Dale J P; Addiction & Mental Hlth-ARF, 33 Russell St, Toronto ON M5S 2S1; Man'08; CCFP; Staff, Centre for Addiction & Mental Health (CAMH) - Russell Street Site; (416)535-8501; Fax. (416)595-6821.

WIEBE, Diana H; 14-1225 Wanyandi Rd NW, Edmonton AB T6M 2W7; Alb'66; Anes. Chief Alternate, Covenant Health - Misericordia Community Hospital; Clin Instructor, University of Alberta; (780)481-3734; Fax. (780)481-3734.

WIEBE, Douglas H; Sunwood Med Clinic, 3000 Lougheed Hwy, Coquitlam BC V3B 1C5; Tor'81; Staff, Work Safety & Insurance Board of BC; (604)464-0345; douglas.wiebe@worksafebc.com.

WIEBE, Edward; University of Alberta Hosp, 2B2 41-8440 112 St NW, Edmonton AB T6G 2B7; Sask'79; FRCPC; DiagRad. Staff Diagnostic Imaging, University of Alberta Hospital; Prog Dir Diagnostic Radiol Residency Prog, University of Alberta; (780)407-1210; Fax. (780)425-5979.

WIEBE, Ellen R; Fairmont Med Bldg, 1013-750 Broadway W, Vancouver BC V5Z 1H9; UBC'75; CCFP; FCFP; Vis Staff, Vancouver General Hospital - Centennial Pavillion; Clin Prof, University of British Columbia; (604)709-5611; Fax. (604)873-8304; ewiebe@interchange.ubc.ca.

WIEBE, Ericka M; Cross Cancer Institute, 11560 University Ave NW, Edmonton AB T6G 1Z2; Wes'06; FRCPC; RadOncol (Medical Oncology). Staff, Cross Cancer Institute; (780)432-8749

WIEBE, Harold J; Abbotsford Reg Hosp & CC, 32900 Marshall Rd, Abbotsford BC V2S 0C2; Man'90; CCFP; CCFP(E.M.); FCFP; Staff, Abbotsford Regional Hospital & Cancer Centre; (604)851-4756

WIEBE, Hazel L J; Eden Mental Health Centre, 1500 Pembina Ave, Winkler MB R6W 1T4; Man'88; FRCPC; Psy;CCFP; Staff, Eden Mental Health Centre; (204)325-4325; Fax. (204)325-8429.

WIEBE, Henry; Northern Lights Reg Health Ctr, 7 Hospital Dr, Fort McMurray AB T9H 1P2; Alb'67; FRCPC; Anes. Staff, Northern Lights Regional Health Centre; (780)791-6161; Fax. (780)791-6029.

WIEBE, Jeffrey L; Kin Place Primary Healthcare, PO Box 28 689 Main St, Oakbank MB R0E 1J0; Man'96; CCFP; (204)444-2227; Fax. (204)444-7851.

WIEBE, Jennifer A; Hope Centre Health Care, 240 Powers St, Winnipeg MB R2W 5L1; Man'85; CCFP; FCFP; Staff, Seven Oaks General Hospital; Med Dir, Hope Centre Health Care Inc.

WIEBE, Kevin M A; Central Alberta Prof Centre, 250-5201 43 St, Red Deer AB T4N 1C7; Sask'98; FRCSC; ObstGyn. Asst Clin Prof, University of Alberta; (403)340-2100; Fax. (403)340-1622.

WIEBE, Kim L; GB248-820 Sherbrooke, Winnipeg MB R3A 1R9; Man'92; IntMed; FRCPC; IntMed; Critical Care Medicine. Staff, Foothills Medical Centre; (204)787-4550; Fax. (204)787-3996; klwiebe@hsc.mb.ca.

WIEBE, Kristopher P; Chilliwack Gen Hosp, 45600 Menholm Rd, Chilliwack BC V2P 1P7; UBC'00; CCFP; CCFP(E.M.); Staff, Chilliwack General Hospital; (604)795-4141

WIEBE, Lawrence P; 206-285 Aurora Cres, Kelowna BC V1X 7N6; Alb'83; Staff, Kelowna General Hospital; (250)765-6767; Fax. (250)765-9015.

WIEBE, Miriam J; East End Commun Health Centre, 1619 Queen St E, Toronto ON M4L 1G4; Tor'94; CCFP; Langs: Spanish; (416)778-5858; Fax. (416)778-5855.

WIEBE, Patricia K; First Nation & Inuit Branch, PL1920B-171 Slater St, Ottawa ON K1A 0L3; Tor'97; FRCPC; Psy.

WIEBE, Russell; Family Med Clinic, PO Box 130 711 Cliff Ave, Enderby BC V0E 1V0; UBC'70; (250)838-0595

WIEBE, Sandra L; Westview Med Centre, 400-2609 Westview Dr, North Vancouver BC V7N 4M2; Man'87; (604)980-0012; wiebemd@axion.net.

WIEBE, Sandra N; Fort St John Med Clinic, 10011 96 St, Fort St. John BC V1J 3P3; Man'09; CCFP; (250)785-6677

WIEBE, Scott C; The Rehabilitation Centre, 1105C-505 Smyth Rd, Ottawa ON K1H 8M2; Ott'03; FRCPC; PhysMed&Rehab (Sports Medicine). Staff, The Ottawa Hospital Rehabilitation Centre; (613)737-7350; Fax. (613)737-9638.

WIEBE, Shannon J; Keewatin Med Clinic, 904 Ottawa St Box 847, Keewatin ON P0X 1C0; Man'04; BSc(Hon); CCFP; Staff, Lake of the Woods District Hospital; Asst Prof, Northern Ontario School of Medicine-Laurentian University; (807)547-2818; Fax. (807)547-3285; shannonwiebe@yahoo.ca.

WIEBE, Shannon N; 5-1116 Mountain Rd, Moncton NB E1C 2T3; UBC'04; FRCSC; GenSurg (Laparoscopic Surgery). Staff, The Moncton Hospital; (506)851-8197; Fax. (506)851-1545.

WIEBE, Sheldon P; MUHC-Montreal Children's Hosp, 2300 rue Tupper, Montreal QC H3H 1P3; Sask'95; LMCC; FRCPC; DiagRad (Pediatric Radiology). Staff, McGill University Health Centre - Montreal Children's Hospital; (514)412-4400

WIEBE, Tannis H; Sterling Lyon Health Centre, 401-1020 Lorimer Blvd, Winnipeg MB R3P 1C7; Man'01; FRCPC; Peds (Developmental Pediatrics).

WIEBE-VELAZQUEZ, Samuel; Foothills Med Centre, C1224-1403 29 St NW, Calgary AB T2N 2T9; Guadalajara (Mexico)'83; FRCPC; Neur (Epilepsy). Staff Neurol, Foothills Medical Centre; Langs: Spanish; (403)944-8535; Fax. (403)944-3465; swiebe@ucalgary.ca.

WIEBENGA, Marjie L; Core Family Health Centre, 825 Richmond St, London ON N6A 3H7; Tor'96; CCFP; (519)318-1015; Fax. (519)963-1880.

WIECKOWSKA, Anna; Ctre Hosp Univ de Laval, 2705 boul Laurier, Quebec QC G1V 4G2; McG'99; Gastroent; Peds (Pediatric Gastroenterology). Staff, Centre Hospitalier Universitaire de Quebec-CHUL; Langs: Polish; French; (418)654-2282; Fax. (418)654-2137.

WIECZOREK, Krzysztof; Primrose Med Clinic, 8436 182 St NW, Edmonton AB T5T 1Y7; Warsaw (Poland)'68; Langs: Ukrainian; Polish; (780)487-7532; Fax. (780)487-8862.

WIECZOREK, Paul M; SMBD Jewish Gen Hosp, A335-3755 Cote-Sainte-Catherin, Montreal QC H3T 1E2; McG'02; FRCPC; Anes. Staff, Sir Mortimer B Davis Jewish General; (514)340-8222 x5701

WIEDER, Jana; Family Practice Associates, 200-6155 North St, Halifax NS B3K 5R3; Purkyne (Czech Republic)'73; Langs: Czech; Russian; (902)453-3511; Fax. (902)454-9010.

WIEDMEYER, Heather M; 301-1678 Bloor St W, Toronto ON M6P 1A9; McG'08; CCFP; (416)975-9300; Fax. (416)975-0314.

WIEDRICK, James E D; Aberdeen Med Centre, 1966 Harrison Way, Kamloops BC V1S 1M9; Alb'98; CCFP; (250)314-5321

WIEHAHN, George J; 200-945 Southill St, Kamloops BC V2B 7Z9; Pretoria (South Africa)'92; LMCC; FRCPC; Psy (General Adult Psychiatry). Clin Dir South Hills, Shuswap Health Services; Clin Dir, Interior Health Authority-Thompson Cariboo; Physician Forensic Psy, Forensic Psychiatric Services Commission-Kamloops; Clin Dir South Hills, Interior Health Authority-Travel & Vaccine Clinic; Teacher Tutor, University of British Columbia; Langs: Afrikaans; Dutch; (250)554-5583

WIELECKI, Sylvia D; William Osler HC-Brampton, 2100 Bovaird Dr E, Brampton ON L6R 3J7; Kansas (USA)'00; Staff, William Osler Health System - Brampton Civic Hospital; (905)494-2120

WIELGOSZ, Andreas T J; The Ottawa Hosp-Gen Campus, 501 Smyth Rd, Ottawa ON K1H 8L6; McM'74; BSc; MSc; PhD; FRCPC; IntMed; Cardiol. Consultant, Pembroke Regional Hospital Inc; Clin Staff Cardiol, The Ottawa Hospital - General Campus; Consultant Cardiol, Civil Aviation Canada; Prof Med, University of Ottawa; Langs: Polish; French; Spanish; (613)737-8153; Fax. (613)737-8918; wielgosz@uottawa.ca.

WIEMAN, Cornelia G; Elm Centre Support Program, 150 Elizabeth St, Toronto ON M5G 0B1; McM'93; BSc(Hons.); MSc; Psy (Aboriginal Health). Staff Elm Centre Support Program, YWCA Toronto; Asst Prof Public Health Services, University of Toronto; (416)260-2000; Fax. (416)961-8106.

WIEMER, Chad C; Central Alberta Med Imaging, 4312 54 Ave, Red Deer AB T4N 4M1; UBC'00; FRCPC; DiagRad. Staff, Red Deer Regional Hospital Centre; (403)343-6172

WIENER, John S; 108-235 St Clair Ave W, Toronto ON M4V 1R4; McG'76; FRCPC; Psy (Psychotherapy). Staff, Centre for Addiction & Mental Health (CAMH) - College Street Site; Lecturer, University of Toronto; (416)944-1061; johnwiener@rogers.com.

WIENS, Andrew S; Royal Ottawa Hlth Care Group, 1145 Carling Ave, Ottawa ON K1Z 7K4; Ott'87; BMedSci; FRCPC; Psy (Geriatric Psychiatry). Staff, The Ottawa Hospital - Civic Campus; Staff, Royal Ottawa Mental Health Centre - Royal Ottawa Health Care Group; Assoc Prof Psy, University of Ottawa; Langs: Bilingual(French/English); (613)722-6521 x6526; Fax. (613)798-2999.

WIENS, Anthony V; Dauphin Med Clinic, 622 3rd St SW, Dauphin MB R7N 1R5; Man'95; CCFP; (204)638-6445; Fax. (204)638-5670.

WIENS, Barry M; Red Deer Reg Hosp Centre, PO Box 5030 Stn Postal Box Ctr 3942 50A Ave, Red Deer AB T4N 6R2; Alb'97; CCFP; FCFP; CCFP(E.M.); Staff Emerg, Red Deer Regional Hospital Centre; (403)343-4444

WIENS, Debra D; 559 6th St, Courtenay BC V9N 1M5; Cal'84; Ac Staff, St Joseph's General Hospital; Staff, Dr Richard T Engman & Dr Debra D Wiens Inc; (250)338-1391; Fax. (250)338-2385.

WIENS, Donald E; 2-14 Lisa St, Brampton ON L6T 4W2; Tor'86; CCFP; Langs: German; (905)460-1762; Fax. (905)460-1981.

WIENS, Doris H; Niagara HS-St Catharines Gen, 142 Queenston St, St Catharines ON L2R 7C6; McM'06; CCFP; Staff, Niagara Health System - St Catharines General Site; Langs: German; (905)684-7271

WIENS, Ernest; 23110 Township Road 520, Sherwood Park AB T8B 1E9; Alb'68; FRCSC; GenSurg. Staff, Royal Alexandra Hospital; Staff, Cross Cancer Institute; Staff Teacher, University of Alberta.

WIENS, H Edward; Associate Med Clinic, 4705 48 Ave, Red Deer AB T4N 3T1; Sask'67; CCFP; Assoc Staff, Red Deer Regional Hospital Centre; Physician, Associate Medical Group; Langs: German; (403)346-2057; Fax. (403)347-2989; hewiens@telusplanet.net.

WIENS, Irene; Circle Med @ Copperfield, 123-15566 McIvor Blvd SE, Calgary AB T2Z 4Y2; Sask'96; CCFP; Staff, Low Risk Maternity Clinic; (403)726-0524; Fax. (403)726-0579.

WIENS, James J; Medical Arts Bldg, 1010-233 Kennedy St, Winnipeg MB R3C 3J5; Sask'81; FRCSC; Ophth (Cornea/External Disease). Staff, Misericordia Health Centre; (204)943-1520; Fax. (204)957-0294.

WIENS, James; Wrinch Mem Doctors Clinic, PO Bag 999, Hazelton BC V0J 1Y0; Man'00; CCFP; Staff, Wrinch Memorial Hospital; Wrinch Memorial Doctors Clinic; (250)842-5234; Fax. (250)842-5065.

WIENS, Joel L; Georgian Bay Gen Hosp, PO Box 760 Stn Main 1112 St Andrews Dr, Midland ON L4R 4P4; Qns'07; CCFP; Staff, Georgian Bay General Hospital - Midland; (705)526-3751; Fax. (416)867-3726.

WIENS, John L; Assiniboine Clinic, M20-2727 Portage Ave, Winnipeg MB R3J 0R2; Sask'74; FRCSC; OrthSurg (Arthroscopy & Knee Ligament Reconstruction). Staff, The Salvation Army Grace Hospital; Site Med Mgr-Surg, Seven Oaks General Hospital; (204)888-5905; Fax. (204)885-9671.

WIENS, Peter J; Prairie Trail Med Centre, 100-1345 Taylor Ave, Winnipeg MB R3M 3Y9; UBC'92; CCFP; FCFP; (204)475-0088

WIENS, Rebecca J; Tom Baker Cancer Centre, 1331 29 St NW, Calgary AB T2N 4N2; Wes'03; CCFP; Staff, Foothills Medical Centre; Staff, Tom Baker Cancer Centre; Staff, Rockyview General Hospital; Staff, Carewest Sarcee Hospice; (403)521-3446

WIENS, Scott W; University of Alberta Hosp, 2D2 32-8440 112 St NW, Edmonton AB T6G 2B7; Alb'05; FRCSC; OrthSurg (Upper Extremity Reconstruction). Staff, University of Alberta Hospital; (780)407-2816; Fax. (780)407-2819.

WIENS, Sharon A; Royal University Hosp, 103 Hospital Dr, Saskatoon SK S7N 0W8; Cal'80; FRCPC; Peds (Cardiovascular Anesthesia); Anes. Ac Staff Anes, Royal University Hospital; Asst Prof, University of Saskatchewan; (306)655-1183; Fax. (306)655-1279.

WIENS, Sheldon E; Sturgeon Community Hosp, 201 Boudreau Rd, St. Albert AB T8N 6C4; Alb'97; CCFP; CCFP(E.M.); Staff, Sturgeon Community Hospital; (780)418-8229; Fax. (780)418-7376.

WIERSTRA, Benjamin T; Pembroke Reg Hosp, 705 Mackay St, Pembroke ON K8A 1G8; Ott'06; CCFP; Staff, Montfort Hospital; Staff, Pembroke Regional Hospital; Staff, Base Hospital-CFB Petawawa; (613)732-3675; Fax. (613)732-9986; benjamin.wierstra@pemreghos.org.

WIERZBICKI, Agnieszka E; Sunpark Professional Centre, 118-40 Sunpark Plaza SE, Calgary AB T2X 3X7; (403)254-4000; Fax. (403)254-1282.

WIERZBICKI, Rafal F; Lakeridge Hlth Corp-Oshawa, 1 Hospital Crt, Oshawa ON L1G 2B9; Poznan (Poland)'74; FRCPC; IntMed; MedOncol. Staff, Lakeridge Health - Oshawa Site; Langs: Polish; French; (905)576-8711 x3283; Fax. (905)721-4741.

WIERZCHOSLAWSKI, Krzysztof; White Eagle Med Clinic, 3-250 Pleasant St, Miramichi NB E1V 1Y5; Poznan (Poland)'88; Att Physician Family Med, Miramichi Regional Hospital; Physician, Miramichi Senior Citizens Nursing Home; Physician Team, Biathlow New Brunswick; Langs: Polish; (506)778-5747; Fax. (506)778-5740.

WIESE, Ben; Health Wise Family Practice, 3-1499 Gordon Dr, Kelowna BC V1Y 9R2; Pretoria (South Africa)'06; MB ChB; Langs: Afrikaans; (778)484-5560; Fax. (778)484-5564.

WIESE, Bonnie S; Vancouver Gen Hosp, 855 12th Ave W, Vancouver BC V5Z 1M9; UBC'02; FRCPC; Psy. Staff, Vancouver General Hospital - Centennial Pavillion; (604)875-4111

WIESE, Lize; Health Wise Family Practice, 3-1499 Gordon Dr, Kelowna BC V1Y 9R2; Pretoria (South Africa)'05; Langs: Afrikaans; (778)484-5560; Fax. (778)484-5564.

WIESENBERG-SMITH, Sara E; PO Box 425, Bragg Creek AB T0L 0K0; McM'81; CCFP; FCFP; (403)949-2457; Fax. (403)949-2424.

WIESENFELD, Lesley A; Mount Sinai Hosp, 918-600 University Ave, Toronto ON M5G 1X5; Tor'98; FRCPC; Psy. Staff, Mount Sinai Hospital; (416)586-4800; Fax. (416)586-8654.

WIESENFELD, Lorne M; The Ottawa Hosp-Civic Campus, 1103-1053 Carling Ave, Ottawa ON K1Y 4E9; McG'92; FACP; MDCM; FRCPC; EmergMed. Att Staff Emerg Dept, The Ottawa Hospital - Civic Campus; Asst Prof Med/Dir Interim Residency Prog, University of Ottawa; Langs: English; French; (613)761-4773

WIESENTHAL, Alain A; Northridge Plaza, 105-265 King George Rd, Brantford ON N3R 6Y1; Man'93; BA; FRCSC; Otol (Head & Neck Surgery)., The Brant Community Healthcare System - Brantford General Hospital Site; Langs: Hebrew; (519)720-0743; Fax. (519)720-0744.

WIESENTHAL, Benjamin D; Rossmere Med Centre, 1046C Henderson Hwy, Winnipeg MB R2K 2M5; Man'82; (204)338-0315

WIESENTHAL, Joshua D; 200-550 West Ave, Kelowna BC V1Y 4Z4; McM'04; FRCSC; Urol. (250)469-7763

WIESENTHAL, Marvin M; 1739 Bathurst St, Toronto ON M5P 3K5; McG'67; (416)483-5468

WIESENTHAL, Stephanie R; Toronto East Gen Hosp Inc, C416-825 Coxwell Ave, Toronto ON M4C 3E7; Tor'02; FRCPC; Psy. Staff, Toronto East General Hospital Inc; (416)469-6580; Fax. (416)469-6179.

WIESENTHAL, Zeph M; Kerrisdale Station Med Clinic, 2077 42 Ave W, Vancouver BC V6M 2B4; Man'84; Staff Med Services Branch &, Northern Medical Unit; Langs: Hebrew; (604)261-9494

WIESINGER, Holly A R; 110-2504 Skaha Lake Rd, Penticton BC V2A 6G1; UBC'05; FRCPC; IntMed; Gastroent. (250)492-3511

WIGGELINKHUIZEN, Nicola; 5001 Anderson WAy, Vernon BC V1T 9V1; Cape Town (South Africa)'91; CCFP; Langs: Afrikaans; Zulu; (250)545-8338

WIGGERS, Joris A J; Nanaimo Reg Gen Hosp, 1200 Dufferin Cres, Nanaimo BC V9S 2B7; Boston,MA (USA)'92; FRCPC; Psy. Staff, Nanaimo Regional General Hospital; (250)755-7691; Fax. (250)716-7747.

WIGGINS, M Christo; Chilliwack Prof Centre, 108-9123 Mary St., Chilliwack BC V2P 4H7; Pretoria (South Africa)'79; MB ChB; FRCSC; GenSurg (Breast Cancer). Staff, Chilliwack General Hospital; Langs: Afrikaans; (604)792-8099; Fax. (604)792-3015; wiggins@telus.net.

WIGHTMAN, Daniela M T; Seven Oaks Gen Hosp, 2300 McPhillips St, Winnipeg MB R2V 3M3; Man'84; AnatPath. Ac Staff, Seven Oaks General Hospital; (204)632-7133 x3252

WIGHTMAN, H Robert; Salvation Army Grace Gen Hosp, 300 Booth Dr, Winnipeg MB R3J 3M7; Man'84; AnatPath. Ac Staff Path, The Salvation Army Grace Hospital; (204)837-8311 x2132

WIGHTMAN, Howard A; Valley Reg Hosp, 150 Exhibition St, Kentville NS B4N 5E3; UBC'82; FACC; FRCPC; IntMed (Clinical Cardiology); Cardiol. Staff, Valley Regional Hospital; (902)678-1411; Fax. (902)679-1250; how@ns.sympatico.ca.

WIGHTMAN, Nancy A; 1-25 Sherbrook St, Winnipeg MB R3C 2B1; Man'86; FRCPC; Psy. Staff, St Boniface General Hospital; Staff, Health Sciences Centre; Consultant Psy, Concordia General Hospital; Consultant, University of Manitoba; (204)788-8114

WIGHTMAN, Patricia A; Psychealth Centre, 771 Bannatyne Ave, Winnipeg MB R3E 3N4; Man'56; FRCPC; Psy. Staff, Psychealth Centre; (204)787-3887; pwightman@exchange.hsc.mb.ca.

WIGINTON, Richard J; Brighton Family Health Team, PO Box 9 170 Main St, Brighton ON K0K 1H0; Qns'87; BSc; (613)475-1555; Fax. (613)475-5556.

WIGLE, Ronald D; Queen's University, 102 Stuart St, Kingston ON K7L 2V6; Qns'65; FRCPC; IntMed (Respirology). Staff, Lennox & Addington County General Hospital; Staff, Kingston General Hospital; Emeritus Prof, Queen's University; (613)548-2384; Fax. (613)549-1459; wigler@post.queensu.ca.

WIGMORE, C Frederick; The Professional Bldg, 107-54 Ominica St W, Moose Jaw SK S6H 1W9; Sask'81; (306)693-1362; Fax. (306)692-8029.

WIGMORE, William M; Nanaimo Reg Gen Hosp, 1200 Dufferin Cres, Nanaimo BC V9S 2B7; Alb'89; CCFP; CCFP(E.M.); Staff, Nanaimo Regional General Hospital; (250)754-2141

WIGNALL, Geoffrey R; 209-1101 2nd Ave E, Owen Sound ON N4K 2J1; Qns'01; AB; FRCSC; Urol (Endocrinology). Staff, Grey Bruce Health Services - Owen Sound; (519)371-1212; Fax. (519)372-0731.

WIGNALL, John B W; Medical Centre, 12-14 West St, Corner Brook NL A2H 2Z1; (England)'76; (709)634-5241; Fax. (709)634-5244.

WIHLBORG, Christel E M; Raymond Med Clinic, PO Box 769 Stn Main 20 Church Ave, Raymond AB T0K 2S0; CCFP; (403)752-3337

WIID, Estelle M; Oasis Med Clinic, 2145 Louie Dr, Westbank BC V4T 3E6; Orange Free State (South Africa)'98; MB ChB; Langs: Afrikaans; (250)768-7656

WIJAY, Shamal N C; Family First Family Health Team, 4270 Innes Rd, Orleans ON K4A 5E6; Tor'89; (613)841-7009; Fax. (613)841-0106.

WIJAYANAYAGAM, Akushla I; A. Wijayanagam Inc, 162-5091 Tsuma-As Dr, Port Alberni BC V9Y 8X9; Mem'99; FRCSC; GenSurg (Breast Surgical Oncology). Staff, West Coast General Hospital; (250)720-2283; Fax. (250)720-2263.

WIJAYANAYAGAM, Yoganandthan; Western Memorial Health Clinic, 3 Herald Ave, Corner Brook NL A2H 4B8; Ceylon (Sri Lanka)'68; MB BS; FRCS(Eng); FRC; FACS; FRCSC; Ophth (Retina Vitreous Surgery). Head Div of Ophth, Western Memorial Regional Hospital; (709)632-2023; Fax. (709)632-2103; drwijay@nf.sympatico.ca.

WIJAYASINGHE, Sheila; Health Centre @ 80 Bond St, 80 Bond St, Toronto ON M5B 1X2; Alb'04; CCFP; Physician, Queen West Community Health Centre; Langs: Spanish; Sinhalese; (416)864-3011

WIJERATNE, H M Rasika; Kingston Gen Hosp, 76 Stuart St, Kingston ON K7L 2V7; Fudan University (Other Foreign)'02; CCFP; Staff, Kingston General Hospital; Teach Staff, Queen's University; (613)549-6666

WIJEWARDENA, Handun; Office of Chief Med Examiner, 210-1 Wesley Ave, Winnipeg MB R3C 4C6.

WIJEYESINGHE, E Cornel R; Royal Inland Hosp, 311 Columbia St, Kamloops BC V2C 2T1; (Sri Lanka)'73; MB BS; FRCP(Lond); MSc(UK); FACP; FRCPC; IntMed; Nephrol. Ac Staff, Royal Inland Hospital; (250)314-2849; Fax. (250)314-2348.

WIJEYSUNDERA, Duminda N; Univ Hlth Network-Toronto Gen, EN3 450-200 Elizabeth St, Toronto ON M5G 2C4; UBC'98; FRCPC; Anes. Staff, Toronto General Hospital - UHN; (416)340-4800 x8981; Fax. (416)340-3698.

WIJEYSUNDERA, Harindra C; Sunnybrook Hlth Sciences Ctre, 209D-2075 Bayview Ave, Toronto ON M4N 3M5; UBC'00; FRCPC; IntMed; Cardiol. Staff, Sunnybrook Health Sciences Centre; (416)480-6100; Fax. (416)480-4527.

WIK, Lori M; 1-25 12th Ave S, Cranbrook BC V1C 2R8; Alb'04; FRCPC; IntMed. (250)426-1995

WILANSKY, Douglas L; William Osler HC-Etobicoke, 101 Humber College Blvd, Etobicoke ON M9V 1R8; Dal'51; FRCPC; IntMed; NuclearMed. Dir Dept of NuclearMed, William Osler Health System - Etobicoke General Hospital; Founder Chief Nuclear Med, Dr Douglas Wilansky Nuclear Medicine Services; (416)747-3478; Fax. (416)747-3609.

WILANSKY, Hannah; 742-118 Eglinton Ave W, Toronto ON M4R 2G4; Mem'86; FRCPC; Psy. (416)929-6931

WILANSKY, Rhonda; Summerville Family Health Team, 5F-101 Queensway W, Mississauga ON L5B 2P7; Mem'82; CCFP; Trillium Health Centre - Mississauga; Lecturer, University of Toronto; (905)272-9700 x2; Fax. (905)272-1416; rwilansky@sympatico.ca.

WILANSKY, Selig; Royal Columbian Hosp, 330 Columbia St E, New Westminster BC V3L 3W7; Mem'93; CCFP; Staff, Royal Columbian Hospital; (604)520-4001

WILBERFORCE, Kevin C; 218 Frederica St W, Thunder Bay ON P7E 3W2; Qns'83; FRCPC; Psy. Staff, Lakehead Psychiatric Hospital - St. Joseph's Care Group; (807)577-3540; Fax. (807)577-3675.

WILBERFORCE, Nicola C; Fort William Clinic, 117 McKellar St S, Thunder Bay ON P7E 1H5; McM'03; BScPT; CCFP; Staff, Thunder Bay Regional Health Sciences Centre; (807)626-1256; Fax. (807)623-2316.

WILCOCK, Alison F; Broadway & Burrard Med Clinic, 1816 Broadway W, Vancouver BC V6J 1Y9; Sheffield (England)'69; MB ChB; CCFP; Locum Tenens, Cowichan District Hospital; Ac Staff, Nanaimo Regional General Hospital; Coroner, Oxford County; Staff, Valleyview Treatment Centre; Aj Prof, University of Western Ontario; (604)736-1888

WILCOCK, Georgina E M; 309-1920 Ellesmere Rd, Scarborough ON M1H 2V6; (Zimbabwe)'86; MB ChB; FRCSC; ObstGyn. Staff, The Scarborough Hospital - General Campus; (416)289-0519; Fax. (416)289-3910.

WILCOX, Carol L; 106-100 Humber College Blvd, Etobicoke ON M9V 5G4; Tor'98; Staff, Baycrest Centre for Geriatric Care; Staff, Peel Public Health; (416)742-9449; Fax. (416)742-6963; wilcoxc@peelregion.ca.

WILCOX, M Elizabeth; Univ Hlth Network-Toronto Western Hosp, McI 2411P-399 Bathurst St, Toronto ON M5T 2S8; Cal'03; FRCPC; IntMed; Critical Care Medicine. Staff, Toronto Western Hospital - University Health Network; (416)719-0008

WILCOX, Neil E; 3821 Peak Dr, Campbell River BC V9H 1M8; Alb'73.

WILCOX, Pearce G; St Paul's Hosp, 8B-1081 Burrard St, Vancouver BC V6Z 1Y6; Qns'80; FRCPC; IntMed (Cystic Fibrosis); Respir. Staff Pacific Lung Health Centre, Providence Health Care - St Paul's Hospital; Assoc Prof, University of British Columbia; (604)806-8818; Fax. (604)806-8839; p.wilcox@providencehealth.bc.ca.

WILCZYNSKI, John S; 3989 Main St, Niagara Falls ON L2G 6B9; Wroclaw (Poland)'83; Langs: Italian; Polish; (905)295-4367; Fax. (905)295-7914.

WILD, Gary E; MUHC-Montreal Gen Hosp, D7 200-1650 av Cedar, Montreal QC H3G 1A4; McG'83; PhD; FRCPC; IntMed; Gastroent (P.Q.). Staff, McGill University Health Centre - Montreal General Campus; (514)934-8309; Fax. (514)934-8531; gary.wild@mcgill.ca.

WILD, Paul J; 969 Queen St E, Sault Ste. Marie ON P6A 2C4; University of Leicester (England)'05; CCFP; Staff, Sault Area Hospital - Sault Ste Marie; (705)759-3434

WILDE, Brent K; St Paul's Hosp, 1702 20th St W, Saskatoon SK S7M 0Z9; Sask'99; FRCPC; GenPath. Staff, St Paul's Hospital (Grey Nuns) of Saskatoon; (306)655-5604; Fax. (306)655-5667.

WILDE, Eric R; 1903 9 Ave S, Lethbridge AB T1J 1W8; Cal'89; FRCPC; IntMed; Respir. Staff, Chinook Regional Hospital; (403)320-0633; Fax. (403)320-0353.

WILDE, James M; Royal Jubilee Hosp, 1952 Bay St, Victoria BC V8R 1J8; Leeds (England)'56; MB ChB; Ac Staff, Victoria General Hospital; Staff Palliative Care, BC Cancer Agency Vancouver Island Centre; Ac Staff, Royal Jubilee Hospital; Victoria Hospice Society; Clin Instructor, University of British Columbia; (250)370-8715; Fax. (250)370-8625.

WILDE, Sean K; Chinook Regional Hosp, 260 19 St S, Lethbridge AB T1J 1W5; Cal'09; CCFP; CCFP(E.M.); Staff, Chinook Regional Hospital; (403)388-6111

WILDEBOER, David W; Mainstreet Med Services, 4929 50 Ave, Lacombe AB T4L 1K3; Mem'94; BMedSci; BSc; MD; CCFP; FCFP; Staff, Lacombe Hospital & Care Centre; Staff/Chief Family Med, Central Zone David Thompson Health Region; (403)782-6717; Fax. (403)782-4240.

WILDENBOER, Wilhelmina H; Rochdale Crossing Med Clinic, 7-5875 Rochdale Blvd, Regina SK S4X 2P9; Pretoria (South Africa)'89; MB ChB; CCFP; Physician, Regina Rehabilitation & Family Medical Clinic; (306)205-8020; Fax. (306)205-8023.

WILDENHAIN, Yvonne D; Guelph Emerg Med Services, 305-73 Delhi St, Guelph ON N1E 6L9; McM'92; CCFP; CCFP(E.M.); Staff, Cambridge Memorial Hospital; (519)837-0133

WILDERDIJK, Margot F; Viking Med Clinic, GD 5301 51 St, Viking AB T0B 4N0; Cal'10; CCFP; (780)336-4780; Fax. (780)336-2020.

WILDERMAN, Igor S; Wilderman Med Clinic, 8054 Yonge St, Thornhill ON L4J 1W3; Tashkent (Russia (Federation))'85; CCFP; Med Dir, Wilderman Medical Clinic; Med Dir, Canadian Centre for Clinical Trials; Med Dir, Chronic Pain Clinic; Langs: Hebrew; Russian; (905)886-1212; Fax. (905)886-0248.

WILDGRUBE, Frank P; Sechelt Med Clinic, GD 5531 Inlet Rd S, Sechelt BC V0N 3A0; Alb'88; Locum Tenens, Shuswap Lake General Hospital; (604)885-2257

WILDGRUBE, Peter D; Coronation Plaza, 202-14310 111 Ave NW, Edmonton AB T5M 3Z7; Alb'88; FRCPC; Anes. Staff, Capital Health Authority; Staff OR, Royal Alexandra Hospital; Staff, Sturgeon Community Hospital; Clin Teacher Anes, University of Alberta; (780)488-2724; Fax. (780)488-2774; wildgp@telusplanet.net.

WILDISH, Julia A; Saint John Reg Hosp, PO Box 2100 Stn Main 3BJ3-400 University Ave, Saint John NB E2L 4L2; Dal'03; BSc; CCFP; Staff, Saint John Regional Hospital; Staff, Hospice Palliative Care Outreach; Lecturer Family Med, Dalhousie University; (506)648-6000; Fax. (506)649-2634.

WILDSCHUT, Jason A; The Hosp for Sick Children, 555 University Ave, Toronto ON M5G 1X8; Queensland (Australia)'97; Fellow Ped Cardiol, The Hospital For Sick Children; (416)813-1500; Fax. (416)813-5711.

WILE, Iona; Hants Community Hosp, 89 Payzant Dr, Windsor NS B0N 2T0; Dal'88; Dip SportMed(SportMed); CCFP; FCFP; Court Staff/Staff Primary Care Chronic Pain Clinic, Hants Community Hospital; Preceptor, Dalhousie University; (902)792-2108

WILEJTO, Marta; The Hosp for Sick Children, BL 9402-555 University Ave, Toronto ON M5G 1X8; Tor'06; FRCPC; Peds (Hematological Oncology). Staff, The Hospital For Sick Children; (416)813-7742

WILEY, Alan M; Albany Med Clinic, 807 Broadview Ave, Toronto ON M4K 2P8; Dublin (Ireland)'49; FRCS(E); MCh; FRCSC; OrthSurg (Upper Extremity & Arthroscopic Surgery). Court Staff, Toronto Western Hospital - University Health Network; Consultant, Workers' Comp Board of ON; Physician, Albany Medical Clinic; Physician, Boniface Park Medical Clinic; (416)461-9471; Fax. (416)461-2710; awiley@cheo.on.ca.

WILEY, J Preston; Sport Med Centre, 2500 University Dr NW, Calgary AB T2N 1N4; Cal'84; BPE; MPE; MD; CCFP; FCFP; Court Staff Family Practice, Foothills Medical Centre; Assoc Prof Kinesiology, University Of Calgary; (403)220-8518; Fax. (403)282-6170.

WILEY, Joseph C; The Hosp for Sick Children, 555 University Ave, Toronto ON M5G 1X8; Tor'10; Staff, The Hospital For Sick Children; (416)813-5310

WILEY, Kate M; LifeMark Health Centre, 2225 MacLeod Trail SE, Calgary AB T2G 5B6; Qns'90; Dip SportMed; CCFP; (403)237-5633; Fax. (403)237-5142.

WILEY, Lauren K; Dr Everett Chalmers Hosp, PO Box 9000 Stn A, Fredericton NB E3B 5N5; McM'09; CCFP; Staff, Dr Everett Chalmers Regional Hospital; (506)452-5400

WILEY, Scott; 108-10 Lamport Ave, Toronto ON M4W 1S6; McM'99; IntMed (Cardiol); (416)442-5600; Fax. (416)510-6870.

WILFORD, Edward H; Nanaimo Reg Gen Hosp, 1200 Dufferin Cres, Nanaimo BC V9S 2B7; UBC'88; CCFP; CCFP(E.M.); FCFP; Staff, Nanaimo Regional General Hospital; (250)754-2141

WILHELM, Andrea; Masset Med Clinic, PO Box 319, Masset BC V0T 1M0; McM'04; CCFP; Physician, Medical Clinic; Physician, Medical Clinic; Langs: Spanish; (250)626-4702; Fax. (250)626-4708.

WILHELM, Julia E; University Downs Fam Practice, 425 University Ave E, Waterloo ON N2K 4C9; Wes'94; BSc(Hon.); CCFP; FCFP; (519)569-8821; Fax. (519)569-8823.

WILHELM-BOYLES, Carrie M; Surrey Mem Hosp, 13750 96 Ave, Surrey BC V3V 1Z2; Man'04; CCFP; CCFP(E.M.); Staff, Peace Arch Hospital; Staff, Surrey Memorial Hospital; (604)581-2211

WILHELMY, Mario; Clinique Med du Luc, 33 rue Saint-Patrice E, Magog QC J1X 5B7; Mon'85; (819)868-2112; Fax. (819)843-7217.

WILK, Andrew; Shoppers Drug Mart Med Clinic, 1-300 Taunton Rd E, Oshawa ON L1G 7T4; Colegio Mayor De Ntra Sra Del Rosario (Colombia)'83; Ac Staff Family Pract & Palliative Care Cons, Lakeridge Health - Oshawa Site; Langs: Polish; Spanish; (905)725-4928; Fax. (905)725-0640.

WILK, Jerry P; Guelph Nuclear Imaging, 105-83 Dawson Rd, Guelph ON N1H 1B1; Tor'79; DABR; FRCPC; DiagRad (Nuclear Medicine). Staff, Guelph Imaging Centre; Staff, Niagara Diagnostic Imaging Centre; (519)767-0550; jwilk@niagarahealth.on.ca.

WILK, Lucie A; Leslie & Gordon Diamond HCC, 8205B-2775 Laurel St, Vancouver BC V5Z 1M9; Ott'99; BSc(Hons); Rheum; IntMed (Family Medicine). Staff, Gordon & Leslie Diamond Health Care Centre; (604)875-8270; Fax. (604)875-5992.

WILKE, Derek R; Nova Scotia Cancer Centre, 2027-5820 University Ave, Halifax NS B3H 1V7; Tor'94; MSc; FRCPC; RadOncol (Prostate Cancer). Asst Prof, Queen Elizabeth II Health Sciences Centre - Victoria General Site; Staff, Nova Scotia Cancer Center; Asst Prof, Dalhousie University; (902)473-6022; Fax. (902)473-7205; derek.wilke@cdha.nshealth.ca.

WILKEN, Waldemar P; Glenbrook Med Clinic, 111-4306 Richmond Rd SW, Calgary AB T3E 4P6; (South Africa)'83; CCFP; Langs: Afrikaans; (403)685-5480; Fax. (403)685-5482.

WILKES, Gordon H; Meadowlark Health Centre, 174 Meadowlark Shopping Ctr NW, Edmonton AB T5R 5W9; Alb'75; FRCSC; PlasSurg (Cosmetic Surgery). Clin Prof Surg, University of Alberta; (780)483-6400; Fax. (780)481-3002.

WILKES, Heidi R; Garneau Prof Centre, 407-11044 51 Ave NW, Edmonton AB T6H 5B4; Alb'00; FRCPC; Psy (Child Psychiatry). Clin Lecturer Psy, University of Alberta; (780)438-6181; Fax. (780)437-3499; hwilkes@childpsychiatry.ca.

WILKES, Peter R H; Univ of Ottawa Heart Institute, 40 Ruskin St, Ottawa ON K1Y 4W7; Cal'90; PhD; FRCPC; Anes; Critical Care Medicine. Clin Associate Ottawa Heart Inst, The Ottawa Hospital - Civic Campus; Staff, University of Ottawa Heart Institute; Clin Associate, University of Ottawa; (613)761-4379; Fax. (613)761-4925.

WILKES, Thomas C R; Foothills Med Centre, 1403 29 St NW, Calgary AB T2N 2T9; Birmingham (England)'76; DCH; MRC; MRCPsy; BSc(Hons); FRCPC; Psy (Adolescent Medicine). Ac Staff Psy, Foothills Medical Centre; Physician, Alberta Mental Health Board; Dir Psy Resindency, University of Calgary; (403)944-2489; Fax. (403)283-1563; wilkes@telusplanet.net.

WILKHU, Gagan D S; W Medical Clinic, 8675 120 St, Delta BC V4C 6R4; St George's (Grenada)'05; (604)596-4222

WILKHU, Gagandeep S; Kwantlen Med Clinic, 1-12818 72 Ave, Surrey BC V3W 2M9; St George's University (Grenada)'05; CCFP; Langs: Punjabi; (604)572-8161

WILKIE, Allan V; Valley Reg Hosp, 150 Exhibition St, Kentville NS B4N 5E3; Dal'95; CCFP; CCFP(E.M.); Staff, Valley Regional Hospital; (902)678-7381; Fax. (902)679-1206.

WILKIE, Catherine L; Women's Health Clinic, 3F-419 Graham Ave, Winnipeg MB R3C 0M3; Qns'77; CCFP; FCFP; (204)947-1517; Fax. (204)944-0223.

WILKIE, David H L; Vancouver Urogyn & Gyn Surg, 300-1338 Broadway W, Vancouver BC V6H 1H2; UBC'78; DObst; RC; FRCSC; ObstGyn (Urological Gynecology). Consultant, BC Children's Hospital; Ac Staff, Vancouver General Hospital - Centennial Pavillion; Assoc Staff, BC Women's Hospital & Health Centre; Clin Assoc Prof ObstGyn, University of British Columbia; (604)736-5404; Fax. (604)736-5424.

WILKIE, John A C; Penticton Reg Hosp, 500 Carmi Ave, Penticton BC V2A 3G6; Man'04; FRCPC; DiagRad. Staff, Penticton Regional Hospital; (204)774-6511

WILKIE, Treena D; Addiction & Mental Hlth-Queen, 3 4-1001 Queen St W, Toronto ON M6J 1H4; Ott'00; FRCPC; Psy. Staff, Centre for Addiction & Mental Health (CAMH) - Queen Site; (416)535-8501

WILKIE, W Clarke; Selkirk Mental Health Centre, PO Box 9600 Stn Main, Selkirk MB R1A 2B5; Man'77; FRCPC; Psy (Cross-Culture Psychiatry). Staff Psy, Selkirk Mental Health Centre; Staff J A Hildes Northern Med Unit, University of Manitoba; (204)482-3810; Fax. (204)482-6390; wc-wilkie@shaw.ca.

WILKIE GILMORE, Andrea; Children's Hosp, 840 Sherbrook St, Winnipeg MB R3A 1S1; Man'05; FRCPC; Peds; PedEmergMed. Staff, Health Sciences Centre; (204)774-8511

WILKIN, Richard P; Rockyview Gen Hosp, 6625-7007 14 St SW, Calgary AB T2V 1P9; Alb'75; BSc; FRCSC; Urol. Ac Staff, Rockyview General Hospital; Ac Staff, Foothills Medical Centre; University of Calgary; (403)943-8991; Fax. (403)943-8993.

WILKINS, Douglas F; The Ottawa Hosp-Civic Campus, 1053 Carling Ave, Ottawa ON K1Y 4E9; Wes'82; BSc; FRCPC; Psy (Consultation-Liaison). Consultant, Royal Ottawa Mental Health Centre - Royal Ottawa Health Care Group; Att Staff, The Ottawa Hospital - Civic Campus; Asst Prof, University of Ottawa; (613)761-4588; Fax. (613)761-4177; dwilkins@ottawahospital.on.ca.

WILKINS, Jean; Hôpital Ste-Justine, 3175 ch Cote-Sainte-Catherine, Montreal QC H3T 1C5; Mon'70; BA; Peds (Adolescent Medicine). Staff, Hôpital Ste-Justine; Prof, Universite de Montreal; Langs: Bilingual(French/English); (514)345-4722; Fax. (514)345-4778; jean_wilkins@ssss.gouv.qc.ca.

WILKINS, Judy A; 203-453A Eglinton Ave W, Toronto ON M5N 1A7; Man'76; FRCPC; Psy. (416)894-8571

WILKINS, Kathryn R; Georgian Prof Centre, 305-125 Bell Farm Rd, Barrie ON L4M 6L2; Qns'88; FRCPC; PhysMed&Rehab (Electromyography). (705)726-7427; Fax. (705)725-7313.

WILKINS, Margaret A; 3-765 Ward St RR 1, Bridgenorth ON K0L 1H0; McM'86; CCFP; FCFP; Staff, Peterborough Regional Health Centre - Hospital Drive; Staff, Peterborough Regional Health Centre - Rogers St Site; (705)292-1991; Fax. (705)292-1995.

WILKINS, Mark A; Mattawa Health Clinic, PO Box 328 Stn Main 310 7th St, Mattawa ON P0H 1V0; Tor'79; CCFP; Staff Chief, Mattawa Hospital; Staff, Algonquin Nursing Home; Staff, Mattawa Health; Langs: English; French; (705)744-5541; Fax. (705)744-4162.

WILKINS, Michael A; Radiology Associates Inc, 1122 Scenic Dr S, Lethbridge AB T1K 7E5; Man'95; FRCPC; DiagRad. Staff, Elk Valley Hospital; Staff, Chinook Regional Hospital; (403)328-1122; michael.wilkins@interiorhealth.ca.

WILKINS, Paul J; 107-121 Dundas St E, Belleville ON K8N 1C3; Qns'95; BSc(LifeSciences); MSc(Path.); CCFP; (613)961-7600; Fax. (613)961-1377.

WILKINS, Warren T; Peterborough Reg Health Centre, 1 Hospital Dr, Peterborough ON K9J 2C6; Wes'75; FRCPC; IntMed. Dir IntMed Program, Peterborough Regional Health Centre - Hospital Drive; (705)740-6871

WILKINS-HO, Michael; Vancouver Gen Hosp, 5F-855 12th Ave W, Vancouver BC V5Z 1M9; UBC'95; FRCPC; Psy (AIDS/HIV). Staff, Providence Health Care - Mount Saint Joseph Hospital; Staff, Vancouver General Hospital - Centennial Pavillion; (604)562-1804

WILKINSON, Anna N; Ottawa Reg Cancer Centre, 503 Smyth Rd, Ottawa ON K1H 1C4; Ott'01; CCFP; Physician, Ottawa Regional Cancer Centre; (613)792-2616

WILKINSON, Diana J; Alberta Prof Bldg, 303-320 23 Ave SW, Calgary AB T2S 0J2; Cal'91; CCFP; (403)686-2150; Fax. (403)209-1299.

WILKINSON, Jane E; Commercial Street Med Centre, 208-311 Commercial St, Milton ON L9T 3Z9; McM'80; FRCSC; ObstGyn (Prenatal Care). (905)875-2280; Fax. (905)875-9172.

WILKINSON, Janet P; PO Box 65094 Rpo North Hill, Calgary AB T2N 4T6; Cal'83.

WILKINSON, John W; 5-1111 Franklin Blvd, Cambridge ON N1R 8B5; Wes'93; BSc; FRCSC; Ophth. Associate, Grand River Hospital - Kitchener/Waterloo Health Centre; Associate, St Mary's General Hospital; Associate, Cambridge Memorial Hospital; (519)623-4333; Fax. (519)622-3313.

WILKINSON, Mark A; 285 Huron St, Stratford ON N5A 5T3; Wes'82; Staff, Stratford General Hospital - Huron Perth Healthcare Alliance; (519)275-2604; Fax. (519)271-9451; drmark@mawmedic.com.

WILKINSON, Michael R; Vancouver 2010 Olympic, 3055 Wesbrook Mall, Vancouver BC V6T 1Z3; Witwatersrand (South Africa)'87; MB ChB; Dir Medical Services/Physician Vancouver Canucks Team/Physician Canadian Rowing Team, Vancouver 2010 Olympics Organizing Committee; Langs: Afrikaans; Dutch; (604)822-3614; Fax. (604)822-9058.

WILKINSON, Ross S; Riverside Prof Centre, 312-1919 Riverside Dr, Ottawa ON K1H 1A2; Ott'87; FRCSC; OrthSurg. (613)523-3245; Fax. (613)733-3651.

WILKINSON, Roy P; PO Box 1301, Jasper AB T0E 1E0; Edinburgh (Scotland)'65; MB ChB; FRCS(Ed); (780)852-4764; Fax. (780)852-2199.

WILKINSON, Sharon I; 407-672 Brant St, Burlington ON L7R 2H3; City Univ N Y Mount Sinai School of Med (USA)'76; FRCPC; Rheum; IntMed. Ac Staff, Joseph Brant Memorial Hospital; (905)632-0607; Fax. (905)632-8810.

WILKINSON, Susan E; 4007-381 Kent St, Ottawa ON K2P 2A8; Sask'79; CCFP; FCFP; (613)238-4123; Fax. (613)238-9393.

WILKINSON, Tandi L; PO Box 1984, Yellowknife NT X1A 2P5; UBC'90; CCFP; CCFP(E.M.); Staff, Kootenay Lake General Hospital.

WILL, Bruno O; Mango Tree Family Health Team, 35 Harvard Rd, Guelph ON N1G 3A2; Wes'66; Langs: German; (519)224-0547

WILL, David R A; 102-9145 82 Ave NW, Edmonton AB T6C 0Z4; Sask'69; FRCSC; Otol (Head & Neck Surgery). (780)469-4704; Fax. (780)469-4920.

WILL, Stephen B; 153 Colborne St W, Orillia ON L3V 2Z4; Mem'95; FRCSC; ObstGyn (Prenatal Care). Associate, Orillia Fertility Associates; (705)325-9503; Fax. (705)325-2385.

WILLAEYS, Veerle R P; Burnaby Ctr for Mental Hlth &, 3405 Willingdon Ave, Burnaby BC V5G 3H4; Antwerp Institute (Belgium)'89; FRCPC; CommunMed (Family Medicine). Staff, Burnaby Centre for Mental Health & Addictions; Langs: Dutch; French; (604)675-3950

WILLAMOWICZ, Anna S; Oshawa Med Arts Bldg, 210-300 King St W, Oshawa ON L1J 2K1; Warsaw (Poland)'88; ABIM; FRCPC; IntMed; Endocrin&Metab. Langs: Polish; (905)723-4330; Fax. (905)723-0204.

WILLANS, Gordon W; 32 First Ave, Orangeville ON L9W 1H8; Alb'66; LMCC; BA(Political Science); FRCPC; IntMed (Consultation). Staff, Headwaters Health Care Centre - Orangeville Site; (519)941-3232; Fax. (519)940-0821; gordwillans@sympatico.ca.

WILLANS, Martin J; AL-568 Christina St N, Sarnia ON N7T 5W6; Alb'61; FRCPC; IntMed (Rheumatology). Ac Staff, Bluewater Health - Norman Site; Ac Staff, Bluewater Health - Mitton Site; Ac Staff, Bluewater Health - Charlotte Eleanor Englehart Hospital; (519)332-1640; Fax. (519)332-2956.

WILLARD, Garry L; Goodfellow Prof Centre, 208-170 McEwan Dr E, Bolton ON L7E 4C8; Qns'63; FRCS(Ed); FACS; FICS; FRCSC; GenSurg (General,Thoracic & Vascular Medicine). (905)951-0555; Fax. (905)951-3698.

WILLARD, Martha J; Red River Family Med Centre, 139 Carmen Ave, Winnipeg MB R2L 0E5; Man'97; AB; MA; BSc; DVM; FCAP; FRCPC; AnatPath.

WILLARD, Peter T; 2H-570 King St, Welland ON L3B 3L2; Wes'89; FRCSC; GenSurg (Minimal Invasive Surgery). Staff, Niagara Health System - Welland Hospital Site; Staff, Niagara Health System - Port Colborne General Site; Teach Staff Health Sciences, McMaster University; Langs: Bilingual(French/English); (905)714-0080; Fax. (905)714-1828.

WILLEMOT, Patrick; MUHC-Royal Victoria Hosp, E2 61-687 av des Pins O, Montreal QC H3A 1A1; McG'00; FRCPC; IntMed. Staff, McGill University Health Centre - Royal Victoria Hospital; (514)934-1934 x31515; Fax. (514)843-1582; patrick.willemot@mail.mcgill.ca.

WILLEMS, Bernard E; CHUM-Hop St-Luc, 1058 rue Saint-Denis, Montreal QC H2X 3J4; Louvain (Belgium)'77; IntMed (P.Q.) (Hepatology). Ac Staff Liver Unit, Centre Hospitalier l'Université De Montréal (CHUM) - Hôpital Saint-luc; Prof Med, Universite de Montreal; Langs: English; French; Dutch; (514)890-8000 x35706; Fax. (514)412-7314; bernard.willems@umontreal.ca.

WILLEMS, Cara L M; William Osler HC-Etobicoke, 101 Humber College Blvd, Etobicoke ON M9V 1R8; Wes'92; FRCPC; NuclearMed. Staff, William Osler Health System - Etobicoke General Hospital; (416)747-3400 x2005; Fax. (416)747-3609.

WILLEMS, David D; Klinic Comm Health Centre, 870 Portage Ave, Winnipeg MB R3G 0P1; Man'92; CCFP; FCFP; (204)784-4090; Fax. (204)784-4013.

WILLEMSE, Pieter; Riding Mountain Surg Clinic, PO Box 606, Dauphin MB R7N 2V4; Pretoria (South Africa)'68; MB ChB; FRCS(Glas); Preceptor, University of Manitoba; Langs: Dutch; Afrikaans; dwillem2@mts.net.

WILLER, Christopher C; St Michael's Hosp, CCW 17-30 Bond St, Toronto ON M5B 1W8; UBC'07; FRCPC; Psy. Staff, St Michael's Hospital; (416)864-6060

WILLETT, Janice A; Doctors Bldg, 215-955 Queen St E, Sault Ste. Marie ON P6A 2C3; Wes'84; FRCSC; ObstGyn. Staff, Sault Area Hospital - Sault Ste Marie; Div Head Clinical Sciences/Section Leader Women's Health, Northern Ontario School of Medicine; (705)946-1332; Fax. (705)946-5113.

WILLETT, Paule; CSSS du Pontiac, 160 Ch de la Chute, Fort-Coulonge QC J0X 1V0; Sher'89; LMCC; CCFP; Staff, CSSS du Pontiac; Langs: Bilingual(French/English); (819)683-3000 x224; Fax. (819)683-2008.

WILLIAM, Anita L; Burntwood Comm Hlth Resource, 50 Selkirk Ave, Thompson MB R8N 0M7; (Other Foreign)'00; CCFP; Staff, Burntwood Regional Health Authority; (204)677-1777

WILLIAM, Hany; 202 Marlborough St N, Cornwall ON K6H 4A2; Cairo (Egypt)'73; MB ChB; CCFP; FCFP; Langs: Arabic; French; (613)933-1841; Fax. (613)933-3892.

WILLIAM, Nihad N; Steinbach Family Med Centre, 10-333 Loewen Blvd, Steinbach MB R5G 0C3; Staff, Thompson General Hospital; (204)326-3401

WILLIAMS, Aaron R; UBC Faculty of Medicine, 2775 Laurel St, Vancouver BC V5Z 1M9; UBC'10; CCFP; Staff, Gordon & Leslie Diamond Health Care Centre; (604)875-4111

WILLIAMS, Albert R; Dartmouth Gen Hosp, 325 Pleasant St, Dartmouth NS B2Y 4G8; Mem'03; CCFP; CCFP(E.M.); Staff, Dartmouth General Hospital; (902)465-8300

WILLIAMS, AnnaMary J; Trillium Med Centre, 306-1062 Ghislain St, Hawkesbury ON K6A 3B2; Alb'69; FAAD; FRCPC; Derm. Consultant Derm, Hawkesbury & District General Hospital; Consultant, Centre Hospitalier d'Argenteuil; Langs: English; French; (613)632-4073; Fax. (613)632-4454; ajwilliams@bellnet.ca.

WILLIAMS, Anne C; Whitehorse Gen Hosp, 5 Hospital Rd, Whitehorse YT Y1A 3H7; Ott'84; CCFP; FCFP; Staff, Whitehorse General Hospital; (867)393-8923; Fax. (867)393-8924.

WILLIAMS, Anne E; Terrace On The Square, 204-8 Rowan St, St. John's NL A1B 2X3; Mem'81; FACC; BMedSci; FRCPC; IntMed (Clinical Cardiology); Cardiol. Ac Staff Cardiol Eastern Health, Health Sciences Centre; Dir, Adult Congenital Cardiac Clinic; Assoc Prof Cardiol, Memorial University Of Newfoundland; (709)738-8883; Fax. (709)738-8898.

WILLIAMS, Anthony; Piper Creek Med Clinic, 200-3215 49 Ave, Red Deer AB T4N 0M8; Alb'81; Ac Staff, Red Deer Regional Hospital Centre; (403)986-7265; Fax. (403)986-7604.

WILLIAMS, Brent A; The Hosp for Sick Children, 555 University Ave, Toronto ON M5G 1X8; Dal'99; FAAP; FRCPC; Peds (Pediatric Hematology Oncology); Hem. Staff, The Hospital For Sick Children; (416)813-1500

WILLIAMS, C Noel; 16-409 Hunters Green NW, Edmonton AB T6R 2Z1; Leeds (England)'60; MRCS; LRCP; FACP; MACG; FRCP; FRCPC; IntMed (Gastroenterology). Staff, University of Alberta Hospital; Emeritus Prof, Dalhousie University; Aj Prof Med, University of Alberta; (780)432-8143; Fax. (780)432-8143.

WILLIAMS, Carole; Hôp Georges L-Dumont, 330 av Universite, Moncton NB E1C 2Z3; Sher'02; FRCSC; ObstGyn (P.Q.); GynOnco. Staff, Centre Hospitalier l'Université de Montréal (CHUM) - Hôpital Notre-Dame; Staff, Dr Georges-L-Dumont University Hospital Centre; (506)862-4000

WILLIAMS, Carole L; 107-2349 Millstream Rd, Victoria BC V9B 3R5; Cal'79; ATLS; ACLS; CCFP; Staff, Sante Spa Bear Mountain; (250)391-7554

WILLIAMS, Carole S; 100-311 McArthur Ave, Vanier ON K1L 8M3; Ott'83; Langs: English; French; (613)749-1414; Fax. (613)749-2007.

WILLIAMS, Cathy L; 5230 Mitch Owens Rd, Manotick ON K4M 1B2; Ott'08; (613)692-2571

WILLIAMS, Chadwick; Saint John Reg Hosp, PO Box 2100 Stn Main 400 University Ave, Saint John NB E2L 4L2; Dal'04; FRCPC; IntMed; Gastroent. Staff, Saint John Regional Hospital; (506)648-6000

WILLIAMS, Charles A; 555 Richmond St, Chatham ON N7M 1R2; Mem'90; FRCSC; Urol. (519)352-5139

WILLIAMS, Christina; BC Women's Hosp & Hlth Ctre, D6-4500 Oak St, Vancouver BC V6H 3N1; Barcelona (Spain)'81; FRCSC; ObstGyn (Gynecological Reproductive Endocrinology). Staff, BC Women's Hospital & Health Centre; Langs: Catalan; Spanish; (604)875-2445; Fax. (604)875-2569; cwilliam@vanhosp.bc.ca.

WILLIAMS, Constance L; McMaster Univ Childrens Hosp, 4F-1280 Main St W, Hamilton ON L8S 4K1; Tor'02; FRCPC; Peds (Neonatal & Perinatal Medicine). Staff, Mount Sinai Hospital; (905)521-2100

WILLIAMS, Dale; McMaster University, 5N 527-1280 Main St W, Hamilton ON L8S 4K1; Dal'02; FRCSC; OrthSurg (Joint Replacement). Staff, Hamilton Health Sciences Centre - Hamilton General Hospital; Asst Prof Surg, McMaster University; (905)527-0271; Fax. (905)577-8235; arner@hhsc.ca.

WILLIAMS, Daphne T; St Joseph's Health Centre, GFE-30 The Queensway, Toronto ON M6R 1B5; McM'96; CCFP; Staff, St Joseph's Health Centre; (416)530-6860; Fax. (416)530-6160; willid@stjoe.on.ca.

WILLIAMS, Dave J; 5-2168 McCallum Rd, Abbotsford BC V2S 6R6; West Indies (Jamaica)'79; MB BS; BSc; MSc; ABIM; FRCPC; IntMed (Critical Care Medicine); Respir. Med Dir, Abbotsford Regional Hospital & Cancer Centre; Clin Preceptor, University of British Columbia; (604)853-9022; Fax. (604)853-0695.

WILLIAMS, David C; University of Alberta Hosp, 2D4 39 WCM-8440 112 St NW, Edmonton AB T6G 2B7; Alb'92; MSc; FRCSC; GenSurg (Surgical Oncology); Public Health & Preventive Med. Staff, University of Alberta Hospital; Staff, Covenant Health - Misericordia Community Hospital; Staff, Cross Cancer Institute; Asst Prof, University of Alberta; (780)407-7815; Fax. (780)407-7817.

WILLIAMS, David C; Thunder Bay Dist Health Unit, 999 Balmoral St, Thunder Bay ON P7B 6E7; Tor'76; MHSc; FRCPC; CommunMed; Public Health & Preventive Med (Sexual Medicine). Med Officer of Hlth, City of Thunder Bay; Langs: Nepali; (807)625-5965; Fax. (807)625-5973; david.williams@tbdhu.com.

WILLIAMS, David; 6914 Early Settler Row, Mississauga ON L5W 1C6; Tor'81; CCFP.

WILLIAMS, David; Medical Arts Bldg, 93 St Vincent St N, Stratford ON N5A 6H5; Dundee (Scotland)'72; MB ChB; Staff FamMed, Stratford General Hospital - Huron Perth Healthcare Alliance; (519)271-5344; Fax. (519)273-7512; lwr@sentex.net.

WILLIAMS, David G; Cross Cancer Institute, 11560 University Ave, Edmonton AB T6G 1Z2; (United Kingdom)'95; Staff, Cross Cancer Institute; (780)995-3402

WILLIAMS, David G; Dr David G Williams Inc, 1569 Eric Rd, Victoria BC V8N 5Y6; UBC'86; CCFP; FCFP; (250)477-1858; Fax. (250)477-7580.

WILLIAMS, David J; Kelowna Gen Hosp, 2268 Pandosy St, Kelowna BC V1Y 1T2; Cal'02; FRCPC; EmergMed. Staff, Kelowna General Hospital; (250)862-4000

WILLIAMS, David R; Southlake Reg Health Centre, 596 Davis Dr, Newmarket ON L3Y 2P9; McG'83; FRCPC; EmergMed (Aeronautical Medicine);CCFP; FCFP; Staff, Southlake Regional Health Centre; Dir McMaster Centre for Medical Robotics, St Joseph's Healthcare - Charlton Campus; Langs: Bilingual(English/French); (905)895-4521; Fax. (905)853-2220.

WILLIAMS, Dorothy L; West Coast Gen Hosp, 3949 Port Alberni Hwy, Port Alberni BC V9Y 4S1; Alb'94; FRCPC; IntMed (Dementia); GeriatricMed. Staff, Royal Jubilee Hospital; Staff, West Coast General Hospital; (250)731-1370 x48112

WILLIAMS, Edward A; Quinte HC Corp-Belleville Gen, 265 Dundas St E, Belleville ON K8N 5A9; Tor'93; FRCPC; Anes. Staff, QHC Belleville General; (613)969-7400 x2448

WILLIAMS, Eldon S V; Healthchoices Centre, 815 College St, Toronto ON M6G 1C9; McG'60; BSc; MDCM; CSPQ; GenSurg (Trauma). Langs: French; Italian; Spanish; Portuguese; (416)533-1145; Fax. (416)533-3918; dresvwilliams@bellnet.ca.

WILLIAMS, Evelyn M; Sunnybrook Hlth Sciences Ctre, KGE31-2075 Bayview Ave, Toronto ON M4N 3M5; UBC'79; CCFP; FCFP; Head Div of Long Term Care, Sunnybrook Health Sciences Centre; Lecturer Family & CommunMed, University of Toronto; (416)480-6100 x3496; Fax. (416)480-5893.

WILLIAMS, Fouche; Rochdale Crossing Med Clinic, 7-5875 Rochdale Blvd, Regina SK S4X 2P9; Pretoria (South Africa)'89; MB ChB; CCFP; Physician, Regina Rehabilitation & Family Medical Clinic; (306)205-8020; Fax. (306)205-8023.

WILLIAMS, Gaynor J; Health Sciences Centre, MS 5-820 Sherbrook St, Winnipeg MB R3A 1R9; Man'83; BSc; PhD; FRCPC; AnatPath (Hematology Pathology). Assoc Prof, University of Manitoba; (204)787-4544

WILLIAMS, Gordon E; 855 Ingersoll Crt, Mississauga ON L5J 2S2; Tor'59; Assoc Staff, Halton Healthcare Services Corporation - Oakville Site; (905)822-9161 Semi-Retired.

WILLIAMS, Harvey R; Professional Bldg, 2100-222 King St E, Bowmanville ON L1C 1P6; Tor'92; BSc; CCFP; Staff, Lakeridge Health - Bowmanville Site; (905)623-0323; Fax. (905)697-0230.

WILLIAMS, Henry S; 106 Silver Stream Ave, Richmond Hill ON L4S 1Z4; London (England)'67; (905)770-2751 Semi-Retired.

WILLIAMS, Howell T; Clinique Med McDermott, 37 av Donegani, Pointe-Claire QC H9R 2V7; Alb'86; (514)697-1410; Fax. (514)697-1411.

WILLIAMS, J David; AMDocs Inc, 77 Main St, Winnipeg MB R3C 2R1; Man'84; BSc; CCFP; FCFP; Med Dir/Chief of Staff, AMDocs Inc; (204)934-1525; Fax. (204)934-1602.

WILLIAMS, James E; Dundas Family Med Group, 201-133 King St W, Hamilton ON L9H 1V3; Cal'75; MD; CCFP; FCFP; Ac Staff, Hamilton Health Sciences Centre - McMaster Children's Hospital; Asst Prof Family Med, McMaster University; (905)628-6355; Fax. (905)628-0664; williamj@mcmaster.ca.

WILLIAMS, Jason G; Queen Elizabeth II HSC-Halifax, 4447-1796 Summer St, Halifax NS B3H 3A7; Dal'00; FRCSC; PlasSurg. Staff, Queen Elizabeth II Health Sciences Centre - Halifax Infirmary Site; (902)473-6315; Fax. (902)473-6296.

WILLIAMS, Jennifer A; Royal Alexandra Hosp, CSC 541-10240 Kingsway NW, Edmonton AB T5H 3V9; McG'05; FRCPC; EmergMed. Staff Emerg Med, University of Alberta Hospital; Staff, Royal Alexandra Hospital; (780)735-5200

WILLIAMS, Jennifer J; 1031 Russet Rd NE, Calgary AB T2E 5L2; Mem'03; FRCPC; IntMed; Gastroent. Staff/Clinical Asst Prof, Rockyview General Hospital; (403)277-7321; Fax. (403)277-7327.

WILLIAMS, John T L; St Clare's Mercy Hosp, 154 Lemarchant Rd, St. John's NL A1C 5B8; Dal'73; FRCPC; Anes. Staff, St Clare's Mercy Hospital; (709)778-3521

WILLIAMS, Julie M; IWK Health Centre, PO Box 9700 Rpo CSC 5850-5980 University Ave, Halifax NS B3K 6R8; Tor'93; LMCC; FRCPC; Anes. Staff, IWK Health Centre; (902)470-8251; Fax. (902)470-7911.

WILLIAMS, Kelly M; Georgetown ED, 1 Princess Anne Dr, Georgetown ON L7G 2B8; Tor'04; CCFP; CCFP(E.M.); (905)873-0111

WILLIAMS, Kenneth B; Terrace on the Square, 8-10 Rowan St Box 13, St. John's NL A1B 2X3; Mem'02; FRCSC; Ophth. (709)726-2075; Fax. (709)726-2027.

WILLIAMS, Kenneth J; Sundridge Med Centre, PO Box 750 5 Park St, Sundridge ON P0A 1Z0; McM'79; Staff, Huntsville District Memorial Hospital - Muskoka Algonquin Healthcare; Med Examiner Aviation, Transport Canada; (705)384-5258; Fax. (705)384-7209.

WILLIAMS, Kiely; Bowmont Med Clinic, 6535 Bowness Rd NW, Calgary AB T3B 0E8; UBC'08; CCFP; (403)247-9797; Fax. (403)247-0014.

WILLIAMS, Kurt E; Royal University Hosp, 103 Hospital Dr, Saskatoon SK S7N 0W8; Cal'80; FRCPC; IntMed; InfectDis. Staff Med, Royal University Hospital; Consultant, St Paul's Hospital (Grey Nuns) of Saskatoon; Consultant, Saskatoon City Hospital; Consultant STD Clinic, Saskatoon Community Health Unit; Assoc Prof Med & Microbiol, University of Saskatchewan; (306)655-1777; Fax. (306)975-0383.

WILLIAMS, Lara J; Queen Elizabeth II HSC, 8 824-1276 South Park St, Halifax NS B3H 2Y9; Wes'03; FRCSC; GenSurg (Colorectal Surgery). Staff, Queen Elizabeth II Health Sciences Centre - Victoria General Site; (902)473-3937; Fax. (902)428-4176; emily.rendell@cdha.nshealth.ca.

WILLIAMS, Leslie G; Saanich Plaza Med Clinic, 3544 Blanshard St, Victoria BC V8X 1W3; Sask'75.

WILLIAMS, Llewelyn K; Laurel Med Centre Ltd, 202-888 8th Ave W, Vancouver BC V5Z 3Y1; UBC'64; BSc; (604)872-5688; Fax. (604)872-7394.

WILLIAMS, Lyle K; Downtown Med Clinic, PO Box 1866, Unity SK S0K 4L0; (306)228-4450; Fax. (306)228-4277.

WILLIAMS, Malcolm B; Western Cardiology Associates, 335-1900 Richmond Ave, Victoria BC V8R 4R2; London (England)'64; MB BS; MRC; FACC; MRCP(UK); FRCPC; IntMed (Interventional Cardiology). Staff, Vancouver Island Health Authority; (250)595-1551; Fax. (250)595-6793.

WILLIAMS, Megan K; Somerset West CHC, 55 Eccles St, Ottawa ON K1R 6S3; Wes'05; CCFP; Staff, Arnprior & District Memorial Hospital; (613)238-1220; Fax. (613)235-2982.

WILLIAMS, Michael D; Grey Bruce HS-Owen Sound, PO Box 1800 Stn Main 1800 8th St E, Owen Sound ON N4K 6M9; McM'91; BSc; AB; FRCPC; EmergMed (Sports Medicine). Staff, Grey Bruce Health Services - Owen Sound; Clin Asst, University of Toronto; (519)376-2121

WILLIAMS, N Ashley; 264-10816 Macleod Trail SE, Calgary AB T2J 5N8; Birmingham (England)'80; MB ChB; Staff, Carepoint Medical Clinic; (403)247-2253; Fax. (403)206-7141.

WILLIAMS, Owen R T; Health Sciences Centre, GB 103-820 Sherbrook St, Winnipeg MB R3A 1R9; Cal'86; BSc; MBA; FRCSC; Neursurg (Spine). Att Staff, Health Sciences Centre; Asst Prof, University of Manitoba; (204)787-7271; Fax. (204)783-7356.

WILLIAMS, Paul A; Trent Hills Family Health Team, 119 Isabella St, Campbellford ON K0L 1L0; Tor'98; CCFP; Chief Medical Staff/Hd CommunMed/Hd FamilyMed, Campbellford Memorial Hospital; (705)653-1801; Fax. (705)653-5483.

WILLIAMS, Paula B; 205-840 Coxwell Ave, Toronto ON M4C 5T2; Tor'75; Staff Family Pract, Toronto East General Hospital Inc; Lecturer Family & Commun Med, University of Toronto; Langs: English; French; (416)465-6301; Fax. (416)465-5754.

WILLIAMS, Pieter; 22313 Selkirk Ave, Maple Ridge BC V2X 2X6; Pretoria (South Africa)'73; MB ChB; Langs: Afrikaans; (604)463-8814; Fax. (604)463-9927.

WILLIAMS, R Christopher; Caroline Family Hlth Team-CMG, 15-3305 Harvester Rd, Burlington ON L7N 3N2; Tor'99; CCFP; Ac Staff, Joseph Brant Memorial Hospital; (905)632-8007; Fax. (905)632-0375.

WILLIAMS, R Geoffrey; 200-5340 1 St SW, Calgary AB T2H 0C8; Cal'85; DAB; FRCSC; Ophth (Retina Vitreous Surgery). Associate, Rockyview General Hospital; Clinical Asst Prof, University of Calgary; (403)286-6802; Fax. (403)286-6819; geoff.williams@calgaryretina.ca.

WILLIAMS, Rachel C; Delta Health Sciences Centre, 202-4515 Harvest Dr, Delta BC V4K 4L1; UBC'07; CCFP; Physician, Delta Health Sciences Centre; (604)946-6411

WILLIAMS, Randall G; Hys Med Centre, 350-11010 101 St NW, Edmonton AB T5H 4B9; Alb'77; FRCPC; IntMed (Echocardiography); Cardiol. Ac Staff, Royal Alexandra Hospital; Consultant, Covenant Health - Grey Nuns Community Hospital; Consultant, University of Alberta Hospital; Clin Prof, University of Alberta; (780)428-3246; Fax. (780)425-0487; randywilliams07@gmail.com.

WILLIAMS, Richard; Victoria Mental Health Centre, 2328 Trent St, Victoria BC V8R 4Z3; London (England)'74; MB BS; MPhil; FRCPC; Psy (Psychiatric Rehabilitation). Dir Schizophrenia Serv/Chief Psychiatric Rehab, Royal Jubilee Hospital; Clin Prof Psy, University of British Columbia; (250)370-8158; Fax. (250)370-8161.

WILLIAMS, Robert C; Ontario Telemedicine Network, A-640 Ross Ave E, Timmins ON P4N 8P2; Wes'75; CCFP; Ac Staff, Timmins & District Hospital; (705)360-7252; Fax. (705)360-1484; rwilliams@tadh.com.

WILLIAMS, Robert D; Glenmore Clinic, 1605 Gordon Dr, Kelowna BC V1Y 3G8; UBC'85; (250)762-2532; Fax. (250)762-4477.

WILLIAMS, Robert E; 15435 Yonge St, Aurora ON L4G 1P3; Tor'69; Sr Staff, Southlake Regional Health Centre; (905)727-1319; Fax. (905)727-4791.

WILLIAMS, Robert; UMF Charles Lemoyne, 201-299 boul Sir Wilfrid-Lauri, Longueuil QC J4R 2L1; Mon'84; CCFP; (450)466-5630; Fax. (450)466-5631.

WILLIAMS, Robert S; Brant Community HS-Willet Site, 238 Grand River St N, Paris ON N3L 2N7; Melbourne (Australia)'73; Ac Staff, The Brant Community Healthcare System - Willett Hospital Site; Ac Staff, The Brant Community Healthcare System - Brantford General Hospital Site; (519)442-7150; Fax. (519)442-3411; r.williams@rogers.com.

WILLIAMS, Robin L; Rogers House, 399 Smyth Rd, Ottawa ON K1H 8L2; Qns'05; FRCPC; Peds. Staff, Montfort Hospital; Langs: Bilingual(English/French); (613)523-6300

WILLIAMS, Russell G; Mental Health & Addictions Ctr, 1440 14 Ave, Vernon BC V1B 2T1; Michigan (USA)'01; FRCPC; Psy. (250)549-5700

WILLIAMS, Ruthanne L; Fort William Clinic, 117 McKellar St S, Thunder Bay ON P7E 1H5; Wes'07; CCFP; Staff, Thunder Bay Regional Health Sciences Centre; (807)626-1234

WILLIAMS, Ryan A; Regional Rehabilitation Centre, 300 Wellington St N, Hamilton ON L8L 0A4; Medical University of the Americas (Other Foreign)'06; FRCPC; PhysMed&Rehab. Staff, Hamilton Health Sciences Centre - Regional Rehabilitation Centre; (905)521-2100; williamsr@hhsc.ca.

WILLIAMS, S Geoffrey; Queen Elizabeth II HSC, 1276 South Park St, Halifax NS B3H 2Y9; Mem'02; FRCPC; IntMed; Gastroent. Staff, Queen Elizabeth II Health Sciences Centre - Victoria General Site; (902)473-4585

WILLIAMS, Sarah L; Broadway Family Physicians, 1801 Broadway Ave, Saskatoon SK S7H 2B6; Sask'01; CCFP; Teach Staff, University of Saskatchewan; (306)652-2632; Fax. (306)652-2637.

WILLIAMS, Stacey P; Queen Elizabeth II HSC-VG Site, 906-1278 Tower Rd, Halifax NS B3H 2Y9; Dal'99; FRCPC; IntMed; Gastroent. Staff, Queen Elizabeth II Health Sciences Centre - Victoria General Site; (902)473-3721; Fax. (902)473-4406.

WILLIAMS, Stephan; CHUM-Hop Notre-Dame, AS 1115-1560 rue Sherbrooke E, Montreal QC H2L 4M1; Mon'98; Anes. Staff, Centre Hospitalier l'Université de Montréal (CHUM) - Hôpital Notre-Dame; (514)890-8000

WILLIAMS, Suzan A; The Hosp for Sick Children, 10414A-555 University Ave, Toronto ON M5G 1X8; Tor'97; BSc; MSc; FRCPC; Peds (Thrombosis). Staff Hem/Oncol, The Hospital For Sick Children; (416)813-7758; Fax. (416)813-5327; suzan.williams@sickkids.ca.

WILLIAMS, Tammy C; Southwood Med Clinic, 1700-2751 Cliffe Ave, Courtenay BC V9N 2L8; Dal'88; (250)334-2212

WILLIAMS, Tanya-Gay M; Rouge Valley Fertility Centre, 309-100 Consilium Place, Scarborough ON M1E 3E3; Tor'88; BA; FRCSC; ObstGyn (Infertility). Court Staff, Rouge Valley Health System - Centenary Health Centre Site; (416)283-5539; Fax. (416)283-1636.

WILLIAMS, Tara M; St Joseph's Health Centre, 30 The Queensway, Toronto ON M6R 1B5; Qns'91; FRCPC; DiagRad. Staff, St Joseph's Health Centre; (416)530-6486 x4486

WILLIAMS, Taryn M; Two Rivers FHT-Hespeler Med Cl, B12-350 Conestoga Blvd, Cambridge ON N1R 7L7; McM'07; CCFP; (519)629-4615; Fax. (519)629-4630.

WILLIAMS, Tina W; Groves Mem Community Hosp, 235 Union St E, Fergus ON N1M 1W3; McG'90; FRCSC; GenSurg. Staff, Groves Memorial Community Hospital; (519)843-2322; Fax. (519)843-2705.

WILLIAMS, Tracey L; C-339 Willow St, Truro NS B2N 5A6; Dal'99; BSc; FRCPC; Peds (Family Medicine). Staff, Colchester East Hants Health Centre; (902)893-5505; Fax. (902)893-3444.

WILLIAMS, V Guy; 219 Main St E, Hawkesbury ON K6A 1A1; London (England)'68; MB BS; LRCP; MRCS; DObstRCOG; Langs: English; French; (613)632-8811; Fax. (613)632-9404.

WILLIAMS, Vivian P; Glen Erin Med & Dental Ctre, 11-2318 Dunwin Dr, Mississauga ON L5L 1C7; Tor'85; BSc; Clin Physician, Regional Peel Healthy Sexuality; (905)828-1145; Fax. (905)828-1144.

WILLIAMS, W Shane; South Muskoka Mem Hosp, 75 Ann St, Bracebridge ON P1L 2E4; Mem'99; BSc(Pharm); FRCPC; IntMed; Cardiol (Critical Care Medicine). Staff, South Muskoka Memorial Hospital - Muskoka Algonquin Healthcare; (705)645-4404

WILLIAMS, Walter S; Williams Cardiology, 2-90 Kimberley Ave, Bracebridge ON P1L 2A4; Mem'99; Staff, South Muskoka Memorial Hospital - Muskoka Algonquin Healthcare; (705)645-4404

WILLIAMS, Wendy C; Thornhill Family Physicians, 35-7700 Bathurst St, Thornhill ON L4J 7Y3; Tor'94; BScPharm; CCFP; FCFP; Staff, Mackenzie Richmond Hill Hospital; (905)881-6510; Fax. (905)881-6513.

WILLIAMS, William L; Univ of Ottawa Heart Institute, 40 Ruskin St, Ottawa ON K1Y 4W7; McG'69; FRCPC; IntMed (Acute Coronary Care); Cardiol. Staff, University of Ottawa Heart Institute; Att Physician, The Ottawa Hospital - Civic Campus; Assoc Prof, University of Ottawa; Langs: English; French; (613)761-5000

WILLIAMSON, David G; Okanagan Plastic Surgery Centr, 401-3320 Richter St, Kelowna BC V1W 4V5; Dal'94; BSc; FACS; MRCS; FRCSC; PlasSurg (Plastic & Reconstructive Surgery). Ac Staff, Kelowna General Hospital; Staff, Summerland Memorial Health Centre; Staff Surgical Floor, Okanagan Plastic Surgery Centre; Dir Skin Care Floor, Okanagan Skin Care Centre; Clin Instructor, University of British Columbia; (250)868-9290; Fax. (250)868-9704.

WILLIAMSON, Donald B; Queensway Med Centre, 125 Queensway E, Simcoe ON N3Y 4M5; Man'98; (519)426-0911; Fax. (519)426-9753.

WILLIAMSON, J Scott; Okanagan Plastic Surgery Centr, 401-3320 Richter St, Kelowna BC V1W 4V5; Qns'89; FACS; FRCSC; PlasSurg. Staff, Kelowna General Hospital; Staff Surgical Floor, Okanagan Plastic Surgery Centre; Dir Skin Care Floor, Okanagan Skin Care Centre; Staff, Okanagan Health Surgical Centre; Teach Staff PlasSurg, University of British Columbia; (250)868-9290; Fax. (250)868-9704.

WILLIAMSON, Jeffrey; Saint John Reg Hosp, PO Box 2100 Stn A, Saint John NB E2L 4L2; Dal'09; CCFP; Staff, Saint John Regional Hospital; (506)648-6000

WILLIAMSON, Kelvin W; Concordia Gen Hosp, 1095 Concordia Ave, Winnipeg MB R2K 3S8; Man'05; FRCPC; Anes. Staff, Brandon Regional Health Centre; Staff, Concordia General Hospital; (204)667-1560

WILLIAMSON, Kimberly A; St Joseph's Healthcare, 50 Charlton Ave E, Hamilton ON L8N 4A6; Wes'80; MCFP(EM); Ac Staff Emerg, St Joseph's Healthcare - Charlton Campus; Assoc Staff Emerg, Halton Healthcare Services Corporation - Oakville Site; Asst Prof Family Med, McMaster University; Langs: English; French; (905)522-4941 x8510; Fax. (905)573-4842.

WILLIAMSON, Owen D; Jim Pattison Outpatient Care, 9750 140 St, Surrey BC V3T 0G9; Melbourne (Australia)'82; MB BS; (604)582-4587

WILLIAMSON, Peter C; London HSC-University Hosp, PO Box 5339 Stn B 10F-339 Windermere Rd, London ON N6A 5A5; Wes'77; FRCPC; Psy (Schizophrenia). Affil Researcher, London Health Sciences Centre - University Hospital; Prof Psy & Neurological Sciences, University of Western Ontario; (519)663-3032; Fax. (519)663-3935.

WILLIAMSON, William D; 100-5791 No. 3 Rd, Richmond BC V6X 2C9; UBC'70; DiagRad. Court Staff, Richmond Hospital; Court Staff, Burnaby Hospital; Physician, Kingsway Medical Plaza Phase III; (604)278-9152; Fax. (604)278-9291.

WILLINSKY, Robert A; Univ Hlth Network-Toronto Western Hosp, 399 Bathurst St, Toronto ON M5T 2S8; Wes'76; FRCPC; DiagRad (Neuro Radiology). Staff, Toronto Western Hospital - University Health Network; (416)603-5981; Fax. (416)603-4257.

WILLIS, Brian D; Edson Med Centre, PO Box 6660 Stn Main, Edson AB T7E 1V1; Belfast (Ireland)'72; MB ChB; Ac Staff, Edson Healthcare Centre; Clin Lecturer, University of Alberta; (780)723-3366; Fax. (780)723-3437.

WILLIS, Kenneth R; Riverside Prof Centre, 414-1919 Riverside Dr, Ottawa ON K1H 1A2; Ott'74; FACP; FCCP; CSPQ; FRCPC; IntMed; Respir. Ac Staff (All Sites), The Ottawa Hospital - General Campus; Ac Staff, Montfort Hospital; Langs: English; French; (613)738-7585; Fax. (613)738-1019.

WILLIS, Marianne I J; Main Street Med Associates, PO Box 489, Oliver BC V0H 1T0; Cape Town (South Africa)'80; MB ChB; CCFP; Staff, BC Children's Hospital; Langs: Afrikaans; (250)498-3411; Fax. (250)498-0233; docsvhf@uniserve.com.

WILLIS, Stephen A; Saint John Med Clinic, 299 Metcalf St, Saint John NB E2K 4P8; Dal'74; CCFP; Ac Staff, Saint John Regional Hospital; Ac Staff, St Joseph's Hospital; Lecturer, Dalhousie University; (506)634-3093; Fax. (506)634-2114.

WILLIS JR., R Baxter; Children's Hosp Eastern Ont, 401 Smyth Rd, Ottawa ON K1H 8L1; Wes'71; FRCSC; OrthSurg. Staff, Children's Hospital of Eastern Ontario (CHEO); (613)737-7600

WILLISCROFT, David M; Lions Gate Hosp, 231 15th St E, North Vancouver BC V7L 2L7; UBC'01; CCFP; CCFP(E.M.); Staff, Lions Gate Hospital; (604)562-1006

WILLISTON, Luke A; Tonquin Med Clinic, PO Box 189 220 First St, Tofino BC V0R 2Z0; UBC'05; CCFP; (250)725-3282; Fax. (250)725-3215.

WILLISTON, Maryse; 247 University Ave, Moncton NB E1C 5K4; Sher'05; FRCPC; IntMed; Respir.

WILLITS, Kevin R; Fowler Kennedy Sports Med Clin, 3M-1151 Richmond St, London ON N6A 3K7; McM'96; FRCSC; OrthSurg (Arthroscopy). (519)661-4121

WILLMORE, Wendy S; Central Health Consultants, 129 Lincoln Rd, Grnd-Falls-Windsor NL A2A 1P3; Qns'02; FRCSC; GenSurg. Staff, Central Newfoundland Regional Health Centre; (709)489-2700

WILLMOTT, Andrew D; Seafield Med Bldg, 3-1179 Seafield Cres, Nanaimo BC V9S 4S1; McM'07; PhysMed&Rehab. (250)741-0755

WILLMOTT, Caroline; West Bowness Shopp Centre, 52-7930 Bowness Rd NW, Calgary AB T3B 0H3; (403)247-1303; Fax. (403)288-6670.

WILLMS, Arthur G; Colebrook Family Practice, 107-15240 56 Ave, Surrey BC V3S 5K7; Cal'74; CCFP; CCFP(E.M.); Ac Staff, Surrey Memorial Hospital; Med Dir, Zion Park Manor; Site Dir Family Practice Residency Prog, University of British Columbia; (778)574-1414; arthur.willms@fraserhealth.ca.

WILLMS, Larry A; Meno Ya Win Health Centre, PO Box 909 1 Meno Ya Win Way, Sioux Lookout ON P8T 1B4; McM'92; CCFP; FCFP; Staff, Sioux Lookout Meno-Ya-Win Health Centre; McMaster University; Langs: Spanish; (807)737-5160

WILLMS, Rhonda L; 4255 Laurel St, Vancouver BC V5Z 2G9; UBC'95; FRCPC; PhysMed&Rehab (Amputee & Orthotics). Staff, G F Strong Rehabilitation Centre; University of British Columbia; (604)714-4113; Fax. (604)737-6251.

WILLOUGHBY, Brian C; Spectrum Health, 702-1080 Howe St, Vancouver BC V6Z 2T1; Wes'73; CCFP; Ac Staff/Member, Providence Health Care - St Paul's Hospital; Clin Assoc Prof Family & Commun Med, University of British Columbia; Langs: Bilingual(English/French); (604)681-1080; Fax. (604)681-0244.

WILLOUGHBY, D Paul; 379 Hunter St, Woodstock ON N4S 4G3; Wes'71; MSc(OccupMed); CCFP; Ac Staff, Woodstock General Hospital; (519)536-0567; Fax. (519)539-2005; pwwillowdon@gmail.com.

WILLOUGHBY, Joanne S; Guelph Medical Place 2, 107-89 Dawson Rd, Guelph ON N1H 1B1; McM'85; FRCPC; Derm. Consultant, Grand River Hospital - Freeport Site; Consultant, Hamilton Health Sciences Centre - McMaster Children's Hospital; Asst Prof, McMaster University; Langs: Bilingual(English/French); (519)836-7326; Fax. (519)763-5440.

WILLOUGHBY, Rodney P N; Sudbury Vascular Laboratory, 345-2140 Regent St, Sudbury ON P3E 5S8; Tor'92; BSc(Hon); MD; FRCS; RVT; FRCSC; VascSurg; GenSurg. Ac Staff, Health Sciences North-Laurentian Site; Asst Prof Surg, Northern Ontario School of Medicine; (705)522-4611; Fax. (705)522-4158; rwilloughby@hrsrh.on.ca.

WILLOUGHBY, Siri A; Wilson Family Med Centre, 1-2185 Wilson Ave, Port Coquitlam BC V3C 6C1; Cal'87; BSc; CCFP; (604)942-7227; Fax. (604)942-7058.

WILLOWS, James R; Seven Oaks Gen Hosp, 2300 McPhillips St, Winnipeg MB R2V 3M3; Man'91; FRCPC; Psy. Staff, Seven Oaks General Hospital; Staff, Selkirk Mental Health Centre; (204)632-7133

WILLOWS, Melanie D; Royal Ottawa Health Care Group, 1145 Carling Ave, Ottawa ON K1Z 7K4; Ott'99; CCFP; Staff Royal Substance Use & Concurrent Disorders Program, Royal Ottawa Mental Health Centre - Royal Ottawa Health Care Group; (613)722-6521; Fax. (613)761-3617.

WILLOX, David L; Associate Med Clinic, PO Box 7590 Stn Main, Peace River AB T8S 1T2; Alb'80; (780)624-2581; Fax. (780)624-4015.

WILLOX, Laurene A; Associate Med Clinic, PO Box 7590 Stn Main, Peace River AB T8S 1T2; Alb'81; (780)624-2581; Fax. (780)624-4015.

WILLS, Lee Ann M; Continuum Med Care, 202-520 17th St, West Vancouver BC V7V 3S8; Wes'87; CCFP; Staff Privil, Lions Gate Hospital; (604)913-8183; Fax. (604)913-8804.

WILLS, Michael C; 202-289 Pinnacle St, Belleville ON K8N 3B3; Tor'75; MSc; DIH; FRCPC; OccupMed;CCFP; (613)966-4114; Fax. (613)966-4130.

WILLSIE, W Robert; 201 Signature Way SW, Calgary AB T3H 2Y2; Qns'70; FRCPC; Anes.

WILLSON, Morgan C; Foothill Med Centre, 1403 29 St NW, Calgary AB T2N 2T9; Cal'06; FRCPC; DiagRad. Staff, Foothills Medical Centre; (403)944-4747; Fax. (403)944-4577.

WILMOT, Kim; Glenmore Landing, D261-1600 90 Ave SW, Calgary AB T2V 5A8; Wes'80; (403)252-8855; Fax. (403)255-1667.

WILNER, Asher P; Allan Memorial Institute, 1025 av des Pins O, Montreal QC H3A 1A1; McM'76; FRCPsy; PABPN; FRCPC; Psy (Consultant Liaison Psychiatry). Staff, Allan Memorial Institute; adj Prof, McGill University; (514)934-1934 x35502; Fax. (514)843-2858; asher.wilner@mcgill.ca.

WILSON, Adriana E; Lacewood Med Clinic, 200-366 Lacewood Dr, Halifax NS B3S 1M7; Man'06; BA; BSc; MEd; FRCPC; Psy (Life Expectancy). Asst Prof Psy, Dalhousie University; Langs: Bilingual(English/French); (902)445-9400; Fax. (902)445-7108.

WILSON, Allan; Royal Ottawa Hlth Care Group, 1145 Carling Ave, Ottawa ON K1Z 7K4; Man'81; Clin Dir Substance Use & Concurrent Disorder Prog, Royal Ottawa Mental Health Centre - Royal Ottawa Health Care Group; Prof, University of Ottawa; Langs: English; French; (613)722-6521 x6508; Fax. (613)722-5048.

WILSON, Andrea S; 161-31 Southridge Dr, Okotoks AB T1S 2N3; Sask'01; CCFP; CCFP(E.M.); Staff, South Calgary Urgent Care Centre; (403)995-5740; Fax. (403)995-5742; asw180@hotmail.com.

WILSON, Anne; Northbrook Med Center, RR 1, Northbrook ON K0H 2G0; Tor'10; CCFP; (613)336-8888

WILSON, Anthony B; Oakridge Centre South Tower, 209-650 41st Ave W, Vancouver BC V5Z 2M9; UBC'78; CCFP; FCFP; Ac Staff, Vancouver General Hospital - Centennial Pavillion; Clinical Asst Prof, University of British Columbia; (604)261-5626; Fax. (604)263-1541.

WILSON, Aze S A; London HSC-Victoria Campus, PO Box 5010 Stn B E1 317-800 Commissioners Rd E, London ON N6A 5W9; Wes'08; IntMed. Staff, London Health Sciences Centre - Victoria Campus; (519)667-6843

WILSON, Benjamin; Clinical Tenant Support Team, 211 Gore Ave, Vancouver BC V6A 0B6; UBC'08; CCFP; (604)660-8859

WILSON, Beverly A; Edmonton Clinic Health Academy, 3 516-11405 87 St NW, Edmonton AB T5B 3M2; Alb'85; FRCPC; Peds (Pediatric Oncology). Staff Stollery Children's Hosp, University of Alberta Hospital; Assoc Prof Peds, University of Alberta; (780)248-5530

WILSON, Bonnie L; Dr Bonnie L Wilson Med Office, GF-458 Maclaren St, Ottawa ON K1R 5K6; McG'88; BSc; MDCM; FRCPC; Psy (Psychotherapy). Consultant Psy, The Ottawa Hospital - General Campus; Lecturer, University of Ottawa; (613)230-0564; Fax. (613)230-9204.

WILSON, Brett P; The Associate Clinic, PO Box 549 1222 Bev McLachlin Dr, Pincher Creek AB T0K 1W0; Cal'10; CCFP; (403)627-3321; Fax. (403)627-2280.

WILSON, Brian D; Fifth Avenue Med Centre, 500-14 Fifth Ave, Orangeville ON L9W 1G2; Tor'86; CCFP; Staff, Dufferin Caledon Health Care Corporation; (519)942-1501; Fax. (519)942-3492.

WILSON, Brianna C; Good Shepherd Health Clinic, 128 Emerald St S, Hamilton ON L8N 2V5; McM'07; CCFP; (905)526-7137; Fax. (905)526-7969.

WILSON, Bruce J; Phoenix Med Centre, 310-2155 10th Ave, Prince George BC V2M 5J6; UBC'90; Staff, University Hospital of Northern British Columbia; (250)564-8219; Fax. (250)564-1674.

WILSON, C Ruth; Family Med Centre, PO Box 8888 Stn Main 220 Bagot St, Kingston ON K7L 5E9; Tor'76; CCFP; FCFP; Prof Family Med, Queen's University; (613)533-6000 x73959; Fax. (613)544-9899; wilsonrw@queensu.ca.

WILSON, Cameron B; Regina Internal Med Specialist, 1821 Rose St, Regina SK S4P 1Z7; Sask'67; FRCPC; IntMed (Nephrology). Dir Hematol Dialysis Unit, Regina General Hospital; Pres, Saskatchewan Nephrology Association; Physician, Regina Internal Medicine Specialists; Assoc Prof Med, University of Saskatchewan; (306)757-6633; Fax. (306)359-1068.

WILSON, Chantelle N; Gore Bay Med Centre, PO Box 219 70 Meredith St, Gore Bay ON P0P 1H0; Ott'00; CCFP; Langs: English; French; (705)282-2262; Fax. (705)282-2370.

WILSON, Christine M; BC Cancer Agency-Vancouver CC, 600 10th Ave W, Vancouver BC V5Z 4E6; Sask'79; FRCPC; DiagRad (Breast Imaging). Staff, BC Cancer Agency Vancouver Centre; (604)877-6098

WILSON, Colin G; Kingston Family Health Team, 403-800 Princess St, Kingston ON K7L 5E4; Dal'06; CCFP; (613)549-0464

WILSON, Collis; Business Bldg, 410-1200 Burrard St, Vancouver BC V6Z 2C7; McG'72; MDCM; Ac Staff, Providence Health Care - St Paul's Hospital; Staff, Bentall 4 Clinic; (604)681-7561; Fax. (604)681-6995.

WILSON, Dale R; Springbank Med Centre, 306-460 Springbank Dr, London ON N6J 0A8; Wes'85; CCFP; CCFP(E.M.); FCFP; Physician, Wortley Village Medical Centre; Clin Lecturer Family Med, University of Western Ontario; (519)661-0047; Fax. (519)661-0917.

WILSON, Dana F; King Street Med Arts Centre, 406-71 King St W, Mississauga ON L5B 4A2; Tor'84; BSc; FRCSC; OrthSurg (Spine Surgery). (905)275-7327; Fax. (905)275-1094.

WILSON, David A K; Medical & Dental Bldg, 510-586 Eglinton Ave E, Toronto ON M4P 1P2; Tor'75; FRCPC; Psy. (416)481-7347; Fax. (416)481-9094; dakwilson@rogers.com.

WILSON, David H; PO Box 368, Shelburne NS B0T 1W0; Glasgow (Scotland)'77; MB ChB; DRCOG; MRC(UK); Staff, Roseway Hospital; (902)875-2457; Fax. (902)875-1468.

WILSON, Diane B; Dr Hennenfent & Dr Wilson Inc, PO Box 1617, Lunenburg NS B0J 2C0; Cal'85; FRCPC; IntMed; Rheum. (902)634-1951; Fax. (902)634-3522.

WILSON, Donald C; BC Cancer Agency-Vancouver CC, 600 10th Ave W, Vancouver BC V5Z 4E6; Sask'89; BSc; FRCPC; NuclearMed; RadOncol. Staff, BC Cancer Agency Vancouver Centre; (604)877-6000 x2681; Fax. (604)877-6278; dowilson@bccancer.bc.ca.

WILSON, Donald G; Oceanview Women's Clinic, 101-1757 Beaufort Ave, Comox BC V9M 1R8; Cal'01; FRCSC; ObstGyn. Langs: French; Creole; (250)339-3114; Fax. (250)339-4186.

WILSON, Donald K; 403-267 O'Connor St, Ottawa ON K2P 1V3; Alb'85; Langs: Bilingual(English/French); (613)567-3904; Fax. (613)567-3917.

WILSON, Donald M; The Ottawa Hosp-Riverside, 1967 Riverside Dr, Ottawa ON K1H 7W9; Ott'79; FRCPC; Anes. Staff, The Ottawa Hospital - Riverside Campus; (613)738-8400

WILSON, Donald W S; Hawkstone Med Clinic, 204-18332 Lessard Rd NW, Edmonton AB T6M 2W8; Alb'86; BSc; Clin Instructor Family Med, University of British Columbia; (780)486-3461; Fax. (780)486-0087.

WILSON, G Andrew C; 55 Highway 118 W PO Box 20001 Rpo IDA Pharmacy, Bracebridge ON P1L 2H6; Qns'69; FRCPC; Psy (Developmental Disability). Ac Staff, South Muskoka Memorial Hospital - Muskoka Algonquin Healthcare; Psychiatrist, Huronia Regional Centre; (705)646-2673; Fax. (705)646-2674.

WILSON, G S Lowen; 12 Wolf Dr, Redwood Meadows AB T3Z 1A3; Belfast (Ireland)'59; MB ChB; BAO; MRCS; LRCP; (403)949-3368; Fax. (403)949-2445.

WILSON, Gordon A; 120-1641 Hillside Ave, Victoria BC V8T 5G1; Alb'76; Ac Staff, Royal Jubilee Hospital; Ac Staff, Victoria General Hospital; (250)592-4212

WILSON, Gregory J; The Hosp for Sick Children, 3128-555 University Ave, Toronto ON M5G 1X8; McM'75; FRCPC; AnatPath (Pediatric Cardiovascular Pathology). Sr Staff Path & Scientist, The Hospital For Sick Children; Prof, University of Toronto; (416)813-5965; Fax. (416)813-7927; gregory.wilson@sickkids.ca.

WILSON, Gregory P; Oakfield Med Clinic, 102-1021 Court Ave, Winnipeg MB R2P 1V7; Man'95; CCFP; (204)388-3062

WILSON, Heather C; 203-3040 Tutt St, Kelowna BC V1Y 2H5; UBC'03; FRCSC; GenSurg. Langs: Bilingual(English/French); (250)763-2226

WILSON, Ian F; William Jackman Mem Hosp, 410 Booth St, Labrador City NL A2V 2K1; Cork (Ireland)'90; MB BCh; Staff, Captain William Jackman Memorial Hospital; (709)944-2632

WILSON, Ian M; Belmont Prof Bldg, 203-564 Belmont Ave W, Kitchener ON N2M 5N6; McM'83; FAAP; FRCPC; Peds. Staff, Grand River Hospital - Kitchener/Waterloo Health Centre; Court Staff, St Mary's General Hospital; Clin Assoc Prof Peds, McMaster University; (519)578-5670; Fax. (519)578-4820.

WILSON, J Galt; College of Phys & Surgs of BC, 300-669 Howe St, Vancouver BC V6C 0B4; UBC'79; FCFP; MScEd; CCFP; FCFP; Staff, University Hospital of Northern British Columbia; Staff, College of Physicians & Surgeons of British Columbia; Clin Prof/Clin Dir Clerkship Northern Med Program, University of British Columbia; (604)733-7758 x2229; Fax. (604)733-3503; galt.wilson@northernhealth.ca.

WILSON, James A; Ultima Med Services, 4440 Stark St, Richmond BC V7B 1A1; UBC'71; CCFP; FCFP; Ac Staff, Richmond Hospital; (604)270-1370; Fax. (604)270-3306.

WILSON, James B; Brockville Gen Hosp, 75 Charles St, Brockville ON K6V 1S8; Dal'98; CCFP; CCFP(E.M.); Staff, Brockville General Hospital - Charles Street; (613)345-5645

WILSON, James W L; EMP 4-76 Stuart St, Kingston ON K7L 2V7; Qns'77; MSc; FACS; BSc(Hon); FRCSC; Urol (Urolithiasis). Staff Urol, Kingston General Hospital; Att Staff, Hotel-Dieu Hospital; Consultant, QHC Prince Edward County Memorial; Assoc Prof Urol, Queen's University; (613)548-2493; Fax. (613)545-1970.

WILSON, Jane; Lethbridge Cancer Centre, 960 19 St S, Lethbridge AB T1J 1W5; UBC'88; FRCPC; RadOncol. Staff, Chinook Regional Hospital; Staff, Tom Baker Cancer Centre; Staff, Lethbridge Cancer Centre; Staff, Jack Ady Cancer Centre; (403)388-6860; Fax. (403)327-2530.

WILSON, Janet H; Clinique Med Roper, 4500 rue Sherbrooke O, Westmount QC H3Z 1E6; Tor'80; CCFP; FCFP; Langs: English; French; (514)937-8000; Fax. (514)937-8884.

WILSON, Janet L; Spingbank Med Centre, 306-460 Springbank Dr, London ON N6J 0A8; Wes'85; MEd; FRCPC; IntMed (Thyroid Diseases). (519)661-0047; Fax. (519)661-0917.

WILSON, Jean-Marie J; Mill Bay Med Centre, 230-2720 Mill Bay Rd RR 1, Mill Bay BC V0R 2P1; Qns'92; BSc; CCFP; CCFP(E.M.); Staff, Cowichan District Hospital; Langs: Bilingual(English/French); (250)743-3211; Fax. (250)743-2800.

WILSON, Jennifer L; Uxbridge Family Health Clinic, B-2 Elgin Park Dr, Uxbridge ON L9P 0B1; McM'97; CCFP; CCFP(E.M.); Ac Staff, Markham Stouffville Hospital - Uxbridge Site; (905)852-1009; Fax. (905)852-3531.

WILSON, Jennifer M; 50-45905 Yale Rd W, Chilliwack BC V2P 2M6; McM'96; MD; BMus; FRCPC; FRCPC; Respir; IntMed (Transplantation). Staff, Gordon & Leslie Diamond Health Care Centre; Staff, Vancouver General Hospital - Centennial Pavillion; University of British Columbia; (604)792-2266; jmwilson@interchange.ubc.ca.

WILSON, John C N; West Coast Gen Hosp, 3949 Port Alberni Hwy, Port Alberni BC V9Y 4S1; London (England)'71; MB BS; CCFP; FCFP; Staff, West Coast General Hospital; (250)731-1370

WILSON, John T; 126-3030 Lincoln Ave, Coquitlam BC V3B 6B4; Edinburgh (Scotland)'56; Ac Staff, Eagle Ridge Hospital & Health Care Centre; Ac Staff, BC Cancer Agency Fraser Valley Centre; Ac Staff, Royal Columbian Hospital; (604)942-4500; Fax. (604)942-4500; jayne.w@telus.net.

WILSON, Jonathan J; 205-1017 Wilson Ave, Toronto ON M3K 1Z1; Tor'77; FACP; FRCPC; IntMed; MedOncol; Hem. Staff, Humber River Regional Hospital - Church Street Site; Court Staff, West Park Healthcare Centre; Court Staff, St Michael's Hospital; University of Toronto; (416)249-4367; jwilson@hrrh.on.ca.

WILSON, Joshua S M; Foothills Med Centre, C229-1403 29 St NW, Calgary AB T2N 2T9; Dal'04; FRCPC; Anes. Staff, Foothills Medical Centre; (403)944-1430; Fax. (403)944-2425.

WILSON, Joslyn V; Lennox & Addington County GH, 8 Richmond Park Dr, Napanee ON K7R 2Z4; Qns'02; CCFP; Staff, Lennox & Addington County General Hospital; (613)354-3301

WILSON, Karen M; MCI The Doctors Office, PO Box 134 LR8-200 Bay St, Toronto ON M5J 2J3; Tor'89; BSc(Hons.); (416)368-6787; Fax. (416)368-7632.

WILSON, Kathleen M; Parkholm Place, 9090 Newman Rd, Chilliwack BC V2P 3Z8; Belfast (Ireland)'73; MB ChB; BAO; (604)703-2012; Fax. (604)792-0262.

WILSON, Keith W; St Joseph's Comm Hlth Ctre, 130 Bayard Dr, Saint John NB E2L 3L6; Mem'99; PhD; CCFP; Asst Prof, Dalhousie University; (506)632-5700; Fax. (506)632-5657; wilkei@reg2.health.nb.ca.

WILSON, Kenneth L; IWK Health Centre, PO Box 9700 Rpo CSC 5850 University Ave, Halifax NS B3K 6R8; Tor'72; PlasSurg (Pediatric Plastic Surgery). Staff, IWK Health Centre; (902)470-8168; Fax. (902)470-7939; kenneth.wilson@iwk.nshealth.ca.

WILSON, Kenneth S; BC Cancer Agency-Vanc Isl Ctr, 2410 Lee Ave, Victoria BC V8R 6V5; Edinburgh (Scotland)'70; MB ChB(Edinburgh); ABMO; FACP(Ed); FRCPE; FRCPC; FRCPC; MedOncol; IntMed (Gastrointestinal Cancer). Staff Oncol, BC Cancer Agency Vancouver Island Centre; Staff, Vancouver Island Health Authority; Clin Prof Med, University of British Columbia; (250)519-5570; Fax. (250)519-2017; kwilson@bccancer.bc.ca.

WILSON, Kerri D; Dingwall Med Group, PO Box 3011 Stn Main 40 Goodall St, Dryden ON P8N 2Z6; Man'06; CCFP; (807)223-2258; Fax. (807)223-4733.

WILSON, Kevin R; Rosedale Med Associates, PO Box 460 200-13009 Rosedale Ave, Summerland BC V0H 1Z0; UBC'90; Staff, Royal Jubilee Hospital; (250)404-4242

WILSON, Kumanan R; The Ottawa Hosp-Civic Campus, 1019-1053 Carling Ave Box 684, Ottawa ON K1Y 4E9; Wes'93; MSc; FRCPC; IntMed. Staff Administrative Services, The Ottawa Hospital - Civic Campus; Scientist, University of Ottawa; (613)798-5555 x17921; Fax. (613)761-5492.

WILSON, Linda J; 201-9775 Fourth St, Sidney BC V8L 2Z8; UBC'92; CCFP; (250)656-4011; Fax. (250)656-4014.

WILSON, Linda L; Ctr for the North Prince Georg, 1215 Lethbridge Ave, Prince George BC V2M 7E9; Qns'98; CCFP; FCFP; Staff, University Hospital of Northern British Columbia; (250)645-7300; doclinda98@hotmail.com.

WILSON, Lisa A; Cottage Med Clinic, PO Box 2140 300 Miette Ave, Jasper AB T0E 1E0; McM'01; CCFP; Staff, Jasper (Seton) Health Centre; (780)852-4885; Fax. (780)852-2199.

WILSON, Lisa A; Mill Bay Med Centre, 230-2720 Mill Bay Rd, Mill Bay BC V0R 2P1; Qns'92; Staff, Cowichan District Hospital; (250)743-3211; Fax. (250)743-2800.

WILSON, Lorne W; Manulife Insurance Co, PO Box 800 Stn C 25 Water St S, Kitchener ON N2G 4Y5; Tor'76; Med Consultant, Manulife Insurance Co; (519)747-7000

WILSON, Lynn M; Family Practice Health Centre, 77 Grenville St, Toronto ON M5S 1B3; Tor'83; CCFP; FCFP; Ac Staff Family Med, St Joseph's Health Centre; Chair, Univerity of Toronto Continuing Education; Chair Family & Community Med, University of Toronto; (416)323-6060

WILSON, M Kaetlen; Morton Comm Healthcare Centre, 01-150 Strickland Rd, Lakefield ON K0L 2H0; McM'90; CCFP; FCFP; Staff, Peterborough Regional Health Centre - Hospital Drive; (705)651-0222; Fax. (705)651-0224.

WILSON, Maithili K; Royal Health Care Centre, PO Box 92 130 Adelaide St W, Toronto ON M5H 3P5; Dal'88; DAB; BSc; FRCPC; Derm (Cosmetic Dermatology). Staff Derm, St Michael's Hospital; Lecturer, University of Toronto; Langs: Tamil; (416)361-6142; Fax. (416)361-1200.

WILSON, Malcolm A G; Huntsville Prof Bldg, 204-348 Muskoka Rd 3 N, Huntsville ON P1H 1H8; Qns'75; FRCPC; IntMed (Pacemaker). Consultant, Huntsville District Memorial Hospital - Muskoka Algonquin Healthcare; Court Staff, South Muskoka Memorial Hospital - Muskoka Algonquin Healthcare; Reg Dir Internal Med East, Northern Ontario School of Medicine; (705)789-1268; Fax. (705)789-9698; mwilson@vianet.on.ca.

WILSON, Marci L; Horizon Family Medicine, 65 Hewlett Park Landing, Red Deer County AB T4S 2J3; McM'02; CCFP; (403)887-0510; Fax. (403)887-0520.

WILSON, Margaret A; The Ottawa Hosp-Gen Campus, 501 Smyth Rd, Ottawa ON K1H 8L6; Ott'10; CCFP; Staff Emerg Med, The Ottawa Hospital - General Campus; (613)722-7000

WILSON, Margo M; Labrador Health Centre, PO Box 7000 Stn C 227 Hamilton River Rd, Happy-Valley-Goose NL A0P 1C0; Ott'07; CCFP; CCFP(E.M.); Staff, Labrador Health Centre; Staff, St Clare's Mercy Hospital; (709)897-2000

WILSON, Marie A Y; Garneau Prof Centre, 335-11044 82 Ave NW, Edmonton AB T6G 0T2; Alb'77; (780)433-1759; Fax. (780)433-2479.

WILSON, Martha E; 203-518 Lake St, Nelson BC V1L 4C6; McM'95; Staff, Kootenay Lake General Hospital; (250)354-4414; Fax. (250)354-1912.

WILSON, Mary L; Sault Area Hosps, 750 Great Northern Rd, Sault Ste. Marie ON P6B 0A8; Ott'95; CCFP; FCFP; Staff, Sault Area Hospital - Sault Ste Marie; (705)759-3434; Fax. (705)759-3815.

WILSON, Mary T; Wellington Dufferin Guelph Pub, 600 Southgate Dr, Guelph ON N1G 4P6; Tor'69; Staff, Wellington-Dufferin-Guelph Public Health South Guelph; (519)846-2715

WILSON, Meghan D; Kingston Gen Hosp, 76 Stuart St, Kingston ON K7L 2V7; Dal'10; CCFP; Staff, Kingston General Hospital; (613)549-6666

WILSON, Michael B; Regional Supervising Coroner, PO Box 4500 Stn P 401A-189 Red River Rd, Thunder Bay ON P7B 6G9; McM'94; CCFP; FCFP; Clin Assoc Prof Family Med, Northern Ontario School of Medicine; Asst Prof Family Med, McMaster University; Langs: German; (807)343-7663; Fax. (807)343-7665.

WILSON, Michael S; Burris Clinic, 300-275 Lansdowne St, Kamloops BC V2C 6J3; Alb'77; BSc; (250)377-3343; Fax. (250)571-3361.

WILSON, Murray B; Bradford Med Walk-In Clinic, PO Box 1601 Stn Main 7 John St, Bradford ON L3Z 2B8; McG'78; Langs: French; Spanish; Portuguese; (905)775-3900; Fax. (905)775-3981.

WILSON, Murray E; WRHA Breast Health Centre, 100-400 Tache Ave, Winnipeg MB R2H 3C3; Man'82; AB; FACR; FRCPC; DiagRad. Staff, St Boniface General Hospital; Staff, Misericordia Health Centre; Physician, Manitoba Breast Screening Program; Lecturer Diagnostic Imaging, University of Manitoba; (204)235-3906

WILSON, Nagwa; MUHC-Montreal Children's Hosp, 2300 rue Tupper, Montreal QC H3H 1P3; Staff, McGill University Health Centre - Montreal Children's Hospital; (514)412-4400

WILSON, Patricia I; 1-95 Hamilton St PO Box 890, Waterdown ON L0R 2H0; McM'82; MSW; BA; CCFP; FCFP; Staff, Joseph Brant Memorial Hospital; (905)689-6134; Fax. (905)689-5665.

WILSON, Paul J; Peterborough Reg HC-Hosp, 1 Hospital Dr, Peterborough ON K9J 7C6; Qns'00; FRCPC; DiagRad. Staff, Peterborough Regional Health Centre - Hospital Drive; (705)743-2121 x5039

WILSON, Paul R; Royal Victoria Hosp, 201 Georgian Dr, Barrie ON L4M 6M2; Qns'83; Staff, Royal Victoria Regional Health Centre; (705)728-9802; Fax. (705)728-5922.

WILSON, Peter S; 3-1133 Lawson Ave, Kelowna BC V1Y 6T8; UBC'82; FACOG; FRCSC; ObstGyn. Teach Staff Southern Med Prog, University of British Columbia; (250)763-0640; Fax. (250)763-0646.

WILSON, Peter S; The Moncton Hosp, 135 MacBeath Ave, Moncton NB E1C 6Z8; Dal'03; FRCPC; Anes. Staff, The Moncton Hospital; (506)857-5520

WILSON, R Douglas; Foothills Med Centre, NT 435-1403 29 St NW, Calgary AB T2N 2T9; UBC'77; DrMedCh; FRCSC; ObstGyn (Reproductive Genetics). Staff ObstGyn, Foothills Medical Centre; Dept Head ObstGyn, University Of Calgary; (403)944-4419; Fax. (403)283-0415; doug.wilson@albertahealthservices.ca.

WILSON, Renald; 444 Parkside Dr, Bathurst NB E2A 1N4; Mon'85.

WILSON, Richard J; Columbia Family Medicine, 302-1101 Dewdney Ave, Trail BC V1R 4T1; UBC'84; Ac Staff, Kootenay Boundary Regional Hospital; (250)368-9394; Fax. (250)368-8281.

WILSON, Richard M; 3609 Nico Wynd Dr, Surrey BC V4P 1J1; Alb'68; (604)538-0014

WILSON, Robert A; Cowichan Dist Hosp, 3045 Gibbins Rd, Duncan BC V9L 1E5; Alb'01; FRCPC; DiagRad. Staff Medical Imaging, Cowichan District Hospital; (250)709-3000; Fax. (250)715-1212.

WILSON, Robert J; 1096 Goyeau St, Windsor ON N9A 1J1; Dal'74; FRCPC; IntMed (Diabetology); Endocrin&Metab. Staff, Windsor Regional Hospital - Tayfour Site; Hôtel-Dieu Grace Hospital; Ac Staff, Windsor Regional Hospital - Metropolitan Site; Staff, Regional Bariatric Assessment & Treatment Centre; (519)258-0718; Fax. (519)258-8936; robwil@mnsi.net.

WILSON, Robert W; Golden Med Clinic, PO Box 1170, Golden BC V0A 1H0; Cal'74; FRCPC; Peds. Med Staff, Golden & District General Hospital; (250)344-2211; Fax. (250)344-7620.

WILSON, Robin T; 303-22112 52 Ave, Langley BC V2Y 2M6; Dal'81; Staff, Langley Memorial Hospital; (604)530-5656; Fax. (604)530-4718.

WILSON, Rodney D; Northend Comm Health Centre, 2165 Gottingen St, Halifax NS B3K 3B7; McM'92; Staff, College of Physicians & Surgeons of Nova Scotia; Langs: English; French; (902)420-0303; Fax. (902)422-0859; rwilson@cpsns.ns.ca.

WILSON, Ronald A; BC Women's Hosp & Health Ctre, F326-4500 Oak St, Vancouver BC V6H 3N1; UBC'78; CCFP; Staff, BC Women's Hospital & Health Centre; Staff, Vancouver General Hospital - Centennial Pavillion; Asst Prof Family Med, University of British Columbia; (604)875-2029; Fax. (604)875-3197; rwilson@interchange.ubc.ca.

WILSON, Ronald H; 208-4235 Sheppard Ave E, Scarborough ON M1S 1T7; Wes'63; FRCPC; Neur (Sleep Medicine). (416)449-2807; Fax. (416)449-0054.

WILSON, Ruth K; 87 Adelaide St N, Lindsay ON K9V 4L4; Wes'06; CCFP; Locum Tenens, Ross Memorial Hospital; (705)324-2561; Fax. (705)328-1816.

WILSON, Sarah E; Public Health Ontario, 300-480 University Ave, Toronto ON M5G 1V2; Tor'05; FRCPC; CommunMed;CCFP; Staff, Ontario Agency for Health; (647)260-7100

WILSON, Scott E R; Health Sciences Centre, 300 Prince Philip Dr, St. John's NL A1B 3V6; Mem'89; CCFP; CCFP(E.M.); Staff, Health Sciences Centre; (709)777-5397; Fax. (709)777-8007.

WILSON, Scott F; 726-10 Discovery Ridge Hills S, Calgary AB T3H 5X2; Alb'94; BSc; FRCPC; Neur. Teach Staff Neurol, University of Calgary; (403)217-1222; Fax. (403)217-1125.

WILSON, Scott N; Marathon Family Health Team, PO Box 399 22 Peninsula Rd, Marathon ON P0T 2E0; Ott'95; CCFP; FCFP; Langs: English; French; (807)229-3243; Fax. (807)229-2672.

WILSON, Scott W J; 5394 Pierres Point Rd, Salmon Arm BC V1E 3A1; UBC'86; FRCSC; GenSurg.

WILSON, Sophie E R; Westmount Med Bldg, 306-77 Westmount Rd, Guelph ON N1H 5J1; McM'00; CCFP; Clin Asst Prof Waterloo Campus, McMaster University; (519)827-1399; Fax. (519)827-1858.

WILSON, Stephanie R; Foothills Med Centre, 1403 29 St NW, Calgary AB T2N 2T9; Alb'70; FRCPC; DiagRad (Ultrasound). Staff Radiol, Foothills Medical Centre; Clin Prof, University of Calgary; (403)944-2680; Fax. (403)944-2790; stephanie.wilson@albertahealthservices.ca.

WILSON, Tania; Happy Valley Family Hlth Team, PO Box 1120 268 Maiden Lane, St Marys ON N4X 1B7; Wes'07; CCFP; Staff, Alexandra Marine & General Hospital; (519)284-3450; Fax. (519)284-4471; twilson@stmmc.ca.

WILSON, Terrance R; The Medical Centre FHT, PO Box 4200 Stn Main 707 Charlotte St, Peterborough ON K9J 7B3; McG'76; Ac Staff, Peterborough Regional Health Centre - Rogers St Site; Ac Staff, Peterborough Regional Health Centre - Hospital Drive; Langs: English; French; (705)743-6222; Fax. (705)743-1449.

WILSON, Theresa M; Highland Family Practice, 107C-1966 Guthrie Rd, Comox BC V9M 3X7; McM'03; CCFP; (250)890-0919; there_sa6@hotmail.com.

WILSON, Thomas R; Hop Jean-Talon, 1385 rue Jean-Talon E, Montreal QC H2E 1S6; Sask'02; FRCPC; IntMed; Respir. Staff, CSSS du Coeur de l'Isle Hôpital Jean-Talon; (514)495-6767

WILSON, Thomas W; Royal University Hosp, 3544-103 Hospital Dr, Saskatoon SK S7N 0W8; Alb'67; MSc(Pharm.); FRCPC; IntMed (Clinical Pharmacology). Ac Staff Med, Royal University Hospital; Prof Med, University of Saskatchewan; (306)966-7967; Fax. (306)966-7970.

WILSON, Tracy L; Big Thunder Orthopaedics, 206-984 Oliver Rd, Thunder Bay ON P7B 7C7; Tor'90; BSc(Hons); FRCSC; OrthSurg (Trauma Adult Reconstructive Surgery). Staff, Thunder Bay Regional Health Sciences Centre; Physician, Big Thunder Orthopaedics; Langs: English; French; (807)344-1123; Fax. (807)344-1166.

WILSON, Trevor G; Dr Trevor G Wilson Inc, 115-12080 Nordel Way, Surrey BC V3W 1P6; Belfast (Ireland)'91; MB ChB; BAO; CCFP; FCFP; (604)543-0888

WILSON, Wendy L; West Parry Sound Hlth Centre, 6 Albert St, Parry Sound ON P2A 3A4; Tor'94; MSc; Asst Prof, Northern Ontario School of Medicine-Laurentian University; (705)746-9321; Fax. (705)773-4054.

WILSON-HAFFENDEN, Cara K; Lonsdale Med Dental Bldg, 108-1940 Lonsdale Ave, North Vancouver BC V7M 2K2; McG'92; BSc; Langs: English; French; (604)987-3347; Fax. (604)987-7624.

WILSON THOMAS SORIAL, Mona; Centre Med Brunswick, 300-955 boul Saint-Jean, Pointe-Claire QC H9R 5K3; Cairo (Egypt)'79; Staff, Centre Hospitalier Rouyn-Noranda; Langs: Bilingual(French/English); (514)459-3433; mona_sorial@hotmail.ca.

WILT, Frances R; 105-1525 8 Ave W, Vancouver BC V6J 1T5; Man'70; FRCPC; Psy (Psychoanalysis). Staff, UBC Hospital - Koerner Pavillion; Clin Assoc Prof Psy, University of British Columbia; (604)733-9737

WILTERS, Petrus; Western Mem Reg Hosp, PO Box 2005 Stn Main 1 Brookfield Ave, Corner Brook NL A2H 6J7; Pretoria (South Africa)'89; MB ChB; Staff, Western Memorial Regional Hospital; (709)637-5000

WILTON, David W; Vancouver Gen Hosp, 3500 JP3N-855 12th Ave W, Vancouver BC V5Z 1M9; Wes'00; CCFP; Staff, Vancouver General Hospital - Centennial Pavillion; (604)822-7121

WILTON, Michael B; Dr Michael Wilton Prof Corp, 5-123 Guildwood Pky, Scarborough ON M1E 4V2; Qns'90; CCFP; FCFP; Staff Family Pract, The Scarborough Hospital - General Campus; Staff Family Pract, Rouge Valley Health System - Centenary Health Centre Site; Teach Staff Family & Commun Med, University of Toronto; (416)269-5088; Fax. (416)261-3112.

WILTON, Stephen B; Health Research Innovation Ctr, TRW GE64-3280 Hospital Dr NW, Calgary AB T2N 4Z6; Tor'01; BSc; FRCPC; IntMed; Cardiol (Electrophysiology). Asst Prof, Foothills Medical Centre; Staff, Health Research Innovation Centre; Langs: French; (403)210-7102; Fax. (403)210-9180.

WILTSHIRE, David G; 100-175 av Stillview, Pointe-Claire QC H9R 4S3; Tor'68; DABOS; CSPQ; FRCSC; OrthSurg (Hand Surgery). Staff, Shriners Hospitals For Children - Canada; Staff, Lakeshore General Hospital - Pointe Claire; Physician Medical Evaluation Office, Ministry of Labour & Solidarite(Quebec); Conférencier Surg, McGill University; Langs: English; French; (514)697-1582; Fax. (514)694-3610.

WILTSHIRE, Jonathan M; Brock Med Clinic, 204-1800 Tranquille Rd, Kamloops BC V2B 3L9; Aberdeen (Scotland)'01; MB ChB; (250)461-7079

WILTSHIRE, Katie M; South Health Campus, 4448 Front St SE, Calgary AB T3M 1M4; Alb'07; Neur. Staff Neurosciences, South Health Campus; (403)956-2445

WILTSHIRE, Marc L; Thunder Bay Reg HSC, 980 Oliver Rd, Thunder Bay ON P7B 6V4; Man'88; CCFP; CCFP(E.M.); Staff, Thunder Bay Regional Health Sciences Centre; Langs: English; French; (807)684-6000

WIN, Lay Lay; Balmoral Med Arts Facility, 301-1366 Yonge St, Toronto ON M4T 3A7; Mandalay Institute of Medicine (Other Foreign)'01; FRCPC; IntMed; Gastroent. Langs: Burmese; (416)926-0262; Fax. (416)926-0936.

WINCKEL, Christopher P; Woodroffe South Med Bldg, 104-1637 Woodroffe Ave, Ottawa ON K2G 1W2; Tor'88; FRCSC; GenSurg. Staff, Queensway Carleton Hospital; (613)228-7772; Fax. (613)228-7776.

WINCOTT, J Leigh; Glenrose Rehabilitation Hosp, 10230 111 Ave, Edmonton AB T5G 0B7; McM'91; BSc(Hons.); FRCPC; Peds. Staff, Glenrose Rehabilitation Hospital; Assoc Prof, University of Alberta; (780)735-7963; Fax. (780)735-7909.

WIND, Stojna T; 238-5780 Cambie St, Vancouver BC V5Z 3A7; UBC'89; Staff Student Health Serv, UBC Hospital - Koerner Pavillion; (604)323-8836

WINDER, Anthony R; Professional Bldg, 200-740 4 Ave S, Lethbridge AB T1J 0N9; Qns'81; FRCPC; Neur (Neuro Otology). Consultant Neurol & NeuroOtol, Lethbridge Cancer Centre; Staff, Elk Valley Hospital; Consultant Med, Alberta Health Services Edmonton; (403)329-6886; Fax. (403)329-6889.

WINDER, Mary J; Westhill Centre, 205-1808 Bowen Rd, Nanaimo BC V9S 5W4; UBC'84; CCFP; Staff, AVI Health Centre; (250)753-6646; Fax. (250)753-6174.

WINDISCH, Louis; Centre Chirurgical de Joliette, 202-222 rue de la Visitation, Joliette QC J6E 4N5; Mon'92; FRCSC; GenSurg. Staff, Centre Hospitalier Régional de Lanaudière; (450)753-7588; Fax. (450)756-6144.

WINDRAM, Jonathan D; United Nurses of Alberta, 2C2 WMC-8440 112 St NW, Edmonton AB T6G 2B7; Glasgow (Scotland)'98; Staff, University of Alberta Hospital; Staff, United Nurses of Alberta; (780)407-3177; Fax. (780)407-6452.

WINDRIM, Rory C; Ontario Power Generation Bldg, 3205-700 University Ave, Toronto ON M5G 1Z5; Dublin (Ireland)'84; MB ChB; FRCSC; ObstGyn (Maternal Fetal Medicine). Staff, Mount Sinai Hospital; (416)586-4800 x7756; Fax. (416)586-8617.

WINDRIM, Sean G; Peterborough Reg HC-Hospital, 1 Hospital Dr, Peterborough ON K9J 7C6; Dublin (Ireland)'82; FRCPC; Anes. Staff, Peterborough Regional Health Centre - Hospital Drive; (705)876-5038; Fax. (705)876-5105.

WINDSOR, Scott J; Aurora Medical & Dental Bldg, 302-372 Hollandview Trail, Aurora ON L4G 0A5; Tor'80; CCFP; FCFP; Ac Staff, Southlake Regional Health Centre; (905)727-6124; Fax. (905)727-6149.

WINDT, Adriaan; West Oaks Med Centre, 310-32700 South Fraser Way, Abbotsford BC V2T 4M5; Witwatersrand (South Africa)'82; MB ChB; Staff, Grimshaw/Berwyn and District Community Health Centre; Staff, Peace River Community Health Centre; Langs: Afrikaans; Dutch; (604)557-9938; adriaan.windt@pchr.ca.

WINE, Eytan; Edmonton Clinic Health Academy, 4 577-11405 87 Ave NW, Edmonton AB T6G 1C9; Tel-Aviv (Israel)'99; Staff, Stollery Children's Hospital; Asst Prof, University of Alberta; (780)248-5420; Fax. (780)248-5627.

WINE, Nina H; Rosedale Heights Plaza, 17-531 Atkinson Ave, Thornhill ON L4J 8L7; Boston (USA)'93; FRCPC; IntMed (Endocrinology); Endocrin&Metab. (905)763-8660; Fax. (905)763-0708; nina.wine@lmc.ca.

WINE, Stanley J; Dermatology Associates, 103-4430 Bathurst St, North York ON M3H 3S3; Tor'65; FRCPC; Derm. Court Staff, Mount Sinai Hospital; Ac Staff, Baycrest Centre for Geriatric Care; Court Staff, North York General Hospital; Langs: Yiddish; (416)638-7226; Fax. (416)638-0765.

WINEGARD, John C; Bluewater Health-CEE Site, 450 Blanche St, Petrolia ON N0N 1R0; McM'76; Staff, Bluewater Health - Charlotte Eleanor Englehart Hospital; (519)882-4325

WINEMAKER, Mitchell J; Hamilton Med Arts Bldg, 708-1 Young St, Hamilton ON L8N 1T8; Tor'91; FRCSC; OrthSurg (Arthroplasty). Staff, Hamilton Health Sciences Centre-Juravinski Site; (905)570-8884; Fax. (905)570-1675.

WINEMAKER, Samantha P; Hamilton CCAC, 310 Limeridge Rd W, Hamilton ON L9C 2V2; McM'01; CCFP; (905)523-8600; Fax. (905)574-6335.

WINER, Daniel A; Univ Hlth Network-Toronto Gen, 11F-200 Elizabeth St, Toronto ON M5G 2C4; Ott'02; FRCPC; AnatPath. Staff, Toronto General Hospital - UHN; (416)340-4800; Fax. (416)340-5517.

WINER, Laura H R; Hassle Free Women's Clinic, 2F-66 Gerrard St E, Toronto ON M5B 1G3; Pennsylvania State University Coll of Me (USA)'86; Med Dir, Hassle Free Women's Clinic; (416)922-0566; Fax. (416)922-2018.

WINFIELD, Doris J; University Downs Fam Practice, 425 University Ave E, Waterloo ON N2K 4C9; Qns'93; CCFP; Med Dir, Chateau Gardens Nursing Home; Med Dir, Twin Oaks Maryhill; (519)569-8821; Fax. (519)569-8823.

WINFIELD, Harvey B; Flesherton Med Clinic, PO Box 220, Flesherton ON N0C 1E0; Qns'87; CCFP; FCFP; (519)924-2012; Fax. (519)924-3828.

WING, Kevin J; Dr Kevin J Wing Inc, 1000-1200 Burrard St, Vancouver BC V6Z 2C7; UBC'94; FRCSC; OrthSurg. (604)629-9265

WING, Peter C; Heather Pavilion, D6-2733 Heather St, Vancouver BC V5Z 1M9; Edinburgh (Scotland)'66; FRCS; FRCSC; OrthSurg (P.Q.) (Arthroplasty). (604)875-5857; Fax. (604)875-5858; peter.wing@vch.ca.

WING, Simon S; M905-687 av des Pins O, Montreal QC H3A 1A1; McG'81; FRCPC; IntMed; Endocrin&Metab. ac Staff, McGill University Health Centre - Royal Victoria Hospital; Prof, McGill University; Langs: Cantonese; French; (514)934-1934 x35623; Fax. (514)982-0825.

WINGATE, Jordan T; Family Physicians Group, PO Box 2170 25B-1121 Main St, Melfort SK S0E 1A0; Sask'96; CCFP; Physician, Family Physicians Group; (306)752-9033; Fax. (306)752-9032.

WINGER, Michael J; Tecumseh Life Center, 114-11811 Tecumseh Rd E, Windsor ON N8N 4M7; Man'82; AB; FRCPC; Neur. Ac Staff Med, Hôtel-Dieu Grace Hospital; Ac Staff, Windsor Regional Hospital - Metropolitan Site; Clin Lecturer Neurological Sciences, University of Western Ontario; (519)739-2157; Fax. (519)739-2160.

WINGERIN, Ruth C; Oakridge Pediatrics, 207-650 41st Ave W, Vancouver BC V5Z 2M9; Cape Town (South Africa)'86; FRCPC; Peds (Developmental Pediatrics). Staff, BC Children's Hospital; (604)266-1874; Fax. (604)266-1583.

WINGNEAN, David; 11807 Jasper Ave NW, Edmonton AB T5K 0N8; UBC'93; CCFP; (780)488-1222; Fax. (780)488-2112.

WINIKOFF, Rochelle; Hôpital Ste-Justine, 3175 ch Cote-Sainte-Catherine, Montreal QC H3T 1C5; McG'95; BSc; MDCM; MSc; Hem; IntMed., Hôpital Ste-Justine; (514)345-4931 x4639; Fax. (514)345-4884.

WINK, Michael J; Calwood Med Clinic, 11432 Groat Rd NW, Edmonton AB T5M 4B7; London (England)'75; BSc(Hons.); MB BS; LRCP; MRCS; Consultant Bioidentical HRT, True Balance; (780)452-4590; Fax. (780)455-3133.

WINKELAAR, Gerrit B; Tawa Centre, 205-3017 66 St NW, Edmonton AB T6K 4B2; Alb'91; BMedSci; MSc; FRCSC; GenSurg; VascSurg. Clinical Asst Prof Surg, University of Alberta; (780)461-6012; Fax. (780)461-5442; gbwinkelaar@surgicorp.ca.

WINKLER, Christoph; Professional Arts Bldg, 403-100 Arden St, Moncton NB E1C 4B7; Heidelberg (Germany)'76; Staff, The Moncton Hospital; (506)857-5993; Fax. (506)857-5905.

WINKLER, Heather D; Yorkview Med Centre, 104-3695 Keele St, North York ON M3J 1N2; Tor'96; BSc; CCFP; Ac Staff Family & Commun Med, Humber River Regional Hospital - Finch Avenue Site; (416)633-3711; Fax. (416)630-7338.

WINKLER, Lawrence H; 515A Campbell St, Nanaimo BC V9R 3G9; Qns'79; FRCPC; IntMed. Staff Internist, Nanaimo Regional General Hospital; (250)754-1055; Fax. (250)754-1053.

WINN, Edward P; West Coast Gen Hosp, 3949 Port Alberni Hwy, Port Alberni BC V9Y 4S1; Wes'83; FRCPC; DiagRad. Staff Radiol, West Coast General Hospital; (250)724-8811 x1157; Fax. (250)724-8801.

WINNICKI, Monika; The Dermatology Group, 302-1448 Lawrence Ave E, North York ON M3B 3B3; Wes'04; FRCPC; Derm. (416)750-8400; Fax. (416)750-1091.

WINNING, J Barry; Ontario Med Imaging, 309-328 Highway 7 E, Richmond Hill ON L4B 3P7; Cape Town (South Africa)'63; FRCPC; DiagRad. Court Staff, Mackenzie Richmond Hill Hospital; Court Staff, Southlake Regional Health Centre; (905)731-4001

WINOGRODZKA, Christina; Birchwood Med Clinic, 2416 Portage Ave, Winnipeg MB R3J 0M8; Wroclaw (Poland)'81; Langs: Polish; (204)888-8712; Fax. (204)889-2279.

WINOGRODZKI, Arthur; Birchwood Med Clinic, 2416 Portage Ave, Winnipeg MB R3J 0M8; Man'05; FRCPC; Psy.

WINQUIST, Eric W; London Health Sciences Centre, 790 Commissioners Rd E, London ON N6A 4L6; Alb'86; FRCPC; IntMed (Head & Neck); MedOncol. Staff, London Health Sciences Centre - Victoria Campus; University of Western Ontario; (519)685-8640 x53346; Fax. (519)685-8624.

WINSBY, Brian K; 104-777 Blanshard St, Victoria BC V8W 2G9; UBC'69; Ac Staff, Victoria General Hospital; (250)388-5577; Fax. (250)382-3240.

WINSLOW, Inge G; 201-22 Richmond St, Richmond Hill ON L4C 3Y1; Copenhagen (Denmark)'74; Langs: German; Danish; Norwegian; Swedish; (905)884-3602; Fax. (905)884-3609.

WINSOR, Craig E; Seiden Health Management Inc, 1400-365 Bloor St E, Toronto ON M4W 3L4; Mem'90; BSc; Staff Emerg, Rouge Valley Health System - Centenary Health Centre Site; Physician Occupational Health Services, Air Canada Medical Clinic; (416)362-8611; Fax. (416)362-6070.

WINSOR, Stephanie H M; McMaster Univ Medical Centre, HSC 4D9-1280 Main St W, Hamilton ON L8S 4L8; Wes'93; FRCSC; ObstGyn (Maternal Fetal Medicine). Staff, Hamilton Health Sciences Centre - McMaster Children's Hospital; Langs: German; Swedish; French; (905)521-2100 x76254; Fax. (905)527-2675.

WINSOR, Wendy A; Queen Elizabeth II HSC-VG Site, 928 VB-1276 South Park St, Halifax NS B3H 2Y9; Mem'02; FRCPC; IntMed; Gastroent. Staff, Queen Elizabeth II Health Sciences Centre - Victoria General Site; (902)473-4979; Fax. (902)473-4406.

WINSTON, Brent W; Calgary Heart Centre, 4C64-3280 Hospital Dr NW, Calgary AB T2N 4Z6; Alb'84; BSc(Hons.); FRCPC; IntMed; Critical Care Medicine; Respir. Assoc Prof Med, University of Calgary; (403)220-4341; Fax. (403)283-1267.

WINSTON, Howard A; Centre For Health & Sports Med, 2790 Bathurst St, North York ON M6B 3A5; Tor'87; Dip SportMed(CASM); CCFP; FCFP; Staff Family & Commun Med, Toronto General Hospital - UHN; Assoc Staff, Rouge Valley Health System - Centenary Health Centre Site; Assoc Staff, Sunnybrook Health Sciences Centre - Holland Orthopaedic & Arthritic Centre; Asst Prof Family & Commun Med, University of Toronto; (416)789-2476; Fax. (416)789-1308; h.winston@chsm.net.

WINSTON, Karin Y; Alberta Children's Hosp, 2888 Shaganappi Trail NW, Calgary AB T3B 6A8; Cal'07; FRCPC; Peds. Staff, Alberta Children's Hospital; (403)955-7301

WINSTON, Paul J; Victoria Med Rehab Consultants, 402-1245 Esquimalt Rd, Victoria BC V9A 3P2; Wes'02; FRCPC; PhysMed&Rehab. Langs: Bilingual(English/French); (250)598-9922

WINSTON, Robert D; BC Cancer Agency-Abbotsford, 32900 Marshall Rd, Abbotsford BC V2S 0C2; North Carolina (USA)'83; FRCPC; IntMed; MedOncol. Physician, Abbotsford Regional Hospital & Cancer Centre; (604)851-4710

WINTEMUTE, Kimberly J; 501-1110 Sheppard Ave E, Toronto ON M2K 2W2; Tor'94; CCFP; Ac Staff, North York General Hospital; University of Toronto; (416)223-0555; Fax. (416)223-0540.

WINTER, A Leo; McMaster Institute of Urology, G339A-50 Charlton Ave E, Hamilton ON L8N 4A6; Tor'77; FRCSC; Urol (Lower Urinary Tract Dysfunction). Ac Staff, St Joseph's Healthcare - Charlton Campus; Court Staff, Hamilton Health Sciences Centre - McMaster University Medical Centre; Staff, McMaster Institute of Urology; Asst Prof Surg, McMaster University; Langs: Hebrew; Polish; (905)522-1155 x2981; Fax. (905)521-1751.

WINTER, Arthur J; Andrew Street Family Hlth Ctre, 16 Andrew St, Kitchener ON N2H 5R2; Wes'09; CCFP; (519)804-9234; Fax. (519)804-2604.

WINTER, Christopher K; Medical Imaging Consultants, MF-11010 101 St NW, Edmonton AB T5H 4B9; Alb'01; FRCPC; DiagRad; NuclearMed. Staff, University of Alberta Hospital; (780)426-1121; Fax. (780)424-7780.

WINTER, Elric D; Ctr Hosp de Verdun, 4000 boul Lasalle, Verdun QC H4G 2A3; Dal'78; FRCPC; IntMed (P.Q.); Cardiol (P.Q.). Staff, Centre Hospitalier de Verdun; (514)632-1000 x2447; Fax. (514)766-6462.

WINTER, I Alexander; 440-75 Bruyere St, Ottawa ON K1N 5C8; Dal'93; CCFP; Chair InfectDis, SCO Health Service - Élisabeth Bruyère Hospital; Dir Medical Services, Royal Ottawa Mental Health Centre - Royal Ottawa Health Care Group; Physician, Austrian Embassy; (613)244-0006; Fax. (613)244-4449.

WINTER, Itta M; 559 6th St, Courtenay BC V9N 1M5; Dal'89; CCFP; FCFP; Langs: German; (250)338-1391

WINTER, Kyle D; South Vancouver Med Clinic, 350 Marine Dr SE, Vancouver BC V5X 2S5; UBC'09; CCFP; (604)323-0077

WINTERBACH, Uys; PO Box 1180, Onoway AB T0E 1V0; (780)967-6477; Fax. (780)967-3700.

WINTERMARK, Pia; MUHC-Montreal Children's Hosp, 2300 rue Tupper, Montreal QC H3H 1P3; Lausanne (Other Foreign)'02; Staff, McGill University Health Centre - Montreal Children's Hospital; (514)412-4400 x23477

WINTERS, Michael J; Kensington Children's Clinic, 6548 Hastings St, Burnaby BC V5B 1S2; Man'98; FRCPC; Peds. Staff, BC Women's Hospital & Health Centre; (604)299-9769; Fax. (604)299-9772.

WINTERS, Sean D; University of Alberta Hosp, 2A2 33-8440 112 St NW, Edmonton AB T6G 2B7; Alb'02; DiagRad. Staff, University of Alberta Hospital; (780)407-6907; Fax. (780)407-1202.

WINTERSTEIN, Jeffrey; Hys Med Centre, 503-11010 101 ST NW, Edmonton AB T5H 4B9; (Netherlands Antilles)'05; (780)496-1390

WINTERTON, Adam C; Chesley Med Clinic, PO Box 68, Chesley ON N0G 1L0; McM'86; CCFP; FCFP; Fam Med, South Bruce Grey Health Services - Chesley Site; Staff, Hanover & District Hospital; Fam Med, South Bruce Grey Health Centre - Walkerton Site; (519)363-3220; Fax. (519)363-0385; awinterton@sbghc.on.ca.

WINTERTON, Victoria D J; 210C-1717 2nd Ave E, Owen Sound ON N4K 6V4; Qns'79; CCFP; FCFP; (519)372-2511; Fax. (519)372-2962.

WINTHROP, Andrea L; Kingston Gen Hosp, B2-76 Stuart St, Kingston ON K7L 2V7; Qns'81; FRCSC; GenSurg; PedGenSurg. Staff, Kingston General Hospital; (613)549-6666

WINTON, Timothy L; University of Alberta Hosp, 2D2 09 WCM-8440 112 St NW, Edmonton AB T6G 2B7; Qns'80; BSc(Hons.); MSc; ThorSurg; GenSurg (Critical Care Medicine). Assoc Prof, University of Alberta Hospital; (780)407-3623; Fax. (780)407-8130; twinton@cha.ab.ca.

WINWOOD, Paul J; Cottage Clinic, 1569 6th Ave, Prince George BC V2L 3N4; London (England)'85; MB BS; FRCPC; IntMed (Gastroenterology). Staff, University Hospital of Northern British Columbia; Staff, Northern Medical Program; (250)562-8002

WINZER, Willie P; AIM Orleans Hlth & Wellness Cl, 3-1605 Orleans Blvd, Orleans ON K1C 7E2; Alb'79; BSc; Langs: English; French; (613)830-6890; Fax. (613)837-6312.

WIRASINGHE, Manoji S; Signal Hill Med Centre, 2-5986 Signal Hill Ctr SW, Calgary AB T3H 3P8; Cal'00; CCFP; (403)240-2660; Fax. (403)242-8390.

WIRCH, M Faye; Canwest Global Place, 18F-201 Portage Ave, Winnipeg MB R3B 3K6; Sask'83; FRCPC; CCFP; Psy (Trauma). (204)233-3304; Fax. (204)926-8501; mfwirch@mb.sympatico.ca.

WIRES, Shannon M; 208-3330 Ritcher St, Kelowna BC V1W 4V5; Tor'05; FRCSC; Peds. (250)762-0466

WIRSIG, Nadine M; Don Valley Med Associates, 330-1333 Sheppard Ave E, North York ON M2J 1V1; Wes'89; CCFP; FCFP; Staff, North York General Hospital; University of Toronto; (416)497-1375; Fax. (416)497-4793; nwirsig@baycrest.org.

WIRTH, Sandra S; PO Box 94, Laird SK S0K 2H0; Qns'79; Teach Staff, University of Saskatchewan.

WIRTZFELD, Deborah A; CancerCare Manitoba, 2044-675 McDermot Ave, Winnipeg MB R3E 0V9; Cal'93; FRCSC; GenSurg. Staff, CancerCare Manitoba; (204)787-2197

WIRZBA, Brian J; 205-9148 23 Ave NW, Edmonton AB T6N 1H9; Alb'94; FRCPC; IntMed (Cardiology). Staff, Covenant Health - Grey Nuns Community Hospital; Clin Prof, University of Alberta; (780)462-3010; Fax. (780)440-2911.

WISE, Daniel J; Credit Valley Imaging Assoc, G02-2300 Eglinton Ave W, Mississauga ON L5M 2V8; Tor'62; FRCPC; DiagRad. Chief DiagRad, The Credit Valley Hospital; (905)828-0653; Fax. (905)828-0765.

WISE, Jack S; 4330 rue Sherbrooke O, Westmount QC H3Z 1E1; McG'69; Ophth. Att Staff, Sir Mortimer B Davis Jewish General; Att Staff, McGill University Health Centre - Montreal Children's Hospital; adj Prof, McGill University; (514)933-3511; Fax. (514)933-8541.

WISE, Katherine E; Kelowna Reg Fertility Centre, 202-1630 Pandosy St, Kelowna BC V1Y 1P7; Wes'93; FRCSC; ObstGyn (Infertility). Staff, Kelowna General Hospital; Med Dir, Kelowna Regional Fertility Centre; (250)861-6811; Fax. (250)861-6814; info@krfc.ca.

WISE, Laura S; Southridge Prof Centre, 5-1224 Strachan Rd SE, Medicine Hat AB T1B 4R2; (South Africa)'05; CCFP; (403)580-3888; Fax. (403)504-1220.

WISE, Mark; The Travel Clinic, 308-3292 Bayview Ave, North York ON M2M 4J5; Tor'75; DTMH(Lond); Ac Staff, North York General Hospital; Staff, The Travel Clinic; Langs: English; French; (416)221-7990; Fax. (416)221-4378; mark.wise@vch.ca.

WISE, Sheldon A; 103-3910 Bathurst St, North York ON M3H 5Z3; Tor'73; FRCPC; Peds. Staff, North York General Hospital; Staff, Women's College Hospital; Staff, St Michael's Hospital; Asst Prof Peds, University of Toronto; Langs: Hebrew; Yiddish; (416)635-5581; Fax. (416)638-5286.

WISE, Talya C; The Hosp for Sick Children, BW 1447-555 University Ave, Toronto ON M5G 1X8; McM'05; FRCPC; Peds; PedEmergMed. Staff, The Hospital For Sick Children; (416)813-1500

WISE, Yishai A; Markham Family Health Team, 101-377 Church St, Markham ON L6B 1A1; Wes'02; CCFP; (905)471-9999; Fax. (905)471-3627.

WISEBORD, Susan R; Inst of Comm & Family Psy, 4333 ch Cote-Sainte-Catherine, Montreal QC H3T 1E4; McG'86; FRCPC; Psy. Staff, Sir Mortimer B Davis Jewish General; (514)340-8210; Fax. (514)340-7507.

WISEMAN, Daniele P; London HSC-Victoria Hosp, PO Box 5010 Stn B 800 Commissioners Rd E, London ON N6A 5W9; Mem'99; FRCPC; DiagRad. Staff, London Health Sciences Centre - Victoria Campus; (519)685-8500

WISEMAN, David G H; Manitoba Clinic, 790 Sherbrook St, Winnipeg MB R3A 1M3; Man'70; BSc(Hon.Chem); BSc(Med.); FRCPC; IntMed (Endocrinology). Staff, Health Sciences Centre; (204)788-5737; Fax. (204)783-6579.

WISEMAN, Eve; Saint John Reg Hosp, PO Box 2100 Stn Main 400 University Ave, Saint John NB E2L 4L2; Kentucky (USA)'80; Staff, Saint John Regional Hospital; (506)648-6000

WISEMAN, Fred; Centre Med Brunswick, 300-955 boul Saint-Jean, Pointe-Claire QC H9R 5K3; Wes'64; Peds (Primary Care). Vis Consultant, McGill University Health Centre - Montreal Children's Hospital; Vis Consultant, Sir Mortimer B Davis Jewish General; Prof Peds, McGill University; Langs: English; French; (514)459-3433; ruesesame@yahoo.com.

WISEMAN, Jeffrey G; MUHC-Royal Victoria Hosp, E2 61-687 av des Pins O, Montreal QC H3A 1A1; McG'76; FRCPC; IntMed. Dir Undergrad Educ & Executive Health Serv/Staff, McGill University Health Centre - Royal Victoria Hospital; Med Advisor, Bank of Montreal; assoc Prof, McGill University; Langs: English; French; (514)843-1515 x31506; Fax. (514)843-1725; jeffrey.wiseman@mcgill.ca.

WISEMAN, Kevin W; 3107 35 Ave, Vernon BC V1T 2T2; UBC'00; FRCSC; GenSurg. (250)545-6443

WISEMAN, Marni C; Dermatology Clinic, 205 Edmonton St, Winnipeg MB R3C 1R4; Man'96; FRCPC; Derm (Skin Cancer). Staff, CancerCare Manitoba; (204)943-4922; Fax. (204)942-4399.

WISEMAN, Nathan E; Winnipeg Children's Hosp, AE 406-840 Sherbrook St, Winnipeg MB R3A 1S1; Man'68; FRCSC; GenSurg; PedGenSurg. Att Staff Div of Ped Surg, Health Sciences Centre; Att Staff, St Boniface General Hospital; Consultant, Ste Amant Centre; Assoc Prof Surg, University of Manitoba; (204)787-2682; Fax. (204)787-2028; nwiseman@exchange.hsc.mb.ca.

WISEMAN, Sam M; St Paul's Hosp, C303-1081 Burrard St, Vancouver BC V6Z 1Y6; Man'95; BSc; FRCSC; GenSurg (Head & Neck). Staff, Providence Health Care - St Paul's Hospital; Asst Prof Surg, University of British Columbia; (604)806-9108; Fax. (604)806-9957.

WISEMAN, Stephen R; St Paul's Hosp, 1081 Burrard St, Vancouver BC V6Z 1Y6; Cal'89; FRCPC; Psy. Staff, Providence Health Care - St Paul's Hospital; (604)812-4827; Fax. (604)222-1926.

WISENBERG, Gerald; London HSC-University Hosp, PO Box 5339 Stn B 339 Windermere Rd, London ON N6A 5A5; Tor'73; MD; FRCPC; IntMed (Cardiac Imaging); Cardiol. Staff, London Health Sciences Centre - University Hospital; (519)663-3083; Fax. (519)663-3084.

WISHART, Ian M; Rockyview Gen Hosp, 7007 14 St SW, Calgary AB T2V 1P9; Alb'87; FRCPC; EmergMed; FamilyMed. Staff, Rockyview General Hospital; (403)541-3450; Fax. (403)943-3220.

WISHART, Robert L; UBC Department of Pediatrics, 4480 Oak St, Vancouver BC V6H 3V4; Monash (Australia)'74; MB BS; FRCP; FRCPC; Peds (Autism). Clinical Asst Prof, University of British Columbia; rwish@telus.net.

WISHLOW, Kevin A; Peace Arch Hosp, 15521 Russell Ave, White Rock BC V4B 2R4; Cal'08; CCFP; CCFP(E.M.); Staff, Peace Arch Hospital; (604)531-5512

WISMARK, Jennine A; Heritage Med Clinic, 105-2841 109 St NW, Edmonton AB T6J 6B7; Alb'00; CCFP; Staff, Covenant Health - Grey Nuns Community Hospital; Chair, Edmonton Southside Primary Care Network; (780)436-3790; Fax. (780)434-8378.

WISMER, David I A; Dr David Wismer Med Prof Crop, 666 Concession St, Hamilton ON L8V 4T9; McM'76; FRCSC; OrthSurg (Arthroplasty). Ac Staff, Hamilton Health Sciences Centre-Juravinski Site; (905)575-3300; Fax. (905)575-5666; drwismersoffice@bellnet.ca.

WISMER, Judy E M; Ancaster Dermatology, 34 Stone Church Rd, Ancaster ON L9K 1S5; McM'88; FRCPC; Derm (Skin Cancer). Head Div of Derm, Hamilton Health Sciences Centre - McMaster Children's Hospital; Consultant, St Joseph's Healthcare - Charlton Campus; Assoc Prof Med & Head, McMaster University; (905)304-1122; Fax. (905)304-3768; judywismer@sympatico.ca.

WISMER, Sandra J; 201-851 Fischer Hallman Rd, Kitchener ON N2M 5N8; McM'83; CCFP; FCFP; (519)743-1011; Fax. (519)743-0041.

WISNIEWSKA, Anna B; Kelowna Gen Hosp, 2268 Pandosy St, Kelowna BC V1Y 1T2; UBC'97; FRCPC; Psy (Clinical Psychiatry). Staff, Kelowna General Hospital; Langs: Polish; (250)862-4000; Fax. (250)862-4026.

WISNIOWSKI, Leon E; Scotia Med Clinic, 961 Bedford Hwy, Bedford NS B4A 1A9; Dal'91; Langs: Polish; French; (902)832-2380; Fax. (902)444-3074.

WISS, Raymond J R; Health Sciences North-Laurenti, 41 Ramsey Lake Rd, Sudbury ON P3E 5J1; McM'93; CCFP; CCFP(E.M.); FCFP; Staff, Health Sciences North-St Joseph's Health Centre; Staff, Health Sciences North-Laurentian Site; Langs: Spanish; French; (705)674-3181

WISTAFF, Robert; CHUM-Hotel-Dieu, 3840 rue Saint-Urbain, Montreal QC H2W 1T8; Mon'89; FRCPC; IntMed. Staff, Centre Hospitalier l'Université de Montréal (CHUM) - Hôtel-Dieu; (514)890-8000 x14444

WITCHER, Janice L; Fairview Med Arts Centre, 203-2200 Fairview St, Burlington ON L7R 4H9; Tor'78; (905)637-0852; Fax. (905)637-0792.

WITHER, Joan E; Univ Hlth Network-Toronto Western Hosp, 1E420 EW-399 Bathurst St, Toronto ON M5T 2S8; Alb'80; PhD; FRCPC; Rheum; IntMed. Sr Scientist, Toronto Western Hospital - University Health Network; Assoc Prof Med, University of Toronto; (416)603-6205; Fax. (416)603-4348; jwither@uhnresearch.ca.

WITHERS, Martin J; 301-1433 London Rd, Sarnia ON N7S 1P6; Wes'87; CCFP; (519)542-0144; Fax. (519)542-0682.

WITHERS, Michelle C; 207-3900 Hastings St, Burnaby BC V5C 6C1; UBC'99; FRCPC; Derm. Staff, Vancouver General Hospital - Centennial Pavillion; (604)299-3110; Fax. (604)299-3140.

WITHERS, Monique J; Deer Valley Family Med Centre, 101-83 Deerpoint Rd SE, Calgary AB T2J 6W5; Alb'82; CCFP; FCFP; Langs: Dutch; (403)271-5123; Fax. (403)225-1276.

WITHERS, Nicholas J; Pacific Reg Surgeon CFH Serv, PO Box 17000 Stn Forces CFB Esquimalt, Victoria BC V9A 7N2; Mem'96; CCFP; FCFP; Staff, Canadian Forces Health Services; (250)363-7067

WITHERS, Trevor M; Fort Saskatchewan Med Clinic, 9421 94 Ave, Fort Saskatchewan AB T8L 1N6; (South Africa)'92; Staff, Fort Saskatchewan Health Centre; (780)998-7757; Fax. (780)998-0636.

WITHERSPOON, Sandra E; 1145 Commercial Dr, Vancouver BC V5L 3X3; Wes'72; CCFP; FCFP; Ac Staff, Providence Health Care - St Paul's Hospital; Court Staff, BC Women's Hospital & Health Centre; Court Staff, BC Children's Hospital; Staff Teacher, University of British Columbia; (604)254-1354; Fax. (604)258-9190; sandi@reachcentre.bc.ca.

WITHINGTON, Davinia E; MUHC-Montreal Children's Hosp, C1119-2300 rue Tupper, Montreal QC H3H 1P3; Southampton (England)'79; FRCA; MRCP; MB; Staff, McGill University Health Centre - Montreal Children's Hospital; assoc Prof, McGill University; Langs: French; Italian; (514)412-4400 x22463; Fax. (514)412-4341; davinia.withington@mcgill.ca.

WITMANS, Manisha B; Synergy Wellness Centre, 201-501 Bethel Dr, Sherwood Park AB T8H 0N2; Sask'97; FAAP; DABPed; DABSM; LRCPS; MD; Peds; FRCPC; FRCPC; Respir; Peds (Pediatric Respiratory Medicine). Staff, University of Alberta Hospital; Staff, Stollery Children's Hospital; Aj Prof, University of Alberta; Langs: Gujarati; (780)800-6906; Fax. (780)800-6907.

WITMER, Michael R; Belgage Med Arts Bldg, 110-525 Belmont Ave, Kitchener ON N2M 5E2; Tor'94; MSc; CCFP; CCFP(E.M.); Staff, Stratford General Hospital - Huron Perth Healthcare Alliance; (519)571-1000; Fax. (519)571-0728.

WITT, Alexandra P; Campbellford Mem Hosp, PO Box 1027 146 Oliver Rd, Campbellford ON K0L 1L0; Alb'08; CCFP; Staff, Campbellford Memorial Hospital; (705)653-1140

WITT, Alvera; 15-1594 Fairfield Rd PO Box 50003, Victoria BC V8S 1G1; UBC'67; FRCPC; Psy (Consultant Liaison Psychiatry). Staff, Eagle Ridge Hospital & Health Care Centre; (604)461-2022

WITT, Jonathan A; Royal University Hosp, 103 Hospital Dr, Saskatoon SK S7N 0W8; Sask'98; CCFP; CCFP(E.M.); FCFP; Staff, Royal University Hospital; (306)655-1364; Fax. (306)655-1011.

WITT, Norbert J; 10816 124 St NW, Edmonton AB T5M 0H3; Alb'79; FRCPC; Neur (Electrodiagnostic). Consultant, Royal Alexandra Hospital; Ac Staff, University of Alberta Hospital; Clin Assoc Prof Med/Aj Prof, University of Alberta; Langs: German; (780)454-3800; Fax. (780)455-7992; neuroadmin@jonoke.com.

WITT, Susan A; Medicine Hat Reg Hosp, 666 5 St SW, Medicine Hat AB T1A 4H6; Alb'87; CCFP; FCFP; Staff, Medicine Hat Regional Hospital; (403)529-8000

WITT-SULLIVAN, Helga B; Hamilton HS-General Site, 424-237 Barton St E, Hamilton ON L8L 2X2; McM'83; BSc(PhysEd); FRCPC; IntMed (Gastroenterology). Ac Staff, Hamilton Health Sciences Centre - Hamilton General Hospital; Assoc Staff, St Joseph's Healthcare - Charlton Campus; McMaster University; Langs: German; (905)528-2564; Fax. (905)527-4126.

WITTEN, Allan D; Rocky Med Clinic, PO Box 99 Stn Main, Rocky-Mtn-Hse AB T4T 1A1; Alb'78; CCFP; (403)845-2815; Fax. (403)845-2177.

WITTEN, Edward J; Associates Med Clinic, 123 10th Ave S, Cranbrook BC V1C 2N1; Alb'80; (250)426-4231; Fax. (250)426-4357.

WITTENBERG, Jean-Victor P; 2402-77 Gerrard St W, Toronto ON M5G 2A1; Tor'71; DCP; FRCPC; Psy. Staff, The Hospital For Sick Children; Assoc Prof Psy, University of Toronto; Langs: English; French; (416)977-1580; Fax. (416)977-5027.

WITTENBERG, Leah A; 200-555 Sixth St, New Westminster BC V3L 5H1; UBC'03; FRCSC; Ophth. Staff, Vancouver General Hospital - Centennial Pavillion; (604)521-4144

WITTER, Tobias; Queen Elizabeth II HSC, 1276 South Park St, Halifax NS B3H 2Y9; (Germany)'99; Staff, Queen Elizabeth II Health Sciences Centre - Victoria General Site; (902)473-2331

WITTERICK, Ian J; Mount Sinai Hosp, 413-600 University Ave, Toronto ON M5G 1X5; Wes'86; FRCSC; Otol (Head & Neck Surgery). Staff, Mount Sinai Hospital; Head Otol, St Joseph's Health Centre; Consultant, Princess Margaret Hospital - University Health Network; Dept Chair Otol Head & Neck Surgery, University of Toronto; (416)586-4800 x8313; Fax. (416)586-8583; iwitterick@mtsinai.on.ca.

WITTES, Robert C; Wits-End Med Clinic, 301-7131 Bathurst St, Thornhill ON L4J 7Z1; McG'78; BA; MSc; LMCC; FRCPC; CommunMed;CCFP; Public Health & Preventive Med. Ac Staff Family Med, Mackenzie Richmond Hill Hospital; Ac Staff Urol, Princess Margaret Hospital - University Health Network; Court Staff, Humber River Regional Hospital - Finch Avenue Site; Prof Parasitology & Epidemiol, McGill University; Langs: French; (905)771-7505; Fax. (905)771-0236; dr.r.wittes@witsendmed.com.

WITTMANN, Rita; Murrayville Health Care Ctre, 205-22112 52 Ave, Langley BC V2Y 2M6; UBC'93; Respir; IntMed. Staff, Langley Memorial Hospital; (604)530-3662; Fax. (604)530-3612.

WITTMEIER, Robert W; Royal Alexandra Hosp, 541 CSB-10240 Kingsway Ave, Edmonton AB T5H 3V9; Cal'98; CCFP; CCFP(E.M.); Staff, Royal Alexandra Hospital; (780)735-4442; Fax. (780)735-4916.

WITTNER-SMITH, Carlissa R; South Side Womens Hlth Ctre, 120-3017 66 St NW, Edmonton AB T6K 4B2; Sask'99; FRCSC; ObstGyn. Staff, Covenant Health - Grey Nuns Community Hospital; (780)461-6220; Fax. (780)461-4197.

WITTY, Melissa J; Royal Victoria Hosp, 201 Georgian Dr, Barrie ON L4M 6M2; Tor'96; CCFP; FCFP; Assoc Staff, Royal Victoria Regional Health Centre; (705)792-3333; Fax. (705)728-4120; mwitty@rogers.com.

WITZKE, Gaynelle J; Athabascan Place, 140-80 Chippewa Rd, Sherwood Park AB T8A 4W6; Cal'80.

WITZKE, Ronald W; Medical Arts Centre, 100-770 6 St SW, Medicine Hat AB T1A 8M7; Man'73; FRCSC; GenSurg (Endoscopic Surgery). Ac Staff/Chief GenSurg, Medicine Hat Regional Hospital; Consultant, Tom Baker Cancer Centre; (403)502-8941; Fax. (403)504-1449; rwwitzke@telusplanet.net.

WIVIOTT, Gerald S; Allan Memorial Institute, 206 9-1025 av des Pins O, Montreal QC H3A 1A1; New York(NY) (USA)'67; FRCPC; Psy. Staff, McGill University Health Centre - Royal Victoria Hospital; (514)934-1934

WIWCHARUK, Gillian L; The Brantford Comm Hlth System, 200 Terrace Hill St, Brantford ON N3R 1G9; McM'08; CCFP; Staff, The Brant Community Healthcare System - Brantford General Hospital Site; (519)751-5510

WIZNURA, Richard A; Links Clinic, 104-11910 111 Ave NW, Edmonton AB T5G 3G6; Alb'82; (780)454-0351; Fax. (780)452-6767.

WLADICHUK, Adrian L; 400-1128 Hornby St, Vancouver BC V6Z 2L4; Qns'07; CCFP; (604)707-2273

WLODARCZYK, Stanislaw R; Family Physician, 238 King St N, Waterloo ON N2J 2Y7; Cracow (Poland)'81; Staff, St Mary's General Hospital; Staff, Grand River Hospital - Kitchener/Waterloo Health Centre; Langs: Polish; (519)747-4770; Fax. (519)747-5231.

WLODARSKI, Martin J; CDK Family Medicine, 175 Princess St, Kingston ON K7L 1A9; UBC'10; CCFP; (613)766-0318

WO, Bi Lan; CHUM-Hopital Saint-Luc, 1058 rue Saint-Denis, Montreal QC H2X 3J4; Mon'04; FRCSC; ObstGyn (Maternal Fetal Medicine). Staff, Centre Hospitalier l'Université De Montréal (CHUM) - Hôpital Saint-luc; (514)890-8000

WOBESER, Wendy L; Queens University, 3009 Etherington Hall, Kingston ON K7L 3N6; Sask'90; MD(Epidemiol.); FRCPC; IntMed (AIDS/HIV); InfectDis. Staff, Kingston General Hospital; Langs: Spanish; (613)533-2978; Fax. (613)533-6304; wlw@queensu.ca.

WODYNSKI, Peter J; 10th Street Medicentre, 75 Tenth St, New Westminster BC V3M 3X4; Qns'67; (604)526-3308; Fax. (604)526-2984.

WOELK, Cornelius J; Dr C W Wiebe Med Corp, 385 Main St, Winkler MB R6W 1J2; Man'86; CCFP; FCFP; Med Dir Palliative Care, Central Manitoba Regional Health Associates; Asst Prof Family Med, University of Manitoba; Langs: German; (204)325-4312; Fax. (204)325-4594; cvwoelk@mts.net.

WOHLGELERNTER, Joseph I O; 201-441 Clark Ave W, Thornhill ON L4J 6W8; Tor'70; DABPN; FRCPC; Psy (Marital Therapy). Langs: Hebrew; Yiddish; (905)882-8103; Fax. (905)882-8549.

WOHLGEMUT, Andrew H; The Boardwalk Prof Centre, 20 Water Street Pky, Charlottetown PE C1A 9M5; Wes'98; CCFP; (902)367-4444

WOHLGEMUT, Joel R P; Alexandra Hosp, 2F-29 Noxon St, Ingersoll ON N5C 1B8; Wes'01; CCFP; Staff, Alexandra Hospital; (519)425-9000; Fax. (519)485-9609.

WOJAKOWSKI, Krystyna H; London Children's Aid Society, 1680 Oxford St, London ON N5Y 5R8; Cracow (Poland)'60; FRCPC; Psy (Child & Adolescent Psychiatry). Langs: Polish; French; Russian; (519)455-9000; Fax. (519)455-4355.

WOJCICKA, Anna M; Toronto Sunnybrook Reg Cancer, 2075 Bayview Ave, Toronto ON M4N 3M5; Bialystok (Poland)'77; FRCPC; RadOncol (Palliative Care). Staff, Sunnybrook Health Sciences Centre; Staff, Southlake Regional Health Centre; Staff, Toronto Sunnybrook Regional Cancer Centre; Langs: Polish; Slovak; (416)480-6100

WOJCICKI, Andre T; Vivian Medical Spa, 6165 Vivian Rd, Mount Albert ON L0G 1M0; Bialystok (Poland)'77; FRCPC; IntMed (Cardiology). Staff, Southlake Regional Health Centre; Staff, Mackenzie Richmond Hill Hospital; Physician, Vivian Medical Spa; Langs: Polish; (905)473-4117; Fax. (905)473-1235; wojcicki@total.net.

WOJCIECHOWSKI, Agnieszka E; Health Plus Med Centre, 1075 Autumnwood Dr, Winnipeg MB R2J 1C6; Cal'04; BSc; CCFP; Staff Family Med Clinic, University of Alberta Hospital; Staff Family Med Clinic, Justik Medical Clinic; (204)594-2100

WOJCIK, John P; Heart Protection Strategies, 207-450 Central Ave, London ON N6B 2E8; Tor'98; BSc; MBA; FRCPC; IntMed (Endocrinology). Clin Asst ICU, Grand River Hospital - Kitchener/Waterloo Health Centre; Clin Asst ICU, St Joseph's Hospital - St Joseph's Health Care; Med Dir London Kincardine Goderich Aylmer & West Lorne, Heart Protection Strategies; Staff Endocrinologist, South Grey Bruce Health Centre; (519)435-0063; Fax. (519)435-0184.

WOJCIK, Joseph; 202-5885 ch Cote-des-Neiges, Montreal QC H3S 2T2; Mem'82; BSc(McGill); MSc; BMedSci; CCFP; Staff, Kateri Memorial Hospital Centre; Staff, Sir Mortimer B Davis Jewish General; (514)342-4522; Fax. (514)342-2441.

WOJCIK, Ronald W; Cdn Forces Hlth Services Centr, PO Box 99000 Stn Forces, Halifax NS B3K 5X5; Dal'85; Staff, Canadian Forces Health Services Centre (Atlantic); (902)721-7844

WOJCIK, Tammy-Lynn; Chilliwack Gen Hosp, 45600 Menholm Rd, Chilliwack BC V2P 1P7; McM'09; CCFP; Staff, Chilliwack General Hospital; (604)795-4141

WOJCIK, Wladyslaw; Glencairn Med & Dental Office, 1600 E Dewdney Ave, Regina SK S4N 4Y5; Stettin (Poland)'69; FRCPC; IntMed (Cardiology). Staff, Regina General Hospital; Physician, Glencairn Medical & Dental Office; Langs: Polish; Russian; Ukrainian; (306)352-6499; Fax. (306)347-7939.

WOJTOWICZ, Jeremy M; Hamilton HS-General Site, 214-237 Barton St E, Hamilton ON L8L 2X2; Cal'05; CCFP; CCFP(E.M.); Staff, Hamilton Health Sciences Centre - Hamilton General Hospital; (905)521-2100; Fax. (905)527-7051.

WOJTOWSKA, Ewa; 5973 Fraser St, Vancouver BC V5W 2Z6; Poznan (Poland)'70; FRCPC; IntMed (Cardiology). Staff, Providence Health Care - Mount Saint Joseph Hospital; Langs: Polish; (604)327-8085; Fax. (604)321-7602.

WOJTYK, Ronald J; Cdn Health Support Unit-HCC, 1745 Alta Vista Dr, Ottawa ON K1A 0K6; Tor'85; PhD; Staff Emerg, Stevenson Memorial Hospital; Staff, Canadian Forces Health Services Centre; Langs: Ukrainian; German; French; (613)945-6661; Fax. (613)945-6668.

WOLAK, Anna L; Broadway-Burrard Med Clinic, 1816 Broadway W, Vancouver BC V6J 1Y9; Adelaide (Australia)'04; MB BS; Physician Diagnostic, Rapid Access Breast Clinic; Clin Instructor, University of British Columbia; Langs: Tagalog; (604)736-1888; Fax. (604)736-5544; anna.tan@alumni.adelaide.edu.au.

WOLANSKI, Renee J; CLSC Rene-Cassin, 500-5800 boul Cavendish, Cote Saint-Luc QC H4W 2T5; McG'94; Langs: English; French; (514)484-7878 x1494; Fax. (514)485-2978.

WOLBER, Robert A; Lions Gate Hosp, 231 15th St E, North Vancouver BC V7L 2L7; Ann Arbor (USA)'84; FRCPC; AnatPath. Staff, Lions Gate Hospital; (604)984-5756; Fax. (604)984-5984; robert.wolber@vch.ca.

WOLCH, Gary R; University of Alberta Hosp, 4T1 09-8440 112 St NW, Edmonton AB T6G 2B7; Alb'93; CCFP; Staff Palliative Care Program, University of Alberta Hospital; (780)407-2840; Fax. (780)407-1394.

WOLCHOK, Garnet R; PO Box 1392, Aldergrove BC V4W 2V1; Tor'72; Ac Staff, Langley Memorial Hospital; (604)308-4732

WOLDE-GIORGHIS, Rahel; McGill Mental Health Centre, 5500-3600 rue McTavish, Montreal QC H3A 0G3; Mon'92; FRCSC; ObstGyn; Psy. (514)398-6019

WOLDER, Thomas; 17 Frank St, Strathroy ON N7G 2R2; Wes'75; Ac Staff, Strathroy Middlesex General Hospital - Middlesex Hospital Alliance; Langs: Dutch; (519)245-1609; Fax. (519)245-6560; drthomaswolder@rogers.com.

WOLDNIK, Mark F; Cumberland Med Clinic, PO Box 719 2765A Dunsmule Ave, Cumberland BC V0R 1S0; Qns'87; BSc(Biology); CCFP; FCFP; (250)336-2208; Fax. (250)336-2237.

WOLEVER, Thomas M S; St Michael's Hosp, 30 Bond St, Toronto ON M5B 1W8; Oxford (England)'80; PhD; Staff, St Michael's Hospital; Prof 1, University of Toronto; (416)978-5556; thomas.wolever@utoronto.ca.

WOLF, M Uri; Baycrest Centre for Geriatric, 4C91-3560 Bathurst St, Toronto ON M6A 2E1; Tor'05; FRCPC; Psy. Staff, Baycrest Centre for Geriatric Care; Staff, Brain Health Clinic; (416)785-2500; Fax. (416)785-2492.

WOLF, Marc A; Douglas Mental Hlth Univ Inst, 6875 boul Lasalle, Verdun QC H4H 1R3; Strasbourg (France)'84; FRCPC; Psy (P.Q.). Staff, Douglas Mental Health University Institute; adj Prof Psy, McGill University; (514)761-6131 x2831; wolmar@douglas.mcgill.ca.

WOLF, Michael; Cariboo Mem Hosp, 517 Sixth Ave N, Williams Lake BC V2G 2G8; Johannes Gutenberg University (Germany)'00; Staff, Cariboo Memorial Hospital and Health Centre; Langs: German; (250)392-4411

WOLF, Michael T; South Health Campus, 4448 Front St E, Calgary AB T3M 1M4; Wes'09; CCFP; CCFP(E.M.); Staff, Peter Lougheed Centre; Staff, South Health Campus; (403)956-1111

WOLFE, Brian K; Cowichan Dist Hosp, 3045 Gibbins Rd, Duncan BC V9L 1E5; Qns'82; FRCPC; DiagRad. Staff, Cowichan District Hospital; (250)746-4141 x4217; Fax. (250)709-3009.

WOLFE, Judith S; St Paul's Hosp, 3MC-1081 Burrard St, Vancouver BC V6Z 1Y6; Wes'95; FRCPC; Peds. Staff, Providence Health Care - St Paul's Hospital; (604)682-2344

WOLFE, Kevin B; St Boniface Gen Hosp, Y3023-409 Tache Ave, Winnipeg MB R2H 2A6; Man'85; FRCPC; IntMed; Cardiol. Staff, St Boniface General Hospital; Staff Cardiol, Health Sciences Centre; Asst Prof Med & Cardiol WRHA Cardiac Sciences Prog Bergen Cardiac Care Centre, University of Manitoba; (204)258-1274; Fax. (204)233-2157.

WOLFE, Marcel; Clinique Troubles de l'humeur, 404-8000 boul Langelier, Saint-Leonard QC H1P 3K2; Mon'68; CSPQ; Psy (P.Q.) (Consultation). ac Staff, Hopital Louis-H Lafontaine; Langs: Bilingual(English/French); (514)323-1617; Fax. (514)323-1569; mwolfe.hlhl@ssss.gouv.qc.ca.

WOLFE, Robert E; 602-790 Bay St PO Box 69, Toronto ON M5G 1N8; Tor'77; FRCPC; IntMed; Cardiol. Staff, Toronto General Hospital - UHN; Staff, Women's College Hospital; Asst Prof, University of Toronto; (416)921-7415; Fax. (416)921-6816.

WOLFE, Scott A D; Health Sciences Centre, AE2-820 Sherbrook St, Winnipeg MB R3A 1R9; Man'01; FRCPC; Anes. Staff Harry Medovy House, Health Sciences Centre; (204)774-6511

WOLFF, Bryan C; North York Gen Hosp, 4001 Leslie St, Toronto ON M2K 1E1; Wes'89; CCFP; CCFP(E.M.); Staff, North York General Hospital; (416)756-6001

WOLFF, Evelyn; 1-23 Dairy Lane, Huntsville ON P1H 1T4; Wes'72; Langs: Dutch; (705)789-9521; Fax. (705)789-9066.

WOLFF, Gerald K; The Rehabilitation Centre, 1105-505 Smyth Rd, Ottawa ON K1H 8M2; Qns'04; CSCN; FRCPC; PhysMed&Rehab. Staff, The Ottawa Hospital Rehabilitation Centre; (613)737-7350 x75598; Fax. (613)737-9638.

WOLFF, Jean-Luc; CHUS-Hop Fleurimont, 3001 12e av N, Sherbrooke QC J1H 5N4; Strasbourg (France)'79; Nephrol (P.Q.) (Kidney Transplantation). Staff, Centre Hospitalier Universitaire de Sherbrooke-Hopital Fleurimont; Prof, Universite de Sherbrooke; (819)564-5221; Fax. (819)564-5369; jean-luc.wolff@usherbrooke.ca.

WOLFISH, Karen R; Riverside Prof Centre, 311-1919 Riverside Dr, Ottawa ON K1H 1A2; Ott'90; FRCSC; ObstGyn. (613)526-0080; Fax. (613)526-9749.

WOLFLI, James N; 227-9148 23 Ave NW, Edmonton AB T6N 1H9; Cal'00; BSc; FRCSC; PlasSurg. Clin Assoc Prof, University of Alberta Hospital; (780)433-1393; Fax. (780)433-8748.

WOLFMAN, Wendy L; Hydro Place Bldg, 8F 712-700 University Ave, Toronto ON M5G 1Z5; Cal'75; FRCOG; ABOG; FRCSC; ObstGyn (Menopause Gynecology). Staff, Mount Sinai Hospital; Assoc Prof ObstGyn, University of Toronto; (416)586-4753; Fax. (416)586-4699; wwolfman@mtsinai.on.ca.

WOLFROM, Brent D; Queens Family Health Team, 115 Clarence St, Petawawa ON K8H 2X3; Sask'04; CCFP; Staff, Base Hospital-CFB Petawawa; (613)533-9303; Fax. (613)544-9899.

WOLFS, Maria E; St Michael's Health Centre, 6113-61 Queen St E, Toronto ON M5C 2T2; Wes'99; FRCPC; IntMed; Endocrin&Metab. (416)867-7424; Fax. (416)867-3654.

WOLFSOHN, Allan L; 750 Peter Morand Cres, Ottawa ON K1G 6S4; Cape Town (South Africa)'94; MB ChB; FRCPC; AnatPath. Ac Staff Path & Lab Med, The Ottawa Hospital - General Campus; Med Dir/Consultant, Gamma-Dynacare Laboratories; Teacher, University of Ottawa; (613)729-0200 x6600; Fax. (613)729-1127; wolfsohna@gamma-dynacare.com.

WOLFSON, Gary S; James Bay Med Centre, 547 Michigan St, Victoria BC V8V 1S5; Tor'78; CCFP; (250)388-6811; Fax. (250)380-0244.

WOLGELERNTER, Sia B; Scarborough Comm Mental Hlth, 12-2425 Eglinton Ave E, Scarborough ON M1K 5G8; Wes'81; (416)755-8301; Fax. (416)755-9220.

WOLINSKA, Justyna M; North York Gen Hosp, 4001 Leslie St, North York ON M2K 1E1; Jagiellonian University (Poland)'07; GenSurg. Staff, North York General Hospital; (416)756-6000

WOLINSKY, Joel L; Scarborough Hosp-General Div, 3050 Lawrence Ave E, Scarborough ON M1P 2V5; Tor'74; Staff, The Scarborough Hospital - General Campus; (416)431-8101

WOLK, Adele M; 2200 Oak Bay Ave PO Box 42063 Rpo Oak Bay, Victoria BC V8R 6T4; Man'75; MPH; CCFP; (250)385-5554; Fax. (250)385-5556.

WOLKOFF, David A; KW Sleep Laboratory, 290-180 King St S, Waterloo ON N2J 1P8; Syracuse(NY) (USA)'96; FRCPC; Psy. Staff, Homewood Health Centre; (519)745-2621; Fax. (519)745-7174.

WOLKOFF, Irvin I; 1-11 Elvina Gardens, Toronto ON M4P 1X7; Tor'76; FRCPC; Psy (Adult Psychiatry). (416)485-2680; Fax. (416)250-7857.

WOLKOVE, Norman; SMBD Jewish Gen Hosp, G203-3755 ch Cote-Sainte-Cathe, Montreal QC H3T 1E2; McG'71; DABIM; FCCP; FRCPC; Respir (Pulmonary Medicine). Ac Staff, Sir Mortimer B Davis Jewish General; adj Prof Med, McGill University; (514)340-8244; Fax. (514)240-7555.

WOLLACH, Barry A; 924 5 Ave N, Lethbridge AB T1H 0M4; Cape Town (South Africa)'83; FRCPC; Anes. Staff, Foothills Medical Centre; (403)471-4115; Fax. (403)382-3579.

WOLLACH, Jeffrey A; Anaesthetic Services, 213-2186 Oak Bay Ave, Victoria BC V8R 1G3; Cape Town (South Africa)'73; MB ChB; DAB; FRCPC; Anes (Cardiovascular Anesthesia). Ac Staff Anes, Royal Jubilee Hospital; Langs: Afrikaans; (250)595-7211; Fax. (250)595-7211.

WOLLIN, Brenda L; 201-5651 Riverbend Rd NW, Edmonton AB T6H 5K4; Sask'89; CCFP; FCFP; (780)438-8844; Fax. (780)436-9511.

WOLLIN, Timothy A; Alberta Urology Institute Inc, 400-11010 101 St NW, Edmonton AB T5H 4B9; Sask'89; FRCSC; Urol (Endocrinology). (780)423-6843; Fax. (780)441-2580.

WOLMAN, Stephen L; Univ Hlth Network-Toronto Gen, 9N 979-200 Elizabeth St, Toronto ON M5G 2C4; Tor'74; BSc; FRCPC; IntMed (Inflammatory Bowel Disease); Gastroent. Staff, Mount Sinai Hospital; Staff, Toronto General Hospital - UHN; Asst Prof Med, University of Toronto; (416)340-3507; Fax. (416)340-4785.

WOLNIK, Monica S; Royal Victoria Hosp, 201 Georgian Dr, Barrie ON L4M 6M2; McM'93; CCFP; CCFP(E.M.); Assoc Staff, Royal Victoria Regional Health Centre; (705)728-9802 x4121; Fax. (705)728-5922.

WOLOSZCZUK, Andrea D; Pickering Urgent Care Fam Ctre, 6B-1450 Kingston Rd, Pickering ON L1V 1C1; (Grenada)'81; Langs: Ukrainian; (905)831-8240; Fax. (905)831-8858.

WOLOVITZ, David M; CBI Medical Clinic, 202-940 Goldstream Ave, Nanaimo BC V9S 2Y4; Stellenbosch (South Africa)'84; MB ChB; Staff, Vancouver Island Health Authority; (250)474-9115; Fax. (250)474-7313.

WOLPERT, Maureen; 405-1240 Bay St, Toronto ON M5R 2A7; Witwatersrand (South Africa)'74; FRCS(Edin); FRCSC; Ophth. Staff Ophth, St Joseph's Health Centre; (416)925-2933; Fax. (416)925-0965.

WOLPERT, Natalie; St Michaels Hosp, 30 Bond St, Toronto ON M5B 1W8; Qns'01; FRCPC; EmergMed. Staff, Mackenzie Richmond Hill Hospital; Staff, St Michael's Hospital; (416)864-5976; Fax. (416)864-5341.

WOLSKI, Darryl M; Pelham Group Health Centre, 204C-245 Pelham Rd, St Catharines ON L2S 1X8; Wes'91; CCFP; FCFP; Staff Family Med, Niagara Health System - St Catharines General Site; Niagara Region-Min of Commun Safety & Correctional Serv., Prov of Ontario; (905)937-8787; Fax. (905)937-8786.

WOLSKI, Piotr S; The Ottawa Hosp-Civic Campus, 1053 Carling Ave, Ottawa ON K1Y 4E9; Academy of Medicine Lublin (Other Foreign)'94; Staff, The Ottawa Hospital - Civic Campus; (613)737-8187

WOLSKI, Winicjusz M; Credit Valley Med Arts Centre, 405-2000 Credit Valley Rd, Mississauga ON L5M 4N4; Tor'06; FRCPC; IntMed; Respir. Langs: Polish; (905)608-2424; Fax. (905)608-2992.

WOLSTENHOLME, Keith R; 300-4309 52 Ave, Red Deer AB T4N 6S4; Cal'04; FRCSC; OrthSurg. (403)309-2001; Fax. (403)358-5808.

WOLTING, Jacqueline; Chilliwack Gen Hosp, 45600 Menholm rd, Chilliwack BC V2P 1P7; Wes'10; CCFP; Staff, Chilliwack General Hospital; (604)795-4141

WOLWERTZ, John; Ctre de Psychiatrie Legal, 500-6555 boul Metropolitain E, Saint-Leonard QC H1P 3H3; Mon'65; Psy (P.Q.). (514)328-7800 x234; Fax. (514)328-9108.

WONG, Aaron W Y; 202-179 Davie St, Vancouver BC V6Z 2Y1; UBC'08; (604)669-7772

WONG, Albert G; Credit Valley Med Arts Centre, 402-2000 Credit Valley Rd, Mississauga ON L5M 4N4; Tor'88; ABIM; ABAI; FRCPC; IntMed (Allergic Disorders); ClinImmunol&Allergy. Court Staff IntMed, The Credit Valley Hospital; (905)828-1077; aw123@rogers.com.

WONG, Albert H C; Addiction & Mental Hlth-Clarke, 711-250 College St, Toronto ON M5T 1R8; Tor'93; PhD; FRCPC; Psy (Clinician Investigator Program). Staff Psy/Rsch Scientist, Centre for Addiction & Mental Health (CAMH) - College Street Site; Assoc Prof Psy/Teach Staff, University of Toronto; (416)535-8501 x4010; Fax. (416)979-6936; albert.wong@utoronto.ca.

WONG, Albert S C; Bay College Med Centre, PO Box 135 C216-777 Bay St, Toronto ON M5G 2C8; Wes'89; Langs: Cantonese; (416)977-8878; Fax. (416)977-0118.

WONG, Albert S H; 797 Broadview Ave, Toronto ON M4K 2P8; Tor'87; Langs: Chinese; (416)463-3228; Fax. (416)463-7868.

WONG, Alex H C; Canadian Sport Medicine, 2424 University Drive NW, Calgary AB T2N 3Y9; UBC'03; CCFP; (403)289-8959; Fax. (403)284-9139.

WONG, Alexander; 4E-1440 14th Ave, Regina SK S4P 0W5; Wes'05; FRCPC; IntMed; InfectDis. Staff InfecDis, Regina General Hospital; (306)766-3915; Fax. (306)766-3995.

WONG, Alice C N; 105-372 Hollandview Trail, Aurora ON L4G 0A5; Ott'98; CCFP; (905)726-8332; Fax. (905)726-9899.

WONG, Alice H M; Royal University Hosp, 103 Hospital Dr, Saskatoon SK S7N 0W8; Man'89; MPH; FRCPC; IntMed; Critical Care Medicine; InfectDis. Staff InfectDis, Royal University Hospital; Langs: Chinese; (306)655-7494; Fax. (306)975-0383.

WONG, Alice S L; B100-5510 Mavis Rd, Mississauga ON L5V 2X5; Tor'81; CCFP; Langs: Chinese; (905)501-6008; Fax. (905)568-3901.

WONG, Allan P G; 211-460 Nanaimo St, Vancouver BC V5L 4W3; Cal'84; BSc(Pharm); FRCPC; Psy (Crisis Intervention). Clin Assoc Prof, University of British Columbia; Langs: Cantonese; Toishan; (604)646-4664

WONG, Allen S; Terwillegar Med Clinic, 101-121 Haddow Close NW, Edmonton AB T6R 3W3; Alb'99; BSc(Med.); CCFP; (780)989-5300; Fax. (780)989-5301.

WONG, Amy H; 18-16945 Leslie St, Newmarket ON L3Y 9A2; New York(N.Y.) (USA)'02; CCFP; Physician, Mackenzie Richmond Hill Hospital; Physician, Park Place Manor Retirement Residence; Physician, Mon Sheong Home for the Aged; Langs: Cantonese; (905)868-8689; Fax. (905)868-9479.

WONG, Amy N; 310-3101 Bloor St W, Etobicoke ON M8X 2W2; Alb'88; CCFP; Langs: Cantonese; Mandarin; (416)231-1111; Fax. (416)231-7947.

WONG, Andrea B; Sundance Med Clinic, 113-31 Sunpark Plaza SE, Calgary AB T2X 3W5; Cal'91; CCFP; (403)254-2030; Fax. (403)254-2929.

WONG, Andrew C H; The Raxlen Clinic, B102-340 College St, Toronto ON M5T 3A9; Tor'81; Langs: Chinese; (416)966-3641; Fax. (416)944-9947.

WONG, Andrew C Y; 303-240 Alton Towers Cir, Scarborough ON M1V 4P3; (Hong Kong)'71; FRCS(Ed); FACS; CCFP; Staff, The Scarborough Hospital - Birchmount Campus; Langs: Chinese; (416)321-1232

WONG, Andrew H K; Surrey Med Arts Bldg, 116-13798 94A Ave, Surrey BC V3V 1N1; UBC'93; FRCSC; GenSurg. Staff Surg, Surrey Memorial Hospital; Langs: Cantonese; (604)588-2388; Fax. (604)588-2389.

WONG, Andrew L; Alberta Children's Hosp, 403A-2888 Shaganappi Trail NW, Calgary AB T3B 6A8; Glasgow (Scotland)'71; MB ChB; FRCS(Glasgow); MSc; FRCSC; GenSurg (Minimal Access Surgery); PedGenSurg. Sec Head Pediatric GenSurg, Alberta Children's Hospital; Prog Dir Pediatric GenSurg/Clin Assoc Prof, University Of Calgary; (403)955-7253; Fax. (403)955-7634; andrewwong@albertahealthservices.ca.

WONG, Andrew P T; Callingwood Family Clinic, 454-6650 177 St NW, Edmonton AB T5T 4J5; Alb'86; (780)487-1223; Fax. (780)444-0974.

WONG, Andy V F; Fairmount Med Clinic, 7811 Fairmount Dr SE, Calgary AB T2H 0X8; Alb'92; (403)242-7300; Fax. (403)242-7302.

WONG, Angela M Y; 2-9640 Bayview Ave, Richmond Hill ON L4C 9P7; (Hong Kong)'74; MRC(UK); DCH(Lond); CCFP; Court Staff, Mackenzie Richmond Hill Hospital; Langs: Chinese; (905)737-0509; Fax. (905)737-4889.

WONG, Angela S C; Bay College Med Centre, PO Box 135 C216-777 Bay St, Toronto ON M5G 2C8; Wes'96; CCFP; FCFP; Langs: Cantonese; (416)977-8878; Fax. (416)977-0118.

WONG, Angela S W; Crosscultural Psy Clinic, 715 12th Ave W, Vancouver BC V5Z 1M9; UBC'95; FRCPC; Psy (Emergency Psychiatry). Staff, Vancouver General Hospital - Centennial Pavillion; Langs: Cantonese; (604)875-4115; Fax. (604)875-5386.

WONG, Anita K; 103-20644 Fraser Hwy, Langley BC V3A 4G5; Man'91; CCFP; Langs: Cantonese; (604)530-4979; Fax. (604)530-2975.

WONG, Anne K; St Joseph's Healthcare, 50 Charlton Ave E, Hamilton ON L8N 4A6; Tor'86; FRCPC; Anes. Staff, St Joseph's Healthcare - Charlton Campus; (905)522-1155; Fax. (905)521-6019.

WONG, Anthony D; St Paul's Hosp, 1081 Burrard St, Vancouver BC V6Z 1Y6; Otago (New Zealand)'66; FRCPC; DiagRad. Staff, Providence Health Care - St Paul's Hospital; (604)682-2344

WONG, Arnold K Y; North Scarborough Prof Centre, 309-3420 Finch Ave E, Scarborough ON M1W 2R6; (Hong Kong)'71; Court Staff, The Scarborough Hospital - Birchmount Campus; Langs: Cantonese; (416)499-1143; Fax. (416)499-4604.

WONG, Asa W; 5026 Joyce St, Vancouver BC V5R 4G6; Alb'92; CCFP; Langs: Cantonese; (604)438-8581; Fax. (604)438-8547.

WONG, Benjamin B L; North York Gen Hosp, 4001 Leslie St, North York ON M2K 1E1; Tor'97; ABAI; FRCPC; IntMed; ClinImmunol&Allergy. Consultant Med, North York General Hospital; Consultant Med, Rouge Valley Health System - Centenary Health Centre Site; Langs: Cantonese; (416)756-6000

WONG, Benjamin C; Reginal Fertility Program, 400-2000 Veteran's Place NW, Calgary AB T3B 4N2; Alb'96; FRCSC; ObstGyn (Reproductive Endocrinology). Att Physician, Alberta Health Services Calgary; Clinical Asst Prof, University of Calgary; Langs: Cantonese; Mandarin; (403)284-9103; Fax. (403)284-9293.

WONG, Bill I; Trillium Hlth Ctr-Mississauga, 100 Queensway W, Mississauga ON L5B 1B8; Man'85; BSc(Med); FRCPC; Anes (Cardiovascular Anesthesia). Staff, Trillium Health Centre - Mississauga; Asst Prof, University of Toronto; (905)848-7100

WONG, Billy R; Hys Med Centre, 510-11010 101 St NW, Edmonton AB T5H 4B9; Alb'96; FRCSC; ObstGyn. Asst Clin Prof, University of Alberta; (780)414-0782; Fax. (780)414-0784.

WONG, Bobby C H; Ridge Meadows Hosp & Hlth CC, 11666 Laity St, Maple Ridge BC V2X 5A3; Tor'92; BSc(Hons.); FRCPC; DiagRad. Staff, Ridge Meadows Hospital & Health Care Centre; Staff, Royal Columbian Hospital; Ac Staff Gen & Emerg, Abbotsford Regional Hospital & Cancer Centre; Langs: Cantonese; (604)463-1853

WONG, Boon L; 230-7360 Westminster Hwy, Richmond BC V6X 1A1; London (England)'90; MB BS; Staff, Richmond Hospital; Clin Instructor, University of British Columbia; Langs: Cantonese; Mandarin; (604)231-9099; Fax. (604)231-9098.

WONG, Brendan J; 204-6440 Royal Oak Ave, Burnaby BC V5H 3P2; Man'08; CCFP; (604)482-6100

WONG, Brian M; Sunnybrook Health Sciences Ctr, H466-2075 Bayview Ave, Toronto ON M4N 3M5; Tor'03; FRCPC; IntMed. Staff, Sunnybrook Health Sciences Centre; (416)480-4290; Fax. (416)480-6777.

WONG, Brian Y L; Four Corners Med Bldg, 205-2009 Long Lake Rd, Sudbury ON P3E 6C3; Qns'95; FRCPC; IntMed (Interventional Cardiology); Cardiol. Staff, Health Sciences North - Memorial Site; Langs: Cantonese; (705)674-8148; Fax. (705)674-8919.

WONG, Bruce M; Victoria Emerg Phys Mgmt Ltd, 325-1627 Fort St, Victoria BC V8R 1H8; UBC'86; FACEP; FRCPC; EmergMed. Staff, Vancouver Island Health Authority; (250)479-1442; Fax. (250)479-1472.

WONG, Byron E; 4825 Dalhousie Dr NW, Calgary AB T3A 6K7; Cal'90; FRCPC; Peds (Acupuncture). Clinical Asst Prof, University of Calgary; Langs: Chinese; (403)239-9333; Fax. (403)208-1648.

WONG, Camilla L; St Michael's Hosp, SW4 002-30 Bond St, Toronto ON M5B 1W8; Tor'03; FRCPC; IntMed; GeriatricMed. Staff, St Michael's Hospital; Langs: Cantonese; (416)864-5015; Fax. (416)864-5735.

WONG, Carrie K; Kingsway Plaza Phase III, 710-4980 Kingsway, Burnaby BC V5H 4K7; Alb'94; BSc(Med.); FRCSC; ObstGyn. Ac Staff, Burnaby Hospital; Langs: Cantonese; (604)433-8900; Fax. (604)433-8506.

WONG, Catherine K; Postgrad Med Education Office, 2F-500 University Ave, Toronto ON M5G 1V7; Dal'07; FRCPC; Anes.

WONG, Chet G; 1910-8171 Ackroyd Rd, Richmond BC V6X 3K1; Qns'07; FRCPC; IntMed; ClinImmunol&Allergy. (604)370-3009

WONG, Chi Mun; Walk-In & Family Practice, 1D-211 Martindale Rd, St Catharines ON L2S 3V7; Ibadan (Nigeria)'86; MB BS; FCFP(SA); CCFP; Langs: Cantonese; Mandarin; (905)688-8222; Fax. (905)688-2022.

WONG, Chong Shun; Sunnybrook Hlth Sciences Ctre, T2-2075 Bayview Ave, Toronto ON M4N 3M5; Tor'80; FRCPC; RadOncol (Gastrointestinal Disorders). Chief RadOncol, Sunnybrook Health Sciences Centre; Head Radiation Treatment Prog, Sunnybrook Health Sciences Centre - Edmond Odette Cancer Centre; Prof RadOncol & Med Biophysics, University of Toronto; (416)480-4619; Fax. (416)480-6002.

WONG, Christopher C K; Thunderbird Family Practice, D114-20159 88 Ave, Langley BC V1M 0A4; UBC'87; Staff, Langley Memorial Hospital; (604)888-6220; Fax. (604)882-1383.

WONG, Christopher K; Keary Med Centre, 203-245 Columbia St E, New Westminster BC V3L 3W4; Sask'63; FRCPC; IntMed (Infectious Diseases). Staff, Royal Columbian Hospital; Langs: Chinese; (604)525-9666; Fax. (604)525-2173.

WONG, Cindy M; Sturgeon Community Hosp, 201 Boudreau Rd, St. Albert AB T8N 6C4; Alb'98; CCFP; CCFP(E.M.); Staff, Sturgeon Community Hospital; (780)418-8229

WONG, Clara K; UBC Dept of Anaesthesiology, 3300-910 10th Ave W, Vancouver BC V5Z 1M9; UBC'08; (604)875-5855

WONG, Clarence K W; Royal Alexandra Hosp, 218-10240 Kingsway Ave, Edmonton AB T5H 3V9; Alb'95; BSc; ABIM; FRCPC; IntMed (Oncology); Gastroent. Staff Community Services Centre, Royal Alexandra Hospital; Att Staff, Cross Cancer Institute; Assoc Prof, University of Alberta; Langs: Cantonese; (780)735-6838; Fax. (780)735-6792.

WONG, Clement K L; Meadowvale Prof Centre, 226-6855 Meadowvale Town Ctre, Mississauga ON L5N 2Y1; Tor'81; Langs: Mandarin; Cantonese; (905)821-2114; Fax. (905)821-1360.

WONG, Clint S; Brandon Reg Health Centre, 150 McTavish Ave E, Brandon MB R7A 2B3; Man'05; FRCPC; Anes. Staff, Brandon Regional Health Centre; (204)578-4000

WONG, Clinton L; St Paul's Hosp, 1081 Burrard St, Vancouver BC V6Z 1Y6; UBC'83; FRCPC; Anes. Staff, Providence Health Care - St Paul's Hospital; Clin Associate Prof, University of British Columbia; (604)806-8337; Fax. (604)806-8487.

WONG, Colin J; Vernon Jubilee Hosp, 2101 32 St, Vernon BC V1T 5L2; UBC'85; FRCPC; Anes. Staff, Vernon Jubilee Hospital; Staff, Pleasant Valley Health Centre; (250)545-2211

WONG, Cynthia S; 2251 Lawrence Ave E, Scarborough ON M1P 2P5; Tor'89; Langs: Cantonese; (416)759-5251; Fax. (416)759-1253.

WONG, Daniel C; 273-5 Fairview Mall Dr, North York ON M2J 2Z1; Ott'01; FRCPC; Neur. Langs: Bilingual(English/French); (416)502-8100; Fax. (416)502-8110.

WONG, Daniel D; 828 Dundas St W, Toronto ON M6J 1V3; Man'68; Langs: Mandarin; Cantonese; Taiwanese; (416)603-9009; Fax. (416)603-7364.

WONG, Daniel G; Royal Columbian Hosp, 330 Columbia St E, New Westminster BC V3L 3W7; UBC'05; CCFP; CCFP(E.M.); Staff, Royal Columbian Hospital; (604)520-4637

WONG, Daniel K C; Haney Prof Bldg, 201-11743 224 St, Maple Ridge BC V2X 6A4; Adelaide (Australia)'71; MB BS; Ac Staff, Ridge Meadows Hospital & Health Care Centre; Clin Instructor, University of British Columbia; Langs: Hakka; Cantonese; Mandarin; (604)467-5525; Fax. (604)467-7382.

WONG, Daniel M T; 204-3410 Sheppard Ave E, Scarborough ON M1T 3K4; (Hong Kong)'79; MRC(UK); ABIM; FRCPC; IntMed (Rheumatology). Staff, The Scarborough Hospital - Birchmount Campus; Langs: Cantonese; Mandarin; (416)293-1978; Fax. (416)293-3528.

WONG, Daniel R; 105-245 Columbia St E, New Westminster BC V3L 3W4; Tor'99; MPH; FRCSC; CardSurg (Aortic Surg). Affil Asst Prof, University of Victoria; Clin Instructor, University of British Columbia; (604)522-6800; cvtsurgery@cvtsurgery.com.

WONG, Danny H K; Crestwood Med & Dental Bldg, 103-6051 Gilbert Rd, Richmond BC V7C 3V3; UBC'80; Langs: Cantonese; (604)278-9555; Fax. (604)278-9556.

WONG, Dave; Cape Breton Hlthcare Complex, 1482 George St, Sydney NS B1P 1P3; Alb'97; BSc(Hon); FRCPC; IntMed (Cardiology). Att Staff, Cape Breton Healthcare Complex; (902)567-7290; Fax. (902)567-7292.

WONG, David A; All Med Health, 1-16880 Yonge St, Newmarket ON L3Y 0A3; Wes'84; CCFP; FCFP; Staff, Southlake Regional Health Centre; Langs: Chinese; (905)895-9777; Fax. (905)895-9720.

WONG, David H W; Associated Anaes Services, M2A-601 Broadway W, Vancouver BC V5Z 4C2; (Hong Kong)'67; MB BS; FRCPC; Anes. Head Neuro Anes, Vancouver General Hospital - Centennial Pavillion; Clin Prof/Dir, University of British Columbia; (604)874-5291; Fax. (604)875-5344.

WONG, David K H; Univ Hlth Network-Toronto Western Hosp, 6B 176-399 Bathurst St, Toronto ON M5T 2S8; Tor'88; MD; FRCP; FRCPC; IntMed (Hepatology). Staff, Toronto Western Hospital - University Health Network; Staff Hepatologist, St Michael's Hospital; Staff Immunodeficiency, Toronto General Hospital - UHN; Staff, Toronto Western Hospital Liver Clinic; Specialized Positive Care Clinic; Staff, Immunodefiency Clinic; (416)603-6234; Fax. (416)603-6281.

WONG, David K W; Yellowknife Hlth & Social Serv, PO Box 608, Yellowknife NT X1A 2N5; Alb'87; Staff, Stanton Territorial Health Authority; Langs: Chinese; (867)920-7777; Fax. (867)920-7711; david_wong@gov.nt.ca.

WONG, David L H; 230-7031 Westminster Hwy, Richmond BC V6X 1A3; Man'90; FRCSC; Otol (Head & Neck Surgery). (604)273-2928; Fax. (604)273-7489.

WONG, David M C; Family Med Clinic, 1200 Lawrence Ave E, Toronto ON M3A 1C1; Tor'92; CCFP; FCFP; Langs: Cantonese; French; (416)391-5155; Fax. (416)391-5286.

WONG, David T W; Univ Hlth Network-Toronto Western Hosp, 6B 176-399 Bathurst St, Toronto ON M5T 2S8; Tor'81; Anes; IntMed. Staff, Halton Healthcare Services Corporation - Oakville Site; Staff, Toronto Western Hospital - University Health Network; Asst Prof, University of Toronto; Langs: Cantonese; (416)603-5118; Fax. (416)603-6494.

WONG, David T W; 801-61 Queen St E, Toronto ON M5C 2T2; Tor'89; MD; ABOph; FRCSC; Ophth (AIDS/HIV). Staff, St Michael's Hospital; University of Toronto; Langs: Cantonese; Chinese; (416)867-3670; Fax. (416)867-3687; wongd@smh.ca.

WONG, David T W; Summerside Med Centre, 101-475 Granville St, Summerside PE C1N 3N9; (Hong Kong)'74; MB BS; FAAP; FRCPC; Peds (Asthma). Chief Peds, Prince County Hospital; Teacher, Dalhousie University; (902)432-8181; Fax. (902)436-9660.

WONG, Davidicus A; Prime Care Med Centre, 202-7315 Edmonds St, Burnaby BC V3N 1A7; UBC'89; Dept Head Family Practice, Burnaby Hospital; Chair Health Authority Med Committee, Fraser Health Authority Corporate Office; Clinical Asst Prof Family Med, University of British Columbia; (604)540-8228

WONG, Delora; Oakdale Med Bldg, 428-2065 Finch Ave W, North York ON M3N 2V7; Wes'93; CCFP; Staff Privil, Humber River Regional Hospital - Finch Avenue Site; Att Physician, Cummer Lodge Home for the Aged; (416)745-3574; Fax. (416)745-9702.

WONG, Denise W; Medical Assoc Of Port Perry, 462 Paxton St, Port Perry ON L9L 1L9; Tor'10; CCFP; (905)985-2895; Fax. (905)985-8521.

WONG, Dennis K; Dennis K K Wong Prof Corp, 253-1623 Centre St NW, Calgary AB T2E 8S7; Cal'84; CCFP; (403)230-3333; Fax. (403)230-1696.

WONG, Dennis S; London Cardiac Institute, 302-256 Pall Mall St, London ON N6A 5P6; Tor'92; FRCPC; IntMed (Cardiology). (519)645-0146; Fax. (519)645-1584; wong@londoncardiac.ca.

WONG, Dennis Y R; Heritage Village Medicentre, 2041 111 St NW, Edmonton AB T6J 4V9; Alb'77; BSc; Langs: Chinese; French; (780)438-2306; Fax. (780)461-2632.

WONG, Derek T H; Children's Hosp of Eastern Ont, 3317-401 Smyth Rd, Ottawa ON K1H 8L1; Wes'02; FRCPC; Peds; Cardiol. Staff, Children's Hospital of Eastern Ontario (CHEO); (613)737-7600; Fax. (613)738-4835.

WONG, Diana; Gemini Health Centre, 2010-6708 48 Ave, Camrose AB T4V 4S3; Alb'98; FRCSC; PlasSurg. Staff, Covenant Health - St Mary's Hospital; Langs: Chinese; (780)672-9886; Fax. (780)672-9104.

WONG, Diane C; Glow Medi Spa, 4F-129 Yorkville Ave, Toronto ON M5R 1C4; McM'96; BSc; CCFP; (416)920-9998

WONG, Eddie W; Kingsway Med Clinic, 4645 Kingsway, Burnaby BC V5H 2B3; Alb'80; Physician, Broadway Station Med Clinic; (604)558-2611

WONG, Eddy K K; AIM Orleans Hlth & Wellness Cl, 1605 Orleans Blvd, Orleans ON K1C 7E2; Ott'76; FAAP; FRCPC; Peds. Ac Staff, Children's Hospital of Eastern Ontario (CHEO); Ac Staff, The Ottawa Hospital - General Campus; Langs: Cantonese; (613)830-6890; Fax. (613)837-6312.

WONG, Edmund K Y; 201-1637 Woodroffe Ave, Nepean ON K2G 1W2; Tor'76; CCFP; FCFP; Langs: Chinese; (613)226-2279; Fax. (613)226-8162.

WONG, Edward W H; The Richmond Hosp, 7000 Westminster Hwy, Richmond BC V6X 1A2; Wes'04; CCFP; Staff, Richmond Hospital; (604)725-3672

WONG, Edward Y C; Danforth & Pape X-Ray, 698 Danforth Ave, Toronto ON M4J 1L1; Tor'63; FRCPC; DiagRad (Ultrasound). Langs: Cantonese; Chinese; (416)463-3011; Fax. (416)463-4651.

WONG, Eileen M; 2302 4th Ave W PO Box 19094 Rpo Fourth Ave, Vancouver BC V6K 4R8; Alb'85; CCFP; CCFP(E.M.); FCFP; (604)263-2822; Fax. (604)263-2822.

WONG, Eric K W; St Joseph's Family Med Centre, 346 Platt's Lane, London ON N6G 1J1; Wes'02; CCFP; Staff, South Huron Hospital Association; Staff, London Health Sciences Centre - Victoria Campus; (519)672-9660; Fax. (519)672-7727.

WONG, Eric P C; Family Physician Med Clinic, 10610 Bayview Ave, Richmond Hill ON L4C 3N8; Tor'76; Staff, Mackenzie Richmond Hill Hospital; Langs: Cantonese; (905)884-4040; Fax. (905)884-2755.

WONG, Eric Y L; University of Alberta Hosp, 2E4 32 WCM-8440 112 St NW, Edmonton AB T6G 2B7; Alb'85; ABIM; FRCPC; IntMed; Respir. Staff, University of Alberta Hospital; Assoc Prof, University of Alberta; Langs: Cantonese; (780)407-7551; Fax. (780)407-6384.

WONG, Fedrick; 8173 Granville St, Vancouver BC V6P 4Z6; UBC'90; Staff, Providence Health Care - Mount Saint Joseph Hospital; Staff, Providence Health Care - St Vincent's Hospital-Heather Site; Langs: Cantonese; (604)321-0015; Fax. (604)327-1037.

WONG, Flora F M; St Luke Family Practice, 5-5761 Glover Rd, Langley BC V3A 8M8; Cal'98; BSc; CCFP; Staff, Langley Memorial Hospital; (604)530-5825; Fax. (604)530-5828; flora_kwan@telus.net.

WONG, Florence S H; Univ Hlth Network-The Toronto, 9N 983-200 Elizabeth St, Toronto ON M5G 2C4; Melbourne (Australia)'78; MB BS; FRACP; FRCPC; IntMed (Hepatology); Gastroent. Att Staff Outdoor Hepatol, St Michael's Hospital; Scientist, Toronto General Hospital - UHN; Prof, University of Toronto; Langs: Chinese; (416)340-3834; Fax. (416)340-5019.

WONG, Frances L W; BC Cancer Agency-Fraser Valley, 13750 96 Ave, Surrey BC V3V 1Z2; UBC'79; FRCPC; RadOncol. Staff, BC Cancer Agency Fraser Valley Centre; Langs: Cantonese; (604)930-4032; Fax. (604)930-4065.

WONG, Frank G; C-309 Commissioners Rd W, London ON N6J 1Y4; Wes'77; CCFP; FCFP; Ac Staff, London Health Sciences Centre - Victoria Campus; Court Staff, St Joseph's Hospital - St Joseph's Health Care; Aj Prof Dept of Family Med, University of Western Ontario; (519)657-5434; Fax. (519)641-7734.

WONG, Frank K L; Wolfedale Plaza, 848 Burnhamthorpe Rd W, Mississauga ON L5C 2S3; (Taiwan)'62; Langs: Cantonese; Mandarin; (905)276-2332; Fax. (905)276-8211.

WONG, Frank S H; ENT Associates, 401-1990 Fort St, Victoria BC V8R 6V4; National (Taiwan)'67; FACS; FRCSC; Otol (Head & Neck Surgery). Staff, Royal Jubilee Hospital; Staff, Victoria General Hospital; Langs: Mandarin; Cantonese; (250)595-7564; Fax. (250)595-2319.

WONG, Franklin T; Seniors Health Centre, 2 Buchan Crt, North York ON M2J 5A3; Qns'93; FRCPC; Psy (Geriatric Psychiatry). Staff, North York General Hospital; University of Toronto; (416)756-6050; Fax. (416)756-1844.

WONG, Fung L; Chalmers Gate Mem Bldg, 207-328 Highway 7 E, Richmond Hill ON L4B 3P7; (Hong Kong)'89; CCFP; FCFP; Langs: Cantonese; (905)763-0311; Fax. (905)763-7459; funglwong@gmail.com.

WONG, Gabriel F Y; 19A-279 Kingston Rd E, Ajax ON L1Z 0K5; Tor'84; Staff, The Scarborough Hospital - General Campus; Staff, Rouge Valley Health System - Ajax & Pickering Health Centre Site; Langs: Chinese; (905)428-2913; Fax. (905)686-1295.

WONG, Gail K; The Hosp for Sick Children, 555 University Ave, Toronto ON M5G 1X8; New South Wales (Australia)'98; Staff, The Hospital For Sick Children; (416)813-5586; Fax. (416)813-7543.

WONG, Garway M V; Thornhill Med Centre, 18 Centre St, Thornhill ON L4J 1E9; McM'08; CCFP; (905)889-3634; Fax. (905)889-3986.

WONG, George A; 221A Mitton St N, Sarnia ON N7T 6H5; Tor'79; FRCSC; OrthSurg. Staff, Bluewater Health - Mitton Site; Staff, Bluewater Health - Norman Site; (519)332-8005; Fax. (519)332-8068.

WONG, George K K; 7875 Riverside Dr E, Windsor ON N8S 1E1; Sydney (Australia)'71; FRCPC; IntMed. (519)974-0005; Fax. (519)974-0008.

WONG, George P L; Keele-Ingram Prof Centre, 306-2221 Keele St, North York ON M6M 3Z5; Tor'81; BASc; MSc; FRCSC; ObstGyn. Staff, Humber River Regional Hospital - Keele Street Site; (416)240-0027; Fax. (416)240-8978.

WONG, Gina S H; Bells Corner Med Group, 103-1956 Robertson Rd, Nepean ON K2H 5B9; Ott'92; BSc(Hons-Genetics); BA(Psychology); (613)596-0911; Fax. (613)596-3162.

WONG, Godfrey L; Finch-Midland Med Centre, 208-4190 Finch Ave E, Scarborough ON M1S 4T7; Wes'74; Ac Staff, The Scarborough Hospital - Birchmount Campus; Ac Staff, North York General Hospital; Ac Staff, Rouge Valley Health System - Centenary Health Centre Site; Langs: Chinese; (416)297-8624; Fax. (416)297-7509.

WONG, Gordon K T; Credit Valley Prof Bldg, 501-2300 Eglinton Ave W, Mississauga ON L5M 2V8; Tor'89; FRCPC; IntMed; Nephrol. Assoc Staff, The Credit Valley Hospital; Langs: Cantonese; (905)820-8770; Fax. (905)820-3703.

WONG, Grace K S; Fifth Avenue Med Centre, 300 14th Ave, Orangeville ON L9W 1G2; Alb'05; CCFP; (519)942-1515; Fax. (519)942-5112.

WONG, Graham C; Gordon & Leslie Diamond HCC, L9-2775 Laurel St, Vancouver BC V5Z 1M9; UBC'95; FRCPC; IntMed; Cardiol. Staff, Gordon & Leslie Diamond Health Care Centre; Dir Coronary Care Unit, Vancouver General Hospital - Centennial Pavillion; Clinical Asst Prof, University of British Columbia; Langs: Bilingual(English/French); (604)875-5735; Fax. (604)875-5736.

WONG, Grover; Elgin Med Centre, 101-2255 Elgin Ave, Port Coquitlam BC V3C 2B4; UBC'92; CCFP; (604)942-7292; Fax. (604)942-9698.

WONG, H C George; Fairmont Med Bldg, 1200-750 Broadway W, Vancouver BC V5Z 1J2; UBC'72; FAAAAI; FRCPC; IntMed (Alternative Medicine); ClinImmunol&Allergy. Ac Staff, Vancouver General Hospital - Centennial Pavillion; Member Medical Review Panel, Workers' Comp Board of BC; Clin Prof, University of British Columbia; Langs: Cantonese; Mandarin; (604)879-8491; Fax. (604)879-8438.

WONG, H H Adriana; Tsawwassen Fam Hlth Centre, 101-5461 12 Ave, Delta BC V4M 2B2; UBC'91; (604)943-3982; Fax. (604)943-8077.

WONG, Harley; Children's Hosp, AE 203-840 Sherbrook St, Winnipeg MB R3A 1S1; Man'80; FRCPC; Anes (Pediatric Anesthesia). Ac Staff Anes, Health Sciences Centre; Asst Prof Anes, University of Manitoba; (204)787-2560; Fax. (204)787-1560.

WONG, Harvey H; 6408 Main St, Vancouver BC V5W 2V4; UBC'81; CCFP; Vis Staff, Providence Health Care - St Paul's Hospital; Vis Staff, Vancouver General Hospital - Centennial Pavillion; Langs: Chinese; (604)322-8881; Fax. (604)322-8690.

WONG, Harvey H; Agincourt Pulmonary Services, 208-240 Alton Towers Cir, Scarborough ON M1V 4P3; McM'05; FRCPC; IntMed; Respir. Staff, St Michael's Hospital; (416)321-2613; Fax. (416)321-6844.

WONG, Helen H L; Markham Stouffville Hosp, PO Box 1800 381 Church St, Markham ON L3P 7P3; Qns'06; FRCPC; Peds. Staff, Markham Stouffville Hospital; (905)472-7000

WONG, Henry C H; 108-2051 McCallum Rd, Abbotsford BC V2S 3N5; UBC'04; FRCPC; IntMed; Nephrol. Langs: Cantonese; (604)870-9886

WONG, Henry D; Quibble Creek Consultants, 203-13798 94a Ave, Surrey BC V3V 1N1; UBC'86; ABIM; FRCPC; IntMed (Gastrointestinal Disorders); Gastroent. Ac Staff, Surrey Memorial Hospital; (604)951-9186; Fax. (604)584-4550; drhdwong@gmail.com.

WONG, Henry K H; 6483 Fraser St, Vancouver BC V5W 3A6; UBC'87; (604)324-4631; Fax. (604)273-9282.

WONG, Henry W F; Bridlewood Prof Centre, 203-3443 Finch Ave E, Scarborough ON M1W 2S1; Tor'79; Staff, The Scarborough Hospital - Birchmount Campus; Staff, The Scarborough Hospital - General Campus; Staff, Rouge Valley Health System - Centenary Health Centre Site; Langs: Chinese; (416)493-4424; Fax. (416)490-8180.

WONG, Herbert F; Valley Med Clinic, 335 Jubilee St, Duncan BC V9L 1W9; UBC'82; (250)748-8151

WONG, Herbert M; Sunnybrook Hlth Sciences Ctre, B621-2075 Bayview Ave, Toronto ON M4N 3M5; Tor'98; MSc; BSc; FRCSC; ObstGyn (Laparoscopic Surgery). Staff, Women's College Hospital; Staff, Sunnybrook Health Sciences Centre; Asst Prof ObstGyn, University of Toronto; (416)480-6780; Fax. (416)480-5159.

WONG, Hoa Leng; Kennedale Shopp Centre, 10-12981 50 St NW, Edmonton AB T5A 3P3; (Singapore)'70; MB BS; Langs: Chinese; (780)478-2710; Fax. (780)475-9804.

WONG, Hon-Wah; 123-8787 Woodbine Ave, Markham ON L3R 9S2; (Hong Kong)'75; Langs: Cantonese; (905)513-8795; Fax. (905)513-9497.

WONG, Howard L; Crest Med Clinic, 8695 10th Ave, Burnaby BC V3N 2S9; Wes'88; (604)525-3828; Fax. (604)525-3829.

WONG, Hubert M C; Rouge Valley HS-Centenary, 2867 Ellesmere Rd, Scarborough ON M1E 4B9; Qns'00; FRCPC; Peds; Nephrol. Staff, Rouge Valley Health System - Centenary Health Centre Site; (416)284-8131

WONG, Ian K Y; Brooke Radiology, 5791 No 3 Rd, Richmond BC V6X 2C9; UBC'03; FRCPC; DiagRad. Staff, Radiology Associates of Regina; (604)278-9151

WONG, Ivan F L; Family Health Centre, 3003 Danforth Ave, Toronto ON M4C 1M9; Tor'87; Langs: Cantonese; Mandarin; (416)694-4343; Fax. (416)694-4241.

WONG, Ivan H; Camp Hill Veteran's Mem Bldg, 2106-5655 Veteran's Memorial L, Halifax NS B3H 2E1; Dal'03; FRCSC; OrthSurg (Arthroscopic Shoulder & Hip). (902)473-7626; Fax. (902)425-3879.

WONG, J Szeman; University of Alberta Hosp, 2C2 WMC-8440 112 St NW, Edmonton AB T6G 2B7; (Hong Kong)'90; FRCSC; IntMed; Cardiol. Staff, University of Alberta Hospital; (780)407-7403; Fax. (780)407-6452.

WONG, Jackson Y W; Edmonton Clinic Health Academy, 529-11405 87 Ave NW, Edmonton AB T6G 1C9; (United Kingdom)'87; MB BS; DCH(UK); FHKAM; Staff, Stollery Children's Hospital; Staff Peds, Edmonton Clinic Health Academy; Asst Prof, University of Alberta; (780)248-5579

WONG, Jacqueline M S; Chesley Med Clinic, PO Box 389 33 2nd St SE, Chesley ON N0G 1L0; Qns'95; CCFP; (519)363-3220; Fax. (519)363-0385.

WONG, James M; Heritage Med Clinic, 950-3803 Calgary Trail NW, Edmonton AB T6J 5M8; Alb'87; CCFP; Langs: Chinese; (780)436-7240; Fax. (780)436-8142.

WONG, James W; Montfort Hosp, 713 Montreal Rd, Ottawa ON K1K 0T2; Ott'06; FRCSC; Urol. Staff, Montfort Hospital; (613)746-4621; Fax. (613)837-5781.

WONG, James Y K; 33 Collingwood St E PO Box 3386 Stn Main, Meaford ON N4L 1A5; Qns'82; Langs: Chinese; (519)538-4222

WONG, Jamie; Hop Maisonneuve-Rosemont, 5415 boul de l'Assomption, Montreal QC H1T 2M4; Boston(MA) (USA)'94; FRCSC; Ophth. Staff, Hopital Maisonneuve-Rosemont; (514)252-3400

WONG, Janice; Vancouver Gen Hosp, 855 12th Ave W, Vancouver BC V5Z 1M9; Tor'08; Staff, Vancouver General Hospital - Centennial Pavillion; (604)875-4111

WONG, Janice; Chinook Reg Hosp, 960 19 St S, Lethbridge AB T1J 1W5; Alb'90; CCFP; CCFP(E.M.); FCFP; Staff, Chinook Regional Hospital; (403)388-6301; Fax. (403)382-6183.

WONG, Janice-Lynn K; Providence HC-St Vincent's Hos, 4F-4650 Oak St, Vancouver BC V6H 4J4; Man'05; CCFP; Staff, Providence Health Care - St Vincent's Hospital-Brock Fahrni Site; Staff, Providence Health Care-Youville Residence; Staff, The Doctor's Office; (604)806-9716; jwong@bcmhs.bc.ca.

WONG, Jason H P; The Court Med Offices, 314-2863 Ellesmere Rd, Scarborough ON M1E 5E9; Qns'94; FRCSC; GenSurg (Advanced Laparoscopic Surgery). Ac Staff, Rouge Valley Health System - Centenary Health Centre Site; Langs: Cantonese; (416)287-8303; Fax. (416)287-3239.

WONG, Jason J; School of Population & Public, 2206 East Mall, Vancouver BC V6J 0A8; Alb'09; CCFP.

WONG, Jason K; Foothills Med Centre, 1403 29 St NW, Calgary AB T2N 2T9; Cal'99; FRCPC; DiagRad. Staff Radiol, Foothills Medical Centre; (403)944-1969; Fax. (403)944-1687.

WONG, Jason W T; Juravinski Cancer Centre, 699 Concession St, Hamilton ON L8V 5C2; McM'97; CCFP; Staff Privil, Hamilton Health Sciences Centre - Hamilton General Hospital; Staff privil, St Joseph's Healthcare - Charlton Campus; Staff, The Juravinski Cancer Centre; (905)387-9495 x64704

WONG, Jean; Univ Hlth Network-Toronto Western Hosp, 399 Bathurst St, Toronto ON M5T 2S8; Man'92; FRCPC; Anes. Staff, Toronto Western Hospital - University Health Network; (416)603-5118; Fax. (416)603-6494.

WONG, Jean M; Links Clinic Office, 104-11910 111 Ave NW, Edmonton AB T5G 3G6; Man'86; (780)454-0351

WONG, Jeanny; 4419 Hastings St, Burnaby BC V5C 2K1; UBC'88; BSc; Staff, Burnaby Hospital; Langs: Mandarin; Cantonese; (604)299-3457; Fax. (604)299-3492.

WONG, Jennifer Y Y; K-W Urgent Care Clinic, 385 Fairway Rd S, Kitchener ON N2C 2N9; Wes'00; CCFP; CCFP(E.M.); (519)748-2327

WONG, Jeremy C; 308-2347 Kennedy Rd, Scarborough ON M1T 3T8; Tor'79; BSc; FRCSC; ObstGyn (Infertility). Staff, North York General Hospital - Branson Division; University of Toronto; Langs: Mandarin; Cantonese; (416)609-3328; jc2001tor@yahoo.ca.

WONG, Jerome C Y; Langley Memorial Hosp, 22051 Fraser Hwy, Langley BC V3A 4H4; Alb'02; FRCPC; DiagRad. Staff, Langley Memorial Hospital; Langs: Cantonese; (604)534-4114

WONG, Jerry; The Doctors' Office, 600-1001 Broadway W, Vancouver BC V6H 4B1; Alb'73; (604)739-4247; Fax. (604)739-4244.

WONG, Jill M; Nova Scotia Rehab Centre, 1341 Summer St, Halifax NS B3H 4K4; Dal'99; FRCPC; IntMed; Rheum. Staff, Nova Scotia Rehabilitation Centre; (902)473-1288

WONG, John H Y; Foothills Med Centre, C1242B-1403 29 St NW, Calgary AB T2N 2T9; Alb'92; FRCSC; Neursurg (Cerebrovascular Surgery). Staff Clinical Neurosciences, Foothills Medical Centre; Asst Prof, University Of Calgary; (403)944-4550; Fax. (403)944-8712.

WONG, John W; Sunnybrook Hlth Sciences Ctre, E4 17-2075 Bayview Ave, Toronto ON M4N 3M5; Tor'85; DrMedCh; ABP; FRCPC; AnatPath (Cytopath). Staff, Women's College Hospital; Staff, Sunnybrook Health Sciences Centre; Langs: Cantonese; (416)480-4013

WONG, Jonathan K; St Boniface Gen Hosp, 409 Tache Ave, Winnipeg MB R2H 2A6; McM'07; FRCPC; IntMed. Staff Palliative Care Program, St Boniface General Hospital; (204)233-8563

WONG, Jonathan Y; High Street House, 311-933 17 Ave SW, Calgary AB T2T 5R6; Cal'05; FRCSC; Ophth. (403)245-3304; Fax. (403)245-9625.

WONG, Jorge A S; Foothills Med Centre, 1403 29 St NW, Calgary AB T2N 2T9; McM'06; FRCSC; IntMed; Cardiol. Staff Electrophysiology, Foothills Medical Centre; (403)944-3282

WONG, Joseph K; Credit Valley Prof Bldg, 401-2300 Eglinton Ave W, Mississauga ON L5M 2V8; Tor'81; ABPS; FRCSC; Otol (Head & Neck Surgery). Court Staff, William Osler Health System - Brampton Civic Hospital; Ac Staff, The Credit Valley Hospital; Court Staff, Trillium Health Centre - West Toronto; Langs: Cantonese; Mandarin; (905)820-8484; Fax. (905)820-7628.

WONG, Joseph P C; Ridge Meadows Hosp & HCC, 11666 Laity St, Maple Ridge BC V2X 5A3; (Hong Kong)'88; MB ChB; FRCPC; Anes. Staff, Ridge Meadows Hospital & Health Care Centre; Langs: Chinese; (604)463-1870

WONG, Joseph S; 301-3410 Sheppard Ave E, Scarborough ON M1T 3K4; Finch University of Health Sciences (USA)'86; FAB(PhysMed&Rehab); FRCPC; PhysMed&Rehab (Musculoskeletal Medicine). Langs: Chinese; (416)293-7333

WONG, Joseph Y K; 134-78 Saint Patrick St, Toronto ON M5T 3K8; Bronx(NY) (USA)'76; BEng; DSc; Langs: Chinese; (416)591-6837; Fax. (416)591-2325.

WONG, Joseph Y S; Toronto Pain & Stress Clinic, 312-1110 Sheppard Ave E, North York ON M2K 2W2; Canton (China)'55; FRCPC; PhysMed&Rehab (Pain Management). Med Dir, Toronto Pain & Stress Clinic; Langs: Cantonese; Mandarin; (416)512-6754; Fax. (416)512-1885; torontopainstress@yahoo.ca.

WONG, Joyce; Peter Lougheed Centre, 3601-3500 26 Ave NE, Calgary AB T1Y 6J4; Alb'82; FRCSC; GenSurg; VascSurg. Med Staff, Peter Lougheed Centre; Med Staff, Foothills Medical Centre; Consultant, Rockyview General Hospital; Asst Clin Prof, University of Calgary; Langs: Chinese; (403)943-5483; Fax. (403)291-2734.

WONG, Judy S Y; 3945 17 Ave SW, Calgary AB T3E 0C3; Alb'07; CCFP; (403)242-8633; Fax. (403)242-8884.

WONG, Justin K F; JJ399-700 William Ave, Winnipeg MB R3E 0Z3; UBC'99; FRCPC; IntMed; Critical Care Medicine. Staff, Health Sciences Centre; Langs: Cantonese; (204)787-3112

WONG, K Judy; Laurel Med Center, 215-888 8th Ave W, Vancouver BC V5Z 3Y1; Man'86; Langs: Mandarin; Cantonese; (604)872-0345

WONG, K S Rebecca; Univ Hlth Network-Princess M, 5-807-610 University Ave, Toronto ON M5G 2M9; Sheffield (England)'84; MB BS; MSc; FRCPC; RadOncol (Telehealth)., Princess Margaret Hospital - University Health Network; Assoc Prof RadOncol, University of Toronto; Langs: Chinese; (416)946-2126; Fax. (416)946-6561; rebecca.wong@rmp.uhn.on.ca.

WONG, K W Rose; 5591 West Boulevard, Vancouver BC V6M 3W6; (Other Foreign)'06; CCFP; (604)558-4633

WONG, Kan Shick; West End Prof Bldg, 201-9509 156 St NW, Edmonton AB T5P 4J5; (Taiwan)'61; PhD; FRCPC; Peds. Court Staff, University of Alberta Hospital; Ac Staff Peds, Covenant Health - Misericordia Community Hospital; Clin Assoc Prof, University of Alberta; Langs: Chinese; (780)489-3339; Fax. (780)483-8172.

WONG, Karen; Zeidler-Ledcor Centre, 130 University Campus NW, Edmonton AB T6G 2X8; Alb'02; FRCPC; IntMed; Gastroent. Staff, University of Alberta Hospital; (780)248-1674; Fax. (780)492-8121.

WONG, Karen; 250-5780 Cambie St, Vancouver BC V5Z 3A7; Alb'04; (604)696-1849

WONG, Karen; Women's College Hosp, 76 Grenville St, Toronto ON M5S 1B2; Alb'00; MD; CCFP; Staff, Women's College Hospital; (416)323-6060 x1; Fax. (416)323-6345.

WONG, Karen W; The Hosp For Sick Children, 5430-555 University Ave, Toronto ON M5G 1X8; Tor'06; FRCSC; PlasSurg. Staff, The Hospital For Sick Children; (416)813-6448

WONG, Kathleen S W; University of Alberta Hosp, 4B1 33-8440 112 St NW, Edmonton AB T6G 2B7; UBC'01; FRCPC; GenPath; HemPath. Staff, University of Alberta Hospital; (780)407-6052; Fax. (780)407-8599.

WONG, Kathleen W F; Scarborough North Med Arts, 207-4040 Finch Ave E, Scarborough ON M1S 4V5; Tor'81; Assoc Staff, The Scarborough Hospital - Birchmount Campus; Langs: Chinese; (416)754-2727; Fax. (416)754-2728.

WONG, Keet Peng; Associate Med Clinic, 2-8720 Franklin Ave, Fort McMurray AB T9H 3K8; Kuala Lumpur (Malaysia)'70; FACOG; ObstGyn. (780)743-8484; Fax. (780)743-9586.

WONG, Keith C K; Hillcrest Clinic, 7381 Hurd St, Mission BC V2V 3H8; UBC'77; MHSc; Clin Instructor Family Pract, University of British Columbia; Langs: Cantonese; (604)826-8345; Fax. (604)826-1930.

WONG, Keith F; Jane-Lessard Med Clinic, 1-727 Jane St, Toronto ON M6N 4B3; London (England)'62; (416)767-7017; Fax. (416)762-1118.

WONG, Keith H; University of Western Ontario, 1151 Richmond St, London ON N6A 5C1; Tor'09; CCFP; (519)661-2019; Fax. (519)850-2492.

WONG, Keith H; Scarborough Prof Centre, 312-1371 Neilson Rd, Scarborough ON M1B 4Z8; Tor'81; FRCPC; Gastroent; IntMed. Consultant, Rouge Valley Health System - Centenary Health Centre Site; Langs: Cantonese; (416)287-8107; Fax. (416)287-0079.

WONG, Kelly D; The Credit Valley Hosp, 2200 Eglinton Ave W, Mississauga ON L5M 2N1; Tor'95; FRCPC; DiagRad;CCFP; CCFP(E.M.); Court Staff, North York General Hospital; Assoc Staff, The Credit Valley Hospital; (905)813-2200; Fax. (905)813-3042.

WONG, Kenneth; Royal Columbian Hosp, 330 Columbia St E, New Westminster BC V3L 3W7; UBC'94; FRCPC; DiagRad. Staff, Royal Columbian Hospital; Staff, Medray Imaging; (604)520-4640; Fax. (604)520-4801.

WONG, Kenny K; IWK Health Centre, PO Box 9700 Rpo CSC 5850 University Ave, Halifax NS B3K 6R8; Alb'98; FRCPC; Peds (Pediatric Cardiology); Cardiol. Staff Ped Cardiol, IWK Health Centre; Asst Prof Peds, Dalhousie University; (902)470-6956; Fax. (902)470-6616.

WONG, Kevin H; Professional Place, 305-2901 Lawrence Ave E, Scarborough ON M1P 2T3; Tor'78; FRCSC; GenSurg (Surgical Oncology). Staff, The Scarborough Hospital - General Campus; Langs: Chinese; (416)264-4600; Fax. (416)264-0656.

WONG, Kevin K; Royal University Hosp, 103 Hospital Dr, Saskatoon SK S7N 0W8; Sask'05; FRCPC; Anes. Staff, Royal University Hospital; (306)655-1183

WONG, Kevin K M; 103-9815 97 St, Grande Prairie AB T8V 8B9; Alb'04; FRCSC; Otol (Head & Neck Surgery). Staff, Queen Elizabeth II Hospital; (780)513-2255; Fax. (780)513-2265.

WONG, Kim T S; Health Sciences North, 41 Ramsey Lake Rd, Sudbury ON P3E 5J1; Ott'06; FRCPC; Anes. Staff, Health Sciences North-Laurentian Site; (705)523-7100

WONG, Lai-Wah; 59-3888 Rupert St, Vancouver BC V5R 6E4; Tor'79; CCFP; Court Staff, Burnaby Hospital; Langs: Chinese; Cantonese; (604)434-2708

WONG, Lawrence H S; 209-4885 Kingsway, Burnaby BC V5H 4T2; Wes'01; FRCPC; IntMed; Cardiol. (604)568-6685

WONG, Leo K H; St Luke Family Practice, 5-5761 Glover Rd, Langley BC V3A 8M8; Qns'98; CCFP; FCFP; Staff, Langley Memorial Hospital; Langs: Cantonese; (604)530-5825; Fax. (604)530-5828.

WONG, Leo T M; Surrey Med Bldg, 200-9656 King George Hwy, Surrey BC V3T 2V5; Alb'88; CCFP; FCFP; Staff, Langley Memorial Hospital; Langs: Chinese; (604)581-4611; Fax. (604)581-2652.

WONG, Lillian; Ministry of Labour, 19F-505 University Ave, Toronto ON M7A 1T7; Tor'78; DIH; FRCPC; OccupMed;CCFP; Physician, Ministry of Labour; (416)326-7879; Fax. (416)326-2988.

WONG, Lillian; Richmond Health Sciences Ctre, 200-6091 Gilbert Rd, Richmond BC V7C 5L9; Wes'97; FRCSC; Otol (Head & Neck Surgery). Ac Staff, Vancouver General Hospital - Centennial Pavillion; Clin Instructor, University of British Columbia; Langs: Cantonese; (604)276-2336; Fax. (604)276-2396.

WONG, Linda Y; 404 Medical Clinic, 46-1111 Davis Dr, Newmarket ON L3Y 8X2; Wes'90; CCFP; FCFP; Staff, Southlake Regional Health Centre; (905)868-8330; Fax. (905)868-8332.

WONG, Lori-Ann; St Mary's Univ Health Services, 923 Robie St, Halifax NS B3H 3C3; Dal'97; BSc; CCFP; Teach Staff, St Mary's University; (902)420-5611; Fax. (902)496-8222; davela@gmail.com.

WONG, Louise L Y; All Med Health, 1-16880 Yonge St, Newmarket ON L3Y 0A3; (Other Foreign)'06; CCFP; (905)895-9777; Fax. (905)895-9720.

WONG, M F Agnes; The Hosp for Sick Children, 555 University Ave, Toronto ON M5G 1X8; McG'94; FRCSC; Ophth (Neuro Ophthalmology). Sr Scientist, The Hospital For Sick Children; Staff Ophth, Toronto Western Hospital - University Health Network; Langs: Cantonese; (416)813-7654 x2642; Fax. (416)813-5159.

WONG, Mandy; Lakeshore Vein & Aesthetics, 101-3293 Lakeshore Rd, Kelowna BC V1W 3S9; Alb'91; BMedSci; Physician, Lakeshore Vein & Aesthetics Clinic Inc; (250)868-9290; Fax. (250)868-9704; mandy@okanaganhealth.ca.

WONG, Marcus G; St Joseph's Health Centre, 30 The Queensway, Toronto ON M6R 1B5; Wes'93; FRCPC; Anes. Staff Anes, St Joseph's Health Centre; (416)530-6090; Fax. (416)530-6300.

WONG, Mark A; Thunder Bay Reg HSC, 980 Oliver Rd, Thunder Bay ON P7B 6V4; Qns'05; FRCPC; IntMed; Nephrol. Staff, Thunder Bay Regional Health Sciences Centre; (807)684-6000

WONG, Martin S; 821B 5 St SW, Medicine Hat AB T1A 4H7; Alb'76; CCFP; Med Staff, Medicine Hat Regional Hospital; (403)529-9252; Fax. (403)529-9662.

WONG, Mary M Y; Pine Seven Med Centre, 175-4600 Highway 7, Woodbridge ON L4L 4Y7; Tor'84; CCFP; Assoc Staff, Humber River Regional Hospital - Finch Avenue Site; Langs: Cantonese; (905)856-3611; Fax. (905)856-3612.

WONG, Matthew G; Abbotsfield Shoppers Mall, 214-3210 118 Ave NW, Edmonton AB T5W 4W1; Alb'01; CCFP; (780)471-2071; Fax. (780)474-8001.

WONG, Maxine Y W; Bayview North Dermatology Clin, 205-3292 Bayview Ave, North York ON M2M 4J5; Belfast (Ireland)'95; MRCP(UK); FRCSC; Derm. Staff, Toronto Western Hospital - University Health Network; Teach Staff, University of Toronto; Langs: Cantonese; Mandarin; (416)222-7546; Fax. (416)221-7546.

WONG, Michael D; Peter Lougheed Centre, 3500 26 Ave NE, Calgary AB T1Y 6J4; Alb'03; FRCPC; IntMed; Hem. Staff, Peter Lougheed Centre; (403)943-5425; Fax. (403)943-4017.

WONG, Michael; Children's & Women's HC of BC, 1Q72-4500 Oak St, Vancouver BC V6H 3N1; UBC'06; FRCPC; Anes. Staff, BC Women's Hospital & Health Centre; (604)875-2158

WONG, Michael T W; One Healthclubs Bldg, 205-2021 Cliff Rd, Mississauga ON L5A 3N7; Tor'93; CCFP; Staff Family Med, Trillium Health Centre - Mississauga; (905)276-0205; Fax. (905)276-8211.

WONG, Michelle P; Surrey Mem Hosp, 13750 96 Ave, Surrey BC V3V 1Z2; UBC'03; FRCPC; HemPath. Staff, Surrey Memorial Hospital; (604)581-2211

WONG, Mildred T W; The Richmond Hosp, 7000 Westminster Hwy, Richmond BC V6X 1A2; Tor'05; CCFP; CCFP(E.M.); Staff, Richmond Hospital; (604)278-9711

WONG, Milton J; 5525 West Boulevard PO Box 223, Vancouver BC V6M 3W6; UBC'63; FRCPC; Neur. Ac Staff, Providence Health Care - St Paul's Hospital; Clin Assoc Prof, University of British Columbia; Langs: Cantonese; (604)874-1141

WONG, Min Min C; Medical Clinic Bldg, 309-89 Humber College Blvd, Etobicoke ON M9V 4B8; Tor'82; FACP; ABIM; FRCPC; IntMed; Endocrin&Metab. (416)740-9663; Fax. (416)740-0827.

WONG, Monique L; Alan Cashmore Centre, 420-1669 Broadway E, Vancouver BC V5N 1V9; UBC'04; FRCPC; Psy. Staff, Richmond Hospital; Langs: Cantonese; (604)675-3996

WONG, Morley P; 1903 9 Ave S, Lethbridge AB T1J 1W8; Cal'93; BSc; FRCPC; IntMed; Nephrol. Staff Internist/Nephrol, Chinook Regional Hospital; (403)320-0633; Fax. (403)320-0353.

WONG, Natalie; St Michael's Hosp, 30 Bond St, Toronto ON M5B 1W8; Tor'98; FRCPC; IntMed; Critical Care Medicine. Staff, St Michael's Hospital; Langs: English; French; (416)864-5431

WONG, Nathan D; Halton HCS Corp-Milton, 7030 Derry Rd, Milton ON L9T 7H6; McM'04; CCFP; Staff, Halton Healthcare Services Corporation - Milton District Hospital; (905)878-2383

WONG, Nick N L; 10010 102A Ave NW, Edmonton AB T5J 0G5; Alb'99; CCFP; (780)422-1302; Fax. (780)427-0777.

WONG, Norman C W; HSC-Faculty of Med, 3330 Hospital Dr NW, Calgary AB T2N 4N1; Cal'80; BSc; MSc; FRCPC; IntMed (Diabetes). Prof Med, University Of Calgary; Langs: Chinese; Cantonese; (403)220-8867; Fax. (403)270-0979.

WONG, Norris A; 126 Kingsway Mall PO Box 34189 Rpo Kingsway, Edmonton AB T5G 3G4; Alb'00; CCFP; Langs: Cantonese; (780)497-5073; Fax. (780)497-5699.

WONG, On Yu; Finch-Midland Med Centre, 312-4190 Finch Ave E, Scarborough ON M1S 4T7; (Hong Kong)'75; MB BS; MRCP(UK); FHKAM(Med.); Court Staff, The Scarborough Hospital - Birchmount Campus; Court Staff Family Med, The Scarborough Hospital - General Campus; Langs: Chinese; (416)321-8302

WONG, Ophelia C Y; 201-9019 Bayview Ave, Richmond Hill ON L4B 3M6; Alb'89; Langs: Cantonese; (905)886-2829; Fax. (905)886-3597.

WONG, Patricia A; Six Points Plaza, 5230 Dundas St W, Etobicoke ON M9B 1A8; Dal'99; CCFP; (416)234-8668; Fax. (416)234-8720.

WONG, Patricia; 1910-8171 Ackroyd Rd, Richmond BC V6X 3K1; UBC'75; Langs: Mandarin; Cantonese; (604)273-5501

WONG, Patrick B Y; The Ottawa Hosp-Gen Campus, CCW 1401-501 Smyth Rd, Ottawa ON K1H 8L6; Qns'06; FRCPC; Anes. Staff, The Ottawa Hospital - General Campus; (613)737-8187; Fax. (613)737-8189.

WONG, Patrick G W; Rockyview Gen Hosp, 7007 14 St SW, Calgary AB T2V 1P9; Cal'87; CCFP; Staff, Rockyview General Hospital; (403)943-3597; Fax. (403)943-8411; wongpa@shaw.ca.

WONG, Patrick; Bay College Med Centre, C216-777 Bay St, Toronto ON M5G 2C8; Sask'10; CCFP; (416)977-8878; Fax. (416)977-0118.

WONG, Paul C H; Com El Med Bldg, 303-2620 Commercial Dr, Vancouver BC V5N 4C4; McG'74; BSc(Hon); MDCM; CCFP; FCFP; Ac Staff, Vancouver General Hospital - Centennial Pavillion; Assoc Staff, Providence Health Care - Mount Saint Joseph Hospital; Court Staff, BC Women's Hospital & Health Centre; Member Board of Director, Society of Clinical Preventive Health Care; Member Board of Directors, British Columbia College of Family Physicians; Member, Society of Obstetrics & Gynecologist of Canada; Clin Prof, University of British Columbia; Langs: Mandarin; French; Cantonese; (604)879-3320; Fax. (604)879-9522; pwong@doctor.com.

WONG, Paul K; PO Box 1385 Stn Main, Edmonton AB T5J 2N2; Alb'80.

WONG, Paul K C; KW 301-650 Sammon Ave, East York ON M4C 5M5; Tor'90; MSc; FRCSC; OrthSurg (Arthroscopy). Staff, Toronto East General Hospital Inc; Staff, One Medical Place Hosp; Lecturer, University of Toronto; Langs: Cantonese; (416)443-3308; Fax. (416)443-3236.

WONG, Peggy P C; BC Children's Hosp, A119-4480 Oak St, Vancouver BC V6H 3V4; Tor'01; FRCPC; Peds; PedHemaOncol. Staff, BC Children's Hospital; Langs: Cantonese; (604)875-2345

WONG, Peter D; Medical Office Bldg, 303-89 Humber College Blvd, Etobicoke ON M9V 4B8; University of West Indies (Jamaica)'82; MB BS; FAAP; MPH; FRCPC; Peds; Cardiol. Staff, William Osler Health System - Etobicoke General Hospital; Asst Prof Peds, University of Toronto; (416)743-6063; Fax. (416)743-0101.

WONG, Peter K H; PO Box 38003 Rpo King Edward M, Vancouver BC V5Z 4L9; McM'75; FRCPC; Neur (Electroencephalography). Dir EEG Dept, BC Children's Hospital; Prof, University of British Columbia; Langs: Cantonese; Mandarin; (604)875-2124; Fax. (604)875-2656.

WONG, Peter K K; 2-3033 Main St, Vancouver BC V5T 3G6; UBC'88; Assoc Staff, Vancouver General Hospital - Centennial Pavillion; Langs: Cantonese; (604)879-8311; Fax. (604)879-8119.

WONG, Peter N; Port Dover Med Centre, 807 St George St Box 1029, Port Dover ON N0A 1N0; Mem'75; BMedSci; Ac Staff, Norfolk General Hospital; Langs: Cantonese; (519)583-0894; Fax. (519)583-2814; peter.wong@reveraliving.com.

WONG, Philip E; Albany Med Clinic, 807 Broadview Ave, Toronto ON M4K 2P8; Tor'77; MD; Ac Staff Family Pract, Toronto East General Hospital Inc; (416)461-9471; Fax. (416)461-2710; pewmd@rogers.com.

WONG, Philip; MUHC-Royal Victoria Hosp, R2 28-687 av des Pins O, Montreal QC H3A 1A1; Sask'94; BScPharm; FRCPC; IntMed (Hepatology); Gastroent. Staff, McGill University Health Centre - Royal Victoria Hospital; Staff Teacher, McGill University; Langs: Bilingual(English/French); (514)934-1934 x31616; Fax. (514)843-1421.

WONG, Phoebus W C; Richmond Laser Skin Care, 2168-3779 Sexsmith Rd, Richmond BC V6X 3Z9; Dublin (Ireland)'89; MB ChB; BAO; Med Dir, Richmond Laser Skin Care & Wellness Centre; Langs: Chinese; (604)279-0081; Fax. (604)279-0031; doctor@drphoebuswong.com.

WONG, Rajalaximi; North Bay Reg Health Centre, 50 College Dr, North Bay ON P1B 0A4; Colombo (Sri Lanka)'79; FFARCSI; LRCP(Lond); MRCS(Eng); FRCPC; Anes. Staff Anes, North Bay Regional Health Centre - Regional Mental Health; Langs: Sinhalese; (705)474-8600

WONG, Ralph P W; St Boniface Gen Hosp, L1 102-409 Tache Ave, Winnipeg MB R2H 2A6; UBC'88; BSc; MD; FRCPC; IntMed; MedOncol. Staff Oncol Administration, St Boniface General Hospital; Asst Prof Med, University of Manitoba; (204)235-3141; Fax. (204)237-6048.

WONG, Rene; Grandin Med Clinic, 1 St Anne St, St. Albert AB T8N 2E8; Alb'80; BSc; CCFP; FCFP; Ac Staff, Sturgeon Community Hospital; (780)459-5581; Fax. (780)458-7515.

WONG, Rene; Univ Hlth Network-Toronto Gen, EN12 217-200 Elizabeth St, Toronto ON M5G 2C4; Dal'98; FRCPC; IntMed; Endocrin&Metab. Staff, Toronto General Hospital - UHN; (416)340-4053; Fax. (416)340-3314.

WONG, Richard L; Meadowbrook Lane Med Centre, 109-4591 Highway 7, Markham ON L3R 1M6; Cal'83; FRCPC; Peds (Developmental Pediatrics). Ac Staff, Markham Stouffville Hospital; Langs: Cantonese; Mandarin; (905)940-0112

WONG, Robert A; Port Credit Med Centre, 374 Lakeshore Rd E, Mississauga ON L5G 1H5; Cape Town (South Africa)'64; MB ChB; IntMed. (905)271-9000; Fax. (905)271-8889.

WONG, Robert M C; 135 Whitefield Dr NE, Calgary AB T1Y 5X1; Alb'95; CCFP; (403)590-9992; Fax. (403)590-9994.

WONG, Roger Y M; 7153-2775 Laurel Street, Vancouver BC V5Z 1M9; Alb'92; FACP; MD; BMedSci; FRCP; FRCPC; IntMed; GeriatricMed. Staff, Gordon & Leslie Diamond Health Care Centre; Staff Geriatric Med, Vancouver General Hospital - Centennial Pavillion; Langs: Cantonese; (604)875-4826; Fax. (604)875-5696.

WONG, Roland C K; LL-287 Spadina Ave, Toronto ON M5T 2E6; Man'82; MSc(Audiology); FRCPC; CommunMed (Occupational Medicine). Staff, St Michael's Hospital; Physician Occup Health, Occupational Clinics for Ontario Workers Inc; Langs: Cantonese; (416)506-8768; Fax. (416)506-8737; wong261@yahoo.com.

WONG, Ronald Y T; 105A-4909 17 Ave SE, Calgary AB T2A 0V5; McG'76; BSc; CCFP; FCFP; (403)272-9731

WONG, S M Simon; Westminster Med Bldg, 606-625 Fifth Ave, New Westminster BC V3M 1X4; UBC'93; FRCPC; Derm. (604)528-3961; Fax. (604)528-3962.

WONG, Sam Ken; Edmonton Clinic Health Academy, 3 520-11405 87 Ave NW, Edmonton AB T6G 1C9; Alb'96; MD; BSc; BEd; FRCPC; Peds. Staff, University of Alberta Hospital; Staff, Edmonton Clinic Health Academy; (780)248-5517; Fax. (780)248-5626.

WONG, Samuel C Y; Golden Mile Med Centre, 153-1880 Eglinton Ave E, Scarborough ON M1L 2L1; Qns'99; CCFP; (416)285-7575; Fax. (416)285-7574.

WONG, Samuel; Davis Drive Med Clinic, 7-291 Davis Dr, Newmarket ON L3Y 2N6; Tor'93; FRCPC; PhysMed&Rehab (Physiology). Ac Staff, Southlake Regional Health Centre; (905)898-5777; Fax. (905)898-7665.

WONG, Sarah H M; Medical Centre, 507-3030 Lawrence Ave E, Scarborough ON M1P 2T7; Cal'02; FRCSC; PlasSurg. (416)289-7100; Fax. (416)289-4256.

WONG, Shek-Leung; 13636 Grosvenor Rd, Surrey BC V3R 5C9; UBC'65; Vice Chief, Surrey Memorial Hospital; Langs: Cantonese; (604)584-6636; Fax. (604)582-8338.

WONG, Shun-Chi; Park Avenue Med Centre, 4F-4634 Park Ave, Terrace BC V8G 1V7; Man'73; Med Staff, Mills Memorial Hospital; Langs: Cantonese; (250)615-5040; Fax. (250)615-5049.

WONG, Sian E; South East Toronto FHT, 1871 Danforth Ave, Toronto ON M4C 1J3; Tor'00; CCFP; Staff, Toronto East General Hospital Inc; (416)699-7775; Fax. (416)699-7776.

WONG, Simon W C; S Wong Medical Inc, 10-1099 Kingsbury Ave, Winnipeg MB R2P 2P9; Tor'83; FRCSC; Urol. Med Staff, Seven Oaks General Hospital; (204)694-7882; Fax. (204)694-0716.

WONG, Simone N; William Osler HS-Brampton Civi, 2100 Bovaird Dr E, Brampton ON L6R 3J7; Tor'07; CCFP; CCFP(E.M.); Staff, William Osler Health System - Brampton Civic Hospital; (905)494-2120

WONG, Siu Hung; Gimli Community Health Centre, 120 6 Ave, Gimli MB R0C 1B0; (Other Foreign)'03.

WONG, Sophia S F; Sunnybrook Hlth Sciences Ctre, M2 200-2075 Bayview Ave, Toronto ON M4N 3M5; Ott'96; FRCPC; Anes. Staff, Sunnybrook Health Sciences Centre; Langs: Cantonese; (416)480-6100; Fax. (416)480-6039; sofan.wong@utoronto.ca.

WONG, Stan G; 13506 127 St NW, Edmonton AB T5L 1B9; Alb'86; CCFP; FCFP; (780)454-0738; Fax. (780)451-6702.

WONG, Stephanie W; 1-2810 Major Mackenzie Dr, Vaughan ON L6A 1R8; Wes'08; CCFP; (905)832-3838; Fax. (905)832-9097.

WONG, Stephen G; John Buhler Research Centre, 803G-715 McDermot Ave, Winnipeg MB R3E 3P4; Man'95; FRCPC; IntMed (Hepatology). Staff, Health Sciences Centre; Asst Prof Hepatology, University of Manitoba; (204)789-3658; Fax. (204)789-3987; s_wong@umanitoba.ca.

WONG, Stephen S; Professional Place, 405-2901 Lawrence Ave E, Scarborough ON M1P 2T3; Tor'69; Langs: Cantonese; Mandarin; (416)267-2444; Fax. (416)267-5586.

WONG, Steven; Crestwood Med & Dental Bldg, 205-6051 Gilbert Rd, Richmond BC V7C 3V3; Cal'94; FRCPC; IntMed (Cardiology). Staff, Richmond Hospital; Physician, Seymour Medical Clinic; Prog Dir Comm IntMed & Technologies in Med, University of British Columbia; (604)278-9116; Fax. (604)207-7757.

WONG, Sunny Y C; Mackenzie Richmond Hill Hosp, 10 Trench St, Richmond Hill ON L4C 4Z3; Tor'02; CCFP; Staff, Mackenzie Richmond Hill Hospital; Langs: Cantonese; (416)883-1212

WONG, Susan Y; Richmond Public Market, 2270-8260 Westminster Hwy, Richmond BC V6X 3Y2; Alb'97; CCFP; Langs: Cantonese; (604)821-1112; Fax. (604)821-1274.

WONG, Susanna S S; 210-3850 Finch Ave E, Scarborough ON M1T 3T6; Tor'85; Langs: Chinese; (416)293-9393

WONG, Suzanne T; St Joseph's Health Centre, 5E 114-30 The Queensway, Toronto ON M6R 1B5; Harvard(MA) (USA)'95; FABOG; FRCSC; ObstGyn. Assoc Staff, St Joseph's Health Centre; University of Toronto; (416)530-6790; Fax. (416)530-6811.

WONG, Sylvia; Oakridge Shopping Ctr, 360-650 41st Ave W, Vancouver BC V5Z 2M9; UBC'91; Staff, Oakridge Centre South Tower; Langs: Cantonese; (604)261-6000

WONG, Tat Hang; Riverdale Med Centre, 455 Carlaw Ave, Toronto ON M4K 3H9; Tor'89; Langs: Chinese; (416)462-3025; Fax. (416)462-0607.

WONG, Tat-Kwan; Grace Health Centre, 402-2830 Keele St, North York ON M3M 3E5; Tor'85; Court Staff, Humber River Regional Hospital - Finch Avenue Site; Langs: Cantonese; (416)633-7337; Fax. (416)633-7337.

WONG, Tat-Ying; Grace Med Centre, 402-2830 Keele St, North York ON M3M 3E5; Tor'85; Court Staff, Humber River Regional Hospital - Finch Avenue Site; Langs: Chinese; (416)633-7337; Fax. (416)633-7337.

WONG, Ted Yee T; 4132 Main St, Vancouver BC V5V 3P7; Edinburgh (England)'85; MB ChB; MRCGPract; CCFP; Langs: Cantonese; (604)876-8414; Fax. (604)876-1012.

WONG, Terry H; The Doctor's Office, 13-205 Marycroft Ave, Woodbridge ON L4L 5X8; Alb'95; CCFP; (905)856-2100; Fax. (905)856-2101.

WONG, Thomas S; Aberdeen Health Centre, 2180-4151 Hazelbridge Way, Richmond BC V6X 4J7; UBC'73; BSc; CCFP; FCFP; Court Staff, Surrey Memorial Hospital; Med Dir, Vancouver Chinese Diabetes Education Centre; Clin Assoc Prof Family Med, University of British Columbia; Langs: Cantonese; Mandarin; (604)233-0068; Fax. (604)233-0078.

WONG, Thomas; AL 0602C LCDC Bldg, 2391C-100 Eglantine Driveway, Ottawa ON K1A 0K9; McG'84; MPH; FRCPC; IntMed;CCFP; Physician, Health Canada; Aj Lecturer, University of Toronto; Aj Prof, University of Ottawa; Langs: English; French; (613)941-7539; Fax. (613)941-9813; tom_wong@hc-sc.gc.ca.

WONG, Thompson K W; 15-7010 Warden Ave, Markham ON L3R 5Y3; Tor'79; Court Staff Family Pract, Trillium Health Centre - West Toronto; Court Staff, Trillium Health Centre - Mississauga; Langs: Mandarin; Cantonese; (905)307-0084

WONG, Titus T T; 1119-899 12 Ave W, Vancouver BC V5Z 1M9; UBC'07; MedMicrobiol. Staff, Vancouver General Hospital - Centennial Pavillion; (604)875-8228

WONG, Tracy T Y; U of Ottawa Health Services, 300-100 Marie Curie Private, Ottawa ON K1N 6N5; Qns'08; CCFP; (613)564-3950

WONG, Tsing San; 506-1221 Algonquin Ave, North Bay ON P1B 4Y3; Colombo (Sri Lanka)'79; MB BS; MRC(UK); LRCP(Lond); MRCS(Eng); FRCSC; ObstGyn. Vis Staff, Temiskaming Hospital; Staff, North Bay Regional Health Centre - Regional Mental Health; Langs: Sinhalese; (705)495-2939; Fax. (705)495-1489.

WONG, Turnly; St Boniface Gen Hosp, C5116-409 Tache Ave, Winnipeg MB R2H 2A6; Man'84; BSc(Med.); ABIM; FRCPC; IntMed. Staff, St Boniface General Hospital; Assoc Prof, University of Manitoba; (204)237-2545; Fax. (204)233-7154.

WONG, Vanessa H; SGH Medical Mall, 507-3030 Lawrence Ave E, Scarborough ON M1P 2T7; Cal'05; FRCSC; PlasSurg. (416)289-3200; Fax. (416)289-3220.

WONG, Vanessa P; Peter Lougheed Centre, 3500 26 Ave NE, Calgary AB T1Y 6J4; Alb'94; FRCPC; Anes. Staff, Peter Lougheed Centre; (403)943-5554; Fax. (403)943-4474.

WONG, Victor C H; Winston Park Family Physicians, 104-2315 Bristol Cir, Oakville ON L6H 6P8; Ott'97; CCFP; FCFP; Langs: Cantonese; (905)829-2826; Fax. (905)829-2846.

WONG, Victor K; Richmond Health Science Ctre, 250-6091 Gilbert Rd, Richmond BC V7C 5L9; UBC'02; FRCPC; IntMed; Gastroent. Langs: Cantonese; (604)273-4447; Fax. (604)273-4254.

WONG, Vincent A; Fairmont Med Bldg, 802-750 Broadway W, Vancouver BC V5Z 1H7; Tor'95; FRCSC; Ophth (Oculo Plastic Surgery). Staff, Providence Health Care - Mount Saint Joseph Hospital; Staff, Delta Hospital; Clin Physician, Providence Health Care - St Paul's Hospital; Langs: Mandarin; Cantonese; (604)681-8963; Fax. (604)681-4963.

WONG, Vincent W; Health Sciences Centre, 1263-300 Prince Philip Dr, St. John's NL A1B 3V6; Mem'90; BSc(BioChem); BMedSci; Staff Human Resources Consulting Services, Health Sciences Centre; (709)777-3170; Fax. (709)777-6595.

WONG, Vivian K; Yonge-Eglinton Med Centre, 204-2401 Yonge St, Toronto ON M4P 3H1; Cal'00; BSc(PhysicalTherapy); CCFP; Langs: Cantonese; (416)485-2222; Fax. (416)485-2276.

WONG, W W Loretta; 409-3420 Finch Ave E, Scarborough ON M1W 2R6; Tor'82; Court Staff, The Scarborough Hospital - General Campus; Court Staff, The Scarborough Hospital - Birchmount Campus; Court Staff, Toronto General Hospital - UHN; Langs: Chinese; (416)502-8222; Fax. (416)502-8405.

WONG, Wai-Ben; Lions Gate Hosp, 231 15th St E, North Vancouver BC V7L 2L7; Qns'06; CCFP; CCFP(E.M.); Staff Emerg Med, Lions Gate Hospital; Langs: Bilingual(English/French); (604)984-5720

WONG, Wellington P; 201-726 Bloor St W, Toronto ON M6G 4A1; West Indies (Jamaica)'78; Court Staff Family Pract, Toronto General Hospital - UHN; (416)532-2211

WONG, Wilfred K K; 103-4235 Sheppard Ave E, Scarborough ON M1S 1T7; Tor'75; BEng; MASc; Court Staff, The Scarborough Hospital - Birchmount Campus; Court Staff, The Scarborough Hospital - General Campus; Langs: Chinese; (416)291-3366; Fax. (416)297-0058.

WONG, Wilfred T; Gain Med Centre, 1199 Austin Ave, Coquitlam BC V3K 3P4; UBC'73; Langs: Cantonese; (604)939-7345; Fax. (604)939-7781.

WONG, William H; 56 Grand Ave N, Cambridge ON N1S 2K9; Tor'79; BMath; Med Staff, Cambridge Memorial Hospital; Langs: Cantonese; (519)622-1577; Fax. (519)622-4606.

WONG, William K W; 6483 Fraser St, Vancouver BC V5W 3A6; UBC'73; Staff, Richmond Hospital; Langs: Chinese; (604)324-4631

WONG, Winnie T; Oak Ridges Med & Urgent Care, 100-13291 Yonge St, Richmond Hill ON L4E 4L6; Tor'03; CCFP; CCFP(E.M.); Staff, Medcan Health Management Inc; (905)773-7759

WONG, Winnie W S; Zeidler Ledcor Centre, 1-130 University Campus NW, Edmonton AB T6G 2X8; Man'89; FRCPC; IntMed (Gastrointestinal Disorders); Gastroent. Staff Gastroent., University of Alberta Hospital; Asst Prof, University of Alberta; Langs: Cantonese; (780)492-8134; Fax. (780)492-1600; wingshan@gpu.srv.ualberta.ca.

WONG, Winston P; Regional Mental HC-St Thomas, PO Box 2004 Stn Main 467 Sunset Dr, St Thomas ON N5P 3V9; Washington(DC) (USA)'70; Staff Psy, Regional Mental Health Care-St Joseph's Health Care; (519)631-8510; Fax. (519)631-2512; winston.wong@sjhc.london.on.ca.

WONG, Winston Y C; Scarborough Hosp-Gen Campus, 3050 Lawrence Ave E, Scarborough ON M1P 2V5; Tor'78; DABA; FRCPC; Anes. Ac Staff Anesthetist, St Joseph's Health Centre; Locum Tenens, Humber River Regional Hospital - Finch Avenue Site; Locum Tenens, Mackenzie Richmond Hill Hospital; Staff, The Scarborough Hospital - General Campus; (416)431-8133

WONG, Xing; Langley Mem Hosp, 22051 Fraser Hwy, Langley BC V3A 4H4; Mem'03; FRCPC; DiagRad. Staff, Langley Memorial Hospital; Langs: Cantonese; (604)534-4114

WONG ARMSTRONG, Susan; Alberta College of Phys & Surg, 370-10403 172 St NW, Edmonton AB T5S 1K9; Staff, College of Family Physicians of Canada-Alberta; (780)488-2395; Fax. (780)488-2396.

WONG-PACK, William K; St Joseph's Healthcare, 50 Charlton Ave E, Hamilton ON L8N 4A6; West Indies (Jamaica)'77; MB BS; AB; FRCPC; DiagRad; NuclearMed. Head Dept of NuclearMed, St Joseph's Healthcare - Charlton Campus; Staff, Women's College Hospital; Staff, Niagara Health System - Ontario Street Site; (905)522-4941; Fax. (905)521-6018.

WONG SHUE, Stephen G; York Prof Bldg, 209-679 Davis Dr, Newmarket ON L3Y 5G8; Tor'91; Dip SportMed; (905)830-1022; Fax. (905)830-1092.

WONG-TING, Joy J Y; 102-17770 56 Ave, Surrey BC V3S 1C7; (Singapore)'72; MB BS; DABPed; FAAP; (604)574-7883

WONG WONG KEET, Annick; CSSS du Suroit, 150 rue Saint-Thomas, Salaber-de-Valleyf QC J6T 6C1; Mon'07; MedOncol; IntMed. Staff, Centre Hospitalier Régional du Suroît; (450)371-9920 x2778

WONKO, Neil A; Royal University Hosp, 103 Hospital Dr, Saskatoon SK S7N 0W8; Sask'91; BSc(Adv); FRCPC; Peds (Neonatal & Perinatal Medicine). Staff Peds, Royal University Hospital; (306)966-8129; Fax. (306)975-3767.

WONNACOTT, J Brian; Kings County Med Centre, PO Box 1169, Montague PE C0A 1R0; Dal'72; BSc(Hon); (902)566-8030; Fax. (902)566-8890.

WONNACOTT, Matthew W T; Loyalist Plaza, 18 Manitou Cres W, Amherstview ON K7N 1S3; Wes'09; CCFP; (613)634-1813; Fax. (613)634-1253.

WOO, Allan K H; Saskatoon Ortho & Sports Med C, 104-311 Ludlow St, Saskatoon SK S7S 1N6; Sask'94; FRCSC; OrthSurg. (306)651-0800; Fax. (306)651-0801.

WOO, Andrea; Royal Alexandra Hosp, 10240 Kingsway NW, Edmonton AB T5H 3V9; UBC'03; CCFP; Staff, Royal Alexandra Hospital; (780)735-4777

WOO, Anna; Univ Hlth Network-Toronto Gen, 4N506-200 Elizabeth St, Toronto ON M5G 2C4; McG'92; MDCM; DABIM; FRCPC; IntMed; Cardiol. Staff, Toronto General Hospital - UHN; Assoc Prof Med, University of Toronto; Langs: English; French; (416)340-5270; Fax. (416)340-3959; anna.woo@uhn.on.ca.

WOO, Casey D; Woo Med Centre, 489 St Mary's Rd, Winnipeg MB R2M 3L1; Man'93; (204)254-2360; cwoo@shaw.ca.

WOO, Connie; Nanaimo Reg Gen Hosp, 1200 Dufferin Cres, Nanaimo BC V9S 2B7; Sask'87; Staff, Nanaimo Regional General Hospital; (250)754-2141

WOO, Daniel C; Valley Reg Hosp, 150 Exhibition St, Kentville NS B4N 5E3; Man'01; FRCPC; IntMed; Cardiol. Staff, Valley Regional Hospital; (902)678-1511; Fax. (902)679-1250.

WOO, Debbie; Hopital de Lachine, 650 16e av, Lachine QC H8S 3N5; McG'04; FRCSC; GenSurg. Staff, McGill University Health Centre - Royal Victoria Hospital; Staff, Centre Hospitalier de Lachine; (514)934-1934; debbie.woo@mail.mcgill.ca.

WOO, Dennis K; Market Village Total Health, PO Box 147 C13B-4392 Steeles Ave E, Markham ON L3R 9V8; Tor'89; Langs: Chinese; (905)477-7880; Fax. (905)477-4656.

WOO, Elaine K J; York-Med Medical Arts Centre, 212-250 Harding Blvd W, Richmond Hill ON L4C 9M7; Sask'89; FRCSC; Ophth (Glaucoma). Lecturer, University of Toronto; (905)883-0338; Fax. (905)883-6109.

WOO, Emile C; Seymour Med Clinic, 200-1530 7th Ave W, Vancouver BC V6J 1S3; UBC'97; FRCSC; GenSurg. Langs: Cantonese; Mandarin; (604)739-5615; Fax. (604)738-2132.

WOO, Francis C M; Humber Valley Med Centre, 6-2630 Kipling Ave, Etobicoke ON M9V 4B9; Tor'76; Ac Staff, William Osler Health System - Etobicoke General Hospital; Ac Staff, Humber River Regional Hospital - Church Street Site; Langs: Cantonese; (416)743-7424; Fax. (416)743-9923.

WOO, George H K; Rosedale Med Centre, 509-600 Sherbourne St, Toronto ON M4X 1W4; UBC'65; FACOG; FRCSC; ObstGyn (Infertility). Ac Staff, Toronto East General Hospital Inc; Langs: Cantonese; Chinese; Mandarin; (416)968-0414

WOO, Glenn M; Trillium Health Care Centre, 150 Sherway Dr, Etobicoke ON M9C 1A5; Man'87; AB; FRCPC; DiagRad. Staff, Trillium Health Centre - West Toronto; Staff, Six Points Radiology Association; (416)521-4047; glennw@allstream.net.

WOO, Henry L; Cross Roads Obst & Gyn, 330-507 Broadwa Ave W, Vancouver BC V5Z 1E6; Tor'91; FRCSC; ObstGyn (Urology). Staff ObstGyn, BC Women's Hospital & Health Centre; Staff ObstGyn, Vancouver General Hospital - Centennial Pavillion; Cross Roads Bladder Health Clinic; Instructor, University of British Columbia; Langs: Cantonese; (604)708-0788

WOO, James K H; Rouge Valley HS-Centenary, 2867 Ellesmere Rd, Scarborough ON M1E 4B9; Wes'05; FRCPC; DiagRad. Staff, Rouge Valley Health System - Centenary Health Centre Site; (416)284-8131

WOO, Joseph C H; St Joseph's Healthcare, 50 Charlton Ave E, Hamilton ON L8N 4A6; Glasgow (Scotland)'73; MB ChB; FRCPC; Anes (Chronic Pain Management). Staff, St Joseph's Healthcare - Charlton Campus; Staff, Hamilton Health Sciences Centre - McMaster University Medical Centre; Clin Assoc Prof Anes, McMaster University; Langs: Cantonese; (905)522-1155 x3853; Fax. (905)521-6019.

WOO, Kenny S; 2933 66 St NW, Edmonton AB T6K 4C1; Alb'75; FACC; FRCPC; Cardiol (Interventional Cardiology); IntMed. Staff, University of Alberta Hospital; Langs: Chinese; (780)485-6669; Fax. (780)485-6835.

WOO, Kin Yee; Hillcroft Med Centre, 6-5 Hillcroft Dr, Markham ON L3S 1R7; Tor'85; Langs: Chinese; (905)477-3232; Fax. (905)477-2782.

WOO, Lenny C Y; Royal Jubilee Hosp, 1952 Bay St, Victoria BC V8R 1J8; UBC'06; CCFP; Staff, Royal Jubilee Hospital; (250)370-8000

WOO, Michael Y; The Ottawa Hosp-Civic Campus, 1053 Carling Ave, Ottawa ON K1Y 4E9; Qns'98; CCFP; CCFP(E.M.); FCFP; Staff, The Ottawa Hospital - Civic Campus; Langs: English; French; (613)761-4621; Fax. (613)761-5088.

WOO, Minna N; 6 114-61 Queen St E, Toronto ON M5C 2T2; Tor'91; FRCPC; IntMed; Endocrin&Metab. Staff, St Michael's Hospital; Langs: Korean; French; (416)867-7424; Fax. (416)867-3696.

WOO, Nobby D; Woo Med Centre, 489 St Mary's Rd, Winnipeg MB R2M 3L1; Man'88; FACS; FRCSC; GenSurg. (204)953-1930; Fax. (204)953-1935.

WOO, Paul C Y; 10610 Bayview Ave, Richmond Hill ON L4C 3N8; Man'70; Ac Staff, Mackenzie Richmond Hill Hospital; Med Dir, Mon Sheong Richmond Hill Long Term Care; Langs: Fukinese; Cantonese; (905)884-4040; Fax. (905)884-2755.

WOO, Stanley K C; Southlake Reg Health Centre, 596 Davis Dr, Newmarket ON L3Y 2P9; Tor'63; FACS; Urol. Court Staff, Southlake Regional Health Centre; Langs: Chinese; (905)895-4521

WOO, Thomas Y; Southland Court Med Clinic, 150-10601 Southport Rd SW, Calgary AB T2W 3M6; Cal'80; FRCPC; Derm. (403)286-6888; Fax. (403)225-2914.

WOO, Tricia K W; St Peter's Hosp, 88 Maplewood Ave, Hamilton ON L8M 1W9; Tor'99; FRCPC; IntMed; GeriatricMed. Staff, Hamilton Health Sciences Centre - St Peter's Hospital; (905)777-3837 x12440; Fax. (905)526-2062.

WOO, Vincent C; Winnipeg Clinic, 425 St Mary Ave, Winnipeg MB R3C 0N2; Man'85; FRCPC; IntMed (Thyroid Diseases); Endocrin&Metab. Dept Head, Health Sciences Centre; University of Manitoba; (204)957-3218; Fax. (204)943-3516; vwoo@hsc.mb.ca.

WOO, Vincent L; Addiction & Mental Health, 4-1001 Queen St W, Toronto ON M6J 1H4; Tor'96; FRCPC; Psy (Psycho Geriatrics). Staff, Centre for Addiction & Mental Health (CAMH) - Queen Site; (416)535-8501 x3235; Fax. (416)583-1272; vincent_woo@camh.net.

WOO, Young-Chi; Royal Oak Med Centre, 103-6440 Royal Oak Ave, Burnaby BC V5H 3P2; McG'70; FRCSC; Urol (Stress Incontinence). Staff, Burnaby Hospital; Langs: Cantonese; Hokkin; (604)433-1823; Fax. (604)433-2612.

WOOD, Ashley; 101-55 Drury Cove Rd, Saint John NB E2H 2Z8; Mem'08; CCFP; Staff, Saint John Regional Hospital; (506)652-3900; Fax. (506)652-7976.

WOOD, Barbara L; Allin Clinic, 10155 120 St NW, Edmonton AB T5K 2A2; Alb'83; CCFP; FCFP; (780)482-7551; Fax. (780)488-2056.

WOOD, Carolyn E; Almonte Gen Hosp, 75 Spring St, Almonte ON K0A 1A0; Ott'04; Staff, Almonte General Hospital; (613)256-2500; Fax. (613)256-8549.

WOOD, Clare M P F; Lansdowne Prof Bldg, 160-1641 Hillside Ave, Victoria BC V8T 5G1; Pretoria (South Africa)'83; MB ChB; FFPsy; DCH; FRCPC; Psy. Langs: Afrikaans; (250)592-3221; Fax. (250)592-3021.

WOOD, Daniel R; Peter Lougheed Centre, 3500 26 Ave NE, Calgary AB T1Y 6J4; Alb'97; FRCPC; Anes;CCFP; FCFP; Staff, Peter Lougheed Centre; (403)943-5554

WOOD, David A; Gordon & Leslie Diamond HCC, L9-2775 Laurel St, Vancouver BC V5Z 1M9; UBC'01; FRCPC; IntMed; Cardiol. Staff, Gordon & Leslie Diamond Health Care Centre; Staff, Vancouver General Hospital - Centennial Pavillion; (604)875-5601

WOOD, David A; Thunder Bay Reg HSC-T-Bay, 980 Oliver Rd, Thunder Bay ON P7B 6V4; Tor'95; MSc(Physiol.); CCFP; CCFP(E.M.); FCFP; Staff, Thunder Bay Regional Health Sciences Centre; (807)684-6000; Fax. (807)684-5828.

WOOD, David C; 1600 Edward St, Halifax NS B3H 3J1; Dal'86; Staff Teacher, Dalhousie University; (902)429-0023; Fax. (902)422-8109.

WOOD, Douglas S; Summit Med Clinic, 4-1380 Summit Dr, Kamloops BC V2C 1T8; UBC'91; (250)374-9800; Fax. (250)374-9876; dswood57@telus.net.

WOOD, Ellen P; IWK Health Centre, PO Box 9700 Rpo CSC K 127-5980 University Ave, Halifax NS B3K 6R8; Dal'80; MSc; FRCP; FRCPC; Peds (Pediatric Neurology); Neur. Staff, IWK Health Centre; Assoc Prof, Dalhousie University; (902)470-8477; Fax. (902)470-8486; ewood@dal.ca.

WOOD, Evan G R; BC Ctr for Excellence in HIV/A, 1081 Burrard St, Vancouver BC V6Z 1Y6; Cal'07; FRCPC; IntMed. Staff, Urban Health Research Initiative; (604)682-2344 x66373

WOOD, Gavin C A; Kingston Gen Hosp, 76 Stuart St, Kingston ON K7L 2V7; Aberdeen (Scotland)'95; OrthSurg. Staff, Kingston General Hospital; (613)549-6666

WOOD, George O; Alberta Health Services, Misericordia Hospital 1N95-16940 87 Ave NW, Edmonton AB T5R 4H5; Alb'83; CRCP; FRCPC; AnatPath; GenPath. Staff, Covenant Health - Misericordia Community Hospital; (780)735-2776; Fax. (780)735-2870; george.wood@albertahealthservices.ca.

WOOD, Gordon G; Victoria Gen Hosp, 1 Hospital Way, Victoria BC V8Z 6R5; Qns'82; FRCPC; Anes; Critical Care Medicine. Staff Anes, Victoria General Hospital; (250)727-4212; gordonwood@hotmail.com.

WOOD, Jeremy R; Queen Elizabeth II HSC-Halifax, 2272-1796 Summer St, Halifax NS B3H 3A7; Dal'80; FRCSC; GenSurg (Vascular Surgery); Cardiovasc&ThorSurg. Staff, Queen Elizabeth II Health Sciences Centre - Victoria General Site; (902)473-2356; Fax. (902)473-4448.

WOOD, John C; Medical Clinic, PO Box 730 Stn Main, Salmon Arm BC V1E 4N8; Glasgow (Scotland)'74; MB ChB; DRCOG; Ac Staff, Shuswap Lake General Hospital; (250)832-6092; Fax. (250)832-5235; johnwood@sunwave.net.

WOOD, Laura J; Sheldon M Shumir Health Centre, 1213 4 St SW, Calgary AB T2R 0X7; Alb'10; CCFP; (403)955-9300

WOOD, Leanne J; 101-250 Dogwood St, Campbell River BC V9W 2X9; UBC'05; GenSurg. (250)850-1104

WOOD, Lori A; Queen Elizabeth II HSC, 1276 South Park St, Halifax NS B3H 2Y9; Qns'92; MSc; FRCPC; IntMed (Genito Urinary Tumors); MedOncol. Staff, Queen Elizabeth II Health Sciences Centre - Victoria General Site; Prof Urology Med, Dalhousie University; (902)473-6106; Fax. (902)473-6186.

WOOD, Lorraine E; The Temmy Latner Centre, 4F-60 Murray St, Toronto ON M5T 3L9; McM'79; CCFP; (416)586-4800 x7884; Fax. (416)586-4804.

WOOD, M Lesley; Park Royal Med Clinic, 560-580 Park Royal N, West Vancouver BC V7T 1H9; UBC'92; Staff, Park Royal Medical Clinic; (604)922-7391

WOOD, Marnie J; Nova Scotia Med Examiner Serv, 51 Garland Ave, Dartmouth NS B3B 0J2; Dal'02; DABPath; FRCPC; AnatPath (Forensic Pathology). Med Examiner, Nova Scotia Medical Examiner Services; Asst Prof Path, Dalhousie University; (902)424-2722; Fax. (902)424-0607.

WOOD, Michael R; 205-5359 Dundas St W, Toronto ON M9B 1B1; London (England)'69; MB BS; FRCS; FRCSC; OrthSurg (Hip & Knee Replacement). Ac Staff, St Joseph's Health Centre; University of Toronto; (416)763-1187; Fax. (416)763-7259.

WOOD, Nancy L; Medical Arts Bldg North Wing, 307-121 Wellington St W, Barrie ON L4N 1L2; Mem'90; CCFP; FCFP; Ac Staff Family Med, Royal Victoria Regional Health Centre; (705)726-1555; Fax. (705)726-0094.

WOOD, Stephen L; Foothills Med Centre, NT 403-1403 29 St NW, Calgary AB T2N 2T9; Qns'90; FRCSC; ObstGyn (Prenatal Care). Staff Obst.Gyn., Foothills Medical Centre; Assoc Prof, University of Calgary; (403)670-2017; Fax. (403)270-4249.

WOOD, Stuart J; Medical Associate Support Cred, 2F-333 Lakeshore Rd W, Mississauga ON L5H 1G9; Tor'82; CCFP; Ac Staff, Trillium Health Centre - Mississauga; Ac Staff, The Credit Valley Hospital; (905)274-7044; Fax. (905)274-0227.

WOOD, Tanya D; Boiestown Health Services, 2-6154 Route 8, Boiestown NB E6A 1M4; Dal'92; CCFP; (506)369-2700; Fax. (506)369-2702.

WOOD, Teresa M B; 37896 3rd Ave, Squamish BC V8B 0R2; UBC'06; CCFP; Langs: Bilingual(English/French); (778)861-1545

WOOD, Victor M; Royal Jubilee Hosp, 1952 Bay St, Victoria BC V8R 1J8; Man'71; FRCPC; EmergMed. Staff, Royal Jubilee Hospital; (250)370-8212

WOOD JR., William C; Lacewood Med Centre, 200-366 Lacewood Dr, Bedford NS B4A 1H5; Mem'76; DABPN; DAB; BMedSci; FRANZCP; FRCPC; Psy (Adult General Psychiatry). Staff Mental Health Prog, South Shore Regional Hospital; Staff, Capital Health District Authority; (902)445-9400

WOODALL, Robert J; Windsor Reg Hosp-Metropolitan, 1995 Lens Ave, Windsor ON N8W 1L9; Tor'96; CCFP; CCFP(E.M.); Staff, Windsor Regional Hospital - Metropolitan Site; (519)254-1661

WOODARD, Aaron F; Preventous Collaborative Healt, 1635 17 Ave SW, Calgary AB T2T 0E5; Sask'94; CCFP; Physician, Sheldon M Chumir Urgent Care Physician Group; (403)229-0129; Fax. (403)398-0193; aaron.woodard@albertahealthservices.ca.

WOODBURN, Bruce D; Trail Bay Med Clinic, PO Box 1760, Sechelt BC V0N 3A0; UBC'80; FRCSC; Ophth. (604)885-5885; Fax. (604)885-5193.

WOODBURN, D Layne; Feltham Medical, 103-1660 Feltham Rd, Victoria BC V8N 2A1; UBC'90; BSc; Staff, Vancouver Island Health Authority; Clin Instructor Family Med, University of British Columbia; (250)477-1858; Fax. (250)477-7580.

WOODBURY-SMITH, Marc R; Hamilton HS-General Division, PO Box 2000 Stn Lcd 1 457-1200 Main St W, Hamilton ON L8N 3Z5; Dundee (Scotland)'93; Staff, Hamilton Health Sciences Centre - McMaster University Medical Centre; (905)521-2100; Fax. (905)387-7714.

WOODEND, Dianne M; Family First Family Health Team, 4270 Innes Dr, Orleans ON K4A 5E6; Ott'06; CCFP; (613)841-7009; Fax. (613)841-0106.

WOODER, E Jeffrey; 203-5325 Cordova Bay Rd, Victoria BC V8Y 2L3; Tor'81; FRCPC; Psy. (250)595-1930

WOODER, Scott D; Health Sciences Bldg, 311-15 Mountain Ave S, Stoney Creek ON L8G 2V6; Tor'85; Asst Prof Family Med, McMaster University; (905)662-4911; Fax. (905)666-1688.

WOODFIELD, Wendy A; Fairmont Med Bldg, 713-750 Broadway W, Vancouver BC V5Z 1H6; Dal'89; Staff Privil, Vancouver General Hospital - Centennial Pavillion; Teach Staff Family Med, University of British Columbia; (604)873-4808; Fax. (604)876-7622.

WOODFORD, Elizabeth S; Western Student Health Service, 11-1151 Richmond St, London ON N6A 3K7; Ott'90; CCFP; (519)661-3030; Fax. (519)661-3380.

WOODFORD, Timothy J; 255 Main St PO Box 1720 Stn Main, Liverpool NS B0T 1K0; Dal'84; (902)354-5727; Fax. (902)354-5875.

WOODHAM, Jeremy D; St Paul's Hosp, 2600-1081 Burrard St, Vancouver BC V6Z 1Y6; Manchester (England)'71; MB ChB; FRCS(England); FRCSC; Otol (Sino Nasal). Staff Eye Ear Nose & Throat Clinic/Prof, Providence Health Care - St Paul's Hospital; Physician, Sea to Sky Walk Clinic; Physician, Whistler Health Care Centre; Staff, Dr Jane Bishop's Medical Office; Clin Prof Surg, University of British Columbia; (604)806-8353; Fax. (604)806-8447; fsahib@providencehealth.bc.ca.

WOODHEAD, Robin V; Delta Health Sciences Centre, 206-4515 Harvest Dr, Delta BC V4K 4L1; UBC'93; FRCSC; GenSurg (Laparoscopic Surgery). Staff, Delta Hospital; Physician, Delta Health Sciences Centre; (604)946-6500; Fax. (604)946-8449; robinw@dccnet.com.

WOODHOUSE, Douglas D; Parry Sound Family Health Team, 15 James St, Parry Sound ON P2A 1T4; Qns'05; CCFP; (705)746-9382

WOODHOUSE, I Dorothy; St Paul's Hosp, 1081 Burrard St, Vancouver BC V6Z 1Y6; Dal'70; FRCPC; Anes (Cardiovascular Anesthesia). Staff, Providence Health Care - St Paul's Hospital; Clin Instructor, University of British Columbia; (604)682-2344

WOODHOUSE, Richard T; Parry Sound Family Health Team, 15 James St, Parry Sound ON P2A 1T4; Birmingham (England)'71; MB ChB; Staff Family Med, West Parry Sound Health Centre; (705)746-9382; Fax. (705)746-7758.

WOODLAND, James P; Beamsville Med Ctr Fam Hlth Team, PO Box 430 4279 Hixon St, Beamsville ON L0R 1B0; Wes'99; CCFP; (905)563-5315; Fax. (905)563-0933.

WOODLAND, K Heather; Major's Path Family Practice, 301-35 Major's Path, St. John's NL A1A 4Z9; Mem'77; CCFP; FCFP; Assoc Staff, St Clare's Mercy Hospital; (709)579-2324; Fax. (709)579-3419.

WOODLAND, Robert C; Major's Path Family Practice, 301-35 Major's Path, St. John's NL A1A 4Z9; Mem'77; CCFP; FCFP; (709)579-2324; Fax. (709)579-3419.

WOODLEY, David G; 1-108 Valhalla Rd, Salt Spring Island BC V8K 2V1; UBC'87; (250)537-4811; Fax. (250)537-1610.

WOODMAN, Grant M J; St Clare's Mercy Hosp, 154 Lemarchant Rd, St. John's NL A1C 5B8; Saba (Netherlands)'11; Clin Associate, Health Sciences Centre; Clin Associate, St Clare's Mercy Hospital; (709)777-5000

WOODROW, Adrian R; Nymark Med Centre, 4839 Leslie St, North York ON M2J 2K8; Cal'82; (416)498-3600; Fax. (416)498-1211.

WOODRUFF, Brian G; Dufferin Orthopaedic Clinic, 1135 Dufferin Cres, Nanaimo BC V9S 2B5; Dundee (Scotland)'67; OrthSurg. Ac Staff, Nanaimo Regional General Hospital; (250)754-3727; Fax. (250)754-1447.

WOODRUFF, Christopher; Centre Hosp de LaSalle, 8585 tsse Champlain, LaSalle QC H8P 1C1; UBC'05; FRCPC; Anes. Staff, Centre Hospitalier de LaSalle; Staff, McGill University Health Centre - Royal Victoria Hospital; (514)362-8000

WOODRUFF, Jerry L; Medical Clinic, PO Box 870, Bow Island AB T0K 0G0; Alb'74; Chief Family Med, Bow Island Health Centre; Langs: English; French; (403)545-2244; Fax. (403)545-2099.

WOODS, Anna K; 3326 Assiniboine Ave, Winnipeg MB R3K 0B1; Belfast (Ireland)'72; FRCPC; Psy (Family Therapy). Langs: Finnish; (204)885-5152; Fax. (204)888-0231.

WOODS, Anne; St Joseph's Healthcare, 50 Charlton Ave E, Hamilton ON L8N 4A6; McM'92; CCFP; FCFP; Staff, St Joseph's Healthcare - Charlton Campus; (905)522-1155 x33529; Fax. (905)521-6108.

WOODS, Anthony C; Lakeridge Hlth Corp-Oshawa Sit, 1 Hospital Dr, Oshawa ON L1G 2B9; Dal'96; FRCPC; IntMed; Hem. Staff, Lakeridge Health - Oshawa Site; (905)576-8711; Fax. (905)721-4741.

WOODS, Brenda T; Don Valley Med Centre, 406-855 Broadview Ave, Toronto ON M4K 3Z1; McG'78; MDCM; FACOG; LMCC; FRCSC; ObstGyn (Colposcopy). Staff ObstGyn, Toronto East General Hospital Inc; Asst Prof Obst/Gyn, University of Toronto; Langs: Yiddish; French; (416)462-9918; Fax. (416)462-3516.

WOODS, Curtis J; Forensic Assessment Services, 26F-10004 104 Ave NW, Edmonton AB T5J 0K1; Alb'97; BSc; FRCPC; Psy (Forensic Psychiatry). Staff Forensic Assessment and Community Services, Alberta Mental Health Board; Staff, Forensic Assesstment & Community Services; (780)342-6400; Fax. (780)426-7272; woods@telusplanet.net.

WOODS, David M; St Joseph's Healthcare, 50 Charlton Ave E, Hamilton ON L8N 4A6; McM'77; FRCPC; DiagRad. Staff, St Joseph's Healthcare - Charlton Campus; (905)521-6009; Fax. (905)521-6116.

WOODS, Donald B; Village Square Mall, 124-2 Poyntz St, Penetanguishene ON L9M 1M2; Qns'73; (705)549-8270; Fax. (705)549-8554.

WOODS, Edward F A; Quinte Health Care, 3-393 Sidney St, Belleville ON K8P 3Z9; Tor'82; FRCSC; Urol (Cancer Options & Management). Staff, Quinte Health Care; (613)967-9797; Fax. (613)967-0525.

WOODS, Eric R; Yarmouth Reg Hosp, 60 Vancouver St, Yarmouth NS B5A 2P5; Dal'84; FRCPC; DiagRad. Staff, Yarmouth Regional Hospital; (902)742-3541; Fax. (902)742-5199.

WOODS, Erin L; Saskatoon Pediatric Consultant, 301A-39 23rd St E, Saskatoon SK S7K 0H6; UBC'03; FRCPC; Peds. (306)653-7741; Fax. (306)653-7743.

WOODS, Georgia J; 2828 Nanaimo St, Victoria BC V8T 4W9; McM'87; CCFP; FCFP; (250)953-3966

WOODS, Ian B; Northside Med Group, 210-1465 Salisbury Ave, Port Coquitlam BC V3B 6J3; UBC'76; Member Med Exec, Royal Columbian Hospital; (604)941-8277; Fax. (604)941-5622.

WOODS, John F; MUHC-Montreal Neurology Inst, 3801 rue University, Montreal QC H3A 2B4; Dublin (Ireland)'61; MB ChB; BAO; MSc(NeuroPhysiol); FRCPC; Neur; Electroenceph (P.Q.). assoc Staff, McGill University Health Centre - Montreal Neurological Hospital; (514)398-8551; Fax. (514)398-2745; ivanwoods@hotmail.com.

WOODS, Kathleen; Oromocto Prof Bldg, 242-66 Broad Rd, Oromocto NB E2V 1C2; McM'00; BScN; CCFP; (506)357-8720; Fax. (506)357-7898; drwoodsoffice@gmail.com.

WOODS, Lauren J; 269 King St W, Dundas ON L9H 1W2; McM'80; CCFP; (905)628-6042; Fax. (905)627-3058.

WOODS, Margaret E C; Thunder Bay Med Centre, 470-63 Algoma St N, Thunder Bay ON P7A 4Z6; McM'81; CCFP; FCFP; (807)344-8475; Fax. (807)344-6323.

WOODS, Murray C; Valley Med Clinic, 335 Jubilee St, Duncan BC V9L 1W9; UBC'87; Med Staff Assoc, Cowichan District Hospital; (250)748-8151; Fax. (250)748-8157.

WOODS, Nancy G; Timmins Family Health Team, 250-123 Third Ave, Timmins ON P4N 1C6; Tor'85; MSc; BA; BPHE; CCFP; FCFP; Site Dir Timmins Family Practice Residency, Northern Ontario School of Medicine; (705)264-1313; Fax. (705)268-7444.

WOODS, Philippe; CSSS du Sud de Lanaudière, 911 montee des Pionniers, Terrebonne QC J6V 2H2; Mon'00; Critical Care Medicine; IntMed. Staff, Centre Hospitalier Pierre le Gardeur; (450)654-7525; Fax. (450)470-2640.

WOODS, Robert A; Royal University Hosp, 2689-103 Hospital Dr, Saskatoon SK S7N 0W8; Sask'02; FRCPC; EmergMed. Staff Emerg Dept, Royal University Hospital; (306)655-1559; Fax. (306)955-3241.

WOODS, Sandra G B; CSSS de la Vallée de l'Or, 725 6e rue, Val-d'Or QC J9P 3Y1; Dublin (Ireland)'76; MB ChB; BAO; FAAP; FRCPC; Peds. Staff, McGill University Health Centre - Montreal Children's Hospital; Consultant Dept of Peds, Centre Hospitalier de Val d'Or; adj Prof, McGill University; Langs: French; Irish; (819)825-6711; Fax. (819)825-5624.

WOODS, Si-Ann H L; The Ottawa Hosp-Civic Campus, A6-1053 Carling Ave, Ottawa ON K1Y 4E9; UBC'98; FRCPC; Psy. Staff, The Ottawa Hospital - Civic Campus; (613)761-4581; Fax. (613)761-5328.

WOODS, Terence C H; Deep River & Dist Hosp, RR 1 117 Banting Dr, Deep River ON K0J 1P0; Dal'06; CCFP; Staff, Deep River & District Hospital; Langs: German; French; (613)584-3333

WOODS, Thomas C H; 1729B Comox Ave, Comox BC V9M 3M2; McM'03; FRCSC; OrthSurg. (250)941-0080

WOODSIDE, D Blake; Univ Hlth Network-Toronto Gen, 8EN 219-200 Elizabeth St, Toronto ON M5G 2C4; Qns'82; FRCPC; Psy (Eating Disorders). Staff, Toronto General Hospital - UHN; Prof Psy, University of Toronto; Langs: English; French; (416)340-4445; Fax. (416)340-4198; b.woodside@utoronto.ca.

WOODSIDE, Scott M; Addiction & Mental Hlth-Queen, 1001 Queen St W, Toronto ON M6J 1H4; McM'92; LLL; FRCPC; Psy (Forensic Psychiatry). Staff Assessment & Triage Unit, Centre for Addiction & Mental Health (CAMH) - Queen Site; Staff, Centre for Addiction & Mental Health (CAMH) - College Street Site; University of Toronto; (416)535-8501; Fax. (416)583-4327.

WOODWARD, Brian J; The Medical Assoc Clinic, 806 Vernon St, Nelson BC V1L 4G5; UBC'96; CCFP; Coord Continuing Med Educ, Kootenay Lake General Hospital; (604)352-6611; Fax. (604)352-6624.

WOODWARD, Kevin S; Charlton Med Centre, 300-25 Charlton Ave E, Hamilton ON L8N 1Y2; McM'04; FRCPC; IntMed; InfectDis. Staff, Hamilton Health Sciences Centre - McMaster Children's Hospital; (905)522-1155; Fax. (905)523-7352.

WOODWARD, Larry E; 39 King St E, Powassan ON P0H 1Z0; Man'80; (705)724-1020; Fax. (705)724-5499.

WOODWARD, Peter S; Northumberland Hills Hosp, 1000 Depalma Dr, Cobourg ON K9A 5W6; Tor'86; Staff, Northumberland Hills Hospital; (905)372-6811

WOODWARD, Roger D; Northumberland Hills Hosp, 1000 Depalma Dr, Cobourg ON K9A 5W6; Tor'96; CCFP; FCFP; Staff, Northumberland Hills Hospital; (905)372-6811

WOOFF, Jill C; Pasqua Hosp, 4101 Dewdney Ave, Regina SK S4T 1A5; Sask'06; FRCPC; AnatPath. Staff, Pasqua Hospital; (306)766-2222

WOOGH, Carolyn M; Kingston Gen Hosp, 76 Stuart St, Kingston ON K7L 2V7; Qns'71; MSc; FRCPC; Psy. Att Staff, Kingston General Hospital; Att Staff, Hotel-Dieu Hospital; Assoc Prof Psy, Queen's University; (613)544-3310; Fax. (613)544-9666; wooghc@post.queensu.ca.

WOOLF, Robert J; 2-564 South Railway St SE, Medicine Hat AB T1A 2V6; Sask'85; CCFP; CCFP(E.M.); FCFP; (403)526-1721; Fax. (403)504-4577.

WOOLFENDEN, Andrew R; Laurel Med Centre Ltd, 208-888 8th Ave W, Vancouver BC V5Z 3Y1; Alb'91; FRCPC; Neur. (604)879-4725; Fax. (604)879-0122.

WOOLFORD, Bernard J; Scarborough Prof Centre, 315-1371 Neilson Rd, Scarborough ON M1B 4Z8; London (England)'61; MB BS; MRCS; LRCP; DCH; FRCSC; OrthSurg (Low Back Pain). Ac Staff, Rouge Valley Health System - Centenary Health Centre Site; Vis Consultant, Rouge Valley Health System - Ajax & Pickering Health Centre Site; (416)282-1507; Fax. (416)282-8064.

WOOLFORD, Bonnie L; Park Royal Village Med Clinic, J2-925 Main St, West Vancouver BC V7T 2Z3; Man'01; CCFP.

WOOLFORD, Lorraine; The Credit Valley Hosp, 2200 Eglinton Ave W, Mississauga ON L5M 2N1; McM'76; MSc; FRCSC; ObstGyn. Staff, The Credit Valley Hospital; Langs: Bilingual(English/French); (905)813-2200

WOOLFREY, Jody A M; Dr Hugh Twomey Health Care Ctr, PO Box 250 25 Twomey Dr, Botwood NL A0H 1E0; Mem'95; CCFP; FCFP; Staff, Dr Hugh Twomey Health Care Centre; (709)257-5282; Fax. (709)257-4687.

WOOLFREY, Karen G H; Sunnybrook Hlth Sciences Ctre, C7 53-2075 Bayview Ave, Toronto ON M4N 3M5; Mem'91; FRCPC; EmergMed. Staff, St Joseph's Healthcare - Charlton Campus; Staff, Sunnybrook Health Sciences Centre; (416)480-6100; Fax. (416)480-6769.

WOOLFREY, Michael R; Brant Community HC-Brantford, 200 Terrace Hill St, Brantford ON N3R 1G9; Mem'91; FRCSC; OrthSurg. Staff, The Brant Community Healthcare System - Brantford General Hospital Site; Staff, St Joseph's Healthcare - Charlton Campus; (519)751-5894

WOOLFREY, Paul G W; Western Mem Reg Hosp, PO Box 2005 Stn Main 1 Brookfield Ave, Corner Brook NL A2H 6J7; Mem'92; FRCPC; PhysMed&Rehab. Clinical Asst Prof Med, Memorial University Of Newfoundland; (709)634-9255; Fax. (709)634-7357.

WOOLFSON, Ian K; Taunton Surgical Centre, 1300 Keith Ross Dr, Oshawa ON L1H 7K4; Tor'82; FRCSC; GenSurg. Staff, Lakeridge Health - Oshawa Site; (905)723-8551; Fax. (905)721-6665.

WOOLFSON, Neil B; Credit Valley Surgical Assoc, 2207 Dunwin Dr, Mississauga ON L5L 1X1; Witwatersrand (South Africa)'85; FRCSC; GenSurg (Oncology). Staff, The Credit Valley Hospital; (905)820-6233; Fax. (905)820-3352.

WOOLGAR, Mary-Jo V; Alexandra Comm Health Centre, 101-1318 Centre St NE, Calgary AB T2E 2R7; Cal'78; CCFP; FCFP; Staff, Foothills Medical Centre; (403)266-2622; Fax. (403)266-2692.

WOOLHOUSE, Susan J; South Riverdale Comm Hlth Ctr, 955 Queen St E, Toronto ON M4M 3P3; Wes'01; CCFP; (416)461-1925; Fax. (416)461-8295.

WOOLLAM, Christopher J; C120-11 King St W, Toronto ON M5H 4C7; Ott'68; Dip SportMed(SportsMed); Member Team Physician, St Michael's Majors; Med Dir, Toronto Marathon; Med Dir, Mississauga Marathon; (416)368-9990; Fax. (416)368-9992; cwoollam@bellnet.ca.

WOOLLAM, Gabriel B; Labrador Grenfell Health, PO Box 7000 Stn C 227 Hamilton River Rd, Happy-Valley-Goose NL A0P 1C0; UBC'06; CCFP; Staff, Labrador Health Centre; (709)897-2000; Fax. (709)777-7913.

WOOLLAM, Robin C; Winston Park Family Physicians, 104-2315 Bristol Cir, Oakville ON L6H 6P8; Ott'76; Staff Addiction & Concurrent Disorder Clinic, The Credit Valley Hospital; Physician, Halton Recovery House; (905)829-2826; Fax. (905)829-2846.

WOOLLARD, Robert F; David Strangway Bldg, 320-5950 University Blvd, Vancouver BC V6T 1Z3; Alb'69; MD; CCFP; FCFP; Vis Staff, Vancouver General Hospital - Centennial Pavillion; Prof, University of British Columbia; (604)827-4168; Fax. (604)827-4184.

WOOLLER, Angela J; Sunpark Prof Centre, 118-40 Sunpark Plaza SE, Calgary AB T2X 3X7; Sask'94; CCFP; (403)254-4000; Fax. (403)254-1282.

WOOLLER, Krista R; The Ottawa Hosp-Civic Campus, CPC 410-1053 Carling Ave, Ottawa ON K1Y 4E9; Sask'03; FRCPC; IntMed. Staff, The Ottawa Hospital - Civic Campus; (613)737-8899

WOOLLEY, Brenda A; Medisys Health Group Inc, 12F-95 St Clair Ave W, Toronto ON M4V 1N6; Wes'76; Staff, Civil Aviation Canada; Sr Consultant Med, Medisys Health Group Inc; (416)926-6464 x2980; Fax. (416)324-7905.

WOOLLISCROFT, David G; LA Medical, 30-5201 50 St, Leduc AB T9E 6T4; London (England)'80; MB BS; MRCGPract; AFOM; DAvMed; (780)986-9600; Fax. (780)986-9732.

WOOLNER, Derek B; Crowfoot West Business Ctre, 225-600 Crowfoot Cres NW, Calgary AB T3G 0B4; Cal'88; FRCPC; Derm. Staff, Peter Lougheed Centre; Clin Instructor, University of Calgary; (403)247-7070; Fax. (403)247-7080.

WOOLNER, Douglas S; Doctors Bldg, 215-955 Queen St E, Sault Ste. Marie ON P6A 2C3; Cal'85; FRCSC; PlasSurg. Staff, Sault Area Hospital - Sault Ste Marie; (705)946-1332; Fax. (705)946-5113; dwoolner@shaw.ca.

WOOLNER, Elisabeth; 224-555 Strathcona Blvd SW, Calgary AB T3H 2Z9; Cal'88; (403)686-2911

WOOLRIDGE, Bryan S; James Paton Mem Hosp, 125 Trans Canada Hwy, Gander NL A1V 1P7; Mem'03; FRCSC; OrthSurg. Staff Orthopaedic Clinic, James Paton Memorial Hospital; (709)256-2500

WOOLSEY, Guy H; University of Alberta Hosp, 8440 112 St NW, Edmonton AB T6G 2B7; Alb'91; CCFP; Staff, University of Alberta Hospital; (780)990-6383

WOOLSEY, Jennifer E; Golden Medical Clinic, PO Box 1170 1030 Denman St, Golden BC V0A 1H0; Cal'07; CCFP; (250)344-2211

WOOLTORTON, Eric J; Civic Family HealthTeam, 210 Melrose Ave, Ottawa ON K1Y 4K7; Qns'99; BSc; MSc; CCFP; Staff, Kemptville District Hospital; Lecturer, University of Ottawa; Langs: English; French; (613)761-4334

WOOSTER, Douglas L; Islington Med Clinic, 1202-1243 Islington Ave, Etobicoke ON M8X 1Y9; Wes'74; FACS; FRCSC; GenSurg (Vascular Ultrasound); VascSurg. Prof, University of Toronto; (416)516-4399; Fax. (416)516-1704; drdwooster@bellnet.ca.

WOOTTON, John C S; Pontiac Hospital Centre, 200 rue Argue, Shawville QC J0X 2Y0; McG'78; MDCM; LMCC; Dir-svcs prof, Pontiac Hospital Centre; Staff, Clinique Medicale de Shawville; adj Prof Family Med, McGill University; Langs: Bilingual(French/English); Portuguese; (819)647-6601; Fax. (819)647-2845; woottonjc@me.com.

WORKENTIN, Kevin M; Southeast Toronto Fam Hlth Team, 105-840 Coxwell Ave, Toronto ON M4C 5T2; Tor'00; BSc; BEd; CCFP; Staff, Toronto East General Hospital Inc; Lecturer Family & Commun Med, University of Toronto; (416)469-6464; Fax. (416)469-6164.

WORKEWYCH, Jaroslaw V; Churchill Family Med Practice, 6750 Winston Churchill Blvd, Mississauga ON L5N 4C4; Tor'84; Ac Staff, The Credit Valley Hospital; Langs: Ukrainian; (905)824-3700; Fax. (905)824-9956.

WORKMAN, C Murray; Paterson Med Centre, 45 Wolsley St, Kenora ON P9N 3W7; Wes'80; Lake of the Woods District Hospital; (807)468-3021; Fax. (807)468-5565.

WORKMAN, Holly K; PO Box 1120, Sparwood BC V0B 2G0; Qns'93; Staff, Sparwood Healthcare Centre; (250)425-4501; Fax. (250)425-4549.

WORKMAN, Stephen R; Queen Elizabeth II HSC, 437-1276 South Park St, Halifax NS B3H 2Y9; Qns'89; MSc; FRCPC; IntMed. Staff, Queen Elizabeth II Health Sciences Centre - Victoria General Site; Staff, IWK Health Centre; (902)473-3961; Fax. (902)473-8430.

WORKUN, Shane A; Foothills Med Centre, 1403 29 St NW, Calgary AB T2N 2T9; Cal'01; CCFP; Staff, Foothills Medical Centre; (403)944-2800

WORLEY, Scott W; Stan Cassidy Centre for Rehab, 800 Priestman St, Fredericton NB E3B 0C7; Cal'02; FRCPC; PhysMed&Rehab (Neurologic Rehab). Hd PhysMed&Rehab, Stan Cassidy Centre for Rehabilitation; Asst Prof, Dalhousie University; (506)474-4578; Fax. (506)447-4749; sarah.piercy@horizonnb.ca.

WORMSBECKER, Anne E; Health Protection & Promotion, 300-480 University Ave, Toronto ON M5G 1V2; Cal'04; FRCPC; Peds. Supt-Fibreline, The Hospital For Sick Children; Staff, Ontario Agency for Health; (647)260-7443

WORMSBECKER, Sean C; Royal Columbian Hosp, 330 Columbia St E, New Westminster BC V3L 3W7; Alb'05; FRCPC; EmergMed. Staff, Royal Columbian Hospital; (604)520-4253

WORNDL, M Michele; 2-210 Lorraine Ave, Kitchener ON N2B 3T4; Wes'86; Staff, St Mary's General Hospital; Staff, Grand River Hospital - Kitchener/Waterloo Health Centre; (519)570-1223; Fax. (519)570-9367.

WORNELL, Philip A; C-339 Willow St, Truro NS B2N 5A6; Dal'00; FRCPC; Peds; Nephrol. Staff, Colchester East Hants Health Centre; (902)893-5505; Fax. (902)893-3444.

WOROBETZ, Lawrence J; Royal University Hosp, 103 Hospital Dr, Saskatoon SK S7N 0W8; Sask'77; FRCPC; Gastroent; IntMed. Prof Med, Royal University Hospital; (306)655-1000; Fax. (306)966-1254.

WORRALL, Graham J; Bonavista Peninsula HCC, PO Box 1, Bonavista NL A0C 1B0; London (England)'70; DRCOG; MRC; CCFP; FCFP; Staff, Bonavista Peninsula Health Care Centre; (709)468-7881

WORRALL, James J; The Ottawa Hosp-Civic Campus, 1053 Carling Ave, Ottawa ON K1Y 4E9; Qns'01; CCFP; CCFP(E.M.); Staff, The Ottawa Hospital - Civic Campus; (613)761-4773

WORRY, Kevin W; Northern Lights Health Region, 7 Hospital St, Fort McMurray AB T9H 1P2; Tor'95; CCFP; CCFP(E.M.); FCFP; Staff, Northern Lights Regional Health Centre; (780)791-6221; Fax. (780)791-6029.

WORSLEY, Daniel F; 899 12th Ave W, Vancouver BC V5Z 1M9; UBC'89; FRCPC; NuclearMed. Staff Nuclear Med, Vancouver General Hospital - Centennial Pavillion; (604)875-4629

WORSLEY, Jennifer J; University Village Med Clinic, 228-2155 Allison Rd, Vancouver BC V6T 1T5; UBC'89; (604)222-2273; Fax. (604)222-3403.

WORSTER, Andrew S; Hamilton HS-Hamilton Gen, 237 Barton St E, Hamilton ON L8L 2X2; Dal'91; MSc; CCFP; CCFP(E.M.); FCFP; Staff Emerg, Hamilton Health Sciences Centre - Hamilton General Hospital; Dir-Research EmergMed, Hamilton Health Sciences Centre - McMaster Children's Hospital; Clinical Asst Prof Med & Clin Epidemiol & Biostat, McMaster University; (905)527-4322

WORTH, Glen G; Medical Arts Bldg, 208-336 Kings Rd, Sydney NS B1S 1A9; Dal'90; Ac Staff, Cape Breton Healthcare Complex; (902)539-9183; Fax. (902)562-3217.

WORTHINGTON, James R; The Ottawa Hosp-Civic Campus, M017-1053 Carling Ave, Ottawa ON K1Y 4E9; Birmingham (England)'71; FRCPC; EmergMed. Sr VP Medical Affairs Quality Patient Safety, The Ottawa Hospital - Civic Campus; Asst Prof., Family Med., University of Ottawa; (613)761-4203; Fax. (613)761-5311.

WORTHY, Robert J; 24 Health Services, PO Box 1000 Stn Forces 8 Wing Trenton, Astra ON K0K 3W0; Ott'08; CCFP; Staff, DND 8 Wing Trenton; (613)392-2811

WORTMAN, James A; First Nations & Inuit Health B, 540-757 Hastings St W, Vancouver BC V6C 3E6; Cal'84; CCFP; Staff, First Nations & Inuit Health Branch-BC Regions; (604)787-0894; Fax. (604)913-2975.

WORTON, Eleanor M; PO Box 91077 Rpo Royal Oak, Calgary AB T3G 5W6; Alb'88.

WORTSMAN, A Jay; North York Gen Hosp, 4001 Leslie St, North York ON M2K 1E1; Tor'79; FRCPC; DiagRad. Staff Diag Imaging, North York General Hospital - Branson Division; Staff, North York General Hospital; (416)756-6444

WORTZMAN, David J; Medcan Health Mgmt Inc, 1500-150 York St, Toronto ON M5H 3S5; Tor'81; FRCPC; EmergMed (Sports Medicine). Staff, Markham Stouffville Hospital; Staff, Medcan Health Management Inc; (416)380-3576; Fax. (416)350-5981.

WOTHERSPOON, Scott D M; Queen Elizabeth Hosp, PO Box 6600 Stn Central 60 Riverside Dr, Charlottetown PE C1A 8T5; Dal'04; FRCSC; OrthSurg. Staff, Queen Elizabeth Hospital; (902)894-2111

WOUDSTRA, Kevin C; 3404 9th St PO Box 670, Houston BC V0J 1Z0; Pretoria (South Africa)'01; Langs: Dutch; Afrikaans; (250)845-2555; Fax. (250)845-2544.

WOUDSTRA, Trudy D; Shawnigan Village Family, PO Box 240 2749 Dundas Lake Rd, Shawnigan Lake BC V0R 2W0; Alb'05; CCFP; (250)743-0793; Fax. (250)743-0754.

WOULFE, John M J; The Ottawa Hosp-Civic Campus, 1053 Carling Ave, Ottawa ON K1Y 4E9; McM'94; FRCPC; NeurPath. Assoc Scientist, The Ottawa Hospital - Civic Campus; (613)798-5555 x13345; Fax. (613)761-4199; jwoulfe@ottawahospital.on.ca.

WOURMS, Vincent P; Univ Hlth Network-Toronto Western Hosp, EC2 046-399 Bathurst St, Toronto ON M5T 2S8; Sask'06; FRCPC; Anes. Staff, Toronto Western Hospital - University Health Network; (416)603-2581

WOUTERLOOT, Johan; Mission Oaks Med Centre, 32136 Lougheed Hwy, Mission BC V2V 1A4; UBC'78; CCFP; FCFP; Ac Staff, Mission Memorial Hospital; Staff, Abbotsford Addiction Centre; Staff, Alouette Addictions Services; (604)826-7111; Fax. (604)826-4467.

WOUTERS, Lilliane S; 515-10333 Southport Rd SW, Calgary AB T2W 3X6; Wes'80; CCFP; Staff, Rockyview General Hospital; (403)252-4410; Fax. (403)252-4674; calvein@veinlase.com.

WOWK, Cory P; 271 Midpark Blvd SE, Calgary AB T2X 1S3; Cal'05; CCFP; Staff, Foothills Medical Centre; Physician, Siksika Health Centre; (403)873-2352; Fax. (403)873-2364.

WOWK-LITWIN, Maria L; Bethesda Hosp Steinbach, 316 Henry St, Steinbach MB R5G 0P9; Man'01; Staff, Bethesda Hospital Steinbach; (204)326-6411; mwowk-litwin@sehealth.mb.ca.

WOYCHUK, Walter; 241 Brebeuf St, Sudbury ON P3C 5H2; Tor'59; CCBOM; (705)522-8592; Fax. (705)673-9537.

WOYCHUK, Wesley F; Plaza 33, PO Box 23122 Rpo Plaza 33, Kelowna BC V1X 7K7; UBC'87; Physician Emerg Med, Kelowna General Hospital; (250)765-5500

WOYTIUK, Harvey P; Associate Med Centre, PO Box 219 4909 50th Ave, St Paul AB T0A 3A0; Alb'72; CCFP; Staff, Associate Medical Centre; (780)645-4411; Fax. (780)645-4566.

WOZNEY, Leonard R; Transcona Med Clinic, 200-701 Regent Ave W, Winnipeg MB R2C 1S3; Man'68; Assoc Staff, Concordia General Hospital; Assoc Staff, St Boniface General Hospital; (204)222-5221; Fax. (204)224-2053.

WOZNIAK, Andrew E; 203-5 Quarry Ridge Rd, Barrie ON L4M 7G1; Szczecin (Poland)'82; Court Staff, Royal Victoria Regional Health Centre; Langs: Polish; (705)728-2618; Fax. (705)728-3813.

WOZNIAK, Ewa A; Royal Victoria Hosp, 201 Georgian Dr, Barrie ON L4M 6M2; Dal'94; BSc(Med.Sci); FRCPC; GenPath (Cytopath). Staff, Royal Victoria Regional Health Centre; Langs: Polish; (705)728-9090; Fax. (705)739-5685.

WOZNIAK, Miranda L; Life Labs MLS, 100 International Blvd, Etobicoke ON M9W 6J6; Ott'06; FRCPC; HemPath. Staff, Life Labs; (416)675-4530; Fax. (416)213-4206.

WOZNIAK, Paul R; 801-60 St Clair Ave E, Toronto ON M4T 1N5; Tor'91; (416)944-0320

WOZNIAK, Peter C; Cambridge Walk-In Clinic, 980 Franklin Blvd, Cambridge ON N1R 8R3; Ott'88; CCFP; FCFP; (519)654-2260; Fax. (519)654-2231.

WOZNY, Diane M; 140-555 Sixth St, New Westminster BC V3L 5H1; Alb'92; (604)523-1166; Fax. (604)523-1722.

WRAY, George I; F-7819 East Saanich Rd, Saanichton BC V8M 2B4; Cal'79; CCFP; (250)652-4313; Fax. (250)652-1256.

WRAY, Heather E; St Joseph's Health Centre, 30 The Queensway, Toronto ON M6R 1B5; Cal'10; CCFP; Staff, St Joseph's Health Centre; (416)530-6000

WRAY, M Brent; Barrhead Healthcare Centre, PO Box 4540 Stn Main 5040 49A St, Barrhead AB T7N 1A4; Alb'74; Staff/Site Chief, Barrhead Healthcare Centre; (780)674-2231; Fax. (780)674-2447; durlingb@shaw.ca.

WRAY, Rebecca S; Medical Associates of Port Per, 462 Paxton St, Port Perry ON L9L 1L9; Qns'07; CCFP; (905)985-2895

WRAY, Richard G; Dr R G Way Med Clinic, 4645 52 St, Olds AB T4H 1E8; Alb'54; (403)556-3355; Fax. (403)556-4154.

WRAY, Roger W; Barrhaven Mall, 900 Greenbank Rd, Nepean ON K2J 1S8; McG'78; Langs: English; French; (613)825-1843

WREN, Colwyn J; 465 Ellis St, Penticton BC V2A 4M1; Witwatersrand (South Africa)'86; MB ChB; (250)490-4862

WREN, Denise M; St Mary's Gen Hosp, 911 Queens Blvd, Kitchener ON N2M 1B2; Wes'77; Chief Hospitalist & Family Med/Ac Staff, St Mary's General Hospital; (519)744-3311

WREN, Patricia L; IWK Health Centre, PO Box 9700 RPO CSC 5980 University Ave, Halifax NS B3K 6R8; Qns'78; FRCPC; Peds (Pediatric Emergency Medicine). Assoc Chief Emerg, IWK Health Centre; Asst Prof, Dalhousie University; (902)470-8823; Fax. (902)470-7248; patricia.wren@iwk.nshealth.ca.

WREZEL, Olga A; MUHC-Montreal Gen Hosp, 1650 av Cedar, Montreal QC H3G 1A4; Wes'09; CCFP; CCFP(E.M.); Staff, McGill University Health Centre - Montreal General Campus; (514)934-1934

WRIGHT, Alison F C; Family Practice Health Centre, 3F-77 Grenville St, Toronto ON M5S 1B3; McM'10; CCFP; Staff, Women's College Hospital; (416)323-6060

WRIGHT, Alistair; IWK Health Centre, PO Box 9700 Rpo CSC 5850-5980 University Ave, Halifax NS B3K 6R8; Dal'05; FRCPC; Anes. Staff, IWK Health Centre; (902)470-2870; Fax. (902)470-7911.

WRIGHT, Barbara E; Sunnybrook Health Sciences Ctr, MG 162-2075 Bayview Ave, Toronto ON M4N 3M5; Sask'71; FRCPC; DiagRad. Staff, Sunnybrook Health Sciences Centre; Asst Prof DiagRad, University Of Toronto; (416)480-6100 x1418

WRIGHT, Brock J; Winnipeg Reg Health Authority, 4F-650 Main St, Winnipeg MB R3B 1E2; Man'84; MBA; BSc; FRCPC; CommunMed (Public Health). Sr VP Clinical Services/Chief Medical Officer, Winnipeg Regional Health Authority; Assoc Dean Clinical Affairs, University of Manitoba; (204)926-8143; Fax. (204)926-8008; bwright@wrha.mb.ca.

WRIGHT, Bruce J; Rockyview Gen Hosp, 7007 14 St SW, Calgary AB T2V 1P9; Cal'87; CCFP; FCFP; Staff, Rockyview General Hospital; Assoc Dean Undergrad Med Educ, University Of Calgary; (403)943-3000; wrightb@ucalgaray.ca.

WRIGHT, C Stewart; Sunnybrook Holland Ortho Arthr, 325-43 Wellesley St E, Toronto ON M4Y 1H1; Mem'75; BMedSci; FRCSC; OrthSurg (Total Joint Replacement & Hand Surgery). Staff Surg, Sunnybrook Health Sciences Centre - Holland Orthopaedic & Arthritic Centre; Asst Prof, University of Toronto; (416)967-7889; Fax. (416)967-8748.

WRIGHT, Cheryl L; Royal Jubilee Hosp, 1952 Bay St, Victoria BC V8R 1J8; Wes'89; FRCPC; AnatPath. Staff Path, Royal Jubilee Hospital; (250)370-8836

WRIGHT, David C; Greene Stone Muskoka, 3571 Muskoka Road 169, Bala ON P0C 1A0; Cal'87; FRCPC; Psy (Personality Disorders). Staff Prog for Traumatic Stress Recovery & Cons Privil, Homewood Health Centre; Consultant Privil, Guelph General Hospital; Staff, Parkwood Hospital - St Joseph's Health Care; Clinical Asst Prof Psy, McMaster University; (877)762-5501; Fax. (705)762-1937.

WRIGHT, Douglas S; Hamilton HS-Hamilton Gen, 237 Barton St E, Hamilton ON L8L 2X2; McM'08; FRCPC; IntMed. Staff, Hamilton Health Sciences Centre - Hamilton General Hospital; (905)521-2100

WRIGHT, Erin D; University of Alberta Hosp, 1E4 WMC-8440 112 St NW, Edmonton AB T6G 2B7; McG'93; BSc(Hon); MEd; ABOtol; FRCSC; Otol (Head & Neck Surgery). Ac Staff, University of Alberta Hospital; Ac Staff, Royal Alexandra Hospital; Dir, Alberta Sinus Centre; Prof, University of Alberta; Langs: Bilingual(English/French); (780)407-7656; Fax. (780)407-7658.

WRIGHT, Frances C; Sunnybrook Hlth Sciences Ctre, T2 016-2075 Bayview Ave, Toronto ON M4N 3M5; Tor'96; FRCSC; GenSurg (Surgical Oncology). Staff Breast Surg & Oncologic Reconstruction, Sunnybrook Health Sciences Centre - Edmond Odette Cancer Centre; (416)480-4329; Fax. (416)480-6002.

WRIGHT, Frederick F; Sudbury Med Centre, 411-65 Larch St, Sudbury ON P3E 1B8; Wes'75; FRCSC; GenSurg. Ac Staff, Health Sciences North-Laurentian Site; Ac Staff, Health Sciences North-St Joseph's Health Centre; Ac Staff, Health Sciences North - Memorial Site; (705)674-2232; Fax. (705)675-2572.

WRIGHT, Heather D L; Packham Avenue Med Clinic, 104-335 Packham Ave, Saskatoon SK S7N 4S1; Sask'00; CCFP; (306)651-7091; Fax. (306)651-7092.

WRIGHT, Ilka Y S; Wentworth Limeridge Med Ctre, 209-849 Upper Wentworth St, Hamilton ON L9A 5H4; Tor'84; BSc; MSc; CCFP; FCFP; Staff, St Joseph's Healthcare - Charlton Campus; Staff, Hamilton Health Sciences Centre-Juravinski Site; Langs: German; (905)389-5212; Fax. (905)389-3152.

WRIGHT, James G; The Hosp for Sick Children, 1254-555 University Avenue, Toronto ON M5G 1X8; Tor'81; MPH; FRCSC; OrthSurg (Pediatric Orthopedics)., The Hospital For Sick Children; Prof Surg Public Health Sciences Health Policy Management & Evaluation, University of Toronto; (416)813-6433 x2; Fax. (416)813-7369; james.wright@sickkids.ca.

WRIGHT, James M; UBC Hospital, 2211 Wesbrook Mall, Vancouver BC V6T 2B5; Alb'68; PhD; IntMed (Clinical Pharmacology). Dir High Blood Pressure Clinic/Head, UBC Hospital - Koerner Pavillion; Prof, University of British Columbia; (604)822-7134; Fax. (604)822-0701.

WRIGHT, James R; The Juravinski Cancer Centre, 699 Concession St, Hamilton ON L8V 5C2; McM'90; FRCPC; RadOncol. Staff, Hamilton Health Sciences Centre - McMaster University Medical Centre; Consultant, The Brant Community Healthcare System - Brantford General Hospital Site; Asst Prof Med, McMaster University; (905)387-9495 x64706; Fax. (905)575-6326; jim.wright@hrcc.on.ca.

WRIGHT, Jamie E; Div of Urologic Sciences, L6-2775 Laurel St, Vancouver BC V5Z 1M9; Alb'66; FRCSC; Urol. Ac Staff, Vancouver General Hospital - Centennial Pavillion; (604)875-5003; Fax. (604)875-5604.

WRIGHT, Janet L; Telus Plaza South, 2700-10020 100 St NW, Edmonton AB T5J 0N3; Cal'82; FRCPC; Psy. Clin Assoc Prof, University of Calgary; (780)969-4940; Fax. (780)420-0651; jlwright@cpsa.ab.ca.

WRIGHT, Janice G; Inspire Health, 200-1330 8 Ave W, Vancouver BC V6H 4A6; McM'96; CCFP; (604)734-7125; Fax. (604)734-7105.

WRIGHT, Joanne L; St Paul's Hosp, 1081 Burrard St, Vancouver BC V6Z 1Y6; Alb'74; FRCPC; AnatPath. Ac Staff, UBC Hospital - Koerner Pavillion; Ac Staff, Providence Health Care - St Paul's Hospital; Prof Path, University of British Columbia; (604)806-8201

WRIGHT, John A; Family Med Practice, 347 10th St W, Owen Sound ON N4K 3R4; Tor'68; Court Staff, Grey Bruce Health Services - Owen Sound; (519)372-2329; Fax. (519)372-0431.

WRIGHT, John R; Scarborough Hosp-Birchmount, 3030 Birchmount Rd, Scarborough ON M1W 3W3; Tor'68; MBA; FRCPC; IntMed; Gastroent. Pres/CEO, The Scarborough Hospital - Birchmount Campus; Assoc Prof, University of Toronto; (416)495-2521; Fax. (416)495-2598; john.wright@uhn.on.ca.

WRIGHT, Kelley M; Kelly Wright Med Prof Corp, 101-489 Essa Rd, Barrie ON L4N 8E4; McM'97; CCFP; Staff, Royal Victoria Regional Health Centre; Staff, Roberta Place Retirement Lodge; Langs: French; (705)739-5262; Fax. (705)739-5263.

WRIGHT, Laura E; Carlisle Family Med Centre, PO Box 311 1493 Centre Rd, Carlisle ON L0R 1H0; McM'10; CCFP; (905)689-3301; Fax. (905)689-5772.

WRIGHT, Leslie C; Medical Clinic Person-Ctred Ps, 403-265 Yorkland Blvd, North York ON M2J 1S5; Wes'93; FRCPC; Psy (Addiction Psychiatry). Ac Staff, Ontario Shores Centre for Mental Health Sciences; Court Staff, Waypoint Centre for Mental Health Care; Staff, The Medical Clinic for Person-Centred Psychotherapy; (416)229-2399; Fax. (416)229-9771.

WRIGHT, Linette; The Fraser Valley Maternity Gr, 33525 Seventh St, Mission BC V2V 2E8; London (England)'00; MB BS; Staff, The Fraser Valley Maternity Group; (604)826-5112

WRIGHT, Martha E; 1508-77 St Clair Ave E, Toronto ON M4T 1M5; McM'77; Psy (Infant Psychiatry). Staff Psy, Centre for Addiction & Mental Health (CAMH) - College Street Site; Lecturer, University of Toronto; (416)960-8775

WRIGHT, Mary A; 205 Mutual St, Toronto ON M5B 2B4; Otago (New Zealand)'66; MB ChB; FRCPC; Psy (Psychoanalysis). (416)964-6174

WRIGHT, Michael D; Wright Incorporated, 9820 101 Ave, Fort St. John BC V1J 2B2; Qns'74; CCFP; FCFP; Staff, Fort St John Hospital & Health Centre; Staff, Wright Incorporated; (250)261-9979; Fax. (250)787-8842; mgjrm@pris.ca.

WRIGHT, Monique D M; Sunnyhill Pediatric Clinic, 200-1632 14 Ave NW, Calgary AB T2N 1M7; Cal'85; BSc; MSc; FRCPC; Peds. Ad Staff Privil, Alberta Children's Hospital; Ad Staff Privil, Foothills Medical Centre; Asst Prof, University of Calgary; (403)284-0001; Fax. (403)284-1593.

WRIGHT, Nicola A M; Alberta Children's Hosp, 4004-2888 Shaganappi Trail NW, Calgary AB T3B 6A8; Cal'97; FRCPC; Peds (Hematology). Staff, Alberta Children's Hospital; (403)955-3035; Fax. (403)955-3055.

WRIGHT, Philip H; Saskatoon Cancer Centre, 20 Campus Dr, Saskatoon SK S7N 4H4; Sask'03; BSc; MSc; FRCPC; RadOncol. Staff RadOncol, Saskatoon Cancer Centre; Clinical Asst Prof Oncol, University of Saskatchewan; (306)655-2740; Fax. (306)655-2639; philip.wright@saskcancer.ca.

WRIGHT, Robert B; Edmonton Clinic Health Academy, 11405 87 Ave NW, Edmonton AB T6G 1C9; Man'95; FRCPC; Peds (Pediatric Emergency Medicine). Staff, University of Alberta Hospital; Staff, Edmonton Clinic Health Academy; Asst Prof Peds, University of Alberta; (780)248-5575; Fax. (888)775-8876.

WRIGHT, Ryan T; Edmonton Clinic, 11400 University Ave, Edmonton AB T6G 1Z1; Alb'03; CCFP; Staff Family Med Clinic, University of Alberta Hospital; Staff, Royal Alexandra Hospital; Surg Asst, Leduc Community Hospital; (780)407-7755; Fax. (780)407-1828; ryanwright@shaw.ca.

WRIGHT, S Elizabeth; Bedford Central Med Clinic, 2F-1650 Bedford Hwy, Bedford NS B4A 4J7; Man'87; CCFP; FCFP; Physician, Canadian Forces Health Services Centre (Atlantic); (902)835-4777; Fax. (902)835-5502.

WRIGHT, Scott R; L5-30 Dupont St E, Waterloo ON N2J 2G9; Wes'99; CCFP; (519)883-8581; Fax. (519)883-7192.

WRIGHT, Stefanie T B; L5-30 Dupont St E, Waterloo ON N2J 2G9; Wes'96; BSc; CCFP; (519)883-8581; Fax. (519)883-7192.

WRIGHT, Stephen J; Lumby Health Centre, PO Box 247 2135 Norris Ave, Lumby BC V0E 2G0; Leicester (England)'86; MB ChB; CCFP; (250)547-2127; drsjwright@yahoo.com.

WRIGHT, Thomas A; Univ Hlth Network-Toronto Western Hosp, 244-399 Bathurst St, Toronto ON M5T 2S8; Tor'56; BSc(Med); FRCSC; OrthSurg (Spine Surgery). Staff, Toronto Western Hospital - University Health Network; Consultant, Health Canada; Asst Prof Surg, University of Toronto; (416)603-5267; Fax. (416)603-3437.

WRIGHT, Timothy G; Care Point Med Clinic, 1123 Davie St, Vancouver BC V6E 1N2; London (England)'72; (604)915-9517

WRIGHT, W D Grant; 426 Bate Cres, Saskatoon SK S7H 3A7; Sask'65; FRCSC; Otol. Ac Staff, St Paul's Hospital (Grey Nuns) of Saskatoon; Ac Staff, Saskatoon City Hospital; (306)221-1270

WRIGHT JR., James R; Diagnostic & Scientific Centre, 9-3535 Research Rd NW, Calgary AB T2L 2K8; Ohio State University (USA)'84; ABP; PhD(Exp Path); MA; Staff Path, Alberta Children's Hospital; Physician, Alberta Health Services; Staff, Calgary Laboratory Services; Dept Head Path & Lab Med/Prof, University Of Calgary; (403)770-3569; Fax. (403)770-3788; jim.wright@cls.ab.ca.

WRIGLEY, Heather L; PO Box 61102 Rpo Kensington, Calgary AB T2N 4S6; Cal'07; CCFP.

WRINCH, John H; Victoria Gen Hosp, 1 Hospital Dr, Victoria BC V8Z 6R5; UBC'63; DiagRad. Ac Staff, Victoria General Hospital; (250)727-4208; Fax. (250)727-4290.

WRITER, Hilary K; Children's Hosp Eastern Ont, 401 Smyth Rd, Ottawa ON K1H 8L1; Dal'89; MD; FRCPC; Peds; Critical Care Medicine. Staff, Children's Hospital of Eastern Ontario (CHEO); (613)737-7600; Fax. (613)738-4287; hwriter@cheo.on.ca.

WRITER, William D; Queen Elizabeth II HSC-VG Site, 1276 South Park St, Halifax NS B3H 2Y9; (United Kingdom)'58; Staff, Queen Elizabeth II Health Sciences Centre - Victoria General Site; (902)473-2331; Fax. (902)423-9454.

WRIXON, Katherine J; St Paul's Hosp, 2N-1081 Burrard St, Vancouver BC V6Z 1Y6; Dal'94; BSc; FRCPC; Psy. Staff Outpatient Dept, Providence Health Care - St Paul's Hospital; Staff, West End Mental Health Team; (604)682-2344 x62133; Fax. (604)806-8714; kwrixon@forensic.bc.ca.

WROBEL, Iwona T; Alberta Children's Hosp, 2888 Shaganappi Trail NW, Calgary AB T3B 6A8; Lublin (Poland),'96; FRCPC; Peds (Pediatric Gastroenterology); Gastroent. Clin Staff Mentor Specialist, Alberta Children's Hospital; Staff, Gastroenterology Clinic; Clinical Asst Prof, University of Calgary; Langs: Polish; (403)955-3071; Fax. (403)955-2922.

WROBLEWSKI, Julius A; Mount St Joseph Hosp, 3080 Prince Edward St, Vancouver BC V5T 3N4; Man'78; AB; MRCPath; FRCP; FRCPC; GenPath; AnatPath. Staff, Providence Health Care - Mount Saint Joseph Hospital; Vis Staff, Providence Health Care - St Paul's Hospital; Langs: Polish; (604)877-8330 x207; Fax. (604)877-8108; jwroblewski@providencehealth.bc.ca.

WROBLEWSKI, Karol C; William Osler Health Centre, 101 Humber College Blvd, Etobicoke ON M9V 1R8; Tor'04; CCFP; CCFP(E.M.); Staff, William Osler Health System - Etobicoke General Hospital; Langs: Polish; (416)494-2120

WROGEMANN, Jens J W; Children's Hosp, 840 Sherbrook St, Winnipeg MB R3A 1S1; Man'98; FRCPC; DiagRad (Pediatric Radiology). Staff, Health Sciences Centre; jwrogemann@hsc.mb.ca.

WROZ, Paul W K; Royal Inland Hosp, 311 Columbia St, Kamloops BC V2C 2T1; Dal'96; CCFP; CCFP(E.M.); Staff, Royal Inland Hospital; (250)314-2533; Fax. (250)314-2333.

WROZ, Thom W; 520 Nicola St, Kamloops BC V2C 2R1; Dal'93; FRCSC; ObstGyn. Langs: Polish; (250)374-4456; Fax. (250)374-4549.

WU, Adam S G; Royal University Hosp, 103 Hospital Dr, Saskatoon SK S7N 0W8; Tor'01; MSc; FRCSC; Neursurg (Surgical Oncology). Staff Neurosurg, Royal University Hospital; (306)966-8023; Fax. (306)966-8140; adam.wu@usask.ca.

WU, Alwin; First Markham Place, 176-3255 Highway 7, Markham ON L3R 3P9; (Hong Kong)'76; CCFP; Langs: Cantonese; Mandarin; (905)940-4820; Fax. (905)940-4821.

WU, Arthur; 1425 Lakeshore Rd E, Oakville ON L6J 1L9; London (England)'69; MB BS; FRCP; FACP; FACG; FRCPC; IntMed (Clinical Research); Gastroent. Affil Staff, Halton Healthcare Services Corporation - Oakville Site; (905)338-2033; Fax. (905)338-3468; arthurwu@sympatico.ca.

WU, Beatrice M Y; Dominion Health Centre, 2383 111 St NW, Edmonton AB T6J 5E5; Alb'02; BMedSci; CCFP; (780)436-0020; Fax. (780)436-0603.

WU, Bennet P Y; Minden Med Clinic, PO Box 700 6 McPherson St, Minden ON K0M 2K0; Tor'76; Langs: Cantonese; (705)286-2001; Fax. (705)286-2022.

WU, Caren M; HSC-Faculty of Med, 1434-3330 Hospital Dr NW, Calgary AB T2N 4N1; Tor'97; MSc; FRCPC; IntMed. (403)220-4504; Fax. (403)283-6151.

WU, Chin Yu; Park Barton Med Group, 78 Barton St W, Hamilton ON L8L 1A6; (Taiwan)'64; Langs: Mandarin; Taiwanese; (905)525-4343; Fax. (905)525-4349.

WU, Cynthia M J; Clinical Sciences Bldg, 4 112-11350 83 Ave, Edmonton AB T6G 2G3; Alb'03; FRCPC; IntMed (Thromboembolism); Hem. Staff, University of Alberta Hospital; (780)407-1584; Fax. (780)407-2680.

WU, Douglas D K Q; Stouffville Med Centre, 2F-34 Civic Ave, Stouffville ON L4A 1H2; UBC'00; (905)640-3100; Fax. (905)640-5346.

WU, Evelyn P S; South Vancouver Med Clinic, 350 Marine Dr SE, Vancouver BC V5X 2S5; UBC'09; CCFP; (604)323-0077

WU, George G; Dr George G Wu Med Prof Corp, 501-2300 Eglinton Ave W, Mississauga ON L5M 2V8; Tor'78; FACP; FRCPC; IntMed; Nephrol. Med Dir Renal Program, The Credit Valley Hospital; Langs: Mandarin; Cantonese; (905)820-8770; Fax. (905)820-3703.

WU, Gilbert K P; Mackenzie Richmond Hill Hosp, 10 Trench St, Richmond Hill ON L4C 4Z3; Cal'02; FRCPC; IntMed; Cardiol. Staff, Mackenzie Richmond Hill Hospital; (905)534-1872; Fax. (905)534-1872.

WU, Grace C Y; Carling-Broadview Med Bldg, 308-770 Broadview Ave, Ottawa ON K2A 3Z3; McM'00; FRCPC; IntMed; Hem. Staff, Queensway Carleton Hospital; (613)725-9374; Fax. (613)725-9195.

WU, H T Tony; Oakville Med Arts Bldg, 18-358 Reynolds St, Oakville ON L6J 3L9; Tor'77; Staff, Halton Healthcare Services Corporation - Oakville Site; Langs: Chinese; (905)845-3415

WU, Harry K C; Belgage Med Arts Bldg, 207-525 Belmont Ave W, Kitchener ON N2M 5E2; Wes'05; FRCPC; IntMed; Gastroent. Staff, Toronto Western Hospital - University Health Network; (519)568-8811; Fax. (519)340-0388.

WU, Henry M W; Hillside Med Centre, 2867 Lawrence Ave E, Scarborough ON M1P 2T2; Tor'75; Langs: Chinese; (416)261-7223; Fax. (416)261-6374.

WU, Howard; Smart Health Med Clinic, 8-4080 Steeles Ave E, Markham ON L3R 4C3; Qns'94; CCFP; Supvr Elective Family Med Student, University of Toronto; Langs: Mandarin; Cantonese; (905)948-9738; Fax. (905)948-9740; howard.wu@utoronto.ca.

WU, Jackson S Y; Tom Baker Cancer Centre, 1331 29 St NW, Calgary AB T2N 4N2; UBC'93; LMCC; FRCPC; RadOncol (Clinical Epidemiology). Staff, Tom Baker Cancer Centre; Staff, Foothills Medical Centre; Clin Assoc Prof, University of Calgary; Langs: Chinese; (403)521-3708; Fax. (403)283-1651.

WU, Jenny; KMH Cardiology & Diagnostic Ct, 109-55 Town Centre Crt, Scarborough ON M1P 4X4; University of Miami (USA)'94; Langs: Mandarin; (905)855-1860; Fax. (416)290-0183.

WU, John K M; Children's & Women's HC of BC, A119-4480 Oak St, Vancouver BC V6H 3V4; (Hong Kong)'80; DAB; MSc; FRCPC; Peds (Pediatric Hematology Oncology); Hem. Staff HemOncol, BC Children's Hospital; Clin Prof, University of British Columbia; Langs: Mandarin; Cantonese; (604)875-2406; Fax. (604)875-2911.

WU, John W Y; 207 8A St NE, Calgary AB T2E 4H9; Ott'72; FAAP; FRCPC; Hem; Peds. Staff, Alberta Children's Hospital; Staff, Foothills Medical Centre; Staff, Peter Lougheed Centre; Clin Assoc Prof, University of Calgary; Langs: Chinese; (403)234-9212; Fax. (403)234-9213.

WU, Johnny J; Burnaby Hosp, 3935 Kincaid St, Burnaby BC V5G 2X6; UBC'05; FRCPC; Psy. Staff, Burnaby Hospital; Staff, Burnaby Mental Health Services; (604)434-4211

WU, Jonn S; BC Cancer Agency-Vancouver CC, 600 10th Ave W, Vancouver BC V5Z 4E6; Alb'93; FRCPC; RadOncol. Staff, BC Cancer Agency Vancouver Centre; (604)877-6000 x2673; Fax. (604)877-0505; jwu@bccancer.bc.ca.

WU, K Y William; Queen Elizabeth II HSC-Halifax, 3021-1796 Summer St, Halifax NS B3H 3A7; Dal'79; Staff, Queen Elizabeth II Health Sciences Centre - Victoria General Site; (902)473-8769; Fax. (902)473-3617.

WU, Louis; Lakeridge Hlth Corp-Oshawa, 1 Hospital Crt, Oshawa ON L1G 2B9; McG'95; FRCPC; DiagRad. Staff, Lakeridge Health - Oshawa Site; Langs: Bilingual(French/English); (905)576-8711; Fax. (905)743-5942.

WU, Melinda Y; Women's College Hosp, 76 Grenville St, Toronto ON M5S 1B2; Tor'09; CCFP; Staff, Women's College Hospital; (416)323-6060; Fax. (416)323-6402.

WU, Nancy P; William Osler HS-Etobicoke, 101 Humber College Blvd, Etobicoke ON M9V 1R8; St George's University (Grenada)'04; Staff, William Osler Health System - Etobicoke General Hospital; (416)747-3400

WU, Paul T K; G14A-1455 Lakeshore Rd, Burlington ON L7S 2J1; Tor'77; FRCSC; ObstGyn. Staff, Joseph Brant Memorial Hospital; Staff, Halton Healthcare Services Corporation - Milton District Hospital; Langs: Chinese; (905)681-1553; Fax. (905)681-1554.

WU, Raymond H C; Unionville Family Med Clinic, 1-8 Cox Blvd, Markham ON L3R 4G1; Dublin (Ireland)'81; MSc(ClinPharmacol); Staff, Markham Stouffville Hospital; Langs: Cantonese; (905)470-6840; Fax. (905)470-6841.

WU, Robert C; Univ Hlth Network-Toronto Gen, 14E 222-200 Elizabeth St, Toronto ON M5G 2C4; Tor'96; FRCPC; IntMed. Staff, Toronto General Hospital - UHN; (416)340-4567; Fax. (416)595-5826.

WU, Sibra S C; 1216 King St W, Toronto ON M6K 1G4; Tor'84; Staff, Toronto Western Hospital - University Health Network; Court Staff, St Joseph's Health Centre; Staff Home for the Aged, City of Toronto; Physician, Yee Hong Centre For Geriatric Care; Langs: Cantonese; Mandarin; (416)531-3337; Fax. (416)531-2051.

WU, Sing Man; Victoria Terrace Med Centre, 203-1448 Lawrence Ave E, North York ON M4A 2V6; Tor'76; MSc; Staff, The Scarborough Hospital - General Campus; Langs: Cantonese; (416)449-7121; Fax. (416)449-7122.

WU, Stephen C K; Langley Mem Hosp, 22051 Fraser Hwy, Langley BC V3A 4H4; UBC'06; FRCPC; Anes. Staff, Langley Memorial Hospital; (604)534-4121

WU, Stephen T W; Dundas Med Centre, 206-220 Dundas St W, Whitby ON L1N 8M7; (Taiwan)'70; CCFP; FCFP; Staff, Lakeridge Health - Whitby Site; Staff, Lakeridge Health - Oshawa Site; Langs: Cantonese; Mandarin; (905)668-3633; Fax. (905)668-3633.

WU, Theresa F; Alberta Children's Hosp, 2888 Shaganappi Trail NW, Calgary AB T3B 6A8; Cal'07; FRCPC; Peds. Staff, Alberta Children's Hospital; (403)671-0114

WU, Vincent M Y; Royal Court Med Centre, 305-1 Quarry Ridge Rd, Barrie ON L4M 7G1; Tor'92; FRCSC; ObstGyn. Staff, Royal Victoria Regional Health Centre; Langs: Chinese; (705)728-5311; Fax. (705)728-5601.

WU, William; 508 15 Ave SW, Calgary AB T2R 0R2; Alb'90; CCFP; FCFP; (403)398-5449; Fax. (403)229-1759.

WU, Yan; Saskatoon Community Clinic, 455 2nd Ave N, Saskatoon SK S7K 2C2; Beijing (China)'84; MB; PhD; CCFP; Physician, Saskatoon Community Health Unit; Langs: Chinese; (306)652-0300; Fax. (306)664-4120.

WU, Yan; Primrose Family Med Centre, 35 Primrose Ave, Ottawa ON K1R 0A1; Mudanjiang Medical College (Other Foreign)'09; CCFP; (613)230-7788

WU, Ying; Centre Hosp de Verdun, 4000 boul Lasalle, Verdun QC H4G 2A3; Shanghai (China)'87; FRCPC; Neur. Staff, Centre Hospitalier de Verdun; (514)362-1000; Fax. (514)765-7314.

WU, Yizheng; Rideau Valley Health Services, 1221 Greenbank Rd, Ottawa ON K2J 5V7; McG'04; CCFP; Langs: Bilingual(English/French); (613)258-8710; Fax. (613)440-3238.

WU, Yue; Royal University Hosp, 103 Hospital Dr, Saskatoon SK S7N 0W8; Staff Path, Royal University Hospital; (306)655-1000

WUDOM, Kofi A; Peel Village Med Centre, 28 Rambler Dr, Brampton ON L6W 1E2; Accra (Ghana)'79; LMCC; MB ChB; CCFP; Langs: Akan; Twi; (905)451-5586; Fax. (905)451-1233.

WULFF, Tanya A; 313-2083 Alma St, Vancouver BC V6R 4N6; Alb'69; FRCPC; Psy;CCFP; (604)222-2083; Fax. (604)222-2045.

WULFFHART, Jeffrey I; St John's Rehab Hosp, 285 Cummer Ave, North York ON M2M 2G1; Witwatersrand (South Africa)'86; CCFP; Court Staff, Sunnybrook Health Sciences Centre; Court Staff, Bridgepoint Health Centre; Staff, St John's Rehabilitation Hospital; Langs: Afrikaans; Hebrew; (416)226-6780

WULFFHART, Zaev A; Newmarket Med Place, 105-712 Davis Dr, Newmarket ON L3Y 8C3; Witwatersrand (South Africa)'84; MB ChB; FACC; FRCPC; IntMed (Electrophysiology); Cardiol. Court Staff, Sunnybrook Health Sciences Centre; Staff, Southlake Regional Health Centre; Court Staff, St Michael's Hospital; Asst Prof, University of Toronto; (905)953-7917; Fax. (905)953-0046.

WUNDER, Jay S; Mount Sinai Hosp, 476-600 University Ave, Toronto ON M5G 1X5; Tor'86; FACS; FRCSC; OrthSurg (Orthopedic Oncology). Ac Staff, Mount Sinai Hospital; Ac Staff, Princess Margaret Hospital - University Health Network; (416)586-4800 x8807; Fax. (416)586-8397.

WURSTER, Charles L; Dartmouth Gen Hosp, 325 Pleasant St, Dartmouth NS B2Y 4G8; Dal'98; CCFP; CCFP(E.M.); Staff, Dartmouth General Hospital; (902)465-8491; Fax. (902)465-8579.

WURTELE, Patika A; 11-525 Highland Rd W, Kitchener ON N2M 5K1; Wes'89; (519)747-2172; Fax. (519)571-1174; wurtele@kw.igs.net.

WURTELE, Paul; 110-2780 av Raymond, Saint-Hyacinthe QC J2S 5W7; Mon'72; DAB; Otol (P.Q.). Staff, Centre Hospitalier Honore-Mercier; (450)773-4322; Fax. (450)773-9474.

WYAND, Anna E H; The Ottawa Hosp-Civic Campus, 1053 Carling Ave Box 249C, Ottawa ON K1Y 4E9; Dal'02; FRCPC; Anes. Staff, The Ottawa Hospital - Civic Campus; Langs: Bilingual(English/French); (613)761-4169; Fax. (613)761-5209.

WYANT, John D; Port Arthur Hlth Centre Inc, 194 Court St N, Thunder Bay ON P7A 4V7; McG'62; DAB; FACS; FRCSC; GenSurg (Skin Diseases). Court Staff, Thunder Bay Regional Health Sciences Centre Port-Arthur; (807)346-1000; Fax. (807)346-6209.

WYANT-CROSSMAN, Kerrie E I; Aikens Street Comm Health Ctre, 601 Aikins St, Winnipeg MB R2W 4J5; Man'99; CCFP; (204)940-2025; Fax. (204)940-2069; kwyant-crossman@wrha.mb.ca.

WYATT, Diana S; Bath Institution, 5775 Bath Rd, Bath ON K0H 1G0; Ott'83; (613)351-8014

WYATT, Emma L; McMaster Univ-Children's Hosp, 3A-1280 Main St W, Hamilton ON L8S 4K1; Western Australia (Australia)'00; Staff, McMaster University; (905)521-2100

WYATT, Judith L; Anaesthesia Associates, 439 Park St, Kitchener ON N2G 1N4; Wes'72; FRCPC; Anes. (519)744-7361

WYATT, Philip R; Mackenzie Richmond Hill Hosp, 10 Trench St, Richmond Hill ON L4C 4Z3; Lexington(KY) (USA)'80; PhD; Consultant, Mackenzie Richmond Hill Hospital; Consultant, Mount Sinai Hospital; (905)883-1212 x7579

WYBENGA, Milton P; Colchester East Hants Hlth Ctr, 600 Abenaki Rd, Truro NS B2N 5A1; Dal'84; FRCPC; Anes (Pain Management). Staff, Colchester East Hants Health Centre; Langs: Dutch; (902)893-4321

WYBOUW, Cedric; Clinique Med Memramcook, PO Box 1560 Stn B 152 rue Centrale, Memramcook NB E4K 3V2; Sher'96; LMCC; CCFP; Staff, Dr Georges-L-Dumont University Hospital Centre; Langs: English; (506)758-2290; Fax. (506)758-2278.

WYCLIFFE-JONES, Keith; Sunridge Family Med Teaching C, 2685 36 St NE, Calgary AB T1Y 5S3; (United Kingdom)'83; CCFP; Assoc Prof Family Med, University Of Calgary; (403)943-5000; Fax. (403)476-8784.

WYCOCO, Danilo A; Grand River Hosp-KW Hlth Ctre, PO Box 9056 Stn C 835 King St W, Kitchener ON N2G 1G3; Manila (Philippines)'72; FRCPC; DiagRad (Interventional Radiology). Chief Medical Imaging, Grand River Hospital - Kitchener/Waterloo Health Centre; Langs: Tagalog; (519)749-4300 x3822; Fax. (519)749-4296.

WYLIE, J Stewart M; Gates Med Centre, 15-300 Kingston Rd, Pickering ON L1V 6Z9; Wes'03; CCFP; (905)509-4595; Fax. (905)509-4597.

WYLIE, James R; First Choice Med Centre, 9-1 Wexford Rd, Brampton ON L6Z 2W1; Glasgow (Scotland)'71; MB ChB; Langs: Vietnamese; Spanish; French; Slovak; (905)451-2220; Fax. (905)970-9076.

WYLIE, Kevin J; Oak Bay Family Physician Ltd, 101-1640 Oak Bay Ave, Victoria BC V8R 1B2; UBC'85; (250)598-6744; Fax. (250)598-6778.

WYLIE, Louise B M; Parkdale Med Tower, 607-1081 Carling Ave, Ottawa ON K1Y 4G2; Ott'87; Langs: Spanish; French; (613)725-3117; Fax. (613)725-3237.

WYLIE, Mark O; Greenwood Family Physicians, PO Box 5, Sundre AB T0M 1X0; Cal'09; CCFP; (403)638-3580; Fax. (403)638-3580.

WYLLIE, Blair F; London Health Sciences Ctre, PO Box 5010 Stn B 800 Commissioners Rd E, London ON N6A 5W9; Wes'01; FRCPC; IntMed; Nephrol. Staff, London Health Sciences Centre - University Hospital; (519)685-8132; Fax. (519)685-8357.

WYMAN, Chester R; 6 Parade St, Yarmouth NS B5A 3A4; Dal'70.

WYMAN, Jennifer J; Medical & Dental Bldg, 712-586 Eglinton Ave E, Toronto ON M4P 1P2; McM'91; BA; CCFP; Staff, Women's College Hospital; Court Staff, Sunnybrook Health Sciences Centre; Lecturer Family & Comm Med, University of Toronto; (416)440-1880; Fax. (416)440-1106.

WYMAN, Roy J; Medical Office, 105-840 Coxwell Ave, Toronto ON M4C 5T2; Tor'94; CCFP; FCFP; Staff, Toronto East General Hospital Inc; Staff, Humber River Regional Hospital - Keele Street Site; Staff, Providence Healthcare; University of Toronto; (416)469-6464; Fax. (416)469-6164.

WYMAN, Tanya; 311-4800 Leslie St, North York ON M2J 2K9; Tor'97; CCFP; Staff Family Med, Mount Sinai Hospital; Staff, North York General Hospital; (416)222-5439; Fax. (416)229-2513.

WYND, Henriette D; Dr H D Wynd Med Office, PO Box 986 Stn Main 203-184 Charlotte St, Peterborough ON K9J 7A5; Qns'66; DCPsy; FRCPC; Psy (Child & Family Psychiatry). Consultant, Peterborough Regional Health Centre - Hospital Drive; (705)743-9654; Fax. (705)743-7669.

WYND, Kimberly P; Peterborough Reg HC-Hosp Dr, 1 Hospital Dr, Peterborough ON K9J 7C6; National (Ireland)'03; FRCPC; Anes. Staff, Peterborough Regional Health Centre - Hospital Drive; (705)743-2121; Fax. (705)876-5120.

WYND, Peter B; 203-184 Charlotte St PO Box 986 Stn Main, Peterborough ON K9J 7A5; Qns'65; FRCPC; Anes. Staff, Peterborough Regional Health Centre - Hospital Drive; Staff, Peterborough Regional Health Centre - Rogers St Site; Staff, Campbellford Memorial Hospital; (705)743-9654

WYNNE, Andrew D; Royal Inland Hosp, 311 Columbia St, Kamloops BC V2C 2T1; Cal'89; CCFP; CCFP(E.M.); Staff, Royal Inland Hospital; (250)374-5111

WYNNE, Elaine J; Pine Free Clinic, 1985 4th Ave W, Vancouver BC V6J 1M7; UBC'77; (604)736-2391; Fax. (604)731-9479.

WYNNE, Linda A; The Ottawa Hosp-Civic Campus, 1053 Carling Ave, Ottawa ON K1Y 4E9; London (England)'78; MB BS; FRCPC; Anes (Pain Management). Court Staff, The Ottawa Hospital - General Campus; Staff, The Ottawa Hospital - Civic Campus; (613)761-4169; Fax. (613)761-5209.

WYNNYCHUK, Lesia A; Sunnybrook Hlth Sciences Ctre, 356-2075 Bayview Ave, Toronto ON M4N 3M5; Alb'85; Consultant Palliative Med, Sunnybrook Health Sciences Centre; Asst Prof Dept of Fam & Comm Med, University of Toronto; (416)480-6100 x7255; Fax. (416)480-5146.

WYNTERS, John; Prairie Med Clinic, 10309 98 St, Grande Prairie AB T8V 2E7; London (England)'64; MB BS; MRCS; Chief Anes. Serv., Queen Elizabeth II Hospital; (780)539-4330

WYNVEEN, William B; West Street Health Centre, 301-216 West St, Simcoe ON N3Y 1S8; Wes'77; Ac Staff, Norfolk General Hospital; Physician, Esso Imperial Oil; (519)426-9082; Fax. (519)426-2812.

WYSE, Carl W; Lynde Centre for Dermatology, 3 Ovida Blvd, Markham ON L3P 7N8; Wes'62; FRCPC; Derm. Staff, Sunnybrook Health Sciences Centre; (905)471-5063; Fax. (905)471-0580.

WYSE, D George; Cardiac Sciences Bldg, GC064-3280 Hospital Dr NW, Calgary AB T2N 4Z6; Cal'74; MSc; PhD; FACP; FACC; FRCPC; IntMed (Clinical Cardiac); Cardiol. Consultant Cardiol, Calgary Regional Health Authority; Emeritus Prof, University Of Calgary; (403)220-2052; Fax. (403)283-8878; dgwyse@ucalgary.ca.

WYSE, J Patrick H; Bow River Prof Centre, 313-4411 16 Ave NW, Calgary AB T3B 0M3; UBC'75; PhD; BSc(Hon.CellBial); FRCSC; Ophth. Clin Assoc Prof Eye Clinic, Rockyview General Hospital; (403)286-3335; Fax. (403)286-3316.

WYSE, Jonathan M; SMBD-Jewish Gen Hosp, G304-3755 ch Cote-Sainte-Cathe, Montreal QC H3T 1E2; McG'02; Gastroent; IntMed. Staff, Sir Mortimer B Davis Jewish General; (514)340-8222 x8286

WYSYNSKI, Anna-Marie; Brant Community HC-Brantford, 200 Terrrace Hill St, Brantford ON N3R 1G9; McM'98; Staff, The Brant Community Healthcare System - Brantford General Hospital Site; (519)751-5507; Fax. (905)751-5570.

WYSZOGRODSKI, Isaac; 202-3400 rue du Marche, Dollard-D-Ormeaux QC H9B 2Y1; McG'78; MSc; PhD; Staff, Sir Mortimer B Davis Jewish General; Conférencier Family Med, McGill University; Langs: English; French; (514)683-1262; Fax. (514)683-5528.

WYTSMA, Julia L; U of T-Family & Community Med, 3F-500 University Ave, Toronto ON M5G 1V7; McM'10; CCFP; (416)946-5938

WYTSMA, Richard D; The Group Health Ctre, 240 McNabb St, Sault Ste. Marie ON P6B 1Y5; Wes'82; (705)759-1234; Fax. (705)541-2226.

XAVIER MATTESCO, Carole F A; Hopital de Hull, 116 boul Lionel-Emond, Gatineau QC J8Y 1W7; Staff, Hull Hospital; (819)966-6038

XENOCOSTAS, Anargyros; A2 401-800 Commissioners Rd E PO Box 5010 Stn B, London ON N6A 5W9; McG'95; FRCPC; IntMed (Hemo Stem Cell Transplantation); Hem. Staff, London Health Sciences Centre - Victoria Campus; Langs: French; Greek; English; (519)685-8500 x56357; Fax. (519)685-8477; anargyros.xenocostas@lhsc.on.ca.

XENODEMETROPOULOS, Theodore T; McMaster University, 2F63-1280 Main St W, Hamilton ON L8S 4K1; Alb'05; FRCPC; Gastroent; IntMed. Staff, Hamilton Health Sciences Centre - McMaster Children's Hospital; Teach Staff, McMaster University; (905)521-2100 x76380; Fax. (905)523-6048.

XENOS, John B; Clinique Med Cite Rive, 107-7095 boul Gouin E, Montreal QC H1E 6N1; McG'63; MDCM; LMCC; hon Staff, Hopital Maisonneuve-Rosemont; Med Consultant, Centre Hospitalier l'Université de Montréal (CHUM) - Hôpital Notre-Dame; Langs: Greek; English; (514)329-4000; Fax. (514)329-9912.

XENOYANNIS, George L; 201C-600 Princess St, Woodstock ON N4S 4H4; Qns'04; FRCPC; OrthSurg. Staff, Queen Elizabeth II Health Sciences Centre - Halifax Infirmary Site; (519)290-2460

XENOYANNIS, Sophia; Carlisle Med Centre, PO Box 311 1493 Centre Rd, Carlisle ON L0R 1H0; Wes'95; CCFP; FCFP; (905)689-3301; Fax. (905)689-5772.

XEROULIS, George J; Baywood Med Centre, 503-95 Bayly St W, Ajax ON L1S 7K8; Wes'02; FRCSC; GenSurg (Laparoscopic Surgery). Staff Surg, Rouge Valley Health System - Ajax & Pickering Health Centre Site; Langs: Greek; (905)427-1718; Fax. (905)427-3827.

XHIGNESSE, Marianne C; CHUS-Hop Fleurimont, 3001 12e av N, Sherbrooke QC J1H 5N4; Sask'83; MD; BA; LMCC; MClSc; Dip Ed; Staff, Centre Hospitalier Universitaire de Sherbrooke-Hopital Fleurimont; Prof Family Med, Universite de Sherbrooke; Langs: Bilingual(French/English); (819)820-6868 x12719; Fax. (819)820-6894; marianne.xhignesse@usherbrooke.ca.

XIANG, Jianxin; Dr George-L. Dumont Reg Hosp, 330 av Universite, Moncton NB E1C 2Z3; Shanghai (China)'83; FRCPC; Anes. Staff, Dr Georges-L-Dumont University Hospital Centre; (506)862-4000

XIDOS, George; Saint John Reg Hosp, PO Box 2100 Stn Main 400 University Ave, Saint John NB E2L 4L2; Mem'87; Staff, Saint John Regional Hospital; Langs: Greek; (506)648-6000; gnxidos@yahoo.com.

XIE, Edward C; Univ Hlth Network-Toronto Gen, 200 Elizabeth St, Toronto ON M5G 2C4; Wes'09; CCFP; CCFP(E.M.); Staff, Toronto General Hospital - UHN; (416)340-3947

XIE, Jane Y; City Square Med Centre, 126-555 12th Ave W, Vancouver BC V5Z 3X7; Shanghai (China)'85; (604)568-8377

XIE, Liya; Sunridge Prof Centre, 201-2675 36 St NE, Calgary AB T1Y 6H6; (China)'82; PhD(Japan); Staff Forensic Psy Inpatient & Outpatient, Peter Lougheed Centre; Clinical Asst Prof Psy, University Of Calgary; Langs: Chinese; Japanese; (403)943-5656 x35616; Fax. (403)219-3521.

XIE, Rong; Ocean Walk Med Centre, 1884 Marine Dr, West Vancouver BC V7V 1J6; Laval'09; CCFP; Staff, Ocean Walk Medical Centre; Langs: Mandarin; French; (604)925-1884

XIE, Ying Chang; Clinique Carrefour Med Laval, 3030 boul Le Carrefour, Laval QC H7T 2P5; Sher'08; CCFP; (450)686-8899

XIN, Aiqun; Sundance West Business Park, 4120-15 Sunpark Plaza SE, Calgary AB T2X 0M5; (Other Foreign)'94; CCFP; (403)910-3990; Fax. (403)910-0449.

XU, Dejun; Carbonear Gen Hosp, 86 Highroad S, Carbonear NL A1Y 1A4; (China)'82; Staff, Carbonear General Hospital; (709)945-5111

XU, Haibo; Haldimand Family Health Team, 334 Broad St W, Dunnville ON N1A 1T1; Beijing Medical University (China)'99; CCFP; Langs: Mandarin; (905)774-7431; Fax. (905)774-4310.

XU, Jie; IWK Health Centre, PO Box 9700 Rpo CSC 5850-5980 University Ave, Halifax NS B3K 6R8; Nanjing (China)'93; Staff, IWK Health Centre; Langs: Chinese; (902)420-6749; Fax. (902)420-6469.

XU, Qiwei; Royal Jubilee Hosp, F5-1952 Bay St, Victoria BC V8R 1J8; Taishan (China)'82; FRCPC; HemPath. Staff Hem Path, Royal Jubilee Hospital; Langs: Chinese; (250)370-8995; Fax. (250)370-8873; qiwei.xu@viha.ca.

XU, Y Sophia; Hamilton HS-McMaster Site, PO Box 2000 Stn Lcd 1 1200 Main St, Hamilton ON L8N 3Z5; McM'08; FRCPC; Peds. Staff, Hamilton Health Sciences Centre - McMaster University Medical Centre; (905)521-2100

XU, Zhaodong; The Ottawa Hosp-Gen Campus, 501 Smyth Rd, Ottawa ON K1H 8L6; China Medical University (China)'91; HemPath. Staff Lab Med, The Ottawa Hospital - General Campus; (613)737-8899

XU, Zhaolin; DJ Mackenzie Bldg, 7F-5788 University Ave, Halifax NS B3H 1V8; Shanghai (China)'82; FCAP; FRCPC; AnatPath (Pulmonary Pathology). Staff, Queen Elizabeth II Health Sciences Centre - Victoria General Site; (902)473-7287; Fax. (902)473-3897.

XUAN, Andrew Y; Bayshore Med Bldg, 203-3029 Carling Ave, Ottawa ON K2B 8E8; Tor'02; FRCPC; IntMed; Gastroent. Langs: Mandarin; (613)216-8650; Fax. (613)216-8651.

XUE, Shuwen; 11 Victoria Ave, Chatham ON N7L 2Z7; Beijing (China)'82; FRCPC; IntMed. Langs: Chinese; (519)397-0684; Fax. (519)397-1817.

XULU, Helen M A; Helma Med Clinic, 103A-9914 Morrison St, Fort McMurray AB T9H 4A4; (South Africa)'03; (780)747-8703; Fax. (780)747-8728.

YABLON, Stuart; Glenrose Rehabilitation Hosp, 10230 111 Ave NW, Edmonton AB T5G 0B7; PhysMed&Rehab. Staff, Glenrose Rehabilitation Hospital; (780)735-7905; Fax. (780)735-6123.

YABLONSKY, Shmuel S; Canora Med Clinic, 14924 Stony Plain Rd NW, Edmonton AB T5P 3X8; McM'00; CCFP; Langs: Hebrew; (780)443-0300; Fax. (780)443-0059.

YACCARINI, Olivier; CHUQ-St-Francois D'Assise, 10 rue de l'Espinay, Quebec QC G1L 3L5; Laval'98; CCFP; CCFP(E.M.); Staff, Centre Hospitalier Universitaire De Québec - Pavillon De St-françois-d'assise; Langs: Spanish; English; (418)525-4444; Fax. (418)525-6338.

YACH, Jeff D; Kingston Gen Hosp, N3 305-76 Stuart St, Kingston ON K7L 2V7; Qns'93; FRCSC; OrthSurg (Spine Surgery). Staff, Kingston General Hospital; Staff, Kingston Orthopaedic & Pain Institute; Asst Prof Orthopaedic Surg, Queen's University; (613)549-6666 x3961; Fax. (613)548-1306; yachj@kgh.kari.net.

YACHNIN, Michael D; Greenboro Family Med Clinic, 25 Tapiola Cres, Ottawa ON K1T 2J7; Tor'83; Staff, The Ottawa Hospital - Riverside Campus; Staff, Children's Hospital of Eastern Ontario (CHEO); Staff, The Ottawa Hospital - General Campus; (613)738-0303

YACK, Mary E; 77 MacLaren St, Ottawa ON K2P 0K5; McM'79; FRCPC; Psy., University of Ottawa; (613)231-4146

YACOUB, Amgad K I; Rouge Valley-Ajax & Pickering, 580 Harwood Ave S, Ajax ON L1S 2J4; Ain Shams (Egypt)'86; FRCPC; Anes. Staff, Rouge Valley Health System - Ajax & Pickering Health Centre Site; (905)683-2320

YACOUB, Ashraf K I; Lorraine Wing Tower C, 201 Deacon St, Pembroke ON K8A 2J6; Ain Shams (Egypt)'84; MB ChB; MRC; FRCSC; ObstGyn. Langs: Arabic; (613)732-3675; Fax. (613)732-6339.

YACOUB, Inas; Campbellton Reg Hosp, PO Box 880 189 Lily Lake Rd, Campbellton NB E3N 3H3; Ain Shams (Egypt)'81; Staff, Hôpital Régional Campbellton; (506)789-5000

YACOUB, Magued F S; Peter Lougheed Centre, 3636-3500 26 Ave NE, Calgary AB T1Y 6J4; Cairo (Egypt)'89; MB BCh; MRCPsy; DPM; DCP; LMCC; FRCPC; Psy (Forensic Psychiatry). Staff Short Stay Unit, Peter Lougheed Centre; Clinical Asst Prof, University of Calgary; Langs: Arabic; (403)943-4904; Fax. (403)943-4815.

YACOUB, Nader S T; Percy E Moore Hosp, PO Box 190, Hodgson MB R0C 1N0; Staff, Percy E Moore Hospital; (204)372-8444

YACOUB, Ninos; Leamington & Area FHT, 197 Talbot St W, Leamington ON N8H 1N8; Ross University (USA)'03; CCFP; Staff, Leamington District Memorial Hospital; (519)322-1100; Fax. (519)322-2055.

YACOUB, Wadieh R; 730-9700 Jasper Ave NW, Edmonton AB T5J 4C3; Alexandria (Egypt)'81; MB ChB; MSc; FRCPC; CommunMed; Public Health & Preventive Med (Aboriginal Health). Clinical Asst Prof Public Health Sciences, University of Alberta; Clinical Asst Prof Community Health Sciences, University Of Calgary; Langs: Arabic; French; (780)495-3391; Fax. (780)495-8070; wadieh_yacoub@hc-sc.gc.ca.

YACOWAR, Mayer; Medcare Jane Finch, 3869 Jane St, North York ON M3N 2K1; McG'94; CCFP; Staff, Southlake Regional Health Centre; Langs: English; French; (416)636-7077; Fax. (416)635-0562.

YACYSHYN, Brian J; Radiology Consultants Assoc, 120A-6707 Elbow Dr SW, Calgary AB T2V 0E3; Alb'86; FRCPC; DiagRad. (403)777-3009; Fax. (403)777-3008.

YACYSHYN, Bruce R; University Hosp of Northern BC, 408-1475 Edmonton St, Prince George BC V2M 1S2; Alb'82; ABIM; FRCPC; IntMed (Inflammatory Bowel Disease); Gastroent. Staff, University Hospital of Northern British Columbia; (250)565-2000

YACYSHYN, Elaine A; Heritage Med Research Ctre, 562-107 University Campus NW, Edmonton AB T6G 2S2; Alb'93; FRCPC; IntMed; Rheum. Staff Heritage Med Research Ctre, University of Alberta Hospital; Staff, Royal Alexandra Hospital; Clin Teacher, University of Alberta; (780)407-7535; Fax. (780)407-6055.

YACYSHYN, Harold P; 3005 33 St, Vernon BC V1T 9X3; Alb'87; FRCPC; IntMed (Respirology). Staff, Vernon Jubilee Hospital; (250)545-9285

YACYSHYN, Vincent J; Cardiovascular Associates, 416-1011 Glenmore Trail SW, Calgary AB T2V 4R6; Alb'89; FRCPC; IntMed (Cardiology). (403)252-1311; Fax. (403)252-1317.

YADAV, Mahesh P; Medical & Dental Bldg, 504-1221 Algonquin Ave, North Bay ON P1B 4Y3; Nagpur (India)'63; MB BS; MS(GenSurg.); DAB; FAAOS; FRCSC; OrthSurg. Staff, North Bay Regional Health Centre - Regional Mental Health; Assoc Prof OrthSurg, Northern Ontario School of Medicine-Laurentian University; Langs: Urdu; Hindi; Marathi; Punjabi; (705)472-0520; Fax. (705)494-8831.

YADAV, Sunil K; Saskatoon Cancer Centre, 20 Campus Dr, Saskatoon SK S7N 4H4; Rajasthan (India)'85; MB BS; Staff, Saskatoon Cancer Centre; (306)655-2662; Fax. (306)655-2910.

YADEGARI, Andrew B; London HSC-University Campus, PO Box 5339 Stn B B6 117B-339 Windermere Rd, London ON N6A 5A5; UBC'07; IntMed (Cardiology). Staff, London Health Sciences Centre - University Hospital; (519)663-3662

YAFAI, Abdul-Aziz; PO Box 160, Kingston NS B0P 1R0; Manchester (England)'75; MB ChB; (902)765-3304; Fax. (902)765-6668.

YAFFE, Barbara A; Toronto Public Health, 5F-277 Victoria St, Toronto ON M5B 1W2; Tor'78; MHSc; FRCPC; CommunMed; Public Health & Preventive Med. Court Staff, Humber River Regional Hospital - Finch Avenue Site; Staff, Toronto Public Health Corporate Office; Aj Prof School of Public Health, University of Toronto; (416)392-7405; Fax. (416)392-0713; byaffe@toronto.ca.

YAFFE, Clifford S; 200-400 Tache Ave, Winnipeg MB R2H 3C3; Man'76; FACS; FRCSC; GenSurg (Gastrointestinal Surgery). Ac Staff, St Boniface General Hospital; Ac Staff, Concordia General Hospital; Ac Staff, Health Sciences Centre; Assoc Prof Surg/Assoc Dean Postgradate Med Education, University of Manitoba; (204)237-2326; cyaffe@sbgh.mb.ca.

YAFFE, Mark J; St Mary's Hosp Centre, 3830 av Lacombe, Montreal QC H3T 1M5; McG'76; MClSc; CCFP; FCFP; Att Médecin Family Med, St Mary's Hospital Centre; Consultant, Sir Mortimer B Davis Jewish General; Staff, St Mary's Hospital Family Medical Centre; assoc Prof, McGill University; Langs: English; French; (514)734-2677; Fax. (514)734-2602; mark.yaffe@mcgill.ca.

YAGER, Jerome Y; Edmonton Clinic Health Academy, 3 469-11405 87 Ave, Edmonton AB T6G 1C9; Man'80; CRCP; FRCPC; Peds (Neonatal Neurology). Ac Staff, University of Alberta Hospital; Prof/Head, University of Alberta; (780)248-5630

YAGHINI, Reza; Blue Mountain Comm Hlth Ctre, PO Box 280 78 King St E, Thornbury ON N0H 2P0; Shaheed Beheshti University (Israel)'92; CCFP; Staff, Grey Bruce Health Services - Meaford Site; (519)538-1311

YAHIA CHÉRIF, Dallel; Centre Med Hochelaga, 9080 rue Hochelaga, Montreal QC H1L 2N9; Ferhat Abbas University (Other Foreign)'02; (514)353-8742

YAHIA CHERIF, Tewfik; Hop Charles Lemoyne, 3120 boul Taschereau, Greenfield Park QC J4V 2H1; Sher'02; CCFP; Staff, Hopital Charles LeMoyne; (450)466-5000

YAHMAD, Nagib Y R; Toronto Memory Program, 400-1 Valleybrook Dr, North York ON M3B 2S7; University of Al Fateh (Libya)'98; FRCPC; Neur. Staff, Sunnybrook Health Sciences Centre; Staff, Toronto Memory Program; Langs: Arabic; (416)386-9761; Fax. (416)386-0458; yahmad@memorydisorders.ca.

YAHYAVI, Pooneh; Mackenzie Richmond Hill Hosp, 10 Trench St, Richmond Hill ON L4C 4Z3; Qns'94; FRCPC; IntMed. Staff, Mackenzie Richmond Hill Hospital; Langs: Farsi; (905)883-1212

YAJNIK, Dushyant K; 8A-4631 rue Sherbrooke O, Westmount QC H3Z 1G2; Minneapolis (USA)'76; Langs: Gujarati; French; Hindi; (514)989-1164

YAKE, Marvin A; Lennox & Addington Gen Hosp, 8 Richmond Park Dr, Napanee ON K7R 2Z4; Qns'75; EmergMed. Ac Staff EmergMed, London Health Sciences Centre - Victoria Campus; Staff, Lennox & Addington County General Hospital; Assoc Staff, St Joseph's Hospital - St Joseph's Health Care; Assoc Staff, London Health Sciences Centre - University Hospital; Clin Assoc Prof, University of Western Ontario; (613)354-3301; marvin.yake@lhsc.on.ca.

YAKEMCHUK, George H; Royal Jubilee Hosp, 1952 Bay St, Victoria BC V8R 1J8; Cal'77; FRCPC; DiagRad; NuclearMed. Staff, Royal Jubilee Hospital; (250)370-8272; Fax. (250)370-8594.

YAKEMCHUK, Valerie N; Hamilton HS-McMaster Site, 1200 Main St W, Hamilton ON L8N 3Z5; Cal'76; FRCPC; DiagRad; NuclearMed. Staff, Hamilton Health Sciences Centre - McMaster University Medical Centre; Staff, Hamilton Health Sciences Centre-Juravinski Site; (905)527-4322

YAKIMETS, Walter J; Meadowlark Surgical Mgmt Corp, 184 Meadowlark Shopping Ctr NW, Edmonton AB T5R 5W9; Alb'88; DAB; FRCSC; GenSurg (Breasts). Ac Staff, Covenant Health - Misericordia Community Hospital; Ac Staff, Royal Alexandra Hospital; Ac Staff, Covenant Health - Grey Nuns Community Hospital; Asst Prof, University of Alberta; (780)484-1122; Fax. (780)489-4121.

YAKIMOV, Margaret C; Interior Health Authority Corp, 1815 Kirschner Rd, Kelowna BC V1Y 4N7; UBC'83; FRCSC; ObstGyn. Staff, Kootenay Boundary Regional Hospital; Staff, Interior Health Authority Kootenay Boundary Health Service; (250)304-9815

YAKOUB, Elvira; 208-2425 Tecumseh Rd E, Windsor ON N8W 1E6; Tiranes (Albania)'94; CCFP; Langs: Albanian; Italian; (519)258-2778; Fax. (519)258-3102.

YAKOUB, Emad I; Grandview Med Ctr Fam Hlth Team, 167 Hespeler Rd, Cambridge ON N1R 3H7; Ain Shams (Egypt)'85; CCFP; Langs: Arabic; (519)623-4200; Fax. (519)623-2546.

YAKOUT, Nesrin; Scenic Acres Med Clinic, 8555 Scurfield Dr NW, Calgary AB T3L 1Z6; (Egypt)'86; CCFP; (403)547-2255; Fax. (403)547-2254.

YAKUB, Abu M; Peel Med Clinic, 475 Charolais Blvd, Brampton ON L6Y 0M2; Dacca (Bangladesh)'81; Staff, Peel Medical Clinic; Langs: Hindi; Bengali; Farsi; (905)454-3347; Fax. (905)454-3288.

YAKUBOVICH, Natalia; McMaster University Med Centre, HSC 3V51-1280 Main St W, Hamilton ON L8S 4K1; UBC'04; FRCPC; IntMed; Endocrin&Metab. Staff, Hamilton Health Sciences Centre - McMaster University Medical Centre; Staff, St Joseph's Healthcare - Charlton Campus; (905)521-2100; Fax. (905)521-4971.

YAKUBOVICH, Svetlana N; PO Box 2075 Stn Terminal, Vancouver BC V6B 3S3; UBC'03; CCFP.

YAKUBOVICH, Tatiana Y; Cannon Clinic, 4-2151 Mccallum Rd, Abbotsford BC V2S 3N9; Grodno (Belarus)'76; Langs: Russian; (604)853-3314; Fax. (604)853-2171.

YAKUNCHIKOV, Dmitry Y; Healthpoint Med Centre, 710-11010 101 St NW, Edmonton AB T5H 4B9; (Russia (Federation))'88; Staff, University of Alberta Hospital; (780)453-5255; Fax. (780)453-9099.

YALE, Jean-Francois; MUHC-Royal Victoria Hosp, 687 av des Pins O, Montreal QC H3A 1A1; Sher'79; FRCPC; Endocrin (P.Q.) (Diabetology); Endocrin&Metab. assoc Staff, McGill University Health Centre - Royal Victoria Hospital; Prof Med, McGill University; Langs: Bilingual(French/English); (514)934-1934 x35576; Fax. (514)843-1706; jean-francois.yale@mcgill.ca.

YALE, Pierre-Paul; Serv Exeterne de Psychiatrie, 230-383 boul du Seminaire N, St-Jean-sur-Richel QC J3B 8C5; Sher'76; Psy. VP, Purkinje Inc; (450)346-2222 x8450; Fax. (514)346-2311; pierre-paul.yale@rrsss16.gouv.qc.ca.

YALTHO, C Mathew; Royal Alexandra Hosp, 10240 Kingsway NW, Edmonton AB T5H 3V9; Kerala (India)'70; MB BS; DPM; DTMH; MRCPsy; FRCPC; Psy (Adult Psychiatry). Consultant Psy., Royal Alexandra Hospital; Clin Prof Med, University of Alberta; Langs: Malayalam; (780)735-4111; Fax. (780)735-4797.

YALTHO, Smitha; MacEwan Med Clinic, 10700 104 Ave NW, Edmonton AB T5J 4S2; (India)'99; CCFP; Staff CSB Weight Wise Program, Royal Alexandra Hospital; (780)497-5699; Fax. (780)497-5073.

YAM, Cecilia S F; Chancellor Medical, 821 9th St, Brandon MB R7A 4B7; Taipei (Taiwan)'73; Med Officer of Hlth, Province of Manitoba; Langs: Chinese; (204)571-6876; Fax. (204)728-1987.

YAM, Charles C T; 225-45 Edenwold Dr NW, Calgary AB T3A 3S8; Cal'78; CCFP; FCFP; (403)239-7111; Fax. (403)241-3505.

YAM, Edric C W; Pinnacle Health Sciences Centr, 2-9651 Yonge St, Richmond Hill ON L4C 1V7; Tor'93; BSc; CCFP; Langs: Cantonese; (905)780-8823 x221; Fax. (905)780-8821.

YAM, Ka-Wai; Laurel Med Centre Ltd, 202-888 8th Ave W, Vancouver BC V5Z 3Y1; UBC'08; CCFP; Langs: Cantonese; Mandarin; (604)872-5688; Fax. (604)872-7394.

YAM, Patrick K; Peace Arch Hosp, 15521 Russell Ave, White Rock BC V4B 2R4; Cal'95; CCFP; Staff, Richmond Hospital; Staff, Peace Arch Hospital; (604)531-5512

YAM, Vincy W S; 225-45 Edenwold Dr NW, Calgary AB T3A 3S8; Cal'99; CCFP; (403)241-2888; Fax. (403)241-3505; vincyyam@hotmail.com.

YAMABE, David L; Associate Med Centre, 5016 48 Ave, Taber AB T1G 1R8; Alb'84; CCFP; FCFP; Staff Chief, Taber Health Centre; (403)223-3525; Fax. (403)223-9020.

YAMADA, Drew C; Fishermen's Mem Hosp, 14 High St, Lunenburg NS B0J 2C0; Dal'07; FRCPC; Peds. Staff, Fishermen's Memorial Hospital; (902)634-8801

YAMAGISHI, Kyle F Y; Gates Med Centre, 15-300 Kingston Rd, Pickering ON L1V 6Z9; Alb'06; CCFP; (905)509-4595; Fax. (905)509-4597.

YAMAMOTO, Brian R; Fairview Med Arts Centre, 208-2200 Fairview St, Burlington ON L7R 4H9; Wes'84; Staff, Joseph Brant Memorial Hospital; (905)632-2542; Fax. (905)632-2617.

YAMAMOTO, Hans Y; Catledowns Medicentre, 120-15277 Castle Downs Rd NW, Edmonton AB T5X 3N5; Alb'87; (780)457-5511; Fax. (780)456-4004.

YAMAMOTO, Kenneth K; Winnipeg Clinic, 425 St Mary Ave, Winnipeg MB R3C 0N2; Alb'76; BMedSci; DABOG; FACOG; FSOGC; FRCSC; ObstGyn (Endometriosis). Ac Staff Women's Hosp, Health Sciences Centre; Ac Staff, Seven Oaks General Hospital; Asst Prof ObstGyn/Clin Lecturer Family Practice, University of Manitoba; (204)957-3209; Fax. (204)943-1900.

YAMAMURA, Deborah L R; Hamilton HSC-Hamilton Gen Hosp, 1 117-237 Barton St E, Hamilton ON L8L 2X2; Qns'92; BSc; ABIM; FRCPC; IntMed; MedMicrobiol; InfectDis. Staff Med Microbiol & InfectDis, Hamilton Health Sciences Centre - Hamilton General Hospital; Staff Med Microbiol & InfectDis, St Joseph's Healthcare - Charlton Campus; Assoc Prof Path & Molecular Med, McMaster University; (905)527-4322; Fax. (905)529-7142.

YAMANAKA, Michael W; Occupational Health Programs, PO Box 9421 Stn Prov Govt, Vancouver BC V6Z 2H2; UBC'95; BSc; MSc; FRCPC; OccupMed. Staff, Workers' Comp Board of BC; Staff, BC Public Service Agency; (250)952-4228

YAMASHIRO, Hirotaka; Pinnacle Health Sciences Centr, 2-9651 Yonge St, Richmond Hill ON L4C 1V7; Tor'93; FRCP; FAAP; FRCPC; Peds (Respirology). Staff, Pinnacle Health Sciences Centre; Lecturer Comm Peds, University of Toronto; Langs: Japanese; (905)780-8823; Fax. (905)780-8821.

YAMASHITA, Cory M; Lawson Health Research Inst, E5 102-268 Grosvenor St, London ON N6A 4V2; Man'01; FRCPC; IntMed; Respir. Staff, London Health Sciences Centre - University Hospital; Staff, Lawson Health Research Institute; (519)646-6000; Fax. (519)646-6404; cory.yamashita@lhsc.on.ca.

YAMASHITA, Kathryn F; Legacy Med Centre, 378 4 Ave S, Lethbridge AB T1J 5E9; Cal'75; CCFP; FCFP; Ac Staff, Chinook Regional Hospital; Ac Staff, Covenant Health - St Michael's Health Centre; (403)320-1504; Fax. (403)329-3778; dryam@telusplanet.net.

YAMKA, Edward M; William Osler HC-Etobicoke, 101 Humber College Blvd, Etobicoke ON M9V 1R8; Tor'64; FRCPC; Anes. Staff, William Osler Health System - Etobicoke General Hospital; (416)747-3554

YAMMINE, Fady G; CSSS Jardins-Roussillons, 200 boul Brisebois, Chateauguay QC J6K 4W8; Beyrouth (Lebanon)'91; Staff, Hôpital Anna-Laberge; (450)699-2425

YAMSUAN, Marlen C; Meadowood Med Centre, 1555 St Mary's Rd, Winnipeg MB R2M 5L9; UP (Philippines)'84; FRCPC; Peds.

YAN, Alexander; 124 Street Med Group, 10839 124 St NW, Edmonton AB T5M 0H4; Alb'83; BMedSci; FRCPC; IntMed; Rheum. Ac Staff, Royal Alexandra Hospital; Ac Staff, Glenrose Rehabilitation Hospital; Clin Assoc Prof, University of Alberta; Langs: Chinese; Cantonese; (780)455-6740; Fax. (780)452-8936.

YAN, Andrew T; St Michael's Hosp, Q6 030-30 Bond St, Toronto ON M5B 1W8; Tor'98; FRCPC; IntMed; Cardiol. Staff Cardiol/Asst Prof Med, St Michael's Hospital; Langs: Cantonese; (416)864-5465

YAN, Brian; London HSC-Victoria Campus, PO Box 5010 Stn B E1 419A-800 Commissioners Rd E, London ON N6A 5W9; Cal'01; BScH; FRCPC; IntMed (Endoscopic Ultrasound); Gastroent. Staff, London Health Sciences Centre - Victoria Campus; Langs: Chinese; (519)667-6582; Fax. (519)667-6820.

YAN, David B; Mount Sinai Hosp, 410-600 University Ave, Toronto ON M5G 1X5; Tor'92; FRCSC; Ophth. Staff, Mount Sinai Hospital; Staff, Ontario Power Generation Inc; Langs: Chinese; (416)586-5151; david.yan@opg.com.

YAN, Hongyun; Thunder Bay Reg HSC, 980 Oliver Rd, Thunder Bay ON P7B 6V4; Hebei Medical College (Other Foreign)'87; CCFP; Staff Hospitalist Program, Thunder Bay Regional Health Sciences Centre; (807)684-6000

YAN, Ilym G; Prime Care Medical, 108-8927 152 St, Surrey BC V3R 4E5; McG'86; CCFP; FCFP; Langs: Cantonese; (604)588-8998; Fax. (604)588-8926.

YAN, Justin W; Four Counties Health Services, 1824 Concession Dr, Newbury ON N0L 1Z0; Wes'09.

YAN, Michael; Ermineskin Med Clinic, 301-2377 111 St NW, Edmonton AB T6J 5E5; Alb'00; CCFP; (780)436-8731; Fax. (780)434-8732.

YAN, Raymond T; Scarborough Prof Centre, 406-1371 Neilson Rd, Scarborough ON M1B 4Z8; Tor'01; FRCPC; IntMed; Cardiol. Staff, St Michael's Hospital; Langs: Chinese; (416)281-9499; Fax. (416)283-5705.

YAN, Sen Rong; Dr Everett Chalmers Hosp, PO Box 9000 Stn A 700 Priestman St, Fredericton NB E3B 5N5; Guangdong (China)'82; FRCPC; AnatPath. Staff, Dr Everett Chalmers Regional Hospital.

YANCHAR, Natalie L; IWK Health Centre, PO Box 9700 Rpo CSC 5850-5980 University Ave, Halifax NS B3K 6R8; Qns'90; MSc; FRCSC; GenSurg; PedGenSurg. Staff Gen Ped/Med Dir IWK Trauma Care Program, IWK Health Centre; Assoc Prof Surg, Dalhousie University; (902)470-8114; Fax. (902)470-7260; natalie.yanchar@iwk.nshealth.ca.

YANCHULA, Catherine A; Windsor Health Centre, 360-1720 Howard Ave, Windsor ON N8X 5A6; McM'96; RN; BScN; BA; CCFP; FCFP; Aj Prof Family Med, University of Western Ontario; (519)977-6458; Fax. (519)977-6471.

YANCHYSHYN, Gordon W; 1106-180 Bloor St W, Toronto ON M5S 2V6; Man'74; FRCPC; Psy. Assoc Prof/Asst Staff, The Hospital For Sick Children; Asst Prof, University of Toronto; (416)960-9129

YANG, Brian P T; 309-233 Nelson's Cres, New Westminster BC V3L 0E4; UBC'05; FRCSC; Urol. Langs: Mandarin; (604)522-1005

YANG, Carol S; Lincoln Heights Med Centre, 201-1305 Richmond Rd, Ottawa ON K2B 7Y4; Tor'82; Langs: American Sign Language; (613)829-3221; Fax. (613)829-6832.

YANG, Christine P; SCOHS-Elisabeth Bruyere Hosp, 43 Bruyere St, Ottawa ON K1N 5C8; Shanghai (China)'85; FRCPC; PhysMed&Rehab (Stroke Rehabilitation). Staff PhysMed& Rehab Services, SCO Health Service - Élisabeth Bruyère Hospital; Asst Prof, University of Ottawa; (613)562-0050; Fax. (613)562-6312; cyang@scohs.on.ca.

YANG, Connie L; Children's & Women's HC of BC, 4480 Oak St, Vancouver BC V6H 3N1; Tor'04; FRCPC; Peds; Respir. Staff, BC Children's Hospital; (604)875-2345

YANG, Elisa Y S; Dr Elisa Yang Med Clinic, 243-2039 Robertson Rd, Nepean ON K2H 8R2; Ott'76; Langs: Chinese; (613)829-3401; Fax. (613)829-1237.

YANG, Heather C; St Joseph's Health Centre, 30 The Queensway, Toronto ON M6R 1B5; Mem'96; FRCPC; Peds. Staff, St Joseph's Health Centre; (416)530-6625; Fax. (416)530-6294.

YANG, Homer Y H; The Ottawa Hosp-Civic Campus, B309-1053 Carling Ave, Ottawa ON K1Y 4E9; Tor'80; FRCPC; Anes;CCFP; Chief, The Ottawa Hospital - Civic Campus; Dir Professionalism/Dept Chair Anes, University of Ottawa; Langs: Chinese; (613)761-4940; Fax. (613)761-5032.

YANG, Hua; Foothills Med Centre, 1403 29 St NW, Calgary AB T2N 2T9; Shanghai (China)'83; FRCPC; AnatPath. Staff Calgary Lab Services, Foothills Medical Centre; (403)944-4056; Fax. (403)944-4748.

YANG, Hui-Min; St Paul's Hosp, 1081 Burrard St, Vancouver BC V6Z 1Y6; Vanderbilt University (USA)'05; Staff, Providence Health Care - St Paul's Hospital; Langs: Mandarin; (604)682-2344

YANG, Huiming; 2202 2 St SW, Calgary AB T2S 3C1; Shanxi (China)'84; FRCPC; CommunMed. Staff, Tom Baker Cancer Centre; (403)698-8122; Fax. (403)355-3289.

YANG, Ilun; Univ of Ottawa, 2044-451 Smyth Rd, Ottawa ON K1H 8M5; Tor'06; FRCSC; GenSurg. Teacher, University of Ottawa.

YANG, Iwan; MCI Medical Clinic, 245 Eglinton Ave E, Toronto ON M4P 3B7; Tor'93; CCFP; (416)488-1455; Fax. (416)488-8846.

YANG, Jerome; 29 Pender St W, Vancouver BC V6B 1R3; UBC'04; CCFP; (604)669-9181

YANG, Jianing; Clinic Source Unique Hawkesbur, 219 Main St E, Hawkesbury ON K6A 1A1; McG'06; MDCM; Langs: Mandarin; English; (613)632-4185

YANG, Jiao; UBC Hosp, S110-2211 Wesbrook Mall, Vancouver BC V6T 2B5; Sask'05; FRCPC; IntMed; Cardiol. Staff, Vancouver General Hospital - Centennial Pavillion; Staff, Gordon & Leslie Diamond Health Care Centre; Staff, UBC Hospital - Koerner Pavillion; (604)822-1747

YANG, Joanne; Crossroads Clinic, 350-507 Broadway W, Vancouver BC V5Z 1E6; Dal'06; CCFP; (204)253-5320; Fax. (204)253-5753.

YANG, John C; Cambridge Mem Hosp, 700 Coronation Blvd, Cambridge ON N1R 3G2; Wes'93; FRCPC; IntMed; GeriatricMed. Staff, Cambridge Memorial Hospital; Asst Prof Med, McMaster University; (519)621-2330 x3390; Fax. (519)740-4942.

YANG, Joseph C; Nordel Crossing Med Clinic, 115-12080 Nordel Way, Surrey BC V3W 1P6; Tor'93; CCFP; (604)543-0888; Fax. (604)543-0231.

YANG, Kwang; Gateway Med Centre, 102-10751 King George Blvd, Surrey BC V3T 2X6; (Taiwan)'69; CCFP; FCFP; Ac Staff, Surrey Memorial Hospital; Teach Staff Alternative Route to Certification in Family Med, British Columbia College of Family Physicians; Facilitator, Diabetic & Viral Hepatitis Teaching Courses; Assoc Prof, University of British Columbia; Langs: Cantonese; Vietnamese; Chinese; Chiuchow; Chowchau; Fukinese; Taiwanese; Hainam; (604)581-2611; Fax. (604)581-5069.

YANG, Lawrence; Gateway Med Centre, 10751 King George Hwy, Surrey BC V3T 2X6; Dominica (Other Foreign)'05; CCFP; (604)588-5988

YANG, Lisa D S; Loch Lomond Med Clinic, 243 Loch Lomond Rd, Saint John NB E2J 1Y6; Mem'97; CCFP; Langs: Bilingual(English/French); (506)648-0606; Fax. (506)652-4284.

YANG, Malissa; William Osler HC-Brampton Civi, 2100 Bovaird Dr E, Brampton ON L6R 3J7; McM'01; Staff, William Osler Health System - Brampton Civic Hospital; Langs: Cantonese; (905)494-2120

YANG, Marjorie L; Winchester Dist Mem Hosp, 566 Louise St, Winchester ON K0C 2K0; Alb'99; CCFP; CCFP(E.M.); Staff, Winchester District Memorial Hospital; (613)774-2422

YANG, Min Kang; City Centre Med Clinic, 203-3420 Hurontario St, Mississauga ON L5B 4A9; Tor'92; Ac Staff, Trillium Health Centre - Mississauga; Langs: Chinese; (905)897-1998; Fax. (905)897-1178.

YANG, Peter B; 475-4789 Kingsway, Burnaby BC V5H 0A3; (Taiwan)'71; Langs: Cantonese; Mandarin; Shanghai; (604)435-4733

YANG, Robert C; St Joseph's Healthcare, 50 Charlton Ave E, Hamilton ON L8N 4A6; Qns'00; FRCPC; IntMed; Nephrol. Staff, St Joseph's Healthcare - Charlton Campus; (905)522-1155

YANG, Sharmila; Gateway Med Centre, 10751 King George Blvd, Surrey BC V3T 2X6; (Other Foreign)'06; CCFP; (604)588-5988

YANG, Theresa L; Peter Lougheed Centre, 3500 26 Ave NE, Calgary AB T1Y 6J4; Cal'93; BSc; FRCPC; Anes. Staff Anes, Peter Lougheed Centre; Clinical Asst Prof, University of Calgary; (403)943-5554; Fax. (403)943-4474.

YANG, Tony; 6290 199 St NW PO Box 73057 Rpo Hampton, Edmonton AB T5T 2K4; Alb'01; CCFP; Member, Alberta Medical Association.

YANG, Tung C; Burrard Health Bldg, 203-1160 Burrard St, Vancouver BC V6Z 2E8; Ott'85; FRCPC; IntMed; MedMicrobiol; InfectDis. Staff, Providence Health Care - St Paul's Hospital; Staff, Providence Health Care - Mount Saint Joseph Hospital; Langs: Chinese; Japanese; (604)689-7200; tcyang@providencehealth.bc.ca.

YANG, Una M C; Brunswick Clinic, 401-955 boul Saint-Jean, Pointe-Claire QC H9R 5K3; McG'97; CCFP; Staff, St Mary's Hospital Centre; (514)426-6677; unayang@hotmail.com.

YANG, Victor X D; Sunnybrook Hlth Sciences Ctre, 2075 Bayview Ave, Toronto ON M4N 3M5; Tor'06; FRCSC; Neursurg. Staff, Sunnybrook Health Sciences Centre; (416)480-6100

YANG, W Y Philip; Bridlewood Med Clinic, 203-3443 Finch Ave E, Scarborough ON M1W 2S1; Tor'78; Court Staff Family Pract, The Scarborough Hospital - Birchmount Campus; Langs: Chinese; (416)493-4424; Fax. (416)490-8180.

YANG, William H; Yang Med Prof Corp, 707-1081 Carling Ave, Ottawa ON K1Y 4G2; National Taiwan University (Taiwan)'72; FAAAI; FRCPC; IntMed (Clinical Immunology & Allergy). Dir Allergy & Asthma Research Centre/Pres, The Ottawa Hospital - Civic Campus; Clinical Asst Prof, University of Ottawa; Langs: Burmese; Chinese; (613)725-2113 x223; Fax. (613)725-0317; wyang@yangmedicine.com.

YANIVKER, Susanna; Hamilson HSC-Hamilton Gen Hosp, 237 Barton St E, Hamilton ON L8L 2X2; Wes'00; Staff, Hamilton Health Sciences Centre - Hamilton General Hospital; Langs: Russian; (416)340-3947; Fax. (416)340-5466.

YANKO, Paul E; Nicola Med Dental Bldg, 200-321 Nicola St, Kamloops BC V2C 6G6; UBC'80; CCFP; FCFP; (250)372-5522; Fax. (250)372-8412.

YANKOVA, Sylvia A; Centre Hosp de LaSalle, 8585 tsse Champlain, LaSalle QC H8P 1C1; Sofia (Bulgaria)'88; CCFP; Staff, Centre Hospitalier de LaSalle; Langs: Bulgarian; (514)362-8000

YANKOVSKY, Alexei E; Health Sciences Centre, GE 543-820 Sherbrook St, Winnipeg MB R3A 1R9; Sverdlovsk State Medical Institute (Other Foreign)'93; FRCPC; Neur. Staff, Health Sciences Centre; (204)774-6511

YANNI, Ahlam H R; Family Practice & Obstetrics, 202-1920 Ellesmere Rd, Scarborough ON M1H 2V6; Cairo (Egypt)'80; Ac Member, The Scarborough Hospital - General Campus; Langs: Arabic; (416)449-6132; Fax. (416)449-6132.

YANOFSKY, Howard; 609-5885 ch Cote-des-Neiges, Montreal QC H3S 2T2; McG'73; FAB; FRCPC; Derm. Langs: English; French; (514)342-2646; Fax. (514)341-9375.

YANOFSKY, Michael J; Beach Clinic, 350 Beech Ave, Toronto ON M4E 3T8; Tor'85; Staff Privil, Toronto East General Hospital Inc; (416)694-1126; Fax. (416)691-5040.

YANOFSKY, Rochelle A; Cancercare Manitoba, 675 McDermot Ave, Winnipeg MB R3E 0V9; Man'77; FRCPC; Peds (Pediatric Hematology Oncology). Ac Staff Ped HemOncol, Health Sciences Centre; Ac Staff Ped HemOncol, CancerCare Manitoba; Assoc Prof Peds/Coord Elective, University of Manitoba; (204)787-4135; Fax. (204)786-0195; rochelle.yanofsky@cancercare.mb.ca.

YANOVER, David F; 1568 Main St W, Hamilton ON L8S 1E7; McM'96; BSc; LLB; CCFP; (905)529-3211; Fax. (905)529-3864.

YANOVER, H Clifford; Chinook Reg Hosp, 960 19 St S, Lethbridge AB T1J 1W5; McM'84; LLB; BA; FRCPC; Anes. Staff, Chinook Regional Hospital; (403)388-6131; Fax. (403)388-6135.

YANSOUNI, Cedric; MUHC-Montreal Gen Hosp, L10 509-1650 av Cedar, Montreal QC H3G 1A4; McG'02; FRCPC; IntMed; MedMicrobiol; InfectDis. Staff, McGill University Health Centre - Montreal General Campus; (514)934-1934 x48049

YAO, Christiana Y; Meadowlands Fam Hlth Ctre, 888 Meadowlands Dr, Ottawa ON K2C 3R2; UBC'97; CCFP; FCFP; Physician, Meadowlands Family Health Centre; (613)228-2882; Fax. (613)228-2856.

YAO, Jennifer K; G F Strong Rehabilitation Ctre, 4255 Laurel St, Vancouver BC V5Z 2G9; UBC'97; BSc(Hon); FRCPC; PhysMed&Rehab (Stroke). Staff, G F Strong Rehabilitation Centre; Clinical Asst Prof, University of British Columbia; Langs: Mandarin; (604)714-4113; Fax. (604)737-6251.

YAO, Louis C H; Westlaw Bldg, 230-1920 Weston Rd, York ON M9N 1W4; Man'78; FRCPC; Cardiol. Staff, Humber River Regional Hospital - Church Street Site; University of Toronto; Langs: Chinese; (416)241-1119; Fax. (416)241-2623.

YAO, Peter Y O; 308-1676 Martin Dr, Surrey BC V4A 6E7; Quezon City (Philippines)'73; FRCSC; OrthSurg. Consultant, Peace Arch Hospital; Langs: Chinese; Mandarin; Tagalog; (604)536-1446; Fax. (604)536-1213.

YAO, Roger; University of Alberta Hosp, 1G1-8440 112 St NW, Edmonton AB T6G 2B7; Alb'92; CCFP; CCFP(E.M.); Staff, University of Alberta Hospital; (780)407-7047

YAO, Shaoyee; 108-2051 McCallum Rd, Abbotsford BC V2S 3N5; UBC'07; FRCPC; IntMed; Nephrol. (604)870-9886

YAO, Shengtao; PO Box 23204 Rpo Prairie Mall, Grande Prairie AB T8V 7G7; Shandong (China)'86; Staff Emerg, Queen Elizabeth II Hospital; Langs: Mandarin; (780)665-2786; Fax. (780)665-2786.

YAO, Yu-Ju; CLSC des Faubourgs, 1250 rue Sanguinet, Montreal QC H2X 3E7; Mon'02; CCFP; Staff, Centre Hospitalier l'Université De Montréal (CHUM) - Hôpital Saint-luc; Langs: Chinese; English; (514)527-2361

YAO, Zhenhai; Mackenzie Richmond Hill Hosp, 10 Trench St, Richmond Hill ON L4C 4Z3; Sun Yat Sen (China)'87; FRCPC; Anes. Staff, Mackenzie Richmond Hill Hospital; Langs: Chinese; (905)883-1212

YAP, Audrey P G; Toronto Rehab Inst-Univ Ctr, 550 University Ave, Toronto ON M5G 2A2; UBC'02; DipABPMR; FRCPC; PhysMed&Rehab (Musculoskeletal Rehabilitation). Staff MSK Physiatry Outpatient Clinic, Toronto Rehabilitation Institute - University Centre; Staff, Lyndhurst Centre; (416)597-3422 x6133; Fax. (416)516-6373; audrey.yap@uhn.ca.

YAP, David T T; 203-3825 Sunset St, Burnaby BC V5G 1T4; Cal'99; ACLS; BSc; FCFP; LMCC; MCFP; FICA; (604)434-9515; Fax. (604)434-5984.

YAP, Hanle O; Jackson Park Health Centre, 150-2475 McDougall Ave, Windsor ON N8X 3N9; UP (Philippines)'94; FRCPC; IntMed; GeriatricMed. Staff, Leamington District Memorial Hospital; Langs: Chinese; Tagalog; (519)252-9861; Fax. (519)252-7787.

YAP, Jason Y K; Edmonton Clinic Health Academy, 4 573-11405 87 Ave NW, Edmonton AB T6G 1C9; Auckland (New Zealand)'96; Staff, Edmonton Clinic Health Academy; (780)248-5420; Fax. (780)248-5627.

YAP, John C P; Royal City Centre, 228B-610 Sixth St, New Westminster BC V3L 3C2; UBC'87; (604)521-8522; Fax. (604)521-8554.

YAP, Keith D; South Richter Prof Bldg, 207-3330 Richter St, Kelowna BC V1W 4V5; Alb'89; FRCSC; Ophth (Pediatric Ophthalmology & Adult Strabismus). (250)868-3866; Fax. (250)868-3858.

YAP, Stanley A; Univ Hlth Network-Princess M, 3 130-610 University Ave, Toronto ON M5G 2M9; Loyola University of Chicago (USA)'04; FRCSC; Urol. Staff, Princess Margaret Hospital - University Health Network; (416)946-2909

YAP, Stephanie T M; Ryerson Med Centre, 350 Victoria St, Toronto ON M5B 2K3; Qns'09; CCFP; (416)979-5070; Fax. (416)979-5073.

YAPHE, Joel S; 293 Rushton Rd, Toronto ON M6C 2X8; Tor'78; FRCPC; EmergMed. Staff, Toronto Western Hospital - University Health Network; (416)654-1865

YAQUB, Syed M T; Millbourne Med Clinic, 115 Millbourne Shopp Ctr NW, Edmonton AB T6K 3L6; Dacca (Bangladesh)'58; (587)521-2022; Fax. (587)521-2023.

YAR, Qasim A; West Haldimand Gen Hosp, 3-75 Parkview Lane, Hagersville ON N0A 1H0; Jabalpur (India)'83; MB BS; Staff, West Haldimand General Hospital; Langs: Hindi; Persian; Pashtu; (905)768-3311

YAR KHAN, Saulat; R J A Medicentres Cnd Inc, 204-10458 Mayfield Rd NW, Edmonton AB T5P 4P4; (780)483-7115; Fax. (780)484-6315.

YARASCAVITCH, Alec J; Northern Ontario School of Med, 935 Ramsey Lake Rd, Sudbury ON P3E 2C6; McM'10; CCFP.

YARASCAVITCH, Blake A; McMaster University, MDCL 3101A-1280 Main St W, Hamilton ON L8S 4K1; McM'08.

YARDE, Muriel V; Bluewater Health-Norman Site, 89 Norman St, Sarnia ON N7T 6S3; West Indies (Other Foreign)'66; MB BS; FRCPC; Anes. Staff, Bluewater Health - Norman Site; Staff, Bluewater Health - Mitton Site; (519)464-4500 x5407

YARDLEY, Nicholas J; Postgrad Med Education Office, 602-500 University Ave, Toronto ON M5G 1V7; Wes'06; FRCSC; OrthSurg.

YARED, Kibar; Rouge Valley Cardiology, 406-1371 Neilson Rd, Scarborough ON M1B 4Z8; McG'01; FRCPC; Cardiol; IntMed. Langs: Arabic; French; (416)281-9499; Fax. (416)283-5705.

YARED, Nada; 3120 boul Taschereau, Greenfield Park QC J4V 2H1; Mon'04; FRCPC; IntMed; InfectDis; MedMicrobiol. Staff, Hopital Charles LeMoyne; (450)466-5000 x2960; Fax. (450)466-5778.

YARED, Zeina; LMC Centre d'endocrinologie, 6363-238 rte Transcanadienne, Saint-Laurent QC H4T 1Z9; Mon'99; FRCPC; IntMed (Diabetology); Endocrin&Metab. Staff, Hôpital du Sacre-Coeur de Montréal; Staff, Institut de Recherches Cliniques de Montreal; Langs: Arabic; English; (514)744-5620

YAREMA, Mark C; Foothills Med Centre, C213-1403 29 St NW, Calgary AB T2N 2T9; UBC'96; FRCPC; EmergMed. Staff Poison & Drug Information, Foothills Medical Centre; (403)944-6900; Fax. (403)944-1472.

YAREMCO, Michael E; Steel Head Med Centre, PO Box 1238 2370 Poutton Ave, Houston BC V0J 1Z0; Alb'75; (250)845-7747; Fax. (250)845-7713.

YAREMKO, Brian P; London Reg Cancer Centre, 790 Commissioners Rd E, London ON N6A 4L6; Alb'00; FRCPC; RadOncol. Staff, London Regional Cancer Center; Langs: Bilingual(English/French); (519)685-8500; Fax. (519)685-8627; brian.yaremko@lhsc.on.ca.

YAREMKO, John F; 4500 rue Sherbrooke O, Westmount QC H3Z 1E6; McG'80; FAAP; FRCPC; Peds (Infectious Diseases). Staff Pt-Time, McGill University Health Centre - Montreal Children's Hospital; adj Prof, McGill University; Langs: English; French; (514)932-4975; Fax. (514)932-9984.

YAREMKO-DOLAN, Marie; 65 av Westminster N, Montreal-Ouest QC H4X 1Y8; McG'77; CCFP; Asst Prof Family Med, McGill University; (514)481-0008; Fax. (514)369-1234.

YAREN, Stanley; Psychealth Centre, PX 362-771 Bannatyne Ave, Winnipeg MB R3E 3N4; Man'72; FRCPC; Psy (Forensic Psychiatry). Ac Staff, Health Sciences Centre; Med Staff Assoc, Regional Psychiatric Centre - Prairies; Dir Adult Forensic Services, Manitoba Health; Assoc Prof, University of Manitoba; (204)787-3887; Fax. (204)945-1112; stanley.yaren@gov.mb.ca.

YARNOLD, Cynthia; St Paul's Hosp, 3F-1081 Burrard St, Vancouver BC V6Z 1Y6; UBC'02; FRCPC; Anes. Staff, Providence Health Care - St Paul's Hospital; (604)875-5855

YARROW, Colin F; Glenmore Clinic, G-1605 Gordon Dr, Kelowna BC V1Y 3G8; UBC'84; CCFP; FCFP; (250)763-4400; Fax. (250)763-4388.

YASEEN, Muhammad; Sunnybrook Hlth Sciences Ctre, 3F-2075 Bayview Ave, Toronto ON M4N 3M5; Punjab University (India)'98; Anes. Staff, Sunnybrook Health Sciences Centre; (416)480-6100

YASEEN, Salma; Foothills Med Centre, 1243-1403 29 St NW, Calgary AB T2N 2T9; (Pakistan)'76; Staff Clinical Neurosciences, Foothills Medical Centre; (403)944-4220; Fax. (403)283-2270.

YASER, Aseel; Langstaff Med Centre, 12B-8401 Weston Rd RR 2, Woodbridge ON L4L 1A6; Baghdad (Iraq)'91; MB ChB; CCFP; Langs: Arabic; (905)856-6142; Fax. (905)856-9824.

YASHPAL, Nina K; Credit Valley Family Health Te, 101-2300 Eglinton Ave W, Mississauga ON L5M 2V8; Tor'08; CCFP; Staff, The Credit Valley Hospital; Aj Prof Part-Time, University of Toronto; Langs: Punjabi; (905)813-3850

YASIN, Nasif I; 303-828 8th Ave W, Vancouver BC V5Z 1E2; Garyunis (Libya)'79; MB ChB; FRCPC; PhysMed&Rehab. Langs: Arabic; (604)877-0807; Fax. (604)877-0507.

YASIN, Saad; Humana Med Clinic, 136-3715 51 St SW, Calgary AB T3E 6V2; (Other Foreign)'98; CCFP; Langs: Urdu; Punjabi; Hindi; (403)686-6967; Fax. (403)686-3736.

YASINIAN, Azadeh Y; Wilson Med Centre, 130 Wilson St, Hamilton ON L8R 1K2; Xavier University School of Medicine (Aruba)'06.

YASMEEN, Naveeda; Professional Arts Bldg, 102-155 James St S, Hamilton ON L8P 3A4; Punjab University (Pakistan)'87; MB BS; CCFP; Langs: Hindi; Urdu; Punjabi; (905)528-8747; Fax. (905)528-9742; drnaveeda@hotmail.com.

YASSA, Mariam; CHUM-Hopital Hotel-Dieu, 3840 rue Saint Urbain, Montreal QC H2W 1T8; Ain Shams (Egypt)'76; RadOncol (P.Q.). assoc Staff, St Mary's Hospital Centre; Staff, Centre Hospitalier l'Université de Montréal (CHUM) - Hôtel-Dieu; Langs: Arabic; French; (514)890-8066

YASSA, Michael; Hop Maisonneuve-Rosemont, 5415 boul de l'Assomption, Montreal QC H1T 2M4; McG'03; FRCPC; RadOncol. Staff, Hopital Maisonneuve-Rosemont; (514)252-3425; Fax. (514)252-3558.

YASSA, Naguib H; Brockville Gen Hosp, 75 Charles St, Brockville ON K6V 1S8; Alexandria (Egypt)'76; FRCPC; GenPath; AnatPath. Chief Lab Mgr, Brockville General Hospital - Charles Street; Langs: Arabic; French; (613)345-5649 x1161; yasna@bgh-on.ca.

YASSA, Samir A R; McConnell Med Centre, 215-820 McConnell Ave, Cornwall ON K6H 4M4; Cairo (Egypt)'63; FRCSC; Urol (Pediatric & Adult). Consultant, Glengarry Memorial Hospital; Staff Urol, Cornwall Community Hospital; Urology, Cornwall Community Hospital - Second Street Site; Langs: Arabic; (613)933-1610; Fax. (613)938-0537.

YASSA, Teraiza S S; The Court Centenary Hosp, 319-2863 Ellesmere Rd, Scarborough ON M1E 5E9; Cairo (Egypt)'83; FRCPC; IntMed; Nephrol. Staff, Rouge Valley Health System - Centenary Health Centre Site; Langs: Arabic; (416)281-3336; Fax. (416)281-8385.

YASSEIN, Hossam; 201 King St W, Oshawa ON L1J 2J5; Qns'86; FRCSC; Ophth. Assoc Staff, Lakeridge Health - Bowmanville Site; Assoc Staff, Lakeridge Health - Oshawa Site; Assoc Staff, Lakeridge Health - Whitby Site; (905)434-1694; Fax. (905)434-6308.

YASSER, Zaid J; Malvern Med Centre, 335-1333 Neilson Rd, Scarborough ON M1B 4Y9; Baghdad (Iraq)'98; FRCSC; GenSurg (Surgical Oncology). Langs: Arabic; (416)724-7774; Fax. (416)724-7752.

YASSI, Annalee; 114-1917 4th Ave W, Vancouver BC V6J 1M7; McM'77; CCBOM; DOHS; FRCPC; CommunMed; OccupMed. Langs: Spanish; French; (604)916-6764

YASUFUKU, Kazuhiro; Univ Hlth Network-Toronto Gen, E9N 957-200 Elizabeth St, Toronto ON M5G 2C4; Chiba Medical University (Japan)'92; PhD; Staff Thoracic Surg, Toronto General Hospital - UHN; Asst Prof, University of Toronto; Langs: Japanese; (416)340-4290; Fax. (416)340-3660.

YATES, Derrick A; 299 Main St N, Callander ON P0H 1H0; McM'03; CCFP; Staff, North Bay Regional Health Centre - Regional Mental Health; (705)752-1004; Fax. (705)752-4507.

YATES, John G; Oakville Health Centre, 208-1060 Speers Rd, Oakville ON L6L 2X4; McM'83; Ac Staff, Halton Healthcare Services Corporation - Oakville Site; Langs: Creole; (905)842-3735; Fax. (905)842-8001.

YATES, Stephen K; Maple Key Clinic Family Hlth Team, D2-1036 Princess St, Kingston ON K7L 1H2; Wes'88; CCFP; FCFP; (613)546-9721

YATES, Thomas H; York Radiology Consultants, 100-1333 Sheppard Ave E, North York ON M2J 1V1; Tor'60; DiagRad. Staff Diag Imaging, North York General Hospital; (416)494-8800; Fax. (416)494-9257.

YATES, Timothy T; Henry Huang Bldg, 320-2204 2 St SW, Calgary AB T2S 3C2; McG'68; DPsy; FRCPC; Psy (Psychodynamic/Psychotherapy). Clin Associate Prof Peds & Psy, University of Calgary; Langs: Bilingual(English/French); (403)244-9962; Fax. (403)255-9340; yatest@telus.net.

YATHAM, Lakshmi N; UBC-Dept of Psychiatry, 0007-2255 Wesbrook Mall, Vancouver BC V6T 2A1; Tirupati (India)'84; MB BS; MRCPsy; FRCPC; Psy. Staff, UBC Hospital - Koerner Pavillion; Langs: Telugu; Kanarese; (604)822-7325; Fax. (604)822-7922; yatham@interchange.ubc.ca.

YATHINDRA, Yashi K; North York Gen Hosp, 4001 Leslie St, North York ON M2K 1E1; Tor'08; CCFP; CCFP(E.M.); Staff Emerg, North York General Hospital; (416)756-6882

YATSCOFF, Michael A; Abbotsford Reg Hosp & CC, 32900 Marshall Rd, Abbotsford BC V2S 0C2; Alb'08; CCFP; CCFP(E.M.); Staff, Abbotsford Regional Hospital & Cancer Centre; (604)851-4752

YATSINA, Alexandre N; Erindale Health Centre, 2-50 Kenderdine Rd, Saskatoon SK S7N 3A1; (Ukraine)'87; Staff, Erindale Health Centre; Langs: Russian; Ukrainian; (306)934-6601; Fax. (306)934-6615; yatsina@sasktel.net.

YATSINA, Oksana Y; Erindale Health Centre, 2-50 Kenderdine Rd, Saskatoon SK S7N 3A1; (Ukraine)'91; CCFP; Physician, Kelsey Trail Health Region; Physician, Nipawin Health Centre; Langs: Ukrainian; Polish; (306)934-6601; Fax. (306)934-6615; yatsina@sasktel.net.

YATSYNOV, Viktor; Rouge Valley HS-Centenary, 2867 Ellesmere Rd, Scarborough ON M1E 4B9; Belarussian State Medical University (Belarus)'91; Staff, Rouge Valley Health System - Centenary Health Centre Site; (416)281-7318

YATSYNOVICH, Viktor; Rouge Valley HS-Centenary, 2867 Ellesmere Rd, Scarborough ON M1E 4B9; Belarussian State Medical University (Belarus)'91; Staff, Rouge Valley Health System - Centenary Health Centre Site; (416)281-7318

YAU, Annie; Carewest Fanning Day Hosp, 722 16th Ave NE, Calgary AB T2E 6V7; Mon'85; MSc; CCFP; Staff, Foothills Medical Centre; Staff, Dr Vernon Fanning Extended Care Centre; Asst Prof, University of Calgary; Langs: Bilingual(English/French); (403)520-2100; Fax. (403)230-6904; ayau@ucalgary.ca.

YAU, Anthony P C; 303-1223 St Clair Ave W, Toronto ON M6E 1B5; Manchester (England)'64; Langs: Italian; Cantonese; (416)654-8864; Fax. (416)654-9446.

YAU, Farrah M; Market Mall Prof Bldg, 329-4935 40 Ave NW, Calgary AB T3A 2N1; Alb'06; FRCSC; PlasSurg. (587)352-3260; Fax. (587)352-9339.

YAU, Frank C O; 1025 Gerrard St E, Toronto ON M4M 1Z6; (Hong Kong)'76; MB BS; Court Staff, Toronto East General Hospital Inc; Langs: Cantonese; Mandarin; (416)461-3539; Fax. (416)461-3530.

YAU, Jaron A; Sault Area Hosp, 750 Great Northern Rd, Sault Ste. Marie ON P6B 0A8; McM'04; FRCPC; DiagRad. Staff, Sault Area Hospital - Sault Ste Marie; (705)759-3434

YAU, Jennifer K W; Central Ottawa Fam Med Assoc, 500-267 O'Connor St, Ottawa ON K2P 1V3; Wes'99; BSc; CCFP; Langs: Cantonese; (613)760-3723; Fax. (613)232-4818.

YAU, Jonathan C; Rockyview Gen Hosp, 7007 14 St SW, Calgary AB T2V 1P9; Alb'78; FRCPC; IntMed; MedOncol. Staff, Rockyview General Hospital; Staff IntMed, Foothills Medical Centre; Langs: Chinese; (403)943-3000

YAU, K Y Steven; 199-4438 10th Ave W, Vancouver BC V6R 4R8; UBC'09; CCFP; (604)255-3151

YAU, Patrick W N; Finch-Midland Med Centre, 402-4190 Finch Ave E, Scarborough ON M1S 4T7; Tor'93; FRCSC; GenSurg (Bariatric Surgery). Ac Staff, The Scarborough Hospital - Birchmount Campus; (416)291-1900; Fax. (416)291-9469.

YAU, Ryan J H; Mitchell Eye Centre, 100-5340 1 St SW, Calgary AB T2H 0C8; Alb'05; BSc; Ophth (Cataract). Clinical Asst Prof, University of Calgary; Langs: Cantonese; (403)258-1773; Fax. (403)258-2704; ryan.yau@mitchelleyecentre.com.

YAU, Terrence M; Univ Hlth Network-The Toronto, 4N 470-200 Elizabeth St, Toronto ON M5G 2C4; McG'88; MSc; BA; DABS; FRCS; CM; FRCSC; GenSurg (Adult Cardiac Surgery); CardSurg. Scientist, Toronto General Hospital - UHN; Teach Staff Surg, University of Toronto; Langs: Cantonese; (416)340-4074; Fax. (416)340-4385; terry.yau@utoronto.ca.

YAU, William Y T; Southside Med Clinic, 104-2603 Hewes Way NW, Edmonton AB T6L 6W6; Alb'88; CCFP; FCFP; Langs: Cantonese; (780)462-1221; Fax. (780)466-4747.

YAU, Yvonne C W; The Hosp for Sick Children, 36 100-555 University Ave, Toronto ON M5G 1X8; Tor'89; MD; FRCPC; MedMicrobiol. Staff, The Hospital For Sick Children; Langs: Chinese; (416)813-7654 x3478

YAXLEY, David T; USTAT/Mental Health Services, 11195 Pembroke St W, Victoria BC V8T 1J3; Ott'81; BSc; FRCPC; Psy. Ac Staff Psy, Vancouver General Hospital - Centennial Pavillion; Consultant, South Vancouver Mental Health Team; Staff, USTAT/Group Mental Health Services; Clin Asst Prof, University of British Columbia; (250)213-4400

YAZDANI, Arash; 8F-481 University Ave, Toronto ON M5G 2E9; Qns'08; FRCPC; IntMed.

YAZDANI, Arjang; London HSC-Victoria Campus, PO Box 5010 Stn B E2 647-800 Commissioners Rd E, London ON N6A 5W9; McM'00; FRCSC; PlasSurg. Staff, London Health Sciences Centre - Victoria Campus; Langs: Farsi; (519)685-8500 x58320

YAZDANI, Ramin; St Clare's Mercy Hosp, S104A-154 LeMarchant Rd, St. John's NL A1C 5B8; University of Tehran (Iran)'92; Staff, St Clare's Mercy Hospital; (709)777-5000

YAZDANI, Shahin; Optimum Healthcare Centre, 3-1339 Stittsville Main St, Stittsville ON K2S 1C6; Tor'96; CCFP; Staff, Queensway Carleton Hospital; Langs: Persian; (613)435-6045; Fax. (613)435-6046.

YAZDANI BOROUJENI, Fereshteh; 203-73 Delhi St, Guelph ON N1E 6L9; Tehran (Iran)'76; Langs: Farsi; (519)826-7937; Fax. (519)826-4319.

YAZDANIAN, Shirin O; Herzl Family Practice Clinic, PH 2F-3755 ch Cote-Sainte-Cath, Montreal QC H3T 1E2; Tor'06; CCFP; Staff, Centre de Medecine Familiale Herzl; (514)340-8256; Fax. (514)340-7579.

YAZER, Erika; Cape Breton Reg Hosp, 1482 George St, Sydney NS B1P 1P3; Dal'09; CCFP; Staff, Cape Breton Healthcare Complex; (902)467-8000

YAZER, Harold; Queen Elizabeth II HSC-Victori, 1276 South Park St, Halifax NS B3H 2Y9; Dal'71; DAB; FRCPC; Anes (Obstetrics Anesthesia). Ac Staff, Queen Elizabeth II Health Sciences Centre - Victoria General Site; Ac Staff, IWK Health Centre; Asst Prof, Dalhousie University; (902)473-4326; Fax. (902)423-9454.

YE, Charles C; Southlake Reg Health Centre, 596 Davis Dr, Newmarket ON L3Y 2P9; Shanghai (China)'83; FCAP; FASCP; FRCPC; GenPath (Hematology Pathology). Staff, Southlake Regional Health Centre; Langs: Mandarin; (905)895-4521; Fax. (905)952-2884; cye@southlakeregional.org.

YE, Jian; St Paul's Hosp, 493-1081 Burrard St, Vancouver BC V6Z 1Y6; Wenzhou (China)'83; MSc; FRCSC; CardSurg (Thoracic Aortic Surgery). Staff Cardiac Surg, Vancouver General Hospital - Centennial Pavillion; Staff Cardiac Surg, Providence Health Care - St Paul's Hospital; Clin Prof, University of British Columbia; Langs: Chinese; (604)806-9349; Fax. (604)806-8375.

YE, Juan; Towne Centre Med Clinic, 201-3603 Highway 7 E, Markham ON L3R 0M3; Shanghai (China)'95; CCFP; Langs: Mandarin; (905)604-5535; Fax. (905)604-7750.

YE, Zhongbo J; The Richmond Hosp, 7000 Westminster Hwy, Richmond BC V6X 1A2; Shen Ya (China)'84; FRCPC; Psy. Staff, Vancouver General Hospital - Centennial Pavillion; Staff, Richmond Hospital; Staff, Richmond Mental Health Team; Staff, Cross Cultural Program Health Centre; Langs: Mandarin; (604)244-5504

YEADON, Carol A M; CHUM-Hop Notre-Dame, 1560 rue Sherbrooke E, Montreal QC H2L 4M1; McG'74; FRCPC; IntMed; Rheum (P.Q.). Consultant, CSSS de Dorval-Lachine-Lasalle; ac Staff, Centre Hospitalier l'Université de Montréal (CHUM) - Hôpital Notre-Dame; assoc Prof, Universite de Montreal; Langs: English; French; (514)890-8000 x28800; Fax. (514)412-7630; carol-anne.yeadon.chum@ssss.gouv.qc.ca.

YEADON, Derek E; Cobequid Commun Health Centre, 40 Freer Lane, Lower Sackville NS B4C 0A2; Dal'73; FRCPC; DiagRad. Head Diagnostic Imaging, Cobequid Community Health Centre; Asst Prof, Dalhousie University; (902)869-6122; Fax. (902)869-6121; derek.yeadon@cdha.nshealth.ca.

YEANDLE-HIGNELL, James; Northern Ontario School of Med, 955 Oliver Rd, Thunder Bay ON P7B 5E1; London (England)'73; MRCS; LRCP; Asst Prof, Northern Ontario School of Medicine-Lakehead University; (807)766-7300; Fax. (807)766-7370.

YEARSLEY, George C; Seafield Eye Clinic, 5-1179 Seafield Cres, Nanaimo BC V9S 4S1; UBC'06; FRCSC; Ophth. (250)753-3323

YEATES, Gillian R; Collingwood Gen & Marine Hosp, 459 Hume St, Collingwood ON L9Y 1W9; Dal'95; BA; FRCSC; ObstGyn. Staff, Collingwood General & Marine Hospital; (705)444-5533; Fax. (705)444-6655.

YEATES, Karen E; Queen's Univ-Etherington Hall, 94 University Ave, Kingston ON K7L 3N5; Qns'97; MPH; FRCPC; IntMed (Public Health); Nephrol. Staff, Kingston General Hospital; Asst Prof, Queen's University; (613)533-6730; Fax. (613)533-3214.

YEATS, Barbara A; 5230 Mitch Owens Rd PO Box 580, Manotick ON K4M 1B2; Wes'85; CCFP; FCFP; (613)692-2571; Fax. (613)820-2462.

YEBOAH, Emmanuel K; Wall Street Med Bldg, 370-140 Wall St, Saskatoon SK S7K 1N4; Accra (Ghana)'76; FRCSC; ObstGyn. Staff, Royal University Hospital; Staff, Saskatoon City Hospital; Clin Prof ObstGyn, University of Saskatchewan; (306)652-4331; Fax. (306)242-4855.

YEBOAH, Ophelia; Univ of Toronto, 602-500 University Ave, Toronto ON M5G 1V7; Tor'07; IntMed.

YECHOURON, Ariane; Ctr Hosp de Verdun, 4000 boul Lasalle, Verdun QC H4G 2A3; McG'84; FRCPC; IntMed; MedMicrobiol; InfectDis. Staff Microbiology Lab, Centre Hospitalier de Verdun; (450)699-2425; Fax. (514)765-7343.

YEE, Adrian S Y; Cook Medical Bldg, 314-1175 Cook St, Victoria BC V8V 4A1; Tor'99; FRCPC; IntMed; Hem. Staff, BC Cancer Agency Vancouver Island Centre; Langs: Cantonese; (250)384-7377; Fax. (250)384-7372; ayee@bccancer.bc.ca.

YEE, Albert J M; Sunnybrook Hlth Sciences Ctre, MG 371B-2075 Bayview Ave, Toronto ON M4N 3M5; Tor'92; FRCSC; OrthSurg. Staff, Sunnybrook Health Sciences Centre; Langs: Chinese; (416)480-6815; Fax. (416)480-5886.

YEE, Allan C N; Humber River Reg Hosp-Finch, 2111 Finch Ave W, North York ON M3N 1N1; Tor'80; DiagRad., Humber River Regional Hospital - Finch Avenue Site; (416)747-3853; Fax. (416)747-3759.

YEE, Allan J; Markham Stouffville Hosp, PO Box 1800 Stn Main 381 Church St, Markham ON L3P 7P3; Tor'91; FRCPC; IntMed. Staff, Markham Stouffville Hospital; Langs: Cantonese; (905)472-7000 x6743; Fax. (905)472-7621.

YEE, Angelina; William Osler Health Centre, 101 Humber College Blvd, Etobicoke ON M9V 1R8; Tor'03; CCFP; (416)747-3500; Fax. (416)747-3698.

YEE, Chok-Ching; 7A-13305 Highway 27 GD, Nobleton ON L0G 1N0; McG'69; Langs: Cantonese; Mandarin; (905)859-1099; Fax. (905)859-8611.

YEE, Daphne P; Lakeshore Gen Hosp, 160 av Stillview, Pointe-Claire QC H9R 2Y2; McG'99; FRCPC; IntMed; Respir. Staff, McGill University Health Centre - Royal Victoria Hospital; Staff, Lakeshore General Hospital - Pointe Claire; (514)630-2225

YEE, David P; Thunder Bay Reg HSC, 980 Oliver Rd, Thunder Bay ON P7B 6V4; McG'88; Staff, Thunder Bay Regional Health Sciences Centre; Langs: Cantonese; (807)684-6000

YEE, Diana A; Valley Ridge Family Physicians, 321-11245 Valley Ridge Dr NW, Calgary AB T3B 5V4; Sask'03; CCFP; (403)282-3806; Fax. (403)284-5601.

YEE, Don; Cross Cancer Institute, 11560 University Ave NW, Edmonton AB T6G 1Z2; Alb'96; FRCPC; RadOncol. Staff RadOncol, Cross Cancer Institute; (780)432-8783; Fax. (780)432-8380; donyee@cancerboard.ab.ca.

YEE, Donna L J; Oakridge Plaza, 238-5780 Cambie St, Vancouver BC V5Z 3A7; Qns'95; BSc; CCFP; Ac Staff, Providence Health Care - St Paul's Hospital; Clin Instructor Family Med, University of British Columbia; Langs: Cantonese; Mandarin; (604)323-8836; Fax. (604)323-8891; donnawinston@telus.net.

YEE, Doreen A; Sunnybrook Hlth Sciences Ctre, M 3200-2075 Bayview Ave, Toronto ON M4N 3M5; Tor'82; MD; MBA; FRCPC; Anes (Trauma). Staff, Sunnybrook Health Sciences Centre; Asst Prof, University of Toronto; Langs: Cantonese; (416)480-4864; Fax. (416)480-6039; doreen.yee@sunnybrook.ca.

YEE, Edgar H; 205-3502 Taylor St E, Saskatoon SK S7H 5H9; West Indies (Jamaica)'78; FAAP; FRCPC; Peds (Clinical Immunology & Allergy). (306)373-8870; Fax. (306)373-8870.

YEE, Ernest; Quinte HC-Belleville Gen Hosp, 412-265 Dundas St E, Belleville ON K8N 5A9; Sher'92; FRCPC; IntMed (Cardiology)., QHC Belleville General; Langs: English; French; (613)969-5511

YEE, Gayle M; Superior Family Health Team, 48-44 Great Northern Rd, Sault Ste. Marie ON P6B 0A8; Wes'96; BSc(Hon.); PhD; CCFP; FCFP; Staff, Sault Area Hospital - Sault Ste Marie; (705)759-3434; Fax. (705)759-3731.

YEE, George E; Medical Labs of Windsor, 1428 Ouellette Ave, Windsor ON N8X 1K4; Man'60; FRCPC; GenPath. Pres, Medical Labs of Windsor; (519)258-1991; Fax. (519)258-9505; mlwpurchasing@wincom.net.

YEE, Gilbert Y M; Centric Health Atria 1, W300-2255 Sheppard Ave E, North York ON M2J 4Y1; Tor'95; FRCSC; OrthSurg. (416)445-4459; Fax. (416)445-9692.

YEE, Gordon; Lasalle Medicale, 200-8190 boul Newman, LaSalle QC H8N 1X9; Sher'85; CCFP; Langs: Chinese; English; (514)368-8666; Fax. (514)368-9477.

YEE, Harris A; Foothills Prof Bldg, 110-1620 29 St NW, Calgary AB T2N 4L7; Tor'97; FRCPC; MedGenetics. (403)571-0450; Fax. (403)571-0455.

YEE, Irvan; Royal Victoria Hosp, 201 Georgian Dr, Barrie ON L4M 6M2; UBC'85; FRCPC; Anes. Staff, Royal Victoria Regional Health Centre; (705)728-9090 x46550; Fax. (705)739-5613.

YEE, Ivan C Y; 2809 Eglinton Ave E, Scarborough ON M1J 2E1; Tor'77; Court Staff, The Scarborough Hospital - General Campus; Court Staff, Rouge Valley Health System - Centenary Health Centre Site; Langs: Chinese; (416)261-2212; Fax. (416)261-3921.

YEE, John C K; 214-2425 Tecumseh Rd E, Windsor ON N8W 1E6; Galway (Ireland)'68; DCH; MRCP(Ire.); Langs: English; French; (519)252-8283; Fax. (519)252-3320; jyeemd@hotmail.com.

YEE, John; Diamond Health Care Centre, 7115-2775 Laurel St, Vancouver BC V5Z 1M9; McG'88; FRCSC; GenSurg (Surgical Oncology); ThorSurg; CardSurg. Langs: French; Cantonese; (604)875-5388; Fax. (604)875-5828.

YEE, John; Centre for Family Medicine, 10B Victoria St S, Kitchener ON N2G 1C5; Wes'96; CCFP; (519)783-0023; Fax. (519)783-0033.

YEE, Karen W L; Univ Hlth Network-Princess M, 5 218-610 University Ave, Toronto ON M5G 2M9; McG'92; FRCPC; IntMed (Leukemia); Hem. Staff, Princess Margaret Hospital - University Health Network; Langs: English; French; (416)946-4495; karen.yee@uhn.on.ca.

YEE, Kenny Y V; 111-3640 Hwy 3 W PO Box 27, Barrington Passage NS B0W 1G0; Adelaide (Australia)'90; MB BS; DObst(Obst.); CCFP; FCFP; Ac Staff, Roseway Hospital; Ac Staff, Yarmouth Regional Hospital; Lecturer, Dalhousie University; Langs: Chinese; Malay; (902)637-3550; Fax. (902)637-3552.

YEE, Lauren L; South Walkerville Med Centre, 300-2224 Walker Rd, Windsor ON N8W 5L7; Tor'87; Associate Family Med, Hôtel-Dieu Grace Hospital; Langs: English; French; (519)971-8874; Fax. (519)971-8672.

YEE, Main Chiong; Chatham-Kent Health Alliance, PO Box 2030 Stn Main 80 Grand Ave W, Chatham ON N7M 5L9; Dal'85; FRCPC; DiagRad. Staff Radiol, Chatham-Kent Health Alliance; (519)352-6400; Fax. (519)437-6039.

YEE, May-Sann; Southlake Reg Health Centre, 596 Davis Dr, Newmarket ON L3Y 2P9; Man'03; FRCPC; Anes. Staff, Southlake Regional Health Centre; (905)895-4521

YEE, Norman; Copeman Health Care Centre, 400-628 12 Ave SW, Calgary AB T2R 0H6; Cal'90; CCFP; FCFP; Ac Staff, Foothills Medical Centre; Asst Prof Family Med, University of Calgary; (403)270-2273; Fax. (403)521-2250; nyee@telusplanet.net.

YEE, Raymond; London HSC-University Hosp, PO Box 5339 Stn B C6 114-339 Windermere Rd, London ON N6A 5A5; Alb'77; FACC; FRCPC; Cardiol. Staff Cardiac Investiation Unit, London Health Sciences Centre - University Hospital; Prof, University of Western Ontario; (519)663-3746; Fax. (519)663-3782.

YEE, Selena L; 182-8720 MacLeod Trail SE, Calgary AB T2H 0M4; Cal'06; CCFP; (403)282-1038; Fax. (403)282-1071.

YEE, Stephen E; Davis Drive Med Clinic, 6-291 Davis Dr, Newmarket ON L3Y 2N6; Tor'95; CCFP; FCFP; (905)836-6609; Fax. (905)830-0483.

YEE, Vernie F; 215 North Town Mall NW, Edmonton AB T5E 6C1; Alb'80; CCFP; (780)475-0502; Fax. (780)473-5493.

YEE, Wendy H; Rockyview Gen Hosp, 63-7007 14 St SW, Calgary AB T2V 1P9; Man'84; FRCPC; Peds (Neonatal & Perinatal Medicine). Staff, Rockyview General Hospital; (403)943-3563; Fax. (403)212-1243.

YEE, William C; Vancouver Gen Hosp, 855 12th Ave W, Vancouver BC V5Z 1M9; Wes'92; FRCPC; DiagRad. Staff, Vancouver General Hospital - Centennial Pavillion; Langs: Cantonese; (604)872-9862; Fax. (604)875-4319; wyue@cmmt.ubc.ca.

YEGAPPAN, Chidambaram; The Ottawa Hosp-Gen Campus, 1303-501 Smyth Rd Box 207, Ottawa ON K1H 8L6; Mem'05; Critical Care Medicine; Anes. Staff, The Ottawa Hospital - General Campus; (613)737-8701

YEGAPPAN, Chidambaram M; St Joseph's Health Care, F512-50 Charlton Av E, Hamilton ON L8N 4A6; Madras(Chennai) (India)'80; MB ChB; FRCP; FACP; FRCPC; Neur (Stroke). Staff Neurol, St Joseph's Healthcare - Charlton Campus; Staff Neurol, Hamilton Health Sciences Centre - Hamilton General Hospital; Assoc Prof Neurol, McMaster University; Langs: Tamil; (905)522-1155 x33546; Fax. (905)521-6144.

YEGAPPAN, Muthulakshmi; Allied Health Centre, 302-5673 North St, Niagara Falls ON L2G 1J4; Madras (India)'79; DGO; MRCOG; MB BS; FRCSC; ObstGyn. Staff, Niagara Health System - Greater Niagara General Site; Langs: Tamil; (905)358-5851; Fax. (905)358-8862; yeg@iaw.on.ca.

YEGHIAYAN, Edouard; St Mary's Hosp Centre, 3830 av Lacombe, Montreal QC H3T 1M5; Alexandria (Egypt)'67; DiagRad (P.Q.). Staff, St Mary's Hospital Centre; (514)734-2620; Fax. (514)734-2659.

YEH, Eluen A; The Hosp for Sick Children, 555 University Ave, Toronto ON M5G 1X8; McM'99; FRCPC; Peds (Neurology). Staff, The Hospital For Sick Children; Assoc Prof, University of Toronto; Langs: Chinese; Japanese; (416)813-6332; Fax. (416)813-7096.

YEH, Jennifer N; Children's & Women's HC of BC, 4480 Oak St, Vancouver BC V6H 3V4; UBC'06; FRCPC; Psy. Staff, BC Children's Hospital; (604)875-4111

YEH, Louis S; Greylawn Med Office, 1943A Victoria Park Ave, Scarborough ON M1R 1V1; Tor'90; Court Staff Family Med, North York General Hospital; (416)445-1754; Fax. (416)445-1754.

YEH, Timothy W; University of Alberta Hosp, 8440 112 St NW, Edmonton AB T6G 2B7; Man'87; Anes. Staff Anes, University of Alberta Hospital; (780)407-8861

YEHYA ALADIN, Jaled W; College Plaza 3, 225-8215 112 St NW, Edmonton AB T6G 2C8; University of Valle (Other Foreign)'01; FRCPC; IntMed; Respir. Staff, Sturgeon Community Hospital; (780)492-0203; Fax. (780)407-3027.

YEKINNI, Idris O; Estevan Med Clinic, 110-1175 Nicholson Rd, Estevan SK S4A 2S7; (306)634-2661; Fax. (306)634-8821.

YELAMANCHILI, Radhika; 201-112 Queenston St, St Catharines ON L2R 2Z4; Andhra (India)'01; FRCPC; IntMed; MedOncol. Staff, Niagara Health System - St Catharines General Site; Staff, The Juravinski Cancer Centre; Langs: Hindi; Telugu; (905)685-8082

YELENBAUGEN, Irina; The Healthy Way, 105-1120 Finch Ave W, North York ON M3J 3H7; Leningrad (Russia (Federation))'74; Staff, The Scarborough Hospital - Birchmount Campus; Langs: Russian; (416)667-8498; Fax. (416)667-8478.

YELLAND, Joel C; Parkridge Centre, 110 Gropper Cres, Saskatoon SK S7M 5N9; Sask'80; Ac Staff, Saskatoon City Hospital; Staff Med, Saskatoon District Health Board; (306)655-3928; Fax. (306)655-3801.

YELLE, Carole-Anne L; Surrey Mem Hosp, 13750 96 Ave, Surrey BC V3V 1Z2; Ott'95; FRCPC; IntMed; Critical Care Medicine; Endocrin&Metab. Staff ICU, Surrey Memorial Hospital; Staff, Richmond Hospital; Langs: Bilingual(English/French); (604)616-3907

YELLE, J P Jean-Denis; The Ottawa Hosp-Civic Campus, CPC 162-1053 Carling Ave, Ottawa ON K1Y 4E9; Mon'81; FACS; FRCSC; GenSurg (Abdominal Surgery). Staff, The Ottawa Hospital - Civic Campus; Langs: Bilingual(French/English); (613)798-5555 x19605; Fax. (613)761-4262.

YELLE, Jean-Pierre; Clinique Med Havre Sante, 521 boul du Havre, Salaber-de-Valleyf QC J6S 4Z5; Mon'71; (450)371-6444; Fax. (450)371-5315.

YELLE, Louise; CHUM-Hop Notre-Dame, 1560 rue Sherbrooke E, Montreal QC H2L 4M1; Mon'79; FRCPC; IntMed; MedOncol; Hem. Staff, Centre Hospitalier l'Université de Montréal (CHUM) - Hôpital Notre-Dame; (514)890-8000 x25381; Fax. (514)412-7572; louise.yelle.chum@ssss.gouv.qc.ca.

YELLE, Robert M; Bridlewood Med Centre, 64 Stonehaven Dr, Kanata ON K2M 2Y2; McG'94; CCFP; FCFP; Staff, The Ottawa Hospital - General Campus; Assoc Prof, University of Ottawa; Langs: English; French; (613)592-0805; Fax. (613)592-0961.

YELLIN, Joel W; Hamilton Commun Health Centre, M1-414 Victoria Ave N, Hamilton ON L8L 5G8; Tor'83; CCFP; FCFP; (905)529-5221; Fax. (905)546-0361.

YEMCHUK, Bohdan R; Thames Valley FHT-W London FH, 200-785 Wonderland Rd S, London ON N6K 1M6; Tor'81; CCFP; FCFP; Med Dir, McCornick Home; Aj Prof Family Med, University of Western Ontario; Langs: Ukrainian; (519)641-6712; Fax. (519)641-6189; byemchuk@uwo.ca.

YEMEN, Brian L; Hamilton HS-Juravinski Site, 711 Concession St, Hamilton ON L8V 1C3; Sask'83; FRCPC; DiagRad (Academic Medicine). Asst Prof, McMaster University; (905)527-4322; Fax. (905)575-2660.

YEMEN, D Jill; Rockyview Gen Hosp, 7007 14 St SW, Calgary AB T2V 1P9; Sask'77; FRCPC; Anes (Clinical Anaesthesia). Staff, Rockyview General Hospital; Teach Staff Quality Improvement, University of Calgary; (403)943-8720; Fax. (403)944-2425.

YEMEN, Gary W; Sunridge Prof Centre, 3-2675 36 St NE, Calgary AB T1Y 6H6; Sask'76; FRCPC; DiagRad (Diagnostic Imaging). (403)291-3315; Fax. (403)291-9308.

YEN, David; Kingston Gen Hosp, D5-76 Stuart St, Kingston ON K7L 2V7; Tor'85; MD; FRCSC; OrthSurg (Spine Surgery). Staff, Kingston General Hospital; Staff, Hotel-Dieu Hospital; Queen's University; (613)548-2545; Fax. (613)548-2518; yend@kgh.kari.net.

YEN, Shiu Kee; Lloydminster Clinic, 75-5120 46 St, Lloydminster AB T9V 2P7; Tokyo (Japan)'61; Staff, Lloydminster Medical Clinic; (780)875-2221; Fax. (780)875-0605.

YEN, Tien; Hys Med Centre, 710-11010 101 St NW, Edmonton AB T5H 4B9; Sask'05; FRCPC; PhysMed&Rehab. Staff, University of Alberta Hospital; (780)453-5255

YEN, Tin-Wing; 11F-1190 Hornby St, Vancouver BC V6Z 2K5; Sask'07; Staff, BC Women's Hospital & Health Centre; (604)682-2344 x66140; tyen@cw.bc.ca.

YEN, Ziny C; CDK Family Medicine, 175 Princess St, Kingston ON K7L 1A9; Qns'09; CCFP; (613)766-0318; Fax. (613)766-0339.

YENDT, Edmund R; Kingston Med Arts Centre, 209-800 Princess St, Kingston ON K7L 5E4; Tor'48; FRCPC; IntMed. Consultant, Kingston General Hospital; Consultant, Hotel-Dieu Hospital; Emeritus Prof Med, Queen's University; (613)547-0303; Fax. (613)547-0312.

YENSON, Paul R; Gordon & Leslie Diamond HCC, 10F-2775 Laurel St, Vancouver BC V5Z 1M9; UBC'02; FRCPC; IntMed; Hem. Staff, Vancouver General Hospital - Centennial Pavillion; Staff, Gordon & Leslie Diamond Health Care Centre; (604)875-5387

YEO, Erik L; Univ Hlth Network-Toronto Gen, 8N 885-200 Elizabeth St, Toronto ON M5G 2C4; Qns'79; FRCPC; IntMed (Hemostasis); Hem. Staff, Toronto General Hospital - UHN; Assoc Prof, University of Toronto; (416)340-4069; Fax. (416)340-3799; erik.yeo@uhn.ca.

YEO, Linda I; Health Sciences Centre, 820 Sherbrook St, Winnipeg MB R3A 1R9; Man'88; FRCPC; DiagRad. Staff, Health Sciences Centre; (204)774-8511

YEO, Thomas A; Hys Med Centre, 202-11010 101 St NW, Edmonton AB T5H 4B9; Man'92; BSc; FRCPC; DiagRad (Neuro Radiology). Staff Radiol, University of Alberta Hospital; (780)426-1121; Fax. (780)425-5979.

YEOMANS, Timothy C; PO Box 400, Gold River BC V0P 1G0; UBC'76; (250)283-2541; Fax. (250)283-7561.

YEOMANS, Wendy R; Vancouver Gen Hosp, JPP 16A-899 12th Ave W, Vancouver BC V5Z 1M9; UBC'87; Ac Staff Palliative Care Unit, Vancouver General Hospital - Centennial Pavillion; Clin Instructor, University of British Columbia; (604)875-4715; Fax. (604)875-4967.

YEP, Timothy C; 290-5255 Richmond Rd SW, Calgary AB T3E 7C4; Alb'01; CCFP; (403)249-3165; Fax. (403)249-3120.

YEPES, Horacio; 1487 George St, Sydney NS B1P 1P2; Instituto de Ciencias de la Salud (Colombia)'88; Staff Orthopedic, Cape Breton Healthcare Complex; Staff, Queen Elizabeth II Health Sciences Centre - Victoria General Site; Dalhousie University; Langs: Spanish; French; (902)539-1150; Fax. (902)539-9846.

YEPES RESTREPO, Natasha; 201-715 Fischer Hallman Rd, Kitchener ON N2E 4E9; Colombia (Colombia)'93; FRCSC; Ophth. Langs: Spanish; (519)745-3690; Fax. (519)745-4856.

YERETSIAN, Sarkis; Clinique Medic-Aide, 10870 av de Bois de Boulogne, Montreal QC H3M 2X1; Beyrouth (Lebanon)'71; FRCSC; GenSurg (P.Q.). Langs: Arabic; French; (514)339-5309; Fax. (514)339-5309.

YERGEAU, Andree; CSSS Vieille Capitale, 55 ch Sainte-Foy, Quebec QC G1R 1S9; Laval'85; Médecin, Centre Hospitalier Universitaire de Québec (CHUQ) - Siege Social; Médecin, CSSS Haute-Ville; Prof Med, Université Laval; Langs: Bilingual(French/English); (418)641-2572 x5305; Fax. (418)522-5437; andree.yergeau@irdpq.qc.ca.

YERGEAU, Stephanie; Centre Hosp Reg de Lanaudiere, 1000 boul Sainte-Anne, Joliette QC J6E 6J2; Mon'07; FRCPC; IntMed. Staff, Centre Hospitalier Régional de Lanaudière; (450)759-8222

YERMAN, Todd J; Surrey Memorial Hosp, 13750 96 Ave, Surrey BC V3V 1Z2; Tor'05; FRCPC; IntMed; Critical Care Medicine. Staff ICU, Surrey Memorial Hospital; (604)588-3306

YERMUS, Joseph A; 5989 av de Verdun, LaSalle QC H4H 1M6; Tor'72; Staff Gen & Family Med, St Mary's Hospital Centre; (514)766-2246; Fax. (514)766-6462; drjyermus@sympatico.ca.

YERMUS, Ryan D; Markham Stoufville Urgent Care, 100-110 Cooper Creek Dr, Markham ON L6B 0P9; Ott'07; CCFP; (905)472-8911

YESLI, Madjid; Clinique Med des Boises, 4670 boul Saint-Martin O, Laval QC H7T 2Y2; (Algeria)'89; (450)687-8585; Fax. (450)687-0203.

YESOVITCH, Rose P; Northwood Med Clinic, 2009 Long Lake Rd, Sudbury ON P3E 6C3; McG'06; MDCM; CCFP; (705)522-3380

YESSAD, Abderahmane; CMSSC de la Mitis, 800 av du Sanatorium, Mont-Joli QC G5H 3L6; Alger (Algeria)'84; Staff Physiatre, CSSS de la Mitis; (418)775-7261; Fax. (418)775-1686.

YEUNG, Adela K T; Rosedale Med Centre, 512-600 Sherbourne St, Toronto ON M4X 1W4; Tor'79; Langs: Cantonese; Mandarin; (416)961-0516; Fax. (416)961-0516.

YEUNG, Albert A C L; Royal Alexandra Hosp, 649 CSC-10240 Kingsway NW, Edmonton AB T5H 3V9; Glasgow (Scotland)'74; MB ChB; MSc; FRCPC; IntMed (Hypertension). Ac Staff Hypertension Lipid Clinic, Royal Alexandra Hospital; Prof Med & Pharmacology, University of Alberta; (780)944-1440; Fax. (780)474-4865; ayeung@ualberta.ca.

YEUNG, Albert; Carefirst Family Health Team, 206-420 Highway 7 E, Richmond Hill ON L4B 3K2; Qns'95; FRCPC; Peds;CCFP; ClinImmunol&Allergy. Staff, Carefirst Family Health Team; Langs: Mandarin; (905)695-1133

YEUNG, Alexander K; Royal Alexandra Hosp, 541 CSC-10240 Kingsway NW, Edmonton AB T5H 3V9; Alb'90; CCFP; CCFP(E.M.); FCFP; Court Staff, Royal Alexandra Hospital; (780)735-4442; Fax. (780)477-4916.

YEUNG, Alfred K; Alberta Children's Hosp, 2888 Shaganappi Trail NW, Calgary AB T3B 6A8; Qns'05; FRCPC; Peds; Gastroent. Staff, Alberta Children's Hospital; (403)955-3071; Fax. (403)955-2922.

YEUNG, Aref; Royal Alexandra Hosp, 10240 Kingsway Dr NW, Edmonton AB T5H 3V9; Cal'03; CCFP; CCFP(E.M.); Staff, Royal Alexandra Hospital; (780)735-4442; Fax. (780)474-4865.

YEUNG, Brian K P; Mackenzie Richmond Hill Hosp, 10 Trench St, Richmond Hill ON L4C 4Z3; Qns'02; FRCPC; DiagRad; NuclearMed. Staff, Mackenzie Richmond Hill Hospital; (905)883-1212

YEUNG, C F Jeffery; McKenzie Towne Medical, 102-620 Mckenzie Towne Dr SE, Calgary AB T2Z 0Y6; Alb'99; CCFP; (403)262-6311; Fax. (403)262-5911.

YEUNG, Carolyn G; Centro Medical, 4610 Main St, Vancouver BC V5V 3R7; Qns'08; CCFP; (604)559-9933

YEUNG, Choi Kit; Gordon & Leslie Diamond HCC, 5F-2775 Laurel St, Vancouver BC V5Z 1M9; (Hong Kong)'73; FRACP; FRCPC; IntMed; Nephrol. Staff, Gordon & Leslie Diamond Health Care Centre; Ac Staff Nephrol, Vancouver General Hospital - Centennial Pavillion; Prof, University of British Columbia; Langs: Cantonese; (604)875-5950; Fax. (604)875-5952.

YEUNG, Christine R; York Health Centre, 302-1650 Elgin Mills Rd, Richmond Hill ON L4S 0B2; McM'09; CCFP; (289)809-3131; Fax. (289)809-3132.

YEUNG, Clement S L; Winnipeg Clinic, 425 St Mary Ave, Winnipeg MB R3C 0N2; Man'74; FRCPC; IntMed (Infectious Diseases). Consultant InfectDis, Victoria General Hospital; Consultant, Concordia General Hospital; Asst Prof, University of Manitoba; Langs: Chinese; (204)957-3340; Fax. (204)943-3516.

YEUNG, Clement W T; 308-4800 Leslie St, North York ON M2J 2K9; Tor'91; BSc(Wisconsin); MSc(Calif.); PhD(CA); Langs: Cantonese; Mandarin; (416)496-0003; Fax. (416)644-0222.

YEUNG, Dan W H; Village Square Med Centre, 2942 Finch Ave E, Scarborough ON M1W 2T4; Tor'91; Langs: Chinese; (416)756-2725; Fax. (416)756-3898.

YEUNG, Danny S C; 402-2830 Keele St, North York ON M3M 3E5; Tor'86; CCFP; FCFP; Assoc Dir Clinical, Institute of Family Living; Langs: Cantonese; (416)633-7337; Fax. (416)633-7337.

YEUNG, Douglas E; 4825 Dalhousie Dr NW, Calgary AB T3A 6K7; Cal'93; BSc; MSc; FRCPC; Peds. Staff, Alberta Children's Hospital; (403)239-9333; Fax. (403)208-1648.

YEUNG, Elaine T; Scarborough Gastroent Assoc, 208-1585 Markham Rd, Scarborough ON M1B 2W1; Tor'01; BA(Chemistry); FRCPC; IntMed (Therapeutic Endoscopy); Gastroent. Ac Staff, The Scarborough Hospital - General Campus; Langs: Chinese; Tagalog; (416)439-9253; Fax. (416)439-3875; elaine.yeung@utoronto.ca.

YEUNG, Emilie N M; 180-7340 Westminster Hwy, Richmond BC V6X 1A1; Glasgow (Scotland)'83; Staff, Richmond Hospital; Staff, UBC Hospital - Koerner Pavillion; (604)270-9751; Fax. (604)270-9705.

YEUNG, Ernest C H; Beddington Med Clinic, 105-8120 Beddington Blvd NW, Calgary AB T3K 2A8; Alb'82; CCFP; (403)292-0160; Fax. (403)275-6263.

YEUNG, Eugene Y C; Rouge Valley-Centenary HC, 2867 Ellesmere Rd, Scarborough ON M1E 4B9; London (England)'78; BSc; FRCR; MRC; FRCPC; DiagRad. Staff Radiol, Rouge Valley Health System - Centenary Health Centre Site; Asst Prof, University of Toronto; (416)284-8131 x4140

YEUNG, Gerald Y L; 5539 Victoria Dr, Vancouver BC V5P 3W2; Alb'93; CCFP; Langs: Cantonese; Mandarin; (604)325-3465; Fax. (604)325-3460.

YEUNG, Gordon K; Cape Breton Reg Hosp, 1482 George St, Sydney NS B1P 1P3; Sask'05; FRCPC; IntMed; Nephrol. Staff, Cape Breton Healthcare Complex; (902)567-8000

YEUNG, Grace W; Mayfair Place, 120-6707 Elbow Dr SW, Calgary AB T2V 0E3; UBC'03; FRCPC; DiagRad.

YEUNG, H Eddie; 3L-507 Broadway W, Vancouver BC V5Z 1E6; UBC'76; (604)568-7229

YEUNG, Helen P; Rockyview Gen Hosp, 7007 14 St SW, Calgary AB T2V 1P9; Alb'03; FRCPC; Psy. Staff, Rockyview General Hospital; (403)943-3808; Fax. (403)212-1234.

YEUNG, Jack K P S Y; Burlington Med Arts Bldg, 761 Brant St, Burlington ON L7R 2H7; National (Ireland)'65; MB ChB; BAO; Langs: Chinese; French; (905)632-0442; Fax. (905)632-2867.

YEUNG, Jacky Y; The Peterborough Clinic, 26 Hospital Dr, Peterborough ON K9J 7C3; Tor'06; FRCSC; Ophth. Langs: Cantonese; Mandarin; (705)740-6837; Fax. (705)740-6811.

YEUNG, James C F; Parker Place Med Clinic, 1550-4380 No 3 Rd, Richmond BC V6X 3V7; Man'73; Langs: Cantonese; (604)273-9899

YEUNG, Jared C C; 8210 109 St PO Box 52176 Rpo Garneau, Edmonton AB T6G 2T5; Cal'03; CCFP; (780)735-4111

YEUNG, Jensen M; Women's College Hosp, 8F-76 Grenville St, Toronto ON M5S 1B2; McM'01; FRCPC; Derm (Melanoma). Clin Associate, Women's College Hospital; Langs: Cantonese; (416)323-7546; Fax. (416)323-6236.

YEUNG, Joanne P; King Edward Pediatrics Clinic, 926 West King Edward, Vancouver BC V5Z 2E2; UBC'07; ClinImmunol&Allergy; Peds. (604)600-7282

YEUNG, Kam-Tong; Seniors Health Centre, 2 Buchan Crt, North York ON M2J 5A3; (Hong Kong)'83; MB BS; MRCP(UK); FCCP; FRCPC; IntMed; GeriatricMed. Staff, North York General Hospital; Lecturer Family & Commun Med, University of Toronto; Langs: Cantonese; (416)756-6050

YEUNG, Karen J; Royal Columbian Hosp, 330 Columbia St E, New Westminster BC V3L 3W7; Alb'93; FRCPC; GenPath. Staff Path, Royal Columbian Hospital; (604)520-4560; Fax. (604)520-4409.

YEUNG, Latifa T F; Galaxy 12 Child & Teen Clinic, 12F-2867 Ellesmere Rd, Scarborough ON M1E 4B9; Tor'95; MSc(ClinEpidem.); FRCPC; Peds (Pediatric Gastroenterology); Gastroent. Staff, Rouge Valley Health System - Centenary Health Centre Site; Teach Staff Peds, University of Toronto; Langs: Cantonese; (416)281-7476; Fax. (416)281-7313.

YEUNG, Margaret M W; 304-7031 Westminster Hwy, Richmond BC V6X 1A3; Alb'86; FRCPC; IntMed. (604)231-9697; Fax. (604)276-9601.

YEUNG, Marianne Y T; The Ottawa Hosp-Civic Campus, 1053 Carling Ave, Ottawa ON K1Y 4E9; Tor'91; CCFP; CCFP(E.M.); FCFP; Staff, Arnprior & District Memorial Hospital; Staff, The Ottawa Hospital - Civic Campus; (613)798-5555

YEUNG, Michael K; 2812 Bayview Ave, North York ON M2K 1E4; Dal'65; DPsy(Psych.); FRCPC; Psy. Langs: Cantonese; Fukinese; Mandarin; (416)222-8836; Fax. (416)222-3330.

YEUNG, Michael M C; 3500 26 Ave NE, Calgary AB T1Y 6J4; Alb'84; FRCPC; Neur (Multiple Sclerosis). Staff, Peter Lougheed Centre; Staff, Alberta Health Services; Clinical Asst Prof, University of Calgary; (403)943-5477; Fax. (403)219-3296.

YEUNG, Peter K; Surrey Med Arts Bldg, 308-13798 94A Ave, Surrey BC V3V 1N1; Tor'74; BSc(Hon); ABOG; FRCSC; ObstGyn (Colposcopy). Consultant Staff, BC Cancer Agency Sindi Ahluwalia Hawkins Centre for the Southern Interior; Consultant, Surrey Memorial Hospital; Langs: Cantonese; (604)585-3313; Fax. (604)585-3316.

YEUNG, Rae S M; The Hosp for Sick Children, 555 University Ave, Toronto ON M5G 1X8; Tor'87; FRCPC; Peds. Scientist, The Hospital For Sick Children; Langs: Chinese; (416)813-8964; Fax. (416)813-8883; rae.yeung@sickkids.ca.

YEUNG, Raymond Y M; Mackenzie Richmond Hill Hosp, 10 Trench St, Richmond Hill ON L4C 4Z3; London (England)'88; MB BS; MRC; FRCPC; Anes. Chief Anes, Mackenzie Richmond Hill Hospital; Lecturer Anes, University of Toronto; (905)883-2110; Fax. (905)883-2122; ryeung@yorkcentral.on.ca.

YEUNG, Robert; Sunnybrook Hlth Sciences Ctr, AG31C-2075 Bayview Ave, Toronto ON M4N 3M5; Tor'01; FRCPC; DiagRad (Neuro Radiology). Staff, Sunnybrook Health Sciences Centre; (416)480-6100

YEUNG, Sonia N; Medical Bldg, 1603-805 Broadway W, Vancouver BC V5Z 1K1; UBC'05; FRCSC; Ophth. Langs: Cantonese; Mandarin; (604)875-8889

YEUNG, T Myriam; Grey Nuns Community Hosp & HC, 1100 Youville Drive West NW, Edmonton AB T6L 5X8; Glasgow (Scotland)'78; DRCOG; Staff, Covenant Health - Grey Nuns Community Hospital; Physician Public Health Services, Alberta Health Services; (780)735-7346; Fax. (780)735-7444.

YEUNG, Timothy T C; Capilano Med Clinic, 7905 106 Ave NW, Edmonton AB T6A 1H7; Alb'04; CCFP; Staff, University of Alberta Hospital; Physician, Westview Health Centre; (780)465-0951; Fax. (780)465-6928.

YEUNG, Titus C; Vancouver Gen Hosp, 855 12th Ave W, Vancouver BC V5Z 1M9; Qns'07; FRCPC; EmergMed. Staff, Vancouver General Hospital - Centennial Pavillion; (604)875-4111

YEUNG, William C Y; Aberdeen Health Centre, 2180-4151 Hazelbridge Way, Richmond BC V6X 4J7; (Hong Kong)'70; LRCP(Lond); MRCS(Eng); MB BS(Hongkong); CCFP; Langs: Cantonese; (604)233-0068; Fax. (604)882-1383.

YEUNG, William H W; Haney Prof Bldg, 104-11743 224 St, Maple Ridge BC V2X 6A4; (Taiwan)'72; DAB; FACOG; FSOGC; FRCSC; ObstGyn. Chief ObstGyn, Ridge Meadows Hospital & Health Care Centre; Langs: Chinese; (604)467-0866; Fax. (604)467-8148.

YEUNG, Wilson T; Abbotsford Reg Hosp & CC, 32900 Marshall Rd, Abbotsford BC V2S 0C2; (Hong Kong)'86; MB BS; FRCPA; FRCPC; HemPath. Staff, Abbotsford Regional Hospital & Cancer Centre; Staff Hematopath, Fraser Health Authority Fraser East Service Abbotsford Public Health Unit; Staff, BC Biomedical Laboratories Ltd; Langs: Cantonese; (604)851-4700; wilson.yeung@faserhealth.ca.

YEUNG-LAI-WAH, John A; Burrard Health Bldg, 401-1160 Burrard St, Vancouver BC V6Z 2E8; Glasgow (Scotland)'77; MB ChB; MRCP(UK); ABIM; FACC; FRCPC; Cardiol (Cardiac Electrophysiology); IntMed. Staff, Providence Health Care - St Paul's Hospital; Consultant, Vancouver General Hospital - Centennial Pavillion; Prof, University of British Columbia; Langs: French; (604)662-7225; Fax. (604)662-7271.

YEWCHUK, Lila K; Children's & Women's HC of BC, 1L56-4480 Oak St, Vancouver BC V6H 3V4; UBC'97; FRCPC; DiagRad. Staff, BC Children's Hospital; (604)875-2131; Fax. (604)875-2367.

YHAP, Margaret C; 5850/5980 University Ave PO Box 9700 Rpo CSC, Halifax NS B3K 6R8; Bristol (England)'73; MB ChB; DObstRCOG; DCH; Peds (Pediatric Oncology). Ac Staff, IWK Health Centre; Asst Prof, Dalhousie University; (902)470-8778; Fax. (902)470-7216; margaret.yhap@iwk.nshealth.ca.

YI, Man; Women's Hosp, WS012-735 Notre Dame Ave, Winnipeg MB R3E 0L8; (China)'92; Staff, Children's Hospital of Winnipeg; (204)787-4218

YIANNAKIS, Georgia; Clinique Med Belanger, 300-3871 rue Belanger, Montreal QC H1X 3M7; Mon'01; (514)722-1166

YIANNOPOULOS, Anna; CHUM-Hop Notre-Dame, H2116 5-1560 rue Sherbrooke E, Montreal QC H2L 4M1; McG'96; ABIM; FRCPC; IntMed (Cardiology); Respir. Staff, Centre Hospitalier l'Université de Montréal (CHUM) - Hôpital Notre-Dame; Langs: Greek; French; (514)890-8000 x25123; Fax. (514)412-7687.

YIK, David K H; London HSC-Victoria Hosp, PO Box 5010 Stn B 800 Commissioners Rd E, London ON N6A 5W9; Tor'08; IntMed. Staff, London Health Sciences Centre - Victoria Campus; (519)685-8500; Fax. (519)685-8127.

YIK, Kwok Yeong; Columbia Med Bldg, 410-301 Columbia St E, New Westminster BC V3L 3W5; Dublin (Ireland)'73; MB ChB; BAO; FRCPC; Gastroent; IntMed. Langs: Cantonese; (604)525-0155; Fax. (604)525-1699.

YILMAZ, Asli; Rockyview Gen Hosp, 7007 14 St SW, Calgary AB T2V 1P9; Ankara (Turkey)'88; FRCPC; AnatPath. Staff Path, Rockyview General Hospital; (403)943-3630; Fax. (403)943-3333.

YILMAZ, Serdar; Foothills Med Centre, 729NT-1403 29 St NW, Calgary AB T2N 2T9; (Turkey)'86; Staff, Foothills Medical Centre; Assoc Prof, University Of Calgary; Langs: Turkish; (403)944-4266; Fax. (403)944-4693.

YIM, Annabella C; Grand River Hosp-KW HC, PO Box 9056 Stn C 835 King St W, Kitchener ON N2G 1G3; Qns'03; FRCPC; DiagRad. Staff, Grand River Hospital - Kitchener/Waterloo Health Centre; (519)749-4600

YIM, Conrad C Y; Trillium Hlth Ctr-Mississauga, 100 Queensway W, Mississauga ON L5B 1B8; Tor'93; FRCPC; Peds (Pediatric Neurology). Staff, Trillium Health Centre - Mississauga; Langs: Cantonese; Mandarin; (905)848-7360; Fax. (905)804-7741.

YIM, Daniel; Finch Medical Centre, 78 Finch Ave E, North York ON M2N 7J5; Tor'88; Langs: Korean; (416)222-3383; Fax. (416)222-8009.

YIM, Gary Y G; South Common Med Centre, 3-2110 Burnhamthorpe Rd W, Mississauga ON L5L 5Z5; Wes'88; (905)820-3209; Fax. (905)820-2576.

YIM-LEE, Famy L; Doctor's on Bayview, 15900 Bayview Ave, Aurora ON L4G 7Y3; Tor'89; Associate, Southlake Regional Health Centre; (905)726-9755; Fax. (905)726-9631.

YIN, Alan Z L; Finch-Midland Med Centre, 309-4190 Finch Ave E, Scarborough ON M1S 4T7; Alb'96; BSc(Hons); CCFP; Langs: Mandarin; (416)335-3308

YIN, Vivian; Univ Hlth Network-Toronto Western Hosp, 7E 405-399 Bathurst St, Toronto ON M5T 2S8; Tor'07; Ophth. Staff, Toronto Western Hospital - University Health Network; (416)603-2581

YING, Ethel; St Michael's Hosp, 15F-30 Bond St, Toronto ON M5B 1W8; Tor'97; FRCPC; Peds (Neonatal & Perinatal Medicine). Staff Peds, North York General Hospital; Dir NICU & Neonatal Follow Up Clinic, St Michael's Hospital; University of Toronto; Langs: Chinese; (416)867-3655; Fax. (416)867-3736.

YING, Irene; Regent Park Comm Health Centre, 465 Dundas St E, Toronto ON M5A 2B2; Tor'08; CCFP; (416)203-4507; Fax. (416)364-0822.

YING, James J; 102-83 Mill St, Georgetown ON L7G 5E9; (Taiwan)'68; Staff, Halton Healthcare Services Corporation - Georgetown Hospital; Langs: Chinese; (905)877-4111; Fax. (905)877-5638.

YING, Luis T J; Brampton Gastroenterology, 11-470 Chrysler Dr, Brampton ON L6S 0C1; Tor'94; FRCPC; IntMed; Gastroent. Staff, William Osler Health System - Brampton Civic Hospital; Langs: Cantonese; Mandarin; Spanish; (905)790-6362; Fax. (905)790-6612.

YING, Raymond; Care Point Med Centre, 711 Pender St W, Vancouver BC V6C 3T2; Dal'00; CCFP; (604)687-4858

YING, Thomas S F; T Ying Medicine Prof Corp, 1792 Liverpool Rd, Pickering ON L1V 4G6; Tor'84; Langs: Cantonese; (905)420-0041; Fax. (905)420-2316.

YING, Wai-Leung; The Moncton Hosp, 135 MacBeath Ave, Moncton NB E1C 6Z8; (Taiwan)'69; ABP; Staff, The Moncton Hospital; (506)857-5317; Fax. (506)857-5312; waying@serha.ca.

YING, Ying; A-8100 boul Taschereau, Brossard QC J4X 1C2; Shanghai (China)'86; CCFP; Langs: Chinese; French; (450)465-5589; Fax. (450)465-0092.

YING, Yvonne; Children's Hosp Eastern Ont, 3363-401 Smyth Rd, Ottawa ON K1H 8L1; Cal'02; FRCSC; PlasSurg. Staff, Children's Hospital of Eastern Ontario (CHEO); (613)737-2568; Fax. (613)738-4840.

YIP, Andrea J; First Care Med Centre, 2590 Commercial Dr, Vancouver BC V5N 4C2; UBC'94; CCFP; (604)871-1535

YIP, Augustine Y L; One World Med Centre, 3575 20 Ave NE, Calgary AB T1Y 6R3; Alb'92; CCFP; Langs: Cantonese; (403)248-7955; Fax. (403)285-5013.

YIP, Barbara Y; 20-1161 The High St, Coquitlam BC V3B 7W3; Alb'90; Langs: Cantonese; Mandarin; (604)945-8368; Fax. (604)945-8328.

YIP, Benson; St Boniface Gen Hosp, Z3041-409 Tache Ave, Winnipeg MB R2H 2A6; Wes'92; FRCSC; GenSurg. Staff, St Boniface General Hospital; (204)233-8563

YIP, Berwin P Y; 12-4465 Sheppard Ave E, Scarborough ON M1S 5H9; Tor'85; Ac Staff, The Scarborough Hospital - Birchmount Campus; (416)297-4077; Fax. (416)297-4077.

YIP, Clarwyn; 507-960 Lawrence Ave W, North York ON M6A 3B5; Tor'94; FRCPC; IntMed (Medical Microbiology); InfectDis. Assoc Staff, Humber River Regional Hospital - Keele Street Site; Langs: Cantonese; (416)782-1536; Fax. (416)782-0595; clarwyn@yahoo.com.

YIP, Daniel L K; 20-1161 The High St, Coquitlam BC V3B 7W3; Alb'90; Langs: Cantonese; (604)945-8368; Fax. (604)945-8328.

YIP, David G; 404 Medical Clinic, 46-1111 Davis Dr, Newmarket ON L3Y 8X2; Tor'91; CCFP; (905)868-8330; Fax. (905)868-8332.

YIP, David K W; Tera Losa Med Centre, 9760 170 St NW, Edmonton AB T5T 5L4; Alb'79; MPH; CCFP; (780)486-3660; Fax. (780)486-3673.

YIP, Florence S; Evergold Centre, 28-3833 Midland Ave, Scarborough ON M1V 5L6; Tor'88; CCFP; FCFP; Langs: Chinese; (416)291-0980; Fax. (416)297-9666.

YIP, Gina T C; Health For All Family Health T, 202-379 Church St, Markham ON L6B 0T1; Tor'09; CCFP; (905)472-2200

YIP, Gordon; Hamilton HS-General Site, 237 Barton St E, Hamilton ON L8L 2X2; McM'95; FRCPC; DiagRad. Staff, Hamilton Health Sciences Centre - Hamilton General Hospital; (905)527-4322; Fax. (905)527-5761.

YIP, Jeanne C; Halton HSC Corp-Oakville, 327 Reynolds St, Oakville ON L6J 3L7; Ott'08; CCFP; Staff, Halton Healthcare Services Corporation - Oakville Site; Langs: Cantonese; (905)845-2571

YIP, Lisa Y; 319-55 Erb St E, Waterloo ON N2J 4K8; Wes'94; FRCPC; IntMed; ClinImmunol&Allergy. (519)885-7037; Fax. (519)885-8197.

YIP, Melissa; Centre Med Via Medica, 3943 boul Saint-Jean, Roxboro QC H9G 1X2; Mon'98; FRCPC; DiagRad. (514)626-5888

YIP, Raymond W; Royal University Hosp, 103 Hospital Dr, Saskatoon SK S7N 0W8; Sask'79; FRCPC; Anes (Cardiovascular Anesthesia). Ac Staff Anes, Royal University Hospital; Head Dept of Anes, University of Saskatchewan; (306)655-1183; Fax. (306)655-1279; yipr@sdh.sk.ca.

YIP, Samuel; Gordon & Leslie Diamond HCC, 8F-2775 Laurel St, Vancouver BC V5Z 1M9; UBC'02; FRCPC; Neur. Staff, Gordon & Leslie Diamond Health Care Centre; Langs: Cantonese; (604)875-5126

YIP, Stephen T; Vancouver Gen Hosp, 899 12 Ave W, Vancouver BC V5Z 1M9; UBC'99; FRCPC; NeurPath (Clinician Investigator Program). Staff, BC Cancer Agency Vancouver Centre; Staff Path & Lab Med, Vancouver General Hospital - Centennial Pavillion; Langs: Cantonese; (604)875-4111 x63968

YIP, T C Kathy; KMH Cardiology & Diagnostic Ct, 2075 Hadwen Rd, Mississauga ON L5K 2L3; Tor'80; BSc; ABNM; FRCPC; NuclearMed; IntMed. Consultant Nuclear Med., KMH Cardiology & Diagnostic Centre; Langs: Chinese; (905)855-1860; Fax. (905)855-1863.

YIP, Todd R; RebalanceMD, 104-3551 Blanshard St, Victoria BC V8Z 0B9; Qns'02; FRCPC; PhysMed&Rehab. Staff, CBI Health Centre; (250)940-4444

YIPP, Bryan G; Foothills Med Centre, E157-1403 29 St NW, Calgary AB T2N 2T9; Cal'05; FRCPC; IntMed; Critical Care Medicine. Staff, Foothills Medical Centre; (403)943-5488; Fax. (403)291-1491.

YIU, Douglas W; 335-3381 Cambie St, Vancouver BC V5Z 4R3; UBC'03; CCFP; Langs: Chinese; (604)218-0947

YIU, Stella H M; The Ottawa Hosp-Gen Campus, 501 Smyth Rd, Ottawa ON K1H 8L6; Tor'01; CCFP; CCFP(E.M.); Staff, The Ottawa Hospital - General Campus; Langs: Cantonese; (613)722-7000

YIU, Verna W Y; Seventh Street Plaza, 14 030-10030 107 St NW, Edmonton AB T5J 3E4; Alb'86; FRCPC; Peds (Pediatric Nephrology); Nephrol. Staff Ped Nephrol, University of Alberta Hospital; Staff, Edmonton Clinic Health Academy; Dean Fac of Med & Dentistry(Interim), University of Alberta; Langs: Cantonese; (780)342-2011; Fax. (780)342-2060; vyiu@cha.ab.ca.

YIU, Wendy W S; 407-131 Bloor St W, Toronto ON M5S 1R1; Alb'92; FRCPC; Psy. Langs: Chinese; (416)923-8838; Fax. (416)923-8820; wyiu@bellnet.ca.

YLANKO, V Heikki; Leaside Health Centre, 795 Eglinton Ave E, East York ON M4G 4E4; Tor'84; BSc; MSc; Staff, North York General Hospital; Langs: Finnish; (416)424-3145; Fax. (416)424-2611; heka.ylanko@rogers.com.

YLANKO, Veli J; Leaside Health Centre, 795 Eglinton Ave E, East York ON M4G 4E4; Turku (Finland)'57; LMCC; CCFP; FCFP; Hon Staff, North York General Hospital; Court Staff, Women's College Hospital; Langs: Finnish; (416)424-3145; Fax. (416)424-2611.

YMERI, Hylkije; Nova Scotia Cancer Centre, 5820 University Ave, Halifax NS B3H 1V7; Tirana University (Other Foreign)'97; Staff, Nova Scotia Cancer Center; (902)473-6185; hylkije.ymeri@cdha.nshealth.ca.

YOGANATHAN, Pradeepa; North Toronto Eye Care, 407-2115 Finch Ave W, North York ON M3N 2V6; Albany (USA)'03; FRCSC; Ophth. (416)748-2020; Fax. (416)748-8582.

YOGAPARAN, Thirumagal; Baycrest Ctr for Geriatric Car, 3560 Bathurst St, North York ON M6A 2E1; Jaffna (Sri Lanka)'89; FRCPC; IntMed; GeriatricMed. Staff, Baycrest Centre for Geriatric Care; Langs: Tamil; (416)785-2500; Fax. (416)785-2683.

YOGESWARAN, Kumaresan; Univ Hlth Network-Toronto Gen, 9N 980-200 Elizabeth St, Toronto ON M5G 2C4; Wes'06; FRCPC; IntMed; Gastroent. Staff, Toronto General Hospital - UHN; Langs: Tamil; (416)340-3893

YOKOYAMA, Benjamin C; 104-32423 Lougheed Hwy, Mission BC V2V 7B8; UBC'91; (604)820-7676

YOLLES, Linda A; 39 Pleasant Blvd, Toronto ON M4T 1K2; Tor'89; BSc; CCFP; FCFP; (416)967-4446; Fax. (416)967-9406.

YONEDA, Bruce T; RebalanceMD, 104-3551 Blanshard St, Victoria BC V8Z 0B9; Alb'72; BSc; FRCSC; OrthSurg (Knee Surgery). Ac Staff, Royal Jubilee Hospital; Ac Staff, Victoria General Hospital; Assoc Staff, Queen Alexandra Centre for Children's Health; Ac Staff, Saanich Peninsula Hospital; (250)940-4444; cadu@shawcable.com.

YONEDA, Janet; University of Alberta Hosp, 8440 112 St NW, Edmonton AB T6G 2B7; Alb'76; CASM; Staff, University of Alberta Hospital; Member, University of Alberta; (780)407-8822

YONEMORI, Peter S; Claresholm Med Centre, PO Box 2050 4215 3rd St W, Claresholm AB T0L 0T0; (Australia)'96; (403)625-3900; Fax. (403)625-3969.

YONEYAMA, Norma J; Dr N Yoneyama Med Prof Corp, 302-372 Hollandview Trail, Aurora ON L4G 0A5; McM'88; CCFP; FCFP; Staff, Southlake Regional Health Centre; (905)727-6600; Fax. (905)750-0085.

YONG, Chu Hua; Shouldice Hosp, 7750 Bayview Ave, Thornhill ON L3T 4A3; (Hong Kong)'57; Staff, Shouldice Hospital; Langs: Chinese; (905)889-1125

YONG, Collin K K; 205-5678 Granville St, Vancouver BC V6M 3C5; Leicester (England)'89; MB ChB; FRCPC; Peds. Staff, Providence Health Care - St Paul's Hospital; Staff, BC Women's Hospital & Health Centre; University of British Columbia; Langs: Hakka; Cantonese; Mandarin; (604)322-9750; Fax. (604)323-2102.

YONG, Elaine; Sunnybrook Health Sciences Cen, HG 60-2075 Bayview Ave, Toronto ON M4N 3M5; Qns'99; Gastroent; IntMed (Family Medicine). Staff, Sunnybrook Health Sciences Centre; (416)480-5910

YONG, Paul C K; 2316 96 St NW, Edmonton AB T6N 1J8; Alb'73; CCFP; FCFP; Staff, Covenant Health - Grey Nuns Community Hospital; Staff, Caritas Health Group-Edmonton; (780)468-5999; Fax. (780)468-5398.

YONG, Paul J; BC Women's Hosp & Health Ctre, F2-4500 Oak St, Vancouver BC V6H 3N1; UBC'06; FRCSC; ObstGyn. Staff, BC Women's Hospital & Health Centre; Staff, BC Women's Centre for Pelvic Pain & Endometriosis; (604)875-2534

YONG, Peter L; Victoria Med Centre, 6239 Victoria Dr, Vancouver BC V5P 3X5; (Singapore)'74; Langs: Chinese; (604)430-3667; Fax. (604)430-1194.

YONG, Sharon H; King Edward Pediatrics Clinic, 926 King Edward Ave, Vancouver BC V5Z 2E2; Alb'08; Peds. (604)600-7282

YONG, Siu-Li; BC Women's Hosp & Health Ctre, C234-4500 Oak St, Vancouver BC V6H 3N1; (Singapore)'69; MB BS; DABPed; FCCMG; MMed; FRCPC; Peds (Medical Genetics). Ac Staff, BC Women's Hospital & Health Centre; Clin Prof Med Genetics, University of British Columbia; (604)875-2157; Fax. (604)875-2376; slyong@cw.bc.ca.

YONG, Yean-Sim; 3-13665 96 Ave, Surrey BC V3V 1Z1; Wes'98; (604)588-8368; Fax. (604)588-3237.

YONG, Yu-Sen; 3-13665 96 Ave, Surrey BC V3V 1Z1; (Taiwan)'61; FRCSC; Urol; GenSurg. Langs: Chinese; (604)588-8368

YONG HING, Charlotte J; BC Cancer Agency, 600 10th Ave W, Vancouver BC V5Z 4E6; Sask'02; FRCPC; DiagRad. Staff Diagnostic Imaging, BC Cancer Agency Vancouver Centre; (604)877-6000

YONG-HING, Ken Yow; Royal University Hosp, 103 Hospital Dr, Saskatoon SK S7N 0W8; Liverpool (England)'68; MB ChB; FRCS(Glas); DABOS; FRCSC; OrthSurg (Spine). Prof OrthSurg, Royal University Hospital; Prof, University of Saskatchewan; (306)966-8200; Fax. (306)966-8196; ken.yong-hing@usask.ca.

YONG-SET, Wrenrick E; William Osler HC-Brampton, 2100 Bovaird Dr E, Brampton ON L6R 3J7; Leeds (England)'71; Staff, William Osler Health System - Brampton Civic Hospital; (905)494-2120

YONT, Karrie R; Rockyview Gen Hosp, 7007 14 St SW, Calgary AB T2V 1P9; Sask'97; FRCPC; Anes. Staff, St Joseph's General Hospital; Staff, Rockyview General Hospital; (403)992-1793

YOO, Carolyn T; Maternal Child Clinic, 130-1402 8 Ave NW, Calgary AB T2N 1B8; Alb'01; CCFP; (403)509-3080

YOO, Jennifer W J; University Down Family Pract, 425 University Ave E, Waterloo ON N2K 4C9; Tor'99; CCFP; Langs: Korean; (519)569-8821; Fax. (519)569-8823.

YOO, John H J; London HSC-Victoria Hosp, PO Box 5010 Stn B B3 433-800 Commissioners Rd E, London ON N6A 5W9; Tor'91; DAB; FACS; FRCSC; Otol (Head & Neck Surgery). Staff, London Health Sciences Centre - Victoria Campus; Staff, St Joseph's Hospital - St Joseph's Health Care; Staff, London Regional Cancer Centre; Dept Chair Otol/Prof, University of Western Ontario; Langs: Korean; (519)685-8457; Fax. (519)685-8567; john.yoo@lhsc.on.ca.

YOO, Shi-Joon; The Hosp For Sick Children, 555 University Ave, Toronto ON M5G 1X8; Seoul (Korea)'77; PhD; FRCPC; DiagRad. Teach Staff, The Hospital For Sick Children; Langs: Korean; (416)813-6037; shi-joon.yoo@sickkids.ca.

YOON, Frederick H; Royal Victoria Hosp, 201 Georgian Dr, Barrie ON L4M 6M2; Wes'05; FRCPC; RadOncol (Genito Urinary Oncology). Staff, Royal Victoria Regional Health Centre; Court Staff Odette Cancer Centre, Sunnybrook Health Sciences Centre; Staff, Simcoe Muskoka Regional Cancer Centre; (705)728-9090; Fax. (705)729-5619.

YOON, Grace; The Hosp for Sick Children, 555 University Ave, Toronto ON M5G 1X8; Dal'98; FRCPC; MedGenetics (Clinical & Metabolic Genetics). Asst Prof Peds Clinical & Metabolic Genetics, The Hospital For Sick Children; Langs: Spanish; French; (416)813-6387; grace.yoon@sickkids.ca.

YOON, Philip W; Royal Columbia Hosp, 330 Columbia St E, New Westminster BC V3L 3W7; Alb'93; CCFP; CCFP(E.M.); FCFP; Staff, Queen Elizabeth II Health Sciences Centre - Halifax Infirmary Site; (604)520-4253

YOON, Ted Tai J; 103-3195 Granville St, Vancouver BC V6H 3K2; UBC'02; CCFP; (604)739-8011

YOON, Yeung-Seu; 105-3950 14th Ave, Markham ON L3R 0A9; Tor'90; FRCPC; Peds. (905)305-1700; Fax. (905)305-1706.

YOONG, K T Thomas; Oshawa Clinic, 117 King St E, Oshawa ON L1H 1B9; Tor'77; Court Staff, Lakeridge Health - Oshawa Site; Langs: Cantonese; (905)723-8551; Fax. (905)721-3557.

YOONG, Kevin; Albany Med Clinic, 807 Broadview Ave, Toronto ON M4K 2P8; McM'09; CCFP; (416)461-9471; Fax. (416)461-2710.

YORK, Daniel C; Phoenix Med Centre, 405-2155 10th Ave, Prince George BC V2M 5J6; Sask'00; CCFP; (250)564-8018; Fax. (250)562-5253.

YORK, Ernest L; Wetaskiwin Lung Laboratory, 5217A 50 St, Wetaskiwin AB T9A 3B8; Witwatersrand (South Africa)'68; MRC(UK); FRCPC; IntMed (Pediatric Respiratory Medicine); Respir. (780)352-7085; Fax. (780)352-7870; eyork@telusplanet.net.

YORK, Graham J; Cameron Med Clinic, 302 Cameron St, Williams Lake BC V2G 1S9; UBC'88; (250)305-1102

YORK, Stephen; British Army Training Unit-Suf, PO BOX 5000 LCD 1, Medicine Hat AB T1A 8K7; Staff, British Army Training Unit-Suffield; (403)544-4108; stephen.york@cubic.com.

YORKE, Alan J; 205-9808 King George Blvd, Surrey BC V3T 2V6; Dublin (Ireland)'74; FRCPC; IntMed (Rheumatology). Consultant Rheum, Surrey Memorial Hospital; (604)581-4446

YORSTON, Janet E; Central Hastings Fam Hlth Team, PO Box 744 52 St Lawrence St E, Madoc ON K0K 2K0; McM'78; CCFP; (613)473-4134; Fax. (613)473-4740.

YOSHIDA, Eric M; Gordon & Leslie Diamond HCC, 5153-2775 Laurel St, Vancouver BC V5Z 1M9; Tor'86; FACP; MHSc; FACG; FRCPC; IntMed; Gastroent. Ac Staff, Vancouver General Hospital - Centennial Pavillion; Staff, Gordon & Leslie Diamond Health Care Centre; Head Div of Gastroent/Prof, University of British Columbia; (604)875-5371; Fax. (604)875-5447; eric.yoshida@vch.ca.

YOSHIDA, Kenneth M; 104-316 George St, Sarnia ON N7T 4P4; Tor'87; FRCPC; IntMed; MedOncol. Chief Internal Med Program/Med Dir Internal Med Program, Bluewater Health - Mitton Site; (519)336-6765; Fax. (519)336-7319.

YOSHIDA, Lianne M; Fenwick Med Centre, 211-5595 Fenwick St, Halifax NS B3H 4M2; McM'97; CCFP; FCFP; (902)423-3323; Fax. (902)442-5593.

YOSHIDA, Owen I; 210-3001 Tutt St, Kelowna BC V1Y 2H4; Alb'82; BSc; FRCSC; ObstGyn. (250)869-1550; Fax. (250)869-1580.

YOSHIDA, Sam S; Windsor Reg Cancer Centre, 2220 Kildare Rd, Windsor ON N8W 2X3; Tor'68; FRCPC; IntMed (Medical Oncology). Ac Staff, Windsor Regional Hospital - Metropolitan Site; Assoc Staff, Hôtel-Dieu Grace Hospital; Internal Medicine, Windsor Regional Hospital - Windsor Regional Cancer Centre; (519)253-5253; sam_yoshida@wrh.on.ca.

YOSHIDA, Sean H; North Shore Med Imaging, 139 16th St W, North Vancouver BC V7M 1T3; UBC'91; FRCPC; DiagRad. (604)987-9729; Fax. (604)984-8395.

YOSHIDA, Winifred R; 4 Burnhamthorpe Rd, Etobicoke ON M9A 5C9; McM'92; CCFP; (416)234-1987; Fax. (416)234-8631.

YOSHITOMI, Kerry M; Peace Arch Hosp, 15521 Russell Ave, White Rock BC V4B 2R4; Qns'86; CCFP; CCFP(E.M.); FCFP; Staff Emergency Med, Peace Arch Hospital; (604)531-5512; Fax. (604)538-4212.

YOSKOVITCH, Adi; Polyclinique Fabreville, 380 boul Cure-Labelle, Laval QC H7P 5L3; Philadelpia(PA) (USA)'96; MSc; FRCS; FRCSC; Otol (Facial Plastic Surgery). Chef Otol, Centre Hospitalier Fleury; (450)628-5800

YOSTOS, Philippe R; Kyrellos Clinic, C4-2901 Eglinton Ave W, Mississauga ON L5M 6J3; Ain Shams (Egypt)'68; MB ChB; CCFP; Langs: Arabic; (905)607-4747; dryostos@yahoo.com.

YOU, Calorine; Headwaters Health Care Centre, 100 Rolling Hills Dr, Orangeville ON L9W 4X9; Tor'08; CCFP; Staff, Headwaters Health Care Centre - Orangeville Site; (519)941-2410

YOU, John J; Hamilton HS-McMaster Site, PO Box 2000 Stn Lcd 1 3V51-1200 Main St W, Hamilton ON L8N 3Z5; Tor'00; FRCPC; IntMed. Staff, Hamilton Health Sciences Centre - McMaster Children's Hospital; (905)521-2100; Fax. (905)521-4971.

YOU, John M S; Corporate Med Centre, 10-78 Corporate Dr, Scarborough ON M1H 3G4; Dal'90; FRCS; FRCSC; GenSurg; VascSurg. Staff, The Scarborough Hospital - General Campus; (416)279-0855; Fax. (416)279-0857; jmyou@yahoo.com.

YOU, Yong Dong; The Richmond Hosp, 7000 Westminster Hwy, Richmond BC V6X 1A2; Dal'03; FRCPC; IntMed. Staff, Richmond Hospital; Langs: Mandarin; (604)278-9711

YOU, Yue; Hotel Dieu Hosp, 382C-166 Brock St, Kingston ON K7L 5G2; Berlin (Germany)'03; Staff, Hotel-Dieu Hospital; (613)544-3310

YOU-TEN, Fung Voon K; Mount Sinai Hosp, 600 University Ave, Toronto ON M5G 1X5; Tor'00; FRCPC; Anes. Staff, Mount Sinai Hospital; Langs: Bilingual(English/French); (416)586-5270; Fax. (416)586-8664.

YOUAKIM, Hany N; Well Point Health Clinic, 303-1 Kingsway Garden Mall NW, Edmonton AB T5G 3A6; (Egypt)'91; MB ChB; CCFP; Langs: Arabic; (780)479-3699; Fax. (780)479-3399.

YOUAKIM, Sami; PO Box 53507 Rpo Broadmead, Victoria BC V8X 5K2; McG'87; FRCPC; OccupMed;CCFP; Staff, Workers' Comp Board of BC; Langs: Bilingual(French/English); (250)858-1559

YOUHNOVSKA, Pavlina; Ctr Hosp de Lachine, 650 16e av, Lachine QC H8S 3N5; Medical Academy of Varna (Other Foreign)'96; Ophth. Staff, Centre Hospitalier de Lachine; (514)637-2351 x77256; pavlina.youhnovska@mail.mcgill.ca.

YOULA, Adama R; PO Box 393, Campbellton NB E3N 3G7; Conakry (Other Foreign)'85; Staff, Hôpital Régional Campbellton; (506)789-5000

YOUMBISSI TCHETAGNI, Joseph; Ctr Hosp Trois-Riv-St-Joseph, 731 rue Sainte-Julie, Trois-Rivieres QC G9A 1Y1; Yaounde (Cameroon)'75; MSc; FRCP; CSPQ; Chef Nephrol, Centre Hospitalier Regional de Trois-Rivieres; Langs: Bilingual(French/English); (819)697-3333; Fax. (819)372-3506.

YOUNAN, Rami J; CHUM-Hop Notre-Dame, 1560 rue Sherbrooke E, Montreal QC H2L 4M1; Laval'97; FRCSC; GenSurg; General Surgical Oncology (P.Q.). Staff, Centre Hospitalier l'Université de Montréal (CHUM) - Hôpital Notre-Dame; (514)890-8000; Fax. (514)412-7821.

YOUNAN, Sawsan I; Credit Valley Med Arts Centre, 210-2000 Credit Valley Rd, Mississauga ON L5M 4N4; Cairo (Egypt)'79; MB ChB; Staff, The Credit Valley Hospital; Medical Officer, Canadian Forces Health Services Group; Langs: Arabic; (905)820-4000; Fax. (905)820-9998.

YOUNAN, Younan-Samy; Lonsdale Med Dental Bldg, 108-1940 Lonsdale Ave, North Vancouver BC V7M 2K2; Ain Shams (Egypt)'65; MB BCh; CCFP; (604)987-3357

YOUNES, Chahine; CSSS De La Haute-Yamaska, 205 boul Leclerc O, Granby QC J2G 1T7; Beirut (Lebanon)'79; FRCSC; OrthSurg (Neuro-Surgery). Staff, Centre Hospitalier de Granby; (450)372-5491; Fax. (450)375-8032.

YOUNES, John K; St Boniface Gen Hosp, 409 Tache Ave, Winnipeg MB R2H 2A6; Man'94; FRCPC; AnatPath. Staff, St Boniface General Hospital; (204)235-3104

YOUNES, Layla; GMF Cote-des-Neiges, 5700 ch Cote-des-Neiges, Montreal QC H3T 2A8; Medical University of Sofia (Other Foreign)'90; CCFP; Langs: Arabic; Bulgarian; French; (514)734-8531; Fax. (514)731-0536.

YOUNG, Aaron M; 401-2020 Richmond Rd, Victoria BC V8R 6R5; UBC'06; FRCPC; IntMed; Respir. (250)995-0211

YOUNG, Alan J; Claro Family Practice, 107-4930 55 Ave, Drayton Valley AB T7A 1W2; (Other Foreign)'01; (780)621-0202; Fax. (780)621-0213.

YOUNG, Alix M; Grandview Med Ctr Fam Hlth Team, 167 Hespeler Rd, Cambridge ON N1R 3H7; McM'81; CCFP; FCFP; Ac Staff, Cambridge Memorial Hospital; Staff, District Health Council; University of Western Ontario; (519)623-4200; Fax. (519)623-2546.

YOUNG, Allan H; Strangway Bldg, 430-5950 University Blvd, Vancouver BC V6T 1Z3; Edinburgh (Scotland)'84; FRCPC; Psy. (604)827-4287; Fax. (604)827-3373.

YOUNG, Barbara M; MUHC Montreal Gen Hosp, 1650 av Cedar, Montreal QC H3G 1A4; McG'98; FRCPC; IntMed. Staff, McGill University Health Centre - Montreal General Campus; Langs: Bilingual(French/English); (514)934-8053; barbara.young@mcgill.ca.

YOUNG, Bernita A; Kipling Heights Med Centre, 2291 Kipling Ave, Etobicoke ON M9W 4L6; Tor'79; CCFP; FCFP; Ac Staff, William Osler Health System - Etobicoke General Hospital; (416)741-4545; Fax. (416)744-1484.

YOUNG, Beverly; Mount Sinai Hosp, 600 University Ave, Toronto ON M5G 1X5; Qns'96; FRCPC; Psy. Staff, Mount Sinai Hospital; Langs: English; French; (416)586-4800 x8419; Fax. (416)586-8654.

YOUNG, Brent C; Prairie Trails Med Clinic, 100-1345 Taylor Ave, Winnipeg MB R3M 3Y9; Man'02; CCFP; (204)475-0088

YOUNG, Brian R; McConnell Med Centre, 128-820 McConnell Ave, Cornwall ON K6H 4M4; Ott'77; (613)936-1564; Fax. (613)936-0174.

YOUNG, Bryan C; Foothills Med Centre, C231-1403 29 St NW, Calgary AB T2N 2T9; Alb'82; FRCPC; EmergMed. Staff Emerg, Foothills Medical Centre; (403)944-1635

YOUNG, Carmen B; Royal Alexandra Hosp, 10240 Kingsway NW, Edmonton AB T5H 3V9; Alb'04; FRCSC; ObstGyn (Maternal Fetal Medicine). Staff Perinatal Clinic, Royal Alexandra Hospital; Staff, Lois Hole Hospital for Women; Staff, Perinatal Clinic; (780)735-4813; Fax. (780)735-4814.

YOUNG, Carmen E; Links Clinic, 104-11910 111 Ave NW, Edmonton AB T5G 3G6; Alb'89; (780)454-0351; Fax. (780)452-6767.

YOUNG, Casey; Lloydminster Hosp, 3820 43rd Ave, Lloydminster SK S9V 1Y5; Sask'07; FRCPC; DiagRad. Staff, Lloydminster Hospital; (306)820-6045; Fax. (306)820-6054.

YOUNG, Claire A; Town Centre Med Clinic, 18-2475 Dobbin Rd, Westbank BC V4T 2E9; Leicester (England)'01; MB ChB; BSc; MRCGPract; (250)768-8315

YOUNG, Dana G; Simcoe Family Med Centre, 301 Blake St, Barrie ON L4M 1K7; Mem'98; BMedSci; CCFP; (705)727-9896; Fax. (705)727-9294.

YOUNG, Darryl K; Nepean Med Centre, 408-1 Centrepointe Dr, Nepean ON K2G 6E2; Mem'03; FRCSC; OrthSurg. Staff, Queensway Carleton Hospital; (613)225-1188; Fax. (613)225-7770.

YOUNG, David C; Seymour Med Clinic, 1530 7th Ave W, Vancouver BC V6J 1S2; Man'72; CCFP; FCFP; (604)738-2151; Fax. (604)738-1487.

YOUNG, David C; IWK Health Centre, PO Box 9700 RPO CSC G2141-5980 University Ave, Halifax NS B3K 6R8; Dal'73; MSc; FRCSC; ObstGyn (Fetal & Maternal Medicine). Staff, IWK Health Centre; (902)470-7491; Fax. (902)425-1125; david.young@iwk.nshealth.ca.

YOUNG, David S F; 33 University Ave, Toronto ON M5J 2S7; Tor'90.

YOUNG, David W; Central Park Medical, 301-1711 Cook St, Victoria BC V8T 3P2; McG'70; DAB; FRCSC; Ophth. Ac Staff, Victoria General Hospital; Ac Staff, Royal Jubilee Hospital; Langs: Bilingual(English/French); (250)385-0811; Fax. (250)385-0877.

YOUNG, Deidre C; Albany Med Clinic, 807 Broadview Ave, Toronto ON M4K 2P8; McG'02; CCFP; Langs: Bilingual(English/French); (416)461-9471; Fax. (416)461-2710.

YOUNG, Donald J; Campbell River & Dist Gen Hosp, 375 2nd Ave, Campbell River BC V9W 3V1; UBC'94; CCFP; FCFP; Staff, Campbell River & District General Hospital; (250)287-7111; Fax. (250)830-6962.

YOUNG, Elizabeth Y F; Pediatric Ambulatory Clinic, 2F-61 Queen St E, Toronto ON M5C 2T2; McM'02; FRCPC; Peds (Developmental Pediatrics). Staff, Holland Bloorview Kids Rehabilitation Hospital; (416)867-3655; Fax. (416)867-3736; eyoung@hollandbloorview.ca.

YOUNG, Eric R; Office of the Prov Health Offi, 4F-1515 Blanshard St, Victoria BC V8W 3C8; Ott'74; MHSc; FRCPC; CommunMed (Public Health);CCFP; Staff Deputy Provincial Health Officer, Ministry Of Health Services; Langs: Bilingual(English/French); (250)592-1330; Fax. (250)592-1362; eric.young@gov.bc.ca.

YOUNG, Frederick N M; Elliot Lake Family Health Team, 31 Nova Scotia Walk, Elliot Lake ON P5A 1Y9; West Indies (Jamaica)'64; Ac Staff, St Joseph's General Hospital Elliot Lake; (705)461-8882; Fax. (705)848-3449.

YOUNG, G Bryan; London HSC-University Hosp, PO Box 5339 Stn B B10-106-339 Windermere Rd, London ON N6A 5A5; Sask'70; FRCPC; Neur (Critical Care Medicine). Staff, London Health Sciences Centre - University Hospital; (519)663-2911; Fax. (519)663-3152; bryan.young@lhsc.on.ca.

YOUNG, Gordon V; PO Box 1090, Pictou NS B0K 1H0; Dal'74; (902)485-6700; Fax. (902)485-4045.

YOUNG, Graeme M; Dr Everett Chalmers Reg Hosp, PO Box 9000 Stn A 700 Priestman St, Fredericton NB E3B 5N5; Mem'92; CCFP; CCFP(E.M.); Staff Emerg, Dr Everett Chalmers Regional Hospital; (506)459-7592; Fax. (506)459-7596.

YOUNG, H Thomas; Manitouwadge Gen Hosp, 1 Health Care Cres, Manitouwadge ON P0T 2C0; Dal'70; CCFP; FCFP; Staff, Manitouwadge General Hospital; (807)826-3251; Fax. (807)826-4216.

YOUNG, Iain D; Kingston Gen Hosp, 76 Stuart St, Kingston ON K7L 2V7; McG'82; FRCPC; AnatPath. Att Staff Path & Molecular Med, Kingston General Hospital; Att Staff Path & Molecular Med, Hotel-Dieu Hospital; Prof Path & Molecular Med, Queen's University; (613)548-3232; Fax. (613)331-6361; young@cliff.path.queensu.ca.

YOUNG, Ian G; Simcoe Family Med Centre, 301 Blake St, Barrie ON L4M 1K7; Mem'03; CCFP; Staff Emerg, Royal Victoria Regional Health Centre; (705)727-9896; Fax. (705)727-9294.

YOUNG, J Edward M; St Joseph's Healthcare, 50 Charlton Ave E, Hamilton ON L8N 4A6; Tor'69; FACS; FRCSC; GenSurg (Head & Neck Surgery). Staff Surg, St Joseph's Healthcare - Charlton Campus; Clin Prof Surg, McMaster University; (905)522-1255; Fax. (905)522-9460; jemyoung@stjosham.on.ca.

YOUNG, J Neil; Terrace Clinic, 204-35 Major's Path, St. John's NL A1A 4Z9; Mem'99; Staff, Waterford Hospital; (709)777-3450

YOUNG, James W; Humber River Reg Hosp-Church, 200 Church St, York ON M9N 1N8; Man'97; FRCPC; Anes. Staff, Humber River Regional Hospital - Church Street Site; (416)249-8111

YOUNG, Janice L; Student Health Services, B106-1280 Main St W, Hamilton ON L8S 4K1; McM'85; FCFP; CCFP; FCFP; Physician, McMaster University; (905)525-9140 x27700; Fax. (905)546-1663; youngjan@mcmaster.ca.

YOUNG, Jeanne; Salvation Army Grace Gen Hosp, 300 Booth Dr, Winnipeg MB R3J 3M7; Qns'97; CCFP; FCFP; Staff, The Salvation Army Grace Hospital; (204)837-8311

YOUNG, Jennifer L; St Joseph's Healthcare, 50 Charlton Ave E, Hamilton ON L8N 4A6; Mem'07; FRCPC; DiagRad. Staff, St Joseph's Healthcare - Charlton Campus; (905)522-4941

YOUNG, Jennifer P; 27 Third St, Collingwood ON L9Y 1K4; Tor'88; CCFP; CCFP(E.M.); Assoc Staff, Collingwood General & Marine Hospital; Assoc Prof Family Med, McMaster University; Langs: Dutch; French; (705)445-4111; Fax. (705)445-8250.

YOUNG, Jennifer S; Mount Sinai Hosp, 600 University Ave, Toronto ON M5G 1X5; West Indies (Other Foreign)'97; Staff, Mount Sinai Hospital; (416)813-6927

YOUNG, Joanne M; 203-1448 Commercial Dr, Vancouver BC V5L 3X9; McM'91; CCFP; FCFP; Staff, Strathcona Mental Health Team; (604)255-6565; Fax. (604)255-6559.

YOUNG, John G; 692 Euclid Ave, Toronto ON M6G 2T9; Tor'82; (416)901-9020

YOUNG, John G; 327 Frank St, Ottawa ON K2P 0X7; Qns'76; Otol (Head & Neck Surgery). Ac Staff, The Ottawa Hospital - Riverside Campus; Langs: Danish; French; (613)234-6615; Fax. (613)230-9416.

YOUNG, Jonathan; MUHC-Royal Victoria Hosp, E4 40-687 av des Pins O, Montreal QC H3A 1A1; McG'04; FRCSC; Otol (Head & Neck Surgery). Staff, McGill University Health Centre - Royal Victoria Hospital; (514)934-1934

YOUNG, Kathleen R; Rideau Med & Dental Centre, 101-1711 4 St SW, Calgary AB T2S 1V8; Qns'07; CCFP; (403)228-3667; Fax. (403)228-3660.

YOUNG, Kay; Strathcona Mental Health Team, 330 Heatley Ave, Vancouver BC V6A 3G3; UBC'84; FRCPC; Psy. Staff, Vancouver General Hospital - Centennial Pavillion; Staff, Strathcona Mental Health Team; (604)253-4401

YOUNG, Kelly A; Alberta Prof Bldg, 300-320 23 Ave SW, Calgary AB T2S 0J2; Alb'80; (403)228-3822; Fax. (403)228-9828.

YOUNG, Kevin J; Orillia Soldiers' Mem Hosp, 170 Colborne St W, Orillia ON L3V 2Z3; Tor'07; GeriatricMed; IntMed. Staff, Orillia Soldiers' Memorial Hospital; (705)325-2201

YOUNG, L Trevor; Addiction & Mental Hlth-Clarke, 835-250 College St, Toronto ON M5T 1R8; Man'83; FRCPC; Psy (Mood Disorders). Staff, Centre for Addiction & Mental Health (CAMH) - College Street Site; Chair Psy, University of Toronto; (416)979-6948; Fax. (416)979-6928.

YOUNG, Louise H; Dr Louise Young Inc, PO Box 1450 Stn A, Comox BC V9M 7Z9; UBC'94; CCFP; CCFP(E.M.); FCFP.

YOUNG, M Christine; 205-4040 Finch Ave E, Scarborough ON M1S 4V5; Tor'80; FRCS(A); AB(Certified); FRCSC; OrthSurg (Arthroplasty). Staff, The Scarborough Hospital - Birchmount Campus; Lecturer, University of Toronto; (416)754-7312; Fax. (416)754-0116; mcyoung@idirect.com.

YOUNG, Malcolm J; Misericordia Comm Hosp & H C, 16940 87 Ave NW, Edmonton AB T5R 4H5; Alb'69; Ac Staff, Covenant Health - Misericordia Community Hospital; (780)735-2819; Fax. (780)735-2966.

YOUNG, Mark R; Assiniboine Clinic, 633 Lodge Ave, Winnipeg MB R3J 0S9; Man'67; Neur. Staff, Health Sciences Centre; Staff, The Salvation Army Grace Hospital.

YOUNG, Maureen A; Foothills Med Centre, G28-1403 29 St NW, Calgary AB T2N 2T9; Cal'03; CCFP; Staff, Foothills Medical Centre; (403)944-2800; Fax. (403)283-7365.

YOUNG, Melanie; Western Mem Reg Hosp, PO Box 2005 Stn Main 1 Brookfield Ave, Corner Brook NL A2H 6J7; Mem'10; CCFP; Locum Tenens, Western Memorial Regional Hospital; (709)637-5000

YOUNG, Michael J; IWK Health Centre, PO Box 9700 Rpo CSC 5850-5980 University Ave, Halifax NS B3K 6R8; Dal'92; FRCPC; Peds. Staff, IWK Health Centre; (902)470-7248; Fax. (902)470-8823; michael_young@gov.nt.ca.

YOUNG, Michelle F; Pearlgate Med Clinic, 18 Gibson Dr, Mount Pearl NL A1N 5K8; Mem'97; CCFP; (709)364-3909; Fax. (709)364-7554; michellefyoung@hotmail.com.

YOUNG, Neil G; Saint John Reg Hosp, PO Box 2100 Stn Main 400 University Ave, Saint John NB E2L 4L2; Ott'92; CCFP; CCFP(E.M.); FCFP; Staff, Sussex Health Centre; Staff, Saint John Regional Hospital; Staff, St Joseph's Hospital; Mgr EmergMed, Dalhousie University; (506)648-6958; Fax. (506)648-6060.

YOUNG, Peter G J; Perfect Reflections Laser Skin, 211 Martindale Rd, St Catharines ON L2S 3V7; Wes'95; FRCSC; PlasSurg. (905)988-6153; Fax. (905)988-6298.

YOUNG, Rebekka B; 23 Marley St, Kingston ON K7M 2M4; Qns'84; BSc(Hons.); MSc(Physiol.); (613)546-4566; Fax. (613)546-0935.

YOUNG, Robert J; Millbrook Mall, 326-2 Herald Ave, Corner Brook NL A2H 4B5; Mem'76; (709)639-9906

YOUNG, Robert S; St Boniface Gen Hosp, 409 Tache Ave, Winnipeg MB R2H 2A6; Man'97; FRCPC; Anes. Staff, St Boniface General Hospital; (204)233-8563

YOUNG, Robert W; College of Phys & Surgs of NL, W100-120 Torbay Rd, St. John's NL A1A 2G8; Dal'58; MDCM; FRCPC; IntMed (Cardiology). Registrar, College of Physicians & Surgeons of Newfoundland & Labrador; Clin Prof Med, Memorial University Of Newfoundland; (709)726-8546; Fax. (709)726-4725.

YOUNG, Ronald M L; 515-10333 Southport Rd SW, Calgary AB T2W 3X6; Sask'81; CCFP; (403)252-4410; Fax. (403)252-4674; calvein@veinlase.com.

YOUNG, Scott D; Northeastern On Reg Cancer Ctr, 41 Ramsey Lake Rd, Sudbury ON P3E 5J1; Tor'93; PhD; FRCPC; IntMed (Breasts); MedOncol. Staff, Health Sciences North-Laurentian Site; Asst Prof, University of Ottawa; (705)522-6237

YOUNG, Scott K; Canadian Forces Base, PO Box 17000 Stn Forces 17 Medical Clinic, Winnipeg MB R3J 3Y5; Man'91; CCFP; FCFP; Staff, Canadian Forces Base; (204)833-2500

YOUNG, Sheila-Mae; Lindsay Prof Bldg, 9-65 Angeline St N, Lindsay ON K9V 5N7; Tor'72; Court Staff, Ross Memorial Hospital; Staff Primary Care Lead-Central East Regional Cancetr Program, Cancer Care Ontario - Provincial Office; (705)324-8212; Fax. (705)324-8223.

YOUNG, Sherylan; Sunnybrook Hlth Sciences Ctre, A102-2075 Bayview Ave, Toronto ON M4N 3M5; Tor'94; CCFP; FCFP; Assoc Staff Privil, Mount Sinai Hospital; Staff Family & Comm Med, Sunnybrook Health Sciences Centre; Asst Prof Family & Commun Med, University of Toronto; (416)480-4931; Fax. (416)480-6038.

YOUNG, Stephanie L; Humber River Reg Hosp-Church, 200 Church St, Toronto ON M9N 1N8; Qns'92; FRCPC; DiagRad. Staff, Humber River Regional Hospital - Church Street Site; Staff, The Scarborough Hospital - General Campus; (416)744-2500

YOUNG, Theron K; Dalla Lana School of Public He, 547-155 College St, Toronto ON M5T 3M7; McG'73; FRCPC; CommunMed. Langs: Chinese; (416)978-6459

YOUNG, Thomas W; Hoy Medical, 402-2155 10th Ave, Prince George BC V2M 5J6; Dal'82; Staff, University Hospital of Northern British Columbia; (250)564-6664; Fax. (250)564-1121.

YOUNG, Todd K; Green Bay Comm Health Ctre, PO Box 280, Springdale NL A0J 1T0; McM'04; CCFP; Staff, Green Bay Community Health Centre; (709)673-3911

YOUNG, Vanessa J; 109-284 Helmcken Rd, Victoria BC V9B 1T2; UBC'92; BSc(Human Performance); Dip SportMed; (250)479-6962; Fax. (250)474-5617.

YOUNG, Vicki; North York Med Arts Bldg, 330-1333 Sheppard Ave E, North York ON M2J 1V1; Tor'90; CCFP; FCFP; Staff, The Scarborough Hospital - Birchmount Campus; (416)494-7533; Fax. (416)497-4793.

YOUNG, Vincent P J; The Ottawa Hosp-Gen Campus, 501 Smyth Rd, Ottawa ON K1H 8L6; Qns'73; FRCPC; Hem (Medical Oncology). Staff Reg Cancer Centre, The Ottawa Hospital - General Campus; Staff MedOncol, Ontario Cancer Foundation; Asst Prof, University of Ottawa; Langs: English; French; (613)737-7700; Fax. (613)247-3511; vyoung@ottawahospital.on.ca.

YOUNG, Wade M; Health Sciences Centre, 300 Prince Philip Dr, St. John's NL A1B 3V6; Mem'00; CCFP; CCFP(E.M.); Staff Emerg Dept, Health Sciences Centre; (709)777-8016

YOUNG, William R; Central Alberta Prof Centre, 250-5201 43 St, Red Deer AB T4N 1C7; Alb'74; FRCSC; ObstGyn. (403)340-2100; Fax. (403)340-1622.

YOUNG TAI, Kin Fan W; Mount Sinai Hosp, 775A-600 University Ave, Toronto ON M5G 1X5; West Indies (Jamaica)'80; MB BS; FRCPC; Peds (Neonatology). Staff, Mount Sinai Hospital; (416)586-4800 x5312; Fax. (416)586-8745; kfyoungtai@mtsinai.on.ca.

YOUNGASH, Ronald W; Victoria Emerg Phys Mgmt Ltd, 325-1627 Fort St, Victoria BC V8R 1H8; Wes'73; FRCPC; EmergMed. (250)479-1442; Fax. (250)479-1472.

YOUNGE, Derek A; Stanton Terr Health Authority, 550 Byrne Rd, Yellowknife NT X1A 2N1; Alb'68; AB; FRCSC; OrthSurg (Hand Surgery). Staff, Stanton Territorial Health Authority; (867)669-4111

YOUNGER, Alastair S E; Vancouver Bone & Joint Clinic, 560-1144 Burrard St, Vancouver BC V6Z 2A5; Aberdeen (Scotland)'85; FRCSC; OrthSurg (Foot & Ankle Surgery). Staff, Providence Health Care - St Paul's Hospital; Physician, Vancouver Bone & Joint Clinic; Staff Teacher, University of British Columbia; (604)683-3585; Fax. (604)683-3464.

YOUNGER, Ritchie A L; Younger Facial Surgery Centre, 105-2025 Broadway W, Vancouver BC V6J 1Z6; Alb'79; AB; AB; FRCSC; Otol (Facial Plastic Surgery). Ac Staff, Vancouver General Hospital - Centennial Pavillion; Ac Staff, Providence Health Care - Mount Saint Joseph Hospital; Ac Staff, Pemberton Health Centre; Clin Prof Surg, University of British Columbia; (604)738-3223; Fax. (604)730-2838; younger@pembertonsurgery.co.uk.

YOUNGER-LEWIS, Catherine J; AL 0701 Health Protection Bldg, 200 Tunney's Pasture Driveway, Ottawa ON K1A 0K9; Qns'77; (613)948-6346; Fax. (613)952-6011.

YOUNGSON, Bruce J; Univ Hlth Network-Toronto Gen, 11E 227-200 Elizabeth St, Toronto ON M5G 2C4; Tor'84; FRCPC; AnatPath. Staff, Toronto General Hospital - UHN; Asst Prof Path, University of Toronto; (416)340-5573; Fax. (416)340-5517.

YOUNIS, Tallal H; Queen Elizabeth II HSC-Halifax, 454-1276 South Park St, Halifax NS B3H 2Y9; Cairo (Egypt)'92; MB BCh; Staff, Queen Elizabeth II Health Sciences Centre - Victoria General Site; Asst Prof, Dalhousie University; (902)473-6054; Fax. (902)473-6186.

YOUNUS, Jawaid; London Reg Cancer Centre, 790 Commissioners Rd E, London ON N6A 4L6; Punjab (Pakistan)'85; MB BS; FRCPC; IntMed; MedOncol. Asst Prof Med & Dentistry, University of Western Ontario; Langs: Urdu; (519)685-8300 x53327; Fax. (519)685-8624.

YOUSEF, George M; St Michael's Hosp, 2 075QW-30 Bond St, Toronto ON M5B 1W8; Zagazig (Egypt)'87; FRCPC; AnatPath. Staff, St Michael's Hospital; Langs: Arabic; (416)864-6060 x6129; Fax. (416)864-5648.

YOUSEF, Jakline M Y; Humber River Reg Hosp-Keele, 2175 Keele St, North York ON M6M 3Z4; University of Mansura (Other Foreign)'92; MB ChB; FRCPC; Psy. Staff, Humber River Regional Hospital - Keele Street Site; Langs: Arabic; (416)249-8111

YOUSEF, Osama A E; Grand River Hosp-KW HC, PO Box 9056 Stn C 835 King St, Kitchener ON N2G 1G3; Al-Fateh (Libya)'97; FRCPC; DiagRad. Staff, Grand River Hospital - Kitchener/Waterloo Health Centre; Langs: Arabic; (519)749-4300

YOUSEFI, Mehrnaz; Westbrook Shopping Centre, 28-1200 37 St SW, Calgary AB T3C 1S2; (Other Foreign)'94; CCFP; (403)264-1895; Fax. (403)264-7015.

YOUSEFI, Rojyar R; City View Family Practice, 2480 Heather St, Vancouver BC V5Z 3H9; UBC'10; CCFP; (604)879-3900

YOUSEFI, Vandad; Vancouver Gen Hosp, 855 12th Ave W, Vancouver BC V5Z 1M9; UBC'04; CCFP; Staff, Vancouver General Hospital - Centennial Pavillion; (604)875-4111

YOUSFIE, Samer; Surrey Mem Hosp, 13750 96 Ave, Surrey BC V3V 1Z2; Damascus (Syria)'01; FRCPC; Peds. Staff, Surrey Memorial Hospital; (604)585-5666 x5530

YOUSIF, Eman J; Gillam Hospital, PO Box 2000 115 Gillam Dr, Gillam MB R0B 0L0; (Other Foreign)'87; CCFP; Staff, Gillam Hospital; (204)652-2600

YOUSIF, Haythem; Queen Elizabeth Hosp, PO Box 6600 Stn Central 60 Riverside Dr, Charlottetown PE C1A 8T5; Staff, Queen Elizabeth Hospital; (902)894-2111

YOUSIF, Mazin A; Yonge Davis Centre, C2B-17480 Yonge St, Newmarket ON L3Y 8A7; University of Al-Mustansiriyah (Iraq)'98; MB ChB; CCFP; (905)898-3700; Fax. (905)898-3738.

YOUSIF, Samad S; Tuscany Med Clinic, 105-9100 Jane St, Vaughan ON L4K 0A4; University of Al-Mustansiriyah (Other Foreign)'97; MB ChB; CCFP; Langs: Arabic; (905)760-1140

YOUSIF, Thair H; North Walkerville Ortho Assoc, 106-2425 Tecumseh Rd E, Windsor ON N8W 1E6; Al-Basrah (Iraq)'82; MB ChB; FRCSC; OrthSurg. Langs: Arabic; Assyrian; (519)254-5763; Fax. (519)254-6356.

YOUSSEF, Elham A A; 170 University Ave W, Waterloo ON N2L 3E9; Al-Fateh (Libya)'01; CCFP; Langs: Arabic; (519)725-1514

YOUSSEF, Ernest A N; Credit River Med Clinic, F001B-6045 Creditview Rd, Mississauga ON L5V 2A8; Alexandria (Egypt)'75; MB ChB; CCFP; Physician, Albina-Thistle Down Clinic; Langs: Arabic; (905)826-6095; Fax. (905)826-9219.

YOUSSEF, Fady; Montfort Hosp, 713 Montreal Rd, Ottawa ON K1K 0T2; Ott'02; CCFP; CCFP(E.M.); Staff, Montfort Hospital; Langs: Arabic; French; German; (613)746-4621

YOUSSEF, George M Y; 906 Brant St, Burlington ON L7R 2J5; Mansura (Egypt)'95; MB ChB; FRCPC; IntMed; Nephrol.

YOUSSEF, Hany A A; Yorkdale Med Clinic, A103-11685 Yonge St, Richmond Hill ON L4E 0K7; (Other Foreign)'93; CCFP; (905)770-9057; Fax. (905)917-0215.

YOUSSEF, Hany M R; Montfort Hosp, 713 Montreal Rd, Ottawa ON K1K 0T2; Ott'05; FRCPC; Anes. Staff, Montfort Hospital; Langs: Bilingual(English/French); (613)746-4621

YOUSSEF, Heba S S; Selkirk Med Centre, 353 Eveline St, Selkirk MB R1A 1N1.

YOUSSEF, Magdy B; Brockville Gen Hosp, 75 Charles St, Brockville ON K6V 1S8; Ein Shams (Egypt)'65; FRCPC; Anes. Ac Staff, Brockville General Hospital - Charles Street; Langs: Arabic; (613)342-7788; Fax. (613)342-7788.

YOUSSEF, Mariam F G; Medica One, 2019 Caroline St, Burlington ON L7R 1L1; Cairo (Egypt)'97; MRCP; CCFP; Langs: Arabic; French; (905)333-0911; Fax. (905)333-0311.

YOUSSEF, Marie D; CSSS de Laval, 1755 boul Rene-Laennec, Laval QC H7M 3L9; Cairo (Egypt)'68; Anes. Staff, Hopital de la Cite de la santé; (450)975-5388

YOUSSEF, Nagy A G; Adult ADHD Clinic, 201-9148 23 Ave NW, Edmonton AB T6N 1H9; Cairo (Egypt)'71; MB ChB; MSc(Psych); FRCPC; Psy (Adult ADHD). Clin Associate Prof, University of Alberta; (780)988-9770; Fax. (780)988-9877.

YOUSSEF, Nancy A B; Sheppard Med Bldg, 101-701 Sheppard Ave E, North York ON M2K 2Z3; Mansura (Egypt)'82; CCFP; (416)221-0451; Fax. (416)221-0282.

YOUSSEF, Nayer M M; Hamilton HS-McMaster Site, PO Box 2000 2 U 2-1200 Main St W, Hamilton ON L8N 3Z5; Ain Shams University (Egypt)'03; Staff, Hamilton Health Sciences Centre - McMaster Children's Hospital; (905)521-2100

YOUSSEF, Nermeen A; Carman Med Group, PO Box 728, Carman MB R0G 0J0; (Other Foreign)'82; CCFP.

YOUSSEF, Sami A; Hôpital Ste-Justine, 3175 ch Cote-Sainte-Catherine, Montreal QC H3T 1C5; Jerusalem (Israel)'62; DAB; PedGenSurg; GenSurg (Emergency Medicine). Ac Staff, Hôpital Ste-Justine; Staff, McGill University Health Centre - Montreal Children's Hospital; Langs: French; (514)345-4879; Fax. (514)345-4964; sami_youssef@hotmail.com.

YOUSSEF, Victor S F; 103-470 Bronte St S, Milton ON L9T 2J4; Cairo (Egypt)'00; CCFP; Langs: Arabic; French; (905)864-3323; Fax. (905)864-1778.

YOUSSEF, Wafaa; Meadowlark Health Centre, 142 Meadowlark Shopping Ctr NW, Edmonton AB T5R 5W9; Cairo (Egypt)'78; MB ChB; Langs: Arabic; (780)486-7777; Fax. (780)486-7747.

YOUSSEF, Youssef M R; Durham Reg Cancer Centre, 1 Hospital Crt, Oshawa ON L1G 2B9; Dal'89; FRCPC; RadOncol (Oncology). Staff, Lakeridge Health - Oshawa Site; Langs: Arabic; German; (905)576-8711; Fax. (905)721-6101.

YOUSSOUFIAN DE PEREZ, Never; Youthdale Treatment Centres, 227 Victoria St, Toronto ON M5B 1T8; Buenos Aires (Argentina)'73; FRCPC; Psy (Child & Adolescent Psychiatry). Court Staff, Waypoint Centre for Mental Health Care; Court Staff, North York General Hospital - Branson Division; Court Staff Psy, Youthdale Psychiatric Crisis Services; Staff Psy, Youthdale Treatment Centres; Langs: Armenian; Spanish; (416)363-3751 x420; Fax. (416)363-7945.

YOUSUF, Junaid A H; Windsor Reg Cancer Centre, 2220 Kildare Rd, Windsor ON N8W 2X3; Ott'05; RadOncol. Staff, Windsor Regional Hospital - Windsor Regional Cancer Centre; (519)253-5253

YOUSUF, Kashif A H; Hotel-Dieu Grace Hosp, 1030 Ouellette Ave, Windsor ON N9A 1E1; McM'06; Anes. Staff, Hôtel-Dieu Grace Hospital; (519)973-4444

YOUSUF, Mohammad; Supermall, 700 St. Peter Ave, Bathurst NB E2A 2Y7; Punjab (Pakistan)'65; MB BS; DABOT; FRCSC; Otol (Head & Neck Surgery). Ac Staff, Hopital Regional Chaleur; Langs: Urdu; (506)546-3500; Fax. (506)544-2440; drsaab@hotmail.com.

YOUWAKIM, Basseem H; Dr Everett Chalmers Reg Hosp, PO Box 9000 Stn A 700 Priestman St, Fredericton NB E3B 5N5; Ain Shams (Egypt)'81; MB ChB; CCFP; Staff, Dr Everett Chalmers Regional Hospital; (506)452-5400

YOVANOVICH, Robert M; 410 Giles Blvd E, Windsor ON N9A 4C6; Wes'70; FRCSC; OrthSurg (Otolaryngology). Consultant, Hôtel-Dieu Grace Hospital; (519)256-1823; Fax. (519)254-3849.

YOW, Desiree S; North Hill Med Centre, 200-1632 14 Ave NW, Calgary AB T2N 1M7; Alb'08; Peds. (403)284-0001

YU, Andrew H; Burnaby Hosp, 3935 Kincaid St, Burnaby BC V5G 2X6; UBC'94; FRCPC; Anes. Staff, Burnaby Hospital; (604)412-6311

YU, B W Daniel; Place du Golf, 400-28 ch du Golf E, Joliette QC J6E 2B4; Laval'05; Ophth. (450)753-9293

YU, Carlos C S; 103-174 Harwood Ave S, Ajax ON L1S 2H6; Wes'87; CCFP; CCFP(E.M.); Staff, Rouge Valley Health System - Ajax & Pickering Health Centre Site; Langs: Mandarin; (905)683-0690; Fax. (905)683-0691.

YU, Catherine H; 7 034-61 Queen St E, Toronto ON M5C 2T2; Tor'02; FRCPC; IntMed; Endocrin&Metab. Staff, St Michael's Hospital; (416)867-7424; Fax. (416)867-3654.

YU, Catherine L; Toronto East Gen & Orth Hosp, 825 Coxwell Ave, East York ON M4C 3E7; Tor'01; CCFP; CCFP(E.M.); Staff, Toronto East General Hospital Inc; Langs: Tagalog; (416)461-8272

YU, Chun Ming; Northfield Med Centre, 206-99 Northfield Dr E, Waterloo ON N2K 3P9; Shanghai Medical University (China)'93; CCFP; (519)744-2592; Fax. (519)744-1197.

YU, Derek; Balmoral Med Arts Facility, 301-1366 Yonge St, Toronto ON M4T 3A7; Tor'05; BSc; FRCPC; IntMed (Hepatology); Gastroent. Staff, Mackenzie Richmond Hill Hospital; Langs: Cantonese; (416)926-0262; Fax. (416)926-0936; drderekyuoffice@gmail.com.

YU, Edward W T; London Reg Cancer Centre, 790 Commissioners Rd E, London ON N6A 4L6; McG'88; PhD(Pharm); FRCPC; RadOncol (Palliative Care). Staff, London Health Sciences Centre - Victoria Campus; Assoc Prof Oncol & Med Biophysics, University of Western Ontario; Langs: Chinese; French; (519)685-8600; Fax. (519)685-8627.

YU, Eric H C; Univ Hlth Network-Toronto Western Hosp, EW5 470-399 Bathurst St, Toronto ON M5T 2S8; Tor'90; DABIM; FACC; MEd; FRCPC; IntMed; Cardiol. Staff, Toronto Western Hospital - University Health Network; Assoc Prof Med, University of Toronto; Langs: Cantonese; French; (416)603-5815; Fax. (416)603-5398.

YU, Grace W; City Square Pediatrics, 495WT-555 12th Ave W, Vancouver BC V5Z 3X7; McG'97; FRCPC; Peds. Staff, BC Children's Hospital; Clin Instructor, University of British Columbia; Langs: Cantonese; French; (604)730-5622; Fax. (604)875-6717.

YU, Herbert D; 406-2299 Dundas St W, Toronto ON M6R 1X7; RCS (Ireland)'78; Langs: Chinese; (416)535-3511; Fax. (416)535-5993.

YU, Hojun; Queen Elizabeth II Hosp, 10409 98 St, Grande Prairie AB T8V 2E8; Staff, Queen Elizabeth II Hospital; (780)538-7100

YU, Horace; Rideau Valley Health Services, 1221 Greenbank Rd, Ottawa ON K2J 5V7; Cal'10; CCFP; (613)258-8710; Fax. (613)440-3238; dr.fish2010@gmail.com.

YU, Jaime C; 301-3295 Lakeshore Rd, Kelowna BC V1W 3S9; Cal'05; FRCPC; PhysMed&Rehab. (250)862-3756

YU, Jane S; 11022 101 St NW, Edmonton AB T5H 2T1; Alb'85; (780)424-5417; Fax. (780)425-8297.

YU, Jasmine M Y; North York Med Arts Bldg, 330-1333 Sheppard Ave E, North York ON M2J 1V1; Tor'09; CCFP; (416)497-6444; Fax. (416)497-4793.

YU, Jen Zhen; City Square Med Centre, 126-555 12th Ave W, Vancouver BC V5Z 3X7; Beijing (China)'83; PhD(Pharm); FRCPC; IntMed. Locum Tenens, Delta Hospital; Locum Tenens, Peace Arch Hospital; Langs: Mandarin; (604)568-8377; jenyu@shaw.ca.

YU, Jessica J; 522-790 Bay St Box 58/59, Toronto ON M5G 1N8; Tor'03; CCFP; (416)571-1222; Fax. (416)541-1227.

YU, Jian Z; Rouge Valley HS-Centenary, 2867 Ellesmere Rd, Scarborough ON M1E 4B9; McG'97; FRCPC; Anes. Staff, Rouge Valley Health System - Centenary Health Centre Site; Langs: Mandarin; (416)284-8131 x4054; Fax. (416)281-7453.

YU, Jinwoo R; Halton HCS Corp-Oakville, 327 Reynolds St, Oakville ON L6J 3L7; Tor'98; FRCPC; DiagRad. Staff, Halton Healthcare Services Corporation - Oakville Site; (905)845-2571

YU, Joanne L; Univ Hlth Network-Princess M, 5 110-610 University Ave, Toronto ON M5G 2M9; Tor'08; FRCPC; IntMed. Staff, Princess Margaret Hospital - University Health Network; (416)946-2000

YU, John C; Montfort Hosp, 713 Montreal Rd, Ottawa ON K1K 0T2; Ott'97; FRCPC; DiagRad. Staff, Montfort Hospital; Staff, The Ottawa Hospital - Civic Campus; Langs: French; Mandarin; (613)746-4621

YU, John T; 206B-1916 Lonsdale Ave, North Vancouver BC V7M 2K1; McG'03; FRCPC; Derm. Langs: Bilingual(English/French); (604)987-0917

YU, Joyce W; Medical Bldg, 1803-805 Broadway W, Vancouver BC V5Z 1K1; McG'99; FRCPC; Peds; ClinImmunol&Allergy. Langs: Chinese; French; (604)876-4433; Fax. (604)876-4431.

YU, Katie; Lindsay Commun Health Clinic, 108 Angeline St S, Lindsay ON K9V 3L5; Tor'09; CCFP; (705)879-4100; Fax. (705)324-8411.

YU, Larry L W; Lemg-Wan's Clinic, 101-3330 Main St, Vancouver BC V5V 3M7; (Taiwan)'63; MB; Langs: Chinese; (604)873-8733; Fax. (604)569-0292.

YU, Ling Pui; Hewes Way Med Clinic, 206-2603 Hewes Way NW, Edmonton AB T6L 6W6; Alb'88; CCFP; FCFP; (780)462-4210; Fax. (780)462-4214.

YU, Maria C Y; 103-174 Harwood Ave, Ajax ON L1S 2H6; Qns'77; BSc; CCFP; Langs: Mandarin; (905)683-0690; Fax. (905)683-1431.

YU, Ming; Carlton Church Medical, 60 Carlton St, Toronto ON M5B 1J2; Cal'10; CCFP; (416)646-1980

YU, Norman B M; Northwood Med Centre, 35 Springbank Ave N, Woodstock ON N4S 7P6; Wes'94; Staff, Woodstock General Hospital; (519)537-6147; Fax. (519)537-2944.

YU, Oriana H Y; Hopital chinois de Montreal, 189 av Viger E, Montreal QC H2X 3Y9; Cal'06; Endocrin&Metab; IntMed. Staff, Hôpital Chinois de Montréal; (514)871-0961

YU, Patrick W W; 150-17475 56 Ave, Surrey BC V3S 2X6; Wes'91; CCFP; FCFP; Staff, Brickyard Medical Clinic; (604)576-7701

YU, Patrick Y H; JPP2 2449-910 10th Ave W, Vancouver BC V5Z 1M9; UBC'84; FRCPC; Anes. Staff, UBC Hospital - Koerner Pavillion; Clin Instructor, University of British Columbia; (604)875-4304; Fax. (604)875-5209.

YU, Philip H F; Philip Yu Medicine Prof Corp, 27-160 Main St S, Brampton ON L6W 2E1; Ott'83; Court Staff, William Osler Health System - Brampton Civic Hospital; Physician Healthy Sexuality Clinic/Med Examiner Civil Aviation, Regional Municipality of Peel; Langs: Cantonese; (905)595-7788; Fax. (905)595-7789.

YU, Richard K W; Surrey Memorial Hosp, 13790 96 Ave, Surrey BC V3V 1Z2; Qns'93; FRCP; FRCPC; GenPath. Staff, Surrey Memorial Hospital; Staff, BC Biomedical Laboratories Ltd; (604)585-5666

YU, Richard S O; St Michael's Hosp, 30 Bond St, Toronto ON M5B 1W8; Wes'81; FACEP; FRCPC; EmergMed;CCFP; CCFP(E.M.); FCFP; Staff Emerg, St Michael's Hospital; Asst Prof, University of Toronto; Langs: Cantonese; (416)864-5094; Fax. (416)864-5493.

YU, S Eugene; Univ Hlth Network-Princess M, 3 959-610 University Ave, Toronto ON M5G 2M9; Tor'96; FRCPC; DiagRad (Neuro Radiology). Staff, Princess Margaret Hospital - University Health Network; (416)946-4501 x4989; Fax. (416)946-6564.

YU, Shihao; 106-15966 108 Ave, Surrey BC V4N 5V6; Shanghai (China)'62; PhD; Langs: Chinese; (604)582-8820

YU, Simon; Kingsway Plaza Phase III, 705-4980 Kingsway, Burnaby BC V5H 4K7; UBC'00; FRCPC; IntMed; MedOncol. Staff, BC Cancer Agency Vancouver Centre; Langs: Cantonese; Mandarin; (604)434-5001; Fax. (604)434-5053.

YU, Stanley S F; Wentworth Limeridge Med Ctre, 403-849 Upper Wentworth St, Hamilton ON L9A 5H4; National (Taiwan)'69; CCFP; FCFP; Langs: Chinese; (905)388-5996; Fax. (905)388-5721.

YU, T C Michael; Lasalle Bldg, 146 Stuart St, Kingston ON K7L 3N6; Tor'79; Staff, Queen's University; (613)533-2506; Fax. (613)533-6740.

YU, Tsai Hsing; 9 Court St, St Catharines ON L2R 4R3; Utkal (India)'76; MB BS; Langs: Hakka; Hindi; Chinese; (905)682-2709; Fax. (905)397-5934.

YU, Weiming; Alberta Children's Hosp, 2888 Shaganappi Trail NW, Calgary AB T3B 6A8; Nantong (China)'78; FRCPC; AnatPath (Cardiovascular Pathology). Staff Path, Alberta Children's Hospital; (403)955-2257; Fax. (403)955-2321.

YU, William Y; 360-5740 Cambie St, Vancouver BC V5Z 3A6; (Hong Kong)'66; FRCSC; OrthSurg. Staff, Providence Health Care - Mount Saint Joseph Hospital; Staff, Providence Health Care - St Vincent's Hospital-Heather Site; Clin Assoc Prof, University of British Columbia; Langs: Chinese; (604)322-1021; Fax. (604)324-8751.

YU, Y W Edward; Lougheed Plaza, 285-9600 Cameron St, Burnaby BC V3J 7N3; Tor'93; FRCSC; Ophth (Cataract & Refractive). Langs: Cantonese; Mandarin; (604)422-8389; Fax. (604)422-8381.

YU-SIAO, Barbara A; Niagara Health System-Niagara, PO Box 1018 Stn Main 5546 Portage Rd, Niagara Falls ON L2E 6X2; Karachi (Pakistan)'96; FRCPC; Psy. Staff, Niagara Health System - Greater Niagara General Site; Langs: Hindi; (905)378-4647

YU-WATSON, Maria C Y; 103-174 Harwood Ave S, Ajax ON L1S 2H6; Wes'94; BSc; CCFP; Staff, Rouge Valley Health System - Ajax & Pickering Health Centre Site; (905)683-0690; Fax. (905)683-1431.

YUAN, G Bernadette; Steveston Med Center, 103-3811 Chatham St, Richmond BC V7E 2Z4; UBC'81; Staff, Richmond Hospital; (604)277-9577; Fax. (604)277-9517.

YUAN, George; St Joseph's Healthcare, 50 Charlton Ave E, Hamilton ON L8N 4A6; Wes'08; FRCPC; IntMed. Staff, St Joseph's Healthcare - Charlton Campus; Staff, Firestone Clinic; (905)522-1155

YUAN, Jane; 507-586 Eglinton Ave E, Toronto ON M4P 1P2; Tor'05; FRCPC; IntMed; Respir. Teach Staff, University of Toronto; Langs: Mandarin; (416)488-6980; Fax. (416)488-3998.

YUAN, Lilian; Public Health Branch, 17250 Yonge St, Newmarket ON L3Y 6Z1; Tor'81; MSc(Epidem.); FRCPC; CommunMed;CCFP; Staff, Regional Municipality of York; Langs: Chinese; (905)830-4444 x2007; Fax. (905)895-3166; lilian.yuan@hc-sc.gc.ca.

YUAN-INNES, Melissa J; Cornwall Community Hosp, 840 McConnell Ave, Cornwall ON K6H 5S5; Wes'00; CCFP; CCFP(E.M.); Staff, Cornwall Community Hospital; Staff, Glengarry Memorial Hospital; (613)938-4240

YUCEL, Yeni H; St Michael's Hosp, 409-30 Bond St, Toronto ON M5B 1W8; Strasbourg (France)'85; FRCPC; NeurPath (Ophthalmology Pathology). Staff, St Michael's Hospital; Prof Ophth, University of Toronto; Langs: Turkish; French; (416)864-6060 x6755; Fax. (416)864-5648; yeni.yucel@utoronto.ca.

YUDIN, Alexandra; Prime Care Family Hlth Team, 206-470 Bronte St S, Milton ON L9T 2J4; Bukovinian State Medical Academy (Other Foreign)'01; CCFP; (905)878-6793

YUDIN, Jovana; McMaster University, 3W11-1280 Main St W, Hamilton ON L8S 4K1; Tor'08; IntMed.

YUDIN, Mark H; 5F-61 Queen St E, Toronto ON M5C 2T2; Tor'95; MD; BA; MSc; FRCSC; ObstGyn. Ac Staff, St Michael's Hospital; Assoc Prof, University of Toronto; (416)867-7480; Fax. (416)867-7478.

YUDIN, Mark; Kelowna Gen Hosp, 2268 Pandosy St, Kelowna BC V1Y 1T2; Tor'01; FRCPC; Anes. Staff, Kelowna General Hospital; (250)863-7375

YUE, Anthony W B; Central Park Medical, 304-1711 Cook St, Victoria BC V8T 3P2; Alb'93; BMedSci; CCFP; Staff, Vancouver Island Health Authority; Langs: Mandarin; Cantonese; (250)361-9616; Fax. (250)360-0084.

YUE, David; Belmont Medicentre, 2903 137 Ave NW, Edmonton AB T5A 5G8; Alb'90; BMedSci; Langs: Cantonese; (780)475-7070; Fax. (780)472-2367.

YUE, Frank W L; 5570 Joyce St, Vancouver BC V5R 4H6; UBC'76; Langs: Cantonese; Mandarin; Shanghai; (604)430-2311; Fax. (604)430-2350.

YUE, Jason K; Rouge Valley HS-Centenary, 2867 Ellesmere Rd, Scarborough ON M1E 4B9; Tor'01; CCFP; CCFP(E.M.); Staff, Rouge Valley Health System - Centenary Health Centre Site; (416)281-7270

YUE, Jenise J W; Fairmont Med Bldg, 915-750 Broadway W, Vancouver BC V5Z 1H8; UBC'94; FRCSC; ObstGyn. Staff, BC Women's Hospital & Health Centre; Assoc Prof, University of British Columbia; Langs: Chinese; (604)877-8688; Fax. (604)877-8611; drjyue@gmail.com.

YUE, Jennifer F W; Summit Centre Family Clinic, 209-200 Boudreau Rd, St. Albert AB T8N 6B9; UBC'00; CCFP; (780)458-7000; Fax. (780)458-8484.

YUE, Jody; Abbotsfield Shoppers Mall, 214-3210 118 Ave NW, Edmonton AB T5W 4W1; Alb'09; CCFP; (780)471-2071

YUE, K Kevin; 5571 Victoria Dr, Vancouver BC V5P 3W2; UBC'82; CCFP; Ac Staff, Providence Health Care - Mount Saint Joseph Hospital; Ac Staff, Providence Health Care - St Vincent's Hospital-Heather Site; Court Staff, BC Women's Hospital & Health Centre; Langs: Cantonese; Mandarin; (604)669-4121; Fax. (604)688-1591.

YUE, Ming Yee; 4904 48 St, Leduc AB T9E 6X4; Alb'91; CCFP; Staff, Leduc Community Hospital; (780)986-2712; Fax. (780)986-0356.

YUE, Paul K; South Lake Reg Health Centre, 596 Davis Dr, Newmarket ON L3Y 2P9; Wes'95; FRCPC; Anes. Staff, Southlake Regional Health Centre; (905)895-4521

YUE, Ping; Foothills Med Centre, 1403 29 St NW, Calgary AB T2N 2T9; (China)'82; Staff, Foothills Medical Centre; (403)944-1157

YUE, Randy S; Southlake Reg Health Centre, 596 Davis Dr, Newmarket ON L3Y 2P9; McM'01; FRCPC; Anes. Staff, Southlake Regional Health Centre; Langs: Cantonese; (905)895-4521

YUE-TANG, Bonnie W M; 110 Beverley St, Toronto ON M5T 1Y2; Tor'78; Court Staff, Toronto Western Hospital - University Health Network; Staff Student Health Services, University of Toronto; Langs: Chinese; (416)340-8989

YUEN, Amy K W; 336-10654 82 Ave NW, Edmonton AB T6E 2A7; Alb'88; CCFP; (780)434-3675; Fax. (780)434-3575.

YUEN, Cham-Wah; 4226 Main St, Vancouver BC V5V 3P9; (Hong Kong)'72; Langs: Mandarin; (604)875-6818; Fax. (604)875-6685.

YUEN, Chui Kin; Cross Roads Ob/Gyn, 330-507 Broadway W, Vancouver BC V5Z 1E6; Man'72; FACOG; FSOGC; FRCSC; ObstGyn. Staff, Health Sciences Centre; University of Manitoba; Langs: Cantonese; Mandarin; (604)872-5484; cyuen@ms.umanitoba.ca.

YUEN, Darana W; EyeMD Institute, 401-7900 Hurontario St, Brampton ON L6Y 0P6; Alb'04; FRCSC; Ophth. Staff, Toronto Western Hospital - University Health Network; (905)456-9500; Fax. (905)456-9508.

YUEN, Darren A; St Michael's Health Centre, 9F-61 Queen St E, Toronto ON M5C 2T2; Tor'02; FRCPC; IntMed; Nephrol. Staff, Mackenzie Richmond Hill Hospital; (416)867-7479

YUEN, Doris E; London HSC-Victoria Campus, PO Box 5010 Stn B D4 202-800 Commissioner's Rd E, London ON N6A 5W9; UBC'88; PhD; FAAP; FRCPC; Peds (Neonatal & Perinatal Medicine). Staff, St Joseph's Hospital - St Joseph's Health Care; Staff, London Health Sciences Centre - Victoria Campus; Langs: Chinese; (519)685-8500

YUEN, Harold J; Southlake Family Health Team, 201-581 Davis Dr, Newmarket ON L3Y 2P6; Qns'07; CCFP; Staff, Markham Stouffville Hospital - Uxbridge Site; Staff, Southlake Regional Health Centre; (905)853-3103; Fax. (905)853-9136.

YUEN, Jasper S Y; The Credit Valley Hosp, 2200 Eglinton Ave W, Mississauga ON L5M 2N1; Wes'03; FRCPC; RadOncol. Staff, The Credit Valley Hospital; (905)813-1100; Fax. (905)813-3962.

YUEN, Jenna L Y B; Women's Health Clinic, 419 Graham Ave, Winnipeg MB R3C 0M3; Man'10; CCFP.

YUEN, K H Peter; Finch-Midland Med Centre, 122-4190 Finch Ave E, Scarborough ON M1S 4T7; (Hong Kong)'75; MB BS; CCFP; FCFP; Staff, Finch-Midland Medical Centre; Langs: Cantonese; Mandarin; (416)321-3228; Fax. (416)291-9844.

YUEN, Kenneth W H; Royal Court Med Bldg, 307-1 Quarry Ridge Rd, Barrie ON L4M 7G1; Tor'93; MD; FRCPC; IntMed (Clinician Investigator Program); Rheum. Langs: Cantonese; (705)792-6593; Fax. (705)792-4325.

YUEN, Michael L F; Evergold Centre, G-3833 Midland Ave, Scarborough ON M1V 5L6; (Hong Kong)'81; FRCPC; DiagRad. Langs: Chinese; (416)321-9243; Fax. (416)321-1650; mlyuen@accessv.com.

YUEN, Michelle K; The Doctor's Office, 101-777 Broadway W, Vancouver BC V5Z 4J7; Wes'09; CCFP; (604)734-8252

YUEN, Owen L; Strathcona Square Shopp Centre, 224-555 Strathcona Blvd SW, Calgary AB T3H 2Z9; Cal'97; MSc; BSc; CCFP; (403)686-2911; Fax. (403)246-7830.

YUEN, Richard H; Thorncliffe Med Centre, 5618 4 St NW, Calgary AB T2K 1B2; Witwatersrand (South Africa)'93; MB ChB; LMCC; Physician, Albert Park Family Medical Centres; Staff, Properties Medical Clinic; Langs: Chinese; Mandarin; (403)295-7666; Fax. (403)295-8960.

YUEN, S Y Sheila; Health for All Family Health T, 202-379 Church St, Markham ON L6B 0T1; Tor'06; CCFP; Staff, Markham Stouffville Hospital; Lecturer, University of Toronto; Langs: Cantonese; (905)472-2200; Fax. (905)472-5662.

YUEN, Sai Yan; Hop Maisonneuve-Rosemont, 5415 boul de l'Assomption, Montreal QC H1T 2M4; Laval'00; FRCPC; IntMed; Rheum. Staff, Hopital Maisonneuve-Rosemont; (514)252-3400

YUEN, Sze-Ming; South Burnaby Mental Hlth Ctre, 3935 Kincaid St, Burnaby BC V5G 2X6; (Hong Kong)'60; DPM(Eng); FRCPC; Psy. Consultant, Burnaby Hospital; Staff, Burnaby Mental Health Services; Langs: Chinese; (604)453-1968

YUEN, Tommy K; Medical Clinic, 8195 120 St, Delta BC V4C 6P7; (Hong Kong)'70; CCFP; Assoc Staff, Surrey Memorial Hospital; Langs: Cantonese; Mandarin; (604)594-8451; Fax. (604)596-4819.

YUEN, Vincent H; Properties Med Clinic, 5102 Rundlehorn Dr NE, Calgary AB T1Y 1C1; Witwatersrand (South Africa)'94; MB ChB; LMCC; Staff, Properties Medical Clinic; Physician, Albert Park Family Medical Centres; (403)280-2700; Fax. (403)285-2641; vincity@hotmail.com.

YUEN, Vivian K; 303-343 Wilson Ave, North York ON M3H 1T1; Tor'04; CCFP; Staff, Sunnybrook Health Sciences Centre; (416)785-8412; Fax. (416)785-8324.

YUFE, Robert S; Medical Clinic Bldg, 208-89 Humber College Blvd, Etobicoke ON M9V 4B8; McG'73; DABPN; FRCPC; Neur. Staff, William Osler Health System - Etobicoke General Hospital; Staff, Mount Sinai Hospital; Asst Prof, University of Toronto; (416)746-1171; Fax. (416)746-1172; robertyufe@yahoo.ca.

YUH, Joseph Y J; Surrey Med Health Centre, 307-2130 Lawrence Ave E, Scarborough ON M1R 1R9; Wes'00; CCFP; Langs: Korean; (416)751-6141; Fax. (416)751-5270.

YUKAWA, Masaru R; Clinical Sciences Bldg, 8 120-152 University Campus NW, Edmonton AB T6G 2G3; UBC'03; FRCPC; Anes. Staff, University of Alberta Hospital; (780)407-8887; Fax. (780)407-3200.

YULE, Joanna E; Queen's Family Health Team, 101-115 Clarence St, Kingston ON K7L 5A3; Qns'10; CCFP; (613)533-9300

YUN, Jennifer M; Medicalwest, 212-3001 Gordon Ave, Port Coquitlam BC V3C 2K7; Mem'92; CCFP; Langs: Korean; (604)944-4077; Fax. (604)944-0677.

YUN, John W S; Richmond Health Science Ctre, 560-6091 Gilbert Rd, Richmond BC V7C 5L9; Mem'88; FRCPC; IntMed; MedOncol. Langs: Korean; (604)273-2747; Fax. (604)214-0602.

YUNG, Chen Fong; Crescent Heights Health Clinic, 107-233 16 Ave NW, Calgary AB T2M 0H5; Mem'10; (403)230-3866; Fax. (403)230-5866.

YUNG, Derek; Univ of Ottawa Heart Institute, 40 Ruskin St, Ottawa ON K1Y 4W7; Ott'05; Cardiol; IntMed. Staff, University of Ottawa Heart Institute; (613)761-5000

YUNG, Francoise; Hôpital Ste-Justine, 3175 ch Cote-Sainte-Catherine, Montreal QC H3T 1C5; Caen (Other Foreign)'00; Staff, Hôpital Ste-Justine; (514)345-4733; Fax. (514)345-4601.

YUNG, Grant S Y; Children's Hosp, 840 Sherbrook St, Winnipeg MB R3A 1S1; Sask'99; FRCPC; Peds. Staff Emerg, Thompson General Hospital; (204)677-2381

YUNG, Jason D K; Dartmouth Gen Hosp, 325 Pleasant St, Dartmouth NS B2Y 4G8; Dal'00; FRCPC; IntMed; Cardiol. Staff, Dartmouth General Hospital; (902)465-8300; Fax. (902)460-4154.

YUNG, Lee; Hôpital régional Chaleur, 1750 Sunset Dr, Bathurst NB E2A 4L7; Sao Polo (Brazil)'01; Staff, Hopital Regional Chaleur; (506)544-3000

YUNG, Manuel M; Humber River Reg Hosp-Finch, 2111 Finch Ave W, North York ON M3N 1N1; Tor'76; FRCPC; Anes. Staff, Humber River Regional Hospital - Finch Avenue Site; (416)744-2500

YUNG, Stephen Y W; 164 McCaul St, Toronto ON M5T 1W4; Emory (USA)'71; Ac Staff, St Joseph's Health Centre; Langs: Chinese; (416)597-0262; Fax. (416)445-1521.

YUNG, Wingko W; Mackenzie Richmond Hill Hosp, 10 Trench St, Richmond Hill ON L4C 4Z3; Tor'84; FRCPC; Anes. Staff Anes, Mackenzie Richmond Hill Hospital; Langs: Chinese; (905)883-2110

YUNG, Yick Shing; Bathurst Medical Dental Clinic, 403-800 Bathurst St, Toronto ON M5R 3M8; Sydney (Australia)'70; MB BS; FRCSC; ObstGyn. Ac Staff, Toronto General Hospital - UHN; Ac Staff, Toronto Western Hospital - University Health Network; University of Toronto; Langs: Cantonese; Fukinese; Mandarin; (416)537-5114; Fax. (416)537-7114.

YUNKER, Peter J; 91 Cornelia St W, Smiths Falls ON K7A 5L3; Tor'77; CCFP; CCFP(E.M.); FCFP; (613)283-0710; Fax. (613)284-8331.

YUNKER, Warren; Alberta Children's Hosp, 2888 Shaganappi Trail NW, Calgary AB T3B 6A8; Alb'05; BSc; PhD; FRCSC; Otol (Pediatric Otolaryngology). Staff, Alberta Children's Hospital; (403)955-2858; Fax. (403)955-7634.

YUONESS, Salem A H; Postgrad Med Education Office, M106-1151 Richmond St, London ON N6A 5C1; Al-Fateh (Libya)'01; NuclearMed.

YURMAN, Edward D; Dixie X-Ray Asociates, 101-2115 Finch Ave W, North York ON M3N 2V6; Tor'68; FRCPC; DiagRad. (416)744-2655; Fax. (416)744-0581.

YUSUF, Aroon Y; SGH Medical Mall, 211-3030 Lawrence Ave E, Scarborough ON M1P 2T7; Tor'03; Staff, The Scarborough Hospital - General Campus; Langs: Hindi; (416)439-5775; Fax. (416)439-2526.

YUSUF, Kamran; Health Sciences Centre, 2273-3330 Hospital Dr NW, Calgary AB T2N 4N1; (Pakistan)'81; Asst Prof, Foothills Medical Centre; Langs: Urdu; Punjabi; (403)210-3930; Fax. (403)283-6151.

YUSUF, Nureni T; 102-290 4th Ave NE, Moose Jaw SK S6H 0C6; (306)693-0925; Fax. (306)693-0927.

YUSUF, Sabah H; Halton HSC Corp-Oakville, 327 Reynolds St, Oakville ON L6J 3L7; McM'04; CCFP; Staff, Halton Healthcare Services Corporation - Oakville Site; (905)845-2571

YUSUF, Salim; Hamilton HS-General Site, C2 119-237 Barton St E, Hamilton ON L8L 2X2; Bangalore (India)'75; MB BS; PhD; FRCP(UK); FACC; FRCPC; Cardiol. Staff M A C Clinic/Staff Population Health Research Institute, Hamilton Health Sciences Centre - Hamilton General Hospital; Dir, Population Health Research Institute; Dir Cardiol/Prof Med, McMaster University; Langs: Hindi; Malayalam; (905)527-7327; Fax. (905)297-3781; yusufs@mcmaster.ca.

YUSWACK, Timothy J; UBC Hospital, M334-2211 Wesbrook Mall, Vancouver BC V6T 2B5; UBC'86; FRCPC; Psy. Staff, UBC Hospital - Koerner Pavillion; (604)822-7689; Fax. (604)822-7889.

YUZAK, Monica J; Mainland Med Clinic, 1061 Hamilton St, Vancouver BC V6B 5G4; Sask'80; (604)683-3973; Fax. (604)683-3809.

YUZDA, Edward S; Community Mental Hlth Services, 3F-55 Union St, Saint John NB E2L 5B7; Cal'97; BSc; MSc; FRCPC; Psy (Adult Psychiatry). Physician, Community Mental Health Services; Asst Prof, Dalhousie University; Asst Prof, Memorial University Of Newfoundland; (506)658-3199; Fax. (506)658-3739; ward.yuzda@grh.ca.

YUZPE, A Albert; Genesis Fertility Centre, 300-1367 Broadway Ave W, Vancouver BC V6H 4A7; Wes'64; FSOGC; MSc; FRCSC; ObstGyn (P.Q.) (Infertility). Consultant, BC Women's Hospital & Health Centre; Emeritus Prof, University of Western Ontario; Clin Prof ObstGyn, University of British Columbia; (604)879-3032; Fax. (604)875-1432; alberty@genesis-fertility.com.

YVORCHUK, Kenneth J; Western Cardiology Associates, 335-1900 Richmond Ave, Victoria BC V8R 4R2; McG'87; FRCPC; IntMed (Echocardiography); Cardiol. Langs: Bilingual(English/French); (250)595-1551; Fax. (250)595-6793.

YWAKIM, Fikry M; 4-305 Baldwin Ave, Cornwall ON K6H 4J6; Assiut (Egypt)'74; MB BS; FRCSC; ObstGyn. Staff, Cornwall Community Hospital; Langs: Arabic; (613)937-3218; Fax. (613)937-4053.

ZAAROUR, Christian E; The Hosp for Sick Children, 555 University Ave, Toronto ON M5G 1X8; Beirut (Lebanon)'93; Staff, The Hospital For Sick Children; Langs: Bilingual(English/French); (416)813-7445; Fax. (416)813-7543.

ZAAYMAN, Melani; Port Hardy Med Associates, 8785 Greg St, Port Hardy BC V0N 2P0; Pretoria (South Africa)'97; MB ChB; Langs: Afrikaans; (250)949-5920

ZAAZOU, Mostafa A F T I; 308-77 Queensway W, Mississauga ON L5B 1B7; Cairo (Egypt)'83; FRCPC; Peds. Staff, Trillium Health Centre - Mississauga; (905)275-4400; Fax. (905)275-4403.

ZABANI, Najla A H I; London HSC-University Hosp, PO Box 5339 Stn B 339 Windermere Rd, London ON N6A 5A5; King Abdul (Saudi Arabia)'03; Nephrol; IntMed. Staff, London Health Sciences Centre - University Hospital; (519)685-8300

ZABEL, Ralph W; Nepean Med Centre, 202-1 Centrepointe Dr, Nepean ON K2G 6E2; Wes'83; Ophth. Langs: German; (613)226-8991; Fax. (613)226-2803.

ZABIAN, Randa; CLSC Chateauguay, 95 av La Verdure, Chateauguay QC J6K 0E8; Damascus (Syria)'85; PhD; CCFP; ac Staff, CSSS Jardins-Roussillon; Langs: Arabic; English; (450)699-3333; Fax. (450)699-2325; randa.zabian@rrsss16.gouv.ca.

ZABIB, Nassr A; Gimli Community Health Centre, 120 Sixth Ave, Gimli MB R0C 1B0; (Other Foreign)'02; CCFP; Staff, Gimli Community Health Centre (Johnson Memorial Hospital); (204)642-5116

ZABOLOTNY, Brent P; Salvation Army Grace Gen Hosp, 300 Booth Dr, Winnipeg MB R3J 3M7; Man'97; FRCSC; GenSurg; General Surgical Oncology. Staff, The Salvation Army Grace Hospital; (204)837-0391

ZABRODSKI, Richard M; Deer Valley Family Med Centre, 101-83 Deerpoint Rd SE, Calgary AB T2J 6W5; Cal'80; CCFP; CCFP(E.M.); Staff, Rockyview General Hospital; (403)271-5123; Fax. (403)225-1276.

ZABTIA, Nazar R; Hamilton HSC-Juravinski Site, 711 Concession St, Hamilton ON L8V 1C3; Al-Fateh (Libya)'00; FRCSC; OrthSurg. Staff, Hamilton Health Sciences Centre-Juravinski Site; Staff, Hamilton Health Sciences Centre - Hamilton General Hospital; Langs: Arabic; (905)521-2100

ZACARIAS, Nancy S; Foothills Med Centre, 924-1403 29 St NW, Calgary AB T2N 2T9; (Philippines)'83; Staff, Foothills Medical Centre; (403)944-1157; Fax. (403)944-2714.

ZACHARIADIS, George P; Don Valley Med Centre, 101-855 Broadview Ave, Toronto ON M4K 3Z1; Alexandria (Egypt)'64; Langs: Arabic; French; Greek; (416)466-6699; Fax. (416)465-6179.

ZACHARIAS, Abe; East Kootenay Reg Hosp, 13 24th Ave N, Cranbrook BC V1C 3H9; Man'63; FRCPC; DiagRad. Head Radiol, East Kootenay Regional Hospital; (250)426-5281; Fax. (250)426-5610.

ZACHARIAS, Gordon W; Esquimalt Treatment Centre, 918 Esquimalt Rd, Victoria BC V9A 3M6; Man'88; CCFP; FCFP; (250)858-1480

ZACHARIAS, Howard J; Agassiz Med Centre, 130-30 Stephen St, Morden MB R6M 2G3; Man'71; CCFP; (204)822-4474; hjzach@sdnet.ca.

ZACHARIAS, James M; Health Sciences Centre, GE644-820 Sherbrook St, Winnipeg MB R3A 1R9; Man'92; BSc(Med.); MSc; FRCPC; IntMed; Nephrol. Staff Internal Med, Health Sciences Centre; Asst Prof, University of Manitoba; (204)787-3863; Fax. (204)787-3453.

ZACHARIAS, Rosemary; Orillia Soldier's Mem Hosp, 170 Colborne St W, Orillia ON L3V 2Z3; McM'99; CCFP; Staff, Orillia Soldiers' Memorial Hospital; (705)323-9800; zachariasrose@hotmail.com.

ZACHARIAS, S Ramesh K; Aim Health Group, 9-6400 Millcreek Dr, Mississauga ON L5N 3E7; Wes'80; FRCSC; GenSurg (Geriatric Medicine). Clinical Asst Prof Anes, McMaster University; (905)858-1368; Fax. (905)858-1399; rzacharias@medemerg.com.

ZACHARIAS, Sherma R; Regina Qu'Applle HR-Regina, 1440 14th Ave, Regina SK S4P 0W5; Sask'01; FRCPC; IntMed; Critical Care Medicine. Staff, Regina General Hospital; (306)766-4444

ZACHARIN, Laura S; U of Toronto-Health Services, 214 College St, Toronto ON M5T 2Z9; McG'84; CCFP; FCFP; Court Staff Family & CommunMed, Women's College Hospital; Langs: French; (416)978-8030; Fax. (416)971-2089.

ZACHOS, Constantine R; Oakridges Med & Urgent Care, 100-13291 Yonge St, Richmond Hill ON L4E 4L6; Tor'91; Staff, Royal Victoria Regional Health Centre; Staff, Ontario Addiction Treatment Centre; Staff, Huronia Urgent Care Clinic; Staff, Barrie Chronic Pain Clinic; Langs: Greek; (905)773-7759 x4; zachosc@sah.on.ca.

ZACHOS, Marianthi; Hamilton HS-McMaster Site, PO Box 2000 Stn Lcd 1 1200 Main St W, Hamilton ON L8N 3Z5; Tor'95; FRCPC; Peds; Gastroent. Staff, Hamilton Health Sciences Centre - McMaster University Medical Centre; Staff, Halton Healthcare Services Corporation - Oakville Site; Staff, Halton Healthcare Services Corporation - Milton District Hospital; Staff, Halton Healthcare Services Corporation - Georgetown Hospital; Langs: Greek; (905)521-2100; Fax. (905)521-2655.

ZACK, Barend N; The Surrey Eye Care Centre, 13490 104 Ave, Surrey BC V3T 1V8; UBC'00; ABOph; FRCSC; Ophth. Surg Staff, Surrey Memorial Hospital; (604)585-6414; Fax. (604)951-8510.

ZACK, Deborah E; Allan Memorial Institute, 1025 av des Pins O, Montreal QC H3A 1A1; McM'75; FRCPC; Psy. Att Staff, McGill University Health Centre - Royal Victoria Hospital; Conférencier Psy, McGill University; (514)934-1934 x36106; Fax. (514)843-1644.

ZACK, Philip S; East Van Med Bldg, 406-1750 10th Ave E, Vancouver BC V5N 5K4; UBC'72; CCFP; FCFP; Ac Staff, Vancouver General Hospital - Centennial Pavillion; (604)872-1672; Fax. (604)872-7032.

ZACKON, David H; 410-2255 Carling Ave, Ottawa ON K2B 7Z5; Ott'77; FRCSC; Ophth (Neuro Ophthalmology). Staff, The Ottawa Hospital - General Campus; Assoc Prof Ophth, University of Ottawa; (613)596-0300; Fax. (613)596-0848.

ZACKON, Harold M; 203-5515 rue St-Jacques, Montreal QC H4A 2E3; McG'71; Respir (P.Q.); IntMed (Pulmonary Medicine). Médecin traitant Respirology, St Mary's Hospital Centre; assoc Prof Med, McGill University; (514)483-9910; Fax. (514)483-9910.

ZACKS, David J; Victoria Gen Hosp, 1 Hospital Way, Victoria BC V8Z 6R5; Cape Town (South Africa)'67; MB ChB; DMRD; FRCR; DiagRad. Staff Med Imaging, Victoria General Hospital; (250)727-4212

ZACKS, Jason A; Six Nations Family Health Team, PO Box 5000 1745 Chiefswood Rd, Ohsweken ON N0A 1M0; Tor'95; CCFP; (519)445-4019; Fax. (519)445-1917.

ZADEH, Teanoosh; Clinique Verite, 1200-1 Car Westmount, Westmount QC H3Z 2P9; Laval'87; FRCSC; GenSurg (Esthetic Plastic Surgery); PlasSurg. Staff, Hôpital Anna-Laberge; adj Prof Plastic Surg, McGill University Health Centre - Montreal General Campus; Staff, Centre Hospitalier l'Université de Montréal (CHUM) - Hôpital Notre-Dame; adj Prof Plastic Surg, McGill University Health Centre - Royal Victoria Hospital; adj Prof Plastic Surg, McGill University Health Centre - Montreal Children's Hospital; adj Prof Plastic Surg, McGill University; Langs: French; Farsi; (514)933-9131; Fax. (514)933-0730; drzadeh@verite-esthetique.com.

ZADHOUSH, Kourosh; Bradford Med Centre, PO Box 207 7-157 Holland St E, Bradford ON L3Z 2A8; Isfahan University (Other Foreign)'98; CCFP; Staff, Newmarket Health Centre; Langs: Farsi; Persian; (905)551-6555; Fax. (905)551-7655.

ZADIK, Robert A; Humber River Reg Hosp-Finch, 2111 Finch Ave W, North York ON M3N 1N1; Wes'98; FRCPC; Anes. Staff, Humber River Regional Hospital - Finch Avenue Site; Langs: Hebrew; (416)744-2500

ZADOR, Katalin; Clinique Med Chemin St-Jean, 675 ch de Saint-Jean, La Prairie QC J5R 2L2; Mon'88; ac Staff, Hôpital du Haut-Richelieu; Langs: Bilingual(English/French); (450)444-2002; Fax. (450)444-4920.

ZADOR, Nicolas M; Plexo-Mediclub, 6100 av du Boise, Montreal QC H3S 2W1; Sher'93; (514)739-5646

ZADOROZNY, Oleg G; CSSSG-Hop de Hull, 116 boul Lionel-Emond, Gatineau QC J8Y 1W7; McG'79; AB; ABIM; FRCPC; IntMed; Rheum. ac Staff, Hull Hospital; Consultant, Centre Hospitalier Gatineau Mémorial; Consultant, CH-CHSLD de Papineau - Pavillon du centre hospitalier; Langs: English; French; (819)777-6664; Fax. (819)777-0138.

ZADRA, Joseph A; Royal Court Med Bldg, 206-1 Quarry Ridge Rd, Barrie ON L4M 7G1; McG'83; FRCS; FRCSC; Urol (Adult & Pediatric Urology). Chief Urol, Royal Victoria Regional Health Centre; Asst Prof, McMaster University; Langs: Italian; Spanish; (705)728-4501; Fax. (705)728-8332; joezadra@rogers.com.

ZADRA, Remo; Newmarket Med Place, 208-712 Davis Dr, Newmarket ON L3Y 8C3; Ott'88; FRCPC; IntMed; Cardiol. Staff, Southlake Regional Health Centre; Langs: Italian; (905)853-2888; Fax. (905)853-6607.

ZADYKO, Jerry; Royal York Med Arts Bldg, 205-1436 Royal York Rd, Etobicoke ON M9P 3A9; Tor'62; CCFP; CCFP(E.M.); FCFP; Ac Staff, St Joseph's Health Centre; Langs: Ukrainian; (416)236-3888; Fax. (416)236-1379.

ZAFAR, Aftab; 201-715 Fischer Hallman Rd, Kitchener ON N2E 4E9; Ott'97; FRCSC; Ophth (Oculo Plastic Surgery). Langs: French; Urdu; (519)745-3690; Fax. (519)745-4856.

ZAFAR, Moiz M; Dr Moiz M Zafar Med Prof Corp, 212-16700 Bayview Ave, Newmarket ON L3X 1W1; Wes'98; BSc; MSc; MD; FRCPC; IntMed; Critical Care Medicine; Respir. Staff, Southlake Regional Health Centre; (905)954-1500; Fax. (905)954-0744.

ZAFAR, Rosy; Trillium Summerville Teaching, 7F-101 Queensway W, Mississauga ON L5B 2P7; Punjab (Pakistan)'91; CCFP; Langs: Urdu; Hindi; Punjabi; (905)272-9900; Fax. (905)272-9977.

ZAFAR, Saira; London HSC-Victoria Campus, PO Box 5010 Stn B E1 311B-800 Commissioners Rd E, London ON N6A 5W9; Punjab (Pakistan)'00; FRCPC; IntMed. Staff, London Health Sciences Centre - Victoria Campus; Staff, London Health Sciences Centre - University Hospital; Langs: Hindi; Punjabi; (519)685-8500

ZAGHLOUL, Emad; C-2309 McCallum Rd, Abbotsford BC V2S 3N7; Cairo (Egypt)'76; MB ChB; MRCPsy(UK); FRCPC; Psy (Child & Adolescent Psychiatry). Staff, Abbotsford Regional Hospital & Cancer Centre; Langs: Arabic; (604)854-3122; Fax. (604)854-3162.

ZAGOZESKI, Cheryl A; Regina Centre Crossing, 172-1621 Albert St, Regina SK S4P 2S5; Sask'83; BSc(Hons.); CCFP; FCFP; Staff Family Med, Regina General Hospital; Assoc Prof, University of Saskatchewan; (306)766-0444

ZAGURY, Gaby; Ellendale Med Bldg, 270-5845 ch Cote-des-Neiges, Montreal QC H3S 1Z4; Sher'76; CCFP; Langs: Bilingual(French/English); (514)735-6639; Fax. (514)735-0244; drgzagury@videotron.ca.

ZAHARATOS, Gerasimos J; SMBD Jewish Gen Hosp, G142 1-3755 Cote-Sainte-Cather, Montreal QC H3T 1E2; McG'95; FRCPC; IntMed; MedMicrobiol; InfectDis. Staff, Sir Mortimer B Davis Jewish General; (514)340-8222 x2933; Fax. (514)340-7578.

ZAHARESCU, Desiree; Centre Med des Generations, 200-465 rue Bibeau, Saint-Eustache QC J7R 0C8; Mon'84; Langs: French; (450)472-1955; Fax. (450)472-1905; dzaharescu@cm25.ca.

ZAHARIA, Florin; CSST-Direction Regionale Montr, CP 3 Succ Pl-desjardins TS-1 Complexe desjardins, Montreal QC H5B 1H1; Mon'75; CSPQ; FRCSC; GenSurg (Industrial Occupational Medicine). Médecin, CSST-Direction Regionale Montreal; Physician, Workmen's Compensation of Quebec; Langs: Romanian; English; (514)906-3671; Fax. (514)906-3531.

ZAHARIA, Francoise; CHUM-Hop St-Luc, 1058 rue Saint-Denis, Montreal QC H2X 3J4; Paris (France)'75; Anes (P.Q.). Staff, Centre Hospitalier l'Université De Montréal (CHUM) - Hôpital Saint-luc; (514)281-2121; Fax. (514)890-8000.

ZAHARIA, Marian-Ananda; Clinique Med l'Assomption, RC10-5345 boul de l'Assomption, Montreal QC H1T 4B3; Bucharest (Romania)'69; FRCSC; Ophth. Prof Ophth, Centre Hospitalier Universitaire de Sherbrooke-Hopital Fleurimont; Consultant, Centre Hospitalier Universitaire de Sherbrooke-Hôpital Hôtel-Dieu; assoc Prof, Universite de Sherbrooke; (514)251-2240

ZAHARIA, Mihai-Cristian; Centre Med Brunswick, 955 boul St Jean, Pointe-Claire QC H9R 5K3; (Other Foreign)'04; CCFP; (514)426-6677; Fax. (514)426-3323.

ZAHARIADIS, George; London HSC-Victoria Campus, PO Box 5010 Stn B B10 119B-800 Commissioners Rd, London ON N6A 5W9; Tor'97; FRCPC; IntMed (AIDS/HIV); MedMicrobiol; InfectDis. Staff, London Health Sciences Centre - Victoria Campus; (519)685-8500

ZAHAVI, Michael A; 17-600 King St E, Oshawa ON L1H 1G6; Tor'89; CCFP; Staff, Lakeridge Health - Oshawa Site; (905)432-1017; Fax. (905)432-0070.

ZAHEDI, Afshan; Bridlewood Prof Centre, 310-3443 Finch Ave E, Scarborough ON M1W 2S1; Tor'95; ABIM; FRCPC; FRCPC; Endocrin&Metab; IntMed. Asst Prof Med, Women's College Hospital; Staff Endocrinologist, The Scarborough Hospital - Birchmount Campus; Asst Prof Med, University of Toronto; Langs: Farsi; (416)495-1830; Fax. (416)495-1389; af.zahedi@utoronto.ca.

ZAHEER, Juveria S; Addiction & Mental Health-Clar, 250 College St, Toronto ON M5T 1R8; Qns'07; FRCPC; Psy. Staff, Centre for Addiction & Mental Health (CAMH) - College Street Site; (416)595-6111

ZAHER, Amjad N; Nineteen-O-Nine Med Centre, A-1909 Tecumseh Rd E, Windsor ON N8W 1C9; Damascus (Syria)'84; FRCPC; Peds. Langs: Arabic; (519)258-7671; Fax. (519)258-9281.

ZAHIRIEH, Alireza; Sunnybrook Hlth Sciences Ctr, A140-2075 Bayview Ave, Toronto ON M4N 3M5; Wes'02; FRCPC; IntMed (AIDS/HIV); Nephrol. Staff, Sunnybrook Health Sciences Centre; (416)480-6100; Fax. (416)480-5270; alireza.zahirieh@sunnybrooke.ca.

ZAHIRNEY, Georgina M; MUHC-Royal Victoria Hosp, 1025 av des Pins O, Montreal QC H3A 1A1; McG'96; FRCPC; Psy. Staff, Hopital Louis-H Lafontaine; Staff, McGill University Health Centre - Royal Victoria Hospital; Médecin, Allan Memorial Institute; Clin Prof Psy, Universite de Montreal; Langs: English; French; (514)934-1934

ZAHLAN, Usama; Lake of the Woods Dist Hosp, RR 1 21 Sylvan St, Kenora ON P9N 3W7; Cluj-Nopoca (Romania)'82; FRCPC; Psy. Staff, Lake of the Woods District Hospital; Staff, Kenora District ACT Team Connection; Langs: Arabic; (807)468-9861 x262; Fax. (807)468-1428; uzahlan@lwdh.on.ca.

ZAHN, Catherine A; Univ Hlth Network-Toronto Western Hosp, WW5-399 Bathurst St, Toronto ON M5T 2S8; Tor'78; FRCPC; Neur. Staff, Toronto General Hospital - UHN; Staff Site VP, Toronto Western Hospital - University Health Network; (416)603-5232; Fax. (416)603-5768.

ZAHN, Karen A; Vancouver Gen Hosp, 855 12th Ave W, Vancouver BC V5Z 1M9; Dal'95; DAB; FRCPC; EmergMed. Staff, Vancouver General Hospital - Centennial Pavillion; (604)875-4700

ZAHRADNIK, Joseph; The Medical Centre, PO Box 4200 Stn Main 707 Charlotte St, Peterborough ON K9J 7B3; Prague (Czech Republic)'74; FRCSC; ObstGyn. Ac Staff, Peterborough Regional Health Centre - Hospital Drive; Ac Staff, Peterborough Regional Health Centre - Rogers St Site; Langs: Czech; Slovak.

ZAHRAN, Ali H M; Hamilton HS-McMaster Site, PO Box 2000 Stn Lcd 1 2U1-1200 Main St W, Hamilton ON L8N 3Z5; Kharkov Medical University (Russia (Federation))'98; Clin Fellow Anes, Hamilton Health Sciences Centre - McMaster University Medical Centre; (905)521-2100

ZAHREBELNY, George R; 1726 Huron Church Rd, Windsor ON N9C 2L4; Tor'80; Ac Staff, Windsor Regional Hospital - Tayfour Site; Ac Staff, Hôtel-Dieu Grace Hospital; Langs: Ukrainian; (519)258-3093; Fax. (519)946-0258.

ZAIB, Jehan; Thunder Bay Reg HSC, 980 Oliver Rd, Thunder Bay ON P7B 6V4; University of Peshawar (Pakistan)'92; CCFP; Staff, Thunder Bay Regional Health Sciences Centre; (807)680-6030

ZAID, Akram A A; Belmore Square, 100-1011 Glenmore Trail SW, Calgary AB T2V 4R6; (Libya)'03; CCFP; (403)663-5974; Fax. (403)663-5979.

ZAIDEL, Patrick A; Burnaby Hosp, 3935 Kincaid St, Burnaby BC V5G 2X6; UBC'93; FRCPC; IntMed. Staff Rapid Access Pain Chest Clinic, Burnaby Hospital; Clin Assoc Prof IntMed & Family Med, University of British Columbia; Langs: Spanish; French; (604)292-9260; Fax. (604)739-6169.

ZAIDI, Hasan A; Oshawa Med Clinic, 117 King St E, Oshawa ON L1H 1B9; Cal'99; BSc; FRCPC; IntMed (Hepatology); Gastroent. Staff Gastroent, Lakeridge Health - Oshawa Site; Staff, Markham Endoscopy; (905)721-7726; Fax. (905)721-4978.

ZAIDI, Houria; Hôpital du Haut-Richelieu, 920 boul du Seminaire N, St-Jean-sur-Richel QC J3A 1B7; Algiers (Algeria)'93; Staff, Hôpital du Haut-Richelieu; (450)359-5000 x5232; Fax. (450)359-5251.

ZAIDI, Mudassir A; 1813 Lasalle Blvd, Sudbury ON P3A 2A3; Dow Medical College (Pakistan)'97; CCFP; (705)560-9422

ZAIDI, Mukarram A; Oasis Med Clinic, 216-8338 18 St SE, Calgary AB T2C 4E4; Dow Medical College (Pakistan)'97; Langs: Hindi; Urdu; (403)236-2344; Fax. (403)236-2383.

ZAIDI, Syed A A; Albert Park Family Med Centre, 3992 Albert St, Regina SK S4S 3R1; (Other Foreign)'87; CCFP; (306)584-3833; Fax. (306)585-3833.

ZAITLEN, Marshall S; WOHC-Brampton Civic Hosp, 2100 Bovaird Dr E, Brampton ON L6R 3J7; Sask'79; FRCPC; Neur. Staff, Chapleau General Hospital - Division of Services de santé de Chapleau Health Services; Staff, Lady Minto Hospital Cochrane; Staff, Bingham Memorial Hospital; Ac Staff, William Osler Health System - Brampton Civic Hospital; (905)459-2000; Fax. (905)459-1293.

ZAITZOW, Michael D; Peace Arch Hosp, 15521 Russell Ave, White Rock BC V4B 2R4; UBC'81; FRCPC; Psy. Staff, Peace Arch Hospital; (604)541-7171; Fax. (604)538-8500.

ZAJACZKOWSKA-KIELSKA, Anna; Morgan Creek Business Ctre, 301A-15252 32 Ave, Surrey BC V3S 0R7; Gdansk (Poland)'72; FRCPC; Peds (Cystic Fibrosis). Staff Cystic Fibrosis Clinic, BC Women's Hospital & Health Centre; Clinical Asst Prof Peds, University of British Columbia; Langs: Polish; (604)875-8750

ZAJC-DALCOURT, Natasha; 3-45 Grist Mill Rd, Holland Landing ON L9N 1M7; Tor'94; CCFP; Ac Staff, Southlake Regional Health Centre; (905)853-8966; Fax. (905)853-2953.

ZAJDLIK, Anne-Marie; Guelph Family Health Team, 21 Yarmouth St, Guelph ON N1H 4G2; McM'88; Staff, Guelph General Hospital; Founder/Dir, Centre for Local-Regional & Global Health-HIV Clinic; Staff, Masai Centre; (519)822-7831; Fax. (519)822-6234.

ZAJDMAN, Michael L; The Southcom Bldg, 301-2227 South Millway, Mississauga ON L5L 3R6; McG'85; FRCPC; Peds. Staff, The Credit Valley Hospital; (905)569-9798; Fax. (905)569-8630; mzajdman@cvh.on.ca.

ZAJNER, Michael W J; South Walkerville Med Bldg, 133-2224 Walker Rd, Windsor ON N8W 5L7; Qns'88; CCFP; FCFP; (519)255-7366; Fax. (519)255-7957.

ZAKARIA, Fozia; Meadowbrook Clinic, 3907 34 St NW, Edmonton AB T6T 1L5; (Other Foreign)'90; CCFP; (780)448-1166; Fax. (780)448-2830.

ZAKARIA, Hanaa; Clinique Med le Plein Ciel, 475 boul de la Cote-Vertu, Saint-Laurent QC H4L 1X7; Ein Shams (Egypt)'82; Staff, Hopital du CSS de la Region de Thetford; (514)337-3171; Fax. (514)337-6023.

ZAKARIA, Joseph D; 101-3335 Dougall Ave, Windsor ON N9E 1S8; Wes'08; CCFP; (519)945-8623; Fax. (519)945-5708.

ZAKARIA, Muhammed; Lakeridge Health-Oshawa Site, 1 Hospital Crt, Oshawa ON L1G 2B9; Dacca (Bangladesh)'76; MB BS; DCH; FRCPC; Psy. Staff, Lakeridge Health - Oshawa Site; Staff, Fairview Lodge; Langs: Bengali; (905)576-8711; Fax. (905)721-4742.

ZAKHAROVA SMIRNOVA, Natalia; Kateri Mem Hosp Centre, PO Box 10, Kahnawake QC J0L 1B0; Sher'10; CCFP; Staff, Kateri Memorial Hospital Centre; (450)638-3930

ZAKHARY, Gamel S; Finchgate Med Centre, 321-40 Finchgate Blvd, Brampton ON L6T 3J1; Cairo (Egypt)'77; FRCPC; Peds. Langs: Arabic; (905)793-7855

ZAKHARY, Jena M I; York Medical, 14800 Yonge St, Aurora ON L4G 1N3; American University of Antigua (Antigua & Barbuda)'10; CCFP.

ZAKHARY, Kristina; Mission Med Clinic, 803-2303 4 St SW, Calgary AB T2S 2S7; McG'99; FRCSC; Otol (Facial Plastic Surgery). (403)450-3759; Fax. (403)450-3789; zakharyclinic@yahoo.com.

ZAKHARY, Liliane H; William Osler Health Centre, 401-100 Humber College Blvd, Etobicoke ON M9V 5G4; Cairo (Egypt)'76; MB ChB; FRCPC; Peds (Respirology). Staff, William Osler Health System - Etobicoke General Hospital; Langs: Arabic; French; (416)747-7122; Fax. (416)747-7122.

ZAKHARY, Mariam R; Brameast Family Health Org, 38-2130 North Park Dr, Brampton ON L6S 0C9; Ain Shams (Egypt)'97; CCFP; Langs: Arabic; French; (905)792-2211; Fax. (905)792-2901.

ZAKHARY, Mourad I S; Reg Mental Health Care-London, PO Box 5532 Stn B 850 Highbury Ave N, London ON N6A 4H1; Assiut (Egypt)'75; CCFP; Staff, Regional Mental Health Care-St Joseph's Health Care; Staff, St Joseph's Hospital - St Joseph's Health Care; Staff, Highbury Medical Clinic; Langs: Arabic; (519)455-5110 x47442; Fax. (519)452-4396.

ZAKI, Amel E; Bison Primacy Med Clinic, 1-80 Bison Dr, Winnipeg MB R3T 4Z7; University of Alexandria (Egypt)'90; CCFP; Staff, DeSalaberry District Health Centre; (204)275-1500

ZAKI, Emad L A; Hamilton HS-McMaster Site, PO Box 2000 Stn Lcd 1 3A55-1200 Main St W, Hamilton ON L8N 3Z5; Ain Shams (Egypt)'88; Staff, Hamilton Health Sciences Centre - McMaster University Medical Centre; Langs: Arabic; (905)521-2100; Fax. (905)308-7548.

ZAKI, Magdy F; Fort Street Med Clinic, 300 Fort St, Winnipeg MB R3C 1E5; Alexandria (Egypt)'78; MB ChB; FRCSC; GenSurg.

ZAKI, Moheb E; Perth Med Clinic, 1-500 East Riverside Dr, Perth-Andover NB E7H 1Z1; Cairo (Egypt)'95; MB BCh; CCFP; (506)273-9544

ZAKI, Nasser A; Lakeshore West Med Centre, 2083 Lakeshore Blvd W, Etobicoke ON M8V 4G2; Ain Shams (Egypt)'91; MB ChB; LMCC; AAFP; CCFP; Staff, Sure Health Medical Centre; Assoc Prof, Schulich School of Medicine-Windsor Campus; Langs: Arabic; French; (416)252-2775; Fax. (416)252-2773.

ZAKI, Sami F; Glenrose Rehab Hosp, 10230 111 Ave NW, Edmonton AB T5G 0B7; Mansura (Egypt)'92; MB BCh; FRCPC; PhysMed&Rehab (Spinal Cord Injury). Staff Adult Rehab, Glenrose Rehabilitation Hospital; Clinical Asst Prof, University of Alberta; (780)735-7999; Fax. (780)735-6018.

ZAKLAMA, Nora; Lakeshore Gen Hosp, 160 av Stillview, Pointe-Claire QC H9R 2Y2; Tor'80; GenPath (P.Q.). Chef Dept of Lab, Lakeshore General Hospital - Pointe Claire; Langs: Arabic; French; (514)630-2225 x5536

ZAKLOS, Mayer M; 207-5655 av du Parc, Montreal QC H2V 4H2; McG'79; CCFP; McGill University; Langs: Yiddish; French; (514)274-4339

ZAKRISON, Tanya L; St Michael's Hosp, 30 Bond St, Toronto ON M5B 1W8; Tor'03; FRCSC; GenSurg. Staff, St Michael's Hospital; Staff, Univerity of Toronto Continuing Education; Langs: Spanish; French; (416)366-6139

ZAKRZEWSKI, Peter A; 201-20434 64 Ave, Langley BC V2Y 1N4; Tor'04; FRCSC; Ophth. (778)387-0900

ZAKRZEWSKI, W Paul; Sundance West Business Park, 4120-15 Sunpark Plaza SE, Calgary AB T2X 0M5; Alb'97; MSc; PhD; CCFP; Staff, Calgary Trail Medicentres; (403)910-3990; Fax. (403)910-0449.

ZALAI, Christian V; Centre Med Ormstown, 24 rue Gale, Ormstown QC J0S 1K0; McG'04; FRCSC; GenSurg. Staff, Barrie Memorial Hospital; (450)829-2331

ZALAM, Mahmoud M M; Children's Hospital, 840 Sherbrook St, Winnipeg MB R3A 1S1; Staff, Health Sciences Centre.

ZALAN, Paul R; 2558 Danforth Ave, Toronto ON M4C 1L3; Tor'74; Assoc Staff, Toronto East General Hospital Inc; Ac Staff, Providence Healthcare; Assoc Staff, St Michael's Hospital; Langs: Hungarian; (416)691-4168

ZALAN, Peter G; Health Sciences North, 41 Ramsey Lake Rd, Sudbury ON P3E 5J1; Tor'71; FRCPC; Anes (Critical Care Medicine). Staff, Health Sciences North-St Joseph's Health Centre; Staff, Health Sciences North-Laurentian Site; (705)522-7100

ZALAN, Robert M; North York Gen Hosp, 8N 809-4001 Leslie St, North York ON M2K 1E1; Wes'03; FRCPC; Psy. Staff, North York General Hospital; (416)756-6695; Fax. (416)756-6671.

ZALESKI, Witold M; London HSC-Victoria Hosp, PO Box 5010 Stn B D1 104-800 Commissioners Rd E, London ON N6A 5W9; Sask'83; FRCPC; DiagRad (Mammography). Ac Staff Radiol, London Health Sciences Centre - Victoria Campus; Asst Prof DiagRad & Nuclear Med, University of Western Ontario; Langs: Polish; French; (519)685-8500 x55006; Fax. (519)667-6771.

ZALEV, Arthur H; St Michael's Hosp, 30 Bond St, Toronto ON M5B 1W8; Tor'70; DABR; FACR; MBA; FRCPC; DiagRad (Gastrointestinal Radiology). Ac Staff, St Michael's Hospital; Consultant, Providence Healthcare; Asst Prof, University of Toronto; (416)864-5740; Fax. (416)864-5380; zaleva@smh.toronto.on.ca.

ZALEWSKI, Pawel G; Lakeridge Hlth Corp-Oshawa, 1 Hospital Crt, Oshawa ON L1G 2B9; Warsaw (Poland)'88; FRCPC; IntMed; MedOncol. Staff Durham Reg Cancer Centre/Staff Oncology Clinic, Lakeridge Health - Oshawa Site; Langs: Polish; Russian; (905)576-8711 x4573; Fax. (905)721-6103; pawel_zalewski@hotmail.com.

ZALMAEV, Evgueni B; Lakeshore Gen Hosp, 160 av Stillview, Pointe-Claire QC H9R 2Y2; Moscow (Russia (Federation))'86; Anes (P.Q.). Staff, Lakeshore General Hospital - Pointe Claire; (514)630-2225

ZALMANOWITZ, Leo I; Rockyview Gen Hosp, 7007 14 St SW, Calgary AB T2V 1P9; Alb'77; FRCPC; EmergMed. Staff EmergMed, Rockyview General Hospital; Teacher, University of Calgary; (403)943-3449

ZALTER, Mark S; Hamilton Commun Health Centre, M1-414 Victoria Ave N, Hamilton ON L8L 5G8; McG'87; Staff Family Med, Hamilton Health Sciences Centre - McMaster University Medical Centre; Langs: English; French; (905)529-5221; Fax. (905)667-1082.

ZALTZ, Arthur P; Sunnybrook Hlth Sciences Ctre, B710-2075 Bayview Ave, Toronto ON M4N 3M5; Tor'82; FRCSC; ObstGyn. Ac Staff, Sunnybrook Health Sciences Centre; Ac Staff, Women's College Hospital; Asst Prof, University of Toronto; (416)480-4789; Fax. (416)480-4839.

ZALTZMAN, Jeffrey S; 9138Q-61 Queen St E, Toronto ON M5C 2T2; McG'85; ABIM; FRCPC; IntMed (Renal Transplant); Nephrol. Staff, St Michael's Hospital; Assoc Prof, University of Toronto; Langs: English; French; (416)867-7444; jeffrey.zaltzman@utoronto.ca.

ZALUNARDO, Nadia Y; Gordon & Leslie Diamond HCC, 5F-2775 Laurel St, Vancouver BC V5Z 1M9; UBC'99; BSc; MSc; FRCPC; IntMed; Nephrol. Staff Clinician Investigator Prog, Gordon & Leslie Diamond Health Care Centre; (604)875-5950; Fax. (604)875-5952.

ZALZAL, Nayla; Port Hope Comm Health Ctre, 99 Toronto Rd, Port Hope ON L1A 3S6; Tor'84; Staff, Lakeridge Health - Whitby Site; Staff, Port Hope Community Centre; Staff, Oshawa Community Health Centre; Langs: Arabic; French; (905)885-2626; Fax. (905)885-2646.

ZALZAL, Paul K; A3-481 North Service Rd W, Oakville ON L6M 2V6; McM'96; FRCSC; OrthSurg. Staff, Halton Healthcare Services Corporation - Oakville Site; Asst Prof Clinical Surg, McMaster University; Langs: Bilingual(English/French); (905)844-7706; Fax. (905)844-7808; pzandbw@hotmail.com.

ZAMAN, Atiq U; PO Box 160, Cross Lake MB R0B 0J0; (Other Foreign)'77.

ZAMAN, Kamruz; Dawes Family Practice & Walk-I, 2772 Danforth Ave, Toronto ON M4C 1L7; Dhaka (Bangladesh)'79; MB BS; CCFP; Langs: Arabic; Bengali; Hindi; Urdu; (416)690-1042; Fax. (416)690-1046; kamruz.zaman14@gmail.com.

ZAMAN, Khawar-Uz; Dartmouth Gen Hosp, 325 Pleasant St, Dartmouth NS B2Y 4G8; Punjab (Pakistan)'87; MB BS; FRCPC; IntMed (Cardiology). Staff, Dartmouth General Hospital; Langs: Urdu; Punjabi; (902)460-4150; Fax. (902)460-4154; thisiszaman@hotmail.com.

ZAMANI, Haseebullah; 214 Med Place, 12F-9909 102 St, Grande Prairie AB T8V 2V4; (Germany)'89; (780)539-3022; Fax. (780)532-0949.

ZAMANPOUR, Kamran; Capilano Med Clinic, 85-935 Marine Dr, North Vancouver BC V7P 1S3; Shiraz (Iran)'94; CCFP; Langs: Farsi; (604)988-3443; Fax. (604)988-3447.

ZAMEL, Noe; Univ Hlth Network-Toronto Western Hosp, 7EW-399 Bathurst St, Toronto ON M5T 2S8; Porto Alegre (Brazil)'58; FRCPC; MedScient(Med). Staff, Toronto Western Hospital - University Health Network; Staff Physician, Mount Sinai Hospital; Staff Physician, Women's College Hospital; Langs: Portuguese; Spanish; (416)603-5767; Fax. (416)603-5501; noe@zamel.ca.

ZAMEL, Rola; Springdale Prof Bldg, 614-2250 Bovaird Dr E, Brampton ON L6R 0W3; (Jordan)'00; FRCPC; IntMed; Endocrin&Metab. Staff, Trillium Health Centre - Mississauga; Langs: Arabic; (905)790-7900; Fax. (905)790-7907.

ZAMFIR, Catalina D; Royal Columbian Hosp, 330 Columbia St E, New Westminster BC V3L 3W7; Bucarest (Romania)'88; CCFP; Staff, Royal Columbian Hospital; Langs: Romanian; (604)520-4253

ZAMMIT-MAEMPEL, Joseph G; McMaster Niagara Fam Hlth Ctr, 22 Ontario St, St Catharines ON L2R 7M3; University of Dundee (Scotland)'84; (905)984-3335; Fax. (905)984-6008.

ZAMONSKY, Corinne G; Richmond Square, 70-3915 51 St SW, Calgary AB T3E 6N1; Sask'88; CCFP; FCFP; (403)229-2273; Fax. (403)246-9688; drczamonsky@aol.com.

ZAMORA, Emil N; 1601 King St E, Hamilton ON L8K 1T5; Qns'60; MSc; MDCM; FRCPC; Psy (Electroconvulsive Therapy). Ac Staff, St Joseph's Healthcare - Charlton Campus; Consultant Matrix Health Serv, Behavioral Medical Centre; Consultant, Odyssey Health Clinic; Clin Assoc Prof Psy, McMaster University; Langs: Ukrainian; Polish; (905)549-8800; Fax. (905)549-4933.

ZAMORA, Jorge E; Kingston Gen Hosp, 76 Stuart St, Kingston ON K7L 2V7; Qns'91; FRCPC; Anes (Thoracic Anesthesia). Staff, Hotel-Dieu Hospital; Staff, Providence Care - Mental Health Services; Staff, Kingston General Hospital; Assoc Prof Anes, Queen's University; Langs: English; French; (613)548-7827; Fax. (613)548-1375.

ZAMORA, Mary M; Trafalgar Med Clinic, 200-1235 Trafalgar Rd, Oakville ON L6H 3P1; Qns'85; CCFP; CCFP(E.M.); FCFP; Ac Staff, Halton Healthcare Services Corporation - Oakville Site; (905)844-3281; Fax. (905)849-1076.

ZAMORSKI, Mark A; Cdn Forces Support Unit-HCC, 2A 210DND-1745 Alta Vista Dr, Ottawa ON K1A 0K6; Detroit(MI) (USA)'89; CCFP; Staff, Canadian Forces Health Services Centre; (613)945-8062; Fax. (613)945-6745.

ZAMPARINI, Adriana M; Downtown Comm Hlth Clinic, 569 Powell St, Vancouver BC V6A 1G8; Cape Town (South Africa)'89; MB ChB; CCFP; Staff, Downtown Community Health Clinic; (604)255-3151; Fax. (604)255-0314.

ZAMPINI, Marisa A; SMBD Jewish Gen Hosp, 3755 ch Cote-Sainte-Catherine, Montreal QC H3T 1E2; McG'05; CCFP; Staff, Sir Mortimer B Davis Jewish General; (514)340-8278; Fax. (514)340-8298; marisa.zampini@mail.mcgill.ca.

ZAN, Nathalie; Hop Maisonneuve Rosemont, 5415 boul de l'Assomption, Montreal QC H1T 2M4; Mon'91; CCFP; Staff, CHSLD de la MRC de Champlain-Centre Saint-Lambert; Staff, Institut Universitaire de Gériatrie de Montréal; Staff, Hopital Maisonneuve-Rosemont; (514)252-3400 x6084; Fax. (514)252-3573; nathalie.zan@rrsss16.gouv.qc.ca.

ZANDER, Dennis R; Trillium Hlth Ctr-West Toronto, 150 Sherway Dr, Etobicoke ON M9C 1A5; Wes'94; FRCPC; DiagRad. Staff, Trillium Health Centre - West Toronto; Staff, Etobicoke Medical Centre Family Health Team; Staff, Radiology Associates Mississauga; Staff, Radiology Associates Clarkson; Staff, Six Points Diagnostic Imaging; (416)259-6671; dennis.zander@stjoe.on.ca.

ZANDIEH, Iman; Medical Arts Bldg, 201-582 Goldstream Ave, Victoria BC V9B 2W7; UBC'02; FRCPC; IntMed; Gastroent. Staff Gastrotent, Royal Jubilee Hospital; Langs: Farsi; French; (250)388-7047; Fax. (250)388-7049.

ZANELLI, Patrizia A C; MUHC-Montreal Gen Hosp, D6 253-1650 av Cedar, Montreal QC H3G 1A4; McG'89; FRCPC; IntMed (Intensive Care); Critical Care Medicine. Staff, McGill University Health Centre - Montreal General Campus; adj Prof, McGill University; Langs: Italian; French; (514)934-1934 x43067; Fax. (514)937-0803; patrizia.zanelli@mcgill.ca.

ZANETTE, Paul A; All-In-One Health Care Clinic, 100-10083 Keele St, Maple ON L6A 3Y8; Wes'97; CCFP; Ac Staff, Mackenzie Richmond Hill Hospital; Langs: Italian; (905)832-4644; Fax. (905)832-7717.

ZANETTI, Fabio G; North Brantford Prof Bldg, LL006-525 Park Rd N, Brantford ON N3R 7K8; Ott'86; FRCSC; Ophth. Langs: Italian; French; (519)752-7978; Fax. (519)752-7452.

ZANGANEH, Shahin; Windsor Allergy & Asthma Assoc, 1407 Ottawa St, Windsor ON N8X 2G1; McG'00; FRCPC; IntMed; ClinImmunol&Allergy. Staff, London Health Sciences Centre - University Hospital; (519)258-4356; Fax. (519)258-3502.

ZANIEWSKI, Gregory A; Peterborough Clinic, 202-26 Hospital Dr, Peterborough ON K9J 7C3; (Other Foreign)'08; CCFP; Langs: Polish; (705)740-6849; Fax. (705)743-4392.

ZANKE, Brent W; The Ottawa Hosp-Gen Campus, 501 Smyth Rd, Ottawa ON K1H 8L6; Man'83; PhD; FRCPC; IntMed (Malignant Lymphoma); MedOncol. Staff, The Ottawa Hospital - General Campus; (613)737-8899

ZANOZIN, Dmitrij; Northern Interior Health Unit, 1444 Edmonton St, Prince George BC V2M 6W5; Moscow (Russia (Federation))'90; CCFP; FCFP; Staff, Sparwood Healthcare Centre; Staff, Northern Health Northern Interior Health Service Prince George; Langs: Russian; (250)565-2666

ZANUSSI, Lauren W; Foothills Med Centre, 704-1403 29 St NW, Calgary AB T2N 2T9; Cal'98; FRCPC; Psy. Staff, Foothills Medical Centre; (403)944-5872; Fax. (403)944-2409.

ZANUSSI, Ursula; Adolescent Day Treatment Prog, 200-2204 2 St SW, Calgary AB T2S 3C2; Cal'04; FRCPC; Psy. (403)802-2265; Fax. (403)244-7964.

ZAPASNIK, Marta; Med Stop Heritage Plaza, 8330 MacLeod Trail SE, Calgary AB T2H 2V2; (Poland)'01; CCFP; (403)238-3000

ZAPASNIK, Romuald; Heritage Family Med Centre, 8330 Macleod Trail SE, Calgary AB T2H 2V2; Krakow (Poland)'76; (403)253-6188

ZAPATA, Myrna B; Bayvalley Med Arts Bldg, 401-145 Queenston St, St Catharines ON L2R 2Z9; Manila (Philippines)'73; FRCPC; Peds. Langs: Ilonggo; Tagalog; (905)688-6650; Fax. (905)688-4551.

ZAPF-GILJE, Margery H; Fairmont Med Bldg, 414-750 Broadway W, Vancouver BC V5Z 1H6; UBC'82; CCFP; FCFP; Vis Physician, Vancouver General Hospital - Centennial Pavillion; Vis Physician, BC Women's Hospital & Health Centre; Vis Physician, BC Children's Hospital; Vis Physician, University of British Columbia; Langs: Norwegian; (604)675-9433; Fax. (604)675-9434; drs.office@shawbiz.ca.

ZAPHIRATOS, Thomas A; 202-7200 rue Hutchison, Montreal QC H3N 1Z2; McG'78; BSc(Chem.); ABIM; MDCM; Staff, Sir Mortimer B Davis Jewish General; Staff, Donald Berman Maimonides Geriatric Centre; Langs: Greek; French; (514)495-2555; Fax. (514)495-7932.

ZAPHIRATOS, Vasiliki V; IWK Health Centre, PO Box 9700 RPO CSC 5850-5980 University Ave, Halifax NS B3K 6R8; Mon'07; FRCPC; Anes. Staff Women's & Obstetrics Anes, IWK Health Centre; (902)470-6627; Fax. (902)470-6626.

ZAPPITELLI, Michael; MUHC-Montreal Children's Hosp, E213-2300 rue Tupper, Montreal QC H3H 1P3; McG'00; Nephrol; Peds. Staff, McGill University Health Centre - Montreal Children's Hospital; (514)412-4400 x22524; Fax. (514)412-4359; mzaprdr@yahoo.ca.

ZARA, Nicolas; Hopital Charles Lemoyne, 3120 boul Taschereau, Longueuil QC J4V 2H1; Laval'07; DiagRad. Staff, Hopital Charles LeMoyne; (450)466-5000

ZARAGOZA, Antonio J; Village Park Med Clinic, 110-937 Fir St, Sherwood Park AB T8A 4N6; Manila (Philippines)'61; (780)467-8886; Fax. (780)467-6763.

ZARB, Marie-Therese A; Hincks-Dellcrest Treatment Ctr, 440 Jarvis St, Toronto ON M4Y 2H4; Ott'98; FRCPC; Psy. (416)924-1164; Fax. (416)924-8208.

ZARE-PARSI, Mojgan; North York Gen Hosp, 4001 Leslie St, North York ON M2K 1E1; Tehran (Iran)'81; FRCPC; Psy. Staff, North York General Hospital - Branson Division; Ac Staff, North York General Hospital; Staff, North York General Hospital Mental Health Clinic; Ac Staff East Metro Connections, Canadian Mental Health Associaton; Langs: Farsi; (416)756-6655; Fax. (416)756-6731.

ZAREEF, Shaista K; Caremedics Kanata Inc, 5357 Fernbank Rd, Stittsville ON K2S 1B6; McG'97; CCFP; FCFP; Langs: Punjabi; Urdu; (613)831-7300; Fax. (613)831-7377.

ZAREMBA, Ewelina; Woodlawn Med Clinic, 92 Main St, Dartmouth NS B2X 1R6; Jagiellonski (Other Foreign)'08; CCFP; (902)434-1500; Fax. (902)434-5011.

ZAREMBA, Janina; Bank Med Centre, 1935 Bank St, Ottawa ON K1V 8A3; Warsaw (Poland)'71; PhD(Endoc); Langs: Polish; French; (613)521-2391; Fax. (613)521-5443.

ZAREMBA, Jozef; Amherst Family Health Clinic, 1000-158 Robert Angus Dr, Amherst NS B4H 4R7; Bialystok (Poland)'79; CCFP; Staff, Cumberland Regional Health Care Center; Langs: Polish; (902)667-1923; Fax. (902)667-1926.

ZAREMBA, Michael G; Woodbridge Fam Practice Ctre, 201-8077 Islington Ave, Woodbridge ON L4L 7X7; Ott'78; CCFP; FCFP; Staff, Dr Langer & Associates; Langs: English; French; (905)851-3996; Fax. (905)851-1139.

ZARETSKY, Ari E; Addiction & Mental Hlth-Clarke, FG 24A-250 College St, Toronto ON M5T 1R8; Tor'88; FRCPC; Psy (Cognitive Therapy). Staff, Centre for Addiction & Mental Health (CAMH) - College Street Site; Att Staff, Sunnybrook Health Sciences Centre; Asst Prof, University of Toronto; Langs: Hebrew; (416)535-8501; Fax. (416)480-5070; ari.zaretsky@sw.ca.

ZARETSKY, Karolyn R; CML Healthcare Inc, 102-71 King St W, Mississauga ON L5B 4A2; Tor'89; FRCPC; DiagRad. (905)276-1022; Fax. (905)897-1146.

ZARETSKY, Yael S; The Credit Valley Hosp, 2200 Eglinton Ave W, Mississauga ON L5M 2N1; Tor'97; FRCPC; IntMed; Hem. Staff, The Credit Valley Hospital; Staff, Peel Regional Cancer Centre; (905)813-1100 x5135; Fax. (905)813-4024.

ZARIFA, Gihane W; Credit Valley Family Health Te, 2300 Eglinton Ave W, Mississauga ON L5M 2V8; Tor'00; MSc; BSc; CCFP; Ac Staff, The Credit Valley Hospital; (905)813-3850; Fax. (905)813-3851.

ZARINEHBAF ASADI, Sanaz; Summeridge Health Centre, 26-8707 Dufferin St, Thornhill ON L4J 0A2; McM'10; CCFP; (905)764-0005

ZARINS, Eric D; Homewood Health Centre, 150 Delhi St, Guelph ON N1E 6K9; Tor'74; FRCPC; Psy. Staff, Homewood Health Centre; (519)824-1010; Fax. (519)767-3537.

ZARKADAS, Peter C; 214-145 15 St W, North Vancouver BC V7M 1R9; UBC'01; FRCSC; OrthSurg. Staff, Lions Gate Hospital; Langs: Greek; French; (604)980-5779

ZARKOVIC, Mirjana; Allan Blair Cancer Centre, 4101 Dewdney Ave, Regina SK S4T 7T1; Staff, Allan Blair Cancer Centre; (306)766-2213; Fax. (306)766-2688.

ZARNETT, Mark E R; The Sports Med Specialists, 5F-150 Eglinton Ave E, Toronto ON M4P 1E8; Tor'83; MSc; FRCSC; OrthSurg (Arthroscopic Surgery). Ac Staff Surg, Humber River Regional Hospital - Church Street Site; (416)636-9965; Fax. (416)636-9119.

ZARNKE, Kelly B; University of Calgary, 1470-3330 Hospital Dr NW, Calgary AB T2N 4N1; Wes'86; MSc(Epidem&Biostat); FRCPC; IntMed (Cardiovascular Disease). Staff, Foothills Medical Centre; Teach Staff, University of Calgary; (403)220-5926; Fax. (403)210-8723.

ZAROUKIAN, Sevag; Pontiac Health Centre, 200 rue Argue, Shawville QC J0X 2Y0; Mon'00; CCFP; Staff, Pontiac Hospital Centre; (819)647-2211; Fax. (819)647-2409.

ZAROWSKY, Christina H A; Clinique Med de Plantagenet, PO Box 305, Plantagenet ON K0B 1L0; McM'85; Staff, Camp Can Aqua; Langs: Ukrainian; French; (613)673-4318; c.zarowsky@nursinghomeratings.ca.

ZARRELLI, Marianna; Hôpital Ste-Justine, 3175 ch Cote-Sainte-Catherine, Montreal QC H3T 1C5; Mon'93; FRCPC; Psy (Pediatric Psychiatry). Staff PedPsy, Hôpital Ste-Justine; Universite de Montreal; Langs: Italian; English; (514)345-4931 x5683; Fax. (514)345-2187.

ZARRUK, Alexandro R L; Centre Med Pierrefonds, 12774 boul Gouin O, Roxboro QC H8Z 1W5; University of Saint Eustatius (Other Foreign)'07; FRCPC; IntMed. (514)684-8460

ZARRUK, Ricardo; Centre Med Pierrefonds, 12774 boul Gouin O, Pierrefonds QC H8Z 1W5; Madrid (Spain)'70; MSc; PhD; ac Staff, Lakeshore General Hospital - Pointe Claire; Langs: Spanish; French; Italian; Portuguese; Arabic; (514)684-8460; Fax. (514)683-0588; zarruk@videotron.ca.

ZARYCHANSKI, Ryan L; CancerCare Manitoba, ON2051-675 McDermot Ave, Winnipeg MB R3E 0V9; Ott'00; FRCPC; IntMed; Critical Care Medicine; Hem. Staff, CancerCare Manitoba; (204)787-2197

ZARZOUR, Zane D S; Rebalance MD, 104-3551 Blanshard St, Victoria BC V8Z 0B9; Wes'94; FRCSC; OrthSurg (Shoulder & Elbow). (250)381-5424; Fax. (250)385-8150.

ZASOWSKI, John J; Thistlewood Prof Centre, 210-8077 Islington Ave, Woodbridge ON L4L 7X7; Tor'85; CCFP; Staff, William Osler Health System - Etobicoke General Hospital; Langs: Polish; (905)264-2888; Fax. (905)264-2549; dr.zasowski@hotmail.com.

ZASSOKO, Roman; Queensway Med Associates, 100-101 Queensway W, Mississauga ON L5B 2P7; Wes'09; CCFP; (905)949-0801; Fax. (905)949-0803.

ZATELNY, Diane L; 206-128 Penetang St, Barrie ON L4M 1V6; Ott'82; IntMed (Endocrinology). Staff Endocrin & IntMed, Royal Victoria Regional Health Centre; (705)734-3888

ZATZMAN, Ian R; Maple Med Centre, 208-955 Major Mackenzie W, Vaughan ON L6A 4P9; Dal'83; Ac Staff, Mackenzie Richmond Hill Hospital; (289)553-7711; Fax. (289)553-7722; medz@rogers.com.

ZATZMAN, Raymond L; All Health Med Centre, 7-180 Steeles Ave W, Thornhill ON L4J 2L1; Dal'84; Ac Staff, North York General Hospital - Branson Division; Court Staff, Mackenzie Richmond Hill Hospital; (905)886-0116; Fax. (905)597-6774.

ZAUGG, Michael; Clinical Sciences Bldg, 8 120-152 University Campus NW, Edmonton AB T6G 2G3; Zurich (Switzerland)'89; Staff/Prof Anes, University of Alberta Hospital; (780)407-3854; Fax. (780)407-3200; michael.zaugg@ualberta.ca.

ZAVAGNIN, Nicole J; Westfort Village Walk-In Clini, 129 Frederica St W, Thunder Bay ON P7E 3V8; NOSM'09; CCFP; Staff, Thunder Bay Regional Health Sciences Centre; Staff, Northern Ontario School of Medicine; (807)473-5410; Fax. (807)285-0266.

ZAVALETA JUSTINIANO, Jannet; CSSS Lac Temiscamingue, 22 rue Notre-Dame N, Ville-Marie QC J9V 1W8; Nacional de Trujillo (Other Foreign)'93; (819)629-2420

ZAVALKOFF, Samara; MUHC-Montreal Children's Hosp, 2300 rue Tupper, Montreal QC H3H 1P3; McG'03; MDCM; FRCPC; Peds; Critical Care Medicine. Staff, McGill University Health Centre - Montreal Children's Hospital; (514)412-4400 x22696

ZAVERY, Oanali T; Lindsay Prof Bldg, 7-65 Angeline St N, Lindsay ON K9V 5N7; Ott'76; ABIM; FRCPC; IntMed (Cardiology). Staff, Ross Memorial Hospital; Langs: Gujarati; (705)328-0461; Fax. (705)328-0462.

ZAVIEH, Kevin; The Moncton Hosp, 135 MacBeath Ave, Moncton NB E1C 6Z8; Ross University (USA)'98; Staff, The Moncton Hospital; (506)857-5111

ZAVODNI, Anna E H; University of Alberta Hosp, 2A2 41WCM-8440 112 St NW, Edmonton AB T6G 2B7; Alb'05; FRCPC; DiagRad. Staff, University of Alberta Hospital; (780)407-8822

ZAVODNI, Louis S; PO Box 30016 Upper James PO, Hamilton ON L9B 0E4; Wes'69; DAB; FAAFP; CCFP; FCFP; Ac Staff, St Joseph's Healthcare - Charlton Campus; Ac Staff, Hamilton Health Sciences Centre - McMaster University Medical Centre; Ac Staff, Hamilton Health Sciences Centre - St Peter's Hospital; Langs: Hungarian; French.

ZAW-TUN, Ni Ni S; 221-339 Aspen Glen Landing SW, Calgary AB T3H 0N6; Alb'78; FRCPC; IntMed. (403)263-7997; Fax. (403)263-7996.

ZAWADA, Annabella; North Shore Family Health Team, PO Box 819 20B Cartier Rd, Terrace Bay ON P0T 2W0; Tor'03; CCFP; Staff, The McCausland Hospital; Coroner, Province of Ontario; Physician, Terrace Bay Medical Group; Langs: Polish; (807)825-3235; Fax. (807)825-3239; dr.bella@gmail.com.

ZAWADOWSKI, Andrew G A; Core Cardiology Services, 215-1060 Speers Rd, Oakville ON L6L 2X4; McM'78; FACC; FESC; FAHA; FRCPC; IntMed (Cardiology). Ac Staff, Halton Healthcare Services Corporation - Oakville Site; Clinical Asst Prof Cardiol, McMaster University; Langs: French; Polish; (905)842-6084; Fax. (905)842-4579.

ZAWADOWSKI, Michael A J; 21st Medical Clinic, 502-402 21st St E, Saskatoon SK S7K 0C3; Jagiellonian University (Poland)'08; IntMed (Cardiology). (306)934-3300; Fax. (306)956-3577.

ZAWAHIR, Mohamed M; Stratford Gen Hosp, 46 General Hospital Dr, Stratford ON N5A 2Y6; Aga Khan University (Other Foreign)'94; Staff, Stratford General Hospital - Huron Perth Healthcare Alliance; Langs: Tamil; Urdu; (519)271-8120

ZAWARYNSKI, Diane M; Tillsonburg Med Centre, 200 Broadway St, Tillsonburg ON N4G 5A7; Wes'98; CCFP; FCFP; (519)842-4231; Fax. (519)842-3793.

ZAYANI, Abdulati; Lessard Med Clinic, 6633 177 St NW, Edmonton AB T5T 4K3; (780)757-7999

ZAYANI, Adeb S M; West End Professional Bldg, M7-9509 156 ST NW, Edmonton AB T5P 4J5; (780)756-3300; Fax. (780)756-3301.

ZAYED, Ekram; Life Labs Med Lab Services, 3201-4464 Markham St, Victoria BC V8Z 7X8; Alexandria (Egypt)'75; MB ChB; FRCPC; HemPath. Consultant Hempath, Life Labs Medical Laboratory Services; Langs: Arabic; (250)881-3111 x2153

ZAYED, Saleh; Appletree Med Group, 2016 Ogilvie Rd, Gloucester ON K1J 7N9; Jordan (Jordan)'82; MB BS; CCFP; Staff, Montfort Hospital; Staff, Canadian Forces Health Services Centre; (613)749-5549; Fax. (613)749-3105.

ZAYED, Tareg; 12620A 132 Ave NW, Edmonton AB T5L 3P9; (Other Foreign)'04; (780)990-1820; Fax. (780)488-0988.

ZAYID, Dina P; Scarborough Prof Centre, 308-1371 Neilson Rd, Scarborough ON M1B 4Z8; Dal'89; Court Staff, Rouge Valley Health System - Centenary Health Centre Site; (416)283-7701; Fax. (416)283-7108.

ZAYID, Omar I; Argus Med Centre, 300-581 Argus Rd, Oakville ON L6J 3J4; Dal'97; BSc; (905)338-9900; Fax. (905)338-9904.

ZAYONC, David A; 101-15451 Russell Ave, White Rock BC V4B 2R5; UBC'09; CCFP; (604)531-5595; Fax. (604)531-9818.

ZAYOUNA, Maher N; Windsor Reg Hosp-Metropolitan, 1995 Lens Ave, Windsor ON N8W 1L9; American University of the Caribbean (St Maarten)'03; Staff, Windsor Regional Hospital - Metropolitan Site; Staff, Health Trush Medical Centre; Langs: Arabic; (519)254-5577

ZAZA, Khaled O A; Southeastern Cancer Ctre, 25 King St W, Kingston ON K7L 5P9; Cairo (Egypt)'89; FRCPC; RadOncol. Staff RadOncol, Kingston General Hospital; (613)544-2631 x4506

ZAZULA, Marian; 3301 Cawthra Rd, Mississauga ON L5A 2X4; Wes'67; Ac Staff, St Joseph's Health Centre; Langs: Ukrainian; Polish; (905)276-7754; Fax. (905)276-8375.

ZAZULAK, Joyce; McMaster Family Practice, A-690 Main St W, Hamilton ON L8S 1A4; McM'94; BSc; MSc; CCFP; FCFP; Staff, Hamilton Health Sciences Centre - Hamilton General Hospital; Staff, St Joseph's Healthcare - Charlton Campus; Assoc Prof Family Med, McMaster University; (905)521-5016; Fax. (905)521-5010; zazulj@mcmaster.ca.

ZBIERANOWSKI, Ingrid J; Sunnybrook Hlth Sciences Ctre, E416-2075 Bayview Ave, Toronto ON M4N 3M5; Tor'83; FRCPC; AnatPath. Staff, Sunnybrook Health Sciences Centre; Assoc Prof Path, University of Toronto; (416)480-6100 x3579; Fax. (416)480-4271.

ZBITNEW, Geoff L; Health Sciences Centre, 300 Prince Philip Dr, St. John's NL A1B 3V6; Alb'00; FRCPC; Anes. Staff, Health Sciences Centre; (709)777-6300

ZBUK, Kevin M; Juravinski Cancer Centre, 699 Concession St, Hamilton ON L8V 5C2; Alb'97; FRCPC; IntMed; MedOncol. Staff, The Juravinski Cancer Centre; (905)387-9495; Fax. (905)575-6326.

ZBUK, Randall S; Toronto East Gen Hosp Inc, 825 Coxwell Ave, Toronto ON M4C 3E7; Alb'06; FRCPC; Psy. Staff, Toronto East General Hospital Inc; (416)461-8272

ZEBROWSKA, Grazyna A; Niagara H System-St Catharines, PO Box 3018 Stn Main, St Catharines ON L2R 7C6; Warsaw (Poland)'78; DABPath; FRCPC; AnatPath (General Pathology). Staff, Niagara Health System - St Catharines General Site; Langs: Polish; (905)684-7271; Fax. (905)984-5578.

ZEBROWSKI, Andrzej; Niagara H System-St Catharines, PO Box 3018 Stn Main, St Catharines ON L2R 7C6; Warsaw (Poland)'78; FRCPC; Psy. Staff, Niagara Health System - St Catharines General Site; Langs: Polish; (905)684-7271; Fax. (905)704-4769.

ZED, Joanna L; Dalhousie Family Medicine, 0265-6960 Mumford Rd, Halifax NS B3L 4P1; Dal'88; CCFP; Court Staff, IWK Health Centre; (902)473-4700; Fax. (902)473-8548; joanna.zed@dal.ca.

ZEDEL, Albert H; Saanich Plaza Med Clinic, 3544 Blanshard St, Victoria BC V8X 1W3; Alb'68; Ac Staff, Royal Jubilee Hospital; Assoc Staff, Victoria General Hospital; (250)475-1101; Fax. (250)475-1157.

ZEDKOVA, Lenka; Alberta Hospital Edmonton, PO Box 307 17480 Fort Rd, Edmonton AB T5J 2J7; Prague (Czech Republic)'96; FRCPC; Psy. Staff, Alberta Hospital Edmonton; (780)342-5539

ZEE, Allen; 908 Royal York Rd, Etobicoke ON M8Y 2V7; Qns'85; Staff, Trillium Health Centre - West Toronto; Langs: Cantonese; (416)239-8896; Fax. (416)239-6507.

ZEGLINSKI, Cathryn M; Northlands Med Clinic, 101-4359 Main St, Whistler BC V0N 1B4; Man'90; Dip SportMed; CCFP; Langs: Bilingual(English/French); (604)932-8362; Fax. (604)932-8363.

ZEGLINSKI, Joie A; Ottawa Anxiety & Trauma Clinic, 202-2277 Riverside Dr, Ottawa ON K1H 7X6; Man'89; Psy (Psychotherapy). Consultant, The Ottawa Hospital - General Campus; Staff Psy, Ottawa Anxiety & Trauma Clinic; Langs: English; French; (613)737-1194; Fax. (613)737-5884.

ZEHR, Patricia A; The Group Health Ctre, 240 McNabb St, Sault Ste. Marie ON P6B 1Y5; McM'87; FRCSC; ObstGyn. (705)759-1234; Fax. (705)759-7466.

ZEIDAN SHWIRI, Tawfiq; The Moncton Hosp, 135 MacBeath Ave, Moncton NB E1C 6Z8; Technion-Israel Institute of Technology (Israel)'00; Staff, The Moncton Hospital; (506)857-5111

ZEIFMAN, Claude; PO Box 5585 Stn Main, Squamish BC V8B 0C2; Athens (Greece)'87.

ZEILER, Frederick; First Street Clinic, PO Box 1360, Beausejour MB R0E 0C0; Man'81; (204)268-3363; Fax. (204)268-2218.

ZEILIG, Lauren V; Keele Ingram Med Centre, 307-2221 Keele St, North York ON M6M 3Z5; Tor'62; Ac Staff, Humber River Regional Hospital - Church Street Site; Ac Staff, Humber River Regional Hospital - Keele Street Site; Langs: Italian; French; (416)785-8889; Fax. (416)785-7844.

ZEINDLER, Peter R; Defence Research Dev Canada, 1133 Sheppard Ave W, North York ON M3K 2B3; Cal'84; BA; MSc; CCBOM; CCFP; FCFP; (416)635-2014

ZEINEDDIN, Maryam; Ambleside Med Centre, 250 16th St, West Vancouver BC V7V 3R5; UBC'03; BSc(Hons); CCFP; Staff, Lions Gate Hospital; Clin Instructor Family Practice Residency, University of British Columbia; Langs: Farsi; Swedish; Spanish; (604)926-1510; Fax. (604)926-6933.

ZEIT, Harry J; Medical Clinic Person-Ctred Ps, 403-265 Yorkland Blvd, North York ON M2J 1S5; Tor'82; DABEM; Staff, The Medical Clinic for Person-Centred Psychotherapy; (416)229-2399 x275; Fax. (416)229-9771; harryzeit@sympatico.ca.

ZEITOUNI, Anthony G; MUHC-Royal Victoria Hosp, E4 41-687 av des Pins O, Montreal QC H3A 1A1; Sher'88; FRCSC; Otol (Head & Neck Surgery). Staff, McGill University Health Centre - Royal Victoria Hospital; (514)842-1231 x34974; Fax. (514)843-1529.

ZEKULIN, Anthony G; Brameast Family Physicians, 38-2130 North Park Dr, Brampton ON L6S 0C9; McG'70; Ac Staff, William Osler Health System - Brampton Civic Hospital; Med Consultant, RBC Travel Insurance Company; Langs: Czech; French; (905)792-2211; Fax. (905)792-2901.

ZELAZO, Jay A; Canada Diagnostic Centres, 1-6020 1A St SW, Calgary AB T2H 0G3; Alb'98; FRCPC; DiagRad. Physician, Canada Diagnostic Centres; (403)253-4666; Fax. (403)253-4669; jzelazo@canadadiagnostics.ca.

ZELCER, Irving; 110-120 Overbrook Place, North York ON M3H 4P8; Tor'68; BSc(Med); CCFP; FCFP; Ac Staff, North York General Hospital - Branson Division; Asst Prof, McMaster University; Asst Prof Family & Commun Med, University of Toronto; Langs: Yiddish; (416)633-4984; Fax. (416)633-4446; irving.zelcer@utoronto.ca.

ZELCER, Shayna M; Westminster Tower, PO Boc 5010 B1 116-800 Commissioners Rd W, London ON N6K 1C2; Tor'96; FRCPC; Peds. (519)685-8494; Fax. (519)685-8384.

ZELDIN, Robert A; Dr Robert A Zeldin Prof Corp, 401K-650 Sammon Ave, East York ON M4C 5M5; Tor'77; FACS; FRCSC; GenSurg (Esophageal Surgery); ThorSurg. Staff Cons, Sunnybrook Health Sciences Centre; Ac Staff, Toronto East General Hospital Inc; Asst Prof Surg, University of Toronto; (416)461-0109; Fax. (416)469-7714; rzeld@tegh.on.ca.

ZELDIN, Susan G; 718-123 Edward St, Toronto ON M5G 1E2; Tor'88; CCFP; FCFP; (416)971-7730; Fax. (416)408-2802.

ZELIGER, Agnes M; 4484 rue Sherbrooke O, Westmount QC H3Z 1E6; Heidelberg (Germany)'59; FRCPC; Peds. Adj Peds, McGill University Health Centre - Montreal Children's Hospital; adj Prof, McGill University; Langs: Hungarian; German; French; (514)933-4490; Fax. (514)933-6934.

ZELIN, Jennifer M; Sherwood Med Centre, 15 Brackley Pt Rd, Charlottetown PE C1A 5P8; Tor'99; CCFP; Ad Staff Privil, Queen Elizabeth Hospital; (902)628-3800; Fax. (902)628-3830; j.zelin@utoronto.ca.

ZELINA, Peter I; 29 Centre St W, Richmond Hill ON L4C 3P3; Padua (Italy)'79; BSc; FRCPC; Psy (Psycho Geriatrics). Chief Psy/Clin Dir Mental Health, Mackenzie Richmond Hill Hospital; Langs: Czech; Italian; Slovak; (905)883-9054; Fax. (905)883-9057.

ZELLER, Jeanne T; St Joseph's Health Centre, 30 The Queensway, Toronto ON M6R 1B5; Rene Descartes Universite (France)'91; Staff Derm, St Joseph's Health Centre; (416)530-6043; Fax. (416)530-6472.

ZELLER, Michelle P; London HSC-Victoria Hosp, PO Box 5010 Stn B A2 401-800 Commissioners Rd E, London ON N6A 5W9; Tor'07; FRCPC; IntMed; Hem. Staff, London Health Sciences Centre - Victoria Campus; (519)685-8500

ZELLER, Reinhard D; The Hosp for Sick Children, S107-555 University Ave, Toronto ON M5G 1X8; Paris (France)'90; FRCSC; OrthSurg (Pediatric Orthopedics). Staff, The Hospital For Sick Children; Langs: German; French; (416)813-6265; Fax. (416)813-6414; sharon.younker@sickkids.ca.

ZELMAN, Mitchell I; Queen Elizabeth Hosp, PO Box 6600 Stn Central 60 Riverside Dr, Charlottetown PE C1A 8T5; McG'86; FRCPC; Peds (Respirology). Staff, Queen Elizabeth Hospital; Med Dir, PA Gill Asthma Education Centre; Chief Deputy Health Officer, Province Of Prince Edward Isand; Langs: Bilingual(French/English); (902)894-2440; Fax. (902)894-2477; mitch@pei.aibn.com.

ZELOVITZKY, Jerahmie L; I C572-585 University Ave, Toronto ON M5G 2N4; Cape Town (South Africa)'63; DiagRad. Staff, Toronto General Hospital - UHN; (416)340-4800

ZELT, David T; Kingston Gen Hosp, V3-76 Stuart St, Kingston ON K7L 2V7; Qns'84; FRCSC; GenSurg; VascSurg. Staff, Kingston General Hospital; Asst Prof, Queen's University; (613)548-2573; Fax. (613)548-6153.

ZELT, Ronald G; 124-100 ch Rockland, Mont-Royal QC H3P 2V9; McG'84; MScEd; FRCSC; PlasSurg. Staff, McGill University Health Centre - Montreal General Campus; Asst Prof Surg, McGill University; (514)933-3449; Fax. (514)564-1010; info@rgzelt.com.

ZEMAN, George J; North Bay Reg Health Centre, 50 College Dr, North Bay ON P1B 0A4; Purkyne (Czech Republic)'58; FACOG; FRCSC; ObstGyn. Head Dept of ObstGyn, North Bay Regional Health Centre - Regional Mental Health; Langs: Czech; German; (705)474-8600 x4036; Fax. (705)495-8454.

ZEMAN, Marilyn V; Hys Med Centre, 310-11010 101 St NW, Edmonton AB T5H 4B9; Cal'02; MSc; FRCPC; IntMed (Hepatology); Gastroent. Staff Gastroent, Royal Alexandra Hospital; Langs: French; (780)421-1029; Fax. (780)425-5533.

ZEMAN, Peter R; Oak Ridges Med Centre, 303-13291 Yonge St, Richmond Hill ON L4E 4L6; Qns'01; FRCPC; IntMed; Cardiol. Staff, Southlake Regional Health Centre; (905)751-2941; Fax. (905)751-0107.

ZEMAN, Robert; Rosedale Med Centre, 306-600 Sherbourne St, Toronto ON M4X 1W4; Komensky (Slovakia)'59; AB; ABIM; FACP; FRCPC; IntMed (Bone Densitometry); Endocrin&Metab; NuclearMed. Staff Endocrin, St Michael's Hospital; Asst Prof, University of Toronto; Langs: Czech; Slovak; Polish; (416)925-1224; robert.zeman@sympatico.ca.

ZEMANS, Marcia S; Child Youth & Family Program, 80 Workman Way, Toronto ON M6J 1H4; Tor'96; FRCPC; Psy. Staff Child Youth & Family Prog, Centre for Addiction & Mental Health (CAMH) - College Street Site; Staff, Centre for Addiction & Mental Health (CAMH) - Queen Site; Staff, Queen West Community Health Centre; Staff, Child Youth & Family Program (CAMH); (416)535-8501

ZEMEK, Roger L; Children's Hosp of Eastern Ont, 401 Smyth Rd, Ottawa ON K1H 8L1; Bogota (Colombia)'99; FRCPC; Peds; PedEmergMed. Staff, Children's Hospital of Eastern Ontario (CHEO); Langs: Spanish; (613)737-2280

ZEMERLI, Fatima Z; Health Park, 308-45 Weatherbee Rd, Mira Road NS B1M 0A1; University of Mentouri Constantine (Algeria)'03; CCFP; (902)567-0660; Fax. (902)270-3236.

ZENER, Shery H K; 1024-790 Bay St PO Box 49, Toronto ON M5G 1N8; Tor'73; BSc; FRCPC; Psy (Geriatric Psychiatry). Staff/Teach Staff, Baycrest Centre for Geriatric Care; Court Staff, North York General Hospital; Lecturer/Staff Psychiatric Clinic, University of Toronto; Langs: Yiddish; (416)925-9982; Fax. (905)475-4082.

ZENG, Janice J; The Credit Valley Hosp, 2200 Eglinton Ave W, Mississauga ON L5M 2N1; McM'98; FRCPC; GenPath. Staff Lab Med, The Credit Valley Hospital; Langs: Mandarin; (905)813-2696; jzeng@cvh.on.ca.

ZENG, Wanzhen; The Ottawa Hosp-Ciivic Campus, 1053 Carling Ave, Ottawa ON K1Y 4E9; Cal'98; FRCPC; NuclearMed. Staff, University of Ottawa Heart Institute; Staff, The Ottawa Hospital - Civic Campus; Langs: Chinese; (613)761-4842; Fax. (613)761-4041.

ZENG, Xing; MUHC-Royal Victoria Hosp, 687 av des Pins O, Montreal QC H3A 1A1; McG'06; MDCM; FRCSC; ObstGyn. Staff, McGill University Health Centre - Royal Victoria Hospital; (514)934-1934

ZENI, Deborah R; Georgetown Med Associates, 199 Princess Anne Dr, Georgetown ON L7G 0E3; Tor'79; CCFP; Staff, Halton Healthcare Services Corporation - Georgetown Hospital; (905)873-3013; Fax. (905)873-0800.

ZENI, Paul J; Georgetown Med Associates, 199 Princess Anne Dr, Georgetown ON L7G 2B8; Tor'79; Ac Staff, Halton Healthcare Services Corporation - Georgetown Hospital; Langs: Italian; Spanish; French; (905)873-3013; Fax. (905)873-0800.

ZENTNER, Alissa S; Continuum Med Care Ltd, 201-520 17th St, West Vancouver BC V7V 3S8; McM'97; BSc; ABIM; FRCPC; IntMed (Cardiology). Staff, Chinook Regional Hospital; Dir IntMed, Continuum Medical Care Clinic; (604)913-8183; Fax. (604)913-8814; zentner@gmail.com.

ZEPEDA GOMEZ, Sergio; Ziedler Ledcor Centre, 120A-130 University Campus NW, Edmonton AB T6G 2X8; Universidad La Salle Escuela (Other Foreign)'96; (780)248-1259; Fax. (780)492-9865.

ZEPIC, Ines; High Park Health Centre, 507-2333 Dundas St W, Toronto ON M6R 3A6; Tor'87; Langs: Bilingual(English/French); (416)766-2718; Fax. (416)766-0196.

ZERAJIC, Sinisa; GAMA Integrated Med Centre, PO Box 2060, Warman SK S0K 4S0; Sask'08; CCFP; (306)382-5554; Fax. (306)382-5567.

ZEREY, Caroline M; 25 Cumberland St, Cornwall ON K6J 4G8; Mon'05; CCFP; Staff, Cornwall Community Hospital; Langs: Bilingual(English/French); (613)938-2552; Fax. (613)938-2559.

ZERGUINI, Amina A; Clinique Med Belanger, 300-3871 rue Belanger, Montreal QC H1X 3M7; Constantine (Turkey)'81; (514)722-1166 x1; Fax. (514)722-6022.

ZERHOUNI ABDOUH, Siham; Canadian Blood Services, 67 College St, Toronto ON M5G 2M1; McG'09; (416)340-4800

ZETARUK, Merrilee N; Legacy Sport Med Clinic, 14-160 Meadowood Dr, Winnipeg MB R2M 5L6; Man'91; FRCPC; Peds. Staff, Health Sciences Centre; (204)787-2496

ZETLER, Peter J; Royal Columbian Hosp, 330 Columbia St E, New Westminster BC V3L 3W7; Cape Town (South Africa)'83; MB ChB; FRCPC; GenPath. Staff, Royal Columbian Hospital; (604)520-4796

ZETTEL, Janet M T; Frederick Street Mall, 20B-385 Frederick St, Kitchener ON N2H 2P2; McM'92; CCFP; FCFP; (519)747-1340; Fax. (519)747-1560.

ZETTEL, Lenore A; West Lincoln Mem Hosp, D2-169 Main St E, Grimsby ON L3M 1P3; McM'95; BSc; MSc; FRCSC; GenSurg (Breasts). Staff, West Lincoln Memorial Hospital; (905)309-5335; Fax. (905)309-6996.

ZETTLE, Randy M; Springdale Complete Med Centre, 15-630 Peter Robertson Blvd, Brampton ON L6R 1T4; Tor'83; BL; FCFP; CCFP; CCFP(E.M.); FCFP; (905)793-8868; Fax. (905)793-8957.

ZETTLER, Michael L; Halton Healthcare Services, 1 Princess Anne Dr, Georgetown ON L7G 2B8; Wes'10; CCFP; Staff, Halton Healthcare Services Corporation - Georgetown Hospital; (905)873-0111

ZEVALLOS, Gonzalo F; Commercial Street Med Centre, 103-311 Commercial St, Milton ON L9T 3Z9; (Costa Rica)'84; Court Staff, Halton Healthcare Services Corporation - Milton District Hospital; Langs: Spanish; (905)876-3881; Fax. (905)876-0794.

ZEVIN, Boris; Sunnybrook Health Science Ctre, 2075 Bayview Ave, Toronto ON M4N 3M5; Tor'08; Staff, Sunnybrook Health Sciences Centre; (416)480-6100; Fax. (416)480-6033.

ZEYL, Thomas; 4413 Ontario St, Beamsville ON L0R 1B5; McM'78; BSc(Hon); CCFP; FCFP; Ac Staff, West Lincoln Memorial Hospital; Med Dir, Bethesda Home for the Mentally Retarded; Langs: Dutch; (905)563-7600; Fax. (905)563-4404.

ZEZNIK, Laura A; Nicola Med Dental Bldg, 303-321 Nicola St, Kamloops BC V2C 6G6; UBC'97; FRCSC; OrthSurg. (250)377-8332; Fax. (250)374-9232.

ZHANG, Chi; Associated Med Specialist, 1555 Second Ave, Trail BC V1R 1M3; Shanghai (China)'92; FRCPC; IntMed; Nephrol. Staff, Kootenay Boundary Regional Hospital; Langs: Chinese; (250)368-3301; Fax. (250)368-5053.

ZHANG, Dajiang; Cross Culture Program Hlth Ctr, 715 12th Ave W, Vancouver BC V5Z 1M9; Bethune (China)'94; FRCPC; Psy. Staff, Vancouver General Hospital - Centennial Pavillion; Staff, Midtown Mental Health Team; Staff, Strathcona Mental Health Team; Langs: Mandarin; (604)875-4115

ZHANG, Irene; St Joseph's Healthcare, 50 Charlton St E, Hamilton ON L8N 4A6; McM'05; FRCSC; Otol. Staff, St Joseph's Healthcare - Charlton Campus; Langs: Mandarin; (905)522-1155

ZHANG, Kenny J; Meadowvale Prof Centre, 102-6855 Meadowvale Town Ctre, Mississauga ON L5N 2Y1; Qns'95; CCFP; Assoc Staff, The Credit Valley Hospital; Langs: Cantonese; Mandarin; Hakka; (905)567-9911; Fax. (905)567-9011; kennyzhang@yahoo.com.

ZHANG, Lianfeng C; Edmundston Reg Hosp, 275 Hebert Blvd, Edmundston NB E3V 4E4; Harbin Medical University (China)'99; Staff, Hôpital regional d'Edmundston; (506)739-2200

ZHANG, Lu; Queen Elizabeth II HSC, 4875-1796 Summer St, Halifax NS B3H 3A7; Peking Univ Health Science Center (China)'87; FRCSC; OrthSurg. Staff, Queen Elizabeth II Health Sciences Centre - Halifax Infirmary Site; (902)473-4035; Fax. (902)473-4490.

ZHANG, Mona M; North Edmonton Health Centre, 14007 50 St NW, Edmonton AB T5A 5E4; Alb'04; FRCPC; Peds. (780)342-4168; Fax. (780)342-4196.

ZHANG, Rong; Victoria Med Bldg, 307-1669 Victoria St, Prince George BC V2L 2L5; (Other Foreign)'09; CCFP; (250)562-8308

ZHANG, Rui; Seymour Med Clinic, 1530 7th Ave W, Vancouver BC V6J 1S3; Shandong (China)'91; CCFP; Langs: Mandarin; (604)739-5615; Fax. (604)738-2132.

ZHANG, Seamus Q; Empire Med Centre, 1-204 Freshwater Rd, St. John's NL A1C 2P5; Wes'97; LMCC.

ZHANG, Siui-Mei; Whitehorse Med Services, 406 Lambert St, Whitehorse YT Y1A 1Z7; Norman Bethune University (China)'86; Staff, Whitehorse General Hospital; Physician, Whitehorse Medical Services Ltd; Staff, Traditional Chinese Medicine; Staff, East & West Health Centre Ltd; Langs: Mandarin; (867)393-6632; Fax. (867)393-6601.

ZHANG, Ting; St Michael's Hosp, 30 Bond St, Toronto ON M5B 1W8; McG'09; Staff Cardiac Surg, St Michael's Hospital; (416)864-5366

ZHANG, Xiaosi; Clinique Metro-Medic, 1538 rue Sherbooke O, Montreal QC H3G 1L5; Mon'07; CCFP; (514)932-2122

ZHANG, Xinyun; Royal Alexandra Hosp, 10240 Kingsway NW, Edmonton AB T5H 3V9; Alb'09; Staff, Royal Alexandra Hospital; (780)735-4442

ZHANG, Y Jackie; 8-9019 Bayview Ave, Richmond Hill ON L4B 3M6; Sun Yat Sen (China)'92; CCFP; Staff Campus Health Centre, Durham College; Langs: Cantonese; Mandarin; (905)889-0062; Fax. (905)889-9685.

ZHANG, Y H Connie; 120-8120 Cook Rd, Richmond BC V6Y 1T9; Shanghai (China)'88; CCFP; Langs: Cantonese; Mandarin; (604)278-5191

ZHANG, Ying; Cachet Family Physicians, 2-9255 Woodbine Ave, Markham ON L6C 1Y9; Wes'04; CCFP; (905)887-2222; Fax. (905)887-3655.

ZHANG, Zhi Ping; CSSS de Laval, 1755 boul Rene-Laennec, Laval QC H7M 3L9; Shen Yang Medical College (China)'85; FRCPC; AnatPath. Staff, Hopital de la Cite de la santé; (450)668-1010

ZHAO, Charles; The Ottawa Hosp-Civic Campus, 1053 Carling Ave, Ottawa ON K1Y 4E9; Ott'01; CCFP; CCFP(E.M.); Staff, Hôtel-Dieu Grace Hospital; Staff Emerg, The Ottawa Hospital - Civic Campus; (519)973-4411

ZHAO, Hong Yun; Rockyview Gen Hosp, 63-7007 14 St SW, Calgary AB T2V 1P9; (China)'89; Staff, Rockyview General Hospital; (403)943-3563

ZHAO, Xiu Chang; Baycrest Centre for Geriatric, 3560 Bathurst St, Toronto ON M6A 2E1; McM'10; CCFP; Staff, Baycrest Centre for Geriatric Care; (416)785-2500

ZHAO, Ying Ying; London HSC-Victoria Campus, PO Box 5010 Stn B 800 Commissioners Rd E, London ON N6A 5W9; Wes'08; FRCPC; IntMed. Staff, London Health Sciences Centre - Victoria Campus; (519)667-6767; Fax. (519)685-8406.

ZHENG, Stanley M; North Scarborough Prof Centre, 304-3420 Finch Ave E, Scarborough ON M1W 2R6; Tor'94; BSc; PhD; CCFP; Staff, The Scarborough Hospital - Birchmount Campus; Dir Cancer & Palliative Care Services, Yee Hong Centre For Geriatric Care; Teacher, University of Toronto; Aj Prof, McMaster University; Langs: Cantonese; Mandarin; (416)497-8818; Fax. (416)497-8848; stanley.zheng@utoronto.ca.

ZHENG, Xueyan; Dr Xue Yan Zheng Med Clinic, 120-8120 Cook Rd, Richmond BC V6Y 1T9; (China)'82; CCFP; Physician, Cambie Plaza Medical Clinic; Langs: Chinese; (604)270-9833; Fax. (604)270-8127.

ZHENG, Zuoyu; Niagara HS-St Catherines Gen, 142 Queenston St, St Catharines ON L2R 7C6; Hunan Medical University (China)'95; FRCPC; GenPath. Staff, Niagara Health System - St Catharines General Site; Langs: Chinese; (905)378-4647

ZHIVKOV, Alexander; Clinique Med de Fort-Coulonge, CP 520 543B rue Baume, Fort-Coulonge QC J0X 1V0; Sofia (Bulgaria)'66; assoc Staff, Pontiac Hospital Centre; Langs: Bulgarian; Russian; French; (819)683-2254; Fax. (819)683-2759; alezhi@renc.igs.net.

ZHONG, Toni; Univ Hlth Network-Toronto Gen, 8N 871EW-200 Elizabeth St, Toronto ON M5G 2C4; Wes'02; FRCSC; PlasSurg (Breast Reconstruction). Staff, Toronto General Hospital - UHN; Staff, Princess Margaret Hospital - University Health Network; Staff, Mount Sinai Hospital; Langs: Mandarin; (416)340-3858; Fax. (416)340-4403; toni.zhong@uhn.on.ca.

ZHOU, Chen Qian; BC Cancer Agency-Vancouver CC, 600 10th Ave W, Vancouver BC V5Z 4E6; (China)'82; FRCPC; AnatPath. Staff, BC Cancer Agency Vancouver Centre; Langs: Chinese; (604)877-6000 x2082

ZHOU, Youwen F; Skin Care Center, 835 10th Ave W, Vancouver BC V5Z 4E8; Tor'95; MSc; PhD; FRCPC; Derm (Laser Dermatology). Consultant, Vancouver General Hospital - Centennial Pavillion; Consultant, BC Cancer Agency Vancouver Centre; Member Medical Review Board, Workers' Comp Board of BC; Asst Prof, University of British Columbia; Langs: Mandarin; (604)875-4682; Fax. (604)873-9919; ywzhou@interchange.ubc.ca.

ZHU, Jiajia; Carefirst Family Health Team, 27-420 Hwy 7, Richmond Hill ON L4B 3K2; Tor'10; CCFP; (905)695-1133; Fax. (905)695-0826; jiajia.zhu@carefirstfht.com.

ZHU, Kang-Min; East Kootenay Reg Hosp, 13 24th Ave N, Cranbrook BC V1C 3H9; Qns'01; FRCPC; DiagRad. Staff, East Kootenay Regional Hospital; Langs: Mandarin; Shanghai; (250)489-6472; Fax. (250)426-5285.

ZHU, Nancy Y; Clinical Hematology Division, 14 112 CSB-11350 83 Ave, Edmonton AB T6G 2G3; Sask'04; FRCPC; IntMed (Myelodysplasia); Hem. Asst Prof, University of Alberta Hospital; (780)407-8450; Fax. (780)407-2680.

ZHUANG, Lihua; Carefirst Family Health Team, 27-420 Highway 7, Richmond Hill ON L4B 3K2; Nantong Medical College (China)'86; CCFP; (905)895-1133; Fax. (905)895-0826; lihua.zhuang@carefirstfht.com.

ZIA, Khalid R; 26-2 Thorncliffe Park Dr, East York ON M4H 1H2; Quaid-E-Azam (Pakistan)'91; MB BS; CCFP; Langs: Hindi; (416)467-7786; Fax. (416)467-9900.

ZIA, Mohammad I; Dr M Zia Medicine Prof Corp, 208-688 Coxwell Ave, Toronto ON M4C 3B7; Cal'02; FRCPC; IntMed; Cardiol. Staff, Sunnybrook Health Sciences Centre; Langs: Hindi; Punjabi; Urdu; (416)406-0101; Fax. (416)406-9951.

ZIA, Peter K Y; Mackenzie Richmond Hill Hosp, 10 Trench St, Richmond Hill ON L4C 4Z3; Tor'97; FRCPC; DiagRad;CCFP; Staff, Mackenzie Richmond Hill Hospital; (905)883-1212

ZIA, Shahzad; Hys Med Centre, 302-11010 101 St NW, Edmonton AB T5H 4B9; Karachi (Pakistan)'90; MB BS; FRCPC; IntMed. Staff, Royal Alexandra Hospital; (780)496-1390; Fax. (780)496-1387.

ZIADA, Mohammed M A; Souris Med Associates, PO Box 400 31 Crescent Ave, Souris MB R0K 2C0; (Other Foreign)'01; (204)333-7808

ZIADA, Zeinab H; Group Health Centre, 240 McNabb St, Sault Ste. Marie ON P6B 1Y5; Cairo (Egypt)'91; CCFP; Langs: Arabic; (705)759-1234

ZIAEI SABA, Shahnaz; Brandon Med Clinic, 620 Dennis St, Brandon MB R7A 5E7; (204)728-4440

ZIAI, Setareh; Univ of Ottawa Eye Institute, 501 Smyth Rd Box 370, Ottawa ON K1H 8L6; Ott'05; FRCSC; Ophth. Staff, University of Ottawa Eye Institute; Langs: Farsi; French; (613)737-8899; Fax. (613)739-6291; setareh@fishermansmarket.com.

ZIBDAWI, Labib A A; Stronach Reg Cancer Centre, 596 Davis Dr, Newmarket ON L3Y 2P9; Ain Shams (Egypt)'83; MB ChB; FRCPC; IntMed; MedOncol. Staff, Southlake Regional Health Centre; Staff, Stronach Regional Cancer Centre; Langs: Arabic; (905)895-4521 x6335; Fax. (905)952-2818.

ZIBDAWI, M Mohamad; University of Alberta Hosp, 3A6 078-8440 112 St NW, Edmonton AB T6G 2B7; Cal'93; FRCPC; IntMed; Critical Care Medicine. Staff Mazankowski Alberta Heart Institute, University of Alberta Hospital; Staff, Covenant Health - Grey Nuns Community Hospital; Staff, Alberta Heart Institute; (780)407-6326; Fax. (780)407-3482.

ZIBIN, Kerry E; Seymour Health Centre, 1530 7th Ave W, Vancouver BC V6J 1S2; UBC'02; CCFP; Staff, Foothills Medical Centre; (604)738-2151

ZICHERMAN, Viviane; SMBD Jewish Gen Hosp, 3755 ch Cote-Sainte-Catherine, Montreal QC H3T 1E2; McG'73; FRCPC; Psy (Hospital Consultation). Dir Consultation-Liason Psy, Sir Mortimer B Davis Jewish General; adj Prof, McGill University; (514)340-7902; Fax. (514)340-8126; lyoung@icfp.jgh.mcgill.ca.

ZIDEL, Brian S; Goreway Med Centre, 7330 Goreway Dr, Mississauga ON L4T 4J2; Tor'83; Staff, William Osler Health System - Etobicoke General Hospital; Langs: English; French; (905)677-4200; Fax. (905)677-0541.

ZIDES, Colin I; SelectMD, 125-589 South Pelham Rd, Welland ON L3C 3C7; Mem'91; Staff, Niagara Health System - Welland Hospital Site; Staff, Pelham Urgent Care; (905)788-1500; Fax. (905)788-1510.

ZIDULKA, Arnold; MUHC-Montreal Gen Hosp, D7 201-1650 av Cedar, Montreal QC H3G 1A4; McG'66; DABIM; AB; IntMed; Respir (P.Q.) (Intensive Care). ac Staff, McGill University Health Centre - Montreal General Campus; ac Staff, McGill University Health Centre - Montreal Chest Institute; ac Staff, McGill University Health Centre - Royal Victoria Hospital; assoc Prof, McGill University; (514)934-8014; Fax. (514)934-8226.

ZIDULKA, Joan R; St Mary's Hosp Centre, 3830 Av Lacombe, Montreal QC H3T 1M5; Bronx(NY) (USA)'70; MedOncol (P.Q.); Hem (Hematological Oncology). Staff Cancer Care Prog, St Mary's Hospital Centre; Staff, McGill University Health Centre - Royal Victoria Hospital; assoc Prof Med, McGill University; Langs: English; French; (514)345-3511; Fax. (514)734-2663.

ZIEBA, Iwona E; Hamilton HS-General Site, 3F-237 Barton St E, Hamilton ON L8L 2X2; McM'01; FRCPC; Anes. Staff, Hamilton Health Sciences Centre - Hamilton General Hospital; (905)527-0271

ZIEDENBERG, Robert W; Victoria Terrace Med Centre, 215-1448 Lawrence Ave E, North York ON M4A 2V6; Tor'70; CCFP; FCFP; Ac Staff, North York General Hospital; (416)757-7027; Fax. (416)757-0090.

ZIEFFLIE, Laura J; 101-4695 Hastings St, Burnaby BC V5C 2K6; McM'05; CCFP; Langs: Bilingual(English/French); (604)298-7201

ZIEGENHORN, Andreas A; CSSS de Saint-Jerome, 290 rue de Montigny, Saint-Jerome QC J7Z 5T3; Humboldt (Other Foreign)'98; Staff, Hôtel-Dieu de Saint-Jérôme; (450)431-8392

ZIEGLER, Cleve; H333 2-5790 ch Cote-des-Neiges, Montreal QC H3S 1Y9; Tor'88; FRCSC; ObstGyn (Gynecological Surgery). Staff, Sir Mortimer B Davis Jewish General; Asst Prof ObstGyn, McGill University; Langs: English; French; (514)340-8222 x3323; Fax. (514)340-7941.

ZIEGLER, Richard D; Deer Valley Med Clinic, 33-1221 Canyon Meadows Dr SE, Calgary AB T2J 6G2; Alb'69; (403)278-2164; Fax. (403)278-3192.

ZIELENIAK, Adam M; Clinique Med de la Cite, 150-175 rue de la Visitation, St-Charles-Brromee QC J6E 4N4; Katowice (Poland)'74; Staff, Centre de Sante Isle-Dieu Matagami; Langs: Polish; English; Spanish; (450)759-1444; Fax. (450)755-2036.

ZIELINSKI, Dawid K; Hop de Montreal pour Enfants, D 380-2300 rue Tupper, Montreal QC H3H 1P3; Man'03; FRCPC; Peds; Respir. Staff, McGill University Health Centre - Montreal Children's Hospital; (514)412-4444

ZIELINSKI, Janice-Marie; Millwoods Family Med Clinic, 104-2551 Hewes Way NW, Edmonton AB T6L 6W6; Alb'96; BSc; CCFP; FCFP; (780)462-2767; Fax. (780)463-7025.

ZIELINSKY, N Ariel; 601-1200 Bay St, Toronto ON M5R 2A5; Buenos Aires (Argentina)'73; FRCPC; Psy (Adult Psychiatry). Staff Pt-Time, St Michael's Hospital; University of Toronto; Langs: Spanish; (416)928-5913; Fax. (416)928-0292.

ZIELKE, Diane B; Red Lake Family Health Team, PO Box 311, Red Lake ON P0V 2M0; Tor'79; Ac Staff, Red Lake Margaret Cochenour Memorial Hospital; Asst Prof, Northern Ontario School of Medicine; (807)727-2617; Fax. (807)727-3122; dzielke@redlakehospital.ca.

ZIELONKA, Lucjan J; Surrey Mental Hlth & Addiction, 13401 108 Ave, Surrey BC V3T 5T3; Wroclaw (Poland)'84; FRCPC; Psy (Geriatric Psychiatry). Staff, Royal Columbian Hospital; Clin Instructor, University of British Columbia; Langs: Polish; Italian; Latin; (604)953-4900

ZIEROTH, Shelley R; St Boniface Gen Hosp, Y3016-409 Tache Ave, Winnipeg MB R2H 2A6; Man'98; FRCPC; IntMed (Heart Failure); Cardiol. Dir Heart Failure & Transplant Clinics, St Boniface General Hospital; (204)237-2744; Fax. (204)233-2157.

ZIESMANN, Manfred; 560-201 Portage Ave, Winnipeg MB R3B 3K6; Man'80; PlasSurg (Cosmetic Surgery). Staff Surg, Health Sciences Centre; Staff, St Boniface General Hospital; Staff, Victoria General Hospital; Assoc Prof, University of Manitoba; (204)942-5070; Fax. (204)942-5200; man3@mymts.net.

ZIFKIN, Benjamin G; 210-1255 Greene Ave, Westmount QC H3Z 2A4; McG'75; AB; FRCPC; Neur (Epilepsy); Electroenceph (P.Q.). Consultant Zeisure Clinic/Consultant EEG Lab, McGill University Health Centre - Montreal Neurological Hospital; Langs: English; French; (514)484-4036

ZIGANTE, Nina; 2 Shaffer Lane, Blackville NB E9B 1P4; Mem'88; CCFP; FCFP; (506)843-2910; Fax. (506)843-2911.

ZIGBY, Jean A; GMF Cote-des-Neiges, 500-5700 ch Cote-Des-Neiges, Montreal QC H3T 2A6; McG'97; CCFP; (514)731-8531; jeanzigby@mac.com.

ZIGMAN, Daniel; MUHC-Montreal Gen Hosp, A2 232-1650 av Cedar, Montreal QC H3G 1A4; McG'06; MDCM; FRCPC; Psy. Staff, McGill University Health Centre - Montreal General Campus; Staff, Royal Ottawa Mental Health Centre - Royal Ottawa Health Care Group; (514)934-1934

ZIGMAN, Michael; 506-5885 ch Cote-des-Neiges, Montreal QC H3S 2T2; McG'73; principale Médecin, Sir Mortimer B Davis Jewish General; Langs: English; French; (514)737-0996; michael.zigman@mail.mcgill.ca.

ZIKMAN, Jerrold M; 4V Clinic McMaster Hosp, 1200 Main St W, Hamilton ON L8N 3Z5; McG'65; BSc; MDCM; FRCSC; Urol. Staff, Hamilton Health Sciences Centre - McMaster University Medical Centre; Staff, McMaster Hospital 4V Clinic; Clin Assoc Prof, McMaster University; Langs: English; French; (905)522-4055; Fax. (905)522-3414; jmzmd@cobeco.ca.

ZIKOS, Eugenia; MUHC-Montreal Gen Hosp, 1025 Pine Ave W, Montreal QC H3A 1A1; Mon'98; FRCPC; Psy. Staff, McGill University Health Centre - Montreal General Campus; Langs: English; French; Greek; Spanish; (514)934-1934 x34475; Fax. (514)843-2858; eugenia.zikos@mail.mcgill.ca.

ZILBER-SHLENSKY, Caren F; Cook Street Vllage Health Cent, 200-1075 Pendergast St, Victoria BC V8V 0A1; Touro University College (USA)'05; CCFP; Langs: Spanish; French; Indonesian; (250)477-5433; Fax. (250)477-5431.

ZILBERT, Arthur W; Dr Arthur W Zilbert Med Clinic, 306-44 Portland St, Dartmouth NS B2Y 1H4; Dal'74; BSc; FACOG; FRCSC; ObstGyn. Ac Staff, IWK Health Centre; Asst Prof, Dalhousie University; (902)465-8700; Fax. (902)465-2279; arthur.zilbert@ns.sympatico.ca.

ZILKA, Sonal D; Timmins & District Hosp, 700 Ross Ave E, Timmins ON P4N 8P2; McM'05; CCFP; CCFP(E.M.); Staff, Timmins & District Hospital; Langs: Gujarati; (705)267-2131; Fax. (705)671-1688.

ZILLER, Matthias G; St Mary's Hosp Centre, 3830 av Lacombe, Montreal QC H3T 1M5; Mon'03; FRCPC; Neur. Staff, St Mary's Hospital Centre; (514)345-6511

ZILLI, Cheryl A; 26 Pine Ridge Dr, London ON N5X 3G7; Wes'82; FRCPC; Psy. (519)660-1795; Fax. (519)660-1795.

ZIMAKAS, George W; 5803 Main St, Niagara Falls ON L2G 5Z6; McG'93; MDCM; DABIM; BA; FRCPC; IntMed. Chief IntMed & Cons, Niagara Health System - Greater Niagara General Site; Langs: English; French; (905)371-1117; Fax. (905)371-9986; george.zimakas@sympatico.ca.

ZIMBALATTI, Carol A; Ferris Med Clinic, 5-41 Lakeshore Dr, North Bay ON P1A 2A1; Tor'04; CCFP; (705)495-4000; Fax. (705)495-4007.

ZIMBLER, Jessica; University Hosp of Northern BC, 1475 Edmonton St, Prince George BC V2M 1S2; McG'09; CCFP; Staff, University Hospital of Northern British Columbia; (250)565-2000

ZIMCIK, Heather L; Toronto Rehab Institute-Lyndhu, 520 Sutherland Dr, Toronto ON M4G 3V9; Tor'06; CCFP; Staff, Toronto Rehabilitation Institute - Lyndhurst Centre; Staff, Toronto Rehabilitation Institute - Queen Elizabeth Centre; (416)597-3422

ZIMM, Abraham J; Adamson Cosmetic Facial Surger, 150 Bloor St W, Toronto ON M5S 2X9; Medical College of Virginia (USA)'95.

ZIMMER, Kenneth W; Psychealth Centre, PZ 202-771 Bannatyne Ave, Winnipeg MB R3E 3N4; Man'80; FRCPC; Psy. Staff, Health Sciences Centre; Assoc Prof, University of Manitoba; (204)787-3970; Fax. (204)787-7480; zimmerk@cc.umanitoba.ca.

ZIMMER, Rachelle C; Royal University Hosp, 241-103 Hospital Dr, Saskatoon SK S7N 0W8; Sask'03; FRCPC; Psy (Child & Adolescent Psychiatry). Staff Child & Youth Psy, Royal University Hospital; (306)966-7531; Fax. (306)966-8250; rachelle.zimmer@saskatoonhealthregion.ca.

ZIMMER, Rudolf A G; Richmond Square Med Centre, 70-3915 51 St SW, Calgary AB T3E 6N1; Wes'87; FRCPC; CommunMed (Environmental Medicine);CCFP; FCFP; Public Health & Preventive Med. Staff, Market Mall Executive Professional Centre; Clinical Asst Prof Community Health Sciences, University of Calgary; (403)229-2273; Fax. (403)246-9688.

ZIMMERING, Linda D; Oak Park Med Clinic, 1-2530 Sixth Line, Oakville ON L6H 6W5; McG'83; (905)257-1006

ZIMMERMAN, Deborah L; The Ottawa Hosp-Riverside, 1967 Riverside Dr, Ottawa ON K1H 7W9; Cal'93; MSc; FRCPC; IntMed; Nephrol. Staff, The Ottawa Hospital - Riverside Campus; Assoc Prof, University of Ottawa; (613)738-8400; Fax. (613)738-8337.

ZIMMERMAN, Harvey S; 203-1223 St Clair Ave W, Toronto ON M6E 1B5; Tor'68; Staff, Mount Sinai Hospital; (416)652-3133; Fax. (416)652-7828.

ZIMMERMAN, Paul R; Mental Health Services, 2F-3 Applewood Dr, Trenton ON K8V 4E3; Qns'91; FRCPC; Psy. Asst Psy, QHC Trenton Memorial; Staff, QHC Belleville General; (613)779-7329; Fax. (613)779-7156.

ZIMMERMANN, Bruce R; Indian Head Med Clinic, PO Box 790, Indian Head SK S0G 2K0; Sask'87; Staff Chief Family Med, Indian Head Hospital; Physician, Indian Head Medical Clinic; (306)695-2276; Fax. (306)695-2732.

ZIMMERMANN, Camilla C U; Univ Hlth Network-Princess M, 16 712-610 University Ave, Toronto ON M5G 2M9; McG'93; FRCPC; IntMed (Palliative Care). Head Palliative Care, Princess Margaret Hospital - University Health Network; Langs: German; English; (416)946-4501 x3477; Fax. (416)946-2866.

ZIMMERMANN, Donald L; Kelowna Gen Hosp, 2268 Pandosy St, Kelowna BC V1Y 1T2; Sask'90; FRCPC; Anes. Staff, Kelowna General Hospital; (250)862-4000

ZIMMERMANN, Gordon A; Kelowna Gen Hosp, 2268 Pandosy St, Kelowna BC V1Y 1T2; Sask'89; FRCPC; Anes. Staff, Kelowna General Hospital; (250)862-4000

ZIMMERMANN, Rodney H; Regina Cardiology Associates, 701-2125 11th Ave, Regina SK S4P 3X3; Sask'88; FACC; FRCPC; IntMed; Cardiol. Physician, Regina Cardiology Associates; (306)781-7944; Fax. (306)781-6997.

ZINCK, Mary S; IWK Health Centre, PO Box 9700 Rpo CSC 5850-5980 University Ave, Halifax NS B3K 6R8; Dal'98; FRCPC; Psy. Staff Maritime Outpatient Psy, IWK Health Centre; Asst Prof Psy, Dalhousie University; Langs: Bilingual(English/French); (902)470-8375; Fax. (902)470-8937.

ZINGA BOLENGE, Roland X; CLSC Saint-Pamphile, 103 rue du Foyer N, Saint-Pamphile QC G0R 3X0; Brussels (Belgium)'92; (418)356-3393; Fax. (418)356-5535; rolandzinga@hotmail.com.

ZINGG, Hans H; MUHC-Royal Victoria Hosp, 687 av des Pins O, Montreal QC H3A 1A1; Basel (Switzerland)'73; PhD; assoc Staff, McGill University Health Centre - Royal Victoria Hospital; Chef Pharmacol & Therapeutics, McGill University; Langs: English; French; (514)398-3621; Fax. (514)398-2045.

ZINI, Armand S; St Mary's Hosp Centre, 2304-3830 av Lacombe, Montreal QC H3T 1M5; McG'89; BSc; FRCSC; Urol (Male Infertility). Chef urologie, St Mary's Hospital Centre; Langs: English; French; (514)345-3511; Fax. (514)734-2718.

ZINKIEW, Kristi; Mill Bay Med Centre, 230-2720 Mill Bay Rd RR 1, Mill Bay BC V0R 2P1; Sask'93; FRCPC; Peds. Staff, Victoria General Hospital; Staff, Cowichan District Hospital; Staff, Shawnigan Village Family Practice; (250)743-3211; Fax. (250)743-2800.

ZINMAN, Bernard; Mount Sinai Hosp, L5024-60 Murray St Box 17, Toronto ON M5T 3L9; McG'68; MDCM; FACP; FRCPC; IntMed; Endocrin (P.Q.). Dir Leadership Sinai Centre for Diabetes, Mount Sinai Hospital; Chair Diabetes, Sam & Judy Pener Family Centre; Sr Scientist, Samuel Lunenfeld Research Institute; Prof, University of Toronto; (416)586-8747; Fax. (416)586-4740; zinman@mshri.on.ca.

ZINMAN, Lorne H; Sunnybrook Health Sciences Ctr, M1 600-2075 Bayview Ave, Toronto ON M4N 3M5; Cal'98; FRCPC; Neur. Staff, Sunnybrook Health Sciences Centre; (416)480-4475; Fax. (416)480-4674.

ZIOMEK, Anna M; College of Phys & Surgs of MB, 1000-1661 Portage Ave, Winnipeg MB R3J 3T7; Gdansk (Poland)'80; Medical Officer Emerg, Concordia General Hospital; Asst Registrar Qualifications & Complaints, College of Physicians & Surgeons of Manitoba; Staff Teacher, University of Manitoba; (204)774-4344

ZIOUZINA, Olga; 330-401 9 Ave SW, Calgary AB T2P 3C5; Man'04; FRCPC; IntMed; Rheum. Staff, Foothills Medical Centre; (403)221-4465; Fax. (403)221-4419; olgaziouzina@hotmail.com.

ZIP, Catherine M; The Dermatology Centre, 124 42 Ave SW, Calgary AB T2S 3B3; Alb'87; FAAD; FRCPC; Derm. Consultant, Alberta Children's Hospital; Consultant, Rockyview General Hospital; Consultant, Foothills Medical Centre; Asst Prof, University of Calgary; (403)299-5840; Fax. (403)299-5844.

ZIPURSKY, Robert B; St Joseph's Mountain Hlth Serv, C114A-100 5th St W, Hamilton ON L8N 3K7; McM'82; FRCPC; Psy (Schizophrenia). Staff, St Joseph's Healthcare - Charlton Campus; Chief Psy, St Joseph's Healthcare Hamilton - West 5th Campus; Chief Psy, Hamilton Health Sciences Centre - Hamilton General Hospital; Prof, McMaster University; (905)522-1155; Fax. (905)381-5633.

ZIPURSKY, Sheldon; The Richmond Hosp, WT 2-7000 Westminster Hwy, Richmond BC V6X 1A2; Man'72; DABPN; FRCPC; Psy (Administration). Dep Head Psy/Med Dir Mental Health & Addiction, Richmond Hospital; Med Dir, Vancouver Community Mental Health Services; Med Dir Mental Health & Addiction/Sr Physician, Richmond Mental Health Child & Adolescent Program; Clin Prof Psy, University of British Columbia; (604)244-5241; Fax. (604)278-4819; sheldon.zipursky@vch.ca.

ZIRADKAR, Jyotsna S; The Doctors Med Walk-In Clinic, 105-641 Commissioners Rd E, London ON N6C 2T9; Bombay (India)'82; MB BS; CCFP; Staff, Highbury Medical Clinic; Staff Student Health Section, University of Western Ontario; Langs: Gujarati; Hindi; (519)963-0232; Fax. (519)963-0233.

ZIRADKAR, Shaliendra Y; South London Urgent Care Clini, 595 Bradley Ave, London ON N6E 3Z8; Bombay (India)'81; MB BS; CCFP; Staff, Doctors Walk-In Clinic; Staff, Highbury Medical Clinic; Langs: Gujarati; Hindi; (519)681-8300; Fax. (519)681-5200.

ZIRK, Harry A; Millwoods Family Med Clinic, 104-2551 Hewes Way NW, Edmonton AB T6L 6W6; Cal'90; CCFP; FCFP; (780)462-2767; Fax. (780)463-7025.

ZIRKLE, Molly S; St Michael's Hosp, 8F-30 Bond St, Toronto ON M5B 1W8; Yale University (USA)'96; FRCSC; Otol (Head & Neck Surgery). Staff, St Michael's Hospital; (416)864-5187; Fax. (416)864-5469.

ZIS, Athanasios P; UBC Hospital, 2211 Wesbrook Mall, Vancouver BC V6T 2B5; Athens (Greece)'69; FRCPC; Psy. Langs: Greek; (604)875-4111 x68294

ZITER, Dale D; Windsor Prof Centre, 200-2462 Howard Ave, Windsor ON N8X 3V6; Wes'82; CCFP; FCFP; Ac Staff, Hôtel-Dieu Grace Hospital; Court Staff, Windsor Regional Hospital - Metropolitan Site; Acad Dir Family Med/Teach Staff, Schulich School of Medicine & Dentistry; (519)258-4143; Fax. (519)258-4456.

ZITER, Paul S; Family Health Centre, 113-2462 Howard Ave, Windsor ON N8X 3V6; Wes'78; Chief FamMed, Hôtel-Dieu Grace Hospital; Langs: Italian; Arabic; (519)258-4334; Fax. (519)258-2169.

ZITNER, David; Public Garden Med Group, 200-5675 Spring Garden Rd, Halifax NS B3J 1H1; Dal'74; CCFP; FCFP; Dir Med Informatics/Prof, Dalhousie University; (902)425-5440; Fax. (902)482-6019; david.zitner@dal.ca.

ZITNEY, Michael I; Headache & Pain Relief Centre, 220-251 Consumers Rd, North York ON M2J 4R3; Tor'85; DAAPM; Dir, Headache & Pain Relief Centre; (416)493-9762; Fax. (416)493-7043; zitney@ica.net.

ZITSOW, Bernard S; Dr B Zitsow & Associates, LL4-1525 Albion Rd, Etobicoke ON M9V 5G5; Man'64; FRCPC; DiagRad. (416)741-5661; Fax. (416)741-6417.

ZITSOW, Jason H; 431 King St E, Toronto ON M5A 1L5; Tor'99; CCFP; CCFP(E.M.); Staff, Humber River Regional Hospital - Finch Avenue Site; (416)368-6304

ZIVIC-DELIU, Ljiljana; Springview Family Practice, 6A-5675 Spring Garden Rd, Halifax NS B3J 1H1; University of Nis (Croatia)'84; CCFP; Langs: Croatian; (902)423-2908; Fax. (902)429-6564.

ZIVKOVIC BURSAC, Slavica; Ctr de Sante de Temiskaming, 180 rue Anvik CP 760, Temiscaming QC J0Z 3R0; Belgrade (Serbia)'85; Staff, Centre de santé de Témiscaming; (819)627-3385; Fax. (819)627-9497.

ZIWENGA, Ophillia; Clinical Sciences Bldg, 8 120-152 University Campus NW, Edmonton AB T6G 2G3; (Zimbabwe)'97; Staff, University of Alberta Hospital; (780)407-8861; Fax. (780)407-3200.

ZIZZO, Angelo J; 201-325 Winterberry Dr, Hamilton ON L8J 0B6; Tor'66; CCFP; FCFP; Ac Staff Family Med, St Joseph's Healthcare - Charlton Campus; Clin Prof Famiy Med, McMaster University; (905)388-1254; Fax. (905)388-1009.

ZIZZO, Dean J; 201-325 Winterberry Dr, Hamilton ON L8J 0B6; Wes'93; BSc; CCFP; FCFP; Staff, St Joseph's Healthcare - Charlton Campus; (905)388-1254; Fax. (905)388-1255; dzizzo@msn.com.

ZIZZO, Richard A; 206-325 Winterberry Dr, Stoney Creek ON L8J 0B6; McM'78; CCFP; FCFP; Court Staff, Hamilton Health Sciences Centre - McMaster University Medical Centre; Ac Staff, St Joseph's Healthcare - Charlton Campus; Asst Prof Family Med, McMaster University; (905)575-9004; Fax. (905)575-9026.

ZLIPKO, Terrance S; St Paul's Hosp, 1702 20th St W, Saskatoon SK S7M 0Z9; Sask'74; Staff, St Paul's Hospital (Grey Nuns) of Saskatoon; Clin Teacher Family Med, University of Saskatchewan; Langs: Ukrainian; (306)655-5113; Fax. (306)655-5963.

ZLOCHOWER, David B; Albany Med Clinic, 807 Broadview Ave, Toronto ON M4K 2P8; Tel Aviv University (Israel)'05; (416)461-9471; Fax. (416)461-2710.

ZLOT, Zoe A; Foothills Med Centre, 2025-1403 29 St NW, Calgary AB T2N 2T9; Alb'90; CCFP; CCFP(E.M.); Staff Emerg, Foothills Medical Centre; (403)944-1315; Fax. (403)249-6183.

ZLOTKIN, Stanley H; The Hosp for Sick Children, 555 University Ave, Toronto ON M5G 1X8; McM'74; PhD; FRCPC; Peds (Nutrition). Assoc Staff, Women's College Hospital; Div Head GI/Nutrition, The Hospital For Sick Children; Prof Peds & Nutritional Sciences, University of Toronto; (416)813-6171; Fax. (416)813-4972; stanley.zlotkin@sickkids.ca.

ZLOTNIK, Gregorio; Clin de la Migraine de Mtl, 420-1600 boul Henri-Bourassa O, Montreal QC H3M 3E2; Buenos Aires (Argentina)'61; Langs: Portuguese; French; Spanish; (514)337-0432; Fax. (514)337-0942.

ZLOTTA, Alexandre R; 60 Murray St Box 19, Toronto ON M5T 3L9; Brussels (Belgium)'89; FRCSC; GenSurg (Urologic Oncology); Urol. Dir Uro-Oncology, Mount Sinai Hospital; Langs: Dutch; French; (416)586-4800; Fax. (416)586-8354.

ZLOTY, David M; Skin Care Centre, 835 10th Ave W, Vancouver BC V5Z 4E8; Alb'89; FRCPC; Derm (Cosmetic Surgery). Staff Dermatologic Surg, Vancouver General Hospital - Centennial Pavillion; Clin Assoc Prof, University of British Columbia; (604)875-4888; Fax. (604)875-4777; david.zloty@vch.ca.

ZLOTY, Richard B; Manitoba Health, 300 Carlton St, Winnipeg MB R3B 3M9; Man'73; FRCPC; Psy. Staff/Consultant Psy Dept of Health & Commun Services-Prov of Manitoba, Manitoba Adolescent Treatment Centre; Asst Prof, University of Manitoba; rzloty@matc.ca.

ZMIJOWSKYJ, Timothy J; Shkagamik-Kwe Health Centre, 161 Applegrove St, Sudbury ON P3C 1N2; Ott'93; CCFP; Staff, Shkagamik-Kwe Health Centre; Staff, Shkagamik-KWE Health Centre; Div Head Clin Sciences, Northern Ontario School of Medicine; (705)675-1596

ZNAJDA, James P; 203-1585 Markham Rd, Scarborough ON M1B 2W1; Qns'62; DAB; FRCSC; Ophth (Surgical & Medical Ophthalmology). Court Staff, The Scarborough Hospital - Birchmount Campus; Court Staff, The Scarborough Hospital - General Campus; Langs: Ukrainian; (416)284-0289; Fax. (416)284-7590.

ZNAJDA, Tamara L; Lakeshore Gen Hosp, 160 av Stillview, Pointe-Claire QC H9R 2Y2; Tor'98; FRCSC; GenSurg; Critical Care Medicine. Staff, Lakeshore General Hospital - Pointe Claire; (514)630-2225; Fax. (514)630-4708.

ZNAMIROWSKI, Anna I M; Cambridge Place, 407-73 Water St N, Cambridge ON N1R 7L6; Ott'81; FRCSC; ObstGyn. Staff, Cambridge Memorial Hospital; Langs: Polish; French; (519)623-0865; Fax. (519)623-2112.

ZNOJKIEWICZ, Kathia; CLSC Parc Extension, 7085 rue Hutchison, Montreal QC H3N 1Y9; Sher'92; Médecin, CLSC Parc Extension; Langs: Polish; Spanish; English; (514)273-9591; Fax. (514)380-8138; kathia.znojkiewicz.dlm@ssss.gouv.qc.ca.

ZNOJKIEWICZ, Maria H; Clinique Pediatrique Beaubien, 2301 rue Belanger, Montreal QC H2G 1C9; Warsaw (Poland)'65; Peds. (514)728-1559; Fax. (514)728-4480.

ZOBERMAN, Lawrence; The Scarborough Hosp-Gen Div, 3050 Lawrence Ave E, Scarborough ON M1P 2V5; Tor'70; CCFP; Ac Staff, The Scarborough Hospital - General Campus; Court Staff, North York General Hospital; Court Staff, Mount Sinai Hospital; Lecturer Family & Commun Med, University of Toronto; Langs: Hebrew; Yiddish; (416)438-2911 x3715; Fax. (416)431-8236.

ZOCCOLILLO, Mark; Clinique Med Roper, 4500 rue Sherbrooke O, Westmount QC H3Z 1E6; Charlottesville(VA) (USA)'80; Psy (P. Q.). (514)937-8000; Fax. (514)937-8884.

ZOCHODNE, Douglas W; Heritage Med Research Centre, 168-3330 Hospital Dr NW, Calgary AB T2N 4N1; Wes'80; FRCPC; Neur (Clinical Neurophysiology). Prof, University of Calgary; (403)220-8831; Fax. (403)283-8731; dzochodn@ucalgary.ca.

ZOFFMANN, Elisabeth; 607-409 Granville St, Vancouver BC V6C 1T2; UBC'86; FRCPC; Psy (Forensic Psychiatry). (604)646-4664; Fax. (604)646-4662.

ZOGHBY, Magdy; Complexe Sante Reine-Elizabeth, 2100 av Marlowe, Montreal QC H4A 3L5; Ein Shams (Egypt)'70; Staff, McGill University Health Centre - Royal Victoria Hospital; Staff, Centre de santé Queen Elizabeth; Langs: Arabic; French; (514)934-8080; Fax. (514)934-8385.

ZOGOPOULOS, George; MUHC-Royal Victoria Hosp, S9 30-687 av des Pins O, Montreal QC H3A 1A1; Tor'02; FRCSC; GenSurg. Staff, McGill University Health Centre - Royal Victoria Hospital; (514)934-1934

ZOHOOR, Arash; St Paul Family Hlth Organizati, 4F-99 Wayne Gretzky Pky, Brantford ON N3S 6T6; Wes'06; CCFP; Langs: Farsi; (519)756-6400

ZOHRAB, Andrew E F; Rouge Valley HS-Ajax/Pickering, 580 Harwood Ave, Ajax ON L1S 2J4; UBC'99; CCFP; Staff, Rouge Valley Health System - Ajax & Pickering Health Centre Site; (905)683-2320

ZOHRAB, W John; Professional Centre, 520-145 17th St W, North Vancouver BC V7M 3G4; Otago (New Zealand)'65; MB ChB; FRCPC; Gastroent. (604)980-5731; Fax. (604)983-8760; wjzohrabmd@shaw.ca.

ZOLEIN, Mohammad M; Penticton Reg Hosp, 550 Carmi Ave, Penticton BC V2A 3G6; Rafsanjan Medical University (Other Foreign)'93; GenPath. Staff Lab Services, Penticton Regional Hospital; Langs: Farsi; (250)492-4000

ZOLFAGHARI, Shahram; Rideau Valley Health Services, 1221 Greenbank Rd, Ottawa ON K2J 5V7; Ghazvin Medical School (Other Foreign)'96; FRCSC; GenSurg (Colorectal Surgery). Staff, The Ottawa Hospital - General Campus; (613)258-8716

ZOLIS, Lynne R; Yonge/York Mills Women's Clinic, 100-36 York Mills Rd, North York ON M2P 2E9; McM'04; FRCSC; ObstGyn. (416)644-1404

ZOLPIS, Edward C A; 202-117 Murray St, Ottawa ON K1N 5M5; Cal'78; FRCPC; Psy (Cognitive Therapy). (613)594-5738

ZONDERVAN, James H; Medical Arts Bldg, 656-750 Spadina Cres E, Saskatoon SK S7K 3H3; Sask'69; FRCSC; PlasSurg. Ac Staff, Royal University Hospital; Ac Staff, Saskatoon City Hospital; Ac Staff, St Paul's Hospital (Grey Nuns) of Saskatoon; Clin Assoc Prof, University of Saskatchewan; (306)244-1333; Fax. (306)244-1334; drzondervan@sasktel.net.

ZOPPA, Robert J M; Selkirk Med Clinic, 353 Eveline St, Selkirk MB R1A 1N1; Man'05; BSc; CCFP; Att Physician, Selkirk & District General Hospital; Co-Med Dir, Betel Personal Care Home; (204)785-8588; Fax. (204)785-1290.

ZORN, Kevin C; 301-235 boul Rene-Levesque E, Montreal QC H2X 1N8; McG'00; FRCSC; Urol. (514)861-0213; Fax. (514)861-3021.

ZORN, Marietta L T; The Court Hlth Centenary Centr, 413-2863 Ellesmere Rd, Scarborough ON M1E 5E9; Ott'78; FRCSC; PlasSurg (General Surgery). Court Staff, The Hospital For Sick Children; Court Staff, The Scarborough Hospital - General Campus; Staff, Rouge Valley Health System - Ajax & Pickering Health Centre Site; Langs: German; French; (416)283-5871; Fax. (416)283-5875.

ZORZELA, Liliane M; University of Alberta Hosp, 8440 112 St NW, Edmonton AB T6G 2B7; (Brazil)'02; Staff, University of Alberta Hospital; (780)407-1673

ZORZITTO, Joanna R; New Vision Family Hlth Team, 421 Greenbrook Dr, Kitchener ON N2M 4K1; Tor'09; CCFP; (519)578-3510

ZORZITTO, Maria L; St Michael's Hosp, SW4 002-30 Bond St, Toronto ON M5B 1W8; McM'76; MSc; BSc(Hon); FRCPC; IntMed (Telehealth); GeriatricMed. Staff, St Michael's Hospital; Asst Prof, University of Toronto; Langs: Italian; French; (416)864-5015; Fax. (416)864-5735; zorzitto@smh.ca.

ZOU, Lenore L; Dundas Family Med Group, 201-133 King St W, Hamilton ON L9H 1V3; Alb'97; CCFP; Langs: Mandarin; (905)628-6355; Fax. (905)628-0664.

ZOU, Limai; Sheppard Med Bldg, 201-701 Sheppard Ave E, North York ON M2K 2Z3; Tor'99; CCFP; Staff, The Scarborough Hospital - Birchmount Campus; Langs: Mandarin; (416)916-6090; Fax. (647)435-6730.

ZOUDIS, Adamantios P; 205-272 Lawrence Ave W, North York ON M5M 4M1; Wes'09; CCFP; (416)787-7516

ZOUROS, Irene A; Brockville Gen Hosp, 75 Charles St, Brockville ON K6V 1S8; Dal'03; CCFP; CCFP(E.M.); Staff, Brockville General Hospital - Charles Street; (613)345-5649

ZOUTMAN, Dick E; Quinte Healthcare Corporation, 265 Dundas St E, Belleville ON K8N 5A9; Man'82; DABIM; FRCPC; IntMed (Infection Control); InfectDis; MedMicrobiol. Chief of Staff, QHC Belleville General; Prof Med, Queen's University; Langs: Dutch; (613)969-7400; Fax. (613)969-0486; zoutmand@kgh.kari.net.

ZOWNIR, Jerry R; St Michael's Hosp, 4 149 ECW-30 Bond St, Toronto ON M5B 1W8; Wes'64; BScPharm; FRCPC; IntMed (Geriatric Medicine). Ac Staff, St Michael's Hospital; Att Staff, Ukrainian Canadian Care Centre; Asst Prof, University of Toronto; Langs: Ukrainian; French; (416)864-5903; Fax. (416)361-1471.

ZRINSCAK, Christine; Crown Point Family Health Ctre, 1-67 Kenilworth Ave N, Hamilton ON L8H 4R6; McM'99; CCFP; (905)525-9140; Fax. (905)546-0805.

ZSIGMOND, Otto; 8B-750 Fortune Dr, Kamloops BC V2B 2L2; Cluj (Romania)'67; Staff, Royal Inland Hospital; Langs: Hungarian; Romanian; (250)376-2366

ZUBAIR, Naeem A; Lakeridge HC-Bowmanville, 47 Liberty St S, Bowmanville ON L1C 2N4; Karachi (Pakistan)'76; DSc; MB BS; Staff Anes, Lakeridge Health - Bowmanville Site; Langs: Urdu; Punjabi; (905)623-3331 x1700; zubairna@yahoo.com.

ZUBEK, Elizabeth M; Westgate Med Clinic, 402-20395 Lougheed Hwy, Maple Ridge BC V2X 2P9; Man'91; BSc; CCFP; Ac Staff Privil, Ridge Meadows Hospital & Health Care Centre; Langs: Bilingual(English/French); (604)465-3900; Fax. (604)465-3990.

ZUBERBIER, Oonagh A; Broadway Plaza Bldg, 902-601 Broadway Ave W, Vancouver BC V5Z 4C2; UBC'02; BA; BGS; FRCPC; Psy (Anxiety Disorder). (604)876-7004

ZUBERBUHLER, Peter C; Baker Clinic, 220-10405 Jasper Ave NW, Edmonton AB T5J 3N4; Alb'76; FRCPC; Peds. Ac Staff, Royal Alexandra Hospital; Assoc Staff, University of Alberta Hospital; (780)421-1990; Fax. (780)944-9599.

ZUBERI, Najeeb A; 115-1856 Ambrosi Rd, Kelowna BC V1Y 4R9; (Dominican Republic)'86; (778)484-5474

ZUBERT, Shelly A; Health Sciences Centre, GF201-820 Sherbrook St, Winnipeg MB R3A 1R9; Man'05; FRCPC; EmergMed; Critical Care Medicine. Staff, Health Sciences Centre; (204)774-8511

ZUBI, Kalfalla M; Eastwood Med Clinic, 7919 118 Ave NW, Edmonton AB T5B 0R5; Altahady (Other Foreign)'99; FRCPC; Peds. (780)756-3666

ZUBIS, John C; Avenida Bonavista Shopp Ctre, 315-12445 Lake Fraser Dr SE, Calgary AB T2J 7A4; Alb'67; (403)723-2453; Fax. (403)723-2463.

ZUBKO, M Grant; 235-2335 162 Ave SW, Calgary AB T2Y 4S6; Cal'74; (403)921-2660; Fax. (403)238-4778.

ZUBOVITS, Judit T; Scarborough Hosp-Birchmount, 3030 Birchmount Rd, Scarborough ON M1W 3W3; Qns'94; FRCPC; AnatPath. Staff, The Scarborough Hospital - Birchmount Campus; Langs: Hungarian; (416)495-2701; Fax. (416)495-2477.

ZUCCARO, Anthony; Anchor Family Medicine, 1450 Waddington Rd, Nanaimo BC V9S 4V9; UBC'94; CCFP; FCFP; Ac Staff, Nanaimo Regional General Hospital; (250)754-5545; Fax. (250)754-5954.

ZUCCONI, Anthony L P; 108-359 Riverside Dr, Sudbury ON P3E 1H5; Tor'94; MSc; CCFP; (705)688-1359; Fax. (705)688-1422.

ZUCHELKOWSKI, Jan S; Millway Med Centre Inc, 7-3200 Erin Mills Pky, Mississauga ON L5L 1W8; Poznan (Poland)'80; CCFP; FCFP; Langs: Polish; (905)607-0017; Fax. (905)607-0078.

ZUCKER, Marc E; Children's Hosp Eastern Ont, 401 Smyth Rd, Ottawa ON K1H 8L1; Qns'95; FRCPC; Peds. Staff, Children's Hospital of Eastern Ontario (CHEO); (613)737-7600 x2571; Fax. (613)738-4878.

ZUCKER, Rosalind M; 207-3410 Sheppard Ave E, Scarborough ON M1T 3K4; Leeds (England)'64; MB ChB; DCH(Glas); BSc(Anat.); Court Staff Family Med, The Scarborough Hospital - Birchmount Campus; Court Staff, North York General Hospital; (416)299-6998; Fax. (416)299-7492.

ZUCKER, Tal; Sturgeon Community Hosp, 201 Boudreau Rd, St. Albert AB T8N 6C4; Tel-Aviv University (Israel)'01; FRCPC; IntMed. Staff, Glenrose Rehabilitation Hospital; Staff, Sturgeon Community Hospital; Staff, Royal Alexandra Hospital; (780)418-8200

ZUCKERMAN, Hanna E; North York Family Health Team, 701-240 Duncan Mill Rd, North York ON M3B 3S6; Tor'76; BSc; CCFP; FCFP; Ac Staff, North York General Hospital; (416)229-6300; Fax. (416)229-6283.

ZUCKIER, Lionel S; The Ottawa Hosp-Gen Campus, 1472-501 Smyth Rd Box 240, Ottawa ON K1H 8L6; Yeshiva University (USA)'82; NuclearMed. Staff, The Ottawa Hospital - General Campus; (613)722-7000

ZUEGE, Danny J; Peter Lougheed Centre, 3500 26 Ave NE, Calgary AB T1Y 6J4; Alb'90; FRCP; FRCPC; IntMed; Critical Care Medicine; Respir. Ad Staff ICU, Peter Lougheed Centre; Ad Staff, Foothills Medical Centre; Clinical Asst Prof Med, University of Calgary; (403)943-4308; Fax. (403)291-1491.

ZUFELT, Kirk W; The Group Health Ctre, 240 McNabb St, Sault Ste. Marie ON P6B 1Y5; McM'93; FRCPC; Peds (Pediatric Cardiology). (705)759-1234; Fax. (705)541-2224.

ZUIDHOF, Aaron; Queen's North Health Centre, PO Box 1004 Stn Main, Minto NB E4B 3Y6; UBC'06; CCFP; Staff, Dr Everett Chalmers Regional Hospital; (506)327-7888; Fax. (506)327-7899.

ZUIJDWIJK, Caroline S; The Hosp For Sick Children, 555 University Ave, Toronto ON M5G 1X8; McM'05; FRCPC; Peds; Endocrin&Metab. Staff, The Hospital For Sick Children; (416)813-7654; Fax. (416)813-8407.

ZUIN, Claudia C; Victoria General Hosp, 1 Hospital Way, Victoria BC V8Z 6R5; Cordoba (Argentina)'86; FRCPC; Peds. Staff, Victoria General Hospital; (250)727-4212

ZUK, Lorne M; 11-36 Riedel St, Fort McMurray AB T9H 3E1; Alb'75; FRCSC; GenSurg. (780)743-5888; Fax. (780)743-1663.

ZUKER, Ronald M; The Hosp for Sick Children, 5416-555 University Ave, Toronto ON M5G 1X8; Tor'69; FACS; FAAP; FRCSC; PlasSurg (Pediatric Plastic Surgery). Staff Surg, The Hospital For Sick Children; Staff, Toronto General Hospital - UHN; Consultant, Mount Sinai Hospital; Prof Surg, University of Toronto; Langs: Spanish; (416)813-6447; Fax. (416)813-6147.

ZUKER-FUCHS, Joyce; Lakeshore Gen Hosp, 160 av Stillview, Pointe-Claire QC H9R 2Y2; McG'80; FRCPC; Anes. Staff, Lakeshore General Hospital - Pointe Claire; (514)630-2225 x2699

ZUKOR, David J; E 003-SMBD Jewish Gen Hosp, 3755 ch Cote-Sainte-Catherine, Montreal QC H3T 1E2; McG'80; FRCS; FRCSC; OrthSurg (Hip & Knee Reconstruction). Chef Dept of OrthSurg, Sir Mortimer B Davis Jewish General; assoc Prof Surg, McGill University; Langs: Hebrew; French; (514)340-8222 x2995; Fax. (514)340-7595; david.zukor@mcgill.ca.

ZULFIQAR, Muhammad; Abbotsford Reg Hosp & CC, 32900 Marshall Rd, Abbotsford BC V2S 0C2; Nishtar (Pakistan)'93; MB; BSc; FRCPC; IntMed; MedOncol. Staff, Abbotsford Regional Hospital & Cancer Centre; Langs: Hindi; Punjabi; Urdu; (604)851-4700

ZULIANI, Preston A; Glenridge Med Bldg, 100-1 Belton Blvd, St Catharines ON L2T 3Y4; Tor'75; CCFP; FCFP; Court Staff, Niagara Health System - St Catharines General Site; (905)688-6460; Fax. (905)687-1855.

ZULYNIAK, Holly J; Signal Hill Med Centre, 2-5986 Signal Hill Ctr SW, Calgary AB T3H 3P8; Sask'05; CCFP; (403)240-2660; Fax. (403)242-8390.

ZULYS, Vytas J; 1888 Steepbank Cres, Mississauga ON L4X 1T8; Tor'78; FRCPC; Anes (Cardiovascular Anesthesia). Langs: Lithuanian; (905)602-9257

ZUMMER, Michel; Hop Maisonneuve-Rosemont, 5415 boul de l'Assomption, Montreal QC H1T 2M4; Laval'81; FRCPC; IntMed; Rheum. Staff, Hopital Maisonneuve-Rosemont; Universite de Montreal; (514)252-3400 x4925; Fax. (514)252-3899.

ZUMMO, Mario; Clinique Les Jardins Dorval, 204-352 av Dorval, Dorval QC H9S 3H8; Mon'80; Staff, CSSS de Dorval-Lachine-Lasalle; Langs: English; (514)631-6086; Fax. (514)631-6691.

ZUMMO, Michel; Centre de Phlebologie, 916 boul Saint-Joseph E, Montreal QC H2J 1K6; Mon'81; BSP(SC); Pres, Congres Mondial-Union Internationale de Phlebologie; Pres, Societe Canadienne de Phlebologie; Member, Societe Francaise de Phlebologie; Langs: English; French; (514)526-8888; Fax. (514)526-2800; phlebodoc@guail.com.

ZUNDER, Ian H L; The Ottawa Hosp-Civic Campus, 249C-1053 Carling Ave, Ottawa ON K1Y 4E9; Ott'86; FRCPC; Anes. Att Staff Anes, The Ottawa Hospital - Civic Campus; Asst Prof Anes, University of Ottawa; Langs: English; French; (613)761-4169; Fax. (613)761-5209.

ZUNG, Hor-Ven A; Saddle Ridge Fam Physicians, 113-600 Saddletowne Cir NE, Calgary AB T3J 5M1; Alb'89; CCFP; FCFP; Ac Staff, Peter Lougheed Centre; (403)280-0179; Fax. (403)280-0216.

ZUNG, Nora P Y; Scarborough North Med Arts, 308-4040 Finch Ave E, Scarborough ON M1S 4V5; Tor'80; CCFP; Staff, The Scarborough Hospital - General Campus; Langs: Cantonese; Mandarin; (416)754-2800; Fax. (647)258-0422.

ZUPNIK, Joseph; York-Finch Med Centre, 216D-2115 Finch Ave W, North York ON M3N 2V6; McG'80; IntMed., Humber River Regional Hospital - Finch Avenue Site; (416)747-9839; Fax. (416)747-7105.

ZUR, Daniel; 4-100 Highland Rd W, Kitchener ON N2M 3B5; Wes'78; (519)576-1910; Fax. (519)576-9791.

ZURAWSKA, Joanna H; Medical Sciences Bldg, 6263-1 King's College Circle, Toronto ON M5S 1A8; Wes'08; FRCPC; IntMed. Teacher, University of Toronto; (416)978-1562

ZURAWSKA, Urszula; Univ Hlth Network-Princess M, 5 110-610 University ave, Toronto ON M5G 2M9; Wes'08; IntMed. Staff, Princess Margaret Hospital - University Health Network; (416)917-9639

ZUROWSKI, Mateusz-Jerzy; Univ Hlth Network-Toronto Western Hosp, 7 403-399 Bathurst St, Toronto ON M5T 2S8; Qns'98; FRCPC; Psy. Staff, Toronto Western Hospital - University Health Network; Langs: Polish; (416)603-5145; Fax. (416)603-5292.

ZUROWSKI, Wojciech J; 112-2238 Dundas St W, Toronto ON M6R 3A9; Warsaw (Poland)'68; Langs: Polish; (416)531-1056; Fax. (416)531-9269.

ZUZIC, Nancy L; Rockyview Gen Hosp, 7007 14 St SW, Calgary AB T2V 1P9; Ott'97; CCFP; CCFP(E.M.); Staff Emerg, Rockyview General Hospital; (403)943-7000; Fax. (403)283-1477.

ZWACK, Rhonda M; Regina Qu'Appelle HR-Regina, 1440 14th Ave, Regina SK S4P 0W5; Sask'96; FRCPC; Anes. Staff, Regina General Hospital; (306)766-4444; Fax. (306)766-4443.

ZWAI, Akram M; Univ of Regina Allied Hlth Ctr, 3737 Wascana Pky, Regina SK S4S 0A2; FRCSC; Neursurg. Staff NeuroSurg, Regina General Hospital; Physician Allied Health Centre, University Of Regina; (306)337-3282; Fax. (306)337-3294.

ZWAIGENBAUM, Lonnie; Glenrose Rehabilitation Hosp, E209-10230 111 Ave NW, Edmonton AB T5G 0B7; Tor'91; FRCPC; Peds (Autism). Staff, Glenrose Rehabilitation Hospital; (780)735-8280; Fax. (780)735-8249.

ZWANE, Mishack P; Humboldt Med Clinic, PO Box 220, Humboldt SK S0K 2A0; (306)682-2618; Fax. (306)682-4499.

ZWANEPOEL, Helen F; South Calgary Med Clinic, 118-40 Sunpark Plaza SE, Calgary AB T2X 3X7; (South Africa)'99; (403)254-4000; Fax. (403)254-1282.

ZWANEPOEL, Ruan; South Calgary Med Clinic, 118-40 Sunpark Plaza SE, Calgary AB T2X 3X7; Kansas (USA)'99; (403)254-4000; Fax. (403)254-1282.

ZWARDON, Michael; Grey Bruce HS-Southampton, 340 High St, Southampton ON N0H 2L0; Jagiellonian University (Poland)'09; CCFP; Staff, Grey Bruce Health Services - Southampton Site; (519)797-3230

ZWECKER, Philip; 304-438 rue Saint-Pierre, Montreal QC H2Y 2M5; McG'10; MDCM; CCFP; Staff, Cree Board of Health & Social Services James Bay; (514)961-8980

ZWICKER, Christine L; RCMP Health Services, 601-1595 Bedford Hwy, Bedford NS B4A 3Y4; Dal'93; CCFP; Staff, RCMP Health Services; Med Advisor, Worker's Compensation Board of NS; (902)426-0812; Fax. (902)426-0510.

ZWICKER, Daniel M; Lunenburg Med Clinic, PO Box 1450, Lunenburg NS B0J 2C0; Dal'75; Staff, Fishermen's Memorial Hospital; (902)634-7299; Fax. (902)634-4944.

ZWICKER, Deborah A; Cape Breton Hlthcare Complex, 1482 George St, Sydney NS B1P 1P3; Dal'94; FRCPC; IntMed (Diabetology); Endocrin&Metab. Internal Medicine, Cape Breton Healthcare Complex; (902)567-8127; Fax. (902)567-8128.

ZWICKER, Holly J; Crossroads Family Practice, 201-5110 St Margarets Bay Rd, Upper Tantallon NS B3Z 1E2; Dal'96; CCFP; (902)826-9096; Fax. (902)820-9399.

ZWICKER, Jocelyn C; The Ottawa Hosp-Civic Campus, C2178-1053 Carling Ave, Ottawa ON K1Y 4E9; Tor'97; FRCPC; Neur (Neuromuscular Diseases). Neurologist, The Ottawa Hospital - Civic Campus; Langs: French; (613)761-5353 x5; Fax. (613)761-5360.

ZWICKER, John W; 5 Beck Blvd, Penetanguishene ON L9M 1C1; Tor'81; BSc; Staff, Georgian Bay General Hospital - Midland; Staff, Waypoint Centre for Mental Health Care; (705)549-4646; Fax. (705)549-1414.

ZWICKER, Kelly A; 495-555 12 Ave W, Vancouver BC V5Z 3X7; Cal'08; FRCPC; Peds. (604)730-5622

ZWIEBEL, Pierre; Hotel-Dieu de Roberval, 450 rue Brassard, Roberval QC G8H 1B9; Strasbourg (France)'90; Psy. Psychiatre, Hotel-Dieu de Roberval; (418)275-0110; Fax. (418)275-4829; pierre.zwiebel@sympatico.ca.

ZWIERS, Karen G; Goldie Zwiers Maternity Clinic, 130-1402 8 Ave NW, Calgary AB T2N 1B8; Alb'97; CCFP; Clin Lecturer, University of Calgary; (403)242-1626; Fax. (403)242-4140.

ZWIMPFER, Thomas J; Gordon & Leslie Diamond HCC, 8109-2775 Laurel St, Vancouver BC V5Z 1M9; Tor'83; PhD(McG); FRCSC; Neursurg (Spine Surgery). Staff NeuroSurg, Vancouver General Hospital - Centennial Pavillion; Staff, Gordon & Leslie Diamond Health Care Centre; Clin Assoc Prof Surg, University of British Columbia; (604)875-5747; Fax. (604)269-3734.

ZWIREWICH, Charles V; Vancouver Gen Hosp, G787-855 12th Ave W, Vancouver BC V5Z 1M9; Wes'85; FRCPC; DiagRad. Assoc Staff, Vancouver General Hospital - Centennial Pavillion; (604)875-4111 x63705; Fax. (604)875-4806.

ZYGUN, David A; University of Alberta Hosp, 3C1 16WMC-8440 112 St NW, Edmonton AB T6G 2B7; Tor'96; FRCPC; IntMed (Critical Care Medicine). Staff, University of Alberta Hospital; Staff, Foothills Medical Centre; (780)407-6755; Fax. (780)407-1228.

ZYLBERGOLD, Arnold; 202-5885 ch Cote-des-Neiges, Montreal QC H3S 1Z1; McG'74; Att Staff, Sir Mortimer B Davis Jewish General; (514)342-4522; Fax. (514)342-2441.

ZYLBERGOLD-SCHONFELD, Betty; 406-5885 ch Cote-des-Neiges, Montreal QC H3S 2T2; McG'76; BSc; MDCM; Peds. Att Staff, McGill University Health Centre - Montreal Children's Hospital; Att Staff, Sir Mortimer B Davis Jewish General; McGill University; Langs: Bilingual(English/French); (514)731-0772; Fax. (514)731-3026.

ZYLBERSZAC, Bernard; 606-987 rue White, Saint-Laurent QC H4M 2Y1; Brussels (Belgium)'57; (514)386-4285

ZYPCHEN, Leslie N; Gordon & Leslie Diamond HCC, 10F-2775 Laurel St, Vancouver BC V5Z 1M9; Ott'97; FRCPC; IntMed; Hem. Staff, Vancouver General Hospital - Centennial Pavillion; Staff, Gordon & Leslie Diamond Health Care Centre; (604)875-4952; Fax. (604)875-4763.

ZYSMAN, Michele A; Don Valley Med Associates, 216-1333 Sheppard Ave E, North York ON M2J 1V1; Tor'07; CCFP; (416)498-9331; Fax. (416)498-3114; mzysman@baycrest.org.

LANGUAGES SPOKEN BY PHYSICIANS

AFRIKAANS

Dr Alan R Abelsohn, Toronto, ON - Family Medicine
Dr Carel W Ackermann, Kamloops, BC - Orthopedic Surgery
Dr Mohamed N Z Adams, Regina, SK - General Practice
Dr Anita Adlam, Terrace, BC - Pediatrics
Dr Hendrik Alberts, Welland, ON - Family Medicine
Dr Albert R Albertyn, Nipawin, SK - General Practice
Dr John E Allen, Winkler, MB - General Practice
Dr P Paul A Anderson, Perth, ON - Orthopedic Surgery
Dr Cecile L Andreas, Cranbrook, BC - General Practice
Dr Richard J Ansell, Okotoks, AB - General Practice
Dr Marius H Aucamp, Vernon, BC - General Practice
Dr Christo Baben, Cambridge, ON - Family Medicine
Dr Karen A Badenhorst, Calgary, AB - Family Medicine
Dr Josias S Badenhorst, Red Deer, AB - General Practice
Dr Frederik J Badenhorst, Selkirk, MB - General Practice
Dr Lynette Badenhorst, Winnipeg, MB - General Practice
Dr Johannes G Badenhorst, Penetanguishene, ON - Family Medicine
Dr Anthony E Barale, Sechelt, BC - Psychiatry
Dr Joanne Barker, Welland, ON - Family Medicine
Dr Frederick Barkhuizen, Penticton, BC - General Practice
Dr Cornel Barnard, Chase, BC - Family Medicine
Dr Isabel H Barnard, Kamloops, BC - Family Medicine
Dr Werner J Barnard, Regina, SK - General Practice
Dr B Norman Barwin, Ottawa, ON - General Practice
Dr Paul J Basson, Chilliwack, BC - General Practice
Dr Pravin Batohi, London, ON - Anesthesia
Dr Ernest P Behm, Terrace, BC - Diagnostic-Radiology
Dr Jacob C Bellingan, Osoyoos, BC - General Practice
Dr Johannes G Benade, Sherwood Park, AB - Family Medicine
Dr Michael G Bendall, Whitehorse, YT - Obstetrics & Gynecology
Dr Brian Berger, Richmond Hill, ON - Family Medicine
Dr Michael Berman, White Rock, BC - Ophthalmology
Dr Neil R Berrington, Winnipeg, MB - General Practice
Dr Belinda A Bester, Jasper, AB - Family Medicine
Dr Stephanus P Bester, Chilliwack, BC - General Practice
Dr Daniel Beytell, Abbotsford, BC - General Practice
Dr Lindsay Bick, Camrose, AB - General Practice
Dr Johann Blignaut, Winkler, MB - General Practice
Dr Lourens P G Blignaut, Regina, SK - General Practice
Dr Linda Bloem, Unity, SK - General Practice
Dr Charl J P Blom, Lloydminster, AB - General Practice
Dr Lourens Blom, Winnipeg, MB - Family Medicine
Dr Christine R Blom, Penetanguishene, ON - Family Medicine
Dr Jeannette Boeke, Williams Lake, BC - General Practice
Dr Erasmus J Bonthuys, Salmon Arm, BC - General Practice
Dr C Francois Booysen, Grande Prairie, AB - General Practice
Dr Johan A Boshoff, Keremeos, BC - Family Medicine
Dr Amanda Bosman, Kamloops, BC - Family Medicine
Dr Nicolaas J Botha, Fairview, AB - Family Medicine
Dr Diederick F Botha, Hardisty, AB - General Practice
Dr Daniel J P Botha, Dawson Creek, BC - Family Medicine
Dr Daniel J Botha, Dawson Creek, BC - General Practice
Dr David Botha, Hope, BC - General Practice
Dr Nicolaas C Botha, Oxbow, SK - General Practice
Dr Daniel P J Bothma, Nanaimo, BC - Family Medicine
Dr Louis B Boucher, Vernon, BC - Family Medicine
Dr Elizma Bouwer, Stettler, AB - Family Medicine
Dr David F Bowler, Comox, BC - Family Medicine
Dr John M W Bradford, Brockville, ON - Psychiatry
Dr Barend J Bredenkamp, Campbell River, BC - Psychiatry
Dr Andries P Bredenkamp, Surrey, BC - Family Medicine
Dr Johann H Brink, Coquitlam, BC - Psychiatry
Dr Bernice Brits, Surrey, BC - Family Medicine
Dr Nico Brits, Saskatoon, SK - Anatomical Pathology
Dr Owen H Brown, Port Alberni, BC - Family Medicine
Dr Candice Browne, Vancouver, BC - General Practice
Dr Karen V Brunner, Didsbury, AB - General Practice
Dr Heinrich D Brussow, High Level, AB - General Practice
Dr Jacques E Brussow, Dawson Creek, BC - General Practice
Dr Sturla E Bruun-Meyer, Toronto, ON - Psychiatry
Dr Anna D B Bruwer, Lethbridge, AB - General Practice
Dr Eduard Buchner, St. Catharines, ON - Family Medicine
Dr Nadine M Bukmuz, Toronto, ON - General Practice
Dr Octaaf S P J Bulterys, Dawson Creek, BC - General Practice
Dr Martin K Bunge, Winnipeg, MB - Diagnostic-Radiology
Dr Leon E Burger, Athabasca, AB - General Practice
Dr Lydia A Burger, Medicine Hat, AB - Family Medicine
Dr Tobias J L Burger, Dawson Creek, BC - General Practice
Dr Stephanus Buys, Quesnel, BC - General Practice
Dr Jaco Calitz, Whitecourt, AB - General Practice
Dr Essop M Cassim, Kingston, ON - General Practice
Dr G Charles Catzavelos, Cornwall, ON - Anatomical Pathology
Dr Andre Celliers, Summerside, PE - General Practice
Dr Michael Chernick, Richmond Hill, ON - Family Medicine
Dr Runjan Chetty, Toronto, ON - General Practice
Dr Anthony J Chinner, Scarborough, ON - General Practice
Dr J Pieter Claasen, Courtenay, BC - Ophthalmology
Dr Andre N Claassen, Swift Current, SK - General Practice
Dr Hendrik A Coetze, Victoria, BC - General Practice
Dr Louis J Coetzee, Bonnyville, AB - General Practice
Dr Maarten J Coetzee, Brooks, AB - General Practice
Dr Corneli M Coetzee, Prince Rupert, BC - General Practice
Dr Gillaume Coetzee, Prince Rupert, BC - General Practice
Dr Louise Coetzer, Vernon, BC - Family Medicine
Dr Celeste Collins, Campbellford, ON - Family Medicine
Dr Johan A Conradie, Calgary, AB - Internal Medicine
Dr Marius Conradie, Calgary, AB - General Practice
Dr Hannes Conradie, Kelowna, BC - Family Medicine
Dr Andrew C Cook, Comox, BC - Anesthesia
Dr Rohan Cornelissen, Prince Albert, SK - General Practice
Dr Karin Liezel Corrigan, Fox Creek, AB - General Practice
Dr John A Croft, Prince Rupert, BC - Family Medicine
Dr David P G Cronje, Miramichi, NB - General Practice
Dr Pierre D Crouse, Calgary, AB - General Practice
Dr Michael R Currin, London, ON - Anesthesia
Dr Anna-Maria Da Silva, Barrie, ON - Family Medicine
Dr Geraldine R Daniel, Surrey, BC - Family Medicine
Dr Terence Davids, Humboldt, SK - General Practice
Dr Omotayo Dawodu, Calgary, AB - Emergency Family Med
Dr Yusuf Dawood-Mohamed, Scarborough, ON - General Practice
Dr Tanja Daws, Courtenay, BC - General Practice
Dr Jan A De Beer, Vernon, BC - Family Medicine
Dr Walter De Bruin, Chilliwack, BC - Ophthalmology
Dr Maria M De Bruin, Terrace, BC - General Practice
Dr Maria E De Bruyn, Calgary, AB - Family Medicine
Dr Lodewyk P De Jager, Courtenay, BC - General Practice
Dr Jacobus F De Jager, Regina, SK - Orthopedic Surgery
Dr Heinrich L De Jongh, Whitecourt, AB - General Practice
Dr Leon De Klerk, Red Deer, AB - General Practice
Dr Matthys J De Kock, Grimshaw, AB - General Practice
Dr Victor E De Kock, Kamloops, BC - Family Medicine
Dr Stefanus F De Nysschen, Cabri, SK - General Practice
Dr Albert De Villiers, Grande Prairie, AB - General Practice
Dr Werner De Vos, Wainwright, AB - General Practice
Dr Peter W De Vos, Vanderhoof, BC - General Practice
Dr Willem E De Vynck, Langley, BC - Emergency Family Med
Dr Derick De Waal, Airdrie, AB - Family Medicine
Dr Johann De Wet, Brooks, AB - Family Medicine
Dr Steyn De Wet, Pincher Creek, AB - General Practice
Dr Susanna A De Wet, Kamloops, BC - General Practice
Dr Rene De Wet, Welland, ON - Family Medicine
Dr Arend A C Delport, Powell River, BC - General Practice
Dr Raubenheimer Denkema, Grande Prairie, AB - General Practice
Dr Judy A Dercksen, Quesnel, BC - Family Medicine
Dr Tania Diener, Regina, SK - General Practice
Dr Celeste Dietrichsen, Lethbridge, AB - General Practice
Dr Johannes Dirkschen Van Schalkwyk, Labrador City, NL - General Practice
Dr Marthinus H Doman, Boyle, AB - General Practice
Dr Allan J Donkin, Powell River, BC - General Practice
Dr Nicolette M Dreyer, Armstrong, BC - General Practice
Dr Christiaan Dreyer, Winkler, MB - General Practice
Dr Marissa Dry, Lloydminster, SK - General Practice
Dr Gert C Du Plessis, Canmore, AB - Emergency Family Med
Dr Mia Du Plessis, Edson, AB - General Practice
Dr Johan Du Plessis, Kelowna, BC - Family Medicine
Dr Pierre Du Plessis, Powell River, BC - Obstetrics & Gynecology
Dr Jean G Du Plessis, Terrace, BC - General Practice
Dr Johan Du Plooy, Brandon, MB - General Practice
Dr Amelia Du Preez, Bonnyville, AB - General Practice
Dr Miranda Du Preez, Kamloops, BC - Family Medicine
Dr Anneline Du Preez, Kimberley, BC - Family Medicine
Dr Joachim J Du Preez, Selkirk, MB - General Practice
Dr Anton E Du Toit, Leduc, AB - Family Medicine
Dr Martha C Du Toit, Ponoka, AB - General Practice
Dr Jacques H Du Toit, Powell River, BC - General Practice
Dr Jacobus J Du Toit, Miramichi, NB - General Practice
Dr Lionel Du Toit, Lloydminster, SK - General Practice
Dr Stefanus E Du Toit, Swift Current, SK - General Practice
Dr Elizabeth J Dubois, Kingston, ON - Family Medicine
Dr Anna Dunhin, North Battleford, SK - General Practice
Dr Farouk A Ebrahim, Brampton, ON - Family Medicine
Dr Darryn J Edmunds, Prince Rupert, BC - Family Medicine
Dr Ben Eksteen, Squamish, BC - Family Medicine
Dr Meandi Els, Williams Lake, BC - General Practice
Dr Stephanus J Engelbrecht, Brandon, MB - General Practice
Dr Jan Engelbrecht, Brandon, MB - General Practice
Dr Frederik H S Engelbrecht, Battleford, SK - Family Medicine
Dr Jacobus F Erasmus, Redwater, AB - General Practice
Dr Magda Erasmus, Redwater, AB - General Practice
Dr Guy R Eriksen, Surrey, BC - Diagnostic-Radiology
Dr Andries G Erlank, Quesnel, BC - Family Medicine
Dr Minette B Erlank, Quesnel, BC - General Practice
Dr Philip G Ettin, Kitchener, ON - General Practice
Dr Beverly-Ann Eysele, Prince Rupert, BC - General Practice
Dr Yousef M S Fakhry, Mississauga, ON - Ophthalmology
Dr Vincent G Falck, Calgary, AB - Anatomical Pathology
Dr Conrad Falkson, Kingston, ON - Radiation Oncology
Dr Terence J Fargher, Parry Sound, ON - Internal Medicine
Dr Hendri Faul, Medicine Hat, AB - Emergency Family Med
Dr John A Fawell, Prince Rupert, BC - General Practice
Dr Sunelle Fawell, Prince Rupert, BC - General Practice
Dr Annette S J Feigenbaum, Toronto, ON - Pediatrics
Dr Franz B Ferraris, Almonte, ON - General Practice
Dr Stephanus C Ferreira, Prince George, BC - Family Medicine
Dr Sidney W Field, White Rock, BC - General Practice
Dr Simon Field, Halifax, NS - Emergency Family Med
Dr John W Fletcher, Victoria, BC - Family Medicine
Dr Jackie A Ford, Georgetown, ON - General Practice
Dr Anna P Fourie, Sexsmith, AB - General Practice
Dr W Jacobus Fourie, Terrace, BC - General Practice
Dr Hendrina H C E Fourie, Terrace, BC - General Practice
Dr Phillip J Fourie, Yorkton, SK - General Practice
Dr Gidon Frame, Burnaby, BC - Family Medicine
Dr Patricia K Francis, Brampton, ON - Family Medicine
Dr Selby A Frank, Vegreville, AB - General Practice
Dr Alister F Frayne, Langley, BC - Family Medicine
Dr Peter-John Frew, Mission, BC - General Practice
Dr Robin I Friedlander, Burnaby, BC - Psychiatry
Dr Ernest W Fullagar, Vancouver, BC - Psychiatry
Dr Joanne P C Fynn, Moose Jaw, SK - General Practice
Dr Laurette Geldenhuys, Halifax, NS - Anatomical Pathology
Dr Dorothy I Gerber, Grande Cache, AB - Family Medicine
Dr Christiaan J F Gerber, Lloydminster, AB - General Practice
Dr Michelle R Gerber, Surrey, BC - General Practice
Dr David Gerber, Toronto, ON - Obstetrics & Gynecology
Dr Bea Gerbrands, Regina, SK - Family Medicine
Dr Werner Gericke, Saskatoon, SK - General Practice
Dr Werner E Gerntholtz, Surrey, BC - Emergency Family Med
Dr Liesel Gillies, Calgary, AB - Family Medicine

Dr Aldo Giovannoni, Fredericton, NB - Family Medicine
Dr Mario R Glas, Medicine Hat, AB - Family Medicine
Dr Andre Goetze, Dawson Creek, BC - General Practice
Dr Kevin M Goldberg, Salmon Arm, BC - General Practice
Dr Pamela R Goldberg, North York, ON - Anesthesia
Dr T Joseph Goso, Grande Prairie, AB - General Practice
Dr Glenwood D Goss, Ottawa, ON - Internal Medicine
Dr Raymond Gottschalk, Hamilton, ON - Internal Medicine
Dr Roelof Gous, Edson, AB - General Practice
Dr Daniel R Gouws, Vancouver, BC - General Practice
Dr Sundren Govender, Victoria, BC - Family Medicine
Dr Gertie Greyling, Abbotsford, BC - General Practice
Dr Johannes C Greyling, Wasaga Beach, ON - General Practice
Dr Ernst L Greyvenstein, Calgary, AB - Family Medicine
Dr Jacobus P D Grobbelaar, Brooks, AB - General Practice
Dr Josias M Grobler, Red Deer, AB - General Practice
Dr Ettiene Groenewald, Camrose, AB - General Practice
Dr Leon C Groenewald, Grande Prairie, AB - General Practice
Dr L Henriette Groenewald, Winnipeg, MB - Family Medicine
Dr Veronica A Gross, North York, ON - General Practice
Dr Christiaan J Grundling, Red Deer, AB - General Practice
Dr Margaret J Grunebaum, North York, ON - General Practice
Dr Michael D Grunow, West Vancouver, BC - Family Medicine
Dr Anita Harding, Saskatoon, SK - Obstetrics & Gynecology
Dr Paul M Harris, Regina, SK - Family Medicine
Dr Michelle Hart, Calgary, AB - General Practice
Dr Riyaan Hassen, Wabasca, AB - General Practice
Dr Evert Hattingh, Whitecourt, AB - General Practice
Dr H Suzanne Hattingh, Saskatoon, SK - General Practice
Dr William M Healley, Calgary, AB - General Practice
Dr John R Hedden, Portage La Prairie, MB - General Practice
Dr Jan-Willem Henning, Calgary, AB - Internal Medicine
Dr Jan L Henning, Owen Sound, ON - Orthopedic Surgery
Dr Maurice H J Hennink, Regina, SK - General Practice
Dr Hendrik D Henstock, Maple Ridge, BC - General Practice
Dr Martin A Herzenberg, Windsor, ON - General Practice
Dr Adriaan Heunis, Salmon Arm, BC - General Practice
Dr Edward W Hillary, Vancouver, BC - Family Medicine
Dr Micheal E Howard-Tripp, Edmonton, AB - Family Medicine
Dr Wouter L Hugo, Camrose, AB - Obstetrics & Gynecology
Dr Charles C Huisamen, Comox, BC - Emergency Family Med
Dr Stanley D Hurwitz, Richmond, BC - Family Medicine
Dr Werner K Ilse, Winnipeg, MB - Internal Medicine
Dr Philip L Immelman, Slave Lake, AB - General Practice
Dr Wessel J Ingram, Vernon, BC - Ophthalmology
Dr Johan J Jacobs, Winnipeg, MB - General Practice
Dr Annelie Janse Van Rensberg, Prince Albert, SK - Family Medicine
Dr Renier Janse Van Rensburg, Nanaimo, BC - Family Medicine
Dr Dawid A Janse Van Rensburg, Terrace, BC - Obstetrics & Gynecology
Dr Nicholas A Jansen Van Rensburg, Beausejour, MB - Family Medicine
Dr Cornelius Jansen Van Vuuren, Daysland, AB - General Practice
Dr Cornelius J Jansen Van Vuuren, Lloydminster, SK - General Practice
Dr Lize Jones, Red Deer, AB - General Practice
Dr Franz A Jonker, Medicine Hat, AB - Family Medicine
Dr Johan L Joubert, Dawson Creek, BC - General Practice
Dr Jan J M Joubert, Prince Rupert, BC - General Practice
Dr Paul F Kantor, Toronto, ON - Cardiology
Dr Magdalena J Kapp, Innisfail, AB - General Practice
Dr Stanley F Karon, Vancouver, BC - Family Medicine
Dr Geoffrey B Kaye, Edmonton, AB - Ophthalmology
Dr Madelene S Kellerman, Lethbridge, AB - General Practice
Dr Adriaan I Kellerman, Lillooet, BC - General Practice
Dr Elizabeth G Kelly, Olds, AB - General Practice
Dr Theo Kemp, Blackfalds, AB - General Practice
Dr Ilse Kemp, Gander, NL - Pediatrics
Dr Michael R Kenyon, Terrace, BC - Internal Medicine
Dr Thomas E Kerlis, Lloydminster, AB - General Practice
Dr Daniel S Kilian, Penticton, BC - General Practice
Dr Rochagne Kilian, Williams Lake, BC - Family Medicine
Dr Sven Kip, Kamloops, BC - Family Medicine
Dr Andre R Kirsten, Nelson, BC - Family Medicine
Dr Pierre J Kirwin, North York, ON - Physical Medicine & Rehab
Dr Douwe Kits, Brooks, AB - General Practice
Dr Arno Kitshoff, Port Alberni, BC - General Practice
Dr Johanna H Klopper, Athabasca, AB - General Practice
Dr Stephanus P Kloppers, Chilliwack, BC - General Practice
Dr Johan F Kritzinger, Dawson Creek, BC - General Practice
Dr Jan Kroeze, Chilliwack, BC - General Practice
Dr Petrus F Kruger, Edmonton, AB - General Practice
Dr Pieter Ernst Kruger, Fort McMurray, AB - General Practice
Dr Stephanus J Kruger, Red Deer, AB - General Practice
Dr Frederick J Kruger, Kamloops, BC - Family Medicine
Dr Fernando H Kuhn, Abbotsford, BC - General Practice
Dr Mari C La Cock, North Battleford, SK - General Practice
Dr Hugo Lambrechts, Pine Falls, MB - General Practice
Dr Gideon P Lamprecht, Vanderhoof, BC - General Practice
Dr Michael L Lang, Regina, SK - Anesthesia
Dr Jan H J Lategan, Westlock, AB - General Practice
Dr Muriel L Laxdal, Biggar, SK - General Practice
Dr Johannes L Le Roux, Airdrie, AB - Family Medicine
Dr Jacobus J Le Roux, Quesnel, BC - Family Medicine
Dr Noelene Le Roux, Prince Albert, SK - General Practice
Dr Carl J Le Roux, Saskatoon, SK - General Practice
Dr Brian P Lee, Wetaskiwin, AB - General Practice
Dr Archie Lee Son, Vancouver, BC - General Practice
Dr Leon B Lerm, Lindsay, ON - Family Medicine
Dr Wilfred Levin, Toronto, ON - Radiation Oncology
Dr Sheila Lewin, Toronto, ON - General Practice
Dr Tersia Lichtenstein, Kelowna, BC - General Practice
Dr Mogamad N Lilla, Chilliwack, BC - Psychiatry
Dr Hilton Ling, Vancouver, BC - Cardiovasc/ThorSurg
Dr Willem S J Lombard, Kitimat, BC - General Surgery
Dr Theodore P Lombard, Brantford, ON - Anesthesia
Dr John W S Longland, Williams Lake, BC - General Practice
Dr Wian H Lotter, La Scie, NL - General Practice
Dr Petrus C Lotz, Terrace, BC - General Practice
Dr Albertus B Lotz, Regina, SK - General Practice
Dr Heloise Lotz, Regina, SK - General Practice
Dr Tracey A Lotze, Prince George, BC - General Practice
Dr Michael Loudon, Teulon, MB - General Practice
Dr Marc Lourens, Salmon Arm, BC - General Practice
Dr Deon F Louw, Calgary, AB - Neurosurgery
Dr Wynand F Louw, Invermere, BC - Family Medicine
Dr Ursula Luitingh, Maple Ridge, BC - General Practice
Dr Eugene W A Magerman, Calgary, AB - General Practice
Dr Johannes J Malan, Calgary, AB - General Practice
Dr Francois A Malan, Lethbridge, AB - General Practice
Dr Stephan P Malan, Provost, AB - General Practice
Dr Johann H Malan, Saskatoon, SK - General Practice
Dr Cilliers Marais, Maple Ridge, BC - General Practice
Dr Lutz Marburg, Edmonton, AB - General Practice
Dr Jean-Pierre Mare, Lac La Biche, AB - Family Medicine
Dr Narinda Maree, Moose Jaw, SK - General Practice
Dr David C Maresky, Toronto, ON - Pediatrics
Dr Ivor J Margolis, Brampton, ON - Pediatrics
Dr Justin R Marillier, Slave Lake, AB - General Practice
Dr Theo Marx, Swan River, MB - General Practice
Dr Michele A Matter, Selkirk, MB - Family Medicine
Dr Colleen Maytham, Invermere, BC - Family Medicine
Dr Peter A N Maytom, Nelson, BC - Ophthalmology
Dr Johannes J McCallaghan, Port Coquitlam, BC - General Practice
Dr Johannes V McDonald, Quesnel, BC - General Practice
Dr Monica McKay, Williams Lake, BC - General Practice
Dr Wilhelm A H C Meerholz, Cochrane, AB - General Practice
Dr Mtimkulu Mehlomakulu, Kingston, ON - Pediatrics
Dr Madeleine E Meiring, Medicine Hat, AB - Family Medicine
Dr Helena J Mentz, Calgary, AB - General Practice
Dr Jan M Meyburg, Terrace, BC - General Practice
Dr Johannes G Meyer, Coaldale, AB - Family Medicine
Dr Petrus S Meyer, Cold Lake, AB - General Practice
Dr Marius G Meyer, Dawson Creek, BC - General Practice
Dr Frederick J T Meyer, Port Alberni, BC - General Practice
Dr Melissa Meyer, Powell River, BC - General Practice
Dr Catharina J Meyer, Carlyle, SK - Family Medicine
Dr Jeffrey Meyerson, Hamilton, ON - Endocrin/Metabolism
Dr Shabir M Mia, Saskatoon, SK - General Practice
Dr Dinesh J Mistry, Golden, BC - Family Medicine
Dr Mohamed Moolla, Regina, SK - General Practice
Dr Johnathan Moolman, Terrace, BC - General Practice
Dr Andre Moolman, Kitchener, ON - Family Medicine
Dr Michele A Moss, Calgary, AB - General Practice
Dr Andreas W Mostert, Revelstoke, BC - Family Medicine
Dr Francois D P Mostert, Winkler, MB - General Practice
Dr Rasheda Motala, Calgary, AB - Family Medicine
Dr Godwin P Mouton, Redwater, AB - Family Medicine
Dr J Stefan Mulder, Nanaimo, BC - General Practice
Dr Diederik J Muller, Shoal Lake, MB - Family Medicine
Dr Andries J Muller, Saskatoon, SK - Family Medicine
Dr Magnus Murphy, Calgary, AB - Obstetrics & Gynecology
Dr Andrew Murray, Nelson, BC - Family Medicine
Dr Willem M Myburgh, Red Deer, AB - Family Medicine
Dr Johannes L Myburgh, Sylvan Lake, AB - General Practice
Dr Karunagaran Naidoo, Lloydminster, AB - General Surgery
Dr Prenilla Naidu, Edmonton, AB - General Practice
Dr Dharmesh J Natha, White Rock, BC - Family Medicine
Dr Bharat C Nathoo, Richmond Hill, ON - Internal Medicine
Dr Adel H Naude, Lloydminster, AB - General Practice
Dr Francois P Naude, Lloydminster, AB - General Practice
Dr Jan J S Naude, Powell River, BC - General Practice
Dr Gert P Nel, Olds, AB - General Practice
Dr Izak B Nel, Port Alberni, BC - General Practice
Dr Philip N Nel, Prince Rupert, BC - General Surgery
Dr Hermann S Nell, Port Alberni, BC - General Practice
Dr Christoffel H Neveling, Dawson Creek, BC - Anesthesia
Dr Michael J Newton, Abbotsford, BC - General Practice
Dr Riaan Nieman, Viking, AB - General Practice
Dr Rudolph E Niemand, Sylvan Lake, AB - General Practice
Dr Stephanus Nieuwoudt, Lacombe, AB - General Practice
Dr Josephus J Nolte, Surrey, BC - Family Medicine
Dr Werner Oberholzer, Radville, SK - Family Medicine
Dr Ana-Maria Oelschig, Okotoks, AB - General Practice
Dr Jean M Oosthuizen, Ottawa, ON - Family Medicine
Dr Christopher P E Outram, Kelowna, BC - General Practice
Dr Nigel A Painter, Prince Albert, SK - General Practice
Dr David M A Paisley, Penticton, BC - General Practice
Dr John Paleta, Hubbards, NS - General Practice
Dr Sandra Pansegrouw, Penticton, BC - Family Medicine
Dr Jhodipraghasen Pather, Lloydminster, SK - General Practice
Dr Margot Patterson, Denwood, AB - General Practice
Dr Motlobeng D Pebane, Indian Head, SK - General Practice
Dr Elaine F Peddie, Vancouver, BC - Family Medicine
Dr Erus J Peens, Rocky-Mtn-Hse, AB - General Practice
Dr Ihsaan C Peer, Abbotsford, BC - Family Medicine
Dr Jeffrey E Peimer, Williams Lake, BC - General Practice
Dr John R H Penhall, Campbell River, BC - Family Medicine
Dr Jose L Pereira, Ottawa, ON - Family Medicine
Dr Jacobus A L Perold, White Rock, BC - Family Medicine
Dr Hein Peters, Winnipeg, MB - Family Medicine
Dr Sonja Pienaar, Calgary, AB - Family Medicine
Dr Colette Pienaar, Burnaby, BC - General Practice
Dr Louise Pienaar, Lantzville, BC - Family Medicine
Dr Marius P Pienaar, Prince Rupert, BC - Obstetrics & Gynecology
Dr Leonie Pieterse, Grande Prairie, AB - General Practice
Dr Shunmoogam W Pillay, Surrey, BC - Geriatric Medicine
Dr Johann D D Pitout, Calgary, AB - General Practice
Dr Stephanus D Potgieter, Stony Plain, AB - Emergency Family Med
Dr Martelle Preller, Calgary, AB - Family Medicine
Dr Juan M Pretorius, Mission, BC - General Practice
Dr Barbara A Pretorius, Smithers, BC - General Practice
Dr Luzelle Pretorius, Steinbach, MB - General Practice
Dr Alexander P Pretorius, Winnipeg, MB - Anesthesia
Dr Marina Pretorius, Lindsay, ON - Family Medicine
Dr Johannes Prins, Lacombe, AB - General Practice
Dr Willem N Prinsloo, Campbell River, BC - Family Medicine
Dr Gerrit C Prinsloo, Williams Lake, BC - General Practice
Dr Abel H Raath, Consort, AB - Family Medicine
Dr Johannes J Raath, New Westminster, BC - Family Medicine
Dr Christiaan S Rabie, Calgary, AB - General Practice
Dr Anton M Raubenheimer, Smoky Lake, AB - General Practice
Dr Stephan Raubenheimer, Smoky Lake, AB - Family Medicine
Dr Johannes N Redelinghuys, Cambridge, ON - Family Medicine

Dr Carolus J Reinecke, Nelson, BC - General Practice
Dr PJ Petrus Retief, Chilliwack, BC - Family Medicine
Dr Gary Richardson, Nanaimo, BC - Family Medicine
Dr Eugene F Ries, Cranbrook, BC - General Practice
Dr Wynne M Rigal, Edmonton, AB - Orthopedic Surgery
Dr Arthur Robinson, Saskatoon, SK - Family Medicine
Dr Frauke Rode, Victoria, BC - General Practice
Dr Kurt R E Roelens, Saskatoon, SK - General Practice
Dr Louisa F Roets, Moosomin, SK - General Practice
Dr Paul C J Rogers, Vancouver, BC - Pediatrics
Dr Lourene A Roode, Calgary, AB - Family Medicine
Dr Estelle L Roos, Calgary, AB - General Practice
Dr David E Rosman, Vaughan, ON - Obstetrics & Gynecology
Dr Vincent E Rossouw, Duncan, BC - General Practice
Dr Pieter A Rossouw, Powell River, BC - Family Medicine
Dr Linell Rossouw, Regina, SK - General Practice
Dr Ettienne Roux, Dawson Creek, BC - General Practice
Dr Jan G Roux, Virden, MB - General Practice
Dr Emile V W Roux, Miramichi, NB - General Practice
Dr Marek A Rozwadowski, Port Alberni, BC - General Practice
Dr Steven Z Rubin, Calgary, AB - General Surgery
Dr Marius J I Saayman, Kamloops, BC - Anesthesia
Dr Herbert W Sacks, Edmonton, AB - Family Medicine
Dr Karen Saperson, Hamilton, ON - Psychiatry
Dr Gavin R Sapsford, Victoria, BC - Anesthesia
Dr Anton Scamvougeras, Vancouver, BC - Psychiatry
Dr W Albrecht Schall, York, ON - Anatomical Pathology
Dr Louis D V Scheepers, Vancouver, BC - Anesthesia
Dr Jan J Scheeres, Barrie, ON - Obstetrics & Gynecology
Dr Kim E Scher, Fort Erie, ON - Family Medicine
Dr Gunther Schlenther, Ponoka, AB - General Practice
Dr Meyer Schoeman, Innisfail, AB - General Practice
Dr Stefan Schoeman, Courtenay, BC - Emergency Family Med
Dr Hendrik N Schoeman, Oshawa, ON - Family Medicine
Dr Mervin Scholtz, Chilliwack, BC - Family Medicine
Dr Martin M Scholtz, Smithers, BC - General Practice
Dr Lindi Scribante, Lloydminster, AB - General Practice
Dr Ivan G Scrooby, Williams Lake, BC - General Practice
Dr P Gareth R Seaward, Toronto, ON - Obstetrics & Gynecology
Dr Isidor Segers, Kelowna, BC - General Practice
Dr Roger C Seldon, Campbell River, BC - Family Medicine
Dr Margaretha A Senekal, St Paul, AB - General Practice
Dr Lance B Setterfield, Victoria, BC - General Practice
Dr Colin M Shapiro, Toronto, ON - Psychiatry
Dr Morris Sherman, Toronto, ON - Internal Medicine
Dr Kevin Shiffman, Whitby, ON - Psychiatry
Dr Gina Shochat, Toronto, ON - Family Medicine
Dr Neal A Shone, Abbotsford, BC - Obstetrics & Gynecology
Dr Desmond Shulman, Red Deer, AB - General Practice
Dr Cecilia Siegling, Prince George, BC - Family Medicine
Dr Jacques Simenhoff, Parksville, BC - General Practice
Dr Gertjan Simons, Cranbrook, BC - General Surgery
Dr Ian W C Simons, Killarney, MB - General Practice
Dr Dharumaraj Singaram, Brampton, ON - Family Medicine
Dr Minesh Singh, Windsor, ON - General Surgery
Dr Wilma L Sirkin, North York, ON - Anatomical Pathology
Dr Willem H Slabbert, Camrose, AB - General Practice
Dr Dalibor E Slavik, Saskatoon, SK - Family Medicine
Dr I A Jeremy Sloan, North York, ON - Anesthesia
Dr Mudi Smit, Calgary, AB - Family Medicine
Dr Louwrens E Smit, Edmonton, AB - Psychiatry
Dr Kenneth H Smit, Lacombe, AB - Family Medicine
Dr Deon F Smit, Chilliwack, BC - General Practice
Dr Andries A Smit, Merritt, BC - General Practice
Dr Johan Smit, Port Alberni, BC - General Practice
Dr Dirk J Smit, Port Alberni, BC - General Practice
Dr Cecile Smit, Port Alberni, BC - General Practice
Dr Jacques-Henri Smit, Prince Rupert, BC - Anesthesia
Dr Morne M Smit, Quesnel, BC - Family Medicine
Dr Nelis Smit, Quesnel, BC - General Practice
Dr Gideon Smit, Vernon, BC - General Practice
Dr Alexander J Smith, Drayton Valley, AB - General Practice
Dr Quentin A Smith, Chilliwack, BC - Family Medicine
Dr Jan D W Smith, Chilliwack, BC - Obstetrics & Gynecology
Dr Erasmus J Smith, Nanaimo, BC - Orthopedic Surgery
Dr Samuel A Smith, Prince Rupert, BC - General Practice
Dr David V B Smith, Princeton, BC - Family Medicine
Dr Helene Smith, Quesnel, BC - General Practice
Dr Louis F Smith, Winnipeg, MB - Family Medicine
Dr Patricia A Smith, Hamilton, ON - Obstetrics & Gynecology
Dr Marianna S Snyman, Chilliwack, BC - General Practice
Dr Marius R Snyman, Penticton, BC - Family Medicine
Dr Adam J Snyman, Toronto, ON - Anesthesia
Dr Barend J Sonnenberg, Edmonton, AB - General Practice
Dr Elias Soumbasis, Calgary, AB - Family Medicine
Dr Edwin B Spence, Ottawa, ON - General Practice
Dr Leonore D Stampa, Olds, AB - Family Medicine
Dr Wayne E Stanley, Lindsay, ON - Family Medicine
Dr Bruce T Starke, Golden, BC - General Practice
Dr Robert D Stecher, Carp, ON - Family Medicine
Dr Stefanie Steel, Nanaimo, BC - Family Medicine
Dr Melane Steenberg, Swift Current, SK - General Practice
Dr Jakobus W Steenkamp, Cut Knife, SK - General Practice
Dr Robert M Steffen, Melfort, SK - Family Medicine
Dr Raymond D Stein, Toronto, ON - Clin Immun/Allergy
Dr Johannes L Steinberg, Chilliwack, BC - Otolaryngology
Dr Ernest F Stephan, Parksville, BC - General Practice
Dr Jolien A Steyl, Williams Lake, BC - General Practice
Dr Morrison F Steyn, Medicine Hat, AB - General Practice
Dr Jacobus H Steyn, Kamloops, BC - General Practice
Dr Marius F Steyn, Lantzville, BC - Family Medicine
Dr Janus Steyn, Vernon, BC - General Practice
Dr Jacobus J Steyn, Brockville, ON - Family Medicine
Dr Mariette Steyn, Brockville, ON - Family Medicine
Dr Chris Steyn, London, ON - Family Medicine
Dr Pierre G Steyn, Ottawa, ON - General Practice
Dr Jacobus A Steyn, Prince Albert, SK - General Practice
Dr Eric E Stockenstrom, Vancouver, BC - General Practice
Dr Christina I Stocks, Lethbridge, AB - General Practice
Dr James G Stopforth, Chilliwack, BC - Family Medicine
Dr Jeanne Stopforth, Chilliwack, BC - General Practice
Dr Caron Strahlendorf, Vancouver, BC - General Practice
Dr Frederik J Strauss, Calgary, AB - General Practice
Dr Jacoba C Strauss, Calgary, AB - General Practice
Dr Pieter Strauss, Abbotsford, BC - Psychiatry
Dr Carin S Strydom, Grande Prairie, AB - Family Medicine
Dr Henriette Strydom, Powell River, BC - General Practice
Dr Jacobus Strydom, Terrace, BC - General Practice
Dr Gerhardus J Strydom, Vancouver, BC - General Practice
Dr Heinre Strydom, Saskatoon, SK - General Practice
Dr Robert L Sutherland, Campbell River, BC - Family Medicine
Dr Abraham C J Swanepoel, Jasper, AB - General Practice
Dr Vandeurs Swart, Calgary, AB - General Practice
Dr Henry C Swart, Summerside, PE - General Practice
Dr Carin Swartz, Wetaskiwin, AB - General Practice
Dr Roxanne L Swiegers, Medicine Hat, AB - Family Medicine
Dr Jonathan Tankel, Edmonton, AB - Obstetrics & Gynecology
Dr Garnett M Tarr, Osoyoos, BC - General Practice
Dr Ivor Teitelbaum, North York, ON - General Practice
Dr Ockert C Terblanche, Edmonton, AB - Anesthesia
Dr Paul C Terlien, Duncan, BC - Family Medicine
Dr Bhavna K Thakersee, Waterdown, ON - Family Medicine
Dr Angela G Thermann, Vancouver, BC - General Practice
Dr Jan J H Theron, Comox, BC - Pediatrics
Dr Karina Theron, Salmon Arm, BC - General Practice
Dr Andrew Travlos, Vancouver, BC - Physical Medicine & Rehab
Dr Shaun K Tregoning, Abbotsford, BC - Obstetrics & Gynecology
Dr Jean J Trollip, Ottawa, ON - Family Medicine
Dr Danel Ungerer, St. Albert, AB - General Practice
Dr Kenneth J Upton, Vernon, BC - Obstetrics & Gynecology
Dr Tharina Uys, Brandon, MB - General Practice
Dr Renier G Van Aardt, Truro, NS - Family Medicine
Dr Lucretia Van Den Berg, Toronto, ON - Internal Medicine
Dr Jan D Van Der Berg, Red Deer, AB - General Practice
Dr Etienne Van Der Linde, Clarenville, NL - General Practice
Dr Hubertus Van Der Lugt, Cranbrook, BC - Psychiatry
Dr Johann V Van Der Merwe, Calgary, AB - General Practice
Dr Phillip W Van Der Merwe, Calgary, AB - Family Medicine
Dr Estie Van Der Merwe, Edson, AB - General Practice
Dr Cornelis M Van Der Merwe, Lloydminster, AB - General Practice
Dr Errol J Van Der Merwe, Merritt, BC - General Practice
Dr Daniel T H Van Der Merwe, Port Alberni, BC - General Practice
Dr Daniel F Van Der Merwe, Port Alberni, BC - General Practice
Dr Johannes M Van Der Merwe, Vancouver, BC - Orthopedic Surgery
Dr Shirley G Van Der Merwe, Vernon, BC - General Practice
Dr Francina J Van Der Merwe, Williams Lake, BC - General Practice
Dr Herman S Van Der Merwe, Elkhorn, MB - Family Medicine
Dr Adam B Van Der Merwe, Saskatoon, SK - General Practice
Dr Susanna M Van Der Vyver, Nelson, BC - General Practice
Dr Izak A Van Der Vyver, Summerland, BC - General Practice
Dr Marthinus J Van Der Vyver, Toronto, ON - Anesthesia
Dr Petrus J Van Der Walt, Cold Lake, AB - General Practice
Dr Johannes C Van Der Walt, Wetaskiwin, AB - General Practice
Dr Louiza Van Der Walt, Welland, ON - Family Medicine
Dr Adriaan D F Van Der Wart, Prince Rupert, BC - Family Medicine
Dr Gabriel J E Van Der Watt, Calgary, AB - General Practice
Dr Leon Van Der Watt, Regina, SK - General Practice
Dr Christiaan L Van Der Westhuizen, Ponoka, AB - Family Medicine
Dr Aletta H Van Dyk, Calgary, AB - General Practice
Dr Frederick P Van Dyk, Quesnel, BC - General Practice
Dr Werner W A Van Dyk, Winnipeg, MB - Emergency Family Med
Dr Johannes H Van Eeden, Vancouver, BC - General Practice
Dr Stephanus F Van Eeden, Vancouver, BC - Internal Medicine
Dr Johannes C Van Heerde, Fort McMurray, AB - General Practice
Dr Alida Van Heerden, Leduc, AB - General Practice
Dr Andre Van Heerden, Kelowna, BC - Family Medicine
Dr Lizaan Van Heerden, Quesnel, BC - General Practice
Dr Gert B Van Heerden, Moose Jaw, SK - General Practice
Dr Aletta J Van Heerden, Moose Jaw, SK - General Practice
Dr Hendrik G Van Heerden, Nipawin, SK - General Practice
Dr Werner D Van Jaarsveldt, Winnipeg, MB - Family Medicine
Dr Izak J M Van Niekerk, Lacombe, AB - General Practice
Dr Dirk J T Van Niekerk, Vancouver, BC - Anatomical Pathology
Dr Esias R Van Rensburg, Vancouver, BC - Pediatrics
Dr Henrietta M Van Rooi, Calgary, AB - Family Medicine
Dr Tersia Van Rooijen, Williams Lake, BC - General Practice
Dr Calin L Van Rooyen, Viking, AB - General Practice
Dr Daniel J Van Schalkwyk, Whitecourt, AB - General Practice
Dr Jacobus J Van Sittert, Comox, BC - Orthopedic Surgery
Dr Lambert W Van Sittert, Welland, ON - Emergency Family Med
Dr Jacobus P L Van Straaten, Lethbridge, AB - General Practice
Dr Andre R Van Wyk, Langley, BC - Family Medicine
Dr Hadriaan S Van Wyk, Williams Lake, BC - General Practice
Dr Audrey Van Zanten, Saskatoon, SK - General Practice
Dr Anneleen Van Zyl, Port Alberni, BC - General Practice
Dr Andre Van Zyl, Port Alberni, BC - Family Medicine
Dr Johannes P Van Zyl, Prince George, BC - Orthopedic Surgery
Dr Maria-Louise Van Zyl, Vernon, BC - Family Medicine
Dr Andre T Van Zyl, Gander, NL - General Practice
Dr Leendert P C Van Zyl, Barrie, ON - General Practice
Dr Lizette Van Zyl, Owen Sound, ON - Family Medicine
Dr Cornelius J Van Zyl, Owen Sound, ON - Emergency Family Med
Dr William P Van Zyl, Scarborough, ON - General Practice
Dr Louis T Van Zyl, Toronto, ON - Psychiatry
Dr Mariam Vania, North York, ON - Psychiatry
Dr Martin Veith, Prince Albert, SK - General Practice
Dr Gerrit C Velthuysen, Quesnel, BC - General Practice
Dr J Christiaan Venter, Wetaskiwin, AB - Family Medicine
Dr Anton Venter, Chetwynd, BC - General Practice
Dr Herman C A Venter, Salmon Arm, BC - General Practice
Dr Jan F Venter, Vancouver, BC - Family Medicine
Dr Hendrik L Venter, Fonthill, ON - Family Medicine
Dr Willem A Viljoen, Calgary, AB - General Practice
Dr Johann H Viljoen, Red Deer, AB - Family Medicine
Dr Rene Viljoen, Red Deer, AB - Family Medicine
Dr Johan Viljoen, St Catharines, ON - Obstetrics & Gynecology
Dr Etienne E Vilonel, North Vancouver, BC - General Practice
Dr Mark D Vincent, London, ON - Internal Medicine

Dr Pieter J Visser, Wainwright, AB - General Practice
Dr Nicolaas C Vlok, Brandon, MB - Family Medicine
Dr Martin V Vogel, Ottawa, ON - General Practice
Dr Mark T R Vooght, Moose Jaw, SK - General Practice
Dr Alewyn P Vorster, Treherne, MB - General Practice
Dr Sarel Vorster, Lindsay, ON - Family Medicine
Dr Johannes J Vorster, Yorkton, SK - General Practice
Dr Dianne L Vosloo, Burnaby, BC - Family Medicine
Dr Johannes M B Wagenaar, Qualicum Beach, BC - General Practice
Dr Marius C Wahl, Kitimat, BC - General Practice
Dr Lukmaan Waja, North Bay, ON - Obstetrics & Gynecology
Dr Malcolm G Walker, Fort McMurray, AB - Family Medicine
Dr Mark B Walker, Quesnel, BC - General Practice
Dr Wilhelm H Warmenhoven, Maple Ridge, BC - General Practice
Dr Marthinus Wasserfall, Vancouver, BC - Family Medicine
Dr Delene Wassermann, Williams Lake, BC - General Practice
Dr Charles D Webb, Vancouver, BC - General Practice
Dr Tanya Weideman, Cochrane, AB - General Practice
Dr Sophie-Anne Weimar, Kamloops, BC - Family Medicine
Dr Mimi B Weldon, Surrey, BC - Family Medicine
Dr Kathryn Wentworth, Cranbrook, BC - General Practice
Dr Johann D Wentzel, Kerrobert, SK - General Practice
Dr Ronald Werb, Vancouver, BC - Internal Medicine
Dr Isabella M Werkman, St Paul, AB - General Practice
Dr Philip H Wessels, Lloydminster, AB - General Practice
Dr Marie-Louise Wessels, Victoria, BC - Family Medicine
Dr Jacques West, Abbotsford, BC - General Practice
Dr Michael J Whitehead, Kamloops, BC - Anesthesia
Dr George J Wiehahn, Kamloops, BC - Psychiatry
Dr Ben Wiese, Kelowna, BC - General Practice
Dr Lize Wiese, Kelowna, BC - General Practice
Dr Nicola Wiggelinkhuizen, Vernon, BC - Family Medicine
Dr M Christo Wiggins, Chilliwack, BC - General Surgery
Dr Estelle M Wiid, Westbank, BC - General Practice
Dr Waldemar P Wilken, Calgary, AB - Family Medicine
Dr Michael R Wilkinson, Vancouver, BC - General Practice
Dr Pieter Willemse Sr, Dauphin, MB - General Practice
Dr Pieter Williams, Maple Ridge, BC - General Practice
Dr Marianne I J Willis, Oliver, BC - Family Medicine
Dr Adriaan Windt, Abbotsford, BC - General Practice
Dr Jeffrey A Wollach, Victoria, BC - Anesthesia
Dr Clare M P F Wood, Victoria, BC - Psychiatry
Dr Kevin C Woudstra, Houston, BC - General Practice
Dr Jeffrey I Wulffhart, North York, ON - Family Medicine
Dr Melani Zaayman, Port Hardy, BC - General Practice
Dr Stefan R de Swardt, Williams Lake, BC - General Practice
Dr Magarietha J du Plooy, Red Deer, AB - General Practice
Dr Petrus J van Niekerk, Terrace, BC - General Practice

AKAN

Dr Theophilus Ampofo, Toronto, ON - General Practice
Dr Ahmed Boachie, Newmarket, ON - Psychiatry
Dr Clarence E Clottey, Oakville, ON - Family Medicine
Dr Nana Graves, Dollard-D-Ormeaux, QC - Pediatrics
Dr Albert Gyimah, Brampton, ON - Psychiatry
Dr Isaac Odame, Toronto, ON - General Practice
Dr Henry I Quaye, Stony Plain, AB - General Practice
Dr Obodai Sai, Scarborough, ON - Psychiatry
Dr Francis B Sam, North York, ON - Obstetrics & Gynecology
Dr Barnaby E A Tamakloe, East York, ON - Psychiatry
Dr David Y Twum-Barima, Oakville, ON - Internal Medicine
Dr Kofi A Wudom, Brampton, ON - Family Medicine

AKLANON

Dr Karen A Gronau, Brampton, ON - Obstetrics & Gynecology

ALBANIAN

Dr Khami Chokani, Prince Albert, SK - General Practice
Dr Enkelejda Delialllisi, Newmarket, ON - General Surgery
Dr Enver Deliu, Halifax, NS - Family Medicine
Dr Juliana Gorja, Whitby, ON - Family Medicine
Dr Delvina Hasimja Saraqini, Ottawa, ON - Internal Medicine
Dr Briseida Mema, Toronto, ON - Pediatrics
Dr Roland Mollanji, North York, ON - Family Medicine
Dr Elvira Yakoub, Windsor, ON - Family Medicine

AMERICAN SIGN LANGUAGE

Dr Christopher A Bauer, Kentville, NS - General Practice
Dr Hartley B Bressler, North York, ON - General Practice
Dr Paul J Daeninck, Winnipeg, MB - Internal Medicine
Dr Linda Gagnon, Dartmouth, NS - Family Medicine
Dr Salvatore J Scala, Toronto, ON - General Practice
Dr Michael R Taylor, Ottawa, ON - Emergency Family Med
Dr Maria Valois, Toronto, ON - Internal Medicine
Dr Carol S Yang, Ottawa, ON - General Practice

AMHARIC

Dr Efrem Alemayehu, Toronto, ON - General Practice
Dr Kebede H Amede, Brandon, MB - General Practice
Dr Getnet A Asrat, Perth, ON - Family Medicine
Dr Berhanu Balcha, Winnipeg, MB - General Practice
Dr Katyg Behesnilian, Toronto, ON - Psychiatry
Dr Ledjalem A Daba, Woodbridge, ON - Cardiology
Dr Tadese F Debretsion, Oakville, ON - Family Medicine
Dr Yidersal Gebeyehu, Kitchener, ON - Family Medicine
Dr Ephrem Gebrechristos, York, ON - General Surgery
Dr Eyob Gebremicael, Oshawa, ON - General Practice
Dr Fikre A Germa, Brantford, ON - Emergency Family Med
Dr Haregua Getu, Toronto, ON - General Practice
Dr Biruk Y Habteselassie, Newmarket, ON - Family Medicine
Dr Helena Haile Meskel, Scarborough, ON - Anatomical Pathology
Dr Yemisrach Hailemeskel, Toronto, ON - Family Medicine
Dr Maru E Hailu, Oshawa, ON - Family Medicine
Dr Tewodros G Mequanent, Grande Prairie, AB - Family Medicine
Dr Cherinet Seid, Deep River, ON - Family Medicine
Dr Makeda Semret, Montreal, QC - Infectious Diseases
Dr Amde M Teferi, Guelph, ON - Psychiatry
Dr Edo Teku, Toronto, ON - Family Medicine
Dr Yoseph Tesfaye, Montreal, QC - General Practice
Dr Edemariam Tsega, Hamilton, ON - Internal Medicine

ARABIC

Dr Fayez Abboud, Gatineau, QC - General Practice
Dr Amel Abdallah, Thunder Bay, ON - Family Medicine
Dr Farid M Abdel Hadi, Whitby, ON - Obstetrics & Gynecology
Dr Abdel M K Abdel Meguid, Brampton, ON - General Practice
Dr Mona A M Abdel-Bary, Richmond Hill, ON - Family Medicine
Dr Mohamed M Abdel-Fattah, North Vancouver, BC - Psychiatry
Dr Mohamed A Abdel-Keriem, Calgary, AB - Psychiatry
Dr Mamdouh Z Abdel-Malak, Thunder Bay, ON - Urology
Dr Maximous Y M Abdel-Malek, Mississauga, ON - Family Medicine
Dr Husam-Eldin M Abdel-Qadir, Toronto, ON - Internal Medicine
Dr Hama S I Abdel-Salam, Espanola, ON - Family Medicine
Dr Abdelgalel Abdelgader, Windsor, ON - Internal Medicine
Dr Mohamed M M S Abdelhaleem, Toronto, ON - Hematological Pathology
Dr Essam A Y Abdelmottal, Kingston, ON - General Practice
Dr Ghanim I Abdelsalam, York, ON - Family Medicine
Dr Hasan Abdessamad, Vancouver, BC - Obstetrics & Gynecology
Dr Ibrahim Abdul-Rahman, Oshawa, ON - Family Medicine
Dr Mohamed H Abdulhadi, Regina, SK - Internal Medicine
Dr Amid K Abdullah, Calgary, AB - General Pathology
Dr Atef A M Abdulsamad, Edmonton, AB - Family Medicine
Dr Esmail Abej, Winnipeg, MB - Family Medicine
Dr Anthony Abela, Montreal, QC - Otolaryngology
Dr Victor Abikhzer, Montreal, QC - General Practice
Dr Oussama A Abla, Toronto, ON - General Practice
Dr Ayman A Aboguddah, Regina, SK - Cardiology
Dr Mirna Abou Abdo, Gatineau, QC - General Practice
Dr Yasser Abou Mourad, Vancouver, BC - Internal Medicine
Dr Edith Abou Said, Ottawa, ON - Family Medicine
Dr Iman Abou-Gareeb, Richmond, BC - Family Medicine
Dr Awni Abou-Nassar, Mississauga, ON - General Practice
Dr Maher K M Abou-Seido, Brampton, ON - Obstetrics & Gynecology
Dr Jamal Aboujamra, Toronto, ON - Family Medicine
Dr Samir Abouna, Mississauga, ON - Family Medicine
Dr Dikran J Abrahamian, Penetanguishene, ON - General Practice
Dr Farid Absi, Trois-Rivieres, QC - Internal Medicine
Dr Anwar H M Abu Dieh, Kanata, ON - Family Medicine
Dr Maysan Abu-Hakima, Calgary, AB - Internal Medicine
Dr Mohamed A Abufayed, Edmonton, AB - Family Medicine
Dr Read M A Abughaduma, Scarborough, ON - Orthopedic Surgery
Dr Tareq S M Abughamja, Toronto, ON - Family Medicine
Dr Ahmed M Abuhelala, Edmonton, AB - General Practice
Dr Ramzi Y Abunassar, Ottawa, ON - Internal Medicine
Dr Madeleine Achkar, Laval, QC - General Practice
Dr Yasser Ad-Dab'bagh, Ottawa, ON - Psychiatry
Dr Niam Adamo, Mississauga, ON - Family Medicine
Dr Moustafa A A Adams, Edmonton, AB - General Practice
Dr Hany A M M Aeta, Orleans, ON - General Practice
Dr Rasheed A E Affifi, Thornhill, ON - General Surgery
Dr Victor A Ahad, Verdun, QC - Internal Medicine
Dr Hala M A Ahmed, Surrey, BC - Family Medicine
Dr Nafeesa Q Ahmed, Oakville, ON - General Practice
Dr Syed T Ahmed, St Thomas, ON - Pediatrics
Dr Abdelaziz A E Ahmed, Windsor, ON - Internal Medicine
Dr Tahira S Ahmed, Windsor, ON - General Practice
Dr Abubaker A Ahmer, Woodstock, ON - Orthopedic Surgery
Dr Youssef AinMelk, Sherbrooke, QC - Obstetrics & Gynecology
Dr Ronald Akhras, Montreal, QC - Family Medicine
Dr Mouafak Al Hadi, Mindemoya, ON - Family Medicine
Dr Mustafa H A Al Maini, Toronto, ON - Clin Immun/Allergy
Dr Osama M Al-Agha, Regina, SK - Anatomical Pathology
Dr Aqeel I M Al-Aqeel, Simcoe, ON - General Surgery
Dr Elias Al-Chaddad, Jonquiere, QC - General Surgery
Dr Haider M Al-Dabbagh, Mississauga, ON - Family Medicine
Dr Firas F Al-Dhaher, Petrolia, ON - Family Medicine
Dr Bassel Al-Farra, Windsor, ON - Urology
Dr Abeer A M Al-Gasim, Toronto, ON - Family Medicine
Dr Saed S Al-Habib, Whitby, ON - General Practice
Dr Khalid E A Al-Harbi, Hamilton, ON - General Surgery
Dr Ibrahim M M Al-Hashmi, Etobicoke, ON - Pediatrics
Dr Abdurrahman O S Al-Hesayen, Toronto, ON - Cardiology
Dr Fatih M W Al-Katib, Saskatoon, SK - General Practice
Dr Nabil M Al-Kayssi, Edmonton, AB - Family Medicine
Dr Suhaib Al-Kurtass, Edmonton, AB - General Practice
Dr Rasha N A Al-Manahi, New Glasgow, NS - General Practice
Dr Nather N Al-Shakarji, Acton, ON - Family Medicine
Dr Hossam M Al-Tatari, Windsor, ON - General Practice
Dr Abdulwahab J Al-Tourah, Surrey, BC - Internal Medicine
Dr Elsayed E Alamelhuda, Windsor, ON - Family Medicine
Dr May A G Alarab, Toronto, ON - General Practice
Dr Mohamed J H Albrbar, Edmonton, AB - Family Medicine
Dr Samer Aldandashi, Edmonton, AB - General Practice
Dr Naji M A Alhulaimi, Edmonton, AB - Cardiology
Dr Fadhil S Ali, Calgary, AB - Family Medicine
Dr Yaser M A Ali, East York, ON - Clin Immun/Allergy
Dr Nihad H Ali-Ridha, Oshawa, ON - Anatomical Pathology
Dr Khaled M A Alnhisi, St Catharines, ON - Family Medicine
Dr Salem O S Alowami, Hamilton, ON - Anatomical Pathology
Dr Mohamed T Alphin, Medicine Hat, AB - Urology
Dr Mohamed-Rida A Alsaden, Windsor, ON - Anesthesia
Dr Heytham K Alsaffar, Ottawa, ON - General Practice
Dr Emad E Amer, Mississauga, ON - Internal Medicine
Dr Maurice Amsellem, Montreal-Nord, QC - General Practice
Dr Jean I Anawati, Sturgeon Falls, ON - General Practice
Dr Donna M Arab-O'Brien, Toronto, ON - Endocrin/Metabolism
Dr Neema A Arafa, Toronto, ON - General Practice
Dr Erfan Arfali, Brantford, ON - Emergency Family Med
Dr Nahla M Aris-Jilwan, Montreal, QC - Endocrinology & Metabolism
Dr Georges Arjane, Verdun, QC - Hematological Pathology
Dr Abdelwahab A Arrazaghi, Scarborough, ON - Cardiology

Dr Elsharif M M Ashater, Thunder Bay, ON - Internal Medicine
Dr Kassem A Ashe, Kitchener, ON - Cardiac Surgery
Dr Dalal M Assaad, Toronto, ON - Anatomical Pathology
Dr Samir R G Assad, Maple, ON - Family Medicine
Dr Manutchehr Assemi, Nepean, ON - Pediatrics
Dr Hazem Assi, Moncton, NB - General Practice
Dr Maher G Y Atalla, Brampton, ON - Family Medicine
Dr Soheir Atalla, Brossard, QC - General Practice
Dr Khaled A Ateer, Edmonton, AB - General Practice
Dr Abdulrazzak O Atiyah, New Waterford, NS - Plastic Surgery
Dr Amany A Y Attalla, Cambridge, ON - Family Medicine
Dr Amine N Attia, Mississauga, ON - Family Medicine
Dr Samia Attia-Galand, Gatineau, QC - Psychiatry
Dr Nabil Attie, Saint-Leonard, QC - Rheumatology
Dr Ezzedine Attig, Riviere-du-Loup, QC - Neurology
Dr Nevine Audi, Ottawa, ON - Emergency Family Med
Dr Imad T Awad, Toronto, ON - General Practice
Dr Sawsan M Awad-El-Kariem, Moose Jaw, SK - General Practice
Dr Suzan Awadde Alla Ghattas, Mississauga, ON - Family Medicine
Dr Misaa M S Ayad, Hamilton, ON - Pediatrics
Dr Raed Azer, New Waterford, NS - Family Medicine
Dr Ahmed T Aziz, Quesnel, BC - Internal Medicine
Dr Dalal A Aziz, Milton, ON - General Surgery
Dr E Michel Azouz, Westmount, QC - Diagnostic-Radiology
Dr Fadi-Boutros Azzi, Hawkesbury, ON - Family Medicine
Dr Mervat A Bacily, Winnipeg, MB - Family Medicine
Dr Entisar M Badi, Vaughan, ON - Obstetrics & Gynecology
Dr Dalal Badlissi, St-Charles-Brromee, QC - Community Medicine
Dr Aida Bairam, Quebec, QC - Pediatrics
Dr Adnan Bajelan, Summerside, PE - Family Medicine
Dr Sameena A Bajwa, Calgary, AB - Family Medicine
Dr Fady K Balaa, Ottawa, ON - General Surgery
Dr Samia M Barakat, Winnipeg, MB - Psychiatry
Dr Rola Baram, Saint-Laurent, QC - General Practice
Dr Zaim Bardakji, Saint-Laurent, QC - General Practice
Dr Maya Barnouti-Calotti, Oakville, ON - Family Medicine
Dr Laith M Barsoom, North York, ON - Family Medicine
Dr Milad K Barsoum, Toronto, ON - Urology
Dr Mounir Bashour, Montreal, QC - Ophthalmology
Dr Fadi Basile, Montreal, QC - Cardiovasc/ThorSurg
Dr Girair Basmadjian, Montreal, QC - Ophthalmology
Dr Hanan A Bassyouni, Calgary, AB - Endocrin/Metabolism
Dr Mourad M Basta, Ottawa, ON - Family Medicine
Dr Nabil R Bechai, North York, ON - Diagnostic-Radiology
Dr Magdy R Bekhit, North York, ON - Family Medicine
Dr Leila Ben Amor, Levis, QC - General Practice
Dr Mansour M Bendago, Scarborough, ON - Plastic Surgery
Dr Sameera Benjamen, Woodbridge, ON - General Practice
Dr Antranik N Benohanian, Montreal, QC - Dermatology
Dr Amal Bensaleh-Ratmi, Moncton, NB - General Practice
Dr Patricia Berbari, Gatineau, QC - Plastic Surgery
Dr Abdullahi A Berih, Etobicoke, ON - Family Medicine
Dr Sanaa S Beshay, Mississauga, ON - Emergency Family Med
Dr Hany Y Beshay, Mississauga, ON - Family Medicine
Dr Redouane Bettahar, Rimouski, QC - General Practice
Dr Hussein K Beydoun, Halifax, NS - Cardiology
Dr Janan F Y Bilbily, Scarborough, ON - Family Medicine
Dr Azhar Bishay, Etobicoke, ON - Pediatrics
Dr Tarek A Bismar, Calgary, AB - General Practice
Dr Atef H K Boctor, Gander, NL - Family Medicine
Dr Wagdy Botros, Kitchener, ON - Psychiatry
Dr Yasser Botros, North York, ON - General Surgery
Dr Charles Bou Farah, Sorel-Tracy, QC - General Practice
Dr Belkacem Bouchek, Amos, QC - General Practice
Dr Aladin E Boulad, Laval, QC - General Practice
Dr Patrick R Boulos, Sherbrooke, QC - Ophthalmology
Dr Ibrahim Bounatiro, Pointe-Claire, QC - General Practice
Dr Asmae Boutaleb, Montreal, QC - General Practice
Dr Hedy N Boutros, Scarborough, ON - Anatomical Pathology
Dr Cecile Boutros, Montreal, QC - General Practice
Dr Hagob A Boyrazian, Scarborough, ON - General Practice
Dr Joseph F Braidy, Longueuil, QC - Critical Care Medicine
Dr Amer M A Burhan, Toronto, ON - Psychiatry
Dr Abdul Mujib A K M Cadili, St. Albert, AB - General Surgery
Dr Edward F E Cattan, Orleans, ON - Psychiatry
Dr Ahmad M A Chaker, Windsor, ON - Family Medicine
Dr Chamoun Chamoun, Ottawa, ON - Cardiology
Dr Jihad Y Chaya, St Thomas, ON - Psychiatry
Dr Walif Chbeir, Gatineau, QC - Diagnostic-Radiology
Dr Mustapha Chelfi, Gatineau, QC - General Practice
Dr Rene Chemaly, Montreal, QC - Obstetrics & Gynecology
Dr Abdallah Chidiac, Saint-Laurent, QC - Pediatrics
Dr Georges N Choueri, Laval, QC - Gastroenterology
Dr Michel Copti, Montreal, QC - Electroencephal
Dr Abdallah S Daar, Toronto, ON - General Surgery
Dr Georges Dadour, Montreal, QC - General Practice
Dr Antoine Daher, Chateauguay, QC - General Practice
Dr Jehad Dahman, Whitby, ON - General Practice
Dr Genevieve Dallaire, St-Jean-Sur-Richel, QC - Emergency Family Med
Dr Ghassan Y Dally, Mississauga, ON - Family Medicine
Dr Mukhaimer H Dani, Miramichi, NB - General Practice
Dr Nicolas Daoud, Chicoutimi, QC - Diagnostic-Radiology
Dr Mahmoud A Darrat, Hamilton, ON - Anesthesia
Dr Dawood G Dawood, Gloucester, ON - Obstetrics & Gynecology
Dr Sylvaine De Plaen, Montreal, QC - Psychiatry
Dr Chaouki Debs, Drummondville, QC - Urology
Dr Hassan Deif, North York, ON - Diagnostic-Radiology
Dr Ashraf Dief, Bradford, ON - Family Medicine
Dr Luay F Dindo, Surrey, BC - General Practice
Dr Mohamed A Diyaeb, Mississauga, ON - Family Medicine
Dr Saleena Djearam, Victoria, BC - Family Medicine
Dr Santosh Dubey, Calgary, AB - General Practice
Dr Ramy EL Zaharna, Ajax, ON - Family Medicine
Dr Manal Ebeid, North York, ON - Family Medicine
Dr Osama Ebesh, Chilliwack, BC - General Practice
Dr Abdurrahman A Eddeb, Toronto, ON - Diagnostic-Radiology
Dr Raouf K A Edward, North York, ON - Psychiatry
Dr Clovis Eid, Moncton, NB - Ophthalmology
Dr Karim E C Eid, Scarborough, ON - General Practice
Dr Jouhaina Eid, Montreal, QC - Nephrology
Dr Ahmed El Alfy, Cambridge, ON - Anesthesia
Dr Abdulhakim A A El Ghamudi, Cambridge, ON - Anesthesia
Dr Enas El Gouhary El Gouhary, Toronto, ON - Pediatrics
Dr Akram M I El Keilani, Windsor, ON - Anatomical Pathology
Dr Nihal El Khouly, Bolton, ON - Family Medicine
Dr William S El Masri, Toronto, ON - Otolaryngology
Dr Mohammed El Saidi, Belleville, ON - Psychiatry
Dr Somaya El Seisi, Richmond Hill, ON - Family Medicine
Dr Mohamed El Shatshat, Arborg, MB - Family Medicine
Dr Basel A El Tawil, Leamington, ON - Internal Medicine
Dr Rabeh M A El Zuway, Niagara Falls, ON - Internal Medicine
Dr Dalia El-Ashry, Mississauga, ON - Gastroenterology
Dr Nemer El-Batnigi, Oshawa, ON - Emergency Family Med
Dr Hossam El-Beheiry, Mississauga, ON - Anesthesia
Dr Mary R R El-Brakey, Kitchener, ON - Anesthesia
Dr Ali Abdel Halim Hussein El-Gayed, Saskatoon, SK - General Practice
Dr Nady A El-Guebaly, Calgary, AB - Psychiatry
Dr May I El-Hajj, Owen Sound, ON - Obstetrics & Gynecology
Dr Hamdy G E H El-Hakim, Edmonton, AB - General Practice
Dr Philippe P El-Helou, Hamilton, ON - Internal Medicine
Dr Hayam H R El-Kateb, Markham, ON - Family Medicine
Dr Hesham El-Madah, Brampton, ON - Family Medicine
Dr Medhat W El-Mallah, Oshawa, ON - Radiation Oncology
Dr Amira El-Messidi, Montreal, QC - Obstetrics & Gynecology
Capt Salman A K El-Sadi, London, ON - Emergency Family Med
Dr Dina El-Sahrigy, Ajax, ON - Anatomical Pathology
Dr Elias El-Salibi, Alexandria, ON - Family Medicine
Dr Gamal I El-Salviti, Woodstock, ON - General Surgery
Dr Reda M El-Sawy, Ottawa, ON - Physical Medicine & Rehab
Dr Samy M El-Sayed, Ottawa, ON - Radiation Oncology
Dr Rawieh El-Sayegh, Mississauga, ON - Family Medicine
Dr Mohamed T El-Sherbiny, Montreal, QC - Urology
Dr Issam K El-Takli, Brampton, ON - Gastroenterology
Dr Bassam El-Tatari, Windsor, ON - Family Medicine
Dr Hala M T El-Zimaity, Toronto, ON - Anatomical Pathology
Dr Ramadan E ElSugy, Brampton, ON - Obstetrics & Gynecology
Dr Abdusalam Elalem, Windsor, ON - General Surgery
Dr Abdurrahim A Elashaal, Toronto, ON - Neurosurgery
Dr Abdelrahman A B Elashaal, Windsor, ON - Orthopedic Surgery
Dr Mustafa M Elbreki, Windsor, ON - Otolaryngology
Dr Azza Eldeiry, Edmonton, AB - General Practice
Dr Ashraf M Elfiky, Sherwood Park, AB - General Practice
Dr Ali Salem B Elfirjani, Ajax, ON - Internal Medicine
Dr Abdulmonem Elghamari, Etobicoke, ON - Family Medicine
Dr Turia A Elghdewi, Lloydminster, AB - Obstetrics & Gynecology
Dr Tamer Elghobary, Mississauga, ON - Cardiac Surgery
Dr Eimad M E Elghol, Edmonton, AB - Family Medicine
Dr Suzan M Elias, Oshawa, ON - Family Medicine
Dr John D Elie, Montreal, QC - Dermatology
Dr Samer Elkassem, Medicine Hat, AB - General Surgery
Dr Saad M A Elkelani, Sarnia, ON - Obstetrics & Gynecology
Dr Omran R Elmanfud, Toronto, ON - Cardiology
Dr Nader Elmayergi, Toronto, ON - Cardiology
Dr Mohamed S Elmusharaf, Fort McMurray, AB - Family Medicine
Dr Carol M M Y Eloskouf, Keswick, ON - Family Medicine
Dr Thaer Elrefai, Ottawa, ON - Family Medicine
Dr Elsaid R Elrify, Ajax, ON - General Practice
Dr Sameer Elsayed, London, ON - Infectious Diseases
Dr Reem Elsobky, Toronto, ON - Internal Medicine
Dr Suha Eltayeb, Ajax, ON - Obstetrics & Gynecology
Dr Ausama H Elyas, Flin Flon, MB - General Practice
Dr Abdul F M Elzawi, Toronto, ON - Internal Medicine
Dr Barry Emara, Windsor, ON - Ophthalmology
Dr Sherif G S Emil, Montreal, QC - General Surgery
Dr Houda A Ergaiey, Kitchener, ON - Gastroenterology
Dr Souad Esadeg, Kitchener, ON - Family Medicine
Dr Monira Eskandar, Toronto, ON - Family Medicine
Dr Ihab Eskander, Kitchener, ON - Family Medicine
Dr Mohyeddin Essabri, Etobicoke, ON - Family Medicine
Dr Hatoon M Ezzat, Vancouver, BC - Hematology
Dr Khalid Fadeel, Scarborough, ON - Family Medicine
Dr Enass Faheim, Mississauga, ON - Family Medicine
Dr Maged I Fahim, Brampton, ON - Family Medicine
Dr Sylvia Fahim, Mississauga, ON - Family Medicine
Dr Simone S I Fahim, Ottawa, ON - Dermatology
Dr Yousef W Fahmy, Mississauga, ON - Family Medicine
Dr Samir A Faidi, Hamilton, ON - General Surgery
Dr Yousef M S Fakhry, Mississauga, ON - Ophthalmology
Dr Isis Fanous, Edmonton, AB - General Practice
Dr Nabil E Fanous, Westmount, QC - Otolaryngology
Dr Rafat Y Faraawi, Kitchener, ON - Internal Medicine
Dr Rose F Farag, Mississauga, ON - Family Medicine
Dr Sameh S Farah, Sault Ste. Marie, ON - Endocrin/Metabolism
Dr Antoine Farah, Gatineau, QC - Nephrology
Dr Christiane Farazli, Ottawa, ON - Gastroenterology
Dr Walid A Farhat, Toronto, ON - Urology
Dr Salaheddin G Farjalla, Windsor, ON - Gastroenterology
Dr Nabil Fawaz, Saint-Leonard, QC - General Practice
Dr Ashraf Fayad, Ottawa, ON - Anesthesia
Dr Ibrahim Fayez, Toronto, ON - Family Medicine
Dr Tharwat A E Fera, Vancouver, BC - Internal Medicine
Dr Majed Fianni, Goderich, ON - Internal Medicine
Dr Naiema M Fiel, Georgetown, ON - Obstetrics & Gynecology
Dr Judith E Finlayson, Victoria, BC - Family Medicine
Dr Ali O Fiture, Richmond Hill, ON - General Surgery
Dr Rasem L Fituri, Windsor, ON - Gastroenterology
Dr Mohamed M R Foda, Leduc, AB - Urology
Dr Magdy A M Fouad, Port Alberni, BC - Obstetrics & Gynecology
Dr Mohamed I Gaber, Belleville, ON - Anatomical Pathology
Dr Yousry Gabrail, Oakville, ON - Family Medicine
Dr Manal Y Gabril, London, ON - Anatomical Pathology
Dr Fathi A Gadhafi, Niagara Falls, ON - Family Medicine
Dr Magdi M A Gaid, Ajax, ON - Anesthesia
Dr Nagy F A E Gallab, Welland, ON - Internal Medicine
Dr Sargon B Gandilo, Nepean, ON - Diagnostic-Radiology
Dr Salah H Gareiw, Hamilton, ON - General Practice
Dr Hassan A M Gargoum, Regina, SK - Cardiology
Dr Khalid Gazala, Oakville, ON - Neurology

Dr Mustafa M Geneve, Winnipeg, MB - Family Medicine
Dr Lillian K F George, Orleans, ON - Family Medicine
Dr Nasim K S Gerges, Etobicoke, ON - Family Medicine
Dr Maha F G Gerges, Milton, ON - Family Medicine
Dr Ayman Gerges, Mississauga, ON - Family Medicine
Dr Nagi N R Ghabbour, Toronto, ON - Psychiatry
Dr Ashraf M Ghali, Burlington, ON - Family Medicine
Dr Samia S K Ghali, Windsor, ON - Nuclear Medicine
Dr Saad Ghali, Delson, QC - General Practice
Dr Gehan R Ghally, Kitchener, ON - Family Medicine
Dr Ezzat G Ghaly, Cornwall, ON - Internal Medicine
Dr Fatemeh Ghannadi, West Vancouver, BC - Family Medicine
Dr Youssef Ghantous, Cornwall, ON - Family Medicine
Dr Shler Gharib, Brantford, ON - Family Medicine
Dr Osama Gharsaa, Oshawa, ON - Orthopedic Surgery
Dr Samir Ghatalia, Ottawa, ON - Anesthesia
Dr Paul B Ghattas, Nepean, ON - General Practice
Dr Khalida K Ghazala, Mississauga, ON - Family Medicine
Dr Boulos A Ghazarian, Point Edward, ON - Obstetrics & Gynecology
Dr Danny M D Ghazarian, Toronto, ON - Anatomical Pathology
Dr Heitham A A Gheriani, Terrace, BC - Otolaryngology
Dr M Ghobrial, Ottawa, ON - Pediatrics
Dr Bassam I A Gholam, Simcoe, ON - Emergency Family Med
Dr Zeina Ghorab, Toronto, ON - General Practice
Dr Magdy R B Gibara, Oakville, ON - Family Medicine
Dr Medhat F Gindi, Mississauga, ON - Community Medicine
Dr Gimiana N Gindi, Mississauga, ON - Family Medicine
Dr Raafat F Gindi, Toronto, ON - General Practice
Dr Samira W A Girgis, Mississauga, ON - Family Medicine
Dr Siham Girgis, Mississauga, ON - Family Medicine
Dr Magdy Girgis, North York, ON - Family Medicine
Dr Mona Girgis, North York, ON - Psychiatry
Dr Adel Girgis, Thornhill, ON - Family Medicine
Dr Gehad G M Gobran, Halifax, NS - Family Medicine
Capt Marcos Gobrial, North York, ON - Family Medicine
Dr Sherif A A E Gordon, Mississauga, ON - Family Medicine
Dr Verkeen S Gorguy, Scarborough, ON - Psychiatry
Dr Hany Guirgis, Thornhill, ON - Otolaryngology
Dr Samir S Guirguis, Etobicoke, ON - General Practice
Dr Dina Guirguis, Mississauga, ON - Family Medicine
Dr Emad S L Guirguis, Oakville, ON - Family Medicine
Dr Ezzat F Guirguis, Orillia, ON - Psychiatry
Dr Adel F Guirguis, Ottawa, ON - General Practice
Dr Hesham S R Guirguis, Sorel-Tracy, QC - Internal Medicine
Dr Emad A Habib, Ottawa, ON - Family Medicine
Dr Bahaa S Habib, Thornhill, ON - Family Medicine
Dr Nader H Habib, Laval, QC - General Practice
Dr Samir Habib, Montreal, QC - Family Medicine
Dr Adel F Habib, Sorel-Tracy, QC - Psychiatry
Dr Magdi Habra, Bois-des-Filion, QC - General Practice
Dr Munir Habra, Greenfield Park, QC - General Practice
Dr Haissam A Haddad, Ottawa, ON - Cardiology
Dr Wael M Haddara, London, ON - Critical Care Medicine
Dr Ghassan M Hadi, Edmonton, AB - General Surgery
Dr Ali Hadi, Burlington, ON - Family Medicine
Dr Hachemi Hadjoudj, Laval, QC - Internal Medicine
Dr Basem K Hafazalla, Brockville, ON - Obstetrics & Gynecology
Dr Kevin Hafez, Calgary, AB - Family Medicine
Dr Hasan Hafiz, Calgary, AB - General Practice
Dr Falih M Hafuth, Guelph, ON - Family Medicine
Dr Esam M S Haider, Owen Sound, ON - Orthopedic Surgery
Dr Youssef Haikal, Longueuil, QC - Otolaryngology
Dr Jean J Hallak, Montreal, QC - Obstetrics & Gynecology
Dr Fawaz Halwani, Ottawa, ON - Anatomical Pathology
Dr Fatin Hamad, North York, ON - Family Medicine
Dr Husein Z Hamandi, Oakville, ON - Family Medicine
Dr Nermeen R I Hamdy, North York, ON - Family Medicine
Dr Hazem A Hamdy, Ottawa, ON - Family Medicine
Dr Ahmed Hamdy, Toronto, ON - Anesthesia
Dr Reggie C A Hamdy, Montreal, QC - Orthopedic Surgery
Dr Azza A W M Hamed, Mississauga, ON - Pediatrics
Dr Hala M F Hamed Abdelazim, Welland, ON - Anesthesia
Dr Fayad Hamideh, Oakville, ON - General Practice
Dr Hachmi Hammami, Salaber-de-Valleyf, QC - Ophthalmology
Dr Souhaila Hammoud, Mississauga, ON - Family Medicine
Dr M Wahbi Hammouda, Brampton, ON - Hematology
Dr Aseel Hamoudi, Hamilton, ON - Obstetrics & Gynecology
Dr Abuobeida Hamour, Prince George, BC - Infectious Diseases
Dr Basma Hanna, Edmonton, AB - Family Medicine
Dr Mary Hanna, Ancaster, ON - Family Medicine
Dr Samer K F Hanna, Brampton, ON - Orthopedic Surgery
Dr Magda W Hanna, Cornwall, ON - Psychiatry
Dr Neveen M Hanna, Etobicoke, ON - Family Medicine
Dr Rafik B A M Hanna, Hamilton, ON - Family Medicine
Dr Rose K F A Hanna, Mississauga, ON - Family Medicine
Dr Nevin-Wadie N Hanna, Mississauga, ON - Family Medicine
Dr Sameh K Hanna, Oakville, ON - Family Medicine
Dr Shoukry Hanna, Richmond Hill, ON - Family Medicine
Dr Magdy M Hanna, Scarborough, ON - Family Medicine
Dr Hany S H Hanna, Thorold, ON - Family Medicine
Dr Amir K Hanna, Toronto, ON - Endocrin/Metabolism
Dr Wedad M Hanna, Toronto, ON - Anatomical Pathology
Dr Linda Hanna, Toronto, ON - Family Medicine
Dr Phebe Hanna, Woodbridge, ON - Family Medicine
Dr Yousri Hanna, Anjou, QC - General Practice
Dr Samer Hanna, Laval, QC - Urology
Dr Sarwat K Hanna Dief, Scarborough, ON - Psychiatry
Dr Fadi Hannouche, Oshawa, ON - Anesthesia
Dr M Georges Hannouche, Montreal, QC - General Practice
Dr Nabil Hannouche, Montreal, QC - Diagnostic-Radiology
Dr Raymond T Harb, St Catharines, ON - Family Medicine
Dr Gamal W Haroun, Brampton, ON - Diagnostic-Radiology
Dr Osama Hasan, Kitchener, ON - Emergency Family Med
Dr Omar N Hasan, Amqui, QC - General Surgery
Dr Maliheh Hasemzadeh-Balouchi, Richmond Hill, ON - Family Medicine
Dr Abdalla A Hassan, Bridgewater, NS - General Surgery
Dr Amal Hassan, Mississauga, ON - Family Medicine
Dr Sameh A Hassan, Toronto, ON - Psychiatry
Dr Durreshahwar Hassan, Roxboro, QC - Obstetrics & Gynecology
Dr Magdy Hassouna, Toronto, ON - Urology
Dr Fatma E Hawash-Mostafa, London, ON - General Practice
Dr Nasr A E Hegazy, Etobicoke, ON - Anesthesia
Dr Ruby S Heikal, Oakville, ON - Family Medicine
Dr Hanna E Hejjaji, Mississauga, ON - Diagnostic-Radiology
Dr Michael E Helewa, Winnipeg, MB - Obstetrics & Gynecology
Dr Sanaa T H A Helmi, Kitchener, ON - Psychiatry
Dr Hussam A Helou, Pointe-Claire, QC - Family Medicine
Dr Emad Henein, London, ON - Family Medicine
Dr John Henein, Oakville, ON - Family Medicine
Dr Raafat Henen, Scarborough, ON - Ophthalmology
Dr Mohsen Henis, Scarborough, ON - Family Medicine
Dr Claire Sadek Hennes, Brampton, ON - Family Medicine
Dr Michel Hereish, Montreal, QC - General Practice
Dr Fadia Hermiz, Windsor, ON - Family Medicine
Dr Wael Hezam, Grande Prairie, AB - General Practice
Dr Ali Abbas M Hilal, Windsor, ON - Otolaryngology
Dr Sharifa A Himidan, Toronto, ON - General Surgery
Dr Hanna M Hinnawi, Etobicoke, ON - General Practice
Dr Khalid J Hirmiz, Windsor, ON - Radiation Oncology
Dr Ahmed Hussein, St. Albert, AB - Infectious Diseases
Dr Evelin Ibrahim, Port Moody, BC - Family Medicine
Dr Adel F A Ibrahim, Winnipeg, MB - Family Medicine
Dr Mahdi K Ibrahim, Bonavista, NL - General Practice
Dr Samia M R Ibrahim, Orleans, ON - General Practice
Dr Hany S H Ibrahim, Scarborough, ON - Family Medicine
Dr Narmin Ibrahim, Saskatoon, SK - Family Medicine
Dr Isaac F Isaac, London, ON - Psychiatry
Dr Magda Ishac, North York, ON - General Practice
Dr Pervez Ishrat Ali Khan, Edmonton, AB - General Practice
Dr Hani Iskandar, Verdun, QC - General Practice
Dr Salah S G Iskander, Winnipeg, MB - Family Medicine
Dr John W Iskander, Georgetown, ON - General Surgery
Dr Alexander W Iskander, North York, ON - General Surgery
Dr Mariam F G Iskander, Thornhill, ON - Family Medicine
Dr Amal K E Iskandir, Mississauga, ON - Family Medicine
Dr Aden A Ismail, London, ON - Psychiatry
Dr Koma D Israel, Hamilton, ON - Family Medicine
Dr Kheirie Issa, Ottawa, ON - Pediatrics
Dr Simon Issid, Saint-Laurent, QC - General Practice
Dr Mohamed S Izzeldin, London, ON - Family Medicine
Dr Mohammad Jaamour, Windsor, ON - General Practice
Dr Mohamed S Jadi, Guelph, ON - Obstetrics & Gynecology
Dr Helen Jazrawy, Thornhill, ON - Diagnostic-Radiology
Dr Mazin K A Jelloo, Whitbourne, NL - Family Medicine
Dr Ibrahim K Jillood, Lethbridge, AB - General Practice
Dr Louai Jony, New Glasgow, NS - Obstetrics & Gynecology
Dr Mohamad G Joundi, Winnipeg, MB - General Practice
Dr M Said Jumaa, Penticton, BC - General Practice
Dr Nuri I M B Kaal, Owen Sound, ON - Internal Medicine
Dr Harry Kadoch, Ormstown, QC - Family Medicine
Dr Albert Kadri, Windsor, ON - Internal Medicine
Dr Raymond N Kahwaji, Vancouver, BC - Anesthesia
Dr Emad H Kamel, Gambo, NL - Family Medicine
Dr Mona K Kamel, Mississauga, ON - Anatomical Pathology
Dr Ibrahim D Kamel, North York, ON - Ophthalmology
Dr Ahmed K Kamouna, Milton, ON - Family Medicine
Dr Jacques Karam, St-Jean-Sur-Richel, QC - Cardiology
Dr Meryem Karzazi, Saint-Georges, QC - Internal Medicine
Dr Hassan Kayssi, Montreal, QC - General Practice
Dr Tarek A Khalefih, Milton, ON - Pediatrics
Dr Mahmoud A Khalifa, Toronto, ON - Anatomical Pathology
Dr Samir Khalife, Montreal, QC - Obstetrics & Gynecology
Dr Ayman M R Khalil, Etobicoke, ON - Family Medicine
Dr Evon W H Khalil, Richmond Hill, ON - Family Medicine
Dr Muhammad A Khan, Sydney, NS - Emergency Family Med
Dr Saadia N Khan, Mississauga, ON - Family Medicine
Dr Somaia A M Khataan, Mississauga, ON - Family Medicine
Dr Kamal Khayat, Saint-Jerome, QC - Pediatrics
Dr Assil I Khelil, Winnipeg, MB - Family Medicine
Dr Lucie M Khouri, Saint-Laurent, QC - Ophthalmology
Dr Shahira S Khoury, North York, ON - Physical Medicine & Rehab
Dr Lara Khoury, Ottawa, ON - Geriatric Medicine
Dr Nabil M Khoury, Bois-des-Filion, QC - General Practice
Dr Samir Khoury, Montreal, QC - Pediatrics
Dr Elie G Khoury, Saint-Laurent, QC - Ophthalmology
Dr Khalil Khoury, Sherbrooke, QC - Endocrinology
Dr Pierre Khouzam, Newmarket, ON - General Practice
Dr Antoine Kibrite, Quebec, QC - General Surgery
Dr Krikor Kichian, Ottawa, ON - Gastroenterology
Dr Ali K A A Kilany, Toronto, ON - Cardiology
Dr Nadim Korban, Montreal, QC - Otolaryngology
Dr Joseph A Korkis, Burlington, ON - Otolaryngology
Dr Claude Kortas, London, ON - Internal Medicine
Dr Dnyanada L Kothare, Regina, SK - General Practice
Dr Mervat N Kozman, Calgary, AB - Psychiatry
Dr Risk Kronfli, Dartmouth, NS - Psychiatry
Dr Hayder S H Kubba, Mississauga, ON - Family Medicine
Dr Rita Kuyumjian, Montreal, QC - Psychiatry
Dr Jirair Kuyumjian, Montreal, QC - General Practice
Dr Edmond Kyrillos, Ottawa, ON - Family Medicine
Dr Maggy G H Kyrollos, Ottawa, ON - General Pathology
Dr Alena Ladki, North Vancouver, BC - Pediatrics
Dr Abdulrahem L A Laftah, Summerside, PE - Family Medicine
Dr Nadine J Lahoud, Lasalle, QC - Internal Medicine
Dr Salim Lahoud, Montreal, QC - Ophthalmology
Dr Hesham M M A Lakosha, Halifax, NS - Ophthalmology
Dr Jean-Baptiste Lattouf, Montreal, QC - Urology
Dr Sasson Lavi, Thornhill, ON - Pediatrics
Dr Nibal Lubbad, Burlington, ON - Family Medicine
Dr Caroline Maamari, Greenfield Park, QC - General Practice
Dr Angelo G Macrodimitris, Winnipeg, MB - Ophthalmology
Dr Lucy N Magharious, North York, ON - Family Medicine
Dr Hayder T Mahdi, Burlington, ON - Family Medicine
Dr Georges Mahfoud, Saint-Leonard, QC - General Practice
Dr Haidar A Mahmoud, Scarborough, ON - Obstetrics & Gynecology
Dr Falah S Majid, Moose Jaw, SK - General Practice
Dr Magdy S I Makar, Orillia, ON - General Surgery
Dr Suzanne Malaab, Val-d'Or, QC - Pediatrics
Dr Fawzi A Mankal, Ottawa, ON - Family Medicine
Dr Mervat F Mankarious, Mississauga, ON - Family Medicine
Dr John J V Manoukian, Montreal, QC - Otolaryngology
Dr Fenar A Mansoor, Scarborough, ON - Family Medicine
Dr Raafat A E Mansour, North York, ON - Family Medicine

Dr Samer Mansour, Montreal, QC - General Practice
Dr Michael Mansour, Montreal, QC - General Practice
Dr Catherine Marks, Orleans, ON - Family Medicine
Dr Razawa F Maroof, Regina, SK - Family Medicine
Dr Sami S Marqus, Scarborough, ON - Internal Medicine
Dr Saida Marrat, Scarborough, ON - Family Medicine
Dr R Albert Y Massabki, Oshawa, ON - Psychiatry
Dr Emad Massoud, Halifax, NS - Otolaryngology
Dr Fadi A Massoud, Montreal, QC - Geriatric Medicine
Dr Elias Matouk, Montreal, QC - Internal Medicine
Dr Adel G Mattar, Chatham, ON - Nuclear Medicine
Dr Kamal Mattar, Niagara Falls, ON - Urology
Dr Nabih Mattar, Simcoe, ON - General Surgery
Dr Edward T Matti, Cambridge, ON - Psychiatry
Dr Hagop K Mazmanian, Welland, ON - Urology
Dr Mohamed A Megahed Gheis, Victoria, BC - Psychiatry
Dr Saly Mekhael, Thornhill, ON - Family Medicine
Dr Mamdouh A H Metrie, Mississauga, ON - Family Medicine
Dr George P Michael, Newmarket, ON - Family Medicine
Dr Antoinette A Michael, Whitby, ON - Family Medicine
Dr Mary F S Michaiel, Calgary, AB - Family Medicine
Dr Azza M Mikail, Mississauga, ON - Family Medicine
Dr Mamdouh T Mikhail, Whitby, ON - Family Medicine
Dr Mina M F Mina, Winnipeg, MB - Otolaryngology
Dr Nahed R Mishriki, Toronto, ON - Family Medicine
Dr Ataher S Mohamed, Edmonton, AB - Family Medicine
Dr El-Fellani A Mohammed, Regina, SK - Endocrin/Metabolism
Dr Samy Stephane Maurice Mohanna, Gatineau, QC - Community Medicine
Dr Mona M Mohareb, Cornwall, ON - General Practice
Dr Ibrahim M M Momenkhan, Regina, SK - Critical Care Medicine
Dr Mohib Morcos, Quebec, QC - General Practice
Dr Roger Morcos, Sherbrooke, QC - Orthopedic Surgery
Dr Aida E Morgan, North York, ON - Family Medicine
Dr Anwar V K Morgan, Toronto, ON - Anesthesia
Dr Sonia Mosaad, Toronto, ON - Family Medicine
Dr Patricia Mouaikel, Nepean, ON - Family Medicine
Dr Elie Mouaikel, Montreal, QC - Hematology
Dr Wasseem M I Moussa, Cornwall, ON - General Surgery
Dr Assanassios Moussa Faltas, Orleans, ON - Family Medicine
Dr Taim A Muayqil, Edmonton, AB - Neurology
Dr Anwar S A Muftah, Regina, SK - Internal Medicine
Dr Abdalla G Muftah, Regina, SK - Internal Medicine
Dr Talib Muhammed, Calgary, AB - General Practice
Dr Jafaar Muhsen, Toronto, ON - Family Medicine
Dr Sukayna Murtada Dite Al-Sayed, Oshawa, ON - Family Medicine
Dr Abdalhakim Mustafa, Windsor, ON - Neurology
Dr Abdurrazag M Mutat, North Vancouver, BC - Neurosurgery
Dr Brian H Muth, Vancouver, BC - General Practice
Dr Adnan Nached, Montreal, QC - General Practice
Dr Ayoub Nahal, Montreal, QC - Anatomical Pathology
Dr Dolly T Nahri, Ottawa, ON - General Practice
Dr Adel L C Nakhla, Mississauga, ON - Family Medicine
Dr Kamil Nasr, Brossard, QC - Ophthalmology
Dr Hamid A Nasser, Guelph, ON - General Surgery
Dr Ishaq M Natsheh, Goulds, NL - General Practice
Dr Sherif P Nessim, Mississauga, ON - General Practice
Dr Firouzeh Niakosari, North York, ON - Anatomical Pathology
Dr Mounir H A Noor, Brampton, ON - Family Medicine
Dr Mohamed Nouh, St Paul, AB - General Practice
Dr Ninos M Oda, Toronto, ON - Orthopedic Surgery
Dr Charles G Orfali, Sherbrooke, QC - Plastic Surgery
Dr Abdessebar Ouasti, St-Jean-Sur-Richel, QC - Psychiatry
Dr Kamaldine Oudjhane, Toronto, ON - General Practice
Dr Apkar Papazian, Saint-Leonard, QC - Urology
Dr Stefanos Patmanidis, Woodbridge, ON - Psychiatry
Dr Kevork Minas Peltekian, Halifax, NS - Gastroenterology
Dr Ernest Z Phillipos, Edmonton, AB - Pediatrics
Dr George S R Philteos, Ajax, ON - Internal Medicine
Dr Samar Raad, Temiscaming, QC - Family Medicine
Dr Faten S Rabie, Kanata, ON - General Practice
Dr Jasim M Radhi, Peterborough, ON - Anatomical Pathology
Dr Farouk Radwan, Montreal, QC - Medical Biochemistry
Dr Ehab A Rafail, Peterborough, ON - Diagnostic-Radiology
Dr Salah R G Ragheb, Richmond, BC - General Practice
Dr Bahaa G Ragheb, Orleans, ON - Family Medicine
Dr Sakina Raj, Calgary, AB - Family Medicine
Dr Said Ramadan, London, ON - Pediatrics
Dr Fauzi Ramadan, Moose Jaw, SK - General Practice
Dr Medhat N Ramzy, Scarborough, ON - Family Medicine
Dr Ahmed Raouf-Alkadhimi, Acton, ON - Family Medicine
Dr Nashed Rashed, Point Edward, ON - Pediatrics
Dr Wagdy E A Rayes, Apsley, ON - General Practice
Dr Jalees M S Razavi, Calgary, AB - Occupational Med
Dr Soha R Rizk, Dartmouth, NS - Family Medicine
Dr Sarah Z Y Hanna Rizk, Bolton, ON - General Practice
Dr Kamilia S Rizkalla, London, ON - Anatomical Pathology
Dr Hoda G Rizkalla, Scarborough, ON - Family Medicine
Dr Nagui A M Ross, Mississauga, ON - Family Medicine
Dr Amr Rostom, Toronto, ON - Family Medicine
Dr Nabil K Saad, Stonewall, MB - General Practice
Dr Salwa Saad, Mississauga, ON - General Practice
Dr Maan H A Saad, Ottawa, ON - Family Medicine
Dr Salwa A Saadaldeen, London, ON - Family Medicine
Dr Mohammad F Sabouba, Hamilton, ON - Family Medicine
Dr Rida A Sabri, Brampton, ON - Family Medicine
Dr Boshra I Sabry, Orleans, ON - General Practice
Dr Ghada-Maria Saddi, Chateauguay, QC - Family Medicine
Dr Irene Sadek, Halifax, NS - Hematological Pathology
Dr Amel H F Sadek, Thorold, ON - Family Medicine
Dr Gamal E Sadek-Botros, London, ON - Psychiatry
Dr Aksam Sadik, Thornhill, ON - Family Medicine
Dr Zaki K Sadik, Vaughan, ON - Family Medicine
Dr Najib N Safieddine, Toronto, ON - General Surgery
Dr Samih S S Salama, Hamilton, ON - Anatomical Pathology
Dr Said S S Salama, Toronto, ON - Anesthesia
Dr Wassim Salamoun, Summerside, PE - General Practice
Dr Hala Saleem, Mississauga, ON - Family Medicine
Dr Wasfy S Saleh, Ottawa, ON - General Surgery
Dr Fatehia Saleh, Chateauguay, QC - Psychiatry
Dr Eman G Salem, Windsor, ON - Anesthesia
Dr Cherien Salem, York, ON - Family Medicine
Dr Jeannette L Salib, Etobicoke, ON - Family Medicine
Dr Michel G Salib, Yorkton, SK - General Practice
Dr Nasri Saliba, Gatineau, QC - Urology
Dr Raafat B Salih, Orangeville, ON - General Surgery
Dr Nabeel B Samad, Halifax, NS - General Practice
Dr Pensee A Sami, Sudbury, ON - General Practice
Dr Magdi H Sami, Montreal, QC - Cardiology
Dr David Samra, Scarborough, ON - Obstetrics & Gynecology
Dr Hassan Sannoufi, Kanata, ON - Emergency Family Med
Dr Rajni Saraf, Sarnia, ON - Obstetrics & Gynecology
Dr Abraham Sasson, Thornhill, ON - General Practice
Dr Hany F S Sawires, East York, ON - General Surgery
Dr Jeannette E Scandar, Cornwall, ON - Family Medicine
Dr Fatiha Seddiki, Laval, QC - Pediatrics
Dr Maged G A Seif, Mississauga, ON - Family Medicine
Dr Zygmunt P Sekula, Halifax, NS - General Practice
Dr Rafi F Setrak, St Catharines, ON - Emergency Family Med
Dr Joseph A Shaban, Windsor, ON - Endocrin/Metabolism
Dr Wael M Shabana, Ottawa, ON - General Practice
Dr Osama M Shabash, Toronto, ON - Family Medicine
Dr Gihad M H Shabib, Ottawa, ON - Obstetrics & Gynecology
Dr Wagih K A Shaheed, London, ON - Pediatrics
Dr Riad M A Shahid, Surrey, BC - Orthopedic Surgery
Dr Hala D S Shakhatreh, St Catharines, ON - Pediatrics
Dr Mohanad J Shalan Al-Gazi, Burlington, ON - Pediatrics
Dr Abdalla R M Shamisa, Windsor, ON - Neurosurgery
Dr Nouri I Shammas, Scarborough, ON - Plastic Surgery
Dr Nagi S A Shams, Brampton, ON - Family Medicine
Dr Raghad Shareef, Oakville, ON - Family Medicine
Dr Nader Sharifi, Surrey, BC - Family Medicine
Dr Abdul Q A Sharkawy, Toronto, ON - Infectious Diseases
Dr Nazar R Sharobim, Ajax, ON - Emergency Family Med
Dr Faiz F A Shasha, Windsor, ON - Family Medicine
Dr Souad M Shatshat, Halifax, NS - Internal Medicine
Dr Melad F R Shawush, Regina, SK - Neurology
Dr Allam A K Shawwa, Halifax, NS - General Pathology
Dr Iman A M Shbash, Hamilton, ON - Pediatrics
Dr Daniel Shedid, Montreal, QC - Neurosurgery
Dr Esther I Shehata, Coquitlam, BC - Family Medicine
Dr Ramez S H Shehata, Cambridge, ON - Anesthesia
Dr Sarwat W M Shehata, Sudbury, ON - Radiation Oncology
Dr Nadine Shehata, Toronto, ON - Hematology
Dr Gul Nawaz Sheikh, Ajax, ON - Internal Medicine
Dr Nancy M S Shenouda, Brampton, ON - Family Medicine
Dr Nazih F Shenouda, Ottawa, ON - Diagnostic-Radiology
Dr Ahmed S O Sherghin, Windsor, ON - Urology
Dr Ali M Shickh, Bowmanville, ON - Internal Medicine
Dr Basil M A Shilash, Brampton, ON - Family Medicine
Dr Laith D Shimon, Sydney, NS - Family Medicine
Dr Abdalrhman A Shnishah, Grande Prairie, AB - Family Medicine
Dr Ahmed S A H Shoker, Saskatoon, SK - Internal Medicine
Dr Phoebe E Shokry, Markham, ON - Anatomical Pathology
Dr Ali T Shoughary, Pembroke, ON - Ophthalmology
Dr Faten S Shoukralla, Richmond Hill, ON - Family Medicine
Dr Muhammad Z Shrayyef, Oakville, ON - General Practice
Dr Wael Shublaq, St. John's, NL - General Practice
Dr Zubaida Siddiqui, Elliot Lake, ON - Family Medicine
Dr Mary H Sidhom, Halifax, NS - Family Medicine
Dr Abdallah Y Sidky, Vancouver, BC - Psychiatry
Dr Maged Sidra Gerges, Winnipeg, MB - Family Medicine
Dr Richard Sioufi, Chateauguay, QC - Urology
Dr Shireen M Sirhan, Cowansville, QC - Hematology
Dr Denis Sirhan, Montreal, QC - Neurosurgery
Dr Esther A M Soccar, Ottawa, ON - Family Medicine
Dr Ehab S Soliman, Stellarton, NS - Family Medicine
Dr Wassim G F Soliman, Brampton, ON - Psychiatry
Dr Gamal M L Soliman, St Catharines, ON - Internal Medicine
Dr Samy Soliman, St Thomas, ON - Internal Medicine
Dr Hany Soliman, Toronto, ON - Radiation Oncology
Dr Maurice Somma, Montreal, QC - Endocrinology
Dr Soliman M Sonbol, Whitby, ON - Psychiatry
Dr Mark Z Sorial, Abbotsford, BC - Pediatrics
Dr Ashraf M G Sorial, Ignace, ON - General Practice
Dr Mary L R Sorial, Newmarket, ON - Family Medicine
Dr Ihab Z N Sorial, Oshawa, ON - Psychiatry
Dr Kamel Souissi, Val-d'Or, QC - General Practice
Dr Fibi B W Sourial, Brampton, ON - Family Medicine
Dr Nabil M Sultan, London, ON - Internal Medicine
Dr Mahmud M T Sultan, St Catharines, ON - Family Medicine
Dr Khalil Sultanem, Montreal, QC - Radiation Oncology
Dr Omar Q M Swadi, Toronto, ON - Anesthesia
Dr Mohamed M M Swenia, Fort McMurray, AB - General Surgery
Dr Gurcharan S Syan, Sudbury, ON - Cardiology
Dr Mohamed A Tabib, Windsor, ON - Diagnostic-Radiology
Dr Sharif W Tadros, Burlington, ON - General Practice
Dr Ibtissam F H Tadros, Mississauga, ON - Family Medicine
Dr Shaheer Tadros, Ottawa, ON - General Surgery
Dr Monir L Tadros, Toronto, ON - Ophthalmology
Dr Latif A A S Tadross, Guelph, ON - Anatomical Pathology
Dr Emmanuel H Tadross, Kitchener, ON - Psychiatry
Dr Zakaria L T Tadrous, Abbotsford, BC - Ophthalmology
Dr Mohammed Tagemouati, Pointe claire, QC - General Practice
Dr Tania Tajirian, Toronto, ON - Family Medicine
Dr Nagwa A Takla, St Catharines, ON - Family Medicine
Dr Samir Taleb, Campbellton, NB - General Practice
Dr Lawrence F Tanious, Pickering, ON - General Practice
Dr Rosemonde E Tannous, Niagara Falls, ON - Cardiology
Dr Waguih N Tannous, Montreal, QC - Family Medicine
Dr Osman A Tarabain, Windsor, ON - Internal Medicine
Dr Ahmad R Tarakji, Yarmouth, NS - Internal Medicine
Dr Fadi Tarazi, Burnaby, BC - Orthopedic Surgery
Dr Wadea M Tarhuni, Moose Jaw, SK - Cardiology
Dr Fouad Tayfour, Windsor, ON - Ophthalmology
Dr Artin M Ternamian, Toronto, ON - Obstetrics & Gynecology
Dr Sherif Tewfik, North York, ON - Psychiatry
Dr Tewfik L Tewfik, Montreal, QC - Otolaryngology
Dr Laila Tewfik Moussa, Chilliwack, BC - Family Medicine
Dr Ali S Thiab, Niagara Falls, ON - Family Medicine
Dr Rabi Tiguert, Quebec, QC - General Practice
Dr Simon Tinawi, Montreal, QC - Physical Medicine & Rehab
Dr Sarah G Toma, Edmonton, AB - General Practice
Dr Tamer S Toma, Dartmouth, NS - Family Medicine
Dr Azhar M Toma, Etobicoke, ON - Family Medicine

Dr Antoun A M Toma, Mississauga, ON - Family Medicine
Dr Mouhieddin Traboulsi, Calgary, AB - Cardiology
Dr Ibrahim M Treki, Windsor, ON - Internal Medicine
Dr Kamaleddin H Tumi, Barrie, ON - Plastic Surgery
Dr Uttam J K Wadhwa, Mississauga, ON - Psychiatry
Dr Rasha G S Wahba, Mississauga, ON - Family Medicine
Dr Odette Z Wahba, Mississauga, ON - Family Medicine
Dr Wahan Wanis, Vancouver, BC - Psychiatry
Dr Mohammed M Warsi, Waterville, NB - General Practice
Dr Atef M Wasfi, Montreal, QC - General Practice
Dr Samia W Wasfy, Mississauga, ON - Family Medicine
Dr Evet A Wasif, Saskatoon, SK - Diagnostic-Radiology
Dr Kawsar K Wassef, Cornwall, ON - Psychiatry
Dr Lamia F F Wassef, Nepean, ON - Family Medicine
Dr Hanaa S N Wassef, Newmarket, ON - Family Medicine
Dr Georgina Wassef, Ottawa, ON - Family Medicine
Dr Hany William, Cornwall, ON - Family Medicine
Dr Magued F S Yacoub, Calgary, AB - Psychiatry
Dr Wadieh R Yacoub, Edmonton, AB - Community Medicine
Dr Ashraf K I Yacoub, Pembroke, ON - Obstetrics & Gynecology
Dr Nagib Y R Yahmad, North York, ON - Neurology
Dr Emad I Yakoub, Cambridge, ON - Family Medicine
Dr Ahlam H R Yanni, Scarborough, ON - General Practice
Dr Kibar Yared, Scarborough, ON - Cardiology
Dr Zeina Yared, Saint-Laurent, QC - Endocrin/Metabolism
Dr Aseel Yaser, Woodbridge, ON - Family Medicine
Dr Nasif I Yasin, Vancouver, BC - Physical Medicine & Rehab
Dr Naguib H Yassa, Brockville, ON - Anatomical Pathology
Dr Samir A R Yassa, Cornwall, ON - Urology
Dr Teraiza S S Yassa, Scarborough, ON - Internal Medicine
Dr Mariam Yassa, Montreal, QC - Radiation Oncology
Dr Zaid J Yasser, Scarborough, ON - General Surgery
Dr Sarkis Yeretsian, Montreal, QC - General Surgery
Dr Philippe R Yostos, Mississauga, ON - Family Medicine
Dr Hany N Youakim, Edmonton, AB - Family Medicine
Dr Sawsan I Younan, Mississauga, ON - General Practice
Dr Layla Younes, Montreal, QC - Family Medicine
Dr Osama A E Yousef, Kitchener, ON - Diagnostic-Radiology
Dr Jakline M Y Yousef, North York, ON - Psychiatry
Dr George M Yousef, Toronto, ON - Anatomical Pathology
Dr Samad S Yousif, Vaughan, ON - Family Medicine
Dr Thair H Yousif, Windsor, ON - Orthopedic Surgery
Dr Wafaa Youssef, Edmonton, AB - General Practice
Dr Magdy B Youssef, Brockville, ON - Anesthesia
Dr Mariam F G Youssef, Burlington, ON - Family Medicine
Dr Victor S F Youssef, Milton, ON - Family Medicine
Dr Ernest A N Youssef, Mississauga, ON - Family Medicine
Dr Youssef M R Youssef, Oshawa, ON - Radiation Oncology
Dr Fady Youssef, Ottawa, ON - Emergency Family Med
Dr Elham A A Youssef, Waterloo, ON - Family Medicine
Dr Fikry M Ywakim, Cornwall, ON - Obstetrics & Gynecology
Dr Randa Zabian, Chateauguay, QC - Family Medicine
Dr Nazar R Zabtia, Hamilton, ON - Orthopedic Surgery
Dr George P Zachariadis, Toronto, ON - General Practice
Dr Emad Zaghloul, Abbotsford, BC - Psychiatry
Dr Amjad N Zaher, Windsor, ON - Pediatrics
Dr Usama Zahlan, Kenora, ON - Psychiatry
Dr Mariam R Zakhary, Brampton, ON - Family Medicine
Dr Gamel S Zakhary, Brampton, ON - Pediatrics
Dr Liliane H Zakhary, Etobicoke, ON - Pediatrics
Dr Mourad I S Zakhary, London, ON - Family Medicine
Dr Nasser A Zaki, Etobicoke, ON - Family Medicine
Dr Emad L A Zaki, Hamilton, ON - General Practice
Dr Nora Zaklama, Pointe-Claire, QC - General Pathology
Dr Nayla Zalzal, Port Hope, ON - General Practice
Dr Kamruz Zaman, Toronto, ON - Family Medicine
Dr Rola Zamel, Brampton, ON - Endocrin/Metabolism
Dr Ricardo Zarruk, Pierrefonds, QC - General Practice
Dr Ekram Zayed, Victoria, BC - Hematological Pathology
Dr Maher N Zayouna, Windsor, ON - General Practice
Dr Zeinab H Ziada, Sault Ste. Marie, ON - Family Medicine
Dr Labib A A Zibdawi, Newmarket, ON - Internal Medicine
Dr Paul S Ziter, Windsor, ON - General Practice
Dr Magdy Zoghby, Montreal, QC - General Practice

ARMENIAN

Dr Dikran J Abrahamian, Penetanguishene, ON - General Practice
Dr Haig Ashikian, Gloucester, ON - Family Medicine
Dr Hovsep Baghdadlian, North York, ON - Infectious Diseases
Dr Arsene J Basmadjian, Montreal, QC - Cardiology
Dr Girair Basmadjian, Montreal, QC - Ophthalmology
Dr Katyg Behesnilian, Toronto, ON - Psychiatry
Dr Antranik N Benohanian, Montreal, QC - Dermatology
Dr Avedis Bogosyan, North York, ON - General Practice
Dr Avidis H Boudakian, Markham, ON - Urology
Dr Karoon C Danayan, Toronto, ON - Pediatrics
Dr Ari Demirjian, Mont-Royal, QC - Dermatology
Dr Chahe B Derghazarian, Saint-Leonard, QC - Hematology
Dr William S El Masri, Toronto, ON - Otolaryngology
Dr Danny M D Ghazarian, Toronto, ON - Anatomical Pathology
Dr Jean J Hallak, Montreal, QC - Obstetrics & Gynecology
Dr Herag Hamboyan, Brampton, ON - Family Medicine
Dr Sevan Hopyan, Toronto, ON - Orthopedic Surgery
Dr Gerard E Huni, Cowansville, QC - Anesthesia
Dr Marina Khatchatourian, North York, ON - Gastroenterology
Dr Lucie M Khouri, Saint-Laurent, QC - Ophthalmology
Dr Elie G Khoury, Saint-Laurent, QC - Ophthalmology
Dr Krikor Kichian, Ottawa, ON - Gastroenterology
Dr Rita Kuyumjian, Montreal, QC - Psychiatry
Dr Jirair Kuyumjian, Montreal, QC - General Practice
Dr Raffi S Kuyumjian, Saint-Hubert, QC - Family Medicine
Dr John J V Manoukian, Montreal, QC - Otolaryngology
Dr Berge Marcarian, Scarborough, ON - Otolaryngology
Dr Hagop K Mazmanian, Welland, ON - Urology
Dr Gregory B Meterissian, Montreal, QC - Psychiatry
Dr Patricia Mouaikel, Nepean, ON - Family Medicine
Dr Arakel Movsesyan, Hamilton, ON - General Practice
Dr Sevan G Ortaaslan, Kirkland, QC - Orthopedic Surgery
Dr Michael S Pandes, Richmond Hill, ON - Internal Medicine
Dr Apkar Papazian, Saint-Leonard, QC - Urology
Dr Kevork Minas Peltekian, Halifax, NS - Gastroenterology
Dr Rafi F Setrak, St Catharines, ON - Emergency Family Med
Dr Jean C Setrakian, Sherbrooke, QC - Internal Medicine
Dr Vahe Sivaciyan, Toronto, ON - Cardiology
Dr Tania Tajirian, Toronto, ON - Family Medicine
Dr Artin M Ternamian, Toronto, ON - Obstetrics & Gynecology
Mr Axel Tosikyan, Montreal, QC - Hematology
Dr Astghik Vartanian, Montreal, QC - General Practice
Dr Wahan Wanis, Vancouver, BC - Psychiatry
Dr Never Youssoufian de Perez, Toronto, ON - Psychiatry

ASHANTI

Dr Ahmed Boachie, Newmarket, ON - Psychiatry

ASSYRIAN

Dr Samir Abouna, Mississauga, ON - Family Medicine
Dr Parvaneh Beheshti, West Vancouver, BC - General Practice
Dr Sameera Benjamen, Woodbridge, ON - General Practice
Dr Sargon B Gandilo, Nepean, ON - Diagnostic-Radiology
Dr Sami S Marqus, Scarborough, ON - Internal Medicine
Dr Edward T Matti, Cambridge, ON - Psychiatry
Dr Ninos M Oda, Toronto, ON - Orthopedic Surgery
Dr Laith D Shimon, Sydney, NS - Family Medicine
Dr Sarah G Toma, Edmonton, AB - General Practice
Dr Thair H Yousif, Windsor, ON - Orthopedic Surgery

AZERI

Dr Kamel Alizadeh-Khiavi, Calgary, AB - Family Medicine
Dr Esmail K Arfai, North York, ON - Psychiatry
Dr Leila Fazeli Chaghoshi, North York, ON - Pediatrics
Dr Akbar Rajabi-Asl, Toronto, ON - Psychiatry

BELEN

Dr Abdullahi A Berih, Etobicoke, ON - Family Medicine

BELGIAN

Dr Ezzedine Attig, Riviere-du-Loup, QC - Neurology
Dr Paul J Jacquemin, Verdun, QC - Respirology

BEMBA

Dr Khami Chokani, Prince Albert, SK - General Practice

BENGALI

Dr Abul B M Ahmed, Milton, ON - Psychiatry
Dr Nazma Akter, Edmonton, AB - General Practice
Dr Tasriqul M Alam, London, ON - Family Medicine
Dr Zeenat Y Alam, Windsor, ON - Internal Medicine
Dr Syed A Ali, Edmonton, AB - General Practice
Dr Nabeel Ali, Montreal, QC - Pediatrics
Dr M Murad Bakht, Brampton, ON - Psychiatry
Dr Tuhin K Bakshi, Wetaskiwin, AB - Family Medicine
Dr Avik U Banerjee, Kitchener, ON - Otolaryngology
Dr Anna Banerji, Toronto, ON - Infectious Diseases
Dr Tapan K Banik, Brampton, ON - Psychiatry
Dr S Mahin Baqi, Etobicoke, ON - Infectious Diseases
Dr Hussam-Ul H Bawa, Calgary, AB - Psychiatry
Dr Rehana Begum, East York, ON - Family Medicine
Dr Ashok Bhagat, Richmond Hill, ON - General Practice
Dr Subramanya Bhagavatula, Sudbury, ON - Psychiatry
Dr Amal Bhattacharyya, Dartmouth, NS - General Practice
Dr Asok K Bhattacharyya, Nepean, ON - General Surgery
Dr Iqbal H Biswas, Cambridge, ON - Anesthesia
Dr Subrata Chakrabarti, London, ON - Anatomical Pathology
Dr Amitava D Chowdhury, Winnipeg, MB - General Practice
Dr Dhiman Chowdhury, Halifax, NS - General Practice
Dr Smriti Chowdhury, Halifax, NS - General Practice
Dr Monidipa Dasgupta, London, ON - Geriatric Medicine
Dr Susmita Datta, Scarborough, ON - General Practice
Dr Jyotirmoy Datta, Saskatoon, SK - General Practice
Dr Nibhas De, Thunder Bay, ON - Pediatrics
Dr Pushpal Desarkar, Toronto, ON - General Practice
Dr Shashi P Devi, North York, ON - Family Medicine
Dr Monika Dutt, Sydney, NS - Community Medicine
Dr Abu T M Firoz, Vaughan, ON - Family Medicine
Dr Satyajit N Ganguli, Brampton, ON - Diagnostic-Radiology
Dr Mahua Ghosh, Edmonton, AB - Endocrin/Metabolism
Dr Indraneel Ghosh, Hamilton, ON - Emergency Family Med
Dr Madhulika A Gupta, London, ON - Family Medicine
Dr Sanjoy Gupta, Thunder Bay, ON - Ophthalmology
Dr Malati Gupta, Toronto, ON - Psychiatry
Dr Hassan R Hakim, Barrie, ON - Psychiatry
Dr Syed M S Haq, Vancouver, BC - Family Medicine
Dr Khurshid Haque, Campbellton, NB - General Practice
Dr S K Mahmud Hasan, Winnipeg, MB - General Practice
Dr Sachin K Hazra, St Catharines, ON - Internal Medicine
Dr M Zahirul Hoque, Fort Saskatchewan, AB - General Practice
Dr Bonnieca F Islam, Edmonton, AB - Pediatrics
Dr Shashikant A Joglekar, Scarborough, ON - General Practice
Dr Aporna Kali, Grande Prairie, AB - Family Medicine
Dr Mandy Karim, Vancouver, BC - General Practice
Dr Mahmood A H Khan, Toronto, ON - Internal Medicine
Dr Kiron C Mallick, Winnipeg, MB - General Practice
Dr Tapas Mondal, Hamilton, ON - Cardiology
Dr Diana Mukherjee, Moncton, NB - General Practice
Dr Golam Murtoza, Brampton, ON - Family Medicine
Dr Monzur Naher, London, ON - Family Medicine
Dr Zahirul Quayyum, Hamilton, ON - Family Medicine
Dr Anusha Raghuraman, North York, ON - Psychiatry
Dr Mohammad M Rahman, Selkirk, MB - General Practice
Dr Dalia Ray, North York, ON - Obstetrics & Gynecology
Dr Sonia Sabir, Markham, ON - Emergency Family Med
Dr Amal K Saha, Halifax, NS - Family Medicine
Dr Indira Sen, Thornhill, ON - General Practice
Dr Natavarlal H Shah, Cornwall, ON - General Practice
Dr Tarun K Shaha, Vancouver, BC - Family Medicine
Dr Nirmal K Shahoo, Ponoka, AB - General Practice
Dr Farrukh B Sheikh, Pickering, ON - General Practice
Dr Nayeema Siddiq, Toronto, ON - General Practice

Dr Tahira Siddiqui, North York, ON - Anesthesia
Dr Roona Sinha, Saskatoon, SK - Pediatric Hematology Oncology
Dr Teesta B Soman, Toronto, ON - General Practice
Dr Shahida Sultana, Markham, ON - Internal Medicine
Dr Monalisa Sur, Hamilton, ON - Anatomical Pathology
Dr Ranjan K Sur, Hamilton, ON - Radiation Oncology
Dr Momtaz H Talukdar, Guelph, ON - Family Medicine
Dr Chiranjib Talukdar, Regina, SK - Pediatrics
Dr Syed M A Tayab, Fort Erie, ON - Internal Medicine
Dr Ma Khin Thida, Vancouver, BC - Family Medicine
Dr A H M Jamal Uddin, Toronto, ON - Internal Medicine
Dr Fatima Uddin, Toronto, ON - Family Medicine
Dr Sankar Vaidyanathan, Brampton, ON - Family Medicine
Dr Prema Vaidyanathan, Etobicoke, ON - Obstetrics & Gynecology
Dr Rajkumar Vajpeyi, Toronto, ON - Anatomical Pathology
Dr Abu M Yakub, Brampton, ON - General Practice
Dr Muhammed Zakaria, Oshawa, ON - Psychiatry
Dr Kamruz Zaman, Toronto, ON - Family Medicine

BERBER

Dr Mustapha Chelfi, Gatineau, QC - General Practice
Dr Kamaldine Oudjhane, Toronto, ON - General Practice

BICOL

Dr Antonio P Carretero Jr, Moose Jaw, SK - Anatomical Pathology
Dr Jiri J Dubec, Surrey, BC - Family Medicine

BILINGUAL(ENGLISH/FRENCH)

Dr Shawn D Aaron, Ottawa, ON - Critical Care Medicine
Dr Edith Abou Said, Ottawa, ON - Family Medicine
Dr Sydney L Abramson, Sudbury, ON - Family Medicine
Dr Josee Adam, Rockland, ON - Family Medicine
Dr Robert Adams, Moncton, NB - Neurosurgery
Dr Ali Adibfar, Toronto, ON - Plastic Surgery
Dr Ejaz Ahmad, Winnipeg, MB - Family Medicine
Dr Frederick L Albert, Prescott, ON - General Practice
Dr Clifford Albert, Montreal, QC - Family Medicine
Dr Martin Albert, Montreal, QC - Critical Care Medicine
Dr Natalie Albert, Quebec, QC - Anesthesia
Dr Jean Joseph Thierry Alcindor, Montreal, QC - Hematology
Dr Andre Allard, Saint-Jerome, QC - Community Medicine
Dr Nathalie Alos, Montreal, QC - General Practice
Dr Justine L Amaro, Ottawa, ON - Emergency Family Med
Dr Rebecca K Amer, Hamilton, ON - Internal Medicine
Dr Dimitrios J Anastakis, Toronto, ON - Plastic Surgery
Dr Jean I Anawati, Sturgeon Falls, ON - General Practice
Dr Aubie Angel, Toronto, ON - Internal Medicine
Dr Gordon A Arbess, Toronto, ON - Family Medicine
Dr Marcel Arcand, Sherbrooke, QC - Family Medicine
Dr Patrice Archambault, Pointe-Claire, QC - Ophthalmology
Dr Jonathan M Archibald, Peterborough, ON - Family Medicine
Dr Stephen Arnold, Cap-aux-Meules, QC - Family Medicine
Dr Alison Arnot, Mississauga, ON - Emergency Family Med
Dr Pradeepan Arulchelvam, Scarborough, ON - Family Medicine
Dr Tony Assouline, LaSalle, QC - Family Medicine
Dr Sarit Assouline, Montreal, QC - Hematology
Dr James A Atkins, Mississauga, ON - Emergency Family Med
Dr Jennifer A Atwood, Thunder Bay, ON - Family Medicine
Dr Anne Aube, Beamsville, ON - Family Medicine
Dr J Claude Aucoin, Cheticamp, NS - General Practice
Dr Marcel D Aucoin, Cheticamp, NS - Family Medicine
Dr Nathalie Audet, Quebec, QC - Otolaryngology
Dr Veronique Auger, Campbell River, BC - Family Medicine
Dr Louise T Auger, Montreal, QC - Pediatrics
Dr Edouard Auger, Quebec, QC - Psychiatry
Dr Brian J Aw, Richmond Hill, ON - Family Medicine
Dr Kim L Ayuen, Toronto, ON - Family Medicine
Dr Patricia C Baass, London, ON - Family Medicine
Dr Karine Badra Quirion, Vancouver, BC - Family Medicine
Dr Anne M Baggley, Ottawa, ON - Family Medicine
Dr Kashif M Baig, Ottawa, ON - Ophthalmology
Dr Elise M J Balaisis, Vancouver, BC - Family Medicine
Dr Penny J D Ballem, Vancouver, BC - Hematology
Dr Richard Balys, Lower Sackville, NS - Otolaryngology
Dr Diane F Bamford, Ottawa, ON - Family Medicine
Dr Devi Banerjee, Montreal, QC - Clin Immun/Allergy
Dr Elizabeth Barbour-Jones, Slocan Park, BC - General Practice
Dr Daniel Barolet, Laval, QC - Dermatology
Mr Peter C Barriga, Montreal, QC - Infectious Diseases
Dr Anise C Barton, Kamloops, BC - General Surgery
Dr Samir J Batarseh, Toronto, ON - Obstetrics & Gynecology
Dr Maureen Baxter, Ottawa, ON - Orthopedic Surgery
Dr Sara Bazinet, Shediac, NB - Family Medicine
Dr Carrie R Beallor, Thornhill, ON - Family Medicine
Dr Lise B Beaubien, Ottawa, ON - Family Medicine
Dr Philippe R Beaudry, Burlington, ON - Cardiology
Dr J Pierre Beaudry, Montreal, QC - Cardiology
Dr Monique Belanger, Sudbury, ON - Family Medicine
Dr Caroline A Beliveau, Burlington, ON - Obstetrics & Gynecology
Dr Robert Beliveau, Montreal, QC - General Practice
Dr Warren R Bell, Salmon Arm, BC - Family Medicine
Dr Liane M Belland, Calgary, AB - Obstetrics & Gynecology
Dr Jean-Francois Bellemare, Montreal, QC - General Surgery
Dr Isabelle A Bence-Bruckler, Ottawa, ON - Hematology
Dr Caroline O Benedek, Vancouver, BC - Family Medicine
Dr Antranik N Benohanian, Montreal, QC - Dermatology
Dr Janna Bentley, Kelowna, BC - Family Medicine
Dr Riva E Berezowski, Owen Sound, ON - Obstetrics & Gynecology
Dr Josee Bernatchez, Dieppe, NB - Pediatrics
Dr Simon Bernatchez, La Sarre, QC - General Practice
Dr Jean-Pierre Bernatchez, Quebec, QC - Psychiatry
Dr Francois P Bernier, Calgary, AB - Medical Genetics
Dr Kenneth Berris, Gatineau, QC - Internal Medicine
Dr Eric Berthelet, Vancouver, BC - Radiation Oncology
Dr Luc R Berthiaume, Calgary, AB - Critical Care Medicine
Dr Marc Berthiaume, Ottawa, ON - Family Medicine
Dr Carl Bertrand, Kanata, ON - General Practice
Dr Monique Bertrand, London, ON - Obstetrics & Gynecology
Dr Marc D Bibeau, Edmonton, AB - Internal Medicine
Dr Sandra R D Biem, Pointe-Claire, QC - Obstetrics & Gynecology
Dr Natasha Bird, Coaticook, QC - General Practice
Dr Shirley Blaichman, Westmount, QC - Pediatrics
Dr Normand Blais, Montreal, QC - Hematology
Dr Jeffrey A Blicker, Vancouver, BC - Ophthalmology
Dr Pierre Blier, Ottawa, ON - General Practice
Dr Alain J Blinn, Meteghan Centre, NS - General Practice
Dr Edith M Blondel-Hill, Kelowna, BC - Infectious Diseases
Dr Earl R Bogoch, Toronto, ON - Orthopedic Surgery
Dr Gilles Boire, Sherbrooke, QC - Internal Medicine
Dr Stephane Bolduc, Quebec, QC - Urology
Dr Richard R Bon, Surrey, BC - Cardiology
Dr Richard A Bonin, Gatineau, QC - Medical Microbiology
Dr Laurier Bouchard, Chicoutimi, QC - Obstetrics & Gynecology
Dr Remi W Bouchard, Quebec, QC - Electroencephal
Dr Pierre Boucher Jr, Longueuil, QC - Emergency Family Med
Dr Nathalie M Boudreau, New Westminster, BC - Family Medicine
Dr Eve M Boudreau, Bathurst, NB - Family Medicine
Dr France P Boudreau, Ottawa, ON - Family Medicine
Dr Richard Boule, Sherbrooke, QC - Family Medicine
Dr Louis-Philippe Boulet, Quebec, QC - Respirology
Dr Luc N Bourgon, Ottawa, ON - Psychiatry
Dr Julie Boyczum, St-Joseph-du-Lac, QC - General Practice
Dr Marc R Boyle, North Vancouver, BC - Orthopedic Surgery
Dr Angele Y Brabant, Sudbury, ON - Internal Medicine
Dr Bernadette Bradbury, Burnaby, BC - Family Medicine
Dr Philippa H Brain, Calgary, AB - Obstetrics & Gynecology
Dr Liza Brassard, Chicoutimi, QC - General Practice
Dr Myriam Brassard, Montreal, QC - Cardiology
Dr Marie-Josee Breau, Moncton, NB - Family Medicine
Dr Barry Breger, Montreal, QC - General Practice
Dr Terence P A Brennan, Osgoode, ON - Family Medicine
Dr Julie Breton-Fortin, Sturgeon Falls, ON - Family Medicine
Dr Malcolm L Brigden, Lethbridge, AB - Hematology
Dr Ronald J Brisebois, Edmonton, AB - General Surgery
Dr Dennis A T Brisson, Windsor, ON - Otolaryngology
Dr Andrea Brkovich, Windsor, ON - Obstetrics & Gynecology
Dr Lise Brochu, Montreal, QC - Psychiatry
Dr Dennis J T Brodie, Burlington, ON - Family Medicine
Dr Alexandra L Brooks-Hill, Whistler, BC - Orthopedic Surgery
Dr Kenneth L B Brown, Vancouver, BC - Orthopedic Surgery
Dr Seymour Brownstein, Ottawa, ON - Ophthalmology
Dr Michele F M Brule, Sudbury, ON - General Surgery
Dr Frank V Buffam, Vancouver, BC - Ophthalmology
Dr Maria Buithieu, Montreal, QC - Pediatrics
Dr Louis Bujold, Dalhousie, NB - Family Medicine
Dr Mark L Burman, Montreal, QC - Orthopedic Surgery
Dr Robert A F Burn, Calgary, AB - Family Medicine
Dr Irving J Burstein, Cote Saint-Luc, QC - General Practice
Dr Nicholas M W Busing, Ottawa, ON - Family Medicine
Dr Richard Bussieres, Quebec, QC - Otolaryngology
Dr Laith A Bustani, Nepean, ON - Family Medicine
Dr H Max Buxton, Calabogie, ON - Emergency Family Med
Dr Diane T Cabana, Mercier, QC - Obstetrics & Gynecology
Dr Chrystella K Calvert, Dundas, ON - Pediatrics
Dr Daniel J Cameron, Ottawa, ON - Family Medicine
Dr Judith M Cameron, Montreal, QC - Dermatology
Dr Douglas M Campbell, Toronto, ON - Pediatrics
Dr Sylvie M D Cantin, Pembroke, ON - Family Medicine
Dr Kenneth Z Cantor, Montreal, QC - Cardiology
Dr Lucille B Carling-Chambers, Burlington, ON - Cardiology
Dr Heidi M Carlson-Reid, Moncton, NB - Pediatrics
Dr Michel Carmel, Sherbrooke, QC - Urology
Dr Marc Carrier, Ottawa, ON - Hematology
Dr Pierre Cartier, Saint-Jerome, QC - Internal Medicine
Dr Michelle Casey, Lansdowne, ON - Family Medicine
Dr Shirley L Caspin, Toronto, ON - Family Medicine
Dr Luc Chagnon, Hawkesbury, ON - Family Medicine
Dr Karen Chambers, Ladysmith, QC - Family Medicine
Dr Jean-Pierre Chanoine, Vancouver, BC - General Practice
Dr Suzanne Charbonneau, Laval, QC - General Practice
Dr Yves G Charette, Val Caron, ON - Family Medicine
Dr Julia C Charles, Thunder Bay, ON - Anesthesia
Dr Anne-Marie Charpentier, Toronto, ON - Radiation Oncology
Dr E Ruth Chaytor, Montreal, QC - Orthopedic Surgery
Dr David Z I Cherney, Toronto, ON - Internal Medicine
Dr Ramasami V Chettiar, Gr-Sault/Gr-Falls, NB - General Practice
Dr Chantal Chiasson, Shediac, NB - Dermatology
Dr Veronic Clair, Vancouver, BC - Community Medicine
Dr Jamieson C Clark, Williams Lake, BC - General Practice
Dr Dale B Clayton, New Westminster, BC - Endocrin/Metabolism
Dr Jennifer E J Clement, Etobicoke, ON - Family Medicine
Dr Isabelle Cochrane, Nelson, BC - Emergency Family Med
Dr Gina S A Coleman, Ottawa, ON - General Practice
Dr Neil C Colman, Montreal, QC - Internal Medicine
Dr Alban L Comeau, Saulnierville, NS - General Practice
Dr Pierre Comte, Lachute, QC - Pediatrics
Dr C Andrew Connely, Edmundston, NB - General Practice
Dr William T Conner, Hamilton, ON - Pediatrics
Dr W Edward S Connolly, Montreal, QC - Ophthalmology
Dr Kevin M Convery, Morden, MB - Family Medicine
Dr David Copeland, Cornwall, ON - Clin Immun/Allergy
Dr Michel Copti, Montreal, QC - Electroencephal
Dr Trevor A Corneil, Kelowna, BC - Community Medicine
Dr Glenn G Corneil, New Liskeard, ON - Family Medicine
Dr André E Corriveau, Edmonton, AB - Community Medicine
Dr Joseph A M A Cote, Ottawa, ON - General Practice
Dr Aurore Cote, Montreal, QC - Pediatrics
Dr Michael E Cotterill, Wawa, ON - Family Medicine
Dr Jason E Coupland, Vancouver, BC - Psychiatry
Capt Cyd Courchesne, Ottawa, ON - General Practice
Dr Olivier Court, Montreal, QC - Critical Care Medicine
Dr Aidlee R Craft, North York, ON - Family Medicine
Dr Jeffrey W H Cranford, St Catharines, ON - General Surgery
Dr Michelle Crawford, Dieppe, NB - General Practice
Dr Jason D Creaghan, Ottawa, ON - Family Medicine
Dr Terrence M Creatchman, Hamilton, ON - Family Medicine
Dr Brigitte A Crepeau, Penticton, BC - Anesthesia
Dr Christopher F Cressey, Palmerston, ON - Family Medicine

Dr Agathe Croteau, Quebec, QC - General Practice
Dr Charles J E Cruise, Mississauga, ON - Anesthesia
Dr Daniel J Cuillerier, London, ON - Anesthesia
Dr Heather T Culbert, Toronto, ON - Family Medicine
Dr Michael J Curran, Ottawa, ON - Anesthesia
Dr Richard A Currie, Salmon Arm, BC - Family Medicine
Dr John J D Curry, Port Coquitlam, BC - General Practice
Dr Kimberley A Curtin, Peterborough, ON - Family Medicine
Dr Meghan M Cusack, Sudbury, ON - Family Medicine
Dr Sharon Cushing, Toronto, ON - Otolaryngology
Dr Robert A Cushman Jr, Ottawa, ON - Community Medicine
Dr Jean-Claude Cutz, Hamilton, ON - Anatomical Pathology
Dr Anthony G Czaharyn, Kirkland, QC - Family Medicine
Dr Barbara A Czerkawski, Kelowna, BC - Internal Medicine
Dr Catherine M D'Amico, Nepean, ON - Family Medicine
Dr A M Michele D'Iorio, Mississauga, ON - Psychiatry
Dr Emilie Daigneault, Orleans, ON - Family Medicine
Dr Julie F Daitchman, Thornhill, ON - Endocrin/Metabolism
Dr Stephane Dallaire, Kingston, ON - Emergency Family Med
Dr Jocelyne M Danais Brown, Winnipeg, MB - Family Medicine
Dr Brigitte L M Dandenault, Moncton, NB - Psychiatry
Dr Ronald Dandurand, Cornwall, ON - Internal Medicine
Dr Jerome Dansereau, Victoria, BC - Obstetrics & Gynecology
Dr Hani Daoud, Virden, MB - General Practice
Dr Justine Dassa, Montreal, QC - Pediatrics
Dr Eric Davenport, Thunder Bay, ON - Critical Care Medicine
Dr Michelle A L Davey, Winchester, ON - General Surgery
Dr James A Davidson, Surrey, BC - Internal Medicine
Dr Lindsay K Davidson, Kingston, ON - Orthopedic Surgery
Dr Alan E Davis, Cornwall, ON - Emergency Family Med
Dr Darryl R Davis, Ottawa, ON - Cardiology
Dr Victoria J Davis, Scarborough, ON - Obstetrics & Gynecology
Dr Beverley M Davis, Toronto, ON - Family Medicine
Dr Soraya Davoudi, Ottawa, ON - Emergency Medicine
Dr Michel De Billy, Whitby, ON - Family Medicine
Dr Louise De Guire, Montreal, QC - General Practice
Dr Sandrine De Ribaupierre, London, ON - General Practice
Dr Joost M De Ruiter, Toronto, ON - Anesthesia
Dr Selwyn X P De Souza, Ottawa, ON - Family Medicine
Dr Robin M Deans, Windsor, ON - Ophthalmology
Dr Shoshanah E C Deaton, Rockland, ON - Family Medicine
Dr Wilber Deck, Gaspe, QC - Community Medicine
Dr Christopher Decker, Parry Sound, ON - General Surgery
Dr Jaime Del Carpio, Montreal, QC - Clin Immun/Allergy
Dr Eugene Delabays, Montreal, QC - Anesthesia
Dr Rejean-Andre Delisle, Chicoutimi, QC
- Medical Microbiology & Infectious Diseases
Dr Raffaele A Dell'Aquila, North Bay, ON - Family Medicine
Dr Marie-Eve Demers, Saint-Hyacinthe, QC - General Practice
Dr Mychele C Deneault, Rockland, ON - Family Medicine
Dr Manon A Denis-LeBlanc, St Isidore, ON - Family Medicine
Dr Greta A Dervish, Ottawa, ON - General Surgery
Dr Pierre Dery, Quebec, QC - Pediatrics
Dr Christiane S Deschenes, Almonte, ON - General Practice
Dr Julie Deschenes, Longueuil, QC - Internal Medicine
Dr Jean-Gaston Descoteaux, Golden, BC - General Surgery
Dr Jean-Haulis R Desimon, Dollard-D-Ormeaux, QC
- General Practice
Dr JP Jean-Pierre Desjardins, Ottawa, ON - Orthopedic Surgery
Dr Marie-Josee Desjardins, Montreal, QC - General Practice
Dr Natale Desrochers, Dunnville, ON - Family Medicine
Dr Marie-Isabelle Desrosiers, Orleans, ON - Family Medicine
Dr Sean J Dickie, Ottawa, ON - Anesthesia
Dr Michael T Dickinson, Miramichi, NB - Pediatrics
Dr Nicole E Didyk, Kitchener, ON - Geriatric Medicine
Dr Robert Diez-d'Aux, Montreal, QC - Family Medicine
Dr Jonathan A Dingle, Hamilton, ON - Anesthesia
Dr Laurent Dinh, Ottawa, ON - Nuclear Medicine
Dr Natalie M Dinovitzer, Ottawa, ON - Family Medicine
Dr Martin Dobkin, Mississauga, ON - General Practice
Dr Peter S Docherty, Moncton, NB - Internal Medicine
Dr Paul L Doiron, Moncton, NB - Anesthesia
Dr Rehana N Dosani, Mississauga, ON - Family Medicine
Dr Monique R Dostaler, Sarnia, ON - Family Medicine
Dr Paul R Doucet, Drummondville, QC
- Obstetrics & Gynecology
Dr Jennifer F Douek, Ottawa, ON - Family Medicine
Dr Karen J Dover, Ottawa, ON - General Practice
Dr James A Downar, Toronto, ON - Critical Care Medicine
Dr Mary-Anne Doyle, Ottawa, ON - Endocrin/Metabolism
Dr Kenneth R Doyle, Montreal, QC - Emergency Medicine
Dr Francois Dubeau, Montreal, QC - Electroencephal
Dr James Ducharme, Mississauga, ON - Emergency Medicine
Dr David Duclos, Gatineau, QC - General Practice
Dr Susie Duff, Ottawa, ON - Internal Medicine
Dr Neil Duggal, London, ON - Neurosurgery
Dr Shauna Duigenan, Ottawa, ON - Diagnostic-Radiology
Dr Marin J Duke, Waterloo, ON - Family Medicine
Dr Rejean Dumais, Sherbrooke, QC - Orthopedic Surgery
Dr Michel Dunberry, St-Charles-Boromee, QC - General Surgery
Dr Eric G Duncan, Mississauga, ON - Neurosurgery
Dr Desiree Dunn, Corner Brook, NL - Family Medicine
Dr Nicolas Dupre, Quebec, QC - Neurology
Dr Jean-Eric J Dupuis, Moose Creek, ON - General Practice
Dr Nicholas Dust, Ottawa, ON - Pediatrics
Dr Peter A Dutchak, Kingston, ON - Nuclear Medicine
Dr Arthur Dworetz, Saint-Sauveur, QC - Psychiatry
Dr Barry Dworkin, Ottawa, ON - Family Medicine
Dr Tamina Eapen, Ottawa, ON - Psychiatry
Dr Brad D Eason, Petawawa, ON - Family Medicine
Dr Christopher J Eaton, Ottawa, ON - Psychiatry
Dr Robert J Eaton, Ottawa, ON - General Practice
Dr Daniel Ebert, Brockville, ON - Emergency Family Med
Dr Sarah J Eckler, Toronto, ON - Family Medicine
Dr Michael W Edgerley, Scarborough, ON - Family Medicine
Dr David R Edmison, Ottawa, ON - Ophthalmology
Dr Gillian Edmonds, Listowel, ON - Family Medicine
Dr Gian Egger, Mississauga, ON - Pediatrics
Dr Pamela D Eisener-Parsche, Ottawa, ON - Family Medicine
Dr Gayle P Ekstrand, Gloucester, ON - Family Medicine
Dr Pauline R Ekwalanga, Calgary, AB - Obstetrics & Gynecology
Dr Salhab el Helou, Hamilton, ON - General Practice
Dr Robert D Elliott, Ottawa, ON - Anesthesia
Dr John D Elltoft, St Catharines, ON - General Practice
Dr Carl P Emond, Montreal, QC - General Surgery
Dr Francois Emond, Quebec, QC - Neurology
Dr Shane English, Ottawa, ON - Critical Care Medicine
Dr Atika Ennaifer, LaSalle, QC - Family Medicine
Dr Nancy E Epstein, Toronto, ON - Ophthalmology
Dr Robert G Esguerra, Kanata, ON - General Practice
Dr Manuel N Esquivel, Toronto, ON - Internal Medicine
Dr Mark Essak, Cobourg, ON - Family Medicine
Dr David Evans, Vancouver, BC - General Surgery
Dr Holly C Evans, Ottawa, ON - Anesthesia
Dr Bruce S Eveleigh, Ottawa, ON - General Practice
Dr Patrice L Eydoux, Vancouver, BC - General Practice
Dr Alison Eyre, Ottawa, ON - Family Medicine
Dr John A Fairfield, Hawkesbury, ON - General Practice
Dr Paul H K Fan-Lun, Whitby, ON - General Practice
Dr Ruth Farey, Ottawa, ON - Family Medicine
Dr Gloria Farhat, Oakville, ON - Family Medicine
Dr Michelle Farine, Toronto, ON - Pediatrics
Dr Catherine A Farrell, Montreal, QC - Critical Care Medicine
Dr Carolyn R Faught, Ottawa, ON - Hematology
Dr Haydarally H Fazal, Markham, ON - Pediatrics
Dr Luke M Fazio, North York, ON - Urology
Dr Robert J Feibel, Ottawa, ON - Orthopedic Surgery
Dr Lori Feigelson, North York, ON - Physical Medicine & Rehab
Dr Rubin M Feldman, Vancouver, BC
- Physical Medicine & Rehab
Dr Shim S I Felsen, North York, ON - Family Medicine
Dr Daphna Fenyves, Montreal, QC - Gastroenterology
Dr Pierre A Ferguson, Hawkesbury, ON - Psychiatry
Dr Lisa F Fettes, North Bay, ON - Anesthesia
Dr Giuseppe Ficara, Montreal, QC - Pediatrics
Dr Stephen K Field, Calgary, AB - Internal Medicine
Dr Aurore Fifi-Mah, Calgary, AB - Internal Medicine
Dr Lucie C Filteau, Ottawa, ON - Anesthesia
Dr Harvey Finkelstein, Ottawa, ON - Dermatology
Dr Susan Finlay, Sudbury, ON - General Practice
Dr Marc Fischer, Hamilton, ON - Urology
Dr Rebecca Fisher, Ottawa, ON - General Practice
Dr Gillian Fisher, Montreal, QC - General Practice
Dr Leona Fishman-Shapiro, North York, ON - Pediatrics
Dr David H Fitchett, Toronto, ON - Cardiology
Dr Carrie L Fitzsimons, Nelson, BC - Pediatrics
Dr Tamar Y Flanders, Toronto, ON - Pediatrics
Dr Nathalie Fleming, Ottawa, ON - Obstetrics & Gynecology
Dr M Dominique Flynn, Ottawa, ON - Family Medicine
Dr Tomas Fogl, Ottawa, ON - Psychiatry
Dr Stephane Foidart, Kenora, ON - Family Medicine
Dr Conchita Fonseca, Ottawa, ON - Emergency Family Med
Dr Amelie Fontaine, Edmonton, AB - Hematology
Dr Elizabeth L Ford-Jones, Toronto, ON - Pediatrics
Dr Lisa Forster, Picton, ON - Family Medicine
Dr Dalilah Fortin, London, ON - General Surgery
Dr Dean J Foti, Vancouver, BC - Neurology
Dr Vasilios A Fragiskos, Hearst, ON - General Practice
Dr Nathan P Frank, Richmond Hill, ON - Family Medicine
Dr Jean-Yves Frappier, Montreal, QC - Pediatrics
Dr Margaret A Fraser, Ottawa, ON - Diagnostic-Radiology
Dr D Leigh Fraser-Roberts, Ottawa, ON - Pediatrics
Dr Marc Frechette, Winnipeg, MB - Family Medicine
Dr Paul P Fredette, Val Caron, ON - Family Medicine
Dr Stephen M Freedman, Toronto, ON - Internal Medicine
Dr Ryan L Freistatter, North Bay, ON - Family Medicine
Dr Gordon J French, Ottawa, ON - Diagnostic-Radiology
Dr Veronique French Merkley, Ottawa, ON - Family Medicine
Dr Thomas P Frenette, Moncton, NB - Family Medicine
Dr Gerald Friedman, Thornhill, ON - Pediatrics
Dr Robert N Friedman, Toronto, ON - Psychiatry
Dr Ian M Frost, Ottawa, ON - Anesthesia
Dr James E D Fullerton, Carleton Place, ON - Family Medicine
Dr Celeste Fung, Ottawa, ON - Family Medicine
Dr Robert P Gabriel, Oakville, ON - General Practice
Dr Helene M Gagne, Nepean, ON - Obstetrics & Gynecology
Dr Kevin R Gagne, North Bay, ON - Anesthesia
Dr Sylvain Gagne, Ottawa, ON - Anesthesia
Dr Rachel M Gagnier, London, ON - Emergency Family Med
Dr Jean-Guy R Gagnon, Sudbury, ON - Psychiatry
Dr Yvon-Rene Gagnon, Vermilion Bay, ON - Family Medicine
Dr Marianne Gagnon, Amos, QC - General Practice
Dr Josee Gagnon, Quebec, QC - Critical Care Medicine
Dr Isabelle Gagnon, St-Jean-sur-Richel, QC - General Practice
Dr Isabelle Gagnon, Whitehorse, YT - General Practice
Dr Pierre Gailloux, Weedon, QC - General Practice
Dr Louise Galarneau, Montreal, QC - Community Medicine
Dr Daniel J Galley, Cornwall, ON - Diagnostic-Radiology
Dr Shital Gandhi, Toronto, ON - Internal Medicine
Dr Bryan Garber, Ottawa, ON - Critical Care Medicine
Dr Claude Garceau, Quebec, QC - Internal Medicine
Dr Donald I Gardiner, Midland, ON - Family Medicine
Dr Bertha Gardner-Maher, Scarborough, ON - Neurology
Dr Sunil Garg, Lachine, QC - Cardiology
Dr Hassan A M Gargoum, Regina, SK - Cardiology
Dr Andrea D Garland, Saint John, NB - Otolaryngology
Dr Philippe M Garzon, Mississauga, ON - General Surgery
Dr Anne M Gaskin, Kingston, ON - Family Medicine
Dr Raymond B Gay, Ottawa, ON - General Surgery
Dr Sharon G Gazeley, Toronto, ON - Family Medicine
Dr David Gee, Oshawa, ON - Family Medicine
Dr Andrew S Gee, Ottawa, ON - Emergency Medicine
Dr Herman Gelber, Scarborough, ON - Psychiatry
Dr Marcel Genest, Burnaby, BC - General Practice
Dr Rene Genest, Quebec, QC - General Practice
Dr Sylvain Genest, Saint-Jerome, QC - General Surgery
Dr Stephanie I Genge, St. John's, NL - Internal Medicine
Dr Paul C Geoffrion, Raymond, AB - Emergency Family Med
Dr Pierre Geoffroy, Aurora, ON - Family Medicine
Dr Caroline M A Gerin-Lajoie, Ottawa, ON - Psychiatry
Dr Louis-Philippe Germain, Gatineau, QC - General Surgery
Dr Michael M Gertler, Whitby, ON - General Practice
Dr Lauren A Gewurz, Toronto, ON - Family Medicine
Dr Maged Ghali, Montreal, QC - Gastroenterology
Dr Sanyukta K Ghoorah, Saskatoon, SK - Internal Medicine
Dr Rishi K Ghosh, Sault Ste. Marie, ON - Critical Care Medicine
Dr A Alan Giachino, Ottawa, ON - Orthopedic Surgery
Dr Sean Gibson, Oshawa, ON - Urology

Dr Rose-Marie A L Gieni, Sault Ste. Marie, ON - General Practice
Dr Steven M Gilberg, Ottawa, ON - Ophthalmology
Dr Kenneth Gilbert, London, ON - Internal Medicine
Dr Lucy Gilbert, Montreal, QC - Obstetrics & Gynecology
Dr Anne M W Gillies, Ottawa, ON - Pediatrics
Dr Judy R M Gillies, Timmins, ON - Family Medicine
Dr Laurent C Gilloteaux, Scarborough, ON - Diagnostic-Radiology
Dr Isabelle Giordano, Kanata, ON - Family Medicine
Dr Stephanie M Girard, Burlington, ON - Diagnostic-Radiology
Dr Anthony E Glanz, Windsor, ON - Cardiology
Dr Verne J Glavin, Cambridge, ON - Infectious Diseases
Dr Francis Glorieux, Montreal, QC - General Practice
Dr Linda Gobessi, Ottawa, ON - Psychiatry
Dr Suzanne Godsoe, Nepean, ON - Emergency Medicine
Dr Phil Gold, Montreal, QC - Clin Immun/Allergy
Dr David S Goldbloom, Toronto, ON - Psychiatry
Dr Mindy R Goldman, Ottawa, ON - Hematology
Dr Marc B Goldstein, Toronto, ON - Internal Medicine
Dr Eric Goldstein, Toronto, ON - Dermatology
Dr Mark Goldszmidt, London, ON - Internal Medicine
Dr Charles L Gomberg, Montreal, QC - Internal Medicine
Dr Natalie N Goodale, Sudbury, ON - Family Medicine
Dr John C Goodall, Ottawa, ON - Dermatology
Dr Robert L Goodman, London, ON - Cardiovasc/ThorSurg
Dr Michelle Gordon, Orillia, ON - Pediatrics
Dr John A Gorfinkel, Toronto, ON - Ophthalmology
Dr Pierre Gosselin, Quebec, QC - General Practice
Dr Alexis Goth, Kapuskasing, ON - Family Medicine
Dr Chloe Gottlieb, Ottawa, ON - Ophthalmology
Dr Elizabeth Gottman, Ottawa, ON - Family Medicine
Dr Mona R Goubran, Ottawa, ON - Family Medicine
Dr Ginette Goulard, Gatineau, QC - Psychiatry
Dr Eric Goyer, Saint-Jerome, QC - Community Medicine
Dr Mark E Gracia, Williams Lake, BC - Emergency Family Med
Dr Pierre Granger, Montreal, QC - General Practice
Dr Valerie Gratton, Ottawa, ON - General Practice
Dr Anne-Marie Gravel, Montreal, QC - Dermatology
Dr Gillian R Graves, Halifax, NS - Obstetrics & Gynecology
Dr Peter S Graves, Nepean, ON - Emergency Family Med
Dr Lisa Graves, Sudbury, ON - Family Medicine
Dr Jonathan D Gray, Ottawa, ON - Psychiatry
Dr Jennifer Green, Toronto, ON - Family Medicine
Dr Ellen M Greenblatt, Toronto, ON - Obstetrics & Gynecology
Dr Sylvie Gregoire, Vanier, ON - Gastroenterology
Dr M M Catherine Grenier, Mississauga, ON - Emergency Medicine
Dr Geoff Grieve, Peterborough, ON - Family Medicine
Dr Patricia E Griffiths, Ottawa, ON - Family Medicine
Dr Gregory B Griffiths, St Catharines, ON - Internal Medicine
Dr Andrea Grin, Toronto, ON - Anatomical Pathology
Dr Rolf Gronas, North York, ON - Anesthesia
Dr Loren D Grossman, Toronto, ON - Endocrin/Metabolism
Dr Douglas Gruner, Ottawa, ON - Family Medicine
Dr Benoit Guay, Ottawa, ON - Otolaryngology
Dr Helene Guay, Amos, QC - General Practice
Dr Dominique Guenard, Levis, QC - General Practice
Dr Charles Guertin, Montreal, QC - Plastic Surgery
Dr Gregory M T Guilcher, Calgary, AB - Hematology
Dr Marie-Claude Guimond, North York, ON - Psychiatry
Dr Benoit Guindon, Cornwall, ON - Ophthalmology
Dr Vydas Gurekas, Temiscaming, QC - General Practice
Dr Andrea Gutauskas, Ottawa, ON - General Surgery
Dr Pierre Guy, Vancouver, BC - Orthopedic Surgery
Dr Eric M Haapala, Bruce Mines, ON - Family Medicine
Dr L Richard Haber, Ste-Anne-de-Bellev, QC - Pediatrics
Dr Sharon L Hackett, Calgary, AB - Dermatology
Dr Dimitri E Haddad, Cambridge, ON - Orthopedic Surgery
Dr Amir Tinouch Haghighat Talab, Gatineau, QC - Cardiology
Dr Christopher W Hall, Oshawa, ON - Family Medicine
Dr Kelly Halliday, Etobicoke, ON - Family Medicine
Dr Sarah M F Halliday, Ottawa, ON - Psychiatry
Dr Patrick Hamel, Montreal, QC - Ophthalmology
Dr Donald J Hamilton, Red Deer, AB - General Surgery
Dr Anne Hamilton, Ottawa, ON - Family Medicine
Dr Dominique Hanna, Sherbrooke, QC - Dermatology
Dr Peter G Hanson, Toronto, ON - General Practice
Dr Patrick G Harris, Montreal, QC - Plastic Surgery
Dr Pierre Harvey, Chicoutimi, QC - General Practice
Dr Omar N Hasan, Amqui, QC - General Surgery
Dr Jean-Louis Hausser, Montreal, QC - General Practice
Dr Jessica Haussmann, Calgary, AB - Gastroenterology
Dr Oliver R Haw For Chin, Calgary, AB - Internal Medicine
Dr Tracy Hayes, Sudbury, ON - Emergency Family Med
Dr Catherine T Haywood, Brampton, ON - Plastic Surgery
Dr Guy J Hebert, Ottawa, ON - Emergency Medicine
Dr Christian-Rene Hebert, Quebec, QC - Family Medicine
Dr C Colette Hegarty, Toronto, ON - Anesthesia
Dr Frederic Helie, Saint-Jerome, QC - Otolaryngology
Dr Martin Heller, North York, ON - Orthopedic Surgery
Dr James M Henderson, Fredericton, NB - Rheumatology
Dr Tamara A Henderson, Kingston, ON - Anesthesia
Dr Graeme A Hendry, Smiths Falls, ON - Family Medicine
Dr Sybil M Henteleff, Delta, BC - General Practice
Dr Pierre Hermans, Verdun, QC - General Surgery
Dr Renee C Hessian, Ottawa, ON - Cardiology
Dr Dean Hickey, Bathurst, NB - Internal Medicine
Dr Michael Hier, Montreal, QC - Otolaryngology
Dr Samantha Hill, Toronto, ON - Cardiac Surgery
Dr Michael S Hirsh, Ottawa, ON - Family Medicine
Dr Tuan Van Hoang, Montreal, QC - General Practice
Dr Elisabeth J Hobden, Ottawa, ON - Emergency Medicine
Dr Chaker A Hobeika, St. John's, NL - Pediatrics
Dr Brian D Hodges, Toronto, ON - Psychiatry
Dr Therese M M Hodgson, Orleans, ON - Family Medicine
Dr John R Hoey, Port Perry, ON - Community Medicine
Dr Megan R Hogan, Oakville, ON - Dermatology
Dr Angela Hogan, Ottawa, ON - Anesthesia
Dr Jacqueline L Holm Jhass, St. Albert, AB - Family Medicine
Dr Debbie F Honickman, Toronto, ON - Family Medicine
Dr Kenneth Hook, Tavistock, ON - Family Medicine
Dr Lawrence C Hookey, Kingston, ON - Gastroenterology
Dr Ruth Horn, Montreal, QC - Infectious Diseases
Dr Patricia A M Horsham, Mississauga, ON - Pediatrics
Dr John Hortop, Ormstown, QC - Cardiology
Dr Sheik N Hosenbocus, Kamloops, BC - Psychiatry
Dr Stefaine Houde, Rossland, BC - Family Medicine
Dr Frederic S Hould, Quebec, QC - General Surgery
Dr Sylvain Houle, Toronto, ON - Nuclear Medicine
Dr Ronald A House, Toronto, ON - Occupational Med
Dr Jane M Howard, North Bay, ON - Psychiatry
Dr Andrew W Howard, Toronto, ON - Orthopedic Surgery
Dr Marck P J Hudon, North Vancouver, BC - General Practice
Dr Bevan G Hughes, Vancouver, BC - Anesthesia
Dr Richard J Huntsman, Saskatoon, SK - Neurology
Dr Byron M Hyde, Ottawa, ON - General Practice
Dr Cam J Inch, Toronto, ON - Emergency Family Med
Dr Mihaela Ionita, Laval, QC - Family Medicine
Dr Marc H Isler, Montreal, QC - Orthopedic Surgery
Dr Laurie L Itcush, Surrey, BC - General Practice
Dr Sheila V Jacob, Montreal, QC - Pediatrics
Dr Raymond G Jacques, Coniston, ON - General Practice
Dr Hilary F Jaeger, Ottawa, ON - General Practice
Dr Anne-France M Jaworski, Brockville, ON - General Practice
Dr Nathalie Jette, Calgary, AB - Neurology
Dr Sanjay K Jindal, Huntsville, ON - Internal Medicine
Dr Ernest B Johnson, Halifax, NS - General Practice
Dr Wendy S W Johnston, Edmonton, AB - Neurology
Dr Edmund F Jones, Kingston, ON - Otolaryngology
Dr Serge P Jothy, Toronto, ON - Anatomical Pathology
Dr David P Joyce, Vancouver, BC - Emergency Family Med
Dr Warren R Julien, Summerland, BC - General Practice
Dr Luc C Jutras, Montreal, QC - Cardiology
Dr Joel H Kailia, Nelson, BC - Family Medicine
Dr Michael J Kalin, Montreal, QC - Family Medicine
Dr Paula J Kebarle, Vancouver, BC - Emergency Family Med
Dr Douglas N Keeling, Quispamsis, NB - Dermatology
Dr Lisa M Kellett, Toronto, ON - Dermatology
Dr Meghan L Kelly, Nanaimo, BC - Family Medicine
Dr Brendan G Kenny, Moncton, NB - Neurosurgery
Dr Pauline E Kerr, Ottawa, ON - Clin Immun/Allergy
Dr May Khairy, Montreal, QC - Pediatrics
Dr Renu Khullar, Gatineau, QC - General Practice
Dr David C Khuon, Ottawa, ON - Family Medicine
Dr Antoine Kibrite, Quebec, QC - General Surgery
Dr Robert F Kidd, Renfrew, ON - General Practice
Dr Andrea F Kirsh, Toronto, ON - Family Medicine
Dr Marie-Josee Klett, Orleans, ON - Family Medicine
Dr Allan Knight, Toronto, ON - Internal Medicine
Dr John B Kortbeek, Calgary, AB - General Surgery
Dr Frank B Kortbeek, Edmonton, AB - Orthopedic Surgery
Dr Clifford A Korzinstone, Oshawa, ON - Ophthalmology
Dr Marjorie E Krabbe, Summerland, BC - Family Medicine
Dr Danielle Kraus, Pointe-Claire, QC - Ophthalmology
Dr Teresa K Kus, Montreal, QC - Cardiology
Dr Frank J LaRue, Gatineau, QC - General Practice
Dr Claude Laberge, Montreal, QC - General Practice
Dr Jean-Martin Laberge, Montreal, QC - General Surgery
Dr Gilles F Labrecque, St-Jean-Port-Joli, QC - General Practice
Dr Diane V Lacaille, Richmond, BC - Internal Medicine
Dr Yves Lacasse, Quebec, QC - Internal Medicine
Dr Jacques E Lacasse, Ste-Anne-des-Monts, QC - Diagnostic-Radiology
Dr Guy Lacombe, Sherbrooke, QC - Geriatric Medicine
Dr Lucie E Lafay-Cousin, Calgary, AB - General Practice
Dr Celine Laferriere, Montreal, QC - Infectious Diseases
Dr Claude Laflamme, Toronto, ON - Anesthesia
Dr Philippe Lageix, Verdun, QC - General Practice
Dr Bernard G Lalonde, Ottawa, ON - General Practice
Dr Robert A Lamarche, Casselman, ON - General Practice
Dr Monique Landry, Montreal, QC - General Practice
Dr Marie-France Langlois, Sherbrooke, QC - Endocrin/Metabolism
Dr Jonathan L Lapin, Toronto, ON - Diagnostic-Radiology
Dr Michael A C Lapner, London, ON - Orthopedic Surgery
Dr Katherine E Lariviere, Ottawa, ON - Family Medicine
Dr Marie Larochelle-Beland, Quebec, QC - Radiation Oncology
Dr Heather A Larton, Waterloo, ON - General Practice
Dr Jonathan F Lasich, Brockville, ON - General Practice
Dr Rowena Lass, Kenora, ON - General Practice
Dr Warren C W Latham, Scarborough, ON - Orthopedic Surgery
Dr Jean Latreille, Greenfield Park, QC - Hematology
Dr Genevieve Lauzon, West Vancouver, BC - General Practice
Dr Gilles Lauzon, Montreal, QC - General Surgery
Dr Ronald F Lavigne, Renfrew, ON - Family Medicine
Dr Guy J Lavoie, Edmonton, AB - Orthopedic Surgery
Dr Josee Lavoie, Montreal, QC - Anesthesia
Dr Colleen E Lawlor, West Vancouver, BC - Family Medicine
Dr Sarah L Lawrence, Ottawa, ON - Pediatrics
Dr Sarah E Lawrence, Ottawa, ON - Endocrin/Metabolism
Dr Louis J Lawton, Ottawa, ON - Orthopedic Surgery
Dr Michel A Le Breton, Dieppe, NB - Orthopedic Surgery
Dr Daniel LeBlond, Lethbridge, AB - Physical Medicine & Rehab
Dr Jacques G Leblanc, Vancouver, BC - Cardiovasc/ThorSurg
Dr Yves Leclerc, Kitchener, ON - Cardiovasc/ThorSurg
Dr Denis G Leduc, Westmount, QC - Pediatrics
Dr Daniel P Lefrancois, Longueuil, QC - Emergency Medicine
Dr Richard Leger, Calgary, AB - Ophthalmology
Dr Chantal S Leger, Vancouver, BC - Hematology
Dr Claude Leger, Salaber-de-Valleyf, QC - Diagnostic-Radiology
Dr Martine Lehoux, Quebec, QC - General Practice
Dr Douglas M Leitner, Penticton, BC - General Practice
Dr Valery Lemelin, Quebec, QC - Gastroenterology
Dr Marie L C Lemire, Cornwall, ON - Family Medicine
Dr Edmond G Lemire, Saskatoon, SK - Medical Genetics
Dr Anik Lepage, Moncton, NB - Dermatology
Dr Denis J B Lepage, Sherbrooke, QC - Psychiatry
Dr Suzanne Lepine, Montreal, QC - Psychiatry
Dr Mark R Lesk, Montreal, QC - Ophthalmology
Dr Ronald R Lett, Vancouver, BC - General Surgery
Dr Liisa K Levasseur, Lively, ON - Family Medicine
Dr Adeera Levin, Vancouver, BC - Internal Medicine
Dr Richard Levin, Montreal, QC - General Practice
Dr Janette I Lindley, Vancouver, BC - Ophthalmology
Dr D Robertson Lloyd-Smith, Vancouver, BC - General Practice
Dr Laurie A Logan, Vancouver, BC - Family Medicine
Dr Marc Lonergan, Montreal, QC - Psychiatry
Dr Mona R Loutfy, Toronto, ON - Infectious Diseases

Dr Jonathan R Love, Calgary, AB - Gastroenterology
Dr Stanley Lubin, Vancouver, BC - Family Medicine
Dr Nathalie Lucas, Montreal, QC - Pediatrics
Dr Daniel E Lusignan, Bourget, ON - Family Medicine
Dr Christopher J Lyons, Vancouver, BC - Ophthalmology
Dr Stephannie M MacDonell, Osgoode, ON - Family Medicine
Dr W Gregory MacDougall, Victoria, BC - Family Medicine
Dr Laura S MacLaren, Kahnawake, QC - Emergency Family Med
Dr Vona MacMillan, Dalhousie, NB - Family Medicine
Dr Jack F Machin, Lac-Megantic, QC - General Practice
Dr Graeme F Magor, Comox, BC - General Practice
Dr Jean-Noel Mahy, Burnaby, BC - General Surgery
Dr Babak Maleki, Halifax, NS - Ophthalmology
Dr Margaret L Manville, Comox, BC - Family Medicine
Dr Marc H Marion, Carleton Place, ON - General Practice
Dr Brenda A Markland, Nanaimo, BC - Orthopedic Surgery
Dr Andrea K Marrin, Oakville, ON - Clin Immun/Allergy
Dr Marilyn C Marshall, Stratford, ON - Psychiatry
Dr Danielle A S Martin, Toronto, ON - Family Medicine
Dr Andre-Guy Martin, Quebec, QC - Radiation Oncology
Dr Pierre Martin, Sorel-Tracy, QC - General Surgery
Dr Daphne R Marussi, Sherbrooke, QC - General Practice
Dr Ariel R Masetto, Sherbrooke, QC - General Practice
Dr Joseph Massad, Toronto, ON - Family Medicine
Dr Joanna L Massam, Toronto, ON - Pediatrics
Dr Yanick N R Masse, Ottawa, ON - Emergency Family Med
Dr Claude J Massicotte, Ottawa, ON - Gastroenterology
Dr Surya Master, Campbellton, NB - General Surgery
Dr Paul G Mathers, Montreal, QC - Emergency Family Med
Dr David M Matheson, Elliot Lake, ON - General Practice
Dr R Brian Mathieu, Roberval, QC - Ophthalmology
Dr Christel C Mathis, Montreal, QC - Diagnostic-Radiology
Dr Douglas G Matsell, Vancouver, BC - Nephrology
Dr Keith L Matthews, Montreal, QC - Urology
Dr Richard May, Montreal, QC - General Practice
Dr James P McAuley, London, ON - Orthopedic Surgery
Dr Simon O McCall, Hawkesbury, ON - General Practice
Dr Anne E McCarthy, Ottawa, ON - Infectious Diseases
Dr Fiona C McConville, Pickering, ON - Obstetrics & Gynecology
Dr David R McCoubrey, Ottawa, ON - Obstetrics & Gynecology
Dr Mark E McLean, Vancouver, BC - Community Medicine
Dr Reid M McLean Wiest, Calgary, AB - Family Medicine
Dr Martin A J McNamara, Midland, ON - Emergency Family Med
Dr Jose H Mejia, London, ON - Psychiatry
Dr Sara J Meltzer, Montreal, QC - Endocrinology
Dr Henri A Menard, Montreal, QC - Rheumatology
Dr Claude Mercier, Montreal, QC - Neurosurgery
Dr Donald G Merrett, Metcalfe, ON - General Practice
Dr Luc L Mertens, Toronto, ON - General Practice
Dr Sarkis H Meterissian, Montreal, QC - General Surgery
Dr Stephanie Metrakos, Kirkland, QC - Pediatrics
Dr Robert A W Miller, Halifax, NS - Dermatology
Dr Catherine A Milne, Montreal, QC - General Surgery
Dr Stephen J G Mintsioulis, Calgary, AB - Family Medicine
Dr John Moini, Verdun, QC - Family Medicine
Dr Gregory J Monkewich, Burnaby, BC - Gastroenterology
Dr Carolyne J Montgomery, Vancouver, BC - Anesthesia
Dr Rami Morcos, Mont-Royal, QC - Electroencephal
Dr Mohib Morcos, Quebec, QC - General Practice
Dr Daniel Moreau, Orleans, ON - Obstetrics & Gynecology
Dr Scott C Morgan, Ottawa, ON - Radiation Oncology
Dr Bernard Morin, Quebec, QC - General Practice
Dr Brenda E Moroz, Montreal, QC - Dermatology
Dr Andree Y Morrison, Sturgeon Falls, ON - Family Medicine
Dr Walter Moscovitz, Calgary, AB - Obstetrics & Gynecology
Dr Brian G Moses, Yarmouth, NS - Internal Medicine
Dr Pinos M Mpiana, Conception-Bay-S, NL - General Practice
Dr Roland J Muise, Yarmouth, NS - General Practice
Dr Marc A Mullie, Mont-Royal, QC - Ophthalmology
Dr Matthew D Mulligan, Ottawa, ON - Internal Medicine
Dr Diane L Munz, Westmount, QC - Pediatrics
Dr Craig S Murray, Vancouver, BC - Emergency Family Med
Dr J Scott Murray, Pembroke, ON - Urology
Dr Gilles Murray, Terrebonne, QC - Medical Microbiology
Dr Gabriel Muruve, Winnipeg, MB - Pediatrics
Dr Miriam Myers, Thornhill, ON - General Practice

Dr Steven P Nadler, Ottawa, ON - Internal Medicine
Dr Leslie A X Nash, St Catharines, ON - Pediatrics
Dr James B Nasmith, Vancouver, BC - Cardiology
Dr Francoise Naud, Quebec, QC - Anatomical Pathology
Dr Douglas D R Naudie, London, ON - Orthopedic Surgery
Dr Najmi Nazerali-Sunderji, Vancouver, BC - Family Medicine
Dr Kara A Nerenberg, Edmonton, AB - Internal Medicine
Dr Peter R Neufeld, Vancouver, BC - Internal Medicine
Dr Nicholas M Newman, Montreal, QC - Orthopedic Surgery
Dr Ngoc-Van Nguyen, Lachine, QC - General Surgery
Dr Lan Chau Nguyen, Saint-Lambert, QC - General Practice
Dr Melissandre Noel, Vancouver, BC - Family Medicine
Dr Sean P Nolan, Vancouver, BC - Psychiatry
Dr Diane M Normandin, Ste-Marthe-S-L-Lac, QC - General Practice
Dr Seamus Norton, Delhi, ON - Pediatrics
Dr William H Novick, Montreal, QC - Otolaryngology
Dr Jacqueline M O'Connell, Richmond, BC - Obstetrics & Gynecology
Dr Catherine S O'Connor, Gloucester, ON - Family Medicine
Dr Cameron R Oishi, Ottawa, ON - Family Medicine
Dr Kamaldine Oudjhane, Toronto, ON - General Practice
Dr Hugue A Ouellette, Vancouver, BC - Diagnostic-Radiology
Dr Rachel E Ouellette, Fredericton, NB - Pediatrics
Dr Sylvie A Ouellette, Moncton, NB - Internal Medicine
Dr Carolyn J Owen, Calgary, AB - Hematology
Dr Catherine M Owen, Scarborough, ON - Obstetrics & Gynecology
Dr Marcella M S Palad, Orangeville, ON - Family Medicine
Dr Max J Palayew, Montreal, QC - Diagnostic-Radiology
Dr Peter H L Pang, Gatineau, QC - General Practice
Dr Gaetan Paradis, Levis, QC - Urology
Dr John E Parsons, Orleans, ON - General Practice
Dr John D Paton-Gay, Edmonton, AB - Critical Care Medicine
Dr John C Pecknold, Westmount, QC - Psychiatry
Dr Tripler Pell, Toronto, ON - Family Medicine
Dr Julien Pelletier, Quebec, QC - Psychiatry
Dr Yael Perez, Mississauga, ON - Neurology
Dr Marty Perlmutar, Toronto, ON - Pediatrics
Dr Christine M Perreault, Vancouver, BC - Pediatrics
Dr Therese Perreault, Montreal, QC - Pediatrics
Dr Odette Perron, Maniwaki, QC - Orthopedic Surgery
Dr Allan D Peterkin, Toronto, ON - Family Medicine
Dr Nick J Petrella, Saint-Leonard, QC - General Practice
Dr Michael A Phillipowsky, Ottawa, ON - General Practice
Dr Dianne K Phillips, Langley, BC - General Practice
Dr Phay Pich, Vancouver, BC - General Practice
Dr Nicholas Pilote, Moncton, NB - Diagnostic-Radiology
Dr France Pinault, Quebec, QC - General Practice
Dr Francisco Pinero-Medina, Sherbrooke, QC - Psychiatry
Dr Johanne Plante, Brossard, QC - General Practice
Dr Diane N F Poilly, Cornwall, ON - Emergency Family Med
Dr Angela M Poirier, Halifax, NS - General Practice
Dr Richard F Poole, Alexandria, ON - General Practice
Dr Barry I Posner, Westmount, QC - Endocrinology
Dr Ronald B Postuma, Montreal, QC - Neurology
Dr Wayne J Potashner, North York, ON - Internal Medicine
Dr Catherine M Pound, Ottawa, ON - Pediatrics
Dr Maryse Power, Vancouver, BC - General Practice
Dr Umesh H Prabhu, Yarmouth, NS - Internal Medicine
Dr Franck G Prat, Richmond, BC - General Practice
Dr David Prchal, Vancouver, BC - Internal Medicine
Dr Ignacio Prieto, Montreal, QC - Cardiovasc/ThorSurg
Dr France Proulx, Montreal, QC - Psychiatry
Dr Josee Provencher, Laval, QC - General Surgery
Dr Simone Provencher, Longueuil, QC - General Practice
Dr Eric S Pugash, New Westminster, BC - Plastic Surgery
Dr Jeffrey W Purkis, White Rock, BC - General Practice
Dr Theodore Rabinovitch, North York, ON - Ophthalmology
Dr Barry Rabinovitch, Montreal, QC - Internal Medicine
Dr Jean-Mathieu Racicot, Amos, QC - Anesthesia
Dr Jamie M Rappaport, Montreal, QC - Otolaryngology
Dr Charles A D Raybaud, Toronto, ON - Diagnostic-Radiology
Dr Linda M Redman, Toronto, ON - Psychiatry
Dr Paolo Renzi, Montreal, QC - Internal Medicine
Dr Louise-Isabelle Rivard, Montreal, QC - Family Medicine

Dr Magali Robert, Calgary, AB - Obstetrics & Gynecology
Dr Alain A Robillard, Montreal, QC - Electroencephal
Dr Paul Robinson, Gatineau, QC - General Practice
Dr Luc J W Rochon, Ottawa, ON - Gastroenterology
Dr William J Rock, Vanier, ON - Ophthalmology
Dr Rejean Rock, North Hatley, QC - General Practice
Dr Maria del Rosario Rodriguez Moya, Montreal, QC - General Practice
Dr Pierre B Roland, Montreal, QC - General Practice
Dr Jean Rosenberg, Huntingdon, QC - General Practice
Dr David S Rosenblatt, Montreal, QC - Med Scientist
Dr B Catherine Ross, Calgary, AB - Critical Care Medicine
Dr Jacques Rouleau, Quebec, QC - Cardiology
Dr Pierre Rousseau, Montreal, QC - Radiation Oncology
Dr Nancy Roy, Gatineau, QC - General Surgery
Dr Isabelle Roy, Montreal, QC - Radiation Oncology
Dr Jean-Francois Roy, Quebec, QC - Orthopedic Surgery
Dr P James A Ruiter, London, ON - General Practice
Dr Paula P Ryan, Salt Spring Island, BC - Family Medicine
Dr M Suzanne Rydzik, Ottawa, ON - General Practice
Dr Emile Saad, Beaver Bank, NS - Family Medicine
Dr Robert Sabbagh, Sherbrooke, QC - Urology
Dr Kenneth B Sabourin, Nepean, ON - Family Medicine
Dr Gulzar P Sachedina, Calgary, AB - Anesthesia
Dr Julie Samson, Timmins, ON - Emergency Family Med
Dr Richard Satin, Montreal, QC - Diagnostic-Radiology
Dr Claude Sauve, Montreal, QC - Cardiology
Dr Alyssa Scheim, Mont-Royal, QC - Family Medicine
Dr Heidi N Schmaltz, Calgary, AB - Geriatric Medicine
Dr David A Schneiderman, Ottawa, ON - Internal Medicine
Dr Stefan P J Schovanek, Comox, BC - Psychiatry
Dr Kevin J Schwartzman, Montreal, QC - Internal Medicine
Dr Christopher J H Sedergreen, Anmore, BC - General Practice
Dr Roanne J Segal, Ottawa, ON - Internal Medicine
Dr Daniel R Seguin, Rockland, ON - Family Medicine
Dr Ernest G Seidman, Montreal, QC - Pediatrics
Dr Laura P Sellers, Ottawa, ON - Family Medicine
Dr William Semaan, Sherbrooke, QC - General Practice
Dr Vyta M Senikas, Ottawa, ON - Obstetrics & Gynecology
Dr Danya A Sereda, West Vancouver, BC - Dermatology
Dr K Briar Sexton, Vancouver, BC - Ophthalmology
Dr Justin A Shah, Victoria, BC - Gastroenterology
Dr Jack Shahin, Scarborough, ON - Otolaryngology
Dr A Allison Shaikh, London, ON - Diagnostic-Radiology
Dr Scott E Shannon, Hamilton, ON - General Practice
Dr Kerrie A Shaw, Mississauga, ON - Family Medicine
Dr Nathan M Sheiner, Montreal, QC - Cardiovasc/ThorSurg
Dr Margaret A Shepherd, Vancouver, BC - Pediatrics
Dr Robert W Shepherd, Victoria, BC - Family Medicine
Dr Frances A Shepherd, Toronto, ON - Hematology
Dr Mark Sherman, Victoria, BC - Family Medicine
Dr Caroline B E Shilhan, Cranbrook, BC - Family Medicine
Dr Lina A Shoppoff, Iroquois Falls, ON - Family Medicine
Dr Craig A Shott, Brantford, ON - Family Medicine
Dr Christian L Shriqui, Quebec, QC - Psychiatry
Dr Laurel G D Shugarman, Richmond Hill, ON - Family Medicine
Dr Hemen P Shukla, Toronto, ON - Family Medicine
Dr Jacqueline M C Shukle, Nepean, ON - Dermatology
Dr Scott M Shulman, North Bay, ON - Gastroenterology
Dr Ian I Sibbald, Rossland, BC - Emergency Family Med
Dr Ian M F Silver, Kingston, ON - Diagnostic-Radiology
Dr Andree-Anne Simard, Montreal, QC - General Practice
Dr Gary A Simatos, Edmonton, AB - Family Medicine
Dr Sarah R Simkin, Pembroke, ON - Family Medicine
Dr Gerald J Simkus, New Westminster, BC - Cardiology
Dr Kiri J M Simms, Victoria, BC - Psychiatry
Dr Judith Simoneau-Roy, Sherbrooke, QC - Endocrin/Metabolism
Dr D Irene Simons, Montreal, QC - Family Medicine
Dr Margaret I Simpson, Calgary, AB - Family Medicine
Dr Gabrielle T Singer, Ottawa, ON - Family Medicine
Dr Vidyanand B Singh, Sarnia, ON - Family Medicine
Dr Sunita K S Singh, Toronto, ON - Internal Medicine
Dr Christian Sirois, Montreal, QC - General Surgery
Dr Wendy R Sissons, Montreal, QC - Dermatology
Dr M Amanda L Skoll, Vancouver, BC - Obstetrics & Gynecology

Dr Asad Sleiman, Granby, QC - General Practice
Dr David I Small, Montreal, QC - Internal Medicine
Dr Peter Small, Montreal, QC - Clin Immun/Allergy
Dr Sydney E H Smart, Toronto, ON - Anatomical Pathology
Dr Michal A N Smialowski, Tatlayoko Lake, BC - Family Medicine
Dr Jenni Smith, North Vancouver, BC - General Surgery
Dr Telisha J Smith-Gorvie, Toronto, ON - Emergency Medicine
Dr James A R Snodgrass, Victoria, BC - Family Medicine
Dr Sumeet K Sodhi, Toronto, ON - Family Medicine
Dr Stephen Sohmer, Campbell River, BC - Orthopedic Surgery
Dr David J Sollazzo, Hamilton, ON - Emergency Family Med
Dr John N Sollazzo, Richmond Hill, ON - Emergency Family Med
Dr M A Andrew Solomon, Ottawa, ON - Psychiatry
Dr Daniel M Somogyi, Thornhill, ON - Family Medicine
Dr Howard H Song, Toronto, ON - Infectious Diseases
Dr Alexander M Sorisky, Ottawa, ON - Endocrin/Metabolism
Dr Caroline Spiers, Beaumont, AB - Family Medicine
Dr Marcia A Spooner, Carleton Place, ON - Family Medicine
Dr Kyna J Squarey, St. John's, NL - Neurology
Dr Nadim Srour, Ottawa, ON - Internal Medicine
Dr Blair A St Martin, Edmonton, AB - Urology
Dr Jason J St-Hilaire, Port Colborne, ON - Family Medicine
Dr Mireille C St-Jean, Ottawa, ON - Family Medicine
Dr Karen L Stancer, Vancouver, BC - Family Medicine
Dr Gerald W Stanimir, Montreal, QC - Obstetrics & Gynecology
Dr Mark A Steeves, Ottawa, ON - Orthopedic Surgery
Dr Thomas D L Steeves, Toronto, ON - Neurology
Dr Mark A Stefan, Laval, QC - Community Medicine
Dr Henry J Stefanison, Barrie, ON - General Surgery
Dr Astrid E Stegaru, Saint-Eustache, QC - Family Medicine
Dr Debra G Stein, Toronto, ON - Psychiatry
Dr Errol Stern, Montreal, QC - Emergency Medicine
Dr Sarah C Stevens, Halifax, NS - Anesthesia
Dr Christiaan S M Stevens, Barrie, ON - Radiation Oncology
Dr Liisa H Stevens, Smiths Falls, ON - Family Medicine
Dr Allen I Steverman, Laval, QC - Family Medicine
Dr James K Stewart, Edmonton, AB - General Surgery
Dr Julia R Stewart, Burnaby, BC - Family Medicine
Dr John D Stewart, North Vancouver, BC - Neurology
Dr Bradley E Stewart, Halifax, NS - General Practice
Dr Andrea K Stewart, Ottawa, ON - Psychiatry
Dr Aviva T Stewart, Pembroke, ON - Emergency Family Med
Dr Jeremie R Stewart, Sudbury, ON - Anesthesia
Dr Andrew P Stiell, Ottawa, ON - Emergency Family Med
Dr Linda J Stirk, North York, ON - Obstetrics & Gynecology
Maj Melville Storrier, Kingston, ON - Family Medicine
Dr Tonja L Stothart, Nepean, ON - Family Medicine
Dr Irena M Straszak, Vancouver, BC - Psychiatry
Dr Jessica S Strike, Ottawa, ON - Family Medicine
Dr Jeremy F G Sturgeon, Montreal, QC - Internal Medicine
Dr Barry J Sullivan, Kelowna, BC - General Surgery
Dr Patrick J Sullivan, Toronto, ON - Family Medicine
Dr James D Sullivan, Montreal, QC - Orthopedic Surgery
Dr Glen L Sumner, Calgary, AB - Cardiology
Dr R Sudhir Sundaresan, Ottawa, ON - General Surgery
Dr Penelope A Sutcliffe, Sudbury, ON - Community Medicine
Dr Aparna Swaminathan, Toronto, ON - Family Medicine
Dr Jean E Swenerton, Vancouver, BC - Anesthesia
Dr Agata Szlanta, Kingston, ON - Family Medicine
Dr Roman G Szumski, Ottawa, ON - General Pathology
Dr Jason E W D Taam, Edmonton, AB - Anesthesia
Dr Thomas K Tabor, London, ON - Family Medicine
Dr Mario Talajic, Montreal, QC - Cardiology
Dr Denise H Tam, Scarborough, ON - Internal Medicine
Dr Patrick B Tan, Brampton, ON - Gastroenterology
Dr Ian F Tannock, Toronto, ON - Internal Medicine
Dr Herbert Tanzer, North York, ON - Ophthalmology
Dr Jean-Claude Tardif, Montreal, QC - Cardiology
Dr Daniel J Tascona, Orillia, ON - Internal Medicine
Dr Robert H Taylor, Vancouver, BC - General Surgery
Dr William H Taylor, Barrie, ON - Anesthesia
Dr Allan J Taylor, Ottawa, ON - Family Medicine
Dr Joel M H Teichman, Vancouver, BC - Urology
Dr Harshad Telang, Thunder Bay, ON - General Surgery
Dr Dominique Tessier, Montreal, QC - Family Medicine
Dr J Francois A Theriault, Kelowna, BC - Ophthalmology
Dr Richard P Thomas, Kingston, ON - Obstetrics & Gynecology
Dr Sophia Thomas, Windsor, ON - Family Medicine
Dr Josyane Thomassin, Kirkland, QC - Family Medicine
Dr David M P Thomson, Montreal, QC - Clin Immun/Allergy
Dr Lisa D Thurgur, Toronto, ON - Emergency Medicine
Dr Mary E L Tidmarsh, Vancouver, BC - Psychiatry
Dr Milvi K Tiislar, Victoria, BC - Family Medicine
Dr Janice A Tijssen, Toronto, ON - Pediatrics
Dr William W Tinmouth, Courtenay, BC - Urology
Dr Jill M Tinmouth, Toronto, ON - Gastroenterology
Dr Lee V Toner, Sudbury, ON - Emergency Family Med
Dr Arman Topakian, Repentigny, QC - Obstetrics & Gynecology
Dr Carlos H Torres, Ottawa, ON - General Practice
Dr Melissa J Torriero, Calgary, AB - Family Medicine
Dr Manon Tougas, Hamilton, ON - Critical Care Medicine
Dr Naji J Touma, Kingston, ON - Urology
Dr Eric S Touzin, Sioux Lookout, ON - General Surgery
Dr Tiffany N Townsend, Vancouver, BC - Neurology
Dr Andrea F Townson, Vancouver, BC - Physical Medicine & Rehab
Dr Carla N Trail, Brockville, ON - Family Medicine
Dr Ninh Ngoc Tran, Hamilton, ON - Community Medicine
Dr Michael D Traynor, Vancouver, BC - Anesthesia
Dr John B Treilhard, Whitby, ON - General Practice
Dr Madeleine D Tremblay, Vancouver, BC - Psychiatry
Dr Ronald Tremblay, Cornwall, ON - General Practice
Dr Catherine Tremblay, Toronto, ON - Obstetrics & Gynecology
Dr Michele Tremblay, Montreal, QC - General Practice
Dr Germain L Trempe, Montreal, QC - Hematological Pathology
Dr J Andrew Trenholm, Halifax, NS - Orthopedic Surgery
Dr Richard L Trenholm, Huntsville, ON - Family Medicine
Dr Daniel C J Trottier, Ottawa, ON - General Surgery
Dr Konia J Trouton, Victoria, BC - Family Medicine
Dr James Truong, Callander, ON - General Practice
Dr Togas Tulandi, Montreal, QC - Obstetrics & Gynecology
Dr Michel Tulin, Chambly, QC - Gastroenterology
Dr Kathrin M Turchin, Toronto, ON - Family Medicine
Dr Michele A Turek, Ottawa, ON - Cardiology
Dr Bruno Turmel, Montreal, QC - General Practice
Dr Bridget K Tutschka, London, ON - Family Medicine
Dr Jennifer R Tynan, Saskatoon, SK - Diagnostic-Radiology
Dr Anne Marie Uhlir, Sainte-Croix, QC - General Practice
Dr Mark A Unger, Mississauga, ON - Family Medicine
Dr Steven R Uttley, Pembroke, ON - Family Medicine
Dr Trina C Uwiera, Edmonton, AB - Otolaryngology
Dr Claude Vaillancourt, Montreal, QC - General Practice
Dr Edith E Valcourt, Orleans, ON - Obstetrics & Gynecology
Dr Chantal Vallee, Greenfield Park, QC - Internal Medicine
Dr Nicole Van Rossum, Sherbrooke, QC - Endocrin/Metabolism
Dr Richard C Van Wylick, Kingston, ON - Pediatrics
Dr Claude Vandal, Levis, QC - Family Medicine
Dr Robert G Varadi, York, ON - Internal Medicine
Dr Philip X Vayalumkal, Brampton, ON - Emergency Family Med
Dr Shelley L Veinish, North York, ON - Geriatric Medicine
Dr Karen M Verbeeten, Toronto, ON - Diagnostic-Radiology
Dr Alan R Vernec, Montreal, QC - General Practice
Dr Jennifer M Vethamuthu, Ottawa, ON - Nephrology
Dr Gilles Vezina, Cookshire, QC - General Practice
Dr Diane Villanyi, Vancouver, BC - Geriatric Medicine
Dr Pierre Villeneuve, Newmarket, ON - Hematology
Dr Patrick J Villeneuve, Ottawa, ON - General Surgery
Dr Michael J Vizel, Etobicoke, ON - General Practice
Dr Slavica Vlahovich, Ottawa, ON - General Practice
Dr Pierre Voisine, Quebec, QC - Cardiac Surgery
Dr Monika Volesky, Montreal, QC - Orthopedic Surgery
Dr Gyula Voros, Oakville, ON - Family Medicine
Dr Stephane M Voyer, Vancouver, BC - Internal Medicine
Dr Erik N Vu, Vancouver, BC - Critical Care Medicine
Dr Mark P Vu, Vancouver, BC - Anesthesia
Dr Guy Waddell, Sherbrooke, QC - Obstetrics & Gynecology
Dr Peter B Waind, Waterloo, ON - Ophthalmology
Dr Richard E Waldolf, Pembroke, ON - Family Medicine
Dr Mathieu A D Walker, Montreal, QC - Cardiology
Dr Jens-Erik Walter, Montreal, QC - Obstetrics & Gynecology
Dr J Mark Walton, Hamilton, ON - General Surgery
Dr Kimberly J Walton, Ottawa, ON - Anesthesia
Dr Christine C Walton, Toronto, ON - Orthopedic Surgery
Dr Hsiu-Li Wang, Waterloo, ON - Community Medicine
Dr Karen Wanger, Vancouver, BC - Emergency Medicine
Dr Glen K Ward, Langley, BC - Pediatrics
Dr Mylene Ward, Guelph, ON - General Surgery
Dr Rosalind A Ward-Smith, Burlington, ON - Family Medicine
Dr Edward M I Wasser, Markham, ON - Family Medicine
Dr Karen N Watanabe Duffy, Ottawa, ON - Internal Medicine
Dr Valerie J Waters, Toronto, ON - Infectious Diseases
Dr Priya N Watson, Toronto, ON - Psychiatry
Dr Peter D Watt, Newmarket, ON - Obstetrics & Gynecology
Dr Suzanne E Watters, Comox, BC - Family Medicine
Dr Robyn J Watts, Richmond, BC - Plastic Surgery
Dr Johanne I Weberpals, Ottawa, ON - Obstetrics & Gynecology
Dr David Weigens, Westmount, QC - Family Medicine
Dr Gabrielle S Weiler, Ottawa, ON - Nephrology
Dr Francine B Wein, Montreal, QC - Ophthalmology
Dr Robert P Weinstein, North York, ON - Psychiatry
Dr S John Weisnagel, Quebec, QC - Endocrin/Metabolism
Dr Margaret D Weiss, Vancouver, BC - Psychiatry
Dr Brian N Weitzman, Ottawa, ON - Emergency Family Med
Dr Tania L Welters, Oakville, ON - Emergency Family Med
Dr Avram D Whiteman, Montreal, QC - Family Medicine
Dr Wilma G Whiting, Oshawa, ON - Anesthesia
Dr J Scott Whittaker, Vancouver, BC - Gastroenterology
Dr David R Williams, Newmarket, ON - Emergency Medicine
Dr Robin L Williams, Ottawa, ON - Pediatrics
Dr Brian C Willoughby, Vancouver, BC - Family Medicine
Dr Joanne S Willoughby, Guelph, ON - Dermatology
Dr Heather C Wilson, Kelowna, BC - General Surgery
Dr Jean-Marie J Wilson, Mill Bay, BC - Emergency Family Med
Dr Adriana E Wilson, Halifax, NS - Psychiatry
Dr Donald K Wilson, Ottawa, ON - General Practice
Dr Paul J Winston, Victoria, BC - Physical Medicine & Rehab
Dr Marcel Wolfe, Saint-Leonard, QC - Psychiatry
Dr Wai-Ben Wong, North Vancouver, BC - Emergency Family Med
Dr Graham C Wong, Vancouver, BC - Cardiology
Dr Daniel C Wong, North York, ON - Neurology
Dr Philip Wong, Montreal, QC - Gastroenterology
Dr Teresa M B Wood, Squamish, BC - Family Medicine
Dr Lorraine Woolford, Mississauga, ON - Obstetrics & Gynecology
Dr Erin D Wright, Edmonton, AB - Otolaryngology
Dr Yizheng Wu, Ottawa, ON - Family Medicine
Dr Anna E H Wyand, Ottawa, ON - Anesthesia
Dr Lisa D S Yang, Saint John, NB - Family Medicine
Dr Brian P Yaremko, London, ON - Radiation Oncology
Dr Timothy T Yates, Calgary, AB - Psychiatry
Dr Annie Yau, Calgary, AB - Family Medicine
Dr Carole-Anne L Yelle, Surrey, BC - Critical Care Medicine
Dr Fung Voon K You-Ten, Toronto, ON - Anesthesia
Dr David W Young, Victoria, BC - Ophthalmology
Dr Eric R Young, Victoria, BC - Community Medicine
Dr Deidre C Young, Toronto, ON - Family Medicine
Dr Hany M R Youssef, Ottawa, ON - Anesthesia
Dr John T Yu, North Vancouver, BC - Dermatology
Dr Kenneth J Yvorchuk, Victoria, BC - Cardiology
Dr Christian E Zaarour, Toronto, ON - General Practice
Dr Katalin Zador, La Prairie, QC - General Practice
Dr Paul K Zalzal, Oakville, ON - Orthopedic Surgery
Dr Cathryn M Zeglinski, Whistler, BC - Family Medicine
Dr Ines Zepic, Toronto, ON - General Practice
Dr Caroline M Zerey, Cornwall, ON - Family Medicine
Dr Laura J Zieffle, Burnaby, BC - Family Medicine
Dr Mary S Zinck, Halifax, NS - Psychiatry
Dr Elizabeth M Zubek, Maple Ridge, BC - Family Medicine
Dr Betty Zylbergold-Schonfeld, Montreal, QC - Pediatrics

BILINGUAL(FRENCH/ENGLISH)

Dr Stacey Ageranioti-Belanger, Montreal, QC - Pediatrics
Dr Christian Ahmarani, Montreal-Nord, QC - Otolaryngology
Dr Najma N Ahmed, Montreal, QC - Pediatrics
Dr Gerald A Ahronheim, Westmount, QC - Medical Microbiology

Dr Jean Alain, Gatineau, QC - Medical Biochemistry
Dr Isabelle Alain, Trois-Rivieres, QC - General Practice
Dr Hughette Alarie, Trois-Rivieres, QC - General Practice
Dr Diane Albert, Rimouski, QC - Family Medicine
Dr Gilles R Albert, Saint-Hubert, QC - Pediatrics
Dr Luce Albert-Daigle, Saint-Jacques, NB - Family Medicine
Dr Ariane Alimenti, Vancouver, BC - General Practice
Dr Denis Allaire, Saint-Jerome, QC - Otolaryngology
Dr Joffre C Allard, Rimouski, QC - Hematology
Dr Denis Allard, Saint-Jerome, QC - Urology
Dr Manon Allard, Westmount, QC - Pediatrics
Dr Julie Almasi, Cote Saint-Luc, QC - Family Medicine
Dr Isabelle Amyot, Montreal, QC - Pediatrics
Dr Marcel A Amyot, Saint-Laurent, QC - Ophthalmology
Dr Sanjiv Anand, Dieppe, NB - Family Medicine
Dr Pamela Anand, Ottawa, ON - Family Medicine
Dr Marylene Anctil, Trois-Rivieres, QC - General Practice
Dr Chantal Anctil, Vaudreuil-Dorion, QC - Family Medicine
Dr Aline Antaki, Repentigny, QC - Pediatrics
Dr Golbarg Araghi, Richmond Hill, ON - Family Medicine
Dr Stephanie Archambault-Leger, Orleans, ON - Family Medicine
Dr M Renee Arnold, Hawkesbury, ON - Family Medicine
Dr Andre M Arsenault, Montreal, QC - Nuclear Medicine
Dr Sarto Arsenault, Saint-Georges, QC - Orthopedic Surgery
Dr Isabelle Arsenault, Saint-Lambert, QC - Family Medicine
Dr Marie-Eve Arsenault, Trois-Rivieres, QC - Neurology
Dr Nadine Arsenault-Samson, Summerside, PE - Family Medicine
Dr David Ashby, Charlottetown, PE - General Surgery
Dr Clement Asselin, Rimouski, QC - Orthopedic Surgery
Dr Hazem Assi, Moncton, NB - General Practice
Dr Philippe Aubin, Maria, QC - Family Medicine
Dr Genevieve Aubin, Sainte-Therese, QC - Pediatrics
Dr Colette Aucoin, Moncton, NB - Psychiatry
Dr Richard Audet, Maria, QC - Internal Medicine
Dr Daniel Audy, Montreal, QC - Anesthesia
Dr Dominique Auger, Gatineau, QC - Family Medicine
Dr Nathalie Auger, Montreal, QC - Community Medicine
Dr Pierre L Auger, Quebec, QC - Hematology
Dr Jean-Marie Auger, Quebec, QC - General Practice
Dr Louis Auger, Victoriaville, QC - General Practice
Dr Guy L Aumais, Montreal, QC - Gastroenterology
Dr Ginette Aumond, Riviere-Rouge, QC - General Practice
Dr Anis Aziz, Sault Ste. Marie, ON - Urology
Dr Khalid Azzouzi, Gatineau, QC - Hematology
Dr Jacinthe Babin, St-Jean-sur-Richel, QC - Internal Medicine
Dr Stephane Bachand, Rimouski, QC - Orthopedic Surgery
Dr Badir Francis Badir, Montreal, QC - Internal Medicine
Dr Dalal Badlissi, St-Charles-Brromee, QC - Community Medicine
Dr Boris Bahoric, Montreal, QC - Radiation Oncology
Dr Georges I Bahsali, Laval, QC - Endocrin/Metabolism
Dr Craig D Baldry, Montreal, QC - Anesthesia
Dr Nikolay Baldzhiyski, Bathurst, NB - General Practice
Dr Shana C Balfour, Moncton, NB - Internal Medicine
Dr Joelle Baril, Longueuil, QC - Dermatology
Dr Chantale Baril, Sept-Iles, QC - Family Medicine
Dr Claude Baril, Victoriaville, QC - General Surgery
Dr Emmanuelle Baron, Saint-Lambert, QC - Family Medicine
Dr Louis-Rene Barrette, Chicoutimi, QC - Urology
Dr Stephane Barrette, Verdun, QC - Hematology
Dr Nancy Bastien, Riviere-du-Loup, QC - General Practice
Dr Linda Beauclair, Montreal, QC - Psychiatry
Dr Nicole Beaudoin, Montreal, QC - Physical Medicine & Rehab
Dr Daniel Beaudry, Moncton, NB - Respirology
Dr Michel F Beaulieu, Orleans, ON - General Practice
Dr Denis Beaulieu, Quebec, QC - General Practice
Dr Andre Beaulieu, Quebec, QC - Rheumatology
Dr Patrice Beauregard, Sherbrooke, QC - Hematology
Dr Eric Beausejour, Greenfield Park, QC - Family Medicine
Dr Fannie Bechard, Nicolet, QC - Family Medicine
Dr Philip R Beck, Montreal, QC - Psychiatry
Dr Eric L Bedard, Edmonton, AB - General Surgery
Dr Anne-Marie Bedard, Quebec, QC - Orthopedic Surgery
Dr Alain Bedard, Quebec, QC - General Practice
Dr Marc Bedard, Saint-Raymond, QC - General Practice
Dr Anna Bedkowska, Verdun, QC - General Practice
Dr Eric V Begin, Gatineau, QC - General Surgery
Dr Jean-Francois Begin, Levis, QC - Orthopedic Surgery
Dr Marie-Lyne Belair, Montreal, QC - Ophthalmology
Dr Marie Beland, Montreal, QC - Pediatrics
Dr Marie Josee Beland, Montreal, QC - Cardiology
Dr Eric C Belanger, Ottawa, ON - Anatomical Pathology
Dr Pierre Belanger, Sept-Iles, QC - Pediatrics
Dr Damien Belisle, Chicoutimi, QC - Internal Medicine
Dr Pierre Belisle, St-Roch-D'Ach, QC - General Practice
Dr Genevieve Beliveau, Boucherville, QC - General Practice
Dr Pierre Beliveau, Quebec, QC - Physical Medicine & Rehab
Dr Samuel Beliveau, Saint-Georges, QC - Internal Medicine
Dr Caroline Bell, Shawinigan, QC - Psychiatry
Dr Ethel Bellavance, Victoriaville, QC - General Practice
Dr Patrice Bellefeuille, Blainville, QC - General Practice
Dr Guy Bellemare, Quebec, QC - Obstetrics & Gynecology
Dr Manon Belliveau, Moncton, NB - Family Medicine
Dr Paul Belliveau, Kingston, ON - General Surgery
Dr Robert Belzile, Gatineau, QC - General Practice
Dr Gabriel Belzile, Montreal, QC - Psychiatry
Dr Francois Benard, Vancouver, BC - Nuclear Medicine
Dr Francois Benard, Montreal, QC - Urology
Dr J D Jacques Bender, St. Eugene, ON - General Practice
Dr Elise Benech-Riopel, Acton Vale, QC - General Practice
Dr Matityahu Beniar, Riviere-du-Loup, QC - General Practice
Dr Marcia D Benjamin, Barrie, ON - Psychiatry
Dr Robert Benoit, Montreal, QC - Endocrinology & Metabolism
Dr Suzie Benoit, Sainte-Julie, QC - General Practice
Dr Eric Bensimon, Montreal, QC - Plastic Surgery
Dr Michael Benzazon, Greenfield Park, QC - Cardiology
Dr Claire Berard, Gatineau, QC - General Practice
Dr Maurice Bergeron, Beauharnois, QC - General Practice
Dr Eric Bergeron, Greenfield Park, QC - General Surgery
Dr Julie Bergeron, Montreal, QC - Hematology
Dr Richard F Bergeron, Montreal, QC - Ophthalmology
Dr Annie-Claude Bergeron, Saint-Eustache, QC - General Practice
Dr Simon Bergman, Montreal, QC - General Surgery
Dr Howard Bergman, Montreal, QC - Family Medicine
Dr Genevieve Bernard, Montreal, QC - Neurology
Dr Maryse Bernard, Montreal, QC - Radiation Oncology
Dr Jeanne Bernardin, Moncton, NB - Obstetrics & Gynecology
Dr Sophie Bernier, Lac-Bouchette, QC - General Practice
Dr Michel Bernier, N-D-Des-Prairies, QC - Family Medicine
Dr Yvan Bernier, N-D-Des-Prairies, QC - Family Medicine
Dr Elise Bernier, Sherbrooke, QC - General Practice
Dr Margaret A Berry, Montreal, QC - Pediatrics
Dr Valerie Bertelle, Sherbrooke, QC - General Practice
Dr Simon Berthelot, Calgary, AB - Emergency Medicine
Dr Georges Berthiaume, Saint-Leonard, QC - General Practice
Dr C Francois Bertrand, Montreal, QC - Emergency Medicine
Dr Robert A Bertrand, Montreal, QC - Otolaryngology
Dr Isabelle Bertrand, Quebec, QC - Emergency Medicine
Dr Alain Berube, Sherbrooke, QC - General Practice
Dr Michel Bessette, Sainte-Adele, QC - General Practice
Dr Lubraine Bien-Aime, Greenfield Park, QC - Family Medicine
Maj Marc Bilodeau, Ottawa, ON - Emergency Family Med
Dr Yvonne Bilodeau, Quebec, QC - General Practice
Dr Jean-Francois Bilodeau, Sherbrooke, QC - Internal Medicine
Dr Christopher Birch, Pointe-Claire, QC - Family Medicine
Dr Anne B Biringer, Toronto, ON - Family Medicine
Dr Marie-Yanouk Blain, Gaspe, QC - Obstetrics & Gynecology
Dr Chantal Blais, Farnham, QC - General Practice
Dr Rene Blais, Quebec, QC - Emergency Medicine
Dr Pierre W Blanchard, Quebec, QC - Pediatrics
Dr Julie Blanchard, Sherbrooke, QC - Family Medicine
Dr Richard Blanchet, Quebec, QC - General Practice
Dr Francois Blanchette, Quebec, QC - Ophthalmology
Dr David W Blank, Montreal, QC - Medical Biochemistry
Dr Julie Blouin, Saint-Hyacinthe, QC - Family Medicine
Dr Marie-Claude Blouin, Sorel-Tracy, QC - Ophthalmology
Dr Mireille Boily, Alma, QC - General Practice
Dr Christine Bois, Port-Cartier, QC - General Practice
Dr Celine Boismenu, Sherbrooke, QC - General Practice
Dr Isabelle Boisvert, Riviere-Du-Loup, QC - Urology
Dr Zeljko Bolesnikov, Fredericton, NB - General Practice
Dr Jocelyne Bonin, Saint-Hyacinthe, QC - Family Medicine
Dr Jeanne Bonnaud, Rosemere, QC - General Practice
Dr Marilyn Bosse, Bathurst, NB - Orthopedic Surgery
Dr J Jacques A Bouchard, Calgary, AB - Orthopedic Surgery
Dr Marie-Claude Bouchard, St. Albert, AB - Family Medicine
Dr Clermont Bouchard, Chateauguay, QC - General Practice
Dr Pierre Bouchard, Jonquiere, QC - General Practice
Dr Marc Bouchard, Quebec, QC - Orthopedic Surgery
Dr Jean-Pierre L Bouchard, Quebec, QC - Neurology
Dr Gilles R Bouchard, Stanstead, QC - General Practice
Dr Marc Bouchard, Verdun, QC - General Practice
Dr Francois-Gilles Boucher, Ottawa, ON - Family Medicine
Dr Catherine Boucher, Charny, QC - Family Medicine
Dr Carl Boucher, Gatineau, QC - Otolaryngology
Dr Jean-Louis Boucher, Levis, QC - Diagnostic-Radiology
Dr Chantale Boucher, Longueuil, QC - Pediatrics
Dr Marc Boucher, Montreal, QC - Obstetrics & Gynecology
Dr Renee-Myriam Boucher, Quebec, QC - Neurology
Dr Martin Boucher, Quebec, QC - Emergency Family Med
Dr Claude Boucher, Quebec, QC - General Practice
Dr Guy Boucher, Rimouski, QC - Cardiology
Dr Marie Boudreau, Quebec, QC - General Practice
Dr Bernard Boudreau, Quebec, QC - Family Medicine
Dr Richard Boudreau, Riviere-du-Loup, QC - Community Medicine
Dr Jocelyn Boulanger, Fermont, QC - General Practice
Dr Jean-Martin Boulanger, Greenfield Park, QC - Neurology
Dr Caroline Boulanger, St-Augustin-D-Desm, QC - General Practice
Dr Patrick R Boulos, Sherbrooke, QC - Ophthalmology
Dr Pierre Bourassa, Ottawa, ON - General Practice
Dr Pierre Bourgeau, Montreal, QC - Neurology
Dr Daniel Bourgouin, Trois-Rivieres, QC - General Surgery
Dr Pierre R Bourque, Ottawa, ON - Neurology
Dr Gilles Bouvier, Saint-Hyacinthe, QC - General Practice
Dr Liette Boyer, Amos, QC - Internal Medicine
Dr Sandra Boyer, Saint-Eustache, QC - Family Medicine
Dr David Bracco, Montreal, QC - Anesthesia
Dr Neil Branch, Bathurst, NB - Orthopedic Surgery
Dr Lucie Brault, Longueuil, QC - Family Medicine
Dr Guy Breault, Dieppe, NB - Urology
Dr Dalius J Briedis, Montreal, QC - Internal Medicine
Dr Annie Brochu, Quebec, QC - Family Medicine
Dr Gaetan Brochu, Quebec, QC - General Surgery
Dr Chantal Brochu, St-Etienne-de Lauz, QC - General Practice
Dr Lyne Brouillette, Baie-Comeau, QC - Family Medicine
Dr Denis Brouillette, Val-d'Or, QC - General Surgery
Col Russell J Brown, St. Albert, AB - Anesthesia
Dr Nathalie Brui, Shawinigan-Sud, QC - Family Medicine
Dr Michel Brulotte, Saint-Jacques, NB - General Practice
Dr Nathalie Bruneau, Cowansville, QC - Orthopedic Surgery
Dr Serge Bruneau, Gatineau, QC - General Practice
Dr Claire-Lucie Brunet, Chelmsford, ON - Family Medicine
Dr Kimberly D Butt, Fredericton, NB - Obstetrics & Gynecology
Dr Sylvie Cadet, Varennes, QC - General Practice
Dr Eva Callary, Ottawa, ON - Community Medicine
Dr Anne-Marie Calva, Saint-Bruno, QC - General Practice
Dr Christian Calvy, Moncton, NB - General Practice
Dr Rejean Cantin, Riviere-du-Loup, QC - Anatomical Pathology
Dr Real Cantin, Sainte-Croix, QC - General Practice
Dr Andre M Cantin, Sherbrooke, QC - Respirology
Dr Annie Carbonneau, Montreal, QC - Radiation Oncology
Dr Simon Carette, Toronto, ON - Internal Medicine
Dr Marie-Eve Carette, Laval, QC - Obstetrics & Gynecology
Dr Sebastien Carignan, Chicoutimi, QC - General Surgery
Dr Benoit Carignan, Sherbrooke, QC - General Practice
Dr Marie-Josee Caron, Montreal, QC - Family Medicine
Dr Maurice Caron, Montreal, QC - General Practice
Dr Renee Caron, Sherbrooke, QC - General Practice
Dr Pierre Carrier, St-Jean-sur-Richel, QC - General Practice
Dr David J Carswell, Harrow, ON - General Practice
Dr Raymond Cartier, Montreal, QC - Cardiovasc/ThorSurg
Dr Pierre Cartwright, Cap-aux-Meules, QC - General Practice
Dr Leanne K Casaubon, Toronto, ON - Neurology
Dr Julie Castilloux, Quebec, QC - Gastroenterology

Dr Jean-Francois Castilloux, Sherbrooke, QC - Hematology
Dr Natalie Cauchon, Bathurst, NB - Family Medicine
Dr Michel Cauchon, Quebec, QC - Family Medicine
Dr Nathalie Cayer, La Malbaie, QC - Family Medicine
Dr Sylvie Cayer, Quebec, QC - Gastroenterology
Dr Chiraz Chaalala, Montreal, QC - Neurosurgery
Dr Denys Chabot, Quebec, QC - Plastic Surgery
Dr Julie V Chabot, Quebec, QC - Family Medicine
Dr Magda Chabot, Thetford Mines, QC - Otolaryngology
Dr Zave H Chad, Gatineau, QC - Clin Immun/Allergy
Dr Sanae Chaer, Saint-Leonard, QC - Pediatrics
Dr Chamoun Chamoun, Ottawa, ON - Cardiology
Dr Pierre Champagne, Quebec, QC - General Practice
Dr Kateri Champagne, Saint-Laurent, QC - Internal Medicine
Dr Isabelle Chapados, Edmonton, AB - Endocrin/Metabolism
Dr Gerard Chaput, Lac-Megantic, QC - General Practice
Dr Melanie Charest, Dieppe, NB - Family Medicine
Dr Dhany T Charest, Moncton, NB - Neurosurgery
Dr Andre Charest, Richmond Hill, ON - Internal Medicine
Dr Stephane Charest, Trois-Rivieres, QC - Electroencephal
Dr Luc Charette, Gatineau, QC - Pediatrics
Dr Simon Charlebois, Montreal, QC - Diagnostic-Radiology
Dr Danielle Charpentier, Montreal, QC - Hematology
Dr Louis Charron, Donnacona, QC - General Practice
Dr Sophie Chartier, Brossard, QC - General Practice
Dr Daniel Chartrand, Montreal, QC - Anesthesia
Dr Jean-Pierre Chartrand, Pointe-Claire, QC - Ophthalmology
Dr Denis Chauret, Ottawa, ON - Internal Medicine
Dr Mustapha Chelfi, Gatineau, QC - General Practice
Dr Elisabeth Chenier, Terrebonne, QC - Dermatology
Dr Jean-Francois Chevalier, Kamloops, BC - Neurosurgery
Dr Line Chevrette, Westmount, QC - Ophthalmology
Dr M Helene Chomienne, Ottawa, ON - Family Medicine
Dr Julie Choquette, Laval, QC - General Practice
Dr Julie Choquette, Rouyn-Noranda, QC - Family Medicine
Dr Lise Choquette, Verdun, QC - General Practice
Dr Guy Chouinard, Montreal, QC - Psychiatry
Dr Rino Cianciulli, Montreal, QC - Plastic Surgery
Dr Marie-Juie Cimon, Quebec, QC - Psychiatry
Dr Alain Cirkovic, Verdun, QC - Orthopedic Surgery
Dr Denis Claveau, Montreal, QC - Psychiatry
Dr Joel Claveau, Quebec, QC - Dermatology
Dr Carole Clavette, Saint-Jacques, NB - General Practice
Dr Manon Clavette, Ottawa, ON - Family Medicine
Dr Shirley-Anne Clements, Campbellton, NB - Family Medicine
Dr Richard J Clermont, Montreal, QC - Gastroenterology
Dr Nathalie Cliche, Montreal, QC - General Practice
Dr Paul Cloutier, Edmundston, NB - General Surgery
Dr Isabelle Cloutier, Gatineau, QC - General Practice
Dr Martin Cloutier, Greenfield Park, QC - Neurology
Dr Nicole Cloutier, Laval, QC - General Practice
Dr Réal Cloutier, Montreal, QC - General Practice
Dr Sonia Cloutier, Quebec, QC - Diagnostic-Radiology
Dr Sophie Cloutier, Saint-Eustache, QC - General Practice
Dr Mireille Cloutier, Saint-Remi, QC - General Practice
Dr Jean-Francois Cloutier, Verdun, QC - Otolaryngology
Dr Martine Cohade, Laval, QC - Family Medicine
Dr Philip F Cohen, North Vancouver, BC - Nuclear Medicine
Dr Shawn L Cohen, Montreal, QC - Ophthalmology
Dr Chantal Cohonner, Laval, QC - General Practice
Dr Tina Comeau, Dieppe, NB - General Surgery
Dr Louise Constantineau, Sherbrooke, QC
- Obstetrics & Gynecology
Dr James R Conway, Smiths Falls, ON - General Practice
Dr Jules Cormier, Dieppe, NB - Family Medicine
Dr Janice Cormier, Moncton, NB - General Practice
Dr Roberta T Cormier, Montreal, QC - General Practice
Dr Louise Corneille, Laval, QC - Nephrology
Dr Paul M Cortin, Campbellton, NB - Ophthalmology
Dr Louis Cossette, Senneterre, QC - Family Medicine
Dr Pierre Cossette, Sherbrooke, QC - Internal Medicine
Dr Marie-Agnes Costisella, Vaudreuil-Dorion, QC - Psychiatry
Dr Bruce H Costom, Montreal, QC - Pediatrics
Dr Suzanne Cote, Brossard, QC - General Practice
Dr Andree Cote, Gatineau, QC - General Practice
Dr Jean Cote, Louiseville, QC - General Practice
Dr France Cote, Matagami, QC - General Practice
Dr Patricia Cote, Mont-Royal, QC - Family Medicine
Dr Annie V Cote, Montreal, QC - Anesthesia
Dr Andreanne Cote, Montreal, QC - General Practice
Dr Mendy Cote, Montreal, QC - General Practice
Dr Benoit Cote, N-D-Des-Prairies, QC - General Practice
Dr Josee Cote, Rimouski, QC - General Practice
Dr Julie Cote, Roberval, QC - General Practice
Dr Elisabeth Cote, Saint-Eustache, QC - Diagnostic-Radiology
Dr Anne-Marie Cote, Sherbrooke, QC - Internal Medicine
Dr Alain Couet, Gatineau, QC - General Practice
Dr Martine Couillard, Levis, QC - General Practice
Dr Denis A Coulombe, Quebec, QC - Cardiology
Dr Julie Cournoyer, Gatineau, QC - General Surgery
Dr Ghislain Cournoyer, Saint-Jerome, QC - Hematology
Dr Pierre E Cousineau, Beaupre, QC - Psychiatry
Dr Pierre A Coutu, Oshawa, ON - General Surgery
Dr Madeleine Couture, La Pocatiere, QC - General Practice
Dr Louis P Couture, Quebec, QC - Internal Medicine
Dr Daniel Couture, Sherbrooke, QC - General Practice
Dr Lise Claudette Couturier, Montreal, QC - General Practice
Dr Jacques M Crepeau, Montreal, QC - Cardiology
Dr Benjamin Croft, Hamilton, ON - Family Medicine
Dr Jean-Charles Crombez, Montreal, QC - Psychiatry
Dr Juanita M Crook, Kelowna, BC - Radiation Oncology
Dr Carl Cummings, Cote Saint-Luc, QC - Pediatrics
Dr Francis Cummings, Laval, QC - General Practice
Dr Ingrid Custeau, Ottawa, ON - Anesthesia
Dr A Adam Cwinn, Ottawa, ON - Emergency Medicine
Dr Luc Cyr, Cap-aux-Meules, QC - General Practice
Dr Louise Cyrenne, Montreal, QC - Anesthesia
Dr Eric Czech, Riviere-Du-Loup, QC - Internal Medicine
Dr Pierre D'Amour, Montreal, QC - Endocrinology
Dr Martin D'Amours, Quebec, QC - Endocrin/Metabolism
Dr Chantal D'Aoust-Bernard, Vanier, ON - Family Medicine
Dr Michel D'Astous, Dieppe, NB - Cardiology
Dr Vassant Dabee, Ottawa, ON - Pediatrics
Dr Thierry Daboval, Ottawa, ON - Pediatrics
Dr Helene Daemen-Darveau, Dorval, QC - General Practice
Dr Michel H Dagenais, Montreal, QC - General Surgery
Dr Nathalie Dagenais, Saint-Hyacinthe, QC - General Practice
Dr Giselle Daher Matta, St-Jean-sur-Richel, QC - Anesthesia
Dr Sylvie Daigle, Dieppe, NB - Family Medicine
Dr Celine Daigneault, Chambly, QC - General Practice
Dr Karl Dalery, Sherbrooke, QC - Cardiology
Dr Robert Dallaire, Armagh, QC - General Practice
Dr Michel Dallaire, Montreal, QC - General Practice
Dr Genevieve Dallaire, St-Jean-Sur-Richel, QC
- Emergency Family Med
Dr Linda Dalpe, Caraquet, NB - Family Medicine
Dr Nicole Daneault, Montreal, QC - Neurology
Dr Michele Danelice, Surrey, BC - Anesthesia
Dr Nha Khanh Dang, Montreal, QC - General Practice
Dr Phu An Dang, Montreal-Nord, QC - General Practice
Dr Jean-Guy Daniels, Asbestos, QC - General Practice
Dr Cyril J E Danjoux, Toronto, ON - Radiation Oncology
Dr Ronald Dansereau, Orleans, ON - General Practice
Dr Luc Dansereau, Cap-aux-Meules, QC - Internal Medicine
Dr Lise Dauphin, Verdun, QC - General Practice
Dr Genevieve Davignon, Orleans, ON - Family Medicine
Dr Jonathan Davine, Hamilton, ON - Family Medicine
Dr Jean De La Chevrotiere, Gatineau, QC - General Practice
Dr Hugues De Lachevrotiere, Repentigny, QC - Family Medicine
Dr Alain De Ladurantaye, Hawkesbury, ON - General Practice
Dr Michele De Margerie, Nepean, ON - Family Medicine
Dr Jean De Serres, Saint-Laurent, QC - Family Medicine
Dr Charles M A Deacon, Sherbrooke, QC - Neurology
Dr J Bruno Debruille, Verdun, QC - Psychiatry
Dr Genevieve Dechene, Verdun, QC - General Practice
Dr Eric Dehoux, Gatineau, QC - Physical Medicine & Rehab
LCol Michel P Deilgat, Ottawa, ON - General Practice
Dr Gilles Delage, Saint-Laurent, QC - Medical Microbiology
Dr Pascale Deland, Mont-Joli, QC - General Practice
Dr Benoit Deligne, Montreal, QC - Internal Medicine
Dr Georges Delisle, Quebec, QC - Cardiology
Dr Francois L Demay, Sorel-Tracy, QC - Ophthalmology
Dr Carole J Dennie, Ottawa, ON - Diagnostic-Radiology
Dr Roma Deroy, Quebec, QC - General Practice
Dr Stephane Dery, Chicoutimi, QC - General Practice
Dr Marie-Claude Dery, Chicoutimi, QC - General Surgery
Dr Sylvain Des Groseilliers, Longueuil, QC - General Surgery
Dr Benoit P Des Roches, Mont-Saint-Hilaire, QC - Psychiatry
Dr Gilles Desaulniers, Montreal, QC - Obstetrics & Gynecology
Dr Denis Desaulniers, Quebec, QC - Cardiovasc/ThorSurg
Dr Alain Desbiens, Alma, QC - General Practice
Dr Isabelle Desbiens, Saint-Hyacinthe, QC
- Physical Medicine & Rehab
Dr Yan Deschaintre, Montreal, QC - Neurology
Dr Elaine Deschenes, Memramcook, NB - Pediatrics
Dr Jacques C Deschenes, Montreal, QC - General Practice
Dr Christian Deschenes, N-D-Des-Prairies, QC - Ophthalmology
Dr Jean-Francois Desgagnes, Saint-Jerome, QC - Dermatology
Dr Isabelle Deshaies, Quebec, QC - General Surgery
Dr Annie Deshaies, Sherbrooke, QC - Orthopedic Surgery
Dr Pierre Deshaies, Warwick, QC - General Practice
Dr Pierre Desjardins, Greenfield Park, QC - Hematology
Dr Caroline Desjardins, Laval, QC - Obstetrics & Gynecology
Dr Colette Deslandres, Montreal, QC - Pediatrics
Dr Daniel Deslauriers, Levis, QC - Medical Biochemistry
Dr Julie Desmarais, Montreal, QC - Psychiatry
Dr Maryse Desmarais, Sainte-Adele, QC - Family Medicine
Dr Paul Desmeules, Chicoutimi, QC - Community Medicine
Dr Yvon Desormeaux, Saint-Hippolyte, QC - General Practice
Dr Lise Despres, McMasterville, QC - General Practice
Dr Chantale Desrochers, Montreal, QC - General Practice
Dr Denis P Desrochers, Quebec, QC - Cardiology
Dr Gilles Desroches, Ottawa, ON - Ophthalmology
Dr Jean V Desroches, Montreal, QC - General Practice
Dr France Desrosiers, Pte-Robichaud, NB - Family Medicine
Dr Sophie Desrosiers, St-Charles-Brromee, QC - Otolaryngology
Dr Louise Dessureault, Montreal-Nord, QC - Family Medicine
Dr Nicole Devost, Oshawa, ON - Family Medicine
Dr Ghislain J Devroede, Sherbrooke, QC - General Surgery
Dr Maryse Dion, Orleans, ON - Psychiatry
Dr Marie-Josee Dion, Rimouski, QC - Internal Medicine
Dr Yves Dion, Sorel-Tracy, QC - Psychiatry
Dr Rejean Dion, Ste-Anne-de-Bellev, QC - General Practice
Dr Richard Dionne, Ottawa, ON - Emergency Family Med
Dr Langis Dionne, Quebec, QC - General Practice
Dr Annie Dionne, Quebec, QC - Neurology
Dr Lan Vinh Do, Dieppe, NB - General Surgery
Dr Valerie Dome, Ottawa, ON - Obstetrics & Gynecology
Dr David J Donath, Montreal, QC - Radiation Oncology
Dr Judy Dorais, Montreal, QC - Gastroenterology
Dr Denis M Doren, Bancroft, ON - General Practice
Dr Pierre Dorion, Quebec, QC - Psychiatry
Dr Guerin Dorval, Saint-Hyacinthe, QC - Clin Immun/Allergy
Dr Gaston Dorval, Thetford Mines, QC
- Obstetrics & Gynecology
Dr Jacques P Dostaler, Orleans, ON - Family Medicine
Dr Sarah Dostie, Saint-Eustache, QC - Obstetrics & Gynecology
Dr Danielle Doucet, Bathurst, NB - Family Medicine
Dr Annie Doucet, Quebec, QC - General Practice
Dr Elizabeth Dougherty, Beloeil, QC - Family Medicine
Dr Jamie Dow, Quebec, QC - General Practice
Dr Daniel Doyle, Quebec, QC - Cardiovasc/ThorSurg
Dr Yvon Doyon, Trois-Rivieres, QC - General Practice
Dr Nicole Drapeau, Pierrefonds, QC - General Practice
Dr Christine Drouin, Levis, QC - Critical Care Medicine
Dr Suzanne E Drouin, Montreal, QC - Diagnostic-Radiology
Dr Pierre Drouin, Montreal, QC - Obstetrics & Gynecology
Dr Jean Drouin, Quebec, QC - General Practice
Dr Regen Drouin, Sherbrooke, QC - Medical Genetics
Dr Johanne Drouin, St-Jean-sur-Richel, QC - Urology
Dr Gilbert Dru, Bathurst, NB - Psychiatry
Dr Marie-Josee Dube, Hamilton, ON - Obstetrics & Gynecology
Dr Christine Dube, Ottawa, ON - Emergency Family Med
Dr Magalie Dube, Ottawa, ON - Diagnostic-Radiology
Dr Helene Dube, Montreal, QC - General Practice
Dr Sylvie Dube, Montreal, QC - Family Medicine
Dr Paule Dube, Quebec, QC - Ophthalmology
Dr Yolande Dube, Quebec, QC - Ophthalmology

Dr Jean Dubuc, Quebec, QC - General Practice
Dr Rene Ducharme, Ottawa, ON - Psychiatry
Dr Martine Ducharme, St-Eustache, QC - General Practice
Dr Paul A Duchastel, York, ON - Family Medicine
Dr Yves J Duchastel, Montreal, QC - Electroencephal
Dr Rachel Duchesne, Gatineau, QC - Family Medicine
Dr Robert Duchesne, Terrebonne, QC - Orthopedic Surgery
Dr Jean Duckett, Montreal, QC - General Practice
Dr Marie Duclos, Montreal, QC - Radiation Oncology
Dr Barbara Duda, Montreal, QC - Endocrin/Metabolism
Dr Suzanne Dufour, Alma, QC - General Practice
Dr Georges Dufour, Shawinigan-Sud, QC - Otolaryngology
Dr Marc L G Dufresne, Chicoutimi, QC - Plastic Surgery
Dr Giselle Dugas, Meteghan Centre, NS - Family Medicine
Dr Isabelle L Dugas, Sydney, NS - Family Medicine
Dr Pierre Duguay, Quebec, QC - Ophthalmology
Dr Denise Duguay Vibert, Lameque, NB - Family Medicine
Dr Alexis Dumais, Longueuil, QC - General Practice
Dr Gaston R J Dumais, Montreal, QC - Dermatology
Dr Jean-Marc Dumas, Brossard, QC - Diagnostic-Radiology
Dr Serge Dumas, Quebec, QC - General Practice
Dr Guillaume Dumont, Sept-Iles, QC - Psychiatry
Dr Andre Dumont, Ste-Anne-des-Monts, QC - General Practice
Dr Carolyn M Dunn, Longueuil, QC - Pediatrics
Dr Jean A Duperre, Montreal, QC - Ophthalmology
Dr Louise Duperron, Mont-Royal, QC - Obstetrics & Gynecology
Dr Stephane Dupont, Granby, QC - Ophthalmology
Dr Michel Dupont, Quebec, QC - General Practice
Dr Raymonde Dupras, Longueuil, QC - General Practice
Dr Annik Dupras, Montreal, QC - Geriatric Medicine
Dr Veronique Dupuis, Lameque, NB - Family Medicine
Dr Paule Dupuis, Longueuil, QC - Otolaryngology
Dr Andre Dupuy, Longueuil, QC - General Practice
Dr Alfred M Duranceau, Longueuil, QC - Ophthalmology
Dr Christian P Durepos, Timmins, ON - Family Medicine
Dr Julie Dutil, Chibougamau, QC - Family Medicine
Dr Renald Dutil, Montreal, QC - General Practice
Dr Richard Duval, Ste Anne, MB - General Practice
Dr Marie-Dominique Dzineku, Sherbrooke, QC - Family Medicine
Dr Nathalie East, Rouyn-Noranda, QC - Obstetrics & Gynecology
Dr Donald J Edde, Montreal, QC - Diagnostic-Radiology
Dr Roula Eid, Ottawa, ON - Family Medicine
Dr David H Eidelman, Montreal, QC - Internal Medicine
Dr Mohamed T El-Sherbiny, Montreal, QC - Urology
Dr Emile Elfassi, Montreal, QC - General Practice
Dr Stephane Elkouri, Montreal, QC - General Surgery
Dr Laurence Eloy, St-Charles-Brromee, QC - General Surgery
Dr John Embil, Winnipeg, MB - Infectious Diseases
Dr Gilles Emond, Saint-Jerome, QC - General Practice
Dr Philip Esper, Drummondville, QC - Ophthalmology
Dr Philippe Esterez, Outremont, QC - General Practice
Dr Roya Etemad-Rezai, London, ON - Diagnostic-Radiology
Dr Brigitte Fanzolato, Saint-Hippolyte, QC - General Practice
Dr David F Farber, Laval, QC - Gastroenterology
Dr Joelle M T Fareau-Weyl, Guelph, ON - Psychiatry
Dr David Farrar, Sherbrooke, QC - General Practice
Dr Francois Fassier, Montreal, QC - Orthopedic Surgery
Dr Line Faucher, Chibougamau, QC - Family Medicine
Dr Jacques Faucher, Ham-Nord, QC - General Practice
Dr Janusz Feber, Ottawa, ON - Pediatrics
Dr Valerie Fedorowicz, Montreal, QC - Psychiatry
Dr Genevieve Ferdais, Verdun, QC - Family Medicine
Dr Alex S Ferenczy, Montreal, QC - General Pathology
Dr Marc-Andre Ferland, Verdun, QC - General Surgery
Dr Katia Ferland-Lavigne, Charlemagne, QC - Psychiatry
Dr Pierre Ferron, Quebec, QC - Otolaryngology
Dr Jacques Filiatrault, Chicoutimi, QC - Nephrology
Dr Santo Filice, Moncton, NB - Radiation Oncology
Dr Edith Filion, Montreal, QC - Radiation Oncology
Dr Serge Filion, St-Jean-Sur-Richel, QC - Internal Medicine
Dr Lucie Filion, Terrebonne, QC - General Practice
Dr Genevieve Filteau, Laval, QC - Family Medicine
Dr Michel Finlay, Gatineau, QC - General Practice
Dr G Allen Finley, Halifax, NS - Anesthesia
Dr Jose Firszt, Montreal, QC - Urology
Dr Danielle Fisch, Canton-De-Hatley, QC - Family Medicine
Dr Amelie Fiset, Drummondville, QC - General Practice
Dr Helene Flageole, Hamilton, ON - General Surgery
Dr Daniel I Flanders, Toronto, ON - Pediatrics
Dr Gilles Fleury, Ottawa, ON - Psychiatry
Dr Marie Florescu, Montreal, QC - Internal Medicine
Dr Philip A Fong Wai Chin, Weyburn, SK - General Practice
Dr Liette Forest, Edmundston, NB - Family Medicine
Dr Robert J Forget, Ottawa, ON - Orthopedic Surgery
Dr Sylvie Forget, Charlemagne, QC - Psychiatry
Dr Marie-Josee Forgues, Plantagenet, ON - Family Medicine
Dr Ghyslain Fortier, Salaber-de-Valleyf, QC - Anesthesia
Dr Pierre Fortin, Kitchener, ON - Radiation Oncology
Dr Luc Fortin, Montreal, QC - Physical Medicine & Rehab
Dr Celine Fortin, Pont-Rouge, QC - Family Medicine
Dr Paul Fortin, Quebec, QC - Internal Medicine
Dr Lucie Fortin, Sainte-Therese, QC - Psychiatry
Dr Lynne Foucault, Gatineau, QC - General Practice
Dr Anne Fournier, Montreal, QC - Cardiology
Dr Denis Fournier, Quebec, QC - General Practice
Dr Sylvie Fournier, Saint-Georges, QC - Family Medicine
Dr Marie-Pierre Founier-Gosselin, Montreal, QC - Neurosurgery
Dr Robert A Fowler, Toronto, ON - Internal Medicine
Dr Susan B Fox, Greenfield Park, QC - Hematology
Dr Anne Fradet, Sherbrooke, QC - Cardiology
Dr Violaine Franchomme-Fosse, Sherbrooke, QC - Family Medicine
Dr Denyse Francis, La Baie, QC - General Practice
Dr Chantal A M Frechette, Ste Anne, MB - General Practice
Dr Robert C Frechette, Hawkesbury, ON - General Practice
Dr Pierre Frechette, Charny, QC - Emergency Medicine
Dr Julie Frechette, Trois-Rivieres, QC - General Practice
Dr Guillaume Frechette, Victoriaville, QC - Psychiatry
Dr Patrick J L Fredette, Ste Anne, MB - General Practice
Dr Remi J Frenette, Beresford, NB - Orthopedic Surgery
Dr Guy Frenette, Cap-Sante, QC - General Practice
Dr Gilles A Frenette, Montreal, QC - Plastic Surgery
Dr Steven Friedman, Toronto, ON - Emergency Family Med
Dr Jack Friedman, Montreal, QC - Pediatrics
Dr Daniel Froment, Montreal, QC - Internal Medicine
Dr Renee Fugere, Montreal, QC - Psychiatry
Dr Louis Gaboury, Montreal, QC - Anatomical Pathology
Dr Alexandra Gagne, Alma, QC - Obstetrics & Gynecology
Dr Jeannine Gagne, Deux-Montagnes, QC - General Practice
Dr Dominique Gagne, Quebec, QC - Internal Medicine
Dr Michel Gagne, St-Eustache, QC - Internal Medicine
Dr Francois Gagnon, Saint-Jacques, NB - General Practice
Dr Marie-Claude Gagnon, Ottawa, ON - Family Medicine
Dr Andre Gagnon, Gatineau, QC - Psychiatry
Dr Alain Gagnon, Longueuil, QC - General Practice
Dr Sonia I Gagnon, Montreal, QC - Obstetrics & Gynecology
Dr Pierre R Gagnon, Quebec, QC - Psychiatry
Dr Genevieve Gagnon, Quebec, QC - Obstetrics & Gynecology
Dr Claudia Gagnon, Quebec, QC - Endocrin/Metabolism
Dr Marie-Therese Gagnon, Quebec, QC - General Practice
Dr Nathalie Gagnon, Riviere-Du-Loup, QC - Urology
Dr Serge Gagnon, Saint-Georges, QC - Orthopedic Surgery
Dr Nathalie Gagnon, Sherbrooke, QC - Emergency Family Med
Dr Elaine Gagnon, St-Augustin-D-Desm, QC - General Practice
Dr Jacques-Eric Gagnon, Verdun, QC - Cardiology
Dr Michel B Gagnon, Victoriaville, QC - Diagnostic-Radiology
Dr Eleni Galanis, Vancouver, BC - Community Medicine
Dr Pierre Galarneau, Entrelacs, QC - General Surgery
Dr France Galarneau, Shawinigan-Sud, QC - General Practice
Dr Genevieve Gallagher, Quebec, QC - Hematology
Dr Bruce Garfield, Montreal, QC - Rheumatology
Dr Jacques Gariepy, Brossard, QC - Neurosurgery
Dr Yvon Garneau, Quebec, QC - Psychiatry
Dr Valerie Garneau, Trois-Rivieres, QC - General Practice
Dr Antoine Gaspard, Salaber-de-Valleyf, QC - Orthopedic Surgery
Dr Rudolph E Gasparelli, Ohsweken, ON - Family Medicine
Dr Matthieu Gaudet, Moncton, NB - Internal Medicine
Dr Martine Gaul, Sainte-Julie, QC - Family Medicine
Dr Jeannot Gauthier, Amqui, QC - General Practice
Dr Serge Gauthier, Laval, QC - Psychiatry
Dr Marie-Sophie Gauthier, Rimouski, QC - Otolaryngology
Dr Serge G Gauthier, Verdun, QC - Neurology
Dr Michel Gauvreau, Quebec, QC - General Practice
Dr Alain Gauvreau, Ste-Anne-des-Monts, QC - General Practice
Dr Lucie M Gelinas, Saint-Constant, QC - General Practice
Dr Louise Gelinas, St-Stanislas-D-Cha, QC - General Practice
Dr M F Liliane Gendreau-Reid, Victoria, BC - Clin Immun/Allergy
Dr Francois Germain, Kelowna, BC - Radiation Oncology
Dr Louis Germain, Lachine, QC - Psychiatry
Dr Richard D Germain, Pointe-Claire, QC - General Practice
Dr Violaine Germain, Quebec, QC - General Practice
Dr Jon M Gerrard, Winnipeg, MB - Pediatrics
Dr Sophie Gervais, Amqui, QC - Family Medicine
Dr Georges Ghattas, Montreal, QC - Gastroenterology
Dr Roger Ghoche, Toronto, ON - Family Medicine
Dr Alain Giard, Ste-Agathe-des-Mts, QC - General Surgery
Dr Julie Gignac, Chicoutimi, QC - General Practice
Dr Eliane Giguere, Orleans, ON - Family Medicine
Dr Marie-Chantal Giguere, St-Jean-sur-Richel, QC - General Practice
Dr Sebastien Gilbert, Ottawa, ON - General Surgery
Dr Stefanie Gingras, Montreal, QC - Family Medicine
Dr Isabelle M Girard, Calgary, AB - General Practice
Dr Michel Girard, Montreal, QC - General Practice
Dr Guylaine Girard, Montreal, QC - General Practice
Dr Ronald Girard, Sherbrooke, QC - General Practice
Dr Gabriel Girouard, Moncton, NB - Infectious Diseases
Dr Nathalie Girouard, LaSalle, QC - General Practice
Dr Yvon Giroux, Laval, QC - Gastroenterology
Dr Diane Giroux, Montreal, QC - General Practice
Dr Josee Giroux, Verdun, QC - General Practice
Dr Kim Gloutney, LaSalle, QC - General Practice
Dr Richard Godbout, Greenfield Park, QC - Diagnostic-Radiology
Dr Veronique Godbout, Montreal, QC - Orthopedic Surgery
Dr Yves-Laurent Godbout, Trois-Rivieres, QC - General Practice
Dr J Mark Godel, Cold Lake, AB - Family Medicine
Dr Maurice Godin, Montreal, QC - Cardiology
Dr Patricia Godon, Lachute, QC - General Practice
Dr David Goldman, St Thomas, ON - Psychiatry
Dr David Goltzman, Montreal, QC - Internal Medicine
Dr Pierre Gonthier, Rimouski, QC - General Practice
Dr Michel Gosselin, Longueuil, QC - General Surgery
Dr Gilbert Gosselin, Montreal, QC - Cardiology
Dr Johanne Gosselin, Vallee-Jonction, QC - General Practice
Dr Francois Gougoux, Cacouna, QC - General Practice
Dr Andre Gougoux, Montreal, QC - Internal Medicine
Dr Jean-Francois Goulard, Bathurst, NB - General Practice
Dr Conrad A Goulet, Victoria, BC - General Practice
Dr Audrey-Anne Goulet, Gatineau, QC - General Practice
Dr Serge Goulet, Saint-Lambert, QC - General Practice
Dr Isabelle Goupil-Sormany, Quebec, QC - Community Medicine
Dr Pierre Goyer, Laval, QC - General Practice
Dr Roger Goyette, Chambly, QC - General Practice
Dr Monique Goyette, Trois-Rivieres, QC - Medical Microbiology
Dr Steve Graham, Montreal-Est, QC - General Practice
Dr Andrew M Grant, Sherbrooke, QC - Medical Biochemistry
Dr Normand Gravel, Verdun, QC - Anesthesia
Dr Serge Gregoire, Baie-Comeau, QC - Family Medicine
Dr Marie-Claude Gregoire, Granby, QC - General Practice
Dr Mireille Gregoire, Quebec, QC - Urology
Dr Jean Gregoire, Quebec, QC - Obstetrics & Gynecology
Dr Louis-Simon Grenier, Jonquiere, QC - Family Medicine
Dr Raynald Grenier, Quebec, QC - Dermatology
Dr Marie-Andree Grenier, Salaber-de-Valleyf, QC - General Practice
Dr Jean-Paul Grenier, Sherbrooke, QC - Otolaryngology
Dr Laval J Grimard, Ottawa, ON - Radiation Oncology
Dr Guy Grimard, Montreal, QC - Orthopedic Surgery
Dr Natalie Grizenko, Verdun, QC - Psychiatry
Dr Danielle Grondin, Ottawa, ON - Pediatrics
Dr Louis Grondin, Gatineau, QC - General Practice
Dr Anne-Marie Grothe, Montreal, QC - Endocrin/Metabolism
Dr Stefan C W Grzybowski, Vancouver, BC - Family Medicine
Dr Louise Guay, Gatineau, QC - Family Medicine
Dr Elizabeth Guay, Terrebonne, QC - Dermatology
Dr Anne-Marie Guerguerian, Toronto, ON - Pediatrics
Dr Raymond Guevin, Montreal, QC - Hematology

Dr Jimmy Guignard, Saint-Antoine, NB - Family Medicine
Dr Valerie Guilbeault, Gatineau, QC - General Practice
Dr Helene Guilbeault, Montreal, QC - Diagnostic-Radiology
Dr Fernand Guillemette, Trois-Rivieres, QC - Pediatrics
Dr Mireille C Hache, Bathurst, NB - Psychiatry
Dr Marilene Hache, Bathurst, NB - Family Medicine
Dr Chantal Hache, Levis, QC - Gastroenterology
Dr Elie Haddad, Montreal, QC - Clin Immun/Allergy
Dr Carine Haggar, Montreal, QC - Emergency Medicine
Dr Caroline Haineault, Chateauguay, QC - Family Medicine
Dr Ugur Halac, Montreal, QC - Gastroenterology
Dr Harvey I Halperin, Vancouver, BC - General Practice
Dr Daphné Hamel-Breault, Longueuil, QC - General Practice
Dr Barbara R Hannach, Toronto, ON - Hematology
Dr Nabil Hannouche, Montreal, QC - Diagnostic-Radiology
Dr Jehan Harissi Dagher, Montreal, QC
- Physical Medicine & Rehab
Dr Carmen Harnois, Quebec, QC - General Practice
Dr JoAnn E Harrold, Ottawa, ON - Pediatrics
Dr Michel Harvey, Chicoutimi, QC - Otolaryngology
Dr Normand Harvey, La Malbaie, QC - General Practice
Dr Richard Harvey, Sherbrooke, QC - Cardiology
Dr Janique Harvey, Verdun, QC - Psychiatry
Dr Marie Hayes, Sherbrooke, QC - Family Medicine
Dr Jocelyne Hebert, Dieppe, NB - General Surgery
Dr Josee Hebert, Chateauguay, QC - Obstetrics & Gynecology
Dr Jean-Pierre Hebert, Huntingdon, QC - General Practice
Dr Nicolas Hebert Croteau, Brockville, ON - Internal Medicine
Dr J A Edouard Hendriks, Miramichi, NB
- Emergency Family Med
Dr Josee Heroux, Granby, QC - Dermatology
Dr Julie Heroux, Rouyn-Noranda, QC - Internal Medicine
Dr Nhung T C Ho, North York, ON - Dermatology
Dr France Hoquet, Saint-Jerome, QC - General Practice
Dr Helene Hottlet, La Sarre, QC - General Practice
Dr Sylvie Houde, Montreal, QC - Neurology
Dr Christine Houde, Quebec, QC - Cardiology
Dr Melanie Hould, Hawkesbury, ON - Family Medicine
Dr Normand Houle, Quebec, QC - Plastic Surgery
Dr Gabriel Houle, Saint-Fabien, QC - General Practice
Dr Claudia Houle, Trois-Rivieres, QC - Medical Microbiology
Dr Michel G Hurtubise, Saint-Bruno, QC - General Practice
Dr Paul A L S Hwang, Toronto, ON - Neurology
Dr Reda Ibrahim, Montreal, QC - Cardiology
Dr Stuart J Iglesias, Bella Bella, BC - General Practice
Dr Sabina P Ijaz, Pine Falls, MB - Family Medicine
Dr A Micheil Innes, Calgary, AB - Medical Genetics
Dr Rinda-Bun H Ith, Laval, QC - General Practice
Dr Helene Jacob, Quebec, QC - General Practice
Dr Avrum I Jacobson, Pointe-Claire, QC - Urology
Dr Valerie Jacques, Quebec, QC - General Practice
Dr Stephanie Jacques, Rouyn-Noranda, QC - Neurology
Dr John F Jarrell, Calgary, AB - Obstetrics & Gynecology
Dr Gabriel Jean, Gaspe, QC - Orthopedic Surgery
Dr Irene Jednak, Westmount, QC - General Practice
Dr Nicolas Jobin, Baie-Comeau, QC - Family Medicine
Dr Marcel R Jodoin, Longueuil, QC - Obstetrics & Gynecology
Dr Claude Johnson, Montreal, QC - Anesthesia
Dr Andre Jolicoeur, Saint-Georges, QC - General Practice
Dr Claude Jolicoeur, Verdun, QC - Psychiatry
Dr Isabelle Jolin, Cowansville, QC - General Practice
Dr Patrick Jolly, Montreal, QC - Urology
Dr Mohamad G Joundi, Winnipeg, MB - General Practice
Dr Jerome-Oliver Jutras, Chateauguay, QC - Family Medicine
Dr Luc C Jutras, Montreal, QC - Cardiology
Dr Serge Jutras, St-Jean-sur-Richel, QC - General Practice
Dr Mathias Kalina, Montreal, QC - Family Medicine
Dr Sherri L Katz, Ottawa, ON - Pediatrics
Dr Mortimer Katz, Ottawa, ON - General Practice
Dr Louis J Kennedy, Kingston, ON - General Practice
Dr Marie-Paule Kerry, Lameque, NB - General Practice
Dr Fiona M Key, Montreal, QC - Pediatrics
Dr Viviane Khoury, Montreal, QC - Diagnostic-Radiology
Dr Jeannette L Kisak-Tomiuk, Lachine, QC - General Practice
Dr Jean-Jacques Klopfenstein, St-Charles-Brromee, QC
- General Surgery
Dr Charles D Knapp, North York, ON - Anesthesia
Dr Kathleen F Knowles, Montreal, QC - Infectious Diseases
Dr Thomas B Kosatsky, Vancouver, BC - Community Medicine
Dr Simon Kouz, St-Charles-Brromee, QC - Cardiology
Dr Thomas A Kovesi, Ottawa, ON - Pediatrics
Dr Robin Kugelmass, Pierrefonds, QC - Pediatrics
Dr Christiane Kuntz, Gloucester, ON - Family Medicine
Dr Elizabeth C Kurien, Calgary, AB - Radiation Oncology
Dr Jirair Kuyumjian, Montreal, QC - General Practice
Dr Maggy G H Kyrollos, Ottawa, ON - General Pathology
Dr Genevieve L'Ecuyer, Laval, QC - General Practice
Dr Vincent L'Ecuyer, Rouyn-Noranda, QC - Family Medicine
Dr Georges L'Esperance, Montreal, QC - Neurosurgery
Dr Helene L'Esperance, Quebec, QC - General Practice
Dr Marie-Claude L'Hebreux, Levis, QC - General Practice
Dr Sophie L'Heureux, Quebec, QC - Psychiatry
Dr Jean Labbe, Quebec, QC - Pediatrics
Dr Sylvain Labbe, Victoriaville, QC - Family Medicine
Dr Pierre-R. Laberge, Sept-Iles, QC - Medical Microbiology
Dr Robert Labine, Saint-Jerome, QC - Psychiatry
Dr Isabelle Labonte, Quebec, QC - Internal Medicine
Dr Claude Labrie, Quebec, QC - General Practice
Dr Michel Lacerte, London, ON - Physical Medicine & Rehab
Dr Marc Lachance, Drummondville, QC - General Practice
Dr Danielle Lachance, LaSalle, QC - General Practice
Dr Alain Lachance, Saint-Georges, QC - Ophthalmology
Dr Nadine Lachance, Saint-Hyacinthe, QC - General Practice
Dr Jean Lachapelle, Montreal, QC - Pediatrics
Dr Louis Lacombe, Quebec, QC - Urology
Dr Marc Lacroix, Quebec, QC - Family Medicine
Dr Remi Lacroix, Quebec, QC - Physical Medicine & Rehab
Dr Marie-Josee Ladora, Vanier, ON - General Practice
Dr Diane Ladouceur, Longueuil, QC - Obstetrics & Gynecology
Dr Noemie Laferte, Shawinigan-Sud, QC - Family Medicine
Dr Melissa Laflamme, Quebec, QC - Orthopedic Surgery
Dr Nathalie Laflamme, Saint-Eustache, QC - Family Medicine
Dr Patrice Laflamme, Sainte-Marie, QC - Community Medicine
Dr Nadia Laflamme, Trois-Rivieres, QC - General Practice
Dr Johanne Lafond, Longueuil, QC - General Practice
Dr Robert E Lafontaine, Timmins, ON - Orthopedic Surgery
Dr Jacques M Laforge, Quebec, QC - Respirology
Dr Mario Laforte, Chicoutimi, QC - Respirology
Dr Chantal Lafortune, Lasalle, QC - Obstetrics & Gynecology
Dr Marie-France Lafreniere, Saint-Jerome, QC - Psychiatry
Dr Catherine Lagace, Terrebonne, QC - Dermatology
Dr Elisabeth Lajoie, Longueuil, QC - Community Medicine
Dr Christine Lajoie, Quebec, QC - General Practice
Dr Francois Lajoie, Sherbrooke, QC - Obstetrics & Gynecology
Dr Denis Laliberte, Quebec, QC - Community Medicine
Dr Isabelle Laliberte, Quebec, QC - Ophthalmology
Dr Anne Laliberte, Saint-Anselme, QC - General Practice
Dr Suzanne Lalonde, Montreal, QC - General Practice
Dr Gilles Lalonde, Quebec, QC - Ophthalmology
Dr Yves Lambert, Longueuil, QC - Family Medicine
Dr Richard Lambert, Montreal, QC - Physical Medicine & Rehab
Dr Diane Lambert, St-J-Chrysostome, QC - General Practice
Dr Danielle Lamer, Montreal, QC - General Practice
Dr Martin Lamontagne, Montreal, QC
- Physical Medicine & Rehab
Dr Bruno Lamothe, Alma, QC - General Practice
Dr Marcel Lamothe, Montreal, QC - General Practice
Dr Marie-Eve Lamy, Shawinigan-Sud, QC - Family Medicine
Dr Lianne Lamy-Monnot, Laval, QC - Family Medicine
Dr Claude Lanctot, Montreal, QC - Dermatology
Dr Rosaire Lanctot, Saint-Remi, QC - General Practice
Dr Guy Lanctot, Salaber-de-Valleyf, QC - Pediatrics
Dr Ivan Landry, Laval, QC - Otolaryngology
Dr Stephanie Landry, Levis, QC - Internal Medicine
Dr Lynda Landry, Mont-Laurier, QC - General Practice
Dr Sarah Landry, Rimouski, QC - Psychiatry
Dr Anny Langevin, Alma, QC - Obstetrics & Gynecology
Dr Pierre L Langevin, Quebec, QC - Electroencephal
Dr Lise Langis, Bouctouche, NB - Family Medicine
Dr Albert Langlais, Sherbrooke, QC - General Practice
Dr Marie-Eve Langlois, Calgary, AB - Family Medicine
Dr Sylvie Langlois, Vancouver, BC - Pediatrics
Dr Patrice Langlois, Ottawa, ON - Anesthesia
Dr Stephanie F Langlois, Renfrew, ON - General Practice
Dr Francois Langlois, Gatineau, QC - General Practice
Dr Melanie Langlois, Quebec, QC - Neurology
Dr Nathalie Langlois, Sherbrooke, QC - Internal Medicine
Dr Danielle Lanoue, Montreal, QC - General Practice
Dr Martin Lanoue, St-Leonard-d'Aston, QC - Family Medicine
Dr Sophie Lapalme, Trois-Rivieres, QC - Neurology
Dr Jean-Guy Lapierre, Montreal, QC - Pediatrics
Dr Claude Lapierre, Montreal, QC - General Practice
Dr Yves Lapierre, Saint-Georges, QC - Psychiatry
Dr Carole S M Lapointe, Thunder Bay, ON - Psychiatry
Dr Real Lapointe, Montreal, QC - General Surgery
Dr Richard H Lapointe, Montreal, QC - Plastic Surgery
Dr Richard Lapointe, Rouyn-Noranda, QC - General Practice
Dr Gerald Lapointe, Varennes, QC - General Practice
Dr Genevieve Laprise, Drummondville, QC - Psychiatry
Dr Chantal Laquerre, Gatineau, QC - Family Medicine
Dr Christian Lareau, Shawville, QC - Diagnostic-Radiology
Dr Pierre Larin, Sorel-Tracy, QC - Cardiology
Dr J Louis R Lariviere, Ottawa, ON - General Practice
Dr Michele Lariviere, Ottawa, ON - General Practice
Dr Anne-Marie Larkin, Baie-Comeau, QC
- Emergency Family Med
Dr Isabel Larochelle, L'Ancienne-Lorette, QC - General Practice
Dr Daniel Larochelle, Longueuil, QC - Otolaryngology
Dr Annick Larochelle, Longueuil, QC - Obstetrics & Gynecology
Dr Pascale Larochelle, Victoriaville, QC - Orthopedic Surgery
Dr Rene Larocque, Grand-Mere, QC - General Practice
Dr Isabelle Larocque, L'Assomption, QC - General Practice
Dr Annie Larocque, Laval, QC - Dermatology
Dr Michel Larose, Montreal, QC - General Practice
Dr Isabelle Larouche, Moncton, NB - Family Medicine
Dr Lucie Larouche, Granby, QC - Obstetrics & Gynecology
Dr Nicole Larouche, Montreal, QC - General Practice
Dr Valerie Larouche, Quebec, QC - Hematology
Dr Jacynthe Larouche, Trois-Rivieres, QC - Gastroenterology
Dr Sandrine Larue, Greenfield Park, QC - Neurology
Dr Marc-Andre Latour, Quebec, QC - Orthopedic Surgery
Dr Louis G Latulippe, Magog, QC - General Practice
Dr Micheline C Lau, Scarborough, ON - General Practice
Dr Jerome R Laufer, Montreal, QC - Nuclear Medicine
Dr John B Laughrea, Quebec, QC - Internal Medicine
Dr Francois Laurendeau, Amos, QC - General Practice
Dr Guy Laurent, Laval, QC - Urology
Dr Marcel Laurion, Laval, QC - General Surgery
Dr Monique Laurion, Quebec, QC - General Practice
Dr Nathalie Lauzier, Montreal, QC - General Practice
Dr Julie L Lauzon, Calgary, AB - Medical Genetics
Dr France Lauzon, Terrebonne, QC - General Practice
Dr Marie-Aimee Lavigne, Rouyn-Noranda, QC - General Practice
Dr Caroline Lavigne, Saint-Eustache, QC - Family Medicine
Dr Eric L Laviolette, Hawkesbury, ON - Emergency Family Med
Dr Martin Lavoie, Edmonton, AB - Community Medicine
Dr Pascal Lavoie, Vancouver, BC - Pediatrics
Dr Denis J Lavoie, Vernon, BC - Urology
Dr Roberto Lavoie, North Bay, ON - Internal Medicine
Dr Raynald Lavoie, Chicoutimi, QC - Otolaryngology
Dr Suzanne Lavoie, Quebec, QC - Physical Medicine & Rehab
Dr Claude A Lavoie, Quebec, QC - Psychiatry
Dr Eric Lavoie, Sherbrooke, QC - Pediatrics
Dr Angeline Law, Ottawa, ON - Cardiology
Dr Lyly H Le, Surrey, BC - Internal Medicine
Dr Tuyet-Diem Le, Montreal, QC - Pediatrics
Dr Annie-Josee Le Bouthillier, Orleans, ON - Family Medicine
Dr Arthur Leader, Ottawa, ON - Obstetrics & Gynecology
Dr Real Lebeau, Montreal, QC - Cardiology
Dr Daniel Lebel, Smooth Rock Falls, ON - General Practice
Dr Alain Lebel, Montreal, QC - Psychiatry
Dr Michel H Lebel, Rimouski, QC - Urology
Dr Sylvie J Leblanc, Moncton, NB - Family Medicine
Dr Michelle Leblanc, Gaspe, QC - General Practice
Dr Benoit Leblanc, Montreal, QC - Plastic Surgery
Dr Jean Leblanc, Montreal, QC - Psychiatry
Dr Jean-Paul M Leblanc, Rimouski, QC - Ophthalmology
Dr Helene Leblond, Montreal, QC - Pediatrics

Dr Anne Lebouthillier, Bathurst, NB - Obstetrics & Gynecology
Dr Andre Lebrun, Saint-Laurent, QC - Hematology
Dr Patrick W Leclair, Orleans, ON - Family Medicine
Dr Jean Leclair, Quebec, QC - General Practice
Dr Pierre J A Leclerc, Gaspe, QC - General Surgery
Dr Jean Leclerc, Montreal, QC - General Practice
Dr Roselyn Leclerc, Nicolet, QC - Family Medicine
Dr Sylvie Leclerc, Quebec, QC - General Practice
Dr Daniel Lecoeur, Trois-Rivieres, QC - General Practice
Dr Caroline Lecomte, Sherbrooke, QC - Emergency Family Med
Dr Catherine Lecours, Quebec, QC - Plastic Surgery
Dr Bernard E Leduc, Montreal, QC - Physical Medicine & Rehab
Dr Warren L Lee, Toronto, ON - Internal Medicine
Dr Guylaine G Lefebvre, Toronto, ON - Obstetrics & Gynecology
Dr Arlette M L Lefebvre, Toronto, ON - Psychiatry
Dr Josee Lefebvre, Verdun, QC - Obstetrics & Gynecology
Dr Louise A Lefort, Ottawa, ON - Emergency Family Med
Dr Daniel P Lefrancois, Longueuil, QC - Emergency Medicine
Dr Katleen Lefrancois, Quebec, QC - General Practice
Dr Veronique Legault, Moncton, NB - Family Medicine
Dr Pierre-Marc B Legault, Toronto, ON - Family Medicine
Dr Louis Legault, Montreal, QC - Psychiatry
Dr Michel Legault, St-Charles-Brromee, QC - General Surgery
Dr Yves A Leger, Moncton, NB - Community Medicine
Dr Francine Leger, Montreal, QC - General Practice
Dr Julie Leger, Sept-Iles, QC - Family Medicine
Dr Celine Legris, St-Jean-sur-Richel, QC - Ophthalmology
Dr David Lemaire, Dieppe, NB - Otolaryngology
Dr Guillaume Lemay, Beloeil, QC - Family Medicine
Dr Frederic Lemay, Sherbrooke, QC - Gastroenterology
Dr Nadia Lemay, Terrebonne, QC - Obstetrics & Gynecology
Dr Myra M Lemelin, Ottawa, ON - Emergency Family Med
Dr Tania Lemelin, Wakefield, QC - Family Medicine
Dr Bruno Lemieux, Montreal, QC - General Practice
Dr Sylvie Lemieux, Sainte-Marie, QC - General Practice
Dr Myriam Lemire, Greenfield Park, QC - Psychiatry
Dr Martine Lemire, Sherbrooke, QC - Clin Immun/Allergy
Dr Michel M Lemoyne, Montreal, QC - Gastroenterology
Dr Pierre J Leouffre, Montreal, QC - Psychiatry
Dr France Lepage, Bathurst, NB - Dermatology
Dr Sylvie Lepage, Campbellton, NB - Family Medicine
Dr Marie-Christine Lepage, Lachute, QC - General Practice
Dr Christiane Lepage, Montreal, QC - General Practice
Dr Patrice Lepage, Saint-Lazare, QC - General Practice
Dr Martin Lepine, Chibougamau, QC - Family Medicine
Dr Manon Leroux, Dieppe, NB - General Practice
Dr Nathalie Leroux, Montreal, QC - Obstetrics & Gynecology
Dr Jean-Francois Leroux, St-Jean-sur-Richel, QC - Otolaryngology
Dr Raphaelle Leroux-Levesque, Saint-Hyacinthe, QC - Emergency Family Med
Dr Valerie Leroyer, St-Alexis-D-Monts, QC - General Practice
Dr Jacques Lesage, Anjou, QC - Psychiatry
Dr Michel Lesage, Joliette, QC - Community Medicine
Dr Alain Lesage, Mont-Laurier, QC - General Practice
Dr Lyne Lessard, Montreal, QC - General Practice
Dr Myriam Lessard, Montreal, QC - Internal Medicine
Dr Julie Lessard, Quebec, QC - Pediatrics
Dr Isabelle Letourneau, St-Charles-Brromee, QC - Internal Medicine
Dr Sylvie Letovanec, St-Jean-Sur-Richel, QC - General Practice
Dr Jean-Pierre Leung, Calgary, AB - Family Medicine
Dr Caroline Levac, St-Lin-Laurentides, QC - General Practice
Dr Dominique Levesque, Montreal, QC - Gastroenterology
Dr Sylvie Levesque, Montreal, QC - Psychiatry
Dr Jacques Levesque, Quebec, QC - Diagnostic-Radiology
Dr Annabelle Levesque-Chouinard, Gatineau, QC - Family Medicine
Dr Gisele Li, Montreal, QC - Ophthalmology
Dr Patrick Liang, Sherbrooke, QC - Internal Medicine
Dr A Moishe Liberman, Montreal, QC - General Surgery
Dr Hung-Ba Lieu, Gatineau, QC - Neurosurgery
Dr Andree Lirette, Moncton, NB - Radiation Oncology
Dr Michel Lizotte, Quebec, QC - General Practice
Dr Denis Lockman, Ottawa, ON - Emergency Family Med
Dr Rolf Loertscher, Pointe-Claire, QC - General Practice
Dr Pierre Loiselle, St-Joseph-Du-Lac, QC - General Practice
Dr Marc Lonergan, Montreal, QC - Psychiatry
Dr Helene Long, Laval, QC - Endocrin/Metabolism
Dr Patricia Lord, Laval, QC - General Practice
Dr Julien Lord, Montreal, QC - Obstetrics & Gynecology
Dr Yvan Lorquet, Edmundston, NB - General Practice
Dr Lise Losier, Tracadie-Sheila, NB - Family Medicine
Dr Katie Luneau, Montreal, QC - Ophthalmology
Dr Colette P Luneau, Sherbrooke, QC - Neurosurgery
Dr Tinh-Nhan Luong, Montreal, QC - Pediatrics
Dr Robert Lussier, Orleans, ON - Obstetrics & Gynecology
Dr J R Yves Lussier, Longueuil, QC - General Practice
Dr David Lussier, Montreal, QC - Geriatric Medicine
Dr Yen Luu, Saint-Jerome, QC - General Surgery
Dr Michel Lynch, Lachute, QC - General Practice
Dr Yolanda Madarnas, Kingston, ON - Internal Medicine
Dr Eric Magnoux, Montreal, QC - General Practice
Dr Peter Mah, Gatineau, QC - Family Medicine
Dr Colin M Mailer, London, ON - Ophthalmology
Dr Philippe Major, Montreal, QC - Neurology
Dr Elizabeth A Malec, Ormstown, QC - Family Medicine
Dr Laurie Malenfant, Edmundston, NB - Internal Medicine
Dr Helene Malenfant, Drummondville, QC - General Practice
Dr Michele Mallet, Lameque, NB - Family Medicine
Dr Yvon Mallette, Sorel-Tracy, QC - General Practice
Dr Natacha Malmedy, Trois-Rivieres, QC - Obstetrics & Gynecology
Dr Jean-Luc Malo, Montreal, QC - Respirology
Dr Romain Mandel, Montreal, QC - General Practice
Dr Helene Mandeville, Montreal, QC - General Practice
Dr Marie-Josee Marceau, Terrebonne, QC - General Practice
Dr Valerie Marchand, Montreal, QC - Gastroenterology
Dr Eric Marchand, Quebec, QC - Geriatric Medicine
Dr Isabelle Marcil, Montreal, QC - Dermatology
Dr Francois Marcotte, Montreal, QC - Cardiology
Dr Jean Marcotte, Quebec, QC - Emergency Family Med
Dr Judith Marcoux, Montreal, QC - Neurosurgery
Dr Howard C Margolese, Montreal, QC - Psychiatry
Dr Pascale Marinier, Montreal, QC - Dermatology
Dr Etienne Marquis, Dieppe, NB - Psychiatry
Dr Solange Marquis, Blainville, QC - General Practice
Dr Francois Marquis, Montreal, QC - Critical Care Medicine
Dr Chantal Marquis, Rimouski, QC - Family Medicine
Dr Isabelle Marquis, Sherbrooke, QC - General Practice
Dr Christopher J C Marriott, Hamilton, ON - Nuclear Medicine
Dr Julie Martel, Drummondville, QC - Psychiatry
Dr Gaetan Martel, Gatineau, QC - General Practice
Dr Alain Y Martel, Quebec, QC - Internal Medicine
Dr Johanne Martial, Brossard, QC - Psychiatry
Dr Josee Martin, Saint-Jacques, NB - Family Medicine
Dr Elise J Martin, Maria, QC - Pediatrics
Dr Paul A Martineau, Montreal, QC - Orthopedic Surgery
Dr Bernard Martineau, Sherbrooke, QC - Family Medicine
Dr Sylvain Masse, Campbellton, NB - General Practice
Dr Eric M Massicotte, Toronto, ON - Neurosurgery
Dr Pierre Masson, Farnham, QC - General Practice
Dr Laurence Masson-Cote, Sherbrooke, QC - Radiation Oncology
Dr Sylvain Mathews, Montreal, QC - Anesthesia
Dr Michel A Mathieu, Blainville, QC - General Practice
Dr Genevieve Mathieu, Longueuil, QC - Internal Medicine
Dr Jean-Pierre Mathieu, Montreal, QC - Rheumatology
Dr Guy Mathieu, Sherbrooke, QC - General Practice
Dr Jean-Francois Mathieu, Verdun, QC - General Practice
Dr Andree Mathieu-Serra, Montreal, QC - Dermatology
Dr Chantal M H Mayer, Vancouver, BC - Obstetrics & Gynecology
Dr Helene Mayrand, Laval, QC - Cardiology
Dr Serge Mayrand, Montreal, QC - Gastroenterology
Dr Isaac B Mbonjo, Gatineau, QC - Family Medicine
Dr Daniel J McBain, Kenora, ON - Family Medicine
Dr John McDermott, Edmonton, AB - Neurology
Dr Nathalie McFadden, Sherbrooke, QC - General Surgery
Dr Neil J McGee, Nepean, ON - Emergency Family Med
Dr Elizabeth A McGraw, Sorel-Tracy, QC - General Practice
Dr Jocelyne M A McKenna, Ottawa, ON - Anesthesia
Dr Danny McKinnon, Quebec, QC - General Practice
Dr Nathalie McLaughlin, Dieppe, NB - Obstetrics & Gynecology
Dr James S McPhee, Winnipeg, MB - Psychiatry
Dr Anne McSween, Sherbrooke, QC - General Practice
Dr Stephane B Meere, Montreal, QC - Ophthalmology
Dr Christopher J M Meilleur, Kapuskasing, ON - Emergency Family Med
Dr Serge B Melancon, Montreal, QC - Medical Genetics
Dr Karen A Melanson, Dieppe, NB - Family Medicine
Dr Nathalie P Menard, Cornwall, ON - Family Medicine
Dr Ginette Menard, Longueuil, QC - General Practice
Dr Sylvain Menard, Saint-Sauveur, QC - General Practice
Dr Charles Menard, Sherbrooke, QC - Gastroenterology
Dr Cathy Menkarios, Montreal, QC - Radiation Oncology
Dr Isabelle Mercier, Thetford Mines, QC - General Practice
Dr Suzanne Mercille, Montreal, QC - Internal Medicine
Dr Marc Merizzi, St-Jean-sur-Richel, QC - General Practice
Dr Michel J Messier, Verdun, QC - Psychiatry
Dr Helene F Meunier, Baie-Comeau, QC - Family Medicine
Dr Jean Michaud, Ottawa, ON - Anatomical Pathology
Dr Raouf E Mikhail, Cowansville, QC - Family Medicine
Dr Yann G Milbeo, Greenfield Park, QC - General Practice
Dr Ashley P Miller, Vancouver, BC - Psychiatry
Dr Jean Miller, Baie-Saint-Paul, QC - General Practice
Dr Heather I Milliken, Halifax, NS - Psychiatry
Dr Francois Milord, Longueuil, QC - Community Medicine
Dr Stephanie Minorgan, Ottawa, ON - Family Medicine
Dr Jan Fredrik Moe, Kinistino, SK - General Practice
Dr Denis Monfette, Laurier-Station, QC - Family Medicine
Dr Guy J P Mongeon, Sudbury, ON - Family Medicine
Dr Livia Montalin, Quebec, QC - Plastic Surgery
Dr Claude Montsion, Gatineau, QC - General Practice
Dr Andrew D Moore, Greenfield Park, QC - Clin Immun/Allergy
Dr Katherine Moore, Quebec, QC - Urology
Dr Marcel F Moreau, Saint-Anselme, QC - General Practice
Dr Pierre Morency, Quebec, QC - General Practice
Dr Mario B Morency, Victoriaville, QC - Psychiatry
Dr Stephen R Morgan, Montreal, QC - General Surgery
Dr Gisele S L Morier, Winnipeg, MB - Psychiatry
Dr Gilles Morin, Asbestos, QC - General Practice
Dr Francois Morin, Quebec, QC - Orthopedic Surgery
Dr Bernard Morin, Quebec, QC - General Practice
Dr Gertrude Morin, Saint-Lambert, QC - General Practice
Dr Luc Morin, Sherbrooke, QC - Psychiatry
Dr Guy Morin, Trois-Rivieres, QC - Gastroenterology
Dr Diane Morissette, Hawkesbury, ON - Psychiatry
Dr Lucie Morissette, Quebec, QC - Diagnostic-Radiology
Dr Lucie Morneau, Saint-Romuald, QC - General Practice
Dr Hugo Morrissette, Levis, QC - Gastroenterology
Dr Roger Morrissette, Maria, QC - Ophthalmology
Dr Sophie Mottard, Montreal, QC - Orthopedic Surgery
Dr Jacinthe Moulin, Quebec, QC - Family Medicine
Dr Roger Mousseau, Montreal, QC - Gastroenterology
Dr Cristin Muecke, Fredericton, NB - Community Medicine
Dr Max N Myara, Montreal, QC - General Practice
Dr Marie-Eve Nadeau, Ste-Anne-des-Monts, QC - General Surgery
Dr Francine Nagy, Montreal, QC - General Practice
Dr Veronique Nally, Montreal, QC - General Practice
Dr Serge Naoum, Cornwall, ON - General Surgery
Dr Lili Nasseri, Coquitlam, BC - Family Medicine
Dr Lorraine R Natho, Calgary, AB - Family Medicine
Dr Stanley Nattel, Montreal, QC - Cardiology
Dr Theodore Nault, Matane, QC - Orthopedic Surgery
Dr Paul Nault, Saint-Laurent, QC - Dermatology
Dr Odette Nazair, Victoriaville, QC - General Practice
Dr Roxane Neron, Montreal, QC - General Practice
Dr Quang Binh Nguyen, Vancouver, BC - General Practice
Dr H Tuong Quan Nguyen, Montreal, QC - General Practice
Dr Ha-Nam P Nguyen, Montreal, QC - Otolaryngology
Dr Mohammad T Niazi, Montreal, QC - Radiation Oncology
Dr Marie-Frederique Noel, Campbell River, BC - Family Medicine
Dr Jean-Francois Noel, Cap-aux-Meules, QC - General Practice
Dr Brooke M E Noftle, London, ON - Family Medicine
Dr Nicolas Noiseux, Montreal, QC - Cardiac Surgery
Dr Pierre Noiseux, Saint-Hyacinthe, QC - General Practice

Dr Christine Nolze, Waterloo, QC - General Practice
Dr David K Nonnenman, Saint-Lambert, QC - Plastic Surgery
Dr Caroline Noory, Rigaud, QC - Family Medicine
Dr Mireille A Norris, Toronto, ON - Geriatric Medicine
Dr Richard Novick, London, ON - Cardiovasc/ThorSurg
Dr Mandiangu Nsungu, Yorkton, SK - General Practice
Dr Kim O'Connor, Quebec, QC - Cardiology
Dr Lisa O'Farrell, Quebec, QC - Family Medicine
Dr Pierre Olivier, Carleton, QC - General Practice
Dr Andre Olivier, Montreal, QC - Neurosurgery
Dr Richard Ostiguy, Montreal, QC - Gastroenterology
Dr Valerie Oudar, Quebec, QC - General Practice
Dr Danielle Ouellet, La Malbaie, QC - General Practice
Dr Caroline Ouellet, Montreal, QC - Pediatric Emergency Medicine
Dr Pierre Ouellet, Quebec, QC - Hematology
Dr Jean-Pascal Ouellet, Sherbrooke, QC - Emergency Medicine
Dr Eve-Marie Ouellet, Terrebonne, QC - General Practice
Dr Erik Ouellette, Orleans, ON - Emergency Family Med
Dr Jean-Paul Ouellette, Orleans, ON - Family Medicine
Dr Alain A Ouimet, Montreal, QC - General Surgery
Dr Denis Ouimet, Montreal, QC - Nephrology
Dr Francine M G Page, Vanier, ON - Psychiatry
Dr Sylvain Palardy, Montreal, QC - Psychiatry
Dr Francois Panaccio, Montreal, QC - Dermatology
Dr Jerome Paquet, Quebec, QC - Neurosurgery
Dr Nadine Paquet, Sainte-Julie, QC - General Practice
Dr Nancy Paquet, Sherbrooke, QC - Nuclear Medicine
Dr Ghislain Paquet, St-Jean-Sur-Richel, QC - General Practice
Dr Suzanne Paquette, Charlemagne, QC - Psychiatry
Dr Michel Paquin, Salaber-de-Valleyf, QC - Obstetrics & Gynecology
Dr Yvon Paquin, Shawinigan, QC - General Practice
Dr Marc Paquin, Ste-Agathe-des-Mts, QC - General Practice
Dr Michel Parayre, Rouyn-Noranda, QC - Family Medicine
Dr Jean-Louis Pare, Moncton, NB - General Practice
Dr Lyne Pare, Saint-Pamphile, QC - General Practice
Dr Yves Parent, Montreal, QC - General Practice
Dr Roger Parent, Quebec, QC - General Practice
Dr Louise Passerini, Greenfield Park, QC - Critical Care Medicine
Dr Ketan N Patel, London, ON - General Practice
Dr J J Francois Patenaude, Montreal, QC - Hematology
Dr Nicolas Patenaude, Sherbrooke, QC - Orthopedic Surgery
Dr Alexander H G Paterson, Calgary, AB - General Practice
Dr Mario Payette, Saint-Bruno, QC - General Practice
Dr Wilhelm B Pellemans, Laval, QC - Plastic Surgery
Dr Marcel J Pelletier, Longueuil, QC - General Practice
Dr Lysanne Pelletier, Rimouski, QC - Endocrin/Metabolism
Dr Suzanne Pelletier, Saint-Bruno, QC - Pediatrics
Dr Caroline Peloquin, Saint-Hyacinthe, QC - Family Medicine
Dr Annie Pepin, Saint-Lambert, QC - General Practice
Dr Michel-Antoine Perrault, Sherbrooke, QC - Anesthesia
Dr Andre Perreault, Montreal, QC - Orthopedic Surgery
Dr Sylvie Perreault, Sherbrooke, QC - General Practice
Dr Caroline Perreault, St-Jean-sur-Richel, QC - General Practice
Dr Christian Perreault, Terrebonne, QC - Ophthalmology
Dr Alban Perrier, Laval, QC - General Practice
Dr Paul Perrotte, Montreal, QC - Urology
Dr Thierry Petry, Gaspe, QC - Anesthesia
Dr Veronique Phan, Montreal, QC - Nephrology
Dr Veronique Phaneuf, Saint-Cesaire, QC - General Practice
Dr Denis C Phaneuf, Terrebonne, QC - Cardiology
Dr Jean-Claude Philibert, Shawinigan, QC - General Practice
Dr Johanne Philippe, Mashteuiatsh, QC - General Practice
Dr Lincoln R Phipps, Leamington, ON - General Practice
Dr Leo Picard, Moncton, NB - Internal Medicine
Dr Claudette Picard, Ottawa, ON - Family Medicine
Dr Jean-Marc Picard, Saint-Romuald, QC - General Practice
Dr Lyne Picard, Verdun, QC - Otolaryngology
Dr Marcel Piche, Lorraine, QC - General Practice
Dr Monique Pichette, Warwick, QC - General Practice
Dr Edith Pigeon, Gatineau, QC - Family Medicine
Dr Nicole Pigeon, Sherbrooke, QC - Pediatrics
Dr Pierre D Pigeon, St-Eustache, QC - General Surgery
Dr Genevieve Pinho, Rouyn-Noranda, QC - General Practice
Dr Jacques Plamondon, Quebec, QC - Psychiatry
Dr Isabelle Plamondon, Quebec, QC - Critical Care Medicine
Dr Daniel Plante, Pembroke, ON - Family Medicine
Dr Annick Plante, Greenfield Park, QC - General Practice
Dr Francois J Plante, Verdun, QC - Respirology
Dr Claudia Plourde, Gaspe, QC - Family Medicine
Dr Diane Plourde, Riviere-Du-Loup, QC - Obstetrics & Gynecology
Dr Isabelle Plourde, Riviere-du-Loup, QC - General Practice
Dr Suzie Plourde, Sherbrooke, QC - General Practice
Dr Suzanne Poirier, Anjou, QC - General Practice
Dr Nancy C Poirier, Montreal, QC - Cardiac Surgery
Dr Brigitte Poirier, Quebec, QC - General Surgery
Dr Jean-Francois Poissant, Shawinigan-Sud, QC - General Surgery
Dr Benoit P Poitras, Montreal, QC - Orthopedic Surgery
Dr Jonathan S Ponesse, Ottawa, ON - Neurology
Dr Clara Popa, Rouyn-Noranda, QC - General Practice
Dr Glenn D Posner, Ottawa, ON - Obstetrics & Gynecology
Dr Sacha Poulin, Montreal, QC - Psychiatry
Dr Marie-Claude Poulin, Quebec, QC - Internal Medicine
Dr Marie-Christine Pouliot, Levis, QC - General Practice
Dr Denis Pouliot, Quebec, QC - Otolaryngology
Dr Bernard Pouliot, Riviere-Du-Loup, QC - Community Medicine
Dr Kevin V Power, Nepean, ON - Urology
Dr Jean-Paul Praud, Sherbrooke, QC - Respirology
Dr David J Price, Hamilton, ON - Family Medicine
Dr Denis Proulx, Beloeil, QC - General Practice
Dr Pierre-Yvon Proulx, Victoriaville, QC - Internal Medicine
Dr Robert Provencher, Montreal, QC - General Practice
Dr Henri Prud'Homme, Donnacona, QC - General Practice
Dr Marie L P Prud'Homme, Windsor, QC - General Practice
Dr William E Pryse-Phillips, St. John's, NL - Neurology
Dr Rosita Punti, Montreal, QC - Psychiatry
Dr Dominique M J Racine, Ottawa, ON - Family Medicine
Dr Francois R J Racine, Ottawa, ON - Physical Medicine & Rehab
Dr Louis Racine, Montreal, QC - Ophthalmology
Dr Len Ralley, Toronto, ON - Psychiatry
Dr Andree Rasquin-Weber, Montreal, QC - Pediatrics
Dr Martine Raymond, Laval, QC - Internal Medicine
Dr Mary Jo Recoskie, Greenfield Park, QC - Nuclear Medicine
Dr Marie-Claude Renaud, Quebec, QC - Gynecologic Oncology
Dr Evelyne Rey, Montreal, QC - Internal Medicine
Dr Caroline Rheaume, Quebec, QC - Family Medicine
Dr Genevieve Ricard, Saint-Jerome, QC - Neurology
Dr Claude Richard, Gr-Sault/Gr-Falls, NB - General Practice
Dr Pierre Richer, Montreal, QC - Anesthesia
Dr Michael J Rieder, London, ON - Pediatrics
Dr Guy Riendeau, Montreal, QC - General Practice
Dr Sheilagh P Riley, Montreal, QC - Pediatrics
Dr Julie Riopel, Quebec, QC - Anatomical Pathology
Dr Gisele Rioux, Saint-Jerome, QC - General Practice
Dr Paul Rivard, Chandler, QC - Psychiatry
Dr Caroline Robert, Granby, QC - Internal Medicine
Dr Louis Robert, Quebec, QC - General Practice
Dr Steve A I Roberts, Grande Prairie, AB - Ophthalmology
Dr A Edwin Roberts, Windsor, ON - Anesthesia
Dr Line Robichaud, Bathurst, NB - General Practice
Dr Martin Robichaud, Moncton, NB - Family Medicine
Dr Jean-Luc Robichaud, Salaber-de-Valleyf, QC - General Practice
Dr Andre Robidoux, Montreal, QC - General Surgery
Dr Lucile C Robillard-McNulty, Ottawa, ON - General Practice
Dr Maxime Robin-Boudreau, Lourdes-d-Bl-Sabl, QC - Family Medicine
Dr Martine Robinson, Asbestos, QC - General Practice
Dr Johane M Robitaille, Halifax, NS - Ophthalmology
Dr France D Rocheleau, Hawkesbury, ON - Psychiatry
Dr Michelle Rochon, Montreal, QC - Psychiatry
Dr Alain Rochon, Sherbrooke, QC - Community Medicine
Dr Peter L Rosenbaum, Hamilton, ON - Pediatrics
Dr Michel Rossignol, Montreal, QC - Community Medicine
Dr Sheri L Roszell, Chatham, ON - Emergency Family Med
Dr Pierre Rouillard, Quebec, QC - Psychiatry
Dr Joelle Rouillard-Lafond, Alma, QC - Pediatrics
Dr Claude A Rouleau, Quebec, QC - General Surgery
Dr Jean-Francois Rouleau, Saint-Jerome, QC - General Practice
Dr Danielle Rouse, Saint-Jerome, QC - General Practice
Dr Andre Rousseau, Levis, QC - Pediatrics
Dr Julie Rousseau, Montreal, QC - Hematology
Dr Claire N Roussel, Fredericton, NB - Family Medicine
Dr Louise Roux, Amos, QC - Neurology
Dr Robert P A Roy, Burnaby, BC - Obstetrics & Gynecology
Dr Melanie Roy, Bathurst, NB - Ophthalmology
Dr Viateur Roy, Candiac, QC - General Practice
Dr Marie-Josee Roy, Longueuil, QC - Pediatrics
Dr Claude C Roy, Montreal, QC - Gastroenterology
Dr Genevieve Roy, Montreal, QC - Obstetrics & Gynecology
Dr Denis Roy, Montreal, QC - Cardiology
Dr Alain Roy, Montreal, QC - Orthopedic Surgery
Dr Roger Roy, Quebec, QC - General Practice
Dr Louis Roy, Quebec, QC - General Practice
Dr Andre Roy, Sainte-Julie, QC - General Practice
Dr Amelia Roy, Sherbrooke, QC - Family Medicine
Dr Alain Roy, St-Joseph-Du-Lac, QC - General Practice
Dr Christelle Royer, Granby, QC - General Practice
Dr Ethan Rubinstein, Winnipeg, MB - General Practice
Dr Louise Ruest, Fredericton, NB - Family Medicine
Dr Greg Ryan, Toronto, ON - Obstetrics & Gynecology
Dr Roger Saadia, Winnipeg, MB - General Practice
Dr Eric Sabbah, Longueuil, QC - Cardiology
Dr Norman Sabin, Montreal, QC - Emergency Family Med
Dr Alexis Sabourin, Saint-Hyacinthe, QC - Endocrin/Metabolism
Dr H Leonard Sadinsky, Etobicoke, ON - General Practice
Dr Claire H Saint-Cyr, Montreal, QC - Pediatrics
Dr Chantal Saint-Dizier, Repentigny, QC - General Practice
Dr Marie Saint-Laurent, Montreal, QC - Psychiatry
Dr Franck J A Sajous, St-Charles-Brromee, QC - Urology
Dr Wassim Salamoun, Summerside, PE - General Practice
Dr Yvan Samson, Montreal, QC - Hematology
Dr Cathie Sanfacon, Levis, QC - Family Medicine
Dr Martin Sasseville, Matagami, QC - General Practice
Dr Denis Sasseville, Montreal, QC - Dermatology
Dr Jean-Francois Saucier, Montreal, QC - Psychiatry
Dr Guylene Savard, Brampton, ON - General Practice
Dr Anne Savard, Quebec, QC - General Practice
Dr Gilles Savard, Riviere-du-Loup, QC - General Practice
Dr Melanie Savard-Cote, St-Joseph-Du-Lac, QC - Family Medicine
Dr Anik Savoie, Dieppe, NB - Family Medicine
Dr Louise Savoie, Montreal, QC - General Practice
Dr Cynthia A Savoy, Dieppe, NB - Family Medicine
Dr Danial M I Schecter, Midland, ON - Family Medicine
Dr Jeffrey Schiff, Toronto, ON - Internal Medicine
Dr Karen A Scott, Sechelt, BC - Family Medicine
Dr Krista S Scott, Vancouver, BC - Ophthalmology
Dr James L Scott, Victoria, BC - Neurology
Dr Bernard Seguin, Chicoutimi, QC - Orthopedic Surgery
Dr Chantal Seguin, Montreal, QC - Hematology
Dr Eric Seguin, Verdun, QC - General Practice
Dr Lynne Senecal, Montreal, QC - Internal Medicine
Dr Sylvie Senechal, Grand Falls, NB - Family Medicine
Dr Charles Serero, Montreal, QC - General Practice
Dr Mylene Sergerie, Laval, QC - General Practice
Dr Danielle Serra, Mont-Tremblant, QC - General Practice
Dr Feryal Sharabyani, Vaudreuil-Dorion, QC - Family Medicine
Dr Sanjeev P Sharma, Ottawa, ON - Orthopedic Surgery
Dr James J Sheridan, Grnd Falls-Windsor, NL - Internal Medicine
Dr Mark H Sherman, Montreal, QC - Endocrin/Metabolism
Dr Marie-Eve Sicard, Trois-Rivieres, QC - Radiation Oncology
Dr Conrad J Sichler, Burlington, ON - Family Medicine
Dr Caroline Simard, Dieppe, NB - General Practice
Dr P Line Simard, Chandler, QC - Diagnostic-Radiology
Dr France Simard, Laval, QC - General Practice
Dr Andree-Anne Simard, Montreal, QC - General Practice
Dr Raymond Simard, Rimouski, QC - Ophthalmology
Dr Jennifer M Simard, St-Charles-Brromee, QC - Family Medicine
Dr Jocelyne Simoneau, Salaber-de-Valleyf, QC - General Pathology
Dr Nathalie Sirois, Sept-Iles, QC - Pediatrics
Dr Alfred Sisto, Nepean, ON - Pediatrics
Dr Susan E Skanes, Dieppe, NB - General Surgery

Dr Nathalie M C Slaney, Sudbury, ON - General Practice
Dr Valerie L Soland, Montreal, QC - Electroencephal
Dr Jill K Solomon, Scarborough, ON - Pediatrics
Dr Martin L Solomon, Montreal, QC - Psychiatry
Dr Eric Soubiran, Saint-Hyacinthe, QC - General Practice
Dr Francois D Soucie, Edmundston, NB - Family Medicine
Dr Cathya Soucy, Rimouski, QC - General Practice
Dr Lyne H Souligny, Hawkesbury, ON - Family Medicine
Dr Julie S Souligny, Orleans, ON - General Practice
Dr Hugo St-Amand, Gatineau, QC - Plastic Surgery
Dr Dominique St-Cyr, Winchester, ON
- Obstetrics & Gynecology
Dr Yvan St-Cyr, Quebec, QC - Orthopedic Surgery
Dr Philippe St-Gelais, Saint-Georges, QC - Ophthalmology
Dr Pascal St-Germain, Quebec, QC - General Surgery
Dr Eve St-Hilaire, Moncton, NB - Hematology
Dr Sophie St-Hilaire, Montreal, QC - Psychiatry
Dr Benoit St-Jean, Ottawa, ON - General Surgery
Dr Edith St-Jean, Saint-Hyacinthe, QC - Endocrin/Metabolism
Dr Renaud St-Laurent, Dorval, QC - General Practice
Dr Nancy St-Pierre, Ottawa, ON - Family Medicine
Dr Frederic St-Pierre, Montmagny, QC - Anesthesia
Dr Robert I Stein, London, ON - Endocrin/Metabolism
Dr Louis-Mathieu Stevens, Montreal, QC - Cardiac Surgery
Dr Elisabeth M Stumpf, Shipshaw, QC - General Practice
Dr Mazen Sultan, Shawinigan-Sud, QC - Ophthalmology
Dr Veronique Susset, Montreal, QC - Physical Medicine & Rehab
Dr Neil B Sweezey, Toronto, ON - Pediatrics
Dr Dominique Synnott, Mont-Royal, QC - General Surgery
Dr Raymond Taillefer, St-Jean-Richelieu, QC - Nuclear Medicine
Dr A Monique Taillon, Fredericton, NB
- Physical Medicine & Rehab
Dr Luminita Tandareanu, Montreal, QC - Family Medicine
Dr David F Tang-Wai, Toronto, ON - Neurology
Dr Agnes M J Tanguay, Ottawa, ON - General Practice
Dr Marie-Claude Tanguay, Longueuil, QC
- Obstetrics & Gynecology
Ms Caroline Tanguay, Montmagny, QC - General Practice
Dr Jean-Francois Tanguay, Montreal, QC - Cardiology
Dr Louise Tardif, Montreal, QC - General Practice
Dr Isabelle Tardif, Montreal, QC - Family Medicine
Dr Chantal Tardif, Victoriaville, QC - General Practice
Dr Francois Teasdale, Montreal, QC - Pediatrics
Dr Robert J Teskey, Saint John, NB - Cardiology
Dr Francine Tessier, Vancouver, BC - Obstetrics & Gynecology
Dr Michel Tessier, Quebec, QC - Nuclear Medicine
Dr Joseph X Thavundayil, Verdun, QC - General Practice
Dr Jean Thellen, Mont-Saint-Hilaire, QC - General Practice
Dr Louis F J Theriault, Dieppe, NB - Psychiatry
Dr Josee Theriault, Sudbury, ON - Critical Care Medicine
Dr A Nathanaelle Theriault, Quebec, QC - Community Medicine
Dr Genevieve Therien, Quebec, QC - Dermatology
Dr Natalie Therriault, Gatineau, QC - Orthopedic Surgery
Dr J Jean A G Therrien, Hawkesbury, ON - General Practice
Dr Sylvie Therrien, Saint-Hyacinthe, QC - General Practice
Dr Elise Thibault, Laval, QC - General Surgery
Dr Manon Thibault, Quebec, QC - Electroencephal
Dr Claude Thibault, Quebec, QC - General Surgery
Dr Suzanne Thibault, Varennes, QC - General Practice
Dr Danny Thibeault, Bathurst, NB - Family Medicine
Dr Claude Thibeault, Brossard, QC - General Practice
Dr Roseline Thibeault, Quebec, QC - Infectious Diseases
Dr Michel E Thibodeau, Hawkesbury, ON - Internal Medicine
Dr Pierre Thibodeau, Lachute, QC - General Practice
Dr Paul Thomas, Longueuil, QC - General Practice
Dr Nancy Thomas, Quebec, QC - Obstetrics & Gynecology
Dr Jean-Pierre Thompson, Sainte-Julie, QC - General Practice
Dr Linda N Thyer, Vancouver, BC - Family Medicine
Dr Camille M L Tittley, Hamilton, ON - General Practice
Dr Nadine J Touma, Orleans, ON - Family Medicine
Dr Thi-My-Linh Tran, Montreal, QC - General Practice
Dr Valerie M C Tremblay, North Bay, ON - Otolaryngology
Dr Marc-Andre Tremblay, Alma, QC - Orthopedic Surgery
Dr Marie-France Tremblay, Blainville, QC - General Practice
Dr Jean-Denis Tremblay, Dolbeau-Mistassini, QC
- General Practice
Dr Sylvie Tremblay, Drummondville, QC - General Practice
Dr Florence Tremblay, Montreal, QC - Family Medicine
Dr Helene Tremblay, Quebec, QC - General Practice
Dr Sylvie Tremblay, Quebec, QC - General Practice
Dr Micheline Tremblay, Quebec, QC - Family Medicine
Dr Michel Tremblay, Saint-Romuald, QC - General Practice
Dr Anouk Tremblay, Trois-Rivieres, QC - Hematology
Dr Chantal Tremblay, Val-d'Or, QC - General Practice
Dr Suzanne Trempe-Gourdeau, Quebec, QC - General Practice
Dr Jean-Pierre Trepanier, Joliette, QC - Community Medicine
Dr Louise Trepanier, Montreal, QC - Family Medicine
Dr Sebastien Trop, Toronto, ON - Cardiac Surgery
Dr J R Guy Tropper, Longueuil, QC - Otolaryngology
Dr Sylvie Trottier, Quebec, QC - Medical Microbiology
Dr Marielle Trottier, Varennes, QC - General Practice
Dr Patrick Trudeau, Chicoutimi, QC - General Surgery
Dr Pierre Trudeau, Laval, QC - General Practice
Dr Sonia Trudeau, Montreal, QC - Psychiatry
Dr Guy Trudel, Ottawa, ON - Physical Medicine & Rehab
Dr Jean-René Trudel, Ottawa, ON - Psychiatry
Dr Francoise Truong, Mississauga, ON - Anatomical Pathology
Dr Patrick D C Truong, Niagara Falls, ON - Anesthesia
Dr Pascale Turbide, Sept-Iles, QC - Ophthalmology
Dr Manon Turbide, Val-d'Or, QC - Obstetrics & Gynecology
Dr Renee Turcotte, Dieppe, NB - General Practice
Dr Robert Turcotte, Montreal, QC - Orthopedic Surgery
Dr Gilles Turcotte, Quebec, QC - Medical Biochemistry
Dr Jean-Francois Turcotte, Quebec, QC - Neurosurgery
Dr Eric Turcotte, Sherbrooke, QC - Nuclear Medicine
Dr Jean Turgeon, Montreal, QC - Pediatrics
Dr Yvan Turmel, St-Anne-Beaup, QC - General Practice
Dr Joan C Tyler, Pembroke, ON - Family Medicine
Dr Natalie Vachon, Chibougamau, QC - Psychiatry
Dr Andre Vachon, La Guadeloupe, QC - General Practice
Dr Roger Vadeboncoeur, Montreal, QC
- Physical Medicine & Rehab
Dr Christian Vaillancourt, Ottawa, ON - Emergency Medicine
Dr Rosaire Vaillancourt, Quebec, QC - Cardiovasc/ThorSurg
Dr Raymonde Vaillancourt, Sherbrooke, QC - Family Medicine
Dr Catherine R Vakil, Kingston, ON - Family Medicine
Dr Noemie Valiquette, Magog, QC - General Practice
Dr Helene Vallee, Saint-Georges, QC - General Practice
Dr Pierre Vallee, Verdun, QC - General Practice
Dr Isabelle Vallieres, Quebec, QC - Radiation Oncology
Dr Nathalie Vallieres, Saint-Lambert, QC - General Practice
Dr Carol Valois, Saint-Lambert, QC - Family Medicine
Dr Chantal Valois, St-Adolphe-D'Howrd, QC - General Practice
Dr Antoinette M Van Den Brekel, Vancouver, BC - Pediatrics
Dr Marie-Josee Van Sterthem, Pincourt, QC - General Practice
Dr Caroline Varga, Terrebonne, QC - Neurology
Dr Jean R Varin, Gatineau, QC - Orthopedic Surgery
Dr Melina Vassiliou, Montreal, QC - General Surgery
Dr Alain Vaugeois, Trois-Rivieres, QC - Family Medicine
Dr Rejean Veillette, Montreal, QC - General Practice
Dr Yves Veillette, Montreal, QC - Anesthesia
Dr Brigitte Veilleux, Beaupre, QC - General Practice
Dr Marie-Christine Veilleux, Gatineau, QC - General Practice
Dr Martin Veilleux, Montreal, QC - Electroencephal
Dr Sophie Venne, Longueuil, QC - Obstetrics & Gynecology
Dr Benoit Verret, Riviere-Du-Loup, QC - Internal Medicine
Dr Sylvie Verrette, Montreal, QC - General Practice
Dr Francois Vezina, Sherbrooke, QC - Orthopedic Surgery
Dr Louise Vidal, Sherbrooke, QC - Family Medicine
Dr Mario Viens, Sherbrooke, QC - General Surgery
Dr Julie Vigeant, Sherbrooke, QC - General Practice
Dr Eric Vigneault, Quebec, QC - Radiation Oncology
Dr Diane Villeneuve, Montreal, QC - General Practice
Dr Natacha Vincent, Richmond, QC - General Practice
Dr Claude P Violette, Bathurst, NB - Internal Medicine
Dr Chantal L Violette, Edmundston, NB - Internal Medicine
Dr Achla R Virmani, Verdun, QC - General Practice
Dr Blair J Voyvodic, Killaloe, ON - General Practice
Dr Thi Thuong T Vu, Montreal, QC - General Practice
Dr Daniel Wagner, Delson, QC - General Practice
Dr Ann D Walling, Montreal, QC - Cardiology
Dr Philippe Walsh, St-Jean-sur-Richel, QC - Urology
Dr Sylvie Watelle, La Sarre, QC - General Practice
Dr John B Watson, Ottawa, ON - Anesthesia
Dr Nancy Watts, Jonquiere, QC - Family Medicine
Dr Helene Watts, Laval, QC - General Practice
Dr Peter M Webster, Toronto, ON - Internal Medicine
Dr Eveline Wecowski, Terrebonne, QC - General Practice
Dr Wieslaw Wegrzycki, Maniwaki, QC - Family Medicine
Dr Jeffrey N Weinberg, Markham, ON - General Practice
Dr Julie H Whalen, Dieppe, NB - Family Medicine
Dr Chantal I Whelan, Ottawa, ON - Psychiatry
Dr Paula M White, Maria, QC - General Practice
Dr Pierre Whitlock, Moncton, NB - Hematology
Dr Andrew S Wiens, Ottawa, ON - Psychiatry
Dr Jean Wilkins, Montreal, QC - Pediatrics
Dr Peter T Willard, Welland, ON - General Surgery
Dr Paule Willett, Fort-Coulonge, QC - Family Medicine
Dr Mona Wilson Thomas Sorial, Pointe-Claire, QC
- General Practice
Dr John C S Wootton, Shawville, QC - General Practice
Dr Louis Wu, Oshawa, ON - Diagnostic-Radiology
Dr Marianne C Xhignesse, Sherbrooke, QC - General Practice
Dr Jean-Francois Yale, Montreal, QC - Endocrin/Metabolism
Dr J P Jean-Denis Yelle, Ottawa, ON - General Surgery
Dr Andree Yergeau, Quebec, QC - General Practice
Dr Sami Youakim, Victoria, BC - Family Medicine
Dr Joseph Youmbissi Tchetagni, Trois-Rivieres, QC
- General Practice
Dr Barbara M Young, Montreal, QC - Internal Medicine
Dr Gaby Zagury, Montreal, QC - Family Medicine
Dr Mitchell I Zelman, Charlottetown, PE - Pediatrics
Dr Michel de Maupeou, La Sarre, QC - General Practice

BISLAMA

Dr Jean-Yves Dupuis, Ottawa, ON - Anesthesia
Dr David F Hepburn, Victoria, BC - General Practice

BRETON

Dr Simon R J Nigen, Montreal, QC - Dermatology

BULGARIAN

Dr Yasser Abou Mourad, Vancouver, BC - Internal Medicine
Dr Lubomir Alexov, Scarborough, ON - General Practice
Dr David Algom, Nepean, ON - Clin Immun/Allergy
Dr Jordanka Angelova, Edmonton, AB - Family Medicine
Dr Nikolay Baldzhiyski, Bathurst, NB - General Practice
Dr Atanas K Dochev, Bridgewater, NS - General Practice
Dr Nevena Dourova, London, ON - Psychiatry
Dr Vlade M Gagovski, North York, ON - General Practice
Dr Margarita Gatchev, North Bay, ON - Family Medicine
Dr William S George, Woodstock, ON - General Practice
Dr Aleksander Georgievski, Thornhill, ON - General Practice
Dr Margarita Gitev, Toronto, ON - Psychiatry
Dr Svetoslav A Gueordjev, Nelson, BC - General Practice
Dr Samir Habib, Montreal, QC - Family Medicine
Dr Velizar A Harizanov, Toronto, ON - General Practice
Dr Elia Huidovici, Windsor, ON - Family Medicine
Dr T N Teodor Ivanov, Pitt Meadows, BC - Family Medicine
Dr Ilko S Karagiozov, Scarborough, ON - Family Medicine
Dr Evguenia L Marinova, Oshawa, ON - Family Medicine
Dr Sergio Mazzadi, Hamilton, ON - General Practice
Dr Roumen Milev, Kingston, ON - Psychiatry
Dr Lili G Mileva, Kingston, ON - Family Medicine
Dr Silvia Pavlova, Beloeil, QC - General Practice
Dr Kalina Popova, Victoria, BC - Anesthesia
Dr Blaga A Stancheva, Vancouver, BC - Family Medicine
Dr Chris P Stefanovich, Etobicoke, ON - Family Medicine
Dr Vasia Stefou, Toronto, ON - General Practice
Dr Christo I Tchervenkov, Montreal, QC - Cardiovasc/ThorSurg
Dr Milka A Tchervenkova, Brossard, QC - General Practice
Dr Krasimir G Todorov, Abbotsford, BC - General Practice
Dr Christo Todorov, Montreal, QC - Psychiatry
Dr Eva E Vozis, Toronto, ON - Anatomical Pathology

Dr Sylvia A Yankova, LaSalle, QC - Family Medicine
Dr Layla Younes, Montreal, QC - Family Medicine
Dr Alexander Zhivkov, Fort-Coulonge, QC - General Practice

BURMESE

Dr Steven K H Aung, Edmonton, AB - General Practice
Dr Marybelle M T Chain-Chang, Brampton, ON - General Practice
Dr Victor Han, London, ON - Pediatrics
Dr Peter T Hwee, Kitchener, ON - General Practice
Dr Tun Zan Maung, Abbotsford, BC - Internal Medicine
Dr Raymond T A Maung, Kamloops, BC - Anatomical Pathology
Dr Khin M Myint, Mississauga, ON - Family Medicine
Dr Lucy K Y Nee, Vancouver, BC - Family Medicine
Dr Christopher M Oung, Woodstock, ON - General Surgery
Dr Chiranjib Talukdar, Regina, SK - Pediatrics
Dr Sou K Thain, Kingston, ON - Radiation Oncology
Dr Ma Khin Thida, Vancouver, BC - Family Medicine
Dr Mohan S Virick, Sydney, NS - General Practice
Dr Lay Lay Win, Toronto, ON - Gastroenterology
Dr William H Yang, Ottawa, ON - Internal Medicine

CANTONESE

Dr Lee-Cyn Ang, London, ON - Neuro-Pathology
Dr Christine W L Applegarth, Vancouver, BC - General Practice
Dr Ambrose S S Au, Brockville, ON - Family Medicine
Dr How Hoong Au, Scarborough, ON - General Surgery
Dr Pauline Champion, Charlottetown, PE - General Practice
Dr John K F Chan, Abbotsford, BC - Family Medicine
Dr Paul Y H Chan, Coquitlam, BC - Family Medicine
Dr Albert W Chan, New Westminster, BC - Cardiology
Dr Philip Chan, North Vancouver, BC - Family Medicine
Dr Edmond S Chan, Vancouver, BC - Clin Immun/Allergy
Dr Jeanie C Chan, Vancouver, BC - General Practice
Dr Cyril F Y Chan, Vancouver, BC - General Practice
Dr Irene M Y Chan, Vancouver, BC - General Practice
Dr Karl K S Chan, Vancouver, BC - General Practice
Dr Ming-Ka Chan, Winnipeg, MB - Pediatrics
Dr Laura H Y Chan, Barrie, ON - Family Medicine
Dr Benjamin T Chan, Espanola, ON - General Practice
Dr Anthony K C Chan, Hamilton, ON - Hematology
Dr David H Chan, Hamilton, ON - Family Medicine
Dr Yvonne Chan, Mississauga, ON - Otolaryngology
Dr Paul C Chan, Mississauga, ON - General Practice
Dr Loh Yen L Chan, Mississauga, ON - Family Medicine
Dr Tommy K C Chan, North York, ON - Orthopedic Surgery
Dr Kwan-Leung Chan, Ottawa, ON - Cardiology
Dr Andrew C S Chan, Peterborough, ON - Gastroenterology
Dr Raymond K H Chan, Richmond Hill, ON - Family Medicine
Dr John F Y Chan, Richmond Hill, ON - General Practice
Dr Gerald C B Chan, Scarborough, ON - Gastroenterology
Dr Gabriel F P Chan, Scarborough, ON - Geriatric Medicine
Dr Lawrence K C Chan, Scarborough, ON - Family Medicine
Dr Paul S H Chan, Scarborough, ON - General Practice
Dr Kwok-Hung Chan, Scarborough, ON - General Practice
Dr Michael C K Chan, Scarborough, ON - General Surgery
Dr Aaron Y Chan, St Catharines, ON - Family Medicine
Dr Richard C W Chan, Toronto, ON - General Practice
Dr Charles K N Chan, Toronto, ON - Internal Medicine
Dr Christopher T M Chan, Toronto, ON - Internal Medicine
Dr Kevin J Chan, Toronto, ON - Pediatric Emergency Medicine
Dr Wing Chow Chan, Toronto, ON - Ophthalmology
Dr David Y K Chan, Toronto, ON - General Practice
Dr Helen S L Chan, Toronto, ON - Pediatrics
Dr Alex T C Chan, Toronto, ON - General Practice
Dr Clara C Chan, Toronto, ON - Ophthalmology
Dr Kenneth L Chan, Greenfield Park, QC - Gynecologic Oncology
Dr Mildred W M Chang, White Rock, BC - Emergency Family Med
Dr Daniel K M Chang, Brampton, ON - Dermatology
Dr C Michael Chang, Oshawa, ON - Urology
Dr Peter P Chang, Toronto, ON - Psychiatry
Dr Kathleen D K Chang, Toronto, ON - Family Medicine
Dr Peter H W Chau, Calgary, AB - General Practice
Dr Laurence K L Chau, Oakville, ON - Internal Medicine
Dr Helen Y Chen, Vancouver, BC - Family Medicine
Dr Jerry C L Chen, Vancouver, BC - General Surgery
Dr Chee Pyn Chen, Barrie, ON - Pediatrics
Dr Connie Chen, Etobicoke, ON - Family Medicine
Dr Jia-De Chen, North York, ON - Internal Medicine
Dr Robert E W Chen, Toronto, ON - Neurology
Dr Jim I Cheng, Sherwood Park, AB - Community Medicine
Dr Henry J C K Cheng, Brampton, ON - Obstetrics & Gynecology
Dr Alice Y Cheng, Mississauga, ON - Endocrin/Metabolism
Dr Anthony Cheng, North York, ON - Internal Medicine
Dr Malcolm H F Cheng, North York, ON - Pediatrics
Dr Michael T W Cheng, Richmond Hill, ON - General Practice
Dr Mary M L Cheng, Scarborough, ON - Obstetrics & Gynecology
Dr Susanna Y Cheng, Toronto, ON - Hematology
Dr Ken Cheung, Calgary, AB - Anesthesia
Dr King Cheung, Edmonton, AB - Diagnostic-Radiology
Dr Humphrey H Cheung, Lethbridge, AB - General Practice
Dr Stephen S K Cheung, Surrey, BC - Cardiology
Dr Francesca T Cheung, Markham, ON - Family Medicine
Dr W C Thomas Cheung, Mississauga, ON - Family Medicine
Dr Patrick C F Cheung, Toronto, ON - Radiation Oncology
Dr Angela M Cheung, Toronto, ON - Internal Medicine
Dr Melody Cheung-Lee, Edmonton, AB - Dermatology
Dr Brian P A Chew, Edmonton, AB - Family Medicine
Dr Sen Chew, Surrey, BC - General Practice
Dr Ben H Chew, Vancouver, BC - Urology
Dr Jesse Chew, Vancouver, BC - Ophthalmology
Dr Gilbert M M Chew, Victoria, BC - General Practice
Dr N M Sheryl Chiang, Edmonton, AB - General Practice
Dr S M Joseph Chien, Scarborough, ON - Internal Medicine
Dr Ying Wai Chin, New Westminster, BC - Geriatric Medicine
Dr Elaine I Chin, North York, ON - General Practice
Dr Karen P Ching, St. Albert, AB - Family Medicine
Dr Emily K Y Ching, Burlington, ON - Gastroenterology
Dr Paul K Chiu, Edmonton, AB - General Practice
Dr John F S Chiu, Edmonton, AB - Family Medicine
Dr Peter L S L Chiu, Edmonton, AB - Internal Medicine
Dr Aaron Chiu, Winnipeg, MB - Pediatrics
Dr Hak M Chiu, Oshawa, ON - Hematology
Dr Arthur K K Chiu, Scarborough, ON - General Surgery
Dr Simon S Chiu, St Thomas, ON - Psychiatry
Dr Priscilla P L Chiu, Toronto, ON - General Surgery
Dr Ann M Chiu, Windsor, ON - Ophthalmology
Dr Helen Y H Cho, Calgary, AB - Family Medicine
Dr Matthew C K Choi, Port Coquitlam, BC - Family Medicine
Dr Peter T Choi, Vancouver, BC - Anesthesia
Dr Antonio M F Choi, Toronto, ON - Family Medicine
Dr Betty L S Choi-Fung, North York, ON - Family Medicine
Dr David L T Chong, Surrey, BC - Emergency Family Med
Dr Paul W C Chong, Richmond Hill, ON - Cardiology
Dr Robert H Chong, Toronto, ON - General Practice
Dr Ivan S Y Choo, Delta, BC - Family Medicine
Dr Darren W K Choo, Vancouver, BC - General Practice
Dr Wee Kei Choong, Delta, BC - General Practice
Dr Mark W H Chor, Oshawa, ON - General Practice
Dr Benjamin Chou, Langley, BC - General Practice
Dr Bill P C Chow, Calgary, AB - Ophthalmology
Dr J Holden Chow, Abbotsford, BC - Family Medicine
Dr Victor D W Chow, North Vancouver, BC - Urology
Dr Stacey A Chow, Surrey, BC - General Practice
Dr Daliah Y L Chow, Ajax, ON - Family Medicine
Dr Kan-Yan Chow, Brampton, ON - Otolaryngology
Dr Mabel Y T Chow, Burlington, ON - Internal Medicine
Dr Andrew Chow, Mississauga, ON - Internal Medicine
Dr Peter H Chow, Sault Ste. Marie, ON - General Practice
Dr Harold H K Chow, Scarborough, ON - General Practice
Dr Kenneth C K Chow, Scarborough, ON - General Practice
Dr Yen Chow, Thunder Bay, ON - Family Medicine
Dr Chi-Ming Chow, Toronto, ON - Cardiology
Dr Chung Wai Chow, Toronto, ON - Internal Medicine
Dr Raphael K T Chow, Toronto, ON - Physical Medicine & Rehab
Dr Y B Dominic Chow, Unionville, ON - Family Medicine
Dr Benjamin S Choy, Markham, ON - Family Medicine
Dr Francis J L Chu, Richmond, BC - General Practice
Dr Mary P H Chu, Richmond, BC - General Practice
Dr Joseph Y C Chu, Etobicoke, ON - Internal Medicine
Dr Melvyn Chu, Richmond Hill, ON - Family Medicine
Dr Norman H Y Chu, Scarborough, ON - Emergency Family Med
Dr James C M Chu, Scarborough, ON - General Practice
Dr Karen L Chu, Toronto, ON - Emergency Family Med
Dr Lica Chui, Vancouver, BC - Ophthalmology
Dr Chin K Chung, North York, ON - Family Medicine
Dr Cynthia Chung, Scarborough, ON - General Practice
Dr Thomas Chung, Thornhill, ON - Ophthalmology
Dr Phuong Dang, Mississauga, ON - Family Medicine
Dr Glenn L Dong, Richmond, BC - Anesthesia
Dr Raymond Dong, Surrey, BC - Cardiology
Dr Aik-Ping Eng, Vancouver, BC - General Practice
Dr Helen W K Eng, White Rock, BC - Family Medicine
Dr Frank Eng, Newmarket, ON - General Surgery
Dr A P N Fam, Sault Ste Marie, ON - Obstetrics & Gynecology
Dr Mei Sum Fok, Edmonton, AB - Family Medicine
Dr Justine H S Fong, Calgary, AB - Family Medicine
Dr George Y Fong, Edmonton, AB - Family Medicine
Dr Chi Wai Fong, Scarborough, ON - General Practice
Dr Katherine W Fong, Toronto, ON - Diagnostic-Radiology
Dr Marshall C Foo, Toronto, ON - General Practice
Dr Weng-Leong Foong, Scarborough, ON - General Practice
Dr Jackie A Ford, Georgetown, ON - General Practice
Dr Gidon Frame, Burnaby, BC - Family Medicine
Dr Joseph S L Fu, Nepean, ON - General Practice
Dr Peter S M Fung, Spruce Grove, AB - Family Medicine
Dr Raymond C Fung, East York, ON - Endocrin/Metabolism
Dr Kee-Wai Fung, Etobicoke, ON - Pediatrics
Dr Kan Ying Fung, Mississauga, ON - General Practice
Dr W L Alan Fung, North York, ON - Psychiatry
Dr Wing-Tai Fung, Scarborough, ON - General Practice
Dr Kenneth P L Fung, Toronto, ON - Psychiatry
Dr Ambrose Y T Fung, Toronto, ON - Family Medicine
Dr Scott Fung, Toronto, ON - Gastroenterology
Dr S W Helen Gan, Vancouver, BC - Family Medicine
Dr Michael Ha, Hamilton, ON - Emergency Medicine
Dr Andrew C T Ha, Toronto, ON - Cardiology
Dr Sheila L Hew, Scarborough, ON - Family Medicine
Dr Kay Ho, Chilliwack, BC - General Practice
Dr Thomas M W Ho, Vancouver, BC - Family Medicine
Dr Vincent C Y Ho, Vancouver, BC - Dermatology
Dr Wei-Ning Ho, Vancouver, BC - General Practice
Dr Kendall Ho, Vancouver, BC - Emergency Medicine
Dr Elinda P L Ho, Vancouver, BC - General Practice
Dr Elaine P L Ho, Bowmanville, ON - Family Medicine
Dr Edward S Ho, Brantford, ON - General Practice
Dr Philip C Ho, Etobicoke, ON - Pediatrics
Dr Victoria Y W Ho, Kitchener, ON - Internal Medicine
Dr Shen-Pang E Ho, Lindsay, ON - General Pathology
Dr Doris S C Ho, London, ON - General Practice
Dr Hon-Lau Ho, Markham, ON - Family Medicine
Dr Yvonne Ho, Mississauga, ON - Diagnostic-Radiology
Dr W M Amy Ho, North York, ON - General Practice
Dr Grant K C Ho, Orillia, ON - Family Medicine
Dr Nancy S K Ho, Richmond Hill, ON - General Practice
Dr Alexander S Ho, Toronto, ON - Anesthesia
Dr Tommy K L Ho, Toronto, ON - Pediatrics
Dr Joanne M Ho, Toronto, ON - Geriatric Medicine
Dr Paul Ho-Tai, Kitchener, ON - Diagnostic-Radiology
Dr Lily M Ho-Tai, Scarborough, ON - Anesthesia
Dr Hilary C Hong, Surrey, BC - Dermatology
Dr Tommy Hong, Mississauga, ON - Family Medicine
Dr Yann J Hsiao, Vancouver, BC - General Practice
Dr Mabel Hsin, Bradford, ON - General Practice
Dr John S C Hsuen, North York, ON - Pediatrics
Dr Patrick O Huang, Richmond, BC - General Practice
Dr Paul B T Huang, Vancouver, BC - Emergency Medicine
Dr Ling Ling Huang, Mississauga, ON - Family Medicine
Dr Pein-Pein Huang, Ottawa, ON - Pediatrics
Dr Louis Huang, Scarborough, ON - Anesthesia
Dr Hilary K Hui, Richmond, BC - General Practice
Dr Ivy Y C Hui, Richmond, BC - Family Medicine
Dr Jacqueline C W Hui, Vancouver, BC - Psychiatry
Dr Catherine C M Hui, Vancouver, BC - Family Medicine
Dr Alphonsus Z Hui, Vancouver, BC - General Practice

Dr Betty M Hum, Toronto, ON - Family Medicine
Dr Tawny W Hung, Vancouver, BC - General Practice
Dr Orlando Hung, Halifax, NS - Anesthesia
Dr Frederico A Hung, Mississauga, ON - General Practice
Dr C Francis Hung, North York, ON - Diagnostic-Radiology
Dr Lick San Hung, Toronto, ON - Anatomical Pathology
Dr Hien Huynh, Edmonton, AB - Pediatrics
Dr Mei L Hwang, Scarborough, ON - General Practice
Dr Angela Hwang, Scarborough, ON - Family Medicine
Dr Christine Hwang, Toronto, ON - General Practice
Dr Paul A L S Hwang, Toronto, ON - Neurology
Dr Edsel B Ing, Toronto, ON - Ophthalmology
Dr Yiu Ban Ip, Surrey, BC - General Practice
Dr Simon C M Iu, North York, ON - General Surgery
Dr Timothy W T Kam, Vancouver, BC - General Practice
Dr Yolanda A Kirkham, Toronto, ON - Obstetrics & Gynecology
Dr Peter Ko, Vancouver, BC - Family Medicine
Dr Jevan Ko, Scarborough, ON - Obstetrics & Gynecology
Dr Waitak Kong, Brampton, ON - Cardiology
Dr Kester Kong, Scarborough, ON - Internal Medicine
Dr Betty K K Koo, North York, ON - Neurology
Dr Rose C Kung, Toronto, ON - Obstetrics & Gynecology
Dr Susan Y L Kwan, Burnaby, BC - Internal Medicine
Dr Bartholomew P Kwan, Brampton, ON - Diagnostic-Radiology
Dr Robert P K F Kwan, Scarborough, ON - General Practice
Dr Lawrence W Kwan, Scarborough, ON - Family Medicine
Dr Yee-Nga Yong Kwee, Surrey, BC - Pediatrics
Dr Jimmy C W Kwok, Calgary, AB - Geriatric Medicine
Dr Ezra Kwok, Richmond, BC - Family Medicine
Dr Eva Kwok, Scarborough, ON - Internal Medicine
Dr Keith Kwok, Scarborough, ON - Cardiology
Dr T Y Paul Kwong, Brampton, ON - General Practice
Dr Jeffrey C Y Kwong, Toronto, ON - Community Medicine
Dr Jatina Lai, North Vancouver, BC - Emergency Family Med
Dr James K Lai, Vancouver, BC - Family Medicine
Dr David K F Lai, Vancouver, BC - Family Medicine
Dr Kenneth K K Lai, Newmarket, ON - General Practice
Dr Albert I Lai, Thornhill, ON - General Practice
Dr Christopher C Lai, Thunder Bay, ON - Cardiology
Dr Anthony K S Lam, Calgary, AB - Family Medicine
Dr K S Kenneth Lam, Calgary, AB - Physical Medicine & Rehab
Dr Charles N H Lam, Nanaimo, BC - General Practice
Dr Simon R Lam, New Westminster, BC - Ophthalmology
Dr Alan J Lam, Squamish, BC - General Practice
Dr C Allan Lam, Vancouver, BC - General Practice
Dr Wai-Arm Lam, Vancouver, BC - General Practice
Dr Joseph K P Lam, Vancouver, BC - Family Medicine
Dr Jasmine C Lam, Vancouver, BC - Family Medicine
Dr Christopher Lam, Victoria, BC - Family Medicine
Dr Yuen-Ming Lam, Exeter, ON - General Practice
Dr Michael Y C Lam, Mississauga, ON - Family Medicine
Dr Vincent Y Y Lam, North York, ON - General Practice
Dr James H C Lam, Orillia, ON - General Practice
Dr Tukien M Lam, Richmond Hill, ON - Internal Medicine
Dr Sheung L L Lam, St Catharines, ON - Anesthesia
Dr Bridget Y C Lang, Vancouver, BC - General Practice
Dr Brenda W Lau, Surrey, BC - Anesthesia
Dr Herman H M Lau, Vancouver, BC
- Physical Medicine & Rehab
Dr Tain Ming Lau, Vancouver, BC - Anesthesia
Dr Amanda W M Lau, Vancouver, BC - Family Medicine
Dr Yan Lau, Winnipeg, MB - Gastroenterology
Dr Agatha Lau, Markham, ON - Gastroenterology
Dr Michael C K Lau, Markham, ON - Anatomical Pathology
Dr David Y M Lau, Scarborough, ON - General Practice
Dr Gary K L Lau, Scarborough, ON - General Practice
Dr Micheline C Lau, Scarborough, ON - General Practice
Dr Eddy C H Lau, Toronto, ON - Pediatrics
Dr Ching Lau, Toronto, ON - Cardiology
Dr Peter P T Lau, Toronto, ON - Family Medicine
Dr William W L Lau, Laval, QC - General Practice
Dr Charles C S Law, Vancouver, BC - General Practice
Dr Francis C H Law, Vancouver, BC - Ophthalmology
Dr Bonnie Law, Vancouver, BC - Family Medicine
Dr Sally S C Law, Vancouver, BC - Family Medicine
Dr Samuel F Law, Toronto, ON - Psychiatry
Dr Calvin H L Law, Toronto, ON - General Surgery
Dr Howe Leam, Lethbridge, AB - Family Medicine
Dr Agnes S Lee, Edmonton, AB - Obstetrics & Gynecology
Dr Tzu-Kuang Lee, Edmonton, AB - Internal Medicine
Dr Herman Lee, Burnaby, BC - Family Medicine
Dr Mona Lee, North Vancouver, BC - Family Medicine
Dr Shui Hing Lee, Richmond, BC - Ophthalmology
Dr Carol K Lee, Vancouver, BC - Anatomical Pathology
Dr Patricia Lee, Vancouver, BC - Otolaryngology
Dr Pui-Kee Lee, Vancouver, BC - Cardiology
Dr Cheng-Han Lee, Vancouver, BC - Anatomical Pathology
Dr Judy K M Lee, Vancouver, BC - General Practice
Dr Rachel N Lee, Vancouver, BC - General Practice
Dr Tom Lee, Vancouver, BC - General Practice
Dr Agnes Y Y Lee, Vancouver, BC - Hematology
Dr Donald D Lee, Vancouver, BC - General Practice
Dr Sandra W Lee, Vancouver, BC - Family Medicine
Dr Peter C K Lee, Dartmouth, NS - Family Medicine
Dr Winifred Lee, Dartmouth, NS - Obstetrics & Gynecology
Dr Edward S C Lee, Ajax, ON - Family Medicine
Dr Patricia P S Lee, Etobicoke, ON - Family Medicine
Dr David S C Lee, London, ON - Pediatrics
Dr Hayvin Lee, Markham, ON - Family Medicine
Dr Kevin A Lee, Markham, ON - Pediatrics
Dr Lap Cheung Lee, North York, ON - General Practice
Dr Joyce W Y Lee, North York, ON - Family Medicine
Dr Victor K G Lee, Peterborough, ON - Gastroenterology
Dr Michael C F Lee, Ridgeway, ON - General Practice
Dr Julietta C T Lee, Scarborough, ON - Internal Medicine
Dr Victor Chee Choon Lee, Scarborough, ON - General Practice
Dr Winnie W S Lee, Toronto, ON - General Practice
Dr Peter Lee, Toronto, ON - Internal Medicine
Dr Liesly Lee, Toronto, ON - Neurology
Dr Bonnie P Y Lee, Windsor, ON - Emergency Family Med
Dr Gary L Lee, Montreal, QC - Emergency Family Med
Dr M Madeleine Lee-Ng, Scarborough, ON - General Practice
Dr Kathy K Y Lee-Son, Vancouver, BC - Nephrology
Dr T C Benny Lei, Winnipeg, MB - General Practice
Dr Eric W H Leong, Toronto, ON - Gastroenterology
Dr Renata M W Leong, Toronto, ON - Family Medicine
Dr Fook Lin Leong-Sit, Edmonton, AB - Ophthalmology
Dr Jean-Pierre Leung, Calgary, AB - Family Medicine
Dr Patrick P Leung, Port Coquitlam, BC - Family Medicine
Dr Jason K Leung, Richmond, BC - Family Medicine
Dr Michael N F Leung, Vancouver, BC - General Practice
Dr Cosmas W M Leung, Vancouver, BC - Emergency Medicine
Dr Henry H K Leung, Vancouver, BC - General Practice
Dr N L Eillen Leung, Vancouver, BC - General Practice
Dr Vicki W K Leung, Vancouver, BC - Pediatrics
Dr Victor Leung, Vancouver, BC - Infectious Diseases
Dr Frederick C C Leung, Ajax, ON - Family Medicine
Dr Nin-Ming Leung, Markham, ON - Family Medicine
Dr Kent K K Leung, Markham, ON - General Practice
Dr Sophia S Y Leung, Mississauga, ON - General Practice
Dr Robert S L Leung, Mississauga, ON - General Practice
Dr Ellen P Leung, Mississauga, ON - Family Medicine
Dr James C K Leung, North York, ON - Family Medicine
Dr Chung-Shan Leung, North York, ON - Anatomical Pathology
Dr Ernest Yuen-Lun Leung, Richmond Hill, ON - Family Medicine
Dr Albert S H Leung, Richmond Hill, ON - Psychiatry
Dr Winnie W C Leung, Scarborough, ON - General Surgery
Dr Bill P Y Leung, St Catharines, ON - General Practice
Dr Karen M C Leung, Toronto, ON - General Practice
Dr Frances Y K Leung, Toronto, ON - Internal Medicine
Dr Richard S T Leung, Toronto, ON - Internal Medicine
Dr Terence L N Leung, Toronto, ON - General Practice
Dr Charles H Li, Vancouver, BC - Hematology
Dr John H S Li, Moncton, NB - General Practice
Dr Siu Hung C Li, Georgetown, ON - General Practice
Dr Bessie P T Li, Markham, ON - Family Medicine
Dr Christopher W H Li, Scarborough, ON - Cardiology
Dr Jason Li, Scarborough, ON - Family Medicine
Dr Alan T W Li, Toronto, ON - General Practice
Dr Christopher K Li, Toronto, ON - Internal Medicine
Dr Howard S H Liang, Vancouver, BC - Pediatrics
Dr Raymond A Liang, Vancouver, BC - Psychiatry
Dr William Liang, Hamilton, ON - General Practice
Dr H Robert Liao, Scarborough, ON - Ophthalmology
Dr Kim L Liew, Vancouver, BC - General Practice
Capt Chiam L Liew, Belleville, ON - Family Medicine
Dr Wing F Lim, Sherwood Park, AB - Family Medicine
Dr Meng Eng Lim, North Vancouver, BC - Psychiatry
Dr May-Ling J Lim, Vancouver, BC - General Practice
Dr Elaine B Ling, Ajax, ON - General Practice
Dr Michael C Ling, Scarborough, ON - Cardiology
Dr Jenny Y Liu, Vancouver, BC - Family Medicine
Dr Mitchell C C Liu, Vancouver, BC - Radiation Oncology
Dr Weldon Liu, Etobicoke, ON - Diagnostic-Radiology
Dr Tony H Lo, Calgary, AB - Psychiatry
Dr Reginald W W Lo, Vancouver, BC - General Practice
Dr Cynthia Y W Lo, Vancouver, BC - Family Medicine
Dr Lydia C L Lo, Brockville, ON - Family Medicine
Dr Jason H T Lo, Markham, ON - Family Medicine
Dr Adrian W Lo, Markham, ON - Family Medicine
Dr Ada Y T Lo, Markham, ON - Family Medicine
Dr Stephen C W Lo, Mississauga, ON - General Practice
Dr Anne Lo, Scarborough, ON - Family Medicine
Dr Christina K Y Lo, Scarborough, ON - Family Medicine
Dr Edmond K W Lo, Scarborough, ON - General Practice
Dr Hung-Tat Lo, Scarborough, ON - Psychiatry
Dr Hanson K C Lo, Whitby, ON - General Practice
Dr George Loh, Vancouver, BC - General Practice
Dr Diana P Y Loh, Vancouver, BC - Psychiatry
Dr Karmen K M Loh, Vancouver, BC - General Practice
Dr Henry T C Lok, Etobicoke, ON - Anesthesia
Dr Wilson W S Loo, Mississauga, ON - Family Medicine
Dr William L Louie, Calgary, AB - Family Medicine
Dr Peter Louie, Vancouver, BC - Pediatrics
Dr Andrew J Louie, Vancouver, BC - General Practice
Dr Shao-Hua Lu, Vancouver, BC - Psychiatry
Dr Annie Lu, Mount Forest, ON - Family Medicine
Dr Robert C Lui, Calgary, AB - General Surgery
Dr Spenser M Y Lui, Richmond, BC - Orthopedic Surgery
Dr Harvey Lui, Vancouver, BC - Dermatology
Dr Alexander Lui, Oakville, ON - General Practice
Dr Kim C Lui, Unionville, ON - General Practice
Dr Tse Li Luk, Winnipeg, MB - General Practice
Dr Edward C H Luke, Vancouver, BC - Emergency Family Med
Dr Edward Lum, Vancouver, BC - General Practice
Dr David W K Lum, St Thomas, ON - Family Medicine
Dr Ian S Ma, Vancouver, BC - General Practice
Dr Tze Y Ma, Mississauga, ON - Pediatrics
Dr Joseph J K Ma, North York, ON - Ophthalmology
Dr Felix Ma, Montreal, QC - Cardiac Surgery
Dr Michael K Mah, Calgary, AB - Family Medicine
Dr Elaine Mah, Langley, BC - Obstetrics & Gynecology
Dr Kam Kong Mak, North York, ON - General Practice
Dr Mabel Mak, Peterborough, ON - Family Medicine
Dr Victor Mak, Richmond Hill, ON - Urology
Dr Kwok-Chu Man, Whitby, ON - Internal Medicine
Dr Anthony Marchie, Richmond Hill, ON - Orthopedic Surgery
Dr Dennis C P Mark, Scarborough, ON - General Practice
Dr Hubert K Marr, Calgary, AB - Family Medicine
Dr Anita B Mo, Scarborough, ON - Obstetrics & Gynecology
Dr Gordon W Moe, Toronto, ON - Cardiology
Dr Hiram L H Mok, Vancouver, BC - Psychiatry
Dr Andrew K C Mok, Montreal, QC - Obstetrics & Gynecology
Dr Jimmy K Y Mui, Oshawa, ON - Radiation Oncology
Dr Philip K Ng, Port Coquitlam, BC - General Practice
Dr Douglas B G Ng, Surrey, BC - General Practice
Dr Wing Hon Ng, Vancouver, BC - General Practice
Dr David C Ng, Vancouver, BC - General Practice
Dr Stephen S Ng, Vancouver, BC - General Practice
Dr Louis H S Ng, Vancouver, BC - General Practice
Dr Ken H M Ng, Markham, ON - General Practice
Dr Stephen Ng, Markham, ON - General Practice
Dr Anthony T H Ng, Richmond Hill, ON - Anesthesia
Dr Esther Ng, Richmond Hill, ON - Obstetrics & Gynecology
Dr Eugene H L Ng, Toronto, ON - Pediatrics
Dr Dominic S K Ng, Toronto, ON - Endocrin/Metabolism
Dr Albert P Ng, Windsor, ON - General Practice
Dr David Ng, Windsor, ON - Family Medicine

Dr Toan D Nhan, Toronto, ON - General Practice
Dr Luis C E Noronha, Toronto, ON - Internal Medicine
Dr Teik Chye Ooi, Ottawa, ON - Internal Medicine
Dr Jeffrey T W Pang, Toronto, ON - Cardiology
Dr Jin-Si Pao, Vancouver, BC - General Surgery
Dr York P C Pei, Toronto, ON - Internal Medicine
Dr Carol Peng, Scarborough, ON - Obstetrics & Gynecology
Dr David W Pi, Vancouver, BC - Hematological Pathology
Dr Lorne Poon, Edmonton, AB - Family Medicine
Dr Mimi M L Poon, Vancouver, BC - General Practice
Dr C C Terry Poon, Markham, ON - Family Medicine
Dr Jimmy C M Poon, Mississauga, ON - Family Medicine
Dr Yin Hun Ian Pun, Scarborough, ON - General Practice
Dr Christine W H Pun, Sudbury, ON - Family Medicine
Dr Stanley K K Seah, Montreal, QC - Internal Medicine
Dr Shawn C W Seit, Markham, ON - General Practice
Dr Francis W C Sem, Toronto, ON - Emergency Family Med
Dr Paul H Seto, Edmonton, AB - General Practice
Dr Angela M Shen, Richmond, BC - Family Medicine
Dr Peter D Shih, Coquitlam, BC - General Practice
Dr Dominic Shiu, Abbotsford, BC - General Practice
Dr Daniel S P Shu, Coquitlam, BC - General Practice
Dr Y W Maggie Shu, North York, ON - Pediatrics
Dr Raymond M Shu, Scarborough, ON - Pediatrics
Dr Paul K Shuen, North York, ON - Obstetrics & Gynecology
Dr Michael S L Shum, Vancouver, BC - General Practice
Dr H T Peter Shum, Mississauga, ON - General Practice
Dr Andrew S C Shum, Toronto, ON - General Practice
Dr David T Shum, Windsor, ON - Anatomical Pathology
Dr Winnie W K Sia, Edmonton, AB - Internal Medicine
Dr Yin Shan Sia, Williams Lake, BC - General Practice
Dr Ying Tung Sia, Alexandria, ON - Cardiology
Dr Angeline C Sia-Venugopal, Chilliwack, BC - General Practice
Dr Philip C Sin, Richmond Hill, ON - General Practice
Dr Michelle Sit, Scarborough, ON - Family Medicine
Dr Marisa Sit, Toronto, ON - Ophthalmology
Dr Sze Wan Sit, Toronto, ON - Family Medicine
Dr May P Siu, Calgary, AB - Family Medicine
Dr Danny W Siu, Coquitlam, BC - General Practice
Dr Connie M Siu, Vancouver, BC - Diagnostic-Radiology
Dr King Fun Siu, Toronto, ON - Family Medicine
Dr Yan P So, Coquitlam, BC - General Practice
Dr Stevenson K F So, Mississauga, ON - General Practice
Dr B H Norman Soo, North York, ON - General Practice
Dr Anna S K Soong, Richmond Hill, ON - General Practice
Dr Donna Sue, Burnaby, BC - General Practice
Dr Edric C H Sum, Mississauga, ON - General Practice
Dr Keith L Sun, New Westminster, BC - Anesthesia
Dr Joyce Sun, Vancouver, BC - Family Medicine
Dr Patrick P W Sung, Vegreville, AB - General Practice
Dr Mabel C Sze, Vancouver, BC - Family Medicine
Dr Kenneth P C Szeto, Markham, ON - General Practice
Dr Isabella W Szeto, Orangeville, ON - Family Medicine
Dr Charles C F Tai, Vancouver, BC - Internal Medicine
Dr Derek Y H Tai, London, ON - Family Medicine
Dr Evelyn K Tai, Mississauga, ON - Family Medicine
Dr Emelda M Tai, Toronto, ON - General Practice
Dr Winston T L Tam, Surrey, BC - Obstetrics & Gynecology
Dr K Felix Tam, Vancouver, BC - General Practice
Dr Wilson W Tam, Vancouver, BC - General Practice
Dr Edwin M Tam, Vancouver, BC - Psychiatry
Dr Daphne C Tam, Vancouver, BC - Family Medicine
Dr Mae Yit M Tam, White Rock, BC - Ophthalmology
Dr Hon-Yin A Tam, Milton, ON - General Practice
Dr Diamond Y F Tam, Mississauga, ON - General Practice
Dr David W Tam, Oakville, ON - Obstetrics & Gynecology
Dr W S Theresa Tam, Ottawa, ON - Infectious Diseases
Dr Paul Y W Tam, Scarborough, ON - Internal Medicine
Dr Christopher K H Tam, Scarborough, ON - General Practice
Dr Robert C Tam, Toronto, ON - General Practice
Dr Wing-Hei Tam, Windsor, ON - Diagnostic-Radiology
Dr B J Nicholas Tan, Golden, BC - General Practice
Dr Brenda P Tan, Richmond, BC - Family Medicine
Dr Michelle W Tan, Richmond, BC - Family Medicine
Dr Jensen C C Tan, North York, ON - General Surgery
Dr Darrell H S Tan, Toronto, ON - Infectious Diseases
Dr Chin Kien Tan, Toronto, ON - General Practice
Dr Seang Lin Tan, Montreal, QC - Obstetrics & Gynecology
Dr Tin-Yan Tang, Vancouver, BC - General Practice
Dr Vincent W Tang, Vancouver, BC - General Practice
Dr Anthony S L Tang, Victoria, BC - Cardiology
Dr Bao Quy Tang, Victoria, BC - General Surgery
Dr Hung-Yip Tang, Richmond Hill, ON - General Practice
Dr Dominic M H Tang, Sault Ste. Marie, ON - General Practice
Dr Gordon L S Tang, Scarborough, ON - Family Medicine
Dr Keng Y Tay, London, ON - Diagnostic-Radiology
Dr M C Matthew Teh, Markham, ON - General Practice
Dr H M Vincent Thai, Edmonton, AB - Family Medicine
Dr Elizabeth Tham, Etobicoke, ON - Family Medicine
Dr Pooi-Lin Tham, London, ON - Family Medicine
Dr Michael P Thirlwell, Montreal, QC - Internal Medicine
Dr Chee Nyok Thong, Vancouver, BC - Otolaryngology
Dr Lancelot K Tin, Mississauga, ON - General Surgery
Dr Agnes S To, Richmond, BC - Psychiatry
Dr Daniel Y Tong, Vancouver, BC - General Practice
Dr Shu Kow Tong, Richmond Hill, ON - General Practice
Dr Ying Lai H Toong, Toronto, ON - General Practice
Dr Adrienne Tors, Scarborough, ON - General Practice
Dr Margaret H M Tran, Vancouver, BC - Family Medicine
Dr Vu-Kiet Tran, Scarborough, ON - Emergency Family Med
Dr Kim L L Truong, Calgary, AB - General Practice
Dr Victor T L Tsang, Vancouver, BC - General Surgery
Dr Peter W K Tsang, Vancouver, BC - Hematology
Dr Teresa S M Tsang, Vancouver, BC - Cardiology
Dr Ian K Tsang, Vancouver, BC - Internal Medicine
Dr John Y C Tsang, Vancouver, BC - Anesthesia
Dr Michael B Tsang, Hamilton, ON - Internal Medicine
Dr W Y Eliza Tsang, Markham, ON - Family Medicine
Dr Bernice Tsang, Newmarket, ON - Cardiology
Dr Raymond W M Tsang, North York, ON - General Practice
Dr Michael S M Tsang, Richmond Hill, ON - Family Medicine
Dr Jennifer L Tsang, Toronto, ON - Critical Care Medicine
Dr Smiley G S Tsao, Unionville, ON - Family Medicine
Dr Luke B S Tse, Prince Rupert, BC - Family Medicine
Dr Geoffrey N W Tse, Surrey, BC - General Surgery
Dr Frances W M Tse, Hamilton, ON - Gastroenterology
Dr Kenneth K Y Tse, Hamilton, ON - Anesthesia
Dr Anthony C H Tse, North York, ON - General Practice
Dr Shirley M L Tse, Toronto, ON - Pediatrics
Dr Karen W Tsin, Scarborough, ON - Family Medicine
Dr Keith S K Tsoi, Hamilton, ON - Gastroenterology
Dr Connie C W Tsui, Vancouver, BC - Family Medicine
Dr Joseph K Tsui, Vancouver, BC - Neurology
Dr Elaine Y L Tsui, Scarborough, ON - Endocrin/Metabolism
Dr Simon Y T Tsui, Scarborough, ON - Internal Medicine
Dr Vincent T Tsui, Toronto, ON - Geriatric Medicine
Dr I L Helen Tsui, Unionville, ON - Pediatrics
Dr K K Stanley Tung, Vancouver, BC - Internal Medicine
Dr Frances Y Tung, Toronto, ON - Family Medicine
Dr Chantelle Y W Ung, North York, ON - Dermatology
Dr Berton Y K Ung, Scarborough, ON - Family Medicine
Dr Victor B C Van, Georgetown, ON - Family Medicine
Dr Thomas T C Van, Scarborough, ON - Family Medicine
Dr Michael A Van Ameringen, Hamilton, ON - Family Medicine
Dr Calvin K N Wan, Kelowna, BC - Cardiac Surgery
Dr John C Wan, Markham, ON - Internal Medicine
Dr Andrew W C Wan, Markham, ON - Family Medicine
Dr Yue Wang, Surrey, BC - Family Medicine
Dr Patrick C W Wat, Stouffville, ON - General Practice
Dr Ho-Yin Wei, Richmond Hill, ON - Family Medicine
Dr Simon S Wing, Montreal, QC - Endocrin/Metabolism
Dr Norman C W Wong, Calgary, AB - Internal Medicine
Dr Benjamin C Wong, Calgary, AB - Obstetrics & Gynecology
Dr Eric Y L Wong, Edmonton, AB - Internal Medicine
Dr Norris A Wong, Edmonton, AB - Family Medicine
Dr Winnie W S Wong, Edmonton, AB - Gastroenterology
Dr Clarence K W Wong, Edmonton, AB - Gastroenterology
Dr Henry C H Wong, Abbotsford, BC - Internal Medicine
Dr Carrie K Wong, Burnaby, BC - Obstetrics & Gynecology
Dr Jeanny Wong, Burnaby, BC - General Practice
Dr Wilfred T Wong, Coquitlam, BC - General Practice
Dr Jerome C Y Wong, Langley, BC - Diagnostic-Radiology
Dr Xing Wong, Langley, BC - Diagnostic-Radiology
Dr Anita K Wong, Langley, BC - Family Medicine
Dr Leo K H Wong, Langley, BC - Family Medicine
Dr Daniel K C Wong, Maple Ridge, BC - General Practice
Dr Bobby C H Wong, Maple Ridge, BC - Diagnostic-Radiology
Dr Keith C K Wong, Mission, BC - General Practice
Dr Victor K Wong, Richmond, BC - Gastroenterology
Dr Lillian Wong, Richmond, BC - Otolaryngology
Dr Thomas S Wong, Richmond, BC - Family Medicine
Dr Boon L Wong, Richmond, BC - General Practice
Dr Danny H K Wong, Richmond, BC - General Practice
Dr Patricia Wong, Richmond, BC - General Practice
Dr Susan Y Wong, Richmond, BC - Family Medicine
Dr Andrew H K Wong, Surrey, BC - General Surgery
Dr Frances L W Wong, Surrey, BC - Radiation Oncology
Dr Shek-Leung Wong, Surrey, BC - General Practice
Dr Shun-Chi Wong, Terrace, BC - General Practice
Dr Ted Yee T Wong, Vancouver, BC - Family Medicine
Dr Peggy P C Wong, Vancouver, BC - Pediatric Hematology Oncology
Dr Vincent A Wong, Vancouver, BC - Ophthalmology
Dr Peter K H Wong, Vancouver, BC - Neurology
Dr Angela S W Wong, Vancouver, BC - Psychiatry
Dr Sylvia Wong, Vancouver, BC - General Practice
Dr Monique L Wong, Vancouver, BC - Psychiatry
Dr Milton J Wong, Vancouver, BC - Neurology
Dr Peter K K Wong, Vancouver, BC - General Practice
Dr Roger Y M Wong, Vancouver, BC - Geriatric Medicine
Dr H C George Wong, Vancouver, BC - Clin Immun/Allergy
Dr Allan P G Wong, Vancouver, BC - Psychiatry
Dr Asa W Wong, Vancouver, BC - Family Medicine
Dr K Judy Wong, Vancouver, BC - General Practice
Dr Lai-Wah Wong, Vancouver, BC - Family Medicine
Dr Fedrick Wong, Vancouver, BC - General Practice
Dr Paul C H Wong, Vancouver, BC - Family Medicine
Dr Frank S H Wong, Victoria, BC - Otolaryngology
Dr Justin K F Wong, Winnipeg, MB - Critical Care Medicine
Dr William H Wong, Cambridge, ON - General Practice
Dr Paul K C Wong, East York, ON - Orthopedic Surgery
Dr Amy N Wong, Etobicoke, ON - Family Medicine
Dr Hon-Wah Wong, Markham, ON - General Practice
Dr Richard L Wong, Markham, ON - Pediatrics
Dr Thompson K W Wong, Markham, ON - General Practice
Dr Frank K L Wong, Mississauga, ON - General Practice
Dr Joseph K Wong, Mississauga, ON - Otolaryngology
Dr Clement K L Wong, Mississauga, ON - General Practice
Dr Gordon K T Wong, Mississauga, ON - Internal Medicine
Dr Amy H Wong, Newmarket, ON - Family Medicine
Dr Tat-Kwan Wong, North York, ON - General Practice
Dr Benjamin B L Wong, North York, ON - Clin Immun/Allergy
Dr Joseph Y S Wong, North York, ON - Physical Medicine & Rehab
Dr Maxine Y W Wong, North York, ON - Dermatology
Dr Victor C H Wong, Oakville, ON - Family Medicine
Dr Eddy K K Wong, Orleans, ON - Pediatrics
Dr Peter N Wong, Port Dover, ON - General Practice
Dr Sunny Y C Wong, Richmond Hill, ON - Family Medicine
Dr Ophelia C Y Wong, Richmond Hill, ON - General Practice
Dr Eric P C Wong, Richmond Hill, ON - General Practice
Dr Fung L Wong, Richmond Hill, ON - Family Medicine
Dr Jason H P Wong, Scarborough, ON - General Surgery
Dr Arnold K Y Wong, Scarborough, ON - General Practice
Dr Cynthia S Wong, Scarborough, ON - General Practice
Dr Keith H Wong, Scarborough, ON - Gastroenterology
Dr Jeremy C Wong, Scarborough, ON - Obstetrics & Gynecology
Dr Daniel M T Wong, Scarborough, ON - Internal Medicine
Dr Stephen S Wong, Scarborough, ON - General Practice
Dr Chi Mun Wong, St Catharines, ON - Family Medicine
Dr Brian Y L Wong, Sudbury, ON - Cardiology
Dr Camilla L Wong, Toronto, ON - Geriatric Medicine
Dr Sophia S F Wong, Toronto, ON - Anesthesia
Dr David M C Wong, Toronto, ON - Family Medicine
Dr Angela S C Wong, Toronto, ON - Family Medicine
Dr M F Agnes Wong, Toronto, ON - Ophthalmology
Dr Roland C K Wong, Toronto, ON - Community Medicine
Dr Albert S C Wong, Toronto, ON - General Practice

Dr Ivan F L Wong, Toronto, ON - General Practice
Dr Daniel D Wong, Toronto, ON - General Practice
Dr David T W Wong, Toronto, ON - Anesthesia
Dr David T W Wong, Toronto, ON - Ophthalmology
Dr Edward Y C Wong, Toronto, ON - Diagnostic-Radiology
Dr John W Wong, Toronto, ON - Anatomical Pathology
Dr Vivian K Wong, Toronto, ON - Family Medicine
Dr Mary M Y Wong, Woodbridge, ON - Family Medicine
Dr Young-Chi Woo, Burnaby, BC - Urology
Dr Emile C Woo, Vancouver, BC - General Surgery
Dr Henry L Woo, Vancouver, BC - Obstetrics & Gynecology
Dr Francis C M Woo, Etobicoke, ON - General Practice
Dr Joseph C H Woo, Hamilton, ON - Anesthesia
Dr Paul C Y Woo, Richmond Hill, ON - General Practice
Dr George H K Woo, Toronto, ON - Obstetrics & Gynecology
Dr John K M Wu, Vancouver, BC - Hematology
Dr Raymond H C Wu, Markham, ON - General Practice
Dr Howard Wu, Markham, ON - Family Medicine
Dr Alwin Wu, Markham, ON - Family Medicine
Dr Bennet P Y Wu, Minden, ON - General Practice
Dr George G Wu, Mississauga, ON - Internal Medicine
Dr Sing Man Wu, North York, ON - General Practice
Dr Sibra S C Wu, Toronto, ON - General Practice
Dr Stephen T W Wu, Whitby, ON - Family Medicine
Dr Ka-Wai Yam, Vancouver, BC - Family Medicine
Dr Edric C W Yam, Richmond Hill, ON - Family Medicine
Dr Alexander Yan, Edmonton, AB - Internal Medicine
Dr Ilym G Yan, Surrey, BC - Family Medicine
Dr Andrew T Yan, Toronto, ON - Cardiology
Dr Peter B Yang, Burnaby, BC - General Practice
Dr Kwang Yang, Surrey, BC - Family Medicine
Dr Malissa Yang, Brampton, ON - General Practice
Dr Ryan J H Yau, Calgary, AB - Ophthalmology
Dr William Y T Yau, Edmonton, AB - Family Medicine
Dr Jennifer K W Yau, Ottawa, ON - Family Medicine
Dr Frank C O Yau, Toronto, ON - General Practice
Dr Terrence M Yau, Toronto, ON - Cardiac Surgery
Dr Anthony P C Yau, Toronto, ON - General Practice
Dr John Yee, Vancouver, BC - Cardiac Surgery
Dr William C Yee, Vancouver, BC - Diagnostic-Radiology
Dr Donna L J Yee, Vancouver, BC - Family Medicine
Dr Adrian S Y Yee, Victoria, BC - Hematology
Dr Allan J Yee, Markham, ON - Internal Medicine
Dr Chok-Ching Yee, Nobleton, ON - General Practice
Dr David P Yee, Thunder Bay, ON - General Practice
Dr Doreen A Yee, Toronto, ON - Anesthesia
Dr Wilson T Yeung, Abbotsford, BC - Hematological Pathology
Dr William C Y Yeung, Richmond, BC - Family Medicine
Dr James C F Yeung, Richmond, BC - General Practice
Dr Peter K Yeung, Surrey, BC - Obstetrics & Gynecology
Dr Choi Kit Yeung, Vancouver, BC - Internal Medicine
Dr Gerald Y L Yeung, Vancouver, BC - Family Medicine
Dr Sonia N Yeung, Vancouver, BC - Ophthalmology
Dr Kam-Tong Yeung, North York, ON - Geriatric Medicine
Dr Clement W T Yeung, North York, ON - General Practice
Dr Danny S C Yeung, North York, ON - Family Medicine
Dr Michael K Yeung, North York, ON - Psychiatry
Dr Jacky Y Yeung, Peterborough, ON - Ophthalmology
Dr Latifa T F Yeung, Scarborough, ON - Gastroenterology
Dr Jensen M Yeung, Toronto, ON - Dermatology
Dr Adela K T Yeung, Toronto, ON - General Practice
Dr Kwok Yeong Yik, New Westminster, BC - Gastroenterology
Dr Conrad C Y Yim, Mississauga, ON - Pediatrics
Dr Luis T J Ying, Brampton, ON - Gastroenterology
Dr Thomas S F Ying, Pickering, ON - General Practice
Dr Augustine Y L Yip, Calgary, AB - Family Medicine
Dr Barbara Y Yip, Coquitlam, BC - General Practice
Dr Daniel L K Yip, Coquitlam, BC - General Practice
Dr Samuel Yip, Vancouver, BC - Neurology
Dr Stephen T Yip, Vancouver, BC - Neuro-Pathology
Dr Clarwyn Yip, North York, ON - Infectious Diseases
Dr Jeanne C Yip, Oakville, ON - Family Medicine
Dr Verna W Y Yiu, Edmonton, AB - Nephrology
Dr Stella H M Yiu, Ottawa, ON - Emergency Family Med
Dr Collin K K Yong, Vancouver, BC - Pediatrics
Dr K T Thomas Yoong, Oshawa, ON - General Practice
Dr Simon Yu, Burnaby, BC - Internal Medicine
Dr Y W Edward Yu, Burnaby, BC - Ophthalmology
Dr Grace W Yu, Vancouver, BC - Pediatrics
Dr Philip H F Yu, Brampton, ON - General Practice
Dr Richard S O Yu, Toronto, ON - Emergency Family Med
Dr Eric H C Yu, Toronto, ON - Cardiology
Dr Derek Yu, Toronto, ON - Gastroenterology
Dr David Yue, Edmonton, AB - General Practice
Dr Frank W L Yue, Vancouver, BC - General Practice
Dr K Kevin Yue, Vancouver, BC - Family Medicine
Dr Anthony W B Yue, Victoria, BC - Family Medicine
Dr Randy S Yue, Newmarket, ON - Anesthesia
Dr Tommy K Yuen, Delta, BC - Family Medicine
Dr Chui Kin Yuen, Vancouver, BC - Obstetrics & Gynecology
Dr Kenneth W H Yuen, Barrie, ON - Internal Medicine
Dr S Y Sheila Yuen, Markham, ON - Family Medicine
Dr K H Peter Yuen, Scarborough, ON - Family Medicine
Dr Yick Shing Yung, Toronto, ON - Obstetrics & Gynecology
Dr Allen Zee, Etobicoke, ON - General Practice
Dr Y H Connie Zhang, Richmond, BC - Family Medicine
Dr Kenny J Zhang, Mississauga, ON - Family Medicine
Dr Y Jackie Zhang, Richmond Hill, ON - Family Medicine
Dr Stanley M Zheng, Scarborough, ON - Family Medicine
Dr Nora P Y Zung, Scarborough, ON - Family Medicine

CATALAN

Dr Jordi Cisa, Sudbury, ON - Orthopedic Surgery
Dr Angeles Garcia, Kingston, ON - Geriatric Medicine
Dr Elena Kasatiya Trevisani, Ottawa, ON - General Practice
Dr Fidel Vila-Rodriguez, Vancouver, BC - Psychiatry
Dr Christina Williams, Vancouver, BC - Obstetrics & Gynecology

CEBUANO

Dr Radzfel A Geonzon, Calgary, AB - Family Medicine
Dr Antonio F Uy Jr, Peterborough, ON - Family Medicine

CHAKMA

Dr Chiranjib Talukdar, Regina, SK - Pediatrics

CHAVACANO

Dr Gilles Lauzon, Montreal, QC - General Surgery

CHICHEWA

Dr Khami Chokani, Prince Albert, SK - General Practice
Dr M Dokiso Nchama, Cornwall, ON - Pediatrics
Dr Edwards D Ndovi, Bonnyville, AB - Internal Medicine

CHINESE

Dr Michael J M Ackermann, Sherbrooke, NS - General Practice
Dr Lee-Cyn Ang, London, ON - Neuro-Pathology
Dr Steven K H Aung, Edmonton, AB - General Practice
Dr Onil Bhattacharyya, Toronto, ON - Family Medicine
Dr Marybelle M T Chain-Chang, Brampton, ON - General Practice
Dr Pauline Champion, Charlottetown, PE - General Practice
Dr Kam Ming Chan, Edmonton, AB - Physical Medicine & Rehab
Dr John K F Chan, Abbotsford, BC - Family Medicine
Dr Alfred T Chan, Vernon, BC - Family Medicine
Dr Anthony K C Chan, Hamilton, ON - Hematology
Dr Winnie W Y Chan, Kitchener, ON - General Pathology
Dr Monica K H Chan, Markham, ON - Family Medicine
Dr W Mun-Kam Chan, Markham, ON - General Practice
Dr John W L Chan, Mississauga, ON - General Practice
Dr Yun Kai Chan, Niagara Falls, ON - Internal Medicine
Dr Eng-Soon Chan, North York, ON - Community Medicine
Dr Victoria M Y Chan, Richmond Hill, ON - Internal Medicine
Dr John Y W Chan, Richmond Hill, ON - General Practice
Dr Wai Lam W Chan, Scarborough, ON - General Practice
Dr Chin K Chan, Thornhill, ON - General Surgery
Dr King-Sun Chan, Toronto, ON - General Practice
Dr Patrick S P Chan, Toronto, ON - Dermatology
Dr Vincent Chan, Vanier, ON - General Practice
Dr W Y Winifred Chan-Lui, Winnipeg, MB - Neurology
Dr Indira Chandran, Brampton, ON - Obstetrics & Gynecology
Dr Lawrence J A Chang, Newmarket, ON - Pediatrics
Dr Hong Chang, Toronto, ON - Hematological Pathology
Dr Peter P Chang, Toronto, ON - Psychiatry
Dr Patricia Y Chang, Toronto, ON - Family Medicine
Dr Paul T Chang, Toronto, ON - Obstetrics & Gynecology
Dr Thomas M S Chang, Montreal, QC - Med Scientist
Dr Claudius T K Che, Fort Erie, ON - General Practice
Dr Adam Y H Chen, Mississauga, ON - Family Medicine
Dr Yen-Fu Chen, Richmond Hill, ON - Physical Medicine & Rehab
Dr Jim I Cheng, Sherwood Park, AB - Community Medicine
Dr Calvino K Cheng, Halifax, NS - Hematological Pathology
Dr Jerry H C Cheng, North York, ON - General Practice
Dr Bai-Sen Cheng, Scarborough, ON - Family Medicine
Dr Richard S S Cheng, Scarborough, ON - General Practice
Dr K M Andrew Cheong, Port Coquitlam, BC - Family Medicine
Dr Anson W C Cheung, Vancouver, BC - Cardiac Surgery
Dr Anthony P Y Cheung, Vancouver, BC - Obstetrics & Gynecology
Dr Lai-Keung Cheung, Winnipeg, MB - General Surgery
Dr Wendy H Cheung, Hamilton, ON - Pediatrics
Dr Tak-Kee Cheung, Harrow, ON - General Practice
Dr Bonnie Cheung, Richmond Hill, ON - General Practice
Dr M C Raphael Cheung, Windsor, ON - Endocrin/Metabolism
Dr Frank W Chi, Elliot Lake, ON - General Practice
Dr Isabelle Chiu, Edmonton, AB - Infectious Diseases
Dr Chung Fok Chiu, North York, ON - General Practice
Dr John H C Chiu, Toronto, ON - Diagnostic-Radiology
Dr Roger K N Cho, Calgary, AB - Orthopedic Surgery
Dr Xin Chong, Niagara Falls, ON - Family Medicine
Dr Shirley H Y Chou, Ottawa, ON - General Surgery
Dr Andrew Chow, Mississauga, ON - Internal Medicine
Dr Judy T Chow, Ottawa, ON - General Practice
Dr Edward L W Chow, Toronto, ON - Radiation Oncology
Dr Chi-Ming Chow, Toronto, ON - Cardiology
Dr Stephen S Chow, Toronto, ON - Internal Medicine
Dr Ping Fun Choy, North York, ON - Family Medicine
Dr Gregory W Choy, Toronto, ON - Internal Medicine
Dr Mary P H Chu, Richmond, BC - General Practice
Dr Kelly K-P Chu, Victoria, BC - General Practice
Dr Joseph Y C Chu, Etobicoke, ON - Internal Medicine
Dr Katherine H C Chu, Scarborough, ON - Obstetrics & Gynecology
Dr Sik On Chu, Scarborough, ON - General Practice
Dr Michael W Chu, Toronto, ON - Family Medicine
Dr Grace L Chua, Maple, ON - Cardiology
Dr Andrew Y W Chung, Scarborough, ON - Family Medicine
Dr Jean P Deong, Brandon, MB - Family Medicine
Dr Ba-Hiep Dinh, Montreal, QC - General Practice
Dr Huu Thanh Duong, Ottawa, ON - General Practice
Dr Marlene T Dytoc, Edmonton, AB - Dermatology
Dr Michael K D Fan, Ajax, ON - General Practice
Dr Luming Feng, Ancaster, ON - Family Medicine
Dr Tse Chen Fong, Calgary, AB - Diagnostic-Radiology
Dr George Y Fong, Edmonton, AB - Family Medicine
Dr Andrew Fong, North York, ON - General Practice
Dr Chi Wai Fong, Scarborough, ON - General Practice
Dr Philip A Fong Wai Chin, Weyburn, SK - General Practice
Dr Marshall C Foo, Toronto, ON - General Practice
Dr Gary W T Fung, Edmonton, AB - General Practice
Dr Kee-Wai Fung, Etobicoke, ON - Pediatrics
Dr Irving C Fung, London, ON - Otolaryngology
Dr Kan Ying Fung, Mississauga, ON - General Practice
Dr Frank Fung, Oshawa, ON - General Practice
Dr Wing-Tai Fung, Scarborough, ON - General Practice
Dr Kenneth P L Fung, Toronto, ON - Psychiatry
Dr Ambrose Y T Fung, Toronto, ON - Family Medicine
Dr Herbert Y Gaisano, Toronto, ON - Gastroenterology
Dr Hudson K H Giang, Lindsay, ON - General Pathology
Dr Lin Rui Guo, London, ON - Cardiovasc/ThorSurg
Dr Anthony Y P Hii, Toronto, ON - General Practice
Dr John Hii, Toronto, ON - Medical Microbiology

Dr Della S W Ho, Calgary, AB - Pediatrics
Dr Clinton Ho, Burnaby, BC - General Pathology
Dr Kay Ho, Chilliwack, BC - General Practice
Dr Hip Wah Ho, Surrey, BC - Internal Medicine
Dr Hoi Shing Ho, Vancouver, BC - General Practice
Dr Kenneth S W Ho, Brampton, ON - Anesthesia
Dr Kwok Fan Ho, Mississauga, ON - General Practice
Dr Gerald C L Ho, Richmond Hill, ON - Pediatrics
Dr Michael S C Ho, Toronto, ON - General Practice
Dr Chia-Sing Ho, Toronto, ON - Diagnostic-Radiology
Dr Helen H Y Ho, Toronto, ON - Obstetrics & Gynecology
Dr Hon-Fai Ho, Toronto, ON - Diagnostic-Radiology
Dr Collin Hong, North York, ON - Plastic Surgery
Dr Frank L Hou, Vancouver, BC - General Practice
Dr Peter Hoy, Terrace, BC - General Practice
Dr G Y Robin Hsiung, Vancouver, BC - Neurology
Dr John S C Hsuen, North York, ON - Pediatrics
Dr Fang Hu, Bradford, ON - Family Medicine
Dr Weimin Hu, Mississauga, ON - Anatomical Pathology
Dr Weei-Yuarn Huang, Halifax, NS - Anatomical Pathology
Dr Eleanor C Y Huang, London, ON - Family Medicine
Dr Virgil Y F Huang, North York, ON - General Practice
Dr Pein-Pein Huang, Ottawa, ON - Pediatrics
Dr K M Nicoletta Huen, Mississauga, ON - Family Medicine
Dr Frederick Hui, North York, ON - Family Medicine
Dr Annie Hum, Markham, ON - General Practice
Dr Paul A L S Hwang, Toronto, ON - Neurology
Dr Peter T Hwee, Kitchener, ON - General Practice
Dr Yiu Ban Ip, Surrey, BC - General Practice
Dr Hongxing Jiang, Edmonton, AB - Orthopedic Surgery
Dr Harry Jim, Keswick, ON - General Practice
Dr Nin Jing, Windsor, ON - Family Medicine
Dr Hsiao-Ming Jung, Toronto, ON - Family Medicine
Dr Wai-On Kan, Richmond, BC - General Practice
Dr Pion Kao, Calgary, AB - Pediatrics
Dr Warren J Ke, Whitby, ON - General Practice
Dr Laval Kon Kam King, Summerside, PE - General Practice
Dr Yolanda A Kirkham, Toronto, ON - Obstetrics & Gynecology
Dr Gordon D Ko, Markham, ON - Emergency Family Med
Dr Dennis T Ko, Toronto, ON - Cardiology
Dr Betty K K Koo, North York, ON - Neurology
Dr Alano Kuan, Surrey, BC - Emergency Family Med
Dr Poh Gin Kwa, St. John's, NL - Pediatrics
Dr Robert P K F Kwan, Scarborough, ON - General Practice
Dr Lawrence W Kwan, Scarborough, ON - Family Medicine
Dr T Y Paul Kwong, Brampton, ON - General Practice
Dr Kai-Fai Lai, Delta, BC - General Surgery
Dr Mark K K Lai, Ajax, ON - General Practice
Dr Eliza P Y Lai, Markham, ON - Family Medicine
Dr Enoch K Y Lai, North York, ON - Diagnostic-Radiology
Dr Raymond P C Lai, Regina, SK - General Practice
Dr Richard P Lam, Calgary, AB - Family Medicine
Dr Simon R Lam, New Westminster, BC - Ophthalmology
Dr Stephen C T Lam, Vancouver, BC - Internal Medicine
Dr Christopher Lam, Victoria, BC - Family Medicine
Dr Andy S C Lam, Grimsby, ON - Internal Medicine
Dr Angela W W Lam, Markham, ON - General Practice
Dr James H C Lam, Orillia, ON - General Practice
Dr Sheung L L Lam, St Catharines, ON - Anesthesia
Dr Wai-Ching Lam, Toronto, ON - Ophthalmology
Dr Harold Y H Lau, Calgary, AB - Radiation Oncology
Dr Chuen-Ping Lau, Burnaby, BC - Internal Medicine
Dr Eunice Lau, Mississauga, ON - Family Medicine
Dr Francis T Y Lau, Mississauga, ON - Family Medicine
Dr Benson P S Lau, Scarborough, ON - General Practice
Dr Man Pang Lau, Scarborough, ON - Psychiatry
Dr Susie K S Lau, Montreal, QC - Gynecologic Oncology
Dr Hugo K C Law, Richmond Hill, ON - General Practice
Dr Teresa H L Law, Montreal, QC - Dermatology
Dr Howe Leam, Lethbridge, AB - Family Medicine
Dr Sammy S H Lee, Richmond, BC - General Practice
Dr Mary Lee, Vancouver, BC - Obstetrics & Gynecology
Dr Francis F W Lee, Winnipeg, MB - Obstetrics & Gynecology
Dr Peter C K Lee, Dartmouth, NS - Family Medicine
Dr Winifred Lee, Dartmouth, NS - Obstetrics & Gynecology
Dr Doris S Lee, Etobicoke, ON - General Practice
Dr David S C Lee, London, ON - Pediatrics
Dr Kwok Ching Lee, North York, ON - Anesthesia
Dr Michael C F Lee, Ridgeway, ON - General Practice
Dr Vansen M Lee, Toronto, ON - General Practice
Dr Liesly Lee, Toronto, ON - Neurology
Dr T C Benny Lei, Winnipeg, MB - General Practice
Dr Philip W T Leong, Vancouver, BC - General Practice
Dr Jean-Pierre Leung, Calgary, AB - Family Medicine
Dr Stephen T Y Leung, Calgary, AB - Family Medicine
Dr Alexander K C Leung, Calgary, AB - Pediatrics
Dr Wing Yee V Leung, Vancouver, BC - General Practice
Dr Man K Leung, Vancouver, BC - General Practice
Dr Kent K K Leung, Markham, ON - General Practice
Dr See-Lap Leung, Mississauga, ON - General Practice
Dr Wilson W S Leung, Niagara Falls, ON - Family Medicine
Dr Kevin M K Leung, Scarborough, ON - General Practice
Dr Daniel P Leung, Strathroy, ON - General Practice
Dr Wilson L Leung, Toronto, ON - General Practice
Dr Bing Li, Edmonton, AB - Family Medicine
Dr Zhi Li, Edmonton, AB - Family Medicine
Dr Judy W S Li, Edmonton, AB - Family Medicine
Dr Qiuyan Li, Kelowna, BC - Anatomical Pathology
Dr Charles H Li, Vancouver, BC - Hematology
Dr John H S Li, Moncton, NB - General Practice
Dr Qinglu Li, Barrie, ON - Family Medicine
Dr Chumei Li, Hamilton, ON - Medical Genetics
Dr Mok-Dock Li, London, ON - Pediatrics
Dr Kong Ching Li, Pembroke, ON - Internal Medicine
Dr Kan Wen Li, Richmond Hill, ON - General Practice
Dr Heung-Wing Li, Scarborough, ON - General Practice
Dr Cheuk-Hon Li, Toronto, ON - General Practice
Dr Janice Y Liao, Edmonton, AB - Dermatology
Dr Lie Ming Lie, North York, ON - Anesthesia
Dr Wing F Lim, Sherwood Park, AB - Family Medicine
Dr Khian-Kok Lim, Lachine, QC - Ophthalmology
Dr Peter J Lin, Scarborough, ON - Family Medicine
Dr Cynthia Littlejohn, Burlington, ON - General Practice
Dr Richard Liu, Edmonton, AB - Otolaryngology
Dr Allen T L Liu, Edmonton, AB - Critical Care Medicine
Dr Bin Liu, Nepean, ON - Internal Medicine
Dr Hwayue Liu, Richmond Hill, ON - Family Medicine
Dr Louis W C Liu, Toronto, ON - Gastroenterology
Dr Jeremy C K Lo, Ottawa, ON - Family Medicine
Dr Edmond K W Lo, Scarborough, ON - General Practice
Dr Tak-Shing Lo, Scarborough, ON - General Practice
Dr Kirk C L Lo, Toronto, ON - Urology
Dr Adrian L H Long, Winnipeg, MB - General Practice
Dr Jian-Qiang Lu, Edmonton, AB - Neuro-Pathology
Dr Spenser M Y Lui, Richmond, BC - Orthopedic Surgery
Dr Alexander Lui, Oakville, ON - General Practice
Dr Derek P K Lui, Woodstock, ON - Ophthalmology
Dr Koon-Hung Luke, Ottawa, ON - Pediatrics
Dr Yigang Luo, Saskatoon, SK - General Surgery
Dr Mang-Ming Ma, Edmonton, AB - Gastroenterology
Dr Gilbert Ma, Vancouver, BC - General Practice
Dr Joanne L C Ma, Scarborough, ON - Obstetrics & Gynecology
Dr Manson M T Mak, Brampton, ON - Emergency Family Med
Dr Kam Kong Mak, North York, ON - General Practice
Dr Mabel Mak, Peterborough, ON - Family Medicine
Dr Victor Mak, Richmond Hill, ON - Urology
Dr Ellen N Mak, Toronto, ON - General Practice
Dr Gregory C K Man, Richmond Hill, ON - Pediatrics
Dr Gary T Mok, North York, ON - General Practice
Dr Kam W Mong, St. John's, NL - Cardiothor Surgery
Dr Mahdi Murti, Toronto, ON - General Practice
Dr Patrick M Nesbitt, West Vancouver, BC - General Practice
Dr John P Y Ng, Vancouver, BC - General Practice
Dr Shang C Ng, Vancouver, BC - General Practice
Dr Grace Ng, Vancouver, BC - General Practice
Dr Raymond Ng, Markham, ON - Otolaryngology
Dr S Y Andrew Ng, Mississauga, ON - Family Medicine
Dr Matilda W Ng, Richmond Hill, ON - Internal Medicine
Dr Sai-Sun Ng, Scarborough, ON - General Practice
Dr David Ng, Scarborough, ON - Family Medicine
Dr Nelly W Ng, Scarborough, ON - General Practice
Dr Eugene H L Ng, Toronto, ON - Pediatrics
Dr Dominic S K Ng, Toronto, ON - Endocrin/Metabolism
Dr Edward H W Ng, Windsor, ON - General Practice
Dr Edward K K Ng Tung Hing, Newmarket, ON
- Internal Medicine
Dr Nhiem Nguyen, Richmond, BC - Dermatology
Dr L Michael Nip, North York, ON - Family Medicine
Dr Howard H Pai, Victoria, BC - Radiation Oncology
Dr Wen-Mei Pan, Pembroke, ON - Anesthesia
Dr Peter H L Pang, Gatineau, QC - General Practice
Dr Philip W Peng, Toronto, ON - Anesthesia
Dr John C P Poon, Calgary, AB - Family Medicine
Dr Wilson H Y Roa, Edmonton, AB - Radiation Oncology
Dr Veronica K L Sam, Calgary, AB - Family Medicine
Dr Ying Suey Seid, Toronto, ON - General Practice
Dr Xi Shan, Brampton, ON - Internal Medicine
Dr Michael Shih, Burlington, ON - General Practice
Dr Mike C M Shih, Woodbridge, ON - General Practice
Dr Patrick K Y Shiu, Surrey, BC - General Practice
Dr Dominique Shum-Tim, Montreal, QC - Cardiothor Surgery
Dr Wee-Lim Sim, Montreal, QC - Obstetrics & Gynecology
Dr Sidney K Siu, London, ON - Occupational Med
Dr Lillian L Y Siu, Toronto, ON - Internal Medicine
Dr Cong Y Stonestreet, Penticton, BC - General Practice
Dr Didacus Su, Ottawa, ON - Family Medicine
Dr Yi-Hui Sun, Calgary, AB - Family Medicine
Dr Jenet H F Sun, Richmond, BC - General Practice
Dr John C Sy, London, ON - General Practice
Dr Peter Y Sy, Mississauga, ON - General Practice
Dr Tuyet Phi Ta, Montreal, QC - General Practice
Dr Chao Tai, Edmonton, AB - Neurology
Dr T H Patricia Tai, Regina, SK - Radiation Oncology
Dr Kin-Hung Tam, Belleville, ON - General Practice
Dr William Y Tam, Hamilton, ON - Psychiatry
Dr Martina Y T Tam, Leamington, ON - General Practice
Dr Thomas W H Tam, London, ON - Family Medicine
Dr Michael C C Tam, North York, ON - Diagnostic-Radiology
Dr Ronald K H Tam, Ottawa, ON - Pediatrics
Dr Sydney P Tam, Toronto, ON - Family Medicine
Dr Jonny H S Tam, Woodstock, ON - General Practice
Dr Chin Chai Tan, St. John's, NL - General Practice
Dr Christopher Y K Tan, Markham, ON - Family Medicine
Dr K W Andre Tan, Napanee, ON - Otolaryngology
Dr Thuang Kim Tan, Toronto, ON - General Practice
Dr Lee Puan Tan, Windsor, ON - Internal Medicine
Dr S C Albert Tang, Ottawa, ON - Family Medicine
Dr Godwin P Y Tang, Richmond Hill, ON - Family Medicine
LCol Homer C Tien, Toronto, ON - General Surgery
Dr K H George Ting, Burlington, ON - Diagnostic-Radiology
Dr Robert H Ting, Scarborough, ON - Internal Medicine
Dr Eng-Tjie Tjan, St. John's, NL - Otolaryngology
Dr Joshua K Tjong, Sault Ste. Marie, ON - Diagnostic-Radiology
Dr Agnes S To, Richmond, BC - Psychiatry
Dr Tony P T Tom, Vancouver, BC - Family Medicine
Dr Kevin L F Tong, Vancouver, BC - General Practice
Dr Xia-Hoe Tran, Montreal, QC - General Practice
Dr Shaun K Tregoning, Abbotsford, BC
- Obstetrics & Gynecology
Dr Kien V Trinh, Ancaster, ON - Family Medicine
Dr K Y Denny Trinh, Toronto, ON - Internal Medicine
Dr Cong Phuc Truong, Louiseville, QC - General Practice
Dr Shian-Yih Tsai, Hamilton, ON - Urology
Dr Ellen Tsai, Ottawa, ON - Pediatrics
Dr Henry H K Tsang, Prince George, BC
- Obstetrics & Gynecology
Dr Joseph W T Tsang, Vancouver, BC - General Practice
Dr Monica C W Tsang, Vancouver, BC - Family Medicine
Dr Jim H C Tsang, Mississauga, ON - General Practice
Dr Ann S Y Tsang, Scarborough, ON - Family Medicine
Dr Albert H Tsang, Toronto, ON - Family Medicine
Dr Kam-Yuen Tsang, Woodbridge, ON - General Practice
Dr Ming-Sound Tsao, Toronto, ON - Anatomical Pathology
Dr H H Steve Tschen, Windsor, ON - General Practice
Dr Joanne S Tse, Calgary, AB - General Practice
Dr Geoffrey N W Tse, Surrey, BC - General Surgery
Dr Chingying Tse, Etobicoke, ON - General Practice
Dr Man Buen Tse, North York, ON - Obstetrics & Gynecology

Dr Wing Kin Tse, Scarborough, ON - General Practice
Dr Leonard W H Tse, Toronto, ON - General Surgery
Dr Thomas T Y Tsin, Woodbridge, ON - Diagnostic-Radiology
Dr Kwan-Cheung Tsui, North York, ON - Diagnostic-Radiology
Dr Tommy H T Tung, Keswick, ON - General Practice
Dr Muoy Ung, Montreal, QC - General Practice
Dr Kevin K S Voon, Burlington, ON - Family Medicine
Dr Li Wang, Calgary, AB - Family Medicine
Dr Bing Wang, Calgary, AB - Anesthesia
Dr Xiaoping Wang, Edmonton, AB - General Practice
Dr Thur Wang, Grande Prairie, AB - General Practice
Dr Xin-Yong Wang, Burnaby, BC - Family Medicine
Dr Jen-Te Wang, Surrey, BC - General Practice
Dr Ay-Ling Wang, Kitchener, ON - Family Medicine
Dr Henry Wang, Newmarket, ON - Endocrin/Metabolism
Dr Don Wang, Ottawa, ON - Anatomical Pathology
Dr Yan Wang, Smiths Falls, ON - Obstetrics & Gynecology
Dr Chen Wang, Toronto, ON - Hematological Pathology
Dr Zhi Wang, Saint-Jerome, QC - Orthopedic Surgery
Dr Man-Joe Watt, Edmonton, AB - Pediatrics
Dr Joyce Wong, Calgary, AB - General Surgery
Dr Norman C W Wong, Calgary, AB - Internal Medicine
Dr Byron E Wong, Calgary, AB - Pediatrics
Dr Diana Wong, Camrose, AB - Plastic Surgery
Dr Kan Shick Wong, Edmonton, AB - Pediatrics
Dr James M Wong, Edmonton, AB - Family Medicine
Dr Hoa Leng Wong, Edmonton, AB - General Practice
Dr Dennis Y R Wong, Edmonton, AB - General Practice
Dr Joseph P C Wong, Maple Ridge, BC - Anesthesia
Dr Christopher K Wong, New Westminster, BC - Internal Medicine
Dr Phoebus W C Wong, Richmond, BC - General Practice
Dr Leo T M Wong, Surrey, BC - Family Medicine
Dr Harvey H Wong, Vancouver, BC - Family Medicine
Dr Lai-Wah Wong, Vancouver, BC - Family Medicine
Dr William K W Wong, Vancouver, BC - General Practice
Dr David K W Wong, Yellowknife, NT - General Practice
Dr Gabriel F Y Wong, Ajax, ON - General Practice
Dr James Y K Wong, Meaford, ON - General Practice
Dr Alice S L Wong, Mississauga, ON - Family Medicine
Dr Edmund K Y Wong, Nepean, ON - Family Medicine
Dr David A Wong, Newmarket, ON - Family Medicine
Dr Tat-Ying Wong, North York, ON - General Practice
Dr Angela M Y Wong, Richmond Hill, ON - Family Medicine
Dr Henry W F Wong, Scarborough, ON - General Practice
Dr Andrew C Y Wong, Scarborough, ON - Family Medicine
Dr Godfrey L Wong, Scarborough, ON - General Practice
Dr Joseph S Wong, Scarborough, ON - Physical Medicine & Rehab
Dr Kathleen W F Wong, Scarborough, ON - General Practice
Dr Kevin H Wong, Scarborough, ON - General Surgery
Dr On Yu Wong, Scarborough, ON - General Practice
Dr Susanna S S Wong, Scarborough, ON - General Practice
Dr W W Loretta Wong, Scarborough, ON - General Practice
Dr Wilfred K K Wong, Scarborough, ON - General Practice
Dr Albert S H Wong, Toronto, ON - General Practice
Dr Andrew C H Wong, Toronto, ON - General Practice
Dr K S Rebecca Wong, Toronto, ON - Radiation Oncology
Dr David T W Wong, Toronto, ON - Ophthalmology
Dr Edward Y C Wong, Toronto, ON - Diagnostic-Radiology
Dr Tat Hang Wong, Toronto, ON - General Practice
Dr Joseph Y K Wong, Toronto, ON - General Practice
Dr Florence S H Wong, Toronto, ON - Gastroenterology
Dr Alice H M Wong, Saskatoon, SK - Critical Care Medicine
Dr Kenny S Woo, Edmonton, AB - Cardiology
Dr Dennis K Woo, Markham, ON - General Practice
Dr Kin Yee Woo, Markham, ON - General Practice
Dr Stanley K C Woo, Newmarket, ON - Urology
Dr George H K Woo, Toronto, ON - Obstetrics & Gynecology
Dr Jackson S Y Wu, Calgary, AB - Radiation Oncology
Dr John W Y Wu, Calgary, AB - Hematology
Dr Vincent M Y Wu, Barrie, ON - Obstetrics & Gynecology
Dr Paul T K Wu, Burlington, ON - Obstetrics & Gynecology
Dr H T Tony Wu, Oakville, ON - General Practice
Dr Henry M W Wu, Scarborough, ON - General Practice
Dr Yan Wu, Saskatoon, SK - Family Medicine
Dr Liya Xie, Calgary, AB - General Practice
Dr Qiwei Xu, Victoria, BC - Hematological Pathology
Dr Jie Xu, Halifax, NS - General Practice
Dr Shuwen Xue, Chatham, ON - Internal Medicine
Dr Cecilia S F Yam, Brandon, MB - General Practice
Dr Alexander Yan, Edmonton, AB - Internal Medicine
Dr Brian Yan, London, ON - Gastroenterology
Dr Raymond T Yan, Scarborough, ON - Cardiology
Dr David B Yan, Toronto, ON - Ophthalmology
Dr Kwang Yang, Surrey, BC - Family Medicine
Dr Tung C Yang, Vancouver, BC - Infectious Diseases
Dr Min Kang Yang, Mississauga, ON - General Practice
Dr Elisa Y S Yang, Nepean, ON - General Practice
Dr Homer Y H Yang, Ottawa, ON - Anesthesia
Dr William H Yang, Ottawa, ON - Internal Medicine
Dr W Y Philip Yang, Scarborough, ON - General Practice
Dr Peter Y O Yao, Surrey, BC - Orthopedic Surgery
Dr Zhenhai Yao, Richmond Hill, ON - Anesthesia
Dr Louis C H Yao, York, ON - Cardiology
Dr Yu-Ju Yao, Montreal, QC - Family Medicine
Dr Hanle O Yap, Windsor, ON - Geriatric Medicine
Dr Jonathan C Yau, Calgary, AB - Internal Medicine
Dr Yvonne C W Yau, Toronto, ON - Medical Microbiology
Dr Jian Ye, Vancouver, BC - Cardiac Surgery
Dr Kenny Y V Yee, Barrington Passage, NS - Family Medicine
Dr Ivan C Y Yee, Scarborough, ON - General Practice
Dr Albert J M Yee, Toronto, ON - Orthopedic Surgery
Dr Gordon Yee, LaSalle, QC - Family Medicine
Dr Eluen A Yeh, Toronto, ON - Pediatrics
Dr William H W Yeung, Maple Ridge, BC - Obstetrics & Gynecology
Dr Clement S L Yeung, Winnipeg, MB - Internal Medicine
Dr Jack K P S Y Yeung, Burlington, ON - General Practice
Dr Elaine T Yeung, Scarborough, ON - Gastroenterology
Dr Dan W H Yeung, Scarborough, ON - General Practice
Dr Rae S M Yeung, Toronto, ON - Pediatrics
Dr James J Ying, Georgetown, ON - General Practice
Dr Ethel Ying, Toronto, ON - Pediatrics
Dr Ying Ying, Brossard, QC - Family Medicine
Dr T C Kathy Yip, Mississauga, ON - Internal Medicine
Dr Florence S Yip, Scarborough, ON - Family Medicine
Dr Douglas W Yiu, Vancouver, BC - Family Medicine
Dr Wendy W S Yiu, Toronto, ON - Psychiatry
Dr Yu-Sen Yong, Surrey, BC - General Surgery
Dr Peter L Yong, Vancouver, BC - General Practice
Dr Chu Hua Yong, Thornhill, ON - General Practice
Dr Theron K Young, Toronto, ON - Community Medicine
Dr Shihao Yu, Surrey, BC - General Practice
Dr Larry L W Yu, Vancouver, BC - General Practice
Dr William Y Yu, Vancouver, BC - Orthopedic Surgery
Dr Joyce W Yu, Vancouver, BC - Clin Immun/Allergy
Dr Stanley S F Yu, Hamilton, ON - Family Medicine
Dr Edward W T Yu, London, ON - Radiation Oncology
Dr Tsai Hsing Yu, St Catharines, ON - General Practice
Dr Herbert D Yu, Toronto, ON - General Practice
Dr Lilian Yuan, Newmarket, ON - Community Medicine
Dr Jenise J W Yue, Vancouver, BC - Obstetrics & Gynecology
Dr Bonnie W M Yue-Tang, Toronto, ON - General Practice
Dr Richard H Yuen, Calgary, AB - General Practice
Dr Sze-Ming Yuen, Burnaby, BC - Psychiatry
Dr Doris E Yuen, London, ON - Pediatrics
Dr Michael L F Yuen, Scarborough, ON - Diagnostic-Radiology
Dr Wingko W Yung, Richmond Hill, ON - Anesthesia
Dr Stephen Y W Yung, Toronto, ON - General Practice
Dr Wanzhen Zeng, Ottawa, ON - Nuclear Medicine
Dr Chi Zhang, Trail, BC - Internal Medicine
Dr Xueyan Zheng, Richmond, BC - Family Medicine
Dr Zuoyu Zheng, St Catharines, ON - General Pathology
Dr Chen Qian Zhou, Vancouver, BC - Anatomical Pathology

CHIUCHOW

Dr Gabriel F P Chan, Scarborough, ON - Geriatric Medicine
Dr Kwang Yang, Surrey, BC - Family Medicine

CHIYAO

Dr Khami Chokani, Prince Albert, SK - General Practice

CHOWCHAU

Dr Kwang Yang, Surrey, BC - Family Medicine

CONCANI

Dr Sylvia B Athaide, North York, ON - General Practice

CREOLE

Dr Jean Joseph Thierry Alcindor, Montreal, QC - Hematology
Dr Antony Alcindor, Montreal, QC - General Pathology
Dr Jean-Claude Armand, Verdun, QC - General Practice
Dr Alezandre Dauphin, Hamilton, ON - Anesthesia
Dr Cecile D Davey, Kitchener, ON - Pediatrics
Dr Jean Claude Decarie, Montreal, QC - Diagnostic-Radiology
Dr Michel C Demers, Quebec, QC - General Practice
Dr Raymond Duperval, Sherbrooke, QC - Internal Medicine
Dr Joelle M T Fareau-Weyl, Guelph, ON - Psychiatry
Dr Janice Y Faulknor, Georgetown, ON - Family Medicine
Dr Marie-Carmel Fernandez, Saint-Leonard, QC - General Practice
Dr Bernard E Ferreira, Point Edward, ON - Obstetrics & Gynecology
Dr Florence Flambert, Quebec, QC - General Practice
Dr Philip A Fong Wai Chin, Weyburn, SK - General Practice
Dr Kara J Gibson, Hamilton, ON - Anesthesia
Dr Geoffrey T Gooding, Thunder Bay, ON - Internal Medicine
Dr Edith M Guntley-Lorimer, Toronto, ON - General Practice
Dr Farook Hossenbux, Ottawa, ON - Internal Medicine
Dr Martine Hudicourt, St-Charles-Brromee, QC - Family Medicine
Dr Philippe Lageix, Verdun, QC - General Practice
Dr Marie-Florence Legros, Montreal-Nord, QC - Family Medicine
Dr Louis-Charles Levros, Montreal, QC - General Practice
Dr Pierre Monpremier, Vanier, ON - Psychiatry
Dr Dolly T Nahri, Ottawa, ON - General Practice
Dr Stanley Norris, La Tuque, QC - Psychiatry
Dr Bossuet Painson, Montreal, QC - General Pathology
Dr J J Pierre Plourde, Winnipeg, MB - Infectious Diseases
Dr Harry Prochette, Repentigny, QC - General Practice
Dr Willine R Rozefort, Verdun, QC - Family Medicine
Dr Mandy Ruthnum, Courtenay, BC - Family Medicine
Dr Serge Saint-Amant, Saint-Antoine, NB - Family Medicine
Dr Irma-Nancy Sully, Ottawa, ON - Family Medicine
Dr Claudette Thomas Fils-Aime, Montreal, QC - General Practice
Dr Jean E Weir, Peterborough, ON - Family Medicine
Dr Donald G Wilson, Comox, BC - Obstetrics & Gynecology
Dr John G Yates, Oakville, ON - General Practice

CROATIAN

Dr Sanja Avdic, Toronto, ON - Pediatrics
Dr Boris Bahoric, Montreal, QC - Radiation Oncology
Dr Hifzija H Bajramovic, Ottawa, ON - Psychiatry
Dr Ivan Barac, Winnipeg, MB - General Practice
Dr Maja Barnard, North York, ON - Anatomical Pathology
Dr Andrea Bezjak, Toronto, ON - Internal Medicine
Dr Nada Bodruzic, Strathmore, AB - General Practice
Dr Ivan Brodarec, Yarmouth, NS - General Practice
Dr Anita Buriloski-Chkipova, Victoria, BC - General Practice
Dr Nick B Cuberovic, Milton, ON - Family Medicine
Dr Srdjan Curuvija, Ottawa, ON - Diagnostic-Radiology
Dr Enver Deliu, Halifax, NS - Family Medicine
Dr Roy R Diklich, Windsor, ON - General Practice
Dr Bojana Djordjevic, Ottawa, ON - Anatomical Pathology
Dr Dubravka Dodig, Toronto, ON - Neurology
Dr Dragoslav Drca, Orleans, ON - General Practice
Dr Frank Drkulec, Windsor, ON - General Practice
Dr Andrew D Duic, Toronto, ON - Pediatrics
Dr Olga Dzever, Etobicoke, ON - Family Medicine
Dr Erik Eryavec, Hamilton, ON - General Practice

Dr Mohyeddin Essabri, Etobicoke, ON - Family Medicine
Dr Zdenko Filakovic, Toronto, ON - Diagnostic-Radiology
Dr Don Z Fulgosi, Toronto, ON - Psychiatry
Dr Desanka Gajic, Toronto, ON - General Practice
Dr Mirjana Garic, Burlington, ON - Family Medicine
Dr Aleksander Georgievski, Thornhill, ON - General Practice
Dr Boris P Gimbarzevsky, Kamloops, BC - General Practice
Dr Andrej J Habjan, Thunder Bay, ON - General Practice
Dr Maja Haslah, Toronto, ON - Family Medicine
Dr Dragan Hercig, Toronto, ON - Psychiatry
Dr Ljiljana Jaksic-Tomanovic, Toronto, ON - Family Medicine
Dr Jadranka A Jambrosic, Etobicoke, ON - Anatomical Pathology
Dr Sanja Karalic, North Vancouver, BC - Family Medicine
Dr Z Branislav Katalinic, Quesnel, BC - General Surgery
Dr Diana Kljenak, Toronto, ON - Psychiatry
Dr Kathy A Knezic, Winnipeg, MB - Family Medicine
Dr Peter A Kokan, Burnaby, BC - Orthopedic Surgery
Dr Tilda Konforte-Vasiljevic, St Stephen, NB - General Practice
Dr Ljiljana Kordic, Delta, BC - Family Medicine
Dr Zlatko Kostic, Lloydminster, AB - Internal Medicine
Dr Jelka-Maria Lujic-Thebaud, Edmonton, AB - General Practice
Dr Dusan Lukic, Hamilton, ON - General Practice
Dr Ana Lulic-Hrvojic, Toronto, ON - Psychiatry
Dr Borislava Mijavec, Orleans, ON - Family Medicine
Dr Ljiljana Miladinovic, Toronto, ON - Family Medicine
Dr Tatjana Muhamedagic, Oakville, ON - Psychiatry
Dr Etela Neumann, Vancouver, BC - Neuro-Pathology
Dr Dijana Oliver, Kingston, ON - Psychiatry
Dr Danica Petrovic, Vancouver, BC - General Practice
Dr Petr Polasek, Kelowna, BC - Cardiology
Dr Mate Poljicak, Montreal, QC - General Surgery
Dr Lillian M Rojnica, Mississauga, ON - Pediatrics
Dr Katarina Rovis, London, ON - Pediatrics
Dr Mladen V Rusnov, Montreal, QC - General Surgery
Dr Mile Savic, Belleville, ON - Family Medicine
Dr Ljubinka Segedi, Kitchener, ON - Family Medicine
Dr Mladen Seidl, Etobicoke, ON - General Practice
Dr Maja M Seidl, Mississauga, ON - Family Medicine
Dr Joseph Sertic, Mississauga, ON - Family Medicine
Dr Jana Sidorov, Prince George, BC - General Practice
Dr Dusan Sijan, Windsor, ON - General Practice
Dr Jovan G Simeon, Vanier, ON - Psychiatry
Dr Ivo Slezic, Mississauga, ON - Diagnostic-Radiology
Dr Stoyan Solarich, North York, ON - General Practice
Dr Rajka Soric, Toronto, ON - Physical Medicine & Rehab
Dr Chris P Stefanovich, Etobicoke, ON - Family Medicine
Dr Snezana Stegnajic, East York, ON - Family Medicine
Dr Dubravka Sturman, Markham, ON - General Pathology
Dr Katica Sumanac, Dundas, ON - Family Medicine
Dr Emile D Svarc, Montreal, QC - Ophthalmology
Dr Tomislav Svoboda, Toronto, ON - Community Medicine
Dr Samir Taleb, Campbellton, NB - General Practice
Dr Cedomirka Todorovic, Port Moody, BC - Family Medicine
Dr Peter M Vignjevic, Hamilton, ON - Dermatology
Dr Maryann Vitaro, Woodbridge, ON - Family Medicine
Dr Josip Vlahovich, Toronto, ON - General Practice
Dr Branislav Vlaovic, East York, ON - General Practice
Dr Laura Voltic, Windsor, ON - Family Medicine
Dr Doris F Vretenar, Vancouver, BC - Anesthesia
Dr Ivica Vucemilo, Mississauga, ON - General Surgery
Dr Neda Vujicic, North York, ON - Family Medicine
Dr Duska Vukojevic, Belleville, ON - General Practice
Dr Milorad Vukovic, Scarborough, ON - Psychiatry
Dr Michael J Walmsley, Mississauga, ON - General Surgery
Dr Ljiljana Zivic-Deliu, Halifax, NS - Family Medicine

CZECH

Dr Mouafak Al Hadi, Mindemoya, ON - Family Medicine
Dr Karolina Altmann, London, ON - General Practice
Dr Daniela Baloun, Toronto, ON - General Practice
Dr Frantisek Beck, Burnaby, BC - Family Medicine
Dr Timea Belej-Rak, Vaughan, ON - Obstetrics & Gynecology
Dr L Jane Berka, North York, ON - Family Medicine
Dr Eva Berman-Wong, Gladstone, MB - Family Medicine
Dr Maria Bertlik, Brampton, ON - Anesthesia
Dr Henry J Bibr, Hamilton, ON - Psychiatry
Dr Jana M Blaskovic, St Thomas, ON - General Practice
Dr Clara J Bohm, Winnipeg, MB - Internal Medicine
Dr Miloslav B Bozdech, Red Deer, AB - Ophthalmology
Dr Helena Buchar, Cranbrook, BC - Family Medicine
Dr Anna Chlebak, Langley, BC - General Practice
Dr Jarmila Chrappa, Corner Brook, NL - Pediatrics
Dr Michelle P Cipera, Kuujjuarapik, QC - Family Medicine
Dr Janina H Dutkiewicz-Stvrtecky, Oakville, ON - General Practice
Dr Vladimir Dzavik, Toronto, ON - Cardiology
Dr Dana Eisner, Etobicoke, ON - General Practice
Dr Bassam El-Tatari, Windsor, ON - Family Medicine
Dr Janusz Feber, Ottawa, ON - Pediatrics
Dr Katarina Fiala, Toronto, ON - Dermatology
Dr Jindrich Fiala, Toronto, ON - Family Medicine
Dr Jiri Frohlich, Vancouver, BC - Medical Biochemistry
Dr Pavel Geier, Ottawa, ON - General Practice
Dr Marie Geizer, Vancouver, BC - Psychiatry
Dr Stanley Z Gertler, Ottawa, ON - Internal Medicine
Dr Yves Giguere, Quebec, QC - Medical Biochemistry
Dr Marketa Gogela-Spehar, Vancouver, BC - Obstetrics & Gynecology
Dr Eva Gomez, Kanata, ON - General Practice
Dr Marie Grabec, Hamilton, ON - General Practice
Dr Paul Gregor, Hamilton, ON - General Surgery
Dr Peter A Gresko, Windsor, ON - General Practice
Dr Paul Grof, Ottawa, ON - Psychiatry
Dr Vit B Gunka, Vancouver, BC - Anesthesia
Dr Pavel Hamet, Montreal, QC - Endocrinology
Dr Didi V Harries, Chilliwack, BC - Pediatrics
Dr Jane Healey, Mississauga, ON - Pediatrics
Dr Barbara Hejdankova, North Vancouver, BC - Family Medicine
Dr Grazyna W Hofner, Truro, NS - Psychiatry
Dr Evelyn M Honsl, Ottawa, ON - General Practice
Dr Stuart Z Horak, North Vancouver, BC - Emergency Family Med
Dr Maria A Horani, North York, ON - General Practice
Dr Stefan Horny, Montreal, QC - General Practice
Dr Irene Hoyer, Calgary, AB - General Practice
Dr Vaclav R Hoyer, Calgary, AB - General Practice
Dr Nadine S Hradsky, Toronto, ON - Dermatology
Dr Joseph Hrncirik, Miramichi, NB - General Practice
Dr Vera Hynie, Ottawa, ON - General Practice
Dr Henry J Jelinek, Etobicoke, ON - General Practice
Dr Milos Jenicek, Hamilton, ON - Community Medicine
Dr Eva M Jokay, Etobicoke, ON - Psychiatry
Dr Hanna Kadanka, North York, ON - General Practice
Dr Helen Karsai, Vancouver, BC - General Practice
Dr Karin M Kausky, Whistler, BC - Family Medicine
Dr Petr Kavan, Montreal, QC - General Practice
Dr Hana Kocandrle, Toronto, ON - General Practice
Dr Victor Kokta, Montreal, QC - Anatomical Pathology
Dr David Kopriva, Regina, SK - General Surgery
Dr Vitezslava V Kozel, Englehart, ON - General Practice
Dr Jana Krajbich, Calgary, AB - Family Medicine
Dr Milos J Krajny, Toronto, ON - Internal Medicine
Dr Lida Kratka, Vanier, ON - General Practice
Dr Antonin Kratky, London, ON - General Practice
Dr Peter Krykorka, Vancouver, BC - Family Medicine
Dr Lenka Kucerova, Sarnia, ON - General Practice
Dr Karol Kuperberg, Montreal, QC - General Practice
Dr Vladimir Kurgansky, Kirkland, QC - Urology
Dr Alena Ladki, North Vancouver, BC - Pediatrics
Dr Radomila Lenz, Ottawa, ON - Psychiatry
Dr Miroslava Lhotsky, Toronto, ON - Family Medicine
Dr Andrea Melicharkova, Peterborough, ON - Gastroenterology
Dr Ladislav Mesensky, Etobicoke, ON - General Practice
Dr Marcella Mesensky, Toronto, ON - General Practice
Dr Bohdan Molckovsky, Mississauga, ON - General Practice
Dr Amira Muncner, Edmonton, AB - General Practice
Dr Etela Neumann, Vancouver, BC - Neuro-Pathology
Dr Viktor Neumann, Vancouver, BC - General Practice
Dr Jana Nigrin, Edmonton, AB - Medical Microbiology
Dr Teresa Oliva, Nepean, ON - Family Medicine
Dr Ondrej Pacin, Winnipeg, MB - Family Medicine
Dr John Paleta, Hubbards, NS - General Practice
Dr Danielle E Pastierovic, Victoria, BC - General Practice
Dr Eva Patocka, Devon, AB - General Practice
Dr Tomas M Pauk, Barrie, ON - Family Medicine
Dr Ivan Petrov, Toronto, ON - General Practice
Dr Imelda S Pilar, Mississauga, ON - Family Medicine
Dr Ludek Podhradsky, Orillia, ON - Family Medicine
Dr Petr Polasek, Kelowna, BC - Cardiology
Dr David Ponka, Ottawa, ON - Emergency Family Med
Dr Marie B Prihoda, Coquitlam, BC - Dermatology
Dr Michal Princ, Devon, AB - General Practice
Dr Jan Prsala, Victoria, BC - General Practice
Dr Vladimir Pucholt, North York, ON - Pediatrics
Dr Rudolf Reindl, Montreal, QC - Orthopedic Surgery
Dr Charles V Rohlicek, Montreal, QC - Cardiology
Dr Otokar J Roob, Fort Saskatchewan, AB - General Practice
Dr George J Rosenkranz, Ponoka, AB - Family Medicine
Dr Jan Rozehnal, Toronto, ON - General Practice
Dr Marcel Ruzicka, Ottawa, ON - Internal Medicine
Dr Jan M Salat, Ottawa, ON - General Practice
Dr Paul Sandor, Toronto, ON - Psychiatry
Dr Suzanne Schuh, Toronto, ON - Pediatrics
Dr Jan I Schulz, Montreal, QC - Clin Immun/Allergy
Dr Miriam Shanks, Edmonton, AB - Cardiology
Dr Raisa Sheftel, Verdun, QC - General Practice
Dr Caroline A Shooner, Queen Charlotte, BC - Family Medicine
Dr Jaroslav J Simice, Comox, BC - Internal Medicine
Dr Yana Simice, Nanaimo, BC - Emergency Family Med
Dr Martin Simonik, North York, ON - General Practice
Dr Dagmar Simonik, North York, ON - General Practice
Dr Karen E Slatkovsky, Guelph, ON - Emergency Family Med
Dr Dalibor E Slavik, Saskatoon, SK - Family Medicine
Dr Iva Smrz, Saint John, NB - Ophthalmology
Dr Vaclav Smula, Toronto, ON - General Practice
Dr Elena Somska, Toronto, ON - General Practice
Dr Dusan Soudek Jr, Dartmouth, NS - General Practice
Dr Stan Z Spacek, Goderich, ON - Emergency Family Med
Dr Kimberly L Spacek, Goderich, ON - Emergency Family Med
Dr Alena M Spacek, Ottawa, ON - Emergency Family Med
Dr Jan Spacek, Sherbrooke, QC - General Practice
Dr Paul J Sperka, Edmonton, AB - Occupational Med
Dr Jitka Stankova, Montreal, QC - General Practice
Dr Pavel F Straka, York, ON - Anesthesia
Dr Milosh S Surka, Richmond, BC - General Practice
Dr Monica Susil, Lively, ON - Family Medicine
Dr Pavol Sventek, Val-d'Or, QC - Family Medicine
Dr Michaela Swekla, Cambridge, ON - General Practice
Dr Edo Teku, Toronto, ON - Family Medicine
Dr Eva Tlusty, Oakville, ON - Diagnostic-Radiology
Dr Vesna Tokic, Vancouver, BC - Family Medicine
Dr Ladislav Tomes, Toronto, ON - Anatomical Pathology
Dr Stanislav Valnicek, Kelowna, BC - Obstetrics & Gynecology
Dr J Nicholas Vanek, North York, ON - General Practice
Dr Irene J Vanek, Toronto, ON - Ophthalmology
Dr Frantisek Vetiska, Oakville, ON - General Practice
Dr Ludmila Vlckova, Abbotsford, BC - General Practice
Dr J Suzanne Vobecky, Montreal, QC - Cardiovasc/ThorSurg
Dr Ludmila Vokac, North York, ON - General Practice
Dr Nandanie Weerasinghe, Edmonton, AB - General Practice
Dr Alan A Weiss, Vancouver, BC - Gastroenterology
Dr Jana Wieder, Halifax, NS - General Practice
Dr Joseph Zahradnik, Peterborough, ON - Obstetrics & Gynecology
Dr Anthony G Zekulin, Brampton, ON - General Practice
Dr Peter I Zelina, Richmond Hill, ON - Psychiatry
Dr George J Zeman, North Bay, ON - Obstetrics & Gynecology
Dr Robert Zeman, Toronto, ON - Endocrin/Metabolism

DANISH

Dr Mary Ann Bramstrup, Nackawic, NB - General Practice
Dr Shyah S Delarom, Victoria, BC - General Practice
Dr Christian Falkenberg-Andersen, Calgary, AB - Family Medicine
Dr Hartley Garfield, Toronto, ON - Pediatrics
Dr Kristin Gisladottir, Toronto, ON - Psychiatry

Dr Ole Hammerberg, London, ON - Medical Microbiology
Dr Bent Hougesen, Hazelton, BC - Community Medicine
Dr Dorrit Klarke, New Westminster, BC - General Practice
Dr Michael F P Madsen, Vancouver, BC - Family Medicine
Dr Jan Fredrik Moe, Kinistino, SK - General Practice
Dr Peter R Olesen, Campbell River, BC - Plastic Surgery
Dr Susie D Pedersen, Calgary, AB - Endocrin/Metabolism
Dr Ole S Rasmussen, Regina, SK - General Practice
Dr Indrojit Roy, Montreal, QC - Anatomical Pathology
Dr Gabrielle K Savard, Calgary, AB - Family Medicine
Dr Peter M Segato, Wolfville, NS - Family Medicine
Dr Paul H B Sorensen, Vancouver, BC - Anatomical Pathology
Dr Martin Svartberg, Toronto, ON - Psychiatry
Dr Ellen N Thompson, Ottawa, ON - Anesthesia
Dr Inge G Winslow, Richmond Hill, ON - General Practice
Dr John G Young, Ottawa, ON - Otolaryngology

DARI

Dr Ahmad S Ashrafi, Surrey, BC - General Surgery
Dr Ziaullah Fahim, Surrey, BC - General Practice
Dr Azim F Juma, Scarborough, ON - Family Medicine
Dr Adam S Kayumi, Mississauga, ON - Family Medicine
Dr Farid A Rahimi, Mission, BC - General Practice
Dr Fareidoon Rezazadah, Langley, BC - General Practice
Dr Merajuddin Shams, Vaughan, ON - Family Medicine

DEAF-MUTE

Dr Helene Mandeville, Montreal, QC - General Practice

DIOULA

Dr Mahamadou Chaibou, Moncton, NB - General Practice

DUTCH

Dr Jan-Martin Albers, Toronto, ON - Family Medicine
Dr Albert R Albertyn, Nipawin, SK - General Practice
Dr P Paul A Anderson, Perth, ON - Orthopedic Surgery
Dr Alastair W J Annan, Enderby, BC - General Practice
Dr Rudolf J Arts, Barrie, ON - Neurology
Dr Mary Ann Beimers, Vancouver, BC - Pediatrics
Dr Harold P Berghuis, Truro, NS - Family Medicine
Dr Marian E Berry, Nelson, BC - Neurology
Dr Jan Jaap Bijlsma, Vancouver, BC - Emergency Medicine
Dr Maurice Blitz, Toronto, ON - General Surgery
Dr Marion C Blouw, Victoria, BC - Family Medicine
Dr Richard H Blouw, Winnipeg, MB - Family Medicine
Dr Maarten Bokhout, Clinton, ON - Family Medicine
Dr Amy J Borkent, Edmonton, AB - General Practice
Dr Geert B Braam, Edmonton, AB - General Practice
Dr Johann H Brink, Coquitlam, BC - Psychiatry
Dr Maryleen Brouw, Quebec, QC - General Practice
Dr Janki Butchey, London, ON - Psychiatry
Dr Irene Cohen, London, ON - Family Medicine
Dr Cornelis De Boer, Truro, NS - Psychiatry
Dr Walter De Bruin, Chilliwack, BC - Ophthalmology
Dr Wilhelmina De Groot, Etobicoke, ON - General Practice
Dr Johannes D De Vries, Calgary, AB - Psychiatry
Dr Willem E De Vynck, Langley, BC - Emergency Family Med
Dr Levinus Albert Dieleman, Edmonton, AB - General Practice
Dr Joan Don, Lindsay, ON - Anesthesia
Dr Jeffrey F T Dresselhuis, Burnaby, BC - General Practice
Dr Marc E Dufour, Sudbury, ON - Obstetrics & Gynecology
Dr R Maarten Egeler, Toronto, ON - General Practice
Dr Catharina H G M Foolen, Sundre, AB - Family Medicine
Dr Bing Siang Gan, London, ON - Plastic Surgery
Dr Edward F H Gentis, Vancouver, BC - General Surgery
Dr David Gerber, Toronto, ON - Obstetrics & Gynecology
Dr Karin G Goddard, Montreal, QC - Psychiatry
Dr Walter H Gotlieb, Montreal, QC - Obstetrics & Gynecology
Dr Peter G Greidanus, Lethbridge, AB - General Practice
Dr Martin P Grypma, Langley, BC - Orthopedic Surgery
Dr Jaap N Hamburger, Vancouver, BC - Cardiology
Dr Rob J Hekkenberg, Barrie, ON - Otolaryngology
Dr Robert P Helt, Midland, ON - General Practice
Dr Maurice H J Hennink, Regina, SK - General Practice
Dr Adriaan Heunis, Salmon Arm, BC - General Practice
Dr Stefan O P Hofer, Toronto, ON - Plastic Surgery
Dr John A Hofhuis, Port Stanley, ON - Family Medicine
Dr Jane M J Hosdil, Rockwood, ON - General Practice
Dr Menno Huikeshoven, Vancouver, BC - General Practice
Dr Louise M Jackson, Courtenay, BC - Anesthesia
Dr Diederick W Jalink, Kingston, ON - General Surgery
Dr Gerard H Jansen, Ottawa, ON - Neuro-Pathology
Dr Dorothy M Janzen, North Vancouver, BC - General Practice
Dr Urvi Joshi, New Westminster, BC - Nuclear Medicine
Dr Johan L Joubert, Dawson Creek, BC - General Practice
Dr Rob J Kamermans, Coe Hill, ON - General Practice
Dr Madelene S Kellerman, Lethbridge, AB - General Practice
Dr Michael R Kenyon, Terrace, BC - Internal Medicine
Dr Robert K Koenekoop, Montreal, QC - Ophthalmology
Dr Pieter Ernst Kruger, Fort McMurray, AB - General Practice
Dr Kai Liang Kwee, White Rock, BC - Orthopedic Surgery
Dr Eugene P Landsbergen, Sundre, AB - General Practice
Dr Guy Jean Laroye, Terrace, BC - General Pathology
Dr Kay I Lie, Toronto, ON - Obstetrics & Gynecology
Dr Daniel T H Liem, Windsor, ON - Internal Medicine
Dr Bernadette Loontjens, St-Charles-Brromee, QC - General Practice
Dr Wynand F Louw, Invermere, BC - Family Medicine
Dr Hilda A Makken, Fort Erie, ON - Pediatrics
Dr Monica McKay, Williams Lake, BC - General Practice
Dr Stephane B Meere, Montreal, QC - Ophthalmology
Dr Catharina J Meyer, Carlyle, SK - Family Medicine
Dr Hilda Moens, Burlington, ON - General Practice
Dr Francois O P Moens, Hamilton, ON - Obstetrics & Gynecology
Dr Andre Moolman, Kitchener, ON - Family Medicine
Dr Paula Nieuwstraten, Toronto, ON - Family Medicine
Dr Bernhard J Olberg, Ottawa, ON - Anatomical Pathology
Dr Danielle M Over, Oakville, ON - General Practice
Dr Peter Palma, Fort McMurray, AB - Emergency Family Med
Dr Harold T Popma, Sackville, NB - Family Medicine
Dr Mary-Ann J Pubben, North York, ON - Family Medicine
Dr Marc Puts, Port Alberni, BC - General Practice
Dr Abel H Raath, Consort, AB - Family Medicine
Dr Michael J Reedijk, Toronto, ON - General Surgery
Dr Martinus Reedyk, Three Hills, AB - General Practice
Dr Hendrik W Reems, Nanaimo, BC - General Practice
Dr Theodora C G Ruijs, Brampton, ON - General Pathology
Dr Herbert W Sacks, Edmonton, AB - Family Medicine
Dr Jan J Scheeres, Barrie, ON - Obstetrics & Gynecology
Dr Stefan Schoeman, Courtenay, BC - Emergency Family Med
Dr Barbara Schogt, Toronto, ON - Psychiatry
Dr Ian D Schokking, Prince George, BC - Family Medicine
Dr Hendrik A Scholtens, Carlisle, ON - Family Medicine
Dr Irma E Schuurman, Surrey, BC - Family Medicine
Dr Niels E Schwarz, Nanaimo, BC - Internal Medicine
Dr Wael M Shabana, Ottawa, ON - General Practice
Dr Raphael F Sharon, Edmonton, AB - General Practice
Dr Kian Gwan Sie, East York, ON - Family Medicine
Dr Bernardus H W G M Smit, White Rock, BC - Orthopedic Surgery
Dr Yves P Starreveld, Calgary, AB - Neurosurgery
Dr Elout Starreveld, Edmonton, AB - Neurology
Dr Robert K Steer, London, ON - Family Medicine
Dr Karen G Stel, Scarborough, ON - Family Medicine
Dr Mary H Stephens, Edmonton, AB - General Surgery
Dr Antony W Steyn, Claremont, ON - Internal Medicine
Dr Pierre G Steyn, Ottawa, ON - General Practice
Dr Vivien V Suttorp, Lethbridge, AB - Family Medicine
Dr Henry C Swart, Summerside, PE - General Practice
Dr Tjien-King Tan, Thornhill, ON - General Practice
Dr Garnett M Tarr, Osoyoos, BC - General Practice
Dr John P T F Taylor, Sarnia, ON - General Surgery
Dr Karel G Ter Brugge, Toronto, ON - Diagnostic-Radiology
Dr Hendrik Ter Keurs, Calgary, AB - Internal Medicine
Dr Bernhard J Toews, Coquitlam, BC - General Practice
Dr Johan L Trapman, North York, ON - General Practice
Dr Shaun K Tregoning, Abbotsford, BC - Obstetrics & Gynecology
Dr Jolanda C Turley, Ottawa, ON - Family Medicine
Dr John E E Van Aerde, Surrey, BC - Pediatrics
Dr Morris Van Andel, Vancouver, BC - Family Medicine
Dr Elsbeth C Van Arkel, Calgary, AB - General Practice
Dr Nicolaas Van As, Sarnia, ON - Emergency Family Med
Dr Paul J Van Boxel, Amherst, NS - General Surgery
Dr Richard H C Van Der Jagt, Ottawa, ON - Hematology
Dr Etienne Van Der Linde, Clarenville, NL - General Practice
Dr Johannes Van Dorp, Wiarton, ON - General Practice
Dr Stan G Van Duyse, Montreal, QC - General Practice
Dr Jacqueline M Van Hees, Cornwall, ON - Emergency Family Med
Dr Vincent L Van Hooydonk, Tillsonburg, ON - General Practice
Dr Cornelia H M Van Ineveld, Winnipeg, MB - Geriatric Medicine
Dr Clara D Van Karnebeek, Vancouver, BC - General Practice
Dr T M Matthew J Van Olm, Calgary, AB - Internal Medicine
Dr Peter R Van Rhijn, Mississauga, ON - General Practice
Dr Stanislaus H M Van Uum, London, ON - Endocrin/Metabolism
Dr Guy Van Vliet, Montreal, QC - Endocrinology
Dr Andre R Van Wyk, Langley, BC - Family Medicine
Dr Sander J Van Zanten, Edmonton, AB - Gastroenterology
Dr Walter J Vanast, Kahnawake, QC - Neurology
Dr John Vanderkooy, Harriston, ON - General Practice
Dr Rudolf Vandersluis, Oshawa, ON - Emergency Family Med
Dr Ronald Vandersluis, Scarborough, ON - Orthopedic Surgery
Dr Gerrit Veenman, Guelph, ON - General Practice
Dr Jacob Veenstra, Brampton, ON - General Practice
Dr Fedde Veenstra, Owen Sound, ON - Emergency Family Med
Dr Keimpe Veldhuis, London, ON - Internal Medicine
Dr Johannes H Verbeek, Timmins, ON - General Pathology
Dr Adrian J E Verburg, Chatham, ON - General Practice
Dr Nicolaas P L G Verhoeff, North York, ON - Psychiatry
Dr Jentien H Vermaat, Scarborough, ON - Pediatrics
Dr Rex E Verschuren, Scarborough, ON - Family Medicine
Dr Henry J Vlaar, Ayr, ON - General Practice
Dr Margaret W M Voorpostel, Newmarket, ON - General Practice
Dr Patrick M Vos, Vancouver, BC - Diagnostic-Radiology
Dr W Robbert Vroom, Vancouver, BC - Emergency Family Med
Dr Johannes L T Vuurmans, New Westminster, BC - General Practice
Dr Malcolm G Walker, Fort McMurray, AB - Family Medicine
Dr Thomas Warkus, Montreal, QC - General Practice
Dr Michael J Weinberg, Mississauga, ON - Plastic Surgery
Dr Isabella M Werkman, St Paul, AB - General Practice
Dr Jacques West, Abbotsford, BC - General Practice
Dr Hendrik H Westenberg, Kingston, ON - General Practice
Dr Djoen Widjanarko, Sudbury, ON - General Practice
Dr George J Wiehahn, Kamloops, BC - Psychiatry
Dr Michael R Wilkinson, Vancouver, BC - General Practice
Dr Veerle R P Willaeys, Burnaby, BC - Community Medicine
Dr Bernard E Willems, Montreal, QC - Internal Medicine
Dr Pieter Willemse Sr, Dauphin, MB - General Practice
Dr Adriaan Windt, Abbotsford, BC - General Practice
Dr Monique J Withers, Calgary, AB - Family Medicine
Dr Thomas Wolder, Strathroy, ON - General Practice
Dr Evelyn Wolff, Huntsville, ON - General Practice
Dr Kevin C Woudstra, Houston, BC - General Practice
Dr Milton P Wybenga, Truro, NS - Anesthesia
Dr Jennifer P Young, Collingwood, ON - Emergency Family Med
Dr Thomas Zeyl, Beamsville, ON - Family Medicine
Dr Alexandre R Zlotta, Toronto, ON - General Surgery
Dr Dick E Zoutman, Belleville, ON - Infectious Diseases
Dr Nathalia H M de Bruin, Calgary, AB - General Practice

EDO

Dr Asiru Abu-Bakare, Thunder Bay, ON - Endocrin/Metabolism
Dr Osamudiamen C Omosigho, Estevan, SK - General Practice

ENGLISH

Dr Fayez Abboud, Gatineau, QC - General Practice
Dr Amal Abdel-Baki, Montreal, QC - Psychiatry
Dr Hamed Abdoulraman, North Vancouver, BC - Psychiatry

Dr Anthony Abela, Montreal, QC - Otolaryngology
Dr Victor Abikhzer, Montreal, QC - General Practice
Dr Mirna Abou Abdo, Gatineau, QC - General Practice
Dr Allan Abramovitch, Scarborough, ON - Urology
Dr Farid Absi, Trois-Rivieres, QC - Internal Medicine
Dr Madeleine Achkar, Laval, QC - General Practice
Dr Khim C Ah-Lan, Saint-Hubert, QC - General Practice
Dr Victor A Ahad, Verdun, QC - Internal Medicine
Dr Marie-Jose Aiello, Greenfield Park, QC - Psychiatry
Dr Youssef AinMelk, Sherbrooke, QC - Obstetrics & Gynecology
Dr Ronald Akhras, Montreal, QC - Family Medicine
Dr Elias Al-Chaddad, Jonquiere, QC - General Surgery
Dr Guylaine Alain, Gatineau, QC - Dermatology
Dr Michel Alary, Quebec, QC - General Practice
Dr Jean-Francois Albert, Trois-Rivieres, QC - Anesthesia
Dr Antony Alcindor, Montreal, QC - General Pathology
Dr Lenny C Alladin, Montreal, QC - General Practice
Mr Andre Allaire, St-Charles-Brromee, QC - Anatomical Pathology
Dr David Allan, Ottawa, ON - Hematology
Dr Denis G Allard, Moncton, NB - Community Medicine
Dr Johane Allard, Toronto, ON - Gastroenterology
Dr Rollande Allard, Longueuil, QC - General Practice
Dr Gaston Allard, St-Felix-de-Valois, QC - General Practice
Dr Kathleen A Allard-Wasajja, Quebec, QC - General Practice
Dr Timothy V Allen, Mississauga, ON - Emergency Medicine
Dr Alexandre Alterescu, North York, ON - General Practice
Dr Maxime Amar, Quebec, QC - General Practice
Dr Myriam N Amimi, Sault Ste. Marie, ON - Obstetrics & Gynecology
Dr Smita Amin, North York, ON - Dermatology
Dr Louis-Philippe Amiot, Montreal, QC - Orthopedic Surgery
Dr Maurice Amsellem, Montreal-Nord, QC - General Practice
Dr Luce Amyot, Laval, QC - General Practice
Dr Suzanne Anctil, Sainte-Therese, QC - Pediatrics
Dr Duncan P Anderson, Vancouver, BC - Ophthalmology
Dr Scott B Anderson, London, ON - Critical Care Medicine
Dr Dawn L Anderson, Montreal, QC - General Surgery
Dr Stella Andonatos, Cote Saint-Luc, QC - General Practice
Dr Debora Andriuk, Cowansville, QC - General Practice
Dr James D Angle, Greenfield Park, QC - Internal Medicine
Dr Rui L Antunes, Cornwall, ON - General Surgery
Dr Andre M April, Gatineau, QC - General Practice
Dr Stella L Arbitman, Thornhill, ON - Family Medicine
Dr Jean-Francois Arcand-Bosse, Trois-Rivieres, QC - Internal Medicine
Dr Lisa M J Archambault, Lasalle, QC - Pediatrics
Dr Maryse Archambault, Quebec, QC - Family Medicine
Dr Christopher Archibald, Ottawa, ON - Community Medicine
Dr Lise Archibald, Quebec, QC - General Practice
Dr Sylvie J Argouarch, Victoria, BC - Psychiatry
Dr Denis A Arguin, Rouyn-Noranda, QC - General Practice
Dr Yasemin Arikan, New Westminster, BC - Internal Medicine
Dr Nahla M Aris-Jilwan, Montreal, QC - Endocrinology & Metabolism
Dr Georges Arjane, Verdun, QC - Hematological Pathology
Dr Jean-Claude Armand, Verdun, QC - General Practice
Dr Barry D Armstrong, Thunder Bay, ON - General Surgery
Dr Ian M F Arnold, Ottawa, ON - General Surgery
Dr Horacio Arruda, Quebec, QC - Community Medicine
Dr Lyne Arsenault, Hawkesbury, ON - Family Medicine
Dr Mylene Arsenault, Laval, QC - Family Medicine
Dr Caroline Arsenault, Longueuil, QC - General Practice
Dr Fernand G Arseneau, Moncton, NB - General Practice
Dr Bryan P Arthurs, Montreal, QC - Ophthalmology
Dr Sylvia L Asa, Toronto, ON - Anatomical Pathology
Dr Adel A Assaf, Montreal, QC - Diagnostic-Radiology
Dr Alfred Assalian, Longueuil, QC - Ophthalmology
Dr Pierre Assalian, Montreal, QC - Psychiatry
Dr Kenneth A Atkinson, New Westminster, BC - Gastroenterology
Dr Henri Atlas, Mont-Royal, QC - General Surgery
Dr Samia Attia-Galand, Gatineau, QC - Psychiatry
Dr Ezzedine Attig, Riviere-du-Loup, QC - Neurology
Lt Sanita Atwal, Edmonton, AB - General Surgery
Dr Michel Aube, Montreal, QC - Electroencephalography
Dr Denise Aube, Quebec, QC - Community Medicine
Dr Michele Aubin, Quebec, QC - Family Medicine
Dr Dominique Aubin, St-Jean-Sur-Richel, QC - Obstetrics & Gynecology
Dr Richard Aubin, Verdun, QC - General Practice
Dr F Kris Aubrey-Bassler, St. John's, NL - Emergency Family Med
Dr Jean R Aubry, North Bay, ON - Family Medicine
Dr Martine Aubry, Victoriaville, QC - Obstetrics & Gynecology
Dr Andre Aucoin, Edmundston, NB - General Surgery
Dr Lyne Audet, Calgary, AB - Family Medicine
Dr Jean-Francois Audet, Quebec, QC - Urology
Dr Helene Audet, Quebec, QC - General Practice
Dr Pierre Audet-Lapointe, Montreal, QC - Obstetrics & Gynecology
Dr Myriam Audette, Mascouche, QC - General Practice
Dr Marie Audy, Donnacona, QC - General Practice
Dr Julie R Auger, Timmins, ON - Family Medicine
Dr Pierre Auger, Levis, QC - Cardiology
Dr Manon Auger, Montreal, QC - Anatomical Pathology
Dr Francois Auger, Quebec, QC - Medical Microbiology
Dr Renee Auger, Quebec, QC - Diagnostic-Radiology
Dr Felix A Ayala Paredes, Sherbrooke, QC - General Practice
Dr Christopher N Ayers, Calgary, AB - Family Medicine
Dr Jose Ayllon Ugarte, Greenfield Park, QC - General Practice
Dr Evans C Ayotte, Joliette, QC - General Practice
Dr Normand J Ayotte, Shawinigan, QC - Obstetrics & Gynecology
Dr Linda Azancot, Montreal, QC - General Practice
Dr Sameh C Azer, Fort Saskatchewan, AB - General Practice
Dr S Yasmin Aziz, Ottawa, ON - Obstetrics & Gynecology
Dr Sandra Babin, Gatineau, QC - Endocrin/Metabolism
Dr Charles E Babin, Huntingdon, QC - General Practice
Dr Monique Bachand, Montreal, QC - General Practice
Dr Carolyn E H Baer, Moncton, NB - Internal Medicine
Dr Chaikou Bah, Laval, QC - Orthopedic Surgery
Dr Robert F Bailey, Montreal, QC - Geriatric Medicine
Dr David Baillargeon, Laval, QC - Orthopedic Surgery
Dr Jean-Martin Baillargeon, Montreal, QC - Diagnostic-Radiology
Dr David Bakish, Ottawa, ON - Psychiatry
Dr Vijayabalan Balasingam, Pointe-Claire, QC - Neurosurgery
Dr A Gordon Balazsi, Mont-Royal, QC - Ophthalmology
Dr James H Ballard, Victoria, BC - General Practice
Dr Gerry A Bally, Ottawa, ON - Family Medicine
Dr Marcel A Baltzan, Cote Saint-Luc, QC - Internal Medicine
Dr Franziska Baltzer, Westmount, QC - Pediatrics
Dr J D Russell Bamford, Whitehorse, YT - Family Medicine
Dr Elisabeth Banon, Montreal, QC - Psychiatry
Dr Dana Baran, Montreal, QC - Internal Medicine
Dr Jean-Jacques Barbeau, Knowlton, QC - General Practice
Dr Claudette L Bardin, Montreal, QC - Pediatrics
Dr Alain Baribeault, Quebec, QC - Physical Medicine & Rehab
Dr Pierre Baril, Quebec, QC - Emergency Medicine
Dr Jeffrey S T Barkun, Montreal, QC - General Surgery
Dr Paul E Barre, Montreal, QC - Internal Medicine
Dr Serge Barrette, Cap-aux-Meules, QC - General Practice
Dr Ian Barrette, Gatineau, QC - Family Medicine
Dr Keith J Barrington, Montreal, QC - Pediatrics
Dr Arsene J Basmadjian, Montreal, QC - Cardiology
Dr Amrik S Bassi, Calgary, AB - General Practice
Dr Pierre Bastien, Mont-Laurier, QC - Obstetrics & Gynecology
Dr Gilles Simon Bastien, Montreal, QC - Family Medicine
Dr Marie-Claude Bastien, Saint-Eustache, QC - General Practice
Dr Yves Bastien, Saint-Jerome, QC - Internal Medicine
Dr Jane S Batten, Ottawa, ON - Family Medicine
Dr Robert Bauer, Toronto, ON - Cardiology
Dr Paul Bayardelle, Montreal, QC - Medical Microbiology
Dr Mark T Bayley, Toronto, ON - Physical Medicine & Rehab
Dr Sylvie Bazin, Quebec, QC - Obstetrics & Gynecology
Dr Brigitte Bazinet, Laval, QC - Physical Medicine & Rehab
Dr Jean-Michel Beau, Malartic, QC - General Practice
Dr Jacques Beauchamp, Laval, QC - General Practice
Dr Gilles Beauchamp, Montreal, QC - General Surgery
Dr Marc Beauchamp, Montreal, QC - Orthopedic Surgery
Dr Suzanne M Beauchemin, Orleans, ON - Family Medicine
Dr Eric Beauchemin, Beaupre, QC - Family Medicine
Dr Pierre Beauchemin, Quebec, QC - General Practice
Dr Marie-Andree Beauchemin, Terrebonne, QC - Psychiatry
Dr Luc M Beauchesne, Ottawa, ON - Cardiology
Dr Christian Beauchesne, Granby, QC - General Practice
Dr Marie-France Beaudet, Quebec, QC - Family Medicine
Dr C Chantal Beaudet-Pleszczynska, Sherbrooke, QC - General Practice
Dr Robert Beaudoin, Montreal, QC - General Practice
Dr Rene Beaudoin, Sherbrooke, QC - Emergency Medicine
Dr Annie Beaudoin, Sherbrooke, QC - Gastroenterology
Dr Catherine Beaudoin, Trois-Rivieres, QC - General Practice
Dr Josianne E Beaudry, Borden, ON - Family Medicine
Dr Michel G Beaudry, Chicoutimi, QC - Electroencephal
Dr Jean-Marc Beaudry, Quebec, QC - Internal Medicine
Dr Pierre-Andre Beaulieu, Moncton, NB - Family Medicine
Dr Rene Beaulieu, Longueuil, QC - General Practice
Dr Jean-Yves Beaulieu, Montreal-Nord, QC - General Practice
Dr Serge Beaulieu, Verdun, QC - Psychiatry
Dr Louis Beaumont, Montreal, QC - Obstetrics & Gynecology
Dr Mona Beaunoyer, Montreal, QC - General Surgery
Dr Andre Beaupre, Montreal, QC - General Surgery
Dr Liette Beauregard, Ottawa, ON - Anesthesia
Dr Marie Beauregard, Montreal, QC - Family Medicine
Dr Catherine Beauregard, Montreal, QC - Endocrin/Metabolism
Dr Michel Beauregard, Ripon, QC - General Practice
Dr Solange Beauregard, Sherbrooke, QC - Dermatology
Dr Charles Beaurivage, Victoriaville, QC - Internal Medicine
Dr Pierre Beausejour, Sherbrooke, QC - Psychiatry
Dr Michel Beauvais, Quebec, QC - Anesthesia
Dr Gloria Becerro Garijo, Campbellton, NB - General Practice
Dr Rafik R Bechbache, Unionville, ON - Family Medicine
Dr Julie Bedard, Quebec, QC - Anesthesia
Dr Diane Bedard, Quebec, QC - Family Medicine
Dr Rejean Bedard, Ste-Agathe-Des-Mts, QC - General Practice
Dr Luc Bedard, Thetford Mines, QC - General Practice
Dr Alicja Bedkowska, Verdun, QC - General Practice
Dr Deegrasjsing S Beeharry, Calgary, AB - General Practice
Dr Micheline Begin, Ottawa, ON - Internal Medicine
Dr Louis R Begin, Montreal, QC - Anatomical Pathology
Dr Thierry Begin, Quebec, QC - Family Medicine
Dr M H Julie Begin, Vaudreuil-Dorion, QC - General Practice
Dr Rama R Behki, Gatineau, QC - Ophthalmology
Dr Marcellus A Behr, Montreal, QC - Infectious Diseases
Dr Jacques D Belair, Saint-Georges, QC - Obstetrics & Gynecology
Dr Helene Beland-Vachon, Longueuil, QC - General Practice
Dr Robert Belanger, Chateauguay, QC - Hematological Pathology
Dr Huguette Belanger, Longueuil, QC - General Practice
Dr Jean-Francois Belanger, Mont-Joli, QC - General Practice
Dr Yvan Belanger, Rimouski, QC - Pediatrics
Dr Guy-Alain Belanger, Sainte-Catherine, QC - General Practice
Dr Helene Belanger-Bonneau, Saint-Jerome, QC - Community Medicine
Dr Robert A Beldavs, Winnipeg, MB - Ophthalmology
Dr Denise Belisle, Montreal, QC - General Practice
Dr James F Beliveau, Kingston, ON - Family Medicine
Dr Lionel Beliveau, Mont-Royal, QC - Psychiatry
Dr Pierre Belle-Isle, Plessisville, QC - General Practice
Dr Louis Bellemare, Amos, QC - Orthopedic Surgery
Dr Emmanuel Belley, Mont-Laurier, QC - Family Medicine
Dr Daniel J Belliveau, Halifax, NS - Ophthalmology
Dr Leila Ben Amor, Levis, QC - General Practice
Dr Arie Benchetrit, Pointe-Claire, QC - General Surgery
Dr Catherine Benes, Toronto, ON - Psychiatry
Dr Jaimes-S. Benhamron, Montreal, QC - Gastroenterology
Dr Philippe Benoit, Saint-Hyacinthe, QC - General Practice
Dr Patricia Berbari, Gatineau, QC - Plastic Surgery
Dr Joanne E Bergens, Edmonton, AB - Family Medicine
Dr Chantal Bergeron, Gatineau, QC - Family Medicine
Dr Marc-Yves Bergeron, Montmagny, QC - General Practice
Dr Celine Bergeron, Montreal, QC - Internal Medicine
Dr Pierre Bergeron, Montreal, QC - Community Medicine
Dr Jean Bergeron, Quebec, QC - Medical Biochemistry
Dr Dan Bergeron, Quebec, QC - Ophthalmology
Dr Rodney M Bergh, Ottawa, ON - Pediatrics
Dr Howard Bergman, Montreal, QC - Family Medicine
Dr Richard G Bergstrom, Edmonton, AB - Anesthesia

Dr Bruno Bernardin, Montreal, QC - Emergency Medicine
Dr Mario F Bernier, Laval, QC - Plastic Surgery
Dr Gilles P Bernier, Montreal, QC - Electroencephal
Dr Denyse Bernier, Quebec, QC - General Practice
Dr Vincent Bernier, Quebec, QC - Anatomical Pathology
Dr Danielle A Bernier, St-Jean-Sur-Richel, QC - Obstetrics & Gynecology
Dr Andre Bernier, Trois-Rivieres, QC - Diagnostic-Radiology
Dr Lucie M Bernier-Lycka, Edmonton, AB - Family Medicine
Dr Marc Berthiaume, Ottawa, ON - Family Medicine
Dr Yves Berthiaume, Montreal, QC - Respirology
Dr Sylvie Berthiaume, Montreal, QC - Family Medicine
Dr Claude Berthiaume, Salaber-de-Valleyf, QC - General Practice
Dr Henri A Bertrand, Maniwaki, QC - General Practice
Dr Michel Bertrand, Montreal, QC - Internal Medicine
Dr Olivier Bertrand, Quebec, QC - General Practice
Dr Michel J A Berube, Cap-aux-Meules, QC - Internal Medicine
Dr Jocelyn Berube, Rimouski, QC - General Practice
Dr Martine Berube, Sherbrooke, QC - Psychiatry
Dr Louis Bessette, Quebec, QC - Internal Medicine
Dr Paul Bessette, Sherbrooke, QC - Obstetrics & Gynecology
Dr Brian G Bexton, Montreal, QC - Psychiatry
Dr Subramanya Bhagavatula, Sudbury, ON - Psychiatry
Dr Luc Bherer, Quebec, QC - General Practice
Dr Antonio U Bianchini, LaSalle, QC - Family Medicine
Dr Daniel Bichet, Montreal, QC - Internal Medicine
Dr Eric Bicrell, Montreal, QC - General Practice
Dr Genevieve Bienvenu, Gatineau, QC - General Practice
Dr Rino Bier, Montreal, QC - Diagnostic-Radiology
Dr Eric Bigelow, Nepean, ON - General Surgery
Dr Jean-Marc Bigonnesse, Sherbrooke, QC - Family Medicine
Dr Jean-Sebastien Billiard, Montreal, QC - Diagnostic-Radiology
Dr David Billings, Southampton, ON - Emergency Family Med
Dr Marc Bilodeau, Montreal, QC - Gastroenterology
Dr Luc Bilodeau, Montreal, QC - Cardiology
Dr Jacques Binet, St-Jean-sur-Richel, QC - General Practice
Dr J Richard F Binette, Peterborough, ON - Family Medicine
Dr Patricia Ę Birk, Winnipeg, MB - Nephrology
Dr Barbara M Birkett, Milton, ON - Dermatology
Dr Debra S Birnbaum, North York, ON - Family Medicine
Dr Robert J Birnbaum, Ottawa, ON - Family Medicine
Dr Daniel Biron, Drummondville, QC - Family Medicine
Dr Clare E Bishop, Ottawa, ON - Family Medicine
Dr Tarek A Bismar, Calgary, AB - General Practice
Dr Cédric Bisson, Montreal, QC - Family Medicine
Dr Louis Bissonnette, Farnham, QC - Family Medicine
Dr Bernard F Bissonnette, Montreal, QC - Internal Medicine
Dr Alain Bissonnette, Quebec, QC - General Practice
Dr Martine Bissonnette, Sherbrooke, QC - General Practice
Dr Daniel O Black, Quebec, QC - Ophthalmology
Dr Philippe Blais, Brossard, QC - General Practice
Dr Francine Blais, Gatineau, QC - Obstetrics & Gynecology
Dr Bernard Blais, Quebec, QC - General Practice
Dr Johanne Blais, Quebec, QC - Family Medicine
Dr Andre Blais, Rimouski, QC - Hematology
Dr Stephanie Blais-Boilard, Cookshire-Eaton, QC - Emergency Family Med
Dr Luc Blanchet, Montreal, QC - Psychiatry
Dr Sylvain Blanchet, Quebec, QC - Family Medicine
Dr Pierre Blanchet, Quebec, QC - Obstetrics & Gynecology
Dr Richard Blanchet, Riviere-Du-Loup, QC - General Surgery
Dr Tania Blanchette, Courcelette, QC - Psychiatry
Dr Suzanne Blanchette, Laval, QC - Pediatrics
Dr France Blanchette, Longueuil, QC - General Practice
Dr David Blanchette, Montreal, QC - Orthopedic Surgery
Dr Christine Blanchette, Roberval, QC - Pediatrics
Dr Pierre J Blanchette, Trois-Rivieres, QC - Hematology
Dr Myles K Blank, Vancouver, BC - Psychiatry
Dr Maria Blanque Martinez, Montreal, QC - General Practice
Dr Marc P Blayney, Sudbury, ON - Pediatrics
Dr Pierre Bleau, Montreal, QC - Psychiatry
Dr Jean Blier, Ottawa, ON - Anesthesia
Dr Rita J M Blom, Parksville, BC - Diagnostic-Radiology
Dr Fernand Blondeau, Quebec, QC - Family Medicine
Dr Gerald G Blunt, Englehart, ON - General Practice
Dr Rebecca Bodok, Bolton, ON - Family Medicine
Dr Marc A Boileau, North Vancouver, BC - Family Medicine
Dr Jacques Boileau, Montreal, QC - Hematological Pathology
Dr Michel Boileau, Montreal, QC - General Practice
Dr Miriam E Boillat, Montreal, QC - Family Medicine
Dr Diane Boisselle, Quebec, QC - General Practice
Dr Mariette Boisvert, Gatineau, QC - Pediatrics
Dr Caroline Boisvert, St-Jerome, QC - General Practice
Dr Jean-François Boivin, Montreal, QC - Community Medicine
Dr Grlica Bolesnikov, Fredericton, NB - General Practice
Dr Raoul I L Bonan, Montreal, QC - Cardiology
Dr Melanie Bonin, London, ON - Family Medicine
Dr Pierre Bonin, Sudbury, ON - Family Medicine
Dr Michel L Bonin, Sudbury, ON - General Pathology
Dr Nathalie Bonneville, Saint-Eustache, QC - General Practice
Dr Yves Bonnier-Viger, Sainte-Marie, QC - Community Medicine
Dr Marie-Josee Bordeleau, Ottawa, ON - Family Medicine
Dr Serge Bordeleau, Quebec, QC - General Practice
Dr Celine Bordeleau, Trois-Pistoles, QC - Family Medicine
Dr Jacinthe Bordeleau, Trois-Pistoles, QC - General Practice
Dr J Andre Borduas, Hawkesbury, ON - Family Medicine
Dr Francois Borgeat, Montreal, QC - Psychiatry
Dr Illya C Boridy, Calgary, AB - Diagnostic-Radiology
Dr Rainer H Borkenhagen, Vancouver, BC - Family Medicine
Dr Charles Bou Farah, Sorel-Tracy, QC - General Practice
Dr Marie Bouchard, Edmundston, NB - General Practice
Dr Francoise Bouchard, Kuujjuaq, QC - Community Medicine
Dr Andre Bouchard, La Malbaie, QC - General Practice
Dr Manon Bouchard, Levis, QC - Neurology
Dr Jacques Bouchard, Longueuil, QC - Psychiatry
Dr Josee Bouchard, Pohenegamook, QC - General Practice
Dr Isabelle Bouchard, Quebec, QC - Pediatrics
Dr Maurice Bouchard, Quebec, QC - Pediatrics
Dr Roger Bouchard, Rimouski, QC - Obstetrics & Gynecology
Dr Belkacem Bouchek, Amos, QC - General Practice
Dr Catherine Boucher, Ottawa, ON - Psychiatry
Dr Julie M Boucher, Longueuil, QC - Family Medicine
Dr Anne Boucher, Montreal, QC - Internal Medicine
Dr Serge S B Boucher, Quebec, QC - Respirology
Dr Francois Boucher, Quebec, QC - Pediatrics
Dr Rejean Boucher, Quebec, QC - General Practice
Dr Marie-Claude Boucher, Saint-Polycarpe, QC - Family Medicine
Dr Emilie Boucher-Gagne, Chandler, QC - General Practice
Dr Richard Boudreau, Riviere-du-Loup, QC - Community Medicine
Dr Isabelle Boudreault, Gatineau, QC - General Practice
Dr Gerald Bouffard, St-Redempteur, QC - Family Medicine
Dr Michael J Bouhadana, Montreal, QC - Family Medicine
Dr Mickael Bouin, Montreal, QC - General Practice
Dr Aladin E Boulad, Laval, QC - General Practice
Dr Jean Boulanger, Quebec, QC - Dermatology
Dr Michel J Boulanger Jr., Edmonton, AB - Emergency Medicine
Dr Daniel Boulet, Quebec, QC - Physical Medicine & Rehab
Dr Patrick R Boulos, Sherbrooke, QC - Ophthalmology
Dr Ibrahim Bounatiro, Pointe-Claire, QC - General Practice
Dr Marie-Claude Bourassa, Granby, QC - Psychiatry
Dr Claude E Bourassa, Mansonville, QC - Family Medicine
Dr Dominique Bourassa, Rimouski, QC - General Practice
Dr Jean Bourbeau, Montreal, QC - Internal Medicine
Dr Christine Bourbonniere, Gatineau, QC - Family Medicine
Dr Andre Bourbonniere, Laval, QC - General Practice
Dr Raymond Bourdages, Levis, QC - Gastroenterology
Dr Danielle Bourdeau, Toronto, ON - Psychiatry
Dr Christian Bourdy, Montreal, QC - General Practice
Dr Klere Bourgault, Verner, ON - Family Medicine
Dr Judith Bourgault, La Tuque, QC - General Practice
Dr Michel Bourgoin, Dieppe, NB - General Surgery
Dr Kevin E Bourke, Halifax, NS - General Practice
Dr Jean-Andre Bourque, Caraquet, NB - General Practice
Dr Berthier Bourque, Saint-Georges, QC - General Practice
Dr Asmae Boutaleb, Montreal, QC - General Practice
Dr Alain Bouthat, Longueuil, QC - General Practice
Dr Jean Bouthillier, Gatineau, QC - General Practice
Dr Renee Bouthillier, Montreal, QC - Pediatrics
Dr Christine Boutin, Montreal, QC - Cardiology
Dr Stefan R Boyle, Petawawa, ON - Family Medicine
Dr William R Bradley, Dartmouth, NS - Family Medicine
Dr Robert W Bradstock, Edmonton, AB - Family Medicine
Dr Jacques Bradwejn, Ottawa, ON - Psychiatry
Dr Michel P Brassard, Quebec, QC - General Practice
Dr Richard Brassard, Sept-Iles, QC - General Practice
Dr Jacques-Christian Brault, Pohenegamook, QC - General Practice
Dr Yves Brault, Quebec, QC - Physical Medicine & Rehab
Dr John C Bray, Pointe-Claire, QC - Obstetrics & Gynecology
Dr Karlina A Breikss, Victoria, BC - Pediatrics
Dr Martin A M Breton, Calgary, AB - Family Medicine
Dr Chantal Breton, Pointe-Claire, QC - Family Medicine
Dr Yvon Bricault, Laval, QC - General Practice
Dr Josee Briere, Beauharnois, QC - General Practice
Dr Claude Brissette, Saint-Jerome, QC - General Practice
Dr Paul Brisson, Orleans, ON - Dermatology
Dr Henri Brisson, Longueuil, QC - Psychiatry
Dr Michel Brisson, Quebec, QC - General Practice
Dr Francois Brochet, Chicoutimi, QC - General Practice
Dr Jocelyne Brochu, Montreal, QC - Ophthalmology
Dr Gordon I Brock, Temiscaming, QC - Family Medicine
Dr Elizabeth J Brodkin, Surrey, BC - Community Medicine
Dr Stephen C Brodovsky, Winnipeg, MB - Ophthalmology
Dr Sorel L Brohovici, Montreal, QC - General Practice
Dr Lisa A Bromley, Ottawa, ON - Family Medicine
Dr Michel Brossard, Thetford Mines, QC - General Practice
Dr Anais Brosseau-Roberge, St-Charles-Brromee, QC - Obstetrics & Gynecology
Dr Michel Brouillet, Sherbrooke, QC - General Practice
Dr Johanne Brouillette, Levis, QC - Psychiatry
Dr France Brouillette, Montreal-Est, QC - General Practice
Dr Maryleen Brouw, Quebec, QC - General Practice
Dr Dean V Brown, West Vancouver, BC - Emergency Family Med
Dr D Stephen Brown, Moncton, NB - General Surgery
Dr Basil S Brown, Digby, NS - Diagnostic-Radiology
Dr C Elizabeth A Brown, Brockville, ON - Emergency Family Med
Dr Pierre Brown, Gatineau, QC - General Practice
Dr Linda D Brown-Thomson, Kingston, ON - Family Medicine
Dr Claude Bruneau, Saint-Redempteur, QC - General Practice
Dr Denis Brunet, Quebec, QC - Neurology
Dr Sylvain Brunet, Saint-Hyacinthe, QC - Internal Medicine
Dr Alessandra Bruns, Sherbrooke, QC - General Practice
Dr Lizabeth A Brydon, Regina, SK - Obstetrics & Gynecology
Dr Wanda T Brzezinski, Westmount, QC - General Practice
Dr Raffaele Bucci, Saint-Leonard, QC - General Practice
Dr Daniela Bucur, Montreal, QC - General Practice
Dr Sharon E Buehner, Sault Ste. Marie, ON - Emergency Family Med
Dr Linh-Khue Bui, Longueuil, QC - Electroencephal
Dr Robert Buie, Dundas, ON - Psychiatry
Dr Marie-Claire Bujold, Orleans, ON - Family Medicine
Dr Yanick Bureau, Ville-Marie, QC - General Practice
Dr Michael Burger, St Catharines, ON - Pediatrics
Dr Susan C Burgess, Vancouver, BC - Family Medicine
Dr Tracy A Burgess, Orleans, ON - Family Medicine
Dr Gerard M Burns, Kanata, ON - General Practice
Dr Kevin D Burns, Ottawa, ON - Internal Medicine
Dr M Shayne Burwell, Saskatoon, SK - Plastic Surgery
Dr Denis Busque, Grand-Mere, QC - General Practice
Dr Alan J Byrne, Oakville, ON - General Surgery
Dr Francois Cabana, Sherbrooke, QC - Orthopedic Surgery
Dr Louise Cabana, Sherbrooke, QC - Family Medicine
Dr Louise Cadoret, Chateauguay, QC - General Practice
Dr Forrest H Caldwell, Guelph, ON - Family Medicine
Dr Todd C R Calhoun, North York, ON - Anesthesia
Dr Terrence S Callanan, St. John's, NL - Psychiatry
Dr Lynn C Calvert, Burlington, ON - General Practice
Dr Peter R Camfield, Halifax, NS - Neurology
Dr Sophie Camire, Bathurst, NB - Family Medicine
Dr Pierre Camire, Montreal, QC - General Practice
Dr Pamela C Campbell, Calgary, AB - Family Medicine
Dr Marcelo Cantarovich, Montreal, QC - Nephrology
Dr Marie-Andree Cantin, Montreal, QC - Orthopedic Surgery
Dr Jerome Cantin, Shawinigan-Sud, QC - Obstetrics & Gynecology
Dr Louise Caouette-Laberge, Montreal, QC - Plastic Surgery

Dr Paul S Cappon, Ottawa, ON - Community Medicine
Dr Bernice M Capusten, Red Deer, AB - Diagnostic-Radiology
Dr Heloise Cardinal, Montreal, QC - Internal Medicine
Dr Jacqueline Carignan, Quebec, QC - Ophthalmology
Dr Maureen T Carlier, Ottawa, ON - Anatomical Pathology
Dr Robert C Carlin, Montreal, QC - Family Medicine
Dr Carole Caron, Alma, QC - Anatomical Pathology
Dr Michel Caron, Gatineau, QC - General Practice
Dr Josee Caron, Montreal, QC - General Surgery
Dr Daniel C Caron, Montreal, QC - Endocrinology
Dr Dominique Caron, Saint-Bruno, QC - Family Medicine
Dr Christine Caron, Saint-Lambert, QC - General Practice
Dr Genevieve Caron-Fauconnier, Saint-Georges, QC - Family Medicine
Dr Marie-Pierre Carpentier, Ottawa, ON - Emergency Family Med
Dr Julie Carrier, Moncton, NB - Family Medicine
Dr Daniel A Carrier, Levis, QC - Family Medicine
Dr Christian Carrier, Trois-Rivieres, QC - Hematology
Dr Jacques Carriere, Quebec, QC - Psychiatry
Dr Katharine D Carson, Ottawa, ON - Family Medicine
Dr Christopher J Carter, Gatineau, QC - Orthopedic Surgery
Dr Marie Cartier, Granby, QC - General Practice
Dr Andre Cartier, Montreal, QC - Respirology
Dr Julie Castonguay, Edmundston, NB - Family Medicine
Dr Richard F H Catchlove, Montreal, QC - General Practice
Dr Florina Cealicu Toma, Gatineau, QC - Psychiatry
Dr Kathlyn Celestin, Montreal, QC - Family Medicine
Dr Maria Cernica, Verdun, QC - General Practice
Dr Francoise Chagnon, Montreal, QC - Otolaryngology
Dr Michel Chagnon, Montreal, QC - General Surgery
Dr Marybelle M T Chain-Chang, Brampton, ON - General Practice
Dr Bachar Chalati, Stewiacke, NS - General Practice
Dr Robert Chalifour, Ottawa, ON - General Practice
Dr Colin H Chalk, Montreal, QC - Neurology
Dr Susan M Chamberlain, Kingston, ON - Obstetrics & Gynecology
Dr Elaine M C Champagne, Cote Saint-Luc, QC - Pediatrics
Dr Francois Champagne, Drummondville, QC - General Practice
Dr Ginette Champagne, Montreal, QC - General Practice
Dr Myriam Champagne, Terrebonne, QC - Emergency Family Med
Dr Adrien M T Chan, Thunder Bay, ON - Internal Medicine
Dr Chan-San H Chan-Tai-Kong, Lloydminster, AB - General Practice
Dr A Joseph Chan-Tai-Kong, Regina, SK - Anesthesia
Dr Gilles R Chaput, Montreal, QC - Ophthalmology
Dr Fabien A Charbonneau, Campbellville, ON - General Practice
Dr Jacques Charbonneau, Gatineau, QC - Dermatology
Dr Jean Charbonneau, Mont-Saint-Hilaire, QC - General Practice
Dr Myriam Charbonneau, Quebec, QC - General Practice
Dr Michel Charest, Montreal, QC - General Practice
Dr Francois G Charette, Longueuil, QC - General Practice
Dr Ali Charghi, Montreal, QC - Urology
Dr Raymond P Charland, Montreal, QC - Cardiology
Dr Pierre Charland, Sorel-Tracy, QC - Diagnostic-Radiology
Dr Marco Charneux, Montreal, QC - Critical Care Medicine
Dr Jean-Claude Chartier, Quebec, QC - General Practice
Dr Raymonde Chartrand, Montreal, QC - Nuclear Medicine
Dr Hughes Chasse, Ottawa, ON - Psychiatry
Dr Sylvie Chateauvert, Quebec, QC - General Practice
Dr Marc J Chayer, Lindsay, ON - General Practice
Dr Mustapha Chelfi, Gatineau, QC - General Practice
Dr Rene Chemaly, Montreal, QC - Obstetrics & Gynecology
Dr Darin P Cherniwchan, Chilliwack, BC - Family Medicine
Dr Tracey M Chesser, Moncton, NB - Emergency Family Med
Dr Philippe Chessex, Montreal, QC - Pediatrics
Dr Vincent S J Cheung, Peterborough, ON - Internal Medicine
Dr Marie-Lise Chiasson, Caraquet, NB - General Practice
Dr Paul Chiasson, Dieppe, NB - Family Medicine
Dr Renelle Chiasson, Tracadie-Sheila, NB - Family Medicine
Dr J Roland Chiasson, Summerside, PE - General Practice
Dr Jean-P. Chiasson, Mont-Royal, QC - General Practice
Dr Renee Chiasson-Basque, Lameque, NB - General Practice
Dr Madeleine Chicha-Dzineku, Montreal, QC - Anesthesia
Dr Margareta Chiorpec-Georgescu, Lachute, QC - General Practice
Dr Andre Chollet, Montreal, QC - Plastic Surgery
Dr Edmond E Chouinard, Cambridge, ON - Internal Medicine
Dr Guy Chouinard, Quebec, QC - General Practice
Dr Sylvain R Chouinard, Quebec, QC - Internal Medicine
Dr David R Chow, Toronto, ON - Ophthalmology
Dr Moy Fee Chow Siet Yam, Brossard, QC - General Practice
Dr Michel Chretien, Ottawa, ON - Endocrin/Metabolism
Dr Janet E Christie-Seely, Nepean, ON - Family Medicine
Dr Joseph Y C Chu, Etobicoke, ON - Internal Medicine
Dr Pierre Chue, Edmonton, AB - Psychiatry
Dr Margaret A Churcher, Calgary, AB - Family Medicine
Dr Mark H C Churman, Haileybury, ON - Family Medicine
Dr Mario V Ciccone, Timmins, ON - Emergency Family Med
Dr Michelle Cinq-Mars, Sorel-Tracy, QC - General Practice
Dr Michelle P Cipera, Kuujjuarapik, QC - Family Medicine
Dr Sharon L Cirone, Toronto, ON - Emergency Family Med
Dr Brenda G Clark, Edmonton, AB - Pediatrics
Dr Leigh L Clarke, Pembroke, ON - General Practice
Dr Terrence Clarke, Gatineau, QC - General Practice
Dr Richard L Claveau, Hearst, ON - Family Medicine
Dr Jacques Claveau, Sorel-Tracy, QC - Obstetrics & Gynecology
Maj Martin Clavet, Quebec, QC - Family Medicine
Dr Paul F Clavette, Edmundston, NB - Internal Medicine
Dr Gerald S Clayden, Carman, MB - General Practice
Dr Pierre Clement, Ottawa, ON - Psychiatry
Dr Marie-Jose Clermont, Montreal, QC - Nephrology
Dr David R Cleveland, Penticton, BC - Internal Medicine
Dr Nancy A Clevette, Ottawa, ON - Family Medicine
Dr Yves J J Clouatre, Penticton, BC - Internal Medicine
Dr Robert Cloutier, Magog, QC - General Practice
Dr Richard Cloutier, Montreal, QC - Psychiatry
Dr Fernand Cloutier, Quebec, QC - General Practice
Dr Guylene Cloutier, Rouyn-Noranda, QC - Psychiatry
Dr Leslie A Cockhill, Vancouver, BC - Psychiatry
Dr Marianne Codsi, Laval, QC - Family Medicine
Dr Alan J H Coffey, Montreal, QC - Ophthalmology
Dr Samantha J Cogan, Etobicoke, ON - Family Medicine
Dr Mark J Cohen, Toronto, ON - Ophthalmology
Dr Stephen S Cohen, Whitby, ON - Family Medicine
Dr Jack Cohen, Montreal, QC - Plastic Surgery
Dr Albert Cohen, Montreal, QC - Gastroenterology
Dr Sandra R A Cohen, Montreal, QC - Hematology
Dr Rolande M Colas, Moncton, NB - General Practice
Dr David C Collins, Orillia, ON - General Practice
Dr Sophie Collins, Montreal, QC - Anesthesia
Dr Nathalie Comeau, Mercier, QC - General Practice
Dr Louise M Comeau, Pte-aux-Trembles, QC - General Practice
Dr Stuart J Connolly, Hamilton, ON - Cardiology
Dr Steven A Connor, Cobourg, ON - General Practice
Dr Nathalie Cook, Ottawa, ON - Pediatrics
Dr Terrance Cooligan, Toronto, ON - Internal Medicine
Dr John F Coombs, Fallbrook, ON - General Practice
Dr Jean M Corbin, New Liskeard, ON - Family Medicine
Dr Serge Corbin, Roxton Pond, QC - General Practice
Dr Francois Corbin, Sherbrooke, QC - Medical Biochemistry
Dr Gilles J Cormier, Dieppe, NB - Ophthalmology
Dr Helene Cormier, Saint-Georges, QC - General Practice
Dr Charline Cormier, Sherbrooke, QC - General Practice
Dr Richard A Cornell, Collingwood, ON - Emergency Family Med
Dr Marc M Corriveau, Montreal, QC - General Surgery
Dr Maria D P Cortes Nino, Montreal, QC - General Practice
Dr Nicole Cossette-Poirier, Levis, QC - Diagnostic-Radiology
Dr Isabelle Cote, Hamilton, ON - Psychiatry
Dr Genevieve L Cote, Orleans, ON - Family Medicine
Dr Jean Cote, Timmins, ON - Family Medicine
Dr Remi Cote, Chambly, QC - General Practice
Dr Annie Cote, Chicoutimi, QC - Family Medicine
Dr Jean R Cote, Mirabel, QC - Dermatology
Dr Nathalie Cote, Montreal, QC - General Practice
Dr Sylvie Cote, Montreal, QC - General Practice
Dr Johanne Cote, Quebec, QC - Internal Medicine
Dr Louise Cote, Quebec, QC - Family Medicine
Dr Isabelle M H Cote, Quebec, QC - Physical Medicine & Rehab
Dr Andre Cote, Riviere-du-Loup, QC - Otolaryngology
Dr Manon Cote, Saint-Laurent, QC - Family Medicine
Dr Michel J Cote, Sherbrooke, QC - Obstetrics & Gynecology
Dr G Thomas Cottreau, Charlottetown, PE - General Surgery
Dr Michael P Coughlin, Windsor, ON - General Surgery
Dr Larry P Coughlin, Dollard-D-Ormeaux, QC - Orthopedic Surgery
Capt Bernard Couillard Jr, Courcelette, QC - Emergency Family Med
Dr Louise A Coulombe, Nepean, ON - General Practice
Dr Gerald Coupal, Saint-Hubert, QC - Psychiatry
Dr Marie Courtemanche, Sherbrooke, QC - General Practice
Dr Pierre Coutu, Montreal, QC - General Practice
Dr Marianne Coutu, Sherbrooke, QC - Cardiac Surgery
Dr Elise Couture, Montreal, QC - Pediatrics
Dr Josee Couture, Montreal, QC - General Practice
Dr Francois Couture, Outremont, QC - Internal Medicine
Dr Francois Couturier, Saint-Lambert, QC - Family Medicine
Dr Nancy V Craig, Edmonton, AB - Family Medicine
Dr Douglas B Craig, Montreal, QC - Anesthesia
Dr Gordon L Crelinsten, Montreal, QC - Cardiology
Dr Rene Crepeau, Montreal, QC - Plastic Surgery
Dr Kenneth Croitoru, Toronto, ON - Gastroenterology
Dr Catherine Cronin, Kelowna, BC - Pediatrics
Dr William G Cross, Cobourg, ON - Family Medicine
Dr Stephane Croteau, Montreal, QC - General Practice
Dr Frederic Croteau, Sherbrooke, QC - Plastic Surgery
LCdr Stephen Crummey, St. John's, NL - Anesthesia
Dr Marie-Jose Cucuzza, Montreal, QC - General Practice
Dr P Maria Cudnoch, Laval, QC - Family Medicine
Dr Kate N Culman, Calgary, AB - Infectious Diseases
Dr Carl Cummings, Cote Saint-Luc, QC - Pediatrics
Dr Ina E Cummings, Dorval, QC - Family Medicine
Dr Suzanne Cummings, Montreal, QC - General Practice
Dr Gregory P Curnew, Hamilton, ON - Cardiology
Dr Jean Cusson, Greenfield Park, QC - Internal Medicine
Dr Daniel Cusson, Laval, QC - General Practice
Dr Lise Cusson, Montreal, QC - Family Medicine
Dr Diane F Cusson, Pintendre, QC - General Practice
Dr Danielle D Cutts, Regina, SK - Family Medicine
Dr Elizabeth Cvejic, Toronto, ON - Psychiatry
Dr Elizabeth Czyziw, Montreal, QC - General Practice
Dr Mario D'Annunzio, St-Eustache, QC - General Practice
Dr H Lina D'Apice, Matagami, QC - General Practice
Dr Christine L D'Arsigny, Kingston, ON - Critical Care Medicine
Dr Jacqueline R D'Eon, Pubnico, NS - General Practice
Dr Derek Da Costa, Dollard-D-Ormeaux, QC - General Practice
Dr Richard A Dabrusin, Cote Saint-Luc, QC - Respirology
Dr Georges Dadour, Montreal, QC - General Practice
Dr Olga Dafniotis, Trois-Rivieres, QC - Orthopedic Surgery
Dr Pierre Dagenais, Montreal, QC - Internal Medicine
Dr Aime Dahan, Pointe-Claire, QC - General Practice
Dr Antoine Daher, Chateauguay, QC - General Practice
Dr Sebastien Daigle, Bathurst, NB - Urology
Dr Samuel Daigle, Bathurst, NB - Family Medicine
Dr Jean-Pierre Daigle, Boucherville, QC - Plastic Surgery
Dr Steve Daigle, Sherbrooke, QC - General Practice
Dr Chrystian Dallaire, Quebec, QC - Gastroenterology
Dr Abdallah Dallal, Saint-Jerome, QC - Psychiatry
Dr Pierre M Daloze, Montreal, QC - General Surgery
Dr Michel H Dalpe-Charron, Cheneville, QC - General Practice
Dr Sharon A Dalrymple, Pointe-Claire, QC - General Surgery
Dr Douglass Dalton, Montreal, QC - Family Medicine
Dr Andrew Daly, Calgary, AB - Hematology
Dr Robin Dancose, Kirkland, QC - General Practice
Dr Dinh Quang Dang, Montreal, QC - General Practice
Dr Gail Dangoor, North York, ON - Family Medicine
Dr Sarah B Danial, Niagara Falls, ON - Psychiatry
Dr Helene Daniel, Lachine, QC - General Practice
Dr Lise Daniels, Sherbrooke, QC - General Practice
Dr Richard Danylewick, Laval, QC - General Surgery
Dr Hong Quyen Dao, Gatineau, QC - General Practice
Dr T Trang Dao, Montreal, QC - Psychiatry
Dr Nicolas Daoud, Chicoutimi, QC - Diagnostic-Radiology
Dr Marleen Daris, Quebec, QC - Obstetrics & Gynecology
Dr A Marc Dauphin, Richelain, QC - General Practice
Dr Marjolaine Daviau, Farnham, QC - Family Medicine
Dr Elizabeth Daviault, Montreal, QC - General Practice
Dr Claude David, Mont-Tremblant, QC - General Practice
Dr Julie David, Montreal, QC - Diagnostic-Radiology

Dr Marc David, Montreal, QC - Radiation Oncology
Dr Joseph K Davidson, Mississauga, ON - Ophthalmology
Dr Jan M Davies, Calgary, AB - Anesthesia
Dr Deborah J Davis, Ottawa, ON - Pediatrics
Dr Dawood G Dawood, Gloucester, ON - Obstetrics & Gynecology
Dr Lesa Dawson, St. John's, NL - Obstetrics & Gynecology
Dr Ainsley E Dawson, Toronto, ON - Endocrinology & Metabolism
Dr David J Dawson, Montreal, QC - Internal Medicine
Dr Ross C De Belle, Longueuil, QC - Pediatrics
Dr Suzanne De Blois, Montreal, QC - Community Medicine
Dr Eric De Broux, Montreal, QC - General Surgery
Dr Remi De Champlain, Gatineau, QC - Family Medicine
Dr Jean-Andre De Groot, Trois-Rivieres, QC - Ophthalmology
Dr Anne De Loppinot, Montreal, QC - General Practice
Dr Anne De Medicis, Farnham, QC - General Practice
Dr Rene De Montigny, St-Germain-D-Grant, QC - General Practice
Dr Alexandra De Pokomandy, Montreal, QC - Family Medicine
Dr Marthe De Serres, St-Gabriel-D-Brand, QC - General Practice
Dr France De Villers, Saint-Jerome, QC - Pediatrics
Dr Cheri L Deal, Montreal, QC - Endocrin/Metabolism
Dr Heather J Dean, Winnipeg, MB - Pediatrics
Dr Chaouki Debs, Drummondville, QC - Urology
Dr Jean Claude Decarie, Montreal, QC - Diagnostic-Radiology
Dr Denise Decarie, Saint-Jerome, QC - General Practice
Dr Mary Delafield, Quebec, QC - General Practice
Dr Perlita Delaney, Kingston, ON - General Practice
Dr Marie-France Delisle, Vancouver, BC - Obstetrics & Gynecology
Dr Caroline Delisle, Greenfield Park, QC - General Practice
Dr Nadia Delle Donne, Pointe-Claire, QC - Emergency Family Med
Dr Chantal Delorme, Cap-aux-Meules, QC - Ophthalmology
Dr Jocelyn Delorme, Montreal, QC - Medical Microbiology & Infectious Diseases
Dr Sophie Delorme, Montreal, QC - Endocrin/Metabolism
Dr Isabelle Delorme, Saint-Hyacinthe, QC - Dermatology
Dr Thomas J Demarco, Whistler, BC - General Practice
Dr Philippe Demers, Cowansville, QC - General Surgery
Dr Louis Demers, Gatineau, QC - General Practice
Dr Sylvie Demers, Gatineau, QC - General Practice
Dr Liliane Demers, Montreal, QC - General Practice
Dr Pierre Demers, Montreal, QC - Ophthalmology
Dr Michel C Demers, Quebec, QC - General Practice
Dr Marcel Denicourt, Mont-Saint-Hilaire, QC - General Practice
Dr Chahe B Derghazarian, Saint-Leonard, QC - Hematology
Dr Renee Dery, Montreal, QC - Diagnostic-Radiology
Dr Veronique Dery, Montreal, QC - Community Medicine
Dr Jean-Pierre Dery, Quebec, QC - Cardiology
Dr Lucie Des Parois, Greenfield Park, QC - Psychiatry
Dr Rene Desautels, Verdun, QC - Psychiatry
Dr Dominique Deschenes, Levis, QC - Internal Medicine
Dr Dominique Deschenes, Quebec, QC - Family Medicine
Dr Isabelle Deschenes, St-Jean-sur-Richel, QC - Internal Medicine
Dr Micheline Desgagne, Caplan, QC - General Practice
Dr Doris Deshaies, Montreal, QC - General Practice
Dr Jean-Francois Deshaies, Sherbrooke, QC - Emergency Family Med
Dr Celine Desjardins, Montreal, QC - Obstetrics & Gynecology
Dr Gisele Desjardins, Montreal, QC - Family Medicine
Dr Alain Desjardins, Montreal, QC - Internal Medicine
Dr Daniel C J Desjardins, Montreal, QC - Ophthalmology
Dr Monique Desjardins, Montreal, QC - Psychiatry
Dr Marco Desjardins, Trois-Rivieres, QC - General Practice
Dr Jean Deslauriers, Quebec, QC - Cardiovasc/ThorSurg
Dr Danielle Desloges, Lemoyne, QC - Orthopedic Surgery
Dr Nicole Desmarais, Hanmer, ON - Family Medicine
Dr Eric Desmarais, Chateauguay, QC - Diagnostic-Radiology
Dr Dominique Desmarais, Saint-Jerome, QC - Pediatrics
Dr Isabelle Desormeau, Laval, QC - Anesthesia
Dr Lise Desormeaux, Cote Saint-Luc, QC - Family Medicine
Dr Cathy Despres, Terrebonne, QC - General Surgery
Dr Real Desranleau, McMasterville, QC - General Practice
Dr Josee Desrochers, Montreal, QC - Family Medicine
Dr Jean-Paul Desrochers, Ste-Agathe-des-Mts, QC - General Practice
Dr Francois Desroches, East Angus, QC - General Practice
Dr Francois Dessureault, Boucherville, QC - General Practice
Dr Josee Dessureault, Quebec, QC - Dermatology
Dr M Michele Dessureault, Trois-Rivieres, QC - Internal Medicine
Dr Dominique Desy, Knowlton, QC - General Practice
Dr Madeleine Desy, Saint-Jerome, QC - Hematology
Dr Meredith Deutsch-Levy, Richmond Hill, ON - Family Medicine
Dr Carole Deveau, Moncton, NB - Family Medicine
Dr Daniela Di Iorio, Montreal, QC - Infectious Diseases
Dr Maria Di Lorenzo, Montreal, QC - Cardiology
Dr Razvan Diaconescu, Montreal, QC - Hematology
Dr Absa Diallo, Montreal, QC - General Practice
Dr Luis Victor Diaz de Bedoya, Quebec, QC - Radiation Oncology
Dr Mijanou Didier, Amqui, QC - General Practice
Dr Dubravka A Diksic, Montreal, QC - Pediatrics
Dr Lisa G Dillon, Winnipeg, MB - Family Medicine
Dr Ronald A Dimentberg, Montreal, QC - Orthopedic Surgery
Dr Emmanuel Dingemans, Saint-Jerome, QC - Anesthesia
Dr Hoang-Diep Dinh, Anjou, QC - General Practice
Dr Gerald Dion, Mistissini, QC - General Practice
Dr Jean D Dion, Mont-Tremblant, QC - General Practice
Dr Dominique Dion, Montreal, QC - General Practice
Dr Yves-Marie Dion, Quebec, QC - General Surgery
Dr Pierre Dion, Quebec, QC - General Practice
Dr Paul G Dionne, Gatineau, QC - Anatomical Pathology
Dr Renee Dionne, Gatineau, QC - Otolaryngology
Dr Michele Dionne, Pointe-Claire, QC - General Practice
Dr Marc Dionne, Quebec, QC - Community Medicine
Dr Quoc-Bao Do, Montreal, QC - Cardiac Surgery
Dr Quynh Huong Doan, Vancouver, BC - Pediatric Emergency Medicine
Dr Ly Huong Doan, Montreal, QC - General Practice
Dr Bernard K Dobovicnik, Trail, BC - General Practice
Dr Otilia-Maria Dobrescu, Montreal, QC - Pediatrics
Dr Marjorie A Docherty, Kelowna, BC - Family Medicine
Dr Anne-Marie Dollois, Pointe-Claire, QC - Family Medicine
Dr Peter J Dolman, Vancouver, BC - Ophthalmology
Dr Johanne Donati, Trois-Rivieres, QC - General Practice
Dr Julie Dorion, Quebec, QC - General Practice
Dr Dominique Dorion, Sherbrooke, QC - Otolaryngology
Dr Clare B Dossetor, Ottawa, ON - Dermatology
Dr Geoffrey E Dougherty, Montreal, QC - Community Medicine
Dr Pierre Douville, Quebec, QC - Medical Biochemistry
Dr Yvan Douville, Quebec, QC - General Surgery
Dr Monique Douville-Fradet, Quebec, QC - Community Medicine
Dr John F C Dove, Moose Factory, ON - Family Medicine
Dr Marion Dove, Montreal, QC - Family Medicine
Dr Guy Doyon, Sherbrooke, QC - Ophthalmology
Dr Marie-Lucie Doyon, Westmount, QC - Diagnostic-Radiology
Dr Anne Draginda, Edmonton, AB - Family Medicine
Dr C Lewis W Draper, Regina, SK - Family Medicine
Dr Danny Dreige, Baie-Comeau, QC - Ophthalmology
Dr Valerie Dreyfuss, St-Jean-sur-Richel, QC - Psychiatry
Dr Celyne Drolet, Montreal, QC - General Practice
Dr Johanne F Drouin, Edmonton, AB - Family Medicine
Dr Yves Drouin, Drummondville, QC - Diagnostic-Radiology
Dr Eric Drouin, Montreal, QC - Gastroenterology
Dr Jean Drouin, Quebec, QC - General Practice
Dr Christian A Drouin, Riviere-Du-Loup, QC - Dermatology
Dr Marietjie Du Plessis, Salmon Arm, BC - General Practice
Dr Bertrand Du Souich, Montreal, QC - General Practice
Dr Chantal J Du Vernet, Smiths Falls, ON - Emergency Family Med
Dr Marc DuPere, Toronto, ON - Plastic Surgery
Dr Pascale Dube, Amos, QC - Ophthalmology
Dr Robert Dube, Quebec, QC - Anatomical Pathology
Dr Rejean Dube, Quebec, QC - Gastroenterology
Dr Francois Dube, Quebec, QC - Internal Medicine
Dr Christian Dube, Rouyn-Noranda, QC - Psychiatry
Dr Suzy Dubois, Chicoutimi, QC - Obstetrics & Gynecology
Dr Chantal Dubois, St-Roch-de-l'Achig, QC - Family Medicine
Dr Marc Dubuc, Montreal, QC - Cardiology
Dr Sylvain Duchaine, Trenton, ON - General Practice
Dr Morency Duchastel, Montreal, QC - General Practice
Dr Line Duchesne, Joliette, QC - Internal Medicine
Dr Andre Duchesne, Longueuil, QC - General Practice
Dr Lucie Duclos, Montreal, QC - Plastic Surgery
Dr Madeleine Duclos, Montreal, QC - Family Medicine
Dr Genevieve M Ducros, Astra, ON - Family Medicine
Dr Emmanuelle M J Dudon, Riviere-Du-Loup, QC - Orthopedic Surgery
Dr Daniel M Dufour, Brockville, ON - Family Medicine
Dr Anne Dufour, Quebec, QC - General Practice
Dr Marcel Dufour, Quebec, QC - Orthopedic Surgery
Dr Maurice J A Dufresne, Ottawa, ON - General Practice
Dr Jean-Claude Dufresne, Laval, QC - General Practice
Dr Roger A Dufresne, Montreal, QC - Psychiatry
Dr Serge Dufresne, Montreal, QC - Family Medicine
Dr Louis R Dufresne, Quebec, QC - Internal Medicine
Dr Diane Dufresne, Roberval, QC - Otolaryngology
Dr Jean Dufresne, Sherbrooke, QC - Hematology
Dr Ludivine Dugas, Mont-Laurier, QC - General Practice
Dr Luc-Antoine Dugas, Rimouski, QC - Orthopedic Surgery
Dr Annie Duguay, Bonaventure, QC - Family Medicine
Dr Robert Dumais, Sudbury, ON - Anesthesia
Dr Francois Dumas, Maria, QC - Pediatrics
Dr Jean F Dumas, Repentigny, QC - General Practice
Dr Guy Dumas, St-Leonard-d'Aston, QC - General Practice
Dr Luiza A A Dumitrescu, Ste-Agathe-Des-Mts, QC - Psychiatry
Dr Julie Dumont, Chicoutimi, QC - Obstetrics & Gynecology
Dr Luc Dumont, Thetford Mines, QC - Orthopedic Surgery
Dr David Dupere, Halifax, NS - Internal Medicine
Dr Raymond Duperval, Sherbrooke, QC - Internal Medicine
Dr Jacinthe Dupont, Quebec, QC - General Practice
Dr Marguerite Dupre, Montreal, QC - Emergency Medicine
Dr Isabelle Dupuis, Ste-Anne-Madawaska, NB - Family Medicine
Dr Jean-Yves Dupuis, Ottawa, ON - Anesthesia
Dr Martine Dupuis, Laval, QC - General Practice
Dr Robert Dupuis, Thetford Mines, QC - Internal Medicine
Dr Emilie Dupuis-Riendeau, Gaspe, QC - Family Medicine
Dr Jacques A Duranceau, Bromont, QC - Physical Medicine & Rehab
Dr Marie-Josee Durand, LaSalle, QC - General Practice
Dr France Durocher, Laval, QC - Obstetrics & Gynecology
Dr Martin Dussault, Baie-Saint-Paul, QC - Psychiatry
Dr Jan P Dutz, Vancouver, BC - Dermatology
Dr Louis-Rene Duval, Sept-Iles, QC - General Practice
Dr Nicolas Duval, Vimont, QC - Orthopedic Surgery
Dr Gary S Dvorkin, Verdun, QC - Neurology
Dr Michael Dworkind, Montreal, QC - Family Medicine
Dr Katrina Eastwood, Kingston, ON - General Practice
Dr Donald Echenberg, Sherbrooke, QC - Internal Medicine
Dr Patrick Eddie, Bathurst, NB - Family Medicine
Dr Chaim Z I Edelstein, Montreal, QC - Ophthalmology
Dr Melvin L Edgar, Vancouver, BC - Family Medicine
Dr Donna F Edwards, North York, ON - Family Medicine
Dr Clovis Eid, Moncton, NB - Ophthalmology
Dr Jouhaina Eid, Montreal, QC - Nephrology
Dr David Eiley, Pointe-Claire, QC - Urology
Dr Mark J Eisenberg, Montreal, QC - Cardiology
Dr Elias El-Salibi, Alexandria, ON - Family Medicine
Dr David A Elias, Grand-Bay-Wesfld, NB - Emergency Family Med
Dr Kathryn D Elie, Lachine, QC - Medical Microbiology
Dr Sonia Eliev, Gracefield, QC - Family Medicine
Dr Denise M Elliott, Ottawa, ON - Family Medicine
Dr Josee Ellyson, Sherbrooke, QC - General Practice
Dr Andrew P Ember, Ottawa, ON - Family Medicine
Dr France Emery, Terrebonne, QC - General Practice
Dr Anne Emond, Montreal, QC - Psychiatry
Dr Natalie Emond, Montreal, QC - Family Medicine
Dr Michael L Engo, Montreal, QC - Emergency Family Med
Dr Catherine M A Entwistle, Ottawa, ON - Ophthalmology
Dr Florence A Erdman, North York, ON - Psychiatry
Dr Julius Erdstein, Pierrefonds, QC - Pediatrics
Dr Patrick L Ergina, Montreal, QC - Cardiothor Surgery
Dr Philippe M Erhard, Winnipeg, MB - Family Medicine
Dr Gary P Ernest, Liverpool, NS - Family Medicine
Dr Francis L C Ervin, Maple Ridge, BC - Internal Medicine
Dr David S Esdaile, Ottawa, ON - Family Medicine

Dr Jean Ethier, Montreal, QC - Internal Medicine
Dr Lisa Evered, Edmonton, AB - Pediatrics
Dr John M Eydt, Gatineau, QC - General Practice
Dr Anne Faber, Quebec, QC - General Practice
Dr Hussein Fadlallah, Montreal, QC - Cardiology
Dr Pierre Falardeau, Montreal, QC - Nephrology
Dr Catherine Falardeau, Rouyn-Noranda, QC - Family Medicine
Dr Rejean Falardeau, Shefford, QC - General Practice
Dr Noreen Fardy, St. John's, NL - Family Medicine
Dr Justine Farley-Deschamps, Montreal, QC - General Practice
Dr Jean-Pierre Farmer, Montreal, QC - Neurosurgery
Dr Afsoon Fathollahzadeh, Oakville, ON - Pediatrics
Dr Lucien L Faucher, Ottawa, ON - Psychiatry
Dr Nacia Faure, Montreal, QC - Endocrinology
Dr Gilles Faust, Sherbrooke, QC - Gastroenterology
Dr Marc B Favreau, Montreal, QC - Internal Medicine
Dr Nabil Fawaz, Saint-Leonard, QC - General Practice
Dr Annie H Fecteau, Toronto, ON - General Surgery
Dr Stephen H Feder, Ottawa, ON - Family Medicine
Dr Erwin Feige, North Bay, ON - Family Medicine
Dr Christopher M S Feindel, Toronto, ON - Cardiovasc/ThorSurg
Dr Liane S Feldman, Montreal, QC - General Surgery
Dr Joseph Feldmann, Toronto, ON - Psychiatry
Dr Vivien Fellegi, Mississauga, ON - General Practice
Dr Jonathan A S Fenton, Richmond, BC - Orthopedic Surgery
Dr Deborah A Ferguson, Calgary, AB - Family Medicine
Dr Craig A Ferguson, Bridgewater, NS - Family Medicine
Dr Karen E Ferguson, Carp, ON - Family Medicine
Dr Gisele M C Ferguson, Saskatoon, SK - Psychiatry
Dr Nanette M Ferguson-Losier, Dartmouth, NS - General Practice
Dr Daniela Ferigutti, Gatineau, QC - Family Medicine
Dr Andre Ferland, Calgary, AB - Internal Medicine
Dr Christian Ferland, Saint-Constant, QC - Family Medicine
Dr John R Fernandes, Hamilton, ON - General Pathology
Dr Marie-Carmel Fernandez, Saint-Leonard, QC - General Practice
Dr Pasquale Ferraro, Montreal, QC - General Surgery
Dr Christian Ferremi, Laval, QC - Ophthalmology
Dr Caroline R Ferris, Surrey, BC - Family Medicine
Dr Marcel Ferron, Saint-Laurent, QC - General Practice
Dr Majed Fianni, Goderich, ON - Internal Medicine
Dr Stephen H Fichman, Montreal, QC - Ophthalmology
Dr Alexandra O Figaro, Windsor, ON - Family Medicine
Dr Lyne Filiatrault, Vancouver, BC - Emergency Medicine
Dr Liliane Filiatrault, Laval, QC - Psychiatry
Dr Denis Filiatrault, Montreal, QC - Diagnostic-Radiology
Dr Alain Filion, Quebec, QC - Hematology
Dr Marie-Josee Filteau, Quebec, QC - Psychiatry
Dr Maria Filyk, Calgary, AB - Psychiatry
Dr Geoffrey M Fine, Mississauga, ON - Emergency Family Med
Dr Allan M Finesilver, Montreal, QC - Otolaryngology
Dr Hillel M Finestone, Ottawa, ON - Physical Medicine & Rehab
Dr Caroll Fiset, Richelain, QC - General Practice
Dr Rowan Fish, Montreal, QC - Dermatology
Dr Christina M Fisher, Toronto, ON - Family Medicine
Dr Charlene D Fitzgerald, Happy-Valley-Goose, NL - Family Medicine
Dr Kelly P Fitzpatrick, Hamilton, ON - Pediatrics
Dr Francois J Flamand, Cambridge, ON - General Surgery
Dr Florence Flambert, Quebec, QC - General Practice
Dr Martine Flament, Ottawa, ON - Psychiatry
Dr Cathy Flanagan, New Westminster, BC - Internal Medicine
Dr John F Flannery, Toronto, ON - Physical Medicine & Rehab
Dr David M Fleiszer, Montreal, QC - General Surgery
Dr Karen E Fleming, Toronto, ON - Family Medicine
Dr Alain Fleury, St-Charles-Brromee, QC - General Surgery
Dr William Flexer, Edmonton, AB - Anesthesia
Dr Alberto L Flores-Vargas, Scarborough, ON - General Practice
Dr Anne-Josee Flynn, Quebec, QC - Family Medicine
Dr Finola M Fogarty, Edmonton, AB - Psychiatry
Dr Curtis S Folkerson, Wakefield, QC - Family Medicine
Dr Jean-Yves Fontaine, Quebec, QC - Obstetrics & Gynecology
Dr John R Foote, Toronto, ON - Emergency Family Med
Dr Daniel Forest, Saint-Jerome, QC - General Practice
Dr Marie-Chantal Forget, Longueuil, QC - Family Medicine
Dr Sylviane Forget, Montreal, QC - Gastroenterology
Dr Melissa A Forgie, Ottawa, ON - Hematology
Dr Bertram Forse, Markham, ON - General Practice
Dr Pierre Fortier, Gatineau, QC - Family Medicine
Dr Suzanne Fortin, Gatineau, QC - General Practice
Dr Anne Fortin, Lasalle, QC - Obstetrics & Gynecology
Dr Claude A Fortin, Lasalle, QC - Obstetrics & Gynecology
Dr Bernard Fortin, Montreal, QC - Radiation Oncology
Dr Isabelle Fortin, Rimouski, QC - Internal Medicine
Dr J B Christian Fortin, Saint-Lambert, QC - Cardiology
Dr Michel R Fortin, Shawinigan-Sud, QC - Otolaryngology
Dr Nathalie Foucault, Drummondville, QC - Pediatrics
Dr Annick V Fournier, Ottawa, ON - Ophthalmology
Dr Karl Fournier, Lemoyne, QC - Orthopedic Surgery
Dr Paul J R Fournier, Montreal, QC - Obstetrics & Gynecology
Dr Renee Fournier, Montreal, QC - Family Medicine
Dr Johanne Fournier, Montreal, QC - Family Medicine
Dr Christiane Fournier, Quebec, QC - Psychiatry
Dr Brigitte Fournier, Sainte-Marie, QC - General Practice
Dr Andre Fournier, St-Jean-Sur-Richel, QC - Otolaryngology
Dr Guy Fournier, Westmount, QC - Orthopedic Surgery
Dr Jonathan R Fox, Fall River, NS - Family Medicine
Dr Catharine Foyle, Calgary, AB - Family Medicine
Dr Vincent Fradet, Quebec, QC - Urology
Dr Jeffrey M Franc-Law, Edmonton, AB - Emergency Family Med
Dr Marie-Josee Francoeur, Greenfield Park, QC - Clin Immun/Allergy
Dr Jacques Francoeur, Quebec, QC - Neurosurgery
Dr Jose M G Francois, Winnipeg, MB - Family Medicine
Dr William D Fraser, Montreal, QC - Obstetrics & Gynecology
Dr Robert Frazer, Sherbrooke, QC - General Practice
Dr France Frechette, Chateauguay, QC - General Practice
Dr Christie L Freeman, Peterborough, ON - Family Medicine
Dr Marc Frenette, Laval, QC - Cardiology
Dr Lucie Frenette, Levis, QC - General Practice
Dr Marie G L Frenette, Quebec, QC - Pediatrics
Dr Jacques Frenette, Quebec, QC - Family Medicine
Dr Michel Frenette, Ste-Agathe-Des-Mts, QC - General Practice
Dr Gad Friedman, Montreal, QC - Gastroenterology
Dr Byron P P Friesen, Hawkesbury, ON - General Surgery
Dr Robert Frongillo, Montreal, QC - General Practice
Dr Lucien-P Fruchtermann, Montreal, QC - General Practice
Dr Bertha Fuchsman, Montreal, QC - Family Medicine
Dr Barbara E Fuller, Kingston, ON - Family Medicine
Dr Deana Funaro, Montreal, QC - Dermatology
Dr Shek Hong Fung, Montreal, QC - Geriatric Medicine
Dr Aicha Gafsi, Rimouski, QC - Internal Medicine
Dr Gilbert Gagne, Mirabel, QC - Family Medicine
Dr Guy Gagne, Quebec, QC - General Practice
Dr Richard Gagne, Rimouski, QC - General Surgery
Dr Nancy Gagne, Sherbrooke, QC - Endocrin/Metabolism
Dr Guy-Paul Gagne, Verdun, QC - Obstetrics & Gynecology
Dr D'Arcy W Gagnon, Toronto, ON - General Practice
Dr Louis Gagnon, Chicoutimi, QC - Emergency Family Med
Dr Alexis Gagnon, Gatineau, QC - Neurology
Dr Sophie Gagnon, Gatineau, QC - Neurology
Dr Marjolaine M Gagnon, Gatineau, QC - Ophthalmology
Dr Serge Gagnon, Gatineau, QC - General Practice
Dr Marie-Josee Gagnon, La Malbaie, QC - Family Medicine
Dr Sylvain Gagnon, Montreal, QC - Orthopedic Surgery
Dr Jacques R Gagnon, Montreal, QC - Psychiatry
Dr Bruno Gagnon, Quebec, QC - General Practice
Dr Isabelle Gagnon, Quebec, QC - Plastic Surgery
Dr Remi Gagnon, Quebec, QC - Clin Immun/Allergy
Dr Pierre Gagnon, Quebec, QC - Gastroenterology
Dr Simon Gagnon, Quebec, QC - Otolaryngology
Dr Francois Gagnon, Riviere-Du-Loup, QC - Internal Medicine
Dr Sylvie Gagnon, Riviere-Du-Loup, QC - Anatomical Pathology
Dr Christine Gagnon, Rouyn-Noranda, QC - General Practice
Dr Jean Gagnon, Trois-Rivieres, QC - Dermatology
Dr Andre F Gagnon, Trois-Rivieres, QC - Electroencephal
Dr Suzanne Gagnon, Vimont, QC - Dermatology
Dr Madeleine Gagnon, Vimont, QC - Dermatology
Dr M Lynne Galipeau, Newmarket, ON - General Practice
Dr Louise Galipeau, Cowansville, QC - General Practice
Dr Denise L Gallant, Dieppe, NB - Family Medicine
Dr Peter W Galley, Pembroke, ON - General Practice
Dr Anik Galley, St-Charles-Brromee, QC - General Practice
Dr Louis Gamache, Chertsey, QC - General Practice
Dr Sylvie Gamache, Rimouski, QC - Pediatrics
Dr Prem Gandham, Rosthern, SK - General Practice
Dr Mark S Gans, Montreal, QC - Ophthalmology
Dr Jacques Garant, Saint-Lambert, QC - Psychiatry
Dr George J Garbe, Regina, SK - Cardiology
Dr Richard Garceau, Moncton, NB - Medical Microbiology
Dr Patrick Garceau, Montreal, QC - Cardiology
Dr Michel Garcia, Ste-Anne-des-Monts, QC - General Practice
Dr Michael A Gardam, Toronto, ON - Infectious Diseases
Dr Edward M Gardiner, Ottawa, ON - Emergency Family Med
Dr Jacques Y Gareau, Saint-Jerome, QC - General Practice
Dr Naveen Garg, Pointe-Claire, QC - Family Medicine
Dr Genevieve Garneau, Saint-Hyacinthe, QC - Emergency Family Med
Dr Jean Garon, Gatineau, QC - Endocrin/Metabolism
Dr Dominique Garrel, Montreal, QC - Endocrinology
Dr Ronald G Garston, Riverside-Albert, NB - Urology
Dr John G Gartner, Winnipeg, MB - Anatomical Pathology
Dr Bernard Gascon, Saint-Jerome, QC - General Practice
Dr Mathieu M Gatien, Ottawa, ON - Emergency Family Med
Dr Christine Gaucher, St-Jean-sur-Richel, QC - General Practice
Dr Pascale Gaudet, Amos, QC - Obstetrics & Gynecology
Dr Daniel Gaudet, Chicoutimi, QC - General Practice
Dr Guylaine P Gaudet, Montreal, QC - Hematology
Dr Louise Gaudet, St-Joseph-Du-Lac, QC - General Practice
Dr Jules Gaudreau, Quebec, QC - General Practice
Dr Pierre Gaudreault, Montreal, QC - Pediatrics
Dr Colette Gaulin, Quebec, QC - General Practice
Dr Louise F Gauthier, Ottawa, ON - Anesthesia
Dr Alain Gauthier, Perth, ON - Family Medicine
Dr Valere Gauthier, Beauharnois, QC - General Practice
Dr Louise Gauthier, Boucherville, QC - General Surgery
Dr Pierre A Gauthier, Laval, QC - Family Medicine
Dr Jules Gauthier, Longueuil, QC - General Practice
Dr Alain Gauthier, Montreal, QC - Anesthesia
Dr Francois Gauthier, Montreal, QC - Family Medicine
Dr Carole Gauthier, Montreal-Nord, QC - General Practice
Dr Gilles Gauthier, Quebec, QC - General Practice
Dr Cajetan M Gauthier Jr, Quebec, QC - Obstetrics & Gynecology
Dr Daniel Gauthier, Saint-Nicephore, QC - Ophthalmology
Dr Pierre Gauthier, St-Charles-Brromee, QC - Otolaryngology
Dr Dominic Gauthier, St-Jean-Sur-Richel, QC - Family Medicine
Dr Celine Gauthier, Trois-Rivieres, QC - General Practice
Dr Johanne Gauthier, Trois-Rivieres, QC - General Practice
Dr Micheline Gauvin, Mont-Royal, QC - General Practice
Dr Joseph Gauze, Montreal, QC - Otolaryngology
Dr Fay E H Gayle, North York, ON - Family Medicine
Dr William O Geisler, Toronto, ON - Internal Medicine
Dr Claude Gelinas, Boucherville, QC - Diagnostic-Radiology
Dr Danielle Gelinas, Gatineau, QC - General Practice
Dr Bernard Gelinas, Gatineau, QC - General Practice
Dr Marie-Christine Gelinas, Sainte-Julie, QC - General Practice
Dr Andre L Gelly, LaSalle, QC - Gastroenterology
Dr Michel Gemme, Saint-Hyacinthe, QC - General Practice
Dr Tina-Louise Gendron, Rimouski, QC - Orthopedic Surgery
Dr Jacques A P R Genest, Ottawa, ON - Radiation Oncology
Dr Isabelle Genest, Quebec, QC - Emergency Medicine
Dr Mathieu Genest, Rimouski, QC - Orthopedic Surgery
Dr Angela L Genge, Montreal, QC - Internal Medicine
Dr Genevieve Geoffrion, Montreal, QC - Dermatology
Dr Lila L Georgevich, Scarborough, ON - Internal Medicine
Dr Richard Germain, Coaticook, QC - General Practice
Dr Guy Germain, Montreal, QC - Internal Medicine
Dr Robert-Paul Gervais, Ottawa, ON - Community Medicine
Dr Robert Gervais, Drummondville, QC - General Practice
Dr Marc H Gervais, Montreal, QC - Nephrology
Dr Jean-Guy Gervais, Plessisville, QC - General Practice
Dr Saad Ghali, Delson, QC - General Practice
Dr Robert Gibeault, Saint-Lambert, QC - General Practice
Dr Susan V Gick, Richmond, ON - Family Medicine
Dr Celine Gigoux, Salaber-de-Valleyf, QC - General Practice
Dr Michel R Gil, Repentigny, QC - Psychiatry

Dr François Gilbert, Kirkland, QC - Endocrinology
Dr Philippe Gilbert, Montreal, QC - Internal Medicine
Dr Jean Gilbert, Montreal, QC - General Practice
Dr Francois Gilbert, Pointe-Claire, QC - Emergency Medicine
Dr Nathalie Gilbert, Quebec, QC - General Surgery
Dr Marc Gingras, Lachute, QC - General Surgery
Dr Caroline Gingras, Saint-Eustache, QC - General Practice
Dr Edmonde Gionet, Bathurst, NB - Family Medicine
Dr Louis C Girard, North York, ON - Family Medicine
Dr J Marc Girard, Montreal, QC - Electroencephal
Dr Marie-France Giron, Dorval, QC - General Practice
Dr Marie-Helene Girouard, Trois-Rivieres, QC - General Surgery
Dr Rosaire Giroux, Cowansville, QC - General Practice
Dr Marc F Giroux, Laval, QC - Neurosurgery
Dr Marie-France Giroux, Montreal, QC - Diagnostic-Radiology
Dr Marc Giroux, Quebec, QC - General Practice
Dr Mario Giroux, Trois-Rivieres, QC - Orthopedic Surgery
Dr Robert R M Glasgow, Edmonton, AB - Orthopedic Surgery
Dr Yvon Glaude, Roberval, QC - Diagnostic-Radiology
Dr Peter R Glazer, Toronto, ON - Emergency Family Med
Dr Joan Glenn, Quebec, QC - General Practice
Dr Vivian P Glenns, North York, ON - Internal Medicine
Dr Shawn W Gmora, North York, ON - Family Medicine
Dr Gabriella Gobbi, Montreal, QC - Psychiatry
Dr Martine Gobeil, Montreal, QC - General Practice
Dr Cynthia Godbout, Montreal, QC - Family Medicine
Dr Bernard Godin, Moncton, NB - Family Medicine
Dr Patricia Goggin, Montreal, QC - General Practice
Dr Mary Susan L B Goheen, Ottawa, ON - Anesthesia
Dr Deborah Golberg, Montreal, QC - Family Medicine
Dr Pamela D Gold, Hanover, ON - Family Medicine
Dr David I Gold, Wakefield, QC - Family Medicine
Dr Eudice Goldberg, Toronto, ON - Pediatrics
Dr Richard B Goldbloom, Halifax, NS - Pediatrics
Dr John N H Goldhar, Toronto, ON - Dermatology
Dr Gail Goldman, Montreal, QC - Internal Medicine
Dr Elliot M Goldner, Vancouver, BC - Psychiatry
Dr Barry Goldsman, Westmount, QC - General Practice
Dr William Goldstein, Ottawa, ON - Cardiovasc/ThorSurg
Dr Alfonso Gomez-Jimenez, Bathurst, NB - Plastic Surgery
Dr Yolanda Gonzalez, Grand-Mere, QC - Family Medicine
Dr Mariel Gonzalez, Laval, QC - General Practice
Dr Luis A Gonzalez Herrera, Rimouski, QC - Neurology
Dr Marni A Goodman, New Minas, NS - Family Medicine
Dr Ian C Gorin, Montreal, QC - General Practice
Dr Sylvie Gosselin, Sherbrooke, QC - Electroencephal
Dr Sophie Gosselin, Sherbrooke, QC - Family Medicine
Dr Francois Gosselin, Ste-Agathe-des-Mts, QC - General Practice
Dr Walter H Gotlieb, Montreal, QC - Obstetrics & Gynecology
Dr Richard Goudie, Barrie, ON - Family Medicine
Dr Constance Goulet, Radisson, QC - General Practice
Dr Helene Gousseau, Trenton, ON - Family Medicine
Dr Sandra Graham, Sainte-Therese, QC - General Practice
Dr Francois Grand'Maison, Greenfield Park, QC - Electroencephal
Dr Maria S Grande, St. Catharines, ON - Family Medicine
Dr Jean Granger, Gatineau, QC - General Practice
Dr Eugenie Granger-Juneau, Quebec, QC - General Practice
Dr Vincent J Grant, Calgary, AB - Pediatrics
Dr Adele Gratton, Toronto, ON - General Practice
Dr Denis H Gravel, Ottawa, ON - Anatomical Pathology
Dr Charles A Gravel, Lemoyne, QC - Orthopedic Surgery
Dr Jean-Pierre Gravel, Quebec, QC - Ophthalmology
Dr Marie-Pascale Gravel, Saint-Eustache, QC - General Practice
Dr Raymond Green, Hope, BC - Family Medicine
Dr Gary H Greenberg, Ottawa, ON - Emergency Medicine
Dr Brian J Greenfield, Montreal, QC - Psychiatry
Dr Edith Gregoire, Cap-aux-Meules, QC - General Practice
Dr Ginette Gregoire, Montreal, QC - Psychiatry
Dr Genevieve Gregoire, Montreal, QC - Internal Medicine
Dr Jocelyn Gregoire, Quebec, QC - Cardiovasc/ThorSurg
Dr Michelle Greiver, North York, ON - Family Medicine
Dr Claude Grenier, Greenfield Park, QC - Psychiatry
Dr Yvan Grenier, Montreal, QC - Anesthesia
Dr Gilles Grenier, St-Jean-sur-Richel, QC - General Practice
Dr Michael Greschner, Moncton, NB - Anesthesia
Dr Joanne M Grevler, Toronto, ON - Family Medicine
Dr Sylvain Grignon, Sherbrooke, QC - General Practice
Dr Stephen H Grodinsky, Nepean, ON - Pediatrics
Dr Tamara C Grodzicky, Montreal, QC - Internal Medicine
Dr Donald R Groenewege, Montreal, QC - Psychiatry
Dr Pierre Grondin, Baie-Comeau, QC - Diagnostic-Radiology
Dr Francois R Grondin, Levis, QC - Cardiology
Dr Ian G Gross, Ottawa, ON - Plastic Surgery
Dr Antoine Groulx, Gaspe, QC - Family Medicine
Dr Andree M R Gruslin, Ottawa, ON - Obstetrics & Gynecology
Dr Francine Guay, Levis, QC - Ophthalmology
Dr Alan Guberman, Ottawa, ON - Neurology
Dr Pierre Guerette, Sherbrooke, QC - Emergency Medicine
Dr Danielle Guerin, Gatineau, QC - General Practice
Dr Lucie C Guerin, Verdun, QC - Internal Medicine
Dr Paul Guilbault, Quebec, QC - General Practice
Dr Edith Guilbert, Quebec, QC - General Practice
Dr Chantal Guillemette, Havre-Saint-Pierre, QC - Family Medicine
Dr Julie Guillemette, Quebec, QC - Obstetrics & Gynecology
Dr Daniel B S Guimaraes, Sherbrooke, QC - Psychiatry
Dr Richard Guimond, Chicoutimi, QC - Obstetrics & Gynecology
Dr Claude Guimond, LaSalle, QC - Cardiology
Dr Jean-Gilles Guimond, Montreal, QC - Critical Care Medicine
Dr Mauril Guimond, Quebec, QC - General Practice
Dr Noemi Guindon, Windsor, ON - General Practice
Dr Hesham S R Guirguis, Sorel-Tracy, QC - Internal Medicine
Dr Neeru Gupta, Toronto, ON - Ophthalmology
Dr Ashvini H Gursahaney, Montreal, QC - Critical Care Medicine
Dr Klaus S Gutfreund, Edmonton, AB - Gastroenterology
Dr Peter Gutmanis, Nanaimo, BC - Orthopedic Surgery
Dr Astrid Guttmann, Toronto, ON - Pediatrics
Dr Randolph P Guzman, Winnipeg, MB - General Surgery
Dr Martin Gyger, Montreal, QC - Hematological Pathology
Dr Nader H Habib, Laval, QC - General Practice
Dr Adel F Habib, Sorel-Tracy, QC - Psychiatry
Dr Munir Habra, Greenfield Park, QC - General Practice
Dr Hachemi Hadjoudj, Laval, QC - Internal Medicine
Dr Richard N Haichin, Montreal, QC - Cardiology
Dr Youssef Haikal, Longueuil, QC - Otolaryngology
Dr M Taghi Hakami, Chicoutimi, QC - General Practice
Dr Ann Mary Hall, Brantford, ON - General Pathology
Dr Trevor L Hall, Cambridge, ON - Family Medicine
Dr Jean J Hallak, Montreal, QC - Obstetrics & Gynecology
Dr Denis Halle, Gatineau, QC - Internal Medicine
Dr Jean-Pierre Halle, Montreal, QC - Endocrinology
Dr James Halvorson, Duncan, BC - Emergency Family Med
Dr Fawaz Halwani, Ottawa, ON - Anatomical Pathology
Dr Reggie C A Hamdy, Montreal, QC - Orthopedic Surgery
Dr Pavel Hamet, Montreal, QC - Endocrinology
Dr John R Hamilton, Antigonish, NS - Ophthalmology
Dr Hachmi Hammami, Salaber-de-Valleyf, QC - Ophthalmology
Dr Robert Hanel, Cap-aux-Meules, QC - Internal Medicine
Dr Yousri Hanna, Anjou, QC - General Practice
Dr Samer Hanna, Laval, QC - Urology
Dr M Georges Hannouche, Montreal, QC - General Practice
Dr Janet E Hantho, Calgary, AB - General Practice
Dr Barbara J Hardt, Calgary, AB - Family Medicine
Dr Jean-Francois Hardy, Montreal, QC - Anesthesia
Dr Mark Hardy, Montreal, QC - General Surgery
Dr Didi V Harries, Chilliwack, BC - Pediatrics
Dr Robert W Harris, Cornwall, ON - Plastic Surgery
Dr Nancy L Harris, Orillia, ON - Family Medicine
Dr Trevor D Harterre, Timmins, ON - Emergency Family Med
Dr Johanne Harvey, Chicoutimi, QC - Pediatrics
Dr Naomi A Hasegawa, Pointe-Claire, QC - Ophthalmology
Dr Raymond Hasel, Pointe-Claire, QC - Anesthesia
Dr Joelle Hassoun, Sherbrooke, QC - Psychiatry
Dr Sharon N Hatcher, Chicoutimi, QC - Family Medicine
Dr Jana B Havrankova, Saint-Lambert, QC - Endocrinology
Dr Toni P Hawkes, Calgary, AB - Family Medicine
Dr David S Hayden, Bridgewater, NS - Plastic Surgery
Dr Francis B Healey, Vernon, BC - General Practice
Dr Paul C Hebert, Ottawa, ON - Critical Care Medicine
Dr Isabelle Hebert, Chandler, QC - Internal Medicine
Dr Michele Hebert, Gatineau, QC - General Practice
Dr Josee Hebert, Montreal, QC - Hematology
Dr Lily T Hechtman, Westmount, QC - Psychiatry
Dr Yanick Hector, Montreal, QC - General Practice
Dr Paul L Heilpern, Montreal, QC - Internal Medicine
Dr Antoine Hejeily, Sorel-Tracy, QC - Urology
Dr Judith Helszajn, Mascouche, QC - General Practice
Dr Christian Hemmings, Montreal, QC - General Practice
Dr Robert Hemmings, Montreal, QC - Obstetrics & Gynecology
Dr Raymond Hendel, Sudbury, ON - General Surgery
Dr Kenneth J Henderson, St. John's, NL - Pediatrics
Dr Rene Hendriks, Quebec, QC - General Practice
Dr Richard Henri, Montreal, QC - Anesthesia
Dr Donna G Henrikson, Toronto, ON - General Practice
Dr Elise Heon, Toronto, ON - Ophthalmology
Dr Jean-Francois Herard, Riviere-du-Loup, QC - General Practice
Dr Gavril Hercz, Toronto, ON - Internal Medicine
Dr Olivia Hernandez-Sanchez, Rouyn-Noranda, QC - General Practice
Dr Timothy A Heron, Montreal, QC - Orthopedic Surgery
Dr Sheldon Hershkop, Mississauga, ON - Family Medicine
Dr Eleanor Hew, Westmount, QC - Family Medicine
Dr John Hii, Toronto, ON - Medical Microbiology
Dr Michael Hill, Calgary, AB - Internal Medicine
Dr Jeanne Hill, Cowansville, QC - General Practice
Dr Harry S Himal, Toronto, ON - General Surgery
Dr Ingrid M Hings, Montreal, QC - Hematology
Dr Andrea Hirscheimer, London, ON - Family Medicine
Dr Michel Hjelkrem, Trail, BC - Orthopedic Surgery
Dr Eugene N Hladky, Montreal, QC - Ophthalmology
Dr Ngoc-Khoi Hoang, Toronto, ON - General Practice
Dr Minh Chau Hoang, Montreal, QC - General Practice
Dr Antoine Hoang, Pointe-Claire, QC - General Practice
Dr William G Hodge, London, ON - Ophthalmology
Dr Matthew J Hodge, Toronto, ON - Community Medicine
Dr George N Honos, Montreal, QC - Cardiology
Dr P Frank Horan, Belleville, ON - Dermatology
Dr John C Hostetler, Victoria, BC - Neurology
Dr Sebastien J Hotte, Hamilton, ON - Internal Medicine
Dr Jean-Luc Houde, Chicoutimi, QC - General Surgery
Dr Danielle Houde, Courcelette, QC - General Practice
Dr Marc Houde, Montreal, QC - Nephrology
Dr Gaetan Houde, Quebec, QC - Cardiology
Dr Richard J Housley, Niagara Falls, ON - Gastroenterology
Dr Erik Howarth, Merrickville, ON - Family Medicine
Dr Todd C Howlett, Dartmouth, NS - Emergency Family Med
Dr Sophia Hrycko, Ottawa, ON - Psychiatry
Dr Claudia H Hubbes, Ottawa, ON - Family Medicine
Dr Marvin Huberman, Coquitlam, BC - General Practice
Dr Martine Hudicourt, St-Charles-Brromee, QC - Family Medicine
Dr Sylvie R Hudon, Ottawa, ON - Family Medicine
Dr Nathalie Hudon, Chicoutimi, QC - General Practice
Dr Claire Hudon, Quebec, QC - Pediatrics
Dr Edward G Hughes, Burlington, ON - Obstetrics & Gynecology
Dr Annie Hum, Markham, ON - General Practice
Dr Susan M Humphrey, Ottawa, ON - Internal Medicine
Dr Gerard E Huni, Cowansville, QC - Anesthesia
Dr David J Huot, Vanier, ON - Pediatrics
Dr Pierre Huot, Ste-Cath-d-l-J-Car, QC - General Practice
Dr Anne Hupe, Mont-Joli, QC - Family Medicine
Dr Chantal Huppe, Gatineau, QC - Family Medicine
Dr Nisarul M Huq, Windsor, ON - Cardiology
Dr Julie M Hurteau, Ottawa, ON - Diagnostic-Radiology
Dr Nadeem A Hussain, London, ON - Gastroenterology
Dr Jean M F Hyacinthe, Montreal, QC - Plastic Surgery
Dr Edgar Ibrahim, Repentigny, QC - General Practice
Dr Claire Infante-Rivard, Montreal, QC - Community Medicine
Dr Alistair J Ingram, Hamilton, ON - Internal Medicine
Dr Adriana Ionescu, Pointe-Claire, QC - Family Medicine
Dr Kashif Irshad, Brampton, ON - General Surgery
Dr Laila Ismail, Pierrefonds, QC - Pediatrics
Dr Robert Issenman, Hamilton, ON - Pediatrics
Dr Joseph J Itovitch, Salaber-de-Valleyf, QC - Urology
Dr Michael J Jacka, Edmonton, AB - Anesthesia
Dr Steven J Jackson, Scarborough, ON - General Surgery
Dr Genevieve Jacob, Montreal, QC - General Practice
Dr Stephen A Jacobson, Montreal, QC - Urology
Dr Francis R M Jacot, Danville, QC - General Practice

Dr Geraldine Jacquemin, Montreal, QC
- Physical Medicine & Rehab
Dr Paul J Jacquemin, Verdun, QC - Respirology
Dr Marc-Andre Jacques, Montreal, QC - General Practice
Dr Rene Jacques, Quebec, QC - General Practice
Dr Frederic Jacques, Quebec, QC - Cardiac Surgery
Dr Maya Jalbert, Greenfield Park, QC - Psychiatry
Dr Bruce M Jamison, Ottawa, ON - Anatomical Pathology
Dr Liesbet M Jansen, Alliston, ON - Family Medicine
Dr Annie F Janvier, Montreal, QC - Pediatrics
Dr Allan M Jarjour, Saint-Lazare, QC - Pediatrics
Dr David Jarman, Courtenay, BC - General Practice
Dr G Eric Jarvis, Montreal, QC - Psychiatry
Dr Francoise Jasserand, Montreal, QC - General Practice
Dr Robert R Javidi, Bathurst, NB - Ophthalmology
Dr Martine A Jaworski, Ottawa, ON - Pediatrics
Dr Catherine Jean, Montreal, QC - Obstetrics & Gynecology
Dr Carlo Jean-Louis, Rimouski, QC - Family Medicine
Dr Hartley F Jeffery, New Liskeard, ON - General Surgery
Dr Kenneth Jenkins, Corner Brook, NL - General Practice
Dr Christopher W B Jensen, Winnipeg, MB - Urology
Dr Gilles Jodoin, Cowansville, QC - Respirology
Dr Joyce E Johansson, Montreal, QC - Orthopedic Surgery
Dr Dawn A Johansson, Montreal, QC - Obstetrics & Gynecology
Dr Nelie C Johnson, Maple Ridge, BC - Family Medicine
Dr Roger J Johnson, Victoria, BC
- Public Health & Preventive Medicine
Dr H Alan Johnston, Ottawa, ON - Family Medicine
Dr Karen M Johnston, Toronto, ON - Neurosurgery
Dr Diane Jolicoeur, Montreal, QC - General Practice
Dr Paul Jolicoeur, Montreal, QC - General Practice
Dr Denis Jolicoeur, Saint-Romuald, QC - General Practice
Dr Isabelle-Sophie Jolin, Gatineau, QC - Family Medicine
Dr Jacqueline L Joly, Kanata, ON - Pediatrics
Dr Jean-Gil Joly, Saint-Jerome, QC - Internal Medicine
Dr Paul-Aime Joncas, Lourdes-D-Bl-Sabl, QC - General Practice
Dr Edward C Jones, Vancouver, BC - Anatomical Pathology
Dr Julie Jones, Winnipeg, MB - Family Medicine
Dr Gwynne Jones, Ottawa, ON - Internal Medicine
Dr Edward A Jones, Regina, SK - Anatomical Pathology
Dr Nicola J Jones-Stokreef, Orillia, ON - Pediatrics
Dr M K Rashid Joomun, Whitewood, SK - General Practice
Dr Sally H Jorgensen, Bridgewater, NS
- Obstetrics & Gynecology
Dr Francois Joubarne, Laval, QC - General Practice
Dr Marie-Suzanne Joyal, Verdun, QC - Family Medicine
Dr Pierre G Juery, Ottawa, ON - Family Medicine
Dr Gilles Julien, Montreal, QC - Pediatrics
Dr Rene Julien, Quebec, QC - General Practice
Dr Jean-Francois Julien, Stoneham, QC - General Practice
Dr Hans W Jung, Ottawa, ON - General Practice
Dr Marie Jutras, Richmond, QC - General Practice
Dr Claire Jutras, Saint-Jerome, QC - General Practice
Dr Isaac-Jacques Kadoch, Montreal, QC - General Practice
Dr Rhoda S Kagan, North York, ON - Clin Immun/Allergy
Dr Christian Y Kako, Richmond Hill, ON - General Practice
Dr Tef Kalaparambath, Etobicoke, ON - Cardiology
Dr Lalit K Kamdar, Edmonton, AB - General Practice
Dr Kami Kandola, Yellowknife, NT - Family Medicine
Dr Nachiketa M Kanungo, Windsor, ON - Diagnostic-Radiology
Dr Morton A Kapusta, Montreal, QC - Internal Medicine
Dr Athanassios Karabatsos, Shawville, QC - Internal Medicine
Dr Gregory J Karaguesian, Haliburton, ON - General Practice
Dr Jacques Karam, St-Jean-Sur-Richel, QC - Cardiology
Dr Constantine G Karnis, Burlington, ON - General Practice
Dr Alan J Karovitch, Ottawa, ON - Internal Medicine
Dr Shelby N Karpman, Edmonton, AB - Family Medicine
Dr Lisa M Karvelas, Winnipeg, MB - Psychiatry
Dr Meryem Karzazi, Saint-Georges, QC - Internal Medicine
Dr Jacinthe Kassab, Calgary, AB - Ophthalmology
Dr Jeannine Kassis, Montreal, QC - Hematology
Dr Murray S Katz, Dollard-D-Ormeaux, QC - General Practice
Dr Edward Katz, Montreal, QC - General Practice
Dr Robert Kaud, Saint-Laurent, QC - Family Medicine
Dr Sanda Kaufman-Clain, Saint-Eustache, QC - General Practice
Dr Dounia Kayal, Montreal, QC - General Practice

Dr Hassan Kayssi, Montreal, QC - General Practice
Dr Michael V Keating, Sault Ste. Marie, ON - General Practice
Dr Nancy B Keesal, Toronto, ON - Internal Medicine
Dr Heather E Keizer, Charlottetown, PE - Psychiatry
Dr John S Kell, Toronto, ON - Urology
Dr Catherine M K Kelly, Toronto, ON - Endocrinology
Dr Anthea G Kelly, Sherbrooke, QC - Medical Biochemistry
Dr Robert A Kemp, Brampton, ON - Family Medicine
Dr Isabelle Kemp, Montreal, QC - Psychiatry
Dr Gerald Kenefick, Burnaby, BC - Family Medicine
Dr James R Kennedy, Vancouver, BC - Internal Medicine
Dr Renee S Kennedy, Saskatoon, SK - Thoracic Surgery
Dr Lorraine M R Kerr, Winnipeg, MB - Pediatrics
Dr Samir Khalife, Montreal, QC - Obstetrics & Gynecology
Dr Manish Khanna, Montreal, QC - Dermatology
Dr Kapil Khatter, Ottawa, ON - Family Medicine
Dr Kamal Khayat, Saint-Jerome, QC - Pediatrics
Dr Lucie M Khouri, Saint-Laurent, QC - Ophthalmology
Dr Nabil M Khoury, Bois-des-Filion, QC - General Practice
Dr Elie G Khoury, Saint-Laurent, QC - Ophthalmology
Dr Khalil Khoury, Sherbrooke, QC - Endocrinology
Dr Pierre Khouzam, Newmarket, ON - General Practice
Dr Teresa M Kieser, Calgary, AB - Cardiovasc/ThorSurg
Dr Debra A Kiez, Richmond Hill, ON - Emergency Family Med
Dr R John Kimoff, Montreal, QC - Internal Medicine
Dr Susan Kimpton, Rimouski, QC - Pediatrics
Dr Arlene King, Toronto, ON - Community Medicine
Dr Andre L Kiss, Vercheres, QC - General Practice
Dr Marc Klasa, Calgary, AB - Family Medicine
Dr Richard J Klasa, Vancouver, BC - Internal Medicine
Dr Jean-Marc Y Klein, Charlottetown, PE - Dermatology
Dr Marina B Klein, Montreal, QC - Infectious Diseases
Dr Kristine E Klubien, Montreal, QC - General Practice
Dr Jacqueline Klvana, Brossard, QC - Family Medicine
Dr Hans Knecht, Sherbrooke, QC - Hematology
Dr Marion D Koch, Wakefield, QC - Psychiatry
Dr Marie-Charlotte Koenig, Kuujjuaq, QC - Family Medicine
Dr Andre Kokis, Montreal, QC - Cardiology
Dr Victor Kokta, Montreal, QC - Anatomical Pathology
Dr Nadim Korban, Montreal, QC - Otolaryngology
Dr Endre L Koritar, Vancouver, BC - Psychiatry
Dr Antonio I Kos, Timmins, ON - Family Medicine
Dr Karen M Kost, Montreal, QC - Otolaryngology
Dr Ekaterine Koutroularas, Montreal, QC - General Practice
Dr Odile Kowalski, Montreal, QC - General Practice
Dr Piotr Koziarz, Welland, ON - General Surgery
Dr Daniel J Kraus, Montreal, QC - Psychiatry
Dr Stuart H Kreisman, Vancouver, BC - Internal Medicine
Dr Richard B Kremer, Montreal, QC - Medical Biochemistry
Dr Preetha Krishnamoorthy, Montreal, QC
- Endocrin/Metabolism
Dr Allison Kukhta, Val-d'Or, QC - Clin Immun/Allergy
Dr Anne C D Kulenkamp, Gaspe, QC - Family Medicine
Dr Joy Kuncheria, Cambridge, ON - Family Medicine
Dr Beverly Kupfert, North York, ON - Pediatrics
Dr Christine Kupsh, Sudbury, ON - Emergency Family Med
Dr Renee Kuska, Saint-Agapit, QC - General Practice
Dr Raffi S Kuyumjian, Saint-Hubert, QC - Family Medicine
Dr Beverley Kyle, Pointe-Claire, QC - Family Medicine
Dr Guy L'Esperance, Levis, QC - Gastroenterology
Dr Monique S La France, Inverness, NS - Family Medicine
Dr Nathalie LaRue, Cowansville, QC - General Surgery
Dr Lionel J Labbe, Vanier, ON - General Practice
Dr Mario Labbe, Clermont, QC - General Practice
Dr Caroline Labbe, Levis, QC - Otolaryngology
Dr Raymond Labbe, Quebec, QC - General Surgery
Dr Jean C Labbe, Trois-Rivieres, QC - General Practice
Dr Eric R Labelle, Timmins, ON - General Surgery
Dr Robert Labelle, Saint-Hyacinthe, QC - General Practice
Dr J Roger Laberge, Chateauguay, QC - General Practice
Dr Renee Laberge, Quebec, QC - General Practice
Dr Caroline Laberge, Quebec, QC - Family Medicine
Dr Jacques Labreche, Drummondville, QC - General Surgery
Dr Isabelle Labrie, Gatineau, QC - General Practice
Dr Christian Labrie, Longueuil, QC - Psychiatry
Dr Christiane Labrie, Windsor, QC - General Practice

Dr Josee L Labrosse, Ottawa, ON - General Practice
Dr Lise Lacasse, Moncton, NB - General Practice
Dr Diane Lacasse, Anjou, QC - General Practice
Dr Louis-Andre Lacasse, Saint-Jerome, QC - Family Medicine
Dr Lori-Ann D Lach, Winnipeg, MB - Family Medicine
Dr Marie-Pierre Lachaine, Gatineau, QC - Family Medicine
Dr Lynda Lachaine, Mont-Laurier, QC - General Practice
Dr Jean-Rene Lachance, Montreal, QC - Gastroenterology
Dr Lucie Lachance, Quebec, QC - General Practice
Dr Jacques R Lachance, St-Jean-Port-Joli, QC
- General Practice
Dr Yves Lacourciere, Quebec, QC - Internal Medicine
Dr Sylvie Lacoursiere, Trois-Rivieres, QC - General Practice
Dr Lianne Lacroix, Kelowna, BC - General Practice
Dr J L Denis Lacroix, Hearst, ON - General Practice
Dr Daniel Lacroix, Moose Creek, ON - General Practice
Dr Thomas B Lacroix, Sarnia, ON - Pediatrics
Dr Jacques Lacroix, Montreal, QC - Pediatrics
Dr Marie-Pierre Laflamme, Montreal, QC - General Practice
Dr Georges Laflamme, Montreal, QC - Orthopedic Surgery
Dr Louis Laflamme, St-Jean-Sur-Richel, QC
- Diagnostic-Radiology
Dr J J Rene Lafleche, Hearst, ON - Family Medicine
Dr Martine Lafleur, Montreal, QC - Geriatric Medicine
Dr Gilles-Philippe Lafond, Quebec, QC - Ophthalmology
Dr Jacques J Laforest, Angus, ON - General Practice
Dr Stephane Laframboise, Toronto, ON
- Obstetrics & Gynecology
Dr Rachel Laframboise, Quebec, QC - Medical Genetics
Dr Rene Lafreniere, Calgary, AB - General Surgery
Dr Ronald T J Lafreniere, Victoria, BC
- Physical Medicine & Rehab
Dr Marc Lagace, Campbellton, NB - General Surgery
Dr Real Lagace, Rimouski, QC - Anatomical Pathology
Dr Louis-Marie Lagace, Ste-Agathe-Des-Mts, QC
- General Practice
Dr Louise Laganiere, Longueuil, QC - General Practice
Dr Normand Lague, Cowansville, QC - General Practice
Dr Salim Lahoud, Montreal, QC - Ophthalmology
Dr Christopher C Lai, Thunder Bay, ON - Cardiology
Dr Andre Lainesse, Trois-Rivieres, QC - Cardiology
Dr Louise Lajoie, Longueuil, QC - General Practice
Dr Yves Lajoie, Sherbrooke, QC - Psychiatry
Dr Daniel Laliberte, Dorval, QC - Family Medicine
Dr Marc-Andre Laliberte, Montreal, QC - Psychiatry
Dr Bernard Laliberte, Quebec, QC - Orthopedic Surgery
Dr Martin Lalinec-Michaud, Quebec, QC - General Practice
Dr Leonora Lalla, Montreal, QC - Family Medicine
Dr Michel Lallier, Montreal, QC - General Surgery
Dr Donald H Lalonde, Saint John, NB - Plastic Surgery
Dr Jocelyne Lalonde, Gatineau, QC - General Practice
Dr Richard G J Lalonde, Montreal, QC - Infectious Diseases
Dr Carole Lalonde, Salaber-de-Valleyf, QC
- Obstetrics & Gynecology
Dr Lise Lalonde, Sherbrooke, QC - Family Medicine
Dr Jean Lalonde, Ville-Marie, QC - General Practice
Dr Y Sophie Lam-Yuk-Tseung, Chandler, QC - Family Medicine
Dr Maurice Lamarche, Shawville, QC - General Practice
Dr Isabella Lamargese, Terrebonne, QC - Internal Medicine
Dr Michel Lambert, Sherbrooke, QC - General Practice
Dr Roch Lambert, St-Lambert-de-Lauz, QC - General Practice
Dr France Lambert, Trois-Rivieres, QC - Nephrology
Dr Robert W Lamont, Scarborough, ON - Anesthesia
Dr Yves Lamontagne, Montreal, QC - Psychiatry
Dr Daniel Lamontagne, Quebec, QC - General Practice
Dr G Albert Lamontagne, Sherbrooke, QC - Electroencephal
Dr Marc Lamothe, Victoriaville, QC - Internal Medicine
Dr Diane Lamoureux, Longueuil, QC - Anatomical Pathology
Dr Christian Lamoureux, Victoriaville, QC - General Practice
Dr Diane Lanciault, Lachute, QC - General Practice
Dr Jean-Claude Landa, Hawkesbury, ON - Family Medicine
Dr Daniel A Landry, Moncton, NB - Family Medicine
Dr Martine Landry, Brossard, QC - Pediatrics
Dr Daniel Landry, Montreal, QC - Obstetrics & Gynecology
Dr Brian A Lang, Scarborough, ON - Family Medicine
Dr Diane Langelier, Sherbrooke, QC - Gastroenterology
Dr Serge Langevin, Sherbrooke, QC - Gastroenterology

Dr Marc V Langill, Ottawa, ON - Family Medicine
Dr Heather I Langille, Ottawa, ON - Emergency Family Med
Dr Denis Langis, Laval, QC - General Practice
Dr Julie Langlois, Bathurst, NB - Family Medicine
Dr Yves Langlois, Montreal, QC - Cardiovasc/ThorSurg
Dr Serge Langlois, Quebec, QC - Internal Medicine
Dr Line Langlois, Sherbrooke, QC - Family Medicine
Dr Michel Langlois, St-Jacques-D-Leeds, QC - General Practice
Dr Pierre J Lanoix, Rockland, ON - Family Medicine
Dr Pierre Lanouette, Varennes, QC - General Practice
Dr Jean-Pierre Lanteigne, Bathurst, NB - General Practice
Dr Luc Laperriere, Mirabel, QC - General Practice
Dr Eric V Laperriere-Nguyen, Verdun, QC - General Practice
Dr Veronique Lapie, Sherbrooke, QC - General Surgery
Dr Bernard Lapierre, Longueuil, QC - General Practice
Dr Yves L Lapierre, Montreal, QC - Neurology
Dr Andre J Lapierre, Montreal, QC - Cardiology
Dr Louis Lapierre, Montreal, QC - Internal Medicine
Dr Patricia Lapierre, Saint-Romuald, QC - General Practice
Dr Richard Laplante, Drummondville, QC - General Surgery
Dr Sophie Laplante, Mont-Royal, QC - Diagnostic-Radiology
Dr Lucie Laplante, Montreal, QC - General Practice
Dr Bernard Laplante, Sept-Iles, QC - General Practice
Dr Pierre Lapointe, Levis, QC - Orthopedic Surgery
Dr Normand Lapointe, Montreal, QC - Pediatrics
Dr Marc-Henry Lapointe, Ville-Marie, QC - Psychiatry
Dr Michel A Lapointe, Westmount, QC - Family Medicine
Dr Pierre Laporte, Boucherville, QC - General Practice
Dr Yanick Larivee, Granby, QC - Otolaryngology
Dr Francois Lariviere, Montreal, QC - Medical Biochemistry
Dr Anne Larkin-Chagnon, Waterloo, QC - General Practice
Dr Robert Laroche, Longueuil, QC - General Practice
Dr Vincent Laroche, Quebec, QC - Hematology
Dr Esther Laroche, Terrebonne, QC - General Practice
Dr Andre Larochelle, Jonquiere, QC - Obstetrics & Gynecology
Dr Denis Larochelle, Levis, QC - Anesthesia
Dr Julie Larochelle, Saint-Romuald, QC - General Practice
Dr Isabelle Larocque, Montreal, QC - General Practice
Dr Robert Larocque, Ste-Agathe-des-Mts, QC - General Practice
Dr Pierre Larose, Greenfield Park, QC - General Surgery
Dr Dominic Larose, Montreal, QC - General Practice
Dr Eric Larose, Quebec, QC - Cardiology
Dr Gontran Larose, Saint-Constant, QC - General Practice
Dr Gilles Larouche, La Baie, QC - General Practice
Dr Pierre Larouche, Salaber-de-Valleyf, QC - General Practice
Dr Alain Larouche, St-Ferreol-L-Neig, QC - General Practice
Dr Marie Larue, Maria, QC - General Surgery
Dr Leo Lasalle, Verdun, QC - General Practice
Dr David A Latter, Toronto, ON - Cardiovasc/ThorSurg
Dr Jean-Baptiste Lattouf, Montreal, QC - Urology
Dr Patricia A Laughrea, Quebec, QC - Ophthalmology
Dr Marc P Launay, Montreal, QC - Endocrinology
Dr Lyne Laurendeau, Saint-Hubert, QC - Family Medicine
Dr Gilles Laurin, Boisbriand, QC - General Practice
Dr Daniel Laurin, Laval, QC - General Practice
Dr Pierre-Michel Laurin, Saint-Jerome, QC - General Practice
Dr Norman R Laurin, Trois-Rivieres, QC - Nuclear Medicine
Dr Christian Lauriston, Montreal, QC - General Practice
Dr Jean G Lauzon, Surrey, BC - General Surgery
Dr Carol L Lavallee, Sudbury, ON - Psychiatry
Dr Yvon-Jacques Lavallee, Chicoutimi, QC - Psychiatry
Dr Jean-Pierre Lavallee, Cowansville, QC - Cardiology
Dr Sophie Lavallee, Mont-Saint-Hilaire, QC - General Practice
Dr Michel Laverdiere, Montreal, QC - Infectious Diseases
Dr Michel-Andre Laverdiere, Montreal, QC - Cardiology
Dr Annie Laverdiere, Trois-Rivieres, QC - Emergency Family Med
Dr Martin Lavigne, Montreal, QC - Orthopedic Surgery
Dr Patrick Lavigne, Montreal, QC - Orthopedic Surgery
Dr Denis Lavigueur, Saint-Eustache, QC - General Practice
Dr Cecile R Lavoie, Bonnyville, AB - General Practice
Dr Susan D Lavoie, Ottawa, ON - Internal Medicine
Dr Bertrand Lavoie, Amos, QC - General Practice
Dr Mona Lavoie, Levis, QC - Anatomical Pathology
Dr Remi Lavoie, Levis, QC - Gastroenterology
Dr Vincent Lavoie, Montreal, QC - Cardiology
Dr Sylvain Lavoie, Quebec, QC - Gastroenterology
Dr Normand Lavoie, Rosemere, QC - General Practice
Dr Pauline Lavoie, Vimont, QC - General Practice
Dr Lionel A Lavoie, Melfort, SK - Family Medicine
Dr Line Lavoie-Dufour, Grand Falls, NB - General Practice
Dr John Lawless, St-Augustin-D-Desm, QC - General Practice
Dr Sofia Lazaridis, Ottawa, ON - Family Medicine
Dr Charles Lazzam, Mississauga, ON - Cardiology
Dr Phuoc-Hai Le, Edmonton, AB - Family Medicine
Dr Binh-Dang Le, Laval, QC - General Practice
Dr Thien Nhan Le, Montreal, QC - General Practice
Dr Thi Qui Le, Montreal, QC - General Practice
Dr Thi Xuan Mai Le, Montreal-Nord, QC - General Practice
Dr Quang Tien Le, Saint-Laurent, QC - General Practice
Dr Catherine A Le Feuvre, Mississauga, ON - Cardiology
Dr Paul Le Guerrier, Montreal, QC - Family Medicine
Dr Jean-Michel Le Melledo, Edmonton, AB - General Practice
Dr Francoise Le Mevel-Moreira, Terrebonne, QC - Psychiatry
Dr Natalie Le Sage, Quebec, QC - Emergency Medicine
Dr Nicole M A Le Saux, Ottawa, ON - Anatomical Pathology
Dr Mai Anh Le Van, Montreal, QC - Emergency Family Med
Dr Guy LeBlanc, Moncton, NB - Urology
Dr Roger P LeBlanc, Montreal, QC - Internal Medicine
Dr Marie-Claude Lebeau, Gaspe, QC - Pediatrics
Dr Pierre Lebel, Montreal, QC - Medical Microbiology
Dr Carole Leblanc, Moncton, NB - Obstetrics & Gynecology
Dr Constance Leblanc, Halifax, NS - Emergency Family Med
Dr Francois Leblanc Jr, Granby, QC - General Practice
Dr Richard Leblanc, Montreal, QC - Hematology
Dr Danielle Leblanc, Montreal, QC - General Practice
Dr Claire Leblanc, Montreal, QC - Pediatrics
Dr Martin Leblond, Greenfield Park, QC - Psychiatry
Dr Pierre F Leblond, Quebec, QC - Hematology
Dr Jean-Louis Leboeuf, Gatineau, QC - General Practice
Dr Rebecca Leboeuf, Montreal, QC - Endocrin/Metabolism
Dr Nathalie J Lebreton, Dieppe, NB - Family Medicine
Dr Mortimer Lechter, Westmount, QC - Neurology
Dr J Robert Leckey, Fredericton, NB - Physical Medicine & Rehab
Dr Claude Leclerc, Baie-Comeau, QC - General Practice
Dr Suzanne Leclerc, Montreal, QC - General Practice
Dr Anne Leclerc, Quebec, QC - General Practice
Dr Celine Leclerc, Quebec, QC - Family Medicine
Dr Michel Leclerc, Riviere-du-Loup, QC - Anesthesia
Dr Michele Leclerc, Saint-Hyacinthe, QC - Ophthalmology
Dr Claude E Leclerc, St-Jean-Sur-Richel, QC - General Practice
Dr Martin Lecompte, Gatineau, QC - Diagnostic-Radiology
Dr Rene Lecours, Montreal, QC - Internal Medicine
Dr Danielle S Leddy, Kitchener, ON - Cardiology
Dr Dean C Leduc, Orleans, ON - Family Medicine
Dr Claude Leduc, Laval, QC - Family Medicine
Dr Line Leduc, Montreal, QC - Obstetrics & Gynecology
Dr Joseph Y Lee, Mississauga, ON - Obstetrics & Gynecology
Dr Yuna Lee, Toronto, ON - Internal Medicine
Dr Marie-Claude Lefebvre, Montreal, QC - Family Medicine
Dr Francine Lefebvre, Quebec, QC - General Practice
Dr Jocelyn Lefebvre, Rouyn-Noranda, QC - General Practice
Dr Marc Lefebvre, St-Charles-Brromee, QC - Psychiatry
Dr Jean-Francois Legare, Halifax, NS - Cardiac Surgery
Dr Lyne Legare, Niagara Falls, ON - Diagnostic-Radiology
Dr Pierre Legault, Laval, QC - General Practice
Dr Danielle Legault, Montreal, QC - Family Medicine
Dr Sylvie Legault, Montreal, QC - Cardiology
Dr Alain Leger, Saint-Tite, QC - General Practice
Dr Francine Leger, St-Jean-sur-Richel, QC - General Practice
Dr Lorraine Legrand Westfall, Ottawa, ON - General Surgery
Dr Marie-Florence Legros, Montreal-Nord, QC - Family Medicine
Dr Francois Lehmann, Verdun, QC - Family Medicine
Dr M Christine Lejtenyi, Montreal, QC - Clin Immun/Allergy
Dr Jane B Lemaire, Calgary, AB - Internal Medicine
Dr Celine Lemaire, Montreal, QC - Radiation Oncology
Dr Michel Lemay, Cowansville, QC - Obstetrics & Gynecology
Dr Andre Lemay, Quebec, QC - Endocrinology
Dr Marianne Lemay, Victoriaville, QC - General Practice
Dr François Lemelin, Levis, QC - Urology
Dr Robert Lemery, Ottawa, ON - Cardiology
Dr Jacques Lemieux, Gatineau, QC - Diagnostic-Radiology
Dr Real Lemieux, Laval, QC - Orthopedic Surgery
Dr Raymond G Lemieux, Magog, QC - Psychiatry
Dr Daniele Lemieux, Montreal, QC - General Practice
Dr Julie Lemieux, Quebec, QC - Hematology
Dr Jacinthe C Lemieux, St-Etienne-Ds-Gres, QC - General Practice
Dr Francois Lemire, Montreal, QC - Cardiology
Dr Isabelle Lemire, Repentigny, QC - Psychiatry
Dr Chantal Lemire, Sherbrooke, QC - Clin Immun/Allergy
Dr Pierre Lemlin, St-Charles-Brromee, QC - Otolaryngology
Dr Marie-Helene Lemoine, Saint-Hyacinthe, QC - Pediatrics
Dr Jean Lemonde, Gatineau, QC - Pediatrics
Dr Eric M Lenczner, Montreal, QC - Orthopedic Surgery
Dr Robert S Lepage, Sudbury, ON - Emergency Family Med
Dr Jean-Marc Lepage, La Prairie, QC - General Practice
Dr Marie-Aline Lepage, Montreal, QC - Anesthesia
Dr Serge Lepage, Sherbrooke, QC - Cardiology
Dr Jean-Marc Lepine, Quebec, QC - Orthopedic Surgery
Dr Mariette Lepine-Martin, Sherbrooke, QC - Hematology
Dr Andre-Marie Leroux, Ottawa, ON - Obstetrics & Gynecology
Dr Genevieve Leroux, Rockland, ON - Family Medicine
Dr Alain D Lesage, Montreal, QC - Psychiatry
Dr Daniel Lesiege, Terrebonne, QC - Medical Biochemistry
Dr Denis Lesieur, Sutton, QC - General Practice
Dr Michel Lessard, Chicoutimi, QC - Anatomical Pathology
Dr Pierre Lessard, Levis, QC - Orthopedic Surgery
Dr Monique Lessard, Montreal, QC - Radiation Oncology
Dr Bernard Lessard, Montreal, QC - Family Medicine
Dr Pascal Lessard, Quebec, QC - General Practice
Dr Lucie Lessard, Quebec, QC - General Practice
Dr Francois Letellier, Longueuil, QC - General Surgery
Dr Elaine Letendre, Montreal, QC - Medical Biochemistry
Dr Francois Letendre, Montreal, QC - Hematology
Dr Richard Letourneau, Montreal, QC - General Surgery
Dr Max Leung, Oshawa, ON - Emergency Family Med
Dr Nathalie M C Leung, Richmond Hill, ON - Endocrin/Metabolism
Dr Marie-France Levac, Cornwall, ON - Endocrin/Metabolism
Dr Francois Levac, Saint-Bruno, QC - General Practice
Dr Chau Levan, Montreal, QC - General Practice
Dr Judith L Levasseur, Oakville, ON - General Practice
Dr Michel P Leveille, Montreal, QC - Internal Medicine
Dr Julie Levesque, Winnipeg, MB - Family Medicine
Dr Yves A Levesque, Beloeil, QC - General Practice
Dr Jean-Marc Levesque, Chateauguay, QC - Orthopedic Surgery
Dr Nancy Levesque, Fortierville, QC - General Practice
Dr Rejean-Yves Levesque, Jonquiere, QC - Diagnostic-Radiology
Dr Christian Levesque, Laval, QC - Occupational Med
Dr Chantale Levesque, Montreal, QC - Family Medicine
Dr Renee Levesque, Montreal, QC - Internal Medicine
Dr Jean-Charles Levesque, Montreal, QC - Anesthesia
Dr Sonia Levesque, Saint-Hyacinthe, QC - General Surgery
Dr Maude Levesque Rouleau, Saint-Jerome, QC - Internal Medicine
Dr Aline Levi, Dollard-D-Ormeaux, QC - General Practice
Dr Sharon S Levine, Ottawa, ON - Psychiatry
Dr Daniel S Levine, Ottawa, ON - Family Medicine
Dr Louis-Charles Levros, Montreal, QC - General Practice
Dr David Levy, Montreal, QC - General Practice
Dr Danielle C Lewington, Halifax, NS - General Practice
Dr Ronald T Lewis, Ottawa, ON - General Surgery
Dr Arthur Leznoff, Toronto, ON - Clin Immun/Allergy
Dr Clare E Liddy, Ottawa, ON - Family Medicine
Dr Anne-Marie Liebich, Montreal, QC - General Practice
Dr Margaret R Lightheart, Hamilton, ON - Obstetrics & Gynecology
Dr Sophie Ligier, Montreal, QC - Internal Medicine
Dr Michel Limoges, Montreal, QC - General Practice
Dr Stan Lipnowski, Winnipeg, MB - Pediatrics
Dr Jennifer B Lipscombe, Mississauga, ON - Internal Medicine
Dr Lee Ha Liu Chen Kiow, Montreal, QC - Family Medicine
Dr Pierre Lizotte, Montreal, QC - General Practice
Dr Katrin Loczy, Quebec, QC - General Practice
Dr Diane M Logan, London, ON - Internal Medicine
Dr Caroline Loignon, Granby, QC - General Practice
Dr Ramesh Lokanathan, Prince George, BC - General Surgery

Dr Daniele Longpre, Montreal, QC - General Practice
Dr Bernadette Loontjens, St-Charles-Brromee, QC - General Practice
Dr Karl J Looper, Montreal, QC - Psychiatry
Dr Isabelle Lopez, Laval, QC - Psychiatry
Dr Jose F Lopez, Saskatoon, SK - Internal Medicine
Dr Benoit Loranger, Saint-Eustache, QC - General Practice
Dr Louise Loranger, Sherbrooke, QC - Dermatology
Dr Marie-Josee Lord, Quebec, QC - Psychiatry
Dr John W Lorimer, Ottawa, ON - General Surgery
Dr Rasmy Loungnarath, Montreal, QC - General Surgery
Dr Robert B Love, Kanata, ON - Otolaryngology
Dr Peter L Loveridge, Glenwood, NS - General Practice
Dr Charles T Low, Brockville, ON - Family Medicine
Dr Nibal Lubbad, Burlington, ON - Family Medicine
Dr Mara S Ludwig, Montreal, QC - Internal Medicine
Dr Diep T Luong, Montreal, QC - General Practice
Dr J R Guy Lupien, Iroquois Falls, ON - Emergency Family Med
Dr G Harvey Lupu, Montreal, QC - Pediatrics
Dr France Lussier, Joliette, QC - General Practice
Dr Marie-Therese Lussier, Laval, QC - Family Medicine
Dr Chinh-Duc Luu, Mercier, QC - General Practice
Dr Joseph-Andre Luyet, Montreal, QC - Psychiatry
Dr Jean Lyonnais, Quebec, QC - Hematology
Dr Caroline Maamari, Greenfield Park, QC - General Practice
Dr Lorraine M Mabon, Calgary, AB - Emergency Medicine
Dr Michele Mabon, Montreal, QC - Ophthalmology
Dr Roderick G G MacArthur, Edmonton, AB - Cardiac Surgery
Dr Kimberly R MacAskill, Kanata, ON - Family Medicine
Dr Patricia L MacCallum, Moncton, NB - Otolaryngology
Dr Ian M MacDonald, Edmonton, AB - Ophthalmology
Dr Susan C MacDonald, Prince George, BC - Family Medicine
Dr Sharon M MacDonald, Winnipeg, MB - Community Medicine
Dr Jennifer L MacDonald, Liverpool, NS - Family Medicine
Dr William A MacDonald, Iqaluit, NU - Family Medicine
Dr Kathryn J MacDonald, Ohsweken, ON - Psychiatry
Dr B Jean MacDonnell, Montreal, QC - Family Medicine
Dr Michael H MacEachern, Moncton, NB - Neurology
Dr Lynne S MacGregor, Ottawa, ON - Physical Medicine & Rehab
Dr Thomas J MacKay, Halifax, NS - Psychiatry
Dr Anthony R MacLean, Calgary, AB - General Surgery
Dr Stephen W MacLean, Halifax, NS - Family Medicine
Dr N Wayne MacLeod, Halifax, NS - Family Medicine
Dr Elizabeth M MacNamara, Montreal, QC - Medical Biochemistry
Dr Douglas W MacPherson, Cheltenham, ON - Internal Medicine
Dr Robert M MacRae, Ottawa, ON - Radiation Oncology
Dr Ruth M MacSween, Kingston, ON - Dermatology
Dr Daniel B Macek, Cowansville, QC - Internal Medicine
Dr Francois Madore, Montreal, QC - Internal Medicine
Dr Andre Mageau, Salaber-de-Valleyf, QC - General Practice
Dr Bryan D Magwood, Winnipeg, MB - Critical Care Medicine
Dr Jaysen Mahadoo, Victoria, BC - General Practice
Dr Usha Maharaj, Sherwood Park, AB - Family Medicine
Dr John T Maher, Peterborough, ON - Psychiatry
Dr Georges Mahfoud, Saint-Leonard, QC - General Practice
Dr Michele Mahone, Montreal, QC - Internal Medicine
Dr Emmanuel Maicas, Moncton, NB - Anatomical Pathology
Dr Jean Mailhot, Grand-Mere, QC - Endocrinology
Dr Suzanne Mailly, Laval, QC - General Practice
Dr Maria J Maingot-Douketis, Scarborough, ON - Family Medicine
Dr Rachel J Maisonneuve, Timmins, ON - Family Medicine
Dr Pierre P Major, Hamilton, ON - Internal Medicine
Dr Ross S Male, Paris, ON - Family Medicine
Dr Michelle Malenfant, Chibougamau, QC - Family Medicine
Dr Dominic Malenfant, Victoriaville, QC - General Practice
Dr Paul M J Malette, Val Caron, ON - General Practice
Dr Stéphanie C Malherbe, Ottawa, ON - Emergency Family Med
Dr Vikram K Malhotra, Saint-Eustache, QC - General Surgery
Dr Marcel Mallet, Moncton, NB - Internal Medicine
Dr Lise Mallette-Tetreault, Mont-Royal, QC - General Practice
Dr Therese Manganas, Montreal, QC - General Practice
Dr Gilles Manhes, Quebec, QC - General Practice
Dr Mervat F Mankarious, Mississauga, ON - Family Medicine
Dr Samer Mansour, Montreal, QC - General Practice
Dr Michael Mansour, Montreal, QC - General Practice
Dr Elias R Maraghi, Hastings, ON - General Practice
Dr Julie P Maranda, Hawkesbury, ON - Family Medicine
Dr Jacques Maranda, Riviere-du-Loup, QC - General Practice
Dr Richard Marchand, Montreal, QC - Internal Medicine
Dr Pierre Marchand, Sherbrooke, QC - General Practice
Dr Louise Marcheterre, Baie-Comeau, QC - Family Medicine
Dr Patrick Marcotte, Moncton, NB - Psychiatry
Dr Luc Marcoux, Montreal, QC - Orthopedic Surgery
Dr Danielle Marcoux, Montreal, QC - Dermatology
Dr Louis-Etienne Marcoux, Quebec, QC - Ophthalmology
Dr Claude Marcoux, Quebec, QC - Internal Medicine
Dr Victoria A Marcus, Montreal, QC - Anatomical Pathology
Dr Gisele Marier, Bridgewater, NS - Family Medicine
Dr Louis Marin, St-Jean-sur-Richel, QC - General Practice
Dr Gilles Marineau, Repentigny, QC - General Practice
Dr Arthur J Markus, Montreal, QC - Pediatrics
Dr Michel Marleau, Lachute, QC - Family Medicine
Dr Errol B Marliss, Montreal, QC - Internal Medicine
Dr Jean-Francois Marquis, Ottawa, ON - Cardiology
Dr Stephanie M Marsan, Montreal, QC - Family Medicine
Dr Gilbert Marsan, Repentigny, QC - General Practice
Dr Kate M A Marshall, York, ON - Family Medicine
Dr Diane B Martel, Granby, QC - General Practice
Dr Julie Martel, Lasalle, QC - Dermatology
Dr Elaine Martel, Longueuil, QC - General Practice
Dr Michel Martel, Longueuil, QC - General Practice
Dr Andre Martel, Mont-Royal, QC - Anesthesia
Dr Elise Martel, St-Charles-Brromee, QC - General Surgery
Dr Jocelyne Martial, Sherbrooke, QC - General Practice
Dr Eric Martin, Rexton, NB - Family Medicine
Dr Lucie C Martin, Ottawa, ON - Diagnostic-Radiology
Dr Andrew J Martin, Thornhill, ON - Family Medicine
Dr Isabelle M C Martin, Gatineau, QC - Family Medicine
Dr Markus C Martin, Montreal, QC - Obstetrics & Gynecology
Dr Louise Martin, Quebec, QC - General Practice
Dr Rene Martin, Sherbrooke, QC - Anesthesia
Dr Susanna M Martin, Saskatoon, SK - Pediatrics
Dr Dawn-Marie L Martin Ward, Lameque, NB - Family Medicine
Dr Mario Martineau, Lavaltrie, QC - General Practice
Dr Jose Luis Martinez Marin, Montreal, QC - General Practice
Dr Valdemar Martinho, Ottawa, ON - General Practice
Dr Joel E Maser, Toronto, ON - Internal Medicine
Dr Orly H Mashal, Dollard-D-Ormeaux, QC - General Practice
Dr Joan E Mason, Brossard, QC - General Practice
Dr Elizabeth A Massarelli, Sackville, NB - Family Medicine
Dr Andre P M Masse, Montreal, QC - Psychiatry
Dr Richard Masse, Montreal, QC - Community Medicine
Dr Jacques Masse, Quebec, QC - Medical Biochemistry
Dr Fadi A Massoud, Montreal, QC - Geriatric Medicine
Dr Surya Master, Campbellton, NB - General Surgery
Dr Nicola Masucci, Chateauguay, QC - General Practice
Dr Tshilay Matand, Regina, SK - General Practice
Dr Jane M Mathew, Gatineau, QC - Critical Care Medicine
Dr John F Mathieu, Chicoutimi, QC - Cardiovasc/ThorSurg
Dr Yves Mathieu, Lyster, QC - General Practice
Dr Elias Matouk, Montreal, QC - Internal Medicine
Dr Hugues Matte, Saint-Hyacinthe, QC - Urology
Dr Jean P Matton, Carleton, QC - General Practice
Dr Andre A Mauffette, Montreal, QC - Psychiatry
Dr Marc L P Mauguin, Ottawa, ON - Psychiatry
Dr Pierre Maurice, Quebec, QC - Community Medicine
Dr Yasmine Mawji, Toronto, ON - Emergency Family Med
Dr J O Jean-Pierre Mayer, Kirkland, QC - Cardiology
Dr Pierre Mayer, Montreal, QC - Internal Medicine
Dr Richard Mazerolle, Chateauguay, QC - General Surgery
Dr Donna E Maziak, Ottawa, ON - General Surgery
Dr Richard H McCall, Hawkesbury, ON - Family Medicine
Dr Jacqueline McClaran, Montreal, QC - General Practice
Dr Donna J McClure, Vancouver, BC - Family Medicine
Dr Sarah D McDonald, Hamilton, ON - Obstetrics & Gynecology
Dr Shelley McFadden, Bouctouche, NB - Family Medicine
Dr Douglas M McGregor, Victoria, BC - General Practice
Dr J Roger McKelvey, Dartmouth, NS - Neurology
Dr John D R McMorran, Vancouver, BC - General Practice
Dr Lisa A McMurray, Ottawa, ON - Psychiatry
Dr T Bruce D McNeely, Kamloops, BC - Anatomical Pathology
Dr P Ruth McPherson, Ottawa, ON - Endocrin/Metabolism
Dr David E McPherson, Westmount, QC - Psychiatry
Dr Suzy Meagher, Laval, QC - General Practice
Dr Bheemdev Meetarbhan, Coquitlam, BC - General Practice
Dr Sanjay Mehta, London, ON - Internal Medicine
Dr Simone A Meikleham, Little Current, ON - Emergency Family Med
Dr Monica Meisels, Courcelette, QC - Family Medicine
Dr Joan M Meitin, Ottawa, ON - Psychiatry
Dr Francois Melancon, Courcelette, QC - General Practice
Dr Eric Melancon, La Malbaie, QC - General Practice
Dr Denis Melancon, Montreal, QC - Diagnostic-Radiology
Dr Claude Menard, Gatineau, QC - Ophthalmology
Dr Jacques G Menard, Gatineau, QC - General Practice
Dr Andre Menard, Repentigny, QC - General Practice
Dr Daniel B Menard, Sherbrooke, QC - Gastroenterology
Dr Claude Menard, Sorel-Tracy, QC - General Practice
Dr Marie-Chantal Menard, St-Jean-Sur-Richel, QC - General Practice
Dr Johanne Menassa, Greenfield Park, QC - Ophthalmology
Dr Jack Mendelson, Montreal, QC - Infectious Diseases
Dr Menhem-Jean Menhem, Saint-Bruno, QC - General Practice
Dr Jay G Mercer, Ottawa, ON - Family Medicine
Dr David Mercier, Baie-Comeau, QC - General Practice
Dr Gilles G Mercier, Pointe-Claire, QC - Obstetrics & Gynecology
Dr Dominique Mercier, Sherbrooke, QC - General Practice
Dr Francine Metcalfe, Saint-Lambert, QC - General Practice
Dr Catherine Meunier, Newmarket, ON - Family Medicine
Dr Nicole Meunier, St-Charles-Brromee, QC - Dermatology
Dr Dominique H Meyer, Quebec, QC - Ophthalmology
Dr Kathleen A Michalski, Orillia, ON - Family Medicine
Dr Jean-Marie C Michel, Shippagan, NB - General Practice
Dr Rene P Michel, Montreal, QC - Anatomical Pathology
Dr Andre L Michon, Sudbury, ON - Family Medicine
Dr Brigitte Migneault, Montreal, QC - Anesthesia
Dr Helena Mihalovits, Hawkesbury, ON - Ophthalmology
Dr Jose L Mijangos-Pelaez, Val-d'Or, QC - General Surgery
Dr John J Milczarek, Fredericton, NB - Physical Medicine & Rehab
Dr Alain Millette, Ottawa, ON - General Practice
Dr C Michelle Milne, Montreal, QC - General Practice
Dr Slobodan Milosevic, Louiseville, QC - General Practice
Dr Marcel Milot, Chicoutimi, QC - Pediatrics
Dr Diane Milot, Montreal, QC - General Practice
Dr Julie Milot, Quebec, QC - Internal Medicine
Dr Martin Milot, Trois-Rivieres, QC - Orthopedic Surgery
Dr Thomas M Milroy, Montreal, QC - Psychiatry
Dr Richard E Mimeault, Ottawa, ON - General Surgery
Dr Genevieve Minville, Chicoutimi, QC - General Practice
Dr Hortensia S Mircescu, Montreal, QC - Endocrin/Metabolism
Dr Gilles Mireault, St-Charles-Brromee, QC - Psychiatry
Dr Asma S Mirza, Trois-Rivieres, QC - General Practice
Dr A Gregor Mitchell, Lachute, QC - Family Medicine
Dr David A Mitchell, Montreal, QC - Hematology
Dr Grant A Mitchell, Montreal, QC - Medical Genetics
Dr Samy Stephane Maurice Mohanna, Gatineau, QC - Community Medicine
Dr Gerard Mohr, Montreal, QC - Neurosurgery
Dr Franck Molin, Quebec, QC - Cardiology
Dr Luigina Mollica, Montreal, QC - Hematology
Dr Francine Molloy, Rouyn-Noranda, QC - General Practice
Dr Frank J Molnar, Ottawa, ON - Geriatric Medicine
Dr M Anne Monahan, Ottawa, ON - Family Medicine
Dr Nathalie Monarque, St-Eustache, QC - General Practice
Dr Jacques Monday, Montreal, QC - Psychiatry
Dr Thomas Mondor, Rawdon, QC - General Practice
Dr Marie-Jose Monette, Laval, QC - Internal Medicine
Dr Diane Monette, Montreal, QC - General Practice
Dr Andre Monette, Salaber-de-Valleyf, QC - Psychiatry
Dr Pascale Monfette, Maniwaki, QC - Family Medicine
Dr Pierre Monpremier, Vanier, ON - Psychiatry
Dr Brigitte M A E Monrose, Markham, ON - Family Medicine
Dr Barbara A Montgomery, Courtice, ON - Family Medicine
Dr Christopher W Montgomery, Oshawa, ON - Pediatrics

Dr Patrice Montminy, Quebec, QC - Orthopedic Surgery
Dr Stephane Montminy-Metivier, Saint-Jerome, QC - Hematology
Dr Madeleine R Montpetit, Ottawa, ON - Family Medicine
Dr Serge Montplaisir, Montreal, QC - Medical Microbiology
Dr Kieran M Moore, Kingston, ON - Emergency Family Med
Dr Daniel H Moquin, Parry Sound, ON - Family Medicine
Dr Jean-Pierre Moquin, Montreal, QC - Hematology
Dr Jose A Morais, Montreal, QC - Geriatric Medicine
Dr Guy Moranville, Quebec, QC - General Practice
Dr Roger Morcos, Sherbrooke, QC - Orthopedic Surgery
Dr Marc J Moreau, Edmonton, AB - Orthopedic Surgery
Dr Monique F Moreau, Alliston, ON - Family Medicine
Dr Michele Moreau, Montreal, QC - General Practice
Dr Anne Moreau, Quebec, QC - Family Medicine
Dr Richard F Morel, Vanier, ON - Psychiatry
Dr Claude Morel, Joliette, QC - General Practice
Dr Rene-Louis Morency, Trail, BC - Ophthalmology
Dr Elizabeth Morency, Quebec, QC - General Practice
Dr Johanne Morency, Quebec, QC - Ophthalmology
Dr Renald Morency, Quebec, QC - Anatomical Pathology
Dr Isabelle Morency, St-Charles-Brromee, QC - General Surgery
Dr Ronaldo Moriconi, Chambly, QC - General Practice
Dr M T Caroline Morin, Calgary, AB - Psychiatry
Dr Evelyn Morin, Anjou, QC - General Practice
Dr Johanne Morin, Longueuil, QC - Emergency Medicine
Dr Jacques Morin, Montmagny, QC - Psychiatry
Dr Suzanne N Morin, Montreal, QC - Internal Medicine
Dr Marie-Eve Morin, Montreal, QC - Family Medicine
Dr Claude Morin, Quebec, QC - Emergency Family Med
Dr Yan Morin, Quebec, QC - Family Medicine
Dr Martine Morin, Sherbrooke, QC - Family Medicine
Dr Louise Morin-Bienvenu, Montreal, QC - General Practice
Dr Marie-Eve Morisset, Baie-Comeau, QC - Family Medicine
Dr Louis G Morissette, Ottawa, ON - Family Medicine
Dr Lucie Morissette, Brossard, QC - General Practice
Dr Louis Morissette, Montreal, QC - Psychiatry
Dr Jean J Morissette, Quebec, QC - Diagnostic-Radiology
Dr Colombe Morneau, Longueuil, QC - General Practice
Dr S Anthony Morris, Red Deer, AB - General Pathology
Dr Steven Morris, Halifax, NS - Plastic Surgery
Dr Brian M Morris, Montreal, QC - Urology
Dr Dennis Morrison, Calgary, AB - Psychiatry
Dr Jean-Pierre P Morrissey, Vanier, ON - General Practice
Dr Sean R Morrissy, Minto, NB - Family Medicine
Dr Dianne P Mosher, Calgary, AB - Internal Medicine
Dr Francois Mosimann, Sherbrooke, QC - General Surgery
Dr Genevieve Moss, St-Jean-sur-Richel, QC - Psychiatry
Dr Christine Motheron, Quebec, QC - Family Medicine
Dr Elie Mouaikel, Montreal, QC - Hematology
Dr Richard Moufarrege, Montreal, QC - Plastic Surgery
Dr Patricia A Moussette, Winchester, ON - Family Medicine
Dr Jean-Marie Moutquin, Montreal, QC - Obstetrics & Gynecology
Dr T Romain Muboyayi, Orleans, ON - Family Medicine
Dr J Jean Muggah, Port Williams, NS - General Practice
Dr Channy Y Muhn, Burlington, ON - Dermatology
Dr Sylvia K Muir, Toronto, ON - Family Medicine
Dr David S Mulder, Montreal, QC - Cardiovasc/ThorSurg
Dr Siobhan M Muldowney, Smiths Falls, ON - Family Medicine
Dr Nancy Murphy, Halifax, NS - Emergency Family Med
Dr Daniel A Muruve, Calgary, AB - Internal Medicine
Dr P Regine Mydlarski, Calgary, AB - Dermatology
Dr Gail A Myhr, Montreal, QC - Psychiatry
Dr Virginia J Myles, Montreal, QC - Family Medicine
Dr Philip M B Myron, North York, ON - Cardiology
Dr Adnan Nached, Montreal, QC - General Practice
Dr Yvon-A. Nadeau, Levis, QC - General Practice
Dr Reginald A Nadeau, Montreal, QC - Cardiology
Dr Sophie Nadeau, Quebec, QC - Pediatrics
Dr Claude Nadeau, Trois-Rivieres, QC - Otolaryngology
Dr Gauri Nadkarni, Gatineau, QC - General Surgery
Dr Laurie J Nadolny, Nepean, ON - Family Medicine
Dr N P Vasavan Nair, Verdun, QC - Psychiatry
Dr Claire Nantel, St-Patr-Beaur, QC - General Practice
Dr Steven A Narod, Toronto, ON - Community Medicine
Dr Constance M Nasello, Chatham, ON - Obstetrics & Gynecology
Dr Emil Nashi, Montreal, QC - Clin Immun/Allergy
Dr Alain Naud, Quebec, QC - Family Medicine
Dr Laurie A Neapole, New Westminster, BC - Obstetrics & Gynecology
Dr David R Nemtean, Saint-Leonard, QC - General Practice
Dr Alain Neveu, Montreal, QC - General Practice
Dr Nathalie A Neveu, Montreal, QC - Endocrin/Metabolism
Dr Marc Neveu, Rouyn-Noranda, QC - Neurology
Dr Lynda K Newkirk, Hamilton, ON - Family Medicine
Dr Trevor M Newton, Langley, BC - Emergency Family Med
Dr Derek Ng, North Bay, ON - Emergency Family Med
Dr Alan Ng Cheng Hin, Ottawa, ON - Family Medicine
Dr Caroline Ng Cheong, Montreal, QC - Family Medicine
Dr Raphael Ng Fuk Chong, L'Ile-Perrot, QC - General Practice
Dr Roland Ng-Thow Hing, Pembroke, ON - General Practice
Dr Dung P Nghiem, Pointe-Claire, QC - General Practice
Dr Cuong Ngo Minh, Ottawa, ON - Family Medicine
Dr Tuyet Thi Nguyen, Belleville, ON - Family Medicine
Dr Thien Huong Nguyen, Belleville, ON - Nuclear Medicine
Dr Ngoc Truong T Nguyen, Oshawa, ON - Family Medicine
Dr Tang-Dong Nguyen, Brossard, QC - General Practice
Dr Tang-Thong Nguyen, Gatineau, QC - Cardiology
Dr Huu Nam Nguyen, Greenfield Park, QC - General Practice
Dr Thi Van Anh Nguyen, Laval, QC - Diagnostic-Radiology
Dr Thi Thanh T Nguyen, Laval, QC - Medical Microbiology
Dr Hoa Hieu Nguyen, Longueuil, QC - General Practice
Dr C L Remy Nguyen, Montreal, QC - Otolaryngology
Dr Bich-Ngoc Nguyen, Montreal, QC - Anatomical Pathology
Dr Van-Hung Nguyen, Montreal, QC - Anatomical Pathology
Dr Khue Huu Nguyen, Montreal, QC - Dermatology
Dr Bich Ngoc Nguyen, Montreal, QC - Psychiatry
Dr Tuong Minh Nguyen, Montreal, QC - Family Medicine
Dr Kim Anh Nguyen, Montreal, QC - General Practice
Dr Ngoc Bich Nguyen, Montreal, QC - Internal Medicine
Dr Doan-Trang Nguyen, Montreal, QC - Internal Medicine
Dr Thao Nguyen, Montreal, QC - Ophthalmology
Dr Mau Hoang Nguyen, Montreal-Nord, QC - General Practice
Dr Tuong-Nam Nguyen, Pointe-Claire, QC - Ophthalmology
Dr Van Hoi Nguyen, Saint-Laurent, QC - Family Medicine
Dr Michel Nguyen, Sherbrooke, QC - Cardiology
Dr Hai Hac Nguyen, St-Jean-sur-Richel, QC - Dermatology
Dr Myvan Nguyen, Verdun, QC - General Practice
Dr Thuy-Tien Nguyen-Dang, Amqui, QC - General Practice
Dr Felix Phuc Nguyen-Tan, Montreal, QC - Radiation Oncology
Dr Anna Niajko, Richelieu, QC - General Practice
Dr Doina Nica-Danes, Montreal, QC - General Practice
Dr Vaughan Nicholls, La Loche, SK - General Practice
Dr Robert M Nicholson, Granby, QC - Anatomical Pathology
Dr Marie-Noelle Nicole, Ottawa, ON - Family Medicine
Dr Alexandru Nicolescu-Zinca, Montreal, QC - Family Medicine
Dr Lynne E Nield, Toronto, ON - Cardiology
Dr Devin R Nielsen, Canmore, AB - Family Medicine
Dr Tara Nigam, Ottawa, ON - Psychiatry
Dr Anil Nigam, Montreal, QC - Cardiology
Dr Cheri L D Nijssen-Jordan, Calgary, AB - Pediatrics
Dr Ana Nikolic, Waterloo, ON - Family Medicine
Dr Jean-Noel Ning, Ottawa, ON - General Practice
Dr Gregoire E Noel, Montreal, QC - Medical Microbiology
Dr Daniel R Noel, Terrebonne, QC - Hematological Pathology
Dr Francoise Noel, Verdun, QC - Ophthalmology
Dr Robert Noiseux, Levis, QC - Psychiatry
Dr Jean-Marc Noiseux, Longueuil, QC - General Practice
Dr Daniel Noiseux, St-Jean-sur-Richel, QC - Endocrin/Metabolism
Dr Kevin J M Nolan, Ottawa, ON - Anesthesia
Dr Linda Nolin, Montreal, QC - Nephrology
Dr Luc Normandin, Montreal, QC - General Practice
Dr Jean-Junior Normandin, Saint-Hubert, QC - Dermatology
Dr Ginette Normandin-Noel, Pte-aux-Trembles, QC - General Practice
Dr Stanley Norris, La Tuque, QC - Psychiatry
Dr Scott A North, Edmonton, AB - Internal Medicine
Dr Fred M Novice, Windsor, ON - Dermatology
Dr Michael Nowlan, Gr-Sault/Gr-Falls, NB - General Practice
Dr Robert W Nugent, Fort Frances, ON - Family Medicine
Dr Shelley O'Blenis Caines, Oromocto, NB - Emergency Family Med
Dr David M O'Brien, Belleville, ON - Obstetrics & Gynecology
Dr Dermot B O'Brien, Hamilton, ON - Ophthalmology
Dr Heather V O'Brien, Sault Ste. Marie, ON - Anesthesia
Dr Mary O'Byrne, Calgary, AB - Pediatrics
Dr Colleen M O'Connell, Fredericton, NB - Physical Medicine & Rehab
Dr John K O'Driscoll, Montreal, QC - Emergency Family Med
Dr Terry A O'Farrell, Kelowna, BC - Orthopedic Surgery
Dr John A O'Neil, Montreal, QC - Psychiatry
Dr P Martin O'Shaughnessy, Gravenhurst, ON - General Practice
Dr Katherine O'Sullivan, Cowansville, QC - General Surgery
Dr Jason A Ohayon, Hamilton, ON - Clin Immun/Allergy
Dr Peter R Olesen, Campbell River, BC - Plastic Surgery
Dr Luc L Oligny, Montreal, QC - General Pathology
Dr Ronald Olivenstein, Montreal, QC - Internal Medicine
Dr Chantal Olivier, Brossard, QC - General Practice
Dr Marlene Olivier, Quebec, QC - General Practice
Dr David Olivier, Shawinigan, QC - Psychiatry
Dr Patrick Olivier, Sherbrooke, QC - Ophthalmology
Dr Narh Omaboe, Trenton, ON - Obstetrics & Gynecology
Dr Ronald M Onerheim, Montreal, QC - Anatomical Pathology
Dr Heather A Onyett, Kingston, ON - Infectious Diseases
Dr Farook N Oosman, Calgary, AB - General Practice
Dr David B Opper, Brantford, ON - Family Medicine
Dr Charles G Orfali, Sherbrooke, QC - Plastic Surgery
Dr Jacqueline Orquin, Montreal, QC - Ophthalmology
Dr Sevan G Ortaaslan, Kirkland, QC - Orthopedic Surgery
Dr John W Osterman, Laval, QC - Community Medicine
Dr Genevieve Ostiguy, Mont-Royal, QC - Family Medicine
Dr Gaston L Ostiguy, Montreal, QC - Internal Medicine
Dr Sylvie Ott-Braschi, Montreal, QC - General Practice
Dr Abdessebar Ouasti, St-Jean-Sur-Richel, QC - Psychiatry
Dr Jean-Albert Ouellet, Montreal, QC - Orthopedic Surgery
Dr Linda Ouellet, Riviere-du-Loup, QC - Pediatrics
Dr Yves Ouellet, Victoriaville, QC - Otolaryngology
Dr Paul Ouellette Jr, Granby, QC - Urology
Dr Denise M A Ouellette, Montreal, QC - General Surgery
Dr Nathalie Ouellette, Pierrefonds, QC - Pediatrics
Dr Michele Ouellette, Saint-Eustache, QC - General Practice
Dr Robert A Ouellette, Ste-Anne-de-Bellev, QC - Psychiatry
Dr Marie-Jo Ouimet, Montreal, QC - General Practice
Dr Denise Ouimet, Rouyn-Noranda, QC - Diagnostic-Radiology
Dr Dominique Ouimet, Saint-Jerome, QC - Cardiology
Dr Karen Oulianine, Montreal, QC - Emergency Family Med
Dr Nadine Packwood, Quebec, QC - General Practice
Dr Charles A Paco, Toronto, ON - Internal Medicine
Dr Michel Page, Dollard-D-Ormeaux, QC - General Practice
Dr Jean-Francois Paillard, Edmundston, NB - Orthopedic Surgery
Dr Bossuet Painson, Montreal, QC - General Pathology
Dr Jorge A Palacios-Boix, Montreal, QC - Psychiatry
Dr Karen S Palayew, Ottawa, ON - Pediatrics
Dr Mark D Palayew, Montreal, QC - Internal Medicine
Dr Louis-Philippe Palerme, Prince George, BC - General Surgery
Dr Linda K Panaro, Ottawa, ON - Community Medicine
Dr Dominique Panet-Raymond, Montreal, QC - Pediatrics
Dr Mitchell S Pantel, Montreal, QC - Family Medicine
Dr Henriette A Panzini, Mississauga, ON - Dermatology
Dr Demetrios Papadatos, Ottawa, ON - Diagnostic-Radiology
Dr Apkar Papazian, Saint-Leonard, QC - Urology
Dr Lisanne Papin, Laval, QC - General Practice
Dr Martin Papineau, Hearst, ON - Family Medicine
Dr Martin Paquet, Sherbrooke, QC - General Practice
Dr Isabelle Paquet, Terrebonne, QC - Internal Medicine
Dr Lise J Paquette, Toronto, ON - Family Medicine
Dr Daniel Paquette, Laval, QC - Community Medicine
Dr Serge Paquette, Laval, QC - General Practice
Dr Isabelle Paquette, Montreal, QC - Psychiatry
Dr Nicole Paquette, Pte-aux-Trembles, QC - Dermatology
Dr Louis Paquette, Saint-Georges, QC - Emergency Family Med
Dr Colette Paquin, Toronto, ON - Dermatology
Dr Rejean Paradis, Ottawa, ON - Community Medicine
Dr Rachelle L Paradis, Sudbury, ON - General Surgery

Dr Yves Paradis, Amos, QC - General Practice
Dr Andre Paradis, Quebec, QC - Family Medicine
Dr Robert Pare, Laval, QC - General Practice
Dr Jocelyne Parent, North York, ON - Pediatrics
Dr Yves Parent, Montreal, QC - General Practice
Dr Josee Parent, Montreal, QC - Gastroenterology
Dr Jean-Guy Parent, Quebec, QC - Respirology
Dr Marie-Josee Parent, Quebec, QC - General Practice
Dr Rene Parent, Quebec, QC - Physical Medicine & Rehab
Dr Andre Parent, Saint-Isidore, QC - General Practice
Dr Mariloue Parent, Vaudreuil-Dorion, QC - General Practice
Dr Chantal Parenteau, Trois-Rivieres, QC - Endocrin/Metabolism
Dr Catherine Paris, Sorel-Tracy, QC - Family Medicine
Dr Gladys Parisien, Shawinigan-Sud, QC - General Pathology
Dr Ian R A Park, Campbellford, ON - General Practice
Dr Joel L Parlow, Kingston, ON - Anesthesia
Dr Andre Pasternac, Westmount, QC - Cardiology
Dr Brian L Patenaude, Gatineau, QC - Ophthalmology
Dr Simon Patry, Quebec, QC - Psychiatry
Dr Michel Patry, Trois-Rivieres, QC - Obstetrics & Gynecology
Dr Judy L Patterson, Ottawa, ON - Family Medicine
Dr Adrien Paul, Amos, QC - Pediatrics
Dr Chantal Paulin, Sherbrooke, QC - Cardiology
Dr Clement Payette, St-Felix-de-Valois, QC - General Practice
Dr Richard Payeur, Maniwaki, QC - Psychiatry
Dr Allen Payne, Montreal, QC - General Practice
Dr Jonathan L Peck, Mississauga, ON - Family Medicine
Dr Caroline Pedneault, Longueuil, QC - Pediatrics
Dr Yousouf A Peerbaye, Toronto, ON - Emergency Medicine
Dr Kevin Pehr, Westmount, QC - Dermatology
Dr Bonavuth Pek, St-Charles-Brromee, QC - Internal Medicine
Dr Stephane Pelet, Quebec, QC - General Practice
Dr Marcel Pelland, St-Gabriel-d-Brand, QC - General Practice
Dr Michel Pellerin, Montreal, QC - Cardiovasc/ThorSurg
Dr Denis P Pelletier, Edmundston, NB - General Practice
Dr Denis Pelletier, La Pocatiere, QC - General Practice
Dr Christine Pelletier, Montreal, QC - General Practice
Dr Jean Pelletier, Montreal, QC - Family Medicine
Dr Michele Pelletier, Montreal, QC - General Practice
Dr Veronique Anne Pelletier, Montreal, QC - Pediatrics
Dr Rene Pelletier, Quebec, QC - Medical Microbiology
Dr Alain Pelletier, Shawinigan-Sud, QC - General Practice
Dr Jean Peloquin, Greenfield Park, QC - Psychiatry
Dr Francois A Peloquin, Montreal, QC - Urology
Dr Jean Peloquin, Quebec, QC - General Surgery
Dr Jacques Peloquin, St-Joseph-du-Lac, QC - General Practice
Dr Kevork Minas Peltekian, Halifax, NS - Gastroenterology
Dr Ancuta Pepelea, Ste-Anne-de-Bellev, QC - General Practice
Dr E Paul Pepin, Mascouche, QC - Neurology
Dr Sylvie Pepin, St-Jean-des-Piles, QC - General Practice
Dr Paul B Percheson, North York, ON - General Practice
Dr Robert B Pereira, Surrey, BC - Family Medicine
Dr Masis Perk, Truro, NS - Internal Medicine
Dr Robert J Perlman, Dorval, QC - General Practice
Dr Louis P Perrault, Montreal, QC - Cardiovasc/ThorSurg
Dr Pierre Perreault, Montreal, QC - Diagnostic-Radiology
Dr Jean-Paul Perreault, Montreal, QC - Urology
Dr Francois Perreault, Ste-Anne-De-Bellev, QC - General Practice
Dr Lyette Perreault, Terrebonne, QC - Diagnostic-Radiology
Dr Guy Perrier, La Sarre, QC - General Practice
Dr Marie-Pascale Perrier, Sherbrooke, QC - Psychiatry
Dr Linda Perron, Quebec, QC - Community Medicine
Dr Patrice Perron, Sherbrooke, QC - Endocrin/Metabolism
Dr Thierry Perron, Sorel-Tracy, QC - General Surgery
Dr Megan A Persson, Montreal, QC - Emergency Family Med
Dr George Peterson, Saint-Hubert, QC - General Practice
Dr Marc Petitclerc, Levis, QC - Electroencephal
Dr Claude Petitclerc, Quebec, QC - Hematology
Dr Xuan H Pham, Ottawa, ON - Nuclear Medicine
Dr Tuong-Vi Pham, Val-d'Or, QC - Family Medicine
Dr Martin Pham-Dinh, Gatineau, QC - Emergency Family Med
Dr Xuan Truong Phan, Montreal, QC - General Practice
Dr Denis Phaneuf, Montreal, QC - Medical Microbiology
Dr Marielle R P Pharand, Vanier, ON - General Practice
Dr Francois Philippon, Quebec, QC - Cardiology
Dr Peter G Phillips, Collingwood, ON - Family Medicine
Dr Claude Picard, Quebec, QC - Neurosurgery
Dr Daniel Picard, Saint-Jerome, QC - Nuclear Medicine
Dr Laura R Piccinin, Sudbury, ON - Emergency Family Med
Dr Daniele Piche, St-Aug-D-Desm, QC - General Practice
Dr Francois Picher, Deschambault, QC - General Practice
Dr Jean-Francois Pidgeon, Thetford Mines, QC - General Surgery
Dr Jean-Rene Pierre, Maniwaki, QC - General Practice
Dr Michel B J Pigeon, Penetanguishene, ON - General Surgery
Dr Josee L Pilon, Ottawa, ON - Family Medicine
Dr Claude Pilon, Montreal, QC - Cardiology
Dr Robert P Pilorge, Montreal, QC - Obstetrics & Gynecology
Dr Nicholas Pilote, Moncton, NB - Diagnostic-Radiology
Dr Louise Pilote, Montreal, QC - Internal Medicine
Dr Marie Pinault, Gatineau, QC - General Practice
Dr Michel Pineau, Lourdes-D-Bl-Sabl, QC - Family Medicine
Dr Christian A Pineau, Montreal, QC - Internal Medicine
Dr Monique Pinsonneault, Longueuil, QC - Internal Medicine
Dr Linda Pinsonneault, Montreal, QC - Community Medicine
Dr Jose M Pires, Ottawa, ON - General Surgery
Dr Cesar Pison, Montreal, QC - Endocrinology
Dr Lino A Pistor, Sault Ste. Marie, ON - Psychiatry
Dr Gilles Plamondon, Montreal, QC - General Practice
Dr Jean-Francois Planet, Ottawa, ON - Otolaryngology
Dr Judith C Plante, Pembroke, ON - Family Medicine
Dr Michel Plante, Montreal, QC - General Practice
Dr Diane Plante, Sherbrooke, QC - General Practice
Dr Ludovic Plante Jr, Sherbrooke, QC - General Practice
Dr Robert P Pless, Ottawa, ON - General Practice
Dr Pierre Plourde, Salaber-de-Valleyf, QC - Internal Medicine
Dr Joseph L Po, Ottawa, ON - Anesthesia
Dr Marc J Poirier, Gatineau, QC - General Practice
Dr Michel Poirier, Granby, QC - General Practice
Dr Claude Poirier, Levis, QC - Cardiology
Dr Charles D Poirier, Montreal, QC - Internal Medicine
Dr Madeleine Poirier, Montreal, QC - General Surgery
Dr Helene Poirier, Montreal, QC - Psychiatry
Dr Jacques Poirier, Repentigny, QC - General Practice
Dr Andre Poisson, Dolbeau-Mistassini, QC - General Practice
Dr Marco Poisson, Victoriaville, QC - General Practice
Dr Marie-Josee Poitras, Dieppe, NB - Family Medicine
Dr Daniel Poitras, Laval, QC - General Practice
Dr Pierre Poitras, Laval, QC - Pediatrics
Dr Gaetan Poitras, Saint-Leonard, QC - General Practice
Dr Ronald P Pokrupa, Kingston, ON - Neurosurgery
Dr Steven A Poleski, Ottawa, ON - Ophthalmology
Dr Denis Poliquin, St-Jean-Sur-Richel, QC - General Surgery
Dr Mate Poljicak, Montreal, QC - General Surgery
Dr Michael N Pollak, Montreal, QC - Internal Medicine
Dr Constantin Polychronakos, Montreal, QC - Endocrinology
Dr Damien Pomerleau, Montreal, QC - Pediatrics
Dr John Pommerville, Victoria, BC - Urology
Dr Eric Pontbriand, Windsor, QC - General Practice
Dr Alexander J Poole, Whitehorse, YT - General Surgery
Dr Mihai Pop, Montreal, QC - Ophthalmology
Dr Laila Popescu-Dumbrava, Sept-Iles, QC - Family Medicine
Dr Geoffrey A Porter, Halifax, NS - General Surgery
Dr Steven D Potoker, Montreal, QC - Dermatology
Dr Jacques A Potvin, Saint-Bruno, QC - Neurosurgery
Dr Jean-Guy Potvin, Saint-Jerome, QC - General Practice
Dr Patrice E E Poubelle, Quebec, QC - Rheumatology
Dr Renald M Poulin, Alma, QC - General Surgery
Dr Chantal Poulin, Montreal, QC - Electroencephal
Dr Jean-Francois Poulin, Quebec, QC - Cardiology
Dr Yves P Poulin, Quebec, QC - Dermatology
Dr Sonya Poulin, Quebec, QC - Internal Medicine
Dr Stephane Poulin, Ste-Agathe-Des-Mts, QC - General Practice
Dr Maurice Poulin, Trois-Rivieres, QC - Occupational Med
Dr Johanne Pouliot, Mascouche, QC - General Practice
Dr Rene Pouliot, Quebec, QC - Internal Medicine
Dr Robert Poupart, Saint-Jerome, QC - Cardiology
Dr Emmanuelle Pourcher, Quebec, QC - Neurology
Dr Kathryn A Powell-Francis, Scarborough, ON - Anesthesia
Dr Alexandre Prat, Montreal, QC - Neurology
Dr Patrick Prefontaine, Ste-Anne-Plai, QC - General Practice
Dr Jean J M Prenovault, Winnipeg, MB - Family Medicine
Dr Lise Prescott, Verdun, QC - Neurology
Dr Guy Preville, Val-David, QC - Anesthesia
Dr Derek Prevost, Surrey, BC - Pediatrics
Dr Francois A Prevost, Inukjuak, QC - General Practice
Dr Sylvain Prevost, Sherbrooke, QC - Nuclear Medicine
Dr Francois J Primeau, Levis, QC - Psychiatry
Dr Navin Prinja, North Bay, ON - Otolaryngology
Dr Harry Prochette, Repentigny, QC - General Practice
Dr Allison B Prokopiak, Stittsville, ON - Family Medicine
Dr Albert Prossin, Montreal, QC - Family Medicine
Dr Guylaine Proulx, Gatineau, QC - Family Medicine
Dr Francois Proulx, Montreal, QC - Critical Care Medicine
Dr Simon-Pierre Proulx, Quebec, QC - General Practice
Dr Reno Proulx, Sherbrooke, QC - General Practice
Dr Edith Provencal, Chateauguay, QC - General Practice
Dr France Provencher, Laval, QC - General Practice
Dr Yves L Provost, Montreal, QC - Diagnostic-Radiology
Dr Denis Prud'Homme, Gatineau, QC - General Practice
Dr Rodrigue Prud'Homme, Gatineau, QC - General Practice
Dr Pramod S Puligandla, Montreal, QC - Critical Care Medicine
Dr Lizy Puri-Alanoly, Vaudreuil-Dorion, QC - General Practice
Dr Adrian Pusca, Lac-Megantic, QC - Internal Medicine
Dr Baqir A Qizilbash, Montreal, QC - Anesthesia
Dr Caroline Quach-Thanh, Montreal, QC - Infectious Diseases
Dr Daniel R Quance, Montreal, QC - Anesthesia
Dr Michael G Quigley, Montreal, QC - Ophthalmology
Dr Brendan P Quinn, Ottawa, ON - Cardiology
Dr M C Diane Quintal, Ottawa, ON - Dermatology
Dr France Quintal, Beloeil, QC - General Practice
Dr Marie Quintal, Gatineau, QC - Psychiatry
Dr Sylvie Quirion, Joliette, QC - Community Medicine
Dr Salman T Qureshi, Montreal, QC - Critical Care Medicine
Dr Irving Rabin, Brossard, QC - Pediatrics
Dr Samuel M Rabinovitch, Scarborough, ON - Diagnostic-Radiology
Dr Mark A Rabinovitch, Westmount, QC - Cardiology
Dr Nicole Racette, Vancouver, BC - Obstetrics & Gynecology
Dr Francois Racette, Saint-Eustache, QC - Internal Medicine
Dr Anita R Rachlis, Toronto, ON - Infectious Diseases
Dr Michel Racine, Laval, QC - Family Medicine
Dr Normand Racine, Montreal, QC - Cardiology
Dr Simon Racine, Quebec, QC - Community Medicine
Dr Mohan Radhakrishna, Montreal, QC - Physical Medicine & Rehab
Dr Victor Radoux, Montreal, QC - Rheumatology
Dr Farouk Radwan, Montreal, QC - Medical Biochemistry
Dr M Rose Rahmani, Toronto, ON - Diagnostic-Radiology
Dr J C Bruno Rainville, Quebec, QC - General Surgery
Dr Janet Rak, Thornhill, ON - Family Medicine
Dr Denis C Ramalho, Trois-Rivieres, QC - General Practice
Dr Mathangi Ramani, Lasalle, QC - Diagnostic-Radiology
Dr Droovnath Ramful, Elk Point, AB - General Practice
Dr R Alec Ramsay, Montreal, QC - Psychiatry
Dr Jacques Ramsay, Montreal, QC - General Practice
Dr Patrice A Ranger, Vancouver, BC - Family Medicine
Dr Wayne M Rankin, Sarnia, ON - General Practice
Dr George Rateb, Sherbrooke, QC - General Practice
Dr Michael B Rath, Langley, BC - Family Medicine
Dr Jack T Ratner, Montreal, QC - Gastroenterology
Dr Neil V Rau, Oakville, ON - Infectious Diseases
Dr Christopher J Rauscher, Vancouver, BC - Geriatric Medicine
Dr Karen E Raymer, Hamilton, ON - Anesthesia
Dr Yves L Raymond, Timmins, ON - Family Medicine
Dr Giles P Raymond, Pierrefonds, QC - Dermatology
Dr Vincent Raymond, Quebec, QC - General Practice
Dr Paul-Emile Raymond, Rimouski, QC - Radiation Oncology
Dr Mark L Reardon, Ottawa, ON - Emergency Family Medicine
Dr Margaretha Rebel, London, ON - Obstetrics & Gynecology
Dr Robert B Reddoch, Cornwall, ON - Emergency Family Med
Dr Wayne M Redmond, St. John's, NL - Otolaryngology
Dr Lynda Redwood-Campbell, Hamilton, ON - Family Medicine
Dr Nittin K Reebye, New Westminster, BC - Physical Medicine & Rehab
Dr Charles E Reed, Guelph, ON - General Practice
Dr Katherine M Reed, Pointe-Claire, QC - General Practice
Dr Leonora J Regenstreif, Hamilton, ON - Family Medicine
Dr Marc Regimbal, Gatineau, QC - General Practice

Dr Laura R J Regnier, Ottawa, ON - Family Medicine
Dr Heather N Reich, Toronto, ON - Internal Medicine
Dr Miles E Reid, Fort McMurray, AB - Diagnostic-Radiology
Dr Barbara A Reid, Cornwall, ON - Anatomical Pathology
Dr Diane E Reid, Hamilton, ON - Otolaryngology
Dr Kenneth R Reid, Kingston, ON - General Surgery
Dr Craig W Reid, Nepean, ON - Anesthesia
Dr Dennis Reid, Ottawa, ON - Anesthesia
Dr Annick Reid, Blainville, QC - General Practice
Dr John J Reisman, Ottawa, ON - Pediatrics
Dr Jean Remillard, Montreal, QC - Physical Medicine & Rehab
Dr Guy M Remillard, Montreal, QC - Electroencephal
Dr Francine Remillard, Sherbrooke, QC - General Practice
Dr Pierre Renaud, Orleans, ON - General Practice
Dr Eric G Renaud, Laval, QC - Orthopedic Surgery
Dr Suzane M Renaud, Verdun, QC - Psychiatry
Dr Johanne Renaud, Verdun, QC - Psychiatry
Dr Paule Renault, Candiac, QC - General Practice
Dr Marcel Reny, Gatineau, QC - General Practice
Dr Alfonso Restrepo, St-Eustache, QC - General Practice
Dr Richard K Reznick, Kingston, ON - General Surgery
Dr Paul L C Rheault, Sudbury, ON - Family Medicine
Dr Teresa A I Rheaume, Beachburg, ON - General Practice
Dr Caroline I Rheaume, Quebec, QC - Obstetrics & Gynecology
Dr Ian N Rhodes, Ottawa, ON - Diagnostic-Radiology
Dr Margarita R Riano Alvarez, LaSalle, QC - Family Medicine
Dr Stephane Ricard, Sherbrooke, QC - Orthopedic Surgery
Dr Norbert S Richard, Moncton, NB - General Practice
Dr Michael T Richard, Ottawa, ON - Neurosurgery
Dr Luc Richard, Forestville, QC - General Practice
Dr Bernard Richard Jr, Salaber-de-Valleyf, QC - General Practice
Dr Claude Richard, Victoriaville, QC - Internal Medicine
Dr Douglas W Richards, Toronto, ON - General Practice
Dr Donald W Richardson, Kingston, ON - Pediatrics
Dr Lawrence Richer, Edmonton, AB - Neurology
Dr Genevieve Richer, Kirkland, QC - General Practice
Dr Kenneth Richter, Montreal, QC - Psychiatry
Dr Pierre-Jacques Ricot, Pointe-Claire, QC - Pediatrics
Dr David Riddell, Cornwall, ON - Anesthesia
Dr Stephane Rinfret, Quebec, QC - Cardiology
Dr Pierre Ringwald, Ottawa, ON - Dermatology
Dr Richard J Riopelle, Kingston, ON - Internal Medicine
Dr Johanne Rioux, Greenfield Park, QC - Psychiatry
Dr Marie-France Rioux, Sherbrooke, QC - Neurology
Dr Janet Ritchie, Montreal, QC - Psychiatry
Dr Charles H Rivard, Montreal, QC - Orthopedic Surgery
Dr Jose A Rivas, St-Jean-sur-Richel, QC - General Practice
Dr Jason Rivers, Vancouver, BC - Dermatology
Dr Denis Rivest, Amos, QC - Family Medicine
Dr Natalie Rivest, Laval, QC - Medical Microbiology
Dr Donald Rivest, Levis, QC - Electroencephal
Dr Martin Rivest, Terrebonne, QC - Emergency Family Med
Dr Andre G Rivet, North Bay, ON - General Practice
Dr Real J F Rivet, Ville-Marie, QC - General Practice
Dr Robert N Rivington, Ottawa, ON - Internal Medicine
Dr Barbara R Roback, Victoria, BC - Family Medicine
Dr Rene R Roberge, Baie-Saint-Paul, QC - Anesthesia
Dr Claude A Roberge, Montreal, QC - Pediatrics
Dr Daniel Roberge, Quebec, QC - General Practice
Dr Danielle Roberge, Saint-Jerome, QC - General Practice
Dr Annie Roberge, Sherbrooke, QC - General Practice
Dr Michael Robern, Nepean, ON - Dermatology
Dr Paul F Robert, St Catharines, ON - Orthopedic Surgery
Dr Monique Robert, Montreal, QC - Pediatrics
Dr Michael C Roberts, Toronto, ON - Family Medicine
Dr Richard D Roberts, Pointe-Claire, QC - Neurology
Dr Lynne H Robertson, Calgary, AB - Dermatology
Dr Dale F Robertson, Canmore, AB - Pediatrics
Dr Nancy L Robertson, Bedford, NS - General Practice
Dr Sylvie Robichaud, Bathurst, NB - Internal Medicine
Dr Delbe J Robichaud, Campbellton, NB - General Practice
Dr Jeffrey M Robichaud, St Catharines, ON - Otolaryngology
Dr Nicole Robillard, Montreal, QC - Ophthalmology
Dr Antoine Robineault, Maria, QC - Pediatrics
Dr Virginia W Robinson, Fernie, BC - Emergency Family Med
Dr Dale K Robinson, Markham, ON - Neurology
Dr Linda A Robinson, Ottawa, ON - Anesthesia
Dr Eric J Robinson, Sudbury, ON - Orthopedic Surgery
Dr Marie-Brigitte Robinson, Sudbury, ON - Otolaryngology
Dr Elizabeth Robinson, Montreal, QC - Community Medicine
Dr E Jean Robison, Toronto, ON - Family Medicine
Dr Daniel Robitaille, Baie-Comeau, QC - Medical Biochemistry
Dr David Robitaille, Longueuil, QC - Psychiatry
Dr Yves Robitaille, Montreal, QC - General Pathology
Dr Nancy Robitaille, Montreal, QC - Hematology
Dr Nancy-Michelle Robitaille, Quebec, QC - Cardiology
Dr Robert J Robson, Elora, ON - Emergency Medicine
Dr Hugh G Robson, Montreal, QC - Internal Medicine
Dr J J C Andre Roch, Sudbury, ON - General Practice
Dr Guillermo Rocha, Brandon, MB - Ophthalmology
Dr Denise T Rochon, Montreal, QC - Psychiatry
Dr Jean Rochon, Montreal, QC - Community Medicine
Dr Marc A Rodger, Ottawa, ON - Hematology
Dr Pierre Y Rodrigue, Gatineau, QC - General Practice
Dr Jean Rodrigue, Quebec, QC - General Practice
Dr Ghislaine Roederer, Montreal, QC - General Practice
Dr Peter Rohan, Montreal, QC - General Practice
Dr Daryl S Roitman, North York, ON - Hematology
Dr Marek Rola-Pleszczynski, Sherbrooke, QC - Clin Immun/Allergy
Dr Ramon Roman, Verdun, QC - Anesthesia
Dr Nancy K Romsa, St Thomas, ON - Emergency Family Med
Dr Allan R Ronald, Winnipeg, MB - Internal Medicine
Dr Chantal Rondeau, Laval, QC - Emergency Family Med
Dr Mark J Ropeleski, Kingston, ON - Gastroenterology
Dr Peter D L Roper, Westmount, QC - Psychiatry
Dr Colin P Rose, Montreal, QC - Cardiology
Dr Nathan A Rosen, Burlington, ON - Dermatology
Dr Dalia S Rosen-Zaidener, Richmond Hill, ON - Family Medicine
Dr Lawrence Rosenberg, Montreal, QC - General Surgery
Dr Ellen E Rosenberg, Montreal, QC - Family Medicine
Dr Andrea Rosenbloom, Scarborough, ON - Cardiology
Dr I Shoel Rosenhek, Windsor, ON - Cardiology
Dr Donald Rosenthal, Hamilton, ON - Dermatology
Dr Gary A Rosenthal, Scarborough, ON - General Surgery
Dr Stephen E Rosenthal, Montreal, QC - Emergency Family Med
Dr Leonard Rosenthall, Montreal, QC - Diagnostic-Radiology
Dr Michael A Rosman, Saint-Leonard, QC - Orthopedic Surgery
Dr Leslie A Rosoph, North Bay, ON - Dermatology
Dr David B Ross, Edmonton, AB - Cardiovasc/ThorSurg
Dr Stephen G Ross, Toronto, ON - Family Medicine
Dr Walter W Rosser, Kingston, ON - Family Medicine
Dr John P Rossiter, Kingston, ON - Neuro-Pathology
Dr Nathan L Roth, Scarborough, ON - Obstetrics & Gynecology
Dr Steven W Rothman, Toronto, ON - Family Medicine
Dr John M Rothschild, Calgary, AB - Cardiovasc/ThorSurg
Dr Gervais Rouillard, Victoriaville, QC - Otolaryngology
Dr Lucie Rouleau, Alma, QC - Obstetrics & Gynecology
Dr Charles D Rouleau, Gatineau, QC - General Practice
Dr Jean-Lucien Rouleau, Montreal, QC - Cardiology
Dr Michel Rouleau, Quebec, QC - Respirology
Dr Timothy W Rourke, Gloucester, ON - General Practice
Dr Genevieve D Rousseau, Ottawa, ON - Obstetrics & Gynecology
Dr Come Rousseau, Chicoutimi, QC - Hematology
Dr Pierre Rousseau, Montreal, QC - Anesthesia
Dr Helene Rousseau, Montreal, QC - Family Medicine
Dr Louise Rousseau, Montreal, QC - Psychiatry
Dr Francois Rousseau, Quebec, QC - Psychiatry
Dr Shelley Ann A Routhier, Hanmer, ON - Family Medicine
Dr Line Routhier, Chandler, QC - General Practice
Dr J J Richard Routhier, Gatineau, QC - General Practice
Dr Marie-Claude Routhier, Quebec, QC - General Practice
Dr Bruce M T Rowat, Toronto, ON - Internal Medicine
Dr Richard Rowland, Kingston, ON - General Practice
Dr Gerald C Rowland, Tillsonburg, ON - General Practice
Dr Maurice J B Roy, Ste Anne, MB - Family Medicine
Dr Maurice P Roy, Grand Falls, NB - General Practice
Dr Daniel J Roy, Saint-Leonard, NB - General Practice
Dr Marc J Roy, Kanata, ON - Family Medicine
Dr Marie L Roy, North York, ON - Occupational Med
Dr Paul D Roy, Ottawa, ON - Psychiatry
Dr Nathalie A L Roy, Sudbury, ON - Family Medicine
Dr Bernadette Roy, Baie-Saint-Paul, QC - General Practice
Dr Martine Roy, Jonquiere, QC - General Practice
Dr Sebastien Roy, Laval, QC - Anesthesia
Dr Nathalie Roy, Levis, QC - Internal Medicine
Dr Denis-Claude Roy, Montreal, QC - Hematology
Dr Diane Roy, Montreal, QC - General Practice
Dr Louis-Edouard Roy, Montreal, QC - Electroencephal
Dr Louise Roy, Montreal, QC - Internal Medicine
Dr Marie-Claude Roy, Quebec, QC - Medical Microbiology
Dr Genevieve Roy, Quebec, QC - Pediatrics
Dr Marie-Christine Roy, Quebec, QC - Obstetrics & Gynecology
Dr Michel Roy, Quebec, QC - Gynecologic Oncology
Dr Helene Roy, Quebec, QC - General Practice
Dr Sylvie Roy, Saint-Eustache, QC - General Practice
Dr Aline Roy, Sherbrooke, QC - General Practice
Dr Suzanne Roy, Trois-Rivieres, QC - General Practice
Dr Anne-Marie Roy-Boulos, Ottawa, ON - Dermatology
Dr Charmaine A Roye, Brantford, ON - Obstetrics & Gynecology
Dr Williine R Rozefort, Verdun, QC - Family Medicine
Dr Heather Rubenstein, Montreal, QC - Family Medicine
Dr Steven E Rubenzahl, North York, ON - General Practice
Dr Mitchell B Rubin, North Vancouver, BC - Family Medicine
Dr Barry B Rubin, Toronto, ON - Vascular Surgery
Dr Gordon Rubin, Montreal, QC - Family Medicine
Dr Nicholas S Ruddock, Guelph, ON - General Practice
Dr Edward J Rumble, North York, ON - Orthopedic Surgery
Dr Lenuta Rus-Serban, Pointe-Claire, QC - General Practice
Dr Ronald Ruskin, Toronto, ON - Psychiatry
Dr Mladen V Rusnov, Montreal, QC - General Surgery
Dr Marianne T Russell, Coquitlam, BC - Family Medicine
Dr Jennifer S W Russell, Fredericton, NB - Family Medicine
Dr Balbina Russillo, Montreal, QC - Family Medicine
Dr Alexandra D Ruszkowski, Oshawa, ON - Plastic Surgery
Dr L Poovendren Ruthnum, Surrey, BC - Pediatrics
Dr Robert D H Rutledge, Halifax, NS - Radiation Oncology
Dr Jacqueline I Ruttenberg, Saint-Hubert, QC - Family Medicine
Dr J Georges Sabourin, Edmonton, AB - Obstetrics & Gynecology
Dr Karine Sabourin, Mont-Laurier, QC - Family Medicine
Dr Gregory C Safar, Brantford, ON - Emergency Family Med
Dr Serge Saint-Amant, Saint-Antoine, NB - Family Medicine
Dr Robert R Saint-Jacques, Saint-Eustache, QC - Dermatology
Dr Daniel Saint-Laurent, Montreal, QC - Psychiatry
Dr Suzanne Saint-Martin, Outremont, QC - General Practice
Dr Jean-Yves Saint-Pierre, Sherbrooke, QC - Psychiatry
Dr Dickens Saint-Vil, Montreal, QC - General Surgery
Dr Michel Sakellarides, Cornwall, ON - General Practice
Dr Gorgin Salami, Montreal, QC - General Practice
Dr Karl H Sales, Kirkland Lake, ON - Ophthalmology
Dr Nasri Saliba, Gatineau, QC - Urology
Dr David A Salisbury, Ottawa, ON - Community Medicine
Dr Gurjinder P Sall, Montreal, QC - General Practice
Dr Nancy E Salter, Toronto, ON - Psychiatry
Dr Ginetta L Salvalaggio, Edmonton, AB - Family Medicine
Dr Linda A Samotis-Tchervenkov, Montreal, QC - Pediatrics
Dr Olivia J Sampson, Vancouver, BC - Family Medicine
Dr Isabelle Samson, Quebec, QC - Family Medicine
Dr Isabelle Samson, Sherbrooke, QC - Community Medicine
Dr Gilles Samson, Thetford Mines, QC - General Practice
Dr Marisol Sanchez, Montreal, QC - Pediatric Emergency Medicine
Dr Andree Sansregret, Montreal, QC - Obstetrics & Gynecology
Dr Josee Sarrazin, Toronto, ON - Diagnostic-Radiology
Dr Gerald Sarrazin, Terrebonne, QC - General Practice
Dr Janik G Sarrazin, Val-d'Or, QC - Family Medicine
Dr Francine Sasseville, Longueuil, QC - General Practice
Dr Philippe Sauthier, Montreal, QC - Gynecologic Oncology
Dr Chantal Sauvageau, Quebec, QC - Community Medicine
Dr Jean-Paul Sauvageau, Riviere-Du-Loup, QC - Pediatrics
Dr Patrick Savard, Quebec, QC - Otolaryngology
Dr Liette Savoie, Amos, QC - Pediatrics
Dr Anne-Marie Savoie, Levis, QC - General Practice
Dr Louis Savoie, St-Mar-des-Carr, QC - General Practice
Dr Bassem Sawan, Sherbrooke, QC - Anatomical Pathology
Dr Renee Sayegh, Verdun, QC - General Practice

Dr Carmen P Scaffidi, Ville-Marie, QC - Family Medicine
Dr Dominique Scarfone, Outremont, QC - Psychiatry
Dr Christine Scarinci, Montreal, QC - Pediatrics
Dr Dimitrios Scarvelis, Ottawa, ON - Hematology
Dr Frederic J Scheid, Terrebonne, QC - Psychiatry
Dr Jacques Scherer, Laval, QC - General Practice
Dr Gilles Scherer, Longueuil, QC - Psychiatry
Dr Ernesto L Schiffrin, Montreal, QC - Internal Medicine
Dr Mitchell J Schipper, Montreal, QC - Family Medicine
Dr Walter Schurch, Montreal, QC - Anatomical Pathology
Dr M J F Lise Scott, Gloucester, ON - Family Medicine
Dr Carol L Scott, Markham, ON - General Practice
Dr Hugh A Scott, Quebec, QC - Emergency Family Med
Dr Rosie Scuccimarri, Montreal, QC - Pediatrics
Dr Fatiha Seddiki, Laval, QC - Pediatrics
Dr Andrew J E Seely, Ottawa, ON - Critical Care Medicine
Dr Eli Segal, Montreal, QC - Emergency Medicine
Dr Marilyn Segal, Montreal, QC - Psychiatry
Dr Bernard A Seguin, Orleans, ON - Family Medicine
Dr Jean J Seguin, Vanier, ON - Family Medicine
Dr Joseph J Y Seguin, Gatineau, QC - Psychiatry
Dr Anick Seguin, Victoriaville, QC - Anesthesia
Dr Jose A C Segura, Chandler, QC - Psychiatry
Dr Houfar Sekhavat, Dieppe, NB - Ophthalmology
Dr Claude Sergerie, Boisbriano, QC - General Practice
Dr Manuel Serrano, Montreal, QC - Psychiatry
Dr Robert N Sers, Antigonish, NS - General Surgery
Dr Francois Sestier, Montreal, QC - Cardiology
Dr Jean C Setrakian, Sherbrooke, QC - Internal Medicine
Dr E Peter Seviour, St. John's, NL - Family Medicine
Dr Anna Sfriso, Levis, QC - Otolaryngology
Dr April A Shamy, Montreal, QC - Hematology
Dr A M James Shapiro, Edmonton, AB - General Surgery
Dr R Jean Shapiro, Vancouver, BC - Internal Medicine
Dr Marla Shapiro, North York, ON - Community Medicine
Dr Robert S Shapiro, Cote Saint-Luc, QC - Otolaryngology
Dr Vijay K Sharma, Miramichi, NB - Ophthalmology
Dr Roberta M Shear, Montreal, QC - Obstetrics & Gynecology
Dr Daniel Shedid, Montreal, QC - Neurosurgery
Dr Raisa Sheftel, Verdun, QC - General Practice
Dr Michael I Shevell, Montreal, QC - Neurology
Dr Claude Shields, Quebec, QC - Hematology
Dr Joseph Shuster, Montreal, QC - Med Scientist
Dr Pascale L R Sibille, Gatineau, QC - General Practice
Dr Jaime Siclait, Boisbriand, QC - Family Medicine
Dr Jean-Guy Sicotte, Magog, QC - General Practice
Dr Zouhair Sidani, Montreal, QC - Otolaryngology
Dr Lucas Sideris, Montreal, QC - General Surgery
Dr Irving J Siegel, Brampton, ON - General Practice
Dr Daniela Sielecka, Mansonville, QC - General Practice
Dr Sergio Sierra-Dupont, Montreal, QC - Otolaryngology
Dr Eric H Sigman, Montreal, QC - Emergency Family Med
Dr Fidelia A Silva, Moncton, NB - Gastroenterology
Dr Sylvain Simard, Chicoutimi, QC - Family Medicine
Dr Normand Simard, Chicoutimi, QC - Psychiatry
Dr Louis Simard, Chicoutimi, QC - Family Medicine
Dr Jacques Simard, Laval, QC - Pediatrics
Dr Sylvain Simard, Quebec, QC - Endocrinology
Dr Genevieve Simard-Racine, Amqui, QC - General Practice
Dr Sonia Simion, Montreal, QC - General Practice
Dr Allyson Simms, Coaticook, QC - General Practice
Dr Jeannine G M Simon, Pointe-Claire, QC - Obstetrics & Gynecology
Dr Mathieu Simon, Quebec, QC - Critical Care Medicine
Dr Santokh Singh, Montreal, QC - Psychiatry
Dr Marsha C Sklar, Montreal, QC - Anatomical Pathology
Dr Barry Slapcoff, Westmount, QC - Family Medicine
Dr Karen E Slatkovsky, Guelph, ON - Emergency Family Med
Dr Jeffrey P E Sloan, Sudbury, ON - Anesthesia
Dr Donald S Smallman, Kingston, ON - Ophthalmology
Dr Lesley J Smith, Edmonton, AB - Pediatrics
Dr Gregory L Smith, Raymond, AB - Family Medicine
Dr W Gary Smith, Orillia, ON - Pediatrics
Dr Kevin D Smith, Ottawa, ON - Ophthalmology
Dr Patricia Smyth, La Pocatiere, QC - General Practice
Dr Peter H Solomon, Gatineau, QC - Anesthesia
Dr Saundra-Lisa Somera, Verdun, QC - General Practice
Dr Maurice Somma, Montreal, QC - Endocrinology
Dr Julio C Soto, Montreal, QC - Community Medicine
Dr Frederique Souchon, Montreal, QC - Electroencephal
Dr F Pierre Soucie, Hawkesbury, ON - General Practice
Dr S Pierre Soucie, Ottawa, ON - Family Medicine
Dr J L Rene Soucy, Ottawa, ON - Family Medicine
Dr Renee Soucy, Chandler, QC - Obstetrics & Gynecology
Dr Jean-Paul Soucy, Montreal, QC - Nuclear Medicine
Dr Michele Soucy, Pointe-Claire, QC - General Practice
Dr Frederic Soucy, Quebec, QC - Urology
Dr Marc Soucy, Sherbrooke, QC - Pediatrics
Dr Fernande Soucy-Hirtle, Quebec, QC - General Practice
Dr Kamel Souissi, Val-d'Or, QC - General Practice
Dr Gilles Soulez, Montreal, QC - Diagnostic-Radiology
Dr Elena Spacek, Montreal, QC - Physical Medicine & Rehab
Dr Linda S Spigelblatt, Montreal, QC - Pediatrics
Dr Gwendoline M Spurll, Montreal, QC - Hematology
Dr Srikala S Sridhar, Toronto, ON - Internal Medicine
Dr Philip D St John, Winnipeg, MB - Geriatric Medicine
Dr Marie St-Amour, Longueuil, QC - Community Medicine
Dr Renald St-Arneault, Boucherville, QC - General Practice
Dr Bernard St-Jean, La Malbaie, QC - Anesthesia
Dr Michel St-Onge, Beloeil, QC - General Practice
Dr Nathalie St-Onge, Sept-Iles, QC - General Practice
Dr Luc St-Pierre, Victoriaville, QC - Obstetrics & Gynecology
Dr Gordon M Stahl, Vancouver, BC - Family Medicine
Dr Valerie I Stanzl, Lethbridge, AB - Obstetrics & Gynecology
Dr Micheline T Ste-Marie, Montreal, QC - Gastroenterology
Dr Louis-Georges Ste-Marie, Montreal, QC - Endocrinology
Dr Marc Steben, Montreal, QC - Family Medicine
Dr Daniel C Steeves, Lethbridge, AB - General Practice
Dr Naomi B Stein, Westmount, QC - Pediatrics
Dr Mitchell H Stendel, Montreal, QC - Emergency Family Med
Dr Robert J Stenstrom, Vancouver, BC - Emergency Family Med
Dr James A Stewart, Montreal, QC - Cardiology
Dr Karen L Stillman, Almonte, ON - Obstetrics & Gynecology
Dr Michael Stumpf, Laval, QC - General Practice
Dr Erika Stumpf, Montreal, QC - Neurology
Dr N Gabriel Suhani, Saint-Eustache, QC - Psychiatry
Dr Daria A Sultan, Montreal, QC - General Practice
Dr Khalil Sultanem, Montreal, QC - Radiation Oncology
Dr Anne Surprenant, Stanstead, QC - General Practice
Dr Ann Sutton, Quebec, QC - Gastroenterology
Dr Jessica C Svitek, Dorval, QC - Family Medicine
Dr Andrew C Swan, Victoria, BC - Family Medicine
Dr Pierre-Luc Sylvain, Matane, QC - General Practice
Dr Gabriel Szabo, Salaber-de-Valleyf, QC - General Practice
Dr Tuyet Phi Ta, Montreal, QC - General Practice
Dr Cherif Tadros, Edmonton, AB - Orthopedic Surgery
Dr Mohammed Tagemouati, Pointe claire, QC - General Practice
Dr Majd Tahan, Salaber-de-Valleyf, QC - Internal Medicine
Dr Michel Taillefer, Saint-Sauveur, QC - General Practice
Dr Joseph E A C Taillon, Thetford Mines, QC - Internal Medicine
Dr Paul A Taillon, Saskatoon, SK - Family Medicine
Dr Jo-Ann Talbot, Saint John, NB - Emergency Medicine
Dr Jacques Talbot, Montreal, QC - Psychiatry
Dr Karine Talbot, Trois-Rivieres, QC - General Practice
Dr Paul Talbot Jr., Quebec, QC - Cardiology
Dr John P Taliano, St Catharines, ON - General Practice
Dr Peter Talko, Shawville, QC - General Practice
Dr Charles E Talon, Longueuil, QC - General Practice
Dr Christine E Tang, Mississauga, ON - Emergency Family Med
Dr Alexander W L Tang, North York, ON - Anesthesia
Dr Alain G Tanguay, Gatineau, QC - Emergency Family Med
Dr Caroline Tanguay, Granby, QC - Family Medicine
Dr David W Tannenbaum, Toronto, ON - Family Medicine
Dr Terry-Nan Tannenbaum, Montreal, QC - Community Medicine
Dr Daniel Tardif, Cantley, QC - General Practice
Dr Michele Tardif, Montreal, QC - Plastic Surgery
Dr Solange Tardy, Montreal, QC - General Practice
Dr Sue R Tatemichi, Fredericton, NB - Family Medicine
Dr Richard H B Tatham, Penticton, BC - Family Medicine
Dr Robert F Tautkus, Brampton, ON - Family Medicine
Dr Franco G Tavazzani, Brampton, ON - Orthopedic Surgery
Dr F Georges Tawagi, Nepean, ON - Obstetrics & Gynecology
Dr James D N Taylor, Victoria, BC - Ophthalmology
Dr John D Taylor, Chapleau, ON - General Practice
Dr J Robert M Taylor, Ottawa, ON - Hematology
Dr Elaine M Taylor, Ottawa, ON - Family Medicine
Dr Bryce R Taylor, Toronto, ON - General Surgery
Dr William J Taylor, Windsor, ON - Anesthesia
Dr Jean I Tchervenkov, Montreal, QC - General Surgery
Dr Lynne D Teasell, Okotoks, AB - General Practice
Dr Nathalie Teboul, Gatineau, QC - Ophthalmology
Dr Eric A Teboul, Saint-Jerome, QC - Psychiatry
Dr Barbara K Teboul, Salaber-de-Valleyf, QC - Ophthalmology
Dr Lori E Teeple, Zurich, ON - Emergency Family Med
Dr Raymond J M Tellier, Calgary, AB - Medical Microbiology
Dr Lyne Tellier, Levis, QC - Obstetrics & Gynecology
Dr Raymond P L Tempier, Ottawa, ON - Psychiatry
Dr Danny S Tenaschuk, Ottawa, ON - Diagnostic-Radiology
Dr Stefan Teolis, Laval, QC - Family Medicine
Dr Jean-Pierre Teolis, Montreal, QC - General Practice
Dr Jamie L Tepper, Oshawa, ON - Clin Immun/Allergy
Dr Jean-Claude Terras, Saint-Quentin, NB - General Practice
Dr Luke M Teskey, Surrey, BC - General Practice
Dr Julie L Tessier, Kingston, ON - Obstetrics & Gynecology
Dr Pierre C Tessier, Ottawa, ON - Family Medicine
Dr Guylaine Tessier, Gatineau, QC - Family Medicine
Dr Lorraine Tessier, Montreal, QC - General Practice
Dr Daniel Tessier, Sherbrooke, QC - Geriatric Medicine
Dr Michael J Tessler, Montreal, QC - Anesthesia
Dr Louise-Marie Tetrault, Ottawa, ON - General Practice
Dr Guy Tetreault, Drummondville, QC - Family Medicine
Dr Susan P L Tha, Vancouver, BC - Anatomical Pathology
Dr An Than Trong, Montreal, QC - General Surgery
Dr Lan Quang Thanh, St-Jean-Sur-Richel, QC - Gastroenterology
Dr Josee Theberge, Val-d'Or, QC - Psychiatry
Dr Francois A J Theoret, Hawkesbury, ON - Family Medicine
Dr M Y Diane Theriault, Dartmouth, NS - Internal Medicine
Dr Gilles Theriault, Montreal, QC - Community Medicine
Dr Lyne Theriault, Princeville, QC - General Practice
Dr J Germain-Michel Theriault, Quebec, QC - General Practice
Dr Serge Therien, Sherbrooke, QC - Pediatrics
Dr Pierre Theroux, Montreal, QC - Cardiology
Dr Anne-Marie Therrien, Gatineau, QC - General Practice
Dr Sylvie Thibaudeau, Paspebiac, QC - General Practice
Dr Johanne Thibaudeau, Terrebonne, QC - General Practice
Dr Nicolas Thibault, Edmonton, AB - Family Medicine
Dr Nicole Thibault, Brossard, QC - General Practice
Dr Caroline Thibault, LaSalle, QC - Family Medicine
Dr Ginette Thibault, Lachute, QC - General Practice
Dr Sebastien Thibault, Trois-Rivieres, QC - General Practice
Dr Daniele Thibodeau, Dieppe, NB - Family Medicine
Dr Jean-Louis Thibodeau, Saint-Jacques, NB - General Practice
Dr Daniel Thibodeau, Sherbrooke, QC - Obstetrics & Gynecology
Dr Gilbert Thiffault, Laval, QC - Orthopedic Surgery
Dr Jocelyne Thiffault, Laval, QC - General Practice
Dr Robert B Thirsk, Longueuil, QC - General Practice
Dr Jean Thisdale, St-Eustache, QC - General Practice
Dr Caroll Thivierge, Quebec, QC - General Practice
Dr Richard P Thomas, Kingston, ON - Obstetrics & Gynecology
Dr Claudette Thomas Fils-Aime, Montreal, QC - General Practice
Dr Michele D Thomasse, Kelowna, BC - Family Medicine
Dr Michael G Thomassin, Montreal, QC - Family Medicine
Dr David K Thompson, Brantford, ON - Family Medicine
Dr Calvin P Thompson, Ottawa, ON - Anesthesia
Dr Tracey A Thompson, Gatineau, QC - Plastic Surgery
Dr Paul Thompson, Montreal, QC - Ophthalmology
Dr Leanne M Thomson, Kincardine, ON - Family Medicine
Dr John G Thomson, Ottawa, ON - Internal Medicine
Dr Larry S Thorsteinson, Sudbury, ON - Emergency Family Med
Dr Amelie Thuot, St-Jean-Sur-Richel, QC - Medical Microbiology
Dr M Lynne Thurling, Fergus, ON - Psychiatry
Dr Peter R Thurston, Ottawa, ON - Orthopedic Surgery
Dr Olimpia M Timar-Banu, Longueuil, QC - Family Medicine
Dr Jean-Robert Timothee, Greenfield Park, QC - Cardiology
Dr Simon Tinawi, Montreal, QC - Physical Medicine & Rehab
Dr Alan T Tinmouth, Ottawa, ON - Hematology
Dr Jean-Marie Tissot, Quebec, QC - General Practice
Dr Sabine P Y Tjia, LaSalle, QC - General Practice

Dr Ian P Toft, St Thomas, ON - Family Medicine
Dr Daniel R Toledano, Toronto, ON - General Practice
Dr Richard D Tombler, Cornwall, ON - Orthopedic Surgery
Dr Eva M Tomiak, Ottawa, ON - Internal Medicine
Dr Christina Tong, Westmount, QC - Family Medicine
Dr Luis Toriz, Saint-Jerome, QC - Orthopedic Surgery
Dr Marie Toscano, Gatineau, QC - Dermatology
Dr Caroline M A Tosoni, Orleans, ON - Family Medicine
Dr Matthieu Touchette, Sherbrooke, QC - Internal Medicine
Dr Michael J Touchie, Ottawa, ON - General Practice
Dr Jacques Toueg, Laval, QC - Orthopedic Surgery
Dr Genevieve Toupin, Levis, QC - Psychiatry
Dr June A D Tourangeau, Toronto, ON - Anesthesia
Dr Richard Tourigny, Quebec, QC - Ophthalmology
Dr Claude P J Tousignant, Toronto, ON - Anesthesia
Dr Michel P Tousignant, Grand-Mere, QC - General Practice
Dr Jean Tousignant, Trois-Rivieres, QC - Anesthesia
Dr M Junie B Toussaint, Toronto, ON - General Practice
Dr Martin Toussaint, Saint-Eugene, QC - General Practice
Dr Carol A Townsley, Toronto, ON - Family Medicine
Dr William Toy, LaSalle, QC - General Practice
Dr Nancy M Tozer, Pointe-Claire, QC - Family Medicine
Dr Daniel P Tozzi, Montreal, QC - General Practice
Dr John Trachtenberg, Toronto, ON - Urology
Dr Golda E Tradounsky, Cote Saint-Luc, QC - Family Medicine
Dr Chaim J Trager, Markham, ON - General Practice
Dr J Simon-Pierre Trahan, Russell, ON - General Practice
Dr S Stanley Tran, Scarborough, ON - Gastroenterology
Dr Boi Anh Tran, Longueuil, QC - General Practice
Dr Xia-Hoe Tran, Montreal, QC - General Practice
Dr Thu-Hang Tran, Montreal, QC - Emergency Family Med
Dr Cuong Tran Ngoc, Mississauga, ON - Diagnostic-Radiology
Dr Nguyen Trang, Arnprior, ON - Family Medicine
Dr John Tranqui, Mississauga, ON - General Practice
Dr Sean A Travers, North Bay, ON - Anesthesia
Dr Lionel D B Traverse, Abbotsford, BC - Pediatrics
Dr Darin J Treleaven, Hamilton, ON - Internal Medicine
Dr Francisco Trelles, Quebec, QC - Gastroenterology
Dr Alain Tremblay, Calgary, AB - Internal Medicine
Dr Pierre-Michel Tremblay, Moncton, NB - General Practice
Dr Michele M Tremblay, Ottawa, ON - Psychiatry
Dr Lorraine N Tremblay, Toronto, ON - General Surgery
Dr Marie-Claude S Tremblay, Boisbriand, QC - General Practice
Dr Pierre Tremblay, Bromont, QC - General Practice
Dr Pascale Tremblay, Jonquiere, QC - General Practice
Dr Richard Tremblay, Laval, QC - Internal Medicine
Dr Gilles R Tremblay, Montreal, QC - Orthopedic Surgery
Dr Robert Tremblay, N-D-Des-Prairies, QC - General Practice
Dr Rene M Tremblay, Quebec, QC - Gastroenterology
Dr Helene Tremblay, Quebec, QC - General Practice
Dr Bruno Tremblay, Quebec, QC - General Practice
Dr Genevieve Tremblay, Quebec, QC - Community Medicine
Dr Roland R Tremblay, Quebec, QC - Endocrinology
Dr Marie-Claude Tremblay, Sainte-Therese, QC - Ophthalmology
Dr Jacques Tremblay, Verdun, QC - General Practice
Dr Fannie Tremblay-Allan, Dolbeau-Mistassini, QC - General Surgery
Dr Nicolas-Olivier Tremblay-Reinhardt, Roberval, QC - General Practice
Dr Jean R Trepanier, Ottawa, ON - General Practice
Dr Line Trepanier, Thetford Mines, QC - General Practice
Dr Mark A Trifiro, Montreal, QC - Internal Medicine
Dr Ba-Truc Trinh, Laval, QC - Otolaryngology
Dr Isabelle Trop, Montreal, QC - Diagnostic-Radiology
Dr Antonio G Trottier, Greenfield Park, QC - Electroencephal
Dr Mylene Trottier, Montreal, QC - General Practice
Dr Sylvie Trottier, Quebec, QC - Medical Microbiology
Dr Michel L Truchon, Bonfield, ON - General Practice
Dr Marc Trudeau, Medicine Hat, AB - Internal Medicine
Dr Luc Trudeau, Montreal, QC - Internal Medicine
Dr Suzanne M Trudel, Toronto, ON - Hematology
Dr Manon Trudel, Chicoutimi, QC - General Practice
Dr Jean-Francois Trudel, Sherbrooke, QC - Psychiatry
Dr Tuyet Lan Truong, Pointe-Claire, QC - General Practice
Dr Willis H Tsai, Calgary, AB - Internal Medicine
Dr Anna Tsakalaki, Gatineau, QC - Family Medicine
Dr Ana-Maria C Tsanaclis, Sherbrooke, QC - General Practice
Dr Marisa A Tucci, Montreal, QC - Pediatrics
Dr Joan M Tucker, North York, ON - Psychiatry
Dr Elrie C Tucker, Montreal, QC - Obstetrics & Gynecology
Dr Raman Tuli, Ottawa, ON - Ophthalmology
Dr Jennifer I L Tupper, Banff, AB - Emergency Family Med
Dr Chantal Turcotte, Montreal, QC - General Practice
Dr Gilles Turcotte, Quebec, QC - Medical Biochemistry
Dr Jean Turcotte, Verdun, QC - General Practice
Dr Mathieu Turcotte-Lagace, Greenfield Park, QC - Emergency Family Med
Dr Francoise Turgeon, Jonquiere, QC - General Practice
Dr Nathalie Turgeon, Quebec, QC - Medical Microbiology
Dr Manon Turgeon, Repentigny, QC - General Practice
Dr Alexis Turgeon-Fournier, Quebec, QC - Anesthesia
Dr David T Turineck, Smooth Rock Falls, ON - General Practice
Dr Yves Turmel, Sherbrooke, QC - General Practice
Dr John D Turnbull, Hamilton, ON - Internal Medicine
Dr Mark O Turner, Surrey, BC - Internal Medicine
Dr D Christopher Turner, Ottawa, ON - Pediatrics
Dr Howard M Turner, Montreal, QC - Internal Medicine
Dr Joel P Turner, Montreal, QC - Emergency Medicine
Dr Thom V Tyson, Ottawa, ON - General Practice
Dr Simeon G Tzeneff, Ottawa, ON - General Practice
Dr Patricia Ugolini, Montreal, QC - Diagnostic-Radiology
Dr Peter A F Uhthoff, Ottawa, ON - General Practice
Dr Lorne N Umemoto, Quebec, QC - Clin Immun/Allergy
Dr Sharon L Unger, Toronto, ON - Pediatrics
Dr Bernard Unger, Montreal, QC - Emergency Family Med
Dr Adrian R M Upton, Hamilton, ON - Neurology
Dr Francois N Urfer, Hawkesbury, ON - General Practice
Dr Mylene J Vachet, Rockland, ON - Family Medicine
Dr Marie-France Vachon, Levis, QC - General Practice
Dr Shailla Vaidya, Toronto, ON - Emergency Family Med
Dr David A Valenti, Montreal, QC - Diagnostic-Radiology
Dr Luc Valiquette, Montreal, QC - Urology
Dr Sophie Vallette, Montreal, QC - Endocrin/Metabolism
Dr M Beth Vallieres, Cambridge, ON - Emergency Family Med
Dr Joyce Valois, Saint-Lambert, QC - Family Medicine
Dr Gerhard Van Der Westhuizen, Calgary, AB - General Practice
Dr Guy Van Vliet, Montreal, QC - Endocrinology
Dr Louise Vanasse, Ottawa, ON - Family Medicine
Dr Catherine Vanasse, Sherbrooke, QC - General Practice
Dr Theodore A Vandenberg, London, ON - Internal Medicine
Dr Ruth E Vander Stelt, Quyon, QC - Family Medicine
Dr Anik R M Vandewaetere, Ottawa, ON - Family Medicine
Dr J Gerald Vangurp, Montreal, QC - General Practice
Dr Stephane Vanier, Montreal, QC - Family Medicine
Dr Astghik Vartanian, Montreal, QC - General Practice
Dr Michele Vartian, Montreal, QC - Pediatrics
Dr Christopher B Varty, Scarborough, ON - Anesthesia
Dr Mariette Varvarikos, Montreal, QC - Emergency Family Med
Dr John R Vary, Rimouski, QC - Urology
Dr Yvonne B Vasilie, Pointe-Claire, QC - Obstetrics & Gynecology
Dr Peter W Vaughan, Bridgewater, NS - General Practice
Dr Line M Vautour, Montreal, QC - Endocrin/Metabolism
Dr A Adriana Veer, Charlottetown, PE - Family Medicine
Dr Sarto Veilleux, Quebec, QC - General Practice
Dr Anna L Veksler, Montreal, QC - Diagnostic-Radiology
Dr Ronald B Vender, Hamilton, ON - Dermatology
Dr Nina E N Venkatarangam, Scarborough, ON - Obstetrics & Gynecology
Dr Josee Verdon, Montreal, QC - Geriatric Medicine
Dr John-Paul Veri, Peterborough, ON - Orthopedic Surgery
Dr Carlo Vernacchia, Montreal, QC - General Practice
Dr Andre Veronneau, Contrecoeur, QC - General Practice
Dr Nina Verreault, Quebec, QC - Clin Immun/Allergy
Dr Jean Verreault, Sherbrooke, QC - Nuclear Medicine
Dr Louis Verret, Quebec, QC - Neurology
Dr Pierre Verrier, Montreal, QC - Psychiatry
Dr Colette Y T B Vervaeck, Didsbury, AB - General Practice
Dr Claude T J Vezina, Timmins, ON - Diagnostic-Radiology
Dr Danielle Vezina, Laval, QC - Internal Medicine
Dr Michel Vezina, Quebec, QC - Community Medicine
Dr Pascale Vezina, Saint-Eustache, QC - Orthopedic Surgery
Dr Leonardo Vieira Neto, Chicoutimi, QC - General Practice
Dr Marcel Vien, Dolbeau-Mistassini, QC - General Practice
Dr Claudette Viens, Les Bergeronnes, QC - General Practice
Dr Huguette Vigeant, Quebec, QC - General Practice
Dr Marie Villeneuve, Montreal, QC - Psychiatry
Dr Patrick Vinay, Montreal, QC - Nephrology
Dr Denis R J Vincent, Edmonton, AB - Family Medicine
Dr Matthieu Vincent, Longueuil, QC - Emergency Medicine
Dr Pierre M Vincent, Quebec, QC - Psychiatry
Dr Annick Vincent, St-Augustin-D-Desm, QC - Psychiatry
Dr Shaun L Visser, Ottawa, ON - Emergency Family Med
Dr Louise Y Vitou, Kitchener, ON - Critical Care Medicine
Dr Anthony C H Vivian, Chilliwack, BC - Internal Medicine
Dr Saul Vizel, Cambridge, ON - Cardiology
Dr Thi Nhu Y Vo, Gatineau, QC - General Practice
Dr Thi Minh D Vo, LaSalle, QC - Family Medicine
Dr Minh Ha Vo, LaSalle, QC - General Practice
Dr Kim-Loan Vo-Doan, Montreal, QC - Otolaryngology
Dr J Suzanne Vobecky, Montreal, QC - Cardiovasc/ThorSurg
Dr Carlos A Vollinoti, Gatineau, QC - Obstetrics & Gynecology
Dr Peter Von Dadelszen, Vancouver, BC - Obstetrics & Gynecology
Dr Michael Vonniessen, Pointe-Claire, QC - Emergency Family Med
Dr Ngoc Dien Vu, Montreal, QC - General Practice
Dr Dung Vu, Montreal, QC - General Practice
Dr Caroline X L Vu-Nguyen, Montreal, QC - General Practice
Dr Raj Waghmare, Aurora, ON - Family Medicine
Dr David M Wagman, Bolton, ON - General Practice
Dr Elisabeth M Wagner, Calgary, AB - Obstetrics & Gynecology
Dr Brenda L M Wagner, Richmond, BC - Obstetrics & Gynecology
Dr J Scott Wakefield, Calgary, AB - Family Medicine
Dr Leslie A Waldron, Kingston, ON - Family Medicine
Dr Jason T Wale, Comox, BC - Emergency Family Med
Dr Jennifer D Walker, North Vancouver, BC - Family Medicine
Dr Janet A Walker, Bathurst, NB - General Surgery
Dr C Robin Walker, London, ON - Pediatrics
Dr Angela J Walker, St-Basile-le-Grand, QC - Family Medicine
Dr Jane M Wall, Toronto, ON - Diagnostic-Radiology
Dr Keith E Walling, Lower Sackville, NS - Otolaryngology
Dr Herve Walti, Sherbrooke, QC - General Practice
Dr Yan Wang, Smiths Falls, ON - Obstetrics & Gynecology
Dr Beatrice Wang, Montreal, QC - Dermatology
Dr Chang Shu Wang, Sherbrooke, QC - General Practice
Dr Michael C T Wansbrough, Toronto, ON - Emergency Family Med
Dr Leanne M Ward, Ottawa, ON - Endocrin/Metabolism
Dr Michelle G K Ward, Ottawa, ON - Pediatrics
Dr Mark A Ware, Montreal, QC - General Practice
Dr Margaret N Warner, Montreal, QC - Hematology
Dr Thomas F Warnock, Stratford, ON - General Practice
Dr Ian M Warrack, Ottawa, ON - Family Medicine
Dr Susan Waserman, Hamilton, ON - Clin Immun/Allergy
Dr Pnina C Wasser, Montreal, QC - Family Medicine
Dr Daniel Watkin, Wasaga Beach, ON - General Practice
Dr Sheila D Watson, Calgary, AB - Obstetrics & Gynecology
Dr William J Watson, Toronto, ON - Family Medicine
Dr James H Watt, St. Albert, AB - Diagnostic-Radiology
Dr Garth B Watt, Halifax, NS - Psychiatry
Dr Menashe B Waxman, Toronto, ON - Internal Medicine
Dr Stacie D Weber, Barrie, ON - Family Medicine
Dr Christopher C Weber, Ottawa, ON - General Practice
Dr Marie E Weber, Montreal, QC - Family Medicine
Dr Andrew S Weeks, Simcoe, ON - Cardiology
Dr Corey N Weigensberg, Scarborough, ON - Anatomical Pathology
Dr Terri E Weinberg, North York, ON - Family Medicine
Dr Robert B Weinberg, Toronto, ON - Family Medicine
Dr Robert D Weinman, Pointe-Claire, QC - Family Medicine
Dr Joy M Weisbloom, Nepean, ON - Family Medicine
Dr Brent A Weiser, Toronto, ON - Ophthalmology
Mr Karl A Weiss, Montreal, QC - Medical Microbiology
Dr Alfred Weksberg, North York, ON - Dermatology
Dr Charles J Weldon, Cowansville, QC - Ophthalmology
Dr Eleanor Wellman, Quebec, QC - Family Medicine
Dr Mary K Wells, St. John's, NL - General Surgery

Dr John D Wells, Hamilton, ON - Neurosurgery
Dr Richard A Wennberg, Toronto, ON - Electroencephal
Dr Denise H Werker, Ottawa, ON - Community Medicine
Dr Michael Westwood, Baie-D'Urfe, QC - Pediatrics
Dr Marvin J Wexler, Montreal, QC - General Surgery
Dr Sylvia A M Whalen, Orleans, ON - Family Medicine
Dr Karen A Whalen-Browne, Kingston, ON - Family Medicine
Dr Christine L White, Ottawa, ON - Family Medicine
Dr Lisa A White, Ottawa, ON - Family Medicine
Dr Richard A White, Peterborough, ON - Pediatrics
Dr M Edward White, Charlottetown, PE - Family Medicine
Dr Sharon E Whiting, Ottawa, ON - Neurology
Dr Susan A Whitley, Ottawa, ON - Family Medicine
Dr N Blair Whittemore, Montreal, QC - Hematology
Dr Sonja C Wicklum, Calgary, AB - Family Medicine
Dr Lorne M Wiesenfeld, Ottawa, ON - Emergency Medicine
Dr Mark A Wilkins, Mattawa, ON - Family Medicine
Dr Bernard E Willems, Montreal, QC - Internal Medicine
Dr AnnaMary J Williams, Hawkesbury, ON - Dermatology
Dr V Guy Williams, Hawkesbury, ON - General Practice
Dr William L Williams, Ottawa, ON - Cardiology
Dr Paula B Williams, Toronto, ON - General Practice
Dr Carole S Williams, Vanier, ON - General Practice
Dr Kimberly A Williamson, Hamilton, ON - General Practice
Dr Kenneth R Willis, Ottawa, ON - Internal Medicine
Dr Rodney D Wilson, Halifax, NS - General Practice
Dr Chantelle N Wilson, Gore Bay, ON - Family Medicine
Dr Scott N Wilson, Marathon, ON - Family Medicine
Dr Allan Wilson, Ottawa, ON - General Practice
Dr Terrance R Wilson, Peterborough, ON - General Practice
Dr Tracy L Wilson, Thunder Bay, ON - Orthopedic Surgery
Dr Janet H Wilson, Westmount, QC - Family Medicine
Dr Cara K Wilson-Haffenden, North Vancouver, BC - General Practice
Dr Marc L Wiltshire, Thunder Bay, ON - Emergency Family Med
Dr David G Wiltshire, Pointe-Claire, QC - Orthopedic Surgery
Dr Willie P Winzer, Orleans, ON - General Practice
Dr Mark Wise, North York, ON - General Practice
Dr Jeffrey G Wiseman, Montreal, QC - Internal Medicine
Dr Fred Wiseman, Pointe-Claire, QC - Pediatrics
Dr Jean-Victor P Wittenberg, Toronto, ON - Psychiatry
Dr Renee J Wolanski, Cote Saint-Luc, QC - General Practice
Dr Thomas Wong, Ottawa, ON - Family Medicine
Dr Natalie Wong, Toronto, ON - Critical Care Medicine
Dr Michael Y Woo, Ottawa, ON - Emergency Family Med
Dr Anna Woo, Toronto, ON - Cardiology
Dr Jerry L Woodruff, Bow Island, AB - General Practice
Dr D Blake Woodside, Toronto, ON - Psychiatry
Dr Eric J Wooltorton, Ottawa, ON - Family Medicine
Dr Roger W Wray, Nepean, ON - General Practice
Dr Cedric Wybouw, Memramcook, NB - Family Medicine
Dr Isaac Wyszogrodski, Dollard-D-Ormeaux, QC - General Practice
Dr Anargyros Xenocostas, London, ON - Hematology
Dr John B Xenos, Montreal, QC - General Practice
Dr Olivier Yaccarini, Quebec, QC - Emergency Family Med
Dr Mayer Yacowar, North York, ON - Family Medicine
Dr Mark J Yaffe, Montreal, QC - Family Medicine
Dr Jianing Yang, Hawkesbury, ON - General Practice
Dr Howard Yanofsky, Montreal, QC - Dermatology
Dr Yu-Ju Yao, Montreal, QC - Family Medicine
Dr Zeina Yared, Saint-Laurent, QC - Endocrin/Metabolism
Dr John F Yaremko, Westmount, QC - Pediatrics
Dr Carol A M Yeadon, Montreal, QC - Internal Medicine
Dr Ernest Yee, Belleville, ON - Internal Medicine
Dr Karen W L Yee, Toronto, ON - Hematology
Dr Lauren L Yee, Windsor, ON - General Practice
Dr John C K Yee, Windsor, ON - General Practice
Dr Gordon Yee, LaSalle, QC - Family Medicine
Dr Robert M Yelle, Kanata, ON - Family Medicine
Dr Vincent P J Young, Ottawa, ON - Hematology
Dr Beverly Young, Toronto, ON - Psychiatry
Dr Randa Zabian, Chateauguay, QC - Family Medicine
Dr Oleg G Zadorozny, Gatineau, QC - Internal Medicine
Dr Florin Zaharia, Montreal, QC - General Surgery
Dr Georgina M Zahirney, Montreal, QC - Psychiatry
Dr Mark S Zalter, Hamilton, ON - General Practice
Dr Jeffrey S Zaltzman, Toronto, ON - Internal Medicine
Dr Jorge E Zamora, Kingston, ON - Anesthesia
Dr Michael G Zaremba, Woodbridge, ON - Family Medicine
Dr Marianna Zarrelli, Montreal, QC - Psychiatry
Dr Joie A Zeglinski, Ottawa, ON - Psychiatry
Dr Brian S Zidel, Mississauga, ON - General Practice
Dr Joan R Zidulka, Montreal, QC - Hematology
Dr Cleve Ziegler, Montreal, QC - Obstetrics & Gynecology
Dr Adam M Zieleniak, St-Charles-Brromee, QC - General Practice
Dr Benjamin G Zifkin, Westmount, QC - Electroencephal
Dr Michael Zigman, Montreal, QC - General Practice
Dr Jerrold M Zikman, Hamilton, ON - Urology
Dr Eugenia Zikos, Montreal, QC - Psychiatry
Dr George W Zimakas, Niagara Falls, ON - Internal Medicine
Dr Camilla C U Zimmermann, Toronto, ON - Internal Medicine
Dr Hans H Zingg, Montreal, QC - General Practice
Dr Armand S Zini, Montreal, QC - Urology
Dr Kathia Znojkiewicz, Montreal, QC - General Practice
Dr Mario Zummo, Dorval, QC - General Practice
Dr Michel Zummo, Montreal, QC - General Practice
Dr Ian H L Zunder, Ottawa, ON - Anesthesia
Dr Michel de Maupeou, La Sarre, QC - General Practice
Dr Daniel de Yturralde, Shediac, NB - Orthopedic Surgery

ESPERANTO

Dr Jean Alain, Gatineau, QC - Medical Biochemistry

ESTONIAN

Dr Roland E Amolins, Oakville, ON - Family Medicine
Dr Allan R Hess, Newmarket, ON - Cardiology
Dr Riho Kalda, Vancouver, BC - Psychiatry
Dr Talvi C Maimets, Toronto, ON - Family Medicine
Dr Jaanus Marley, Toronto, ON - General Practice
Dr Leili Pede, Brampton, ON - Family Medicine
Dr Ago Peters, York, ON - General Practice
Dr Peeter A Poldre, Toronto, ON - Hematology
Dr Juri Rand, Peterborough, ON - General Practice
Dr Ann K Rebane, Toronto, ON - Family Medicine
Dr Jaak T Reichmann, Barrie, ON - Psychiatry
Dr Mai Liis Riives, Dartmouth, NS - General Practice
Dr George Rungi, Port Colborne, ON - Family Medicine
Dr Toomas P Sauks, Owen Sound, ON - General Practice
Dr Jakov Shlik, Ottawa, ON - General Practice
Dr Alan H Tallmeister, Scarborough, ON - Anesthesia
Dr Ingrid Tein, Toronto, ON - Pediatrics
Dr Peter Tinits, Stratford, ON - Anesthesia
Dr Ants Toi, Toronto, ON - Diagnostic-Radiology
Dr Reet Vanaselja, Toronto, ON - Family Medicine
Dr Hillar Vellend, Toronto, ON - Infectious Diseases
Dr David W Wallik, Burlington, ON - Family Medicine

EWE

Dr Setorme A Tsikata, Spruce Grove, AB - Family Medicine

FANTI

Dr J Oluwagbenga Ajayi-Obe, Sarnia, ON - Family Medicine
Dr Essandoh K Dankwa, St Anthony, NL - Anatomical Pathology
Dr Nana Graves, Dollard-D-Ormeaux, QC - Pediatrics
Dr Francis B Sam, North York, ON - Obstetrics & Gynecology
Dr Setorme A Tsikata, Spruce Grove, AB - Family Medicine

FARSI

Dr Babak Abadi, Toronto, ON - Psychiatry
Dr Amid K Abdullah, Calgary, AB - General Pathology
Dr Mohammed M Abed, Regina, SK - Obstetrics & Gynecology
Dr Oveis Adl Golchin, The Pas, MB - General Practice
Dr Mansour Adle, Westmount, QC - General Surgery
Dr Mohsen Agharazii, Quebec, QC - Internal Medicine
Dr Saeed Ahmadinejad, Edmonton, AB - Family Medicine
Dr Faria Ajamian, Edmonton, AB - General Practice
Dr Shahrzad Akhtari, Richmond Hill, ON - Family Medicine
Dr Javad Alaghband-Rad, Halifax, NS - General Practice
Dr Kamel Alizadeh-Khiavi, Calgary, AB - Family Medicine
Dr Neda Amani, Ottawa, ON - General Practice
Dr Hossein Amani, Toronto, ON - Physical Medicine & Rehab
Dr Farnaz Amoozegar, Calgary, AB - Neurology
Dr Mehran Anvari, Hamilton, ON - General Surgery
Dr Farnaz Ardeshiri, North York, ON - Pediatrics
Dr Esmail K Arfai, North York, ON - Psychiatry
Dr M Anwar Asady, Mississauga, ON - General Practice
Dr Khalil Asayesh, Brampton, ON - Psychiatry
Dr Manutchehr Assemi, Nepean, ON - Pediatrics
Dr Ardavan Assemi, Ottawa, ON - Family Medicine
Dr Abbas G Azadian, Thornhill, ON - Psychiatry
Dr Maryam Baghbannazary, Vancouver, BC - Family Medicine
Dr Mohammad Bahasadri, Etobicoke, ON - General Surgery
Dr Farhad Bakezadeh, Saint John, NB - General Practice
Dr Hamid S Banijamali, Calgary, AB - Cardiology
Dr Peyvand A Basti, North York, ON - Family Medicine
Dr Parvaneh Beheshti, West Vancouver, BC - General Practice
Dr Mojtaba N Beheshti, Brampton, ON - Urology
Dr Sharareh Behmanesh, North Vancouver, BC - Family Medicine
Dr Abdollah Behzadi, Mississauga, ON - General Surgery
Dr Nemat A Daraei, Orillia, ON - Family Medicine
Dr Mojgan Davallou, Toronto, ON - Anesthesia
Dr Parham Davoudpour, Newmarket, ON - Emergency Family Med
Dr Payman Dehghani-Mohammadabidi, Scarborough, ON - Emergency Family Med
Dr Shyah S Delarom, Victoria, BC - General Practice
Dr Maryam Eftekhari, Richmond Hill, ON - Family Medicine
Dr Ali Eslami, Surrey, BC - General Practice
Dr Haydeh F Esmaili, Comox, BC - General Practice
Dr Roya Etemad-Rezai, London, ON - Diagnostic-Radiology
Dr Ziba Fadavi, Orillia, ON - Anatomical Pathology
Dr Mehrnoosh Faghih, Burlington, ON - Obstetrics & Gynecology
Dr Ziaullah Fahim, Surrey, BC - General Practice
Dr Keyghobad Farid Araki, Toronto, ON - Psychiatry
Dr Afsoon Fathollahzadeh, Oakville, ON - Pediatrics
Dr Toghra GhaemMaghami, North York, ON - Psychiatry
Dr Maryam Ghaffar-Sedeh, Pickering, ON - Family Medicine
Dr Seyed M Ghafouri, North York, ON - Internal Medicine
Dr Fatemeh Ghannadi, West Vancouver, BC - Family Medicine
Dr Mahshid Gharedaghi, West Vancouver, BC - Family Medicine
Dr Abbas Ghavam-Rassoul, Toronto, ON - Family Medicine
Dr Mohammed T Ghazavi, Scarborough, ON - Orthopedic Surgery
Dr M Reza Ghobadian, Whitby, ON - Family Medicine
Dr Farnaz Ghorbani, Richmond Hill, ON - Family Medicine
Dr Mojdeh Gonabady Namadon, West Vancouver, BC - General Practice
Dr Masoud Goodarzi, Niagara Falls, ON - Internal Medicine
Dr Mehri Habibi, York, ON - Anesthesia
Dr Sonia Habibian, West Vancouver, BC - Family Medicine
Dr Keyvan Hadad, Vancouver, BC - Pediatrics
Dr Abbas H Hadian, North York, ON - General Practice
Dr Rod Hafezi, Saskatoon, SK - Internal Medicine
Dr Sara Hafezi Bakhtiari, Toronto, ON - Anatomical Pathology
Dr Falih M Hafuth, Guelph, ON - Family Medicine
Dr Amir Tinouch Haghighat Talab, Gatineau, QC - Cardiology
Dr Roya Hajy Aghaei, North York, ON - Family Medicine
Dr M Taghi Hakami, Chicoutimi, QC - General Practice
Dr Farzad Hariri, Etobicoke, ON - General Surgery
Dr Omar N Hasan, Amqui, QC - General Surgery
Dr Maliheh Hasemzadeh-Balouchi, Richmond Hill, ON - Family Medicine
Dr Shahin Hatami, Maple, ON - Family Medicine
Dr Ali Hazrati, North York, ON - Family Medicine
Dr Reza Heidarpour Meymeh, Barrie, ON - Family Medicine
Dr Mojgan Hodaie, Toronto, ON - Neurosurgery
Dr Freydoun Homayounfar, Shawville, QC - General Practice
Dr Siavash Jafari, Vancouver, BC - General Practice
Dr Parveen F Jahandar, Edmonton, AB - Psychiatry
Dr Mohammad R Jahandardoost, Medicine Hat, AB - Internal Medicine

Dr Manouchehr Javidan, Vancouver, BC - Neurology
Dr Nasir Jetha, Vancouver, BC - Pediatrics
Dr Shamin Jetha, Vancouver, BC - Family Medicine
Dr Azim F Juma, Scarborough, ON - Family Medicine
Dr Shadan Kabiri-Abyaneh, West Vancouver, BC - Family Medicine
Dr Sahar Kajbaf, Brampton, ON - Internal Medicine
Dr Saeed Kalantari, North York, ON - Family Medicine
Dr Rozmin F Kamani, Vancouver, BC - Family Medicine
Dr Mahshid Kamyab, Coquitlam, BC - Family Medicine
Dr Leila Kasrai, Etobicoke, ON - Plastic Surgery
Dr Mandana Kaviani, Vancouver, BC - Clin Immun/Allergy
Dr Ali-Reza Kazemi, North Vancouver, BC - General Practice
Dr Gholamreza Keshavarzi, North Vancouver, BC - Family Medicine
Dr Mohammad Keshoofy, Alliston, ON - General Surgery
Dr Leila Keyvani, Prince George, BC - Gastroenterology
Dr Mark Khalili, Port Coquitlam, BC - Family Medicine
Dr Firouz Khamsi, Toronto, ON - Internal Medicine
Dr Afshin Khazei, Vancouver, BC - Emergency Medicine
Dr Kasra Khorasani, Toronto, ON - Psychiatry
Dr Narges Khoshnood, Toronto, ON - Family Medicine
Dr Steven L Kirzner, Vancouver, BC - Ophthalmology
Dr Rizwana Lilani, Maple, ON - Family Medicine
Dr Mahnaz Mahmoodi, Newmarket, ON - Family Medicine
Dr Rowja Malek, Scarborough, ON - Family Medicine
Dr Mohammad R Maleki-Yazdi, Toronto, ON - Internal Medicine
Dr Bahera Mali, Regina, SK - Medical Biochemistry
Dr Mahnaz Maneshgar, Edmonton, AB - Family Medicine
Dr Fereshteh Mazloom, Etobicoke, ON - Family Medicine
Dr Ali-Reza Milani, Calgary, AB - General Practice
Dr Saman Miremadi, Surrey, BC - Psychiatry
Dr Mehrnoush Mirhosseini, Edmonton, AB - Family Medicine
Dr Patricia A Mirwaldt, Vancouver, BC - Family Medicine
Dr Yazdan Mirzanejad, Surrey, BC - Infectious Diseases
Dr Ehsan Mohammadi, Sault Ste. Marie, ON - Emergency Family Med
Dr Maryam Mohammady, North York, ON - Family Medicine
Dr Kam Mohaseb, North Vancouver, BC - Ophthalmology
Dr Hadi Mohsenibod, Toronto, ON - General Practice
Dr Arsalan Monavvari, Toronto, ON - Family Medicine
Dr Amir A Mortazavi, North York, ON - Cardiology
Dr Roksana Mottahedi, Kanata, ON - Family Medicine
Dr Lili Naghdi, Maple, ON - Family Medicine
Dr Roya Najafi, West Vancouver, BC - Family Medicine
Dr Ehsaneddin Nasirzadeh, Mississauga, ON - Family Medicine
Dr Firouzeh Niakosari, North York, ON - Anatomical Pathology
Dr Keyvan Pazuki, North York, ON - General Practice
Dr Ahmad Poostizadeh, Kelowna, BC - Cardiac Surgery
Dr Reza Pourvali, Vancouver, BC - Emergency Family Med
Dr Farid A Rahimi, Mission, BC - General Practice
Dr Mohammad Rassouli-Rashti, Barrie, ON - Internal Medicine
Dr Yasmin Rehemtula, Mississauga, ON - General Practice
Dr Fareidoon Rezazadah, Langley, BC - General Practice
Dr Kourosh Sabri, Hamilton, ON - General Practice
Dr Daryoush Sadri, Aurora, ON - Family Medicine
Dr Soheil Saeedi-Tabar, Mississauga, ON - Family Medicine
Dr Sina Sajed, Gananoque, ON - Family Medicine
Dr Khashayar Sanandaji, Vaughan, ON - Family Medicine
Dr Javad Sattarian, Scarborough, ON - Orthopedic Surgery
Dr Alireza Semsar, Springhill, NS - General Practice
Dr Pooneh Seyed Akhavan, Toronto, ON - Internal Medicine
Dr Roshan S Shafai-Sarshar, Newmarket, ON - Internal Medicine
Dr Marzieh Shafie, Burnaby, BC - Family Medicine
Dr Bahram Shahi, Fort Frances, ON - General Surgery
Dr Aram Shahparaki, Burnaby, BC - Internal Medicine
Dr Masoud Shahrokhi, West Vancouver, BC - Family Medicine
Dr Roya Shaikholeslami, Cambridge, ON - General Practice
Dr Merajuddin Shams, Vaughan, ON - Family Medicine
Dr Mehrnoosh Shamsi, Port Moody, BC - Family Medicine
Dr Elham Shamsian, Ottawa, ON - Family Medicine
Dr Hossein Shayan, Vancouver, BC - Cardiac Surgery
Dr Maryam Shayesteh Alam, Barrie, ON - Dermatology
Dr Hassan Shenassa, Ottawa, ON - Obstetrics & Gynecology
Dr Mohammad B Shokravi, North Vancouver, BC - Dermatology
Dr Sayed M A Shourideh-Ziabari, Barrie, ON - Family Medicine
Dr Mohammad Tabari, Scarborough, ON - General Surgery
Dr Farshid Tabloie, Scarborough, ON - Orthopedic Surgery
Dr Mojgan Taremi, Newmarket, ON - Radiation Oncology
Dr Bahman Torkian-Valashani, Oshawa, ON - Family Medicine
Dr Rushad T Udwadia, New Westminster, BC - General Surgery
Dr Aref Vaezi, Toronto, ON - Family Medicine
Dr Francis H Vala, North Vancouver, BC - Family Medicine
Dr Mojgan Vaziri, North Vancouver, BC - Anatomical Pathology
Dr P Ariana Verdizad, Pitt Meadows, BC - Family Medicine
Dr Pooneh Yahyavi, Richmond Hill, ON - Internal Medicine
Dr Abu M Yakub, Brampton, ON - General Practice
Dr Arjang Yazdani, London, ON - Plastic Surgery
Dr Fereshteh Yazdani Boroujeni, Guelph, ON - General Practice
Dr Teanoosh Zadeh, Westmount, QC - General Surgery
Dr Kourosh Zadhoush, Bradford, ON - Family Medicine
Dr Afshan Zahedi, Scarborough, ON - Endocrin/Metabolism
Dr Kamran Zamanpour, North Vancouver, BC - Family Medicine
Dr Iman Zandieh, Victoria, BC - Gastroenterology
Dr Mojgan Zare-Parsi, North York, ON - Psychiatry
Dr Maryam Zeineddin, West Vancouver, BC - Family Medicine
Dr Setareh Ziai, Ottawa, ON - Ophthalmology
Dr Arash Zohoor, Brantford, ON - Family Medicine
Dr Mohammad M Zolein, Penticton, BC - General Pathology

FINNISH

Dr Anne Duvall, Barrie, ON - Family Medicine
Dr Kevin Hafez, Calgary, AB - Family Medicine
Dr Pentti A Joutsi, Newmarket, ON - Obstetrics & Gynecology
Dr Gary W Kivinen, Sudbury, ON - Internal Medicine
Dr Ken Kontio, Ottawa, ON - Orthopedic Surgery
Dr Lawrence J Kotkas, Lethbridge, AB - Psychiatry
Dr Jouni P Kraft, Thunder Bay, ON - General Practice
Dr Talvi C Maimets, Toronto, ON - Family Medicine
Dr Paivi M H Miettunen, Calgary, AB - Pediatrics
Dr Kimmo T T Murto, Ottawa, ON - Anesthesia
Dr Ervin T Oinonen, St Catharines, ON - General Practice
Dr Anthony A Papp, Vancouver, BC - Plastic Surgery
Dr Ross E Phillips, Whitehorse, YT - Family Medicine
Dr Anne M Sepanmaa-Lund, Edmonton, AB - General Practice
Dr Olli M Sovio, Abbotsford, BC - Orthopedic Surgery
Dr Eija M Valikangas, Toronto, ON - Diagnostic-Radiology
Dr Harry M Voogjarv, Timmins, ON - Critical Care Medicine
Dr Anna K Woods, Winnipeg, MB - Psychiatry
Dr V Heikki Ylanko, East York, ON - General Practice
Dr Veli J Ylanko, East York, ON - Family Medicine

FLEMISH

Dr Madelene S Kellerman, Lethbridge, AB - General Practice
Dr Wynand F Louw, Invermere, BC - Family Medicine
Dr Francois O P Moens, Hamilton, ON - Obstetrics & Gynecology
Dr Renier G Van Aardt, Truro, NS - Family Medicine
Dr John E E Van Aerde, Surrey, BC - Pediatrics
Dr Etienne Van Der Linde, Clarenville, NL - General Practice
Dr Vincent L Van Hooydonk, Tillsonburg, ON - General Practice
Dr Paul-Robert V Vanhoutte, Saint John, NB - Family Medicine

FOOCHOW

Dr James F K Hii, Vancouver, BC - General Practice
Dr Peter L Ting, Vancouver, BC - General Practice

FOOKIEN

Dr Aik-Ping Eng, Vancouver, BC - General Practice
Dr Margaret C Gan-Gaisano, Scarborough, ON - Pediatrics
Dr James F K Hii, Vancouver, BC - General Practice
Dr Pein-Pein Huang, Ottawa, ON - Pediatrics
Dr Charles C S Law, Vancouver, BC - General Practice
Dr Meng Eng Lim, North Vancouver, BC - Psychiatry
Dr David C Lim, Toronto, ON - General Practice
Dr David T Lin, Vancouver, BC - Ophthalmology
Dr Liang Ng, West Vancouver, BC - General Practice
Dr Dennis D Ong, Saskatoon, SK - Anesthesia
Dr Milton C Po, Surrey, BC - Radiation Oncology
Dr Michelle W Tan, Richmond, BC - Family Medicine
Dr Clementine Tang, Vancouver, BC - Pediatrics
Dr Smiley G S Tsao, Unionville, ON - Family Medicine
Dr Edgardo Y Wee, Vancouver, BC - General Practice

FRENCH

Dr Bruce V Abbey, Guelph, ON - General Practice
Dr Amel Abdallah, Thunder Bay, ON - Family Medicine
Dr Hama S I Abdel-Salam, Espanola, ON - Family Medicine
Dr Hamed Abdoulraman, North Vancouver, BC - Psychiatry
Dr Aboobaker Aboo, Ottawa, ON - General Practice
Dr Dikran J Abrahamian, Penetanguishene, ON - General Practice
Dr Allan Abramovitch, Scarborough, ON - Urology
Dr Forough Abtahi, Cornwall, ON - General Practice
Dr Maysan Abu-Hakima, Calgary, AB - Internal Medicine
Dr Michael J M Ackermann, Sherbrooke, NS - General Practice
Dr Yael Acre, Montreal, QC - Family Medicine
Dr Christian Adam, Fredericton, NB - Obstetrics & Gynecology
Dr Edward I Adelson, Montreal, QC - Cardiology
Dr Mansour Adle, Westmount, QC - General Surgery
Dr Rasheed A E Affifi, Thornhill, ON - General Surgery
Dr Ravi Agarwala, St. Catharines, ON - Internal Medicine
Dr Khim C Ah-Lan, Saint-Hubert, QC - General Practice
Dr Paul D Ahlgren, Montreal, QC - Internal Medicine
Dr S Zareen Ahmad, Toronto, ON - Internal Medicine
Dr Alexandra H Ahmet, Ottawa, ON - Endocrin/Metabolism
Dr Joseph Aicher, Saint John, NB - Psychiatry
Dr Fatih M W Al-Katib, Saskatoon, SK - General Practice
Dr Michel Albert, Thunder Bay, ON - Emergency Family Med
Dr Darren L Albert, Montreal, QC - Ophthalmology
Dr Krystyna A Albin-Cook, Etobicoke, ON - General Practice
Dr David Algom, Nepean, ON - Clin Immun/Allergy
Dr Karima M Ali, Calgary, AB - Family Medicine
Dr Lenny C Alladin, Montreal, QC - General Practice
Dr David Allan, Ottawa, ON - Hematology
Dr Johane Allard, Toronto, ON - Gastroenterology
Dr Timothy V Allen, Mississauga, ON - Emergency Medicine
Dr Gillian B Allen, Toronto, ON - General Practice
Dr Federico A Allodi, Toronto, ON - Psychiatry
Dr Deborah Alper, Montreal, QC - Family Medicine
Dr Alexandre Alterescu, North York, ON - General Practice
Dr A Nanette Alvarez, Calgary, AB - Cardiology
Dr Gonzalo G Alvarez, Ottawa, ON - Internal Medicine
Dr Fernando Alvarez, Montreal, QC - General Practice
Dr Neda Amani, Ottawa, ON - General Practice
Dr Maxime Amar, Quebec, QC - General Practice
Dr Myriam N Amimi, Sault Ste. Marie, ON - Obstetrics & Gynecology
Dr Smita Amin, North York, ON - Dermatology
Dr Evangelia-Lila Amirali, Montreal, QC - Psychiatry
Dr Roland E Amolins, Oakville, ON - Family Medicine
Dr Jean I Anawati, Sturgeon Falls, ON - General Practice
Dr Duncan P Anderson, Vancouver, BC - Ophthalmology
Dr M Catherine Anderson, Fergus, ON - Family Medicine
Dr Scott B Anderson, London, ON - Critical Care Medicine
Dr Dawn L Anderson, Montreal, QC - General Surgery
Dr Stella Andonatos, Cote Saint-Luc, QC - General Practice
Dr Veronica Andrenyi, Montreal, QC - Diagnostic-Radiology
Dr James D Angle, Greenfield Park, QC - Internal Medicine
Dr Chantal D Ansell, Saskatoon, SK - Family Medicine
Dr Natalie E Antonenko, Selkirk, MB - General Practice
Dr John Antoniou, Montreal, QC - Orthopedic Surgery
Dr Andre R Anzarut, Vancouver, BC - Neurology
Dr Luis C Appeltauer, Montreal, QC - General Practice
Dr Stella L Arbitman, Thornhill, ON - Family Medicine
Dr Julio E Arboleda-Florez, Belleville, ON - Psychiatry
Dr Lisa M J Archambault, Lasalle, QC - Pediatrics
Dr Christopher Archibald, Ottawa, ON - Community Medicine
Dr Patricia M Arenas, Casselman, ON - General Practice
Dr Sylvie J Argouarch, Victoria, BC - Psychiatry
Dr Yasemin Arikan, New Westminster, BC - Internal Medicine
Dr David Armstrong, Hamilton, ON - Gastroenterology

Dr Barry D Armstrong, Thunder Bay, ON - General Surgery
Dr Ian M F Arnold, Ottawa, ON - General Surgery
Dr Bryan P Arthurs, Montreal, QC - Ophthalmology
Dr A Neil Arya, Kitchener, ON - Family Medicine
Dr Sylvia L Asa, Toronto, ON - Anatomical Pathology
Dr Haig Ashikian, Gloucester, ON - Family Medicine
Dr Alfred Assalian, Longueuil, QC - Ophthalmology
Dr Pierre Assalian, Montreal, QC - Psychiatry
Dr Manutchehr Assemi, Nepean, ON - Pediatrics
Dr Ardavan Assemi, Ottawa, ON - Family Medicine
Dr Soheir Atalla, Brossard, QC - General Practice
Dr Kenneth A Atkinson, New Westminster, BC - Gastroenterology
Dr Amany A Y Attalla, Cambridge, ON - Family Medicine
Lt Sanita Atwal, Edmonton, AB - General Surgery
Dr Heather-Jane Au, Edmonton, AB - Internal Medicine
Dr F Kris Aubrey-Bassler, St. John's, NL - Emergency Family Med
Dr Jean R Aubry, North Bay, ON - Family Medicine
Dr Nevine Audi, Ottawa, ON - Emergency Family Med
Dr Julie R Auger, Timmins, ON - Family Medicine
Dr Pierre Auger, Levis, QC - Cardiology
Dr Manon Auger, Montreal, QC - Anatomical Pathology
Dr Christopher N Ayers, Calgary, AB - Family Medicine
Dr Jean-Pierre M Ayoub, Montreal, QC - Internal Medicine
Dr Sameh C Azer, Fort Saskatchewan, AB - General Practice
Dr Raed Azer, New Waterford, NS - Family Medicine
Dr Dalal A Aziz, Milton, ON - General Surgery
Dr Fadi-Boutros Azzi, Hawkesbury, ON - Family Medicine
Dr Charles E Babin, Huntingdon, QC - General Practice
Dr Eric M Babins, Calgary, AB - Family Medicine
Dr John H Backler, Westmount, QC - Family Medicine
Dr Carolyn E H Baer, Moncton, NB - Internal Medicine
Dr Philip A Baer, Scarborough, ON - Internal Medicine
Dr Hovsep Baghdadlian, North York, ON - Infectious Diseases
Dr Chaikou Bah, Laval, QC - Orthopedic Surgery
Dr Gillian F Bailey, Halifax, NS - General Practice
Dr Robert F Bailey, Montreal, QC - Geriatric Medicine
Dr Jean-Martin Baillargeon, Montreal, QC - Diagnostic-Radiology
Dr Sangeeta Bajaj, Brampton, ON - Internal Medicine
Dr Kevin R Baker, Ottawa, ON - Obstetrics & Gynecology
Dr David Bakish, Ottawa, ON - Psychiatry
Dr A Gordon Balazsi, Mont-Royal, QC - Ophthalmology
Dr Gerry A Bally, Ottawa, ON - Family Medicine
Dr Marcel A Baltzan, Cote Saint-Luc, QC - Internal Medicine
Dr J D Russell Bamford, Whitehorse, YT - Family Medicine
Dr Edith Bandi, Montreal, QC - Anesthesia
Dr Elisabeth Banon, Montreal, QC - Psychiatry
Dr Dana Baran, Montreal, QC - Internal Medicine
Dr Norma Barbieri, Abbotsford, BC - Psychiatry
Dr Zaim Bardakji, Saint-Laurent, QC - General Practice
Dr Claudette L Bardin, Montreal, QC - Pediatrics
Dr Genevieve Baril-Guerard, Nelson, BC - General Practice
Dr Ronald G Barr, Vancouver, BC - Pediatrics
Dr Ian Barrette, Gatineau, QC - Family Medicine
Dr Stephane Barrette, Verdun, QC - Hematology
Dr Keith J Barrington, Montreal, QC - Pediatrics
Dr Colin A Barry, Saint John, NB - Cardiology
Dr Milad K Barsoum, Toronto, ON - Urology
Dr Peter G Barss, Salmon Arm, BC - Community Medicine
Dr Ola J Barter, St. John's, NL - Critical Care Medicine
Dr Roger Bashala, Campbellton, NB - Family Medicine
Dr Mounir Bashour, Montreal, QC - Ophthalmology
Dr Arsene J Basmadjian, Montreal, QC - Cardiology
Dr Girair Basmadjian, Montreal, QC - Ophthalmology
Dr Gilles Simon Bastien, Montreal, QC - Family Medicine
Dr Jane S Batten, Ottawa, ON - Family Medicine
Dr Robert Bauer, Toronto, ON - Cardiology
Dr Stephanie A Baxter, Kingston, ON - Ophthalmology
Dr Maureen Baxter, Ottawa, ON - Orthopedic Surgery
Dr Mark T Bayley, Toronto, ON - Physical Medicine & Rehab
Dr Aude Beauchamp, New Westminster, BC - Obstetrics & Gynecology
Dr Marc Beauchamp, Montreal, QC - Orthopedic Surgery
Dr Suzanne M Beauchemin, Orleans, ON - Family Medicine
Dr Luc M Beauchesne, Ottawa, ON - Cardiology
Dr Annie Beaudoin, Sherbrooke, QC - Gastroenterology
Dr Lucie M Beaupre, Ottawa, ON - General Practice
Dr Catherine Beauregard, Montreal, QC - Endocrin/Metabolism
Dr Pierre Beausejour, Sherbrooke, QC - Psychiatry
Dr Rafik R Bechbache, Unionville, ON - Family Medicine
Dr Gail M Beck, Ottawa, ON - Psychiatry
Dr Julie Bedard, Quebec, QC - Anesthesia
Dr Luc Bedard, Thetford Mines, QC - General Practice
Dr Vanessa Bedard, Saskatoon, SK - Pediatrics
Dr Deegrasjsing S Beeharry, Calgary, AB - General Practice
Dr Louis R Begin, Montreal, QC - Anatomical Pathology
Dr M H Julie Begin, Vaudreuil-Dorion, QC - General Practice
Dr Parvaneh Beheshti, West Vancouver, BC - General Practice
Dr Rama R Behki, Gatineau, QC - Ophthalmology
Dr Marcellus A Behr, Montreal, QC - Infectious Diseases
Dr Abdollah Behzadi, Mississauga, ON - General Surgery
Dr Darren T Beiko, Kingston, ON - Urology
Dr Mary Ann Beimers, Vancouver, BC - Pediatrics
Dr Mario Bejerman, Montreal, QC - General Surgery
Dr Robert A Beldavs, Winnipeg, MB - Ophthalmology
Dr James F Beliveau, Kingston, ON - Family Medicine
Dr Laura P Bell, Courtenay, BC - Family Medicine
Dr Lorraine E Bell, Montreal, QC - Nephrology
Dr Steven J Y R Bellemare, Ottawa, ON - Pediatrics
Dr Daniel J Belliveau, Halifax, NS - Ophthalmology
Dr Arie Benchetrit, Pointe-Claire, QC - General Surgery
Dr Oleg D Bendz, Toronto, ON - General Practice
Dr Catherine Benes, Toronto, ON - Psychiatry
Dr Alice Benjamin, Montreal, QC - Obstetrics & Gynecology
Dr Carmen L Benkoczi, Lethbridge, AB - Family Medicine
Dr Brien G Benoit, Ottawa, ON - Neurosurgery
Dr Marie-Jose Benoit, Ottawa, ON - General Practice
Dr Amal Bensaleh-Ratmi, Moncton, NB - General Practice
Dr Susanne Benseler, Toronto, ON - General Practice
Dr Frances C Berard, Notre-Dame-Lr, MB - Family Medicine
Dr Joanne E Bergens, Edmonton, AB - Family Medicine
Dr Pierre Bergeron, Montreal, QC - Community Medicine
Dr Marco Bergevin, Laval, QC - Infectious Diseases
Dr Rodney M Bergh, Ottawa, ON - Pediatrics
Dr Richard G Bergstrom, Edmonton, AB - Anesthesia
Col J Jean-Robert S Bernier, Ottawa, ON - General Practice
Dr Denyse Bernier, Quebec, QC - General Practice
Dr Danielle A Bernier, St-Jean-Sur-Richel, QC - Obstetrics & Gynecology
Dr Lucie M Bernier-Lycka, Edmonton, AB - Family Medicine
Dr Mark L Bernstein, Halifax, NS - Hematology
Dr Mark Bernstein, Toronto, ON - Neurosurgery
Dr Robert L Bernstein, Dorval, QC - General Practice
Dr Bruno Bernucci, Saint-Leonard, QC - General Practice
Dr Marian E Berry, Nelson, BC - Neurology
Dr Marc Berthiaume, Ottawa, ON - Family Medicine
Dr Claude Berthiaume, Salaber-de-Valleyf, QC - General Practice
Dr Hugo A R Bertozzi, Grande Prairie, AB - Family Medicine
Dr Helene Bertrand, North Vancouver, BC - Family Medicine
Dr Henri A Bertrand, Maniwaki, QC - General Practice
Dr Michel J A Berube, Cap-aux-Meules, QC - Internal Medicine
Dr Denis Berube, Montreal, QC - Pediatrics
Dr Markus Besemann, Ottawa, ON - Physical Medicine & Rehab
Dr Catherine Besner, Gatineau, QC - Family Medicine
Dr Benoit J Bessette, Ottawa, ON - Orthopedic Surgery
Dr Isabelle Bessette, St-Charles-Brromee, QC - Family Medicine
Dr Ricardo Bessoudo, Saint John, NB - Cardiology
Dr Andrea Bezjak, Toronto, ON - Internal Medicine
Dr Michael Bezuhly, Halifax, NS - Plastic Surgery
Dr Sanjiv K Bhalla, Edmonton, AB - Diagnostic-Radiology
Dr Nadeem H Bhanji, Calgary, AB - Psychiatry
Dr Onil Bhattacharyya, Toronto, ON - Family Medicine
Dr Luc Bherer, Quebec, QC - General Practice
Dr Fernando A Bianchi, Hamilton, ON - Internal Medicine
Dr Antonio U Bianchini, LaSalle, QC - Family Medicine
Dr Lindsay Bick, Camrose, AB - General Practice
Dr H Jay Biem, Pointe-Claire, QC - Internal Medicine
Dr Eric Bigelow, Nepean, ON - General Surgery
Dr Jean-Marc Bigonnesse, Sherbrooke, QC - Family Medicine
Dr Jan Jaap Bijlsma, Vancouver, BC - Emergency Medicine
Dr Jean-Sebastien Billiard, Montreal, QC - Diagnostic-Radiology
Dr Robin C Billick, Montreal, QC - Dermatology
Dr Kendall Billick, Pointe-Claire, QC - Infectious Diseases
Dr David Billings, Southampton, ON - Emergency Family Med
Dr Birubi R Biman, Thunder Bay, ON - Internal Medicine
Dr Jacques Binet, St-Jean-sur-Richel, QC - General Practice
Dr J Richard F Binette, Peterborough, ON - Family Medicine
Dr Natasha Bird, Coaticook, QC - General Practice
Dr Patricia E Birk, Winnipeg, MB - Nephrology
Dr Barbara M Birkett, Milton, ON - Dermatology
Dr Debra S Birnbaum, North York, ON - Family Medicine
Dr Robert J Birnbaum, Ottawa, ON - Family Medicine
Dr Marilena Biscotti, Beamsville, ON - Family Medicine
Dr Laila D Bishara, Markham, ON - Endocrin/Metabolism
Dr Clare E Bishop, Ottawa, ON - Family Medicine
Dr Hany E Bissada, Ottawa, ON - Psychiatry
Dr Louis Bissonnette, Farnham, QC - Family Medicine
Dr Bindu Bittira, Sudbury, ON - Cardiac Surgery
Dr Martin Bitzan, Montreal, QC - General Practice
Dr Piotr A Blachut, Vancouver, BC - Orthopedic Surgery
Dr Daniel O Black, Quebec, QC - Ophthalmology
Dr Guy R Blais, Edmonton, AB - Family Medicine
Dr Robert J D Blais, Gatineau, QC - Family Medicine
Dr Basil A Blanchard, Rogersville, NB - General Practice
Dr German Blando, Dieppe, NB - General Practice
Dr Myles K Blank, Vancouver, BC - Psychiatry
Dr Marc P Blayney, Sudbury, ON - Pediatrics
Dr Jean Blier, Ottawa, ON - Anesthesia
Dr Anna A Blinkina, Cornwall, ON - Family Medicine
Dr Steve Blitzer, Thornhill, ON - General Practice
Dr Rita J M Blom, Parksville, BC - Diagnostic-Radiology
Dr Robert A Bluman, Vancouver, BC - Family Medicine
Dr Herbert M Blumer, Montreal, QC - Clin Immun/Allergy
Dr Gerald G Blunt, Englehart, ON - General Practice
Dr Armour I Boake, Thunder Bay, ON - Internal Medicine
Dr A Barbara Bodmer, Montreal, QC - Obstetrics & Gynecology
Dr Rebecca Bodok, Bolton, ON - Family Medicine
Dr R Dan Boghen, Montreal, QC - Neurology
Dr Avedis Bogosyan, North York, ON - General Practice
Dr Marc A Boileau, North Vancouver, BC - Family Medicine
Dr Miriam E Boillat, Montreal, QC - Family Medicine
Dr Caroline Boisvert, St-Jerome, QC - General Practice
Dr Maarten Bokhout, Clinton, ON - Family Medicine
Dr Pierre Bonin, Sudbury, ON - Family Medicine
Dr Michel L Bonin, Sudbury, ON - General Pathology
Dr Francine M Bonnet, Ottawa, ON - Family Medicine
Dr Timothy W Bood, Halifax, NS - General Practice
Dr Serge Bordeleau, Quebec, QC - General Practice
Dr Illya C Boridy, Calgary, AB - Diagnostic-Radiology
Dr Rainer H Borkenhagen, Vancouver, BC - Family Medicine
Dr Pierre Bornais, Amqui, QC - General Practice
Dr David Borts, Brampton, ON - Cardiology
Dr Francis M Boston, Montreal, QC - Diagnostic-Radiology
Dr Sarah Bouchard, Montreal, QC - General Surgery
Dr Julie A Boucher, Kapuskasing, ON - Family Medicine
Dr Francois Boucher, Quebec, QC - Pediatrics
Dr Eric Bouffet, Toronto, ON - Pediatrics
Dr Julie Boulanger, Les Escoumins, QC - Family Medicine
Dr Michel J Boulanger Jr., Edmonton, AB - Emergency Medicine
Dr Pauline Boulos, Hamilton, ON - Internal Medicine
Dr Patrick R Boulos, Sherbrooke, QC - Ophthalmology
Dr Helen L A Bouman, Bragg Creek, AB - Family Medicine
Dr Christine Bourbonniere, Gatineau, QC - Family Medicine
Dr Danielle Bourdeau, Toronto, ON - Psychiatry
Dr Christian Bourdy, Montreal, QC - General Practice
Dr Robert F Bourgault, Ottawa, ON - General Practice
Dr Louise A Bourgault, Ottawa, ON - General Practice
Dr Klere Bourgault, Verner, ON - Family Medicine
Dr Ronald L J Bourgeois, Moncton, NB - Cardiology
Dr Daniel J Bourgeois, Peterborough, ON - Diagnostic-Radiology
Dr Kevin E Bourke, Halifax, NS - General Practice
Dr Jean-Andre Bourque, Caraquet, NB - General Practice
Dr Robert G Bourrier, Ottawa, ON - Family Medicine
Dr Renda Bouzayen, Halifax, NS - Obstetrics & Gynecology
Dr Stefan R Boyle, Petawawa, ON - Family Medicine
Dr Patrick Boyle, Sarnia, ON - Family Medicine
Dr William R Bradley, Dartmouth, NS - Family Medicine

Dr Robert W Bradstock, Edmonton, AB - Family Medicine
Dr Jacques Bradwejn, Ottawa, ON - Psychiatry
Dr Luis H P Braga, Hamilton, ON - General Practice
Dr Evan J Brahm, Montreal, QC - Psychiatry
Dr Joseph F Braidy, Longueuil, QC - Critical Care Medicine
Dr Jack S Brandes, Toronto, ON - Psychiatry
Dr Alain Brassard, Edmonton, AB - Dermatology
Dr Ioana Bratu, Edmonton, AB - General Surgery
Dr John C Bray, Pointe-Claire, QC - Obstetrics & Gynecology
Dr Carol M J Brebion, LaSalle, QC - Psychiatry
Dr Laurie T Breger, Pointe-Claire, QC - Family Medicine
Dr Karlina A Breikss, Victoria, BC - Pediatrics
Dr Martin A M Breton, Calgary, AB - Family Medicine
Dr Chantal Breton, Pointe-Claire, QC - Family Medicine
Dr Johnny D Brisebois, Kanata, ON - Family Medicine
Dr Paul Brisson, Orleans, ON - Dermatology
Dr Henri Brisson, Longueuil, QC - Psychiatry
Dr Heather F Britten, Windsor, ON - Family Medicine
Dr Gordon I Brock, Temiscaming, QC - Family Medicine
Dr Elizabeth J Brodkin, Surrey, BC - Community Medicine
Dr Stephen C Brodovsky, Winnipeg, MB - Ophthalmology
Dr Lisa A Bromley, Ottawa, ON - Family Medicine
Dr Michal Broniewski, Calgary, AB - General Practice
Dr Edward Brook, Ottawa, ON - General Practice
Dr Laurene J Brooks, Edmonton, AB - Family Medicine
Dr Michel Brouillet, Sherbrooke, QC - General Practice
Dr Maryleen Brouw, Quebec, QC - General Practice
Dr Dean V Brown, West Vancouver, BC - Emergency Family Med
Dr D Stephen Brown, Moncton, NB - General Surgery
Dr Basil S Brown, Digby, NS - Diagnostic-Radiology
Dr C Elizabeth A Brown, Brockville, ON - Emergency Family Med
Dr Kenneth E Brown, Verdun, QC - Family Medicine
Dr Anita Marie Brown-Johnson, Montreal, QC - Family Medicine
Dr Linda D Brown-Thomson, Kingston, ON - Family Medicine
Dr Sylvie M Brule, Rockland, ON - Emergency Family Med
Dr Giovanni F Bruno, Alliston, ON - Diagnostic-Radiology
Dr Lizabeth A Brydon, Regina, SK - Obstetrics & Gynecology
Dr Wojciech S Brzezinski, Medicine Hat, AB - General Surgery
Dr Wanda T Brzezinski, Westmount, QC - General Practice
Dr Zoheir Bshouty, Winnipeg, MB - Internal Medicine
Dr Raffaele Bucci, Saint-Leonard, QC - General Practice
Dr Suzanne C Buchanan, Scarborough, ON - Family Medicine
Dr Balint L Budai, Vancouver, BC - Family Medicine
Dr Sharon E Buehner, Sault Ste. Marie, ON - Emergency Family Med
Dr Ralf R Buhrmann, Ottawa, ON - Ophthalmology
Dr Robert Buie, Dundas, ON - Psychiatry
Dr Marie-Claire Bujold, Orleans, ON - Family Medicine
Dr Yury Bulaev, Edmonton, AB - General Practice
Dr Emily M Bulanski, Cambridge, ON - Family Medicine
Dr George M Burden, Elmsdale, NS - General Practice
Dr Michael Burger, St Catharines, ON - Pediatrics
Dr Susan C Burgess, Vancouver, BC - Family Medicine
Dr Tracy A Burgess, Orleans, ON - Family Medicine
Dr Mairi Burnett, Niverville, MB - General Practice
Dr Christopher J Burnett, Niverville, MB - General Practice
Dr Miguel N Burnier, Montreal, QC - General Practice
Dr A George Burns, Louisbourg, NS - Family Medicine
Dr Gerard M Burns, Kanata, ON - General Practice
Dr Kevin D Burns, Ottawa, ON - Internal Medicine
Dr Jeffrey R Burton, Edmonton, AB - Cardiology
Dr M Shayne Burwell, Saskatoon, SK - Plastic Surgery
Dr Sonia D Buttar, Surrey, BC - General Practice
Dr Andreana M Butter, London, ON - General Surgery
Dr Alan J Byrne, Oakville, ON - General Surgery
Dr Anna M Byszewski, Ottawa, ON - Geriatric Medicine
Dr Anthony E Cabrera, St Catharines, ON - Ophthalmology
Dr Margherita O Cadeddu, Hamilton, ON - General Surgery
Dr Eric Cadesky, Vancouver, BC - Family Medicine
Dr Louise Cadoret, Chateauguay, QC - General Practice
Dr Martin Cadorette, Trois-Rivieres, QC - General Practice
Dr Forrest H Caldwell, Guelph, ON - Family Medicine
Dr Todd C R Calhoun, North York, ON - Anesthesia
Dr Terrence S Callanan, St. John's, NL - Psychiatry
Dr Lynn C Calvert, Burlington, ON - General Practice
Dr Colin J Cameron, Brockville, ON - Psychiatry
Dr Glenn G Cameron, Penetanguishene, ON - Family Medicine
Dr Peter R Camfield, Halifax, NS - Neurology
Dr Roberto M Campanaro, Atikokan, ON - General Practice
Dr Pamela C Campbell, Calgary, AB - Family Medicine
Dr Duncan A Campbell, Edmonton, AB - Internal Medicine
Dr Alan J Campbell-Moscrop, Hamilton, ON - Plastic Surgery
Dr Denise L Campbell-Scherer, Edmonton, AB - Family Medicine
Dr Pablo O Cano, Sudbury, ON - Internal Medicine
Dr Marcelo Cantarovich, Montreal, QC - Nephrology
Dr Paul S Cappon, Ottawa, ON - Community Medicine
Dr Bernice M Capusten, Red Deer, AB - Diagnostic-Radiology
Dr Manuel R Cardoso, Montreal, QC - Internal Medicine
Dr Peter L Carlen, Toronto, ON - Neurology
Dr Maureen T Carlier, Ottawa, ON - Anatomical Pathology
Dr Robert C Carlin, Montreal, QC - Family Medicine
Dr Catherine M Caron, Ottawa, ON - Family Medicine
Dr Noah H Carpenter, Brandon, MB - General Surgery
Dr David C Carpenter, Ottawa, ON - General Practice
Dr Jacques Carriere, Quebec, QC - Psychiatry
Dr John K Carsley, Vancouver, BC - Community Medicine
Dr Katharine D Carson, Ottawa, ON - Family Medicine
Dr Jan K Carstoniu, Toronto, ON - Anesthesia
Dr Christopher J Carter, Gatineau, QC - Orthopedic Surgery
Dr Nicola Casacalenda, Montreal, QC - Psychiatry
Dr Bruce W Case, Montreal, QC - Anatomical Pathology
Dr Richard F H Catchlove, Montreal, QC - General Practice
Dr Edward F E Cattan, Orleans, ON - Psychiatry
Dr Pablo Cervantes, Montreal, QC - Psychiatry
Dr Francoise Chagnon, Montreal, QC - Otolaryngology
Dr Leopoldo Chagoya, Toronto, ON - Psychiatry
Dr Marybelle M T Chain-Chang, Brampton, ON - General Practice
Dr Bachar Chalati, Stewiacke, NS - General Practice
Dr Colin H Chalk, Montreal, QC - Neurology
Dr Tara S Chalmers-Nixon, Calgary, AB - Gastroenterology
Dr Susan M Chamberlain, Kingston, ON - Obstetrics & Gynecology
Dr Elaine M C Champagne, Cote Saint-Luc, QC - Pediatrics
Dr Ginette Champagne, Montreal, QC - General Practice
Dr Benjamin T Chan, Espanola, ON - General Practice
Dr Ariane C Chan, Newmarket, ON - General Practice
Dr Adrien M T Chan, Thunder Bay, ON - Internal Medicine
Dr Christopher T M Chan, Toronto, ON - Internal Medicine
Dr Kevin J Chan, Toronto, ON - Pediatric Emergency Medicine
Dr Kenneth L Chan, Greenfield Park, QC - Gynecologic Oncology
Dr Chan-San H Chan-Tai-Kong, Lloydminster, AB - General Practice
Dr A Joseph Chan-Tai-Kong, Regina, SK - Anesthesia
Dr Lambros N Chaniotis, Pointe-Claire, QC - Cardiology
Dr Fabien A Charbonneau, Campbellville, ON - General Practice
Dr Ali Charghi, Montreal, QC - Urology
Dr Marco Charneux, Montreal, QC - Critical Care Medicine
Dr Martin Charron, Toronto, ON - Nuclear Medicine
Dr Jane Charters, Oakville, ON - General Practice
Dr Prosanto K Chaudhury, Montreal, QC - General Surgery
Dr Rameshchandra P Chauhan, Ottawa, ON - Orthopedic Surgery
Dr Laurel A Chauvin-Kimoff, Montreal, QC - Pediatrics
Dr Ashis K Chawla, Toronto, ON - Urology
Dr Jihad Y Chaya, St Thomas, ON - Psychiatry
Dr Marc J Chayer, Lindsay, ON - General Practice
Dr Walif Chbeir, Gatineau, QC - Diagnostic-Radiology
Dr Mustapha Chelfi, Gatineau, QC - General Practice
Dr Benjamin H Chen, Napanee, ON - Family Medicine
Dr Robert J B Chen, Toronto, ON - Anesthesia
Dr Calvino K Cheng, Halifax, NS - Hematological Pathology
Dr Donna A G Cherniak, Sherbrooke, QC - Family Medicine
Dr Darin P Cherniwchan, Chilliwack, BC - Family Medicine
Dr Tracey M Chesser, Moncton, NB - Emergency Family Med
Dr Philippe Chessex, Montreal, QC - Pediatrics
Dr Vincent S J Cheung, Peterborough, ON - Internal Medicine
Dr James A Chiarotto, Scarborough, ON - Internal Medicine
Dr J Roland Chiasson, Summerside, PE - General Practice
Dr Abdallah Chidiac, Saint-Laurent, QC - Pediatrics
Dr Charles Chocron, Montreal, QC - General Practice
Dr Shirley H Y Chou, Ottawa, ON - General Surgery
Dr Georges N Choueri, Laval, QC - Gastroenterology
Dr Edmond E Chouinard, Cambridge, ON - Internal Medicine
Dr David R Chow, Toronto, ON - Ophthalmology
Dr Jarmila Chrappa, Corner Brook, NL - Pediatrics
Dr Michel Chretien, Ottawa, ON - Endocrin/Metabolism
Dr Janet E Christie-Seely, Nepean, ON - Family Medicine
Dr Nicolas V Christou, Saint-Laurent, QC - General Surgery
Dr Wendy M Chrusch, Regina, SK - Physical Medicine & Rehab
Dr Bernard Chrysler, Montreal, QC - Internal Medicine
Dr Karen L Chu, Toronto, ON - Emergency Family Med
Dr Margaret A Churcher, Calgary, AB - Family Medicine
Dr Michael J Churchill-Smith, Montreal, QC - Internal Medicine
Dr Mark H C Churman, Haileybury, ON - Family Medicine
Dr Tatiana Chypchar, Cambridge, ON - Family Medicine
Dr Mario V Ciccone, Timmins, ON - Emergency Family Med
Dr Claudio S Cina, North York, ON - General Surgery
Dr Michelle P Cipera, Kuujjuarapik, QC - Family Medicine
Dr Sharon L Cirone, Toronto, ON - Emergency Family Med
Dr Jordi Cisa, Sudbury, ON - Orthopedic Surgery
Dr Felipe Cisternas, Vancouver, BC - Family Medicine
Dr Wojtek P Ciszak, Vancouver, BC - General Practice
Dr Sergiu Ciubotaru, Medicine Hat, AB - Family Medicine
Dr Brenda G Clark, Edmonton, AB - Pediatrics
Dr Leigh L Clarke, Pembroke, ON - General Practice
Dr Terrence Clarke, Gatineau, QC - General Practice
Dr Richard L Claveau, Hearst, ON - Family Medicine
Dr Gerald S Clayden, Carman, MB - General Practice
Dr W Robert L Clemmey, Yellowknife, NT - Psychiatry
Dr David R Cleveland, Penticton, BC - Internal Medicine
Dr Nancy A Clevette, Ottawa, ON - Family Medicine
Dr Jean-Pierre Cliche, Toronto, ON - Nuclear Medicine
Dr Richard Cloutier, Montreal, QC - Psychiatry
Dr Edward G Coates, Vancouver, BC - Pediatrics
Dr C David C Coates, Amherstburg, ON - General Practice
Dr Pamela J K Coates, Mississauga, ON - Pediatrics
Dr Leslie A Cockhill, Vancouver, BC - Psychiatry
Dr Alan J H Coffey, Montreal, QC - Ophthalmology
Dr Samantha J Cogan, Etobicoke, ON - Family Medicine
Dr Antonio Cogliano, London, ON - Family Medicine
Dr Harry Cohen, North York, ON - General Practice
Dr Dan A D Cohen, North York, ON - Family Medicine
Dr Mark J Cohen, Toronto, ON - Ophthalmology
Dr Howard R Cohen, Toronto, ON - Obstetrics & Gynecology
Dr Stephen S Cohen, Whitby, ON - Family Medicine
Dr Jeffrey J Cohen, Windsor, ON - General Practice
Dr Jack Cohen, Montreal, QC - Plastic Surgery
Dr Albert Cohen, Montreal, QC - Gastroenterology
Dr Martin A Cohen, Pointe-Claire, QC - Internal Medicine
Dr Claire I Coire, Mississauga, ON - Anatomical Pathology
Dr Susan J Coish, Thornhill, ON - General Practice
Dr Alice Cojocaru, Edmonton, AB - Psychiatry
Dr Rolande M Colas, Moncton, NB - General Practice
Dr Donald C Cole, Toronto, ON - Community Medicine
Dr Martin G Cole, Montreal, QC - Psychiatry
Dr David C Collins, Orillia, ON - General Practice
Dr Sharon C Collins, Renfrew, ON - Internal Medicine
Dr Stuart J Connolly, Hamilton, ON - Cardiology
Dr Steven A Connor, Cobourg, ON - General Practice
Dr Alina D Constantin, Canmore, AB - Family Medicine
Dr Nicolas Constas-Costopoulos, Montreal, QC - General Practice
Dr Brian Conway, Vancouver, BC - Internal Medicine
Dr Nathalie Cook, Ottawa, ON - Pediatrics
Dr Terrance Cooligan, Toronto, ON - Internal Medicine
Dr John F Coombs, Fallbrook, ON - General Practice
Dr E Alexander Cooper, Quebec, QC - Family Medicine
Dr Joseph E Copeland, Vancouver, BC - Emergency Family Med
Dr Michael A Copland, Vancouver, BC - Internal Medicine
Dr Juan L Cordova, Winnipeg, MB - General Practice
Dr Yvon F Cormier, Quebec, QC - Respirology
Dr Richard A Cornell, Collingwood, ON - Emergency Family Med
Dr Anne M J Cornet, Ottawa, ON - Pediatrics
Dr Gary A Costain, Saint John, NB - Internal Medicine
Dr Paolo Costi, Montreal, QC - Cardiology
Dr Isabelle Cote, Hamilton, ON - Psychiatry
Dr Peter B Cote, Manitouwadge, ON - Family Medicine
Dr Jean Cote, Timmins, ON - Family Medicine

Dr G Thomas Cottreau, Charlottetown, PE - General Surgery
Dr Michael P Coughlin, Windsor, ON - General Surgery
Dr Larry P Coughlin, Dollard-D-Ormeaux, QC - Orthopedic Surgery
Capt Bernard Couillard Jr, Courcelette, QC - Emergency Family Med
Dr Louise A Coulombe, Nepean, ON - General Practice
Dr Jean-Francois Courval, LaSalle, QC - Anesthesia
Dr Jafna L Cox, Halifax, NS - Cardiology
Dr Nancy V Craig, Edmonton, AB - Family Medicine
Dr Douglas B Craig, Montreal, QC - Anesthesia
Dr Joseph H Cramer, Scarborough, ON - Obstetrics & Gynecology
Dr Timothy S Cran, Calgary, AB - Family Medicine
Dr Gordon L Crelinsten, Montreal, QC - Cardiology
Dr Kenneth Croitoru, Toronto, ON - Gastroenterology
Dr Catherine Cronin, Kelowna, BC - Pediatrics
Dr William G Cross, Cobourg, ON - Family Medicine
LCdr Stephen Crummey, St. John's, NL - Anesthesia
Dr Nick B Cuberovic, Milton, ON - Family Medicine
Dr Kate N Culman, Calgary, AB - Infectious Diseases
Dr Carl Cummings, Cote Saint-Luc, QC - Pediatrics
Dr Ina E Cummings, Dorval, QC - Family Medicine
Dr Charles Cuncins, North Bay, ON - General Practice
Dr Gregory P Curnew, Hamilton, ON - Cardiology
Dr George R Curnew, Verdun, QC - Anesthesia
Dr Srdjan Curuvija, Ottawa, ON - Diagnostic-Radiology
Dr Steven L Cusimano, Hamilton, ON - Family Medicine
Dr Robert J Cusimano, Toronto, ON - Cardiovasc/ThorSurg
Dr Michael D Cusimano, Toronto, ON - Neurosurgery
Dr Jean Cusson, Greenfield Park, QC - Internal Medicine
Dr Daniel Cusson, Laval, QC - General Practice
Dr Danielle D Cutts, Regina, SK - Family Medicine
Dr Elizabeth Cvejic, Toronto, ON - Psychiatry
Dr Elizabeth Czyziw, Montreal, QC - General Practice
Dr Christine L D'Arsigny, Kingston, ON - Critical Care Medicine
Dr Darryl I D'Costa, Collingwood, ON - General Practice
Dr Jacqueline R D'Eon, Pubnico, NS - General Practice
Dr Derek Da Costa, Dollard-D-Ormeaux, QC - General Practice
Dr Vasco F Da Silva, Ottawa, ON - Neurosurgery
Dr Richard A Dabrusin, Cote Saint-Luc, QC - Respirology
Dr Georges Dadour, Montreal, QC - General Practice
Dr Olga Dafniotis, Trois-Rivieres, QC - Orthopedic Surgery
Dr Michael H Dahan, Montreal, QC - Obstetrics & Gynecology
Dr Robert J P Daigle, Fredericton, NB - General Practice
Dr Peter G Daignault, Pointe-Claire, QC - General Practice
Dr Abdallah Dallal, Saint-Jerome, QC - Psychiatry
Dr Pierre M Daloze, Montreal, QC - General Surgery
Dr Sharon A Dalrymple, Pointe-Claire, QC - General Surgery
Dr Douglass Dalton, Montreal, QC - Family Medicine
Dr Andrew Daly, Calgary, AB - Hematology
Dr Leslie R Damude, London, ON - General Practice
Dr Ratna Dan, Ajax, ON - Diagnostic-Radiology
Dr Silvia L C Dancea, Sudbury, ON - Anatomical Pathology
Dr Adrian B Dancea, Montreal, QC - Cardiology
Dr Robin Dancose, Kirkland, QC - General Practice
Dr Virgil Danescu, Abbotsford, BC - Family Medicine
Dr Dinh Quang Dang, Montreal, QC - General Practice
Dr Gail Dangoor, North York, ON - Family Medicine
Dr Mukhaimer H Dani, Miramichi, NB - General Practice
Dr Sarah B Danial, Niagara Falls, ON - Psychiatry
Dr Shevanta G Daniel, Ajax, ON - Family Medicine
Dr Lise Daniels, Sherbrooke, QC - General Practice
Dr Frederic J Dankoff, Montreal, QC - Family Medicine
Dr Richard Danylewick, Laval, QC - General Surgery
Dr Tien Trong Dao, Laval, QC - Diagnostic-Radiology
Dr Allison B Dart, Winnipeg, MB - Nephrology
Dr Andre Dascal, Montreal, QC - Infectious Diseases
Dr Monidipa Dasgupta, London, ON - Geriatric Medicine
Dr Faiz Daudi, Etobicoke, ON - General Surgery
Dr Alexandre Dauphin, Hamilton, ON - Anesthesia
Dr Christiane Dauphinais, Toronto, ON - Family Medicine
Dr William J Davenport, Calgary, AB - Neurology
Dr Sheila J David, North York, ON - General Practice
Dr Joseph K Davidson, Mississauga, ON - Ophthalmology
Dr William Davidson, Mississauga, ON - Pediatrics
Dr Jan M Davies, Calgary, AB - Anesthesia
Dr E Colin Davies, Saint John, NB - Anesthesia
Dr Michael G Davis, North York, ON - Dermatology
Dr Deborah J Davis, Ottawa, ON - Pediatrics
Dr Keith Granger Dawson, Vancouver, BC - Endocrin/Metabolism
Dr Lesa Dawson, St. John's, NL - Obstetrics & Gynecology
Dr David J Dawson, Montreal, QC - Internal Medicine
Dr Ross C De Belle, Longueuil, QC - Pediatrics
Maj Thomas De Boeck, Midland, ON - Family Medicine
Dr Farideh De Bosset, Toronto, ON - Psychiatry
Dr Gilles De La Salle, Kemptville, ON - Anesthesia
Dr Rene De Montigny, St-Germain-D-Grant, QC - General Practice
Dr Sylvaine De Plaen, Montreal, QC - Psychiatry
Dr Michael De Roode, Burks Falls, ON - Family Medicine
Dr Lara De Salaberry, Ottawa, ON - Family Medicine
Dr J Paul De Young, Cornwall, ON - Endocrin/Metabolism
Dr Franco DeNardi, St. Catharines, ON - Anatomical Pathology
Dr Cheri L Deal, Montreal, QC - Endocrin/Metabolism
Dr John M Dean, Vancouver, BC - Clin Immun/Allergy
Dr Heather J Dean, Winnipeg, MB - Pediatrics
Dr Hassan Deif, North York, ON - Diagnostic-Radiology
Dr Dario F Del Rizzo, Woodbridge, ON - Cardiothor Surgery
Dr Johnny Y Deladoey, Montreal, QC - General Practice
Dr Mary Delafield, Quebec, QC - General Practice
Dr John Deliakis, Toronto, ON - Family Medicine
Dr Isabelle M G Delisle, Dartmouth, NS - Obstetrics & Gynecology
Dr Max Della Zazzera, Ottawa, ON - General Practice
Dr Liliane Demers, Montreal, QC - General Practice
Dr Nestor N Demianczuk, Edmonton, AB - Obstetrics & Gynecology
Dr Ari Demirjian, Mont-Royal, QC - Dermatology
Dr Ian Dempsey, Dartmouth, NS - Otolaryngology
Dr Judah Denburg, Hamilton, ON - Hematology
Dr Chahe B Derghazarian, Saint-Leonard, QC - Hematology
Dr Geoff Dervin, Ottawa, ON - Orthopedic Surgery
Dr H Zihni Dervish, Ottawa, ON - General Surgery
Dr Renee Dery, Montreal, QC - Diagnostic-Radiology
Dr Veronique Dery, Montreal, QC - Community Medicine
Dr Jean-Pierre Dery, Quebec, QC - Cardiology
Dr Larissa A Derzko-Dzulynsky, Etobicoke, ON - Ophthalmology
Dr Jean-Pierre DesGroseilliers, Ottawa, ON - Dermatology
Dr Vikas R Desai, Kamloops, BC - Emergency Family Med
Dr Nathalie A Desbois, Carlisle, ON - Family Medicine
Dr Dominique Deschenes, Levis, QC - Internal Medicine
Dr Joanne Desjardins, Plantagenet, ON - Family Medicine
Dr Nicole Desmarais, Hanmer, ON - Family Medicine
Dr Joelle Desparmet, Montreal, QC - Anesthesia
Dr Real Desranleau, McMasterville, QC - General Practice
Dr Michel Desrosiers, Montreal, QC - General Practice
Dr Carole Deveau, Moncton, NB - Family Medicine
Dr Jaswinder S Dhillon, Brantford, ON - Emergency Family Med
Dr Indra M C Dhunnoo, Edmonton, AB - Pediatrics
Dr Giovanni A Di Costanzo, Markham, ON - Urology
Dr Giuseppina Di Meglio, Westmount, QC - Pediatrics
Dr Vincenzo Di Nicola, Montreal, QC - Psychiatry
Dr Andrea B L Di Paolo, Renfrew, ON - Family Medicine
Dr Anthony P Di Pierdomenico, Toronto, ON - Obstetrics & Gynecology
Dr Luigia G A Di Primio, Ottawa, ON - Diagnostic-Radiology
Dr Tania Di Renna, Ottawa, ON - Anesthesia
Dr Nicholas E Diamant, Kingston, ON - Internal Medicine
Dr Yenge Diambomba, Toronto, ON - Pediatrics
Dr Ana M Diaz De Molnar, Toronto, ON - General Practice
Dr James Dickson, Ottawa, ON - Anesthesia
Dr Christine Diekmeyer, Ottawa, ON - Family Medicine
Dr Levinus Albert Dieleman, Edmonton, AB - General Practice
Dr Dubravka A Diksic, Montreal, QC - Pediatrics
Dr Lisa G Dillon, Winnipeg, MB - Family Medicine
Dr Ronald A Dimentberg, Montreal, QC - Orthopedic Surgery
Dr John L Dimock, Nepean, ON - Psychiatry
Dr Anh T T Dinh, Edmonton, AB - General Practice
Dr Claudia G Dinu, West Vancouver, BC - Family Medicine
Dr Isabelle Dion, Oshawa, ON - Family Medicine
Dr Yves-Marie Dion, Quebec, QC - General Surgery
Dr Michel Dionne, Ottawa, ON - Anatomical Pathology
Dr Paul G Dionne, Gatineau, QC - Anatomical Pathology
Dr David C Diosy, London, ON - Neurology
Dr Peter Dirks, Toronto, ON - Neurosurgery
Dr Martha H Dirks, Montreal, QC - Gastroenterology
Dr Marino J Discepola, Mont-Royal, QC - Ophthalmology
Dr Kemal Divanli, Edmundston, NB - General Practice
Dr Marjorie Dixon, North York, ON - Obstetrics & Gynecology
Dr Bernard K Dobovicnik, Trail, BC - General Practice
Dr Herbert Dobrinski, Montreal, QC - General Practice
Dr Marek Dobrowolski, Lourdes-D-Bl-Sabl, QC - General Practice
Dr Marjorie A Docherty, Kelowna, BC - Family Medicine
Dr Ahmed R Docrat, Calgary, AB - Family Medicine
Dr Dubravka Dodig, Toronto, ON - Neurology
Dr Geoffrey P Doherty, Ottawa, ON - Diagnostic-Radiology
Dr Daniel Doiron, Ottawa, ON - Psychiatry
Dr Suzan Dojeiji, Ottawa, ON - Physical Medicine & Rehab
Dr Hisham Dokainish, Hamilton, ON - Cardiology
Dr Janet Dollin, Ottawa, ON - Family Medicine
Dr Anne-Marie Dollois, Pointe-Claire, QC - Family Medicine
Dr Peter J Dolman, Vancouver, BC - Ophthalmology
Dr Joan Don, Lindsay, ON - Anesthesia
Dr Maurice H J Dongier, Verdun, QC - Psychiatry
Dr Alicia Donohue, Ottawa, ON - Family Medicine
Dr Marie-Denise Donovan, Moncton, NB - Community Medicine
Dr Gordon Donsky, Toronto, ON - Pediatrics
Dr Marcel Dore, Guelph, ON - General Practice
Dr Seema Dosaj, Pickering, ON - Family Medicine
Dr Clare B Dossetor, Ottawa, ON - Dermatology
Dr Rehan Dost, Paris, ON - Neurology
Dr Geoffrey E Dougherty, Montreal, QC - Community Medicine
Dr Alan B Douglass, Ottawa, ON - Psychiatry
Dr James D Douketis, Hamilton, ON - Internal Medicine
Dr Monique Douville-Fradet, Quebec, QC - Community Medicine
Dr John F C Dove, Moose Factory, ON - Family Medicine
Dr Marion Dove, Montreal, QC - Family Medicine
Dr Anthony H Dowell, Pointe-Claire, QC - Family Medicine
Dr Jonathan Downar, Toronto, ON - Psychiatry
Dr Anne Draginda, Edmonton, AB - Family Medicine
Dr C Lewis W Draper, Regina, SK - Family Medicine
Dr Jonathan Dreyer, London, ON - Emergency Medicine
Dr Johanne F Drouin, Edmonton, AB - Family Medicine
Dr Michel A Drouin, Quebec, QC - Clin Immun/Allergy
Dr Chantal J Du Vernet, Smiths Falls, ON - Emergency Family Med
Dr Mark R Dube, Sudbury, ON - Emergency Family Med
Dr Ruth Dubin, Kingston, ON - Family Medicine
Dr Jacques H Dubins, North York, ON - General Practice
Dr Isser L Dubinsky, Toronto, ON - Emergency Family Med
Dr Marc Dubuc, Montreal, QC - Cardiology
Dr Sylvia P Ducceschi, Vancouver, BC - Family Medicine
Dr Sylvain Duchaine, Trenton, ON - General Practice
Dr Helena L Duchowska, Richmond, BC - General Practice
Dr Genevieve M Ducros, Astra, ON - Family Medicine
Dr Jacalyn M Duffin, Kingston, ON - Hematology
Dr Daniel M Dufour, Brockville, ON - Family Medicine
Dr Maurice J A Dufresne, Ottawa, ON - General Practice
Dr Louis R Dufresne, Quebec, QC - Internal Medicine
Dr Alison K Dugan, Ottawa, ON - Internal Medicine
Dr Robert Dumais, Sudbury, ON - Anesthesia
Dr Huu Thanh Duong, Ottawa, ON - General Practice
Dr David Dupere, Halifax, NS - Internal Medicine
Dr Audrey Dupere, Chicoutimi, QC - Dermatology
Dr Liam V Durcan, Montreal, QC - Neurology
Dr Manon Dusablon, Blainville, QC - General Practice
Dr Monika Dutt, Sydney, NS - Community Medicine
Dr Jan P Dutz, Vancouver, BC - Dermatology
Dr Gary S Dvorkin, Verdun, QC - Neurology
Dr Michael Dworkind, Montreal, QC - Family Medicine
Dr Irving M Dylewski, Montreal, QC - Internal Medicine
Dr Joe S Dylewski, Montreal, QC - Internal Medicine
Dr Katrina Eastwood, Kingston, ON - General Practice
Dr Martin S Eckhart, Peace River, AB - Family Medicine
Dr Anizor Ede, Edmonton, AB - Psychiatry
Dr Chaim Z I Edelstein, Montreal, QC - Ophthalmology

Dr Earl Edelstein, Montreal, QC - General Practice
Dr Melvin L Edgar, Vancouver, BC - Family Medicine
Dr Donna F Edwards, North York, ON - Family Medicine
Dr E Patricia Egerszegi, Montreal, QC - Plastic Surgery
Dr Karim E C Eid, Scarborough, ON - General Practice
Dr Jouhaina Eid, Montreal, QC - Nephrology
Dr David Eiley, Pointe-Claire, QC - Urology
Dr Eric L Eisenberg, Mississauga, ON - Dermatology
Dr Mark J Eisenberg, Montreal, QC - Cardiology
Dr William S El Masri, Toronto, ON - Otolaryngology
Dr Nady A El-Guebaly, Calgary, AB - Psychiatry
Dr May I El-Hajj, Owen Sound, ON - Obstetrics & Gynecology
Dr Hamdy G E H El-Hakim, Edmonton, AB - General Practice
Dr Philippe P El-Helou, Hamilton, ON - Internal Medicine
Dr Amira El-Messidi, Montreal, QC - Obstetrics & Gynecology
Dr Reda M El-Sawy, Ottawa, ON - Physical Medicine & Rehab
Dr Samy M El-Sayed, Ottawa, ON - Radiation Oncology
Dr Mohammed Elahi, Etobicoke, ON - Family Medicine
Dr Mohammed Elahi, North York, ON - Otolaryngology
Dr Graham M Elder, Sault Ste. Marie, ON - Orthopedic Surgery
Dr Tamer Elghobary, Mississauga, ON - Cardiac Surgery
Dr David A Elias, Grand-Bay-Wesfld, NB - Emergency Family Med
Dr Kathryn D Elie, Lachine, QC - Medical Microbiology
Dr John D Elie, Montreal, QC - Dermatology
Dr Thomas G Elliott, Vancouver, BC - Endocrin/Metabolism
Dr Denise M Elliott, Ottawa, ON - Family Medicine
Dr Carol M M Y Eloskouf, Keswick, ON - Family Medicine
Dr Suha Eltayeb, Ajax, ON - Obstetrics & Gynecology
Dr Andrew P Ember, Ottawa, ON - Family Medicine
Dr Sherif G S Emil, Montreal, QC - General Surgery
Dr Frank Eng, Newmarket, ON - General Surgery
Dr Andre Engel, Ottawa, ON - Pediatrics
Dr Marc Engfield, Gatineau, QC - Internal Medicine
Dr Michael L Engo, Montreal, QC - Emergency Family Med
Dr Angela C Enright, Victoria, BC - Anesthesia
Dr Catherine M A Entwistle, Ottawa, ON - Ophthalmology
Dr Siegfried R Erb, Vancouver, BC - Internal Medicine
Dr Florence A Erdman, North York, ON - Psychiatry
Dr Julius Erdstein, Pierrefonds, QC - Pediatrics
Dr Patrick L Ergina, Montreal, QC - Cardiothor Surgery
Dr Philippe M Erhard, Winnipeg, MB - Family Medicine
Dr Gary P Ernest, Liverpool, NS - Family Medicine
Dr Francis L C Ervin, Maple Ridge, BC - Internal Medicine
Dr Bernd A Esche, Ottawa, ON - Radiation Oncology
Dr Sandra I Escoredo, Edmonton, AB - General Practice
Dr Juan L Escudero, Ottawa, ON - General Practice
Dr David S Esdaile, Ottawa, ON - Family Medicine
Dr Vidal Essebag, Montreal, QC - Cardiology
Dr Jean-Luc Ethier, Timmins, ON - Otolaryngology
Dr Dardye Eugene, Quebec, QC - Endocrin/Metabolism
Dr Lisa Evered, Edmonton, AB - Pediatrics
Dr T David Ewing-Bui, Sudbury, ON - Thoracic Surgery
Dr John M Eydt, Gatineau, QC - General Practice
Dr Anca Facy, Toronto, ON - Family Medicine
Dr Sylvia Fahim, Mississauga, ON - Family Medicine
Dr Simone S I Fahim, Ottawa, ON - Dermatology
Dr Pierre Falardeau, Montreal, QC - Nephrology
Dr Carlo A Fallone, Montreal, QC - Gastroenterology
Dr Nabil E Fanous, Westmount, QC - Otolaryngology
Dr Antoine Farah, Gatineau, QC - Nephrology
Dr Christiane Farazli, Ottawa, ON - Gastroenterology
Dr Noreen Fardy, St. John's, NL - Family Medicine
Dr Julio Faria, Montreal, QC - General Surgery
Dr Dan Farine, Toronto, ON - Obstetrics & Gynecology
Dr Jean-Pierre Farmer, Montreal, QC - Neurosurgery
Dr James A Farquhar, Verdun, QC - Psychiatry
Dr C F Cristina Fasie-Neagoe, Pointe-Claire, QC - Family Medicine
Dr Afsoon Fathollahzadeh, Oakville, ON - Pediatrics
Dr Lucien L Faucher, Ottawa, ON - Psychiatry
Dr Marie E Faughnan, Toronto, ON - Internal Medicine
Dr Karima Fazal Karim, Montreal, QC - Family Medicine
Dr Annie H Fecteau, Toronto, ON - General Surgery
Dr Stephen H Feder, Ottawa, ON - Family Medicine
Dr Erwin Feige, North Bay, ON - Family Medicine
Dr Christopher M S Feindel, Toronto, ON - Cardiovasc/ThorSurg
Dr Imre B Fejer, Scarborough, ON - General Practice
Dr Joseph Feldmann, Toronto, ON - Psychiatry
Dr Vivien Fellegi, Mississauga, ON - General Practice
Dr Nicolette K Fellegi, Ottawa, ON - Family Medicine
Dr Roger F Fenster, Montreal, QC - General Surgery
Dr Jonathan A S Fenton, Richmond, BC - Orthopedic Surgery
Dr John A Fenton, Sudbury, ON - General Surgery
Dr Jae-Marie Ferdinand, Montreal, QC - Pediatrics
Dr Deborah A Ferguson, Calgary, AB - Family Medicine
Dr Craig A Ferguson, Bridgewater, NS - Family Medicine
Dr Karen E Ferguson, Carp, ON - Family Medicine
Dr Gisele M C Ferguson, Saskatoon, SK - Psychiatry
Dr Nanette M Ferguson-Losier, Dartmouth, NS - General Practice
Dr John R Fernandes, Hamilton, ON - General Pathology
Dr Julio C Fernandes, Montreal, QC - Orthopedic Surgery
Dr Robert Ferrari, Edmonton, AB - Internal Medicine
Dr Christian Ferremi, Laval, QC - Ophthalmology
Dr Catherine Ferrier, Montreal, QC - Family Medicine
Dr Caroline R Ferris, Surrey, BC - Family Medicine
Dr Ernst Fibich, Prince George, BC - General Practice
Dr Giuseppe Ficara, Montreal, QC - Pediatrics
Dr Stephen H Fichman, Montreal, QC - Ophthalmology
Dr Michael P Fielden, Calgary, AB - Ophthalmology
Dr Allan G Fielding, Montreal, QC - Psychiatry
Dr Alexandra O Figaro, Windsor, ON - Family Medicine
Dr Indira C Figueiredo, Toronto, ON - General Practice
Dr Lyne Filiatrault, Vancouver, BC - Emergency Medicine
Dr Alain Filion, Quebec, QC - Hematology
Dr Daniel L Filipini, Montreal, QC - General Practice
Dr Maria Filyk, Calgary, AB - Psychiatry
Dr Geoffrey M Fine, Mississauga, ON - Emergency Family Med
Dr Barnet Fine, Saint-Georges, QC - General Practice
Dr Allan M Finesilver, Montreal, QC - Otolaryngology
Dr David L Finestone, Ottawa, ON - Family Medicine
Dr Hillel M Finestone, Ottawa, ON - Physical Medicine & Rehab
Dr Philip Fingrut, North York, ON - General Practice
Dr Theodore Fischbacher, Alliston, ON - General Practice
Dr Rowan Fish, Montreal, QC - Dermatology
Dr Christina M Fisher, Toronto, ON - Family Medicine
Dr William D Fisher, Montreal, QC - Orthopedic Surgery
Dr Charlene D Fitzgerald, Happy-Valley-Goose, NL - Family Medicine
Dr John D Fitzpatrick, Courtenay, BC - General Practice
Dr Kelly P Fitzpatrick, Hamilton, ON - Pediatrics
Dr Francois J Flamand, Cambridge, ON - General Surgery
Dr Martine Flament, Ottawa, ON - Psychiatry
Dr Cathy Flanagan, New Westminster, BC - Internal Medicine
Dr John F Flannery, Toronto, ON - Physical Medicine & Rehab
Dr Kenneth M Flegel, Montreal, QC - Internal Medicine
Dr David M Fleiszer, Montreal, QC - General Surgery
Dr Karen E Fleming, Toronto, ON - Family Medicine
Dr Mark A Fletcher, Dartmouth, NS - Emergency Family Med
Dr Philip B Fleuriau-Chateau, Ottawa, ON - Orthopedic Surgery
Dr William Flexer, Edmonton, AB - Anesthesia
Dr Pierre Flor-Henry, Edmonton, AB - Psychiatry
Dr Anne-Josee Flynn, Quebec, QC - Family Medicine
Dr Mohamed M R Foda, Leduc, AB - Urology
Dr Myrosia M Foga, Mississauga, ON - Diagnostic-Radiology
Dr Finola M Fogarty, Edmonton, AB - Psychiatry
Dr Eva Foldes, Montreal, QC - Internal Medicine
Dr Curtis S Folkerson, Wakefield, QC - Family Medicine
Dr John R Foote, Toronto, ON - Emergency Family Med
Dr Patricia A Forbes, Montreal, QC - Pediatrics
Dr Anthony E A Ford-Jones, Burlington, ON - Pediatrics
Dr Sylviane Forget, Montreal, QC - Gastroenterology
Dr Melissa A Forgie, Ottawa, ON - Hematology
Dr Frank Fornasier, Burlington, ON - Family Medicine
Dr Bertram Forse, Markham, ON - General Practice
Dr Raymond A Forse, Ottawa, ON - General Surgery
Dr Milena F Forte, Toronto, ON - Family Medicine
Dr Denis C J Fortier, Notre-Dame-Lr, MB - Family Medicine
Dr Bernard Fortin, Montreal, QC - Radiation Oncology
Dr Paul J R Fournier, Montreal, QC - Obstetrics & Gynecology
Dr Renee Fournier, Montreal, QC - Family Medicine
Dr Jonathan R Fox, Fall River, NS - Family Medicine
Dr Allan J Fox, Toronto, ON - Diagnostic-Radiology
Dr Catharine Foyle, Calgary, AB - Family Medicine
Dr Jeffrey M Franc-Law, Edmonton, AB - Emergency Family Med
Dr Marie-Josee Francoeur, Greenfield Park, QC - Clin Immun/Allergy
Dr T Emmett Francoeur, Westmount, QC - Pediatrics
Dr William D Fraser, Montreal, QC - Obstetrics & Gynecology
Dr Robert Frazer, Sherbrooke, QC - General Practice
Dr Mark S Freedman, Ottawa, ON - Neurology
Dr David M Freedman, Thornhill, ON - Cardiology
Dr Christie L Freeman, Peterborough, ON - Family Medicine
Dr Carolyn R Freeman, Montreal, QC - Radiation Oncology
Dr Anatoli Freiman, North York, ON - Dermatology
Dr Anthony J French, Vancouver, BC - General Practice
Dr Nadine French, Orangeville, ON - Family Medicine
Dr Jacques Frenette, Quebec, QC - Family Medicine
Dr George Freundlich, Matheson, ON - Family Medicine
Dr Oded P Fried, North York, ON - General Practice
Dr Veronika A Fried, Toronto, ON - Family Medicine
Dr Gad Friedman, Montreal, QC - Gastroenterology
Dr Jan Oliver Friedrich, Toronto, ON - Critical Care Medicine
Dr Matthias G W Friedrich, Montreal, QC - Cardiology
Dr Byron P P Friesen, Hawkesbury, ON - General Surgery
Dr Abraham Friesner, Toronto, ON - General Practice
Dr Michael P V Froeschl, Ottawa, ON - Cardiology
Dr Robert Frongillo, Montreal, QC - General Practice
Dr Lucien-P Fruchtermann, Montreal, QC - General Practice
Dr Roland P J Fuca, Ottawa, ON - General Practice
Dr Maria Fuks, Cote Saint-Luc, QC - General Practice
Dr Barbara E Fuller, Kingston, ON - Family Medicine
Dr Deana Funaro, Montreal, QC - Dermatology
Dr Shek Hong Fung, Montreal, QC - Geriatric Medicine
Dr Gabriel G C Fuoco, Peterborough, ON - Otolaryngology
Dr Christoph Fusch, Hamilton, ON - Pediatrics
Dr Christian J M Gagne, Hawkesbury, ON - Family Medicine
Dr Alain Gagnon, Vancouver, BC - Obstetrics & Gynecology
Dr Patricia Gagnon, Orleans, ON - General Practice
Dr Serge Gagnon, Gatineau, QC - General Practice
Dr Jacques R Gagnon, Montreal, QC - Psychiatry
Dr Jean Gagnon, Trois-Rivieres, QC - Dermatology
Dr Carol B Gailey, New Westminster, BC - Cardiology
Dr M Lynne Galipeau, Newmarket, ON - General Practice
Dr Jocelyn F Galipeau, North Bay, ON - General Practice
Dr Denise L Gallant, Dieppe, NB - Family Medicine
Dr Michel Gallant, Ottawa, ON - Plastic Surgery
Dr Stephen H Gallay, Ajax, ON - Orthopedic Surgery
Dr Shelly Galler, Toronto, ON - Psychiatry
Dr Peter W Galley, Pembroke, ON - General Practice
Dr Nathalie Gamache, Gatineau, QC - Obstetrics & Gynecology
Dr Soma Ganesan, Vancouver, BC - Psychiatry
Dr Eric W Gangbar, Richmond Hill, ON - Cardiology
Dr Satyajit N Ganguli, Brampton, ON - Diagnostic-Radiology
Dr Mark S Gans, Montreal, QC - Ophthalmology
Dr Andres Gantous, Toronto, ON - Otolaryngology
Dr George J Garbe, Regina, SK - Cardiology
Dr Gary E Garber, Ottawa, ON - Infectious Diseases
Dr Angeles Garcia, Kingston, ON - Geriatric Medicine
Dr Michael A Gardam, Toronto, ON - Infectious Diseases
Dr Edward M Gardiner, Ottawa, ON - Emergency Family Med
Dr Jacques Y Gareau, Saint-Jerome, QC - General Practice
Dr Natasha Garfield, Montreal, QC - Endocrin/Metabolism
Dr Sylvia G Garnis-Jones, Welland, ON - Dermatology
Dr Ronald G Garston, Riverside-Albert, NB - Urology
Dr John G Gartner, Winnipeg, MB - Anatomical Pathology
Dr Joseph Gasser, Toronto, ON - Ophthalmology
Dr Margarita Gatchev, North Bay, ON - Family Medicine
Dr Mathieu M Gatien, Ottawa, ON - Emergency Family Med
Dr Colette Gaulin, Quebec, QC - General Practice
Dr Louise F Gauthier, Ottawa, ON - Anesthesia
Dr Alain Gauthier, Perth, ON - Family Medicine
Dr Francois Gauthier, Montreal, QC - Family Medicine
Dr Micheline Gauvin, Mont-Royal, QC - General Practice
Dr Joseph Gauze, Montreal, QC - Otolaryngology
Dr Adam Gavsie, Montreal, QC - Family Medicine
Dr Fay E H Gayle, North York, ON - Family Medicine

Dr William O Geisler, Toronto, ON - Internal Medicine
Dr Stephen G Gelber, North York, ON - Psychiatry
Dr Christine E Gemeinhardt, Delta, BC - Family Medicine
Dr Angela L Genge, Montreal, QC - Internal Medicine
Dr Michael A Geoghegan, Calgary, AB - General Practice
Dr Lila L Georgevich, Scarborough, ON - Internal Medicine
Dr Nina J Georgiadis, Hamilton, ON - General Practice
Dr Stanley Z Gertler, Ottawa, ON - Internal Medicine
Dr Pierre Gfeller, Mont-Laurier, QC - General Practice
Dr Gissou S Ghadirian, Etobicoke, ON - Family Medicine
Dr Ezzat G Ghaly, Cornwall, ON - Internal Medicine
Dr Youssef Ghantous, Cornwall, ON - Family Medicine
Dr Abbas Ghavam-Rassoul, Toronto, ON - Family Medicine
Dr Gabriela Ghitulescu, Montreal, QC - General Surgery
Dr M Ghobrial, Ottawa, ON - Pediatrics
Dr Zeina Ghorab, Toronto, ON - General Practice
Dr Roberto A Giaccone, Nepean, ON - Neurology
Dr Tony Giantomaso, Calgary, AB - Physical Medicine & Rehab
Dr William T Gibson, Vancouver, BC - Medical Genetics
Dr Michelle C Gibson, Kingston, ON - Family Medicine
Dr Susan V Gick, Richmond, ON - Family Medicine
Dr Gordon R Giddings, Windsor, ON - Family Medicine
Dr Lucia G Giglia, Hamilton, ON - Pediatrics
Dr Chantal M Giguere, Montreal, QC - Otolaryngology
Dr Rodica Gilca, Quebec, QC - General Practice
Dr Norbert Gilmore, Montreal, QC - General Practice
Dr Marc Gingras, Lachute, QC - General Surgery
Dr Caroline Gingras, Saint-Eustache, QC - General Practice
Dr Donald Ginsberg, Montreal, QC - Family Medicine
Dr Hernan Giraldo, Chateauguay, QC - Pediatrics
Dr Louis C Girard, North York, ON - Family Medicine
Dr Adel Girgis, Thornhill, ON - Family Medicine
Dr Marie-France Giron, Dorval, QC - General Practice
Dr Peter K Girschek, Toronto, ON - Ophthalmology
Dr Rudolph Gittens, Ottawa, ON - Orthopedic Surgery
Dr Antonio Giulivi, Ottawa, ON - Hematological Pathology
Dr Brook W Glanville, Salmon Arm, BC - Family Medicine
Dr Robert R M Glasgow, Edmonton, AB - Orthopedic Surgery
Dr Peter R Glazer, Toronto, ON - Emergency Family Med
Dr Vivian P Glenns, North York, ON - Internal Medicine
Dr James D Glezos, New Westminster, BC - Internal Medicine
Dr Rafael S Glikstein, Ottawa, ON - Diagnostic-Radiology
Dr Shawn W Gmora, North York, ON - Family Medicine
Dr Cynthia Godbout, Montreal, QC - Family Medicine
Dr Karin G Goddard, Montreal, QC - Psychiatry
Dr Charles M Godfrey, Toronto, ON - Physical Medicine & Rehab
Dr Sanjeev Goel, Brampton, ON - Family Medicine
Dr Vivek Goel, Toronto, ON - Community Medicine
Dr Aashish Goela, London, ON - Diagnostic-Radiology
Dr Mary Susan L B Goheen, Ottawa, ON - Anesthesia
Dr M Ilhami Gokcen, Scarborough, ON - Psychiatry
Dr Deborah Golberg, Montreal, QC - Family Medicine
Dr Ileana-Maria Gold, Brampton, ON - Anesthesia
Dr Pamela D Gold, Hanover, ON - Family Medicine
Dr Jewel Gold, Toronto, ON - Cardiology
Dr Phil Gold, Montreal, QC - Clin Immun/Allergy
Dr Chaim J Goldberg, Scarborough, ON - Ophthalmology
Dr Eudice Goldberg, Toronto, ON - Pediatrics
Dr Richard B Goldbloom, Halifax, NS - Pediatrics
Dr John N H Goldhar, Toronto, ON - Dermatology
Dr Mindy R Goldman, Ottawa, ON - Hematology
Dr Gail Goldman, Montreal, QC - Internal Medicine
Dr Elliot M Goldner, Vancouver, BC - Psychiatry
Dr Barry Goldsman, Westmount, QC - General Practice
Dr William J Goldsmith, Montreal, QC - Obstetrics & Gynecology
Dr William Goldstein, Ottawa, ON - Cardiovasc/ThorSurg
Dr Victor Gomel, Vancouver, BC - Obstetrics & Gynecology
Dr Eva Gomez, Kanata, ON - General Practice
Dr Julius E S Gomolin, Montreal, QC - Ophthalmology
Dr Hernan Gonzalez, Edmonton, AB - Pediatrics
Dr Gonzalo Gonzalez-Amaya, Sherbrooke, QC - General Surgery
Dr Marni A Goodman, New Minas, NS - Family Medicine
Dr Devdass Goojha, Saskatoon, SK - General Practice
Dr Ann Gordon, Kentville, NS - Internal Medicine
Dr Robert G Gordon, Etobicoke, ON - Orthopedic Surgery
Dr Randy D Gordon, North York, ON - General Practice
Dr Ian C Gorin, Montreal, QC - General Practice
Dr Peter B C Gorman, Moncton, NB - Neurosurgery
Dr Todd E Gorman, Quebec, QC - Critical Care Medicine
Dr Richard Goudie, Barrie, ON - Family Medicine
Dr Francois W Gougeon, High River, AB - General Surgery
Dr Helene Gousseau, Trenton, ON - Family Medicine
Dr Claudia J Grabner, Brantford, ON - General Practice
Dr Gail E Graham, Ottawa, ON - Medical Genetics
Dr Lyla M Graham, Ottawa, ON - Family Medicine
Dr Maria S Grande, St. Catharines, ON - Family Medicine
Dr Nathalie Granger, Chateauguay, QC - Internal Medicine
Dr Vincent J Grant, Calgary, AB - Pediatrics
Dr Adele Gratton, Toronto, ON - General Practice
Dr Denis H Gravel, Ottawa, ON - Anatomical Pathology
Dr Charles A Gravel, Lemoyne, QC - Orthopedic Surgery
Dr Robert A Greco, Sudbury, ON - Diagnostic-Radiology
Dr Raymond Green, Hope, BC - Family Medicine
Dr Stefanie L Green, Victoria, BC - Family Medicine
Dr David J M Green, St Stephen, NB - General Practice
Dr Lawrence Green, Cambridge, ON - General Surgery
Dr Gary H Greenberg, Ottawa, ON - Emergency Medicine
Dr Brian J Greenfield, Montreal, QC - Psychiatry
Dr Mark Greenwald, North York, ON - Pediatrics
Dr Michelle Greiver, North York, ON - Family Medicine
Dr Claude Grenier, Greenfield Park, QC - Psychiatry
Dr Michael Greschner, Moncton, NB - Anesthesia
Dr Peter A Gresko, Windsor, ON - General Practice
Dr Joanne M Grevler, Toronto, ON - Family Medicine
Dr Leslie B Griffin, Halifax, NS - Family Medicine
Dr Haralambos B Grillas, Lachine, QC - Anesthesia
Dr Stephen H Grodinsky, Nepean, ON - Pediatrics
Dr Donald R Groenewege, Montreal, QC - Psychiatry
Dr Louis Grondin, Calgary, AB - General Practice
Dr Sean C Grondin, Calgary, AB - General Surgery
Dr Marie M S Gross, Edmonton, AB - Family Medicine
Dr Ian G Gross, Ottawa, ON - Plastic Surgery
Dr Gil Gross, Toronto, ON - Pediatric Cardiology
Dr James M Gruber, Montreal, QC - Internal Medicine
Dr Andree M R Gruslin, Ottawa, ON - Obstetrics & Gynecology
Dr Alan Guberman, Ottawa, ON - Neurology
Dr Enza-Josie Gucciardi, Orangeville, ON - Emergency Family Med
Dr Lyn C C Guenther, London, ON - Dermatology
Dr F John Guilfoyle, Sioux Lookout, ON - Family Medicine
Dr Noemi Guindon, Windsor, ON - General Practice
Dr Hany Guirgis, Thornhill, ON - Otolaryngology
Dr Samir S Guirguis, Etobicoke, ON - General Practice
Dr Ezzat F Guirguis, Orillia, ON - Psychiatry
Dr Adel F Guirguis, Ottawa, ON - General Practice
Dr Hesham S R Guirguis, Sorel-Tracy, QC - Internal Medicine
Dr Roxan M Guise, Niagara Falls, ON - Family Medicine
Dr Edith M Guntley-Lorimer, Toronto, ON - General Practice
Dr Seema Gupta, Guelph, ON - Family Medicine
Dr Sanjoy Gupta, Thunder Bay, ON - Ophthalmology
Dr Neeru Gupta, Toronto, ON - Ophthalmology
Dr Namta Gupta, Montreal, QC - Family Medicine
Dr Ashvini H Gursahaney, Montreal, QC - Critical Care Medicine
Dr Jose Gutauskas, Ottawa, ON - General Surgery
Dr Klaus S Gutfreund, Edmonton, AB - Gastroenterology
Dr Peter Gutmanis, Nanaimo, BC - Orthopedic Surgery
Dr Astrid Guttmann, Toronto, ON - Pediatrics
Dr Roger G Guy, Montreal, QC - General Practice
Dr Randolph P Guzman, Winnipeg, MB - General Surgery
Dr Alice Gwyn, Norris Point, NL - Family Medicine
Dr Martin Gyger, Montreal, QC - Hematological Pathology
Dr Katalin Gyomorey, Thunder Bay, ON - Psychiatry
Dr Andrew F Gyopar, Chateauguay, QC - General Surgery
Dr Erika Haase, Edmonton, AB - General Surgery
Dr Flavio Habal, Toronto, ON - Gastroenterology
Dr Samir Habib, Montreal, QC - Family Medicine
Dr Magdi Habra, Bois-des-Filion, QC - General Practice
Dr Keyvan Hadad, Vancouver, BC - Pediatrics
Dr Haissam A Haddad, Ottawa, ON - Cardiology
Dr Cecil D A Hahn, Toronto, ON - Neurology
Dr Margaret K Hahn, Toronto, ON - Psychiatry
Dr Richard N Haichin, Montreal, QC - Cardiology
Dr Laura N Haiek, Westmount, QC - Family Medicine
Dr Donald Haigh, Halifax, NS - General Practice
Dr James S J Haight, Toronto, ON - Otolaryngology
Dr Katerina K Haka-Ikse, Toronto, ON - Pediatrics
Dr Jack Hakoun, Toronto, ON - General Practice
Dr Ilona Hale, Kimberley, BC - Family Medicine
Dr Ann Mary Hall, Brantford, ON - General Pathology
Dr Trevor L Hall, Cambridge, ON - Family Medicine
Dr James Halvorson, Duncan, BC - Emergency Family Med
Dr Fawaz Halwani, Ottawa, ON - Anatomical Pathology
Dr Trevor J Ham, Owen Sound, ON - Pediatrics
Dr Herag Hamboyan, Brampton, ON - Family Medicine
Dr Fayad Hamideh, Oakville, ON - General Practice
Dr John R Hamilton, Antigonish, NS - Ophthalmology
Dr Philip P Hamilton, Gatineau, QC - Anesthesia
Dr D Ian Hammond, Ottawa, ON - Diagnostic-Radiology
Dr M Wahbi Hammouda, Brampton, ON - Hematology
Dr Michael Hancock, Edmonton, AB - General Practice
Dr B J Hancock, Winnipeg, MB - Critical Care Medicine
Dr Dan J Hancu, North York, ON - Family Medicine
Dr Richard S Handfield-Jones, Ottawa, ON - Family Medicine
Dr Sameh K Hanna, Oakville, ON - Family Medicine
Dr Wedad M Hanna, Toronto, ON - Anatomical Pathology
Dr Janet E Hantho, Calgary, AB - General Practice
Dr Andrei Harabor, Calgary, AB - Pediatrics
Dr Raymond T Harb, St Catharines, ON - Family Medicine
Dr Martha Harczy, Nepean, ON - Internal Medicine
Dr Peter W Harding, Gloucester, ON - Ophthalmology
Dr Barbara J Hardt, Calgary, AB - Family Medicine
Dr Mark Hardy, Montreal, QC - General Surgery
Dr Gregory B Hariton, Hamilton, ON - General Practice
Dr Kelly M Harper, Ajax, ON - General Practice
Dr Robert W Harris, Cornwall, ON - Plastic Surgery
Dr Nancy L Harris, Orillia, ON - Family Medicine
Dr Trevor D Harterre, Timmins, ON - Emergency Family Med
Dr Naomi A Hasegawa, Pointe-Claire, QC - Ophthalmology
Dr Raymond Hasel, Pointe-Claire, QC - Anesthesia
Dr Ezat Hashim, Montreal, QC - Plastic Surgery
Dr Durreshahwar Hassan, Roxboro, QC - Obstetrics & Gynecology
Dr Magdy Hassouna, Toronto, ON - Urology
Dr Sharon N Hatcher, Chicoutimi, QC - Family Medicine
Dr Jo Hauser, Ottawa, ON - Family Medicine
Dr Toni P Hawkes, Calgary, AB - Family Medicine
Dr Huguette S Hayden, Langley, BC - Psychiatry
Dr David S Hayden, Bridgewater, NS - Plastic Surgery
Dr Paul R Hayes, Saskatoon, SK - General Surgery
Dr Francis B Healey, Vernon, BC - General Practice
Dr Jeffrey S Healey, Hamilton, ON - Cardiology
Dr Paul C Hebert, Ottawa, ON - Critical Care Medicine
Dr Lily T Hechtman, Westmount, QC - Psychiatry
Dr George A W Heckman, Kitchener, ON - Geriatric Medicine
Dr Michael D Hefferon, Kingston, ON - Pediatrics
Dr Michael J Heiber, Scarborough, ON - Emergency Family Med
Dr Paul L Heilpern, Montreal, QC - Internal Medicine
Dr John A Heine, Calgary, AB - General Surgery
Dr Katja Heineck, Toronto, ON - Family Medicine
Dr Michael E Helewa, Winnipeg, MB - Obstetrics & Gynecology
Dr Hussam A Helou, Pointe-Claire, QC - Family Medicine
Dr Robert Hemmings, Montreal, QC - Obstetrics & Gynecology
Dr Raymond Hendel, Sudbury, ON - General Surgery
Dr Kenneth J Henderson, St. John's, NL - Pediatrics
Dr Raafat Henen, Scarborough, ON - Ophthalmology
Dr Claire Sadek Hennes, Brampton, ON - Family Medicine
Dr Alexandre R Henri-Bhargava, North York, ON - Neurology
Dr Donna G Henrikson, Toronto, ON - General Practice
Dr Elise Heon, Toronto, ON - Ophthalmology
Dr Gavril Hercz, Toronto, ON - Internal Medicine
Dr Fadia Hermiz, Windsor, ON - Family Medicine
Dr Orly Hermon, Pierrefonds, QC - Family Medicine
Dr Paul Hernandez, Halifax, NS - Internal Medicine
Dr Timothy A Heron, Montreal, QC - Orthopedic Surgery
Dr Sheldon Hershkop, Mississauga, ON - Family Medicine
Dr Valerie Hetu, St-Charles-Brromee, QC - Obstetrics & Gynecology
Dr Eleanor Hew, Westmount, QC - Family Medicine

Dr Kamran Heydarzadeh-Azar, Fort St. John, BC - Anatomical Pathology
Dr Marsha R Heyman, Montreal, QC - Psychiatry
Dr Marc P Hickeson, Montreal, QC - Nuclear Medicine
Dr Tracy E Hicks, Langley, BC - Orthopedic Surgery
Dr John Hii, Toronto, ON - Medical Microbiology
Dr Ali Abbas M Hilal, Windsor, ON - Otolaryngology
Dr Michael Hill, Calgary, AB - Internal Medicine
Dr Vivian E Hill, Calgary, AB - Ophthalmology
Dr David J Hill, North York, ON - General Practice
Dr Mariana G Hill, North York, ON - Psychiatry
Dr Andrew B Hill, Ottawa, ON - General Surgery
Dr Harry S Himal, Toronto, ON - General Surgery
Dr Valerie Hindle, Ottawa, ON - Family Medicine
Dr Ingrid M Hings, Montreal, QC - Hematology
Dr Khalid J Hirmiz, Windsor, ON - Radiation Oncology
Dr Andrea Hirscheimer, London, ON - Family Medicine
Dr Denton Hirsh, Surrey, BC - Pediatrics
Dr Holger Hirte, Hamilton, ON - Internal Medicine
Dr Michel Hjelkrem, Trail, BC - Orthopedic Surgery
Dr Quang Nhan Ho, Montreal, QC - General Surgery
Dr T Boi-Ngoc Hoang, Hamilton, ON - Obstetrics & Gynecology
Dr Ngoc-Khoi Hoang, Toronto, ON - General Practice
Dr William G Hodge, London, ON - Ophthalmology
Dr Matthew J Hodge, Toronto, ON - Community Medicine
Dr Victor Hoffstein, Toronto, ON - Respirology
Dr Corinne M Hohl, Vancouver, BC - Emergency Medicine
Dr Anthony J C Holland, Port Alberni, BC - Anesthesia
Dr Gary R Hollingworth, Ottawa, ON - Family Medicine
Dr Russell J Hollins, Kingston, ON - Otolaryngology
Dr Freydoun Homayounfar, Shawville, QC - General Practice
Dr P Frank Horan, Belleville, ON - Dermatology
Dr Eric M Horlick, Toronto, ON - Cardiology
Dr Stefan Horny, Montreal, QC - General Practice
Dr John C Hostetler, Victoria, BC - Neurology
Dr Sebastien J Hotte, Hamilton, ON - Internal Medicine
Dr Jill S Hoube, Vancouver, BC - Pediatrics
Dr Leslie S Housefather, North York, ON - Family Medicine
Dr Richard J Housley, Niagara Falls, ON - Gastroenterology
Dr Kathleen G Howard, Espanola, ON - General Practice
Dr Erik Howarth, Merrickville, ON - Family Medicine
Dr Todd C Howlett, Dartmouth, NS - Emergency Family Med
Dr Joseph Hrncirik, Miramichi, NB - General Practice
Dr Sophia Hrycko, Ottawa, ON - Psychiatry
Dr Henry Y Huang, Ajax, ON - Otolaryngology
Dr Allen R Huang, Ottawa, ON - Geriatric Medicine
Dr Felicia Huang, Whitehorse, YT - General Surgery
Dr Claudia H Hubbes, Ottawa, ON - Family Medicine
Dr Marvin Huberman, Coquitlam, BC - General Practice
Dr George E Huculak, Whitby, ON - General Practice
Dr Edward G Hughes, Burlington, ON - Obstetrics & Gynecology
Dr John B Hughes, Westmount, QC - General Practice
Dr Otto H Huhn, Banff, AB - General Pathology
Dr Elia Huidovici, Windsor, ON - Family Medicine
Dr Annie Hum, Markham, ON - General Practice
Dr Susan M Humphrey, Ottawa, ON - Internal Medicine
Dr Peter Humphreys, Ottawa, ON - Neurology
Dr David R Huneault, Sudbury, ON - Obstetrics & Gynecology
Dr Georgia C Hunt, Vancouver, BC - Family Medicine
Dr Ryan D Hunt, Montreal, QC - Emergency Family Med
Dr Alasdair G W Hunter, Ottawa, ON - Medical Genetics
Dr David J Huot, Vanier, ON - Pediatrics
Dr Nasimul S Huq, Niagara Falls, ON - Plastic Surgery
Dr Nisarul M Huq, Windsor, ON - Cardiology
Dr Andre L Hurtubise, New Liskeard, ON - Family Medicine
Dr Regina Husa, Montreal, QC - Cardiology
Dr Ali M A Husain, Dieppe, NB - Plastic Surgery
Dr Nadeem A Hussain, London, ON - Gastroenterology
Dr Irene Hussain-Autenried, Etobicoke, ON - General Practice
Dr Christine Hwang, Toronto, ON - General Practice
Dr Adel F A Ibrahim, Winnipeg, MB - Family Medicine
Dr Samia M R Ibrahim, Orleans, ON - General Practice
Dr Alfred W Illescas, Montreal, QC - General Practice
Dr Werner K Ilse, Winnipeg, MB - Internal Medicine
Dr Alistair J Ingram, Hamilton, ON - Internal Medicine
Dr Alan I Iny, Ottawa, ON - Family Medicine
Dr Fauzia Irshad, Mississauga, ON - Family Medicine
Dr Lisa A Isaac, Toronto, ON - Anesthesia
Dr Hani Iskandar, Verdun, QC - General Practice
Dr Anna M Issakoff-Meller, Guelph, ON - General Practice
Dr Robert Issenman, Hamilton, ON - Pediatrics
Dr Simon Issid, Saint-Laurent, QC - General Practice
Dr Joseph J Itovitch, Salaber-de-Valleyf, QC - Urology
Dr Karin Jablonowski, Thornhill, ON - Psychiatry
Dr Michael J Jacka, Edmonton, AB - Anesthesia
Dr Steven J Jackson, Scarborough, ON - General Surgery
Dr Genevieve Jacob, Montreal, QC - General Practice
Dr Stephen A Jacobson, Montreal, QC - Urology
Dr Francis R M Jacot, Danville, QC - General Practice
Dr Edgar T Jaeggi, Toronto, ON - Pediatrics
Dr Neelesh K Jain, North York, ON - General Surgery
Dr Difat E Jakubovicz, Toronto, ON - Family Medicine
Dr Neil T Jamensky, Scarborough, ON - Anesthesia
Dr J Walter James, Toronto, ON - Pediatrics
Dr Bruce M Jamison, Ottawa, ON - Anatomical Pathology
Dr Liesbet M Jansen, Alliston, ON - Family Medicine
Dr Kurt A Jansen, Montreal, QC - Family Medicine
Dr Dorothy M Janzen, North Vancouver, BC - General Practice
Dr Allan M Jarjour, Saint-Lazare, QC - Pediatrics
Dr David Jarman, Courtenay, BC - General Practice
Dr Carl W Jarvis, Halifax, NS - Emergency Family Med
Dr Ingrid M Jarvis, Toronto, ON - Dermatology
Dr G Eric Jarvis, Montreal, QC - Psychiatry
Dr Peter F Jarzem, Montreal, QC - Orthopedic Surgery
Dr Martine A Jaworski, Ottawa, ON - Pediatrics
Dr Roman Jednak, Montreal, QC - Urology
Dr Hartley F Jeffery, New Liskeard, ON - General Surgery
Dr Milos Jenicek, Hamilton, ON - Community Medicine
Dr Kenneth Jenkins, Corner Brook, NL - General Practice
Dr Christopher W B Jensen, Winnipeg, MB - Urology
Dr Alexandra Jevremovic, Richmond Hill, ON - Cardiology
Dr Christopher P Jinot, Bruce Mines, ON - Family Medicine
Dr Klaus Jochem, Montreal, QC - General Practice
Dr Joyce E Johansson, Montreal, QC - Orthopedic Surgery
Dr Patricia L Johansson, Montreal, QC - General Practice
Dr Dawn A Johansson, Montreal, QC - Obstetrics & Gynecology
Dr Nelie C Johnson, Maple Ridge, BC - Family Medicine
Dr Roger J Johnson, Victoria, BC - Public Health & Preventive Medicine
Dr H Alan Johnston, Ottawa, ON - Family Medicine
Dr Karen M Johnston, Toronto, ON - Neurosurgery
Dr Jacqueline L Joly, Kanata, ON - Pediatrics
Dr Edward C Jones, Vancouver, BC - Anatomical Pathology
Dr Julie Jones, Winnipeg, MB - Family Medicine
Dr Donald P Jones, Mississauga, ON - General Surgery
Dr Gwynne Jones, Ottawa, ON - Internal Medicine
Dr Pamela L Jones, Kirkland, QC - Orthopedic Surgery
Dr Edward A Jones, Regina, SK - Anatomical Pathology
Dr Nicola J Jones-Stokreef, Orillia, ON - Pediatrics
Dr M K Rashid Joomun, Whitewood, SK - General Practice
Dr Sally H Jorgensen, Bridgewater, NS - Obstetrics & Gynecology
Dr Urvi Joshi, New Westminster, BC - Nuclear Medicine
Dr C Mark Joyce, Calgary, AB - Family Medicine
Dr Marek A Jung, Calgary, AB - Internal Medicine
Dr Hans W Jung, Ottawa, ON - General Practice
Dr Shadan Kabiri-Abyaneh, West Vancouver, BC - Family Medicine
Dr Isaac-Jacques Kadoch, Montreal, QC - General Practice
Dr Harry Kadoch, Ormstown, QC - Family Medicine
Dr Andrew Kaegi, Whitehorse, YT - Hematology
Dr H Wilfried S Kaethler, Steinbach, MB - Family Medicine
Dr Henryk P Kafka, Belleville, ON - Cardiology
Dr Rhoda S Kagan, North York, ON - Clin Immun/Allergy
Dr Raymond N Kahwaji, Vancouver, BC - Anesthesia
Dr Christian Y Kako, Richmond Hill, ON - General Practice
Dr Malgorzata E Kaminska, Calgary, AB - Family Medicine
Dr Kami Kandola, Yellowknife, NT - Family Medicine
Dr Harbhajan S Kang, Montreal, QC - Internal Medicine
Dr Hussein D Kanji, Vancouver, BC - Emergency Medicine
Dr Nachiketa M Kanungo, Windsor, ON - Diagnostic-Radiology
Dr Harvey Kaplovitch, Toronto, ON - Family Medicine
Dr Videsh Kapoor, Richmond, BC - Family Medicine
Dr Vimal S Kapoor, Markham, ON - Community Medicine
Dr Suneil Kapur, Nepean, ON - Internal Medicine
Dr Morton A Kapusta, Montreal, QC - Internal Medicine
Dr Gregory J Karaguesian, Haliburton, ON - General Practice
Dr Pierre Karakiewicz, Montreal, QC - Urology
Dr Christos Karatzios, Montreal, QC - Infectious Diseases
Dr Nicolas Karellis, Laval, QC - General Practice
Dr Megan M F Karnis, Burlington, ON - Obstetrics & Gynecology
Dr Alan J Karovitch, Ottawa, ON - Internal Medicine
Dr Craig Karpilow, Hamilton, ON - Family Medicine
Dr Martin E Karpinski, Winnipeg, MB - Internal Medicine
Dr Jolanta A M Karpinski, Ottawa, ON - Internal Medicine
Dr Shelby N Karpman, Edmonton, AB - Family Medicine
Dr Cengiz H Karsli, Toronto, ON - Anesthesia
Dr Lisa M Karvelas, Winnipeg, MB - Psychiatry
Dr Elena Kasatiya Trevisani, Ottawa, ON - General Practice
Dr Jacinthe Kassab, Calgary, AB - Ophthalmology
Dr Brian M Katchan, North York, ON - Internal Medicine
Dr Athanasios Katsarkas, Montreal, QC - Otolaryngology
Dr John Katsounakis, Westmount, QC - Family Medicine
Dr Murray S Katz, Dollard-D-Ormeaux, QC - General Practice
Dr Edward Katz, Montreal, QC - General Practice
Dr Robert Kaud, Saint-Laurent, QC - Family Medicine
Dr Conrad Kavalec, Montreal, QC - Ophthalmology
Dr Walter F Kean, Hamilton, ON - Internal Medicine
Dr Michael V Keating, Sault Ste. Marie, ON - General Practice
Dr Nancy B Keesal, Toronto, ON - Internal Medicine
Dr Heather E Keizer, Charlottetown, PE - Psychiatry
Dr John S Kell, Toronto, ON - Urology
Dr Adrian P Kelly, Sackville, NB - Family Medicine
Dr Brian F Kelly, Kitchener, ON - General Practice
Dr Catherine M K Kelly, Toronto, ON - Endocrinology
Dr Anthea G Kelly, Sherbrooke, QC - Medical Biochemistry
Dr Yasmine S Kelton, Richmond Hill, ON - Family Medicine
Dr Ilse Kemp, Gander, NL - Pediatrics
Dr Robert A Kemp, Brampton, ON - Family Medicine
Dr Gerald Kenefick, Burnaby, BC - Family Medicine
Dr Richard J Kennedy, Calgary, AB - Internal Medicine
Dr James R Kennedy, Vancouver, BC - Internal Medicine
Dr Karen M Kennedy, Orillia, ON - Family Medicine
Dr Renee S Kennedy, Saskatoon, SK - Thoracic Surgery
Dr Lorraine M R Kerr, Winnipeg, MB - Pediatrics
Dr Peter J Kertes, Toronto, ON - Ophthalmology
Dr Jalal Keshmirian, London, ON - Family Medicine
Dr R. John R Keyserlingk, Montreal, QC - General Surgery
Dr Manish Khanna, Montreal, QC - Dermatology
Dr Kapil Khatter, Ottawa, ON - Family Medicine
Dr Katayoun S Khorrami, Calgary, AB - Family Medicine
Dr Lara Khoury, Ottawa, ON - Geriatric Medicine
Dr Samir Khoury, Montreal, QC - Pediatrics
Dr Rosy Khurana, Mistissini, QC - Family Medicine
Dr Krikor Kichian, Ottawa, ON - Gastroenterology
Dr Teresa M Kieser, Calgary, AB - Cardiovasc/ThorSurg
Dr Debra A Kiez, Richmond Hill, ON - Emergency Family Med
Dr Frances T Kilbertus, Ottawa, ON - Family Medicine
Dr Dyan Kimia, Westmount, QC - Pediatrics
Dr R John Kimoff, Montreal, QC - Internal Medicine
Dr Arlene King, Toronto, ON - Community Medicine
Dr Laval Kon Kam King, Summerside, PE - General Practice
Dr Erle J Kirby, Wawa, ON - Family Medicine
Dr Irina Kirtsman, Cornwall, ON - Pediatrics
Dr Robert J Klaassen, Ottawa, ON - Hematology
Dr Stephanie Klam, Montreal, QC - Obstetrics & Gynecology
Dr Marc Klasa, Calgary, AB - Family Medicine
Dr Richard J Klasa, Vancouver, BC - Internal Medicine
Dr Jean-Marc Y Klein, Charlottetown, PE - Dermatology
Dr Jack Klein, Kirkland, QC - General Practice
Dr Marina B Klein, Montreal, QC - Infectious Diseases
Dr Max Kleinman, North York, ON - Physical Medicine & Rehab
Dr Izabela Klosowski, Saint-Bruno, QC - Family Medicine
Dr Kristine E Klubien, Montreal, QC - General Practice
Dr Lawrence Knight, Westmount, QC - Internal Medicine
Dr Frank D Knoefel, Ottawa, ON - Family Medicine
Dr Marion D Koch, Wakefield, QC - Psychiatry
Dr Robert K Koenekoop, Montreal, QC - Ophthalmology

Dr David A Koff, Hamilton, ON - Diagnostic-Radiology
Dr Peter Koopmann, Cowansville, QC - Hematology
Dr Marguerite M Kopaniak, Toronto, ON - Family Medicine
Dr Eleonor Kopylenko, Newmarket, ON - Family Medicine
Dr Miroslav Kordich, Montreal, QC - General Surgery
Dr Endre L Koritar, Vancouver, BC - Psychiatry
Dr Joseph B Kornacki, Verdun, QC - Orthopedic Surgery
Dr Claude Kortas, London, ON - Internal Medicine
Dr Antonio I Kos, Timmins, ON - Family Medicine
Dr Karen M Kost, Montreal, QC - Otolaryngology
Dr David P Kostiuk, Montreal, QC - Cardiology
Dr Lawrence J Kotkas, Lethbridge, AB - Psychiatry
Dr Susan V B Kovacs, Toronto, ON - Pediatrics
Dr Lajos B Kovacs, Montreal, QC - Pediatrics
Dr Piotr Koziarz, Welland, ON - General Surgery
Dr Lida Kratka, Vanier, ON - General Practice
Dr Daniel J Kraus, Montreal, QC - Psychiatry
Dr Stuart H Kreisman, Vancouver, BC - Internal Medicine
Dr Richard B Kremer, Montreal, QC - Medical Biochemistry
Dr Mark Krieger, Toronto, ON - General Practice
Dr Preetha Krishnamoorthy, Montreal, QC - Endocrin/Metabolism
Dr Risk Kronfli, Dartmouth, NS - Psychiatry
Dr Lech Krotecki, Ormstown, QC - Family Medicine
Dr Maria H Krzywicka, Calgary, AB - General Practice
Dr Allison Kukhta, Val-d'Or, QC - Clin Immun/Allergy
Dr Joy Kuncheria, Cambridge, ON - Family Medicine
Dr Karol Kuperberg, Montreal, QC - General Practice
Dr Beverly Kupfert, North York, ON - Pediatrics
Dr Christine Kupsh, Sudbury, ON - Emergency Family Med
Dr Vladimir Kurgansky, Kirkland, QC - Urology
Dr Robin A Kuritzky, New Westminster, BC - Cardiology
Dr Beverley Kyle, Pointe-Claire, QC - Family Medicine
Dr Edmond Kyrillos, Ottawa, ON - Family Medicine
Dr Monique S La France, Inverness, NS - Family Medicine
Dr Lino P LaGrotteria, Hamilton, ON - Family Medicine
Dr Nathalie LaRue, Cowansville, QC - General Surgery
Dr Eric R Labelle, Timmins, ON - General Surgery
Dr Roger E Labonte, Sudbury, ON - Cardiology
Dr Josee L Labrosse, Ottawa, ON - General Practice
Dr Louis-Andre Lacasse, Saint-Jerome, QC - Family Medicine
Dr James D Lacey, Kanata, ON - Plastic Surgery
Dr Lori-Ann D Lach, Winnipeg, MB - Family Medicine
Dr Daniel Lacroix, Moose Creek, ON - General Practice
Dr Linda A M Lacroix, Ottawa, ON - Hematology
Dr Thomas B Lacroix, Sarnia, ON - Pediatrics
Dr Luc-Phillippe J Lacroix, Gatineau, QC - Family Medicine
Dr Mylene H Lacroix, Quebec, QC - Family Medicine
Dr Julie B D Lacuna, Vancouver, BC - Family Medicine
Dr Louis Laflamme, St-Jean-Sur-Richel, QC - Diagnostic-Radiology
Dr J J Rene Lafleche, Hearst, ON - Family Medicine
Dr Jacques J Laforest, Angus, ON - General Practice
Dr Stephane Laframboise, Toronto, ON - Obstetrics & Gynecology
Dr Karen F Laframboise, Saskatoon, SK - Critical Care Medicine
Dr Rene Lafreniere, Calgary, AB - General Surgery
Dr Ronald T J Lafreniere, Victoria, BC - Physical Medicine & Rehab
Dr Leda C Lagrotteria, Hamilton, ON - Family Medicine
Dr Nadine J Lahoud, Lasalle, QC - Internal Medicine
Dr Ginette Lajoie, Brampton, ON - Anatomical Pathology
Dr Danielle Lajoie, St-J-Chrysostome, QC - General Practice
Dr Michelle Lajzerowicz, Wakefield, QC - Family Medicine
Dr Martin Lalinec-Michaud, Quebec, QC - General Practice
Dr Rosemarie N Lall, Scarborough, ON - Family Medicine
Dr Leonora Lalla, Montreal, QC - Family Medicine
Dr Fiore R Lalla, Pointe-Claire, QC - Psychiatry
Dr Donald H Lalonde, Saint John, NB - Plastic Surgery
Dr Richard G J Lalonde, Montreal, QC - Infectious Diseases
Dr Pierre Lalonde, Montreal, QC - Psychiatry
Dr Michelle A Lamarre, Sudbury, ON - Family Medicine
Dr David C Lambert, Brossard, QC - Orthopedic Surgery
Dr Cecilia Lamenza, Toronto, ON - Pediatrics
Dr Robert W Lamont, Scarborough, ON - Anesthesia
Dr Yves Lamontagne, Montreal, QC - Psychiatry
Dr Andre Lamy, Hamilton, ON - Cardiothor Surgery
Dr Stephan J Landis, Guelph, ON - Internal Medicine
Dr Daniel A Landry, Moncton, NB - Family Medicine
Dr Jennifer S Landry, Montreal, QC - Critical Care Medicine
Dr Eugene P Landsbergen, Sundre, AB - General Practice
Dr Brian A Lang, Scarborough, ON - Family Medicine
Dr Sam Lang Hang Yee, Burnaby, BC - Family Medicine
Dr Marc V Langill, Ottawa, ON - Family Medicine
Dr Heather I Langille, Ottawa, ON - Emergency Family Med
Dr David Langleben, Montreal, QC - Cardiology
Dr E Anne Langlois, Toronto, ON - Family Medicine
Dr Marcelo Lannes, Montreal, QC - Anesthesia
Dr Pierre J Lanoix, Rockland, ON - Family Medicine
Dr Gabor Lantos, Toronto, ON - General Practice
Dr Yves L Lapierre, Montreal, QC - Neurology
Dr Manfred Lapner, Ottawa, ON - Pediatrics
Dr Peter L C Lapner, Ottawa, ON - Orthopedic Surgery
Dr Pierre Lapointe, Levis, QC - Orthopedic Surgery
Dr Marc Laporta, Montreal, QC - Psychiatry
Dr Albert Larbrisseau, Montreal, QC - Neurology
Dr E Sheila Laredo, Toronto, ON - Endocrin/Metabolism
Dr Yanick Larivee, Granby, QC - Otolaryngology
Dr Bruno Laroche, Quebec, QC - Urology
Dr Roger E J Larochelle, Spanish, ON - General Practice
Dr Leon Larouche, La Baie, QC - General Practice
Dr Richard Larouche, Montreal, QC - General Practice
Dr Guy Jean Laroye, Terrace, BC - General Pathology
Dr Marie Larue, Maria, QC - General Surgery
Dr Wojciech Laskowski, Ottawa, ON - General Practice
Dr David A Lasry, Montreal, QC - Emergency Family Med
Dr Jennifer Latella, Thunder Bay, ON - Internal Medicine
Dr David A Latter, Toronto, ON - Cardiovasc/ThorSurg
Dr William W L Lau, Laval, QC - General Practice
Dr Ulrich S Lauf, Calgary, AB - Family Medicine
Dr Brian Laufer, Montreal, QC - Critical Care Medicine
Dr Marc P Launay, Montreal, QC - Endocrinology
Dr Michel A Laurin, Saint-Hyacinthe, QC - Anatomical Pathology
Dr Jean G Lauzon, Surrey, BC - General Surgery
Dr Carol L Lavallee, Sudbury, ON - Psychiatry
Dr Lee-Anne Laverty, Trail, BC - Orthopedic Surgery
Dr Patrick Lavigne, Montreal, QC - Orthopedic Surgery
Dr Cecile R Lavoie, Bonnyville, AB - General Practice
Dr Susan D Lavoie, Ottawa, ON - Internal Medicine
Dr Mona Lavoie, Levis, QC - Anatomical Pathology
Dr Lionel A Lavoie, Melfort, SK - Family Medicine
Dr David Lawee, Toronto, ON - Family Medicine
Dr Sofia Lazaridis, Ottawa, ON - Family Medicine
Dr Juris Lazovskis, Sydney, NS - General Practice
Dr Charles Lazzam, Mississauga, ON - Cardiology
Dr Frank T Lazzara, LaSalle, QC - General Practice
Dr Quynh M T Le, Brampton, ON - Obstetrics & Gynecology
Dr Khoa-Anh Le, Markham, ON - Internal Medicine
Dr Chu Quang Le, Toronto, ON - General Practice
Dr Roger E Le Bel, Pointe-Claire, QC - Otolaryngology
Dr Catherine A Le Feuvre, Mississauga, ON - Cardiology
Dr Jean-Michel Le Melledo, Edmonton, AB - General Practice
Dr Nicole M A Le Saux, Ottawa, ON - Anatomical Pathology
Dr Linda M LeBlanc, Moncton, NB - Radiation Oncology
Dr Roger P LeBlanc, Montreal, QC - Internal Medicine
Dr Patrick J Leahy, Kemptville, ON - Family Medicine
Dr Marc Lebeau, Toronto, ON - Family Medicine
Dr Pierre Lebel, Montreal, QC - Medical Microbiology
Dr Paulette M Leblanc, Moncton, NB - General Practice
Dr Constance Leblanc, Halifax, NS - Emergency Family Med
Dr Claire Leblanc, Montreal, QC - Pediatrics
Dr Mortimer Lechter, Westmount, QC - Neurology
Dr Nadine S Lecuyer, Winnipeg, MB - Family Medicine
Dr Danielle S Leddy, Kitchener, ON - Cardiology
Dr Jose Ledezma, Quispamsis, NB - General Practice
Dr Dean C Leduc, Orleans, ON - Family Medicine
Dr Mao-Cheng Lee, Edmonton, AB - Internal Medicine
Dr John O Lee, Kanata, ON - Family Medicine
Dr Joseph Y Lee, Mississauga, ON - Obstetrics & Gynecology
Dr Kwok Ching Lee, North York, ON - Anesthesia
Dr Gary L Lee, Montreal, QC - Emergency Family Med
Dr M Madeleine Lee-Ng, Scarborough, ON - General Practice
Dr Carole Legare, Ottawa, ON - Family Medicine
Dr Teisha Legault, Winchester, ON - Family Medicine
Dr Celine N Leger-Nolet, New Liskeard, ON - Internal Medicine
Dr Janice M Legere, Brantford, ON - General Practice
Dr Christine M Legler, Montreal, QC - Internal Medicine
Dr Lorraine Legrand Westfall, Ottawa, ON - General Surgery
Dr M Christine Lejtenyi, Montreal, QC - Clin Immun/Allergy
Dr Jane B Lemaire, Calgary, AB - Internal Medicine
Dr Marie-Claude Lemieux, Montreal, QC - Obstetrics & Gynecology
Dr Sylvie Lemieux, Sainte-Marie, QC - General Practice
Dr Eric M Lenczner, Montreal, QC - Orthopedic Surgery
Dr Vittorio Lentini, Scarborough, ON - General Practice
Dr Sylvie Leone, Mississauga, ON - Obstetrics & Gynecology
Dr Eric W H Leong, Toronto, ON - Gastroenterology
Dr Fook Lin Leong-Sit, Edmonton, AB - Ophthalmology
Dr Robert S Lepage, Sudbury, ON - Emergency Family Med
Dr Bram Lermer, Richmond, BC - Family Medicine
Dr Michel Lessard, Chicoutimi, QC - Anatomical Pathology
Dr M Lucie Lessard, Montreal, QC - Otolaryngology
Dr Pascal Lessard, Quebec, QC - General Practice
Dr Max Leung, Oshawa, ON - Emergency Family Med
Dr Nathalie M C Leung, Richmond Hill, ON - Endocrin/Metabolism
Dr Judith L Levasseur, Oakville, ON - General Practice
Dr Joseph I Leventhal, Toronto, ON - Family Medicine
Dr Chantale Levesque, Montreal, QC - Family Medicine
Dr Aline Levi, Dollard-D-Ormeaux, QC - General Practice
Dr Daniel P Levin, Winnipeg, MB - Nuclear Medicine
Dr Sharon S Levine, Ottawa, ON - Psychiatry
Dr Daniel S Levine, Ottawa, ON - Family Medicine
Dr Danielle C Lewington, Halifax, NS - General Practice
Dr Ronald T Lewis, Ottawa, ON - General Surgery
Dr John R Lewis, Montreal, QC - Emergency Family Med
Dr Arthur Leznoff, Toronto, ON - Clin Immun/Allergy
Dr Michael D Libman, Montreal, QC - Infectious Diseases
Dr Clare E Liddy, Ottawa, ON - Family Medicine
Dr Nathania R Liem, Windsor, ON - Physical Medicine & Rehab
Dr Trina X Liew, Scarborough, ON - Family Medicine
Dr Margaret R Lightheart, Hamilton, ON - Obstetrics & Gynecology
Dr Sophie Ligier, Montreal, QC - Internal Medicine
Dr Khian-Kok Lim, Lachine, QC - Ophthalmology
Dr David T Lin, Vancouver, BC - Ophthalmology
Dr Karen W Lin, Scarborough, ON - General Practice
Dr Jorin M Lindensmith, Dartmouth, NS - Internal Medicine
Dr Rebecca J Lindley, Pemberton, BC - Family Medicine
Dr Susan K Lindley, Montreal, QC - Ophthalmology
Dr Daniel J Lindsay, Selkirk, MB - Diagnostic-Radiology
Dr Stan Lipnowski, Winnipeg, MB - Pediatrics
Dr Jennifer B Lipscombe, Mississauga, ON - Internal Medicine
Dr Lorraine L Lipscombe, Toronto, ON - Endocrin/Metabolism
Dr Charles Listgarten, Woodbridge, ON - Internal Medicine
Dr John M Little, Montreal, QC - Ophthalmology
Dr Richard Liu, Edmonton, AB - Otolaryngology
Dr Lee Ha Liu Chen Kiow, Montreal, QC - Family Medicine
Dr E Lock, Amherst, NS - Psychiatry
Dr Diane M Logan, London, ON - Internal Medicine
Dr Nick F Logarakis, Scarborough, ON - Urology
Dr Caroline A Lohrisch, Vancouver, BC - Internal Medicine
Dr Ramesh Lokanathan, Prince George, BC - General Surgery
Dr M Hossen Lokhat, Ottawa, ON - General Surgery
Dr Rocco A Lombardi, Bowmanville, ON - Emergency Family Med
Dr Elgin M Loney, Lions Head, ON - General Practice
Dr Karl J Looper, Montreal, QC - Psychiatry
Dr Isabelle Lopez, Laval, QC - Psychiatry
Dr Louise Loranger, Sherbrooke, QC - Dermatology
Dr C Gabriella Lorenzon, Vancouver, BC - General Practice
Dr John W Lorimer, Ottawa, ON - General Surgery
Dr Donna C Lougheed, Ottawa, ON - Psychiatry
Dr Robert B Love, Kanata, ON - Otolaryngology
Dr Peter L Loveridge, Glenwood, NS - General Practice
Dr Steven L Low, Coaldale, AB - Family Medicine
Dr Charles T Low, Brockville, ON - Family Medicine
Dr Deborah M Loyer, Pierrefonds, QC - Pediatrics

Dr Andres M Lozano, Toronto, ON - Neurosurgery
Dr Paul A Lubitz, Canmore, AB - Dermatology
Dr Simon J Lucy, Winnipeg, MB - Anesthesia
Dr Mara S Ludwig, Montreal, QC - Internal Medicine
Dr Jelka-Maria Lujic-Thebaud, Edmonton, AB - General Practice
Dr David W K Lum, St Thomas, ON - Family Medicine
Dr Fernando A Luna, Gatineau, QC - General Practice
Dr J R Guy Lupien, Iroquois Falls, ON - Emergency Family Med
Dr G Harvey Lupu, Montreal, QC - Pediatrics
Dr John K Luther, Regina, SK - General Practice
Dr Paul Lysy, Westmount, QC - Family Medicine
Dr Felix Ma, Montreal, QC - Cardiac Surgery
Dr Lorraine M Mabon, Calgary, AB - Emergency Medicine
Dr Michele Mabon, Montreal, QC - Ophthalmology
Dr Roderick G G MacArthur, Edmonton, AB - Cardiac Surgery
Dr Kimberly R MacAskill, Kanata, ON - Family Medicine
Dr Patricia L MacCallum, Moncton, NB - Otolaryngology
Dr Alexander MacCordick, Gatineau, QC - Psychiatry
Dr Ian M MacDonald, Edmonton, AB - Ophthalmology
Dr Susan C MacDonald, Prince George, BC - Family Medicine
Dr Sharon M MacDonald, Winnipeg, MB - Community Medicine
Dr Jennifer L MacDonald, Liverpool, NS - Family Medicine
Dr William A MacDonald, Iqaluit, NU - Family Medicine
Dr Russell D MacDonald, Mississauga, ON - Emergency Medicine
Dr Kathryn J MacDonald, Ohsweken, ON - Psychiatry
Dr Suzanne F MacDonald, Montreal, QC - Pediatrics
Dr B Jean MacDonnell, Montreal, QC - Family Medicine
Dr Michael H MacEachern, Moncton, NB - Neurology
Dr Lynne S MacGregor, Ottawa, ON - Physical Medicine & Rehab
Dr Thomas J MacKay, Halifax, NS - Psychiatry
Dr Sarah J MacKinnon, Sundridge, ON - Family Medicine
Dr Anthony R MacLean, Calgary, AB - General Surgery
Dr Stephen W MacLean, Halifax, NS - Family Medicine
Dr Alan J MacLean, Montreal, QC - Internal Medicine
Dr Anne-Marie MacLellan, Montreal, QC - Pediatrics
Dr N Wayne MacLeod, Halifax, NS - Family Medicine
Dr Suzanne M MacMillan, Ottawa, ON - Internal Medicine
Dr Elizabeth M MacNamara, Montreal, QC - Medical Biochemistry
Dr Douglas W MacPherson, Cheltenham, ON - Internal Medicine
Dr Robert M MacRae, Ottawa, ON - Radiation Oncology
Dr Ruth M MacSween, Kingston, ON - Dermatology
Dr Daniel B Macek, Cowansville, QC - Internal Medicine
Dr Mary E Machamer, Toronto, ON - General Practice
Dr J William Mackie, Vancouver, BC - Family Medicine
Dr Richard J Mackler, Montreal, QC - Endocrinology
Dr Angelo G Macrodimitris, Winnipeg, MB - Ophthalmology
Dr Ilana Magder, Toronto, ON - Pediatrics
Dr Sheldon A Magder, Montreal, QC - Cardiology
Dr Lucia B Magnani, Pierrefonds, QC - Pediatrics
Dr John A C Maguire, Vancouver, BC - Anatomical Pathology
Dr Bryan D Magwood, Winnipeg, MB - Critical Care Medicine
Dr Michael K Mah, Calgary, AB - Family Medicine
Dr Jaysen Mahadoo, Victoria, BC - General Practice
Dr Usha Maharaj, Sherwood Park, AB - Family Medicine
Dr John T Maher, Peterborough, ON - Psychiatry
Dr Trudy L Mahood, Thunder Bay, ON - Family Medicine
Dr David D Mai, Ottawa, ON - Family Medicine
Dr Emmanuel Maicas, Moncton, NB - Anatomical Pathology
Dr Alain Maillette, Trois-Rivieres, QC - Urology
Dr Maria J Maingot-Douketis, Scarborough, ON - Family Medicine
Dr Rachel J Maisonneuve, Timmins, ON - Family Medicine
Dr Pierre P Major, Hamilton, ON - Internal Medicine
Dr Kami L Makar, Lethbridge, AB - Emergency Family Med
Dr Suzanne Malaab, Val-d'Or, QC - Pediatrics
Dr Ross S Male, Paris, ON - Family Medicine
Dr Roy A Male, Toronto, ON - Family Medicine
Dr Paul M J Malette, Val Caron, ON - General Practice
Dr Garnet J M Maley, Milton, ON - General Practice
Dr Vikram K Malhotra, Saint-Eustache, QC - General Surgery
Dr Naseem Malleck, Swift Current, SK - Obstetrics & Gynecology
Dr Joseph Mamazza, Ottawa, ON - General Surgery
Dr Joy E Mangel, London, ON - Hematology
Dr Thomas Maniatis, Montreal, QC - Internal Medicine
Dr Alaudin E Manji, Delta, BC - Family Medicine
Dr Mervat F Mankarious, Mississauga, ON - Family Medicine
Dr Gary M Mann, Thornhill, ON - General Practice
Dr John J V Manoukian, Montreal, QC - Otolaryngology
Dr Valerie I Mantle, Sudbury, ON - Family Medicine
Dr Elias R Maraghi, Hastings, ON - General Practice
Dr Julie P Maranda, Hawkesbury, ON - Family Medicine
Dr Dominic Marando, LaSalle, QC - General Practice
Dr Maya Marc, Chateauguay, QC - Pediatrics
Dr Berge Marcarian, Scarborough, ON - Otolaryngology
Dr Deborah J Marchand, Port Hawkesbury, NS - General Practice
Dr Anthony Marchie, Richmond Hill, ON - Orthopedic Surgery
Dr Loretta Marcon, Montreal, QC - Obstetrics & Gynecology
Dr René Marcotte, Laval, QC - General Practice
Dr Victoria A Marcus, Montreal, QC - Anatomical Pathology
Dr Howard C Margolese, Montreal, QC - Psychiatry
Dr Gisele Marier, Bridgewater, NS - Family Medicine
Dr Alina Marin, Kingston, ON - General Practice
Dr Gilles Marineau, Repentigny, QC - General Practice
Dr Alexander Marks, Toronto, ON - General Practice
Dr Arthur J Markus, Montreal, QC - Pediatrics
Dr Errol B Marliss, Montreal, QC - Internal Medicine
Dr Joseph E V Marmina, Pickering, ON - General Practice
Dr Gerald Marquette, Vancouver, BC - Obstetrics & Gynecology
Dr Saida Marrat, Scarborough, ON - Family Medicine
Dr Joseph G Marsan, Ottawa, ON - Otolaryngology
Dr Stephanie M Marsan, Montreal, QC - Family Medicine
Dr Kate M A Marshall, York, ON - Family Medicine
Dr Janet A Marta, Toronto, ON - Psychiatry
Dr Stuart Martin, Hamilton, ON - Plastic Surgery
Dr Lucie C Martin, Ottawa, ON - Diagnostic-Radiology
Dr Andrew J Martin, Thornhill, ON - Family Medicine
Dr James G Martin, Montreal, QC - Respirology
Dr Markus C Martin, Montreal, QC - Obstetrics & Gynecology
Dr Stephen C Martin, Westmount, QC - Family Medicine
Dr Susanna M Martin, Saskatoon, SK - Pediatrics
Dr Jose A Martinez, Terrebonne, QC - Otolaryngology
Dr Jose Luis Martinez Marin, Montreal, QC - General Practice
Dr Humberto Martinho, Ottawa, ON - Family Medicine
Dr Valdemar Martinho, Ottawa, ON - General Practice
Dr Joel E Maser, Toronto, ON - Internal Medicine
Dr Orly H Mashal, Dollard-D-Ormeaux, QC - General Practice
Dr Joan E Mason, Brossard, QC - General Practice
Dr R Albert Y Massabki, Oshawa, ON - Psychiatry
Dr Elizabeth A Massarelli, Sackville, NB - Family Medicine
Dr Ephraim G Massey, Montreal, QC - General Practice
Dr Emad Massoud, Halifax, NS - Otolaryngology
Dr Surya Master, Campbellton, NB - General Surgery
Dr Nicola Masucci, Chateauguay, QC - General Practice
Dr Tshilay Matand, Regina, SK - General Practice
Dr Jane M Mathew, Gatineau, QC - Critical Care Medicine
Dr Nicolas Mathieu, Riviere-Rouge, QC - General Practice
Dr Elias Matouk, Montreal, QC - Internal Medicine
Dr Michele A Matter, Selkirk, MB - Family Medicine
Dr Marc L P Mauguin, Ottawa, ON - Psychiatry
Dr Cleo A Mavriplis, Ottawa, ON - Family Medicine
Dr Yasmine Mawji, Toronto, ON - Emergency Family Med
Dr E Linda Maxwell, Markham, ON - Otolaryngology
Dr Cynthia V Maxwell, Toronto, ON - Obstetrics & Gynecology
Dr Barbara J A Mayr, West Vancouver, BC - General Practice
Dr Patricia J Mayr, Guelph, ON - General Practice
Dr Bruce D Mazer, Montreal, QC - Clin Immun/Allergy
Dr Donna E Maziak, Ottawa, ON - General Surgery
Dr Stanley T Maziarz, Gatineau, QC - Family Medicine
Dr Hagop K Mazmanian, Welland, ON - Urology
Dr Eric D Mazoff, Pointe-Claire, QC - Family Medicine
Dr Guiseppe Mazza, Montreal, QC - General Practice
Dr Mark Mazzarelli, LaSalle, QC - General Practice
Dr Denis B Mbanza, Regina, SK - General Practice
Dr Felicien K M Mbuyi, Calgary, AB - General Practice
Dr Simon McBride, London, ON - General Practice
Dr Richard H McCall, Hawkesbury, ON - Family Medicine
Dr Robert McCallum, Cambridge, ON - Family Medicine
Dr Jacqueline McClaran, Montreal, QC - General Practice
Dr Donna J McClure, Vancouver, BC - Family Medicine
Dr Todd A McConnell, Montreal, QC - Internal Medicine
Dr Catherine C McCuaig, Montreal, QC - Dermatology
Dr Sarah D McDonald, Hamilton, ON - Obstetrics & Gynecology
Dr James W McGillivray, Hearst, ON - General Surgery
Dr Douglas M McGregor, Victoria, BC - General Practice
Dr Alyson M McGregor-Shaw, Ottawa, ON - Pediatrics
Dr R Philip McGuire, Midland, ON - Emergency Family Med
Dr L Lynn McIntyre, Calgary, AB - Community Medicine
Dr Mary E McIntyre, Chatham, ON - General Practice
Dr J Roger McKelvey, Dartmouth, NS - Neurology
Dr Rowen A McLellan, Fredericton, NB - Urology
Dr John D R McMorran, Vancouver, BC - General Practice
Dr Lisa A McMurray, Ottawa, ON - Psychiatry
Dr T Bruce D McNeely, Kamloops, BC - Anatomical Pathology
Dr P Daniel McNeely, Halifax, NS - Neurosurgery
Dr P Ruth McPherson, Ottawa, ON - Endocrin/Metabolism
Dr David E McPherson, Westmount, QC - Psychiatry
Dr Suzy Meagher, Laval, QC - General Practice
Dr Timothy W Meagher, Montreal, QC - Internal Medicine
Dr Barbara D Mederski, North York, ON - Internal Medicine
Dr Bheemdev Meetarbhan, Coquitlam, BC - General Practice
Dr Sanjay Mehta, London, ON - Internal Medicine
Dr Simone A Meikleham, Little Current, ON - Emergency Family Med
Dr Joan M Meitin, Ottawa, ON - Psychiatry
Dr Jose H Mejia, London, ON - Psychiatry
Dr Gilles G J Melanson, Ottawa, ON - Psychiatry
Dr Ekaterina Melcuk, Montreal, QC - Pediatrics
Dr Donald Meldrum, Calgary, AB - Cardiology
Dr Calvin A Melmed, Montreal, QC - Neurology
Dr Lydia C Melnyk, Montreal, QC - Family Medicine
Dr Nejat Memiche, Bathurst, NB - Gastroenterology
Dr Reshat Memiche, Bathurst, NB - Gastroenterology
Dr Jacques G Menard, Gatineau, QC - General Practice
Dr Jack Mendelson, Montreal, QC - Infectious Diseases
Dr Tilak Mendis, Ottawa, ON - Neurology
Dr Robert D Menzies, Vancouver, BC - Family Medicine
Dr Jay G Mercer, Ottawa, ON - Family Medicine
Dr Gregory B Meterissian, Montreal, QC - Psychiatry
Dr P Peter Metrakos, Montreal, QC - General Surgery
Dr Michelle M Mezei, Vancouver, BC - Neurology
Dr Antoinette A Michael, Whitby, ON - Family Medicine
Dr Kathleen A Michalski, Orillia, ON - Family Medicine
Dr Rene P Michel, Montreal, QC - Anatomical Pathology
Dr Andre L Michon, Sudbury, ON - Family Medicine
Dr Catalin Mihalcioiu, Montreal, QC - Internal Medicine
Dr Elena Mihu, Kinmount, ON - Family Medicine
Dr Jose L Mijangos-Pelaez, Val-d'Or, QC - General Surgery
Dr Janina Milanska, Ottawa, ON - Pediatrics
Dr John J Milczarek, Fredericton, NB - Physical Medicine & Rehab
Dr Wilson Miller, Montreal, QC - General Practice
Dr Lisa T Millstein, North York, ON - Family Medicine
Dr C Michelle Milne, Montreal, QC - General Practice
Dr Slobodan Milosevic, Louiseville, QC - General Practice
Dr Thomas M Milroy, Montreal, QC - Psychiatry
Dr Richard E Mimeault, Ottawa, ON - General Surgery
Dr Paul H Minc, Acton, ON - Family Medicine
Dr Klaus K Minde, Montreal, QC - Psychiatry
Dr Thomas Minde, Ste-Cecile-de-Mash, QC - Family Medicine
Dr Cristina S Mindru, Montreal, QC - Internal Medicine
Dr Genevieve Minville, Chicoutimi, QC - General Practice
Dr Gabriel R Minz, Dorval, QC - Family Medicine
Dr Hortensia S Mircescu, Montreal, QC - Endocrin/Metabolism
Dr Joaquim A Miro, Montreal, QC - Cardiology
Dr Andrew A Mis, Winnipeg, MB - Ophthalmology
Dr Nahed R Mishriki, Toronto, ON - Family Medicine
Dr Rebecca S Mitchell, Edmonton, AB - Endocrin/Metabolism
Dr A Gregor Mitchell, Lachute, QC - Family Medicine
Dr David A Mitchell, Montreal, QC - Hematology
Dr Grant A Mitchell, Montreal, QC - Medical Genetics
Dr Nikolina Mizdrak, Toronto, ON - Family Medicine
Dr Henry F Mizgala, Vancouver, BC - Cardiology
Dr Sophia Mobilos, Toronto, ON - Family Medicine
Dr Hilda Moens, Burlington, ON - General Practice

Dr Francois O P Moens, Hamilton, ON - Obstetrics & Gynecology
Dr Vivian M Moir, Keswick, ON - Family Medicine
Dr Andrew K C Mok, Montreal, QC - Obstetrics & Gynecology
Dr Henry J Moller, Toronto, ON - Psychiatry
Dr Frank J Molnar, Ottawa, ON - Geriatric Medicine
Dr Nicolae Molotiu, Strathroy, ON - Anesthesia
Dr M Anne Monahan, Ottawa, ON - Family Medicine
Dr Arsalan Monavvari, Toronto, ON - Family Medicine
Dr Jacques Monday, Montreal, QC - Psychiatry
Dr Brigitte M A E Monrose, Markham, ON - Family Medicine
Dr Julio S G Montaner, Vancouver, BC - Internal Medicine
Dr Manuel M Montero Odasso, London, ON - Geriatric Medicine
Dr Valentina C Montessori, Vancouver, BC - Infectious Diseases
Dr Barbara A Montgomery, Courtice, ON - Family Medicine
Dr Christopher W Montgomery, Oshawa, ON - Pediatrics
Dr Silvia Monti De Flores, Montreal, QC - Psychiatry
Dr Richard Montoro, Montreal, QC - Psychiatry
Dr David R Montoya, Ottawa, ON - Emergency Medicine
Dr Madeleine R Montpetit, Ottawa, ON - Family Medicine
Dr Serge Montplaisir, Montreal, QC - Medical Microbiology
Dr Ronit Mooallem, Dollard-D-Ormeaux, QC - Family Medicine
Dr Kieran M Moore, Kingston, ON - Emergency Family Med
Dr Peter Moosbrugger, Comox, BC - Family Medicine
Dr Daniel H Moquin, Parry Sound, ON - Family Medicine
Dr Marc J Moreau, Edmonton, AB - Orthopedic Surgery
Dr Monique F Moreau, Alliston, ON - Family Medicine
Dr Anne Moreau, Quebec, QC - Family Medicine
Dr Richard F Morel, Vanier, ON - Psychiatry
Dr Rene-Louis Morency, Trail, BC - Ophthalmology
Dr Suzanne N Morin, Montreal, QC - Internal Medicine
Dr Guy Morin, Trois-Rivieres, QC - Gastroenterology
Dr Marie-Eve Morisset, Baie-Comeau, QC - Family Medicine
Dr S Anthony Morris, Red Deer, AB - General Pathology
Dr Steven Morris, Halifax, NS - Plastic Surgery
Dr David Morris, Montreal, QC - Endocrinology
Dr Brian M Morris, Montreal, QC - Urology
Dr Dennis Morrison, Calgary, AB - Psychiatry
Dr Sean R Morrissy, Minto, NB - Family Medicine
Dr Amir A Mortazavi, North York, ON - Cardiology
Dr Matthew L Morton, Toronto, ON - Obstetrics & Gynecology
Dr Gregory J Mosdossy, London, ON - Emergency Medicine
Dr Edith K Moser, Vancouver, BC - Family Medicine
Dr Dianne P Mosher, Calgary, AB - Internal Medicine
Dr Christine Motheron, Quebec, QC - Family Medicine
Dr Nasima S Mottiar, Hamilton, ON - Family Medicine
Dr Patricia Mouaikel, Nepean, ON - Family Medicine
Dr Alain Moukheiber, Rouyn-Noranda, QC - Otolaryngology
Dr Patricia A Moussette, Winchester, ON - Family Medicine
Dr Christopher Mpofu, Saskatoon, SK - Pediatrics
Dr Jean-Thadee Muambi-Kabongo, Saint John, NB - General Practice
Dr Thierry M Muanza, Montreal, QC - Psychiatry
Dr Elizabeth K Mueller, Cambridge, ON - Family Medicine
Dr Daniel J Mueller, Toronto, ON - General Practice
Dr J Jean Muggah, Port Williams, NS - General Practice
Dr Channy Y Muhn, Burlington, ON - Dermatology
Dr David S Mulder, Montreal, QC - Cardiovasc/ThorSurg
Dr Siobhan M Muldowney, Smiths Falls, ON - Family Medicine
Dr Hellmuth A Muller Delgado, Winnipeg, MB - Orthopedic Surgery
Dr Christina Mundi, Ottawa, ON - Family Medicine
Dr Rajeev H Muni, Toronto, ON - Ophthalmology
Dr Letitia V Muresan, Dollard-D-Ormeaux, QC - Electroencephal
Dr Nancy Murphy, Halifax, NS - Emergency Family Med
Dr Daniel A Muruve, Calgary, AB - Internal Medicine
Dr P Regine Mydlarski, Calgary, AB - Dermatology
Dr Gail A Myhr, Montreal, QC - Psychiatry
Dr Virginia J Myles, Montreal, QC - Family Medicine
Dr Philip M B Myron, North York, ON - Cardiology
Dr Miklos Nadasdi, North York, ON - General Practice
Dr Paul O Nadeau, Quebec, QC - Orthopedic Surgery
Dr Claude Nadeau, Trois-Rivieres, QC - Otolaryngology
Dr Norman J Nadler, Montreal, QC - Internal Medicine
Dr Laurie J Nadolny, Nepean, ON - Family Medicine
Dr Roland G Nador, Vancouver, BC - General Practice
Dr Alexander G Nagy, Vancouver, BC - General Surgery
Dr Shamsia M Nainar, Hamilton, ON - Family Medicine
Dr N P Vasavan Nair, Verdun, QC - Psychiatry
Dr Adel L C Nakhla, Mississauga, ON - Family Medicine
Dr Steven A Narod, Toronto, ON - Community Medicine
Dr Constance M Nasello, Chatham, ON - Obstetrics & Gynecology
Dr Emil Nashi, Montreal, QC - Clin Immun/Allergy
Dr Louise L Nasmith, Vancouver, BC - Family Medicine
Dr Kamil Nasr, Brossard, QC - Ophthalmology
Dr Hamid A Nasser, Guelph, ON - General Surgery
Dr Joaquin X R Navarro, Ottawa, ON - Psychiatry
Dr Laurie A Neapole, New Westminster, BC - Obstetrics & Gynecology
Dr Joachim F Neffgen, Drumheller, AB - General Practice
Dr Juan C Negrete, Montreal, QC - Psychiatry
Dr Lori L Neily, Oromocto, NB - General Practice
Dr Gregory Neiman, Montreal, QC - Internal Medicine
Dr Roxana Nemes Bratis, Longueuil, QC - General Practice
Dr Joe Nemeth, Montreal, QC - Emergency Family Med
Dr David R Nemtean, Saint-Leonard, QC - General Practice
Dr Lynda K Newkirk, Hamilton, ON - Family Medicine
Dr Jack Newman, North York, ON - Pediatrics
Dr Trevor M Newton, Langley, BC - Emergency Family Med
Dr Derek Ng, North Bay, ON - Emergency Family Med
Dr David Ng, Windsor, ON - Family Medicine
Dr Alan Ng Cheng Hin, Ottawa, ON - Family Medicine
Dr Caroline Ng Cheong, Montreal, QC - Family Medicine
Dr Edward K K Ng Tung Hing, Newmarket, ON - Internal Medicine
Dr Roland Ng-Thow Hing, Pembroke, ON - General Practice
Dr Dung P Nghiem, Pointe-Claire, QC - General Practice
Dr Minh Hien Nguyen, Burnaby, BC - Family Medicine
Dr Nhiem Nguyen, Richmond, BC - Dermatology
Dr Viem Chung Nguyen, Vancouver, BC - Physical Medicine & Rehab
Dr Tuyet Thi Nguyen, Belleville, ON - Family Medicine
Dr The-Huy Nguyen, Brampton, ON - General Practice
Dr Lam Van Nguyen, Hamilton, ON - General Practice
Dr The-Minh Nguyen, Ottawa, ON - Neurology
Dr San Duy Nguyen, Toronto, ON - Psychiatry
Dr Quang V K Nguyen, Toronto, ON - Family Medicine
Dr Huu Nam Nguyen, Greenfield Park, QC - General Practice
Dr Van-Hung Nguyen, Montreal, QC - Anatomical Pathology
Dr Mau Hoang Nguyen, Montreal-Nord, QC - General Practice
Dr Phong Nguyen-Ho, Peterborough, ON - Cardiology
Dr Vaughan Nicholls, La Loche, SK - General Practice
Dr Robert M Nicholson, Granby, QC - Anatomical Pathology
Dr Olu-Kayode Nicol, Mississauga, ON - General Practice
Dr Bruno S Nicoletti, Nepean, ON - Family Medicine
Dr Lynne E Nield, Toronto, ON - Cardiology
Dr Devin R Nielsen, Canmore, AB - Family Medicine
Dr Tara Nigam, Ottawa, ON - Psychiatry
Dr Anil Nigam, Montreal, QC - Cardiology
Dr Cheri L D Nijssen-Jordan, Calgary, AB - Pediatrics
Dr Ana Nikolic, Waterloo, ON - Family Medicine
Dr Andreas Nikolis, Montreal, QC - Plastic Surgery
Dr Jean-Noel Ning, Ottawa, ON - General Practice
Dr Steven Nitzkin, North York, ON - General Practice
Dr S A Trefor Nodwell, Ottawa, ON - Plastic Surgery
Dr Daniel R Noel, Terrebonne, QC - Hematological Pathology
Dr Robert Noiseux, Levis, QC - Psychiatry
Dr Kevin J M Nolan, Ottawa, ON - Anesthesia
Dr Scott A North, Edmonton, AB - Internal Medicine
Dr Mohamed Nouh, St Paul, AB - General Practice
Dr Fred M Novice, Windsor, ON - Dermatology
Dr Malgorzata J M Nowaczyk, Hamilton, ON - Pediatrics
Dr Mark J J Nowaczynski, Toronto, ON - Family Medicine
Dr Michael Nowlan, Gr-Sault/Gr-Falls, NB - General Practice
Dr Robert W Nugent, Fort Frances, ON - Family Medicine
Dr Claire M Nunes-Vaz, Toronto, ON - Family Medicine
Dr Bulangu L(Gregoire) Nyomba, Winnipeg, MB - General Practice
Dr Carole Patricia O'Beirne, Toronto, ON - Pediatrics
Dr Shelley O'Blenis Caines, Oromocto, NB - Emergency Family Med
Dr Barra F O'Briain, Vancouver, BC - Family Medicine
Dr David M O'Brien, Belleville, ON - Obstetrics & Gynecology
Dr Dermot B O'Brien, Hamilton, ON - Ophthalmology
Dr Heather V O'Brien, Sault Ste. Marie, ON - Anesthesia
Dr Mary O'Byrne, Calgary, AB - Pediatrics
Dr Colleen M O'Connell, Fredericton, NB - Physical Medicine & Rehab
Dr John K O'Driscoll, Montreal, QC - Emergency Family Med
Dr Terry A O'Farrell, Kelowna, BC - Orthopedic Surgery
Dr John G O'Kelly, Edmonton, AB - Psychiatry
Dr John A O'Neil, Montreal, QC - Psychiatry
Dr Ailbhe E O'Riordan, London, ON - Diagnostic-Radiology
Dr P Martin O'Shaughnessy, Gravenhurst, ON - General Practice
Dr Eoghan B O'Shea, Ottawa, ON - Family Medicine
Dr Anthony M Ocana, West Vancouver, BC - Family Medicine
Dr Joel J Oger, Vancouver, BC - Neurology
Dr Jason A Ohayon, Hamilton, ON - Clin Immun/Allergy
Dr Henry G Olders, Westmount, QC - Psychiatry
Dr Peter R Olesen, Campbell River, BC - Plastic Surgery
Dr Teresa Oliva, Nepean, ON - Family Medicine
Dr Ronald Olivenstein, Montreal, QC - Internal Medicine
Dr Wojciech P Olszynski, Saskatoon, SK - Internal Medicine
Dr Narh Omaboe, Trenton, ON - Obstetrics & Gynecology
Dr Osamudiamen C Omosigho, Estevan, SK - General Practice
Dr Ronald M Onerheim, Montreal, QC - Anatomical Pathology
Dr Lindsay Ong-Tone, Regina, SK - Ophthalmology
Dr Heather A Onyett, Kingston, ON - Infectious Diseases
Dr Farook N Oosman, Calgary, AB - General Practice
Dr David B Opper, Brantford, ON - Family Medicine
Dr Alexandru A F Opris, Toronto, ON - General Practice
Dr Charles G Orfali, Sherbrooke, QC - Plastic Surgery
Dr Amy E Ornstein, Halifax, NS - Pediatrics
Dr Luis H Ospina, Montreal, QC - General Practice
Dr John W Osterman, Laval, QC - Community Medicine
Dr Jean-Albert Ouellet, Montreal, QC - Orthopedic Surgery
Dr Jean-Yves Ouellet, St-Charles-Brromee, QC - Diagnostic-Radiology
Dr Denise M A Ouellette, Montreal, QC - General Surgery
Dr Nathalie Ouellette, Pierrefonds, QC - Pediatrics
Dr Christopher M Oung, Woodstock, ON - General Surgery
Dr David P Owers, New Westminster, BC - Family Medicine
Dr Charles A Paco, Toronto, ON - Internal Medicine
Dr Sarah Paikin, North York, ON - General Practice
Dr Nicholas V J Pairaudeau, North York, ON - Obstetrics & Gynecology
Dr Jorge A Palacios-Boix, Montreal, QC - Psychiatry
Dr Karen S Palayew, Ottawa, ON - Pediatrics
Dr Mark D Palayew, Montreal, QC - Internal Medicine
Dr Louis-Philippe Palerme, Prince George, BC - General Surgery
Dr Paula M Paley, Saskatoon, SK - Family Medicine
Dr Linda K Panaro, Ottawa, ON - Community Medicine
Dr Luigia M Pancaro, York, ON - General Practice
Dr A M Chelvi Pandian, Gatineau, QC - Family Medicine
Dr Mitchell S Pantel, Montreal, QC - Family Medicine
Dr Henriette A Panzini, Mississauga, ON - Dermatology
Dr Demetrios Papadatos, Ottawa, ON - Diagnostic-Radiology
Dr Apostolos Papageorgiou, Montreal, QC - Pediatrics
Dr Vasilios W Papanastasiou, Westmount, QC - Plastic Surgery
Dr George Papatheodorou, Toronto, ON - Psychiatry
Dr Martin Papineau, Hearst, ON - Family Medicine
Dr Vasiliki Papukna, London, ON - General Practice
Dr Lise J Paquette, Toronto, ON - Family Medicine
Dr Serge Paquette, Laval, QC - General Practice
Dr Colette Paquin, Toronto, ON - Dermatology
Dr Christian Paradis, St Thomas, ON - Family Medicine
Dr Rachelle L Paradis, Sudbury, ON - General Surgery
Dr Steven Paraskevas, Montreal, QC - General Surgery
Dr Jocelyne Parent, North York, ON - Pediatrics
Dr Lorne J Parent, Ottawa, ON - Family Medicine
Dr Yves Parent, Montreal, QC - General Practice
Dr Ian R A Park, Campbellford, ON - General Practice
Dr Joel L Parlow, Kingston, ON - Anesthesia
Dr Jillian N Parsons, St. John's, NL - Family Medicine
Dr Dante U Pascali, Nepean, ON - Obstetrics & Gynecology
Dr Sergio G Pasian, Quebec, QC - General Practice
Dr Danielle E Pastierovic, Victoria, BC - General Practice
Dr Natalia M Pastuszewska, Brantford, ON - Internal Medicine

Dr Brian L Patenaude, Gatineau, QC - Ophthalmology
Dr Stefanos Patmanidis, Woodbridge, ON - Psychiatry
Dr Katherine E Paton, Vancouver, BC - Ophthalmology
Dr Judy L Patterson, Ottawa, ON - Family Medicine
Dr Andrew R Patterson, Stouffville, ON - General Practice
Dr Michael D Paul, St. John's, NL - Internal Medicine
Dr Alan V Pavilanis, Montreal, QC - Family Medicine
Dr Elio Pavone, Oshawa, ON - Gastroenterology
Dr Brooke E Pearson, Brantford, ON - Pediatrics
Dr F Griffith Pearson, Mansfield, ON - General Surgery
Dr Jonathan L Peck, Mississauga, ON - Family Medicine
Dr Yousouf A Peerbaye, Toronto, ON - Emergency Medicine
Dr Kevin Pehr, Westmount, QC - Dermatology
Dr Denisse Pella Fernandez, Ottawa, ON - Family Medicine
Dr Michel Pellerin, Montreal, QC - Cardiovasc/ThorSurg
Dr Rene Pelletier, Quebec, QC - Medical Microbiology
Dr Alain Pelletier, Shawinigan-Sud, QC - General Practice
Dr Jean Peloquin, Quebec, QC - General Surgery
Dr Kevork Minas Peltekian, Halifax, NS - Gastroenterology
Dr Tessa M Penrod, Beaumont, AB - Family Medicine
Dr Paul Pepin, Verdun, QC - Anesthesia
Dr Paul B Percheson, North York, ON - General Practice
Dr Jose L Pereira, Ottawa, ON - Family Medicine
Dr Masis Perk, Truro, NS - Internal Medicine
Dr Robert J Perlman, Dorval, QC - General Practice
Dr Jeffrey M Pernica, Hamilton, ON - Infectious Diseases
Dr Louis P Perrault, Montreal, QC - Cardiovasc/ThorSurg
Dr Lyette Perreault, Terrebonne, QC - Diagnostic-Radiology
Dr Thomas L Perry Jr, Vancouver, BC - Internal Medicine
Dr Megan A Persson, Montreal, QC - Emergency Family Med
Dr Richard Perusse, Sherbrooke, QC - Family Medicine
Dr Lynne S Peters, Montreal, QC - Psychiatry
Dr Teresa Petraglia, Montreal, QC - Family Medicine
Dr Guy C Petroz, Toronto, ON - General Practice
Dr Christine Anh Ngoc Pham, Calgary, AB - Diagnostic-Radiology
Dr Anne-Marie Pham, Mississauga, ON - Family Medicine
Dr Martin Pham-Dinh, Gatineau, QC - Emergency Family Med
Dr T H I Dang Phan, Montreal, QC - Family Medicine
Dr Diane A Philipp, Toronto, ON - Psychiatry
Dr Debbie J Phillips, Vernon, BC - Emergency Family Med
Dr Peter G Phillips, Collingwood, ON - Family Medicine
Dr Perry Phillips, Toronto, ON - Obstetrics & Gynecology
Dr Ross E Phillips, Whitehorse, YT - Family Medicine
Dr Laura R Piccinin, Sudbury, ON - Emergency Family Med
Dr Joyce L Pickering, Montreal, QC - Internal Medicine
Dr Jean-Francois Pidgeon, Thetford Mines, QC - General Surgery
Dr Josee L Pilon, Ottawa, ON - Family Medicine
Dr Michel Pineau, Lourdes-D-Bl-Sabl, QC - Family Medicine
Dr Christian A Pineau, Montreal, QC - Internal Medicine
Dr Dana Pintea, Burlington, ON - Family Medicine
Dr Joao L P Pippi-Salle, Toronto, ON - Urology
Dr Arthur E Pires, Quebec, QC - Psychiatry
Dr Lino A Pistor, Sault Ste. Marie, ON - Psychiatry
Dr Andre Piver, Slocan Park, BC - Family Medicine
Dr Judith C Plante, Pembroke, ON - Family Medicine
Dr Virginie Plante, St-Charles-Brromee, QC - Family Medicine
Dr Robert P Pless, Ottawa, ON - General Practice
Dr Markus Ploesser, Vancouver, BC - General Practice
Dr J J Pierre Plourde, Winnipeg, MB - Infectious Diseases
Dr Pierre Plourde, Salaber-de-Valleyf, QC - Internal Medicine
Dr Joseph L Po, Ottawa, ON - Anesthesia
Dr Marc J Poirier, Gatineau, QC - General Practice
Dr Charles D Poirier, Montreal, QC - Internal Medicine
Dr Lucille J Poisson, Ottawa, ON - Family Medicine
Dr Daniel Poitras, Laval, QC - General Practice
Dr Ronald P Pokrupa, Kingston, ON - Neurosurgery
Dr Vivian A Polak, Drayton, ON - Psychiatry
Dr Steven A Poleski, Ottawa, ON - Ophthalmology
Dr Denis Poliquin, St-Jean-Sur-Richel, QC - General Surgery
Dr Michael N Pollak, Montreal, QC - Internal Medicine
Dr Robert C Polomeno, Westmount, QC - Ophthalmology
Dr Herbert A Polson, Dorval, QC - General Surgery
Dr John Pommerville, Victoria, BC - Urology
Dr David Ponka, Ottawa, ON - Emergency Family Med
Dr Alexander J Poole, Whitehorse, YT - General Surgery
Dr Ahmad Poostizadeh, Kelowna, BC - Cardiac Surgery
Dr Marc Pope, Mississauga, ON - General Surgery
Dr Stephanie A Popiel, Perth, ON - Family Medicine
Dr Ilija Popovic, Calgary, AB - General Practice
Dr Jerzy Poray-Wybranowski, Longueuil, QC - Family Medicine
Dr S Joseph Porepa, North York, ON - Pediatrics
Dr Geoffrey A Porter, Halifax, NS - General Surgery
Dr Steven D Potoker, Montreal, QC - Dermatology
Dr Kevin C Pottie, Ottawa, ON - Family Medicine
Dr Maurice Poulin, Trois-Rivieres, QC - Occupational Med
Dr David N Poulin, Saskatoon, SK - Emergency Family Med
Dr Elena Poulos, Etobicoke, ON - Dermatology
Dr Kathryn A Powell-Francis, Scarborough, ON - Anesthesia
Dr J E J Michel Prefontaine, London, ON - Obstetrics & Gynecology
Dr Zorana Prelevic, Montreal, QC - Psychiatry
Dr Jean J M Prenovault, Winnipeg, MB - Family Medicine
Dr Lise Prescott, Verdun, QC - Neurology
Dr Derek Prevost, Surrey, BC - Pediatrics
Dr Michel R Prevost, Almonte, ON - Obstetrics & Gynecology
Dr Navin Prinja, North Bay, ON - Otolaryngology
Dr Allison B Prokopiak, Stittsville, ON - Family Medicine
Dr Evan J Propst, Toronto, ON - Otolaryngology
Dr Albert Prossin, Montreal, QC - Family Medicine
Dr Normand L Proulx, Gatineau, QC - Internal Medicine
Dr Jean Proulx, St-Charles-Brromee, QC - Nephrology
Dr John Provatopoulos, Sudbury, ON - Obstetrics & Gynecology
Dr France Provencher, Laval, QC - General Practice
Dr Gerald J Prud'Homme, Toronto, ON - Anatomical Pathology
Dr Jose A Prudencio, Waterloo, ON - Otolaryngology
Dr David R Prupas, Pierrefonds, QC - General Practice
Dr Krystyna Prutis-Misterska, North York, ON - Physical Medicine & Rehab
Dr Pramod S Puligandla, Montreal, QC - Critical Care Medicine
Dr Marc Puts, Port Alberni, BC - General Practice
Dr M Shafiq Qaadri, Toronto, ON - General Practice
Dr Baqir A Qizilbash, Montreal, QC - Anesthesia
Dr Daniel R Quance, Montreal, QC - Anesthesia
Dr J A Jean Quevillon, Ottawa, ON - Cardiology
Dr Michael G Quigley, Montreal, QC - Ophthalmology
Dr Brendan P Quinn, Ottawa, ON - Cardiology
Dr M C Diane Quintal, Ottawa, ON - Dermatology
Dr Elsa S Quiros-Calinoiu, Montreal, QC - Obstetrics & Gynecology
Dr Salman T Qureshi, Montreal, QC - Critical Care Medicine
Dr Samar Raad, Temiscaming, QC - Family Medicine
Dr Faten S Rabie, Kanata, ON - General Practice
Dr Irving Rabin, Brossard, QC - Pediatrics
Dr Jed Rabinovitch, Scarborough, ON - Ophthalmology
Dr Samuel M Rabinovitch, Scarborough, ON - Diagnostic-Radiology
Dr Mark A Rabinovitch, Westmount, QC - Cardiology
Dr Nicole Racette, Vancouver, BC - Obstetrics & Gynecology
Dr Anita R Rachlis, Toronto, ON - Infectious Diseases
Dr Mohan Radhakrishna, Montreal, QC - Physical Medicine & Rehab
Dr George Rado, North York, ON - Physical Medicine & Rehab
Dr Jerry M Radziuk, Ottawa, ON - Med Scientist
Dr Stephan C Ragaz, Peterborough, ON - Family Medicine
Dr Bahaa G Ragheb, Orleans, ON - Family Medicine
Dr Roya Rahimpour, Mississauga, ON - General Practice
Dr M Rose Rahmani, Toronto, ON - Diagnostic-Radiology
Dr Faisal S Raja, Kitchener, ON - Diagnostic-Radiology
Dr Janet Rak, Thornhill, ON - Family Medicine
Dr Pawan K Ram, Surrey, BC - General Practice
Dr Denis C Ramalho, Trois-Rivieres, QC - General Practice
Dr Mathangi Ramani, Lasalle, QC - Diagnostic-Radiology
Dr Antonio Rambaldi, Varennes, QC - General Practice
Dr Droovnath Ramful, Elk Point, AB - General Practice
Dr Rajendranath Ramgoolam, Winnipeg, MB - General Practice
Dr Oswaldo C Ramirez, Alliston, ON - Family Medicine
Dr Alnoor Ramji, Vancouver, BC - Gastroenterology
Dr R Alec Ramsay, Montreal, QC - Psychiatry
Dr Jacques Ramsay, Montreal, QC - General Practice
Dr Suzanne E Ramsey, Halifax, NS - Pediatrics
Dr Rosemarie Ramsingh, Timmins, ON - Community Medicine
Dr Patrice A Ranger, Vancouver, BC - Family Medicine
Dr Alastair S Rankin, Edmonton, AB - Family Medicine
Dr Myurathy Rao, Toronto, ON - Internal Medicine
Dr Scott C Rappard, Dartmouth, NS - Internal Medicine
Dr Eugenio A Rasio, Montreal, QC - Endocrinology
Dr Michael Rasminsky, Montreal, QC - Neurology
Dr Michael B Rath, Langley, BC - Family Medicine
Dr Jack T Ratner, Montreal, QC - Gastroenterology
Dr Neil V Rau, Oakville, ON - Infectious Diseases
Dr Dietmar E Raudzus, Vancouver, BC - Family Medicine
Dr Christopher J Rauscher, Vancouver, BC - Geriatric Medicine
Dr Manisha Raut, Brossard, QC - General Practice
Dr Tarsem S Ravi, Mississauga, ON - Family Medicine
Dr Shashi K Rawal, Lemoyne, QC - General Practice
Dr Wagdy E A Rayes, Apsley, ON - General Practice
Dr Karen E Raymer, Hamilton, ON - Anesthesia
Dr Michele Raymond, Ottawa, ON - Family Medicine
Dr Yves L Raymond, Timmins, ON - Family Medicine
Dr Vincent Raymond, Quebec, QC - General Practice
Dr Felix C Re Martinez, St Catharines, ON - General Practice
Dr Mark L Reardon, Ottawa, ON - Emergency Medicine
Dr Mary-Lynne Reardon, Ottawa, ON - General Practice
Dr Margaretha Rebel, London, ON - Obstetrics & Gynecology
Dr Robert B Reddoch, Cornwall, ON - Emergency Family Med
Dr Wayne M Redmond, St. John's, NL - Otolaryngology
Dr Lynda Redwood-Campbell, Hamilton, ON - Family Medicine
Dr Nittin K Reebye, New Westminster, BC - Physical Medicine & Rehab
Dr Pratibha N Reebye, Vancouver, BC - Psychiatry
Dr Charles E Reed, Guelph, ON - General Practice
Dr Katherine M Reed, Pointe-Claire, QC - General Practice
Dr Leonora J Regenstreif, Hamilton, ON - Family Medicine
Dr Bouchra Reggad, St-Charles-Brromee, QC - Emergency Family Med
Dr Marc Regimbal, Gatineau, QC - General Practice
Dr Laura R J Regnier, Ottawa, ON - Family Medicine
Dr Heather N Reich, Toronto, ON - Internal Medicine
Dr Miles E Reid, Fort McMurray, AB - Diagnostic-Radiology
Dr Barbara A Reid, Cornwall, ON - Anatomical Pathology
Dr Diane E Reid, Hamilton, ON - Otolaryngology
Dr Kenneth R Reid, Kingston, ON - General Surgery
Dr Craig W Reid, Nepean, ON - Anesthesia
Dr Dennis Reid, Ottawa, ON - Anesthesia
Dr Annick Reid, Blainville, QC - General Practice
Dr Rudolf Reindl, Montreal, QC - Orthopedic Surgery
Dr John J Reisman, Ottawa, ON - Pediatrics
Dr Pierre Renaud, Orleans, ON - General Practice
Dr Leo P Renaud, Ottawa, ON - Med Scientist
Dr Clayton Reynolds, Victoria, BC - Internal Medicine
Dr Parisa Rezaiefar, Ottawa, ON - Family Medicine
Dr Richard K Reznick, Kingston, ON - General Surgery
Dr Paul L C Rheault, Sudbury, ON - Family Medicine
Dr Elise Rheault, Quebec, QC - General Practice
Dr Teresa A I Rheaume, Beachburg, ON - General Practice
Dr Ian N Rhodes, Ottawa, ON - Diagnostic-Radiology
Dr Flora Ricciuti, North York, ON - Family Medicine
Dr Norbert S Richard, Moncton, NB - General Practice
Dr Michael T Richard, Ottawa, ON - Neurosurgery
Dr Douglas W Richards, Toronto, ON - General Practice
Dr Donald W Richardson, Kingston, ON - Pediatrics
Dr J Donald Richardson, London, ON - Psychiatry
Dr Lawrence Richer, Edmonton, AB - Neurology
Dr Anne-Katrin Richter, Montreal, QC - Family Medicine
Dr Kenneth Richter, Montreal, QC - Psychiatry
Dr Pierre-Jacques Ricot, Pointe-Claire, QC - Pediatrics
Dr David Riddell, Cornwall, ON - Anesthesia
Dr R Markus Rieckenberg, Orillia, ON - Anatomical Pathology
Dr Daniel G Riegert, Toronto, ON - Anesthesia
Dr Claudio Rigatto, Winnipeg, MB - Internal Medicine
Dr Pierre Ringwald, Ottawa, ON - Dermatology
Dr Richard J Riopelle, Kingston, ON - Internal Medicine
Dr Janet Ritchie, Montreal, QC - Psychiatry
Dr Jose A Rivas, St-Jean-sur-Richel, QC - General Practice
Dr Linda Riven, Westmount, QC - Psychiatry
Dr Luis Rivero Pinelo, Shawville, QC - Family Medicine
Dr Jason Rivers, Vancouver, BC - Dermatology
Dr Martin Rivest, Terrebonne, QC - Emergency Family Med

Dr Andre G Rivet, North Bay, ON - General Practice
Dr Robert N Rivington, Ottawa, ON - Internal Medicine
Dr Soha R Rizk, Dartmouth, NS - Family Medicine
Dr Sarah Z Y Hanna Rizk, Bolton, ON - General Practice
Dr Barbara R Roback, Victoria, BC - Family Medicine
Dr Kerryn L Roberge, Calgary, AB - Family Medicine
Dr Roger M J Roberge, Moncton, NB - General Surgery
Dr Michael Robern, Nepean, ON - Dermatology
Dr Paul F Robert, St Catharines, ON - Orthopedic Surgery
Dr Nasreen Roberts, Kingston, ON - Psychiatry
Dr Michael C Roberts, Toronto, ON - Family Medicine
Dr Richard D Roberts, Pointe-Claire, QC - Neurology
Dr Lynne H Robertson, Calgary, AB - Dermatology
Dr Dale F Robertson, Canmore, AB - Pediatrics
Dr Barbara J Robertson, White Rock, BC - Anesthesia
Dr Nancy L Robertson, Bedford, NS - General Practice
Dr Delbe J Robichaud, Campbellton, NB - General Practice
Dr Jeffrey M Robichaud, St Catharines, ON - Otolaryngology
Dr Joan L Robillard, Vancouver, BC - General Practice
Dr Lise-Anne Robillard, Ottawa, ON - General Practice
Dr Pierre Robillard, Joliette, QC - Community Medicine
Dr Nicole Robillard, Montreal, QC - Ophthalmology
Dr Virginia W Robinson, Fernie, BC - Emergency Family Med
Dr Dale K Robinson, Markham, ON - Neurology
Dr Linda A Robinson, Ottawa, ON - Anesthesia
Dr Eric J Robinson, Sudbury, ON - Orthopedic Surgery
Dr Marie-Brigitte Robinson, Sudbury, ON - Otolaryngology
Dr Elizabeth Robinson, Montreal, QC - Community Medicine
Dr E Jean Robison, Toronto, ON - Family Medicine
Dr David Robitaille, Longueuil, QC - Psychiatry
Dr Yves Robitaille, Montreal, QC - General Pathology
Dr Robert J Robson, Elora, ON - Emergency Medicine
Dr Hugh G Robson, Montreal, QC - Internal Medicine
Dr J J C Andre Roch, Sudbury, ON - General Practice
Dr Guillermo Rocha, Brandon, MB - Ophthalmology
Dr Marie Rochette, Quebec, QC - Community Medicine
Dr Denise T Rochon, Montreal, QC - Psychiatry
Dr Celia J Rodd, Montreal, QC - Endocrin/Metabolism
Dr Marc A Rodger, Ottawa, ON - Hematology
Dr Irwin J Rodier, Montreal, QC - General Practice
Dr Americo V F Rodrigues, Ottawa, ON - General Practice
Dr Joseph Rodriguez, Montreal, QC - General Surgery
Dr Cleo C Rogakou, Newmarket, ON - Orthopedic Surgery
Dr Judith A Roger, Vancouver, BC - General Surgery
Dr M Bryson Rogers, Edmonton, AB - Dermatology
Dr Peter Rohan, Montreal, QC - General Practice
Dr Charles V Rohlicek, Montreal, QC - Cardiology
Dr Daryl S Roitman, North York, ON - Hematology
Dr Sandra Romain, Brampton, ON - Family Medicine
Dr Nancy K Romsa, St Thomas, ON - Emergency Family Med
Dr Juan J Ronco, Vancouver, BC - Internal Medicine
Dr Chantal Rondeau, Laval, QC - Emergency Family Med
Dr Mark J Ropeleski, Kingston, ON - Gastroenterology
Dr Peter D L Roper, Westmount, QC - Psychiatry
Dr Colin P Rose, Montreal, QC - Cardiology
Dr David C Rosen, Mississauga, ON - General Practice
Dr Joel Rosen, Montreal, QC - Ophthalmology
Dr Dalia S Rosen-Zaidener, Richmond Hill, ON - Family Medicine
Dr Lawrence Rosenberg, Montreal, QC - General Surgery
Dr Ellen E Rosenberg, Montreal, QC - Family Medicine
Dr Andrea Rosenbloom, Scarborough, ON - Cardiology
Dr I Shoel Rosenhek, Windsor, ON - Cardiology
Dr Donald Rosenthal, Hamilton, ON - Dermatology
Dr Gary A Rosenthal, Scarborough, ON - General Surgery
Dr Stephen E Rosenthal, Montreal, QC - Emergency Family Med
Dr Leonard Rosenthall, Montreal, QC - Diagnostic-Radiology
Dr Michael A Rosman, Saint-Leonard, QC - Orthopedic Surgery
Dr Leslie A Rosoph, North Bay, ON - Dermatology
Dr David B Ross, Edmonton, AB - Cardiovasc/ThorSurg
Dr Stephen G Ross, Toronto, ON - Family Medicine
Dr Walter W Rosser, Kingston, ON - Family Medicine
Dr John P Rossiter, Kingston, ON - Neuro-Pathology
Dr Maryam Rostami, Hamilton, ON - Family Medicine
Dr Nathan L Roth, Scarborough, ON - Obstetrics & Gynecology
Dr Steven W Rothman, Toronto, ON - Family Medicine
Dr Ann Rothman, Montreal, QC - Family Medicine
Dr John M Rothschild, Calgary, AB - Cardiovasc/ThorSurg
Dr Robert S Rothwell, New Westminster, BC - Internal Medicine
Dr Charles D Rouleau, Gatineau, QC - General Practice
Dr Jean-Lucien Rouleau, Montreal, QC - Cardiology
Dr Paul Roumeliotis, Cornwall, ON - Pediatrics
Dr Timothy W Rourke, Gloucester, ON - General Practice
Dr Louise Rousseau, Montreal, QC - Psychiatry
Dr Shelley Ann A Routhier, Hanmer, ON - Family Medicine
Dr J J Richard Routhier, Gatineau, QC - General Practice
Dr Marie-Claude Routhier, Quebec, QC - General Practice
Dr Larissa Roux, Richmond, BC - Family Medicine
Dr Bruce M T Rowat, Toronto, ON - Internal Medicine
Dr Richard Rowland, Kingston, ON - General Practice
Dr Gerald C Rowland, Tillsonburg, ON - General Practice
Dr Martine N Roy, Edmonton, AB - Obstetrics & Gynecology
Dr Maurice P Roy, Grand Falls, NB - General Practice
Dr Marc J Roy, Kanata, ON - Family Medicine
Dr Marie L Roy, North York, ON - Occupational Med
Dr Paul D Roy, Ottawa, ON - Psychiatry
Dr Nathalie A L Roy, Sudbury, ON - Family Medicine
Dr Denis Roy, Sudbury, ON - Internal Medicine
Dr Carmella A Roy, Montreal, QC - Psychiatry
Dr Indrojit Roy, Montreal, QC - Anatomical Pathology
Dr Genevieve Roy, Quebec, QC - Pediatrics
Dr Anne-Marie Roy-Boulos, Ottawa, ON - Dermatology
Dr Charmaine A Roye, Brantford, ON - Obstetrics & Gynecology
Dr Gundars E Roze, Richmond Hill, ON - Anesthesia
Dr Willine R Rozefort, Verdun, QC - Family Medicine
Dr Jan Rozehnal, Toronto, ON - General Practice
Dr Eva Rozenfarb, Repentigny, QC - Dermatology
Dr Heather Rubenstein, Montreal, QC - Family Medicine
Dr Steven E Rubenzahl, North York, ON - General Practice
Dr Mitchell B Rubin, North Vancouver, BC - Family Medicine
Dr Barry B Rubin, Toronto, ON - Vascular Surgery
Dr Gordon Rubin, Montreal, QC - Family Medicine
Dr Nicholas S Ruddock, Guelph, ON - General Practice
Dr Leona C Rudinskas, York, ON - Hematology
Dr Marc Ruel, Ottawa, ON - Cardiac Surgery
Dr Donato A Ruggiero, Toronto, ON - General Practice
Dr Edward J Rumble, North York, ON - Orthopedic Surgery
Dr Meera Ruparelia, Brockville, ON - Family Medicine
Dr Ronald Ruskin, Toronto, ON - Psychiatry
Dr Marianne T Russell, Coquitlam, BC - Family Medicine
Dr Jennifer S W Russell, Fredericton, NB - Family Medicine
Dr Barbara L Russell-Mahoney, Sioux Lookout, ON - Family Medicine
Dr Balbina Russillo, Montreal, QC - Family Medicine
Dr Mandy Ruthnum, Courtenay, BC - Family Medicine
Dr L Poovendren Ruthnum, Surrey, BC - Pediatrics
Dr Robert D H Rutledge, Halifax, NS - Radiation Oncology
Dr Edward A J Ryan, Etobicoke, ON - Obstetrics & Gynecology
Dr Salwa Saad, Mississauga, ON - General Practice
Dr Maan H A Saad, Ottawa, ON - Family Medicine
Dr Genevieve S Saad, Windsor, ON - Family Medicine
Dr Roland Sabbagh, Ottawa, ON - Cardiology
Dr Charles N J Sabbagh, Ottawa, ON - Gastroenterology
Dr I Morris Sabin, Montreal, QC - Obstetrics & Gynecology
Dr Mitchell Sabloff, Ottawa, ON - Internal Medicine
Dr J Georges Sabourin, Edmonton, AB - Obstetrics & Gynecology
Dr Marcel J L Sabourin, Ottawa, ON - Ophthalmology
Dr Boshra I Sabry, Orleans, ON - General Practice
Dr Eugene G Sacevich, Thunder Bay, ON - General Practice
Dr Ghada-Maria Saddi, Chateauguay, QC - Family Medicine
Dr Irene Sadek, Halifax, NS - Hematological Pathology
Dr Zaki K Sadik, Vaughan, ON - Family Medicine
Dr John T S Sadler, Hamilton, ON - Orthopedic Surgery
Dr Perie A Saeed, Niagara Falls, ON - General Practice
Dr Gregory C Safar, Brantford, ON - Emergency Family Med
Dr Patrick Safieh, North York, ON - Emergency Family Med
Dr Raphael Saginur, Ottawa, ON - Internal Medicine
Dr Uri Sagman, Toronto, ON - Internal Medicine
Dr Demetrios D J Sahlas, Hamilton, ON - Neurology
Dr Hani N I Sahyoun, Scarborough, ON - Psychiatry
Dr Beatriz M Sainz, Oromocto, NB - Family Medicine
Dr Rajni Saksena, Montreal, QC - Family Medicine
Dr Said S S Salama, Toronto, ON - Anesthesia
Dr Miriam Salamon, Ottawa, ON - Family Medicine
Dr Gary C Salasidis, Kitchener, ON - Cardiothor Surgery
Dr Jan M Salat, Ottawa, ON - General Practice
Dr Juan R Salcedo, Nepean, ON - Cardiology
Dr Wasfy S Saleh, Ottawa, ON - General Surgery
Dr Cherien Salem, York, ON - Family Medicine
Dr Valerie Sales, Markham, ON - Infectious Diseases
Dr David A Salisbury, Ottawa, ON - Community Medicine
Dr Irving E Salit, Toronto, ON - Internal Medicine
Dr Gurjinder P Sall, Montreal, QC - General Practice
Dr Rosaline Salo, Stratford, ON - Psychiatry
Dr Marc E J Saltel, Ottawa, ON - Urology
Dr Nancy E Salter, Toronto, ON - Psychiatry
Dr Ginetta L Salvalaggio, Edmonton, AB - Family Medicine
Dr Natacha Samedy, L'Assomption, QC - General Practice
Dr Magdi H Sami, Montreal, QC - Cardiology
Dr Karoon Samikian, Amherstview, ON - Family Medicine
Dr Linda A Samotis-Tchervenkov, Montreal, QC - Pediatrics
Dr David Samra, Scarborough, ON - Obstetrics & Gynecology
Dr Isabelle Samson, Sherbrooke, QC - Community Medicine
Dr Steve E S Samuel, North York, ON - Plastic Surgery
Dr Charles Samuel, Montreal, QC - General Practice
Dr Federico J Sanchez, Etobicoke, ON - Family Medicine
Dr Millaray Sanchez, Ottawa, ON - Family Medicine
Dr Adolfo Sanchez, Toronto, ON - Psychiatry
Dr Emilio Sanchez-Arroyo, Pointe-Claire, QC - Diagnostic-Radiology
Dr Franco Sandrin, Kirkland, QC - Cardiology
Dr Mahendra B S Sangani, Greenfield Park, QC - General Practice
Dr Hemalata J B Sangani, Greenfield Park, QC - General Practice
Dr Claudia Santos, Toronto, ON - Critical Care Medicine
Dr Tarek M Sardana, Orleans, ON - General Practice
Dr S Kemal Sartekin, Port Coquitlam, BC - Family Medicine
Dr David W Saslove, Markham, ON - General Practice
Dr Gary H Satenstein, Wakefield, QC - Family Medicine
Dr Janet L Saunderson, Toronto, ON - Pediatrics
Dr Peter Sauret, Toronto, ON - General Practice
Dr Nathalie Sauriol, Thornbury, ON - Family Medicine
Dr Anny Sauvageau, Edmonton, AB - Anatomical Pathology
Dr Michel D Sauve, Fort McMurray, AB - Critical Care Medicine
Dr Gabrielle K Savard, Calgary, AB - Family Medicine
Dr Pascal Savard, Boisbriand, QC - Dermatology
Dr Elyse Savaria, Owen Sound, ON - General Practice
Dr Nellina Saveriano, Hamilton, ON - Dermatology
Dr Mary-Lynn Savoie, Calgary, AB - Hematology
Dr Bassem Sawan, Sherbrooke, QC - Anatomical Pathology
Dr Stephanie C Sbrocchi, Sudbury, ON - Family Medicine
Dr Carmen P Scaffidi, Ville-Marie, QC - Family Medicine
Dr Jeannette E Scandar, Cornwall, ON - Family Medicine
Dr Andrew G Scarfe, Edmonton, AB - Internal Medicine
Dr Peter G H Schaal, Toronto, ON - General Surgery
Dr Joyce Schachter, Nepean, ON - Obstetrics & Gynecology
Dr Debbie C Schachter, Toronto, ON - Psychiatry
Dr Erick Schampaert, Montreal, QC - Cardiology
Dr Theodor H Schapira, Concord, ON - General Practice
Dr Lorne H Scharf, Cornwall, ON - Emergency Family Med
Dr Ariah J Schattner, Oshawa, ON - Hematology
Dr Louis J Scheinman, Etobicoke, ON - General Practice
Dr Duncan A Schellenberg, Montreal, QC - General Practice
Dr Christian H Schenk, Vancouver, BC - Psychiatry
Dr Marianne Schenker, Ottawa, ON - General Practice
Dr Gerald N Schep, Newmarket, ON - Gastroenterology
Dr Nita Scherer, Ottawa, ON - Otolaryngology
Dr Robert M Schertzer, Vancouver, BC - Ophthalmology
Dr Stephen J Schertzer, Vancouver, BC - Psychiatry
Dr Benjamin Z Schiff, Montreal, QC - Family Medicine
Dr Alicia Schiffrin, Montreal, QC - Endocrinology
Dr Mitchell J Schipper, Montreal, QC - Family Medicine
Dr Hyman M Schipper, Montreal, QC - Neurology
Dr Peter E H Schmalfuss, Bolton, ON - General Practice
Dr Howard Schneider, North York, ON - Family Medicine
Dr Gerd Schneider, Ottawa, ON - Family Medicine
Dr Ian D Schokking, Prince George, BC - Family Medicine
Dr Irving B Schonfeld, Montreal, QC - Clin Immun/Allergy

Dr Gil J Schreier, London, ON - Family Medicine
Dr Maria-Louise Schroeder, Winnipeg, MB - Pediatrics
Dr Michael J Schull, Toronto, ON - Emergency Medicine
Dr Deborah R Schuller, Toronto, ON - Psychiatry
Dr Jan I Schulz, Montreal, QC - Clin Immun/Allergy
Dr Stacey A Schwartz, Halifax, NS - Pediatrics
Dr Roslyn T Schwartz, Kingston, ON - Family Medicine
Dr Michael L Schwartz, Toronto, ON - Neurosurgery
Dr Thomas Schwartz, Cote Saint-Luc, QC - Endocrin/Metabolism
Dr Niels E Schwarz, Nanaimo, BC - Internal Medicine
Dr Gaston Schwarz, Montreal, QC - Plastic Surgery
Dr Jorge A Schwarz, Westmount, QC - Plastic Surgery
Dr Franzjosef Schweiger, Moncton, NB - Gastroenterology
Dr Morris Schweitzer, Montreal, QC - Endocrinology
Dr Lynne I Schwertfeger, Timmins, ON - Family Medicine
Dr Gregory T Scott, Kingston, ON - Family Medicine
Dr Carol L Scott, Markham, ON - General Practice
Dr Douglas F Scott, Nipigon, ON - Family Medicine
Dr Elizabeth M Scott, Ottawa, ON - General Practice
Dr John F Scott, Ottawa, ON - General Practice
Dr Robert H Scott, Toronto, ON - General Practice
Dr Hugh A Scott, Quebec, QC - Emergency Family Med
Dr Rosie Scuccimarri, Montreal, QC - Pediatrics
Dr Michael V Scully, Rossland, BC - General Practice
Dr Mary-Frances Scully, St. John's, NL - Hematology
Dr Hugh E Scully, Toronto, ON - Cardiovasc/ThorSurg
Dr Stanley K K Seah, Montreal, QC - Internal Medicine
Dr Edward R Seale, Orleans, ON - Emergency Family Med
Dr Janet E Seale, Ottawa, ON - Family Medicine
Dr Leah V Seaman, Inuvik, NT - Family Medicine
Dr Ronald D Seegobin, Kingston, ON - Anesthesia
Dr Jean M Seely, Ottawa, ON - Diagnostic-Radiology
Dr Mary V Seeman, Toronto, ON - Psychiatry
Dr Eli Segal, Montreal, QC - Emergency Medicine
Dr Marilyn Segal, Montreal, QC - Psychiatry
Dr Gerald L Seguin, Plantagenet, ON - General Practice
Dr Robert W Seguin, Sudbury, ON - General Practice
Dr Anick Seguin, Victoriaville, QC - Anesthesia
Dr Jose A C Segura, Chandler, QC - Psychiatry
Dr Dashminder Sehdev, Hamilton, ON - Emergency Family Med
Dr Yogi Sehgal, Fredericton, NB - Family Medicine
Dr Christine Seidler, South River, ON - Family Medicine
Dr Sheryl G Seidman, Toronto, ON - Family Medicine
Dr Ernest G Seidman, Montreal, QC - Pediatrics
Dr Oliver Seifert, Edmonton, AB - General Practice
Dr Eric C Seltzer, Whitby, ON - General Practice
Dr Nazia Selzner-Malekkiani, Toronto, ON - General Practice
Dr Makeda Semret, Montreal, QC - Infectious Diseases
Dr Alp Sener, London, ON - Urology
Dr Edward S Sennett, Val-d'Or, QC - Emergency Family Med
Dr Lisa M Sennewald Teskey, Surrey, BC - General Practice
Dr Mary K Senterman, Ottawa, ON - Anatomical Pathology
Dr Richard E Seppala, Ottawa, ON - Diagnostic-Radiology
Dr Didier M Serero, Montreal, QC - Emergency Family Med
Dr Consolato Sergi, Edmonton, AB - General Practice
Dr Robert N Sers, Antigonish, NS - General Surgery
Dr E Peter Seviour, St. John's, NL - Family Medicine
Dr Rosann E Seviour, St. John's, NL - Community Medicine
Dr Patricia F Seymour, Duncan, BC - Family Medicine
Dr Steven B Shadowitz, Toronto, ON - Internal Medicine
Dr Mark R Shaffer, North York, ON - Family Medicine
Dr Natalie Shaffer, Longueuil, QC - Dermatology
Dr Rajiv R Shah, Toronto, ON - Obstetrics & Gynecology
Dr Riad M A Shahid, Surrey, BC - Orthopedic Surgery
Dr Rita M Shahin, Toronto, ON - Community Medicine
Dr David R Shahin, Cote Saint-Luc, QC - General Practice
Dr Edmond B N Shahin, Cote Saint-Luc, QC - Clin Immun/Allergy
Dr Amina J Shamsie, Ottawa, ON - Family Medicine
Dr April A Shamy, Montreal, QC - Hematology
Dr Michael E Shannon, Ottawa, ON - General Practice
Dr Janet L Shannon, Saskatoon, SK - Anesthesia
Dr A M James Shapiro, Edmonton, AB - General Surgery
Dr R Jean Shapiro, Vancouver, BC - Internal Medicine
Dr Joanna L Shapiro, Etobicoke, ON - Family Medicine
Dr Thomas E Shapiro, Kanata, ON - General Practice
Dr Marla Shapiro, North York, ON - Community Medicine
Dr Stanley A Shapiro, Sudbury, ON - General Practice
Dr Solomon M Shapiro, Toronto, ON - Psychiatry
Dr Robert S Shapiro, Cote Saint-Luc, QC - Otolaryngology
Dr Abdul Q A Sharkawy, Toronto, ON - Infectious Diseases
Dr Vijay K Sharma, Miramichi, NB - Ophthalmology
Dr Arunabh B Sharma, Oshawa, ON - Internal Medicine
Dr Kamal Sharma, Ottawa, ON - Cardiology
Dr Charles S Shaver, Ottawa, ON - Internal Medicine
Dr Jinny J Shaw, Ottawa, ON - Family Medicine
Dr Thomas A W Shaw-Stiffel, Ottawa, ON - Gastroenterology
Dr Roberta M Shear, Montreal, QC - Obstetrics & Gynecology
Dr John K Shearman, Ottawa, ON - Family Medicine
Dr Ramez S H Shehata, Cambridge, ON - Anesthesia
Dr Amber Z Sheikh, Niagara Falls, ON - Ophthalmology
Dr Glenn S Sheiner, North York, ON - Emergency Family Med
Dr Sam D Shemie, Montreal, QC - Critical Care Medicine
Dr Robert L Shenker, Waterloo, ON - Plastic Surgery
Dr Nazih F Shenouda, Ottawa, ON - Diagnostic-Radiology
Dr Lois E Shepherd, Kingston, ON - Hematological Pathology
Dr Richard J Sheppard, Montreal, QC - Cardiology
Dr Nykola Sheshko, Ottawa, ON - Family Medicine
Dr Michael I Shevell, Montreal, QC - Neurology
Dr Judy Y Shiau, Ottawa, ON - Internal Medicine
Dr Henry R Shibata, Montreal, QC - General Surgery
Dr Michael E Shinder, Brossard, QC - General Practice
Dr Janet Shinder, Montreal, QC - Obstetrics & Gynecology
Dr Judith A Shindman, Toronto, ON - General Practice
Dr Joseph F Shine, Montreal, QC - Obstetrics & Gynecology
Dr Susan Shinoff, Etobicoke, ON - Obstetrics & Gynecology
Dr Caroline A Shooner, Queen Charlotte, BC - Family Medicine
Dr S Ronald Shorser, Toronto, ON - General Practice
Dr Ian Shrier, Montreal, QC - General Practice
Dr Raymond M Shu, Scarborough, ON - Pediatrics
Dr Samuel Shuldiner, Montreal, QC - General Practice
Dr Barbara Shulman, Vancouver, BC - Psychiatry
Dr Dominique Shum-Tim, Montreal, QC - Cardiothor Surgery
Dr Michael Shupak, Toronto, ON - General Practice
Dr Michael Shuster, Banff, AB - Emergency Medicine
Dr Joseph Shuster, Montreal, QC - Med Scientist
Dr Ying Tung Sia, Alexandria, ON - Cardiology
Dr Joanne E Sicard, Ottawa, ON - Family Medicine
Dr Dolores A Sicheri, Thunder Bay, ON - Internal Medicine
Dr Jaime Siclait, Boisbriand, QC - Family Medicine
Dr Jean-Guy Sicotte, Magog, QC - General Practice
Dr Abdallah Y Sidky, Vancouver, BC - Psychiatry
Dr Lee F Siebert, London, ON - Ophthalmology
Dr Irving J Siegel, Brampton, ON - General Practice
Dr Deborah G Siemiatycki, North York, ON - Pediatrics
Dr Ronald J Sigal, Calgary, AB - Endocrin/Metabolism
Dr Eric H Sigman, Montreal, QC - Emergency Family Med
Dr Karen G Sigman, Montreal, QC - Clin Immun/Allergy
Dr Theodore N Siller, Scarborough, ON - Orthopedic Surgery
Dr Enrique Silva, Pembroke, ON - Anatomical Pathology
Dr Michael Silver, Scarborough, ON - Obstetrics & Gynecology
Dr Barry L Silver, Dorval, QC - Ophthalmology
Dr Alexis S W Silverberg, Peterborough, ON - General Practice
Dr Mark S Silverman, Ottawa, ON - Endocrin/Metabolism
Dr Howard J Silverman, Ottawa, ON - Plastic Surgery
Dr Melvin Silverman, Toronto, ON - Internal Medicine
Dr Ezra A Silverstein, Toronto, ON - Orthopedic Surgery
Dr Fanny Silviu-Dan, Montreal, QC - Clin Immun/Allergy
Dr Quan-Yong Sim, Ottawa, ON - Family Medicine
Dr Emmanuel Simantirakis, Ottawa, ON - Diagnostic-Radiology
Dr Jovan G Simeon, Vanier, ON - Psychiatry
Dr Jeannine G M Simon, Pointe-Claire, QC - Obstetrics & Gynecology
Dr Andrew A Simone, Etobicoke, ON - Dermatology
Dr Martin Simonik, North York, ON - General Practice
Dr E Rand Simpson, North York, ON - Ophthalmology
Dr Richard B Simpson, Toronto, ON - Psychiatry
Dr Christopher H Sims, Calgary, AB - Anesthesia
Dr Richard H Sims, Toronto, ON - Obstetrics & Gynecology
Dr Thomas M Sinclair, Canmore, AB - Plastic Surgery
Dr William Singer, East York, ON - Internal Medicine
Dr Debrah G C Singer, Thornhill, ON - Endocrin/Metabolism
Dr Michael I Singer, Pointe-Claire, QC - Dermatology
Dr Jonathan Singerman, Montreal, QC - Emergency Family Med
Dr Harpal Singh, Burlington, ON - Family Medicine
Dr Sheila K Singh, Hamilton, ON - Neurosurgery
Dr Kunwar K Singh, Sarnia, ON - Pediatrics
Dr Parul Singh, Toronto, ON - Emergency Family Med
Dr Santokh Singh, Montreal, QC - Psychiatry
Dr Anna Barbara Sinsky, Terrebonne, QC - Diagnostic-Radiology
Dr Richard Sioufi, Chateauguay, QC - Urology
Dr Shireen M Sirhan, Cowansville, QC - Hematology
Dr Denis Sirhan, Montreal, QC - Neurosurgery
Dr Giovanna Sirianni, Toronto, ON - Family Medicine
Dr Mehmet R Sirman, York, ON - Psychiatry
Dr M M Jeanne Sirois, Gatineau, QC - General Practice
Dr Marcia Sirota, Toronto, ON - Psychiatry
Dr Jeffrey Sirzyk, Hawkesbury, ON - Emergency Family Med
Dr Sze Wan Sit, Toronto, ON - Family Medicine
Dr Vahe Sivaciyan, Toronto, ON - Cardiology
Dr Marco L A Sivilotti, Kingston, ON - Emergency Medicine
Dr Patrick J Skalenda, Toronto, ON - Family Medicine
Dr Christopher R R Skinner, Ottawa, ON - Internal Medicine
Dr Marsha C Sklar, Montreal, QC - Anatomical Pathology
Dr Anna K Skorzewska, Toronto, ON - Psychiatry
Dr Monica J Skrukwa, Calgary, AB - Family Medicine
Dr Barry Slapcoff, Westmount, QC - Family Medicine
Dr Jonathan D Slater, Kelowna, BC - Pediatrics
Dr David N Slaughter, York, ON - Internal Medicine
Dr Marie N Slegr, Toronto, ON - Internal Medicine
Dr Peter D Slinger, Toronto, ON - Anesthesia
Dr David A Sliwowicz, Ajax, ON - General Practice
Dr Jeffrey P E Sloan, Sudbury, ON - Anesthesia
Dr Allan R Slomovic, Toronto, ON - Ophthalmology
Dr Jane E Sly, Ottawa, ON - General Practice
Dr Allison M Small, Huntsville, ON - Family Medicine
Dr Lorne N Small, Mississauga, ON - Infectious Diseases
Dr Donald S Smallman, Kingston, ON - Ophthalmology
Dr Christina A Smeja, Eastmain, QC - General Practice
Dr Helen Smeja, Pierrefonds, QC - General Practice
Dr Charlene R Smelsky, Winnipeg, MB - Family Medicine
Dr Mark Smilovitch, Montreal, QC - Cardiology
Dr Lesley J Smith, Edmonton, AB - Pediatrics
Dr Gregory L Smith, Raymond, AB - Family Medicine
Dr M C Patricia Smith, Hearst, ON - Family Medicine
Dr Bryan V Smith, Kanata, ON - Internal Medicine
Dr David P Smith, Kitchener, ON - Pediatrics
Dr Crystal A Smith, Markham, ON - Orthopedic Surgery
Dr W Gary Smith, Orillia, ON - Pediatrics
Dr Kevin D Smith, Ottawa, ON - Ophthalmology
Dr Daniel N Smith, Ottawa, ON - Family Medicine
Dr C Douglas Smith, Ottawa, ON - Internal Medicine
Dr Oakley D Smith, Toronto, ON - Otolaryngology
Dr Roger M L Smith, Toronto, ON - General Practice
Dr Donald A Smith, Toronto, ON - Family Medicine
Dr Graham H R Smith, Toronto, ON - Family Medicine
Dr Edward J Smith, Vanier, ON - General Practice
Dr Julia A Smith, Windsor, ON - Anesthesia
Dr Jacqueline A Smith-Auguste, North York, ON - Orthopedic Surgery
Dr Alma J Smitheringale, North York, ON - Otolaryngology
Dr David J Smosarski, Hamilton, ON - General Practice
Dr Galina Smushkin, Victoria, BC - General Practice
Dr Michael G B Smylie, Edmonton, AB - Internal Medicine
Dr Harley S Smyth, Mississauga, ON - Neurosurgery
Dr Catherine E Smyth, Ottawa, ON - Anesthesia
Dr Wayne R Snook, Orleans, ON - General Practice
Dr Esther A M Soccar, Ottawa, ON - Family Medicine
Dr Steven J Socransky, Sudbury, ON - Emergency Medicine
Dr Adrian B T Sohn, Guelph, ON - Family Medicine
Dr Avrum A Soicher, Brampton, ON - Internal Medicine
Dr Dina R Sokoloff, Ottawa, ON - Family Medicine
Dr Robert S Solomon, Toronto, ON - Dermatology
Dr Leslie J Solomon, Cote Saint-Luc, QC - Family Medicine
Dr Peter H Solomon, Gatineau, QC - Anesthesia
Dr Daniel Solonyna, Pointe-Claire, QC - Psychiatry
Dr George I M Soltys, Greenfield Park, QC - Internal Medicine
Dr Susan Solymoss, Montreal, QC - Hematology

Dr Peter J Somerville, Guelph, ON - Internal Medicine
Dr Hillel M Sommer, Winnipeg, MB - Physical Medicine & Rehab
Dr Elena Somska, Toronto, ON - General Practice
Dr Michael J Sonea, Montreal, QC - Dermatology
Dr Anne Song, Ottawa, ON - Family Medicine
Dr Deepa Soni, Mississauga, ON - Emergency Family Med
Dr Alok Pal Sood, Toronto, ON - Family Medicine
Dr Shawn J Soon, Scarborough, ON - Urology
Dr Curtis J Sorgini, Sudbury, ON - Ophthalmology
Dr Alain G Sotto, Brampton, ON - General Practice
Dr Jean-Pierre Souaid, Ottawa, ON - Otolaryngology
Dr Elaine Soucy, Mississauga, ON - Internal Medicine
Dr J L Rene Soucy, Ottawa, ON - Family Medicine
Dr Renee Soucy, Chandler, QC - Obstetrics & Gynecology
Dr Luis Souhami, Montreal, QC - Radiation Oncology
Dr Fibi B W Sourial, Brampton, ON - Family Medicine
Dr Myra Sourkes, Toronto, ON - Electroencephal
Dr Joaquin F Sousa-Poza, Galiano, BC - Psychiatry
Dr Silvana Spadafora, Sault Ste. Marie, ON - Internal Medicine
Dr Joseph J Spano, Sarnia, ON - General Practice
Dr Richard C Spees, Ottawa, ON - Psychiatry
Dr Martin H Spencer, Nanaimo, BC - Ophthalmology
Dr Jon R L Spencer, North Bay, ON - Ophthalmology
Dr Helen R Spenser, Vanier, ON - Family Medicine
Dr Stanley Spier, Thornhill, ON - Dermatology
Dr Linda S Spigelblatt, Montreal, QC - Pediatrics
Dr John S Spika, Ottawa, ON - General Practice
Dr Rachel F Spitzer, Toronto, ON - Obstetrics & Gynecology
Dr Gwendoline M Spurll, Montreal, QC - Hematology
Dr Philip J R Squires, Stratford, ON - Pediatrics
Dr Srikala S Sridhar, Toronto, ON - Internal Medicine
Dr Philip D St John, Winnipeg, MB - Geriatric Medicine
Dr John E M St Rose, Peterborough, ON - General Practice
Dr Marc A St-Amand, London, ON - Anesthesia
Dr Eric St-Amour, Gatineau, QC - Family Medicine
Dr Julie St-Cyr, Montreal, QC - Anatomical Pathology
Dr Maurice St-Martin, Sudbury, ON - General Practice
Dr Sabrina M Stables, Toronto, ON - General Practice
Dr Gordon M Stahl, Vancouver, BC - Family Medicine
Dr Jonathan M S Standley, Bath, ON - General Practice
Dr Timothy R Stanford, Barrie, ON - Family Medicine
Dr Michael A Stanger, Victoria, BC - Orthopedic Surgery
Dr Valerie I Stanzl, Lethbridge, AB - Obstetrics & Gynecology
Dr Janet A Star, Toronto, ON - Pediatrics
Dr Philippe E Starosta, Kanata, ON - Family Medicine
Dr Michael R Starr, Pointe-Claire, QC - Internal Medicine
Dr Ronald F Starra, Gatineau, QC - Internal Medicine
Dr Ferdinand M Stasiak, North Vancouver, BC - General Practice
Dr Ewa M Stasiak, Montreal, QC - General Practice
Dr Christa Staudenmaier, St-Jean-Sur-Richel, QC - Ophthalmology
Dr Micheline T Ste-Marie, Montreal, QC - Gastroenterology
Dr Louis-Georges Ste-Marie, Montreal, QC - Endocrinology
Dr Liora R Steele, Mitchell, ON - Family Medicine
Dr Daniel C Steeves, Lethbridge, AB - General Practice
Dr Rodica Stefaniu, York, ON - Psychiatry
Dr Snezana Stegnajic, East York, ON - Family Medicine
Dr Nolan-Paul A Stein, Toronto, ON - General Practice
Dr Barry L Stein, Montreal, QC - General Surgery
Dr Michael A Stein, Montreal, QC - Internal Medicine
Dr Naomi B Stein, Westmount, QC - Pediatrics
Dr Jeffrey C Stein, Saskatoon, SK - Internal Medicine
Dr George Steiner, Toronto, ON - Internal Medicine
Dr Warren Steiner, Montreal, QC - Psychiatry
Dr Daniel K Steinitz, Belleville, ON - Orthopedic Surgery
Dr Tracy L F Steinitz, Belleville, ON - Emergency Family Med
Dr Martin W Steinruck, Kelowna, BC - Family Medicine
Dr Michael Steirman, Markham, ON - Diagnostic-Radiology
Dr Karen G Stel, Scarborough, ON - Family Medicine
Dr Josef Stelzer, Winnipeg, MB - General Practice
Dr Ashleigh D Stelzer-Chilton, Vancouver, BC - Family Medicine
Dr Christopher J Stemerdink, Guelph, ON - Family Medicine
Dr James E Stempien, Saskatoon, SK - Emergency Family Med
Dr Robert J Stenstrom, Vancouver, BC - Emergency Family Med
Dr Paul K Stephenson, Montreal, QC - Orthopedic Surgery
Dr Carlo Sterlin, Montreal, QC - Psychiatry
Dr Hartley S Stern, Montreal, QC - General Surgery
Dr Jerry Stern, Montreal, QC - Diagnostic-Radiology
Dr David A Steven, London, ON - Neurosurgery
Dr Samuel D Stevens, Brockville, ON - Ophthalmology
Dr Katrina G Stevens, Kingston, ON - General Practice
Dr Colin G Stevenson, Hamilton, ON - Family Medicine
Dr Robert F Stevenson, Sault Ste. Marie, ON - Ophthalmology
Dr Lindsay C Stewart, Nepean, ON - Emergency Family Med
Dr John P Stewart, Orleans, ON - General Practice
Dr David J Stewart, Ottawa, ON - Internal Medicine
Dr Duncan J Stewart, Ottawa, ON - Cardiology
Dr James A Stewart, Montreal, QC - Cardiology
Dr Simona Stiharu, Pierrefonds, QC - Family Medicine
Dr Janet E Still, Ottawa, ON - General Practice
Dr Karen L Stillman, Almonte, ON - Obstetrics & Gynecology
Dr John M Stimac, Hamilton, ON - Cardiology
Dr Kent Stobart, Edmonton, AB - Pediatrics
Dr Susan R Stock, Montreal, QC - Community Medicine
Dr Jayson M Stoffman, Winnipeg, MB - Hematology
Dr Cynthia Stolovitz, Montreal, QC - Emergency Family Med
Dr Katherine J Stoltz, St Catharines, ON - Internal Medicine
Dr Susan J V Stone, North York, ON - Family Medicine
Dr David G W Storey, Langley, BC - Anesthesia
Dr Brian R Stotland, Newmarket, ON - Gastroenterology
Dr Antonio P Strafella, Toronto, ON - Neurology
Dr Maurice Strasfeld, New Glasgow, NS - General Practice
Dr Marina A Straszak-Suri, Nepean, ON - Obstetrics & Gynecology
Dr Philip A T Stratford, Cobourg, ON - Family Medicine
Dr Hanka H E A Stratmann, Woodbridge, ON - Family Medicine
Dr Stephen Strigler, Toronto, ON - Family Medicine
Dr Helene G Strobach, Montreal, QC - General Practice
Dr Roger D Stronell, Kitchener, ON - Diagnostic-Radiology
Dr Philip F Stuart, North York, ON - Medical Microbiology
Dr Howard R Stuart, Montreal, QC - Emergency Family Med
Dr Lucille Stuart, Whitehorse, YT - Family Medicine
Dr Shelly Sud, Ottawa, ON - Family Medicine
Dr Tamar Sudai, North York, ON - Family Medicine
Dr Jean C Suk, Ottawa, ON - Pediatrics
Dr Irma-Nancy Sully, Ottawa, ON - Family Medicine
Dr Soraya G S Sultan, Montreal, QC - Psychiatry
Dr Omar Sultan, Regina, SK - Cardiology
Dr Manickavasagam Sundaram, Oshawa, ON - Family Medicine
Dr Dorothy J Sunderland, Collingwood, ON - Family Medicine
Dr Diann J Superina-Bell, Toronto, ON - Pediatrics
Dr Rita Suri, Montreal, QC - Internal Medicine
Dr Monica Susil, Lively, ON - Family Medicine
Dr Jonathan Sussman, Hamilton, ON - Family Medicine
Dr Emile D Svarc, Montreal, QC - Ophthalmology
Dr Pavol Sventek, Val-d'Or, QC - Family Medicine
Dr William J Svihovec, Longueuil, QC - General Practice
Dr Ganesh Swamy, Calgary, AB - Orthopedic Surgery
Dr Andrew C Swan, Victoria, BC - Family Medicine
Dr Margaret E Sweet, Thunder Bay, ON - Neurology
Dr Robert C G Sweet Jr, Montreal, QC - Otolaryngology
Dr J Robert Swenson, Ottawa, ON - Psychiatry
Dr Richard O Swieca, Salaber-de-Valleyf, QC - Ophthalmology
Dr Jacques P E Sylvain, Ottawa, ON - Obstetrics & Gynecology
Dr Michael J Sylvester, Kingston, ON - Family Medicine
Dr Colin W Syme, Ajax, ON - General Practice
Dr Anne R Synnes, Vancouver, BC - Pediatrics
Dr Michael S Szabo, Toronto, ON - Emergency Family Med
Dr Eileen M Szabo, Saskatoon, SK - Internal Medicine
Dr Blazej I Szczygielski, Kuujjuaq, QC - Emergency Family Med
Dr Peter L Szego, Montreal, QC - Gastroenterology
Dr Tibor J Sziklas, Montreal, QC - General Practice
Dr Andrew Szilagyi, Montreal, QC - Gastroenterology
Dr Nadia Szkrumelak, Montreal, QC - Psychiatry
Dr Isaac I E Szpindel, Toronto, ON - General Practice
Dr Ewa F Szumacher, Toronto, ON - Radiation Oncology
Dr Wanda M Szymonowicz, Mississauga, ON - Pediatrics
Dr Roger J Tabah, Montreal, QC - General Surgery
Dr Cherif Tadros, Edmonton, AB - Orthopedic Surgery
Dr Sharif W Tadros, Burlington, ON - General Practice
Dr Shaheer Tadros, Ottawa, ON - General Surgery
Dr Emmanuel H Tadross, Kitchener, ON - Psychiatry
Dr Mohammed Tagemouati, Pointe claire, QC - General Practice
Dr Majd Tahan, Salaber-de-Valleyf, QC - Internal Medicine
Dr Michel Taillefer, Saint-Sauveur, QC - General Practice
Dr Paul A Taillon, Saskatoon, SK - Family Medicine
Dr Nagwa A Takla, St Catharines, ON - Family Medicine
Dr Jo-Ann Talbot, Saint John, NB - Emergency Medicine
Dr John P Taliano, St Catharines, ON - General Practice
Dr Peter Talko, Shawville, QC - General Practice
Dr Chiranjib Talukdar, Regina, SK - Pediatrics
Dr Edwin M Tam, Vancouver, BC - Psychiatry
Dr Ronald K H Tam, Ottawa, ON - Pediatrics
Dr Sydney P Tam, Toronto, ON - Family Medicine
Dr Domenica Tambasco, Toronto, ON - Family Medicine
Dr Robert Tambay, Ottawa, ON - Gastroenterology
Dr Charles C Tan, Richmond Hill, ON - General Practice
Dr Darrell H S Tan, Toronto, ON - Infectious Diseases
Dr Seang Lin Tan, Montreal, QC - Obstetrics & Gynecology
Dr Christine E Tang, Mississauga, ON - Emergency Family Med
Dr Alexander W L Tang, North York, ON - Anesthesia
Dr Joanne A Tannenbaum, Ottawa, ON - Family Medicine
Dr David W Tannenbaum, Toronto, ON - Family Medicine
Dr Terry-Nan Tannenbaum, Montreal, QC - Community Medicine
Dr Anita D Tannis, West Vancouver, BC - Family Medicine
Dr Rosemonde E Tannous, Niagara Falls, ON - Cardiology
Dr Waguih N Tannous, Montreal, QC - Family Medicine
Dr Lisa H Taras, Ottawa, ON - Family Medicine
Dr Fadi Tarazi, Burnaby, BC - Orthopedic Surgery
Dr Gaetan Tardif, Toronto, ON - Physical Medicine & Rehab
Dr Daniel Tardif, Cantley, QC - General Practice
Dr Sue R Tatemichi, Fredericton, NB - Family Medicine
Dr Richard H B Tatham, Penticton, BC - Family Medicine
Dr Philippa J Tattersall, Hamilton, ON - General Practice
Dr Fabiano A S Taucer, Ottawa, ON - Diagnostic-Radiology
Dr Robert F Tautkus, Brampton, ON - Family Medicine
Dr Franco G Tavazzani, Brampton, ON - Orthopedic Surgery
Dr F Georges Tawagi, Nepean, ON - Obstetrics & Gynecology
Dr James D N Taylor, Victoria, BC - Ophthalmology
Dr Gretta Taylor, Halifax, NS - Family Medicine
Dr John D Taylor, Chapleau, ON - General Practice
Dr Michael R Taylor, Ottawa, ON - Emergency Family Med
Dr J Robert M Taylor, Ottawa, ON - Hematology
Dr Elaine M Taylor, Ottawa, ON - Family Medicine
Dr John P T F Taylor, Sarnia, ON - General Surgery
Dr Bryce R Taylor, Toronto, ON - General Surgery
Dr William J Taylor, Windsor, ON - Anesthesia
Dr Sophia B Tchervenkov, Montreal, QC - Obstetrics & Gynecology
Dr Jean I Tchervenkov, Montreal, QC - General Surgery
Dr Christo I Tchervenkov, Montreal, QC - Cardiovasc/ThorSurg
Dr Milka A Tchervenkova, Brossard, QC - General Practice
Dr Lynne D Teasell, Okotoks, AB - General Practice
Dr Nathalie Teboul, Gatineau, QC - Ophthalmology
Dr Eric A Teboul, Saint-Jerome, QC - Psychiatry
Dr Barbara K Teboul, Salaber-de-Valleyf, QC - Ophthalmology
Dr Susan E Tector, Ottawa, ON - Emergency Family Med
Dr Lori E Teeple, Zurich, ON - Emergency Family Med
Dr Ingrid Tein, Toronto, ON - Pediatrics
Dr Peter S Teitelbaum, Ottawa, ON - General Practice
Dr Raymond J M Tellier, Calgary, AB - Medical Microbiology
Dr Adam H Telner, East York, ON - Endocrin/Metabolism
Dr Abdelkader Temkit, Gatineau, QC - General Practice
Dr Danny S Tenaschuk, Ottawa, ON - Diagnostic-Radiology
Dr Lionel Tenby, Richmond, BC - General Practice
Dr Jamie L Tepper, Oshawa, ON - Clin Immun/Allergy
Dr Hendrik Ter Keurs, Calgary, AB - Internal Medicine
Dr Artin M Ternamian, Toronto, ON - Obstetrics & Gynecology
Dr Yoseph Tesfaye, Montreal, QC - General Practice
Dr Luke M Teskey, Surrey, BC - General Practice
Dr Julie L Tessier, Kingston, ON - Obstetrics & Gynecology
Dr Pierre C Tessier, Ottawa, ON - Family Medicine
Dr Guylaine Tessier, Gatineau, QC - Family Medicine
Dr Michael J Tessler, Montreal, QC - Anesthesia
Dr Louise-Marie Tetrault, Ottawa, ON - General Practice
Dr Tewfik L Tewfik, Montreal, QC - Otolaryngology
Dr Susan P L Tha, Vancouver, BC - Anatomical Pathology
Dr Bernard C F Thebaud, Edmonton, AB - Pediatrics

Dr Lilly Thenganatt, East York, ON - Family Medicine
Dr John S Theodoropoulos, Toronto, ON - Orthopedic Surgery
Dr Francois A J Theoret, Hawkesbury, ON - Family Medicine
Dr M Y Diane Theriault, Dartmouth, NS - Internal Medicine
Dr Caroline Thibault, LaSalle, QC - Family Medicine
Dr Jean-Louis Thibodeau, Saint-Jacques, NB - General Practice
Dr Celeste J Thirlwell, Toronto, ON - Psychiatry
Dr Michael P Thirlwell, Montreal, QC - Internal Medicine
Dr Robert B Thirsk, Longueuil, QC - General Practice
Dr Roger E Thomas, Calgary, AB - Family Medicine
Dr Mary Ann Thomas, Calgary, AB - Medical Genetics
Dr Roger H Thomas, Richmond, BC - Ophthalmology
Dr Richard P Thomas, Kingston, ON - Obstetrics & Gynecology
Dr Michele D Thomasse, Kelowna, BC - Family Medicine
Dr Michael G Thomassin, Montreal, QC - Family Medicine
Dr Thomas R Thompson, Winnipeg, MB - Psychiatry
Dr David K Thompson, Brantford, ON - Family Medicine
Dr Calvin P Thompson, Ottawa, ON - Anesthesia
Dr Tracey A Thompson, Gatineau, QC - Plastic Surgery
Dr Leanne M Thomson, Kincardine, ON - Family Medicine
Dr John G Thomson, Ottawa, ON - Internal Medicine
Dr Larry S Thorsteinson, Sudbury, ON - Emergency Family Med
Dr M Lynne Thurling, Fergus, ON - Psychiatry
Dr Peter R Thurston, Ottawa, ON - Orthopedic Surgery
Dr Maria-Elena Tiboni, Hamilton, ON - Internal Medicine
Dr Brian Ticoll, Markham, ON - Psychiatry
Dr Lorenzo P Tincoca, Sorel-Tracy, QC - Internal Medicine
Dr Alan T Tinmouth, Ottawa, ON - Hematology
Dr Marion A Tipple, Vancouver, BC - Pediatric Cardiology
Dr Rossana M Tirado, Orleans, ON - Pediatrics
Dr Jacques G Tittley, Hamilton, ON - General Surgery
Dr Christo Todorov, Montreal, QC - Psychiatry
Dr Ian P Toft, St Thomas, ON - Family Medicine
Dr Daniel R Toledano, Toronto, ON - General Practice
Dr Richard D Tombler, Cornwall, ON - Orthopedic Surgery
Dr Eva M Tomiak, Ottawa, ON - Internal Medicine
Dr Heather A Tomlin, Toronto, ON - Diagnostic-Radiology
Dr Thanh-Thao Ton-Nu, St-Charles-Brromee, QC - Cardiology
Dr Quoc-Huy Ton-That, Montreal, QC - Emergency Family Med
Dr Daniel Y Tong, Vancouver, BC - General Practice
Dr Christina Tong, Westmount, QC - Family Medicine
Dr Nestor E Torres Martinez, Brockville, ON - Family Medicine
Dr Caroline M A Tosoni, Orleans, ON - Family Medicine
Dr Adam A Toth, Etobicoke, ON - Otolaryngology
Dr Joseph Toth, Montreal, QC - Diagnostic-Radiology
Dr Andre P Touchburn, Moncton, NB - Emergency Family Med
Dr Michael J Touchie, Ottawa, ON - General Practice
Dr Claire E Touchie, Ottawa, ON - Infectious Diseases
Dr June A D Tourangeau, Toronto, ON - Anesthesia
Dr Claude P J Tousignant, Toronto, ON - Anesthesia
Dr Michel P Tousignant, Grand-Mere, QC - General Practice
Dr Jean Tousignant, Trois-Rivieres, QC - Anesthesia
Dr M Junie B Toussaint, Toronto, ON - General Practice
Dr Carol A Townsley, Toronto, ON - Family Medicine
Dr William Toy, LaSalle, QC - General Practice
Dr John W Toye, Orillia, ON - Plastic Surgery
Dr Nancy M Tozer, Pointe-Claire, QC - Family Medicine
Dr John Trachtenberg, Toronto, ON - Urology
Dr Chaim J Trager, Markham, ON - General Practice
Dr J Simon-Pierre Trahan, Russell, ON - General Practice
Dr T G Joe Tran, Mississauga, ON - General Practice
Dr Van Nham Tran, Mississauga, ON - General Practice
Dr Bernie B C Tran, North York, ON - General Practice
Dr Viet Tan Tran, Ottawa, ON - Urology
Dr Vu-Kiet Tran, Scarborough, ON - Emergency Family Med
Dr Teresa B C Tran, Vaughan, ON - Family Medicine
Dr Van-Dung Tran, Montreal, QC - General Practice
Dr John Tranqui, Mississauga, ON - General Practice
Dr Sean A Travers, North Bay, ON - Anesthesia
Dr Darin J Treleaven, Hamilton, ON - Internal Medicine
Dr Alain Tremblay, Calgary, AB - Internal Medicine
Dr Pierre-Michel Tremblay, Moncton, NB - General Practice
Dr Michele M Tremblay, Ottawa, ON - Psychiatry
Dr Lorraine N Tremblay, Toronto, ON - General Surgery
Dr Gilles R Tremblay, Montreal, QC - Orthopedic Surgery
Dr Marie-Claude Tremblay, Sainte-Therese, QC - Ophthalmology
Dr Jacques Tremblay, Verdun, QC - General Practice
Dr Jean R Trepanier, Ottawa, ON - General Practice
Dr Stephane N Treyvaud, Oakville, ON - Psychiatry
Dr Mark A Trifiro, Montreal, QC - Internal Medicine
Dr Thomas Q N Trinh, Langley, BC - Family Medicine
Dr Ngoc Chau Trinh, Gatineau, QC - General Practice
Dr Nathalie Trinh, Montreal, QC - Otolaryngology
Dr Maria G Trivieri, Toronto, ON - Internal Medicine
Dr Daria A Trojan, Montreal, QC - Physical Medicine & Rehab
Dr A Karen Trollope, Hamilton, ON - Family Medicine
Dr Myron Troster, Stratford, ON - Anatomical Pathology
Dr Kiril Trpkov, Calgary, AB - Anatomical Pathology
Dr Margaret B Truchan, Saskatoon, SK - Internal Medicine
Dr Michel L Truchon, Bonfield, ON - General Practice
Dr Marc Trudeau, Medicine Hat, AB - Internal Medicine
Dr Chantal D Trudeau, Moncton, NB - Cardiology
Dr Suzanne M Trudel, Toronto, ON - Hematology
Dr Pauline T Truong, Victoria, BC - Radiation Oncology
Dr Dang-Toan Truong, Nepean, ON - Diagnostic-Radiology
Dr Cong Phuc Truong, Louiseville, QC - General Practice
Dr Willis H Tsai, Calgary, AB - Internal Medicine
Dr Ellen Tsai, Ottawa, ON - Pediatrics
Dr Victor T L Tsang, Vancouver, BC - General Surgery
Dr W Y Eliza Tsang, Markham, ON - Family Medicine
Dr Jonathan R Tsao, Mississauga, ON - Radiation Oncology
Dr Leonard W H Tse, Toronto, ON - General Surgery
Dr Georges Tsoukas, Montreal, QC - Endocrinology
Dr Christos M Tsoukas, Montreal, QC - Internal Medicine
Dr Joan M Tucker, North York, ON - Psychiatry
Dr Nancy A Tucker, Toronto, ON - Ophthalmology
Dr Elrie C Tucker, Montreal, QC - Obstetrics & Gynecology
Dr Izolda L Tuhan Mirza Baranowski, Timmins, ON - Psychiatry
Dr Raman Tuli, Ottawa, ON - Ophthalmology
Dr Jennifer I L Tupper, Banff, AB - Emergency Family Med
Dr Astrid E Tupper, Calgary, AB - Family Medicine
Dr Jean-Francois Turcotte, Quebec, QC - Neurosurgery
Dr Nathalie Turgeon, Quebec, QC - Medical Microbiology
Dr David T Turineck, Smooth Rock Falls, ON - General Practice
Dr Jolanda C Turley, Ottawa, ON - Family Medicine
Dr John D Turnbull, Hamilton, ON - Internal Medicine
Dr Mark O Turner, Surrey, BC - Internal Medicine
Dr D Christopher Turner, Ottawa, ON - Pediatrics
Dr Howard M Turner, Montreal, QC - Internal Medicine
Dr Joel P Turner, Montreal, QC - Emergency Medicine
Dr Lucy M Turnham, Vancouver, BC - General Practice
Dr Victoria E Tuvivovich, Salaber-de-Valleyf, QC - General Practice
Dr Thom V Tyson, Ottawa, ON - General Practice
Dr Simeon G Tzeneff, Ottawa, ON - General Practice
Dr Sameena Uddin, Mississauga, ON - General Surgery
Dr Peter A F Uhthoff, Ottawa, ON - General Practice
Dr Sylvia Uhthoff Munro, Ottawa, ON - General Practice
Dr Gintaras T Uleckas, North York, ON - Family Medicine
Dr Jurate K Uleckas, Laval, QC - Ophthalmology
Dr Lorne N Umemoto, Quebec, QC - Clin Immun/Allergy
Dr Chantelle Y W Ung, North York, ON - Dermatology
Dr Berton Y K Ung, Scarborough, ON - Family Medicine
Dr Sharon L Unger, Toronto, ON - Pediatrics
Dr Bernard Unger, Montreal, QC - Emergency Family Med
Dr Linda M Uniat, Edmonton, AB - Ophthalmology
Dr Adrian R M Upton, Hamilton, ON - Neurology
Dr Jean-Luc C P Urbain, Brantford, ON - Nuclear Medicine
Dr R Pierre Urbanski, Lasalle, QC - Pediatrics
Dr H Richard Uretsky, Edmonton, AB - Obstetrics & Gynecology
Dr Jean-Philippe Vaccani, Ottawa, ON - Otolaryngology
Dr Mylene J Vachet, Rockland, ON - Family Medicine
Dr Gabriel A Vadasz, Toronto, ON - Family Medicine
Dr Shailla Vaidya, Toronto, ON - Emergency Family Med
Dr Peter Vaktor, Montreal, QC - General Practice
Dr David A Valenti, Montreal, QC - Diagnostic-Radiology
Dr Pamela Valentino, Toronto, ON - Gastroenterology
Dr Nicholas Valettas, Hamilton, ON - Cardiology
Dr Bhavna Valia, Ottawa, ON - Family Medicine
Dr M Beth Vallieres, Cambridge, ON - Emergency Family Med
Dr Maria Valois, Toronto, ON - Internal Medicine
Dr John E E Van Aerde, Surrey, BC - Pediatrics
Dr Gerhard Van Der Westhuizen, Calgary, AB - General Practice
Dr Johannes Van Dorp, Wiarton, ON - General Practice
Dr Stan G Van Duyse, Montreal, QC - General Practice
Dr Jacqueline M Van Hees, Cornwall, ON - Emergency Family Med
Dr T M Matthew J Van Olm, Calgary, AB - Internal Medicine
Dr Walter J Vanast, Kahnawake, QC - Neurology
Dr Theodore A Vandenberg, London, ON - Internal Medicine
Dr Anik R M Vandewaetere, Ottawa, ON - Family Medicine
Dr J Gerald Vangurp, Montreal, QC - General Practice
Dr Paul-Robert V Vanhoutte, Saint John, NB - Family Medicine
Dr Jean-Marie Vantelon, Moncton, NB - General Practice
Dr Marica Varga, Toronto, ON - Geriatric Medicine
Dr Devesh K Varma, Mississauga, ON - Ophthalmology
Dr Christopher B Varty, Scarborough, ON - Anesthesia
Dr John R Vary, Rimouski, QC - Urology
Dr Gabriela Vasile, Port Moody, BC - Family Medicine
Dr Denise M Vasiliou, East York, ON - Internal Medicine
Dr Demetra Vassiliou, Ottawa, ON - Obstetrics & Gynecology
Dr Michael Vassilyadi, Ottawa, ON - Neurosurgery
Dr Peter W Vaughan, Bridgewater, NS - General Practice
Dr Line M Vautour, Montreal, QC - Endocrin/Metabolism
Dr Silvano R Vecchio, Edmonton, AB - General Practice
Dr Michael J Vecchio, North York, ON - General Practice
Dr A Adriana Veer, Charlottetown, PE - Family Medicine
Dr Valmiki Veerapen, Campbell River, BC - Family Medicine
Dr Anna L Veksler, Montreal, QC - Diagnostic-Radiology
Dr Keimpe Veldhuis, London, ON - Internal Medicine
Dr Pamela Velos, North York, ON - Ophthalmology
Dr Lea S Velsher, North York, ON - Pediatrics
Dr Ronald B Vender, Hamilton, ON - Dermatology
Dr Nina E N Venkatarangam, Scarborough, ON - Obstetrics & Gynecology
Dr Sunita Venkateswaran, Ottawa, ON - Neurology
Dr Mario R Ventresca, Port Colborne, ON - Ophthalmology
Dr Josee Verdon, Montreal, QC - Geriatric Medicine
Dr Nicolaas P L G Verhoeff, North York, ON - Psychiatry
Dr John-Paul Veri, Peterborough, ON - Orthopedic Surgery
Dr Shailendra Verma, Ottawa, ON - Internal Medicine
Dr Neil Verma, Richmond Hill, ON - Emergency Family Med
Dr Rex E Verschuren, Scarborough, ON - Family Medicine
Dr George E Vertes, Scarborough, ON - Cardiology
Dr Colette Y T B Vervaeck, Didsbury, AB - General Practice
Dr Phyllis-Marie Vetere, Montreal, QC - General Practice
Dr Antonio Vettese, Mississauga, ON - Ophthalmology
Dr Claude T J Vezina, Timmins, ON - Diagnostic-Radiology
Dr Stephen Vida, Montreal, QC - Psychiatry
Dr Lucy M Vieira, Pointe-Claire, QC - Neurology
Dr Antonio A L Vigano, Montreal, QC - General Practice
Dr Monique Villanueva Arquint, Markham, ON - General Pathology
Dr Matthieu Vincent, Longueuil, QC - Emergency Medicine
Dr Annick Vincent, St-Augustin-D-Desm, QC - Psychiatry
Dr Julie F Vinette-Azzi, Gloucester, ON - Family Medicine
Dr Shaun L Visser, Ottawa, ON - Emergency Family Med
Dr Louise Y Vitou, Kitchener, ON - Critical Care Medicine
Dr Bennedetto B Vitullo, Charlottetown, PE - Pediatrics
Dr Anthony C H Vivian, Chilliwack, BC - Internal Medicine
Dr Saul Vizel, Cambridge, ON - Cardiology
Dr Helen Vlachos, Sherbrooke, QC - Pediatrics
Dr Thoi Hen Vo, Toronto, ON - General Practice
Dr Tan Tai Vo, Val-d'Or, QC - Anatomical Pathology
Dr Peter Von Dadelszen, Vancouver, BC - Obstetrics & Gynecology
Dr Michael Vonniessen, Pointe-Claire, QC - Emergency Family Med
Dr Harry M Voogjarv, Timmins, ON - Critical Care Medicine
Dr Arnold J Voth, Edmonton, AB - Internal Medicine
Dr T A John Vu, Courtice, ON - General Practice
Dr David D V Vu, Toronto, ON - General Practice
Dr Ngoc Dien Vu, Montreal, QC - General Practice
Dr The-Hung Vu, Montreal, QC - General Practice
Dr Oswald F Wachtler, Calgary, AB - General Practice
Dr Atma S Wadhwa, Sturgeon Falls, ON - Internal Medicine
Dr Raj Waghmare, Aurora, ON - Family Medicine
Dr David M Wagman, Bolton, ON - General Practice
Dr Elisabeth M Wagner, Calgary, AB - Obstetrics & Gynecology

Dr Brenda L M Wagner, Richmond, BC - Obstetrics & Gynecology
Dr J Scott Wakefield, Calgary, AB - Family Medicine
Dr Robert W Wald, Toronto, ON - Cardiology
Dr Ron Wald, Toronto, ON - Internal Medicine
Dr Lyle H Waldman, Montreal, QC - General Practice
Dr Leslie A Waldron, Kingston, ON - Family Medicine
Dr James B Waldron, Westmount, QC - Ophthalmology
Dr Jason T Wale, Comox, BC - Emergency Family Med
Dr Jennifer D Walker, North Vancouver, BC - Family Medicine
Dr Janet A Walker, Bathurst, NB - General Surgery
Dr C Robin Walker, London, ON - Pediatrics
Dr Peter Walker, Ottawa, ON - Endocrinology
Dr Angela J Walker, St-Basile-le-Grand, QC - Family Medicine
Dr Jane M Wall, Toronto, ON - Diagnostic-Radiology
Dr Avi Wallerstein, Montreal, QC - Ophthalmology
Dr Keith E Walling, Lower Sackville, NS - Otolaryngology
Dr Julie Walsh, Donnacona, QC - Family Medicine
Dr Xin-Yong Wang, Burnaby, BC - Family Medicine
Dr Beatrice Wang, Montreal, QC - Dermatology
Dr Zhi Wang, Saint-Jerome, QC - Orthopedic Surgery
Dr Michael C T Wansbrough, Toronto, ON - Emergency Family Med
Dr Leanne M Ward, Ottawa, ON - Endocrin/Metabolism
Dr Michelle G K Ward, Ottawa, ON - Pediatrics
Dr Mark A Ware, Montreal, QC - General Practice
Dr Margaret N Warner, Montreal, QC - Hematology
Dr Thomas F Warnock, Stratford, ON - General Practice
Dr Ian M Warrack, Ottawa, ON - Family Medicine
Dr Kevin A Waschke, Montreal, QC - Gastroenterology
Dr Susan Waserman, Hamilton, ON - Clin Immun/Allergy
Dr Atef M Wasfi, Montreal, QC - General Practice
Dr Samia W Wasfy, Mississauga, ON - Family Medicine
Dr Evet A Wasif, Saskatoon, SK - Diagnostic-Radiology
Dr Gregory D Waslen, Calgary, AB - Plastic Surgery
Dr Georgina Wassef, Ottawa, ON - Family Medicine
Dr Ramses Wassef, Montreal, QC - General Surgery
Dr Pnina C Wasser, Montreal, QC - Family Medicine
Dr Daniel Watkin, Wasaga Beach, ON - General Practice
Dr Sheila D Watson, Calgary, AB - Obstetrics & Gynecology
Dr Michael W B Watson, Edmonton, AB - General Practice
Dr William J Watson, Toronto, ON - Family Medicine
Dr James H Watt, St. Albert, AB - Diagnostic-Radiology
Dr Garth B Watt, Halifax, NS - Psychiatry
Dr Menashe B Waxman, Toronto, ON - Internal Medicine
Dr Ashley D Wazana, Montreal, QC - Psychiatry
Dr Louis E P Weatherhead, Ottawa, ON - Dermatology
Dr Stacie D Weber, Barrie, ON - Family Medicine
Dr Christopher C Weber, Ottawa, ON - General Practice
Dr Marie E Weber, Montreal, QC - Family Medicine
Dr Joy Y M Wee, Kingston, ON - Physical Medicine & Rehab
Dr Andrew S Weeks, Simcoe, ON - Cardiology
Dr Corey N Weigensberg, Scarborough, ON - Anatomical Pathology
Dr Howard P Wein, Montreal, QC - Electroencephal
Dr Michael J Weinberg, Mississauga, ON - Plastic Surgery
Dr Terri E Weinberg, North York, ON - Family Medicine
Dr Robert B Weinberg, Toronto, ON - Family Medicine
Dr Robert D Weinman, Pointe-Claire, QC - Family Medicine
Dr Joy M Weisbloom, Nepean, ON - Family Medicine
Dr Brent A Weiser, Toronto, ON - Ophthalmology
Dr Alan A Weiss, Vancouver, BC - Gastroenterology
Dr Helen M Weiss, Vancouver, BC - General Practice
Dr Issie S Weissglas, Montreal, QC - General Surgery
Dr Alfred Weksberg, North York, ON - Dermatology
Dr Charles J Weldon, Cowansville, QC - Ophthalmology
Dr Eleanor Wellman, Quebec, QC - Family Medicine
Dr Mary K Wells, St. John's, NL - General Surgery
Dr John D Wells, Hamilton, ON - Neurosurgery
Dr Richard A Wennberg, Toronto, ON - Electroencephal
Dr Denise H Werker, Ottawa, ON - Community Medicine
Dr Steven J Wesley, Hamilton, ON - Psychiatry
Dr Anna Wesolkowska, Sydney, NS - General Practice
Dr Ewa B Wesolowska, Montreal, QC - Medical Biochemistry
Dr Hendrik H Westenberg, Kingston, ON - General Practice
Dr John A R Westerlund, St-Charles-Brromee, QC - Medical Biochemistry
Dr Michael Westwood, Baie-D'Urfe, QC - Pediatrics
Dr Wolfgang H Wetzer, Saanichton, BC - General Practice
Dr Marvin J Wexler, Montreal, QC - General Surgery
Dr Mark G Whalen, Campbellton, NB - Internal Medicine
Dr Sylvia A M Whalen, Orleans, ON - Family Medicine
Dr Karen A Whalen-Browne, Kingston, ON - Family Medicine
Dr Ian S White, Invermere, BC - Family Medicine
Dr Christine L White, Ottawa, ON - Family Medicine
Dr Lisa A White, Ottawa, ON - Family Medicine
Dr Richard A White, Peterborough, ON - Pediatrics
Dr M Edward White, Charlottetown, PE - Family Medicine
Dr Debrah L White, Westmount, QC - General Practice
Dr Natalie M Whiting, Victoria, BC - Family Medicine
Dr Sharon E Whiting, Ottawa, ON - Neurology
Dr Susan A Whitley, Ottawa, ON - Family Medicine
Dr N Blair Whittemore, Montreal, QC - Hematology
Dr Sonja C Wicklum, Calgary, AB - Family Medicine
Dr Anna Wieckowska, Quebec, QC - Gastroenterology
Dr Andreas T J Wielgosz, Ottawa, ON - Cardiology
Dr Rafal F Wierzbicki, Oshawa, ON - Internal Medicine
Dr Lorne M Wiesenfeld, Ottawa, ON - Emergency Medicine
Dr Mark A Wilkins, Mattawa, ON - Family Medicine
Dr Veerle R P Willaeys, Burnaby, BC - Community Medicine
Dr Bernard E Willems, Montreal, QC - Internal Medicine
Dr Hany William, Cornwall, ON - Family Medicine
Dr AnnaMary J Williams, Hawkesbury, ON - Dermatology
Dr V Guy Williams, Hawkesbury, ON - General Practice
Dr William L Williams, Ottawa, ON - Cardiology
Dr Paula B Williams, Toronto, ON - General Practice
Dr Eldon S V Williams, Toronto, ON - General Surgery
Dr Carole S Williams, Vanier, ON - General Practice
Dr Kimberly A Williamson, Hamilton, ON - General Practice
Dr Kenneth R Willis, Ottawa, ON - Internal Medicine
Dr Donald G Wilson, Comox, BC - Obstetrics & Gynecology
Dr Rodney D Wilson, Halifax, NS - General Practice
Dr Murray B Wilson, Bradford, ON - General Practice
Dr Chantelle N Wilson, Gore Bay, ON - Family Medicine
Dr Scott N Wilson, Marathon, ON - Family Medicine
Dr Allan Wilson, Ottawa, ON - General Practice
Dr Terrance R Wilson, Peterborough, ON - General Practice
Dr Tracy L Wilson, Thunder Bay, ON - Orthopedic Surgery
Dr Janet H Wilson, Westmount, QC - Family Medicine
Dr Cara K Wilson-Haffenden, North Vancouver, BC - General Practice
Dr Stephen B Wilton, Calgary, AB - Cardiology
Dr Marc L Wiltshire, Thunder Bay, ON - Emergency Family Med
Dr David G Wiltshire, Pointe-Claire, QC - Orthopedic Surgery
Dr Simon S Wing, Montreal, QC - Endocrin/Metabolism
Dr Stephanie H M Winsor, Hamilton, ON - Obstetrics & Gynecology
Dr Willie P Winzer, Orleans, ON - General Practice
Dr Mark Wise, North York, ON - General Practice
Dr Jeffrey G Wiseman, Montreal, QC - Internal Medicine
Dr Fred Wiseman, Pointe-Claire, QC - Pediatrics
Dr Leon E Wisniowski, Bedford, NS - General Practice
Dr Raymond J R Wiss, Sudbury, ON - Emergency Family Med
Dr Davinia E Withington, Montreal, QC - General Practice
Dr Jean-Victor P Wittenberg, Toronto, ON - Psychiatry
Dr Robert C Wittes, Thornhill, ON - Community Medicine
Dr Krystyna H Wojakowski, London, ON - Psychiatry
Dr Ronald J Wojtyk, Ottawa, ON - General Practice
Dr Renee J Wolanski, Cote Saint-Luc, QC - General Practice
Dr Dennis Y R Wong, Edmonton, AB - General Practice
Dr Paul C H Wong, Vancouver, BC - Family Medicine
Dr Thomas Wong, Ottawa, ON - Family Medicine
Dr David M C Wong, Toronto, ON - Family Medicine
Dr Natalie Wong, Toronto, ON - Critical Care Medicine
Dr Michael Y Woo, Ottawa, ON - Emergency Family Med
Dr Minna N Woo, Toronto, ON - Endocrin/Metabolism
Dr Anna Woo, Toronto, ON - Cardiology
Dr Jerry L Woodruff, Bow Island, AB - General Practice
Dr Terence C H Woods, Deep River, ON - Family Medicine
Dr Brenda T Woods, Toronto, ON - Obstetrics & Gynecology
Dr Sandra G B Woods, Val-d'Or, QC - Pediatrics
Dr D Blake Woodside, Toronto, ON - Psychiatry
Dr Eric J Wooltorton, Ottawa, ON - Family Medicine
Dr Roger W Wray, Nepean, ON - General Practice
Dr Kelley M Wright, Barrie, ON - Family Medicine
Dr James R Wylie, Brampton, ON - General Practice
Dr Louise B M Wylie, Ottawa, ON - General Practice
Dr Isaac Wyszogrodski, Dollard-D-Ormeaux, QC - General Practice
Dr Anargyros Xenocostas, London, ON - Hematology
Dr Rong Xie, West Vancouver, BC - Family Medicine
Dr Wadieh R Yacoub, Edmonton, AB - Community Medicine
Dr Mayer Yacowar, North York, ON - Family Medicine
Dr Mark J Yaffe, Montreal, QC - Family Medicine
Dr Dushyant K Yajnik, Westmount, QC - General Practice
Dr Howard Yanofsky, Montreal, QC - Dermatology
Dr Kibar Yared, Scarborough, ON - Cardiology
Dr John F Yaremko, Westmount, QC - Pediatrics
Dr Naguib H Yassa, Brockville, ON - Anatomical Pathology
Dr Mariam Yassa, Montreal, QC - Radiation Oncology
Dr Annalee Yassi, Vancouver, BC - Community Medicine
Dr Carol A M Yeadon, Montreal, QC - Internal Medicine
Dr John Yee, Vancouver, BC - Cardiac Surgery
Dr Ernest Yee, Belleville, ON - Internal Medicine
Dr Karen W L Yee, Toronto, ON - Hematology
Dr Lauren L Yee, Windsor, ON - General Practice
Dr John C K Yee, Windsor, ON - General Practice
Dr Robert M Yelle, Kanata, ON - Family Medicine
Dr Horacio Yepes, Sydney, NS - General Practice
Dr Sarkis Yeretsian, Montreal, QC - General Surgery
Dr Jack K P S Y Yeung, Burlington, ON - General Practice
Dr John A Yeung-Lai-Wah, Vancouver, BC - Cardiology
Dr Anna Yiannopoulos, Montreal, QC - Internal Medicine
Dr Ying Ying, Brossard, QC - Family Medicine
Dr Grace Yoon, Toronto, ON - Medical Genetics
Dr Layla Younes, Montreal, QC - Family Medicine
Dr Jennifer P Young, Collingwood, ON - Emergency Family Med
Dr John G Young, Ottawa, ON - Otolaryngology
Dr Vincent P J Young, Ottawa, ON - Hematology
Dr Beverly Young, Toronto, ON - Psychiatry
Dr Mariam F G Youssef, Burlington, ON - Family Medicine
Dr Victor S F Youssef, Milton, ON - Family Medicine
Dr Fady Youssef, Ottawa, ON - Emergency Family Med
Dr Sami A Youssef, Montreal, QC - General Surgery
Dr Joyce W Yu, Vancouver, BC - Clin Immun/Allergy
Dr Grace W Yu, Vancouver, BC - Pediatrics
Dr Edward W T Yu, London, ON - Radiation Oncology
Dr John C Yu, Ottawa, ON - Diagnostic-Radiology
Dr Eric H C Yu, Toronto, ON - Cardiology
Dr Yeni H Yucel, Toronto, ON - Neuro-Pathology
Dr George P Zachariadis, Toronto, ON - General Practice
Dr Laura S Zacharin, Toronto, ON - Family Medicine
Dr Teanoosh Zadeh, Westmount, QC - General Surgery
Dr Oleg G Zadorozny, Gatineau, QC - Internal Medicine
Dr Aftab Zafar, Kitchener, ON - Ophthalmology
Dr Desiree Zaharescu, Saint-Eustache, QC - General Practice
Dr Georgina M Zahirney, Montreal, QC - Psychiatry
Dr Patrick A Zaidel, Burnaby, BC - Internal Medicine
Dr Mariam R Zakhary, Brampton, ON - Family Medicine
Dr Liliane H Zakhary, Etobicoke, ON - Pediatrics
Dr Nasser A Zaki, Etobicoke, ON - Family Medicine
Dr Nora Zaklama, Pointe-Claire, QC - General Pathology
Dr Mayer M Zaklos, Montreal, QC - Family Medicine
Dr Tanya L Zakrison, Toronto, ON - General Surgery
Dr Witold M Zaleski, London, ON - Diagnostic-Radiology
Dr Mark S Zalter, Hamilton, ON - General Practice
Dr Jeffrey S Zaltzman, Toronto, ON - Internal Medicine
Dr Nayla Zalzal, Port Hope, ON - General Practice
Dr Jorge E Zamora, Kingston, ON - Anesthesia
Dr Iman Zandieh, Victoria, BC - Gastroenterology
Dr Patrizia A C Zanelli, Montreal, QC - Critical Care Medicine
Dr Fabio G Zanetti, Brantford, ON - Ophthalmology
Dr Thomas A Zaphiratos, Montreal, QC - General Practice
Dr Janina Zaremba, Ottawa, ON - General Practice
Dr Michael G Zaremba, Woodbridge, ON - Family Medicine
Dr Peter C Zarkadas, North Vancouver, BC - Orthopedic Surgery
Dr Christina H A Zarowsky, Plantagenet, ON - General Practice

Dr Ricardo Zarruk, Pierrefonds, QC - General Practice
Dr Louis S Zavodni, Hamilton, ON - Family Medicine
Dr Andrew G A Zawadowski, Oakville, ON - Internal Medicine
Dr Joie A Zeglinski, Ottawa, ON - Psychiatry
Dr Lauren V Zeilig, North York, ON - General Practice
Dr Anthony G Zekulin, Brampton, ON - General Practice
Dr Agnes M Zeliger, Westmount, QC - Pediatrics
Dr Reinhard D Zeller, Toronto, ON - Orthopedic Surgery
Dr Marilyn V Zeman, Edmonton, AB - Gastroenterology
Dr Paul J Zeni, Georgetown, ON - General Practice
Dr Alexander Zhivkov, Fort-Coulonge, QC - General Practice
Dr Setareh Ziai, Ottawa, ON - Ophthalmology
Dr Brian S Zidel, Mississauga, ON - General Practice
Dr Joan R Zidulka, Montreal, QC - Hematology
Dr Cleve Ziegler, Montreal, QC - Obstetrics & Gynecology
Dr Benjamin G Zifkin, Westmount, QC - Electroencephal
Dr Michael Zigman, Montreal, QC - General Practice
Dr Jerrold M Zikman, Hamilton, ON - Urology
Dr Eugenia Zikos, Montreal, QC - Psychiatry
Dr Caren F Zilber-Shlensky, Victoria, BC - Family Medicine
Dr George W Zimakas, Niagara Falls, ON - Internal Medicine
Dr Hans H Zingg, Montreal, QC - General Practice
Dr Armand S Zini, Montreal, QC - Urology
Dr Gregorio Zlotnik, Montreal, QC - General Practice
Dr Alexandre R Zlotta, Toronto, ON - General Surgery
Dr Anna I M Znamirowski, Cambridge, ON - Obstetrics & Gynecology
Dr Magdy Zoghby, Montreal, QC - General Practice
Dr Marietta L T Zorn, Scarborough, ON - Plastic Surgery
Dr Maria L Zorzitto, Toronto, ON - Geriatric Medicine
Dr Jerry R Zownir, Toronto, ON - Internal Medicine
Dr David J Zukor, Montreal, QC - Orthopedic Surgery
Dr Michel Zummo, Montreal, QC - General Practice
Dr Ian H L Zunder, Ottawa, ON - Anesthesia
Dr Jocelyn C Zwicker, Ottawa, ON - Neurology
Dr Michel de Maupeou, La Sarre, QC - General Practice
Dr Joseph A de Nanassy, Ottawa, ON - Anatomical Pathology
Dr Sandra K de la Ronde, Ottawa, ON - Obstetrics & Gynecology
Dr Raquel del Carpio, Montreal, QC - Diagnostic-Radiology

FUKINESE

Dr Emily T Dy Pac, Toronto, ON - Psychiatry
Dr Shen-Pang E Ho, Lindsay, ON - General Pathology
Dr Wing F Lim, Sherwood Park, AB - Family Medicine
Dr Liang Ng, West Vancouver, BC - General Practice
Dr Charles C Tan, Richmond Hill, ON - General Practice
Dr Grace Y Tanhuanco-Kho, Victoria, BC - Anatomical Pathology
Dr Kevin L F Tong, Vancouver, BC - General Practice
Dr Jason Y S Tsai, North York, ON - General Practice
Dr Paul C Y Woo, Richmond Hill, ON - General Practice
Dr Kwang Yang, Surrey, BC - Family Medicine
Dr Michael K Yeung, North York, ON - Psychiatry
Dr Yick Shing Yung, Toronto, ON - Obstetrics & Gynecology

GA

Dr Clarence E Clottey, Oakville, ON - Family Medicine
Dr Diana B Mills-Tettey, North York, ON - Pediatrics
Dr Isaac Odame, Toronto, ON - General Practice
Dr Obodai Sai, Scarborough, ON - Psychiatry
Dr Francis B Sam, North York, ON - Obstetrics & Gynecology
Dr Barnaby E A Tamakloe, East York, ON - Psychiatry
Dr Setorme A Tsikata, Spruce Grove, AB - Family Medicine

GAELIC

Dr John Burke, Winchester, ON - General Practice
Dr James F A Fahy, Midland, ON - Internal Medicine
Dr Michael D Hefferon, Kingston, ON - Pediatrics
Dr David J Hill, North York, ON - General Practice
Dr Brendan G Kenny, Moncton, NB - Neurosurgery
Dr Kenneth J MacRitchie, North York, ON - Psychiatry
Dr William R Mackle, Kelowna, BC - General Practice
Dr Peter F O'Donohoe, Sudbury, ON - General Practice
Dr John G O'Kelly, Edmonton, AB - Psychiatry
Dr Michael J O'Malley, Prince George, BC - Family Medicine
Dr Eoghan B O'Shea, Ottawa, ON - Family Medicine
Dr Edward A J Ryan, Etobicoke, ON - Obstetrics & Gynecology
Dr James J Sheridan, Grnd Falls-Windsor, NL - Internal Medicine
Dr John T Street, Vancouver, BC - General Practice
Dr Michael D Teehan, Halifax, NS - Psychiatry
Dr John L Veale, Ajax, ON - Pediatrics
Dr Joseph Walker, Nanaimo, BC - Psychiatry
Dr Mary G A Walsh, Toronto, ON - Psychiatry

GERMAN

Dr Michael J M Ackermann, Sherbrooke, NS - General Practice
Dr Charlotte Alabaster, Calgary, AB - Family Medicine
Dr Elsayed E Alamelhuda, Windsor, ON - Family Medicine
Dr Jan-Martin Albers, Toronto, ON - Family Medicine
Dr Julius Alexy, Selkirk, MB - General Practice
Dr Nabeel Ali, Montreal, QC - Pediatrics
Dr Gillian B Allen, Toronto, ON - General Practice
Dr Eric W Amann, Toronto, ON - General Practice
Dr Annette Anderson, Waterville, NB - General Practice
Dr Martin R Ankenbauer, Castlegar, BC - General Practice
Dr David Armstrong, Hamilton, ON - Gastroenterology
Dr Gerd Asche, Hope, BC - Family Medicine
Dr Ahmad S Ashrafi, Surrey, BC - General Surgery
Dr M Susan L Aubin, Ottawa, ON - Obstetrics & Gynecology
Dr Frank G H Baillie, Hamilton, ON - General Surgery
Dr Barbara J Ballermann, Edmonton, AB - Internal Medicine
Dr Franziska Baltzer, Westmount, QC - Pediatrics
Dr Edith Bandi, Montreal, QC - Anesthesia
Dr Alan N G Barkun, Montreal, QC - Gastroenterology
Dr Jeffrey S T Barkun, Montreal, QC - General Surgery
Dr Isabel H Barnard, Kamloops, BC - Family Medicine
Dr S Alexander Bartel, Chilliwack, BC - General Practice
Dr Doris B A Barwich, Surrey, BC - Family Medicine
Dr Oliver F Bathe, Calgary, AB - General Surgery
Dr Christopher A Bauer, Kentville, NS - General Practice
Dr Heiko Baunemann, Thunder Bay, ON - Obstetrics & Gynecology
Dr Raphael Beck, Victoria, BC - Pediatrics
Dr Mary Ann Beimers, Vancouver, BC - Pediatrics
Dr Johannes G Benade, Sherwood Park, AB - Family Medicine
Dr Bruno G Benfey, Montreal, QC - General Practice
Dr Susanne Benseler, Toronto, ON - General Practice
Dr Claude M Benton, Parksville, BC - General Practice
Dr Irene C Bergh, Kelowna, BC - Family Medicine
Dr Brant E Bergstrome, Penetanguishene, ON - Psychiatry
Dr Reinhold Bernat, Surrey, BC - General Practice
Dr Markus Besemann, Ottawa, ON - Physical Medicine & Rehab
Dr Rakesh Bhandari, London, ON - Anesthesia
Dr H Jay Biem, Pointe-Claire, QC - Internal Medicine
Dr Jean-Pierre Bienvenu, Greenfield Park, QC - Psychiatry
Dr Jan Jaap Bijlsma, Vancouver, BC - Emergency Medicine
Dr Robert J Birnbaum, Ottawa, ON - Family Medicine
Dr Markus Bischoff, Milton, ON - Orthopedic Surgery
Dr Cédric Bisson, Montreal, QC - Family Medicine
Dr Martin Bitzan, Montreal, QC - General Practice
Dr Piotr A Blachut, Vancouver, BC - Orthopedic Surgery
Dr Karen J L Black, Halifax, NS - Pediatrics
Dr Dirk E Bock, London, ON - General Practice
Dr Gene R Boehme, Lethbridge, AB - General Practice
Dr Jean-François Boivin, Montreal, QC - Community Medicine
Dr Maarten Bokhout, Clinton, ON - Family Medicine
Dr Zeljko Bolesnikov, Fredericton, NB - General Practice
Dr Peter Bolli, St Catharines, ON - General Practice
Dr Rainer H Borkenhagen, Vancouver, BC - Family Medicine
Dr Peter W Boronowski, Inuvik, NT - Family Medicine
Dr Daniel P J Bothma, Nanaimo, BC - Family Medicine
Dr Belkacem Bouchek, Amos, QC - General Practice
Dr Mickael Bouin, Montreal, QC - General Practice
Dr David Bracco, Montreal, QC - Anesthesia
Dr Florian G A Braig, Belleville, ON - Otolaryngology
Dr E Lorne Brandt, Richmond, BC - Family Medicine
Dr Martin E Braun, Vancouver, BC - Emergency Family Med
Dr Erwin A Braun, Winnipeg, MB - Family Medicine
Dr Karlina A Breikss, Victoria, BC - Pediatrics
Dr Christine Brenckmann, Prince George, BC - Family Medicine
Dr Ernst G Brenken, Toronto, ON - Psychiatry
Dr Arthur Breward, Bowmanville, ON - Anesthesia
Dr Bernice Brits, Surrey, BC - Family Medicine
Dr Ivan Brodarec, Yarmouth, NS - General Practice
Dr Reinhard Brunner, Hamilton, ON - Family Medicine
Dr Heinrich D Brussow, High Level, AB - General Practice
Dr Zoheir Bshouty, Winnipeg, MB - Internal Medicine
Dr Kenneth P W Buchholz, Annapolis Royal, NS - Family Medicine
Dr Margret Budzianowska-Kwiatkowski, Port Coquitlam, BC - Family Medicine
Dr Ralf R Buhrmann, Ottawa, ON - Ophthalmology
Dr Martin K Bunge, Winnipeg, MB - Diagnostic-Radiology
Dr Simona C Burs, Calgary, AB - Internal Medicine
Dr Erhard W Busse, Milton, ON - Psychiatry
Dr Abdul Mujib A K M Cadili, St. Albert, AB - General Surgery
Dr Eva Callary, Ottawa, ON - Community Medicine
Dr Louis Camirand, Rouyn-Noranda, QC - General Practice
Dr Denise L Campbell-Scherer, Edmonton, AB - Family Medicine
Dr Paul S Cappon, Ottawa, ON - Community Medicine
Dr David C Carpenter, Ottawa, ON - General Practice
Dr J Ann Carter, Williams Lake, BC - General Practice
Dr Luigi A Castagna, Scarborough, ON - Pediatrics
Dr E Rosemary Christinck, Petawawa, ON - Family Medicine
Dr Dae-Gyun Chung, North York, ON - Diagnostic-Radiology
Dr Jolanda Cibere, Richmond, BC - Internal Medicine
Dr W Robert L Clemmey, Yellowknife, NT - Psychiatry
Dr Alexandra K U Collins, Meaford, ON - General Practice
Dr Brigitte V Cote, Montreal, QC - Community Medicine
Dr Manon Cote, Saint-Laurent, QC - Family Medicine
Dr Michael P Coughlin, Windsor, ON - General Surgery
Dr Dorothy M Craig, Quesnel, BC - Family Medicine
Dr Natascha Crispino, Toronto, ON - Family Medicine
Dr Loris Cristante, Winnipeg, MB - General Practice
Dr David P G Cronje, Miramichi, NB - General Practice
Dr William J Cunningham, Duncan, BC - Emergency Family Med
Dr Johann Cunningham, Victoria, BC - General Surgery
Dr Erik Cunningham, Victoria, BC - Family Medicine
Dr Rita M Dahlke, Calgary, AB - Family Medicine
Dr Scott Dammermann, Maple, ON - General Practice
Dr A Michael Damus, Uxbridge, ON - Family Medicine
Dr Karen Dang, Etobicoke, ON - Family Medicine
Dr A Marc Dauphin, Richelain, QC - General Practice
Dr Till Davy, Toronto, ON - Pediatrics
Dr Keith Granger Dawson, Vancouver, BC - Endocrin/Metabolism
Maj Thomas De Boeck, Midland, ON - Family Medicine
Dr Cornelis De Boer, Truro, NS - Psychiatry
Dr Eric Degen, Toronto, ON - Family Medicine
Dr Eva C Dekany, Toronto, ON - Ophthalmology
Dr Johnny Y Deladoey, Montreal, QC - General Practice
Dr Thomas J Demarco, Whistler, BC - General Practice
Dr Eberhard H Diehl, Kamloops, BC - Anesthesia
Dr Levinus Albert Dieleman, Edmonton, AB - General Practice
Dr Klaus Dittberner, Winnipeg, MB - General Practice
Dr Bernard K Dobovicnik, Trail, BC - General Practice
Dr Michael Doepner, Gatineau, QC - Otolaryngology
Dr David C Doerksen, Windsor, ON - Anesthesia
Dr Erroll R Doermer, Winnipeg, MB - General Practice
Dr Brigitte H M T Dohm, Powell River, BC - General Practice
Dr Gordon Donsky, Toronto, ON - Pediatrics
Dr Michael F Dorsch, Edmonton, AB - General Practice
Dr Marion Dove, Montreal, QC - Family Medicine
Dr C Lewis W Draper, Regina, SK - Family Medicine
Dr Christiaan Dreyer, Winkler, MB - General Practice
Dr Christian A Drouin, Riviere-Du-Loup, QC - Dermatology
Dr Andrew D Duic, Toronto, ON - Pediatrics
Dr Jan P Dutz, Vancouver, BC - Dermatology
Dr Gordon H Dyck, Steinbach, MB - General Practice
Dr Gordon Dzieciol, Etobicoke, ON - General Practice
Dr Martin S Eckhart, Peace River, AB - Family Medicine
Dr Thomas G Ehlen, Vancouver, BC - Obstetrics & Gynecology
Dr Helga Ehrlich, Ottawa, ON - Family Medicine
Dr Jouhaina Eid, Montreal, QC - Nephrology

Dr Bernhard Eigl, Vancouver, BC - Internal Medicine
Dr Nihal El Khouly, Bolton, ON - Family Medicine
Dr Thomas G Elliott, Vancouver, BC - Endocrin/Metabolism
Dr Christine Elser, Toronto, ON - General Practice
Dr Marc Engfield, Gatineau, QC - Internal Medicine
Dr Siegfried R Erb, Vancouver, BC - Internal Medicine
Dr Heidrun Y Erb, Kitchener, ON - General Practice
Dr Gunnar D Erhardt, New Westminster, BC - General Practice
Dr Bernd A Esche, Ottawa, ON - Radiation Oncology
Dr Roya Etemad-Rezai, London, ON - Diagnostic-Radiology
Dr Werner A Fabian, Barrie, ON - General Practice
Dr Kornelia Falkenberg, Regina, SK - Psychiatry
Dr Janusz Feber, Ottawa, ON - Pediatrics
Dr Barbara C Fehlau, Comox, BC - Family Medicine
Dr Michael Fehlings, Toronto, ON - Neurosurgery
Dr Martina M Feierabend, Scarborough, ON - Anesthesia
Dr Imre B Fejer, Scarborough, ON - General Practice
Dr Mathias O Fellenz, Vernon, BC - Ophthalmology
Dr Conrad V Fernandez, Halifax, NS - Pediatrics
Dr Ernst Fibich, Prince George, BC - General Practice
Dr Michael P Fielden, Calgary, AB - Ophthalmology
Dr Guido Filler, London, ON - Pediatrics
Dr Judith E Finlayson, Victoria, BC - Family Medicine
Dr Bettina G Fleige-Zahradka, Duncan, BC - Obstetrics & Gynecology
Dr Philip B Fleuriau-Chateau, Ottawa, ON - Orthopedic Surgery
Dr Traudl E Flock, Whitby, ON - Family Medicine
Dr Alberto L Flores-Vargas, Scarborough, ON - General Practice
Dr Eva Foldes, Montreal, QC - Internal Medicine
Dr Catharina H G M Foolen, Sundre, AB - Family Medicine
Dr Lutz Forkert, Kingston, ON - Respirology
Dr Phillip J Fourie, Yorkton, SK - General Practice
Dr Thomas P Francis, Oliver, BC - Family Medicine
Dr R Bernard Franklin, Sudbury, ON - Obstetrics & Gynecology
Dr Andreas P Freitag, Hamilton, ON - Internal Medicine
Dr Anthony J French, Vancouver, BC - General Practice
Dr Susan H Freter, Halifax, NS - Geriatric Medicine
Dr George Freundlich, Matheson, ON - Family Medicine
Dr Michael G Frey, Richmond, BC - General Practice
Dr Jan Oliver Friedrich, Toronto, ON - Critical Care Medicine
Dr Matthias G W Friedrich, Montreal, QC - Cardiology
Dr Reinhard Friesen, Peterborough, ON - Family Medicine
Dr Christian Fritsch, Ladysmith, BC - General Practice
Dr Emanuel Fritsch, Ladysmith, BC - General Practice
Dr Sandra Froeschl, Ottawa, ON - Internal Medicine
Dr Michael P V Froeschl, Ottawa, ON - Cardiology
Dr Joachim Fuchs, Duncan, BC - General Practice
Dr Sigrid Fuchs-Garcia, Cornwall, ON - General Practice
Dr Eva B Furesz, Ottawa, ON - General Practice
Dr Christoph Fusch, Hamilton, ON - Pediatrics
Dr Jerzy Gajewski, Halifax, NS - Urology
Dr Elizabeth Galanter, Oakville, ON - Pediatrics
Dr Bing Siang Gan, London, ON - Plastic Surgery
Dr Pierre A Gauthier, Laval, QC - Family Medicine
Dr William O Geisler, Toronto, ON - Internal Medicine
Dr Christine E Gemeinhardt, Delta, BC - Family Medicine
Dr Isabelle Genest, Quebec, QC - Emergency Medicine
Dr Michael A Geoghegan, Calgary, AB - General Practice
Dr Sabine R George, Etobicoke, ON - Pediatrics
Dr William S George, Woodstock, ON - General Practice
Dr Alan H Gerulath, Toronto, ON - Obstetrics & Gynecology
Dr K Christopher Giede, Saskatoon, SK - Gynecologic Oncology
Dr François Gilbert, Kirkland, QC - Endocrinology
Dr Peter K Girschek, Toronto, ON - Ophthalmology
Dr Rodney Glynn-Morris, Vancouver, BC - Family Medicine
Dr Charles M Godfrey, Toronto, ON - Physical Medicine & Rehab
Dr Gabriela Gohla, Hamilton, ON - Anatomical Pathology
Dr William J Goldsmith, Montreal, QC - Obstetrics & Gynecology
Dr Walter H Gotlieb, Montreal, QC - Obstetrics & Gynecology
Dr Claudia J Grabner, Brantford, ON - General Practice
Dr Waldemar Grandwilewski, Hamilton, ON - General Practice
Dr Pierre Granger, Montreal, QC - General Practice
Dr Andrew M Grant, Sherbrooke, QC - Medical Biochemistry
Dr Hartmut Graseman, Toronto, ON - General Practice
Dr Alexandra Greenhill, Vancouver, BC - Family Medicine
Dr Leon C Groenewald, Grande Prairie, AB - General Practice
Dr Marie M S Gross, Edmonton, AB - Family Medicine
Dr Lars Grosse-Wortmann, Toronto, ON - General Practice
Dr Karin H Grubner, Toronto, ON - General Practice
Dr Astrid Guttmann, Toronto, ON - Pediatrics
Dr Sandor Gyomorey, Etobicoke, ON - Orthopedic Surgery
Dr Katalin Gyomorey, Thunder Bay, ON - Psychiatry
Dr Mathias Gysler, Mississauga, ON - Obstetrics & Gynecology
Dr Erika Haase, Edmonton, AB - General Surgery
Dr Hasan Hafiz, Calgary, AB - General Practice
Dr Kenneth A Hahlweg, Winnipeg, MB - Family Medicine
Dr Cecil D A Hahn, Toronto, ON - Neurology
Dr James S J Haight, Toronto, ON - Otolaryngology
Dr Ilona Hale, Kimberley, BC - Family Medicine
Dr Adolf Hamann, Corner Brook, NL - General Practice
Dr Carroll D Harder, St Thomas, ON - Emergency Family Med
Dr Hans E Harlos, Elmvale, ON - General Practice
Dr Didi V Harries, Chilliwack, BC - Pediatrics
Dr Michael C Hartwig, Surrey, BC - General Practice
Dr Peter A Hawrylyshyn, Toronto, ON - Obstetrics & Gynecology
Dr Heinz B Heese, Winnipeg, MB - General Practice
Dr Wolfgang W F Heidenreich, Winnipeg, MB - General Practice
Dr Katja Heineck, Toronto, ON - Family Medicine
Dr Hartmut Henning, Vancouver, BC - Internal Medicine
Dr Adriaan Heunis, Salmon Arm, BC - General Practice
Dr Vivian E Hill, Calgary, AB - Ophthalmology
Dr Ingrid M Hings, Montreal, QC - Hematology
Dr Gabriel H Hirsch, Vancouver, BC - Physical Medicine & Rehab
Dr Andrei E Hirsch, Scarborough, ON - General Practice
Dr Holger Hirte, Hamilton, ON - Internal Medicine
Dr Johann K Hitzler, Toronto, ON - Hematology
Dr Volker S Hocke, London, ON - Psychiatry
Dr Karen H Hofmann, Sherwood Park, AB - Diagnostic-Radiology
Dr Corinne M Hohl, Vancouver, BC - Emergency Medicine
Dr Helmut Hollenhorst, Halifax, NS - Radiation Oncology
Dr G Stephen Holzapfel, Toronto, ON - Family Medicine
Dr Stefan Horny, Montreal, QC - General Practice
Dr Kathleen G Howard, Espanola, ON - General Practice
Dr Claudia H Hubbes, Ottawa, ON - Family Medicine
Dr Helmut T Huebert, Winnipeg, MB - Orthopedic Surgery
Dr Otto H Huhn, Banff, AB - General Pathology
Dr Tilman F Humpl, Toronto, ON - General Practice
Dr Ryan D Hunt, Montreal, QC - Emergency Family Med
Dr Irene Hussain-Autenried, Etobicoke, ON - General Practice
Dr Harold G Hynscht, Port Dover, ON - General Practice
Dr Sabina P Ijaz, Pine Falls, MB - Family Medicine
Dr Philip L Immelman, Slave Lake, AB - General Practice
Dr Osman S Ipsiroglu, Vancouver, BC - General Practice
Dr Marlis E Jabs, Winnipeg, MB - Family Medicine
Dr George A Jaciw, Whitby, ON - General Practice
Dr Thomas B Jacobs, Port Coquitlam, BC - General Practice
Dr Edgar T Jaeggi, Toronto, ON - Pediatrics
Dr Fred H Janke, Sylvan Lake, AB - Family Medicine
Dr Gerard H Jansen, Ottawa, ON - Neuro-Pathology
Dr Kurt A Jansen, Montreal, QC - Family Medicine
Dr Ernest P Janzen, Lethbridge, AB - Internal Medicine
Dr Peter F Jarzem, Montreal, QC - Orthopedic Surgery
Dr S Vanita Jassal, Toronto, ON - Internal Medicine
Dr Alphonse Jeanneret-Grosjean, Montreal, QC - Internal Medicine
Dr Peter Jechel, Perth, ON - Emergency Family Med
Dr Klaus Jochem, Montreal, QC - General Practice
Dr Janice Journeau, Salmon Arm, BC - General Surgery
Dr C Mark Joyce, Calgary, AB - Family Medicine
Dr Tibor Juda, Toronto, ON - Urology
Dr Ursula Jurt, Brampton, ON - Cardiology
Dr Andrew Kaegi, Whitehorse, YT - Hematology
Dr H Wilfried S Kaethler, Steinbach, MB - Family Medicine
Dr Frieder Kaethler, Markdale, ON - General Practice
Dr Pierre Karakiewicz, Montreal, QC - Urology
Dr Athanasios Katsarkas, Montreal, QC - Otolaryngology
Dr Madelene S Kellerman, Lethbridge, AB - General Practice
Dr Karen M Kennedy, Orillia, ON - Family Medicine
Dr Thomas E Kerlis, Lloydminster, AB - General Practice
Dr M Ibrahim Khan, Regina, SK - General Practice
Dr Gerhard N Kiefer, Calgary, AB - Orthopedic Surgery
Dr Norman G Kienitz, Kamloops, BC - Emergency Family Med
Dr Katharina E Kieser, Halifax, NS - Obstetrics & Gynecology
Dr Gunther Klein, Campbell River, BC - Family Medicine
Dr Hans Knecht, Sherbrooke, QC - Hematology
Dr Randolph P Knipping, Palgrave, ON - Family Medicine
Dr Frank D Knoefel, Ottawa, ON - Family Medicine
Dr Martin R J Kolb, Hamilton, ON - General Practice
Dr Christian Kollmannsberger, Vancouver, BC - Internal Medicine
Dr V Gary Koop, Lively, ON - General Practice
Dr Peter Koopmann, Cowansville, QC - Hematology
Dr Claudia A Korwan, Ajax, ON - Diagnostic-Radiology
Dr Walter Koslowski, Milton, ON - General Practice
Dr Kalman T Kovacs, Toronto, ON - Anatomical Pathology
Dr James K H Krahn, Winnipeg, MB - Family Medicine
Dr Adam Krajewski, North York, ON - Geriatric Medicine
Dr Milos J Krajny, Toronto, ON - Internal Medicine
Dr Andreas H Kramer, Calgary, AB - Critical Care Medicine
Dr Hans J Kreder, Toronto, ON - Orthopedic Surgery
Dr Ian T Kroll, Calgary, AB - Psychiatry
Dr Pieter Ernst Kruger, Fort McMurray, AB - General Practice
Dr Fernando H Kuhn, Abbotsford, BC - General Practice
Dr Anne C D Kulenkamp, Gaspe, QC - Family Medicine
Dr Christiane Kuntz, Gloucester, ON - Family Medicine
Dr Karol Kuperberg, Montreal, QC - General Practice
Dr Raffi S Kuyumjian, Saint-Hubert, QC - Family Medicine
Dr Gilles-Philippe Lafond, Quebec, QC - Ophthalmology
Dr Real Lagace, Rimouski, QC - Anatomical Pathology
Dr Louise Lajoie, Longueuil, QC - General Practice
Dr Eugene P Landsbergen, Sundre, AB - General Practice
Dr H Benno Lang, Upper Tantallon, NS - Family Medicine
Dr Manfred Lapner, Ottawa, ON - Pediatrics
Dr Gilles Larouche, La Baie, QC - General Practice
Dr Guy Jean Laroye, Terrace, BC - General Pathology
Dr Maria J Laschuk, Windsor, ON - Anesthesia
Dr Steve Lassey, Pictou, NS - General Practice
Dr Micheline C Lau, Scarborough, ON - General Practice
Dr Ulrich S Lauf, Calgary, AB - Family Medicine
Dr Juris Lazovskis, Sydney, NS - General Practice
Dr Jean L Lette, Montreal, QC - Nuclear Medicine
Dr Man K Leung, Vancouver, BC - General Practice
Dr Mark A Levstik, London, ON - Internal Medicine
Dr Elisabeth Lewke-Bogle, Milk River, AB - Family Medicine
Dr Christoph P B Licht, Toronto, ON - Nephrology
Dr Lie Ming Lie, North York, ON - Anesthesia
Dr Kay I Lie, Toronto, ON - Obstetrics & Gynecology
Dr Daniel T H Liem, Windsor, ON - Internal Medicine
Dr Aukse T Lingys, Mississauga, ON - General Practice
Dr Charles Listgarten, Woodbridge, ON - Internal Medicine
Dr M Christine Loepp, Winnipeg, MB - Family Medicine
Dr Rolf Loertscher, Pointe-Claire, QC - General Practice
Dr Mary L Loewen, Vancouver, BC - General Practice
Dr Jens Lohser, Vancouver, BC - Anesthesia
Dr Adrian L H Long, Winnipeg, MB - General Practice
Dr Eva M Lonn, Hamilton, ON - Cardiology
Dr Juliana Losier, Mayne, BC - Family Medicine
Dr Jelka-Maria Lujic-Thebaud, Edmonton, AB - General Practice
Dr Alexander MacCordick, Gatineau, QC - Psychiatry
Dr Gisela L P MacPhail, Calgary, AB - Infectious Diseases
Dr Jack F Machin, Lac-Megantic, QC - General Practice
Dr Richard J Mackler, Montreal, QC - Endocrinology
Dr Vera V Madison, Toronto, ON - General Practice
Dr Saadet Mahmutoglu, Toronto, ON - General Practice
Dr Trudy L Mahood, Thunder Bay, ON - Family Medicine
Dr Peter C Maier, North York, ON - Family Medicine
Dr Colin M Mailer, London, ON - Ophthalmology
Dr Kenneth G Makus, Edmonton, AB - Neurology
Dr Johann H Malan, Saskatoon, SK - General Practice
Dr Garnet J M Maley, Milton, ON - General Practice
Dr Katharina M Manassis, Toronto, ON - Psychiatry
Dr Valerie I Mantle, Sudbury, ON - Family Medicine
Dr Lutz Marburg, Edmonton, AB - General Practice
Dr Alina Marin, Kingston, ON - General Practice
Dr Karl H Mascher, Lillooet, BC - General Practice
Dr Ephraim G Massey, Montreal, QC - General Practice
Dr Barbara J A Mayr, West Vancouver, BC - General Practice

Dr Patricia J Mayr, Guelph, ON - General Practice
Dr Heinz George Mayr, London, ON - General Practice
Dr Colleen Maytham, Invermere, BC - Family Medicine
Dr Annette L McCall, North Vancouver, BC - Family Medicine
Dr James W McGillivray, Hearst, ON - General Surgery
Dr H M Rosemary Meier, Toronto, ON - Psychiatry
Dr Michael H Mengel, Edmonton, AB - General Practice
Dr Robert D Menzies, Vancouver, BC - Family Medicine
Dr Ladislav Mesensky, Etobicoke, ON - General Practice
Dr Hans A Messner, Toronto, ON - Internal Medicine
Dr Ronit Mesterman, Hamilton, ON - Neurology
Dr Daniel L Metzger, Vancouver, BC - Endocrin/Metabolism
Dr Ulrike Meyer, Dawson Creek, BC - Family Medicine
Dr Catharina J Meyer, Carlyle, SK - Family Medicine
Dr Melitta Mezody, Toronto, ON - General Practice
Dr Jean-Marie C Michel, Shippagan, NB - General Practice
Dr Jorg E Michels, Victoria, BC - General Practice
Dr Cornelia I Mielke, Hamilton, ON - Family Medicine
Dr Paivi M H Miettunen, Calgary, AB - Pediatrics
Dr Richard W Milde, Nelson, BC - General Practice
Dr M Martin Milewski, Maple Ridge, BC - General Practice
Dr Paul H Minc, Acton, ON - Family Medicine
Dr Klaus K Minde, Montreal, QC - Psychiatry
Dr Thomas Minde, Ste-Cecile-de-Mash, QC - Family Medicine
Dr Thankamma Modi, Hamilton, ON - General Practice
Dr Jan Fredrik Moe, Kinistino, SK - General Practice
Dr Gerard Mohr, Montreal, QC - Neurosurgery
Dr Vivian M Moir, Keswick, ON - Family Medicine
Dr Henry J Moller, Toronto, ON - Psychiatry
Dr Andre Moolman, Kitchener, ON - Family Medicine
Dr Peter Moosbrugger, Comox, BC - Family Medicine
Dr Henry Morgentaler, Toronto, ON - General Practice
Dr Jacques Morin, Montmagny, QC - Psychiatry
Dr David Morris, Montreal, QC - Endocrinology
Dr Wojciech Morzycki, Halifax, NS - Internal Medicine
Dr Edith K Moser, Vancouver, BC - Family Medicine
Dr Francois Mosimann, Sherbrooke, QC - General Surgery
Dr Olga Moukhortova-Von Lipinski, Vancouver, BC - Obstetrics & Gynecology
Dr Peter Mucalov, Keswick, ON - General Practice
Dr Caroline P Mueller, Richmond, BC - Obstetrics & Gynecology
Dr Elizabeth K Mueller, Cambridge, ON - Family Medicine
Dr Daniel J Mueller, Toronto, ON - General Practice
Dr Ingrid Mueller-Wilm, Toronto, ON - General Practice
Dr Mahdi Murti, Toronto, ON - General Practice
Dr Reginald A Nadeau, Montreal, QC - Cardiology
Dr Stanley Nattel, Montreal, QC - Cardiology
Dr Joachim F Neffgen, Drumheller, AB - General Practice
Dr Joe Nemeth, Montreal, QC - Emergency Family Med
Dr Bernd R Neu, North York, ON - Plastic Surgery
Dr Etela Neumann, Vancouver, BC - Neuro-Pathology
Dr Peter T Newton, London, ON - Anesthesia
Dr Anna Niajko, Richelieu, QC - General Practice
Dr Paula Nieuwstraten, Toronto, ON - Family Medicine
Dr Brooke M E Noftle, London, ON - Family Medicine
Dr Robert A W Northey, Ottawa, ON - Psychiatry
Dr Richard Novick, London, ON - Cardiovasc/ThorSurg
Dr Barry Nuechterlein, Charlottetown, PE - Anesthesia
Dr Ailbhe E O'Riordan, London, ON - Diagnostic-Radiology
Dr Anthony M Ocana, West Vancouver, BC - Family Medicine
Dr Erwin N Oechslin, Toronto, ON - Cardiology
Dr Denise Ouimet, Rouyn-Noranda, QC - Diagnostic-Radiology
Dr Danielle M Over, Oakville, ON - General Practice
Dr Henry F Pabst, Edmonton, AB - Pediatrics
Dr Peter Palma, Fort McMurray, AB - Emergency Family Med
Dr Hans Pasterkamp, Winnipeg, MB - Pediatrics
Dr Andrew R Patterson, Stouffville, ON - General Practice
Dr Ernest J Pauls, Abbotsford, BC - Family Medicine
Dr Alan V Pavilanis, Montreal, QC - Family Medicine
Dr F Griffith Pearson, Mansfield, ON - General Surgery
Dr Sumithra A Peeris, Waterford, ON - General Practice
Dr Stephane Pelet, Quebec, QC - General Practice
Dr Deborah Pestell, Halifax, NS - Family Medicine
Dr Guy C Petroz, Toronto, ON - General Practice
Dr Sabine I Pfeifer, Kitchener, ON - Family Medicine
Dr Thuy-Nga Tia Pham, East York, ON - Family Medicine
Dr Lincoln R Phipps, Leamington, ON - General Practice
Dr Helena Piccinini, Halifax, NS - Family Medicine
Dr Robert P Pilorge, Montreal, QC - Obstetrics & Gynecology
Dr Johanne Plante, Brossard, QC - General Practice
Dr Markus Ploesser, Vancouver, BC - General Practice
Dr Bernhard Pohlmann-Eden, Halifax, NS - General Practice
Dr J Anne W Pollett, Mississauga, ON - Anesthesia
Dr Manfred E Popke, Edmonton, AB - General Practice
Dr Ilija Popovic, Calgary, AB - General Practice
Dr Barbara M Powell, Kanata, ON - Family Medicine
Dr Alexandre Prat, Montreal, QC - Neurology
Dr Jutta K Preiksaitis, Edmonton, AB - Internal Medicine
Dr Jacqueline S Purtzki, Vancouver, BC - Physical Medicine & Rehab
Dr Arif S Qureshi, Listowel, ON - Family Medicine
Dr Michael A Raabe, Winnipeg, MB - Cardiac Surgery
Dr Stephan C Ragaz, Peterborough, ON - Family Medicine
Dr Farid A Rahimi, Mission, BC - General Practice
Dr Alastair S Rankin, Edmonton, AB - Family Medicine
Dr Felix Ratjen, Toronto, ON - Pediatrics
Dr Frank T Rauch, Montreal, QC - General Practice
Dr Dietmar E Raudzus, Vancouver, BC - Family Medicine
Dr Theodore D Redekop, Winnipeg, MB - Community Medicine
Dr Henrike Rees, Saskatoon, SK - Anatomical Pathology
Dr Agnes E Reicher, North York, ON - Dermatology
Dr Darren K Reimer, Steinbach, MB - Family Medicine
Dr Rudolf Reindl, Montreal, QC - Orthopedic Surgery
Dr David J Reinhardt, Kitchener, ON - Family Medicine
Dr Regina R Rempel, Winnipeg, MB - Pediatrics
Dr Elfrieda Rempel, Georgetown, ON - General Practice
Dr Regina-Maria A K Renner, Nanaimo, BC - Obstetrics & Gynecology
Dr Eberhard L Renner, Toronto, ON - Gastroenterology
Dr Christine Renz, Calgary, AB - General Practice
Dr Melinde Richards, Victoria, BC - Family Medicine
Dr Anne-Katrin Richter, Montreal, QC - Family Medicine
Dr R Markus Rieckenberg, Orillia, ON - Anatomical Pathology
Dr H Volker Rininsland, Moose Jaw, SK - Family Medicine
Dr Kerryn L Roberge, Calgary, AB - Family Medicine
Dr Heidi C Roberts, Toronto, ON - Diagnostic-Radiology
Dr Judith A Roger, Vancouver, BC - General Surgery
Dr M Bryson Rogers, Edmonton, AB - Dermatology
Dr Elke H Roland, Vancouver, BC - Neurology
Dr Gabriel M Ronen, Hamilton, ON - Neurology
Dr Wayne S Rosen, Calgary, AB - General Surgery
Dr Linell Rossouw, Regina, SK - General Practice
Dr Julia E Rouget, Edmonton, AB - Internal Medicine
Dr Jan G Roux, Virden, MB - General Practice
Dr Jan Rozehnal, Toronto, ON - General Practice
Dr Ethan Rubinstein, Winnipeg, MB - General Practice
Dr Christian J Rucker, Vancouver, BC - Family Medicine
Dr William Warren H Rudd, Toronto, ON - General Surgery
Dr Greg Ryan, Toronto, ON - Obstetrics & Gynecology
Dr S Vahid Sahiholnasab, Richmond, BC - Internal Medicine
Dr Jan M Salat, Ottawa, ON - General Practice
Dr John T Salvendy, Toronto, ON - Psychiatry
Dr Steve E S Samuel, North York, ON - Plastic Surgery
Dr Shubhayan Sanatani, Vancouver, BC - Cardiology
Dr Michael S Sanatani, London, ON - Internal Medicine
Dr Pablo E R F Sanhueza Luco, North Bay, ON - Psychiatry
Dr Tarek M Sardana, Orleans, ON - General Practice
Dr Dioscoro D C Sarile, Toronto, ON - General Practice
Dr David W Saslove, Markham, ON - General Practice
Dr Peter G H Schaal, Toronto, ON - General Surgery
Dr David F Schaeffer, Vancouver, BC - Anatomical Pathology
Dr Helga T Schafer-MacDonald, North Vancouver, BC - Family Medicine
Dr W Albrecht Schall, York, ON - Anatomical Pathology
Dr Joseph Schatzker, Toronto, ON - Orthopedic Surgery
Dr Markus Schatzmann, Milton, ON - Family Medicine
Dr J Christian Schaub, Winnipeg, MB - Psychiatry
Dr Katrin Scheinemann, Hamilton, ON - General Practice
Dr Duncan A Schellenberg, Montreal, QC - General Practice
Dr Robert J Schemmer, Barrie, ON - Dermatology
Dr Christian H Schenk, Vancouver, BC - Psychiatry
Dr Marianne Schenker, Ottawa, ON - General Practice
Dr Frank J Scheuermeyer, Vancouver, BC - Emergency Family Med
Dr Peter W Scheufler, Mississauga, ON - Obstetrics & Gynecology
Dr Robert Schlagintweit, Port Coquitlam, BC - General Practice
Dr Gunther Schlenther, Ponoka, AB - General Practice
Dr Michael G Schlossmacher, Ottawa, ON - Neurology
Dr Peter E H Schmalfuss, Bolton, ON - General Practice
Dr Johannes S J Schneider, Salmon Arm, BC - General Surgery
Dr Gerd Schneider, Ottawa, ON - Family Medicine
Dr Bernie W Schopf, Abbotsford, BC - General Surgery
Dr Maria-Louise Schroeder, Winnipeg, MB - Pediatrics
Dr Heidemarie Schroter, Calgary, AB - Pediatrics
Dr Holger J Schuenemann, Hamilton, ON - Internal Medicine
Dr Andre C Schuh, Toronto, ON - Hematology
Dr Jan I Schulz, Montreal, QC - Clin Immun/Allergy
Dr Gerhard Schumacher, Kamloops, BC - Family Medicine
Dr Albert J Schumacher, Windsor, ON - General Practice
Dr Walter Schurch, Montreal, QC - Anatomical Pathology
Dr Martin Schuster, Cambridge, ON - Family Medicine
Dr Monika E Schwab-Lang, Burlington, ON - Family Medicine
Dr Gerry K Schwalfenberg, Edmonton, AB - Family Medicine
Dr Rosemarie R Schwarz, Mississauga, ON - Internal Medicine
Dr Peter R Schwarz, Sault Ste. Marie, ON - Family Medicine
Dr Bogdan L Schwarz-Michorowski, Guelph, ON - Cardiology
Dr Franzjosef Schweiger, Moncton, NB - Gastroenterology
Dr Eckhart H C Schweihofer, Toronto, ON - General Practice
Dr Rolf J Sebaldt, Hamilton, ON - Internal Medicine
Dr Said Secerbegovic, Watson Lake, YT - General Practice
Dr Oliver Seifert, Edmonton, AB - General Practice
Dr Nazia Selzner-Malekkiani, Toronto, ON - General Practice
Dr Eric A Semlacher, Edmonton, AB - Gastroenterology
Dr Consolato Sergi, Edmonton, AB - General Practice
Dr Andrea C Seufert, Calgary, AB - Family Medicine
Dr Riad M A Shahid, Surrey, BC - Orthopedic Surgery
Dr Wajid A Shaikh, Scarborough, ON - Pediatrics
Dr Raphael F Sharon, Edmonton, AB - General Practice
Dr Charles S Shaver, Ottawa, ON - Internal Medicine
Dr Alexander I Shenderey, Brampton, ON - Anesthesia
Dr Carolin H Shepherd, Seaforth, ON - General Practice
Dr David C R Sheppard, Denwood, AB - General Practice
Dr Arthur A Shier, Delta, BC - General Practice
Dr Jaroslav O Shklar, Etobicoke, ON - General Practice
Dr Vidur Shyam, Kingston, ON - Anesthesia
Dr Jana Sidorov, Prince George, BC - General Practice
Dr Ezra A Silverstein, Toronto, ON - Orthopedic Surgery
Dr William Singer, East York, ON - Internal Medicine
Dr Sheila K Singh, Hamilton, ON - Neurosurgery
Dr Anna Barbara Sinsky, Terrebonne, QC - Diagnostic-Radiology
Dr Dalibor E Slavik, Saskatoon, SK - Family Medicine
Dr Alexander J Smith, Drayton Valley, AB - General Practice
Dr Joyce So, Oshawa, ON - Medical Genetics
Dr Christian M Soder, Halifax, NS - Anesthesia
Dr Rex B Sokolies, Winnipeg, MB - Family Medicine
Dr T Drew Sommerfeldt, Lethbridge, AB - Family Medicine
Dr Elena Somska, Toronto, ON - General Practice
Dr G Werner Spangehl, White Rock, BC - General Practice
Dr Martin H Spencer, Nanaimo, BC - Ophthalmology
Dr Alexander J Spudas, North York, ON - General Practice
Dr Randolf A Staab, Mississauga, ON - Psychiatry
Dr Leonore D Stampa, Olds, AB - Family Medicine
Dr Jitka Stankova, Montreal, QC - General Practice
Dr Wayne E Stanley, Lindsay, ON - Family Medicine
Dr Christa Staudenmaier, St-Jean-Sur-Richel, QC - Ophthalmology
Dr Carolyn R Steinberg, Richmond, BC - Psychiatry
Dr Meir Steiner, Hamilton, ON - Psychiatry
Dr Daniel K Steinitz, Belleville, ON - Orthopedic Surgery
Dr Martin W Steinruck, Kelowna, BC - Family Medicine
Dr Hans J Stelzer, Peterborough, ON - Internal Medicine
Dr Ashleigh D Stelzer-Chilton, Vancouver, BC - Family Medicine
Dr Glenn E Stelzl, Squamish, BC - General Practice
Dr Harold E Stephany, Langley, BC - General Practice
Dr Duncan J Stewart, Ottawa, ON - Cardiology
Dr Karl E Stobbe, St. Catharines, ON - Emergency Family Med
Dr Gerda S Stockler-Ipsiroglu, Vancouver, BC - Neurology

Dr Robert Stopainig, Edmonton, AB - Family Medicine
Dr Hanka H E A Stratmann, Woodbridge, ON - Family Medicine
Dr Hans D Strauss, Mississauga, ON - Cardiology
Dr Claudia T Strehlke, Grande Prairie, AB - Internal Medicine
Dr Lucille Stuart, Whitehorse, YT - Family Medicine
Dr Agnes Z Supala-Berger, Toronto, ON - Neurology
Dr Jonathan Sussman, Hamilton, ON - Family Medicine
Dr Steven D I Sutcliffe, Vancouver, BC - Internal Medicine
Dr Vivien V Suttorp, Lethbridge, AB - Family Medicine
Dr Henry C Swart, Summerside, PE - General Practice
Dr Carin Swartz, Wetaskiwin, AB - General Practice
Dr Michaela Swekla, Cambridge, ON - General Practice
Dr Imre Z Szilvassy, Hamilton, ON - General Practice
Dr Alan H Tallmeister, Scarborough, ON - Anesthesia
Dr Tjien-King Tan, Thornhill, ON - General Practice
Dr Timothy R Tatzel, Thorold, ON - Family Medicine
Dr Raymond P L Tempier, Ottawa, ON - Psychiatry
Dr Lionel Tenby, Richmond, BC - General Practice
Dr Hendrik Ter Keurs, Calgary, AB - Internal Medicine
Dr Gerald J M Tevaarwerk, Victoria, BC - Endocrin/Metabolism
Dr B L Linda The, North York, ON - Obstetrics & Gynecology
Dr Bernard C F Thebaud, Edmonton, AB - Pediatrics
Dr Lilly Thenganatt, East York, ON - Family Medicine
Dr Angela G Thermann, Vancouver, BC - General Practice
Dr Roger E Thomas, Calgary, AB - Family Medicine
Dr Roger H Thomas, Richmond, BC - Ophthalmology
Dr Lilian U Thorpe, Saskatoon, SK - Psychiatry
Dr Roger H Tiede, Cranbrook, BC - General Practice
Dr Alfred E Tober, Vancouver, BC - Emergency Medicine
Dr Bernhard J Toews, Coquitlam, BC - General Practice
Dr Ronald P Toews, Kitchener, ON - Family Medicine
Dr Allan G Toguri, Scarborough, ON - Urology
Dr Heather A Tomlin, Toronto, ON - Diagnostic-Radiology
Dr Victor A Toran, York, ON - Otolaryngology
Dr Andre P Touchburn, Moncton, NB - Emergency Family Med
Dr Johan L Trapman, North York, ON - General Practice
Dr Stephane N Treyvaud, Oakville, ON - Psychiatry
Dr H H Steve Tschen, Windsor, ON - General Practice
Dr Astrid E Tupper, Calgary, AB - Family Medicine
Dr Peter G Turner, Burlington, ON - Psychiatry
Dr Kaspars B Tuters, Toronto, ON - Psychiatry
Dr Felix J Tyndel, Scarborough, ON - Internal Medicine
Dr Sylvia Uhthoff Munro, Ottawa, ON - General Practice
Dr Doris B Ullman, Brantford, ON - Family Medicine
Dr Waldemar G Unger, Vancouver, BC - Obstetrics & Gynecology
Dr H Richard Uretsky, Edmonton, AB - Obstetrics & Gynecology
Dr Francois N Urfer, Hawkesbury, ON - General Practice
Dr Mikas A Valadka, Toronto, ON - General Practice
Dr John E E Van Aerde, Surrey, BC - Pediatrics
Dr Jan D Van Der Berg, Red Deer, AB - General Practice
Dr Daniel T H Van Der Merwe, Port Alberni, BC - General Practice
Dr Hendrik G Van Heerden, Nipawin, SK - General Practice
Dr T M Matthew J Van Olm, Calgary, AB - Internal Medicine
Dr Peter R Van Rhijn, Mississauga, ON - General Practice
Dr Stanislaus H M Van Uum, London, ON - Endocrin/Metabolism
Dr Andre R Van Wyk, Langley, BC - Family Medicine
Dr Irene J Vanek, Toronto, ON - Ophthalmology
Dr David W Vas, Pointe-Claire, QC - Emergency Family Med
Dr Inge Vasovich, Hamilton, ON - General Practice
Dr Martin B Veall, Midland, ON - Family Medicine
Dr Otto F Veidlinger, Toronto, ON - Neurology
Dr Keimpe Veldhuis, London, ON - Internal Medicine
Dr Yvonne D Verbeeten, Toronto, ON - Family Medicine
Dr Nicolaas P L G Verhoeff, North York, ON - Psychiatry
Dr Thomas R Verny, Stratford, ON - Psychiatry
Dr Monique Villanueva Arquint, Markham, ON - General Pathology
Dr Gisela H Vischer, North Vancouver, BC - Anatomical Pathology
Dr Thilo E Vollrath, Ottawa, ON - Psychiatry
Dr Bernhard A Volz, Beamsville, ON - Family Medicine
Dr Herbert P Von Schroeder, Toronto, ON - Orthopedic Surgery
Dr Arnold J Voth, Edmonton, AB - Internal Medicine
Dr Oswald F Wachtler, Calgary, AB - General Practice
Dr Malcolm G Walker, Fort McMurray, AB - Family Medicine
Dr Michael J Walmsley, Mississauga, ON - General Surgery
Dr Kai-Yun Wang, Toronto, ON - General Practice
Dr Theodore E Warkentin, Hamilton, ON - Hematology
Dr Thomas Warkus, Montreal, QC - General Practice
Dr Gordon Warme, Toronto, ON - Psychiatry
Dr Gregory D Waslen, Calgary, AB - Plastic Surgery
Dr Delene Wassermann, Williams Lake, BC - General Practice
Dr Michael W B Watson, Edmonton, AB - General Practice
Dr Otto Weiglein, Burlington, ON - Plastic Surgery
Dr Rudolf A Weitemeyer, New Westminster, BC - General Surgery
Dr Thomas Wendel, Cranbrook, BC - General Practice
Dr Wilfred Wendland, 100 Mile House, BC - General Practice
Dr Larry M Wengle, Toronto, ON - General Practice
Dr Thomas R Wenske, London, ON - General Practice
Dr Isabella M Werkman, St Paul, AB - General Practice
Dr Monica J Werner, Edmonton, AB - General Practice
Dr Frank Wernicke, Comox, BC - General Practice
Dr Trevor Wesson, Montreal, QC - General Practice
Dr Hendrik H Westenberg, Kingston, ON - General Practice
Dr Wolfgang H Wetzer, Saanichton, BC - General Practice
Dr Ian S White, Invermere, BC - Family Medicine
Dr Carl H B Wiebe, Vancouver, BC - Psychiatry
Dr H Edward Wiens, Red Deer, AB - Family Medicine
Dr Donald E Wiens, Brampton, ON - Family Medicine
Dr Doris H Wiens, St Catharines, ON - Family Medicine
Dr Bruno O Will, Guelph, ON - General Practice
Dr Michael B Wilson, Thunder Bay, ON - Family Medicine
Dr Inge G Winslow, Richmond Hill, ON - General Practice
Dr Stephanie H M Winsor, Hamilton, ON - Obstetrics & Gynecology
Dr Itta M Winter, Courtenay, BC - Family Medicine
Dr Norbert J Witt, Edmonton, AB - Neurology
Dr Helga B Witt-Sullivan, Hamilton, ON - Internal Medicine
Dr Cornelius J Woelk, Winkler, MB - Family Medicine
Dr Ronald J Wojtyk, Ottawa, ON - General Practice
Dr Michael Wolf, Williams Lake, BC - General Practice
Dr Terence C H Woods, Deep River, ON - Family Medicine
Dr Ilka Y S Wright, Hamilton, ON - Family Medicine
Dr Youssef M R Youssef, Oshawa, ON - Radiation Oncology
Dr Fady Youssef, Ottawa, ON - Emergency Family Med
Dr Ralph W Zabel, Nepean, ON - Ophthalmology
Dr Agnes M Zeliger, Westmount, QC - Pediatrics
Dr Reinhard D Zeller, Toronto, ON - Orthopedic Surgery
Dr George J Zeman, North Bay, ON - Obstetrics & Gynecology
Dr Camilla C U Zimmermann, Toronto, ON - Internal Medicine
Dr Marietta L T Zorn, Scarborough, ON - Plastic Surgery
Dr Joseph A de Nanassy, Ottawa, ON - Anatomical Pathology

GHANAIAN

Dr J Oluwagbenga Ajayi-Obe, Sarnia, ON - Family Medicine
Dr Ama De Graft-Johnson, Hamilton, ON - Anesthesia
Dr Thomas E Forson, Cornwall, ON - General Practice
Dr Albert Gyimah, Brampton, ON - Psychiatry
Dr Horace D Laryea, Pointe-Claire, QC - Internal Medicine

GREEK

Dr Stacey Ageranioti-Belanger, Montreal, QC - Pediatrics
Dr Maria Alexiadis, Halifax, NS - General Practice
Dr Iakovina Alexopoulou, Hamilton, ON - Anatomical Pathology
Dr Evangelia-Lila Amirali, Montreal, QC - Psychiatry
Dr Lefkos Anastasiades, Winnipeg, MB - Internal Medicine
Dr Stella Andonatos, Cote Saint-Luc, QC - General Practice
Dr Charalambos Andreou, Surrey, BC - Urology
Dr E Roseann Andreou, Toronto, ON - Hematology
Dr John Antoniou, Montreal, QC - Orthopedic Surgery
Dr Constantine Apostolides, Halifax, NS - Family Medicine
Dr Peter Assimakopoulos, Montreal, QC - Endocrin/Metabolism
Dr George N Assuras, Winnipeg, MB - General Surgery
Dr Sofia Bazios, Toronto, ON - Family Medicine
Dr Michael J Bazos, Toronto, ON - General Practice
Dr Christos Boulias, Toronto, ON - Physical Medicine & Rehab
Dr Pauline Boulos, Hamilton, ON - Internal Medicine
Dr Ilias Cagiannos, Ottawa, ON - Urology
Dr Lambros N Chaniotis, Pointe-Claire, QC - Cardiology
Dr Georges N Choueri, Laval, QC - Gastroenterology
Dr George T Christakis, Toronto, ON - Cardiovasc/ThorSurg
Dr John T Christakis, Toronto, ON - Ophthalmology
Dr Nicolas V Christou, Saint-Laurent, QC - General Surgery
Dr Nicolas Constas-Costopoulos, Montreal, QC - General Practice
Dr Zafiris Daskalakis, Toronto, ON - Psychiatry
Dr Rina Daskalopoulos, Cobourg, ON - Family Medicine
Dr Dawood G Dawood, Gloucester, ON - Obstetrics & Gynecology
Dr John Deliakis, Toronto, ON - Family Medicine
Dr Francois Dessureault, Boucherville, QC - General Practice
Dr Indra M C Dhunnoo, Edmonton, AB - Pediatrics
Dr Nicholas E Diamant, Kingston, ON - Internal Medicine
Dr Pantelis Diamantouros, London, ON - Cardiology
Dr Dimitrios P Dimitrakoudis, Toronto, ON - Neurology
Dr Dimitrios Divaris, Kitchener, ON - General Pathology
Dr Gus Dotsikas, Oshawa, ON - Diagnostic-Radiology
Dr James D Douketis, Hamilton, ON - Internal Medicine
Dr Anastasios T Dracopoulos, Toronto, ON - Family Medicine
Dr Demetrios A Drakos, Brantford, ON - Plastic Surgery
Dr Peter Dzongowski, London, ON - Family Medicine
Dr Effie Fanaras, Kingston, ON - Internal Medicine
Dr Ioannis Felemegos, Cornwall, ON - Family Medicine
Dr Tharwat A E Fera, Vancouver, BC - Internal Medicine
Dr Panayiotis N Fountas, Toronto, ON - Cardiology
Dr Agoritsa T Foussias, Toronto, ON - Psychiatry
Dr George Foussias, Toronto, ON - Psychiatry
Dr Panayiotis E Frangou, Calgary, AB - Family Medicine
Dr Eleni Galanis, Vancouver, BC - Community Medicine
Dr Dimitrios Giannoulias, Toronto, ON - Obstetrics & Gynecology
Dr Nick T Giftochristos, Keswick, ON - Family Medicine
Dr Haralambos B Grillas, Lachine, QC - Anesthesia
Dr Anastasia Hadjiyannakis, Ottawa, ON - Endocrin/Metabolism
Dr Katerina K Haka-Ikse, Toronto, ON - Pediatrics
Dr Athanasios Harmantas, Toronto, ON - General Surgery
Dr Stamatina Kappos, Bracebridge, ON - Family Medicine
Dr Charalabos B Karabatsos, Brampton, ON - Orthopedic Surgery
Dr Athanassios Karabatsos, Shawville, QC - Internal Medicine
Dr Peter Karalis, Toronto, ON - General Practice
Dr Stavros Karanicolas, Toronto, ON - Internal Medicine
Dr Anastassios Karantonis, Toronto, ON - General Practice
Dr Christos Karatzios, Montreal, QC - Infectious Diseases
Dr Nicolas Karellis, Laval, QC - General Practice
Dr Constantine G Karnis, Burlington, ON - General Practice
Dr John P Karvelas, Winnipeg, MB - Urology
Dr Athanasios Katsarkas, Montreal, QC - Otolaryngology
Dr John Katsounakis, Westmount, QC - Family Medicine
Dr William Kavouris, Etobicoke, ON - General Practice
Dr Lisa M Kellett, Toronto, ON - Dermatology
Dr Spiros Konstantatos, Toronto, ON - Emergency Family Med
Dr Akateneny Kontsiotis, Regina, SK - Family Medicine
Dr Claude Kortas, London, ON - Internal Medicine
Dr Evangelos P Kouros, Welland, ON - General Practice
Dr Chrisostomos Kouroukis, Hamilton, ON - Hematology
Dr Ekaterine Koutroularas, Montreal, QC - General Practice
Dr Georgios Koutsoukos, Toronto, ON - Psychiatry
Dr Demetrios J Kutsogiannis, Edmonton, AB - Internal Medicine
Dr Margarita Lam Antoniades, Toronto, ON - Family Medicine
Dr Steven Larigakis, Surrey, BC - Emergency Family Med
Dr Haralambos Liaconis, Brantford, ON - General Surgery
Dr Rania I Lingas, Toronto, ON - Internal Medicine
Dr Nick F Logarakis, Scarborough, ON - Urology
Dr Lotfullah Lotfi-Seysan, Petawawa, ON - Family Medicine
Dr Andrew D Lukaris, Prince George, BC - Ophthalmology
Dr Caroline Maamari, Greenfield Park, QC - General Practice
Dr Angelo G Macrodimitris, Winnipeg, MB - Ophthalmology
Dr Angelo H Mailis, Toronto, ON - Physical Medicine & Rehab
Dr Therese Manganas, Montreal, QC - General Practice
Dr Thomas Maniatis, Montreal, QC - Internal Medicine
Dr Theodore K Marras, Toronto, ON - Internal Medicine
Dr Cleo A Mavriplis, Ottawa, ON - Family Medicine

Dr Louie Mavrogiannis, Toronto, ON - Family Medicine
Dr P Peter Metrakos, Montreal, QC - General Surgery
Dr Michael Michailidis, Newmarket, ON - Anesthesia
Dr Sophia Mobilos, Toronto, ON - Family Medicine
Dr Patricia A Mousmanis, Richmond Hill, ON - Family Medicine
Dr Savvakis Nicolaou, Vancouver, BC - Diagnostic-Radiology
Dr Andreas Nikolis, Montreal, QC - Plastic Surgery
Dr Luc L Oligny, Montreal, QC - General Pathology
Dr Konstantino P Panagiotopoulos, North Vancouver, BC - Orthopedic Surgery
Dr Panayiotis Panayides, Red Deer, AB - General Surgery
Dr Apostolos Papageorgiou, Montreal, QC - Pediatrics
Dr Alexandra Papaioannou, Hamilton, ON - Geriatric Medicine
Dr Vasilios W Papanastasiou, Westmount, QC - Plastic Surgery
Dr George Papatheodorou, Toronto, ON - Psychiatry
Dr Vasiliki Papukna, London, ON - General Practice
Dr Emilyos Paras, Saint John, NB - Pediatrics
Dr Steven Paraskevas, Montreal, QC - General Surgery
Dr Irene Patelis-Siotis, Hamilton, ON - Psychiatry
Dr Stefanos Patmanidis, Woodbridge, ON - Psychiatry
Dr John R H Penhall, Campbell River, BC - Family Medicine
Dr Constantine S Petrou, Scarborough, ON - Pediatrics
Dr Peter Photopoulos, Toronto, ON - Family Medicine
Dr Andreas Pierratos, Toronto, ON - Internal Medicine
Dr Eugenia Piliotis, Toronto, ON - Hematology
Dr Christina Plaskos, St Catharines, ON - General Practice
Dr Irene Polidoulis, Scarborough, ON - Family Medicine
Dr Constantin Polychronakos, Montreal, QC - Endocrinology
Dr Spiro Polyhronopoulos, Langley, BC - Emergency Family Med
Dr George S Porfiris, Toronto, ON - Emergency Family Med
Dr Vassilios Poulopoulos, Orillia, ON - Internal Medicine
Dr Elena Poulos, Etobicoke, ON - Dermatology
Dr John Provatopoulos, Sudbury, ON - Obstetrics & Gynecology
Dr Cleo C Rogakou, Newmarket, ON - Orthopedic Surgery
Dr Paul Roumeliotis, Cornwall, ON - Pediatrics
Dr Demetrios D J Sahlas, Hamilton, ON - Neurology
Dr Gary C Salasidis, Kitchener, ON - Cardiothor Surgery
Dr Georgoulla Savvidou, East York, ON - General Practice
Dr Dimitrios Scarvelis, Ottawa, ON - Hematology
Dr David J Segal, Vancouver, BC - General Practice
Dr Athanasios T Shizas, Oshawa, ON - General Practice
Dr Lucas Sideris, Montreal, QC - General Surgery
Dr John Sigalas, Scarborough, ON - Endocrin/Metabolism
Dr Pantelis Simantirakis, Oshawa, ON - Anesthesia
Dr Emmanuel Simantirakis, Ottawa, ON - Diagnostic-Radiology
Dr Jovan G Simeon, Vanier, ON - Psychiatry
Dr Maria Skarpathiotakis, Toronto, ON - Diagnostic-Radiology
Dr Nicholas Skouras, Toronto, ON - Ophthalmology
Dr Monica J Skrukwa, Calgary, AB - Family Medicine
Dr Christos Soulios, Toronto, ON - Psychiatry
Dr Elias Soumbasis, Calgary, AB - Family Medicine
Dr Christos Spirou, Tecumseh, ON - Family Medicine
Dr Chrissoula S Stavrakaki, Nepean, ON - Psychiatry
Dr Vasia Stefou, Toronto, ON - General Practice
Dr Victoria Stergiopoulos, Toronto, ON - Psychiatry
Dr Andreas Tassis, Richmond Hill, ON - General Surgery
Dr John S Theodoropoulos, Toronto, ON - Orthopedic Surgery
Dr Achilleas Thoma, Hamilton, ON - Plastic Surgery
Dr Mary Thomas, Toronto, ON - Family Medicine
Dr Konstantinos Tirovolas, Mississauga, ON - Psychiatry
Dr Apostolus Titis, Oshawa, ON - Family Medicine
Dr Apostolos A Tountas, North York, ON - Orthopedic Surgery
Dr Andrew Travlos, Vancouver, BC - Physical Medicine & Rehab
Dr Mark Triantafillou, Charlottetown, PE - General Practice
Dr Leonidas Trigazis, Bolton, ON - Family Medicine
Dr Anna Tsakalaki, Gatineau, QC - Family Medicine
Dr Theodoros Tsakiridis, Hamilton, ON - Radiation Oncology
Dr Nickoli Tsandelis, Kitchener, ON - Obstetrics & Gynecology
Dr Eleftheria Tsatsaronis, Toronto, ON - General Practice
Dr John Tsihlias, Etobicoke, ON - Urology
Dr Georges Tsoukas, Montreal, QC - Endocrinology
Dr Christos M Tsoukas, Montreal, QC - Internal Medicine
Dr Katina Tzanetos, Toronto, ON - Internal Medicine
Dr Nicholas Valettas, Hamilton, ON - Cardiology
Dr Marica Varga, Toronto, ON - Geriatric Medicine
Dr Mariette Varvarikos, Montreal, QC - Emergency Family Med
Dr Denise M Vasiliou, East York, ON - Internal Medicine
Dr Demetra Vassiliou, Ottawa, ON - Obstetrics & Gynecology
Dr Michael Vassilyadi, Ottawa, ON - Neurosurgery
Dr George Vavougios, Aurora, ON - Family Medicine
Dr James Vavougios, Toronto, ON - Family Medicine
Dr Harry R Vedelago, Guelph, ON - Family Medicine
Dr George D Veenhuyzen, Calgary, AB - Cardiology
Dr James L Velianou, Hamilton, ON - Cardiology
Dr Pamela Velos, North York, ON - Ophthalmology
Dr Dimitrios Vergidis, Thunder Bay, ON - Hematology
Dr George A Vilos, London, ON - Obstetrics & Gynecology
Dr Helen Vlachos, Sherbrooke, QC - Pediatrics
Dr Donna S Vlahos, Scarborough, ON - Family Medicine
Dr George Voineskos, Toronto, ON - Psychiatry
Dr Nicholas C Voudouris, Thornhill, ON - General Practice
Dr Anastasios Vourlas, East York, ON - Diagnostic-Radiology
Dr Emorphea Voutsilakos, Vancouver, BC - Psychiatry
Dr Constantin G Vozis, Toronto, ON - General Practice
Dr Socrates A Vozoris, York, ON - Cardiology
Dr Anargyros Xenocostas, London, ON - Hematology
Dr John B Xenos, Montreal, QC - General Practice
Dr George J Xeroulis, Ajax, ON - General Surgery
Dr George Xidos, Saint John, NB - General Practice
Dr Anna Yiannopoulos, Montreal, QC - Internal Medicine
Dr George P Zachariadis, Toronto, ON - General Practice
Dr Marianthi Zachos, Hamilton, ON - Gastroenterology
Dr Constantine R Zachos, Richmond Hill, ON - General Practice
Dr Thomas A Zaphiratos, Montreal, QC - General Practice
Dr Peter C Zarkadas, North Vancouver, BC - Orthopedic Surgery
Dr Eugenia Zikos, Montreal, QC - Psychiatry
Dr Athanasios P Zis Sr, Vancouver, BC - Psychiatry

GUJARATI

Dr Mustafa H Abdulhusein, Brampton, ON - General Practice
Dr Abbas G Abdulhusein, Garson, ON - General Practice
Dr Alnoor Abdulla, Vancouver, BC - Cardiology
Dr Alykhan S Abdulla, Manotick, ON - Family Medicine
Dr Ismail Y Aboo, Owen Sound, ON - General Practice
Dr Meenaxi S Acharya, Bay l'Argent, NL - Physical Medicine & Rehab
Dr Virbala C Acharya, Ottawa, ON - Anatomical Pathology
Dr Tasneem Adenwala, Bolton, ON - Family Medicine
Dr Iram F Ahmed, Niagara Falls, ON - General Practice
Dr Karima M Ali, Calgary, AB - Family Medicine
Dr Yasmin Ali, Coquitlam, BC - Family Medicine
Dr Shabbir M H Alibhai, Toronto, ON - Geriatric Medicine
Dr Shabbir F Amin, Fort Saskatchewan, AB - Family Medicine
Dr Dinyar H Amrolia, Calgary, AB - General Practice
Dr Nafisa J Aptekar, Brampton, ON - Family Medicine
Dr Shiraz F Aziz, Surrey, BC - General Practice
Dr Ashraf M Bandali, Brampton, ON - General Practice
Dr Asifa Bawangoanwala, Mississauga, ON - Family Medicine
Dr Nadeem H Bhanji, Calgary, AB - Psychiatry
Dr Nazmudin M F Bhanji, Vancouver, BC - Pediatrics
Dr Gunvantrai J Bhatt, Windsor, ON - General Practice
Dr Fatima Bhetasi, Welland, ON - Pediatrics
Dr Paramjit S Bhui, Surrey, BC - Pediatrics
Dr Pargat S Bhurji, Surrey, BC - Pediatrics
Dr Essop M Cassim, Kingston, ON - General Practice
Dr Jayshree Chanchlani, Brampton, ON - General Practice
Dr Prafulchandra C Chandarana, London, ON - Psychiatry
Dr Jayantilal J Changela, Saskatoon, SK - Family Medicine
Dr Upesh C Chauhan, Innisfail, AB - Family Medicine
Dr Rameshchandra P Chauhan, Ottawa, ON - Orthopedic Surgery
Dr Harvinder K Chawla, Brockville, ON - Pediatrics
Dr Mukesh Chhanabhai, Surrey, BC - General Pathology
Dr Nazim F Damji, Etobicoke, ON - Hematology
Dr Alkarim Damji, Etobicoke, ON - Family Medicine
Dr Mehboob Damji, Stoney Creek, ON - General Practice
Dr Shahnaz Dar, Scarborough, ON - Pediatrics
Dr Abdulsultan A Datoo, Richmond Hill, ON - Anesthesia
Dr Kishorchandra M Dave, Toronto, ON - Family Medicine
Dr Mohamed N Daya, Etobicoke, ON - Family Medicine
Dr Salim H Daya, Mississauga, ON - Obstetrics & Gynecology
Dr Naeema C Degani, Mississauga, ON - General Practice
Dr Cassim T Degani, Mississauga, ON - General Surgery
Dr Harsha V Dehejia, Ottawa, ON - Internal Medicine
Dr Fareed M Denath, Windsor, ON - Diagnostic-Radiology
Dr Sunil Desai, Edmonton, AB - Pediatrics
Dr Satish S Desai, Parksville, BC - General Practice
Dr Jagdish Desai, Brantford, ON - General Practice
Dr Nimesh Desai, Cambridge, ON - Ophthalmology
Dr Dushyant Desai, Kitchener, ON - Cardiology
Dr Rashmikant J Desai, Mississauga, ON - Urology
Dr Milind G Desai, North York, ON - Gastroenterology
Dr Shalini Desai, Toronto, ON - Infectious Diseases
Dr Devanshu Desai, Toronto, ON - Psychiatry
Dr Hiren B Desai, Windsor, ON - Neurology
Dr Shashi P Devi, North York, ON - Family Medicine
Dr Fatima Dhalla, Ottawa, ON - Family Medicine
Dr Aminmohamed Dhalla, Scarborough, ON - General Practice
Dr Mohsin N Dhalla, Stoney Creek, ON - Family Medicine
Dr Al-Noor Dhanani, Mississauga, ON - Neurology
Dr Pankaj M Dhawan, Vancouver, BC - Physical Medicine & Rehab
Dr Roshan M Dheda, Bradford, ON - Family Medicine
Dr Farouk Dindar, Scarborough, ON - Neurology
Dr Murtaza A Diwan, Guelph, ON - Otolaryngology
Dr Ariz A Engineer, Toronto, ON - General Practice
Dr Sleem Feroze, Oakville, ON - Obstetrics & Gynecology
Dr Tina D Gai, Grimsby, ON - Obstetrics & Gynecology
Dr Karamchand J Gandhi, Bridgewater, NS - General Practice
Dr Asmitha Gangani, Aurora, ON - Family Medicine
Dr Prakash S Gangdev, London, ON - General Practice
Dr Anil Garach, Sarnia, ON - Orthopedic Surgery
Dr Shiva K Gaur, Scarborough, ON - General Practice
Dr Lalji R Gohill, Calgary, AB - General Practice
Dr Sandhya Gokhale, Kitchener, ON - Family Medicine
Dr Jairaj J Govan, North York, ON - Pediatrics
Dr Sajadhussein S Gulamhusein, Edmonton, AB - Cardiology
Dr Murtaza Gulamhussein, Grimsby, ON - General Practice
Dr Rekha Gupta, Halifax, NS - Anatomical Pathology
Dr Shaukat Hasan, Oshawa, ON - Family Medicine
Dr Parviz M Hasham, Brampton, ON - General Practice
Dr Mahjabeen Hussain, Calgary, AB - Family Medicine
Dr Shabnam Hussain, Ottawa, ON - Family Medicine
Dr Shiraz H Ismail, North York, ON - General Practice
Dr Naaznin K Jaffer, Scarborough, ON - General Practice
Dr Hem C Jain, Cambridge, ON - Dermatology
Dr Dawood I Jamal, Toronto, ON - General Practice
Dr Sherally K Jamani, Hamilton, ON - General Practice
Dr Aarti Jani, Prince George, BC - Psychiatry
Dr Amin R Javer, Vancouver, BC - Otolaryngology
Dr Adam M Jeeva, High River, AB - General Practice
Dr Shamim Jessa, Calgary, AB - General Practice
Dr Nasir Jetha, Vancouver, BC - Pediatrics
Dr Bhiku Jethalal, Scarborough, ON - Internal Medicine
Dr Arvind K N Jethwa, London, ON - General Practice
Dr Gulnaz B Jiwa, Edmonton, AB - Obstetrics & Gynecology
Dr Abdulkarim M Jiwa, Vancouver, BC - Psychiatry
Dr Azim H Jiwani, West Vancouver, BC - Family Medicine
Dr Krishna Jokhani, Vancouver, BC - Psychiatry
Dr Mini G Joshipura, Etobicoke, ON - Geriatric Medicine
Dr Azim F Juma, Scarborough, ON - Family Medicine
Dr Rozmin F Kamani, Vancouver, BC - Family Medicine
Dr Allaudin A S Kamani, Vancouver, BC - Anesthesia
Dr Azadali A Kamani, Vancouver, BC - General Practice
Dr Hussein D Kanji, Vancouver, BC - Emergency Medicine
Dr Narendra K Karia, Calgary, AB - General Practice
Dr Nasim A Karim, Calgary, AB - General Practice
Dr Mohamed A Karmali, Toronto, ON - Medical Microbiology
Dr Shameela S F Karmali-Rawji, Calgary, AB - Family Medicine
Dr Narmin Kassam, Edmonton, AB - Internal Medicine
Dr Hement K Katarey, Oakville, ON - Family Medicine
Dr Arvind D Khambhla, Toronto, ON - Obstetrics & Gynecology
Dr Mahmuda B Khan, Scarborough, ON - Family Medicine
Dr Dnyanada L Kothare, Regina, SK - General Practice
Dr Mohanlal Lad, Hamilton, ON - General Practice
Dr Anis H Lakha, North Vancouver, BC - General Practice
Dr Naznin Lalani, Scarborough, ON - Family Medicine

Dr Rakesh K Lamba, Abbotsford, BC - Psychiatry
Dr Rizwana Lilani, Maple, ON - Family Medicine
Dr Gulshan Lodhi, St Jacobs, ON - General Practice
Dr Shashi Lota, Calgary, AB - General Practice
Dr Deviani Maher, West Vancouver, BC - Geriatric Medicine
Dr Surya Master, Campbellton, NB - General Surgery
Dr Al-Karim Mawani, Stouffville, ON - Family Medicine
Dr Nazlin K McAlister, Whitby, ON - Family Medicine
Dr Shahbegum A Meghji, Edmonton, AB - General Practice
Dr Pravinsagar G Mehta, Winnipeg, MB - Family Medicine
Dr Tushar Mehta, Brampton, ON - Family Medicine
Dr Labhshanker S Mehta, St Catharines, ON - Diagnostic-Radiology
Dr Sanjay V Mehta, Toronto, ON - Pediatric Emergency Medicine
Dr Suryakant D Mehta, Toronto, ON - General Practice
Dr Dilipkumar H Mehta, Toronto, ON - Pediatrics
Dr Damini Mehta, Woodbridge, ON - Family Medicine
Dr Shamsh Y Merali, Milton, ON - Family Medicine
Dr Pradeep Merchant, Ottawa, ON - Pediatrics
Dr Amirudin A M Mewa, Toronto, ON - Internal Medicine
Dr Dinesh J Mistry, Golden, BC - Family Medicine
Dr Prabhudas N Mistry, Langley, BC - Psychiatry
Dr Dalpatbhai B Mistry, Oshawa, ON - Psychiatry
Dr Pyarali A Mitha, Calgary, AB - General Practice
Dr Akber H Mithani, Vancouver, BC - General Practice
Dr Nashila N Mohamed, Etobicoke, ON - Family Medicine
Dr Parbhoo Morar, Scarborough, ON - General Practice
Dr Rasheda Motala, Calgary, AB - Family Medicine
Dr Manisha M Mulgund, Burlington, ON - Internal Medicine
Dr Rajeev H Muni, Toronto, ON - Ophthalmology
Dr Ashnoor Nagji, Vancouver, BC - Family Medicine
Dr Rohit S Nagpal, Brampton, ON - Family Medicine
Dr A Ali Najarali, Brampton, ON - General Practice
Dr Shamim G Najarali, Brampton, ON - Anesthesia
Dr Gulammohamed G V Nanji, Calgary, AB - Anesthesia
Dr Dharmesh J Natha, White Rock, BC - Family Medicine
Dr Bharat C Nathoo, Richmond Hill, ON - Internal Medicine
Dr Karim B Nazarali, Mississauga, ON - Otolaryngology
Dr Sudhir D Pandya, Calgary, AB - Emergency Medicine
Dr Anand H Pandya, Brampton, ON - Critical Care Medicine
Dr Sudhir P Pandya, Oakville, ON - Gastroenterology
Dr Praful K Parekh, Calgary, AB - Internal Medicine
Dr Kalavati B Patel, Wetaskiwin, AB - General Practice
Dr Bhasker M Patel, Wetaskiwin, AB - Family Medicine
Dr Kirit K Patel, St. John's, NL - General Practice
Dr Rupa Patel, Kingston, ON - Family Medicine
Dr Ketan N Patel, London, ON - General Practice
Dr Ila M Patel, Mississauga, ON - Family Medicine
Dr Vishnu K Patel, Orleans, ON - General Practice
Dr Naresh R Patel, Tilbury, ON - Family Medicine
Dr Hasmukh G Patel, Windsor, ON - Anesthesia
Dr Prakash C Patel, Regina, SK - Internal Medicine
Dr Rajnikant L Patel, Regina, SK - General Practice
Dr Chakrabarty L Pole, Surrey, BC - Psychiatry
Dr Hemraj R Porwal, Niagara Falls, ON - Family Medicine
Dr Ally K P H Prebtani, Hamilton, ON - Endocrin/Metabolism
Dr Yasmeen A B Punjani, Scarborough, ON - Internal Medicine
Dr Dinshaw K Punthakee, Hamilton, ON - Orthopedic Surgery
Dr Nimishchandra N Purohit, Burlington, ON - Psychiatry
Dr Kiran Rabheru, Ottawa, ON - Family Medicine
Dr Yasmin H Rahim, Newmarket, ON - Hematology
Dr Sultaneih S P Rajabali, New Westminster, BC - General Practice
Dr Hasmukhlal R Rajani, Edmonton, AB - Pediatrics
Dr Kantilal R Rajani, Winnipeg, MB - Pediatrics
Dr Priya K Rajani, Oakville, ON - Family Medicine
Dr Mohamed G V Rajani, Toronto, ON - General Practice
Dr Moizali A Ramji, Sherwood Park, AB - General Practice
Dr Ranjit N Ranawaya, Calgary, AB - Neurology
Dr Sudesh Rayner, Burlington, ON - General Practice
Dr Ranjodh S Rehal, Winnipeg, MB - General Practice
Dr Yasmin Rehemtula, Mississauga, ON - General Practice
Dr El-Karim F J Rhemtulla, St Catharines, ON - Ophthalmology
Dr Meera Ruparelia, Brockville, ON - Family Medicine
Dr Vasant C Ruparelia, Manotick, ON - General Practice
Dr Surendra P Ruparelia, Oshawa, ON - General Practice

Dr Gulzar P Sachedina, Calgary, AB - Anesthesia
Dr Bashirudin Sachedina, Brampton, ON - Gastroenterology
Dr Fakhruddin Sadikali, St Catharines, ON - Internal Medicine
Dr Dhun S Sadry, Toronto, ON - Family Medicine
Dr Amirali M Samji, Toronto, ON - General Practice
Dr Mahendra B S Sangani, Greenfield Park, QC - General Practice
Dr Hemalata J B Sangani, Greenfield Park, QC - General Practice
Dr Eshratbanu Sayani, Scarborough, ON - Family Medicine
Dr Ebrahim Sayed, Welland, ON - General Practice
Dr Vir Bhushan Sennik, Mississauga, ON - Orthopedic Surgery
Dr Chirag R Shah, Calgary, AB - Ophthalmology
Dr Sachit P Shah, Surrey, BC - Family Medicine
Dr Natavarlal H Shah, Cornwall, ON - General Practice
Dr Jay K Shah, Hamilton, ON - Pediatrics
Dr Bharatkumar K Shah, North York, ON - General Practice
Dr Sheila Shah, North York, ON - General Practice
Dr Meera Shah, Scarborough, ON - Emergency Family Med
Dr Amit P Shah, St Thomas, ON - Emergency Family Med
Dr Pravin C Shah, Strathroy, ON - Anatomical Pathology
Dr Hemant A Shah, Toronto, ON - Gastroenterology
Dr Rajiv R Shah, Toronto, ON - Obstetrics & Gynecology
Dr Prakeshkumar S Shah, Toronto, ON - Pediatrics
Dr Vibhuti S Shah, Toronto, ON - Pediatrics
Dr Vinod H Shah, Welland, ON - General Practice
Dr Bashirunnisa A Shaikh, Etobicoke, ON - General Practice
Dr Bashiruddin N Shaikh, Toronto, ON - Urology
Dr Farid M Shamji, Ottawa, ON - Cardiovasc/ThorSurg
Dr Shiraz B K Shariff, Brampton, ON - General Practice
Dr Shivani Sharma, Markham, ON - General Practice
Dr Maqbool K Sheriff, Nanaimo, BC - Internal Medicine
Dr Tej N Sheth, Hamilton, ON - Cardiology
Dr Tarang N Sheth, Mississauga, ON - Diagnostic-Radiology
Dr Nikita T Sheth, Oakville, ON - Family Medicine
Dr Hinal Sheth, Toronto, ON - Family Medicine
Dr Pravin J Shukle, Nepean, ON - Internal Medicine
Dr Nandini J Singh, Calgary, AB - Psychiatry
Dr Mansurali R Somani, Mission, BC - Family Medicine
Dr Sohel Somani, Brampton, ON - Ophthalmology
Dr Deepa Soni, Mississauga, ON - Emergency Family Med
Dr Permjit S Suri, Nepean, ON - Internal Medicine
Dr Bhadreshchandra V Surti, London, ON - Psychiatry
Dr Adarsh Tailor, Barrie, ON - Internal Medicine
Dr Ashnoor S Talib, Vaughan, ON - Family Medicine
Dr Mharukh Y Tamboli, Ottawa, ON - General Practice
Dr Gemini V Tanna, Toronto, ON - Internal Medicine
Dr Shamim J Tejpar, Stratford, ON - Pediatrics
Dr Bhavna K Thakersee, Waterdown, ON - Family Medicine
Dr Kirit V Thakkar, Mississauga, ON - General Practice
Dr Harilal Thakorlal, Vancouver, BC - General Practice
Dr Mansukhlal L Thakrar, Calgary, AB - General Practice
Dr Yasmin Thobani, Mississauga, ON - General Practice
Dr Sushila M Treasurer, North York, ON - General Practice
Dr Juzer M Tyebkhan, Edmonton, AB - Pediatrics
Dr Bhikubhai D Unarket, Calgary, AB - General Practice
Dr Amitkumar S Upadhyay, Aurora, ON - Family Medicine
Dr Gunjan M Vador, Scarborough, ON - Internal Medicine
Dr Himat Vaghadia, Vancouver, BC - Anesthesia
Dr M Tariq Vakani, Mississauga, ON - Cardiology
Dr Bhavna Valia, Ottawa, ON - Family Medicine
Dr Pravesh K Vallabh, Edmonton, AB - Family Medicine
Dr Mariam Vania, North York, ON - Psychiatry
Dr Azim M Velji, Niagara Falls, ON - Family Medicine
Dr Azizadin S Vellani, Vancouver, BC - General Practice
Dr Pramod K Verma, Edmonton, AB - Obstetrics & Gynecology
Dr Mumtaz A Virji, Vancouver, BC - Pediatrics
Dr Harshala P Vora, Hamilton, ON - Family Medicine
Dr Mukul N Vyas, Vancouver, BC - Internal Medicine
Dr Yasmin J Wadia, White Rock, BC - General Practice
Dr Shiraz A Walji, Calgary, AB - General Practice
Dr Zulfikarali A Wallani, Markham, ON - Psychiatry
Dr Manisha B Witmans, Sherwood Park, AB - Pediatrics
Dr Dushyant K Yajnik, Westmount, QC - General Practice
Dr Oanali T Zavery, Lindsay, ON - Internal Medicine

Dr Sonal D Zilka, Timmins, ON - Emergency Family Med
Dr Jyotsna S Ziradkar, London, ON - Family Medicine
Dr Shaliendra Y Ziradkar, London, ON - Family Medicine

HAINAM

Dr Kwang Yang, Surrey, BC - Family Medicine

HAKKA

Dr Wee Kei Choong, Delta, BC - General Practice
Dr Aik-Ping Eng, Vancouver, BC - General Practice
Dr Jacques S How, Montreal, QC - Endocrin/Metabolism
Dr Charles C S Law, Vancouver, BC - General Practice
Dr Lap Cheung Lee, North York, ON - General Practice
Dr Victor Chee Choon Lee, Scarborough, ON - General Practice
Dr Fook Lin Leong-Sit, Edmonton, AB - Ophthalmology
Dr Kan Wen Li, Richmond Hill, ON - General Practice
Dr Peter H L Pang, Gatineau, QC - General Practice
Dr Min Sen Phang, Vancouver, BC - Pediatrics
Dr Vincent V S Thien, Scarborough, ON - Gastroenterology
Dr Chee Nyok Thong, Vancouver, BC - Otolaryngology
Dr Luke B S Tse, Prince Rupert, BC - Family Medicine
Dr Daniel K C Wong, Maple Ridge, BC - General Practice
Dr Collin K K Yong, Vancouver, BC - Pediatrics
Dr Tsai Hsing Yu, St Catharines, ON - General Practice
Dr Kenny J Zhang, Mississauga, ON - Family Medicine

HAUSA

Dr Megeri Ede, Ottawa, ON - Internal Medicine
Dr Paul O Oladipo, St Catharines, ON - Family Medicine
Dr Adrian B T Sohn, Guelph, ON - Family Medicine

HEBREW

Dr Victor Abikhzer, Montreal, QC - General Practice
Dr Awni Abou-Nassar, Mississauga, ON - General Practice
Dr Ramzi Y Abunassar, Ottawa, ON - Internal Medicine
Dr Deena E Ages, North York, ON - General Practice
Dr David Algom, Nepean, ON - Clin Immun/Allergy
Dr Doron Almagor, Toronto, ON - Psychiatry
Dr Eitan Amir, Toronto, ON - General Practice
Dr Andre R Anzarut, Vancouver, BC - Neurology
Dr Grygory Aronshtam, Vancouver, BC - Family Medicine
Dr Ronnie Aronson, Toronto, ON - Endocrin/Metabolism
Dr Raphael Beck, Victoria, BC - Pediatrics
Dr Howard P Berger, Toronto, ON - General Practice
Dr Jason N Berman, Halifax, NS - Pediatrics
Dr Jeffrey J Bernholtz, Richmond Hill, ON - General Practice
Dr Martin Bitzan, Montreal, QC - General Practice
Dr Harvey Blankenstein, North York, ON - Family Medicine
Dr Steve Blitzer, Thornhill, ON - General Practice
Dr Rebecca Bodok, Bolton, ON - Family Medicine
Dr Michael J Bouhadana, Montreal, QC - Family Medicine
Dr Jack S Brandes, Toronto, ON - Psychiatry
Dr Francine Brill, Newmarket, ON - Psychiatry
Dr Yoav Brill, Toronto, ON - Obstetrics & Gynecology
Dr Pnina W Bross, Thornhill, ON - Family Medicine
Dr Zoheir Bshouty, Winnipeg, MB - Internal Medicine
Dr Rena Buckstein, Toronto, ON - Hematology
Dr Nadine M Bukmuz, Toronto, ON - General Practice
Dr Peter L Carlen, Toronto, ON - Neurology
Dr David A Chitayat, Toronto, ON - Medical Genetics
Dr Paul Claman, Ottawa, ON - Obstetrics & Gynecology
Dr Irene Cohen, London, ON - Family Medicine
Dr Shawn L Cohen, Montreal, QC - Ophthalmology
Dr Joseph H Cramer, Scarborough, ON - Obstetrics & Gynecology
Dr Eugene Crystal, Toronto, ON - Cardiology
Dr Aime Dahan, Pointe-Claire, QC - General Practice
Dr Cyril J E Danjoux, Toronto, ON - Radiation Oncology
Dr Jonathan Davine, Hamilton, ON - Family Medicine
Dr Judah Denburg, Hamilton, ON - Hematology
Dr Meredith Deutsch-Levy, Richmond Hill, ON - Family Medicine

Dr Aubie J Diamond, Thornhill, ON - General Practice
Dr Zeev M Diena, North York, ON - Family Medicine
Dr Ronald A Dlin, Edmonton, AB - General Practice
Dr Anatoly Dobrousin, Edmonton, AB - Family Medicine
Dr David Dorenbaum, Toronto, ON - Pediatrics
Dr Yigal Dror, Toronto, ON - Hematology
Dr Isser L Dubinsky, Toronto, ON - Emergency Family Med
Dr David W Eisen, Etobicoke, ON - Family Medicine
Dr Doron A Eisen, Pickering, ON - Family Medicine
Dr Mark J Eisenberg, Montreal, QC - Cardiology
Dr Andre Engel, Ottawa, ON - Pediatrics
Dr David Engelberg, Toronto, ON - Family Medicine
Dr Julius Erdstein, Pierrefonds, QC - Pediatrics
Dr Hanna J Erez, Mississauga, ON - Pediatrics
Dr Dan Farine, Toronto, ON - Obstetrics & Gynecology
Dr Faith P Feinberg, Thornhill, ON - Family Medicine
Dr Jacob Feldman, York, ON - Pediatrics
Dr Philip Fingrut, North York, ON - General Practice
Dr Yaron Finkelstein, Toronto, ON - General Practice
Dr Lawrence Fishman, Winnipeg, MB - Otolaryngology
Dr Raphael Ralph Folman, Mississauga, ON - Pediatrics
Dr Noah A Forman, North York, ON - Family Medicine
Dr Leandra M Forman, Thornhill, ON - Family Medicine
Dr Allan J Fox, Toronto, ON - Diagnostic-Radiology
Dr Gidon Frame, Burnaby, BC - Family Medicine
Dr Jonathan E Freedhoff, Nepean, ON - Family Medicine
Dr Orit C Freedman, Oshawa, ON - Internal Medicine
Dr Mark S Freedman, Ottawa, ON - Neurology
Dr Oded P Fried, North York, ON - General Practice
Dr Eve L M Fried, Woodbridge, ON - Obstetrics & Gynecology
Dr Yael Friedman, Mississauga, ON - Neurology
Dr Jerry A Friedman, Toronto, ON - Psychiatry
Dr Tsvi Gallant, North York, ON - General Practice
Dr Lee Ann Gallant, North York, ON - Pediatrics
Dr Shelly Galler, Toronto, ON - Psychiatry
Dr Beth D Gamulka, Scarborough, ON - Pediatrics
Dr Colin H Geft, North York, ON - Pediatrics
Dr Marvin A Gelkopf, North York, ON - Family Medicine
Dr Elyahu E Gilad, Calgary, AB - General Practice
Dr Stephen A Glazer, North York, ON - Critical Care Medicine
Dr Ileana-Maria Gold, Brampton, ON - Anesthesia
Dr Jewel Gold, Toronto, ON - Cardiology
Dr Chaim J Goldberg, Scarborough, ON - Ophthalmology
Dr Lesley P Goldenberg, Toronto, ON - Psychiatry
Dr Leslie Goldenberg, Toronto, ON - Geriatric Medicine
Dr Sheldon W Goldhar, Scarborough, ON - Ophthalmology
Dr Faye A Goldman, Ottawa, ON - Family Medicine
Dr John I Goldsand, Toronto, ON - Family Medicine
Dr Sol J Goldstein, North York, ON - Psychiatry
Dr Warren C Goldstein, Richmond Hill, ON - Neurology
Dr Benjamin I Goldstein, Toronto, ON - Psychiatry
Dr Julius E S Gomolin, Montreal, QC - Ophthalmology
Dr Michael Gordon, North York, ON - Geriatric Medicine
Dr Olga Gorodetsky, Newmarket, ON - Family Medicine
Dr Fabian P Gorodzinsky, London, ON - Pediatrics
Dr Walter H Gotlieb, Montreal, QC - Obstetrics & Gynecology
Dr Bernard M Green, North York, ON - General Practice
Dr Joseph Greenbaum, Hamilton, ON - Clin Immun/Allergy
Dr Manuel S Greenberg, Thornhill, ON - Pediatrics
Dr David E Greenberg, Toronto, ON - General Practice
Dr Mark A Greenberg, Toronto, ON - Family Medicine
Dr Mark Greenwald, North York, ON - Pediatrics
Dr Kenneth J Greenwald, Toronto, ON - Family Medicine
Dr Gil Gross, Toronto, ON - Pediatric Cardiology
Dr Liuba Grossman, North York, ON - General Practice
Dr Dinah C Gruber, North York, ON - Pediatrics
Dr Batya N Grundland, Toronto, ON - Family Medicine
Dr Eyal Grunebaum, Toronto, ON - General Practice
Dr Juda Habot, Newmarket, ON - Cardiology
Dr Jack Hakoun, Toronto, ON - General Practice
Dr Stewart B Harris, London, ON - Family Medicine
Dr Alexander Hartman, Thornhill, ON - Diagnostic-Radiology
Dr Yaniv Hason, Mississauga, ON - General Practice
Dr Naomi Himel, Toronto, ON - Family Medicine
Dr Leslie S Housefather, North York, ON - Family Medicine
Dr Alan I Iny, Ottawa, ON - Family Medicine

Dr Koma D Israel, Hamilton, ON - Family Medicine
Dr Howard Jacobs, Markham, ON - General Practice
Dr Edward L Jacobson, Oakville, ON - General Practice
Dr Difat E Jakubovicz, Toronto, ON - Family Medicine
Dr Aaron Jesin, North York, ON - General Practice
Dr Tibor Juda, Toronto, ON - Urology
Dr Harry Kadoch, Ormstown, QC - Family Medicine
Dr Allan D Kagal, Concord, ON - Internal Medicine
Dr Yigal Kaikov, Vancouver, BC - Pediatrics
Dr Richard S Kaminker, Scarborough, ON - Orthopedic Surgery
Dr David Kantor, Etobicoke, ON - Psychiatry
Dr David M Kaplan, North York, ON - Family Medicine
Dr Harvey Kaplovitch, Toronto, ON - Family Medicine
Dr Stanley F Karon, Vancouver, BC - Family Medicine
Dr Shelby N Karpman, Edmonton, AB - Family Medicine
Dr Brian M Katchan, North York, ON - Internal Medicine
Dr Dan G Katz, Ajax, ON - Physical Medicine & Rehab
Dr Ron Keren, Toronto, ON - Psychiatry
Dr Ayman M R Khalil, Etobicoke, ON - Family Medicine
Dr Rita M Kharonsky, North York, ON - Family Medicine
Dr Dyan Kimia, Westmount, QC - Pediatrics
Dr Albert J Kirshen, Toronto, ON - Geriatric Medicine
Dr Alla Kirshner, Winnipeg, MB - Psychiatry
Dr Pierre J Kirwin, North York, ON - Physical Medicine & Rehab
Dr Dmitry D Kisselgoff, Thunder Bay, ON - General Practice
Dr Laz V Klein, North York, ON - General Surgery
Dr Max Kleinman, North York, ON - Physical Medicine & Rehab
Dr Gideon Koren, Toronto, ON - Med Scientist
Dr Ilan Lashevsky, Toronto, ON - General Practice
Dr Sasson Lavi, Thornhill, ON - Pediatrics
Dr Sylvie Leone, Mississauga, ON - Obstetrics & Gynecology
Dr Ilona Levin, Lethbridge, AB - General Practice
Dr David Levy, Montreal, QC - General Practice
Dr Leora R Lewittes, Toronto, ON - Family Medicine
Dr Alisa B Lipson, Vancouver, BC - Pediatrics
Dr Jeffrey H Lipton, Toronto, ON - Internal Medicine
Dr Eva M Lonn, Hamilton, ON - Cardiology
Dr G Harvey Lupu, Montreal, QC - Pediatrics
Dr Ilana Magder, Toronto, ON - Pediatrics
Dr Gary M Mann, Thornhill, ON - General Practice
Dr David C Maresky, Toronto, ON - Pediatrics
Dr Howard C Margolese, Montreal, QC - Psychiatry
Dr Ivor J Margolis, Brampton, ON - Pediatrics
Dr Alexander Matz, Lindsay, ON - General Surgery
Dr Bruce D Mazer, Montreal, QC - Clin Immun/Allergy
Dr Yehiel C Meghory, Bolton, ON - Family Medicine
Dr Daniel Melamedov, Thornhill, ON - General Surgery
Dr Harold Merskey, London, ON - Psychiatry
Dr Ronit Mesterman, Hamilton, ON - Neurology
Dr Yoram Minnes, Vancouver, BC - Psychiatry
Dr Allan L Moll, Thornhill, ON - Family Medicine
Dr Ronit Mooallem, Dollard-D-Ormeaux, QC - Family Medicine
Dr Matthew L Morton, Toronto, ON - Obstetrics & Gynecology
Dr Adam Moscovitch, North York, ON - Psychiatry
Dr Ophyr Mourad, Toronto, ON - Internal Medicine
Dr Rami S Mozes, Toronto, ON - General Practice
Dr Stanley Nattel, Montreal, QC - Cardiology
Dr Gil B Nimni, Richmond Hill, ON - Emergency Family Med
Dr Michael Ostro, Mississauga, ON - General Practice
Dr Sam Ozersky, North York, ON - Psychiatry
Dr Eddy H Pakes, North York, ON - Psychiatry
Dr Isaac Perlman, Vancouver, BC - General Practice
Dr Kusiel Perlman, Toronto, ON - Pediatrics
Dr Neora Pick, Vancouver, BC - Internal Medicine
Dr Galina G Portnoi, Thornhill, ON - Family Medicine
Dr Waldemar Pruzanski, Toronto, ON - Internal Medicine
Dr Harold I Reiter, Hamilton, ON - Radiation Oncology
Dr Ayala Revah, North York, ON - Obstetrics & Gynecology
Dr Irwin J Rodier, Montreal, QC - General Practice
Dr Chaim M Roifman, Toronto, ON - Med Scientist
Dr Inna Roitberg, Thornhill, ON - Family Medicine
Dr David S Rootman, Toronto, ON - Ophthalmology
Dr David S Rosenblatt, Montreal, QC - Med Scientist
Dr Rebeccah M Rosenblum, Edmonton, AB - Emergency Medicine
Dr David M Rosenstein, Toronto, ON - Emergency Family Med

Dr Robert M Rosenthal, North York, ON - General Practice
Dr Steven Z Rubin, Calgary, AB - General Surgery
Dr Ethan Rubinstein, Winnipeg, MB - General Practice
Dr Rachel Rubinstein-Schipper, Montreal, QC - Dermatology
Dr Abraham Rudnick, Victoria, BC - Psychiatry
Dr Herbert W Sacks, Edmonton, AB - Family Medicine
Dr Evgeny A Sadikov, Regina, SK - General Practice
Dr Linda S Saffer, Thornhill, ON - Psychiatry
Dr Mark D Saffer, Thornhill, ON - Psychiatry
Dr Eliyhoo A Sagi, Oshawa, ON - Psychiatry
Dr Uri Sagman, Toronto, ON - Internal Medicine
Dr John T Salvendy, Toronto, ON - Psychiatry
Dr David Samra, Scarborough, ON - Obstetrics & Gynecology
Dr Steve E S Samuel, North York, ON - Plastic Surgery
Dr Oded Samuel, North York, ON - Emergency Family Med
Dr Marina Sapozhnikov, Tofield, AB - General Practice
Dr Esther Sarid, North York, ON - Psychiatry
Dr Abraham Sasson, Thornhill, ON - General Practice
Dr Ariah J Schattner, Oshawa, ON - Hematology
Dr Hyman M Schipper, Montreal, QC - Neurology
Dr Kathleen C Schneider, Toronto, ON - Psychiatry
Dr Gil J Schreier, London, ON - Family Medicine
Dr Martin B Schwartz, Toronto, ON - General Practice
Dr Thomas Schwartz, Cote Saint-Luc, QC - Endocrin/Metabolism
Dr Michael J Schweitzer, Stoney Creek, ON - Emergency Family Med
Dr Dennis Scolnik, Toronto, ON - Pediatrics
Dr Allan M Seidenfeld, Toronto, ON - Hematology
Dr Sheryl G Seidman, Toronto, ON - Family Medicine
Dr Ernest G Seidman, Montreal, QC - Pediatrics
Dr Didier M Serero, Montreal, QC - Emergency Family Med
Dr J Zevi Shainhouse, Scarborough, ON - Internal Medicine
Dr Marcia H Shapir Kahan, Toronto, ON - Psychiatry
Dr Joanna L Shapiro, Etobicoke, ON - Family Medicine
Dr Stanley A Shapiro, Sudbury, ON - General Practice
Dr Yaron Shargall, Hamilton, ON - Thoracic Surgery
Dr Sharon Sharir, North York, ON - Urology
Dr Raphael F Sharon, Edmonton, AB - General Practice
Dr Randi C Shaul, Toronto, ON - General Practice
Dr Robert L Shenker, Waterloo, ON - Plastic Surgery
Dr Franklin W Sheps, Thornhill, ON - Emergency Family Med
Dr Zoia Sherman, Windsor, ON - General Practice
Dr Mark H Sherman, Montreal, QC - Endocrin/Metabolism
Dr T Miriam Shichor, Hamilton, ON - General Practice
Dr Yehudi P Shields, Toronto, ON - General Practice
Dr Kevin Shiffman, Whitby, ON - Psychiatry
Dr Eran Shlomovitz, Toronto, ON - Diagnostic-Radiology
Dr Doron Shmorgun, Ottawa, ON - Obstetrics & Gynecology
Dr Elliot H Shub, North York, ON - General Practice
Dr David L Shulman, North York, ON - Family Medicine
Dr Michael Shupak, Toronto, ON - General Practice
Dr Carol S Silverstein, North York, ON - Family Medicine
Dr Raymond Singer, Winnipeg, MB - Family Medicine
Dr Debrah G C Singer, Thornhill, ON - Endocrin/Metabolism
Dr Jonathan R Singer-Jordan, Etobicoke, ON - Diagnostic-Radiology
Dr Lorne N Small, Mississauga, ON - Infectious Diseases
Dr Abraham Snaiderman, Toronto, ON - Psychiatry
Dr Niv Sne, Hamilton, ON - General Surgery
Dr Dina R Sokoloff, Ottawa, ON - Family Medicine
Dr M Charles Solnik, Mississauga, ON - General Practice
Dr Natalia Solomon, Edmonton, AB - Medical Microbiology
Dr Hillel M Sommer, Winnipeg, MB - Physical Medicine & Rehab
Dr Doron D Sommer, Hamilton, ON - Otolaryngology
Dr Leeor Z Sommer, Toronto, ON - Emergency Family Med
Dr Sanford M Spiegel, East York, ON - Diagnostic-Radiology
Dr Rachel F Spitzer, Toronto, ON - Obstetrics & Gynecology
Dr Arthur Staroselsky, Thornhill, ON - Family Medicine
Dr Meir Steiner, Hamilton, ON - Psychiatry
Dr Josef Stelzer, Winnipeg, MB - General Practice
Dr Cynthia Stolovitz, Montreal, QC - Emergency Family Med
Dr Roger D Stronell, Kitchener, ON - Diagnostic-Radiology
Dr Esther R W Sturm, North York, ON - Family Medicine
Dr Heshy Sturm, Thornhill, ON - Pediatrics
Dr Tamar Sudai, North York, ON - Family Medicine

Dr Edison Susman, Scarborough, ON - General Practice
Dr Emile D Svarc, Montreal, QC - Ophthalmology
Dr Keith Symon, Burnaby, BC - General Practice
Dr Julio Szmuilowicz, Toronto, ON - Psychiatry
Dr Isaac I E Szpindel, Toronto, ON - General Practice
Dr David T Tal, Toronto, ON - Geriatric Medicine
Dr Itamar E Tamari, Etobicoke, ON - Family Medicine
Dr Joanne A Tannenbaum, Ottawa, ON - Family Medicine
Dr Bryan S Taylor, North York, ON - Family Medicine
Dr Jesse D Teitel, North York, ON - Family Medicine
Dr Ivor Teitelbaum, North York, ON - General Practice
Dr Joseph Telch, Markham, ON - Pediatrics
Dr D Jonathan Tobin, Ottawa, ON - Family Medicine
Dr Victoria E Tuvivovich, Salaber-de-Valleyf, QC - General Practice
Dr H Richard Uretsky, Edmonton, AB - Obstetrics & Gynecology
Dr Murray B Urowitz, Toronto, ON - Internal Medicine
Dr Shoshana Urson, Richmond Hill, ON - Psychiatry
Dr Sharonie S Valin, North York, ON - Family Medicine
Dr Michael Varenbut, Richmond Hill, ON - Family Medicine
Dr David W Vas, Pointe-Claire, QC - Emergency Family Med
Dr Lea S Velsher, North York, ON - Pediatrics
Dr Danielle L Vicus, Toronto, ON - General Practice
Dr Zohar Waisman, North York, ON - Psychiatry
Dr Ron Wald, Toronto, ON - Internal Medicine
Dr Avi Wallerstein, Montreal, QC - Ophthalmology
Dr Leonard C Warner, Thornhill, ON - Internal Medicine
Dr Ellen Warner, Toronto, ON - Internal Medicine
Dr Avi Wasserman, Windsor, ON - Internal Medicine
Dr Jordan J Weinstein, Toronto, ON - Internal Medicine
Dr Michael S Weinstock, Toronto, ON - General Practice
Dr Jeffrey M Weissberger, Markham, ON - Family Medicine
Dr Antoinette Wertman, North York, ON - Emergency Family Med
Dr Zeph M Wiesenthal, Vancouver, BC - General Practice
Dr Alain A Wiesenthal, Brantford, ON - Otolaryngology
Dr Igor S Wilderman, Thornhill, ON - Family Medicine
Dr A Leo Winter, Hamilton, ON - Urology
Dr Sheldon A Wise, North York, ON - Pediatrics
Dr Joseph I O Wohlgelernter, Thornhill, ON - Psychiatry
Dr Jeffrey I Wulffhart, North York, ON - Family Medicine
Dr Shmuel S Yablonsky, Edmonton, AB - Family Medicine
Dr Robert A Zadik, North York, ON - Anesthesia
Dr Ari E Zaretsky, Toronto, ON - Psychiatry
Dr Lawrence Zoberman, Scarborough, ON - Family Medicine
Dr David J Zukor, Montreal, QC - Orthopedic Surgery

HINDI

Dr Mustafa H Abdulhusein, Brampton, ON - General Practice
Dr Ismail Y Aboo, Owen Sound, ON - General Practice
Dr Thoppil M Abraham, Welland, ON - Psychiatry
Dr Meenaxi S Acharya, Bay l'Argent, NL - Physical Medicine & Rehab
Dr Tasneem Adenwala, Bolton, ON - Family Medicine
Dr Anil Agarwal, Guelph, ON - Internal Medicine
Dr Naresh K Aggarwal, Brampton, ON - Family Medicine
Dr Ram K Aggarwal, Woodbridge, ON - Internal Medicine
Dr Vandana Ahluwalia, Brampton, ON - Internal Medicine
Dr Amar K Ahluwalia, St Catharines, ON - General Practice
Dr Aijaz Ahmad, Medicine Hat, AB - General Practice
Dr Ejaz Ahmad, Winnipeg, MB - Family Medicine
Dr Abul B M Ahmed, Milton, ON - Psychiatry
Dr Nafeesa Q Ahmed, Oakville, ON - General Practice
Dr Bashir Ahmed, Ottawa, ON - General Practice
Dr Syed T Ahmed, St Thomas, ON - Pediatrics
Dr Shafiq F Akbar, Edmonton, AB - Internal Medicine
Dr Zaubaria Akbar, Surrey, BC - General Practice
Dr Haider M Al-Dabbagh, Mississauga, ON - Family Medicine
Dr Tasriqul M Alam, London, ON - Family Medicine
Dr Zeenat Y Alam, Windsor, ON - Internal Medicine
Dr Syed A Ali, Edmonton, AB - General Practice
Dr Yasmin Ali, Coquitlam, BC - Family Medicine
Dr Iqbal Ali, Surrey, BC - Internal Medicine
Dr Liaqat Ali, Barrie, ON - Psychiatry
Dr Pervez Ali, North York, ON - Orthopedic Surgery
Dr Fahim H Ali, Port Perry, ON - Family Medicine
Dr Shabbir F Amin, Fort Saskatchewan, AB - Family Medicine
Dr Shilpa Amin, Burlington, ON - Obstetrics & Gynecology
Dr Afsari B Amjad, Ottawa, ON - Psychiatry
Dr Dinyar H Amrolia, Calgary, AB - General Practice
Dr Neeru Anand, Delta, BC - Family Medicine
Dr Sundaram Anand, North York, ON - General Surgery
Dr Mohinder K Angl, Courtice, ON - General Practice
Dr Saira Ansari, Scarborough, ON - Anatomical Pathology
Dr A Hashsham Ansari, Scarborough, ON - Family Medicine
Dr Saju Antony, Chilliwack, BC - Psychiatry
Dr Nafisa J Aptekar, Brampton, ON - Family Medicine
Dr Nawaz Arora, Brantford, ON - Family Medicine
Dr Sunder S Arora, Ottawa, ON - Psychiatry
Dr Amit Arya, Brampton, ON - Family Medicine
Dr A Neil Arya, Kitchener, ON - Family Medicine
Dr Ahmad S Ashrafi, Surrey, BC - General Surgery
Dr Vijaykumar V Ashtekar, Swift Current, SK - General Practice
Dr Paramjit S Aulakh, Surrey, BC - General Practice
Dr Lakyntiew P S Aulakh, Sudbury, ON - General Practice
Dr Abdul Aziz, Lethbridge, AB - General Practice
Dr Shiraz F Aziz, Surrey, BC - General Practice
Dr Harry S Badhan, Brampton, ON - General Practice
Dr Jagdeep S Badhesha, Calgary, AB - Family Medicine
Dr Amit Bagga, Windsor, ON - Internal Medicine
Dr Jatinder S Baidwan, Victoria, BC - Family Medicine
Dr Sangeeta Bajaj, Brampton, ON - Internal Medicine
Dr Harpreet S Bajaj, Brampton, ON - General Practice
Dr Parvesh Bajaj, Nepean, ON - General Practice
Dr Sameena A Bajwa, Calgary, AB - Family Medicine
Dr Gurjit Bajwa, Etobicoke, ON - General Practice
Dr Tuhin K Bakshi, Wetaskiwin, AB - Family Medicine
Dr Harmeet K Bami, Brampton, ON - Psychiatry
Dr Amrik S Bassi, Calgary, AB - General Practice
Dr Nandita Batchra, Burlington, ON - Otolaryngology
Dr Navdeep Bath, Mississauga, ON - Family Medicine
Dr Alice Benjamin, Montreal, QC - Obstetrics & Gynecology
Dr Ashok Bhagat, Richmond Hill, ON - General Practice
Dr Subramanya Bhagavatula, Sudbury, ON - Psychiatry
Dr Kapil M Bhagirath, Surrey, BC - Cardiology
Dr Chander P Bhagirath, Niagara Falls, ON - Pediatrics
Dr Sanjiv K Bhalla, Edmonton, AB - Diagnostic-Radiology
Dr Dinesh Bhalla, Moncton, NB - Psychiatry
Dr Rakesh Bhandari, London, ON - Anesthesia
Dr Dalip K Bhangu, Etobicoke, ON - Obstetrics & Gynecology
Dr Raminder K Bhangu, Windsor, ON - Psychiatry
Dr Nazmudin M F Bhanji, Vancouver, BC - Pediatrics
Dr Nirmala Bharatwal, Toronto, ON - Physical Medicine & Rehab
Dr Asha Bhardwaj, London, ON - Physical Medicine & Rehab
Dr Manoj Bhargava, Etobicoke, ON - Orthopedic Surgery
Dr Someshwar Bhargava, Orleans, ON - Pediatrics
Dr Rakesh K Bhargava, Oshawa, ON - Cardiology
Dr Rashmi Bhargava, Regina, SK - Obstetrics & Gynecology
Dr Sunil K Bhatt, Vancouver, BC - Family Medicine
Dr Gunvantrai J Bhatt, Windsor, ON - General Practice
Dr Amal Bhattacharyya, Dartmouth, NS - General Practice
Dr Virinder S Bhatti, Maple Ridge, BC - General Practice
Dr Balbir C Bhatti, Surrey, BC - Family Medicine
Dr Renu Bhayana, Winnipeg, MB - General Practice
Dr Fatima Bhetasi, Welland, ON - Pediatrics
Dr Laila Bhimani, Surrey, BC - Family Medicine
Dr Jaswant S Bhopal, Richmond, BC - Psychiatry
Dr Paramjit S Bhui, Surrey, BC - Pediatrics
Dr Vipul K Bhupal, York, ON - General Practice
Dr Pargat S Bhurji, Surrey, BC - Pediatrics
Dr Vinita Bindlish, Kitchener, ON - Family Medicine
Dr Iqbal H Biswas, Cambridge, ON - Anesthesia
Dr Shabab Boparai, Scarborough, ON - Family Medicine
Dr Parminder S Brar, St Catharines, ON - Pediatrics
Dr Santosh A Britto, Salmon Arm, BC - General Surgery
Dr Mary Chacko, Scarborough, ON - Family Medicine
Dr Usha Chada, North York, ON - General Practice
Dr Rati Chadha, Calgary, AB - Obstetrics & Gynecology
Dr Jayshree Chanchlani, Brampton, ON - General Practice
Dr Pavanjeet Chand, Windsor, ON - Family Medicine
Dr Ranjit K Chandra, Mississauga, ON - Pediatrics
Dr Indira Chandran, Brampton, ON - Obstetrics & Gynecology
Dr Vinod Chandran, Toronto, ON - General Practice
Dr Vikram Chandurkar, St. John's, NL - Endocrin/Metabolism
Dr Jayantilal J Changela, Saskatoon, SK - Family Medicine
Dr Laura M Chapman, Victoria, BC - Psychiatry
Dr Vinjamuri R Chari, Hamilton, ON - Physical Medicine & Rehab
Dr Prabhat K Chaturvedi, Glace Bay, NS - General Surgery
Dr Mohammad I Chaudhary, Mississauga, ON - Family Medicine
Dr Sajjad A Chaudhry, Toronto, ON - Anesthesia
Dr Sukarno N Chaudhry, Windsor, ON - Internal Medicine
Dr Upesh C Chauhan, Innisfail, AB - Family Medicine
Dr Rakesh K Chawla, Hammonds Plains, NS - General Practice
Dr Harvinder K Chawla, Brockville, ON - Pediatrics
Dr Satish K Chawla, Niagara Falls, ON - Anatomical Pathology
Dr Ashis K Chawla, Toronto, ON - Urology
Dr Gulzar S Cheema, Surrey, BC - Family Medicine
Dr Waqar M Cheema, Brampton, ON - Family Medicine
Dr Vinnie Chengapa, Halifax, NS - Psychiatry
Dr Samir R Chhabra, Oshawa, ON - Orthopedic Surgery
Dr Khami Chokani, Prince Albert, SK - General Practice
Dr Jagdish C Chopra, Oshawa, ON - General Practice
Dr Sushil Choudhry, Brampton, ON - Family Medicine
Dr Amitava D Chowdhury, Winnipeg, MB - General Practice
Dr Prem K Chugh, Dartmouth, NS - General Practice
Dr Krishna V Chunduri, North York, ON - Family Medicine
Dr Nolda M D'Cunha, Toronto, ON - Family Medicine
Dr Ryan D'Souza, Waterloo, ON - Family Medicine
Dr Shilpa Dabholkar, Coquitlam, BC - Family Medicine
Dr Alkarim Damji, Etobicoke, ON - Family Medicine
Dr Mehboob Damji, Stoney Creek, ON - General Practice
Dr Sujith K Dandina, Surrey, BC - General Practice
Dr Amathul A Danial, Edmonton, AB - General Practice
Dr Bahauddin H Danial, Mississauga, ON - Internal Medicine
Dr A Rashid Dar, London, ON - Radiation Oncology
Dr Madhavan S Das, Edmonton, AB - General Practice
Dr Abdulsultan A Datoo, Richmond Hill, ON - Anesthesia
Dr Jyotirmoy Datta, Saskatoon, SK - General Practice
Dr Faiz Daudi, Etobicoke, ON - General Surgery
Dr Asfa Daudi, Mississauga, ON - Family Medicine
Dr Kanta B Dave, Calgary, AB - General Practice
Dr Malini G Dave, North York, ON - Pediatrics
Dr Kishorchandra M Dave, Toronto, ON - Family Medicine
Dr Meenakshi Dawar, Vancouver, BC - Community Medicine
Dr Shamim Dawood, Oakville, ON - Family Medicine
Dr Nibhas De, Thunder Bay, ON - Pediatrics
Dr Naeema C Degani, Mississauga, ON - General Practice
Dr Cassim T Degani, Mississauga, ON - General Surgery
Dr Harsha V Dehejia, Ottawa, ON - Internal Medicine
Dr Roya F Dehghani-Yar, Hamilton, ON - Family Medicine
Dr Satish S Desai, Parksville, BC - General Practice
Dr Jagdish Desai, Brantford, ON - General Practice
Dr Dushyant Desai, Kitchener, ON - Cardiology
Dr Milind G Desai, North York, ON - Gastroenterology
Dr Devanshu Desai, Toronto, ON - Psychiatry
Dr Hiren B Desai, Windsor, ON - Neurology
Dr Smeeta Desai-Ranchod, Richmond, BC - General Practice
Dr Pushpal Desarkar, Toronto, ON - General Practice
Dr Ashish Deshpande, Windsor, ON - Pediatrics
Dr Manik Devane, Niagara Falls, ON - General Practice
Dr Asha K Devanesen, Mississauga, ON - General Practice
Dr Sudarshan Devanesen, Mississauga, ON - Family Medicine
Dr Chikkahanumaiah Devaraj, Mississauga, ON - Geriatric Medicine
Dr Bijayalaxmi Devi, Ajax, ON - Psychiatry
Dr Shashi P Devi, North York, ON - Family Medicine
Dr Harbhajan S Dhaliwal, Winnipeg, MB - General Practice
Dr Amarinder S Dhaliwal, Brampton, ON - General Practice
Dr Preet B K Dhaliwal, LaSalle, ON - Family Medicine
Dr Fatima Dhalla, Ottawa, ON - Family Medicine
Dr Mohsin N Dhalla, Stoney Creek, ON - Family Medicine
Dr Kavita P Dhamanaskar, Hamilton, ON - Diagnostic-Radiology
Dr Karan S Dhami, Ottawa, ON - Emergency Family Med
Dr Dharminder S Dhanda, New Westminster, BC - Ophthalmology
Dr Avtar S Dhanoa, Mississauga, ON - General Practice
Dr Jag Mohan Dhar, Sarnia, ON - Internal Medicine
Dr Anil Dhar, Windsor, ON - Critical Care Medicine

Dr Nishi Dhawan, Vancouver, BC - Family Medicine
Dr Pankaj M Dhawan, Vancouver, BC - Physical Medicine & Rehab
Dr Baldev S Dhillon, Delta, BC - Family Medicine
Dr Manu Dhillon, Brampton, ON - General Practice
Dr Jaswinder S Dhillon, Brantford, ON - Emergency Family Med
Dr Ripple Dhillon, Oshawa, ON - Family Medicine
Dr Karamvir K Dhillon, Oshawa, ON - Family Medicine
Dr Indra M C Dhunnoo, Edmonton, AB - Pediatrics
Dr Kushal J Dighe, Toronto, ON - Cardiology
Dr Shamoon Din, Mississauga, ON - General Practice
Dr Murtaza A Diwan, Guelph, ON - Otolaryngology
Dr Sanjay Dixit, Burlington, ON - Internal Medicine
Dr Saleena Djearam, Victoria, BC - Family Medicine
Dr Arun K Dosaj, Madoc, ON - General Practice
Dr Seema Dosaj, Pickering, ON - Family Medicine
Dr Varinder Dua, London, ON - Psychiatry
Dr Sampurnanand Dube, Grande Prairie, AB - General Practice
Dr Santosh Dubey, Calgary, AB - General Practice
Dr Sidharth Dutta, Brampton, ON - Family Medicine
Dr Reena E Eapen-John, Mississauga, ON - Family Medicine
Dr Farouk A Ebrahim, Brampton, ON - Family Medicine
Dr Saibishkumar Elantholi Parameswaran, Toronto, ON - Radiation Oncology
Dr Ariz A Engineer, Toronto, ON - General Practice
Dr Rajeev Erry, Pickering, ON - General Practice
Dr Shruthi Eswar, Surrey, BC - Psychiatry
Dr Ziaullah Fahim, Surrey, BC - General Practice
Dr Mohammad Fahim, New Glasgow, NS - General Practice
Dr Shireen Fahim, Etobicoke, ON - Family Medicine
Dr Muna I Farooqi, Guelph, ON - Family Medicine
Dr Najla Fasih, Ottawa, ON - General Practice
Dr Shabeena Fazhulla, Calgary, AB - Family Medicine
Dr Alcantro B Fernandez, Stoney Creek, ON - General Practice
Dr Naila Furqan, Mississauga, ON - Family Medicine
Dr Priya Gaba, Ottawa, ON - Family Medicine
Dr Tina D Gai, Grimsby, ON - Obstetrics & Gynecology
Dr Puneeta Gambhir, Hamilton, ON - Family Medicine
Dr Indu B Gambhir, Ottawa, ON - General Practice
Dr Gobi R Ganapathy, London, ON - Neurology
Dr Satnam S Gandham, Richmond, BC - General Practice
Dr Vinod K Gandhi, Delta, BC - Family Medicine
Dr Amita Gandhi, Delta, BC - Psychiatry
Dr Karamchand J Gandhi, Bridgewater, NS - General Practice
Dr Shruti Gandhi, Etobicoke, ON - Medical Biochemistry
Dr Sonal Gandhi, Toronto, ON - Internal Medicine
Dr Asmitha Gangani, Aurora, ON - Family Medicine
Dr Prakash S Gangdev, London, ON - General Practice
Dr Vinod K Gangolli, Kitchener, ON - Psychiatry
Dr Rohan Ganguli, Toronto, ON - Psychiatry
Dr Anil Garach, Sarnia, ON - Orthopedic Surgery
Dr Hari N Garbharran, Markham, ON - Psychiatry
Dr Arun K Garg, New Westminster, BC - Medical Biochemistry
Dr Narinder K Garg, Brampton, ON - Family Medicine
Dr Divya Garg, St Thomas, ON - Family Medicine
Dr Naveen Garg, Pointe-Claire, QC - Family Medicine
Dr Shiva K Gaur, Scarborough, ON - General Practice
Dr Mohammed A Gauri, Fort Saskatchewan, AB - General Practice
Dr Susan George, Cambridge, ON - Family Medicine
Dr Susan R George, Toronto, ON - Internal Medicine
Dr Sandeep Ghai, Toronto, ON - General Practice
Dr Sangeet Ghai, Toronto, ON - General Practice
Dr Ikram Ghani, Mississauga, ON - General Practice
Dr Hemant B Ghate, Windsor, ON - Anesthesia
Dr Sameera Ghaznavi, Oakville, ON - Family Medicine
Dr Mahua Ghosh, Edmonton, AB - Endocrin/Metabolism
Dr Indraneel Ghosh, Hamilton, ON - Emergency Family Med
Dr Ali T Ghouse, Hamilton, ON - Physical Medicine & Rehab
Dr Jaspinder Ghuman, Surrey, BC - Emergency Family Med
Dr Hamid J Gilani, Guelph, ON - General Practice
Dr Paramjit Gill, Mississauga, ON - General Practice
Dr Vikramjit S Gill, Mississauga, ON - General Practice
Dr Randeep S Gill, Nepean, ON - General Practice
Dr Joginder S Gill, Niagara Falls, ON - Family Medicine
Dr Gurpreet S Gill, Niagara Falls, ON - Internal Medicine
Dr Kulwant S Gill, Sudbury, ON - Hematological Pathology
Dr Satpal S Girgla, Oakville, ON - Psychiatry
Dr Devendra P Goel, Burnaby, BC - General Surgery
Dr Sanjeev Goel, Brampton, ON - Family Medicine
Dr Reena Goel, Brampton, ON - Family Medicine
Dr Sadan K Goel, Brampton, ON - General Surgery
Dr Sunita Goel, Burlington, ON - Family Medicine
Dr Aashish Goela, London, ON - Diagnostic-Radiology
Dr Rupinder K Gogia, Hamilton, ON - Family Medicine
Dr Lalji R Gohill, Calgary, AB - General Practice
Dr Sandhya Gokhale, Kitchener, ON - Family Medicine
Dr Hirekatur V Gopinath, Maple Ridge, BC - Psychiatry
Dr Rupashi Goswami, Welland, ON - Family Medicine
Dr Kempe Gowda, Saskatoon, SK - Internal Medicine
Dr Supriya M Goyal, Calgary, AB - Family Medicine
Dr Kimmy Goyal, Brampton, ON - Family Medicine
Dr Kharak S Grewal, Brampton, ON - General Practice
Dr Manavdeep Grewal, Brampton, ON - Family Medicine
Dr Kamal P Grewal, Brampton, ON - Family Medicine
Dr Puneet Grewal, Burlington, ON - Family Medicine
Dr Simarjot K Grewal, East York, ON - Family Medicine
Dr Rajdeep Grewal, Hamilton, ON - Emergency Family Med
Dr Rajwant K Grewal, Mississauga, ON - General Practice
Dr Deepak Grover, Chilliwack, BC - Orthopedic Surgery
Dr Arvinder Grover, Mississauga, ON - Cardiology
Dr Sanjiv K Gulati, Brockville, ON - General Practice
Dr Brij B Gulati, Lindsay, ON - General Practice
Dr Geetha Gupta, Langley, BC - Family Medicine
Dr Madhu Gupta, Vancouver, BC - Obstetrics & Gynecology
Dr Chander K Gupta, Winnipeg, MB - Obstetrics & Gynecology
Dr Daya K Gupta, Winnipeg, MB - Ophthalmology
Dr Rekha Gupta, Halifax, NS - Anatomical Pathology
Dr Rohit Gupta, Bracebridge, ON - General Surgery
Dr Ram Gupta, Brampton, ON - Family Medicine
Dr Milan Gupta, Brampton, ON - Cardiology
Dr Seema Gupta, Guelph, ON - Family Medicine
Dr Madhulika A Gupta, London, ON - Family Medicine
Dr Aditya K Gupta, London, ON - Dermatology
Dr Anil Gupta, Mississauga, ON - Cardiology
Dr Sanjeev Gupta, Mississauga, ON - General Practice
Dr Asha Gupta, Mississauga, ON - Family Medicine
Dr Hemi Gupta, Sault Ste. Marie, ON - Family Medicine
Dr Inder P Gupta, Sault Ste. Marie, ON - Cardiology
Dr Sanjoy Gupta, Thunder Bay, ON - Ophthalmology
Dr Abha A Gupta, Toronto, ON - Pediatrics
Dr Vikas Gupta, Toronto, ON - General Practice
Dr Samir Gupta, Toronto, ON - Internal Medicine
Dr Malati Gupta, Toronto, ON - Psychiatry
Dr Rasna Gupta, Windsor, ON - General Practice
Dr Namta Gupta, Montreal, QC - Family Medicine
Dr Kiran Guru, Mississauga, ON - General Practice
Dr Jaswant Guzder, Montreal, QC - Psychiatry
Dr Naiyer Habib, Abbotsford, BC - Internal Medicine
Dr Kamil Haider, Etobicoke, ON - Family Medicine
Dr Raju Hajela, Calgary, AB - Family Medicine
Dr Usha Harikumar, Scarborough, ON - Obstetrics & Gynecology
Dr Upninderjit S Harrad, Surrey, BC - Psychiatry
Dr Yasmin Harrison, Toronto, ON - Family Medicine
Dr Shaukat Hasan, Oshawa, ON - Family Medicine
Dr Sadiq Hasan, Whitby, ON - Psychiatry
Dr Haron Hassan, Surrey, BC - Family Medicine
Dr Tariq Hassan, Kingston, ON - General Practice
Dr Sachin K Hazra, St Catharines, ON - Internal Medicine
Dr Daljit S Herar, Surrey, BC - General Pathology
Dr Naushad Hirani, Calgary, AB - Internal Medicine
Dr S Baqir Husain, Prince Albert, SK - Psychiatry
Dr Mahjabeen Hussain, Calgary, AB - Family Medicine
Dr Shabnam Hussain, Ottawa, ON - Family Medicine
Dr Kashif Irshad, Brampton, ON - General Surgery
Dr Jaya M Islur, Toronto, ON - Pediatrics
Dr Shiraz H Ismail, North York, ON - General Practice
Dr Arif M A Ismaili, Kitchener, ON - Gastroenterology
Dr V Chandy Jacob, Winkler, MB - General Surgery
Dr Naaznin K Jaffer, Scarborough, ON - General Practice
Dr Rajesh Jaidka, Brampton, ON - General Practice
Dr Sajal Jain, Burnaby, BC - Internal Medicine
Dr Leena Jain, New Westminster, BC - Geriatric Medicine
Dr Nita Jain, Vancouver, BC - Pediatrics
Dr Narendra K Jain, Winnipeg, MB - General Practice
Dr Shalini Jain, Amherstview, ON - Family Medicine
Dr Hem C Jain, Cambridge, ON - Dermatology
Dr Subhash C Jain, London, ON - Psychiatry
Dr Neelesh K Jain, North York, ON - General Surgery
Dr Rachna Jain, Ottawa, ON - General Practice
Dr Mahendra K Jain, Scarborough, ON - General Practice
Dr Preeti Jain, Toronto, ON - Pediatrics
Dr Umesh Jain, Toronto, ON - Urology
Dr Aarti Jani, Prince George, BC - Psychiatry
Dr Balvinder S Jassar, Edmonton, AB - Family Medicine
Dr Amin R Javer, Vancouver, BC - Otolaryngology
Dr Ajantha Jayabarathan, Halifax, NS - Family Medicine
Dr Jyothi Jayaraman, Vancouver, BC - Family Medicine
Dr Shamim Jessa, Calgary, AB - General Practice
Dr Nasir Jetha, Vancouver, BC - Pediatrics
Dr Shamin Jetha, Vancouver, BC - Family Medicine
Dr Bhiku Jethalal, Scarborough, ON - Internal Medicine
Dr Kailash K Jindal, Edmonton, AB - Internal Medicine
Dr Azim H Jiwani, West Vancouver, BC - Family Medicine
Dr Anvita S Joglekar, North York, ON - Psychiatry
Dr Shashikant A Joglekar, Scarborough, ON - General Practice
Dr Malkit K Johal, Toronto, ON - Family Medicine
Dr Verghese John, Scarborough, ON - Psychiatry
Dr Krishna Jokhani, Vancouver, BC - Psychiatry
Dr Mala Joneja, Kingston, ON - Internal Medicine
Dr Javed Joseph, Regina, SK - General Practice
Dr Changulanda M Joshi, New Glasgow, NS - Obstetrics & Gynecology
Dr Manohar L Joshi, Etobicoke, ON - General Practice
Dr Atul Joshi, Orangeville, ON - Internal Medicine
Dr Suhas B Joshi, St Catharines, ON - Anatomical Pathology
Dr Mini G Joshipura, Etobicoke, ON - Geriatric Medicine
Dr Yajna Jugdave, Waterloo, ON - General Practice
Dr Azim F Juma, Scarborough, ON - Family Medicine
Dr Meghna P Juta, St. Albert, AB - Family Medicine
Dr Umang B Kachroo, North York, ON - Family Medicine
Dr Desikan R Kadambi, Winnipeg, MB - Ophthalmology
Dr Baldev S Kahlon, Delta, BC - General Practice
Dr Soumini Kaiprath, New Glasgow, NS - Family Medicine
Dr Karna C Kale, Mississauga, ON - Family Medicine
Dr Aporna Kali, Grande Prairie, AB - Family Medicine
Dr Bharat B Kalra, Scarborough, ON - General Practice
Dr Allaudin A S Kamani, Vancouver, BC - Anesthesia
Dr Azadali A Kamani, Vancouver, BC - General Practice
Dr Palinder Kamra, St. John's, NL - Pediatrics
Dr Arvind Kang, North Vancouver, BC - Psychiatry
Dr Parmjit S Kang, Surrey, BC - Endocrin/Metabolism
Dr G Shimi Kang, Vancouver, BC - Psychiatry
Dr Amrit K Kang, Toronto, ON - Internal Medicine
Dr Rani Kanthan, Saskatoon, SK - Anatomical Pathology
Dr Videsh Kapoor, Richmond, BC - Family Medicine
Dr Vimal S Kapoor, Markham, ON - Community Medicine
Dr Pankaj V Kapoor, Windsor, ON - General Practice
Dr Nishitha Kapur, Scarborough, ON - Family Medicine
Dr Narendra K Karia, Calgary, AB - General Practice
Dr Shameela S F Karmali-Rawji, Calgary, AB - Family Medicine
Dr Vikas V Karnik, Windsor, ON - General Practice
Dr Savita Karol, Fredericton, NB - Family Medicine
Dr Laila Karwa, Surrey, BC - Anesthesia
Dr Rajendra P Kashyap, Scarborough, ON - General Practice
Dr Hement K Katarey, Oakville, ON - Family Medicine
Dr Arvind A Kati, Winnipeg, MB - General Practice
Dr Balaraju B Katta, Richmond, BC - Psychiatry
Dr Satinder Kaur, Kitchener, ON - Family Medicine
Dr Swarsha Kaushik, Guelph, ON - Family Medicine
Dr Adam S Kayumi, Mississauga, ON - Family Medicine
Dr Soofia L Kazi, London, ON - Family Medicine
Dr Huma Kazmie, Windsor, ON - Pediatrics
Dr Arvind D Khambhla, Toronto, ON - Obstetrics & Gynecology
Dr Safeer A Khan, Calgary, AB - General Practice
Dr Naeem A H Khan, Etobicoke, ON - Psychiatry
Dr Rita R Khan, Kitchener, ON - General Practice

Dr Arshad Khan, Kitchener, ON - Psychiatry
Dr M Viqar Khan, Oakville, ON - Family Medicine
Dr Shajia Khan, Ottawa, ON - Internal Medicine
Dr Razia Khan, Scarborough, ON - General Practice
Dr Shagufta U Khan, Toronto, ON - Endocrin/Metabolism
Dr Mahmood A H Khan, Toronto, ON - Internal Medicine
Dr M Sohail Khattak, Whitby, ON - Pediatrics
Dr Surinder S Khinda, Fort McMurray, AB - Internal Medicine
Dr Anil K Khithani, Scarborough, ON - Family Medicine
Dr Sarjiwan Khullar, Devon, AB - General Practice
Dr J Sevena Khunkhun, Vancouver, BC - Family Medicine
Dr Ajay P S Khural, Carbonear, NL - General Practice
Dr Mona Khurana, Toronto, ON - Family Medicine
Dr Rosy Khurana, Mistissini, QC - Family Medicine
Dr Vishwas M Kini, Brampton, ON - Family Medicine
Dr Abbas A Kohja, Steinbach, MB - General Practice
Dr Sukhdev S Kooner, Windsor, ON - Internal Medicine
Dr Arvind Koshal, Edmonton, AB - Cardiovasc/ThorSurg
Dr Dnyanada L Kothare, Regina, SK - General Practice
Dr Murali Krishnan, Barrie, ON - Internal Medicine
Dr Ramaiyer Krishnaswamy, Fredericton, NB - Pediatrics
Dr Asha Kukreti, Scarborough, ON - General Practice
Dr Vishal Kukreti, Toronto, ON - Hematology
Dr Ramesh Kulkarni, North Bay, ON - Obstetrics & Gynecology
Dr Swati Kulkarni, Windsor, ON - Internal Medicine
Dr Saroj Kumar, Delta, BC - General Practice
Dr Ragbir S Kumar, Cambridge, ON - Internal Medicine
Dr Ganraj Kumar, Scarborough, ON - Internal Medicine
Dr Rajender Kumar, Sudbury, ON - Psychiatry
Dr C L Prasanna Kumar, Toronto, ON - Obstetrics & Gynecology
Dr Krishna Kumar, Regina, SK - Neurosurgery
Dr P Karunakaran Kutty, Brampton, ON - Gastroenterology
Dr Mohanlal Lad, Hamilton, ON - General Practice
Dr Bahubali D Lagare, Mississauga, ON - Family Medicine
Dr Prem P Lakra, Calgary, AB - General Practice
Dr Kartar Lal, Grande Prairie, AB - General Practice
Dr Akbar V Lalani, New Westminster, BC - Cardiology
Dr Rakesh K Lamba, Abbotsford, BC - Psychiatry
Dr Manisha Lamba, Ottawa, ON - General Pathology
Dr Natasha B Leighl, Toronto, ON - Internal Medicine
Dr Hwayue Liu, Richmond Hill, ON - Family Medicine
Dr Shashi Lota, Calgary, AB - General Practice
Dr Richa P Love, Calgary, AB - Family Medicine
Dr Sanjeev S Luthra, Brampton, ON - Pediatrics
Dr Meera Luthra, Hamilton, ON - Endocrin/Metabolism
Dr Gyaandeo S Maharajh, Ottawa, ON - Cardiac Surgery
Dr Raj K Mahay, Winnipeg, MB - General Practice
Dr Nizar N Mahomed, Toronto, ON - Orthopedic Surgery
Dr Manish Maingi, Mississauga, ON - Cardiology
Dr Bharat Maini, Peterborough, ON - Anesthesia
Dr Rajesh R Mainra, North Vancouver, BC - Critical Care Medicine
Dr Sarah Makhdoom, High River, AB - Family Medicine
Dr Tilak R Malhotra, Prince Albert, SK - Pediatrics
Dr Rita K Maliakkal, Calgary, AB - Family Medicine
Dr Anupam Malik, Brampton, ON - General Practice
Dr Anjna A Malik, Ottawa, ON - General Practice
Dr Harinath Mallavarapu, Surrey, BC - Psychiatry
Dr Raman Manchanda, Surrey, BC - Family Medicine
Dr Avdhut R Manerkar, Miramichi, NB - General Practice
Dr Ashok Manga, Delta, BC - Family Medicine
Dr Sandeep Mangat, Placentia, NL - Family Medicine
Dr Baljinder Mann, Calgary, AB - Family Medicine
Dr Tejinder K Mann, New Westminster, BC - General Practice
Dr Satish K Mann, Prince George, BC - Family Medicine
Dr Shalini Manucha, North York, ON - General Practice
Dr Zahida Masood, Mississauga, ON - Family Medicine
Dr Surya Master, Campbellton, NB - General Surgery
Dr Chaudhry F Masud, Brampton, ON - Family Medicine
Dr Mathen K Mathen, Winnipeg, MB - Ophthalmology
Dr Biju Mathew, Maple Ridge, BC - Psychiatry
Dr Baboo M Mathew, Burin, NL - Endocrin/Metabolism
Dr John Mathews, Windsor, ON - Internal Medicine
Dr Arun K Mathur, Oshawa, ON - Urology
Dr Vinod K Mathur, Sault Ste. Marie, ON - Family Medicine
Dr Shahbegum A Meghji, Edmonton, AB - General Practice
Dr Labhshanker S Mehta, St Catharines, ON - Diagnostic-Radiology
Dr Suryakant D Mehta, Toronto, ON - General Practice
Dr Anilkumar S Menon, Brampton, ON - Cardiology
Dr Rajashree K Menon, Cornwall, ON - General Surgery
Dr Gopinath T Menon, Hamilton, ON - General Surgery
Dr Shamsh Y Merali, Milton, ON - Family Medicine
Dr Saba M Merchant, Maple, ON - Pediatrics
Dr Pradeep Merchant, Ottawa, ON - Pediatrics
Dr M Mohan Merchea, London, ON - Ophthalmology
Dr A Nadeem Mian, Edmonton, AB - Pediatrics
Dr Vishal M Midha, Brampton, ON - Family Medicine
Dr Tarun Misra, Calgary, AB - Gastroenterology
Dr Shaila Misri, Vancouver, BC - Psychiatry
Dr Dinesh J Mistry, Golden, BC - Family Medicine
Dr Prabhudas N Mistry, Langley, BC - Psychiatry
Dr Dalpatbhai B Mistry, Oshawa, ON - Psychiatry
Dr Akber H Mithani, Vancouver, BC - General Practice
Dr Vidushi Mittra-Melrose, Powell River, BC - Family Medicine
Dr Deepshikha Modi, Vancouver, BC - Family Medicine
Dr Ami N Mody, Mississauga, ON - Internal Medicine
Dr Nashila N Mohamed, Etobicoke, ON - Family Medicine
Dr Naveed S Mohammad, Etobicoke, ON - General Practice
Dr Naufal Mohammed, Hamilton, ON - Internal Medicine
Dr Rajesh Mohan, Etobicoke, ON - General Practice
Dr Mahendranath D Moharir, Toronto, ON - General Practice
Dr Sonali A Mohile, Uxbridge, ON - Pediatrics
Dr Afshan Mohsin, Orangeville, ON - Internal Medicine
Dr Tapas Mondal, Hamilton, ON - Cardiology
Dr Mohamed Moolla, Regina, SK - General Practice
Dr Malek B Moosa, Surrey, BC - Family Medicine
Dr Naeem H Muhammad, London, ON - Family Medicine
Dr Atreyi Mukherji, Hamilton, ON - Internal Medicine
Dr Manisha M Mulgund, Burlington, ON - Internal Medicine
Dr Udaya K K Mulpuri, Vancouver, BC - General Practice
Dr Amitha J Mundenchira, Oakville, ON - Family Medicine
Dr Rajeev H Muni, Toronto, ON - Ophthalmology
Dr Autar K Munshi, Sydney, NS - Psychiatry
Dr Ravi Murthy, Toronto, ON - General Practice
Dr Ashnoor Nagji, Vancouver, BC - Family Medicine
Dr Rohit S Nagpal, Brampton, ON - Family Medicine
Dr Anil K Nagpal, Kitchener, ON - Internal Medicine
Dr Ranjana Nagpurkar, Brampton, ON - Psychiatry
Dr Renuka S Naidu, Sarnia, ON - Critical Care Medicine
Dr Latha D Naik, Saskatoon, SK - Internal Medicine
Dr Shamsia M Nainar, Hamilton, ON - Family Medicine
Dr Girish M Nair, Ottawa, ON - Cardiology
Dr Meenakshi Nanda, Calgary, AB - Family Medicine
Dr Sunita Nandy, Scarborough, ON - General Practice
Dr Arif Naqvi, Scarborough, ON - Cardiology
Dr Satinder P S Narang, Surrey, BC - Psychiatry
Dr Chitra Narayanan, Scarborough, ON - General Practice
Dr Bharat C Nathoo, Richmond Hill, ON - Internal Medicine
Dr Shah Nawaz, Sudbury, ON - Cardiology
Dr Anuradha Nayar, Vancouver, BC - General Practice
Dr Saiyed M Nazar-Ul-Iman, Winnipeg, MB - General Practice
Dr Harish K Neelakant, Vancouver, BC - Psychiatry
Dr Nazia S Niazi, Surrey, BC - General Practice
Dr Srishti P Nigam, Edmonton, AB - General Pathology
Dr Veena Nikore, Brantford, ON - General Practice
Dr Abraham Ninan, Saskatoon, SK - Pediatrics
Dr Amarjit S Nirwan, Victoria, BC - Family Medicine
Dr Naushad A Noorani, Brampton, ON - Psychiatry
Dr Kamal K S Ohson, St. John's, NL - Dermatology
Dr Ravinderpal S Ohson, Hamilton, ON - Family Medicine
Dr Shakkeela Padanilathu Kunjummar, Newmarket, ON - Family Medicine
Dr Rajbir S Pahil, Sydney, NS - General Practice
Dr Raveen S Pal, Kingston, ON - Cardiology
Dr Suniti Pande, Nepean, ON - Psychiatry
Dr Anil K Pandey, Thompson, MB - Psychiatry
Dr A Shekhar Pandey, Cambridge, ON - Cardiology
Dr Hemant M Pandhi, Mississauga, ON - General Practice
Dr A M Chelvi Pandian, Gatineau, QC - Family Medicine
Dr Vikas Pandith, Burlington, ON - Internal Medicine
Dr Sudhir D Pandya, Calgary, AB - Emergency Medicine
Dr Anand H Pandya, Brampton, ON - Critical Care Medicine
Dr Sudhir P Pandya, Oakville, ON - Gastroenterology
Dr Dilkhush D Panjwani, Etobicoke, ON - Psychiatry
Dr Sooraja P Papneja, Mississauga, ON - General Practice
Dr Manoj Parameshwar, Penticton, BC - General Practice
Dr Sujata H Parashar, Windsor, ON - Family Medicine
Dr Sheela Parihar, Vancouver, BC - General Practice
Dr Jasneet K Parmar, Edmonton, AB - General Practice
Dr Malvinder S Parmar, Timmins, ON - Internal Medicine
Dr Baynazir Parray, Oshawa, ON - Family Medicine
Dr Naeem Parvez, Regina, SK - General Practice
Dr Deepti Pasricha, Markham, ON - Family Medicine
Dr Suvercha Pasricha, Toronto, ON - Psychiatry
Dr Kalavati B Patel, Wetaskiwin, AB - General Practice
Dr Bhasker M Patel, Wetaskiwin, AB - Family Medicine
Dr Ila M Patel, Mississauga, ON - Family Medicine
Dr Vishnu K Patel, Orleans, ON - General Practice
Dr Naresh R Patel, Tilbury, ON - Family Medicine
Dr Hasmukh G Patel, Windsor, ON - Anesthesia
Dr Shaila Patodia, Oakville, ON - Internal Medicine
Dr Ashalatha Paul, Calgary, AB - General Practice
Dr Daisy R Pavri, London, ON - Pediatrics
Dr Patricia S R Pawaroo, Ajax, ON - Family Medicine
Dr Sushama R Pendharkar, Mississauga, ON - Psychiatry
Dr Chakrabarty L Pole, Surrey, BC - Psychiatry
Dr Hemraj R Porwal, Niagara Falls, ON - Family Medicine
Dr Vilas S Prabhu, Penticton, BC - Otolaryngology
Dr Yasmeen A B Punjani, Scarborough, ON - Internal Medicine
Dr Punnamkuzhil C Punnen, North York, ON - Urology
Dr Dinshaw K Punthakee, Hamilton, ON - Orthopedic Surgery
Dr Bhupinder S Purewal, Scarborough, ON - General Practice
Dr Nimishchandra N Purohit, Burlington, ON - Psychiatry
Dr M Shafiq Qaadri, Toronto, ON - General Practice
Dr Mussarrat K Qaadri, Toronto, ON - Obstetrics & Gynecology
Dr Shehla Qadeer, Whitby, ON - Family Medicine
Dr Khalida Qazi, Milton, ON - Family Medicine
Dr M Salim Quraishi, London, ON - General Practice
Dr Irfan T Qureshi, Fort McMurray, AB - Orthopedic Surgery
Dr Azra Qureshi, Scarborough, ON - General Practice
Dr Rita H Rabheru, London, ON - Family Medicine
Dr Rania N Rabie, Newmarket, ON - Gastroenterology
Dr Afshan Rafay, Mississauga, ON - Family Medicine
Dr Fizza Z Rafiq, Calgary, AB - Family Medicine
Dr Abdul Rahman, Calgary, AB - Psychiatry
Dr Sultaneih S P Rajabali, New Westminster, BC - General Practice
Dr Shabnam S Rajani, Brampton, ON - General Pathology
Dr Chellappa Rajgopal, London, ON - General Surgery
Dr Manjulata Rajguru, Cambridge, ON - Pediatrics
Dr Mahesh Raju, Saint John, NB - Internal Medicine
Dr Shoba Raju, Saint John, NB - General Practice
Dr Surender K Ralh, North York, ON - General Practice
Dr Pawan K Ram, Surrey, BC - General Practice
Dr Veer Ramakrishna, Hamilton, ON - Family Medicine
Dr Nithyakalyani Ramani, Surrey, BC - Family Medicine
Dr Rajendranath Ramgoolam, Winnipeg, MB - General Practice
Dr Babra M Rana, Burnaby, BC - Psychiatry
Dr Ranjit S Rana, Scarborough, ON - General Practice
Dr Ranjit N Ranawaya, Calgary, AB - Neurology
Dr Chitra Rao, Hamilton, ON - General Pathology
Dr Shanti E Rao, Windsor, ON - Family Medicine
Dr Shalini Rastogi, Thornhill, ON - Family Medicine
Dr Rajinder S Rathee, North York, ON - Ophthalmology
Dr Seema R Rathee, Toronto, ON - Family Medicine
Dr Manisha Raut, Brossard, QC - General Practice
Dr Tarsem S Ravi, Mississauga, ON - Family Medicine
Dr Grama D Ravi, Sudbury, ON - Cardiology
Dr Shashi K Rawal, Lemoyne, QC - General Practice
Dr Brijendra K Rawat, Edmonton, AB - Diagnostic-Radiology
Dr Dalia Ray, North York, ON - Obstetrics & Gynecology
Dr Sudesh Rayner, Burlington, ON - General Practice
Dr Nayyar K Razvi, Toronto, ON - Family Medicine
Dr Pratibha N Reebye, Vancouver, BC - Psychiatry
Dr Bajinder S Reen, Brampton, ON - Internal Medicine
Dr Mehar S Reen, Cornwall, ON - Physical Medicine & Rehab
Dr Ranjodh S Rehal, Winnipeg, MB - General Practice

Dr Yasmin Rehemtula, Mississauga, ON - General Practice
Dr Waseema Rehman, Glace Bay, NS - Family Medicine
Dr Mujeeb U Rehman, Mississauga, ON - Psychiatry
Dr El-Karim F J Rhemtulla, St Catharines, ON - Ophthalmology
Dr Kulwant S Riar, Vancouver, BC - Psychiatry
Dr Rakesh K Rikhye, Etobicoke, ON - General Practice
Dr Syed M H Rizvi, Windsor, ON - General Practice
Dr Madan M Roy, Hamilton, ON - Pediatrics
Dr Meera Ruparelia, Brockville, ON - Family Medicine
Dr Vasant C Ruparelia, Manotick, ON - General Practice
Dr Surendra P Ruparelia, Oshawa, ON - General Practice
Dr Krishan K Sachdeva, Oshawa, ON - Urology
Dr Fakhruddin Sadikali, St Catharines, ON - Internal Medicine
Dr Dhun S Sadry, Toronto, ON - Family Medicine
Dr Niloufer Saeed, Cambridge, ON - Hematological Pathology
Dr Tariq M Saeed, Mississauga, ON - Family Medicine
Dr Arshad Saeed, Ottawa, ON - Family Medicine
Dr Bal Makund Sahay, Sarnia, ON - Internal Medicine
Dr Ramesh L Sahjpaul, North Vancouver, BC - Neurosurgery
Dr Tejinder Sainbhee, Camrose, AB - General Practice
Dr Parampreet Sainbhee, Camrose, AB - Family Medicine
Dr Rajeev Saincher, Surrey, BC - General Practice
Dr Mukesh C Saini, Brampton, ON - General Practice
Dr Joginder K Saini, Kanata, ON - General Practice
Dr Preeti Saini, Markham, ON - Family Medicine
Dr Asim Salim, Brantford, ON - Pediatrics
Dr Imran Samad, Burnaby, BC - Otolaryngology
Dr Nabeel B Samad, Halifax, NS - General Practice
Dr Amirali M Samji, Toronto, ON - General Practice
Dr Khashayar Sanandaji, Vaughan, ON - Family Medicine
Dr Gurpal S Sandha, Edmonton, AB - Gastroenterology
Dr Parminder K Sandhu, Calgary, AB - Family Medicine
Dr Jatinder S Sandhu, Surrey, BC - Psychiatry
Dr Sukhbir S Sandhu, Dauphin, MB - Psychiatry
Dr Jasbir K Sandhu, Brampton, ON - General Practice
Dr Mahendra B S Sangani, Greenfield Park, QC - General Practice
Dr Hemalata J B Sangani, Greenfield Park, QC - General Practice
Dr Baldev S Sanghera, Burnaby, BC - Family Medicine
Dr Gurinder P Sanghera, Toronto, ON - Ophthalmology
Dr Rajni Saraf, Sarnia, ON - Obstetrics & Gynecology
Dr Didar S Sarai, Brampton, ON - Family Medicine
Dr Michael K Sarin, Toronto, ON - Internal Medicine
Dr Brij M Sarup, London, ON - General Practice
Dr Jinka R Sathya, St. John's, NL - Radiation Oncology
Dr Ravinder P S Sawhney, Surrey, BC - Internal Medicine
Dr Gulshan Sawhney, Milton, ON - Internal Medicine
Dr Onkar N Saxena, Lanigan, SK - General Practice
Dr Anurag Saxena, Saskatoon, SK - Anatomical Pathology
Dr Manoj K Sayal, Oakville, ON - Critical Care Medicine
Dr Eshratbanu Sayani, Scarborough, ON - Family Medicine
Dr M A Raffath Sayeed, Lloydminster, SK - General Practice
Dr Jaishree Sehgal, Kitchener, ON - General Practice
Dr Narinder S Sehravat, Etobicoke, ON - Family Medicine
Dr Peter L Selby, Toronto, ON - Family Medicine
Dr Rita Selby, Toronto, ON - Hematology
Dr Indira Sen, Thornhill, ON - General Practice
Dr Vir Bhushan Sennik, Mississauga, ON - Orthopedic Surgery
Dr Aditya Seth, Salmon Arm, BC - Ophthalmology
Dr Arun K Seth, Toronto, ON - General Practice
Dr Asha L Seth, Toronto, ON - General Practice
Dr Shilpa Sethi, Middle Musquodoboi, NS - General Practice
Dr Jagmeet Sethi, Cayuga, ON - Internal Medicine
Dr Baldev R Sethi, Stittsville, ON - General Practice
Dr Yatish N Setty, Owen Sound, ON - General Practice
Dr Chirag R Shah, Calgary, AB - Ophthalmology
Dr Natavarlal H Shah, Cornwall, ON - General Practice
Dr Jay K Shah, Hamilton, ON - Pediatrics
Dr Bharatkumar K Shah, North York, ON - General Practice
Dr Sheila Shah, North York, ON - General Practice
Dr Pravin C Shah, Strathroy, ON - Anatomical Pathology
Dr Prakeshkumar S Shah, Toronto, ON - Pediatrics
Dr Vibhuti S Shah, Toronto, ON - Pediatrics
Dr Vinod H Shah, Welland, ON - General Practice
Dr Shahzad Z Shahmalak, Cambridge, ON - General Practice
Dr Nirmal K Shahoo, Ponoka, AB - General Practice
Dr Nasir Shaikh, Winnipeg, MB - General Practice
Dr Bashirunnisa A Shaikh, Etobicoke, ON - General Practice
Dr S Yasmin Shaikh, North York, ON - Family Medicine
Dr Wajid A Shaikh, Scarborough, ON - Pediatrics
Dr Bashiruddin N Shaikh, Toronto, ON - Urology
Dr Sadia Shakil, Edmonton, AB - General Practice
Dr Lalitha Shankar, Toronto, ON - Diagnostic-Radiology
Dr Kanwal Shankardass, Dundas, ON - General Practice
Dr Sapna Sharan, London, ON - General Practice
Dr Sumit Sharan, Sudbury, ON - Anesthesia
Dr Rajeshvar K Sharda, Hamilton, ON - Ophthalmology
Dr Shiraz B K Shariff, Brampton, ON - General Practice
Dr Aftab M Shariff, Ottawa, ON - Pediatrics
Dr Pankaj Sharma, Surrey, BC - Family Medicine
Dr Sushil K Sharma, Truro, NS - Family Medicine
Dr Shikhi Sharma, Truro, NS - Family Medicine
Dr Niti Sharma, Barrie, ON - Family Medicine
Dr Shreekant Sharma, Brantford, ON - Psychiatry
Dr Poonam Sharma, Brantford, ON - Psychiatry
Dr Sangita Sharma, Burlington, ON - Emergency Medicine
Dr Maheshwar D Sharma, Ingersoll, ON - Internal Medicine
Dr Ashok Sharma, Kitchener, ON - General Practice
Dr Vinod K Sharma, Kitchener, ON - Gastroenterology
Dr Ajay Sharma, London, ON - Pediatrics
Dr Verinder Sharma, London, ON - Psychiatry
Dr Rajrishi Sharma, London, ON - Orthopedic Surgery
Dr Manas Sharma, London, ON - General Practice
Dr Shivani Sharma, Markham, ON - General Practice
Dr Subhash C Sharma, Newbury, ON - Family Medicine
Dr Amar D Sharma, Oakville, ON - General Practice
Dr Kamal Sharma, Ottawa, ON - Cardiology
Dr Meena P Sharma, Ottawa, ON - General Practice
Dr Bal Krishan Sharma, Sarnia, ON - Family Medicine
Dr Vijay Sharma, Scarborough, ON - Anesthesia
Dr Monika Sharma, Strathroy, ON - Family Medicine
Dr Shakti Sharma, Thornhill, ON - Dermatology
Dr Shiv R Sharma, Toronto, ON - Family Medicine
Dr Kawal J Sharma, Toronto, ON - Obstetrics & Gynecology
Dr Satyendra Sharma, Toronto, ON - Physical Medicine & Rehab
Dr Malika Sharma, Toronto, ON - Internal Medicine
Dr Madan G Sharman, Regina, SK - General Practice
Dr Gul Nawaz Sheikh, Ajax, ON - Internal Medicine
Dr Amber Z Sheikh, Niagara Falls, ON - Ophthalmology
Dr Vasanti N Shende, Guelph, ON - Internal Medicine
Dr Rajeev Sheoran, Penticton, BC - Psychiatry
Dr Jitendra B Sheshgiri, Mississauga, ON - Emergency Family Med
Dr Charudutt D Shete, Langley, BC - General Surgery
Dr Nikita T Sheth, Oakville, ON - Family Medicine
Dr Nahid K Shethwala, Guelph, ON - Pediatrics
Dr Rathnakar B Shetty, St Catharines, ON - Obstetrics & Gynecology
Dr Geeta R Shetty, St Catharines, ON - Anesthesia
Dr Karunakara N Shetty, Charlottetown, PE - Internal Medicine
Dr Hemant R Shirali, Markham, ON - Orthopedic Surgery
Dr Sanam S Shorey, Brampton, ON - Endocrin/Metabolism
Dr Satish Shrikhande, Victoria, BC - Psychiatry
Dr Avanish K Shukla, St Catharines, ON - Psychiatry
Dr Hrishikesh Shukla, Windsor, ON - Family Medicine
Dr Sushama Shukla, Saskatoon, SK - General Practice
Dr Zia A Sial, Etobicoke, ON - Family Medicine
Dr Sanjay Siddhartha, Miramichi, NB - General Practice
Dr Nilofar Siddiqi, Owen Sound, ON - Family Medicine
Dr Muzaffar M Siddiqui, Edmonton, AB - Neurology
Dr Mughina A Siddiqui, Antigonish, NS - General Practice
Dr Zubaida Siddiqui, Elliot Lake, ON - Family Medicine
Dr Tahira Siddiqui, North York, ON - Anesthesia
Dr Nishat A Siddiqui, Ottawa, ON - General Practice
Dr Naveed T Siddiqui, Toronto, ON - General Practice
Dr Parmjit K Sidhu, Abbotsford, BC - Psychiatry
Dr Rabinder S Sidhu, Surrey, BC - Family Medicine
Dr Surinder S Sidhu, Brampton, ON - General Practice
Dr Gurmeet Sidhu, Brampton, ON - Family Medicine
Dr Gurpreet S Sidhu, Brantford, ON - General Practice
Dr Gurpreet S Sidhu, London, ON - Psychiatry
Dr Raj K Sidhu, Mississauga, ON - Family Medicine
Dr Shabana Sikander, Mississauga, ON - Family Medicine
Dr Sujata S Sikka, Mississauga, ON - Anesthesia
Dr Rajneesh Sikri, Etobicoke, ON - Family Medicine
Dr Ram K Singal, Thornhill, ON - General Surgery
Dr Sewa R Singal, Toronto, ON - Internal Medicine
Dr Rajiv K Singal, Toronto, ON - Urology
Dr Nandini J Singh, Calgary, AB - Psychiatry
Dr Ram R Singh, Calgary, AB - Internal Medicine
Dr Paramvinder Singh, Calgary, AB - Family Medicine
Dr Vijay P Singh, Edmonton, AB - Psychiatry
Dr Jitendra Singh, Red Deer, AB - Internal Medicine
Dr Amar Singh, Red Deer, AB - General Practice
Dr Jit J Singh, Delta, BC - General Practice
Dr Gurwant Singh, Surrey, BC - Neurology
Dr Kanwarjit Singh, Surrey, BC - General Practice
Dr Avash J Singh, Vancouver, BC - Pediatrics
Dr Gurdayal Singh, Vancouver, BC - Internal Medicine
Dr Kulbir I Singh, Vancouver, BC - Psychiatry
Dr Jaspal Singh, Kentville, NS - Obstetrics & Gynecology
Dr Jagmohan K Singh, Truro, NS - Internal Medicine
Dr Jogindra Singh, Ajax, ON - Physical Medicine & Rehab
Dr Amarendra N Singh, Belleville, ON - Psychiatry
Dr Padamjit M Singh, Bowmanville, ON - Obstetrics & Gynecology
Dr Shiv P Singh, Brampton, ON - Family Medicine
Dr Narendra Singh, Brampton, ON - Cardiology
Dr Parvinder Singh, Brampton, ON - Family Medicine
Dr Amandeep Singh, Brampton, ON - General Practice
Dr Harleen Singh, Brampton, ON - Family Medicine
Dr Baljit Singh, Chatham, ON - Obstetrics & Gynecology
Dr Inderjit Singh, Hamilton, ON - Family Medicine
Dr Barinder Singh, Kingston, ON - Family Medicine
Dr Manbir Singh, Kitchener, ON - Psychiatry
Dr Ram N Singh, London, ON - Critical Care Medicine
Dr Abhay K Singh, London, ON - Psychiatry
Dr Anita D Singh, London, ON - Family Medicine
Dr Ravinder Singh, North Bay, ON - General Surgery
Dr Rajiva R Singh, Point Edward, ON - Urology
Dr Kunwar K Singh, Sarnia, ON - Pediatrics
Dr Tejinder P Singh, Scarborough, ON - Family Medicine
Dr Simron Singh, Toronto, ON - Internal Medicine
Dr Parul Singh, Toronto, ON - Emergency Family Med
Dr Jitendra K Singh, Whitby, ON - Internal Medicine
Dr Minesh Singh, Windsor, ON - General Surgery
Dr Arvind G Singh, Summerside, PE - Psychiatry
Dr Kanwerjit Singh Aujla, Calgary, AB - Family Medicine
Dr Rashmi Singhai, Delta, BC - General Practice
Dr Nalini Singhal, Calgary, AB - Pediatrics
Dr Nishma Singhal, Hamilton, ON - Infectious Diseases
Dr Sanjeev Singwi, Orangeville, ON - General Practice
Dr Amita Singwi, Toronto, ON - Family Medicine
Dr Sachchida N Sinha, Winnipeg, MB - Internal Medicine
Dr Dinesh P Sinha, Halifax, NS - General Practice
Dr Rajinder K Sippy, Brampton, ON - Family Medicine
Dr Parmjit S Sohal, Surrey, BC - Family Medicine
Dr Anand Sohla, Tillsonburg, ON - General Practice
Dr Teesta B Soman, Toronto, ON - General Practice
Dr Mansurali R Somani, Mission, BC - Family Medicine
Dr Jitin Sondhi, Ingersoll, ON - Family Medicine
Dr Asha P Sondhi, Newmarket, ON - Family Medicine
Dr Ramesh K Soni, Burlington, ON - General Practice
Dr Prabhu Sonpar, Leduc, AB - Family Medicine
Dr Brijendra Sood, Calgary, AB - General Practice
Dr Alok Sood, Abbotsford, BC - Family Medicine
Dr Balbhadar D Sood, Etobicoke, ON - Psychiatry
Dr Gautam R Soparkar, Sarnia, ON - Internal Medicine
Dr Amuchou S Soraisham, Calgary, AB - Pediatrics
Dr Jami Sridhar, Campbellton, NB - General Practice
Dr Thangamani Subramanian, Hamilton, ON - Family Medicine
Dr Anantasivan Subramanian, Niagara Falls, ON - General Surgery
Dr Shelly Sud, Ottawa, ON - Family Medicine
Dr Shiraz Suleman, Brampton, ON - Obstetrics & Gynecology
Dr Ghazala Sultan, Chatham, ON - Family Medicine
Dr Omar Sultan, Regina, SK - Cardiology
Dr Sumeet K Suneja, Brampton, ON - Internal Medicine

Dr Pal S Sunerh, Etobicoke, ON - General Practice
Dr Priya Suppal, Brampton, ON - Family Medicine
Dr Smeeksha S Sur, Brampton, ON - Pediatrics
Dr Monalisa Sur, Hamilton, ON - Anatomical Pathology
Dr Ranjan K Sur, Hamilton, ON - Radiation Oncology
Dr Hemchand Surajballi, The Pas, MB - Family Medicine
Dr Sabiha M Surangiwala, Mississauga, ON - Family Medicine
Dr Ramakrishna R Surapaneni, Kitchener, ON - Psychiatry
Dr Permjit S Suri, Nepean, ON - Internal Medicine
Dr Bhadreshchandra V Surti, London, ON - Psychiatry
Dr Shveta Suryavanshi, Sarnia, ON - Family Medicine
Dr Rajeev K Suryavanshi, Sarnia, ON - General Surgery
Dr Sam Swaminath, Chatham, ON - Psychiatry
Dr Suresh Syal, Concord, ON - General Practice
Dr Swaran K Syan, Sudbury, ON - Family Medicine
Dr Gurcharan S Syan, Sudbury, ON - Cardiology
Dr Abdul R Syed, Barrie, ON - General Practice
Dr Ali A Syed, Etobicoke, ON - Anesthesia
Dr Abu A Syed, Lindsay, ON - Internal Medicine
Dr Saadat A S Syed, North York, ON - Family Medicine
Dr A Shaista Syed, North York, ON - Family Medicine
Dr Nazia Syed, Richmond Hill, ON - Internal Medicine
Dr Yasmeen Syed, Scarborough, ON - General Practice
Dr Uzma Syed, Scarborough, ON - Internal Medicine
Dr Khalid A Syed, Toronto, ON - Orthopedic Surgery
Dr Laeeq A Tahir, Moncton, NB - Psychiatry
Dr Pramil Tahlan, Woodstock, ON - Psychiatry
Dr Jatinder Takhar, London, ON - Psychiatry
Dr Chiranjib Talukdar, Regina, SK - Pediatrics
Dr P Aravind Talwalkar, Mississauga, ON - General Practice
Dr Puneeta Tandon, Edmonton, AB - Gastroenterology
Dr Vikas Tandon, Hamilton, ON - Cardiology
Dr Anu Tandon, Toronto, ON - Internal Medicine
Dr Ravi Taneja, London, ON - Anesthesia
Dr Minakshi S Taparia, Edmonton, AB - General Practice
Dr Khalida P Tariq, Edmonton, AB - Family Medicine
Dr Muhammad Tasneem, Mississauga, ON - Family Medicine
Dr Mangi N Tauh, Edmonton, AB - Obstetrics & Gynecology
Dr Syeda N Tauqir Naqvi, Woodstock, ON - Anatomical Pathology
Dr Nazia Tauseef, Courtice, ON - Obstetrics & Gynecology
Dr Narsimhachary Telikicharla Kandala, Terrace, BC - General Practice
Dr Sou K Thain, Kingston, ON - Radiation Oncology
Dr Bhavna K Thakersee, Waterdown, ON - Family Medicine
Dr Elizabeth Thakkar, Calgary, AB - General Practice
Dr Kirit V Thakkar, Mississauga, ON - General Practice
Dr Harilal Thakorlal, Vancouver, BC - General Practice
Dr Smita V Thatte, Ottawa, ON - Psychiatry
Dr Ma Khin Thida, Vancouver, BC - Family Medicine
Dr Yasmin Thobani, Mississauga, ON - General Practice
Dr Mukund B Tinguria, Brantford, ON - Anatomical Pathology
Dr Lubna T Tirmizi, Pickering, ON - Family Medicine
Dr Dalvinder S Toor, Vancouver, BC - Family Medicine
Dr Sushila M Treasurer, North York, ON - General Practice
Dr Andrew W Trevor, Brantford, ON - General Practice
Dr Davender K Tripathi, Newmarket, ON - Gastroenterology
Dr A Karen Trollope, Hamilton, ON - Family Medicine
Dr Padmini N Turlapati, Markham, ON - Pediatrics
Dr Ram S Ubhi, Calgary, AB - General Practice
Dr Surinder K Ubhi, Calgary, AB - Family Medicine
Dr Jagdeep S Ubhi, New Westminster, BC - Obstetrics & Gynecology
Dr Verjinderpal S Ubhi, Mississauga, ON - Family Medicine
Dr Sameena Uddin, Mississauga, ON - General Surgery
Dr A H M Jamal Uddin, Toronto, ON - Internal Medicine
Dr Rushad T Udwadia, New Westminster, BC - General Surgery
Dr Huma Z Ul Haq, Shelburne, ON - Family Medicine
Dr Farid Ullah, Kelowna, BC - General Practice
Dr Samira Ummat, Vancouver, BC - Physical Medicine & Rehab
Dr Sunil K Ummat, Vancouver, BC - Otolaryngology
Dr Bhikubhai D Unarket, Calgary, AB - General Practice
Dr Rajat Upadhyay, Calgary, AB - Emergency Family Med
Dr Amitkumar S Upadhyay, Aurora, ON - Family Medicine
Dr Harpreet K Upneja, Windsor, ON - Internal Medicine
Dr Sonia Uppal, Abbotsford, BC - Psychiatry
Dr Rakesh Uppal, Brampton, ON - General Practice
Dr Gayatri Uppal, Ottawa, ON - Family Medicine
Dr Jaishree Uppal, Sarnia, ON - General Practice
Dr Gunjan M Vador, Scarborough, ON - Internal Medicine
Dr Himat Vaghadia, Vancouver, BC - Anesthesia
Dr Seemin A Vahidy, Edmonton, AB - General Practice
Dr Sangeeta Vaideswaran, London, ON - Family Medicine
Dr Sankar Vaidyanathan, Brampton, ON - Family Medicine
Dr Prema Vaidyanathan, Etobicoke, ON - Obstetrics & Gynecology
Dr Rajkumar Vajpeyi, Toronto, ON - Anatomical Pathology
Dr M Tariq Vakani, Mississauga, ON - Cardiology
Dr Pravesh K Vallabh, Edmonton, AB - Family Medicine
Dr Sreelatha P Varapravan, London, ON - Psychiatry
Dr Divya J Varma, Dartmouth, NS - Family Medicine
Dr Devesh K Varma, Mississauga, ON - Ophthalmology
Dr Prem K Varma, Ottawa, ON - General Practice
Dr Gokuldas R Varma, Toronto, ON - General Practice
Dr Shashi Vashisht, Vancouver, BC - General Practice
Dr Akshya Vasudev, London, ON - General Practice
Dr Mudalodu V Vasudevan, Windsor, ON - General Practice
Dr Varadaraj R Velamoor, Guelph, ON - Psychiatry
Dr Azim M Velji, Niagara Falls, ON - Family Medicine
Dr Manhar L B N Verma, Calgary, AB - Anesthesia
Dr Pramod K Verma, Edmonton, AB - Obstetrics & Gynecology
Dr Kumud Verma, Delta, BC - Family Medicine
Dr Narpendra Verma, Lisle, ON - General Practice
Dr Shailendra Verma, Ottawa, ON - Internal Medicine
Dr Vinod K Verma, Scarborough, ON - General Practice
Dr Prem A Verma, Charlottetown, PE - General Practice
Dr Ashok K Verma, Regina, SK - Diagnostic-Radiology
Dr Kamla R Verma, Regina, SK - Psychiatry
Dr Kartar S Vig, London, ON - General Surgery
Dr Raj Vijay, Mississauga, ON - Family Medicine
Dr Meeta Vijh, Brampton, ON - Family Medicine
Dr Mirza R Virani, Markham, ON - General Practice
Dr Manjit S Virdee, Brampton, ON - Family Medicine
Dr Mohan S Virick, Sydney, NS - General Practice
Dr Mumtaz A Virji, Vancouver, BC - Pediatrics
Dr Achla R Virmani, Verdun, QC - General Practice
Dr Asha D Vohra, Burlington, ON - General Practice
Dr Sukh C Vohra, Burlington, ON - General Practice
Dr Harshala P Vora, Hamilton, ON - Family Medicine
Dr Sachi M Voruganti, Hamilton, ON - Radiation Oncology
Dr Lakshmi N P Voruganti, Oakville, ON - Psychiatry
Dr Mukul N Vyas, Vancouver, BC - Internal Medicine
Dr Uttam J K Wadhwa, Mississauga, ON - Psychiatry
Dr Atma S Wadhwa, Sturgeon Falls, ON - Internal Medicine
Dr Yasmin J Wadia, White Rock, BC - General Practice
Dr Waqar Waheed, Calgary, AB - Psychiatry
Dr Shobha Wahi, Hamilton, ON - Pediatrics
Dr Tamana Walia, Abbotsford, BC - General Practice
Dr Shiraz A Walji, Calgary, AB - General Practice
Dr Ihsan U Waraich, Brampton, ON - Family Medicine
Dr Qasim H Wasti, Maple Ridge, BC - Family Medicine
Dr Tehmina Q Wasti, Maple Ridge, BC - Family Medicine
Dr Mahesh P Yadav, North Bay, ON - Orthopedic Surgery
Dr Dushyant K Yajnik, Westmount, QC - General Practice
Dr Abu M Yakub, Brampton, ON - General Practice
Dr Qasim A Yar, Hagersville, ON - General Practice
Dr Saad Yasin, Calgary, AB - Family Medicine
Dr Naveeda Yasmeen, Hamilton, ON - Family Medicine
Dr Radhika Yelamanchili, St Catharines, ON - Internal Medicine
Dr Tsai Hsing Yu, St Catharines, ON - General Practice
Dr Barbara A Yu-Siao, Niagara Falls, ON - Psychiatry
Dr Salim Yusuf, Hamilton, ON - Cardiology
Dr Aroon Y Yusuf, Scarborough, ON - General Practice
Dr Saira Zafar, London, ON - Internal Medicine
Dr Rosy Zafar, Mississauga, ON - Family Medicine
Dr Mukarram A Zaidi, Calgary, AB - General Practice
Dr Kamruz Zaman, Toronto, ON - Family Medicine
Dr Khalid R Zia, East York, ON - Family Medicine
Dr Mohammad I Zia, Toronto, ON - Cardiology
Dr Jyotsna S Ziradkar, London, ON - Family Medicine
Dr Shaliendra Y Ziradkar, London, ON - Family Medicine
Dr Muhammad Zulfiqar, Abbotsford, BC - Internal Medicine

HINDKO

Dr Imran Samad, Burnaby, BC - Otolaryngology

HOKKIN

Dr John Hii, Toronto, ON - Medical Microbiology
Dr Charles C S Law, Vancouver, BC - General Practice
Dr Richard Lee, Vancouver, BC - Diagnostic-Radiology
Dr Teik Chye Ooi, Ottawa, ON - Internal Medicine
Dr Min Sen Phang, Vancouver, BC - Pediatrics
Dr Angeline C Sia-Venugopal, Chilliwack, BC - General Practice
Dr Michelle W Tan, Richmond, BC - Family Medicine
Dr H M Vincent Thai, Edmonton, AB - Family Medicine
Dr Peter L Ting, Vancouver, BC - General Practice
Dr Young-Chi Woo, Burnaby, BC - Urology

HUNGARIAN

Dr Edith Abou Said, Ottawa, ON - Family Medicine
Dr Julius Alexy, Selkirk, MB - General Practice
Dr Veronica Andrenyi, Montreal, QC - Diagnostic-Radiology
Dr Steve J Angyalfi, Calgary, AB - Radiation Oncology
Dr Istvan S Bacskai, Ottawa, ON - General Practice
Dr Julianna E K Balaton, Saskatoon, SK - Family Medicine
Dr A Gordon Balazsi, Mont-Royal, QC - Ophthalmology
Dr Berhanu Balcha, Winnipeg, MB - General Practice
Dr Alexander G Balogh, Calgary, AB - Radiation Oncology
Dr Peter A Batay-Csorba, Richmond Hill, ON - General Practice
Dr Timea Belej-Rak, Vaughan, ON - Obstetrics & Gynecology
Dr Irene C Bergh, Kelowna, BC - Family Medicine
Dr Maria M Blass, Windsor, ON - General Practice
Dr Gilda A Bowdridge, Halifax, NS - Family Medicine
Dr Balint L Budai, Vancouver, BC - Family Medicine
Dr Judith I Bus, Vancouver, BC - General Practice
Dr Bernard Chrysler, Montreal, QC - Internal Medicine
Dr Christine M Cserti-Gazdewich, Toronto, ON - Hematology
Dr Andrea Z Csordas, Hamilton, ON - General Practice
Dr Andreea Cupsa, Kanata, ON - Family Medicine
Dr Andreas Cziffer, Sault Ste Marie, ON - General Practice
Dr Andrew E Debreceni, Oakville, ON - Otolaryngology
Dr Eva C Dekany, Toronto, ON - Ophthalmology
Dr Paul Devenyi, North York, ON - Internal Medicine
Dr Robert A Dicker, North York, ON - General Practice
Dr Diane J Donat, Toronto, ON - Endocrin/Metabolism
Dr E Patricia Egerszegi, Montreal, QC - Plastic Surgery
Dr Zoltan J Egri, North York, ON - Cardiology
Dr Andre Engel, Ottawa, ON - Pediatrics
Dr Ivan G Fantus, Toronto, ON - Endocrin/Metabolism
Dr Imre B Fejer, Scarborough, ON - General Practice
Dr Piroska R Fejes, Barrie, ON - General Practice
Dr Katherine J Feleki, Kingston, ON - Family Medicine
Dr John L Felix, Toronto, ON - General Practice
Dr Nicolette K Fellegi, Ottawa, ON - Family Medicine
Dr Erika Feuerstein, Toronto, ON - Family Medicine
Dr Katarina Fiala, Toronto, ON - Dermatology
Dr Eva Foldes, Montreal, QC - Internal Medicine
Dr George Freundlich, Matheson, ON - Family Medicine
Dr Veronika A Fried, Toronto, ON - Family Medicine
Dr John C Fulop, Ottawa, ON - Cardiology
Dr Tamas Fulop, Sherbrooke, QC - Geriatric Medicine
Dr Eva B Furesz, Ottawa, ON - General Practice
Dr Judit M Gaal, Whitby, ON - General Practice
Dr Robert Z Gabor, Barrie, ON - Family Medicine
Dr Zsuzsanna Gabor, Scarborough, ON - General Practice
Dr Anna E Gergely, Courtice, ON - Family Medicine
Dr Haregua Getu, Toronto, ON - General Practice
Dr Fatemeh Ghannadi, West Vancouver, BC - Family Medicine
Dr Andrew J Gomori, Winnipeg, MB - Neurology
Dr Zuzana Gross, Thornhill, ON - General Practice
Dr Reka Z Gustafson, Vancouver, BC - Community Medicine
Dr Gabor T Gyenes, Edmonton, AB - General Practice
Dr Sandor Gyomorey, Etobicoke, ON - Orthopedic Surgery
Dr Katalin Gyomorey, Thunder Bay, ON - Psychiatry
Dr Andrew F Gyopar, Chateauguay, QC - General Surgery
Dr Peter Hacker, Montreal, QC - Dermatology

Dr Kevin Hafez, Calgary, AB - Family Medicine
Dr Martha Harczy, Nepean, ON - Internal Medicine
Dr Tibor A Harmathy, Orillia, ON - Family Medicine
Dr Alexander Hartman, Thornhill, ON - Diagnostic-Radiology
Dr Gavril Hercz, Toronto, ON - Internal Medicine
Dr Andrei E Hirsch, Scarborough, ON - General Practice
Dr George N Honos, Montreal, QC - Cardiology
Dr Ladislav Horak, North York, ON - General Practice
Dr Ingrid M Jarvis, Toronto, ON - Dermatology
Dr Elizabeth V M Jeney, Hamilton, ON - Otolaryngology
Dr Christa M Jeney, Toronto, ON - Family Medicine
Dr Tibor Juda, Toronto, ON - Urology
Dr Zsuzsanna Kaszas, Kinmount, ON - Family Medicine
Dr Leslie Kelen, Cote Saint-Luc, QC - General Practice
Dr Peter J Kertes, Toronto, ON - Ophthalmology
Dr Leslie T Kiraly, Toronto, ON - Psychiatry
Dr Zelma H T Kiss, Calgary, AB - Neurosurgery
Dr Erzsebet B Kiss, Barrie, ON - Family Medicine
Dr Eva B Kitagawa, Spirit River, AB - Family Medicine
Dr Charles D Knapp, North York, ON - Anesthesia
Dr Andrew Korda, York, ON - Family Medicine
Dr Endre L Koritar, Vancouver, BC - Psychiatry
Dr Judit Korosi, Langley, BC - Internal Medicine
Dr Kalman T Kovacs, Toronto, ON - Anatomical Pathology
Dr Susan V B Kovacs, Toronto, ON - Pediatrics
Dr Julie A J Kovacs, Toronto, ON - Internal Medicine
Dr Jean-Claude Landa, Hawkesbury, ON - Family Medicine
Dr Gabor Lantos, Toronto, ON - General Practice
Dr Diana C Laza, Etobicoke, ON - Family Medicine
Dr Eva Lorber, Toronto, ON - General Practice
Dr Peter C Maier, North York, ON - Family Medicine
Dr Ana Marias-Radu, Lac-Megantic, QC - Family Medicine
Dr Frank Markus, Woodbridge, ON - General Practice
Dr Eva S Mate, Toronto, ON - Respirology
Dr John Mazurka, Hamilton, ON - Obstetrics & Gynecology
Dr Michelle M Mezei, Vancouver, BC - Neurology
Dr Melitta Mezody, Toronto, ON - General Practice
Dr Helena Mihalovits, Hawkesbury, ON - Ophthalmology
Dr Elena Mihu, Kinmount, ON - Family Medicine
Dr Geza B Molnar, Brampton, ON - General Practice
Dr Izabella Morava-Protzner, Calgary, AB - Anatomical Pathology
Dr Adam Moscovitch, North York, ON - Psychiatry
Dr Gregory J Mosdossy, London, ON - Emergency Medicine
Dr Istvan Mucsi, Montreal, QC - Nephrology
Dr Christina Mundi, Ottawa, ON - Family Medicine
Dr Paul Munk, Toronto, ON - Pediatrics
Dr Miklos Nadasdi, North York, ON - General Practice
Dr Roland G Nador, Vancouver, BC - General Practice
Dr Alexander G Nagy, Vancouver, BC - General Surgery
Dr Maria Nagy, Toronto, ON - General Practice
Dr Joe Nemeth, Montreal, QC - Emergency Family Med
Dr Etela Neumann, Vancouver, BC - Neuro-Pathology
Dr Melinda Nichols, Penticton, BC - Psychiatry
Dr Janos J Pataki, Mississauga, ON - Internal Medicine
Dr Claudia Petrescu, North York, ON - General Practice
Dr Agnes Por-Somfai, North York, ON - Diagnostic-Radiology
Dr Kalman Protzner, Saint John, NB - Anatomical Pathology
Dr George Rado, North York, ON - Physical Medicine & Rehab
Dr Agnes E Reicher, North York, ON - Dermatology
Dr Peter Rosenthal, Winnipeg, MB - Psychiatry
Dr Lenuta Rus-Serban, Pointe-Claire, QC - General Practice
Dr Richard G A Safranyos, St Catharines, ON - Geriatric Medicine
Dr S Vahid Sahiholnasab, Richmond, BC - Internal Medicine
Dr Ildiko M Sajo, Scarborough, ON - General Practice
Dr John T Salvendy, Toronto, ON - Psychiatry
Dr Steve E S Samuel, North York, ON - Plastic Surgery
Dr Oded Samuel, North York, ON - Emergency Family Med
Dr Zsuzsanna S Sandor, Etobicoke, ON - Psychiatry
Dr George K B Sandor, Toronto, ON - Plastic Surgery
Dr Paul Sandor, Toronto, ON - Psychiatry
Dr Mark E Saul, Wakefield, QC - Family Medicine
Dr Marianne Schenker, Ottawa, ON - General Practice
Dr Agnes M Schlanger, Etobicoke, ON - General Practice
Dr Kathleen C Schneider, Toronto, ON - Psychiatry
Dr Thomas Schwartz, Cote Saint-Luc, QC - Endocrin/Metabolism
Dr Istvan Sekely, Mississauga, ON - Family Medicine
Dr Theodore N Siller, Scarborough, ON - Orthopedic Surgery
Dr Leslie V Solomon, Hamilton, ON - Family Medicine
Dr Ildiko E Solyom, Vancouver, BC - Psychiatry
Dr Thomas Stefopulos, Lindsay, ON - General Practice
Dr Alex Stern, Ajax, ON - Family Medicine
Dr Robert J Stern, Woodstock, ON - General Practice
Dr Agnes Z Supala-Berger, Toronto, ON - Neurology
Dr Leslie Suranyi, Cornwall, ON - Neurology
Dr Barbara E Suranyi-Cadotte, Verdun, QC - Psychiatry
Dr Elod Z Szabo, Toronto, ON - Anesthesia
Dr Eileen M Szabo, Saskatoon, SK - Internal Medicine
Dr Esther A Szaky, Richmond Hill, ON - Internal Medicine
Dr Istvan L Szarka, Hamilton, ON - Family Medicine
Dr John Szasz, Woodstock, ON - Ophthalmology
Dr Peter L Szego, Montreal, QC - Gastroenterology
Dr Eva M Szentgyorgyi, Toronto, ON - Anatomical Pathology
Dr Tibor J Sziklas, Montreal, QC - General Practice
Dr Andrew Szilagyi, Montreal, QC - Gastroenterology
Dr Imre Z Szilvassy, Hamilton, ON - General Practice
Dr Tibor Z Szirmay-Kalos, Stratford, ON - Obstetrics & Gynecology
Dr Laszlo N Takats, Edmonton, AB - Internal Medicine
Dr Maria T Torok, Dartmouth, NS - Pediatrics
Dr Julius L R Toth, Newmarket, ON - Critical Care Medicine
Dr Joseph Toth, Montreal, QC - Diagnostic-Radiology
Capt Andrea Tuka, Victoria, BC - Psychiatry
Dr Peter Vadas, Toronto, ON - Clin Immun/Allergy
Dr Agnes Vago, Toronto, ON - Anatomical Pathology
Dr Peter Vaktor, Montreal, QC - General Practice
Dr Lajos Valyi, Ajax, ON - Emergency Family Med
Dr David W Vas, Pointe-Claire, QC - Emergency Family Med
Dr Otto F Veidlinger, Toronto, ON - Neurology
Dr George E Vertes, Scarborough, ON - Cardiology
Dr Stephen Vida, Montreal, QC - Psychiatry
Dr Miklos I Vilaghy, Toronto, ON - General Practice
Dr Allen J Wahby, Windsor, ON - General Practice
Dr Robert W Wald, Toronto, ON - Cardiology
Dr Avi Wallerstein, Montreal, QC - Ophthalmology
Dr Thomas Weinberger, Scarborough, ON - General Practice
Dr Jeffrey M Weissberger, Markham, ON - Family Medicine
Dr Janet I Weisz, Burlington, ON - Pediatrics
Dr Paul R Zalan, Toronto, ON - General Practice
Dr Louis S Zavodni, Hamilton, ON - Family Medicine
Dr Agnes M Zeliger, Westmount, QC - Pediatrics
Dr Otto Zsigmond, Kamloops, BC - General Practice
Ms Judit T Zubovits, Scarborough, ON - Anatomical Pathology
Dr Joseph A de Nanassy, Ottawa, ON - Anatomical Pathology

IBIBIO

Dr Emmanuel U J Udoeyop, Cornwall, ON - Obstetrics & Gynecology

IBO

Dr Megeri Ede, Ottawa, ON - Internal Medicine
Dr Norbert I Ekeh, Scarborough, ON - Obstetrics & Gynecology
Dr Ngozi Ikeji, Whitehorse, YT - General Practice
Dr Uduma O Kalu, Sudbury, ON - Internal Medicine
Dr Innocent C Okafor, Brampton, ON - Family Medicine
Dr Godwin O Okolo, Edmonton, AB - General Practice
Dr Herbert O Onwudiwe, Strathmore, AB - General Practice
Dr Oluyomi A Sobowale, Peterborough, ON - Obstetrics & Gynecology
Dr Sylvester O Ukabam, Regina, SK - General Practice
Dr Jude I Umeh, Orangeville, ON - Obstetrics & Gynecology

ICELANDIC

Dr Hallgrimur Benediktsson, Calgary, AB - Anatomical Pathology
Dr Kristin Gisladottir, Toronto, ON - Psychiatry

ILICAN

Dr Rodolfo C Gallardo, Etobicoke, ON - General Practice

ILONGGO

Dr Enrico F Cabigon, Regina, SK - Anatomical Pathology
Dr Myrna B Zapata, St Catharines, ON - Pediatrics

INDONESIAN

Dr Linda Hondubrata, Cambridge, ON - Family Medicine
Dr Gitta K N Kindle, Ottawa, ON - General Practice
Dr Charles C S Law, Vancouver, BC - General Practice
Dr Kay I Lie, Toronto, ON - Obstetrics & Gynecology
Dr Daniel T H Liem, Windsor, ON - Internal Medicine
Dr Mahdi Murti, Toronto, ON - General Practice
Dr Kian Gwan Sie, East York, ON - Family Medicine
Dr Tjien-King Tan, Thornhill, ON - General Practice
Dr B L Linda The, North York, ON - Obstetrics & Gynecology
Dr Chee Nyok Thong, Vancouver, BC - Otolaryngology
Dr Anindita Tjahjadi, Ottawa, ON - Pediatrics
Dr Eugenie U Tjan, Mississauga, ON - General Practice
Dr Joshua K Tjong, Sault Ste. Marie, ON - Diagnostic-Radiology
Dr Ming-Sound Tsao, Toronto, ON - Anatomical Pathology
Dr Lianti Widjanarko, Sudbury, ON - Anatomical Pathology
Dr Djoen Widjanarko, Sudbury, ON - General Practice
Dr Caren F Zilber-Shlensky, Victoria, BC - Family Medicine

IRISH

Dr Joseph Dooley, Sioux Lookout, ON - Family Medicine
Dr F John Guilfoyle, Sioux Lookout, ON - Family Medicine
Dr Peter I M Moran, Mississauga, ON - Psychiatry
Dr Mary H O'Brien, St. John's, NL - Critical Care Medicine
Dr Peter J O'Malley, Prince George, BC - Family Medicine
Dr Ailbhe E O'Riordan, London, ON - Diagnostic-Radiology
Dr Greg Ryan, Toronto, ON - Obstetrics & Gynecology
Dr Mary-Frances Scully, St. John's, NL - Hematology
Dr James J Sheridan, Grnd Falls-Windsor, NL - Internal Medicine
Dr Joseph Walker, Nanaimo, BC - Psychiatry
Dr Sandra G B Woods, Val-d'Or, QC - Pediatrics

ITALIAN

Dr Oussama A Abla, Toronto, ON - General Practice
Dr Aboobaker Aboo, Ottawa, ON - General Practice
Dr Marie-Jose Aiello, Greenfield Park, QC - Psychiatry
Dr Ariane Alimenti, Vancouver, BC - General Practice
Dr Gillian B Allen, Toronto, ON - General Practice
Dr Federico A Allodi, Toronto, ON - Psychiatry
Dr Alexandre Alterescu, North York, ON - General Practice
Dr Maxime Amar, Quebec, QC - General Practice
Dr Jean I Anawati, Sturgeon Falls, ON - General Practice
Dr Francesco A Anello, Cambridge, ON - Family Medicine
Dr Mark P Angelini, Etobicoke, ON - Orthopedic Surgery
Dr Julio E Arboleda-Florez, Belleville, ON - Psychiatry
Dr Antonio A Armani, Toronto, ON - General Practice
Dr Michael A Arsenault, Montreal, QC - Pediatrics
Dr Gerd Asche, Hope, BC - Family Medicine
Dr Boris Bahoric, Montreal, QC - Radiation Oncology
Dr Adrian M Baranchuk, Kingston, ON - Neurology
Dr Zaim Bardakji, Saint-Laurent, QC - General Practice
Dr Davide D Bardana, Kingston, ON - Orthopedic Surgery
Dr Francesco Barnabi, Belleville, ON - General Surgery
Dr Tony Barozzino, Toronto, ON - Pediatrics
Dr Giuliano Barrettara, Oshawa, ON - General Practice
Dr Giampiero Bartolucci, Hamilton, ON - Psychiatry
Dr Michael Bartucci, Markham, ON - Family Medicine
Dr Luigi A Battel, Kingston, ON - Family Medicine
Dr Renaldo N Battista, Montreal, QC - Community Medicine
Dr Robert Bauer, Toronto, ON - Cardiology
Dr Marc Beauchamp, Montreal, QC - Orthopedic Surgery
Dr Rene Beaulieu, Longueuil, QC - General Practice
Dr Thierry Begin, Quebec, QC - Family Medicine

Dr Agostino M Bellissimo, Toronto, ON - Emergency Family Med
Dr Bernard Benard, Greenfield Park, QC - Endocrinology
Dr Antranik N Benohanian, Montreal, QC - Dermatology
Dr Bruno Bernucci, Saint-Leonard, QC - General Practice
Dr Hugo A R Bertozzi, Grande Prairie, AB - Family Medicine
Dr Vince Bertucci, Woodbridge, ON - Dermatology
Dr Hussein K Beydoun, Halifax, NS - Cardiology
Dr Andrea Bezjak, Toronto, ON - Internal Medicine
Dr Fernando A Bianchi, Hamilton, ON - Internal Medicine
Dr Antonio U Bianchini, LaSalle, QC - Family Medicine
Dr Eric Bicrell, Montreal, QC - General Practice
Dr Rino Bier, Montreal, QC - Diagnostic-Radiology
Dr Rosetta Bilotta, Woodbridge, ON - Community Medicine
Dr Marilena Biscotti, Beamsville, ON - Family Medicine
Dr Cédric Bisson, Montreal, QC - Family Medicine
Dr Bernard F Bissonnette, Montreal, QC - Internal Medicine
Dr Alain Bolduc, Moncton, NB - Dermatology
Dr Zeljko Bolesnikov, Fredericton, NB - General Practice
Dr Raoul I L Bonan, Montreal, QC - Cardiology
Dr Sergio M Borgia, Brampton, ON - Infectious Diseases
Dr Eric Bouffet, Toronto, ON - Pediatrics
Dr Ivan A Bracalenti, Stoney Creek, ON - Family Medicine
Dr David Bracco, Montreal, QC - Anesthesia
Dr Rosa M Braga-Mele, Toronto, ON - Ophthalmology
Dr Frank Bravo, Whitby, ON - Otolaryngology
Dr Francois Brochet, Chicoutimi, QC - General Practice
Dr Sorel L Brohovici, Montreal, QC - General Practice
Dr Renato Brun Del Re, Mississauga, ON - General Practice
Dr Claude Bruneau, Saint-Redempteur, QC - General Practice
Dr Giovanni F Bruno, Alliston, ON - Diagnostic-Radiology
Dr Alessandra Bruns, Sherbrooke, QC - General Practice
Dr Wojciech S Brzezinski, Medicine Hat, AB - General Surgery
Dr Raffaele Bucci, Saint-Leonard, QC - General Practice
Dr George P Buldo, Oshawa, ON - Internal Medicine
Dr Anthony E Cabrera, St Catharines, ON - Ophthalmology
Dr Margherita O Cadeddu, Hamilton, ON - General Surgery
Dr Daniele Camazzola, Richmond Hill, ON - Orthopedic Surgery
Dr Milena K Campbell, Abbotsford, BC - Family Medicine
Dr Louis F Canella, Toronto, ON - Psychiatry
Dr Paul G Cantarutti, Newmarket, ON - Family Medicine
Dr Paul S Cappon, Ottawa, ON - Community Medicine
Dr Heloise Cardinal, Montreal, QC - Internal Medicine
Dr Nicola Casacalenda, Montreal, QC - Psychiatry
Dr Maria Casale, Guelph, ON - Family Medicine
Dr Luigi Casella, Toronto, ON - Internal Medicine
Dr Luigi A Castagna, Scarborough, ON - Pediatrics
Dr Mario F Castelli, Toronto, ON - Internal Medicine
Dr John S Castiglione, Toronto, ON - General Practice
Dr Joseph Castrodale, North York, ON - General Practice
Dr Tamara Catona, Surrey, BC - Psychiatry
Dr Edward F E Cattan, Orleans, ON - Psychiatry
Dr Alfonso Ceccherini-Nelli, Edmonton, AB - General Practice
Dr Lambros N Chaniotis, Pointe-Claire, QC - Cardiology
Dr Larry S Chapman, Guelph, ON - Internal Medicine
Dr Jean-Pierre Chartrand, Pointe-Claire, QC - Ophthalmology
Dr James A Chiarotto, Scarborough, ON - Internal Medicine
Dr Madeleine Chicha-Dzineku, Montreal, QC - Anesthesia
Dr Albino Chiodo, East York, ON - Otolaryngology
Dr Michael J Churchill-Smith, Montreal, QC - Internal Medicine
Dr Michael Cianfrone, North York, ON - General Practice
Dr G Adrian Cianfrone, North York, ON - General Practice
Dr Claudio S Cina, North York, ON - General Surgery
Dr Sergiu Ciubotaru, Medicine Hat, AB - Family Medicine
Dr Nicholas S Ciurria, Toronto, ON - General Practice
Dr Antonio Cogliano, London, ON - Family Medicine
Dr Patricia C Colangelo, Toronto, ON - Pediatrics
Dr James P Cooper, Toronto, ON - Psychiatry
Dr Juan L Cordova, Winnipeg, MB - General Practice
Dr Marc M Corriveau, Montreal, QC - General Surgery
Dr Leonardo Cortese, Windsor, ON - Psychiatry
Dr Paolo Costi, Montreal, QC - Cardiology
Dr Natascha Crispino, Toronto, ON - Family Medicine
Dr Loris Cristante, Winnipeg, MB - General Practice
Dr Marie-Jose Cucuzza, Montreal, QC - General Practice
Dr Robert Curridor, North York, ON - General Practice
Dr Steven L Cusimano, Hamilton, ON - Family Medicine
Dr Robert J Cusimano, Toronto, ON - Cardiovasc/ThorSurg
Dr Michael D Cusimano, Toronto, ON - Neurosurgery
Dr Raffaele D'Agrosa, Toronto, ON - Family Medicine
Dr Enzo D'Alessandro, Toronto, ON - Psychiatry
Dr Joan W D'Andrea, Concord, ON - Family Medicine
Dr Anthony J D'Angelo, Whitby, ON - General Practice
Dr H Lina D'Apice, Matagami, QC - General Practice
Dr Giuseppe D'Ignazio, Dollard-d-Ormeaux, QC - General Practice
Dr George F D'Onofrio, York, ON - General Practice
Dr Vincent D'Ovidio, Toronto, ON - General Practice
Dr Anthony D D'Urzo, Toronto, ON - Family Medicine
Dr Arianna Dal Cin, Hamilton, ON - Plastic Surgery
Dr Rosemary P Danielli, Guelph, ON - Family Medicine
Dr Joseph Dattilo, Windsor, ON - General Practice
Dr Faiz Daudi, Etobicoke, ON - General Surgery
Dr A Marc Dauphin, Richelain, QC - General Practice
Dr Elizabeth Daviault, Montreal, QC - General Practice
Dr Ainsley E Dawson, Toronto, ON - Endocrinology & Metabolism
Dr Dan De Angelis, Mississauga, ON - Ophthalmology
Dr Debra A De Rubeis, Hamilton, ON - Neurology
Dr Andrea De Rubeis, Hamilton, ON - Family Medicine
Dr Anne De Silva, Toronto, ON - General Practice
Dr Franco DeNardi, St. Catharines, ON - Anatomical Pathology
Dr Matthew A Deangelis, Nepean, ON - Psychiatry
Dr Jaime Del Carpio, Montreal, QC - Clin Immun/Allergy
Dr Lisa Maria Elisabeth Del Giudice, Toronto, ON - Family Medicine
Dr Rolando Del Maestro, Montreal, QC - Neurosurgery
Dr Dario F Del Rizzo, Woodbridge, ON - Cardiothor Surgery
Dr Diego H Delgado, Toronto, ON - General Practice
Dr Max Della Zazzera, Ottawa, ON - General Practice
Dr Nadia Delle Donne, Pointe-Claire, QC - Emergency Family Med
Dr Jocelyn Delorme, Montreal, QC - Medical Microbiology & Infectious Diseases
Dr Walter Delpero, Ottawa, ON - Ophthalmology
Dr Thomas J Demarco, Whistler, BC - General Practice
Dr Jacques E Des Marchais, Montreal, QC - Orthopedic Surgery
Dr Joelle Desparmet, Montreal, QC - Anesthesia
Dr Francois Dessureault, Boucherville, QC - General Practice
Dr Domenico Di Carlo, North York, ON - General Practice
Dr Robert Di Cecco, London, ON - Obstetrics & Gynecology
Dr Giovanni A Di Costanzo, Markham, ON - Urology
Dr Daniela Di Iorio, Montreal, QC - Infectious Diseases
Dr Maria Di Lorenzo, Montreal, QC - Cardiology
Dr Antoinette Di Maria, Woodbridge, ON - Family Medicine
Dr Giuseppina Di Meglio, Westmount, QC - Pediatrics
Dr Luciano S Di Nardo, Woodbridge, ON - Family Medicine
Dr Vincenzo Di Nicola, Montreal, QC - Psychiatry
Dr Bruno L Di Paolo, Hamilton, ON - General Practice
Dr Andrea B L Di Paolo, Renfrew, ON - Family Medicine
Dr Fernando G Di Pierdomenico, Amherstburg, ON - General Practice
Dr Anthony P Di Pierdomenico, Toronto, ON - Obstetrics & Gynecology
Dr Luigia G A Di Primio, Ottawa, ON - Diagnostic-Radiology
Dr Claudio D Di Prizito, Mississauga, ON - Internal Medicine
Dr Tania Di Renna, Ottawa, ON - Anesthesia
Dr Razvan Diaconescu, Montreal, QC - Hematology
Dr Absa Diallo, Montreal, QC - General Practice
Dr Louis R Diraimo, Ottawa, ON - General Practice
Dr Marino J Discepola, Mont-Royal, QC - Ophthalmology
Dr Hisham Dokainish, Hamilton, ON - Cardiology
Dr Sylvia P Ducceschi, Vancouver, BC - Family Medicine
Dr Andrew D Duic, Toronto, ON - Pediatrics
Dr Nicolas Dupre, Quebec, QC - Neurology
Dr William S El Masri, Toronto, ON - Otolaryngology
Dr Abdul F M Elzawi, Toronto, ON - Internal Medicine
Dr Irvin Epstein, Toronto, ON - Psychiatry
Dr Juan L Escudero, Ottawa, ON - General Practice
Dr Daniel Ezekiel, Vancouver, BC - General Practice
Dr Hussein Fadlallah, Montreal, QC - Cardiology
Dr Carlo A Fallone, Montreal, QC - Gastroenterology
Dr James A Farquhar, Verdun, QC - Psychiatry
Dr Leonardo A Farrauto, Hamilton, ON - Physical Medicine & Rehab
Dr Nabil Fawaz, Saint-Leonard, QC - General Practice
Dr Frank Fazzari, North Bay, ON - Pediatrics
Dr Mario A Febbraro, Sault Ste. Marie, ON - General Practice
Dr Guiliana M Federici, Burlington, ON - Pediatrics
Dr Paolo Federico, Calgary, AB - Neurology
Dr Daniela Ferigutti, Gatineau, QC - Family Medicine
Dr Nestor D P Fernandez, Toronto, ON - General Practice
Dr Robert Ferrari, Edmonton, AB - Internal Medicine
Dr Bernard E Ferreira, Point Edward, ON - Obstetrics & Gynecology
Dr Valter Feyles, London, ON - Obstetrics & Gynecology
Dr Giuseppe Ficara, Montreal, QC - Pediatrics
Dr Philip Fingrut, North York, ON - General Practice
Dr Loretta Fiorillo, Edmonton, AB - Dermatology
Dr Godfrey T Fiorini, Toronto, ON - General Practice
Dr Alberto L Flores-Vargas, Scarborough, ON - General Practice
Dr Alexander E Forcina, Toronto, ON - Family Medicine
Dr Frank Fornasier, Burlington, ON - Family Medicine
Dr Victor Fornasier, Scarborough, ON - General Pathology
Dr Luis R Fornazzari, Toronto, ON - Neurology
Dr Milena F Forte, Toronto, ON - Family Medicine
Dr Louis Francescutti, Edmonton, AB - Community Medicine
Dr Sante J Fratesi, Sault Ste. Marie, ON - General Surgery
Dr Claudio G Fregonas, Toronto, ON - Pediatrics
Dr Marc Frenette, Laval, QC - Cardiology
Dr Matthias G W Friedrich, Montreal, QC - Cardiology
Dr Gabriel G C Fuoco, Peterborough, ON - Otolaryngology
Dr Menuccia Gagliardi, Sidney, BC - Family Medicine
Dr Tsvi Gallant, North York, ON - General Practice
Dr Lee Ann Gallant, North York, ON - Pediatrics
Dr Satyajit N Ganguli, Brampton, ON - Diagnostic-Radiology
Dr Andres Gantous, Toronto, ON - Otolaryngology
Dr Bertha Garcia, London, ON - Anatomical Pathology
Dr Rudolph E Gasparelli, Ohsweken, ON - Family Medicine
Dr Fred Gentili, Toronto, ON - Neurosurgery
Dr Roberto A Giaccone, Nepean, ON - Neurology
Dr Rosella Giammarco, Hamilton, ON - Neurology
Dr Lina Giancola, Toronto, ON - Family Medicine
Dr Tony Giantomaso, Calgary, AB - Physical Medicine & Rehab
Dr Louis R Giavedoni, Toronto, ON - Ophthalmology
Dr Lucia G Giglia, Hamilton, ON - Pediatrics
Dr Chantal M Giguere, Montreal, QC - Otolaryngology
Dr Francois Gilbert, Pointe-Claire, QC - Emergency Medicine
Dr Louis C Girard, North York, ON - Family Medicine
Dr Caroline Girouard, Montreal, QC - Hematology
Dr Antonio Giulivi, Ottawa, ON - Hematological Pathology
Dr Giuseppe Giustino, Surrey, BC - Internal Medicine
Dr May L Go, Scarborough, ON - General Practice
Dr Gabriella Gobbi, Montreal, QC - Psychiatry
Dr Chaim J Goldberg, Scarborough, ON - Ophthalmology
Dr Sol J Goldstein, North York, ON - Psychiatry
Dr Victor Gomel, Vancouver, BC - Obstetrics & Gynecology
Dr Armando Gonzalez, Toronto, ON - General Practice
Dr Randy D Gordon, North York, ON - General Practice
Dr Juliana Gorja, Whitby, ON - Family Medicine
Dr Maria S Grande, St. Catharines, ON - Family Medicine
Dr Robert A Greco, Sudbury, ON - Diagnostic-Radiology
Dr Ginette Gregoire, Montreal, QC - Psychiatry
Dr Maria C Grignano, Woodbridge, ON - Family Medicine
Dr Michelle Grinman, Toronto, ON - Internal Medicine
Dr Karen A Gronau, Brampton, ON - Obstetrics & Gynecology
Dr Giuseppe Guaiana, St Thomas, ON - General Practice
Dr Enza-Josie Gucciardi, Orangeville, ON - Emergency Family Med
Dr Ezzat F Guirguis, Orillia, ON - Psychiatry
Dr Flavio Habal, Toronto, ON - Gastroenterology
Dr James S J Haight, Toronto, ON - Otolaryngology
Dr Robert Hamel, Montreal, QC - General Practice
Dr Hachmi Hammami, Salaber-de-Valleyf, QC - Ophthalmology
Dr M Wahbi Hammouda, Brampton, ON - Hematology
Dr Dan J Hancu, North York, ON - Family Medicine
Dr Gervais A Harry, Etobicoke, ON - Urology
Dr David J Hill, North York, ON - General Practice
Dr Victor Hoffstein, Toronto, ON - Respirology

Dr Nadine S Hradsky, Toronto, ON - Dermatology
Dr Irene Hussain-Autenried, Etobicoke, ON - General Practice
Dr Biagio Iannantuono, Bracebridge, ON - General Surgery
Dr Edgar Ibrahim, Repentigny, QC - General Practice
Dr Alfred W Illescas, Montreal, QC - General Practice
Dr Hani Iskandar, Verdun, QC - General Practice
Dr Aden A Ismail, London, ON - Psychiatry
Dr Anna M Issakoff-Meller, Guelph, ON - General Practice
Dr Wesley D Jackson, Calgary, AB - Family Medicine
Dr J Walter James, Toronto, ON - Pediatrics
Dr Peter F Jarzem, Montreal, QC - Orthopedic Surgery
Dr Alphonse Jeanneret-Grosjean, Montreal, QC - Internal Medicine
Dr Sunny V Johnson, Mississauga, ON - Psychiatry
Dr Donald P Jones, Mississauga, ON - General Surgery
Dr Pamela L Jones, Kirkland, QC - Orthopedic Surgery
Dr Yigal Kaikov, Vancouver, BC - Pediatrics
Dr Athanassios Karabatsos, Shawville, QC - Internal Medicine
Dr Elena Kasatiya Trevisani, Ottawa, ON - General Practice
Dr Walter F Kean, Hamilton, ON - Internal Medicine
Dr Michael R Kenyon, Terrace, BC - Internal Medicine
Dr Elie G Khoury, Saint-Laurent, QC - Ophthalmology
Dr Pierre Khouzam, Newmarket, ON - General Practice
Dr Bob B Kiaii, London, ON - Cardiac Surgery
Dr Teresa M Kieser, Calgary, AB - Cardiovasc/ThorSurg
Dr Max Kleinman, North York, ON - Physical Medicine & Rehab
Dr Hans Knecht, Sherbrooke, QC - Hematology
Dr Sharon H Kreidstein, North York, ON - Internal Medicine
Dr Karol Kuperberg, Montreal, QC - General Practice
Dr Robin A Kuritzky, New Westminster, BC - Cardiology
Dr Ignazio La Delfa, Toronto, ON - Internal Medicine
Dr Lino P LaGrotteria, Hamilton, ON - Family Medicine
Dr Renee Laberge, Quebec, QC - General Practice
Dr Peter Labruzzo, Woodstock, ON - General Practice
Dr Linda A M Lacroix, Ottawa, ON - Hematology
Dr Marie-Pierre Laflamme, Montreal, QC - General Practice
Dr Martine Lafleur, Montreal, QC - Geriatric Medicine
Dr Gilles-Philippe Lafond, Quebec, QC - Ophthalmology
Dr Leda C Lagrotteria, Hamilton, ON - Family Medicine
Dr Ginette Lajoie, Brampton, ON - Anatomical Pathology
Dr Fiore R Lalla, Pointe-Claire, QC - Psychiatry
Dr Isabella Lamargese, Terrebonne, QC - Internal Medicine
Dr Cecilia Lamenza, Toronto, ON - Pediatrics
Dr Marcelo Lannes, Montreal, QC - Anesthesia
Dr Michel A Lapointe, Westmount, QC - Family Medicine
Dr Marc Laporta, Montreal, QC - Psychiatry
Dr Francois Lariviere, Montreal, QC - Medical Biochemistry
Dr Pierre Larouche, Salaber-de-Valleyf, QC - General Practice
Dr Ilan Lashevsky, Toronto, ON - General Practice
Dr Benjamin H Lasko, Etobicoke, ON - General Practice
Dr Steve Lassey, Pictou, NS - General Practice
Dr Jennifer Latella, Thunder Bay, ON - Internal Medicine
Dr Micheline C Lau, Scarborough, ON - General Practice
Dr David Lawee, Toronto, ON - Family Medicine
Dr Frank T Lazzara, LaSalle, QC - General Practice
Dr Vittorio Lentini, Scarborough, ON - General Practice
Dr Ercole F Leone, Vancouver, BC - Urology
Dr Rosa Leone, North York, ON - General Practice
Dr Alain D Lesage, Montreal, QC - Psychiatry
Dr William Liang, Hamilton, ON - General Practice
Dr Anne M Liberatore, Burlington, ON - General Practice
Dr Samuel Librach, Toronto, ON - Obstetrics & Gynecology
Dr Rosanna V Lima, Vancouver, BC - Family Medicine
Dr Charles Listgarten, Woodbridge, ON - Internal Medicine
Dr Rocco A Lombardi, Bowmanville, ON - Emergency Family Med
Dr Luciano P Lombardi, Scarborough, ON - General Practice
Dr Pietro Lombardi, Toronto, ON - Family Medicine
Dr C Gabriella Lorenzon, Vancouver, BC - General Practice
Dr Suzanne F MacDonald, Montreal, QC - Pediatrics
Dr Anne-Marie MacLellan, Montreal, QC - Pediatrics
Dr Keith A MacLellan, Shawville, QC - General Practice
Dr Richard J Mackler, Montreal, QC - Endocrinology
Dr Yolanda Madarnas, Kingston, ON - Internal Medicine
Dr J Robert Madronich, Concord, ON - Plastic Surgery
Dr Lucia B Magnani, Pierrefonds, QC - Pediatrics
Dr Vincent Maida, Toronto, ON - Family Medicine
Dr Garnet J M Maley, Milton, ON - General Practice
Dr Mario L Malizia, London, ON - General Practice
Dr Joseph Mamazza, Ottawa, ON - General Surgery
Dr Maria P Manno, Oakville, ON - Family Medicine
Dr Dominic Marando, LaSalle, QC - General Practice
Dr Alex S Marazzi, Mission, BC - Emergency Family Med
Dr Paul J Marchetti, Milton, ON - Neurology
Dr Catherine A Marchetti, Mississauga, ON - Emergency Family Med
Dr Loretta Marcon, Montreal, QC - Obstetrics & Gynecology
Dr Marilena Marignani, London, ON - Plastic Surgery
Dr Joseph E V Marmina, Pickering, ON - General Practice
Dr Joseph G Marsan, Ottawa, ON - Otolaryngology
Dr Elise J Martin, Maria, QC - Pediatrics
Dr Stephen C Martin, Westmount, QC - Family Medicine
Dr Frank A Martino, Brampton, ON - Emergency Family Med
Dr Adelmo E Martoglio, Toronto, ON - Obstetrics & Gynecology
Dr Antony Masellis, Markham, ON - General Practice
Dr Mario Masellis, Toronto, ON - Neurology
Dr Ralph Masi, North York, ON - Family Medicine
Dr Caterina Mastrogiacomo, Scarborough, ON - Family Medicine
Dr Frank F Mastrogiacomo, Toronto, ON - Orthopedic Surgery
Dr Guiseppe Mazza, Montreal, QC - General Practice
Dr Sergio Mazzadi, Hamilton, ON - General Practice
Dr Mark Mazzarelli, LaSalle, QC - General Practice
Dr Catherine C McCuaig, Montreal, QC - Dermatology
Dr Caterina McGuire, Vancouver, BC - Family Medicine
Dr Maria F Melchior, Etobicoke, ON - Obstetrics & Gynecology
Dr Victor L Mele, North York, ON - General Practice
Dr Briseida Mema, Toronto, ON - Pediatrics
Dr Catherine Meunier, Newmarket, ON - Family Medicine
Dr Josee Michaud, Sudbury, ON - Cardiology
Dr Michael J Mindel, Montreal, QC - Diagnostic-Radiology
Dr Marie-Jose F Miron, Montreal, QC - Internal Medicine
Dr Yazdan Mirzanejad, Surrey, BC - Infectious Diseases
Dr Rino P Moccia, Vancouver, BC - General Practice
Dr Luigina Mollica, Montreal, QC - Hematology
Dr Ilaria Moneta, Westmount, QC - Pediatrics
Dr Walter J Montanera, Toronto, ON - Diagnostic-Radiology
Dr Manuel M Montero Odasso, London, ON - Geriatric Medicine
Dr Valentina C Montessori, Vancouver, BC - Infectious Diseases
Dr Liliana L Monti, Hamilton, ON - Psychiatry
Dr Corrado G Morana, Scarborough, ON - Family Medicine
Dr Henry Morgentaler, Toronto, ON - General Practice
Dr Ronaldo Moriconi, Chambly, QC - General Practice
Dr Luciano F Moro, Malton, ON - General Practice
Dr Pasqualino Morra, Oshawa, ON - Internal Medicine
Dr David Morris, Montreal, QC - Endocrinology
Dr Lia M Mortellaro, Richmond Hill, ON - Family Medicine
Dr Mario A Moscarello, Toronto, ON - General Practice
Dr Daniel J Mueller, Toronto, ON - General Practice
Dr Frank V Muia, London, ON - General Practice
Dr Diana Mukherjee, Moncton, NB - General Practice
Dr Marie Munoz, Montreal, QC - General Practice
Dr Maria Muraca, North York, ON - Family Medicine
Dr Letitia V Muresan, Dollard-D-Ormeaux, QC - Electroencephal
Dr Mafalda S Musacchio, Vancouver, BC - Psychiatry
Dr John G Muscedere, Kingston, ON - Internal Medicine
Dr Saverio Naccarato, Vancouver, BC - General Practice
Dr Alexander G Nagy, Vancouver, BC - General Surgery
Dr Kamil Nasr, Brossard, QC - Ophthalmology
Dr Renato Natale, London, ON - Obstetrics & Gynecology
Dr Doina Nica-Danes, Montreal, QC - General Practice
Dr Bruno S Nicoletti, Nepean, ON - Family Medicine
Dr Frank Nigro, Thunder Bay, ON - Cardiology
Dr Steven Nitzkin, North York, ON - General Practice
Dr Luis C E Noronha, Toronto, ON - Internal Medicine
Dr Richard Novick, London, ON - Cardiovasc/ThorSurg
Dr Yvonne A V Opalinski, Newmarket, ON - General Practice
Dr Alexandru A F Opris, Toronto, ON - General Practice
Dr Denise M A Ouellette, Montreal, QC - General Surgery
Dr Nicholas V J Pairaudeau, North York, ON - Obstetrics & Gynecology
Dr Luigia M Pancaro, York, ON - General Practice
Dr Fulvio Paolucci, Kingston, ON - General Practice
Dr Osvaldo Papini, Woodbridge, ON - Family Medicine
Dr Dante U Pascali, Nepean, ON - Obstetrics & Gynecology
Dr Andre Pasternac, Westmount, QC - Cardiology
Dr Margot Patterson, Denwood, AB - General Practice
Dr Elio Pavone, Oshawa, ON - Gastroenterology
Dr Denis Pelletier, La Pocatiere, QC - General Practice
Dr Rosana Pellizzari, Peterborough, ON - Community Medicine
Dr Gavino Perez, Hamilton, ON - Internal Medicine
Dr Vincenzo Peschisolido, Etobicoke, ON - General Practice
Dr Teresa Petraglia, Montreal, QC - Family Medicine
Dr Nick J Petrella, Saint-Leonard, QC - General Practice
Dr Ivan Petrov, Toronto, ON - General Practice
Dr Donato Pezzutto, London, ON - General Practice
Dr Lucia Pezzutto, London, ON - Family Medicine
Dr Perry Phillips, Toronto, ON - Obstetrics & Gynecology
Dr Helena Piccinini, Halifax, NS - Family Medicine
Dr Roberto L G Piemontesi, Nanaimo, BC - Ophthalmology
Dr Monique Piersanti, Mississauga, ON - Endocrin/Metabolism
Dr Antonio Pignatiello, Toronto, ON - Psychiatry
Dr Angelo Pinto, Bolton, ON - General Practice
Dr Lucina M Pinto, Toronto, ON - General Practice
Dr Antonio Pinto, Montreal, QC - General Practice
Dr Lucille J Poisson, Ottawa, ON - Family Medicine
Dr Vivian A Polak, Drayton, ON - Psychiatry
Dr Joseph O Polimeni, Winnipeg, MB - Psychiatry
Dr Robert C Polomeno, Westmount, QC - Ophthalmology
Dr Gregory M Polyakov, Vancouver, BC - General Surgery
Dr Galdino E Pontarini, Mississauga, ON - General Practice
Dr Michelle G Ponti-Sgargi, London, ON - Pediatrics
Dr Mihai Pop, Montreal, QC - Ophthalmology
Dr Frank A Potestio, Thunder Bay, ON - Obstetrics & Gynecology
Dr Antonio F Preto, North Vancouver, BC - Orthopedic Surgery
Dr Adele F Preto, Salmon Arm, BC - General Practice
Dr Francois J Primeau, Levis, QC - Psychiatry
Dr Ralph Profetto, Stoney Creek, ON - Family Medicine
Dr Krystyna Prutis-Misterska, North York, ON - Physical Medicine & Rehab
Dr Serge Querin, Montreal, QC - Internal Medicine
Dr Dominic L F Raco, Brampton, ON - Cardiology
Dr F Emilio Raimondo, St Catharines, ON - Internal Medicine
Dr Francesco Ramadori, Montreal, QC - Anesthesia
Dr Antonio Rambaldi, Varennes, QC - General Practice
Dr Gloria M Rambaldini, Thornhill, ON - Endocrin/Metabolism
Dr Oswaldo C Ramirez, Alliston, ON - Family Medicine
Dr Eugenio A Rasio, Montreal, QC - Endocrinology
Dr Felix C Re Martinez, St Catharines, ON - General Practice
Dr Dennis A G Reich, Sudbury, ON - Family Medicine
Dr Morton J Reingold, North York, ON - General Practice
Dr Elio E Ricci, Hamilton, ON - General Practice
Dr Luigi T Ricciardi, Virgil, ON - Family Medicine
Dr Flora Ricciuti, North York, ON - Family Medicine
Dr Claudio Rigatto, Winnipeg, MB - Internal Medicine
Dr Santos Rijo, Woodbridge, ON - General Practice
Dr Linda Riven, Westmount, QC - Psychiatry
Dr Nicholas A Rizzo, Hamilton, ON - Family Medicine
Dr Adriano Rocci, Oakville, ON - Family Medicine
Dr Carlos H Rodriguez, Toronto, ON - Internal Medicine
Dr Joseph Rodriguez, Montreal, QC - General Surgery
Dr Maria A Rogano, North York, ON - General Practice
Dr Chaim M Roifman, Toronto, ON - Med Scientist
Dr Marek Rola-Pleszczynski, Sherbrooke, QC - Clin Immun/Allergy
Dr Norbert J Rose, Toronto, ON - General Practice
Dr Joel Rosen, Montreal, QC - Ophthalmology
Dr Frank W Rosenberg, Etobicoke, ON - Dermatology
Dr Miriam F. Rossi, Toronto, ON - Pediatrics
Dr Peter A Rostas, North York, ON - General Practice
Dr Jan Rozehnal, Toronto, ON - General Practice
Dr Donato A Ruggiero, Toronto, ON - General Practice
Dr Mladen V Rusnov, Montreal, QC - General Surgery
Dr Hani N I Sahyoun, Scarborough, ON - Psychiatry
Dr Robert R Saint-Jacques, Saint-Eustache, QC - Dermatology
Dr Paul Salcicciolí, Brampton, ON - Family Medicine
Dr Patricia Sammarelli, Victoria, BC - Family Medicine
Dr Federico J Sanchez, Etobicoke, ON - Family Medicine
Dr Arturo Sanchez, Toronto, ON - Pediatrics

Dr Franco Sandrin, Kirkland, QC - Cardiology
Dr Pablo E R F Sanhueza Luco, North Bay, ON - Psychiatry
Dr Claudia Santos, Toronto, ON - Critical Care Medicine
Dr Dioscoro D C Sarile, Toronto, ON - General Practice
Dr Abraham Sasson, Thornhill, ON - General Practice
Dr Peter Sauret, Toronto, ON - General Practice
Dr Nellina Saveriano, Hamilton, ON - Dermatology
Dr Katherine M Savoia, Calgary, AB - Family Medicine
Dr Stephanie C Sbrocchi, Sudbury, ON - Family Medicine
Dr Salvatore J Scala, Toronto, ON - General Practice
Dr Jim N Scali, Thunder Bay, ON - Family Medicine
Dr Nicola Scampoli, Mississauga, ON - Emergency Family Med
Dr Dante G Scanga, Edmonton, AB - Family Medicine
Dr Dominique Scarfone, Outremont, QC - Psychiatry
Dr Alicia Schiffrin, Montreal, QC - Endocrinology
Dr Vanna Schiralli, Toronto, ON - Family Medicine
Dr Peter E H Schmalfuss, Bolton, ON - General Practice
Dr Gerd Schneider, Ottawa, ON - Family Medicine
Dr Holger J Schuenemann, Hamilton, ON - Internal Medicine
Dr Walter Schurch, Montreal, QC - Anatomical Pathology
Dr Carmela Sciarra, Hamilton, ON - Obstetrics & Gynecology
Dr Douglas F Scott, Nipigon, ON - Family Medicine
Dr Paul S Scotton, Orangeville, ON - General Practice
Dr David Sedran, North York, ON - Family Medicine
Dr Consolato Sergi, Edmonton, AB - General Practice
Dr Stefano Serra, Toronto, ON - General Practice
Dr Anna Sfriso, Levis, QC - Otolaryngology
Dr James J Sheridan, Grnd Falls-Windsor, NL - Internal Medicine
Dr Sandy E Shulman, North York, ON - Family Medicine
Dr Dolores A Sicheri, Thunder Bay, ON - Internal Medicine
Dr Andrew A Simone, Etobicoke, ON - Dermatology
Dr Angelo M Simone, Mississauga, ON - Endocrin/Metabolism
Dr Carmine Simone, Toronto, ON - Thoracic Surgery
Dr William Singer, East York, ON - Internal Medicine
Dr Surjeet S Sira, Malton, ON - General Surgery
Dr Giovanna Sirianni, Toronto, ON - Family Medicine
Dr Salvatore Sirna, Toronto, ON - General Practice
Dr Jeffrey Sirzyk, Hawkesbury, ON - Emergency Family Med
Dr Marco L A Sivilotti, Kingston, ON - Emergency Medicine
Dr Robert L Sleightholm, Brampton, ON - Plastic Surgery
Dr Harley S Smyth, Mississauga, ON - Neurosurgery
Dr Elisabeth K Sochocka, Milton, ON - General Practice
Dr Lorne W Sokol, Toronto, ON - Family Medicine
Dr Vito A Sorrento, Woodbridge, ON - Emergency Family Med
Dr Jan Spacek, Sherbrooke, QC - General Practice
Dr Peter J Spadafora, Guelph, ON - Family Medicine
Dr Silvana Spadafora, Sault Ste. Marie, ON - Internal Medicine
Dr Joseph J Spano, Sarnia, ON - General Practice
Dr Giuseppe Spano Greco, Toronto, ON - General Practice
Dr Amerigo D Sparanese, Victoria, BC - Family Medicine
Dr Donato Spensieri, Woodbridge, ON - General Practice
Dr Filippo M Staibano, Stoney Creek, ON - Family Medicine
Dr Gerda S Stockler-Ipsiroglu, Vancouver, BC - Neurology
Dr Antonio P Strafella, Toronto, ON - Neurology
Dr Diann J Superina-Bell, Toronto, ON - Pediatrics
Dr Vincenzo R Susini, Geraldton, ON - General Practice
Dr Emile D Svarc, Montreal, QC - Ophthalmology
Dr Saadat A S Syed, North York, ON - Family Medicine
Dr Wanda M Szymonowicz, Mississauga, ON - Pediatrics
Dr Domenica Tambasco, Toronto, ON - Family Medicine
Dr Robert Tambay, Ottawa, ON - Gastroenterology
Dr Donatella Tampieri, Montreal, QC - Diagnostic-Radiology
Dr Gino Tancon, Courtenay, BC - General Practice
Dr Tanya J Tarshis, Toronto, ON - General Practice
Dr Giuseppe P Tarulli, Toronto, ON - Diagnostic-Radiology
Dr Fabiano A S Taucer, Ottawa, ON - Diagnostic-Radiology
Dr Peter S Teitelbaum, Ottawa, ON - General Practice
Dr Stefan Teolis, Laval, QC - Family Medicine
Dr Jean-Pierre Teolis, Montreal, QC - General Practice
Dr Kristin A Terenzi, Woodbridge, ON - Family Medicine
Dr Maria-Elena Tiboni, Hamilton, ON - Internal Medicine
Dr Brian Ticoll, Markham, ON - Psychiatry
Dr Nadia D Toffoli-Zadra, Vaughan, ON - Family Medicine
Dr Denny Toffolo, Hamilton, ON - General Practice
Dr Robert Tommasini, Toronto, ON - Family Medicine
Dr Marie Toscano, Gatineau, QC - Dermatology
Dr Jacques Toueg, Laval, QC - Orthopedic Surgery
Dr Daniel P Tozzi, Montreal, QC - General Practice
Dr Stephane N Treyvaud, Oakville, ON - Psychiatry
Dr Maria Triassi Asper, Woodbridge, ON - Clin Immun/Allergy
Dr Anthony L J Tripodi, Etobicoke, ON - Diagnostic-Radiology
Dr Maria G Trivieri, Toronto, ON - Internal Medicine
Dr Margaret B Truchan, Saskatoon, SK - Internal Medicine
Dr Marisa A Tucci, Montreal, QC - Pediatrics
Dr Eldon R Tunks, Hamilton, ON - Psychiatry
Dr Alfredo Tura, Comox, BC - Family Medicine
Dr Jean-Philippe Vaccani, Ottawa, ON - Otolaryngology
Dr Gabriel A Vadasz, Toronto, ON - Family Medicine
Dr Maria Valente, Thunder Bay, ON - General Practice
Dr Alissia R Valentinis, Toronto, ON - Family Medicine
Dr Pamela Valentino, Toronto, ON - Gastroenterology
Dr Anthony M Vannelli, London, ON - Anesthesia
Dr Marica Varga, Toronto, ON - Geriatric Medicine
Dr Fabio Varlese, North York, ON - Geriatric Medicine
Dr Gokuldas R Varma, Toronto, ON - General Practice
Dr Manuel O Vasquez, York, ON - General Practice
Dr John A Vecchiarelli, North York, ON - General Practice
Dr Silvano R Vecchio, Edmonton, AB - General Practice
Dr Michael J Vecchio, North York, ON - General Practice
Dr Nadia Venchiarutti, Vaughan, ON - Family Medicine
Dr Elisa A Venier, Toronto, ON - General Practice
Dr Mario R Ventresca, Port Colborne, ON - Ophthalmology
Dr Carlo Vernacchia, Montreal, QC - General Practice
Dr Mauro Verrelli, Winnipeg, MB - Internal Medicine
Dr Phyllis-Marie Vetere, Montreal, QC - General Practice
Dr Antonio Vettese, Mississauga, ON - Ophthalmology
Dr Antonio A L Vigano, Montreal, QC - General Practice
Dr Giovanni Villella, Windsor, ON - Psychiatry
Dr Diana E Visentin, Barrie, ON - Internal Medicine
Dr Bennedetto B Vitullo, Charlottetown, PE - Pediatrics
Dr Angelo A Vivona, Markham, ON - General Surgery
Dr The-Hung Vu, Montreal, QC - General Practice
Dr Howard P Wein, Montreal, QC - Electroencephal
Dr Gerald I Weisbrod, North York, ON - General Practice
Dr Laura L Whiteacre, North York, ON - General Surgery
Dr John S Wilczynski, Niagara Falls, ON - General Practice
Dr Eldon S V Williams, Toronto, ON - General Surgery
Dr Davinia E Withington, Montreal, QC - General Practice
Dr Elvira Yakoub, Windsor, ON - Family Medicine
Dr Anthony P C Yau, Toronto, ON - General Practice
Dr Joseph A Zadra, Barrie, ON - Urology
Dr Remo Zadra, Newmarket, ON - Cardiology
Dr Patrizia A C Zanelli, Montreal, QC - Critical Care Medicine
Dr Paul A Zanette, Maple, ON - Family Medicine
Dr Fabio G Zanetti, Brantford, ON - Ophthalmology
Dr Marianna Zarrelli, Montreal, QC - Psychiatry
Dr Ricardo Zarruk, Pierrefonds, QC - General Practice
Dr Lauren V Zeilig, North York, ON - General Practice
Dr Peter I Zelina, Richmond Hill, ON - Psychiatry
Dr Paul J Zeni, Georgetown, ON - General Practice
Dr Lucjan J Zielonka, Surrey, BC - Psychiatry
Dr Paul S Ziter, Windsor, ON - General Practice
Dr Maria L Zorzitto, Toronto, ON - Geriatric Medicine
Dr Raquel del Carpio, Montreal, QC - Diagnostic-Radiology

JAPANESE

Dr Ryojo Akagami, Vancouver, BC - Neurosurgery
Dr Eriko Aota, Vancouver, BC - Family Medicine
Dr Eull N Aum, Thornhill, ON - Anesthesia
Dr Naoki Chiba, Guelph, ON - Gastroenterology
Dr Mutsuko Emond, Montreal, QC - Psychiatry
Dr Margarita K Hojyo Tomoka, Etobicoke, ON - General Practice
Dr Akiko N Hosokawa, North York, ON - Family Medicine
Dr John S C Hsuen, North York, ON - Pediatrics
Dr Roland M Ikuta, Lethbridge, AB - Geriatric Medicine
Dr Shinya Ito, Toronto, ON - Pediatrics
Dr Xiaoyan Jia, Langley, BC - Pediatrics
Dr Steven L Kirzner, Vancouver, BC - Ophthalmology
Dr Jean L Lette, Montreal, QC - Nuclear Medicine
Dr Man K Leung, Vancouver, BC - General Practice
Dr Jian-Qiang Lu, Edmonton, AB - Neuro-Pathology
Dr John A D Miller, Victoria, BC - General Practice
Dr Robert T Miyagishima, Vancouver, BC - Cardiovasc/ThorSurg
Dr Richard M Nakamura, Port Moody, BC - General Practice
Dr Joyce L Pickering, Montreal, QC - Internal Medicine
Dr Henry R Shibata, Montreal, QC - General Surgery
Dr Tomoko Takano, Montreal, QC - General Practice
Dr Sachiko Takaya, Saskatoon, SK - Infectious Diseases
Dr Asae Tanaka, Richmond, BC - Family Medicine
Dr Yoko Tarumi, Edmonton, AB - General Practice
Dr Marion A Tipple, Vancouver, BC - Pediatric Cardiology
Dr Allan G Toguri, Scarborough, ON - Urology
Dr Maorong Tong, Thunder Bay, ON - Family Medicine
Dr Shian-Yih Tsai, Hamilton, ON - Urology
Dr H H Steve Tschen, Windsor, ON - General Practice
Dr Juhn A Wada, Vancouver, BC - Neurology
Dr Eiko Waida, Vernon, BC - Pediatrics
Dr Liya Xie, Calgary, AB - General Practice
Dr Hirotaka Yamashiro, Richmond Hill, ON - Pediatrics
Dr Tung C Yang, Vancouver, BC - Infectious Diseases
Dr Kazuhiro Yasufuku, Toronto, ON - General Practice
Dr Eluen A Yeh, Toronto, ON - Pediatrics

KACCHI

Dr Alykhan S Abdulla, Manotick, ON - Family Medicine
Dr Shiraz F Aziz, Surrey, BC - General Practice
Dr Abdulsultan A Datoo, Richmond Hill, ON - Anesthesia
Dr Salim H Daya, Mississauga, ON - Obstetrics & Gynecology
Dr Al-Noor Dhanani, Mississauga, ON - Neurology
Dr Murtaza Gulamhussein, Grimsby, ON - General Practice
Dr Parviz M Hasham, Brampton, ON - General Practice
Dr Alim Hirji, Prince George, BC - Internal Medicine
Dr Shiraz H Ismail, North York, ON - General Practice
Dr Amin R Javer, Vancouver, BC - Otolaryngology
Dr Shamin Jetha, Vancouver, BC - Family Medicine
Dr Rozmin F Kamani, Vancouver, BC - Family Medicine
Dr Allaudin A S Kamani, Vancouver, BC - Anesthesia
Dr Abdul Malik, Brampton, ON - Family Medicine
Dr Shamsh Y Merali, Milton, ON - Family Medicine
Dr Akber H Mithani, Vancouver, BC - General Practice
Dr M Muni Nazerali-Sunderji, New Westminster, BC - Internal Medicine
Dr Suleman S Remtulla, Mississauga, ON - Family Medicine
Dr Farid M Shamji, Ottawa, ON - Cardiovasc/ThorSurg
Dr Shiraz B K Shariff, Brampton, ON - General Practice
Dr Mohamed R Suleman, Kitchener, ON - Diagnostic-Radiology
Dr Shahida Surmawala, Edmonton, AB - Family Medicine
Dr Ashnoor S Talib, Vaughan, ON - Family Medicine
Dr Shamim J Tejpar, Stratford, ON - Pediatrics
Dr Mumtaz A Virji, Vancouver, BC - Pediatrics
Dr Shiraz A Walji, Calgary, AB - General Practice

KANARESE

Dr K Rama Bhat, Richmond Hill, ON - General Surgery
Dr Santosh A Britto, Salmon Arm, BC - General Surgery
Dr Nolda M D'Cunha, Toronto, ON - Family Medicine
Dr Chikkahanumaiah Devaraj, Mississauga, ON - Geriatric Medicine
Dr Kempe Gowda, Saskatoon, SK - Internal Medicine
Dr Jaya M Islur, Toronto, ON - Pediatrics
Dr Jyothi Jayaraman, Vancouver, BC - Family Medicine
Dr Changulanda M Joshi, New Glasgow, NS - Obstetrics & Gynecology
Dr Desikan R Kadambi, Winnipeg, MB - Ophthalmology
Dr Dattatri L Keshav, St Thomas, ON - Psychiatry
Dr Ramesh Kulkarni, North Bay, ON - Obstetrics & Gynecology
Dr U Sujana Kumar, London, ON - Family Medicine
Dr Bahubali D Lagare, Mississauga, ON - Family Medicine
Dr Ramachandra N Moorthy, Richmond, BC - Psychiatry
Dr Munithanamma J Mysore, Winnipeg, MB - Psychiatry
Dr Sankar N Prakash, Windsor, ON - General Practice
Dr Jayasimha M Rao, London, ON - Psychiatry
Dr Shanti E Rao, Windsor, ON - Family Medicine
Dr Grama D Ravi, Sudbury, ON - Cardiology
Dr Pushpa Sathya, St. John's, NL - Pediatrics

Dr Jinka R Sathya, St. John's, NL - Radiation Oncology
Dr Yatish N Setty, Owen Sound, ON - General Practice
Dr Aftab M Shariff, Ottawa, ON - Pediatrics
Dr Ravishankar T Shenava, Windsor, ON - Psychiatry
Dr Jitendra B Sheshgiri, Mississauga, ON - Emergency Family Med
Dr Panduranga Y Shetty, Sarnia, ON - Internal Medicine
Dr Rathnakar B Shetty, St Catharines, ON - Obstetrics & Gynecology
Dr Geeta R Shetty, St Catharines, ON - Anesthesia
Dr Karunakara N Shetty, Charlottetown, PE - Internal Medicine
Dr Hindupuram V Sriharsha, Orillia, ON - Internal Medicine
Dr Vasundhara Srinivasan, Etobicoke, ON - Psychiatry
Dr Arun N E Sundaram, Toronto, ON - Neurology
Dr Sam Swaminath, Chatham, ON - Psychiatry
Dr Guruswamy N Swamy, London, ON - Psychiatry
Dr Mudalodu V Vasudevan, Windsor, ON - General Practice
Dr Lakshmi N Yatham, Vancouver, BC - Psychiatry

KANKANI

Dr Umesh H Prabhu, Yarmouth, NS - Internal Medicine

KASHMIRI

Dr Jag Mohan Dhar, Sarnia, ON - Internal Medicine
Dr Anil Dhar, Windsor, ON - Critical Care Medicine
Dr Surendar K Kilam, Lethbridge, AB - General Surgery
Dr Autar K Munshi, Sydney, NS - Psychiatry
Dr Baynazir Parray, Oshawa, ON - Family Medicine
Dr Ravinder P S Sawhney, Surrey, BC - Internal Medicine
Dr Gul Nawaz Sheikh, Ajax, ON - Internal Medicine
Dr Inderjit Singh, Hamilton, ON - Family Medicine

KHMER

Dr Rith Chea, Edmonton, AB - Internal Medicine
Dr Rajni Saksena, Montreal, QC - Family Medicine

KIKONGO

Dr Mandiangu Nsungu, Yorkton, SK - General Practice

KISWAHILI

Dr S Amadala, Calgary, AB - Psychiatry
Dr Shahnaz Dar, Scarborough, ON - Pediatrics
Dr Nasir Jetha, Vancouver, BC - Pediatrics
Dr Azim H Jiwani, West Vancouver, BC - Family Medicine
Dr Allaudin A S Kamani, Vancouver, BC - Anesthesia
Dr Surya Master, Campbellton, NB - General Surgery
Dr Akber H Mithani, Vancouver, BC - General Practice
Dr Stanley K Muwanguzi, Camrose, AB - Emergency Family Med
Dr Gulammohamed G V Nanji, Calgary, AB - Anesthesia
Dr Anuradha Nayar, Vancouver, BC - General Practice
Dr Sudhir P Pandya, Oakville, ON - Gastroenterology
Dr Fakhruddin Sadikali, St Catharines, ON - Internal Medicine
Dr Mohamed A Salyani, Maple, ON - General Practice
Dr Maqbool K Sheriff, Nanaimo, BC - Internal Medicine

KONKANI

Dr Santosh A Britto, Salmon Arm, BC - General Surgery
Dr Anne De Silva, Toronto, ON - General Practice
Dr Indira C Figueiredo, Toronto, ON - General Practice
Dr Avdhut R Manerkar, Miramichi, NB - General Practice

KOREAN

Dr Eull N Aum, Thornhill, ON - Anesthesia
Dr Mijin Brown, Brampton, ON - Pediatrics
Dr Diana M Chang, Vancouver, BC - Emergency Family Med
Dr Jung Hoon Chee, Scarborough, ON - Internal Medicine
Dr James Choe, Etobicoke, ON - General Practice
Dr Richard F Y Choi, Toronto, ON - Cardiology
Dr Samuel S S Chun, Dartmouth, NS - Urology
Dr Wan M Chung, Edmonton, AB - General Practice
Dr Minjeong Eom, Ottawa, ON - Family Medicine
Dr Elizabeth Y H Glowczewski-Park, Scarborough, ON - Family Medicine
Dr Andrew Ha, Hamilton, ON - Cardiology
Dr June H Hahn-Lee, Windsor, ON - Pediatrics
Dr Caroline C Huh, Scarborough, ON - Obstetrics & Gynecology
Dr Tae-Bin T Im, Brantford, ON - General Practice
Dr Stephen S Im, Toronto, ON - Obstetrics & Gynecology
Dr H L Nancy Kim, Calgary, AB - Diagnostic-Radiology
Dr Brian Kim, Calgary, AB - Family Medicine
Dr Seung Kim, Burnaby, BC - Clin Immun/Allergy
Dr James S J Kim, Brampton, ON - General Practice
Dr Myung-Gi Kim, Fort Erie, ON - General Practice
Dr Don Kim, Mississauga, ON - Internal Medicine
Dr Justin Kim, Mississauga, ON - Family Medicine
Dr M Marie Kim, Mississauga, ON - Pediatrics
Dr Hae Ryong Kim, North York, ON - Psychiatry
Dr Rak Hay Kim, North York, ON - Endocrin/Metabolism
Dr Young-In Kim, Toronto, ON - Gastroenterology
Dr Dennis D H Kim, Toronto, ON - General Practice
Dr Steven L Kirzner, Vancouver, BC - Ophthalmology
Dr Seung S Ko, Scarborough, ON - Family Medicine
Dr John J Kwak, Surrey, BC - Otolaryngology
Dr D Dae-Won Lee, North Vancouver, BC - Endocrin/Metabolism
Dr Victoria E H Lee, Vancouver, BC - Community Medicine
Dr Christine H C Lee, Hamilton, ON - Infectious Diseases
Dr John O Lee, Kanata, ON - Family Medicine
Dr Mark H Lee, Richmond Hill, ON - General Surgery
Dr Yuna Lee, Toronto, ON - Internal Medicine
Dr Douglas S Y Lee, Toronto, ON - Cardiology
Dr Peter S H Lim, North Vancouver, BC - Psychiatry
Dr Angela Y Nguan, Vancouver, BC - Family Medicine
Dr Dennis E Oh, Coquitlam, BC - Family Medicine
Dr Joseph Park, Hamilton, ON - Anesthesia
Dr Vincent Park, Mississauga, ON - Family Medicine
Dr Joonseong Park, Mississauga, ON - General Practice
Dr Esther M Park, Toronto, ON - Obstetrics & Gynecology
Dr Paul M U Ra, Windsor, ON - Anatomical Pathology
Dr Athanasius S K Ro, Oshawa, ON - Ophthalmology
Dr Doo Ho Shin, Surrey, BC - Anatomical Pathology
Dr Anne Y Shin, Richmond Hill, ON - Internal Medicine
Dr Whun Yong Shin, Toronto, ON - General Practice
Dr Donald D H Sin, Vancouver, BC - Internal Medicine
Dr Young S Suh, Langley, BC - Family Medicine
Dr Gregory T H Um, Markham, ON - General Practice
Dr Yun-Lin Wang, Toronto, ON - General Practice
Dr Minna N Woo, Toronto, ON - Endocrin/Metabolism
Dr Daniel Yim, North York, ON - General Practice
Dr John H J Yoo, London, ON - Otolaryngology
Dr Shi-Joon Yoo, Toronto, ON - Diagnostic-Radiology
Dr Jennifer W J Yoo, Waterloo, ON - Family Medicine
Dr Joseph Y J Yuh, Scarborough, ON - Family Medicine
Dr Jennifer M Yun, Port Coquitlam, BC - Family Medicine
Dr John W S Yun, Richmond, BC - Internal Medicine

KURDISH

Dr Hoshiar Abdollah, Kingston, ON - Cardiology
Dr Amid K Abdullah, Calgary, AB - General Pathology
Dr Erfan Arfali, Brantford, ON - Emergency Family Med
Dr Adnan Bajelan, Summerside, PE - Family Medicine
Dr Shler Gharib, Brantford, ON - Family Medicine
Dr Omar N Hasan, Amqui, QC - General Surgery
Dr Kawa M A Ibrahiem, Cambridge, ON - Family Medicine
Dr Mahdi K Ibrahim, Bonavista, NL - General Practice
Dr Narmin Ibrahim, Saskatoon, SK - Family Medicine
Dr Koma D Israel, Hamilton, ON - Family Medicine
Dr Razawa F Maroof, Regina, SK - Family Medicine
Dr Khashayar Sanandaji, Vaughan, ON - Family Medicine

LATIN

Dr Khami Chokani, Prince Albert, SK - General Practice
Dr Robert Ferrari, Edmonton, AB - Internal Medicine
Dr Colin M Mailer, London, ON - Ophthalmology
Dr James J Sheridan, Grnd Falls-Windsor, NL - Internal Medicine
Dr Lucjan J Zielonka, Surrey, BC - Psychiatry

LATVIAN

Dr Maris Andersons, Toronto, ON - Family Medicine
Dr Andris Blokmanis, Vancouver, BC - Otolaryngology
Dr Charles Cuncins, North Bay, ON - General Practice
Dr George N Djaiani, Toronto, ON - Anesthesia
Dr Margrieta Edels, London, ON - General Practice
Dr Sylvia G Garnis-Jones, Welland, ON - Dermatology
Dr Ralph Grinberg, Conestogo, ON - Anesthesia
Dr Voldemars Gulens, Toronto, ON - Psychiatry
Dr Peter Gutmanis, Nanaimo, BC - Orthopedic Surgery
Dr Larisa I Hausmanis, Toronto, ON - Family Medicine
Dr Lauma A Kalins, North York, ON - General Practice
Dr Klara Koblents, Woodbridge, ON - General Practice
Dr Juris Lazovskis, Sydney, NS - General Practice
Dr Janis G Lusis, Brampton, ON - General Practice
Dr Egils Mierins, Ottawa, ON - Internal Medicine
Dr Gundars E Roze, Richmond Hill, ON - Anesthesia
Dr Andris A Rubenis, Scarborough, ON - General Practice
Dr Peter Sakuls, Toronto, ON - Family Medicine
Dr Roland Skrastins, Toronto, ON - Internal Medicine
Dr Anita D Tannis, West Vancouver, BC - Family Medicine
Dr Kaspars B Tuters, Toronto, ON - Psychiatry
Dr Richard L Upenieks, Kitchener, ON - Family Medicine

LEBANESE

Dr Hussein Fadlallah, Montreal, QC - Cardiology
Dr Antoine Farah, Gatineau, QC - Nephrology
Dr Antoine Hejeily, Sorel-Tracy, QC - Urology
Dr Samir Khoury, Montreal, QC - Pediatrics
Dr Richard Moufarrege, Montreal, QC - Plastic Surgery
Dr Alain Moukheiber, Rouyn-Noranda, QC - Otolaryngology

LINGALA

Dr Roger Bashala, Campbellton, NB - Family Medicine
Dr Christopher J Burnett, Niverville, MB - General Practice
Dr Khami Chokani, Prince Albert, SK - General Practice
Dr T Romain Muboyayi, Orleans, ON - Family Medicine
Dr Mandiangu Nsungu, Yorkton, SK - General Practice

LITHUANIAN

Dr Aras J Balsys, York, ON - Internal Medicine
Dr Edward Bekeris, Toronto, ON - General Practice
Dr Dalius J Briedis, Montreal, QC - Internal Medicine
Dr Liuba Grossman, North York, ON - General Practice
Dr Jose Gutauskas, Ottawa, ON - General Surgery
Dr Anne N N E Josiukas, Collingwood, ON - Psychiatry
Dr Rita M Kharonsky, North York, ON - Family Medicine
Dr Herbert I Khosid, Thornhill, ON - General Practice
Dr Philip J Klemka, Edmonton, AB - General Practice
Dr Aukse T Lingys, Mississauga, ON - General Practice
Dr Larissa M Matukas, Toronto, ON - Infectious Diseases
Dr Daiva L Norkus, Etobicoke, ON - Family Medicine
Dr Alan V Pavilanis, Montreal, QC - Family Medicine
Dr Rima Petroniene, Barrie, ON - Internal Medicine
Dr Sara Pliamm, North York, ON - General Practice
Dr Leona C Rudinskas, York, ON - Hematology
Dr Stanley J Salkauskis, North York, ON - Emergency Family Med
Dr Ramunas F J Saplys, Mississauga, ON - Orthopedic Surgery
Dr Danguole Sileikiene, Red Deer, AB - Anatomical Pathology
Dr Gailius J Skrinskas, North York, ON - Internal Medicine
Dr Alexander J Spudas, North York, ON - General Practice
Dr Romas V Stas, Ajax, ON - General Practice
Dr Rima G Styra, Toronto, ON - Psychiatry
Dr Sharif W Tadros, Burlington, ON - General Practice
Dr Gintaras T Uleckas, North York, ON - Family Medicine
Dr Jurate K Uleckas, Laval, QC - Ophthalmology

Dr Saulius M Valadka, Oakville, ON - Diagnostic-Radiology
Dr Mikas A Valadka, Toronto, ON - General Practice
Dr Algis P J Valiulis, Oakville, ON - General Surgery
Dr Vytas J Zulys, Mississauga, ON - Anesthesia

LUGANDA

Dr Joseph E Buwembo, Regina, SK - Neurosurgery
Dr Stanley K Muwanguzi, Camrose, AB - Emergency Family Med
Dr Saturday N A Nsisi, Lethbridge, AB - General Practice

LUNDA

Dr Dereck Maseka, Drumheller, AB - Family Medicine

MACEDONIAN

Dr Hifzija H Bajramovic, Ottawa, ON - Psychiatry
Dr Steven T Elia, North York, ON - Anesthesia
Dr Vlade M Gagovski, North York, ON - General Practice
Dr Desanka Gajic, Toronto, ON - General Practice
Dr Aleksander Georgievski, Thornhill, ON - General Practice
Dr Danny Givelas, North York, ON - Pediatrics
Dr Steven Litsas, Woodbridge, ON - Family Medicine
Dr Juliana Losier, Mayne, BC - Family Medicine
Dr Constantine Mallin, Grand Valley, ON - Family Medicine
Dr Christina Plaskos, St Catharines, ON - General Practice
Dr Henry I Quaye, Stony Plain, AB - General Practice
Dr Jovan G Simeon, Vanier, ON - Psychiatry
Dr Thomas C Stavro Sholdoff, Scarborough, ON - General Practice
Dr Chris P Stefanovich, Etobicoke, ON - Family Medicine
Dr Thomas Stefopulos, Lindsay, ON - General Practice
Dr Vasia Stefou, Toronto, ON - General Practice
Dr Nick Strumas, Hamilton, ON - Plastic Surgery
Dr Kiril Trpkov, Calgary, AB - Anatomical Pathology
Dr Constantin G Vozis, Toronto, ON - General Practice

MALAY

Dr Ganesan Annamala, Toronto, ON - General Practice
Dr Bhavani Arumugam, Burlington, ON - Family Medicine
Dr Mary Chacko, Scarborough, ON - Family Medicine
Dr Wee Kei Choong, Delta, BC - General Practice
Dr Santhi P P Da Samy, Chatham, ON - Otolaryngology
Dr Jeyapandy T Dason, Guelph, ON - Family Medicine
Dr Avtar S Dhanoa, Mississauga, ON - General Practice
Dr Aik-Ping Eng, Vancouver, BC - General Practice
Dr Sheila L Hew, Scarborough, ON - Family Medicine
Dr John Hii, Toronto, ON - Medical Microbiology
Dr Mohamed H Irfan, Port au Choix, NL - Family Medicine
Dr Kai Liang Kwee, White Rock, BC - Orthopedic Surgery
Dr Charles C S Law, Vancouver, BC - General Practice
Dr Sammy S H Lee, Richmond, BC - General Practice
Dr Richard Lee, Vancouver, BC - Diagnostic-Radiology
Capt Chiam L Liew, Belleville, ON - Family Medicine
Dr Thurairajan Light, Cambridge, ON - Family Medicine
Dr Frank F S Lim, Maple Ridge, BC - General Practice
Dr Meng Eng Lim, North Vancouver, BC - Psychiatry
Dr M Firdaus M Mydeen, Westlock, AB - Family Medicine
Dr Douglas B G Ng, Surrey, BC - General Practice
Dr Liang Ng, West Vancouver, BC - General Practice
Dr Hari K Ondiveeran, Saint John, NB - Critical Care Medicine
Dr Gayathri P Shyamal, Toronto, ON - Family Medicine
Dr Angeline C Sia-Venugopal, Chilliwack, BC - General Practice
Dr Amar Singh, Red Deer, AB - General Practice
Dr Michelle W Tan, Richmond, BC - Family Medicine
Dr Chin Chai Tan, St. John's, NL - General Practice
Dr Chee Nyok Thong, Vancouver, BC - Otolaryngology
Dr Peter L Ting, Vancouver, BC - General Practice
Dr Kenny Y V Yee, Barrington Passage, NS - Family Medicine

MALAYALAM

Dr Thoppil M Abraham, Welland, ON - Psychiatry
Dr Geeta Achyuthan, Regina, SK - General Practice
Dr Saju Antony, Chilliwack, BC - Psychiatry
Dr Pradeep Balakrishnan, Guelph, ON - Psychiatry
Dr Mary J Chakkalackal, North York, ON - General Practice
Dr Indira Chandran, Brampton, ON - Obstetrics & Gynecology
Dr Vinod Chandran, Toronto, ON - General Practice
Dr Kavitha Chandrasenan, Edmonton, AB - Family Medicine
Dr Alice T Cherian, Scarborough, ON - Pediatrics
Dr Madhavan S Das, Edmonton, AB - General Practice
Dr Malini G Dave, North York, ON - Pediatrics
Dr Mary T Devassy, North York, ON - General Practice
Dr Saleena Djearam, Victoria, BC - Family Medicine
Dr Reena E Eapen-John, Mississauga, ON - Family Medicine
Dr Leelamma J Elavathil, Hamilton, ON - Anatomical Pathology
Dr Puthenkalathil P George, Kentville, NS - Psychiatry
Dr Rosamma George, Mississauga, ON - Anatomical Pathology
Dr Elizabeth George, Scarborough, ON - General Practice
Dr Susan R George, Toronto, ON - Internal Medicine
Dr Usha Harikumar, Scarborough, ON - Obstetrics & Gynecology
Dr R Padmanabhan Iyer, Chatham, ON - Internal Medicine
Dr Thomas John, Oshawa, ON - Physical Medicine & Rehab
Dr Verghese John, Scarborough, ON - Psychiatry
Dr Suni J Johnson, Owen Sound, ON - Internal Medicine
Dr Mary Joseph, Canning, NS - General Practice
Dr Mariamma G Joseph, London, ON - General Pathology
Dr Anil P Joseph, Sudbury, ON - Psychiatry
Dr Mini G Joshipura, Etobicoke, ON - Geriatric Medicine
Dr Soumini Kaiprath, New Glasgow, NS - Family Medicine
Dr Ramaiyer Krishnaswamy, Fredericton, NB - Pediatrics
Dr P Karunakaran Kutty, Brampton, ON - Gastroenterology
Dr George Mathai, Cambridge, ON - Internal Medicine
Dr Biju Mathew, Maple Ridge, BC - Psychiatry
Dr Baboo M Mathew, Burin, NL - Endocrin/Metabolism
Dr Beena Mathew, Sudbury, ON - Psychiatry
Dr John Mathews, Windsor, ON - Internal Medicine
Dr Anilkumar S Menon, Brampton, ON - Cardiology
Dr Rajashree K Menon, Cornwall, ON - General Surgery
Dr Thankamma Modi, Hamilton, ON - General Practice
Dr Naufal Mohammed, Hamilton, ON - Internal Medicine
Dr Amitha J Mundenchira, Oakville, ON - Family Medicine
Dr Girish M Nair, Ottawa, ON - Cardiology
Dr Shah Nawaz, Sudbury, ON - Cardiology
Dr Abraham Ninan, Saskatoon, SK - Pediatrics
Dr Shakkeela Padanilathu Kunjummar, Newmarket, ON - Family Medicine
Dr Ashalatha Paul, Calgary, AB - General Practice
Dr Chinnamma Punnen, Burlington, ON - Anesthesia
Dr Punnamkuzhil C Punnen, North York, ON - Urology
Dr Lizy Puri-Alanoly, Vaudreuil-Dorion, QC - General Practice
Dr Chitra Rao, Hamilton, ON - General Pathology
Dr Thangamani Subramanian, Hamilton, ON - Family Medicine
Dr Elizabeth Thakkar, Calgary, AB - General Practice
Dr Joseph X Thavundayil, Verdun, QC - General Practice
Dr Lilly Thenganatt, East York, ON - Family Medicine
Dr C Kuncheria Thomas, Espanola, ON - Emergency Family Med
Dr Valsa Thomas, London, ON - General Practice
Dr Boji Varghese, Sudbury, ON - Endocrin/Metabolism
Dr Gokuldas R Varma, Toronto, ON - General Practice
Dr Antony J Vayalumkal, Hamilton, ON - Ophthalmology
Dr C Mathew Yaltho, Edmonton, AB - Psychiatry
Dr Salim Yusuf, Hamilton, ON - Cardiology

MALTESE

Dr Godfrey T Fiorini, Toronto, ON - General Practice
Dr Marion Frendo, Virgil, ON - General Pathology
Dr Anthony M Galea, Etobicoke, ON - General Practice

MANDARIN

Dr Lee-Cyn Ang, London, ON - Neuro-Pathology
Dr Onil Bhattacharyya, Toronto, ON - Family Medicine
Dr H Jay Biem, Pointe-Claire, QC - Internal Medicine
Dr Lily S L Cha, North York, ON - Obstetrics & Gynecology
Dr John K F Chan, Abbotsford, BC - Family Medicine
Dr Paul Y H Chan, Coquitlam, BC - Family Medicine
Dr Cyril F Y Chan, Vancouver, BC - General Practice
Dr Karl K S Chan, Vancouver, BC - General Practice
Dr Wee Shian Chan, Vancouver, BC - Internal Medicine
Dr Paul C Chan, Mississauga, ON - General Practice
Dr Raymond K H Chan, Richmond Hill, ON - Family Medicine
Dr Gerald C B Chan, Scarborough, ON - Gastroenterology
Dr Gabriel F P Chan, Scarborough, ON - Geriatric Medicine
Dr Lawrence K C Chan, Scarborough, ON - Family Medicine
Dr Richard C W Chan, Toronto, ON - General Practice
Dr Wing Chow Chan, Toronto, ON - Ophthalmology
Dr David Y K Chan, Toronto, ON - General Practice
Dr C C Nancy Chang, Markham, ON - Family Medicine
Dr Peter P Chang, Toronto, ON - Psychiatry
Dr Patricia Y Chang, Toronto, ON - Family Medicine
Dr Paul T Chang, Toronto, ON - Obstetrics & Gynecology
Dr Peter H W Chau, Calgary, AB - General Practice
Dr Julie L Chen, Calgary, AB - Family Medicine
Dr Charlie C Chen, New Westminster, BC - Family Medicine
Dr Simon I Chen, Vancouver, BC - Emergency Family Med
Dr Helen Y Chen, Vancouver, BC - Family Medicine
Dr Jerry C L Chen, Vancouver, BC - General Surgery
Dr Chi Nan Chen, Vancouver, BC - Psychiatry
Dr Andy Y H Chen, Mississauga, ON - General Practice
Dr Adam Y H Chen, Mississauga, ON - Family Medicine
Dr Benjamin H Chen, Napanee, ON - Family Medicine
Dr Jia-De Chen, North York, ON - Internal Medicine
Dr Danny K Chen, Richmond Hill, ON - Infectious Diseases
Dr Grant I Chen, Scarborough, ON - Gastroenterology
Dr Eric Chen, Toronto, ON - Internal Medicine
Dr Charles Y Y Cheng, Vancouver, BC - General Practice
Dr Malcolm H F Cheng, North York, ON - Pediatrics
Dr Michael T W Cheng, Richmond Hill, ON - General Practice
Dr Mary M L Cheng, Scarborough, ON - Obstetrics & Gynecology
Dr Michael J C Cheng, St Thomas, ON - Urology
Dr Francesca T Cheung, Markham, ON - Family Medicine
Dr W C Thomas Cheung, Mississauga, ON - Family Medicine
Dr Bonnie Cheung, Richmond Hill, ON - General Practice
Dr Melody Cheung-Lee, Edmonton, AB - Dermatology
Dr Brian P A Chew, Edmonton, AB - Family Medicine
Dr Sen Chew, Surrey, BC - General Practice
Dr N M Sheryl Chiang, Edmonton, AB - General Practice
Dr Christopher K C Chiang, Brampton, ON - Family Medicine
Dr Paul K Chiu, Edmonton, AB - General Practice
Dr Arthur K K Chiu, Scarborough, ON - General Surgery
Dr Ann M Chiu, Windsor, ON - Ophthalmology
Dr Sophia S H Chong, Vancouver, BC - General Practice
Dr Xin Chong, Niagara Falls, ON - Family Medicine
Dr Darren W K Choo, Vancouver, BC - General Practice
Dr Wee Kei Choong, Delta, BC - General Practice
Dr Benjamin Chou, Langley, BC - General Practice
Dr Jenny W Chou, Surrey, BC - Pediatrics
Dr Shirley H Y Chou, Ottawa, ON - General Surgery
Dr Daliah Y L Chow, Ajax, ON - Family Medicine
Dr Chi-Ming Chow, Toronto, ON - Cardiology
Dr Benjamin S Choy, Markham, ON - Family Medicine
Dr Francis J L Chu, Richmond, BC - General Practice
Dr Mary P H Chu, Richmond, BC - General Practice
Dr Joseph Y C Chu, Etobicoke, ON - Internal Medicine
Dr Melvyn Chu, Richmond Hill, ON - Family Medicine
Dr Norman H Y Chu, Scarborough, ON - Emergency Family Med
Dr James C M Chu, Scarborough, ON - General Practice
Dr Katherine H C Chu, Scarborough, ON - Obstetrics & Gynecology
Dr Lica Chui, Vancouver, BC - Ophthalmology
Dr Bruce T W Chung, Durham, ON - General Practice
Dr Pin Chung, Keswick, ON - Family Medicine
Dr Thomas Chung, Thornhill, ON - Ophthalmology
Dr Raymond Dong, Surrey, BC - Cardiology
Dr Christian Falkenberg-Andersen, Calgary, AB - Family Medicine
Dr A P N Fam, Sault Ste Marie, ON - Obstetrics & Gynecology

Dr Xueping Fang, Hamilton, ON - General Practice
Dr Ann Qian Feng, Vancouver, BC - Pediatrics
Dr Chi Wai Fong, Scarborough, ON - General Practice
Dr Marshall C Foo, Toronto, ON - General Practice
Dr Johan R Friesen, Calgary, AB - Family Medicine
Dr Peter S M Fung, Spruce Grove, AB - Family Medicine
Dr Kan Ying Fung, Mississauga, ON - General Practice
Dr W L Alan Fung, North York, ON - Psychiatry
Dr Wing-Tai Fung, Scarborough, ON - General Practice
Dr Kenneth P L Fung, Toronto, ON - Psychiatry
Dr Scott Fung, Toronto, ON - Gastroenterology
Dr S W Helen Gan, Vancouver, BC - Family Medicine
Dr Margaret C Gan-Gaisano, Scarborough, ON - Pediatrics
Dr Zu-Hua Gao, Montreal, QC - Anatomical Pathology
Dr Shian Gu, Burnaby, BC - General Practice
Dr Sheila L Hew, Scarborough, ON - Family Medicine
Dr Ting H Hii, Trail, BC - General Practice
Dr James F K Hii, Vancouver, BC - General Practice
Dr Thomas M W Ho, Vancouver, BC - Family Medicine
Dr Vincent C Y Ho, Vancouver, BC - Dermatology
Dr Wei-Ning Ho, Vancouver, BC - General Practice
Dr Kendall Ho, Vancouver, BC - Emergency Medicine
Dr Philip C Ho, Etobicoke, ON - Pediatrics
Dr Shen-Pang E Ho, Lindsay, ON - General Pathology
Dr Hon-Lau Ho, Markham, ON - Family Medicine
Dr H Henry Ho, North York, ON - Family Medicine
Dr Ru-Chie Ho, Oshawa, ON - Otolaryngology
Dr Michael S C Ho, Toronto, ON - General Practice
Dr Tommy K L Ho, Toronto, ON - Pediatrics
Dr Yann J Hsiao, Vancouver, BC - General Practice
Dr Wayne W Y Hsieh, Scarborough, ON - Family Medicine
Dr Mabel Hsin, Bradford, ON - General Practice
Dr Katherine Hsu, Burnaby, BC - General Surgery
Dr John S C Hsuen, North York, ON - Pediatrics
Dr Brian C Huang, Calgary, AB - Family Medicine
Dr Amy Y Huang, Burnaby, BC - General Practice
Dr Ling Ling Huang, Mississauga, ON - Family Medicine
Dr Virgil Y F Huang, North York, ON - General Practice
Dr Qingli L Huang, Oakville, ON - Endocrin/Metabolism
Dr Louis Huang, Scarborough, ON - Anesthesia
Dr Hilary K Hui, Richmond, BC - General Practice
Dr Ivy Y C Hui, Richmond, BC - Family Medicine
Dr Alphonsus Z Hui, Vancouver, BC - General Practice
Dr C Francis Hung, North York, ON - Diagnostic-Radiology
Dr Lick San Hung, Toronto, ON - Anatomical Pathology
Dr Mei L Hwang, Scarborough, ON - General Practice
Dr Angela Hwang, Scarborough, ON - Family Medicine
Dr Paul A L S Hwang, Toronto, ON - Neurology
Dr Xiaoyan Jia, Langley, BC - Pediatrics
Dr Hsiao-Ming Jung, Toronto, ON - Family Medicine
Dr Timothy W T Kam, Vancouver, BC - General Practice
Dr Pion Kao, Calgary, AB - Pediatrics
Dr John T S Kao, Markham, ON - Plastic Surgery
Dr Yolanda A Kirkham, Toronto, ON - Obstetrics & Gynecology
Dr Peter Ko, Vancouver, BC - Family Medicine
Dr Sandy S K Koe, Edmonton, AB - General Practice
Dr Clarissa B K Koh, Winnipeg, MB - Family Medicine
Dr Betty K K Koo, North York, ON - Neurology
Dr Janet V Kushner Kow, Vancouver, BC - Geriatric Medicine
Dr Susan Y L Kwan, Burnaby, BC - Internal Medicine
Dr Yee-Nga Yong Kwee, Surrey, BC - Pediatrics
Dr Eva Kwok, Scarborough, ON - Internal Medicine
Dr Keith Kwok, Scarborough, ON - Cardiology
Dr Albert I Lai, Thornhill, ON - General Practice
Dr Anthony K S Lam, Calgary, AB - Family Medicine
Dr Charles N H Lam, Nanaimo, BC - General Practice
Dr Wai-Arm Lam, Vancouver, BC - General Practice
Dr Joseph K P Lam, Vancouver, BC - Family Medicine
Dr Michael Y C Lam, Mississauga, ON - Family Medicine
Dr Vincent Y Y Lam, North York, ON - General Practice
Dr Sam Lang Hang Yee, Burnaby, BC - Family Medicine
Dr Michael C K Lau, Markham, ON - Anatomical Pathology
Dr Micheline C Lau, Scarborough, ON - General Practice
Dr Ching Lau, Toronto, ON - Cardiology
Dr Peter P T Lau, Toronto, ON - Family Medicine
Dr William W L Lau, Laval, QC - General Practice

Dr Francis C H Law, Vancouver, BC - Ophthalmology
Dr Sally S C Law, Vancouver, BC - Family Medicine
Dr Samuel F Law, Toronto, ON - Psychiatry
Dr Howe Leam, Lethbridge, AB - Family Medicine
Dr Mao-Cheng Lee, Edmonton, AB - Internal Medicine
Dr Tzu-Kuang Lee, Edmonton, AB - Internal Medicine
Dr Herman Lee, Burnaby, BC - Family Medicine
Dr Howard C Lee, Port Hardy, BC - General Practice
Dr Shui Hing Lee, Richmond, BC - Ophthalmology
Dr Pui-Kee Lee, Vancouver, BC - Cardiology
Dr Rachel N Lee, Vancouver, BC - General Practice
Dr Tom Lee, Vancouver, BC - General Practice
Dr Kenny Lee, Vancouver, BC - General Practice
Dr Winifred Lee, Dartmouth, NS - Obstetrics & Gynecology
Dr David S C Lee, London, ON - Pediatrics
Dr Lap Cheung Lee, North York, ON - General Practice
Dr Justin T Lee, Richmond Hill, ON - General Surgery
Dr Victor Chee Choon Lee, Scarborough, ON - General Practice
Dr Winnie W S Lee, Toronto, ON - General Practice
Dr Mary C Y Lee, Toronto, ON - Internal Medicine
Dr M Madeleine Lee-Ng, Scarborough, ON - General Practice
Dr Renata M W Leong, Toronto, ON - Family Medicine
Dr Sher-Ping Leung, Nanaimo, BC - General Surgery
Dr Patrick P Leung, Port Coquitlam, BC - Family Medicine
Dr N L Eillen Leung, Vancouver, BC - General Practice
Dr Vicki W K Leung, Vancouver, BC - Pediatrics
Dr Kent K K Leung, Markham, ON - General Practice
Dr Sophia S Y Leung, Mississauga, ON - General Practice
Dr Robert S L Leung, Mississauga, ON - General Practice
Dr Ellen P Leung, Mississauga, ON - Family Medicine
Dr Albert S H Leung, Richmond Hill, ON - Psychiatry
Dr Frances Y K Leung, Toronto, ON - Internal Medicine
Dr Terence L N Leung, Toronto, ON - General Practice
Dr Wei Li, Burnaby, BC - Family Medicine
Dr Charles H Li, Vancouver, BC - Hematology
Dr Xin-Min Li, Winnipeg, MB - Psychiatry
Dr Gene S J Li, Brampton, ON - Family Medicine
Dr Bessie P T Li, Markham, ON - Family Medicine
Dr Jason Li, Scarborough, ON - Family Medicine
Dr Alan T W Li, Toronto, ON - General Practice
Dr Calvin T Lian, Toronto, ON - Emergency Family Med
Dr Howard S H Liang, Vancouver, BC - Pediatrics
Dr Raymond A Liang, Vancouver, BC - Psychiatry
Dr William Liang, Hamilton, ON - General Practice
Dr H Robert Liao, Scarborough, ON - Ophthalmology
Dr Kim L Liew, Vancouver, BC - General Practice
Dr Wing F Lim, Sherwood Park, AB - Family Medicine
Dr Princeton H Lim, Burnaby, BC - General Practice
Dr Frank F S Lim, Maple Ridge, BC - General Practice
Dr Meng Eng Lim, North Vancouver, BC - Psychiatry
Dr Larry F T Lim, Pitt Meadows, BC - General Practice
Dr David C Lim, Toronto, ON - General Practice
Dr Cassie W Lin, New Westminster, BC - Gastroenterology
Dr I C John Lin, Vancouver, BC - General Practice
Dr Karen W Lin, Scarborough, ON - General Practice
Dr Richard Liu, Edmonton, AB - Otolaryngology
Dr Peter P Liu, Ottawa, ON - Cardiology
Dr Vivian W Liu, Toronto, ON - Family Medicine
Dr Edmond K W Lo, Scarborough, ON - General Practice
Dr Hung-Tat Lo, Scarborough, ON - Psychiatry
Dr George Loh, Vancouver, BC - General Practice
Dr Diana P Y Loh, Vancouver, BC - Psychiatry
Dr Karmen K M Loh, Vancouver, BC - General Practice
Dr Henry T C Lok, Etobicoke, ON - Anesthesia
Dr Thomas S Lu, Richmond, BC - Orthopedic Surgery
Dr Shao-Hua Lu, Vancouver, BC - Psychiatry
Dr Spenser M Y Lui, Richmond, BC - Orthopedic Surgery
Dr Kim C Lui, Unionville, ON - General Practice
Dr Edward C H Luke, Vancouver, BC - Emergency Family Med
Dr Edward Lum, Vancouver, BC - General Practice
Dr Marian C Ma, Elkford, BC - Family Medicine
Dr Gilbert Ma, Vancouver, BC - General Practice
Dr Ian S Ma, Vancouver, BC - General Practice
Dr Tze Y Ma, Mississauga, ON - Pediatrics
Dr Joseph J K Ma, North York, ON - Ophthalmology
Dr Joanne L C Ma, Scarborough, ON - Obstetrics & Gynecology

Dr Manson M T Mak, Brampton, ON - Emergency Family Med
Dr Kam Hong Mak, North York, ON - General Practice
Dr Kwok-Chu Man, Whitby, ON - Internal Medicine
Dr Gordon W Moe, Toronto, ON - Cardiology
Dr Hiram L H Mok, Vancouver, BC - Psychiatry
Dr Andrew K C Mok, Montreal, QC - Obstetrics & Gynecology
Dr Jimmy K Y Mui, Oshawa, ON - Radiation Oncology
Dr Douglas B G Ng, Surrey, BC - General Practice
Dr Wing Hon Ng, Vancouver, BC - General Practice
Dr Louis H S Ng, Vancouver, BC - General Practice
Dr Liang Ng, West Vancouver, BC - General Practice
Dr Toan D Nhan, Toronto, ON - General Practice
Dr Richard Novick, London, ON - Cardiovasc/ThorSurg
Dr Sharon Rose Y Ong, Surrey, BC - General Surgery
Dr Che-Wei R Ou, Richmond Hill, ON - Obstetrics & Gynecology
Dr Howard H Pai, Victoria, BC - Radiation Oncology
Dr Jin-Si Pao, Vancouver, BC - General Surgery
Dr York P C Pei, Toronto, ON - Internal Medicine
Dr Milton C Po, Surrey, BC - Radiation Oncology
Dr Yin Hun Ian Pun, Scarborough, ON - General Practice
Dr Francis W C Sem, Toronto, ON - Emergency Family Med
Dr Richard H Shao, East York, ON - Internal Medicine
Dr K Y Kevin Sheu, Burnaby, BC - Family Medicine
Dr Dawn D Shi, Toronto, ON - Family Medicine
Dr Robert H Shih, Etobicoke, ON - Family Medicine
Dr Aaron C T Shih, Etobicoke, ON - Family Medicine
Dr Paul K Shuen, North York, ON - Obstetrics & Gynecology
Dr Andrew S C Shum, Toronto, ON - General Practice
Dr Yin Shan Sia, Williams Lake, BC - General Practice
Dr Philip C Sin, Richmond Hill, ON - General Practice
Dr Michelle Sit, Scarborough, ON - Family Medicine
Dr Danny W Siu, Coquitlam, BC - General Practice
Dr King Fun Siu, Toronto, ON - Family Medicine
Dr Stevenson K F So, Mississauga, ON - General Practice
Dr Quintin R Son-Hing, Vancouver, BC - Plastic Surgery
Dr Wei-Yi Song, Victoria, BC - Psychiatry
Dr Helen B Song, Guelph, ON - Family Medicine
Dr B H Norman Soo, North York, ON - General Practice
Dr Shawn J Soon, Scarborough, ON - Urology
Dr Christine Soong, Toronto, ON - Family Medicine
Dr Jason W S Su, Pickering, ON - Family Medicine
Dr Andy G Suk, Mississauga, ON - Endocrin/Metabolism
Dr Edric C H Sum, Mississauga, ON - General Practice
Dr Joyce Sun, Vancouver, BC - Family Medicine
Dr John C L Sun, Victoria, BC - Neurosurgery
Dr Patrick P W Sung, Vegreville, AB - General Practice
Dr William Y Sy, Scarborough, ON - Psychiatry
Dr Mabel C Sze, Vancouver, BC - Family Medicine
Dr Kenneth P C Szeto, Markham, ON - General Practice
Dr Isabella T W Tai, Vancouver, BC - Gastroenterology
Dr Evelyn K Tai, Mississauga, ON - Family Medicine
Dr R W Melissa Tai, North York, ON - Obstetrics & Gynecology
Dr Lucas Tai, Toronto, ON - General Practice
Dr Emelda M Tai, Toronto, ON - General Practice
Dr Winston T L Tam, Surrey, BC - Obstetrics & Gynecology
Dr K Felix Tam, Vancouver, BC - General Practice
Dr Wilson W Tam, Vancouver, BC - General Practice
Dr Daphne C Tam, Vancouver, BC - Family Medicine
Dr Christopher K H Tam, Scarborough, ON - General Practice
Dr Thomas C Tam, Toronto, ON - General Practice
Dr Wing-Hei Tam, Windsor, ON - Diagnostic-Radiology
Dr B J Nicholas Tan, Golden, BC - General Practice
Dr Michelle W Tan, Richmond, BC - Family Medicine
Dr Chin Kien Tan, Toronto, ON - General Practice
Dr Allan Tan, Toronto, ON - Family Medicine
Dr Seang Lin Tan, Montreal, QC - Obstetrics & Gynecology
Dr Tin-Yan Tang, Vancouver, BC - General Practice
Dr Vincent W Tang, Vancouver, BC - General Practice
Dr Clementine Tang, Vancouver, BC - Pediatrics
Dr Shangguo Tang, Hamilton, ON - Anatomical Pathology
Dr Hung-Yip Tang, Richmond Hill, ON - General Practice
Dr Lan Tang, Vaughan, ON - General Practice
Dr Sha Tao, Edmonton, AB - General Practice
Dr Keng Y Tay, London, ON - Diagnostic-Radiology
Dr M C Matthew Teh, Markham, ON - General Practice
Dr Johnny C Teoh, Edmonton, AB - Pediatrics

Dr H M Vincent Thai, Edmonton, AB - Family Medicine
Dr Pooi-Lin Tham, London, ON - Family Medicine
Dr Lancelot K Tin, Mississauga, ON - General Surgery
Dr John U L Ting, Surrey, BC - General Practice
Dr Peter L Ting, Vancouver, BC - General Practice
Dr Helen C I Ting, Vancouver, BC - Family Medicine
Dr Robert H Ting, Scarborough, ON - Internal Medicine
Dr Joshua K Tjong, Sault Ste. Marie, ON - Diagnostic-Radiology
Dr Agnes S To, Richmond, BC - Psychiatry
Dr Daniel Y Tong, Vancouver, BC - General Practice
Dr Kevin L F Tong, Vancouver, BC - General Practice
Dr Maorong Tong, Thunder Bay, ON - Family Medicine
Dr Ying Lai H Toong, Toronto, ON - General Practice
Dr Margaret H M Tran, Vancouver, BC - Family Medicine
Dr Vance C Tsai, Abbotsford, BC - Otolaryngology
Dr Jason Y S Tsai, North York, ON - General Practice
Dr Ellen Tsai, Ottawa, ON - Pediatrics
Dr Ian K Tsang, Vancouver, BC - Internal Medicine
Dr W Y Eliza Tsang, Markham, ON - Family Medicine
Dr Michael S M Tsang, Richmond Hill, ON - Family Medicine
Dr Smiley G S Tsao, Unionville, ON - Family Medicine
Dr Luke B S Tse, Prince Rupert, BC - Family Medicine
Dr Geoffrey N W Tse, Surrey, BC - General Surgery
Dr Frances W M Tse, Hamilton, ON - Gastroenterology
Dr Anthony C H Tse, North York, ON - General Practice
Dr George W Tseng, Vancouver, BC - Emergency Family Med
Dr Joseph K Tsui, Vancouver, BC - Neurology
Dr Elaine Y L Tsui, Scarborough, ON - Endocrin/Metabolism
Dr I L Helen Tsui, Unionville, ON - Pediatrics
Dr David T Tu, Vancouver, BC - Family Medicine
Dr Geming S Tu, London, ON - General Practice
Dr K K Stanley Tung, Vancouver, BC - Internal Medicine
Dr Kenneth S H Tung, Scarborough, ON - General Practice
Dr Berton Y K Ung, Scarborough, ON - Family Medicine
Dr Calvin K N Wan, Kelowna, BC - Cardiac Surgery
Dr Andrew W C Wan, Markham, ON - Family Medicine
Dr Wenjie Wang, Calgary, AB - Internal Medicine
Dr Haili Wang, Edmonton, AB - General Surgery
Dr Shao-Hua Wang, Edmonton, AB - Cardiac Surgery
Dr Caroline Y M Wang, Richmond, BC - General Practice
Dr Yue Wang, Surrey, BC - Family Medicine
Dr Clayton J Wang, Vancouver, BC - Family Medicine
Dr Shaoli Wang, Vancouver, BC - Family Medicine
Dr Wen-Shan Wang, London, ON - General Practice
Dr Yongjin Wang, Mississauga, ON - Radiation Oncology
Dr Angela J Wang, Petrolia, ON - Family Medicine
Dr Robert Y Wang, Richmond Hill, ON - Orthopedic Surgery
Dr Cheng T Wang, Toronto, ON - Family Medicine
Dr Yun-Lin Wang, Toronto, ON - General Practice
Dr Benjamin C Wong, Calgary, AB - Obstetrics & Gynecology
Dr Jeanny Wong, Burnaby, BC - General Practice
Dr Daniel K C Wong, Maple Ridge, BC - General Practice
Dr Thomas S Wong, Richmond, BC - Family Medicine
Dr Boon L Wong, Richmond, BC - General Practice
Dr Patricia Wong, Richmond, BC - General Practice
Dr Vincent A Wong, Vancouver, BC - Ophthalmology
Dr Peter K H Wong, Vancouver, BC - Neurology
Dr H C George Wong, Vancouver, BC - Clin Immun/Allergy
Dr K Judy Wong, Vancouver, BC - General Practice
Dr Paul C H Wong, Vancouver, BC - Family Medicine
Dr Frank S H Wong, Victoria, BC - Otolaryngology
Dr Amy N Wong, Etobicoke, ON - Family Medicine
Dr Richard L Wong, Markham, ON - Pediatrics
Dr Thompson K W Wong, Markham, ON - General Practice
Dr Frank K L Wong, Mississauga, ON - General Practice
Dr Joseph K Wong, Mississauga, ON - Otolaryngology
Dr Clement K L Wong, Mississauga, ON - General Practice
Dr Joseph Y S Wong, North York, ON - Physical Medicine & Rehab
Dr Maxine Y W Wong, North York, ON - Dermatology
Dr Jeremy C Wong, Scarborough, ON - Obstetrics & Gynecology
Dr Daniel M T Wong, Scarborough, ON - Internal Medicine
Dr Stephen S Wong, Scarborough, ON - General Practice
Dr Chi Mun Wong, St Catharines, ON - Family Medicine
Dr Ivan F L Wong, Toronto, ON - General Practice
Dr Daniel D Wong, Toronto, ON - General Practice
Dr Emile C Woo, Vancouver, BC - General Surgery
Dr George H K Woo, Toronto, ON - Obstetrics & Gynecology
Dr John K M Wu, Vancouver, BC - Hematology
Dr Chin Yu Wu, Hamilton, ON - General Practice
Dr Howard Wu, Markham, ON - Family Medicine
Dr Alwin Wu, Markham, ON - Family Medicine
Dr George G Wu, Mississauga, ON - Internal Medicine
Dr Jenny Wu, Scarborough, ON - General Practice
Dr Sibra S C Wu, Toronto, ON - General Practice
Dr Stephen T W Wu, Whitby, ON - Family Medicine
Dr Rong Xie, West Vancouver, BC - Family Medicine
Dr Haibo Xu, Dunnville, ON - Family Medicine
Dr Andrew Y Xuan, Ottawa, ON - Gastroenterology
Dr Ka-Wai Yam, Vancouver, BC - Family Medicine
Dr Peter B Yang, Burnaby, BC - General Practice
Dr Brian P T Yang, New Westminster, BC - Urology
Dr Hui-Min Yang, Vancouver, BC - General Practice
Dr Jianing Yang, Hawkesbury, ON - General Practice
Dr Shengtao Yao, Grande Prairie, AB - General Practice
Dr Peter Y O Yao, Surrey, BC - Orthopedic Surgery
Dr Jennifer K Yao, Vancouver, BC - Physical Medicine & Rehab
Dr Frank C O Yau, Toronto, ON - General Practice
Dr Zhongbo J Ye, Richmond, BC - Psychiatry
Dr Juan Ye, Markham, ON - Family Medicine
Dr Charles C Ye, Newmarket, ON - General Pathology
Dr Donna L J Yee, Vancouver, BC - Family Medicine
Dr Chok-Ching Yee, Nobleton, ON - General Practice
Dr Gerald Y L Yeung, Vancouver, BC - Family Medicine
Dr Sonia N Yeung, Vancouver, BC - Ophthalmology
Dr Clement W T Yeung, North York, ON - General Practice
Dr Michael K Yeung, North York, ON - Psychiatry
Dr Jacky Y Yeung, Peterborough, ON - Ophthalmology
Dr Albert Yeung, Richmond Hill, ON - Clin Immun/Allergy
Dr Adela K T Yeung, Toronto, ON - General Practice
Dr Conrad C Y Yim, Mississauga, ON - Pediatrics
Dr Alan Z L Yin, Scarborough, ON - Family Medicine
Dr Luis T J Ying, Brampton, ON - Gastroenterology
Dr Barbara Y Yip, Coquitlam, BC - General Practice
Dr Collin K K Yong, Vancouver, BC - Pediatrics
Dr Yong Dong You, Richmond, BC - Internal Medicine
Dr Simon Yu, Burnaby, BC - Internal Medicine
Dr Y W Edward Yu, Burnaby, BC - Ophthalmology
Dr Jen Zhen Yu, Vancouver, BC - Internal Medicine
Dr Maria C Y Yu, Ajax, ON - Family Medicine
Dr Carlos C S Yu, Ajax, ON - Emergency Family Med
Dr John C Yu, Ottawa, ON - Diagnostic-Radiology
Dr Jian Z Yu, Scarborough, ON - Anesthesia
Dr Jane Yuan, Toronto, ON - Internal Medicine
Dr Frank W L Yue, Vancouver, BC - General Practice
Dr K Kevin Yue, Vancouver, BC - Family Medicine
Dr Anthony W B Yue, Victoria, BC - Family Medicine
Dr Richard H Yuen, Calgary, AB - General Practice
Dr Tommy K Yuen, Delta, BC - Family Medicine
Dr Cham-Wah Yuen, Vancouver, BC - General Practice
Dr Chui Kin Yuen, Vancouver, BC - Obstetrics & Gynecology
Dr K H Peter Yuen, Scarborough, ON - Family Medicine
Dr Yick Shing Yung, Toronto, ON - Obstetrics & Gynecology
Dr Janice J Zeng, Mississauga, ON - General Pathology
Dr Y H Connie Zhang, Richmond, BC - Family Medicine
Dr Rui Zhang, Vancouver, BC - Family Medicine
Dr Dajiang Zhang, Vancouver, BC - Psychiatry
Dr Irene Zhang, Hamilton, ON - Otolaryngology
Dr Kenny J Zhang, Mississauga, ON - Family Medicine
Dr Y Jackie Zhang, Richmond Hill, ON - Family Medicine
Dr Siui-Mei Zhang, Whitehorse, YT - General Practice
Dr Stanley M Zheng, Scarborough, ON - Family Medicine
Dr Toni Zhong, Toronto, ON - Plastic Surgery
Dr Youwen F Zhou, Vancouver, BC - Dermatology
Dr Kang-Min Zhu, Cranbrook, BC - Diagnostic-Radiology
Dr Lenore L Zou, Hamilton, ON - Family Medicine
Dr Limai Zou, North York, ON - Family Medicine
Dr Nora P Y Zung, Scarborough, ON - Family Medicine

MARATHI

Dr Tasneem Adenwala, Bolton, ON - Family Medicine
Dr Vijaykumar V Ashtekar, Swift Current, SK - General Practice
Dr Asifa Bawangoanwala, Mississauga, ON - Family Medicine
Dr Nirmala Bharatwal, Toronto, ON - Physical Medicine & Rehab
Dr Paramjit S Bhui, Surrey, BC - Pediatrics
Dr Pargat S Bhurji, Surrey, BC - Pediatrics
Dr Vikram Chandurkar, St. John's, NL - Endocrin/Metabolism
Dr Shilpa Dabholkar, Coquitlam, BC - Family Medicine
Dr Harsha V Dehejia, Ottawa, ON - Internal Medicine
Dr Sanjeev Deodhare, Mississauga, ON - Anatomical Pathology
Dr Milind G Desai, North York, ON - Gastroenterology
Dr Hiren B Desai, Windsor, ON - Neurology
Dr Ashish Deshpande, Windsor, ON - Pediatrics
Dr Manik Devane, Niagara Falls, ON - General Practice
Dr Tina D Gai, Grimsby, ON - Obstetrics & Gynecology
Dr Karamchand J Gandhi, Bridgewater, NS - General Practice
Dr Prakash S Gangdev, London, ON - General Practice
Dr Vinod K Gangolli, Kitchener, ON - Psychiatry
Dr Hemant B Ghate, Windsor, ON - Anesthesia
Dr Sandhya Gokhale, Kitchener, ON - Family Medicine
Dr Anvita S Joglekar, North York, ON - Psychiatry
Dr Suhas B Joshi, St Catharines, ON - Anatomical Pathology
Dr Karna C Kale, Mississauga, ON - Family Medicine
Dr Arvind D Khambhla, Toronto, ON - Obstetrics & Gynecology
Dr Anil K Khithani, Scarborough, ON - Family Medicine
Dr Dnyanada L Kothare, Regina, SK - General Practice
Dr Ramesh Kulkarni, North Bay, ON - Obstetrics & Gynecology
Dr Bahubali D Lagare, Mississauga, ON - Family Medicine
Dr Avdhut R Manerkar, Miramichi, NB - General Practice
Dr Saba M Merchant, Maple, ON - Pediatrics
Dr Pradeep Merchant, Ottawa, ON - Pediatrics
Dr Mahendranath D Moharir, Toronto, ON - General Practice
Dr Sonali A Mohile, Uxbridge, ON - Pediatrics
Dr Manisha M Mulgund, Burlington, ON - Internal Medicine
Dr Sachin R Pendharkar, Calgary, AB - Internal Medicine
Dr Chakrabarty L Pole, Surrey, BC - Psychiatry
Dr Hemraj R Porwal, Niagara Falls, ON - Family Medicine
Dr Vilas S Prabhu, Penticton, BC - Otolaryngology
Dr Dhun S Sadry, Toronto, ON - Family Medicine
Dr Hemalata J B Sangani, Greenfield Park, QC - General Practice
Dr Peter L Selby, Toronto, ON - Family Medicine
Dr Rita Selby, Toronto, ON - Hematology
Dr Jay K Shah, Hamilton, ON - Pediatrics
Dr Vibhuti S Shah, Toronto, ON - Pediatrics
Dr Bashiruddin N Shaikh, Toronto, ON - Urology
Dr Meena P Sharma, Ottawa, ON - General Practice
Dr Vasanti N Shende, Guelph, ON - Internal Medicine
Dr Jitendra B Sheshgiri, Mississauga, ON - Emergency Family Med
Dr Charudutt D Shete, Langley, BC - General Surgery
Dr Nikita T Sheth, Oakville, ON - Family Medicine
Dr Rathnakar B Shetty, St Catharines, ON - Obstetrics & Gynecology
Dr Geeta R Shetty, St Catharines, ON - Anesthesia
Dr Hemant R Shirali, Markham, ON - Orthopedic Surgery
Dr Satish Shrikhande, Victoria, BC - Psychiatry
Dr Nandini J Singh, Calgary, AB - Psychiatry
Dr Arvind G Singh, Summerside, PE - Psychiatry
Dr Anantasivan Subramanian, Niagara Falls, ON - General Surgery
Dr Sabiha M Surangiwala, Mississauga, ON - Family Medicine
Dr P Aravind Talwalkar, Mississauga, ON - General Practice
Dr Narsimhachary Telikicharla Kandala, Terrace, BC - General Practice
Dr Smita V Thatte, Ottawa, ON - Psychiatry
Dr Gunjan M Vador, Scarborough, ON - Internal Medicine
Dr Harshala P Vora, Hamilton, ON - Family Medicine
Dr Mahesh P Yadav, North Bay, ON - Orthopedic Surgery

MONTAGNAIS

Dr Danny Dreige, Baie-Comeau, QC - Ophthalmology

NEPALI

Dr Davey Y M Gin, Surrey, BC - Family Medicine
Dr David J M Green, St Stephen, NB - General Practice
Dr Klaus Jochem, Montreal, QC - General Practice
Dr Meghna P Juta, St. Albert, AB - Family Medicine
Dr Rosana Pellizzari, Peterborough, ON - Community Medicine
Dr Nabeel B Samad, Halifax, NS - General Practice
Dr Ian D Schokking, Prince George, BC - Family Medicine
Dr Kamal Sharma, Ottawa, ON - Cardiology
Dr Prakash T Shrestha, Hazelton, BC - Family Medicine
Dr Rajat Upadhyay, Calgary, AB - Emergency Family Med
Dr David C Williams, Thunder Bay, ON - Community Medicine

NIGERIAN

Dr J Oluwagbenga Ajayi-Obe, Sarnia, ON - Family Medicine
Dr Felix S Odaibo, Grande Prairie, AB - Pediatrics

NORWEGIAN

Dr Francis M Boston, Montreal, QC - Diagnostic-Radiology
Dr Leif-Erik Bredesen, Camrose, AB - General Practice
Dr Britt Bright, Maple Ridge, BC - Psychiatry
Dr Sturla E Bruun-Meyer, Toronto, ON - Psychiatry
Dr Leon C Groenewald, Grande Prairie, AB - General Practice
Dr Ingrid A Harle, Kingston, ON - Family Medicine
Dr Jan Fredrik Moe, Kinistino, SK - General Practice
Dr A Barbro Normann, Burlington, ON - General Practice
Dr Kerryn L Roberge, Calgary, AB - Family Medicine
Dr James L Scott, Victoria, BC - Neurology
Dr Martin Svartberg, Toronto, ON - Psychiatry
Dr Anne R Synnes, Vancouver, BC - Pediatrics
Dr Peter S Teitelbaum, Ottawa, ON - General Practice
Dr Ellen N Thompson, Ottawa, ON - Anesthesia
Dr Kristin Udjus Teitelbaum, Ottawa, ON - Diagnostic-Radiology
Dr Phyllis-Marie Vetere, Montreal, QC - General Practice
Dr Lloyd Westby, Penticton, BC - Family Medicine
Dr Inge G Winslow, Richmond Hill, ON - General Practice
Dr Margery H Zapf-Gilje, Vancouver, BC - Family Medicine

NZIMA

Dr Kwame E Badoe, Guelph, ON - Psychiatry

ORIYA

Dr Bijayalaxmi Devi, Ajax, ON - Psychiatry
Dr Jami Sridhar, Campbellton, NB - General Practice

OROMO

Dr Berhanu Balcha, Winnipeg, MB - General Practice

OTHER LANGUAGE

Dr Rand A Askalan, Toronto, ON - Neurology
Dr Richard J McCammon, Winnipeg, MB - Family Medicine

PASHTU

Dr Ahmad S Ashrafi, Surrey, BC - General Surgery
Dr Ismat Z Dost, Brantford, ON - Pediatrics
Dr Ziaullah Fahim, Surrey, BC - General Practice
Dr Kazi A Hameed, Winnipeg, MB - Internal Medicine
Dr Nageen Hameed, Oakville, ON - Internal Medicine
Dr Mohammad A Khan, Melfort, SK - General Practice
Dr M Sohail Khattak, Whitby, ON - Pediatrics
Dr Khalida Qazi, Milton, ON - Family Medicine
Dr Merajuddin Shams, Vaughan, ON - Family Medicine
Dr Syed A R Sherazi, Abbotsford, BC - General Practice
Dr Qasim A Yar, Hagersville, ON - General Practice

PERSIAN

Dr Syed T H Abedi, Scarborough, ON - Anatomical Pathology
Dr Forough Abtahi, Cornwall, ON - General Practice
Dr Nahid Afshari-Azad, Ottawa, ON - Geriatric Medicine
Dr Bashir Ahmed, Ottawa, ON - General Practice
Dr Faria Ajamian, Edmonton, AB - General Practice
Dr Javad Alaghband-Rad, Halifax, NS - General Practice
Dr Liaqat Ali, Barrie, ON - Psychiatry
Dr Ahmad S Ashrafi, Surrey, BC - General Surgery
Dr Abdul Aziz, Lethbridge, AB - General Practice
Dr Maziar Badii, Vancouver, BC - Internal Medicine
Dr Mohammad Bahasadri, Etobicoke, ON - General Surgery
Dr Farhad Bakezadeh, Saint John, NB - General Practice
Dr Hamid S Banijamali, Calgary, AB - Cardiology
Dr Nazmudin M F Bhanji, Vancouver, BC - Pediatrics
Dr Samieh Chavoshi, Burlington, ON - Anesthesia
Dr Navid Dehghani, Vancouver, BC - Pediatric Emergency Medicine
Dr Roya F Dehghani-Yar, Hamilton, ON - Family Medicine
Dr Kourosh Dinyari, Edmonton, AB - General Practice
Dr Ziba Fadavi, Orillia, ON - Anatomical Pathology
Dr Ziaullah Fahim, Surrey, BC - General Practice
Dr Mahmood Fazl, Toronto, ON - Neurosurgery
Dr Farin Foroodi, Oakville, ON - Family Medicine
Dr Gissou S Ghadirian, Etobicoke, ON - Family Medicine
Dr Maryam Ghaffar-Sedeh, Pickering, ON - Family Medicine
Dr Hournaz Ghandehari, Toronto, ON - Diagnostic-Radiology
Dr M Reza Ghobadian, Whitby, ON - Family Medicine
Dr Ali T Ghouse, Hamilton, ON - Physical Medicine & Rehab
Dr Ejaz A Ghumman, Leamington, ON - General Surgery
Dr Shahpar Grouhi, Richmond Hill, ON - General Practice
Dr Amir Tinouch Haghighat Talab, Gatineau, QC - Cardiology
Dr Roya Hajy Aghaei, North York, ON - Family Medicine
Dr Fawaz Halwani, Ottawa, ON - Anatomical Pathology
Dr Hormoz Hamrahi, Toronto, ON - Family Medicine
Dr Omar N Hasan, Amqui, QC - General Surgery
Dr Ali Hazrati, North York, ON - Family Medicine
Dr Kamran Heydarzadeh-Azar, Fort St. John, BC - Anatomical Pathology
Dr Rahmatullah Ishaqzay, Milton, ON - Family Medicine
Dr Siavash Jafari, Vancouver, BC - General Practice
Dr Naaznin K Jaffer, Scarborough, ON - General Practice
Dr Shamin Jetha, Vancouver, BC - Family Medicine
Dr Fariba Kaboli, Vancouver, BC - Occupational Med
Dr Alireza Kachooie, Scarborough, ON - Physical Medicine & Rehab
Dr Saeed Kalantari, North York, ON - Family Medicine
Dr Reza Kazemi, Dunnville, ON - General Practice
Dr Leila Keyvani, Prince George, BC - Gastroenterology
Dr Aliasghar Khadem, Winnipeg, MB - General Practice
Dr Amir A H Khadir, Terrebonne, QC - Medical Microbiology
Dr Marina Khatchatourian, North York, ON - Gastroenterology
Dr Katayoun S Khorrami, Calgary, AB - Family Medicine
Dr Bob B Kiaii, London, ON - Cardiac Surgery
Dr Negin Liaghati-Nasseri, Richmond Hill, ON - Family Medicine
Dr Lotfullah Lotfi-Seysan, Petawawa, ON - Family Medicine
Dr Kourosh Mastali, Collingwood, ON - General Practice
Dr Fereshteh Mazloom, Etobicoke, ON - Family Medicine
Dr Flora Z Mehrmanesh, Brampton, ON - Pediatrics
Dr S Jamaluddin Mirmiran, Vancouver, BC - Psychiatry
Dr Mehran Mogharrabi, Sault Ste. Marie, ON - General Practice
Dr Behrooz H Mohammadzadeh Yaghchi, Guelph, ON - Anesthesia
Dr John Moini, Verdun, QC - Family Medicine
Dr Massood Molavi, North Vancouver, BC - Internal Medicine
Dr Homayoon Moosavi, Kitchener, ON - General Practice
Dr Ayoob Mossanen, North York, ON - Neurology
Dr Sam Naghibi, Newmarket, ON - Family Medicine
Dr Houshang Naimi, Beaconsfield, QC - General Practice
Dr Ali Nia, Simcoe, ON - Internal Medicine
Dr Keyvan Pazuki, North York, ON - General Practice
Dr Zahirul Quayyum, Hamilton, ON - Family Medicine
Dr A Quddus Qureshi, Calgary, AB - Family Medicine
Dr Ziaur-Rehman T Qureshi, Calgary, AB - Family Medicine
Dr Roya Rahimpour, Mississauga, ON - General Practice
Dr Katayoun Rahnavardi, Dartmouth, NS - Family Medicine
Dr Akbar Rajabi-Asl, Toronto, ON - Psychiatry
Dr Moizali A Ramji, Sherwood Park, AB - General Practice
Dr Pasteur Rasuli, Ottawa, ON - Diagnostic-Radiology
Dr Parisa Rezaiefar, Ottawa, ON - Family Medicine
Dr Kevin Rod, North York, ON - Family Medicine
Dr Maryam Rostami, Hamilton, ON - Family Medicine
Dr Farzad Saberi, Burnaby, BC - Internal Medicine
Dr S Vahid Sahiholnasab, Richmond, BC - Internal Medicine
Dr Morad K Sarraf, North York, ON - Obstetrics & Gynecology
Dr Atih Seif-Zadeh, Richmond Hill, ON - Psychiatry
Dr Houfar Sekhavat, Dieppe, NB - Ophthalmology
Dr Farshad Sepandj, Calgary, AB - Internal Medicine
Dr Pooneh Seyed Akhavan, Toronto, ON - Internal Medicine
Dr Nasim Shahbazi, Thunder Bay, ON - Internal Medicine
Dr Bahram Shahi, Fort Frances, ON - General Surgery
Dr Pegah Shahriaree, Scarborough, ON - Family Medicine
Dr Masoud Shahrokhi, West Vancouver, BC - Family Medicine
Dr S Yasmin Shaikh, North York, ON - Family Medicine
Dr Riaz Shariff, Ajax, ON - General Practice
Dr Hassan Shenassa, Ottawa, ON - Obstetrics & Gynecology
Dr Zubaida Siddiqui, Elliot Lake, ON - Family Medicine
Dr Mohammad K Sohail, Whitby, ON - Psychiatry
Dr Mohammad Tabari, Scarborough, ON - General Surgery
Dr Aref Tabarsi, Campbell River, BC - General Pathology
Dr Farshid Tabloie, Scarborough, ON - Orthopedic Surgery
Dr Tahmouresse Toussi, Montreal, QC - Pediatrics
Dr Aref Vaezi, Toronto, ON - Family Medicine
Dr Ramamohan Veluri, Sudbury, ON - Psychiatry
Dr Mirza R Virani, Markham, ON - General Practice
Dr Qasim A Yar, Hagersville, ON - General Practice
Dr Shahin Yazdani, Stittsville, ON - Family Medicine
Dr Kourosh Zadhoush, Bradford, ON - Family Medicine

PIDGIN

Dr J Oluwagbenga Ajayi-Obe, Sarnia, ON - Family Medicine

POLISH

Dr Barbara H Agopsowicz, Edmonton, AB - General Practice
Dr Krystyna A Albin-Cook, Etobicoke, ON - General Practice
Dr Janusz Aleksiejuk, Welland, ON - General Practice
Dr Ilona L Amstutz, Fort St. John, BC - General Practice
Dr Lucyna J Anderson, Kanata, ON - Obstetrics & Gynecology
Dr Adam K Andronowski, Sudbury, ON - Radiation Oncology
Dr Wojciech Aniol, Red Lake, ON - General Practice
Dr Iwona A Auer-Grzesiak, Calgary, AB - Anatomical Pathology
Dr Malgorzata A Bak, Delhi, ON - General Practice
Dr Lidia M Bartosik, Mississauga, ON - Anesthesia
Dr Alicja Bedkowska, Verdun, QC - General Practice
Dr Nadia M Belsky, Etobicoke, ON - General Practice
Dr L Jane Berka, North York, ON - Family Medicine
Dr Jerzy Bialczak, Edmonton, AB - Family Medicine
Dr Halina Bienkowski, Amherst, NS - General Practice
Dr Peter Bienkowski, Ottawa, ON - Orthopedic Surgery
Dr Miroslaw Bilski-Piotrowski, Halifax, NS - Psychiatry
Dr Alexander Birnbaum, Toronto, ON - Neurology
Dr Piotr A Blachut, Vancouver, BC - Orthopedic Surgery
Dr Maria E Bleszynski, Surrey, BC - Obstetrics & Gynecology
Dr Dariuz Bochinski, Edmonton, AB - Urology
Dr Derek D Borowka, Edmonton, AB - General Practice
Dr Jeanie Shkimba Brezina, Toronto, ON - General Practice
Dr Michal Broniewski, Calgary, AB - General Practice
Dr Jerzy T Brzeski, Calgary, AB - General Practice
Dr Wojciech S Brzezinski, Medicine Hat, AB - General Surgery
Dr Wanda T Brzezinski, Westmount, QC - General Practice
Dr Malgorzata J Buczek, Ottawa, ON - Family Medicine
Dr Andrzej K Buczkowski, Vancouver, BC - General Surgery
Dr Margret Budzianowska-Kwiatkowski, Port Coquitlam, BC - Family Medicine
Dr Margaret B Bugdahn, Unionville, ON - Family Medicine
Dr Bernard P Bukala, Stratford, ON - Urology
Dr Emily M Bulanski, Cambridge, ON - Family Medicine
Dr Katherine D Bury, Etobicoke, ON - General Surgery
Dr Janki Butchey, London, ON - Psychiatry

Dr Anna M Byszewski, Ottawa, ON - Geriatric Medicine
Dr Barbara A Cenkowski, Winnipeg, MB - Family Medicine
Dr Helena Chekina, North York, ON - General Practice
Dr Svitlana Cheshenchuk, Regina, SK - Family Medicine
Dr Sy-Hua Chiu, Edmonton, AB - General Practice
Dr Anna K Chodyra, Port Moody, BC - Family Medicine
Dr Zbigniew P Chrzanowski, Edmonton, AB - General Practice
Dr Malgorzata Cieslak, New Westminster, BC - General Practice
Dr Zenon Cieslak, New Westminster, BC - Pediatrics
Dr P Maria Cudnoch, Laval, QC - Family Medicine
Dr Joseph B Cybulski, Barrys Bay, ON - Family Medicine
Dr Wlodzimierz Czarnecki, Winnipeg, MB - Cardiology
Dr Andrew Czarnecki, Toronto, ON - Cardiology
Dr Gregory Jan Czarnota, Toronto, ON - Radiation Oncology
Dr Z Charles Czarnowski, Ottawa, ON - Family Medicine
Dr Wojciech Czernikiewicz, Hamilton, ON - Psychiatry
Dr Anna A Czok, Etobicoke, ON - Physical Medicine & Rehab
Dr Elizabeth Czolpinska, Thunder Bay, ON - Psychiatry
Dr Thaddeus R Czolpinski, Thunder Bay, ON - Internal Medicine
Dr Arkadiusz M Daniel, Nepean, ON - Family Medicine
Dr Irena B Darczewski, Winnipeg, MB - Family Medicine
Dr Maria Daszkiewicz-Recizac, Maple Ridge, BC - Psychiatry
Dr Aneta Dauksza, Ottawa, ON - Family Medicine
Dr Grace Debosz-Szczerbowski, London, ON - General Practice
Dr Christine M Derzko, Toronto, ON - Obstetrics & Gynecology
Dr Larissa A Derzko-Dzulynsky, Etobicoke, ON - Ophthalmology
Dr Aleksander I Dias, North York, ON - General Practice
Dr Isabella Dobek, Chester, NS - General Practice
Dr Wojciech B Dobkowski, London, ON - Anesthesia
Dr Andrzej Dobosiewicz, St Catharines, ON - Obstetrics & Gynecology
Dr Julian Dobranowski, Hamilton, ON - Diagnostic-Radiology
Dr Marek Dobrowolski, Lourdes-D-Bl-Sabl, QC - General Practice
Dr Malgorzata M S Dobson, North Vancouver, BC - General Practice
Dr Zbigniew Downar-Zapolski, Ottawa, ON - General Practice
Dr Lukasz Drzymala, Etobicoke, ON - Cardiology
Dr Helena L Duchowska, Richmond, BC - General Practice
Dr Malgorzata Dudek, York, ON - Psychiatry
Dr Janusz R Dukszta, Toronto, ON - Psychiatry
Dr Miroslaw Dutczak, Toronto, ON - General Practice
Dr Janina H Dutkiewicz-Stvrtecky, Oakville, ON - General Practice
Dr Andrew S C Dworak, Newmarket, ON - Family Medicine
Dr Vladimir Dzavik, Toronto, ON - Cardiology
Dr Margaret Dziedzic, Etobicoke, ON - Physical Medicine & Rehab
Dr B Dziewaltowska-Gintowt, Halifax, NS - Family Medicine
Dr Stanley A Dziurdzy, Burlington, ON - Psychiatry
Dr Peter Dzongowski, London, ON - Family Medicine
Dr Christine M Erlich, North York, ON - Ophthalmology
Dr Romana Fagan, Toronto, ON - General Practice
Dr Janusz Feber, Ottawa, ON - Pediatrics
Dr Roman Fedyna, Oshawa, ON - General Practice
Dr Roman Feigel, Ottawa, ON - Obstetrics & Gynecology
Dr Danuta Z Fenner, Toronto, ON - Psychiatry
Dr W Adam Filipowicz, Milton, ON - General Practice
Dr Alicja D Fishell, Toronto, ON - Psychiatry
Dr Raphael Ralph Folman, Mississauga, ON - Pediatrics
Dr Derek Ford, Toronto, ON - Plastic Surgery
Dr Ihor Gadacz, Etobicoke, ON - General Practice
Dr Jerzy Gajewski, Halifax, NS - Urology
Dr Martin Gajewski, Waterloo, ON - Family Medicine
Dr Elizabeth Galanter, Oakville, ON - Pediatrics
Dr John A P Gapski, Mississauga, ON - Internal Medicine
Dr Marek J Gawel, Toronto, ON - Neurology
Dr Janusz D Gawlik, Ottawa, ON - Psychiatry
Dr Nina J Georgiadis, Hamilton, ON - General Practice
Dr Adam R Glowacki, Windsor, ON - Obstetrics & Gynecology
Dr Malgorzata Gluszynski, Ottawa, ON - Family Medicine
Dr Marketa Gogela-Spehar, Vancouver, BC - Obstetrics & Gynecology
Dr Bronislaw L Golda, Hamilton, ON - General Practice
Dr Agata A Golosinski, Vernon, BC - Obstetrics & Gynecology
Dr Margaret A Gorecki, Calgary, AB - Anatomical Pathology
Dr Arthur Grabowski, Ajax, ON - Urology
Dr Waldemar Grandwilewski, Hamilton, ON - General Practice
Dr Peter A Gresko, Windsor, ON - General Practice
Dr Margaret A Gronska, North York, ON - Family Medicine
Dr Alicja N Gruder, Lanark, ON - Family Medicine
Dr Beata K Grygowski, Etobicoke, ON - Obstetrics & Gynecology
Dr Stefan C W Grzybowski, Vancouver, BC - Family Medicine
Dr Ewa Gwardjan, Hamilton, ON - General Practice
Dr Andrzej J Gwardjan, Hamilton, ON - Physical Medicine & Rehab
Dr Katarzyna M Gwiazda, Mississauga, ON - Pediatrics
Dr Mary Gwizdal, Belleville, ON - Obstetrics & Gynecology
Dr Krzysztof Habdank-Kossowski, Welland, ON - Diagnostic-Radiology
Dr Violetta A Hadlaw, Port Williams, NS - Internal Medicine
Dr Margaret K Hahn, Toronto, ON - Psychiatry
Dr M Lynn Hamilton, Toronto, ON - Internal Medicine
Dr Christopher A Hawling, Toronto, ON - Anesthesia
Dr Richard B Hladkowicz, Ottawa, ON - Anesthesia
Dr Eugene N Hladky, Montreal, QC - Ophthalmology
Dr Victor Hoffstein, Toronto, ON - Respirology
Dr Grazyna W Hofner, Truro, NS - Psychiatry
Dr Sophie L R Hofstader, Scarborough, ON - Dermatology
Dr Barbara J Hoppe, St. John's, NL - General Practice
Dr Stefan Horny, Montreal, QC - General Practice
Dr Zenona M I Hrabar, Surrey, BC - General Practice
Dr Tomasz W Hruczkowski, Edmonton, AB - Cardiology
Dr Malgorzata Humnicka-Szott, Saskatoon, SK - Family Medicine
Dr Janusz M Idzior, Stephenville, NL - General Practice
Dr Andrew P Ignaszewski, Vancouver, BC - Cardiology
Dr Dorothy Igras-Kulach, Calgary, AB - Obstetrics & Gynecology
Dr Magdalena I Ilcewicz-Klimek, Vancouver, BC - Psychiatry
Dr George A Jaciw, Whitby, ON - General Practice
Dr Allan W Jackiewicz, Niagara Falls, ON - Obstetrics & Gynecology
Dr Grazyna Jackiewicz, Niagara Falls, ON - Pediatrics
Dr Jerry Jakibchuk, St Catharines, ON - General Practice
Dr Andrew T Jakubowski, Richmond, BC - Cardiology
Dr Marek J Jakubowski, Parry Sound, ON - Internal Medicine
Dr Zygmunt Jancelewicz, Etobicoke, ON - Internal Medicine
Dr Alicja W Janicka, Edmonton, AB - Pediatrics
Dr Andrew M Janikowski, Picton, ON - Emergency Family Med
Dr Mariola S Januszewska, Surrey, BC - Family Medicine
Dr Arkadiusz N Jaroni, Camrose, AB - Family Medicine
Dr Anna M Jaroszynska, Burlington, ON - Internal Medicine
Dr Grzegorz C Jaroszynski, Burlington, ON - Orthopedic Surgery
Dr Jacek P Jastrzebski, Vancouver, BC - Internal Medicine
Dr Jerzy S Jaworski, Surrey, BC - Physical Medicine & Rehab
Dr Roman Jednak, Montreal, QC - Urology
Dr Eva M Jokay, Etobicoke, ON - Psychiatry
Dr Marek A Jung, Calgary, AB - Internal Medicine
Dr Pawel Juralowicz, Parksville, BC - Psychiatry
Dr Ewa Jussak-Kiellerman, Victoria, BC - General Practice
Dr Piotr Juszkiewicz, Campbell River, BC - General Surgery
Dr Henryk P Kafka, Belleville, ON - Cardiology
Dr Andrzej J Kajetanowicz, Sydney, NS - General Practice
Dr Danuta M Kajetanowicz, Sydney, NS - General Practice
Dr Leszek Kalinowski, Vancouver, BC - General Practice
Dr Maria T Kalisiak, Toronto, ON - General Practice
Dr Elzbieta A Kaminska, Calgary, AB - Internal Medicine
Dr Malgorzata E Kaminska, Calgary, AB - Family Medicine
Dr Irena Kaminska, St George, NB - General Practice
Dr Pierre Karakiewicz, Montreal, QC - Urology
Dr Marek E Karolak, Kelowna, BC - General Practice
Dr Martin E Karpinski, Winnipeg, MB - Internal Medicine
Dr Jolanta A M Karpinski, Ottawa, ON - Internal Medicine
Dr Danuta Katarzyniak-Kunysz, Lebel-s-Quevillon, QC - General Practice
Dr Andrew J Kiellerman, Victoria, BC - General Practice
Dr Anna J Kizior-Hajduk, Guelph, ON - Family Medicine
Dr Christopher L Klajn, Edmonton, AB - General Practice
Dr Marek G Klimek, Halifax, NS - General Practice
Dr Oleg Klipitch, Etobicoke, ON - Family Medicine
Dr Slawomir M Klodas, Toronto, ON - General Practice
Dr Maria-Teresa Klonowska, Dartmouth, NS - General Practice
Dr Izabela Klosowski, Saint-Bruno, QC - Family Medicine
Dr Pawel M Kluczynski, Sherwood Park, AB - General Practice
Dr Z Marek Knott, Sydney Mines, NS - General Practice
Dr Irene Kolabinski, Picton, ON - General Practice
Dr Alexander W Kolodziej, Ottawa, ON - Psychiatry
Dr Ewa M Konieczna, Toronto, ON - General Practice
Dr Marguerite M Kopaniak, Toronto, ON - Family Medicine
Dr Kinga T Koprowicz, Kirkfield, ON - Family Medicine
Dr Svetlana Korkuczanska, Vancouver, BC - Psychiatry
Dr Joseph B Kornacki, Verdun, QC - Orthopedic Surgery
Dr Tadeusz Kosalka, North York, ON - Obstetrics & Gynecology
Dr M H Kostolowski-Kondysar, Surrey, BC - Psychiatry
Dr Vitezslava V Kozel, Englehart, ON - General Practice
Dr Piotr Koziarz, Welland, ON - General Surgery
Dr Adam Krajewski, North York, ON - Geriatric Medicine
Dr Elizabeth Krause, Edmonton, AB - General Practice
Dr Michael Krawetz, Bala, ON - General Practice
Dr Tadeusz J Kroczak, Winnipeg, MB - General Practice
Dr Jozef Krop, Mississauga, ON - General Practice
Dr Lech Krotecki, Ormstown, QC - Family Medicine
Dr Maria H Krzywicka, Calgary, AB - General Practice
Dr Monika K Krzyzanowska, Toronto, ON - Internal Medicine
Dr Danuta Ksiazek, Trail, BC - Internal Medicine
Dr Agnes Kucharska, Milton, ON - Family Medicine
Dr Karol Kuperberg, Montreal, QC - General Practice
Dr Teresa K Kus, Montreal, QC - Cardiology
Dr Boleslaw Lach, Hamilton, ON - Anatomical Pathology
Dr Jolanta M Lalik, St Stephen, NB - General Practice
Dr Stephan J Landis, Guelph, ON - Internal Medicine
Dr Barbara E Laskowska, Ottawa, ON - General Practice
Dr Wojciech Laskowski, Ottawa, ON - General Practice
Dr Waldemar Lazowski, Souris, PE - Family Medicine
Dr Mykhaylo V Levinskyy, Edmonton, AB - General Practice
Dr Magdalena M Lipowska, North Vancouver, BC - Anesthesia
Dr Elena Lisiak, Vancouver, BC - Psychiatry
Dr Adrian L H Long, Winnipeg, MB - General Practice
Dr Hanna Lotocka-Reysner, Burnaby, BC - Pediatrics
Dr Ala Z Lozinski, Stoney Creek, ON - Dermatology
Dr Krzysztof Lubkiewicz, Pointe-Claire, QC - Pediatrics
Dr Michael Lucewicz, Edmonton, AB - General Practice
Dr Katarzyna E Lukomska, North Bay, ON - Family Medicine
Dr Teresa M Machel, Windsor, NS - Internal Medicine
Dr Wieslaw J Machel, Windsor, NS - General Practice
Dr Zuzanna M Majewski, St Jacobs, ON - General Practice
Dr Pawel A Makarewicz, Powell River, BC - General Surgery
Dr Anna J Malanowska, Edmonton, AB - Pediatrics
Dr Krzysztof W Malicki, Mississauga, ON - General Practice
Dr Ben A Malinowski, Edmonton, AB - Pediatrics
Dr Danuta J Malinowski, Mississauga, ON - General Practice
Dr Krystyna Mandelman, North York, ON - Psychiatry
Dr Zbigniew J Manowski, Mississauga, ON - Anatomical Pathology
Dr Leszek A Marchow, Toronto, ON - General Practice
Dr Zbigniew A Marciniak, Toronto, ON - General Practice
Dr Alexander Marks, Toronto, ON - General Practice
Dr Maria M Marszal, Cobourg, ON - Family Medicine
Dr Grzegorz P Martinka, Richmond, BC - Critical Care Medicine
Dr Magdalena Martinka, Vancouver, BC - Anatomical Pathology
Dr Teresa P Maryniarczyk, Toronto, ON - Family Medicine
Dr Aleksander Maslowski, Pickering, ON - Family Medicine
Dr Stanley T Maziarz, Gatineau, QC - Family Medicine
Dr Zdzislaw R Mech, Brampton, ON - Psychiatry
Dr Barbara D Mederski, North York, ON - Internal Medicine
Dr Lucja U Meier, Calgary, AB - Anatomical Pathology
Dr Andrzej J Michalski, Toronto, ON - General Practice
Dr Janina Milanska, Ottawa, ON - Pediatrics
Dr Andrew A Mis, Winnipeg, MB - Ophthalmology
Dr Joanna Mish, Calgary, AB - Family Medicine
Dr Jacek E Misterski, Guelph, ON - Cardiology
Dr Henry F Mizgala, Vancouver, BC - Cardiology
Dr Eva J M Mocarski, Toronto, ON - Obstetrics & Gynecology
Dr W Hanna Moore, Woodbridge, ON - General Practice
Dr Joanna Morawska-Jablonska, Nepean, ON - Pediatrics
Dr Henry Morgentaler, Toronto, ON - General Practice
Dr Grazyna Morton, Ottawa, ON - Psychiatry
Dr Wojciech Morzycki, Halifax, NS - Internal Medicine
Dr Ihor R Mota, Vancouver, BC - Family Medicine
Dr Gary S Nakhuda, Vancouver, BC - General Practice

LANGUAGES SPOKEN

Dr Etela Neumann, Vancouver, BC - Neuro-Pathology
Dr Anna Neumann, Halifax, NS - Family Medicine
Dr Anna Niajko, Richelieu, QC - General Practice
Dr Violetta Niesobska, Brampton, ON - Family Medicine
Dr Daiva L Norkus, Etobicoke, ON - Family Medicine
Dr Malgorzata J M Nowaczyk, Hamilton, ON - Pediatrics
Dr Mark J J Nowaczynski, Toronto, ON - Family Medicine
Dr Agata M Nowak, Calgary, AB - Family Medicine
Dr Jozef E Nowak, Kelowna, BC - Physical Medicine & Rehab
Dr Zbigniew J Nowak, Miramichi, NB - General Practice
Dr Aleksandra Nowicki, London, ON - Psychiatry
Dr Dorota J Nowodworski, Ottawa, ON - Emergency Family Med
Dr Edward M Nykiforuk, Saskatoon, SK - General Practice
Dr Peter A Nynkowski, Toronto, ON - Psychiatry
Dr Wieslaw J Oczkowski, Hamilton, ON - Neurology
Dr Bohdan Olearczyk, Toronto, ON - General Practice
Dr Wayne Olsheski, Toronto, ON - General Practice
Dr Ewa P Olszynski, Saskatoon, SK - Family Medicine
Dr Wojciech P Olszynski, Saskatoon, SK - Internal Medicine
Dr Yvonne A V Opalinski, Newmarket, ON - General Practice
Dr Eugenia Ostapkowicz, Vancouver, BC - General Practice
Dr Krystyna I Ostrowska, Mississauga, ON - Infectious Diseases
Dr Mirek Otremba, Toronto, ON - Internal Medicine
Dr Anthony G Otto, Vancouver, BC - General Practice
Dr Natalia M Pastuszewska, Brantford, ON - Internal Medicine
Dr Mariusz T Paszkiewicz, Weyburn, SK - General Practice
Dr Elzbieta Pater, Maple Ridge, BC - General Practice
Dr Piotr C Pater, Powell River, BC - General Practice
Dr Jerzy Pawlak, Winnipeg, MB - General Practice
Dr Dariusz P Piatek, Mississauga, ON - General Practice
Dr Tadeusz A Pierscianowski, Ottawa, ON - Dermatology
Dr Mary D S Pietraszek, Etobicoke, ON - General Practice
Dr Barbara A Pilarski, Etobicoke, ON - Family Medicine
Dr Andre Piver, Slocan Park, BC - Family Medicine
Dr Henryk Pluta, Abbotsford, BC - Internal Medicine
Dr Ewa M Pniak, Fredericton, NB - General Practice
Dr Ilona C Polis, Ottawa, ON - Psychiatry
Dr Jerzy Poray-Wybranowski, Longueuil, QC - Family Medicine
Dr Bozena Praglowski, Etobicoke, ON - General Practice
Dr Roman Z Preobrazenski, Hamilton, ON - Family Medicine
Dr Krystyna Prutis-Misterska, North York, ON - Physical Medicine & Rehab
Dr Waldemar Pruzanski, Toronto, ON - Internal Medicine
Dr Maria J Raczynska, Mississauga, ON - General Practice
Dr John S Radwan, Mississauga, ON - Radiation Oncology
Dr Jerry M Radziuk, Ottawa, ON - Med Scientist
Dr Miroslaw Rajda, Halifax, NS - Cardiology
Dr Anna E Rogers, Sault Ste. Marie, ON - Psychiatry
Dr Ludwika Rogozinska, Winnipeg, MB - Obstetrics & Gynecology
Dr Elizabeth T Rokosh, Edmonton, AB - Critical Care Medicine
Dr Marek Rola-Pleszczynski, Sherbrooke, QC - Clin Immun/Allergy
Dr Walter W Romatowski, St Catharines, ON - Gastroenterology
Dr Malgorzata D Rowicka, Halifax, NS - General Practice
Dr Eva Rozenfarb, Repentigny, QC - Dermatology
Dr Marek A Rozwadowski, Port Alberni, BC - General Practice
Dr Alexandra D Ruszkowski, Oshawa, ON - Plastic Surgery
Dr Anna Rutkowska-Rokosz, Pte-aux-Trembles, QC - General Practice
Dr Eva J Rychter, Calgary, AB - General Practice
Dr Edward J J Rzadki, Etobicoke, ON - Psychiatry
Dr Waldemar P Rzepka, Oakville, ON - General Practice
Dr Ghada-Maria Saddi, Chateauguay, QC - Family Medicine
Dr Krystyna Salach-Markiewicz, Mississauga, ON - General Practice
Dr Andrew J Sarne, Toronto, ON - Family Medicine
Dr Joanna T Sasal, Toronto, ON - Internal Medicine
Dr Bozena Schaefer-Zieleniak, St-Charles-Brromee, QC - General Practice
Dr Joseph Schatzker, Toronto, ON - Orthopedic Surgery
Dr Bogdan L Schwarz-Michorowski, Guelph, ON - Cardiology
Dr Mary V Seeman, Toronto, ON - Psychiatry
Dr Zygmunt P Sekula, Halifax, NS - General Practice
Dr Miroslav V Semczyszyn, Hamilton, ON - Family Medicine
Dr Pawel A Serowka, Victoria, BC - Anesthesia
Dr Raisa Sheftel, Verdun, QC - General Practice
Dr Jaroslav O Shklar, Etobicoke, ON - General Practice
Dr Wael Shublaq, St. John's, NL - General Practice
Dr Zia A Sial, Etobicoke, ON - Family Medicine
Dr Jacqueline B C Siedlecki, Midland, ON - Family Medicine
Dr Michal M Siekierski, Hamilton, ON - Psychiatry
Dr Daniela Sielecka, Mansonville, QC - General Practice
Dr Robert Sikorski, Thunder Bay, ON - Anesthesia
Dr M M Jeanne Sirois, Gatineau, QC - General Practice
Dr George W Skocylak, Toronto, ON - General Practice
Dr Robert Skomro, Saskatoon, SK - Internal Medicine
Dr Yoanna K Skrobik, Montreal, QC - Internal Medicine
Dr Jacek Slatnik, Edmonton, AB - Anatomical Pathology
Dr Marek J Smieja, Hamilton, ON - Infectious Diseases
Dr Barbara M A Smiltnieks, Etobicoke, ON - Pediatrics
Dr Marek A Smolarkiewicz, Stephenville, NL - General Practice
Dr Wojciech W Sobkowski, Welland, ON - Internal Medicine
Dr Elisabeth K Sochocka, Milton, ON - General Practice
Dr Anna M Sokolowska, Ottawa, ON - Psychiatry
Dr Danuta Sokolowski, Winnipeg, MB - General Practice
Dr Henry L Solow, Markham, ON - Internal Medicine
Dr Elena Somska, Toronto, ON - General Practice
Dr Mark K Sosnowski, Calgary, AB - Family Medicine
Dr Christopher J Sosnowski, Napanee, ON - Family Medicine
Dr Jan B Splawinski, Vernon, BC - Orthopedic Surgery
Dr Robert B J Stachula, Toronto, ON - General Practice
Dr Teresa M Stalinska, Toronto, ON - General Practice
Dr Ferdinand M Stasiak, North Vancouver, BC - General Practice
Dr Ewa M Stasiak, Montreal, QC - General Practice
Dr Lilianna Stefanczyk-Sapieha, Hamilton, ON - Family Medicine
Dr Henry T Stelfox, Calgary, AB - Critical Care Medicine
Dr Jerzy Sternadel, Welland, ON - Obstetrics & Gynecology
Dr Marina A Straszak-Suri, Nepean, ON - Obstetrics & Gynecology
Dr Lukasz Struzik, Georgetown, ON - Family Medicine
Dr Joanna Z Stuchly, Calgary, AB - General Practice
Dr Milosh S Surka, Richmond, BC - General Practice
Dr Leszek J Swica, Swift Current, SK - Anesthesia
Dr Janusz S Swierczek, Etobicoke, ON - Psychiatry
Dr Peter K Switakowski, Toronto, ON - Emergency Family Med
Dr Ewa Swoboda, Toronto, ON - Psychiatry
Dr Anna M Sylwestrowicz, Victoria, BC - Anesthesia
Dr Thomas A Sylwestrowicz, Saskatoon, SK - Internal Medicine
Dr Marie B Syty-Golda, Hamilton, ON - General Practice
Dr Violetta I Szachnowska, Parksville, BC - Family Medicine
Dr Stanley Szajkowski, Winnipeg, MB - General Practice
Dr Istvan L Szarka, Hamilton, ON - Family Medicine
Dr Blazej I Szczygielski, Kuujjuaq, QC - Emergency Family Med
Dr Marek A Szelag, Barrie, ON - Family Medicine
Dr Joanna T Szelazek, Winnipeg, MB - Psychiatry
Dr Leszek P Szkup, Saskatoon, SK - Diagnostic-Radiology
Dr Mikolaj D Szpakowicz, Surrey, BC - Emergency Family Med
Dr Monika A Szpejda, St Catharines, ON - Pediatrics
Dr Witold J Szpejda, St Catharines, ON - Anesthesia
Dr Michael Szpilberg, Montreal, QC - General Practice
Dr Teresa M Sztukowski, Calgary, AB - Family Medicine
Dr Ewa A Szudek, Halifax, NS - Pediatrics
Dr Elizabeth K Szulc, Brampton, ON - General Practice
Dr Ewa F Szumacher, Toronto, ON - Radiation Oncology
Dr Aleksandra Szymanska, Smithers, BC - Family Medicine
Dr Waldemar A Szymanski, Edmonton, AB - Pediatrics
Dr Wanda M Szymonowicz, Mississauga, ON - Pediatrics
Dr Iwona R Tarasiewicz, Hamilton, ON - Family Medicine
Dr Gretta Taylor, Halifax, NS - Family Medicine
Dr Sophia B Tchervenkov, Montreal, QC - Obstetrics & Gynecology
Dr Alicja Tesiorowski, North Vancouver, BC - Family Medicine
Dr Anna I Tomanek, Cochrane, AB - Family Medicine
Dr Anna B Tomczak-Bojarski, Sudbury, ON - Anatomical Pathology
Dr Edward A Torbicki, Kitchener, ON - Anesthesia
Dr Maria T Torok, Dartmouth, NS - Pediatrics
Dr Elizabeth M Trojanowski, Markham, ON - General Practice
Dr Margaret B Truchan, Saskatoon, SK - Internal Medicine
Dr Anna A Trzcieniecka, Delhi, ON - Family Medicine
Dr Izolda L Tuhan Mirza Baranowski, Timmins, ON - Psychiatry
Dr Hanna M Tuszynska, Hamilton, ON - Anesthesia
Dr R Pierre Urbanski, Lasalle, QC - Pediatrics
Dr Frantisek Vetiska, Oakville, ON - General Practice
Dr Ireneusz Wachowski, Edmonton, AB - Anesthesia
Dr Marcin Wasowicz, Toronto, ON - General Practice
Dr Janusz Wawrzyszyn, Sydney, NS - General Practice
Dr Anna Wesolkowska, Sydney, NS - General Practice
Dr Ewa B Wesolowska, Montreal, QC - Medical Biochemistry
Dr Marta A Wesolowski, Peterborough, ON - General Practice
Dr Beata A Wiatrowska, Ottawa, ON - Anatomical Pathology
Dr Witold J Widajewicz, Coquitlam, BC - Psychiatry
Dr Anna Wieckowska, Quebec, QC - Gastroenterology
Dr Krzysztof Wieczorek, Edmonton, AB - General Practice
Dr Andreas T J Wielgosz, Ottawa, ON - Cardiology
Dr Rafal F Wierzbicki, Oshawa, ON - Internal Medicine
Dr Krzysztof Wierzchoslawski, Miramichi, NB - General Practice
Dr John S Wilczynski, Niagara Falls, ON - General Practice
Dr Andrew Wilk, Oshawa, ON - General Practice
Dr Anna S Willamowicz, Oshawa, ON - Endocrin/Metabolism
Dr Christina Winogrodzka, Winnipeg, MB - General Practice
Dr A Leo Winter, Hamilton, ON - Urology
Dr Anna B Wisniewska, Kelowna, BC - Psychiatry
Dr Leon E Wisniowski, Bedford, NS - General Practice
Dr Stanislaw R Wlodarczyk, Waterloo, ON - General Practice
Dr Krystyna H Wojakowski, London, ON - Psychiatry
Dr Anna M Wojcicka, Toronto, ON - Radiation Oncology
Dr Andre T Wojcicki, Mount Albert, ON - Internal Medicine
Dr Wladyslaw Wojcik, Regina, SK - Internal Medicine
Dr Ewa Wojtowska, Vancouver, BC - Internal Medicine
Dr Winicjusz M Wolski, Mississauga, ON - Internal Medicine
Dr Ewa A Wozniak, Barrie, ON - General Pathology
Dr Andrew E Wozniak, Barrie, ON - General Practice
Dr Iwona T Wrobel, Calgary, AB - Gastroenterology
Dr Julius A Wroblewski, Vancouver, BC - Anatomical Pathology
Dr Karol C Wroblewski, Etobicoke, ON - Emergency Family Med
Dr Thom W Wroz, Kamloops, BC - Obstetrics & Gynecology
Dr Oksana Y Yatsina, Saskatoon, SK - Family Medicine
Dr Anna Zajaczkowska-Kielska, Surrey, BC - Pediatrics
Dr Witold M Zaleski, London, ON - Diagnostic-Radiology
Dr Pawel G Zalewski, Oshawa, ON - Internal Medicine
Dr Emil N Zamora, Hamilton, ON - Psychiatry
Dr Gregory A Zaniewski, Peterborough, ON - Family Medicine
Dr Jozef Zaremba, Amherst, NS - Family Medicine
Dr Janina Zaremba, Ottawa, ON - General Practice
Dr John J Zasowski, Woodbridge, ON - Family Medicine
Dr Annabella Zawada, Terrace Bay, ON - Family Medicine
Dr Andrew G A Zawadowski, Oakville, ON - Internal Medicine
Dr Marian Zazula, Mississauga, ON - General Practice
Dr Grazyna A Zebrowska, St Catharines, ON - Anatomical Pathology
Dr Andrzej Zebrowski, St Catharines, ON - Psychiatry
Dr Robert Zeman, Toronto, ON - Endocrin/Metabolism
Dr Adam M Zieleniak, St-Charles-Brromee, QC - General Practice
Dr Lucjan J Zielonka, Surrey, BC - Psychiatry
Dr Anna I M Znamirowski, Cambridge, ON - Obstetrics & Gynecology
Dr Kathia Znojkiewicz, Montreal, QC - General Practice
Dr Jan S Zuchelkowski, Mississauga, ON - Family Medicine
Dr Mateusz-Jerzy Zurowski, Toronto, ON - Psychiatry
Dr Wojciech J Zurowski, Toronto, ON - General Practice

PORTUGUESE

Dr Aboobaker Aboo, Ottawa, ON - General Practice
Dr Jordanka Angelova, Edmonton, AB - Family Medicine
Dr Rui L Antunes, Cornwall, ON - General Surgery
Dr Adilson A M Araujo, Mississauga, ON - General Practice
Dr Julio E Arboleda-Florez, Belleville, ON - Psychiatry
Dr Horacio Arruda, Quebec, QC - Community Medicine
Dr Luis C Baptista, Edmonton, AB - General Practice
Dr Adrian M Baranchuk, Kingston, ON - Neurology
Dr Peter G Barss, Salmon Arm, BC - Community Medicine
Dr Marc Beauchamp, Montreal, QC - Orthopedic Surgery
Dr Marie Beauregard, Montreal, QC - Family Medicine
Dr Mario Bejerman, Montreal, QC - General Surgery
Dr Rino Bier, Montreal, QC - Diagnostic-Radiology
Dr German Blando, Dieppe, NB - General Practice

Dr Yves Bonnier-Viger, Sainte-Marie, QC - Community Medicine
Dr Patrick R Boulos, Sherbrooke, QC - Ophthalmology
Dr Luis H P Braga, Hamilton, ON - General Practice
Dr Rosa M Braga-Mele, Toronto, ON - Ophthalmology
Dr Alessandra Bruns, Sherbrooke, QC - General Practice
Dr Miguel N Burnier, Montreal, QC - General Practice
Dr Melanie G Caetano, Etobicoke, ON - Obstetrics & Gynecology
Dr Manuel Carcao, Toronto, ON - Hematology
Dr Manuel R Cardoso, Montreal, QC - Internal Medicine
Dr Raul A J Carvalho, Richmond, BC - General Practice
Dr Saulo Castel, Toronto, ON - Psychiatry
Dr Clarence E Clottey, Oakville, ON - Family Medicine
Dr Carmen M Colaco, Oakville, ON - General Practice
Dr Rohan Cornelissen, Prince Albert, SK - General Practice
Dr Leodante B Da Costa Jr, Toronto, ON - General Practice
Dr Anna-Maria Da Silva, Barrie, ON - Family Medicine
Dr Orlando P Da Silva, London, ON - Pediatrics
Dr Vasco F Da Silva, Ottawa, ON - Neurosurgery
Dr Arianna Dal Cin, Hamilton, ON - Plastic Surgery
Dr Tirone David, Toronto, ON - Cardiovasc/ThorSurg
Dr Antonia F De Figueiredo, Toronto, ON - Family Medicine
Dr Delta M De Ponte, Etobicoke, ON - General Practice
Dr Anne De Silva, Toronto, ON - General Practice
Dr Marcelino De Souza, Sherwood Park, AB - General Practice
Dr Fructuoso M De Souza, Mississauga, ON - Otolaryngology
Dr Jaime Del Carpio, Montreal, QC - Clin Immun/Allergy
Dr Diego H Delgado, Toronto, ON - General Practice
Dr Vincenzo Di Nicola, Montreal, QC - Psychiatry
Dr Ana M Diaz De Molnar, Toronto, ON - General Practice
Dr Rejane F Dillenburg, Hamilton, ON - Cardiology
Dr Patricia Disperati, Toronto, ON - Hematology
Dr Vidal Essebag, Montreal, QC - Cardiology
Dr William G Etzkorn, Toronto, ON - Family Medicine
Dr Arthur M Eugenio, Cambridge, ON - Family Medicine
Dr Julio Faria, Montreal, QC - General Surgery
Dr Cristina Fayet, Toronto, ON - Family Medicine
Dr Julio C Fernandes, Montreal, QC - Orthopedic Surgery
Dr Artur J D B Fernandes, Sherbrooke, QC - Rheumatology
Dr Geraldo A J Fernandes, North Battleford, SK - General Practice
Dr Nestor D P Fernandez, Toronto, ON - General Practice
Dr Jose G P Ferraz, Calgary, AB - General Practice
Dr Nelson D B Ferreira, North York, ON - General Practice
Dr Ivone M Ferreira, Toronto, ON - Internal Medicine
Dr Indira C Figueiredo, Toronto, ON - General Practice
Dr Alberto L Flores-Vargas, Scarborough, ON - General Practice
Dr Stephen H Gallay, Ajax, ON - Orthopedic Surgery
Dr Daniel Garros, Edmonton, AB - General Practice
Dr David R Gomes, Strathroy, ON - Internal Medicine
Dr Jose G S Gomide, Cannington, ON - General Practice
Dr M Joana Goncalves, Toronto, ON - General Practice
Dr Armando Gonzalez, Toronto, ON - General Practice
Dr Karin H Grubner, Toronto, ON - General Practice
Dr Daniel B S Guimaraes, Sherbrooke, QC - Psychiatry
Dr Gervais A Harry, Etobicoke, ON - Urology
Dr Jacques Harton, Murdochville, QC - General Practice
Dr Yasmine S Kelton, Richmond Hill, ON - Family Medicine
Dr Andre Kokis, Montreal, QC - Cardiology
Dr Marcelo Lannes, Montreal, QC - Anesthesia
Dr Gabor Lantos, Toronto, ON - General Practice
Dr Mary C Y Lee, Toronto, ON - Internal Medicine
Dr Rosanna V Lima, Vancouver, BC - Family Medicine
Dr Adrian L H Long, Winnipeg, MB - General Practice
Dr Michele Mabon, Montreal, QC - Ophthalmology
Dr Humberto Martinho, Ottawa, ON - Family Medicine
Dr Daphne R Marussi, Sherbrooke, QC - General Practice
Dr John C Masgoret, Toronto, ON - Family Medicine
Dr Aldina C S Matos, Hamilton, ON - General Practice
Dr Pierre Maurice, Quebec, QC - Community Medicine
Dr Sergio Mazzadi, Hamilton, ON - General Practice
Dr John M Mendes, Toronto, ON - Pediatrics
Dr Stephen D Miller, Calgary, AB - Orthopedic Surgery
Dr Patricia B Mills, Vancouver, BC - Physical Medicine & Rehab
Dr Jose A Morais, Montreal, QC - Geriatric Medicine
Dr Richard Moufarrege, Montreal, QC - Plastic Surgery
Dr Juan E Munoz, Hamilton, ON - Family Medicine
Dr A Ali Najarali, Brampton, ON - General Practice
Dr Juan C Negrete, Montreal, QC - Psychiatry
Dr Mark W Nelham, Exeter, ON - General Practice
Dr Marcelo T Nicolela, Halifax, NS - Ophthalmology
Dr Gregoire E Noel, Montreal, QC - Medical Microbiology
Dr Luis C E Noronha, Toronto, ON - Internal Medicine
Dr Isabel M A Nunes, Fonthill, ON - General Practice
Dr Claire M Nunes-Vaz, Toronto, ON - Family Medicine
Dr Ana-Maria Oelschig, Okotoks, AB - General Practice
Dr Victor N Onwukwe, Fort McMurray, AB - General Practice
Dr Sergio G Pasian, Quebec, QC - General Practice
Dr Margot Patterson, Denwood, AB - General Practice
Dr Jose L Pereira, Ottawa, ON - Family Medicine
Dr Any Z Pfeiffer, Milton, ON - General Practice
Dr Helena Piccinini, Halifax, NS - Family Medicine
Dr J Vicente Pinilla, Toronto, ON - General Practice
Dr Lucina M Pinto, Toronto, ON - General Practice
Dr Joao L P Pippi-Salle, Toronto, ON - Urology
Dr Jose M Pires, Ottawa, ON - General Surgery
Dr Arthur E Pires, Quebec, QC - Psychiatry
Dr Eulalia Rech, Edmonton, AB - General Practice
Dr Marciano D Reis, Toronto, ON - Hematological Pathology
Dr Rona G Ribeiro, Sherwood Park, AB - Family Medicine
Dr Claudio Rigatto, Winnipeg, MB - Internal Medicine
Dr Sandro B Rizoli, Toronto, ON - General Surgery
Dr Arthur F Rodrigues, Brampton, ON - General Practice
Dr Americo V F Rodrigues, Ottawa, ON - General Practice
Dr Carlos H Rodriguez, Toronto, ON - Internal Medicine
Dr Joseph Rodriguez, Montreal, QC - General Surgery
Dr Aristides Rodriguez Naranjo, Battleford, SK - General Practice
Dr Luis A Salgado De Leon, Regina, SK - General Practice
Dr Adolfo Sanchez, Toronto, ON - Psychiatry
Dr Arturo Sanchez, Toronto, ON - Pediatrics
Dr Pablo E R F Sanhueza Luco, North Bay, ON - Psychiatry
Dr Claudia Santos, Toronto, ON - Critical Care Medicine
Dr Peter Sauret, Toronto, ON - General Practice
Dr Monica Z Scalco, Toronto, ON - Psychiatry
Dr Andreia Z Scalco, Toronto, ON - Psychiatry
Dr Anabel M Scaranelo, Toronto, ON - General Practice
Dr Lidia M Schuster, Kelowna, BC - Psychiatry
Dr Marcia H Shapir Kahan, Toronto, ON - Psychiatry
Dr Marcelo C Shibata, Edmonton, AB - General Practice
Dr Nayeema Siddiq, Toronto, ON - General Practice
Dr Douglas M Sider, Toronto, ON - Community Medicine
Dr Sergio Sierra-Dupont, Montreal, QC - Otolaryngology
Dr Fidelia A Silva, Moncton, NB - Gastroenterology
Dr Jose M A D Silveira, Toronto, ON - Psychiatry
Dr Richard H Sims, Toronto, ON - Obstetrics & Gynecology
Dr Claudio D N Soares, Hamilton, ON - Psychiatry
Dr Julio C Soto, Montreal, QC - Community Medicine
Dr Luis Souhami, Montreal, QC - Radiation Oncology
Dr Fernando A C Spencer Netto, Toronto, ON - General Surgery
Dr Leila F Srour, Vancouver, BC - Community Medicine
Dr Nina R Stein, Hamilton, ON - General Practice
Dr Aravind Subramanian, Calgary, AB - General Practice
Dr Diann J Superina-Bell, Toronto, ON - Pediatrics
Dr Julio Szmuilowicz, Toronto, ON - Psychiatry
Dr Wanda M Szymonowicz, Mississauga, ON - Pediatrics
Dr Isabella T W Tai, Vancouver, BC - Gastroenterology
Dr Philippa J Tattersall, Hamilton, ON - General Practice
Dr Joseph Telch, Markham, ON - Pediatrics
Dr Dominique Tessier, Montreal, QC - Family Medicine
Dr Arawn A A Therrien, Gananoque, ON - Family Medicine
Dr Jean Thisdale, St-Eustache, QC - General Practice
Dr Kevin L F Tong, Vancouver, BC - General Practice
Dr Ana-Maria C Tsanaclis, Sherbrooke, QC - General Practice
Dr Percy G Urback, Toronto, ON - Internal Medicine
Dr Jose A Vasconcelos, Brandon, MB - Psychiatry
Dr Lucy M Vieira, Pointe-Claire, QC - Neurology
Dr Leonardo Vieira Neto, Chicoutimi, QC - General Practice
Dr Giselle C P Villar, Vancouver, BC - Anesthesia
Dr Larry M Wengle, Toronto, ON - General Practice
Mrs Christiane C F Werneck, Mississauga, ON - General Practice
Dr Eldon S V Williams, Toronto, ON - General Surgery
Dr Murray B Wilson, Bradford, ON - General Practice
Dr John C S Wootton, Shawville, QC - General Practice
Dr Noe Zamel, Toronto, ON - Med Scientist
Dr Ricardo Zarruk, Pierrefonds, QC - General Practice
Dr Gregorio Zlotnik, Montreal, QC - General Practice

PUNJABI

Dr Mustafa H Abdulhusein, Brampton, ON - General Practice
Dr Naresh K Aggarwal, Brampton, ON - Family Medicine
Dr Ram K Aggarwal, Woodbridge, ON - Internal Medicine
Dr Vandana Ahluwalia, Brampton, ON - Internal Medicine
Dr Mohinderjit S Ahluwalia, Mississauga, ON - General Practice
Dr Amar K Ahluwalia, St Catharines, ON - General Practice
Dr Aijaz Ahmad, Medicine Hat, AB - General Practice
Dr Ejaz Ahmad, Winnipeg, MB - Family Medicine
Dr Sheikh N Ahmed, Abbotsford, BC - Radiation Oncology
Dr Shafiq F Akbar, Edmonton, AB - Internal Medicine
Dr Zaubaria Akbar, Surrey, BC - General Practice
Dr Saima Amjad, Mississauga, ON - Family Medicine
Dr Afsari B Amjad, Ottawa, ON - Psychiatry
Dr Neeru Anand, Delta, BC - Family Medicine
Dr Mohinder K Angl, Courtice, ON - General Practice
Dr A Hashsham Ansari, Scarborough, ON - Family Medicine
Dr Nawaz Arora, Brantford, ON - Family Medicine
Dr Sunder S Arora, Ottawa, ON - Psychiatry
Dr Amit Arya, Brampton, ON - Family Medicine
Dr Rajinder K Atwal, North York, ON - Family Medicine
Dr Prince S S Aujla, Richmond Hill, ON - Internal Medicine
Dr Paramjit S Aulakh, Surrey, BC - General Practice
Dr Lakyntiew P S Aulakh, Sudbury, ON - General Practice
Dr Tariq M Awan, Calgary, AB - Family Medicine
Dr Abdul Aziz, Lethbridge, AB - General Practice
Dr S Yasmin Aziz, Ottawa, ON - Obstetrics & Gynecology
Dr Harry S Badhan, Brampton, ON - General Practice
Dr Jagdeep S Badhesha, Calgary, AB - Family Medicine
Dr Charanjit S Bageria, North York, ON - Family Medicine
Dr Jatinder S Baidwan, Victoria, BC - Family Medicine
Dr Puneet Bains, North Vancouver, BC - Internal Medicine
Dr Jason D Bains, Surrey, BC - Family Medicine
Dr Harpreet S Bajaj, Brampton, ON - General Practice
Dr Parvesh Bajaj, Nepean, ON - General Practice
Dr Renu Bajaj, Waterloo, ON - Emergency Family Med
Dr Sameena A Bajwa, Calgary, AB - Family Medicine
Dr Gurjit Bajwa, Etobicoke, ON - General Practice
Dr Harmeet K Bami, Brampton, ON - Psychiatry
Dr Raghmeet Basati, Calgary, AB - Family Medicine
Dr Khalid Bashir, Prince George, BC - Internal Medicine
Dr Amrik S Bassi, Calgary, AB - General Practice
Dr Nandita Batchra, Burlington, ON - Otolaryngology
Dr Navdeep Bath, Mississauga, ON - Family Medicine
Dr Sue K Batth, Nepean, ON - Psychiatry
Dr Hussam-Ul H Bawa, Calgary, AB - Psychiatry
Dr Bhupinder S Bedi, Winnipeg, MB - General Practice
Dr Subramanya Bhagavatula, Sudbury, ON - Psychiatry
Dr Kapil M Bhagirath, Surrey, BC - Cardiology
Dr Chander P Bhagirath, Niagara Falls, ON - Pediatrics
Dr Dinesh Bhalla, Moncton, NB - Psychiatry
Dr Dalip K Bhangu, Etobicoke, ON - Obstetrics & Gynecology
Dr Raminder K Bhangu, Windsor, ON - Psychiatry
Dr Asha Bhardwaj, London, ON - Physical Medicine & Rehab
Dr Ranbir S Bhatia, Nepean, ON - General Practice
Dr Rajinder S Bhatti, Abbotsford, BC - General Practice
Dr Virinder S Bhatti, Maple Ridge, BC - General Practice
Dr Balbir C Bhatti, Surrey, BC - Family Medicine
Dr Jaswant S Bhopal, Richmond, BC - Psychiatry
Dr Paramjit S Bhui, Surrey, BC - Pediatrics
Dr Pargat S Bhurji, Surrey, BC - Pediatrics
Dr Harjinder J S Bining, Richmond, BC - Diagnostic-Radiology
Dr Shabab Boparai, Scarborough, ON - Family Medicine
Dr Darshan S Brar, Calgary, AB - General Practice
Dr Parminder S Brar, St Catharines, ON - Pediatrics
Dr Sonia D Buttar, Surrey, BC - General Practice
Dr Usha Chada, North York, ON - General Practice
Dr Rati Chadha, Calgary, AB - Obstetrics & Gynecology
Dr Jeevyn K Chahal, Kamloops, BC - Family Medicine
Dr Jayshree Chanchlani, Brampton, ON - General Practice
Dr Pavanjeet Chand, Windsor, ON - Family Medicine

Dr Ranjit K Chandra, Mississauga, ON - Pediatrics
Dr Mohammad I Chaudhary, Mississauga, ON - Family Medicine
Dr Mobina A Chaudhry, Fort McMurray, AB - Family Medicine
Dr Sajjad A Chaudhry, Toronto, ON - Anesthesia
Dr Sukarno N Chaudhry, Windsor, ON - Internal Medicine
Dr Rakesh K Chawla, Hammonds Plains, NS - General Practice
Dr Harvinder K Chawla, Brockville, ON - Pediatrics
Dr Satish K Chawla, Niagara Falls, ON - Anatomical Pathology
Dr Ashis K Chawla, Toronto, ON - Urology
Dr Gulzar S Cheema, Surrey, BC - Family Medicine
Dr Waqar M Cheema, Brampton, ON - Family Medicine
Dr Amarjit S Cheema, Mississauga, ON - Clin Immun/Allergy
Dr Rakesh S Chehil, Surrey, BC - General Practice
Dr Samir R Chhabra, Oshawa, ON - Orthopedic Surgery
Dr Jagdish C Chopra, Oshawa, ON - General Practice
Dr Ashwani Choudhry, Mississauga, ON - Cardiology
Dr Prem K Chugh, Dartmouth, NS - General Practice
Dr Amathul A Danial, Edmonton, AB - General Practice
Dr A Rashid Dar, London, ON - Radiation Oncology
Dr Shahnaz Dar, Scarborough, ON - Pediatrics
Dr Milind G Desai, North York, ON - Gastroenterology
Dr Shashi P Devi, North York, ON - Family Medicine
Dr Harjinder S Dhaliwal, Burnaby, BC - Ophthalmology
Dr Harmanpreet V Dhaliwal, Surrey, BC - Family Medicine
Dr Harbhajan S Dhaliwal, Winnipeg, MB - General Practice
Dr Amarinder S Dhaliwal, Brampton, ON - General Practice
Dr Jagtaran S Dhaliwal, Brampton, ON - Psychiatry
Dr Preet B K Dhaliwal, LaSalle, ON - Family Medicine
Dr Yadvinder S Dhaliwal, Mississauga, ON - General Practice
Dr Karan S Dhami, Ottawa, ON - Emergency Family Med
Dr Dharminder S Dhanda, New Westminster, BC - Ophthalmology
Dr Permjeet S Dhanjal, Winnipeg, MB - Family Medicine
Dr Avtar S Dhanoa, Mississauga, ON - General Practice
Dr Nishi Dhawan, Vancouver, BC - Family Medicine
Dr Pankaj M Dhawan, Vancouver, BC - Physical Medicine & Rehab
Dr Avtar S Dhillon, Delta, BC - Internal Medicine
Dr Baldev S Dhillon, Delta, BC - Family Medicine
Dr Pawandeep K Dhillon, Surrey, BC - Family Medicine
Dr Manu Dhillon, Brampton, ON - General Practice
Dr Jatinder S Dhillon, Brantford, ON - General Practice
Dr Jaswinder S Dhillon, Brantford, ON - Emergency Family Med
Dr Rajwinder S Dhillon, Niagara Falls, ON - Internal Medicine
Dr Ripple Dhillon, Oshawa, ON - Family Medicine
Dr S Paul Dhiman, Surrey, BC - Emergency Family Med
Dr Navraj S Dhiraj, Milton, ON - Family Medicine
Dr John M Dickson, Surrey, BC - Otolaryngology
Dr Shamoon Din, Mississauga, ON - General Practice
Dr Arun K Dosaj, Madoc, ON - General Practice
Dr Seema Dosaj, Pickering, ON - Family Medicine
Dr Ismat Z Dost, Brantford, ON - Pediatrics
Dr Rehan Dost, Paris, ON - Neurology
Dr Varinder Dua, London, ON - Psychiatry
Dr Santosh Dubey, Calgary, AB - General Practice
Dr Mohammed Elahi, Etobicoke, ON - Family Medicine
Dr Mohammed Elahi, North York, ON - Otolaryngology
Dr Rajeev Erry, Pickering, ON - General Practice
Dr Steven M Evans, Oliver, BC - General Practice
Dr Shireen Fahim, Etobicoke, ON - Family Medicine
Dr Mohammed Farooq, Sydney, NS - General Practice
Dr Najla Fasih, Ottawa, ON - General Practice
Dr Sleem Feroze, Oakville, ON - Obstetrics & Gynecology
Dr Puneeta Gambhir, Hamilton, ON - Family Medicine
Dr Indu B Gambhir, Ottawa, ON - General Practice
Dr Satnam S Gandham, Richmond, BC - General Practice
Dr Prem Gandham, Rosthern, SK - General Practice
Dr Vinod K Gandhi, Delta, BC - Family Medicine
Dr Amita Gandhi, Delta, BC - Psychiatry
Dr Shruti Gandhi, Etobicoke, ON - Medical Biochemistry
Dr Narinder K Garg, Brampton, ON - Family Medicine
Dr Naveen Garg, Pointe-Claire, QC - Family Medicine
Dr Shiva K Gaur, Scarborough, ON - General Practice
Dr Mohammed A Gauri, Fort Saskatchewan, AB - General Practice
Dr Abdul Ghaffar, Brampton, ON - Pediatrics
Dr Sandeep Ghai, Toronto, ON - General Practice
Dr Ikram Ghani, Mississauga, ON - General Practice
Dr Jaspinder Ghuman, Surrey, BC - Emergency Family Med
Dr Ejaz A Ghumman, Leamington, ON - General Surgery
Dr Sadia Gilani, Hamilton, ON - Psychiatry
Dr Satvir Gill, Edmonton, AB - Family Medicine
Dr Manmohanjit S Gill, Abbotsford, BC - General Practice
Dr Karamjit K Gill, Surrey, BC - Hematology
Dr Navdip S Gill, Surrey, BC - Family Medicine
Dr Paramjit Gill, Brampton, ON - Critical Care Medicine
Dr Aneeqa A Gill, London, ON - Family Medicine
Dr Paramjit Gill, Mississauga, ON - General Practice
Dr Vikramjit S Gill, Mississauga, ON - General Practice
Dr Randeep S Gill, Nepean, ON - General Practice
Dr Joginder S Gill, Niagara Falls, ON - Family Medicine
Dr Gurpreet S Gill, Niagara Falls, ON - Internal Medicine
Dr Kulwant S Gill, Sudbury, ON - Hematological Pathology
Dr Davinder S Gill, Windsor, ON - Diagnostic-Radiology
Dr Satpal S Girgla, Oakville, ON - Psychiatry
Dr Devendra P Goel, Burnaby, BC - General Surgery
Dr Rupinder K Gogia, Hamilton, ON - Family Medicine
Dr Manjit Gosal, Abbotsford, BC - General Practice
Dr Rupashi Goswami, Welland, ON - Family Medicine
Dr Supriya M Goyal, Calgary, AB - Family Medicine
Dr Kimmy Goyal, Brampton, ON - Family Medicine
Dr Sarbjit S Grewal, Calgary, AB - General Practice
Dr Kharak S Grewal, Brampton, ON - General Practice
Dr Manavdeep Grewal, Brampton, ON - Family Medicine
Dr Kamal P Grewal, Brampton, ON - Family Medicine
Dr Puneet Grewal, Burlington, ON - Family Medicine
Dr Rajdeep Grewal, Hamilton, ON - Emergency Family Med
Dr Rajwant K Grewal, Mississauga, ON - General Practice
Dr Rasveg S Grewal, Nepean, ON - Cardiology
Dr Anita Grewal, Oakville, ON - Family Medicine
Dr Deepak Grover, Chilliwack, BC - Orthopedic Surgery
Dr Arvinder Grover, Mississauga, ON - Cardiology
Dr Sanjiv K Gulati, Brockville, ON - General Practice
Dr Brij B Gulati, Lindsay, ON - General Practice
Dr Madhu Gupta, Vancouver, BC - Obstetrics & Gynecology
Dr Chander K Gupta, Winnipeg, MB - Obstetrics & Gynecology
Dr Daya K Gupta, Winnipeg, MB - Ophthalmology
Dr Rekha Gupta, Halifax, NS - Anatomical Pathology
Dr Rohit Gupta, Bracebridge, ON - General Surgery
Dr Ram Gupta, Brampton, ON - Family Medicine
Dr Milan Gupta, Brampton, ON - Cardiology
Dr Anil K Gupta, Etobicoke, ON - Family Medicine
Dr Sanjeev Gupta, Mississauga, ON - General Practice
Dr Jagdeep S Gupta, North York, ON - Family Medicine
Dr Hemi Gupta, Sault Ste. Marie, ON - Family Medicine
Dr Vikas Gupta, Toronto, ON - General Practice
Dr Rasna Gupta, Windsor, ON - General Practice
Dr Karmdeep Guram, Mississauga, ON - Diagnostic-Radiology
Dr Kanan Gutgutia, Toronto, ON - General Practice
Dr Jaswant Guzder, Montreal, QC - Psychiatry
Dr Syed Y A Haider, Markham, ON - Orthopedic Surgery
Dr Saima Haleem, Sydney, NS - Family Medicine
Dr Kazi A Hameed, Winnipeg, MB - Internal Medicine
Dr Saadia Hameed, London, ON - Family Medicine
Dr Narpinder Hans, Edmonton, AB - Family Medicine
Dr Iftikhar U Haq, Thunder Bay, ON - Neurosurgery
Dr Upninderjit S Harrad, Surrey, BC - Psychiatry
Dr Sadiq Hasan, Whitby, ON - Psychiatry
Dr Ali Hassan, Brantford, ON - General Practice
Dr Navraj S Heran, New Westminster, BC - Neurosurgery
Dr Manraj K S Heran, Vancouver, BC - Diagnostic-Radiology
Dr Daljit S Herar, Surrey, BC - General Pathology
Dr Mahjabeen Hussain, Calgary, AB - Family Medicine
Dr Syed S Hussain, Saskatoon, SK - Family Medicine
Dr Mohammed A Ibrahim, Brampton, ON - Urology
Dr Mohammad S Ijaz, Regina, SK - General Practice
Dr Kashif Irshad, Brampton, ON - General Surgery
Dr Fauzia Irshad, Mississauga, ON - Family Medicine
Dr Rahmatullah Ishaqzay, Milton, ON - Family Medicine
Dr Pervez Ishrat Ali Khan, Edmonton, AB - General Practice
Dr Muhammad U Islam, Abbotsford, BC - Diagnostic-Radiology
Dr Arif M A Ismaili, Kitchener, ON - Gastroenterology
Dr Rajesh Jaidka, Brampton, ON - General Practice
Dr Sajal Jain, Burnaby, BC - Internal Medicine
Dr Leena Jain, New Westminster, BC - Geriatric Medicine
Dr Nita Jain, Vancouver, BC - Pediatrics
Dr Hem C Jain, Cambridge, ON - Dermatology
Dr Umesh Jain, Toronto, ON - Urology
Dr S Vanita Jassal, Toronto, ON - Internal Medicine
Dr Balvinder S Jassar, Edmonton, AB - Family Medicine
Dr Nasir Jetha, Vancouver, BC - Pediatrics
Dr Kailash K Jindal, Edmonton, AB - Internal Medicine
Dr Azim H Jiwani, West Vancouver, BC - Family Medicine
Dr Malkit K Johal, Toronto, ON - Family Medicine
Dr Krishna Jokhani, Vancouver, BC - Psychiatry
Dr Mala Joneja, Kingston, ON - Internal Medicine
Dr Manohar L Joshi, Etobicoke, ON - General Practice
Dr Baldev S Kahlon, Delta, BC - General Practice
Dr Bharat B Kalra, Scarborough, ON - General Practice
Dr Yamuna Kalyanpur, Vancouver, BC - Obstetrics & Gynecology
Dr Palinder Kamra, St. John's, NL - Pediatrics
Dr Arvind Kang, North Vancouver, BC - Psychiatry
Dr Parmjit S Kang, Surrey, BC - Endocrin/Metabolism
Dr G Shimi Kang, Vancouver, BC - Psychiatry
Dr Amrit K Kang, Toronto, ON - Internal Medicine
Dr Harbhajan S Kang, Montreal, QC - Internal Medicine
Dr Vimal S Kapoor, Markham, ON - Community Medicine
Dr Pankaj V Kapoor, Windsor, ON - General Practice
Dr Nishitha Kapur, Scarborough, ON - Family Medicine
Dr Narendra K Karia, Calgary, AB - General Practice
Dr Savita Karol, Fredericton, NB - Family Medicine
Dr Sukhvinder S Kasbia, Kanata, ON - Family Medicine
Dr Rajendra P Kashyap, Scarborough, ON - General Practice
Dr Hement K Katarey, Oakville, ON - Family Medicine
Dr Satinder Kaur, Kitchener, ON - Family Medicine
Dr Munaa Khaliq-Kareemi, Calgary, AB - Gastroenterology
Dr Safeer A Khan, Calgary, AB - General Practice
Dr Rita R Khan, Kitchener, ON - General Practice
Dr Mahmuda B Khan, Scarborough, ON - Family Medicine
Dr Mohammad A Khan, Melfort, SK - General Practice
Dr M Sohail Khattak, Whitby, ON - Pediatrics
Dr Surinder S Khinda, Fort McMurray, AB - Internal Medicine
Dr Sarjiwan Khullar, Devon, AB - General Practice
Dr J Sevena Khunkhun, Vancouver, BC - Family Medicine
Dr Ajay P S Khural, Carbonear, NL - General Practice
Dr Mona Khurana, Toronto, ON - Family Medicine
Dr Vishwas M Kini, Brampton, ON - Family Medicine
Dr Abbas A Kohja, Steinbach, MB - General Practice
Dr Sukhdev S Kooner, Windsor, ON - Internal Medicine
Dr Saroj Kumar, Delta, BC - General Practice
Dr Rajender Kumar, Sudbury, ON - Psychiatry
Dr Kartar Lal, Grande Prairie, AB - General Practice
Dr Rakesh K Lamba, Abbotsford, BC - Psychiatry
Dr Shazia Latif, Milton, ON - Family Medicine
Dr Natasha B Leighl, Toronto, ON - Internal Medicine
Dr Nirvair K Levitt, Vancouver, BC - Family Medicine
Dr Rizwana Lilani, Maple, ON - Family Medicine
Dr Shashi Lota, Calgary, AB - General Practice
Dr Tahir S Lucman, Winnipeg, MB - Internal Medicine
Dr Sanjeev S Luthra, Brampton, ON - Pediatrics
Dr Meera Luthra, Hamilton, ON - Endocrin/Metabolism
Dr Gyaandeo S Maharajh, Ottawa, ON - Cardiac Surgery
Dr Raj K Mahay, Winnipeg, MB - General Practice
Dr Neelam Mahil, Edmonton, AB - Psychiatry
Dr Shazia T Mahmood, Regina, SK - General Practice
Dr S Asad Mahmud, Moncton, NB - Psychiatry
Dr Bharat Maini, Peterborough, ON - Anesthesia
Dr Arshad Majeed, Oshawa, ON - Psychiatry
Dr Sarah Makhdoom, High River, AB - Family Medicine
Dr Tilak R Malhotra, Prince Albert, SK - Pediatrics
Dr Abdul Malik, Brampton, ON - Family Medicine
Dr Anupam Malik, Brampton, ON - General Practice
Dr Raman Manchanda, Surrey, BC - Family Medicine
Dr Ashok Manga, Delta, BC - Family Medicine
Dr Sandeep Mangat, Placentia, NL - Family Medicine
Dr Alaudin E Manji, Delta, BC - Family Medicine
Dr Baljinder Mann, Calgary, AB - Family Medicine

Dr Tejinder K Mann, New Westminster, BC - General Practice
Dr Satish K Mann, Prince George, BC - Family Medicine
Dr Chaudhry F Masud, Brampton, ON - Family Medicine
Dr M Mohan Merchea, London, ON - Ophthalmology
Dr A Nadeem Mian, Edmonton, AB - Pediatrics
Dr Ahmed R Mian, Toronto, ON - Emergency Family Med
Dr Vishal M Midha, Brampton, ON - Family Medicine
Dr Bilal T Mir, Victoria, BC - Emergency Family Med
Dr Naveed S Mohammad, Etobicoke, ON - General Practice
Dr Solomon Mohammed, Burnaby, BC - General Practice
Dr Rajesh Mohan, Etobicoke, ON - General Practice
Dr Sonali A Mohile, Uxbridge, ON - Pediatrics
Dr Malek B Moosa, Surrey, BC - Family Medicine
Dr Jawaid I Mughal, Mississauga, ON - General Practice
Dr Maqbool A Mughal, Mississauga, ON - General Practice
Dr Naeem H Muhammad, London, ON - Family Medicine
Dr Iffat A Muhammad, Regina, SK - General Practice
Dr Ravi Murthy, Toronto, ON - General Practice
Dr Harpinder S Nagi, Vancouver, BC - Internal Medicine
Dr Rohit S Nagpal, Brampton, ON - Family Medicine
Dr Anil K Nagpal, Kitchener, ON - Internal Medicine
Dr Syed M Najfi, Gander, NL - General Surgery
Dr Bikramjit S Nanar, Mississauga, ON - General Practice
Dr Meenakshi Nanda, Calgary, AB - Family Medicine
Dr Satinder P S Narang, Surrey, BC - Psychiatry
Dr Anuradha Nayar, Vancouver, BC - General Practice
Dr Saiyed M Nazar-Ul-Iman, Winnipeg, MB - General Practice
Dr Nazia S Niazi, Surrey, BC - General Practice
Dr Pravjot K Nijjar, Burnaby, BC - Family Medicine
Dr Veena Nikore, Brantford, ON - General Practice
Dr Amarjit S Nirwan, Victoria, BC - Family Medicine
Dr Lachman D Oad, Wetaskiwin, AB - General Surgery
Dr Kamal K S Ohson, St. John's, NL - Dermatology
Dr Ravinderpal S Ohson, Hamilton, ON - Family Medicine
Dr Rajbir S Pahil, Sydney, NS - General Practice
Dr A Shekhar Pandey, Cambridge, ON - Cardiology
Dr Hemant M Pandhi, Mississauga, ON - General Practice
Dr Sudhir P Pandya, Oakville, ON - Gastroenterology
Dr Dilkhush D Panjwani, Etobicoke, ON - Psychiatry
Dr Sooraja P Papneja, Mississauga, ON - General Practice
Dr Sujata H Parashar, Windsor, ON - Family Medicine
Dr Gurdeep Parhar, Vancouver, BC - General Practice
Dr Jasneet K Parmar, Edmonton, AB - General Practice
Dr Malvinder S Parmar, Timmins, ON - Internal Medicine
Dr Naeem Parvez, Regina, SK - General Practice
Dr Ila M Patel, Mississauga, ON - Family Medicine
Dr Sukhbinderjit K Powar, Oakville, ON - Family Medicine
Dr Punnamkuzhil C Punnen, North York, ON - Urology
Dr Bhupinder S Purewal, Scarborough, ON - General Practice
Dr Mussarrat K Qaadri, Toronto, ON - Obstetrics & Gynecology
Dr Khalida Qazi, Milton, ON - Family Medicine
Dr M Salim Quraishi, London, ON - General Practice
Dr A Quddus Qureshi, Calgary, AB - Family Medicine
Dr Ziaur-Rehman T Qureshi, Calgary, AB - Family Medicine
Dr Irfan T Qureshi, Fort McMurray, AB - Orthopedic Surgery
Dr Azra Qureshi, Scarborough, ON - General Practice
Dr Bushra Qureshy, Toronto, ON - General Practice
Dr Mubeen F Rafay, Winnipeg, MB - General Practice
Dr Afshan Rafay, Mississauga, ON - Family Medicine
Dr Fizza Z Rafiq, Calgary, AB - Family Medicine
Dr Abdul Rahman, Calgary, AB - Psychiatry
Dr Sakina Raj, Calgary, AB - Family Medicine
Dr Faisal S Raja, Kitchener, ON - Diagnostic-Radiology
Dr Shabnam S Rajani, Brampton, ON - General Pathology
Dr Surender K Ralh, North York, ON - General Practice
Dr Pawan K Ram, Surrey, BC - General Practice
Dr Babra M Rana, Burnaby, BC - Psychiatry
Dr Ranjit S Rana, Scarborough, ON - General Practice
Dr Kavita Randhawa, North York, ON - Family Medicine
Dr Mohsin Rashid, Halifax, NS - Pediatrics
Dr Tarsem S Ravi, Mississauga, ON - Family Medicine
Dr Jalees M S Razavi, Calgary, AB - Occupational Med
Dr Bajinder S Reen, Brampton, ON - Internal Medicine
Dr Mehar S Reen, Cornwall, ON - Physical Medicine & Rehab
Dr Ranjodh S Rehal, Winnipeg, MB - General Practice
Dr Waseema Rehman, Glace Bay, NS - Family Medicine
Dr Mujeeb U Rehman, Mississauga, ON - Psychiatry
Dr Ziaur Rehman, Regina, SK - Neurology
Dr Kulwant S Riar, Vancouver, BC - Psychiatry
Dr Rakesh K Rikhye, Etobicoke, ON - General Practice
Dr Syed M H Rizvi, Windsor, ON - General Practice
Dr Jasdip S Sachdeva, Brampton, ON - Internal Medicine
Dr Krishan K Sachdeva, Oshawa, ON - Urology
Dr Arshad Saeed, Ottawa, ON - Family Medicine
Dr Ramesh L Sahjpaul, North Vancouver, BC - Neurosurgery
Dr Saroj Saigal, Hamilton, ON - Pediatrics
Dr Tejinder Sainbhee, Camrose, AB - General Practice
Dr Parampreet Sainbhee, Camrose, AB - Family Medicine
Dr Rajeev Saincher, Surrey, BC - General Practice
Dr Mukesh C Saini, Brampton, ON - General Practice
Dr Joginder K Saini, Kanata, ON - General Practice
Dr Kuljit K Sajjan, Vancouver, BC - Family Medicine
Dr Baljinder S Salh, Vancouver, BC - Gastroenterology
Dr Asim Salim, Brantford, ON - Pediatrics
Dr Imran Samad, Burnaby, BC - Otolaryngology
Dr Gurpal S Sandha, Edmonton, AB - Gastroenterology
Dr Amonpreet K Sandhu, Calgary, AB - Pediatrics
Dr Parminder K Sandhu, Calgary, AB - Family Medicine
Dr Gary G Sandhu, Delta, BC - General Practice
Dr Manbir S Sandhu, New Westminster, BC - General Practice
Dr Jatinder S Sandhu, Surrey, BC - Psychiatry
Dr Dalip S Sandhu, Surrey, BC - General Practice
Dr Sukhbir S Sandhu, Dauphin, MB - Psychiatry
Dr Jasbir K Sandhu, Brampton, ON - General Practice
Dr Satinder K Sanghe, Surrey, BC - Family Medicine
Dr Parminder S Sanghe, Surrey, BC - Family Medicine
Dr Baldev S Sanghera, Burnaby, BC - Family Medicine
Dr Gurinder P Sanghera, Toronto, ON - Ophthalmology
Dr Sheetal Sapra, Oakville, ON - Dermatology
Dr Didar S Sarai, Brampton, ON - Family Medicine
Dr Michael K Sarin, Toronto, ON - Internal Medicine
Dr Brij M Sarup, London, ON - General Practice
Dr Ravinder P S Sawhney, Surrey, BC - Internal Medicine
Dr Gulshan Sawhney, Milton, ON - Internal Medicine
Dr Manoj K Sayal, Oakville, ON - Critical Care Medicine
Dr Dashminder Sehdev, Hamilton, ON - Emergency Family Med
Dr Parmila Sehgal, Etobicoke, ON - General Practice
Dr Jaishree Sehgal, Kitchener, ON - General Practice
Dr Narinder S Sehravat, Etobicoke, ON - Family Medicine
Dr Vir Bhushan Sennik, Mississauga, ON - Orthopedic Surgery
Dr Aditya Seth, Salmon Arm, BC - Ophthalmology
Dr Arun K Seth, Toronto, ON - General Practice
Dr Asha L Seth, Toronto, ON - General Practice
Dr Shilpa Sethi, Middle Musquodoboi, NS - General Practice
Dr Jagmeet Sethi, Cayuga, ON - Internal Medicine
Dr Rajiv Sethi, Etobicoke, ON - Gastroenterology
Dr Chirag R Shah, Calgary, AB - Ophthalmology
Dr Zafar A Shah, London, ON - General Surgery
Dr Muhammad Shahbaz, Calgary, AB - Family Medicine
Dr Sundeep Shahi, Kitchener, ON - Radiation Oncology
Dr Muhammad Shahnawaz, Prince George, BC - Family Medicine
Dr Karina Shahzad, Orangeville, ON - Family Medicine
Dr Bashirunnisa A Shaikh, Etobicoke, ON - General Practice
Dr S Yasmin Shaikh, North York, ON - Family Medicine
Dr Sadia Shakil, Edmonton, AB - General Practice
Dr Kanwal Shankardass, Dundas, ON - General Practice
Dr Sunil Sharad, Waterloo, ON - Internal Medicine
Dr Rajeshvar K Sharda, Hamilton, ON - Ophthalmology
Dr Mohammad S Sharif, Surrey, BC - General Surgery
Dr Pankaj Sharma, Surrey, BC - Family Medicine
Dr Anu K Sharma, Vancouver, BC - General Practice
Dr Sushil K Sharma, Truro, NS - Family Medicine
Dr Shreekant Sharma, Brantford, ON - Psychiatry
Dr Poonam Sharma, Brantford, ON - Psychiatry
Dr Maheshwar D Sharma, Ingersoll, ON - Internal Medicine
Dr Ajay Sharma, London, ON - Pediatrics
Dr Verinder Sharma, London, ON - Psychiatry
Dr Manas Sharma, London, ON - General Practice
Dr Shivani Sharma, Markham, ON - General Practice
Dr Amar D Sharma, Oakville, ON - General Practice
Dr Bal Krishan Sharma, Sarnia, ON - Family Medicine
Dr Vijay Sharma, Scarborough, ON - Anesthesia
Dr Shiv R Sharma, Toronto, ON - Family Medicine
Dr Kawal J Sharma, Toronto, ON - Obstetrics & Gynecology
Dr Malika Sharma, Toronto, ON - Internal Medicine
Dr Om Prakash Sharma, Toronto, ON - Orthopedic Surgery
Dr Madan G Sharman, Regina, SK - General Practice
Dr Anees A Shehzad, Sydney, NS - Family Medicine
Dr Farrukh B Sheikh, Pickering, ON - General Practice
Dr Tasnim K Sheikh, Scarborough, ON - Anatomical Pathology
Dr Khalid M Sheikh, Estevan, SK - General Practice
Dr Syed A R Sherazi, Abbotsford, BC - General Practice
Dr Charudutt D Shete, Langley, BC - General Surgery
Dr Nikita T Sheth, Oakville, ON - Family Medicine
Dr Zia A Sial, Etobicoke, ON - Family Medicine
Dr Zaeem A Siddiqi, Edmonton, AB - General Practice
Dr Nilofar Siddiqi, Owen Sound, ON - Family Medicine
Dr Muzaffar M Siddiqui, Edmonton, AB - Neurology
Dr Mughina A Siddiqui, Antigonish, NS - General Practice
Dr Zubaida Siddiqui, Elliot Lake, ON - Family Medicine
Dr Naveed T Siddiqui, Toronto, ON - General Practice
Dr Parmjit K Sidhu, Abbotsford, BC - Psychiatry
Dr Jiwan S Sidhu, Surrey, BC - Family Medicine
Dr Rabinder S Sidhu, Surrey, BC - Family Medicine
Dr Fulroop Sidhu, Vancouver, BC - General Practice
Dr Tejinder K Sidhu, Victoria, BC - General Practice
Dr Surinder S Sidhu, Brampton, ON - General Practice
Dr Gurmeet Sidhu, Brampton, ON - Family Medicine
Dr Gurpreet S Sidhu, Brantford, ON - General Practice
Dr Gurpreet S Sidhu, London, ON - Psychiatry
Dr Raj K Sidhu, Mississauga, ON - Family Medicine
Dr Kuldeep S Sidhu, North York, ON - Emergency Family Med
Dr Shabana Sikander, Mississauga, ON - Family Medicine
Dr Rajneesh Sikri, Etobicoke, ON - Family Medicine
Dr Mona Singal, Vancouver, BC - Critical Care Medicine
Dr Ram K Singal, Thornhill, ON - General Surgery
Dr Sewa R Singal, Toronto, ON - Internal Medicine
Dr Harjot K Singh, Calgary, AB - General Practice
Dr Ram R Singh, Calgary, AB - Internal Medicine
Dr Paramvinder Singh, Calgary, AB - Family Medicine
Dr Amar Singh, Red Deer, AB - General Practice
Dr Jit J Singh, Delta, BC - General Practice
Dr Kanwal K Singh, Delta, BC - General Practice
Dr Gurwant Singh, Surrey, BC - Neurology
Dr Kanwarjit Singh, Surrey, BC - General Practice
Dr Lakhbir Singh, Vancouver, BC - Family Medicine
Dr Avash J Singh, Vancouver, BC - Pediatrics
Dr Gurdayal Singh, Vancouver, BC - Internal Medicine
Dr Kulbir I Singh, Vancouver, BC - Psychiatry
Dr Ichpal Singh, Bonavista, NL - General Practice
Dr Jaspal Singh, Kentville, NS - Obstetrics & Gynecology
Dr Jagmohan K Singh, Truro, NS - Internal Medicine
Dr Jogindra Singh, Ajax, ON - Physical Medicine & Rehab
Dr Padamjit M Singh, Bowmanville, ON - Obstetrics & Gynecology
Dr Shiv P Singh, Brampton, ON - Family Medicine
Dr Parvinder Singh, Brampton, ON - Family Medicine
Dr Amandeep Singh, Brampton, ON - General Practice
Dr Harleen Singh, Brampton, ON - Family Medicine
Dr Jagdeep Singh, Brampton, ON - Internal Medicine
Dr Baljit Singh, Chatham, ON - Obstetrics & Gynecology
Dr Inderjit Singh, Hamilton, ON - Family Medicine
Dr Barinder Singh, Kingston, ON - Family Medicine
Dr Manbir Singh, Kitchener, ON - Psychiatry
Dr Ravinder Singh, North Bay, ON - General Surgery
Dr S Sony Singh, Ottawa, ON - Obstetrics & Gynecology
Dr Kunwar K Singh, Sarnia, ON - Pediatrics
Dr Tejinder P Singh, Scarborough, ON - Family Medicine
Dr Simron Singh, Toronto, ON - Internal Medicine
Dr Ravinderpal Singh, Toronto, ON - General Practice
Dr Arvind G Singh, Summerside, PE - Psychiatry
Dr Kanwerjit Singh Aujla, Calgary, AB - Family Medicine
Dr Rajinder K Sippy, Brampton, ON - Family Medicine
Dr Surjeet S Sira, Malton, ON - General Surgery
Dr Naila Siraj, Aurora, ON - Family Medicine
Dr Parmjit S Sohal, Surrey, BC - Family Medicine
Dr Avtar S Sohal, Hamilton, ON - Internal Medicine

Dr Barjinder S Sohal, Toronto, ON - Family Medicine
Dr Ravinder K Sohi, Mississauga, ON - Family Medicine
Dr Herpreet S Sohi, North York, ON - General Surgery
Dr Mansurali R Somani, Mission, BC - Family Medicine
Dr Jitin Sondhi, Ingersoll, ON - Family Medicine
Dr Asha P Sondhi, Newmarket, ON - Family Medicine
Dr Ramesh K Soni, Burlington, ON - General Practice
Dr Brijendra Sood, Calgary, AB - General Practice
Dr Alok Sood, Abbotsford, BC - Family Medicine
Dr Balbhadar D Sood, Etobicoke, ON - Psychiatry
Dr Baldev S Soodan, Cornwall, ON - Internal Medicine
Dr Ghazala Sultan, Chatham, ON - Family Medicine
Dr Sumeet K Suneja, Brampton, ON - Internal Medicine
Dr Pal S Sunerh, Etobicoke, ON - General Practice
Dr Sohail Sunner, Brampton, ON - Family Medicine
Dr Priya Suppal, Brampton, ON - Family Medicine
Dr Smeeksha S Sur, Brampton, ON - Pediatrics
Dr Monalisa Sur, Hamilton, ON - Anatomical Pathology
Dr Manindar Surbey, Delta, BC - General Practice
Dr Permjit S Suri, Nepean, ON - Internal Medicine
Dr Shahida Surmawala, Edmonton, AB - Family Medicine
Dr Shveta Suryavanshi, Sarnia, ON - Family Medicine
Dr Rajeev K Suryavanshi, Sarnia, ON - General Surgery
Dr Suresh Syal, Concord, ON - General Practice
Dr Swaran K Syan, Sudbury, ON - Family Medicine
Dr Gurcharan S Syan, Sudbury, ON - Cardiology
Dr Saadat A S Syed, North York, ON - Family Medicine
Dr A Shaista Syed, North York, ON - Family Medicine
Dr Yasmeen Syed, Scarborough, ON - General Practice
Dr Zakaria L T Tadrous, Abbotsford, BC - Ophthalmology
Dr Laeeq A Tahir, Moncton, NB - Psychiatry
Dr Surriya J Tahirkheli, Ottawa, ON - Psychiatry
Dr Jatinder Takhar, London, ON - Psychiatry
Dr Vikas Tandon, Hamilton, ON - Cardiology
Dr Ravi Taneja, London, ON - Anesthesia
Dr Khalida P Tariq, Edmonton, AB - Family Medicine
Dr Muhammad Tasneem, Mississauga, ON - Family Medicine
Dr Kiran D K Tatlay, Windsor, ON - Family Medicine
Dr Syeda N Tauqir Naqvi, Woodstock, ON - Anatomical Pathology
Dr Nazia Tauseef, Courtice, ON - Obstetrics & Gynecology
Dr Kirit V Thakkar, Mississauga, ON - General Practice
Dr Vijay K Thapar, Edmonton, AB - Family Medicine
Dr Lubna T Tirmizi, Pickering, ON - Family Medicine
Dr Dalvinder S Toor, Vancouver, BC - Family Medicine
Dr Davender K Tripathi, Newmarket, ON - Gastroenterology
Dr Hardeep S Tumber, Surrey, BC - General Practice
Dr P Paul S Tumber, Toronto, ON - Anesthesia
Dr Ram S Ubhi, Calgary, AB - General Practice
Dr Surinder K Ubhi, Calgary, AB - Family Medicine
Dr Perminder S Ubhi, Calgary, AB - Physical Medicine & Rehab
Dr Jagdeep S Ubhi, New Westminster, BC - Obstetrics & Gynecology
Dr Verjinderpal S Ubhi, Mississauga, ON - Family Medicine
Dr Mandeep S Ubhi, Saskatoon, SK - Internal Medicine
Dr Rushad T Udwadia, New Westminster, BC - General Surgery
Dr Huma Z Ul Haq, Shelburne, ON - Family Medicine
Dr Farid Ullah, Kelowna, BC - General Practice
Dr Samira Ummat, Vancouver, BC - Physical Medicine & Rehab
Dr Harpreet K Upneja, Windsor, ON - Internal Medicine
Dr Sonia Uppal, Abbotsford, BC - Psychiatry
Dr Rakesh Uppal, Brampton, ON - General Practice
Dr Gayatri Uppal, Ottawa, ON - Family Medicine
Dr Abida Usman, Thornhill, ON - General Practice
Dr Himat Vaghadia, Vancouver, BC - Anesthesia
Dr Seemin A Vahidy, Edmonton, AB - General Practice
Dr Sankar Vaidyanathan, Brampton, ON - Family Medicine
Dr Rajkumar Vajpeyi, Toronto, ON - Anatomical Pathology
Dr Jarnail S Vanvat, Brampton, ON - Family Medicine
Dr Amrit B Varma, Winnipeg, MB - Otolaryngology
Dr Shashi Vashisht, Vancouver, BC - General Practice
Dr Akshya Vasudev, London, ON - General Practice
Dr Manhar L B N Verma, Calgary, AB - Anesthesia
Dr Pramod K Verma, Edmonton, AB - Obstetrics & Gynecology
Dr Kumud Verma, Delta, BC - Family Medicine
Dr Subhash C Verma, Stephenville-Cross, NL - General Practice
Dr Narpendra Verma, Lisle, ON - General Practice
Dr Neil Verma, Richmond Hill, ON - Emergency Family Med
Dr Prem A Verma, Charlottetown, PE - General Practice
Dr Ashok K Verma, Regina, SK - Diagnostic-Radiology
Dr Kamla R Verma, Regina, SK - Psychiatry
Dr Kartar S Vig, London, ON - General Surgery
Dr Meeta Vijh, Brampton, ON - Family Medicine
Dr Manjit S Virdee, Brampton, ON - Family Medicine
Dr Mohan S Virick, Sydney, NS - General Practice
Dr Achla R Virmani, Verdun, QC - General Practice
Dr Asha D Vohra, Burlington, ON - General Practice
Dr Sukh C Vohra, Burlington, ON - General Practice
Dr Pradeep Wadhwa, Calgary, AB - General Practice
Dr Uttam J K Wadhwa, Mississauga, ON - Psychiatry
Dr Atma S Wadhwa, Sturgeon Falls, ON - Internal Medicine
Dr Waqar Waheed, Calgary, AB - Psychiatry
Dr Tamana Walia, Abbotsford, BC - General Practice
Dr Manjit S Walia, Kitchener, ON - Pediatrics
Dr Ihsan U Waraich, Brampton, ON - Family Medicine
Dr Qasim H Wasti, Maple Ridge, BC - Family Medicine
Dr Tehmina Q Wasti, Maple Ridge, BC - Family Medicine
Dr Gagandeep S Wilkhu, Surrey, BC - Family Medicine
Dr Mahesh P Yadav, North Bay, ON - Orthopedic Surgery
Dr Nina K Yashpal, Mississauga, ON - Family Medicine
Dr Saad Yasin, Calgary, AB - Family Medicine
Dr Naveeda Yasmeen, Hamilton, ON - Family Medicine
Dr Kamran Yusuf, Calgary, AB - General Practice
Dr Saira Zafar, London, ON - Internal Medicine
Dr Rosy Zafar, Mississauga, ON - Family Medicine
Dr Khawar-Uz Zaman, Dartmouth, NS - Internal Medicine
Dr Shaista K Zareef, Stittsville, ON - Family Medicine
Dr Mohammad I Zia, Toronto, ON - Cardiology
Dr Naeem A Zubair, Bowmanville, ON - General Practice
Dr Muhammad Zulfiqar, Abbotsford, BC - Internal Medicine

ROMANIAN

Dr Aboobaker Aboo, Ottawa, ON - General Practice
Dr Elsayed E Alamelhuda, Windsor, ON - Family Medicine
Dr Alexandre Alterescu, North York, ON - General Practice
Dr Edith Bandi, Montreal, QC - Anesthesia
Dr Carmen L Benkoczi, Lethbridge, AB - Family Medicine
Dr Patricia Berbari, Gatineau, QC - Plastic Surgery
Dr Adriana N Berbece, Toronto, ON - Internal Medicine
Dr R Dan Boghen, Montreal, QC - Neurology
Dr Gilda A Bowdridge, Halifax, NS - Family Medicine
Dr Ioana Bratu, Edmonton, AB - General Surgery
Dr Sorel L Brohovici, Montreal, QC - General Practice
Dr Daniela Bucur, Montreal, QC - General Practice
Dr Simona C Burs, Calgary, AB - Internal Medicine
Dr Gheorghe V Capusan, La Tuque, QC - General Practice
Dr Tamara Catona, Surrey, BC - Psychiatry
Dr Florina Cealicu Toma, Gatineau, QC - Psychiatry
Dr Maria Cernica, Verdun, QC - General Practice
Dr Margareta Chiorpec-Georgescu, Lachute, QC - General Practice
Dr Sergiu Ciubotaru, Medicine Hat, AB - Family Medicine
Dr Yves J J Clouatre, Penticton, BC - Internal Medicine
Dr Alice Cojocaru, Edmonton, AB - Psychiatry
Dr Gina S A Coleman, Ottawa, ON - General Practice
Dr Alina D Constantin, Canmore, AB - Family Medicine
Dr Cristina Constantinescu, Montreal, QC - Family Medicine
Dr Ioana R Costin, Cambridge, ON - Family Medicine
Dr Andreea Cupsa, Kanata, ON - Family Medicine
Dr Delia Curea, North York, ON - Family Medicine
Dr Silvia L C Dancea, Sudbury, ON - Anatomical Pathology
Dr Adrian B Dancea, Montreal, QC - Cardiology
Dr Virgil Danescu, Abbotsford, BC - Family Medicine
Dr Septimiu C Danescu, Tillsonburg, ON - General Practice
Dr Andre Dascal, Montreal, QC - Infectious Diseases
Dr Razvan Diaconescu, Montreal, QC - Hematology
Dr Mariana Diaconita, North York, ON - Family Medicine
Dr Claudia G Dinu, West Vancouver, BC - Family Medicine
Dr Otilia-Maria Dobrescu, Montreal, QC - Pediatrics
Dr Luiza A A Dumitrescu, Ste-Agathe-Des-Mts, QC - Psychiatry
Dr Nemer El-Batnigi, Oshawa, ON - Emergency Family Med
Dr Anca Facy, Toronto, ON - Family Medicine
Dr C F Cristina Fasie-Neagoe, Pointe-Claire, QC - Family Medicine
Dr Gabriela Franklin, Richmond Hill, ON - Family Medicine
Dr George Freundlich, Matheson, ON - Family Medicine
Dr Anna E Gergely, Courtice, ON - Family Medicine
Dr Camelia M Gheorghe, Richmond Hill, ON - Family Medicine
Dr Gabriela Ghitulescu, Montreal, QC - General Surgery
Dr Rodica Gilca, Quebec, QC - General Practice
Dr Ileana-Maria Gold, Brampton, ON - Anesthesia
Dr Tatiana Golu, Guelph, ON - Family Medicine
Dr Emil-Vasile Grigore, West Lorne, ON - General Practice
Dr Dan J Hancu, North York, ON - Family Medicine
Dr Andrei Harabor, Calgary, AB - Pediatrics
Dr Orly Hermon, Pierrefonds, QC - Family Medicine
Dr Mariana G Hill, North York, ON - Psychiatry
Dr Andrei E Hirsch, Scarborough, ON - General Practice
Dr Gabriela A Horvath, Vancouver, BC - Pediatrics
Dr Elia Huidovici, Windsor, ON - Family Medicine
Dr Diana Ionescu, Vancouver, BC - Anatomical Pathology
Dr Adriana Ionescu, Pointe-Claire, QC - Family Medicine
Dr Claudiu Iordache, Lamont, AB - General Practice
Dr Rodica F Janz, Nelson, BC - Family Medicine
Dr Louai Jony, New Glasgow, NS - Obstetrics & Gynecology
Dr Dan G Katz, Ajax, ON - Physical Medicine & Rehab
Dr Sanda Kaufman-Clain, Saint-Eustache, QC - General Practice
Dr Erzsebet B Kiss, Barrie, ON - Family Medicine
Dr Claude Kortas, London, ON - Internal Medicine
Dr Carmen Kun, Scarborough, ON - General Practice
Dr Vladimir Lafkovici, Digby, NS - Family Medicine
Dr Mihaela F Lapuste, Vancouver, BC - Family Medicine
Dr Diana C Laza, Etobicoke, ON - Family Medicine
Dr Eva M Lonn, Hamilton, ON - Cardiology
Dr Mihai A Manicatide, Toronto, ON - General Practice
Dr Niculina M Margulies, Toronto, ON - Gastroenterology
Dr Ana Marias-Radu, Lac-Megantic, QC - Family Medicine
Dr Alina Marin, Kingston, ON - General Practice
Dr Lavinia M Mascan, Richmond Hill, ON - Family Medicine
Dr Adriana E Mechetiuc, Hamilton, ON - Family Medicine
Dr Elena Mihu, Kinmount, ON - Family Medicine
Dr Jonel Miklea, Hamilton, ON - Family Medicine
Dr Cristina S Mindru, Montreal, QC - Internal Medicine
Dr Hortensia S Mircescu, Montreal, QC - Endocrin/Metabolism
Dr Adina A Moldoveanu, Markham, ON - General Practice
Dr Carmen V Molgat, Kamloops, BC - Psychiatry
Dr Nicolae Molotiu, Strathroy, ON - Anesthesia
Dr Rami S Mozes, Toronto, ON - General Practice
Dr Letitia V Muresan, Dollard-D-Ormeaux, QC - Electroencephal
Dr Marius C Naghiu, London, ON - Family Medicine
Dr Roxana Nechifor, Red Deer, AB - Family Medicine
Dr Roxana Nemes Bratis, Longueuil, QC - General Practice
Dr Doina Nica-Danes, Montreal, QC - General Practice
Dr Melinda Nichols, Penticton, BC - Psychiatry
Dr Alexandru Nicolescu-Zinca, Montreal, QC - Family Medicine
Dr Mihaela Nicula, Oshawa, ON - Geriatric Medicine
Dr Alexandru A F Opris, Toronto, ON - General Practice
Dr Vasiliki Papukna, London, ON - General Practice
Dr Ileana C Parlea, Kitchener, ON - Family Medicine
Dr Silvia Pavlova, Beloeil, QC - General Practice
Dr Ancuta Pepelea, Ste-Anne-de-Bellev, QC - General Practice
Dr Claudia Petrescu, North York, ON - General Practice
Dr Dana Pintea, Burlington, ON - Family Medicine
Dr Mihai Pop, Montreal, QC - Ophthalmology
Dr Cornelia Popa, Dawson Creek, BC - Family Medicine
Dr Brindusa M Popa, Caledon East, ON - Family Medicine
Dr Clara Popa, Rouyn-Noranda, QC - General Practice
Dr Marc Pope, Mississauga, ON - General Surgery
Dr Elena Pope, Toronto, ON - Pediatrics
Dr Oana-Eugenia Popescu, Vancouver, BC - Anatomical Pathology
Dr Adriana L Popescu, Guelph, ON - Family Medicine
Dr Laila Popescu-Dumbrava, Sept-Iles, QC - Family Medicine
Dr Ilija Popovic, Calgary, AB - General Practice
Dr Adrian Pusca, Lac-Megantic, QC - Internal Medicine
Dr Carina G Pusca, Lac-Megantic, QC - General Practice
Dr Morel Rubinger, Winnipeg, MB - Hematology

Dr Rodica Rudner, North York, ON - General Practice
Dr Lenuta Rus-Serban, Pointe-Claire, QC - General Practice
Dr Sina Sajed, Gananoque, ON - Family Medicine
Dr Adrian G Savin, Etobicoke, ON - Family Medicine
Dr Theodor H Schapira, Concord, ON - General Practice
Dr Herawaty Sebajang, Montreal, QC - General Surgery
Dr Zoia Sherman, Windsor, ON - General Practice
Dr Fanny Silviu-Dan, Montreal, QC - Clin Immun/Allergy
Dr Sonia Simion, Montreal, QC - General Practice
Dr John Slanina, Lamont, AB - General Practice
Dr Elionora P Sofronova, Waterloo, ON - Family Medicine
Dr Michael J Sonea, Montreal, QC - Dermatology
Dr Diana C Stancu, West Vancouver, BC - Family Medicine
Dr Rodica Stefaniu, York, ON - Psychiatry
Dr Simona Stiharu, Pierrefonds, QC - Family Medicine
Dr Cristina-Delia Suciu, Brantford, ON - Anesthesia
Dr N Gabriel Suhani, Saint-Eustache, QC - Psychiatry
Dr Daria A Sultan, Montreal, QC - General Practice
Dr Gabriel Szabo, Salaber-de-Valleyf, QC - General Practice
Dr Wanda M Szymonowicz, Mississauga, ON - Pediatrics
Dr Luminita Tandareanu, Montreal, QC - Family Medicine
Dr Anca F Tapardel, Edmonton, AB - Internal Medicine
Dr Olimpia M Timar-Banu, Longueuil, QC - Family Medicine
Dr Ioana Tita, Caledon East, ON - Family Medicine
Dr Lily Toma, Calgary, AB - Family Medicine
Dr Alina Toma, Toronto, ON - Critical Care Medicine
Dr Nicola Toma, Montreal, QC - General Practice
Dr Camelia A Trambitas, Oshawa, ON - Family Medicine
Dr Cristina Tulai, Ottawa, ON - General Practice
Dr Liliana Ulic, Newmarket, ON - Psychiatry
Dr Bogdan-Christian I Ulic, Toronto, ON - Psychiatry
Dr Marica Varga, Toronto, ON - Geriatric Medicine
Dr Gabriela Vasile, Port Moody, BC - Family Medicine
Dr Ovidiu Vasilescu, North York, ON - Family Medicine
Dr Yvonne B Vasilie, Pointe-Claire, QC - Obstetrics & Gynecology
Dr Aneta Veisman, Toronto, ON - Psychiatry
Dr Corina M Velehorschi, Windsor, ON - Psychiatry
Dr Alexa P Veresezan, London, ON - Psychiatry
Dr Avi Wallerstein, Montreal, QC - Ophthalmology
Dr Florin Zaharia, Montreal, QC - General Surgery
Dr Catalina D Zamfir, New Westminster, BC - Family Medicine
Dr Otto Zsigmond, Kamloops, BC - General Practice

RUSSIAN

Dr Farid M Abdel Hadi, Whitby, ON - Obstetrics & Gynecology
Dr Anwar H M Abu Dieh, Kanata, ON - Family Medicine
Dr Alexander L Agranovich, Surrey, BC - Radiation Oncology
Dr Diana R Ahmed, Brantford, ON - Family Medicine
Dr Moses A Alatishe, Moncton, NB - Psychiatry
Dr David Algom, Nepean, ON - Clin Immun/Allergy
Dr Alexander Antonenko, North York, ON - Family Medicine
Dr Grygory Aronshtam, Vancouver, BC - Family Medicine
Dr Taras Babiak, Toronto, ON - Neuro-Pathology
Dr Akerke T Baibergenova, Toronto, ON - Dermatology
Dr Nikolay Baldzhiyski, Bathurst, NB - General Practice
Dr Benjamin Barankin, North York, ON - Dermatology
Dr Tatyana Barankin, North York, ON - Psychiatry
Dr Nadia M Belsky, Etobicoke, ON - General Practice
Dr Svetlana Belyavskaya, Thornhill, ON - General Practice
Dr Oleg D Bendz, Toronto, ON - General Practice
Dr L Jane Berka, North York, ON - Family Medicine
Dr Michael Bezuhly, Halifax, NS - Plastic Surgery
Dr Anna A Blinkina, Cornwall, ON - Family Medicine
Dr Alexandre P Bohdanowicz, Dorchester, ON - General Practice
Dr Hagob A Boyrazian, Scarborough, ON - General Practice
Dr Jeanie Shkimba Brezina, Toronto, ON - General Practice
Dr Mark B Brodsky, North York, ON - General Practice
Dr Michal Broniewski, Calgary, AB - General Practice
Dr Wanda T Brzezinski, Westmount, QC - General Practice
Dr Malgorzata J Buczek, Ottawa, ON - Family Medicine
Dr Margret Budzianowska-Kwiatkowski, Port Coquitlam, BC - Family Medicine
Dr Karina Bukhanov, Toronto, ON - Diagnostic-Radiology
Dr Yury Bulaev, Edmonton, AB - General Practice
Dr Barbara A Cenkowski, Winnipeg, MB - Family Medicine
Dr Elena G Charapova, Ottawa, ON - Family Medicine
Dr Helena Chekina, North York, ON - General Practice
Dr William Chernenkoff, Saskatoon, SK - Family Medicine
Dr Svitlana Cheshenchuk, Regina, SK - Family Medicine
Dr Wojtek P Ciszak, Vancouver, BC - General Practice
Dr Eugene Crystal, Toronto, ON - Cardiology
Dr Shevanta G Daniel, Ajax, ON - Family Medicine
Dr Irena B Darczewski, Winnipeg, MB - Family Medicine
Dr Grace Debosz-Szczerbowski, London, ON - General Practice
Dr George N Djaiani, Toronto, ON - Anesthesia
Dr Victoria Dmitrieva, Maple Ridge, BC - Psychiatry
Dr Andrzej Dobosiewicz, St Catharines, ON - Obstetrics & Gynecology
Dr Anatoly Dobrousin, Edmonton, AB - Family Medicine
Dr Atanas K Dochev, Bridgewater, NS - General Practice
Dr Alex A Donskoy, North York, ON - General Practice
Dr Vadim Dreyzin, Etobicoke, ON - Family Medicine
Dr Helena L Duchowska, Richmond, BC - General Practice
Dr Emmanuelle M J Dudon, Riviere-Du-Loup, QC - Orthopedic Surgery
Dr Elena Dyachuk, Astra, ON - Family Medicine
Dr Roman Elinson, Toronto, ON - Family Medicine
Dr Thaer Elrefai, Ottawa, ON - Family Medicine
Dr Ekaterina P Erendzhinova, Vancouver, BC - Pediatrics
Dr Romana Fagan, Toronto, ON - General Practice
Dr Leandra M Forman, Thornhill, ON - Family Medicine
Dr Gidon Frame, Burnaby, BC - Family Medicine
Dr David M Freedman, Thornhill, ON - Cardiology
Dr Anatoli Freiman, North York, ON - Dermatology
Dr Maria Fuks, Cote Saint-Luc, QC - General Practice
Dr Basheva Furer, North York, ON - General Practice
Dr Priya Gaba, Ottawa, ON - Family Medicine
Dr Ruben Gagarin, Scarborough, ON - Psychiatry
Dr Vlade M Gagovski, North York, ON - General Practice
Dr Elizabeth Galanter, Oakville, ON - Pediatrics
Dr Lena Galimova, Winnipeg, MB - Physical Medicine & Rehab
Dr Asmitha Gangani, Aurora, ON - Family Medicine
Dr Leila Gibson, Saskatoon, SK - General Practice
Dr Rodica Gilca, Quebec, QC - General Practice
Dr Frina Gofman, North York, ON - General Practice
Dr Peter D Golin, Vancouver, BC - General Practice
Dr Olga Gorodetsky, Newmarket, ON - Family Medicine
Dr Galina Gotesman, North York, ON - Geriatric Medicine
Dr Igor Goussev, Ajax, ON - General Surgery
Dr Julia Grebenyuk, Vaughan, ON - Diagnostic-Radiology
Dr Natalie Grizenko, Verdun, QC - Psychiatry
Dr Zuzana Gross, Thornhill, ON - General Practice
Dr Liuba Grossman, North York, ON - General Practice
Dr Svetoslav A Gueordjev, Nelson, BC - General Practice
Dr Pavel Hamet, Montreal, QC - Endocrinology
Dr Velizar A Harizanov, Toronto, ON - General Practice
Dr Omar N Hasan, Amqui, QC - General Surgery
Dr Victor Hoffstein, Toronto, ON - Respirology
Dr Grazyna W Hofner, Truro, NS - Psychiatry
Dr Sophie L R Hofstader, Scarborough, ON - Dermatology
Dr Stefan Horny, Montreal, QC - General Practice
Dr Tetyana Y Hurmatov, St Catharines, ON - General Practice
Dr Vadim B Ilivitsky, Ottawa, ON - Psychiatry
Dr Jeewani Irfan, Port au Choix, NL - General Practice
Dr T N Teodor Ivanov, Pitt Meadows, BC - Family Medicine
Dr Marek A Jung, Calgary, AB - Internal Medicine
Dr Leszek Kalinowski, Vancouver, BC - General Practice
Dr Ilko S Karagiozov, Scarborough, ON - Family Medicine
Dr John Kargbo, Sault Ste. Marie, ON - Emergency Family Med
Dr Maryna Karpiyevich, Spruce Grove, AB - Family Medicine
Dr Larissa Kasianik, Kincardine, ON - Family Medicine
Dr Danuta Katarzyniak-Kunysz, Lebel-s-Quevillon, QC - General Practice
Dr Petr Kavan, Montreal, QC - General Practice
Dr Rita M Kharonsky, North York, ON - Family Medicine
Dr Yaariv Khaykin, Newmarket, ON - Cardiology
Dr Herbert I Khosid, Thornhill, ON - General Practice
Dr Natan L Khotianov, North York, ON - Family Medicine
Dr Alla Kirshner, Winnipeg, MB - Psychiatry
Dr Irina Kirtsman, Cornwall, ON - Pediatrics
Dr Dmitry D Kisselgoff, Thunder Bay, ON - General Practice
Dr Oleg Klipitch, Etobicoke, ON - Family Medicine
Dr Klara Koblents, Woodbridge, ON - General Practice
Dr Izabella Kogan, Alliston, ON - Family Medicine
Dr Eva Kogan, Markham, ON - Endocrin/Metabolism
Dr Maxim V Kondrashov, Regina, SK - Family Medicine
Dr Eleonor Kopylenko, Newmarket, ON - Family Medicine
Dr Svetlana Korkuczanska, Vancouver, BC - Psychiatry
Dr Michael Kounine, Whitby, ON - Psychiatry
Dr Vitezslava V Kozel, Englehart, ON - General Practice
Dr Marina Krasnopolsky, North York, ON - General Practice
Dr Andrei Krassioukov, Vancouver, BC - Physical Medicine & Rehab
Dr Jozef Krop, Mississauga, ON - General Practice
Dr Karol Kuperberg, Montreal, QC - General Practice
Dr Jirair Kuyumjian, Montreal, QC - General Practice
Dr Abdulrahem L A Laftah, Summerside, PE - Family Medicine
Dr Vladimir Lakher, Coquitlam, BC - General Practice
Dr Galina Langer, Thornhill, ON - Cardiology
Dr Waldemar Lazowski, Souris, PE - Family Medicine
Dr Ilona Levin, Lethbridge, AB - General Practice
Dr Alexander L Levin, Vancouver, BC - Psychiatry
Dr Mykhaylo V Levinskyy, Edmonton, AB - General Practice
Dr Vitaly A Liashko, Moncton, NB - Psychiatry
Dr Hanna Lotocka-Reysner, Burnaby, BC - Pediatrics
Dr Nibal Lubbad, Burlington, ON - Family Medicine
Dr Krzysztof Lubkiewicz, Pointe-Claire, QC - Pediatrics
Dr Michael Lucewicz, Edmonton, AB - General Practice
Dr Nikita A Makretsov, Vancouver, BC - Anatomical Pathology
Dr Ekatherena V Maltseva, North York, ON - Family Medicine
Dr Edward Margolin, Toronto, ON - Ophthalmology
Dr Aleksander Maslowski, Pickering, ON - Family Medicine
Dr Alexander Matz, Lindsay, ON - General Surgery
Dr Stanley T Maziarz, Gatineau, QC - Family Medicine
Dr Daniel Melamedov, Thornhill, ON - General Surgery
Dr Ekaterina Melcuk, Montreal, QC - Pediatrics
Dr Ellen Melton, Thunder Bay, ON - Internal Medicine
Dr Ladislav Mesensky, Etobicoke, ON - General Practice
Dr Yuri L Metelitsa, Calgary, AB - General Practice
Dr Roumen Milev, Kingston, ON - Psychiatry
Dr Slobodan Milosevic, Louiseville, QC - General Practice
Dr Yuri Moltyaner, Brampton, ON - Internal Medicine
Dr W Hanna Moore, Woodbridge, ON - General Practice
Dr Wojciech Morzycki, Halifax, NS - Internal Medicine
Dr Ihor R Mota, Vancouver, BC - Family Medicine
Dr Olga Moukhortova-Von Lipinski, Vancouver, BC - Obstetrics & Gynecology
Dr Anushi T Mousa, London, ON - Family Medicine
Dr Arakel Movsesyan, Hamilton, ON - General Practice
Dr Basdeo Nankissoor, Edmonton, AB - Family Medicine
Dr Daiva L Norkus, Etobicoke, ON - Family Medicine
Dr Richard Novick, London, ON - Cardiovasc/ThorSurg
Dr Malgorzata J M Nowaczyk, Hamilton, ON - Pediatrics
Dr Zbigniew J Nowak, Miramichi, NB - General Practice
Dr Bohdan Olearczyk, Toronto, ON - General Practice
Dr Beatrice K Osoro, Keswick, ON - Family Medicine
Dr Vladislav L Ovchinnikov, East York, ON - Cardiology
Dr Mariusz T Paszkiewicz, Weyburn, SK - General Practice
Dr Katerina Pavenski, Toronto, ON - Hematology
Dr Silvia Pavlova, Beloeil, QC - General Practice
Dr Irina E Payne, North Vancouver, BC - Family Medicine
Dr Vsevolod S Perelman, Toronto, ON - Emergency Family Med
Dr Paul Perlon, Richmond Hill, ON - Emergency Family Med
Dr Rima Petroniene, Barrie, ON - Internal Medicine
Dr Elena Petrov, Calgary, AB - Psychiatry
Dr Sara Pliamm, North York, ON - General Practice
Dr Henryk Pluta, Abbotsford, BC - Internal Medicine
Dr Gregory M Polyakov, Vancouver, BC - General Surgery
Dr Galina G Portnoi, Thornhill, ON - Family Medicine
Dr Emmanuelle Pourcher, Quebec, QC - Neurology
Dr Viachislav Prigozhikh, North York, ON - General Practice
Dr Waldemar Pruzanski, Toronto, ON - Internal Medicine
Dr Samar Raad, Temiscaming, QC - Family Medicine
Dr Valentyna B Rembez, Vancouver, BC - Family Medicine
Dr Maria Richardson, Toronto, ON - Family Medicine
Dr Alex S Rivlin, North York, ON - General Practice

Dr Inna Roitberg, Thornhill, ON - Family Medicine
Dr Ella A Ross, Vanier, ON - Ophthalmology
Dr Larissa Roux, Richmond, BC - Family Medicine
Dr Roman R Rozencwaig, Montreal, QC - General Practice
Dr Eugene G Sacevich, Thunder Bay, ON - General Practice
Dr Evgeny A Sadikov, Regina, SK - General Practice
Dr Amal K Saha, Halifax, NS - Family Medicine
Dr Krystyna Salach-Markiewicz, Mississauga, ON - General Practice
Dr Hassan Sannoufi, Kanata, ON - Emergency Family Med
Dr Marina Sapozhnikov, Tofield, AB - General Practice
Dr Oleg A Savenkov, Hamilton, ON - Psychiatry
Dr Jan I Schulz, Montreal, QC - Clin Immun/Allergy
Dr Bogdan L Schwarz-Michorowski, Guelph, ON - Cardiology
Dr Mladen Seidl, Etobicoke, ON - General Practice
Dr Zygmunt P Sekula, Halifax, NS - General Practice
Dr Manivannan Selvananthan, Scarborough, ON - Family Medicine
Dr Tatyana Selyanina, Mississauga, ON - Family Medicine
Dr Senthe S Senthelal, Mississauga, ON - Radiation Oncology
Dr Danielle Sergeeva, Maple Ridge, BC - Family Medicine
Dr Shilpa Sethi, Middle Musquodoboi, NS - General Practice
Dr Yakov Shapiro, Edmonton, AB - Psychiatry
Dr Sergey Shapiro, Toronto, ON - Psychiatry
Dr Raisa Sheftel, Verdun, QC - General Practice
Dr Zoia Sherman, Windsor, ON - General Practice
Dr Ludmila A Shimanovsky, Vaughan, ON - Family Medicine
Dr Jaroslav O Shklar, Etobicoke, ON - General Practice
Dr Jakov Shlik, Ottawa, ON - General Practice
Dr Doron Shmorgun, Ottawa, ON - Obstetrics & Gynecology
Dr Lesya M Shuba, Halifax, NS - Ophthalmology
Dr Evelyn K Shukin, Surrey, BC - General Practice
Dr Jana Sidorov, Prince George, BC - General Practice
Dr Danguole Sileikiene, Red Deer, AB - Anatomical Pathology
Dr Christopher R R Skinner, Ottawa, ON - Internal Medicine
Dr Robert Skomro, Saskatoon, SK - Internal Medicine
Dr Nataliya Skuridina, North Vancouver, BC - Public Health & Preventive Medicine
Dr Anna Slavina, North York, ON - Family Medicine
Dr Dagmar Smatanova, Victoria, BC - Family Medicine
Dr Marek A Smolarkiewicz, Stephenville, NL - General Practice
Dr Galina Smushkin, Victoria, BC - General Practice
Dr Elisabeth K Sochocka, Milton, ON - General Practice
Dr Elionora P Sofronova, Waterloo, ON - Family Medicine
Dr Elena A Sokolova, Thunder Bay, ON - General Practice
Dr Natalia Solomon, Edmonton, AB - Medical Microbiology
Dr Elena Somska, Toronto, ON - General Practice
Dr Janna Soubbotina, Langley, BC - Family Medicine
Dr Elena A Sourovtseva, Oakville, ON - Family Medicine
Dr Jan Spacek, Sherbrooke, QC - General Practice
Dr Blaga A Stancheva, Vancouver, BC - Family Medicine
Dr Jitka Stankova, Montreal, QC - General Practice
Dr Arthur Staroselsky, Thornhill, ON - Family Medicine
Dr Vasia Stefou, Toronto, ON - General Practice
Dr Galina Strovskaia, Surrey, BC - Family Medicine
Dr Semion Strovski, Surrey, BC - Family Medicine
Dr Emile D Svarc, Montreal, QC - Ophthalmology
Dr Oleksandr I Svystonyuk, Newmarket, ON - Obstetrics & Gynecology
Dr Ewa Swoboda, Toronto, ON - Psychiatry
Dr Michael Szpilberg, Montreal, QC - General Practice
Dr Ewa F Szumacher, Toronto, ON - Radiation Oncology
Dr Waldemar A Szymanski, Edmonton, AB - Pediatrics
Dr Inaa A Tcherenkova, La Loche, SK - Family Medicine
Dr Andrei G Tchernov, Thornhill, ON - Family Medicine
Dr Milka A Tchervenkova, Brossard, QC - General Practice
Dr Alexander Tischenko, Winnipeg, MB - Cardiology
Dr Paul J Tkalych, Calgary, AB - General Practice
Dr Christo Todorov, Montreal, QC - Psychiatry
Dr Janny Tomashpolskaya, Etobicoke, ON - Diagnostic-Radiology
Dr Anna A Toptchieva, East York, ON - Anesthesia
Dr Anna A Trzcieniecka, Delhi, ON - Family Medicine
Dr Oleg Tugalev, Woodstock, ON - Physical Medicine & Rehab
Dr Elena Tugaleva, London, ON - Anatomical Pathology
Dr Victoria E Tuvivovich, Salaber-de-Valleyf, QC - General Practice
Dr Shoshana Urson, Richmond Hill, ON - Psychiatry
Dr Michael Varenbut, Richmond Hill, ON - Family Medicine
Dr Astghik Vartanian, Montreal, QC - General Practice
Dr Nataliya V Vasylevych, Oakville, ON - Family Medicine
Dr Albina Veltman, Hamilton, ON - Psychiatry
Dr Frantisek Vetiska, Oakville, ON - General Practice
Dr Nataliya V Vostretsova, Richmond, BC - Family Medicine
Dr Zohar Waisman, North York, ON - Psychiatry
Dr Wahan Wanis, Vancouver, BC - Psychiatry
Dr Ewa B Wesolowska, Montreal, QC - Medical Biochemistry
Dr Jana Wieder, Halifax, NS - General Practice
Dr Igor S Wilderman, Thornhill, ON - Family Medicine
Dr Krystyna H Wojakowski, London, ON - Psychiatry
Dr Wladyslaw Wojcik, Regina, SK - Internal Medicine
Dr Tatiana Y Yakubovich, Abbotsford, BC - General Practice
Dr Susanna Yanivker, Hamilton, ON - General Practice
Dr Alexandre N Yatsina, Saskatoon, SK - General Practice
Dr Irina Yelenbaugen, North York, ON - General Practice
Dr Pawel G Zalewski, Oshawa, ON - Internal Medicine
Dr Dmitrij Zanozin, Prince George, BC - Family Medicine
Dr Alexander Zhivkov, Fort-Coulonge, QC - General Practice

RUTOORO

Dr Saturday N A Nsisi, Lethbridge, AB - General Practice

SERBIAN

Dr Sanja Avdic, Toronto, ON - Pediatrics
Dr Hifzija H Bajramovic, Ottawa, ON - Psychiatry
Dr Ivan Barac, Winnipeg, MB - General Practice
Dr Nada Bodruzic, Strathmore, AB - General Practice
Dr Svetlana Cakarevic, Ottawa, ON - Family Medicine
Dr Nebojsa Denic, St. John's, NL - Anatomical Pathology
Dr Roy R Diklich, Windsor, ON - General Practice
Dr Bojana Djordjevic, Ottawa, ON - Anatomical Pathology
Dr Milla Djuricic, Orleans, ON - Family Medicine
Dr Aleksandra Dlacic, North York, ON - Anesthesia
Dr Marijana Drandic, Ajax, ON - Psychiatry
Dr Dragoslav Drca, Orleans, ON - General Practice
Dr Milutin Drobac, North York, ON - Cardiology
Dr Olga Dzever, Etobicoke, ON - Family Medicine
Dr Petar Erdeljan, Scarborough, ON - Urology
Dr Nenad Gagic, Hamilton, ON - General Surgery
Dr Vlade M Gagovski, North York, ON - General Practice
Dr Desanka Gajic, Toronto, ON - General Practice
Dr Mirjana Garic, Burlington, ON - Family Medicine
Dr Aleksander Georgievski, Thornhill, ON - General Practice
Dr Filip Gilic, Trenton, ON - Emergency Family Med
Dr Ljubica Gulan-Vujnovic, Toronto, ON - General Practice
Dr Velizar A Harizanov, Toronto, ON - General Practice
Dr Ljiljana Jaksic-Tomanovic, Toronto, ON - Family Medicine
Dr Alexandra Jevremovic, Richmond Hill, ON - Cardiology
Dr Sanja Karalic, North Vancouver, BC - Family Medicine
Dr Djordje Kljajic, Vancouver, BC - General Practice
Dr Diana Kljenak, Toronto, ON - Psychiatry
Dr Tilda Konforte-Vasiljevic, St Stephen, NB - General Practice
Dr Ljiljana Kordic, Delta, BC - Family Medicine
Dr Karol Kuperberg, Montreal, QC - General Practice
Dr Dusan Lukic, Hamilton, ON - General Practice
Dr Borislava Mijavec, Orleans, ON - Family Medicine
Dr Mirko Miladinovic, North York, ON - Anatomical Pathology
Dr Ljiljana Miladinovic, Toronto, ON - Family Medicine
Dr Svetlana Milenkovic, Toronto, ON - Psychiatry
Dr Slobodan Milosevic, Louiseville, QC - General Practice
Dr Nikolina Mizdrak, Toronto, ON - Family Medicine
Dr Dijana Oliver, Kingston, ON - Psychiatry
Dr Jelena Pekez, Edmonton, AB - Family Medicine
Dr Danica Petrovic, Vancouver, BC - General Practice
Dr Petr Polasek, Kelowna, BC - Cardiology
Dr Stanislav Popovic, Toronto, ON - Internal Medicine
Dr Jelena Popovic, Toronto, ON - Pediatrics
Dr Zorana Prelevic, Montreal, QC - Psychiatry
Dr Nikola Preradovic, Oakville, ON - Family Medicine
Dr Djordje G Radisic, Edmonton, AB - Pediatrics
Dr Dubravka Rakic, Calgary, AB - Family Medicine
Dr Miodrag A Ristic, Windsor, ON - General Surgery
Dr George Sakotic, North York, ON - Anesthesia
Dr Mile Savic, Belleville, ON - Family Medicine
Dr Ljubinka Segedi, Kitchener, ON - Family Medicine
Dr Dusan Sijan, Windsor, ON - General Practice
Dr Jovan G Simeon, Vanier, ON - Psychiatry
Dr Dino Smiljic, Banff, AB - Family Medicine
Dr Bojana Solaric, Toronto, ON - Anesthesia
Dr Stoyan Solarich, North York, ON - General Practice
Dr Rajka Soric, Toronto, ON - Physical Medicine & Rehab
Dr Aleksandra Stefanovic, Vancouver, BC - Infectious Diseases
Dr Chris P Stefanovich, Etobicoke, ON - Family Medicine
Dr Snezana Stegnajic, East York, ON - Family Medicine
Dr Katica Sumanac, Dundas, ON - Family Medicine
Dr Emile D Svarc, Montreal, QC - Ophthalmology
Dr Ratka Timarac, Hamilton, ON - General Practice
Dr Cedomirka Todorovic, Port Moody, BC - Family Medicine
Dr Inge Vasovich, Hamilton, ON - General Practice
Dr Peter M Vignjevic, Hamilton, ON - Dermatology
Dr Josip Vlahovich, Toronto, ON - General Practice
Dr Peter D Vlaovic, East York, ON - Urology
Dr Branislav Vlaovic, East York, ON - General Practice
Dr Neda Vujicic, North York, ON - Family Medicine
Dr Predrag Vujnovic, Toronto, ON - General Practice
Dr Snezana Vukmirovic-Popovic, Hamilton, ON - Anatomical Pathology
Dr Duska Vukojevic, Belleville, ON - General Practice
Dr Ljubomir Vukovic, Kingston, ON - Otolaryngology
Dr Milorad Vukovic, Scarborough, ON - Psychiatry

SERBO-CROATIAN

Dr Zeljko Bolesnikov, Fredericton, NB - General Practice
Dr Grlica Bolesnikov, Fredericton, NB - General Practice
Capt Katarina Bozic, Edmonton, AB - Family Medicine
Dr Velizar A Harizanov, Toronto, ON - General Practice
Dr Diana Kljenak, Toronto, ON - Psychiatry
Dr Jonel Miklea, Hamilton, ON - Family Medicine
Dr Amira Muncner, Edmonton, AB - General Practice
Dr Dragana Pilavdzic, Montreal, QC - Anatomical Pathology
Dr Ilija Popovic, Calgary, AB - General Practice
Dr Jelena Popovic, Toronto, ON - Pediatrics
Dr Henry I Quaye, Stony Plain, AB - General Practice
Dr Said Secerbegovic, Watson Lake, YT - General Practice
Dr Vesna Tokic, Vancouver, BC - Family Medicine
Dr Peter M Vignjevic, Hamilton, ON - Dermatology
Dr Darija Vujosevic, St Catharines, ON - Family Medicine
Dr Duska Vukojevic, Belleville, ON - General Practice

SHANGHAI

Dr Peter P Chang, Toronto, ON - Psychiatry
Dr Jim I Cheng, Sherwood Park, AB - Community Medicine
Dr Ying Lai H Toong, Toronto, ON - General Practice
Dr Smiley G S Tsao, Unionville, ON - Family Medicine
Dr Yue Wang, Surrey, BC - Family Medicine
Dr Peter B Yang, Burnaby, BC - General Practice
Dr Frank W L Yue, Vancouver, BC - General Practice
Dr Kang-Min Zhu, Cranbrook, BC - Diagnostic-Radiology

SHONA

Dr Christopher Mpofu, Saskatoon, SK - Pediatrics

SIGN LANGUAGE

Dr Marcia D Benjamin, Barrie, ON - Psychiatry
Dr Lori R Coman-Wood, Mississauga, ON - General Practice
Dr E Lock, Amherst, NS - Psychiatry

SINDHI

Dr Jayshree Chanchlani, Brampton, ON - General Practice
Dr Anil K Khithani, Scarborough, ON - Family Medicine
Dr Kartar Lal, Grande Prairie, AB - General Practice

Dr Abdul Malik, Brampton, ON - Family Medicine
Dr Lachman D Oad, Wetaskiwin, AB - General Surgery
Dr Rita Selby, Toronto, ON - Hematology

SINHALESE

Dr Chitralekha R Abeysinghe, Markham, ON - Family Medicine
Dr Jeyaranee Aloysius, Halifax, NS - Family Medicine
Dr Sukeshini Amarasekera, Scarborough, ON - Pediatrics
Dr Pradeepan Arulchelvam, Scarborough, ON - Family Medicine
Dr Bhamini Balachandra, Edmonton, AB - Psychiatry
Dr Thambirajah Balachandra, Winnipeg, MB - Anatomical Pathology
Dr B Leonard Chandrarajan, Kingston, ON - Family Medicine
Dr Ranjith D Chandrasena, Chatham, ON - Psychiatry
Dr Chandima Chandrasena, Ottawa, ON - Family Medicine
Dr Shyamali Damboragama, Brantford, ON - Family Medicine
Dr Shevanta G Daniel, Ajax, ON - Family Medicine
Dr Sudarshan Devanesen, Mississauga, ON - Family Medicine
Dr Sivakumaran Devarajan, Chatham, ON - Psychiatry
Dr Mohamed B H Faizer, Cornwall, ON - General Surgery
Dr Joseph Fernando, Edmonton, AB - General Practice
Dr F Priyalal Fernando, Windsor, ON - Psychiatry
Dr M Lakshman Fernando, Woodstock, ON - Psychiatry
Dr Victor J Figurado, Mississauga, ON - General Practice
Dr Sujeewa D Fonseka, Milton, ON - Family Medicine
Dr Ajantha Gnanabaskaran, Dawson Creek, BC - Family Medicine
Dr Sangarapillai Gnanabaskaran, Dawson Creek, BC - General Practice
Dr Kandiah P Gnanendran, Windsor, ON - Anesthesia
Dr Aiyathurai Gnaneswaran, Oshawa, ON - Psychiatry
Dr Selvaratnam Gunaratnam, Georgetown, ON - Obstetrics & Gynecology
Dr S Yamuna Gunawardena, Richmond Hill, ON - Pediatrics
Dr Milanthi Hapuarachchi, Milton, ON - Family Medicine
Dr Dimithra N Hippola, Vancouver, BC - Family Medicine
Dr Manel R Imbulgoda, Waterdown, ON - Family Medicine
Dr Mohamed H Irfan, Port au Choix, NL - Family Medicine
Dr Jeewani Irfan, Port au Choix, NL - General Practice
Dr D Sushila Jayasuriya, Ottawa, ON - Psychiatry
Dr Coomarasamy Kirupananthan, Scarborough, ON - Obstetrics & Gynecology
Dr Dayananda Kodagoda, Sydney, NS - Family Medicine
Dr Sandhya Kurukula Arachchi, London, ON - Family Medicine
Dr Sujatha M Lena, Ottawa, ON - Pediatrics
Dr Varagunan Mahadevan, Uxbridge, ON - Family Medicine
Dr Gnanindra N Manawadu, Mississauga, ON - Family Medicine
Dr William A D Mather, Scarborough, ON - Family Medicine
Dr Tilak Mendis, Ottawa, ON - Neurology
Dr Roubiya S Mohamed, Scarborough, ON - Family Medicine
Dr Anushi T Mousa, London, ON - Family Medicine
Dr Arumairajah Muhunthan, Sarnia, ON - General Surgery
Dr Jothimalar Muhunthan, Sarnia, ON - Neurology
Dr Rock R X Mylvaganam, Ottawa, ON - Psychiatry
Dr Sivakumar Nagamuttu, Markham, ON - Family Medicine
Dr Nirmaladevi Ollegasagrem, Saskatoon, SK - Family Medicine
Dr W Malathi D Pereira, Mississauga, ON - Internal Medicine
Dr Thurairajasingham Ponnampalam, Scarborough, ON - Family Medicine
Dr Thusitha Premachandra, Ottawa, ON - General Practice
Dr Savithiri Ratnapalan, Toronto, ON - Pediatrics
Dr Umesh Rayar, Brampton, ON - Pediatrics
Dr Mallika M Samarasena, St. John's, NL - General Practice
Dr Niranjala Satkunam, Edmonton, AB - General Pathology
Dr Manivannan Selvananthan, Scarborough, ON - Family Medicine
Dr Savitri C Senaratne, Edmonton, AB - Internal Medicine
Dr Senthe S Senthelal, Mississauga, ON - Radiation Oncology
Dr Sashikala Senthelal, Mississauga, ON - Psychiatry
Dr Sockalingam Senthillmohan, Cleveland, NS - General Practice
Dr Krishanthy Shu, London, ON - Family Medicine
Dr Ponnuthurai Sivaji, Scarborough, ON - Internal Medicine
Dr Panchasheila Sivakumar, Scarborough, ON - Family Medicine
Dr Kalawathy Sivarajah, Bathurst, NB - Anatomical Pathology
Dr Ramanan Sivasundaram, Regina, SK - Family Medicine
Dr Sukumar D Solomon, Mississauga, ON - General Practice
Dr Subramanian Sothilingam, Brampton, ON - Family Medicine
Dr Shanthini Sundareswaran, Mississauga, ON - Family Medicine
Dr Niththialuxmy Thamotharam, Scarborough, ON - Family Medicine
Dr Jeyasakthy J Thayaparan, Richmond Hill, ON - Internal Medicine
Dr Vakeesan Thirugnanasampanthapillai, Brampton, ON - Family Medicine
Dr Arulanandam Varadarasa, Brampton, ON - Internal Medicine
Dr Veeragathy Vasanthan, Clarenville, NL - General Practice
Dr Visvalingam Vijayaratnam, Toronto, ON - Gastroenterology
Dr Franklyn A Vincent, Halifax, NS - Family Medicine
Dr Piyal L Walpola, Pickering, ON - Family Medicine
Dr Nandanie Weerasinghe, Edmonton, AB - General Practice
Dr Senani D Wickramasinghe, Cornwall, ON - Pediatrics
Dr Sheila Wijayasinghe, Toronto, ON - Family Medicine
Dr Rajalaximi Wong, North Bay, ON - Anesthesia
Dr Tsing San Wong, North Bay, ON - Obstetrics & Gynecology

SLAVIC

Dr Jeanie Shkimba Brezina, Toronto, ON - General Practice

SLOVAK

Dr Julius Alexy, Selkirk, MB - General Practice
Dr Karolina Altmann, London, ON - General Practice
Dr Frantisek Beck, Burnaby, BC - Family Medicine
Dr Timea Belej-Rak, Vaughan, ON - Obstetrics & Gynecology
Dr Branislav Belovic, Oakville, ON - Dermatology
Dr L Jane Berka, North York, ON - Family Medicine
Dr Fred R Besik, Mississauga, ON - General Practice
Dr Anna Chlebak, Langley, BC - General Practice
Dr Jarmila Chrappa, Corner Brook, NL - Pediatrics
Dr Sonia M Cruickshanks, Newmarket, ON - Psychiatry
Dr Janina H Dutkiewicz-Stvrtecky, Oakville, ON - General Practice
Dr Vladimir Dzavik, Toronto, ON - Cardiology
Dr Bassam El-Tatari, Windsor, ON - Family Medicine
Dr Romana Fagan, Toronto, ON - General Practice
Dr Angelica M Fargas-Babjak, Hamilton, ON - Anesthesia
Dr Katarina Fiala, Toronto, ON - Dermatology
Dr Jarmila E Fiser, Oshawa, ON - Anatomical Pathology
Dr Alexander Gabor, Newmarket, ON - General Practice
Dr Joseph Gasser, Toronto, ON - Ophthalmology
Dr Marie Grabec, Hamilton, ON - General Practice
Dr Paul Gregor, Hamilton, ON - General Surgery
Dr Peter A Gresko, Windsor, ON - General Practice
Dr Zuzana Gross, Thornhill, ON - General Practice
Dr Yemisrach Hailemeskel, Toronto, ON - Family Medicine
Dr Mario A Halenar, West Vancouver, BC - General Practice
Dr Peter W Harding, Gloucester, ON - Ophthalmology
Dr Emilia Hlusek, North Bay, ON - Psychiatry
Dr Evelyn M Honsl, Ottawa, ON - General Practice
Dr Ladislav Horak, North York, ON - General Practice
Dr Stefan Horny, Montreal, QC - General Practice
Dr Vaclav R Hoyer, Calgary, AB - General Practice
Dr Joseph Hrncirik, Miramichi, NB - General Practice
Dr Eva M Jokay, Etobicoke, ON - Psychiatry
Dr Tibor Juda, Toronto, ON - Urology
Dr Marianna M Kapala, Mississauga, ON - General Surgery
Dr Helen Karsai, Vancouver, BC - General Practice
Dr Jana Krajbich, Calgary, AB - Family Medicine
Dr Milos J Krajny, Toronto, ON - Internal Medicine
Dr Igor Krizan, Corner Brook, NL - General Practice
Dr Elena Lisiak, Vancouver, BC - Psychiatry
Dr Eva Lorber, Toronto, ON - General Practice
Dr Stanley T Maziarz, Gatineau, QC - Family Medicine
Dr Bohdan Molckovsky, Mississauga, ON - General Practice
Dr Amira Muncner, Edmonton, AB - General Practice
Dr Etela Neumann, Vancouver, BC - Neuro-Pathology
Dr Viktor Neumann, Vancouver, BC - General Practice
Dr Jana Nigrin, Edmonton, AB - Medical Microbiology
Dr Michael Olah, Etobicoke, ON - General Practice
Dr Robert P Paulovic, Oshawa, ON - Family Medicine
Dr Ivan Petrov, Toronto, ON - General Practice
Dr Otokar J Roob, Fort Saskatchewan, AB - General Practice
Dr Norbert J Rose, Toronto, ON - General Practice
Dr Jan Rozehnal, Toronto, ON - General Practice
Dr Viera Saly, Victoria, BC - Neurology
Dr Paul Sandor, Toronto, ON - Psychiatry
Dr Raymond B Sawkiw, Sudbury, ON - Family Medicine
Dr Ljubinka Segedi, Kitchener, ON - Family Medicine
Dr Mathew Sermer, Toronto, ON - Obstetrics & Gynecology
Dr Miriam Shanks, Edmonton, AB - Cardiology
Dr Martin Simonik, North York, ON - General Practice
Dr Dagmar Simonik, North York, ON - General Practice
Dr Ann Maria T Sirek, Guelph, ON - Internal Medicine
Dr Karen E Slatkovsky, Guelph, ON - Emergency Family Med
Dr Dagmar Smatanova, Victoria, BC - Family Medicine
Dr Lenka Snajdrova, Richards Landing, ON - Emergency Family Med
Dr Elena Somska, Toronto, ON - General Practice
Dr Elena Spacek, Montreal, QC - Physical Medicine & Rehab
Dr Jan Spacek, Sherbrooke, QC - General Practice
Dr Paul J Sperka, Edmonton, AB - Occupational Med
Dr Martin Strban, Kitchener, ON - Internal Medicine
Dr Milosh S Surka, Richmond, BC - General Practice
Dr Pavol Sventek, Val-d'Or, QC - Family Medicine
Dr Michaela Swekla, Cambridge, ON - General Practice
Dr Victor A Toran, York, ON - Otolaryngology
Dr Peter Toth, Mississauga, ON - Emergency Family Med
Dr Mario Voros, Peterborough, ON - Diagnostic-Radiology
Dr Stefan Vrablik, Thunder Bay, ON - General Practice
Dr Ewa B Wesolowska, Montreal, QC - Medical Biochemistry
Dr Anna M Wojcicka, Toronto, ON - Radiation Oncology
Dr James R Wylie, Brampton, ON - General Practice
Dr Joseph Zahradnik, Peterborough, ON - Obstetrics & Gynecology
Dr Peter I Zelina, Richmond Hill, ON - Psychiatry
Dr Robert Zeman, Toronto, ON - Endocrin/Metabolism

SLOVENIAN

Dr Andrej J Habjan, Thunder Bay, ON - General Practice
Dr Maya Marc, Chateauguay, QC - Pediatrics
Dr Mladen Seidl, Etobicoke, ON - General Practice
Dr Ana-Sabina Sladic, Kingston, ON - Family Medicine

SOMALI

Dr Ali I Hersi, Hamilton, ON - Emergency Medicine
Dr Aden A Ismail, London, ON - Psychiatry

SOTHO

Dr Jacobus J Du Toit, Miramichi, NB - General Practice
Dr W Jacobus Fourie, Terrace, BC - General Practice
Dr Mtimkulu Mehlomakulu, Kingston, ON - Pediatrics
Dr Stanley K Muwanguzi, Camrose, AB - Emergency Family Med
Dr Motlobeng D Pebane, Indian Head, SK - General Practice
Dr Edwin B Spence, Ottawa, ON - General Practice

SPANISH

Dr Oussama A Abla, Toronto, ON - General Practice
Dr Aboobaker Aboo, Ottawa, ON - General Practice
Dr Luis A Acevedo Mendez, Bay Roberts, NL - General Practice
Dr Yael Acre, Montreal, QC - Family Medicine
Dr Niam Adamo, Mississauga, ON - Family Medicine
Dr Mansour Adle, Westmount, QC - General Surgery
Dr Ravi Agarwala, St. Catharines, ON - Internal Medicine
Dr Ronald Akhras, Montreal, QC - Family Medicine
Dr Charlotte Alabaster, Calgary, AB - Family Medicine
Dr Jean Joseph Thierry Alcindor, Montreal, QC - Hematology
Dr Lubomir Alexov, Scarborough, ON - General Practice
Dr Ariane Alimenti, Vancouver, BC - General Practice
Dr Federico A Allodi, Toronto, ON - Psychiatry
Dr A Nanette Alvarez, Calgary, AB - Cardiology
Dr Carlos A Alvarez, New Glasgow, NS - General Surgery

Dr Gonzalo G Alvarez, Ottawa, ON - Internal Medicine
Dr Fernando Alvarez, Montreal, QC - General Practice
Dr Cesar E Alvarez Bernal, Longueuil, QC - General Practice
Dr Ruben E Alvaro, Winnipeg, MB - General Practice
Dr Maxime Amar, Quebec, QC - General Practice
Dr Pablo Hernán Amigo, Edmonton, AB - General Practice
Dr Maurice Amsellem, Montreal-Nord, QC - General Practice
Dr M Catherine Anderson, Fergus, ON - Family Medicine
Dr Salvador J Andres, Saskatoon, SK - General Practice
Dr Christopher G Andrew, Winnipeg, MB - General Surgery
Dr Jordanka Angelova, Edmonton, AB - Family Medicine
Dr Natalie E Antonenko, Selkirk, MB - General Practice
Dr Andre R Anzarut, Vancouver, BC - Neurology
Dr Luis C Appeltauer, Montreal, QC - General Practice
Dr Hector O Arbillaga, Calgary, AB - General Practice
Dr Ruben Arbitman, North York, ON - Psychiatry
Dr Stella L Arbitman, Thornhill, ON - Family Medicine
Dr Julio E Arboleda-Florez, Belleville, ON - Psychiatry
Dr Lisa M J Archambault, Lasalle, QC - Pediatrics
Dr Maryse Archambault, Quebec, QC - Family Medicine
Dr Edgard A Arcia-Bravo, London, ON - General Practice
Dr Jesus A Ardila-Romero, LaSalle, QC - Pediatrics
Dr Abdelwahab A Arrazaghi, Scarborough, ON - Cardiology
Dr Andre M Arsenault, Montreal, QC - Nuclear Medicine
Dr A Neil Arya, Kitchener, ON - Family Medicine
Dr Haig Ashikian, Gloucester, ON - Family Medicine
Dr Richard Aubin, Verdun, QC - General Practice
Dr Marie Audy, Donnacona, QC - General Practice
Dr Francois Auger, Quebec, QC - Medical Microbiology
Dr Samuel Auron, Hamilton, ON - Psychiatry
Dr Monica Avendano Alvarez, Toronto, ON - Internal Medicine
Dr Arsenio J Avila Insambergth, Toronto, ON - Anesthesia
Dr M Angelica Ayala Arevalo, Sainte-Therese, QC - Psychiatry
Dr Felix A Ayala Paredes, Sherbrooke, QC - General Practice
Dr Jose Ayllon Ugarte, Greenfield Park, QC - General Practice
Dr Normand J Ayotte, Shawinigan, QC - Obstetrics & Gynecology
Dr Jean-Pierre M Ayoub, Montreal, QC - Internal Medicine
Dr Samir Azzaria, Quebec, QC - Family Medicine
Dr Harpreet S Bajaj, Brampton, ON - General Practice
Dr Luis C Baptista, Edmonton, AB - General Practice
Dr Jack Barabtarlo, Richmond Hill, ON - Psychiatry
Dr Adrian M Baranchuk, Kingston, ON - Neurology
Dr Norma Barbieri, Abbotsford, BC - Psychiatry
Dr Genevieve Baril-Guerard, Nelson, BC - General Practice
Dr Ana-Maria Barrenechea, Toronto, ON - Psychiatry
Dr Rolando A Barrios, Vancouver, BC - Community Medicine
Dr Peter G Barss, Salmon Arm, BC - Community Medicine
Dr Peter A Batay-Csorba, Richmond Hill, ON - General Practice
Dr Renaldo N Battista, Montreal, QC - Community Medicine
Dr Robert Beaudoin, Montreal, QC - General Practice
Dr Josianne E Beaudry, Borden, ON - Family Medicine
Dr Michel G Beaudry, Chicoutimi, QC - Electroencephal
Dr Marie Beauregard, Montreal, QC - Family Medicine
Dr Solange Beauregard, Sherbrooke, QC - Dermatology
Dr Vanessa Bedard, Saskatoon, SK - Pediatrics
Dr Natan Behar, Cornwall, ON - General Practice
Dr Beatriz M R Behar, Toronto, ON - Psychiatry
Dr Mario Bejerman, Montreal, QC - General Surgery
Dr Jean-Francois Belanger, Mont-Joli, QC - General Practice
Dr Antonio A Belda, London, ON - Pediatrics
Dr Denise Belisle, Montreal, QC - General Practice
Dr Nadia M Belsky, Etobicoke, ON - General Practice
Dr Oscar R Benavente, Vancouver, BC - Neurology
Dr Jaimes-S. Benhamron, Montreal, QC - Gastroenterology
Dr Antonio Benitez-Gomez, Surrey, BC - Family Medicine
Dr Jose M Benitez-Lazo, Surrey, BC - General Practice
Dr Marcia D Benjamin, Barrie, ON - Psychiatry
Dr Brian R Bennett, Edmonton, AB - General Practice
Dr Bruno Benzaquen, Montreal, QC - Cardiology
Dr Brenda A Bergeron, Greenfield Park, QC - Family Medicine
Dr Marco Bergevin, Laval, QC - Infectious Diseases
Dr Guillermo R Beristain, Courtenay, BC - Urology
Dr Bruno Bernardin, Montreal, QC - Emergency Medicine
Dr Gilles P Bernier, Montreal, QC - Electroencephal
Dr Helene Bertrand, North Vancouver, BC - Family Medicine
Dr Robert A Bertrand, Montreal, QC - Otolaryngology
Dr Martine Berube, Sherbrooke, QC - Psychiatry
Dr Ricardo Bessoudo, Saint John, NB - Cardiology
Dr Leoncio M Best, St. John's, NL - Urology
Dr Onil Bhattacharyya, Toronto, ON - Family Medicine
Dr Susan Biali, West Vancouver, BC - General Practice
Dr Eric Bicrell, Montreal, QC - General Practice
Dr Kendall Billick, Pointe-Claire, QC - Infectious Diseases
Dr Robert J Birnbaum, Ottawa, ON - Family Medicine
Dr Piotr A Blachut, Vancouver, BC - Orthopedic Surgery
Dr Stephanie Blais-Boilard, Cookshire-Eaton, QC - Emergency Family Med
Dr Pierre Blanchet, Quebec, QC - Obstetrics & Gynecology
Dr Richard Blanchet, Riviere-Du-Loup, QC - General Surgery
Dr David Blanchette, Montreal, QC - Orthopedic Surgery
Dr German Blando, Dieppe, NB - General Practice
Dr Maria Blanque Martinez, Montreal, QC - General Practice
Dr Robert A Bluman, Vancouver, BC - Family Medicine
Dr Armour I Boake, Thunder Bay, ON - Internal Medicine
Dr Peter M Bogaty, Montreal, QC - Cardiology
Dr Anibal F Bohorquez, Vancouver, BC - Physical Medicine & Rehab
Dr Caroline Boisvert, St-Jerome, QC - General Practice
Dr Alain Bolduc, Moncton, NB - Dermatology
Dr Jocelyne Bonin, Saint-Hyacinthe, QC - Family Medicine
Dr Francois Bonneau, Montreal-Nord, QC - Family Medicine
Dr Yves Bonnier-Viger, Sainte-Marie, QC - Community Medicine
Dr Timothy W Bood, Halifax, NS - General Practice
Dr Ian Bookman, Toronto, ON - Gastroenterology
Dr Jacinthe Bordeleau, Trois-Pistoles, QC - General Practice
Dr Sergio M Borgia, Brampton, ON - Infectious Diseases
Dr Claudio M Borgono, Toronto, ON - General Practice
Dr Manon Bouchard, Levis, QC - Neurology
Dr Maurice Bouchard, Quebec, QC - Pediatrics
Dr Emilie Boucher-Gagne, Chandler, QC - General Practice
Dr Julie Boulanger, Les Escoumins, QC - Family Medicine
Dr Patrick R Boulos, Sherbrooke, QC - Ophthalmology
Dr Frank Bravo, Whitby, ON - Otolaryngology
Dr Riina I Bray, Maple, ON - Family Medicine
Dr Josee Briere, Beauharnois, QC - General Practice
Dr Rosario Briones-Urbina, Toronto, ON - Endocrin/Metabolism
Dr Johnny D Brisebois, Kanata, ON - Family Medicine
Dr Michal Broniewski, Calgary, AB - General Practice
Dr Laurene J Brooks, Edmonton, AB - Family Medicine
Dr Anais Brosseau-Roberge, St-Charles-Bromee, QC - Obstetrics & Gynecology
Dr Merrilee G Brown, Port Perry, ON - Family Medicine
Dr Anita Marie Brown-Johnson, Montreal, QC - Family Medicine
Dr Suzanne C Buchanan, Scarborough, ON - Family Medicine
Dr Balint L Budai, Vancouver, BC - Family Medicine
Dr Yanick Bureau, Ville-Marie, QC - General Practice
Dr Miguel N Burnier, Montreal, QC - General Practice
Dr Anthony E Cabrera, St Catharines, ON - Ophthalmology
Dr Eric Cadesky, Vancouver, BC - Family Medicine
Dr Pedro Camacho Maldonado, Comox, BC - Internal Medicine
Dr Colin J Cameron, Brockville, ON - Psychiatry
Dr Roberto M Campanaro, Atikokan, ON - General Practice
Dr Alfredo Campos, Summerside, PE - Otolaryngology
Dr Luis A Canadas, Winnipeg, MB - General Practice
Dr Pablo O Cano, Sudbury, ON - Internal Medicine
Dr Marcelo Cantarovich, Montreal, QC - Nephrology
Dr Jerome Cantin, Shawinigan-Sud, QC - Obstetrics & Gynecology
Dr Manuel R Cardoso, Montreal, QC - Internal Medicine
Dr Reynaldo Cardoso, Regina, SK - Obstetrics & Gynecology
Dr Dominique Caron, Saint-Bruno, QC - Family Medicine
Dr Marie-Pierre Carpentier, Ottawa, ON - Emergency Family Med
Dr Paul J Carroll, Montreal, QC - Family Medicine
Dr Marie Cartier, Granby, QC - General Practice
Dr Maria Casale, Guelph, ON - Family Medicine
Dr Luigi Casella, Toronto, ON - Internal Medicine
Dr Oscar G Casiro, Victoria, BC - Pediatrics
Dr Fernando Casses, West Vancouver, BC - General Surgery
Dr Alberto Casses, Barrie, ON - Orthopedic Surgery
Dr Luigi A Castagna, Scarborough, ON - Pediatrics
Dr Eliana Castillo, Calgary, AB - Internal Medicine
Dr Laura Catz-Biro, Toronto, ON - Family Medicine
Dr Emmanuel Cauchois, Verdun, QC - Psychiatry
Dr Pablo Cervantes, Montreal, QC - Psychiatry
Dr Susan M J Chafe, Edmonton, AB - Radiation Oncology
Dr Leopoldo Chagoya, Toronto, ON - Psychiatry
Dr Chamoun Chamoun, Ottawa, ON - Cardiology
Dr Myriam Champagne, Terrebonne, QC - Emergency Family Med
Dr Benjamin T Chan, Espanola, ON - General Practice
Dr C Michael Chang, Oshawa, ON - Urology
Dr B Cecilia Chaparro Mutis, Toronto, ON - General Practice
Dr Francois G Charette, Longueuil, QC - General Practice
Dr Pierre Charland, Sorel-Tracy, QC - Diagnostic-Radiology
Dr Luc Chausse, L'Assomption, QC - General Practice
Dr Mustapha Chelfi, Gatineau, QC - General Practice
Dr Helene Chenard, Laval, QC - General Practice
Dr Donna A G Cherniak, Sherbrooke, QC - Family Medicine
Dr Renelle Chiasson, Tracadie-Sheila, NB - Family Medicine
Dr Hector L Chiavaro, Mississauga, ON - Pediatrics
Dr Abdallah Chidiac, Saint-Laurent, QC - Pediatrics
Dr Juan C L Chirgwin, Montreal, QC - Family Medicine
Dr Charles Chocron, Montreal, QC - General Practice
Dr Julie Choquet, Verdun, QC - Family Medicine
Dr Michelle Cinq-Mars, Sorel-Tracy, QC - General Practice
Dr Jordi Cisa, Sudbury, ON - Orthopedic Surgery
Dr Nestor F Cisneros, Winnipeg, MB - Clin Immun/Allergy
Dr Felipe Cisternas, Vancouver, BC - Family Medicine
Dr Wojtek P Ciszak, Vancouver, BC - General Practice
Dr W Robert L Clemmey, Yellowknife, NT - Psychiatry
Dr Edward G Coates, Vancouver, BC - Pediatrics
Dr Dan A D Cohen, North York, ON - Family Medicine
Dr Jeffrey J Cohen, Windsor, ON - General Practice
Dr Sandra R A Cohen, Montreal, QC - Hematology
Dr Donald C Cole, Toronto, ON - Community Medicine
Dr Sophie Collins, Montreal, QC - Anesthesia
Dr J Robert Colorado, St. Catharines, ON - Family Medicine
Dr Paulette Comeau, Red Deer, AB - General Practice
Dr Nicolas Constas-Costopoulos, Montreal, QC - General Practice
Dr Carlos E Contreras, Etobicoke, ON - Pediatrics
Dr Juan L Cordova, Winnipeg, MB - General Practice
Dr Charline Cormier, Sherbrooke, QC - General Practice
Dr Maria D P Cortes Nino, Montreal, QC - General Practice
Dr Leonardo Cortese, Windsor, ON - Psychiatry
Dr Peter B Cote, Manitouwadge, ON - Family Medicine
Dr Brigitte V Cote, Montreal, QC - Community Medicine
Dr Sylvie Cote, Montreal, QC - General Practice
Dr Michael P Coughlin, Windsor, ON - General Surgery
Dr Josee Couture, Montreal, QC - General Practice
Dr Juanita M Crook, Kelowna, BC - Radiation Oncology
Dr Madelaine Cruz de Pazos, Devon, AB - General Practice
Dr Geoffrey W Cundiff, Vancouver, BC - Plastic Surgery
Dr Orlando P Da Silva, London, ON - Pediatrics
Dr Vasco F Da Silva, Ottawa, ON - Neurosurgery
Dr Michael H Dahan, Montreal, QC - Obstetrics & Gynecology
Dr Aime Dahan, Pointe-Claire, QC - General Practice
Dr Christopher J Dainton, Toronto, ON - Emergency Family Med
Dr Genevieve Dallaire, St-Jean-Sur-Richel, QC - Emergency Family Med
Dr A Michael Damus, Uxbridge, ON - Family Medicine
Dr Ratna Dan, Ajax, ON - Diagnostic-Radiology
Dr Silvia L C Dancea, Sudbury, ON - Anatomical Pathology
Dr Mary Danylak, Toronto, ON - General Practice
Dr Nidal Darwish, Calgary, AB - Family Medicine
Dr Sheila J David, North York, ON - General Practice
Dr Suzanne De Blois, Montreal, QC - Community Medicine
Dr J Lance De Foa, Wawa, ON - General Practice
Dr Francis S De Marco, Windsor, ON - General Practice
Dr Jorge De Maria, Hamilton, ON - Urology
Dr Sylvaine De Plaen, Montreal, QC - Psychiatry
Dr Michael De Roode, Burks Falls, ON - Family Medicine
Dr Lara De Salaberry, Ottawa, ON - Family Medicine
Dr France De Villers, Saint-Jerome, QC - Pediatrics
Dr John M Dean, Vancouver, BC - Clin Immun/Allergy
Dr J C Martin Del Campo, Toronto, ON - Internal Medicine
Dr Jaime Del Carpio, Montreal, QC - Clin Immun/Allergy

Dr Alfonso P Del Valle Rebeil, Etobicoke, ON - Obstetrics & Gynecology
Dr Maria Del Valle-Pison, Montreal, QC - Pediatrics
Dr Perlita Delaney, Kingston, ON - General Practice
Dr Diego H Delgado, Toronto, ON - General Practice
Dr Gisell Delgado Rodriguez, Gloucester, ON - Family Medicine
Dr Rejean-Andre Delisle, Chicoutimi, QC - Medical Microbiology & Infectious Diseases
Dr Thomas J Demarco, Whistler, BC - General Practice
Dr Philippe Demers, Cowansville, QC - General Surgery
Dr Huguette Demers, Montreal, QC - Community Medicine
Dr Ari Demirjian, Mont-Royal, QC - Dermatology
Dr Chahe B Derghazarian, Saint-Leonard, QC - Hematology
Dr Dominique Deschenes, Quebec, QC - Family Medicine
Dr Pierre Deshaies, Sainte-Marie, QC - Community Medicine
Dr Isabelle Desormeau, Laval, QC - Anesthesia
Dr Jean-Paul Desrochers, Ste-Agathe-des-Mts, QC - General Practice
Dr Giuseppina Di Meglio, Westmount, QC - Pediatrics
Dr Vincenzo Di Nicola, Montreal, QC - Psychiatry
Dr Claudio D Di Prizito, Mississauga, ON - Internal Medicine
Dr Razvan Diaconescu, Montreal, QC - Hematology
Dr Absa Diallo, Montreal, QC - General Practice
Dr Pedro E Diaz, Lower Sackville, NS - General Practice
Dr Luis Victor Diaz de Bedoya, Quebec, QC - Radiation Oncology
Dr Julio F Diaz-Bobadilla, Kelowna, BC - Psychiatry
Dr Pablo Diaz-Hermosillo, Toronto, ON - Psychiatry
Dr Francisco Diaz-Mitoma, Sudbury, ON - Medical Microbiology
Dr Manuel Dibildox Gonzalez, Toronto, ON - General Practice
Dr Shamoon Din, Mississauga, ON - General Practice
Dr Emmanuel Dingemans, Saint-Jerome, QC - Anesthesia
Dr Patricia Disperati, Toronto, ON - Hematology
Dr Marjorie Dixon, North York, ON - Obstetrics & Gynecology
Dr Hisham Dokainish, Hamilton, ON - Cardiology
Dr Joan Don, Lindsay, ON - Anesthesia
Dr Suzanne C Donaldson, Surrey, BC - Family Medicine
Dr Marcel Dore, Guelph, ON - General Practice
Dr David Dorenbaum, Toronto, ON - Pediatrics
Dr Jonathan Downar, Toronto, ON - Psychiatry
Dr Christian A Drouin, Riviere-Du-Loup, QC - Dermatology
Dr Bertrand Du Souich, Montreal, QC - General Practice
Dr Marc DuPere, Toronto, ON - Plastic Surgery
Dr Mark R Dube, Sudbury, ON - Emergency Family Med
Dr Ruth Dubin, Kingston, ON - Family Medicine
Dr Jacques H Dubins, North York, ON - General Practice
Dr Morency Duchastel, Montreal, QC - General Practice
Dr Jocelyn Dumatol-Sanchez, Winnipeg, MB - Family Medicine
Dr Kathryn J E Dundas, Calgary, AB - General Practice
Dr Nicolas Dupre, Quebec, QC - Neurology
Dr Emilie Dupuis-Riendeau, Gaspe, QC - Family Medicine
Dr Hector A Duque-Rendon, Hanover, ON - General Surgery
Dr Marie-Josee Durand, LaSalle, QC - General Practice
Dr Monika Dutt, Sydney, NS - Community Medicine
Dr Donald Echenberg, Sherbrooke, QC - Internal Medicine
Dr Eric L Eisenberg, Mississauga, ON - Dermatology
Dr Sonia Eliev, Gracefield, QC - Family Medicine
Dr John Embil, Winnipeg, MB - Infectious Diseases
Dr Angela C Enright, Victoria, BC - Anesthesia
Dr Santiago Ensenat, Edmonton, AB - General Practice
Dr Julius Erdstein, Pierrefonds, QC - Pediatrics
Dr Jaime M Escallon, Toronto, ON - General Surgery
Dr Sandra I Escoredo, Edmonton, AB - General Practice
Dr Juan L Escudero, Ottawa, ON - General Practice
Dr John E Esmond, Mississauga, ON - Family Medicine
Dr Vidal Essebag, Montreal, QC - Cardiology
Dr Gabriel Fabreau, Calgary, AB - Internal Medicine
Dr Anne Fadin, Cowansville, QC - Obstetrics & Gynecology
Dr Hussein Fadlallah, Montreal, QC - Cardiology
Dr Mohammad Fahim, New Glasgow, NS - General Practice
Dr Catherine Falardeau, Rouyn-Noranda, QC - Family Medicine
Dr Joelle M T Fareau-Weyl, Guelph, ON - Psychiatry
Dr Dean Favot, Windsor, ON - General Practice
Dr Karima Fazal Karim, Montreal, QC - Family Medicine
Dr Carlos R Featherston, Ottawa, ON - Psychiatry
Dr Victor M Feder, North York, ON - Psychiatry
Dr Harry L Felcenbuch-Dachis, Newmarket, ON - Psychiatry
Dr Jordan Feld, Toronto, ON - Gastroenterology
Dr Craig A Ferguson, Bridgewater, NS - Family Medicine
Dr Nestor D P Fernandez, Toronto, ON - General Practice
Dr Marie-Carmel Fernandez, Saint-Leonard, QC - General Practice
Dr Jose Fernandez de Lara Nieto, St. Albert, AB - Family Medicine
Dr Robert Ferrari, Edmonton, AB - Internal Medicine
Dr Catherine Ferrier, Montreal, QC - Family Medicine
Dr Alvaro Figueredo, Hamilton, ON - Internal Medicine
Dr Lyne Filiatrault, Vancouver, BC - Emergency Medicine
Dr Daniel L Filipini, Montreal, QC - General Practice
Dr Marie-Josee Filteau, Quebec, QC - Psychiatry
Dr Philip B Fleuriau-Chateau, Ottawa, ON - Orthopedic Surgery
Dr Alejandro A Floh, Toronto, ON - Cardiology
Dr Pierre Flor-Henry, Edmonton, AB - Psychiatry
Dr Luis A Flores, Niagara Falls, ON - Orthopedic Surgery
Dr Alberto L Flores-Vargas, Scarborough, ON - General Practice
Dr Frank Fornasier, Burlington, ON - Family Medicine
Dr Luis R Fornazzari, Toronto, ON - Neurology
Dr Guy Fournier, Westmount, QC - Orthopedic Surgery
Dr Vincent Fradet, Quebec, QC - Urology
Dr Slobodan E Franic, Perth, ON - Diagnostic-Radiology
Dr France Frechette, Chateauguay, QC - General Practice
Dr Carolyn R Freeman, Montreal, QC - Radiation Oncology
Dr Tatiana Freire-Lizama, Toronto, ON - Obstetrics & Gynecology
Dr Anthony J French, Vancouver, BC - General Practice
Dr Marie G L Frenette, Quebec, QC - Pediatrics
Dr Jan Oliver Friedrich, Toronto, ON - Critical Care Medicine
Dr Sigrid Fuchs-Garcia, Cornwall, ON - General Practice
Dr Aldo A Furlani, Red Deer, AB - General Practice
Dr Aicha Gafsi, Rimouski, QC - Internal Medicine
Dr Gilbert Gagne, Mirabel, QC - Family Medicine
Dr Guy Gagne, Quebec, QC - General Practice
Dr D'Arcy W Gagnon, Toronto, ON - General Practice
Dr Sophie Gagnon, Gatineau, QC - Neurology
Dr Bruno Gagnon, Quebec, QC - General Practice
Dr Carol B Gailey, New Westminster, BC - Cardiology
Dr Paz A Gajardo, Toronto, ON - Family Medicine
Dr Eleni Galanis, Vancouver, BC - Community Medicine
Dr Andres Gantous, Toronto, ON - Otolaryngology
Dr Patrick Garceau, Montreal, QC - Cardiology
Dr Bertha Garcia, London, ON - Anatomical Pathology
Dr Andrea Garcia, Mississauga, ON - Family Medicine
Dr Michel Garcia, Ste-Anne-des-Monts, QC - General Practice
Dr Idania Garcia Del Sol, Laval, QC - General Practice
Dr Angeles Garcia, Kingston, ON - Geriatric Medicine
Dr Juan A Garcia-Rodriguez, Calgary, AB - Community Medicine
Dr Raul Garcia-Salinas, Regina, SK - Ophthalmology
Dr Genevieve Garneau, Saint-Hyacinthe, QC - Emergency Family Med
Dr Maria Garrido-Russo, Quebec, QC - Endocrinology
Dr Daniel Garros, Edmonton, AB - General Practice
Dr Lynn Gaudreault, Montreal, QC - Otolaryngology
Dr Adam Gavsie, Montreal, QC - Family Medicine
Dr Barrington A Gayle, North York, ON - Internal Medicine
Dr Silvia R M Gaytan-Graham, Sudbury, ON - Anatomical Pathology
Dr M F Liliane Gendreau-Reid, Victoria, BC - Clin Immun/Allergy
Dr Edward F H Gentis, Vancouver, BC - General Surgery
Dr Talha I Ghadai, Newmarket, ON - Family Medicine
Dr Gissou S Ghadirian, Etobicoke, ON - Family Medicine
Dr Gabriela Ghitulescu, Montreal, QC - General Surgery
Dr William T Gibson, Vancouver, BC - Medical Genetics
Dr Chantal M Giguere, Montreal, QC - Otolaryngology
Dr Jean Gilbert, Montreal, QC - General Practice
Dr Hernan Giraldo, Chateauguay, QC - Pediatrics
Dr Jacques E Girard, Quebec, QC - Community Medicine
Dr Linda Giroux, Fortierville, QC - General Practice
Dr Marie-France Giroux, Montreal, QC - Diagnostic-Radiology
Dr Rudolph Gittens, Ottawa, ON - Orthopedic Surgery
Dr Brook W Glanville, Salmon Arm, BC - Family Medicine
Dr George R Gleisner II, Milton, ON - General Practice
Dr Rafael S Glikstein, Ottawa, ON - Diagnostic-Radiology
Dr Elizabeth Y H Glowczewski-Park, Scarborough, ON - Family Medicine
Dr Martine Gobeil, Montreal, QC - General Practice
Dr Charles M Godfrey, Toronto, ON - Physical Medicine & Rehab
Dr Patricia Goggin, Montreal, QC - General Practice
Dr David I Gold, Wakefield, QC - Family Medicine
Dr H Brian Goldman, Toronto, ON - General Practice
Dr Sol J Goldstein, North York, ON - Psychiatry
Dr Victor Gomel, Vancouver, BC - Obstetrics & Gynecology
Dr Jose-Daniel Gomez, Winnipeg, MB - Anatomical Pathology
Dr E G Enrique Gomez, Port Colborne, ON - General Practice
Dr Jose A Gomez Lemus, London, ON - Anatomical Pathology
Dr Alfonso Gomez-Jimenez, Bathurst, NB - Plastic Surgery
Dr M Joana Goncalves, Toronto, ON - General Practice
Dr Hernan Gonzalez, Edmonton, AB - Pediatrics
Dr Armando Gonzalez, Toronto, ON - General Practice
Dr Yolanda Gonzalez, Grand-Mere, QC - Family Medicine
Dr Mariel Gonzalez, Laval, QC - General Practice
Dr Luis A Gonzalez Herrera, Rimouski, QC - Neurology
Dr Roberto Gonzalez-Almeyda, Leamington, ON - Family Medicine
Dr Gonzalo Gonzalez-Amaya, Sherbrooke, QC - General Surgery
Dr Maria C Gonzalez-Porras, Welland, ON - Anesthesia
Dr Andres E Gordillo, Ajax, ON - Obstetrics & Gynecology
Dr Robert G Gordon, Etobicoke, ON - Orthopedic Surgery
Dr Fabian P Gorodzinsky, London, ON - Pediatrics
Dr Pierre Gosselin, Quebec, QC - General Practice
Dr Francois Gosselin, Ste-Agathe-des-Mts, QC - General Practice
Dr Sidney O Gottlieb, Collingwood, ON - General Practice
Dr Francois W Gougeon, High River, AB - General Surgery
Dr Claudia J Grabner, Brantford, ON - General Practice
Dr Sandra Graham, Sainte-Therese, QC - General Practice
Dr Francois Grand'Maison, Greenfield Park, QC - Electroencephal
Dr Eugenie Granger-Juneau, Quebec, QC - General Practice
Dr Jean-Pierre Gravel, Quebec, QC - Ophthalmology
Dr Michael E Green, Kingston, ON - Family Medicine
Dr Alexandra Greenhill, Vancouver, BC - Family Medicine
Dr Michelle Grinman, Toronto, ON - Internal Medicine
Dr Louis Grondin, Calgary, AB - General Practice
Dr James M Gruber, Montreal, QC - Internal Medicine
Dr Karin H Grubner, Toronto, ON - General Practice
Dr Francine Guay, Levis, QC - Ophthalmology
Dr Lyn C C Guenther, London, ON - Dermatology
Dr Enrique C Guerra, Leamington, ON - Internal Medicine
Dr Chantal Guillemette, Havre-Saint-Pierre, QC - Family Medicine
Dr Daniel B S Guimaraes, Sherbrooke, QC - Psychiatry
Dr S Yamuna Gunawardena, Richmond Hill, ON - Pediatrics
Dr Jose Gutauskas, Ottawa, ON - General Surgery
Dr Andrea Gutauskas, Ottawa, ON - General Surgery
Dr Jaime Guzman, Vancouver, BC - Physical Medicine & Rehab
Dr D Antonio Guzman, Ottawa, ON - Electroencephal
Dr Venus B Guzman, Toronto, ON - General Practice
Dr Juan Guzman Orduz, Hamilton, ON - Internal Medicine
Dr Alice Gwyn, Norris Point, NL - Family Medicine
Dr Vladimir Hachinski, London, ON - Neurology
Dr Rod Hafezi, Saskatoon, SK - Internal Medicine
Dr Ernest M Hahn, Kitchener, ON - Emergency Family Med
Dr Laura N Haiek, Westmount, QC - Family Medicine
Dr Trevor J Ham, Owen Sound, ON - Pediatrics
Dr Adolf Hamann, Corner Brook, NL - General Practice
Dr Herag Hamboyan, Brampton, ON - Family Medicine
Dr Dan J Hancu, North York, ON - Family Medicine
Dr Gregory B Hariton, Hamilton, ON - General Practice
Dr Donald R H Harris, Nepean, ON - General Practice
Dr Gervais A Harry, Etobicoke, ON - Urology
Dr Ezat Hashim, Montreal, QC - Plastic Surgery
Dr Larisa I Hausmanis, Toronto, ON - Family Medicine
Dr Yanick Hector, Montreal, QC - General Practice
Dr Katja Heineck, Toronto, ON - Family Medicine
Dr Khati L Hendry, Summerland, BC - Family Medicine
Dr Richard Henri, Montreal, QC - Anesthesia
Dr Alexandre R Henri-Bhargava, North York, ON - Neurology
Dr Armando Heredia, Whitehorse, YT - General Practice
Dr Olivia Hernandez-Sanchez, Rouyn-Noranda, QC - General Practice
Dr Mariana L N Herskovitz, Ottawa, ON - General Practice

Dr Kamran Heydarzadeh-Azar, Fort St. John, BC - Anatomical Pathology
Dr David J Hill, North York, ON - General Practice
Dr Valerie Hindle, Ottawa, ON - Family Medicine
Dr H Henry Ho, North York, ON - Family Medicine
Dr Mojgan Hodaie, Toronto, ON - Neurosurgery
Dr Margarita K Hojyo Tomoka, Etobicoke, ON - General Practice
Dr Jill S Hoube, Vancouver, BC - Pediatrics
Dr Jean-Luc Houde, Chicoutimi, QC - General Surgery
Dr Stanley C Houston, Edmonton, AB - Infectious Diseases
Dr Sylvie R Hudon, Ottawa, ON - Family Medicine
Dr Ryan D Hunt, Montreal, QC - Emergency Family Med
Dr Jean M F Hyacinthe, Montreal, QC - Plastic Surgery
Dr G M Denise Hyland, St. John's, NL - General Practice
Dr Alfred W Illescas, Montreal, QC - General Practice
Dr Claire Infante-Rivard, Montreal, QC - Community Medicine
Dr Paula L Iriarte, Vancouver, BC - Family Medicine
Dr Anna M Issakoff-Meller, Guelph, ON - General Practice
Dr Geraldine Jacquemin, Montreal, QC - Physical Medicine & Rehab
Dr Marc-Andre Jacques, Montreal, QC - General Practice
Dr Frederic Jacques, Quebec, QC - Cardiac Surgery
Dr Alejandro R Jadad Bechara, Toronto, ON - General Practice
Dr J Walter James, Toronto, ON - Pediatrics
Dr Annie F Janvier, Montreal, QC - Pediatrics
Dr Carlo Jean-Louis, Rimouski, QC - Family Medicine
Dr Alphonse Jeanneret-Grosjean, Montreal, QC - Internal Medicine
Dr Anthony F Jeraj, Medicine Hat, AB - Family Medicine
Dr Christopher P Jinot, Bruce Mines, ON - Family Medicine
Dr Pamela J Johnson, Thunder Bay, ON - Psychiatry
Dr Victor L Jordan, Campbell River, BC - Emergency Family Med
Dr Javed Joseph, Regina, SK - General Practice
Dr Janice Journeau, Salmon Arm, BC - General Surgery
Dr Ramon Eduardo Jovel, Winnipeg, MB - General Practice
Dr France Joyal, Montreal, QC - Internal Medicine
Dr Marie-Suzanne Joyal, Verdun, QC - Family Medicine
Dr H Wilfried S Kaethler, Steinbach, MB - Family Medicine
Dr Rob J Kamermans, Coe Hill, ON - General Practice
Dr Sanja Karalic, North Vancouver, BC - Family Medicine
Dr Craig Karpilow, Hamilton, ON - Family Medicine
Dr Elena Kasatiya Trevisani, Ottawa, ON - General Practice
Dr Dounia Kayal, Montreal, QC - General Practice
Dr Nancy B Keesal, Toronto, ON - Internal Medicine
Dr Lisa M Kellett, Toronto, ON - Dermatology
Dr Isabelle Kemp, Montreal, QC - Psychiatry
Dr Ilmar J Kents, Brantford, ON - General Practice
Dr Amir A H Khadir, Terrebonne, QC - Medical Microbiology
Dr Zarin P Khan, Medicine Hat, AB - General Surgery
Dr Lucie M Khouri, Saint-Laurent, QC - Ophthalmology
Dr Samir Khoury, Montreal, QC - Pediatrics
Dr Frances T Kilbertus, Ottawa, ON - Family Medicine
Dr Erle J Kirby, Wawa, ON - Family Medicine
Dr Andre L Kiss, Vercheres, QC - General Practice
Dr Paula Klurfan, Hamilton, ON - General Practice
Dr Jacqueline Klvana, Brossard, QC - Family Medicine
Dr Marie-Charlotte Koenig, Kuujjuaq, QC - Family Medicine
Dr David P Kogon, Moncton, NB - Obstetrics & Gynecology
Dr Nadim Korban, Montreal, QC - Otolaryngology
Dr Yves A Korcaz, Montreal, QC - Obstetrics & Gynecology
Dr Miroslav Kordich, Montreal, QC - General Surgery
Dr Judit Korosi, Langley, BC - Internal Medicine
Dr C Marcelo M Kremenchutzky, London, ON - Neurology
Dr Mark Krieger, Toronto, ON - General Practice
Dr Agnes Kucharska, Milton, ON - Family Medicine
Dr Karol Kuperberg, Montreal, QC - General Practice
Dr Edmond Kyrillos, Ottawa, ON - Family Medicine
Dr Jean-Martin Laberge, Montreal, QC - General Surgery
Dr Caroline Laberge, Quebec, QC - Family Medicine
Dr Jose Labrador Febles, Meadow Lake, SK - General Practice
Dr Diane Lacasse, Anjou, QC - General Practice
Dr Linda A M Lacroix, Ottawa, ON - Hematology
Dr Mylene H Lacroix, Quebec, QC - Family Medicine
Dr Gilles-Philippe Lafond, Quebec, QC - Ophthalmology
Dr Philippe Lageix, Verdun, QC - General Practice
Dr Carmen Lalanda, Charlemagne, QC - General Practice
Dr Michel Lallier, Montreal, QC - General Surgery
Dr Donald H Lalonde, Saint John, NB - Plastic Surgery
Dr Michelle A Lamarre, Sudbury, ON - Family Medicine
Dr David C Lambert, Brossard, QC - Orthopedic Surgery
Dr Cecilia Lamenza, Toronto, ON - Pediatrics
Dr Marc Lamothe, Victoriaville, QC - Internal Medicine
Dr Michel Lamoureux, Embrun, ON - General Practice
Dr Diane Lamoureux, Longueuil, QC - Anatomical Pathology
Dr Joseph Langer, Belleville, ON - Orthopedic Surgery
Dr Marcelo Lannes, Montreal, QC - Anesthesia
Dr Gabor Lantos, Toronto, ON - General Practice
Dr Eric V Laperriere-Nguyen, Verdun, QC - General Practice
Dr Albert Larbrisseau, Montreal, QC - Neurology
Dr E Sheila Laredo, Toronto, ON - Endocrin/Metabolism
Dr Oscar Larios, Calgary, AB - Infectious Diseases
Dr Anne Larkin-Chagnon, Waterloo, QC - General Practice
Dr Roger E J Larochelle, Spanish, ON - General Practice
Dr Andre Larochelle, Jonquiere, QC - Obstetrics & Gynecology
Dr Isabelle Larocque, Montreal, QC - General Practice
Dr Ramiro A Larrazabal, Hamilton, ON - General Practice
Dr Brian Laufer, Montreal, QC - Critical Care Medicine
Dr Michel A Laurin, Saint-Hyacinthe, QC - Anatomical Pathology
Dr Pierre-Michel Laurin, Saint-Jerome, QC - General Practice
Dr Christian Lauriston, Montreal, QC - General Practice
Dr Marcel C Lavanchy, Westbank, BC - Family Medicine
Dr Vincent Lavoie, Montreal, QC - Cardiology
Dr Francoise Le Mevel-Moreira, Terrebonne, QC - Psychiatry
Dr Mai Anh Le Van, Montreal, QC - Emergency Family Med
Dr Nathalie J Lebreton, Dieppe, NB - Family Medicine
Dr Martin Lecompte, Gatineau, QC - Diagnostic-Radiology
Dr Jose Ledezma, Quispamsis, NB - General Practice
Dr Mao-Cheng Lee, Edmonton, AB - Internal Medicine
Dr Kenny Lee, Vancouver, BC - General Practice
Dr Natasha B Leighl, Toronto, ON - Internal Medicine
Dr Marie-Helene Lemoine, Saint-Hyacinthe, QC - Pediatrics
Dr Roberto Leon, Kelowna, BC - Obstetrics & Gynecology
Dr Sylvie Leone, Mississauga, ON - Obstetrics & Gynecology
Dr Marie-Aline Lepage, Montreal, QC - Anesthesia
Dr Bernard Lessard, Montreal, QC - Family Medicine
Dr Francois Letellier, Longueuil, QC - General Surgery
Dr Elaine Letendre, Montreal, QC - Medical Biochemistry
Dr Jean L Lette, Montreal, QC - Nuclear Medicine
Dr Michel P Leveille, Montreal, QC - Internal Medicine
Dr Christian Levesque, Laval, QC - Occupational Med
Dr Richard Levin, Montreal, QC - General Practice
Dr Michael C Lewin, Collingwood, ON - Family Medicine
Dr John R Lewis, Montreal, QC - Emergency Family Med
Dr Calvin T Lian, Toronto, ON - Emergency Family Med
Dr Anne-Marie Liebich, Montreal, QC - General Practice
Dr Suzanne J Lilker, Toronto, ON - Anesthesia
Dr Rosanna V Lima, Vancouver, BC - Family Medicine
Dr Marina J Lizon, Saskatoon, SK - Psychiatry
Dr Miguel A Llano-Ferro, Toronto, ON - General Practice
Dr Caroline A Lohrisch, Vancouver, BC - Internal Medicine
Dr Rocco A Lombardi, Bowmanville, ON - Emergency Family Med
Dr Luciano P Lombardi, Scarborough, ON - General Practice
Dr Adrian L H Long, Winnipeg, MB - General Practice
Dr Elena Lopez, Vancouver, BC - Medical Genetics
Dr Isabelle Lopez, Laval, QC - Psychiatry
Dr Jose F Lopez, Saskatoon, SK - Internal Medicine
Dr Marie-Josee Lord, Quebec, QC - Psychiatry
Dr Armando J Lorenzo, Toronto, ON - Urology
Dr Hanna Lotocka-Reysner, Burnaby, BC - Pediatrics
Dr Andres M Lozano, Toronto, ON - Neurosurgery
Dr Nathalie Lucas, Montreal, QC - Pediatrics
Dr Fernando A Luna, Gatineau, QC - General Practice
Dr G Harvey Lupu, Montreal, QC - Pediatrics
Dr Michele Mabon, Montreal, QC - Ophthalmology
Dr Christie A MacCallum, Toronto, ON - General Practice
Dr Alexander MacCordick, Gatineau, QC - Psychiatry
Dr Michele E MacLean, Kennetcook, NS - Family Medicine
Dr Yolanda Madarnas, Kingston, ON - Internal Medicine
Dr Vera V Madison, Toronto, ON - General Practice
Dr Mariam Maestre Mendoza, Maniwaki, QC - Family Medicine
Dr Patrick M Magloire, Hamilton, ON - General Practice
Dr Peter Mah, Gatineau, QC - Family Medicine
Dr Colin M Mailer, London, ON - Ophthalmology
Dr Alain Maillette, Trois-Rivieres, QC - Urology
Dr Roy A Male, Toronto, ON - Family Medicine
Dr Stéphanie C Malherbe, Ottawa, ON - Emergency Family Med
Dr Krzysztof W Malicki, Mississauga, ON - General Practice
Dr Dante E Manyari, Surrey, BC - Cardiology
Dr Loretta Marcon, Montreal, QC - Obstetrics & Gynecology
Dr Danielle Marcoux, Montreal, QC - Dermatology
Dr Alejandra I Marin Arellano, Rockwood, ON - Family Medicine
Dr Janet A Marta, Toronto, ON - Psychiatry
Dr Rafael Martell, London, ON - Internal Medicine
Dr Stuart Martin, Hamilton, ON - Plastic Surgery
Dr Jose A Martinez, Terrebonne, QC - Otolaryngology
Dr Jose Luis Martinez Marin, Montreal, QC - General Practice
Dr Jose C Martinez Motta, Cambridge, ON - General Practice
Dr Adelmo E Martoglio, Toronto, ON - Obstetrics & Gynecology
Dr John C Masgoret, Toronto, ON - Family Medicine
Dr Ephraim G Massey, Montreal, QC - General Practice
Dr Eva S Mate, Toronto, ON - Respirology
Dr Nicolas Mathieu, Riviere-Rouge, QC - General Practice
Dr Pierre Maurice, Quebec, QC - Community Medicine
Dr Marina Mauro, Orangeville, ON - Internal Medicine
Dr Pierre Mayer, Montreal, QC - Internal Medicine
Dr Richard Mazerolle, Chateauguay, QC - General Surgery
Dr Fereshteh Mazloom, Etobicoke, ON - Family Medicine
Dr Jorge A Mazza, London, ON - Internal Medicine
Dr Sergio Mazzadi, Hamilton, ON - General Practice
Dr Daniel J McBain, Kenora, ON - Family Medicine
Dr Simon McBride, London, ON - General Practice
Dr Maureen McCall, Red Deer, AB - General Practice
Dr James W McGillivray, Hearst, ON - General Surgery
Dr L Lynn McIntyre, Calgary, AB - Community Medicine
Dr Mary E McIntyre, Chatham, ON - General Practice
Dr Timothy W Meagher, Montreal, QC - Internal Medicine
Dr Jeannine Mechaly-Chokron, Lachine, QC - Ophthalmology
Dr G Alexandra Medellin-Kowalewski, Calgary, AB - Diagnostic-Radiology
Dr Barbara D Mederski, North York, ON - Internal Medicine
Dr Stephane B Meere, Montreal, QC - Ophthalmology
Dr Monica Meisels, Courcelette, QC - Family Medicine
Dr Jose H Mejia, London, ON - Psychiatry
Dr Andrea Melicharkova, Peterborough, ON - Gastroenterology
Dr Hector Mendez Tejada, North York, ON - General Practice
Dr Anselmo Mendez-Fernandez, Hanover, ON - Family Medicine
Dr Roberto Mendoza-Londono, Toronto, ON - General Practice
Dr Gopinath T Menon, Hamilton, ON - General Surgery
Dr David Mercier, Baie-Comeau, QC - General Practice
Dr Dominique Mercier, Sherbrooke, QC - General Practice
Dr Nicole Meunier, St-Charles-Brromee, QC - Dermatology
Dr Jose L Mijangos-Pelaez, Val-d'Or, QC - General Surgery
Dr Paul H Minc, Acton, ON - Family Medicine
Dr Joaquim A Miro, Montreal, QC - Cardiology
Dr Sheona M Mitchell, Vancouver, BC - General Practice
Dr Wade R Mitchell, Collingwood, ON - Family Medicine
Dr Franck Molin, Quebec, QC - Cardiology
Dr Allan L Moll, Thornhill, ON - Family Medicine
Dr Ilaria Moneta, Westmount, QC - Pediatrics
Dr Marie-Jose Monette, Laval, QC - Internal Medicine
Dr Juan C Monge, Toronto, ON - Cardiology
Dr Felix M Monroy-Cuadros, Calgary, AB - General Practice
Dr Julio S G Montaner, Vancouver, BC - Internal Medicine
Dr Jose Montes, Montreal, QC - Neurosurgery
Dr Silvia Monti De Flores, Montreal, QC - Psychiatry
Dr Richard Montoro, Montreal, QC - Psychiatry
Dr David R Montoya, Ottawa, ON - Emergency Medicine
Dr Mark S Moores, Wingham, ON - Family Medicine
Dr Peter Moosbrugger, Comox, BC - Family Medicine
Dr Carmen M Morales, Winnipeg, MB - General Pathology
Dr Dora Morales, Perth-Andover, NB - Family Medicine
Dr Jose J Morales, Perth-Andover, NB - General Surgery
Dr Alvaro Morales, Kingston, ON - Urology
Dr Karen M Moran De Muller, Winnipeg, MB - General Practice
Dr Isabelle Morency, St-Charles-Brromee, QC - General Surgery
Dr Marie-Josee Morier, Rouyn-Noranda, QC - General Practice
Dr Carlos A Morillo, Hamilton, ON - General Practice

Dr Luis E Morillo, Hamilton, ON - Neurology
Dr Marie-Eve Morin, Montreal, QC - Family Medicine
Dr Martine Morin, Sherbrooke, QC - Family Medicine
Dr Jean J Morissette, Quebec, QC - Diagnostic-Radiology
Dr Colombe Morneau, Longueuil, QC - General Practice
Dr David N Moskovitz, North York, ON - Gastroenterology
Dr Richard Moufarrege, Montreal, QC - Plastic Surgery
Dr Hellmuth A Muller Delgado, Winnipeg, MB - Orthopedic Surgery
Dr Flor M Muniz Rodriguez, Hamilton, ON - Physical Medicine & Rehab
Dr Juan E Munoz, Hamilton, ON - Family Medicine
Dr Marie Munoz, Montreal, QC - General Practice
Dr Letitia V Muresan, Dollard-D-Ormeaux, QC - Electroencephal
Dr M Madeleine H Murphy, Gloucester, ON - Family Medicine
Dr Reginald A Nadeau, Montreal, QC - Cardiology
Dr Daniel P Nagel, Whitby, ON - Family Medicine
Dr Basdeo Nankissoor, Edmonton, AB - Family Medicine
Dr Louise L Nasmith, Vancouver, BC - Family Medicine
Dr Alain Naud, Quebec, QC - Family Medicine
Dr Joaquin X R Navarro, Ottawa, ON - Psychiatry
Dr Oscar M Navarro Kunstmann, Toronto, ON - General Practice
Dr Juan C Negrete, Montreal, QC - Psychiatry
Dr Nathalie A Neveu, Montreal, QC - Endocrin/Metabolism
Dr Jack Newman, North York, ON - Pediatrics
Dr Quang V K Nguyen, Toronto, ON - Family Medicine
Dr Tuan Quynh T Nguyen, Montreal, QC - Ophthalmology
Dr C L Remy Nguyen, Montreal, QC - Otolaryngology
Dr Thuy-Tien Nguyen-Dang, Amqui, QC - General Practice
Dr Marcelo T Nicolela, Halifax, NS - Ophthalmology
Dr Steven Nitzkin, North York, ON - General Practice
Dr Gregoire E Noel, Montreal, QC - Medical Microbiology
Dr Eleazar H Noriega, Toronto, ON - Pediatrics
Dr Luis C E Noronha, Toronto, ON - Internal Medicine
Dr Stanley Norris, La Tuque, QC - Psychiatry
Dr Francisco J D Noya, Montreal, QC - Clin Immun/Allergy
Dr Barra F O'Briain, Vancouver, BC - Family Medicine
Dr Anthony M Ocana, West Vancouver, BC - Family Medicine
Dr Robert V Ogilvie, North York, ON - Otolaryngology
Dr John Olarte, Mississauga, ON - Family Medicine
Dr Peter R Olesen, Campbell River, BC - Plastic Surgery
Dr Luc L Oligny, Montreal, QC - General Pathology
Dr Marlene Olivier, Quebec, QC - General Practice
Dr David Olivier, Shawinigan, QC - Psychiatry
Dr Patrick Olivier, Sherbrooke, QC - Ophthalmology
Dr Wayne Olsheski, Toronto, ON - General Practice
Dr Edwin R Orellana-Jordan, Medicine Hat, AB - General Practice
Dr Jacqueline Orquin, Montreal, QC - Ophthalmology
Dr Eliseo Orrantia, Marathon, ON - Family Medicine
Dr Oliva Ortiz-Alvarez, Antigonish, NS - Pediatrics
Dr Luis H Ospina, Montreal, QC - General Practice
Dr Julian A Ospina-Ordonez, Vancouver, BC - Family Medicine
Dr Robert A Ouellette, Ste-Anne-de-Bellev, QC - Psychiatry
Dr Marie-Jo Ouimet, Montreal, QC - General Practice
Dr Denise Ouimet, Rouyn-Noranda, QC - Diagnostic-Radiology
Dr Dominique Ouimet, Saint-Jerome, QC - Cardiology
Dr Karen Oulianine, Montreal, QC - Emergency Family Med
Dr Ruth B Pacis, Dartmouth, NS - Family Medicine
Dr Julio R Padilla, North Vancouver, BC - Neurosurgery
Dr Nicholas V J Pairaudeau, North York, ON - Obstetrics & Gynecology
Dr Jorge A Palacios-Boix, Montreal, QC - Psychiatry
Dr Dominique Panet-Raymond, Montreal, QC - Pediatrics
Dr Lisanne Papin, Laval, QC - General Practice
Dr Martin Paquet, Sherbrooke, QC - General Practice
Dr Rejean Paradis, Ottawa, ON - Community Medicine
Dr Maryse Pare, Montreal, QC - Psychiatry
Dr Jaime P Paredes, Burnaby, BC - Psychiatry
Dr Josee Parent, Montreal, QC - Gastroenterology
Dr Andre Pasternac, Westmount, QC - Cardiology
Dr Danielle E Pastierovic, Victoria, BC - General Practice
Dr Katherine E Paton, Vancouver, BC - Ophthalmology
Dr Andrew R Patterson, Stouffville, ON - General Practice
Dr Alan V Pavilanis, Montreal, QC - Family Medicine
Dr Caroline Pedneault, Longueuil, QC - Pediatrics
Dr Sumithra A Peeris, Waterford, ON - General Practice
Dr Abraham Peliowski, Edmonton, AB - Pediatrics
Dr Arie Peliowski, Toronto, ON - Anesthesia
Dr Denisse Pella Fernandez, Ottawa, ON - Family Medicine
Dr Christine Pelletier, Montreal, QC - General Practice
Dr Rosana Pellizzari, Peterborough, ON - Community Medicine
Dr Jean Peloquin, Quebec, QC - General Surgery
Dr Jose R Perdomo, Calgary, AB - General Practice
Dr F Eduardo Perez, Etobicoke, ON - General Practice
Dr Gavino Perez, Hamilton, ON - Internal Medicine
Dr Edgardo L Perez, St. Catharines, ON - Psychiatry
Dr Anahi Perlas Fontana, Toronto, ON - Anesthesia
Dr Danielle Perreault, Montreal, QC - General Practice
Dr Therese Perreault, Montreal, QC - Pediatrics
Dr Marie-Pascale Perrier, Sherbrooke, QC - Psychiatry
Dr Linda Perron, Quebec, QC - Community Medicine
Dr Thomas L Perry Jr, Vancouver, BC - Internal Medicine
Dr George Peterson, Saint-Hubert, QC - General Practice
Dr Claude Petitclerc, Quebec, QC - Hematology
Dr Christine Anh Ngoc Pham, Calgary, AB - Diagnostic-Radiology
Dr Debbie J Phillips, Vernon, BC - Emergency Family Med
Dr Lincoln R Phipps, Leamington, ON - General Practice
Dr Jean-Rene Pierre, Maniwaki, QC - General Practice
Dr Robert P Pilorge, Montreal, QC - Obstetrics & Gynecology
Dr Marie Pinault, Gatineau, QC - General Practice
Dr Ernesto Pineda-Selva, Calgary, AB - General Practice
Dr Francisco Pinero-Medina, Sherbrooke, QC - Psychiatry
Dr J Vicente Pinilla, Toronto, ON - General Practice
Dr Julio Pintin-Quezada, Winnipeg, MB - General Surgery
Dr Jorge L Pinzon, Calgary, AB - Pediatrics
Dr Joao L P Pippi-Salle, Toronto, ON - Urology
Dr Cesar Pison, Montreal, QC - Endocrinology
Dr Andre Piver, Slocan Park, BC - Family Medicine
Dr Michel Plante, Montreal, QC - General Practice
Dr Ludovic Plante Jr, Sherbrooke, QC - General Practice
Dr David R Playfair, Cardston, AB - Family Medicine
Dr Charles E Pless, Montreal, QC - Family Medicine
Dr Gaetan Poitras, Saint-Leonard, QC - General Practice
Dr Vivian A Polak, Drayton, ON - Psychiatry
Dr Damien Pomerleau, Montreal, QC - Pediatrics
Dr Eric Pontbriand, Windsor, QC - General Practice
Dr Carlos M Ponton-Beltran, Amherst, NS - Emergency Family Med
Dr Stephanie A Popiel, Perth, ON - Family Medicine
Dr Ilija Popovic, Calgary, AB - General Practice
Dr Kevin C Pottie, Ottawa, ON - Family Medicine
Dr Renald M Poulin, Alma, QC - General Surgery
Dr Emmanuelle Pourcher, Quebec, QC - Neurology
Dr J E J Michel Prefontaine, London, ON - Obstetrics & Gynecology
Dr Guy Preville, Val-David, QC - Anesthesia
Dr Francois A Prevost, Inukjuak, QC - General Practice
Dr Ignacio Prieto, Montreal, QC - Cardiovasc/ThorSurg
Dr Gerry D Prince, Medicine Hat, AB - Family Medicine
Dr M Jane Pritchard, East York, ON - Family Medicine
Dr Guylaine Proulx, Gatineau, QC - Family Medicine
Dr Edith Provencal, Chateauguay, QC - General Practice
Dr Jose A Prudencio, Waterloo, ON - Otolaryngology
Dr Serge Querin, Montreal, QC - Internal Medicine
Dr Ricardo Quesada, Portage La Prairie, MB - Family Medicine
Dr Marie Quintal, Gatineau, QC - Psychiatry
Dr Elsa S Quiros-Calinoiu, Montreal, QC - Obstetrics & Gynecology
Dr Jed Rabinovitch, Scarborough, ON - Ophthalmology
Dr Nicole A Radziminski, Vancouver, BC - Pediatrics
Dr J C Bruno Rainville, Quebec, QC - General Surgery
Dr Francesco Ramadori, Montreal, QC - Anesthesia
Dr Antonio Rambaldi, Varennes, QC - General Practice
Dr Oswaldo C Ramirez, Alliston, ON - Family Medicine
Dr Saby E M Ramirez Moreno, Powell River, BC - Psychiatry
Dr Rosemarie Ramsingh, Timmins, ON - Community Medicine
Dr Kavita Randhawa, North York, ON - Family Medicine
Dr Michele Raymond, Ottawa, ON - Family Medicine
Dr Felix C Re Martinez, St Catharines, ON - General Practice
Dr Robert M Rehaluk, North York, ON - Psychiatry
Dr Morton J Reingold, North York, ON - General Practice
Dr Marciano D Reis, Toronto, ON - Hematological Pathology
Dr Ricardo A Rendon, Halifax, NS - Urology
Dr Alfonso Restrepo, St-Eustache, QC - General Practice
Dr Enrique G Reyes, Barrie, ON - Obstetrics & Gynecology
Dr Clayton Reynolds, Victoria, BC - Internal Medicine
Dr Margarita R Riano Alvarez, LaSalle, QC - Family Medicine
Dr Carlos S Ribas, Hamilton, ON - General Practice
Dr Rona G Ribeiro, Sherwood Park, AB - Family Medicine
Dr Annette Richard, London, ON - Family Medicine
Dr Luc Richard, Forestville, QC - General Practice
Dr Richard L Richards, North York, ON - General Practice
Dr Anne-Katrin Richter, Montreal, QC - Family Medicine
Dr R Markus Rieckenberg, Orillia, ON - Anatomical Pathology
Dr Santos Rijo, Woodbridge, ON - General Practice
Dr Juan A Rivera, Montreal, QC - Endocrin/Metabolism
Dr Luis Rivero Pinelo, Shawville, QC - Family Medicine
Dr Luis G Riveros Neira, Miramichi, NB - General Practice
Dr Donald Rivest, Levis, QC - Electroencephal
Dr Sandro B Rizoli, Toronto, ON - General Surgery
Dr Roger M J Roberge, Moncton, NB - General Surgery
Dr Rene R Roberge, Baie-Saint-Paul, QC - Anesthesia
Dr Daniel Roberge, Quebec, QC - General Practice
Dr David Robitaille, Longueuil, QC - Psychiatry
Dr Guillermo Rocha, Brandon, MB - Ophthalmology
Dr Alain Rochon, Sherbrooke, QC - Community Medicine
Dr Felisa L Rochwerger, Toronto, ON - Psychiatry
Dr Irwin J Rodier, Montreal, QC - General Practice
Dr Sylvia L Rodriguez, Guelph, ON - Ophthalmology
Dr Carlos H Rodriguez, Toronto, ON - Internal Medicine
Dr Maria del Rosario Rodriguez Moya, Montreal, QC - General Practice
Dr Aristides Rodriguez Naranjo, Battleford, SK - General Practice
Dr Emilio Rodriguez-Marin, Mississauga, ON - Diagnostic-Radiology
Dr Luna S Roher, Thornhill, ON - Psychiatry
Dr Hector A Roldan, Huntsville, ON - General Surgery
Dr Luis O Roldan Lozano, North York, ON - Psychiatry
Dr Ramon Roman, Verdun, QC - Anesthesia
Dr Juan J Ronco, Vancouver, BC - Internal Medicine
Dr Rosa H Rosario, Winnipeg, MB - General Practice
Dr David C Rosen, Mississauga, ON - General Practice
Dr Lea M Rossiter, Toronto, ON - Family Medicine
Dr Ann Rothman, Montreal, QC - Family Medicine
Dr Paul Roumeliotis, Cornwall, ON - Pediatrics
Dr Helene Rousseau, Montreal, QC - Family Medicine
Dr Pierre Rousseau, Montreal, QC - Radiation Oncology
Dr Marc J Roy, Kanata, ON - Family Medicine
Dr Jean A Roy, Ottawa, ON - Family Medicine
Dr Denis Roy, Sudbury, ON - Internal Medicine
Dr Carmella A Roy, Montreal, QC - Psychiatry
Dr Helene Roy, Quebec, QC - General Practice
Dr Suzanne Roy, Trois-Rivieres, QC - General Practice
Dr Willine R Rozefort, Verdun, QC - Family Medicine
Dr Dominador B Rubio, Belleville, ON - General Practice
Dr David N Rush, Winnipeg, MB - Internal Medicine
Dr Nene O S Rush, Winnipeg, MB - Family Medicine
Dr Robert S Russell, Saskatoon, SK - General Practice
Dr Barbara L Russell-Mahoney, Sioux Lookout, ON - Family Medicine
Dr Edward A J Ryan, Etobicoke, ON - Obstetrics & Gynecology
Dr Najib N Safieddine, Toronto, ON - General Surgery
Dr Patrick Safieh, North York, ON - Emergency Family Med
Dr Beatriz M Sainz, Oromocto, NB - Family Medicine
Dr Juan R Salcedo, Nepean, ON - Cardiology
Dr Karl H Sales, Kirkland Lake, ON - Ophthalmology
Dr Luis A Salgado De Leon, Regina, SK - General Practice
Dr Magdi H Sami, Montreal, QC - Cardiology
Dr Patricia Sammarelli, Victoria, BC - Family Medicine
Dr Arnaud Samson, Baie-Comeau, QC - General Practice
Dr Isabelle Samson, Quebec, QC - Family Medicine
Dr Sheri L Samuels, Edmonton, AB - Family Medicine
Dr Federico J Sanchez, Etobicoke, ON - Family Medicine
Dr Millaray Sanchez, Ottawa, ON - Family Medicine
Dr Adolfo Sanchez, Toronto, ON - Psychiatry
Dr Arturo Sanchez, Toronto, ON - Pediatrics

Dr Marisol Sanchez, Montreal, QC - Pediatric Emergency Medicine
Dr Emilio Sanchez-Arroyo, Pointe-Claire, QC - Diagnostic-Radiology
Dr Pablo E R F Sanhueza Luco, North Bay, ON - Psychiatry
Dr Claudia Santos, Toronto, ON - Critical Care Medicine
Dr Gustavo Saposnik, Toronto, ON - Neurology
Dr Alicia Sarabia, Mississauga, ON - Infectious Diseases
Dr Dioscoro D C Sarile, Toronto, ON - General Practice
Dr Harvey B Sarnat, Calgary, AB - Neurology
Dr Silvia E M Sas, Kanata, ON - General Practice
Dr Mark E Saul, Wakefield, QC - Family Medicine
Dr Peter Sauret, Toronto, ON - General Practice
Dr Michel D Sauve, Fort McMurray, AB - Critical Care Medicine
Dr Gabrielle K Savard, Calgary, AB - Family Medicine
Dr Christine Scarinci, Montreal, QC - Pediatrics
Dr Beatrice M Schamberger-Keren, Toronto, ON - Psychiatry
Dr Erick Schampaert, Montreal, QC - Cardiology
Dr Christian H Schenk, Vancouver, BC - Psychiatry
Dr Ernesto L Schiffrin, Montreal, QC - Internal Medicine
Dr Alicia Schiffrin, Montreal, QC - Endocrinology
Dr Suzan Schneeweiss, Toronto, ON - Pediatrics
Dr Johannes S J Schneider, Salmon Arm, BC - General Surgery
Dr Deborah C Schwartz, Vancouver, BC - Psychiatry
Dr Gaston Schwarz, Montreal, QC - Plastic Surgery
Dr Jorge A Schwarz, Westmount, QC - Plastic Surgery
Dr Robert H Scott, Toronto, ON - General Practice
Dr Michael V Scully, Rossland, BC - General Practice
Dr Jean M Seely, Ottawa, ON - Diagnostic-Radiology
Dr Jose A C Segura, Chandler, QC - Psychiatry
Dr Houfar Sekhavat, Dieppe, NB - Ophthalmology
Dr Erick F Sell Marucco, Ottawa, ON - General Practice
Dr Lisa M Sennewald Teskey, Surrey, BC - General Practice
Dr Didier M Serero, Montreal, QC - Emergency Family Med
Dr Manuel Serrano, Montreal, QC - Psychiatry
Dr Brian A Shamess, Sault Ste. Marie, ON - General Practice
Dr Marcia H Shapir Kahan, Toronto, ON - Psychiatry
Dr Thomas A W Shaw-Stiffel, Ottawa, ON - Gastroenterology
Dr Megan E Sherwood, Vancouver, BC - Psychiatry
Dr Marcelo C Shibata, Edmonton, AB - General Practice
Dr Robert H Shih, Etobicoke, ON - Family Medicine
Dr Prakash T Shrestha, Hazelton, BC - Family Medicine
Dr Michael Shuster, Banff, AB - Emergency Medicine
Dr Pascale L R Sibille, Gatineau, QC - General Practice
Dr Sergio Sierra-Dupont, Montreal, QC - Otolaryngology
Dr Jaime E Silva, Hamilton, ON - Neurology
Dr Mariana Silva, Kingston, ON - Pediatrics
Dr Enrique Silva, Pembroke, ON - Anatomical Pathology
Dr Andree-Anne Simard, Montreal, QC - General Practice
Dr Genevieve Simard-Racine, Amqui, QC - General Practice
Dr Andrew A Simone, Etobicoke, ON - Dermatology
Dr William Singer, East York, ON - Internal Medicine
Dr Christine B Singh, Vancouver, BC - Family Medicine
Dr Marcia Sirota, Toronto, ON - Psychiatry
Dr Yoanna K Skrobik, Montreal, QC - Internal Medicine
Dr Helen Smeja, Pierrefonds, QC - General Practice
Dr Donald A Smith, Toronto, ON - Family Medicine
Dr Jacqueline A Smith-Auguste, North York, ON - Orthopedic Surgery
Dr Steven J Socransky, Sudbury, ON - Emergency Medicine
Dr Alfonso J Solimano, Vancouver, BC - Pediatrics
Dr Jordan B Solmon, North York, ON - Family Medicine
Dr Jorge Soni, Toronto, ON - Psychiatry
Dr Alok Pal Sood, Toronto, ON - Family Medicine
Dr Julio C Soto, Montreal, QC - Community Medicine
Dr Grace G Soto De Machat, Vaughan, ON - Family Medicine
Dr Frederique Souchon, Montreal, QC - Electroencephal
Dr Luis Souhami, Montreal, QC - Radiation Oncology
Dr Joaquin F Sousa-Poza, Galiano, BC - Psychiatry
Dr Richard C Spees, Ottawa, ON - Psychiatry
Dr J David Spence, London, ON - Internal Medicine
Dr Martin H Spencer, Nanaimo, BC - Ophthalmology
Dr Christopher D Stabler, Kamloops, BC - Gastroenterology
Dr Jonathan M S Standley, Bath, ON - General Practice
Dr Marc Steben, Montreal, QC - Family Medicine
Dr Aleksandra Stefanovic, Vancouver, BC - Infectious Diseases
Dr Nolan-Paul A Stein, Toronto, ON - General Practice
Dr Patrick R Stel, Victoria, BC - General Practice
Dr Josef Stelzer, Winnipeg, MB - General Practice
Dr Carlo Sterlin, Montreal, QC - Psychiatry
Dr D Greg Stewart, Huntsville, ON - General Practice
Dr Rosemary A Stogre, Cobourg, ON - General Practice
Dr Philip A T Stratford, Cobourg, ON - Family Medicine
Dr Hanka H E A Stratmann, Woodbridge, ON - Family Medicine
Dr Philip F Stuart, North York, ON - Medical Microbiology
Dr Lina M Suazo Hidalgo, Calgary, AB - Family Medicine
Dr Aravind Subramanian, Calgary, AB - General Practice
Dr I F H James Sugiyama, Toronto, ON - General Practice
Dr Omar Sultan, Regina, SK - Cardiology
Dr Shanthini Sundareswaran, Mississauga, ON - Family Medicine
Dr Patrick P W Sung, Vegreville, AB - General Practice
Dr Diann J Superina-Bell, Toronto, ON - Pediatrics
Dr Manindar Surbey, Delta, BC - General Practice
Dr Brigit A Swenson, North York, ON - Family Medicine
Dr Ikramuddin Syed, Etobicoke, ON - Family Medicine
Dr Pierre-Luc Sylvain, Matane, QC - General Practice
Dr Julio Szmuilowicz, Toronto, ON - Psychiatry
Dr Sharon Szmuilowicz, Toronto, ON - Psychiatry
Dr Wanda M Szymonowicz, Mississauga, ON - Pediatrics
Dr Mary-Margaret Taabazuing, London, ON - Internal Medicine
Dr Mohamed A Tabib, Windsor, ON - Diagnostic-Radiology
Dr Takeshi Takahashi Monroy, Windsor, ON - General Surgery
Dr Charles E Talon, Longueuil, QC - General Practice
Dr Domenica Tambasco, Toronto, ON - Family Medicine
Dr Robert Tambay, Ottawa, ON - Gastroenterology
Dr Darrell H S Tan, Toronto, ON - Infectious Diseases
Dr Lisa H Taras, Ottawa, ON - Family Medicine
Dr Michele Tardif, Montreal, QC - Plastic Surgery
Dr Gretta Taylor, Halifax, NS - Family Medicine
Dr Michael R Taylor, Ottawa, ON - Emergency Family Med
Dr Joseph Telch, Markham, ON - Pediatrics
Dr Jose F Tellez-Zenteno, Saskatoon, SK - General Practice
Dr Lionel Tenby, Richmond, BC - General Practice
Dr Carlos Tesler-Mabe, Vancouver, BC - Psychiatry
Dr Pierre C Tessier, Ottawa, ON - Family Medicine
Dr Daniel Tessier, Sherbrooke, QC - Geriatric Medicine
Dr Patrick Theriault, Ottawa, ON - Family Medicine
Dr Nicolas Thibault, Edmonton, AB - Family Medicine
Dr Jocelyne Thiffault, Laval, QC - General Practice
Dr Celeste J Thirlwell, Toronto, ON - Psychiatry
Dr Claudette Thomas Fils-Aime, Montreal, QC - General Practice
Dr Thomas R Thompson, Winnipeg, MB - Psychiatry
Dr Jannette J Thompson, North York, ON - Family Medicine
Dr Ian B Thompson, Schreiber, ON - Family Medicine
Dr Maria-Elena Tiboni, Hamilton, ON - Internal Medicine
Dr Brian Ticoll, Markham, ON - Psychiatry
Dr Rossana M Tirado, Orleans, ON - Pediatrics
Dr Kevin L F Tong, Vancouver, BC - General Practice
Dr Luis Toriz, Saint-Jerome, QC - Orthopedic Surgery
Dr Monica Torres Jimenez, Goderich, ON - General Practice
Dr Nestor E Torres Martinez, Brockville, ON - Family Medicine
Dr Jean Tousignant, Trois-Rivieres, QC - Anesthesia
Dr John W Toye, Orillia, ON - Plastic Surgery
Dr Daniel Z Traub-Werner, Toronto, ON - Psychiatry
Dr Lionel D B Traverse, Abbotsford, BC - Pediatrics
Dr Jacques Tremblay, Verdun, QC - General Practice
Dr Nicolas-Olivier Tremblay-Reinhardt, Roberval, QC - General Practice
Dr Isabelle Trop, Montreal, QC - Diagnostic-Radiology
Dr Barbara E Trott, Vancouver, BC - General Practice
Dr Ana-Maria C Tsanaclis, Sherbrooke, QC - General Practice
Dr Georges Tsoukas, Montreal, QC - Endocrinology
Dr Francoise Turgeon, Jonquiere, QC - General Practice
Dr Jolanda C Turley, Ottawa, ON - Family Medicine
Dr Lucy M Turnham, Vancouver, BC - General Practice
Dr Hanna M Tuszynska, Hamilton, ON - Anesthesia
Dr Jurate K Uleckas, Laval, QC - Ophthalmology
Dr Andres B Umoquit, Scarborough, ON - General Practice
Dr Raul C Urtasun, Edmonton, AB - Radiation Oncology
Dr Gabriel A Vadasz, Toronto, ON - Family Medicine
Dr Sander J Van Zanten, Edmonton, AB - Gastroenterology
Dr Michele Vartian, Montreal, QC - Pediatrics
Dr Mariette Varvarikos, Montreal, QC - Emergency Family Med
Dr Jose A Vasconcelos, Brandon, MB - Psychiatry
Dr Raul A Vasquez, Belleville, ON - Family Medicine
Dr Manuel O Vasquez, York, ON - General Practice
Dr John A Vecchiarelli, North York, ON - General Practice
Dr Michael J Vecchio, North York, ON - General Practice
Dr Juan M Velasquez Malvehy, St Catharines, ON - Internal Medicine
Dr Ricardo J Velazquez, Duncan, BC - Orthopedic Surgery
Dr Gloria C Velez, Mississauga, ON - Family Medicine
Dr Enrique C G Ventureyra, Ottawa, ON - Neurosurgery
Dr V Antonio Vera Silva, North York, ON - Family Medicine
Dr N Alfonso Verdejo-Aguilar, Vancouver, BC - Internal Medicine
Dr Nicolaas P L G Verhoeff, North York, ON - Psychiatry
Dr Neil Verma, Richmond Hill, ON - Emergency Family Med
Dr Bertha C R B Vidal Peralta, Toronto, ON - Psychiatry
Dr Claudette Viens, Les Bergeronnes, QC - General Practice
Dr Antonio A L Vigano, Montreal, QC - General Practice
Dr Milagro C Viguera Salazar, Lucan, ON - Family Medicine
Dr Fidel Vila-Rodriguez, Vancouver, BC - Psychiatry
Dr Diego Villa Restrepo, Vancouver, BC - Internal Medicine
Dr Monique Villanueva Arquint, Markham, ON - General Pathology
Dr Denis R J Vincent, Edmonton, AB - Family Medicine
Dr Julie F Vinette-Azzi, Gloucester, ON - Family Medicine
Dr Fernando A Visbal Amador, Welland, ON - Pediatrics
Dr Bennedetto B Vitullo, Charlottetown, PE - Pediatrics
Dr Carlos A Vollinoti, Gatineau, QC - Obstetrics & Gynecology
Dr W Robbert Vroom, Vancouver, BC - Emergency Family Med
Dr J Arturo Wadgymar, Mississauga, ON - Internal Medicine
Dr Lyle H Waldman, Montreal, QC - General Practice
Dr Joseph Walker, Nanaimo, BC - Psychiatry
Dr Wahan Wanis, Vancouver, BC - Psychiatry
Dr Gregory D Waslen, Calgary, AB - Plastic Surgery
Dr Terrence S Waters, Vancouver, BC - Anesthesia
Dr Ashley D Wazana, Montreal, QC - Psychiatry
Dr Sara Weinstock-Goldberg, North York, ON - Family Medicine
Dr Jennie L Wells, London, ON - Geriatric Medicine
Dr Larry M Wengle, Toronto, ON - General Practice
Dr Lori J West, Edmonton, AB - Pediatrics
Dr Miriam J Wiebe, Toronto, ON - Family Medicine
Dr Samuel Wiebe-Velazquez, Calgary, AB - Neurology
Dr Andreas T J Wielgosz, Ottawa, ON - Cardiology
Dr Sheila Wijayasinghe, Toronto, ON - Family Medicine
Dr Andrea Wilhelm, Masset, BC - Family Medicine
Dr Andrew Wilk, Oshawa, ON - General Practice
Dr Christina Williams, Vancouver, BC - Obstetrics & Gynecology
Dr Eldon S V Williams, Toronto, ON - General Surgery
Dr Larry A Willms, Sioux Lookout, ON - Family Medicine
Dr Murray B Wilson, Bradford, ON - General Practice
Dr Raymond J R Wiss, Sudbury, ON - Emergency Family Med
Dr Wendy L Wobeser, Kingston, ON - Infectious Diseases
Dr James R Wylie, Brampton, ON - General Practice
Dr Louise B M Wylie, Ottawa, ON - General Practice
Dr Olivier Yaccarini, Quebec, QC - Emergency Family Med
Dr Annalee Yassi, Vancouver, BC - Community Medicine
Dr Horacio Yepes, Sydney, NS - General Practice
Dr Natasha Yepes Restrepo, Kitchener, ON - Ophthalmology
Dr Luis T J Ying, Brampton, ON - Gastroenterology
Dr Grace Yoon, Toronto, ON - Medical Genetics
Dr Never Youssoufian de Perez, Toronto, ON - Psychiatry
Dr Joseph A Zadra, Barrie, ON - Urology
Dr Patrick A Zaidel, Burnaby, BC - Internal Medicine
Dr Tanya L Zakrison, Toronto, ON - General Surgery
Dr Noe Zamel, Toronto, ON - Med Scientist
Dr Ricardo Zarruk, Pierrefonds, QC - General Practice
Dr Maryam Zeineddin, West Vancouver, BC - Family Medicine
Dr Roger L Zemek, Ottawa, ON - Pediatric Emergency Medicine
Dr Paul J Zeni, Georgetown, ON - General Practice
Dr Gonzalo F Zevallos, Milton, ON - General Practice
Dr Adam M Zieleniak, St-Charles-Brromee, QC - General Practice
Dr N Ariel Zielinsky, Toronto, ON - Psychiatry
Dr Eugenia Zikos, Montreal, QC - Psychiatry
Dr Caren F Zilber-Shlensky, Victoria, BC - Family Medicine
Dr Gregorio Zlotnik, Montreal, QC - General Practice

Dr Kathia Znojkiewicz, Montreal, QC - General Practice
Dr Ronald M Zuker, Toronto, ON - Plastic Surgery
Dr Daniel de Yturralde, Shediac, NB - Orthopedic Surgery
Dr Raquel del Carpio, Montreal, QC - Diagnostic-Radiology

SWAHILI

Dr Alnoor Abdulla, Vancouver, BC - Cardiology
Dr S Amadala, Calgary, AB - Psychiatry
Dr Shiraz F Aziz, Surrey, BC - General Practice
Dr Roger Bashala, Campbellton, NB - Family Medicine
Dr Gunvantrai J Bhatt, Windsor, ON - General Practice
Dr Raul A J Carvalho, Richmond, BC - General Practice
Dr Abdallah S Daar, Toronto, ON - General Surgery
Dr Alkarim Damji, Etobicoke, ON - Family Medicine
Dr Mehboob Damji, Stoney Creek, ON - General Practice
Dr Shahnaz Dar, Scarborough, ON - Pediatrics
Dr Vincent De Sa, Thunder Bay, ON - Pediatrics
Dr Levinus Albert Dieleman, Edmonton, AB - General Practice
Dr Peter R Durie, Toronto, ON - Pediatrics
Dr Alcantro B Fernandez, Stoney Creek, ON - General Practice
Dr Sleem Feroze, Oakville, ON - Obstetrics & Gynecology
Dr Shiraz H Ismail, North York, ON - General Practice
Dr Amin R Javer, Vancouver, BC - Otolaryngology
Dr Shamin Jetha, Vancouver, BC - Family Medicine
Dr Azim F Juma, Scarborough, ON - Family Medicine
Dr Yamuna Kalyanpur, Vancouver, BC - Obstetrics & Gynecology
Dr Narendra K Karia, Calgary, AB - General Practice
Dr Arvind A Kati, Winnipeg, MB - General Practice
Dr Mahmuda B Khan, Scarborough, ON - Family Medicine
Dr Gulshan Lodhi, St Jacobs, ON - General Practice
Dr Alaudin E Manji, Delta, BC - Family Medicine
Dr Suryakant D Mehta, Toronto, ON - General Practice
Dr Shamsh Y Merali, Milton, ON - Family Medicine
Dr Amirudin A M Mewa, Toronto, ON - Internal Medicine
Dr Sheona M Mitchell, Vancouver, BC - General Practice
Dr Akber H Mithani, Vancouver, BC - General Practice
Dr Nashila N Mohamed, Etobicoke, ON - Family Medicine
Dr Maqbool A Mughal, Mississauga, ON - General Practice
Dr Stanley K Muwanguzi, Camrose, AB - Emergency Family Med
Dr Stanley N M Muwonge, Grande Prairie, AB - Family Medicine
Dr M Muni Nazerali-Sunderji, New Westminster, BC - Internal Medicine
Dr Beatrice K Osoro, Keswick, ON - Family Medicine
Dr Vincent M Osundwa, Edmonton, AB - Clin Immun/Allergy
Dr George W Otto, North York, ON - General Practice
Dr Sudhir D Pandya, Calgary, AB - Emergency Medicine
Dr Kirit K Patel, St. John's, NL - General Practice
Dr Ila M Patel, Mississauga, ON - Family Medicine
Dr Naresh R Patel, Tilbury, ON - Family Medicine
Dr Hasmukh G Patel, Windsor, ON - Anesthesia
Dr Sultaneih S P Rajabali, New Westminster, BC - General Practice
Dr Moizali A Ramji, Sherwood Park, AB - General Practice
Dr Alnoor Ramji, Vancouver, BC - Gastroenterology
Dr Ranjodh S Rehal, Winnipeg, MB - General Practice
Dr El-Karim F J Rhemtulla, St Catharines, ON - Ophthalmology
Dr Luigi T Ricciardi, Virgil, ON - Family Medicine
Dr Fakhruddin Sadikali, St Catharines, ON - Internal Medicine
Dr Amirali M Samji, Toronto, ON - General Practice
Dr Mahendra B S Sangani, Greenfield Park, QC - General Practice
Dr Riaz Shariff, Ajax, ON - General Practice
Dr Shiv R Sharma, Toronto, ON - Family Medicine
Dr Maliha A H Sherman, Hamilton, ON - Family Medicine
Dr Brijendra Sood, Calgary, AB - General Practice
Dr Permjit S Suri, Nepean, ON - Internal Medicine
Dr Saadat A S Syed, North York, ON - Family Medicine
Dr Verjinderpal S Ubhi, Mississauga, ON - Family Medicine
Dr Himat Vaghadia, Vancouver, BC - Anesthesia
Dr Mirza R Virani, Markham, ON - General Practice
Dr Manjit S Walia, Kitchener, ON - Pediatrics
Dr Shiraz A Walji, Calgary, AB - General Practice

SWAZI

Dr Dereck Maseka, Drumheller, AB - Family Medicine
Dr Motlobeng D Pebane, Indian Head, SK - General Practice

SWEDISH

Dr Hallgrimur Benediktsson, Calgary, AB - Anatomical Pathology
Dr Anne B Biringer, Toronto, ON - Family Medicine
Dr Francis M Boston, Montreal, QC - Diagnostic-Radiology
Dr Christine Brenckmann, Prince George, BC - Family Medicine
Dr Malin K Clark, Saskatoon, SK - Psychiatry
Dr Sandra R A Cohen, Montreal, QC - Hematology
Dr Suliman Gardee, Kanata, ON - General Practice
Dr Michael J Heiber, Scarborough, ON - Emergency Family Med
Dr Eva E Hemmerich, Comox, BC - Family Medicine
Dr Steven G Hobson, Mission, BC - General Practice
Dr Anthony J C Holland, Port Alberni, BC - Anesthesia
Dr Lawrence J Kotkas, Lethbridge, AB - Psychiatry
Dr A Christin Lundgren, Calgary, AB - Family Medicine
Dr Carina M Majaesic, Edmonton, AB - Pediatrics
Dr Michele A Matter, Selkirk, MB - Family Medicine
Dr Paivi M H Miettunen, Calgary, AB - Pediatrics
Dr Jan Fredrik Moe, Kinistino, SK - General Practice
Dr Juri Rand, Peterborough, ON - General Practice
Dr Jonas L Sandstrom, Rossland, BC - Family Medicine
Dr Markus Schatzmann, Milton, ON - Family Medicine
Dr Anne M Sepanmaa-Lund, Edmonton, AB - General Practice
Dr Martin Svartberg, Toronto, ON - Psychiatry
Dr Eva E Thomas, Vancouver, BC - Medical Microbiology
Dr Ellen N Thompson, Ottawa, ON - Anesthesia
Dr Inge G Winslow, Richmond Hill, ON - General Practice
Dr Stephanie H M Winsor, Hamilton, ON - Obstetrics & Gynecology
Dr Maryam Zeineddin, West Vancouver, BC - Family Medicine

TAGALOG

Dr Lea M Amog-Kerr, Cambridge, ON - General Practice
Dr Romulo F Anastasio Jr, Hamilton, ON - General Practice
Dr Mario R Andres, Toronto, ON - Internal Medicine
Dr Salvador J Andres, Saskatoon, SK - General Practice
Dr Emmanuel P B Aquino, Dartmouth, NS - General Practice
Dr Rufino B Balmaceda, Ottawa, ON - Psychiatry
Dr Maria Dulce B Bismonte, Etobicoke, ON - Psychiatry
Dr Emilia M Bordalba, Vancouver, BC - General Practice
Dr Darshan S Brar, Calgary, AB - General Practice
Dr Antonio D Bueno, Vancouver, BC - General Practice
Dr Antonio A Buzon, Scarborough, ON - Urology
Dr Moises D Cabatu, Fredericton, NB - General Practice
Dr Enrico F Cabigon, Regina, SK - Anatomical Pathology
Dr Gerardo G Calderon, Scarborough, ON - General Practice
Dr S Rhona B Capisonda, Lethbridge, AB - General Practice
Dr Antonio P Carretero Jr, Moose Jaw, SK - Anatomical Pathology
Dr Melanio G Catre, East York, ON - Orthopedic Surgery
Dr M Lourdes M Celis, Calgary, AB - Family Medicine
Dr Rolando T Corpus, North York, ON - General Surgery
Dr Geraldine Z V Cruz, Mississauga, ON - Family Medicine
Dr Caridad M Cruz, Scarborough, ON - Psychiatry
Dr Norman M Cruz, Stratford, ON - General Practice
Dr Mary Lou Dancel, Peterborough, ON - Psychiatry
Dr Eleazar W David, Surrey, BC - Family Medicine
Dr Madeline Dayot-Venida, Peterborough, ON - Psychiatry
Dr Ruby L De Guzman, Ottawa, ON - Anatomical Pathology
Dr Filemon De Jesus Jr., Ottawa, ON - Urology
Dr Josephine De La Torre, Guelph, ON - Family Medicine
Dr Maria A De Villa, Toronto, ON - Cardiology
Dr Silvino M Decena, North York, ON - Family Medicine
Dr Daniel S Del Rosario, Scarborough, ON - General Practice
Dr M C Armellie Dela Cruz, Penticton, BC - Obstetrics & Gynecology
Dr Jiri J Dubec, Surrey, BC - Family Medicine
Dr Jocelyn Dumatol-Sanchez, Winnipeg, MB - Family Medicine
Dr Marlene T Dytoc, Edmonton, AB - Dermatology
Dr Froilan N Espiritu, North York, ON - General Practice
Dr Engracia D Eusebio-Torres, Mississauga, ON - Psychiatry
Dr Alfredo F Formoso, Nepean, ON - Diagnostic-Radiology
Dr Francisco C Francisco, Etobicoke, ON - General Practice
Dr Herbert Y Gaisano, Toronto, ON - Gastroenterology
Dr Rodolfo C Gallardo, Etobicoke, ON - General Practice
Dr Margaret C Gan-Gaisano, Scarborough, ON - Pediatrics
Dr Patricio B Garces, Scarborough, ON - Diagnostic-Radiology
Dr Yasmin M A Garcia, Nelson, BC - Family Medicine
Dr Cesar P Garcia, Newmarket, ON - Psychiatry
Dr Rose Marie E Geonzon, Calgary, AB - Family Medicine
Dr Radzfel A Geonzon, Calgary, AB - Family Medicine
Dr Masoud Goodarzi, Niagara Falls, ON - Internal Medicine
Dr Marinett R Gutierrez, Bathurst, NB - General Practice
Dr Venus B Guzman, Toronto, ON - General Practice
Dr Cristina A Kiai, North Vancouver, BC - Family Medicine
Dr Atilano G Lacson, Edmonton, AB - Neuro-Pathology
Dr U Elsa O Lapena, Oshawa, ON - Family Medicine
Dr Hilario S Lapena, Oshawa, ON - Family Medicine
Dr Moises S Lasaleta, Calgary, AB - General Practice
Dr Christina J Ledesma-Cadhit, East York, ON - Family Medicine
Dr Ofelia Legaspi, Langley, BC - General Practice
Dr David C Lim, Toronto, ON - General Practice
Dr Aimee J V Mabini, Oakville, ON - Otolaryngology
Dr Joyce M Magnaye, Moose Jaw, SK - General Practice
Dr Edilberto A Malabanan, Winnipeg, MB - General Practice
Dr Lita L Malig, Mississauga, ON - Family Medicine
Dr Magdalena Marcelo-Macalino, North Battleford, SK - General Practice
Dr Roberto B Matta, North York, ON - General Practice
Dr Maribel B Mendoza, Milton, ON - Family Medicine
Dr Gloria S Meneses, Scarborough, ON - Family Medicine
Dr Maira Obnamia, Etobicoke, ON - General Practice
Dr Sharon Rose Y Ong, Surrey, BC - General Surgery
Dr Larry S Ong, Vancouver, BC - Psychiatry
Dr Dennis D Ong, Saskatoon, SK - Anesthesia
Dr Ruth B Pacis, Dartmouth, NS - Family Medicine
Dr Ben L Pangilinan Jr, Thornhill, ON - Family Medicine
Dr Gelasio F Parlan Jr, Mississauga, ON - General Practice
Dr Joan S Pascual, Fredericton, NB - General Practice
Dr Rossali Pilapil-Lee, Vancouver, BC - Family Medicine
Dr Roel C Poblete, Niagara Falls, ON - Cardiology
Dr Michael G Rayel, Clarenville, NL - General Practice
Dr Larina M Reyes-Smith, Surrey, BC - Family Medicine
Dr Reynaldo P Robes, Scarborough, ON - Internal Medicine
Dr Zenia A Sanchez, Mississauga, ON - General Practice
Dr Milagros F Saraza, Brampton, ON - General Practice
Dr Dioscoro D C Sarile, Toronto, ON - General Practice
Dr Pascualito A Seminiano, Langley, BC - Psychiatry
Dr Hermenegildo-Rommel R Seno, Regina, SK - Anatomical Pathology
Dr Paterno C Serezo, Wallaceburg, ON - General Practice
Dr Coeliflor D Silva, Toronto, ON - General Practice
Dr Romulo M Sinajon, Brampton, ON - General Practice
Dr John C Sy, London, ON - General Practice
Dr Peter Y Sy, Mississauga, ON - General Practice
Dr William Y Sy, Scarborough, ON - Psychiatry
Dr Romeo B Tan, North York, ON - Family Medicine
Dr Lee Puan Tan, Windsor, ON - Internal Medicine
Dr Vilma S Tan-Jarvis, Woodbridge, ON - Family Medicine
Dr Clementine Tang, Vancouver, BC - Pediatrics
Dr Grace Y Tanhuanco-Kho, Victoria, BC - Anatomical Pathology
Dr Christel M Tayag, Windsor, ON - Family Medicine
Dr Shaun K Tregoning, Abbotsford, BC - Obstetrics & Gynecology
Dr Andres B Umoquit, Scarborough, ON - General Practice
Dr Antonio F Uy Jr, Peterborough, ON - Family Medicine
Dr Danilo R Vargas, Surrey, BC - Otolaryngology
Dr Laing P Velicaria, White River, ON - General Practice
Dr Clarita S Vianzon, Winnipeg, MB - General Practice
Capt Daisy M Vianzon Edora, Victoria, BC - Family Medicine
Dr Maselle G Virey, Mississauga, ON - Psychiatry
Dr Edgardo Y Wee, Vancouver, BC - General Practice
Dr Anna L Wolak, Vancouver, BC - General Practice
Dr Danilo A Wycoco, Kitchener, ON - Diagnostic-Radiology
Dr Peter Y O Yao, Surrey, BC - Orthopedic Surgery
Dr Hanle O Yap, Windsor, ON - Geriatric Medicine

Dr Elaine T Yeung, Scarborough, ON - Gastroenterology
Dr Catherine L Yu, East York, ON - Emergency Family Med
Dr Myrna B Zapata, St Catharines, ON - Pediatrics
Dr Rodrigo P de Luna, Peterborough, ON - Family Medicine

TAISHANESE

Dr Frances Y K Leung, Toronto, ON - Internal Medicine
Dr Raymond A Liang, Vancouver, BC - Psychiatry

TAIWANESE

Dr Charlie C Chen, New Westminster, BC - Family Medicine
Dr Simon I Chen, Vancouver, BC - Emergency Family Med
Dr Charles Y Y Cheng, Vancouver, BC - General Practice
Dr Michael J C Cheng, St Thomas, ON - Urology
Dr Aik-Ping Eng, Vancouver, BC - General Practice
Dr Hans C T Guo, Scarborough, ON - Family Medicine
Dr Yann J Hsiao, Vancouver, BC - General Practice
Dr Henry Y Huang, Ajax, ON - Otolaryngology
Dr Harvey Y Huang, Ajax, ON - Anesthesia
Dr Ling Ling Huang, Mississauga, ON - Family Medicine
Dr Louis Huang, Scarborough, ON - Anesthesia
Dr Charles C S Law, Vancouver, BC - General Practice
Dr Mao-Cheng Lee, Edmonton, AB - Internal Medicine
Dr Cheng-Han Lee, Vancouver, BC - Anatomical Pathology
Dr H Robert Liao, Scarborough, ON - Ophthalmology
Dr Edward C H Luke, Vancouver, BC - Emergency Family Med
Dr Douglas B G Ng, Surrey, BC - General Practice
Dr Milton C Po, Surrey, BC - Radiation Oncology
Dr Richard H Shao, East York, ON - Internal Medicine
Dr K Y Kevin Sheu, Burnaby, BC - Family Medicine
Dr Robert H Shih, Etobicoke, ON - Family Medicine
Dr Aaron C T Shih, Etobicoke, ON - Family Medicine
Dr Lucas Tai, Toronto, ON - General Practice
Dr Charles C Tan, Richmond Hill, ON - General Practice
Dr Kevin L F Tong, Vancouver, BC - General Practice
Dr Jason Y S Tsai, North York, ON - General Practice
Dr Smiley G S Tsao, Unionville, ON - Family Medicine
Dr Kenneth S H Tung, Scarborough, ON - General Practice
Dr Angela J Wang, Petrolia, ON - Family Medicine
Dr Daniel D Wong, Toronto, ON - General Practice
Dr Chin Yu Wu, Hamilton, ON - General Practice
Dr Kwang Yang, Surrey, BC - Family Medicine

TAMIL

Dr Chitralekha R Abeysinghe, Markham, ON - Family Medicine
Dr Thoppil M Abraham, Welland, ON - Psychiatry
Dr Jeyaranee Aloysius, Halifax, NS - Family Medicine
Dr Antony S J Amaladoss, Burlington, ON - General Practice
Dr Elancheliyan Ambalavanar, Scarborough, ON - Family Medicine
Dr Ganesan Annamala, Toronto, ON - General Practice
Dr Pradeepan Arulchelvam, Scarborough, ON - Family Medicine
Dr Bhavani Arumugam, Burlington, ON - Family Medicine
Dr Kiritharan Arunasalam, Orangeville, ON - Internal Medicine
Dr Bhamini Balachandra, Edmonton, AB - Psychiatry
Dr Thambirajah Balachandra, Winnipeg, MB - Anatomical Pathology
Dr Alice Benjamin, Montreal, QC - Obstetrics & Gynecology
Dr Subramanya Bhagavatula, Sudbury, ON - Psychiatry
Dr Ericka L Britto, Salmon Arm, BC - Psychiatry
Dr Santosh A Britto, Salmon Arm, BC - General Surgery
Dr Mary Chacko, Scarborough, ON - Family Medicine
Dr Sandrasegaram Chandrakumar, Mississauga, ON - Geriatric Medicine
Dr Indira Chandran, Brampton, ON - Obstetrics & Gynecology
Dr B Leonard Chandrarajan, Kingston, ON - Family Medicine
Dr Akila P Chandrasekaran, Scarborough, ON - Family Medicine
Dr Nolda M D'Cunha, Toronto, ON - Family Medicine
Dr Santhi P P Da Samy, Chatham, ON - Otolaryngology
Dr Amathul A Danial, Edmonton, AB - General Practice
Dr Shevanta G Daniel, Ajax, ON - Family Medicine
Dr Madhavan S Das, Edmonton, AB - General Practice
Dr Jeyapandy T Dason, Guelph, ON - Family Medicine
Dr Malini G Dave, North York, ON - Pediatrics
Dr Sudarshan Devanesen, Mississauga, ON - Family Medicine
Dr Sivakumaran Devarajan, Chatham, ON - Psychiatry
Dr Sudharshan Dharmalingam, Brampton, ON - Endocrin/Metabolism
Dr Therese S Edward-Chandran, Victoria, BC - Psychiatry
Dr Majella Emmanuel, Toronto, ON - Emergency Family Med
Dr Mohamed B H Faizer, Cornwall, ON - General Surgery
Dr Shabeena Fazhulla, Calgary, AB - Family Medicine
Dr Victor J Figurado, Mississauga, ON - General Practice
Dr Patricia K Francis, Brampton, ON - Family Medicine
Dr Sugantha Ganapathy, London, ON - Anesthesia
Dr Gobi R Ganapathy, London, ON - Neurology
Dr Asmitha Gangani, Aurora, ON - Family Medicine
Dr Elizabeth George, Scarborough, ON - General Practice
Dr Ajantha Gnanabaskaran, Dawson Creek, BC - Family Medicine
Dr Sangarapillai Gnanabaskaran, Dawson Creek, BC - General Practice
Dr Kandiah P Gnanendran, Windsor, ON - Anesthesia
Dr Aiyathurai Gnaneswaran, Oshawa, ON - Psychiatry
Dr Balaji Gopidasan, Niagara Falls, ON - Psychiatry
Dr Sita Gourishankar, Edmonton, AB - Internal Medicine
Dr Selvaratnam Gunaratnam, Georgetown, ON - Obstetrics & Gynecology
Dr Usha Harikumar, Scarborough, ON - Obstetrics & Gynecology
Dr Srinivasan Harish, Hamilton, ON - Diagnostic-Radiology
Dr Anita S Hunt, Mississauga, ON - Family Medicine
Dr Mohamed H Irfan, Port au Choix, NL - Family Medicine
Dr Jeewani Irfan, Port au Choix, NL - General Practice
Dr R Padmanabhan Iyer, Chatham, ON - Internal Medicine
Dr Ajantha Jayabarathan, Halifax, NS - Family Medicine
Dr Francia G Jayarajah, Scarborough, ON - Family Medicine
Dr Jyothi Jayaraman, Vancouver, BC - Family Medicine
Dr Komathy Jayashankar, Markham, ON - Family Medicine
Dr Rajadurai Jegatheeswaran, Scarborough, ON - Obstetrics & Gynecology
Dr Manjula Jeyapragasan, Toronto, ON - Family Medicine
Dr A Richard Jeyaranjan, North York, ON - Internal Medicine
Dr Thomas John, Oshawa, ON - Physical Medicine & Rehab
Dr Manamohan Johnson, Mississauga, ON - Psychiatry
Dr Changulanda M Joshi, New Glasgow, NS - Obstetrics & Gynecology
Dr Desikan R Kadambi, Winnipeg, MB - Ophthalmology
Dr Soumini Kaiprath, New Glasgow, NS - Family Medicine
Dr Rani Kanthan, Saskatoon, SK - Anatomical Pathology
Dr Kumudhini Karunakaran, Regina, SK - Internal Medicine
Dr Coomarasamy Kirupananthan, Scarborough, ON - Obstetrics & Gynecology
Dr Dayananda Kodagoda, Sydney, NS - Family Medicine
Dr Narayanan Krishnan, Lindsay, ON - Internal Medicine
Dr Ramaiyer Krishnaswamy, Fredericton, NB - Pediatrics
Dr U Sujana Kumar, London, ON - Family Medicine
Dr P Karunakaran Kutty, Brampton, ON - Gastroenterology
Dr Thurairajan Light, Cambridge, ON - Family Medicine
Dr Varagunan Mahadevan, Uxbridge, ON - Family Medicine
Dr Sathiyapooma Manoharan, Scarborough, ON - Family Medicine
Dr Grace I Mariampillai, North York, ON - Obstetrics & Gynecology
Dr William A D Mather, Scarborough, ON - Family Medicine
Dr Roubiya S Mohamed, Scarborough, ON - Family Medicine
Dr Arumairajah Muhunthan, Sarnia, ON - General Surgery
Dr Jothimalar Muhunthan, Sarnia, ON - Neurology
Dr Nageswary Muraleetharan, Scarborough, ON - Family Medicine
Dr Ravi Murthy, Toronto, ON - General Practice
Dr Karuppan C Muthiah, Perth-Andover, NB - General Practice
Dr M Saravana Muthu, Dartmouth, NS - Psychiatry
Dr M Firdaus M Mydeen, Westlock, AB - Family Medicine
Dr Rock R X Mylvaganam, Ottawa, ON - Psychiatry
Dr Sumathi Nadarajah, Mississauga, ON - Pediatrics
Dr Sivakumar Nagamuttu, Markham, ON - Family Medicine
Dr Girish M Nair, Ottawa, ON - Cardiology
Dr Sriranjinee S Namburi, Ancaster, ON - Family Medicine
Dr Narayanan Nandagopal, Scarborough, ON - Plastic Surgery
Dr S Selvi Nanthakumar, Vancouver, BC - General Pathology
Dr Sujaatha Narayanan, Vancouver, BC - General Practice
Dr Chitra Narayanan, Scarborough, ON - General Practice
Dr Dhanapal Natarajan, Regina, SK - Psychiatry
Dr Viji Nathan, Windsor, NS - Family Medicine
Dr Nirmaladevi Ollegasagrem, Saskatoon, SK - Family Medicine
Dr Hari K Ondiveeran, Saint John, NB - Critical Care Medicine
Dr Shakkeela Padanilathu Kunjummar, Newmarket, ON - Family Medicine
Dr A M Chelvi Pandian, Gatineau, QC - Family Medicine
Dr Thurairajasingham Ponnampalam, Scarborough, ON - Family Medicine
Dr Varagur M Prabhakaran, London, ON - Medical Biochemistry
Dr Jegathesan Pushpapalan, Ajax, ON - Internal Medicine
Dr Varadarajan Raghuraman, North York, ON - Psychiatry
Dr Idumban A Rajan, Windsor, ON - Psychiatry
Dr Jegapathy Rajendra, Scarborough, ON - Psychiatry
Dr Chellappa Rajgopal, London, ON - General Surgery
Dr Veer Ramakrishna, Hamilton, ON - Family Medicine
Dr Krishnan Ramanathan, Vancouver, BC - Cardiology
Dr Nithyakalyani Ramani, Surrey, BC - Family Medicine
Dr Rajamannar Ramasubbu, Calgary, AB - Psychiatry
Dr Kuppuchipalayam K Ramesh, Surrey, BC - Pediatrics
Dr Surianarayanan Rammohan, Niagara Falls, ON - General Surgery
Dr Narasimhan Ranganathan, Toronto, ON - Internal Medicine
Dr Ebenezer V Ranjit, Windsor, ON - General Practice
Dr Koshela Ranjith, Stirling, ON - Family Medicine
Dr Chitra Rao, Hamilton, ON - General Pathology
Dr Myurathy Rao, Toronto, ON - Internal Medicine
Dr Kingsley V J Ratnanather, North York, ON - Psychiatry
Dr Savithiri Ratnapalan, Toronto, ON - Pediatrics
Dr Ann Meera Ravichander, Saskatoon, SK - Obstetrics & Gynecology
Dr Girija Ravindran, Peterborough, ON - Psychiatry
Dr Umesh Rayar, Brampton, ON - Pediatrics
Dr Dhanakodi Rengan, Edmonton, AB - General Practice
Dr Sayanthan Sabanathan, Mission, BC - Family Medicine
Dr Sinnadurai S Sangaralingham, Oshawa, ON - Internal Medicine
Dr Vadivelu Santhakumar, Mississauga, ON - Family Medicine
Dr Kathiraveloo Santher, Niagara Falls, ON - Psychiatry
Dr Marutha Sathiamoorthy, Thompson, MB - General Practice
Dr Niranjala Satkunam, Edmonton, AB - General Pathology
Dr M A Raffath Sayeed, Lloydminster, SK - General Practice
Dr Ganeshan Sayuchchiyadevan, Sudbury, ON - Ophthalmology
Dr Manivannan Selvananthan, Scarborough, ON - Family Medicine
Dr Selliah Selvanayagarajah, Richmond Hill, ON - Family Medicine
Dr Prrasonna Selvarajah, Oshawa, ON - Family Medicine
Dr Senthe S Senthelal, Mississauga, ON - Radiation Oncology
Dr Sashikala Senthelal, Mississauga, ON - Psychiatry
Dr Sockalingam Senthillmohan, Cleveland, NS - General Practice
Dr Chanthirasekaram Seyone, Toronto, ON - Psychiatry
Dr Lalitha Shankar, Toronto, ON - Diagnostic-Radiology
Dr Ranganayaky Shivakumar, Sudbury, ON - Internal Medicine
Dr Krishanthy Shu, London, ON - Family Medicine
Dr Gayathri P Shyamal, Toronto, ON - Family Medicine
Dr Aynharan Sinnarajah, Calgary, AB - Family Medicine
Dr Karthika Sithamparanathan, Scarborough, ON - Family Medicine
Dr Arumugam Sivaganesanathan, Scarborough, ON - Anesthesia
Dr Nirmala Sivaji, Scarborough, ON - Anesthesia
Dr Ponnuthurai Sivaji, Scarborough, ON - Internal Medicine
Dr Panchasheila Sivakumar, Scarborough, ON - Family Medicine
Dr Thevaki Sivakumaran, Cambridge, ON - Internal Medicine
Dr Paramalingam Sivalingam, Edmonton, AB - General Practice
Dr Kalawathy Sivarajah, Bathurst, NB - Anatomical Pathology
Dr Ramanan Sivasundaram, Regina, SK - Family Medicine
Dr Sukumar D Solomon, Mississauga, ON - General Practice
Dr Thuraisamy Sooriabalan, Scarborough, ON - Psychiatry
Dr Thangarajah Sornarajah, Peterborough, ON - Anatomical Pathology
Dr Subramanian Sothilingam, Brampton, ON - Family Medicine
Dr Thushiyanthy Sriharan, Scarborough, ON - Family Medicine
Dr Hindupuram V Sriharsha, Orillia, ON - Internal Medicine

Dr Anuradha Srinivasan, Richmond Hill, ON - General Practice
Dr Janaki Srinivasan, Toronto, ON - Psychiatry
Dr Ramani Srirangarajan, Cleveland, NS - Family Medicine
Dr Maheswaran Srivamadevan, Richmond Hill, ON - Cardiology
Dr Aravind Subramanian, Calgary, AB - General Practice
Dr Thangamani Subramanian, Hamilton, ON - Family Medicine
Dr Anantasivan Subramanian, Niagara Falls, ON - General Surgery
Dr Nirmala Sundaralingam, Whitby, ON - Psychiatry
Dr Shanthini Sundareswaran, Mississauga, ON - Family Medicine
Dr Nagappan Suppiah, St. John's, NL - Anesthesia
Dr Sam Swaminath, Chatham, ON - Psychiatry
Dr Ganesh Swamy, Calgary, AB - Orthopedic Surgery
Dr Sou K Thain, Kingston, ON - Radiation Oncology
Dr Niththialuxmy Thamotharam, Scarborough, ON - Family Medicine
Dr Arulanantham Thangaroopan, Ajax, ON - Psychiatry
Dr Arulnmozhy Thangaroopan, Newmarket, ON - Cardiology
Dr Yasho Tharmaratnam, Scarborough, ON - Family Medicine
Dr Uma M Tharmaratnam, Toronto, ON - Anesthesia
Dr Jeyasakthy J Thayaparan, Richmond Hill, ON - Internal Medicine
Dr Kayalvili Thevathasan, Guelph, ON - General Practice
Dr Pandaram Thillainadarajah, Surrey, BC - Psychiatry
Dr Subarna Thirugnanam, Markham, ON - Critical Care Medicine
Dr Vakeesan Thirugnanasampanthapillai, Brampton, ON - Family Medicine
Dr Senthil K Thiyagarajan, Welland, ON - Anesthesia
Dr Rajeswary Thurairajah, Mississauga, ON - Obstetrics & Gynecology
Dr Indranee Thurairajah, Toronto, ON - Psychiatry
Dr Padmini N Turlapati, Markham, ON - Pediatrics
Dr Sama P Usha, Whitby, ON - Psychiatry
Dr Sangeeta Vaideswaran, London, ON - Family Medicine
Dr Sankar Vaidyanathan, Brampton, ON - Family Medicine
Dr Prema Vaidyanathan, Etobicoke, ON - Obstetrics & Gynecology
Dr Chandraprabha Vaidyanathan, Ottawa, ON - Pediatrics
Dr Rajani Vairavanathan, East York, ON - Emergency Family Med
Dr Kandiah Vaithianathan, Scarborough, ON - Family Medicine
Dr Sivaraji Vakeesan, Brampton, ON - Family Medicine
Dr Arulanandam Varadarasa, Brampton, ON - Internal Medicine
Dr Veeragathy Vasanthan, Clarenville, NL - General Practice
Dr Varadaraj R Velamoor, Guelph, ON - Psychiatry
Dr Rhenugadevi Velmurugiah, Edmonton, AB - Family Medicine
Dr Lakshmi Venkat Raghavan, Toronto, ON - Anesthesia
Dr Bogeswari Venkatesan, London, ON - Psychiatry
Dr Varagur M Venkatesan, London, ON - Radiation Oncology
Dr Thiruganasam Venkatesh, Ottawa, ON - Emergency Family Med
Dr Sunita Venkateswaran, Ottawa, ON - Neurology
Dr Dilini P Vethanayagam, Edmonton, AB - Internal Medicine
Dr Raj Vijay, Mississauga, ON - Family Medicine
Dr Kandiah Vijayakanthan, Sudbury, ON - Obstetrics & Gynecology
Dr Visvalingam Vijayaratnam, Toronto, ON - Gastroenterology
Dr Franklyn A Vincent, Halifax, NS - Family Medicine
Dr Manohary Vipulananthan, Brandon, MB - Psychiatry
Dr Maithili K Wilson, Toronto, ON - Dermatology
Dr Chidambaram M Yegappan, Hamilton, ON - Neurology
Dr Muthulakshmi Yegappan, Niagara Falls, ON - Obstetrics & Gynecology
Dr Thirumagal Yogaparan, North York, ON - Geriatric Medicine
Dr Kumaresan Yogeswaran, Toronto, ON - Gastroenterology
Dr Mohamed M Zawahir, Stratford, ON - General Practice

TELUGU

Dr Afsari B Amjad, Ottawa, ON - Psychiatry
Dr Subramanya Bhagavatula, Sudbury, ON - Psychiatry
Dr Ericka L Britto, Salmon Arm, BC - Psychiatry
Dr Jayshree Chanchlani, Brampton, ON - General Practice
Dr Vinjamuri R Chari, Hamilton, ON - Physical Medicine & Rehab
Dr Krishna V Chunduri, North York, ON - Family Medicine
Dr Venkata S V B Hota, Napanee, ON - General Surgery
Dr R Padmanabhan Iyer, Chatham, ON - Internal Medicine
Dr Balaraju B Katta, Richmond, BC - Psychiatry
Dr Manohar Keesari, Oshawa, ON - Psychiatry
Dr M Viqar Khan, Oakville, ON - Family Medicine
Dr C L Prasanna Kumar, Toronto, ON - Obstetrics & Gynecology
Dr N Rao Malempati, Windsor, ON - Psychiatry
Dr Harinath Mallavarapu, Surrey, BC - Psychiatry
Dr Udaya K K Mulpuri, Vancouver, BC - General Practice
Dr Renuka S Naidu, Sarnia, ON - Critical Care Medicine
Dr Harish K Neelakant, Vancouver, BC - Psychiatry
Dr Chellappa Rajgopal, London, ON - General Surgery
Dr Mahesh Raju, Saint John, NB - Internal Medicine
Dr Shoba Raju, Saint John, NB - General Practice
Dr Veer Ramakrishna, Hamilton, ON - Family Medicine
Dr Suseela Reddy, Burnaby, BC - General Pathology
Dr Jinka R Sathya, St. John's, NL - Radiation Oncology
Dr Shakti Sharma, Thornhill, ON - Dermatology
Dr Pratibhasri A Sharma, Toronto, ON - General Practice
Dr Kunwar K Singh, Sarnia, ON - Pediatrics
Dr Jami Sridhar, Campbellton, NB - General Practice
Dr Hindupuram V Sriharsha, Orillia, ON - Internal Medicine
Dr Vasundhara Srinivasan, Etobicoke, ON - Psychiatry
Dr Ramakrishna R Surapaneni, Kitchener, ON - Psychiatry
Dr Sam Swaminath, Chatham, ON - Psychiatry
Dr Narsimhachary Telikicharla Kandala, Terrace, BC - General Practice
Dr Sou K Thain, Kingston, ON - Radiation Oncology
Dr Padmini N Turlapati, Markham, ON - Pediatrics
Dr M Rao Vallabhaneni, Toronto, ON - Psychiatry
Dr Mudalodu V Vasudevan, Windsor, ON - General Practice
Dr Ramamohan Veluri, Sudbury, ON - Psychiatry
Dr Sachi M Voruganti, Hamilton, ON - Radiation Oncology
Dr Lakshmi N P Voruganti, Oakville, ON - Psychiatry
Dr Lakshmi N Yatham, Vancouver, BC - Psychiatry
Dr Radhika Yelamanchili, St Catharines, ON - Internal Medicine

TEOCHEW

Dr Aik-Ping Eng, Vancouver, BC - General Practice
Dr Wai-Arm Lam, Vancouver, BC - General Practice
Dr Liang Ng, West Vancouver, BC - General Practice
Dr Michelle W Tan, Richmond, BC - Family Medicine

THAI

Dr Vera Chiamvimonvat, Oakville, ON - Cardiology
Dr Somchai Jiaravuthisan, Oshawa, ON - Neurology
Dr Emelda M Tai, Toronto, ON - General Practice

TIGRIGNA

Dr Efrem Alemayehu, Toronto, ON - General Practice
Dr Abdullahi A Berih, Etobicoke, ON - Family Medicine
Dr Tadese F Debretsion, Oakville, ON - Family Medicine
Dr Ephrem Gebrechristos, York, ON - General Surgery
Dr Amde M Teferi, Guelph, ON - Psychiatry
Dr Abedom Tekle, Langley, BC - General Practice
Dr Yoseph Tesfaye, Montreal, QC - General Practice

TOISHAN

Dr Stacey A Chow, Surrey, BC - General Practice
Dr Gary L Lee, Montreal, QC - Emergency Family Med
Dr Robert S L Leung, Mississauga, ON - General Practice
Dr Edward Lum, Vancouver, BC - General Practice
Dr Wing Hon Ng, Vancouver, BC - General Practice
Dr Allan P G Wong, Vancouver, BC - Psychiatry

TURKISH

Dr Mansour Adle, Westmount, QC - General Surgery
Dr Berna Akcakir, Ottawa, ON - Family Medicine
Dr Sueda Akkor, Vancouver, BC - Ophthalmology
Dr Fatih M W Al-Katib, Saskatoon, SK - General Practice
Dr Nihad H Ali-Ridha, Oshawa, ON - Anatomical Pathology
Dr Kamel Alizadeh-Khiavi, Calgary, AB - Family Medicine
Dr Yasemin Arikan, New Westminster, BC - Internal Medicine
Dr Cigdem Arkuran, Richmond, BC - Obstetrics & Gynecology
Dr Natan Behar, Cornwall, ON - General Practice
Dr Avedis Bogosyan, North York, ON - General Practice
Dr Hagob A Boyrazian, Scarborough, ON - General Practice
Dr H Zihni Dervish, Ottawa, ON - General Surgery
Dr Kemal Divanli, Edmundston, NB - General Practice
Dr Mahshid Gharedaghi, West Vancouver, BC - Family Medicine
Dr M Ilhami Gokcen, Scarborough, ON - Psychiatry
Dr Victor Gomel, Vancouver, BC - Obstetrics & Gynecology
Dr Shahpar Grouhi, Richmond Hill, ON - General Practice
Dr Hasan Hafiz, Calgary, AB - General Practice
Dr Jean J Hallak, Montreal, QC - Obstetrics & Gynecology
Dr Osman S Ipsiroglu, Vancouver, BC - General Practice
Dr Siavash Jafari, Vancouver, BC - General Practice
Dr Cengiz H Karsli, Toronto, ON - Anesthesia
Dr Rita Kuyumjian, Montreal, QC - Psychiatry
Dr Jirair Kuyumjian, Montreal, QC - General Practice
Dr Saadet Mahmutoglu, Toronto, ON - General Practice
Dr Nejat Memiche, Bathurst, NB - Gastroenterology
Dr Reshat Memiche, Bathurst, NB - Gastroenterology
Dr Ozgur Mete, Toronto, ON - General Practice
Dr Amir A Mortazavi, North York, ON - Cardiology
Dr Ezel F Orfi, Richmond Hill, ON - Diagnostic-Radiology
Dr Dudu A Pallie, St Catharines, ON - General Practice
Dr Emilyos Paras, Saint John, NB - Pediatrics
Dr Pasteur Rasuli, Ottawa, ON - Diagnostic-Radiology
Dr Yuksel Sadak, Brampton, ON - Internal Medicine
Dr S Kemal Sartekin, Port Coquitlam, BC - Family Medicine
Dr Alp Sener, London, ON - Urology
Dr Mehmet R Sirman, York, ON - Psychiatry
Dr Vahe Sivaciyan, Toronto, ON - Cardiology
Mr Axel Tosikyan, Montreal, QC - Hematology
Dr Gonul Vardar, Toronto, ON - General Practice
Dr P Ariana Verdizad, Pitt Meadows, BC - Family Medicine
Dr Serdar Yilmaz, Calgary, AB - General Practice
Dr Yeni H Yucel, Toronto, ON - Neuro-Pathology

TWI

Dr Kwame E Badoe, Guelph, ON - Psychiatry
Dr Nana Graves, Dollard-D-Ormeaux, QC - Pediatrics
Dr Diana B Mills-Tettey, North York, ON - Pediatrics
Dr Setorme A Tsikata, Spruce Grove, AB - Family Medicine
Dr Kofi A Wudom, Brampton, ON - Family Medicine

UKRAINIAN

Dr Barbara H Agopsowicz, Edmonton, AB - General Practice
Dr Jennifer L Andruchow, St. Albert, AB - General Surgery
Dr Oleh M Antonyshyn, Toronto, ON - Plastic Surgery
Dr Taras Babiak, Toronto, ON - Neuro-Pathology
Dr Natalie Baziuk, Oshawa, ON - Ophthalmology
Dr George H H Beiko, St Catharines, ON - Ophthalmology
Dr Nadia M Belsky, Etobicoke, ON - General Practice
Dr Oleg D Bendz, Toronto, ON - General Practice
Dr Lesia R Boychuk, Edmonton, AB - Infectious Diseases
Dr Christine Brezden-Masley, Toronto, ON - Internal Medicine
Dr Jeanie Shkimba Brezina, Toronto, ON - General Practice
Dr Mark B Brodsky, North York, ON - General Practice
Dr Janki Butchey, London, ON - Psychiatry
Dr Helena Chekina, North York, ON - General Practice
Dr Patricia A Chernesky, Nipawin, SK - General Practice
Dr Svitlana Cheshenchuk, Regina, SK - Family Medicine
Dr William T Chimich, Edmonton, AB - Family Medicine
Dr Norman N Chychota, Taber, AB - General Practice
Dr Tatiana Chypchar, Cambridge, ON - Family Medicine
Dr Irene J Cybulsky, Hamilton, ON - Cardiovasc/ThorSurg
Dr Myron I Cybulsky, Toronto, ON - Anatomical Pathology
Dr Anne Czemerynski, Toronto, ON - Family Medicine
Dr Elizabeth Czyziw, Montreal, QC - General Practice
Dr Irena B Darczewski, Winnipeg, MB - Family Medicine
Dr Nestor N Demianczuk, Edmonton, AB - Obstetrics & Gynecology
Dr Arkadiy Demianczuk, Vancouver, BC - Plastic Surgery
Dr Peter Derkach, Toronto, ON - General Practice

Dr Lydia A L Derzko, Nelson House, MB - General Practice
Dr Christine M Derzko, Toronto, ON - Obstetrics & Gynecology
Dr Larissa A Derzko-Dzulynsky, Etobicoke, ON - Ophthalmology
Dr Robert Dmytryshyn, Toronto, ON - Family Medicine
Dr Anatoly Dobrousin, Edmonton, AB - Family Medicine
Dr Anthony Drohomyrecky, Bracebridge, ON - Urology
Dr William A Dymon, Etobicoke, ON - Emergency Family Med
Dr Ernest J Ewaschuk, Mississauga, ON - Obstetrics & Gynecology
Dr Romana Fagan, Toronto, ON - General Practice
Dr Taras D Fecycz, North York, ON - General Practice
Dr Roman Fedyna, Oshawa, ON - General Practice
Dr Borys Flak, Vancouver, BC - Diagnostic-Radiology
Dr Myrosia M Foga, Mississauga, ON - Diagnostic-Radiology
Dr Ihor Gadacz, Etobicoke, ON - General Practice
Dr Lena Galimova, Winnipeg, MB - Physical Medicine & Rehab
Dr Leila Gibson, Saskatoon, SK - General Practice
Dr Boris P Gimbarzevsky, Kamloops, BC - General Practice
Dr Peter A Gresko, Windsor, ON - General Practice
Dr Tamara C Grodzicky, Montreal, QC - Internal Medicine
Dr Myron Haluk, Mississauga, ON - Emergency Family Med
Dr Eugene N Hladky, Montreal, QC - Ophthalmology
Dr Maria J Hohol, Toronto, ON - Neurology
Dr Adrian A Hornich, Hamilton, ON - Family Medicine
Dr B Hoshowsky, Calgary, AB - Otolaryngology
Dr Zenona M I Hrabar, Surrey, BC - General Practice
Dr O M Irene Hramiak, London, ON - Endocrin/Metabolism
Dr William M Hryniuk, Toronto, ON - Med Scientist
Dr George E Huculak, Whitby, ON - General Practice
Dr Tetyana Y Hurmatov, St Catharines, ON - General Practice
Dr George A Jaciw, Whitby, ON - General Practice
Dr Peter Jacyk, Etobicoke, ON - General Practice
Dr Jerry Jakibchuk, St Catharines, ON - General Practice
Dr Andrew J Jarema, Edmonton, AB - General Practice
Dr Roman Jednak, Montreal, QC - Urology
Dr Roman D Jovey, Mississauga, ON - General Practice
Dr Allan R Kaban, Nanaimo, BC - Family Medicine
Dr Marianna M Kapala, Mississauga, ON - General Surgery
Dr William M Kapusta, Oshawa, ON - General Practice
Dr Stephanie O Keeling, Edmonton, AB - Internal Medicine
Dr Veronica N H Kekosz, Toronto, ON - Physical Medicine & Rehab
Dr Oleg Klipitch, Etobicoke, ON - Family Medicine
Dr Luba N V Komar, Toronto, ON - Pediatrics
Dr Peter M Kondra, Hamilton, ON - Psychiatry
Dr Eleonor Kopylenko, Newmarket, ON - Family Medicine
Dr Stephen E Kosar, Sudbury, ON - Ophthalmology
Dr Michael A M Kowbel, Kamloops, BC - Anesthesia
Dr Joseph H Kozak, Toronto, ON - Family Medicine
Dr Markijan W Kramarchuk, Mississauga, ON - Family Medicine
Dr Michael Krawetz, Bala, ON - General Practice
Dr Andrew Kuchtaruk, Sudbury, ON - Family Medicine
Dr Rodion A W Kunynetz, Barrie, ON - Dermatology
Dr R Walter W Kutcher, Barrie, ON - Internal Medicine
Dr Bohdan Laluck Jr, Toronto, ON - Internal Medicine
Dr Galina Langer, Thornhill, ON - Cardiology
Dr Mykhaylo V Levinskyy, Edmonton, AB - General Practice
Dr Vitaly A Liashko, Moncton, NB - Psychiatry
Dr Michael Lucewicz, Edmonton, AB - General Practice
Dr Ihor I Mayba, Winnipeg, MB - General Surgery
Dr John I Mayba, Winnipeg, MB - General Practice
Dr Stanley T Maziarz, Gatineau, QC - Family Medicine
Dr Wolodymyr Medwidsky, Toronto, ON - Dermatology
Dr Lydia C Melnyk, Montreal, QC - Family Medicine
Dr Lilly J Miedzinski, Edmonton, AB - Internal Medicine
Dr Paul J Moroz, Ottawa, ON - Orthopedic Surgery
Dr Ihor R Mota, Vancouver, BC - Family Medicine
Dr Michael M Myckatyn, Richmond, BC - General Practice
Dr Boris Nahornick, Drumheller, AB - General Practice
Dr Edward M Nykiforuk, Saskatoon, SK - General Practice
Dr Bohdan Olearczyk, Toronto, ON - General Practice
Dr Mariusz T Paszkiewicz, Weyburn, SK - General Practice
Dr Katerina Pavenski, Toronto, ON - Hematology
Dr Walter Pawliwec, Brantford, ON - General Surgery
Dr Vsevolod S Perelman, Toronto, ON - Emergency Family Med
Dr Peter Petrosoniak, Lindsay, ON - General Practice
Dr Bohdan O Pich, Etobicoke, ON - General Practice
Dr Gregory M Polyakov, Vancouver, BC - General Surgery
Dr Galina G Portnoi, Thornhill, ON - Family Medicine
Dr Serge Puksa, Hamilton, ON - Internal Medicine
Dr George B Pylypchuk, Saskatoon, SK - Internal Medicine
Dr Valentyna B Rembez, Vancouver, BC - Family Medicine
Dr George Rewa, Toronto, ON - Cardiology
Dr Walter R Salmaniw, Victoria, BC - General Practice
Dr Raymond B Sawkiw, Sudbury, ON - Family Medicine
Dr Alexandra Schepansky, Edmonton, AB - Obstetrics & Gynecology
Dr Miroslav V Semczyszyn, Hamilton, ON - Family Medicine
Dr Sergey Shapiro, Toronto, ON - Psychiatry
Dr Nykola Sheshko, Ottawa, ON - Family Medicine
Dr David J Shumka, Newmarket, ON - Anesthesia
Dr Walter B Silecky, Oshawa, ON - Internal Medicine
Dr Stephen W Siomra, Oshawa, ON - Otolaryngology
Dr Peter M Sirko, Hamilton, ON - Anesthesia
Dr George W Skocylak, Toronto, ON - General Practice
Dr Orest W I Skrypuch, Brantford, ON - Ophthalmology
Dr Nataliya Skuridina, North Vancouver, BC - Public Health & Preventive Medicine
Dr Paul T Slavchenko, Oshawa, ON - Anesthesia
Dr Vladimir S Sluzar, Mississauga, ON - Cardiology
Dr Robert Snihura, Toronto, ON - Internal Medicine
Dr Arthur Staroselsky, Thornhill, ON - Family Medicine
Dr William P Steciuk, St Thomas, ON - General Practice
Dr Oksana Suchowersky, Edmonton, AB - Neurology
Dr Oleksandr I Svystonyuk, Newmarket, ON - Obstetrics & Gynecology
Dr Ivanna V Tataryn, Edmonton, AB - Obstetrics & Gynecology
Dr Yuriy M Tatuch, North York, ON - Family Medicine
Dr Mary I Terepa, Saskatoon, SK - Family Medicine
Dr Raymond P Tesluk, Port Hope, ON - Family Medicine
Dr Alexander Tischenko, Winnipeg, MB - Cardiology
Dr Paul J Tkalych, Calgary, AB - General Practice
Dr Alexander C Tokarewicz, London, ON - Ophthalmology
Dr Anna A Toptchieva, East York, ON - Anesthesia
Dr Daria A Trojan, Montreal, QC - Physical Medicine & Rehab
Dr Oleg Tugalev, Woodstock, ON - Physical Medicine & Rehab
Dr Elena Tugaleva, London, ON - Anatomical Pathology
Dr Victoria E Tuvivovich, Salaber-de-Valleyf, QC - General Practice
Dr Wayne J Tymchak, Edmonton, AB - Cardiology
Dr Linda M Uniat, Edmonton, AB - Ophthalmology
Dr Peter M Vignjevic, Hamilton, ON - Dermatology
Dr Nataliya V Vostretsova, Richmond, BC - Family Medicine
Dr Oleh R Waler, St Catharines, ON - General Practice
Dr Peter Walkovich, Scarborough, ON - General Surgery
Dr Roman Y Wasylyk, Mississauga, ON - Emergency Family Med
Dr Robert S Werhun, Niagara Falls, ON - Internal Medicine
Dr Krzysztof Wieczorek, Edmonton, AB - General Practice
Dr Wladyslaw Wojcik, Regina, SK - Internal Medicine
Dr Ronald J Wojtyk, Ottawa, ON - General Practice
Dr Andrea D Woloszczuk, Pickering, ON - General Practice
Dr Jaroslaw V Workewych, Mississauga, ON - General Practice
Dr Oksana Y Yatsina, Saskatoon, SK - Family Medicine
Dr Alexandre N Yatsina, Saskatoon, SK - General Practice
Dr Bohdan R Yemchuk, London, ON - Family Medicine
Dr Jerry Zadyko, Etobicoke, ON - Emergency Family Med
Dr George R Zahrebelny, Windsor, ON - General Practice
Dr Emil N Zamora, Hamilton, ON - Psychiatry
Dr Christina H A Zarowsky, Plantagenet, ON - General Practice
Dr Marian Zazula, Mississauga, ON - General Practice
Dr Terrance S Zlipko, Saskatoon, SK - General Practice
Dr James P Znajda, Scarborough, ON - Ophthalmology
Dr Jerry R Zownir, Toronto, ON - Internal Medicine

URDU

Dr Mustafa H Abdulhusein, Brampton, ON - General Practice
Dr Alnoor Abdulla, Vancouver, BC - Cardiology
Dr Syed T H Abedi, Scarborough, ON - Anatomical Pathology
Dr Ismail Y Aboo, Owen Sound, ON - General Practice
Dr Tasneem Adenwala, Bolton, ON - Family Medicine
Dr Aliya Adil, Whitby, ON - Family Medicine
Dr Vandana Ahluwalia, Brampton, ON - Internal Medicine
Dr Aijaz Ahmad, Medicine Hat, AB - General Practice
Dr Ejaz Ahmad, Winnipeg, MB - Family Medicine
Dr S Nizamuddin Ahmed, Edmonton, AB - Neurology
Dr Sheikh N Ahmed, Abbotsford, BC - Radiation Oncology
Dr Abul B M Ahmed, Milton, ON - Psychiatry
Dr Uzma Ahmed, Mississauga, ON - Pediatrics
Dr Iram F Ahmed, Niagara Falls, ON - General Practice
Dr Nafeesa Q Ahmed, Oakville, ON - General Practice
Dr Bashir Ahmed, Ottawa, ON - General Practice
Dr Syed T Ahmed, St Thomas, ON - Pediatrics
Dr Najma A Ahmed, Toronto, ON - Critical Care Medicine
Dr Tahira S Ahmed, Windsor, ON - General Practice
Dr Shahid Ahmed, Saskatoon, SK - Internal Medicine
Dr Shafiq F Akbar, Edmonton, AB - Internal Medicine
Dr Zaubaria Akbar, Surrey, BC - General Practice
Dr Muhammad F Alam, St. John's, NL - Neurology
Dr Tasriqul M Alam, London, ON - Family Medicine
Dr Zeenat Y Alam, Windsor, ON - Internal Medicine
Dr Karima M Ali, Calgary, AB - Family Medicine
Dr Syed A Ali, Edmonton, AB - General Practice
Dr Yasmin Ali, Coquitlam, BC - Family Medicine
Dr Iqbal Ali, Surrey, BC - Internal Medicine
Dr Liaqat Ali, Barrie, ON - Psychiatry
Dr Durya Ali, Bowmanville, ON - Family Medicine
Dr Pervez Ali, North York, ON - Orthopedic Surgery
Dr Fahim H Ali, Port Perry, ON - Family Medicine
Dr Vasima Ali, Scarborough, ON - General Practice
Dr Asim Ali, Toronto, ON - Ophthalmology
Dr Shabbir F Amin, Fort Saskatchewan, AB - Family Medicine
Dr Parsa F Amin, Brampton, ON - Family Medicine
Dr Saima Amjad, Mississauga, ON - Family Medicine
Dr Afsari B Amjad, Ottawa, ON - Psychiatry
Dr Dinyar H Amrolia, Calgary, AB - General Practice
Dr Neeru Anand, Delta, BC - Family Medicine
Dr Mohinder K Angl, Courtice, ON - General Practice
Dr Ziaul B Ansari, Wetaskiwin, AB - General Practice
Dr Saira Ansari, Scarborough, ON - Anatomical Pathology
Dr A Hashsham Ansari, Scarborough, ON - Family Medicine
Dr Sunder S Arora, Ottawa, ON - Psychiatry
Dr Amit Arya, Brampton, ON - Family Medicine
Dr M Anwar Asady, Mississauga, ON - General Practice
Dr Ahmad S Ashrafi, Surrey, BC - General Surgery
Dr Sylvia B Athaide, North York, ON - General Practice
Dr Tariq M Awan, Calgary, AB - Family Medicine
Dr Adeel Azam, Medicine Hat, AB - Internal Medicine
Dr Abdul Aziz, Lethbridge, AB - General Practice
Dr Harry S Badhan, Brampton, ON - General Practice
Dr Jagdeep S Badhesha, Calgary, AB - Family Medicine
Dr Jatinder S Baidwan, Victoria, BC - Family Medicine
Dr M Naseer Baig, Mississauga, ON - Anesthesia
Dr Harpreet S Bajaj, Brampton, ON - General Practice
Dr Parvesh Bajaj, Nepean, ON - General Practice
Dr Sameena A Bajwa, Calgary, AB - Family Medicine
Dr Harmeet K Bami, Brampton, ON - Psychiatry
Dr Khalid Bashir, Prince George, BC - Internal Medicine
Dr Amrik S Bassi, Calgary, AB - General Practice
Dr Navdeep Bath, Mississauga, ON - Family Medicine
Dr Hussam-Ul H Bawa, Calgary, AB - Psychiatry
Dr Asifa Bawangoanwala, Mississauga, ON - Family Medicine
Dr Ashok Bhagat, Richmond Hill, ON - General Practice
Dr Subramanya Bhagavatula, Sudbury, ON - Psychiatry
Dr Dalip K Bhangu, Etobicoke, ON - Obstetrics & Gynecology
Dr Balbir C Bhatti, Surrey, BC - Family Medicine
Dr Fatima Bhetasi, Welland, ON - Pediatrics
Dr Laila Bhimani, Surrey, BC - Family Medicine
Dr Vipul K Bhupal, York, ON - General Practice
Dr Pargat S Bhurji, Surrey, BC - Pediatrics
Dr Usha Chada, North York, ON - General Practice
Dr Rati Chadha, Calgary, AB - Obstetrics & Gynecology
Dr Haji I Chalchal, Regina, SK - General Practice
Dr Ranjit K Chandra, Mississauga, ON - Pediatrics
Dr Mohammad I Chaudhary, Mississauga, ON - Family Medicine
Dr Mobina A Chaudhry, Fort McMurray, AB - Family Medicine
Dr Sajjad A Chaudhry, Toronto, ON - Anesthesia

Dr Sukarno N Chaudhry, Windsor, ON - Internal Medicine
Dr Gulzar S Cheema, Surrey, BC - Family Medicine
Dr Waqar M Cheema, Brampton, ON - Family Medicine
Dr Jagdish C Chopra, Oshawa, ON - General Practice
Dr Krishna V Chunduri, North York, ON - Family Medicine
Dr Nolda M D'Cunha, Toronto, ON - Family Medicine
Dr Amathul A Danial, Edmonton, AB - General Practice
Dr Bahauddin H Danial, Mississauga, ON - Internal Medicine
Dr Shahnaz Dar, Scarborough, ON - Pediatrics
Dr Faiz Daudi, Etobicoke, ON - General Surgery
Dr Asfa Daudi, Mississauga, ON - Family Medicine
Dr Cassim T Degani, Mississauga, ON - General Surgery
Dr Milind G Desai, North York, ON - Gastroenterology
Dr Shashi P Devi, North York, ON - Family Medicine
Dr Harbhajan S Dhaliwal, Winnipeg, MB - General Practice
Dr Preet B K Dhaliwal, LaSalle, ON - Family Medicine
Dr Fatima Dhalla, Ottawa, ON - Family Medicine
Dr Mohsin N Dhalla, Stoney Creek, ON - Family Medicine
Dr Jag Mohan Dhar, Sarnia, ON - Internal Medicine
Dr Manu Dhillon, Brampton, ON - General Practice
Dr Karamvir K Dhillon, Oshawa, ON - Family Medicine
Dr Shamoon Din, Mississauga, ON - General Practice
Dr Murtaza A Diwan, Guelph, ON - Otolaryngology
Dr Ismat Z Dost, Brantford, ON - Pediatrics
Dr Rehan Dost, Paris, ON - Neurology
Dr Shehla Ebrahim, North Vancouver, BC - Family Medicine
Dr Mohammed Elahi, Etobicoke, ON - Family Medicine
Dr Mohammed Elahi, North York, ON - Otolaryngology
Dr Mohammad Fahim, New Glasgow, NS - General Practice
Dr Shireen Fahim, Etobicoke, ON - Family Medicine
Dr Shazia Faisal, Windsor, ON - Family Medicine
Dr Mohammed Farooq, Sydney, NS - General Practice
Dr Muna I Farooqi, Guelph, ON - Family Medicine
Dr Najla Fasih, Ottawa, ON - General Practice
Dr Sharmeen H Feerasta, Toronto, ON - Pediatrics
Dr Imre B Fejer, Scarborough, ON - General Practice
Dr Sleem Feroze, Oakville, ON - Obstetrics & Gynecology
Dr Naila Furqan, Mississauga, ON - Family Medicine
Dr Shruti Gandhi, Etobicoke, ON - Medical Biochemistry
Dr Narinder K Garg, Brampton, ON - Family Medicine
Dr Shiva K Gaur, Scarborough, ON - General Practice
Dr Mohammed A Gauri, Fort Saskatchewan, AB - General Practice
Dr Talha I Ghadai, Newmarket, ON - Family Medicine
Dr Abdul Ghaffar, Brampton, ON - Pediatrics
Dr Ikram Ghani, Mississauga, ON - General Practice
Dr Sameera Ghaznavi, Oakville, ON - Family Medicine
Dr Ali T Ghouse, Hamilton, ON - Physical Medicine & Rehab
Dr Ejaz A Ghumman, Leamington, ON - General Surgery
Dr Hamid J Gilani, Guelph, ON - General Practice
Dr Sadia Gilani, Hamilton, ON - Psychiatry
Dr Aneeqa A Gill, London, ON - Family Medicine
Dr Paramjit Gill, Mississauga, ON - General Practice
Dr Vikramjit S Gill, Mississauga, ON - General Practice
Dr Joginder S Gill, Niagara Falls, ON - Family Medicine
Dr Satpal S Girgla, Oakville, ON - Psychiatry
Dr Kharak S Grewal, Brampton, ON - General Practice
Dr Kamal P Grewal, Brampton, ON - Family Medicine
Dr Puneet Grewal, Burlington, ON - Family Medicine
Dr Arvinder Grover, Mississauga, ON - Cardiology
Dr Sajadhussein S Gulamhusein, Edmonton, AB - Cardiology
Dr Madhu Gupta, Vancouver, BC - Obstetrics & Gynecology
Dr Ram Gupta, Brampton, ON - Family Medicine
Dr Milan Gupta, Brampton, ON - Cardiology
Dr Sanjeev Gupta, Mississauga, ON - General Practice
Dr Vikas Gupta, Toronto, ON - General Practice
Dr Larry O J Gustafson, Surrey, BC - General Practice
Dr Syed W Habib, Edmonton, AB - General Practice
Dr Naiyer Habib, Abbotsford, BC - Internal Medicine
Dr Shujauddin F Hafiz, Mississauga, ON - Pediatrics
Dr Mukhtar Haidar, Wetaskiwin, AB - Family Medicine
Dr Umar Haider, Halifax, NS - Family Medicine
Dr Kamil Haider, Etobicoke, ON - Family Medicine
Dr Syed Y A Haider, Markham, ON - Orthopedic Surgery
Dr Aamir Haider, Oakville, ON - Dermatology
Dr Erum Haider, Whitby, ON - Family Medicine
Dr Raju Hajela, Calgary, AB - Family Medicine
Dr Saima Haleem, Sydney, NS - Family Medicine
Dr Kazi A Hameed, Winnipeg, MB - Internal Medicine
Dr Saadia Hameed, London, ON - Family Medicine
Dr Nageen Hameed, Oakville, ON - Internal Medicine
Dr Iftikhar U Haq, Thunder Bay, ON - Neurosurgery
Dr Rashida Haq, Toronto, ON - Internal Medicine
Dr Khurshid Haque, Campbellton, NB - General Practice
Dr Upninderjit S Harrad, Surrey, BC - Psychiatry
Dr Shabih U Hasan, Calgary, AB - Pediatrics
Dr Shaukat Hasan, Oshawa, ON - Family Medicine
Dr Sadiq Hasan, Whitby, ON - Psychiatry
Dr Haider Hasnain, Tecumseh, ON - Family Medicine
Dr Haron Hassan, Surrey, BC - Family Medicine
Dr Ali Hassan, Brantford, ON - General Practice
Dr Durreshahwar Hassan, Roxboro, QC - Obstetrics & Gynecology
Dr Daljit S Herar, Surrey, BC - General Pathology
Dr Naushad Hirani, Calgary, AB - Internal Medicine
Dr Kiran Humayun, Regina, SK - Family Medicine
Dr Mansoor Husain, Toronto, ON - Cardiology
Dr S Baqir Husain, Prince Albert, SK - Psychiatry
Dr Mahjabeen Hussain, Calgary, AB - Family Medicine
Dr Nadeem A Hussain, London, ON - Gastroenterology
Dr Shabnam Hussain, Ottawa, ON - Family Medicine
Dr Mohammed T Hussain, Windsor, ON - Family Medicine
Dr Syed S Hussain, Saskatoon, SK - Family Medicine
Dr Mohammed A Ibrahim, Brampton, ON - Urology
Dr Mohammad S Ijaz, Regina, SK - General Practice
Dr Kashif Irshad, Brampton, ON - General Surgery
Dr Fauzia Irshad, Mississauga, ON - Family Medicine
Dr Rahmatullah Ishaqzay, Milton, ON - Family Medicine
Dr Pervez Ishrat Ali Khan, Edmonton, AB - General Practice
Dr Muhammad U Islam, Abbotsford, BC - Diagnostic-Radiology
Dr Omar S Islam, Kingston, ON - Diagnostic-Radiology
Dr Shiraz H Ismail, North York, ON - General Practice
Dr Arif M A Ismaili, Kitchener, ON - Gastroenterology
Dr Rajesh Jaidka, Brampton, ON - General Practice
Dr Sajal Jain, Burnaby, BC - Internal Medicine
Dr Leena Jain, New Westminster, BC - Geriatric Medicine
Dr Shalini Jain, Amherstview, ON - Family Medicine
Dr Umesh Jain, Toronto, ON - Urology
Dr Dawood I Jamal, Toronto, ON - General Practice
Dr Amin R Javer, Vancouver, BC - Otolaryngology
Dr Nasir Jetha, Vancouver, BC - Pediatrics
Dr Shamin Jetha, Vancouver, BC - Family Medicine
Dr Azim H Jiwani, West Vancouver, BC - Family Medicine
Dr Manohar L Joshi, Etobicoke, ON - General Practice
Dr Azim F Juma, Scarborough, ON - Family Medicine
Dr Baldev S Kahlon, Delta, BC - General Practice
Dr Karna C Kale, Mississauga, ON - Family Medicine
Dr Bharat B Kalra, Scarborough, ON - General Practice
Dr Azadali A Kamani, Vancouver, BC - General Practice
Dr Parmjit S Kang, Surrey, BC - Endocrin/Metabolism
Dr Fauzia K Kareemi, Calgary, AB - Family Medicine
Dr Shahzad S Karim, New Westminster, BC - Cardiac Surgery
Dr Shameela S F Karmali-Rawji, Calgary, AB - Family Medicine
Dr Savita Karol, Fredericton, NB - Family Medicine
Dr Rajendra P Kashyap, Scarborough, ON - General Practice
Dr Adam S Kayumi, Mississauga, ON - Family Medicine
Dr Soofia L Kazi, London, ON - Family Medicine
Dr Huma Kazmie, Windsor, ON - Pediatrics
Dr Manohar Keesari, Oshawa, ON - Psychiatry
Dr Munaa Khaliq-Kareemi, Calgary, AB - Gastroenterology
Dr Safeer A Khan, Calgary, AB - General Practice
Dr Zarin P Khan, Medicine Hat, AB - General Surgery
Dr Muhammad A Khan, Sydney, NS - Emergency Family Med
Dr A Ghaffar Khan, Cornwall, ON - Psychiatry
Dr Naeem A H Khan, Etobicoke, ON - Psychiatry
Dr Rita R Khan, Kitchener, ON - General Practice
Dr Arshad Khan, Kitchener, ON - Psychiatry
Dr Mohammed A H Khan, Kitchener, ON - General Practice
Dr Shahida R Khan, Markham, ON - Pediatrics
Dr Saadia N Khan, Mississauga, ON - Family Medicine
Dr M Viqar Khan, Oakville, ON - Family Medicine
Dr Shajia Khan, Ottawa, ON - Internal Medicine
Dr Mahmuda B Khan, Scarborough, ON - Family Medicine
Dr Razia Khan, Scarborough, ON - General Practice
Dr Omar D M Khan, St Catharines, ON - Physical Medicine & Rehab
Dr Shagufta U Khan, Toronto, ON - Endocrin/Metabolism
Dr Baseer U Khan, Vaughan, ON - Ophthalmology
Dr Mohammad A Khan, Melfort, SK - General Practice
Dr Hasnain Khandwala, Etobicoke, ON - Endocrin/Metabolism
Dr M Sohail Khattak, Whitby, ON - Pediatrics
Dr Jawad B Khokhar, Ajax, ON - Family Medicine
Dr Bakhtiar J Kidwai, Halifax, NS - General Practice
Dr Abbas A Kohja, Steinbach, MB - General Practice
Dr Asha Kukreti, Scarborough, ON - General Practice
Dr Vishal Kukreti, Toronto, ON - Hematology
Dr Rajender Kumar, Sudbury, ON - Psychiatry
Dr Bahubali D Lagare, Mississauga, ON - Family Medicine
Dr Kartar Lal, Grande Prairie, AB - General Practice
Dr Shazia Latif, Milton, ON - Family Medicine
Dr Rizwana Lilani, Maple, ON - Family Medicine
Dr Richa P Love, Calgary, AB - Family Medicine
Dr Tahir S Lucman, Winnipeg, MB - Internal Medicine
Dr Sanjeev S Luthra, Brampton, ON - Pediatrics
Dr Gyaandeo S Maharajh, Ottawa, ON - Cardiac Surgery
Dr Shazia T Mahmood, Regina, SK - General Practice
Dr Ghias U Mahmud, Calgary, AB - General Practice
Dr S Asad Mahmud, Moncton, NB - Psychiatry
Dr Nizar N Mahomed, Toronto, ON - Orthopedic Surgery
Dr Arshad Majeed, Oshawa, ON - Psychiatry
Dr Sarah Makhdoom, High River, AB - Family Medicine
Dr Tilak R Malhotra, Prince Albert, SK - Pediatrics
Dr Rita K Maliakkal, Calgary, AB - Family Medicine
Dr Saira Malik, Dartmouth, NS - General Practice
Dr Abdul Malik, Brampton, ON - Family Medicine
Dr Ashok Manga, Delta, BC - Family Medicine
Dr Baljinder Mann, Calgary, AB - Family Medicine
Dr Zahida Masood, Mississauga, ON - Family Medicine
Dr Khaja M Masood, Thunder Bay, ON - Internal Medicine
Dr Chaudhry F Masud, Brampton, ON - Family Medicine
Dr Mahmood M Mazhar, Burlington, ON - General Practice
Dr Shahbegum A Meghji, Edmonton, AB - General Practice
Dr Shamsh Y Merali, Milton, ON - Family Medicine
Dr Saba M Merchant, Maple, ON - Pediatrics
Dr M Mohan Merchea, London, ON - Ophthalmology
Dr A Nadeem Mian, Edmonton, AB - Pediatrics
Dr Bilal T Mir, Victoria, BC - Emergency Family Med
Dr S Jamaluddin Mirmiran, Vancouver, BC - Psychiatry
Dr Patricia A Mirwaldt, Vancouver, BC - Family Medicine
Dr Rida K Mirza, London, ON - Psychiatry
Dr Akber H Mithani, Vancouver, BC - General Practice
Dr Nashila N Mohamed, Etobicoke, ON - Family Medicine
Dr Naveed S Mohammad, Etobicoke, ON - General Practice
Dr Solomon Mohammed, Burnaby, BC - General Practice
Dr Rajesh Mohan, Etobicoke, ON - General Practice
Dr Afshan Mohsin, Orangeville, ON - Internal Medicine
Dr Mohamed Moolla, Regina, SK - General Practice
Dr Malek B Moosa, Surrey, BC - Family Medicine
Dr Rasheda Motala, Calgary, AB - Family Medicine
Dr Jawaid I Mughal, Mississauga, ON - General Practice
Dr Maqbool A Mughal, Mississauga, ON - General Practice
Dr Amin A Muhammad, Mississauga, ON - Psychiatry
Dr Iffat A Muhammad, Regina, SK - General Practice
Dr Autar K Munshi, Sydney, NS - Psychiatry
Dr Ravi Murthy, Toronto, ON - General Practice
Dr Waqar Nabi, Mississauga, ON - Family Medicine
Dr Sam Naghibi, Newmarket, ON - Family Medicine
Dr Ashnoor Nagji, Vancouver, BC - Family Medicine
Dr Shamsia M Nainar, Hamilton, ON - Family Medicine
Dr A Ali Najarali, Brampton, ON - General Practice
Dr Shamim G Najarali, Brampton, ON - Anesthesia
Dr Syed M Najfi, Gander, NL - General Surgery
Dr Arif Naqvi, Scarborough, ON - Cardiology
Dr Satinder P S Narang, Surrey, BC - Psychiatry
Dr Muhammad A Naseer, Calgary, AB - General Practice
Dr Shah Nawaz, Sudbury, ON - Cardiology
Dr Ahmad Nawaz, Timmins, ON - General Practice
Dr Saiyed M Nazar-Ul-Iman, Winnipeg, MB - General Practice

Dr Firouzeh Niakosari, North York, ON - Anatomical Pathology
Dr Nazia S Niazi, Surrey, BC - General Practice
Dr Amarjit S Nirwan, Victoria, BC - Family Medicine
Dr Mahmood J Nizam, Edmonton, AB - Family Medicine
Dr Naushad A Noorani, Brampton, ON - Psychiatry
Dr Lachman D Oad, Wetaskiwin, AB - General Surgery
Dr A Shekhar Pandey, Cambridge, ON - Cardiology
Dr Hemant M Pandhi, Mississauga, ON - General Practice
Dr Vikas Pandith, Burlington, ON - Internal Medicine
Dr Dilkhush D Panjwani, Etobicoke, ON - Psychiatry
Dr Sooraja P Papneja, Mississauga, ON - General Practice
Dr Baynazir Parray, Oshawa, ON - Family Medicine
Dr Naeem Parvez, Regina, SK - General Practice
Dr Patricia S R Pawaroo, Ajax, ON - Family Medicine
Dr Khalid Pervaiz, Regina, SK - Family Medicine
Dr Munir A Pirzada, Winnipeg, MB - General Practice
Dr Amrah Pirzada, St. John's, NL - General Practice
Dr Yasmeen A B Punjani, Scarborough, ON - Internal Medicine
Dr Bhupinder S Purewal, Scarborough, ON - General Practice
Dr Nimishchandra N Purohit, Burlington, ON - Psychiatry
Dr M Shafiq Qaadri, Toronto, ON - General Practice
Dr Mussarrat K Qaadri, Toronto, ON - Obstetrics & Gynecology
Dr Shehla Qadeer, Whitby, ON - Family Medicine
Dr Khalida Qazi, Milton, ON - Family Medicine
Dr Ata-Ur-Rehman Quraishi, Halifax, NS - General Practice
Dr M Salim Quraishi, London, ON - General Practice
Dr A Quddus Qureshi, Calgary, AB - Family Medicine
Dr Ziaur-Rehman T Qureshi, Calgary, AB - Family Medicine
Dr Irfan T Qureshi, Fort McMurray, AB - Orthopedic Surgery
Dr Azra Qureshi, Scarborough, ON - General Practice
Dr Bushra Qureshy, Toronto, ON - General Practice
Dr Shahida N Rabbani, Saint-Hubert, QC - Obstetrics & Gynecology
Dr Mubeen F Rafay, Winnipeg, MB - General Practice
Dr Afshan Rafay, Mississauga, ON - Family Medicine
Dr Fizza Z Rafiq, Calgary, AB - Family Medicine
Dr Abdul Rahman, Calgary, AB - Psychiatry
Dr Mohammad M Rahman, Selkirk, MB - General Practice
Dr Sakina Raj, Calgary, AB - Family Medicine
Dr Faisal S Raja, Kitchener, ON - Diagnostic-Radiology
Dr Sultaneih S P Rajabali, New Westminster, BC - General Practice
Dr Babra M Rana, Burnaby, BC - Psychiatry
Dr Ranjit S Rana, Scarborough, ON - General Practice
Dr Mohsin Rashid, Halifax, NS - Pediatrics
Dr Zaihan Rashid, Bowmanville, ON - General Surgery
Dr Tarsem S Ravi, Mississauga, ON - Family Medicine
Dr Shashi K Rawal, Lemoyne, QC - General Practice
Dr Sudesh Rayner, Burlington, ON - General Practice
Dr Jalees M S Razavi, Calgary, AB - Occupational Med
Dr Nayyar K Razvi, Toronto, ON - Family Medicine
Dr Bajinder S Reen, Brampton, ON - Internal Medicine
Dr Yasmin Rehemtula, Mississauga, ON - General Practice
Dr Waseema Rehman, Glace Bay, NS - Family Medicine
Dr Faisal Rehman, London, ON - Internal Medicine
Dr Mujeeb U Rehman, Mississauga, ON - Psychiatry
Dr Ziaur Rehman, Regina, SK - Neurology
Dr El-Karim F J Rhemtulla, St Catharines, ON - Ophthalmology
Dr Kulwant S Riar, Vancouver, BC - Psychiatry
Dr Syed M H Rizvi, Windsor, ON - General Practice
Dr Nasreen Roberts, Kingston, ON - Psychiatry
Dr Mohamed Sabir, Fort Saskatchewan, AB - General Surgery
Dr Krishan K Sachdeva, Oshawa, ON - Urology
Dr Dhun S Sadry, Toronto, ON - Family Medicine
Dr Ayesha L Saeed, Calgary, AB - Family Medicine
Dr Niloufer Saeed, Cambridge, ON - Hematological Pathology
Dr Tariq M Saeed, Mississauga, ON - Family Medicine
Dr Arshad Saeed, Ottawa, ON - Family Medicine
Dr Mukesh C Saini, Brampton, ON - General Practice
Dr Azra K Saleem, London, ON - Psychiatry
Dr Asim Salim, Brantford, ON - Pediatrics
Dr Mohamed A Salyani, Maple, ON - General Practice
Dr Imran Samad, Burnaby, BC - Otolaryngology
Dr Osman Samad, Surrey, BC - General Practice
Dr Arif Samad, Halifax, NS - Ophthalmology
Dr Nabeel B Samad, Halifax, NS - General Practice
Dr Parminder K Sandhu, Calgary, AB - Family Medicine
Dr Gurinder P Sanghera, Toronto, ON - Ophthalmology
Dr Rajni Saraf, Sarnia, ON - Obstetrics & Gynecology
Dr Didar S Sarai, Brampton, ON - Family Medicine
Dr Michael K Sarin, Toronto, ON - Internal Medicine
Dr Brij M Sarup, London, ON - General Practice
Dr Eshratbanu Sayani, Scarborough, ON - Family Medicine
Dr Ebrahim Sayed, Welland, ON - General Practice
Dr M A Raffath Sayeed, Lloydminster, SK - General Practice
Dr Ian D Schokking, Prince George, BC - Family Medicine
Dr Jaishree Sehgal, Kitchener, ON - General Practice
Dr Narinder S Sehravat, Etobicoke, ON - Family Medicine
Dr Vir Bhushan Sennik, Mississauga, ON - Orthopedic Surgery
Dr Arun K Seth, Toronto, ON - General Practice
Dr Asha L Seth, Toronto, ON - General Practice
Dr Shilpa Sethi, Middle Musquodoboi, NS - General Practice
Dr Rajiv Sethi, Etobicoke, ON - Gastroenterology
Dr Baldev R Sethi, Stittsville, ON - General Practice
Dr Muhammad Shafiq, Red Deer, AB - General Practice
Dr Zafar A Shah, London, ON - General Surgery
Dr Pravin C Shah, Strathroy, ON - Anatomical Pathology
Dr Muhammad Shahbaz, Calgary, AB - Family Medicine
Dr Azmeh Shahid, Toronto, ON - General Practice
Dr Shahzad Z Shahmalak, Cambridge, ON - General Practice
Dr Karina Shahzad, Orangeville, ON - Family Medicine
Dr Nasir Shaikh, Winnipeg, MB - General Practice
Dr Bashirunnisa A Shaikh, Etobicoke, ON - General Practice
Dr S Yasmin Shaikh, North York, ON - Family Medicine
Dr Wajid A Shaikh, Scarborough, ON - Pediatrics
Dr Sadia Shakil, Edmonton, AB - General Practice
Dr Safia Shamim, Oakville, ON - Emergency Family Med
Dr Rajeshvar K Sharda, Hamilton, ON - Ophthalmology
Dr Mohammad S Sharif, Surrey, BC - General Surgery
Dr Riaz Shariff, Ajax, ON - General Practice
Dr Pankaj Sharma, Surrey, BC - Family Medicine
Dr Sushil K Sharma, Truro, NS - Family Medicine
Dr Shikhi Sharma, Truro, NS - Family Medicine
Dr Shreekant Sharma, Brantford, ON - Psychiatry
Dr Maheshwar D Sharma, Ingersoll, ON - Internal Medicine
Dr Vijay Sharma, Scarborough, ON - Anesthesia
Dr Shiv R Sharma, Toronto, ON - Family Medicine
Dr Kawal J Sharma, Toronto, ON - Obstetrics & Gynecology
Dr Om Prakash Sharma, Toronto, ON - Orthopedic Surgery
Dr Anees A Shehzad, Sydney, NS - Family Medicine
Dr Gul Nawaz Sheikh, Ajax, ON - Internal Medicine
Dr Amber Z Sheikh, Niagara Falls, ON - Ophthalmology
Dr Adnan M Sheikh, Ottawa, ON - General Practice
Dr Farrukh B Sheikh, Pickering, ON - General Practice
Dr Tasnim K Sheikh, Scarborough, ON - Anatomical Pathology
Dr Khalid M Sheikh, Estevan, SK - General Practice
Dr Jitendra B Sheshgiri, Mississauga, ON - Emergency Family Med
Dr Charudutt D Shete, Langley, BC - General Surgery
Dr Nahid K Shethwala, Guelph, ON - Pediatrics
Dr Sajid Shukoor, Windsor, ON - Anatomical Pathology
Dr Zia A Sial, Etobicoke, ON - Family Medicine
Dr Sanjay Siddhartha, Miramichi, NB - General Practice
Dr Zaeem A Siddiqi, Edmonton, AB - General Practice
Dr Nilofar Siddiqi, Owen Sound, ON - Family Medicine
Dr Muzaffar M Siddiqui, Edmonton, AB - Neurology
Dr Iqbal M Siddiqui, Langley, BC - Family Medicine
Dr Mughina A Siddiqui, Antigonish, NS - General Practice
Dr Farhan Siddiqui, Bolton, ON - Emergency Family Med
Dr Zubaida Siddiqui, Elliot Lake, ON - Family Medicine
Dr Tahira Siddiqui, North York, ON - Anesthesia
Dr Nishat A Siddiqui, Ottawa, ON - General Practice
Dr Nausheen F Siddiqui, Toronto, ON - Internal Medicine
Dr Parmjit K Sidhu, Abbotsford, BC - Psychiatry
Dr Surinder S Sidhu, Brampton, ON - General Practice
Dr Gurmeet Sidhu, Brampton, ON - Family Medicine
Dr Shabana Sikander, Mississauga, ON - Family Medicine
Dr Ram K Singal, Thornhill, ON - General Surgery
Dr Sewa R Singal, Toronto, ON - Internal Medicine
Dr Ram R Singh, Calgary, AB - Internal Medicine
Dr Paramvinder Singh, Calgary, AB - Family Medicine
Dr Jit J Singh, Delta, BC - General Practice
Dr Kanwarjit Singh, Surrey, BC - General Practice
Dr Kulbir I Singh, Vancouver, BC - Psychiatry
Dr Parvinder Singh, Brampton, ON - Family Medicine
Dr Amandeep Singh, Brampton, ON - General Practice
Dr Harleen Singh, Brampton, ON - Family Medicine
Dr Baljit Singh, Chatham, ON - Obstetrics & Gynecology
Dr Inderjit Singh, Hamilton, ON - Family Medicine
Dr Kunwar K Singh, Sarnia, ON - Pediatrics
Dr Tejinder P Singh, Scarborough, ON - Family Medicine
Dr Rajinder K Sippy, Brampton, ON - Family Medicine
Dr Naila Siraj, Aurora, ON - Family Medicine
Dr Mohammad K Sohail, Whitby, ON - Psychiatry
Dr Muriel G Solomon, Calgary, AB - Family Medicine
Dr Alok Sood, Abbotsford, BC - Family Medicine
Dr Balbhadar D Sood, Etobicoke, ON - Psychiatry
Dr Baldev S Soodan, Cornwall, ON - Internal Medicine
Dr Ghazala Sultan, Chatham, ON - Family Medicine
Dr Omar Sultan, Regina, SK - Cardiology
Dr Sumeet K Suneja, Brampton, ON - Internal Medicine
Dr Pal S Sunerh, Etobicoke, ON - General Practice
Dr Smeeksha S Sur, Brampton, ON - Pediatrics
Dr Sabiha M Surangiwala, Mississauga, ON - Family Medicine
Dr Permjit S Suri, Nepean, ON - Internal Medicine
Dr Shahida Surmawala, Edmonton, AB - Family Medicine
Dr Bhadreshchandra V Surti, London, ON - Psychiatry
Dr Rajeev K Suryavanshi, Sarnia, ON - General Surgery
Dr Sam Swaminath, Chatham, ON - Psychiatry
Dr Abdul R Syed, Barrie, ON - General Practice
Dr Ali A Syed, Etobicoke, ON - Anesthesia
Dr Ikramuddin Syed, Etobicoke, ON - Family Medicine
Dr Abu A Syed, Lindsay, ON - Internal Medicine
Dr Jaffer A Syed, London, ON - Cardiology
Dr Sumairah A Syed, Markham, ON - Family Medicine
Dr Arif M Syed, Mississauga, ON - Psychiatry
Dr Saadat A S Syed, North York, ON - Family Medicine
Dr A Shaista Syed, North York, ON - Family Medicine
Dr Yasmeen Syed, Scarborough, ON - General Practice
Dr Uzma Syed, Scarborough, ON - Internal Medicine
Dr Zareen Syed, Scarborough, ON - Internal Medicine
Dr Khalid A Syed, Toronto, ON - Orthopedic Surgery
Dr Fakhruddin Taher, Etobicoke, ON - Internal Medicine
Dr Laeeq A Tahir, Moncton, NB - Psychiatry
Dr Surriya J Tahirkheli, Ottawa, ON - Psychiatry
Dr Anita A Taj, Prince Albert, SK - General Practice
Dr Chiranjib Talukdar, Regina, SK - Pediatrics
Dr Khalida P Tariq, Edmonton, AB - Family Medicine
Dr Muhammad Tasneem, Mississauga, ON - Family Medicine
Dr Syeda N Tauqir Naqvi, Woodstock, ON - Anatomical Pathology
Dr Vijay K Thapar, Edmonton, AB - Family Medicine
Dr Ma Khin Thida, Vancouver, BC - Family Medicine
Dr Lubna T Tirmizi, Pickering, ON - Family Medicine
Dr Dalvinder S Toor, Vancouver, BC - Family Medicine
Dr Tanveer E Towheed, Kingston, ON - Internal Medicine
Dr Ram S Ubhi, Calgary, AB - General Practice
Dr Surinder K Ubhi, Calgary, AB - Family Medicine
Dr Sameena Uddin, Mississauga, ON - General Surgery
Dr A H M Jamal Uddin, Toronto, ON - Internal Medicine
Dr Huma Z Ul Haq, Shelburne, ON - Family Medicine
Dr Hidayat Ullah, Calgary, AB - General Practice
Dr Farid Ullah, Kelowna, BC - General Practice
Dr Faiza Upal, Georgetown, ON - Family Medicine
Dr Sonia Uppal, Abbotsford, BC - Psychiatry
Dr Rakesh Uppal, Brampton, ON - General Practice
Dr Abida Usman, Thornhill, ON - General Practice
Dr Seemin A Vahidy, Edmonton, AB - General Practice
Dr M Tariq Vakani, Mississauga, ON - Cardiology
Dr Pramod K Verma, Edmonton, AB - Obstetrics & Gynecology
Dr Mirza R Virani, Markham, ON - General Practice
Dr Manjit S Virdee, Brampton, ON - Family Medicine
Dr Mohan S Virick, Sydney, NS - General Practice
Dr Mumtaz A Virji, Vancouver, BC - Pediatrics
Dr Achla R Virmani, Verdun, QC - General Practice
Dr Uttam J K Wadhwa, Mississauga, ON - Psychiatry
Dr Waqar Waheed, Calgary, AB - Psychiatry
Dr Shobha Wahi, Hamilton, ON - Pediatrics

Dr Ihsan U Waraich, Brampton, ON - Family Medicine
Dr Mohammed M Warsi, Waterville, NB - General Practice
Dr Mohammed A Warsi, Hamilton, ON - Psychiatry
Dr Zahid Wasti, Kelowna, BC - Psychiatry
Dr Qasim H Wasti, Maple Ridge, BC - Family Medicine
Dr Tehmina Q Wasti, Maple Ridge, BC - Family Medicine
Dr S Fasahat H Wasty, St Thomas, ON - General Pathology
Dr Mahesh P Yadav, North Bay, ON - Orthopedic Surgery
Dr Saad Yasin, Calgary, AB - Family Medicine
Dr Naveeda Yasmeen, Hamilton, ON - Family Medicine
Dr Jawaid Younus, London, ON - Internal Medicine
Dr Mohammad Yousuf, Bathurst, NB - Otolaryngology
Dr Kamran Yusuf, Calgary, AB - General Practice
Dr Aftab Zafar, Kitchener, ON - Ophthalmology
Dr Rosy Zafar, Mississauga, ON - Family Medicine
Dr Mukarram A Zaidi, Calgary, AB - General Practice
Dr Khawar-Uz Zaman, Dartmouth, NS - Internal Medicine
Dr Kamruz Zaman, Toronto, ON - Family Medicine
Dr Shaista K Zareef, Stittsville, ON - Family Medicine
Dr Mohamed M Zawahir, Stratford, ON - General Practice
Dr Mohammad I Zia, Toronto, ON - Cardiology
Dr Naeem A Zubair, Bowmanville, ON - General Practice
Dr Muhammad Zulfiqar, Abbotsford, BC - Internal Medicine

VIETNAMESE

Dr Linh-Khue Bui, Longueuil, QC - Electroencephal
Dr T Bich Dao Can, Sorel-Tracy, QC - Internal Medicine
Dr Karl K S Chan, Vancouver, BC - General Practice
Dr Kim Hang Chu, Montreal, QC - General Practice
Dr Phuong Dang, Mississauga, ON - Family Medicine
Dr Bach-Tuyet T Dang, Toronto, ON - General Practice
Dr Tommy Dang, Windsor, ON - Neurosurgery
Dr Dinh Thien V Dang, Montreal, QC - General Practice
Dr Angela N Dang, Montreal, QC - Family Medicine
Dr Hong Quyen Dao, Gatineau, QC - General Practice
Dr Tien Trong Dao, Laval, QC - Diagnostic-Radiology
Dr T Trang Dao, Montreal, QC - Psychiatry
Dr Anh T T Dinh, Edmonton, AB - General Practice
Dr Hoang-Diep Dinh, Anjou, QC - General Practice
Dr Ba-Hiep Dinh, Montreal, QC - General Practice
Dr Anh Phuong Do, Toronto, ON - Pediatrics
Dr Quoc-Bao Do, Montreal, QC - Cardiac Surgery
Dr Quynh Huong Doan, Vancouver, BC - Pediatric Emergency Medicine
Dr Ly Huong Doan, Montreal, QC - General Practice
Dr Dung Ngoc Duong, Concord, ON - Family Medicine
Dr Nhan Hoang Duong, Ottawa, ON - Family Medicine
Dr Huu Thanh Duong, Ottawa, ON - General Practice
Dr Nguyen H Duong, Toronto, ON - General Practice
Dr T David Ewing-Bui, Sudbury, ON - Thoracic Surgery
Dr Soma Ganesan, Vancouver, BC - Psychiatry
Dr Hudson K H Giang, Lindsay, ON - General Pathology
Dr Nhung T C Ho, North York, ON - Dermatology
Dr Quang Nhan Ho, Montreal, QC - General Surgery
Dr T Boi-Ngoc Hoang, Hamilton, ON - Obstetrics & Gynecology
Dr Minh Chau Hoang, Montreal, QC - General Practice
Dr Antoine Hoang, Pointe-Claire, QC - General Practice
Dr Hien Huynh, Edmonton, AB - Pediatrics
Dr Chau Cong Huynh, Concord, ON - Family Medicine
Dr Quoc Hung P Huynh, North York, ON - General Surgery
Dr Huu Hung Huynh, Longueuil, QC - Internal Medicine
Dr Julie B D Lacuna, Vancouver, BC - Family Medicine
Dr Ngoc Nga Lam, Montreal, QC - General Practice
Dr Grace Le, Calgary, AB - Family Medicine
Dr Thanh Long Le, Calgary, AB - General Practice
Dr Phuoc-Hai Le, Edmonton, AB - Family Medicine
Dr Lyly H Le, Surrey, BC - Internal Medicine
Dr Quynh M T Le, Brampton, ON - Obstetrics & Gynecology
Dr Khoa-Anh Le, Markham, ON - Internal Medicine
Dr Tien Dung Le, Ottawa, ON - Gynecologic Oncology
Dr Brian B Le, Scarborough, ON - Internal Medicine
Dr Chu Quang Le, Toronto, ON - General Practice
Dr Hoang Yen Le, Toronto, ON - Pediatrics
Dr Binh-Dang Le, Laval, QC - General Practice
Dr Thien Nhan Le, Montreal, QC - General Practice
Dr Thi Qui Le, Montreal, QC - General Practice
Dr Thi Xuan Mai Le, Montreal-Nord, QC - General Practice
Dr Tam Le Duc, Longueuil, QC - Respirology
Dr Chau Levan, Montreal, QC - General Practice
Dr Loan T Luong, Kemptville, ON - Family Medicine
Dr Diep T Luong, Montreal, QC - General Practice
Dr Chinh-Duc Luu, Mercier, QC - General Practice
Dr David D Mai, Ottawa, ON - Family Medicine
Dr Thi Minh H Ngo, Saint-Laurent, QC - General Practice
Dr Bao Thoai H Nguyen, Calgary, AB - Family Medicine
Dr Xuandieu T Nguyen, Calgary, AB - Family Medicine
Dr De Nguyen, Edmonton, AB - General Practice
Dr Lynda P Nguyen, Edmonton, AB - Family Medicine
Dr Minh Hien Nguyen, Burnaby, BC - Family Medicine
Dr Nhiem Nguyen, Richmond, BC - Dermatology
Dr Viem Chung Nguyen, Vancouver, BC - Physical Medicine & Rehab
Dr Vi Liet Nguyen, Vancouver, BC - General Practice
Dr N P Julie Nguyen, Vancouver, BC - Family Medicine
Dr Lien Hoang Nguyen, Winnipeg, MB - General Practice
Dr Tuyet Thi Nguyen, Belleville, ON - Family Medicine
Dr The-Huy Nguyen, Brampton, ON - General Practice
Dr Lam Van Nguyen, Hamilton, ON - General Practice
Dr Ngoc Truong T Nguyen, Oshawa, ON - Family Medicine
Dr The-Minh Nguyen, Ottawa, ON - Neurology
Dr Van Tuong Nguyen, Toronto, ON - General Practice
Dr Phuongbich Nguyen, Toronto, ON - General Practice
Dr San Duy Nguyen, Toronto, ON - Psychiatry
Dr Anh Tuan Nguyen, Toronto, ON - General Practice
Dr Nam Anh Nguyen, Toronto, ON - Family Medicine
Dr Quang V K Nguyen, Toronto, ON - Family Medicine
Dr Huy Thanh V Nguyen, Charlottetown, PE - Family Medicine
Dr Tang-Dong Nguyen, Brossard, QC - General Practice
Dr Quy Don Nguyen, Chateauguay, QC - Cardiology
Dr Hieu Dinh Nguyen, Gatineau, QC - General Practice
Dr Tang-Thong Nguyen, Gatineau, QC - Cardiology
Dr Ngoc-Van Nguyen, Lachine, QC - General Surgery
Dr Thi Van Anh Nguyen, Laval, QC - Diagnostic-Radiology
Dr Thi Thanh T Nguyen, Laval, QC - Medical Microbiology
Dr Hoa Hieu Nguyen, Longueuil, QC - General Practice
Dr Tuan Quynh T Nguyen, Montreal, QC - Ophthalmology
Dr T Thanh Tra Nguyen, Montreal, QC - Family Medicine
Dr C L Remy Nguyen, Montreal, QC - Otolaryngology
Dr Bich-Ngoc Nguyen, Montreal, QC - Anatomical Pathology
Dr Van-Hung Nguyen, Montreal, QC - Anatomical Pathology
Dr Duy Nguyen, Montreal, QC - General Practice
Dr Khue Huu Nguyen, Montreal, QC - Dermatology
Dr Ha-Nam P Nguyen, Montreal, QC - Otolaryngology
Dr Minh Hanh Nguyen, Montreal, QC - General Practice
Dr Bich Ngoc Nguyen, Montreal, QC - Psychiatry
Dr Tuong Minh Nguyen, Montreal, QC - Family Medicine
Dr Ngoc Bich Nguyen, Montreal, QC - Internal Medicine
Dr Doan-Trang Nguyen, Montreal, QC - Internal Medicine
Dr Thao Nguyen, Montreal, QC - Ophthalmology
Dr Van Hoi Nguyen, Saint-Laurent, QC - Family Medicine
Dr Thi Ngoc L Nguyen, Saint-Leonard, QC - Family Medicine
Dr Michel Nguyen, Sherbrooke, QC - Cardiology
Dr Hai Hac Nguyen, St-Jean-sur-Richel, QC - Dermatology
Dr Uyen Ly Nguyen Do, Saint-Leonard, QC - Family Medicine
Dr Thuy-Tien Nguyen-Dang, Amqui, QC - General Practice
Dr Quynh-Lang Nguyen-Giang, Oakville, ON - Family Medicine
Dr Phong Nguyen-Ho, Peterborough, ON - Cardiology
Dr Felix Phuc Nguyen-Tan, Montreal, QC - Radiation Oncology
Dr Toan D Nhan, Toronto, ON - General Practice
Dr Christine Anh Ngoc Pham, Calgary, AB - Diagnostic-Radiology
Dr Quynh N Pham, Brampton, ON - General Surgery
Dr Trai Ngoc Pham, Concord, ON - Family Medicine
Dr Thuy-Nga Tia Pham, East York, ON - Family Medicine
Dr Chien Pham, Mississauga, ON - Family Medicine
Dr Anne-Marie Pham, Mississauga, ON - Family Medicine
Dr Xuan H Pham, Ottawa, ON - Nuclear Medicine
Dr Tuong-Vi Pham, Val-d'Or, QC - Family Medicine
Dr T H I Dang Phan, Montreal, QC - Family Medicine
Dr Xuan Truong Phan, Montreal, QC - General Practice
Dr Minh Duc Quan, Mississauga, ON - Family Medicine
Dr Hien Minh Ta, Richmond Hill, ON - Anesthesia
Dr Tuyet Phi Ta, Montreal, QC - General Practice
Dr Thi Ngoc T Than, Mississauga, ON - Family Medicine
Dr An Than Trong, Montreal, QC - General Surgery
Dr Lan Quang Thanh, St-Jean-Sur-Richel, QC - Gastroenterology
Dr Nam Thuat, Edmonton, AB - Family Medicine
Dr Dinh Vu To, Dartmouth, NS - Family Medicine
Dr Toan Bao To, Etobicoke, ON - Cardiology
Dr Thanh-Thao Ton-Nu, St-Charles-Brromee, QC - Cardiology
Dr Quoc-Huy Ton-That, Montreal, QC - Emergency Family Med
Dr Nhan Thien Tong, North York, ON - General Practice
Dr Khai Minh Tram, Toronto, ON - Internal Medicine
Dr Phu Manh Tran, Langley, BC - Emergency Family Med
Dr Quoc Hung Tran, Chatham, ON - Internal Medicine
Dr Anh T N Tran, Concord, ON - Family Medicine
Dr Kham Quang Tran, East York, ON - Critical Care Medicine
Dr T G Joe Tran, Mississauga, ON - General Practice
Dr Van Nham Tran, Mississauga, ON - General Practice
Dr Bernie B C Tran, North York, ON - General Practice
Dr Diem Thu T Tran, Ottawa, ON - Anesthesia
Dr Viet Tan Tran, Ottawa, ON - Urology
Dr S Stanley Tran, Scarborough, ON - Gastroenterology
Dr Van-Chung Tran, Toronto, ON - Family Medicine
Dr D Jeffrey Tran, Toronto, ON - Infectious Diseases
Dr P P Peter Tran, Toronto, ON - Psychiatry
Dr Teresa B C Tran, Vaughan, ON - Family Medicine
Dr Boi Anh Tran, Longueuil, QC - General Practice
Dr Van-Dung Tran, Montreal, QC - General Practice
Dr Thu-Hang Tran, Montreal, QC - Emergency Family Med
Dr Cuong Tran Ngoc, Mississauga, ON - Diagnostic-Radiology
Dr Nhung Tran-Davies, Calmar, AB - Family Medicine
Dr Nguyen Trang, Arnprior, ON - Family Medicine
Dr Thomas Q N Trinh, Langley, BC - Family Medicine
Dr L Hang Bich Trinh, Mississauga, ON - Family Medicine
Dr K Y Denny Trinh, Toronto, ON - Internal Medicine
Dr Ngoc Chau Trinh, Gatineau, QC - General Practice
Dr Ba-Truc Trinh, Laval, QC - Otolaryngology
Dr Nathalie Trinh, Montreal, QC - Otolaryngology
Dr Do Huu Truong, Calgary, AB - General Practice
Dr Kim L L Truong, Calgary, AB - General Practice
Dr Barney T H Truong, Calgary, AB - Family Medicine
Dr Tinh Dinh Truong, Vancouver, BC - General Practice
Dr Pauline T Truong, Victoria, BC - Radiation Oncology
Dr Dang-Toan Truong, Nepean, ON - Diagnostic-Radiology
Dr Cong Phuc Truong, Louiseville, QC - General Practice
Dr Tuyet Lan Truong, Pointe-Claire, QC - General Practice
Dr Thomas T C Van, Scarborough, ON - Family Medicine
Dr Tuyet Bach Vo, North York, ON - General Pathology
Dr Khanh Hong Vo, North York, ON - Family Medicine
Dr H D David Vo, North York, ON - Family Medicine
Dr Thoi Hen Vo, Toronto, ON - General Practice
Dr Thi Nhu Y Vo, Gatineau, QC - General Practice
Dr Thi Minh D Vo, LaSalle, QC - Family Medicine
Dr Minh Ha Vo, LaSalle, QC - General Practice
Dr Tan Tai Vo, Val-d'Or, QC - Anatomical Pathology
Dr Lan Vo Nguyen, New Westminster, BC - Anesthesia
Dr Kim-Loan Vo-Doan, Montreal, QC - Otolaryngology
Dr Trung K Vu, Calgary, AB - Family Medicine
Dr Trevor T C Vu, Edmonton, AB - General Practice
Dr Manh Huu Vu, Hamilton, ON - Diagnostic-Radiology
Dr N Q Wayne Vu, London, ON - Family Medicine
Dr David D V Vu, Toronto, ON - General Practice
Dr Binh Thien Vu, Woodstock, ON - General Practice
Dr The-Hung Vu, Montreal, QC - General Practice
Dr Dung Vu, Montreal, QC - General Practice
Dr Quynh-Phuong Vu Ngoc, Longueuil, QC - Diagnostic-Radiology
Dr Caroline X L Vu-Nguyen, Montreal, QC - General Practice
Dr James R Wylie, Brampton, ON - General Practice
Dr Kwang Yang, Surrey, BC - Family Medicine

WARAY

Dr Enrico F Cabigon, Regina, SK - Anatomical Pathology

WELSH

Dr Dafydd G Bebb, Calgary, AB - Internal Medicine
Dr J Richard Daniel, Gravenhurst, ON - General Practice
Dr D Richard R Thomas, Vancouver, BC - Dermatology
Dr Sally J Watson, Powell River, BC - General Practice

XHOSA

Dr Anthony J Chinner, Scarborough, ON - General Practice
Dr Louis J Coetzee, Bonnyville, AB - General Practice
Dr T Joseph Goso, Grande Prairie, AB - General Practice
Dr Aggrey P Madikiza, Scarborough, ON - Pediatrics
Dr Mtimkulu Mehlomakulu, Kingston, ON - Pediatrics
Dr Nigel A Painter, Prince Albert, SK - General Practice

YIDDISH

Dr Edward I Adelson, Montreal, QC - Cardiology
Dr Jerald Bain, North York, ON - Endocrin/Metabolism
Dr W Barrett Benny, Vancouver, BC - Hematology
Dr Hershl Berman, Toronto, ON - Internal Medicine
Dr Abraham Born, Toronto, ON - Internal Medicine
Dr Izzie Boxen, Brampton, ON - Nuclear Medicine
Dr Edward Brown, Toronto, ON - Psychiatry
Dr Harry Cohen, North York, ON - General Practice
Dr Murray Davidson, Toronto, ON - Internal Medicine
Dr Judah Denburg, Hamilton, ON - Hematology
Dr David Dorenbaum, Toronto, ON - Pediatrics
Dr Maurice N Druck, Mississauga, ON - Cardiology
Dr Michael Dworkind, Montreal, QC - Family Medicine
Dr Isaac Dwosh, Toronto, ON - Internal Medicine
Dr Earl Edelstein, Montreal, QC - General Practice
Dr Robert J Fingerote, Richmond Hill, ON - Gastroenterology
Dr Sam A Friedlander, Toronto, ON - Gastroenterology
Dr Abraham Friesner, Toronto, ON - General Practice
Dr Seymour Frydrych, Toronto, ON - Family Medicine
Dr Abraham Fuks, Montreal, QC - Clin Immun/Allergy
Dr Henry M Gallay, North York, ON - Psychiatry
Dr Eric W Gangbar, Richmond Hill, ON - Cardiology
Dr Marvin A Gelkopf, North York, ON - Family Medicine
Dr Phil Gold, Montreal, QC - Clin Immun/Allergy
Dr Benjamin Goldberg, London, ON - Psychiatry
Dr Chaim J Goldberg, Scarborough, ON - Ophthalmology
Dr Sol J Goldstein, North York, ON - Psychiatry
Dr Julius E S Gomolin, Montreal, QC - Ophthalmology
Dr Fabian P Gorodzinsky, London, ON - Pediatrics
Dr Walter H Gotlieb, Montreal, QC - Obstetrics & Gynecology
Dr Albert H Green, North York, ON - General Practice
Dr Joseph Greenbaum, Hamilton, ON - Clin Immun/Allergy
Dr Liuba Grossman, North York, ON - General Practice
Dr Dinah C Gruber, North York, ON - Pediatrics
Dr Juda Habot, Newmarket, ON - Cardiology
Dr Harvey I Halperin, Vancouver, BC - General Practice
Dr Abraham I Hirsz, Toronto, ON - Family Medicine
Dr Aaron Jesin, North York, ON - General Practice
Dr Tibor Juda, Toronto, ON - Urology
Dr Brian M Katchan, North York, ON - Internal Medicine
Dr Herbert I Khosid, Thornhill, ON - General Practice
Dr Albert J Kirshen, Toronto, ON - Geriatric Medicine
Dr Benjamin H Lasko, Etobicoke, ON - General Practice
Dr Bram Lermer, Richmond, BC - Family Medicine
Dr Sheila Lewin, Toronto, ON - General Practice
Dr Charles Listgarten, Woodbridge, ON - Internal Medicine
Dr Howard C Margolese, Montreal, QC - Psychiatry
Dr Calvin A Melmed, Montreal, QC - Neurology
Dr Matthew L Morton, Toronto, ON - Obstetrics & Gynecology
Dr Stanley Nattel, Montreal, QC - Cardiology
Dr Michael Ostro, Mississauga, ON - General Practice
Dr Sarah Paikin, North York, ON - General Practice
Dr Abraham Peliowski, Edmonton, AB - Pediatrics
Dr Irving B Rosen, Toronto, ON - General Surgery
Dr Frank W Rosenberg, Etobicoke, ON - Dermatology
Dr Rachel Rubinstein-Schipper, Montreal, QC - Dermatology
Dr Hyman M Schipper, Montreal, QC - Neurology
Dr Gerald Schneiderman, Toronto, ON - Psychiatry
Dr Rochelle S Schwartz, Concord, ON - Family Medicine
Dr Yehudi P Shields, Toronto, ON - General Practice
Dr Gina Shochat, Toronto, ON - Family Medicine
Dr Kenneth I Shulman, Toronto, ON - Psychiatry
Dr Michael Shupak, Toronto, ON - General Practice
Dr Ezra A Silverstein, Toronto, ON - Orthopedic Surgery
Dr Neville L Sischy, North York, ON - General Practice
Dr David A Sliwowicz, Ajax, ON - General Practice
Dr Stanley Spier, Thornhill, ON - Dermatology
Dr Maurice Strasfeld, New Glasgow, NS - General Practice
Dr Edison Susman, Scarborough, ON - General Practice
Dr Julio Szmuilowicz, Toronto, ON - Psychiatry
Dr Isaac I E Szpindel, Toronto, ON - General Practice
Dr Lionel Tenby, Richmond, BC - General Practice
Dr Myron Troster, Stratford, ON - Anatomical Pathology
Dr Avi Wallerstein, Montreal, QC - Ophthalmology
Dr Ellen Warner, Toronto, ON - Internal Medicine
Dr Harold A E Weizel, Toronto, ON - General Surgery
Dr Solomon M Werb, Toronto, ON - General Practice
Dr Stanley J Wine, North York, ON - Dermatology
Dr Sheldon A Wise, North York, ON - Pediatrics
Dr Joseph I O Wohlgelernter, Thornhill, ON - Psychiatry
Dr Brenda T Woods, Toronto, ON - Obstetrics & Gynecology
Dr Mayer M Zaklos, Montreal, QC - Family Medicine
Dr Irving Zelcer, North York, ON - Family Medicine
Dr Shery H K Zener, Toronto, ON - Psychiatry
Dr Lawrence Zoberman, Scarborough, ON - Family Medicine

YORUBA

Dr Mofoluwaso A Abolarin, Calgary, AB - Family Medicine
Dr Motunrayo J Adetola, Ottawa, ON - Family Medicine
Dr M Oluwafemi Agbayewa, Burnaby, BC - Psychiatry
Dr J Oluwagbenga Ajayi-Obe, Sarnia, ON - Family Medicine
Dr Olaniyi F Ajisafe, North York, ON - Family Medicine
Dr Amos A Akinbiyi, Regina, SK - Obstetrics & Gynecology
Dr Florence O Akindele, St Paul, AB - General Practice
Dr Idowu C Akinjise, Fort McMurray, AB - Family Medicine
Dr Moses A Alatishe, Moncton, NB - Psychiatry
Dr Babatunde A Awakan, Camrose, AB - Family Medicine
Dr Olufemi R Ayeni, Hamilton, ON - Orthopedic Surgery
Dr R Oluwafemi Ayeni, Kapuskasing, ON - General Surgery
Dr Ogunroti Ayibiowu, Hamilton, ON - Family Medicine
Dr Gbade A Ayoade, Etobicoke, ON - Obstetrics & Gynecology
Dr Omotayo Dawodu, Calgary, AB - Emergency Family Med
Dr Olugbenga O Dehinbo, Cornwall, ON - Obstetrics & Gynecology
Dr Megeri Ede, Ottawa, ON - Internal Medicine
Dr Olanrewaju Y Egbeyemi, Prince Albert, SK - Family Medicine
Dr Adebola Fagbola, Mississauga, ON - Family Medicine
Dr Oluwarotimi Fashoranti, Pugwash, NS - Family Medicine
Dr Ande L Karimu, The Pas, MB - General Practice
Dr Olayiwola A Kassim, Parry Sound, ON - Anatomical Pathology
Dr Lawrence A Marcus, Calgary, AB - Psychiatry
Dr Felix S Odaibo, Grande Prairie, AB - Pediatrics
Dr Oluwole David Odugbemi, Edmonton, AB - Family Medicine
Dr Adebola O Odulana-Ogundimu, Sudbury, ON - Pediatrics
Dr Funmi A Oguntoyinbo, North York, ON - Psychiatry
Dr Innocent C Okafor, Brampton, ON - Family Medicine
Dr Paul O Oladipo, St Catharines, ON - Family Medicine
Dr A Ajike Oladoyin, Calgary, AB - Family Medicine
Dr Oloruntoba J Oluboka, Calgary, AB - Psychiatry
Dr Samuel A Oluwadairo, Calgary, AB - Psychiatry
Dr Olufemi O Omiwole, Bowmanville, ON - Family Medicine
Dr Olutoyese O Oyelese, West Kelowna, BC - Family Medicine
Dr Olusegun Oyewole, North Battleford, SK - General Practice
Dr L Kola Oyewumi, Markham, ON - Psychiatry
Dr Akinlolu O Peluola, Saskatoon, SK - Psychiatry
Dr Kudirat F Pepple, Calgary, AB - General Practice
Dr Oluyomi A Sobowale, Peterborough, ON - Obstetrics & Gynecology
Dr S Kolawole Sogbein, North Bay, ON - Urology
Dr Modupe O J Tunde-Byass, North York, ON - Obstetrics & Gynecology
Dr Emmanuel U J Udoeyop, Cornwall, ON - Obstetrics & Gynecology

YUGOSLAVIAN

Dr Marijana Drandic, Ajax, ON - Psychiatry
Dr Ljubica Gulan-Vujnovic, Toronto, ON - General Practice
Dr Diana Kljenak, Toronto, ON - Psychiatry
Dr Tamara Spaic, London, ON - Endocrin/Metabolism
Dr Ratka Timarac, Hamilton, ON - General Practice
Dr Inge Vasovich, Hamilton, ON - General Practice
Dr Peter M Vignjevic, Hamilton, ON - Dermatology
Dr Predrag Vujnovic, Toronto, ON - General Practice

ZULU

Dr Hendrik Alberts, Welland, ON - Family Medicine
Dr Pravin Batohi, London, ON - Anesthesia
Dr Nicolaas C Botha, Oxbow, SK - General Practice
Dr Martin K Bunge, Winnipeg, MB - Diagnostic-Radiology
Dr Rohan Cornelissen, Prince Albert, SK - General Practice
Dr Sundren Govender, Victoria, BC - Family Medicine
Dr Gertie Greyling, Abbotsford, BC - General Practice
Dr Adriaan Heunis, Salmon Arm, BC - General Practice
Dr Pravesh Jugnundan, Aurora, ON - Family Medicine
Dr Meghna P Juta, St. Albert, AB - Family Medicine
Dr Michael R Kenyon, Terrace, BC - Internal Medicine
Dr Pieter Ernst Kruger, Fort McMurray, AB - General Practice
Dr Fernando H Kuhn, Abbotsford, BC - General Practice
Dr Aggrey P Madikiza, Scarborough, ON - Pediatrics
Dr Eugene W A Magerman, Calgary, AB - General Practice
Dr Jean-Pierre Mare, Lac La Biche, AB - Family Medicine
Dr Dereck Maseka, Drumheller, AB - Family Medicine
Dr Mtimkulu Mehlomakulu, Kingston, ON - Pediatrics
Dr Shabir M Mia, Saskatoon, SK - General Practice
Dr Johnathan Moolman, Terrace, BC - General Practice
Dr Prenilla Naidu, Edmonton, AB - General Practice
Dr Oluwole David Odugbemi, Edmonton, AB - Family Medicine
Dr Motlobeng D Pebane, Indian Head, SK - General Practice
Dr Alexander P Pretorius, Winnipeg, MB - Anesthesia
Dr Jan G Roux, Virden, MB - General Practice
Dr Ebrahim Sayed, Welland, ON - General Practice
Dr Bhavna K Thakersee, Waterdown, ON - Family Medicine
Dr Pravesh K Vallabh, Edmonton, AB - Family Medicine
Dr Shirley G Van Der Merwe, Vernon, BC - General Practice
Dr Nicola Wiggelinkhuizen, Vernon, BC - Family Medicine

SECTION 2 — PHYSICIANS BY GEOGRAPHIC LOCATION

GENERAL PRACTITIONERS AND FAMILY PHYSICIANS OF CANADA

ALBERTA

AIRDRIE

Abdelmalak, Ehab M T.
Adegbulu, Adekunie K., FamilyMed
Adewale, Oluwayemisi O.
Alfalah, Ibrahim M., FamilyMed
Alhaddad, Mohamed O.
Alvi, Fozia S., FamilyMed
Botha, Deon
Carson, Joseph M.
De Waal, Philip F., FamilyMed
De Waal, Philip F.
Desnoyers, Elaine M., FamilyMed
Gautama, Sadhana K., FamilyMed
Geleidi, Aladdin, FamilyMed
Giesbrecht, Sunshine J., FamilyMed
Gye, Emmanuel A.
Hislop, Alan John
Kazatchenko, Lioubov N., FamilyMed
Khumree, Altaf
Kravchenko, Olena
Kyne, Julian A., FamilyMed
Le Roux, Johannes L., FamilyMed
Lupul, Sheri, FamilyMed
MacLachlan, Donald A.
Marzouk, Nariman Z R., FamilyMed
McSorley, John J.
Morrison, Sandra L., FamilyMed
Odubanjo, Oladipo O., FamilyMed
Paulgaard, Tammy M., FamilyMed
Raghavji, Allatif A.
Raza, Shaheen, FamilyMed
Shonubi, Adeyemi O., FamilyMed
Siddiqui, Adil F., FamilyMed
Smith, Patricia R., FamilyMed
Thapar, Tania, FamilyMed
Vakil, Ankitkumar P.
Van Rooyen, Elizabeth E M.
Voros, Sandor
Vorosova, Gertruda
White, Neil G., FamilyMed

ALHAMBRA

McBain, Adina M., FamilyMed

ALSIKE

Muscat, Colin J., FamilyMed

ATHABASCA

Burger, Leon E.
Burger, Michael B.
Buys, Lecia
Esterhuizen, Andries J.
Klopper, Johanna H.
Mol, Adrianus
Smith, Michael J W.

BANFF

Bartley, Simon D K., FamilyMed(EM)
Blaney, Nancy C., FamilyMed
Bossert, Kerri L., FamilyMed(EM)
Chambers, Danaze G.
Fowke, Jane S.
Gauthier, Charles E., FamilyMed(EM)
Irving, Christopher J., FamilyMed
MacDonald, Ian R.
Marriott, M. Lynne, FamilyMed
McLean, Joy E.
Mergler, Sandra G., FamilyMed(EM)
Patterson, Harry S.
Selvanandan, Vamini K., FamilyMed
Shepherd, S. Lance, FamilyMed(EM)
Shigeishi, Stephen A., FamilyMed
Smiljic, Dino, FamilyMed
Tupper, Jennifer I L., FamilyMed(EM)
Turner, Christopher B., FamilyMed(EM)
Watchorn, Adam T S., FamilyMed(EM)

BARRHEAD

Abdulhafid, Adel H.
Azzi, Wadih B., FamilyMed
Bernes, Kent R., FamilyMed
De Waal, Egbertus B.
Gurges, Ramy
Hankinson, Jeffrey J., FamilyMed
Hassan, Fathi T B.
Kallal, E. Timothy
Tawfik, Abdeldaim M.
Velji, Iman
Velmurugiah, Velupillai
Wepener, Frederik J.
Wepener, Liezl
Wray, M. Brent

BASHAW

Mucciarone, Antonio

BASSANO

Alawiye, Alaba A.
Richards, James C., FamilyMed

BEAUMONT

Black, Sandra E.
Bogoch, Ruth E.
Corrigan, Jason R., FamilyMed
Detorakis, Anna
Lund, Christine L., FamilyMed
Penrod, Tessa M., FamilyMed
Riske, David M.
Roberts, Stacey K.
Sails, Alison
Soehn, Scott A., FamilyMed
Spiers, Anne-Marie C.
Spiers, Caroline, FamilyMed
Stewart, Darryl S.

BEAVERLODGE

Balouch, Hamid M.
Clow, Erin C., FamilyMed
Hunter, John R., FamilyMed
Miller, David P., FamilyMed

BEISEKER

Lavens, M. Timothy, FamilyMed(EM)

BELLEVUE

Garbutt, Allan S., FamilyMed
Garland, Leslie A.
McKernan, Peter S.
Sara, William B.

BLACK DIAMOND

Bishop, Jill M., FamilyMed
Branch, Jacques V M., FamilyMed
Congdon, Valerie M., FamilyMed
Doran, Brian J., FamilyMed
Dowdall, Timothy J., FamilyMed
Grisdale, Noel W., FamilyMed
Hembroff, Tristan, FamilyMed
Jablonski, Eric V., FamilyMed
Ray, Gary J., FamilyMed
Schuck, Matthew J., FamilyMed
Siray, Brian L., FamilyMed
Van Aerde, Arne, FamilyMed

BLACKFALDS

Kemp, Theo

BLAIRMORE

Botha, Andries J.
Couto Chuquer, Maria B.
Maritz, J. Johannes
Sudbury, Ian D., FamilyMed

BONNYVILLE

Baburam, Ashokchand
Coetzee, Louis J.
De Freitas, Leonard
Du Preez, Amelia
Gouws, Willem J.
Kritzinger, Irma E.
Lamoureux, Guy A., FamilyMed
Lavoie, Cecile R.
Loge, John M., FamilyMed
Muller, Jacobus M., FamilyMed
Murphy, John D.
Turenne, Annette Y M.
Van Deventer, Tharine
van der Walt, Petrus J.
Van der Watt, Sharne
van der Watt, Hendrik H.
van Rooyen, Marthinus B.

BOW ISLAND

Aniagu, Charles A.
Edwards, Lynn, FamilyMed
Woodruff, Jerry L.

BOYLE

Doman, Marthinus H.
Fourie, Jan G.

BRAGG CREEK

Bouman, Helen L A., FamilyMed
Cameron, Paul E.
Cunning, Leslie R., FamilyMed
McGuire, Jennifer J., FamilyMed
Sargent, Kimberley D., FamilyMed
Wiesenberg-Smith, Sara E., FamilyMed

BRETON

Girard, Procter R M.

BROOKS

Ally, Muhammad S C.
Botting, Catherine E., FamilyMed
Coetzee, Maarten J.
De Wet, Johann, FamilyMed
Elgersma, Vincent V., FamilyMed
Folton, Kenneth L.
Fouche, Nanette
Grobbelaar, Jacobus P D.
Hancke, Petrus
Hendriks, Johannes
Kits, Douwe
Meyer, George R.
Moolman, Johannes Z.
Muller, Thian
Prozesky, Benjamin V M.
Snyman, Gertie P.
Thomson, Mari-Lynn
van der Linde, Erich P., FamilyMed

CALGARY

Abdel-Hafez, Mohammed S., FamilyMed
Abidi, Shuayb M., FamilyMed
Abolarin, Mofoluwaso A., FamilyMed
Abukhadir, Sofian
Acharya, Anish P., FamilyMed
Achtymichuk, Audrey, FamilyMed
Adams, Brendan D., FamilyMed
Adams, Hilary, FamilyMed
Adatia, Sadruddin, FamilyMed
Addleman, Benjamin, FamilyMed
Adeagbo, Bamidele A.
Adebayo, Ayodele L.
Adekeye, Olufemi A., FamilyMed
Adib Azad, Hamid, FamilyMed
Adriano, Alvin, FamilyMed
Aggarwal, Jagan N.
Aghajafari, Fariba, FamilyMed
Agoha, Victor K., FamilyMed
Agwaze, Agatha E.
Ahamed, Zahra S., FamilyMed
Akanayeva, Alnura
Al-Awad, Essa H.
Alabaster, Charlotte, FamilyMed
Aladi, Flora O.
Albayram, Mehmet S.
Albuquerque, Sandra, FamilyMed
Aldridge, Leonard L.
Ali, Alaa H.
Ali, Fadhil S., FamilyMed
Ali, Karima M., FamilyMed
Alikhani, Katayoun
Alizadeh-Khiavi, Kamel, FamilyMed
Alladina, Salima J A., FamilyMed(EM)
Allaire, Sandra L.
Alonso, Wilfred J., FamilyMed
Amendy, Ulrich
Amin, Zahir S., FamilyMed
Amrolia, Dinyar H.
Anders, Karl H.
Anderson, D. Richard
Anderson, Daphne L., FamilyMed(EM)
Anderson, Keith J.
Andersson, Paul O., FamilyMed
Anderton, Adrian G.
Anker, Chad H., FamilyMed
Annandale, Francois C., FamilyMed
Arbillaga, Hector O.
Arcega, Rossana V., FamilyMed
Armson, Heather A., FamilyMed
Armstrong, Ian G., FamilyMed
Arthur, Simon G., FamilyMed
Asher, Ayesha, FamilyMed
Asif, Nusrat, FamilyMed
Askin, W. Joseph, FamilyMed
Aspe Ayer, Diana M., FamilyMed
Auclair, Nathalie, FamilyMed
Aucoin, Michael W., FamilyMed
Audet, Lyne, FamilyMed
Aufricht, Margaret L P., FamilyMed
Aul, Madhurima, FamilyMed
Auld, Ian J.
Auld, Lindsay K., FamilyMed
Awan, Tariq M., FamilyMed
Awosika, Ebi
Awosika, Olukayode O.
Ayad, Hani I.
Ayers, Christopher N., FamilyMed
Aytour, Ibrahim M.
Babins, Eric M., FamilyMed
Backlin, Samuel A., FamilyMed(EM)
Badenhorst, Bartholomeus L., FamilyMed
Badenhorst, Este
Badenhorst, Karen A., FamilyMed
Badenhorst, Stefanus M.
Badhesha, Jagdeep S., FamilyMed
Bahlis, Nizar J.
Bain, Caroline E C., FamilyMed
Bajwa, Sameena A., FamilyMed
Baker, Katarzyna, FamilyMed
Baker, Laurie-Ann, FamilyMed(EM)
Bakshi, Darshan R.
Ballantine, Jane E.
Balzun, Margaret A., FamilyMed
Banage, Christine L N.
Bansal, Deepak
Barg, Stefani S N., FamilyMed
Barlow, Karen M.
Barnard, Corlia E.
Barr, George W., FamilyMed
Barrow, John L., FamilyMed
Barsky, Jacob B., FamilyMed(EM)
Bartha, Lillian J.
Basati, Raghmeet, FamilyMed
Basinger, Marilyn R., FamilyMed
Baskin, Leland B.
Bassi, Amrik S.
Bates, Sarah L., FamilyMed
Baxter, Heather A., FamilyMed
Beach, Scott F., FamilyMed
Beairsto, Susan E., FamilyMed
Bedi, Jasbir S.
Beecroft, Pearl R.
Beeharry, Deegrasjsing S.
Beeharry, Emmattee R.
Beerens, Madelain
Behie, Andrea, FamilyMed
Bekhit, Emil T., FamilyMed
Belenky, Michael
Bell, B. Curtis, FamilyMed
Bell, Kathleen E.
Bell, Stephen J., FamilyMed
Bello-Espinosa, Luis E.
Ben Milud Jalutha, Bashir
Benedictson, Michele S.
Bennion, Laura, FamilyMed
Bensler, Ernest C.
Bensler, Evan A., FamilyMed
Benson, Brian W., FamilyMed
Berg, Cindy L., FamilyMed
Bergh, Anton E.
Bergman, June S., FamilyMed
Berlin, Randall J., FamilyMed
Bernbaum, Stanley, FamilyMed(EM)
Bertsch, Kristine L., FamilyMed
Bester, Johan C.
Bethune, Donald J., FamilyMed(EM)
Bezuidenhout, Leon M.
Bhandal, Samarjeet K.
Bhanwath, Gokul
Bhardwaj, Rajan, FamilyMed
Bhatla, Sanjeev, FamilyMed
Bhullar, Gurdit S.
Biala, Soliman E A.
Billinghurst, Katherine A., FamilyMed
Binsted, Anthony H.
Bismar, Tarek A.
Bissoondath, Rohan S., FamilyMed
Blakely, Reta M., FamilyMed
Bland, Elaine, FamilyMed
Blench, Tanis A.
Bockmuehl, P. Christoph, FamilyMed
Bogle, Lee B., FamilyMed
Bohorquez Cardenas, Diogenes A.
Boissoneau, Mary-Lee
Bolduc, Richard D., FamilyMed
Borghesan, Penelope J., FamilyMed
Bornemisza, Susan A., FamilyMed
Boser, Stacey R., FamilyMed
Boswell, Valerie L.
Botha, Daniel J N.
Botha, Maria M.
Botha, Vincenzo
Bouchard, Thomas P., FamilyMed
Bowen, Steven E., FamilyMed
Bowman, Denise M., FamilyMed
Boyar, M. Avis, FamilyMed
Boyd, Brian K.
Boyko, Mark J., FamilyMed(EM)
Bozdech, Lumir
Bradley, John S., FamilyMed
Brake, Heather L., FamilyMed(EM)
Brandon, Jennifer E., FamilyMed
Brandon, Teresa E., FamilyMed
Brar, Anmol
Brar, Avneet S., FamilyMed
Brar, Darshan S.
Braun, Theodore C., FamilyMed
Breton, Martin A M., FamilyMed
Brett, Kelly R.
Brewerton, Conway N.
Broniewski, Michal
Brooks-Lim, Elizabeth W L.
Brown, Elwyn J., FamilyMed
Brown, Meagan L., FamilyMed

Bryden, Patricia A M.
Brydon, Marni E., FamilyMed
Brzeski, Jerzy T.
Buchhalter, Jeffrey R.
Burke, Judith L., FamilyMed
Burke, Peggy
Burn, Robert A F., FamilyMed
Caine, J. Douglas, FamilyMed
Cairncross, Sarah W., FamilyMed
Calder, Tammy R., FamilyMed
Cameron, Jane L.
Campbell, Deanna L., FamilyMed
Campbell, Malcolm S.
Campbell, Pamela C., FamilyMed
Campbell, Patricia M.
Campbell, William G., FamilyMed
Carey, Colleen M., FamilyMed(EM)
Caro Galvis, Luisa F.
Carter, John R H., FamilyMed
Carter, Julia H G., FamilyMed
Carter, Kerryn J.
Casey, Robin E.
Cebuliak, David N A., FamilyMed(EM)
Cedeno Rojas, Mary Y., FamilyMed
Celis, M. Lourdes M., FamilyMed
Cerny, Kristina G., FamilyMed
Chacko, Sunita, FamilyMed
Chad, Anthony F., FamilyMed(EM)
Chan, Danial L A.
Chan, Jonathan S., FamilyMed(EM)
Chan, Leslie F., FamilyMed
Chan, Trevor H., FamilyMed
Chan, Zoe, FamilyMed
Chandler, Colin R.
Chandler, Vania J J., FamilyMed
Chang, B. Wayne, FamilyMed
Chapman, Allison G., FamilyMed
Chappell, Nicola R., FamilyMed
Charbonneau, Shannon, FamilyMed
Chau, Jaime K., FamilyMed
Chau, Peter H W.
Chaudhary, Mihaela, FamilyMed
Chaudhry, M. Ahsan R.
Cheema, Navbir K., FamilyMed
Chen, Julie L., FamilyMed
Chengalath, Premkumar
Cheung, Candy M W., FamilyMed
Cheung, Chung-Ling, FamilyMed
Chew, Julian I H., FamilyMed
Chia, Shirline S L., FamilyMed
Chin, Andy S W., FamilyMed
Chin, Kwanling
Chiu, Anthony S K., FamilyMed
Cho, Helen Y H., FamilyMed
Cho, Jane, FamilyMed
Choi, Karen E., FamilyMed
Choluj, Agnieszka, FamilyMed
Chow, Pan Chun, FamilyMed
Chrisohou, Ramona G., FamilyMed
Christie, Michael L., FamilyMed
Chu, Catherine S., FamilyMed
Chu, Joyce C., FamilyMed
Chu, Monica M H., FamilyMed
Chuah, S L. Joanna, FamilyMed
Chuang, Ryan
Churcher, Margaret A., FamilyMed
Claasen, Izak E.
Clain, Sheryl A., FamilyMed
Clark, Jodie A.
Clark, Steven M., FamilyMed(EM)
Clarke, Ian M C.
Clemett, Dawn M., FamilyMed
Coakley, Annalee, FamilyMed
Coddington, Douglas A.
Cody, Kenneth D., FamilyMed
Coffey, Lisa A H., FamilyMed
Cohen, Robert I., FamilyMed
Cole, Dale L., FamilyMed
Cole, Robert D., FamilyMed
Colegrave, Craig E.
Collett, F. Dean
Collett, James D., FamilyMed(EM)
Collins, Neil D., FamilyMed(EM)
Conly, Carly A., FamilyMed
Connelly, Michael S.
Connick, Patricia L., FamilyMed
Conradie, Marius
Cooke, Breda
Cooper, Stephen C.
Coppola, Giovanni E., FamilyMed
Corcoran, Erin L.
Coulter, Lesley A., FamilyMed
Courtney, Keith
Courvoisier-Grzywacz, Ewa B., FamilyMed(EM)
Cowie, Robert L.
Craddock, Marcy L., FamilyMed
Cran, Timothy S., FamilyMed
Croft, Lorraine S., FamilyMed
Crouse, Pierre D.
Crowshoe, Lynden F J., FamilyMed
Crutcher, Rodney A., FamilyMed(EM)
Cullingham, Andrea F L., FamilyMed
Cully, Gregory P.
Culos, Donald A., FamilyMed(EM)
Cunes, Jill, FamilyMed
Cunningham, Diana M., FamilyMed
Cunningham, Frank N.
Curtis, Glenn H., FamilyMed
Cutbill, John W., FamilyMed
Da Silva, Stefan G., FamilyMed(EM)
Dahlke, Rita M., FamilyMed
Daniel, Antia O., FamilyMed
Dargie, Robin L., FamilyMed
Darragh, E. Anne, FamilyMed
Darwish, Nidal, FamilyMed
Das, Jiban
Daud, Aamir
Dave, Kanta B.
David, Oliver A.
David, Saloma
Davids, Peter, FamilyMed(EM)
Davies, J. Bradley, FamilyMed
Davies, Martin E., FamilyMed
Davies, Stacy J., FamilyMed
Davis, Melinda
Davis, Paul T.
Davison, Michael J., FamilyMed
Davitt, K. Patrick
Dawes, Simon N., FamilyMed
Dawodu, Omotayo, FamilyMed(EM)
Dawson, Janet E., FamilyMed
de Bruin, Nathalia H M.
De Bruyn, Jeremy, FamilyMed
De Bruyn, Johan H., FamilyMed
De Bruyn, Maria E., FamilyMed
De Fina, Rachel A., FamilyMed
De Robles, Paula A.
De Sanctis, Olga J.
Del Castilho, Colin, FamilyMed(EM)
Demong, Paige M., FamilyMed
Denesuk, Allison, FamilyMed
Derakhshan, Mina, FamilyMed
Dettman, Leah, FamilyMed
Devi, Vimla
Deyholos, Michelle
Dhaliwal, Harinder S.
Dhanji, Sadrudin, FamilyMed
Dharmawardene, Marisa L., FamilyMed
Dhillon, Arunbir
Dhillon, Rajvir, FamilyMed
Dhillon, Ramninder, FamilyMed
Di Palma, Remo A P.
Dickinson, James A., FamilyMed
Dickson, Robert, FamilyMed
Dike, Nwamara
Dischinger, Heidi
Dixon, Susan, FamilyMed
Dobereiner, Elisabeth F A.
Docksteader, Mark J., FamilyMed
Docrat, A. Rashid, FamilyMed
Doherty, Olanrewaju J., FamilyMed
Dong, Dennis N.
Dong, Jay, FamilyMed(EM)
Dorjee, Tsering
Dottridge, Andrew H., FamilyMed(EM)
Dougherty, Stephen H., FamilyMed
Downes, Heather F., FamilyMed
Downie, Elizabeth J., FamilyMed
Drever, Clint, FamilyMed(EM)
Drybrough, Marjolein C., FamilyMed
Du Plessis, Lienki
Du Plessis, Stephan J.
Dubey, Santosh
Dufresne, Geneil, FamilyMed
Duggan, Keltie, FamilyMed
Dundas, Caroline-Ann C., FamilyMed
Dundas, Kathryn J E.
Dunham, Peter B.
Dunn, Charlene R., FamilyMed
Dutton, Patricia M., FamilyMed
Dvorakova, Marie
Dyason, Claire G., FamilyMed
Dyck, David F., FamilyMed(EM)
Eddy, Andrew, FamilyMed
Edwards, John G., FamilyMed
Eek, Judy D., FamilyMed
Eesa, Muneer
Eisner, James R., FamilyMed
Ejaz, Naila
Eksteen, Johannes A.
Eley, Judy M.
Elford, Dwayne R., FamilyMed
Elia, Bashar J.
Eliason, Darrel G.
Eliason, Heather L., FamilyMed
Elkabir, Nabil
Ellestad, Leslie I., FamilyMed
Ellis, Connie L., FamilyMed
Eloff, Arnolda G.
Elumir, Lizette L M., FamilyMed
Elzinga, Christine L., FamilyMed
Emery, William A.
Engelbrecht, William M.
Enns, Echo-Marie E., FamilyMed
Erasmus, Elizabeth A., FamilyMed
Ersh, Gita, FamilyMed
Erum, Uzma
Evans, Kenneth W., FamilyMed
Evans, Laura D., FamilyMed
Evans, Mark, FamilyMed
Evans, Sarah, FamilyMed
Ewa, I. Vivian, FamilyMed
Ewasechko, M. Gail, FamilyMed
Ezaydi, Murad A., FamilyMed
Fadayomi, Victor T., FamilyMed
Faisal, Uzma, FamilyMed
Fajardo, Carlos
Falk, David W., FamilyMed
Falkenberg-Andersen, Chris, FamilyMed
Falodun, Oladeji, FamilyMed
Farhat, Mohamed J K.
Farquharson, Scott, FamilyMed(EM)
Faul, John H., FamilyMed
Fauteux, Jasmin, FamilyMed(EM)
Fazhulla, Shabeena, FamilyMed
Fedwick, Jason, FamilyMed(EM)
Fegler, John G.
Fell, Heidi E., FamilyMed
Feng, Xiaolan
Ferguson, Deborah A., FamilyMed
Fernandes, John L., FamilyMed
Ferrao, Matthew J J.
Ferraz, Jose G P.
Ferri De Barros, Fabio
Feturi, Elaref S.
Ficek, Henrietta
Filyk, Zoe, FamilyMed
Fincati, Maria
Findlay, C. Edward, FamilyMed
Finke, Stefan, FamilyMed
Finvers, Kimberley A., FamilyMed
Fitzgerald, Gregory J.
Fleck, David L.
Fletcher, Christine G.
Flynn, Ethan
Fodil-Cherif, Yamina
Fong, Justine H S., FamilyMed
Fong, Linda D., FamilyMed
Forsyth, Scott C., FamilyMed
Foss, Sandra E., FamilyMed
Fothergill, Marnie, FamilyMed
Fowler, William C.
Foyle, Catharine, FamilyMed
Frangou, Panayiotis E., FamilyMed
Freeman, Adele T.
Fridhandler, Indira, FamilyMed
Friedland, Lisa B., FamilyMed
Friesen, Johan R., FamilyMed
Frizzell, J B. Haldane
Fu, Stanley, FamilyMed
Fung, Thomas K H., FamilyMed
Fyhn, Melissa A., FamilyMed
Galloway, Lyle D., FamilyMed
Gamble, Mardelle H., FamilyMed
Garber, Susan E., FamilyMed
Garlich, Fiona M.
Garnett, Ronald T., FamilyMed(EM)
Gash, Todd G.
Gawlinski, Mary J., FamilyMed
Genge, Leah M., FamilyMed
Geoghegan, Michael A.
Geonzon, Radzfel A., FamilyMed
Geonzon, Rose Marie E., FamilyMed
George, Mini, FamilyMed
Gerard, Marisa A., FamilyMed(EM)
Geremia, Brian
Gerull, Brenda
Getting, Philip R.
Ghobrial, Mohab, FamilyMed
Ghossi-Maragheh, Nazanine, FamilyMed
Gibson, Christine L., FamilyMed
Gierl, Paul
Gilad, Elyahu E.
Gill, David A.
Gillespie, John D N.
Gillies, Liesel, FamilyMed
Gillis, Judith L.
Gingrich, Emerson, FamilyMed
Ginzer, Matthew E., FamilyMed
Girard, Isabelle M.
Girgenti, Kaylene M., FamilyMed
Gladman, Donald J.
Gladman, Paul D., FamilyMed
Glendinning, Karan R.
Glimpel, Perry B., FamilyMed
Glofcheskie, B A. Ron
Glover, Janice A., FamilyMed
Goel, Seema, FamilyMed
Gofton, Jeffery
Gohel, Bhavini
Gohill, Lalji R.
Gohill, Lori B., FamilyMed
Goranson, Sandra L., FamilyMed
Gorrie, Christopher J., FamilyMed
Goswami, Anurag
Gould, Glenn D., FamilyMed
Goyal, Supriya M., FamilyMed
Grabenstetter, Christine L.
Graham, Shelley M., FamilyMed
Grainger, Diana, FamilyMed
Grainger, Mark R.
Gray, Christine E., FamilyMed
Greeff, Leon L.
Green, Francis
Greenfield, Gavin J., FamilyMed(EM)
Greidanus, Margriet, FamilyMed(EM)
Gretton, Adrian R., FamilyMed
Grewal, Damanpreet S., FamilyMed
Grewal, Sarbjit S.
Greyvenstein, Ernst L., FamilyMed
Grisaru, Silviu
Grondin, Louis
Grover, Maya, FamilyMed
Grunberg, Sabetai
Gudeon, Nina
Gui, Xianyong
Guilfoyle, Shoshauna E., FamilyMed
Gupta, Priya
Gurevich, Lev, FamilyMed
Habashy, Suzane F., FamilyMed
Habibi, Hamid R.
Hadley, David L., FamilyMed(EM)
Hafez, Kevin, FamilyMed
Hafiz, Hasan
Haggblad, John S., FamilyMed
Hague, Jayne L A., FamilyMed
Haider, Seemab
Hajela, Raju, FamilyMed
Hakes, Jacqueline J., FamilyMed
Halasa, L. Nicole, FamilyMed
Halasa, M. Christine, FamilyMed
Hall, Matthew, FamilyMed(EM)
Hall, William G., FamilyMed
Halliday, William R S., FamilyMed
Halliwell, Oliver T.
Hames, J. Danelle, FamilyMed
Hamidi, Bijan
Hamilton, Trevor
Han, John, FamilyMed
Hanna, Rania
Hanrahan, Kevin M., FamilyMed(EM)
Hantho, Janet E.
Hardin, Barry E., FamilyMed
Hardt, Barbara J., FamilyMed
Hardy, Christopher D.
Harji, Fayaz G., FamilyMed(EM)
Harper, Robert I., FamilyMed
Harris, Elaine M.
Harris, Eleanor J.
Hart, Michelle
Hartwig, Karen S.
Harvey, Martin C.
Hassan, Shabbir, FamilyMed
Hatcher, Ronagh J., FamilyMed
Hawegi, Tarek H., FamilyMed
Hawkes, Toni P., FamilyMed
Hayer, Kuldip S., FamilyMed
Hayes, Aubrey C.
Healley, William M.
Heard, Patricia M., FamilyMed
Heath, Jennifer
Heaton, Catherine J., FamilyMed
Hecht, Kristian K., FamilyMed(EM)
Hedges, Bruce M.
Heeg, J. Christopher, FamilyMed
Heimbach, Catherine E., FamilyMed
Heldzinger, Derek, FamilyMed
Helleur, Katherine A., FamilyMed
Hellman, Karyn J., FamilyMed
Henegan, Charles P.
Henen, Manal F Y.
Herget, Robert J.
Hessenthaler, Doris M., FamilyMed
Hickie, John P., FamilyMed
Hicks, Heather A.
Hill, Douglas A., FamilyMed
Hiscock, Carrie, FamilyMed(EM)
Hitchcock, Deborah J., FamilyMed
Hla, Nan Htwe
Hnatiuk, Melanie L., FamilyMed
Ho, Chester
Ho, Daniel T.
Hoang, Tina Y H., FamilyMed
Hoffman, Bruce O.
Hoffmann, Renee A.
Hogben, Reed M.
Hong, Julie, FamilyMed
Horan, Vanessa T., FamilyMed
Horton, Joan M., FamilyMed
Horton, Sheryl
Houbi, Yasin, FamilyMed
Howarth, Barbara J., FamilyMed
Hoy, Monica
Hoy, Wayne K F., FamilyMed
Hoyer, Irene
Hoyer, Vaclav R.
Hsu, H. Chia-Hao
Huang, Brian C., FamilyMed
Hudy, Simon M P., FamilyMed
Hughes, Jennifer G., FamilyMed(EM)
Hughes, Shannon M., FamilyMed(EM)
Huhn, Karen M M.
Hui, Creighton, FamilyMed(EM)
Hunter, Graham N.
Hunter, J. Bradley
Hurley, Janette A., FamilyMed
Hussain, Mahjabeen, FamilyMed
Hussan, Naila N.
Hutton, Stewart A., FamilyMed
Hwang, Liana L A., FamilyMed
Hyndman, Lucy T., FamilyMed
Iacucci, Marietta
Iampen, Corrina, FamilyMed
Ilnicki, Teresa M., FamilyMed(EM)
Imoukhuede, Unuigboje
Imran, Ayesha, FamilyMed
Iurasco, Vladislav
Iyer, Natasha, FamilyMed
Jablonski, Theodore J., FamilyMed
Jackson, Wesley D., FamilyMed
Jahns, Krystyna M.
Jain, Evelyn, FamilyMed
Jalil, Rabiya, FamilyMed
James, Mary E., FamilyMed
Jamieson, Peter C., FamilyMed
Jespersen, Bruce W.
Jessa, Shamim
Jim, Jean S., FamilyMed
Joanis, Vincent, FamilyMed(EM)
Johns, Daniel G., FamilyMed
Johns, Katharine L., FamilyMed(EM)
Johnson, Charles F., FamilyMed
Johnson, David W.
Johnson, Kevin N., FamilyMed(EM)
Johnson, Richard R.
Johnson, Steven D W L.
Johnston, Aaron, FamilyMed(EM)
Jones, Lanice K., FamilyMed
Jones, Tera
Jorgensen, Gayleen, FamilyMed
Joseph, Jeffrey T.

Joyce, C. Mark, FamilyMed
Jung, Jacob D., FamilyMed
Jurgens, Dewald
Kabila, Mbongani, FamilyMed
Kaiser, Grant A., FamilyMed
Kalmanovitch, William A., FamilyMed(EM)
Kalsi, Jarnail, FamilyMed
Kam, Cindy L S., FamilyMed
Kamaluddeen, Majeeda S B.
Kamel, Jean-Pierre
Kaminska, Malgorzata E., FamilyMed
Kamran, Abdul Q., FamilyMed
Kanani, Suresh R.
Kandola, Rajdeep R., FamilyMed
Kao, Yolanda M., FamilyMed
Karamdad, Nargis
Karan, Tulika S., FamilyMed
Kareemi, Fauzia K., FamilyMed
Karia, Narendra K.
Karim, Nasim A.
Karmali-Rawji, Shameela S F., FamilyMed
Kassam, Nizar I F., FamilyMed
Kasumu, Yetunde, FamilyMed
Kaur, Balvindar
Kaur, Harmeet
Keashly, Dena, FamilyMed
Keegan, David A., FamilyMed(EM)
Keegan, Philippa A.
Kennedy, Charlene M., FamilyMed
Kennedy, Grant C., FamilyMed(EM)
Kenney, Michael P., FamilyMed(EM)
Kenny, Kathryn
Kers, Albert A.
Kerwin, Stephanie A., FamilyMed
Khan, Ahmar, FamilyMed
Khan, Safeer A.
Khan, Sameena A., FamilyMed
Khan, Syma, FamilyMed(EM)
Khatami Toussi, Mohammad
Khorrami, Katayoun S., FamilyMed
Khosla, Indu
Khosla, Megan A.
Kidd, Monica G., FamilyMed
Kilian, Lu-Inge, FamilyMed
Kim, Brian, FamilyMed
Kim, W. James
Kingston, Susan J., FamilyMed
Kinnie, Brent R., FamilyMed
Kinnie, Susan M., FamilyMed
Kish, Marilyn Y., FamilyMed
Kitwanda, Lawrence H.
Klasa, Marc, FamilyMed
Klassen, Margaret L., FamilyMed
Klassen, Michelle M B.
Klonowski, Paul W.
Knight, B. Joan
Ko, Sang Wook, FamilyMed
Kobel, Martin
Koch, Marcus Werner
Kooiman, Edith D H., FamilyMed
Koonar, Harvir S., FamilyMed(EM)
Korzeniewski, Alexandra
Kozlowska, Marta D., FamilyMed
Kozlowska, Urszula M., FamilyMed
Kozma, Stephanie A C., FamilyMed
Krajbich, Jana, FamilyMed
Krake, Shelley M., FamilyMed(EM)
Krause, Kevin L., FamilyMed(EM)
Kreptul, Dennis W., FamilyMed
Kreutzer, Donovan R A.
Kriel, Wessel J C.
Kroeker, Leanne C M., FamilyMed
Kroetsch, Michael D., FamilyMed
Kropyvnytskyy, Ivan
Kruger, Gita, FamilyMed
Kruger, Jaco, FamilyMed
Krzywicka, Maria H.
Ksienski, Asaph E., FamilyMed
Kubik, Stephanie J M., FamilyMed
Kung, Lina, FamilyMed
Kunneman, Sara F.
Kurian, Susannah
Kurwa, Habib A.
Kutskyy, Orest, FamilyMed
Kuzyk, Cathryn J., FamilyMed
Kyi, Nyunt Nyunt, FamilyMed
Kyle, Pamela J., FamilyMed
Kyle, Sharisse E L., FamilyMed(EM)
La Borde, Heather Y., FamilyMed
LaBrie, Nicole, FamilyMed
Laatsch, A. Keith
Labrecque, Paul A., FamilyMed(EM)
Labrie, Martin J., FamilyMed
Lafay-Cousin, Lucie E.
Lafreniere, Robert W.
Lai, Patrick C W.
Lai, Yew H.
Lakra, Prem P.
Lakra, Roopa K S., FamilyMed
Lalonde, Louise, FamilyMed
Lam, Anthony K S., FamilyMed
Lam, Richard P., FamilyMed
Lam, Sheung-Ying S., FamilyMed
Lambert, Linda A., FamilyMed
Lambert, Lynn A C.
Lambros, George A., FamilyMed
Lamond, Shawna M., FamilyMed
Landero, Jennifer L.
Landy, Cynthia J., FamilyMed
Lane, Carolyn A., FamilyMed
Langlois, Marie-Eve, FamilyMed
Lansing, Barbara E., FamilyMed
Lardner, David R R.
Larsen, Bjorn R., FamilyMed
Larson, Bonnie, FamilyMed
Lasaleta, Moises S.
Lassila, Laura L., FamilyMed
Lategan, Johannes C.
Latman, Irit-Irina, FamilyMed
Lauf, Ulrich S., FamilyMed
Law, Graham R., FamilyMed(EM)
Lawrence, Kim C.
Le, Grace, FamilyMed
Le, Thanh Long
Le Roux, Cindy-Anne
Lea-Makenny, Susan J., FamilyMed
Lebeuf, Christine, FamilyMed
Lee, Aimee W., FamilyMed
Lee, Ann E., FamilyMed
Lee, Clifton R., FamilyMed
Lee, Diana W K., FamilyMed
Lee, Jung Hwa, FamilyMed
Lee, Marilyn
Lee, Michael R., FamilyMed
Lee, Patrick F T., FamilyMed
Lee, Sonya M., FamilyMed
Lefebre, Harry J.
Lefebvre, Charlotte, FamilyMed
Leggett, Alison A., FamilyMed
Lehmann, Carmen, FamilyMed
Leung, Jean-Pierre, FamilyMed
Leung, Kenneth K Y., FamilyMed
Leung, Miriam M L., FamilyMed
Leung, Stephen T Y., FamilyMed
Lewis, Jacqueline E., FamilyMed
Lewis, Valerie K., FamilyMed
Lewis, Victor A.
Li, Xiao Y., FamilyMed
Libin, Michael A., FamilyMed
Lichon, Marek
Liggett, Brian A., FamilyMed
Lightbody, Peter, FamilyMed(EM)
Lim, Ronald T H., FamilyMed
Lind, Daren B., FamilyMed(EM)
Liserani, P. Donna M.
Liu, Edmond K H.
Liu-Tertil, Limin
Livingstone, William D., FamilyMed
Lo, Henry, FamilyMed
Lodha, Abhay K.
Loehr, Jane M., FamilyMed
Loewen, David A J., FamilyMed
Logan, R. Brent
Logsetty, Niraja, FamilyMed
Lombard, Jeane
Long-Innes, Malcolm C.
Lopez, Roehl P F.
Loree, Scott B., FamilyMed
Lota, Shashi
Louie, Donald L.
Louie, William L., FamilyMed
Louw, Andries P., FamilyMed
Love, Nancy E., FamilyMed
Love, Richa P., FamilyMed
Lovo, Lana M., FamilyMed
Luelo, Christine A., FamilyMed
Luft, Wendy A., FamilyMed
Lui, Alwin, FamilyMed
Lumby, Pollie S., FamilyMed
Lun, Victor M Y., FamilyMed
Lundgren, A. Christin, FamilyMed
Luntley, Jeremy B.
Lynch, Anthony
Lysack, Elizabeth J., FamilyMed
Ma, Eileen A., FamilyMed
Mabunda, Nella G.
MacArthur, Angela M.
MacAulay, Christy J., FamilyMed
MacLean, Glenda J., FamilyMed
MacQueen, Allison J., FamilyMed
Macdonald, D. Ross
Madrilejos, Jose C B.
Magerman, Eugene W A.
Magerman, Moira P Z.
Maguire, Nancy S., FamilyMed
Mah, Johnny P., FamilyMed
Mah, Michael K., FamilyMed
Mah, Stephanie G., FamilyMed
Mahlase, Ephraim M.
Mahmood, Nighat, FamilyMed
Mahmud, Ghias U.
Mahomed, Ahmed E.
Mahomed, Malini M.
Majeed, Yasmin T., FamilyMed
Makan, Narendra K., FamilyMed
Malagon Barrera, Maria F., FamilyMed
Malan, Johannes J.
Malcolm, Gordon, FamilyMed
Malhotra, Veronica, FamilyMed
Maliakkal, Rita K., FamilyMed
Malik, Rashid, FamilyMed
Maloka, Nabil, FamilyMed
Malus, Dale A., FamilyMed
Manderson, Robert W.
Mangat, Rupinder K., FamilyMed
Mann, Baljinder, FamilyMed
Manocha, Anoop, FamilyMed(EM)
Mare, Rulene
Marlinga, Jazmin C., FamilyMed
Marr, Hubert K., FamilyMed
Martin, Isabel, FamilyMed
Martin, Tara D., FamilyMed
Masson, Robin K.
Masurkar, Swapna, FamilyMed
Mathur, Harshi, FamilyMed
Matta, Vivian T Y., FamilyMed
Mayer, Stanley P., FamilyMed(EM)
Mayhew, W. James, FamilyMed(EM)
Mayrhofer, Ronald
Mbuyi, Felicien K M.
McAlduff, David E., FamilyMed
McAllister, Elisabeth F A.
McBrien, Kerry, FamilyMed
McCabe, P. Kevin, FamilyMed
McCowan, Conrad W.
McDougall, J. David, FamilyMed
McDougall, Jacqueline Y., FamilyMed
McFarlane, Kari, FamilyMed(EM)
McFee, Ingrid J., FamilyMed
McGinnis, Randall P C., FamilyMed
McIntyre, Rebecca E.
McKenna, Catherine, FamilyMed
McKernan, Corinne G.
McLaughlin, Kevin J.
McLean, Astrid E., FamilyMed
McLean, Lynn E., FamilyMed
McLean, Margot L.
McLean Wiest, Reid M., FamilyMed
McLellan, James L., FamilyMed(EM)
McLeman, Elizabeth R., FamilyMed(EM)
McMurren, Jaime L., FamilyMed
McPhee, Nancy, FamilyMed
McWhirter, Jason R., FamilyMed
Mcluckie, Chantal A.
Meeuwisse, Willem H.
Mehta, Karishma, FamilyMed
Meiring, Peter de Vos
Meldrum, Joan M., FamilyMed
Melenchuk, Ronald S., FamilyMed
Melling, Gordon W.
Meloche, Eryn N., FamilyMed
Menhem, Zoulficar H.
Menon, Bijoy
Mentz, Helena J.
Mercer, Shauna L., FamilyMed
Merchant, Sameena, FamilyMed
Mercuur, Lester G., FamilyMed(EM)
Meshesha, Belayneh
Metelitsa, Yuri L.
Metherell, Leslie S.
Michaiel, Mary F S., FamilyMed
Midgley, Julian P.
Milani, Ali-Reza
Miles, Brendan
Millar, Cassandra B., FamilyMed
Mills, Gerald P., FamilyMed
Milne, Lois A., FamilyMed
Mintsioulis, Stephen J G., FamilyMed
Mir, Asad
Mish, Joanna, FamilyMed
Miskew, Linda D., FamilyMed
Miszkiewicz, Paul, FamilyMed
Mitchell, Cynthia L., FamilyMed
Mitha, Pyarali A.
Mofford, Linda M., FamilyMed(EM)
Mogus, Tally M., FamilyMed
Mohamed, Mahmod S., FamilyMed
Mohammed, Joseph
Moharib, Nabil S., FamilyMed
Monaghan, Elizabeth M., FamilyMed
Monkman, Norman D.
Monroy-Cuadros, Felix M.
Montgomery, Carla M., FamilyMed
Montgomery, Helen F., FamilyMed
Montgomery, Lori S., FamilyMed
Moorhouse-Herx, Leonie, FamilyMed
Moorjani, Vijay
Morales, Hilda A., FamilyMed
Morden, Carla R., FamilyMed
Morgan, Melanie M M., FamilyMed
Morris, Leigh J., FamilyMed(EM)
Morris, Richard D., FamilyMed(EM)
Morrison, Lisa D., FamilyMed
Morse, Christopher R., FamilyMed
Morys, Stephen J., FamilyMed
Moss, Michele A.
Motala, Rasheda, FamilyMed
Muftee, Naqsh, FamilyMed
Mugarab-Samedi, Veronica
Muggli, Jessica B., FamilyMed
Muhammed, Talib
Mukiibi, Herbert K.
Mullin, Stephanie E., FamilyMed
Mulvey, Jamin M.
Munn, Matthew B., FamilyMed(EM)
Muotoh, Ikegwuonu C., FamilyMed
Murfin, Lynne, FamilyMed
Murphy, Lindy, FamilyMed
Murray, Alison J., FamilyMed
Murray, Maureen A., FamilyMed
Murynka, Tania M., FamilyMed
Musah, Christopher A., FamilyMed
Muselius, Brenda H., FamilyMed(EM)
Mushi, Sophia
Myers, Nicholas
Myhre, Douglas L., FamilyMed
Myles, Jeremy D., FamilyMed
Nadori, Attila B., FamilyMed
Nahas, Mirna, FamilyMed
Naidoo, Chitraleka, FamilyMed
Naidoo, Sharmilla, FamilyMed
Nakashima, Brenda, FamilyMed
Nanda, Meenakshi, FamilyMed
Nandi, Dilip K.
Nandi, Jayashri K.
Naqvi, Khadija, FamilyMed
Narang, Kapila
Narendran, Aru Mugavadivel
Narine, Rajkishan K.
Naseer, Muhammad A.
Nasir, Fareeha
Nasser, Ali M., FamilyMed
Natha, Rajivkumar P C.
Natho, Lorraine R., FamilyMed
Naylor, Margaret J., FamilyMed
Neary, Peter A.
Nesbitt, John A.
Neu, S. Randall
Neumann, William C., FamilyMed
Neweduk, Peter M., FamilyMed
Nguyen, Bao Thoai H., FamilyMed
Nguyen, Van Thuy, FamilyMed
Nguyen, Xuandieu T., FamilyMed
Ni, Hongyu
Nichol, Rowland T., FamilyMed
Nickerson, Kenneth R.
Niemczewski, Pawel, FamilyMed
Nixdorff, M. Faith
Nixon, Lara L., FamilyMed
Nkemdirim, Makela E., FamilyMed
Noiles, Mary A., FamilyMed
Noordin, Nadia
Noori Lahroud, Marziyeh
Northcott, Janet E., FamilyMed
Novak, Michele Y L D., FamilyMed
Nowak, Agata M., FamilyMed
Nowak, Peter S., FamilyMed
Nowry, Carolyn E., FamilyMed
Nwachukwu, Izunwanne U.
O'Beirne, Maeve, FamilyMed
O'Connor, Daniel J., FamilyMed(EM)
O'Keefe, Stephen J., FamilyMed
O'Neill, Laura A., FamilyMed
Obianyor, Florence, FamilyMed
Odunze, Salome C., FamilyMed
Ogundipe, Tony B.
Oladoyin, A. Ajike, FamilyMed
Olowu, Sunday
Ooi, Althea L., FamilyMed
Oosman, Farook N.
Orr, Jessica N., FamilyMed
Ortiz Bedoya, Clara L.
Osei-Tutu, Davida, FamilyMed
Osei-Tutu, Kannin, FamilyMed
Oshry, Ronald, FamilyMed
Oyebanji, Olubunmi B., FamilyMed
Oyekanmi, Oyekunle A.
Oyeyemi, Joseph O., FamilyMed
Pabbies, Ashesh K., FamilyMed
Packer, Karen E., FamilyMed
Page, Anne-Marie J.
Palencia Angulo, Joaquin A., FamilyMed
Palmer, Robert D., FamilyMed(EM)
Pandya, Ambrish R.
Panich, Nicole E., FamilyMed
Parker, Nur
Pashniak, Paul A., FamilyMed
Patel, Hasmukh J.
Patel, Jay
Patel, Shantilal M., FamilyMed
Paterson, Alexander H G.
Patient, Steven P.
Patton, Marie B., FamilyMed
Paul, Ashalatha
Pawlik, Sara K., FamilyMed
Payne, Rodney A.
Peacock, Sandra C., FamilyMed
Pearce, Paula A.
Pearson, Dawn M.
Pecharsky, Larry J.
Pedersen, Brian A., FamilyMed
Peiravi, Haleh, FamilyMed
Pelletier, Jerry F., FamilyMed
Peniston, Neil T.
Penkman, Michael A., FamilyMed
Penner, E. Roseanne, FamilyMed
Penner, Lisa F., FamilyMed
Penney, Vicki J., FamilyMed
Pentelichuk, Tanya K., FamilyMed
Pepple, Kudirat F.
Perdomo, Jose R.
Pereira, John X., FamilyMed
Pereles, Lauretta R., FamilyMed
Perry, Rebecca J.
Peterson, Todd M., FamilyMed(EM)
Pezarro, Christine E., FamilyMed
Pfeiffer, Shannon L., FamilyMed
Phillips, Vandana A., FamilyMed
Pickering, Tara L., FamilyMed
Pienaar, Sonja, FamilyMed
Pineda-Selva, C. Ernesto
Pinilla, James F E.
Pitout, Johann D D.
Pivnick, Jeffrey S., FamilyMed
Place, Rodney C., FamilyMed
Poirier, Carmen M., FamilyMed
Poon, John C P., FamilyMed
Poon, Susan F L., FamilyMed
Poothencheri, Sreeja N., FamilyMed
Popov, Serghei
Popovic, Ilija
Popowich, Kenneth R., FamilyMed
Popsor, Emilia
Posadas Calleja, Juan G.
Potts, Lana R., FamilyMed
Pour-Ahmadi, Omid
Pow, David G., FamilyMed
Pow, Randall F.
Powell, Colin
Prediger, Lanette A., FamilyMed(EM)
Preller, Martelle, FamilyMed

Prystajecky, Maria S., FamilyMed(EM)
Przybojewski, Stefan J.
Puddy, Jennifer J., FamilyMed(EM)
Pujara, Bakulesh K P.
Putnam, Debra C., FamilyMed
Quail, Patrick B., FamilyMed
Quartero, Marsha A., FamilyMed
Quinn, Francis R.
Qureshi, A. Quddus, FamilyMed
Qureshi, Sameer
Qureshi, Ziaur-Rehman T., FamilyMed
Rabie, Christiaan S.
Rader, Jeffrey J., FamilyMed
Radinskaia, Dina, FamilyMed
Raedler, Thomas Joseph
Rafiq, Fizza Z., FamilyMed
Rafiq, Zahid, FamilyMed
Rahman, Muhammad Z.
Rahman, Samina M., FamilyMed
Raissi, Behirokh, FamilyMed
Raj, Sakina, FamilyMed
Rajadurai, Sivaseelan, FamilyMed
Rajan, Feroza
Rajput, Sobia I., FamilyMed
Rakic, Dubravka, FamilyMed
Ramanna, Venita, FamilyMed
Ramji, Zulfikar
Ramsay, Donald R.
Ratti, Jillian M., FamilyMed
Ravani, Pietro
Rawling, Jean M., FamilyMed
Rebus, Christopher D., FamilyMed(EM)
Reddy, M. Rita
Regehr, Sonya M., FamilyMed
Regnault, R. Scott, FamilyMed
Rehill, Anjali, FamilyMed
Remmers, John E.
Renchko, Patrick A., FamilyMed
Rennebohm, Robert M.
Renz, Christine
Retzer, Elisabeth C., FamilyMed(EM)
Reynolds, Janet G G., FamilyMed
Reynolds, Kathleen A., FamilyMed
Rho, Jong Min
Rich, Thomas, FamilyMed(EM)
Richardson, Karyn P., FamilyMed
Rigby, Ross S., FamilyMed
Rizwan, Sara
Roberge, Kerryn L., FamilyMed
Rodriguez-Mateo, Jean, FamilyMed
Rogers, Janet L., FamilyMed
Rohatinsky, Delee M.
Roman, Bassem A W., FamilyMed
Roode, Lourene A., FamilyMed
Roos, Estelle L.
Rose, Stuart C., FamilyMed(EM)
Ross, Laurie M., FamilyMed
Ross, Marilyn J., FamilyMed
Rotzinger, Deborah L., FamilyMed
Russell, James A.
Rychter, Eva J.
Sachdeva, Ashok K., FamilyMed
Sadiq, Shahnaz
Sadler, D. James
Saeed, Ayesha L., FamilyMed
Safran, Jaclyn E., FamilyMed
Sahni, Paramjit P., FamilyMed
Sahota, Gurpreet S., FamilyMed
Sahota, Surjit S.
Saieed, Kamila H., FamilyMed
Salazar, Anastasio
Saleh, Ahmed S M S., FamilyMed(EM)
Saleh, Naji, FamilyMed
Salem, Wesam, FamilyMed
Salmi de Watman, Silvia C.
Sam, Veronica K L., FamilyMed
Samii, Leyla, FamilyMed
Samis, Scott O.
Samuels, Charles H., FamilyMed
Sandhu, Parminder K., FamilyMed
Santana Mendez, Sergio
Sargious, Monica M., FamilyMed
Savard, Gabrielle K., FamilyMed
Savoia, Katherine M., FamilyMed
Sawa, Russell J., FamilyMed
Sawatsky, Katrina A., FamilyMed
Sayeed, Asma, FamilyMed
Scantlebury, Morris H.
Schinstine, Malcolm
Schmeling, Heinrike
Schneider, Prism
Schnell, Frank N., FamilyMed(EM)
Schwartz, Owen D.
Scotland, Catherine M., FamilyMed
Scott, Mark A., FamilyMed(EM)
Scott, Sheila G., FamilyMed
Scurfield, Barbara J., FamilyMed
Searles, Lynne E., FamilyMed
Sefcik, T. Wayne
Segedi, Therese T N.
Seigel, Karen J., FamilyMed
Semaka, Frank D., FamilyMed
Semaka, Shirley D., FamilyMed
Sengar, Sarit K.
Seow, Cynthia H.
Sethi, Asha D.
Seto, Mei Fun
Seufert, Andrea C., FamilyMed
Shahbaz, Muhammad, FamilyMed
Shaker, Shameem
Shamanna, Dilip K., FamilyMed
Sharif, Jibran, FamilyMed(EM)
Sharkey, Skye, FamilyMed
Sharma, Rajeev D., FamilyMed
Shaw, Diane E.
Shemilt, Ann Marie, FamilyMed
Shergill, Amarpreet S., FamilyMed
Shergill, Amninder K., FamilyMed
Shillington, John R., FamilyMed
Shivji, Farzana, FamilyMed
Shovkivska, Iryna
Shyleyko, Romuald J.
Shymchyk, Michael
Siauw, Christina L Y., FamilyMed
Siddique, Yaseen
Silvester, Lois E., FamilyMed
Simmons, Kyra E.
Simmons, T. Britt, FamilyMed
Simpson, Margaret I., FamilyMed
Sin Yan Too, Natalie M., FamilyMed
Singh, Harjot K.
Singh, Paramvinder, FamilyMed
Singh Aujla, Kanwerjit, FamilyMed
Sinha, Dave R., FamilyMed
Sinnarajah, Aynharan, FamilyMed
Sirianni, Faye E., FamilyMed
Sit, Grace K., FamilyMed
Siu, May P., FamilyMed
Sivakumar, Chandrasekaran
Skinner, Gregory J., FamilyMed
Skovsbo, Vivian, FamilyMed
Skrukwa, Monica J., FamilyMed
Skulsky, Marina R., FamilyMed
Slaba, Ingrid
Slemko, Scott F., FamilyMed
Slipp, Shanda B., FamilyMed
Slocombe, Linda M.
Sloper, Kirsty R., FamilyMed
Smeltzer, Wendy L., FamilyMed
Smit, Mudi, FamilyMed
Smith, Garth W., FamilyMed(EM)
Smuts, Elvira T.
Smyth, Barbara J., FamilyMed
Soin, Jasminder P., FamilyMed
Solomon, Muriel G., FamilyMed
Sood, Brijendra
Soolsma, Serge J., FamilyMed
Soriano Grondin, Jeannette
Sosnowski, Mark K., FamilyMed
Soumbasis, Elias, FamilyMed
Spady, Michael J., FamilyMed
Spanswick, Christopher C.
Sparkes, David M.
Spence, Brian J., FamilyMed
Spence, Norma L., FamilyMed
Sproule, Julie S.
Squires, Edward M.
Stanhope, Alan L.
Stanich, Warren R.
Staniland, Terri L., FamilyMed
Stapon, Elaine S.
Stassen, Kobus C., FamilyMed(EM)
Stefanek, Wendy L., FamilyMed
Steiger, Roberta A., FamilyMed
Steinhauer, Elizabeth L.
Steininger, Jodi L., FamilyMed
Stelmaschuk, Myron E., FamilyMed
Stevenson, C. Marie
Stevenson, Lisa M., FamilyMed
Stewart, Brian D., FamilyMed(EM)
Stewart, Bruce G., FamilyMed
Stinton, Donald A K., FamilyMed
Stojanovic, Mileva, FamilyMed
Stokes, Shelley M., FamilyMed
Storek, Jan
Storr, Martin A.
Strauss, Frederik J.
Strauss, Jacoba C.
Straza, Lorne D., FamilyMed
Strother, Douglas
Strother, Ralph T., FamilyMed
Stuchly, Joanna Z.
Sturgeon, Mary-Ellen
Stys, Anna M., FamilyMed
Su, Michael C T., FamilyMed(EM)
Suazo Hidalgo, Lina M., FamilyMed
Subramanian, Aravind
Sun, Yi-Hui, FamilyMed
Sung, Deborah H., FamilyMed
Sunkara, Madhava R.
Surani, Karim S., FamilyMed
Suresh, Hemalatha, FamilyMed
Suresh, Mulluvila R K.
Suri, Reena, FamilyMed
Sutton, Susan K., FamilyMed
Swart, Vandeurs
Swirsky, Jacqueline E., FamilyMed
Sy, Magdalena G.
Syeda, Naheed G.
Syrnyk, Jeffrey A., FamilyMed
Szabo, S C. Mary, FamilyMed(EM)
Szabo, Thomas F., FamilyMed(EM)
Sztuczka, Waldemar J.
Sztukowski, Teresa M., FamilyMed
Tackaberry, Kelly M J., FamilyMed
Tadros, Ayman E., FamilyMed
Tagliabue, Giovanni
Tam, Christopher W M., FamilyMed
Tam, Thomas T M., FamilyMed
Tan, Siew-Wan, FamilyMed
Tancon, Scott M A., FamilyMed(EM)
Tanjour, Mazen
Tappay, Joel K., FamilyMed
Tarazona Ramirez, Angela M., FamilyMed
Taub, Dina S., FamilyMed
Taylor, Ardythe E., FamilyMed
Taylor, Heather L., FamilyMed
Teman, Carolin J.
Teman, Paul T.
Teschke, M. Jill
Thakkar, Elizabeth
Thakrar, Mansukhlal L.
Thakur, Nathan, FamilyMed
Thomas, Roger E., FamilyMed
Thompson, Agnes J.
Thompson, Melanie L., FamilyMed
Thompson, Pamela J., FamilyMed
Thomson, Julie J., FamilyMed
Thorne, James D., FamilyMed
Thornton, Peter N., FamilyMed
Thorson, J. Douglas
Thull-Freedman, Jennifer D.
Tillim, Jeremy D., FamilyMed(EM)
Tink, Wendy L H., FamilyMed
Tkalych, Paul J.
Todd, David M., FamilyMed
Todd, Leslie A., FamilyMed
Toma, Lily, FamilyMed
Tompkins, Beverly A.
Toor, Gurdev S.
Topham, Darren J., FamilyMed
Topps, David A., FamilyMed
Topps, Maureen H., FamilyMed
Torfason, Lois A.
Torriero, Melissa J., FamilyMed
Toye, Paul L.
Traiforos, Eirene R., FamilyMed(EM)
Tran, Mai Tuyet, FamilyMed
Traynor, Shirley M M.
Treherne, Kerri A D., FamilyMed
Tretiakov, Michael
Trinh, Tony
Trinh, Trevor, FamilyMed
Truong, Barney T H., FamilyMed
Truong, Do Huu
Truong, Kim L L.
Truong, Theresa, FamilyMed
Tse, Helen S., FamilyMed
Tse, Janet L., FamilyMed
Tse, Joanne S.
Tsoi, Michael T., FamilyMed
Tsujikawa, Ronald K.
Tung, Parampal P., FamilyMed
Tupper, Astrid E., FamilyMed
Turner, Caroline A., FamilyMed
Turner, Diana L., FamilyMed
Ubhi, Ram S.
Ubhi, Surinder K., FamilyMed
Ugarte Torres, Alejandra
Ullah, Hidayat
Unarket, Bhikubhai D.
Undseth, Audrey L., FamilyMed
Ung-Datta, Sheila M L., FamilyMed
Unger, Barbara E.
Upadhyay, Rajat, FamilyMed(EM)
Utigard, Dale K., FamilyMed
Vacy-Lyle, Mark J.
Vaidya, Ann R., FamilyMed
Valdecanas, Georgina G., FamilyMed
Van Arkel, Elsbeth C.
Van Der Merwe, Dirk J.
Van Der Merwe, Johann V.
Van Der Merwe, Phillip W., FamilyMed
Van Der Watt, Gabriel J E.
Van Der Westhuizen, Gerhard
Van Der Westhuizen, Marinus
Van Dyk, Aletta H.
Van Essen, Krista M., FamilyMed
Van Goor, John H.
Van Olm, John M J.
Van Raay, Michelle S., FamilyMed
Van Rooi, Henrietta M., FamilyMed
Van Rooyen, Frederick C.
Van Tonder, Cornelius P.
Van Vuuren, Marius J., FamilyMed
Van Wyk, Mariette
Vant, Thomas E., FamilyMed
Vantanajal, Jimmy S., FamilyMed
Vaughan, Brendan G., FamilyMed
Vaze, Medini, FamilyMed
Venter, Wikus, FamilyMed
Verkley, Elspeth C., FamilyMed
Vettergreen, Frances M., FamilyMed
Vig, Rattanjeet S., FamilyMed
Viljoen, Willem A.
Vipond, Joseph C F., FamilyMed(EM)
Virani, Noordin
Visvanatha, Lakshmi V.
Vitug, Gene A S., FamilyMed
Vo-Tigley, Emilie T., FamilyMed
Von Engelbrechten, Heidi D., FamilyMed
Vu, Trung K., FamilyMed
Wachowich, Donna M., FamilyMed
Wachtler, Oswald F.
Wade, Andrew
Wadhera, Sanjay K., FamilyMed
Wadhwa, Pradeep
Wakefield, J. Scott, FamilyMed
Walji, Shahebina, FamilyMed
Walji, Shiraz A.
Walker, George W.
Walker, Ian W., FamilyMed(EM)
Walls, Lori A., FamilyMed
Walsh, Marie-Jeanne L., FamilyMed
Walsh, Suzanne L., FamilyMed
Wang, Dan-Bing, FamilyMed
Wang, Li, FamilyMed
Wang, Yinong
Ward, Natalie H., FamilyMed
Ward, Richard A., FamilyMed
Warner, Tyson S., FamilyMed
Warness, Richard S S.
Wasylenko, Eric A.
Watkins, Nicola J., FamilyMed
Watman, Silvia C.
Watson, Stephen B., FamilyMed
Watt, Denise A., FamilyMed(EM)
Watt, Natalie A M., FamilyMed
Watty, Margaret R., FamilyMed
Waymouth, Patricia L., FamilyMed
Weber, Therese T H., FamilyMed
Wei, Xingchang
Weir, E. Ruth, FamilyMed
Wertzler, William F., FamilyMed(EM)
Westib, Andreas
Wheeler, Bruce H., FamilyMed
Whitehead, Cheryl L., FamilyMed
Whittaker, Brianne J., FamilyMed
Wickett, Claire F., FamilyMed
Wicklum, Sonja C., FamilyMed
Wiens, Irene, FamilyMed
Wiens, Rebecca J., FamilyMed
Wierzbicki, Agnieszka E.
Wiley, J. Preston, FamilyMed
Wiley, Kate M., FamilyMed
Wilken, Waldemar P., FamilyMed
Wilkinson, Diana J., FamilyMed
Wilkinson, Janet P.
Williams, Kiely, FamilyMed
Williams, N. Ashley
Willmott, Caroline
Wilmot, Kim
Wirasinghe, Manoji S., FamilyMed
Withers, Monique J., FamilyMed
Wolf, Michael T., FamilyMed(EM)
Wong, Alex H C., FamilyMed
Wong, Andrea B., FamilyMed
Wong, Andy V F.
Wong, Dennis K., FamilyMed
Wong, Judy S Y., FamilyMed
Wong, Patrick G W., FamilyMed
Wong, Robert M C., FamilyMed
Wong, Ronald Y T., FamilyMed
Wood, Laura J., FamilyMed
Woodard, Aaron F., FamilyMed
Woolgar, Mary-Jo V., FamilyMed
Wooller, Angela J., FamilyMed
Woolner, Elisabeth
Workun, Shane A., FamilyMed
Worton, Eleanor M.
Wouters, Lilliane S., FamilyMed
Wowk, Cory P., FamilyMed
Wright, Bruce J., FamilyMed
Wright Jr., James R.
Wrigley, Heather L., FamilyMed
Wu, William, FamilyMed
Wycliffe-Jones, Keith, FamilyMed
Xie, Liya
Xin, Aiqun, FamilyMed
Yakout, Nesrin, FamilyMed
Yam, Charles C T., FamilyMed
Yam, Vincy W S., FamilyMed
Yaseen, Salma
Yasin, Saad, FamilyMed
Yau, Annie, FamilyMed
Yee, Diana A., FamilyMed
Yee, Norman, FamilyMed
Yee, Selena L., FamilyMed
Yep, Timothy C., FamilyMed
Yeung, C F. Jeffery, FamilyMed
Yeung, Ernest C H., FamilyMed
Yilmaz, Serdar
Yip, Augustine Y L., FamilyMed
Yoo, Carolyn T., FamilyMed
Young, Kathleen R., FamilyMed
Young, Kelly A.
Young, Maureen A., FamilyMed
Young, Ronald M L., FamilyMed
Yousefi, Mehrnaz, FamilyMed
Yue, Ping
Yuen, Owen L., FamilyMed
Yuen, Richard H.
Yuen, Vincent H.
Yung, Chen Fong
Yusuf, Kamran
Zabrodski, Richard M., FamilyMed(EM)
Zacarias, Nancy S.
Zaid, Akram A A., FamilyMed
Zaidi, Mukarram A.
Zakrzewski, W. Paul, FamilyMed
Zamonsky, Corinne G., FamilyMed
Zapasnik, Marta, FamilyMed
Zapasnik, Romuald
Zhao, Hong Yun
Ziegler, Richard D.
Zlot, Zoe A., FamilyMed(EM)
Zubis, John C.
Zubko, M. Grant
Zulyniak, Holly J., FamilyMed
Zung, Hor-Ven A., FamilyMed
Zuzic, Nancy L., FamilyMed(EM)
Zwanepoel, Helen F.
Zwanepoel, Ruan
Zwiers, Karen G., FamilyMed

CALMAR

Davies, Grant, FamilyMed
Tran-Davies, Nhung, FamilyMed

CAMROSE

Awakan, Babatunde A., FamilyMed
Bick, Lindsay
Bredesen, Leif-Erik
Cook, Dennis J A., FamilyMed
Corrigan, T. Michael
Du Plessis, Magda
El Khatib, Adel A M.
Gori-Nachnani, Maya D.
Groenewald, Ettiene
Hilderman, Ernest D.
Horn, Pieter W.
Iriogbe, Itua G.
Jaroni, Arkadiusz N., FamilyMed
Labbaf, Saeed
Lechelt, David P., FamilyMed(EM)
Letley, Kevyn
McNair, Nora L., FamilyMed
Morrow, Donna M., FamilyMed
Muwanguzi, Stanley K., FamilyMed(EM)
Nichol, Christopher S., FamilyMed
Ninian, Gregory M.
Otto, Johan F.
Peters, Diana M.
Portwig, Georg H.
Sainbhee, Parampreet, FamilyMed
Sainbhee, Tejinder
Singh, Baldev
Slabbert, Willem H.
Smith, Valerie F., FamilyMed
Snyman, Ernst R.
Tober, Gerald P.
Torok-Both, George A., FamilyMed

CANMORE

Acton, Lise-Marie, FamilyMed
Acton, Saskia E., FamilyMed
Amarakone, Inoka D.
Armstrong, N. Jean
Baergen, James G., FamilyMed
Balharry, Richard C.
Barber, Darren C A., FamilyMed
Bicek, Gregory S., FamilyMed(EM)
Bryson, Thomas W.
Constantin, Alina D., FamilyMed
De Caigny-Bicek, Catherine, FamilyMed
Du Plessis, Gert C., FamilyMed(EM)
Duggleby, Gerald E., FamilyMed
Edgar, Patricia A.
Eeles, Ruth
Hawkins, Mark G., FamilyMed
Hendry, James N., FamilyMed(EM)
Hinds, Catharine A., FamilyMed
Kirk, Andrew T.
Kusmirek, Dorothy J., FamilyMed(EM)
Lee, Patricia H., FamilyMed
Lourens, M. Elizabeth, FamilyMed
McLaughlin, Kyle A., FamilyMed(EM)
McPherson, Christa L., FamilyMed
Meronek, Deborah M.
Michalyshyn, John G.
Millard, Matthew J R., FamilyMed(EM)
Mitchell, Joanne E., FamilyMed
Mylrea, Cynthia B., FamilyMed
Nielsen, Devin R., FamilyMed
O'Gorman, Monica M., FamilyMed
Palme, Leif M., FamilyMed
Quinlan, Michael W., FamilyMed
Reed, Andrew R., FamilyMed
Sargent, Randall W., FamilyMed
Sullivan, Peter J., FamilyMed
Thomson, Tracy C., FamilyMed
Westmacott, Clare W M., FamilyMed
Wickham, Michael R., FamilyMed(EM)

CARDSTON

Bester, Daniel J.
Clarke, Lloyd T., FamilyMed
Crawford, Robert B., FamilyMed
Cunningham, Sandy, FamilyMed
Low, D. Brian
Playfair, David R., FamilyMed
Taylor, Kimball J.

CARSTAIRS

Smit, Niel F.

CASTOR

Hanton, David A., FamilyMed
McMillan, James C D.
Wezelman, John

CHESTERMERE

Anozie, Amaraegbulam, FamilyMed
Johnston, K. Ross
Ovakporaye, Moses O I., FamilyMed
Swart, Johan J.
Vermaak, David M.

CLARESHOLM

Al-Yousif, Bahn H H.
Gish, George J., FamilyMed
Jones, Jeffrey K., FamilyMed(EM)
Leishman, Fraser T., FamilyMed
Mitchell, Barry A.
Smith, Scott T., FamilyMed
Stubbs, J. Mark
Yonemori, Peter S.

COALDALE

Baby, Miriam T.
Covert, Earle L.
Geers, Johannes A S M., FamilyMed
Kingston, Robert
Low, Steven L., FamilyMed
Luykenaar, Vincent J.
Meyer, Johannes G., FamilyMed

COCHRANE

Ali, Habeeb T.
Corley, James B.
Corrales, Jennifer, FamilyMed
Cote, Richard V J., FamilyMed(EM)
Foster, Michael J., FamilyMed
Fundytus, Dennis E., FamilyMed
Gill, Andrew J.
Hanlon, William M., FamilyMed
Hayes, Dennis W.
Higgin, Douglas M., FamilyMed(EM)
Howk, Shelley D., FamilyMed
Hucal, Sandie G., FamilyMed
Lahey, Sandra K.
Leonard, Rebecca L., FamilyMed
Lindsay, Shelagh S.
Maharaj, Jaimala
McLaughlin, Robert J C., FamilyMed
Meerholz, Wilhelm A H C.
Nelson, Dwight A.
Nicholson, Katrina M., FamilyMed
O'Neil, David, FamilyMed
Olesen, Sarah A H., FamilyMed
Schoombee, Glenda G D.
Schoombee, Willem
Tomanek, Anna I., FamilyMed
Torrie, Julie C., FamilyMed
Weideman, Tanya

COLD LAKE

Botha, Andre J.
Dekker, Jakob J.
Ellison, Jason J., FamilyMed
Godel, J. Mark, FamilyMed
Gupta, Chander
Heydenrych, Siegfriedt L., FamilyMed
Meyer, Petrus S.
Morrell, Rachel A., FamilyMed
Prinsloo, Yolanda
Richard, Jerry M.
Singh, Nitin K.
Siu, Tung, FamilyMed
Smith, Erin E., FamilyMed
Stander, Joseph M.
Van Der Walt, Petrus J.
van Jaarsveld, Anshia

COLEMAN

Penner, Kristy J., FamilyMed

CONSORT

Eljaoudi, Abdurraouf, FamilyMed
Raath, Abel H., FamilyMed
Usher, Olive E.

CORONATION

McKenzie, Lynne M., FamilyMed
Thompson, Michael A.
Tolmie, Johan, FamilyMed

COWLEY

Anderson, Bruce M.

CROSSFIELD

Collingridge, Robert L., FamilyMed

DARWELL

Plimbley, W. Roger

DAYSLAND

Jansen Van Vuuren, Cornelius
Niemann, Andries J., FamilyMed
Van Veenhuyzen, Eleanor J.

DE WINTON

Gold, Beverly L., FamilyMed
Kendal, Ian K., FamilyMed
Smith, Aidan C.
Watson, Misty A E.

DENWOOD

Gabel, Jesse D., FamilyMed
Noppers, Willem H., FamilyMed
Patterson, Margot
Sheppard, David C R.

DEVON

Amien, Bashrat A.
Cruz de Pazos, Madelaine
Ghali, Kamil, FamilyMed
Kerby, Karmen H., FamilyMed
Khatib, Aisha N., FamilyMed(EM)
Khullar, Chander M.
Khullar, Sarjiwan
Klay, Donna M., FamilyMed
Myles-Ferguson, Joyce M.
Patocka, Eva
Princ, Michal
Sivalingam, Kanchana

DIDSBURY

Adewale, Adesegun A., FamilyMed
Brunner, Karen V.
Jackson, Andrew D.
Playfair, David A.
Smith, Dianne E., FamilyMed
Stoyko, Larry E.
Vervaeck, Colette Y T B.

DRAYTON VALLEY

Ali, Rafaqat
Beacom, Rosalind M.
Bealer, Rodney E.
Belcher, David L.
Botes, Roelof J.
Gigg, Anthony C., FamilyMed
Gossmann, Antoinette
Le Roux, Johannes M.
Peyton, Michael A.
Shoaib, Muhammad
Smith, Alexander J.
Srikisson, Nirupa
Van Der Merwe, Abraham J.
Young, Alan J.

DRUMHELLER

Dayo, Akinkunmi A.
Graham, Robert E.
Khoza, Phumelelo H J.
Kuschke, Johann M.
Maseka, Dereck, FamilyMed
Miller, David D.
Moshood, Ibrahim A., FamilyMed
Nahornick, Boris
Neffgen, Joachim F.
Olfert, Lawrence A., FamilyMed
Poulsen, P. Dorothea, FamilyMed
Racz, Elizabeth M., FamilyMed
Sykes, Glen C.
Tlhape, Daniel R.

EDMONTON

Abbasi, Marjan, FamilyMed
Abdalla, Anwer, FamilyMed
Abdel-Galil, Ramzy, FamilyMed
Abdellatif, Dalia M A., FamilyMed
Abdukadr, Almuez A K.
Abdullah, Ubaidullah
Abesamis, Gregorio R.
Aboelnour, Mustafa S., FamilyMed
Abood, Saifee
Abuderbala, Najat M.
Abufayed, Mohamed A., FamilyMed
Abuhamed, Kusai
Abuhamed, Louai
Abuhelala, Ahmed M.
Adams, Moustafa A A.
Adebayo, Adeleye A M., FamilyMed
Agopsowicz, Barbara H.
Ahmad, Rubeena M., FamilyMed
Ahmadinejad, Saeed, FamilyMed
Ahmed, Ghalib, FamilyMed
Ahmed, Matin A.
Ahmed, Moheddin M B A.
Aitchison, Katherine J.
Ajamian, Faria
Akabutu, John J.
Aklilu, Fasika, FamilyMed(EM)
Akter, Nazma
Al Jahash, Ibrahim M A.
Al-Adra, David P.
Al-Agha, Rany B.
Al-Amodi, Hussein A O.
Al-Izzi, Saif S A L.
Al-Kayssi, Nabil M., FamilyMed
Al-Kurtass, Suhaib
Alaklabi, Mohammed
Alarape, Akadri A.
Alatrash, Akrem K M.
Albrbar, Mohamed J H., FamilyMed
Aldandashi, Samer
Algariani, Tarek G M.
Alhaj Imhmed, Hasan A M.
Ali, Fatima
Ali, Maqsood
Ali, Rizwan
Ali, Samana
Ali, Syed A.
Alima, Limor H., FamilyMed
Alizadehranjbar, Keysun
Aljadi, Alhadi A M., FamilyMed
Allan, G. Michael, FamilyMed
Almaden-Camacho, Emily A., FamilyMed
Alonso, Erik J., FamilyMed(EM)
Alshgagi, Husameddin A.
Altayeb, Samee A.
Altmeyer, Ronald C., FamilyMed
Aman, Ijaz
Amato, Victor, FamilyMed
Ameen, Rukhsana
Amigo, Pablo H.
Anderson, Jarrod R., FamilyMed(EM)
Anderson, Tyler J., FamilyMed(EM)
Andrew, Deborah K., FamilyMed
Andriashek, Diana M.
Andruchow, Marshall F.
Angelova, Jordanka, FamilyMed
Annawi, Hane A., FamilyMed
Ansarian, Mohammad B.
Antoniolli, Lisa, FamilyMed
Antoniuk, Mark J., FamilyMed
Antunes, Marcia O.
Arent, Robin
Ariano, David M., FamilyMed(EM)
Armstrong, Fraser W., FamilyMed
Armstrong, Gavin A.
Armstrong, P. Mark D., FamilyMed
Armstrong, W. Douglas
Arnold, Paul A.
Ashton, Deirdre A.
Askar, Majdi R.
Ateer, Khaled A.
Au, Lillian L C., FamilyMed
Aung, Steven K H.
Ausford, Allen E G., FamilyMed
Aye, Lwin M.
Aziz-Few, Carolyn F.
Baergen, Kathleen G., FamilyMed
Baise, Taryn
Baker, Jane L., FamilyMed
Bakshi, Neeja
Balakrishnan, Leela G.
Bananda Shambu, Sunil
Banerji, Kunal, FamilyMed
Baptista, Luis C.
Barer, Daniel J.
Barnett, Carly A., FamilyMed
Barr, Cameron, FamilyMed
Barrios, Albaro
Barry, Keith R., FamilyMed
Barton, Ronald T.
Baxter, W L. Miranda, FamilyMed
Beaudoin, Angele C.
Becher, Harald H H.
Bector, Neeraj S., FamilyMed
Bedard, Alice M., FamilyMed
Behiels, Stewart J.
Bell, Neil R., FamilyMed
Bell, Peter E., FamilyMed
Bellerose, Sheri A., FamilyMed
Bello, Aminu
Benard, Magali A., FamilyMed
Bennett, Brian R.
Beran, Maud
Berdusco, Edward T M., FamilyMed(EM)
Berendt, Daniel R., FamilyMed
Berg, Angela W Y., FamilyMed
Bergens, Joanne E., FamilyMed
Bernadas, Sue Anne, FamilyMed
Bernier-Lycka, Lucie M., FamilyMed
Bertagnolli-Hansen, Alexa
Bestilny, Allan D.
Bhayat, Qudsiyyah, FamilyMed
Bhimji, Arif M., FamilyMed
Bialczak, Jerzy, FamilyMed
Bidniak, Karen K., FamilyMed
Bilal, Shaukat
Birdi, Ravdeep S., FamilyMed(EM)
Biron, Vincent
Bishop, Brian P.
Bitangcol, John C., FamilyMed(EM)
Blais, Guy R., FamilyMed
Blais, Mark R.
Bleviss, Morley
Bly, Jared D., FamilyMed(EM)
Bodmer, Madeleine
Bokenfohr, Grace M.
Bond, David W.
Borger, Margaret A.
Borkent, Amy J.
Borkent, Herman A., FamilyMed
Borowka, Derek D.
Bowden, Helen G.
Bowland, M. Anne, FamilyMed

Boyko, Boris W., FamilyMed
Bozic, Katarina, FamilyMed
Braam, Geert B.
Bradstock, Robert W., FamilyMed
Brahim, Asad
Brar, Amandeep S., FamilyMed
Brar, Nirmala K.
Braun, Theodore J., FamilyMed(EM)
Bray, Thomas B.
Bremness, Andrew B.
Brenneis, Fraser R., FamilyMed
Briggs, Robert P., FamilyMed
Broniewska, Marta
Brooks, Laurene J., FamilyMed
Brouwer, Grace J., FamilyMed
Brownoff, Rene, FamilyMed
Brox, Dianne E., FamilyMed
Buchholz, Holger W.
Bucholtz, Ann
Bui, Tam Cong
Bulaev, Yury
Bulawka, Craig
Bunn, Steven E.
BurTon-Macleod, Sarah M., FamilyMed
Burchett, Glenn M.
Burchett, Lisa K.
Burling, William W., FamilyMed
Buttenschoen, Klaus
Butzelaar, Joris Y.
Byrne, Kelly P A.
Cadsky, Otakar
Cahill, Gabriel T.
Cameron, James P.
Campbell, Curtis, FamilyMed(EM)
Campbell, Grant K.
Campbell, Susan L.
Campbell, William G.
Campbell-Scherer, Denise L., FamilyMed
Candler, David C.
Canham, Hal B., FamilyMed(EM)
Cardinal, Katharina B., FamilyMed
Carli Buttenschoen, Brigitte D.
Carlson, Christopher G., FamilyMed
Carter, Robert T M., FamilyMed
Castillo Abadia, Maria D.
Caulfield, Joanne H., FamilyMed
Cave, Andrew J., FamilyMed
Cave, Dean B.
Cave, Donna M.
Ceccherini-Nelli, Alfonso
Cembrowski, George S.
Chambers, Steven W.
Chan, Donald R., FamilyMed
Chan, Kitty Y., FamilyMed
Chan, Tiffany S., FamilyMed
Chana, Hari S., FamilyMed
Chandrasenan, Kavitha, FamilyMed
Chang, Alanna M., FamilyMed
Chang, Jason H S., FamilyMed(EM)
Chang, Mui Khoon
Charles, Lesley A., FamilyMed
Charleton, Edmond D.
Chen, Grace Y C.
Chen, Henry J L.
Cheng, Florence J.
Cheng, Judy A.
Cheng, Nancy L., FamilyMed
Cheslock, Carole, FamilyMed
Chetty, Vanessa
Cheung, Garvin L., FamilyMed
Cheung, Joseph Y., FamilyMed
Cheung, Kar Wing, FamilyMed
Cheung, Raymond W., FamilyMed
Chew, Brian P A., FamilyMed
Chiam, Tow-Foon, FamilyMed
Chiang, N M. Sheryl
Chin, Justin
Chisholm, Mary E., FamilyMed
Chiu, Allan Y L.
Chiu, Janet W C.
Chiu, John F S., FamilyMed
Chiu, Paul K.
Chiu, Sy-Hua
Chmelicek, John T., FamilyMed
Cho, Victoria Y W.
Chonko, Douglas M.
Chou, Ming Convir
Chronopoulos, Julia V., FamilyMed
Chrzanowski, Zbigniew P.
Chua, Therese A L.
Chung, Wan M.
Clark, Marc, FamilyMed
Colliton, Irene E.
Connick, Carol D.
Cooney, Judy-Diane, FamilyMed
Corby, Debora J., FamilyMed
Cottier, William A.
Coulden, Richard A R.
Coupland, Nicholas J.
Covenden, Sivalingham
Craig, Janet E., FamilyMed
Craig, Nancy V., FamilyMed
Craven, Michelle D., FamilyMed
Crawley, Cinzia U.
Cromwell, Korwin R., FamilyMed(EM)
Crowther, Sean M.
Cuddihy, Helene L., FamilyMed
Cull, Corine L., FamilyMed
Cunniffe, Aidan M., FamilyMed(EM)
Cunningham, Randolph M., FamilyMed(EM)
Cvetkovic, Igor, FamilyMed(EM)
Danforth, Jay A.
Danial, Amathul A.
Das, Madhavan S.
Dasgupta, Bonnie, FamilyMed
Datta, Suvomoy, FamilyMed(EM)
Davis, Peter V., FamilyMed
Dawson, Wendy L M., FamilyMed
De Kock, Ingrid H.
De Lima, Leslie J.
De Souza, Nilceia L.
Dean, Naeem
Deane, John A.
Delaney, Peter, FamilyMed(EM)
Dempsey, Rose E M.
Dent, Cynthia H., FamilyMed
Deol, Janjeevan S., FamilyMed(EM)
Der, Linda M., FamilyMed
Dhaliwal, Navdeep, FamilyMed
Dhliwayo, Harold K A.
Dhunnoo, Krish
Dieleman, Levinus A.
Dietrich, Jaclyn N., FamilyMed
Dillane, Derek
Dimitry, Raouf
Dinh, Anh T T.
Dinyari, Kourosh
Dlin, Ronald A.
Dobrousin, Anatoly, FamilyMed
Dodd, Roger F.
Donald, Marion, FamilyMed
Donoff, Michel G., FamilyMed
Doran, Shandra A.
Dorsch, Michael F.
Draginda, Anne, FamilyMed
Drouin, Johanne F., FamilyMed
Du Toit, Nadia
Dua, Mini
Duff, Melissa S., FamilyMed
Duia, Sheela, FamilyMed
Dujon, Leighton D., FamilyMed
Duke, Douglas C.
Durand, Lorraine, FamilyMed
Durar, Mahmud
Ebaij, Ali M A., FamilyMed
Edani, Shakibeh A., FamilyMed
Edgecumbe, Boyd M S., FamilyMed(EM)
Eid, Iyad
Ekanem, Aquaeno E.
El Sayed, Jihan M.
El dagni, Mohamed W M M.
El-Fakharany, Fawzia
El-Gouhary, Inas, FamilyMed
El-Hakim, Hamdy G E H.
El-Hawrani, Amged
Eldeiry, Azza
Eledrisi, Fadel
Elforti, Nabil, FamilyMed
Elfourtia, Abdelmunem, FamilyMed
Elghol, Eimad M E., FamilyMed
Elgrigni, Hassan R.
Elhajemhmed, Abdalla
Ellis, Barry J., FamilyMed(EM)
Els, Charl
Elsawiniya, Abdelbaset A.
Elsiddeig, Awatif H E.
Ensenat, Santiago
Escoredo, Sandra I.
Eskharoun, Magdoline
Esmail, Aashif, FamilyMed
Evans, Deborah J., FamilyMed
Faccenda, Kathryne A.
Faily, Joan, FamilyMed
Fainsinger, Robin L., FamilyMed
Fairgrieve-Park, S. Michelle, FamilyMed
Fallis, Shari L., FamilyMed
Fanous, Isis
Farag, Hayam S M.
Farrah, Daniela T., FamilyMed
Fateis, Aimen
Fathalla, Hala H.
Faulder, Douglas G.
Ferdinandis, Talpe G H C.
Ference, Jean L M.
Fernandes, Brian R F.
Fernando, Joseph
Fields, David W., FamilyMed
Fillion, Mariette, FamilyMed
Finzer, Alan
Finzer, John K.
Fiorino, Michael
Flanagan, Sean D.
Flanagan, Thomas F.
Flanagan, Wayne H.
Flath, Travis R., FamilyMed
Flook, Nigel W., FamilyMed
Flynne, Paul R.
Fok, Mei Sum, FamilyMed
Follett, Michael S.
Fong, George Y., FamilyMed
Fonteyne, Douglas C.
Forster, D. Ian M.
Foster, Kevin J., FamilyMed(EM)
Fours, Suliman A A.
Franc-Law, Jeffrey M., FamilyMed(EM)
Francescutti, Louis, FamilyMed
Franke, Amy B., FamilyMed
Frauenstein, Giesela H.
Friesen, Colleen A., FamilyMed
Fung, Gary W T.
Gaas, Masoud Ali
Gainer, Anita L.
Galbraith, Lorri J.
Game, Melaku M.
Garcea, Cristina, FamilyMed(EM)
Garcia Guerra, Gonzalo
Gardener, Kenneth J., FamilyMed
Garros, Daniel
Gawley, Emily, FamilyMed(EM)
Gazala, Sayf
Germain, Carlie, FamilyMed
Gessner, Alessandra
Ghaffari, Mojgan
Ghani, Sayeeda S.
Gheissari, Saeid
Ghitter-Mannes, Sandra
Ghredish, Tareg
Giang, Clarence, FamilyMed
Gilbert, Rebekah
Gill, Anne-Marie, FamilyMed
Gill, Richdeep
Gill, Satvir, FamilyMed
Gillanders, Brian S., FamilyMed
Gingles, Carmen R., FamilyMed
Giuliani, Fabrizio
Goebel, Gary R.
Goez, Rachel H.
Gokul, Adhikar B., FamilyMed
Golbabaei, Mehdi
Goldstuck, Norman D.
Gonzalez-Romero, Luis M.
Gounden, Ranjeeta, FamilyMed
Govender, Bhagwathee
Govender, Sivalingum J.
Grade, A C. Roxane, FamilyMed
Graff, Michael, FamilyMed
Graham, Timothy A D., FamilyMed(EM)
Graham, Tracy-Jean M., FamilyMed
Green, James S E.
Green, Lee
Greenspan, Stanley
Gregg, Randall J.
Gregson, John C., FamilyMed
Grewal, T. Paul S.
Grieve, Catharine D., FamilyMed
Griffith, Philip S.
Grimsrud, Karen
Gritter, Roy A.
Gross, M. Shirley
Gross, Marie M S., FamilyMed
Gross, Zeev Zvi
Grynoch, Roberta E., FamilyMed
Gupta, Vinesh
Gurtu, Rachita, FamilyMed
Gusdal, Jeffrey D., FamilyMed
Gushaty, Leonard N., FamilyMed
Gyenes, Gabor T.
Habib, Syed W.
Haggerty, Mary E.
Hailu, Tesfu
Hajar, Khaled
Halinen, Lea I.
Hall, Jennifer L., FamilyMed
Hamadeh, Mohamad
Hamid, Haroon, FamilyMed
Hamilton, Michael J., FamilyMed
Hamm, Jason S., FamilyMed
Hammerlindl, Donna M A.
Hancock, Michael
Hanelt, Richard R., FamilyMed
Hanna, Basma, FamilyMed
Hanna, Viola
Hans, Narpinder, FamilyMed
Haque, Shelby, FamilyMed(EM)
Haraphongse, Yada, FamilyMed
Hardy, Dean W.
Haroon, Aroosa, FamilyMed
Harris, Kevin J., FamilyMed(EM)
Hartman, Darrell J.
Hartt, Donald J., FamilyMed
Hartt, Marcia R., FamilyMed
Hasal, Simona
Hasan, Bushra F., FamilyMed
Hasan, Khalid H A.
Hasinoff, David A., FamilyMed
Hastings, Donna, FamilyMed
Haubrich, Jay M., FamilyMed
Heisler, Terry L., FamilyMed
Henderson, John E S.
Henning, Slavica
Hetland, Ray K D.
Hiebert, Gayle D.
Hinton, Joan M.
Hirji, Jamil, FamilyMed
Hnydyk, William S.
Ho, Duncan T H., FamilyMed
Hobbs, Sandra E., FamilyMed
Hodlevskyy, Oleksandr
Hogan, Michael S N.
Holmes, Edward S.
Hong, Diana, FamilyMed
Hopkins, Kathleen D.
Hoshizaki, David K.
Hossain, Rana Md Iftekhar
Howard, Raymond
Howard-Tripp, Micheal E., FamilyMed
Hryciuk, Laura E.
Huber, Douglas R., FamilyMed
Huber, Keith D., FamilyMed
Hughes, Sheila L.
Hum, Peter C M., FamilyMed
Humphries, Paul W A., FamilyMed
Huot, Ann, FamilyMed
Hurlburt, Mary E., FamilyMed
Husain, Rafi A.
Hussain, Munawar, FamilyMed
Hussain, Safdar
Hutchison, Susan J.
Huynh, Suong Ngoc
Hyderi, Abbas
Ibrahim, Hisham
Ighema, Mohamed R.
Imlah, Shona M., FamilyMed
Inwood, Matthew J., FamilyMed(EM)
Ip, Hui Yun V.
Irani, Carla A.
Ishrat Ali Khan, Pervez
Ismael, Mahmoud
Ispas, Cristina L.
Izevbaye, Iyare E.
Jabbari-Zadeh, Shahram, FamilyMed
Jackman, Kevin F M.
Jaffray, Fiona K.
Jaglalsingh, L. Harry
Jamal, Kishwar
Janse van Vuuren, Christoffel J.
Jansma, L. Lee-Anne, FamilyMed
Jarema, Andrew J.
Jassar, Balvinder S., FamilyMed
Jassat, Zaheera E.
Jeffery, Glenn J.
Jeh, Jusli P.
Jelani, Anwar D.
Johnston, Andrew G.
Johnston, Colleen G., FamilyMed
Johnston, Joan M., FamilyMed
Jorundson, Edward R.
Joseph, Steven R., FamilyMed
Journi, Amein
Juby, Angela G.
Kaasa, Roderick B., FamilyMed
Kaber, Asem S.
Kaliandasani, Bina
Kalluri, Meena
Kamdar, Lalit K.
Kamitakahara, Holly K., FamilyMed
Kammerer, Hubert, FamilyMed
Karnik, Nachiket S., FamilyMed
Karpman, Shelby N., FamilyMed
Kasavan, Devan S.
Kasha, Katherine A., FamilyMed
Kassiri, Janani
Kasumovic, Janna M., FamilyMed
Kattar, Mireille M.
Kavanagh, Sandra T.
Keeble, William
Kelly, Allan J.
Keough, Gregory G.
Khan, Farhan I A.
Khan, Uzma A Z., FamilyMed
Khanna, Madhur S.
Khder, Jabbar A S.
Khera, A. Sheny, FamilyMed
Khetani, Karim
Khoo, Nee Scze
Khoshkish, Reza
Khosrodad, Nasim, FamilyMed
Kiggundu, Fredrick
Kijewski, Raegan L., FamilyMed
Kiltz, Michael R., FamilyMed
Kim, Lina B., FamilyMed
King, Dolores
Kirkwood, Jessica E M., FamilyMed
Kivi, Paul, FamilyMed
Klajn, Christopher L.
Klein, Douglas J., FamilyMed
Klemka, Philip J.
Kobaisy, Omaima, FamilyMed
Koe, Sandy S K.
Kohler, Andrew J., FamilyMed
Kohler, Anneliese M., FamilyMed
Kolodenko, Yuliya, FamilyMed
Kolotyluk, Timothy D., FamilyMed
Konkin, D. Jill, FamilyMed
Koppula, Sudha, FamilyMed
Korownyk, Christina S., FamilyMed
Korzenowski, Donald W.
Krause, Elizabeth
Kretschmann, Richard J., FamilyMed
Krinke, Valerie, FamilyMed
Kruger, Petrus F.
Kruhlak, Robert T.
Krysa, Clifford J.
Kumar, Amit
Kumar, Manoj
Kumar, Ramneek
Kumaran, Vazhkudai S.
Kumpula, Joseph V., FamilyMed
Kundra, Manu
Kureshi, Jamila
Kutash, Anola L., FamilyMed
Kwan, Peter O.
Kwon, Sabrina
Lakis, Nicolaos
Lal, Moti, FamilyMed
Lalonde, Maryse H., FamilyMed
Lam, Kenneth H M., FamilyMed
Lam, Tong V.
Lamoureux, Robin A J., FamilyMed
Langille, Morgan A.
Langley, Jean E., FamilyMed
Larsen, Carmen H., FamilyMed
Latif, Zahid
Laverty, H K. Kay, FamilyMed
Le, Phuoc-Hai, FamilyMed
Le Melledo, Jean-Michel
Lebrun, Constance M., FamilyMed
Lee, Ann S O., FamilyMed

Lee, Carol, FamilyMed
Lee, Lawrence C H.
Lee, Raymond S Y.
Lee, Stephen
Lee Pong, Noella M I., FamilyMed
Lehmann, Ordan J.
Leon Ardila, Hernando
Leong-Sit, Philip P., FamilyMed
Letwin, Nadine M., FamilyMed
Leung, D. Man-Sun, FamilyMed
Leung, Peter M P.
Levinskyy, Mykhaylo V.
Lewicke, Shannon M., FamilyMed
Leyland, Steven, FamilyMed
Li, Bing, FamilyMed
Li, Judy W S., FamilyMed
Li, Yang
Li, Zhi, FamilyMed
Lilic, Nenad
Lim, Maileen M., FamilyMed
Lindskoog, Ross T.
Linklater, David M., FamilyMed
Liyanaarachchi, Ravini, FamilyMed
Lo, George Y K., FamilyMed
Loeffler, Kimberly N., FamilyMed
Loewen, George
Loewen, Theodore E.
Lohlun, Graham B.
Loiselle, Rhea M., FamilyMed
Long, Brenda M., FamilyMed
Long, Malcolm J., FamilyMed(EM)
Lopaschuk, Catharine C., FamilyMed
Lord, Christopher J., FamilyMed
Lott, Bettina, FamilyMed
Lou, Samuel, FamilyMed
Louie, Karen D., FamilyMed
Lounsbury, David S., FamilyMed
Low, Gavin W Y.
Low, Susan E., FamilyMed
Lowe, Sonya S., FamilyMed
Lucewicz, Michael
Lucyk, Chad M., FamilyMed(EM)
Lucyk, Scott
Lujic-Thebaud, Jelka-Maria
Lukey, Judith G T.
Lung, Gilbert G., FamilyMed(EM)
Luyckx, Valerie
Lyubetska, Valeria, FamilyMed
Ma, Lai Man, FamilyMed
Ma, Warren K.
MacDonald, Anne-Marie H.
MacDonald, Randal J., FamilyMed(EM)
MacGregor, Marguerite A.
MacKenzie, Mark A., FamilyMed(EM)
MacLean, Scott B A., FamilyMed
Maciejewski, Conrad C.
Maciver, Allison H.
Magnan, Michel C E.
Magnus, Kenneth G.
Magsi, Noorullah
Maguire, Anne-Marie D.
Maguire, Thomas
Mah, Nancy E.
Mah, Stanley W., FamilyMed
Mahajan, Sushma, FamilyMed
Maheshwari, Perkash, FamilyMed
Mahmood, Muhammad N.
Makarla, Prakash B.
Makhdoom, Safana A.
Malhotra, Gaurav S., FamilyMed
Mallett, Aaron G.
Mami, Mustafa G A., FamilyMed
Manca, Donna P., FamilyMed
Manchikanti, Srinivasa M., FamilyMed
Maneshgar, Mahnaz, FamilyMed
Manley, W. Arnold
Mannarino, Marco G., FamilyMed
Manouchehri, Namdar
Mansy, Diaa A Y.
Mar, Serena G.
Marburg, Lutz
Marin, Alexandra, FamilyMed
Marner, Paul A T.
Martel, Alison E., FamilyMed
Mason, Andrew L.
Mateo-Rodriguez, Patrocinio C.
Mausolf, Susanne
May, Janice L., FamilyMed
Mazurek, Gordon G., FamilyMed(EM)
Mazurek, Karen A., FamilyMed
McAlpine, Brian D.
McBeath, Kim L., FamilyMed
McCallum, Janis G., FamilyMed
McCallum, Ryan C., FamilyMed
McCarthy, Mairin
McCarty, Douglas M.
McDonald, James
McDonald, Terrence J., FamilyMed
McGaw, W. Timothy
McInroy, Gordon
McLaren, Sherry L.
McNally, Dermot M.
McNeilly, Nancy E.
McPeak, Brian K., FamilyMed
McPhedran, Margaret, FamilyMed
McPherson, Isla L., FamilyMed
Meador, Karine L., FamilyMed
Meghji, Shahbegum A.
Meier, Donald D.
Meier, Kathleen R.
Meleshko, Sarah A., FamilyMed(EM)
Mengel, Michael H.
Mensour, M'Hamed
Mentz, Ricardo A., FamilyMed
Meza-Junco, Judith
Michalska, Elzbieta
Michel, Shawkat S.
Michelakis, Evangelos
Miksa, Ray A., FamilyMed
Millard, Debbie, FamilyMed
Milliken, Douglas R F.
Milne-Epp, Andrea M., FamilyMed
Minion, Daurel
Minnett, Seana K., FamilyMed
Minsos, Jennifer R., FamilyMed
Mirhosseini, Mehrnoush, FamilyMed
Mirza, Aisha, FamilyMed(EM)
Mistry, Aneeta J., FamilyMed(EM)
Mitha, Hamza, FamilyMed
Mittelsteadt, Lyle B.
Miu, Daniela I.
Mkhabela, Sikhumbuzo G.
Mocanu, Adriana, FamilyMed
Modi, Monica, FamilyMed
Modi, Renuca, FamilyMed
Mohamed, Ataher S., FamilyMed
Mohammed, Fateh
Mohler, Jeffrey A.
Mohsen, Yosra M K M.
Mohydeen, Shwan S.
Mok, Gloria M C.
Mokrzanowski, Andrew D.
Mokrzanowski, Elizabeth, FamilyMed
Molberg, Warren R., FamilyMed(EM)
Moledina, Mohamed T A.
Moniuszko, Monika B.
Montano-Loza, Aldo J.
Moores, David G., FamilyMed
Moran, Martin B., FamilyMed
Mori-Torres, Elisea M., FamilyMed
Morley, Ellise C., FamilyMed
Morros, Michelle P., FamilyMed
Mosaico, Francesco, FamilyMed
Moshurchak, Kim M., FamilyMed
Moss, Morton G., FamilyMed(EM)
Mota, Jodi E., FamilyMed
Mouhammed, Samir I., FamilyMed
Mousa Ahmadi, Elaheh
Moussa, Sahar, FamilyMed
Mowat, Gordon
Moyo, Jabulani
Mrochuk, May, FamilyMed(EM)
Mueller, Edrise M.
Mueller, Thomas F.
Muhammad, Mustafa, FamilyMed
Muncner, Amira
Muratoglu, Mikael S.
Murji, Salma B., FamilyMed
Murphy, Katie E., FamilyMed
Murray, Allen R.
Murtha, William J.
Muwais, Osama W., FamilyMed
Muzyka, Raymond A., FamilyMed
Muzyka, William R., FamilyMed
Nafis, Anjum S.
Nahab, Reem
Naib, Ravinder
Naidoo, Oshadhesa, FamilyMed
Naidu, Prenilla
Naidu, Veyantiz J., FamilyMed
Naiker, Randy, FamilyMed
Nair, Govindan K.
Naismith, Angela D., FamilyMed(EM)
Namaruish, Osama A A., FamilyMed
Namusuubo-Kachope, Jane P.
Nankissoor, Basdeo, FamilyMed
Narula, Amarjit S., FamilyMed
Nazir, Talat M.
Neilson, Darren W.
Neilson, Kevin D.
Nelson, Christopher G., FamilyMed
Neuls, Rick A J., FamilyMed
Newman, Stephen C., FamilyMed
Ng, David K K., FamilyMed
Ngan, Michael L M.
Nguyen, De
Nguyen, Lau K., FamilyMed(EM)
Nguyen, Lynda P., FamilyMed
Nichols, Darren N., FamilyMed(EM)
Nickerson, Leigh, FamilyMed
Nishiwaki, Maya, FamilyMed
Nizam, Mahmood J., FamilyMed
Noga, Tom
Nordli, Tania C., FamilyMed
Nulliah, Shirdi, FamilyMed
O'Brien, Kristina G., FamilyMed(EM)
O'Callaghan, Kieran P.
Obeidat, Motaz A.
Obst, Jennifer M., FamilyMed
Odugbemi, O. David, FamilyMed
Ogundiya, Ayodeji L., FamilyMed
Ohlhauser, Larry R.
Okolo, Godwin O.
Oladele, Oluseyi S., FamilyMed
Olijnik, Helen, FamilyMed
Oliva, Maria A.
Olsen, Terry M., FamilyMed
Olughor, Jerome O.
Omar, Assad B., FamilyMed
Ondro, Milena
Ondrus, Peter
Oneschuk, Doreen M., FamilyMed
Oskin, O. Alec
Osman, Ebtihal, FamilyMed
Otto, Catherine E., FamilyMed
Owen, Richard J T.
Ozelsel, Timur J.
Palmer, Jessica L A., FamilyMed
Paludet, Paul P.
Papp, Edward W., FamilyMed
Paquette, Ross N.
Parameswaran, Charmaine D., FamilyMed
Parmar, Jasneet K.
Parrish, Adam A.
Pasiorowski, Michal P.
Patel, Dipak, FamilyMed
Patel, Vimal H.
Pathan, Aarif A., FamilyMed
Patidar, Jayprakash V.
Pattison-Bacon, Manuela, FamilyMed
Patton, William R., FamilyMed(EM)
Pawluski, Kerence P.
Peerani, Nargis N.
Pekez, Jelena, FamilyMed
Pelman, Aaron M., FamilyMed
Peng, Hongwei J., FamilyMed
Pennock, Kevin, FamilyMed
Percy, Maria T.
Perez, Prudencio G.
Pernisie, Laurie D., FamilyMed
Perry, Douglas
Perry, Grace W K.
Peters, Catherine J., FamilyMed
Peters, Rudolf T.
Peterson, Colin L., FamilyMed(EM)
Peterson, Keir M., FamilyMed(EM)
Pezeshki, Bijan, FamilyMed
Phul, Rishi T., FamilyMed
Pickle, David A., FamilyMed
Pidde, Richard J.
Plageman, Maxwell G.
Plucinska, Hanna M., FamilyMed
Poitras, Michael P., FamilyMed
Polushin, Margaret M.
Poon, Lorne, FamilyMed
Popke, Manfred E.
Poplawski, Stanley A.
Potter, Terri
Poukhovski, Andrei
Powell, Mareli
Preston, Leslie J., FamilyMed
Qadry, Syed M S., FamilyMed(EM)
Quek, Kar Chi
Radwell, Jyl, FamilyMed(EM)
Raggi, Paolo
Rahaman, Omar S., FamilyMed
Rai, Avtar S.
Rai, Santoch S.
Rajab, Khaled A M., FamilyMed
Rajput, Romi, FamilyMed
Ramadan, Ziad F B., FamilyMed
Ramer, William D.
Ramsay, Glenna L., FamilyMed
Ramsey, Una P., FamilyMed
Ranieri, Thomas R., FamilyMed
Rankin, Alastair S., FamilyMed
Rao, Namita, FamilyMed
Rashid, Yasmin
Raslan, Tark M E.
Rawani, David A K.
Rebus, Lisa M., FamilyMed
Rech, Eulalia
Redding, Rebecka G.
Reed, Kathy E., FamilyMed
Reese, Heather L.
Rehman, Mujeeb
Reid, Branden P.
Reid, David A.
Reid, James D., FamilyMed
Reid, Natisha D., FamilyMed
Reilly, James G., FamilyMed
Rengan, Dhanakodi
Reynolds, Stuart F., FamilyMed(EM)
Rgei, Mahmoud
Riaz, Asifa, FamilyMed
Ribeiro, Ricardo A., FamilyMed(EM)
Rico, Michelle A., FamilyMed(EM)
Riess, Jennifer A., FamilyMed
Ritchie, Brian D., FamilyMed
Ritchie, John D.
Rizk, Nabil M R.
Rizvi, Qaiser R., FamilyMed
Robinson, Jeffery M., FamilyMed
Robinson, Karen M., FamilyMed
Robson, Nancy B A., FamilyMed
Roche, Anne L.
Rode, Melvin C.
Rohachuk, Kenneth H P., FamilyMed
Rohloff, Jacqueline M M., FamilyMed
Rojas-Vasquez, Marta I.
Romano, Kenneth R S.
Rose, Matthew D B., FamilyMed
Rosenstock, Carl B.
Ross, Betty L., FamilyMed
Ross, David J., FamilyMed
Ross, Mark R., FamilyMed
Rowand, Deborah C.
Rowe, Brian H., FamilyMed(EM)
Rudolph, Florian P.
Ryan, Daniel R., FamilyMed
Sachs, Helen K.
Sacks, Herbert W., FamilyMed
Safranovich, Colin E.
Saieed, Nabil H., FamilyMed
Saint-Martin, Marc, FamilyMed
Sajwani, Tasneem, FamilyMed
Salopek, Anthony P.
Salvalaggio, Ginetta L., FamilyMed
Sameny, Alireza, FamilyMed
Sametz, Joan M., FamilyMed
Samuels, Sheri L., FamilyMed
Samycia, Gary M.
San Agustin, D. Patrick, FamilyMed(EM)
Sandhu, Roopinder K.
Sarlieve, Philippe P.
Sarria, Ricardo
Saunders, Rebecca R., FamilyMed
Savitsky, Trisha A., FamilyMed
Sawicki, Zbigniew A.
Sawisky, Grant R., FamilyMed
Sayani, Ali, FamilyMed
Scanga, Dante G., FamilyMed
Scheirer, Gregg D., FamilyMed(EM)
Schick, Elizabeth L., FamilyMed
Schick, Judith E.
Schimpf, James, FamilyMed
Schipper, Shirley A., FamilyMed
Schmolzer, Georg M.
Schuldhaus, Dianne E., FamilyMed
Schuster, Ernst P., FamilyMed
Schwalfenberg, Gerry K., FamilyMed
Scott, Andrea D., FamilyMed
Secter, Barbara A.
Seibel, Donald G.
Seifert, Oliver
Semeniuk, Deborah D., FamilyMed
Semeniuk, Ross C., FamilyMed
Semenjuk, Michelle A., FamilyMed
Senior, Peter A.
Sepanmaa-Lund, Anne M.
Sereda, Brian D., FamilyMed
Sereda, Daniel D.
Sergi, Consolato
Seto, Paul H.
Shah, Aanand
Shaik, Mehaboob S.
Shaker, Emil, FamilyMed
Shaker, Marian, FamilyMed
Shakespeare, Timothy J.
Shakil, Sadia
Shalaby, Ashraf M K., FamilyMed
Shandro, M. Tami-Lee, FamilyMed
Sharafaddinzadeh, Naser
Sharek, Christine E., FamilyMed
Sharma, Arya M.
Sharma, Leneela, FamilyMed(EM)
Sharma, Rameshwar
Sharon, Raphael F.
Sher, Andrew K., FamilyMed
Sherlock, Jo-Ann I., FamilyMed
Sherman, Rajnish K., FamilyMed(EM)
Shibany, Ashraf G S S., FamilyMed
Shibata, Marcelo C.
Shibata, Mariko A., FamilyMed
Shibil, Majid
Shimizu, Jed, FamilyMed
Shmoorkoff, Jeffrey F., FamilyMed
Shumborski, Terry G.
Shute, Ronald D., FamilyMed
Siddiqi, Zaeem A.
Siddiqui, Farhat
Siderson, Miriam A., FamilyMed
Sidhu, Gurdip S., FamilyMed
Sidhu, Harkirat S., FamilyMed
Silvano, Mary J.
Simatos, Gary A., FamilyMed
Simon, Sandra S., FamilyMed
Singal, Mayank, FamilyMed
Singh, Ashwani K., FamilyMed
Singh, Rondeep, FamilyMed(EM)
Sinn, Barbara A.
Sinn, Ralph D.
Sivalingam, Paramalingam
Slade, Debra J., FamilyMed
Slatnik, Irena
Smeida, Khaled S M.
Smith, Bryar E., FamilyMed
Smith, Christopher J., FamilyMed
Smith, Cornel
Smith, Dana R.
Smith, Faye E., FamilyMed
Smith, Linda L., FamilyMed
Smith, M. Robin, FamilyMed
Smith, Shelley D B., FamilyMed
So, William I., FamilyMed
Solarte Thomas, Carlos E.
Sollereder, Gordon J.
Soneff, Cynthia M., FamilyMed
Soni, Rekha, FamilyMed
Sonnenberg, Barend J.
Soong, Elaine E., FamilyMed
Souster, Matthew
Sowa, Bernard
Spak, Andrew C D., FamilyMed
Sperber, Gregory
Spooner, G. Richard, FamilyMed
Sreenivasan, Bobby, FamilyMed
Stagg, Andrew P., FamilyMed(EM)
Starke, Carola G., FamilyMed
Starko, Michael J J.
Steblecki, Lisa J., FamilyMed
Stepanko, Rosemarie, FamilyMed
Sternberg, Harvey H., FamilyMed
Stetsko, Terry P.
Stewart, Tara L.
Stockburger, Dena L., FamilyMed
Stopainig, Robert, FamilyMed
Strilchuk, Douglas A J.
Stromberg, Lana M., FamilyMed
Strong, Grant C.
Strydom, Marthinus
Suen, Wai Yeung W.

Sultana, Samar, FamilyMed
Sun, W. David, FamilyMed
Sung, Hyun J., FamilyMed
Surmawala, Shahida, FamilyMed
Sutanto, Ian H., FamilyMed
Swaih, Omar M O., FamilyMed
Taeeb, Hussein A A., FamilyMed
Taher, Zaki A.
Takacs, Ernest S.
Talbot-Jones, Robert
Talibi, Tal Talip
Talwar, Shalin R., FamilyMed
Tam, Sandy W., FamilyMed
Tan, Amy Y Y., FamilyMed
Tang, Julian W.
Tao, Sha
Taparia, Minakshi S.
Tariq, Khalida P., FamilyMed
Tarumi, Yoko
Taylor, John C.
Thai, H M. Vincent, FamilyMed
Tham, Edythe B.
Thambiraj, Joshua R.
Thapar, Vijay K., FamilyMed
Theman, M. Allison, FamilyMed
Theron, Ronelle
Thibault, Nicolas, FamilyMed
Thibodeau, James A., FamilyMed
Thuat, Nam, FamilyMed
Toal, Kevin F.
Toal, Stephen, FamilyMed
Toane, E. Benjamin
Toderovich, Eugene
Toma, Sarah G.
Tomi, Salem S.
Tomkiewicz, Robert P.
Tousignant, Michelle M., FamilyMed(EM)
Tran, Anthony L., FamilyMed
Tran, Tanya, FamilyMed
Trifis, Mokhtar H M.
Triscott, Jean A C., FamilyMed
Tsang, Bonnie
Tse, Jennifer E., FamilyMed
Tse, Jennifer E., FamilyMed
Tseng, Jui-Teng
Turner, Justine M.
Turner, Mary Ann S.
Turner, Robert L., FamilyMed
Turner, Simon R.
Twomey, Ciaran F.
Ulan, Susan R., FamilyMed
Unwala, Fatima E.
Urschel, Simon
Ushko, Allan W., FamilyMed(EM)
Vahidy, Seemin A.
Valji, Shairose, FamilyMed
Valtuille, Lucas S.
Van Den Heever, Zacharias A N.
Van Der Merwe, Gerrit F.
Van Zyl, Stephanus D.
Vasanji, Adil N., FamilyMed
Vaselenak, Sharon A., FamilyMed
Vecchio, Silvano R.
Velmurugiah, Rhenugadevi, FamilyMed
Vernon, Errol E.
Verones, Patricia M., FamilyMed
Vetsch, Elizabeth A., FamilyMed
Vicaruddin, Omair, FamilyMed
Vicaruddin, Zehra, FamilyMed
Vincent, Denis R J., FamilyMed
Vliagoftis, Harissios
Voeuk, Anna, FamilyMed
Voldeng, Jason S., FamilyMed
Volkovinskaia, Tamara, FamilyMed
Vu, Trevor T C.
Waclawski, Eugene
Wagg, Adrian S.
Wagner, Michael B., FamilyMed
Wahba, Inas A A.
Walker, Allan F.
Walker, Jennifer L., FamilyMed
Wang, Xiaoping
Wanigaratne, Mihiri M.
War, Leonora B.
Ward, Bryan D., FamilyMed
Wash, Walter F.
Wasilenko, Lotje, FamilyMed
Wat, Stephen W., FamilyMed
Watrich, Deanne G., FamilyMed(EM)
Watson, Michael W B.
Weerasinghe, Nandanie
Weinberg, Mitchell L.
Werner, Monica J.
Wesner, Marni-Lyn, FamilyMed
Wheeler, Devon S., FamilyMed(EM)
White, Amie M., FamilyMed
White, Patrick J.
Whittaker, R. Bryn, FamilyMed
Wieczorek, Krzysztof
Williams, David G.
Wilson, Donald W S.
Wilson, Marie A Y.
Windram, Jonathan D.
Wine, Eytan
Wingnean, David, FamilyMed
Wink, Michael J.
Winterstein, Jeffrey
Wismark, Jennine A., FamilyMed
Wittmeier, Robert W., FamilyMed(EM)
Wiznura, Richard A.
Wolch, Gary R., FamilyMed
Wollin, Brenda L., FamilyMed
Wong, Allen S., FamilyMed
Wong, Andrew P T.
Wong, Dennis Y R.
Wong, Hoa Leng
Wong, Jackson Y W.
Wong, James M., FamilyMed
Wong, Jean M.
Wong, Matthew G., FamilyMed
Wong, Nick N L., FamilyMed
Wong, Norris A., FamilyMed
Wong, Paul K.
Wong, Stan G., FamilyMed
Wong Armstrong, Susan
Woo, Andrea, FamilyMed
Wood, Barbara L., FamilyMed
Woolsey, Guy H., FamilyMed
Wright, Ryan T., FamilyMed
Wu, Beatrice M Y., FamilyMed
Yablonsky, Shmuel S., FamilyMed
Yakunchikov, Dmitry Y.
Yaltho, Smitha, FamilyMed
Yamamoto, Hans Y.
Yan, Michael, FamilyMed
Yang, Tony, FamilyMed
Yao, Roger, FamilyMed(EM)
Yap, Jason Y K.
Yaqub, Syed M T.
Yar Khan, Saulat
Yau, William Y T., FamilyMed
Yee, Vernie F., FamilyMed
Yeung, Alexander K., FamilyMed(EM)
Yeung, Aref, FamilyMed(EM)
Yeung, Jared C C., FamilyMed
Yeung, T. Myriam
Yeung, Timothy T C., FamilyMed
Yip, David K W., FamilyMed
Yoneda, Janet
Yong, Paul C K., FamilyMed
Youakim, Hany N., FamilyMed
Young, Carmen E.
Young, Malcolm J.
Youssef, Wafaa
Yu, Jane S.
Yu, Ling Pui, FamilyMed
Yue, David
Yue, Jody, FamilyMed
Yuen, Amy K W., FamilyMed
Zakaria, Fozia, FamilyMed
Zaugg, Michael
Zayani, Abdulati
Zayani, Adeb S M.
Zayed, Tareg
Zepeda Gomez, Sergio
Zhang, Xinyun
Zielinski, Janice-Marie, FamilyMed
Zirk, Harry A., FamilyMed
Ziwenga, Ophillia
Zorzela, Liliane M.

EDSON

Donkin, Monia
Du Plessis, Mia
Gous, Roelof
Kamedien, Rabiah
Knight, Alison J., FamilyMed
Naidu, Phnendren
Oishi, Roderick L., FamilyMed
Robinson, Jo-Ann, FamilyMed
Sheik, Nasreen
Sood, Rajesh K.
Van Der Merwe, Estie
White, Robert J.
Willis, Brian D.

ELK POINT

Oyebode, Ayobami O., FamilyMed
Ramful, Droovnath

EVANSBURG

Murphy, Michael R.

FAIRVIEW

Andreiuk, John R., FamilyMed
Botha, Nicolaas J., FamilyMed
Claasen, Cornelis J., FamilyMed
Irvine, Harley R.

FALHER

Alshigagi, Emadalden A.

FALLIS

Stroud, Richard R., FamilyMed

FORT MACLEOD

Beekman, Steven G., FamilyMed
Parvanov, Tzvetan V., FamilyMed
Simpson, Robert J., FamilyMed
Uwalaka, Anne N.

FORT MCMURRAY

Akinjise, Idowu C., FamilyMed
Al-Naami, Ghassan
Ambrosano, Lorella
Aniki, Yahaya Y.
Anyalebechi, Obinna
Arruj, Nasim
Baldonado, Narciso
Benade, Maria N.
Benade, Spinnler L.
Bouwer, Johannes C.
Bowman, Jonathan R., FamilyMed
Buni, Reeda
Chaudhry, Mobina A., FamilyMed
Corbett, Elizabeth A S.
Covarrubia, Kelimar C.
Denga, Edward T., FamilyMed
Dufresne, Brian E., FamilyMed(EM)
Elesin, Fayisayo, FamilyMed
Elmsallati, Taher
Elmusharaf, Mohamed S., FamilyMed
Fawole, Olukayode A.
Gaisbichler, Wolfgang H.
Griffin, William
Hibbitts, Erin D., FamilyMed
Ibach, Richard J., FamilyMed(EM)
Kazembe, V. Gertrude
Killick, David G., FamilyMed(EM)
Koranteng, Samuel
Kosick, Thomas M.
Kruger, Pieter Ernst
Largoza, Josef P.
Lee, Loretta E., FamilyMed
McCarthy, Lauren O., FamilyMed
McCombe, Padraic S C., FamilyMed
Nicholson, Allan J B.
Nwaka, Bernard C., FamilyMed
Nyati, Lindiwe L.
O'Connor, John A.
Ogunsina, Olurotimi O.
Onwukwe, Victor N.
Osegbue, Emmanuel U.
Palma, Peter, FamilyMed(EM)
Phiri, Young W.
Rhemtula, Haroun A.
Sheppard, Jeffrey B., FamilyMed
Suleiman, Ali M.
Taiwo, Olumide A., FamilyMed
Tutuncuoglu, Suleyman O.
Van Heerde, Johannes C.
Walker, Malcolm G., FamilyMed
Worry, Kevin W., FamilyMed(EM)
Xulu, Helen M A.

FORT SASKATCHEWAN

Amin, Shabbir F., FamilyMed
Antoniuk, Craig D., FamilyMed
Azer, Sameh C.
Borstlap, Jeanne
Carter, Linda J., FamilyMed
Cervantes, Jaime
Dutt, Purnima
Fung, Gordon C.
Gauri, Mohammed A.
Guzik, Elaine C., FamilyMed
Harrison, Kenneth F.
Hoque, M. Zahirul
Hult, Keith W., FamilyMed
Kumar, Sandeep
Kumari, Amita
Kumleben, Mark A.
Pfeifer, Linda M., FamilyMed
Roob, Otokar J.
Stecyk, Robert W.
Withers, Trevor M.

FORT VERMILION

Breen, Carson F.
De Klerk, Barend J.
Erasmus, Daniel J E.
Le Roux, Marius N.
Van Heerden, Pieter W.
Van Rooyen, Hendrik M.
Verdoorn, Marius

FOX CREEK

Algundi, Abdullah A Y.
Corrigan, Karin Liezel
Olivier, Barend G.

GIBBONS

Botha, Johannes
Oyama, Sonnie E.

GLEICHEN

McNeely, Joni M., FamilyMed

GLENDON

Mannion, Vincent L., FamilyMed

GRANDE CACHE

Barnard, Esther
Darcel, Keith R., FamilyMed
Gerber, Dorothy I., FamilyMed
Gillett, John A.
Noordman, Annelies H.
Walton, Christina R., FamilyMed

GRANDE PRAIRIE

Adham, Tamer M H.
Akintola, D. Raphael, FamilyMed(EM)
Al Masoudi, Faisal K H.
Andrews, Eleanor J., FamilyMed
Ayanrino, Femi B.
Aylward, Darroch L.
Barreth, C. Angela, FamilyMed
Bartie, Darryl C.
Bellamy, Deanna D., FamilyMed
Berhe, Tzeggai
Bertozzi, Hugo A R., FamilyMed
Block, Erwin
Booysen, C. Francois
Campbell, Elroy S.
Campbell, Garth L.
Darif, Suzan Darif Aribi
De Villiers, Albert
Denkema, Raubenheimer
Du Plessis, Nicolaas
Dube, Sampurnanand
Duta, Valentin, FamilyMed
Easwara Murthi, Manjula
Echavarria Cano, Maria
Echezona, Anthony O.
Elbeshti, Essam A M., FamilyMed
Eraghubi, Milad
Erasmus, Marilise
Faltaous, El Sherif I M S.
Folscher, Werner
Goso, T. Joseph
Groenewald, Leon C.
Hackenberg, Libusa
Hattingh, Jacolette
Hezam, Wael
Kafi, Ayotunde O.
Kali, Aporna, FamilyMed
Khan Afridi, Obaid T.
Kloub, Oxana
Lal, Kartar
Lewis, Cledwyn E.
Lindsay, Peter K., FamilyMed
Lyddell, Christopher
Malik, Aasim N.
Martin, Brad W.
Martin, Richard A., FamilyMed
Martin, Riley T., FamilyMed
McEvoy, Patricia L.
McGovern, Peter D A.
Mendis, M M D. Calista, FamilyMed
Mequanent, Tewodros G., FamilyMed
Millar, Brenda J., FamilyMed
Minic, Sanja, FamilyMed
Molnar, Szilamer Z A.
Mumert, Donna J., FamilyMed
Musa, Khalid M S K., FamilyMed
Muwonge, Stanley N M., FamilyMed
Narnaware, Avisha
Noga, Alexandra E., FamilyMed
Norris, Barry K., FamilyMed
Nyachwo, Caroline B., FamilyMed
Obiajulu, Anthony C.
Okonta, Henry I.
Owadally, Bilaal A.
Piepgrass, Brent L.
Pieterse, Leonie
Pillay, Paramesha
Pope, A. James D., FamilyMed
Read, James H.
Renfree, Paul I., FamilyMed
Senekal, Daniel
Shnishah, Abdalrhman A., FamilyMed
Singhal, Rishi K.
Somani, Shelyn
Staples, Robert K.
Stevenson, William T.
Strydom, Carin S., FamilyMed
Tayyeb, Tahir
Vos, Eugene P.
Wang, Thur
Wessels, Wynand
Wynters, John
Yao, Shengtao
Yu, Hojun
Zamani, Haseebullah

GRIMSHAW

Botha, Andries N.
Coetzee, Anka
De Kock, Matthys J.
Louw, Alexander M.

HANNA

Gainer, C. Jane
Hanna, Emad S A., FamilyMed
Mdawe, Isaac M.
Walters, Nicolaas J.

HARDISTY

Botha, Diederick F.

HIGH LEVEL

Brussow, Heinrich D.
Du Plooy, Daniel
Essop, Ridwana
Forder, Mark A.
Marfo, Elijah A.
Strydom, Hendrik G.
Walsh, Paul F., FamilyMed

HIGH PRAIRIE

Armstrong, Glen L E O.
Du Toit, Daniel M.
Edwards, Pamela V.
Laughlin, Robert
Sheopershad, Yuktesh
Swart, Matthys L.
van der Westhuizen, Frans W.

HIGH RIVER

Andruski, Benjamin, FamilyMed
Bagdan, Bonnie L., FamilyMed
Bell-Dingwall, Sarah, FamilyMed
Bozyk, Kevin S.
Finnegan, Stephen J., FamilyMed
Fortin, William J.
Gorsche, Ronald G., FamilyMed
Hagens, John E., FamilyMed
Jeeva, Adam M.
Jeeva, Ashref, FamilyMed
Jensen, Brian W., FamilyMed
Makhdoom, Sarah, FamilyMed
Mercer, Dennis F.
Norheim, Jennifer K., FamilyMed
Ogoke, Valentine C.
Powell, Christopher C., FamilyMed(EM)
Roper, Nicole, FamilyMed
Smillie, Mark A., FamilyMed
Spackman, Keith E.
Vyse, Adam D.
Vyse, Nancy A., FamilyMed
Walsh, Kevin J., FamilyMed

HINTON

Allan, Margaret C., FamilyMed
Armstrong, J. Bradford, FamilyMed
Binette, Brett A J., FamilyMed
Button, Erica A., FamilyMed
Caffaro, Michael J., FamilyMed
Corser, Noel B., FamilyMed
Corser, Sarah A., FamilyMed
Cote, Erin C., FamilyMed
Dreyer, Francois
Faid, Carol E., FamilyMed
Hawkwood, Joseph N H., FamilyMed
Jones, Lee D T., FamilyMed
Lansing, Davina R J., FamilyMed
Rahn, Andrea R., FamilyMed
Schneider, Wolfgang E., FamilyMed
Sorenson, Katherine J., FamilyMed
Stockburger, J. Mark, FamilyMed

HYTHE

Crowe, Robert F G., FamilyMed
Dressler, Jason D T., FamilyMed

INNISFAIL

Barker, Edmund A.
Chauhan, Upesh C., FamilyMed
Damgaard, H. Neils, FamilyMed
Davies, Nigel C M.
Hrdlicka, Adam J., FamilyMed
Kapp, Magdalena J.
Maree, Mattheus
Meding, Gerald C.
Miller, Gerald A.
Rees, Susan C.
Schoeman, Meyer
Short, Leo F N., FamilyMed

JASPER

Addison, Mark J W.
Bester, Belinda A., FamilyMed
Murphy, Melanie J., FamilyMed
Slack, Stephen J.
Swanepoel, Abraham C J.
Unsworth, Declan P., FamilyMed
Wilkinson, Roy P.
Wilson, Lisa A., FamilyMed

KILLAM

Hanton, Timothy E., FamilyMed
Ogbeide, Samuel O.
Weighman, Maurice A T.

LA CRETE

Ghargoum, Abdussalam M H.
Lajili, Fathi Abdalla

LAC LA BICHE

Ackermann, Wendy C.
Birkill, Richard S., FamilyMed
Claassens, Coenraad F.
Coetzee, Fanie
Coetzee, Michelle
Crum, Serena N D., FamilyMed
De Ridder, Handre, FamilyMed
Dehlen, Magdalena D.
Groenewald, Wendy C.
Lippolt, Gordon B.
Mare, Jean-Pierre, FamilyMed
Steyn, Frederik M.

LACOMBE

Darnell, Timothy S., FamilyMed
Elliott, Brian D.
Ethier, Dennis R.
Geates, Barry
Keller, Ronald E.
Kinash, Barbara L.
McKibbin, Cecil S.
Nieuwoudt, J. Stephan
Nischuk, Leighton L.
Olivier, Antoinette
Orr, Suzanne A.
Prins, Johannes
Smit, Kenneth H., FamilyMed
Unger, Kathy D., FamilyMed
Unger, Matthew R., FamilyMed
Van Niekerk, Izak J M.
Wildeboer, David W., FamilyMed

LAKE LOUISE

Page, Brian C.
Page, Douglas B., FamilyMed

LAMONT

El-Hajj, Eyad O.
Iordache, Claudiu
Mohamed, Zainool A., FamilyMed
Namit, Jaime W.
Slanina, John

LEDUC

Abel, Katherine J M., FamilyMed
Balko, Justin P., FamilyMed
Byers, Trevor J., FamilyMed
Chaudhry, Shazia, FamilyMed
Chen, Jieli, FamilyMed
De Freitas, Teresa, FamilyMed
Dinsa, Gurpreet S., FamilyMed
Du Toit, Anton E., FamilyMed
Dulai, Gurjeet, FamilyMed
Gault, Michael H.
Gouda, Amira F B., FamilyMed
Hetherington, D. Maxine, FamilyMed
Holden, Jana P., FamilyMed(EM)
Lee, Christopher T., FamilyMed
Lo, Freda H F., FamilyMed
Low, Jason D., FamilyMed
Majeed Mohammed, Asma'a, FamilyMed
Naidoo, Dadi B.
Oberg, Colin E., FamilyMed
Orth, Michael J., FamilyMed(EM)
Paras, Dwight J.
Rankin, Jason K., FamilyMed
Simard, Robert J., FamilyMed
Smith, Johannes L A D.
Smyth, David J E., FamilyMed
Sonpar, Prabhu, FamilyMed
Sprague, Nancy L.
Taylor, Marian R.
Tran, David V B., FamilyMed
Trofimuk, J. Timothy, FamilyMed
Van Heerden, Alida
Woolliscroft, David G.
Yue, Ming Yee, FamilyMed

LETHBRIDGE

Aborawi, Abdelbasat
Abrahamson, Carrie N., FamilyMed
Allen, Raymond B., FamilyMed
Amatto, Michael J.
Annavukadavu, Abdul S.
Appleton, Erin E., FamilyMed
Aronson, Howard L., FamilyMed(EM)
Aziz, Abdul
Banmann, Daniel H., FamilyMed(EM)
Benkoczi, Carmen L., FamilyMed
Bennett, Ian
Billett, Alan T., FamilyMed
Bishel, Gerald R., FamilyMed
Bly, Eric B., FamilyMed
Boehme, Gene R.
Braithwaite, Philip
Browne, Philip M., FamilyMed
Bruwer, Anna D B.
Buck, Richard M., FamilyMed(EM)
Burton, Wayne P., FamilyMed
Byers, Susan D., FamilyMed
Cahill, Mark K., FamilyMed
Capisonda, S. Rhona B.
Cassis, Mona, FamilyMed
Cheung, Humphrey H.
Collins, Timothy R.
Coma, Aaron L., FamilyMed
Crawford, Stephen G S.
Cronje, J. Stephen, FamilyMed(EM)
De Waal, Willem P.
Derman, Ryan
Devraj-Kizuk, Rozemin P E., FamilyMed
Dietrichsen, Celeste
El-Gehani, Faraj E.
Engelbrecht, Adele
Ericksen, Marty L., FamilyMed
Frick, Kenneth G., FamilyMed
Galbraith, Robert M.
Garden, Dana L., FamilyMed
Gibb, Donald R., FamilyMed
Gillis, Lisa A., FamilyMed
Godwin, Elaine I., FamilyMed
Goicea, Daniela
Gonsalvez, Antony K.
Greidanus, Peter G.
Haberman, John J R.
Haig, Charlotte E., FamilyMed
Hamilton, Nicolas, FamilyMed(EM)
Hardin, Evelyn
Harvey, Janice
Herbert, Linda T.
Hiebert, Mervin P J., FamilyMed(EM)
Horne, Mark R.
Inglis, Edward K.
Ireland, Brenda J., FamilyMed
Jillood, Ibrahim K.
Jonker, Garland P., FamilyMed
Karpakis, Janine
Kellerman, Madelene S.
Kennedy, Dorcas D., FamilyMed
Kennedy, Jennifer R., FamilyMed
Kiared, Ahmed
Koegler, Peter A., FamilyMed
Kozan, James R., FamilyMed
Kremenik, Terri L., FamilyMed
Kwan, Peter, FamilyMed(EM)
Lasore, Olufunmi O.
Leam, Howe, FamilyMed
Levin, Ilona
Lewis, Paul J., FamilyMed(EM)
Lisztwan, Magdalena, FamilyMed(EM)
Lohrenz, Keith S., FamilyMed
Longair, Terrence L., FamilyMed
MacLean, A. Vanessa M., FamilyMed(EM)
Mackey, Duncan S., FamilyMed(EM)
Makar, Kami L., FamilyMed(EM)
Malan, Francois A.
Malpica Vera, Carlos
McLuckie, Duncan A.
McPherson, Alan L.
Meller, David F., FamilyMed
Mueller, Eric M., FamilyMed(EM)
Murray, R. David, FamilyMed(EM)
Musk, Mark C., FamilyMed
Narula, Rajesh K.
Nsisi, Lazarus M.
Nsisi, Saturday N A.
Oishi, Arlene S., FamilyMed
Orr, Darin C., FamilyMed
Orr, Wesley D L., FamilyMed(EM)
Pahulje, Bernadette F., FamilyMed
Palma, Alberto
Piercey, Karen-Lynne, FamilyMed
Plotnyk, Eugene, FamilyMed
Raphael, Julian M C.
Robertson, Karen P., FamilyMed
Simpson, Maurice F., FamilyMed(EM)
Smith, Julie E., FamilyMed(EM)
Sommerfeldt, T. Drew, FamilyMed
Steed, Merrill D., FamilyMed
Steel, W. Dale, FamilyMed
Steeves, Daniel C.
Stewart, Calvin M., FamilyMed
Stewart, David C., FamilyMed
Stewart, Hugh V.
Stocks, Christina I.
Storey, Elaine A.
Strank, Robert L., FamilyMed
Suttorp, Vivien V., FamilyMed
Tupper, Janet K., FamilyMed
Ukrainetz, Owen M., FamilyMed
Van Der Poll, Annerien M.
Van Der Poll, Corneil X.
Van Straaten, Jacobus P L.
Walsh, Colin K., FamilyMed
Walsh, Dionne M., FamilyMed
Watke, Christine A.
Weaver, Joel H., FamilyMed
Westheuser, Susan L., FamilyMed
White, Andrea A., FamilyMed
White, Roger T., FamilyMed
Wicentovich, Lana M., FamilyMed
Wilde, Sean K., FamilyMed(EM)
Wong, Janice, FamilyMed(EM)
Yamashita, Kathryn F., FamilyMed

LLOYDMINSTER

Bilan, Margaret A.
Blom, Charl J P.
Cavanagh, Thomas L., FamilyMed
Chan-Tai-Kong, Chan-San H.
Chapelski, Mark B E., FamilyMed(EM)
Du Plooy, Rian
Gerber, Christiaan J F.
Govender, Kevin
Isaiah, Joel H.
Kenyon, Jolene C., FamilyMed
Kerlis, Thomas E A.
Lakins, Jill E.
Naidoo, Vernon
Naude, Adel H.
Naude, Francois P.
Reddy, Dhanasagren S.
Scribante, Lindi
Snyman, Annamarie
Swart, Wayne
Swart, Werner
Van Der Merwe, Cornelis M.
Wessels, Philippus H.
Yen, Shiu Kee

MAGRATH

Dahl, Kenneth E., FamilyMed
Regehr, Jack C., FamilyMed
Tollestrup, Jonathon B., FamilyMed

MANNING

Turner, Richard H., FamilyMed

MAYERTHORPE

Aird, Mary M.
Bernier, Robert G J.
Jamal, Zahirali, FamilyMed
Lowe, Jeffrey K.
Mwanza, Jonathan
Naicker, Sivalingam S.

MCLENNAN

Butcher, Shaun S.
De Wet, Pieter W.
Eriki, Simon P.
Isiguzo, Obinna F.

MEDICINE HAT

Ahmad, Aijaz
Augustine, Anita, FamilyMed
Bekker, Antoinette
Bennett, Ogonda A.
Boodhoo, Jean A.
Booyens, Barend M J., FamilyMed
Bratvold, Jeffrey S., FamilyMed
Burger, Lydia A., FamilyMed
Burgess, John D.
Cameron-Ross, Lorien
Ciubotaru, Sergiu, FamilyMed
Clugston, Timothy P.
Correia, Amelia T., FamilyMed
Cowtan, Edgar R., FamilyMed(EM)
Currah, Ryan E., FamilyMed(EM)
Devi, Minati
Di Ninno, Vincent L., FamilyMed
Dirker, Caren
Dolatabadi, Amir
Duke, Sandra M., FamilyMed
Durand, Barend J., FamilyMed
Elkink, Meghan S., FamilyMed
Faul, Hendrik J., FamilyMed(EM)
Filanti, Bernardo I.
Foley, Joshua F., FamilyMed
Gangji, Alnoor
Gebhardt, Ian N., FamilyMed
Glas, Mario R., FamilyMed
Greeff, Wessel
Gripp, Mark J.
Grobler, Gert J.
Hall, Dennis K., FamilyMed
Harrison, Sidney W., FamilyMed
Hirsch, Byron D., FamilyMed
Hoffmann, Kristin M I.
Hoogeveen, Larry G.
Horsman, Catherine A., FamilyMed
Hrdlicka, Ash T., FamilyMed
Jaffer, Ashif S., FamilyMed
Jensen, Bryant J., FamilyMed
Jeraj, Anthony F., FamilyMed
Jonker, Franz A., FamilyMed
Josephson, Brian R., FamilyMed
Joubert, Jan G., FamilyMed(EM)
Keshvara, A. Muru, FamilyMed
Kopp, Justin E J., FamilyMed(EM)
Kriel, Adriaan P., FamilyMed
Lee, Judy S M.
Lee, Michael R.
Lintott, Dale N.
Mastel, Douglas G., FamilyMed
Meiring, Madeleine E., FamilyMed

PHYSICIANS BY PROVINCE

Mi, Lei, FamilyMed
Mohanraj, Thomas M., FamilyMed
Northcott, Richard D., FamilyMed
Nunweiler, Donovan E S., FamilyMed
Opperman, Estelle M.
Orellana-Jordan, Edwin R.
Pasternak, John L.
Phelps, Ian J., FamilyMed(EM)
Pirwany, Imran R.
Prince, Gerry D., FamilyMed
Riaz, Salman
Rinaldi, Fredrykka D., FamilyMed
Rinholm, Larry E., FamilyMed
Ruzycki, William A., FamilyMed
Saujani, Virendra S.
Schneider, Matthias
Shrives, Heloise
Sissons, Joy L.
Smith, Anthony A.
Stewart, Christopher J.
Steyn, Morrison F.
Stuart, Andrew J.
Swiegers, Roxanne L., FamilyMed
Thorogood, Mark D., FamilyMed
Van Der Westhuizen, Solomon H., FamilyMed
Van Niekerk, Jozef W.
Venumbaka, Abaya
Venumbaka, S. Anand
Viljoen, Johan A., FamilyMed
Villanueva, Alvin P.
Wanner, Nicoelle R E., FamilyMed
Whitfield, Bobbi-Jo, FamilyMed
Wise, Laura S., FamilyMed
Witt, Susan A., FamilyMed
Wong, Martin S., FamilyMed
Woolf, Robert J., FamilyMed(EM)
York, Stephen

MILK RIVER

Lewke-Bogle, Elisabeth, FamilyMed

NANTON

Alam, Mohammad S.
Mamogobo, Charmaine M.
Tenove, R. John

OKOTOKS

Anderson, Douglas M., FamilyMed
Ansell, Richard J.
Berry, Dale C., FamilyMed
Byam, R. Flayne
Coetzee, Jacoba I.
Collar, Colleen A., FamilyMed
Gordon, Tracey A.
Hart, Stephanie E., FamilyMed
Hill, Monica L., FamilyMed
Hill, N. Grant
Ho, Gilian C., FamilyMed
James, Simon T.
Jansen Van Rensburg, Stella-Amore
Khan, Ashraf, FamilyMed
Lavender, S. Jo Anne
Mazloum, Gloria M., FamilyMed
McCracken, James M.
Nel, Anton J.
Oelschig, Ana-Maria
Ramlall, Jacintha, FamilyMed
Schneider, Alexia
Simmons, Grace
Spice, Ronald N., FamilyMed
Teasell, Lynne D.
Van Tonder, Janna
Walsh, John A., FamilyMed
Wilson, Andrea S., FamilyMed(EM)

OLDS

Auret, Marnel
Cox, Sinclair P.
Craven, Shauna C L., FamilyMed
Duong, Du Ton, FamilyMed
Dykin, Kimberly, FamilyMed
Hoeve, Allan J., FamilyMed
Hoffman, Jaco
Hoffman, Maria E.
Ingles, Martha G C., FamilyMed
Kelly, Elizabeth G.
Nel, Gert P.
Onsongo, Foose M.
Stampa, Leonore D., FamilyMed
Turner, Steven L., FamilyMed
Van Der Vyver, Johannes D., FamilyMed
Vorster, Deon J., FamilyMed
Wray, Richard G.

ONOWAY

Kozakiewicz, Richard
Winterbach, Uys

OYEN

Muller, Petra

PEACE RIVER

Barco, Cynthia C., FamilyMed
De Graad, Gerben J.
Eckhart, Martin S., FamilyMed
Greidanus, Robert I., FamilyMed
Kolber, Michael R., FamilyMed
Lundgard, Karen A H., FamilyMed
May, Tyler B., FamilyMed
McKeown, G. Thomas
Potvin, Nadine S., FamilyMed
Potvin, Nicholas A., FamilyMed
Redman, Kathryn H.
Sequeira, Richard
Unger, Jason B A., FamilyMed
Welch, David S., FamilyMed
Willox, David L.
Willox, Laurene A.

PICTURE BUTTE

Leishman, William R., FamilyMed
Mohamed, Riyaz S E.

PINCHER CREEK

Burton, Beverly A., FamilyMed
Burton, Tracy L., FamilyMed
Cameron, Robert A.
De Wet, Steyn
Derie-Gillespie, Lena, FamilyMed
Gelber, Tobias N M., FamilyMed
Irving, Antony M., FamilyMed
Parker, Gavin G., FamilyMed
Rottger, P. John
Scrimshaw, Catherine L., FamilyMed
Van Bussel, Jared J., FamilyMed
Wilson, Brett P., FamilyMed

PONOKA

Alcaraz-Limcangco, Yolanda, FamilyMed
Bunting, Brendan J.
Campbell, T. Malcolm
Chan, Gregory K., FamilyMed
Currie, Blair M.
Day, Jeremiah B.
Day, Nathaniel, FamilyMed
Du Toit, Martha C.
Girgis, Ehab S S.
Goosen, Hilgard
Greyling, Schalk J.
Halse, Robert A.
Janicki, Tomasz
Jayasuriya, Joseph C.
Kumar, Vilas
Kwan, Stephen C K.
McKinnon, Terry J.
McMillan, Patrick R., FamilyMed
Memon, Abdulaziz
O'Croinin, Feargus
Rosborough, Amy M., FamilyMed
Rosenkranz, George J., FamilyMed
Schlenther, Gunther
Shahoo, Nirmal K.
Van Der Westhuizen, Christiaan L., FamilyMed
Van Der Westhuizen, Izak J., FamilyMed
Visser, Francois C., FamilyMed

PROVOST

De Flamingh, Willem J.
Erasmus, Deon E.
Malan, Stephan P.

RAYMOND

Baker, Eric C., FamilyMed
Geoffrion, Paul C., FamilyMed(EM)
Smith, Gregory L., FamilyMed
Smith, Terrence C.
Steed, Clayne A.
Steed, Regan C., FamilyMed
Tollestrup, Wallace R.
Wihlborg, Christel E M., FamilyMed

RED DEER

Achebe, Ifeoma F.
Amanullah, Syed F.
Apantaku, Olushola M., FamilyMed
Atchison, Katherine E., FamilyMed
Badenhorst, Josias S.
Bakken, Maureen P.
Basson, Nicol, FamilyMed
Benoit, Joseph S.
Benson, Bruce D., FamilyMed
Beshai, Safa
Bester, Charles J.
Bilston, Anne E., FamilyMed
Boorman, David W.
Bouch, Peter J., FamilyMed
Braganza, John A C.
Bromley, John E., FamilyMed
Catherall, Malcolm S.
Church, Wayne F., FamilyMed
Colebrook, John M., FamilyMed(EM)
Comeau, Paulette
Cooper, Robert C., FamilyMed
Costigan, Norman P.
Cowie, Betty S., FamilyMed
Daniel, Kamal M., FamilyMed
Darby, Mark C., FamilyMed
Davidson, Robert G., FamilyMed(EM)
De Klerk, Leon
Dembinski, Brian, FamilyMed
Derouin, Kim, FamilyMed
Devereaux, Emily F., FamilyMed
du Plooy, Magarietha J.
Duffy, Deirdre A., FamilyMed(EM)
Dukeshire, Lauralee, FamilyMed
Eleason, Sheila M., FamilyMed
Elliot, David C., FamilyMed
Ellis, John G.
Flegal, Collette A., FamilyMed(EM)
Foerster, Steven G., FamilyMed(EM)
Ford, Anthony J.
Forgeron, Robert J., FamilyMed(EM)
Furlani, Aldo A.
Gain, Robert H.
Gellner, Darcie L., FamilyMed(EM)
Grabe, Willem A., FamilyMed
Greig, Bradley
Grimbeek, Francois N.
Grobler, Josias M.
Grundling, Christiaan J.
Hermanutz, Katie E., FamilyMed
Hildebrandt, Walter H.
Hindle, Hugh R., FamilyMed(EM)
Hjertaas, Kenneth R.
Hogarth, Walter D., FamilyMed(EM)
Holmes, Colin L.
Hopfner, Joseph
Hovan, Shirley
Hulyk, Raymond, FamilyMed
Hyde, Mandy M., FamilyMed
Johnstone, Kerri L.
Jones, Lize
Julyan-Gudgeon, John, FamilyMed
Keen, Brian D.
Koen, Johannes C.
Konynenbelt, Susan
Kotze, Annegret
Kritzinger, Johan J., FamilyMed(EM)
Kruger, Stephanus J.
Ligate, Lora V.
Logachev, Evgeny
Lundall, Evan
Mah, Peter
McCall, Maureen
McIntyre, James A., FamilyMed
Meikle, Gregg M., FamilyMed(EM)
Menezes, Antonio A C.
Metcalfe, Charles G.
Moffatt, Richard A., FamilyMed
Mulder, Jeffrey D., FamilyMed
Mulder, Robert J.
Murray, Sandy J., FamilyMed
Myburgh, Johannes L., FamilyMed
Myburgh, Willem M., FamilyMed
Nechifor, Roxana, FamilyMed
Neil, Gordon F.
Neira, Rodrigo
Nel, Stephen O., FamilyMed
Nogareda, Jorge G.
Odendaal, Morne L., FamilyMed
Ohanjanians, Edward
Ollewagen, Ferdinand J.
Parrington, Barry D.
Phillpot, C. Aimee, FamilyMed
Pienaar, LeRoy C.
Rattan, Nav P S., FamilyMed
Rautenbach, Derick A.
Rawlek, Peter J.
Reynolds, Walter J F.
Rossouw, Jacques
Rudolph, Kathrin S.
Shafiq, Muhammad
Sharma, Sanjeev K.
Shulman, Desmond
Singh, Amar
Stearn, Donovan
Stewart, Neil A.
Swanepoel, Richard D.
Swarts, Petrus J E.
Taiwo, Tolulola O., FamilyMed
Taylor, Sara B., FamilyMed
Tetz, Rhonda L M.
Thain, Michael J.
Thomas, Lyle S., FamilyMed(EM)
Thompson, Erin E., FamilyMed
Valmana, Anton
Van Der Berg, Jan D.
Van Wyk, Gregory D.
Viljoen, Johann H., FamilyMed
Viljoen, Rene, FamilyMed
Webb, David A.
Wiens, Barry M., FamilyMed(EM)
Wiens, H. Edward, FamilyMed
Williams, Anthony

RED DEER COUNTY

Chacon-Andrade, Hernando E.
Comeau, Raymond R., FamilyMed
Lampard, J. Robert
Schnepf, Trevor
Swainson, Stephen J., FamilyMed
Wilson, Marci L., FamilyMed

REDWATER

Erasmus, Jacobus F.
Erasmus, Magda
Mouton, Godwin P., FamilyMed
Van Der Walt, Marthinus

REDWOOD MEADOWS

Wilson, G S. Lowen

RIMBEY

Adzich, Kim P.
Boorman, Michael G.
De Bruyn, Jurie H., FamilyMed
Ellis, Christine J., FamilyMed
Nawrot, Mitchell R D.
Wickland-Weller, Monica L.

ROCKY MOUNTAIN HOUSE

Aasman, Edward J., FamilyMed
Berjat, Vanessa E I., FamilyMed
Bredenoord, Steven, FamilyMed
Bristow, Stanley G.
Brown, Gordon W., FamilyMed
Game, Kathleen E., FamilyMed
Garrett, Kyle J., FamilyMed
Kendall, Chris J., FamilyMed
Kirstein, Dolen D., FamilyMed
Peens, Erus J.
Peters, Johannes
Robinson, Gregg
Rogers, Kimberly A., FamilyMed
Roth, Harold G.
Saunders, James J., FamilyMed
Van Zyl, Stephanus A.
Witten, Allan D., FamilyMed

SADDLE LAKE

Leivo, Raymond D.

SEDGEWICK

Meer, Ahmed

SEXSMITH

Fourie, Anna P.
Oosthuizen, Jacobus F.
Van Zyl, Matheus C.

SHERWOOD PARK

Adams, James R.
Adams, Mohamed M.
Ahmed, Imran
Algu, Kemchand, FamilyMed
Ali, Hira
Anderson-Hill, Kimberly, FamilyMed
Aradi, Abdussalam M M.
Begalke, Annette D., FamilyMed
Benade, Johannes G., FamilyMed
Binns, Marichal A., FamilyMed
Brown, David J L.
Cahill, Eugene J.
Chiu, Michael S.
Cloete, Pieter D.
Collins, Paul H., FamilyMed
Daniels, Robert W.
De Souza, Marcelino
Denson, Stephen M A.
Dusang, Trent S.
Elfiky, Ashraf M.
Elliott, Vance W., FamilyMed
Emsalem, Ahmed M K M., FamilyMed
Farrell, Patti M., FamilyMed
Fisher, D. Scott
Fisher, Steven W W., FamilyMed(EM)
Ganjizadeh Zavareh, Farahnaz
Gee, Edward
Govender, Indhri, FamilyMed
Guhle, Mark E., FamilyMed
Hatfield, Richard H., FamilyMed
Heard, Neil M., FamilyMed
Ho, Allan
Jansen Van Vuuren, Stephanus J.
Johnson, Paul M., FamilyMed
Katz, Jerry C., FamilyMed
Khatter, Manishi, FamilyMed
Kluczynski, Pawel M.
Lasner, Brian R W.
Lee, Patricia A., FamilyMed

Lim, Wing F., FamilyMed
Mah, Kevin A., FamilyMed
Maharaj, Usha, FamilyMed
Mann Hosford, Lorraine E., FamilyMed
Mansell, Graham L., FamilyMed
Maraj, Reena
Olson, Cynthia I.
Patterson, Christina J., FamilyMed
Ramji, Moizali A.
Rezansoff, Natalie A., FamilyMed
Ribeiro, Rona G., FamilyMed
Robles, Melanie A., FamilyMed
Ruman, Tanya A., FamilyMed
Salgado Benavides, Carlos E., FamilyMed
Seto, Gordon W J., FamilyMed
Shaikh, Sharmeen
Siha, Hany H K.
Soyege, Oyebanjo A., FamilyMed
Stansberry, Patricia E.
Swinton, Andrew A., FamilyMed
Visconti, Vincenzo
Witzke, Gaynelle J.
Zaragoza, Antonio J.

SIKSIKA

Hewton-Backfat, Latisha, FamilyMed
Makokis, James A.

SLAVE LAKE

Caffaro, Paul A.
Du Toit, Petrus
Hamdan, Loai M K.
Hirawan, Natasha
Immelman, Philip L.
Keaveny, John A., FamilyMed
Marillier, Justin R.
Martin, Keith O., FamilyMed
O'Keeffe, Teresa
Payne, Daniel H.
Powell, Kara A., FamilyMed
Sheopershad, Vitesh
Skein, Willem

SMOKY LAKE

Du Toit, Dirk L.
Fatokun, Olumide J.
Raubenheimer, Anton M.
Raubenheimer, Stephan, FamilyMed

SPIRIT RIVER

Kitagawa, Eva B., FamilyMed
Phillips, Thomas J.
Spruyt, O. Wilhelm

SPRUCE GROVE

Abduelmula, Kamal A A.
Al-Shibani, Abdelmagid S M.
Ali, Amna
Bailey, Allan L., FamilyMed
Bergh, Nikoletta, FamilyMed
Currie, Melanie T., FamilyMed
Datar, Sunil
Dunbar, Ross H., FamilyMed
Erian, Ragaee S., FamilyMed
Erickson, Timothy N.
Fatima, Qamar, FamilyMed
Fetouri, Fawzi M., FamilyMed
Fung, Daisy, FamilyMed
Fung, Peter S M., FamilyMed
Gamra, Tarek A R.
Genge, A. Gaylene, FamilyMed
Gordillo, Chris G., FamilyMed
Janmohamed, Jamil, FamilyMed
Janschitz, Kristien N., FamilyMed
Karpiyevich, Maryna, FamilyMed
Khurram, Sabahat, FamilyMed
Kibria, Shawkat Z., FamilyMed
Kroeker, Stanley G., FamilyMed
Laidlaw, Carla S., FamilyMed
Malik, Samreen S., FamilyMed
McArdle, Mary P.
McNicol, Keith L.
Morrison, Matthew K.
Oduwole, Olusesan O.
Perry, Corinne A., FamilyMed
Piebiak-Patterson, Krista K., FamilyMed
Quinn, Matthew T., FamilyMed
Rai, Inderpreet S., FamilyMed
Sadiq, Ammara I.
Schulte, Conrad
Shaftar, Osama
Somani, Parviz N.
Somani, Salim
Soto Molina, Juan A., FamilyMed
Squires, Suzanne R., FamilyMed
Thompson, Elisabeth J., FamilyMed
Tsikata, Setorme A., FamilyMed
Van Slyke, Tiffany, FamilyMed

ST ALBERT

Al-Shami, Mohamad-Rakan
Anderson, Ronald R., FamilyMed
Arya, Neehar
Ayyobi, Amir
Bennett, Krista L., FamilyMed
Bennett, Matthew A., FamilyMed(EM)
Boman, Robert B.
Bouchard, Marie-Claude, FamilyMed
Brocken, Arno A L.
Buhr, Lori A., FamilyMed
Chehimi, Abdul-Hamid, FamilyMed
Ching, Karen P., FamilyMed
Clarke, Deirdre M., FamilyMed
Clarke, John E., FamilyMed
Cyngiser, Frances F.
Daloise, Robert A.
Daviduck, Wayne J., FamilyMed
De Witt, Schalk J., FamilyMed
Deane, Brian C M.
Dixon, Elizabeth, FamilyMed
Dromey, Edel, FamilyMed(EM)
Fahoum, Abdulmajid
Fairfield, Finlay M.
Fischer, Barbara L., FamilyMed
Gannon, Celine M., FamilyMed
Ghiassi-Razavi, Rezvan
Hauptman, Robert S.
Hayden, Brian C., FamilyMed
Hilner, Jon S., FamilyMed
Holm Jhass, Jacqueline L., FamilyMed
Hryciuk, Daniel J.
Jacobs, W F. Gerhardus
Johnston, Ian R.
Juta, Meghna P., FamilyMed
Kassam, Jacqueline C., FamilyMed
Kiraly, Dennis A.
Klassen, Sheri A., FamilyMed
Kralt, Douglas, FamilyMed(EM)
Kuc, Zenia N., FamilyMed
Lalic, Vesna
Lefebvre, Leon A J.
Lidkea, Marlene R., FamilyMed
Maclver, Douglas W., FamilyMed
Maclver, Shaunalee J.
Macedo, B A. Ben, FamilyMed
Mair, Walter M J.
Mangan, Kevin J., FamilyMed(EM)
Marcu, Maria, FamilyMed
Mason, Alicia A J., FamilyMed
McDonald, Allan A., FamilyMed
McDonald, Norman A.
McKague, Jeffrey
Morison, Nicholas J.
Mulder, John-Derek
Muncner, Peter
Mung, Dennis G.
Newnham, Peter J., FamilyMed
Palmer, Janet M.
Panesar, Bhavlene K.
Payne, Arthur A., FamilyMed(EM)
Pon, Freddy A.
Poon, Connie K H.
Pratt, Marielle E., FamilyMed
Pungur, Judit
Pungur Farrell, Erzsi
Rajoo, S. Nischal, FamilyMed
Rawoot, Ashfaq
Riaz, Sarah, FamilyMed
Rokosh, Jacquelyne L.
Ross, Scott A., FamilyMed(EM)
Sainsbury, Joanna B., FamilyMed(EM)
Schaffter, Margaret L.
Schubert, John D.
Shaker, Vajdiyeh
Shields, Stewart D., FamilyMed(EM)
Shukri Alalous, Nidaa
Singh, Sarab M.
Stewart, Darryl F.
Strytveen, Charly A., FamilyMed
Taparia, Sanjay
Toeg, Abraham
Ungerer, Danel
Wiens, Sheldon E., FamilyMed(EM)
Wong, Cindy M., FamilyMed(EM)
Wong, Rene, FamilyMed
Yue, Jennifer F W., FamilyMed

ST PAUL

Adebayo, Francis O.
Ahmad, Iftikhar
Akindele, Florence O.
Amusan, Isaac O.
Botha, Noreen M.
Ellaurie, Isphara
Gordon, Hester A.
Harmse, Albert C., FamilyMed
Nouh, Mohamed
Oosthuizen, Petrus P E.
Senekal, Margaretha A.
Werkman, Isabella M.
Woytiuk, Harvey P., FamilyMed

STAND OFF

Christenson, Susan A.
Tailfeathers, Esther E.

STETTLER

Agwaze, Monday M., FamilyMed
Bouwer, Elizma, FamilyMed
Bouwer, Pieter A., FamilyMed
Drummond, Alasdair R.
Du Toit, Francois J.
Heaven, Charles G.
Lockhat, Hassan S.
Vogel, Philip L.

STONY PLAIN

Abdullah, Ali R.
Bhardwaj, Sanjeev, FamilyMed
Boughen, Gregory C.
Butler, Gary C., FamilyMed(EM)
Chow, Samuel K K., FamilyMed(EM)
Crawford, Brent W E., FamilyMed(EM)
Du Preez, Johannes C., FamilyMed(EM)
Ehlers, Leo G.
Fuchs, C. Christian
Iwashkiw, Boris M.
Jansen, Paul J.
Jones, Anthony H D.
Le Roux, Jolene
Linehan, Patrick T., FamilyMed(EM)
Meeuwissen, Matthew J., FamilyMed(EM)
Nixon, Donald W.
Odugbemi, Olabisi O.
Oland, Ryan C., FamilyMed(EM)
Pattison-Bacon, James N., FamilyMed(EM)
Polack, Zenith E.
Potgieter, Stephanus D., FamilyMed(EM)
Quaye, Henry I.
Savard, Michael M.
Stonehocker, John L., FamilyMed(EM)

STRATHMORE

Avramenko, Victor W., FamilyMed
Bodruzic, Nada
Clarke, Alison M., FamilyMed
Damji, Rahim, FamilyMed
Emery, William T., FamilyMed
Fanning, J. Ward, FamilyMed
Gooden, Heather M., FamilyMed
Lavallee, Melvyn R.
Lobay, Lori A.
McColl, Mary E., FamilyMed
Muller, Samuel J., FamilyMed
Onwudiwe, Herbert O.
Piesas, David J., FamilyMed
Sader, Benjamin J., FamilyMed

SUNDRE

Barnsdale, Christopher A., FamilyMed
Foolen, Catharina H G M., FamilyMed
Irvine, Harland S., FamilyMed
Kowalsky, Glenn D.
Landsbergen, Eugene P.
Reid, Fiona
Reid, Katie
Rowntree, Carol I., FamilyMed
Souster, Timothy P W., FamilyMed
Ward, William J.
Warren, Robert G., FamilyMed
Warren, Vesta M., FamilyMed
Warwick, Simon P.
Wylie, Mark O., FamilyMed

SWAN HILLS

Elharathi, Hythum

SYLVAN LAKE

Bahler, Brad R., FamilyMed
Begley, Gareth
Fugler, Stephen R.
Hernberger, Julie A., FamilyMed
Janke, Fred H., FamilyMed
Kauchali, Muti-Ullah
Larue, Jordan M., FamilyMed
Mulholland, Michael G.
Myburgh, Johannes L.
Nel, Wilhelmina E.
Ngeth, Sereyrath, FamilyMed
Niemand, Rudolph E.
Sorensen, Donna J., FamilyMed
Taylor, Ieleen S., FamilyMed
Van Schalkwyk, Matthys C.

TABER

Beckie, Gerald V., FamilyMed
Chychota, Norman N.
Demontigny, Jillian, FamilyMed
Hargrove, Andrea L., FamilyMed
Hughes, Jeffrey R., FamilyMed
Rasmussen, Derek J., FamilyMed
Steed, Wade B.
Steed, Wesley B.
Torrie, Ryan D., FamilyMed
Wedel, Robert J., FamilyMed
Yamabe, David L., FamilyMed

THREE HILLS

Adebisi, Timothy A., FamilyMed
Dada, Daniel O., FamilyMed
Husain, Navaid
Reedyk, Martinus
Savage, Luke C., FamilyMed

TOFIELD

Hackett, Richard J.
Sapozhnikov, Marina

TROCHU

Calhoun, Erin, FamilyMed
Chari, Anish S., FamilyMed
Jaiyesimi, Olufemi B.

TWO HILLS

Hassan, Waseem
Satar, Abdul M A.
Van Wyk, Louis

VALLEYVIEW

Human, David S.
Schwegmann, LLewellyn
Swart, Ignatius
Verburg, Lucas, FamilyMed

VEGREVILLE

Edgcumbe, Daniel P.
Frank, Helen
Frank, Selby A.
Labuschagne, Pieter Willem
Strydom, David P J.
Sung, Patrick P W.

VERMILION

Bhuiyan, Omor F.
Duvenage, Jan Charles
Louw, Andre J.
Maulud, Awatef
Stewart-Hunter, George C.

VIKING

Gibney, Eugene
Hagen, Margarietha J.
Nieman, Riaan
Potgieter, Hermanus H J., FamilyMed
Van Rooyen, Calin L.
Welman, Johannes
Wilderdijk, Margot F., FamilyMed

VULCAN

Al-Samak, Sofian M A., FamilyMed(EM)
Ayers, Ian B., FamilyMed
Gausvik, Amy L., FamilyMed
Hudson, Sharlene M., FamilyMed
Sun, Gavin R., FamilyMed
Wade, Leonard R., FamilyMed
Webster, R. Shawn, FamilyMed

WABASCA

Hassen, Riyaan
Schofield, Grant M.
Uyirwoth, Gabriel

WAINWRIGHT

Anderson, Gordon S.
Bredenkamp, Thomas L.
Brilz, Beverly V., FamilyMed
De Vos, Werner
Hay, Kevin M., FamilyMed
Payne, Wendy J.
Ramsahoye, J W. Maximilian, FamilyMed
Samuel, John P.
Venter, Ruan F.
Visser, Pieter J.

WESTLOCK

Arps, Gina M., FamilyMed
Chakravarty, Subrata
Coulson, Pamela C., FamilyMed
Da Cunha, Noel A., FamilyMed
Finney, Trevor A.
Fourie, Johannes L., FamilyMed
Keay, James S., FamilyMed
Lategan, Jan H J.
Mydeen, M. Firdaus M., FamilyMed
Patel, Shashikant C.
Rekieh, Kassim M., FamilyMed
Simpson, Noemi S.
Spangenberg, Benjamin
Steyn, Daniela
Sun, J. Jianhang
Van Jaarsveldt, Hendrik S M.

WETASKIWIN

Adebisi, Omoniyi Y., FamilyMed
Ansari, Ziaul B.
Argals, Ivars J., FamilyMed
Bakshi, Tuhin K., FamilyMed
Brand, Johannes E., FamilyMed
De Wet, Lourens J C.
Dippenaar, Helgardt
Drolet, Terrence A., FamilyMed
Erwee, Franle
Gagnon, Bernard P.
Haidar, Mukhtar, FamilyMed
Hendriks, William L J., FamilyMed
Jeffery, Deborah A., FamilyMed
Johnson, Erik P., FamilyMed
Kirwan, Michael C.
Lee, Brian P.
Moolla, Yunus E.
Patel, Bhasker M., FamilyMed
Patel, Kalavati B.
Sikder, Mohammed Z.
Stassen, Leanda
Surgenor, Colum J.
Swartz, Carin
Tam, John K W.
Van Den Berg, Daniel J H.
Van Der Walt, Johannes C.
Venter, J. Christiaan, FamilyMed
Ward, Simon P.

WHITECOURT

Aleker, Junaid
Bablitz, Harvey A.
Bainbridge, J. Andrew
Basson, Ronel C.
Calitz, Jaco
De Jongh, Heinrich L.
Hattingh, Evert
Hodgson, Craig D., FamilyMed
Kulak, Larry M.
Laurence, Craig
Ojedokun, Jane O., FamilyMed
Ojedokun, Joseph O.
Train, Anthony D.
Van Schalkwyk, Daniel J.
Venter, Lizanne

BRITISH COLUMBIA

100 MILE HOUSE

Burton, Jennifer
Dickey, Rod G.
Klopper, Leila
Lubbe, Gerald W., FamilyMed
Mah, Franky, FamilyMed
Nicolson, R. Bruce
Ramorasata Ranaivonar, David H.
Street, Donald G.
Vithalal, Neetha, FamilyMed
Wendland, Wilfred

108 MILE RANCH

Hutchinson, Gordon B., FamilyMed(EM)

ABBOTSFORD

Agbahove, Onome T.
Ainsworth, Erin A E., FamilyMed
Alibhai, Haneef N., FamilyMed
Arham, Muhammad N.
Arnott, Alec H.
Bale, Michael
Barnard, Johan J H.
Beyers, Cornelia
Beytell, Daniel
Bhargavan, Odayoth K., FamilyMed
Bhatti, Harleen K.
Bhatti, Rajinder S.
Bhugra, Hardeep S.
Bjerke, Thomas L., FamilyMed
Blane, Shale
Brown, Stuart M.
Burns, Jonathan A., FamilyMed(EM)
Burrows, Simon L M.
Campbell, Michael D.
Campbell, Milena K., FamilyMed
Cappon, Ian D.
Chafe, Alfred, FamilyMed
Chan, John K F., FamilyMed
Chan, William Y F.., FamilyMed
Chaudhry, Yash
Chow, J. Holden, FamilyMed
Cochlin, Joseph L.
Codio, Circe, FamilyMed
Collingridge, H. Glenn, FamilyMed
Danescu, Virgil, FamilyMed
Dayananda, Narayanappa
De Beer, Johannes J.
De Jager, Eduard J., FamilyMed(EM)
De Leeuw, Charles B.
Driedger, Brian D.
Dueck, Kenneth, FamilyMed
Egolf, Richard J.
Fischer, Barbara J.
Fluit, Paul, FamilyMed
Forrester, Robert D.
Fourie, Clasina E.
Froese, David F.
Gill, Manmohanjit S.
Golshan, Ashkan, FamilyMed(EM)
Gosal, Manjit
Greyling, Gertie
Grover, Gagan C., FamilyMed
Gurjal, Anagha
Haque, Zia-Ul
Harder, Arthur
Hart, Greg C., FamilyMed
Heath, Andrea M., FamilyMed
Heffner, Gary I.
Henderson, Douglas M.
Hilliard, Neil K.
Htun, Ye
Husband, Daniel M.
Jaffri, Syed N.
Jan, Farida
Kahlon, Kuldip S.
Kaler, Harpreet
Khan, Shah F.
Khattak, Abid S.
Kinahan, Consuelo A P.
Konkin, Thomas M.
Kuhn, Fernando H.
Lail, Harajit S., FamilyMed
Landsiedel, Trevor M.
Loewen, Trenton D., FamilyMed
Maharaj, Damien D., FamilyMed
Mangat, Ramanjot K., FamilyMed
Martin, Ian, FamilyMed(EM)
Mbenza, Wenta L.
McConnell, C. Maureen, FamilyMed
McKenzie, Danica R., FamilyMed
Meloche, Leslie N., FamilyMed
Mia, Raziya, FamilyMed
Milne, Daniel, FamilyMed
Minovi, Moshkoo
Mitchell, Gerald O F., FamilyMed
Moodley, Clifford
Moodley, Nateeran P.
Moodley, Zenobia
Moore, Alan W.
Morrison, Ian R.
Muthayan, Dayananden V., FamilyMed(EM)
Neilipovitz, Catherine J., FamilyMed
Newton, Michael J.
Nickel, Murray, FamilyMed(EM)
Nyvall, Mary K., FamilyMed
Park, Andrew J., FamilyMed(EM)
Parkin, Henry N.
Patel, Sayera
Pauls, Ernest J., FamilyMed
Pawlovich, John P., FamilyMed
Pawlovich, Sarah L., FamilyMed
Peer, Ihsaan C., FamilyMed
Peters, Reginald L., FamilyMed(EM)
Rahal, Kamaljit, FamilyMed
Randhawa, Bawa S.
Ross, Donald A., FamilyMed
Saloojee, Farzana
Sartor, Jason R., FamilyMed(EM)
Scaman, Donald R., FamilyMed
Schriefers, Harald M.
Selina, Paul G.
Serelo, Larry G.
Shaikh, M. Asif
Shariff, Tahara J T.
Shaw, Cinthia F., FamilyMed
Shaw, Philip M., FamilyMed(EM)
Sherazi, Syed A R.
Shiu, Dominic
Skanthan, Sithamparanathan
Sood, Alok, FamilyMed
Street, Harry W.
Tan, Ann
Todorov, Krasimir G.
Turchen, Barry J.
Vaish, Saurabh, FamilyMed
Van Der Merwe, Christina J.
Van Tonder, Petrus J., FamilyMed(EM)
Vlckova, Ludmila
Walia, Tamana
Warkentin, James P B., FamilyMed
Watt, Elizabeth J., FamilyMed
Welsh, Richard M., FamilyMed
West, Jacques
White, Carole B T., FamilyMed
Whitley, Carol L.
Whittington, Christine A., FamilyMed
Wiebe, Harold J., FamilyMed(EM)
Windt, Adriaan
Yakubovich, Tatiana Y.
Yatscoff, Michael A., FamilyMed(EM)

AGASSIZ

Beaulieu, Marcella J., FamilyMed
Martins, Ivo P.
Phimister, Wayne, FamilyMed

AIYANSH

Arthur, Thomas D., FamilyMed
Estey, Ronald H., FamilyMed

ALDERGROVE

Ciavarella, Anthony L.
Gill, Sukhdev
Hirowatari, Sandra, FamilyMed
MacDonald, John J.
Tharani, Yasmin
Wolchok, Garnet R.

ALERT BAY

Booth, Susan A.
Ham, Clayton L.

ANMORE

Sedergreen, Christopher J H.

ARMSTRONG

Clement, Maureen A., FamilyMed
Dreyer, Nicolette M.
Kutsche, Reta A., FamilyMed
Lewin, R. Simon
McClellan, Kira, FamilyMed
Rutherford, Philip S., FamilyMed
Sandrik, Hana, FamilyMed
Schofield, John E.
Sherwin, Richard D., FamilyMed
Viljoen, Jean-Pierre

ASHCROFT

Kitshoff, Antoinette

ATLIN

Fast, Richard B.

BANK KELOWNA

Warren, Peter W., FamilyMed

BARRIERE

Clare, Terence P.
Marais, Ilke

BELLA BELLA

Iglesias, Stuart J.
Ikemura, Maki, FamilyMed
Rojeab, Farghad B Y.

BELLA COOLA

Anderson, Nancy J., FamilyMed
Cheng, Erika, FamilyMed
Lodge, Andrew M.

BLIND BAY

Johnston, Mary T.

BOWEN ISLAND

Schloegl, Susanne C.

BRENTWOOD BAY

Davidson, Graham M.
Forster, James H., FamilyMed
Morrice, Lora M., FamilyMed
Morton, David H.
Trottershaw, Terralene L.

BURNABY

Aiken, Paula A.
Alex, Erica S., FamilyMed
Anderson, Stephanie G., FamilyMed
Appleby, Kenneth J.
Apps, David A., FamilyMed
Arora, Amritpal S., FamilyMed
Avinashi, Ramesh K., FamilyMed
Baird, Rosemary D.
Baker, Raymond P., FamilyMed
Baldelli, Robert J., FamilyMed
Basco, Debbie E.
Baxendale, Gary R., FamilyMed(EM)
Beck, Frantisek, FamilyMed
Best, C. Dale, FamilyMed
Bitonti, Rosa M., FamilyMed
Bradbury, Bernadette, FamilyMed
Bradford, Moira
Buie, Anne E.
Byman, Vickie A., FamilyMed(EM)
Cameron, Ian B.
Chang, Kim S.
Chen, Kim W T., FamilyMed
Chiu, Doris, FamilyMed
Chomin, Gary L.
Chong, Elizabeth C., FamilyMed
Chorn, Michael
Choy, Wesley H.
Cochien, Eileen D C., FamilyMed
Collette, Ronald S.
Craigmyle, John W.
Cubra, Satnam S.
Curry, Donald J., FamilyMed
Dave, Mala, FamilyMed
Davey, E. Bruce
Demarchi, Ronald F.
Dhami, Randeep S., FamilyMed(EM)
Dharamsi, Altaf, FamilyMed
Doyle, Gordon L.
Dresselhuis, Jeffrey F T.
Dyment, David B., FamilyMed
Dyment, Lana W., FamilyMed
Earmme, Christine S Y., FamilyMed
Ebrahim, Karim
Ebrahim, Salim K.
Edmeston, John T., FamilyMed
Eichhorst, Nicolas O., FamilyMed
Farnan, Paul A., FamilyMed
Foo, S. Jo Ling, FamilyMed
Frame, Gidon, FamilyMed
Frank, Eleanor M.
Froese, Daniel W.
Fung, Clement, FamilyMed
Genest, Marcel
Germain, Susan T.
Goldberger, Michael H.
Grewal, Jeevan K., FamilyMed
Gu, Shian
Gupta, Vishal

Hanam, Philip J., FamilyMed
Harmer, Andrea L., FamilyMed
Hillier, Mark R.
Hillier, Stephen F.
Holman, Joan L., FamilyMed
Hruby, Lorna E., FamilyMed
Huang, Amy Y.
Jaffer, Perhez, FamilyMed
Jamal, Aliff, FamilyMed
Janzen, Derek S., FamilyMed
Jay, Jack C.
Jensen, Laura A.
Johar, H. Paul, FamilyMed(EM)
Jones, David W.
Kagan, Mary L., FamilyMed
Kam, Joan S., FamilyMed
Kan, Lorna C H., FamilyMed
Kan, Victor C.
Keegan-Henry, M. Jeanne, FamilyMed
Kenefick, Gerald, FamilyMed
Kenney, Gordon W., FamilyMed(EM)
Killick, Geoffrey W.
Klippenstein, Jodine R., FamilyMed
Koorjee, Rajabali G.
Krajina, Vladimir P J.
Kugyelka, Janet, FamilyMed
Ladhani, Azim, FamilyMed
Lai, Ming
Lang Hang Yee, Sam, FamilyMed
Lee, Herman, FamilyMed
Lee, Lawrence C F., FamilyMed(EM)
Legge, Rebecca J., FamilyMed
Lemke, Marvin G.
Leong, Yuen-Moi
Leonor, Rosario S., FamilyMed
Levis, Nicole D., FamilyMed
Li, Wei, FamilyMed
Lim, Princeton H.
Lim, Yen L., FamilyMed
Lin, Betty P., FamilyMed
Loewen, E. Nadine
Look, J. Michael
Lough, David D.
Lui, Albert K H.
Lui, Charlene L.
Lunderville, Peggy R.
MacDonald, Leah M., FamilyMed
MacKie, Susan J.
Malhi, Rajvinder K.
Martinez, Raul R.
McAnulty, Gregory J., FamilyMed
McCaffrey, Lindsay D., FamilyMed
McNeill, Colin A.
Miletto, Giovanni J., FamilyMed
Millar, Hamish S., FamilyMed(EM)
Mitha, Karime
Mohammed, Solomon
Monk, Tracy L.
Monks, Brian J.
Moore, Jennifer E.
Moseley, Douglas M.
Ng, Brian E., FamilyMed
Nguyen, Minh Hien, FamilyMed
Nijjar, Pravjot K., FamilyMed
Niou, Wayne P., FamilyMed
Oh, Charles S.
Oosterholt, Adrian G H.
Orng, Kanitha, FamilyMed
Parker, Salim, FamilyMed
Patel, Surekha G.
Perera, Arjuna R A., FamilyMed
Phan, Khai, FamilyMed
Pienaar, Colette
Radovic, Tatjana, FamilyMed
Rakhra, Ronbir S., FamilyMed
Rasool, Meenaz H A.
Rauh, Juergen R.
Ressl, Waqar-Un-Nissa, FamilyMed
Reznek, Stephen, FamilyMed
Rideout, John A.
Rife, William J., FamilyMed
Robinson, Jennifer M.
Ross, Shelley N., FamilyMed
Rowell-Wong, Joanne L., FamilyMed(EM)
Sakian, Nima, FamilyMed
Sam, Janie L.
Samaroo, Leslie L.
Sanghera, Baldev S., FamilyMed
Seethapathy, Vijayakumar
Shafie, Marzieh, FamilyMed
Sharp, Stephen A., FamilyMed
Sheu, K Y. Kevin, FamilyMed
Silverthorne, Clifford H.
Skinner, Sarah J.
Smith, Peter J.
Stewart, Julia R., FamilyMed
Sue, Donna
Sun, Anna K., FamilyMed
Symon, Keith
Tabarmanaf, Tofigh, FamilyMed
Takaro, Timothy K.
Tan, Lisa L Y., FamilyMed
Tanyous, Manal S R., FamilyMed
Te-Juatco, Lillien
Thauli, Gulraj
Therrien, Guenievre, FamilyMed
Ticea, Marilena C., FamilyMed
Tien, Teri C Y., FamilyMed
Toma, Cristian, FamilyMed
Tseng, Nora C.
Tsui, On Shun
Vasquez, Arthur R.
Verma, A. Tony, FamilyMed
Virani, Shaheena
Vorobeychik, Helena, FamilyMed
Vosloo, Dianne L., FamilyMed
Wang, Xin-Yong, FamilyMed
Wardill, Karen J.
Wong, Brendan J., FamilyMed
Wong, Davidicus A.
Wong, Eddie W.
Wong, Howard L.
Wong, Jeanny
Yang, Peter B.
Yap, David T T.
Zieffle, Laura J., FamilyMed

BURNS LAKE

Graetz, Michael A., FamilyMed
Hill, Alan M.
Norman, Gregory S., FamilyMed

CAMPBELL RIVER

Arnold, Robert C.
Auger, Veronique, FamilyMed
Baerg, Kerry J.
Beselt, Jeffrey K., FamilyMed(EM)
Brown, Paul K.
Byron, Kevin, FamilyMed
Carswell, Brian A.
Chan, Kong
Clark, Philip A H., FamilyMed
Coetzee, Jan Adriaan, FamilyMed
Daniels, Peter H.
Davis, Bre'el, FamilyMed
De Bruin, Louis D.
Dhansay, Aadil
Douglas, Duncan R., FamilyMed
Du Plooy Shuel, Sian, FamilyMed
Friderichs, Peter A., FamilyMed
Frost, Craig C., FamilyMed
Ghosh, Debasish
Gill, Shawn, FamilyMed
Gnawali, Meghraj
Grace, James C A.
Heath, V. Ann
Hinds, Philip R.
Jacobs, Gerhardus C., FamilyMed
Jensen, John M.
Jordan, Victor L., FamilyMed(EM)
Kask, Jennifer A., FamilyMed
Kennedy, Ian
Kindy, Anna O T.
Klein, Gunther, FamilyMed
Lan, Steven C., FamilyMed(EM)
Laxdal, Grant M., FamilyMed(EM)
Lebeuf, Stephen J., FamilyMed
Leslie, Jasmine J T., FamilyMed
MacNeill, Phillip
Marsh, Ian A.
McFadden, Caitlin, FamilyMed
Meckin, Michael C.
Morrison, Anne B., FamilyMed
Nelson, Joseph F., FamilyMed
Ness, Larry M., FamilyMed
Noel, Marie-Frederique, FamilyMed
Penhall, John R H., FamilyMed
Phipps, William H G.
Pocock, Rosemary F., FamilyMed
Prinsloo, Willem N., FamilyMed
Proctor, James S., FamilyMed
Ralston, Robert N.
Ramsey, Catherine O M V., FamilyMed
Ramsey, Robert T., FamilyMed
Ricketson, Jeffrey C., FamilyMed(EM)
Rowe, Patrick D., FamilyMed
Seldon, Roger C., FamilyMed
Stubbs, Esther R., FamilyMed(EM)
Sullivan, Liezl, FamilyMed
Sutherland, Kathleen M.
Sutherland, Robert L., FamilyMed
Veerapen, Valmiki, FamilyMed
Walker, Jonathan S D M.
Wilcox, Neil E.
Young, Donald J., FamilyMed

CASSIDY

Walmsley, Roger M., FamilyMed(EM)

CASTLEGAR

Ankenbauer, Martin R.
Bullock, David, FamilyMed
Clemans-Gibbon, Tracey M.
Jensen, Meghan B., FamilyMed
Larocque, David J., FamilyMed(EM)
Lesperance, M. Jose O., FamilyMed
Merritt, Keith E., FamilyMed
Smart, Ellen F.
Streich, Robert J.
Taylor, Megan M., FamilyMed
Vasil, Lisa, FamilyMed

CHASE

Barnard, Cornel, FamilyMed
Gill, Gursharan, FamilyMed
Sharma, Sandeep K., FamilyMed

CHEMAINUS

Archdekin, Murray W., FamilyMed
Broere, James J., FamilyMed
Gee, Douglas F.
Manhas, Prithpal S., FamilyMed
Morris, Tanis G W., FamilyMed

CHETWYND

De Jager, Johannes, FamilyMed
Roux, Pieter G V D.
Schreve, Siegfried E.
Venter, Anton

CHILLIWACK

Almas, Naveed
Bajwa, Amarjit S.
Bakker, Scott R., FamilyMed
Banta, Gregory A., FamilyMed
Bartel, S. Alexander
Basson, Paul J.
Bester, Stephanus P.
Boshoff, Johannes C.
Bright, Howard L., FamilyMed(EM)
Bright, Julia M., FamilyMed
Brink, Anette
Brodie, Brian D.
Bull, Ronald K.
Cambridge, Rosemarie T P.
Cambridge, Sean L O.
Chang, Ruoh-Yeng, FamilyMed
Cherniwchan, Darin P., FamilyMed
Chow, John C.
Chris, Chantal E., FamilyMed
Clarke, William E J.
Cormier, M. Alana, FamilyMed
Dibski, Daniel, FamilyMed
Dodds, Martin T.
Du Toit, Jacobus J J.
Dueck, Bradley J., FamilyMed
Ebesh, Osama
Enns, Gordon B.
Fitzpatrick, David J., FamilyMed
Fox, Robert G., FamilyMed
Goddard, Gwyllyn, FamilyMed
Graham, Paul A., FamilyMed
Greidanus, Marc, FamilyMed(EM)
Gupta, Kapil
Hall, Jeremy, FamilyMed
Hamilton, John A., FamilyMed
Harder, Kenneth K., FamilyMed
Henry, Alison, FamilyMed
Hirst, Kenneth R.
Ho, Kay
Hopkins, Thomas M.
Insanally, S S A. Reza
Jones, Ralph W M.
Kennedy, Jessica A., FamilyMed
Kishi, Ian G.
Kloppers, Stephanus P.
Krakower, Sharlene B., FamilyMed
Kroeze, Jan
Larsen, Sean S., FamilyMed
Laughland, Lori A., FamilyMed
LeGresley, Lisa B.
Lee, Shelter S., FamilyMed(EM)
Leyen, Heather A.
Lippa, Jodie L., FamilyMed
Lothian, Tara J., FamilyMed
Low, Ling Ling
Lynch, Erin C., FamilyMed
MacIntosh, Lachlan M., FamilyMed
MacKenzie, Mark S., FamilyMed(EM)
MacKenzie, Megan S., FamilyMed
Madill, Melanie L., FamilyMed
Mallam, Paul W., FamilyMed(EM)
Markey, Scott T., FamilyMed
Mummery, Martin R., FamilyMed(EM)
Mussell, Broncyn, FamilyMed
Nagdee, Muhammed Z.
Noble, Vello K.
Nyirenda, Vera R., FamilyMed
Olson, Joshua, FamilyMed(EM)
Oostenbrink, Jacob
Page, David A., FamilyMed
Parekh, Ritesh
Perkins, Laurie K.
Pleydell-Pearce, Julian S.
Prins, Mark R., FamilyMed
Quayle, Alandra N., FamilyMed
Quinn, E. Alan
Rawstron, Brock P., FamilyMed
Retief, PJ. Petrus, FamilyMed
Rose, Chantal E.
Ross, Cameron C., FamilyMed
Salter, Allison E., FamilyMed
Scholtz, Mervin, FamilyMed
Sia-Venugopal, Angeline C.
Singh, Anurag
Smit, Deon F.
Smith, Quentin A., FamilyMed
Snyman, Marianna S.
Stopforth, James G., FamilyMed
Stopforth, Jeanne
Swann, Lauren, FamilyMed
Szezepaniak, Theresa M S.
Ta, Thuan C., FamilyMed
Tewfik Moussa, Laila, FamilyMed
Van Der Watt, Morne J., FamilyMed(EM)
Van Rooyen, Renske
Van Wyk, Elmo
Van Wyk, Schalk S., FamilyMed
Viljoen, Lourens J.
Voth, Bevan R., FamilyMed
Weatherston, Philip M.
Wiebe, Bradley K.
Wiebe, Kristopher P., FamilyMed(EM)
Wilson, Kathleen M.
Wojcik, Tammy-Lynn, FamilyMed
Wolting, Jacqueline, FamilyMed

CHRISTINA LAKE

Lewis, Robert J., FamilyMed
Merry, David A., FamilyMed

CLEARWATER

Soles, John A.

COBBLE HILL

De Beer, Louis N.
Kardera, Edward P.

COMOX

Anderson, Douglas J., FamilyMed
Angus, Robert J.
Austin, Tanya, FamilyMed
Benson, Lissa D., FamilyMed
Bohonis, Dianne H., FamilyMed
Bowler, David F., FamilyMed
Bowler, Jannice, FamilyMed
Brailey, David A.
Bullock, Colin A J., FamilyMed
Burgess, Stephen M., FamilyMed
Calman, Arla S.
Chifor, Daniela P.
Colgan, Simon, FamilyMed
Cortez, Jennifer A., FamilyMed
Dan, Wai Ling, FamilyMed
Davyduke, Daria C., FamilyMed
Dawadi, Sudhakar R.
Esmaili, Haydeh F.
Fehlau, Barbara C., FamilyMed
Fockler, Donald F.
Galway, Carol S., FamilyMed
Graves, Carl O., FamilyMed
Gregory, Erin L., FamilyMed
Harris, Bradley J., FamilyMed
Hemmerich, Eva E., FamilyMed
Houlgrave, Albert W., FamilyMed(EM)
Howard, Edward W., FamilyMed
Huisamen, Charles C., FamilyMed(EM)
Jones, Shannon L., FamilyMed
Luke, Philip B., FamilyMed(EM)
Magor, Graeme F.
Manville, Margaret L., FamilyMed
Moosbrugger, Peter, FamilyMed
Neufeld, Michael J., FamilyMed
Ostry, Carol J.
Potter-Cogan, Rickard M., FamilyMed
Shoesmith, Trevor W., FamilyMed
Stocks, Alison M., FamilyMed
Tura, Alfredo, FamilyMed
Wainberg, Daniel, FamilyMed
Wale, Jason T., FamilyMed(EM)
Watters, Suzanne E., FamilyMed
Wernicke, Frank
Wilson, Theresa M., FamilyMed
Young, Louise H., FamilyMed(EM)

COQUITLAM

Ableman, Darryl J.
Agranovich, Natalie V.
Ali, Yasmin, FamilyMed
Behbahani, Mojgan, FamilyMed
Bergman, Henry S.
Bromilow, Sarah L., FamilyMed
Brumwell, Anne K.
Carkner, Robert M.
Carlson, Brian D.
Chan, Paul Y H., FamilyMed
Charkhsaz, Marjan, FamilyMed
Chek, Vanroeung
Choo Fone, Alan B.
Dabholkar, Shilpa, FamilyMed
Eddy, Donald, FamilyMed
Edwards, Ralph K.
Edworthy, John D., FamilyMed
Fox, Hyman I.
Fyfe, Jennifer M., FamilyMed
Gill, K. Kevin S.
Grootendorst, Martin W J., FamilyMed
Haines, Barbara J.
Hayes, Gary W.
Hediger, Marcel
Hirzer, Robert, FamilyMed
Ho Yuen, Diana E.
Huberman, Marvin

PHYSICIANS BY PROVINCE

Hutchinson, Angela, FamilyMed
Jawanda, Manindar
Kahwaji, Daniel
Kamyab, Mahshid, FamilyMed
Kelly, Dominick T.
Kim, Juan, FamilyMed
Kriik, Vivian H.
Lakher, Vladimir
Landy, Gerald J.
Lane, James E.
Lyon, Michael R.
Meetarbhan, Bheemdev
Merth, Kevin D M.
Moore, David W.
Naiker, Erushka
Nasseri, Lili, FamilyMed
Ng, Kwok Kuen
Oh, Dennis E., FamilyMed
Olson, James G.
Pang, G. Hannah, FamilyMed
Pfefferkorn, Carol R.
Read, Douglas E.
Rosenfeld, Michael W., FamilyMed
Ross, Kathleen M F.
Russell, Marianne T., FamilyMed
Saleeb, Ashraf H S., FamilyMed
Saunier, Dennis E.
Shadmani, Ramak, FamilyMed
Shehata, Esther I., FamilyMed
Shih, Peter D.
Shu, Abigail C.
Shu, Daniel S P.
Siu, Danny W.
Sivucha, Walter J.
So, Yan P.
Steinson, David S., FamilyMed
Stogryn, Dale A G., FamilyMed
Stogryn, Joan R., FamilyMed
Sundvick, Sharon M.
Toews, Bernhard J.
Tomaszewski, Christopher
Tosefsky, Merrick
Van Buuren, John C.
Warner, David W., FamilyMed
Wiebe, Douglas H.
Wilson, John T.
Wong, Wilfred T.
Yip, Barbara Y.
Yip, Daniel L K.

COURTENAY

Bakshi, Amitabh, FamilyMed
Barker, Katherine L K.
Bell, Laura P., FamilyMed
Blacklock, Donald M.
Brown, Ronald T.
Bryant, J. Scott, FamilyMed
Burry, Dana L., FamilyMed
Chow, Maria S M.
Crowe, D. Wayne
Davies, Michael J.
Daws, Tanja
De Jager, Lodewyk P.
Emmott, Kirsten B.
Fitzpatrick, John D.
Froese, Danielle K., FamilyMed
Galik, Marika Y., FamilyMed
Gee, Peter, FamilyMed
Green, Janet E., FamilyMed
Helmer, Richard P.
Herselman, Paul J., FamilyMed(EM)
Ho, Minnie M W., FamilyMed
Hunter, Susan J., FamilyMed
Ingrey, James R., FamilyMed
Jarman, David
Kenny, David J., FamilyMed
Konway, Desmond C.
Kosick, Kevin B.
Lamykina, Olga, FamilyMed
Langhans, J. Marcus, FamilyMed
Law, John O.
Matous, J. Stephen N., FamilyMed
McFadden, Nancy A., FamilyMed
McFarlane, Lori A., FamilyMed
McLaughlin, Janice A.
Murphy, Patricia M., FamilyMed(EM)
Musgrave, David P.
Nishio, Karen R.
Reggler, Jonathan G., FamilyMed
Robertson, Matthew A., FamilyMed
Roessel, Mary
Ruthnum, Mandy, FamilyMed
Sandwith, Sara A M., FamilyMed
Schoeman, Stefan, FamilyMed(EM)
Scruton, Joan H.
Stewart, Megan S.
Swanson, Kevin J., FamilyMed
Tancon, Gino
Thompson, Adam M., FamilyMed
Wiens, Debra D.
Williams, Tammy C.
Winter, Itta M., FamilyMed

CRANBROOK

Ackermann, Frank P., FamilyMed(EM)
Andreas, Cecile L.
Andreas, Gregory S.
Barnard, Alan D., FamilyMed
Bezuidenhout, Jakobus, FamilyMed
Bowden, William F., FamilyMed(EM)
Brown, Kenneth S., FamilyMed
Buchar, Helena, FamilyMed
Casselman, Charles W., FamilyMed
Chesney, Sarah A., FamilyMed
Coetzee, Dorothea
Cutler, Robert L.
Davis, Liesl H.
Dawe, Shawna J., FamilyMed
Dawson, D. Ross
de Villiers, Annalize
Falz, Stefanie, FamilyMed(EM)
Fourie, Hendrina, FamilyMed
Giobbe, Stefania
Heilman, James, FamilyMed(EM)
Hochart, Laurent
Ingram, Andrea D.
Joubert, P. Renier
Khosroshahy, Reza
Kilfoil, John E.
Lenz, David G.
Louw, Hendrik B.
Lowden, Keith G.
Macdonald, Stuart D.
Marlatt, Wanda J., FamilyMed
McIver, Glen R.
McIver, Kevin R., FamilyMed
Mistry, Sheela B., FamilyMed
Niedermayer, Robert W.
O'Brien, Robert L.
Oosthuizen, Madeline
Parnell, Tracey A.
Pienaar, Christopher T.
Pieterse, Wilhelm S.
Pont, Karen
Ries, Eugene F.
Rolandi, Joseph R., FamilyMed
Scheibenstock, Elisabeth A., FamilyMed
Sheffield, Robert I.
Shilhan, Caroline B E., FamilyMed
Shope, Kayode O.
Smith, Linda Y M., FamilyMed
Solcova, Silvia, FamilyMed
Suh, Huhn Soo
Thorne, Mary J., FamilyMed
Tiede, Roger H.
Turner, Jodie R., FamilyMed(EM)
Van Rensburg, Deon R.
Van Rietschoten, Walter A., FamilyMed
Wendel, Thomas
Wentworth, Kathryn
Witten, Edward J.

CRESTON

Blackbeard, Rosalind
Campbell, Crystal R., FamilyMed
Elemuo, Raphael E.
Ewing, Erin, FamilyMed
Griffioen, John P H., FamilyMed
Guthrie, Tara E.
Hoffmann, Daile R., FamilyMed
Hopkins, Suzanne E., FamilyMed
Le Roux, Kriegler, FamilyMed
MacKay, Faye D., FamilyMed
O'Halloran, Elizabeth
Persad, Atma, FamilyMed
Persad, Karen N., FamilyMed
Troughton, Timothy
Walker, Shawn T K.
Weaver, Andrew R., FamilyMed

CUMBERLAND

Hopwood, Marie-Clare
Hubner, Rurik, FamilyMed
Woldnik, Mark F., FamilyMed

DAWSON CREEK

Aganaba, Tari L.
Ashwell, Stephen P., FamilyMed
Aylward, Bedford Z.
Botha, Daniel J.
Botha, Daniel J P., FamilyMed
Brussow, Jacques E.
Bulterys, Octaaf S P J.
Burger, Tobias J L.
Clark, Margaret A.
Fletcher, Matthew D.
Gnanabaskaran, Ajantha, FamilyMed
Gnanabaskaran, Sangarapillai
Goetze, Andre
Hargreaves, James A., FamilyMed
Hellyar, Andrew G.
Joubert, Johan L.
Kritzinger, Johan F.
Larsen, Charles J.
Malik, Saira, FamilyMed
Meyer, Marius G.
Meyer, Ulrike, FamilyMed
Pilgrim, Michael A., FamilyMed
Pillay, Anandhan
Popa, Cornelia, FamilyMed
Roux, Ettienne
Sridhar, Shrikant K.
Verster, Servaas W D.

DEASE LAKE

Beaulieu, David S., FamilyMed

DELTA

Adam, Larry J.
Anand, Neeru, FamilyMed
Balakumar, Mahadeva
Barclay, John W., FamilyMed
Bird, Gordon S., FamilyMed(EM)
Boxer, Jack
Buckley, Heather, FamilyMed
Burger, Jasper G W., FamilyMed
Cameron, Marilyn J., FamilyMed
Cheng, Calvin W K., FamilyMed
Choo, Ivan S Y., FamilyMed
Choong, Wee Kei
Clarke, Robert J.
Commerford, Kathleen C.
Covaser, Florin, FamilyMed
Crossley, John F A.
Curry, Michael, FamilyMed(EM)
Dang, Norman K., FamilyMed
Davidson, Ronald
Dhillon, Baldev S., FamilyMed
El Karsh, Ashraf, FamilyMed
Enns, Heather-Anne S., FamilyMed(EM)
Eustace, A. Veronica, FamilyMed
Eustace, Dominic, FamilyMed
Fleming, Marcia M.
Fletcher, Judith E.
Gandhi, Vinod K., FamilyMed
Gemeinhardt, Christine E., FamilyMed
Gilchrist, Angus, FamilyMed(EM)
Henderson, Sylvia, FamilyMed
Henteleff, Sybil M.
Hoffman, Dale H M.
Hollinger, Horst
Hossack, Karen J., FamilyMed
Hsia, David
James, Richard H B.
Kahlon, Baldev S.
Kaliray, Jagdeepak
Kason, David V., FamilyMed
Kason, Deborah A., FamilyMed
Kason, Jason S., FamilyMed
Kordic, Ljiljana, FamilyMed
Krawchuk, Margaret
Kumar, Saroj
Lafleur, Jacques O J., FamilyMed(EM)
Lai, Ken K K.
Langner, Sabine M., FamilyMed
Lau, Edward T.
Lebel, Laureen D., FamilyMed
Ledsome, John R.
Lee, Colleen M Y M.
Lerner, Edward C.
Long, Rex
Low-Beer, Sophie C., FamilyMed(EM)
Manga, Ashok, FamilyMed
Manji, Alaudin E., FamilyMed
Martin, Craig W.
Martin, Thomas C.
McCuaig, Randall E., FamilyMed
McGrath, Frances C., FamilyMed
Mehraein, Nahid, FamilyMed(EM)
Mitchell, Ian L.
Mullard, David P.
Ng, Eddy H C., FamilyMed
Nicholson, Ashley, FamilyMed
Noble, Stewart J.
Panesar, Jarnail S.
Park, James N.
Porter, Robin B A.
Rai, Jagtar S.
Rai, Kuljinder K.
Rampersaud, Rai V S., FamilyMed
Ray, Martin L.
Revitt, David R.
Riesling, Micheal J., FamilyMed
Rogerson, Jennifer E., FamilyMed
Rubin, Daniel J.
Sachdev, Bhupinder S.
Sandhu, Gary G.
Sandhu, Ravinder S.
Scott, Michael D., FamilyMed
Shah, Inayat A.
Shier, Arthur A.
Sidhu, Kanwarinder S., FamilyMed
Sidhu, Shani
Sidhu, Shivinder S.
Singh, Baghat S., FamilyMed
Singh, Jit J.
Singh, Kanwal K.
Singhai, Rashmi
Surbey, Manindar
Talento, Riccoh R.
Tang, Keith Y K., FamilyMed
Turnbull, Ruth L.
Turner, Bradley J.
Vajravelu, Pavithra
Verma, Kumud, FamilyMed
Vipler, Christopher J., FamilyMed
Wilkhu, Gagan D S.
Williams, Rachel C., FamilyMed
Wong, H H. Adriana
Yuen, Tommy K., FamilyMed

DENMAN ISLAND

Malthouse, Stephen C.
Tetz, Doreen J., FamilyMed

DENNY ISLAND

Arnold, David H., FamilyMed

DUNCAN

Adnams, Michael B.
Avenant, Christiaan R J.
Barr, Susan L., FamilyMed
Bass, Bryan C.
Booth, Shannon
Conrad, Michael J., FamilyMed(EM)
Cunningham, Valorie L., FamilyMed(EM)
Cunningham, William J., FamilyMed(EM)
Cutt, Lorna E., FamilyMed
Eberhard, Juliette A.
Elliott, Teresa C., FamilyMed
Faulkner, Stephen J.
Fazil, Mohammad A.
Fuchs, Joachim
Gallagher, Lawrence P., FamilyMed(EM)
Gilbert, Howard R., FamilyMed
Griffin, Jonathan P M.
Grimes, Richard
Halvorson, James, FamilyMed(EM)
Harris, J. Kent, FamilyMed
Ibrahim, Mohammud S.
Ismail, Michelle M.
Jackson, Lauren E., FamilyMed
Jahnke, Natalie Ann, FamilyMed
Layher, Corrie R., FamilyMed
Lowther, Glen M.
MacGregor, Suilven R., FamilyMed
Malherbe, Jan A., FamilyMed
Martin, Rachael D., FamilyMed
McDonald, Stacey L., FamilyMed
McIntyre, Karen L., FamilyMed
Pascoe, Lynette A.
Pearce, Derek J., FamilyMed(EM)
Pearce, Nicolette S., FamilyMed
Philippson, Daniel O S.
Pullan, Rhoda Z., FamilyMed
Reimer, Harwood L., FamilyMed
Rimmer, Arthur T., FamilyMed
Rimmer, Isabel N., FamilyMed(EM)
Robertson, Nadine L.
Robinson, Daphne, FamilyMed
Robinson, Glenn P.
Rossouw, Vincent E.
Roy, Leonard W., FamilyMed
Sanders, Mark D L., FamilyMed
Scott, Dion, FamilyMed
Scott Ehle, Michelle L., FamilyMed
Seymour, Patricia F., FamilyMed
Swann, Frederick W.
Szabo, Angelika F.
Terlien, Paul C., FamilyMed
Thompson, Ann E.
Thompson, Robert J.
Thomson, Diane R L., FamilyMed
Toth, Gary A., FamilyMed(EM)
Turpin, Galina, FamilyMed
Van Schalkwyk, Johanna M.
Watson, Norman
Watt, Maggie J., FamilyMed
Wong, Herbert F.
Woods, Murray C.

ELKFORD

Klippenstein, Wanda Y L., FamilyMed
Ma, Marian C., FamilyMed
Sugden, Stuart R.

ENDERBY

Annan, Alastair W J.
Millar, Jeffrey H.
Wiebe, Russell

FERNIE

Clark, Ronald R.
Forrest, Shelley L., FamilyMed
Gadsden, Lori J.
Geddis, Rodney H.
Gray, Stephen J.
Loewen, Todd A., FamilyMed
McBeath, David J., FamilyMed(EM)
Michal, Paul T., FamilyMed
Robinson, Virginia W., FamilyMed(EM)
Rodrigue, Annick, FamilyMed
Rohn, Susan E., FamilyMed
Soetaert, Shayne C J., FamilyMed
Tessler, Lisa S., FamilyMed

FORT NELSON

Kassa, A. Ayalew
Lupu, Ioana, FamilyMed
Mostert, Marius, FamilyMed
Nickson, Lisa, FamilyMed

PHYSICIANS BY PROVINCE

FORT ST JAMES

Stent, Paul A.

FORT ST JOHN

Abdalla, Abdallah H.
Ali, Parveen S.
Amstutz, Ilona L.
Badenhorst, Charl J.
Barker, Charles P G.
Brand, Engela
Brand, Lukas J.
Brussow, Waldemar H.
Coatta, Erik S J., FamilyMed
De Bruyn, Jana
De Bruyn, Jesaias P.
Du Preez, Quinton
Esterhuizen, Stefanus C.
Hattingh, Jozua F.
Jamieson, Bruce H D., FamilyMed
Leeuwner, Isabel
Mackey, Paul V., FamilyMed
Moody, Richard G., FamilyMed
Page, Kevin B.
Parker, Jennifer A., FamilyMed
Pelser, Lorraine A.
Potgieter, Petrus D.
Romey, Juliyana, FamilyMed
Shoesmith, David R., FamilyMed
Sieberhagen, Janine A.
Temple, Becky A., FamilyMed
Thomson, Mark F.
Van Eeden, Jean L.
Van Rensburg, Benjamin W.
Watt, William G.
Wiebe, Sandra N., FamilyMed
Wright, Michael D., FamilyMed

FRASER LAKE

Douglas, Shannon, FamilyMed
MacLean, Joanna E., FamilyMed

FRUITVALE

Behrens, Ralph
Dalla Lana, Eric J.
Dryden, Fiona A., FamilyMed
Edge, Kristen, FamilyMed
McCoid, Elizabeth A.
Neil, Cynthia L.

GABRIOLA

Bosman, Francois M.
Brooks, David A.
Secord, Jonathan B., FamilyMed
Smith, Verne P.
Thorne, Tracey E., FamilyMed

GARIBALDI HIGHLANDS

Fisher, Gillian, FamilyMed

GIBSONS

Berinstein, Edward F., FamilyMed
Gupta, Rahul K., FamilyMed
Hourigan, John F.
Lehman, Robert M., FamilyMed
McFarland, James D., FamilyMed
Murphy, Paul E.
Paetkau, Carla
Petzold, James E.
Sparrow, Nicholas R., FamilyMed
Spithoff, Daren, FamilyMed
Stinson, Andrea H., FamilyMed

GILLIES BAY

Black, J. Kevin

GOLD RIVER

Durante, Kathleen M., FamilyMed
Ney, Patrick M B., FamilyMed
Yeomans, Timothy C.

GOLDEN

Clark, Virginia J., FamilyMed
Drysdale, Robert A.
Guy, Meghan L., FamilyMed
Larsen Soles, Trina M.
McCarroll, Kathryn E., FamilyMed
McKnight, Bruce E., FamilyMed
Mistry, Dinesh J., FamilyMed
Starke, Bruce T.
Tan, B J. Nicholas
Woolsey, Jennifer E., FamilyMed

GRAND FORKS

Coleshill, Geoffrey G.
Dalla Lana, Nathan G., FamilyMed
Sebastian, Robert D., FamilyMed

HAGENSBORG

Low Ah Kee, Julia, FamilyMed
Thommasen, Harvey V., FamilyMed

HALFMOON BAY

Newman, Robert W.

HAZELTON

Cummings, Michael R.
Eckfeldt, Charles T., FamilyMed
Kim, Mi Hwa, FamilyMed
Lee, Jenny, FamilyMed
Shrestha, Prakash T., FamilyMed
Shrestha, Sherry K., FamilyMed
Wiens, James, FamilyMed

HOPE

Adams, Rebecca A., FamilyMed
Asche, Gerd, FamilyMed
Asche-Quint, Ursula, FamilyMed
Botha, David
Christie, Susanne C., FamilyMed
Demian, Momen, FamilyMed
Green, Raymond, FamilyMed
Greggain, Joshua, FamilyMed
Kehler, Larry D., FamilyMed
Nanton, Ertha A., FamilyMed
Singleton, David B.
Switzer, Rosanna M., FamilyMed

HORNBY ISLAND

Chalfin, Laura
Chapman, John L.

HOUSTON

Chandler, Christopher J., FamilyMed(EM)
Morkel, Floris J.
Vestvik, Sandra
Woudstra, Kevin C.
Yaremco, Michael E.

INVERMERE

Arif, Stephen G., FamilyMed
De Klerk, Tania
Dibb, Maria, FamilyMed
Fleet, Jane A., FamilyMed
Gooch, Christopher E.
Johnson, Bruce B.
Louw, Wynand F., FamilyMed
Mannheimer, Gareth J.
Maytham, Colleen, FamilyMed
Olmesdahl, Arthur B.
Page, Shannon
Ross, Theresa A., FamilyMed
Walsh, Michael J.
White, Ian S., FamilyMed

KALEDEN

MacLean, Kenneth D.

KAMLOOPS

Anders, Benjamin, FamilyMed
Anderson, Julie A., FamilyMed
Bantock, Ivan M G.
Barnard, Isabel H., FamilyMed
Birdi, Parvinder K.
Borthwick, Murray J., FamilyMed(EM)
Bosman, Amanda, FamilyMed
Botha, Idelette
Boughton, Keith G., FamilyMed
Bradley, Krista A., FamilyMed
Brink, Christiaan, FamilyMed
Brown, William S.
Burris, H. Alan
Bushra, Ambreen
Cattaneo, Matteo, FamilyMed
Chahal, Sukhjiwan K., FamilyMed
Chow, Stephen
Chung, Allison N., FamilyMed
Davidson, R. Bruce, FamilyMed(EM)
De Kock, Hancke
De Kock, Victor E., FamilyMed
De Wet, Susanna A.
Del Begio, Grant R.
Desai, Vikas R., FamilyMed(EM)
Dodd, Graham A A., FamilyMed(EM)
Dong, Wayne A., FamilyMed
Du Preez, Miranda, FamilyMed
Dundas, Timothy, FamilyMed
Ewart, Elizabeth J., FamilyMed
Farrell, Jerome K.
Farrell, Richard P.
Farren, Ruth P.
Fike, Stanley D.
Filek, Brian J., FamilyMed
Gabriel, Alexandra
Gimbarzevsky, Boris P.
Gorman, Peter, FamilyMed
Hamilton, Douglas B.
Hornbeck, Tiffany K., FamilyMed
Howie, James F.
Huang, Alice
Hussain, Chaudry L.
Hutchison, S. Keith
Iqbal, Mudassir
Janz, Christopher B.
Kienitz, Norman G., FamilyMed(EM)
Kilpatrick, Bruce T.
Kip, Sven, FamilyMed
Klassen, Rodney H., FamilyMed(EM)
Koochin, Harvey L.
Kruger, Frederick J., FamilyMed
Langford, Mark E., FamilyMed(EM)
Laupland, Brenda R., FamilyMed
Lawrie, Selena, FamilyMed
Loland, Peter, FamilyMed
Mahmood, Arshad
Malan, Jacobus F.
Manak-Muhr, Mandy K.
Marke, Charles J.
Mawdsley, Caitlin S.
McLaren, Roderick C., FamilyMed
Meredith, Samantha J., FamilyMed
Montalbetti, Kraig C., FamilyMed
Montgomery, Scott B.
Nair, Suresh R.
Newmarch, Bruce G.
O'Connell, Jason C.
Oakes, Jennifer A.
Odubote, Oladele O.
Olabiyi, Bamidele O.
Passerin, Orlando, FamilyMed
Patch, J. Randall, FamilyMed
Patterson, Theresa M A.
Poelzer, Brian J.
Prelypchan, Christopher J., FamilyMed(EM)
Pretorius, Lennard
Rainier-Pope, Nicholas D., FamilyMed(EM)
Reid, John B.
Ring, Todd J., FamilyMed(EM)
Ritenburg, David L.
Ritenburg, Hannelore
Rollheiser, Steven P.
Russell, Edward S.
Schroeder, Adele M., FamilyMed
Schumacher, Gerhard, FamilyMed
Sigalet, J. Phillip
Smillie, Tracey C., FamilyMed
Sommerville, Andrew I.
Steele, Lisa M J.
Stefanyk, Harold N., FamilyMed
Steyn, Jacobus H.
Stinson, R. William
Stoltze, David A., FamilyMed
Sunder, Ravi K B., FamilyMed(EM)
Swart, Servaas D K.
Sze, Shirley W M., FamilyMed
Tevendale, Suzi
Thomas, Jennifer L.
Thomasse, Robert L.
Tsuchiya, Shauna C., FamilyMed
Van Dyk, Johannes B.
Van Heerden, Johannes A W.
Van Zyl, Hendrik P., FamilyMed(EM)
Vlahos, Susan D.
Vukusic, Alan V., FamilyMed(EM)
Waller, Julian R L.
Weimar, Sophie-Anne, FamilyMed
Wiedrick, James E D., FamilyMed
Wilson, Michael S.
Wiltshire, Jonathan M.
Wood, Douglas S.
Wroz, Paul W K., FamilyMed(EM)
Wynne, Andrew D., FamilyMed(EM)
Yanko, Paul E., FamilyMed
Zsigmond, Otto

KASLO

Thibodeau, Denis L.

KELOWNA

Adam, Derek L., FamilyMed
Allardyce, Pamela J., FamilyMed
Allison, James M.
Andrews, Christopher D., FamilyMed(EM)
Andruchow, Angela A., FamilyMed
Appleby, Michael B.
Atrens-Sharko, Maureen, FamilyMed(EM)
Baillie, Mark S M., FamilyMed
Balfour, Nicholas J B., FamilyMed(EM)
Bentley, Janna, FamilyMed
Bergh, Irene C., FamilyMed
Bhatt, Manish, FamilyMed(EM)
Blinkhorn, Nina A.
Bobyn, Larry
Bobyn, Michael P.
Boshoff, Hendrik C.
Brears, Sarah L., FamilyMed
Broome, E. Alan
Brown, Jeffrey K., FamilyMed
Bunten, Earle R.
Burgess, Terrance D., FamilyMed(EM)
Butterworth, Peter J.
Buzatu, Liliana
Canning, K. Alexander
Carver, Rachel D.
Chamberlain, Grant W., FamilyMed
Cheyne, William J., FamilyMed
Chirayath, Haiju
Claremont, Shari L., FamilyMed
Clark, Linden A., FamilyMed
Clark, Mark L.
Conchie, Robert M., FamilyMed(EM)
Conradie, Johannes L., FamilyMed
Cosmann, Peter C.
Cridland, Ronald G., FamilyMed
Crippen, Craig A., FamilyMed
Crittenden, Roger K.
Dawson, John A., FamilyMed
De Pieri, Andrew P., FamilyMed
De Villiers, Frederik U.
Deliyannides, Alexandra, FamilyMed
Dessens, Peter N.
Docherty, Henry V., FamilyMed
Docherty, Marjorie A., FamilyMed
Dortaj Rabori, Mohammad A.
Du Plessis, Johan, FamilyMed
Dusik, Laureen A.
Eliason, Barry K.
Emslie, R. Jim
Erasmus, Dorethea S., FamilyMed
Ertel, Michael J., FamilyMed(EM)
Etheridge, John-Paul B., FamilyMed
Etherington, Jeremy, FamilyMed(EM)
Evans, Janet A., FamilyMed
Fergusson, Sheila M., FamilyMed
Figurski, Michael R.
Fisher, Janis M., FamilyMed
Fitzpatrick, Aaron, FamilyMed(EM)
Fromberg, P. Mark
Fyles, Gillian M.
Garrett, Gerry
Godsell, Sally J.
Golbey, Michael J.
Goldberg, David J.
Gore, Ron
Graham, Dianne, FamilyMed
Graham, Louise, FamilyMed
Greeff, Herman, FamilyMed
Green, Daphne E., FamilyMed
Griswold, Dean A., FamilyMed
Gustavsson, Eric S.
Halpenny, Robert
Hamm, Darrell A., FamilyMed
Hancock, Larry G.
Hart, Paul J.
Hawker, Linda J., FamilyMed
Hayward, Clyde
Henry, Alison, FamilyMed
Hignell, Allen B., FamilyMed
Hopman, Michael, FamilyMed
Hopp, Marilyn H.
Hudson, Gregory N.
Hughes, Adrian M.
Hull, Constance L., FamilyMed
Huxtable, Leslie J.
Imrie, Diana M G.
Jackson, Martin R., FamilyMed
Jameson, Cathy Ann.
Johnston, Terry G.
Jones, Glynn C., FamilyMed
Joshua, Rodney S., FamilyMed
Kanerva, Kevin J., FamilyMed(EM)
Karolak, Marek E.
Ketch, James E., FamilyMed(EM)
Khan, Obaid-Ur-Rahman
Kipnis, Christopher
Klammer, Gayle M., FamilyMed
Koehle, Shawna L., FamilyMed
Kolkind, Kristie-Ann, FamilyMed
Korzan, Gregory J.
Koss, Michael A., FamilyMed
Krznaric, Joseph, FamilyMed
Lacroix, Lianne
Lai, Wayne W.
Lange, Alden W., FamilyMed(EM)
Lichtenstein, Tersia
Linden, Paul N., FamilyMed(EM)
Livingston, Christopher
Loken, John D.
Lypchuk, Lauren C., FamilyMed
MacDonald, Jennifer L.
Mace, Jeanne R., FamilyMed
Mackle, William R.
Maritz, Leonie
Martin, Heather S., FamilyMed
McCloskey, Gregory T.
McDonald, Heather M W., FamilyMed
McGinness, Clare A.
McIntosh, Jan K., FamilyMed
McKee, I. Bruce F.
McLellan, Marie-Carolyne, FamilyMed
McLoughlin, Ravana-Sue

PHYSICIANS BY PROVINCE

McNern, John K., FamilyMed
Medynski, Susan C., FamilyMed
Mirchandani, Deepu
Monteleone, Bradley J., FamilyMed
Morgan, Marianne N.
Morris, Adrian C B., FamilyMed
Murray, Michael J., FamilyMed(EM)
Nash, L W. Sandy
Neufeld, Dennis R.
Nottebrock, Douglas H., FamilyMed
O'Neill, Linda J., FamilyMed(EM)
Obedkoff, Daniel P., FamilyMed
Omelchuk, Alex, FamilyMed
Outram, Christopher P E.
Pagdin, Grant, FamilyMed
Parker, Julie L., FamilyMed
Pasenau, Allison M., FamilyMed
Pavan, Luigi A., FamilyMed
Penner, Peter R.
Perri, Elizabeth M.
Plecash, B. Gail, FamilyMed
Podavin, Joey N., FamilyMed
Price, Jonathan P M., FamilyMed
Purdon, Michael A J.
Reeves, Hien Nguyen
Reynolds, M. Lynn, FamilyMed
Richardson, Dellmari, FamilyMed
Rishi, B. Jane, FamilyMed
Sarbit, M. Danielle, FamilyMed
Scheffler, Erika J., FamilyMed
Schnurr, Joseph A.
Schriemer, Ronnald
Scott, Peter D M.
Sebulsky, Tara L G., FamilyMed
Segers, Isidor
Shaw, Laura K., FamilyMed
Shepherd, Michael A.
Smith, Scott, FamilyMed
Stasiak, Lidia M., FamilyMed
Steinruck, Martin W., FamilyMed
Stevenson, J. Milton
Suciu, Valentin S., FamilyMed
Swart, Rosalie D., FamilyMed
Taylor, Thomas G., FamilyMed
Tereposky, Lynne M., FamilyMed
Thomasse, Michele D., FamilyMed
Thomson, Alexandra E., FamilyMed
Ullah, Farid
Van Heerden, Andre, FamilyMed
Van Heerden, Auret H.
Verdurmen, Maria T., FamilyMed
Wall, Cara L E., FamilyMed
Wall, Mary T.
Warrender, A. Brian
Watson, Andrew F., FamilyMed
White, Keith J.
White, Philip, FamilyMed
Whiting, David A., FamilyMed
Wickstrom, Wendy L., FamilyMed
Wiebe, Lawrence P.
Wiese, Ben
Wiese, Lize
Williams, Robert D.
Wong, Mandy
Woychuk, Wesley F.
Yarrow, Colin F., FamilyMed
Zuberi, Najeeb A.

KEREMEOS

Boshoff, Johan A., FamilyMed
Louw, Marina
Partridge, Gerald W.

KIMBERLEY

Du Preez, Anneline, FamilyMed
Haiduk, Michael J., FamilyMed
Hale, Ilona, FamilyMed
Keyzer, Yvonne J., FamilyMed
Lunge, Ryan J., FamilyMed
Nash, Ronald A.
Van Zyl, Shaun

KITIMAT

Carstens, Derek J.
Craven, Kenneth
Huang, Li Ming.
Kay, Sabina
Mills, Howard J P.
Van Der Westhuyzen, Willem J.
Van Schalkwyk, Andries S., FamilyMed
Van Wyk, Bernize
Wahl, Marius C.

LADYSMITH

Britton-Foster, Timothy S., FamilyMed
Brockley, Graham H., FamilyMed(EM)
Fritsch, Christian
Fritsch, Emanuel
Igbinosa, Christine
Kennedy, Fergus J.
Kilvert, Vivan M., FamilyMed
Lisinski, Julian T., FamilyMed
Potts, John D.
Steeves, Emily N.
Swamy, Pramod, FamilyMed

LAKE COWICHAN

Kerswell, Philip
Postuk, Peter C., FamilyMed

LANGLEY

Adamson, Maureen E., FamilyMed
Afzal, Ayesha N.
Ajayi, Raphael O., FamilyMed
Alaaraji, Yassir
Altman, Yevgeni, FamilyMed(EM)
Ambulgekar, Shivaji M., FamilyMed
Aspinall, Hugh
Astrein, Alexey
Baby, Benjamin J., FamilyMed
Baldock, Robert L.
Bhartia, Sanjay M.
Blackmore, Richard G.
Blankstein, Kenneth C.
Borg, Mary Josephine.
Bowling, Sheila D., FamilyMed
Brown, Windy M., FamilyMed
Brynjolfson, John R.
Budau, Heinz E.
Chapman, David B.
Chin, May K M.
Chitsaz, Niloofar, FamilyMed
Chlebak, Anna
Chou, Benjamin
Cilliers, Philip
Clayton, Russell P., FamilyMed
Cooper, H. Douglas
Coulter, William G.
Day, Stephen C.
De Vynck, Willem E., FamilyMed(EM)
Delair, Leonard C.
Demian, Ruth A.
Desai, Shailesh M., FamilyMed
Du Plessis, Catharina H.
Dutchyn, Shannon L., FamilyMed
Esmail, Mansurali H M.
Fagan, Mitchell
Fasihy, Elham, FamilyMed
Follows, Jonathan M.
Frayne, Alister F., FamilyMed
Gerhart, Stanley
Ghazali, Jufri, FamilyMed
Ghohari, Foroozan, FamilyMed
Gill, Prabhjot, FamilyMed
Gulka, Mark O.
Gupta, Geetha, FamilyMed
Hansen, Steven G.
Haq, Farhan
Heller, Brian W.
Higginson, Judy J., FamilyMed(EM)
Hitchman, Derek W.
Hsu, David H J., FamilyMed
Hsu, Richard C., FamilyMed(EM)
Jhameel, Rafet
Khan, Anwar A., FamilyMed
Khan, Muniba M., FamilyMed
Koorts, Sybil, FamilyMed(EM)
Legaspi, Ofelia
Lirenman, Michael A., FamilyMed(EM)
MacIntosh, W. Daniel
Martin, Brendan E., FamilyMed
Mason, Cheryl R.
Mason, Karen E.
Matthews, Ronald B.
McCann, Michael A.
McDonald, Don G.
McQuarrie, Lucinda J., FamilyMed
Methven, Peter G.
Miller, Mark W.
Morgan, Brian J., FamilyMed
Myers, Nigel T B., FamilyMed
Nataros, Gary S.
Newton, Trevor M., FamilyMed(EM)
Ng, Kenneth K-H.
Ojaghi, Elham, FamilyMed
Park, Thomas J H., FamilyMed
Phillips, Dianne K.
Plante, Jeffrey L., FamilyMed
Polyhronopoulos, Spiro, FamilyMed(EM)
Pushie, Mary K.
Rath, Michael B., FamilyMed
Rees, John D.
Rezazadah, Fareidoon
Rich, Barry W.
Richardson, David R.
Rosenczweig, Carolyn C., FamilyMed
Sank, Leslie G.
Shore, Stephen M.
Siddiqui, Iqbal M., FamilyMed
Simkus, Raymond
Singh, Sonia A., FamilyMed
Smith, Cameron D.
Smith, Robert M.
Somani, Rizwan
Soni, Anil T., FamilyMed
Soubbotina, Janna, FamilyMed
Stephany, Harold E.
Stepney, Sandra K.
Suh, Young S., FamilyMed
Tekle, Abedom
Thompson, Jeannine M., FamilyMed
Tran, Phu Manh, FamilyMed(EM)
Trinh, Thomas Q N., FamilyMed
Van Schagen, Carolyn M., FamilyMed
Van Wyk, Andre R., FamilyMed
Vivier, Hester C., FamilyMed
Wagar, Donald B.
Waiz, Richard L.
Watt, Beth C.
Wilson, Robin T.
Wong, Anita K., FamilyMed
Wong, Christopher C K.
Wong, Flora F M., FamilyMed
Wong, Leo K H., FamilyMed

LANTZVILLE

Grace, Francine S.
Jones, Keith W.
Mark, Patricia H.
Niles, Clarence, FamilyMed
Pienaar, Louise, FamilyMed
Steyn, Marius F., FamilyMed
Stronge, David M., FamilyMed
Torrie, Kathleen A.
Westwood, David M., FamilyMed

LAZO

Christiansen, Gary R.
Hemmerich, David
Minkley, Aaron A D., FamilyMed

LILLOOET

Humber, Nancy L., FamilyMed
Kellerman, Adriaan I.
Mascher, Karl H.
Miller, Terrence R.
Routley, Ian G.

LIONS BAY

Angus, Eric E., FamilyMed(EM)

LOGAN LAKE

Sheik, Uzair

LUMBY

Barss, Alex
Wheeldon, P. John
Wright, Stephen J., FamilyMed

LYTTON

Hoffe, Charles D.

MACKENZIE

Card, James, FamilyMed
Kabongo, Jean-Pierre
MacKenzie, James C., FamilyMed

MALAHAT

Krieger, Michael P.

MAPLE RIDGE

Bartel, Douglas W., FamilyMed(EM)
Bhatti, Virinder S.
Botha, Francois
Botting, Douglas A.
Burns, Kenneth J.
Chapman, Dennis R.
Connor, Marla E.
Dawson, Keith, FamilyMed
De Klerk, Anton B.
Dhaliwal, Shannon
Du Toit, Petrus J J.
Dugdale, Ian P.
Edwards, Wesley J.
Fernandes, Clarence R.
Fetaz, Louise K M.
Gounden, Kandasamy, FamilyMed
Grist, Robert D.
Haider, Syed N.
Harrison, Robert G.
Hatlelid, Leonard W.
Henstock, Hendrik D.
Hyams, Ian A.
Johnson, Nelie C., FamilyMed
Karmali, Alkarim N K.
Kelly, Laura J., FamilyMed(EM)
Khan, Hafshah, FamilyMed
Kim, Don Wook, FamilyMed(EM)
Lam, James S M., FamilyMed(EM)
Lim, Fong-Suan
Little, Michelle J.
Loch, Simone R M., FamilyMed
Louise, Gina, FamilyMed
Luitingh, Ursula
Lytle, Craig R.
Marais, Cilliers
Mawani, Shiraz H L.
Mentz, Hendrik
Milewski, M. Martin
Moore, Deborah C.
Moore, Randall W., FamilyMed
Nadella, Rajasree
Naidoo, Salendra D.
Neufeld, Allen V.
Pater, Elzbieta
Patidar, Deepakkumar V.
Pattinson, Catherine S.
Perry, Theresa
Rak, Viktoria
Richards, Willem J.
Robson, Kathleen E.
Russell, Averil E., FamilyMed
Samimi, Mehran, FamilyMed
Sauder, David A., FamilyMed
Sergeeva, Danielle, FamilyMed
Sidhu, Satinderpal
Sindhar, Tanbir K.
Swanepoel, Wilhelm A.
Swift, Margaret E., FamilyMed
Tinney, Ward T.
Tong, Raymond Q L.
Van Gend, Richard F.
Verbonac, Garth S J., FamilyMed
Verrico, Howard J.
Villasenor, Fernando M., FamilyMed
Walton, Lorne A.
Warmenhoven, Wilhelm H.
Wasti, Qasim H., FamilyMed
Wasti, Tehmina Q., FamilyMed
Williams, Pieter
Wong, Daniel K C.
Zubek, Elizabeth M., FamilyMed

MASSET

Leslie, Michele I., FamilyMed
Rempel, Peter T.
Wilhelm, Andrea, FamilyMed

MAYNE

Losier, Juliana, FamilyMed

MCBRIDE

Jackson, Michael H.
Owega, Josef, FamilyMed

MERRITT

Bester, Urbanus F., FamilyMed
McLeod, Donald M.
Ross, Duncan A.
Simon, Paul B.
Smit, Andries A.
Van Der Merwe, Errol J.

MILL BAY

Decker, Robert F., FamilyMed
Galbraith, L. Dawn, FamilyMed
Grymaloski, Kim, FamilyMed
Hartford, Lesley A., FamilyMed
Klopper, Laurens F.
Laurence, Jennifer, FamilyMed(EM)
Reynolds, William J.
Wilson, Jean-Marie J., FamilyMed(EM)
Wilson, Lisa A.

MISSION

Arnott, Gail L.
Barnsdale, Emily R.
Barnsdale, Peter H., FamilyMed
Bhatt, Manjunath K., FamilyMed
Blackwood, C. Matthew, FamilyMed
Campbell, Morgan R.
De Klerk, Willem A.
Frew, Peter-John
Hobson, Steven G.
Jackson, Robin M.
Johnson, Andrew A., FamilyMed
Kornelsen, Jeffrey L., FamilyMed
Mansingh, Sohan
Marazzi, Alex S., FamilyMed(EM)
Nemanishen, Gerald, FamilyMed
Patel, Parinkumar S., FamilyMed
Pomeroy, Carol A K.
Potter, Lynne M.
Pretorius, Juan M.
Quan, Alyson D.
Rahimi, Farid A.
Rossiter, Liesl C., FamilyMed
Sabanathan, Sayanthan, FamilyMed
Siemens, Gwendolyn B J., FamilyMed
Siemens, Randolph W.
Smith, Jean-Marc C., FamilyMed
Somani, Mansurali R., FamilyMed
Theron, Paul S.
Welsh, Lawrence, FamilyMed
Wong, Keith C K.
Wouterloot, Johan, FamilyMed
Wright, Linette
Yokoyama, Benjamin C.

NAKUSP

Goranson, David C., FamilyMed(EM)
Kelland, Diana M., FamilyMed
Lea, Norman, FamilyMed
Subzwari, Sayed, FamilyMed

NANAIMO

Allison, Simon M., FamilyMed
Babuin, Peter P E.
Baird, Andrew C., FamilyMed
Balfour, Clive H.
Beerman, Stephen B., FamilyMed
Belisle, Melanie, FamilyMed(EM)
Bland, Jonathan D.
Bodenstab, Robert A.
Boshoff, Pieter
Bothma, Daniel P J., FamilyMed
Bradley, Douglas L.
Bruce-Houle, Gwen G.
Bucksteg, Ute
Calvin, Brian C., FamilyMed
Cancade, Edward M., FamilyMed
Carruthers, Robert J.
Chan, Francis M Y C., FamilyMed
Chen, Dalton T., FamilyMed
Cline, John C.
Coates, Kerry J.
Colborne, William H.
Collins, Christopher A., FamilyMed
Cone, Richard L., FamilyMed
Cooper, Carley N., FamilyMed(EM)
Culp, Gregory
Da Silva, Sandy C., FamilyMed
Davies, Thomas J.
De Paoli, Lorne E., FamilyMed(EM)
Dickinson, Lara, FamilyMed
Digney, Andrew
Dorran, Thomas J., FamilyMed(EM)
Dunne, Michel I P., FamilyMed(EM)
Dunstan-Adams, Elizabeth E.
Edwards, Christopher G., FamilyMed
Ehman, William J.
Elekiaby, Amr Saad
Feick, Elizabeth A.
Filanovsky, Yevgeny I., FamilyMed(EM)
Findlay, Sheila J.
Flesher, Michael F.
Forrester, James C., FamilyMed
Francis, James E., FamilyMed
Gooch, Peter A.
Goodall, R. Lorne, FamilyMed
Grabher, John J., FamilyMed(EM)
Grantner, Eric W.
Guzder, Rustom N.
Harkness, Debra L., FamilyMed
Hatchwell, Anthony R.
Hepburn, Beth
Ho, Ben, FamilyMed(EM)
Houghton, Kelvin T.
Humphries, Alexander, FamilyMed
Huska, Linda A., FamilyMed
Igbinosa, Osayuwame
Irvine, Lorne G.
Janse Van Rensburg, Renier, FamilyMed
Janssen, Nicolaas J C., FamilyMed
Javaheri, Erfan
Jonker, Jacobus M.
Kaban, Allan R., FamilyMed
Kao, K. Jesse, FamilyMed(EM)
Karrel, Abram I G., FamilyMed
Kazanowski, Davina A.
Kelly, Meghan L., FamilyMed
King, Kathryn A., FamilyMed
King, Peter A C.
Kingsley, Justin J., FamilyMed
Kotze, Charlene, FamilyMed
Kulla, Steven B., FamilyMed
Kurytnik, Ryan D., FamilyMed
Lam, Charles N H.
Lane, Anthony P., FamilyMed
Lanfear, Paul C., FamilyMed
Love, Robin R R., FamilyMed
Luttrell, Kerry S S.
Mander, Jatinder S., FamilyMed
Mann, Kenneth F.
Marback, Randolph M.
Mark, Helmut W.
Marshall, L. Maureen
Marwood, Daniel C.
McIlwaine, Margaret C.
McNie, R. Scott
Metrowich, Peter J., FamilyMed(EM)
Miller, Luella M., FamilyMed
Mitchell, L. Andrew
Montgomery, Ian D.
Moonsamy, Chrisen
Moonsamy, Prunella
Moore, Derrick D., FamilyMed(EM)
Morris, Michael J., FamilyMed
Mulder, Josef S.
Njalsson, Thorstein, FamilyMed
Nuamah, Francis N.
O'Farrell, Jennifer A C., FamilyMed
Oberholster, Melissa
Olivier, Johannes C.
Oluyede, Kehinde B.
Otte, Jessica A., FamilyMed
Pace, Beverly A., FamilyMed
Paris, Marc R.
Pereira, Miguel
Phillips, R. Keith, FamilyMed
Pillay, Leanne
Pillay, Leveshen
Poteryko, Derek, FamilyMed
Propp, Donald J., FamilyMed(EM)
Quinn, Fiona S., FamilyMed
Raynor, Lianne R.
Redpath, William L.
Reems, Hendrik W.
Richardson, Gary, FamilyMed
Rodriguez-Sarmiento, Juan G., FamilyMed(EM)
Roe, Richard C.
Rogers, Neil R., FamilyMed
Schulson, Nicholas G.
Sheppard, George F., FamilyMed(EM)
Simice, Yana, FamilyMed(EM)
Spry, Geoffrey A.
Steel, Stefanie, FamilyMed
Stewart, Robin K., FamilyMed(EM)
Steyn, Frederick W.
Syed, Husnain
Teixeira, Marc A., FamilyMed(EM)
Uchman, Dubravka, FamilyMed
Van Aerde, Lisa, FamilyMed
Van Aerde, Tim, FamilyMed(EM)
Van Der Goes, Theresa A., FamilyMed
Vaney, Dagny L., FamilyMed
Vaughan, Gerrard A.
Visser, Hermann B., FamilyMed
Voetmann, Susanne
Walker, Colin M.
Weisenburger, Earle F.
White, Brian A.
Wigmore, William M., FamilyMed(EM)
Wilford, Edward H., FamilyMed(EM)
Winder, Mary J., FamilyMed
Wolovitz, David M.
Woo, Connie
Zuccaro, Anthony, FamilyMed

NARAMATA

Louw, Perold J., FamilyMed

NELSON

Baril-Guerard, Genevieve
Bassingthwaighte, Mary
Boyd, Jeanette E., FamilyMed
Bridger, Keith C., FamilyMed
Cochrane, Christopher H.
Cochrane, Isabelle, FamilyMed(EM)
Dale, John R.
de Koker, Annemarie
Garcia, Yasmin M A., FamilyMed
Grymonpre, Ilona M A.
Gueordjev, Svetoslav A.
Hand, Gregory R F.
Janz, Rodica F., FamilyMed
Janz, Trevor W.
Kailia, Joel H., FamilyMed
Khosla, Rahul, FamilyMed(EM)
Kirsten, Andre R., FamilyMed
Kobayashi, Robert B., FamilyMed
Lee, Sharon J.
Lindsay, A. Morgan, FamilyMed
Link, Margot
MacIntyre, Margaret A., FamilyMed
MacKay, Lee D M., FamilyMed
McIntyre, Katherine V., FamilyMed
McKechnie, Kevin A., FamilyMed
Milde, Richard W.
Moulson, Brian C.
Murray, Andrew, FamilyMed
Musaji, Shelina, FamilyMed
Noiles, James R., FamilyMed
Reinecke, Carolus J.
Rodgers, Laurren K.
Sawyer, Elisabeth M., FamilyMed
Simms, Robin M., FamilyMed
Sonnichsen, David G.
Taylor, Robert A.
Van Der Vyver, Susanna M.
Wachtel, Sean L., FamilyMed
Wilson, Martha E.
Woodward, Brian J., FamilyMed

NEW DENVER

Burkholder, Charles L., FamilyMed
Hughes, Miranda C.
Magier, Michael G., FamilyMed

NEW WESTMINSTER

Akbar-Zadeh, Ali, FamilyMed
Al-Jawadi, Omar, FamilyMed
Albrecht, Ana-Ruth
Albrecht, John E.
Ali Majid, Nadia
Amariei, I. Camelia
Appleton, Brent E.
Arcadi, Sonia
Aung, Stephanie
Baranoff, Oleg
Barclay, Neil G., FamilyMed(EM)
Bawa, Yusuf E.
Berman, Kevin
Boudreau, Nathalie M., FamilyMed
Bradley, Joelle M., FamilyMed
Braunstein, Jonathan, FamilyMed(EM)
Buchan, Susan M., FamilyMed
Chen, Charlie C., FamilyMed
Chorny, Irina
Cieslak, Malgorzata
Cioata, Liliana, FamilyMed
Coleman, Douglas S.
Cornish, Bruce M.
Cottle, Margaret S M.
Croitoru, Kendra L A., FamilyMed
Cybula, Tomasz
De Couto, John L.
Drummond, Douglas, FamilyMed
Erhardt, Gunnar D.
Esau, David J., FamilyMed
Eshafi, Kourosh, FamilyMed
Essak, Alexander F.
Essak, Zafar M.
Finding, Diane
Fisher, Nigel R.
Freedman, David
Fry, Karen J.
Gabriel, Patricia S., FamilyMed
Gall, Brent D., FamilyMed
Gayed, Alaa M M., FamilyMed
Geisler, Arthur E M., FamilyMed
Hadid, David
Hedges, Donald G.
Hogarth, Teresa K.
Hudani, Sayeeda A.
Hudlicky, Ivo J., FamilyMed
Javer, Akbar K.
John, Lal
Jones, Kathryn G.
Kasteel, Kelly A., FamilyMed(EM)
Keszthelyi, Eniko J., FamilyMed(EM)
Khanbadr, Daryoush, FamilyMed
Klarke, Dorrit
Klein, Bernhard E.
LeMaitre, John P.
Leon, Magda M., FamilyMed
MacKay, Rory C.
MacKenzie, Andrew J.
MacNab, Jessica M., FamilyMed
MacPhail, Iain A., FamilyMed(EM)
Mann, Tejinder K.
Mathew, Jinu J., FamilyMed
McLennan, James A.
Metzak, Daniel J.
Miki, Kenneth K.
Milgrom, Michael
Milne, Stephen M.
Mudie, Dayna L., FamilyMed
Nagaria, Mohammad H.
Natarajan-Kailley, Anita, FamilyMed
Nguyen, Huy T S.
O'Brien, Julie
Owers, David P., FamilyMed
Paletta, Michael J.
Pawlik, Michal, FamilyMed
Payten, Susan A.
Petropolis, Nicholas P., FamilyMed
Pollock, Neil L.
Raath, Johannes J., FamilyMed
Rahnema, Nazanine, FamilyMed(EM)
Rajabali, Sultaneih S P.
Rajora, Manisha, FamilyMed
Rebeyka, Walter P.
Reynolds, Julia C.
Rodriguez, Richie-Ann, FamilyMed
Sandhu, Manbir S.
Segal, Mikel K., FamilyMed
Shearer, Carl T.
Siu, Kevin D., FamilyMed
Sobey, Paul W H., FamilyMed
Stamm, Holly A., FamilyMed
Sun, Rosemarie H L., FamilyMed
Sung, Emily E K C., FamilyMed
Sy, Candice, FamilyMed
Tan, Weiping, FamilyMed
Tang, S P. Allan
Totounchian, Fatemeh
Tully, Shawn A., FamilyMed
Tung, Julie, FamilyMed
Voon, Victor B H.
Vuurmans, Johannes L T.
Wilansky, Selig, FamilyMed
Wodynski, Peter J.
Wong, Daniel G., FamilyMed(EM)
Wozny, Diane M.
Yap, John C P.
Yoon, Philip W., FamilyMed(EM)
Zamfir, Catalina D., FamilyMed

NORTH SAANICH

Brink, Rosemary L.
Burke, John H.
Miles, Gary E.

NORTH VANCOUVER

Adair, John D.
Akhavein, Katayoon, FamilyMed
Ambrozic, Laura K., FamilyMed
Andolfatto, Gary, FamilyMed(EM)
Bard, Leon, FamilyMed(EM)
Barnett, Diane L.
Baron, Deneen D.
Bayfield, Sofia T., FamilyMed
Bazilli, Catherine J.
Behmanesh, Sharareh, FamilyMed
Bell-Irving, Kathleen A., FamilyMed
Bergstrom, Craig L.
Bertrand, Helene, FamilyMed
Bieg, Ralph P., FamilyMed
Boileau, Marc A., FamilyMed
Bovard, James A P.
Brache, M. Lou-Jacques, FamilyMed
Brisco, E. Bertha
Brisco, Eric J.
Broker, Hayley M., FamilyMed
Bruchet, Melvin R.
Bugeja, Francis X.
Byman, Andrea L.
Campling, M. Ruth
Cassidy, Brighid, FamilyMed(EM)
Chaboyer, Raymond, FamilyMed
Chakraborty, Tapash
Chalmers, George R.
Chan, Patrick F.
Chan, Philip, FamilyMed
Cheng, Andrew M.
Cheng, Dawn M L., FamilyMed
Chestnut, Shannon G., FamilyMed(EM)
Chow, Susan T.
Clark, Alison R.
Clark, Cynthia L., FamilyMed
Class, Sabrina F M.
Clement, Siobhan P., FamilyMed
Colwell, Katie, FamilyMed
Compagna, Thomas, FamilyMed(EM)
Conly, Maureen, FamilyMed
Corcoran, Louise A., FamilyMed
Cormack, Maura A.
Crawford, John G., FamilyMed
Crossen, Nancy P.
Davidson, Michael H.
Dobson, Malgorzata M S.
Doeksen, Corwin N D., FamilyMed
Dommann, Steven C.
Donnelly, S. Jane
Dunn, Michael P.
Early, Anita M.
Ebrahim, Shehla, FamilyMed
Edmonds, William
Edmunds, Peter M.
Evans, David, FamilyMed
Florakas, Christine, FamilyMed
Fowler, Jacqueline M., FamilyMed
Gaede, Lisa A., FamilyMed
Galloway, Emma, FamilyMed
Galt, Elaine L.
Geddes, Ross, FamilyMed(EM)
Goodman, Joseph
Haaf, Dana J., FamilyMed
Harrison, Linda M.
Hasinoff, Erin A., FamilyMed
Hayton, Peter M.
Hayward, James M., FamilyMed
Hazlett, David L., FamilyMed
Hejdankova, Barbara, FamilyMed
Henry, Elizabeth A., FamilyMed
Holmes, Kathryn J.
Horak, Stuart Z., FamilyMed(EM)
Howard, Paisley G., FamilyMed
Hudon, Marck P J.
Iro, Chinedu J.
Janzen, Dorothy M.
Joo, Daniel A., FamilyMed(EM)
Jurenka, Blanka, FamilyMed
Karalic, Sanja, FamilyMed
Karimirad, Helen, FamilyMed
Kazemi, Ali-Reza
Keshavarzi, Gholamreza, FamilyMed
Kiai, Cristina A., FamilyMed
Kroll, Edward S.
Lahiffe, Brian F., FamilyMed(EM)
Lai, Jatina, FamilyMed(EM)
Lakha, Anis H.
Lawson, Laurie E M., FamilyMed
Lea, John N.
Lebrun, John B.
Lee, David S.
Lee, Mona, FamilyMed
Lee Kim Koon, Andrew C.
Lees, Sharon A.
Loveless, Wendy J., FamilyMed
Lupton, Richard D.
Malon, Paul A.
Maree, Gert
Marshall, Michael T.
Martin, Kim, FamilyMed
Maynard, John E.
McCall, Annette L., FamilyMed
McGrogan, Jonathan, FamilyMed(EM)
McLeod, Heather A., FamilyMed
McShane, Lucy M., FamilyMed
McWhinney, Murray A.
Miller, Philip Y., FamilyMed(EM)
Montemuro, Paul T.
Morgenstern, Katherine V., FamilyMed
Moric, Mary A G.
Murray, Gail A.
Naran, Mineshbhai
Norton, Bryan R.
O'Connor, Brian A.
O'Neil, Michael B., FamilyMed(EM)
Ortynsky, Garry B., FamilyMed
Park, Hazel S., FamilyMed(EM)
Payne, Irina E., FamilyMed

PHYSICIANS BY PROVINCE

Penner, Ramona C.
Penner, Raymond C.
Phillips, Jennifer M., FamilyMed
Puddicombe, Robert E.
Purvis, Alison
Quirke, David B.
Rai, Kulwant
Read, Brandi L., FamilyMed(EM)
Reineking, Samantha J., FamilyMed
Reynolds, Vernon L.
Richards, Peter V.
Ritchie, Alec H., FamilyMed(EM)
Robertson, Mary L.
Robinson, Claire E., FamilyMed
Roeck, Kyra D., FamilyMed
Rowthorn, Leanne M., FamilyMed(EM)
Rubin, Mitchell B., FamilyMed
Russenes, Rune T., FamilyMed
Sambor, Krystine E., FamilyMed
Samborski, Rockford W., FamilyMed
Satake, Ken, FamilyMed
Schafer-MacDonald, Helga T., FamilyMed
Schwarz, Peter J., FamilyMed(EM)
Seger, Mark R.
Seliske, Maureen E., FamilyMed
Shams Tabrizi, Shahram, FamilyMed
Shaw, Jennifer J.
Sikhakhane, Arnold M., FamilyMed
Sojat, Alexander J.
Stager, Andrew C., FamilyMed(EM)
Staniforth, Sean M., FamilyMed(EM)
Stasiak, Ferdinand M.
Surgenor, Hannah
Sutherland, Katrine C.
Tang, Judy M., FamilyMed
Taylor, Gordon
Tekano, Kenneth J.
Tesiorowski, Alicja, FamilyMed
Thompson, Franklin C.
Tikhonova, Elina, FamilyMed
Trebell, Joanne R.
Vala, Francis H., FamilyMed
Vegsund, Bjorn C., FamilyMed(EM)
Village, Ronald S.
Vilonel, Etienne E.
Walker, Jennifer D., FamilyMed
Walton-Knight, Nicola A., FamilyMed
Waterson, Lydia
Watt, Anne M., FamilyMed(EM)
Wiebe, Sandra L.
Williscroft, David M., FamilyMed(EM)
Wilson-Haffenden, Cara K.
Wong, Wai-Ben, FamilyMed(EM)
Younan, Younan-Samy, FamilyMed
Zamanpour, Kamran, FamilyMed

OKANAGAN FALLS

Robertson, Andrew P., FamilyMed
Robertson, James G J.

OLIVER

De Vries, Ansunette
Entwistle, Peter B.
Evans, Steven M.
Francis, Thomas P., FamilyMed
Hamilton, A. Mark
Johnston, C. Stuart, FamilyMed
Myslek, Margaret A.
Rooke, Catherine A., FamilyMed
Ruddiman, Alan W.
Shaw, David R., FamilyMed
Willis, Marianne I J., FamilyMed

OSOYOOS

Bellingan, Jacob C.
De Vries, Matthys A.
de Witt, Elzaan
Kane, Lorraine A., FamilyMed
Tarr, Garnett M.

PARKSVILLE

Bell, Bradley D.
Benton, Claude M.
Desai, Satish S.
Fridriksson, Thor
Hancock, Ronald J.
Henderson, Richard J.
Hickey Somerville, Julia M.
Jayaraman, Vadula
Lipsey, Philip, FamilyMed
Loughead, Garth T., FamilyMed
MacCari, Robert J.
McClure, Lawrence H., FamilyMed
Morris, Mark W., FamilyMed
Noble, H. Stephen
Simenhoff, Jacques
Stephan, Ernest F.
Sulz, Carey J.
Szachnowska, Violetta I., FamilyMed
Waite, Robert P.
White, Graham E., FamilyMed

PEACHLAND

Brinkerhoff, John, FamilyMed
Chetty, Praven

PEMBERTON

Coward, Jeremy
Fisher, Hugh S.
Hays, Luke, FamilyMed
Ho Chen, Anthony
Jones, David R L., FamilyMed
Lindley, Rebecca J., FamilyMed
Patterson, Danielle E.

PENDER ISLAND

Moore, Gerald D., FamilyMed
Thompson, Michael R.

PENTICTON

Agbodo, Johnson C L.
Anderson, Donella, FamilyMed
Atkins, Barbara R.
Ayling, Geraldine Z.
Barkhuizen, Frederick
Bobart, Vonda A S.
Burgoyne, Glen D., FamilyMed
Calitz, Johannes J.
Caskey, William A.
Cobbin, Paul L., FamilyMed
Collyer, Steven J.
Congram, Sandra P.
Connolly, Trevor W., FamilyMed(EM)
De Kock, Johannes L.
Dutchman, David A J.
Frasinski, Alicja
Fullard, Ginevra A M H.
Gatenby, Allan D., FamilyMed(EM)
Gill, Carl A.
Gray, Stanley W.
Harries, Jeffrey K.
Harries, Leona T.
Harrold, Brent D., FamilyMed(EM)
Hooper, R. Allen, FamilyMed
Hughes, John M.
Ingram, Heidi M., FamilyMed
Johnston, James W.
Jumaa, M. Said
Kennedy, John C., FamilyMed
Kilian, Daniel S.
Kooy, Jacobus, FamilyMed
Landecker, Elizabeth A M.
Lawrie, W. Mark
Leitner, Douglas M.
Maier, Vivian R.
Main, Barbara A., FamilyMed
Main, Blair F., FamilyMed
McIntosh, Robert E.
McMillan, Morag J., FamilyMed(EM)
Nixon, Alan J., FamilyMed
O'Neil, Ross L.

Paisley, David M A.
Pansegrouw, Sandra, FamilyMed
Parameshwar, Manoj
Phillips, Timothy M.
Pugachev, Alexander, FamilyMed
Raison, Bradford W., FamilyMed(EM)
Ross, Wendy J.
Samoyloff, Stephan D., FamilyMed(EM)
Seipp, Timothy T.
Selinger, Gregory E., FamilyMed
Sheehan, Mary C., FamilyMed
Sit, Lindsay A., FamilyMed
Sloan, Michael J.
Snyman, Marius R., FamilyMed
Stonestreet, Cong Y.
Stothart, Danielle C.
Surkan, David L.
Surkan, John M.
Surkan, Michael W., FamilyMed
Tatham, Richard H B., FamilyMed
Toneff, Christopher J.
Ward, Christopher R.
Watters, Elizabeth C.
Westby, Lloyd, FamilyMed
Wren, Colwyn J.

PITT MEADOWS

Dodds, Christopher A.
Ivanov, T N. Teodor, FamilyMed
Jessop, Darrell J.
Lim, Larry F T.
Prem-Smith, Melodie R., FamilyMed
Sommi, Kevin J B.
Verdizad, P. Ariana, FamilyMed

PORT ALBERNI

Brown, Owen H., FamilyMed
Craven, Charles P.
De Pape, Gregory E., FamilyMed
De Witt, Andries J.
Fadeyi, Oludare S.
Feyi, Kennedy K K.
Fraser, Alan B.
Grant, James M.
Johnsen, Wendy A., FamilyMed
Kandiah, Anushiya
Khabbaz, Samir, FamilyMed
Kitshoff, Arno
Longman, Shane A., FamilyMed
Lund, R. Daryl
Marie, Simona G.
Martin, Diane C., FamilyMed
Meyer, Frederick J T.
Meyer, John P.
Morris, Chester N.
Muehlenberg, Bernd A.
Nel, Izak B.
Nell, Hermann S.
Puts, Marc
Rozwadowski, Marek A.
Sander, Donald A.
Smit, Cecile
Smit, Dirk J.
Smit, Johan
Sutcliffe, Graham V.
Van Der Merwe, Daniel F.
Van Der Merwe, Daniel T H.
Van Zyl, Andre, FamilyMed
Van Zyl, Anneleen
White, Damian F A., FamilyMed
Wilson, John C N., FamilyMed

PORT ALICE

Hubler, Dana G., FamilyMed
MacKenzie, Ian M., FamilyMed

PORT COQUITLAM

Arntsen, Helen M.
Barron, Stephen R., FamilyMed
Boon, Peter J.
Brown, Margaret A.

Budzianowska-Kwiatkowski, Margret, FamilyMed
Cheong, K M. Andrew, FamilyMed
Choi, Matthew C K., FamilyMed
Chung, Ngai Sang P.
Clutterham, Suzanne M., FamilyMed
Cordoni, Teresa, FamilyMed
Crothers, Ivan S.
Cullen, Angela K., FamilyMed
Curry, John J D.
D'Archangelo, Eugene S.
Ducholke, Linda M., FamilyMed
Farag, Hanan, FamilyMed
Flynn, Paula S., FamilyMed
Hacquebard, Simone M A.
Hasham, Amin M.
Henderson, Allison M., FamilyMed
Hildebrand, Mary M.
Hume, Laura J.
Jacobs, Thomas B.
Khalili, Mark, FamilyMed
Khangura, Seema S., FamilyMed
Kochendorfer, Robert L.
Leung, Patrick P., FamilyMed
Malley, Laura K.
Maunsell, Jonathan B.
McCallaghan, Johannes J.
McCarthy, Martha A.
Mortil, Nanette
Ng, Philip K.
Payne, Elizabeth E.
Sartekin, S. Kemal, FamilyMed
Schlagintweit, Robert
Sclater, Kevin W.
Shaw, Clifford A.
Shaw, Kimberly A., FamilyMed
Soltani-Khorshidi, Nazila, FamilyMed
Spooner, G. Robin
Thomson, Veronica M.
Van Der Westhuizen, Lucas C.
Wasswa-Kintu, Jemima J.
Willoughby, Siri A., FamilyMed
Wong, Grover, FamilyMed
Woods, Ian B.
Yun, Jennifer M., FamilyMed

PORT HARDY

De Wit, Andre J., FamilyMed
Douglas, Datonye D O.
Lee, Howard C.
Zaayman, Melani

PORT MCNEILL

Armogam, Preianathan, FamilyMed
Avery, Granger R.
Blackburn, Graham A., FamilyMed
Clelland, M. Jane, FamilyMed
Maheswaran, Charuka V.
Scragg, Richard
Whittaker, David

PORT MOODY

Andrucson, Victor M.
Belton, Kenneth W.
Bever, Klaus
Chodyra, Anna K., FamilyMed
Eddy, M. Joan, FamilyMed
Farhangpour, Erfan, FamilyMed
Ibrahim, Evelin, FamilyMed
Ibrahim, Ihab I S.
Lim, Nathan E., FamilyMed(EM)
McInnis, Joseph B.
Morley, Julia C.
Nair, Kieran, FamilyMed
Nakamura, Richard M.
Penn, Caroline M G., FamilyMed
Shamsi, Mehrnoosh, FamilyMed
Sumar, Shahirose
Todorovic, Cedomirka, FamilyMed
Tognotti, Darin M T., FamilyMed(EM)
Ungar, Clifford N.
Vasile, Gabriela, FamilyMed
Warneboldt, Jean A., FamilyMed

POWELL RIVER

Addison, Cynthia A.
Andreae, Martin E.
Bonsor, Claire N.
Bremner, Kyla
Burechailo, Leta R., FamilyMed
Burns, Stephen R., FamilyMed
Chao, Te Wei
Delport, Arend A C.
Dohm, Brigitte H M T.
Donkin, Allan J.
Du Toit, Jacques H.
Head, Robert B., FamilyMed(EM)
Hobson, Bruce C.
Horsfall, Susan J., FamilyMed
Krowitz, Jason K., FamilyMed
Lynskey, Jeffrey W., FamilyMed
Maguire, Anna-Marie L.
Mann, David L., FamilyMed(EM)
Maree, Tamlyn
May, David J.
McDonald, Barrie M.
Meyer, Melissa
Mittra-Melrose, Vidushi, FamilyMed
Morwood, Christopher D C., FamilyMed
Naude, Jan J S.
Pater, Piotr C.
Rossouw, Pieter A., FamilyMed
Schweitzer, Bradley H., FamilyMed
Strydom, Henriette
Toole, Douglas R.
Watson, Sally J.
White, Nicholas

PRINCE GEORGE

Akhtar, Muhammad
Ames, Janet E., FamilyMed
Ashraf, Nazia, FamilyMed
Asquith, Philip R., FamilyMed
Attia, Tammy, FamilyMed
Bamgbade, Olumuyiwa A.
Belda, Patricia, FamilyMed
Bond, Donald G., FamilyMed
Botha, Johannes J., FamilyMed(EM)
Brenckmann, Christine, FamilyMed
Burg, Jan B.
Cameron, Elizabeth A., FamilyMed
Carlson, Erin P V., FamilyMed
Chang, Steven, FamilyMed(EM)
Closson, Keri L., FamilyMed
Collins, Courtney L C., FamilyMed
Cook, Laurence M.
Cosio, Ingrid, FamilyMed
Crompton, Daniel, FamilyMed(EM)
Crompton, Stephanie L., FamilyMed
Cunniffe, Kathleen A., FamilyMed(EM)
Curran, Shelia, FamilyMed
Dabbs, Ronald H.
Daskarev, Albena M.
Daskarev, Zlatin L.
Dhadly, Pritam P S.
Ducharme, J M. Pierre
El Gendi, Amina
Eselle, Emmanuel N.
Fabriel-Leclerc, Christin A., FamilyMed
Faraz, Muniba
Ferreira, Stephanus C., FamilyMed
Fibich, Ernst
Fraser, Garnet D., FamilyMed
Gillis, Melissa C., FamilyMed(EM)
Goodman, Trisha A., FamilyMed
Graham, Candida R.
Grobbelaar, Barend, FamilyMed
Groot, Marcel C.
Hadi, Haidar M.
Hagen, Barry A.
Hagen, Catherine A., FamilyMed(EM)
Haley, George F.
Higgins, William E.
Hillhouse, Brian, FamilyMed
Horvat, Daniel
Hundal, Prabhjot
Hunsinger, Leigh A., FamilyMed(EM)
Hunter, Meredith D., FamilyMed
Jabbar, Faiza
Jabbar, Faraz

Janzen, Matthew, FamilyMed(EM)
Javed, Arshad, FamilyMed
Javed, Khalid, FamilyMed
Johnson, Amy E., FamilyMed
Joss, Kasandra, FamilyMed
Kelly, Albert S.
Key, Siobhan L., FamilyMed(EM)
Khan, Iftkhar H.
Khare, Umesh
Knoll, Susan E., FamilyMed
Kozlovski, Christopher H.
Kwantes, Lindsay N., FamilyMed
Lakhani, Amin
Lakhoo, Parbhoobhai
Lamb, Sandra I.
Lotze, Tracey A.
MacDonald, Susan C., FamilyMed
MacEoin, Colin
MacNicol, Melanie L., FamilyMed
Mah, John F., FamilyMed
Makadiama-Bantsimba, Yvon
Mann, Satish K., FamilyMed
Manraj, Lea H.
Marquis, Edward J.
McGhee, Rachel A., FamilyMed
McGlynn, James, FamilyMed
McLeod, Denise C., FamilyMed
Mehmood, Shehzad
Merritt, Kyle D., FamilyMed
Morgan, David W.
Murad, Nazar J.
Murray, Paul M.
Nadeem, Muhammad B., FamilyMed
Neary, Ann P.
Nowlan, Ruth G.
O'Brien, Anita M., FamilyMed
O'Malley, Kathleen, FamilyMed
O'Malley, Michael J., FamilyMed
O'Malley, Peter J., FamilyMed
Okorie, Eugene
Osei, William D.
Oyeye, Grant
Plouffe, Daniel T., FamilyMed
Powell, Ruth M., FamilyMed
Preston, Anthony J.
Prigmore, Gerrard T., FamilyMed
Raymond, Richard J., FamilyMed(EM)
Reddy, Devan
Reddy, Inbakumaran
Redenbach, Zoe, FamilyMed(EM)
Riome-York, Sasha A., FamilyMed
Rowe, Patrick D., FamilyMed(EM)
Ryan, John C., FamilyMed(EM)
Saadeddin, Abdulrahman
Schokking, Ian D., FamilyMed
Schulzkump, Linda
Seshia, Jyoti B., FamilyMed
Shahnawaz, Muhammad, FamilyMed
Shea, Theresa M., FamilyMed(EM)
Shier, Edward C., FamilyMed
Sidorov, Jana L.
Siegling, Cecilia, FamilyMed
Sinawan, Riaz A.
Smith, Heather, FamilyMed
Smith, Michael M., FamilyMed(EM)
Snadden, David, FamilyMed
Spooner, Devin A., FamilyMed(EM)
St Rose, Auton D F., FamilyMed
Textor, Catherine, FamilyMed(EM)
Turner, S. Patrick D., FamilyMed(EM)
Turski, Edgar R., FamilyMed
Veale, Kimberly D., FamilyMed
Waqar, Mohsin
Weisgerber, Kim J.
Wilson, Bruce J.
Wilson, Linda L., FamilyMed
York, Daniel C., FamilyMed
Young, Thomas W.
Zanozin, Dmitrij, FamilyMed
Zhang, Rong, FamilyMed
Zimbler, Jessica, FamilyMed

PRINCE RUPERT

Belgardt, Gerald R.
Brocker, Johann F.
Coburn, Harris C.
Coetzee, Corneli M.
Coetzee, Gillaume
Croft, John A., FamilyMed
Edmunds, Darryn J., FamilyMed
Eysele, Beverly-Ann
Fawell, John A.
Fawell, Sunelle
Gayda, Edward X.
Ikari, Michael Y., FamilyMed
Joubert, Jan J M.
Klapstein, Kim F., FamilyMed
Kloppers, Amor
Mothelesi, Ronald R.
Ryeburn, Michael V.
Smith, Samuel A.
Tse, Luke B S., FamilyMed
Van Der Wart, Adriaan D F., FamilyMed
Watson, George K.

PRINCETON

Adams, John M., FamilyMed
Idanwekhai, Evaristus, FamilyMed
Robb, Clive B., FamilyMed
Smith, David V B., FamilyMed

QUALICUM BEACH

Bartlett, Penelope
Biglow, Clair E.
Biro, Andrew J., FamilyMed
Dalla Lana, John C.
Fletcher, K A. Hugh
Gubbins, W. Beresford G.
Gushulak, Brian D.
Haslett, Peter J.
Johnson, J. Edward
Martin, Kevin J F.
Papo, Khomotso
Swart, Pieter D.
Van Der Weyde, Marlene P., FamilyMed
Wagenaar, Johannes M B.

QUATHIASKI COVE

Graham, Keith
Kellerhals, Erika K S., FamilyMed

QUEEN CHARLOTTE

Chrones, James P., FamilyMed
Horner, Gordon, FamilyMed
Lake, Peter R., FamilyMed
Morton, Tracy L., FamilyMed
Shooner, Caroline A., FamilyMed

QUESNEL

Bond, Stephen D.
Buys, Stephanus
Craig, Dorothy M., FamilyMed
Dercksen, Judy A., FamilyMed
Eksteen, Hendrik
Ellison, Anthony K.
Erlank, Andries G., FamilyMed
Erlank, Minette B.
Fine, Jonathan P H.
Furstenburg, Dietrich
Grapes, Gavin P.
Havens, John R., FamilyMed
Jacobsohn, Friedrich G.
Kozic, Jennifer R.
Le Roux, Jacobus J., FamilyMed
Maile, John K C.
Martins, Grace L., FamilyMed
McDonald, Johannes V.
McFetridge, Gerald P., FamilyMed
Scheepers, Eugene
Sear, Andrew I., FamilyMed
Slabbert, Pieter H.
Smit, Morne M., FamilyMed
Smit, Nelis
Smith, George A.
Smith, Helen L.
Smith, Helene
Stals, Roelof L.
Van Dyk, Frederick P.
Van Heerden, Lizaan
Velthuysen, Gerrit C.
Walker, Mark B.

REVELSTOKE

Brown, Sara, FamilyMed
Farrugia, Alexandra A E., FamilyMed
Gornall, Annie, FamilyMed
Hunt, Travis L., FamilyMed
Jarmula, Bartosz M., FamilyMed
Leslie, Neil G., FamilyMed
MacDonald, Christopher, FamilyMed
MacLeod, A. Cameron, FamilyMed
Molder, Cameron J., FamilyMed
Mostert, Andreas W., FamilyMed
O'Connor, Kathleen M., FamilyMed
Rennie, Courtney, FamilyMed

RICHMOND

Abou-Gareeb, Iman, FamilyMed
Adams, Nigel J., FamilyMed
Ahmad, Khawaja M N.
Alexiadis, Alexandros
Austin, Nancy E., FamilyMed(EM)
Avina-Zubieta, Juan A.
Baker, Robert A.
Bertram, Katherine J., FamilyMed
Booth, Esther G., FamilyMed
Brandt, E. Lorne, FamilyMed
Brown, Leslie N.
Bulger, Maureen A.
Cabrera, Maria Linda T.
Carruthers, D. Barry, FamilyMed
Carvalho, Gustavo J.
Carvalho, Raul A J.
Chan, Denise W., FamilyMed
Chan, Richard K., FamilyMed(EM)
Chang, Adam, FamilyMed
Chang, Jacqueline, FamilyMed
Chang, Peter F E.
Chang, Stanley S.
Chao, Kelvin C.
Cheah, Andrew, FamilyMed
Chee, Peter M Y., FamilyMed
Chen, Patrick Q H., FamilyMed(EM)
Cheung, Anita S P., FamilyMed
Chin, Dennis
Chiu, Frank K K.
Chow, Kenmau
Chu, Francis J L.
Chu, Mary P H.
Cohen, Leslie S.
Coppin, James A.
Cutforth, Dauna R.
David, Morton J.
Desai-Ranchod, Smeeta
Dhingra, Danny
Dodd, Sharon, FamilyMed
Donaldson, Jane, FamilyMed(EM)
Duchowska, Helena L.
Duncan, Barbara R.
Eckland Jetzer, Shelly, FamilyMed
Faulkner, Donald E.
Fedder, Steven A., FamilyMed(EM)
Foo, Violet L Y., FamilyMed
Forsyth, Sara J., FamilyMed
Frey, Michael G.
Fung, Julian, FamilyMed
Gandham, Satnam S.
Garrison, Scott R.
Ghobassy, Bahar, FamilyMed
Goodman, Earl L.
Gordon, Morris
Griffiths, Robert A.
Hambleton, Corey R., FamilyMed
Hamza, Essam, FamilyMed
Hau, Cheryl S., FamilyMed
Ho, Terrence T L.
Horii, Allan H.
Howie, Sebastian, FamilyMed
Hsu, Justin W., FamilyMed
Hu, John H W., FamilyMed
Huang, Patrick O.
Hui, Hilary K.
Hui, Ivy Y C., FamilyMed
Hung, James
Hung, Violet W T., FamilyMed(EM)
Hurwitz, Stanley D., FamilyMed
Ip, Vincent K L.
Jiang, Charles C Y.
Johal, Kashmir S.
Kagee, Rafeeq
Kallas, Alari
Kan, Wai-On
Kapoor, Videsh, FamilyMed
Khazamipour, Kazem
Kim, Ki Sun
Kliman, Jacob J.
Koss, Gary M.
Kudo, Patricia A., FamilyMed
Kung, Tania Y L., FamilyMed
Kuo, Susan, FamilyMed
Kwok, Ezra, FamilyMed
Kwok, Matthew M K., FamilyMed(EM)
Kwok, Stephen T F., FamilyMed
Lai, Grace H K.
Lam, Augustine S K.
Lau, Andrew H C., FamilyMed
Lee, Cindy W., FamilyMed
Lee, Sammy S H.
Lee, Tracy Y., FamilyMed
Lee-Chen, Beverley, FamilyMed
Lejay, P. Sue
Leong-Sit, Kee Sheen
Lermer, Bram, FamilyMed
Leung, Jason K., FamilyMed
Leung, Paul M K.
Leung, Tamara J.
Lew, Jason W L., FamilyMed
Li, David W., FamilyMed
Li, Hui-Wah, FamilyMed
Ling, Chee K.
Liu, Tanya
Lu, James D.
Lum, Jeffrey H., FamilyMed(EM)
MacDonald, Helene E., FamilyMed
McCreary, A. James R.
McKenzie, Robert, FamilyMed
Moffat, Stephanie M., FamilyMed
Mondor, Frances L., FamilyMed(EM)
Morrell, Robert W.
Morris, Sheldon R., FamilyMed
Myckatyn, Michael M.
Nagle, Cheryl Y.
Newman, David G., FamilyMed
Ng, Vienna K Y., FamilyMed
Ngai, Henry C P., FamilyMed
O'Driscoll, Mary-Louise, FamilyMed
O'Neal, Erica L.
Pinkhasik, Paul
Prat, Franck G.
Quelch, Peter C.
Ragheb, Salah R G.
Remer, Samuel T.
Riyat, Sharan
Romashin, Stanislav, FamilyMed
Roosma, Jennifer E.
Rothfels, Peter L.
Roux, Larissa, FamilyMed
Ruthe, Keri S.
Sagorin, Richard A., FamilyMed
Segal, Basil, FamilyMed
Sharma, Sandhya K.
Sharma Aucone, Rachila, FamilyMed
Shen, Angela M., FamilyMed
Shiu, Simon S.
Sigismund, John G.
Singhal, Manoj K., FamilyMed
Singhal, Manoj
Smith, Dean G., FamilyMed(EM)
Sourisseau, Louise A.
Stitt, James C., FamilyMed(EM)
Stokes, Erika L.
Sun, Jenet H F.
Surka, Milosh S.
Tan, Brenda P., FamilyMed
Tan, Michelle W., FamilyMed
Tanaka, Asae, FamilyMed
Tenby, Lionel
Tomson, William G.
Tong, Norman T.
Tsang, Allan Y.
Tucker, Devin, FamilyMed
Vellani, Zahir S., FamilyMed
Viegas, Desmond S I.
Vostretsova, Nataliya V., FamilyMed
Wang, Amy R Y., FamilyMed
Wang, Caroline Y M.
Watts, Eric D J.
Weaver, Robert G.
West, William, FamilyMed(EM)
Wilson, James A., FamilyMed
Wong, Boon L.
Wong, Danny H K.
Wong, Edward W H., FamilyMed
Wong, Mildred T W., FamilyMed(EM)
Wong, Patricia
Wong, Phoebus W C.
Wong, Susan Y., FamilyMed
Wong, Thomas S., FamilyMed
Yeung, Emilie N M.
Yeung, James C F.
Yeung, William C Y., FamilyMed
Yuan, G. Bernadette
Zhang, Y H. Connie, FamilyMed
Zheng, Xueyan, FamilyMed

ROSSLAND

Bazley, Kynan P.
Fisher, Janet H., FamilyMed(EM)
Goodison, Karin L.
Grey, Jane
Houde, Stefaine, FamilyMed
Jenkins, Andrea N., FamilyMed
Kerby, Lilli D., FamilyMed
McCarroll, Kirk P., FamilyMed
O'Flanagan, Brian
Purssell, J. Eileen
Sandstrom, Jonas L., FamilyMed
Scully, Michael V.
Sibbald, Ian I., FamilyMed(EM)
Trenholme, Brenda J.

SAANICHTON

Bosenberg, Marc H.
Bosman, Jan C.
Chadha, Randeep K R., FamilyMed(EM)
Crisci, Elisabeth M V.
Davies, T H P. Ashley
De Mott, Wayne T.
Du Toit, Andre, FamilyMed
Harper, Telen T.
Irvine, Brendon R., FamilyMed(EM)
Kennedy, Richard, FamilyMed
Lovely, Donald S.
Meadows, Terence F.
Michel, Alison J., FamilyMed
Shehata, Nadia, FamilyMed
Tam, Terence K Y., FamilyMed(EM)
Tetley, Christopher D., FamilyMed(EM)
Thicke, Steven C.
Unger, Jeffrey J., FamilyMed(EM)
Wetzer, Wolfgang H.
Whyte, Jennifer A., FamilyMed
Wray, George I., FamilyMed

SALMO

Dixon-Warren, Nattana B L., FamilyMed
Inniss, Michael W.

SALMON ARM

Aitchison, Juliann M., FamilyMed
Bell, Warren R., FamilyMed
Black, Colleen L., FamilyMed
Bonthuys, Erasmus J.
Bratty, Joan E M., FamilyMed
Breugem, Dirk J., FamilyMed(EM)
Brighouse, M. Ruth
Currie, Richard A., FamilyMed
De Wet, Guy A.
Drury, Megan B.
Du Plessis, Marietjie
Edmondson, Victoria J.
Glanville, Brook W., FamilyMed
Goldberg, Kevin M.
Gow, Alan L.
Grieve, Kimberley A., FamilyMed
Hepburn, Keith G., FamilyMed(EM)
Hepburn, Laura D., FamilyMed
Heunis, Adriaan
Howatt, Alison L., FamilyMed
Kirkman, Stacey D., FamilyMed
Kirkpatrick, J. Nicole, FamilyMed(EM)

PHYSICIANS BY PROVINCE

Levins, James P., FamilyMed
Lorenz, Darren A., FamilyMed
Lourens, Marc
Malinowski, Cindy E.
McCallum, Grant
McDonald, Ross M., FamilyMed
McLellan, Fiona J.
Megyesi, Amy E., FamilyMed
Newell, Philip G.
Ostby, Randi A., FamilyMed(EM)
Plessis, Angela D.
Preto, Adele F.
Rose, Andrea L., FamilyMed
Skubiak, Michael J.
Sonmor, Frederick S.
Theron, Karina
Trow, Rory M.
Venter, Herman C A.
Ward, Simon D.
Weicker, Christopher R., FamilyMed
Welder, Clayton A., FamilyMed
Wood, John C.

SALT SPRING ISLAND

Barclay, Shane B.
Beaver, David J F., FamilyMed
Berg, Karen M.
Cole, Candace C.
Crichton, Robert T., FamilyMed
Edmonds, Colleen L.
Gummeson, Ian D., FamilyMed
Reznick, Ronald R.
Ryan, Paula P., FamilyMed
Sadouski, Maria M., FamilyMed
Slakov, Holly A., FamilyMed
Woodley, David G.

SCOTCH CREEK

Bates, Janet M.
Bates, Kenneth R J., FamilyMed

SECHELT

Bishop, Jane M., FamilyMed
Bryson, Malcolm J.
Cairns, Alan J.
Farrer, John P.
Fogarty, Doris C., FamilyMed
Forgie, Karen E., FamilyMed
Gibbons, Jeannette M., FamilyMed
Hughan, Isabelle C.
Jaschinski, Joerg
Lasuta, Sarah A M., FamilyMed
Marton, Monica E., FamilyMed
McDowell, Timothy J., FamilyMed
Moodie, Sarah M., FamilyMed
Mundy, Ronald J T.
Myhill-Jones, Brian J., FamilyMed
Reznick, Simon, FamilyMed
Robinson, Bruce T.
Rogers, Denis
Scott, Karen A., FamilyMed
Westlake, Alice G., FamilyMed
Wildgrube, Frank P.

SHAWNIGAN LAKE

Dhanoa, Ravijindera S.
Howie, Graham M.
Moulaison, William G.
Woudstra, Trudy D., FamilyMed

SICAMOUS

Beech, Jack H.
Kelsall, Rosemary

SIDNEY

Beller, Albert M.
Brown, Robert H., FamilyMed
Byrne, Aidan P., FamilyMed
Cadger, Ewan M.
Coleman, Fiona M.
Cowan, Cornelius C.
Cowan, Valerie Y.
Cruz, Sean M.
Evans, Katharine, FamilyMed
Gagliardi, Menuccia, FamilyMed
Gallins, Kelly, FamilyMed(EM)
Gallins, Shannon, FamilyMed(EM)
George, Eric J., FamilyMed
Hartrick, Terrance R., FamilyMed
Henderson, Gordon T.
Hosie, Andrew D.
James, Christopher M.
Jovic, Draga, FamilyMed
Keith, Paul E., FamilyMed
Lewis, Andrea P.
Lorenzo, Thomas
Marsh, Ambrose A.
Naismith, Amanda E.
Orr, Thomas
Potter, Tracy C.
Rhoades, Elizabeth H.
Ritonja, Laura M., FamilyMed
Spencer, George R.
Sweeney, Maureen F.
Tamboline, Colin R.
Walsh, Patric B.
Wilson, Linda J., FamilyMed

SLOCAN PARK

Barbour-Jones, Elizabeth
Piver, Andre, FamilyMed

SMITHERS

Bastian, Elizabeth J.
Blouw, Karin J.
Flynn, D. Justin, FamilyMed
Froese, Nicole L., FamilyMed
Haskins, Marlowe, FamilyMed
Jakubec, Darren M., FamilyMed
Knight, Mary, FamilyMed
Miles, Susan L.
Page, Crystal, FamilyMed
Preto, Jodi, FamilyMed
Pretorius, Barbara A.
Pretorius, Isaac G V.
Scholtz, Martin M.
Smith, Sheila C., FamilyMed
Szymanska, Aleksandra, FamilyMed

SOOKE

Anderson, Jennifer E.
Forsberg, Tracy L., FamilyMed
Pocock, Jeffrey L., FamilyMed
Rabien, Anton, FamilyMed
Saunders, Robin D.
Vally, Tomas, FamilyMed

SORRENTO

Paterson, Donald C.

SPARWOOD

Higgins, Derek A., FamilyMed
Pigott, Tara G., FamilyMed
Workman, Holly K.

SQUAMISH

Becker, Lev A., FamilyMed(EM)
Bohn, A. David, FamilyMed
Cranston, James G., FamilyMed
Cudmore, Richard H., FamilyMed
Davies, Anne-Marie, FamilyMed
Eksteen, Ben, FamilyMed
Fothergill, Judith
Hlynsky, Julia A., FamilyMed
Illingworth, Meghan, FamilyMed
Jamieson, James D.
Kelly, Rachel S., FamilyMed
Klein, Lawrence W.
Kranz, T. Robert
Lam, Alan J.
Malherbe, Gerhardus J., FamilyMed
Martin, Louise A., FamilyMed
Masselink, William S.
Morum, David R G.
Nagase, Daniel Y., FamilyMed(EM)
Quiring, David J.
Read, Rua L., FamilyMed
Rivers, Angela S., FamilyMed
Schellenberg, Kenneth L.
Stelzl, Glenn E.
Stevenson, Skai F J., FamilyMed
Swope, Sheila A.
Tavares, Grace E E., FamilyMed
Wood, Teresa M B., FamilyMed
Zeifman, Claude

STEWART

Kawerninski, Michael S., FamilyMed

SUMMERLAND

Bannerman, Alistair R E.
Bennett, Peter W., FamilyMed
Brown, Denis R C., FamilyMed
Guenther, Neil V.
Harrold, Catherine G., FamilyMed
Hendry, Khati L., FamilyMed
Julien, Warren R.
Krabbe, Marjorie E., FamilyMed
Lebel, Martine
Manders, Terence P.
Richardson, Wendy L.
Severide, Susan P., FamilyMed
Stevens, Kyle D., FamilyMed
Van Der Vyver, Izak A.
Venkataraman, Murali
Wilson, Kevin R.

SURREY

Abraham, Ronnie P.
Acheson, Todd M.
Ahmed, Hala M A., FamilyMed
Akbar, Zaubaria
Ali, Tahmeena T., FamilyMed
Amankwe, Isaac O., FamilyMed
Ambrose, Laura E., FamilyMed
Anderson, David K.
Anderson, Patricia C.
Araki, Michael T.
Arnold, Todd W., FamilyMed
Athwal, Bali
Aulakh, Paramjit S.
Aziz, Shiraz F.
Baasch, Erik J., FamilyMed
Bains, Jason D., FamilyMed
Baker, Wayne K., FamilyMed
Balakrishna, Rangappa, FamilyMed
Barrio, Sally E., FamilyMed
Barwich, Doris B A., FamilyMed
Benitez-Gomez, Antonio, FamilyMed
Benitez-Lazo, Jose M.
Bernat, Reinhold
Bhatt, Arun, FamilyMed
Bhatti, Balbir C., FamilyMed
Bhimani, Laila, FamilyMed
Blackshaw, Patricia M P., FamilyMed
Blackshaw, W. Roy
Blinkhorn, Mark T.
Bourke, Michael A E.
Bredenkamp, Andries P., FamilyMed
Brits, Bernice, FamilyMed
Brock, Jonathan H., FamilyMed(EM)
Brookstone, Alan J.
Buttar, Sonia D.
Byrne, Brendan J O.
Chan, Kelvin, FamilyMed
Cheema, Gulzar S., FamilyMed
Chehil, Rakesh S.
Chemerika, Philip J V.
Chen, Szu-Yang
Cheung, Christian S G., FamilyMed
Chew, Sen
Chong, David L T., FamilyMed(EM)
Chow, Stacey A.
Claire, Daljit T S.
Cooner, Manpreet K., FamilyMed
Cox, Christopher J.
Crisp, Barbara J.
Dandina, Sujith K.
Daniel, Geraldine R., FamilyMed
Dave, Hemang J.
David, Eleazar W., FamilyMed
Dawkins, Christopher J.
Deernsted, Eric A.
Derkach, Sandra E., FamilyMed
Dhaliwal, Harmanpreet V., FamilyMed
Dhillon, Pawandeep K., FamilyMed
Dhiman, S. Paul, FamilyMed(EM)
Di Cesare, Marie
Dindo, Luay F.
Dindo, Rashad F.
Donaldson, Suzanne C., FamilyMed
Dosanjh, Ramneek K., FamilyMed
Dubec, Jiri J., FamilyMed
Durnin-Goodman, Eithne M., FamilyMed
Dyer, David W., FamilyMed
Eadie, Carmen N., FamilyMed
Ellis, Olga F.
Eslami, Ali
Fahim, Ziaullah
Ferris, Caroline R., FamilyMed
Finley, Scott G., FamilyMed(EM)
Forsyth, Robert D., FamilyMed(EM)
Frankel, Michael
Fransen, Donald A.
Frobb, Mark K., FamilyMed
Fujiwara, Joan R.
Garry, Benedict M., FamilyMed
Garvin, Robin W.
Gaucher, Anita L.
Gerber, Michelle R.
Gerntholtz, Werner E., FamilyMed(EM)
Ghanipour Farahani, Ali, FamilyMed
Ghuman, Jaspinder, FamilyMed(EM)
Ghura, Parminder S.
Gibbings, Grant W J., FamilyMed
Giles, Catherine E.
Gill, Navdip S., FamilyMed
Gin, Davey Y M., FamilyMed
Golden, Jonathan G., FamilyMed(EM)
Goldie, Morag E.
Green, Mark C.
Gustafson, Larry O J.
Gutteridge, Tim J., FamilyMed
Guy, David J.
Hainc, Milan
Hair, Amarjit S.
Hari, Krishna S P.
Haribhai, Jayshree C.
Hartwig, Michael C.
Hassan, Haron, FamilyMed
Henderson, David M.
Hepburn, Robert W A., FamilyMed
Herbert, Melodie, FamilyMed
Hrabar, Zenona M I.
Hussain, Ijaz
Icton, Carolyn D., FamilyMed
Ip, Yiu Ban
Itcush, Laurie L.
Iwama, Tom T., FamilyMed
Jackson, Elaine E.
Januszewska, Mariola S., FamilyMed
Jassal, Harinder
Jassal, Inderjit S., FamilyMed
Jawanda, Madhumeet K., FamilyMed
Jiwa, Karima, FamilyMed
Johnson, Sharon B.
Johnston, Jeremy V W.
Joseph, Anu Bala
Kalsi, Gursharan S.
Kanagaratnam, Christina N., FamilyMed
Kara, Sukaina, FamilyMed
Kashif, Muhammad
Khalsa, Kesar S.
Khalsa, Satwant K.
Khan, Liaquat H.
Khan, Muhammad N.
Khan, Shereena, FamilyMed
Khandelwal, Sanjay
Kim, Anne M., FamilyMed
King, Charles D.
King, Pamela A.
King, Timothy R.
Kirkpatrick, Janice M.
Koseff, Howard D.
Kothari, Kasiyal, FamilyMed
Krishan, Vivek T.
Kuan, Alano, FamilyMed(EM)
Laifer, Elizabeth
Lal, Smita J.
Lam, Mayda
Lammerse, Christine, FamilyMed
Larigakis, Steven, FamilyMed(EM)
Lau, Juliet Y., FamilyMed
Laubenstein, Susan
Lawrie, Susan L.
Lebl, Martin G., FamilyMed
Lee, Michael D.
Lee, Susan, FamilyMed
Lei, K K. Lourenco
Leifso, Lowell R.
Leon, Malcolm, FamilyMed
Leung, Bess
Lim, Rosemary Dy.
Lin, Hong, FamilyMed
Lockhart, Alexander S.
Lockhart, Pamela J.
Loke, Mei Woei, FamilyMed
Louw, Johannes
Low, Anthony C L.
Low, Bligh K W.
Low, Edmond C M.
Low, Louise J Y., FamilyMed
Lowe, Derek W., FamilyMed
Lu, Yvette C., FamilyMed
Luk, W T. David
Ma, Alan S.
MacCharles, George R.
Mahungu Longo-Kitoko, P.
Major, Andrew F., FamilyMed
Manchanda, Raman, FamilyMed
Manji, Rahimali, FamilyMed
Mann, Jotinder S., FamilyMed
Mann, Ramandeep, FamilyMed
Martens, Jay D.
Masuda, Judith M.
Mattu, Gurdial S.
McClelland, Janet M.
McCormack, Philip C.
McDonald, Angus C., FamilyMed
Meek, Grant P., FamilyMed
Melamed, Jennifer B.
Mendoza, Paul J., FamilyMed
Mercer, Jean A.
Mergens, Joseph E.
Minhas, Shikha, FamilyMed
Mittermaier, Barbara M E., FamilyMed
Mittermaier, Michael E R., FamilyMed(EM)
Moosa, Malek B., FamilyMed
Mugisha, James K.
Mukheibir, Peter, FamilyMed
Muncey, Joy A., FamilyMed
Murphy, Alan S.
Nagra, Riffat S.
Naidoo, Erin C.
Nakai, Harumi
Narod, Mairi M.
Narwal, Anita S.
Nelson, Elena, FamilyMed
Neufeld, William P.
Ng, Chan-Poh
Ng, Douglas B G.
Ng, Susanna S N.
Niazi, Nazia S.
Nolte, Josephus J., FamilyMed
Nordli, Charlene M.
O'Brien, Fiona J., FamilyMed
O'Brien, John I.
O'Brien-Bell, John
O'Dwyer, Niall P., FamilyMed
O'Halloran, Richard G.
Omelchenko, Victor
Ozolins, Laura N., FamilyMed
Pabani, Anizmohamed S.
Parikh, Ameet
Park, Grace H., FamilyMed
Parsons, Thomas D., FamilyMed
Patel, Kaleena, FamilyMed(EM)
Pather, Jhodipraghasen
Patricelli, Charissa J., FamilyMed
Peace, Janice L.

Peach, Stephen C., FamilyMed
Pereira, Robert B., FamilyMed
Petrovic, Sean
Peyvandi, Banafsheh, FamilyMed
Phillips, Jonathan D.
Picton, Avis R., FamilyMed
Pollock, Andrea E., FamilyMed
Prentice, Bryan R.
Pretty, James A., FamilyMed
Prevost, Jay, FamilyMed
Raffle, Valerie J.
Rai, Pardeep S.
Ram, Pawan K.
Ramani, Nithyakalyani, FamilyMed
Rauniyar, Pooja, FamilyMed
Rayavarapu, Beaulah, FamilyMed
Raza, Hammad
Reyes-Smith, Larina M., FamilyMed
Riskalla, Frey F F., FamilyMed
Rostvig, L. Jeffrey, FamilyMed
Rouhana, Elisson, FamilyMed
Ruffo, Connie J.
Ryan, Andrea C., FamilyMed
Rykszynski, Cathy M., FamilyMed
Sabados, Wade A., FamilyMed(EM)
Sahota, Perminder S.
Sahota, Preena S., FamilyMed
Saincher, Rajeev
Samad, Osman
Samoil, Darryl P., FamilyMed(EM)
Sandhar, Ajit, FamilyMed
Sandhu, Dalip S.
Sanghe, Parminder S., FamilyMed
Sanghe, Satinder K., FamilyMed
Sangster, Joan E., FamilyMed
Sawhney, Sandeep, FamilyMed
Schuurman, Irma E., FamilyMed
Scott, Jeremy G., FamilyMed
Sennewald Teskey, Lisa M.
Shah, Sachit P., FamilyMed
Sharif, Omar, FamilyMed
Sharifi, Nader, FamilyMed
Sharma, Pankaj, FamilyMed
Shiu, Patrick K Y.
Shukin, Evelyn K.
Sidhu, Jiwan S., FamilyMed
Sidhu, Mandeep K., FamilyMed
Sidhu, Rabinder S., FamilyMed
Singh, Kanwarjit
Singh, Sukhwinder, FamilyMed
Smit, Martina
Smit, Willem J E.
Smith, Deirdre D., FamilyMed
Sohal, Parmjit S., FamilyMed
Sommerfeld, Martin R., FamilyMed
Starke, Victor A.
Stephens, John D.
Strauts, Zigurts
Strijack, Bradford J.
Strovskaia, Galina, FamilyMed
Strovski, Semion, FamilyMed
Stuart, Katherine A., FamilyMed
Suh, Sung-Hee, FamilyMed
Suleiman, Thomas, FamilyMed
Sutherland, Michelle
Szpakowicz, Mikolaj D., FamilyMed(EM)
Tadros, William I.
Tallos, Peter B.
Tan-Tam, Clara C H.
Tang, Howard H L.
Taub, Nadine S., FamilyMed
Tawar, Vinod C., FamilyMed
Taylor, Dale B.
Teskey, Luke M.
Ting, John U L.
Tom, Roger W J.
Towill, Garry A., FamilyMed
Trinder, Tammy C., FamilyMed
Tu, Kimphry M., FamilyMed(EM)
Tumber, Hardeep S.
Tung, Amrik S.
Tyrell, Benjamin D.
Uyeda, Linda E.
Van Aardt, Jan A N.
Van Buynder, Paul
Van Donkersgoed, Lubbertus, FamilyMed
Vanukuru, Venkata R., FamilyMed
Villalon, Reynaldo D M.
Vinnitsky, Leonid
Vipler, Sharon K., FamilyMed
Wadge, Richard
Wagner, Brent G.
Wagner, Christine M., FamilyMed
Walter, Phillip C.
Wang, Jen-Te
Wang, Yue, FamilyMed
Warrington, Cara L E.
Warshawski, Patricia A.
Watson, Ann E.
Webb, Margot A.
Weiler, Kathleen A., FamilyMed
Weldon, Mimi B., FamilyMed
West, Susan M.
Wilhelm-Boyles, Carrie M., FamilyMed(EM)
Wilkhu, Gagandeep S., FamilyMed
Williamson, Owen D.
Willms, Arthur G., FamilyMed(EM)
Wilson, Richard M.
Wilson, Trevor G., FamilyMed
Wong, Leo T M., FamilyMed
Wong, Shek-Leung
Wong-Ting, Joy J Y.
Yan, Ilym G., FamilyMed
Yang, Joseph C., FamilyMed
Yang, Kwang, FamilyMed
Yang, Lawrence, FamilyMed
Yang, Sharmila, FamilyMed
Yong, Yean-Sim
Yu, Patrick W W., FamilyMed
Yu, Shihao

TAKLA LANDING

Pawlovich, John P., FamilyMed

TATLAYOKO LAKE

Smialowski, Michal A N., FamilyMed

TELKWA

Laskowski, Alfred E., FamilyMed

TERRACE

Appleton, Geoffrey M.
Barton, Nicola A.
Bowering, David
Brauer, Barbara J.
Brown, Lennox N.
De Bruin, Maria M.
De Wit, Christiaan C.
Du Plessis, Jean G.
Fourie, Hendrina H C E.
Fourie, W. Jacobus
Hoy, Peter
Iyayi, Ehinomen A., FamilyMed
Jardine, Ivan
Linton, Gregory J., FamilyMed
Lotz, Petrus C.
Meyburg, Jan M.
Moolman, Johnathan
Olorunfemi, Ayodele O.
Strydom, Jacobus
Telikicharla Kandala, Narsimhachary
van Niekerk, Petrus J.
Wong, Shun-Chi

TOFINO

Armstrong, John
Frazee, Pamela J.
Killins, Brian A.
Stogryn, Krista M., FamilyMed
Williston, Luke A., FamilyMed

TRAIL

Aiken, Trevor C., FamilyMed
Benzer, Susan D.
Cameron, Stephanie A., FamilyMed
Campbell, Gwen A M.
Cochran, Jennifer J D., FamilyMed
De Greef, Andre
Dobovicnik, Bernard K.
Fawcett, Bruce M.
Forman, Katherine C.
Gill, Tara M., FamilyMed(EM)
Grey, Robert G.
Hii, Ting H.
Hume, Cheryl A., FamilyMed
Hussey, Jeffrey A., FamilyMed(EM)
Jacobsen, Marnie
Knox, Corinne E L., FamilyMed
Krampl, Peter, FamilyMed(EM)
Latendresse, Myriam, FamilyMed(EM)
Lum, Derek W., FamilyMed
Paul, Leslie V.
Phillips, Rowland L.
Pratt, Adele, FamilyMed
Segal, Samantha
Smith, Miles J C., FamilyMed
Spencer, Steven
Stanley, Blair D., FamilyMed
Toews, Gertrude J.
Tucker, Sarah A., FamilyMed
Von Dehn, Stephanie K., FamilyMed
Wilson, Richard J.

TUMBLER RIDGE

Bredenkamp, Lynne
Helm, Charles W., FamilyMed
Louw, Chrisman J.

UCLUELET

Marshall, Carrie
O'Brien, John M., FamilyMed

VALEMOUNT

Keyter, Herman P., FamilyMed
Markham, Ray J., FamilyMed

VANCOUVER

Abbey, Mark D., FamilyMed
Abbott, David F.
Abdel-Barr, Sara J.
Abrahams, Ronald R., FamilyMed
Abu Sharar, Ziad
Ackland, Susan
Aghanajafi, Effat, FamilyMed
Agulnik, David B., FamilyMed(EM)
Ahamad, Keith R.
Ahmed, Shaheen
Ali, Naved A., FamilyMed
Alimenti, Ariane
Allaye-Chan, Louise T.
Amin, Prakash A.
Anderson, Carol P.
Anderson, Cheryl D.
Andrew, Rodney F., FamilyMed
Aota, Eriko, FamilyMed
Aparicio, Catriona L.
Apostle, Nicole A., FamilyMed
Applegarth, Christine W L.
Armstrong, Kristy A., FamilyMed
Arnold, Barbra J., FamilyMed
Arnold, Karen P., FamilyMed
Aronshtam, Grygory, FamilyMed
Atkinson, Kathryn J., FamilyMed
Avinashi, Sanja, FamilyMed
Ayling, Grant R.
Badra Quirion, Karine, FamilyMed
Baggoo, Darlene M., FamilyMed
Baghbannazary, Maryam, FamilyMed
Bailey, Anthony J.
Baird, Lawson D.
Bakonyi, Judit, FamilyMed
Balaisis, Elise M J., FamilyMed
Baldwin, Caroline L., FamilyMed
Balog, Stephanie A., FamilyMed
Baranyi, Katherine A.
Barber, George P.
Barbour, Kathryn A.
Baria, Niloofer, FamilyMed
Barnes, Lisa M., FamilyMed
Barrett, Thomas A.
Barrigar, Diana, FamilyMed
Bartlett, Sarah K B., FamilyMed
Barzelai, Laurence P., FamilyMed
Bassett, Kenneth L.
Basson, Rosemary J.
Bates, Joanna M., FamilyMed
Batt, Nathan
Bauman, Gary T.
Bedell, Richard A.
Behra, Tasniem
Behroozi, Dara, FamilyMed
Bell, Georgina L., FamilyMed
Bell, Jeffrey H., FamilyMed
Benedek, Caroline O., FamilyMed
Bergman, Arthur, FamilyMed
Bergson, Victor S.
Beveridge, Paul M., FamilyMed
Bhatt, Sunil K., FamilyMed
Bhola-Reebye, Stacy C., FamilyMed
Bienert, Tasha N., FamilyMed
Birch, J. Andrew
Bishop, Paul B.
Black, Charlyn D.
Blackman, Douglas H., FamilyMed
Blaney, Gregory P.
Blaxland, Joanne B.
Bluman, Robert A., FamilyMed
Boey, Gerald E.
Bojanowska-Moore, Czeslawa
Bootsman, Laurie B.
Boparai, Gurdev S.
Boraston, Suni E.
Bordalba, Emilia M.
Borkenhagen, Rainer H., FamilyMed
Botting, Emily F., FamilyMed
Bowlsby, Glenn O.
Bowlsby, Jeffrey K.
Brands, Ralph H.
Brar, Harinderpal S.
Braun, Martin E., FamilyMed(EM)
Brcic, Vanessa E.
Bregman, Isaiah D., FamilyMed
Brison, Meghan L.
Britton, Brian H.
Broady, Raewyn C.
Brooks, Paul A.
Broughton, Steven A.
Brown, Deborah S.
Brown, Roy A.
Browne, Candice
Browning, David P.
Bruyere, Helene A T.
Budai, Balint L., FamilyMed
Bueno, Antonio D.
Buhler, Karen I., FamilyMed
Burak, A. John, FamilyMed
Burgess, Susan C., FamilyMed
Burlin, Robert M.
Burns, Graham B.
Burns, Michael A.
Burrill, Joshua H P.
Bus, Judith I.
Butt, Donald F., FamilyMed
Butt, John C.
Byczko, Beata J.
Cadenhead, Kathleen, FamilyMed
Cadesky, Eric, FamilyMed
Calam, Betty, FamilyMed
Campbell, Christina S F., FamilyMed
Canderle, Frank, FamilyMed
Cardoso, Tatiana, FamilyMed
Carter, Michael G R.
Casey, Brett M.
Cassidy, Myles J A.
Chadha, Neil K.
Chadha, Rashmi, FamilyMed
Chalmers, Paula D., FamilyMed
Chambers, Gordon K.
Chan, Andy
Chan, Cynthia S Y., FamilyMed
Chan, Cyril F Y.
Chan, Irene M Y.
Chan, Jeanie C.
Chan, Jessica W., FamilyMed
Chan, Kai-Sun
Chan, Karl K S.
Chan, Kenneth H., FamilyMed
Chan, S H. Sandy
Chan, Sherry, FamilyMed
Chan-Yan, Sharon J., FamilyMed
Chandna, Divi
Chang, Bruce H.
Chang, Cindy C H.
Chang, Diana M., FamilyMed(EM)
Chang, Heather A.
Chang, Terence A.
Chanoine, Jean-Pierre
Chao, Hubert Y.
Chapman, Sharon, FamilyMed
Chau, Anthony
Chen, Chih-Chien
Chen, Helen Y., FamilyMed
Chen, James C.
Chen, Simon I., FamilyMed(EM)
Cheng, A. Lawrence, FamilyMed(EM)
Cheng, Charles Y Y.
Cherkezoff, Alexander N., FamilyMed
Cherneski, Heather M., FamilyMed
Chete, Edwin O.
Cheung, Andrea, FamilyMed
Chew, Sander J L.
Chilvers, Mark A.
Chin, Christopher A.
Chiu, Peter C H.
Chiu, Wing-Gay
Cho, Kenneth M C., FamilyMed
Choi, W M. Joyce, FamilyMed
Chong, Henry K H.
Chong, Sophia S H.
Chong, Tiffany L., FamilyMed
Choo, Darren W K.
Chow, Faye H.
Chow, Raymond
Chu, Stephanie W., FamilyMed
Chung, Kalyani, FamilyMed
Cinarli, Bahar, FamilyMed
Cisternas, Felipe, FamilyMed
Ciszak, Wojtek P.
Clark, Peter D.
Clarke, Andrew L.
Clarke, B. Jean
Clarke, Sophie
Clarke, Teresa Anne.
Clarren, Sterling Keith
Clelland, Catherine A., FamilyMed
Cline, Leah L A.
Coburn, M. Ellen
Coleman, Jeffrey R.
Collins, Deborah L., FamilyMed
Comay, Susan E.
Comeau, Gisele M.
Condon, Caroline D.
Connell, Ian D.
Connolly, Allan K.
Cooper, Donald A.
Cooper, Jacqueline M., FamilyMed
Copeland, Joseph E., FamilyMed(EM)
Corvalan-Grossling, Veronica, FamilyMed
Coschizza, Rose-Marie, FamilyMed
Cottick, Kimberley R., FamilyMed
Covert, Cristina
Craggs, Rachael T.
Creba, Aran S., FamilyMed
Cresswell, Silke
Culham, Tania L., FamilyMed
Dadachanji, Shiroy, FamilyMed
Dahlmanns, Matthias
Dalgarno, S. Michelle, FamilyMed
Dann, Kathleen K., FamilyMed
Das, Ananya
David, Ivo
Davis, Jeffrey H.
De Vlaming, Stanley C.
De Wet, Joseph J., FamilyMed
Dhawan, Nishi, FamilyMed
Dick, Robert N B.
Dicus, Jennifer, FamilyMed
Dionne, Karla
Dlin, Arnold D.
Dodek, Daniel Y., FamilyMed
Doig, Pamela A., FamilyMed
Donaldson, Beth L., FamilyMed
Donaldson Bramley, Lauren M., FamilyMed
Donnellan, Fergal
Doran, Una, FamilyMed(EM)
Dossa, Fahreen A., FamilyMed
Dubland, Edward J.
Dubord, Janet Y.
Ducceschi, Sylvia P., FamilyMed
Duncan, Fiona C., FamilyMed

PHYSICIANS BY PROVINCE

Dunn, Barbara L.
Dunn, Celina T., FamilyMed
Dunne, Caitlin
Durkin, Chris
Dwyer, Desmond P., FamilyMed
Eberdt, Caroline T., FamilyMed(EM)
Edamura, Arthur
Edgar, Adrian
Edgar, Melvin L., FamilyMed
Edmonds, Kenneth R., FamilyMed(EM)
Edwards, Geoffrey B L.
Elliot, Eleanor K.
Elliott, Stacy L.
Ellison, C. Andrew, FamilyMed
Eng, Aik-Ping
Esler, David J., FamilyMed(EM)
Etches, Duncan J., FamilyMed
Etches, Nora J M., FamilyMed
Evans, C. James
Eydoux, Patrice L.
Ezekiel, Daniel
Faiers, Selena
Fairweather, Tanya, FamilyMed
Falk, Annemarie L., FamilyMed
Fang, Karen Y Y., FamilyMed
Faraday, Trent K.
Farmer, Michael J.
Farrales, Lynn L., FamilyMed
Fay, Heather E.
Fay, Sean Leo
Feinstadt, Garry, FamilyMed
Ferguson, Janis A.
Fernandez, Renee, FamilyMed
Fieschi, Isabelle A., FamilyMed
Findlay, Timothy, FamilyMed(EM)
Fineman, Lauren, FamilyMed
Fisher, Mark M.
Fisher, Teri V., FamilyMed
Fitzmaurice, Michael J., FamilyMed
Fitzpatrick, Tania E., FamilyMed
Fleming, Ian M.
Fofie, Monica
Fong, Keng Lao
Fong, Sharon Y C., FamilyMed
Foster, Nicholas K.
Franiek, Janet N., FamilyMed
French, Anthony J.
Friesen, Graham, FamilyMed
Friesen, Janet M.
Fritz, Bradley A.
Fry, Nicholas J.
Fu, Anita
Fu, Remedios T.
Fung, Daniel Y W.
Fung, Kenneth K.
Gaerber, Shari J.
Gagne, Ann A.
Gallagher, Romayne, FamilyMed
Galloway, Meriel A., FamilyMed
Gan, S W. Helen, FamilyMed
Gardner, Jillian, FamilyMed
Garrett, Cynthia A.
Gatto, Joan
Geddes, Valerie, FamilyMed
Gee, Brian, FamilyMed
Genot, Roxane, FamilyMed
Georgilas, Mary
Gerretsen, Martin
Gerring, David R.
Ghahary, Ali
Gharapetian, Angineh
Gibson, Bruce A., FamilyMed
Gibson, G. Thomas C., FamilyMed
Giles, Ann M W., FamilyMed
Gilmore, Andrew
Giovannetti, Brian L.
Gisslow, Mary T.
Glanzberg, Monte M., FamilyMed
Glasner, Carly S., FamilyMed
Glotman, C. Stephanie
Glynn-Morris, Rodney, FamilyMed
Goldie, Craig, FamilyMed
Golin, Peter D.
Gonzalez-Romulus, Marie-Christina, FamilyMed
Gordon, Danielle M., FamilyMed
Gordon, Marla, FamilyMed
Gordon, Rhona M.
Gore, Bing Quon.
Gouws, Daniel R.
Govender, Priya
Graham, Nicholas R., FamilyMed
Grant, Nasha E., FamilyMed
Greenberg, Ronald B.
Greenhill, Alexandra, FamilyMed
Grewal, Navdeep K., FamilyMed(EM)
Griffin, Barbara S., FamilyMed
Gross, Paul, FamilyMed
Grunau, Brian, FamilyMed(EM)
Grzybowski, Stefan C W., FamilyMed
Gudgeon, Avery M., FamilyMed
Guillemi, Silvia
Gunn, Chit-Chan
Gunn, Harold D.
Gutman, Samuel J., FamilyMed(EM)
Hahn, Peter J., FamilyMed
Haji Pavlou, Christopher
Hall, Carolyn M., FamilyMed
Hall, David R A., FamilyMed
Hall, Lacresha L.
Hall, Renee N., FamilyMed
Halperin, Harvey I.
Ham, Kevin
Hameer, Taslim
Hamid, Samina
Hansson, Ann M., FamilyMed
Haq, Syed M S., FamilyMed
Hardial, Janine L., FamilyMed
Harmon, Thomas P.
Harpur, R. Arthur
Harris, Devin R., FamilyMed(EM)
Harris, Marianne, FamilyMed
Harrison, David W., FamilyMed(EM)
Harvey, Catherine A., FamilyMed
Hassam, Imtiaz K.
Hasson, Victor
Hathorn, John F.
Hatlelid, Keith
Hay, Richard C.
Hayward, Judith E.
Heffernan, Mary C.
Henderson, Garry
Henderson, Laura J W., FamilyMed
Henderson, Lemay E., FamilyMed
Henning, Christopher, FamilyMed
Henry, Willa J., FamilyMed
Hii, James F K.
Hillary, Edward W., FamilyMed
Himelfarb, Erite
Hinchliffe, Mary J., FamilyMed
Hippola, Dimithra N., FamilyMed
Ho, Alice K Y., FamilyMed
Ho, Elinda P L.
Ho, Hoi Shing
Ho, Thomas M W., FamilyMed
Ho, Wei-Ning
Ho-Asjoe, Marianne P K., FamilyMed
Hocking, Deborah A.
Hodgson, Christopher J.
Hoeberg, Debbie J.
Holan, Jan
Hollenberg, Susan L.
Holloway, Michael A., FamilyMed(EM)
Horn, Marilyn J.
Horner, Richard H.
Horricks, Colin H., FamilyMed
Horton, Lesley, FamilyMed
Horvath, Gary P., FamilyMed
Hou, Daniel J.
Hou, Frank L.
House, W. Peter
Howard, Sheldon
Howitt, Patricia A.
Hsiao, Yann J.
Hsu, David H.
Hsu, Pei-Ti, FamilyMed
Huang, Gloria W S.
Hubinette, Maria M., FamilyMed
Huff, C. Lynn, FamilyMed
Hui, Alphonsus Z.
Hui, Catherine C M., FamilyMed
Huikeshoven, Menno
Humphries, R. Keith
Hung, Peggy, FamilyMed
Hung, Tawny W.
Hunt, Christopher G E.
Hunt, Georgia C., FamilyMed
Hunter, John M.
Hunter, Kenneth C.
Iloreta, Aileen, FamilyMed
Ip, Janet L., FamilyMed
Ipsiroglu, Osman S.
Iriarte, Paula L., FamilyMed
Irwin, Joanne L., FamilyMed
Ismaily, Nasreen S., FamilyMed
Izen, Randi J., FamilyMed
Jacobsen, Craig A.
Jacoby, Colin S.
Jafari, Siavash
James, Nicola D.
Jamieson, Jean L.
Jando, Linda J., FamilyMed
Jansen, Kara A., FamilyMed
Jayaraman, Chitra, FamilyMed
Jayaraman, Jyothi, FamilyMed
Jenkins, Heather D., FamilyMed
Jetha, Shamin, FamilyMed
Joe, Ronald S.
Joffe, Beth E., FamilyMed
Joffe, John B.
Johnson, Krista M., FamilyMed
Johnson, Laura B.
Johnston, Olwyn
Johnston, Williard P.
Joyce, David P., FamilyMed(EM)
Jue, Perpetua
Kalinowski, Leszek
Kalla, Daniel M., FamilyMed(EM)
Kam, Sau Shun, FamilyMed
Kam, Timothy W T.
Kamani, Azadali A.
Kamani, Rozmin F., FamilyMed
Kang, Maria, FamilyMed
Karim, Mandy
Karon, Stanley F., FamilyMed
Karsai, Helen
Kebarle, Paula J., FamilyMed(EM)
Keenan, Maureen P., FamilyMed
Kei, Olivia C Y., FamilyMed
Kendal, Wendy M.
Kennedy, Russell G.
Kenny, Erin K., FamilyMed(EM)
Kernahan, Jill, FamilyMed
Kestler, Mary H.
Ketene, Atila H.
Khan, Karim
Khan, Mohamed K.
Khara, Milan, FamilyMed
Khunkhun, J. Sevena, FamilyMed
Kilpatrick, Nevin, FamilyMed
Kim, Rozaliya, FamilyMed
King, David S., FamilyMed
Kirk, Peter J., FamilyMed
Kirker, Jennifer M., FamilyMed(EM)
Kirkham, Colleen M., FamilyMed
Klass, Darren
Klassen, Julie A., FamilyMed
Klassen, Vicki J., FamilyMed
Klein, Michael C., FamilyMed
Kljajic, Djordje
Knebel, Laura C., FamilyMed
Kneifel, Dorle G.
Knell, Eva, FamilyMed
Ko, Peter, FamilyMed
Ko, Simon C C.
Koczapski, Andrzej B A., FamilyMed
Koehle, Michael S., FamilyMed
Koehn, Martha E.
Koelink, Anthony F C., FamilyMed
Kolesar, Sharlene E., FamilyMed
Kollmann, Tobias
Koo, Howan
Koo, Jonathan J.
Kozoriz, Kelsey D M., FamilyMed
Krausz, Samuel E., FamilyMed
Kruse, Karen P.
Krykorka, Peter, FamilyMed
Kuhl, David R.
Kurdyak, Stephen A., FamilyMed
Kwan, Raymond S H.
Kwong, Juliet, FamilyMed
Laban, Premakanthie R.
Lacuna, Julie B D., FamilyMed
Lai, Andrea S L P., FamilyMed
Lai, David K F., FamilyMed
Lai, James K., FamilyMed
Lai, Roxanne, FamilyMed
Lakey, William H.
Lam, C. Allan
Lam, Jasmine C., FamilyMed
Lam, Joseph K P., FamilyMed
Lam, Pei-Yoong
Lam, Wai-Arm
Lamb, Tasha H., FamilyMed
Lamont, A. Margaret, FamilyMed
Lang, Bridget Y C.
Lange, Lisa M M., FamilyMed
Lanphear, Nancy E.
Lapuste, Mihaela F., FamilyMed
Laramee, Jani, FamilyMed
Lau, Amanda W M., FamilyMed
Law, Bonnie, FamilyMed
Law, Charles C S.
Law, Sally S C., FamilyMed
Lawrence, Julie B H., FamilyMed
Lawrence, Michael R., FamilyMed
Lee, Angela Y M.
Lee, Anita K., FamilyMed
Lee, Calvin
Lee, Catherine M., FamilyMed
Lee, Donald D.
Lee, Douglas J.
Lee, Judy K M.
Lee, Ka Yiu.
Lee, Kenny
Lee, Michael C., FamilyMed
Lee, Rachel N.
Lee, Sandra W., FamilyMed
Lee, Virginia
Lee, William
Lee Son, Archie
Legg, Karen K.
Leong, Philip W T.
Lepard, Linda
Lepard, Timothy
Leung, Constant H., FamilyMed
Leung, Helen K.
Leung, Henry H K.
Leung, Man K.
Leung, Michael N F.
Leung, Ngar-Lin
Leung, Wing Yee V.
Levitt, Nirvair K., FamilyMed
Levy, Lyall A.
Lewis, Marion E S.
Li, Jiwei, FamilyMed
Liew, Kim L.
Lim, Bin-Keng, FamilyMed(EM)
Lim, Elizabeth S., FamilyMed
Lim, May-Ling J.
Lim, Wi-Guan
Lima, Rosanna V., FamilyMed
Lin, I C. John
Lindsay, Krystaleah
Linekin, Michelle J., FamilyMed
Lipkowitz, Lana G.
Liu, Jenny Y., FamilyMed
Livingstone, Verity H., FamilyMed
Lloyd-Smith, D. Robertson
Lo, Cynthia C Y.
Lo, Cynthia Y W., FamilyMed
Lo, Reginald W W.
Loewen, Mary L.
Logan, Laurie A., FamilyMed
Loh, George
Loh, Karmen K M.
Lorenzon, C. Gabriella
Lorne, Jennifer G W., FamilyMed
Loubert, Lise E.
Louie, Andrew J.
Love, Robert J.
Lovett, Katrin A., FamilyMed
Low, Rhonda S., FamilyMed
Lubin, Stanley, FamilyMed
Lucky, Cindy-Ann, FamilyMed(EM)
Luke, Edward C H., FamilyMed(EM)
Lukowska, Irena
Lum, Edward
Lusina, Jillian B., FamilyMed
Lutsky, Peter M., FamilyMed
Luu, Thanh, FamilyMed
Ma, Gilbert
Ma, Ian S.
Ma, Raymond L T.
Ma, Roderick K C., FamilyMed
MacCarthy, Daniel D.
MacDonald, D. Scott
MacDonald, Donald C.
MacDonald, Malcolm K.
MacDonald, Stephen J H., FamilyMed
MacGowan, Nori A.
MacInnes, Alison M., FamilyMed
MacInnis, Benjamin F., FamilyMed
MacIver, Suzanne A., FamilyMed
MacLeod, Jeanne Z., FamilyMed(EM)
Mackie, J. William, FamilyMed
Madsen, Michael F P., FamilyMed
Mah, Peter G.
Mah, Venetia S J., FamilyMed
Mail, W. John, FamilyMed
Maiter, Nasrin
Majeed, Haseena, FamilyMed
Maki, Ron S.
Malhotra, Unjali, FamilyMed
Malleson, Rosemary M.
Man, Denise I., FamilyMed
Manes, Arturo S., FamilyMed
Mangal, Sunil K., FamilyMed(EM)
Mann, Ranbir S.
Manning, E. David, FamilyMed
March, Roderick J.
Marhin, Wilson W., FamilyMed
Maric-Plavsic, Jelena, FamilyMed
Maroo, Sanjay V.
Marr, Peter J.
Marsden, John J., FamilyMed(EM)
Martin, Ruth E., FamilyMed
Martz, Laurie B.
Mason, Melanie P., FamilyMed
Masri, Rola
Masuhara, E. Joy, FamilyMed
Mate, Gabor
Mathew, Silvy M., FamilyMed
Mathias, Cathleen P., FamilyMed
Matsyk, Jacqueline B.
Mattheis, Kelly G.
Mazowita, Garey B M., FamilyMed
Mazzarella, Angelo A., FamilyMed
McAleer, Katherine A., FamilyMed
McCallum, Catherine L.
McClure, Donna J., FamilyMed
McConville, Raymond J.
McCracken, Rita K., FamilyMed
McDermid, Cheryl E.
McDonald, William R.
McGillivray, Lee W., FamilyMed
McGillivray, William G.
McGregor, Margaret, FamilyMed
McGuire, Caterina, FamilyMed
McIlrath, H. Ruth
McIver, Ian Garth.
McKechnie, M. Paula
McKenzie, Donald C.
McKeown, Janet C.
McKnight, David W G., FamilyMed
McLachlan, Donna L., FamilyMed
McMorran, John D R.
McNestry, Ailve M., FamilyMed
Mead, Annabel J.
Meckler, Garth D.
Medvedev, Nadia
Meher, Abu F M A.
Mehta, Paras B., FamilyMed
Mendelson, Mitchell N.
Menzies, Robert D., FamilyMed
Mercereau, Paul
Mereu, Adriana-Iona
Merkli, Kimberly A., FamilyMed
Merriman, Sarah L., FamilyMed
Messier, Helen M V., FamilyMed
Metcalfe, Sonja J., FamilyMed
Meyer, Maxwell W., FamilyMed
Miles, Brandt D.
Miller, Duncan R.
Miller, Lisa J.
Miller, Milton C.
Mirwaldt, Patricia A., FamilyMed
Mitchell, Sheona M.
Mitchner, Leslie K., FamilyMed
Mithani, Akber H.
Moccia, Patrizia
Moccia, Rino P.
Modi, Deepshikha, FamilyMed
Mohammed, Shelliza N., FamilyMed
Montgomery, Brian F.
Moore, Eva M.
Moore, Simon G D., FamilyMed
Moreau, Arja E., FamilyMed
Morris, Dorian V.
Morris, Tracey M., FamilyMed
Morrison, A. Bruce, FamilyMed(EM)
Morrison, Andrew B.
Morrison, Heather M D.
Morton, Pol G D., FamilyMed

PHYSICIANS BY PROVINCE

Morwen-Smith, Jennifer A.
Moser, Edith K., FamilyMed
Moss, Margaret E M.
Mota, Ihor R., FamilyMed
Mudaliar, Adi K M., FamilyMed
Mulpuri, Udaya K K.
Mulzet, Darlana L., FamilyMed
Murphy, Carol M.
Murphy, John P E.
Murphy, Kirk J.
Murray, Craig S., FamilyMed(EM)
Murschell, Warren D., FamilyMed(EM)
Musial, Alexander J.
Muth, Brian H.
Naccarato, Saverio
Nacht, Irwin J L.
Nador, Roland G.
Nagji, Ashnoor, FamilyMed
Nakhuda, Gary S.
Namazi, Mojgan
Narang, Gurpreet K.
Narayanan, Sujaatha
Narvas, David E., FamilyMed
Nasmith, Louise L., FamilyMed
Nathanson, Sheldon R.
Naus, Gregory J.
Nayar, Anuradha
Nayar, Kiran, FamilyMed
Nazerali-Sunderji, Najmi, FamilyMed
Nedd, Kaiyo S., FamilyMed
Nedd, Kenford W.
Nee, Lucy K Y., FamilyMed
Nelson, Marna J., FamilyMed
Nette, Hannah E., FamilyMed
Neumann, Viktor
Newton, Christie A., FamilyMed
Ng, David C.
Ng, Grace
Ng, John P Y.
Ng, Louis H S.
Ng, Shang C.
Ng, Simon, FamilyMed
Ng, Stephen S H.
Ng, Wing Hon
Nguan, Angela Y., FamilyMed
Ngui, Daniel K F., FamilyMed
Ngui, Simon F P.
Nguyen, Duc Tung, FamilyMed
Nguyen, Huan Dinh.
Nguyen, N P. Julie, FamilyMed
Nguyen, Quang Binh
Nguyen, Vi Liet
Nichol, Erin J., FamilyMed
Noble, A. Bruce
Noel, Melissandre, FamilyMed
Nolan, John F.
Nolan, Kevin R.
Nolten, Audrey E.
Nordahl, Karen M.
Norman, Wendy V., FamilyMed
Norrie, Fraser R., FamilyMed
Nouch, Susan L., FamilyMed
Nunez, Carlos E.
Nussbaumer, Gary R.
O'Briain, Barra F., FamilyMed
O'Keefe, Megan N.
Oda, Joanna J., FamilyMed
Oetter, Heidi M.
Ogilvie, Gina S., FamilyMed
Olson, Sarah E., FamilyMed
Omura, John D., FamilyMed
Oppel, Lloyd B., FamilyMed(EM)
Ospina-Ordonez, Julian A., FamilyMed
Ostapkowicz, Eugenia
Otto, Antoni G.
Oviedo, Angelica
Owusu-Ansah, Kevin
Padda, Roop-Preet K., FamilyMed
Paraskevopoulos, Elena Z., FamilyMed
Pare, Daniel F., FamilyMed
Parhar, Gurdeep
Parihar, Sheela
Parnes, Maria
Paul, Vivian F., FamilyMed
Pauls, Roberta
Pavlovich, Peter, FamilyMed
Pawa, Baljit
Peddie, Elaine F., FamilyMed
Pederson, Karla J., FamilyMed
Peel, Cordell H., FamilyMed
Penner, Jeremy, FamilyMed
Penner, Lynnette E., FamilyMed
Pereira, Michelle M., FamilyMed
Perlman, Isaac
Peters, H. Thomas
Peterson, Robert G.
Petrovic, Danica
Phillips, Sheilagh J.
Pho, Mark, FamilyMed
Phord-Toy, Mark S.
Pich, Phay
Piercey, Maureen L.
Pike, Judith A.
Pilapil-Lee, Rossali, FamilyMed
Pilar, Saul
Pirbhai, Nureen, FamilyMed
Pires, Serena, FamilyMed
Ploesser, Markus
Polay, Michael D.
Poon, Mimi M L.
Porten, Wendy R.
Porter, Kathryn G., FamilyMed
Pourvali, Reza, FamilyMed(EM)
Power, Maryse
Prabhakar, Kristin, FamilyMed(EM)
Prasad, Navin
Prestidge, Timothy D.
Primiani, Nadia S., FamilyMed(EM)
Pulfrey, Simon M., FamilyMed(EM)
Pus, Jacqueline G., FamilyMed
Qayumi, Abdul K.
Quan, Lan Phuong., FamilyMed
Rabbani, F. Nima
Racic, Anita R.
Rahemtulla, Amir
Raine, Todd A., FamilyMed(EM)
Ramji, Farah, FamilyMed
Ramsey, Damon, FamilyMed
Randhawa, Roop S.
Ranger, Patrice A., FamilyMed
Raudzus, Dietmar E., FamilyMed
Rawson, Claire G.
Reeves, Terrence L., FamilyMed
Rehmus, Wingfield E.
Reilkoff, Catherine R.
Rembez, Valentyna B., FamilyMed
Rev, Marianne, FamilyMed
Rich, Kira E., FamilyMed(EM)
Ridley, John A C., FamilyMed
Rieb, Launette M., FamilyMed
Riskin, Ashley E., FamilyMed
Robbertse, Machiel J., FamilyMed
Roberts, Stephen A., FamilyMed
Robillard, Joan L.
Robinson, Anthony H.
Robinson, John
Rondeau, Malcolm R V.
Ross, Elizabeth K.
Ross, Naomi
Ross, Simon A.
Rossi, Lilah R N., FamilyMed
Rucker, Christian J., FamilyMed
Rusnak, Conrad N., FamilyMed
Russell, Joy K., FamilyMed
Russell, Paula M., FamilyMed
Rutherford, Kimberly J., FamilyMed
Ryan, Christopher J.
Ryan, Jacqueline O.
Ryan, Kenneth J., FamilyMed
Ryder, Gerald B.
Rydz, Emilia, FamilyMed(EM)
Sadr, Aida, FamilyMed
Sajjan, Kuljit K., FamilyMed
Sakakibara, Todd K., FamilyMed
Sakaluk, Timothy J., FamilyMed
Salloum, Sharon E., FamilyMed
Salvino, Luigi A., FamilyMed
Salzman, James R.
Sampson, Olivia J., FamilyMed
Samson, Jonah A., FamilyMed
Sangha, Romaine, FamilyMed
Santerre, Marsha J., FamilyMed
Saona, Robert R., FamilyMed(EM)
Saretsky, Lori A.
Savchuk, Yuriy, FamilyMed
Scheuermeyer, Frank J., FamilyMed(EM)
Schmalz, Ruth I.
Schneck, Christopher R., FamilyMed(EM)
Scholtens, Martina, FamilyMed
Schreiber, William E.
Schubert, Harold E.
Schultz, Kirk
Schutz, Christian G.
Schwab, Shirley A.
Segal, David J.
Segal, Samuel
Sehmer, John M.
Senra, Poornima, FamilyMed
Sent, Lorna, FamilyMed
Sestak, Philip M., FamilyMed
Shabbir, Hamid
Shah, Rita, FamilyMed
Shaha, Tarun K., FamilyMed
Sharma, Anil R.
Sharma, Anu K.
Sharma, Ashima, FamilyMed
She, Alex K., FamilyMed
Shearer, Lauri-Ann, FamilyMed
Shereck, Evan B.
Sherwin, Elizabeth D.
Sheth, Sachiv
Shi, Kevin, FamilyMed(EM)
Shintani, Jessica M., FamilyMed
Shivdasani, Kumar, FamilyMed
Shklanka, Karen P., FamilyMed
Shoichet, Arnold J.
Shukla Mohan, Ruchika, FamilyMed
Shum, Michael S L.
Sidhu, Fulroop
Sidhu, Rupinder, FamilyMed
Simmons, Deanna L., FamilyMed
Singh, Christine B., FamilyMed
Singh, Lakhbir, FamilyMed
Sinha, Neel S.
Skinner, William A.
Skrenes, Bryan D.
Slater, Jay M., FamilyMed
Slutsky, Morley
Smith, Cassandra A., FamilyMed(EM)
Smith, Kevin R.
Smith, Lorie A., FamilyMed
Sneath, Jason R.
Sniderman, Jacob B., FamilyMed
Sobol, Isaac H., FamilyMed
Solmundson, Kara P., FamilyMed
Song, Sue Chiat, FamilyMed
Spooner, Lorinda G., FamilyMed
Spring, Beverly F.
Squire, Pamela L., FamilyMed
Stahl, Gordon M., FamilyMed
Stancer, Karen L., FamilyMed
Stancheva, Blaga A., FamilyMed
Stanley, Robert N., FamilyMed
Stein, Jeffrey R.
Steinberg, Malcolm H.
Stelzer-Chilton, Ashleigh D., FamilyMed
Stenstrom, Robert J., FamilyMed(EM)
Stevenson, Lindsay J., FamilyMed
Stewart, Donald W.
Stewart, Justine N., FamilyMed
Stewart-Patterson, Christopher
Stimpson, Rochelle L M., FamilyMed
Stockenstrom, Eric E.
Stone, Sarah J., FamilyMed
Story, Carol L., FamilyMed
Strahlendorf, Caron
Stratis, Anna K., FamilyMed
Street, John T.
Stringer, L. Judith
Stromberg, Susan J., FamilyMed(EM)
Struthers, Graham D N., FamilyMed
Strydom, Gerhardus J.
Strydom, Nardia
Styffe, Philip T.
Su, Winnie, FamilyMed
Sun, I-Chia W., FamilyMed
Sun, Joyce, FamilyMed
Sunshine, Stanley L., FamilyMed
Sutherland, Christy I., FamilyMed
Sweeny, Margo J., FamilyMed
Sze, Mabel C., FamilyMed
Sze, Michael M K., FamilyMed(EM)
Taddeucci, Sean
Tai, Linda C L.
Talbot, Claire F.
Tam, Daphne C., FamilyMed
Tam, K. Felix
Tam, Wilson W.
Tan-Hogg, Wan-Cheng
Tang, Ian
Tang, Tin-Yan
Tang, Vincent W.
Taunton, Jack E.
Taylor, Richard W., FamilyMed
Tejpar, Ismet
Thakorlal, Harilal
Thermann, Angela G.
Thiagarajah, Arjuna
Thida, Ma Khin, FamilyMed
Thompson, Anne M., FamilyMed
Thompson, John L.
Thomson, David B., FamilyMed
Thorsteinson, V. James, FamilyMed
Thrasher, Sarah M.
Thyer, Linda N., FamilyMed
Tiller, Barbara A., FamilyMed
Ting, Helen C I., FamilyMed
Ting, Justin W., FamilyMed
Ting, Lucy P.
Ting, Peter L.
Ting, Sherwin C., FamilyMed
Tobert, Gregory J., FamilyMed
Tokic, Vesna, FamilyMed
Tom, Tony P T., FamilyMed
Tong, Daniel Y.
Tong, Jennifer Y., FamilyMed
Tong, Kevin L F.
Tong, Vicki M., FamilyMed
Tong, Vince, FamilyMed
Toor, Dalvinder S., FamilyMed
Townsend, Marria M., FamilyMed
Tran, Margaret H M., FamilyMed
Tran, Quoc Tan
Trnka, Peter
Trott, Barbara E.
Trudeau, Jacqueline D.
Truong, Tinh Dinh
Tsang, Joseph W T.
Tsang, Monica C W., FamilyMed
Tsang Cheng, Joyce S S., FamilyMed
Tseng, George W., FamilyMed(EM)
Tsui, Connie C W., FamilyMed
Tsung, David
Tsze, Kwok-Khin
Tu, David T., FamilyMed
Tucker, Lori V.
Tukker, Roderick P., FamilyMed
Tung, Guat Khim, FamilyMed
Turgeon, Susie A., FamilyMed
Turnham, Lucy M.
Unger, David A., FamilyMed
Van Andel, Morris, FamilyMed
Van Den Biggelaar, Jane C., FamilyMed(EM)
Van Den Elzen, Peter
Van Der Meer, Isabelle R.
Van Eeden, Johannes H.
Van Karnebeek, Clara D.
Van Wyk, Karen
Vanderfluit, Rhonda L., FamilyMed
Vashisht, Shashi
Vassel, Jennifer L., FamilyMed
Vastardis, Alexander D., FamilyMed
Vellani, Azizadin S.
Venter, Jan F., FamilyMed
Verma, Rishi, FamilyMed
Verma, Serena, FamilyMed
Viljoen, Mark I.
Vogler, Rachel A., FamilyMed
Voigt, Robert F.
Vroom, W. Robbert, FamilyMed(EM)
Waldman, Deborah J., FamilyMed
Wang, Clayton J., FamilyMed
Wang, Shaoli, FamilyMed
Warf, Curren W.
Warren, James M., FamilyMed
Wasserfall, Marthinus, FamilyMed
Watanabe, Wei, FamilyMed
Watterson, Timothy J., FamilyMed
Webb, Charles D.
Weckworth, Mary F.
Wee, Edgardo Y.
Weiss, Helen M.
Weng, Andrew P.
Wenner, Gail R.
Wesa, Mina
Whitelegg, Geraldine M.
Whittaker, John S.
Whynot, Elizabeth M., FamilyMed
Whyte, Simon D.
Wickman, Marlene S., FamilyMed
Wickremasinghe, Lalya S.
Wiebe, Ellen R., FamilyMed
Wiesenthal, Zeph M.
Wilcock, Alison F., FamilyMed
Wilkinson, Michael R.
Williams, Aaron R., FamilyMed
Williams, Llewelyn K.
Willoughby, Brian C., FamilyMed
Wilson, Anthony B., FamilyMed
Wilson, Benjamin, FamilyMed
Wilson, Collis
Wilson, J. Galt, FamilyMed
Wilson, Ronald A., FamilyMed
Wilton, David W., FamilyMed
Wind, Stojna T.
Winter, Kyle D., FamilyMed
Witherspoon, Sandra E., FamilyMed
Wladichuk, Adrian L., FamilyMed
Wolak, Anna L.
Wong, Aaron W Y.
Wong, Asa W., FamilyMed
Wong, Clara K.
Wong, Eileen M., FamilyMed(EM)
Wong, Fedrick
Wong, Harvey H., FamilyMed
Wong, Henry K H.
Wong, Janice
Wong, Janice-Lynn K., FamilyMed
Wong, Jason J., FamilyMed
Wong, Jerry
Wong, K. Judy
Wong, K W. Rose, FamilyMed
Wong, Karen
Wong, Lai-Wah, FamilyMed
Wong, Paul C H., FamilyMed
Wong, Peter K K.
Wong, Sylvia
Wong, Ted Yee T., FamilyMed
Wong, William K W.
Woodfield, Wendy A.
Woollard, Robert F., FamilyMed
Worsley, Jennifer J.
Wortman, James A., FamilyMed
Wright, Janice G., FamilyMed
Wright, Timothy G.
Wu, Evelyn P S., FamilyMed
Wynne, Elaine J.
Xie, Jane Y.
Yakubovich, Svetlana N., FamilyMed
Yam, Ka-Wai, FamilyMed
Yang, Hui-Min
Yang, Jerome, FamilyMed
Yang, Joanne, FamilyMed
Yau, K Y. Steven, FamilyMed
Yee, Donna L J., FamilyMed
Yen, Tin-Wing
Yeomans, Wendy R.
Yeung, Carolyn G., FamilyMed
Yeung, Gerald Y L., FamilyMed
Yeung, H. Eddie
Ying, Raymond, FamilyMed
Yip, Andrea J., FamilyMed
Yiu, Douglas W., FamilyMed
Yong, Peter L.
Yoon, Ted Tai J., FamilyMed
Young, David C., FamilyMed
Young, Joanne M., FamilyMed
Yousefi, Rojyar R., FamilyMed
Yousefi, Vandad, FamilyMed
Yu, Larry L W.
Yue, Frank W L.
Yue, K. Kevin, FamilyMed
Yuen, Cham-Wah
Yuen, Michelle K., FamilyMed
Yuzak, Monica J.
Zack, Philip S., FamilyMed
Zamparini, Adriana M., FamilyMed
Zapf-Gilje, Margery H., FamilyMed
Zhang, Rui, FamilyMed
Zibin, Kerry E., FamilyMed

VANDERHOOF

Batchelor, Bret E., FamilyMed
Campbell, Suzanne M., FamilyMed
Coetzee, Douwette
De Vos, Peter W.
Dhillon, Davy, FamilyMed
Ebert, Nicole, FamilyMed

Ebert, Sean P., FamilyMed
Ho, Shu Fung, FamilyMed
Janssen, Rebecca S., FamilyMed
Klopper, Lukas C.
Lamprecht, Gideon P.
Makin, Michael D., FamilyMed
Muir, Karen Y.
Obayashi, Jeffery T., FamilyMed

VERNON

Arnold, David W., FamilyMed
Aucamp, Marius H.
Ballauf, Frank P., FamilyMed(EM)
Barnard, Johannes M., FamilyMed(EM)
Bintley, Timothy N.
Blyth, Christine G., FamilyMed
Borchert, George H., FamilyMed
Botha, Benjamin J A S., FamilyMed
Boucher, Louis B., FamilyMed
Brown, Cathryn M., FamilyMed
Brox, Anya C., FamilyMed
Butters, Stacey L.
Byrnes, Jennifer R., FamilyMed
Carey, Paul D.
Chan, Alfred T., FamilyMed
Coetzer, Louise, FamilyMed
Concannon, Michael J., FamilyMed(EM)
Croft, Joan D., FamilyMed(EM)
Cunningham, Christopher R., FamilyMed(EM)
De Beer, Jan A., FamilyMed
De Bella, Steven A.
Deetlefs, Francois
Dhaliwal, Rajinder, FamilyMed
Dippenaar, Francois J L.
Dougan, H. Sharon, FamilyMed
Dyck, Frederick G.
Fair, William A.
Fellenz, Lora G., FamilyMed
Flanagan, Margaret J., FamilyMed
Fourie, Annerie, FamilyMed
Fourie, Johan-Andre V., FamilyMed(EM)
French, Margaret E.
Friesen, D. Jon, FamilyMed(EM)
Friesen, Stephen D., FamilyMed
Gilhooly, Timothy R., FamilyMed
Harper, Richard
Hayward, Lindsey
Healey, Francis B.
Heidt, Lisa K., FamilyMed(EM)
Henley, Jeanette L.
Henley, Peter A.
Hewitt, Mathew, FamilyMed(EM)
Hillis, Robert A.
Hodelet, Nicola
Jackson, Craig S.
Jolly, Elizabeth M., FamilyMed
Kraubner, Davina, FamilyMed(EM)
Le Roux, Jacobus F.
Lemiski, William M.
Lepage, Philippe A., FamilyMed
Long, S. Ronald
Mandreck, Larrie H.
Manji, Aisha, FamilyMed
Mann, John R.
McKnight, Margaret J.
Meyer, Allan B.
Middelkamp, Lydia, FamilyMed
Mori, Richard Y.
Murphy, Michael J., FamilyMed
Perrier, Kenneth R., FamilyMed
Pestridge, Andrew D.
Peters, Calvin N., FamilyMed
Phillips, Debbie J., FamilyMed(EM)
Philp, Ian J., FamilyMed
Picken, Barbara R.
Pontifex, Alison T., FamilyMed
Poulin, Brett W., FamilyMed
Pretorius, Francois
Pritchett, Lindsay B.
Rankin, Allison A., FamilyMed
Raupach, Heinz-Dieter, FamilyMed
Rawlek-Stone, Barbara M.
Redelinghuys, Tanja P., FamilyMed
Sanders, April D., FamilyMed
Sanders, William D., FamilyMed
Sawatzky, Robert J.
Schuch, Werner, FamilyMed
Sharma, Ramesh K.
Smart, Gavin W.
Smit, Gideon
Smith, Donald H.
Smithers, Denise L., FamilyMed
Steward, Wayne W.
Steyn, Janus
Van Der Merwe, Shirley G.
Van Zyl, Maria-Louise, FamilyMed
Vincent, Anjali L S., FamilyMed
Waldron, Ross R., FamilyMed
Wiggelinkhuizen, Nicola, FamilyMed

VICTORIA

Abed, Abeer K E., FamilyMed
Adey, Frances M.
Adilman, Stephen M.
Aiken, Jonathan, FamilyMed
Al-Mahmudi, Maha
Amundsen, Susan, FamilyMed
Anderson, John F.
Anzarut, Jody E., FamilyMed
Ariana, Anahita, FamilyMed(EM)
Arnason, Jo Ann V.
Atchison, Amy, FamilyMed
Attwell, A. David
Bachynsky, Theodore J., FamilyMed
Backus, Richard D H.
Baidwan, Jatinder S., FamilyMed
Bailey, Thomas M., FamilyMed
Ballard, James H.
Banks, Kent D., FamilyMed
Barefoot, Judith A.
Barnard, D. Kelly
Barry, David M., FamilyMed
Battershill, Peter M.
Becker, Erin B.
Beeston, S. William
Bekker, Ian S., FamilyMed
Bell, David E., FamilyMed
Bennett-Boutilier, Nicole H., FamilyMed
Berg, Jason M.
Bertoia, Mauro
Bester, Charlotte
Bianco, Rodolfo
Bindra, Heera S., FamilyMed
Black, Fraser, FamilyMed
Blair, David J., FamilyMed
Blom, Phillip P., FamilyMed
Blouw, Marion C., FamilyMed
Boe, Corene D.
Bos, David C., FamilyMed
Boughen, Paul F.
Boylan, Maureen F., FamilyMed
Boyle, Neil G H., FamilyMed
Braithwaite, Debra, FamilyMed
Bridger, Ian M.
Brigel, Paul H., FamilyMed
Brook, David R., FamilyMed
Brothers, Alexander B., FamilyMed(EM)
Brown, Murray C., FamilyMed
Buie, Daniel A.
Bullock, William R.
Buriloski-Chkipova, Anita
Cairns, Heather M.
Callegari, Peter R.
Campbell, Karin M A., FamilyMed
Carlson, Catherine A., FamilyMed
Carr, Brendan S J., FamilyMed(EM)
Carruthers, Joan M.
Cassim, Nasreen
Cavers, William J R., FamilyMed
Cavilla, Benjamin, FamilyMed
Chana, Mundeep S., FamilyMed
Chang, Ernest J.
Cheek, Tyler, FamilyMed
Chew, Gilbert M M.
Childs, Aaron L., FamilyMed
Chkipov, Hristo G.
Chlysta, Dana O., FamilyMed
Chlysta, Terry S.
Chow, Walter K.
Christie, Gordon A.
Critchley, Sarah L., FamilyMed
Chu, Kelly K.
Church, James B., FamilyMed
Clements, Donna V M.
Clinton-Baker, David
Coburn, Christina M., FamilyMed
Coburn, John A., FamilyMed
Coetze, Hendrik A.
Colella, Paul V., FamilyMed(EM)
Conway, Barry P.
Cook, Alan F.
Cotterell, Darren S.
Coutts, Joyce V., FamilyMed
Crofton, Neil
Cross, Charles H T.
Crow, Patricia A M., FamilyMed
Cruickshank, Catherine J., FamilyMed
Cuddeford, Cheryl M.
Cunningham, Erik, FamilyMed
Dabrus, Kathy
Dake, Lauren A.
Dalziel, Christine E.
Dans, Jody-Lynn, FamilyMed
Davis, T. Vernon
De Jager, Jacobus
Delarom, Shyah S.
Dil, Pierre G., FamilyMed
Djearam, Saleena, FamilyMed
Dobyns, Edward, FamilyMed
Domke, Herbert L.
Domovitch, Edward
Donaldson, Ranald R.
Dougall, Alexander
Down, Hugh E., FamilyMed
Down, Karin, FamilyMed
Downing, G. Michael
Doyle, Donna L W.
Dupuis, Kaitlin C., FamilyMed
Dyble, Barbara J., FamilyMed
Dyson, William H.
Eby, John R., FamilyMed
Edmunds, Nevenka, FamilyMed
Edora, Felipe T., FamilyMed
Edwards, Susan L.
Egan, Francis G.
Ehasoo, Valerie A., FamilyMed
Emerson, Brian P.
Erickson, Allan M.
Erwin, Desmond H.
Fairhurst, Nicholas P A., FamilyMed
Farrell, Brian, FamilyMed(EM)
Farrow, James M.
Fast, Eunice M.
Felhaber, Taryl A., FamilyMed
Felix, James, FamilyMed
Fenske, Larry E.
Ferg, Allison, FamilyMed
Fill, Ian H.
Finlayson, Judith E., FamilyMed
Finn, Alexander
Fletcher, John W., FamilyMed
Foley, Mark, FamilyMed
Fontaine, Daphne H.
Forghani, Kamran
Forster, Dwight G.
Foster, Kimberley, FamilyMed
Fougere, Garnet A., FamilyMed
Francis, Dennis R.
Fraser, Brock R.
Fraser, Christopher R R.
Freigang, Dolores D., FamilyMed
French, Derek L.
Fretz, Michele T A., FamilyMed
Friesen, Caspar Z W., FamilyMed
Fry, Jessica, FamilyMed
Fyfe, Mary-Lyn R.
Galanos, Christopher J.
Garside, Kevin, FamilyMed
Gershman, Stuart M.
Glazier, Lee
Gleave, Danica A.
Glen, David R.
Goodchild, Steven R.
Gooderham, Virginia A., FamilyMed
Gordon, Steven C.
Gough, Lisa S.
Goulding, James F.
Goulet, Conrad A.
Govender, Sundren, FamilyMed
Grant, Elizabeth L.
Gray, Catharina A., FamilyMed
Gray, Stephen J., FamilyMed
Green, Stefanie L., FamilyMed
Green-Starr, Iris R.
Greenwood, Michael T., FamilyMed
Grewal, S. Tony, FamilyMed
Grimwood, H. Russell
Ham, Sharon A., FamilyMed
Hamilton, Dorothy J., FamilyMed
Hammell, Darlene M S., FamilyMed
Hammett, Tess, FamilyMed
Hammond, Diana R., FamilyMed
Hancock, Trevor G.
Harmon, Heather C., FamilyMed
Harris, David P.
Hartford, Samuel D.
Hastings, Peter C.
Hauser, Ronda J.
Hawkins, Lindsay, FamilyMed
Hayes, K. Oona, FamilyMed
Healy, Jane
Heaney, Michael J P.
Henderson, David L.
Henry, J. Paul
Henry, Sean, FamilyMed(EM)
Hepburn, David F.
Hiebert, Ron M., FamilyMed
Hinkle, Molli E.
Hoogewerf, Simon E C., FamilyMed(EM)
Houghton, Peter G H.
Houston, James G.
How, Benjamin K.
How, Richard K.
Howey, Jeannine I.
Hudson, Richard E K., FamilyMed
Huggett, Philip M.
Humphreys, Shaun W.
Hunter, Brad C.
Hwang, Naomi, FamilyMed
Inman, Geoffrey A B., FamilyMed
Innes, C. Peter
Isaacs, Gwenyth F.
Janicki, Robert T.
Jenken, Carol L.
Johnsson, Karen E., FamilyMed
Jollymore, John S.
Jones, Christine N., FamilyMed
Jones, Judith L., FamilyMed
Jones, Michael B.
Jong, Anthony K.
Jussak-Kiellerman, Ewa
Kachan, Paul S., FamilyMed
Karwowski, Andrzej S., FamilyMed
Keeler, Steven W.
Kelly, John L.
Kelly, Philip
Khorrami-Arani, Nivmand
Kiellerman, Andrew J.
Kirkpatrick, James R.
Klingenberg, Karen J., FamilyMed
Kluge, Hagen F N., FamilyMed
Kobierski, B. Lynn, FamilyMed
Kolodziejczyk, M. Dean, FamilyMed
Kotb, Rami
Krawciw, Donald, FamilyMed
Kryskow, Pamela A., FamilyMed
L'Esperance, Monica
Laing, James A.
Lam, Christopher, FamilyMed
Lane, Martin P.
Leduc, Eugene R J., FamilyMed
Lee, Jennifer L., FamilyMed
Leggatt, Suzanne, FamilyMed
Lenser, Rose E., FamilyMed
Leong, L. Anthony, FamilyMed
Leslie, Allan S.
Lewans, Raymond L.
Liebscher, Josephine S., FamilyMed
Liebscher, Ryan S., FamilyMed
Lindsay, Mary E.
Lintern, David
Little, Richard H., FamilyMed(EM)
Lobsinger, Meghan P., FamilyMed
Losie, Keith T., FamilyMed
Luckhurst, Geoffrey W M., FamilyMed
Luco, Gerald G.
Lush, Jennifer D., FamilyMed
Lypourlis, Katherine
MacDougall, W. Gregory, FamilyMed
MacKenzie, J. Stephen, FamilyMed
MacMillan, Kier L.
MacNaughton, David J.
MacPherson, Andrew I., FamilyMed(EM)
MacPherson, John K F., FamilyMed
MacSweeney, Orla, FamilyMed(EM)
Madill, David W.
Mah, Larry K.
Mah, Weiling G., FamilyMed
Mahadoo, Jaysen
Maier Phillips, Laura, FamilyMed
Mak, Janet, FamilyMed
Malo, J. Pierre C.
Manklow, Jennifer K., FamilyMed
Manning, Fiona F., FamilyMed
Marshall, Stuart A., FamilyMed
Marthyman, Azaria M.
Martin, Steven E.
Masata, Hana S., FamilyMed
Maskey, Jean M., FamilyMed
Mason, Anna J., FamilyMed
Mathes, Edward J.
Matthews, Susan B., FamilyMed
Mawdsley, J. Michael G., FamilyMed
Mazgani, Mona
McAdam, Donald W.
McCluskey, Walter T P., FamilyMed
McDonald, Andrew J., FamilyMed
McGregor, Douglas M.
McGuire, Michael I.
McKay, W. Ross
McKeen, Katharine I., FamilyMed
McLaughlin, Mark F., FamilyMed
McLeod, Nancy J.
McQueen, Keith R.
Medhurst, Charles W.
Meir, David
Melling, James N.
Mentz, Monica, FamilyMed
Merali, Nazmuddin
Meyer, Peter B.
Michels, Jorg E.
Mickelson, Allan S.
Mihalynuk, Tracy M., FamilyMed
Miles, Michael H.
Milkovich, Daniel J.
Miller, John A D.
Milliken, Megan P E., FamilyMed
Ming, Vivian H C., FamilyMed
Minish, Kelley L., FamilyMed(EM)
Mir, Bilal T., FamilyMed(EM)
Modi, Amita V., FamilyMed
Mogentale, Tara L., FamilyMed
Moher, Matthew J., FamilyMed
Montemuro, Suzanne M.
Morgan, David C.
Morin, Claude M.
Morrow, Christopher C., FamilyMed(EM)
Most, Carole
Muller, Francois
Muller, Marlene
Muniswamappa Sampath, Nagendra
Murray, Bryan H.
Mursell, Charlotte H., FamilyMed
Myette, T. Larry
Naaykens, William E., FamilyMed
Nadra, Imad J.
Naismith, James R A.
Napier, Jolene M.
Nehra, Paul, FamilyMed
Nelson, John C., FamilyMed
Nelson, Michelle L., FamilyMed
Nero, Brook A.
Nezil, Frank A.
Ng, Carol S C., FamilyMed
Nicholls, Pamela J H.
Nicoll, Robert D.
Nielsen, Anthony E.
Nielsen, Darcy L.
Nielsen, Gary K.
Nirwan, Amarjit S., FamilyMed
Norgrove, Leah V A., FamilyMed
Norris, Jill R., FamilyMed
Nuttall, Richard N., FamilyMed
O'Connell, Daniel F.
Olsen, Patricia N., FamilyMed
Ottley, Linda L.
Pai, Emily, FamilyMed
Papp, A. Jane
Partridge, Colin H., FamilyMed
Pastierovic, Danielle E.
Pasula, Brian J.

Patel, Meeta
Patterson, Douglas S.
Pengilly, Christopher J., FamilyMed
Penman, John
Pepler, Pierre-Francois
Pereira, Paul C.
Perera, Anoma K.
Perry, Wayne J., FamilyMed
Phillips, Henry D.
Pillay, Baven
Potiuk, Dustin J., FamilyMed
Pound, Brian S.
Power, Alicia M.
Prendergast, Philip R.
Price, Morgan T., FamilyMed
Prinsloo, Lodewyk, FamilyMed(EM)
Prsala, Jan
Puhky, Ronald S.
Purdon, Derek H.
Putland, Michael S., FamilyMed
Rachapalli, Satish M R.
Ray, Janet E.
Reid, Linda M., FamilyMed
Richards, Melinde, FamilyMed
Riddler, Colin R.
Ripley, David K.
Roback, Barbara R., FamilyMed
Roberts, Deanne M.
Robinson, Anna C.
Robinson, Simon D.
Robinson Power, Alicia M., FamilyMed
Rockerbie, Neil R., FamilyMed
Rode, Frauke
Roome, Stephen W.
Roque, Elmer A., FamilyMed
Rosenthal, Gillian A.
Ross, Jennifer A., FamilyMed
Rutherford, Beverly E., FamilyMed
Saffrey, James A., FamilyMed
Saiger, Gail F., FamilyMed
Salmaniw, Walter R.
Sammarelli, Patricia, FamilyMed
Saunders, Derek E.
Sayad, George R., FamilyMed
Schecter, Bayla E.
Schulz, Jeffrey D., FamilyMed
Sealey, Robert A D.
Sears, Catherine M., FamilyMed
Setterfield, Lance B.
Shafonsky, Eric W.
Shaw, Lynne M.
Sheikh, Osmaan, FamilyMed
Shepherd, Robert W., FamilyMed
Sherman, Mark, FamilyMed
Sherwood, Margaret L.
Shoichet, William N.
Sidhu, Tejinder K.
Simcoff, Micah A., FamilyMed
Skinnarland, Ellen M.
Skinnider, Marie T.
Smardon, Roy A.
Smatanova, Dagmar, FamilyMed
Smith, Dereck A.
Smith, Kenneth D., FamilyMed
Smith, Larry W.
Smith, Margaret G.
Smushkin, Galina
Snodgrass, James A R., FamilyMed
Snozyk, Patricia T., FamilyMed
Sparanese, Amerigo D., FamilyMed
Sparks, George W., FamilyMed
Spencer, Brian P.
Spink, Amy W A., FamilyMed
Spratt, Laura L M., FamilyMed
Stanwood, Murray D.
Starr, Stephen H.
Stel, Patrick R.
Stevens, David C L.
Stockdill, James D., FamilyMed
Strumpfer, Talita, FamilyMed
Sturmwind, Jakob, FamilyMed
Swan, Andrew C., FamilyMed
Taylor, Sandra L.
Templeton, W. Robert
Tessaro, Mark J., FamilyMed
Thackeray, Sharron J., FamilyMed
Thibodeau, Melina J M., FamilyMed
Thiessen, Mark D.
Thompson, Elizabeth, FamilyMed
Thorpe, Dominic J.
Tierney, Shauna L., FamilyMed
Tiislar, Milvi K., FamilyMed
Tranmer, Jennifer E., FamilyMed
Trerice, Deborah A., FamilyMed
Trouton, Konia J., FamilyMed
Ty, Patricia L.
Urban, George S.
Uzaraga, Isabella M.
Vadeboncoeur, Bonita A.
Van Der Linden, Marjorie A., FamilyMed
Van Es, Caroline M.
Vaughan, Michael W.
Veres, Lisa
Verhulst, Lorne A.
Vianzon Edora, Daisy M., FamilyMed
Vizsolyi, Peter T., FamilyMed
Vlachaki, Maria T.
Voon, Frederick H S., FamilyMed(EM)
Wale, Martin C J.
Wardle, Nancy E.
Warner, Anne-Marie
Warnock, David L.
Watt, Christopher J.
Webber, Patina D., FamilyMed(EM)
Wessels, Marie-Louise, FamilyMed
Wheeler, Martin M., FamilyMed
Wheeler, Stephen J.
White, J. Patrick
Whiting, Natalie M., FamilyMed
Whittaker, Stuart J., FamilyMed
Wickens, Jennifer K., FamilyMed
Wilde, James M.
Williams, Carole L., FamilyMed
Williams, David G., FamilyMed
Williams, Leslie G.
Wilson, Gordon A.
Winsby, Brian K.
Withers, Nicholas J., FamilyMed
Wolfson, Gary S., FamilyMed
Wolk, Adele M., FamilyMed
Woo, Lenny C Y., FamilyMed
Woodburn, D. Layne
Woods, Georgia J., FamilyMed
Wylie, Kevin J.
Young, Vanessa J.
Yue, Anthony W B., FamilyMed
Zacharias, Gordon W., FamilyMed
Zedel, Albert H.
Zilber-Shlensky, Caren F., FamilyMed

WEST KELOWNA

Banwell, Michael A., FamilyMed
Brower, Annette A.
Donlevy, Mary J., FamilyMed
Hautala, Bronwyn R.
Oyelese, Olutoyese O., FamilyMed
Reid, Douglas B.

WEST VANCOUVER

Anderson, Juanita M.
Barre, Nicole M., FamilyMed
Beheshti, Parvaneh
Biali, Susan
Brousson, Michelle A., FamilyMed
Brown, Dean V., FamilyMed(EM)
Carlson, Robert F.
Corey, John S.
Dawson, Siobhan M.
Di Lalla, Andrea L.
Dinu, Claudia G., FamilyMed
Ghannadi, Fatemeh, FamilyMed
Gharedaghi, Mahshid, FamilyMed
Gonabady Namadon, Mojdeh
Grunow, Michael D., FamilyMed
Habibian, Sonia, FamilyMed
Halenar, Mario A.
Hislop, Jonathan A., FamilyMed
Jiwani, Azim H., FamilyMed
Kabiri-Abyaneh, Shadan, FamilyMed
Kelpin, Bryce
Knight, Michael C.
Langley, Suzanne M.
Larsen, Joanne H.
Lauzon, Genevieve
Lawlor, Colleen E., FamilyMed
MacDonald, Myron K.
Mayr, Barbara J A.
McCaffrey, Janis A.
Najafi, Roya, FamilyMed
Nesbitt, Patrick M.
Ng, Liang
Ocana, Anthony M., FamilyMed
Pawlowski, Susan M.
Phillips, Gregory L.
Richardson, J. Ian
Salzman, Deborah A.
Scott, Robert J., FamilyMed
Sebba, Richard J.
Shahrokhi, Masoud, FamilyMed
Smith, Wayne M.
Sperling, Zdenka
Stancu, Diana C., FamilyMed
Stevenson, Thomas H., FamilyMed
Sugar, Paul S.
Tannis, Anita D., FamilyMed
Thomsen, Anne Marie
Tichy, Danusa
Van Aggelen, Debra J.
Walton, Nigel G., FamilyMed
Weber, Amy E., FamilyMed
Wills, Lee Ann M., FamilyMed
Wood, M. Lesley
Woolford, Bonnie L., FamilyMed
Xie, Rong, FamilyMed
Zeineddin, Maryam, FamilyMed

WESTBANK

Bystrom, Ryan S., FamilyMed
Gossier, Suzanne M.
Hawkins, David F.
Hugo, Andre
Lavanchy, Marcel C., FamilyMed
Lewke, Bernard O., FamilyMed
Maroney, Roy T.
Muendel, Hans-Christoph
Sorestad, Mark A., FamilyMed
Spiess, Andre J.
Verster, Gerhardus H J., FamilyMed
Verwey, Drikus
Wiid, Estelle M.
Young, Claire A.

WHALETOWN

Kristensen, John W., FamilyMed

WHISTLER

Burgess, Robert D.
Carr, Janice D.
Collins, Marisa B., FamilyMed
Demarco, James A.
Demarco, Thomas J.
Glen, Silvia P.
Johnston, Kristin M., FamilyMed
Kausky, Karin M., FamilyMed
Kendall, T P. Adam, FamilyMed
Lewis, Renata Y.
Mohr, Bruce P., FamilyMed(EM)
Rempel, Monika E., FamilyMed(EM)
Shaw, Lauren M., FamilyMed
Stanley, Ronald L.
Tamplin, Richard E I.
Tripodi, Deanna, FamilyMed(EM)
Von Der Porten, Fern W., FamilyMed(EM)
Walden, Paul D., FamilyMed
Wallman, Daniel A.
Zeglinski, Cathryn M., FamilyMed

WHITE ROCK

Anderson, David M.
Anderson, Glenn P J., FamilyMed
Aulakh, Jasdeep S.
Bassett, Michael C.
Beegan, Daniel, FamilyMed
Bright, Rachel E., FamilyMed
Bunting, Hal G.
Chang, Mildred W M., FamilyMed(EM)
Cheyne, Robert D.
Chin, Wendy W S., FamilyMed
Chong, Joseph M.
Crickmer, Sean D., FamilyMed(EM)
Darby, Lawrence B.
Darby, Niamh M.
Duncan, Sharon A., FamilyMed
Eng, Helen W K., FamilyMed
Fell, Marilyn L.
Field, Sidney W.
Goldie, Sheena
Grunau, Esther S., FamilyMed(EM)
Harper, Debra L.
Hefford, Brenda C.
Hendry, Jerrod, FamilyMed(EM)
Hoshizaki, Dale K., FamilyMed(EM)
Jimenez, Edgar M.
Johal, Manraj S., FamilyMed
Johnson, Fiona
Lamprecht, Albertus J., FamilyMed(EM)
Mangat, Rajeev, FamilyMed
McKnight, Robyn C.
Natha, Dharmesh J., FamilyMed
O'Leary, Denis F.
Parr, Mary G., FamilyMed
Paton, Walter M.
Perold, Jacobus A L., FamilyMed
Purkis, Jeffrey W.
Rahiminejad, Farhad, FamilyMed
Roberts, Gerald K.
Schuman, Leanne E., FamilyMed
Singh, Sonia, FamilyMed
Spangehl, G. Werner
Stevenson, Carolynn, FamilyMed
Tan, Melissa C Y., FamilyMed(EM)
Tavaria, Ashdin
Timothy, Toma J., FamilyMed
Varughese, Elizabeth A.
Veldhuis, Kim A., FamilyMed
Wadia, Yasmin J.
Wishlow, Kevin A., FamilyMed(EM)
Yam, Patrick K., FamilyMed
Yoshitomi, Kerry M., FamilyMed(EM)
Zayonc, David A., FamilyMed

WILLIAMS LAKE

Bannerman, S. Judith
Boeke, Jeannette
Carter, J. Ann
Clark, Jamieson C.
de Swardt, Stefan R.
Els, Meandi
Engelbrecht, Roland
Engelbrecht, Werner
Fedor, Glenn A.
Garrard, Michael J., FamilyMed
Gracia, Mark E., FamilyMed(EM)
Hicks, Roger A G.
Johnson, Robert E., FamilyMed(EM)
Kilian, Rochagne, FamilyMed
Labossiere, Emil J.
Longland, John W S.
Magnuson, Paul H.
McKay, Monica
McMahen, J. Ivor
Neufeld, J. Douglas
Peimer, Jeffrey E.
Prinsloo, Gerrit C.
Rees, Walter J.
Roux, Josua P.
Ruane, Bernard J., FamilyMed
Scrooby, Ivan G.
Sia, Yin Shan
Steyl, Jolien A.
Van Der Merwe, Francina J.
Van Rooijen, Tersia
Van Wyk, Hadriaan S.
Wassermann, Delene
Whitman, Richard J.
Wolf, Michael
York, Graham J.

WINFIELD

Loucks, Ellen J.
Martin, Brian D.
Murphy, Timothy A., FamilyMed
Nickerson, J. Paul, FamilyMed
Oswald, Kevin M., FamilyMed
Penney, Michael R., FamilyMed
Sokol, Denis S.

PHYSICIANS BY PROVINCE

MANITOBA

ALTAMONT

Donnelly, J. Patrick

ALTONA

Ali, Tehmina K.
Bueddefeld, H. Dieter, FamilyMed
Kliewer, Kenneth L., FamilyMed
Prinsloo, Jochemus J.

ARBORG

El Shatshat, Mohamed, FamilyMed
Gerges, Michael M M., FamilyMed
Siddiqui, Issar

ASHERN

Faltas, Samy R N.
Rawoof, Ragad H.
Roets, Willem G.
Warnakulasooriya, Riviraj, FamilyMed

BALDUR

Deegan, Michael F.

BEAUSEJOUR

Askarifar, Rasool
Campbell, Garth
Jansen Van Rensburg, Nicholas A., FamilyMed
Khan, Sadiqa J.
Kohanek, Frances L.

Partyka, Joseph W., FamilyMed
Schmidt, Daphne M A., FamilyMed
Zeiler, Frederick

BOISSEVAIN

Nell, Antonie M.
Pirvu, Adriana M., FamilyMed

BRANDON

Abell, William R.
Ahweng, Andrew G C.
Alshami, Haider A A.
Amede, Kebede H.
Azer, Nivine N Z.
Beeston, Chris, FamilyMed(EM)
Benning, Harjit S.
Beshara, Eren, FamilyMed
Blyth, Scott W.
Butler, Nicolaas M J., FamilyMed
Caplan, Deborah C., FamilyMed
Davis, Michael O.
De Bruyn, Anna C., FamilyMed(EM)
De Muelenaere, Philip F.
De Wet, Johannes M J.
DeCosse, Jillian L., FamilyMed
Decter, Diarmuid
Deong, Jean P., FamilyMed
Du Plooy, Johan
Duncan, S. Jay
Edward, Girgis, FamilyMed
Engelbrecht, Jan
Engelbrecht, Stephanus J.
Fourie, Theo, FamilyMed
Gauthier, Shaun W., FamilyMed(EM)
Ghebrial, Maged S N., FamilyMed
Glenn, David M.
Gray, Catharina, FamilyMed
Grobb, Jacie, FamilyMed
Groves, Lawrence E.
Halka, Hany H I., FamilyMed
Hanna, Michael Y G.
Hechler, Peter, FamilyMed
Heibesh, Suzy G F.
Jones, Cristen D.
Kaiser, Carina, FamilyMed
Kelleher, Barbara E.
Kitz, Stacey L., FamilyMed(EM)
Large, Gregory W.
Levin, Iwan
Loader, Kenneth R.
Maier, Joanne C., FamilyMed
Megalli Basali, Sherif F., FamilyMed
Meredith, Melanie J., FamilyMed
Mikhail, Antoinette
Mikhail, Samy N F., FamilyMed
Moller, Erika
Moller, Liesel
Nasr, Nagwa Y I., FamilyMed
Norman, Charles
Ramaya, Savitri
Rodriguez Marrero, Ildegul
Samoil, Mary F S.
Samuels, Lewis
Santdasani, Sanjay K H.
Sarli, Ricardo
Seitz, Andrew R.
Shunmugam, Revendren
Skead, Lennard
Smith, Dalene, FamilyMed
Soliman, Magdi F L.
St John, Valerie E.
Tamayo Mendoza, Jesus
Tawadros, Mamdouh B E.
Tissera, Ponsuge A D.
Uys, Tharina
Van Rensburg, Pieter D J.
Velthuysen, Elsa, FamilyMed
Velthuysen, Johann
Visser, Gerhardt
Vlok, Nicolaas C., FamilyMed
Wahba Hanna, Talaat W S.
White, Sandra L.
Yam, Cecilia S F.
Ziaei Saba, Shahnaz

BROCHET

Lines, Alfred J.

CARBERRY

Basta, Ayman F., FamilyMed
Forouzandeh, Fariba
Ward, Susan J., FamilyMed

CARMAN

Abdalla, Shaza E E., FamilyMed
Carter, Robin G., FamilyMed
Clayden, Gerald S.
Hunt, Daniel, FamilyMed
Kruk, Robert D., FamilyMed
Memon, Ghulam F.
Memon, Rukhsana F., FamilyMed
Youssef, Nermeen A., FamilyMed

CHURCHILL

Delabie, Ludovic
Tolton, Alexander D., FamilyMed

CROSS LAKE

Jamal, Shabana
Pelletier, Manon M A., FamilyMed
Zaman, Atiq U.

CRYSTAL CITY

Khoury, Marzouk, FamilyMed
Sodhi, Vijay

DAUPHIN

Bretecher, Gilbert J.
Clark, Mark A., FamilyMed
Clark, Sandra G., FamilyMed
Du Toit, Linda
Fjeldsted, Fredrik H., FamilyMed
Johnston, Anna L., FamilyMed
Kish, Scott L., FamilyMed
Lofgren, Sandra R., FamilyMed
Lopez Gardner, Leonora L., FamilyMed
Lulashnyk, Ben J., FamilyMed
Malik, Bittoo S.
Marah, Muhaned A.
Marais, Francois
Mathison, Trina L., FamilyMed
Menard, Sheila M.
Monkman, Lisa M., FamilyMed
Penrose, Michael G., FamilyMed
Potoski, J. Paul
Rauch, Johan F.
Scott, Jason, FamilyMed
Scott, Sara A., FamilyMed
Scott, Thomas J P.
Smith, Riley A L., FamilyMed
Ungarian, Jillian L R., FamilyMed
Van Alstyne, Murray A., FamilyMed
Vuksanovic, Milos
Warrian, William G., FamilyMed
Wiens, Anthony V., FamilyMed
Willemse, Pieter

DELORAINE

Ali, Molud A.
Brackenreed, Nolan L E., FamilyMed
Shahzad, Seema

EAST ST PAUL

Boroditsky, Mark A., FamilyMed
Brar, Kanwaljit S., FamilyMed
Choy, Stephen C., FamilyMed
Fotti, Christopher, FamilyMed
Glazner, Kathryn, FamilyMed
Lafournaise, Carrie L., FamilyMed
Law, Jaimie R., FamilyMed
Olivier, Erin P., FamilyMed
Patenaude, Amanda F.

EASTERVILLE

Boyang, Winston F.

ELIE

Girgis, Hossam, FamilyMed
Malmstrom, Jennifer K., FamilyMed

ELKHORN

Van Der Merwe, Herman S., FamilyMed

EMERSON

Kolakowski, Anna A.

ERIKSDALE

Arara, Mohammed E.

FLIN FLON

El Masry, Amir
Elyas, Ausama H.
Fahim, Galal Z.
Intwala, Chaitasi R.
Kucparic, Peter S.
Mahdi, Tahseen
Sethi, Krishan, FamilyMed
Siddiqi, Nargis
Thwala, Andrea B.

GILLAM

El Sabawy, Mary, FamilyMed
Yousif, Eman J., FamilyMed

GIMLI

Chapnick, Cary N.
Gera, Rakesh M.
Patel, Ramanbhai C.
Patel, Sunilkumar V.
Wong, Siu Hung
Zabib, Nassr A., FamilyMed

GLADSTONE

Berman-Wong, Eva, FamilyMed
Kilada, Baher F N., FamilyMed
Mansour, Samir
Paul, Niranjan C.

GLENBORO

Khan, Sadia N.
Swanepoel, Walter E.
White, Graham D., FamilyMed

GRAND RAPIDS

Ismail, Ibrahim T., FamilyMed

GRANDVIEW

Elliott, Jacobi, FamilyMed
Kanwal, Jaswinder S.

HAMIOTA

Abd El Mesih, Sameh A B M N.
Ajabor, Kenneth U.
Breneman, Christopher D., FamilyMed
Juce, Karen L., FamilyMed
Kristjanson, David N., FamilyMed
Ranson, Allan D., FamilyMed
Shariati, Majid

HODGSON

Abood, Muhanned F.
Malik, Abid I.
Mayes, Camisha, FamilyMed
Paracha, Muhammad S.
Rehsia, Navneet, FamilyMed
Yacoub, Nader S T.

KILLARNEY

Graice, Renee A M F.
Hewett, Fraser G., FamilyMed
Khan, Arshya F., FamilyMed
Nighat, Nazia, FamilyMed
Pio, Anton, FamilyMed
Simons, Ian W C.

LA BROQUERIE

Thiessen, Myron N., FamilyMed

LA SALLE

Hanna, Irin S F., FamilyMed

LAC DU BONNET

Bruneau, Michel R., FamilyMed
Kadirsahib, Sadhak
Papetti, Selena J., FamilyMed

LEAF RAPIDS

Haji, Salah A.

LORETTE

Assaad, Hoda M A., FamilyMed

LUNDAR

Burnet, Neil M.

LYNN LAKE

Vermaak, Christoffel J.

MCCREARY

Hanna, Michael H.

MELITA

Ahmed, Munir
Dizon, Aquilino M.

MINNEDOSA

Bishay, Fekry S., FamilyMed
Frykoda, Amy H., FamilyMed
Hussain, Saad A.
Khandelwal, Ajai S.
Onyshko, Daniel
Roche, Gavin J., FamilyMed
Sulaiman, Mahabat H A.

MORDEN

Armas Enriquez, Ana T., FamilyMed
Azer, Nivin F T., FamilyMed
Bergman, Amanda D., FamilyMed
Botha, Adriana, FamilyMed
Braun, Jeanelle F., FamilyMed
Convery, Kevin M., FamilyMed
Duff, Brian D., FamilyMed
Earl, Kevin D., FamilyMed
Holmes, Carol D., FamilyMed
Mansour, H. Mansour S.
Martens, David B., FamilyMed
Menzies, Robert J., FamilyMed
Nause, Leanne N., FamilyMed
Persson, Enok D., FamilyMed
Zacharias, Howard J., FamilyMed

MORRIS

Fraser, Michael B.
Gharagozloo, Mehrdad
Loewen, Ann E., FamilyMed
Manness, Robert C.

NEEPAWA

Krzyzaniak, Kelly M.
Milligan, Brian E., FamilyMed
Nasralla, George A T., FamilyMed
Ong, George H E.
Poettcker, Robert J., FamilyMed
Rosing, Kim, FamilyMed
Tariq, Muhammad
Tiab, George A.
White, Owen J.

NELSON HOUSE

Derzko, Lydia A L.

NIVERVILLE

Burnett, Christopher J.
Burnett, Mairi

NORWAY HOUSE

Aery, Navrup
Edye-Rowntree, James, FamilyMed
Malekalkalami, Azadeh
Roos, Paul J.

NOTRE DAME DE LOURDES

Berard, Frances C., FamilyMed
Fortier, Denis C J., FamilyMed
Hamilton, Holly D M., FamilyMed
Muhammad, Afzal, FamilyMed

OAKBANK

Dueck, Darrin, FamilyMed
Kowaluk, Bruce A.
Lacerte, Martina M., FamilyMed
Saffari, Hamideh
Shenouda, Nader N S., FamilyMed
Wiebe, Jeffrey L., FamilyMed

PINAWA

Hanna, Nermeen S., FamilyMed
Manzar, Asma

PINE FALLS

Elkhemri, Abdulgader
Essa, Reda A A., FamilyMed
Hashem, Fathi
Ijaz, Sabina P., FamilyMed
Lambrechts, Hugo

PORTAGE LA PRAIRIE

Finney, Brett, FamilyMed
Ghoneim, Mostafa S A F., FamilyMed
Gray, Michael G.
Hedden, John R.
Hunter, Christopher, FamilyMed
Kim, Hae-Kwan J., FamilyMed
Kinnear, David W H P., FamilyMed
Lewis, Anthony B., FamilyMed
MacKlem, Alan K., FamilyMed
Mand, Ravinder P., FamilyMed(EM)
Omichinski, L. Michael, FamilyMed
Parker, Kenneth R., FamilyMed
Price, James B., FamilyMed
Quesada, Ricardo, FamilyMed
Rice, Patrick O., FamilyMed
Rizk, Abdalla M A., FamilyMed
Siyih, Mahysin
St Goddard, Jennifer M., FamilyMed
Tan, Edward, FamilyMed
Thess, Bernard A J.

PUKATAWAGAN

Spring, Lawrence R., FamilyMed

RIVERS

Dhaliwal, Mandeep S.
Nowosad, Heather D., FamilyMed
Vermaak, Anita

RIVERTON

Gerges, Hanan

ROBLIN

Aziz, Aziz N N.
Eskandar-Gergies, Shokry
Rezk, Emad
Tawfik Helmy, Safaa, FamilyMed
Tresoor, Tracy L., FamilyMed

ROSSBURN

Roos, Matthys

RUSSELL

Almalky, Ammar
Erfanfar, Alireza
Fagbemigun, Ayokunle, FamilyMed

SELKIRK

Alexy, Julius
Ansar, Roomana
Antonenko, Natalie E.
Atalla, Niveen
Badenhorst, Frederik J.
BenShaban, Lamin Ra
Csupak, Elaine M., FamilyMed
Demsas, Habtu
Du Preez, Joachim J.
Elbardisy, Nozahy N., FamilyMed
Emerson, Yvette, FamilyMed
Fuchs, Graham R.
Kaldas, Nahed N R.
Komosky, Judy A.
Lindenschmidt, Richard B., FamilyMed
Lindenschmidt, Richard R., FamilyMed
Lopez, Mirtha I.
Matter, Michele A., FamilyMed
Meller, Jack B.
Montoedi, Jacqueline I., FamilyMed(EM)
Prematilake, Suraj
Rahman, Mohammad M.
Randunne, Ayodya S., FamilyMed
Ryckman, Bruce A.
Sakla, Mary S S., FamilyMed
Shaker, Marian R.
Speer, Margaret L., FamilyMed
Stacey, Brett, FamilyMed
Youssef, Heba S S.
Zoppa, Robert J M., FamilyMed

SHILO

Ceponis, Peter J M., FamilyMed
Dickinson, Peter W., FamilyMed
Lindsay, Gary M., FamilyMed
Muggaberg, Sheri G., FamilyMed
Paquin, Isabelle, FamilyMed

SHOAL LAKE

Lall, Frank R.
Muller, Diederik J., FamilyMed
Venter, Hendrik J.

SNOW LAKE

MacLeod, Neil F.
Rhoma, Salahalden

SOMERSET

Vakilha, Mehrdad

SOURIS

Cram, David H., FamilyMed
Stone, Jasper D.
Wasef, Nagy S R., FamilyMed
Weiss, Elise C., FamilyMed
Ziada, Mohammed M A.

SOUTH INDIAN LAKE

Ashton, Martin

ST CLAUDE

Tarun, A S M. Noorullah, FamilyMed
Viens, Gisele, FamilyMed

ST JEAN BAPTISTE

Ahmadi Torshizi, Omid, FamilyMed

ST PIERRE JOLYS

Migally, Samir E B., FamilyMed
Sidhom, Cherine R., FamilyMed

STE ANNE

Bissonnette, Arcel
Chatel, Nadine L., FamilyMed
De Moissac, Paul C.
Duval, Richard
Frechette, Chantal A M.
Fredette, Patrick J L.
James, Keleigh J A., FamilyMed
Lemoine, Gabriel J G.
Roy, Maurice J B., FamilyMed

STE ROSE DU LAC

Gudmundson, Catherine A., FamilyMed
O'Hagan, David B., FamilyMed

STEINBACH

Barkman, Jayson M J., FamilyMed
Bullock Pries, Karen R., FamilyMed(EM)
Duerksen, Mark T., FamilyMed
Dyck, Gordon H.
Earle, Lisa, FamilyMed
Famouri, Sanaz
Ghebray, Tesfay M., FamilyMed
Gingerich, Roger L.
Gumber, Rhythmpal S., FamilyMed
Hoff, Mark, FamilyMed
Ibrahim, Magdy L A.
Ilchyna, Daniel C., FamilyMed
Kaethler, H. Wilfried S., FamilyMed
Kohja, Abbas A.
Krahn, Curtis D N., FamilyMed
Minnaar, Johannes C H., FamilyMed(EM)
Mokate, Lionel M., FamilyMed
Nguyen, Tai Van
Pretorius, Luzelle
Raza, Irfan
Reimer, Darren K., FamilyMed
Roberts, Janice D.
Shoukry, Sahar S.
Toews, Karen A., FamilyMed
Trinh, Hang Kim T., FamilyMed
Van Der Byl, Gwynneth L.
Warkentin, Ray E., FamilyMed
Widdifield, Hillary E.
William, Nihad N.
Wowk-Litwin, Maria L.

STONEWALL

Aguilar, Rodolfo P.
Annakkage, Rannulu D.
Balhaj, Abdelaati A.
Graham, Kerr
Hall, Barbara
Mohamdee, John F., FamilyMed
Pannu, Fazeelat A., FamilyMed
Pinniger, Gregory W.
Saad, Nabil K.
Venter, Dirk J.
Weebedda, Upali S K., FamilyMed

SWAN LAKE

Desmond, Gerard H., FamilyMed

SWAN RIVER

Le Roux, Pieter C.
Marx, Theodore
Mikhaiel, Sameh A B.
Salib, Wagdi
Singh, Mohinder
Theodore, Gene M.

TEULON

Gill, Balwinder S.
Loudon, Michael
Pillay, Pooventhran G.

THE PAS

Adl Golchin, Oveis
Doulatyariazar, Haleh
Ehlers, Marianne, FamilyMed
Karimu, Ande L.
Nahvi, Shahab, FamilyMed
Noel, Colin T., FamilyMed
Noel, Marie L., FamilyMed
Oliaei, Alireza, FamilyMed
Pinder, Michael
Surajballi, Hemchand, FamilyMed

THOMPSON

Abou-Khamis, Rami
Ahmed, Shehla
Ajao, Olarenwaju O., FamilyMed
Al-Kadhaly, Mothafar
Alam, Mohammad S., FamilyMed
Amadu, Adam A., FamilyMed(EM)
Anid, Gabriel A.
Chaudhry, Nadeem A.
Duggal, Kishan
El-Bawab, Najwa
Kania, Jadwiga
Kassem, Wail A.
Kumbharathi, Ravi B.
Leary, Courtney C.
Llanos, Romeo B.
Martinez-Giron, Fernando
Mohajerani, Seyed-Alireza
Ratnayake, Aluthwala D V S P., FamilyMed
Rich, Alan D.
Sarker, Arun, FamilyMed
Sathiamoorthy, Marutha
Sivananthan, Kamalanayani
Storm, Hendrik W.
Tahira, Shamim, FamilyMed
Tassi, Hisham H.
William, Anita L., FamilyMed

TREHERNE

Dixon, Shannon C., FamilyMed
MacTavish, James W E., FamilyMed
Vorster, Alewyn P.

VIRDEN

Ali Nejad, Shahrokh
Daoud, Hani
Fitzgerald, Michael
Hammell, Jennifier, FamilyMed
Pieterse, Wickus, FamilyMed
Roux, Jan G.
Uwabor, Wisdom O.
Van Niekerk, Adria R.

VITA

Muhammed, Khalid A E.

WAWANESA

Abell, Margaret E.
Lee, Della D., FamilyMed

WHITEMOUTH

Tawfik, Viola L.

WINKLER

Abbu, Ganesan P., FamilyMed
Allen, John E.
Basson, Anel
Basson, Hendrik J.
Blignaut, Johann
Booy, Harold, FamilyMed
Brett, Matthew J M., FamilyMed
Caswill, Melissa E., FamilyMed
Day, Marilyn H., FamilyMed
Dixon, Nancy L J., FamilyMed
Dreyer, Christiaan
Greyling, Louw De Lange
Hesom, Margaret S.
Holland-Muter, Elizabeth M.
Klassen, Donald H., FamilyMed
Lane, Eric S., FamilyMed
Le Roux, Carinca, FamilyMed
Lehmann, Heather C., FamilyMed
Lines, Jolyon B., FamilyMed(EM)
Mostert, Francois D P.
Pather, Adashnee Y.
Reimer, Murray B., FamilyMed
Reyneke, Anna M E.
Roberts, Kris A., FamilyMed
Schellenberg, John D.
Van Niekerk, Etienne
Woelk, Cornelius J., FamilyMed

WINNIPEG

Abazid, Nizar R.
Abbott, Burton B., FamilyMed
Abdulrehman, Abdulhamid S.
Abej, Esmail, FamilyMed
Adam, Christopher J E., FamilyMed
Adam-Sdrolias, Heather, FamilyMed
Ahluwalia, Rajpal S.
Ahmad, Ejaz, FamilyMed
Ahmad, Suffia N., FamilyMed
Ahsanuddin, Arshad N.
Akena, Charles
AlJafari, AlHassan K., FamilyMed
Albak, Russell E., FamilyMed
Ali, Ebtihal A.
Almiski, Muhamed S A F.
Alvaro, Ruben E.
Amin, Bita
Amoah-Gyampoh, Maxwell
Anashara, Fouad H., FamilyMed(EM)
Ansari, Muhammad Z.
Anton, Annepa
Appel, Karen A., FamilyMed
Appendino, Juan P.
Araneda, M. Carolina
Arnott, Peter C.
Arrezaghi, Mohamed
Ashfaq, Bushra, FamilyMed
Asskar, Ramzi R., FamilyMed
Atwal, Jasdeep, FamilyMed
Awad, Jaklin A J., FamilyMed
Babick, Terry R.
Bacily, Mervat A., FamilyMed
Badenhorst, Lynette
Bahrami, Tahmoures, FamilyMed
Baidwan, Saminder K.
Bal, Simerpreet S.
Balcha, Berhanu
Balko, George V., FamilyMed
Ball, Fred, FamilyMed
Banach, Theodore M.
Banmann, Darin S., FamilyMed
Barac, Ivan
Barker, Sharon L., FamilyMed
Barnes, William R., FamilyMed
Barodia, Rajiv P.
Baydock, Bradley M S., FamilyMed
Beaudette, Roxanne M., FamilyMed
Bedder, Phyllis M.
Bedi, Bhupinder S.
Bello, Ahmed B.
Bennett, Diana R., FamilyMed
Benningen, R. Grant
Bereznay, Oliver H A., FamilyMed
Bergen, Jerry M., FamilyMed
Bergman, Elin K., FamilyMed
Bergmann, Terence
Bergner, Anahy
Berrington, Neil R.
Bertsch, Angelica R.
Bhanot, Pradeep, FamilyMed
Bhayana, Rajinder K.
Bhayana, Renu
Bhayana, Veena
Bhuiyan, Nazman N.
Bialy, Peter C., FamilyMed
Bibi, Mariam, FamilyMed
Biedermann, Alyson J.
Billinkoff, Errol N.
Bilos, Richard J.
Bishay, Wagdy W S., FamilyMed
Bisson, Danny S., FamilyMed
Blank, Arthur K.
Blom, Lourens, FamilyMed
Blondin, David, FamilyMed(EM)
Blouw, Richard H., FamilyMed
Bohemier, Robert J P., FamilyMed(EM)
Borrett, George F J.
Bosma, Peter A., FamilyMed
Boszko, Michael A., FamilyMed(EM)
Botha, Daniel J.
Bowman, Thomas M.

PHYSICIANS BY PROVINCE

Boyd, Karen L.
Boyd, R. Bruce, FamilyMed
Boyd, R. James, FamilyMed
Bradshaw, Candace D., FamilyMed
Braun, Erwin A., FamilyMed
Braun, Karen Y., FamilyMed
Breckman, David K.
Breckman, Gillian L F.
Broda, Russell J.
Brown, Heather J.
Brown, Jodie S B., FamilyMed
Bryski, Lisa M., FamilyMed(EM)
Buchel, Albert M., FamilyMed(EM)
Buchel, Christine R., FamilyMed
Buchel, Edward W.
Buchel, Tamara L., FamilyMed
Buenafe, Jay R., FamilyMed
Buffo Sequeira, Ilan
Bullen, Sandra, FamilyMed
Burke, Morris E., FamilyMed
Buss, Mandy R.
Butt, Sheldon L., FamilyMed
Bynkoski, Stacey A.
Calderon-Grande, Henry E.
Campbell, Judith M., FamilyMed
Canadas, Luis A.
Caners, Dennis T., FamilyMed
Caron-Boulet, Nicole M., FamilyMed
Cattani, Lynnsey A., FamilyMed
Cavers, Kenneth J., FamilyMed
Cavett, Teresa D., FamilyMed
Cenkowski, Barbara A., FamilyMed
Chakraborty, Amiya R.
Chan, Eliza K., FamilyMed(EM)
Chan, Eng Lyan
Chan, Jennifer M., FamilyMed
Chan, Joseph J.
Chan, Timothy
Chandler, Cara J., FamilyMed
Chernish, Gregory M.
Chittal, Dervla, FamilyMed
Chochinov, Paul
Choptiany, Robert B W.
Chow, Candace S., FamilyMed
Chow, Chi-leng
Chow, Herman, FamilyMed
Chowdhury, Amitava D.
Chubaty, Roman A.
Chudasama, Sushil
Chung, Louis, FamilyMed
Ciecierski, Danuta W.
Clark, Donna L.
Clark, Susan M., FamilyMed
Clarke, Ian S.
Coates, Kevin R., FamilyMed
Condon, Amanda J S., FamilyMed
Connelly, Peter, FamilyMed
Connor, Graham T.
Consunji-Araneta, Raquel
Coodin, Michael G., FamilyMed
Cook, Catherine, FamilyMed
Cordova, Juan L.
Cordova Perez, Francisco
Cosman, Mitchell A.
Coyle, Stephen J.
Craton, Neil
Crawford, David J., FamilyMed
Crawford, Garnet C., FamilyMed
Cristante, Loris
Cross, Robert
Crow, Fiona M.
Cummings, M. Lee, FamilyMed
Cymbalisty, Christopher D., FamilyMed(EM)
Cyr-Hornick, Annie, FamilyMed
Czaplinski, Kazimierz L.
Czarnecka, Monika
Da Silva, Hermano P B.
Da Silva, Laurindo M.
Dakshinamurti, Sowmya S.
Dalling, Gordon N., FamilyMed
Danais Brown, Jocelyne M., FamilyMed
Dandekar, Anand, FamilyMed
Dang, Tai Huu
Darczewski, Irena B., FamilyMed
Davis, Martin H.
Daymont, Carrie B.
de Cabo, Cecilia
De Gussem, Els Maria
De Klerk, Ronel
Delli Pizzi, Andy T., FamilyMed
Demers, Chantale, FamilyMed
Derksen, Angela S L., FamilyMed(EM)
Dhaliwal, Harbhajan S.
Dhanjal, Permjeet S., FamilyMed
Dias, Ernesto M.
Dillon, Lisa G., FamilyMed
Dillon, Michael, FamilyMed
Dissanayake, Dilani T K.
Dittberner, Klaus
Do, Kiet, FamilyMed
Doan, Quy Xuan, FamilyMed
Doermer, Erroll R.
Domke, Heather L.
Domke, Sheila L.
Doucet, Paul M., FamilyMed(EM)
Dowhanik, Monica A.
Dowhanik, Paul B J.
Doyle, Judith I M.
Drain, Brighid, FamilyMed
Drexler, Jaroslav
Du Plessis, Marlie, FamilyMed
Duerksen, Carl D., FamilyMed
Dumatol-Sanchez, Jocelyn, FamilyMed
Duprat, Christine C., FamilyMed
Durcan, Anne M., FamilyMed
Dyck, Clayton H., FamilyMed
Ebbeling-Treon, Lori R., FamilyMed
El-Matary, Wael M M.
El-Sayed, Yasser N E M.
Elias, Kamelia Y R., FamilyMed
Elkams, Sameh, FamilyMed
Elkin, Jonathan A., FamilyMed
Elkin, Mark S., FamilyMed
Emery, Christopher
Eng, Stanley L., FamilyMed
Erhard, Philippe M., FamilyMed
Eshghi Esfahani, Farid
Eskarous, Soad B H., FamilyMed
Evans, Michele J., FamilyMed
Fainman, Shane E.
Farmer, R. Charles
Fatoye, Adetunji, FamilyMed
Finlayson, Nolan A., FamilyMed
Fisher, I. Morag J.
Flattery, Paula M.
Fletcher, Colin W.
Foda, Abdelmonem, FamilyMed
Fogel, Martin L., FamilyMed
Folk, David M., FamilyMed
Fontigny, Nadine J., FamilyMed
Frame, Heather A., FamilyMed
Francois, Jose M G., FamilyMed
Frechette, Marc, FamilyMed
Frechette, Sharon, FamilyMed
Friesen, Kevin L., FamilyMed(EM)
Gabriel, Maila J., FamilyMed
Gall, Perry, FamilyMed
Garland, Allan B.
Geneve, Mustafa M., FamilyMed
George, Ronald, FamilyMed(EM)
Gerber, John D W.
Gibson, Ian
Giesbrecht, J. Elizabeth, FamilyMed
Gill, Daljit S.
Glacken, Robert P., FamilyMed
Glew, Wade B., FamilyMed
Goeke, Fredrick J., FamilyMed(EM)
Goldberg, Grant M., FamilyMed
Goldman, Barbara L., FamilyMed
Goldstine, Ian J., FamilyMed
Gooi, Teong Hean
Goulet, Sara, FamilyMed
Gowda, Sweta, FamilyMed
Grace, Kevin J., FamilyMed
Grass, Stephen B., FamilyMed
Graves, Darren F., FamilyMed
Gray, Donovan O N., FamilyMed(EM)
Greene, Richard E., FamilyMed(EM)
Gregan, Ida-Lynn, FamilyMed
Griggs, Gordon B., FamilyMed
Gripp, Karen E.
Grobler, Wilhelmus P.
Groenewald, L. Henriette, FamilyMed
Grogan, J. Anthony
Grzybowski, Michelle M., FamilyMed
Guindi, Nizar S., FamilyMed
Guindy, Sherine M., FamilyMed
Gujral, Paramjeet, FamilyMed
Gupta, Melanie, FamilyMed
Gupta, Ravi
Gustafson, Robert L.
Gwozdecki, Taras M.
Haggard, Gian, FamilyMed
Hahlweg, Kenneth A., FamilyMed
Haleis, Ahmed R.
Haligowski, David J.
Halmarson, Erica B., FamilyMed
Haque, Farah N.
Harati, Osama, FamilyMed
Harel, Shai, FamilyMed(EM)
Harlos, Michael S., FamilyMed
Hartley, Duane M., FamilyMed
Hartry, A. Shane, FamilyMed(EM)
Hartry, Zoa, FamilyMed
Hasan, S K. Mahmud
Hasdan, Galit, FamilyMed
Haseeb, Sabiha
Hashmi, Sajjad, FamilyMed
Hauch, Susan G., FamilyMed
Hayward, Rowland J., FamilyMed
Heese, Heinz B.
Hegdekar, Mona, FamilyMed(EM)
Heidenreich, Wolfgang W F.
Heinrichs, Kristin, FamilyMed
Henry, Douglas, FamilyMed
Herd, Anthony, FamilyMed(EM)
Hicks, Cynthia D A.
Hildahl, Craig R., FamilyMed
Hildahl, Wayne
Hilderman, Lorraine
Hitchcock, William G., FamilyMed
Hlas, Lucie
Hlynka, Anthony, FamilyMed
Hobbs, Cheryl L.
Hochman, Michael, FamilyMed
Holder, Fryderyk
Holowenko, Dedeshya S., FamilyMed(EM)
Honiball, James, FamilyMed
Horvath, Jeffrey F., FamilyMed
Howatt, Jesse, FamilyMed
Hoy, Gerald J F., FamilyMed
Hudgel, David W.
Hughes, Philip M.
Hulsbosch, Hanna, FamilyMed
Husarewycz, Stephen
Ibbitt, Christopher J.
Ibrahim, Adel F A., FamilyMed
Idiong, N. Daniel
Imam, Isam E D B., FamilyMed
Ip, Angel H.
Iqbal, Irum, FamilyMed
Ireland, Laurie F., FamilyMed
Isaac, Carey D., FamilyMed
Iskander, Salah S G., FamilyMed
Iskander, Suzan F., FamilyMed
Issaivanan, Magimairajan
Jabs, Marlis E., FamilyMed
Jacobs, Johannes J.
Jaeger, Claire P., FamilyMed
Jain, Madhuri
Jain, Narendra K.
Jamieson, Mary J., FamilyMed
Janjua, Meer M., FamilyMed
Jensen, Derrek M., FamilyMed
Johnson, Darcy E., FamilyMed
Johnson, Robert G., FamilyMed
Jones, Julie, FamilyMed
Joshua, Julian M.
Joundi, Mohamad G.
Jovel, Ramon E.
Jowett, Andrew G.
Kaldas, Rhoda M., FamilyMed
Kalturnyk, Blake P.
Kati, Arvind A.
Katz, Alan, FamilyMed
Kaushal, Ravi D.
Kearns, Katherine, FamilyMed
Keijzer, Richard
Kemkaran, Kenneth P F.
Kennedy, Maureen F., FamilyMed
Kesselman, Edward W.
Keynan, Yoav
Khadem, Aliasghar
Khan, Noor M.
Khanahmadi, Shahab
Khangura, Davinder S., FamilyMed
Khelil, Assil I., FamilyMed
Kim, Dennis
Kimelman, Allen L.
Kisil, Kathryn E., FamilyMed
Klaponski, John R., FamilyMed(EM)
Klassen, Norma F.
Klassen, Orla R.
Kloppers, Anton
Klym, Karen L., FamilyMed
Knezic, Kathy A., FamilyMed
Koczanski, Roman P.
Koh, Clarissa B K., FamilyMed
Kojori, Fatemeh
Komenda, Ben W.
Kong, Anne M C., FamilyMed
Konrad, Gerald P., FamilyMed
Kosowan, Marisa R., FamilyMed
Kotecha, Yatish J.
Kousonsavath, Ratana L.
Koven, Sheldon J.
Kowal, Caroline, FamilyMed(EM)
Krahn, James K H., FamilyMed
Kredentser, Sarah E., FamilyMed
Kreml, John A.
Kress, Stephan G., FamilyMed(EM)
Kristjanson, Mark R., FamilyMed
Kroczak, Tadeusz J.
Kuegle, Peter F X., FamilyMed
Kujath, Magdalena
Kuo, Carey P.
Kvern, Brent L., FamilyMed
Kyeremateng, Doris, FamilyMed
La Rue, Leonard B.
Labiyaratne, W W. Chamindra P., FamilyMed
Lach, Lori-Ann D., FamilyMed
Lage, Karen L., FamilyMed
Lagowski, Michael C.
Lam, Charles C K.
Lam, David S C.
Lamb, Julie A., FamilyMed
Lamba, Geetinder K.
Lang, Clement
Langan, John T.
Langridge, James K., FamilyMed
Lau, Yiu-Keung
Lavallee, Barry D A., FamilyMed
Laycock, Tyler M., FamilyMed(EM)
Lazarus, Arie
Lecuyer, Nadine S., FamilyMed
Lee, Sandra S L., FamilyMed
Lei, T C. Benny
Leloka, Clare M.
Lerner, Moe, FamilyMed(EM)
Letkeman, Richard L., FamilyMed
Leung Shing, Louis P.
Levesque, Julie, FamilyMed
Lewis, Jennifer J., FamilyMed
Leylek, Ahmet S.
Lipinski, Grazyna B.
Lobato De Faria, Ricardo J L.
Lobley, Jarrett
Lockman, Leonard E., FamilyMed
Loepp, M. Christine, FamilyMed
Loewen, Sylvia R., FamilyMed
Long, Adrian L H.
Lowden, Cameron S., FamilyMed
Lu, Paul B., FamilyMed
Luk, Tse Li.
Lukie, Brian J.
Lynch, Joanna M., FamilyMed
Lyons, Michael J., FamilyMed
MacKay, Michael J.
MacLeod, Bruce A., FamilyMed
MacMillan, Michael B., FamilyMed
Macaulay, Alexander W., FamilyMed
Macek, Ralf K W., FamilyMed(EM)
Maharaj, Gunness R., FamilyMed
Maharaj, Ian G.
Mahay, Raj K.
Maier, Ronald J C.
Maiti, Soubhik, FamilyMed
Malabanan, Edilberto A.
Malek Marzban, Peiman
Malhi, Arfan M.
Mallick, Kiron C.
Mammen, Thomas
Mancer, Jasdeep K., FamilyMed
Mancini, Enrico V., FamilyMed
Mare, Abraham C W.
Marsh, David W.
Martens, Raymond L.
Martens-Barnes, Carolyn
Martin, Bruce D., FamilyMed
Martin, Francis, FamilyMed
Mason, Christa
Matthews, Christopher M., FamilyMed
Maxwell, Brenda S R., FamilyMed
Mayba, John I.
Mazhari Ravesh, Amir H., FamilyMed
McCammon, Richard J., FamilyMed
McCormack, M. Terry, FamilyMed
McFee, Colin D., FamilyMed
McGregor, Gregor, FamilyMed
McGregor, Jyoti M.
McIntosh, Leslie A., FamilyMed
McKenzie, C. Ann
McKenzie, Thomas, FamilyMed(EM)
McKeown, Iris, FamilyMed
McQuarrie, Shauna L., FamilyMed
McTaggart, Dawn-Lynn M., FamilyMed
Mehta, Asita
Mehta, Pravinsagar G., FamilyMed
Mekhail, Ashraf S H., FamilyMed
Mellon, Aaron M., FamilyMed
Mendis, Maleen R., FamilyMed
Mercier, Nicole
Meyer, Anthon M., FamilyMed
Meza Vargas, Maria S.
Mian, M. Tariq
Mihalchuk, Ainslie J., FamilyMed
Milambiling, Ernesto M.
Milambiling, Ligaya C.
Miller, Donald M.
Mills, Barry J.
Minish, Kimberley J., FamilyMed
Mink, Steven N.
Miskiewicz, Laura M.
Moawad, Victor F F., FamilyMed
Mohammed, Ismail
Moncek, John A., FamilyMed
Monteiro, Gerard E.
Moosa, Alisha B.
Moran De Muller, Karen M.
Morham, Anthony R., FamilyMed
Morris, Andrew L.
Morris, Glenn S., FamilyMed
Morrow, Adrienne, FamilyMed
Mouton, Robert W.
Mowat, Grenville S., FamilyMed(EM)
Mukty, Mahmuda A., FamilyMed
Munsamy, Gonasagran K., FamilyMed
Murray, J. David, FamilyMed
Mymin, David
Nadeem, Yasmin N., FamilyMed
Naidoo, Jenisa
Naidoo, Shireen P.
Nair, Unni K.
Narasimhan, Sowmya
Nasr, Michel R.
Nates, Wayne
Nawrocka, Dorothy
Nazar-Ul-Iman, Saiyed M.
Nemeth, Peter W.
Nepomuceno, Jean R., FamilyMed
Nepon, Jack
Neufeld, Gregory M.
Neufeld, Hertha, FamilyMed
Newman, Suzanne, FamilyMed
Nguetsop, Martin
Nguyen, Lien Hoang
Nguyen, Minh Hung
Nguyen, Xuan-Tung
Niraula, Saroj
Njionhou Kemeni, Marie M., FamilyMed
Noack, Laura A., FamilyMed
Nyomba, Bulangu L.
Oble, Darryl D A.
Ochonska, W. Margaret
Ogaranko, Christopher P., FamilyMed
Oliver, Afsaneh, FamilyMed
Oliver, Zoe J., FamilyMed(EM)
Olson, Robyn L., FamilyMed
Olson, Shanna M., FamilyMed
Olujohungbe, Adebayo B K.
Olynyk, Frederick T.
Omah-Maharajh, Dave A.
Onoferson, Brian K.
Ormiston, John D.
Osei-Bonsu, Adelaide
Pachal, Cindy A.
Pacin, Alojz
Pacin, Ondrej, FamilyMed

Padeanu, Florin, FamilyMed
Pan, Janice M W., FamilyMed
Panaskevich, Tatiana, FamilyMed
Pandian, Alagarsamy
Pang, Eileen G., FamilyMed
Paskvalin, Mario
Patek, Susan
Patel, Jayshree
Patel, Neesha, FamilyMed
Patel, Prafulchandra C., FamilyMed(EM)
Pauls, Merril A., FamilyMed(EM)
Pawlak, Jerzy K.
Peled, Elia
Penner, Kurt, FamilyMed(EM)
Pepelassis, Dionissios
Perez, Margarita J., FamilyMed
Permack, Sheldon M., FamilyMed
Perry, Anamrija M.
Perry, Kyle D.
Peters, Harold O.
Peters, Hein, FamilyMed
Peters, Richard J.
Peters, Ruth E.
Peters, Sheila M., FamilyMed(EM)
Peterson, Cameron G., FamilyMed(EM)
Peterson, John D.
Pettigrew, Norman M.
Pettinger, Cary S., FamilyMed
Pickard, Kathleen J A., FamilyMed
Pidsadny, Shelly, FamilyMed
Pilat, Edward J., FamilyMed
Pinchuk, David M., FamilyMed(EM)
Pinette, Gilles D., FamilyMed
Pinnick, Suzy A O.
Pirzada, Munir A.
Pittman, Patricia G., FamilyMed
Polimeni, Christine J., FamilyMed
Pollet, Virginie
Pollock, Deborah G.
Popplow, James R.
Postolow, Fabiana A.
Potter, Jennifer L., FamilyMed
Prenovault, Jean J M., FamilyMed
Price, Shandis, FamilyMed
Prodan, Orest
Pukay, Gregory
Qureshi, Bilquis, FamilyMed
Qureshi, Rizwan
Racette-Le Neveu, Therese J., FamilyMed
Rados, Lawrence R., FamilyMed
Rafay, Mubeen F.
Raimondi, Christina J., FamilyMed
Ramgoolam, Rajendranath
Randunne, Avanthi, FamilyMed
Raubenheimer, Johannes P., FamilyMed
Ravula, Niroop R.
Reda, John E., FamilyMed
Reda, Margaret M.
Rehal, Ranjodh S.
Reinecke, Marina, FamilyMed
Reynolds, James L., FamilyMed
Ridah, Dekrayat H., FamilyMed
Riese, Nichole M M., FamilyMed
Ripstein, Ira T.
Ritchie, Janet, FamilyMed
Robillard, Susan C., FamilyMed
Roman, Manal, FamilyMed
Roman, Nader S F S., FamilyMed
Rosario, Rosa H.
Ross, David A., FamilyMed
Ross, Frances K., FamilyMed
Ross, Frederick J.
Rothova, Anna
Roy, Danielle M., FamilyMed
Rubinstein, Ethan
Rumbolt, Brian R.
Rusen, Jack B.
Rush, Nene O S., FamilyMed
Rusk, Richard, FamilyMed
Saadia, Roger
Sabzi Mobarakeh, Afshin
Saint-Hilaire, Melanie L., FamilyMed
Saleem, Ashfaq, FamilyMed
Salem, Fayez F S.
Salman, Michael S.
Salter-Oliver, Belynda, FamilyMed
Sami, Sahar, FamilyMed
Saran, Kanwal D S., FamilyMed
Sasse, Sara G.
Saunders, Kevin K., FamilyMed
Sawatzky, Cynthia K., FamilyMed
Sawchuk, J. Paul, FamilyMed
Sawka, Sandra E.
Schellenberg, Donald W.
Schellenberg, William C.
Schifke, William G.
Schneider, Mark, FamilyMed(EM)
Schroeder, Alvin N.
Scrapneck, Ronald A.
Scurfield, Carol M., FamilyMed
Seifer, Colette
Sekiguchi, Debora R.
Sen, Robin
Senderewich, Elizabeth C.
Seshia, Mary M K.
Sewell, Gary M.
Shah, Ashvin, FamilyMed
Shah, Bharat
Shaikh, Nasir
Sharda, Priti, FamilyMed
Sharkey, J. Brian, FamilyMed
Shaw, Sandra A., FamilyMed(EM)
Shell, Melanie D C., FamilyMed
Shenoda, Kamal L M., FamilyMed
Shenouda, Mervat E F G., FamilyMed
Shenouda, Phebe F S., FamilyMed
Shiffman, Frank H.
Shnider, Maurice
Shrom, Jerry B.
Shum, Kum Cheung
Sickert, Helga G.
Sidra Gerges, Maged, FamilyMed
Sikora, Felix J.
Silagy, Stewart J.
Silhova, Dasa, FamilyMed
Silver, Carla D., FamilyMed
Simard-Chiu, Leslie A., FamilyMed
Simkin, Ruth E., FamilyMed
Simons, Frances E.
Simonson, Donald W.
Singer, Alexander G., FamilyMed
Singer, Marilyn C., FamilyMed
Singer, Raymond, FamilyMed
Singh, Amarjit
Sisler, Jeffrey J., FamilyMed
Skakum, Ruth G H., FamilyMed
Slutchuk, Marvin
Slutchuk, Sean C.
Smal, Samuel J.
Smart, J R. Alexander
Smelsky, Charlene R., FamilyMed
Smil, Eva
Smith, Erik R., FamilyMed(EM)
Smith, John R M.
Smith, Louis F., FamilyMed
Smith, Roy W., FamilyMed
Smith, Wendy L., FamilyMed
Snovida, Lioubov
Sobowale, Opeyemi A., FamilyMed
Sokal, John E M., FamilyMed(EM)
Sokolies, Rex B., FamilyMed
Sokolowski, Danuta
Solbrig, Marylou V.
Sookhoo, Siuchan
Soylu, Hanifi
Srinivasan, Ganesh
St Godard, Edward E., FamilyMed
St Vincent, Anthony M.
St-Laurent, Carol A., FamilyMed
Stacey, Campbell A., FamilyMed
Stachowicz, Tyler, FamilyMed(EM)
Stefanyshen, Grant S., FamilyMed
Stelzer, Josef
Stenhouse, James K.
Stephensen, Michael C., FamilyMed
Storoschuk, Gregory W.
Strachan, Ritchie J.
Strank, Roydon K., FamilyMed
Stroescu, Daniela V.
Sud, Anil K.
Sultana, Roksana
Suss, Roger G., FamilyMed(EM)
Susser, M. Marc
Sutherland, James G.
Swain, Valerie J.
Sweetland, Robert J.
Szajkowski, Stanley
Szajkowski, Terrence P., FamilyMed
Teo, Swee L., FamilyMed
Thomas, Shawn T., FamilyMed
Thompson, Ryan M., FamilyMed
Thomson, Brent R J., FamilyMed
Thorlakson, Derek P.
Thorlakson, Ian J.
Thottingal, Antony P.
Titus, Roselin T., FamilyMed
Todary Fahmy, Yvette P., FamilyMed
Tomy, Kerry L.
Tomy, R. Halim, FamilyMed(EM)
Torossi, Gregory A.
Trajano, Janet D.
Tran, Thi Cuc P.
Tretiak, Wendy D., FamilyMed
Tse, Wai Ching, FamilyMed
Unger, Bertram J.
Vadysinghe, Amal
Vakilitahami, Habib
Van De Mosselaer, Gregory J., FamilyMed
Van Dyk, Werner W A., FamilyMed(EM)
Van Horne, Wayne A., FamilyMed
Van Jaarsveldt, Werner D., FamilyMed
Van Rensburg, Corne J., FamilyMed
Van Rooyen, Marthinus L.
Van Tongel, Alexander G C.
Van Vliet, Michael, FamilyMed
Varma, Neel B.
Vattheuer, Annabel G.
Venditti, Marcello W., FamilyMed
Veres, Agnes I.
Verity, Shawn D., FamilyMed
Vianzon, Clarita S.
Vignudo, Silvia, FamilyMed
Visch, Shawn H R., FamilyMed
Vo, Minh Nhat
Volpe, Michael S A., FamilyMed
Wahl, Patrick D., FamilyMed
Walker, Arlene A.
Wall, Donna A.
Wallace, Sharon E.
Warraich, Naseer A., FamilyMed
Wasef, Mervat S R., FamilyMed
Waters, Marnie M., FamilyMed
Watts, Jacqueline
Wawrykow, Teresa M J., FamilyMed(EM)
Weinberg, Eytan N.
Welch, Gilbert J C.
Werier, Jonathon G.
Whetter, Ian C., FamilyMed
Whittaker, Elizabeth I.
Whyte, Stanley L.
Wiatrowski, Joe F K., FamilyMed(EM)
Wiebe, Jennifer A., FamilyMed
Wiens, Peter J., FamilyMed
Wiesenthal, Benjamin D.
Wijewardena, Handun
Wilkie, Catherine L., FamilyMed
Willems, David D., FamilyMed
Williams, J. David, FamilyMed
Wilson, Gregory P., FamilyMed
Winogrodzka, Christina
Wirch, M. Faye, FamilyMed
Wojciechowski, Agnieszka E., FamilyMed
Woo, Casey D.
Wozney, Leonard R.
Wyant-Crossman, Kerrie E I., FamilyMed
Yi, Man
Young, Brent C., FamilyMed
Young, Jeanne, FamilyMed
Young, Scott K., FamilyMed
Yuen, Jenna L Y B., FamilyMed
Zaki, Amel E., FamilyMed
Zalam, Mahmoud M M.
Ziomek, Anna M.

WINNIPEGOSIS

Johnson, Errol

NEW BRUNSWICK

ATHOLVILLE

Beshay, Basem

BAIE-SAINTE-ANNE

Losier, Arthur J.

BAS-CARAQUET

Blanchard, Gilbert, FamilyMed
Boucher, Carl, FamilyMed
Hynes, William, FamilyMed
Lanteigne, Solange, FamilyMed
Martin, Anne-Marie, FamilyMed
Pelletier, Anick, FamilyMed
Robichaud, Johanne, FamilyMed

BATH

Lockhart, Bruce F.
Lockhart, Colin E.

BATHURST

Akbarinejad Moosavi, Seyed M.
Al-Khatib, Dina, FamilyMed
Al-Rejjal, Rafat
Alagbe, Sylvie
Arsenault, Marie-Andree, FamilyMed
Arseneau, Jean-Pierre, FamilyMed
Baldzhiyski, Nikolay
Barnhill, Byron B.
Bouchard, Ariane, FamilyMed
Boudreau, Eve M., FamilyMed
Camire, Sophie, FamilyMed
Cauchon, Natalie, FamilyMed
Chettiar, Nataraj V.
Cormier, Pascal
Daigle, Samuel, FamilyMed
Dion, Michelle, FamilyMed(EM)
Doucet, Danielle, FamilyMed
Doucet, Marc-Andre, FamilyMed
Ducharme, Louis-Albert
Dugas, Anna-Viola M.
Eddie, Patrick, FamilyMed
Fondop, Jean-Jacques
Gionet, Edmonde, FamilyMed
Godin, Dominique, FamilyMed
Goguen, Frederic, FamilyMed
Goli, Harish
Goulard, Jean-Francois
Gutierrez, Marinett R.
Hache, Marilene, FamilyMed
Kamba, E. Francine
Kamba, Samuel
Khider, Mehdi
Laflamme-Fillion, Annie, FamilyMed
Lagacé, Anne-Renée, FamilyMed
Langlois, Julie, FamilyMed
Lanteigne, Jean-Pierre
Larocque, Monique, FamilyMed
Loubani, Mahmoud M.
Loubani, Sara A H.
Maltais, Cathrine, FamilyMed
Martineau, Francis
Matsui, Irene
Millet, Richard F.
Ostashko, Sergiy
Peterson, Karina
Reddy, U. Stanislaus
Richard, Raymond
Risdon, James
Robichaud, Line
Sadaf, Arifa
Shabani, Faryala K.
Shoham-Hazon, Nir
Struthers, Andrew W.
Swati, Ismatun
Theriault, Martine, FamilyMed
Theriault, Maryse, FamilyMed
Thibeault, Danny, FamilyMed
Tremblay, Pierre
Ventura, Karyna
Wade, David A.
Weka-Lungunga, Charles, FamilyMed
White, Robert J.
Wilson, Renald
Yung, Lee

BELLEDUNE

Levesque, Josée, FamilyMed

BERESFORD

Hanzal, Djilali

BLACKVILLE

Zigante, Nina, FamilyMed

BOCABEC

Bartlett, Robert L.

BOIESTOWN

Wood, Tanya D., FamilyMed

BOUCTOUCHE

Fontaine, Ronald J A.
Langis, Lise, FamilyMed
McFadden, Shelley, FamilyMed

BOUDREAU-OUEST

Allanach, R. William

CAMBRIDGE-NARROWS

Stackhouse, Dianne L.

CAMPBELLTON

Aldea, Michael S.
Alsaghir, Abdullah
Andonov, Igor
Anwar, Mariam
Attia-Alla, Ayman
Aumeerally, Farouk L.
Bajwa, Harjeet
Bashala, Roger, FamilyMed
Becerro Garijo, Gloria
Benghida, Riad
Benoit, Catherine, FamilyMed
Clements, Shirley-Anne, FamilyMed
Fuzesi, Gabor
Ghauri, Sabira
Haberer, Marie-Pierre
Haque, Khurshid
Holly, Ralph
Holly, Tania M.
Jahangir, Mubeen
Jamil, Khalid
Khatib, Ahmad
Laevski, Lefter M.
Lamour, Dominique
Landry, Steeve, FamilyMed
Laporte, Bertrand
Lebelle Dejario, Nadine
Lepage, Sylvie, FamilyMed
MacDonald, D. Christopher, FamilyMed
Masse, Caroline
Masse, Sylvain
Matthews, Nicole
Mbala-Katanda, Sylvie
Oni, Oluwole
Robichaud, Delbe J.
Saxena, Saket
Shenoy, Pradeep
Sinha, Prabhat
Sridhar, Jami
Srivastava, Swati
Taleb, Samir
Voges-Martinez, Armando
Wang, Wei
Yacoub, Inas
Youla, Adama R.

CARAQUET

Boucher, Daniel
Bourque, Jean-Andre
Caron, Olivier, FamilyMed
Chiasson, Marie-Lise
Dalpe, Linda, FamilyMed
Dugas, Lise S., FamilyMed
Frenette, E. Ina F.
Leblanc, Jean, FamilyMed
Mallet, Jacques L., FamilyMed
Mea, Demetrio M.
Morissette, Celine
Nardini, Robert, FamilyMed
Schoeffner, Wolfgang V.
Selosse, Bruno M R J.

CHARLO

Barriault, Ronald J., FamilyMed

CHIPMAN

Prendergast, John A., FamilyMed
Tran, Peter, FamilyMed

CLAIR

Carrier, Yves C.
Lang, Roger L.

COCAGNE

Dupuis, Hubert

DALHOUSIE

Adjahoto, Etsé
Benning, Gurpal
Bigras, Magali, FamilyMed
Bujold, Louis, FamilyMed
Calugaroiu, Dariu
Furlong, Dennis J.
Kalim, Myrlène
MacMillan, Vona, FamilyMed
Pelletier, Adrien
Singh, Dharm R.
Tolba, Marwan, FamilyMed
Verdejo Arancibia, Adriana A.

DIEPPE

Anand, Sanjiv, FamilyMed
Arsenault, Chantal, FamilyMed
Babin, Lise M., FamilyMed
Barrieau, Andre, FamilyMed
Bazinet, Emilie, FamilyMed
Benoit, Melanie, FamilyMed
Blando, German
Boissonnault, Pierre, FamilyMed
Boucher-Robichaud, Micheline, FamilyMed
Brideau, Jean-Rene, FamilyMed
Chami, Nidal
Charest, Melanie, FamilyMed
Chiasson, Paul, FamilyMed
Chouinard, Philippe, FamilyMed
Cormier, Jules, FamilyMed
Crawford, Michelle
Daigle, Pierrette, FamilyMed
Daigle, Sylvie, FamilyMed
Desilets, Alice, FamilyMed
Gagnon, Annie, FamilyMed
Gallant, Denise L., FamilyMed
Gallant, Joanne
Gautreau, Renelle, FamilyMed
Landry, Jacques, FamilyMed
Landry, Michel, FamilyMed
Leblanc, Jean-Bernard
Leblanc, Veronique, FamilyMed
Lebreton, Nathalie J., FamilyMed
Leroux, Manon
Melanson, Karen A., FamilyMed
Melanson, Vincent
Moffitt, Julie, FamilyMed
Nadeau, Marie-Josee, FamilyMed
Poirier, Carole D., FamilyMed
Poitras, Marie-Josee, FamilyMed
Robichaud, J. Victor, FamilyMed
Robichaud, Monique, FamilyMed
Roy, Katie, FamilyMed
Roy, Marcel, FamilyMed
Roy, Nadine, FamilyMed
Saulnier, Nancy, FamilyMed
Savoie, Anik, FamilyMed
Savoy, Cynthia A., FamilyMed
Simard, Caroline
Simpson, Janelle D., FamilyMed
St-Pierre, Nicole Y M.
Thibodeau, Daniele, FamilyMed
Turcotte, Renee
Whalen, Julie H., FamilyMed

DOAKTOWN

Chow, Heman

EDMUNDSTON

Akinfolarin, Josephine
Andersen, Michelle
Aouida, Mohamed
Barbosa, Rubens
Baz, Rami
Begum, Rukhsana
Benlamlih, Mohamed
Blier, E. Ludger
Bouchard, Marie
Castonguay, Julie, FamilyMed
Connely, C. Andrew
Cote-Berube, Janik, FamilyMed
Cyr, Anne, FamilyMed
Dada, Azad
Dallaire, Dominic, FamilyMed
Dimachki, Saadedine
Dion, Bertrand R.
Divanli, Kemal
Dumont, Jocelyn
Efoe, Anani
Forest, Liette, FamilyMed
Gibbs, Gaetan, FamilyMed
Haq Choudhuri, Akm Ziaul
Kabwe, Kazadi N.
Kapur, Shiv
Lavoie, Maryse, FamilyMed
Leblanc, Joanne, FamilyMed
Levasseur, Eric, FamilyMed
Lorquet, Yvan
Marino, Nalini
Martin, Pierre
Mayrand, Luc P.
Meddoun, Mamoun
Michaud, Michele D., FamilyMed
Nguimfack Mbodie, Pierre C.
Pelletier, Denis P.
Perkins, Philippe
Poitras, Liette, FamilyMed
Poitras, Nathalie, FamilyMed
Rahbaoui, Ahmed
Roy, Fabienne
Rusu, Viorel-George
Samhan, Omar
Samson, Yves
Sbeity, Samer
Soucie, Francois D., FamilyMed
Soucy, Marina, FamilyMed
Tasovac-Babic, Radmila, FamilyMed
Theriault, Luce, FamilyMed
Tobin, John A.
Transue, Sarah
Virgili, Philippe C.
Zhang, Lianfeng C.

FLORENCEVILLE

Marco, Clayton V., FamilyMed
Tooley, Camilla M.

FREDERCTN-JCT

Richardson, John D.

FREDERICTON

Al-Halimi, Maha, FamilyMed
Al-Sharief, Khaled, FamilyMed
Allen, Genevieve, FamilyMed
Armitage, Michael E., FamilyMed
Aslam, Zeeshan
Athar, Saira, FamilyMed
Banic, Zlatko
Barry, Thomas J., FamilyMed
Barton, Jeffrey D., FamilyMed
Beal, John R.
Bekele, Yilma
Beland, Jacques
Benaya, Sebastian
Bock, Philip W., FamilyMed
Bolesnikov, Grlica
Bolesnikov, Zeljko
Boone, Bonita L., FamilyMed
Broad, Karyn D.
Broeren, Wilma M J.
Bruce, Calvin D.
Cabatu, Moises D.
Cameron, Kelsey
Chen, Yu
Christie, Kevin M., FamilyMed
Cleary, Eilish
Colpitts, Anne F., FamilyMed
Cruz, Leo M P.
Daigle, Robert J P.
Davis, Michael, FamilyMed(EM)
Dempsey-Mckim, Susan R.
Dickinson, Andrew, FamilyMed
Digby, Aaron G., FamilyMed
Digby, Jennifer, FamilyMed
Durrer, Jane K., FamilyMed
Fisher, Michael G.
Flower, David G.
Gallick, David
Galwa, Ram
Giovannoni, Aldo, FamilyMed
Goodyear, Jillian D., FamilyMed
Gowan, Debra
Hadley, Katherine E.
Haene, Roger
Haines, Gregory C., FamilyMed
Harvey, Kathleen
Hauman, Helena, FamilyMed
Hayter, Michael, FamilyMed
Hebb, Linda M., FamilyMed(EM)
Henderson, William R., FamilyMed
Hickey, Andrea E.
Irrinki, Anand, FamilyMed
Jackson, Lori
Karol, Savita, FamilyMed
Keddy, John W., FamilyMed
Kerr, Paul B., FamilyMed
Keschtkar, Nicholas
King, Russell H T., FamilyMed
Lambropoulos, Cristos, FamilyMed
Lemboye, Adeola
Logan, Heather
Luntao, Yuri M A.
MacDonald, Ian M., FamilyMed
MacDougall, Frances J K.
MacKinnon, Brian J.
Majerovich, Jo Ann, FamilyMed
Makary, Hala
Manzar, Khalid
Marisette, Stephen R., FamilyMed
Martin, Alban
McDonald, Gordon, FamilyMed
McGinn, Rebecca, FamilyMed
McIntosh, Shiona M., FamilyMed
McKim, James C.
Murphy, Ronald J.
Njoku, Anthony
Ozumba, Obioma
Pascual, Joan S.
Plant, Louise A., FamilyMed
Plummer, A. Gordon
Pniak, Ewa M.
Pond, Achla
Pond, Stephen D.
Qureshi, Shujauddin
Randall, Troy D.
Raza, Muhammad S.
Reid, Brian J., FamilyMed
Relja, Malgorzata
Robertson, R. Scott
Roussel, Claire N., FamilyMed
Ruest, Louise, FamilyMed
Rushton, Cheryl, FamilyMed
Russell, Jennifer S W., FamilyMed
Sehgal, Yogi, FamilyMed
Shahid, Raheel A.
Shawesh, Salim M.
Simonyi-Gindele, Samuel, FamilyMed
Smith, Patricia J., FamilyMed
Smith, R. Stephen, FamilyMed
Smith, Susan E.
Srinivasan, Kalyani, FamilyMed
Stuart, Carmen M., FamilyMed
Swan, Amber C., FamilyMed
Tatemichi, Sue R., FamilyMed
Thorpe, B. Patricia
Tingley, Brenda M.
Tingley, Erin M., FamilyMed
Touchie, Jane E.
Van Middlesworth, Karen E., FamilyMed
Varty, T. Douglas, FamilyMed
Vayani, Haji A.
White, Naomi, FamilyMed
Wiley, Lauren K., FamilyMed
Young, Graeme M., FamilyMed(EM)
Youwakim, Basseem H., FamilyMed

GRAND BAY WESTFIELD

Elias, David A., FamilyMed(EM)
Scott, Daniel G.
Webb, G. Robert
Webb, Robert J.

GRAND FALLS

Blunston, Shawn D., FamilyMed
Bosembo Ilondjo, Maurice
Lavoie-Dufour, Line
Luttfy, Ghyda
Morin, Maryse, FamilyMed
Roy, Maurice P.
Senechal, Sylvie, FamilyMed

GRAND MANAN

Aliabadi, Hossein
Cairns, Anne, FamilyMed
Heir, Jatinder

GRAND SAULT/ GRAND FALLS

Chettiar, Ramasami V.
Khenissi, Zeineb
Nowlan, Michael
Richard, Claude

HAMPTON

Adeyeye, Adeola, FamilyMed
Carson, Margaret E.
Collings, James C.
Fairman-Wright, Micaela P., FamilyMed
Fisher, Robert, FamilyMed
Hall, J. Douglas, FamilyMed
Jansen, Ann P., FamilyMed
Salgado, David

HANWELL

Carmichael, Paula A., FamilyMed

HARTLAND

Ghanem, Sara
Stocek, Rudolph F.

HARVEY STATION

Fletcher, Daniel, FamilyMed
MacDougall, Joseph A.
Olmstead, David

HILLSBOROUGH

Dykeman, Winston R., FamilyMed

KEDGWICK

Bouchard, Jean-Guy

LAMEQUE

Chiasson-Basque, Renee
Duguay Vibert, Denise, FamilyMed
Dupuis, Veronique, FamilyMed
Kerry, Marie-Paule
Luyela, Asunta
Mallet, Michele, FamilyMed
Martin Ward, Dawn-Marie L., FamilyMed
Santerre, Mylène, FamilyMed

MEMRAMCOOK

Cote, Genevieve M., FamilyMed
Wybouw, Cedric, FamilyMed

MINTO

Haynes, Gordon R.
Morrissy, Sean R., FamilyMed
Ramsey, Patricia A.
Zuidhof, Aaron, FamilyMed

MIRAMICHI

Adoubali, Abdurahman
Ahmed, Najneen
Ahmed, Salim
Ahmed, Syed S., FamilyMed
Balasingham, Prabaharan
Begam, Maksuda
Bent, Stephen
Binedell, Walter
Boulay, Robert M., FamilyMed
Carter, Allister W.
Cohen, Sébastien
Cole, Roy V.
Cronje, David P G.
Dani, Mukhaimer H.
Du Toit, Jacobus J.
Haddad, Camille
Hans, Jeffrey P.
Harebottle, Ronald R.
Henderson, John, FamilyMed
Hendriks, J A. Edouard, FamilyMed(EM)
Hossain, Muhammad
Hrncirik, Joseph
Hudson, Carl R., FamilyMed
Hudson, Linda G.
Keating, Paula M., FamilyMed
Kpogo, Amos L., FamilyMed
Kruger, Schalk
Lehnert, Thomas B., FamilyMed
Losier, Gerard B.
Lubin, Alexandre S.
MacGillivray, William
MacKnight, Roxanne E., FamilyMed
Manerkar, Avdhut R.
Martin, Christopher J., FamilyMed
Martin, William J., FamilyMed
McCann, John A., FamilyMed
McQuaid, Melissa C., FamilyMed
Miah, Mohammad
Morales, Eduardo
Murray, Michele L., FamilyMed(EM)
Nemec, Edith
Nowak, Zbigniew J.
Rai, Vasanth
Rambaran, Totaram M.
Riveros Neira, Luis G.
Roux, Emile V W.
Schaefer, Tanya D.
Siddhartha, Sanjay
Slorach, J. Ninian
Spartaco, Navaro
Vonkeman, Hermen
Wannenburg, Johan
Watts, Jill A.
Weyers, Hendrik
Wierzchoslawski, Krzysztof

MONCTON

Abdel Samad, Nizar
Abdelsalam, Mahmoud
Adenuga, Olugbenga A., FamilyMed
Alame-Assi, Saada
Albert, Jacques, FamilyMed(EM)
Albert, Paul, FamilyMed(EM)
Anthony, Rozario
Arseneau, Fernand G.
Arseneault, Tania, FamilyMed(EM)
Assi, Hazem
Assi, Hussein
Bandyayera, Etienne, FamilyMed
Basque-Arsenault, Lorraine
Beaulieu, Pierre-Andre, FamilyMed
Bedard, Nadia, FamilyMed
Belliveau, Manon, FamilyMed
Benjelloun, Ali
Bensaleh-Ratmi, Amal
Bhalla, Jaswinder, FamilyMed
Blanchard, Marie-Eve, FamilyMed
Bond, Anthony C.
Bonnell Allanach, Camille, FamilyMed
Bouffard, Karine, FamilyMed
Bourque, Stephane, FamilyMed
Breau, Marie-Josee, FamilyMed
Brennan, Amy M., FamilyMed
Burry, Andrea F., FamilyMed
Burton, Corey, FamilyMed
Calvy, Christian
Carrier, Julie, FamilyMed
Chaibou, Mahamadou
Chesser, Tracey M., FamilyMed(EM)
Chesser, W. Gary, FamilyMed
Colas, Rolande M.
Comstock, Ravneet, FamilyMed
Conrod, Michelle A., FamilyMed
Cormier, Blandine, FamilyMed
Cormier, Janice
Crouse, Susan, FamilyMed
Cyr, Nathalie, FamilyMed
Cyr, Valerie-Anne
Dahan, Marc-Albert, FamilyMed
Despres, Mylene, FamilyMed
Deveau, Carole, FamilyMed
Deware, Kimberley J., FamilyMed
Dionne, Natasha P., FamilyMed
Donald, Gregory, FamilyMed
Doucet, Paul G J.
Dufour, Karlyne L., FamilyMed
Duguay, Gary, FamilyMed(EM)
Enright, Jody, FamilyMed
Eros, Eva M., FamilyMed
Frenette, Thomas P., FamilyMed
Gallant, Christopher R., FamilyMed
Geddes, Murray
Ghedira, Monia
Godbout, Jacques-Andre
Godin, Bernard, FamilyMed
Godin, Danny, FamilyMed(EM)
Habib, Adnan
Hache, Rachelle, FamilyMed
Hall-Losier, Suzanne M., FamilyMed
Harb, Mohammed
Harper, William B., FamilyMed
Huntsman, Jennifer C., FamilyMed(EM)
Jamal, Wael E.
Jean, Isabelle
Jean, Renee
Joshi, Ashwini K.
Kelly, Heather L., FamilyMed
Kenney, Stephen W., FamilyMed
Khaleduzzaman, Mohammad
Kwan, Tammi Y., FamilyMed
Lacasse, Lise
Landry, Daniel A., FamilyMed
Landry, Patrice, FamilyMed
Landry, Rachelle, FamilyMed
Landry, Serge M., FamilyMed
Larouche, Isabelle, FamilyMed
Laughlin, Thomas A., FamilyMed
LeBlanc, Karine, FamilyMed
Leblanc, Karine, FamilyMed
Leblanc, Paulette M.
Leblanc, Sylvie J., FamilyMed
Legault, Veronique, FamilyMed
Leger, Roger J.
Levesque, Christopher B.
Li, John H S.
Lord, Frank R.
Losier, Christopher L., FamilyMed(EM)
MacDonald, Angus, FamilyMed
MacDonald, Gerald R C., FamilyMed
Maher-Laporte, Valerie, FamilyMed
Mahmud-Sultan, Farhat
Mansfield, Pamela, FamilyMed
Marrero, Alier
Martin, Yolande, FamilyMed
Matchett, Michael, FamilyMed
McCaw, Elizabeth, FamilyMed
McCrea, John C.
McGraw, Marie-Josee, FamilyMed(EM)
McKenna, Paul G.
McNeill, Jeanne M.
Meagher, John M A.
Melanson, Stephanie, FamilyMed
Melanson-Candela, Denise
Menasria, Ali
Mitton, Kenneth A., FamilyMed
Moghrabi, Bashar S.
Morrison, Elivia
Mukherjee, Diana
Munroe, Alan R., FamilyMed
Nembo Nouangue, Joseph
Northorp, Sharon M E., FamilyMed
O'Hanley, Peter H.
Olatunde, Oluwasayo, FamilyMed
Ouellette, Rodney J.
Oussedik, Youcef
Paradiso, Guillermo
Pare, Jean-Louis
Park, John C S.
Peters, Michael S.
Phelan, Patrick J., FamilyMed
Power, Alison, FamilyMed
Power, Guy, FamilyMed(EM)
Reddin, Katharine P., FamilyMed
Richard, Lise, FamilyMed
Richard, Megan J., FamilyMed
Richard, Norbert S.
Robertson, Jennifer L., FamilyMed
Robichaud, Eric, FamilyMed
Robichaud, Martin, FamilyMed
Robichaud, Martine, FamilyMed
Ross, David, FamilyMed
Sadiq, Syed Z.
Salloum, Sadek R.
Savoie, Antonin, FamilyMed
Schofield, Aurel J., FamilyMed
Searle, Lisa C., FamilyMed
Sheehan, Natalie A., FamilyMed
Silver, Karen L., FamilyMed
Sinclair, Jennifer, FamilyMed
Skanes, Susan M., FamilyMed
Smith, Luella M P., FamilyMed(EM)
St-Coeur, Rachelle, FamilyMed(EM)
Stewart, James G.
Stoddard, Peter C., FamilyMed
Taylor, Ross, FamilyMed
Taylor, William J., FamilyMed
Teakles, Joseph, FamilyMed
Telfer, Christine J., FamilyMed
Touchburn, Andre P., FamilyMed(EM)
Tremblay, Pierre-Michel
Urbain, Melanie, FamilyMed
Vantelon, Jean-Marie
Vardy, Pamela Y., FamilyMed
Verger, Pierre
Walsh, Pamela J.
Ward, Randy R., FamilyMed
Wickrama, Thamara
Winkler, Christoph
Ying, Wai-Leung
Zavieh, Kevin
Zeidan Shwiri, Tawfiq

NACKAWIC

Bramstrup, Mary Ann
McKay, Laura-Lea M., FamilyMed

NEGUAC

Duguay-Picard, Lauza, FamilyMed
Melanson, Adrien L.

NEW MARYLAND

Ginson, Deborah

OROMOCTO

Brown, Kristen, FamilyMed
Charlebois, Sarah, FamilyMed
Escanlar, Vincent
Fraser, Peter K.
Gilbride, Patrick, FamilyMed
Hanson, Everette M.
Higgs, Jillian, FamilyMed
Landry, Daniel, FamilyMed
MacDonald, Michael, FamilyMed
Nason, Gregory M., FamilyMed
Neily, Lori L.
O'Blenis Caines, Shelley, FamilyMed(EM)
O'Halloran, James A., FamilyMed
Paulin, Stephane, FamilyMed
Prosser, Robert G.
Roxborough, Vaughan S.
Sainz, Beatriz M., FamilyMed
Snell, Timothy G., FamilyMed
Stairs, Heather J.
Weber, Keith, FamilyMed
White, Jeffrey A.
Woods, Kathleen, FamilyMed

PARLEEVILLE

Braun, Raymond I., FamilyMed

PERTH-ANDOVER

Bell, David W., FamilyMed
Houshmand, Henry
Jacob, Phillip
Kennedy, Allison T., FamilyMed
Kennedy, Andrew, FamilyMed
Moore, Peter G B., FamilyMed
Morales, Dora, FamilyMed
Muthiah, Karuppan C.
Newton-Moore, Allison M., FamilyMed
Zaki, Moheb E., FamilyMed

PETITCODIAC

Carlos, Mary Anne
Morton, Richard I.
Nayak, Lakhbir R.

PLASTER ROCK

Davilmar, Paule
Litz, Henry A R.

POINT LA NIM

Quintal, Bernard, FamilyMed
Quintal, Jean-Claude, FamilyMed

POINTE ROBICHAUD

Basque, Eric J Y., FamilyMed
Desrosiers, France, FamilyMed

QUISPAMSIS

Ledezma, Jose

REXTON

Allain, Melanie, FamilyMed
Arsenault, Melanie, FamilyMed
Boucher, Andre J.
Leblanc, Michelle M., FamilyMed
Martin, Eric, FamilyMed
McCleave, John J.

RICHIBUCTO

Robichaud, Rene, FamilyMed
Sirois, Josee, FamilyMed

RIVERSIDE-ALBERT

Morcom, Richard

RIVERVIEW

Fitch, William M., FamilyMed
Forbes, Robert A., FamilyMed
Hiltz, David W., FamilyMed
James, Heidi K., FamilyMed

ROGERSVILLE

Blanchard, Basil A.

ROTHESAY

Andrew, Donald M., FamilyMed
Caines, Sarah R., FamilyMed
Dykeman, F. Bruce, FamilyMed
Fellows, Joanne, FamilyMed
Hollway, Gordon, FamilyMed
MacNeil, M. Graham, FamilyMed
Maloney, Patrick, FamilyMed
McLaughlin, Joseph H.
Poirier, Robert F., FamilyMed
Rombaut, Allan J., FamilyMed
Rombaut, Karen R., FamilyMed
Ross, Alexandra, FamilyMed
Sutherland, Lisa J C., FamilyMed

SACKVILLE

Dysart, Andrew A.
Johnston, A. Catherine
Kelly, Adrian P., FamilyMed
Long, Cory S., FamilyMed
Massarelli, Elizabeth A., FamilyMed
Milne, Beatrice D., FamilyMed
Murray, John M.
Popma, Harold T., FamilyMed
Robichaud, Veronique, FamilyMed
Stewart, Graeme G R.
Thomas, G. Ross, FamilyMed
Wall, Andrea E., FamilyMed

SAINT-ANTOINE

Bourdages, Marie-Claude, FamilyMed
Frenette, Stephanie, FamilyMed
Guignard, Jimmy, FamilyMed
Saint-Amant, Serge, FamilyMed

SAINT-JACQUES

Albert-Daigle, Luce, FamilyMed
Brulotte, Michel
Clavette, Carole
Cormier, Renaud
Frenette, Luc, FamilyMed
Gagnon, Francois
Martin, Josee, FamilyMed
Roy, Jean-Philippe, FamilyMed
Thibodeau, Jean-Louis
Tran Huu, Yen

SAINT JOHN

Acar, Behram
Adisesh, Linganatha A.
Akinloye, Olusegun
Aladetoyinbo, Adenike
Aladetoyinbo, Kehinde
Allaby, Leslie
Aly, Hazem M.
Anyaegbuna, Okechukwu
Apantaku-Olajide, Babatunde
Ashfield, Jane G., FamilyMed
Atkinson, Paul R.
Bakezadeh, Farhad
Bakota, Martin, FamilyMed
Behram, Acar
Brien, Erin, FamilyMed
Brunsdon, Peta L.
Bungash, Arif
Canty, Andrea A., FamilyMed
Comeau, Laurel A., FamilyMed
Cook, Alana, FamilyMed
Corless, William J A.
Craig, Brian
Craig, Donald E.
Davies, Christine E., FamilyMed
De Sousa, Natasha, FamilyMed(EM)
Delavarkhan, Morteza
Doherty, Edward J.
Dorey, Sania
El-Bailey, Mohamed
Faridi, Anjum
Flick, James T.
Foster, Mark B.
Fostey, Alan
French, James
Garland, Brian E.
Gedmintas, Audra
Giffin, Scott C.
Godsoe, Deborah E.
Goodfellow, Mary E., FamilyMed

Grabove, Matthew A., FamilyMed(EM)
Grant, Ian M.
Gray, Susan J.
Greer, Matthew, FamilyMed(EM)
Guimond Hemmings, Jessica, FamilyMed
Hall, Jennifer L., FamilyMed
Hannigan, Jay, FamilyMed(EM)
Hannigan, Jennifer, FamilyMed
Hanson, Sonya, FamilyMed(EM)
Hill-Elias, Rachel
Howlett, Michael K., FamilyMed(EM)
Hull, Stephen
Ingersoll, Ruth E.
Irving, William E.
Jarratt, Mary E.
Jurgens, Sabine C., FamilyMed
Kanji, Rajandra
Keating, Michael P., FamilyMed
Keith, Ian C.
Keyes, G. Elizabeth
Keyes, Paul D., FamilyMed(EM)
Keyes, Sean A.
Keyes, Sean J.
Koppert, Theresa M., FamilyMed
Kothapalli, Anil
Kristoffersen, Arthur N.
Kumar, S. Eshwar
Kuriakose, Renju
Lamschtein, Claudia
Le Roux, Andries
Leblanc-Hidebrand, Julie
Lee, Winston
Lewis, David
Lowney, Mark J.
MacCallum, Margaret T., FamilyMed
Mekwan, Jayanand
Middleton, Joanna R., FamilyMed(EM)
Milner Gero, Heidi O., FamilyMed
Misik, Karl K A.
Mohiuddin, M D
Monterrosa, Luis
Muambi-Kabongo, Jean-Thadee
Naseemuddin, Ather
Naz, Farah
O'Brien, Christopher P., FamilyMed
Omotoso, Patrick
Page, Paul D., FamilyMed(EM)
Palmer, Erin, FamilyMed
Parascan, Oana S., FamilyMed
Patterson, William H.
Pishe, Tushar, FamilyMed(EM)
Postuma, Paul, FamilyMed(EM)
Rahmeh, Tarek
Rajappannair, Lakshmi
Raju, Shoba
Ramrattan, Brian
Sallam, Sallam A.
Sarkisian, Anthony
Sealy, Sasha L., FamilyMed
Serb, Abdusalam M.
Shamsuddin, Syed
Sheehan, Wayne F., FamilyMed
Simon, L. Michael, FamilyMed
Smith, R. Vaughn, FamilyMed
Smitheram, Amanda
Smolinski, Walter J.
Stephenson, Linda A.
Sukosd, Eva
Sutherland, Donald F., FamilyMed
Szymanski, Jan F.
Thomas, Sajni S.
Thornhill, George M.
Toal, Satish C.
Tracey, Joshua, FamilyMed
Turner, Lisa A., FamilyMed
Ugabi, Solomon
Umar, Imran
Vaillancourt, Christopher A., FamilyMed(EM)
Vanhoutte, Paul-Robert V., FamilyMed
Verheul, Glenn R., FamilyMed(EM)
Wildish, Julia A., FamilyMed
Williamson, Jeffrey, FamilyMed
Willis, Stephen A., FamilyMed
Wilson, Keith W., FamilyMed
Wiseman, Eve
Wood, Ashley, FamilyMed
Xidos, George
Yang, Lisa D S., FamilyMed
Young, Neil G., FamilyMed(EM)

SAINT-LEONARD

Roy, Daniel J.

SAINT LOUIS DE KENT

Collette, Stephane, FamilyMed

SAINT-QUENTIN

Aubut, Stephanie, FamilyMed
Dupere, Melissa, FamilyMed
Faucher, Helene, FamilyMed
Terras, Jean-Claude
Turcotte, Jessie, FamilyMed

SHEDIAC

Auffrey, Jean-Marie, FamilyMed
Bazinet, Sara, FamilyMed
Boudreau, Rheal, FamilyMed
Charest-Leblanc, Mireille, FamilyMed
Grant, Nathalie, FamilyMed
Landry, Elaine
Legresley, Conrad

SHIPPAGAN

Gauthier, Louis-Marie
Michel, Jean-Marie C.

ST ANDREWS

Desmond, John V., FamilyMed
Peer, Brian R., FamilyMed

ST GEORGE

Anderson, Vance E., FamilyMed
Kaminska, Irena
Natarajan, Meenakshi, FamilyMed

ST MARTINS

Le, Luan B., FamilyMed
Maloney, Gerald P.

ST STEPHEN

Acheson, Donald K.
Ataellahi, Mobin
Debertin, Manfred W.
Green, David J M.
Hamid, Zinia
Konforte-Vasiljevic, Tilda
Lalik, Jolanta M.
Lister, Norman A., FamilyMed
Pinder, Lesley J.
Spencer, Perry W., FamilyMed
Stewart, John S.

STANLEY

Lacey, Kendrick R., FamilyMed

STE ANNE MADAWASKA

Dupuis, Isabelle, FamilyMed

SUSSEX

Gilmore, Kendra, FamilyMed
Green, W. Scott
Haslett, Michael
Kokje, Aron Eduard
MacMillan, David J., FamilyMed
MacMullin, Sunita
McCutcheon, Sharon E., FamilyMed
O'Neill, Brian, FamilyMed
Phillips, M. Elizabeth
Sullivan, Patrick D.
Symington, David J.

TRACADIE-SHEILA

Aucoin, Marc, FamilyMed
Benga-Malulu, Francine
Caron, Sandrine, FamilyMed
Chiasson, Renelle, FamilyMed
Darveau, Stephane, FamilyMed
Dion, Marie-Claude, FamilyMed
Fernandez-Cattelat, Patrice, FamilyMed
Hache, Louise, FamilyMed
Losier, Lise, FamilyMed
Mbangi-Bontolo, Faustin
McGraw, Serge, FamilyMed
Musemba, Justine
Rousselle, Rejeanne, FamilyMed
Saade, Antoine
Smith, Malcolm W.

WATERVILLE CARLETON

Al-Sharief, Alaa, FamilyMed
Anderson, Annette
Bathina, Sudheer
Fisk, Henry J.
Gangodawila, Shantha, FamilyMed
Ivantchev, Sergei, FamilyMed
Jurgeleit, Herbert
MacElwain, Dale A., FamilyMed
Musa, Ihsan M., FamilyMed(EM)
Tadross, Alphonse
Warsi, Mohammed M.

WELSHPOOL

Kay, Philip W., FamilyMed

WOODSTOCK

Alborg, Frances J., FamilyMed
Atmuri, Nagasree, FamilyMed
Beatty, Gary L., FamilyMed
Boyle, Allison M.
Chandra, Michael M., FamilyMed
Dow, Heather, FamilyMed
Goodine, Frederick S., FamilyMed
Gunatilake, K. Deepthi
McGrath, Colm R., FamilyMed
Mutrie, William M.
O'Leary, Deborah G., FamilyMed
Perley, Michael P., FamilyMed
Sinha, Nachiketa
Tubetti-Goodine, Roseanne, FamilyMed

NEWFOUNDLAND AND LABRADOR

ARNOLDS COVE

Fowlow, Geoffrey N., FamilyMed

AVONDALE

Lake, H. Russell

BAIE VERTE

de Wet, Francois B., FamilyMed
Osborne, Perry

BAY BULLS

McCarthy, Annette M., FamilyMed
McCarthy, Rodney P., FamilyMed
Mercer, C. Wade, FamilyMed

BAY L'ARGENT

Acharya, Surendra D P.

BAY ROBERTS

Acevedo Mendez, Luis A.
Dawson, P. Colette, FamilyMed
Humber, Robert E.
Powell, Calvin N., FamilyMed
Shandera, Raymond H.

BELL ISLAND

Al-Mulla Hummadi, Yasmin K A.
Laurie, Alexa M M., FamilyMed
Tucker, S. Walter

BISHOPS FALLS

Bruce, Helen E.
Ismeal, Ali K., FamilyMed

BONAVISTA

Abdulkareem, Ali Ihsan
Al-Khazraji, Wassan S K.
Beithoon, Ziad, FamilyMed
Ibrahim, Mahdi K.
Larsen, David P F.
Paul, Allister R.
Singh, Ichpal
Worrall, Graham J., FamilyMed

BOTWOOD

Aderinto, Rasheedah A., FamilyMed
Barnes, Peter B J., FamilyMed
Goodfellow, Alfred, FamilyMed
McKay, Timothy D., FamilyMed
Woolfrey, Jody A M., FamilyMed

BROOKFIELD

Ghazi-Mirsaeed, Sayedeh-Bahareh
Imana, Mohammed M.
Khorshidi, Amirmohsen
Liaghati-Nasseri, Omid
Mahdy, Ibtihaj
Rofeal, Michael N H.

BUCHANS

Erfan Ezzat, Omar

BURGEO

Roxin, Gheorghe S.
Roxin, Sara

BURIN

Abdulhussein, Salam N.
Alchalabi, Karam R A.
Ali, Taghreed H., FamilyMed
Amissah-Arthur, Justice B.
Aras, Ziya
Cremin, Denis
De Andres Oterino, Jose A.
Kean, H R. Wade
Khalif, Marwan, FamilyMed
Khan, Razaullah
McCarthy, Jeremiah
Newman, David E.
Ogunsina, Ayodeji O.
Saunders, Stacey C., FamilyMed

BURIN BAY ARM

Mayo, Edgar P., FamilyMed
Power, Lynette M., FamilyMed

CARBONEAR

Alewan, Salem, FamilyMed
Aravindakshan, Kenatingal S.
Augla, Salman H.
Azaghdani, Abdulhamid M.
Baker, Gary T.
Becker, Regina, FamilyMed
Belgasem, Nizar
Chilopora, Garvey C.
Coetzee, Barend
Drover, Aidan
Fifield, Frank
Gayapershad, Thasvir K., FamilyMed
Howse, G. Dawn
Ignaszewski, Wojciech M.
Ismat-Raheem, Alia
Jabor, Ammar K A.
Jamil, Fawaz H., FamilyMed
Jerudi, Maher
Karunanithy, Anusha
Khan, Kamran Z.
Khural, Ajay P S.
Lefeuvre, Philip A.
Patey, Christopher P., FamilyMed
Peacock, Ingrid V.
Peddle, Christopher J.
Ramjohn, Zaid O A.

Ringer, Kenneth
Sullivan, Thomas J.
Valkova, Vanelia V.
Xu, Dejun

CATALINA

Dumka, Evelyn

CHANNEL-PAB

Mosawe, Mothafar A.

CHURCHILL FALLS

Kiahosseini, Shirin

CLARENVILLE

Akinsola, Sunday A.
Altaweel, Ziyad E K.
Altitanchy, Hadeel
Austin, Stephen J.
Barakji, Nazir
Barnhill, John A., FamilyMed
Borja, Enrique
Brannan, Mark A.
Brentnall, David M., FamilyMed
Chaytor, Janet B., FamilyMed
Crewe, Harold J.
Hanna, Samim Y., FamilyMed
Khan, Saad M.
Klipin, Louise P.
Mahdi, Rafid, FamilyMed
Meneses, Gayzelle A.
Mohamad, May J., FamilyMed
Nel, Jacobus W A.
O'Reilly, Alan G.
Okafor, Rosemary E I., FamilyMed
Pearce, Blaine F.
Pye, Paula M.
Rayel, Michael G.
Salomon, Paul S., FamilyMed
Saluja, Jasjeet
Samson, Nancy L., FamilyMed
Sharaf El-Dean, Mouhammad Z.
Sheikh, Shoaib I.
Smith, Kelley R., FamilyMed
Van Der Linde, Etienne
Van West, Cornel P.
Vasanthan, Veeragathy
Verster, Ryno J.

CLARKES BEACH

Jones, Emmanuel E.

CONCEPTION BAY SOUTH

Acevedo Mendez, Francisco E.
Aguilar, Eslier G., FamilyMed
Bannister, Elizabeth A G.
Brien, Thomas A.
Cooper, R. Roxanne, FamilyMed
Fraser, James B G.
Garber, Gayle D.
Hardy, John J.
Jardine, Frederick F., FamilyMed
Krisdaphongs, Michoke
Loveys, Annabeth J., FamilyMed
Mpiana, Pinos M.
O'Brien, Wayne J.
Phillips, Danielle M., FamilyMed
Pittman, Jennifer M., FamilyMed
Sheppard, James A G., FamilyMed
Sutton, Gregory, FamilyMed
Verge, Jacqueline L.

CORNER BROOK

Abbasi, Qamar A.
Ahmad, Khalil
Al-Shamam, Ali O.
Aleykina, Natalya O., FamilyMed
Angel, Melissa S., FamilyMed(EM)
Awad, Rita T S.
Ballouk, Fayez
Barker, Nancy, FamilyMed
Battcock, Natalie R., FamilyMed
Bazeley, Peter A., FamilyMed
Bolous, Nagy
Boushra, Rasha G I.
Callahan, Peter J., FamilyMed
Chaulk, Donald A.
Coleman, David A., FamilyMed
Cousens, Christopher W W.
Culliton, Margaret L., FamilyMed
Dunn, Desiree, FamilyMed
Ennis, Robert
Fidel, Jeffrey
Gingrich, Ruth A., FamilyMed
Griffin, Timohty, FamilyMed
Gunson, Kimberly A., FamilyMed
Hamann, Adolf
Ismail, Yahya A.
Jenkins, Kenneth
John, Cyriac
Kathirgamanathan, Mylvaganam
Kazerouni, Abdul H.
Kennedy, Christine A S., FamilyMed
Kevu, Joseph E.
King, Roger B., FamilyMed
Krizan, Igor
Lafferty, Kathleen B., FamilyMed
Luer, Andrew Z.
Mahmood, Nasir
Mahrugh, Abdouraman A M.
Morris, Philip J.
Neil, Paul R.
O'Brien, Melissa A., FamilyMed
O'Connor, Julia E.
O'Driscoll, Robert P., FamilyMed
Obeid, Issam S., FamilyMed
Pasha, Tahir
Penney, Nicola J., FamilyMed
Phillips, Karen A.
Power, Lorena M., FamilyMed
Rashleigh, Dennis, FamilyMed
Reid, Andrea S.
Ryan, Michael E., FamilyMed
Safi, Sohail, FamilyMed
Shaikh, Abdul R.
Simpson, Ian M., FamilyMed
Smallwood, Erin J C., FamilyMed
Smallwood, Mark D., FamilyMed
Sparrow, Carl D., FamilyMed
Szarvas, Szilvia
Talpur, Jehanara
Thistle, Brent E., FamilyMed
Tierney, James J.
Ullyatt, Kim J.
Van Gelder, Jacob R.
Van Niekerk, Christopher
Van Wijk, Jan E.
Vermooten, Carel A.
Wadhwa, Birender P S., FamilyMed
Wasmeier, Torsten E.
Westby, John C.
White, Gavin J.
Wignall, John B W.
Wilters, Petrus
Young, Melanie, FamilyMed
Young, Robert J.

COW HEAD

Watts, Harold R.

COXS COVE

Brake, Robert J.

DEER LAKE

Campbell, Louise
Fay, Nicholas
Kielty, John P., FamilyMed
Maher, Terrence M.

EASTPORT

Patil, Dattu G.

FERRYLAND

Kassem, Manal H M., FamilyMed

FLOWERS COVE

Abulomrain, Ghalib A I.
Al-Baaj, Tholfkar M H.
Mahmood, Bann N.

FOGO

Abulbida, Tarik A.
Agireb, Ahmed E A.
Benissa, Issa A.

FORTEAU

Bulambo Yogolelo, Willy
Ghazal, Zaid

GAMBO

Kamel, Emad H., FamilyMed

GANDER

Abdulla, Safwat S A.
Abulaeha, Rida M A.
Ahmad, Ishtiaq
Al-Shammaa, Ameer K A.
Askar, Wanda M K.
Awad, Nagy S H.
Blackie, Peter B., FamilyMed
Blundell, Krista J M., FamilyMed
Boctor, Atef H K., FamilyMed
Boktor, Basem W H., FamilyMed
Booysen, Johan T.
Brahmbhatt, Rajmayur
Button, Eric G., FamilyMed
Casey, Carmel, FamilyMed
Culleton, Nancy, FamilyMed
Djuric, Miroslav
Dutta, Prasannajit
Farag, Mariam
Forward, Roland
Gabriel, Anthony M., FamilyMed
Hanna, Enas
Johnson, Phyllis J.
Madu, Ikechukwu S.
Magrabi, Hamdi H.
Malak Doss, Sherlene S., FamilyMed
Maritz, Jaco J.
Maritz, Jacobus C.
Matthews, Peter J.
Saad, Ehab, FamilyMed
Sebbi, Esmael M H.
St Croix, Eileen M.
Taj, Amer J.
Tiller, Shawn R., FamilyMed
Ugwoke, Ethelbert T C.
Van Wyk, Stephanie
Van Zyl, Andre T.

GLOVERTOWN

Simpson, Nancy C., FamilyMed

GOOSE BAY

Horwood, Karen L., FamilyMed

GOULDS

Hillman, Alison J.
Natsheh, Ishaq M.

GRAND BANK

Ali, Ghassan H.
Beckley, Sunmolu A.
Chhatwal, Gurpreet S.
Chhatwal, Jasjeet K.
Kobah, Saif D.

GRAND FALLS WINDSOR

Ajiboye, P. Ayodele
Al Anee, Bassam I M.
Alawsi, Sarwah A A A.
Anis, Hanaa N.
Bautista, Elizabeth M., FamilyMed
Beshara, Rafik A S.
Boodhun, Mohamed S.
Butler, Jared J., FamilyMed
Butler, Robert F.
Campbell, John A., FamilyMed(EM)
Campbell, Susan M., FamilyMed
Cohen, Michael T.
Combden, Steven, FamilyMed(EM)
Dalwadi, Bela
Dogar, Ghulam
Higgins, Gina, FamilyMed
Hodder, Donald G.
Jim, King T.
Kabisios, Theodoros
Kalombo, Augustin N.
Khan, Haroon
King, James F., FamilyMed
Kolawole, Rebecca O.
Leon Rey-Sanchez, Raul A.
Minhas, Gurmit S.
Moretti, Justin S.
Poole, Thomas E.
Powell, T. Lynette, FamilyMed
Ralph, Samuel J., FamilyMed
Ravinuthala, Saradadevi
Roberts, Elizabeth A.
Selemani, Salumu
Sheahan, Deirdre C.
Shenouda, Nashwa T M., FamilyMed
Short, R. Keith, FamilyMed
Sullivan, Shelley E., FamilyMed
Walker, Margaret A., FamilyMed

HAMPDEN

Wasef, Mourkus, FamilyMed

HAPPY VALLEY GOOSE BAY

Adeagbo, Francis
Datar, Suhasini
Fitzgerald, Charlene D., FamilyMed
Forsey, Robert G P., FamilyMed
Hosseininejad, Mir M.
Jong, Michael K K., FamilyMed
Karaivanov, Yordan S., FamilyMed
Law, Joyce S., FamilyMed
Morris, Alison J., FamilyMed
Ophel, Judith M., FamilyMed
Patterson, Jeffrey D., FamilyMed
Rawluk, Wieslaw M., FamilyMed
Wilson, Margo M., FamilyMed(EM)
Woollam, Gabriel B., FamilyMed

HARBOUR BRETON

Ben Hamed, Salah R S.
Beshir, Marian
Thind, Charanjit K.

HARBOUR GRACE

Button, Lonzel, FamilyMed
Power, Gerald A.

HERMITAGE

Hoca, Asim
Sohi, Kultar S.

HOLYROOD

Mercer, I. David
Walsh, Paul E.
Whitty, Wanda S., FamilyMed

JACKSON'S ARM

Moawad, Medhat M M G.

JEFFREY'S

Taha, Hussam A A., FamilyMed

LA SCIE

Lotter, Wian H.

LABRADOR CITY

Akinbiyi, Tolulola T A A.
Amoo, Kazeem O.
Arsenault, William E., FamilyMed
Dirkschen Van Schalkwyk, Johannes
Gonzalez Hernandez, Roberto L.
Hans, Harninder P.
Pullela, Visweswara
Sawh, Veejai D.
Sawwan, Ahmad K H.
Thomas, Gene F.
Wilson, Ian F.

LEWISPORTE

Al-Tikriti, Bakir Y D.
Amin, Hussein M N., FamilyMed
Collins, Wayne B.
Kadhem, Rasheed H.
Penney, Brenda A.
Taher, Ismail T A.
Tahir, Ismail T A., FamilyMed

LOURDES

Mercer, Gregory P., FamilyMed

MARYSTOWN

Moulton, William B.
Roberts, Bernard C.

MOUNT PEARL

Desai, Ghanshyam R.
Essaji, Fakhruddin K.
Fitzgerald, Janice, FamilyMed
Halley, Kathleen M.
Hamlyn, Margaret O., FamilyMed
Hatcher, Lydia B., FamilyMed
Hogan, Darryl R., FamilyMed
Horwood, Paula L.
Ivany, Linda E.
Janes, John C.
Keeping, Virginia A.
McGrath, Sheilagh M.
O'Keefe, Dennis
Riche, Cyril R.
Rideout, Gary M., FamilyMed
Rossiter, Andrew M., FamilyMed
Smith, Randell J.
Young, Michelle F., FamilyMed

NEW HARBOUR TB

Bonisteel, Stephen P., FamilyMed

NORRIS POINT

Bowen, James D.
Gwyn, Alice, FamilyMed
Walton, Mark, FamilyMed

OLD PERLICAN

Abu-Almaali, Abeer, FamilyMed
Al-Safar, Anmar S.
Nel, Gert
Rassam, Ammar F.

PARADISE

Chaulk, Domino R.
Furlong, Stephen B., FamilyMed
Furlong, Susan M.
Ledrew, Ruth L J.
Ng, Sheau C., FamilyMed
Parsons, Trent E., FamilyMed
Sheppard, Gillian A., FamilyMed(EM)
White, Jeffrey V., FamilyMed

PLACENTIA

Albir, Yousra Y.
Bulk, Mahamed A., FamilyMed
Mangat, Birender S., FamilyMed
Mangat, Sandeep, FamilyMed
Penney, H. Ross
Rockel, Anthony J.

POLLARDS POINT

Abdel Shahid, Raafat A A.

PORT AU CHOIX

Irfan, Jeewani
Irfan, Mohamed H., FamilyMed

PORT-AUX-BASQUES

Al Nabbot, Salah E E.
Bhalla, Jaideep
Bhalla, Kiran
Blecher, David M., FamilyMed
Brake, Heidi D., FamilyMed
Butler, Matthew R., FamilyMed
Graham, Wendy R., FamilyMed
Husni, Tawfik, FamilyMed
Thomas, David M., FamilyMed

PORT CV-ST PHIL

McDonald, Bethany D., FamilyMed
McKim, Aaron L.
Murthy, Santhi K., FamilyMed

PORT SAUNDERS

Carroll, John R.
Sarfraz, Jawaria

RODDICKTON

Al Suwaih, Addnan R.
Salman, Bashar M.

SOUTH RIVER

Crosbie, Douglas R.

SPANIARDS BAY

Efford, Jason R., FamilyMed

SPRINGDALE

Clancy, Sarah D., FamilyMed
Farhat, Fawzi E S.
Hicks, Frank S., FamilyMed
Young, Todd K., FamilyMed

ST ALBANS

Diebes, Ragaie E.
Shasha, Faris F., FamilyMed

ST ANTHONY

Agbi, Adejumoke A.
Alrezaq, Abdalla, FamilyMed
Alshahabi, Qussay J L., FamilyMed
Buitendag, Ernest
Caro Guzman, Alexis H., FamilyMed
Chipeta, Daniel C.
Fahmy, Hany, FamilyMed
Ibude, Bose E.
Krupski, Malgorzata H.
Kulandaivelu, Murugesan
O'Keefe, Mary G., FamilyMed
Pealing, Vivien
Penney, Catherine J., FamilyMed
Roopram, Devicka J.
Vatturi, Ravi S.

ST GEORGES

Porter, Barry J.

ST JOHN'S

Abbott, Beverly J., FamilyMed
Abd Halim, Siti R.
Abdulkhaliq, Anas, FamilyMed
Adams, Lorne W.
Alteen, Caroline A S H.
Alteen, Lawrence W.
Angus, Karen E., FamilyMed(EM)
Anwar, Shahgul
Au, Jana B., FamilyMed
Aubrey-Bassler, Christine M., FamilyMed
Aubrey-Bassler, F. Kris, FamilyMed(EM)
Avery, Susan M., FamilyMed
Azher, Tanweer
Azher, Zaira, FamilyMed
Aziz, Mohammed A G A., FamilyMed
Bains, Paramjot
Barter, Richard B.
Bennett, Erin A., FamilyMed
Bethune, Cheri E H., FamilyMed
Bishop, Joanne E., FamilyMed
Bobby, Rebecca J., FamilyMed(EM)
Bradbury, Catherine M.
Broderick, Vina L., FamilyMed
Brown, Christina A.
Brown, Gregory S., FamilyMed(EM)
Brown-Brake, Sonya L., FamilyMed
Browne, Noel J., FamilyMed
Brushett, Frederick J., FamilyMed
Bugden, Gena N., FamilyMed(EM)
Butler, Roger G., FamilyMed
Button, Walter W.
Callahan, Elizabeth A., FamilyMed
Callahan-Dyer, Deborah M., FamilyMed
Cantwell, Lorraine M.
Carew, Heidi E., FamilyMed
Carlson, Barbara A.
Carrim, Ebrahim
Chaytor, Kathy L., FamilyMed
Cheeseman, Neil R., FamilyMed(EM)
Chehadi, Abdel-Kareem
Chitsike, Rufaro S.
Colbourne, Danielle N., FamilyMed
Coleman, Amanda C., FamilyMed
Collingwood, John M., FamilyMed
Comerford, Carrie A.
Compton, Amanda Y D., FamilyMed
Crocker, Percy R., FamilyMed
Darcy, Stephen, FamilyMed
Dawe, Christiane M.
Dawson, Celine M., FamilyMed
Delaney, Ronald K.
Deshpandey, Akhil
Donovan, Catherine A.
Doulton, Bruce C., FamilyMed
Drover, H. Blair
Duggan, Norah A T., FamilyMed
Duke, Pauline S., FamilyMed
Dunne, M. Maureen
Dwyer, Lynn E.
Eaton, William H., FamilyMed
Echendu, Wegbo
Elli, Eric R.
Elliott, Jacqueline M., FamilyMed
Ennis, Sandra E., FamilyMed
Enriquez, Carlos E.
Fardy, Noreen, FamilyMed
Farrell, Gerard
Fitzgerald, Laura C., FamilyMed
Fleming, Blair
Fogwill, Terence R., FamilyMed
Gibbons, Maria T.
Godwin, N. Marshall S., FamilyMed
Gough, David W.
Grandy, Barbara, FamilyMed
Grant, William F.
Greene, Mabel T.
Greene, Marian E.
Gullipalli, Ravindra
Hart, David G.
Hart, Randy
Hasnain, Mehrul
Hayes, Megan, FamilyMed
Hayward, Lori, FamilyMed
Heyn, Sujiva, FamilyMed(EM)
Hickey, James P., FamilyMed
Higgins, Gordon A., FamilyMed
Ho, Cosmas V J.
Hollett, Bruce, FamilyMed
Hollohan, Brendan T.
Hoppe, Barbara J.
Howell, Oscar J.
Humes, R. Trevor, FamilyMed(EM)
Hutton, Andrew S., FamilyMed
Hyland, G M. Denise
Ilango, Sumathy
Inkpen, Linda L.
Jackman, Paul D.
Javed, Farrukh
Jewer, Carolyn M., FamilyMed
Joller, Petra, FamilyMed
Jones, Megan G C.
Joseph, Christy S.
Kassim, Ali A K.
Keating-Power, Dianne, FamilyMed
Kennedy, Michael J.
Khan, Yasir H., FamilyMed
Kieley, Lisa A., FamilyMed
King, Susan M.
Kirby, Colleen V., FamilyMed
Kogilwaimath, Siddhath
Lacelle, Johanne, FamilyMed
Lake, Karen F., FamilyMed
Lane, Joanne E L., FamilyMed
LeGrow, Jennifer L., FamilyMed
Lear, N. Adrian
Lee, Norman J., FamilyMed
Lee, Stephen G., FamilyMed
Leonard, Deanne M., FamilyMed
Lilly, Roy A., FamilyMed
Luscombe, Sandra J.
MacDonald, Susan M., FamilyMed
MacIntyre, D. Joanne
MacK, Martin D., FamilyMed(EM)
MacLean, Catherine A., FamilyMed
Major, Stephen R M., FamilyMed
Malone, Daniel J.
Mankaeva, Soussa, FamilyMed
Marshall, Ian M.
Mate, Elizabeth A., FamilyMed
Mathieson, Sarah, FamilyMed(EM)
Matthews, Angela C., FamilyMed
McCarthy, Jason J J., FamilyMed
McIsaac, J. Craig
McVicker, Charles R., FamilyMed(EM)
Mekawy, Mohamed
Metcalfe, Brian D., FamilyMed(EM)
Miller, Robert T., FamilyMed
Mirolo, Hugh
Moffatt, Scott M., FamilyMed
Morgan, David W., FamilyMed(EM)
Morley, John E., FamilyMed
Morry, Peter J.
Mouland, Sylvia P., FamilyMed
Mullins, Eugene
Mumtaz, Shariq
Nafisi, Sepideh, FamilyMed
Noble, E. Keith
Noel, Peter J., FamilyMed
Noseworthy, Melanie A., FamilyMed
O'Dea, Marie T F.
O'Keefe, Danielle, FamilyMed
O'Maonaigh, Conleth E., FamilyMed
O'Shea, Ciaran P.
O'Shea, Fiona
O'Shea, Patrick M., FamilyMed
Ohson, Kamal K S., FamilyMed
Oosthuizen, James H.
Ozerkan, Ebru
Parsons, Ean J., FamilyMed
Parsons, Jillian N., FamilyMed
Parsons, Michael H., FamilyMed(EM)
Parsons, Robert W J.
Parsons, Wanda L., FamilyMed
Patel, Kirit K.
Patel, Vinod K.
Peckham, Deborah C.
Pendergast, Amanda L., FamilyMed
Penton, Mercedes D., FamilyMed
Picco, Bridget M., FamilyMed
Pike Au, Krysta L., FamilyMed
Pirzada, Amrah
Pollock, Cheryl, FamilyMed(EM)
Porter, Mark C., FamilyMed
Porter, Robert N., FamilyMed(EM)
Price, Susanne F G., FamilyMed
Pushpanathan, Anita, FamilyMed
Ramjattan, Brian R.
Rector, Tara J., FamilyMed(EM)
Renouf, Tia, FamilyMed(EM)
Rideout, Debbie
Rideout, Gregory S., FamilyMed
Rideout-Vivian, Susan, FamilyMed
Ripley, Sharon A.
Rizvi, Syed A.
Robbins, Megan, FamilyMed
Robbins, Peter S., FamilyMed
Rogers, Lori A., FamilyMed(EM)
Rogers, Louise
Rogers, Peter J., FamilyMed(EM)
Rolfe, Anthony R.
Rourke, James T B., FamilyMed(EM)
Rourke, Leslie L., FamilyMed
Rudland, Rand B.
Saeed, Khawer
Saldanha, Carla N., FamilyMed
Samarasena, Mallika M.
Sampson, Monica, FamilyMed
Saunders, Kathleen B., FamilyMed
Schaefers, Hans-Joachim D., FamilyMed
Scott, Amanda S., FamilyMed
Seviour, E. Peter, FamilyMed
Shublaq, Wael
Singleton, Andrea M., FamilyMed
Skirving, Paul D.
Smith, Andrew J., FamilyMed(EM)
Smith, Anna J., FamilyMed
Smith, Dee Ann M., FamilyMed
Smith, Megan E., FamilyMed(EM)
Snow, Pamela A., FamilyMed
Somasundaram, Uthayakumaran, FamilyMed
Squires, Tina E., FamilyMed
Stender, Jennifer S.
Stratton, Faith
Stringer, Katherine C., FamilyMed
Tahaineh, Sakher M H.
Tan, Chin Chai
Tarhoni, Mohamed M.
Tarrant, Gary M., FamilyMed
Tau, Mahlodi E.
Taylor-Furey, Allison N., FamilyMed
Thomas, Charlene H., FamilyMed
Thorburn, James P., FamilyMed
Tilley, Joy, FamilyMed
Torres, Frank X.
Udechukwu, Maurice U.
Uthman, Elmonttasir M.
Vaughan-Jackson, Julian D.
Wadden, Robert A.
Wagoner, Michelle L.
Walker, Stephen A J.
Walsh, Paula M., FamilyMed
Watson, Mary E D., FamilyMed
Whelan, Wendy E.
Wilson, Scott E R., FamilyMed(EM)
Wong, Vincent W.
Woodland, K. Heather, FamilyMed
Woodland, Robert C., FamilyMed
Woodman, Grant M J.
Yazdani, Ramin
Young, J. Neil
Young, Wade M., FamilyMed(EM)
Zhang, Seamus Q.

ST LAWRENCE

Haddud, Ahmed
Raphael, Malik
Samour, Fathe M A.

ST MARYS

Suliman, Asem S M.

STEPHENVILLE

Attwood, Zachary P., FamilyMed
Beaumont, Charl G.
Bruff, Karl J., FamilyMed
Chyla, Andrew
Dennis, John T.
Diedericks, Adriaan G.
Hayat, Sikandar
Hough, Henry
Idzior, Janusz M.
Jaber, Wisam M A.
Khan, Fayyaz
Kranenka, Joan
Lamswood, F. Scott S.
Lewis, Sheila M., FamilyMed
McComiskey, Alan J.
Smolarkiewicz, Marek A.
Triki, Msod A M., FamilyMed

STEPHENVILLE CROSSING

Parsons, Edwin L.
Verma, Subhash C.

SUMMERFORD

Hewitt, Daniel C., FamilyMed

TERRENCEVILLE

Al-Badoosh, Auday M A.

TORBAY

Collis, Ernest L., FamilyMed
Drover, Alison C., FamilyMed
Hall, Thomas A., FamilyMed

TREPASSEY

McGarry, Thomas G.

TWILLINGATE

Hunt, Andrew J., FamilyMed
Keough, Michael, FamilyMed
Newman, Colin D., FamilyMed
Ravalia, Mohamed I., FamilyMed
White, Craig P., FamilyMed

WABUSH

Costello, Thomas G., FamilyMed

WAREHAM-CTVLE

Cutler, Michael G., FamilyMed

WESTERN BAY

Khural, Simrit K.
Sturge, Cecil C.

WHITBOURNE

Abdulkhaliq, Taha, FamilyMed
Abumeess, Ahmed A R., FamilyMed
Jelloo, Mazin K A., FamilyMed
Ragnauth, D. Reginald
Savaya, Savaya
Squibb, Stephanie A., FamilyMed

WINTERTON

Leung, Fung

NORTHWEST TERRITORIES

FORT SIMPSON

Pegg, Anne-Marie, FamilyMed

INUVIK

Boronowski, Peter W., FamilyMed
Falk, Ryan G., FamilyMed
Seaman, Leah V., FamilyMed
Virk, Roohina, FamilyMed

YELLOWKNIFE

Banner, Laara, FamilyMed
Coad, Dwayne E., FamilyMed(EM)
Farrell, Theresa, FamilyMed
Galler, Pamela H., FamilyMed
Kandola, Kami, FamilyMed
Lacombe, Christina, FamilyMed
Mansouri, Shireen M., FamilyMed(EM)
McLean, John J., FamilyMed
Reid, Anna C.
Terlingen, Melissa M., FamilyMed
Wilkinson, Tandi L., FamilyMed(EM)
Wong, David K W.

NOVA SCOTIA

AMHERST

Abdul Kadir, Najeeb A.
Abeysekera, Rathnayake M M S.
Arora, Gagan
Atia, John N A.
Bienkowski, Halina
Bienkowski, Krzysztof W.
Bobadilla-Martinez, Julio C., FamilyMed
Ferguson, G. Brian
Frizzle, Tena Ann, FamilyMed
Fynn, John K.
Gradstein, Janneke S., FamilyMed
Harrison, Dean R., FamilyMed
Hydorn, Thomas G.
Kirmani, Saleem
Krol-Lass, Justyna
McCrossin, J. Murray, FamilyMed
Morris, Kelly A., FamilyMed
Osinowo, Adegboyega O.
Ponton-Beltran, Carlos M., FamilyMed(EM)
Rubio-Reyes, Carlos A., FamilyMed
Semenov, Igor
Umar, Amir
White, Celina D.
Zaremba, Jozef, FamilyMed

ANNAPOLIS ROYAL

Barkwell, Robert G., FamilyMed
Bonnington, Simon P., FamilyMed
Buchholz, Kenneth P W., FamilyMed
Conyers, Roop, FamilyMed
Cram, Jennifer, FamilyMed
Gibson, Julia, FamilyMed
Hancock, Caroline A., FamilyMed

ANTIGONISH

Allan, Patricia L.
Allen, Maureen A., FamilyMed(EM)
Booth, A. William, FamilyMed
Brennan, Elizabeth B.
Cameron, Jean M.
Chiasson, John D.
Clifton, Neil A.
Cooper, Phillip W.
Cudmore, David, FamilyMed
El-Halees, Walid
Felderhof, Richard P.
Fuhrmann, Marlene B.
Gallant, Steven J., FamilyMed
Gallivan, Glenn G.
Gorman, Mary C., FamilyMed
Hickey, John S., FamilyMed
Hillyard, Jeremy W.
Howard, Jane A., FamilyMed(EM)
Jurga, Milan, FamilyMed(EM)
Krawczyk, John G.
MacDonald, Karen A., FamilyMed
MacInnis, Maude D., FamilyMed
MacKenzie, Michael A.
McKenna, Patricia J.
Menard, Patricia
Murphy, Michele P G.
Raafat, Sawsan
Rahman, Faisal
Ruggles, Lesley A.
Sadler, Margot C., FamilyMed
Salameh, Muwaffaq
Siddiqui, Mughina A.
Steeves, Brian R.
Sturmy, S. Paul, FamilyMed
Sutherland, George R.

ARICHAT

Babin, Martina, FamilyMed
Boudreau, Daniel, FamilyMed(EM)
Deroche, Steven, FamilyMed
MacNeil, M. Lawrence, FamilyMed

AYLESFORD

Goddard, Peter

BADDECK

Chow, Carlyle S H A.
Garcia Del Busto Cano, Elena, FamilyMed
Genge, Roland J.
Heughan, David, FamilyMed
Holmes, Andrew I., FamilyMed

BARRINGTON PASSAGE

Blair, W. Hunter
Germanus, Faten
Premachandra, Palliyage M.
Yee, Kenny Y V., FamilyMed

BASS RIVER

Ewing, Karen D., FamilyMed

BEAVER BANK

Saad, Emile, FamilyMed

BEDFORD

Ashton, Brian D., FamilyMed
Carroll, Cathie W.
Ciach, Michelle, FamilyMed
Clory, Michael B., FamilyMed(EM)
Deshwal, Natasha A., FamilyMed
Gallagher, Kathleen M.
Griffin, Lisa J., FamilyMed
Haddad, Susan J P., FamilyMed
Jabeen, Shaifta, FamilyMed
Johnstone, James E., FamilyMed
Kapilan, Priyadharsini M., FamilyMed
Khalil, Tarek H Y.
Langley, Christine E.
Lutwick, Renee E., FamilyMed(EM)
MacDonald, Ildiko L., FamilyMed
MacLean, Moira J., FamilyMed
MacNeil, David R.
McAllister, Amy L., FamilyMed
Michael, Liliane F F., FamilyMed
Mong, Irene E.
Mullan, Terence J G.
Newcomb, Paulette F., FamilyMed
Pickett, Bryan M., FamilyMed
Pickett, Wayne E., FamilyMed(EM)
Reynolds, Jason H., FamilyMed
Robertson, Nancy L.
Shaw, Erin R., FamilyMed
Singh, Sarban
Sneddon, Kadre A K., FamilyMed
Swift, Elena R., FamilyMed
Wisniowski, Leon E.
Wright, S. Elizabeth, FamilyMed
Zwicker, Christine L., FamilyMed

BERWICK

Bustin, Robin G., FamilyMed
George, Shaun R.
Jiwani, Almas A., FamilyMed
Langille, Kenneth R.
MacEachern, John R.
Mercer, Christina L., FamilyMed
Stubeda, Yury V.

BRIDGETOWN

King, Elizabeth A.

BRIDGEWATER

Anjorin, Adeyemi G.
Armstrong, Duncan S.
Barss, David H., FamilyMed
Colwell, J. Randolph, FamilyMed(EM)
D'Entremont, Julite, FamilyMed
Dabbour, Islam O.
Dochev, Atanas K.
Du Toit, Daniel J.
Eden, Silke C.
Edmonds, Diane E., FamilyMed
Ferguson, Craig A., FamilyMed
Fortuna, Teresa
Gandhi, Karamchand J.
Ghaffari, Seyed R.
Guptill, Elizabeth, FamilyMed
Jansen, Gregory W.
Johnson, Heather O., FamilyMed
Kalyan, Sangeeta
Kydd, Richard W.
Lennox, Arthur S.
Livingstone, James B.
Marier, Gisele, FamilyMed
Mathisen, Brit L.
Morse, Ewart A., FamilyMed
Newton, Paul X.
O'Neill, Carmen A C., FamilyMed
Parker, Kerry J M., FamilyMed
Pugh, J. Christian, FamilyMed(EM)
Rahman, Diruba
Riding, Timothy J., FamilyMed
Robertson, Heather E.
Sullivan, John M.
Tennant, Sarah C., FamilyMed
Vaughan, Peter W.
Weagle, Everett D E.

BROOKFIELD

Masoumi-Ravandi, Mashallah, FamilyMed
Pugsley, Donald C G.

BROOKSIDE

Ellis, Catherine L.

CALEDONIA

Benne, K M. Tobias, FamilyMed
Benne, Margaret E., FamilyMed
Rafferty, James L., FamilyMed

CANNING

Joseph, Mary

CHESTER

Cox, Karen A., FamilyMed
Dobek, Isabella
Finnamore, Ryan E., FamilyMed
Jollymore, George C.
LaValley, J. William

CHETICAMP

Aucoin, J. Claude
Aucoin, Marcel D., FamilyMed
Chiasson, Michel T., FamilyMed
Sonier, Paul W., FamilyMed

CLEVELAND

Senthillmohan, Sockalingam
Srirangarajan, Ramani, FamilyMed

DARTMOUTH

Adams, J. Henry W.
Ahmad, Khalil
Alrayes, Zeyad
Alyami, Fahad
Alzrighe, Mohamed, FamilyMed
Aquino, Emmanuel P B.
Ascurra De Ortiz, Ana Maria, FamilyMed
Atkinson, Christina M., FamilyMed
Avery, Chandra M., FamilyMed(EM)
Aziz, Sahar, FamilyMed
Banks, John V.
Belliveau, Adele M., FamilyMed
Bhan, Neelma
Bhattacharyya, Amal
Bloom, Nancy A., FamilyMed
Bloom, Seth A., FamilyMed
Botrous, Mary, FamilyMed
Boudreau, Andre D.
Bradley, William R., FamilyMed
Busahmen, Waleed E.
Cameron, Kenneth M., FamilyMed
Cameron, Marianne C., FamilyMed
Campbell, Donald M.
Campbell, Genevieve M., FamilyMed
Carter, John E., FamilyMed(EM)
Carter, Lorna J., FamilyMed
Champion, Jeffrey A.

PHYSICIANS BY PROVINCE

Cheng, Natalie Y., FamilyMed
Chugh, Prem K.
Cooper-Rosen, Ethel, FamilyMed
Creighton, David A.
Crowell, Denise, FamilyMed(EM)
Cruz, Arturo M.
Damacen Soplin, Harvey I.
Dubinsky, Leslie
Eisener, Beverley M.
Entaifa, Hussein
Ferguson-Losier, Nanette M.
Figueroa Perez, Mayelin
Filliter, Bruce D.
Fletcher, Mark A., FamilyMed(EM)
Fraser, Zachary R., FamilyMed
Gagnon, Linda, FamilyMed
Gibson, Richard J., FamilyMed
Gillis, John M., FamilyMed(EM)
Ginn, John L.
Goodwin, Janice R.
Gordon, Alfred
Gregus, Vojtech
Hall, Stephanie, FamilyMed
Harley, Stephen L., FamilyMed
Hart, Renee S., FamilyMed
Hassan, Sameh
Hebb, A. Michael O., FamilyMed(EM)
Holland, Stewart H.
Hopkins, Gary W., FamilyMed
Howard, Janet L.
Howlett, Todd C., FamilyMed(EM)
Izzard, J. Brad, FamilyMed
Joy, Andrea E., FamilyMed
Kinnear, Hilary A., FamilyMed
Klonowska, Maria-Teresa
Lafleur, Edith P., FamilyMed
Laskowski, Derek, FamilyMed
Lawless, Jill, FamilyMed(EM)
Lee, Peter C K., FamilyMed
Lee, William R., FamilyMed(EM)
Lewis, Lorraine N., FamilyMed
Lymburner, Dana L.
MacAulay, Peter M., FamilyMed
MacDonald, Carla K., FamilyMed
MacDonald, John W., FamilyMed
MacLennan, Martin T., FamilyMed
MacPherson, Rayma D.
MacQuarrie, Donald C., FamilyMed(EM)
Mahaney Jr., Gordon R.
Malak, Emad Y W., FamilyMed
Malik, Saira
Mann, Otto
McCormick, Kathleen M., FamilyMed
McMahon, Lynne E., FamilyMed(EM)
McMullen, Mark A., FamilyMed(EM)
Mershati, Abdelwahab K., FamilyMed
Milne, P. Ronald, FamilyMed
Minodin, Mike O.
Mont, Erik
Moriarty, Mary F., FamilyMed
Mozzon, Jeremy B., FamilyMed
Mullins, Rosalind, FamilyMed
Murray, Kim P.
Nagiah, Theepa S., FamilyMed
Nicholson, John D., FamilyMed
O'Connor, John F., FamilyMed
Oliver, Robert A., FamilyMed
Orlik, Jason R., FamilyMed(EM)
Ozere, Christopher P.
Pacis, Ruth B., FamilyMed
Parkash, Ravi, FamilyMed(EM)
Peres, Amos, FamilyMed
Ponnambalam, Chris, FamilyMed
Rahnavardi, Katayoun, FamilyMed
Raiche-Marsden, Michelle D.
Rastikerdar, Ali, FamilyMed
Reid, Daniel S.
Riives, Mai Liis
Rizk, Soha R., FamilyMed
Ross, Edward C.
Roy, Gregory L.
Russell, David
Sanders, David H.
Saric, Djemso, FamilyMed
Sawler, Margaret R., FamilyMed
Schlosser, Gisela E., FamilyMed
Scovil, Susan J., FamilyMed
Seaman, Sarah J., FamilyMed
Setayesh, Ahmad R., FamilyMed
Soudek Jr, Dusan
Stacey, Cooper B., FamilyMed
Steele, Ann-Leone, FamilyMed
Stevens, John A.
Stone, Catherine M.
Stryde, Peter C.
Sulyman, Mutiat O.
Taylor, Jonathan
To, Dinh Vu, FamilyMed
Toma, Tamer S., FamilyMed
Varma, Divya J., FamilyMed
Wadden, Ann M.
Warren, Richard C., FamilyMed
Watson, Andrew
Watson, Matthew T., FamilyMed
Wiebe, Alison W., FamilyMed
Williams, Albert R., FamilyMed(EM)
Wurster, Charles L., FamilyMed(EM)
Zaremba, Ewelina, FamilyMed

DIGBY

Bander, Marek S.
Black, J. Douglas
Lafkovici, Vladimir, FamilyMed
Matsusaki, Ronald

EASTERN PASSAGE

Nowlan, Claire N., FamilyMed

ELMSDALE

Burden, George M.
Farrahi, Siavash
Fraser, Mary-Anne
Harvey, William L G., FamilyMed
MacNeil, Iain P., FamilyMed
Montgomerie, H. Stewart
Montgomery, G. Bruce E.

ESKASONI

Khan, Fareeha S., FamilyMed
Todd, Robert J., FamilyMed

FALL RIVER

Cepica Angel, Denisa, FamilyMed
Fleming, Michael J., FamilyMed
Forbes, Cynthia A., FamilyMed
Fox, Jonathan R., FamilyMed
Kapur, Farah, FamilyMed
MacFarlane, Amy E., FamilyMed
MacIntyre, Lisa A.
McNab, John W., FamilyMed
Peters, Laura M.

GLACE BAY

Boutilier-Thomas, Carol M.
Cadegan, Perry K., FamilyMed
Dias, E. Bernice
Dias, Esther
Ellerker, Mark R., FamilyMed
Ellerker, Stephanie, FamilyMed
Fairfield, Sonia L., FamilyMed
Gallivan, Michael P J.
MacKay, Rose, FamilyMed
MacLachlan, Diane
MacLean, James D C., FamilyMed
O'Brien, Brian J.
Rehman, Waseema, FamilyMed
Soussou, David
Spencer, Gordon J.

GLENWOOD

Loveridge, Peter L.

GRAND PRE

Goddard, Thomas A., FamilyMed(EM)

GREENWOOD

Allan, Mark A.
Ar-Rushdi, Muna, FamilyMed
Laforce, Paul C.
Lorette, Jason G., FamilyMed
Morgan, Paul F.
Trueman, Gillian M.
Vallee, Isabelle, FamilyMed
Vats, Arun R.

GUYSBOROUGH

Ayoub, Haifa H.
Bell, Barbara A., FamilyMed
Foley, Anita A., FamilyMed
Mahendrarajah, Ranjini, FamilyMed

HALIFAX

Abu-Wasel, Bassam
Achenbach, Jillian M., FamilyMed
Adediran, T. Peter
Afzal, Samina
Agaibi, Samuel M.
Ahmed, Shabbeer
Aikman, Peter J., FamilyMed
Al Kharouf, Esam J.
Al-Dhamin, Ammar S S.
Al-Howary, Ala A.
Alaghband-Rad, Javad
Alam, Mahmood
Alexiadis, Maria
Alghamdi, Hassan U.
Aliter, Hashem F.
Aljehani, Yasser
Allen, Douglas L.
Allen, Michael J.
Aloysius, Jeyaranee, FamilyMed
Alwayn, Ian P J.
Anderson, Karen E.
Andrea, Glenn C.
Apostolides, Constantine, FamilyMed
Archibald, Gregory C., FamilyMed
Archibald, J. Fredric, FamilyMed
Archibald, Shauna M., FamilyMed
Askari, Sussan
Aspin, John D.
Atherton, Francis
Atkinson, Susan M., FamilyMed
Azim, Abdul
Bailey, Gillian F.
Barclay, Justin L.
Basta, Magdy N.
Baxter, Edith M., FamilyMed
Bell, Marilynne L., FamilyMed
Beresford, J. Patricia
Bergin, Fiona A., FamilyMed
Bethune, Graeme H G., FamilyMed
Blanchard, Mark C., FamilyMed
Blaszkow-Poranek, Barbara
Bolleddula, Prasad
Bood, Timothy W.
Botten, David L., FamilyMed
Bourke, Kevin E.
Bowdridge, Gilda A., FamilyMed
Brennan, Peter G.
Brokenshire, James, FamilyMed(EM)
Brosky, Gerald M., FamilyMed
Brown, Donald C.
Brown, Robert L.
Brydie, Sarah E., FamilyMed
Burge, Frederick I., FamilyMed
Burnstein, Matthew D.
Burton, Elizabeth A., FamilyMed
Buschmann, Donald K., FamilyMed
Bussey, Lynn-Ann, FamilyMed
Cajee, Ismail, FamilyMed(EM)
Calnen, Charlotte A., FamilyMed
Cameron, Stewart M., FamilyMed
Campbell, Glenn R., FamilyMed
Campbell, Samuel G., FamilyMed(EM)
Carbyn, Kevin M.
Celiker, Mahmut Y.
Cerny, Vladimir
Chao, Eric D., FamilyMed
Charania, Hameeda
Chatrath, Vikram
Cheah, Kee Saik
Chiasson, Darrell E., FamilyMed(EM)
Childs, Christopher M., FamilyMed
Chow, Linda Y.
Chowdhury, Dhiman
Chowdhury, Smriti
Church, Rhonda L.
Cimen, Sertac
Clarke, Barry S., FamilyMed
Connell, Cathy A., FamilyMed
Connidis, Stephanie A.
Conter, Howard S.
Cook, Jolene M., FamilyMed
Couture, Sophie M., FamilyMed
Covington, Nancy I.
Cox, Christopher P.
Crooks, Bruce N A.
D'Anjou, Catherine M., FamilyMed
D'Arcy, Diane L., FamilyMed
Dahn, Uwe
Das, Bijon, FamilyMed(EM)
Davies, Kay M.
Davis, Mary L.
Davis, Philip J.
Dawood, Isis M., FamilyMed
Dayananda, Naresh
De Coste, Rebecca L., FamilyMed
Deliu, Enver, FamilyMed
Desrosiers, Jacques G.
Devins, Mary
Dingle, Margaret
Doane, Frank R.
Doane, Paul H.
Drysdale-Buhr, Carolyn L.
Dziewaltowska-Gintowt, B., FamilyMed
El Nagar, Islam
El-Naggar, Walid I M H.
Elliott, David
Evans, Dafydd
Fay, Donald F.
Ferguson, James
Field, Simon, FamilyMed(EM)
Fraser, John R., FamilyMed
Gao, Dongsheng
Gass, David A., FamilyMed
Gazit, Vered
Gerges, Maged, FamilyMed
Gibbon, Stephen B.
Gillis, Amy E., FamilyMed
Glazebrook, Katherine M., FamilyMed
Gobran, Gehad G M., FamilyMed
Gold, Elisabeth, FamilyMed
Good, Richard I S.
Gow, Nina M.
Gowan, Susan E., FamilyMed
Grada, Atef
Gradstein, Roetka, FamilyMed
Graham, Christopher H D.
Graham, Johanna H.
Grant, D. Augustus, FamilyMed
Graven, Michael A.
Gregoire, Trixie L., FamilyMed
Griffin, Leslie B., FamilyMed
Guerin, John M.
Hadzimurezic, Dzenita
Haider, Umar, FamilyMed
Haigh, Donald
Haislip, Heidi L.
Hajek, Tomas
Hamilton, Gillian R., FamilyMed
Hanna, Adala, FamilyMed
Hanna, Mary H G.
Haque, Nargis
Hatfield, Peter W., FamilyMed
Hayes, Vonda, FamilyMed
Heede, Santa
Henneberry, Ryan, FamilyMed(EM)
Hennen, Brian K E., FamilyMed
Hering, Ramm, FamilyMed
Hickcox, Samuel E., FamilyMed
Higgins, Terrance F.
Horrey, Kathleen A., FamilyMed
Horton, Robert P., FamilyMed
Hosein, Jalal
Hosseini, Mona
Houstoun, Anne L.
Humphrey, Andrew B.
Irwin, Mandi R., FamilyMed
Jack, Zita, FamilyMed
Jain, Sherry, FamilyMed
Jarvie, Andrew
Jarvis, Carl W., FamilyMed(EM)
Jayabarathan, Ajantha, FamilyMed
Johnson, Ernest B.
Johnson, J. Kenneth
Johnson, John K.
Johnston, Christopher A M., FamilyMed
Jones, Bronwen A., FamilyMed
Jones, Christopher T.
Kahwash, Eiad
Kain, Danielle A., FamilyMed
Kawchuk, Terry P.
Keenan, Robert J.
Khan, Kamran A.
Khan, M. Naeem
Khanna, Vijay
Khorovets, Andrei
Kidwai, Bakhtiar J.
King, David P.
King, Meghan A., FamilyMed
Kinley, Cecil E.
Kirby, Jeffrey C.
Kishta, Waleed E M.
Kitamura, Kelly M., FamilyMed
Klimek, Marek G.
Komatsu, Teruya
Kubow, Janusz
Kumar, Shree
Kuznetsov, Fiodar
Kwapisz, Myron M.
Lacas, Alethea D., FamilyMed
Lambeth, Michelle A., FamilyMed
Langille, Donald B.
Leblanc, Constance, FamilyMed(EM)
Lee, George T W.
Leighton, Margaret M., FamilyMed
Lepage, Veronik, FamilyMed
Lewington, Danielle C.
Lewington, Richard B.
Lewis, Valerie, FamilyMed
Lewitzka, Ute
Lindener, Margo
Lo, Frank L.
Logan, Karl John
Lorenz, Konstantin
Love, Michael P.
Lowe, William M., FamilyMed
Luqman, Zubair
MacDonald, Karen A.
MacDonald, Theresa M.
MacDougall, Catherine E., FamilyMed
MacGregor, Janice M.
MacKinnon, Heather A.
MacLachlan, Richard A., FamilyMed
MacLean, Rhonda A., FamilyMed
MacLean, Stephen W., FamilyMed
MacLeod, N. Wayne, FamilyMed
MacNeill, Judith L., FamilyMed
MacPherson, Kathleen M.
Macanovic, Mladen
Maciel-Miranda, Jesus A.
Mader, Judith A., FamilyMed
Maggio, Frederick J.
Mahdi, Gamal E M.
Maianski, Irit
Maianski, Ziv
Malcolm, Scott F., FamilyMed
Maldonado Gonzalez, David F.
Malik, Rizwan
Mallory, Amy E., FamilyMed
Malloy, Susan J., FamilyMed
Mancha, Mirko
Mankavil Kovil Veetil, Aneesh K.
Mann, Karen
Marche, Janet E.
Marsh, Lorne A.
Marshall, Gena M., FamilyMed
Mateos-Corral, Dimas
Matheson, Hugh B.
Matheson, Leslie J.
Matheson, Timothy, FamilyMed
McBride, Graeme N., FamilyMed
McCallum, Alison M.
McCann, D. Burton, FamilyMed
McCarron, M. Janet, FamilyMed
McDonald, Andrea J., FamilyMed
McGrath, Fiona M M., FamilyMed
McIntyre, Paul F., FamilyMed
McKenna, Christine J., FamilyMed
McNeil, Karen A., FamilyMed
McPherson, John, FamilyMed

Meehan, Catheryne N D., FamilyMed
Midgen, Craig A.
Migas, Maria, FamilyMed
Miller, Stephen G., FamilyMed(EM)
Mishra, Harsh V., FamilyMed
Mistry, Dipan N.
Mitchell, Victoria P., FamilyMed
Mohsin, Hina
Molinari, Michele
Montgomery, Katherine P.
Morash, Angela H., FamilyMed
Morgan, Kenneth P.
Morris, David P.
Mosharraf, Syed
Mosher, Pamela J.
Muir, Sarah A., FamilyMed
Murphy, Nancy, FamilyMed(EM)
Murray, Jock A G., FamilyMed(EM)
Myatt, Gerald L.
Nabi, Naeem U.
Nadeem, Syed M N A.
Natarajan, Monika N., FamilyMed
Nejat, Amir M.
Nejmeddin Jalal, Dleer
Neu, Rolf-Dieter
Neumann, Anna, FamilyMed
O'Hearn, Bruce M.
O'Neil, Leonard S., FamilyMed
O'Neill, Mary C.
Ortiz-Dominguez, Tania A.
Pajer, Kathleen A.
Park, Diane H., FamilyMed
Parsons, Arthur H.
Patil, Nikhilesh G.
Patriquin, Maria J., FamilyMed
Pearce, Patricia A., FamilyMed
Pencle, Franz
Pestell, Deborah, FamilyMed
Petropolis, Peter N.
Phillips, Gosia E.
Photopoulos, Spiro
Piccinini, Helena, FamilyMed
Plaxton, E. Kim, FamilyMed
Pohlmann-Eden, Bernhard
Poirier, Angela M.
Portugal Aires, Liana M., FamilyMed
Pottle, M. Kent
Poulos, Robert K.
Power, Michael T., FamilyMed
Premsagar, Sarojadevi R., FamilyMed
Price, Victoria E.
Propper, Lukas
Propperova, Iva, FamilyMed
Quraishi, Ata-Ur-Rehman
Rainbow, Sandra M., FamilyMed
Renault, Paul S.
Rideout, Andrea N., FamilyMed
Ridha, Mahmoud H., FamilyMed
Ripley, Susan M., FamilyMed
Robinson, Juan
Robinson, Katherine A B., FamilyMed
Romao, Rodrigo L P.
Ross, Valerie A., FamilyMed(EM)
Rowicka, Malgorzata D.
Saha, Amal K., FamilyMed
Salih, Rasha, FamilyMed
Samad, Nabeel B.
Sampson, Maria T., FamilyMed
Savvopoulos, Stavros, FamilyMed
Sawaqed, Fadi S.
Sawatzky, K. David
Scheffler, Matthias G.
Schmit, Pierre J M.
Scott, Jeanette M.
Sekula, Zygmunt P.
Selegean, Sorin M.
Shahin Azar, Massoud
Shamout, Zaki
Shankar, Jai Jai S.
Sharkia, Mohamad
Sharma, Rajat
Sheehan, Stephen D A.
Shelton, Rhidian J.
Shukla, Shashi P.
Sidhom, Mary H., FamilyMed
Silburt, Bruce S., FamilyMed
Simpson, D. Lee, FamilyMed
Singleton, Kathleen M., FamilyMed
Sinha, Dinesh P.
Smigas, Halina
Smith, Cheryl D.
Smith, Preston A., FamilyMed
Smith, Shane A., FamilyMed
Snow, D. Martyn
Sobh, Donia M A K.
Sobh, Hoda M.
Somers, Patrick A., FamilyMed
Sommers, Jack G., FamilyMed
Sorhaindo, Mark A G.
Sparavalo, Nebojsa
Spicer, Finlay R.
Sproule, James
St Peters, Craig B., FamilyMed
Stalker, Robert E.
Stecum, Ronald E., FamilyMed
Steele, Curtis A.
Stender, Mark W., FamilyMed
Stewart, Andrew
Stewart, Bradley E.
Strong, Julie K.
Stubeda, Iryna
Subhani, Khaja N.
Swift, Alexander B., FamilyMed(EM)
Swinamer, Deanna L., FamilyMed
Talballa, Hala A H.
Taylor, Gretta, FamilyMed
Teodorescu, Otilia, FamilyMed
Thomson, Carolyn J., FamilyMed
Tilley, David L.
Toplack, Christina M., FamilyMed
Trager, Morris E.
Trenholm, Arthur D.
Veinot-Nash, Janet L., FamilyMed
Veldhuyzen Van Zanten, Sander J O.
Venkatachalam, Viswanathan C.
Verma, Bharti, FamilyMed
Vician, Michael
Vincent, Franklyn A., FamilyMed
Vlatten, Arnim
Wadiwalla, Shamim
Wang, Cheng
Watson, Adrienne N., FamilyMed
Watson, Mary-Lynn, FamilyMed(EM)
Welch, John P.
White, Maureen E., FamilyMed
White, Rosemary A.
Whyte, Tanya R.
Wieder, Jana
Wilson, Rodney D.
Witter, Tobias
Wojcik, Ronald
Wong, Lori-Ann, FamilyMed
Wood, David C.
Writer, William D.
Wu, K Y. William
Xu, Jie
Ymeri, Hylkije
Yoshida, Lianne M., FamilyMed
Younis, Tallal H.
Zed, Joanna L., FamilyMed
Zitner, David, FamilyMed
Zivic-Deliu, Ljiljana, FamilyMed

HAMMONDS PLAINS

Almighairbi, Adel M S., FamilyMed
Burns Lachance, Jennifer L., FamilyMed
Chawla, Rakesh K.

HANTSPORT

Canete, Yuri C., FamilyMed
Price, Judy M., FamilyMed

HATCHET LAKE

Coles, Joyce K T., FamilyMed
Colp, Jeffrey N.
Crooks, Harris G.

HD ST MARGARET BAY

Couper, Janet A.

HUBBARDS

Jarvis, Jolene E., FamilyMed
McLean, James R B., FamilyMed
Paleta, John

INVERNESS

Bennett, Mark S., FamilyMed
Egar, Susanne E., FamilyMed
La France, Monique S., FamilyMed
Lok, Raymond T., FamilyMed
MacDonald, Rhea C., FamilyMed
MacLachlan, Jean M., FamilyMed
MacLean, C. Bernard
Pillai, N. Gopalakrishna G.

KENNETCOOK

MacLean, Michele E., FamilyMed

KENTVILLE

Barry, Anne E.
Bauer, Christopher A.
Beresford, Philip D.
Cogswell, Esther M S., FamilyMed
Grant, David A.
Gunn, Robert F., FamilyMed
Kanagasabai, Sivakumar
King, Yvonne M.
McMillan, Merle K A., FamilyMed
Miller, Robert A., FamilyMed(EM)
Mishra, Achal
Mullan, Robert D., FamilyMed
Nunn, David J., FamilyMed
Opitz, Silke A.
Opthof, Nick P., FamilyMed
Price, Nancy A.
Ranji, Mostafa
Rao, Nasa S K.
Seaman, Donald M.
Seaman, James G.
Sinclair, Michael G., FamilyMed
Singh, Anurita
Sivananth, Ponnampalam, FamilyMed
Somasekaram, Gnanasekaram
Sommer, Markus
Sundararajan, Kanchanamala
Swain, Ann E., FamilyMed
Targett, Matthew M., FamilyMed
Veasey, Duncan A.
Verryn-Stuart, Ian T.
Wadden, Michael R., FamilyMed
Wilkie, Allan V., FamilyMed(EM)

KINGSTON

Ainamo, Jyri S.
McGuire, Paul B.
Yafai, Abdul-Aziz

L'ARDOISE

Pealing, Robert D.

LAKESIDE

Dobek, Luke

LAWRENCETOWN

Goodine, Grant A D.

LIVERPOOL

Blackadar, Andrew M., FamilyMed
Doucet, Albert D., FamilyMed
Ernest, Gary P., FamilyMed
Gunn, David E., FamilyMed
MacDonald, Jennifer L., FamilyMed
Mogan, Norah, FamilyMed
Morash, Garry W.
Thorne, Susan F., FamilyMed
Woodford, Timothy J.

LOUISBOURG

Burns, A. George, FamilyMed
Patel, Navinchandra M.

LOWER SACKVILLE

Awalt, Erin J., FamilyMed
Best, Robert A., FamilyMed(EM)
Carey, Aidan G., FamilyMed
Chui, S T. Thomas
Cloney, Jacqueline F.
Croskerry, Patrick
Davey, Colin F.
Diaz, Pedro E.
Drake, Wendy T., FamilyMed
English, Keltie
Fitzgerald, James M.
Fragoso Alvarez, Zaida, FamilyMed
Gebre-Heywot, Tsedale, FamilyMed
Killeen, Ronald A., FamilyMed
Knight, Jennifer W H.
Lappin, Susan F.
Leckey, Naida L.
Leverman, Jennifer, FamilyMed(EM)
Marshall, Cindy L., FamilyMed
Pein, Cho-Yee
Rivas Hernandez, Juan-Hector
Seetharamdoo, Patrick S.
Spiess, Steven D.
Taylor, Lindsay E.
Taylor, Rosemarie A.

LUNENBURG

Abriel, David L.
Badi, Fathi A.
Beaton, Blaine G., FamilyMed
Conrad, Sarah L., FamilyMed
Hennenfent, Brett W.
Jenkins, John T., FamilyMed
Kelly, Catherine L.
Martell, David R., FamilyMed
Morse, David W.
Zwicker, Daniel M.

MAHONE BAY

Abud, Lely, FamilyMed
McAuley, Paul
Steeves, Alexander L., FamilyMed
Watson, Krista P., FamilyMed(EM)

METEGHAN CENTRE

Blinn, Alain J.
D'Entremont, Lionel J.
Dow, Michelle M., FamilyMed
Dugas, Giselle, FamilyMed

MIDDLE MUSQUODOBOIT

Fewer, Karen A., FamilyMed
Giffin, Barry D., FamilyMed
Hawes, Violet C.
Sethi, Shilpa
Snair, Patti J., FamilyMed

MIDDLETON

Balser, Eric F., FamilyMed
Brooks, Jane C D., FamilyMed
Burgess, Lorraine T.
Craswell, Donald F., FamilyMed
Drysdale, John D., FamilyMed
Lelacheur, Ruth C.
MacLean, Paul D.
McCormick, S. Ashley, FamilyMed
Moore, Irene T.
Salsman, Kenneth R., FamilyMed
Saxon, Patricia M., FamilyMed

MINEVILLE

Nagaiah, Theepa S.
Nicholson, Daniel J.
Oluyede, Olumayokun
Smith, John D.

MIRA ROAD

Asim, Hammad
Bisson, Gail M.
Bulajic, Ranka
Critchley, Carol A., FamilyMed
MacDougall, Steven G., FamilyMed
MacKillop, James H., FamilyMed
Myatt, Gregory A., FamilyMed(EM)
Oei, Ien T.
Ritcey, Susan G.
Sampson, Mark E., FamilyMed(EM)
Sebastian, Antonypillai R., FamilyMed
Zemerli, Fatima Z., FamilyMed

MOUNT UNIACKE

Bhanot, Raj
Harding, Roy A.

MUSQUODOBOIT HARBOUR

Abdulhameed, Abdulnasser N.
Bass, Stephanie J., FamilyMed
Bonang, Lisa M., FamilyMed
Brown, Wayne C.
Kumarasamy, Jeyakumar
Rehan, Fouzia Q., FamilyMed

NEILS HARBOUR

Buffett, Bernard R.
Jacobs, Robert J.
Murray, Kenneth R., FamilyMed

NEW GLASGOW

Al-Manahi, Rasha N A.
Al-Nassar, Rafid S.
Boutilier, Nicole A., FamilyMed
Craig, Patricia A., FamilyMed
Cutler, Susan E., FamilyMed
Elliott, Christopher R., FamilyMed
Ezema, Enyinnaya
Fahim, Mohammad
Farrell, Gerald E.
Flusk, David
Goldchtaub, Valeri
Graham, David J.
Jala, Vikram R.
Jeans-Mingo, L. Aulayne
Kaiprath, Soumini, FamilyMed
Kormos, Arpad I.
Kwasnik-Krawczyk, Anne M., FamilyMed
Larkin, Tara L., FamilyMed
Laskowski, Alexandra
Lee, Peter T C.
MacCara, Melanie L., FamilyMed
MacLean, Gregor W.
Malan, Jean E.
O'Sullivan, Colleen M.
Ogunsona, Adeoluwa O.
Okafor, Livinus
Park, Thomas R.
Perchik, Robert Aslan.
Reddy, Sudhakar D.
Rowicka, Monika M., FamilyMed
Sava, Cristina, FamilyMed
Schnare, Kevin P K.
Strasfeld, Maurice
Straub, Deborah L., FamilyMed(EM)

NEW MINAS

Fleckenstein, Martin H.
Goodman, Marni A., FamilyMed
McAdoo, Keri K., FamilyMed
Todd, Crystal F., FamilyMed

NEW WATERFORD

Azer, Raed, FamilyMed
Farrell, Edward S.
Hanspal, Rajvinder, FamilyMed
Haq, Sheira, FamilyMed
Lange, Jennifer, FamilyMed
Littlejohn, Peter W.
Lowry, Brigittie H., FamilyMed
Lynk, Mary E.

NEWPORT

Cussen, Michael J.
Kazimirski, Judith C.
Mountford, Catherine, FamilyMed

NOEL

O'Neil, Barbara A., FamilyMed
Stewart, Graham M.

NORTH SYDNEY

Bhattacharjee, Debabrata B.
Coish, Charles T., FamilyMed
Dobson, Diana C.
Ghenea, Irina, FamilyMed
Hickey, D. Paul
Hutchison, Mary E.
Kirkpatrick, John H., FamilyMed
Langley, Stephanie A., FamilyMed
MacDonald, William M.
MacIntosh, Bernard H W., FamilyMed
O'Grady, Patrick G.
Salah, Joan C., FamilyMed
Wawer, Andrew R.

OXFORD

Rondeau, Ronald L.

PARRSBORO

Baghaee, Jalal
Dauphinee-Bentley, Patricia K.
Donkervoort, Laura, FamilyMed
Ettehad Dabagh, Mojgan
Howe, David, FamilyMed

PICTOU

Burrill, Randy S.
Cooper, Robert J., FamilyMed
Douglas, Andrew, FamilyMed
Felderhof, Catharina A L.
Ghanem, Yazan, FamilyMed
Lassey, Steve
MacCara, A. Shirley
MacLachlan, A. James
Young, Gordon V.

PORT HAWKESBURY

Boucher, C. Benjamin
Collins, James A., FamilyMed
Marchand, Deborah J.
Pluta, Paul L.

PORT MOUTON

Mulherin, Michael T., FamilyMed

PORT WILLIAMS

Bowden, Lois, FamilyMed
Mindrum, Christa R., FamilyMed
Muggah, J. Jean
Ross, Barbara J., FamilyMed
Taylor Clarke, Rebecca J., FamilyMed

PORTERS LAKE

Merritt, Robert B.
Raghavan, Sai L., FamilyMed

PUBNICO

D'Eon, Jacqueline R.
Rohland, Terry A.

PUGWASH

Blaikie, Peter G.
Fashoranti, Oluwarotimi, FamilyMed
Forshner, David
McFarlane, Brian A E., FamilyMed
Rezvani, M. Kazem

SAULNIERVILLE

Comeau, Alban L.
Van Onselen, Eugene, FamilyMed

SHEET HARBOUR

Antony, Savarimuthiusosai
Atkinson, Bradley C.
MacDonald, Donald G., FamilyMed

SHELBURNE

Chaloner, Wouna M., FamilyMed
Keeler, John E.
O'Sullivan, Eoghan, FamilyMed
Riley, Mark E.
Wambulwa, Charles R.
Wilson, David H.

SHERBROOKE

Ackermann, Michael J M.
Cameron, Ian A., FamilyMed

SHUBENACADIE

Adams, Helika D.
Hindler, Lionel R.
Pelley, Lorraine V J., FamilyMed
Philpott, Stephanie L., FamilyMed
Sheehy, David N.

SPRINGHILL

Alas Lopez, Juan P., FamilyMed
Begin, Paul A.
Kappagantula, Mythri, FamilyMed
Karivelil, Joshy, FamilyMed
Semsar, Alireza
Shakib, Alireza

ST PETERS

Nault, Yvonne D M.

STELLARTON

Ibrahim, Wael F.
Jazrawi, Bashar, FamilyMed
Kirk, D. Grant, FamilyMed
MacDonald, H. Paul
MacDonald, Marion N.
Makhan, Winston M.
Soliman, Ehab S., FamilyMed

STEWIACKE

Chalati, Bachar
Wells, Philip J.

SYDNEY

Abel, Rachel D., FamilyMed
Abu Shullaih, Zaki Omar
Akinlaja, Adeola B.
Akinlaja, Ayodeji O.
Ali, Syed Z.
Annamalai, Sivakumar
Ansari, Shoaib R.
Archibald, John M.
Brodie, Lauren, FamilyMed
Buhariwalla, Farokh R., FamilyMed(EM)
Cameron, Estelle E A.
Campbell, Mary-Anne
Coakley, Arthur G., FamilyMed(EM)
Cohen, Robert E.
Crosbie, Stephen H.
Crosby, Jean D.
Doyle, Mary A.
Dugas, Isabelle L., FamilyMed
Dutt, Monika, FamilyMed
Espinal Montoya, Victor
Farooq, Mohammed
Fashir, Baroudi
Forouzesh, Bahram
Fraser, Margaret
Gammell, Lisa, FamilyMed
Giorno, Andrew, FamilyMed
Glasgow, Daniel F G.
Glaude, Simon-Pierre, FamilyMed
Gracie, Glenn A., FamilyMed
Guy, Trevor, FamilyMed(EM)
Habiba, Ayman A.
Haleem, Saima, FamilyMed
Harless, William
Hasan, Azra
Hussein, Mohamed R.
Jackson, Peter D.
Kajetanowicz, Andrzej J.
Kajetanowicz, Danuta M.
Karanwal, Derek A.
Khan, Muhammad A., FamilyMed(EM)
Khodadad, Kian
Kodagoda, Dayananda, FamilyMed
Lawal, Waheed O.
Lawand, Christopher, FamilyMed(EM)
Lazovskis, Juris
Lopez Blanco, Alejandra V.
MacKenzie, Robert J., FamilyMed
MacLeod, Susan E., FamilyMed
MacNeil, Dorothy E.
MacVicar, G. Neil, FamilyMed(EM)
Mahmoud-Ahmed, Ashraf S.
Mansoor, Samina
Milburn, Christopher R., FamilyMed
Murphy, Paul F., FamilyMed
Naeem, Mehmooda, FamilyMed
Ogah, Oshiomeghe K.
Orrell, Liam F M.
Pahil, Rajbir S.
Parminder, Ranjit K.
Petersen, Agnieszka
Prinsloo, Etienne
Puppala, Venkata Karthik Rao
Rawal, Punam S., FamilyMed
Raza, Syed A.
Ritter, John A., FamilyMed
Roxburgh, Brian
Sardiwalla, Ismail
Sayadi, Hassan
Scherbarth, Sandra E., FamilyMed
Shehzad, Anees A., FamilyMed
Shrafat, Nadeem
Smith, Murdock A., FamilyMed
Sseguya-Lwanga, David
Stokes, Robert, FamilyMed(EM)
Tobin, Cheryl L., FamilyMed
Uhoegbu, Chimdi U.
Usman, Muhammad U.
Virick, Mohan S.
Wawrzyszyn, Janusz
Wesolkowska, Anna
Whyte, Laura M., FamilyMed
Worth, Glen G.
Yazer, Erika, FamilyMed
Yepes, Horacio

SYDNEY MINES

Ignacio, Eugene E., FamilyMed
Knott, Z. Marek
Kohlsmith, Douglas J.
MacCormick, Elizabeth C.
McKeough, Michel F., FamilyMed

TATAMAGOUCHE

Bush, Robert P., FamilyMed
Carsley, Holly H.
Glasgow, Michael J.
MacDonald, Daniel J., FamilyMed
Moss, Christopher J.

TIMBERLEA

Scovil, Robert J.

TRENTON

Barclay, Spencer L.

TRURO

Abdelaty, Amr Nour E.
Abraham, Suma R.
Altenkirk, Gary B., FamilyMed(EM)
Bell, Helen F.
Berghuis, Harold P., FamilyMed
Blois, Beau, FamilyMed
Bower, Neil L.
Brown, Wanda G G.
Cook, Christopher T., FamilyMed
Cook, Steven T.
Ellis, Stephen D., FamilyMed
Feltmate, Mary F.
Ferguson, Linda M., FamilyMed
Ferguson, Murdo E R., FamilyMed(EM)
Field, Deanna J., FamilyMed
Gadir, Yousif, FamilyMed
Graham, Robert D., FamilyMed
Henderson, J. David, FamilyMed
Jones-Locke, Diana C.
Locke, Trevor A.
Loshaj, Ryve, FamilyMed
MacAulay, Andria J., FamilyMed
Makkar, Nina, FamilyMed
McCarthy, Stephen C P., FamilyMed
McLernon, S. Lynn, FamilyMed(EM)
Meadows-Younger, Malcolm D., FamilyMed
Munroe, Tanya M., FamilyMed(EM)
Murray, Michael R., FamilyMed
Murray, Roya R., FamilyMed
Nadour, Jalaa
Phillips, Bruce A., FamilyMed
Rafiq, Suraiya, FamilyMed
Rowe, Donald G.
Sharma, Shikhi, FamilyMed
Sharma, Sushil K., FamilyMed
Shen, Khaled A., FamilyMed
Singh, Sarbjit
Slipp, Frank E., FamilyMed
Smith, Cortney M., FamilyMed
Sommers, Janet M., FamilyMed(EM)
Sommers, Ryan B., FamilyMed
Srivatsa, Kousthub K.
Van Aardt, Renier G., FamilyMed
Vohra, Manoj, FamilyMed

UPPER TANTALLON

Anderson, Charles C.
Crosby, Amanda R., FamilyMed
Herman, Shauna P., FamilyMed
Jones, Lori, FamilyMed
Jones, Sarah D., FamilyMed
Lang, H. Benno, FamilyMed
Lang, Maria T.
O'Connell, Jennifer, FamilyMed
Robertson, Jill D., FamilyMed
Sadler, Laura K., FamilyMed
Thompson, Krista L., FamilyMed
Zwicker, Holly J., FamilyMed

WAGMATCOOK

MacCormick, Shaun A., FamilyMed

WESTVILLE

Forbes, John G.
Jota, Jose M.
MacDougall, Bradley, FamilyMed
Smith, Aaron C., FamilyMed
Stevenson, W. Rodney

WEYMOUTH

Westby, Donald M.

WHYCOCOMAGH

Sutherland, William E.

WINDSOR

Ahmad, Amer R.
Buckley, C. Niall J.
Enright, William M.
Grandy, Elwood C.
Kazimirski, Mark, FamilyMed
Kilcollins, Calvin T., FamilyMed
Leahy, James R.
Machel, Wieslaw J.
Nathan, Viji, FamilyMed
Premsagar, Vickesh, FamilyMed(EM)
Smith, Cathryn L.
Veasey, Jack B., FamilyMed
Wile, Iona, FamilyMed

WOLFVILLE

Dearman, Lisa M.
Doran, William A L., FamilyMed
Hamilton, Roger D.
Hergett, Susan C.
MacNaughton, Janet E.
McNally, Catherine E., FamilyMed
Mossman, Andrea L., FamilyMed
Murray, Jonathan
Pennell, Mark L.
Phillips, Wayne L., FamilyMed
Salazar, Sacha R., FamilyMed
Segato, Peter M., FamilyMed
Wellwood, Alison M., FamilyMed
Wellwood, Heather M.

YARMOUTH

Boudreau, Cindy L.
Brodarec, Ivan
Cain, Michelle R.
Chandler, Julie E.
Cottreau, Alison M.
Dhawan, Bal Chandra
Edgar, Philip A.
Friel, Patrick H.
Gillespie, Laurie
Hemani, Razi
Hublall, Ronald V.
Hussein, Abir H.
Iqbal, Mirza N.
Kysela, Alenia R., FamilyMed
Leahey, Shelagh M.
Legere, Paul W.
Lyons, Brian J.
Maher, Lauren H., FamilyMed
Marais, Abraham J.

Mare, Frans
Mohamed, Ahmed A R.
Muise, Roland J.
Muise, Thomas A.
Murphy, Karma N., FamilyMed
Ntambazi, Matthew
Oguntade, John A.
Pollock, Jenni P.
Rahman, Zia U.
Ramessar, Elena
Ramessar, John A S.
Randell, L. Christopher, FamilyMed
Safakish Kashanifard, Kyarash
Shettar, Channabasav B.
Soto-Moreno, Lourdes
Vandana, Neeraj
Wajeeh, Mohammed
Webster, David M.
Wertlen, Winston G., FamilyMed
Wyman, Chester R.

NUNAVUT

IQALUIT

Barrington, Michelle R.
Cole, Madeleine S C., FamilyMed
De Maio, Patricia A., FamilyMed
Kraft, Claudia S., FamilyMed
Kraus, Steven J., FamilyMed
MacDonald, William A., FamilyMed

ONTARIO

ACTON

Al-Shakarji, Nather N., FamilyMed
Jayalath, Arachchige D., FamilyMed
Minc, Paul H., FamilyMed
Raouf-Alkadhimi, Ahmed, FamilyMed

AILSA CRAIG

Furtado, Norman, FamilyMed
McIver, Donald J L.

AJAX

Ahmad, Marium F., FamilyMed
Ahmed, Bedri U., FamilyMed
Al-Ward, Harith H A., FamilyMed
Alazhari, Khalid E A., FamilyMed(EM)
Amamoo, Adwoa B., FamilyMed
Atkinson, Joan M.
Baker, Norma A.
Brown, J. Terence
Cait, Ted A., FamilyMed
Chacko, Saji A.
Chow, Daliah Y L., FamilyMed
Chuang, Evelyn Y., FamilyMed(EM)
Condon, Richard A.
Daniel, Shevanta G., FamilyMed
Donaghue, C. Scott, FamilyMed
EL Zaharna, Ramy, FamilyMed
Edwards, Neil W.
Elrify, Elsaid R.
Fan, Michael K D.
Gad, Nadia, FamilyMed
Ganeshram, Tharini, FamilyMed
Gove, Anne E.
Hancock, David J.
Harper, Kelly M.
Hoffman, Alan S.
Izzeldin, Abuelgasim, FamilyMed
James, Michael J.
Jun, Martin C., FamilyMed
Kempenaar, Jacob W.
Kerr, Leanne A., FamilyMed
Khan, Mansoor A.
Khokhar, Jawad B., FamilyMed
Kuo, Eugene E C., FamilyMed
Lai, Alvin Y W., FamilyMed
Lai, Mark K K.
Lee, Edward S C., FamilyMed
Lee, John P L., FamilyMed
Leung, Frederick C C., FamilyMed
Li, Donna R., FamilyMed
Ling, Brian M Y.
Ling, Elaine B.
Liu, Li, FamilyMed
Lo, Ronnie Y K.
Lo, Vivian K W.
Mensinkai, Suchitra
Nag, Sanjita, FamilyMed
Nicholas, Seetha D., FamilyMed
Parkinson, Lillian M.
Pawaroo, Patricia S R., FamilyMed
Phillips, Mark R.
Puodziukas, L. Edward
Robertson, Daniel K F.
Shafir, Roslyn S.
Shariff, Riaz
Sharobim, Monica W., FamilyMed
Sharobim, Nazar R., FamilyMed(EM)
Sin, J H. Leo, FamilyMed
Sliwowicz, David A.
Smith, Camala A., FamilyMed
Stas, Romas V.
Stern, Alex, FamilyMed
Stern, Stephen J.
Syme, Colin W.
Thayaparen, Yasotha, FamilyMed
Valyi, Lajos, FamilyMed(EM)
Watson, Ian J., FamilyMed
Wong, Gabriel F Y.
Yu, Carlos C S., FamilyMed(EM)
Yu, Maria C Y., FamilyMed
Yu-Watson, Maria C Y., FamilyMed
Zohrab, Andrew E F., FamilyMed

ALEXANDRIA

Adams, Robert F., FamilyMed
El-Salibi, Elias, FamilyMed
Kilmartin, Patrick E.
Lajoie, Lucie, FamilyMed
Marleau, J G. Ghislain
Millman, Christine G., FamilyMed
Nadkarni, Ashok B.
Poole, Richard F.
Power, Ellen M.
Ross, Anatoly D.
Sasseville, Rachel, FamilyMed

ALLISTON

Affoo, Clifford L., FamilyMed
Ambreen, Shazia, FamilyMed
Farrugia, Michael D P.
Fischbacher, Theodore
Gray, Ian A.
Hassan, Hanadi, FamilyMed
Hendrick, A. Corbin, FamilyMed
Jansen, Liesbet M., FamilyMed
Khalil, Ihab A B., FamilyMed
Kogan, Izabella, FamilyMed
Lawson, Glasine O.
Lo, James W., FamilyMed
Momin, Rizwanali, FamilyMed
Moreau, Monique F., FamilyMed
Myatt, Matthew, FamilyMed
Neami, Khaldon A., FamilyMed
Omylanowski, Diana
Ozon, Pierre J., FamilyMed
Palao, France A., FamilyMed
Park, Jong Bum, FamilyMed
Ramirez, Oswaldo C., FamilyMed
Safar, Modar A., FamilyMed
Swarbreck, Brian S.
Tomini, Stephen R.

ALMONTE

Abramenko, Heather M.
Blaine, William C., FamilyMed
Deschenes, Christiane S.
Ferraris, Franz B.
Forbes-Hoskins, Eleanor, FamilyMed
McGarry, Ursula M.
McKillop, Graeme J., FamilyMed
Miller, Katherine J., FamilyMed
Murphy, Francis A.
Murray, Jody L., FamilyMed
Oldfield, M. Anne
Quackenbush, Suzie J., FamilyMed
Rouf, Rehana K., FamilyMed
Rytwinski, Z. Cecil S., FamilyMed
Turcotte, Karen E., FamilyMed
Wood, Carolyn E.

AMHERSTBURG

Coates, C. David C.
Di Pierdomenico, Fernando G.
Lan-Hing-Ming, Rose-Marie
Lovell, Richard E.
O'Callahan, Timothy S.
Oswald, Angus

AMHERSTVIEW

Connor, Calvin W.
De Jong, Jennifer, FamilyMed
Gazendam, Mary Kate, FamilyMed
Glassco, M. Jane, FamilyMed
Goldstein, Ronald, FamilyMed
Jain, Shalini, FamilyMed
MacKinnon, Laura E., FamilyMed
McCullough, Wendy M.
Pettis, Craig A., FamilyMed
Samikian, Karoon, FamilyMed
Wonnacott, Matthew W T., FamilyMed

ANCASTER

Antoniuk, Karen M., FamilyMed
Boutin, Helene A., FamilyMed
Digregorio, Roland C., FamilyMed
Ellabib, Mohamed
Fahmy, Nader, FamilyMed
Feng, Luming, FamilyMed
Ford, Peter T., FamilyMed
Goebel, Cindy R., FamilyMed
Hanna, Mary, FamilyMed
Loewith, Brenda B.
McCallum, Kimberley C., FamilyMed
McMillan, Sharon K., FamilyMed
Namburi, Sriranjinee S., FamilyMed
Nash, E. Lynn I., FamilyMed
Nelson, John
Phillips, Karen E.
Piccinin, Susan S., FamilyMed
Slack, Irene S., FamilyMed
Stephenson, Michael J., FamilyMed
Trinh, Kien V., FamilyMed
Watters, William B.

ANGUS

Laforest, Jacques J.
Petts, Leslie A.
Seward, E. Glenn

ANNAN

Caulfeild, Roddy T., FamilyMed
Harada, Glenn K.

APSLEY

Rayes, Wagdy E A.
Slattery, Margaret A S.

ARKONA

Beattie, Robert A.
Johnson, Wayne D.

ARNPRIOR

Al Harbi, Faiz M F.
Ali, Asser A A., FamilyMed
Becker, Jennifer C., FamilyMed
Boersma, J. Robert
Borzecki, Mark P., FamilyMed(EM)
Carver, Glenn E.
Gordon, W. Earl
Kurian, Susan, FamilyMed
Massoud, Reza
McCarthy, Susanna M., FamilyMed
Morrison, Cynthia M., FamilyMed
Patterson, Andrew J., FamilyMed
Rivington, Jennifer H., FamilyMed
Robson, Mark G., FamilyMed
Schriver, Christine M., FamilyMed
Suzuki, Aya, FamilyMed
Trang, Nguyen, FamilyMed

ARTHUR

Bon, Lynton S.
Landoni, Thomas A.

ARVA

Doucette, Jacquelyn M.

ASTORVILLE

Seguin, John P., FamilyMed

ASTRA

Casey-Campbell, Mildred, FamilyMed
Ducros, Genevieve M., FamilyMed
Dyachuk, Elena, FamilyMed
Laird, Philip R., FamilyMed
Leon, Sebastian B.
Moreau, Kristina, FamilyMed
Welsh, Melissa E., FamilyMed
Worthy, Robert J., FamilyMed

ATHENS

Dodds, Mark, FamilyMed
Stobo, R. Benjamin, FamilyMed

ATIKOKAN

Barkman, Carla N., FamilyMed
Campanaro, Roberto M.
Clinton, Theresa F.
Fotheringham, John M., FamilyMed
Spencer, Joanne
Van Der Loo, Sara E., FamilyMed
Varty, Kimberly M., FamilyMed

AURORA

Bates, Carol E., FamilyMed
Berns, Trevor A., FamilyMed
Bhardwaj, Gaurav, FamilyMed
Boulanger, Maude, FamilyMed
Boulos, Shahira, FamilyMed
Bromberg, Rudy M., FamilyMed
Burstein, Lili M., FamilyMed
Chao, Sonia Y., FamilyMed(EM)
Chapnik, Victor H., FamilyMed
Chugh, Taher, FamilyMed
Curtis, Ronald D., FamilyMed
Fetherston, William H.
Gangani, Asmitha, FamilyMed
Garcia, Yelian, FamilyMed

Geoffroy, Pierre, FamilyMed
Hamilton, Michael J A., FamilyMed
Hicks, Todd D., FamilyMed
Hindocha, Sandeep P., FamilyMed
Idami, Wilson O., FamilyMed
Jugnundan, Pravesh, FamilyMed
Klassen, Lisa A., FamilyMed
Lea, Janice F C., FamilyMed
Leung, Kevin K., FamilyMed
Ma, Mona K S., FamilyMed
Maaskant, Lori M.
Matthew, Keith A.
Nabata, Elaine S.
Nicholas, Timothy G.
Russell, Elizabeth L., FamilyMed
Sadri, Daryoush, FamilyMed
Siraj, Naila, FamilyMed
Tanaka, Karen R., FamilyMed
Tanaka, Roderick T., FamilyMed
Tung, Amy S L., FamilyMed
Upadhyay, Amitkumar S., FamilyMed
Vant Voort, M. Joan, FamilyMed
Vavougios, George, FamilyMed
Waghmare, Raj, FamilyMed
Welchner, E. Jonathan
Williams, Robert E.
Windsor, Scott J., FamilyMed
Wong, Alice C N., FamilyMed
Yim-Lee, Famy L.
Yoneyama, Norma J., FamilyMed
Zakhary, Jena M I., FamilyMed

AYLMER

Botschner, Monika K.
Graham, David M., FamilyMed
Howe, B. Anne, FamilyMed
Sinclair, Duncan W.
Toogood, Jillian A.
Toth, Michael L., FamilyMed
Vivoda, Edward E., FamilyMed
Washburn, Robert M., FamilyMed

AYR

Jakda, Almas
Kurtzer, Barry D.
Page, Christopher R W.
Parker, Elaine, FamilyMed
Vlaar, Henry J.

AZILDA

Huneault, J. Gaetan O.

BALA

Krawetz, Michael
Patrick, David G., FamilyMed

BANCROFT

Brown, Carolyn J., FamilyMed
Calder, Douglas
Christiansen, Henrik S.
Cooper, Gregory R., FamilyMed
Doren, Denis M.
Fransky, Melissa K., FamilyMed
Gauthier, M. Todd, FamilyMed
Griffin, Steven R., FamilyMed
McEnery, Peter J., FamilyMed
Smith, Barry J., FamilyMed

BARRIE

Advent, Donald A.
AlAsaad, Hani G M.
Ali, Kevin, FamilyMed
Andersen, Lee K., FamilyMed
Armstrong, Thomas M.
Bailey, Joseph
Bajwa, Riffet R.
Baker, Blair, FamilyMed
Bauman, Shannon, FamilyMed
Baxter, Kenneth L.
Beecroft, D. John, FamilyMed
Belau, Marianne R., FamilyMed
Bickle, Robert, FamilyMed(EM)
Bilawski, Darlene, FamilyMed
Boba, Lukasz, FamilyMed(EM)
Bond, Geoffrey H., FamilyMed
Boushy, David, FamilyMed(EM)
Burghardt, Margaret, FamilyMed
Chan, Laura H Y., FamilyMed
Chaudhry, Shamsuddin, FamilyMed(EM)
Chen, William C Y.
Churchill, Gale A.
Clark, Carl I., FamilyMed
Cohen, Joanne P.
Collins, Douglas B., FamilyMed
Collins, Margaret J.
Cooney, Paul R H., FamilyMed
Cooper, Sari D., FamilyMed
Cousineau, Natalie J., FamilyMed(EM)
Crampton, Susan Y., FamilyMed
Cutbush, Wesley S., FamilyMed
Da Costa, Michael S.
Da Silva, Anna-Maria, FamilyMed
Dalziel, Peter
Davidson, Shannon, FamilyMed
Dickson, Colin
Doorly, Patrick
Duvall, Anne, FamilyMed
Elsey, Brent
Emerson, Kelly J., FamilyMed
Fabian, Werner A.
Farooq, Tarik A., FamilyMed
Fejes, Piroska R.
Fischer, Krista L., FamilyMed
Friesen, Nelson D.
Gabor, Robert Z., FamilyMed
Gebien, Darryl
Giorshev, Chris, FamilyMed(EM)
Goudie, Richard, FamilyMed
Grant, Andrew N., FamilyMed(EM)
Haig, Cynthia L., FamilyMed
Haines, Alexander M.
Handley, David
Harman, John K., FamilyMed
Harris, Wendy M.
Heidarpour Meymeh, Reza, FamilyMed
Hoogeveen, Paul, FamilyMed(EM)
Howard, Douglas J., FamilyMed(EM)
Howard, Paul L., FamilyMed(EM)
Iraji, Mandana, FamilyMed
Johnson, Sandra M.
Karasmanis, George N., FamilyMed(EM)
Kargel, Caroline S., FamilyMed(EM)
Khatami, Kian, FamilyMed
Kiss, Erzsebet B., FamilyMed
Kizoff, Peter
Koifman, Rolan, FamilyMed
Korkola, Darrell
Kostenuik, Marcia A., FamilyMed
Krieger, Howard M.
Ku, James L Y.
Kumar, Rajat
Lalik, Christopher A., FamilyMed
Lee, Edward Y., FamilyMed
Levine, Gerald M., FamilyMed
Lewis-Watts, Robert J., FamilyMed
Li, Qinglu, FamilyMed
Lin, Jackson M K., FamilyMed
Lindsay, D. Ian
Lopez-Alonso, Jose O., FamilyMed
MacLean, Tanya M., FamilyMed
Mackesy, J T. Derek
Malik, Nazir A.
Mall, Omar, FamilyMed
Martin, Deborah L., FamilyMed(EM)
Maxwell, Robert I.
May, Andre B., FamilyMed(EM)
McConvey, Michael J., FamilyMed
McKee, John D., FamilyMed
McNally, Linda J., FamilyMed
McNaughton, Jennifer L., FamilyMed
McTurk, Bruce E.
Merry, Graham F.
Mills, Thomas P D.
Moldes, Andrea P., FamilyMed
Morin, Brent D., FamilyMed
Morris, Brian A P., FamilyMed
Mossman, Kerstin, FamilyMed
Mozaffari, Babak, FamilyMed
Murdoch, Stuart A., FamilyMed
Northcott, Rosemary D E., FamilyMed(EM)
Olynyk, Kimberley A., FamilyMed
Onlock, Stephen G., FamilyMed(EM)
Ozimok, Daniel
Parbtani, Anwar, FamilyMed
Pattison, Leslie D.
Pauk, Tomas M., FamilyMed
Poonja, Zahir, FamilyMed
Rampton, Joey V., FamilyMed(EM)
Rapson, Valerie E., FamilyMed
Ruddock, David G S., FamilyMed
Sachar, Seerat
Sacksen, Alain J B., FamilyMed
Schulze, Richard H.
Seaman, Kenneth L.
Sharma, Niti, FamilyMed
Shaver, James H., FamilyMed
Shaver, Laurie E., FamilyMed
Shourideh-Ziabari, Sayed M A., FamilyMed
Skory, Leah M., FamilyMed
Slivko, Tatiana, FamilyMed
Smith, Frederick B.
Springle, Stephen W.
Stanford, Timothy R., FamilyMed
Steciuk, Paige E., FamilyMed
Steffens, Gregory M., FamilyMed
Stewart, Christine E., FamilyMed
Strangway, James F.
Syed, Abdul R.
Szelag, Marek A., FamilyMed
Tanton, Robert L., FamilyMed
Taylor, William L.
Thompson, Carly A., FamilyMed(EM)
Trimble, Nancy E., FamilyMed
Tyler, James B.
Van Volkingburgh, David R.
Van Zyl, Leendert P C.
Vanderwater, Charles L.
Waterman, Heather L., FamilyMed(EM)
Weber, Stacie D., FamilyMed
Whyne, Mitchell S.
Wilson, Paul R.
Witty, Melissa J., FamilyMed
Wolnik, Monica S., FamilyMed(EM)
Wood, Nancy L., FamilyMed
Wozniak, Andrew E.
Wright, Kelley M., FamilyMed
Young, Dana G., FamilyMed
Young, Ian G., FamilyMed

BARRYS BAY

Coulas, Denise P., FamilyMed
Cybulski, Joseph B., FamilyMed
Dawes, C. Raymond S., FamilyMed
MacGillivray, Patrick S., FamilyMed
Malinowski, Jason R J., FamilyMed

BATH

Standley, Jonathan M S.
Wyatt, Diana S.

BAYFIELD

Curtis, Michael A., FamilyMed
Schmitz, Carmen J., FamilyMed
Wallace, Charles J.

BEACHBURG

Daniel, Angus, FamilyMed
Rheaume, Teresa A I.

BEAMSVILLE

Aliu, Teuta, FamilyMed
Aube, Anne, FamilyMed
Biscotti, Marilena, FamilyMed
Habing, David K., FamilyMed
Ireland, Ronald M., FamilyMed
Laverdiere, Ginette M B., FamilyMed
MacEwen, Melissa D., FamilyMed
Martin, Christopher G., FamilyMed
Morrison, Douglas
Peters, William B., FamilyMed
Pillay, Nemi N., FamilyMed
Reed, Cari L., FamilyMed
Savatteri, Michael, FamilyMed
Stacpoole, Rebecca A., FamilyMed
Taylor, Stephen A., FamilyMed
Volz, Bernhard A., FamilyMed
Wall, Leah K., FamilyMed
Woodland, James P., FamilyMed
Zeyl, Thomas, FamilyMed

BEAVERTON

Laudanski, Gerald J.
McCordic, D. Frances
Vinden, G. Dickson

BELLE RIVER

Abdul Hameed, Saleema, FamilyMed
Jezdic, Dusanka D.
Li Wan Po, James Y L.
MacKinnon, Peter M.

BELLEVILLE

Agoston, Hanga, FamilyMed
Allen, Katherine P., FamilyMed
Allin, Jeffrey C.
Bates, Robert
Bates, William F.
Bell, Allan C., FamilyMed(EM)
Bolton, Craig J., FamilyMed(EM)
Bonacci, Giuseppe, FamilyMed
Boyce, Frank G.
Brearley, Donald T.
Brown, Ciara E., FamilyMed
Brown, Marty H., FamilyMed
Bryson, Julie C., FamilyMed
Charriere, Norma M E., FamilyMed
Coady, John E., FamilyMed
Cunningham, William L.
Devins, Robert L.
Dobbs, Ryan C., FamilyMed
Dolan, James
Esperanzate, Patrick, FamilyMed
Forbes, Andrew J., FamilyMed
Goddard-Hill, Alban C., FamilyMed
Goodall, Robert J.
Gray, Peter, FamilyMed
Hamilton, John G., FamilyMed
Hamilton-Irving, Jonathan, FamilyMed(EM)
Hayes, William A.
Holder, Chanse L., FamilyMed
Holton, Gordon R., FamilyMed
Istead, Jannice M.
Kerr, Jonathan R., FamilyMed
Knarr, Nadia K., FamilyMed
Liew, Chiam L., FamilyMed
Lisowski, David F J.
Livingstone, Christopher J., FamilyMed
Lodhen, Tenzin, FamilyMed
Low, Catherine M.
Lynch, Jennifer A., FamilyMed
MacLean, James E W.
MacLeod, Kim S., FamilyMed
Manderville, Eugene A., FamilyMed
Maraj, Ramsarran
Mason, James I A., FamilyMed
McDonald, Lois M., FamilyMed(EM)
McPhail, Janice E.
Miron, M. Michele, FamilyMed(EM)
Nguyen, Tuyet Thi, FamilyMed
Noronha, Osborne I.
Nyholt, Noranda, FamilyMed
Pincock, Robert J., FamilyMed
Reid, James N., FamilyMed
Rubio, Dominador B.
Savic, Mile, FamilyMed
Sherlock, Donald R., FamilyMed
Shipley, William F., FamilyMed
Simmons, Maureen L., FamilyMed
Sloan, Ryan W.
Smith, Eric W., FamilyMed
Sorensen, Kyla M., FamilyMed
Steinitz, Tracy L F., FamilyMed(EM)
Tam, Kin-Hung
Truman, Tony L., FamilyMed
Vasquez, Raul A., FamilyMed
Vukojevic, Duska
Walsh, Ronald J.
Weatherall, Paul I.
Webster, Jennifer D., FamilyMed
Webster, W. Robert W., FamilyMed
Whelan, Jennifer, FamilyMed
Wilkins, Paul J., FamilyMed

BINBROOK

Juriansz, Brian D.

BLENHEIM

Clendenning, Martha K., FamilyMed
Morrison, Allan F.
Perkin, Thomas R., FamilyMed
Sherwin, Elizabeth A., FamilyMed
Wheeler, James K., FamilyMed

BLIND RIVER

Barnes, Christopher H.
Bradford, Marc S.
Deverell, Mark A V.
Fowler, Mark A.
Panabaker, J. Paul
Peer, Ismail G M.
Shamas, Mary E., FamilyMed

BOBCAYGEON

Oldridge, Stephen C., FamilyMed
Snarr, M. Michelle, FamilyMed

BOLTON

Adam, Abbas F Y., FamilyMed
Adenwala, Tasneem, FamilyMed
Ames, Robert P E.
Birnie, Stuart A.
Black, Jason T., FamilyMed
Bodok, Rebecca, FamilyMed
El Khouly, Nihal, FamilyMed
Francis, Amira, FamilyMed
Gagnon, Michael P., FamilyMed
Kacer, Milan R R.
Kankaria, Pratibha, FamilyMed
Khan, Fariha S., FamilyMed
Madonik, Michael L.
Meghory, Yehiel C., FamilyMed
Niedoba, Joseph E.
Peirce, Karen L., FamilyMed
Pinto, Angelo
Quint, Saul
Rafiqi, Wajahat H., FamilyMed
Rizk, Sarah Z Y H.
Romanescu, Craita A., FamilyMed
Schmalfuss, Peter E H.
Siddiqui, Farhan, FamilyMed(EM)
Simmons, James D.
Smullen, Merril J.
Takhar, Amitoj K., FamilyMed
Trigazis, Leonidas, FamilyMed
Wagman, David M.
Weicker, Constance M., FamilyMed

BONFIELD

Truchon, Michel L.

BORDEN

Andrews Alexander, Amy L E., FamilyMed
Bass, Catherine J., FamilyMed
Beaudry, Josianne E., FamilyMed
Benninger, Shawn J., FamilyMed
Britt-Cote, Maxime S R., FamilyMed
Brooks, Tyler D P., FamilyMed
Casault, David J R., FamilyMed
Culic, Cherie A., FamilyMed
Currie, Andrew B.
Lyte, Kristina, FamilyMed
MacDonald, Lorraine A., FamilyMed
Marshall, Luke A., FamilyMed
Morin, Richard H., FamilyMed
Newnham, Darlene J., FamilyMed

BOURGET

Lusignan, Daniel E., FamilyMed

BOWMANVILLE

Ahmed, Ishtiaq, FamilyMed
Ali, Durya, FamilyMed
Azi, Adaku M., FamilyMed
Belfon, Ahmad E.
Bharucha, Pheroze, FamilyMed
Bisset, Lindsay J., FamilyMed(EM)
Boskovic, Radinka R., FamilyMed
Brown-Shreves, Danielle N., FamilyMed
Burke, Howard M., FamilyMed
Calhoun, Kevin W.
Chou, Angela, FamilyMed
Cioata Tomsa, Elena, FamilyMed
Corpus, Teofilo, FamilyMed
Dye, Audrey A., FamilyMed
Fuller, Benjamin R., FamilyMed(EM)
Ho, Elaine P L., FamilyMed
Ho, Vincent W K., FamilyMed
Hollander, Andree L., FamilyMed(EM)
Hoy, Paul J., FamilyMed
Irish, Leon D.
Ladak, Rahim A., FamilyMed
Lennox, Catherine L., FamilyMed
Lombardi, Rocco A., FamilyMed(EM)
Lottering, Wilraad, FamilyMed(EM)
Majeed, Sonilla, FamilyMed
Mazengia, Getachew, FamilyMed
Moolla, Riaz, FamilyMed
Nijmeh, Larry J., FamilyMed
Omiwole, Olufemi O., FamilyMed
Osborne, Edward J., FamilyMed
Palencar-Frost, Adriana, FamilyMed
Quadir, Shamima S., FamilyMed
Rundle, John D.
Sivapalan, Shivajan, FamilyMed
Stone, Anthony B., FamilyMed
Subramaniam, Tharani, FamilyMed
Ward, Michael A., FamilyMed
Williams, Harvey R., FamilyMed
Zubair, Naeem A.

BRACEBRIDGE

Adamson, Sandra C., FamilyMed
Bawa, Faizal I., FamilyMed
Bridle, H. Terrance
Brokenshire, Jennifer S., FamilyMed(EM)
Cross, Keith R., FamilyMed
Daabak, Abdulghani M., FamilyMed
Dechert, K. Victoria
Griffioen, Timothy
Harmon, Christopher G., FamilyMed
Hemens, William D., FamilyMed
Holman, Terry G.
Hotson, Kenneth E., FamilyMed
Hutchinson, Vivien
Kappos, Stamatina, FamilyMed
Kent, David C., FamilyMed
Kents, Kersti, FamilyMed(EM)
Kirstein, Florian P., FamilyMed
Liao, Liang Ying
Martin, Karen A.
McGregor, David B.
Mitchell, Barry A., FamilyMed
Petrie, Matthew D., FamilyMed(EM)
Phillips, Kent M., FamilyMed
Richardson, Christopher W., FamilyMed
Richardson, John W., FamilyMed
Riddle, Gordon E., FamilyMed
Sansom, Robert M., FamilyMed
Shearing, Anthony D., FamilyMed
Weaver, William G.
Williams, Walter S.

BRADFORD

Barcza, Lawrence Z.
Dheda, Roshan M., FamilyMed
Dief, Ashraf, FamilyMed
Hsin, Mabel
Hu, Fang, FamilyMed
Kuzmyk, Susan M., FamilyMed
Shah, Himanshu H., FamilyMed
Taylor, Brian V.
Tsang, Andy H K.
Wilson, Murray B.
Zadhoush, Kourosh, FamilyMed

BRAMPTON

Abdel Meguid, Abdel M K.
Abdul Hadi, Deema S O., FamilyMed
Abdulhusein, Mustafa H.
Abidi, Rabbiya N., FamilyMed
Abraham, Gary C.
Abu-Abed, Mohamed I., FamilyMed
Agarwal, Sanjay, FamilyMed(EM)
Aggarwal, Anita, FamilyMed(EM)
Aggarwal, Naresh K., FamilyMed
Ali, Salah-Eddin, FamilyMed
Alikhan, Riyaaz, FamilyMed(EM)
Amin, Parsa F., FamilyMed
Ananthan, Jean P., FamilyMed
Aptekar, Nafisa J., FamilyMed
Arora, Rajeev K., FamilyMed
Arya, Amit, FamilyMed
Asekomhe, Ikhimhaigie F., FamilyMed
Aspin, Derek G.
Atalla, Maher G Y., FamilyMed
Atcha, Farida, FamilyMed
Attalla, Mona S G., FamilyMed
Badhan, Harry S.
Baily, Mark I.
Bajaj, Harminder P S.
Bajaj, Harpreet S.
Bandali, Ashraf M.
Banerjee, Lopita, FamilyMed
Bansal, Praveen, FamilyMed
Bariana, Sam S., FamilyMed
Bath, Parvinder S., FamilyMed
Baumander, Donald
Beard, Lisa L., FamilyMed
Bennett, Alison M., FamilyMed
Bernard, Afiya, FamilyMed
Bernard, Carrie D., FamilyMed
Best, Adrienne, FamilyMed(EM)
Bhayana, Satinder K., FamilyMed
Bhyat, Rashaad, FamilyMed
Blachford, Patricia
Blechschmidt, Donald R., FamilyMed
Borkar-Aggarwal, Monica D., FamilyMed
Bose, Tarun K., FamilyMed
Bradford, Steven R.
Brar, Harpreet S., FamilyMed
Bruner, Harvey
Budhiraja, Inderpreet S., FamilyMed
Bunn, Roger C., FamilyMed
Butcher, Douglas S.
Byrne, Paul J.
Caplan, Jason A., FamilyMed
Carabott, Paul
Chain-Chang, Marybelle M T.
Chakravarti, Neetu, FamilyMed
Chanchlani, Jayshree
Chandra, Prakash
Chatterjee, Kali S.
Chaudhry, Sapna, FamilyMed
Cheema, Kiran J., FamilyMed
Cheema, Waqar M., FamilyMed
Chen, John S C., FamilyMed(EM)
Chen, Wendell E., FamilyMed
Cherepacha, Douglas L., FamilyMed
Cheskes, Sheldon, FamilyMed(EM)
Cheung, Simon S., FamilyMed
Chiang, Christopher K C., FamilyMed
Chou, George C., FamilyMed
Choudhry, Sushil, FamilyMed
Chowdhury, Ruma, FamilyMed
Chowdry, Seema, FamilyMed
Chuang, Ching C.
Chudnow, Gloria
Clarke, Natasha C T., FamilyMed
Collins, Caroline P., FamilyMed
Cooper, Judith A.
Cox, Ronald H.
Crewson, Marolyn M., FamilyMed
Crystal, Sam
D'Souza, Sameer D., FamilyMed
Davids, Jonathan W., FamilyMed
De Groot, Grant G., FamilyMed
Dennis, Stephen M.
Devon, Joshua G.
Dhadwar, Achinder K., FamilyMed
Dhaliwal, Amarinder S.
Dhaliwal, Jaskaren K., FamilyMed
Dhillon, Anureet, FamilyMed
Dhillon, Manu
Diamond, Catherine, FamilyMed
Dobson, Peter E., FamilyMed
DuBois, Denise M.
Dutta, Sidharth, FamilyMed
Earle, Harry T.
Ebrahim, Farouk A., FamilyMed
El-Madah, Hesham, FamilyMed
Fahim, Maged I., FamilyMed
Farooq, Bushra, FamilyMed
Fatima, Anis
Ferlisi, Mary-Claire, FamilyMed
Forbes, Frederick B T.
Francis, Patricia K., FamilyMed
Garay, Michael E., FamilyMed(EM)
Garg, Narinder K., FamilyMed
Gin, Christopher S W., FamilyMed
Girgis, Ireen, FamilyMed
Glass, Lisa B.
Glover, John
Gnanatissa, Asha S., FamilyMed
Goel, Reena, FamilyMed
Goel, Sanjeev, FamilyMed
Gohil, J. Girishdhai
Gohil, Jyotsna
Goldberg, Norman V.
Gopinath, Malar, FamilyMed
Goyal, Kimmy, FamilyMed
Graham, John D., FamilyMed(EM)
Grainger, Fredric R., FamilyMed
Greenspoon, Mark B.
Greenwood, Eric D.
Grewal, Kamal P., FamilyMed
Grewal, Kharak S.
Grewal, Manavdeep, FamilyMed
Gupta, Anjalee, FamilyMed
Gupta, Nikhil
Gupta, Ram, FamilyMed
Hamboyan, Herag, FamilyMed
Handler, Jeffrey D., FamilyMed(EM)
Hanna, Ivan W.
Hasham, Parviz M.
Hawass, Ammar N.
Hayward, Susan L., FamilyMed
Heffernan, Patrick A T., FamilyMed
Hennes, Claire S., FamilyMed
Herman, Bruce A., FamilyMed
Ho, Adrian W J.
Hoornweg, Karen L., FamilyMed
Hurdle, Maureen, FamilyMed
Husain, Juhi
Hussain, Riaz, FamilyMed
Ibrahim, Sarwat, FamilyMed
Jacobson, Perry A.
Jaidka, Rajesh
Jailall, Davindra N.
Jamieson, Donald M.
Jeevanandam, Sivagami
Jivan, Verandra P., FamilyMed
Johnson, Andrew N., FamilyMed
Joza, Eva V.
Juneja, Romi, FamilyMed
Kaiser, William J., FamilyMed
Kamawi, Malalai, FamilyMed
Kapoor, Vikram J., FamilyMed
Kassam, Hassanali A.
Kaur, Navpreet, FamilyMed
Kaveri Selvan, Kaveri M., FamilyMed
Kazdan, David M., FamilyMed
Kelly, Alvin G.
Kelly, J. Calvin
Kemp, Robert A., FamilyMed
Keogh, J. Thomas, FamilyMed
Khan, Farhana A., FamilyMed
Khan, Mujtaba A., FamilyMed
Khasimuddin, Syed A.
Khawaja, Noumaan, FamilyMed
Kidy, A. Razak
Kim, James S J.
Kini, Vishwas M., FamilyMed
Kivlichan, Robert M.
Kostopoulos, Elen, FamilyMed
Kristof, Lorand
Kular, Kuldip S.
Kwong, Jennifer M., FamilyMed(EM)
Kwong, T Y. Paul
Langer, Lorne J.
Lee, Julia, FamilyMed
Lee, Khong-Yam
Lee, Robin
Leggatt, W. Ker, FamilyMed
Leibovitz, Neil V., FamilyMed
Levine, Noah C., FamilyMed
Li, Gene S J., FamilyMed
Lielmanis, Andris, FamilyMed
Lily, Muriel, FamilyMed
Lobo, Louella S., FamilyMed
Lodhi, Shariq J., FamilyMed
Logan, David A.
Loka, Safaa G T., FamilyMed
Lucas, William J.
Lui, Frederick C C.
Lusis, Janis G.
Luu, Lien Ngoc, FamilyMed
MacDonald, Steven J.
Madan, Pooja
Mak, Manson M T., FamilyMed(EM)
Malam, Faiz G., FamilyMed
Malhotra, Verinder
Malik, Abdul, FamilyMed
Malik, Anupam
Manacki, Leonard A., FamilyMed
Manning, Hubert
Manson, Nadine E F., FamilyMed
Martino, Frank A., FamilyMed(EM)
Masood, Asim
Master, Suketu
Masterson, Grainne M., FamilyMed
Masud, Chaudhry F., FamilyMed
Mathew, Roy K T., FamilyMed
Matta, Ihab
Maynard, Judith A., FamilyMed
McCaffrey, Michael J.
McCallion, Alexander
McClure, Christine J.
McCurdy, John
McQuibban, George A.
Mehta, Chetan, FamilyMed
Mehta, Tushar, FamilyMed
Merker, Darren L., FamilyMed
Merker, Donald S.
Midha, Vishal M., FamilyMed
Mikhail, Boutros B., FamilyMed
Millar, Barbara J., FamilyMed
Millar, David C S.
Milner, Maurice F J.
Mistry, Ritesh K H., FamilyMed
Mitchell, Jacqueline R., FamilyMed
Molnar, Geza B.
Moody, Jeremy W.
Morris, Lauralee R., FamilyMed
Murtoza, Golam, FamilyMed
Myat, Khin M., FamilyMed
Nadeem, Taj G., FamilyMed
Nagpal, Rohit S., FamilyMed
Najarali, A. Ali
Nelles, C. Ruth M.
Nguyen, The-Huy
Niece, Donald P.
Niesobska, Violetta, FamilyMed
Nixon, Jane E M.
Noor, Mounir H A., FamilyMed
O'Neill, Patrick S.
Okafor, Innocent C., FamilyMed
Ortiz-Singh, Janice
Palmer, Dale P.
Palombo, Alessandra D., FamilyMed
Parbhakar, Samir R.
Paribello, Carlo
Pede, Leili, FamilyMed
Peoples, Brian J.
Pereira, Jeffery
Persaud, Jeeshan, FamilyMed
Phalpher, Prashant, FamilyMed(EM)
Piche, Janelle R M., FamilyMed(EM)
Pirzada, Kashif S., FamilyMed(EM)
Poitier, Myles R., FamilyMed
Poon, Jackson C., FamilyMed
Qaisy, Yehia S., FamilyMed
Rajarathna, Mallika P A., FamilyMed
Rao, Geetha, FamilyMed
Rasheed, Nida H., FamilyMed
Ratnasingam, Ranjith K., FamilyMed
Rattan, Simran K., FamilyMed
Rayar, Anusha D., FamilyMed
Rodrigues, Arthur F.
Rogers, Kieran A.
Romain, Sandra, FamilyMed
Rossnagel, Arthur P.
Russell, Alan L.
Sabri, Rida A., FamilyMed
Saggar, Barjinder, FamilyMed
Saha, Sudip K.
Saini, Mukesh C.
Salciccioli, Paul, FamilyMed
Salehi, Leila, FamilyMed(EM)
Sandhu, Jasbir K.
Sandhu, Parampal S., FamilyMed
Sandhu, Roop K., FamilyMed
Sarai, Didar S., FamilyMed
Saraza, Milagros F.
Saroya, Satinder K., FamilyMed
Sasan, Amritpal S.
Savard, Guylene
Sebastian, Anthony R.
Sediq, Aimal, FamilyMed
Sequeira, Donovan S.
Shah, Sameer, FamilyMed
Shaheen, Nighat, FamilyMed
Shaikh, Vaquas M., FamilyMed
Shams, Nagi S A., FamilyMed
Shariff, Shiraz B K.
Sharma, Ashu T.
Sharma, Sanjeev, FamilyMed
Shehata, Ester N E., FamilyMed
Shenouda, Nancy M S., FamilyMed
Shilash, Basil M A., FamilyMed
Sidhu, Gurmeet, FamilyMed
Sidhu, Surinder S.
Siegel, Irving J.
Sinajon, Romulo M.
Singaram, Dharumaraj, FamilyMed
Singh, Amandeep
Singh, Harleen, FamilyMed
Singh, Navpreet, FamilyMed
Singh, Parvinder, FamilyMed
Singh, Shiv P., FamilyMed
Sippy, Rajinder K., FamilyMed
Siyam, Sheima A M M., FamilyMed
Snape, Clive
Sohn, Melanie, FamilyMed(EM)
Song, John J., FamilyMed
Sothilingam, Subramanian, FamilyMed

PHYSICIANS BY PROVINCE

Sotto, Alain G.
Sourial, Fibi B W., FamilyMed
Sues-McKay, Heather A., FamilyMed(EM)
Sunner, Sohail, FamilyMed
Suppal, Priya, FamilyMed
Syslak, Paul H., FamilyMed
Szulc, Elizabeth K.
Tariq, Hanzla, FamilyMed
Tautkus, Robert F., FamilyMed
Teape-Humphrey, Lorna T., FamilyMed
Teper, Shane H., FamilyMed(EM)
Theobald, Geoffrey M.
Thicke, Brian C.
Thirugnanasampanthapillai, Vakeesan, FamilyMed
Toman, John D.
Tracey, John P., FamilyMed
Tynan, Maebh E., FamilyMed
Uppal, Rakesh
Vaidyanathan, Sankar, FamilyMed
Vakeesan, Sivaraji, FamilyMed
Vanlerberghe, Kenneth R., FamilyMed
Vanvat, Jarnail S., FamilyMed
Varughese, Jobin
Vayalumkal, Philip X., FamilyMed(EM)
Veenema, Christopher T., FamilyMed
Veenstra, Jacob
Vijh, Meeta, FamilyMed
Virdee, Manjit S., FamilyMed
Visvanatha, Susmita A., FamilyMed
Wadehra, Davinder B S.
Waitschies, Elfriede G.
Wali, Dilip
Waraich, Ihsan U., FamilyMed
Whitney, J. David
Wielecki, Sylvia D.
Wiens, Donald E., FamilyMed
Wong, Simone N., FamilyMed(EM)
Wudom, Kofi A., FamilyMed
Wylie, James R.
Yakub, Abu M.
Yang, Malissa
Yong-Set, Wrenrick E.
Yu, Philip H F.
Zakhary, Mariam R., FamilyMed
Zekulin, Anthony G.
Zettle, Randy M., FamilyMed(EM)

BRANTFORD

Ahmed, Diana R., FamilyMed
Alagic, Emer, FamilyMed
Allen, Donna B., FamilyMed
Arfali, Erfan, FamilyMed(EM)
Arora, Nawaz, FamilyMed
Auchinachie, Keith T.
Bahra, Parminder S., FamilyMed(EM)
Baker, Alison D., FamilyMed
Bannister, Leslie R., FamilyMed
Benoit, Jean-Marc, FamilyMed(EM)
Busche, Karen L., FamilyMed(EM)
Cameron, David A., FamilyMed
Charlton, Scott T., FamilyMed
Chipman, Nancy L.
Cicoria, Eugenio
Colborne, Brian J., FamilyMed(EM)
Collins, Carola J D., FamilyMed
Comley, Rebecca A., FamilyMed(EM)
Connelly, Anne Marie., FamilyMed
Damboragama, Shyamali, FamilyMed
Desai, Jagdish
Dhillon, Jaswinder S., FamilyMed(EM)
Dhillon, Jatinder S.
Douglas, Anne E., FamilyMed
Dwyer, Kevin C J J.
Elliott, Lori T., FamilyMed(EM)
Elliott, Scott H., FamilyMed
Frey, Lisa, FamilyMed
Galliver, Robert
Germa, Fikre A., FamilyMed(EM)
Gharib, Shler, FamilyMed
Gladstone, Julie A., FamilyMed
Gorcsi, Mary Ann, FamilyMed
Goscimski, Jacqueline, FamilyMed
Grabner, Claudia J.
Gregoire, Lucie H.
Hadley, John D., FamilyMed
Hall, Gregory S., FamilyMed(EM)
Hanley, Catherine L.
Hassan, Ali
Hilsden, Shannon, FamilyMed
Ho, Edward S.
Holmes, Alan R., FamilyMed
Hsiao, Jerry L C.
Ilo, Mary P., FamilyMed(EM)
Im, Tae-Bin T.
Irvine, James E., FamilyMed(EM)
Jarrell, Eugene G., FamilyMed(EM)
Jocic, D. Anna, FamilyMed(EM)
Kents, Ilmar J.
Khan, Raza M., FamilyMed
Kramer, Larry P.
Langton, E. Michelle, FamilyMed
Lavelle, Peter R.
Leach, Leslie A., FamilyMed
Lee, W. Leslie
Legere, Janice M.
Lock, Malcolm S.
Locke, Carolynne
Lowcock, Donald G., FamilyMed
MacIntyre, John D.
Manning, Jeff A., FamilyMed
McNeil, Bernadette
McQueen, Jodi L., FamilyMed(EM)
Minos, Nick, FamilyMed
Montour, Laura, FamilyMed
Murray, Michael R., FamilyMed
Nikore, Veena
Opper, David B., FamilyMed
Plant, Sandi L., FamilyMed
Prowse, Sheryl L.
Quinlan, Paul J.
Quinn, Gerard, FamilyMed
Rahman, K M. Anisur, FamilyMed
Raja, Mohan K., FamilyMed
Rajpura, Anjum, FamilyMed
Rowlands, Donna R., FamilyMed(EM)
Safar, Gregory C., FamilyMed(EM)
Scott, Kirk J I., FamilyMed
Shcherbatykh, Ivan Y., FamilyMed
Shott, Craig A., FamilyMed
Sidhu, Gurpreet S.
Singh, Ruby, FamilyMed
Spaxman, Thomas L., FamilyMed
Spicer, Dwight L., FamilyMed
Stahlbrand, Erik A.
Stone, James M.
Story, Betty-Anne, FamilyMed
Suszek, J. Jeffrey G., FamilyMed(EM)
Swan, Donald W.
Thompson, David K., FamilyMed
Thompson, Elizabeth B.
Trevor, Andrew W.
Tsuchida, William S.
Ullman, Doris B., FamilyMed
Unger, Andrea G., FamilyMed(EM)
Vincent, David C., FamilyMed
Wells, Stephen C.
Wiwcharuk, Gillian L., FamilyMed
Wysynski, Anna-Marie
Zohoor, Arash, FamilyMed

BRECHIN

Brand, Christopher P., FamilyMed
Jamal, Zeeya, FamilyMed

BRESLAU

Schaman, John P.

BRIDGENORTH

Bell, Thomas W G., FamilyMed
Motyer, Michael I S., FamilyMed
Rutledge, David F., FamilyMed
Shannon, William R., FamilyMed
Wilkins, Margaret A., FamilyMed

BRIGHTON

Cohen, Michelle J., FamilyMed
Larmer, James, FamilyMed
MacIntyre, M. Arlene, FamilyMed
Twiddy, Ronald R.
Wiginton, Richard J.

BROCKVILLE

Argue, Donald R.
Ashe, Gerald P., FamilyMed
Au, Ambrose S S., FamilyMed
Audet, William M.
Barton, Douglas G., FamilyMed(EM)
Beattie, David, FamilyMed
Best, Sandra J.
Brambilla, Christa C., FamilyMed
Brooks, Donald G.
Brown, C. Elizabeth A., FamilyMed(EM)
Damji, Zumil, FamilyMed(EM)
Davis, Lestrod A.
Dufour, Daniel M., FamilyMed
Ebert, Daniel, FamilyMed(EM)
Everett, Andrew, FamilyMed(EM)
Gill, Sarbjit S.
Gulati, Sanjiv K.
Haywood-Farmer, Eric, FamilyMed(EM)
Hodgson, Todd R., FamilyMed
Holmes, David N P.
Irvine, Rebecca E., FamilyMed
Jaworski, Anne-France M.
Jordan, Andrew
Jordan, David D.
Kolbe, George A., FamilyMed
Lasich, Jonathan F.
Lauf, Walter W.
Lee, Hoi Kwan
Lo, Lydia C L., FamilyMed
Low, Charles T., FamilyMed
Mansworth, M. Colman
McFeely, Neil H.
McMurray, Stephen J., FamilyMed(EM)
Pajot, Denise M., FamilyMed
Redekopp, Alan W.
Riyaz, Samreen H., FamilyMed
Ruparelia, Meera, FamilyMed
Shenfield, Leisa J., FamilyMed(EM)
Slowey, Alistair
Slowey, Patricia I.
Steacie, Adam D., FamilyMed
Steyn, Mariette, FamilyMed
Thomas, Andrew J., FamilyMed
Tolton, Rani G., FamilyMed
Torres Martinez, Nestor E., FamilyMed
Trail, Carla N., FamilyMed
Van Jaarsveld, Barend P., FamilyMed
Wagg, Brian D., FamilyMed
Wilson, James B., FamilyMed(EM)
Zouros, Irene A., FamilyMed(EM)

BROOKLIN

Cairns, Brenda D.
Derrick, Susan M., FamilyMed
Libby, T. Phillip, FamilyMed
McAllister, Caroline D., FamilyMed
Roy, William A.
Turek, Caroline A.

BRUCE MINES

Haapala, Eric M., FamilyMed
Jinot, Christopher P., FamilyMed
McLeod, Janet A., FamilyMed

BUCKHORN

Ferrier, C J. Scott
Mallory, Jonathan G., FamilyMed

BURFORD

Mohammed, Nurhull H.
Ozog-Bartlett, Joanne L., FamilyMed
Quinlan, Philip L.

BURKS FALLS

Albert, Andrew, FamilyMed
Apramian, David A., FamilyMed
De Roode, Michael, FamilyMed
Dempster, David W.
Vohra, Rajat, FamilyMed

BURLINGTON

Abdelhussein, Hussein S., FamilyMed
Abuelalaa, Enas, FamilyMed
Ahmed, Sabera, FamilyMed
Ahmed, Sadaf K., FamilyMed
Ali Al-Kazely, Luay H., FamilyMed
Amaladoss, Antony S J.
Archibald, Susy R., FamilyMed
Arshat, Daoud J D., FamilyMed
Arumugam, Bhavani, FamilyMed
Aziz, Samir B., FamilyMed(EM)
Barker, Leslie K.
Barry, Patricia E., FamilyMed
Beasley, Debra E., FamilyMed
Boucher, Michael, FamilyMed
Bradford, John P.
Brodie, Dennis J T., FamilyMed
Calvert, Lynn C.
Cameron, Brian W., FamilyMed
Candia, Pascual R., FamilyMed
Carruthers, Benjamin C.
Chalklin, Lori W., FamilyMed
Charman, Sandra M., FamilyMed
Chemparathy, Joseph V., FamilyMed
Chemparathy, Sheela J., FamilyMed
Chiu, Brendan B S.
Chow, Maria C., FamilyMed
Cobus, Peter A.
Comeau, B. Keith, FamilyMed
Conners, Jennifer A.
Costin, Thomas B.
Cuddy, Timothy J., FamilyMed
Daniel, Alan B., FamilyMed
Davis, Amie, FamilyMed
De Santis, Teresa A., FamilyMed(EM)
Diamond, Carolyn K., FamilyMed
Duncan, G. Stephen, FamilyMed
Durcan, Thomas J G., FamilyMed
Echlin, Paul S., FamilyMed
Elliott, Wade C., FamilyMed
Evans, William T.
Faulkner, Paul E., FamilyMed(EM)
Fornasier, Frank, FamilyMed
Foster, Michael J.
Gallaccio, Alicia A., FamilyMed
Galloway, Victoria A., FamilyMed
Garic, Mirjana, FamilyMed
Garland, Marie S., FamilyMed
Ghali, Ashraf M., FamilyMed
Goel, Sunita, FamilyMed
Grewal, Puneet, FamilyMed
Grzeslo, Adam G Z., FamilyMed
Gupta, Anjali
Hack, Arshad, FamilyMed
Hadi, Ali, FamilyMed
Hajcsar, Elizabeth M., FamilyMed
Hajcsar, Ernest E., FamilyMed
Hanna Sarsam, Haithem S., FamilyMed
Hannon, Patricia J.
Hargot, Leonard
Harricharan, Tanujaa, FamilyMed
Hogarth, Margaret T., FamilyMed
Holmes, John J.
Huang, Ann C., FamilyMed(EM)
Ireland, Kim L.
Jerome, Amanda L., FamilyMed
Jhirad, Reuven R., FamilyMed
Johnson, Thomas E., FamilyMed
Kalia, Samir, FamilyMed
Karnis, Constantine G.
Khaled, Mohamed B., FamilyMed
Khan, Shahida, FamilyMed
Khodawandi, Kurosch A., FamilyMed
Kollek, Daniel, FamilyMed(EM)
Konigsberg, Esther
Kovacs, James F.
Kraemer, James M., FamilyMed
Kuskowski, Agnes A.
Kwong, Edward K B., FamilyMed
Lamb, Gregory B., FamilyMed
Lamoureux, Alain G.
Lee, Deborah, FamilyMed
Liberatore, Anne M.
Litteljohn, Cynthia
Lubbad, Nibal, FamilyMed
Ma, Judy P.
Mah, Leevin, FamilyMed
Mahdi, Hayder T., FamilyMed
Mander, Charanjeet
Mann, George H.
Mathur, Arpana C., FamilyMed
Mazhar, Mahmood M.
McDonald, Jane E.
McGillivray, Janis L.
Middlebrook, Shelia M., FamilyMed
Moens, Hilda
Moghaddam-Abrishami, Katayoon, FamilyMed
Moore, Beryl M., FamilyMed
Murdoch, Jason E E.
Murtaugh, Karen E., FamilyMed
Naidoo, Soobramani
Nayar, Anoop
Normann, A. Barbro
Numair, Huma N., FamilyMed
Olsen, Kristina L., FamilyMed
Panabaker, Robert D.
Pegado, V. Vance, FamilyMed
Pintea, Dana, FamilyMed
Plach, Nadia R., FamilyMed
Powers, Bruce N.
Priestner, Ann Marie, FamilyMed
Procter, William C.
Ragonetti, Christopher H., FamilyMed
Rahimpour, Raoufeh
Raja, Sumaira Jamal, FamilyMed
Ramsaywak, Peggy C., FamilyMed
Rana, Amit M., FamilyMed
Rayner, Sudesh
Reimer, Wesley J., FamilyMed
Reiser, Wendy M.
Rivers, Barbara
Rizk, Dalia A S., FamilyMed
Robinson, Matthew G., FamilyMed
Rogers, Carolyn, FamilyMed
Saeed, Lina
Saleem, Asifa K., FamilyMed
Salter, Timothy J., FamilyMed
Samarasinghe, Dewanmina A., FamilyMed
Samuel, Maged Y N., FamilyMed
Sandino, Ximena A., FamilyMed
Sansome, David E.
Saravanabavananthan, Savithri, FamilyMed
Schwab-Lang, Monika E., FamilyMed
Shih, Michael
Sichler, Conrad J., FamilyMed
Simpson, Cheryl L., FamilyMed
Singh, Harpal, FamilyMed
Singh, Kishore, FamilyMed
Smuczek, Joseph A., FamilyMed
Sokar-Todd, Hanan B., FamilyMed
Soni, Ramesh K.
Stempien, Matthew W., FamilyMed(EM)
Stevens, Gillian T.
Strang, John D.
Strome, Janet E., FamilyMed
Sturgeon, Simon
Swan, Kathryn M., FamilyMed
Swanson, J. Graham, FamilyMed
Tadros, Sharif W.
Tam, Christina
Taylor, John A.
Thibodeau, Alfred E.
Thomson, Katherine A., FamilyMed
Turliuk, Robert C.
Van Baardwijk, S. Charles
Vohra, Angeli, FamilyMed
Vohra, Asha D.
Vohra, Sukh C.
Voon, Kevin K S., FamilyMed
Wallik, David W., FamilyMed
Wallington, Marion C.
Walsh, Kimberley A., FamilyMed
Wania, Hormuzshaw J., FamilyMed
Ward-Smith, Rosalind A., FamilyMed
Welch, Barbara K.
Williams, R. Christopher, FamilyMed
Witcher, Janice L.

Yamamoto, Brian R.
Yeung, Jack K P S Y.
Youssef, Mariam F G., FamilyMed

CALABOGIE

Buxton, H. Max, FamilyMed(EM)
Davis, Kristian A M.

CALEDON EAST

Popa, Brindusa M., FamilyMed
Tita, Ioana, FamilyMed

CALEDON VILLAGE

Ponke, Jeffrey, FamilyMed

CALEDONIA

Bottega, Remo, FamilyMed
Cloete, Nicolas G F., FamilyMed
Gunning, Alan L., FamilyMed
Lapsley, Peter K.
Robertson, Marilyn S., FamilyMed

CALLANDER

Lam, Terena P T.
Percival, Timothy A.
Riley, Sheryl A.
Truong, James
Yates, Derrick A., FamilyMed

CAMBRIDGE

Achiume, J. Kirkwood
Achtymichuk, Gerald W.
Alavi, Shazia, FamilyMed
Albrecht, Craig, FamilyMed
Amog-Kerr, Lea M.
Anello, Francesco A., FamilyMed
Arora, Harpreet S.
Arora, Shefali D.
Ashton, Russell W., FamilyMed
Attalla, Amany A Y., FamilyMed
Baben, Christo, FamilyMed
Baker, Jay W., FamilyMed
Bal, Sharon, FamilyMed
Benjamin, Prabhu, FamilyMed
Bennett, Kathryn M., FamilyMed
Birss, John C.
Brown, W. Mark, FamilyMed
Bulanski, Emily M., FamilyMed
Callaghan, Siobhan, FamilyMed
Cameron, Clare R A., FamilyMed
Cary, Paul S.
Cekan, Daniel F., FamilyMed
Chamberlain, Debbie M.
Cherniak, Victor
Chypchar, Tatiana, FamilyMed
Clarke, Richard K., FamilyMed(EM)
Costin, Ioana R., FamilyMed
Covalcic, Catalina
Davidson, Carolyn J., FamilyMed
Davis, Randolph J., FamilyMed
Dissanayake, Chaminda, FamilyMed
Eugenio, Arthur M., FamilyMed
Foote, Margaret J G.
Frape, Norwynne F., FamilyMed
Geddes, Jay, FamilyMed
George, Susan, FamilyMed
Gevorkyan, Rafael, FamilyMed
Gonzalez Lejarza, Rogelio
Gupta, Sunjay
Hall, Trevor L., FamilyMed
Halligan, Rachael, FamilyMed
Hankinson, Keith, FamilyMed
Harvey, P. Robert
Holling, Tamara L.
Hollowell, Jill S., FamilyMed
Hondubrata, Linda, FamilyMed
Hughes, Tracy, FamilyMed
Humphrey, Diane B., FamilyMed
Ibrahiem, Kawa M A., FamilyMed
Kamath, Amisha T.
Kavanagh, James M.
Klomfass, Matthias T., FamilyMed
Kolk, Sarah J., FamilyMed
Kumanan, Mekalai, FamilyMed
Kuncheria, Joy, FamilyMed
Lachman, Matthew
Lalla, Angela, FamilyMed
Lanktree, Bruce B.
Larke, David P., FamilyMed(EM)
Lawrie, Michael E., FamilyMed
Leung, Tin-Chung
Light, Thurairajan, FamilyMed
Lim, Michael D., FamilyMed
MacNabb, Nancy J., FamilyMed
Maheshwari, Anil K.
Main, Jeffrey S., FamilyMed
Mann, Rick R S., FamilyMed
Martinez Motta, Jose C.
Mathai, Shyla R., FamilyMed
Matsuda, Maria T., FamilyMed
Mazerolle, Maryse F., FamilyMed
McCallum, Robert, FamilyMed
Miller, Harold B.
Monkhouse, Alan K., FamilyMed
Morar, Champaklal, FamilyMed
Morar, Shaheen, FamilyMed
Morgan, Kathryn R., FamilyMed
Mueller, Elizabeth K., FamilyMed
Narula, Archna, FamilyMed
Oey, Audrey, FamilyMed
Pandey, Annada K.
Poon, Derek I., FamilyMed(EM)
Redelinghuys, Johannes N., FamilyMed
Reinders, Sabrina M L., FamilyMed
Reizgys, Katerina L., FamilyMed
Renner, David F.
Rowe, Andrea
Roy, Gilles J., FamilyMed
Russek, Richard P., FamilyMed
Sa, Grace A Y., FamilyMed
Sabieh, Sadia
Samolczyk, Janet L., FamilyMed
Samolczyk, Thomas A.
Schurter, Melissa L., FamilyMed
Schuster, Martin, FamilyMed
Shafir, Mark, FamilyMed
Shahmalak, Shahzad Z.
Shaikholeslami, Roya
Siddall, Laura S., FamilyMed
Sims, Louise E., FamilyMed
Skillman, Jean L., FamilyMed
Snyder, D. Bruce
Springate, Russell P., FamilyMed
Sublett, Stirling F.
Swekla, Michaela
Takhar, Baldeep
Tandon, Naveen
Thomson, Valerie R.
Tibbo, Perry M.
Trudel, Philippe J H.
Tysdale, Kim G., FamilyMed
Vallieres, M. Beth, FamilyMed(EM)
Voros, Gabor D., FamilyMed
Wahid, Salman
Wang, Jodie L M C.
Webb, Ronald B., FamilyMed
Whan, Deborah E., FamilyMed
Williams, Taryn M., FamilyMed
Wong, William H.
Wozniak, Peter C., FamilyMed
Yakoub, Emad I., FamilyMed
Young, Alix M., FamilyMed

CAMPBELLFORD

Bain, James B., FamilyMed
Barbero, Joseph
Bartlett, Norman R., FamilyMed(EM)
Collins, Celeste, FamilyMed
Gibson, Glenn, FamilyMed
Henderson, Robert W., FamilyMed
MacKlem, P. Douglas, FamilyMed(EM)
Park, Ian R A.
Parsons-Sheldrake, Jeffrey, FamilyMed
Pritchard, Neil G.
Williams, Paul A., FamilyMed
Witt, Alexandra P., FamilyMed

CAMPBELLVILLE

Charbonneau, Fabien A.
Vona, Frank G.

CANNINGTON

Gomide, Jose G S.
Manfredi, Victoria E., FamilyMed

CARAMAT

Wesley, Shannon J., FamilyMed

CARDINAL

Peters, Geoffrey A.

CARLETON PLACE

Buckley, Gillian L., FamilyMed(EM)
Champagne, Allyson H., FamilyMed
Courchene, Robert J.
Doobay, Jaya, FamilyMed(EM)
Drake, Roger S.
Ferguson, Donald H., FamilyMed
Fernandez, Christina D.
Fullerton, James E D., FamilyMed
Gray, Janice, FamilyMed
Higham, M. Scott, FamilyMed
Ivanovich, Den M.
Jamieson, Erin L., FamilyMed
Johnston, Mary E., FamilyMed(EM)
Kungurov, Maria, FamilyMed
Laskey, Jennifer D., FamilyMed
Lenny, David B.
Marion, Marc H.
Potvin, William R., FamilyMed
Spooner, Marcia A., FamilyMed
Tai, Christine J Y., FamilyMed
Walker, Stephen W.
White, Martin N.

CARLISLE

Bzonek, Peter, FamilyMed
Desbois, Nathalie A., FamilyMed
McMeekin, Barbara L., FamilyMed
Scholtens, Hendrik A., FamilyMed
Wright, Laura E., FamilyMed
Xenoyannis, Sophia, FamilyMed

CARP

Adams, Rachael E., FamilyMed
Bruce, Barry W., FamilyMed
Bruce, Carol E.
Ciechanska, Ewa, FamilyMed
Connell, Amanda E., FamilyMed
Dionne, Jeanette A C., FamilyMed
Ferguson, Karen E., FamilyMed
Fraser, Mark A., FamilyMed
Lawler, Michelle C., FamilyMed
McBride, Kathryn L., FamilyMed
Rosenkrantz, Alicia H., FamilyMed
Stecher, Robert D., FamilyMed
Tonon, Kristen A., FamilyMed
Vigneron, Eugene A., FamilyMed

CARRYING PLACE

Vaughan, R L. Robert, FamilyMed

CASSELMAN

Arenas, Patricia M.
Bastianon, Todd M., FamilyMed
Lamarche, Robert A.

CAYUGA

Bulger, William J.

CHAPLEAU

Huggins, David G.
Saari, Kendra A., FamilyMed
Saari, Stephen J., FamilyMed
Taylor, John D.

CHATHAM

Ade-Conde, Adetunji J.
Adegboyega-Conde, Omotola
Anees, Farah
Bailey, Kathryn A., FamilyMed
Balasubramaniam, Balaji
Balasundaram, Manjula
Bay, Dennis, FamilyMed(EM)
Boekhoud, John W F G.
Boettcher, Allen
Chandrasena, Samantha H.
Chawla, Lalit K., FamilyMed
Da Silva, Sean L.
Denys, Jason A., FamilyMed
Dixon, Anthony R J., FamilyMed
Evans, David
Faruqi, Perves Z.
Galbraith, Jack W.
Gamble, Brian, FamilyMed
Gletsu, Stephen K., FamilyMed(EM)
Goad, Ralph F.
Hastings, Donald
Huffman, David A W., FamilyMed
Karatela, Kamran
Khan, Mateen A.
Khan, Saima W., FamilyMed
Lees, Martin G J.
Leigh, John D.
MacDonald, Avril M.
MacKinnon, Jennifer A., FamilyMed
MacLean, Ian J.
Macher, Ted W., FamilyMed
Matsusaki, Dean I.
McIntyre, Mary E.
Milkovic, Heather J.
Milkovic, Zeke, FamilyMed
Miller, Claire L M., FamilyMed
Morand, Allison R., FamilyMed(EM)
Munro, Susan L., FamilyMed
Narayanan, Kanna R S., FamilyMed
Newell, Michael R., FamilyMed(EM)
Parambil, Sumitha, FamilyMed
Parry, Park W.
Roszell, Sheri L., FamilyMed(EM)
Sheldrick, Peter G.
Stronks, John E., FamilyMed
Sullivan, David B., FamilyMed
Sultan, Ghazala, FamilyMed
Tomen, Mark E.
Verburg, Adrian J E.
Watterud, Donna L., FamilyMed

CHELMSFORD

Brunet, Claire-Lucie, FamilyMed
Merotto, Robert A.

CHESLEY

Egles, Diane E., FamilyMed
Ispahany, M. Mehdi, FamilyMed
Sanborn, Margaret D., FamilyMed
Schipper, Kristine M., FamilyMed
Thompson, A. Ian, FamilyMed
Winterton, Adam C., FamilyMed
Wong, Jacqueline M S., FamilyMed

CLARKSBURG

Elkhuizen, Carola E., FamilyMed
Euler, Karin E.

CLINTON

Bokhout, Maarten, FamilyMed
Cameron, Nancy E.
Hay, J. Keith, FamilyMed
Salsbury, Peter G., FamilyMed
Seevaratnam, Loretta M., FamilyMed
Smith, Anna J M., FamilyMed
Van, Ngoc Binh

COBALT

Sears, Steven T., FamilyMed

COBDEN

Purdon, Carey D.

COBOCONK

Warsi, Shabaz M.

COBOURG

Amin, Jayshree
Barnard-Thompson, Kathleen, FamilyMed
Barrie, Michael A., FamilyMed
Bayer, Judith L., FamilyMed
Bayer, Michael W., FamilyMed(EM)
Broderick, David J.
Caldwell, J. Paul, FamilyMed
Cheung, Teresa P C., FamilyMed
Connor, Steven A.
Cross, William G., FamilyMed
Dahle, Colin T., FamilyMed
Daskalopoulos, Rina, FamilyMed
Emery, Andrew N.
Essak, Mark, FamilyMed
Hakim, Sania
Hameed, Asiya
Haukioja, Ari H O.
Haunts, Kirk, FamilyMed
Jennings, Stacey L., FamilyMed
Jones, Michael W.
Kondejewski, Richard J.
Kwok, Carson C C.
MacPherson, Jeffrey D., FamilyMed(EM)
Marszal, Maria M., FamilyMed
Michalski, Warren C., FamilyMed
Mule, Francesco
Nearing, James P.
Pepper, Erin R., FamilyMed
Plue, Gordon F.
Reynolds, Teresa B.
Sharma, Anuja
Shuman, Earl M.
Simon, Christine J., FamilyMed
Stogre, Rosemary A.
Stratford, Philip A T., FamilyMed
Van Dusen, Diane S., FamilyMed
Vaughan, Matthew M.
Webster, Wanda J.
Woodward, Peter S.
Woodward, Roger D., FamilyMed

COCHRANE

Affleck, Rita M., FamilyMed
Derome, Gaetane
Li, Xiaobin, FamilyMed
McPherrin, Lawrence, FamilyMed
Ross, James A.
Tremblay, Joey E J., FamilyMed

COE HILL

Kamermans, Rob J.

COLBORNE

Hearnden, Trevor A.
Noland, Iris R.

COLDWATER

Ives, Michael S.
Stone, O. Evans

COLLINGWOOD

Arthur, Marion F.
Baird, David F., FamilyMed
Bolton, Gregg M., FamilyMed
Bosman, Kylie A., FamilyMed(EM)
Bouchard, Raymond D., FamilyMed
Bowman, John L.
Clarke, Janet H., FamilyMed
Cornell, Richard A., FamilyMed(EM)
D'Costa, Darryl I.
Debono, Alaine M., FamilyMed
Di Stefano, Joseph M., FamilyMed
Edgar, Allison C., FamilyMed
Enright, Mark L., FamilyMed(EM)
Fraser, Mary, FamilyMed
Furtado, Richard J.
Gottlieb, Sidney O.
Green, Nicole, FamilyMed
Guscott, Jesse R., FamilyMed
Langford, Stephen W., FamilyMed
Lewin, Michael C., FamilyMed
Lowe, David G.
Mastali, Kourosh
McCall, John G.
McLachlin, Lauren K., FamilyMed
Mitchell, Wade R., FamilyMed
Moran, Catherine T.
Moran, Geoffrey
O'Halloran, Harry M.
Phillips, Peter G., FamilyMed
Poyner, Matthew D.
Quigg, T. Mark, FamilyMed
Rowlinson, F. Anthony
Savage, D. Peter
Smith, Jonathan G., FamilyMed
Sunderland, Dorothy J., FamilyMed
Weisbrod, Matthew J.
Wells, Peter B., FamilyMed
Young, Jennifer P., FamilyMed(EM)

COMBER

Anderson, Raymond C.

CONCORD

Brown, Sheryl E Z.
D'Andrea, Joan W., FamilyMed
Duong, Dung Ngoc, FamilyMed
Huynh, Chau Cong., FamilyMed
Lichtman, Sharla F., FamilyMed
Misho, Rita R H., FamilyMed
Pham, Trai Ngoc, FamilyMed
Ponrajah, Sakunthala, FamilyMed
Sandhu, Janmeet
Schapira, Theodor H.
Schwartz, Rachel S., FamilyMed
Syal, Suresh
Tran, Anh T N., FamilyMed

CONISTON

Jacques, Raymond G.

COPPER CLIFF

Martin, Paul B.

CORNWALL

Abtahi, Forough
Alexis, Michele L.
Amer, Amal A M M., FamilyMed
Antunes, Paulo R M., FamilyMed
Behar, Natan
Belanger, Marie S G., FamilyMed(EM)
Bergeron, Pierre, FamilyMed(EM)
Blach, Peter H O.
Blinkina, Anna A., FamilyMed
Bourcier, Joanne D., FamilyMed(EM)
Brassard, Danielle
Briere, Luc F., FamilyMed
Carson, Derek L.
Cook, Ashley G., FamilyMed
Davis, Alan E., FamilyMed(EM)
Davis, Neil L.
Ducas, Dean F.
Edgar, John P.
Felemegos, Ioannis, FamilyMed
Foley, Garrett V M.
Forson, Agatha A.
Forson, Thomas E.
Fuchs-Garcia, Sigrid
Ghantous, Youssef, FamilyMed
Heseltine, N. Geoffrey, FamilyMed
Ibrahim, Jawahir I A., FamilyMed
Jacobson, Elliot S., FamilyMed(EM)
Leigh, Clara P., FamilyMed
Lemire, Marie L C., FamilyMed
Menard, Nathalie P., FamilyMed
Mohareb, Mona M.
Nanji, Amirali M., FamilyMed
Patel, Subhash C., FamilyMed
Poilly, Diane N F., FamilyMed(EM)
Randlett, Mary Jane
Reavely-Diaz, Sheridan
Reddoch, Robert B., FamilyMed(EM)
Rizk, Magdy G A.
Rosenbloom, Alan M., FamilyMed
Sakellarides, Michel
Scandar, Jeannette E., FamilyMed
Scharf, Lorne H., FamilyMed(EM)
Schindler, David L.
Shah, Natavarlal H.
Smar, Mary C., FamilyMed
Tremblay, Roger T., FamilyMed
Tremblay, Ronald
Van Hees, Jacqueline M., FamilyMed(EM)
Watson, Andrew C.
William, Hany, FamilyMed
Young, Brian R.
Yuan-Innes, Melissa J., FamilyMed(EM)
Zerey, Caroline M., FamilyMed

CORUNNA

Borek, Robert J.
O'Mahony, William F.
Wakely, Kathryn A.
Wakely, Peter A.

COURTICE

Albert, Michelle S., FamilyMed
Ali, Michael, FamilyMed
Angl, Mohinder K.
Ballard, Betty L H.
Brankston, Edwin R., FamilyMed(EM)
Edirisinghe, Mayuri M., FamilyMed
Fitzpatrick, David J., FamilyMed
Gergely, Ana E., FamilyMed
James, Debra J.
Lesser, Sharolyn R., FamilyMed
Lurie, Arnold
Marcoux, A. William, FamilyMed
Montgomery, Barbara A., FamilyMed
Nowak-Hariasz, Daria J., FamilyMed
Palinka, Sandra J., FamilyMed
Pang, Wei-Hsi, FamilyMed
Ross, Stacey A., FamilyMed
Samson, Elizabeth A., FamilyMed
Swift, Valerie A., FamilyMed
Toyonaga, Vernon M.
Vaughan, Michele L., FamilyMed
Vu, T A. John

COURTRIGHT

Threndyle, Kenneth L.

CREEMORE

Bowle-Evans, Jo Ann
Engell, Anne, FamilyMed
Houston, Scott A W., FamilyMed
Nichols, J. Bradley, FamilyMed

CRYSLER

Dadjo-Guewa, B. Stephane, FamilyMed

DEEP RIVER

Ben Amor, Hanene, FamilyMed
Bushby, Barbara J., FamilyMed
Greenfield, Thomas
McVey, J. Terrence
Noulty, Elizabeth J., FamilyMed
Park, Donald
Seid, Cherinet, FamilyMed
Woods, Terence C H., FamilyMed

DELHI

Bak, Malgorzata A.
Chan, Ka Lam, FamilyMed
Coelho, Ryan M., FamilyMed
Graham, Susan F B., FamilyMed
Nunn, Paul
Thorogood, William D., FamilyMed
Trzcieniecka, Anna A., FamilyMed

DESERONTO

Reynolds, Robert B.

DORCHESTER

Bohdanowicz, Alexandre P.
MacNeil, Gerard M.

DOWNSVIEW

Burman, Dmitriy K.

DRAYTON

Donald, Christopher R., FamilyMed
Kam, Michael S., FamilyMed
Norman, Tanya L., FamilyMed
Peterkin, Christine E A., FamilyMed
Sun, Hao

DRESDEN

Ng Wong Hing, France
Payne, John C., FamilyMed
Thompson, David C., FamilyMed

DRYDEN

Cook, Bruce H O., FamilyMed
Cortens, Michael, FamilyMed
Dahmer, Mark R., FamilyMed
Goulet, David J., FamilyMed
Jollymore, Kory G., FamilyMed
Kehler, Faye E., FamilyMed
Mazurski, Karen L., FamilyMed
Moir, Adam, FamilyMed
Sherman, Gregory P., FamilyMed
Turcotte, Marie L.
Vann, Patricia M., FamilyMed
Viherjoki, Stephen, FamilyMed
Whittaker, Mark E., FamilyMed
Wilson, Kerri D., FamilyMed

DUNDAS

Chan, Shermeen S M., FamilyMed
Crombie, Carrie
Eisener, Barbara A., FamilyMed
Holland, Lind G., FamilyMed
James, Neil E., FamilyMed
Johns, David G., FamilyMed
Kane-Corriveau, Sandra P., FamilyMed
Kronenwald, Alexander
McMillan, James D.
Nash, W. Scott, FamilyMed
Sender, Rachelle R., FamilyMed
Shankardass, Kanwal
Shott, Paula L., FamilyMed
Steinnagel, Brenda L., FamilyMed
Sumanac, Katica, FamilyMed
Turner, Holtby M., FamilyMed
Turner, J. Patricia, FamilyMed
West, Michael J., FamilyMed
Woods, Lauren J., FamilyMed

DUNNVILLE

Bernard, Dalia A., FamilyMed
Blake, Elizabeth K., FamilyMed
Desrochers, Natale, FamilyMed
Falco-Kazemi, Barbara R.
Kazemi, Reza
McMichen, Iain K S.
Michiels, John F., FamilyMed
Reddy, Nagaram J., FamilyMed
Scallan, Francis
Smith, M. Josephine
Xu, Haibo, FamilyMed

DUNROBIN

Montgomery, Hugh J.

DURHAM

Boniolo, Hernan, FamilyMed
Chung, Bruce T W.
Denyer, Andrew G.
Lakhani, Zubair, FamilyMed
Martins Gorrindo, Anahi, FamilyMed
Pillisch, Mary L., FamilyMed
Walley, David T.

DUTTON

Campbell, Donald C.
Sharman, Peter E., FamilyMed

EAR FALLS

Antonissen, Ludovieus
Khan, Y. Aaron

EAST GWILLIMBURY

Huang, Yu Lun, FamilyMed

EAST YORK

Begum, Rehana, FamilyMed
Cader, Shifaya, FamilyMed
Clarkson, Blaise D., FamilyMed
Doupe, Lisa M.
Fallis, George W B., FamilyMed(EM)
Grewal, Simarjot K., FamilyMed
Guest, R. Gerald
Heyding, Robert K.
Huband, Louisa A., FamilyMed
Issar, Ajay
Ledesma-Cadhit, Christina J., FamilyMed
Ouellette, Michael K., FamilyMed
Pham, Thuy-Nga Tia., FamilyMed
Pollock, I. David
Pritchard, M. Jane, FamilyMed
Rasaratnam, Asvini, FamilyMed
Roqueyya, Rubina, FamilyMed
Rudnick, Alexander
Savvidou, Georgoulla
Scott, Roy
Sie, Kian Gwan, FamilyMed
Stefanski, Katherine E., FamilyMed(EM)
Stegnajic, Snezana, FamilyMed
Thenganatt, Lilly, FamilyMed
Vairavanathan, Rajani, FamilyMed(EM)
Vlaovic, Branislav
Vojdani, O. Kyle A., FamilyMed(EM)
Waxman, Mark L.
Ylanko, V. Heikki
Ylanko, Veli J., FamilyMed
Yu, Catherine L., FamilyMed(EM)
Zia, Khalid R., FamilyMed

EGANVILLE

Petrini, Michael J.

ELIZABETHTOWN

Neeson, George B.

ELLIOT LAKE

Britton-Foster, Michael B.
Chi, Frank W.
De Bortoli, Timothy P.
Groh, Catherine D., FamilyMed
Long, W. John
Margetts, David J.
Matheson, David M.
McLean, Patrick R.
Prescott, Christopher R F.
Purzner, Andrew A., FamilyMed
Siddiqui, Zubaida, FamilyMed
Wannan, Barry W.
Young, Frederick N M.

ELMIRA

Craig, John C.
Jones, Gareth W.
Morlock, J. Scott, FamilyMed(EM)
Norris, I. Michael
Onuska, Frank P.

ELMVALE

Harlos, Hans E.

ELORA

Beamish, Stephen R., FamilyMed(EM)
Brault, David, FamilyMed
Connelly, Ian H., FamilyMed
Incitti, Filomena, FamilyMed
McPhedran, Peter D., FamilyMed
Petrov, Nicole M., FamilyMed
Pridham, Cheryl J., FamilyMed
Ray, Julie A., FamilyMed
Roach, Douglas W., FamilyMed
Simpson, Robert A.

EMBRUN

Brunet, Jacques R.
Gagnon, Antoine, FamilyMed
Lamoureux, J. Michel
Lockman, Julie M I.

EMERYVILLE

Cole, Christopher P.

EMO

Krampetz, Ingrid K.
Meyers, Kimberly L., FamilyMed
Whatley, Philip L.

EMSDALE

Knight, R. William

ENGLEHART

Blunt, Gerald G.
Holwell, James P., FamilyMed
Kozel, Vitezslava V.
Lacasse, Marie-Lynn, FamilyMed
Mbuva, Regina N., FamilyMed(EM)
Shokri, Sharareh, FamilyMed

ERIN

Anderson, Peter R., FamilyMed
Bull, Duncan, FamilyMed
Daly, Laura, FamilyMed
Lennox, Carla
Sasaki, Sharon E.
Thomas, Nell, FamilyMed

ESPANOLA

Abdel-Salam, Hama S I., FamilyMed
Bertrand, Raymond J.
Chan, Benjamin T.
Howard, Kathleen G.
Knox, W F. John
Perlin, Kimberley A., FamilyMed
Thomas, C. Kuncheria, FamilyMed(EM)

ESSEX

Child, Dumaresq M.
Kirwan, Katharine E.
Luciani, Lee M., FamilyMed
Sheehan, Ciaran

ETOBICOKE

Agbayani, Regina N., FamilyMed
Aghazaman Kashani, Soudabeh, FamilyMed
Ahmad, Semina
Ahmed, Salah O., FamilyMed
Akotoye, Christian K., FamilyMed
Albin-Cook, Krystyna A.
Alghalyini, Baraa M K., FamilyMed
Ananthan, Yasotha D.
Anderson, Kenneth E.
Anifowoshe, Akeem B., FamilyMed
Ashley, Jeffrey M.
Bajwa, Gurjit
Bawa, Jameet, FamilyMed
Belsky, Nadia M.
Berih, Abdullahi A., FamilyMed
Boivin, Michelle F.
Bokore, Wasira G., FamilyMed
Boorany, Yusuf
Brankovic, Aleksandra, FamilyMed
Bridge, Kathleen E G.
Brown, Kevin P., FamilyMed
Brunton, James E.
Butt, Shyla Imdad
Byrne, John, FamilyMed(EM)
Caplan, David J., FamilyMed
Chakraborty, Krishna, FamilyMed
Chari, Seshadri M.
Chaudhry, Ijaz-Ahmed, FamilyMed
Chen, Connie, FamilyMed
Chiang, James B.
Chiang, Lisa A.
Choe, James
Ciomyk, Robert
Clement, Jennifer E J., FamilyMed
Cogan, Samantha J., FamilyMed
Cohane, Shannon A., FamilyMed
Cole, G. Denise
Colvin, Rolland G.
Cooray, Anurad R., FamilyMed
Crawley, Margaret G.
Crivat, C. Mirela, FamilyMed
Daien, David, FamilyMed
Damji, Alkarim, FamilyMed
Dang, Karen, FamilyMed
Davey, Darlene G., FamilyMed
Daya, Mohamed N., FamilyMed
De Goias, Albert R.
De Groot, Wilhelmina
De Mello, A. Joseph
De Paoli, Maria A.
De Paoli Jr., John A.
De Ponte, Delta M.
Deitcher, Carol, FamilyMed
Deitcher, Joseph
Donsky, Carolyn, FamilyMed
Doss, Roshan A.
Drab, Stephen A.
Dreyzin, Vadim, FamilyMed
Dyke, Marion E M B.
Dymon, William A., FamilyMed(EM)
Dzever, Olga, FamilyMed
Dzieciol, Gordon
Edney, Rachel E., FamilyMed
Egbert, Alwyn M.
Egier, Stuart
Einstoss, Howard S.
Eisen, David W., FamilyMed
Eisner, Dana
Elahi, Mohammed, FamilyMed
Elahi, Sofia B., FamilyMed
Elghamari, Abdulmonem, FamilyMed
English, Nicole M., FamilyMed
Essabri, Mohyeddin, FamilyMed
Estanbul, Fatuma A.
Fahim, Shireen, FamilyMed
Finkelstein, Sheldon
Fisch, Laura N., FamilyMed
Fisch, Paul
Flowitt, Catherine, FamilyMed
Francisco, Francisco C.
Gadacz, Ihor
Galea, Anthony M.
Gallardo, Rodolfo C.
Gerges, Nasim K S., FamilyMed
Ghadirian, Gissou S., FamilyMed
Gideon, Salva, FamilyMed
Gill, Jasdeep S., FamilyMed
Goldfarb, Peter
Green, Cheryl L.
Green, Stephen C.
Grossman, Robert
Guirguis, Samir S.
Gupta, Anil K., FamilyMed
Gutman, Mory M.
Haider, Kamil, FamilyMed
Halliday, Kelly, FamilyMed
Hanna, Neveen M., FamilyMed
Hasic, Aida, FamilyMed
Hassan, Ahmed, FamilyMed(EM)
Hatlapa, Karolina
Hawass, Oubada, FamilyMed
Henderson, K. Muriel
Herman, Jaclyn, FamilyMed(EM)
Hinnawi, Hanna M.
Ho-A-Shoo, Deanne P., FamilyMed
Hojyo Tomoka, Margarita K.
Huggins, Mary-Anne, FamilyMed
Hussain, Ayesha, FamilyMed
Hussain, Mohammed F I.
Hussain-Autenried, Irene
Iordache, Irina-Liliana, FamilyMed
Isenstein, Norman G.
Iwanchyshyn, George J.
Jacyk, Peter
Jelinek, Henry J.
Johnston, Hariclia, FamilyMed
Joshi, Manohar L.
Jugloff, Lisa S., FamilyMed
Kanani, Subodh D., FamilyMed
Kapusta, Donald J.
Kates, Martin L., FamilyMed
Katsuta, Tsuyoshi
Kavouris, Vasilios
Kayilasanathan, Suganthan, FamilyMed
Kessel, Brian R.
Kessie, Atiemo, FamilyMed(EM)
Khalil, Ayman M R., FamilyMed
Khan, Farhana A.
Khan, Hashmat U., FamilyMed
Khoja, Murtuza, FamilyMed
Klair, Rajbir S., FamilyMed
Klipitch, Oleg, FamilyMed
Knapp, Harvey K.
Kocmur, Elizabeth
Kostovic, Biljana
Kovaleva, Maria
Kreder, Marion R., FamilyMed
Kruger, Alan M.
Kuhlmann, John C.
Kumra, Rajiv
Kushner, Arthur M.
Lacko, Cyril J.
Lal, Justiene, FamilyMed
Lam, Clement W C.
Lappa-Walker, Tracy A., FamilyMed
Laraya, Nadine, FamilyMed
Lasko, Benjamin H.
Laza, Diana C., FamilyMed
Lee, Allan
Lee, Doris S.
Lee, Patricia P S., FamilyMed
Lee, William W.
Leknickas, Liuda R.
Leneman, Michal, FamilyMed
Leong, John C S.
Leong-Poi, Brian C.
Lim, Benito C.
Lindholm, James N T K., FamilyMed
Litman, Melvin
Liu-P'Ng, Tina T S., FamilyMed
Lock O'Brien, Jodi, FamilyMed
Lyznyk, Roman G.
Makhan, Bernard A., FamilyMed
Malik, Puja, FamilyMed
Malisic, Dragoljub, FamilyMed
Maloney, Tshai Nkasi
Mand, Gurpal S.
Mandel, Ronald M., FamilyMed
Martinez, Lionel G.
Martosh, Anita M.
Matthews, Tina R., FamilyMed
Mazaheri, Arash, FamilyMed
Mazloom, Fereshteh, FamilyMed
McIntyre, Sigmund O., FamilyMed
McKinney, Kevin G., FamilyMed
Meffe, Filippa, FamilyMed
Merrick, Bruce W.
Mesensky, Ladislav
Mistry, G. Gavin
Mohamed, Nashila N., FamilyMed
Mohammad, Naveed S.
Mohan, Rajesh
Mokhtari, Makan, FamilyMed
Moodley, Vasse T.
Moses, Ruth M.
Murray, Alastair M.
Nambiar, Sindhu
Nandy, Ranendu
Navaratne, N K. Pradeep, FamilyMed
Nehra, Lollita J.
Ng, Matthew, FamilyMed
Niculae, Natalia
Norkus, Daiva L., FamilyMed
Noza, Assefa F., FamilyMed
Obnamia, Maira
Oczachowski, Caroline
Odumah, Godwin
Ogueri, Emmanuel, FamilyMed
Olah, Marketa, FamilyMed
Olah, Michael J., FamilyMed
Olah, Michael
Omoto, Daniel M., FamilyMed
Oza, Pari U., FamilyMed
Panturescu, Michael J.
Patel, Deepen M., FamilyMed
Patel, Falguni, FamilyMed
Patterson, Frederick
Pazionis, Gregorios
Peckham, Kenneth A.
Pereira, Derek J.
Perez, F. Eduardo
Perry, Scott R.
Peschisolido, Vincenzo
Pich, Bohdan O.
Pietraszek, Mary D S.
Pilarski, Barbara A., FamilyMed
Pinto, Christopher
Popadynec, Ihor V.
Pope, Octavian C.
Praglowski, Bozena
Preston, Gordon L.
Price, David H., FamilyMed
Prokopetz, Sonia A., FamilyMed
Pylypiak, Daria C., FamilyMed
Quigley, Ciara J., FamilyMed
Raddatz, Eric, FamilyMed
Rana, Fakhara N., FamilyMed
Reece, Cadi M., FamilyMed
Render-Teixeira, Caroline L., FamilyMed
Rikhye, Rakesh K.
Rubin, Sharon R.
Rumm, Michael J.
Russell, William
Sadinsky, H. Leonard
Salib, Jeannette L., FamilyMed
Sanchez, Federico J., FamilyMed
Sandhu, Guninder B S.
Sankat, Olivia M.
Savin, Adrian G., FamilyMed
Scheinman, Louis J.
Schlanger, Agnes M.
Sehgal, Parmila
Sehravat, Narinder S., FamilyMed
Seidl, Mladen
Seredycz, Larissa I., FamilyMed
Shaikh, Bashirunnisa A.
Shapiro, Joanna L., FamilyMed
Shih, Aaron C T., FamilyMed
Shih, Robert H., FamilyMed
Shklar, Jaroslav O.
Shore, Frederica D.
Sial, Zia A., FamilyMed
Sikri, Rajneesh, FamilyMed
Skeete, Jason R., FamilyMed
Smith, Arnold I.
Smolkin, Mark A., FamilyMed
Sookhai, Nicole K., FamilyMed
Sosiak, Theodore S.
Stefanik, Paula L., FamilyMed(EM)
Stefanovich, Chris P., FamilyMed
Stephens, Janine W., FamilyMed
Stevens, Howard
Strom, Brian S.
Stroz, Edward S., FamilyMed
Sukerman, Darren J.
Sukhai, Natasha P., FamilyMed
Sun, Christopher K., FamilyMed
Sunerh, Pal S.
Syed, Ikramuddin, FamilyMed
Tamari, Itamar E., FamilyMed
Tapp, Carly A., FamilyMed
Tecimer, Sandy N., FamilyMed
Thai, Wayne, FamilyMed
Tham, Elizabeth, FamilyMed
Toma, Azhar M., FamilyMed
Tse, Chingying
Upenieks, John A.
Upenieks, Maria, FamilyMed
Vaithilingam, Dushandhan S.
Vizel, Michael J.
Von Schlegell, Ahmad S.
Wang, Paul P Y.
Wilcox, Carol L.
Wong, Amy N., FamilyMed
Wong, Patricia A., FamilyMed
Woo, Francis C M.
Wroblewski, Karol C., FamilyMed(EM)
Wu, Nancy P.
Yee, Angelina, FamilyMed
Yoshida, Winifred R., FamilyMed
Young, Bernita A., FamilyMed
Zadyko, Jerry, FamilyMed(EM)
Zaki, Nasser A., FamilyMed
Zee, Allen

EXETER

Bueno Patino, Mario, FamilyMed
Dilworth, Neil, FamilyMed
Farrell, Maureen E., FamilyMed(EM)
Fatum, Krista L., FamilyMed
Jadd, Jerome L.
Kelly, Emily R., FamilyMed
Lam, Yuen-Ming
Mussani, Yasmin
Nelham, Mark W.
Pereira, Jaime M., FamilyMed
Ryan, Sean, FamilyMed(EM)
Steele, Linda G M., FamilyMed

FALLBROOK

Coombs, John F.

FENELON FALLS

Allin, R. Bruce
Gallagher, Patrick F.
McLaren, David J., FamilyMed

FENWICK

Bester, Michiel A N.
Hope, Sarah J.

FERGUS

Anderson, M. Catherine, FamilyMed
Bismilla, Fasel A.
Brown, Brittany J., FamilyMed
Easterbrook, Mark D., FamilyMed
Ewen, W M. John
Gergovich, Richard M.
Gower, Sarah K., FamilyMed
Jafferjee, Juzar, FamilyMed
Kamminga, Amanda M., FamilyMed
Lund, Christopher U., FamilyMed
Mottiar, Yousuff
Norrie, Robert G., FamilyMed
Oh, Eric J., FamilyMed
Orkin, Aaron M., FamilyMed
Otto, Patrick W., FamilyMed
Rose-Janes, Nancy, FamilyMed
Stickney, John R.
Sugamori, Mark E., FamilyMed
Wagler, Amanda M., FamilyMed
Westendorp, Matthew W., FamilyMed

FISHERVILLE

Mead, Timothy G.

FLESHERTON

Power, Brian M., FamilyMed
Winfield, Harvey B., FamilyMed

FONTHILL

Duncan, Charles G.
Nunes, Isabel M A.
Ola, Foluso A., FamilyMed
Oliverio, Paolo
Pelser, Duane D., FamilyMed
Sarides, Constantine A.
Venter, Hendrik L., FamilyMed

FOREST

Berney, Richard T.
Burgel, Sonja H., FamilyMed
Hickey, Michael C., FamilyMed
Oates, D. Julian, FamilyMed
Walker, Kenneth J., FamilyMed

FORT ERIE

Aksoy, Davut E.
Che, Claudius T K.
Csanadi, Michael A.
Frech, Robert J.
Gleeson, Peter F.
Henry, David G.
Jayawardene, Nishan C., FamilyMed
Kamatovic, Ralph J., FamilyMed
Kim, Myung-Gi
Leung, Cho Yau
Marchi, Nicholas, FamilyMed
Mitchell, Hugh J.
Scher, Kim E., FamilyMed
Spencer, Paul S.

FORT FRANCES

Algie, Robert I., FamilyMed
Jenks, Lorena L., FamilyMed
Johnstone, Brian T., FamilyMed
Moorhouse, Cameron W., FamilyMed
Nelson, John N., FamilyMed
Nugent, Robert W., FamilyMed
Saliba, Cynthia H., FamilyMed
Shack, Jason A., FamilyMed

GANANOQUE

Hart, Brian, FamilyMed
Maitland, Alexander J M., FamilyMed
Malevich, Victoria N., FamilyMed
Sajed, Sina, FamilyMed
Therrien, Arawn A A., FamilyMed
Tunnicliffe, Brian W.
Whatley, Darren, FamilyMed

GARSON

Abdulhusein, Abbas G.

GEORGETOWN

Abdel Malek, Wafik F., FamilyMed
Abraham, Hany G., FamilyMed
Aheer, Mukhtiar S., FamilyMed
Alam, Nadia, FamilyMed
Amin, Shaista, FamilyMed
Bartlett, Krista, FamilyMed
Bourns, Robert E., FamilyMed
Busse, Justin E., FamilyMed(EM)
Carson, B G. Craig, FamilyMed
Cheema, Amarpreet S., FamilyMed
Cherla, Kiran U., FamilyMed
Chin, Terrence B., FamilyMed
Chow, Peter M.
Chu, Robert W X., FamilyMed
Cooper, Matthew R., FamilyMed
Darling, Colleen
Deichert, Kenneth
Farragos, Anthony, FamilyMed
Faulknor, Janice Y., FamilyMed
Ferguson, Sarah, FamilyMed
Ford, Jackie A.
Furness, Alexander
Halparin, Elliot, FamilyMed
Jabbar, Yasmeen, FamilyMed
Khanna, Rama J., FamilyMed
Kumar, Naresh, FamilyMed
Li, Siu Hung C.
Mah, Norman A., FamilyMed
Ming Fok, Judy, FamilyMed
Nandra, Sukhjeen K., FamilyMed
Ockley, Carla, FamilyMed
Parimoo, Sabina A., FamilyMed
Phipps, Nigel M.
Poonah, Muhammad F., FamilyMed
Rai, Gurinder S., FamilyMed
Razvi, Yasar S., FamilyMed
Regmi, Dybesh, FamilyMed
Rempel, Elfrieda
Sethi, Ritu, FamilyMed
Stefanac, Mile, FamilyMed(EM)
Struzik, Lukasz, FamilyMed
Sutherland, Jeffrey, FamilyMed
Trant, Donald F., FamilyMed
Upal, Faiza, FamilyMed
Van, Victor B C., FamilyMed
Van Bendegem, Jacobus P.
Vlahovich, Alexandra R., FamilyMed
Williams, Kelly M., FamilyMed(EM)
Ying, James J.
Zeni, Deborah R., FamilyMed
Zeni, Paul J.
Zettler, Michael L., FamilyMed

GERALDTON

Depetrillo, Santino, FamilyMed
Hamilton, Andrew W., FamilyMed
Hargassner, Edward
Iskhakova, Maria A., FamilyMed
Laine, Roy E.
Susini, Vincenzo R.

GLEN HURON

Cowen, Robert P.

GLOUCESTER

Anderson, James G.
Ashikian, Haig, FamilyMed
Baker, Janet D., FamilyMed
Bellefeuille, Julie, FamilyMed
Biro, John E.
Delgado Rodriguez, Gisell, FamilyMed
Ekstrand, Gayle P., FamilyMed
Hemings, David J.
Hussein, Wissam M., FamilyMed
Kuntz, Christiane, FamilyMed
Leduc, David A.
Linney, Louise M., FamilyMed(EM)
Matuk, Naeema B.
McFarland, Kathryn J E.
Miller-Shewchuk, Allison, FamilyMed
Nordin, Christopher E.
O'Connor, Catherine S., FamilyMed
Oroz, Budimka, FamilyMed
Pullan, Wendy M.
Rice, Maryanne S.
Rourke, Timothy W.
Scott, M J F. Lise, FamilyMed
Sharma, Anil B., FamilyMed
Udoeyop, Victoria I., FamilyMed
Vinette-Azzi, Julie F., FamilyMed
Whittaker, Stephen, FamilyMed
Zayed, Saleh, FamilyMed

GODERICH

Appavoo, Samuel D., FamilyMed(EM)
Chan, Charlton C W.
Dawson, Michael J., FamilyMed
Gorguy, Nermine, FamilyMed
Hollingworth, James L., FamilyMed
Koudra, Fahamia, FamilyMed
Lal, Rekha B.
Milne, William K., FamilyMed(EM)
Natuik, Shannon A., FamilyMed
Neal, Donald O., FamilyMed
Noel, Daniel A., FamilyMed
Radan, Aleksandar, FamilyMed
Spacek, Kimberly L., FamilyMed(EM)
Spacek, Stan Z., FamilyMed(EM)
Torres Jimenez, Monica
Watson, Hilary A., FamilyMed

GORE BAY

Hamilton, Robert J.
McRae, Shelagh M., FamilyMed
Wilson, Chantelle N., FamilyMed

GRAND BEND

Englert, Peter S., FamilyMed
Hammond, Michael, FamilyMed
Marshall, P. Iris
O'Connor, William F.
Renaud, Monique M., FamilyMed
Waters, Deborah A., FamilyMed

GRAND VALLEY

Mallin, Constantine, FamilyMed

GRAVENHURST

Daniel, J. Richard
Forester, Kimberley A., FamilyMed
Gair, Graeme A.
Gleeson, Joseph T., FamilyMed
Hillyard, David, FamilyMed
Humble, Richard G.
Irvine, Thomas E., FamilyMed
Jones, Kristen S., FamilyMed
MacLennan, Adam B., FamilyMed
O'Shaughnessy, P. Martin

GREELY

O'Connell, Louis S., FamilyMed
Roy, Alexandra, FamilyMed

GRIMSBY

Abram, Nancy L., FamilyMed
Benson, Gary L., FamilyMed
Charbonneau, Danielle L., FamilyMed
Deegan, Donald M., FamilyMed
Donaghy, Seamus, FamilyMed(EM)
Fernandes, David, FamilyMed(EM)
Gulamhussein, Murtaza
Ibrahim, Nurain, FamilyMed
Johnson, Troy G., FamilyMed
Lawson, Andrea L., FamilyMed
Marshall, Denise I., FamilyMed
Mullen, Glen E.
O'Dea, Mary J.
Pierce, Glenn D., FamilyMed
Roelfsema, Heather J., FamilyMed
Samuels, Peter M., FamilyMed
Scott, Richard T., FamilyMed
Shoemaker, Elisabeth A., FamilyMed
Smith, Donald G.
Timko, Julie B., FamilyMed
Weatherdon, Derek S., FamilyMed
White, Bonnie L., FamilyMed

GUELPH

Abbey, Bruce V.
Albrecht, Gaylord D., FamilyMed
Alexopoulos, Karen N., FamilyMed
Ali, Humaira H., FamilyMed
Arkilander, Adrianna, FamilyMed(EM)
Armour, Pauline D., FamilyMed
Austin, Monica L., FamilyMed
Badalato, Heather A., FamilyMed
Bailey, Jason P., FamilyMed
Beland, Renee L., FamilyMed
Bell, Courtney J., FamilyMed
Bier, Anthony B., FamilyMed(EM)
Bluhm, Melanie, FamilyMed
Braun, Jennifer L., FamilyMed
Brodovsky, Sidney A., FamilyMed
Bueckert, Hartmut, FamilyMed(EM)
Caldwell, Forrest H., FamilyMed
Cameron, Mary M., FamilyMed(EM)
Casale, Maria, FamilyMed
Caspers, Jennifer M., FamilyMed
Chan, Benedict S., FamilyMed
Chan, Lucille S Y., FamilyMed
Chang, Li-Hsin, FamilyMed(EM)
Chittle, Andrea D., FamilyMed
Choi, Ellen H., FamilyMed
Choong, Douglas K M., FamilyMed
Chung, Edward Y C.
Clarke, Stephen C., FamilyMed
Cockburn, Lucas C., FamilyMed(EM)
Corbett, Barbara, FamilyMed
Cranmer, David J., FamilyMed
Danescu, Liviu G.
Danielli, Rosemary P., FamilyMed
Dason, Jeyapandy T., FamilyMed
Davis, Richard C., FamilyMed
De La Torre, Josephine, FamilyMed
Digby, Ian J., FamilyMed(EM)
Dippel, Ruth G A., FamilyMed
Doell, Brian, FamilyMed
Dore, Marcel
Farooqi, Muna I., FamilyMed
Ferguson, Alexander H., FamilyMed(EM)
Fewster, Robert, FamilyMed
Fraser, R. Blair
Friars, Douglas G., FamilyMed
Gaiardo, Robert R.
Ganapathy, Anusoumya
Gat, E. Douglas
Gawron, Stephen J.
Gibson, Malcolm A S., FamilyMed
Gilani, Hamid J.
Goldsmith, Robert, FamilyMed
Goldsmith, William O., FamilyMed
Golu, Tatiana, FamilyMed
Gray, Danielle R., FamilyMed
Gupta, Seema, FamilyMed
Hafuth, Falih M., FamilyMed
Harmantas, Nikolaos, FamilyMed
Hasulo, Lori A., FamilyMed
Helyar, Richard G., FamilyMed
Hendrie, Peter M., FamilyMed
Henry-Ganesh, Brenda P., FamilyMed
Hood, David T., FamilyMed
Hutton, Shannon K., FamilyMed
Huyer, Dirk W.
Issakoff-Meller, Anna M.
Jawahir, George A.
Karl, Paul A.
Kaushik, Swarsha, FamilyMed
Kirby, Sandra J., FamilyMed
Kizior-Hajduk, Anna J., FamilyMed
Kizis, Jeffrey J., FamilyMed(EM)
Kotalik, Thomas, FamilyMed
Laird, John L.
Lamont, Samantha J., FamilyMed
Landy, Philip J., FamilyMed
Levytsky, Adrian A., FamilyMed(EM)
Librach, Kevin S., FamilyMed
Lightle, Angela N., FamilyMed
Little, Kyrie A., FamilyMed
Lostracco, Robert, FamilyMed
MacKenzie, Liliana
MacKie, Carl C., FamilyMed
MacPhee, Ian J., FamilyMed
Madan, Nipun M L., FamilyMed
Martin, Barry M.
May, John D.
Mayr, Michael S G., FamilyMed
Mayr, Patricia J.
McGhee, Donald J., FamilyMed
McPhedran, Amy M., FamilyMed
Mendonca, Paul V., FamilyMed
Millman, John M., FamilyMed
Moodley, Suseelan H., FamilyMed
Morrison, M. Grace
Muller, Florian L., FamilyMed
Naidoo, Denisha, FamilyMed
Nairn, Janet C.
Near, E. John A., FamilyMed
Neilson, Shane D., FamilyMed
Nimetz, Natalie A., FamilyMed(EM)
Noble, Heather L., FamilyMed
Noonan, Karen M., FamilyMed
Oakton, Suzannah E., FamilyMed
Parent, Marcel P F., FamilyMed
Parent, Nancie, FamilyMed
Parker, Alice E.
Pasion, Stella R., FamilyMed
Pavanel, M. Ellen
Peirson, Mary C., FamilyMed
Pervez, Yasmin
Phelps, James H., FamilyMed
Pinksen, Donald A., FamilyMed
Popescu, Luminita A., FamilyMed
Potter, Miriam, FamilyMed
Rahil, Preetinder S., FamilyMed
Reed, Charles E.
Reid-Rafla, Heather J., FamilyMed
Reinhart, Steven J.
Richards, J. Gordon L., FamilyMed
Robinson, Deborah L., FamilyMed
Rosebush, David J., FamilyMed
Ruddock, Nicholas S.
Ruddock, William D J., FamilyMed
Sahay, Sidharth, FamilyMed(EM)
Sandhu, Rupinder K., FamilyMed
Schieck, David O., FamilyMed
Schuurman, Joy C., FamilyMed
Schwartz, Lisa C.
Scullion, P. Gabriel, FamilyMed
Seybold, H. Elizabeth, FamilyMed
Shafir, Cary, FamilyMed
Singh, Farid
Slatkovsky, Karen E., FamilyMed(EM)
Smith, Aaron G., FamilyMed(EM)
Smith-Pellettier, I. Carolyn
Sohn, Adrian B T., FamilyMed
Song, Helen B., FamilyMed
Spadafora, Peter J., FamilyMed
Stemerdink, Christopher J., FamilyMed
Stephenson, Susan L.
Talukdar, Momtaz H., FamilyMed
Thevathasan, Kayalvili
Thomas, Shira, FamilyMed
Thomson, Carol A., FamilyMed
Tobin, Thomas E., FamilyMed
Tolmie, Wendy I.
Trainor, W. Brian, FamilyMed
Traplin, Steven J.
Tudor, Manuela G., FamilyMed
Turvey, Erin A., FamilyMed
Vedelago, Harry R., FamilyMed
Veenman, Gerrit
Vogel, Christine P., FamilyMed
Wallace, Garry E., FamilyMed
Wildenhain, Yvonne D., FamilyMed(EM)
Will, Bruno O.
Wilson, Mary T.
Wilson, Sophie E R., FamilyMed
Yazdani Boroujeni, Fereshteh
Zajdlik, Anne-Marie

HAGERSVILLE

Doroszkiewicz, Nicholas W., FamilyMed
Drijber, F L I. Philip, FamilyMed
Drijber, Shirley E.
Mitchell, Theodore W.
Muirhead, Margaret A., FamilyMed(EM)
Phillips, Katherine G., FamilyMed
Rahimi, Abdulwali S.
Yar, Qasim A.

HAILEYBURY

Churman, Mark H C., FamilyMed
Hutten-Czapski, Peter A., FamilyMed
McDermott, Thomas M., FamilyMed
Olokodana, Femi A., FamilyMed
Roedde, M. Gretchen
Smith, Phillip J., FamilyMed

HALIBURTON

Armstrong, Bryan M., FamilyMed
Bottum, Norman E., FamilyMed
Coles, Scott R., FamilyMed
Conway, Aoife M., FamilyMed
Cossons, Nandini H., FamilyMed
Dawson, Jeffrey A., FamilyMed
Ferracuti, Stephen
Gammon, Kristy L., FamilyMed
Hartwick, Karl R., FamilyMed
Heyes, Robert H., FamilyMed
Isaacs, Theodore R.
Karaguesian, Gregory J.
Stephenson, Christina A.
Varty, Barbara F.

HAMILTON

Abbas, Wassan
Abdel Malak, Nagy M., FamilyMed
Abdul Wahab, Muzafar G.
Adams, Cherie-Lee
Aderibigbe, Taiwo A A., FamilyMed
Agarwal, Ragini, FamilyMed
Agarwal, Vikas, FamilyMed
Aguanno, Jonathan J., FamilyMed
Aiken, Caroline L M., FamilyMed
Akhtar, Shazia, FamilyMed
Akladios, Hala N., FamilyMed
Al Haddad, Wael J T.
Al Shabanah, Hasan A H.
Al-Harbi, Hatem H J A.
Ali, Adib S., FamilyMed
Alipio, Al D S., FamilyMed
Aliu-Berisha, Shpresa, FamilyMed
Allaby, Cheryl L., FamilyMed
Alnassar, Mu'taz M A.
Altokhais, Tariq I S.
Alton, Bryan J., FamilyMed
Alvarez, Elizabeth, FamilyMed
Amin, Faizan Z.
Anaspure, Rahul S.

Anastasio, Romulo F.
Anchala, Krishnapriya
Apriasz, Izabela
Archibald, Marilyn, FamilyMed
Arora, Roopa D., FamilyMed
Athreya, Sriharsha
Atrie, Damon
Attisha, Reneen F.
Ayeni, Olawale O., FamilyMed
Ayibiowu, Ogunroti, FamilyMed
Azzam, Khalid M.
Badawi, Osama K.
Baird, Judy L., FamilyMed
Bane, Anita L.
Bankay, Clarence D C.
Barker, Kimberly L., FamilyMed(EM)
Barkley, Sarah E., FamilyMed
Barnett, Harold B., FamilyMed
Baronia, Benedicto
Barton, Michele C.
Basford, Tavis J., FamilyMed
Beaufield, Gary S.
Belostotsky, Vladimir
Bercik, Premysl
Bertothy, Michele
Bibic, Desa, FamilyMed
Bielecki, Barbara, FamilyMed
Black, Morry, FamilyMed
Black, Richard D., FamilyMed
Blau, Elaine M., FamilyMed
Blew, Laura J., FamilyMed
Book, Robert J.
Bourgeois, James
Boylan, Colm E.
Boyle, Anne B., FamilyMed
Bracken, Keyna J., FamilyMed
Bradfield, Jane G.
Braga, Luis H P.
Braga, Manoela F B.
Bridge, Margaret Ann., FamilyMed
Brozek, Jan Ludwik
Bruinsma, David, FamilyMed(EM)
Bruma, Cleopatra V., FamilyMed
Brunner, Reinhard, FamilyMed
Bullock, Lana, FamilyMed
Bullock, R. Wayne, FamilyMed(EM)
Burgess, Kenneth G., FamilyMed(EM)
Callaghan, Denis J.
Calvo Ballesteros, M. Eugenia
Cameron, Lauren M., FamilyMed
Carol, Angela M., FamilyMed
Casale, Joseph A., FamilyMed
Chan, Audrey S., FamilyMed
Chan, David H., FamilyMed
Chan, H M. Norman
Chan, Teresa M.
Chelvana, Anushya
Cheng, June J., FamilyMed
Cheng, Lucille L T.
Cherian, Joe, FamilyMed(EM)
Chesebrough, John N.
Chin, Stephen J.
Chopra, Sachin S.
Chu, P C. Peter, FamilyMed
Chudasama, Siddharaj
Chung, Leonard C., FamilyMed
Cividino, Maureen E P., FamilyMed
Clarke, Ellen D R., FamilyMed
Clouthier, Sarah, FamilyMed
Copps, Brenda E., FamilyMed
Coren, Lee Anne H., FamilyMed
Coret, Alexander
Coret-Simon, Judit
Corsini, Giovanni J.
Coull, Derek J., FamilyMed
Craigie, Pamela M.
Craven, Marilyn A., FamilyMed
Creatchman, Terrence M., FamilyMed
Cree, David, FamilyMed
Croft, Benjamin, FamilyMed
Crombie, Fionnella S S., FamilyMed
Cronin, Christopher P., FamilyMed
Crosthwaite, Aida I., FamilyMed
Crowson, Jonathan B.
Csordas, Andrea Z.
Cusimano, Steven L., FamilyMed
Dada, Olayinka, FamilyMed
Dao, Chung
Dashti, Behnoosh
Davine, Jonathan, FamilyMed
Davis, Meghan C., FamilyMed
De Rubeis, Andrea, FamilyMed
Dehghani-Yar, Roya F., FamilyMed
Del Bel, Nicole, FamilyMed(EM)
Derrington-Fraser, Danielle, FamilyMed
Desai, Heena Y.
Di Paolo, Bruno L.
Dickson, Robert C., FamilyMed
Divakara Menon, Syamkumar
Dobson, B. Jane, FamilyMed
Donovan, Kelly, FamilyMed
Duong, Mylinh
Eden, David S.
el Helou, Salhab
El Rabaa, Hoda, FamilyMed
Elder, Beverly A.
Emili, Anna-Marie, FamilyMed
English, Kerri E., FamilyMed(EM)
Epstein, Ralph, FamilyMed
Eryavec, Erik
Everson, Jennifer, FamilyMed
Falletta, Joseph S A.
Fang, Xueping
Fletcher, Mary, FamilyMed
Foley, Finola H.
Forero Mantilla, Carlos M.
Fowler, Nancy C., FamilyMed
Frey, Benicio N.
Frey, Michael C., FamilyMed
Fried, Joseph A.
Frotten, Erin M., FamilyMed
Fugere, Christina, FamilyMed
Fulthorpe, Gordon H.
Fundamenski, Marta A., FamilyMed
Gambhir, Puneeta, FamilyMed
Ganame, Javier
Gareiw, Salah H.
Gastaldo, Fernando
Georgiadis, Nina J.
Ghosh, Indraneel, FamilyMed(EM)
Gilani, Ammar
Gill, Rajinder S., FamilyMed
Gogia, Rupinder K., FamilyMed
Golda, Bronislaw L.
Goodacre, Margaret E., FamilyMed
Grabec, Marie
Grafham, Mark R G.
Grandwilewski, Waldemar
Greenspoon, Allen
Greenspoon, Todd T., FamilyMed
Grewal, Rajdeep, FamilyMed(EM)
Griffiths, Melanie
Gudelis, Susan, FamilyMed
Guenter, C. Dale, FamilyMed
Gunnarsson, Thorsteinn
Gwardjan, Ewa
Hadcock, Steven J., FamilyMed
Halder, Smita L S.
Hanel, Erich, FamilyMed(EM)
Hanna, Rafik B A M., FamilyMed
Hariton, Gregory B.
Hart, Paul M.
Harvey, Janice A., FamilyMed
Hattersley, Beverly A., FamilyMed
Heikkila, Andew J.
Henderson, Robert J., FamilyMed
Hernandez Murcia, Lizeth A.
Hindson, Judith M., FamilyMed
Holdway, Geoffrey M.
Holek, Arlene R.
Hope, L. Anna, FamilyMed
Hornich, Adrian A., FamilyMed
Hosseini, Seyed H.
Huang, Lennox
Hui, Melody, FamilyMed
Hutchinson, Debra L., FamilyMed(EM)
Ifabiyi, Godwin O., FamilyMed
Irazuzta, Jorge O E., FamilyMed
Isaza-Zapata, Gloria M.
Israel, Koma D., FamilyMed
Ivanyi, Katalin E., FamilyMed
Jamani, Sherally K.
Jansen, Jan W.
Jaskot, Thomas P.
Jesmin, Rownak S., FamilyMed
Jimenez Fiedler, Waldo G.
Jollymore, Gary E.
Jones, Allen S., FamilyMed
Jowett, Jonathan E., FamilyMed(EM)
Juergens, Rosalyn A.
Junaid, Amjad, FamilyMed(EM)
Junker-Andersen, Lorna R., FamilyMed(EM)
Juta, Dhanesh, FamilyMed
Juta, Manikant M.
Karpilow, Craig, FamilyMed
Kavalsky, Dennis M., FamilyMed
Keeler, H S. Grant
Keeton, Linda H.
Kehinde, Olasunkanmi, FamilyMed
Keith, Nabil T.
Keller, Emily
Kelly, Stephen R.
Kennedy, William E., FamilyMed
Kenny-Scherber, A. Claire, FamilyMed
Kerr, D. Robert, FamilyMed(EM)
Khakshaee, Amir H., FamilyMed
Khera, Joginder S., FamilyMed
Kinzie, Sarah C., FamilyMed
Klinghoffer, Oded, FamilyMed
Klurfan, Paula
Kolb, Martin R J.
Koole, Janice J., FamilyMed
Kopyto, Allan A., FamilyMed
Koziak, Steven J., FamilyMed
Kraftcheck, Daniel J J., FamilyMed
Krizmanich, William J., FamilyMed(EM)
Krol-Szpakowski, Margaret
Kulasingham, Shaneka
LaGrotteria, Lino P., FamilyMed
Labib, Noura A M E.
Lace de Almeida, Claudia
Lad, Mohanlal
Lagrotteria, Leda C., FamilyMed
Lamb, Sheilah B., FamilyMed
Langmann, Caillin
Lapinsky, Anne S.
Lapinsky, J. Gerald
Larche, Margaret J.
Larrazabal, Ramiro A.
Lavis, John N.
Laws, Anthony R E.
Le, De Quang, FamilyMed
Le Lievre, Christine M., FamilyMed
LeBlanc, Guy, FamilyMed
Lee, Nancy B., FamilyMed
Leggett, Peter J., FamilyMed
Leontiadis, Grigorios I.
Levitt, Cheryl A., FamilyMed
Levy, David R., FamilyMed
Levy, Mark E.
Levy, Richard M., FamilyMed
Lewis, Maxine A.
Liang, William
Lim, Henry, FamilyMed
Lin, Daren, FamilyMed(EM)
Lloyd, Stephen R.
Louis, Lenus S.
Lukic, Dusan
Lummack, Keith F.
MacDougall, Paul J., FamilyMed(EM)
MacKinnon, Judith A W., FamilyMed
Macaluso, Salvatore E., FamilyMed
Magloire, Patrick M.
Mannethu, Anne E., FamilyMed
Mantle, Edward R., FamilyMed
Markose, George
Matanovic-Todorovic, Dragana
Matos, Aldina C S.
Mayer, Perry V., FamilyMed
Mazza-Whelan, Angela M., FamilyMed
Mazzadi, Sergio
McCarty, Tracey S., FamilyMed
McInnis, James E R., FamilyMed
McLeod, David S., FamilyMed
McLeod, Ryan M., FamilyMed
McMillan, John K., FamilyMed
Mechetiuc, Adriana E., FamilyMed
Mercante, Nadia F., FamilyMed
Mertz, Dominik
Metcalfe, Ian L.
Mielke, Cornelia I., FamilyMed
Miklea, Jonel, FamilyMed
Mills, Michael J., FamilyMed
Milroy, Connie L., FamilyMed
Modi, Thankamma
Mohatarem, Afshan, FamilyMed
Moore, Ainsley E., FamilyMed
Moran, Judith C., FamilyMed(EM)
Morgan, Nancy
Moriarity, Tracey A T., FamilyMed
Morillo, Carlos A.
Morriello, Florence F.
Morris, Catherine, FamilyMed
Mottiar, Nasima S., FamilyMed
Movsesyan, Arakel
Mullens, Jean L., FamilyMed
Munoz, Juan E., FamilyMed
Murthy, Prashanth
Nainar, Shamsia M., FamilyMed
Nalezny, Stephan J., FamilyMed
Nandagopal, Meena
Nantha-Aree, Manyart
Narine, Rishi A., FamilyMed
Nathanson, Barbara A., FamilyMed
Nathoo, Sameer B.
Neighbour, Helen
Neimanis, Ieva M., FamilyMed
Newkirk, Lynda K., FamilyMed
Ng, David, FamilyMed(EM)
Ng, Kelvin K K.
Nguyen, Lam Van
Noad, Donald V.
Noad, Garth
Noronha, Marie G.
O'Neill, John M D.
O'Toole, Danielle M., FamilyMed
Ohson, Ravinderpal S., FamilyMed
Okorie, Chidimna I., FamilyMed
Oliver, Douglas M., FamilyMed
Opie, J. Anthony, FamilyMed
Opie, John W., FamilyMed(EM)
Ostapenko, Elena, FamilyMed
Otero Fuentes, Carmen G.
Ow, Emily J., FamilyMed
Owen, Julian J.
Owsianik, Walter D J., FamilyMed
Packer, Richard T., FamilyMed
Packer, Tamar W., FamilyMed
Pampalon, Federico
Pang, Benjamin, FamilyMed
Parachin, Deborah C., FamilyMed
Parveen, Kazi S.
Patel, Bhavin B., FamilyMed
Patel, Tejal, FamilyMed
Pek, Barbora M., FamilyMed(EM)
Penderell, Adrienne D., FamilyMed
Petrosoniak, Andrew M.
Piessens, Eva A.
Pinthus, Jehonathan H.
Pinto, Victoria J M., FamilyMed
Pizzale, Stephen
Popuri, Preeti, FamilyMed
Potter, Geraldine D.
Prangley, Catherine A., FamilyMed
Pray, Michael J.
Predescu, Dragos
Premi, Nora J., FamilyMed
Preobrazenski, Roman Z., FamilyMed
Price, David J., FamilyMed
Profetto, Jason R., FamilyMed
Puttappa, Sandesh K.
Pyper, Sheelagh M., FamilyMed
Pysklywec, Michael W., FamilyMed(EM)
Quayyum, Zahirul, FamilyMed
Rabideau, Sparrow L., FamilyMed
Ramakrishna, Veer, FamilyMed
Rana, Alia W., FamilyMed
Razack, Vanessa A.
Rechner, Shelley J., FamilyMed
Reddy, Deven, FamilyMed
Redwood-Campbell, Lynda, FamilyMed
Regenstreif, Leonora J., FamilyMed
Ribas, Carlos S.
Ricci, Elio E.
Risdon, Catherine L., FamilyMed
Ritchie, Laura C., FamilyMed
Rizzo, Nicholas A., FamilyMed
Robinson, David C G., FamilyMed
Rochwerg, Bram N.
Rodriguez, Amadeo R.
Rosenblo, Ehud
Rosenbloom, Ehud
Ross, Angela M., FamilyMed
Rostami, Maryam, FamilyMed
Rudge, Sara K., FamilyMed
Russell, Sharon A M D.
Rutledge, Gregory J., FamilyMed(EM)
Sabouba, Mohammad F., FamilyMed
Sabri, Kourosh
Sachdeva, Nandini
Samaan, Muder C.
Samaan, Zainab A.
Samuel, Justin V.
Sassi, Roberto B.
Schabort, Ingeborg, FamilyMed
Scheinemann, Katrin
Seeley, Richard A M.
Sehdev, Dashminder, FamilyMed(EM)
Selwyn, B. Karen, FamilyMed
Semczyszyn, Miroslav V., FamilyMed
Sergeant, Myles D., FamilyMed
Seth, Puneet, FamilyMed
Sewchand, Lionel S.
Shannon, Scott E.
Shaw, Anne E.
Shaw, Elizabeth A., FamilyMed
Shea, Philip E P., FamilyMed
Sherman, Maliha A H., FamilyMed
Shichor, T. Miriam
Shoemaker, Christopher A.
Simpson, Diane L., FamilyMed(EM)
Singh, Inderjit, FamilyMed
Sischek, Stephanie E.
Siu, Henry Y H., FamilyMed
Sivapalan, Sivaseelan, FamilyMed
Sky, Anastasia
Slaven, Marissa
Smosarski, David J.
Sollazzo, David J., FamilyMed(EM)
Solomon, Leslie V., FamilyMed
Soreni, Noam
Spratt, Elizabeth E.
St Amand, Ruth A O., FamilyMed
Stanborough, Jack R., FamilyMed(EM)
Steen, Rebecca E., FamilyMed
Stefanczyk-Sapieha, Lilianna, FamilyMed
Stein, Nina R.
Stevenson, Colin G., FamilyMed
Stuart, Gary A.
Subramanian, Thangamani, FamilyMed
Sweeney, Clodagh M.
Switchuk, Marianna
Syty-Golda, Marie B.
Szarka, Istvan L., FamilyMed
Szereszewski, Abraham, FamilyMed
Szilvassy, Imre Z.
Szpakowski, Pawel P., FamilyMed
Takrouri, Heba S R.
Taniguchi, Alan
Tarasiewicz, Iwona R., FamilyMed
Tataryn, Brian L., FamilyMed(EM)
Tattersall, Philippa J.
Taylor, Amanda B., FamilyMed
Taylor, J. Grant
Teal, Barbara A., FamilyMed
Thompson, Pamela A., FamilyMed
Timarac, Ratka
Tittley, Camille M L.
Toffolo, Denny
Torres-Trejo, Alejandro
Trollope, A. Karen, FamilyMed
Tulving, Linda, FamilyMed
Tuttle, Irene M.
Tytus, Richard H., FamilyMed
Vadera, Rajiv, FamilyMed(EM)
Van Baardwijk, Susan L.
Varma, Shanta, FamilyMed
Vas, Antonio B L.
Vasovich, Inge
Von Hanna, Silvia G.
Vora, Harshala P., FamilyMed
Wakefield, Jacqueline S G., FamilyMed
Walker, John P.
Walker, Kathleen J., FamilyMed
Walsh, Allyn E., FamilyMed
Wang, Yongdong
Waters, Heather M., FamilyMed
Webb, Irma A S., FamilyMed
Weston, William M.
Williams, James E., FamilyMed
Williamson, Kimberly A.
Wilson, Brianna C., FamilyMed
Winemaker, Samantha P., FamilyMed
Wojtowicz, Jeremy M., FamilyMed(EM)
Wong, Jason W T., FamilyMed

PHYSICIANS BY PROVINCE

Woodbury-Smith, Marc R.
Woods, Anne, FamilyMed
Worster, Andrew S., FamilyMed(EM)
Wright, Ilka Y S., FamilyMed
Wu, Chin Yu
Wyatt, Emma L.
Yanivker, Susanna
Yanover, David F., FamilyMed
Yarascavitch, Blake A.
Yasinian, Azadeh Y.
Yasmeen, Naveeda, FamilyMed
Yellin, Joel W., FamilyMed
Young, Janice L., FamilyMed
Youssef, Nayer M M.
Yu, Stanley S F., FamilyMed
Zahran, Ali H M.
Zaki, Emad L A.
Zalter, Mark S.
Zavodni, Louis S., FamilyMed
Zazulak, Joyce, FamilyMed
Zizzo, Angelo J., FamilyMed
Zizzo, Dean J., FamilyMed
Zou, Lenore L., FamilyMed
Zrinscak, Christine, FamilyMed

HANMER

Desmarais, Nicole, FamilyMed
Routhier, Shelley Ann A., FamilyMed

HANOVER

Abell, Nicholas A., FamilyMed
Basilij, Robert, FamilyMed
Boron, Susan P., FamilyMed
Clark, Kerr W.
Dworkin, Rochelle L., FamilyMed
Edington, R. Bruce, FamilyMed
Gold, Pamela D., FamilyMed
Heerema, Timothy, FamilyMed(EM)
Mendez-Fernandez, Anselmo, FamilyMed
Montag, Randy J J., FamilyMed
Stretch, Neal C., FamilyMed

HARRISTON

Calarco, Mary Jo
Vanderkooy, John

HARROW

Blanchard, Matthew G., FamilyMed
Carswell, David J.
Cheung, Tak-Kee
Goyeau, Francis
Handscomb, Sheina E W.
Lindberg, Alexandra L., FamilyMed
Nwapa, Sylvia I.

HASTINGS

Maraghi, Elias R.

HAWKESBURY

Arnold, M. Renee, FamilyMed
Arsenault, Lyne, FamilyMed
Auger, Marie-Claude, FamilyMed
Azzi, Fadi-Boutros, FamilyMed
Bielinski, Raphael, FamilyMed(EM)
Borduas, J. Andre, FamilyMed
Branco, Joao, FamilyMed
Chagnon, Luc, FamilyMed
Courchesne, Mathieu, FamilyMed
De Ladurantaye, Alain
Fairfield, John A.
Frechette, Robert C.
Gagne, Christian J M., FamilyMed
Hould, Melanie, FamilyMed
King, George W., FamilyMed(EM)
Lajoie, Claude
Landa, Jean-Claude, FamilyMed
Laviolette, Eric L., FamilyMed(EM)
Lemieux, Anne-Marie
Mainville, Barbara J.
Maranda, Julie P., FamilyMed
Markowski, Michael P.
Maxwell, Thomas E.
McCall, Richard H., FamilyMed
McCall, Simon O.
Pung, Carolyne H.
Quenneville, Michel L.
Robert, Johanne, FamilyMed
Rossbach, Valery M J., FamilyMed
Saher, Fouad
Schirmer, Nicholas, FamilyMed(EM)
Sirzyk, Jeffrey, FamilyMed(EM)
Soucie, F. Pierre
Souligny, Lyne H., FamilyMed
Su, Xiao Y., FamilyMed
Teetaert, Matthew A., FamilyMed
Theoret, Francois A J., FamilyMed
Therrien, J. Jean A G.
Urfer, Francois N.
Williams, V. Guy
Yang, Jianing

HEARST

Claveau, Richard L., FamilyMed
Fragiskos, Vasilios A.
Giles, Sarah M., FamilyMed
Jomphe, Michele, FamilyMed
Lacroix, J L. Denis
Lafleche, J J. Rene, FamilyMed
Papineau, Martin, FamilyMed
Smith, M C. Patricia, FamilyMed

HOLLAND LANDING

Ghorayeb, Sahar H., FamilyMed
Lawlis, Catherine M., FamilyMed
Olech, Victoria M., FamilyMed
Zajc-Dalcourt, Natasha, FamilyMed

HORNELL HEIGHTS

Rogers, Kristin D., FamilyMed

HORNEPAYNE

Cameron, Reid S., FamilyMed
Crawford, William F.

HUNTSVILLE

Baechler, Marion G., FamilyMed
Bastedo, Paul A., FamilyMed
Bozek, Nancy L., FamilyMed
Branigan, Sheena M., FamilyMed
Brown, Andrew R., FamilyMed
Dempster, Helen, FamilyMed
Eastmure, John J., FamilyMed
Forestell, Gerald P., FamilyMed(EM)
Gzik, Danusia J., FamilyMed
Harrold, Deborah L., FamilyMed
Herr, Steven J., FamilyMed(EM)
Hill, Stephen D., FamilyMed
Jindal, Catherine M.
Kwiatkowski, Christopher J., FamilyMed(EM)
Lewis, Laura C., FamilyMed
MacDonald, James A., FamilyMed(EM)
MacMillan, Andrew R., FamilyMed
Mar, Melanie C., FamilyMed
Mathies, David J., FamilyMed
McDermott, Pamela D., FamilyMed
McLinden, David N., FamilyMed
McPherson, Ewan C.
Mensour, Mark S., FamilyMed(EM)
Mikhail, G. Pierre, FamilyMed(EM)
Morton, Dann
Munro, Diane E.
Rea, John C., FamilyMed(EM)
Simpson, John A., FamilyMed
Small, Allison M., FamilyMed
Smyth, Thomas J.
Stephenson, Megan A., FamilyMed
Stewart, D. Greg
Trenholm, Richard L., FamilyMed
Varieur, Stephen P., FamilyMed(EM)
Whaley, Robert S.
Wolff, Evelyn

IGNACE

Sorial, Ashraf M G.

ILDERTON

Brubacher, Lloyd, FamilyMed
Burke, Clarissa, FamilyMed
Hoch, N. Charles W.
Howard, Jessica C., FamilyMed
Meredith, A. Ray
Nancekievill, Garry W.
Naylor, Nancy L., FamilyMed
Van Dam, Darren J., FamilyMed

INGERSOLL

Abushawish, Ghassan, FamilyMed
Anthireya-Kakani, Sophia, FamilyMed
Bruce, Lori E.
Chawla, Punkuj, FamilyMed
Frye, Helen, FamilyMed
Hiemstra, Robert, FamilyMed
Matsuo, Jill M., FamilyMed(EM)
Mayberry, Thomas R.
Pariser, Marc R., FamilyMed
Sondhi, Jitin, FamilyMed
Wohlgemut, Joel R P., FamilyMed

INGLESIDE

Coolican, Paul J., FamilyMed
Jacques, Graham A.
Rivington, Elizabeth G.

INNISFIL

Bedard, Andre V., FamilyMed
Hankey, Arthur V.
Poole, Robert T., FamilyMed

IROQUOIS FALLS

Bargh, Gordon J M., FamilyMed
Boyle, Michael
Chiang, Stephen C., FamilyMed
Lupien, J R. Guy, FamilyMed(EM)
Shoppoff, Lina A., FamilyMed

JARVIS

Miller, Mark L.

JORDAN STATION

Manjos, Michael A.
McAuley, Barbara C.

JOYCEVILLE

Leacy, James W B.

KANATA

Abu Dieh, Anwar H M., FamilyMed
Beardsley, Robin M., FamilyMed
Bertrand, Carl
Biggs, Eileen M.
Bihun, Julia A P., FamilyMed
Bowles, Norm R.
Boyd, Barbara J., FamilyMed
Brisebois, Johnny D., FamilyMed
Brown, Elizabeth A., FamilyMed
Burns, Gerard M.
Caskey, Elizabeth R B., FamilyMed
Ceapchi, Nora C., FamilyMed
Chan, Wai Sun
Clersaint, Guyrlaine, FamilyMed
Colpitts, Deanna K.
Condrut, George M.
Connelly, Brendan B., FamilyMed
Cregan, Timothy R., FamilyMed
Crooks Teron, Louisa L C., FamilyMed
Cupsa, Andreea, FamilyMed
Daverne, Heather L., FamilyMed
Dawson, Susan P., FamilyMed
Dobenko, Sheryl N., FamilyMed
Eden-Walker, Michael
Edirisinghe, Manorie, FamilyMed
Esguerra, Robert G.
Fennell, Susan D.
Frankovich, Renata J., FamilyMed
Fraser, Anne L., FamilyMed
Fullerton, Merrilee K.
Gardee, Suliman
Giordano, Isabelle, FamilyMed
Gomez, Eva
Goulet, Kristian B.
Hall, Ronald L.
Hamilton, Wendy, FamilyMed
Hegmann, Erik J., FamilyMed
Jaffer, Salina
Jilkina, Tatiana A., FamilyMed
John, A. Roxane, FamilyMed
Kasbia, Sukhvinder S., FamilyMed
Khulbe, Suman S., FamilyMed
Krupa, Andrea M E., FamilyMed
Kujavsky, Andrew S., FamilyMed
Lacy, Richard A.
Lee, John O., FamilyMed
Lunney, James L., FamilyMed(EM)
MacAskill, Kimberly R., FamilyMed
MacEachern, M. Shauna
MacKenzie, Jonathan A.
Madill, Robert W D.
Main, Alayne J M.
Malaviarachchi, Krishangi, FamilyMed
Matys, Gail L., FamilyMed
McBride, Michelle A., FamilyMed
McNab, Brian R.
Meszaros, C. Michele, FamilyMed
Mottahedi, Roksana, FamilyMed
Motz, Catherine M., FamilyMed
O'Neil, Cathy
Paliga, Andrzej H.
Powell, Barbara M., FamilyMed
Rabie, Faten S.
Rae, Maureen P., FamilyMed
Roy, Marc J., FamilyMed
Saini, Joginder K.
Sannoufi, Hassan, FamilyMed(EM)
Sas, Silvia E M.
Shapiro, Thomas E.
Smith, Paula C., FamilyMed
Starosta, Philippe E., FamilyMed
Wheatley, Brian
White, Gail M C., FamilyMed
Yelle, Robert M., FamilyMed

KAPUSKASING

Boucher, Julie A., FamilyMed
Cheung, Roderick T F., FamilyMed
Goth, Alexis, FamilyMed
Meilleur, Christopher J M., FamilyMed(EM)
Ng-A-Fook, Robert A.
Power, Michael G.

KEEWATIN

Kroeker, Joel S., FamilyMed
Sawatzky, Vernon W.
Wehner, Timothy M., FamilyMed
Wiebe, Shannon J., FamilyMed

KEMPTVILLE

Abdel Malek, Mira G K., FamilyMed
Aggarwal, Neera, FamilyMed
Blaine, Donald D P.
Chung, Wilfred W.
Conway, Emily R D., FamilyMed
Evans, John F.
Jones, David A R., FamilyMed
Kirby, Christopher E., FamilyMed
Leahy, Patrick J., FamilyMed
Leonard, Gregory J., FamilyMed
Lewin, Gabriela A., FamilyMed
Luong, Loan T., FamilyMed
McCallan, Tara L., FamilyMed
Rathwell, Jonathan M., FamilyMed
Rutherford, Suzanne, FamilyMed
Sentongo, Colin, FamilyMed
Wanes Hana, Maha R., FamilyMed

KENORA

Anderson, Kerry A., FamilyMed
Arthurs, James R.
Beveridge, James E.
Bowerman, Brian
Burron, Ian S., FamilyMed
Carlisle, Maxine A., FamilyMed
Czajka-Fedirchuk, Cynthia P., FamilyMed
Daly, Bruce G.
Diamond, Rhonda, FamilyMed
Foidart, Stephane, FamilyMed
Habermehl, Lisa M., FamilyMed
Hammett, D. Clayton, FamilyMed
Hammett, John, FamilyMed
Harris, Kristin R., FamilyMed
Kyle, David W., FamilyMed
Lass, Rowena
Loewen, A. Waldemar
McBain, Daniel J., FamilyMed
Parsons, Susan G.
Pedersen, Sven A., FamilyMed
Retson, Jillie E M., FamilyMed
Sas, Sandra L., FamilyMed
Scaife, Christopher R.
Scatliff, Robert M., FamilyMed
Snyder, Laurel J., FamilyMed(EM)
Spencer, Mandy L., FamilyMed
Thomas, Michelle L., FamilyMed
Vaudry, John S.
Walters, Dana M.
Walters, Daniel J.
Workman, C. Murray

KESWICK

Alter, Larry S., FamilyMed
Chung, Pin, FamilyMed
Cosmin, Nicoleta D., FamilyMed
Eloskouf, Carol M M Y., FamilyMed
Giftochristos, Nick T., FamilyMed
Jim, Harry
Kakavand, Farid, FamilyMed
Lynagh, Niall J.
Moir, Vivian M., FamilyMed
Mucalov, Peter
Osoro, Beatrice K., FamilyMed
Strawbridge, Peter W.
Strelioff, George D.
Tung, Tommy H T.
Wakulich, Joanne A., FamilyMed

KILLALOE

Joo, G. Pil, FamilyMed
Tiedje, I E. Henry, FamilyMed
Voyvodic, Blair J.

KINCARDINE

Denobriga, Lisa M.
Duwyn, Rejean, FamilyMed(EM)
Emond, Michael, FamilyMed
Engle, John
Gurbin, Gary M.
Kasianik, Larissa, FamilyMed
Knox, William H.
Poirier, Steven F j., FamilyMed
Roth, Lisa R., FamilyMed
Scott, Lisa C A., FamilyMed
Taylor, Donna K.
Thomson, Leanne M., FamilyMed
Wiebe, Arthur G., FamilyMed

KING CITY

Leifer, Randy J.
Pearl, Stephen
Randall, Paul T., FamilyMed

KINGSTON

Abdelmottal, Essam A Y.
Abduljalil, Nabil, FamilyMed
Adelman, Karin A E., FamilyMed
Al Saati, Basem
Anweiler, Laura L., FamilyMed
Arber, John W., FamilyMed
Arrowsmith, Sarah C., FamilyMed
Aspy, William J., FamilyMed
Bagnall, Eric G.
Banh, Tu Van, FamilyMed
Baran, Gregory P., FamilyMed
Barber, David T S., FamilyMed
Barber, Neil K., FamilyMed
Barr, Charlie
Battel, Luigi A., FamilyMed
Beck, William J., FamilyMed(EM)
Beckett, Linda A., FamilyMed
Beliveau, James F., FamilyMed
Bernes, Carolyn, FamilyMed
Billing, Suzanne, FamilyMed
Birenbaum, Adina M., FamilyMed
Birtwhistle, Richard, FamilyMed
Bonham-Carter, Charles Riva, FamilyMed
Borins, Carolyn A., FamilyMed
Bradbury, Penelope A.
Brick, R. Andrew, FamilyMed(EM)
Bright, Hugh G J.
Brown, D O. Chester
Brown, Glenn, FamilyMed(EM)
Brown, Robyn, FamilyMed
Brown-Thomson, Linda D., FamilyMed
Browne, Moira M A., FamilyMed
Burget, Nancy E., FamilyMed(EM)
Cabrera-Abreu, Casimiro J.
Callaghan, Maximilian, FamilyMed
Campbell, Barbara E., FamilyMed
Carpenter, Jennifer L., FamilyMed
Cassim, Essop M.
Casson, R. Ian, FamilyMed(EM)
Cervenko, Paul R., FamilyMed
Chandrarajan, B. Leonard, FamilyMed
Chaparro Gomez, Luis
Cheng, Vivian K., FamilyMed
Clarke, Heather E.
Cooke, Kristy A M., FamilyMed
Cristoveanu, Nicholas J., FamilyMed
Cupido, Tracy
Dallaire, Stephane, FamilyMed(EM)
Daneshmend, Deanna J., FamilyMed(EM)
Danforth, Leonard R., FamilyMed
Day, Michael E C.
De La Roche, Michael R P., FamilyMed
Deacon, James E., FamilyMed
Defoort, Ericka N., FamilyMed(EM)
Delaney, Perlita M S.
Di Quinzio, Laura, FamilyMed
Dockrill, Mark B.
Dubin, Ruth, FamilyMed
Dubois, Elizabeth J., FamilyMed
Eastwood, Katrina
El-Adl, Mamdouh
Emrich, H. Walter, FamilyMed
Farnell, Brian J.
Feakins, Martin J.
Feleki, Katherine J., FamilyMed
Frank, Christopher C., FamilyMed
French, Robert J., FamilyMed
Fuller, Barbara E., FamilyMed
Galvin, Imelda M.
Gaskin, Anne M., FamilyMed
Geddes, John A., FamilyMed
Gerlach, Rebecca M.
Gibson, Michelle C., FamilyMed
Graham, Karen L., FamilyMed(EM)
Grant, Anna, FamilyMed
Gray, Aileen A., FamilyMed
Green, Michael E., FamilyMed
Grier, Elizabeth, FamilyMed
Griffiths, Jane M., FamilyMed
Hacking, Jennifer J., FamilyMed
Hall Barber, Karen, FamilyMed
Hammad, Nazik H M.
Hassan, Tariq
Hataley, Joy M., FamilyMed
Hinton, Stephen W., FamilyMed
Hodgetts, P. Geoffrey, FamilyMed
Hoffman, Kerri-Lyn, FamilyMed
Holdsworth, Judith A.
Howse, Kelly L., FamilyMed
Hurst, David W.
Ilan, Roy
Irwin, William F.
Iverson, Gregory C.
Joynt, Margaret S K.
Kain, Brian F., FamilyMed
Karn, Heather A., FamilyMed
Kennedy, Louis J.
Kenny, William F.
Khalid-Khan, Sarosh
Khandelwal, Surbhi, FamilyMed
Kilpatrick, Katherine L., FamilyMed
Klein, Anna E., FamilyMed
Knight, Drew A., FamilyMed
Kondor, Natalie M., FamilyMed
Kozanitis, Chris D., FamilyMed
Lacoursiere, Joan E., FamilyMed
Langley, Hugh G., FamilyMed
Larabie, Lynn M.
Lavoie, Marie-Andree, FamilyMed
Lawlor, Cindy J.
Lawrence, Elizabeth L., FamilyMed
Lee, Ellen F F., FamilyMed
Legnini, Veronica M G., FamilyMed
Lockington, Kathryn, FamilyMed
Lotfallah, Talaat K., FamilyMed
Loughlin, Kevin F., FamilyMed
Lu, Diane J., FamilyMed
MacDonald, Susan E., FamilyMed
MacGillis, Diane R.
MacKenzie, Ewen J M.
MacKenzie, Meredith A., FamilyMed
MacNaughton, Jane M.
MacPherson, David A., FamilyMed
Maksymec, Marta S., FamilyMed
Marcassa, David A., FamilyMed
Marin, Alina
Maskerine, Courtney R., FamilyMed
McBride, Allen R., FamilyMed
McCall, Margaret A., FamilyMed
McCauley, Gordon F.
McIlquham, W. Ross, FamilyMed
McLeod, Valerie L., FamilyMed
Michael, Kevin
Mileva, Lili G., FamilyMed
Miller, Christine, FamilyMed
Milner, Richard G., FamilyMed
Mitchell, Jessica S., FamilyMed
Mohr, Veronica R., FamilyMed
Molson, Jenny L., FamilyMed
Monahan, Michael P.
Moore, Kathryn, FamilyMed
Morison, Jay W., FamilyMed
Munshi, Tariq A.
Murray, Eric J., FamilyMed
Nadkarni, Pallavi S.
Naoum, Susanne, FamilyMed
Neder Serafini, Jose A.
Newbigging, Joseph L., FamilyMed(EM)
Newman, Adam I S S., FamilyMed
Nicholson, Elizabeth J., FamilyMed
Nowak, Justyna M M., FamilyMed
Nuttall, S. John, FamilyMed
O'Connor, Linda A.
O'Donnell, Patricia M E., FamilyMed
Osborne, Gary, FamilyMed
Ostic, Heather A., FamilyMed
Overington, Nancy L., FamilyMed
Paolucci, Fulvio
Parker, Barbara E., FamilyMed
Patel, Rupa, FamilyMed
Patey, Gregory M., FamilyMed
Pearson, D. Mary
Pepin, Celine
Petrof, Elaine O.
Phillips, Susan P., FamilyMed
Pilecki, Maciej W.
Pinkerton, David H., FamilyMed
Poce, Frank R M.
Porter, Sara L., FamilyMed
Priesnitz, Alisha A., FamilyMed
Pritchard, Kenneth B., FamilyMed
Purkey, Eva N., FamilyMed
Quigg, Joseph M., FamilyMed(EM)
Quinlan, Christina W., FamilyMed
Rae, Jennifer A.
Rahmani, Armita, FamilyMed(EM)
Ramachandran, Sanjay, FamilyMed(EM)
Reid, Nancy C., FamilyMed
Ren, Haifeng
Robinson, Catherine A., FamilyMed
Rodgman, M. Susan
Ross, Andrew M.
Rosser, Walter W., FamilyMed
Rowland, Mary J., FamilyMed
Rowland, Richard
Rubenstein, Elizabeth J., FamilyMed(EM)
Saeed, Khalid
Sangers, Caroline A., FamilyMed
Sangster-Gibson, Susan
Schultz, Karen W., FamilyMed
Schwartz, Roslyn T., FamilyMed
Scott, Gregory T., FamilyMed
Sempowski, Ian P., FamilyMed(EM)
Seymour, Lesley K.
Sharma, Susan M., FamilyMed
Shephard, Suzanne D., FamilyMed(EM)
Simpson, Matthew T W., FamilyMed
Simpson, Mia B., FamilyMed
Singh, Barinder, FamilyMed
Singh, Stephen B., FamilyMed
Skinner, Roger P., FamilyMed(EM)
Sladic, Ana-Sabina, FamilyMed
Smallman, Julia L.
Smith, David R.
Stacey, Matthew D G., FamilyMed(EM)
Stassen, C. Frederik
Stevens, Katrina G.
Stewart, G. Ivan
Storrier, Melville, FamilyMed
Susanto, Aida T.
Sylvester, Michael J., FamilyMed
Szlanta, Agata, FamilyMed
Takhar, Amandeep, FamilyMed
Taylor, David R.
Thomson, Robert J.
Trickey, Brian H.
Tyler, Melissa J., FamilyMed
Vaga, Kristin H., FamilyMed(EM)
Vakil, Catherine R., FamilyMed
Valliant, Lew H., FamilyMed
Vartic-Iftene, Felicia
Viola, Raymond A., FamilyMed
Wakeham, Julia C., FamilyMed
Waldron, Leslie A., FamilyMed
Walsh, Penelope E.
Watson, Shayna L., FamilyMed
Watt, Janet A., FamilyMed
Webb, Katie A D., FamilyMed
Webb, Timothy R.
Webster, Colleen A., FamilyMed
West, Robert D.
Westenberg, Hendrik H.
Weston, W. Fenton D.
Whalen-Browne, Karen A., FamilyMed
White, Carol A., FamilyMed
Wijeratne, H M. Rasika, FamilyMed
Wilson, C. Ruth, FamilyMed
Wilson, Colin G., FamilyMed
Wilson, Meghan D., FamilyMed
Wlodarski, Martin J., FamilyMed
Yates, Stephen K., FamilyMed
Yen, Ziny C., FamilyMed
You, Yue
Young, Rebekka B.
Yu, T C. Michael
Yule, Joanna E., FamilyMed

KINGSVILLE

Chowdhry, Atif
Kelton, Peter M.
McNeilly, Kenneth A.
Osborn, David D.

KINMOUNT

Kaszas, Zsuzsanna, FamilyMed
Mihu, Elena, FamilyMed

KIRKFIELD

Koprowicz, Kinga T., FamilyMed

KIRKLAND LAKE

Doelman, William, FamilyMed
Durocher, William
Ek, Nathan
Hart, Paul L.
Henderson, Nadene D., FamilyMed
Hunt, Edgar W.
Jordan, Edward H.
Kitty, Darlene J., FamilyMed
Kruszelnicki, Daniel J., FamilyMed
Kyritsis, Dimitrios, FamilyMed
McPherson, Brian K., FamilyMed
Ooi, See Wei, FamilyMed
Sokolic, Larry J.
Spiller, Mark A.

KITCHENER

Abdalla, Mohamed E., FamilyMed
Adler, Ruth I.
Al Shaar, Wasan, FamilyMed
Alarakhia, Mohamed, FamilyMed
Almanfud, Abdullah A A.
Arnold, Rosemary J.
Arya, A. Neil, FamilyMed
Astawan, Leanne, FamilyMed
Bahadur, Randy, FamilyMed
Baskerville, Leon
Bauman, Kent, FamilyMed
Bausmer, Tracy A., FamilyMed
Baxter, P. Janine
Beaver, David J., FamilyMed(EM)
Bednarska, Elzbieta I., FamilyMed
Bedrosian, Kathleen E.
Bell, Brian D., FamilyMed(EM)
Bhatty, Shahzad A., FamilyMed
Bindlish, Vinita, FamilyMed
Bitonti, David, FamilyMed
Bloomfield, Brian G.
Bodkin, R. Norman
Bordman, John M.
Borys, Thomas J.
Boyd, Stephanie, FamilyMed(EM)
Bright, Phillip A.
Brodie-Brown, William F.
Bruce, Rodney R., FamilyMed
Bryant, William H., FamilyMed
Butris, Jaclin, FamilyMed
Cameron, Karen A., FamilyMed
Campbell, John A.
Carothers, Melanie
Casey, Michael J., FamilyMed
Cescon, Amelio O., FamilyMed
Chan, Steven Y T., FamilyMed
Chapin, Margaret E T.
Chapman, Bryanne L., FamilyMed
Charkow, Steven H.
Colpitts, Lorraine R., FamilyMed
Conte, Paul D., FamilyMed
Cosma, Rodica, FamilyMed
Crowe, Anne R., FamilyMed
Cruickshank, R. Blaine
Curtis, Michael W., FamilyMed(EM)
Day, Leigh A., FamilyMed
De Carolis, Mary L.
Deen, Shajahan
Denbeigh, Paul, FamilyMed
Dignam, Jennifer, FamilyMed
Dixon, Corinne E., FamilyMed
Dixon, Heather L., FamilyMed
Dowdell, Christine J.
Dundon, John, FamilyMed
Dunning, Shelley
Dusseault, Laurie, FamilyMed
Ensing, Dianne, FamilyMed(EM)
Erb, Heidrun Y.
Esadeg, Souad, FamilyMed
Eskander, Ihab, FamilyMed
Ettin, Philip G.
Farooqi, Abdulzahir S.
Fielder, Brian J., FamilyMed
Fikry, Sameh A A., FamilyMed
Findlay, Douglas E., FamilyMed
Freedman, Joel H.
Fuss, Carolyn, FamilyMed
Garrett, J. Daniel
Gartner, Sean, FamilyMed
Gebeyehu, Yidersal, FamilyMed
Ghali, Robert J., FamilyMed
Ghally, Gehan R., FamilyMed
Gingell-Potts, Ruth, FamilyMed
Ginn, Jeffery, FamilyMed(EM)
Gokhale, Sandhya, FamilyMed
Good, Angela M., FamilyMed(EM)
Hahn, Ernest M., FamilyMed(EM)
Hasan, Osama, FamilyMed(EM)
Hickman, Donald N., FamilyMed
Hunter, Robert R T.
Huth, Brian J., FamilyMed
Hwee, Peter T.
Irvine, Thomas R., FamilyMed
Irwin, Susan, FamilyMed
Jaber, Zaid M A., FamilyMed(EM)
Jagas, Ivan F.
Jakda, Ahmed I., FamilyMed
Jiwa, Ashifa, FamilyMed
Johnston, Eamon F.
Johnston, James D.
Kalirai, Baljit S., FamilyMed(EM)
Kane, Martin D., FamilyMed
Kaphengst, Karla
Kaur, Satinder, FamilyMed
Keleher, Stephen T., FamilyMed
Kelly, Brian F.
Kelly, Larry J.
Kennel, E. Ross, FamilyMed
Kennel, Richard L., FamilyMed
Khan, Mohammed A H.
Khan, Rita R.
Kim, Joe, FamilyMed
King, Jeffrey A.
Kitzul, Robert D.
Knibutat, Darren B.
Koke, Michael J., FamilyMed(EM)
Kolbasnik, Alexandr, FamilyMed
Kordish, Paul L.
Korsheed, Shvan, FamilyMed
Kuhnert, Peter E., FamilyMed
Kulkarni, Jyothi, FamilyMed
Lamothe, Francis
Lee, F. Joseph, FamilyMed
Lee, Linda L W., FamilyMed
Lee-Poy, Michael F., FamilyMed
Lehan, Anne E., FamilyMed
Leveck, David E., FamilyMed
Lubitz, Rebecca J., FamilyMed
Luce, Kiersten A., FamilyMed
MacGregor, Stephen A.
MacLeod, Hugh M., FamilyMed
Mahesan, Dhakshana
Maidment, Julie L., FamilyMed
Malon, Catherine R., FamilyMed
Malon, Peter H.
Maric, Peter
Martin, Jane E L., FamilyMed
Mather, J. Frederick, FamilyMed
McFarlane, Lisa A., FamilyMed
McKee, Ryan W C., FamilyMed
McTavish, Wyatt, FamilyMed
Mee, David W.
Meenan, John J.
Mehan, Upender K., FamilyMed
Mensah Kwesi, Albert, FamilyMed
Metcalfe, Shelley E., FamilyMed
Meyer, Caroline M., FamilyMed
Milio, Hany S., FamilyMed
Miller, George B., FamilyMed
Milligan, James D., FamilyMed
Mingiardi, Anne Marie, FamilyMed
Mirza, Nazneen S., FamilyMed
Mitrana, Irene, FamilyMed(EM)
Moolman, Andre, FamilyMed
Moosavi, Homayoon
Mountjoy, Margo L., FamilyMed
Mourcos, Ashraf F Z., FamilyMed
Murji, Amin, FamilyMed
Mutrie, John H.
Nantes, Stephen H., FamilyMed

Nasri, Masood A.
Nedimovic, Ljubica, FamilyMed
Nguyen, Bao Hoang
Nguyen, Thi Ngoc Dang, FamilyMed
Nicholson, Raymond F.
Nurse, William E.
O'Brien, Thomas J., FamilyMed
Owens, Erinn L., FamilyMed
Parekh, Shrenik P.
Parlea, Ileana C., FamilyMed
Patel, Divyesh M.
Patel-Christopher, Abha
Pearce, N. Glenn, FamilyMed
Pefanis, John, FamilyMed
Pendergast, Sara R., FamilyMed(EM)
Pfeifer, Sabine I., FamilyMed
Pienaar, Johannes J., FamilyMed
Poel, Margaret A M., FamilyMed
Pope, John D., FamilyMed
Purohit, Jigna R., FamilyMed
Quartermain, Melanie A., FamilyMed
Raco, Lina C., FamilyMed
Reimer, Wendy J.
Reinhardt, David J., FamilyMed
Renaud, Matthew J., FamilyMed(EM)
Rhodes, Donald A.
Richardson, Donald B.
Sacchini, Clara
Sahsi, Rupinder S.
Saluja, Inderpal S., FamilyMed(EM)
Sandor, Catherine C.
Sawyer, Marc R., FamilyMed
Sayar, Mirwais A., FamilyMed
Schumilas, Harry B., FamilyMed
Schwarz, Duncan K., FamilyMed
Seagrist, W. Scott
Segedi, Ljubinka, FamilyMed
Sehgal, Jaishree
Sehl, John J.
Sellers, Laurene R., FamilyMed
Seyler, Susan J S., FamilyMed
Shadd, Violet W A.
Sharma, Ashok
Shecter, Adam C., FamilyMed(EM)
Smith, Marnie L., FamilyMed
Smith, Patricia E., FamilyMed
Snyder, Douglas R., FamilyMed
Stewart, John M.
Stobie, Shannon B., FamilyMed
Szozda, Timothy J P., FamilyMed
Tan, Lana S., FamilyMed
Taylor, Martha L., FamilyMed
Taylor, Steven J.
Tiegs, Richard G.
Timmons, Pauline M., FamilyMed
Toews, Ronald P., FamilyMed
Tong, Xiaoxing C., FamilyMed(EM)
Turner, Frances N., FamilyMed
Upenieks, Richard L., FamilyMed
Varano, Kristopher, FamilyMed
Vojdani, Merle A.
Waldbillig, David K., FamilyMed(EM)
Wang, Alex C., FamilyMed
Wang, Ay-Ling, FamilyMed
Ward, Donna M., FamilyMed
Warren, E. Janet, FamilyMed
Watson, Alan F.
Whitby, Peter L., FamilyMed
Wickett, Robert G., FamilyMed(EM)
Wilson, Lorne W.
Winter, Arthur J., FamilyMed
Wismer, Sandra J., FamilyMed
Witmer, Michael R., FamilyMed(EM)
Wong, Jennifer Y Y., FamilyMed(EM)
Worndl, M. Michele
Wren, Denise M.
Wurtele, Patika A.
Yee, John, FamilyMed
Zettel, Janet M T., FamilyMed
Zorzitto, Joanna R., FamilyMed
Zur, Daniel

LAKEFIELD

Arthur, Laverne S., FamilyMed
Bailey, Christopher J.
Hughes, Brendan J., FamilyMed
Munoz, Michael A., FamilyMed
Senior, Steven L., FamilyMed
Wilson, M. Kaetlen, FamilyMed

LANARK

Gruder, Alicja N., FamilyMed
Wahay, Leigh R., FamilyMed
Walsh, Gregory J., FamilyMed(EM)

LANSDOWNE

Casey, Michelle, FamilyMed
Erb, John B., FamilyMed
Gitterman, J. Lawrence

LASALLE

Dhaliwal, Preet B K., FamilyMed

LATCHFORD

Hardie, Brenda J., FamilyMed

LEAMINGTON

Chalhoub, Sarkis
Gonzalez-Almeyda, Roberto, FamilyMed
Gorrell, Gerald J.
Greenwood, Julian D., FamilyMed
Heys, Luther, FamilyMed
Holloway, Randy W.
Horen, Sheila A., FamilyMed
Imasogie, Ngozi
Leung, Gregory H Y.
McCoy, Stephen N.
Moncur, Ross, FamilyMed
Oduwole, Queenette
Park, Rachel C., FamilyMed
Phipps, Lincoln R.
Russell, Alan D.
Sabga, Frederick H.
Sarfraz, Saad, FamilyMed
Simpson, Robert C.
Stapleton, Robert J., FamilyMed
Swedan, Ahmed M., FamilyMed(EM)
Tam, Martina Y T.
Tokarewicz, John P M., FamilyMed
Tracy, Susanne
Yacoub, Ninos, FamilyMed

LEVACK

Kealy, Walter W.
Laski, Jennifer B., FamilyMed

LINDSAY

Anderson, Peter L., FamilyMed
Batten, Brian K.
Bothwell, Stuart M., FamilyMed
Brenchley, Reginald
Carruthers, Angela M., FamilyMed(EM)
Chandra, Mark J., FamilyMed(EM)
Chapman, Kathryn A.
Chayer, Marc J.
Dafoe, Joan M., FamilyMed
Dickson, Paul J.
Drury, Robert
Ecob, Naomi A.
Evans, Keith M.
Fagan, Brian
Francis, Michael J D., FamilyMed
Francis, Sara-Lynn D., FamilyMed
Gulati, Brij B.
Hainer, Steven C., FamilyMed
Hayman, Kellie, FamilyMed(EM)
Hussein, Mohammed H., FamilyMed
Jackson, Christopher A.
Jackson, Rosalie J.
Joynt, Meileen, FamilyMed
Katakkar, Jyoti, FamilyMed
Klein, David W.
Knox, John R A., FamilyMed
Konyer, Alan T.
Lerm, Leon B., FamilyMed
Lindsay, J E. Gordon
Loeb, Graham J., FamilyMed
MacMillan, Brent M.
Nancekievill, Ivan W.
Nicholson, Naomi L., FamilyMed
Petrosoniak, Peter
Pretorius, Marina, FamilyMed
Rainkie, Kristopher D., FamilyMed
Ready, Eric, FamilyMed
Reid, Dawn K., FamilyMed(EM)
Roberts, Kristine J., FamilyMed
Rutherford, Debra L.
Sears, Ronald S R.
Stanley, Wayne E., FamilyMed
Stefopulos, Thomas
Stone, Mark C., FamilyMed
Stone, Mervyn A., FamilyMed
Summers, Leslie B.
Ursel, Peter G.
Vorster, Sarel, FamilyMed
Wilson, Ruth K., FamilyMed
Young, Sheila-Mae
Yu, Katie, FamilyMed

LIONS HEAD

Appleton, Alison E., FamilyMed
Loney, Elgin M.
Shoush, Suzanne, FamilyMed
Thomas, Jonathan B., FamilyMed
Thomson, David M., FamilyMed

LISLE

Verma, Narpendra

LISTOWEL

Annis, Robert W K., FamilyMed
Conners, John S.
Edmonds, Gillian, FamilyMed
Latuskie, Russell H K., FamilyMed
Matthews, Barbara A.
Neable, Barry W.
Qureshi, Arif S., FamilyMed
Ramsewak, Ravi D.
Rutherford, Paul
Suggitt, Terry E., FamilyMed
Warren, Rex C.
Westen, Evelyn C.

LITTLE CURRENT

Allen, David M., FamilyMed(EM)
Barss, Kenneth A., FamilyMed
Cooper, Stephen, FamilyMed
Jeffery, Roy D., FamilyMed
Keenan, Tiffany J., FamilyMed
Meikleham, Simone A., FamilyMed(EM)
Poenn, Dieter, FamilyMed
Quackenbush, Benjamin R H., FamilyMed
Renwick, Sherri A., FamilyMed

LIVELY

Bayly, Peter L.
Carscadden, Terence R.
Cox, Jane E., FamilyMed
Duncan, Sarah L H., FamilyMed
Koop, V. Gary
Levasseur, Liisa K., FamilyMed
Richardson, Katherine M., FamilyMed
Susil, Monica, FamilyMed

LONDON

Abdel Malek, Gihan F K., FamilyMed
Aggarwal, Shilpa, FamilyMed
Ahluwalia, Ravjit S., FamilyMed
Ahmed, Shajan, FamilyMed
Ahmed, Syed K S., FamilyMed
Akhtar, Nadeem
Alam, Huma A., FamilyMed
Alam, M. Mumtaz, FamilyMed
Alam, Muhammad M.
Alam, Tasriqul M., FamilyMed
Alghamdi, Khalid H S.
Alija, Agron, FamilyMed
Allen, Julie K., FamilyMed
Altamirano Diaz, Luis A.
Altmann, Karolina
Andrade, Jennifer M., FamilyMed
Andrews, Catriona H.
Annen, A. Albert, FamilyMed
Arabi, Nezhat
Arbeau, Ryan P.
Arcia-Bravo, Edgard A.
Armogan, Edward D., FamilyMed
Armstrong, Robert D., FamilyMed
Armstrong, Sarah A.
Arthur, Frederick E., FamilyMed(EM)
Asem, Kevin D., FamilyMed
Ashok, Dhandapani
Assuras, John W.
Atta, Imran, FamilyMed
Awde, J. Douglas
Awde, Murray G., FamilyMed
Baass, Patricia C., FamilyMed
Baig, Mirza M W., FamilyMed(EM)
Bainbridge, Monica T., FamilyMed
Baker, Leslie A.
Baker, Sharon L.
Balaska, Yasmina, FamilyMed
Baldwin, Clark, FamilyMed
Bali, Amardeep K.
Ballantyne, Patricia K., FamilyMed
Barr, David B.
Bates, W. Paul, FamilyMed
Bax, Kevin
Beal, Timothy
Behme, Nancy A., FamilyMed
Belyea, Melita, FamilyMed
Bendheim, Henry, FamilyMed
Benn, Ruth L., FamilyMed
Bhaduri, Mousumi
Bhalla, Rashmi, FamilyMed
Bhamjee, Hassen
Bhayana, Bhooma, FamilyMed
Bhella, Vishal S., FamilyMed
Bhimani, Munsif, FamilyMed(EM)
Bialik, Sean J.
Bigham, Gerald L.
Birch, David R.
Biro, Antal
Bock, Dirk E.
Bodkin, Andrew C., FamilyMed
Bodkin, E. Anne, FamilyMed
Bonin, Melanie, FamilyMed
Briskin, Alexander
Brookes, Jonathan
Brown, Nadia K.
Brown, Peter J.
Brownscombe, Annette M.
Bruckschwaiger, Christian, FamilyMed
Bruckschwaiger, Dieter, FamilyMed
Bruckschwaiger, Mary L H.
Bryk, Caroline M., FamilyMed
Buconjic, Tomislav
Burneo De Las Casas, Jorge G.
Butchey, Maurice R S.
Cahalan, Alan D., FamilyMed
Campbell, James
Carter, Robert M.
Cavanaugh, David V.
Cejic, Sonny S., FamilyMed
Chaddah, Sasha S D.
Chan, Nelson N S., FamilyMed
Chawla, Virendra S.
Chernick, Elisheva H.
Clarke, Julie L., FamilyMed(EM)
Clayden, Wesley, FamilyMed
Clement, John S.
Cogliano, Antonio, FamilyMed
Cohen, Irene, FamilyMed
Collins, Ronald W., FamilyMed
Consul, Megha
Coome, Grant E A., FamilyMed(EM)
Corrin, Murray D.
Cumberland, Penny K.
Cumming, Jane A K.
Cunningham, Karen N., FamilyMed
Damude, Leslie R.
Daoud, Hani I K.
Dave, Sumit
De Ribaupierre, Sandrine
De Silva, Lande B P., FamilyMed
De Vrijer, Barbra
Debosz-Szczerbowski, Grace
Delaney, Catherine
Delport, Johannes
Despard, Caroline, FamilyMed
Dickie, Gordon, FamilyMed
Dickie, Paul M.
Dixon, David, FamilyMed
Donworth, Michael
Drosdowech, Catriona H., FamilyMed
Dulay, Jaspal, FamilyMed
Dunkerley, Heather, FamilyMed
Dunkerley, Robert
Dymon, Diane A., FamilyMed
Dzongowski, Peter, FamilyMed
Eaton, Jo-Ann
Eberhard, Thomas S C.
Edels, Margrieta
El-Sadi, Salman A K., FamilyMed(EM)
El-Zein, Mohamad A K.
Elepano, Patricia, FamilyMed
Elia, Mario F., FamilyMed
Ellyatt, William G., FamilyMed
Faulds, Catherine, FamilyMed
Feagan, Nancy J., FamilyMed
Feightner, John W., FamilyMed
Ferguson, Keith
Fernandes, Christopher M B.
Finger, Elizabeth
Fischer, Lisa K., FamilyMed
Fleming, Michaele S.
Fodemesi, Frank J.
Fox, Paul
Foxcroft, Laura C., FamilyMed(EM)
Frederick, Catherine E., FamilyMed
Freeman, Jeffrey M., FamilyMed(EM)
Freeman, Thomas, FamilyMed
Gagnier, Rachel M., FamilyMed(EM)
Gangdev, Prakash S.
Gannon, Kathleen, FamilyMed
Garfat, Ronald E.
Garg, Pallav
George, M. Catherine
Gerrie, Alexandra, FamilyMed
Gill, Aneeqa A., FamilyMed
Gillis, Gregory F., FamilyMed
Gilpin, Sharon D.
Gladwell, Heather E., FamilyMed(EM)
Grace, Archie N., FamilyMed
Gracey, Janel L., FamilyMed
Gunaratnam, Lakshman
Gutoski, Donald R.
Hameed, Saadia, FamilyMed
Hamilton, Kirk, FamilyMed
Hammond, Jo-Anne S., FamilyMed
Harmar, Heather C.
Harris, Donald J F.
Harris, Stewart B., FamilyMed
Hawash-Mostafa, Fatma E.
Hawthorne, Diane W., FamilyMed
Henein, Emad, FamilyMed
Henning, Beth M., FamilyMed
Herbert, Carol P., FamilyMed
Herman, Dorli, FamilyMed(EM)
Hernandez Alejandro, Roberto
Hickey, Kristin M., FamilyMed
Hilsden, Richard, FamilyMed
Hirscheimer, Andrea, FamilyMed
Ho, Doris S C.
Hoben, Lionel E.
Hodder, David M.
Hollis, Brian A.
Horne, Jonathan B.
Horne, Pamela E.
Hosseini Moghaddam, Syed M.
Hostetler, Jason L., FamilyMed
Huang, Eleanor C Y., FamilyMed
Hull, M. Louise
Hunter-Orange, Jessica M., FamilyMed
Hussain, Nabil, FamilyMed
Imran, Aatika, FamilyMed
Iyer, Hariharan S.
Izzeldin, Mohamed S., FamilyMed
Jeje, Oluyemi M.
Jethwa, Arvind K N.
Jevremovic, Tatiana, FamilyMed(EM)

Jones, David H D.
Jordan, John M., FamilyMed
Joshi, Shelendra
Judson, Martyn, FamilyMed
Kakani, Nirma K.
Kamath, Vranda S., FamilyMed
Kanji, Zainul A A.
Katsios, Zaharo, FamilyMed
Kazi, Soofia L., FamilyMed
Keast, David H., FamilyMed
Kelland, Jeffrey M., FamilyMed
Kelly, Frances M.
Kernaghan, Gillian A J., FamilyMed
Keshmirian, Jalal, FamilyMed
Khamidbayev, Timur, FamilyMed
Khan, Shahzia, FamilyMed
Kharal, Aysha, FamilyMed
Kim, George P., FamilyMed
Kinigakis, Tracey D., FamilyMed
Klein, Klara P., FamilyMed
Komar, Ronald R.
Koudys, Deborah, FamilyMed
Krakofsky, Sheldon L.
Kratky, Antonin
Kumar, U. Sujana, FamilyMed
Kurukula Arachchi, Sandhya, FamilyMed
Labranche, Rachelle S., FamilyMed
Laity, Alan H., FamilyMed
Langer, Pearl S., FamilyMed
Lavi, Ronit
Lavi, Shahar
Lazo Langner, Alejandro
Lee, Betty H., FamilyMed
Lee, Kenneth W.
Lees, Nicholas M., FamilyMed
Lent, Barbara P., FamilyMed
Leung, Christopher P.
Levy, Michelle H., FamilyMed
Liabotis, Stephanie A., FamilyMed
Liaschko, Alexander A.
Lo, Karen K W., FamilyMed
Lockhart, Michelle A., FamilyMed
Loubani, Mohammed M., FamilyMed(EM)
Loubani, Tarek M., FamilyMed(EM)
Louzada, Martha D L.
Lovesey, Natalie J., FamilyMed
Luke, Seema, FamilyMed
Luton, Robert G.
Lyons, Laura M., FamilyMed
MacDonald, Christine A., FamilyMed(EM)
MacLaren, Susan I.
MacLean, James R L.
MacLean, Susan E., FamilyMed
Mackey, Jennifer E.
Maddeford, William R.
Maharaj, Deonarine
Maharaj, Siobhan C., FamilyMed
Mahmoud, Mohamed A S., FamilyMed
Makar Abdel Messih, Inas H.
Makhdoom, Sohail
Malik, Rubina, FamilyMed
Malik, Shiraz, FamilyMed
Malizia, Mario L.
Mall, Austin, FamilyMed
Malone, Sonya M., FamilyMed
Mann, G. Richard, FamilyMed
Marczuk, Dorota, FamilyMed
Martin, Joie C., FamilyMed
Martin, Rene F., FamilyMed
Martyniak, Dawid, FamilyMed
Mawhinney, Leah A., FamilyMed
Mawji, Altaf S J.
Mayr, Heinz G.
McBride, Simon
McCabe, Philip C., FamilyMed
McCarty, David
McCully, E. Kathleen, FamilyMed
McDonagh, Mary, FamilyMed
McDonagh, Thomas H M., FamilyMed
McDowall, Moira L.
McKay, Janet E., FamilyMed(EM)
McKay, Scott D., FamilyMed
McKee, Kandice A., FamilyMed
McKeough, Nancy, FamilyMed
McKeough, William P., FamilyMed
McLellan, Kenneth C., FamilyMed
McNair, Susan M., FamilyMed
McNeil, Ceara J., FamilyMed(EM)
Mekhaeil, Nermin M E., FamilyMed
Melville, Rhona D S.
Mok, Andrea H., FamilyMed
Mok, C. Albert
Mok, Lesley J., FamilyMed
Monforton, Anne-Marie, FamilyMed
Moore, Dana L., FamilyMed
Morrison, Gavin C.
Morrison, James C.
Moser, Nancy M.
Moulin, Jana M., FamilyMed
Mousa, Anushi T., FamilyMed
Muhammad, Naeem H., FamilyMed
Muia, Frank V.
Munro, David
Mura, Marco
Murchison, Sylvia A., FamilyMed
Myers, William D.
Naghiu, Marius C., FamilyMed
Naher, Monzur, FamilyMed
Nair, Vineet K., FamilyMed
Nelson, John A., FamilyMed
Neumann, Gary R., FamilyMed
Neumann, Laura V.
Nicholls, Eric, FamilyMed
Niesner, Claudia C F., FamilyMed
Nizami, Tariq F., FamilyMed
Noftle, Brooke M E., FamilyMed
Noorani, Shamidah, FamilyMed
Norrie, Deborah L., FamilyMed
Odegaard, Paul R.
Ogunmodede, O. David, FamilyMed
Orsini, Silvia A., FamilyMed
Osborne, Cynthia A.
Ouellet, Tracy Lara., FamilyMed
Owen, Richard John
Owens, Jennifer L., FamilyMed
Paddon, Robert C., FamilyMed
Pamula, Andrea, FamilyMed
Papukna, Vasiliki
Parent, Maria M., FamilyMed
Parry, Matthew T., FamilyMed
Patel, J. Susan, FamilyMed
Patel, Ketan N.
Paterson, Ian R.
Pawelec-Brzychczy, Anna, FamilyMed
Paylor, Dascha L.
Payne, William L., FamilyMed
Peckan, Catherine M., FamilyMed
Pelipyagina, Tetyana O., FamilyMed
Pellar, Karen E.
Persaud, Ganeshwar, FamilyMed
Peterson, Daniel R.
Petrella, Robert J., FamilyMed
Petrlich, Steve T., FamilyMed
Pezzutto, Donato
Pezzutto, Lucia, FamilyMed
Phillips, David D., FamilyMed
Piche, Lawrence C.
Pietrus, Henryk C.
Pietrus, Teresa
Pillon, Sylvia M., FamilyMed
Polsinelli, Kristina, FamilyMed
Pop, Anca, FamilyMed
Potter, C. Peter
Quraishi, M. Salim
Rabheru, Rita H., FamilyMed
Rahman, Shafiur
Rai, Amendeep S.
Rai, Sharadindu, FamilyMed
Rajagopa, Aarthi
Ralley, Fiona E.
Rauch, Ralf
Rayman, Reiza
Reddy, Ramesh, FamilyMed(EM)
Regan, Kelly A., FamilyMed(EM)
Reichert, Sonja-Maria, FamilyMed
Richard, Annette, FamilyMed
Richardson, Christine A., FamilyMed(EM)
Rigby, Megan C.
Rivest, Candice D., FamilyMed
Robinson, Helena M., FamilyMed
Roebotham, Roy W., FamilyMed(EM)
Rooney, Hugh
Rose, David L.
Rouhani, Nassim
Rouhani, Shiva, FamilyMed
Rrafshi, Lulzim, FamilyMed
Rubaiyyat, Tania, FamilyMed
Ruiter, P. James A.
Saadaldeen, Salwa A., FamilyMed
Salmon, Gretchen J.
Saly, Anthony J., FamilyMed
Sandejas, Mario F.
Sangster, John F., FamilyMed
Sargolzaei, Fatemeh, FamilyMed
Sarup, Brij M.
Schacter, Gordon B., FamilyMed
Schaefer, Rachel I., FamilyMed
Schleich, Martin J., FamilyMed
Schmidt, Lawrence G., FamilyMed
Schreier, Gil J., FamilyMed
Sereda, Andrea M., FamilyMed(EM)
Sexton, Frederick G.
Shadd, Joshua D., FamilyMed
Sharan, Sapna
Sharif, Nadder, FamilyMed(EM)
Sharma, Manas
Shaw, James E.
Shearer, Robin S., FamilyMed
Sheppard, Miranda E., FamilyMed
Shin, Frank, FamilyMed
Shmuilovich, Olga
Shu, Krishanthy, FamilyMed
Singh, Anita D., FamilyMed
Smith, Pamela A T., FamilyMed
Smith, Ryan S.
Smith, Stanley G., FamilyMed
Smits, Cheryl L., FamilyMed
Sohal, Jasdeep S., FamilyMed
Soo, Victoria, FamilyMed
Souter, Anne L., FamilyMed
Spano, Frank A., FamilyMed
Spence, Ann K., FamilyMed
Spence, Jeffrey D., FamilyMed
Starok, Carina N., FamilyMed
Steer, Robert K., FamilyMed
Steyn, Chris, FamilyMed
Subraman, Priya
Sukhera, Javeed I.
Sunderji, Salim H J., FamilyMed
Swift, John E., FamilyMed
Swinamer, Stuart A.
Sy, John C.
Tabor, Thomas K., FamilyMed
Taheri, Sepideh
Tai, Derek Y H., FamilyMed
Tallevi, Christie L., FamilyMed
Tallon, Stephen G., FamilyMed
Tam, Thomas W H., FamilyMed
Tambakis, Maria L., FamilyMed
Tanaka, Peter M., FamilyMed(EM)
Taylor-Wall, Suzanne E M., FamilyMed
Tetelbaum, Maria, FamilyMed
Tham, Pooi-Lin, FamilyMed
Theakston, Karl D.
Thomas, Valsa
Thomas, Wendy M., FamilyMed
Thompson, Keith A., FamilyMed
Thurgood, Elaine N.
Trenker, David C.
Tripp, Julie A., FamilyMed
Tse Hing Yuen, Stephanie, FamilyMed
Tu, Geming S.
Tupper, Vashti E., FamilyMed
Tutschka, Bridget K., FamilyMed
Upfold, Jane A., FamilyMed(EM)
Vaideswaran, Sangeeta, FamilyMed
Valiquet, Stacey K., FamilyMed(EM)
Vasudev, Akshya
Vasudev, Kamini
Vigna, Victor
Vladars, Josef M A., FamilyMed
Vockentanz, Birgit M.
Vopicka, Avaleen A., FamilyMed(EM)
Vu, N Q. Wayne, FamilyMed
Wainwright, Ruth E H.
Walker, Tara L.
Walsh, Catherine M., FamilyMed
Walsh, Claire M.
Wang, Wen-Shan
Watkins, Drew B.
Welisch, Eva
Wells, Mark C.
Wenske, Thomas R.
Wetmore, Stephen J., FamilyMed
Whelan, Barbara L.
Whynot, Andrew S., FamilyMed(EM)
Wickens, Courtney M., FamilyMed
Wickett, Jamie A E., FamilyMed
Wiebe, Amanda J., FamilyMed
Wiebenga, Marjie L., FamilyMed
Wilson, Dale R., FamilyMed(EM)
Wong, Eric K W., FamilyMed
Wong, Frank G., FamilyMed
Wong, Keith H., FamilyMed
Woodford, Elizabeth S., FamilyMed
Yemchuk, Bohdan R., FamilyMed
Zakhary, Mourad I S., FamilyMed
Ziradkar, Jyotsna S., FamilyMed
Ziradkar, Shaliendra Y., FamilyMed

LUCAN

Anderson, E. James
Bowler, W. Blake
Lock, Walter A.
Peterson, Michael, FamilyMed
Viguera Salazar, Milagro C., FamilyMed

LUCKNOW

Shubat, J. Michael
Sleeth, Sean P., FamilyMed

LYNDEN

Picketts, Darrell K.

MADOC

Dosaj, Arun K.
Dullege, Suzanne, FamilyMed
Stewart, Adam M., FamilyMed
Webb, Janet L., FamilyMed
Yorston, Janet E., FamilyMed

MALTON

Moro, Luciano F.

MANITOUWADGE

Cote, Peter B., FamilyMed
MacTavish, James C., FamilyMed(EM)
Petersen, Karin, FamilyMed
Young, H. Thomas, FamilyMed

MANITOWANING

Bedard, Michael

MANOTICK

Abdulla, Alykhan S., FamilyMed
Asselstine, Robert C.
Berghuis-Hummel, Wendy D., FamilyMed
Hovey, Jeffrey T., FamilyMed
Jetty, Mandip K., FamilyMed
Kent, Lenore J., FamilyMed
Lal, Shirin B., FamilyMed
Nguyen, John T., FamilyMed
Ozard, Jennifer G., FamilyMed
Puxty, Gillian M.
Ruparelia, Vasant C.
Schnurr, Clare M., FamilyMed
Ting Malone, Christina M Y., FamilyMed
Williams, Cathy L.
Yeats, Barbara A., FamilyMed

MAPLE

Abdel-Malek, Nada, FamilyMed
Agate, William A., FamilyMed(EM)
Assad, Samir R G., FamilyMed
Bray, Riina I., FamilyMed
Castiglione, Alberto, FamilyMed
Chen, Robert C C., FamilyMed
Dammermann, Scott
Di Santo, Loredana, FamilyMed
Ferlisi, Anthony J.
Ferlisi, James R F.
Gillmore, Trevor A.
Hatami, Shahin, FamilyMed
Hussain, Tabassum M., FamilyMed
Kassam, Salma, FamilyMed
Krystolovich, Leonard W.
Levy, Michelle R., FamilyMed
Lieberman, Esther J., FamilyMed
Lilani, Rizwana, FamilyMed
Mak, Ian, FamilyMed
Naghdi, Lili, FamilyMed
Perera, Ethige S C., FamilyMed
Salamon, Lisa, FamilyMed(EM)
Salyani, Mohamed A.
Zanette, Paul A., FamilyMed

MARATHON

Brunskill, Megen, FamilyMed
Fitch, Nancy K., FamilyMed
Kent, Rebecca, FamilyMed
Newbery, Sarah-Lynn, FamilyMed
Orrantia, Eliseo, FamilyMed
Purcell, Daniel M., FamilyMed
Sturwold, Nichole M., FamilyMed
Wilson, Scott N., FamilyMed

MARKDALE

Al-Tukmachi, Ahmad M S.
Kaethler, Frieder
McIntosh, Sandra L.
Morel, Linda D.
Murphy, Charles W.

MARKHAM

Abba, Zaheera, FamilyMed
Abeysinghe, Chitralekha R., FamilyMed
Adams, Amanda J., FamilyMed
Ahmed, Youmna
Albert, Maha A.
Alexander, Michelle L., FamilyMed
Alikhan, Neetan, FamilyMed(EM)
Alvarez, Isabel F., FamilyMed
Ananth, Shobana, FamilyMed(EM)
Arcand, Andrew S., FamilyMed(EM)
Balinson, Alex P.
Bartucci, Michael, FamilyMed
Beca, Sorin G.
Boisvenue, Marc André, FamilyMed
Byrne, Tara, FamilyMed(EM)
Caturay, Michael J., FamilyMed
Chan, Macky M K., FamilyMed
Chan, Monica K H., FamilyMed
Chan, W. Mun-Kam
Chang, Annisa, FamilyMed
Chang, C C. Nancy, FamilyMed
Chapman, Kelly S.
Chen, Lily F., FamilyMed
Cheng, Joan F., FamilyMed(EM)
Cheung, Alicia K F., FamilyMed
Cheung, Francesca T., FamilyMed
Cheung, Hym D.
Chiu, Patrick, FamilyMed
Choy, Benjamin S., FamilyMed
Chrystoja, Walter A.
Craig, Cecil B., FamilyMed
Currie, Heather J., FamilyMed
Dharamshi, Arif
El-Kateb, Hayam H R., FamilyMed
Empey, Karen E., FamilyMed
Esterbauer, Ronald G., FamilyMed
Feng, Z S. Chris, FamilyMed
Feuer, Catherine F.
Filosa, Thomas M., FamilyMed
Forse, Bertram
Gannage, John M., FamilyMed
Goldstein, Mark, FamilyMed
Goodfellow, Anne F., FamilyMed
Gorman, James A.
Greenwald, Ilana, FamilyMed(EM)
Grill, Allan K., FamilyMed

Gupta, Chantal R.
Haw, Peter M., FamilyMed
Himmel, Susan
Ho, Hon-Lau, FamilyMed
Hood, Roberta, FamilyMed
Hum, Annie
Hum, Teresa Y K., FamilyMed
Ibrahim, Magdy, FamilyMed
Iseman, Wendy E., FamilyMed(EM)
Jacob, Abraham J., FamilyMed
Jacobs, Howard
Jang, Douglas K., FamilyMed
Jayashankar, Komathy, FamilyMed
Kandasamy, Gengatharan
Kane, Jennifer J., FamilyMed
Kanetos, Emmanuel, FamilyMed
Kazandji, Dalal, FamilyMed
Khan, Waheed
King, Barbara J., FamilyMed(EM)
Kirubaharan, Rajaratnam, FamilyMed
Kwan, Irene K W.
Lai, Crystal Y C., FamilyMed
Lai, Eliza P Y., FamilyMed
Lam, Angela W W.
Lam, Emilie Y., FamilyMed
Lee, Hayvin, FamilyMed
Leu, Eric D H.
Leung, Andy W C.
Leung, Kent K K.
Leung, Nin-Ming, FamilyMed
Li, Bessie P T., FamilyMed
Li, Janice C Y., FamilyMed
Lo, Ada Y T., FamilyMed
Lo, Adrian W., FamilyMed
Lo, Jason H T., FamilyMed
Loganathan, Rajeswary, FamilyMed
Lougheed, Daryl B., FamilyMed
Lougheed, Eileen M., FamilyMed
Mai, Daryl W.
Makhlouf, Samia M., FamilyMed
Martin, Eva
Masellis, Antony
Maxted, John M., FamilyMed
McLaren, Stephen T., FamilyMed
McLean, Patsy L.
Meinig, Elaine M.
Mingie, Lorraine O.
Minster, Richard
Mitelman, Bernice, FamilyMed(EM)
Moldoveanu, Adina A.
Monrose, Brigitte M A E., FamilyMed
Morgenstern, Justin, FamilyMed(EM)
Morris, Gail A., FamilyMed
Mudrik, Kevin P., FamilyMed(EM)
Nagamuttu, Sivakumar, FamilyMed
Newton, William H., FamilyMed
Ng, David C K.
Ng, Ken H M.
Ng, Stephen
Nicholson, Marcia A., FamilyMed
Nowak, Michael A.
Obney, Jeannette
Pang, Wei-Mei, FamilyMed
Pararajasingam, Thevaki
Pasricha, Deepti, FamilyMed
Philpott, Jane P., FamilyMed
Poon, C C. Terry, FamilyMed
Popa, Christina C., FamilyMed(EM)
Poppen, Jacquline, FamilyMed
Ravindranath, Pathmanathan, FamilyMed
Rawof, Salma, FamilyMed
Rotstein, J R. Jennifer N., FamilyMed
Rudnikoff, Jordana S., FamilyMed
Sabir, Sonia, FamilyMed(EM)
Saini, Preeti, FamilyMed
Saslove, David W.
Sathiaseelan, Seyon, FamilyMed
Scott, Carol L.
Seit, Shawn C W.
Shapero, Gary A., FamilyMed
Sharma, Shivani
Singh, Paramjeet, FamilyMed
Siu, Winnie W., FamilyMed
Sivasubramaniam, Tharsika, FamilyMed
Sjodin, Astrid D., FamilyMed
Strauss, Barry I., FamilyMed
Suchak, Nayana A., FamilyMed
Sue, Sammy C W., FamilyMed(EM)
Syed, Sumairah A., FamilyMed
Syed, Tahniat S.
Szeto, Kenneth P C.
Tam, Alvin H., FamilyMed
Tan, Christopher Y K., FamilyMed
Taylor, Michael J., FamilyMed(EM)
Teh, M C. Matthew
Thangasamy, Rajasekaran
Timol, Shehnaz, FamilyMed
Tjon, Peter E., FamilyMed
Tohme, Juliette, FamilyMed
Trager, Chaim J.
Trinh, Grace H., FamilyMed
Trinh, Hue Co
Trojanowski, Elizabeth M.
Tsang, W Y. Eliza, FamilyMed
Um, Gregory T H.
Vandenberg, Alison P.
Virani, Mirza R.
Wan, Andrew W C., FamilyMed
Wang, Jeffry B., FamilyMed
Wasser, Edward M I., FamilyMed
Weinberg, Jeffrey N.
Weissberger, Jeffrey M., FamilyMed
West, Amanda L., FamilyMed
Wise, Yishai A., FamilyMed
Wong, Hon-Wah
Wong, Thompson K W.
Woo, Dennis K.
Woo, Kin Yee
Wu, Alwin, FamilyMed
Wu, Howard, FamilyMed
Wu, Raymond H C.
Ye, Juan, FamilyMed
Yermus, Ryan D., FamilyMed
Yip, Gina T C., FamilyMed
Yuen, S Y. Sheila, FamilyMed
Zhang, Ying, FamilyMed

MARMORA

Holowaty, Melissa N., FamilyMed
Muscat, Anne H., FamilyMed

MARTINTOWN

Toop, Jo-Ann D.

MASSEY

Cherian, S. Rachael, FamilyMed
Garland, Allan R.

MATHESON

Freundlich, George, FamilyMed
Razack, Tamazadeene, FamilyMed

MATTAWA

Gushe, Leonard D.
Redhead, Clint A.
Wilkins, Mark A., FamilyMed

MAXVILLE

Jaggassar, Theo A., FamilyMed

MEAFORD

Collins, Alexandra K U.
Logan, Renee C., FamilyMed
Lyon, Ronald G.
Weiss, William V.
Wong, James Y K.

MERRICKVILLE

Howarth, Erik, FamilyMed
McGregor, Penelope K., FamilyMed
Mooney, Kevin K., FamilyMed
Saunders-Reuvers, Cynthia B.

METCALFE

Merrett, Donald G.

MIDHURST

Nesdoly, Derek S.
Smith, Susan L M., FamilyMed

MIDLAND

Archer, Robert A., FamilyMed
Bayfield, David J., FamilyMed(EM)
Beeston, Jeffery P., FamilyMed
Besley, Robert H.
Blake, McKenzie M., FamilyMed
Cameron, Peter P G.
Chabikuli, Sibomana S., FamilyMed(EM)
Coutts, Richard A., FamilyMed
De Boeck, Thomas, FamilyMed
Donald, Douglas N.
Fox, William R.
Gannon, Anne B., FamilyMed
Gardiner, Donald I., FamilyMed
Golisky, Bruno J., FamilyMed
Golisky, Jeffrey M., FamilyMed(EM)
Grundmanis, Mark A., FamilyMed
Helt, Robert P.
Hyslop, Douglas R.
Jilesen, Herman C.
Jones, Andrea K., FamilyMed(EM)
Karson, Stanley J., FamilyMed
Kentner, Taryn, FamilyMed
Lau, Ian T., FamilyMed
Lee, Daniel K., FamilyMed(EM)
Loiskandl, Barbara J.
Loiskandl, Rainer H W.
MacSween, Moira A., FamilyMed(EM)
McCutcheon, N. Larry
McGuire, R. Philip, FamilyMed(EM)
McNamara, Martin A J., FamilyMed(EM)
Mossanda Chabikuli, Kenyabu C., FamilyMed
Nel, Andre J.
Pinto, Natasha, FamilyMed
Ralhan, Vikram, FamilyMed
Schecter, Danial M I., FamilyMed
Siedlecki, Jacqueline B C., FamilyMed
Thomas, Richard D., FamilyMed
Van Rooyen, Gert I., FamilyMed
Veall, Martin B., FamilyMed
Wagg, Ian D., FamilyMed
Wiens, Joel L., FamilyMed

MILDMAY

James, Philip B.

MILLBROOK

Liston, James P., FamilyMed
Van Loon, J. David, FamilyMed

MILTON

Abrahim, Mohammed, FamilyMed
Amir, Mohammad F.
Asif, Anjum, FamilyMed
Badawi, Arieg Z E., FamilyMed
Bains, Rajdeep, FamilyMed
Bickhram, Mahendra, FamilyMed
Bird Pyper, Cynthia J., FamilyMed
Boxall, Janice M., FamilyMed(EM)
Chan, H B. Tony, FamilyMed
Chung, Kin Lok
Cuberovic, Nick B., FamilyMed
Dag-Ellams, Ugonwa, FamilyMed
Deans, A. Michael, FamilyMed
Dhiraj, Navraj S., FamilyMed
Easo, James, FamilyMed
Filipowicz, W. Adam
Fonseka, Sujeewa D., FamilyMed
Gerges, Maha F G., FamilyMed
Gilbert, Michael R., FamilyMed
Gleisner, George R.
Goonetillake, Piyanthi, FamilyMed
Gowda, Shruthi, FamilyMed
Hajas, Adriana, FamilyMed
Hapuarachchi, Milanthi, FamilyMed
Hassan, Paul, FamilyMed(EM)
Hunter, Ivan A.
Ishaqzay, Rahmatullah, FamilyMed
Kamouna, Ahmed K., FamilyMed
Kamouna, Mustafa K., FamilyMed
Kathuria, Chanchal, FamilyMed
Khalid, Salman, FamilyMed(EM)
Kiaira, Mary K.
King, Marion J., FamilyMed
Koslowski, Waldemar
Kucharska, Agnes, FamilyMed
Kunica, Richard D.
Lakhanpal, Neeraj, FamilyMed
Latif, Shazia, FamilyMed
Little, Janet G., FamilyMed
Malec, Carolyn L., FamilyMed
Maley, Garnet J M.
Mathew, Beena, FamilyMed
Mathews, Nicole M., FamilyMed
Mendoza, Maribel B., FamilyMed
Merali, Shamsh Y., FamilyMed
Middlestadt, Laurie A.
Moodley, Prabashnee, FamilyMed
Patroi, Anca, FamilyMed
Paulsen, Tennille D S., FamilyMed
Peers, Glenn A.
Peiris, Malwattage J P., FamilyMed
Pfeiffer, Any Z.
Qazi, Khalida, FamilyMed
Robinson, Lynne E.
Sadera, Abhimanyu J S., FamilyMed
Sandhu, Amarpreet S., FamilyMed
Saxena, Pradeep, FamilyMed
Schachter, Sam S.
Schatzmann, Markus, FamilyMed
Shedletzky, Abraham
Sochocka, Elisabeth K.
Stircu, Cristina E., FamilyMed
Tadros, Mina, FamilyMed
Tam, Hon-Yin A.
Tawadross, Sherif M S., FamilyMed
Tooming, Vello E T.
Truong, Catherine, FamilyMed(EM)
Umer, Hafiz M., FamilyMed(EM)
Watada, Brian H., FamilyMed
Wong, Nathan D., FamilyMed
Youssef, Victor S F., FamilyMed
Yudin, Alexandra, FamilyMed
Zevallos, Gonzalo F.

MILVERTON

Birch, Corey T., FamilyMed
Hodes, Peter K.

MINDEMOYA

Al Hadi, Mouafak, FamilyMed
Jeeves, Nicholas G.
O'Connor, Kevin P., FamilyMed
Reade, Maurianne K., FamilyMed(EM)
Stadnyk, Andrew M.

MINDEN

Fiddler, David
Fiddler, Douglas
Helt, Bruno R., FamilyMed
Lingertat, John R., FamilyMed
Wu, Bennet P Y.

MISSISSAUGA

Abdel-Malek, Maximous Y M., FamilyMed
Abou-Nassar, Awni
Abouna, Samir, FamilyMed
Abramson, Norman
Abu Haleeqa, Khaled E M E.
Abu Setteh, Nihad M A., FamilyMed
Adamo, Niam, FamilyMed
Adamson, Margaret E M.
Afsar, Afsaneh
Afshar, Maryam
Agarwal, Shashi
Ahluwalia, Ajit K.
Ahluwalia, Mohinderjit S.
Ahluwalia, Usha
Ahmad, Zafar D., FamilyMed(EM)
Airia, Parisa, FamilyMed
Ajisebutu, Tewogbola S., FamilyMed
Al-Dabbagh, Haider M., FamilyMed
Al-Hamid, Sameer M.
Al-Jazrawi, Nadir, FamilyMed
Alam, Mohammed S., FamilyMed
Alvi, Ruby M., FamilyMed
Amin, Sheikh N U., FamilyMed
Amjad, Saima, FamilyMed
Ammad, Mahjabeen, FamilyMed
Anderson, Manfred E.
Andruko, Brent I.
Ang, Chrizette T.
Anvari, Linda, FamilyMed
Araujo, Adilson A M.
Arnot, Alison, FamilyMed(EM)
Aronnilakkara, Priya P., FamilyMed
Asady, M. Anwar
Asaro, Rosalinda, FamilyMed
Asham-Youssef, Amal A., FamilyMed
Athey, Robert A.
Atkins, James A., FamilyMed(EM)
Attalla, Hani F., FamilyMed
Attalla, Mireille G., FamilyMed
Attia, Amine N., FamilyMed
Attia, Elham B., FamilyMed
Aujla, Ramandeep S., FamilyMed
Awadde Alla Ghattas, Suzan, FamilyMed
Azer, Eman A M., FamilyMed
Baird, Wycliffe H.
Bakker, G. Willemien, FamilyMed
Bansal, Sundeep K.
Banwatt, Sundeep S., FamilyMed
Barwell, Jean, FamilyMed
Bashagha, Ahmed, FamilyMed
Baswick, Brenda, FamilyMed
Bath, Navdeep, FamilyMed
Baugniet, Jessica L., FamilyMed
Bautista, Filomena M., FamilyMed
Bawangoanwala, Asifa, FamilyMed
Beard, Jonathan D.
Bector, Neel S.
Behiya, Ziad H., FamilyMed(EM)
Belchetz, Lance A., FamilyMed(EM)
Beretta, Jennifer A.
Berezowskyj, Alexandra I., FamilyMed
Beshay, Hany Y., FamilyMed
Beshay, Sanaa S., FamilyMed(EM)
Besik, Ferdinand R.
Bhalla, Indu B.
Bharat, Winston S P., FamilyMed
Bielawska, Hanna, FamilyMed(EM)
Biro, Laurence, FamilyMed
Black, Jennifer P.
Black, Ronald W.
Black, Steven M.
Bluemke, Alice M., FamilyMed
Bolland, Mary F., FamilyMed
Bolland, Peter G., FamilyMed
Bollozos, Rene P.
Botros, Mary, FamilyMed
Boule, Christopher J., FamilyMed(EM)
Boules, Isaac, FamilyMed
Bowers, Richard J.
Boyko, Robert M., FamilyMed(EM)
Brereton, Sheila M.
Brooks, David H.
Brown, Simon E.
Brun Del Re, Renato
Buchstein, Miriam L.
Budhoo, Salesh K S., FamilyMed
Bugada, Nadia, FamilyMed
Bui, J. Thuc Thuan, FamilyMed
Calder, M. Suzanne
Campbell, Alan D.
Campbell, Thomas
Cauchi, Mario M.
Chalvardjian, Peter G.
Chan, John W L.
Chan, Juanita Y., FamilyMed
Chan, Loh Yen L., FamilyMed
Chan, Paul C.

Chang, Danny T L.
Charal, John M.
Charboneau, Joan M., FamilyMed
Chaudhary, Mohammad I., FamilyMed
Chaudhry, Uzma S., FamilyMed
Chellew, Matthew G., FamilyMed(EM)
Chen, Adam Y H., FamilyMed
Chen, Andy Y H.
Chen, Richard Y Y., FamilyMed
Chen, Tsai I., FamilyMed(EM)
Chen, Victoria Y S., FamilyMed
Cheung, Paul K., FamilyMed
Cheung, Vera K F., FamilyMed
Cheung, W C. Thomas, FamilyMed
Chew, John K H.
Chin, Peter M C., FamilyMed
Chin Cham, Martin, FamilyMed
Choi, H. David, FamilyMed
Choudhury, Anil
Choy, Henry M T.
Chu, Shiron C Y.
Chu, W K. William
Chung, Michael H., FamilyMed(EM)
Clarkson, David G., FamilyMed
Cohen, M. Geoffrey, FamilyMed
Cohen, Michael R., FamilyMed(EM)
Collins-Williams, Donald J., FamilyMed
Coman-Wood, Lori R.
Connelly, Ruth A., FamilyMed
Corkum, Casey G., FamilyMed
Cousins-Caranci, Frances, FamilyMed
Cruz, Geraldine Z V., FamilyMed
Cytowski, P. Lorraine, FamilyMed
D'Sa, Alfred J.
Dally, Ghassan Y., FamilyMed
Dang, Phuong, FamilyMed
Daudi, Asfa, FamilyMed
Daya, Farahnaz, FamilyMed
Daya, Nazim F.
De Marchi, W. Gregory
Degani, Naeema C.
Deppisch, Linda M., FamilyMed
Desai, Parag
Devanesen, Asha K.
Devanesen, Sudarshan, FamilyMed
Dhaliwal, Yadvinder S.
Dhanoa, Avtar S.
Din, Shamoon
Diyaeb, Mohamed A., FamilyMed
Dobkin, Martin
Dosani, Rehana N., FamilyMed
Duerksen, Anthony J., FamilyMed(EM)
Dunstall, Joanne M., FamilyMed
Eapen-John, Reena E., FamilyMed
Eisen, Joel M.
El-Sayegh, Rawieh, FamilyMed
Epstein, Norman L., FamilyMed(EM)
Esmond, John E., FamilyMed
Everson, Jennifer M., FamilyMed
Ewert, Robert D.
Fagbola, Adebola, FamilyMed
Faheim, Enass, FamilyMed
Fahim, Sylvia, FamilyMed
Fahmy, Yousef W., FamilyMed
Farag, Rose F., FamilyMed
Fellegi, Vivien
Fenty, Pauline L.
Figurado, Victor J.
Findlay, Peter M., FamilyMed
Fine, Geoffrey M., FamilyMed(EM)
Finn, Stephanie K., FamilyMed
Forrester, Dennis H G., FamilyMed
Forster-Gibson, Cynthia
Fowler, Stephen G.
Franklin, Angus L R., FamilyMed
Franklin, LeRoy D.
Fung, Kan Ying.
Furqan, Naila, FamilyMed
Galbraith, Beverley D.
Garcia, Andrea, FamilyMed
Gerges, Ayman, FamilyMed
Ghani, Ikram
Ghazala, Khalida K., FamilyMed
Gill, Paramjit
Gill, Vikramjit S.
Gindi, Gimiana N., FamilyMed
Girgis, Samira W A., FamilyMed
Girgis, Siham, FamilyMed
Gitterman, Michael M., FamilyMed(EM)
Goodman, Jesse B.
Goolam Hussain, M. Rashid, FamilyMed
Gordon, Sherif A A E., FamilyMed
Gorwill, Susan M.
Goyal, Sohal V., FamilyMed
Graham, Debra G.
Graham, Lawrie J., FamilyMed
Graham, Melissa, FamilyMed
Grava-Gubins, Inese
Gray, Gail L., FamilyMed
Grewal, Rajwant K.
Griffin, Wendy A., FamilyMed
Guirguis, Dina, FamilyMed
Guirguis, Isis K., FamilyMed
Gupta, Asha, FamilyMed
Gupta, Renu
Gupta, Sanjeev
Guru, Kiran
Gustafsson, Jan C.
Gutkin, Calvin L., FamilyMed(EM)
Gyongyossy, Edward A.
Halperin, Michael
Haluk, Myron, FamilyMed(EM)
Hammoud, Souhaila, FamilyMed
Hanna, Mary M., FamilyMed
Hanna, Nevin-Wadie N., FamilyMed
Hanna, Rose K F A., FamilyMed
Harild, Laura D., FamilyMed
Hashim, Shahzad
Hason, Yaniv
Hassan, Amal, FamilyMed
Hathout, Deana, FamilyMed(EM)
Hershkop, Sheldon, FamilyMed
Hester, Valerie L.
Hewitt, Cheryl A W., FamilyMed
Hickey, Bruce M.
Hindoosh, Raghad A N A., FamilyMed
Ho, Kwok Fan
Ho, Vincent W S., FamilyMed
Hong, Tommy, FamilyMed
Howard, Craig R.
Huang, Ling Ling., FamilyMed
Hudson, Jean E., FamilyMed
Huen, K M. Nicoletta, FamilyMed
Humniski, Anne-Marie P., FamilyMed(EM)
Hung, Frederico A.
Hunt, Anita S., FamilyMed
Hussain, Tasneem, FamilyMed
Huynh, Xinh
Hyles, Rudolph S.
Iftikhar, Asma, FamilyMed
Irshad, Fauzia, FamilyMed
Iskandir, Amal K E., FamilyMed
Ivankovic, Maria N., FamilyMed(EM)
Jakovcic, Carmela M., FamilyMed
Jamal, Hafeez L., FamilyMed
Javier, Romulo E.
Jawad, Luma R., FamilyMed
Jivanji, Nisreen, FamilyMed
Joshi, Sushma
Jovey, Roman D.
Kale, Karna C., FamilyMed
Kates, Michael D., FamilyMed
Kathiravelu, Anusha, FamilyMed
Kayser, Rebecca J., FamilyMed(EM)
Kayumi, Adam S., FamilyMed
Kebede, Daniel, FamilyMed
Kent, Kimberley, FamilyMed
Kerr, Sarah K., FamilyMed(EM)
Keshavjee, Karim, FamilyMed
Khalid, Hasan F., FamilyMed
Khan, Ruhi A., FamilyMed
Khan, Saadia N., FamilyMed
Khanna, Rajiv
Khataan, Somaia A M., FamilyMed
Kieffer, Marilyn A., FamilyMed
Kim, Ji Hyun, FamilyMed
Kim, Justin, FamilyMed
Kingston, June, FamilyMed
Koch, Joan L.
Koltin, Dror
Kozerawski, Waldemar J.
Kraftcheck, Erin R., FamilyMed
Kramarchuk, Markijan W., FamilyMed
Krizaj-Kapljic, Davorka
Kroll, Michael M., FamilyMed(EM)
Krop, Jozef
Kubazky, Valerie T., FamilyMed
Kubba, Hayder S H., FamilyMed
Kujtan, Peter W.
Kundapur, Mirja
Lagare, Bahubali D., FamilyMed
Lahnsteiner, Eric P., FamilyMed
Lai, Ho-Yin, FamilyMed
Lai, Paul F S., FamilyMed
Laidlaw, Susan M., FamilyMed(EM)
Lam, Michael Y C., FamilyMed
Lane, Judith I., FamilyMed
Lau, Eunice, FamilyMed
Lau, Francis T Y., FamilyMed
Lau, Wayne C., FamilyMed
Lawrence-Patel, Giselle M T., FamilyMed
Lazare, Samuel J.
Lee, Mark K., FamilyMed(EM)
Lemire, Francine L., FamilyMed
Leung, Ellen P., FamilyMed
Leung, Robert S L.
Leung, See-Lap
Leung, Sophia S Y.
Leveille, Kimberley L., FamilyMed
Leveille, Rheal J.
Lewis, David A R.
Ligon, Inocencio R.
Lim, Raymond T., FamilyMed(EM)
Lin, Yeou J J.
Lingys, Auksuole T.
Lo, Eddie S.
Lo, Stephen C W.
Loo, Wilson W S., FamilyMed
Lu, Charles C.
Lyons, Anthony W., FamilyMed
MacDonald, Linda D.
MacKintosh, Alasdair J., FamilyMed
Mah, Douglas W.
Maharajh, Sastri N., FamilyMed
Mahendira, Chanmugam S S., FamilyMed
Majid, Nadine, FamilyMed
Malicki, Krzysztof W.
Malig, Lita L., FamilyMed
Malinowski, Danuta J.
Mallette-Edwards, Shelley A., FamilyMed
Manawadu, Gnanindra N., FamilyMed
Mang, Fan-Wah, FamilyMed
Mankarious, Mervat F., FamilyMed
Marchetti, Catherine A., FamilyMed(EM)
Marko, Jana
Marshall, Karen L., FamilyMed
Martin, Brenda L.
Masood, Zahida, FamilyMed
Mathe, C. Thomas
Matheson, Jeffrey R H.
McConnell, Laura L., FamilyMed
McCuaig, Kenneth O.
McIntyre, Keith R.
McLaren, Jesse T T., FamilyMed(EM)
Meharchand, Mervyn M.
Mehmi, Sanghamitra A.
Meola, Carlo
Metrie, Mamdouh A H., FamilyMed
Mikail, Azza M., FamilyMed
Mistry, Ramesh V.
Mohamed Lamine, Mohamed H.
Mok, S. Simon
Molckovsky, Bohdan
Molnar, Paula C., FamilyMed
Moore, Grant E., FamilyMed(EM)
Moore, James W.
Morehouse, Scott P.
Morningstar, Gary L., FamilyMed
Mosam, Bashir A.
Mouldey, Peter G.
Mughal, Jawaid I.
Mughal, Maqbool A.
Musngi, Cristina B., FamilyMed
Myint, Khin Maung, FamilyMed
Nabi, Waqar, FamilyMed
Nada-Rajah, Shantha S., FamilyMed
Nakhla, Adel L C., FamilyMed
Nanar, Bikramjit S.
Narang, Chander K.
Nasirzadeh, Ehsaneddin, FamilyMed
Neelam, Satbir S., FamilyMed
Nemtean, Theodore S.
Nessim, Sherif P.
Newton, Barbara J.
Ng, C S. Rodney
Ng, S Y. Andrew, FamilyMed
Ngo, Thi Ngoc T., FamilyMed
Nguyen, Hoanh Khoi
Nicol, Olu-Kayode L V.
Ochocinski, Jerzy R.
Ochocinski, Pawel P.
Olarte, John, FamilyMed
Olufemi, Ademola O., FamilyMed
Olurin, Olubunmi I., FamilyMed
Ostro, Michael
Palad, Catalino G.
Palmer, David D., FamilyMed
Palumbo, Nicole M., FamilyMed
Pandhi, Hemant M.
Papneja, Sooraja P.
Park, Jane, FamilyMed
Park, Joonseong
Park, Randy, FamilyMed(EM)
Park, Vincent, FamilyMed
Parlan, Gelasio F.
Patel, Ila M., FamilyMed
Peck, Jonathan L., FamilyMed
Peddle, Ronald C.
Peer, Syed M A.
Pencharz, James N., FamilyMed
Pereira, Christine, FamilyMed
Perera, Jaspreet
Perera, Ruwan T.
Persad, Vashti C., FamilyMed
Pham, Anne-Marie, FamilyMed
Pham, Chien V., FamilyMed
Philbrook, Paul S., FamilyMed
Piacentino, Angelo, FamilyMed
Piatek, Dariusz P.
Pickersgill, Sara M., FamilyMed(EM)
Pilar, Imelda S., FamilyMed
Pinto, Joyce F., FamilyMed
Podell, Marc J.
Pontarini, Galdino E.
Poon, Jimmy C M., FamilyMed
Quan, Minh Duc., FamilyMed
Rabzel, Martina, FamilyMed
Racanelli, V. Saverio, FamilyMed
Race, Karen J., FamilyMed
Raczynska, Maria J.
Rafay, Afshan, FamilyMed
Rafla, Miriam, FamilyMed
Rahimpour, Roya
Ramadan, Samir I., FamilyMed
Raoof, Shariqa
Ravi, Tarsem S., FamilyMed
Rawji, Anik, FamilyMed(EM)
Reece, Susan E., FamilyMed
Rehemtula, Yasmin
Remtulla, Suleman S., FamilyMed
Richman, Jack, FamilyMed
Ritchie, Andrew C.
Rivlin, Leon, FamilyMed(EM)
Rizos, John D., FamilyMed(EM)
Robarts, Simon T T., FamilyMed(EM)
Rosen, David C.
Rosenfeld, S. Allan, FamilyMed
Ross, Katherine M., FamilyMed
Ross, Nagui A M., FamilyMed
Rousseau, Erella, FamilyMed
Rughubir, Nirvashni, FamilyMed
Saad, Salwa
Sabetti, Linda M., FamilyMed
Sachdeva, Ashok
Saeed, Tariq M., FamilyMed
Saeedi-Tabar, Soheil, FamilyMed
Saha, Sandipan
Sahheed, Wade W., FamilyMed
Sajid, Saima
Salach-Markiewicz, Krystyna
Saleem, Hala, FamilyMed
Salib, Shadwa S E., FamilyMed
Sanchez, Zenia A.
Sankat, Nadya, FamilyMed
Santhakumar, Vadivelu, FamilyMed
Sardana, Varun
Sato, Naomi I.
Sauls, Robert J., FamilyMed(EM)
Sayed, Qasim R., FamilyMed
Scala, G. Basil, FamilyMed
Scampoli, Nicola, FamilyMed(EM)
Schulman, Judy L.
Schwartz, Gwynne A., FamilyMed
Sebastian, Geron C.
Seib, Deborah L., FamilyMed
Seidl, Maja M., FamilyMed
Seif, Maged G A., FamilyMed
Seif, Mona F M., FamilyMed
Sekely, Istvan, FamilyMed
Selyanina, Tatyana, FamilyMed
Sequeira, Errol J., FamilyMed
Sertic, Joseph, FamilyMed
Sethi, Monica, FamilyMed
Sharma, Manisha, FamilyMed
Shasha, Farkad F A., FamilyMed
Shaw, Kerrie A., FamilyMed
Shehata-Fouad, Seham Z., FamilyMed
Sheppard, Ricki M.
Sheshgiri, Jitendra B., FamilyMed(EM)
Shievitz, Alan L., FamilyMed(EM)
Shum, H T. Peter
Sidhu, Raj K., FamilyMed
Sikander, Shabana, FamilyMed
Silver, Sheldon
Singh, Jeffrey M., FamilyMed(EM)
Singh, Neena L.
Small, Lynda A.
Smith, Shelley M., FamilyMed
Snyder, Nathan A., FamilyMed
So, Dominic C Y., FamilyMed
So, Stevenson K F.
Sohi, Ravinder K., FamilyMed
Solnik, M. Charles
Solomon, Sukumar D.
Somersall, Allan C.
Somersall, Lee-Anne A., FamilyMed
Soni, Deepa, FamilyMed(EM)
St Amant, Krista M., FamilyMed
Stapper Buitrago, Ingrid S., FamilyMed
Stephen, J. Daniel, FamilyMed
Stevanovski, Peter, FamilyMed
Strickler, Albert C.
Sue, Michelle T., FamilyMed
Sula, Sharon L., FamilyMed
Sum, Edric C H.
Sundareswaran, Shanthini, FamilyMed
Surangiwala, Sabiha M., FamilyMed
Surma, Beata
Sy, Peter Y.
Syed, Zohair H., FamilyMed
Tadros, Ibtissam F H., FamilyMed
Tai, Evelyn K., FamilyMed
Talwalkar, P. Aravind
Tam, Diamond Y F.
Tamari, Erez
Tan, James, FamilyMed(EM)
Tang, Christine E., FamilyMed(EM)
Tang, Joanna W., FamilyMed
Tarek, Shaul Y., FamilyMed(EM)
Targonsky, Elisha D., FamilyMed(EM)
Tasneem, Muhammad, FamilyMed
Taylor, Andrea C., FamilyMed
Taylor, Gerald M J., FamilyMed
Taylor, Rhonda V., FamilyMed(EM)
Tazkarji, M. Bachir, FamilyMed
Temins, Carol A., FamilyMed
Thakkar, Kirit V.
Than, Thi Ngoc T., FamilyMed
Thobani, Yasmin
Thompson, Diana P G., FamilyMed
Thomson, June A K.
Thorneloe, W. David, FamilyMed
Thorner, Richard S., FamilyMed
Tiu, Stephen S., FamilyMed(EM)
Tjan, Eugenie U.
Toma, Antoun A M., FamilyMed
Toth, Peter, FamilyMed(EM)
Tran, T G. Joe
Tran, Van Nham
Tranqui, John
Trinh, L. Hang Bich, FamilyMed
Tsang, Jim H C.
Tyrrell, Allison O.
Ubhi, Verjinderpal S., FamilyMed
Unger, Mark A., FamilyMed
Van Rhijn, Peter R.
Velez, Gloria C., FamilyMed
Venturi, David B.
Vera Mac, Vanessa I.
Vickers, Janet A., FamilyMed(EM)
Vijay, Raj, FamilyMed
Virdy, Kiran, FamilyMed

Wahba, Odette Z., FamilyMed
Wahba, Rasha G S., FamilyMed
Walk, Brian P.
Walling, Marvlyn A., FamilyMed
Wasfy, Samia W., FamilyMed
Wassef, Shadia, FamilyMed
Wasylyk, Roman Y., FamilyMed(EM)
Welland, Francis A.
Werneck, Christiane C F.
Whitmore, Christine A., FamilyMed
Whitney, Nermin A., FamilyMed
Wilansky, Rhonda, FamilyMed
Williams, David, FamilyMed
Williams, Gordon E.
Williams, Vivian P.
Wong, Alice S L., FamilyMed
Wong, Clement K L.
Wong, Frank K L.
Wong, Michael T W., FamilyMed
Wood, Stuart J., FamilyMed
Workewych, Jaroslaw V.
Yang, Min Kang.
Yashpal, Nina K., FamilyMed
Yim, Gary Y G.
Yostos, Philippe R., FamilyMed
Younan, Sawsan I.
Youssef, Ernest A N., FamilyMed
Zafar, Rosy, FamilyMed
Zarifa, Gihane W., FamilyMed
Zassoko, Roman, FamilyMed
Zazula, Marian
Zhang, Kenny J., FamilyMed
Zidel, Brian S.
Zuchelkowski, Jan S., FamilyMed

MITCHELL

Diotallevi, Mark J., FamilyMed
Kenyon, Gregory J., FamilyMed
Lappano, Sergio, FamilyMed
Powell, Mark R., FamilyMed
Schieldrop, Philip J., FamilyMed(EM)
Steele, Liora R., FamilyMed
Tsafnat, Tamar, FamilyMed
Turner, M. Dawn, FamilyMed
Turner, Maria D., FamilyMed

MOOSE CREEK

Dupuis, Jean-Eric J.
Lacroix, Daniel

MOOSE FACTORY

Barkman, Frederick, FamilyMed
Bond, Andrew J., FamilyMed
Dove, John F C., FamilyMed
Gibson, Michael, FamilyMed
Keeling, Patricia
Nevins, Tara A., FamilyMed
Nicoara, Lucia V., FamilyMed
Petconi, Anca V., FamilyMed
Ringrose, Heather M., FamilyMed
Sewell, Louise M.
Waddell, John M.

MORRISBURG

Abbud, Saad L., FamilyMed
Crabtree, Marilyn J.
Domanko, Wayne B.
Ingram-Crooks, Jennifer L., FamilyMed
Salja Halili, Elvira, FamilyMed

MOUNT ALBERT

Firestone, Gail F.

MOUNT BRYDGES

Copeland, Julie A., FamilyMed
Dalal, Vikram, FamilyMed(EM)
Kopechanski, Lauren, FamilyMed
Osmun, William E., FamilyMed

Parr, Jennifer L., FamilyMed
Turkstra, Ian, FamilyMed

MOUNT FOREST

Babey, Kenneth
Goodall, Simon C P.
Lu, Annie, FamilyMed
Mir, Kamran, FamilyMed
Perrin, Hugh M.
Reaume, John K., FamilyMed(EM)
Rowley, Christopher J., FamilyMed

MOUNT HOPE

Lalli, Eleonora C.

MUNCEY

Vreugdenhil, Michael J., FamilyMed

NAIRN CENTRE

Borsato, Stephanie A., FamilyMed

NAPANEE

Alkenbrack, J. Douglas
Andrawis, Mamdouh N R., FamilyMed
Bayoumi, Imaan M., FamilyMed
Beattie, Erin D., FamilyMed
Boon, Linda A.
Chadha, Ashok K.
Chen, Benjamin H., FamilyMed
Connery, Mervin A.
Cook, W. Douglas
Curran, Daniel E H., FamilyMed(EM)
Gonu, Crystal J.
Hadley, Brian P.
Hota, Valli L B., FamilyMed
Kenny, Paul E., FamilyMed
Lee, Carl H., FamilyMed(EM)
Little, Albert W.
Mahoney, Brian A., FamilyMed
Marin, Scott, FamilyMed
Martin, Matthew B., FamilyMed
Morris, Madeline, FamilyMed
Morrison, Kimberley, FamilyMed
Ollson, Gary L.
Simpson, Craig A., FamilyMed(EM)
Singh, Gurpreet
Sloan, Jeffrey R., FamilyMed
Sosnowski, Christopher J., FamilyMed
Touzel, Elizabeth L., FamilyMed
Touzel, Thomas A.
Waldron, Mark A., FamilyMed(EM)
White, Stephen F., FamilyMed(EM)
Wilson, Joslyn V., FamilyMed

NEPEAN

Abiscott, Joshua, FamilyMed
Adams, Jennifer H., FamilyMed
Al-Houssan, Walid, FamilyMed
Armstrong, Jennifer M.
Bajaj, Parvesh
Belanger, Jeannette E., FamilyMed
Bhatia, Ranbir S.
Blair, Mary-Louise, FamilyMed
Bowles, Alan K.
Boyden, Sheri N., FamilyMed
Bustani, Laith A., FamilyMed
Capello-Desjardins, Nancy, FamilyMed(EM)
Chan, Irene O L., FamilyMed
Chan, Wing-Shing
Charania, Hanif, FamilyMed(EM)
Charania, Sahira H., FamilyMed
Christie-Seely, Janet E., FamilyMed
Coulombe, Louise A.
Creaser, Kimberley J., FamilyMed(EM)
D'Amico, Catherine M., FamilyMed
Daniel, Arkadiusz M., FamilyMed

De Margerie, Michele, FamilyMed
De Souza, Eleanor M L.
Dobson, Clifford L., FamilyMed
Earle, John M.
Falconer, Andrew T., FamilyMed(EM)
Freedhoff, Jonathan E., FamilyMed
Fu, Joseph S L.
Gauvreau, Robert
Ghattas, Paul B.
Gill, Randeep S.
Gopalan, Bhaskar S., FamilyMed(EM)
Grace, S. Maureen, FamilyMed
Graves, Peter S., FamilyMed(EM)
Guy, Donald A.
Hacker, Paul L.
Harris, Donald R H.
Hashimoto, Mariko M.
Hockin, James C.
Isserlin, Jonathan
Jassam, Jabir M., FamilyMed
Joe, Barbara A., FamilyMed
Johnson, Beverly A.
Josseau, Melanie J C., FamilyMed(EM)
Kaprielian, Anoush A., FamilyMed
Kee, Gordon A., FamilyMed(EM)
Khatiwada, Bikalpa, FamilyMed(EM)
Leahy, Martin F., FamilyMed(EM)
Lemmex, Byron W G.
Leonard, Allison M., FamilyMed
MacLean, Richard S., FamilyMed
MacLoghlin, Cynthia J., FamilyMed(EM)
Malakieh, Amira L., FamilyMed
Malhotra, Jana L., FamilyMed
Manca, Georgina, FamilyMed(EM)
McGee, Neil J., FamilyMed(EM)
McIsaac, J. Hugh, FamilyMed
Mohamdee, M N. Hassan
Mouaikel, Patricia, FamilyMed
Musca, Claudia E.
Nadolny, Laurie J., FamilyMed
Nagpal, Sandeep K.
Natarajan, Nagamani C.
Newman, Helen B.
Nicholson, Miriam L.
Nicoletti, Bruno S., FamilyMed
Oliva, Teresa, FamilyMed
Oliver, Ian C., FamilyMed
Patel, Daksha N., FamilyMed
Pietrobon, Gianfranco
Pollock, Sandy C.
Popescu, Ligia M., FamilyMed
Raichura, Kalpesh A.
Regimbal, Sara M., FamilyMed
Rodgers, Margaret S.
Rossman, Lloyd H., FamilyMed
Sabourin, Kenneth B., FamilyMed
Sanderson-Guy, Catherine L.
Shortt, Samuel E D., FamilyMed
Shouldice, Elizabeth H., FamilyMed(EM)
Silva, Harini G., FamilyMed
Smith, Erin S.
Spencer, Nigel J.
Stewart, Lindsay C., FamilyMed(EM)
Stothart, Tonja L., FamilyMed
Tee, Rodney K.
Trecarten, Mark A., FamilyMed(EM)
Walker, M. Louise, FamilyMed
Wassef, Lamia F F., FamilyMed
Weisbloom, Joy M., FamilyMed
Westley, Elizabeth A., FamilyMed
Wong, Edmund K Y., FamilyMed
Wong, Gina S H.
Wray, Roger W.
Yang, Elisa Y S.

NEW HAMBURG

Cameron, David J.
Erling, J. Thomas, FamilyMed
Irvine, Richard A.
Schnore, Stephen K., FamilyMed

NEW LISKEARD

Blount, Christopher
Bowles, M. Jean, FamilyMed

Corbin, Jean M., FamilyMed
Corneil, Glenn G., FamilyMed
Davies, Colleen E., FamilyMed
Davies, Donald, FamilyMed
Desilets, Stacy A., FamilyMed
Fong, Jadine H.
Hurtubise, Andre L., FamilyMed
Logan, Patrick A.
Pace, Peter J., FamilyMed
Percy, Glen H., FamilyMed
Spruyt, Marlene E., FamilyMed

NEWBORO

Shiozaki, Ian K.

NEWBURGH

Koester, Catherine, FamilyMed
McDonald, Joanna E., FamilyMed

NEWBURY

Hull, Christopher M., FamilyMed
Keller, Jeremy H., FamilyMed
Papastergiou, Thanos, FamilyMed
Parnell, Robert H A., FamilyMed
Sharma, Subhash C., FamilyMed
Yan, Justin W.

NEWCASTLE

Brunton, Gillian M., FamilyMed
Campbell, John D.
Jefferson, Debra L., FamilyMed
Kassirer, Aubrey G., FamilyMed
Stewardson, Julie A., FamilyMed

NEWMARKET

Adams, Lorna, FamilyMed
Alsahli, Mazen
Baguio, Arnell, FamilyMed
Barbetta, Timothy P.
Bell, Ian R.
Bocknek, Amber L., FamilyMed
Bollano, Enkelejda, FamilyMed
Bourne, Mary, FamilyMed
Boyle, James C., FamilyMed
Brandon, Nicholas C., FamilyMed
Brown, John K.
Cantarutti, Paul G., FamilyMed
Carter, Norma C., FamilyMed
Cavalier, Lisa L.
Chan, Ariane C.
Chan, Edward S M., FamilyMed(EM)
Charnish, Michael B., FamilyMed(EM)
Climpson-Kennedy, L. Gayle
Cluff, Stephen J., FamilyMed(EM)
Colapinto, David A., FamilyMed
Davoudpour, Parham, FamilyMed(EM)
Dawson, Michael P.
Doherty, Robert
Dool, Nancy M.
Douville, Linda A., FamilyMed(EM)
Dukesz, Yitzchok
Dworak, Andrew S C., FamilyMed
Eisenberg, Howard E.
Falk, Jason P.
Flindall, Stephen, FamilyMed(EM)
Fry, Margaret A., FamilyMed
Gabor, Alexander
Galipeau, M. Lynne
Gannage, Christopher, FamilyMed(EM)
Ghadai, Talha I., FamilyMed
Gorodetsky, Olga, FamilyMed
Gupta, Jacqueline P., FamilyMed
Habteselassie, Biruk Y., FamilyMed
Hall, M. Jeremy
Heitzner, Maureen C.
Henein, Sam
Hess, Lembi M., FamilyMed
Iankova, Vesselina, FamilyMed
James, Kristin D.

Jeffery, Andrew H.
Kalyniuk, Jo-Anne
Kalyniuk, Judith A.
Kalyniuk, Norman J.
Kazmi, Samina
Kenworthy, Christopher P., FamilyMed
Khajehdehi, Ali A., FamilyMed
Khouzam, Pierre
Kiehn, Lana, FamilyMed
Kopylenko, Eleonor, FamilyMed
Kritzinger, Philip M., FamilyMed
Kumar, David
Kutsukake, Paul M.
Kuzmina, Alona, FamilyMed
Lai, Kenneth K K.
Lau, Paul P L., FamilyMed
Lee, Helen H K., FamilyMed
Lee, Raymond, FamilyMed(EM)
Leger, Paul S., FamilyMed
Leung, Alfred K.
Liang, Kenneth K C.
Liedeman, Mandy
Lulja, Nevila, FamilyMed
MacKinnon, Kevin M.
Mahmoodi, Mahnaz, FamilyMed
Makary, David, FamilyMed
Mand, Gurpreet T., FamilyMed
Mark, Larry K W.
Masri, Rogy O., FamilyMed
McLean, J. Lynda, FamilyMed
Merrow, Nancy M., FamilyMed
Meunier, Catherine, FamilyMed
Michael, George P., FamilyMed
Naghibi, Sam, FamilyMed
Nasrulla, M. Omar
Nijhawan, Monica, FamilyMed
Opalinski, Yvonne A V.
Oprea, Petra, FamilyMed
Padanilathu Kunjummar, Shakkeela, FamilyMed
Palermo, Eligio, FamilyMed(EM)
Pantano, Alfredo A.
Plow-Jarvis, Lisa G.
Ramdass, Chitra, FamilyMed
Richardson, Martha V., FamilyMed
Roopnarian, Indra P N., FamilyMed
Safavi, Mahsa, FamilyMed
Salehi Baidokhti, Saghi, FamilyMed
Samaha, Samar, FamilyMed
Shreeve, Joanne P.
Shum, Andrew J H S., FamilyMed(EM)
Silverstein, Jay M.
Skory, Gerald M.
Smith, Karen L.
So, Cindy H., FamilyMed
Sondhi, Asha P., FamilyMed
Sorial, Mary L R., FamilyMed
Srour, David, FamilyMed
Tikkanen, Kaarina V., FamilyMed
Voorpostel, Margaret W M.
Wassef, Hanaa S N., FamilyMed
Watson, Keith E.
Whatley, Shawn D., FamilyMed(EM)
Wong, Amy H., FamilyMed
Wong, David A., FamilyMed
Wong, Linda Y., FamilyMed
Wong, Louise L Y., FamilyMed
Wong Shue, Stephen G.
Yee, Stephen E., FamilyMed
Yip, David G., FamilyMed
Yousif, Mazin A., FamilyMed
Yuen, Harold J., FamilyMed

NIAGARA FALLS

Abrahim, Ken S I., FamilyMed
Abu Shahma, Mohamed S., FamilyMed
Adrewi, Hosen S., FamilyMed
Ahmed, Ghazanfar
Ahmed, Iram F.
Aidoo, Rosemond, FamilyMed
Al-Jarrah, Dirgham, FamilyMed
Alfayadh, Ridhab A B R., FamilyMed(EM)
Armstrong, Kenneth T.
Bassil, Brian
Chong, Xin, FamilyMed

Costello, Lawrence M.
Dargavel, Danny A., FamilyMed
Dec, David A., FamilyMed
Devane, Manik
Dhillon, Kirandeep
Dobbin, Stafford, FamilyMed
Farhat, Musbah S., FamilyMed(EM)
Gadhafi, Fathi A., FamilyMed
Gibney, Patrick F., FamilyMed
Gill, Joginder S., FamilyMed
Girard, Drew, FamilyMed
Goodwin, D. Michael
Guise, Roxan M., FamilyMed
Halliday, Fiona
Hill, Joanna E.
Howe, William A.
Javaly, Kedarnath
Kaptein, Sylvia, FamilyMed
Karim, Sadiqa
Krass, Melvin E., FamilyMed
Leung, Wilson W S., FamilyMed
Lum, Julie K., FamilyMed
MacTavish, Alison J., FamilyMed
Marshall, Julia L., FamilyMed
Masood, Syed F.
McGarry, Philip A.
Morin, Jason M., FamilyMed
Munkley, Douglas P.
Nadeau, Gary J M., FamilyMed
Nagel, Michael G., FamilyMed
Nicholson, C. David
Palmer, John T.
Pang, Patrick K K., FamilyMed
Porwal, Hemraj R., FamilyMed
Raizman, Alla
Reka, Altin, FamilyMed
Roman, Raymond M.
Rosa, David A., FamilyMed
Saeed, Perie A.
Seifred, Grant P.
Shaikh, Omer S.
Singh, Artaj, FamilyMed
Singh, Judith M., FamilyMed
Thiab, Ali S., FamilyMed
Torigian, Michael A., FamilyMed
Velji, Azim M., FamilyMed
Waisglass, Barry R.
Wassif, Ehab B A E., FamilyMed
Wilczynski, John S.

NIAGARA ON THE LAKE

Bastedo, Timothy P., FamilyMed
Berti, Karen E., FamilyMed
Frendo, Jennifer S., FamilyMed
Horning, C E. Maxwell
Reimer, David, FamilyMed
Smith, Andrew A N., FamilyMed
Viviers, George F., FamilyMed

NIPIGON

Bond, Rebecca M., FamilyMed
Jackson-Hughes, John F., FamilyMed
Janhunen, David R., FamilyMed
Marquardt, Hans R., FamilyMed
Scott, Douglas F., FamilyMed
Warbeck, Paul J., FamilyMed

NOBLETON

Yee, Chok-Ching

NORTH BAY

Abeysinghe, Nilanga M., FamilyMed
Alldred, J. Byron, FamilyMed
Arthurs, Michael J.
Atapattu, Vidura I., FamilyMed
Aubry, Jean R., FamilyMed
Aylett, Alan A A.
Birosh, Barry A.
Brill, Stephanie, FamilyMed(EM)
Buck, Erica A M., FamilyMed
Buckley, Brian J.
Carter, W. Joel, FamilyMed
Cathers, Christopher R., FamilyMed
Cowan, Ian G., FamilyMed
Cuncins, Charles
Delisle, Richard J J., FamilyMed
Dell'Aquila, Raffaele A., FamilyMed
Dellandrea, David A.
Eckler, Howard
Feige, Erwin, FamilyMed
Freistatter, Ryan L., FamilyMed
Galema, Chris J.
Galipeau, Jocelyn F.
Gatchev, Margarita, FamilyMed
Graham, Wendy, FamilyMed
Guderian, Angela, FamilyMed
Haist, David W.
Hoirch, Adam R., FamilyMed
Jinnah, Inez F., FamilyMed
Keith, Arthur L.
Khan, Ghulam Z.
King, Rebekah M., FamilyMed
Kolb, Elena
Leckie, Michael
Lowry, Peter
Lukomska, Katarzyna E., FamilyMed
Mah, Gordon K., FamilyMed(EM)
Main, James T D.
Makuch, Patricia A.
Mantle, Nancy G.
McKercher, H. Grant, FamilyMed
Meek, Murray D., FamilyMed
Ng, Derek, FamilyMed(EM)
Nodwell, Allison C., FamilyMed
O'Grady, Melanie D., FamilyMed
Oyeniran, Idowu, FamilyMed
Phillipson, Wayne G.
Preston, Paul R.
Prins, Nicholas S.
Rankin, Linda, FamilyMed
Rivet, Andre G.
Rotondo, Terrence G.
Saltstone, Scot P., FamilyMed
Senior, Richard W.
Shaw, Brian M., FamilyMed
Shemilt, Roderick J., FamilyMed
Sheppard, Matthew G L., FamilyMed
Slatarof, Youssef A.
Spencer, Andrew
Steinberg, Steven G.
Stewart, James T., FamilyMed
Stewart, James W., FamilyMed
Trenker, Richard S.
Vaughan, Edward D.
Vigars, James S.
Zimbalatti, Carol A., FamilyMed

NORTH YORK

Aarons, Gilbert H.
Abboud, Rana, FamilyMed
Abrams, H. Joel
Adam, George A., FamilyMed
Adams, Kenneth W.
Adatia, Almas M.
Adelstein, Mitchell
Ages, Deena E.
Ahmad, Fuad, FamilyMed
Ajisafe, Olaniyi F., FamilyMed
Akbari-Nasab, Ardalan
Akhlaghi-Kakroudi, Fatereh, FamilyMed
Al-Saigh, Basil B.
Ali, Azra, FamilyMed(EM)
Ali, Haider, FamilyMed
Allen, Richard E., FamilyMed(EM)
Alloo, Javed A., FamilyMed
Alterescu, Alexandre
Aly, Hoda M M., FamilyMed
Anagnostopoulos, Nikolaos, FamilyMed
Angilletta, Bruno
Antonenko, Alexander, FamilyMed
Aquino, John M., FamilyMed
Ash, Marla R., FamilyMed
Asmal, Mohammed Z D., FamilyMed
Athaide, Sylvia B.
Attersley, Edward M.
Atwal, Kanwaldip S., FamilyMed(EM)
Atwal, Rajinder K., FamilyMed
Awad, Ayman T R A., FamilyMed
Awad, Lucy, FamilyMed
Bafundi, Peter, FamilyMed
Bageria, Charanjit S., FamilyMed
Bakhshi Kahnamouei, Manijeh, FamilyMed
Banach, Ryan L., FamilyMed
Bapat, Archana
Barrett, David J.
Barsoom, Laith M., FamilyMed
Bart, John L.
Barth, Bernard A.
Basta, Sally, FamilyMed
Basti, Peyvand A., FamilyMed
Baum, Sol, FamilyMed
Baxter, Colin H.
Becker, Harold, FamilyMed
Bekhit, Magdy R., FamilyMed
Bell, Alan, FamilyMed
Bell, Lisa, FamilyMed
Belluzzo, Neal, FamilyMed
Berenbaum, Brian
Berg, Marina, FamilyMed
Berka, L. Jane, FamilyMed
Berlin, Seymour, FamilyMed
Bernstein, Ira, FamilyMed
Bernstein, Stanley K.
Birnbaum, Debra S., FamilyMed
Blankenstein, Harvey, FamilyMed
Blinick, Cheryl
Bodasing, Dhawmanie
Bogosyan, Avedis
Bolaji, Yemisi I., FamilyMed
Brcic, Branimir, FamilyMed
Bressler, Hartley B.
Brock, Carol A.
Brodsky, Mark B.
Brown, Allan, FamilyMed
Brown, Bethel
Brown, Edward M., FamilyMed(EM)
Brown, Harry
Brown, James C.
Buchman, Ellen J., FamilyMed
Bunston, Sarah, FamilyMed
Burko, Thomas
Caine, Sean P., FamilyMed(EM)
Caplan, Shari G., FamilyMed
Carr, Jonathan D., FamilyMed
Caruso, Andrew
Castrodale, Joseph
Chada, Usha
Chakkalackal, Mary J.
Champagne, Jean-Pierre, FamilyMed(EM)
Chan, Tak Keung
Chang, W C. Iris
Chekina, Helena
Cheng, Jerry H C.
Chernin, Jeffrey M.
Chin, Elaine I.
Chin, Jeffrey M.
Chin, Maxwell I.
Chiu, Chung Fok.
Chiu, Edward S., FamilyMed
Chiu, Elizabeth M.
Choe, Seong Dong.
Choi, D. Young
Choi-Fung, Betty L S., FamilyMed
Choptiany, Philip J., FamilyMed
Chou, Linda H.
Choy, Ping Fun., FamilyMed
Chris, Stephen D.
Christidis, Nickolas
Chu, Man-Hon, FamilyMed
Chunduri, Krishna V., FamilyMed
Chung, Chin K., FamilyMed
Chuong, Roselynn, FamilyMed
Cianfrone, Fausto M.
Cianfrone, G. Adrian
Citron, Sidney P.
Cloth, Martin I., FamilyMed
Cohen, Dan A D., FamilyMed
Cohen, Harry
Cohen, Rebecca A W., FamilyMed
Cohen-Gelfand, Sara N., FamilyMed
Colla, Simon
Conran, Michelle B.
Corpus, Todd R., FamilyMed
Coutinho, Jude J T.
Craft, Aidlee R., FamilyMed
Cronin, Karen L., FamilyMed
Curea, Delia, FamilyMed
Curridor, Robert
D'Angelo, Peter D.
D'Arcy, Francis D.
D'Souza, Irene C.
Dangoor, Gail, FamilyMed
Das, Pavani R.
David, Sheila J.
Dawe, Elizabeth M., FamilyMed
Decena, Silvino M., FamilyMed
Delva, M. Dianne, FamilyMed
Devassy, Mary T.
Devi, Shashi P., FamilyMed
Di Carlo, Domenico
Diaconita, Mariana, FamilyMed
Dias, Aleksander I.
Dicker, Robert A.
Diena, Zeev M., FamilyMed
Djuric, Vladimir
Dobkin, Earl F.
Donskoy, Alex A.
Doucet, Lorenne, FamilyMed
Driman, Naomi M., FamilyMed
Dubins, Jacques H.
Dwosh, Adam A., FamilyMed
Ebeid, Manal, FamilyMed
Edwards, Donna F., FamilyMed
Ein, Arnold L A.
Elepano, Suzanne M., FamilyMed
Erdelyi, Barbara, FamilyMed
Espiritu, Froilan N.
Evans, Frank W.
Evans, Melissa, FamilyMed
Fecycz, Taras D.
Fegelman, Alan
Feld, S. Michael
Feldman, Risa C., FamilyMed
Feldman, Sidney I D., FamilyMed
Feldman-Glaser, Perle, FamilyMed
Felsen, Shim S I., FamilyMed
Ferreira, Nelson D B.
Fidal, Samuil W., FamilyMed
Fingrut, Philip
Finkelman, Shayna R., FamilyMed
Finkelstein, Ian, FamilyMed
Fong, Andrew
Fong, Harvey O.
Forbes, Geoffrey G A.
Forman, Noah A., FamilyMed
Fouda, Omayma, FamilyMed
Fraleigh, Warren C.
Freedman, Michelle R.
Freedman, Paul E., FamilyMed
Freeman, Risa F., FamilyMed
Fric-Shamji, Elana C., FamilyMed
Fried, Oded P.
Friedberg, A. Martin
Furer, Basheva
Gabay, Jose
Gagovski, Vlade M.
Gallant, Tsvi
Gamble, Kenneth
Garber, Peter N., FamilyMed
Gelkopf, Marvin A., FamilyMed
Gelman, Gregory D., FamilyMed
Gerstein, Betty F., FamilyMed
Gerstein, Francine H., FamilyMed
Gilman, Michael L.
Girard, Louis C., FamilyMed
Girgis, Magdy H., FamilyMed
Gladstone, Joan S.
Gmora, Shawn W., FamilyMed
Gobrial, Marcos, FamilyMed
Gofman, Frina
Goldenberg, Teresa, FamilyMed
Goldfarb, Ludmilla
Goldstein, David I., FamilyMed
Goldstein, Howard J.
Goldstein, Mark L., FamilyMed
Gordon, Randy D.
Gorlick, Steven Z.
Gottesman, Maureen C., FamilyMed
Gottesman, Steven P., FamilyMed
Grant, Kelly E., FamilyMed
Green, Albert H.
Green, Bernard M.
Greig, Anita R A., FamilyMed
Greiver, Michelle, FamilyMed
Grewal, Jaspreet S., FamilyMed
Grodecki, Richard G., FamilyMed
Gronska, Margaret A., FamilyMed
Gross, Veronica A.
Grossman, Daphna L., FamilyMed(EM)
Grossman, Liuba
Grover, Leonard F L., FamilyMed
Grunebaum, Margaret J.
Gupta, Jagdeep S., FamilyMed
Gutierrez, Carlos A.
Hack, Muhammad U., FamilyMed
Hadian, Abbas H.
Hajy Aghaei, Roya, FamilyMed
Hamad, Fatin, FamilyMed
Hamdy, Nermeen R I., FamilyMed
Hancu, Dan J., FamilyMed
Hart, Michelle, FamilyMed
Heath, Diana S., FamilyMed
Helman, Anton D., FamilyMed(EM)
Herman, Leon
Herschorn, Andrea, FamilyMed
Hershenfield, Karen R., FamilyMed
Hew, Amy
Hill, David J.
Himmel, Walter M., FamilyMed(EM)
Ho, Catherine K Y., FamilyMed(EM)
Ho, H. Henry, FamilyMed
Ho, Herbert K K.
Ho, W M. Amy
Hoh, Lydia O K.
Honein, Charles F.
Hong, Angie S., FamilyMed
Hood, Nancy A.
Hooks, Rosalie J., FamilyMed
Horak, Ladislav
Horani, Maria A.
Horvath, Anna M B., FamilyMed
Horvath, Robert D., FamilyMed
Hosokawa, Akiko N., FamilyMed
Hotz, Aaron, FamilyMed
Housefather, Leslie S., FamilyMed
Hsu, David M., FamilyMed
Huang, Virgil Y F.
Huggins, Joseph E.
Hui, Adrian W Y.
Hui, Edith W Y., FamilyMed
Hui, Frederick, FamilyMed
Hunter, Jennifer M.
Hussain, Amna
Ilk, Lisa A., FamilyMed
Inandan, Elnora S.
Ingber, Neil J., FamilyMed
Isaac, Sandra L., FamilyMed
Ishac, Magda
Iskander, Nagi M., FamilyMed
Ismail, Shiraz H.
Jackson, Mervyn M., FamilyMed
Jain, Padma
Jairath, Ashok K.
James, Aisha N P., FamilyMed
James, Stephen R.
Jaskolka, Kenneth M.
Jayarajan, Meera, FamilyMed(EM)
Jesin, Aaron
Jesin, Edward C.
Jin, Eddy Y H., FamilyMed(EM)
Jin, Sheila Y M.
Johnston, Elizabeth L.
Johnston, Karen E., FamilyMed
Jonathan, Stanley R.
Joshi, Virat, FamilyMed(EM)
Joyce, Susan M., FamilyMed
Kaasa, Benjamin M., FamilyMed
Kachroo, Umang B., FamilyMed
Kadanka, Hanna
Kahane, Steven G., FamilyMed
Kakzanov, Vered V., FamilyMed
Kalantari, Saeed, FamilyMed
Kalins, Lauma A.
Kamenskaia, Vera
Kaminski, Michael
Kan, F. Dana
Kaplan, David M., FamilyMed
Karmy, Grigory
Karr, Suzanne M., FamilyMed
Katz, Sheldon
Kauffman-Schenker, Tammy, FamilyMed
Kavazanjian, Hratch
Kay, Marvin S.
Kelley, Catherine L., FamilyMed(EM)
Keltz, Irwin, FamilyMed
Ker, Katherine J., FamilyMed
Keshavjee, Fatehalli C.

Keshavjee, Hassenali C.
Khan, Akbar N.
Kharonsky, Rita M., FamilyMed
Khotianov, Natan L., FamilyMed
Kimelman, Harold S.
Kirstine, Ileana B.
Kodsi, Sherif S.
Koffman, Allyson E.
Koffman, Gerald A.
Kopolovic, Shirley, FamilyMed
Kornhauser, Danny S., FamilyMed
Kosar, Katherine J., FamilyMed
Krasnopolsky, Marina
Krievins, Matthew C., FamilyMed(EM)
Krulewitz, Janet B., FamilyMed
Kumar, Brinda C P.
Kurtz, Sonia
Kustka, Sonja S.
Kwan, Christina Y., FamilyMed
Kwan, Manbun, FamilyMed
Kyanzadeh, Fareiborz, FamilyMed
Laham, Robert S.
Lai, Kevin C Y., FamilyMed
Laine-Gossin, Joanne, FamilyMed
Lakdawalla, Fakhrudin
Lalani, Fereshte N., FamilyMed
Lam, Jennifer K., FamilyMed
Lam, Vincent Y Y.
Lau, Ming-Jarm
Law, Michael K.
Le, David
Lear, Naomi D., FamilyMed
Lee, Eunice
Lee, Joyce W Y., FamilyMed
Lee, Lap Cheung.
Leith, Diane B.
Leone, Rosa
Leung, Allan H H.
Leung, Desmond D., FamilyMed
Leung, James C K., FamilyMed
Levitt, David S.
Levitt, Ralph
Levy, Sharon L., FamilyMed
Levy, Todd
Lewi, Renee, FamilyMed
Lho, Hyoung-Zin, FamilyMed(EM)
Li, Ann L., FamilyMed
Lofsky, Stanley, FamilyMed
Loung, Kenneth C.
MacDonald, Matthew H., FamilyMed
Mackenzie, Richard B., FamilyMed
Madonik, Bonnie H.
Magee, C J. Bruce
Magharious, Lucy N., FamilyMed
Mah, Phillip, FamilyMed
Maier, Peter C., FamilyMed
Mak, Kam Kong
Malayil, Nina B., FamilyMed
Maltseva, Ekatherena V., FamilyMed
Mandel, O. Jack, FamilyMed
Manis, Danielle, FamilyMed
Mansour, Raafat A E., FamilyMed
Manucha, Shalini
Maragh, Dev K., FamilyMed
Marcovitz, Leora
Marie, Julianne, FamilyMed
Markovic, Saira
Marks, Cyril P.
Marzouk, A. Georgi
Masi, Raffaele, FamilyMed
Masters, Susan A.
Mati, Neil M., FamilyMed
Matsenko, Oksana
Matta, Roberto B.
Mayer, Kevin D., FamilyMed
Mazzoli, Paolo, FamilyMed(EM)
McConnell, H. Dianne, FamilyMed
McQuiston, Terence
Meda, Stephen J.
Meglis, Gus, FamilyMed
Mekael, Hany R R., FamilyMed
Melamed, Penina, FamilyMed
Melbourne, Byron A.
Mele, Victor L.
Mendez Tejada, Hector
Meranda, Clara, FamilyMed
Merbaum, Allyson M., FamilyMed
Mertens, Donald J.
Mihic, Alan J.
Mills, Jeffrey K.
Millstein, Lisa T., FamilyMed
Mohammady, Maryam, FamilyMed
Mok, Gary T.
Molder, Susan V.
Mollanji, Roland, FamilyMed
Moody, Sandra
Moore, Nicholas J.
Morgan, Aida E., FamilyMed
Motlani, Faisal
Mula, David E., FamilyMed
Muraca, Maria, FamilyMed
Nadasdi, Miklos
Nadel, Orli Y., FamilyMed
Nahon, Dahlia R.
Naiman, Alisa B., FamilyMed
Nashi, Saad, FamilyMed
Nasso, Domenic
Nath, Rovindra R., FamilyMed
Nathan, Nicole S., FamilyMed
Nazal, Faris A., FamilyMed
Nejad Ghaffar, Shahrokh, FamilyMed
Newman, Barbara J., FamilyMed
Newman, Peter R., FamilyMed
Ng, Cindy K W., FamilyMed
Nguyen, Chinh
Nguyen, Tram Anh Thi, FamilyMed
Nguyen, Truong Van, FamilyMed
Nip, L. Michael, FamilyMed
Nitzkin, Steven D.
Nusinowitz, Sidney, FamilyMed
O'Donnell, Trishia J., FamilyMed
O'Mara, Meghan M., FamilyMed
O'Riordan, Matthew
Oda, Jenny W N., FamilyMed
Ostroff, Shirley J.
Otto, George W.
Paikin, Sarah
Pankowski, Dahlia K., FamilyMed
Pare, Michael F.
Parikh, Munjal S.
Parker, Susan E.
Parris, Clark J.
Parrish, James D., FamilyMed
Parsons, Patricia M., FamilyMed
Patel, Meeta, FamilyMed(EM)
Patodia, Sanjay K., FamilyMed
Pazuki, Kasra
Pazuki, Keyvan
Peck, Ronnie
Penciner, Richard D., FamilyMed(EM)
Percheson, Paul B.
Perry, David A.
Petrescu, Claudia
Pfaff, James R.
Phillipson, Ronald A., FamilyMed
Pliamm, Lew, FamilyMed
Pliamm, Naomi, FamilyMed
Pliamm, Sara
Pohani, Gina, FamilyMed
Poldes, Anu, FamilyMed
Poon, Vincent H K., FamilyMed
Pop, Cristina A., FamilyMed
Posen, David, FamilyMed
Poznan, Zoltan
Prigozhikh, Viachislav
Pu, Yunlong
Pubben, Mary-Ann J., FamilyMed
Pugen, Gregory L.
Pupko, Harold
Pyper, Anne M.
Quinton, Jill A., FamilyMed
Rachlis, Val, FamilyMed
Rajan, Gerald Instep.
Rajmohamed, Afzal E., FamilyMed
Ralh, Surender K.
Rampersad, O'Hara E S., FamilyMed
Ramphal, Premdath J.
Ramprasad, Harrinorine
Randhawa, Kavita, FamilyMed
Rapoport, David, FamilyMed
Rashid, Shahid
Reicheld, Susan M.
Reichman, William
Reingold, Morton J.
Reingold, Terence M.
Reinhartz, Abraham D.
Ricciuti, Flora, FamilyMed
Richards, Gail J E.
Richards, Richard L.
Riddle, Robert J., FamilyMed(EM)
Rifkind, Naomi D., FamilyMed
Rivlin, Alex S.
Rizkalla, Michel
Robinson, Donna L., FamilyMed(EM)
Rod, Kevin, FamilyMed
Rogano, Maria A.
Rohald, Sharon, FamilyMed
Rosen, Gili, FamilyMed
Rosen, Noel A., FamilyMed
Rosenberg, Jodine L., FamilyMed
Rosenberg, Lara M., FamilyMed
Rosenthal, Robert M.
Rosset, Jennifer E., FamilyMed
Rostas, Peter A.
Rotstein, Stephen I., FamilyMed
Rotundo, Mark J., FamilyMed
Rowan, J. Peter, FamilyMed(EM)
Rozen, Dima
Rubenzahl, Steven E.
Rudner, Rodica
Rudnick, Martin
Rustad, Jennifer A., FamilyMed
Rutledge, Timothy F., FamilyMed(EM)
Sacks, Jordana B., FamilyMed
Safieh, Patrick, FamilyMed(EM)
Sager, Mark J., FamilyMed
Saibil, Romy B., FamilyMed
Saito, Robert K.
Salib, Ashraf E A., FamilyMed
Salkauskis, Stanley J., FamilyMed(EM)
Samuel, Oded, FamilyMed(EM)
Sarca, Dana, FamilyMed
Saul, David G.
Saunders, Linda C.
Sax, Lawrence M.
Schacter, Milton W.
Schneider, Howard, FamilyMed
Schwartz, E. Michael, FamilyMed(EM)
Scullion, Catherine M.
Sedran, David, FamilyMed
See, Hilario, FamilyMed
Segal, Russel S., FamilyMed(EM)
Segal, Shaun M., FamilyMed
Senderovich, Helena M.
Shack, Martin N., FamilyMed
Shafer, Robyn T., FamilyMed(EM)
Shaffer, Mark R., FamilyMed
Shah, Bharatkumar K.
Shah, Sheila
Shaikh, S. Yasmin, FamilyMed
Shapero, Stephen E., FamilyMed
Sheiner, Glenn S., FamilyMed(EM)
Shemtov, Oren M., FamilyMed(EM)
Shetty, Niren, FamilyMed
Shub, Elliot H.
Shuldiner, Sarit L., FamilyMed
Shulman, David L., FamilyMed
Shulman, Sandy E., FamilyMed
Siddiqui, Sanam F., FamilyMed
Sidhu, Kuldeep S., FamilyMed(EM)
Sidlofsky, Richard N., FamilyMed
Silverstein, Carol S., FamilyMed
Simonik, Dagmar
Simonik, Martin
Singer, Melissa C., FamilyMed
Sinukoff, Warren E.
Sischy, Neville L.
Slavina, Anna, FamilyMed
Slyfield, David G M.
Small, Debra S., FamilyMed
Solarich, Stoyan
Solmon, Jordan B., FamilyMed
Sonshine, Jodi E., FamilyMed
Soo, B H. Norman
Spencer, Louis R.
Spudas, Alexander J.
Stefansson, Donald A.
Steinberg, Jeffrey M.
Stern, Andrea, FamilyMed(EM)
Stoddard, Douglas W.
Stoller, Rebecca A., FamilyMed
Stone, Susan J V., FamilyMed
Strasberg, Jessica E., FamilyMed
Strasberg, Suzanne R., FamilyMed
Stuckey, Paul Mitchell.
Sturm, Esther R W., FamilyMed
Stutz, Eric M., FamilyMed
Sudai, Tamar, FamilyMed
Sussman, Jack W.
Sweeney, Mila
Swenson, Brigit A., FamilyMed
Syed, A. Shaista, FamilyMed
Syed, Saadat A S., FamilyMed
Tan, Romeo B., FamilyMed
Tanzer, Russell S.
Tarshis, W. Lisa, FamilyMed
Tatuch, Yuriy M., FamilyMed
Taylor, Bryan S., FamilyMed
Teitel, Jesse D., FamilyMed
Teitelbaum, Ivor
Teitelbaum, Stanley, FamilyMed
Teixeira, Frederick A.
Thiem, Sasha C., FamilyMed
Thompson, Jannette J., FamilyMed
Tick, Heather S., FamilyMed
Todd, Judith M., FamilyMed
Tolhurst, Elizabeth A., FamilyMed(EM)
Tomlin Procyk, Jennifer L T., FamilyMed(EM)
Tong, Nhan Thien
Train, Harriet P.
Tran, Bernie B C.
Trapman, Johan L.
Treasurer, Haren M., FamilyMed
Treasurer, Sushila M.
Tsai, Jason Y S.
Tsang, Raymond W M.
Tse, Anthony C H.
Uleckas, Gintaras T., FamilyMed
Urback, Robert K., FamilyMed
Valin, Sharonie S., FamilyMed
Van Der Hout, David M., FamilyMed
Van Lierop, Muriel J.
Vanderspek, Susan C., FamilyMed
Vanek, J. Nicholas
Vasilescu, Ovidiu, FamilyMed
Vecchiarelli, John A.
Vecchio, Michael J.
Vera Silva, V. Antonio, FamilyMed
Vo, H D. David, FamilyMed
Vo, Khanh Hong, FamilyMed
Vokac, Ludmila
Vujicic, Neda, FamilyMed
Wagner, Sheldon I.
Wainberg, Sara J., FamilyMed
Waldman, Murray L., FamilyMed(EM)
Walsh, Philip
Weinberg, Terri E., FamilyMed
Weinroth, H. Judith
Weinstock-Goldberg, Sara, FamilyMed
Weir, Tara G., FamilyMed
Weisbrod, Gerald I.
Wen, Chuck K., FamilyMed
Wertman, Antoinette, FamilyMed(EM)
White, David G., FamilyMed(EM)
Whyte, James F H., FamilyMed
Winkler, Heather D., FamilyMed
Winston, Howard A., FamilyMed
Wirsig, Nadine M., FamilyMed
Wise, Mark
Wong, Delora, FamilyMed
Wong, Tat-Kwan
Wong, Tat-Ying
Woodrow, Adrian R.
Wu, Sing Man
Wulffhart, Jeffrey I., FamilyMed
Wyman, Tanya, FamilyMed
Yacowar, Mayer, FamilyMed
Yathindra, Yashi K., FamilyMed(EM)
Yelenbaugen, Irina
Yeung, Clement W T.
Yeung, Danny S C., FamilyMed
Yim, Daniel
Young, Vicki, FamilyMed
Youssef, Nancy A B., FamilyMed
Yu, Jasmine M Y., FamilyMed
Yuen, Vivian K., FamilyMed
Zeilig, Lauren V.
Zeindler, Peter R., FamilyMed
Zeit, Harry J.
Zelcer, Irving, FamilyMed
Ziedenberg, Robert W., FamilyMed
Zitney, Michael I.
Zou, Limai, FamilyMed
Zoudis, Adamantios P., FamilyMed
Zuckerman, Hanna E., FamilyMed
Zysman, Michele A., FamilyMed

NORTHBROOK

Brereton, Teresa
Elliott, Alan
Tam, Peter
Tobia, Bernard Z.
Wilson, Anne, FamilyMed

NORWICH

Hofer, Michael, FamilyMed
Jeffries, Jennifer F.
Wendling, Lisa C.

NORWOOD

Keogh, Brendan G.

NOTTAWA

MacDougall, Lorna J.

OAKVILLE

Abawi, Shakker
Abbasi, Khawar M., FamilyMed
Abdel-Malak, Maher N M., FamilyMed
Abdul-Razzak, Amane, FamilyMed
Aggarwal, Sandeep K., FamilyMed
Ahluwalia, Nalin K., FamilyMed(EM)
Ahmed, Nafeesa Q.
Alawsi, Maysarah, FamilyMed
Aldridge, E. Jane, FamilyMed
Alexander, Mary E., FamilyMed
Amer, Tehmina
Amolins, Roland E., FamilyMed
Annis, Robert V.
Anosike, Jide E., FamilyMed
Antowan, Samir M., FamilyMed
Arani, Arash M., FamilyMed
Atif, Rabia, FamilyMed
Backo-Shannon, Mirjana, FamilyMed
Badowski, Deborah
Bahmutan, Ana S., FamilyMed
Banerjee, Prasenjit, FamilyMed(EM)
Barnouti-Calotti, Maya, FamilyMed
Bebawy, Amany, FamilyMed
Benjamin, Lynne A.
Beshay, Samy A Y., FamilyMed
Bhullar, Sundeep, FamilyMed
Blair, Cynthia L., FamilyMed
Bloch, Peter
Boktor, Fekri, FamilyMed
Breen, Corinne H L., FamilyMed
Bremermann, R. Danielle M., FamilyMed
Butler, Jeremy R.
Byrne, Doris M.
Cairns, Bonnie J., FamilyMed
Carlson, Britt I., FamilyMed(EM)
Castonguay, Leslie A.
Castura, Christina, FamilyMed
Cawkwell, Margaret E., FamilyMed
Chambers, Michael T.
Charters, Jane
Chauhan, Rebecca A.
Cheng, M F. Frederick, FamilyMed
Choi, Steve C S.
Chong, Dennis K.
Clottey, Clarence E., FamilyMed
Colaco, Carmen M.
Collett, Kenneth A.
Cooper, Carol L., FamilyMed
Curran-Blaney, Nora, FamilyMed
Da Silva, Terence R.
Dawood, Shamim, FamilyMed
De Bolster, C. Leonard, FamilyMed
Debretsion, Tadese F., FamilyMed
Deen, Hurara, FamilyMed
Deeth, Karen L., FamilyMed(EM)
Denby, John D.
Dhawan, Shalini
Dobson, William M., FamilyMed
Dodge, Gregory T., FamilyMed(EM)
Duguid, Murray P.
Dutkiewicz-Stvrtecky, Janina H.
Eddenden, Peter W.
Farhat, Gloria, FamilyMed
Feldman, Debra C., FamilyMed
Fiorini, Cynthia M.
Fong, Harmon, FamilyMed(EM)

Foroodi, Fraindokht, FamilyMed
Found, Margaret H., FamilyMed
Fox, Joanne M.
Gabrail, Yousry, FamilyMed
Gabriel, Robert P.
Ghaznavi, Sameera, FamilyMed
Gibara, Magdy R B., FamilyMed
Ginty, Alexandra C., FamilyMed(EM)
Glover, Rodger M., FamilyMed
Graham, Martha B., FamilyMed
Grapko-Mysak, Deborah A., FamilyMed
Gray, Katherine A.
Grewal, Anita, FamilyMed
Guirguis, Emad S L., FamilyMed
Guirguis, Suzy, FamilyMed
Hamandi, Husein A J., FamilyMed
Hamideh, Fayad
Hanna, Noha, FamilyMed
Hanna, Sameh K., FamilyMed
Healey, Paul D., FamilyMed(EM)
Heikal, Ruby S., FamilyMed
Hemans, Clover A., FamilyMed
Henein, John, FamilyMed
Higgs, Stewart I L., FamilyMed
Hirsch, Steven L., FamilyMed
House, Sheilagh J.
Hussain, Saba
Hussain, Yasmine E., FamilyMed
Inamdar, Mangesh, FamilyMed(EM)
Ing, Sabrina Y., FamilyMed
Inkster, John R.
Isaak, Verner H.
Jacobson, Edward L.
Jamal, Hanif N., FamilyMed
Jeffries, Gregory A., FamilyMed
Jirjis, Luma M., FamilyMed
Jolly, Rajnee K., FamilyMed
Jones, Robert G.
Kadic-Mucevic, Edina, FamilyMed
Kaloni, Rita, FamilyMed
Kamara, Hawa, FamilyMed
Kanaganayakam, Shankary, FamilyMed
Kassis, Lorette B., FamilyMed
Katarey, Hement K., FamilyMed
Katarey, Mamta, FamilyMed
Keeton, Michael
Kelford, Alison M., FamilyMed
Kerr, Roderick G., FamilyMed
Khan, M. Viqar, FamilyMed
Khan, Shahbaz, FamilyMed
Khanna, Rahul, FamilyMed
Kho, Julian, FamilyMed
Knott, David C., FamilyMed(EM)
Koladich, Carol J.
Krishnar, Kannan, FamilyMed
Ku, Nancy S N.
Lapp, Jonathan F., FamilyMed(EM)
Lee, Allan K L., FamilyMed
Levasseur, Judith L.
Lindner, Kirsten K V., FamilyMed
Lui, Y W. Alex
MacDougall, Ian A T., FamilyMed
MacGregor, Katherine E., FamilyMed
MacKay, M. Jane, FamilyMed
MacKenzie, David P.
MacPherson, Gail L., FamilyMed
Madhvani, Seema N., FamilyMed(EM)
Madon, Shilpa, FamilyMed
Mahn, Joanna, FamilyMed(EM)
Makar, Amany S H., FamilyMed
Manno, Maria P., FamilyMed
Martin, Keith L., FamilyMed(EM)
Martin, Lorne W., FamilyMed(EM)
Martiniuk Kingdon, Kris, FamilyMed
Martinovic, Laurie A., FamilyMed
Martyn, Lori E T.
Mascarin, Robert, FamilyMed(EM)
Massoud, Farid H., FamilyMed
Mastrangelo, E. Armando
Matthews, Rita, FamilyMed(EM)
May, Michael J., FamilyMed
McCann, Thomas J.
McCourt, Francine D., FamilyMed
McDowell, Anthony D.
McGibbon, Dianne L C.
Mian, Zafer, FamilyMed
Milloy, Douglas R.
Mirander, Lennox G., FamilyMed
Morris, Geoffrey S.
Mundenchira, Amitha J., FamilyMed
Murton, Andrew G., FamilyMed(EM)
Nahirny, Taras, FamilyMed
Nguyen-Giang, Quynh-Lang, FamilyMed
Noori, Mahir A., FamilyMed
Norman, Lynne M., FamilyMed(EM)
Nuica, Alina D., FamilyMed
O'Brien, Dennis F.
O'Sullivan, Fiona E.
Opyr, Oksana, FamilyMed
Over, Danielle M.
Pao, Peter S.
Parikh, Samir S., FamilyMed
Park, K. Young
Partridge, Jonathan A., FamilyMed(EM)
Patel, Umeshbhai, FamilyMed(EM)
Patodia, Krishan K., FamilyMed
Petrea, Constantin
Plaxton, Patricia A., FamilyMed
Posen, David B.
Powar, Sukhbinderjit K., FamilyMed
Preradovic, Nikola, FamilyMed
Pyle, Helen A.
Qanungo, Muhammed T., FamilyMed
Quadir, Ambereen, FamilyMed
Rajani, Priya K., FamilyMed
Ramos, Edna V., FamilyMed
Rana, Shabana, FamilyMed
Rennie, James S.
Reynolds, David R.
Rezvani-Khorassani, Massoud
Riley, G. Terence
Rizk, Nada N A., FamilyMed
Rocci, Adriano, FamilyMed
Ross, Anthony L., FamilyMed
Rouse, Frank V.
Rzepka, Waldemar P.
Sahota, Vickram S., FamilyMed
Salahuddin, Afroze, FamilyMed
Samuel, Christopher V., FamilyMed(EM)
Sandhu, Nimani, FamilyMed
Schooling, David G.
Shamim, Safia, FamilyMed(EM)
Shareef, Raghad, FamilyMed
Sharma, Amar D.
Sheth, Nikita T., FamilyMed
Shrayyef, Muhammad Z.
Sidhu, Parbaljit S., FamilyMed
Skendaj, Evis, FamilyMed
Skupsky, Gerald
Slinger, Katherine A.
Smith, Deborah L.
Soliman, Sherine S R., FamilyMed
Sourovtseva, Elena A., FamilyMed
Southey, R. George H., FamilyMed
Springle, Milan A.
St James, Sarah A., FamilyMed
Stanton, W. Thomas H., FamilyMed
Stern, Solomon B.
Strang, Lucy J., FamilyMed
Surbey, Glenn D., FamilyMed
Thomson, Gregory W.
Tram, B V. Jenny, FamilyMed
Tziougras, Petra
Van Straalen, Rosemary T.
Vasylevych, Nataliya V., FamilyMed
Vaz, Reena F.
Vetiska, Frantisek
Viegas, Aiza E., FamilyMed
Vincent, Lisa G., FamilyMed
Voros, Gyula, FamilyMed
Welters, Tania L., FamilyMed(EM)
Wheler, R. James
Wong, Victor C H., FamilyMed
Woollam, Robin C.
Wu, H T. Tony
Yates, John G.
Yip, Jeanne C., FamilyMed
Yusuf, Sabah H., FamilyMed
Zamora, Mary M., FamilyMed(EM)
Zayid, Omar I.
Zimmering, Linda D.

OHSWEKEN

East, Andrea J.
Gasparelli, Rudolph E., FamilyMed
Hill, Karen, FamilyMed
Zacks, Jason A., FamilyMed

OMEMEE

Clay, Jane E.
Ludwig, John J.
Sobrian, Jules

ORANGEVILLE

Ahmed, Somaiah, FamilyMed
Akula, Hari P., FamilyMed
Bailey, Jillian C., FamilyMed
Candusso, Cathryn A.
Chong, Sylvia L., FamilyMed
Cino, Peter J., FamilyMed
Colley, Theresa A.
Cormier, David R., FamilyMed
Davenport, Anna M.
Derksen, Kenneth J., FamilyMed
Donaldson, Craig, FamilyMed(EM)
Emini, Neim N., FamilyMed
French, Nadine, FamilyMed
Gucciardi, Enza-Josie, FamilyMed(EM)
Horvat, Amy M K., FamilyMed
Jamal, Dried E., FamilyMed
Josephson, David A J., FamilyMed
Kim, Joon-Han J., FamilyMed(EM)
Knox, David W., FamilyMed
Leddy, Maire
Malhotra, Gurpreet S., FamilyMed
Malik, Saeed A., FamilyMed(EM)
Marien, Leslie R.
Matava, Rachelle K., FamilyMed(EM)
Matzov, Aviram
Mills, Carol E., FamilyMed
Milone, Stephanie M L., FamilyMed
Milone, Stephen, FamilyMed
Miyata, Kenji S., FamilyMed
Mori, Michael K., FamilyMed
Murphy, Mark E F., FamilyMed
Nadarajah, Senthilraj
Okoli, Chukwuemeka V., FamilyMed
Ostrowski, Leisha N., FamilyMed
Palad, Marcella M S., FamilyMed
Price, William H F.
Reesor, David G.
Riddell, D. Alexander
Riekenbrauck, Neal W., FamilyMed(EM)
Sandhu, Karen A P., FamilyMed
Scotton, Paul S.
Shahzad, Karina, FamilyMed
Singwi, Sanjeev
Sood, Rickesh
Soor, Gursharan S., FamilyMed
Stenning, David L., FamilyMed
Stuckey, Erin Fran.
Szeto, Isabella W., FamilyMed
Vasudeva, Pratibha R.
Watts, Barbara E L., FamilyMed
Wilson, Brian D., FamilyMed
Wong, Grace K S., FamilyMed
You, Calorine, FamilyMed

ORILLIA

Aggarwal, Ravinder K., FamilyMed
Aguilar, Karenina, FamilyMed
Armstrong, J. Gregory, FamilyMed
Atkinson, Donald H., FamilyMed
Babcock, Lea J., FamilyMed
Barnett, Aaron D., FamilyMed(EM)
Bates, J. Wayne
Beshay, Nabil M S., FamilyMed
Brewster, C. Francis, FamilyMed
Cambridge, Mary J., FamilyMed
Cambridge, Robert M., FamilyMed
Catford, Erika A., FamilyMed
Chong, Daniel N F.
Collins, David C.
Daniel, Peter, FamilyMed
Daraei, Nemat A., FamilyMed
De Piero, Steven A., FamilyMed(EM)
Deimling, J. Peter, FamilyMed
Dharssi, Karim, FamilyMed
El Gwaidy, Nivine A F., FamilyMed
Fagan, Stephen, FamilyMed
Francis, Michael L.
Gagnon, Antoine, FamilyMed
Gallagher, Julie A., FamilyMed
Gile, David S., FamilyMed(EM)
Haak, Diane S., FamilyMed
Halbert, Cyril
Hall, Henry J E., FamilyMed
Harmathy, Tibor A., FamilyMed
Harris, Nancy L., FamilyMed
Ho, Grant K C., FamilyMed
Italiano, Marc A., FamilyMed
Kapeluto, Daniel, FamilyMed
Kee, Norman G., FamilyMed
Kennedy, Karen M., FamilyMed
Lam, James H C.
Lobsinger, Thomas R., FamilyMed
Lowry, Josiah B., FamilyMed
Markle, Craig D., FamilyMed(EM)
McComb, Wendy M., FamilyMed
McIntosh, Kimberley A., FamilyMed
McNaull, Benjamin B A., FamilyMed
McNaull, M. Elizabeth, FamilyMed
Michalski, Kathleen A., FamilyMed
Mitchell, Ryan W K., FamilyMed
Murphy, Bernadine S., FamilyMed
Odlozinski, Michael P., FamilyMed
Parna, Laura M H., FamilyMed
Perrigo, Bradley E., FamilyMed
Peysar, Gerhard W., FamilyMed
Pitcher, Jeff, FamilyMed
Podhradsky, Ludek, FamilyMed
Porter, Justin M J., FamilyMed
Reid, Anthony J., FamilyMed
Reinders, Maarthen, FamilyMed
Rosati, Mark E., FamilyMed
Rowhani-Seki, Neda, FamilyMed
Sangster, Donald E F., FamilyMed
Sochaniwskyj, Orest T., FamilyMed
Stokreef, G. John C.
Stong, Martha M J.
Strickland, Carol A., FamilyMed
Taher, Karim, FamilyMed
Tazzeo, James I., FamilyMed
Tigchelaar, Sandra R., FamilyMed
Tigchelaar, Timothy C., FamilyMed(EM)
Tillmann, William D., FamilyMed
Van Iersel, Rebecca I., FamilyMed
Zacharias, Rosemary, FamilyMed

ORLEANS

Aeta, Hany A M M.
Archambault-Leger, Stephanie, FamilyMed
Aubin, Raymond F.
Baars, Cornelius M., FamilyMed
Balla, Agneta, FamilyMed
Beauchemin, Suzanne M., FamilyMed
Beaulieu, J J. Michel F.
Bidari, Imane, FamilyMed
Biscay, Caroline, FamilyMed
Bonacci, Giovanni, FamilyMed
Brown, David E.
Bruce, Jane
Bujold, Marie-Claire, FamilyMed
Burgess, Tracy A., FamilyMed
Cain, Patricia R M J., FamilyMed
Charette, Marie-Christine I., FamilyMed
Chiamvimonvat, Kanchana
Coll, Linda B.
Cote, Genevieve L., FamilyMed
Daigneault, Emilie, FamilyMed
Dansereau, Ronald
Davignon, Genevieve, FamilyMed
Deslauriers, J A. Jean
Desrosiers, Marie-Isabelle, FamilyMed
Djuricic, Milla, FamilyMed
Dostaler, Jacques P., FamilyMed
Drca, Dragoslav
Duchesne, J. Luc L.
Dufresne, Genevieve D., FamilyMed
Gagnon, M A. Patricia
George, Lillian K F., FamilyMed
Giguere, Eliane, FamilyMed
Grainger, Sharon L.
Hamilton, Danielle, FamilyMed
Hodgson, Therese M M., FamilyMed
Ibrahim, Samia M R.
Jokinen, Donna L.
Kelly, Kathleen E., FamilyMed
Klett, Marie-Josee, FamilyMed
Kozyra, Lesia M A., FamilyMed(EM)
L'Heureux, Pierre R., FamilyMed
Landriault, Eric, FamilyMed
Lane, Keith M.
Le Bouthillier, Annie-Josee, FamilyMed
Leclair, Patrick W., FamilyMed
Leduc, Dean C., FamilyMed
Leung, Robert O.
Levenstadt, Jeremy S., FamilyMed
Liang, Stephen
Lortie, Mélissa S., FamilyMed
Marks, Catherine, FamilyMed
McCarthy, F. Paul
Meehan, Anne R., FamilyMed
Mellick, Zohra H.
Menard, Alain L.
Mijavec, Borislava, FamilyMed
Mitchell, Paul A.
Mobayed, Georges N E., FamilyMed
Moise, Josiane
Morson, B. Elizabeth, FamilyMed
Moss, Judy M., FamilyMed
Moussa Faltas, Assanassios, FamilyMed
Muboyayi, T. Romain, FamilyMed
Murty, Hima T., FamilyMed
Mwanz, K. Joseph, FamilyMed
Neal, Ronald J.
Nichols, Erwin B.
Northey, Karen, FamilyMed
Ouellette, Erik, FamilyMed(EM)
Ouellette, Jean-Paul, FamilyMed
Parsons, John E.
Patel, Vishnu K.
Pearce, Llewellyn, FamilyMed
Poirier-Groulx, M C. Lise, FamilyMed
Polan, Kerstin M.
Polan, William F.
Ragheb, Bahaa G., FamilyMed
Renaud, Pierre
Rodrigue, Julie M.
Ryan, J. Wilbay M.
Sabry, Boshra I.
Samrai, Gurinder S., FamilyMed
Sardana, Tarek M.
Saville, Leyana R., FamilyMed
Seale, Edward R., FamilyMed(EM)
Seguin, Bernard A., FamilyMed
Snook, Wayne R.
Souligny, Julie S.
Stewart, John P.
Tosoni, Caroline M A., FamilyMed
Touma, Nadine J., FamilyMed
Trenholm, E. Jo-Anne, FamilyMed
Wahalawatta, Punsara D.
Watt, Gordon L D.
Whalen, Sylvia A M., FamilyMed
Wijay, Shamal N C.
Winzer, Willie P.
Woodend, Dianne M., FamilyMed

OSGOODE

Brennan, Brenda, FamilyMed
Brennan, Terence P A., FamilyMed
Devin, Brian, FamilyMed
Faruqui, Ferrukh I., FamilyMed
MacDonell, Stephannie M., FamilyMed

OSHAWA

Abdul-Rahman, Ibrahim, FamilyMed
Akef, Reza, FamilyMed
Al-Atassi, Talal
Alexieva, Nedalina K., FamilyMed
Barker, David J., FamilyMed
Barrettara, Giuliano
Bhargava, Mukesh
Bisessar, Ahailya S., FamilyMed
Blecher, Peter M.
Bolger, J. Grant W., FamilyMed
Brooks, Marni A., FamilyMed
Callow, John A., FamilyMed
Chahal, Mangeet K.
Chan, Tak-Leung, FamilyMed
Chopra, Jagdish C.

PHYSICIANS BY PROVINCE

Chor, Mark W H.
Conley, Douglas W., FamilyMed
Corless, Kevin J.
Coulby, G. Duncan
Devost, Nicole, FamilyMed
Dhillon, Karamvir K., FamilyMed
Dhillon, Ripple, FamilyMed
Dion, Isabelle, FamilyMed
Drury, Kathryn J., FamilyMed
Dukic, Helena, FamilyMed
El-Batnigi, Nemer, FamilyMed(EM)
Elias, Suzan M., FamilyMed
Fedyna, Roman
Fernando, Anna, FamilyMed
Finch, Graham C.
Fung, Frank
Gebremicael, Eyob
Gee, David, FamilyMed
Gepraegs, Tobi, FamilyMed
Ginsburg, M. Neale, FamilyMed
Girdhari, Rajesh P., FamilyMed
Giroux, Richard P.
Green, Kevin H I., FamilyMed
Hailu, Maru E., FamilyMed
Hall, Christopher W., FamilyMed
Hanna, Albert H H., FamilyMed
Hasan, Shaukat, FamilyMed
Hunchak, John F.
Irwin, S. Patrick
Jain, Sanjive, FamilyMed
Jeyaraj, Hamilton, FamilyMed
John, Usha S., FamilyMed
Kapusta, William M.
Kennedy, Joel N D., FamilyMed
Kennedy, Michael G., FamilyMed
Kingsman, Ronald N.
Kondapaneni, Satyam
Koziar, Mary L., FamilyMed
Kung, Elizabeth Y L., FamilyMed
Ladak, Shenif
Lapena, Hilario S., FamilyMed
Lapena, U. Elsa O., FamilyMed
Leahy, Natalie C., FamilyMed
Lettner, Deborah M., FamilyMed
Leung, Max, FamilyMed(EM)
Lewicki, Mark
Li, Chien-Chuang, FamilyMed
Lindsay, R. Alexander
Linett, Lauren J., FamilyMed
Lockner, Charlene A., FamilyMed
Luces, Kevin F.
Luck, Geoffrey M., FamilyMed
MacDonald, Faith
Mar, Warren J., FamilyMed
Marinova, Evguenia L., FamilyMed
Mathur, Soania, FamilyMed
McIntosh, Douglas C., FamilyMed
McLelland, Edwin N.
McNeill, David G.
Mekonnen Tizazu, Girma, FamilyMed
Milankov, Kosta, FamilyMed
Moffat, Murray J.
Mohammadi, Lida, FamilyMed
Mullin, Roger A.
Murtada Dite Al-Sayed, Sukayna, FamilyMed
Musat, Laura, FamilyMed
Nantheeswarar, Chithakan, FamilyMed
Nasarullah, Fareeha, FamilyMed
Neffati, Abdurrahman A L.
Ngo, T K N. Caroline, FamilyMed
Nguyen, Ngoc Truong T., FamilyMed
Nitoiu, Daniela V., FamilyMed
Noble, Peter C., FamilyMed
Oketch, Consolata, FamilyMed
Paidra, Erik J.
Pakijavan, Abdolreza P., FamilyMed(EM)
Panowyk, Timothy J., FamilyMed
Papadopoulos, Yasmin A., FamilyMed
Parray, Baynazir, FamilyMed
Paul, John T.
Paulovic, Robert P., FamilyMed
Pedretti, Luigi T., FamilyMed
Quinn, Leo P.
Qureshi, Omar, FamilyMed
Raheel, Erum, FamilyMed
Raviele, Anelia K.
Rosen, Charles T.
Ruparelia, Surendra P.
Sadiq, Najemus, FamilyMed
Salam, Abdul, FamilyMed
Schlosser, Alexandra Y., FamilyMed
Schoeman, Hendrik N., FamilyMed
Selvarajah, Prrasonna, FamilyMed
Sharma, Manisha, FamilyMed
Shipley, James H., FamilyMed(EM)
Shizas, Athanasios T.
Singarayer, Chandrakumar
Sivaharan, Ajantha
Smith, Judith M A., FamilyMed
Snider-Adler, Melissa A., FamilyMed
Sorensen, Anne K., FamilyMed
Stephen, Lorne J.
Stuparyk, Robert M., FamilyMed(EM)
Sundaram, Manickavasagam, FamilyMed
Thassanapaff, Vatinee
Thow, David P., FamilyMed
Titis, Apostolus, FamilyMed
Torkian-Valashani, Bahman, FamilyMed
Trambitas, Camelia A., FamilyMed
Verdonk, Robert D., FamilyMed
Vieira, Rose-Anne P., FamilyMed
Voinov, Valentin
Weir, Martina J E., FamilyMed
Whitsitt, Paul F.
Wilk, Andrew
Yoong, K T. Thomas
Zahavi, Michael A., FamilyMed

OTTAWA

Abboud, Jeffrey
Abdulkarim, Emad H.
Aboo, Aboobaker
Abou Said, Edith, FamilyMed
Abtahi, Maryam
Abuswider, Samer A.
Addleman-Frankel, Sarah, FamilyMed(EM)
Adetola, Motunrayo J., FamilyMed
Aggarwal, Rohit, FamilyMed
Ahmad, Rukshanda
Ahmed, Bashir
Ahmed, Muhammad E.
Ahmed, Sarwat M., FamilyMed
Aiello, Michael J., FamilyMed
Ainsworth, Leslie A.
Aizenman, Allan I.
Akcakir, Berna, FamilyMed
Al Faris, Jamila A H.
AlAwadhi, Maryam A Z E.
Alassaf, Hossam A M.
Aldridge, Lisa, FamilyMed
Ali, Iftikhar
Allart, Annemarie
Alsaffar, Heytham K.
Amani, Neda
Amarakone, Samudrika H G., FamilyMed
Amaro, Justine L., FamilyMed(EM)
Amini, Zarlasht
Amjad, Asma, FamilyMed
Amyot, Shawn R., FamilyMed
Anand, Pamela, FamilyMed
Anawati, Michelle L., FamilyMed
Anderson, Josdalyne, FamilyMed
Anstee, Grizel C., FamilyMed
Arnold, Ian, FamilyMed
Arora, Monil, FamilyMed
Arora, Sarvsheel, FamilyMed
Assemi, Ardavan, FamilyMed
Atkinson, Carolyn R., FamilyMed
Audi, Nevine, FamilyMed(EM)
Auer, Joseph M.
Auguste, Ulrick
Bacskai, Istvan S.
Baggley, Anne M., FamilyMed
Bailliu, Leslie-Ann, FamilyMed
Bajramovic, Fersada B.
Ballou, Stephen G., FamilyMed
Bally, Gerry A., FamilyMed
Bamford, Diane F., FamilyMed
Baranick, Peter
Barnabe, Patrick
Barnes, Belinda, FamilyMed
Barnes, Christopher, FamilyMed
Barron-Klauninger, Kathryn, FamilyMed
Bartlett, Lynsey E., FamilyMed
Barwin, B. Norman
Basta, Mourad M., FamilyMed
Batten, Jane S., FamilyMed
Bayne, J. Laura, FamilyMed
Beaubien, Lise B., FamilyMed
Beaudet, Nathalie
Beaudette, Katherine N., FamilyMed
Beaulieu, Claude A.
Beaupre, Lucie M.
Beck, Iain V., FamilyMed
Belanger, Mathieu, FamilyMed
Bell, Timothy G.
Bellack, Allan G., FamilyMed
Belmili, Naima A., FamilyMed
Benjelloun, Abdelhaq
Benoit, Marie-Jose
Berardi, Lyndsay M., FamilyMed
Bercier, Jean-Philippe, FamilyMed
Berkman, Frances A., FamilyMed
Bernier, J. Jean-Robert S.
Berolo, Helen M., FamilyMed
Berringer, Ross G.
Berthiaume, Marc, FamilyMed
Bettolli, Marcos
Bhimji, Khadija, FamilyMed
Bigue, Caroline
Bilodeau, Andre, FamilyMed
Bilodeau, Marc, FamilyMed(EM)
Birkett, Nicholas J.
Birnbaum, Robert J., FamilyMed
Bishop, Clare E., FamilyMed
Biyani, Mohan B.
Biyong, Issack
Bjerre, Lise M.
Blake, Patrick A.
Blattel, Ronald A., FamilyMed
Blier, Pierre
Blonde, Yvonne M., FamilyMed
Bloom, Leonard, FamilyMed
Boet, Sylvain
Boivin Riveros, Marie Claire, FamilyMed
Bonnet, Francine M., FamilyMed
Bordeleau, Marie-Josee, FamilyMed
Bosiljcic-Stojanovic, Svetlana, FamilyMed
Bostwick, Joanna, FamilyMed(EM)
Boucher, Francois-Gilles, FamilyMed
Boudreau, France P., FamilyMed
Bould, Matthew
Bourassa, Marie-Lyne
Bourassa, Pierre
Bourgault, Louise A.
Bourgault, Robert F.
Bourrier, Robert G., FamilyMed
Boushey, Edward, FamilyMed(EM)
Bowen, Debra S., FamilyMed
Boyd, Bryan A.
Boyer, Micheline, FamilyMed
Bradley, Lindsay A., FamilyMed
Braidwood, Danielle, FamilyMed
Brewer, John T., FamilyMed
Brewer, Monica P., FamilyMed
Brigham, Sarah I., FamilyMed
Bright, Priscilla M.
Brittain, Rodney W., FamilyMed
Brockway, Wade, FamilyMed
Brodeur, Jennifer F., FamilyMed
Bromley, Lisa A., FamilyMed
Brook, Edward
Brownlee, Carolyn J., FamilyMed
Brunet, Anne-Marie, FamilyMed
Buczek, Malgorzata J., FamilyMed
Budge, Stephen F., FamilyMed
Bursey, Brandy R., FamilyMed(EM)
Burt, David W.
Bush, Shirley H.
Busing, Nicholas M W., FamilyMed
Butler, Jessica M., FamilyMed
Cain, Michael H., FamilyMed
Cakarevic, Svetlana, FamilyMed
Callahan, Justine E., FamilyMed
Cameron, Daniel J., FamilyMed
Campbell, Alisha H., FamilyMed
Campbell, Catherine W.
Campbell, Gregory J., FamilyMed
Capello, Timothy A.
Cappon, Paul S., FamilyMed
Caron, Catherine M., FamilyMed
Carpenter, David C.
Carpentier, Marie-Pierre, FamilyMed(EM)
Carr, Lindsay A., FamilyMed(EM)
Carson, Katharine D., FamilyMed
Carter, Kevin C A., FamilyMed
Cassam, Humaira
Cattran, Meeka L., FamilyMed
Caytak, Joseph, FamilyMed(EM)
Ceresia, Patrick J.
Chagnon, Nicolas L R., FamilyMed(EM)
Chakrabo, Santanu
Chakraborty, Santanu
Chalifour, Robert
Chamia, Nabil J.
Chan, Grace S., FamilyMed
Chan, Kelvin H., FamilyMed
Chan, Raphael L., FamilyMed
Chandrasena, Chandima, FamilyMed
Charapova, Elena G., FamilyMed
Charles, Marie-Muriel, FamilyMed(EM)
Chartrand, Serge
Chasen, Martin R.
Cheff, T. Gail, FamilyMed
Chen, Long
Chesine, Stephen M., FamilyMed
Chestnut, Heidi A., FamilyMed
Cheung, Denis K T., FamilyMed
Chew, Jennifer P S., FamilyMed
Chin, Ami J., FamilyMed
Chomienne, M. Helene, FamilyMed
Chouinard, J A. Jean
Chow, Janet A., FamilyMed
Chow, Judy T.
Chow, Laura C., FamilyMed
Cinanni, Joseph
Clark, Carolyn M., FamilyMed
Clarke, Joseph
Clavette, Manon, FamilyMed
Clermont, Dawn C.
Clevette, Nancy A., FamilyMed
Cloutier, M. Sylvie
Clow, Jennifer E., FamilyMed(EM)
Cockburn, John E., FamilyMed(EM)
Cohen, Howard R., FamilyMed
Coleman, Gina S A.
Comeau, Benjamin M., FamilyMed(EM)
Comerton, Aileen, FamilyMed
Comerton, Mary E., FamilyMed
Condon, Elana M., FamilyMed
Contreras Dominguez, Vladimir
Cooper, Krista A., FamilyMed
Corkery, Douglas L J A.
Corkum, Cheryl D., FamilyMed
Cornell, Lilly K.
Corrales Medina, Vincente F.
Cote, Joseph A M A.
Cotter, Jill E., FamilyMed
Cottrill, Ruth A.
Courchesne, Cyd
Crabtree, Paul O E., FamilyMed
Creaghan, Jason D., FamilyMed
Cucan, Elissa, FamilyMed
Curtis, Shirley L B P.
Czarnowski, Z. Charles, FamilyMed
Daniel, James K.
Dauksza, Aneta J., FamilyMed
Davidson, David, FamilyMed(EM)
Davila Acosta, Jorge H.
Davison, Peter D.
Dawson, John E.
De, Aloke, FamilyMed
De Grace, Michel C., FamilyMed
De Salaberry, Lara, FamilyMed
De Souza, Selwyn X P., FamilyMed
DeLong, Rachel, FamilyMed(EM)
Degani, Aqeel, FamilyMed
Deilgat, Michel P.
Della Zazzera, Massimiliano
Dennison, Heather D., FamilyMed
Dermer, Mark, FamilyMed
Deutsch, Margaret J., FamilyMed
Deveau, Joey, FamilyMed
Dewan, Ambika, FamilyMed
Dhalla, Fatima, FamilyMed
Dhami, Karan S., FamilyMed(EM)
Dhanani, Sonny
DiMarzo, Laura, FamilyMed
Dick, Brian D., FamilyMed
Diekmeyer, Christine, FamilyMed
Dinovitzer, Natalie M., FamilyMed
Dionne, Matthew L., FamilyMed
Dionne, Richard, FamilyMed(EM)
Diraimo, Louis R.
Docking, Annie E., FamilyMed(EM)
Doherty, Dermot R.
Dollin, Janet, FamilyMed
Donohue, Alicia, FamilyMed
Dorland, Katherine E., FamilyMed
Dos Santos, Marlise P.
Doss, Chrishanthini M., FamilyMed
Douek, Jennifer F., FamilyMed
Douglass, Rebecca J., FamilyMed
Douyon De Azevedo, Mario, FamilyMed
Dover, Karen J.
Downar-Zapolski, Zbigniew
Drodge, Karen H., FamilyMed
Dubarsky, Howard B., FamilyMed
Dube, Christine, FamilyMed(EM)
Duchesne, Catherine J., FamilyMed(EM)
Dufresne, Maurice J A.
Duggan, Ann, FamilyMed
Duong, Alex K., FamilyMed
Duong, Huu Thanh
Duong, Nhan Hoang, FamilyMed
Dworkin, Barry, FamilyMed
Dy, Hans A., FamilyMed
Eaton, Robert J.
Edwards, Elizabeth F.
Ehrlich, Helga, FamilyMed
Eid, Roula, FamilyMed
Eipe, Naveen
Eisener-Parsche, Pamela D., FamilyMed
El-Gaddafi, Walid F A.
El-Khodary, Mohamed A I.
Elkin, Eric N.
Elliott, Denise M., FamilyMed
Elmistekawy, El Sayed M.
Elrefai, Thaer, FamilyMed
Ember, Andrew P., FamilyMed
Enright, Paula D., FamilyMed
Eom, Minjeong, FamilyMed
Escudero, Juan L.
Esdaile, David S., FamilyMed
Evans-Olders, Rebecca, FamilyMed
Eveleigh, Bruce S.
Eyre, Alison, FamilyMed
Eyre, Dean P.
Fahim, Raouf M.
Faloon, Thomas, FamilyMed
Farey, Ruth, FamilyMed
Farncombe, Margaret L.
Fasih, Najla
Faught, Andrea L.
Feberova, Jana
Feder, Stephen H., FamilyMed
Fellegi, Nicolette K., FamilyMed
Fernando, Mary L.
Finestone, David L., FamilyMed
Fisher, Rebecca
Fisher, Stephen, FamilyMed
Fisher, Susan C., FamilyMed
Fitzgibbon, Edward, FamilyMed
Flanagan, Amanda, FamilyMed(EM)
Fletcher, Kenneth J.
Flynn, M. Dominique, FamilyMed
Fonseca, Conchita, FamilyMed(EM)
Forestier, Colleen A., FamilyMed
Fox, Eric, FamilyMed
Freeman, Jeffrey
French Merkley, Veronique, FamilyMed
Fuca, Roland P J.
Fung, Celeste, FamilyMed
Fung, Sarah, FamilyMed
Furesz, Eva B.
Gaba, Priya, FamilyMed
Gagnon, Marie-Claude, FamilyMed
Gale-Rowe, Margaret A.
Gambhir, Indu B.
Gardiner, Dennis
Gardiner, Edward M., FamilyMed(EM)
Garinther, Ross
Gatien, Mathieu M., FamilyMed(EM)
Gauthier, Kathryn, FamilyMed

Geffen, Allison S., FamilyMed
Geier, Pavel
Geller, Carol A., FamilyMed
Gervais-Fagnou, Danielle D., FamilyMed
Ghali, Atef M S., FamilyMed
Ghemlas, Ibrahim A M.
Gibson, Rebecca D., FamilyMed
Giovinazzo, George A.
Given, John P.
Glassman, Steven J.
Glenn, John W., FamilyMed
Glinski, Robert G., FamilyMed(EM)
Gluszynski, Malgorzata, FamilyMed
Goindi, Reena, FamilyMed
Goldman, Faye A., FamilyMed
Goldstein, Aubrey
Gonsalves, Violet, FamilyMed
Gostimirovic, Milka, FamilyMed
Gottman, Elizabeth, FamilyMed
Goubran, Mona R., FamilyMed
Graham, Lindsay A.
Graham, Lyla M., FamilyMed
Gratton, Valerie
Griffiths, Patricia E., FamilyMed
Gruner, Douglas, FamilyMed
Grymala, John P.
Guerra, Luis A.
Guirguis, Adel F.
Gunnink, Sara E., FamilyMed
Gupta, Ashish
Habib, Emad A., FamilyMed
Hack, Anna T., FamilyMed
Hall, Elaine J., FamilyMed
Hall, Philippa, FamilyMed
Hall, Trudy M., FamilyMed
Halliday, David M.
Hamdy, Hazem A., FamilyMed
Hamilton, Anne, FamilyMed
Handfield-Jones, Richard S., FamilyMed
Hansen, Mark G., FamilyMed
Harman, Lisa M., FamilyMed
Harmsen, Merril A.
Harrison, Christine E., FamilyMed
Harvey, David
Hasham, Aliya, FamilyMed
Hauser, Joseph, FamilyMed
Hayfron-Benjamin, Jonathan
Haziza, Philippe
Henry, Mary A., FamilyMed(EM)
Herskovitz, Mariana L N.
Hicks, Susan B., FamilyMed
Hilborn, David J.
Hindle, Valerie, FamilyMed
Hiremath, Swapnil
Hirsh, Michael S., FamilyMed
Hodge, Eleanor A.
Hodgins, Michael B., FamilyMed
Hogg, Donald W.
Hollands, Ralph T., FamilyMed
Hollingworth, Gary R., FamilyMed
Holt, Martha, FamilyMed
Honsl, Evelyn M.
Hostland, Sara, FamilyMed(EM)
Hubbes, Claudia H., FamilyMed
Hudon, Sylvie R., FamilyMed
Hughes, Owen P., FamilyMed
Huq, Rokaiya, FamilyMed
Hussain, Shabnam, FamilyMed
Hyde, Byron M.
Hynie, Vera
Iancu, Daniela-Elena
Inacio, Joao M S R.
Iny, Alan I., FamilyMed
Irani, Farhad
Jabouin, Serge
Jackson, Bethany J., FamilyMed
Jacoby, Lynn M.
Jaeger, Hilary F.
Jain, Anil
Jain, Rachna
Jamshaid, Mamoona, FamilyMed
Janna, Peter A., FamilyMed
Jeanes, C. William
Jee, Katie H., FamilyMed
Jenner, Julie A., FamilyMed
Jewer, D. Lemont
Jeyaraj, Leo
Jimenez Rivera, Carolina D.
Joanisse, John A.
John, Miroslava
Johns, Christine R., FamilyMed(EM)
Johns, Karen
Johnson Mora, Ben H.
Johnston, H. Alan, FamilyMed
Johnston, Sharon E., FamilyMed
Jones, Brent D., FamilyMed
Jones, Kenneth D.
Jovanovic, Radmila
Juery, Pierre G., FamilyMed
Jull, Laura A., FamilyMed
Jung, Hans W.
Jurencak, Roman
Kabir, Atif, FamilyMed
Kagan, Hershel H B., FamilyMed
Kahale, Justin A., FamilyMed(EM)
Kale, Rajendra D.
Kalin, H. David, FamilyMed
Kaplan-Myrth, Nili, FamilyMed
Kappagantula, Usha R., FamilyMed
Karas, Philip, FamilyMed
Kasatiya Trevisani, Elena
Katz, Mortimer
Kaushik, Aneel, FamilyMed
Kehoe, Anne, FamilyMed
Kelly, Francis B.
Kelly, Kathleen J., FamilyMed
Kendall, Claire E., FamilyMed
Kennedy, Ryan P., FamilyMed
Kent, Lara C., FamilyMed
Keren, Arieh
Khan, Seema N.
Khandaker, Masud H.
Khatter, Kapil, FamilyMed
Khuon, David C., FamilyMed
Kilbertus, Frances T., FamilyMed
Kilby, Donald L P.
Kindle, Gitta K N.
Kindle, John E.
Kirby, Emily K., FamilyMed
Kissick, James S., FamilyMed
Knight, Caroline A., FamilyMed
Knoefel, Frank D., FamilyMed
Kobewka, Carlynne J., FamilyMed
Koldewey, Natalia, FamilyMed
Koujok, Khaldoun
Kozar, Walter J., FamilyMed(EM)
Kozminski, Mary T., FamilyMed
Kurtz, Stuart F., FamilyMed
Kwan, Helen H., FamilyMed
Kyrillos, Edmond, FamilyMed
L'Ecuyer, Michel A., FamilyMed
Labrosse, Josee L.
Lacaze-Masmonteil, Thierry
Lacroix, Julie D M., FamilyMed
Lad, Shilpa V.
Lafleche, Claire M., FamilyMed
Lalonde, Bernard G.
Lalonde, Lisa M.
Lambert, Wendy C L., FamilyMed
Lamont, Jennifer, FamilyMed
Lang, Sandra R.
Langill, Marc V., FamilyMed
Langille, Heather I., FamilyMed(EM)
Lariviere, J. Louis R.
Lariviere, Katherine E., FamilyMed
Lariviere, Michele
Laskowska, Barbara E.
Laskowski, Wojciech
Latimer, Bradley R.
Laughton, Angela F., FamilyMed
Lavoie, Curtis F., FamilyMed(EM)
Lawlor, Peter G., FamilyMed
Lazaridis, Sofia, FamilyMed
Le, Tung Trong, FamilyMed
Le Gal, Gregoire
Leblanc, P. Nicole, FamilyMed
Lebrun, Paul J.
Leclair, Jason M., FamilyMed
Leduc, Bernard, FamilyMed
Lee, Pi Kay, FamilyMed
Lefort, Louise A., FamilyMed(EM)
Legare, Carole, FamilyMed
Leger, J E. Roland
Leiva, Rene A., FamilyMed
Lemelin, Jacques, FamilyMed
Lemelin, Myra M., FamilyMed(EM)
Leppard, Jennifer L A., FamilyMed(EM)
Lesley, Peter A.
Levine, Daniel S., FamilyMed
Levitan, Riva E., FamilyMed
Lewin, Laura L., FamilyMed
Lezack, Lisa J., FamilyMed
Liddy, Clare E., FamilyMed
Lim, Sen-Mei, FamilyMed
Ling, Audrey L H., FamilyMed(EM)
Litwin, Shlomo, FamilyMed
Lo, Jeremy C K., FamilyMed
Lo, W. Alex
Loemba, Hugues D., FamilyMed
Lofaro, Anthony D., FamilyMed
Lozano, Marina, FamilyMed
Lyen, Catherine L., FamilyMed
Lynn, Brian W.
MacBride, Ajana P., FamilyMed(EM)
MacDonald, Janeen M.
MacEachern, Lisa K., FamilyMed
MacIsaac, Jennifer L., FamilyMed
MacLeod, G. Stuart, FamilyMed
MacMillan, David J., FamilyMed
MacNeil, Hugh A K., FamilyMed
Maher, Daniel T.
Mahrouche Belbachir, Lilia, FamilyMed
Mai, Andrew D., FamilyMed
Mai, David D., FamilyMed
Malek, Michael L., FamilyMed
Malherbe, Stéphanie C., FamilyMed(EM)
Malik, Anjna A.
Maloley, Jeffrey W.
Maloney, Justin P., FamilyMed(EM)
Mankal, Fawzi A., FamilyMed
Mansour, Riad A., FamilyMed
Manzig, Gloria B I., FamilyMed
Marchington, Katie L., FamilyMed
Marriott, Jason J A., FamilyMed
Martin, Sylvie
Martinho, Humberto, FamilyMed
Martinho, Valdemar
Masse, Yanick N R., FamilyMed(EM)
Matin, Roozbeh, FamilyMed
Mavriplis, Cleoniki A., FamilyMed
McBean, Nora M., FamilyMed
McDougall, Donald C., FamilyMed
McGuire, Abigail, FamilyMed
McGuire, Shaun N., FamilyMed
McIntosh, Karen L., FamilyMed
McKim, Susanne E D., FamilyMed
McKinnon, Michelle P., FamilyMed
McLaren, Meaghan E., FamilyMed
McMahon, James D R.
McNaughton-Filion, M. Louise, FamilyMed(EM)
Mehta, Bella, FamilyMed
Mercer, Jay G., FamilyMed
Mes, Tom A E J.
Metz, Gila S., FamilyMed
Michon, Alain, FamilyMed(EM)
Mickelson, R. Ross
Migicovsky, Valerie R., FamilyMed
Mikhail, Mary Y D.
Millar, David R., FamilyMed
Miller, Barbara C., FamilyMed(EM)
Miller, Elka
Miller, Sebastian J.
Millette, Alain
Mills, Heather E., FamilyMed(EM)
Mills, Sian E.
Minorgan, Stephanie, FamilyMed
Mo, Fan D., FamilyMed
Mohammed, Samah A., FamilyMed
Molot, John M., FamilyMed
Monahan, M. Anne, FamilyMed
Montague, Michael, FamilyMed
Montpetit, Madeleine R., FamilyMed
Moore, Joanna D., FamilyMed
Moore, Leonard J., FamilyMed
Moore, Lisa J., FamilyMed
Moores, Daisy E., FamilyMed
Moreau, Natalie, FamilyMed
Moretti, Felipe M.
Morin, Carl G.
Morissette, Louis G., FamilyMed
Morley, Daniel, FamilyMed
Morneau, Kathryn A., FamilyMed
Morris, Barbara D., FamilyMed
Morris, Patricia E., FamilyMed
Morris, William F.
Mossman, Hilary R L., FamilyMed
Motamedi, Farhad, FamilyMed
Mount-Bastianelli, Heather
Mucha, Mary Ann J., FamilyMed
Muggah, Elizabeth A., FamilyMed
Mullan, Michael J.
Mundi, Christina, FamilyMed
Munro, Camille, FamilyMed
Murley, Vanessa R., FamilyMed
Murphy, Jeffrey B., FamilyMed
Murray, Carolyn, FamilyMed
Murray, Jodie
Murtaza, Atif, FamilyMed
Murthy, Vaani V., FamilyMed
Murty, Manoranjan P., FamilyMed
Nadon, F. Vincent G.
Nahas, Richard, FamilyMed
Nahri, Dolly T.
Nasser, Kasim R., FamilyMed
Nassim, Mark, FamilyMed
Nath, Avik, FamilyMed(EM)
Nawrocka, Joanna
Neira Aragon, Victor M.
Nery, Pablo B.
Neskovic, Svetlana, FamilyMed
Neufeld, Troy M., FamilyMed
Ng, Jonathan M., FamilyMed
Ng Cheng Hin, Alan, FamilyMed
Ngo Minh, Cuong, FamilyMed
Nguan, Oliver Y C., FamilyMed
Nguyen, Tung Thanh C., FamilyMed
Nickerson, Katelyn E., FamilyMed
Nicole, Marie-Noelle, FamilyMed
Ning, Jean-Noel
Noel De Tilly, France
Norman, Lawrence I., FamilyMed(EM)
Northoff, Georg F.
Nowodworski, Dorota J., FamilyMed(EM)
Nussbaum, Christopher J., FamilyMed(EM)
Nuth, Janet E., FamilyMed(EM)
Nzau, Duncun M M.
O'Byrne, W L. Gray, FamilyMed
O'Connor, Helene L., FamilyMed
O'Connor, Madeline, FamilyMed
O'Connor, Mary E.
O'Donnell, Shawn M., FamilyMed
O'Shea, Eoghan B., FamilyMed
Oishi, Cameron R., FamilyMed
Oliva, Jiri
Oliver, Sarah J., FamilyMed
Oosthuizen, Jean M., FamilyMed
Orbeck, Kenneth W.
Ostiguy, Nadine P., FamilyMed
Ott, Monica S., FamilyMed(EM)
Ou, Chuhua, FamilyMed
Ouellet, Yanick, FamilyMed(EM)
Owen, Diana C., FamilyMed(EM)
Pageau, Paul G., FamilyMed(EM)
Pagtakhan, Arlene L., FamilyMed
Paidra, Astrid
Paiement, Francois L., FamilyMed
Parbhakar, Meenakshi, FamilyMed
Parent, Lorne J., FamilyMed
Parker, Jacqueline M., FamilyMed(EM)
Parkhill, Nancy L., FamilyMed
Parsons, Elizabeth P., FamilyMed
Patterson, Judy L., FamilyMed
Pegu, Satyaranjan
Pella Fernandez, Denisse, FamilyMed
Peltz, Julie E.
Pena Fernandez, Elena
Pereira, Jose L., FamilyMed
Perrin, Mark J.
Perry, Jeffrey J., FamilyMed(EM)
Perttula, Edward A.
Peters, Karina M., FamilyMed
Pfeiffer, David, FamilyMed
Phelan, Cynthia C., FamilyMed
Phillipowsky, Michael A.
Picard, Claudette, FamilyMed
Pickersgill, Heather M., FamilyMed
Pierce, Jennifer L., FamilyMed
Pilon, Josee L., FamilyMed
Pilon, M M. Louise
Pipe, Andrew L.
Pitre, Lyne, FamilyMed
Pless, Robert P.
Pohl, Daniela
Poisson, Lucille J., FamilyMed
Poitras, Jacqueline E H., FamilyMed
Ponka, David, FamilyMed(EM)
Poplove, Steven H.
Pottie, Kevin C., FamilyMed
Premachandra, Thusitha
Premji, Kamila, FamilyMed
Prince, Renee, FamilyMed
Purdy, Ceilidh L., FamilyMed
Quach, Dieu Hoa, FamilyMed
Racine, Dominique M J., FamilyMed
Ragan, Edward
Rahal, Hussain A.
Rambert, Julian J.
Ramin, Brodie, FamilyMed
Ramphal, Raveena
Rangwala, Sohil, FamilyMed
Raymond, Barbara J.
Raymond, Michele, FamilyMed
Raza, Danyaal, FamilyMed
Reardon, Mary-Lynne
Redpath, Calum J.
Redpath, Stephanie
Reducka, Kathryn G.
Regnier, Laura R J., FamilyMed
Renaud, Claude A., FamilyMed
Ressler, Ladislaus J.
Rezaiefar, Parisa, FamilyMed
Ribchinsky, Sofia, FamilyMed
Ricard, Jacques P J.
Rice, Jill L., FamilyMed
Rice, Sarah C., FamilyMed
Richardson, Ian D., FamilyMed
Riff, Shena R., FamilyMed(EM)
Ritsma, Lindsay R., FamilyMed
Rivet, Christine C., FamilyMed(EM)
Robertson, Helen M., FamilyMed
Robertson, Julia S.
Robillard, Lise-Anne
Robillard-McNulty, Lucile C.
Rochon, Marie-Helene, FamilyMed
Rochowski, Andrzej
Rodrigue, Andree C M., FamilyMed
Rodrigues, Americo V F.
Rogers, Neil J.
Romanowska, Karinka I.
Rose, Edward J., FamilyMed
Rosenberg, Hans, FamilyMed(EM)
Rosenbloom, Arlene R., FamilyMed
Rotaru, Carmen
Roth, Johannes
Rothstein, Sheila
Routhier, J O. Richard
Rouvinez Bouali, Nicole G.
Rowan, Robert A.
Roy, Jean A., FamilyMed
Rusimovic, Lynn, FamilyMed
Russell, Grant
Russell, Jocelyn M., FamilyMed
Ryan, T. Lerato, FamilyMed
Ryding, S. Louise, FamilyMed
Rydzik, M. Suzanne
Saad, Maan H A., FamilyMed
Saar, John E., FamilyMed
Sabatino, Assunta C., FamilyMed
Saeed, Arshad, FamilyMed
Saeed, Maheen
Salamon, Miriam, FamilyMed
Salat, Jan M.
Sampaio, Marcos
Sanchez, Millaray, FamilyMed
Saunders, Christine E., FamilyMed
Savage, Erin C., FamilyMed(EM)
Sawyers, Elizabeth A., FamilyMed
Scandiffio, Ralph J.
Schatz, Jennifer R., FamilyMed
Schenker, Marianne
Schnare, Ted D., FamilyMed
Schneider, Gerd, FamilyMed
Schussle, Olivier
Schwartz, Caitlin J., FamilyMed
Schwartz, Morton L.
Scott, Elizabeth M.
Scott, John F.
Scott-Thomas, Nancy L E., FamilyMed(EM)
Seale, Janet E., FamilyMed
Sekhon, Harmanjatinder S.
Sell Marucco, Erick F.
Sellers, Laura P., FamilyMed
Sethuram, D. Tony, FamilyMed
Shabana, Wael M.
Shadbolt, Nicole S., FamilyMed

Shamji, Salima, FamilyMed
Shamsian, Elham, FamilyMed
Shamsie, Amina J., FamilyMed
Shannon, Michael E.
Sharma, Meena P.
Shaw, Jinny J., FamilyMed
Shearman, John K., FamilyMed
Sheikh, Adnan M.
Sheppard, Matthew J.
Sheridan, Jay T., FamilyMed
Sheshko, Nykola, FamilyMed
Shin, Alice J., FamilyMed
Shlik, Jakov
Shore, Donna A., FamilyMed
Sicard, Joanne E., FamilyMed
Siddiqui, Nishat A.
Sim, Quan-Yong, FamilyMed
Singer, Gabrielle T., FamilyMed
Skillings, Robert L.
Skjenna, Olaf W.
Sloan, Lisa L., FamilyMed
Sly, Jane E.
Smith, Daniel N., FamilyMed
Smith, Douglas W., FamilyMed
Smith, Karlene I., FamilyMed
Smith, Scott A., FamilyMed
Smolkin, Robert D.
Soccar, Esther A M., FamilyMed
Sokoloff, Dina R., FamilyMed
Sollars, Susan J.
Soltys, Katherine M.
Song, Anne, FamilyMed
Soni, Naveen K., FamilyMed
Soni, Nisha, FamilyMed
Soucie, S. Pierre, FamilyMed
Soucy, J L. Rene, FamilyMed
Souter, Francis C G.
Spacek, Alena M., FamilyMed(EM)
Spacek, Katerina B., FamilyMed
Spence, Edwin B.
Spika, John S.
Sproule, James R., FamilyMed(EM)
St-Jean, Mireille C., FamilyMed
St-Pierre, Nancy, FamilyMed
Staples, Kristy L.
Steffenhagen, Nikolai E A.
Stewart, I. Maureen
Stewart, P. David, FamilyMed(EM)
Steyn, Pierre G.
Stiell, Andrew P., FamilyMed(EM)
Still, Janet E.
Stoddart, Karen L., FamilyMed
Stone, Erin K., FamilyMed
Strike, Jessica S., FamilyMed
Stringer, Vernon M.
Su, Didacus, FamilyMed
Sullivan, Tracy
Sully, Irma-Nancy, FamilyMed
Sun, Louise Y P.
Sun, Xiaoli
Sutherland, Eleanor W.
Swami, Kamla A.
Syposz, Benedykt S., FamilyMed
Szczepanik, Dorota M., FamilyMed
Tamboli, Mharukh Y.
Tang, S C. Albert, FamilyMed
Tanguay, Agnes M J.
Tannenbaum, Joanne A., FamilyMed
Tanner, Erika L., FamilyMed
Taras, Lisa H., FamilyMed
Taylor, Allan J., FamilyMed
Taylor, Elaine M., FamilyMed
Taylor, J. Robert D.
Taylor, Mary M.
Taylor, Michael R., FamilyMed(EM)
Taylor, Taryn-Lise, FamilyMed
Tector, Susan E., FamilyMed(EM)
Teitelbaum, Peter S.
Tessier, Pierre C., FamilyMed
Tetrault, Louise-Marie
Theriault, Patrick, FamilyMed
Thompson, Bridget E., FamilyMed
Tobin, D. Jonathan, FamilyMed
Torres, Carlos H.
Torrie, Ian D.
Tostowaryk, Karen J.
Touchie, Michael J.
Townsend, Philip A.
Trabelsi, Asma, FamilyMed
Tracey, Scott J., FamilyMed
Trant, Alison M S.
Trepanier, Jean R.
Trollip, Jean J., FamilyMed
Trottier, Yolaine
Tsang, Philip, FamilyMed
Tulai, Cristina
Turley, Jolanda C., FamilyMed
Twemlow, Diane W., FamilyMed
Tyson, Thom V.
Tzeneff, Simeon G.
Uhthoff, Peter A F.
Uhthoff Munro, Sylvia
Ujjainwalla, Mark H.
Ullmark, Nicole P., FamilyMed
Uppal, Gayatri, FamilyMed
Valia, Bhavna, FamilyMed
Vanasse, Marie-Antoinette A L., FamilyMed
Vandewaetere, Anik R M., FamilyMed
Varma, Prem K.
Venkatesh, Thiruganasam, FamilyMed(EM)
Vernooy, Catherine M., FamilyMed
Vidyasankar, Gokul
Viner, Gary S., FamilyMed
Viner, Norman M.
Virmani, Vivek
Visentin, Laura M., FamilyMed
Visser, Shaun L., FamilyMed(EM)
Vlahovich, Slavica
Vogel, Martin V.
Vyvey, Melissa L., FamilyMed
Wade, Jessica L., FamilyMed
Walker, Alfredo E.
Walker, Carolyn E.
Walker, Robert M C., FamilyMed
Ward, Robert A.
Warrack, Ian M., FamilyMed
Warraich, Kanwarjit, FamilyMed
Wassef, Georgina, FamilyMed
Waters, Eugenie F., FamilyMed
Watkins, William T., FamilyMed
Way, Daniel O., FamilyMed
Weatherhead, Debra J., FamilyMed(EM)
Webber, Gail C., FamilyMed
Weber, Christopher C.
Webster, Michael C., FamilyMed
Weiner, Lorne S., FamilyMed
Weiss, Ronald S., FamilyMed
Wheatley-Prince, Paul F.
White, Christine L., FamilyMed
White, Lisa A., FamilyMed
White, Margaret A., FamilyMed
Whitehead, Kristine M., FamilyMed
Whitley, Susan A., FamilyMed
Wilkinson, Anna N., FamilyMed
Wilkinson, Susan E., FamilyMed
Williams, Megan K., FamilyMed
Willows, Melanie D., FamilyMed
Wilson, Allan
Wilson, Donald K.
Wilson, Margaret A., FamilyMed
Winter, I. Alexander, FamilyMed
Wojtyk, Ronald J.
Wolski, Piotr S.
Wong, Tracy T Y., FamilyMed
Woo, Michael Y., FamilyMed(EM)
Wooltorton, Eric J., FamilyMed
Worrall, James J., FamilyMed(EM)
Wu, Yan, FamilyMed
Wu, Yizheng, FamilyMed
Wylie, Louise B M.
Yachnin, Michael D.
Yang, Carol S.
Yao, Christiana Y., FamilyMed
Yau, Jennifer K W., FamilyMed
Yeung, Marianne Y T., FamilyMed(EM)
Yiu, Stella H M., FamilyMed(EM)
Younger-Lewis, Catherine J.
Youssef, Fady, FamilyMed(EM)
Yu, Horace, FamilyMed
Zamorski, Mark A., FamilyMed
Zaremba, Janina
Zhao, Charles, FamilyMed(EM)

OWEN SOUND

Aboo, Ismail Y.
Barfoot, Alison H., FamilyMed
Chaddah, Vijay K.
Connelly, Kerry L.
Dyke, Debra R., FamilyMed
Eby, Donald H., FamilyMed(EM)
Edwards, Gordon L.
Emsalem, Abdurahman M.
Evoy, Andrea M., FamilyMed
Fleming, Ann P., FamilyMed
Gibbons, Maria K., FamilyMed(EM)
Grant-Hall, Susan C., FamilyMed
Hay, Peter J., FamilyMed
Huff, Hildegard R., FamilyMed
Iqbal, Bland
Kapalanga, Nyolima J B.
Krasovec, Barbara M., FamilyMed
Lackner, Colin R., FamilyMed(EM)
Lebel, Tania C., FamilyMed
Lindsay, John S.
Lukasik, Mark H., FamilyMed(EM)
Lynn, Hazel R., FamilyMed
Marsden, Robert J.
McArthur, Anne-Louise A., FamilyMed
Mehta, Sunil P., FamilyMed(EM)
Mulroy, Brendan J., FamilyMed
Myers, Leslie A., FamilyMed(EM)
Nwebube, Nkiruka I.
Petrie, Alison C R A., FamilyMed
Petrie, Ian B.
Qawi, Huma
Robbins, Anthony J., FamilyMed
Sandhu, Indermohan
Sauks, Toomas P.
Savaria, Elyse
Setty, Yatish N.
Siddiqi, Nilofar, FamilyMed
Stanners, Bruce K., FamilyMed
Sutherland, Kenneth S.
Thomson, Merrin M.
Tweedie, T. Cameron, FamilyMed(EM)
Van Alphen, Katarina M., FamilyMed
Van Zyl, Cornelius J., FamilyMed(EM)
Van Zyl, Lizette, FamilyMed
Veenstra, Fedde, FamilyMed(EM)
Whittle, Daniel J.
Winterton, Victoria D J., FamilyMed
Wright, John A.

PAKENHAM

Kiskis, John
Vilis, Donna M.

PALGRAVE

Knipping, Randolph P., FamilyMed

PALMERSTON

Cressey, Christopher F., FamilyMed
Semelhago, Gavin R.

PARIS

Male, Ross S., FamilyMed
McDonald, John W.
Piercy, Gregory M.
Tamale, John R., FamilyMed(EM)
Williams, Robert S.

PARKHILL

Thorpe, William R.

PARRY SOUND

Brennan, John P., FamilyMed
Clarke, David N., FamilyMed
Cook, Sidney D.
Donevan, Robert H., FamilyMed
Gehrels, Corrine M., FamilyMed
George, W. Derek M., FamilyMed
Gray, Phebe, FamilyMed
Hardie, David P.
Higgins, Thomas J., FamilyMed
Honsinger, Philip, FamilyMed
Hunkin, John B.
Ibey, Christopher C.
Ibey, Margaret M.
Moquin, Daniel H., FamilyMed
Moquin, Kathleen M., FamilyMed
Redmond, Timothy Y., FamilyMed(EM)
Shaw, Stuart J., FamilyMed
Smith, Willard A D., FamilyMed
Stern, Dennis J.
Stevens, Rob F., FamilyMed
Thompson, Maureen E.
Thwin, Noreen
Warwick, Kimberly A., FamilyMed
Wilson, Wendy L.
Woodhouse, Douglas D., FamilyMed
Woodhouse, Richard T.

PEFFERLAW

Marchuk, Patricia M.

PEMBROKE

Baddar, Faisal, FamilyMed
Baxter, Brian
Cantin, Sylvie M D., FamilyMed
Castillo, Heather M., FamilyMed
Clarke, Leigh L.
Coleman, Lomie J.
Corriveau, Michael R A.
Davies, John T., FamilyMed
Forfar, Katie, FamilyMed
Galley, Peter W.
Gerbis, Christine, FamilyMed
Gilbert, Rosemarie G.
Hurley, Thomas C., FamilyMed(EM)
Laliberte, Serge A.
Lavigne, Paul A., FamilyMed
MacPherson, Colin A.
Moeck, Lori S., FamilyMed
Mottiar, Farouk
Ng-Thow Hing, Roland
Owens, Thomas R.
Plante, Daniel, FamilyMed
Plante, Judith C., FamilyMed
Quirion, Charles-Antoine J., FamilyMed(EM)
Rainville, Ginette D M., FamilyMed
Ratnayake, Wasantha P., FamilyMed
Ren, Yubo, FamilyMed
Savoie, Anne-Marie, FamilyMed
Simkin, Sarah R., FamilyMed
Stewart, Aviva T., FamilyMed(EM)
Thomas, Jennifer E., FamilyMed
Tyler, Joan C., FamilyMed
Uttley, Steven R., FamilyMed
Waldolf, Richard E., FamilyMed
Ward, Joel W., FamilyMed
Weatherston, Evelyn J.
Wierstra, Benjamin T., FamilyMed

PENETANGUISHENE

Abrahamian, Dikran J.
Akintan, Abosede
Badenhorst, Johannes G., FamilyMed
Blom, Christine R., FamilyMed
Blomberg, Ann L., FamilyMed
Bolton, James E.
Egbewunmi, Adeyemi T.
Gaffney, Gregory M.
Johnson, Jennifer K., FamilyMed
Moran, Peter D., FamilyMed
Nel, Louis J., FamilyMed(EM)
Olisa, Obidike M., FamilyMed
Stubbins, Robert I.
Uwaifo, Victor O.
Wells, Laurie L., FamilyMed
Woods, Donald B.
Zwicker, John W.

PERTH

Asrat, Getnet A., FamilyMed
Bartleman, Anne-Pascale, FamilyMed
Chaudry, Bushra, FamilyMed(EM)
Cunniffe, Peter J., FamilyMed
Drummond, Alan J., FamilyMed(EM)
Ehrat, Caroline B., FamilyMed(EM)
Gauthier, Alain, FamilyMed
Jechel, Peter, FamilyMed(EM)
Joannou, Manuela H E., FamilyMed(EM)
Kennie, Robin C., FamilyMed
McKinnon, Maxine E.
McLean, Ross R., FamilyMed
Moxon, Richard D.
Popiel, Stephanie Y S A., FamilyMed
Turner, Paul V., FamilyMed
Tweedie, James W.
Tyrrell, Derek J.
Van Noppen, Beth-Anne, FamilyMed
Van Noppen, Boudewyn J., FamilyMed

PETAWAWA

Boyle, Stefan R., FamilyMed
Carriere, Christopher G.
Christinck, E. Rosemary, FamilyMed
Coker, David A., FamilyMed
Crouzat, Michael G., FamilyMed
Davenport, Ethan M., FamilyMed
Dooley, Patrick J.
Eason, Brad D., FamilyMed
Espina, Melanie R., FamilyMed
Fraser, Holly C., FamilyMed
Harrigan, Erin K., FamilyMed
Kucherepa, Nadia N A., FamilyMed
Lane, Lynsay R., FamilyMed
Lloyd, Ronald M.
Lotfi-Seysan, Lotfullah, FamilyMed
Mintz, Randall R., FamilyMed
Murphy, Leah C., FamilyMed
Praught, Jeffery C., FamilyMed
Purdy, Jennifer L., FamilyMed
Rodgman, Graeme M.
Rossi, Carlo, FamilyMed
Rowan, Declan M., FamilyMed
Sakanovic, Alenko, FamilyMed
Schoonbaert, Ian C., FamilyMed
Truong, Long P T., FamilyMed
Weisgerber, Christopher A., FamilyMed
Wolfrom, Brent D., FamilyMed

PETERBOROUGH

Aasheim, Lise H., FamilyMed
Abrahamse, Cornelis J.
Ahee, Richard E M., FamilyMed
Anderson, Mary Lynn
Archibald, Jonathan M., FamilyMed
Arcieri-Piersanti, Vincenzo, FamilyMed(EM)
Armour, Paul W.
Armstrong, Judith-Anne, FamilyMed
Auyeung, Grace C Y., FamilyMed
Beamish, John J., FamilyMed
Berg, Gary R., FamilyMed
Binette, J. Richard F., FamilyMed
Black, Raymond, FamilyMed
Blouin, Lucie M.
Boyce, Debra E., FamilyMed
Boyd, Cameron L.
Brar, Deepinderjit S.
Brown, Carolyn E., FamilyMed
Burns, Brenda R., FamilyMed
Cameron, Bruce C., FamilyMed
Carr, G. David A., FamilyMed(EM)
Clark, Peter A.
Comerford, Mary L., FamilyMed
Courtney, Susan D.
Curtin, Kimberley A., FamilyMed
Darling, Jennifer L., FamilyMed(EM)
De Francesco, Nicole J., FamilyMed(EM)
de Luna, Rodrigo P., FamilyMed
Dickie, Margaret J., FamilyMed
Dillon, Kirk F.
Eldridge, Karen-Lee, FamilyMed
Elliott, Robert M., FamilyMed
Feroze, Nicholas, FamilyMed
Flynn, Kathleen M., FamilyMed

Freeman, Christie L., FamilyMed
Friesen, Dale C.
Friesen, Reinhard, FamilyMed
Gibson, Kevin F., FamilyMed
Gillis-Doyle, Jennifer A., FamilyMed
Gleeson, Susan E., FamilyMed
Goodge, John
Gow, Barbara L., FamilyMed
Greiner, Karin, FamilyMed
Grieve, Geoff, FamilyMed
Gulati, Meena
Hameed, Faiza
Hicks, Lisa K., FamilyMed
Hill, Gary V.
Himann, Joan E., FamilyMed
Holmes, Roger G.
Houpt, Daniel R., FamilyMed
Hsu, Chia-Wen, FamilyMed
Hudson, Neil C., FamilyMed
Jacka, Robert M., FamilyMed
Jeffery, Anthony J.
Jilani, Amer M.
Joyce, Joan E., FamilyMed
Kathirav, Satheesh
Kelly, Janet M., FamilyMed
Kerr, Larry C.
Kerr, Thomas A W.
Khan, Sandra M., FamilyMed
Kilmartin, Patrick J M.
Lencses, Kathy A., FamilyMed
Lindsay, Brian G., FamilyMed
Lokanathan, Vanita, FamilyMed
Lunn, H R. Darlene
M'Cwabeni, Constantine T., FamilyMed(EM)
MacIntosh, F. Douglas, FamilyMed
Magliocco, Maria
Mak, Mabel, FamilyMed
Maltman, Craig J., FamilyMed
May, Terrence A., FamilyMed(EM)
McDonald, Maureen M., FamilyMed
McGorman, James G., FamilyMed(EM)
Messervey, Elizabeth A., FamilyMed
Millar, Thomas
Miller, Thomas, FamilyMed
Morrison, Robert G.
Neville, Jeffrey S., FamilyMed
Neville, Robert J., FamilyMed
Newport, David A., FamilyMed
Peters, Grant M.
Post, Ellen E., FamilyMed
Powell, Gordon W W., FamilyMed
Ragaz, Stephan C., FamilyMed
Rand, Juri
Revel, Lillian C.
Rice, Brenda L.
Richard, Thomas C., FamilyMed
Rodgers, Allen J.
Romanowski, Andrew, FamilyMed
Sexton, Patrick H.
Shaikh, Muhammed
Silverberg, Alexis S W.
Smith, Sheena M H.
Sokolon, Daryl G.
Spink Jr., Donald R., FamilyMed
St Rose, John E M.
Stoker, D. Brent, FamilyMed
Swales, William C.
Syed, Naseeruddin
Thompson, Donald S.
Troughton, K. Mark, FamilyMed(EM)
Turner, R. Douglas
Uy, Antonio F., FamilyMed
Vajid, Muhammad A.
Van Der Kamp, Nicholas H., FamilyMed
Van Dorsser, John G.
Van Leeuwen, Jennifer F., FamilyMed
Vanhoof, Ronald A.
Vilcini, Michelle M., FamilyMed
Webster, James, FamilyMed
Weir, Jean E., FamilyMed
Welch, Robert J.
Wesolowski, Marta A.
Whatley, Richard J., FamilyMed
Wheeler, Jesse J F., FamilyMed
White, Nancy A., FamilyMed(EM)
Wilson, Terrance R.
Zaniewski, Gregory A., FamilyMed

PETROLIA

Al-Dhaher, Firas F., FamilyMed
Butler, John S., FamilyMed
Daniel, Enoch S., FamilyMed
Li Wan Po, Ah-King
MacDonald, Walter A C.
Mather, Susan A., FamilyMed
Ng, Victor K H., FamilyMed(EM)
Riedl, Frank W.
Wang, Angela J., FamilyMed
Winegard, John C.

PICKERING

Ah Now, Walter, FamilyMed
Alidina, Diamond F H.
Alidina, Parviz D F.
Alidina, Zahra, FamilyMed
Boorman, Lyn D., FamilyMed
Charania, Diamondali K.
Chartier, Brenda A.
Chow, Jane, FamilyMed
Chung, Sun Yung., FamilyMed
De Sa, Michelle, FamilyMed
Dosaj, Seema, FamilyMed
Eisen, Doron A., FamilyMed
Erry, Rajeev
Farber, Bernard, FamilyMed
Fischer, C. Richard, FamilyMed
Ghaffar-Sedeh, Maryam, FamilyMed
Hall, Gordon W.
Ho-Kim, Thu-Lan, FamilyMed
Hughes, David A.
Jagota, Ajay, FamilyMed
Jones, Nicole A., FamilyMed
Kurtz, Martin J.
Marmina, Joseph E V.
Maslowski, Aleksander, FamilyMed
McLean, Chris A., FamilyMed
Mehta, Arun K.
Mohammed, Isa K., FamilyMed
Persaude, Darshini D., FamilyMed
Petroff, Howard L., FamilyMed(EM)
Potter, Eleanor R A., FamilyMed
Ram, John R., FamilyMed
Razzaq, Mahreen A.
Semoff, Michael
Shah, Mruna M., FamilyMed
Sheikh, Farrukh B.
Sinha, Jayaditya J., FamilyMed
Stephen, David H.
Su, Jason W S., FamilyMed
Tanious, Lawrence F.
Tirmizi, Lubna T., FamilyMed
Vela, Kanna J.
Walpola, Piyal L., FamilyMed
Woloszczuk, Andrea D.
Wylie, J. Stewart M., FamilyMed
Yamagishi, Kyle F Y., FamilyMed
Ying, Thomas S F.

PICTON

Beach, David A., FamilyMed
Blanchard, Stephen F., FamilyMed
Burke, Graham H.
Christie, Elizabeth A., FamilyMed
Colby, Joshua, FamilyMed(EM)
Connell, Norah D.
Forster, Lisa, FamilyMed
French, John A.
Haigh, Kim D., FamilyMed
Hayward-Stewart, Amber, FamilyMed
Higgins, Greg, FamilyMed
Janikowski, Andrew M., FamilyMed(EM)
Johannsson, Peter W.
Kolabinski, Irene
Koval, Donald C., FamilyMed
Lett, Darren A., FamilyMed(EM)
McDonald, John A.
Nancekievill, Elizabeth A., FamilyMed
Rice, Clifford G., FamilyMed
Russell, Lois E., FamilyMed
Seybold, William D., FamilyMed
Tromp, Margaret M., FamilyMed

PLANTAGENET

Desjardins, Joanne, FamilyMed
Fadaz, Annissa, FamilyMed
Forgues, Marie-Josee, FamilyMed
Lyons, Paul H., FamilyMed
Seguin, Gerald L.
Zarowsky, Christina H A.

POINT EDWARD

Aviles, Alberto J.
Buckton, William A., FamilyMed
Duggal, Anil
Garrett, Rex M.
Monk, Charles M.
Nedic, Igor, FamilyMed
Prendiville, William G M.
Stubbs, Peter J S.

PORT BURWELL

Leatherdale, Charles L.

PORT CARLING

Burns, Paulette E.

PORT COLBORNE

Bell, Amanda L., FamilyMed
Dewar, James D.
Gomez, E G. Enrique
King, Jason J.
Kuhn, Craig J., FamilyMed
Remington, Jeffrey S., FamilyMed(EM)
Rivers, Derek W., FamilyMed
Rungi, George, FamilyMed
St-Hilaire, Jason J., FamilyMed
Wayda, Charlene E.
West, William J H.
Whitehall, Jeffrey D., FamilyMed

PORT DOVER

Beaver, Julia A L.
Hadi, Mohammed, FamilyMed
Hall, John D.
Hynscht, Harold G.
Wong, Peter N.

PORT ELGIN

Brown, Deirdre K., FamilyMed
Gundrum, Susan, FamilyMed
Hollohan, Kirk G., FamilyMed(EM)
Marriott, Michael A., FamilyMed(EM)
McCulloch, Donald F.
Somerville, Tara L., FamilyMed

PORT HOPE

Azzopardi, Mark J A.
Banerjee, Tapas
Durante, Lino M.
Hazell, Paul M.
Knackstedt, Jeffrey V.
Levinson, Steven D.
Long, Michelle
Routh, John M C.
Tesluk, Raymond P., FamilyMed
Tesluk, W. Anne, FamilyMed
Torok, Kim M., FamilyMed
Zalzal, Nayla

PORT PERRY

Adams, Richard M., FamilyMed
Ali, Fahim H., FamilyMed
Allin, Robert C., FamilyMed
Armstrong, Ankelly L M., FamilyMed
Best, Kerri L., FamilyMed
Brown, Anthony L.
Brown, Merrilee G., FamilyMed
Casella, Tesha E., FamilyMed
Chiella, Antonietta A., FamilyMed
Clendenning, Robert D., FamilyMed(EM)
Cull, Sonya M., FamilyMed
Dayal, Amita, FamilyMed
Ferguson, Kimberley A., FamilyMed
Gilmour, Michael M., FamilyMed
Homer, Ivy M., FamilyMed
Hyshka, Sandra A.
Kazarian, Nancy, FamilyMed
Mercer, Gordon R., FamilyMed
Nguyen, Hong Chau, FamilyMed
Pawley, Amanda C., FamilyMed
Puckrin, Paul H.
Ross, Jessica N., FamilyMed
Russell, Elizabeth M.
Russell, Steven B.
Shepherd, Susan E., FamilyMed
Smith, Kevin G.
Stewart, John I.
Stewart, Martin C., FamilyMed
Tse, Brian L., FamilyMed
Tuck, James A.
Westbrook, Christopher J., FamilyMed
Wong, Denise W., FamilyMed
Wray, Rebecca S., FamilyMed

PORT ROWAN

Dukelow, Robert H.
Johnston, Sarah J., FamilyMed

PORT STANLEY

Hofhuis, John A., FamilyMed
Keenleyside, Joel H., FamilyMed

PORTLAND

Evans, Jennifer B.
Laforty, Jack M.
MacKey, Thomas D.

POWASSAN

Houghton, Scott D.
Runciman, Kenneth A C., FamilyMed
Tuck, Sarah E., FamilyMed
Woodward, Larry E.

PRESCOTT

Albert, Frederick L.
Bhatt, Gunvant S.
Bhatt, Nikhil, FamilyMed
Kellam, George W., FamilyMed

RAINY RIVER

Singleton, John D., FamilyMed

RAVENNA

Bryans, Franklin C.

RED LAKE

Aniol, Wojciech
Chu, Marcella, FamilyMed
Isenberg, Jonathan R., FamilyMed
Moreno, Agustin A., FamilyMed
Orth, Peter M R., FamilyMed
Parker, Richard C.
Polle, Mark R., FamilyMed
Tong, Jennifer N., FamilyMed
Zielke, Diane B.

RENFREW

Appleyard, Craig E., FamilyMed
Arcand, Jennifer L., FamilyMed
Bodig, Jessica E., FamilyMed
Caza, Gregoire F., FamilyMed
Clarke, Allison J., FamilyMed
Collins, John A.
Di Paolo, Andrea B L., FamilyMed
Duggan, Robert M.
Kemp, Donald G.
Kidd, Robert F.
Langlois, Stephanie F.
Lavigne, Ronald F., FamilyMed
MacDonald, Catherine A., FamilyMed
Matosh, John
Mickus, V. Alexander
Pinard, Philippe, FamilyMed
Radke, Steven, FamilyMed
Strader, Bruce E.
Varrin, Angela E., FamilyMed
Wang, Noreen B., FamilyMed(EM)

RICHARDS LANDING

Avery, Ross A., FamilyMed
Booth, Karen L., FamilyMed(EM)
MacKay, Ian E., FamilyMed
Snajdrova, Lenka, FamilyMed(EM)

RICHMOND

Gick, Susan V., FamilyMed
Rabb, H. Roderick
Rabb, Lucy M.

RICHMOND HILL

Abdel-Bary, Mona A M., FamilyMed
Akhtari, Shahrzad, FamilyMed
Ameen, Sakeenah, FamilyMed
Anwar Masih, Tahreem S., FamilyMed
Araghi, Golbarg, FamilyMed
Asefi, Shirin, FamilyMed
Aw, Brian J., FamilyMed
Batay-Csorba, Peter A.
Berger, Brian, FamilyMed
Bernholtz, Jeffrey J.
Bhagat, Ashok
Birbrager, David B I.
Boozary, Majid
Borenstein, David A., FamilyMed(EM)
Bose, Teertha J.
Brown, Jordan S I.
Bukmuz, Rica
Cernat, Geta, FamilyMed
Chan, Alex S L., FamilyMed(EM)
Chan, Bonnie F., FamilyMed
Chan, John F Y.
Chan, John Y W.
Chan, Joseph C Y., FamilyMed
Chan, Raymond K H., FamilyMed
Chen, Anthony C., FamilyMed
Cheng, Michael T W.
Cheng, Michelle, FamilyMed
Chernick, Michael, FamilyMed
Cheung, Bonnie
Chong, Esther, FamilyMed
Chu, Melvyn, FamilyMed
Chu, Patrick
Contractor, Masuma M., FamilyMed
Cordos, Mihaela C., FamilyMed
Currid, John M.
Daiter, Jeffrey, FamilyMed
Dawson, John, FamilyMed
Derakhshan, Afrooz, FamilyMed
Deutsch-Levy, Meredith, FamilyMed
Dholasania, Rozina N., FamilyMed
Dumitrescu, Corina, FamilyMed
Eftekhari, Maryam, FamilyMed
El Seisi, Somaya, FamilyMed
Ferguson, Errol
Fortier, Christopher, FamilyMed(EM)
Frank, Nathan P., FamilyMed
Franklin, Gabriela, FamilyMed
Fremont, Larry E.
Fu, Ping, FamilyMed(EM)

PHYSICIANS BY PROVINCE

Fung, Michael G., FamilyMed
Gheorghe, Camelia M., FamilyMed
Ghorbani, Farnaz, FamilyMed
Gill, Harmander S., FamilyMed
Ginzburg, Val E., FamilyMed
Goldstein-Colman, Lisa J., FamilyMed
Gortler, Judith R., FamilyMed
Greenwald, Iris C., FamilyMed
Grossman, Steven M.
Grouhi, Shahpar
Haghighat, Kasra
Handa, Pooja
Hanna, Shoukry, FamilyMed
Hasemzadeh-Balouchi, Maliheh, FamilyMed
Hayami, John A.
Hirano, David Y.
Hirji, Rahim, FamilyMed
Hirtenfeld, Adi
Ho, Nancy S K.
Hormozdi, Homa, FamilyMed
Javanmard, Mahgol, FamilyMed
Kako, Christian Y.
Kalpin, Allen O.
Kanjee, Anjum S., FamilyMed
Kaplan, Alan G., FamilyMed(EM)
Karenkova, Natalia
Kaushal, Anu, FamilyMed
Kelton, Yasmine S., FamilyMed
Khalil, Evon W H., FamilyMed
Khan, Shahnaz
Kiez, Debra A., FamilyMed(EM)
Kliman, Lorne D.
Ko, Evan K Y.
Kwee, Roy T G.
Kwong, Eugene C K., FamilyMed
Lai, Henry H C., FamilyMed(EM)
Lam, Michael C., FamilyMed
Lau, H K. Henry
Law, Hugo K C.
Leader, Susan M A., FamilyMed
Lee, Christina L Y.
Lee, Young M.
Leung, Ernest Y L., FamilyMed
Leventis, Anastasios, FamilyMed
Li, Kan Wen
Li, Xiao Qing, FamilyMed
Liaghati-Nasseri, Negin, FamilyMed
Liang, Charles
Liu, Fay F V.
Liu, Hwayue, FamilyMed
Liu, Suzy S V.
Lusher, Brandon E., FamilyMed
Lyew, Winston J.
Makinde, Oluwatomilola O., FamilyMed
Mandel, Drue H., FamilyMed
Marinosyan, Mari H., FamilyMed
Mascan, Lavinia M., FamilyMed
Mashouf-Fard, Mahsa, FamilyMed
Mauceri, Nella, FamilyMed(EM)
Meghji, Mohamed H., FamilyMed
Mehta, Susan E.
Mikhail, Ashraf S., FamilyMed
Mortellaro, Lia M., FamilyMed
Mousmanis, Patricia A., FamilyMed
Mutukistna, Indren
Nachim, Ilan, FamilyMed
Nagahara, Brian M.
Nesterenko, Maria, FamilyMed
Ng, Victor K., FamilyMed
Nimni, Gil B., FamilyMed(EM)
Notarandrea, Edoardo, FamilyMed(EM)
Paisley, J. Kenneth
Pardis, Bijan, FamilyMed
Partridge, Michael A C., FamilyMed(EM)
Perlon, Paul, FamilyMed(EM)
Rastogi, Sanjay, FamilyMed
Rauchwerger, David R., FamilyMed(EM)
Rhee, Kunuk, FamilyMed
Rosen-Zaidener, Dalia S., FamilyMed
Rosenthal, Eva E., FamilyMed
Safir, Irina, FamilyMed
Salamat, Amirreza, FamilyMed
Samuel, Joyce M., FamilyMed
Selick, Avram Z.
Selvakone, Meera, FamilyMed
Selvanayagarajah, Selliah, FamilyMed
Sennikov, Alexei
Sheffield, Brian
Shoukralla, Faten S., FamilyMed
Shugarman, Laurel G D., FamilyMed
Simkhovitch, Peter, FamilyMed
Sin, Philip C.
Sithamparanathan, Kasthuri, FamilyMed
Sollazzo, John N., FamilyMed(EM)
Soong, Anna S K.
Srinivasan, Anuradha
Sull, Thomas J., FamilyMed(EM)
Swartz, David S., FamilyMed(EM)
Taheri-Anaraki, Atousa, FamilyMed
Tan, Charles C.
Tang, Godwin P Y., FamilyMed
Tang, Hung-Yip
Tasharofi Kia, Mina, FamilyMed
Taub, Sherry J.
Teng, Sophia C.
Tharmaratnam, Thadsha, FamilyMed(EM)
Tobias, Guy, FamilyMed
Tong, Shu Kow
Tsang, Michael S M., FamilyMed
Upitis, Jennifer A.
Varenbut, Michael, FamilyMed
Verma, Neil, FamilyMed(EM)
Wadhwa, Mandeep, FamilyMed
Wasan, Tina, FamilyMed
Wei, Ho-Yin, FamilyMed
Williams, Henry S.
Winslow, Inge G.
Wong, Angela M Y., FamilyMed
Wong, Eric P C.
Wong, Fung L., FamilyMed
Wong, Ophelia C Y.
Wong, Sunny Y C., FamilyMed
Wong, Winnie T., FamilyMed(EM)
Woo, Paul C Y.
Wyatt, Philip R.
Yam, Edric C W., FamilyMed
Yeung, Christine R., FamilyMed
Youssef, Hany A A., FamilyMed
Zachos, Constantine R.
Zhang, Y. Jackie, FamilyMed
Zhu, Jiajia, FamilyMed
Zhuang, Lihua, FamilyMed

RIDGETOWN

Button, John R.
Prins, Claire A., FamilyMed
Prins, Leonard M., FamilyMed
Simmons, Rachel A., FamilyMed
Tariq, Marium, FamilyMed

RIDGEWAY

Lee, Michael C F.

ROCKLAND

Adam, Josee, FamilyMed
Bissonnette, Mélanie, FamilyMed
Brule, Sylvie M., FamilyMed(EM)
Deaton, Shoshanah E C., FamilyMed
Deneault, Mychele C., FamilyMed
Lanoix, Pierre J., FamilyMed
Lefebvre, Yves A., FamilyMed(EM)
Leroux, Genevieve, FamilyMed
Lilly, Erica J., FamilyMed
Mills, Natalie S., FamilyMed
Noel, Kendall A., FamilyMed
Pelletier, J. Steve N., FamilyMed
Seguin, Daniel R., FamilyMed
Vachet, Mylene J., FamilyMed

ROCKWOOD

Hosdil, Jane M J.
Khan, Rabia N., FamilyMed
Marin Arellano, Alejandra I., FamilyMed
Samson, Kevin

RODNEY

Tenki, Michael C.

RUSSELL

Archibald, S B. Wallace, FamilyMed
De Banne, Danielle M., FamilyMed
Heymans, Gerry A., FamilyMed
Menard, Darrell C.
Trahan, J. Simon-Pierre

SARNIA

Ajayi-Obe, J. Oluwagbenga, FamilyMed
Al-Janabi, Hasan
Arnold, Cynthia E., FamilyMed(EM)
Austin, Marc R., FamilyMed
Barnett, Kimberly A.
Bartlett, John M.
Barwitzki, Gary W., FamilyMed(EM)
Bhandal, Harleen G.
Bhargava, Vandana, FamilyMed
Boyle, Patrick, FamilyMed
Campbell, Ian G., FamilyMed
Canning, Aidan W N.
Cheong, Richard A.
Chilvers, Martyn J.
Cooper, Alan J.
Crozier, Melanie A., FamilyMed
Dostaler, Monique R., FamilyMed
Fayad, Hamideh
Gamble, Eamon N.
Gannon, William
Grochowski, James, FamilyMed(EM)
Hirst, Jason O., FamilyMed(EM)
Hislop, Robert I., FamilyMed(EM)
Kanaan, Hassan D.
Kim, David
Kolano, Lori L., FamilyMed
Kucerova, Lenka
Lau, Alvin W W.
Lising, Jean B C.
Maddison, Glen J.
Mangel, Ryan, FamilyMed
McGregor, Clare-Louise, FamilyMed
Mountain, G. Brett, FamilyMed(EM)
Naik, Anjana T.
O'Leary, Brendan P.
O'Mahony, John C., FamilyMed
O'Mahony, Michael F J.
O'Sullivan, P. Niall
Pasqualucci, Renato, FamilyMed(EM)
Peterson, Sean R D., FamilyMed(EM)
Putter, J. Dirk, FamilyMed(EM)
Rahalkar, Mangal R., FamilyMed
Rankin, Wayne M.
Rockwell, Helen A., FamilyMed
Rogan, Heather M.
Saeed, Akhter
Saeed, Muhammad A.
Schlebusch, Gert H G., FamilyMed
Sharma, Bal Krishan, FamilyMed
Singh, Joy R., FamilyMed
Singh, Vidyanand B., FamilyMed
Soeder, Samantha P., FamilyMed
Spano, Joseph J.
Stoesser, Michael J P.
Suryavanshi, Shveta, FamilyMed
Teel, Warren D.
Uppal, Jaishree
Van As, Nicolaas, FamilyMed(EM)
Vornberger, William J.
Vouriot, Daniel D., FamilyMed(EM)
Withers, Martin J., FamilyMed

SAULT STE MARIE

Adebowale, Akinade O.
Antoine, Louis B.
Apostle, Peter D.
Avery, Patricia K.
Balogh, Arpad
Barbeau, Brynlea, FamilyMed
Beck, David A V., FamilyMed
Beduhn, Eitel E R.
Benedek, Linda J., FamilyMed
Bodnar, Michael, FamilyMed(EM)
Bondar, Steven M.
Bonder, Lauren, FamilyMed
Bowen, Nadia, FamilyMed
Bragaglia, Pauline J.
Brooks, Douglas
Bruni, Christopher A., FamilyMed
Buehner, Sharon E., FamilyMed(EM)
Catania, Philip J J.
Center, Richard P.
Chow, Peter H.
Chung, Win Yan
Clarke, John A.
Curran, James A., FamilyMed
Cziffer, Andreas
Dawson, Katharine L., FamilyMed
Dopp, Philip, FamilyMed
Edwards, Mark
Febbraro, Mario A.
Fera, David J.
Fraser, Ronald
Fritz, Daniel R., FamilyMed
Garniss, Derek, FamilyMed(EM)
Gieni, Rose-Marie A L.
Grosso, William T.
Hackett, Michael A.
Hemy, Melissa D., FamilyMed
Hiron, Peter
Hirvi, Edward, FamilyMed
Ianni, Frank A., FamilyMed
Ip, Andrew P., FamilyMed(EM)
Jablanczy, Alexander J N.
Kargbo, John, FamilyMed(EM)
Kargbo, Natalia V., FamilyMed
Keating, Michael V.
Kobelka, Charlotte R.
Kuntz, Carolyn J., FamilyMed
Kuntz, M. Eleanor
Kuntz, Michael P.
Lane, John
Leahy, Marilyn T., FamilyMed
Lee, M. Anne F., FamilyMed
MacIntosh, Donald S L., FamilyMed(EM)
MacMichael, Gordon K.
Maione, Pietro F.
Maloney, Robert J.
McLean, Alan
Meligrana, Peter D.
Mogharrabi, Mehran
Mohammadi, Ehsan, FamilyMed(EM)
O'Brien, Lewis J., FamilyMed
Opryszczko, Krzysztof, FamilyMed
Owen, James E L.
Patterson, Jennifer K., FamilyMed
Pearson, John C.
Poitevin, David G.
Robertson, Julia A., FamilyMed
Rossi, Christine M., FamilyMed
Schamp, Adrianna E., FamilyMed
Schwarz, Peter R., FamilyMed
Shah, Abker, FamilyMed
Shamess, Brian A.
Sharp, Lorraine F., FamilyMed
Smith, Stephen A., FamilyMed
Stewart, Jodie P., FamilyMed
Suppes, Robert J., FamilyMed
Tang, Dominic M H.
Trusdale, Paisley W., FamilyMed(EM)
Tull, Russell G., FamilyMed
Turgeon, Eugene W T., FamilyMed
Wacker, Kevin P.
Wakegijig, Annelind D V., FamilyMed
Wallace, Wendy C., FamilyMed
Waymouth, William E W.
Wild, Paul J., FamilyMed
Wilson, Mary L., FamilyMed
Wytsma, Richard D.
Yee, Gayle M., FamilyMed
Ziada, Zeinab H., FamilyMed

SCARBOROUGH

Abdulhussein, Rahim, FamilyMed
Abounaja, Mohamed A., FamilyMed
Abrahams, Pauline E., FamilyMed
Ahooja, Vineeta
Akbarali, Nurjehan, FamilyMed
Akriotis, Van J., FamilyMed
Al-Odhayb, Sami
Al-Shami, Eman
Alcock, Carl J.
Alexander-Williams, Karen A.
Alexov, Lubomir
Alfred, Premini C P., FamilyMed
Ali, Vasima
Alkon Mintsopoulos, Sultana
Allan, Scott M., FamilyMed
Allen, Joseph A.
Allibhai, Sophia, FamilyMed
Amarasekera, D. Vimal S., FamilyMed
Ambalavanar, Elancheliyan, FamilyMed
Ansari, A. Hashsham, FamilyMed
Arif, Abu S M., FamilyMed
Arnold, Robin A V.
Arulchelvam, Pradeepan, FamilyMed
Asirwatham, Ramesh I., FamilyMed
Ayesha, Qanta, FamilyMed
Azam, Afshan
Azer, Salwa, FamilyMed
Bacher, Larry, FamilyMed
Bacher, Thomas S.
Baciowski, Chris K.
Baker, Lawrence
Balkissoon, Mahadeo
Bangee, Misbah
Bari, Basel
Bavakutty Mohammed, Sheeja, FamilyMed
Beamish, Gregory H., FamilyMed
Belchetz, Brett, FamilyMed
Bilbily, Janan F Y., FamilyMed
Bing-Wo, Sandra, FamilyMed
Bluthardt, Thomas R.
Bongard, Alexandra, FamilyMed(EM)
Boparai, Shabab, FamilyMed
Bordman, Joel S.
Bordman, Risa B., FamilyMed
Boyrazian, Hagob A.
Brodie, Richard J., FamilyMed
Brooks, Lisa H.
Brooymans, Corinne A M., FamilyMed
Broughton, Catherine M.
Buchanan, Suzanne C., FamilyMed
Butchey, Joseph K., FamilyMed(EM)
Butt, Debra A., FamilyMed
Calderon, Gerardo G.
Carlos, Joseph M.
Caulford, Paul G., FamilyMed
Cerkvenik, Majda
Chacko, Mary, FamilyMed
Chakrabarty, Lina S., FamilyMed(EM)
Chan, Brian A.
Chan, Erin T W., FamilyMed
Chan, Kwok-Hung
Chan, Lawrence K C., FamilyMed
Chan, Paul S H.
Chan, Peter K.
Chan, Peter S K.
Chan, Roy K., FamilyMed
Chan, Suk K.
Chan, Thomas T., FamilyMed(EM)
Chan, Wai Lam W.
Chan, William W L.
Chandrasekaran, Akila P., FamilyMed
Charlton, Ronald W R.
Charyk, Rafael, FamilyMed
Chen, Jacky S L., FamilyMed
Cheng, Bai-Sen, FamilyMed
Cheng, Kiu-Sing
Cheng, Richard S S.
Chin, Anthony W.
Chin, Gregory J.
Ching, Daniel H T.
Chinner, Anthony J.
Chiu, Bobby T L., FamilyMed
Chiu, Simon K H., FamilyMed
Chiu, Victor W.
Chow, Harold H K.
Chow, Kenneth C K.
Chow, Sheung C.
Chu, Agnes M C., FamilyMed
Chu, James C M.
Chu, Norman H Y., FamilyMed(EM)
Chu, Sik On
Chua, Caroline L., FamilyMed
Chung, Andrew Y W., FamilyMed
Chung, Cynthia
Chung, Justin A., FamilyMed(EM)

PHYSICIANS BY PROVINCE

Clark, Andrew T., FamilyMed
Cramer, Paul R.
Daniels, Nelson J.
Datta, Susmita
Davies, Ceri J., FamilyMed
Dawood-Mohamed, Yusuf
De Souza, Aloysius P G C.
Dehghani-Mohammadabidi, Payman, FamilyMed(EM)
Del Rosario, Daniel S.
Devon, Jennifer L., FamilyMed(EM)
Dhalla, Aminmohamed
Direnfeld, Leonard, FamilyMed
Drutz, Randall A., FamilyMed
Dulay, Navdesh K., FamilyMed
Edgerley, Michael W., FamilyMed
Eid, Karim E C.
Eisner, Rhonda B.
Erlick, Lawrence S., FamilyMed
Esbin, E L B. Bobby
Esser, David
Etaleb, Osmaa, FamilyMed
Fadeel, Khalid, FamilyMed
Farrington, Bruce
Fashho, Ousama
Fejer, Imre B.
Flood, Joan, FamilyMed
Flores-Vargas, Alberto L.
Fong, Chi Wai.
Foong, Weng-Leong
Forbes, Shauna E., FamilyMed
Franczak, Edwin J., FamilyMed
Friedman, Jonathan, FamilyMed
Fung, Susanna W S., FamilyMed
Fung, Wing-Tai
Gabor, Zsuzsanna
Gaur, Shiva K.
Gelman, Marc L.
George, Elizabeth
Ghotra, Harpreet S.
Gliklich, Ian, FamilyMed
Glowczewski-Park, Elizabeth Y H., FamilyMed
Go, May L.
Goldberg, Bernard
Goldman, Gerald N.
Goldstein, Irwin H.
Gopal, Vanita, FamilyMed
Graham, Kevin P.
Grant, Andrew A., FamilyMed
Grant, James R., FamilyMed
Greenwood, I. Ronald, FamilyMed
Gretsinger, Paula C C.
Guirguis, Emad F T., FamilyMed
Guo, Hans C T., FamilyMed
Hamid, Muhammad A.
Hanna, Magdy M., FamilyMed
Heiber, Michael J., FamilyMed(EM)
Henis, Mohsen, FamilyMed
Hew, Sheila L., FamilyMed
Hirsch, Andrei E.
Hirshfeld, Steven M.
Hsieh, Wayne W Y., FamilyMed
Hu, William
Huebel, Stephen C.
Huynh, Nhu Nguyet, FamilyMed
Hwang, Angela, FamilyMed
Hwang, Mei L.
Ibrahim, Hany S H., FamilyMed
Ibrahim, Maged S H., FamilyMed
Ibrahim, Salwa N K., FamilyMed
Ing, Horne D.
Ingber, Linda G.
Iracleous, Panayiotis, FamilyMed
Irvine Chamberlain, Leanne B., FamilyMed(EM)
Iwasa, Carolyn T.
Jacob, Anu
Jacob, Punnaran, FamilyMed
Jacobs, Susan
Jacobson, Paul D M., FamilyMed(EM)
Jaffer, Naaznin K.
Jagan, Gavin S., FamilyMed
Jain, Mahendra K.
James, David H C.
Jang, Eddy
Jattan, Sarla, FamilyMed
Jay, Howard
Jayarajah, Francia G., FamilyMed
Jegatheeswaran, Dharmavathy
Jeu, Joan P., FamilyMed
Jindal, Vinay K., FamilyMed
Joglekar, Shashikant A.
Jose, Peter F.
Joseph, Marcia
Joshi, Vishal
Juma, Azim F., FamilyMed
Jyu, Christopher A., FamilyMed(EM)
Kalnins, Richard E B.
Kalra, Bharat B.
Kambli, Kamini C., FamilyMed
Kan, John Y C.
Kapur, Nishitha, FamilyMed
Karagiozov, Ilko S., FamilyMed
Kashyap, Rajendra P.
Kassam, Tasneem M., FamilyMed
Katz, Liliana
Kaziuka, Eric N.
Kelton, Timothy J., FamilyMed(EM)
Kerlow, Thomas N., FamilyMed
Keshavjee, Al-Noor M., FamilyMed
Khan, Mahmuda B., FamilyMed
Khan, Nadim A.
Khan, Nusrat U., FamilyMed
Khan, Razia
Khanna, Anuradha, FamilyMed
Khithani, Anil K., FamilyMed
Kirsh, David M., FamilyMed
Kirsh, Gerald L.
Kita, Paul M., FamilyMed
Kleiman, James E B.
Ko, Seung S., FamilyMed
Koifman, Nimrod K., FamilyMed(EM)
Korn, Sheryl F.
Kovacs, Eva
Kramer, Steven
Krishantha, Mahadeva
Kukreti, Asha
Kun, Carmen
Kung, F L. Frank
Kurtz, J. Aube
Kurunathan, Devayani, FamilyMed
Kwan, Lawrence W., FamilyMed
Kwan, Robert P K F.
Kwok, Jason W., FamilyMed
Kwok, Raphael M B., FamilyMed
Kwong, Charles K F.
Kwong, Sher P B.
Lalani, Naznin, FamilyMed
Lall, Rosemarie N., FamilyMed
Lam, David D W., FamilyMed
Lambotharan, Aruna, FamilyMed
Lambotharan, Ramanathan, FamilyMed
Lang, Brian A., FamilyMed
Lathia, Anita, FamilyMed
Latowsky, Mark L.
Lau, Benson P S.
Lau, David Y M.
Lau, Gary K L.
Lau, Micheline C.
Lavorato, Amy
Law, David T S., FamilyMed
Leanoff, Dimitri
Ledger, J. Douglas, FamilyMed
Lee, Chiu-Ying
Lee, Randall T., FamilyMed
Lee, Victor C C.
Lee Cheong, Noel L.
Lee-Ng, M. Madeleine
Lentini, Vittorio
Lerner, Lawrence, FamilyMed
Leung, Ceta M Y.
Leung, James K H.
Leung, Kam Kong
Leung, Kevin M K.
Lewis, Ruby S., FamilyMed
Li, Bernard Y T., FamilyMed
Li, Heung-Wing
Li, Jason, FamilyMed
Li, Olga, FamilyMed
Liang, Lorna L K.
Liew, Trina X., FamilyMed
Lim, Diane
Lim, Hilda H., FamilyMed
Lin, Karen W.
Lin, Peter J., FamilyMed
Linzon, Ernest K., FamilyMed
Lipson, David
Liu, Chin Kee
Liu, Yi, FamilyMed
Lo, Anne O Y., FamilyMed
Lo, Christina K Y., FamilyMed
Lo, Edmond K W.
Lo, Tak-Shing
Lombardi, Luciano P.
Louli, Sami
Low, Aaron A L.
Luk, Alan L., FamilyMed
Lyons, Jerome A.
Mahesan, Glory S., FamilyMed
Mahesan, Sivagnanam, FamilyMed
Maingot-Douketis, Maria J., FamilyMed
Majeed, Abeer A., FamilyMed
Makki, Mehdi
Malek, Rowja, FamilyMed
Malik, Khalid S., FamilyMed
Malkin, Lilia, FamilyMed(EM)
Manasseh, Petrona M.
Manoharan, Sathiyapooma, FamilyMed
Manokara, Kamini
Mansoor, Fenar A., FamilyMed
Mansukhani, Tarun
Marcus, Sandra A.
Mark, Dennis C P.
Mark, Douglas J.
Marrat, Saida, FamilyMed
Mason, Robin L D.
Mastrogiacomo, Caterina, FamilyMed
Mather, William A D., FamilyMed
Matlis, Steven, FamilyMed
McDonald, Jennifer K., FamilyMed
McGarragle, James G.
McKenzie, W G. Mark
McLellan, Kenneth G., FamilyMed
McNiece, Lynne C.
Medina, Xavier V.
Mehta, Avnish C., FamilyMed
Mendelssohn, Krisanne E., FamilyMed
Meneses, Gloria S., FamilyMed
Milgram, Mark Z.
Mitchell, David A., FamilyMed(EM)
Moffatt, Alexander J.
Mohamed, Roubiya S., FamilyMed
Mohammed, Sheeja B.
Moran, Kevin C.
Morana, Corrado G., FamilyMed
Morar, Parbhoo
Morris, Walter G.
Moss, Farley D., FamilyMed
Moss, Miriam A., FamilyMed
Moussa, Raffy, FamilyMed
Muallim, Carol, FamilyMed
Muraleetharan, Nageswary, FamilyMed
Muthalaly, Koshy
Nacua, Judith B.
Nandy, Sunita
Narayanan, Chitra
Nebhwani, Neetu V.
Neumann, Jeffrey L.
Newman, Caroline G.
Ng, Nelly W.
Ng, Sai-Sun
Nguyen, An-Huy
Niel, Ullanda, FamilyMed
Nijmeh, Paul, FamilyMed
Nofech-Mozes, Yehuda
Nord, Peter W., FamilyMed
Novakovic, Petar, FamilyMed(EM)
O'Brien, Paul F.
Oliver, Susan L.
Organek, Andrew J., FamilyMed(EM)
Orner, Abraham I., FamilyMed
Oryema, John U.
Otoo, Andrew A.
Oza, Sangeeta A., FamilyMed
Palcu, Sorin, FamilyMed
Pang, Natalie, FamilyMed
Pang, Peter S.
Pape, Gavin M.
Paramanathan, Thalayasingam, FamilyMed
Parker, Frederick A.
Patel, Ramesh
Patel, Tara J.
Peerbaye, G. Hussein
Peters, Alexander P.
Pham, Dzu Quang, FamilyMed
Pinto, Robin, FamilyMed
Pitt, Paul L., FamilyMed
Plant, Howard M.
Poggemiller, Gertrude A.
Polidoulis, Irene, FamilyMed
Ponnampalam, Thurairajasing, FamilyMed
Prabhakaran, Sivashankary Y., FamilyMed
Press, Cyril I.
Pringle, Allan C.
Prowse, Gordon G., FamilyMed
Pun, Yin Hun Ian.
Purewal, Bhupinder S.
Qureshi, Azra
Rahman, Sana, FamilyMed
Rajakumar, Gwendoline S., FamilyMed
Rajasingham, Rajanathan, FamilyMed
Rajesan, Ratheishan, FamilyMed
Rajeswaran, Srirani, FamilyMed
Ramkissoon, Sachin, FamilyMed(EM)
Ramzy, Medhat N., FamilyMed
Rana, Ranjit S.
Ringnalda, Jacqueline, FamilyMed
Rizkalla, Hoda G., FamilyMed
Rockman, Gerald L.
Rofaiel, Basma P., FamilyMed
Rotbard, Morris, FamilyMed
Rotman, Laurie S.
Rubenis, Andris A.
Rundle, Margaret A., FamilyMed
Ruparelia, Raj, FamilyMed
Saandar, Namjilmaa
Sajo, Ildiko M.
Samagh, Manjot K., FamilyMed(EM)
Sang, Ian T M.
Sarabia, Vivian E., FamilyMed
Sayani, Eshratbanu, FamilyMed
Selvananthan, Manivannan, FamilyMed
Shah, Meera, FamilyMed(EM)
Shaul, Richard A.
Shier, Donald J.
Shogilev, Howard P.
Simmons, Malcolm C.
Singh, Dilmohan C.
Singh, Tejinder P., FamilyMed
Sinnadurai, Sriharan, FamilyMed
Sit, Michelle, FamilyMed
Sithamparanathan, Karthika, FamilyMed
Sivakumar, Panchasheila, FamilyMed
Skuy, Beth J., FamilyMed
Slizheuski, Siarhei
Smith, Jennifer L.
Soberman, Dov D., FamilyMed(EM)
Somer, Jerry A.
Sriharan, Thushiyanthy, FamilyMed
Stait-Gardner, Lia Z., FamilyMed
Stavro Sholdoff, Thomas C.
Steinman, Raymond W.
Stel, Karen G., FamilyMed
Stephan, G. Paul
Stern, Eben L.
Studniberg, Allan P.
Sue-A-Quan, Penelope A.
Susman, Edison
Syed, Yasmeen
Tam, Christopher K H.
Tang, Gordon L S., FamilyMed
Taylor, Susan M.
Teelucksingh, George D.
Teplinsky, Avery L., FamilyMed
Thamotharam, Niththialuxmy, FamilyMed
Tharmaratnam, Yasho, FamilyMed
Thompson, Caroline J., FamilyMed(EM)
Thouin, Susan K., FamilyMed(EM)
Tillotson, Edward C.
Tors, Adrienne
Tran, Vu-Kiet, FamilyMed(EM)
Tsang, Ann S Y., FamilyMed
Tse, Anna, FamilyMed
Tse, Wing Kin.
Tsin, Karen W., FamilyMed
Tulk, Stephen E., FamilyMed
Tung, Kenneth S H.
Tuori, Christopher T.
Umoquit, Andres B.
Ung, Berton Y K., FamilyMed
Vaithianathan, Kandiah, FamilyMed
Van, Thomas T C., FamilyMed
Van Zyl, William P.
Vania, Shera
Vellathottam, Andrew G., FamilyMed
Verma, Vinod K.
Verschuren, Rex E., FamilyMed
Vlahos, Donna S., FamilyMed
Vohra, Geeta B., FamilyMed
Vorps, Harry M.
Vupputuri, Sujana K.
Weinberg, Erica L.
Weinberger, Thomas
Weiss, Janice M., FamilyMed
Weiss, Mark
Wheler, David S., FamilyMed
Wilton, Michael B., FamilyMed
Wolgelernter, Sia B.
Wolinsky, Joel L.
Wong, Andrew C Y., FamilyMed
Wong, Arnold K Y.
Wong, Cynthia S.
Wong, Godfrey L.
Wong, Henry W F.
Wong, Kathleen W F.
Wong, On Yu
Wong, Samuel C Y., FamilyMed
Wong, Stephen S.
Wong, Susanna S S.
Wong, W W. Loretta
Wong, Wilfred K K.
Wu, Henry M W.
Wu, Jenny
Yang, W Y. Philip
Yanni, Ahlam H R.
Yatsynov, Viktor
Yatsynovich, Viktor
Yee, Ivan C Y.
Yeh, Louis S.
Yeung, Dan W H.
Yin, Alan Z L., FamilyMed
Yip, Berwin P Y.
Yip, Florence S., FamilyMed
Yue, Jason K., FamilyMed(EM)
Yuen, K H. Peter, FamilyMed
Yuh, Joseph Y J., FamilyMed
Yusuf, Aroon Y.
Zayid, Dina P.
Zheng, Stanley M., FamilyMed
Zoberman, Lawrence, FamilyMed
Zucker, Rosalind M.
Zung, Nora P Y., FamilyMed

SCHOMBERG

Ateyah, Wameed, FamilyMed
Glinski-Oomen, Margaret B.

SCHREIBER

Hurst, David E.
Quinn, Danielle M., FamilyMed
Thompson, Ian B., FamilyMed

SEAFORTH

Datema, Jason, FamilyMed
Eickmeier, Daniel J., FamilyMed
Eshaghian, Farhang
Kluz, Agnieszka M., FamilyMed
Kluz, Andrzej T., FamilyMed
Percival, Heather A., FamilyMed
Rooyakkers, Daniel J.
Shepherd, Carolin H.

SEELEYS BAY

Briggs, Deborah E., FamilyMed
O'Connor, Emily M., FamilyMed
Stewart, Marilyn J., FamilyMed

SHARBOT LAKE

Bell, Peter W., FamilyMed

SHEDDEN

Robinson, Constance L.

SHELBURNE

MacMillan, James R.
Ul Haq, Huma Z., FamilyMed
van Hoogenhuize, William H.

SIMCOE

Beaver, John
Bobby, Bradley T.
Demian, Hany, FamilyMed
Edwards, Bonnie L.
Gabel, Nancy A.
Ghesquiere, Mark H., FamilyMed
Gholam, Bassam I A., FamilyMed(EM)
Johnston, James G.
Kursell, Paul H., FamilyMed
Luyt, Nathan J R., FamilyMed
Martin-Godelie, Robin S., FamilyMed
McConnell, Natalie R.
Medve, Paul W.
Mohomed, Dave A.
Muhsin, Munir K., FamilyMed
Nagrani, Pritam-Lala
Randazzo, Mary E.
Rich, Peter
Sinkowski, Kerry L.
Theng, Pei Shih
Tschirhart, Jeffrey D.
Weber, Gary G.
Williamson, Donald B.
Wynveen, William B.

SIOUX LOOKOUT

Antone, N. Irwin, FamilyMed
Balderson, Jeffrey O., FamilyMed
Barnes, Ekow N B., FamilyMed
Barthel, Jennifer E., FamilyMed
Billie, Christine, FamilyMed
Chase, Claudette, FamilyMed
Cook, Marlyn A., FamilyMed
Coupland, R. Steven, FamilyMed
Dooley, Joseph, FamilyMed
Fry, Joanne, FamilyMed
Gerber Finn, Lianne, FamilyMed
Giles, Christopher A., FamilyMed
Guilfoyle, F. John, FamilyMed
Hancock, Lindsay E., FamilyMed
Hervieux, Matyas, FamilyMed
Jakubow, Andre N., FamilyMed
Kelly, Leonard, FamilyMed
Kinsner, Kathleen J., FamilyMed
Kirlew, Michael L., FamilyMed
Koval, Marilyn R., FamilyMed
Lennox, Harriet A., FamilyMed
Letkemann, K. Lisa, FamilyMed
Lown, Peter W., FamilyMed
Madden, Sharen N., FamilyMed
Martin, Gregory J., FamilyMed
Minty, Robert, FamilyMed
Mokone, M. Christina, FamilyMed
Morgan, Jonathon, FamilyMed(EM)
Nguyen, Chieu H T., FamilyMed
O'Driscoll, Teresa, FamilyMed
Pouteau, Kathleen M., FamilyMed
Robinson, Anne M., FamilyMed
Russell-Mahoney, Barbara L., FamilyMed
Tilbrook, Devon S J., FamilyMed
Willms, Larry A., FamilyMed

SMITHS FALLS

Burden, Julia K., FamilyMed
Conway, James R.
Du Vernet, Chantal J., FamilyMed(EM)
Hamilton, Jeanette M., FamilyMed
Hendry, Graeme A., FamilyMed
Horsey, Michael W., FamilyMed
Mercer, Christopher M., FamilyMed
Miller, Paul C.
Muldowney, Siobhan M., FamilyMed
Patasi, Beata, FamilyMed
Penney, Brian J., FamilyMed
Shew, Raphael E., FamilyMed
Spencer, Lesley M., FamilyMed
Stevens, Liisa H., FamilyMed
Toth, Agnes, FamilyMed
Yunker, Peter J., FamilyMed(EM)

SMITHVILLE

Bellaire, Joan, FamilyMed
Bender, Kimberley M., FamilyMed
Cano, Paul B., FamilyMed
Davidson, Martha B., FamilyMed
Marrone, Amanda D., FamilyMed
Noble-Wohlgemut, Matthew, FamilyMed
Smith, Shannon E., FamilyMed
Suhadolc, Thomas G., FamilyMed

SMOOTH ROCK FALLS

Lebel, Daniel
Turineck, David T.

SOUTH MOUNTAIN

Adamson, Charles R., FamilyMed
Naciuk, Mary E., FamilyMed

SOUTH PORCUPINE

Houston, David M., FamilyMed(EM)
Vaithilingam, Sudhama S.

SOUTH RIVER

Pessotto, Daniele A., FamilyMed
Seidler, Christine, FamilyMed

SOUTHAMPTON

Billings, David, FamilyMed(EM)
Burkhart, Chadwick T., FamilyMed
Cipolletti, Adriana A., FamilyMed
Dickie, Nadine R., FamilyMed
Dyke, A. Keith, FamilyMed
Glass, David H., FamilyMed
Gowan, Amy J., FamilyMed
Higgins, Louise J., FamilyMed
Leblanc, Robert E M.
Leung, Jessica E., FamilyMed
MacKinnon, Stephen M., FamilyMed
Suke, Ralph, FamilyMed
Zwardon, Michael, FamilyMed

SPANISH

Larochelle, Roger E J.

SPENCERVILLE

Bauermeister, Senta

ST CATHARINES

Ahluwalia, Amar K.
Alazragh, Waled A., FamilyMed
Ali, Karim F.
Alnhisi, Khaled M A., FamilyMed
Arvinte, Galina, FamilyMed
Atkins, Kenneth W.
Atkinson, Elaine L., FamilyMed
Attallah, Gabriel N., FamilyMed
Balasuriya, Rajiv
Bayley, Valerie A., FamilyMed
Beecroft, James M., FamilyMed(EM)
Belgasem, Muftah A., FamilyMed
Bennett, Barbara F., FamilyMed
Bertolo, Monica, FamilyMed
Bertothy, Christine M.
Boily, Raynald C.
Bolli, Peter
Bonifacio, Antonino
Brook, J. Roger, FamilyMed
Brooks, James S.
Buchner, Eduard, FamilyMed
Buetow, Candice L.
Burk-Vassallo, Jane L., FamilyMed
Chan, Aaron Y., FamilyMed
Chauhan, Jitendra
Child, Jeremy R., FamilyMed
Chow, Jonathan S.
Collins, Rhonda L., FamilyMed
Colorado, J. Robert, FamilyMed
Crowe, Adrian C., FamilyMed(EM)
Cucciniello, Sandro, FamilyMed
Cutler, Paul
Derksen, Brent, FamilyMed
Dobson, Tracey
Dooler, Deborah, FamilyMed
Ellingham, Diana, FamilyMed
Elltoft, John D.
Facey-Crowther, Lee-Anne G.
Fallis, Robert R., FamilyMed
Fitzpatrick, George F.
Fung, Carl A.
Fung, Nancy M., FamilyMed
Grande, Maria S., FamilyMed
Grant, Darrell W., FamilyMed(EM)
Greavette, Thomas, FamilyMed
Gregg, John S.
Greenway, Matthew, FamilyMed
Gunawardena, Dishani
Harb, Raymond T., FamilyMed
Henry, David A.
Henry, James A C.
Hildebrand, B. Mark, FamilyMed
Hoosen, Naushad, FamilyMed
Hurmatov, Tetyana Y.
Hutchinson, Janine M., FamilyMed
Hyatt, Peter J., FamilyMed
Jakibchuk, Jerry
Jansen Van Rensburg, Nicolaas M., FamilyMed
Jei Almdhem, Mohamed Y., FamilyMed
Jonas, Krista M.
Kanungo, Tarit K., FamilyMed(EM)
Keeley, Paul J., FamilyMed
Kelada-Sedra, Ibtisam P.
Kerley, Brian K., FamilyMed
Khaleifa, Ali O., FamilyMed
Kimacovich, Richard G., FamilyMed(EM)
Kirmani, Waheed-Ud-Din, FamilyMed
Kopp, Michael, FamilyMed
Kowalchuk, Glenn
Leibfried, Bryan L., FamilyMed
Lennox, Joanne S.
Leung, Bill P Y.
Listoe, Gregory B., FamilyMed
Lorenzen, David
Luce, John T.
Lucey, William F.
Lynch, Ciara M R.
Lynett, Christopher P., FamilyMed
MacKay, R. Fraser
Malaguti, Santina M.
Malak, Ziad, FamilyMed
Mazzone, Thomas
McAuley, John T., FamilyMed(EM)
McMillan, Robert E.
Meshrki, Hanan S D., FamilyMed
Milkovic, Joseph S., FamilyMed
Murray, Timothy I.
Neary, Elizabeth L., FamilyMed
Nour, Emad I., FamilyMed(EM)
O'Reilly, Elaine, FamilyMed
O'Reilly, Philip J., FamilyMed
Oelofse, Wouter, FamilyMed
Oinonen, Ervin T.
Oladipo, Paul O., FamilyMed
Pallie, Dudu A.
Paolone, John A.
Patel, Dharmendra
Petrocci, Michael C., FamilyMed(EM)
Pinto, Martin
Plaskos, Christina
Prince, Timothy D P.
Proulx, Christian A., FamilyMed
Provost, Viviane, FamilyMed
Quart, Reginald D J., FamilyMed
Qureshi, Shahab
Ramanauskas, John V., FamilyMed
Rammohan, Gnanaprabha M., FamilyMed
Ravindran, Mathura P., FamilyMed
Re Martinez, Felix C.
Redman, John A.
Riddle, Christopher, FamilyMed(EM)
Roberts, Mark A.
Rose, Roger C S.
Rosenberg, Bruce N.
Rosloski, Joseph M.
Rungi, Arne A., FamilyMed
Rusnak, Jane A M., FamilyMed
Saeed, Haider A., FamilyMed
Schultz, John A.
Senechal, Melanie L., FamilyMed(EM)
Setrak, Rafi F., FamilyMed(EM)
Shaglouf, Hamdi I., FamilyMed
Shaikh, Maria-Estrella V., FamilyMed
Siddiqui, Sameerah
Singh, Jagdeep, FamilyMed(EM)
St Amand, Timothy A., FamilyMed(EM)
Stark, David G.
Stobbe, Karl E., FamilyMed(EM)
Suk, Allison L., FamilyMed
Sultan, Mahmud M T., FamilyMed
Swayze, Kathleen A., FamilyMed
Takla, Nagwa A., FamilyMed
Taliano, John P.
Taylor, Kenneth N.
Teague, Paul E R., FamilyMed
Teodorini, Irving K.
Thomas, Mary C., FamilyMed
Van Essen, Suzanne N., FamilyMed(EM)
Vujosevic, Darija, FamilyMed
Waler, Oleh R.
Walser-Jebb, Dianne M., FamilyMed
Wan, David A., FamilyMed
Wan, Vera A., FamilyMed
Whitty, C. Dennis
Wiens, Doris H., FamilyMed
Wolski, Darryl M., FamilyMed
Wong, Chi Mun, FamilyMed
Yu, Tsai Hsing
Zammit-Maempel, Joseph G.
Zuliani, Preston A., FamilyMed

ST CHARLES

Kolari, Charis K., FamilyMed

ST EUGENE

Bender, J D. Jacques

ST GEORGE BRANT

Hedges, James D.
Hutton, Timothy, FamilyMed

ST ISIDORE

Clement, J C. Luc, FamilyMed
Denis-LeBlanc, Manon A., FamilyMed
Pomerleau, Marjorie, FamilyMed

ST JACOBS

Gupta, Hansa M., FamilyMed
Lodhi, Gulshan
Majewski, Zuzanna M.
Simpson, J. Thomas, FamilyMed
Stewart, Donald J.

ST MARYS

Davis, Robert W., FamilyMed
Gatfield, Charles T.
Gilmour, Kimberly E., FamilyMed(EM)
Hiscock, Susan L., FamilyMed
Jewson, Frederick A.
Johnston, Peter S.
Komorowski, Laurie A., FamilyMed
Lee, Barbara A.
Partridge, Lindsay A F., FamilyMed
Pook, John J.
Schiedel, Jonathan J., FamilyMed(EM)
Thornton, Tanya H., FamilyMed
Tomlinson, R. Bruce
Wilson, Tania, FamilyMed

ST THOMAS

Ballard, Andrew M., FamilyMed
Balsdon, Jeffrey L.
Balsdon, Lewis A.
Barrett, Scott R.
Beach, Craig
Bishop, Andrew G., FamilyMed(EM)
Blaskovic, Jana M.
Bryans, John
Charlton, Kenneth J., FamilyMed
Dayus, Lisa E., FamilyMed
Dougherty, David J.
Emrich, A. George
Evans, Terry, FamilyMed(EM)
Faulds, Thomas R., FamilyMed(EM)
Floyd, Robert J.
Fox, William P., FamilyMed
Gallinaro, Brian J., FamilyMed
Garg, Divya, FamilyMed
Goodhew, Rick T., FamilyMed
Gregory, David A.
Guaiana, Giuseppe
Haney, Elizabeth, FamilyMed(EM)
Harder, Carroll D., FamilyMed(EM)
Head, James A.
Hertwig, Brian K., FamilyMed
Hollingsworth, Christopher W., FamilyMed(EM)
Hug, Martin B., FamilyMed(EM)
Janzen, Thomas
Johnson, Melissa A., FamilyMed
Jones, Kelly O.
Jones, Robert A.
Khodaei, Minoo, FamilyMed
Kraemer, Geoffrey T., FamilyMed
Krause, Richard A.
Lum, David W K., FamilyMed
Mai, Joseph A.
McCabe, Amelia, FamilyMed
McIntosh, Scott L A., FamilyMed
Menlove, James F., FamilyMed(EM)
Mills, Geoffrey C R., FamilyMed(EM)
Morrison, Kenneth P.
Olorunsola, Kehinde, FamilyMed
Paradis, Christian, FamilyMed
Romsa, Nancy K., FamilyMed(EM)
Scott, Kellie D., FamilyMed
Shah, Amit P., FamilyMed(EM)
Steciuk, William P.
Telford, Edward, FamilyMed
Thomas, Robert S.
Toft, Ian P., FamilyMed
Van Daalen, Erica, FamilyMed(EM)
Vandeyar, Thivian, FamilyMed(EM)
Vaughan, Derek J., FamilyMed(EM)
Warsh, Franklin H., FamilyMed
Wong, Winston P.

STAYNER

Gandhi, M. Suhail
Hutchings, Leslie A., FamilyMed
Lane, James G A., FamilyMed
Marshall, Bryan D., FamilyMed
Recoskie, Bryan, FamilyMed

STIRLING

Mahadeva, Ranjith, FamilyMed
Noronha, Lionel J., FamilyMed
Ranjith, Koshela, FamilyMed

STITTSVILLE

Balon, Jeffrey W., FamilyMed
Evans, Stephen D.
Lazare, Nancy M.
Prokopiak, Allison B., FamilyMed
Romero-Sierra, Cesar P.
Sethi, Baldev R.
Snelling, Carolyn M H., FamilyMed
Watson, Iain S.
Whalen, Brien A.
Yazdani, Shahin, FamilyMed
Zareef, Shaista K., FamilyMed

STONEY CREEK

Allega, Rossano L., FamilyMed
Ambis, Christopher J., FamilyMed
Ambis, Robert J S.
Andrus, Paul G L.
Bombin, Victoria E., FamilyMed
Boutros, Jacqueline L., FamilyMed
Bracalenti, Ivan A., FamilyMed
Damji, Mehboob
De Benedetti, Monica C., FamilyMed
De Tina, Donald S.
Dhalla, Mohsin N., FamilyMed
Fernandez, Alcantro B.
Fraser, Frederick, FamilyMed
Jones, Jennifer K., FamilyMed
Khambalia, Bashir, FamilyMed
Kwok, Trevor P H., FamilyMed
Leong, Baldwin J., FamilyMed
McAndie, Catherine M., FamilyMed
Profetto, Ralph, FamilyMed
Prost, William J.
Razzaque, Asad, FamilyMed
Schweitzer, Michael J., FamilyMed(EM)
Staibano, Filippo M., FamilyMed
Wooder, Scott D.
Zizzo, Richard A., FamilyMed

STOUFFVILLE

Alkhalaf, Sarah G A., FamilyMed
Brodie, Douglas W., FamilyMed
Grant, Paul H H.
Izso, Peter
Ladak, Yasmin, FamilyMed
Mawani, Al-Karim, FamilyMed
Mirtorabi, Nima, FamilyMed
Nunan-Barclay, Sarah J., FamilyMed
Patterson, Andrew R.
Rasul, Zahara, FamilyMed
Sampson, Gweneth L., FamilyMed
Smith, Donald H.
Wat, Patrick C W.
Wu, Douglas D K Q.

STRATFORD

Bandey, Karl
Ben Mansour, El Hassan
Blaine, Sean, FamilyMed(EM)
Brooks, Peter J., FamilyMed
Carrier, Heather N., FamilyMed(EM)
Carstensen, H. Michael
Chahal, Ramandeep S.
Cruz, Norman M.
Edwards, Shawn, FamilyMed
Gobburu, Ram M.
Heisz, Erin M., FamilyMed
Jimenez, Tomas Y., FamilyMed(EM)
Kara, Alnoor F.
Kaura, Amit
Klassen, Miriam
Langford, Grace M., FamilyMed
MacIsaac, Michael G., FamilyMed(EM)
Marchie, Augustine
Martin, Anne J., FamilyMed
Mayer, Anna M., FamilyMed(EM)
McArthur, James N.
Mehrain, Shirin, FamilyMed(EM)
Moore, Laurel E., FamilyMed
Nguyen, Hanh T H.
Parratt, David W.
Parsons, G. Wayne
Pellizzari, Michael P., FamilyMed
Peters, Leanne M., FamilyMed
Snider, Stacey L., FamilyMed
Spiers, S. John
Stewart, Philippe J.
Sylvester, Heather A., FamilyMed
Thomas, Eric K.
Thompson, Douglas J., FamilyMed
Tomlinson, Donna A.
Van Boekel, Patricia E., FamilyMed(EM)
Warnock, Thomas F.
Weir, Paul T.
Wilkinson, Mark A.
Williams, David
Zawahir, Mohamed M.

STRATHROY

Buma, Nicolaas H.
Chaudhary, Omer A., FamilyMed
Crowley, David
Grushka, Daniel H., FamilyMed(EM)
Gunasingam, Padumanithi, FamilyMed
Lam, David L.
Leger, Daniel, FamilyMed
Leung, Daniel P.
MacDonald, Timothy L., FamilyMed
Marcou, John R., FamilyMed(EM)
Marr, Alison J.
Marshall, Ann T., FamilyMed
Marshall, J. Neil, FamilyMed
Mithoowani, Mohamed H A.
Morgan, Moheb, FamilyMed
Perkin, Gary
Puente, Sara C., FamilyMed
Sharma, Monika, FamilyMed
Vanderzwan, Jonas B., FamilyMed
Vandewalle, Philip L., FamilyMed
Wolder, Thomas

STURGEON FALLS

Anawati, Jean I.
Beaucage, Jennifer K., FamilyMed
Behamdouni, Andre
Breton-Fortin, Julie, FamilyMed
Deschene, Jane M.
Ferguson, Gordon
Henstridge, David G., FamilyMed(EM)
Katsuno, Richard M.
Morrison, Andree Y., FamilyMed
Nguyen, Quy Duong, FamilyMed

SUDBURY

Abramson, Sydney L., FamilyMed
Ajueze, Peter C.
Allan, Melissa, FamilyMed(EM)
Anawati, Alexandre G., FamilyMed(EM)
Andersen, Joel E A., FamilyMed
Aniol, Michael J., FamilyMed
Aulakh, Lakyntiew P S.
Bakker, Gerald J J.
Baldisera, Tara, FamilyMed
Bech-Hansen, Kay
Belanger, Monique, FamilyMed
Bonin, Pierre, FamilyMed
Bourdon, Christopher, FamilyMed(EM)
Buttoo, Ajit S.
Caruso, Andrew, FamilyMed(EM)
Ceaser, Jack, FamilyMed
Centis, Tajana M.
Cervin, Catherine K., FamilyMed
Charette, Yannick A., FamilyMed
Chau, James T O., FamilyMed
Chen, Christine M., FamilyMed
Chow, Ting-Bong
Christie, Tyler, FamilyMed(EM)
Clendenning, Christine R.
Connolly, Julie A M., FamilyMed
Costa Vitali, Atilio E.
Cote, Simon, FamilyMed
Crichton, Thomas P., FamilyMed
Cudmore, Stephen, FamilyMed
Cusack, Meghan M., FamilyMed
De Blacam, Killian J., FamilyMed
Dhatt, Deepinderjit R., FamilyMed
Dressler, Brian B.
Dube, Mark R., FamilyMed(EM)
Fairman, Paul M.
Falconi, David R.
Finlay, Susan
Franklyn, Michael T.
Garrioch, Gregory
Gauthier, Michel D J., FamilyMed
Gibb, Paul S., FamilyMed
Goodale, Natalie N., FamilyMed
Graves, Lisa, FamilyMed
Hayes, Tracy, FamilyMed(EM)
Henderson, Ann E., FamilyMed
Henry, Tracy, FamilyMed
Hepting, Kristin L., FamilyMed
Hey, Amanda J., FamilyMed
Holub, Jacob A.
Jacobi, Nicole
Jakelski, Klaus D.
Jones, J H. Lloyd
Khomani, Abderrahim
Knight, Andrew C.
Koka, H. Pavan K., FamilyMed(EM)
Koka, Suman K., FamilyMed
Krawczuk, Daniel M., FamilyMed
Kresan, Patricia J.
Krishna, Popuri M.
Kuchtaruk, Andrew, FamilyMed
Kupsh, Christine, FamilyMed(EM)
Kusnierczyk, John, FamilyMed(EM)
Lamarre, Michelle A., FamilyMed
Laniel, Christian, FamilyMed
Leary, Tara J., FamilyMed
Lepage, Robert S., FamilyMed(EM)
Logan, Louise C., FamilyMed(EM)
Long, Bradley F.
MacCallum, Eoin D.
Mahoney, Sean R., FamilyMed(EM)
Mailloux, Caroline, FamilyMed
Maki, John D.
Mantle, Valerie I., FamilyMed
Marchadier, Virginie, FamilyMed(EM)
Marks De Chabris, Lionel, FamilyMed(EM)
Marsh, David C C.
Masih, Robert J.
McDonald, Anne J., FamilyMed
McKay, James S., FamilyMed
McMillan, Duncan
McMullen, William J M M., FamilyMed(EM)
Messenger, Megan E., FamilyMed
Michon, Andre L., FamilyMed
Middaugh, Jeffrey A., FamilyMed(EM)
Mirka, Theresa M., FamilyMed
Mitchell, Lesley A., FamilyMed
Mongeon, Guy J P., FamilyMed
Morrow, Walter G.
Mulloy, John V.
Najgebauer, Edward J.
Nizzero, Christopher J L., FamilyMed
Notman, Emily B H., FamilyMed
O'Connor, Deborah
O'Donohoe, Peter F.
Olivier, Kary G., FamilyMed
Oommen, Samuel P., FamilyMed(EM)
Pabani, Shehnaz, FamilyMed
Pastre, Robert J., FamilyMed
Pella, Tracy L., FamilyMed
Piccinin, Laura R., FamilyMed(EM)
Pineau, Robert W., FamilyMed(EM)
Prince, Douglas
Prpic, Jason C., FamilyMed(EM)
Pun, Christine W H., FamilyMed
Reich, Dennis A G., FamilyMed
Rheault, Paul L C., FamilyMed
Roch, J J C. Andre
Roy, Nathalie A L., FamilyMed
Sami, Pensee A.
Sawkiw, Raymond B., FamilyMed
Sbrocchi, Stephanie C., FamilyMed
Seguin, Robert W.
Shapiro, Stanley A.
Shine, Robert M.
Singh, Ravi P., FamilyMed
Sivers, David R.
Slaney, Nathalie M C.
Smith, Deborah L., FamilyMed
Spencer, G. Todd, FamilyMed
Squarzolo, Melanie A M., FamilyMed(EM)
St-Martin, Maurice
Stirrett, Glenna M., FamilyMed
Stone, Samuel B., FamilyMed(EM)
Strasser, Roger P.
Syan, Swaran K., FamilyMed
Symington, Ian R., FamilyMed
Tenhunen, Linda M.
Terada, Sharon L., FamilyMed
Thakrar, Sheena, FamilyMed
Thorsteinson, Larry S., FamilyMed(EM)
Tissot, Brian D., FamilyMed(EM)
Toner, Lee V., FamilyMed(EM)
Tujik, Karla L., FamilyMed(EM)
Urban, Thomas M., FamilyMed
Vanderbeck, R. Lindsay, FamilyMed
Widjanarko, Djoen
Wiss, Raymond J R., FamilyMed(EM)
Woychuk, Walter
Yarascavitch, Alec J., FamilyMed
Yesovitch, Rose P., FamilyMed
Zaidi, Mudassir A., FamilyMed
Zmijowskyj, Timothy J., FamilyMed
Zucconi, Anthony L P., FamilyMed

SUNDERLAND

Schurter, Matthew J., FamilyMed

SUNDRIDGE

MacKinnon, Sarah J., FamilyMed
Williams, Kenneth J.

SUTTON WEST

Burrows, George M., FamilyMed
Hall, John S., FamilyMed
MacIntyre, Douglas W.
Stapleton, Andrew J.

SWASTIKA

Hacking, Frederick J.

SYDENHAM

Dietrich, Jeanette L., FamilyMed
Ingo, Steven K.
Raleigh, John P., FamilyMed(EM)

TAMWORTH

Cowan, Sandra L.
Hobbs, R. Neil, FamilyMed
McFadzean, I. Laing

TAVISTOCK

Bartlett, R. Paul, FamilyMed
Card, Bradley D., FamilyMed
Cowing, Barbara L., FamilyMed
Hook, Kenneth, FamilyMed
Stewart, Gregory E., FamilyMed

TECUMSEH

Azam, Almas L., FamilyMed
Bilibajkich, Juliana, FamilyMed
Bilibajkich, Mara M., FamilyMed
Hasnain, Haider, FamilyMed
Rivetna, Roxanna
Spirou, Christos, FamilyMed

TEESWATER

Gear, Marie

TEMAGAMI

Goddard, Stephen P T., FamilyMed

TERRACE BAY

McLeod, Lindsay E C., FamilyMed
Zawada, Annabella, FamilyMed

THAMESVILLE

Jones, D. Stephen R., FamilyMed

THEDFORD

Gibbs, Laurence H S.

THESSALON

Blois, Heather S., FamilyMed
Keating, Frances M., FamilyMed
Ogston, Nigel G.

THORNBURY

Klages, Naomi E., FamilyMed
Remillard, Timothy G., FamilyMed
Sauriol, Nathalie, FamilyMed
Yaghini, Reza, FamilyMed

THORNDALE

Chapeskie, Henry H., FamilyMed

THORNHILL

Arbitman, Stella L., FamilyMed
Ascher, Ilana S.
Barsoum, Randa M K., FamilyMed
Bartfeld, Naama, FamilyMed
Beallor, Carrie R., FamilyMed
Belyavskaya, Svetlana
Blachowitz, Roy, FamilyMed
Blitzer, Andrey, FamilyMed
Blitzer, Steve
Bloom, Tara R., FamilyMed
Blumenfeld, Renee, FamilyMed
Bornstein, Ronald J.
Boxer, Alvin A.
Braude, Paul R.
Braverman, Aliza S.
Bross, Pnina W., FamilyMed
Brown, Jeffrey M.
Cheah, David, FamilyMed
Cheung, Colleen K Y., FamilyMed
Chong, Nancy L.
Coish, Susan J.
Dalgleish, P. Douglas
Diamond, Aubie J.
Dixit, Radhika, FamilyMed
Eckler, Nettie M.
Eisenberg, Morty, FamilyMed
Emami, S. Sean, FamilyMed
Farkas, Noemi, FamilyMed
Feinberg, Faith P., FamilyMed
Fields, Louis
Fink, Alan D.
Forman, Leandra M., FamilyMed
Forman, Paul, FamilyMed
Galter, Meri K.
Georgievski, Aleksander
Girgis, Adel, FamilyMed
Goldberg Jacob, Nesya F F., FamilyMed
Goodbaum, Mark
Griesman, Helene C.
Gross, Zuzana
Habert, Jeffrey S., FamilyMed
Habib, Bahaa S., FamilyMed
Hwang, Irene I L., FamilyMed
Illamperuma Arachchige, Dilum C., FamilyMed

PHYSICIANS BY PROVINCE

Illamperuma Arachchige, Lasith R., FamilyMed
Isen, Susan J C., FamilyMed
Iskander, Mariam F G., FamilyMed
Katz, Shirley, FamilyMed
Khosid, Herbert I.
Kirzner, Michael P., FamilyMed
Konstantinou, Chris
Koopmans, Veronica D., FamilyMed
Kukreja, Tarvinder K., FamilyMed
Lai, Albert I.
Lai, Stephen I H., FamilyMed
Lakhani, Shahnavaz
Lam, Roger H C.
Lao, Victor K C.
Larsen, Darren A., FamilyMed
Lefkowitz, Jacob M., FamilyMed
Leitner, Fredric S., FamilyMed
Libman, Esther R., FamilyMed
Lipszyc, Eli
Litner, Michelle S., FamilyMed
Livshin, Oleg
Lukin, Svitlana
Magee, Gary L., FamilyMed
Maharaj, Ashwin R.
Mahrous, Nevine A., FamilyMed
Mandel, Lisa F., FamilyMed
Mann, Gary M.
Martin, Andrew J., FamilyMed
McAlister, Kenneth R.
Mekhael, Saly, FamilyMed
Mezhericher-Shenderey, Inna, FamilyMed
Milad, M. Naguib
Moll, Allan L., FamilyMed
Morse, Janet L., FamilyMed
Myers, Miriam
Nauth-Misir, Dayanti, FamilyMed
Nelson, Michael G., FamilyMed
Pangilinan, Ben L., FamilyMed
Park, Ingrid
Pellow, M. Robin, FamilyMed(EM)
Perry, Judith A.
Petcho, Yves G., FamilyMed
Poon, K C. Pat
Portnoi, Galina G., FamilyMed
Prabhu, Pooja D.
Rak, Janet, FamilyMed
Rapoport-Glick, Susan, FamilyMed
Rastogi, Shalini, FamilyMed
Raveendran, Arulanantham, FamilyMed
Rittenberg, Kevin M., FamilyMed
Robicsek, Leslie
Roitberg, Inna, FamilyMed
Rona, Zoltan P.
Rosen, Robin J., FamilyMed
Rouzati, Amir
Sadik, Aksam, FamilyMed
Sandhu, Harmanjit S., FamilyMed
Sang, Richard T M.
Sasson, Abraham
Scholes, Michelle L., FamilyMed
Schwartz, Mandy S., FamilyMed
Segal, Galit R., FamilyMed
Sen, Indira
Shariff, Fahrin B., FamilyMed
Shear, Robin J., FamilyMed
Sheps, Franklin W., FamilyMed(EM)
Shiffman, Howard N., FamilyMed
Shouldice, Earle B.
Slater, Keith S.
Somogyi, Daniel M., FamilyMed
Spier, Phyllis
Staroselsky, Arthur, FamilyMed
Tan, Tjien-King
Tchernov, Andrei G., FamilyMed
Tushinski, Morris, FamilyMed
Usman, Abida
Voudouris, Nicholas C.
Weinberg, Elissa J., FamilyMed
Weingarten, David
Whitney, Brenda J., FamilyMed
Wilderman, Igor S., FamilyMed
Williams, Wendy C., FamilyMed
Wong, Garway M V., FamilyMed
Yong, Chu Hua
Zarinehbaf Asadi, Sanaz, FamilyMed
Zatzman, Raymond L.

THOROLD

Feller, Andrea E.
Hanna, Hany S H., FamilyMed
Jaeger, Valerie A., FamilyMed
Kandasamy, Gerald R., FamilyMed
Miller, Howard J.
Overholt, Todd M.
Pringle, Peter S.
Ralph, Douglas G.
Sadek, Amel H F., FamilyMed
Sinton, Geoffrey, FamilyMed
Tatzel, Timothy R., FamilyMed

THUNDER BAY

Abdallah, Amel, FamilyMed
Adams, Michael W H.
Addison, Kirsten, FamilyMed
Affleck, Andrew W., FamilyMed(EM)
Albert, Michel, FamilyMed(EM)
Allison, Roy C.
Almond, Richard G., FamilyMed
Anthes, David L.
Arnold, Kenneth L.
Atkinson, Mary L., FamilyMed
Atwood, Jennifer A., FamilyMed
Balec, Raymond J., FamilyMed
Beaton, Jessica J., FamilyMed
Behse, Joseph H.
Bentz, Peter E., FamilyMed
Bhuiyan, Nihat Z.
Block, Stephanie K., FamilyMed
Bradley, Jeffrey
Bryan, Susan C.
Bukovy, Brent E.
Cannon, Crystal E., FamilyMed
Cappello, Marie L., FamilyMed
Capricci, Arlene P.
Carfagnini, Gregory P., FamilyMed(EM)
Chang, Michael E., FamilyMed(EM)
Chen, Hillary J., FamilyMed
Chow, Yen Gee., FamilyMed
Chung, Corinna R., FamilyMed
Clark, Sarah A R., FamilyMed
Colquhoun, James T.
Coulombe, Rene C., FamilyMed(EM)
Coulson, David B.
Croll, G. Blair
Davis, Geoffrey B.
De Bakker, Paul F.
Denson, Frank G.
Dhaliwal, Ravinder, FamilyMed
Dignan, Thomas A.
Doiron, Maryjo, FamilyMed
Dupuis, Paul, FamilyMed(EM)
Ek, Daniel M., FamilyMed
ElSherif, Hanan E L A.
Everall, Cheryl H., FamilyMed
Exley, Graham D., FamilyMed
Facca, Sarah J., FamilyMed
Feldstein, N. Aaron, FamilyMed
Franchi, Donald B.
Francis, Gregory J., FamilyMed(EM)
Fulford, Jennifer
Gillen, Lorna E R.
Goertzen, James, FamilyMed
Green, Steven A., FamilyMed(EM)
Habjan, Andrej J.
Hales, Kristine E., FamilyMed
Hartford, Brian
Hassan, Ayman
Hassan Abdelmotleb, Hassa A.
Hindle, Peter R.
Hoffman, Shayna E., FamilyMed(EM)
Humphrey, Wayne A., FamilyMed(EM)
Jacobson, Bradley A., FamilyMed(EM)
Johnsen, Bonnie L., FamilyMed
Johnsen, Jon H., FamilyMed
Johnson, David
Johnson, Ross W., FamilyMed
Juvshik, Alexander K., FamilyMed
Kald, Anne-Ly
Kennedy, M. Stewart, FamilyMed
Kibiuk, Laurie A M., FamilyMed
Kim, Arnold F.
Kisselgoff, Dmitry D.
Klassen, Ruby A., FamilyMed
Klassen, Steven B., FamilyMed
Kraft, Jouni P.
Krupa, Norman K.
Kurban, Henry M.
Labib, Yasser M A.
Lailey, Jennifer A., FamilyMed
Lawson, Jennifer J., FamilyMed(EM)
Leishman, Donald M.
Lower, Gary D.
MacGregor, William G., FamilyMed(EM)
Magee-Adams, Kelly M A., FamilyMed
Mahood, Trudy L., FamilyMed
Mangatal, Moira C., FamilyMed
Martel, Patrick, FamilyMed(EM)
Masood, Ali K.
McGillivray, Cameron J., FamilyMed(EM)
McGillivray, Margaret J., FamilyMed(EM)
McLean, Heather L., FamilyMed
Mehta, Darshana J., FamilyMed
Michano-Stewart, Tracy L., FamilyMed
Migay, Andrew S., FamilyMed
Migay, Marcia M., FamilyMed
Miller, Kevin F., FamilyMed
Moulson, Robert A L., FamilyMed
Mulligan, Patrick K., FamilyMed
Mutrie, David E., FamilyMed(EM)
Mymko, Morris, FamilyMed
Naqi, Hadia, FamilyMed
Narine, Tamara K., FamilyMed
Neilipovitz, William A.
Nelson, Delene J., FamilyMed
Noetzel, Harry A.
Noy, Janet L., FamilyMed
Oukachbi, Salima, FamilyMed
Powlowski, Marcus T.
Pratt, S. Lynn
Primmer, Janet J., FamilyMed
Probizanski, David C., FamilyMed
Rao, Pramila, FamilyMed
Reid, James A.
Reid, Kristin S., FamilyMed
Sacevich, Eugene G.
Sarrazin, Frederic, FamilyMed(EM)
Scali, Jim N., FamilyMed
Scott, Kane A.
Shepard, Andrea L., FamilyMed
Silliman, M. Lee
Simpson, Kathleen L., FamilyMed
Slivchak, Jane A M., FamilyMed
Sokolova, Elena A.
Spicer, Tara L., FamilyMed
St Jacques, Nicole S., FamilyMed
Stamler, James M., FamilyMed
Sweet, H. Bruce
Thacker, Kenneth E J., FamilyMed
Tong, Maorong, FamilyMed
Toppin, James L.
Trochimchuk, Teegan M., FamilyMed
Trusdale, Terry N W., FamilyMed
Turner, Shelley A M., FamilyMed
Twelker, Sunny S., FamilyMed(EM)
Valente, Maria
Vanderburgh, J. David H., FamilyMed(EM)
Vasiliu, Irene M.
Vrablik, Stefan
Wasielewski, Joseph F.
Webster, Edwin G.
Wentzell, Scott A.
Wilberforce, Nicola C., FamilyMed
Williams, Ruthanne L., FamilyMed
Wilson, Michael B., FamilyMed
Wiltshire, Marc L., FamilyMed(EM)
Wood, David A., FamilyMed(EM)
Woods, Margaret E C., FamilyMed
Yan, Hongyun, FamilyMed
Yeandle-Hignell, James
Yee, David P.
Zaib, Jehan, FamilyMed
Zavagnin, Nicole J., FamilyMed

TILBURY

Bryan, Colin F.
Engels, Holger
Limbombe, Basunga
Patel, Naresh R., FamilyMed

TILLSONBURG

Abdalla, Mohamed A A.
Andrew, John I., FamilyMed
Arif, Muhammad
Butchey, Robert, FamilyMed
Cheng, Willoon W M., FamilyMed
Chowdhury, Bikash K., FamilyMed
Cluett, James A G., FamilyMed
Dalby, Lisa A., FamilyMed
Danescu, Septimiu C.
Dockx, Daniel J A.
Hainer, Tammy L., FamilyMed
Hevenor, Robert D.
Holowachuk, Brian M., FamilyMed
Khan, Asif A.
Lamb, Howard F.
Michalik, Edward J.
O'Sullivan, Sean J.
Roth, Barry A.
Rowland, Gerald C.
Simpson, J. David
Sohla, Anand
Van Hooydonk, Vincent L.
Zawarynski, Diane M., FamilyMed

TIMMINS

Armstrong, Karen L., FamilyMed
Armstrong, Paul D., FamilyMed
Arnold, Douglas J., FamilyMed
Auger, Julie R., FamilyMed
Beauvais, Nicole L., FamilyMed
Brain, Daryl A., FamilyMed
Bronson, David W.
Catton, Lienne L., FamilyMed(EM)
Champion, J A. Gerard, FamilyMed
Chisholm, John A., FamilyMed
Ciccone, Mario V., FamilyMed(EM)
Clark, K. Christopher, FamilyMed
Cohen, Stephen G., FamilyMed
Coholic, Andrea A., FamilyMed
Cooper, Alfred J.
Cote, Jean, FamilyMed
Coutts, Stephen M.
Critchley, Patrick P., FamilyMed
Durepos, Christian P., FamilyMed
Gillies, Judy R M., FamilyMed
Griffiths, Lesley A., FamilyMed
Harterre, Trevor D., FamilyMed(EM)
Hopkins, Tammy M H., FamilyMed
Kaczmarek, Susan E., FamilyMed
Kanya-Forstner, Nicholas G., FamilyMed
Kim, Jun-Nyun, FamilyMed(EM)
Kos, Antonio I., FamilyMed
Kvas, Richard G., FamilyMed
Lax, Steven A., FamilyMed
Lim, Ka-Chee
Loreto, Chris J., FamilyMed(EM)
Maisonneuve, Rachel J., FamilyMed
Malo, Laurence G., FamilyMed(EM)
Morgan, Stephen, FamilyMed
Nawaz, Ahmad
Paquette, Eric R., FamilyMed
Paupst, Elizabeth A., FamilyMed
Pelletier, Annette M., FamilyMed
Raymond, Yves L., FamilyMed
Samson, Julie, FamilyMed(EM)
Schwertfeger, Lynne I., FamilyMed
Touw, Andrew J., FamilyMed
Ucar, Colin D., FamilyMed
Williams, Robert C., FamilyMed
Woods, Nancy G., FamilyMed
Zilka, Sonal D., FamilyMed(EM)

TOBERMORY

Harpur, George D., FamilyMed

TORONTO

Aazami, Pejman, FamilyMed
Abdul Razak, Albiruni R.
Abdulmajid Al Hamami, Ihsan, FamilyMed
Abells, Yoel B., FamilyMed
Abelsohn, Alan R., FamilyMed
Abla, Oussama A.
Aboujamra, Jamal, FamilyMed
Abrams, Jason A., FamilyMed
Abrams, Jonathan C., FamilyMed
Abriel Keren, Avital
Abu-Assi, Rammy
Abualross, Hani S.
Abughamja, Tareq S M., FamilyMed
Acsai, Megan S., FamilyMed
Adam, Rogelia F R.
Adcock, Lesley, FamilyMed
Adelstein, Raquel, FamilyMed
Adler Nevo, Gili W.
Adno, Brian
Advani, Andrew
Agid, Ofer
Aguayo, Pablo V., FamilyMed
Ah-Sue, Sheri L., FamilyMed
Ahmad, Tahani M T K.
Ahmado, Hend O I.
Ahmed, Samar M S.
Ahsan, Sania
Ailon, Jonathan I.
Akhtar, Sabrina N., FamilyMed
Akindele, Olufunmi O.
Akinfemiwa, Omotayo B., FamilyMed
Akiyama, Tomoyuki
Al Harbi, Nasser S T.
Al Shelleh, Sameeha
Al-Arabi, Ayman M A., FamilyMed
Al-Gasim, Abeer A M., FamilyMed
Al-Jeffri, Abdulla
Al-Kudmani, Basheer S B.
Al-Mejal, Zahra
Al-Naimi, Amal
Al-Qutub, Salma T A.
AlDaoud, Abdullah M A.
AlYousif, Mohammad A S.
Alarab, May A G.
Albers, Jan-Martin, FamilyMed
Aldridge, Christopher, FamilyMed
Alegre, Hugo T.
Alemayehu, Efrem
Alexander, Alexander M.
Alexander, Sarah W.
Ali, Muhammad
Allen, Edward C., FamilyMed
Allen, Gillian B.
Alleyne, Julia M K., FamilyMed
Almasi, Behzad, FamilyMed
Alonso Esteve, Angela
Alsharaf, Zuhair M A.
Altaweel, Alawi A M.
Altman, David L., FamilyMed
Alves, Cristina
Amann, Eric W.
Amaral, Andre C K.
Amaral, Joao G P V.
Amariyen, Dawi H M.
Amir, Eitan
Ampofo, Theophilus
An, Pamela H., FamilyMed
Anderson, Geoffrey M.
Andersons, Maris, FamilyMed
Andrade, Danielle M D.
Ang, Vivienne
Angelini, Paola
Annamala, Ganesan
Anraku, Masaki
Antao, Viola, FamilyMed
Appelby, Mark E., FamilyMed
Arafa, Neema A.
Arbess, Gordon A., FamilyMed
Armani, Antonio A.
Armstrong, Janice P.
Arnaudon, Daniel H J.
Arndt, Talitha A T., FamilyMed
Arnold, Paul F.
Arvanitis, Jennifer M., FamilyMed
Arzola Villalobos, Gracian C.
Asbell, Irwin J., FamilyMed
Ashamalla, Alison K., FamilyMed
Asim, Muhammad
Aslam, Nadeem
Asner, Sandra A H.
Au, Daniel T S.
Au, Susan J L.

Avila, Maria L.
Avila-Casado, Maria del Carmen
Avinoam-Dar, Galit
Avitzur, Yaron
Aw, James J.
Awad, Imad T.
Awerbuck, Jonathan A., FamilyMed
Axler, John T., FamilyMed
Axler, Theodore
Ayow, Michael K., FamilyMed(EM)
Ayuen, Kim L., FamilyMed
Aziz, Alnoor
Aziz, Nevine A.
Babiuk, Danielle
Babwah, Jesse P.
Bacher, Janice K., FamilyMed
Badali, Mary A., FamilyMed(EM)
Bahal, Maglin N., FamilyMed
Baimel, Evelyne, FamilyMed
Baimel, Melanie S., FamilyMed(EM)
Baker, Jason B., FamilyMed(EM)
Balki, Mrinalini S.
Ballinger, Lisa M.
Balmain, Sean
Baloun, Daniela
Banack, Alan D.
Bandyopadhyay, Subrata, FamilyMed
Banerjee, Susitna T., FamilyMed
BaniHani, Rudaina I H.
Banks, Diana, FamilyMed
Bansal, Vikas K., FamilyMed
Barker, Kimberley, FamilyMed
Barman, Mira, FamilyMed
Barmania, Yacoob E.
Barreca, Peter A., FamilyMed
Barrie, William J.
Barrientos, Lorena, FamilyMed
Bartels, Ute K.
Bartlett, Eric S.
Baryla, Yuliya, FamilyMed
Basinski, Antoni
Bastarrika Aleman, Gorka
Batejko, Oksana
Bateman, William A.
Bates, J. Terence, FamilyMed
Batty, Helen P., FamilyMed
Bazios, Sofia, FamilyMed
Bazos, Michael J.
Beach, Anne E.
Beach, Renee A.
Beairsto, W. Art D., FamilyMed
Bearss, Erin, FamilyMed(EM)
Bearss, Luke, FamilyMed(EM)
Bedrossian, Diane M., FamilyMed
Beharry, Rajendra
Behki, Subita
Beintema, Christena
Bekeris, Edward
Belanger, Anais L., FamilyMed
Bellaire, Jacqueline D., FamilyMed
Bendz, Oleg D.
Bennett, Margaret H., FamilyMed
Benseler, Susanne
Bentov, Yaakov H.
Beraldo, Vanessa J., FamilyMed
Berger, Howard P.
Berger, Kenneth J I., FamilyMed(EM)
Berger, Lisa, FamilyMed
Berger, Philip B., FamilyMed
Berger, Sheldon
Bergman, Samuel
Berliner, Yaniv, FamilyMed(EM)
Berman, Hal Kenneth
Bernard, Kelvin J R., FamilyMed
Bernstein, Robert, FamilyMed
Berntson, Laura C.
Berry, Raymond E., FamilyMed
Bertram, Jonathan R.
Beyers, Leslie A., FamilyMed
Bezanson, Kevin, FamilyMed
Bhattacharyya, Onil, FamilyMed
Biagioni, Edward J.
Biancucci, Christina M., FamilyMed
Bichai, Iman G.
Bingham, Katherine D., FamilyMed(EM)
Bir, Amnit S., FamilyMed
Bir, Karen
Biringer, Anne B., FamilyMed
Birmingham, Bradley W C.
Bissessar, Ramnaraise
Biswas, Tuhina, FamilyMed
Black, Dola
Black, Jennifer, FamilyMed
Black, William P G., FamilyMed
Blakeney, Jill
Blanco Alemany, Esther
Bloch, Gary, FamilyMed
Block, Wendell L., FamilyMed
Bloom, Jeff, FamilyMed
Bobiarski, Jerzy J.
Bobrowski, Jacob
Bocking, Natalie D., FamilyMed
Borgono, Claudio M.
Borgundvaag, Bjug, FamilyMed(EM)
Borins, Melvin, FamilyMed
Boroujerdi, Mehrnaz
Borowski, Irwin F M.
Borschel, Debaroti M.
Borschel, Gregory H.
Boruch, Nadia, FamilyMed
Bottenheim, Olivia, FamilyMed
Bourns, Amy E., FamilyMed
Bovett, Geoffrey P.
Bowdin, Sarah C C.
Bowry, Ashna D K., FamilyMed
Boyd, Jennifer A., FamilyMed
Bradley, Timothy J.
Brail, Jerrald N.
Brandao, Leonardo R.
Branigan, Monica A.
Branson, Helen M.
Brar, Pawandeep K., FamilyMed
Bratch, Anita N.
Brezina, Jeanie Shkimba.
Britton, Emmanuelle, FamilyMed
Brooks, Ruth E., FamilyMed
Brosh-Katz, Nirit
Brown, David S L.
Brown, Irving H.
Brown, Vivien P., FamilyMed
Brown, Wendy
Browne, Janis L., FamilyMed
Brunetta, Jason M., FamilyMed
Brunt, Susan, FamilyMed
Brzezinski, Jack J.
Buchman, Stephen, FamilyMed
Buckridan, Al-Beruni S.
Bui, Duong X.
Bukczynski, Jacob M., FamilyMed
Bukmuz, Nadine M.
Bulatovic-Stajkovic, Sladjana
Bunting, Howard
Burchill, Luke
Burge, Jonathan A.
Burns, Anthony S.
Burt, Christiana C.
Buruiana, Manole
Butler, Marcus O.
Bystrin, Irina
Callaghan, Sarah
Cameron, Catherine, FamilyMed
Campbell, Catherine J M., FamilyMed
Campbell, Fiona A.
Canton, Toni J.
Cantor, Elliott J F., FamilyMed
Caraiscos, Valerie B., FamilyMed
Caravaggio, Robert J.
Carmichael, Catherine A., FamilyMed
Carmichael, Richard W.
Carr, David, FamilyMed(EM)
Carroll, June C., FamilyMed
Carvalhal, Adriana S.
Caspin, Shirley L., FamilyMed
Cass, J. Charles
Castiglione, John S.
Castro, Denise A.
Cataudella, Julia A., FamilyMed
Catz-Biro, Laura, FamilyMed
Cavacuiti, Christopher A., FamilyMed
Cellarius, Victor, FamilyMed
Ceresne, Lance A., FamilyMed
Cerskus, Timothy R.
Cha, Charlie Y K.
Chada, Reena R., FamilyMed
Chakraborty, Anita R., FamilyMed
Chan, Alex T C.
Chan, Alvin
Chan, Arlene S L., FamilyMed
Chan, Bowen, FamilyMed
Chan, David Y K.
Chan, Eugene Y C.
Chan, Florence, FamilyMed
Chan, Katherine Y.
Chan, King-Sun
Chan, Richard C W.
Chandola, Rahul
Chandran, Lavan, FamilyMed
Chandran, Vinod
Chandranipapongse, Weerawadee
Chang, Benny H S., FamilyMed
Chang, Boon H., FamilyMed(EM)
Chang, Derrick, FamilyMed(EM)
Chang, Gao-Nan
Chang, Kathleen D K., FamilyMed
Chang, Maria Y., FamilyMed
Chang, Patricia Y., FamilyMed
Chang, Richard, FamilyMed
Chaparro Mutis, B. Cecilia
Chari, Rachna A., FamilyMed
Charlebois, Alison L., FamilyMed
Charles, Jocelyn E., FamilyMed
Charusripan, Paninee
Chaturvedi, Rajiv R.
Chau, Edmond H L.
Chavhan, Govind B.
Che, Priscilla M., FamilyMed
Cheema, Sohail E.
Cheifetz, Arielle, FamilyMed
Chen, Betty H., FamilyMed
Chen, Edmund C F., FamilyMed
Chen, Howard C H., FamilyMed
Chen, Kenneth K O.
Cheng, Elaine V., FamilyMed
Chepesiuk, William N.
Chernin, Trudy R., FamilyMed
Chernoff, Ian W., FamilyMed(EM)
Chesney, Alden E.
Chetty, Runjan
Cheung, Ngai Hoi.
Chien, Karen, FamilyMed
Chin, Francis L.
Chinnapp, Vinod
Chiu, But-Yau
Cho, Kevin Y.
Choi, Antonio M F., FamilyMed
Choi, James H., FamilyMed
Chong, Donald T.
Chong, Robert H.
Chou, Roger
Chow, Esther H., FamilyMed
Chow, Tiffany W.
Chow, Vivian W.
Chowdhury, Muna, FamilyMed
Chu, Karen L., FamilyMed(EM)
Chu, Margaret, FamilyMed
Chu, Michael W., FamilyMed
Chuen, Luan L.
Chui, Sze Wing
Chung, Jim J., FamilyMed(EM)
Chung, Shari A., FamilyMed
Church, Paige T.
Cirone, Sharon L., FamilyMed(EM)
Ciurria, Nicholas S.
Clair, Kiran D K., FamilyMed
Clarfield, Michael D.
Clark, Laura B., FamilyMed
Cleiman, Paula F., FamilyMed(EM)
Cogan, Farrell S., FamilyMed
Coghlan, Matthew A.
Cohen, Abraham
Cohen, C. Ian, FamilyMed
Cohen, Ira T.
Cohen, Joanne, FamilyMed
Cohen, Michal
Cohen, Tracey, FamilyMed
Cohn, Ronald D.
Colledge, Eleanor M., FamilyMed
Connelly, Kim A.
Conway, Denis M.
Cook, Sarah E., FamilyMed
Cooper, Robert A., FamilyMed
Copeland, Laura L.
Cord, Stephen M., FamilyMed(EM)
Cordovani, Daniel
Cornelson, Brian M., FamilyMed
Corrigan, Mark A.
Corrin, Lesley S.
Cotterill, Paul C.
Crean, Andrew M.
Creek, Kristen L B., FamilyMed
Crispino, Natascha, FamilyMed
Crouzat, Frederic B., FamilyMed
Crowcrof, Natasha S.
Cruise, Lora J H., FamilyMed
Crummey, James M., FamilyMed
Cruz, E. Laura, FamilyMed
Crystal, Pavel
Cuffe, Sinead D.
Culbert, Alison J., FamilyMed
Culbert, Heather T., FamilyMed
Culligan, Christopher J., FamilyMed
Curtis, Tyler J., FamilyMed
Cuthbert, Brian H.
Cypel, Marcelo
Cypel, Tatiana
Czemerynski, Anne, FamilyMed
D'Agrosa, Raffaele, FamilyMed
D'Cunha, Nolda M., FamilyMed
D'Ovidio, Vincent
D'Souza, Mark, FamilyMed(EM)
D'Urzo, Anthony D., FamilyMed
Da Costa Jr, Leodante B.
Dacre, Roger I., FamilyMed
Dainton, Christopher J., FamilyMed(EM)
Daly, Meghan , FamilyMed
Dandekar, Masumi, FamilyMed
Dang, Bach-Tuyet T.
Danylak, Maria D.
Daoud, Eyad S A Q.
Das, Paul J., FamilyMed
Das, Sunit
Das, Tilak
Dash, Satya
Dattilo, Giovanni A., FamilyMed
Daunt, Stephen W., FamilyMed
Dauphinais, Christiane, FamilyMed
Dave, Kishorchandra M., FamilyMed
David, Andrea, FamilyMed
Davies, Simon J C.
Davis, Beverley M., FamilyMed
Davis, Jayne L., FamilyMed
De Alwis, Amila
De Carvalho, Elda E B P.
De Figueiredo, Antonia F., FamilyMed
De Lasa, Cristina, FamilyMed
De Los Santos, Christina J., FamilyMed
De Luca, Vincenzo
De Mestral, Charles
De Silva, Anne
De Souza, Kimberley, FamilyMed(EM)
De Souza, Melissa P A., FamilyMed
DeRocher, Mary Elizabeth, FamilyMed
Deering, Susan A., FamilyMed
Degen, Eric, FamilyMed
Del Giudice, Lisa M E., FamilyMed
Del Junco, Maria
Del Pozo, Rolando
Del Sorbo, Lorenzo
Delgado, Diego H.
Deliakis, John, FamilyMed
Derkach, Peter
Desai, Devdatta M.
Desarkar, Pushpal
Deshpand, Poorva P.
Deshpande, Amol
Desson, Sheana, FamilyMed
Destrade Sosa, Lief, FamilyMed
Dew, Bernard, FamilyMed(EM)
Dey, Chris
Di Paola, Francesca A., FamilyMed
Diamond, Ivan
Diaz De Molnar, Ana M.
Dibildox Gonzalez, Manuel
Dickhout, Janet S., FamilyMed
Dillon, David A.
Dimitrakoudis, Helena M., FamilyMed
Dinicolo, Lisa, FamilyMed(EM)
Dixon, Kirsten
Dmytryshyn, Robert, FamilyMed
Doidge, Mark S.
Domb, Sharon, FamilyMed
Dong, Alice
Doria, Andrea S.
Doukas, Kathleen, FamilyMed
Dowsling, Janet L.
Dracopoulos, Anastasios T., FamilyMed
Dragomir, Camelia C., FamilyMed
Draper, Haley, FamilyMed
Dreckmann, Robert H.
Dreyzin, Ilona, FamilyMed
Dubinsky, Isser L., FamilyMed(EM)
Dubord, Gregoire M.
Dunn, Sheila, FamilyMed(EM)
Dunraj, Vishay, FamilyMed
Duong, Nguyen H.
Dushenski, David G., FamilyMed(EM)
Dutczak, Miroslaw
Dutrisac, Renaud, FamilyMed(EM)
Dyment, Stuart Z.
Eckler, Sarah J., FamilyMed
Edelist, Darren, FamilyMed
Eder, Lihi
Edney, James A., FamilyMed
Edwards, James N.
Edwards, Susan A., FamilyMed
Egeler, R. Maarten
Eisen, David
Elbaroun, Basem A O N.
Elinson, Roman, FamilyMed
Elliott, Carl M., FamilyMed
Ellison, Philip, FamilyMed
Elman, Debra R., FamilyMed
Elmekkawi Mohamed, Amir E A.
Elser, Christine
Emmanuel, Majella, FamilyMed(EM)
Emmenegger, Urban
Eng, Henry S.
Engelberg, David, FamilyMed
Engineer, Ariz A.
Epstein, Shirley
Erenrich, Hedi M., FamilyMed
Eskandar, Monira, FamilyMed
Etoom, Yousef A T.
Etzkorn, William G., FamilyMed
Euverman, Rachel M., FamilyMed
Evans, Arthur
Evans, Robyn M., FamilyMed
Everett, Tobias C.
Facy, Anca, FamilyMed
Fagan, Romana
Faiers, Alan A.
Falcioni, Michael K., FamilyMed
Farquharson, Patricia A.
Fayet, Cristina, FamilyMed
Fayez, Ibrahim, FamilyMed
Feiner, Hannah L R., FamilyMed
Feldberg, Melissa R., FamilyMed
Feldman, Kimberley, FamilyMed
Feldman, Sandra H., FamilyMed
Felix, Janos L.
Fenton, Peter M.
Fenton, Stanley S A.
Fernandez, Nestor D P.
Ferreira, M. Thomas D.
Feuerstein, Erika, FamilyMed
Fiala, Jindrich, FamilyMed
Fidler, Lee M.
Figueiredo, Indira C.
Finan, Emer A.
Finkelstein, Murray M., FamilyMed
Finkelstein, Yaron
Fiorini, Godfrey T.
Fischer, Erica G L.
Fischer, Jason W J.
Fischer, Sandra
Fisher, Christina M., FamilyMed
Fisher, Deborah T., FamilyMed
Fisher, Harold N.
Flamer, Cara, FamilyMed
Fleming, Karen E., FamilyMed
Fleming, Sarah, FamilyMed
Flomen, Marcy S., FamilyMed
Fogel, Bernard, FamilyMed
Foley, Frank J., FamilyMed
Foley, Karen A.
Foo, Marshall C.
Foo, Suan-Seh
Foote, John R., FamilyMed(EM)
Forcina, Alexander E., FamilyMed
Forte, Milena F., FamilyMed
Fortin, Christian D.
Fox, Susan H.
Francis, Robert
Frank, William
Franke, Norman A.
Frecker, Richard
Freedman, Amy K., FamilyMed
Freedman, Fred A., FamilyMed
Freeman, Laura M.
Freke, Sarah J.
Fried, Steven E M.

PHYSICIANS BY PROVINCE

Fried, Veronika A., FamilyMed
Friedber, Mark K.
Friedman, Aaron A.
Friedman, Steven, FamilyMed(EM)
Friedman, Susan R., FamilyMed
Friedman, Zeev Z.
Friesner, Abraham
Friz, B. Hansjorg, FamilyMed(EM)
Frydrych, Seymour, FamilyMed
Fujii, Hisaki
Fulton, Jessica, FamilyMed
Fung, Ambrose Y T., FamilyMed
Fung, Gerald
Fung, Leslie C., FamilyMed
Furlan, Andrea D.
Gagnon, D'Arcy W.
Gajardo, Paz A., FamilyMed
Gajic, Desanka
Gallimore, Ian C G.
Garavaglia, Marco M.
Gardner-Nix, Jacqueline S.
Gassas, Adam
Gazeley, Sharon G., FamilyMed
Gebara, Nadine, FamilyMed
Geleff, John S.
George, Anthony G.
Germain, Jennifer M., FamilyMed
Gerstein, Samuel M.
Gerth, Sjaan C., FamilyMed
Getu, Haregua
Gevorgya, Artur
Gewurz, Lauren A., FamilyMed
Ghai, Sandeep
Ghai, Sangeet
Ghavam-Rassoul, Abbas, FamilyMed
Ghoche, Roger, FamilyMed
Gholami, Amir S.
Ghorab, Zeina
Giancola, Lina, FamilyMed
Gibson, Craig R.
Gibson, Douglas S.
Gibson, John W., FamilyMed
Giddens, J. David, FamilyMed(EM)
Gidwani, Andy J.
Gilbert, Barry L R., FamilyMed
Gill, Satinderpal S., FamilyMed
Gindi, Raafat F.
Glazer, Peter R., FamilyMed(EM)
Glazier, Richard H., FamilyMed
Glazman, Bernard G.
Glazman, Trevor N.
Gledhill, N. Scott, FamilyMed
Go, Cristina
Goel, Ritika, FamilyMed
Goldberg, Orli D., FamilyMed
Goldberg, Robert J.
Goldhar, Steven M.
Goldman, H. Brian
Goldman, Howard H., FamilyMed
Goldman, Russell, FamilyMed
Goldman, Ruth A., FamilyMed
Goldsand, John I., FamilyMed
Goldstein, Susan R., FamilyMed
Goncalves, M. Joana
Gonsalves, Patrick M., FamilyMed
Gonska, Tanja Y.
Gonzalez, Armando
Gonzalez Pupo, Rafael
Goodall, Douglas J., FamilyMed
Goodhew, John E.
Goodman, Melvin P., FamilyMed
Gora, Irving, FamilyMed
Gordon, Gayle S.
Gordon, Lloyd P.
Gore, Stanley
Gorfinkel, Iris
Gosevitz, J. Bernard, FamilyMed
Gosset, Brian D.
Gould, Wendy M.
Graff Guerrero, Ariel
Graham, John
Graner, Jerry L.
Grant, A. Leigh, FamilyMed
Grantcharov, Teodor P.
Graseman, Hartmut
Gratton, Adele
Gray, P. Ainslie
Grbac, Leonard, FamilyMed(EM)
Green, Jennifer, FamilyMed
Green, Laurie K., FamilyMed(EM)
Greenberg, David E.

Greenberg, H. Joseph
Greenberg, Mark A., FamilyMed
Greenwald, Kenneth J., FamilyMed
Greenwald, Marci R., FamilyMed
Greer, Mary-Louise C.
Grell, Natashia G K., FamilyMed
Grevler, Joanne M., FamilyMed
Griffin, Virginia M., FamilyMed
Grosett, Oswald W.
Grosse-Wortmann, Lars
Grosser, Norman
Grubner, Karin H.
Grundland, Batya N., FamilyMed
Grunebaum, Eyal
Grunfeld, Eva, FamilyMed
Guerriere, Michael
Guest, Joan E.
Guiang, Charlie B., FamilyMed
Gulan-Vujnovic, Ljubica
Guntley-Lorimer, Edith M.
Guo, Ray
Gupta, K. Kashyap, FamilyMed
Gupta, Vikas
Gutgutia, Kanan
Gutman, I. Edward, FamilyMed
Guzman, Venus B.
Ha, Valerie, FamilyMed
Haas, Yvonne M., FamilyMed
Haddad, Margaret M.
Hailemeskel, Yemisrach, FamilyMed
Hakoun, Jack
Halikowski, Marvin J.
Hall, William A.
Hamani, Clement
Hamedanchi, Reza, FamilyMed
Hamilton, Julia E., FamilyMed
Hamlet, Bevin A., FamilyMed
Hamrahi, Hormoz, FamilyMed
Handford, Curtis D., FamilyMed
Hanet, Stephen H., FamilyMed
Hanlon, Brian A.
Hanna, Linda, FamilyMed
Hanna, Sameh
Hannam, Paul D., FamilyMed(EM)
Hans, Laura M., FamilyMed(EM)
Hansen, Shandi M.
Hanson, Peter G.
Haq, Aamir, FamilyMed
Haq, Farzana, FamilyMed
Harizanov, Velizar A.
Haroon, Nigil
Harrison, Kenneth J.
Harrison, Susan A L., FamilyMed
Harrison, Yasmin, FamilyMed
Harte, Susannah E.
Harvey, Paula
Haslah, Maja, FamilyMed
Hasson, Paul K.
Hatashita, Eric, FamilyMed
Hausmanis, Larisa I., FamilyMed
Hawkins, Paul
Hayman, Coryn, FamilyMed
Healey, Kathryn L., FamilyMed
Hebert, Philip C., FamilyMed
Hedgcock, Malcolm A., FamilyMed
Hedley, David W.
Heineck, Katja, FamilyMed
Heisey, Ruth E., FamilyMed
Henrikson, Donna G.
Henry, Patrick D G.
Herman, Rebecca C., FamilyMed
Hermant, Tammy G., FamilyMed
Hershberg, Melissa B., FamilyMed
Hii, Anthony Y P.
Himel, Naomi, FamilyMed
Hind, Sharon A., FamilyMed
Hirsz, Abraham I., FamilyMed
Ho, C. John, FamilyMed
Ho, Charmaine S., FamilyMed
Ho, Christopher T M.
Ho, Karen C T., FamilyMed(EM)
Ho, Michael S C.
Hoang, Ngoc-Khoi
Hodge, Matthew J., FamilyMed(EM)
Hoffmann, Susan M., FamilyMed
Hogg, Susan C.
Holmes, Candice N., FamilyMed
Holzapfel, G. Stephen, FamilyMed
Honickman, Debbie F., FamilyMed
Honjo, Osami
Hopkins, John P.

Hopkins, Peter D., FamilyMed
Hose, Patricia M., FamilyMed
Howe, Marnie L., FamilyMed
Howell, Jane C., FamilyMed
Hsiang, Diana, FamilyMed
Hsiao, Marvin M.
Hu, Lin Aung (Rex), FamilyMed
Hughes, Carol M E., FamilyMed
Hui, Jacqueline Y., FamilyMed
Hujic, Nirvana, FamilyMed
Hum, Betty M., FamilyMed
Humpl, Tilman F.
Hunchak, Cheryl L., FamilyMed(EM)
Huryn, Mark J., FamilyMed
Husain, Amna F., FamilyMed
Husain, Shahid
Hussain, Farha, FamilyMed
Hussein, Elysha, FamilyMed
Hussein, Shaukat N.
Hussein, Sohaileh
Hussman, Edward A.
Hussman, M. Ruth, FamilyMed
Huston, Marcy A.
Hwang, Christine
Ibrahim, Hisham G E M.
Iglar, Karl T., FamilyMed
Ikizler, Yasemin, FamilyMed
Incardona, Nadia K., FamilyMed
Inch, Cameron J A., FamilyMed(EM)
Irons, Shawna M., FamilyMed
Isaac, Richard G.
Isayama, Tetsuya
Isenberg, Gerald N.
Ivers, Noah, FamilyMed
Jaakkimainen, R. Liisa, FamilyMed
Jackson, A. Beverley, FamilyMed
Jaconello, Paul P.
Jadad Bechara, Alejandro R.
Jafrudy, Russell H., FamilyMed
Jaipargas, Charles C.
Jaksic-Tomanovic, Ljiljana, FamilyMed
Jakubovicz, Difat E., FamilyMed
Jamal, Alykhan M., FamilyMed
Jamal, Dawood I.
Jamal, John, FamilyMed(EM)
Jamal, Shamir M.
Jamal, Zahra, FamilyMed
James, Adrian L.
Janakiram, Praseedha, FamilyMed
Jang, Hyun-Jung
Jang, Karen Y K., FamilyMed
Janjua, Sadiq A.
Jankov, Robert P.
Janmohamed, Anisa, FamilyMed
Janssen, Henricus L A.
Jansz, Gwenderlyn F., FamilyMed
Javanmard, Mahan, FamilyMed(EM)
Jayaraman, Jai
Jeney, Christa M., FamilyMed
Jessamy, Nalya T., FamilyMed
Jewell, Kristyn S., FamilyMed
Jeyapragasan, Manjula, FamilyMed
Jha, Muneesh, FamilyMed
Jha, Prabhat K S.
Jha, Sapna, FamilyMed
Jhaveri, Kartik S.
Jimenez Juan, Laura
Jimenez Zepeda, Victor H.
Jin, Jing, FamilyMed
Joarder, Mohammad Z H.
Joffe, Robert, FamilyMed(EM)
Johal, Malkit K., FamilyMed
John, Rohan
Johnson, Kim C., FamilyMed
Johnson, L. Stephen
Johnson, Sonia C.
Johnston, Erin L., FamilyMed
Johnstone, Saralaine S., FamilyMed
Jonathan, Ernest R.
Joneja, Anu, FamilyMed
Jones, Ernest R.
Jones, Wentworth W.
Joshi, Ramona, FamilyMed
Joshua, Anthony M.
Ju, Hui
Judah, Eli
Jugovic, Pieter J., FamilyMed
Jung, Hsiao-Ming, FamilyMed
Jussaume, Richard L.
Kagan, Jennifer L., FamilyMed

Kahan, Meldon M., FamilyMed
Kalisiak, Maria T.
Kamath Patel, Binita M.
Kamens, Cathy A., FamilyMed
Kampf, N. Noreen, FamilyMed
Kanagaratnam, Sivaruban
Kanhai, Neil A., FamilyMed(EM)
Kanjeekal, Santosh S R., FamilyMed(EM)
Kannu, Peter
Kaplovitch, Harvey, FamilyMed
Kapoor, Aarti, FamilyMed
Kapoor, Monika, FamilyMed(EM)
Kara, Zulfikar S., FamilyMed
Karabegovic, Amna, FamilyMed(EM)
Karalis, Peter
Karamchandani, Jason R P.
Karantonis, Anastassios
Karim, Ruhin
Karlinsky, Audrey L., FamilyMed
Katis, Peter G., FamilyMed(EM)
Katyal, Sonia, FamilyMed
Kaufman, Adam J., FamilyMed(EM)
Kaufman, Jennifer C.
Kaufmann, I. Michael, FamilyMed
Kaya, Ebru
Kee, Barbara E.
Keen, Susan L.
Keller, John R.
Kelley, Simon P.
Keltz, Maurice
Kendal, David
Kennedy, Joseph D., FamilyMed
Kennedy, Josephine A.
Kerametlian, Vatche
Kerin, Noel A.
Kerr, Ernest
Kerr, Kathleen J.
Kestenbaum, Deborah S., FamilyMed
Keunen, Johannes E G M.
Khan, Nadira S., FamilyMed
Khan, Ruhe S., FamilyMed
Khan, Swaleha
Khatri, Prateek
Khoshnood, Narges, FamilyMed
Khoumais, Nuha A O.
Khoury, Michael A.
Khurana, Mona, FamilyMed
Khurshid, Faiza
Kim, Alexandra V.
Kim, Celine C.
Kim, Dennis D H.
Kim, Florence A., FamilyMed
Kim, Hyon Chung, FamilyMed
Kim, Jin Hee, FamilyMed
Kim, Matthew C Y.
Kim, Richard S J., FamilyMed(EM)
Kim, Sarah, FamilyMed
Kim, Susie, FamilyMed
King, Bertram W.
King, Charles B.
Kingsley, Simon J., FamilyMed(EM)
Kingstone, Robert A.
Kingstone, Sheldon I.
Kiraly, Jane M.
Kiran, Tara, FamilyMed
Kirsh, Andrea F., FamilyMed
Kirsh, Jerry J.
Kitai, Carol, FamilyMed
Kitto, Kimberley A., FamilyMed
Klajner, Felix, FamilyMed
Klapecki, Karyn C., FamilyMed
Klapwyk, Linda A., FamilyMed
Klar, Michael
Klar, Michael, FamilyMed
Klein, H. Alexander
Kline, Harvey
Klinghofer, Irvin L.
Klodas, Slawomir M.
Knowles, Holly K E., FamilyMed
Ko, Hyang Mi
Ko, Karen, FamilyMed
Koblic, Paul M., FamilyMed(EM)
Kocandrle, Hana
Kohut, Ludmila B.
Kohut, Nitsa
Kohut, Vera M., FamilyMed
Kokoski, Richard J., FamilyMed
Kolosowska-Rydlewski, Anna
Kong Ting, Margaret C.
Konieczna, Ewa M.

Konstantatos, Spiros, FamilyMed(EM)
Kopaniak, Marguerite M., FamilyMed
Korda, Ryan N., FamilyMed
Kota, Suzanne E.
Kotzer, Eric J.
Kozak, Joseph H., FamilyMed
Krakowsky, Harry W.
Krantz, Roselynn A.
Krema, Muhammed H A A.
Krieger, Mark
Krigstein, Esther S.
Krishnamurthy, Ashok B., FamilyMed
Krivy, Joel L.
Kruger, Tamara L., FamilyMed
Krym, Valerie F., FamilyMed(EM)
Kryshtalskyj, Nina, FamilyMed
Kucharski, Edward A., FamilyMed
Kukreti, Vinay
Kuld, Arvo
Kulkarni, Supriya R.
Kumar, Rakesh, FamilyMed(EM)
Kumar, Rohini, FamilyMed
Kuruganty, Sailaja, FamilyMed
Kusenthiran, Sri Kasthuri
Kuszewski, Maciej J.
Kuutan, Toivo
Kuwahara, Leonard S.
Kuzmar, Dusko N.
Kuzmin, Yulia, FamilyMed
Kwan, Janice L.
Kwok, Bruce C., FamilyMed
Kwok, Juanita W.
Kycia, Katarzyna, FamilyMed
Laffey, John G.
Lai, Alice M.
Lai, Godwin, FamilyMed
Lai, Michael W K.
Lai, Samuel, FamilyMed
Lai, Wendy A., FamilyMed(EM)
Lake, Rae G., FamilyMed
Lakhoo, Sheila, FamilyMed
Lal, Anita
Lam, Andrew J Y W., FamilyMed
Lam, Andrew W K., FamilyMed
Lam, Irina C Y.
Lam, Jennifer K., FamilyMed
Lam, Kenneth W K.
Lam, Richard P.
Lam, Robert E., FamilyMed
Lam, Vincent H C., FamilyMed
Lam Antoniades, Margarita, FamilyMed
Landes, Megan, FamilyMed(EM)
Langford, E. Robert
Langlois, E. Anne, FamilyMed
Lantos, Gabor
Lapointe-Shaw, Lauren
Lara Corrales, Irene
Larochelle, Catherine A.
Lashevsky, Ilan
Lathwell, Margaret J S.
Lau, Albert, FamilyMed(EM)
Lau, Peter P T., FamilyMed
Laussen, Peter C.
Lauwers, Albert E., FamilyMed
Law, Marcus, FamilyMed
Lawee, David, FamilyMed
Lazier, Kate, FamilyMed(EM)
Le, Chu Quang
Le, Minh Van
Lebeau, Marc, FamilyMed
Leber, Wolfgang A.
Lee, C T. Andy
Lee, Connie N., FamilyMed(EM)
Lee, Dennis
Lee, Edward T.
Lee, Kit Shan, FamilyMed
Lee, Lawrence L M.
Lee, Lorraine P H., FamilyMed
Lee, Oscar I.
Lee, Shirley, FamilyMed(EM)
Lee, Stella, FamilyMed
Lee, Vansen M.
Lee, Winnie W S.
Lee-Sing, Richard A.
Leece, Pamela N., FamilyMed
Lefebvre, Lisa G., FamilyMed
Legault, Pierre-Marc B., FamilyMed
Lei, Calvin Z H.
Leibel, Sandra L.
Leibel, Sydney A.

Leitenberg, Samuel, FamilyMed
Lem, Melissa M P., FamilyMed
Lemieux, Camille M., FamilyMed
Lemos, Vivienne M., FamilyMed
Lenauskas, Daiva A., FamilyMed
Lenkov, Pamela L., FamilyMed
Leong, Renata M W., FamilyMed
Leser, Michael
Lester, Michael D.
Leucht, Stephan T.
Leung, Cheryl S Y., FamilyMed
Leung, Chi Tak
Leung, Deborah K B., FamilyMed(EM)
Leung, F. Edmund, FamilyMed
Leung, Karen M C.
Leung, Kelvin W.
Leung, Mark, FamilyMed
Leung, Terence L N.
Leung, Wilson L.
Leventhal, Joseph I., FamilyMed
Levitan, Deborah E., FamilyMed
Levy, Sheldon L.
Levy, Shirley, FamilyMed
Lewin, Sheila
Lewis, Douglas C.
Lewis, Jillian M.
Lewis, Michael E., FamilyMed
Lewittes, Leora R., FamilyMed
Ley, Sebastian
Lhotsky, Miroslava, FamilyMed
Li, Alan T W.
Li, Cheuk-Hon
Li, Dominic W.
Li, Francis
Lian, Calvin T., FamilyMed(EM)
Libman, Robert N., FamilyMed
Librach, S. Lawrence, FamilyMed
Likwornik, Gunilla
Lim, Bill Y B.
Lim, David C.
Limaye, Navika P., FamilyMed
Lin, Susy
Linden, Ronald O., FamilyMed
Linder, Mark R., FamilyMed
Ling, Rosalind L L.
Ling, Simon C.
Lipcsei, Julie A., FamilyMed
Lipsitz, Jeffrey J.
Lipson, Martin H.
Liptay, Christine M., FamilyMed
Lipton, R. Myles
Litner, Geoffrey M., FamilyMed
Liu, H K. Kenneth
Liu, Pamela Y., FamilyMed
Liu, Shi-Kai
Liu, Vivian W., FamilyMed
Llano-Ferro, Miguel A.
Llewellyn, M. Evan, FamilyMed
Lo, Marco C., FamilyMed
Loach, David W.
Lobo, Andrea N., FamilyMed
Lockyer, Michelle A., FamilyMed
Lofchy, A. Norman
Lofters, Aisha K., FamilyMed
Logue, Kenneth J M.
Lombardi, Pietro, FamilyMed
Long, Shane B.
Longley, Catherine D., FamilyMed(EM)
Loo, Tip Wah
Look Kin, Karen T., FamilyMed
Lorber, Eva
Lorde, Ingrid L A., FamilyMed
Loritz, Frank L J.
Lou, Allison S., FamilyMed
Lou, T Y. Justin, FamilyMed
Loukides, Nicholas E.
Lowe, David A., FamilyMed
Lowe, Julia M.
Lower, Darlene P., FamilyMed
Luetkehoelter, Jonathan
Luey, Lai-Lane
Luftspring, Lawrence
Luginbuehl, Igor A.
Lui, Andrew B., FamilyMed(EM)
Lui, Jaime, FamilyMed
Lukenda, Michael A., FamilyMed
Lum, Grant, FamilyMed
Lunney, M. Claire, FamilyMed
Lupovici, Ninia M.
Lutynski, Andrzej

Luvisotto, Terri L., FamilyMed
Lyon, W. Kirk, FamilyMed
Lywood, Allegra, FamilyMed
Ma, Grace C M., FamilyMed
Ma, Lingli, FamilyMed(EM)
MacCallum, Christie A.
MacDonald, Mary Rose
MacDonald, Matthew J., FamilyMed
MacKay, Helen
MacKinnon, David J., FamilyMed(EM)
MacLeod, John D., FamilyMed
MacMillan, Lindsay E., FamilyMed
Machamer, Mary E.
Madan, Monika K., FamilyMed
Madison, Vera V.
Maehle, Waldemar M.
Mah, Richard
Maheshwari, Ekta
Mahmood, Tariq
Mahmoud, Sarah, FamilyMed
Mahmoud, Shireen F A H.
Mahmutoglu, Saadet
Mahtani, Ramona, FamilyMed
Maida, Vincent, FamilyMed
Maimets, Talvi C., FamilyMed
Majeed, Faiza A., FamilyMed
Mak, Ellen N.
Mak, S C. Ernie, FamilyMed
Maker, Dara, FamilyMed
Malcolm, Brendan P., FamilyMed
Malcolm, Jennifer P., FamilyMed
Male, Roy A., FamilyMed
Malek, Anna M., FamilyMed
Malhotra, Sonia, FamilyMed
Malick, Arfa K.
Malkin, Mendl, FamilyMed
Mallouh, Suzy Z., FamilyMed
Mamalias, Nikolaos, FamilyMed(EM)
Mamen, Natalie K., FamilyMed(EM)
Man, Thomas M., FamilyMed
Mandel, Howard, FamilyMed
Mangat, Amardeep S.
Manicatide, Mihai A.
Mansfield, Robert W., FamilyMed
Mansoor, Dana R., FamilyMed
Manzig, Loraine A., FamilyMed
Marchow, Leszek A.
Marciniak, Zbigniew A.
Marcus, Jonathan M., FamilyMed
Marcus-Mand, Nufar
Margarido, Clarita
Mark, Pamela A., FamilyMed
Marks, Alexander
Marley, Jaanus
Marmoreo, Jean E., FamilyMed
Marques, Joseph R.
Marrocco, Angela M P., FamilyMed(EM)
Marsden, Philip A.
Marshall, Judith A., FamilyMed
Marshall, Lynn M.
Martin, Danielle A S., FamilyMed
Martiniuk, Shauna O C., FamilyMed(EM)
Martins, Rui F O., FamilyMed
Maryniarczyk, Teresa P., FamilyMed
Mascarenhas, Lyndon
Masgoret, John C., FamilyMed
Mason, Lou E., FamilyMed
Massad, Joseph, FamilyMed
Masson, Sharonah R., FamilyMed
Matava, Cliade T.
Mattas, Shawn P., FamilyMed
Matthews, Michael K., FamilyMed
Mavrogiannis, Louie, FamilyMed
Mawji, Yasmine, FamilyMed(EM)
Maynes, Jason T.
Mazzotta, Paolo, FamilyMed
McAuliffe, D. Noel
McCabe, Jennifer L., FamilyMed
McCann, Maureen
McCarvill, Erin M., FamilyMed
McCurrach, Anne E G.
McDermid, Brian J.
McDonnell, Conor G.
McDowell, Brenda J., FamilyMed
McElroy, Rosheen T., FamilyMed(EM)
McFadden, Erin L., FamilyMed
McFarlane, Virginia J., FamilyMed
McGee, Allison J., FamilyMed(EM)
McGowan, Carolyn, FamilyMed

McIntosh, Evan M., FamilyMed(EM)
McIntosh, Garfield G G.
McIntyre, Julie J., FamilyMed
McIntyre-Stewart, Sarah M.
McIsaac, Warren J., FamilyMed
McKellar, Robert G.
McKenna-Boot, Patricia E.
McKenzie, Kwame J.
McKeown, Elizabeth M.
McKinley, Marianne, FamilyMed
McKneally, Martin F.
McKnight, J E. Arlene
McLean, Shelley M., FamilyMed
McMillan, Stephen J., FamilyMed
McNally, Catherine M., FamilyMed
McNally, James W.
McNamara, G. Patrick, FamilyMed
McNamara, Patrick J.
McPhail, Marianne A., FamilyMed
Mehta, Suryakant D.
Meineri, Massimiliano
Melady, Donald L., FamilyMed(EM)
Melemis, Steven M.
Melnitzer, Melissa D., FamilyMed
Mendoza-Londono, Roberto
Merali, Sara, FamilyMed
Merkley, Barry D.
Mertens, Luc L.
Mesensky, Marcella M.
Messner, Sandra J., FamilyMed
Mete, Ozgur
Metser, Ur
Meuser, James C., FamilyMed
Meyn, M. Stephen
Mezody, Melitta
Mian, Ahmed R., FamilyMed(EM)
Michalski, Andrzej J.
Miladinovic, Ljiljana, FamilyMed
Mildon, C. Anne
Miller, Rivian S.
Millers, Anna, FamilyMed
Milot, Laurent
Mingo, Nancy S., FamilyMed
Minkovich, Leonid L.
Mintz, Sharon, FamilyMed
Mirchandani, Natasha, FamilyMed
Mireskandari, Kamiar
Mishriki, Nahed R., FamilyMed
Mital, Seema
Mitri, Mira, FamilyMed
Mitwally, Mohamed F M.
Mizdrak, Nikolina, FamilyMed
Mizrahi, Romina
Moaveni, Azadeh, FamilyMed
Mobilos, Sophia, FamilyMed
Moffatt, Michael H.
Mohabir, Nadira N., FamilyMed
Mohamed, Adel A A.
Mohamed, Iman D., FamilyMed
Mohan, Kanayalal D.
Mohareb, Michael M.
Moharir, Mahendranath D.
Mohindra, Ruchi N., FamilyMed(EM)
Mohsenibod, Hadi
Moloney, Michael A.
Monavvari, Arsalan, FamilyMed
Moody, Frederick J.
Moore, Jennifer
Moran, Andrew
Moran, Bryan C., FamilyMed
Morch, S. Ellen, FamilyMed
Morgentaler, Henry
Morin, Mario Y.
Moro, Elena
Morris, Sylvia
Morrow, A. Meyer
Mosaad, Sonia, FamilyMed
Moscarello, Mario A.
Moser, Andrea L., FamilyMed
Moulton, Carol-Anne E.
Mouzaki, Marialena
Mozes, Rami S.
Mueller, Daniel J.
Mueller, Wilhelm
Mueller-Wilm, Ingrid
Mugford, Johanna L., FamilyMed
Muhsen, Jafaar, FamilyMed
Muir, Sylvia K., FamilyMed
Mukherjee, Sutapa
Mulligan, Anna M.
Mungara, Sunil K., FamilyMed

Munk, Marla R., FamilyMed
Murata, Ariana M A., FamilyMed(EM)
Murji-Merali, Karim S.
Murphy, M. Claire C., FamilyMed
Murthy, Ravi
Murti, Mahdi
Myers, Jeffrey W., FamilyMed
Naghi, Alexandru
Nagji, Noorbegum
Nagy, Maria
Naidoo, Radhakrishnan P.
Naimer, Michelle S., FamilyMed
Nair, Krishnakumar
Naqvi, Raza M.
Naqvi, Syed M A.
Naraghi, Ali M F.
Narang, Indra
Naughton, Finola M.
Navarro, Christine, FamilyMed
Navarro Kunstmann, Oscar M.
Nawab, Naveed A., FamilyMed
Nazareth, A. John
Nevin, Robert D.
Nevo, Ori
Newman, Alice A.
Newman, Dana E., FamilyMed
Ng, Anita D., FamilyMed
Ng, Lung K.
Ng, Stephen, FamilyMed
Ng Fuk Chong, Nicholas, FamilyMed
Nguyen, Anh Tuan
Nguyen, Nam Anh, FamilyMed
Nguyen, Phuongbich
Nguyen, Quang V K., FamilyMed
Nguyen, Sy Hoang
Nguyen, Van Tuong
Nhan, Toan D.
Nicholson, James K.
Nickell, Leslie A., FamilyMed
Nieuwstraten, Paula, FamilyMed
Nijhawan, Rajni
Nikolsky, Victor, FamilyMed
Nikore, Vineet, FamilyMed(EM)
Nimjee, Tasleem M., FamilyMed
Nitti, Nicole M., FamilyMed(EM)
Nofech-Mozes, Sharon
Nohara, Naomi J., FamilyMed
Norris, Donald H.
Norwich, Kenneth H.
Novak, Marta
Novak, Tomas, FamilyMed(EM)
Nowaczynski, Mark J J., FamilyMed
Nunes-Vaz, Claire M., FamilyMed
Nutik, Melissa R., FamilyMed
O'Donoghue, Rory, FamilyMed
O'Halpin, Helen
O'Leary, James D.
Oandasan, Ivy F., FamilyMed
Obaji, Hind I A B.
Obaji, James, FamilyMed
Odame, Isaac
Offringa, Martin
Ola, Ebele I., FamilyMed
Olearczyk, Bohdan
Oliveira, Katia F.
Oliver, Catherine L.
Olsheski, Wayne R.
Omotani, Sandra
Opris, Alexandru A F.
Orbinski, James J.
Ordean, Alice, FamilyMed
Ossa Alemparte, Juan
Ostrow, Olivia A.
Ouchterlony, David P., FamilyMed
Ouchterlony, M. Donna, FamilyMed
Oudjhane, Kamaldine
Ovens, Howard J., FamilyMed(EM)
Owen, James R M., FamilyMed
Pagnoux, Christian
Pahuta, Zenon
Palmay, Christine A., FamilyMed
Palmert, Mark R.
Pampe, J. Robert
Pandya, Seema R.
Pannell, Dylan G., FamilyMed
Papadopoulos, Faez
Papanou, Alex
Papneja, Purti, FamilyMed
Paquette, Lise J., FamilyMed
Pariser, Pauline C., FamilyMed
Parnandi, Vandana N., FamilyMed

Parra, Dimitri A A.
Parshuram, Christopher S.
Parthab, Omkar, FamilyMed(EM)
Pascoe, Michael I.
Pasternak, Harvey S.
Pastia, Cristina I., FamilyMed(EM)
Patel, Anish, FamilyMed
Patkar, Shabari, FamilyMed
Patricio, Rodolfo V.
Patsios, Demetris A.
Paulaitis, Christina M M., FamilyMed
Paupst, James C.
Pawlowski, M. Danuta
Pearl, Monica C., FamilyMed
Pearlman, Jennifer B., FamilyMed
Peirovy, Javed
Pell, Tripler, FamilyMed
Peller, Andrew A.
Peranson, Judith S., FamilyMed
Perelman, Vsevolod S., FamilyMed(EM)
Perlin, Shawna F., FamilyMed
Perri, Giulia-Anna, FamilyMed
Persaud, Navindra, FamilyMed
Peters, Myta, FamilyMed
Petrov, Ivan
Petroz, Guy C.
Pham, Nam, FamilyMed
Phillips, Shauna D., FamilyMed
Philp, Lorraine B., FamilyMed
Photopoulos, George J., FamilyMed
Photopoulos, Peter, FamilyMed
Pieczonka, Rosalind M., FamilyMed
Piekos, Anna M., FamilyMed
Pietraszek, Bogdan Z.
Pietucha, Przemyslaw A., FamilyMed
Pilon, Edward W., FamilyMed(EM)
Pimlott, Nicholas J G., FamilyMed
Pinilla, J. Vicente
Pinter, Arnold
Pinto, Anthony J.
Pinto, Ivette R.
Pinto, Lucina M.
Piper, Dominique, FamilyMed
Platnick, Howard A.
Platzker, Daniel, FamilyMed
Podnieks, Mary Jane
Pollard, Alan
Pomer, Edward S.
Poon, Wendell Y C.
Porfiris, George S., FamilyMed(EM)
Porter, Bonita M., FamilyMed
Porter, Stephen C.
Porter, W. Ronald
Portugal, Francisco S.
Porwit, Anna
Pospisil, Caroline S.
Pothier, David D.
Potter, Jennifer A., FamilyMed
Pound, Jeremy I., FamilyMed
Powles, Kristina E., FamilyMed
Prabhudesai, Vikramaditya
Prewal, Hardeep K., FamilyMed
Price, Jason W B.
Pripstein, Laura P., FamilyMed
Proctor, Wendey R., FamilyMed
Provan, David C., FamilyMed
Puetz, Joel A., FamilyMed(EM)
Pulido, Analene F., FamilyMed
Pun, Cynthia, FamilyMed
Puri, Gaurav, FamilyMed(EM)
Pushie, Harold D H.
Qaadri, M. Shafiq
Qi, Victoria Z., FamilyMed
Queen, Daniel S., FamilyMed
Quejada, Michael J., FamilyMed
Quilter, Catherine M.
Quirante-Flora, Fe N.
Qureshy, Bushra
Rackal, Julia M., FamilyMed
Raddatz, Elaine, FamilyMed
Radhakrishnan, Arun K., FamilyMed
Rahim, Alya, FamilyMed
Raiman, Julian A J.
Rajamanickam, Sendhan
Rajani, Mohamed G V.
Rajaram, Nikhil, FamilyMed
Rakhshani, Nasimeh, FamilyMed
Ramji, Nasreen, FamilyMed
Ramji, Noor N W., FamilyMed
Rampes, Hagen

Ramroopsingh, Rickey B.
Rapson, Linda M.
Rashid, Meb, FamilyMed
Rathee, Seema R., FamilyMed
Raut, Abhishek, FamilyMed
Raveendran, Raviraj
Rawal, Shail
Ray, Morris N., FamilyMed
Razack, Jameel K I., FamilyMed
Razak, Fahad
Razavi, Amir H.
Razik, Roshan A.
Razvi, Nayyar K., FamilyMed
Read, James A., FamilyMed(EM)
Rebane, Ann K., FamilyMed
Redington, Andrew N.
Reece-Mills, Michelle N.
Reeve, Kate C., FamilyMed
Reich, Erin J., FamilyMed
Reid, Sarah J., FamilyMed
Rene, Sylvain A.
Reubeni-Zaltz, Renat, FamilyMed
Reynolds, Megan A., FamilyMed(EM)
Rezmovitz, Jeremy J., FamilyMed
Rhee, Steven J.
Ribeiro, Marcos
Richards, Douglas W.
Richardson, Janet A., FamilyMed(EM)
Richardson, Maria, FamilyMed
Richmond, Leslie
Ridley, Julia Z., FamilyMed
Rigamont, Andrea
Rindlisbacher, Timothy J.
Roberts, Michael C., FamilyMed
Robinson, Trevor I.
Robison, E. Jean, FamilyMed
Robson, Scott M., FamilyMed
Rocha, Tristana M., FamilyMed
Roche, Susan L.
Roche-Nagle, Michael G.
Rockman, Patricia F., FamilyMed
Rodrigues, M. Susana B.
Roehrl, Michael H A.
Rogalla, Patrik
Roscoe, Andrew J.
Rose, Norbert J.
Rose, Terence J.
Rose, Velene D.
Rose Sel, Winsley
Rosenberg, J. Joel
Rosenstein, David M., FamilyMed(EM)
Ross, Joel E., FamilyMed(EM)
Ross, Stephen G., FamilyMed
Rossiter, Lea M., FamilyMed
Rostom, Amr, FamilyMed
Rothman, Steven W., FamilyMed
Rouleau, Katherine D., FamilyMed
Roy, Eric, FamilyMed
Rozehnal, Jan
Rubenfeld, Gordon D.
Rubenstein, Warren H., FamilyMed
Rubin, Evelyn T., FamilyMed
Rubin, Gary M.
Rubino, Mary, FamilyMed
Ruderman, James, FamilyMed
Rudner, Howard L., FamilyMed
Ruggiero, Donato A.
Rumack, Eric R., FamilyMed
Rupert, Raymond H.
Sabra, Sally M M H.
Sachdeva, Preeti, FamilyMed
Sackin, H. David
Sadry, Dhun S., FamilyMed
Safar Zadeh, Elika
Sakiyama, Christine M., FamilyMed
Sakoor, Ahmed
Sakuls, Peter, FamilyMed
Salter, Michael
Samji, Amirali M.
Samokhvalov, Andriy V.
Sanchez-Guerrero, Francisco G.
Sandhu, Sharron
Sankey, Christopher L., FamilyMed(EM)
Santo, William D P., FamilyMed
Sarile, Dioscoro D C.
Sarma, Dipanka
Sarne, Andrew J., FamilyMed
Satei, Vali, FamilyMed
Sathi, Nandini, FamilyMed
Satok, David A., FamilyMed
Satok, Peter M.
Saunders, Megan A., FamilyMed
Sauret, Peter
Sawadsky, Bruce V., FamilyMed(EM)
Sayal, Arun K., FamilyMed(EM)
Scala, Salvatore J.
Scappatura, F. Philip
Scaranelo, Anabel M.
Schechter-Fi, Tal Tova
Schiralli, Giovanna M., FamilyMed
Schleifer, Maria R., FamilyMed
Schofield, Lee M., FamilyMed
Schofield, Michel M E.
Schram, Carrie A., FamilyMed
Schulze, Andreas H.
Schwandt, Michael, FamilyMed
Schwartz, Brian I., FamilyMed(EM)
Schwartz, Earl J.
Schwartz, Jacqueline R., FamilyMed
Schwartz, Martin B.
Schweihofer, Eckhart H C.
Scott, Elizabeth A F., FamilyMed
Scott, Robert H.
Seccareccia, Dori-Lynn M., FamilyMed(EM)
Seed, Michael T M.
Segal, Orit, FamilyMed
Segbefia, Catherine I.
Segel, George B.
Segel, Lawrence L.
Seid, Ying Suey
Seiden, Howard S., FamilyMed
Seidman, Sheryl G., FamilyMed
Selby, Peter L., FamilyMed
Selzner, Markus
Selzner-Malekkiani, Nazia
Sem, Francis W C., FamilyMed(EM)
Serra, Stefano
Seruga, Bostjan
Seth, Arun K.
Seth, Asha L.
Shabash, Osama M., FamilyMed
Shabsove, Harold B.
Shafir, M. Sharon, FamilyMed
Shahid, Azmeh
Shapiro, Gary
Shapiro, Jennifer S., FamilyMed
Sharma, Pratibhasri A.
Sharma, Shiv R., FamilyMed
Sharman, Suneel, FamilyMed
Sharpe, Sally A.
Shaul, Randi C.
Shaw, Sarah N., FamilyMed
Shechtman, Grant L., FamilyMed
Shedletzky, Carolyn S., FamilyMed
Sheiner, Jamie B., FamilyMed
Sheldon, Karyn R., FamilyMed
Shelley, A S. Douglas
Shelton, Dominick M., FamilyMed(EM)
Shen, Kay, FamilyMed
Shepherd, Susan M., FamilyMed
Sheps, Jordana L., FamilyMed
Sheps, Rachel L., FamilyMed(EM)
Sheth, Hinal, FamilyMed
Shetty, Rakshay
Shi, Dawn D., FamilyMed
Shields, Yehudi P.
Shin, Whun Yong
Shindman, Judith A.
Shochat, Gina, FamilyMed
Shojania, Kaveh G.
Shorser, S. Ronald
Showler, Adrienne J.
Shrott, Barry H.
Shuchman, Miriam
Shukla, Hemen P., FamilyMed
Shum, Andrew S C.
Shuman, Mira R., FamilyMed
Shupak, Michael
Shyamal, Gayathri P., FamilyMed
Siddall, Hugh A.
Siddiq, Nayeema
Siddiqui, Naveed T.
Sieminowski, Tammy E., FamilyMed
Silva, Coeliflor D.
Silver, Brian
Silver, David M., FamilyMed
Silver, Eric S., FamilyMed
Silver, Jeffrey S., FamilyMed
Silverman, Mark J., FamilyMed
Simmonds, Wrensford F.
Simpson, Alexander I F.
Sinclair, Douglas E., FamilyMed(EM)
Sinclair Mills, Christa, FamilyMed
Singh, Birinder, FamilyMed
Singh, Kirandeep
Singh, Parul, FamilyMed(EM)
Singh, Ravinderpal
Singh, Sandhya K V.
Singwi, Amita, FamilyMed
Siren, Kenneth P J., FamilyMed(EM)
Sirianni, Giovanna, FamilyMed
Siriwardena, Komudi P.
Sirna, Salvatore
Sit, Sze Wan, FamilyMed
Siu, King Fun, FamilyMed
Sivananthan, Shankar
Sivapalasingam, Nihilarani
Skalenda, Patrick J., FamilyMed
Skarratt, Kevin H., FamilyMed(EM)
Skeate, Robert C.
Skelton, Geoffrey G., FamilyMed
Skocylak, George W.
Slessarev, Marat
Sliwin, Fay R., FamilyMed
Sliwowicz, Kevin, FamilyMed(EM)
Slodkowska, Elzbieta
Slutsky, Arthur S.
Small, Elizabeth A.
Smart, Victoria M S., FamilyMed
Smile, Sharon C.
Smith, Andrew J K.
Smith, Beverley J., FamilyMed
Smith, David R F., FamilyMed
Smith, Donald A., FamilyMed
Smith, Graham H R., FamilyMed
Smith, Ira A., FamilyMed
Smith, Kiara K., FamilyMed
Smith, Patricia L., FamilyMed
Smith, Roger M L.
Smula, Vaclav
Smylie, Janet K., FamilyMed
Snider, Bernice E.
Snow, Debbie G., FamilyMed
So, Boris, FamilyMed
Soare, C. Alexander, FamilyMed
Sobers, Godfrey
Soboloff, Michael J., FamilyMed
Sodhi, Sumeet K., FamilyMed
Sohal, Barjinder S., FamilyMed
Sokol, Lorne W., FamilyMed
Solano Salazar, Tanya G.
Solway, Eric W., FamilyMed
Somaiah, Nayana T., FamilyMed
Soman, Teesta B.
Somers, Andrea D., FamilyMed(EM)
Somers, Gino R.
Somerville, Susan E.
Sommer, Leeor Z., FamilyMed(EM)
Somska, Elena
Soneji, Prachi, FamilyMed
Soni, Ebrahim, FamilyMed
Soo, Stephanie M., FamilyMed
Sood, Alok Pal, FamilyMed
Sood, Danesh, FamilyMed
Sood, Priya D., FamilyMed
Sooknanan, Avita, FamilyMed
Soong, Christine, FamilyMed
Spaner, Donna-Mary S., FamilyMed
Spano Greco, Giuseppe
Sparrow, Andrew K., FamilyMed
Spence, Catherine A.
Spithoff, Sheryl M., FamilyMed
Spring, Elise S.
Srinivas, Sathish
Srivastava, Anita, FamilyMed
Stables, Sabrina M.
Stachon, Andrea C.
Stachula, Robert B J.
Stalinska, Teresa M.
Staunton, Marie
Steele, Leah S., FamilyMed
Stefou, Vasia
Stein, Nolan-Paul A.
Steinberg, Hedy, FamilyMed
Steinberg, Leah J., FamilyMed
Steinegg, Cathleen M.
Steinegger, Cathleen M.
Steinhart, Norman S.
Stendardo, Vincenzo R., FamilyMed
Stephenson, Elizabeth A.
Stephenson, Jenny P.
Stewart, Ann M., FamilyMed
Stoller, Jacqueline S., FamilyMed
Stone, Laura D., FamilyMed
Strank, Randall T., FamilyMed
Strigler, Stephen, FamilyMed
Stubbs, Barbara E., FamilyMed
Stulberg, Jennifer R., FamilyMed
Sud, Abhimanyu, FamilyMed
Sue-A-Quan, Andrew I., FamilyMed(EM)
Sugiyama, I F H. James
Sukkar, Ghassan A A.
Sullivan, Patrick J., FamilyMed
Sullivan, William F., FamilyMed
Sullovey, Carl A., FamilyMed
Sulyma, Lelia Y L.
Sun, Clement K.
Sundaram, Sujatha, FamilyMed
Sung, Yong Kyung
Sutton, Neal S.
Svoboda, Tomislav, FamilyMed
Swaminathan, Aparna, FamilyMed
Swaminathan, Sunita, FamilyMed(EM)
Swartz, David A.
Swirsky, Karen N., FamilyMed
Switakowski, Peter K., FamilyMed(EM)
Sykes, Lucinda J.
Syms, Jonathan B., FamilyMed(EM)
Szabo, Michael S., FamilyMed(EM)
Szilagyi, Alison J., FamilyMed
Szpindel, Isaac I E.
Szul, J. Michael, FamilyMed
Tabassum, Farah J., FamilyMed
Tabori, Uri Y.
Tai, Emelda M.
Tai, Lucas
Tajirian, Tania, FamilyMed
Tam, Robert C.
Tam, Sydney P., FamilyMed
Tam, Thomas C.
Taman, Sara M., FamilyMed
Tambasco, Domenica, FamilyMed
Tan, Allan, FamilyMed
Tan, Chin Kien
Tan, Teng Hin
Tan, Thuang Kim
Tannenbaum, David W., FamilyMed
Tarman, Vera I., FamilyMed
Tarshis, Tanya J.
Taylor, James, FamilyMed
Taylor, Katherine L.
Taylor, Martin
Taylor, Ronald W.
Taylor, Shira G., FamilyMed
Teku, Edo, FamilyMed
Telner, Deanna E., FamilyMed
Teo, Astra L., FamilyMed
Teo, Su-Ting, FamilyMed
Teplitsky, Yoella, FamilyMed
Tepper, Joshua D., FamilyMed
Tepper, Stephen J., FamilyMed
Ter Kuile, Sonia A., FamilyMed
Theman, Kirsten D., FamilyMed
Therapondos, Georgios P.
Thomas, Christin, FamilyMed
Thomas, Jill M., FamilyMed
Thomas, Mary, FamilyMed
Thompson, Gregory K.
Thompson, Judith A., FamilyMed
Thyagu, Santhosh
Ticktin, Stephen J.
Tiedemann, Rodger E.
Tilley, David A.
Tillmann, Mary P., FamilyMed
Tirkos, S. Sam, FamilyMed
Tisher, Carolyn R., FamilyMed
To, Howard K H., FamilyMed
To, K H. Kent, FamilyMed
Toledano, Daniel R.
Tomlinson, Robert C K.
Tommasini, Robert, FamilyMed
Toofani, Roya
Toong, Ying Lai H.
Topp, Bruce R., FamilyMed
Torbin, Lauren B.
Torlakovic, Emina
Toubassi, Diana, FamilyMed
Touma, Zahi N.
Toussaint, M. Junie B.
Townsley, Carol A., FamilyMed
Trambakoulos, Dimitra, FamilyMed
Tran, Van-Chung, FamilyMed
Trinos, Baieruss M., FamilyMed
Truscott, Bruce O.
Tsang, Albert H., FamilyMed
Tsatsaronis, Eleftheria
Tsui, Andrew K W., FamilyMed
Tsuneyos, Hiroshi
Tu, Karen, FamilyMed
Tung, Frances Y., FamilyMed
Tunzi, Christina R., FamilyMed
Turchin, Kathrin M., FamilyMed
Turk, Allison H., FamilyMed
Turner, Suzanne D., FamilyMed
Tzakas, Peter, FamilyMed
Uddin, Fatima, FamilyMed
Uetrecht, Jack P.
Uhlig, Eric L P.
Uxa, Amar K.
Vadasz, Gabriel A., FamilyMed
Vaezi, Aref, FamilyMed
Vaidya, Shailla, FamilyMed(EM)
Vaidyanathan, Sammy, FamilyMed(EM)
Valadka, Mikas A.
Vale, Noah A., FamilyMed
Valentinis, Alissia R., FamilyMed
Van Assche, Gert A A.
Van Dyk, Jessie
Van Praet, Oliver M., FamilyMed(EM)
Van Schoor, J. Tinie, FamilyMed
Van den Akker, Machiel T.
Vanaselja, Reet, FamilyMed
Vardar, Gonul
Vari, Barbara J., FamilyMed
Varma, Gokuldas R.
Varner, Catherine E., FamilyMed(EM)
Varney, Ian G., FamilyMed
Vasa, Priya P., FamilyMed
Vavougios, James, FamilyMed
Venier, Elisa A.
Verbeeten, Yvonne D., FamilyMed
Verduyn, Ashley M., FamilyMed
Verduyn, Robin F., FamilyMed
Verma, Manisha, FamilyMed
Verma, Sarita, FamilyMed
Verrilli, David V., FamilyMed
Vicus, Danielle L.
Vilaghy, Miklos I.
Vira, Farzana
Vizhul, Andrey I.
Vlahovich, Josip
Vo, Thoi Hen
Voaden, M E. Carol
Voigtlander-Bolz, Julia I M.
Vowinckel, Erika A M., FamilyMed
Vozis, Constantin G.
Vu, David D V.
Vujnovic, Predrag
Waern, Bryn F.
Wagner, Cheryl A., FamilyMed
Wai, Amy C K., FamilyMed
Waks, Joshua A., FamilyMed
Wallace, Anne A E., FamilyMed
Walman, Noah, FamilyMed
Walters, Anupama A., FamilyMed
Walters, Lawrence T., FamilyMed
Walters, Lawrence T., FamilyMed
Walters, Thomas D.
Wang, Kai-Yun
Wang, Yun-Lin
Wansbrough, Michael C T., FamilyMed(EM)
Ward, Richard
Warden, Sarah J., FamilyMed
Warren, Bethel F., FamilyMed
Wasowicz, Marcin
Wassenaar, Willem
Wasserman, Jonathan D.
Watson, William J., FamilyMed
Watts, Kingsley F., FamilyMed
Waxman, Marvin, FamilyMed
Weatherhead, Michael F.
Weber, Linda J., FamilyMed
Weinberg, Robert B., FamilyMed
Weinstein, Gary S.
Weinstock, Michael S.
Weisbaum, Harry
Weisdorf, Thea M., FamilyMed

Weiss, Andrea M., FamilyMed
Wells, Anthony R.
Weltman, Glen L., FamilyMed
Wengle, Larry M.
Wentlandt, Kirsten, FamilyMed
Werb, Solomon M.
Westlake, Susan J., FamilyMed
Weyman, Karen R., FamilyMed
Wheatcroft, Mark D.
Whelan, Ciara M., FamilyMed
White, Juliet, FamilyMed
White, Laurie J.
Whitehead, Cynthia R., FamilyMed
Whitehead, Katherine E A., FamilyMed(EM)
Whitlock, James A.
Whitten-Stovall, Richard F.
Whylie, Barbara
Wideman, Anne, FamilyMed
Widjaja, Elysa
Widman, Jody K., FamilyMed
Wiebe, Dale J P., FamilyMed
Wiebe, Miriam J., FamilyMed
Wiedmeyer, Heather M., FamilyMed
Wiesenthal, Marvin M.
Wijayasinghe, Sheila, FamilyMed
Wildschut, Jason A.
Wiley, Joseph C.
Williams, Daphne T., FamilyMed
Williams, Evelyn M., FamilyMed
Williams, Paula B.
Wilson, Karen M.
Wilson, Lynn M., FamilyMed
Winer, Laura H R.
Winsor, Craig E.
Wintemute, Kimberly J., FamilyMed
Wolever, Thomas M S.
Wolff, Bryan C., FamilyMed(EM)
Wong, Albert S C.
Wong, Albert S H.
Wong, Andrew C H.
Wong, Angela S C., FamilyMed
Wong, Daniel D.
Wong, David M C., FamilyMed
Wong, Diane C., FamilyMed
Wong, Gail K.
Wong, Ivan F L.
Wong, Joseph Y K.
Wong, Karen, FamilyMed
Wong, Keith F.
Wong, Patrick, FamilyMed
Wong, Philip E.
Wong, Sian E., FamilyMed
Wong, Tat Hang
Wong, Vivian K., FamilyMed
Wong, Wellington P.
Wood, Lorraine E., FamilyMed
Woolhouse, Susan J., FamilyMed
Woollam, Christopher J.
Woolley, Brenda A.
Workentin, Kevin M., FamilyMed
Wozniak, Paul R.
Wray, Heather E., FamilyMed
Wright, Alison F C., FamilyMed
Wu, Melinda Y., FamilyMed
Wu, Sibra S C.
Wyman, Jennifer J., FamilyMed
Wyman, Roy J., FamilyMed
Wynnychuk, Lesia A.
Wytsma, Julia L., FamilyMed
Xie, Edward C., FamilyMed(EM)
Yang, Iwan, FamilyMed
Yanofsky, Michael J.
Yap, Stephanie T M., FamilyMed
Yasufuku, Kazuhiro
Yau, Anthony P C.
Yau, Frank C O.
Yeung, Adela K T.
Ying, Irene, FamilyMed
Yolles, Linda A., FamilyMed
Yoong, Kevin, FamilyMed
Young, David S F.
Young, Deidre C., FamilyMed
Young, Jennifer S.
Young, John G.
Young, Sherylan, FamilyMed
Yu, Herbert D.
Yu, Jessica J., FamilyMed
Yu, Ming, FamilyMed
Yue-Tang, Bonnie W M.
Yung, Stephen Y W.
Zaarour, Christian E.
Zachariadis, George P.
Zacharin, Laura S., FamilyMed
Zalan, Paul R.
Zaman, Kamruz, FamilyMed
Zeldin, Susan G., FamilyMed
Zeller, Jeanne T.
Zepic, Ines
Zerhouni Abdouh, Siham
Zevin, Boris
Zhang, Ting
Zhao, Xiu Chang, FamilyMed
Zimcik, Heather L., FamilyMed
Zimm, Abraham J.
Zimmerman, Harvey S.
Zitsow, Jason H., FamilyMed(EM)
Zlochower, David B.
Zurowski, Wojciech J.

TOTTENHAM

Carroll, Cory J., FamilyMed
D'Addario, Denise
Hurst, Margaret M.
Lussier, Dominique
Nishikawa, Richard A., FamilyMed
Robson, Michael
Ward, Alan E.

TRENTON

Blackmore, Elizabeth J.
Bonn, John M.
Bowler, Adrian P.
Chahine, Danielle A., FamilyMed
Cooke, Donald W.
Duchaine, Sylvain
Feltham, Ian C., FamilyMed
Gerred, R. Kent
Gilic, Filip, FamilyMed(EM)
Gousseau, Helene, FamilyMed
Griffin, Glenn H., FamilyMed
Gugliotta, Donato
Hayman, Christopher, FamilyMed
Healy, Conor M.
Iny, Robert, FamilyMed
Kaladeen, Stephen M.
Mahmood, Adeel, FamilyMed
Perera, Ransri F., FamilyMed(EM)
Prasad, Sharada
Reynolds, Kenneth J.
Shirriff, Michael D.

TWEED

Moher, Kelly L B., FamilyMed
Quinn, Andrew R., FamilyMed

UNIONVILLE

Andrews, D. Katheen
Bechbache, Rafik R., FamilyMed
Bugdahn, Margaret B., FamilyMed
Carson, James D., FamilyMed
Chow, Y B. Dominic, FamilyMed
Gill, Kimberlee D., FamilyMed
Kara-Shariff, Shain
Lodenquai, Jeffrey W.
Lui, Kim C.
Nowak, Mary B., FamilyMed
Oda, Ronald G., FamilyMed
Tsao, Smiley G S., FamilyMed

UXBRIDGE

Bryon, Terry F.
Damus, A. Michael, FamilyMed
Doobay, Calesh D., FamilyMed
Doobay, Dharmeandra, FamilyMed
Husain, Aisha T., FamilyMed
Jensen, Carlye A., FamilyMed(EM)
Mahadevan, Varagunan, FamilyMed
Marlow, Bernard A., FamilyMed
Porter, Gail S.
St John, A. Brian
Suh, Daniel, FamilyMed
Wilson, Jennifer L., FamilyMed(EM)

VAL CARON

Charette, Yves G., FamilyMed
Fredette, Paul P., FamilyMed
Malette, Paul M J.
Nkut, Alfred, FamilyMed

VANIER

Adamowski, Susan
Bouffard, J P. Michel
Caddigan, Deborah M.
Chan, Vincent
D'Aoust-Bernard, Chantal, FamilyMed
Gauthier, Andre L., FamilyMed
Kratka, Lida
Labbe, Lionel J.
Ladora, Marie-Josee
Lafleche, Francois E J., FamilyMed
Lee, Mabel M F., FamilyMed
Morrissey, Jean-Pierre P.
Pelletier, Anne-Marie, FamilyMed
Pharand, Marielle R P.
Poliquin, Sophie A., FamilyMed
Roy, Carolyne D., FamilyMed
Seguin, Jean J., FamilyMed
Smith, Edward J.
Williams, Carole S.

VAUGHAN

Abdulali, Mufaddal
Alo, Nadin, FamilyMed
Bercuson, Judith M., FamilyMed
Buu, Michael M., FamilyMed
Douglas, Simone A., FamilyMed
Firoz, Abu, FamilyMed
Garces, Luis M., FamilyMed
Iskander, Mamdouh A S., FamilyMed
Jespersen, Denise M., FamilyMed
Moussadji, Jack S., FamilyMed
Nakamura, Liane S.
Parkin, Doriana M., FamilyMed
Sadik, Zaki K., FamilyMed
Sanandaji, Khashayar, FamilyMed
Seegobin, Ramesh, FamilyMed
Sen, Roger I.
Shams, Merajuddin, FamilyMed
Shimanovsky, Ludmila A., FamilyMed
Small, Stephen J., FamilyMed
Soto De Machat, Grace G., FamilyMed
Talib, Ashnoor S., FamilyMed
Tang, Lan
Toffoli-Zadra, Nadia D., FamilyMed
Tran, Teresa B C., FamilyMed
Uljanitski, Sofia, FamilyMed
Venchiarutti, Nadia, FamilyMed
Wein, Cheryl R., FamilyMed
Wong, Stephanie W., FamilyMed
Yousif, Samad S., FamilyMed
Zatzman, Ian R.

VERMILION BAY

Gagnon, Yvon-Rene, FamilyMed

VERNER

Bourgault, Klere, FamilyMed

VERONA

Dempsey, Laurel J.
Oglaza, Piotr P., FamilyMed

VIRGIL

Adams, Julian F.
Jimoh, Olubukola, FamilyMed
Manser, Courtney A., FamilyMed
Ricciardi, Luigi T., FamilyMed

WALKERTON

Al Qaseer, Ziad N F., FamilyMed
Bajurny, Gary
Creighton, Robert J.
Gill, T. Michael D.
McArthur, H. Susan, FamilyMed
McArthur, Paul E., FamilyMed
Ponesse, David

WALLACEBURG

Atoe, Dennis E., FamilyMed
Belbin, Donald E., FamilyMed
Dudley, Emer M.
Mayo, Robert E., FamilyMed
McElligott, Michael A., FamilyMed
Pepper, Dale J.
Saxena, Will
Serezo, Paterno C.

WASAGA BEACH

Amundson, Heather J., FamilyMed
Bowman, Caroline, FamilyMed
Boyd, Alyssa, FamilyMed
Brakel, Gillian, FamilyMed
Greyling, Johannes C.
Holloway, Peter J., FamilyMed
Kitai, Therasa A., FamilyMed
Monte, Myrna M., FamilyMed
Prebble, Brenda L., FamilyMed
Singh, Amardip, FamilyMed
Van Der Merwe, Marius
Watkin, Daniel

WATERDOWN

Boyd, Hugh F., FamilyMed
Brunton, Jane A., FamilyMed
Cross, Randolph G., FamilyMed
Faught, James W., FamilyMed
Graham, Janet E., FamilyMed
Greiner, Violetta, FamilyMed
Imbulgoda, Manel R., FamilyMed
Jones, Angela M., FamilyMed
McCord, Phyllis A., FamilyMed
Smart, John E.
Thakersee, Bhavna K., FamilyMed
Wilson, Patricia I., FamilyMed

WATERFORD

Abbott, Laura L., FamilyMed
Callery, Christopher J.
Ezeanya, Mary Angeleen, FamilyMed
Millar-Book, Wendy D., FamilyMed
Peeris, Sumithra A.

WATERLOO

Amin, Surendra, FamilyMed
Anderson, Mary C.
Bain, John
Bajaj, Renu, FamilyMed(EM)
Ballantyne, Robert H., FamilyMed
Bates, Douglas R., FamilyMed
Bell, Ruth E.
Benedet, Lynda, FamilyMed
Bennett, Angus
Burk, Keith W.
Chand, Pankaj P., FamilyMed(EM)
Chettimada, A. Kumar S., FamilyMed
Chow, Theresa C B.
D'Souza, Ryan, FamilyMed
Dawood, M. Farouk, FamilyMed
Duke, Marin J., FamilyMed
Gajewski, Martin, FamilyMed
Garboll, G. Michael
Grant, David R.
Guzar, Rebecca L., FamilyMed
Hoh, Erin S Y., FamilyMed
Jhaveri, Faeza, FamilyMed
Jugdave, Yajna
Keefe, Kathrene M A.
Kugler, Pierre E A., FamilyMed
Landy, Patrick M P M., FamilyMed
Lang, Francis K L.
Larton, Heather A.
Leask, Barbara E.
Lee, Robert K W.
MacMillan, Douglas G.
McLaughlin, Lois Y., FamilyMed
Milne, Darryl D.
Muirhead, William M., FamilyMed
Neary, John M., FamilyMed
Nikolic, Ana, FamilyMed
Pannozzo, Gino
Papastergiou, Derek L., FamilyMed
Parry, Debra J., FamilyMed
Peckan, Karen M., FamilyMed
Peet, Jonathan M., FamilyMed
Pitre, Theresa J., FamilyMed
Proschek, Richard
Quinn, Dana L., FamilyMed
Rainham, David C.
Robinson, R. Jane, FamilyMed
Rondilla, F. Michael A., FamilyMed
Roy, Deborah, FamilyMed
Rueffer, Peter K.
Saban, Shireen S.
Sandhu, Navneet K.
Schaffenburg, Jocelyn E R., FamilyMed
Schumacher, Barbara D I.
Sehl, Michael J.
Singh, Harneet
Sofronova, Elionora P., FamilyMed
Stecho, Terence J.
Takacs, Jennifer M L., FamilyMed
Wilhelm, Julia E., FamilyMed
Winfield, Doris J., FamilyMed
Wlodarczyk, Stanislaw R.
Wright, Scott R., FamilyMed
Wright, Stefanie T B., FamilyMed
Yoo, Jennifer W J., FamilyMed
Youssef, Elham A A., FamilyMed
Yu, Chun Ming, FamilyMed

WAWA

Berger, Samuel
Cotterill, Michael E., FamilyMed
De Foa, J. Lance
Kirby, Erle J., FamilyMed
Murray, John A., FamilyMed
Oberai, Anjali, FamilyMed
Stamler, Christopher J., FamilyMed
Thomas, Anthony D.
Weinstein, Julie L., FamilyMed

WELLAND

Al-Husari, Muhanad A J., FamilyMed
Alberts, Hendrik, FamilyMed
Alberts, Melissa, FamilyMed
Aleksiejuk, Janusz
Ali, Mohamed
Arif, Beenish, FamilyMed
Bak, David M.
Balhous, Wassim, FamilyMed
Barker, Joanne, FamilyMed
Braithwaite-Walton, Heather J., FamilyMed
Brown, Nancy-Shira E., FamilyMed
De Wet, Rene, FamilyMed
De Wit, Christoffel, FamilyMed
Fakim, Abid
Gibbons Gomez, Paul, FamilyMed
Goswami, Rupashi, FamilyMed
Grant, K. Gordon J., FamilyMed(EM)
Hogg, L. Craig
Iyer, Sugantha P.
James, David M., FamilyMed(EM)
Keffer, Glen W.
Kouros, Evangelos P.
Kundi, Anjali, FamilyMed
Kundi, Kusum, FamilyMed
Kundi, Pran J., FamilyMed
Lamb, David J.
Lawrence, Stephen S.
Lovegrove, Michael A.
Luterman, Maynard, FamilyMed
Magee, Robert A.

Malak, Monzer, FamilyMed
Mueller, Jennifer L., FamilyMed
Nova, Natalie, FamilyMed
O'Donnell, John T.
Pauls, C. John, FamilyMed
Rana, Shreyas K., FamilyMed
Sayed, Ebrahim
Shah, Vinod H.
Sulikowski, Angelina, FamilyMed
Van Der Walt, Louiza, FamilyMed
Van Sittert, Lambert W., FamilyMed(EM)
Zides, Colin I.

WELLESLEY

Finn, Brian R., FamilyMed
Luscott, Kathleen S J., FamilyMed
Moore, Kimberly
Snider, Hannah L., FamilyMed
Van Heiningen, Willem P J., FamilyMed

WELLINGTON

Cluett, Helen C., FamilyMed
Scrivens, Blair A., FamilyMed

WEST LORNE

Grigore, Emil-Vasile
MacDonald, K. Yvonne, FamilyMed
Mardell, Kevin, FamilyMed

WESTON

Rodgerson, James S.

WHEATLEY

Eaton, David F.

WHITBY

Adil, Aliya, FamilyMed
Al-Habib, Saed S.
Alem, Atalay E.
Bardai, Sadrudin
Bhatia, Jaspreet K., FamilyMed
Bock, Allan R.
Boulos, Youssef R., FamilyMed
Burwell, G. Scott, FamilyMed
Cecutti, William A.
Chang, Walter W K.
Charania, Naveen N., FamilyMed
Chaudhari, Prashant A.
Cohen, Stephen S., FamilyMed
Copeland, Charles L H., FamilyMed
D'Angelo, Anthony J.
Dahman, Jehad
Daiter, Kenneth A., FamilyMed
Davis, Donna N.
De Billy, Michel, FamilyMed
De Croos, J. Annson B.
Durrani, Ahmad I., FamilyMed
Eapen, Lisbi P J V.
Fan-Lun, Paul H K.
Firouzabadi-Dashti, Roya, FamilyMed
Flock, Traudl E., FamilyMed
Gaal, Judit M.
Gertler, Michael M.
Ghobadian, M. Reza, FamilyMed
Girlan, Larisa, FamilyMed
Gorja, Juliana, FamilyMed
Haider, Erum, FamilyMed
Hsieh, Daniel T T.
Huculak, George E.
Ibsen, David G B., FamilyMed
Jaciw, George A.
Jagan, Nigel N.
Jauhari, Vinod, FamilyMed
Jefremova, Ljudmilla, FamilyMed
Ke, Warren J.
Kwan, Francis S Y.
Laroche, P A. Paul, FamilyMed
Lee, John S., FamilyMed
Lee Sang, Ivan A.
Lee Sang, Katherine A.
Liu, Chongen, FamilyMed
Lo, Hanson K C.
Lubczynski, Celina M., FamilyMed
MacLennan, Virginia L.
Major, M. Gregory, FamilyMed
Malek, Batu
McAlister, Nazlin K., FamilyMed
McIntosh, Glenda J., FamilyMed
McKechnie, Catherine M., FamilyMed
McMaster, Robert G.
Mendonca, Janet A., FamilyMed
Michael, Antoinette A., FamilyMed
Mikhail, Mamdouh T., FamilyMed
Naassan, Natalie C., FamilyMed
Nagel, Daniel P., FamilyMed
Nathoo, Munir F A.
Parmar, Varinderjit S.
Percy, William G.
Pileggi, Lee A.
Pinto, Artur C F., FamilyMed
Qadeer, Shehla, FamilyMed
Randhawa, Manjinder S.
Reed, Brian A.
Reichman, Peeter H.
Seltzer, Eric C.
Szendrey, James J., FamilyMed
Tahir, Ferhana, FamilyMed(EM)
Taylor, Pamela L., FamilyMed
Teodorescu, I. Valentina, FamilyMed
Treilhard, John B.
Wu, Stephen T W., FamilyMed

WHITE RIVER

Velicaria, Laing P.

WHITNEY

Krawczyk, Jan W., FamilyMed

WIARTON

Barker, Eric J., FamilyMed
Barrett, Jeffrey R., FamilyMed
Grewal, Shiv Pal, FamilyMed
Grigg, Megan J., FamilyMed
Lothstein, Daniel B., FamilyMed
McNamara, Laura A., FamilyMed(EM)
Uffen, Kenneth F., FamilyMed
Van Dorp, Johannes
Van Dorp, Nelvia M D., FamilyMed

WINCHESTER

Bailey, Jason M., FamilyMed
Bhagirath, Vikas C., FamilyMed
Burke, John
Darbyshire, Katherine R., FamilyMed
Flowers, David J.
Gil, Lucas, FamilyMed
Kaethler, Yvonne E., FamilyMed
Legault, Teisha, FamilyMed
Moussette, Patricia A., FamilyMed
Prins, Henry B., FamilyMed
Spencer, Kevin D., FamilyMed
Steele, Bart E., FamilyMed
Su, Charles H., FamilyMed(EM)
Yang, Marjorie L., FamilyMed(EM)

WINDSOR

Aboobaker, Suleman
Abu-Rashed, Kamal A.
Adekoya, David A., FamilyMed(EM)
Aggarwal, Seema, FamilyMed
Ahmed, Tahira S.
Aktas, Murat
Al-Tatari, Hossam M.
Alamelhuda, Elsayed E., FamilyMed
Albus, Wayne W., FamilyMed
Amster, Solomon L.
Anand, Sondekere K.
Andary, Leesha Y.
Aoun, Lawrence, FamilyMed
Athar, Humera
Atton, A. Lance
Atwood, Lenisa J., FamilyMed(EM)
Azad, Jason K., FamilyMed
Azharuddin, Tahera, FamilyMed
Azuh, Victor I.
Bacon, Mark J., FamilyMed
Barisic, Dusan
Barnard, Thomas, FamilyMed(EM)
Basker, Rajasekar
Bastianon, William A.
Basur, Roshan L.
Beattie, Beverly A.
Bekasiak, P. Antoni
Berecz, Steven J.
Bhatt, Gunvantrai J.
Bhullar, Harbir S., FamilyMed
Blass, Maria M.
Bleyendaal, Argia, FamilyMed
Blue, Christopher, FamilyMed
Boismier, Jenny L., FamilyMed
Boyer, David K., FamilyMed(EM)
Bradford, Paul, FamilyMed(EM)
Bricker, David J., FamilyMed
Bridgeo, David B., FamilyMed
Britten, Heather F., FamilyMed
Brown, Lanying
Bugwandin, Suria K.
Butler, Geoffrey W.
Cameron, Robert
Cargill, Darren C., FamilyMed
Carlini, Ryan J., FamilyMed
Carom, Donald P.
Chaker, Ahmad M A., FamilyMed
Chan, Wayne W K.
Chand, Pavanjeet, FamilyMed
Chevalier, Marguerite B., FamilyMed
Choppa, Sailaja, FamilyMed
Chopra, Raj K.
Chow, Roxana S.
Chung For Yuen, Kim F.
Clarke, Henry C N.
Coates, John R G., FamilyMed
Cohen, Jeffrey J.
Cox, John O., FamilyMed
Dattilo, Joseph
Day, John C., FamilyMed
De Marco, Francis S.
Dedumets, Paul
Dennison, Jeffrey, FamilyMed
Diklich, Roy R.
Doyle, Sharon, FamilyMed
Draisey, Rebecca M.
Drake, Robert, FamilyMed
Drkulec, Frank
Echlin, Thomas H., FamilyMed
El-Fakharany, Mohamed M.
El-Tatari, Bassam, FamilyMed
Evoy, Olga L., FamilyMed
Faisal, Shazia, FamilyMed
Farago, Peter J.
Favot, Dean
Fedoruk, James
Ferasol, Jairie D., FamilyMed
Figaro, Alexandra O., FamilyMed
Fisher, David T.
Fortuna, Henry, FamilyMed
Gall, James M., FamilyMed
Gallow, Mark D.
Ghafoor, Akmal
Gibb, Robert A.
Giddings, Gordon R., FamilyMed
Greenaway, John R., FamilyMed
Gresko, Peter A.
Guindon, Noemi
Gupta, Rasna
Halonen, Mark A.
Hamdan, Helena, FamilyMed
Hammer, Antony
Hammond, Lynda C., FamilyMed
Hanson, B. Margaret
Hanson, Paul R.
Hawkeswood, Michael L.
Heimann, G. Allen
Hermiz, Fadia, FamilyMed
Herzenberg, Martin A.
Hoffman, Thomas M., FamilyMed
Huidovici, Elia, FamilyMed
Hurst, Jody L., FamilyMed
Hurst, Randall R.
Hussain, Mohammed T., FamilyMed
Ing, Gary
Irwin, Michael E., FamilyMed
Issley, Steven B., FamilyMed
Jaamour, Mohammad
Jaco, Jennifer M., FamilyMed
Jansen, Lisa E., FamilyMed
Jasey, Kathleen A., FamilyMed
Jing, Nin, FamilyMed
Johnston, Charlene F., FamilyMed
Joshi, Harshad P.
Kanjeekal, S. Rajh
Kapoor, Pankaj V.
Karnik, Vikas V.
Kassas, Emad
Keshavjee, Yasmin, FamilyMed
Kinaia, Ban M., FamilyMed
Kirk, Gary M.
Kisiel, Ursula
Kizis, Saulius J.
Klassen, Reginald A.
Koo, Catherine Y.
Koobair, Sandhya, FamilyMed
Koutelas, Nikolaos, FamilyMed
Koutras, Nicholas P.
Krayacich, Nicholas C.
Kruba, Richard
Kuhlmann, Peter A.
Kupeyan, Kristen A., FamilyMed
Kuprowski, Gary N.
Laba-Kaczmarec, Jessica A.
Lall, Vipin, FamilyMed
Lamont, J. Barry
Lee, Bonnie P Y., FamilyMed(EM)
Leung, Michael C C., FamilyMed
Levy, Donald M., FamilyMed(EM)
Liang, Hsien-Cheng, FamilyMed
Lo, Michael K K.
Loaring, Jaimie M., FamilyMed
Loebach, Paul M., FamilyMed
Logan, Charlotte A.
Lubanski, Martin S.
MacKinnon, Michael A.
Makinde, Olumide A., FamilyMed
Maples, Gail A., FamilyMed
Maraj, Vikesh, FamilyMed
Marchuk, Yuri
Markovic, Ruth E.
McCaffrey, Lisa M., FamilyMed
McFarlane, Charles A.
McKay, Robert G R., FamilyMed
McLeod, Ian D.
Mehta, Rashi J., FamilyMed
Meriano, Antonio L., FamilyMed(EM)
Milrod, Elise G., FamilyMed
Minardi, John
Misra, Sabeena
Mohan, Franklin S C., FamilyMed
Morvay, Leslie C., FamilyMed
Musgrove, G. Roy, FamilyMed
Naaman, Saad
Naidoo, Kouslai, FamilyMed
Naidoo, Niren
Naidu, Padmaja R.
Narewal, Mondeep, FamilyMed
Naylor, Scott G.
Ndubisi, Chukwulo C.
Nerga, Alicja B.
Ng, Albert P.
Ng, David, FamilyMed
Ng, Edward H W.
Ng, Rose Ann L O.
Ninkovich, Snezana, FamilyMed(EM)
Nisbet, Colin G.
Nour, Rabih
Novena, Angela R., FamilyMed(EM)
Nurae, Khalid A., FamilyMed
O'Neill, Donald L., FamilyMed
Oozeer, Yusuf
Ozols, Dina Y., FamilyMed
Page, Robert J., FamilyMed
Parashar, Sujata H., FamilyMed
Paterson, David J., FamilyMed
Penava, Laura M., FamilyMed
Perry, Jowan M R., FamilyMed
Persaud, David H.
Peterson, Darin C., FamilyMed
Pignanelli, Biaggio
Posloski, William G.
Pozzi, Anthony C., FamilyMed(EM)
Pradko, Jacqueline A., FamilyMed
Pradko, James F., FamilyMed
Prakash, Sankar N.
Price, Jeffrey J., FamilyMed
Rai, Veena P K.
Rajan, Andrew I.
Rajaraman, Selva R.
Ranjit, Ebenezer V.
Rao, Shanti E., FamilyMed
Rasool, Kashif G.
Rattan, Nitasha
Ray, Reema, FamilyMed
Renaud, Joseph A.
Rizvi, Syed M H.
Robinson, Derek A., FamilyMed
Rosen, Clifford A.
Ruel, Daniel R., FamilyMed
Ryan, Peter W.
Ryglewicz, Kamila J., FamilyMed
Saad, Genevieve S., FamilyMed
Samoila, John P.
Sayed-Ali, Adham A., FamilyMed
Scarfone, David J.
Scarfone, Peter J., FamilyMed
Schincariol, Holly P., FamilyMed
Scholl, Matthew L., FamilyMed
Schumacher, Albert J.
Schwartz, Paul S.
Scott, Roger
Sekhon, Rajinder S., FamilyMed(EM)
Seski, Robert D.
Shasha, Faiz F A., FamilyMed
Shaw, John F., FamilyMed
Shaw, Matthew F., FamilyMed(EM)
Sherman, Zoia
Shobola, Oladayo D.
Shukla, Hrishikesh, FamilyMed
Siddall, Tamara D.
Sijan, Dusan
Smith, Patrick X.
Soong, Patrick Y., FamilyMed
St-Amour, Nicole D., FamilyMed
State, Jonathon P., FamilyMed
Steen, Andrea R., FamilyMed
Stresman, Elaine J., FamilyMed
Stroker, Claire
Sweet, Susan M., FamilyMed
Tak, Farzana Y.
Tatlay, Kiran D K., FamilyMed
Tayag, Christel M., FamilyMed
Tbakhi, Abdelghani I A.
Thamilvaanan, Paramanathan, FamilyMed(EM)
Thamilvaanan, Shanthi, FamilyMed
Thomas, Sophia, FamilyMed
Torne-Perez, Montserrat
Traill, Larisa M.
Tschen, H H. Steve
Tsui, Alice S Y., FamilyMed(EM)
Vail, Gordon R., FamilyMed(EM)
Varsava, Michael E.
Vasey, Kirsten N., FamilyMed
Vasudevan, Mudalodu V.
Voltic, Laura, FamilyMed
Wahby, Allen J.
Walgama, B G. Shiromi D., FamilyMed
Warwaruk, Joslyn A.
Wasil, Bushra I., FamilyMed
Weisenbacher, Arthur
Woodall, Robert J., FamilyMed(EM)
Yakoub, Elvira, FamilyMed
Yanchula, Catherine A., FamilyMed
Yee, John C K.
Yee, Lauren L.
Zahrebelny, George R.
Zajner, Michael W J., FamilyMed
Zakaria, Joseph D., FamilyMed
Zayouna, Maher N.
Ziter, Dale D., FamilyMed
Ziter, Paul S.

WINGHAM

Antoniadis, Gregory A., FamilyMed
Cramer, Christine R., FamilyMed
Marshall, Bonnie L., FamilyMed
Marshall, Shaun A., FamilyMed
Moores, Mark S., FamilyMed

Shuffield, James W., FamilyMed
Vander Klippe, Stephen W., FamilyMed

WOODBRIDGE

Accardo, Marco A.
Bardai, Zahra, FamilyMed
Benjamen, Sameera
Bhardwaj, Ajay K.
Bortnick, Jessica E., FamilyMed
Ceolin-Wietfeldt, Sandra, FamilyMed
Chen, Frederick H.
Chiozza, Stefano, FamilyMed
Chmiel, Peter K.
Chong, Laura J.
Chopra, Justin A., FamilyMed
Chow, Barry L., FamilyMed
Dakhil, Christina M., FamilyMed
Dev, David A.
Di Cecco, David A.
Di Maria, Antoinette, FamilyMed
Di Nardo, Luciano S., FamilyMed
Greig, Jean M M.
Grignano, Maria C., FamilyMed
Hanna, Phebe, FamilyMed
Hobdari, Ilda, FamilyMed
Hughes, Patricia-Lynn M., FamilyMed
Kelly, Patricia E.
Khadim, Hamid Ahmadzai.
Khan, Ehsan U., FamilyMed
Khan, Farah Y., FamilyMed
Klar, Brian D., FamilyMed
Koblents, Klara
Kouvelos, Kallie L.
Kowalewski, Jerzy L.
Leung, Daniel L.
Litsas, Steven, FamilyMed
Louvaris, James H.
Maggisano, Stephanie N., FamilyMed
Mahoney, Donna G., FamilyMed
Markus, Frank
McNabb, Trudy C., FamilyMed
Mehta, Damini, FamilyMed
Mikelova, Lynda K., FamilyMed
Moore, Wieslawa H.
Nadalini, Mary G., FamilyMed
Navaratnarajah, Prashanthini, FamilyMed
Navaratnarajah, Vaanathy, FamilyMed
Nield, Antony S.
Papini, Osvaldo, FamilyMed
Patgunarajah, Anushi
Petrini, Mariano
Pizzuto, Michael
Polemidiotis, George J., FamilyMed
Rijo, Santos
Rosenber, Jacob J.
Shih, Mike C M.
Siddiqui, Adnan S., FamilyMed
Siddiqui, Sadia, FamilyMed
Sidenberg, Lorne H.
Sorrento, Vito A., FamilyMed(EM)
Soutar, W. Blake
Spensieri, Donato
Stratmann, Hanka H E A., FamilyMed
Tan-Jarvis, Vilma S., FamilyMed
Tennenhouse, Ronald S., FamilyMed
Terenzi, Kristin A., FamilyMed
Tesler, Janet, FamilyMed
Thimm, Andreas J.
Tran, Preston T P., FamilyMed
Tsang, Kam-Yuen
Vachhani, Luv, FamilyMed
Vitaro, Maryann, FamilyMed
Waite, Patricia L., FamilyMed
Weinberger, Allen N.
Wong, Mary M Y., FamilyMed
Wong, Terry H., FamilyMed
Yaser, Aseel, FamilyMed
Zaremba, Michael G., FamilyMed
Zasowski, John J., FamilyMed

WOODSTOCK

Aggarwal, Anita
Andersen-Kay, Michelle L., FamilyMed(EM)
Bennett, Nicholas
Bonnett, Jennifer E., FamilyMed
Briggs, Paul S.
Brioux, Joseph E.
Brockway, Andrew G.
Domenicone, Rosaria, FamilyMed
Fryer, Karen E., FamilyMed(EM)
Fuller, Donald, FamilyMed
George, William S.
Green, Kristy-Jill, FamilyMed(EM)
Hamilton, James J A.
Heaton, Kenneth
Khanna, Rokesh K.
Kocsis, Pongrac, FamilyMed
Korvemaker, Michelle L., FamilyMed
Labruzzo, Peter
Liu, Dong Feng
Marcin, Judi D.
Miettinen, Donald A.
Neal, Douglas
Nichols, Jeffrey L., FamilyMed
Onishenko, Donna K., FamilyMed
Pederson, Glen I., FamilyMed(EM)
Reddick, Richard D.
Robins, Ronald N F., FamilyMed(EM)
Stern, Robert J.
Swart, Maritza
Tam, Jonny H S.
Tompkins, Brock J F., FamilyMed
Urbantke, Elizabeth A., FamilyMed(EM)
Vu, Binh Thien.
Willoughby, D. Paul, FamilyMed
Yu, Norman B M.

WOODVILLE

Bingham, J. Lee, FamilyMed
Cescon, Maria A., FamilyMed

YORK

Abdelsalam, Ghanim I., FamilyMed
Bhupal, Vipul K.
Chaudhri, Arif R.
Cohen, Mark D.
Costaris, Angelos, FamilyMed
D'Onofrio, George F.
Dharamshi, Shafik S N.
Dorar, Jabril A., FamilyMed
Duchastel, Paul A., FamilyMed
Herzog, Melvin
Jones, Alexander E.
Kahansky, Leonard M., FamilyMed
Korda, Andrew, FamilyMed
Lu, William H Y.
Marshall, Kate M A., FamilyMed
Matthews, Paul W.
McMillin, Robert S., FamilyMed
Naidu, P R. Paul
Nguyen, Van Hanh, FamilyMed
Onyett-Jeffries, Katherine A G., FamilyMed
Pancaro, Luigia M.
Peachey, David K.
Pegg, William C., FamilyMed
Peracchia, Gabriele
Peters, Ago
Salama, Magdy G A., FamilyMed
Salem, Cherien, FamilyMed
Shergold, David J.
Stephenson, Michael C., FamilyMed
Toyota, Jane C.
Turner, Sheldon A., FamilyMed
Vasquez, Manuel O.

ZURICH

Hurley, Michael
Schreader, Alicia G., FamilyMed
Teeple, Lori E., FamilyMed(EM)

PRINCE EDWARD ISLAND

ALBERTON

Hansen, Philip R., FamilyMed
Naqvi, Syed E.

BEDEQUE

Molyneaux, Lloyd J.

CHARLOTTETOWN

Abdulrahman Alansari, Nabeel M M.
Alansari, Nabeel M.
Ayanbadejo, Clement, FamilyMed
Bader, Jean-Francois, FamilyMed(EM)
Barkhouse, Lana B., FamilyMed
Beck, Gordon
Boswall, Margaret
Brandon, J. Bradley, FamilyMed
Bronaugh, Thomas
Burke-Perry, Rosemary
Cabilio, Nora, FamilyMed
Carruthers, George H., FamilyMed
Champion, Pauline
Champion, Stacy
Chaudhury, Derek
Clark, Barry L.
Coady, Kenneth W., FamilyMed
Cooke, Raymond H.
Corney, Paul R., FamilyMed
Cunniffe, Jill J., FamilyMed
Curtis, M. Shannon, FamilyMed
Cusack, Paul
Ellis Ghiz, Katherine, FamilyMed
Flanagan, M. Barbara
Grimes, Gil
Hoffman, Christine, FamilyMed
Hooley, Peter J D., FamilyMed
Jain, Trevor, FamilyMed(EM)
Kassner, Rachel
Keizer, W. Stirling, FamilyMed
Kelley, Robert J., FamilyMed
Khan, Faraz
Kizilbash, Kamran
Kon Kam King, Christopher A., FamilyMed
Lantz, Christopher J.
Lantz, J. Brodie
Lea, Denise A., FamilyMed
Lecours, Mireille, FamilyMed
Ling, T. Donald
Lowey, John
MacDonald, K. Anne
MacDonald, Linda A.
MacKenzie, David E.
MacKinnon, Randy J., FamilyMed
MacLaren, Angela, FamilyMed
Malhotra, Sanjay
Mark, Suzanne C.
Matheson, A. Grant
McGinn, M. Joanne
McNally, Katherine, FamilyMed
Meek, Douglas H., FamilyMed
Miller, Megan E., FamilyMed
Molyneaux, Shelly D., FamilyMed
Morais, J. Alfred, FamilyMed
Morrison, Heather, FamilyMed(EM)
Morrisson, Heather
Neily, Donald R.
Newman, S. Lewis
Newson, Kristy A., FamilyMed
Nguyen, Huy Thanh V., FamilyMed
O'Brien, Stephen R., FamilyMed
O'Hanley, G. Marie
O'Neill, Kiley J., FamilyMed
Peacock, Edith M., FamilyMed
Peterson, Jocelyn, FamilyMed
Reck, Mona, FamilyMed
Reid, David B., FamilyMed
Rogerson, Janet, FamilyMed
Sampson, John E., FamilyMed(EM)
Saunders, George H.
Saunders, Kristopher D., FamilyMed
Scantlebury, William
Shea, Dawn M.
Slysz, Garth W., FamilyMed
Spears, Benjamin
Stephens, Donald S.
Thompson, James M., FamilyMed(EM)
Triantafillou, Mark
Tweel, Douglas K H.
Veale, A. Christine
Veer, A. Adriana, FamilyMed
Verma, Prem A.
Wedge, Richard
Whalen, Ronald V., FamilyMed(EM)
White, M. Edward, FamilyMed
Wohlgemut, Andrew H., FamilyMed
Yousif, Haythem
Zelin, Jennifer M., FamilyMed

CORNWALL

Stewart, David I., FamilyMed

CRAPAUD

Visser, Hendrik A.

HUNTER RIVER

Friedrich, Carl E., FamilyMed
Jewers, Paul C.

KENSINGTON

MacKean, Peter R., FamilyMed
MacNearney, P. Christine
Phelan, Paul
Reisch, Helga, FamilyMed

MONTAGUE

Bruce, Cameron
Campbell, David S., FamilyMed
Fancy, Nicole D., FamilyMed
Hambly, David
Holland, Bernard
Johnston, Geraldine
MacLeod, Andrew G., FamilyMed
Magennis, W. Terrence
Wonnacott, James B.

NORTH RUSTICO

Pineau, F. Edwin

O'LEARY

Dewar, Charles M., FamilyMed
Dickieson, Herbert P.
Hameed, Babar

SOURIS

Berrow, Paul J.
Henbest, Ronald, FamilyMed
Kennedy, Ambrose
Lazowski, Waldemar, FamilyMed
Morgan, David

SUMMERSIDE

Al Salih, Hala
Arsenault-Samson, Nadine, FamilyMed
Austin, Heather A., FamilyMed
Bajelan, Adnan, FamilyMed
Bannon, David
Cameron, Scott L.
Celliers, Andre
Chiasson, J. Roland
Christensen, Paul E L.
Duffy, Charles H., FamilyMed(EM)
Estey, Frank P., FamilyMed
Harnois, Bryan D., FamilyMed
Johnston, Julie A., FamilyMed
Kapalanga, Joachim
Kelly, Paul B., FamilyMed
King, Laval K K.
Laftah, Abdulrahem L A., FamilyMed
Lakshmi, Santhosh
MacCausland, Owen
MacNeill, R. Steven, FamilyMed(EM)
McNeill, Monica L.
McRae, Harold P.
Molyneaux, Harold W.
Moyse, Cyril A., FamilyMed
Muhammad, Ishtiaq
Nicholson, Ronald D., FamilyMed
O'Neil, Steven D.
Salamoun, Wassim
Sharpe, Jonathan, FamilyMed
Stewart, Trina L., FamilyMed
Stultz, Timothy
Swart, Henry C.
Vickerson, Donald G.

TYNE VALLEY

Abdelmalek, Ihab
Madigane, Joyce
Montgomery, W. Roy

VERNON BRIDGE

De Marsh, John G., FamilyMed

QUÉBEC

ACTON VALE

Benech-Riopel, Elise
Gallant, Marc
Labreque, Luc
Mayette, Richard
Miclette, Sylvie

ALBANEL

Dallaire, Real

ALMA

Audet, Sarah, FamilyMed(EM)
Bechamp-Theberge, Marie-Pier
Blackburn, Robert Y.
Boily, Mireille
Bouchard, Claude
Bouffard, Odette
Bussiere, Marc-Alain
Dery, Francine, FamilyMed
Desbiens, Alain
Drolet, Renald
Du Tremblay, Renee
Dufour, Suzanne
Dumont, Marc
Fleury, Andre
Fleury, Rejean
Foltz, Anne-Marie
Fortin, Luc
Fournier, Charles
Fournier, Jessica
Guay, Michel, FamilyMed
Harvey, Amelie
Hebert, Mireille
Lamothe, Bruno
Lapointe, Helene, FamilyMed
Lavoie, Regis
Levesque, Michel
Mantha, Gaston
Morel, Annie
Neault, Daniel
Peloquin, Francois
Plourde, Andree-Anne
Rodrigue Verhelst, Ariane
Samson, Marie
Saucier, Marie-Claude
Saucier, Maude
Savard, Gilbert
Tremblay, Alain
Tremblay, Suzanne
Veillette, Bruno
Verreault, Guy
Villemure, Philippe, FamilyMed
Villeneuve, Audrey
Villeneuve, Georges-Henri

ALOUETTE

Descoteaux, Chantal, FamilyMed
Plante, Jean-Luc, FamilyMed
Robichaud, Michele, FamilyMed

AMOS

Allard, Nicole
Aubry, Sylvain
Beaulieu, Claude, FamilyMed
Beaulieu, Pierre
Beliveau, Pierre
Bouchek, Belkacem
Boutet, Jean-Yves
Charest, Louise, FamilyMed
Cormier, Nathalie
Darcy, Eve, FamilyMed
Demers, Josiane
Dubois, Alain
Eid, Joseph
Favreault, Luce
Gagnon, Marianne
Gagnon, Sonia, FamilyMed
Garant, Dominique
Guay, Helene
Lamontagne, Serge, FamilyMed
Landry, Chantal
Landry, Diane
Landry, Lyse
Laurendeau, Francois
Lavoie, Bertrand
Lavoie Coutu, Christine
Letendre, Micheline, FamilyMed
Levesque, Lise
Menard, Danielle
Michael, Samer
Michael Awad, Roula
Noel Beau, Noemie
Paradis, Yves
Picard, France
Prisecariu Mocanu, Daniela
Quirion, Karen, FamilyMed
Rivest, Denis, FamilyMed
Robitaille, Isabelle, FamilyMed
Samuel-Thomassin, Véronique
Sauvageau, Yolaine, FamilyMed
Terrault, Stephane
Tran, Yasuo
Tulandi, Thomas
Turgeon, Frederic, FamilyMed

AMQUI

Aboussafy, Andre
Audet, Alexandra, FamilyMed
Blanchette, Melanie
Bornais, Pierre
Boucher, Denis N., FamilyMed
Brochu, Isabelle, FamilyMed
Charland, Patrick
D'Amours, Sonia-Sandra
Didier, Mijanou
Dumais, Marie-Eve, FamilyMed
Gagnon, Yves, FamilyMed(EM)
Gauthier, Jeannot
Gervais, Sophie, FamilyMed
Laddada, Kherdine
Landry, Philip
Lauzon, Guylaine
Marquis, Annie, FamilyMed
Martin, Jean
Nguyen-Dang, Thuy-Tien
Pascot, Agnes, FamilyMed
Poirier, Catherine
Simard-Racine, Genevieve
St-Amant, Manon
Turbide, Pierre, FamilyMed
Vallee, Jacynthe

ANJOU

Arseneault, Denis
Diec, Kien-Quan
Dinh, Hoang-Diep
Fournier, Carl
Hanna, Yousri
Hoang, Ngoc Vinh
Lacasse, Diane
Lavigueur, Michel
Leclair, Marcel, FamilyMed
Martin, Real
Morin, Evelyn
Nguyen, Hoang-Thi
Poirier, Suzanne
Subai, Ziad
Vezina, Paul

ARMAGH

Dallaire, Robert

ASBESTOS

Bilodeau, Francoise
Blanchard, Denis
Daniels, Jean-Guy
Daniels, Michel
Fryer, Veronique, FamilyMed
Landry, Rene, FamilyMed
Lapointe, Richard
Leger, Yves, FamilyMed
Martel, Sonia
Morin, Gilles
Paquette, Amelie
Robinson, Martine
Roy, Nathalie

BAIE-COMEAU

Barnard, Louis
Bazin, Marc
Bosse, Danielle
Boudreau, Pierre-Olivier
Brouillette, Lyne, FamilyMed
Camire, Laurent
Caron, Stephane
Chasse, Daniel
Chretien, Pierre
Claracq, Marine, FamilyMed
Cliche, Marcel
Cloutier, Michele
Cloutier, Raynald
Dallaire, Mario C.
Deschenes, Marie-Andree, FamilyMed
Du Tremblay, Jean
Dube, Roger
Gagnon, Emilie, FamilyMed
Gagnon, Jean-Paul
Garneau, Melanie
Garneau, Sara, FamilyMed
Gingras, Manon
Gitlan, Iulia
Gregoire, Serge, FamilyMed
Grenier, Robert
Jacob, Gaetan
Jerjian, Yacoub
Jobin, Nicolas, FamilyMed
Knap, Michel
Lajeunesse, Judith, FamilyMed
Lamontagne, Roland
Larkin, Anne-Marie, FamilyMed(EM)
Leclerc, Claude
Lee, David, FamilyMed
Levesque, Martine
Louchi, Abdellatif
Marchand, Julie, FamilyMed
Marcheterre, Louise, FamilyMed
Mercier, David
Meunier, Helene F., FamilyMed
Morisset, Marie-Eve, FamilyMed
Naud, Simon, FamilyMed(EM)
Nguyen, Quang D., FamilyMed
Ouellet, Didier
Ouimet, Veronique, FamilyMed
Popova, Margarita, FamilyMed
Richard-Chapleau, Felix, FamilyMed
Rivest, Genevieve
Rivest, Genevieve, FamilyMed
Rotari-Ghidirim, Nadejda, FamilyMed
Roussel, Marc, FamilyMed
Ruelland, Simon
Samson, Arnaud
Somyk, Kostiantyn I., FamilyMed
Trépanier, David, FamilyMed
Vo, Thuy-Quynh

BAIE-SAINT-PAUL

Boivin, Gilles
Cloutier, Jacques
Cote, Marie-Eve, FamilyMed
Dallaire, Gaetan
Deschenes, Catherine, FamilyMed
Dorval, Julie
Drouin, Jacques
Gilbert, Jasmine
Laflamme, Sebastien, FamilyMed
Lemay, Julie, FamilyMed
Marcotte Lupien, Lucie, FamilyMed
Miller, Jean
Paquet, Jean-Denis
Reed, Ann
Roy, Bernadette
Simard, Chantal
Simard, Jean-Francois

BEACONSFIELD

Naimi, Houshang

BEAUCEVILLE

Cornet-Toussaint, Edwine
Cyr, Andreanne, FamilyMed
Fillion, Linda
Guay, Celine
Roy, Bruno
Trudeau, Pierre

BEAUHARNOIS

Aberman, Arnold B.
Bergeron, Maurice
Briere, Josee
Brunet, Richard
Dignard, Eric
Dufresne, Chantelle
Gauthier, Valere
Leblond, Marie-Josee

BEAUPRE

Beauchemin, Eric, FamilyMed
Begin, Claude
Boutet, Pierre
Cadrin, Robert
Cote, Gaston
De Beaumont, Jean-Rene
Drouin, Richard
Kochuyt, Caroline P R.
Lavoie, Alain
Lemay, Christine, FamilyMed
Mercier, Marie-Josee
Pepin, Michele
Tremblay, Jean-Philippe
Vallee, Rene
Veilleux, Brigitte

BECANCOUR

Bouvet, Luc
Chaine, Claude
Deveault, Alain
Girard, Luc
Hebert, Jocelyn
Langlois, Guillaume, FamilyMed
Lessard, Gerard
Pouliot, Louis
St-Arnaud, Nancy, FamilyMed
Toussaint, Simon

BEDFORD

Beaulieu, Pascale
Bouchard, Jean-Simon
Leger, Christian
Morin, France
Nadeau, Maryse, FamilyMed
Peck, Jean-Philippe
Raymond, Bernard, FamilyMed

BELOEIL

Beaudoin, Michel
Bolduc, Sabrina, FamilyMed
Cournoyer, Isabelle
Desrosiers, Catherine
Dougherty, Elizabeth, FamilyMed
Douville, Jocelyn
Doyon, Bernard
Garnier, Pascale
Gauthier, Jean-Guy
Gosselin, Emile
Grenier, Lise
Houde, Julie, FamilyMed
Laneuville, Louis
Lavoie, Julie
Leduc, Jean-Sebastien
Legault, Louis
Lemay, Guillaume, FamilyMed
Lemieux, Marc-Andre
Levesque, Yves A.
Marceau, Stephane
Marsolais, Marcel
Martel, Christiane
Moursy, Asmat, FamilyMed
Pavlova, Silvia
Poulin, Jean-Pierre
Prevost, Pierre
Proulx, Denis
Proulx, Ginette
Provost, Marcel, FamilyMed(EM)
Quidoz, Amelie
Quintal, France
Simard, Ginette
St-Onge, Michel
Ste-Marie, Lise

BERTHIERVILLE

Corriveau, Louise
Denis, Bernard
Dessureault, Jacques
Gendron, Olivier M.
Simard, Martine
Theriault, Serge
Turcotte, Bernard

BLAINVILLE

Agoues, Isabelle
Auger, Pascale
Bedard, Brigitte
Belanger, Pascale
Belisle, Christian
Bellefeuille, Patrice
Belzil, Yves, FamilyMed
Daneault, Helene
Dusablon, Manon
Dutil, Christian
Helie, Genevieve
Kretz, Patrice
Lapointe, Marie
Laurore, Yardley, FamilyMed
Lavoie, Sebastien, FamilyMed
Leblanc, Marie-Andree, FamilyMed
Leclaire, Luc
Makhoulian, Natalie, FamilyMed
Marquis, Solange
Mathieu, Michel A.
Mercier, Nicole
Morin, Eric
Nicolet, Jannick M L., FamilyMed
Nissaire, Robert
Pelletier, Anne-Marie
Pelletier, Diane
Reid, Annick
Rozon, Jacques
Saulnier, Catherine
Savaria, Jean-Pierre
Tremblay, Marie-France
Vuillermet, Denise

BOIS-DES-FILION

Dabbagh, Sufian, FamilyMed
Fequiere, Maguie, FamilyMed
Habra, Magdi
Khoury, Nabil M.
Moisan, Martin

BOISBRIAND

Aumais, Christian
Lafontaine, Danielle
Laurin, Gilles
Lebel, Jocelyn J.
Lesperance, Sylvie, FamilyMed
Martin, Jacques
Phaneuf, Claude
Siclait, Jaime, FamilyMed
Tremblay, Marie-Claude S.

BOISBRIANO

Sergerie, Claude

BONAVENTURE

Duguay, Annie, FamilyMed
Pitre, Jean-Marie

BOUCHERVILLE

Barrette, Michelle
Beausoleil, Caroline
Beliveau, Genevieve
Bissonnette, Lucie
Bosse, Elizabeth
Brossard, Claude F.
Chabot, Marianne
Courchesne, Charles
Courchesne, Josee
Dansereau, Jean-Marc
Demers, Annie
Dessureault, Francois
Dumas, Alain
Fortin, Carole, FamilyMed
Gagne, Michelle
Grosjean-Nicloux, Francine, FamilyMed
Laporte, Pierre
Lavoie, Valerie
Lopez Agudelo, Jose E.
Nicloux, Nathalie, FamilyMed
Perreault, Julie
Racicot, Paolo
Rheaume, Pierre M.
Richard, Karine, FamilyMed
Saillant, Catherine
Sauve, Marie-Lou
Savard, Serge
St-Arneault, Renald
Tetreault, Martine
Tremblay, Louise
Trepanier, Marie C.

BOUCHERVULLE

Page, Francoise

BROMONT

Auger, Alain
Bouthillier, Catherine, FamilyMed
Cousineau, Antoine-Francois
Ferdais, Francois
Parissier, Adrien
Pauze, Genevieve
Racine, Elizabeth
Tremblay, Pierre

BROSSARD

Ahmed, Sabrina, FamilyMed
Atalla, Soheir
Baril, Nicole
Baril-Graham, Suzanne
Blais, Philippe
Charron, Nicole
Chartier, Sophie
Chatelois, Yves
Chatterjee, Manjula
Chow Siet Yam, Moy Fee
Cote, Suzanne
Crepeau, Michel
Dang, My Hue
Demanche, Sylvie
Desaulniers, Gerald
Dragin, Natacha, FamilyMed
Duong, Tuyet Minh
Dupont, Micheline
Gaudet, Rachel
Gouda, Zinab, FamilyMed
Guilmain-Maurice, Micheline
Jette-Grenier, Marie
Klvana, Jacqueline, FamilyMed
Krywulak-Rizzo, Natalia
Langlois, Louis-Charles
Laroche, Chantal
Laurendeau, Louis
Mac, Van Trong
Mailhot, Annie-Claude, FamilyMed
Marotte, Rachel
Mason, Joan E.
Michaud, Francois
Michel, Pierre
Mikhail, Genevieve, FamilyMed
Morissette, Lucie
Nguyen, Huan Truong
Nguyen, Mong Thuy.
Nguyen, Tang-Dong
Olivier, Chantal
Ouellet, Anne
Oumet, Lucie
Plante, Johanne
Raut, Manisha
Shinder, Michael E.
St-Andre, Carmen
Tchervenkova, Milka A.
Thibault, Nicole
Thibeault, Claude
To, Tuyet Anh
Tremblay, Luc
Truong, Quyen
Villeneuve, Suzanne
Ying, Ying, FamilyMed

CABANO

Briand, Claude
Cote, Guildo
Massicotte, Guy
Morissette, Jacqueline

CACOUNA

Gougoux, Francois
Royer, Nicole

CAMPBELL'S BAY

Mutchmore, Lucie, FamilyMed(EM)

CANDIAC

Breton, Robert, FamilyMed
Gravel, Andre
Larochelle, Julie
Noel, Marie-France
Provinciali, Beatrice
Renault, Paule
Riverin, Karine, FamilyMed
Rochon, Lucie
Roy, Christiane
Roy, Viateur
Trudel, Guillaume
Venne, Danielle

CANTLEY

Tardif, Daniel

CANTON DE HATLEY

Fisch, Danielle, FamilyMed

CAP-CHAT

Bouchard, Michel

CAP-SAINT-IGNACE

Boulanger, Michelle
Letourneau, Annie
Proulx, Clement

CAP-SANTE

Frenette, Guy

CAP-AUX-MEULES

Arnold, Stephen, FamilyMed
Barrette, Serge
Bernier-Dutrisac, Anne-Marie, FamilyMed
Boiteau, Étienne
Boshouwers, Marie-Louise
Cartwright, Pierre
Chouinard, Alexandre
Couture, Marcel
Cyr, Luc
Deraspe, Mylene
Fortier, Ychelle
Gagne, Pierre-Thomas
Gregoire, Caroline
Gregoire, Edith
Harvey, Claudette
Hubert, Amelie, FamilyMed
Labrecque, Josee
Landry, Aline, FamilyMed
Lessard, Steve
McNicoll, Annie, FamilyMed
Moreau-Richard, Rosalie
Noel, Jean-Francois
Papillon, Marianne, FamilyMed
Paquet, Christine
Parent, Marc-Antoine
Patry, Rose-Marie, FamilyMed

CAPLAN

Bazinet, Stephan
Benguerel, Robert
Desgagne, Micheline

CARIGNAN

Masse, Lyne

CARLETON

Bernier, Philippe
Matton, Jean P.
Olivier, Pierre

CHAMBLY

Cote, Remi
Daigneault, Celine
Dumais, Marion, FamilyMed
Gagnon, Luc
Goyette, Roger
Labelle, Pierre
Lai, The Hung
Lapie, Frederique
Mailloux, Michel
Moriconi, Ronaldo
Nanini, Bianca
Rheault, Nathalie

CHAMBORD

Berube, Suzanne

CHANDLER

Abrous, Fariza
Anamaria, Isabelle
Boucher-Gagne, Emilie
Breault, Marie D., FamilyMed(EM)
Cherisol, Remy, FamilyMed
Dandois, Maxime G.
David, Donald
Demers, Bernard
Drapeau, Sylvain
Ferland, Stephanie
Fredette, Simon
Gauthier, Julie
Khima, Chahrazed
Lam-Yuk-Tseung, Y. Sophie, FamilyMed
Larocque Laplante, Sylvie
Mercier, Claude
Ouedraogo, Eva, FamilyMed
Routhier, Line
Smith, Audrey
Thibault, Audrey
Tremblay-Tanguay, Charles, FamilyMed
Trudel, Sylvain, FamilyMed(EM)

CHAPAIS

Lafond, Chantal
Leclerc, Martin
Lord, Claire, FamilyMed
Saint-Louis, Nathalie M M.

CHARLEMAGNE

Lalanda, Carmen

CHARLESBOURG

Caron, Renee

CHARNY

Barbeau, Mathilde
Beaulieu, Yohan, FamilyMed(EM)
Boucher, Catherine, FamilyMed
Carrier, Julie
Cloutier, Michele
Lessard, Sylvain, FamilyMed
Nadeau, Michel
Patry, Danielle
Rouleau, Yves

CHATEAU-RICHER

Verreault, Denis

CHATEAUGUAY

Amyot, Karyne
Archambault, Dominique, FamilyMed
Arguin, Frederic, FamilyMed
Beaudin, Genevieve, FamilyMed
Beausejour, Linda
Biron, Marie-Helene, FamilyMed(EM)
Boisvert, Pierre
Bouchard, Clermont
Boudreault, Dorice
Bourassa-Fulop, Caroline, FamilyMed(EM)
Cadoret, Louise
Caron, Elaine
Cassar, Louis J.
Chiry, Samah, FamilyMed
Chretien, Valerie, FamilyMed
Couture, Louis
Daher, Antoine
Dufresne, Sylvie
Dulude, Francois
Fiset, Nathalie
Frechette, France
Gibeault, Audrey, FamilyMed
Gravel, Louis
Haineault, Caroline, FamilyMed
Hamel, Catherine, FamilyMed
Herrera, Pedro
Ibrahim, Nancy, FamilyMed
Jeican, Brandusa R.
Jette, Julie
Jutras, Jerome-Oliver, FamilyMed
Laberge, J. Roger
Laberge, Julie, FamilyMed
Laberge, Sophie, FamilyMed
Labrie, Vincent, FamilyMed(EM)
Lacoste, Lucie, FamilyMed
Landry, Cynthia
Leccia, Jean-Dominique
Lemay, Michele, FamilyMed
Letendre, Marie
Levesque-Halimi, Carole
Loyer, Michel
Maalouf-Sfeir, Nada
Marchand, Celine
Masucci, Nicola
Maynard, Sidney
Nanhou Djomo, Alice, FamilyMed
Nguyen Duong, Y. Nhu, FamilyMed
Normandin, Olivier
Parent, Jean-Philippe, FamilyMed
Pelletier, Marie-France, FamilyMed
Perreault, Chantal
Pinard-Saint-Pierre, Vanessa, FamilyMed(EM)
Prevost, Sylvie, FamilyMed
Primeau, Alain W.
Provencal, Edith
Quach, Sophie M.
Richard, Alex
Saddi, Ghada-Maria, FamilyMed
Simard, Marie-Helene
Smith, Philippe, FamilyMed
Thanh, Christine
Vachon, Mario
Yammine, Fady G.
Zabian, Randa, FamilyMed

CHENEVILLE

Dalpe-Charron, Michel H.

CHERTSEY

Asselin, Michel
Gamache, Louis
Roberge, Paul

CHIBOUGAMAU

Brassard, Josee, FamilyMed
Chabot, Bertrand, FamilyMed
Deschamps, Julie, FamilyMed
Dion, Karine, FamilyMed
Dutil, Julie, FamilyMed
Faucher, Line, FamilyMed
Gagnon, Marie-Anne
Garneau, Jocelyn, FamilyMed
Gauthier, Josee, FamilyMed
Gironne, Claude, FamilyMed
Guillemette, Helene, FamilyMed
Henri, Marcel
Laforge, Marlene, FamilyMed
Lapointe, Jessica, FamilyMed
Lemay, Chantal, FamilyMed
Lemay, Gilbert
Lemoyne, Jean
Lepine, Martin, FamilyMed
Letourneau, Joel
Malenfant, Michelle, FamilyMed
Paquet, Stephanie, FamilyMed
Tremblay Trempe, Renee, FamilyMed

CHICOUTIMI

Allard, Sylvain
Arsenault, Francois
Arsenault, Marie-Claude, FamilyMed
Aubin, Donald
Auger, Caroline
Barabas, Dezso
Baron, Marie-Helene
Beaudet, Pierre
Beaumont, Nancy
Bellefleur, Stephanie, FamilyMed(EM)
Belley, Sylvie
Bergeron, Andre
Bergeron, Ann
Bergeron, Serge B.
Berube, Claude

Berube, Jean-D.
Betala Belinga, Jean-Francois
Bettez, Nathalie, FamilyMed
Blondeau, Jean-Philippe
Blouin, Marie, FamilyMed
Bouchard, Genevieve
Bouchard, Julien, FamilyMed(EM)
Boudana, David A.
Boudreault, Pascal
Boulard-Gondolff, Annick
Boule, Francine, FamilyMed
Brassard, Liza
Brochet, Francois
Cantin, Julie, FamilyMed(EM)
Chamberland, Guy, FamilyMed
Cieza Lara, Tomas A.
Cimon-Carufel, Janie, FamilyMed(EM)
Claveau, Laval
Collard, Stephanie, FamilyMed
Corneau, Richard
Cote, Annie, FamilyMed
Cote, Genevieve
Cote, Lise
Couture, Eva M., FamilyMed
De Oliveira, Marcelo M.
Dery, Stephane
Des Landes, Lysanne, FamilyMed(EM)
Desrochers, Charles
Desrosiers, Dominique
Desy, Marie-Andree, FamilyMed
Drouin, Sylvie
Dube, Melissa
Ferdjoui, Zoheir
Fortin, Martin, FamilyMed
Fortin, Stephane
Fortin, Veronique
Gagnon, Helene
Gagnon, Olivier
Gambu, Helene, FamilyMed(EM)
Gaudet, Daniel
Gaudreault, Gaetan
Gaudreault, Marc
Gaudreault, Mauril D.
Gauthier, Aline
Gignac, Julie
Gilbert, Vanessa, FamilyMed
Godoy Pimenta, Newton J.
Grenier, Chantal, FamilyMed
Guern, Claude
Hakami, M. Taghi
Harvey, Pierre
Hatcher, Sharon N., FamilyMed
Herman-Lemelin, Antoine, FamilyMed(EM)
Hudon, Catherine, FamilyMed
Hudon, Martin
Hudon, Nathalie
Kanza Epunza, Rene
Lachance, Marie-Josee
Lalancette, Christian
Lamarre, Jean
Landry, Marlene
Lapierre, Nathalie
Lapointe, Marie
Lapointe, Mario
Lavoie, Catherine
Leblanc, Marie-Josee, FamilyMed
Leclerc, Marc-Yves
Lefebvre, Sebastien, FamilyMed(EM)
Lemieux, Martin, FamilyMed
Lemieux, Sylvie
Leroux, Claudie, FamilyMed
Leroux, Karine
Lessard, Andréa, FamilyMed
Levesque, Marise, FamilyMed
Lovisi Neto, Bianca
Martin, Caroline I., FamilyMed(EM)
Michaud, Julie
Michaud, Real
Minville, Genevieve
Monette, Jocelyne
Morin, Helene
Ouellet, Andre-Denis
Ouellet, Louise
Paradis, Clement, FamilyMed(EM)
Paradis, Marie-Renee
Parent, Bernard
Patry, Luc
Pelletier, Kathleen
Perron-Cote, Anne-Louise, FamilyMed(EM)
Pion, Kim, FamilyMed(EM)
Poisson, Mireille, FamilyMed
Potvin, Christelle, FamilyMed
Potvin, Johanne
Prive, Annie-Claude
Raffa, Hacene
Richard, Lorraine
Rivard, Sophie
Royer, Sandrine, FamilyMed(EM)
Savoie, Marie-France, FamilyMed
Simard, Louis, FamilyMed
Simard, Sylvain, FamilyMed
St-Cyr, Michel
Stagg, Marie-France
Tardif, Frederic
Thibault, Jean
Tnani, Amel K.
Tremblay, Chantale
Tremblay, Melissa, FamilyMed(EM)
Tremblay, Paul-Benoit
Trudel, Manon
Verreault, France
Vieira Neto, Leonardo
Voyer, Isabelle, FamilyMed

CHISASIBI

Beauce, Catherine, FamilyMed
Contant, Éric, FamilyMed
Copley, James, FamilyMed
Deschesnes, Dimitrios E., FamilyMed(EM)
Gervais, Vanessa, FamilyMed
Holody, Erik A J., FamilyMed(EM)
Lefson, Michael A., FamilyMed
Moschona, Penelope, FamilyMed
Orr, Alexandra R., FamilyMed
Pouteau, Dawn C., FamilyMed
Sabella, Olivier, FamilyMed
Selim, Adrien, FamilyMed
Strakacz, Marta, FamilyMed(EM)
Talbot-Bolduc, Anne-France, FamilyMed
Waterman, Nadia J., FamilyMed(EM)

CLERMONT

Baril, Francois
Blouin, Denis, FamilyMed
Gagnon, Robert
Labbe, Mario
Sauve, Marie-Josee

COATICOOK

Banfill, Suzanne, FamilyMed
Bartlett, Steven, FamilyMed
Beaulieu, Josee
Bird, Natasha
Dussault, Louise
Frenette, Bernard
Frenette, Bertrand
Germain, Richard
Landry, Patricia, FamilyMed
Landry, Sonia
Levasseur, Louis-Bernard
Mainville, Nathalie
Margarit, Marius L., FamilyMed
Monette, Steven
Simms, Allyson

CONTRECOEUR

Boisvert, Anne-Marie
Gauthier, Claude
Peloquin, Sophie, FamilyMed
Veronneau, Andre

COOKSHIRE

Lessard, Marie-Eve, FamilyMed
Parent, Robert
Varin, Ginette
Vezina, Gilles

COOKSHIRE-EATON

Blais, Danielle
Blais-Boilard, Stephanie, FamilyMed(EM)
Martel, Sophie, FamilyMed
Payeur, Helene

COTE SAINT-LUC

Abcarius, Fredericka N., FamilyMed
Almasi, Julie, FamilyMed
Aly, Nahla Y S., FamilyMed
Amdursky, David, FamilyMed
Andonatos, Stella
Benjamin, Ilan, FamilyMed
Borten, Odelia, FamilyMed
Burstein, Irving J.
Desormeaux, Lise, FamilyMed
Fuks, Maria
Goldfarb, Janice
Kelen, Leslie
Khadoury, Adeline, FamilyMed
Klein, Linda, FamilyMed
Levitz, Suzanne F., FamilyMed
Lubarsky, Robert
Luger, Sherry
Majda, Jolanta
Melameth, Regine, FamilyMed
Romano, Marilisa, FamilyMed
Rosenberg, Resa, FamilyMed
Shahin, David R.
Solomon, Leslie J., FamilyMed
Tradounsky, Golda E., FamilyMed
Tremblay, Sonia, FamilyMed
Wolanski, Renee J.

COURCELETTE

Aziez, Abdelaâziz, FamilyMed
Belanger, Andre
Benzaid, El Mostafa, FamilyMed
Bernier, Serge
Bouchard, Annie
Couillard Jr, Bernard, FamilyMed(EM)
Coulombe, Remy
Deslandes, Jean-Luc
Eyestone, G. Russell, FamilyMed
Gagne, Genevieve, FamilyMed
Gauthier, Jean, FamilyMed
Hazzi, Cherine
Hebert, Real, FamilyMed
Houde, Danielle
Langevin, Julie, FamilyMed
Meisels, Monica, FamilyMed
Melancon, Francois
Pepper, Jonathan, FamilyMed
Theodorescu, Paul, FamilyMed

COURCELLES

Hamann, Richard

COWANSVILLE

Adam, Genevieve
Andriuk, Debora
Begin, Veronique
Bonneau, Veronique, FamilyMed
Boudreau, Marie-Claude
Bourbeau, Sophie
Bériault, Karine, FamilyMed
Chagnon, Marie-Noel
Cosman, Catherine E.
Dauth, Pierre
Davoine, Emilie, FamilyMed(EM)
Desmeules, Jean
Fujioka, Robert
Galipeau, Louise
Garant, Jean-Philippe
Gill, Julie, FamilyMed
Giroux, Rosaire
Giugovaz, Sophie
Grand'Maison, Genevieve, FamilyMed
Guichaoua, Yves
Hill, Jeanne
Iny, Karen, FamilyMed
Jolin, Isabelle
Joyal, Renee
Lafond, Elaine
Lague, Normand
Lalla, Daniel E., FamilyMed
Lanctot, Jean-Luc, FamilyMed
Leblanc, Emilie
Lemay-Gervais, Francois, FamilyMed
Lemyre, Reine, FamilyMed
Lesage, David
Macek, Adrian S., FamilyMed
Malo, Jean
Mikhail, Raouf E., FamilyMed
Millette, Julie, FamilyMed
Mout, Julie
Nicolas, Isabelle, FamilyMed
Nolin, Karine, FamilyMed
Ouimet, Myriam H., FamilyMed
Perreault, Etienne
Phillips, Allen, FamilyMed
Rivest, Louise
Rouleau, Anne
Roy, Sophie
Sorge, Raymond, FamilyMed(EM)

DANVILLE

Boutin, Guy
Jacot, Francis R M.
Roy, Regent

DAVELUYVILLE

Rene, Francois
Talbot, Nathalie
Vinette, Christian, FamilyMed

DEGELIS

Lavoie, Bernadette
Soucy, Marieke, FamilyMed

DELSON

Ghali, Saad
L'Épicier, Marilou, FamilyMed
Neron, Anne C., FamilyMed
Papageorges, Jean
Wagner, Daniel

DESCHAMBAULT

Picher, Francois

DEUX-MONTAGNES

Carpentier, Louis
Duclos, Elizabeth
Gagne, Jeannine
Hudon, Paul-Andre
Labonte, Pierre
Savard, Chantal
Trudeau, Michel
Valiquette, Alain

DISRAELI

Cote, Lucie
Dion, Susan
Martineau, France, FamilyMed
Taillon, Jean-Paul

DOLBEAU-MISTASSINI

Allard, Genevieve
Audet, Marc
Audet, Marie-Christine, FamilyMed
Bedard, Robert
Benoit, Celine
Blais, Claude-Francois
Castonguay, Andre
Chabot, Serge
Chettaoui, Olfa
De La Boissiere, Martin
Delaunais, Daniel
Doucet, Audree, FamilyMed
Fortin, Frederick, FamilyMed
Gaudreault, Melina, FamilyMed
Germain, Caroline, FamilyMed
Grenier, Alain
Hinse, Michel
Lacasse, Jacqueline
Leclerc, Lucie
Lessard, Charles
Ouellet, Andre
Poisson, Andre
Proulx, Sylvain
Robitaille, Sylvie
Sasseville, Richard
Savard, Normand
Tremblay, Bianca
Tremblay, Jean-Denis
Vien, Marcel
Villiard, Jean-Sebastien

DOLLARD DES ORMEAUX

Behelak, Youssef
Braha-Wyszogrodski, Linda
Da Costa, Derek
Desimon, Jean-Haulis R.
D'Ignazio, Giuseppe
Djeredjian, Jessica, FamilyMed
Finkelberg, Susan, FamilyMed(EM)
Frank, Agnes, FamilyMed
Gauthier, Michel
Ghazigian, Taline, FamilyMed
Gorzalka, Frances
Kaplan-Krasny, Wendy
Katz, Murray S.
Levi, Aline
Luterman, Rosalind A., FamilyMed
MacGeachy, Fiona J.
Mashal, Orly H.
Mimran, Gracia
Mooallem, Ronit, FamilyMed
Page, Michel
Patel, Harilal B.
Poplawski, Daniel H.
Rioux, Marie-Claude
Wyszogrodski, Isaac

DONNACONA

Audy, Marie
Charron, Louis
Dussault, Marie-Claude
Frenette, Johanne
Girard, Linda
Giroux, Lina
Lavallee, Lucie
Leboeuf, Andreanne
Prud'Homme, Henri
Walsh, Julie, FamilyMed

DORVAL

Andre, Liliane
Bernstein, Robert L.
Cummings, Ina E., FamilyMed
Daemen-Darveau, Helene
Giron, Marie-France
Godin, Marie-Christine, FamilyMed
Laliberte, Daniel, FamilyMed
Lam, Thu Loan, FamilyMed
Lefebvre, Chantal
Minz, Gabriel R., FamilyMed
Perlman, Robert J.
Ross, Peter K.
Rouette, Daniel
Sairam, Ashwin M., FamilyMed
St-Laurent, Renaud
Svitek, Jessica C., FamilyMed
Zummo, Mario

DRUMMONDVILLE

Allard, Marc-Andre
Amyot, Diane
Arevalo Centeno, Ruben D.
Aubin, Lydia, FamilyMed
Beaulieu, Linda
Beaulieu-Denault, Camille, FamilyMed
Benoit, Andree
Bilodeau, Alain
Biron, Daniel, FamilyMed
Boukhalfa, Amokrane
Boyer, Francois
Brouillette, Nancy
Camire, Valerie, FamilyMed
Campeau, Gilles
Cavanagh, Marie-Pier, FamilyMed
Cayouette, Marie-Claude, FamilyMed
Champagne, Francois
Charron, Claire
Chasse, Genevieve
Cloutier, Anne-Marie, FamilyMed
Cote, Andre
Cote, Sylvain
Courchesne, Sophie
Croteau, Myriane, FamilyMed
Daneault, Mathieu
Doyon, Linda, FamilyMed
Durand, Nancy, FamilyMed
Fiset, Amelie
Fontaine, Karine
Forcier, Jean-Francois, FamilyMed
Gagne, Annie-Claude, FamilyMed
Gailloux, Tom, FamilyMed
Gervais, Benoit
Gervais, Robert
Giguere, Nicole
Gingras, Andre
Godin, Isabelle
Gousse-Matte, Olivier
Hebert, Julie
Hebert-Semco, Genevieve, FamilyMed
Jutras, Marcel
Khalil, Sylvia, FamilyMed
L'Heureux, Christian
Lachance, Marc
Lachance, Nicole
Lacroix, Ghyslain
Lafleur, Daniel, FamilyMed
Lague, Guylaine, FamilyMed
Larrivee, Mathieu, FamilyMed
Lemaire, Daniel
Lemaire, Julie, FamilyMed
Malenfant, Helene
Masse, Lyne
Montminy, Gilles
Moreau, Caroline
Morin, Anne-Marie, FamilyMed
Nguyen, Michel C K.
Otis, Daniel
Otis, Gilles, FamilyMed
Ouellet, Gilles
Picotte, Marie-Eve, FamilyMed(EM)
Plamondon, Catherine
Proteau, Caroline
Roy, Christine
Simard, Vincent, FamilyMed
Soucy, Francois C.
St-Onge, Chantal
Tetreault, Guy, FamilyMed
Tetreault, Sylvie
Thibault, Julie
Tran, Jean-Cao P., FamilyMed
Tremblay, Sylvie
Viens, Gilles
Vigneault, Marc
Villeneuve, Michel

DUHAMEL-OUEST

Barbeau, Paul-Emile
Watelle, Hubert

DUNHAM

Magnan, Renee

EAST ANGUS

Branch, Robert G.
Desroches, Francois
Habel, Jean-Paul
Soulard, Mario

EAST BROUGHTON

Grenier, Lucien

EASTMAIN

Smeja, Christina A.

FARNHAM

Biron, Linda
Bissonnette, Louis, FamilyMed
Blais, Chantal
Bourbonnais, Anne, FamilyMed
Cotton, Patrick, FamilyMed
Daviau, Marjolaine, FamilyMed
De Medicis, Anne
Fafard, Bruno
Gamache, Stephan
Jannelle, Jean-Pierre, FamilyMed
Masson, Pierre
Messier, Maryse, FamilyMed
Patenaude-Chagnon, Sophie, FamilyMed

FERME-NEUVE

Comtois, Pierre

FERMONT

Boulanger, Jocelyn
Dubuc, Sebastien
Labourdette, Claudine
Magny, Jacqueline
Mercier, Christian
Pilon, Raynald
Pinard, Josiane
Samson, Isabelle, FamilyMed
St-Gelais, Line

FLEURIMONT

Thuot, Pierre

FORESTVILLE

Drouin, Michel
Picard, Marie
Richard, Luc
Salvetti, Yvan, FamilyMed
Tremblay, Serge

FORT-COULONGE

Bazile, Marie Y., FamilyMed
Benfey, Martin C.
Guillotte, Eve, FamilyMed
Willett, Paule, FamilyMed
Zhivkov, Alexander

FORTIERVILLE

Allen Demers, Catherine
Cantin, Mireille
Davidson, Marie-Helene
Drouin-Berube, Nicolas, FamilyMed
Gagnon, Steeve
Giroux, Linda
Heroux, Isabelle, FamilyMed
Laliberte, Audrey
Laliberte, Josette
Langlois, Jean
Lessard, Marie-Claude
Levesque, Nancy
Roy, Christine, FamilyMed

FRAMPTON

Moreau, Marc-Andre

GASPE

Alberton, Bruno G., FamilyMed
Belanger Ducharme, Frederique, FamilyMed
Bernier, Christian
Bernier, Mathieu, FamilyMed
Berthelot, Eva, FamilyMed
Blais-Morin, Catherine, FamilyMed
Bourque, Sonia, FamilyMed
Cote, Serge
Desjardins, Michel, FamilyMed
Drouin, Guy, FamilyMed
Ducharme, Marie
Duguay, Annick, FamilyMed
Dupuis-Riendeau, Emilie, FamilyMed
Emery, Marie-Lou, FamilyMed(EM)
Eugène, Alain
Forest, France L.
Galarneau, Yolaine
Gaudry, Stefane, FamilyMed
Gauthier, Gilles
Groulx, Antoine, FamilyMed
Heroux, Michelle, FamilyMed
Jacob-Goudreau, Ariane
Judd, Lyne
Kulenkamp, Anne C D., FamilyMed
Lachance-Fortin, Geraldine, FamilyMed
Lacombe, Jean-Guy
Landry, Esther
Leblanc, Michelle
Lefebvre, Andreanne, FamilyMed
Lefebvre, Jean-Francois, FamilyMed
Levesque, Jacques P.
Loiselle, Denis
Mainville, Christian, FamilyMed(EM)
Ouellet, Louis-Olivier, FamilyMed
Phaneuf, Simon, FamilyMed(EM)
Picard, Chantal, FamilyMed
Plourde, Claudia, FamilyMed
Plourde, Isabelle, FamilyMed
Poulin, Michael, FamilyMed
Poulin, Michel
Rheault, Isabelle, FamilyMed
Robichaud, Annie, FamilyMed
Romero Castro, Mario E.
Rousseau, Stephane
Skene, Patsy
Therrien, Mylene, FamilyMed

GATINEAU

Abboud, Fayez
Abdel-Sayed, Farid I.
Abdelhalim-Amdiss, Fatima
Abou Abdo, Mirna
Adams, David
Andraos, Noel H., FamilyMed
April, Andre M.
Archambault, Claude R.
Arvisais, Nadine, FamilyMed
Attignon, Ablavi S H N.
Aube, Gilles, FamilyMed
Aubry, Mark J.
Auger, Dominique, FamilyMed
Ayoub, Paul
Babineau, Gaetan
Babiuk, Olga
Barrette, Ian, FamilyMed
Becotte, Therese
Bedard, Nicholas
Belanger, Sylvie
Belzile, Robert
Berard, Claire
Bergeron, Chantal, FamilyMed
Bergeron, Solange
Besner, Catherine, FamilyMed
Bienvenu, Genevieve
Bisson, Robert
Blais, Robert J D., FamilyMed
Boily, Jean-Claude, FamilyMed
Bonenfant, Guy, FamilyMed
Bonneville, Peter
Bouchard, Suzanne, FamilyMed
Boucher, Serge
Boudreault, Isabelle
Bourassa, Helene, FamilyMed
Bourbonniere, Christine, FamilyMed
Bourgeois, Patrick
Bourque, Marie-Claude
Bouthillier, Jean
Brochu, Richard
Brousseau, Gilles D.
Brown, Pierre
Bruneau, Serge
Bureau, Anne-Marie
Bureau, Helene
Bussieres, Josee
Cadivy, Alexandre
Caffin, Pierre-Yves
Cardinal, Michel
Caron, Michel
Caron, Valerie, FamilyMed
Carriere, Isabelle, FamilyMed
Cazeaux, Myriam
Charland, Nancy
Chelfi, Mustapha
Cimon, Philippe
Clarke, Terrence
Cloutier, Isabelle
Comeau, Marie-Josee, FamilyMed
Constantineau, Genevieve, FamilyMed
Coquet-Le Pape, Bernadette
Cote, Andree
Cote, Denis J P.
Couet, Alain
Couillard, Serge A J.
Coupal, Jean F.
Croteau, Sylvain, FamilyMed
Cyr, Andre
Daigle, Christine
Damphousse, Andreanne, FamilyMed
Dao, Hong Quyen
Daoust, Marguerite
De Champlain, Remi, FamilyMed
De La Chevrotiere, Jean
Demers, Louis
Demers, Sylvie
Desjardins, Francine C.
Desormeaux, Julie, FamilyMed
Desrosiers, Marie-Helene, FamilyMed
Dionne, Christal
Dube, Jean-Marie
Duchesne, Rachel, FamilyMed
Duclos, David
Dupont, Helene
Dussault, Lucie, FamilyMed
Duval, Johanne
Eydt, John M.
Fares, Oussama, FamilyMed
Faullem, Ingrid, FamilyMed
Ferigutti, Daniela, FamilyMed
Finlay, Michel
Foccroulle, Ann-Stephane
Forest, Sophie
Fortier, Pierre, FamilyMed
Fortin, Gilles W.
Fortin, Suzanne
Foucault, Lynne
Gagnon, Genevieve, FamilyMed
Gagnon, Isabelle
Gagnon, Michel
Gagnon, Serge
Galipeau, Jean-Luc
Gallant, Marie-Josee
Gareau, Pierre
Gelinas, Bernard
Gelinas, Danielle
Gendron, Robert
Gervais, Anne, FamilyMed
Gervaise, Amelie
Gillot, Nicolas P M.
Girard, Marie-Eve, FamilyMed
Godbout, Jean
Godin, Johanne, FamilyMed
Gosselin, Kim
Goulet, Audrey-Anne
Gouriou, Dominique
Granger, Jean
Gregory, Alfred J.
Grondin, Louis
Guay, Genevieve
Guay, Louise, FamilyMed
Guerin, Danielle
Guilbault, Marcel
Guilbeault, Valerie
Guirguis, Nancy
Hachemi, Latifa, FamilyMed
Han, Lily, FamilyMed
Hebert, Michele
Huppe, Chantal, FamilyMed
Hurik, Ilona
Iakoub, Elena, FamilyMed
Jbala, Moulay A., FamilyMed
Jean-Francois, Herve G.
Jolin, Isabelle-Sophie, FamilyMed
Khullar, Renu
Kindeki-Luzingu, Pierrette
Kocaefe, Burcu, FamilyMed
Kuate, Xaviere C.
L'Hereault, Sylvie
LaRue, Frank J.
Laberge, Louise, FamilyMed
Labrie, Isabelle
Labrie, Marie-Claude
Lacasse, Martin
Lacasse, Melanie, FamilyMed
Lachaine, Marie-Pierre, FamilyMed
Lacombe, Danyele
Lacroix, Luc-Phillippe J., FamilyMed
Lai, Sio Mei, FamilyMed
Lalonde, Jean-Serge
Lalonde, Jocelyne
Lalonde, Stephanie, FamilyMed(EM)
Lalonde-Kontio, Ginette, FamilyMed
Lamontagne, Lysanne, FamilyMed
Langlois, Alexis, FamilyMed
Langlois, Francois
Lapointe, Marc
Lapointe, Veronique, FamilyMed
Laquerre, Chantal, FamilyMed
Laramee, Delphine, FamilyMed
Lasalle-Folot, Marie-Helene
Laviolette, Genevieve, FamilyMed
Law, Tommy, FamilyMed
Leblanc, Germain
Leboeuf, Jean-Louis
Lecault, Melanie
Leclerc, Claude
Lemay, Guy
Levesque-Chouinard, Annabelle, FamilyMed
Likavcanova, Elena, FamilyMed
Luna, Fernando A.
Mah, Peter, FamilyMed
Mailhot, Philippe
Manseau, Danielle I M., FamilyMed
Marceau, Danielle, FamilyMed
Martel, Gaetan
Martin, Isabelle M C., FamilyMed
Matte, Pierre
Maziarz, Stanislaw T., FamilyMed
Mbonjo, Isaac B., FamilyMed
McConnery, Carol, FamilyMed
Melancon, Genevieve, FamilyMed
Meliji, Zineb, FamilyMed
Menard, Jacques G.
Michaud, Marie-Noelle
Miquelon, Marianne, FamilyMed
Mitton, Jennifer M., FamilyMed
Moamai, Javad
Montsion, Claude
Moorjani, Mira
Moreau, Andre G.
Morissette, Guy
Mourad, Mustapha
Mulaja Wa Mulaja, Aubin, FamilyMed
Nadon, Joel, FamilyMed
Naim, Maurice
Nappert, Rejean A.
Nguyen, Hieu Dinh
Nguyen, Thi Anh T.
Nguyen The, My
Nimpagaritse, Rosalie
Olariu, Carmen, FamilyMed
Ouedraogo, Yacine B., FamilyMed
Pandian, A M. Chelvi, FamilyMed
Pang, Peter H L.
Paquet, J A. Ronald
Paquet, Louis F.
Paradis-Robert, Nina, FamilyMed
Pelissier, Lise
Perello, Andrea S.
Perez, Barbara, FamilyMed
Pham-Dinh, Martin, FamilyMed(EM)
Pigeon, Edith, FamilyMed

PHYSICIANS BY PROVINCE

Pilon, Jacques, FamilyMed
Pilon, Richard A.
Pinault, Marie
Platero Miranda, Hugo E., FamilyMed
Poirier, Marc J.
Poitras, Daniel
Proulx, Guylaine, FamilyMed
Prud'Homme, Denis
Prud'Homme, Rodrigue
Quesnel, Vanessa, FamilyMed
Ranev, Dimitre, FamilyMed
Ratte, Richard R.
Regimbal, Marc
Remillard, Elizabeth
Reny, Marcel
Ridgeway, Kimberly, FamilyMed
Roberge, Elise, FamilyMed(EM)
Robinson, Paul
Rodrigue, Pierre Y.
Rollin, Marie-France
Rooke, J. Louise
Rouleau, Charles D.
Routhier, J J. Richard
Roy, Ghyslain
Rushenas, Alexandre
Saint-Georges, Pierre J., FamilyMed
Salloum, Alexandre
Savard-Woods, Catherine
Savoie, Veronique, FamilyMed(EM)
Seguin, Marie-France
Sergerie, Pascale
Shaw, Julia, FamilyMed
Sibille, Pascale L R.
Simard, Eric
Simonyi-Poirier, Marianne, FamilyMed
Sirois, M M. Jeanne
St-Amour, Eric, FamilyMed
Sylvestre, Andre
Tanguay, Alain G., FamilyMed(EM)
Temkit, Abdelkader
Tessier, Guylaine, FamilyMed
Theilliez, Boris
Theriault, Guylene, FamilyMed
Therrien, Anne-Marie
Tiret, Bertrand-Philippe
Titri Zaibak, Nabyla
To, My Lan
Tozlovanu-Paskal, Viorika, FamilyMed
Tremblay-Bouchard, Emilie, FamilyMed
Trinh, Ngoc Chau
Tsakalaki, Anna, FamilyMed
Tshibumbu, Josiane M., FamilyMed
Vachon, Louise
Vallieres, Andree, FamilyMed
Veilleux, Marie-Christine
Villemaire, Pierre A.
Vo, Thi Nhu Y.
Vu-Khanh, Anh-Thu, FamilyMed
Xavier Mattesco, Carole F A.

GORE

Dufour, Daniel

GRACEFIELD

Eliev, Sonia, FamilyMed

GRANBY

Aleksic, Slavica
Allard, Nathalie, FamilyMed
Beauchesne, Christian
Beaudoin, Denise
Beaulieu, Genevieve, FamilyMed
Beaumier, Isabelle
Beaumont, Nathalie
Bellamy, Danielle
Bergeron, Dino
Bergeron, Jacques
Bernier, Rose-Alexie
Blais, Marianne
Bradette, Isabelle, FamilyMed(EM)
Brault, Suzanne
Cartier, Marie
Cauchon, Guy
Cavanagh, Annik
Charbonneau, Benoit
Cote, Isabelle
Coulombe, Nicole
Dallaire, Louise C.
De Broux, Marie, FamilyMed
Deschamps, Charles
Deschenes, Christian
Dube, Marie-Pier, FamilyMed
Dubuc, Marie-Eve, FamilyMed
Dufour, Serge
Dufour, Stefanie
Dugre, Colette
Dussault, Isabelle, FamilyMed
Favreau, Joel
Fay, Didier
Fortin, Michel-Andre
Foucault, Josee
Fryer, Sonia
Gagnon, Nadya
Gariepy, Philippe, FamilyMed
Geadah, Christian, FamilyMed
Gelinas, Melanie
Gosselin, Richard
Gregoire, Marie-Claude
Grou, Evelyne
Guertin, Paul
Hebert, Francois
Hill, Christine
Lacoste, Sophie
Laplante, Patrick
Larkin, Emilie
Lasnier, Luc
Latulippe, Isabelle, FamilyMed(EM)
Le Gresley, Jovain
Leblanc, Francois
Leblanc, Nadine
Lebrun, Natalie
Leduc, Yves
Lefebvre, Stephane
Loignon, Caroline
Lorquet, Annie
Malo-Poirier, Ann-Claude
Martel, Diane B.
Maynard, Olivier
Mayrand, Isabel, FamilyMed
Mayrand, Sophie, FamilyMed(EM)
Menard, Rejean, FamilyMed
Messier, Mario
Monfette, Benoit
Montel, Catherine
Morin, Marie-Josee, FamilyMed
Ouellet, Gilles
Ouellet, Marie-France
Ouellette, Chantal
Pellerin, Gabriel
Pelletier, J E. Claude
Perusse, Isabelle
Poirier, Michel
Quirion, Andre
Risler, Marie-Claude
Rodrigue, Lise
Roy, Lucie
Royer, Christelle
Saint-Michel, Patrick, FamilyMed(EM)
Sleiman, Asad
Tanguay, Caroline, FamilyMed
Tanguay, Elisabeth
Thibaudeau, Sylvain

GRAND-MERE

Beaulieu Jr., David
Boilard-Lamontagne, Catherine, FamilyMed
Busque, Denis
Cadorette, Sebastien, FamilyMed
Gagnon, Maude
Gonzalez, Yolanda, FamilyMed
Jacques, Andre, FamilyMed
Larocque, Rene
Lefebvre, Jean
Robert, Diane
Rousseau, Frederic
Sylvain-Lucien, Joseph
Tousignant, Michel P.
Trottier, Marc
Trudel, Jocelyn

GRANDE-RIVIERE

Gamache, Germain

GRANDE-VALLEE

Arcouet, Celine
Des Aulniers, Evelyne, FamilyMed
Pacuraru, Jean-Pierre, FamilyMed
Simon, Daniel, FamilyMed

GREENFIELD PARK

Akbaraly, Tasnime
Ayllon Ugarte, Jose
Barbarese, Gabrielle, FamilyMed
Beaulieu, Julie, FamilyMed
Beausejour, Eric, FamilyMed
Bedard, Anne-Marie
Beliveau, Johanne A.
Bergeron, Brenda A., FamilyMed
Bien-Aime, Lubraine, FamilyMed
Boisvert, Nathalie
Boudreau, Serge, FamilyMed
Brodeur, Marie-Claude, FamilyMed(EM)
Bussieres, Nicolas, FamilyMed(EM)
Cayer, Julie
Corazza, Bernard
Crich, Alexandre S., FamilyMed(EM)
Dallaire, Ghyslain
De Angelis, Flavia
Delisle, Caroline
Dupras, Louise
Fiset, Caroline
Fluet, Jocelyne
Gareau, Julie, FamilyMed
Gauthier, Alain
Genot, Veronique
Habra, Munir
Lalonde, Jacques
Lanctot, Jean-Francois, FamilyMed(EM)
Lefebvre, Patrick
Lemaire, Frédéric B., FamilyMed(EM)
Lemay, Gerard
Loranger, Martin, FamilyMed(EM)
Lussier, Bruno
Maamari, Caroline
Maniere, Thibault
Marcil, Brigitte
McCaughey, David F., FamilyMed(EM)
Milbeo, Yann G.
Miot, Robert C.
Mital, Bernard
Moreira Bacha, Omar
Namen, Samia, FamilyMed
Nguyen, Huu Nam
Nik-Akhtar, Tanaz
Nizard, Jacques H V.
O'Doherty, Michael, FamilyMed(EM)
Pilote, Nathalie, FamilyMed
Plante, Annick
Prady, Catherine C.
Proulx, Veronique
Quevillon, Nadine, FamilyMed
Rhein, Stephane, FamilyMed(EM)
Roy, Julie, FamilyMed
Sangani, Hemalata J B.
Sangani, Mahendra B S.
Tetreault, Stephane, FamilyMed(EM)
Turcotte-Lagace, Mathieu, FamilyMed(EM)
Turgeon, Genevieve
Vanier, Laurent, FamilyMed(EM)
Yahia Cherif, Tewfik, FamilyMed

HAM-NORD

Faucher, Jacques

HAMPSTEAD

Bass, Shana, FamilyMed

HAVRE-SAINT-PIERRE

Baillargeon, Claude
Bellemare, Monique
Bernier, Marie-France, FamilyMed
Cote, Pierre G.
Guillemette, Chantal, FamilyMed
Lavoie, Mireille
Monnier, Audrey, FamilyMed
Moore, Pierre
Morin, Elodie, FamilyMed
Paquet, Marc, FamilyMed
Samson, Mimi

HEBERTVILLE

Girard, Jean-Baptiste
Paradis, Serge

HUBERDEAU

Rondeau, Guy

HUDSON

Hryniowski, Ronald G., FamilyMed
Leclair, Marie Ann.
Welik, Leonard J.

HUNTINGDON

Babin, Charles E.
Hebert, Jean-Pierre
Lemieux, Raymond
Rosenberg, Jean

INUKJUAK

Marchand, Marie-Hélène
Prevost, Francois A.

JOLIETTE

Arteau-Gauthier, Myreille
Ayotte, Evans C.
Beaudry, Luce
Boudreault-Larochelle, Samuel, FamilyMed
Bourassa, Sylvie
Boyer, Philippe L.
Breault, Christiane, FamilyMed
Briere, Claude
Daoust, Danielle
Desilets, Joane
Desjardins, Julie, FamilyMed
Dufresne, Normand
Harnois, Pierre A.
Jolicoeur, Sylvie
Khorsi, Sonia R.
Lafarge, Muriel
Laliberte, Carmen
Lussier, France
Martin, Martine
Mazur, Sophie
Mongeon, Mikael
Morel, Claude
Roy, Luc
Stanojlovic, Snezana
Therrien, Michel
Tremblay, Chantal
Villeneuve, Carolyne, FamilyMed

JONQUIERE

Baribeau, Genevieve
Barrette, Andree
Beaulieu, Andree
Belanger, Martin
Bilodeau, Carl
Bilodeau, Marc
Bilodeau, Serge
Blackburn, David
Blanchet, Caroline, FamilyMed
Boisselle, Jacques
Bouchard, Isabelle, FamilyMed
Bouchard, Lucie
Bouchard, Lucie, FamilyMed
Bouchard, Patrick
Bouchard, Pierre
Bouchard, Remi
Boulanger, Emilie
Boulianne, Donald
Carmichael, Rejean
De Champlain, France, FamilyMed
Dery, Claude
Dionne, Jacynthe
Dionne, Jonathan, FamilyMed(EM)
Donais, Guy
Dubois, Mario
Dubois, Marion
Fortier, Gerald
Fortin, Christian
Fortin, Marc
Gagne, Alexandra
Gagne, Caroline
Gagnon, Claude
Gagnon, Roger
Gauthier, Nadia
Gilbert, France
Godin, Marie-Eve, FamilyMed
Gosselin, Johanne
Grenier, Louis-Simon, FamilyMed
Houde, Catherine, FamilyMed
Jolin, Diane
Lapointe, Joris
Lapointe, Romuald
Lavoie, Guylaine
Lecomte, Veronique, FamilyMed
Mansaray, Helene
Michaud, Guillaume
Muslemani, Ali, FamilyMed
Paradis, Jean-Michel
Pedneault, Melodie, FamilyMed(EM)
Perron, Mylene
Roy, Martine
Savard, Catherine
Simard, Frederic, FamilyMed
Simard, Marie C.
Simard, Mylene
Tremblay, Madeleine
Tremblay, Pascale
Turgeon, Francoise
Voyer, Patricia
Watts, Nancy, FamilyMed

KAHNAWAKE

Bruemmer, Aurel T.
Eniojukan, Rachael, FamilyMed
Horn, Ojistoh, FamilyMed
Jones, Suzanne, FamilyMed
MacLaren, Laura S., FamilyMed(EM)
Ross, Andrea J., FamilyMed
Tehranifar, Mitra
Zakharova Smirnova, Natalia, FamilyMed

KAWAWACHIK-AMACH

Lafortune, Claude
Larochelle, Josee

KINGSEY FALLS

Bernier, Manon
Lemieux, Isabelle
Ouellette, Audrey

KIRKLAND

Cholette, Pierre M.
Cohen, Howard S., FamilyMed
Cote, Serge H.
Czaharyn, Anthony G., FamilyMed
Dancose, Robin
Klein, Jack
Levesque, Gilles
Moin-Darbari, Djavad

Normandin, Alexander, FamilyMed
Papageorgakopoulos, P., FamilyMed
Piechota, Paul S., FamilyMed
Richer, Genevieve
Thomassin, Josyane, FamilyMed
Trinh, Bich Hang

KNOWLTON

Barakett, William, FamilyMed
Barbeau, Jean-Jacques
Desy, Dominique
Gendron, Marie-Danielle, FamilyMed
Giannangelo, Dominique, FamilyMed

KUUJJUAQ

Boulanger, Nathalie, FamilyMed
Bourque, Rachel, FamilyMed
Campbell, Latoya L., FamilyMed
Cherradi, Siham, FamilyMed
Desjardins, Julie, FamilyMed
Koenig, Marie-Charlotte, FamilyMed
Mbaye, Saliou D., FamilyMed
Popencu, Madalina, FamilyMed
Souissi, Hassen, FamilyMed
Szczygielski, Blazej I., FamilyMed(EM)

KUUJJUARAPIK

Cipera, Michelle P., FamilyMed
Duong, Van Tinh

L'ANCIENNE-LORETTE

Beauchesne, Andre
Berthelot, Gilles
Berube, Michele
Blouin, Pierre
Grenier, Lise
Jutras, Maryse
Larochelle, Isabel
Larochelle, Real
Pare, Bruno
Tetu, Christian

L'ANGE-GARDIEN

Landry, Michel E.

L'ANSE-SAINT-JEAN

Dumais, Michelle

L'ASSOMPTION

Boucher, Andree-Anne
Bourgoin-Couillard, Sylvie
Cadoret, Pierre
Chausse, Luc
Cyr, Helene
Daigneault, Julie
De Meyer, Philippe
Diotte, Magali
Khim, Hong-Ly
Lachance, Sabrina
Lafortune, Donald
Lafrance, Justine
Larocque, Isabelle
Pare, Gregoire
Pilon, Michel
Roy, Yvan
Samedy, Natacha
Toupin, Jacques R.

L'EPIPHANIE

Rebolledo, Lina, FamilyMed

L'ILE-PERROT

Carrier, Guyta, FamilyMed
Ng Fuk Chong, Raphael
Payer, Pierre

L'ISLETVILLE

Grondin, Louis
Lavallee, Lucie

LA BAIE

Belliveau, Anne C.
Bergeron, Sophie
Boily, Anik
Bouchard, Normand
Boudreault, Melanie, FamilyMed
De Varennes, Maryline, FamilyMed
Duchaine, Denise
Dufresne, Charles
Fortin, Veronique
Francis, Denyse
Gagnon, Dominique
Gagnon, Marie-Elaine, FamilyMed
Gagnon, Sonia
Gauthier, Marcel
Harvey, Annie
Larouche, Gilles
Larouche, Leon
Lefaivre, Robert
Mallet, Veronique
Marceau, Jacinthe
Nadeau, Martine
Potvin, Sandra, FamilyMed
Roy, Danny, FamilyMed
Sergerie, Keven, FamilyMed

LA BALEINE

Ethier, Marcel

LA GUADELOUPE

Cote, Chantal
Hebert, Annie
Legendre, Robert
Michaud, Carole
Vachon, Andre

LA MACAZA

Thibodeau, Jacques, FamilyMed

LA MALBAIE

Bernier, Marie-Jose
Bouchard, Andre
Bouchard, Jacques
Carrier, Pierre
Cayer, Nathalie, FamilyMed
Dupuis, Jean-Luc
Filteau, Chantal, FamilyMed
Gagnon, Marie-Josee, FamilyMed
Gonthier, Danielle
Harvey, Normand
Huppe, Xavier, FamilyMed
Lupien, Nicolas, FamilyMed
Melancon, Eric
Ouellet, Danielle
Plesu, Ioana, FamilyMed
Prie, Veronique
Trudeau, Robert

LA PATRIE

Beliveau, Serge
Brochu, Michele

LA POCATIERE

Caron, Serge
Clapperton, Véronique, FamilyMed
Couture, Madeleine
Deguire, Richard, FamilyMed
Gagnon, Catherine, FamilyMed
Gelinas, Catherine, FamilyMed
Hudon, Jean
La Rochelle, Pierre
Larose, Milie-Ève
Lepage, Dominique
Martin, Lucile
Ouellet, Claudine
Pelletier, Denis
Pelletier, Isabelle
Poulin, Fernand
Rancourt, Claudine, FamilyMed
Rousseau, Josee, FamilyMed
Roux, Christian, FamilyMed
Simard, Melanie, FamilyMed
Smyth, Patricia
St-Louis, Pia

LA PRAIRIE

Aouadi, Adila
Belefqih, Mounia
Boily, Isabelle
Bourdeau, Line, FamilyMed
Boutet, Jacques
Brochu, Gilles B.
Lepage, Jean-Marc
Longtin, Richard
Losa-Vazquez, Jesus
Martel, Francois, FamilyMed
Zador, Katalin

LA SARRE

Aboubzou, Nour-Eddine
Bedoya-Mejia, Juan, FamilyMed
Belanger, Louis
Bernatchez, Simon
Bonicard, Pierre-Alexandre, FamilyMed
Bulai, Bianca A., FamilyMed
Champagne, Nathalie
Charbonneau, Chantal, FamilyMed
Cherif Slimane, Safia, FamilyMed
Clement, Christine
Constant, Yvon
de Maupeou, Michel
Dignard, Mario
Duchesne, Manon
Faille, Christiane
Farah Andrawes, Wafik
Ferhat, Ferroudja
Gauthier, Dominic, FamilyMed
Hottlet, Helene
Langlois, Janick, FamilyMed
Larrivee, Claude
Lebel, Rejean, FamilyMed
Leclerc, Rachel, FamilyMed
Marcoux, Isabelle A., FamilyMed
Masse, Isabelle
Ouertani, Sofiane
Paradis, Sabrina, FamilyMed
Perrier, Guy
Plante, Christine
Schifirnet, Diana E., FamilyMed
Seide, Rony, FamilyMed
St-Jean, Catherine, FamilyMed
Tran, Tri Minh, FamilyMed
Treigys, Darius
Verville, Marcel
Watelle, Sylvie

LA TUQUE

Abbas, Mohammad A.
Albert, Francois
Angers, Daniel
Barthelemy, Bernard F.
Blais, Annie
Bouchard, Claude A.
Bourgault, Judith
Capusan, Gheorghe V.
Dorcély, Amos
Fadois, Emerson
Gauthier, Emmanuelle
Gingras, Guy
Habel, Pierre-David
Jospitre, Joseph-Marie L.
Lacombe, Marc-Andre
Lakrouf, El-Hadi
Morin, Annie
Roberge, Laurence, FamilyMed
Villeneuve, Pierre

LABELLE

Noel, Jean-Marc

LAC-BEAUPORT

Tremblay, Jean

LAC-BOUCHETTE

Bernier, Sophie

LAC-DES-AIGLES

Lemieux, Ghislain

LAC-DROLET

Cote, Jean-F

LAC-ETCHEMIN

Belzil, Simon-Pierre, FamilyMed
Boudreault, Nicolas
Bureau-Morin, Marie-Helene
Dion, Sylvain
Dubuc, Eric
Duguay, Veronique, FamilyMed
Fecteau, Line
Gilbert, Reynald
Gosselin, Guylaine
Guillot-Hardy, Denise
Labbe, Paule
Lamer, Mark
Landry, Caroline
Michaud, Christian
Roy, Marie-Lou, FamilyMed

LAC-MEGANTIC

Bolduc, Nadia, FamilyMed
Brochu, Daniel
Chaput, Gerard
Chouinard, Daniel, FamilyMed
Dulac, Kathleen
Gelinas, Bernard
Giroux, Geraldine
Labrecque, Katherine
Laframboise, Patrice, FamilyMed
Machin, Jack F.
Marias-Radu, Ana, FamilyMed
Michel, Florence, FamilyMed
Nogue, Marc-Rene
Pusca, Carina G.
Rochon, Micheline

LACHENAIE

Vincent, Guy

LACHINE

Audet, Neil
Barezpour, Mohammad Reza, FamilyMed
Baribeau, Sylvia
Beaudry, Daniel
Berube, Elaine
Boskovic Petrovic, Jasmina, FamilyMed
Carreiro, Stephen R., FamilyMed
Daignault, Monique
Daniel, Helene
Daudelin, Luc
Elshobary, Hanan M.
Garon, Claire
Hachachena, Fatima
Khalil, Andrew, FamilyMed(EM)
Kisak-Tomiuk, Jeannette L.
Kurzencwyg, David
Lauzon, Pierre P E.
Masson, Guylaine
Moyal, Yoel, FamilyMed(EM)
Munoz, Carlos A.
Musgrave, John M.
Parent, France
Parsons, William D., FamilyMed(EM)
Rousseau, Daniel
Saba, Paul J.
Saoud, Fahimy, FamilyMed
Tam-Quyen, Marie-Therese, FamilyMed
Theroux, Julie
Vegiard, Chantal

LACHUTE

Cantin, Caroline, FamilyMed
Chiorpec-Georgescu, Margareta
Desbiens, France
Du Sault, Karine, FamilyMed
Durocher, Gilles
Fermini, Richard
Gasiorowska, Paulina, FamilyMed(EM)
Godon, Patricia
Hassanalizadeh, Hamid
Kiderchah, Rabi
Lanciault, Diane
Lepage, Marie-Christine
Lynch, Michel
Madani, Daniel L.
Marleau, Michel, FamilyMed
Mitchell, A. Gregor, FamilyMed
Moutran, Joseph
Poirier, Marie-Andree, FamilyMed
Poulin, Claude
Sabourin, Julie, FamilyMed
Soulard, Caroline, FamilyMed
St-Pierre, France
Talbot, Jessica, FamilyMed
Thibault, Ginette
Thibodeau, Pierre
Trudel, Francois

LADYSMITH

Chambers, Karen, FamilyMed

LAMBTON

Lefebvre, Richard T.
Malenfant, Suzanne
Mercier, Christian

LASALLE

Aina, Judy
Assouline, Tony, FamilyMed
Barette, Marie
Bascaron, Marie-Eve, FamilyMed
Benaim, Daniel
Berlim, Marcelo T.
Bertolo, Luigia
Bianchini, Antonio U., FamilyMed
Blais, P. Clifford
Bourque, Andre
Brouillette, Gilles
Castonguay, J D. Gilles
Charette, Geneviève
Chaufour, Cecile
Colavincenzo, Vincenzo A.
Cote-Pare, Jonathan
Dagenais, Valerie
Dahan, Karen, FamilyMed
Desroches, Valerie, FamilyMed
Duchesne-Panisset, Manon
Duong, Catherine M H N., FamilyMed
Durand, Marie-Josee
Ennaifer, Atika, FamilyMed
Fichman, Anna, FamilyMed
Gagnon, Helene
Gaillardetz, Eveline
Gailloux, Benoit

Gardner, Marieke, FamilyMed
Gervais, Coralie, FamilyMed
Giard, Chantale, FamilyMed
Girouard, Nathalie
Gloutney, Kim
Hajjar, Edward, FamilyMed
Hamel, Jean-Pierre
Hebert, Nathalie
Heinegg, Jennifer
Heneman, Anaïs
Khazandar, Fatimah, FamilyMed
Laberge, Christiane
Labuda, Zuzanna, FamilyMed
Lachance, Danielle
Lajoie, Luce
Lazzara, Frank T.
Marando, Dominic
Martineau Corbeil, Elise
Mazzarelli, Mark
Meagher, Caroline, FamilyMed(EM)
Montbazet, A X. Anne, FamilyMed
Monty, Anne
Negrete, Sebastian, FamilyMed
Papillon, Daphne, FamilyMed
Pavlov, Ivan, FamilyMed
Riano Alvarez, Margarita R., FamilyMed
Rompre, Dominique, FamilyMed
Sanjab, Charbel, FamilyMed
Scott-Fleury, Marie-Helene
Stuckey, Valerie A., FamilyMed
Tabbane, Karim
Teodorescu, Cristina, FamilyMed
Thibault, Caroline, FamilyMed
Thibert, Jean-Francois, FamilyMed(EM)
Tjia, Sabine P Y.
Toupin, M A M. Carole
Toy, William
Turcot, Catherine, FamilyMed
Turqui, Farida, FamilyMed
Vinh, Chuong
Vo, Minh Ha
Vo, Thi Minh D., FamilyMed
Yankova, Sylvia A., FamilyMed
Yee, Gordon, FamilyMed
Yermus, Joseph A.

LATERRIERE

Theriault, Eric, FamilyMed

LAURENTIDES

Dugas, Gisele

LAURIER-STATION

Beaudry, Louise, FamilyMed
Bourgoin, Yves
Cimon, Isabelle, FamilyMed
Gagne, Elaine
Labonte, Chantal
Levesque, Julie
Maranda, Helene
Monfette, Denis, FamilyMed
Routhier, Brigitte
Roy, Michel G.

LAVAL

Achkar, Madeleine
Adem, Doris
Allard Riopel, Miriame
Allison, Francois
Amyot, Luce
Archambault, Claude
Archambault, Denis
Archambault, Martin
Arsenault, Marie-Eve
Arsenault, Mylene, FamilyMed
Asselin, Marcel
Aubin, Marie
Audet, Nicole, FamilyMed
Bakalem-Louli, Radia, FamilyMed
Bazinet, Lucie
Beauchamp, Jacques
Beauchemin, Francine
Beaudoin, Karine
Beaudry, Gaetan
Beaudry, Line, FamilyMed
Bechard, Elisabeth
Bedard, Catherine, FamilyMed
Bedard, Denis
Begin, Pierre, FamilyMed
Belanger, Bruno L.
Belanger, Jacques
Ben Ali, Henda
Bergman, Bonnie R., FamilyMed
Bertrand, Nathalie
Bessette, Isabelle
Blais, Jacques
Blouin, Carole
Blouin, Sylvie
Boies, R. Robert
Boisvert, Wilfrid
Bolduc, Gerard-Raymond
Bonneau, Andre, FamilyMed
Boucher, Mario
Boulad, Aladin E.
Bourbonniere, Andre
Breton, Michel
Bricault, Yvon
Brisson, Guy
Brizard, Martin
Brockman, Angie, FamilyMed
Broughton Wilkinson, Vanessa, FamilyMed
Brouillard, Gaetan
Cardinal, Bernard
Cardinal, Stephanie
Carmel, Luc
Caron, Matthieu
Castaneda-Bucci, Cristina, FamilyMed
Caza, France
Chabane-Chaouch, Nacera, FamilyMed
Chabrol-Joseph, Elsy
Champoux, Jean-J.
Chaoulli, Jacques
Charbonneau, Suzanne
Chenard, Helene
Chenier, Martin
Chesnay, Marylene
Choquette, Julie
Cloutier, Nicole
Coche, Edgar
Codsi, Marianne, FamilyMed
Cohade, Martine, FamilyMed
Cohonner, Chantal
Cotchikian, Rita, FamilyMed
Cote, Alain
Cote, Catherine
Cote, Guy
Courteau, Claire
Couture, Pauline
Croteau, Christian
Croteau, Isabelle
Cudnoch, P. Maria, FamilyMed
Cummings, Francis
Cusson, Daniel
Côté, Geneviève, FamilyMed
Dambreville, Etzer
Dashkovsky, Marina, FamilyMed
David, Jacqueline
De Carufel, France
De Minico, Carlo, FamilyMed
De Sanctis, Norman
Del Grande, Gabriella
Deneault-Lombart, Emmanuelle, FamilyMed(EM)
Depot, Rene
Desfosses, Annik
Desgroseilliers, Denise
Desjardins, Jacques
Desmarais, Jean-Anthony
Desnoyers, Pierre G.
Desruisseaux, Annie
Domingue, Claude
Dufour, Jerome
Dufresne, Jean-Claude
Dumont, Karine
Dupuis, Martine
Duval, Eve
Enache, Lucian, FamilyMed
Filteau, Genevieve, FamilyMed
Fleurent, Suzanne
Fontaine, Francis, FamilyMed
Forget, Andre
Fournier, Jacques, FamilyMed
Franco-Barredo, Francisco
Frappier, Guy
Frechette, Claude, FamilyMed
Gagnon, Ginette
Gagnon, Jean
Gagnon, Maurice
Garcia Del Sol, Idania
Gardiner, Fritz A.
Gauthier, Helene
Gauthier, Louise F.
Gauthier, Pierre A., FamilyMed
Gendron, Stephane
Gobeil, Annie-Emmanuelle
Godue, Francois
Gonzalez, Mariel
Gosselin, Marc-Andre
Goudreau, Alain
Goyer, Pierre
Gratton, Nicole
Gravel, Diane
Grenier, Louis-Philippe
Guay, Raynald
Guillet, Suzanne
Guirguis, Suzette K., FamilyMed
Habib, Nader H.
Hached Baitiche, Leila
Hagopian, Salpi, FamilyMed
Haineault, Rejean
Hakim, Samira
Hardy, Christine
Harris, Denis
Hassan, Sarah, FamilyMed
Henry Ebeid, Jacqueline, FamilyMed
Hoang, Dinh Le, FamilyMed(EM)
Hoang, Le Uyen
Hobden, Christian
Houde, Josee
Huot, Richard
Injoyan, Rita, FamilyMed
Internoscia, Karine, FamilyMed
Ionita, Mihaela, FamilyMed
Ith, Rinda-Bun H.
Jacques, Martin
Jodoin, Lyne, FamilyMed
Joly, Christine
Joubarne, Francois
Juteau, Louis-Christopher, FamilyMed
Karellis, Nicolas
Keryakes, Hany
Kim, Willy S., FamilyMed
Kochenburger-Belanger, S.
Kortbaoui, Alain
Kurdyla, Margaret T.
L'Ecuyer, Genevieve
L'Heureux, Bruno
Labelle, Jacquelin
Lacombe, Francois
Lafleur, Jean-Marc
Lagace, Gilles
Lalonde, Andre
Lalonde, Gilles
Lamarre, Edmond
Lamy-Monnot, Lianne, FamilyMed
Lanctot, Francine
Langis, Denis
Langlois, Isabelle
Laplante, Lise
Lau, William W L.
Laurin, Daniel
Lauzon, Francine
Lavigne, Marie-Claude
Le, Binh-Dang
Le, Nhan Trung
Le Corff, Joelle
Lebel, Roseline
Leblanc, Melanie, FamilyMed
Leduc, Claude, FamilyMed
Leduc, Pierre
Lefebvre, Jonathan, FamilyMed
Lefebvre, Manon
Legault, Pierre
Leroux, Robert
Lessard, Nicole
Levesque, Ghislain
Levin, Moses, FamilyMed
Liboiron, Gilles, FamilyMed
Liboiron, Pierre, FamilyMed
Lopez Osorio, Isabel, FamilyMed
Lord, Patricia
Lortie, Carole
Lussier, Marie-Therese, FamilyMed
Lynch, Sebastien, FamilyMed
Magnan, Johanne
Mai, Nghia Trung
Mailly, Suzanne
Major, Sophie
Malcolm, Dennis
Marceau, Julie
Marcotte, René
Marsolais, Anne-Sophie
Martel, Yvan
Martin, Gerald
Martin, Normand
Martineau, Andre
Martineau, Marie S.
Matte, Lise
Meagher, Suzy
Megie, Marie-Francoise
Merrett, Patrick, FamilyMed
Messier, Pierre
Mezrahi, Michel
Millette, Bernard A., FamilyMed
Minassian, Viken
Miron, Eric
Montpetit, Guy
Moreau, Anne
Morel, Johanne
Morin, Stephanie
Murphy, Patricia
Nadeau, Lynne
Naqvi, Damian D N.
Newman, Leslie
Nguyen, Diem Hong
Nguyen, Giao-Chi
Nguyen, Therese N H M., FamilyMed
Nguyen, Tu Anh, FamilyMed
Nicolas, Hanna, FamilyMed
Noiseux, Isabelle
Nolet, Bernard
Ocasiones, Carmencita
Padureanu, Magdalena
Papin, Lisanne
Paquette, Jean-Pierre
Paquette, Serge
Paquin, Michel
Paradis, Jacques
Pare, Robert
Parise, Patrick
Patry, Louise
Pearson, Margaret, FamilyMed
Pelland, Lynne, FamilyMed
Pelletier, Carole
Penes, Mihai C.
Perrier, Alban
Perron, Robert
Pham, Ngoc Huynh U.
Phaneuf, Louise, FamilyMed
Pilon, Maurice M.
Podaru, Elena-Ioana
Poitras, Daniel
Poitras, Rejean
Pontbriand, Robert
Porchetta, Simon, FamilyMed(EM)
Poulin, Marie-Josee
Poulin, Pascale
Pouliot, Kathleen
Prefontaine, Odette
Proulx, Andre
Proulx, Michele
Proulx, Pierre J L.
Provencher, France
Provost, Francois
Provost-Manseau, Suzanne
Pucella, Elisa, FamilyMed
Pung, Evelyne H., FamilyMed
Quan, T. Diem-Mai, FamilyMed
Racine, Michel, FamilyMed
Ranger, Jacques
Rheault, Diane
Ricard, Christyne
Richer-Comisso, Adriana, FamilyMed
Rioux, Andre
Rioux, Julie
Rivard, Marie-Chantale, FamilyMed
Robitaille, Sylvie A.
Rolland, Pascale
Rondeau, Chantal, FamilyMed(EM)
Rouleau, Brigitte
Royer-Laval, Joanie
Saey, Anne-Marie, FamilyMed
Samoisette, Andre
San, Vong-Virienne
Saucier, Claude
Scherer, Jacques
Sergerie, Mylene
Simard, France
Souliere, Danielle
St-Amour, Jeanne
St-Georges, Marc J E.
St-Hilaire, Jean
St-Hilaire, Lyette
St-Jean, Gilles
St-Laurent, Michel
St-Pierre, Richard
St-Yves, Chantal
Steverman, Allen I., FamilyMed
Stumpf, Michael
Sylvestre, Pierre-Alexandre
Taillefer, Normand
Taillon, Pierre
Talbot, Marie-Pier
Tarakdjian, Megerditch
Tardif, Michel
Tardif, Patrick
Teolis, Stefan, FamilyMed
Tessier, Genevieve
Thibault, Louise
Thiffault, Jocelyne
Torres Rojas, Gisset D L C., FamilyMed
Touchette, Michel
Tran, Nguyen X D.
Trudeau, Pierre
Trudel, Odile
Trudelle, Louis
Turcotte, Alain
Turcotte, Martine
Ulysse, Marc-Andre
Uong Dinh, Bich Thao, FamilyMed
Vachon, Francois
Vaillancourt, Yvon
Vaillant, Nathalie
Vanier, Rejean
Vartazarmian, Raphael
Vincent, Hubert
Vinet, Pierre
Voyer, Danielle
Watts, Helene
Xie, Ying Chang, FamilyMed
Yesli, Madjid

LAVALTRIE

Barcelo Rodriguez, Enrique, FamilyMed
Bedard, Gerry
Bisson, Maude, FamilyMed
Bourgeois, Gilles
Hervieux, David
Hurens, Cindy, FamilyMed
Jalbert, Marc
Laporte-Proulx, Joanie
Martineau, Mario
Metivier, Annie
Plante, Danielle
Senechal, Marie-Claude
Turenne, Francois

LEBEL-S-QUEVILLON

Bergeron, Paule
Chabot, Christian
Julien, Stephane
Katarzyniak-Kunysz, Danuta
Lafontaine, Gilles, FamilyMed

LEMOYNE

Rawal, Shashi K.
Therrien, Michel

LES BERGERONNES

Viens, Claudette

LES CEDRES

Turmel, Serge

LES EBOULEMENTS

Poupart, Normand

LES ESCOUMINS

Bolduc, Francois
Boulanger, Julie, FamilyMed
Chagnon-Lessard, Marie, FamilyMed
Chebil, Samir
Dang-Tran, Khue-My
Denault, Jacinthe, FamilyMed
Gaumond, Marjolaine, FamilyMed
Leger, Claude
Lieke, Anau
Lord, Guillaume
Mercier, Remi, FamilyMed

LEVIS

Arbic, Diane
Arseneault, Daniel
Aumond, Francois, FamilyMed
Baby, Marie-Claire, FamilyMed(EM)
Beaudoin, Julie
Beaulieu, Catherine, FamilyMed(EM)
Begin, Serge A.
Belanger, Julie
Belley, Richard J.
Ben Amor, Leila
Bernard, Nicolas, FamilyMed(EM)
Blanchet, Catherine, FamilyMed
Boilard, Christiane, FamilyMed
Boivin, Frederic, FamilyMed
Bouchard, Michele
Boucher, Maryse, FamilyMed
Bourget, Sandrine, FamilyMed(EM)
Breton, Janie
Brisson, Fernand
Buteau, Dominique
Careau, Dominique
Carrier, Daniel A., FamilyMed
Champagne, Eric, FamilyMed
Chevrette, Evelyne
Cote, Mario, FamilyMed(EM)
Couillard, Martine
Cusson, Diane
D'Astous, Helene, FamilyMed(EM)
Dallaire, Luc
Desrosiers, Anne-Edith
Doucet Jr., Robert J., FamilyMed(EM)
Dropinski, Jean-Pierre
Ducharme, Diane
Dumont, Catherine
Dumont, Serge
Faucher, Jacques
Fleet, Richard, FamilyMed(EM)
Frenette, Lucie
Gagne, Johanne, FamilyMed
Gagnon, Jacques
Gagnon, Johanne
Gilbert, Monica
Gingras, Claude R.
Gosselin, Christine
Grou-Leclerc, Etienne, FamilyMed
Guay, Micheline
Guenard, Dominique
Habel, Maryline, FamilyMed
Hamann, Steven
Jean, Catherine
Kronstrom, Jean
L'Hebreux, Marie-Claude
Labbe, Gilles
Laflamme, David
Lambert-Perrault, Anne-Marie, FamilyMed
Lanthier, Annie, FamilyMed
Larochelle, Leandre
Larue, Louis
Legendre, Eric, FamilyMed(EM)
Levesque, Andre
Loiselle, Luc-Aurele
Madore, Gervais
Mailhot, Marie-Christine, FamilyMed
Malenfant, Jean-Guy
Marceau-Gauvin, Nathalie
Marot, Jean-Paul
Martin, Catherine, FamilyMed
Martineau, Genevieve, FamilyMed(EM)
Mercier, Guylaine
Nadeau, Yvon-A.
Normand, Marie
Ouezzani, Salma
Paquet, Suzanne, FamilyMed
Pelletier, Marie
Pouliot, Marie-Christine
Ratte, Francois, FamilyMed(EM)
Roman, Miriam
Ruest, Ann
Sanfacon, Cathie, FamilyMed
Savoie, Anne-Marie
Shink, Christine
Shink, Daniel
St-Arnaud, Daniel, FamilyMed(EM)
St-Martin, Annie
St-Pierre, Katie
Tanguay, Alain
Theriault, Denise
Therrien, Gaston J E.
Thomassin, David, FamilyMed(EM)
Turcot, Olivier, FamilyMed(EM)
Turcotte, Maryse
Vachon, Marie-France
Vandal, Claude, FamilyMed
Vermette, M. Gabrielle
Vezina, Julie
Villeneuve, Andre, FamilyMed(EM)
Vincent, Serge

LONGUEUIL

Ag Bazet, Albaka, FamilyMed
Allard, Rollande
Alvarez Bernal, Cesar E.
Amyot, Luce S.
Argouin, Isabelle
Arihan, Oguz
Arsenault, Caroline
Arsenault, Claude
Badra, Riad
Beaudin, Julie
Beaulieu, Rene
Beauvolsk, Paul
Beland-Vachon, Helene
Belanger, Huguette
Benmessaoud, Noura
Benoit, Simon
Berdnikoff, Andre
Bergeron, Christine
Bergeron, Maryse
Bigaouette, Andre
Blain, Stephanie
Blanchette, France
Boisvert, Laurent
Boivin, Antoine, FamilyMed
Bordeleau, Gilles
Bouchard, Michel R.
Boucher, Julie M., FamilyMed
Boucher, Michele E.
Boucher, Pierre, FamilyMed(EM)
Boudreau, Janice
Boudreau, Marc
Bougard, Jean
Boulet-Roussin, Genevieve
Bourbeau, Michel
Bourdua, Mathilde, FamilyMed
Bourgouin, Pierre T.
Bouthat, Alain
Boyer, Suzanne
Brasseur, Yves
Brault, Lucie, FamilyMed
Brissette, Sylvie
Brouillet, Louise
Brunelle, Marylene
Brunet, Gilles
Bui, Ngoc Yen G., FamilyMed
Bustros-Lussier, Genevieve, FamilyMed
Carnois, Isabelle
Cesaire, J. Jacques
Charette, Francois G.
Charette, Guy
Charland, Vanessa, FamilyMed
Chenier, Andre
Choquette, Claude
Chouinard, Helene
Cloutier, Annie
Cloutier, Helene
Cloutier, Yvan
Colbert, Mariam
Courchesne, Pierre
Dauphin, Linda
De Guire, Martine
Decarie, Michel
Deguire, Henri, FamilyMed
Delisle, Gilles
Delisle, Sandra
Demers, Donald
Desautels, Lyne
Desjardins, Marie-France
Deslandes, Isabelle, FamilyMed
Desmarais, Elaine
Desmeules, Julie, FamilyMed
Desrochers, Suzon
Desrosiers, Jean-Francois
Dix, Marie D., FamilyMed
Do, Binh Minh
Dragon, Sylvie, FamilyMed(EM)
Dubois, Marie-Josee
Dubuc, Michel
Ducharme, Brigitte, FamilyMed
Duchesne, Andre
Dufour, Emilie, FamilyMed(EM)
Dumais, Alexis
Dumais, Daniel
Dupras, Raymonde
Dupuy, Andre
Dussault, Michele
Emond, Joanne
Evans, Celyne
Favreau, Diane
Favreau, Marie-Helene
Favron, Helene
Filion, Annie-Joelle, FamilyMed(EM)
Fleurant, Micheline
Forget, Judith
Forget, Marie-Chantal, FamilyMed
Forget, Pierre
Fournier, Isabelle
Fournier, Pierre
Fronteddu, Mavi
Gagnon, Alain
Gagnon, Caroline
Gagnon, Sylvie
Gauthier, Chantal
Gauthier, Jules
Gauthier, Michel J.
Geoffroy, Marie-Helene, FamilyMed
Gilbert, Linda
Giroux, Monique
Gleize-Emphoux, Sandrine
Godoy Dalboni de Lima, Renato
Gosselin, Genevieve
Gouin, Jean-Pierre
Goyer, Marie-Eve
Grondin, Jerome
Groulx, Stephane, FamilyMed
Guillet, France
Guimond, Isabelle
Hamel-Breault, Daphné
Hebert, Amelie
Ho, Thi Nhu M.
Hotte, Marie-Josee
Houle, Claude
Houle, Serge
Huynh, Thi Phuong T.
Janelle, France
Kenney, France
Labelle, Jean-Philippe, FamilyMed
Lachance, Marie-Noelle
Lachapelle, Michel
Laflamme, Benoit
Lafleur, Julie
Lafond, Johanne
Lafontaine, Laurie, FamilyMed(EM)
Laganiere, Louise
Lahens, Roger
Lajoie, Louise
Lam Poyuen, Hian Kow
Lamanque, Pascal
Lambert, Louise
Lambert, Yves, FamilyMed
Lamoureux-Robert, Marie-Josee, FamilyMed
Langlois, Veronique
Lapierre, Bernard
Lapierre, Claudie
Laroche, Robert
Larsen-Passe, Marie-Andree
Larue, Bertrand
Laurence, Michel
Lavoie, Gaetan
Le Blanc, Elsa
Le Quoc, Thuy Linh, FamilyMed
Leboeuf, Gilles
Leduc, Yolande
Lee Mei Si, Sylvana
Levac, Eric
Levesque, Jennifer
Lortie, Richard
Lussier, J R. Yves
Mailloux, Martine
Mallette-Gratton, Veronique, FamilyMed
Martel, Elaine
Martel, Jean-Marie
Martel, Michel
Martel, Pierre
Massicotte, Josee
Mazza, Myriam, FamilyMed
Mecarbane, Rose-Marie
Menard, Ginette
Menard, Yvon
Morin, Genevieve
Morneau, Colombe
Morotti, Linda
Nemes Bratis, Roxana
Nguyen, Hoa Hieu
Nguyen, Ngoc Quynh N.
Nguyen, Quynh Nhu.
Nguyen, Thanh Long
Nguyen, Thi Binh M.
Nguyen, Thien-Hoa, FamilyMed
Nguyen, Xuan Trinh
Nicole, Patricia
Noiseux, Jean-Marc
Ostiguy, Mario
Ouellet, Chantal, FamilyMed
Ouimet, France
Paquin, Isabelle
Patry, Manon
Paulhus-Gosselin, Eve, FamilyMed
Pecko, Krystyna
Pelletier, Marcel J.
Pepin, Jean-Francois
Perron, Lina
Pham, Mailan
Picard, Josee
Pierrat, Audrey, FamilyMed
Pilotte, Michele
Poitras, Guy
Poray-Wybranowski, Jerzy, FamilyMed
Prevost, Anne-Patricia, FamilyMed
Prevost, Yvon M.
Provencher, Simone
Ricard, Jacques
Richard, Caroline
Risi, Catherine
Rivard, Claude, FamilyMed
Rivest, Michele, FamilyMed
Ross, Dave
Rousseau, Danny
Rousseau, Sophie
Roy, Elise
Roy, Stephane
Sader, Paul E., FamilyMed
Saint-Amant, Gilles
Sasseville, Francine
Sayegh, Nabil
Seguin, Marie-Claudel
Sirois, Serge, FamilyMed
Smail, Kahina, FamilyMed(EM)
St-Cerny, Jose
St-Germain, Antoine, FamilyMed
Svihovec, William J.
Taillon, David
Talon, Charles E.
Tannir, Hassan
Tardif, Isabelle, FamilyMed
Thai, Minh-Thu, FamilyMed
Thirsk, Robert B.
Thomas, Paul
Thomere, Serge H J.
Timar-Banu, Olimpia M., FamilyMed
Ton, Sau Nu Thi
Toye, Julie
Tran, Boi Anh
Tran, Cao Phanh
Tran, Nguu Tu
Tremblay, Christine
Tremblay, Florence
Tremblay, Serge Y.
Tu, Khue
Vandycke, Laurent
Williams, Robert, FamilyMed

LORRAINE

Choiniere, Daniel
Forest, Natacha
Lamarre, Claude
Larouche, Nathalie
Lauzon, Lucie
Martineau, Jean-Pierre, FamilyMed
Ouellette, Pierre
Piche, Marcel

LOUISEVILLE

Boilard, Jessy, FamilyMed
Cote, Jean
Dambry, Thierry B R.
Dube, Denis
Gregoire Champagne, Samuel, FamilyMed
Grenier, Guy
Hebert, Paulin
Meziane, Hyjr
Milosevic, Slobodan
Ricard, Paul
Truong, Cong Phuc

LOURDES DU BLANC SABLON

Dery, Richard
Dobrowolski, Marek
Ducharme-Dery, Suzanne
Joncas, Paul-Aime
Lasnier, Frederic, FamilyMed
Paradis, Elisabeth
Pineau, Michel, FamilyMed
Quach, Huu-Nghi
Robin-Boudreau, Maxime, FamilyMed

LYSTER

Mathieu, Yves

MAGOG

Arcand, Yves
Arseneau, Jean-Louis
Bellemare, Sarah, FamilyMed
Berger, Lucie
Bernier, Karine, FamilyMed
Brodeur, Isabelle
Brosseau, Marie-Bri, FamilyMed
Cloutier, Robert
Dang, Marilyne
Dufort, Louis
Dufour, Marc
Dugas, Andre
Emond, Karine, FamilyMed
Gaouette, Christian, FamilyMed
Garant, Dorothee
Gauthier, Anne-Genevieve
Gauthier, Benoit
Gauthier, Michel
Gravel, Claude
Guerin, Helene
Jeannotte, Jean-Pierre
Lafleche, Robert A.
Langlais, Caroline
Larrivee, Luc
Latulippe, Louis G.
Marchand, Lucie

Masse, Robert
Mignault, Charles
Ostiguy, Therese
Panet, Diane
Paris, Raphael, FamilyMed
Pelletier, Gaston
Pelletier, Pierre
Poitras, Francois
Riopel, Mathieu, FamilyMed
Royer, Paule
Samson, Karine, FamilyMed
Seguin, Andre M.
Sicotte, Jean-Guy
Trudel, Jacques
Valiquette, Noemie
Wilhelmy, Mario

MALARTIC

Beau, Jean-Michel
Pigeon, Julie
Saib, Rachid

MANIWAKI

Alvarez, Fresnel J., FamilyMed
Amahzoune, Mohamed
Bertrand, Audrey, FamilyMed
Bertrand, Henri A.
Charbonneau, Guillaume, FamilyMed
Cuneo, Jorge L.
Duplessis, Veronique, FamilyMed
Legault, Jean-Pierre J G.
Maestre Mendoza, Mariam, FamilyMed
Mahinrad-Nateghi, Jinoos
Monfette, Pascale, FamilyMed
Nateghi, Vafa
Paradis, Jacinthe
Patzev, Edi, FamilyMed
Pierre, Jean-Rene
Soulama, Yamatien, FamilyMed
Therrien, Andre
Tinh-Phu, Audrey
Wegrzycki, Wieslaw, FamilyMed

MANSONVILLE

Bourassa, Claude E., FamilyMed
Sielecka, Daniela

MAPLE GROVE

Couture, Sylvain, FamilyMed

MARIA

Ammar, Ahmed
Aubin, Philippe, FamilyMed
Beauchamp, Martine, FamilyMed
Bedard, Marie-Lene
Belanger, Chantale
Blais, Eric
Boivin, Andrée, FamilyMed
Boivin, Julie
Bordeleau, Josée
Bouffard, Audrey, FamilyMed
Brouillette, Marie-Helene, FamilyMed
Chapados, Denyse, FamilyMed
Cormier, Jean-Pierre
Ferron, Michel
Gagnon, Sophie-Genevieve
Guenette-Lemieux, Marie, FamilyMed
Hade-Hetu, Sebastien, FamilyMed
Laliberte, Christian
Landry, David
Landry, Helene
Lessard, Marquis
Levac, Sylvain, FamilyMed(EM)
Marcil, Josee, FamilyMed
Masson, Martine
Mathieu, Isabelle
McNeil, Marie-Sophie
Menard, Lyne, FamilyMed
Papineau, Alain, FamilyMed
Pelletier, Gilles, FamilyMed
Prevost, Simon
Sexton, Emilie
St-Laurent, Johanne
Sylvestre, Amélie
Thibault, Marc
Touma, Georges
Tremblay-Gonthier, Elise, FamilyMed
White, Paula M.

MARIEVILLE

Lavoie, Andre
Poirier, Henri W.

MASCOUCHE

Aube, Katherine
Audette, Myriam
Benoit, Daniel
Blais, Sophie, FamilyMed
Blanchard, Marie-Eve
Boulay, Jacques A.
Briard, Raymond
Cabana, Caroline, FamilyMed
Cloutier, Julie, FamilyMed
Desilets, Monique
Dion, Paul
Durnin, Isabelle
Helszajn, Judith
Kaced, Nadia
L'Ecuyer, Serge
Lupien, Melanie
Pouliot, Johanne
Robitaille, Elisabeth
Valois, Lucie, FamilyMed
Vignola Pigeon, Laurie

MASHTEUIATSH

Philippe, Johanne

MASKINONGE

Gelinas, Leonce
Lambert, Luc
Martin, Fabienne

MATAGAMI

Cote, France
D'Apice, H. Lina
Deschambault, Jean
Deschenes, Francois
Sasseville, Martin

MATANE

Banville, Francois
Bergeron, Marie-Eve, FamilyMed
Bernard, Marie, FamilyMed
Blouin, Rejean
Caron, Catherine
D'Amours, Renee
Drouin, Charles
Elyabroudi, William
Fournier, Pascale
Gagnon, Renee, FamilyMed(EM)
Kadri, Nadjla
Lamoureux, Claude
Landry, Serge
Lapointe, Pierre
Larose, Robert
Lavoie, Annie
Lemaitre, Jean-Luc
Pinel-Tremblay, Diane
Rivest, Marie-Christine
Santerre, Denis
St-Germain, Lorraine
St-Sauveur, David, FamilyMed
Sylvain, Pierre-Luc
Tremblay, Hugues
Tremblay, Patrice

MATAPEDIA

Beaulieu, Guylaine
Leblanc, Louis-Paul
Picard, Luce, FamilyMed

MCMASTERVILLE

Despres, Lise
Desranleau, Real

MERCIER

Comeau, Nathalie
Lavoie, Johanne
Luu, Chinh-Duc
Villiard, Paule, FamilyMed

METABETCHOUAN LAC A LA CROIX

Charron, Robert
Duchaine, Claude
Fortin, Marcel
Marchand, Audree, FamilyMed
Tran, Emmanuelle

MIRABEL

Belanger, Richard
Bosse, Paul-Aime
Duquette, France
Gagne, Gilbert, FamilyMed
Garant, Marie-Claude
Gonzalez Lorenzo, Anabel, FamilyMed
Laperriere, Luc
Lavoie, Daniel C G.
Perreault, Mariano
Tellier, Guy
Thibault, Roger

MISTISSINI

Dion, Gerald
Gosal, Kaviraj, FamilyMed
Jiang, Xiao Lei
Khurana, Rosy, FamilyMed
Laforest, Carole
Perreault, Helene

MONT-JOLI

Beaumont, Denis
Belanger, Jean-Francois
Brisson, Jacynthe
Collins, Genevieve
Compera-Rouaud, Claire
Coulombe, Valerie
Deland, Pascale
Dery, Richard L.
Descoteaux, Isabelle
Deslauriers, Louis
Dumaresq, Cynthia
Hupe, Anne, FamilyMed
Julien, Caroline, FamilyMed
Lagace, Dannie, FamilyMed
Lamarre, Caroline
Leger-Bernier, Monique, FamilyMed
Lemelin, Pierre-Paul
Lemieux, Maryse D.
Michaud, Julie
Moreau, Daphne, FamilyMed
Poulin, Genevieve
Samson, Julie
St-Pierre, Louis
Tran, Hieu Duc
Yessad, Abderahmane

MONT-LAURIER

Bahsoun, Rabih
Barbarosie, Teodor P., FamilyMed
Bayle, Marie-Noelle
Belley, Emmanuel, FamilyMed
Bertrand, Charles
Boisvert, Martin-Pierre, FamilyMed
Boury-Simoes, Delphine
Calabrese, Stephane
Cobos Vega, Haydee A.
Dansereau, Michelle, FamilyMed
Dube, Benoit, FamilyMed
Dugas, Ludivine
Fortin, Sylvie
Gfeller, Pierre
Guindon, Myriam
Kouider El Ouahed, Ali
Labelle, Sylvain
Lacaille, Marie-Claude
Lachaine, Lynda
Lagueux, Viviane
Landry, Lynda
Latulippe, Richard
Laurin, Luc
Le Du, Sylvain
Lebel, Suzanne
Lecompte, Brigitte
Lesage, Alain
Marcotte, Yvan
Masse, Michel
McMahon, Patrick, FamilyMed
Neault, Robert
Paquette, Charles
Paquette, Jean-Levy
Paradis, Pierre J.
Poulin, Kathleen, FamilyMed
Roy, Pierre-Olivier
Sabourin, Karine, FamilyMed

MONT-ROYAL

Chamoun, Alain
Chiasson, Jean-P.
Cote, Patricia, FamilyMed
Doss, Sabine
Gagnon, Daniel
Gauvin, Micheline
Glaser, Stuart R., FamilyMed
Lapierre, Luc, FamilyMed
Lapointe, Caroline
Mallette-Tetreault, Lise
Ostiguy, Genevieve, FamilyMed
Ruest, Andree
Scheim, Alyssa, FamilyMed
Sicard, Eric
Taras, Fernand J.
Vitou, Constantine K., FamilyMed

MONT-SAINT-HILAIRE

Charbonneau, Jean
Denicourt, Marcel
Harvey, Daniel G.
Lavallee, Sophie
Masse, Lise
Morasse, Daniel
Perreault, Stephanie, FamilyMed
Thellen, Jean
Trottier, Patrice

MONT-TREMBLANT

Champagne, Jean
Curtis, David
David, Claude
Dion, Jean D.
Gagnon, Marie-Eve
Guilbault, Mathieu
Leonard, Celine
Makuza, Aimable, FamilyMed
Pilon, Pierre
Reid, Alain
Rheaume-Lanoie, Myriam
Serra, Danielle

MONTMAGNY

Auger, Martin
Bergeron, Marc-Yves
Blouin, Patrick
Carle, Jean
Carpentier, Frederic
Doiron, Andre
Fortin, Gilles
Fortin, Raymond
Gaudreau, Mario
Guimont, Marie-Christine
Labrecque, Eric
Labrie, Robert
Leclerc, Andre, FamilyMed(EM)
Lemieux, Claire
Lepage, Ghislain
Martel, Pierre
Mercier, Annie
Mercier, Caroline, FamilyMed
Mercier, Mathieu
Pelletier, Martin
Poirier, Dominique
Poulin, Marie-Helene
Rancourt, Jean-Francois
Roy, Louise
Tanguay, Caroline
Tremblay, Annie

MONTPELLIER

Rioux, Marie-Claude, FamilyMed

MONTREAL

Aalamian, Armand, FamilyMed
Abadie, Pascale
Abadir, Sylvia
Abdelnour, Dona, FamilyMed
Abdelnour, Miriam, FamilyMed
Abergel, Heidi A., FamilyMed
Abikhzer, Myriam, FamilyMed
Abikhzer, Victor
Abikhzer, Yael, FamilyMed
Abrahams, Heather R., FamilyMed
Achim, Michel
Achir, Sanaa
Ackaoui, Elias G.
Acre, Yael, FamilyMed
Adjami, Adele
Aggarwal, Sanjay, FamilyMed
Agier, Jean-Maurice
Ahmad, Imran
Ahronheim, Sara R.
Ait Hamouda, Karima, FamilyMed
Akhras, Ronald, FamilyMed
Alaily, Hana
Alam, Mohammad N., FamilyMed(EM)
Alarie, Pierre
Albadine, Roula
Albert, Clifford, FamilyMed
Alcindor, M C. Michele
Alladin, Lenny C.
Allard, Sylvie
Allegrucci, Philippe
Alos, Nathalie
Alper, Deborah, FamilyMed
Alper, Jennifer, FamilyMed(EM)
Alvarez, Fernando
Ames, Christina M., FamilyMed(EM)
Ammara, Yasmina
Andriamampionona, Francis A.
Angers, Suzanne
Anidjar, Maurice
Ansaldo, Carlos M.
Antonescu, Serban M.
Aouinati, Sophia, FamilyMed
Appeltauer, Luis C.
Arbour, Christiane
Arbour, Maurice H.
Arcand, Andre
Arcand, Lyne
Arcelin, Andre
Arcelin, Katia, FamilyMed
Archambault, Stéphanie, FamilyMed
Archer, Jessie
Arel, Roxanne, FamilyMed
Artho, Giovanni P.
Aspler, Aviva L., FamilyMed
Assal, Michel G.
Assayag, Jacob G.
Assedou, Aaron, FamilyMed(EM)

Assef, Richard, FamilyMed
Asselah, Jamil
Asselin, Francine
Asselin, Marc-A
Aubin, Emmanuelle, FamilyMed
Audibert, Francois M.
Auger, Danielle
Authier, Louise, FamilyMed
Avital, Ofer A.
Ayotte, Louise
Ayoub, Patricia, FamilyMed
Azancot, Linda
Azran, Danielle
Azuelos, Alan, FamilyMed(EM)
Azuelos, Elisabeth
Bachand, Monique
Bachir, Ayda
Bah, Abdoulaye
Baiche, Nadia
Baird, Nicole
Baldini, Gabriele
Baltazar, Carmen, FamilyMed
Banh, Van-Ty
Barbeau, David
Barbier, Alexandre
Bardagi, Victor
Baril, Jean-Guy
Barrette, Real
Barrieau, Louise
Barrier, Alain
Barrier, France
Barsauskas, Algis J.
Bastien, Gilles Simon., FamilyMed
Bates, Susan J.
Baylis, Penny Jane, FamilyMed
Bazzo, Jean-Pierre
Beardsley, Jennifer K., FamilyMed
Beauchamp, Yvon, FamilyMed
Beaudin, Gabriel
Beaudoin, Eddy
Beaudoin, Guylaine
Beaudoin, Robert
Beaudry, Veronique, FamilyMed(EM)
Beaulieu, Marie-D., FamilyMed
Beaulieu, Yves
Beauregard, Marie, FamilyMed
Becker, Giuliano
Bedard, Caroline, FamilyMed
Beique, Caroline, FamilyMed
Bekhechi, Samir E., FamilyMed
Beland, Therese
Belanger, Marcel A.
Belanger, Rene-Maurice
Belanger, Serge
Belhachmi, Samuel S.
Belisle, Denise
Beliveau, Robert
Belizaire-Da Costa, Lise
Belkhous, Nacera, FamilyMed
Bell, Patricia, FamilyMed
Belleau, Luc
Belzile, Catherine
Ben Jmaa, Wissal
Ben Smaine, Nacera K.
Ben Sta, Amor
Ben-Shoshan, Moshe
Benbiga, Loubna
Benfey, Bruno G.
Benhamron, Elias S.
Benkelfat, Chawki
Benoit, Michel
Benrimoh, Daniel
Benslimane, Benaoumeur
Bensouda, Brahim
Bereza, Eugene, FamilyMed
Bergeron, Julie, FamilyMed
Bergeron, Marie
Berjat, B. Maria
Bernard, Sophie
Bernasconi, Andrea G.
Berner, Mark, FamilyMed(EM)
Bernier, Roch, FamilyMed
Berthiaume, Sylvie, FamilyMed
Besrour, Sadok
Bessette, Luc
Beuzeron-Mangina, J. Helene
Bhereur, Anne, FamilyMed
Biagini Cury, Fabio L.
Bichai, W. Michel
Bicrell, Eric
Bier, Michele

Billard, Marc, FamilyMed
Billinghurst, M. Robert, FamilyMed
Binda, Jean
Birckel, Pierre
Birdi, Kirandeep, FamilyMed
Bisaillon, Luc
Bisson, Cédric, FamilyMed
Bitchoka, Joseph
Bittencourt, Henrique
Bitzan, Martin
Bizgu, Victoria
Black, Barbara A., FamilyMed
Black, Hans P.
Bladou, Franck
Blais, Catherine
Blanchette, Claudine
Blanque Martinez, Maria
Blondin, Renee
Blouin, Nathalie
Blusanovics, Peter, FamilyMed
Boileau, Elisabeth, FamilyMed(EM)
Boileau, Michel
Boillat, Miriam E., FamilyMed
Boissonnault, Michel
Boissonneault, Josee
Boissy, Benoit
Bollee, Guillaume
Bordeleau, Daniel
Borod, Manuel, FamilyMed
Borreman, Stephane, FamilyMed(EM)
Bosisio, Bruno
Bouallegue, Abdelkader
Boubekeur, Fadila
Bouchard, Sylvie
Bouchard-Arslanian, Celine
Boucher, Gilberte
Boucher, Karine
Boucher, Pierre R.
Boudreau, Guy
Bouhadana, Michael J., FamilyMed
Bouhrour, Souad, FamilyMed
Bouilly, Michel
Bouin, Mickael
Bouisset, Jeanne, FamilyMed
Boulay, Danielle
Boulet, Sylvie, FamilyMed
Boulianne, Sylvie, FamilyMed
Boulva, Geneviève, FamilyMed
Bourassa, François, FamilyMed
Bourdy, Christian
Bourget, Gaetan
Bourgouin, Jean
Bourkas, Angelo E., FamilyMed
Bouron Dal Soglio, Dorothee
Bourque, Suzanne
Bourret, Andre
Bourret, Danielle
Boutaleb, Asmae
Bouth, Jean-Claude
Bouthillier, Annie
Boutros, Cecile
Boyer, Helene
Boyer, J. Andre
Boyer, Julie, FamilyMed(EM)
Brabant, Michel R.
Bracka, Michel C., FamilyMed
Braverman, Nancy
Breger, Barry
Brenhouse, Michelle, FamilyMed
Brenner, Rudy H., FamilyMed
Brewer, Timothy F.
Bridges, Eileen J.
Briere, Dominique
Briere, Nicole
Brind'Amour, Thomas, FamilyMed
Brissette, Alain
Brissette, Suzanne
Brisson, Pierre
Brisson, Suzanne
Brisson-Joseph, Andre
Brochu, Jean E.
Brodeur, Benoit, FamilyMed
Brodeur-Girard, Sophie
Brohovici, Sorel L.
Bronet, Sandra
Brossard, Martin, FamilyMed
Brouillette, Robert T.
Brown, Bruce P., FamilyMed(EM)
Brown, Richard N.
Brown-Johnson, Anita Marie., FamilyMed

Bruckert, Barbara A., FamilyMed
Brum, Virginia
Bruneau, Anne
Bruneau, Anne, FamilyMed
Bruneau, Danielle, FamilyMed
Bruneau, Genevieve, FamilyMed
Bruneau, Johanne
Bruneau, Julie
Brunelle, Genevieve
Brunelle, Jacques
Brunet, Nadine
Brunier, Jean-Louis
Brunner, Roger, FamilyMed(EM)
Buch, Mark, FamilyMed(EM)
Buckett, William
Bucur, Daniela
Bui, T D N. Dominique
Bulota, Veronique
Burnier, Miguel N.
Bustamante, Helene
Busuioc, Ruxandra, FamilyMed
Bwenge, Alexandra S., FamilyMed
Cabrera-Aleksandrova, Tatiana
Caglar, Derin
Caire Fon, Nathalie M T., FamilyMed
Cajal, Stefan I.
Caldareri, Carmelo, FamilyMed
Camire, Pierre
Can Thi, Bich Ngoc
Cape, Steven D.
Cardin, Michel
Cardinal, Celine
Cardinal, Nadine, FamilyMed
Cardona, Caroline A., FamilyMed
Cardoso, Marguerite
Caricevic, Bogdan
Carlin, Robert C., FamilyMed
Caron, Joanna M., FamilyMed
Caron, Marie-Josee, FamilyMed
Caron, Maurice
Caron, Paul L J.
Carranza, Ruben G.
Carret, Anne-Sophie
Carrier, Gaetan
Carroll, Paul J., FamilyMed
Cartier, Kim
Cassiani, Nadine
Castano, Roberto
Castel, Helene
Castonguay, Danny, FamilyMed
Catchlove, Richard F H.
Cecere, Assunta
Celestin, Kathlyn, FamilyMed
Cernea, Carmen D., FamilyMed
Chabot, Carol
Chami, Rose
Champagne, Ginette
Champagne, Richard S.
Champoux, Nathalie, FamilyMed
Chan-Wai-Ling, Nicolas, FamilyMed(EM)
Chaoual, Mongi
Chaput, Genevieve, FamilyMed
Charbonneau, Anne-Marie, FamilyMed
Charbonneau, Pierre
Charbonneau, Richard
Charbonneau, Yves
Charest, Louise
Charest, Michel
Charghi, Parissa, FamilyMed
Charles, Guy G.
Charron, Marc-Andre, FamilyMed
Charron, Yan
Chartrand, Bernard
Chartrand, Jean-Claude
Chatelier, Alex, FamilyMed
Chatterjee, Surjit, FamilyMed(EM)
Chau, Fannie T., FamilyMed
Chayestemehr, Sacha
Chedeville, Gaelle R S.
Chen, Marie-Luce, FamilyMed
Chen-Tournoux, Annabel A.
Cheng, Gemma L.
Cheng, Yves I B.
Cherigui, Saïda
Chinks, Joshua, FamilyMed(EM)
Chira, Ruxandra I., FamilyMed
Chirgwin, Juan C L., FamilyMed
Chirgwin-Campos, Jerman E., FamilyMed(EM)

Chocron, Charles
Chouinard, Diane, FamilyMed
Chrigui, Abdelaziz
Chu, Kim Hang
Ciuntu, Ioana, FamilyMed
Clark, Gregory, FamilyMed(EM)
Claveau, J. Andre
Clement, Annie, FamilyMed
Clement, Jacques
Clement, Louise
Cliche, Nathalie
Cloutier, Jean
Cloutier, Réal
Co, Ha Thanh, FamilyMed
Coeugniet, Edouard R.
Cohen, Janice M.
Coiteux, Carl C.
Colmegna, Ines
Colpron, Louise
Comtois, Amelie
Comtois, Pierre
Constantinescu, Cristina, FamilyMed
Constas-Costopoulos, Nicolas
Contant, Denys
Coombs, Robin R., FamilyMed
Cordahi, Ghassan
Cordeau, Chantal
Cormier, Roberta T.
Corriveau, Pierre
Cortes Nino, Maria D P.
Cosma, Yann
Costisella, Olivier
Cote, Andreanne
Cote, Laurent
Cote, Mendy
Cote, Nathalie
Cote, Pierre
Cote, Sylvie
Cotran, Marc E., FamilyMed
Courtemanche, Luc
Coutu, Pierre
Couture, Josee
Couturier, Lise Claudette.
Cracower, Jill, FamilyMed
Crerar, Anita, FamilyMed(EM)
Cristache, Aurelian
Croteau, Francois
Croteau, Stephane
Crowe-Bourbonnais, Celine
Cruvellier, Paul E., FamilyMed
Cruz, Javier
Cruz-Santiago, Diane, FamilyMed
Cuchurean, Paul
Cucuzza, Marie-Jose
Cummings, Suzanne
Cusson, Lise, FamilyMed
Cyr, Claude
Czitrom, Jean-Paul
Czyziw, Elizabeth
D'Amico, Josiane, FamilyMed
D'Aoust, Louis-Xavier, FamilyMed
D'Errico, Jean
Dabo, Sambou
Dadour, Georges
Dagenais, Louis J., FamilyMed
Dagher, Eric
Daginawala, Khatija
Dahan, Karen, FamilyMed
Dahdouh, Elias
Daher, Samer
Daigneault, Linda
Dal Pozzo Nizard, Sonia
Dallaire, Michel
Dalton, Douglass, FamilyMed
Dam, Hoa Van
Dang, Angela N., FamilyMed
Dang, Dinh Quang
Dang, Dinh Thien V.
Dang, Nha Khanh
Dang, Thuy Nhien
Dang, Yen Nhi
Daniel, Marie-Florence
Danino, Michel A.
Dankoff, Frederic J., FamilyMed
Dannenbaum, David A., FamilyMed
Dansereau, Pierre
Danson, A. Jeffrey
Dao, Ba Ngoc, FamilyMed
Dao, Thomas T H.
Daskalopoulou, Styliani S.
Davari, Sara, FamilyMed

Daviault, Elizabeth
David, Andree
De Foy, Lise
De Grandpre, Fernand
De Grandpre, Nathalie
De Guire, Louise
De Loppinot, Anne
De Luca, Angelo, FamilyMed
De Margerie, Gilles J B.
De Pauw, Anna, FamilyMed
De Pokomandy, Alexandra, FamilyMed
De Smet, Jan L.
De Vette, Aad
Decker Goano, Adriana, FamilyMed
Decobellis, Tania, FamilyMed
Decoeur, Isabelle, FamilyMed
Defay, J. Yves
Delaby, Liliane
Deladoey, Johnny Y.
Delage, Bastien, FamilyMed
Delisle, Emilie, FamilyMed
Delisle, Robert F.
Delorme, Celine
Demanins-Towers, Anna M., FamilyMed
Demers, Annie
Demers, Daniel
Demers, Liliane
Demers, Mireille, FamilyMed
Demers, Vincent, FamilyMed
Demirtas, Ezgi
Deneault, Melanie, FamilyMed
Dequoy, Genevieve
Deraspe, Amelie, FamilyMed
Des Marais, Lison
Deschamps, Benoit J.
Deschenes, Jacques C.
Deschenes, Mario
Descoings, Benedicte
Descoteaux, Marc I.
Deshaies, Doris
Desilets, Marie-Eve
Desire, Farah, FamilyMed
Desjardins, Gisele, FamilyMed
Desjardins, Marie-Josee
Deslandes, Pierre
Desmarais, Jean-Luc
Desmarais, Marc
Desmarais, Marie
Desmarais, Marie-Claude, FamilyMed
Desrochers, Chantale
Desrochers, Josee, FamilyMed
Desroches, Jean V.
Desrosiers, Michel
Dessau, Jean-Claude
Diallo, Absa
Diaz- Sanchez, Liliana, FamilyMed
Diep, Bich Ngoc
Diez-d'Aux, Robert, FamilyMed
Dinh, Ba-Hiep
Dinh, Le Thu
Dinh, Ngoc Thuy
Dinh, Thi-Kien-Hoa
Dion, Dominique
Dion, J. Harold, FamilyMed
Dion-Cloutier, Philippe
Ditommaso, Stephen N., FamilyMed
Djillali-Berkane, Nacera, FamilyMed
Do, Doan Trang
Doan, Ly Huong
Dobrinski, Herbert
Dolbec, Julie, FamilyMed
Donoso, Fernando
Dore, Francois-Guy
Doucet, Alison M., FamilyMed
Dove, Marion, FamilyMed
Doyle, D. Maureen, FamilyMed
Doyon, Lucie P.
Doyon-Gamache, Noemie
Drali, Ratiba, FamilyMed
Drivod, Marie-Laure, FamilyMed
Drolet, Celyne
Drummond, Robert, FamilyMed(EM)
Du Souich, Bertrand
Dube, Helene
Dube, Sylvie, FamilyMed
Dubois, Alain
Dubrovsky, Bernardo O.
Duchastel, Morency
Duchesneau, Helene

Duckett, Jean
Duclos, Madeleine, FamilyMed
Duffie, Anne F.
Dufort, Jean-Pierre
Dufresne, Chantal
Dufresne, Serge, FamilyMed
Dugas, Ruth
Dugre, Helene
Duguay, Francois
Duguet, Nathalie
Duhaime, Jean-Daniel, FamilyMed(EM)
Dulude, Serge
Dumas-Pilon, Maxine, FamilyMed
Dumbrava, Daniela, FamilyMed
Dumont, Serge
Dumont-Mackay, Vincent, FamilyMed
Duniewicz, Magdalena, FamilyMed(EM)
Duong, Hong-Huy
Duong, Thuy Long
Duplan, Edgard
Dupont, Daniele
Dupont, Serge
Dupont-Girard, Michele
Dupras, Marie-Claude, FamilyMed
Dupriez, Anne-Frederique, FamilyMed
Duquette, Stephane
Dutil, Renald
Dworkind, Michael, FamilyMed
Edelstein, Earl
Eibock, Danielle
El Fouladi, Nadia
El Mezouar, Zineb, FamilyMed
Elbaz, Armand
Elbaz, Audrey, FamilyMed
Elfassi, Emile
Elkabas, Oren S.
Elman, Elyssa R., FamilyMed
Elman, Sheldon, FamilyMed
Emond, Natalie, FamilyMed
Engo, Michael L., FamilyMed(EM)
Estevez, Wendy, FamilyMed
Ethier, Jean-Leon
Ethier, Julie
Ethier, Marie-Pascale, FamilyMed
Fainsilber, Toby, FamilyMed
Fairbairn, James, FamilyMed
Fallenbaum, Fany, FamilyMed
Famil-Dardachti, Djahanguir
Fantini, Fiorella
Farah, Rita, FamilyMed
Farah-Lajoie, Claude
Farand, Lambert
Farley-Deschamps, Justine
Fazal Karim, Karima, FamilyMed
Fazekas, Arpad G.
Ferland, Miren
Fernandez-Llamazares, Carmen
Ferrarotto, Domenic, FamilyMed
Ferri, Patricia
Ferrier, Catherine, FamilyMed
Filipini, Daniel L.
Finestone, Debra S.
Fisher, Gillian
Flamand, Helene, FamilyMed
Florea, Adrian, FamilyMed
Florival, Albert
Fontela, Patricia S.
Fontg-Walmsley, Jorge A., FamilyMed(EM)
Forbes, Peter J A.
Forgeot D'Arc, Baudouin
Fortier, David, FamilyMed
Fortin, Ann
Fortin, Benoit
Fortin, Daniele
Fortin, Jean-Claude
Fortin, Louise
Fortin, Marquis
Fortin, Stephanie, FamilyMed(EM)
Fortin, Yvan
Fournier, Claire
Fournier, Johanne, FamilyMed
Fournier, Renee, FamilyMed
Frechette, Denise, FamilyMed
Friedman, Jason, FamilyMed
Froehlich, Patrick
Frongillo, Robert
Fruchtermann, Lucien-P
Fuchsman, Bertha, FamilyMed

Fugere, Louise
Gagne, Claire
Gagne, Gaston
Gagne, Ginette
Gagne, Marc
Gagnon, Eric
Gagnon, Judith
Gagnon, Louis
Gagnon, Louise
Gagnon, Lucie
Gagnon, Nathalie
Gaiptman, Jack H.
Galarneau, Sophie, FamilyMed
Galperin, Ilana, FamilyMed
Gamache, Jean
Garand, M T. Linda, FamilyMed
Garcia Gonthier, Maite
Gardie, Juan, FamilyMed
Gariepy, Ursule
Garoufalis, Evgenia, FamilyMed
Gasse, Tiffany, FamilyMed(EM)
Gaudreau, Marie-Josee
Gaul, Neil, FamilyMed
Gauthier, Francois, FamilyMed
Gauthier, Julie, FamilyMed
Gauthier-Bizier, Sabrina, FamilyMed
Gauvreau-Gadoua, Louise
Gavsie, Adam, FamilyMed
Gelinas, France
Gelinas, Ginette
Gelinas, Manon
Geoffroy, Normand
Gerin, Camille, FamilyMed
Gerin-Lajoie, Michele
Gervais, Chantal, FamilyMed
Gervais, Yves, FamilyMed
Ghinea, Mircea D.
Ghoprial-Ghali, Marcelle
Ghosh, Shuvo
Ghoubril, Suzette
Giannakis, Andreas
Giannelis, Taxiarhoula
Giasson Jr., Carl
Giguere, Gaetan
Gilbert, Andree
Gilbert, Jean
Gillman, Marcia L., FamilyMed
Gilmore, Norbert
Gingras, Pierre
Gingras, Stefanie, FamilyMed
Ginsberg, Donald, FamilyMed
Giorgi, Conrado
Giraldeau-Belanger, Sarah-Emilie, FamilyMed
Girard, Guylaine
Girard, Jean-Francois
Girard, Michel
Girard, Michel
Giroux, Charles, FamilyMed
Giroux, Diane
Giroux, Julie
Giroux, Pierre F.
Giuristante, Frank A.
Gladu, Francois-Pierre, FamilyMed
Glorieux, Francis
Gobeil, Martine
Godbout, Cynthia, FamilyMed
Godin, Jean
Godin, Louis
Goggin, Patricia
Golberg, Deborah, FamilyMed
Goldberg, Erwin H.
Goldsmith, Lindsay, FamilyMed
Goldstein, Howard, FamilyMed
Gologan, Adrian
Gore, Brian
Gorin, Ian C.
Gormley, Lynda, FamilyMed
Gougoux-Tremblay, Stephanie
Goulet, Francois, FamilyMed(EM)
Goulet, Genevieve, FamilyMed(EM)
Goulet, Marie-Claude, FamilyMed
Goyal, Michelle S., FamilyMed
Goyette, Maxime
Grad, Roland, FamilyMed
Grandmont, Danielle
Granger, Micheline
Granger, Pierre
Gratton, Celine
Gravel, Evelyne, FamilyMed(EM)
Gravel, Jacques

Greenberg, Michael
Greenberg, Stephen H.
Grenier, Isabelle, FamilyMed
Grenon, Lorraine
Grigorian, Anahid
Grodzicky, Roman V.
Groleau, Maroussia
Grunbaum, Beatrice
Gruner, Carole
Guay, Jean-Pierre
Guay, Martine
Guertin, Ghislaine O.
Guigui, Jean-Yves
Guillaume, Eddy
Guimond, Claude
Guimond, Gerard
Guimond, Jean-Pierre, FamilyMed
Guimond, Jean-Victor
Guizani, Sinda, FamilyMed(EM)
Gunn, C. Robin, FamilyMed
Gupta, Geeta, FamilyMed
Gupta, Namta, FamilyMed
Guy, Roger G.
Habel, Michel
Habib, Samir, FamilyMed
Haf Gagne, Valerie, FamilyMed
Hagshi, Judy L., FamilyMed
Hajjar, Eliane, FamilyMed
Hallman, Melissa J., FamilyMed
Hamel, Louise
Hamel, Robert
Hanna, Claudine
Hannouche, M. Georges
Haouara, Fatiha
Harper, Samuel A., FamilyMed
Harrold, A. John, FamilyMed
Hasswani, Samer, FamilyMed
Hausser, Jean-Louis
Haxuan, Sandra, FamilyMed
Hayton, Barbara C., FamilyMed
Hazan, Ariel
Hebert, Helene
Hebert, Hugo
Hebert, Isabelle, FamilyMed
Hebert, Yves
Hector, Yanick
Hejazi, Banafcheh, FamilyMed
Hemmings, Christian
Hereish, Jean-Pierre
Hereish, Michel
Herskovitz, Steven, FamilyMed(EM)
Hersson-Edery, Fanny
Hirtle, Ann, FamilyMed
Ho, Thi Kim, FamilyMed
Ho, Thi Nguyet
Hoang, Minh Chau
Hoang, Tuan Van
Hobden, Roger
Holzer, Gideon
Hope, Paula, FamilyMed
Horny, Stefan
Hotte, Dominique, FamilyMed
Houlachi, Jean-Pascal
Houle, Gaetan
Houle, Michele
Huard, Verilibe, FamilyMed(EM)
Hubert, Christophe
Huchet, Emmanuelle
Hughes, Margaret H., FamilyMed
Huglo, Evelyne
Hunt, Ryan D., FamilyMed(EM)
Huot, Caroline
Hurteloup, Valerie
Huynh, Nam Phuong T., FamilyMed
Ibrahim, Julie, FamilyMed
Ifergan, Nathalie, FamilyMed
Illescas, Alfred W.
Ince-Cushman, Daniel, FamilyMed
Ionescu, Loretta V., FamilyMed
Iordachescu, Andrei, FamilyMed
Irani, Nabil
Irani, Zeubin
Ishak-Boushaki, Fatma-Zohra
Iskandar, Evette
Jabado, Nada
Jacob, Genevieve
Jacques, Andre J., FamilyMed
Jacques, Marc-Andre
Jafarian, Fatemeh
Jagodzinski, Daniel
Jagoe, Robert T.

Jansen, Kurt A., FamilyMed
Jantchou Mbakop, Prevost
Jaquier, Catherine
Jardon, Kris
Jarry, Marie-Claude, FamilyMed
Jarvis, Catherine A., FamilyMed
Jasmin, Christiane L.
Jasmin, Francois
Jasserand, Francoise
Jast, Zygmunt M.
Jean, Suzanne
Jean-Destin, Marie N.
Jilwan, Antoine R.
Jimenez, Vania J., FamilyMed
Jipa, George
Jipa, Ileana, FamilyMed
Jochem, Klaus
Jodoin, Valerie
Johansson, Patricia L.
Johnson, Caroline, FamilyMed
Johnson, Kirsten N., FamilyMed(EM)
Johnson, Martine
Jolicoeur, Diane
Jolicoeur, Isabelle
Jolicoeur, Paul
Jolin, Cathy
Joly, Edith
Jourdenais, Emmanuelle, FamilyMed(EM)
Joyal, Claude
Julien, Isabelle
Jung, Sungmi
Junod, Patrice
Juras, Audrey M.
Kabangu, Emman-Tshiamang, FamilyMed
Kadoch, Isaac-Jacques
Kahwajian, Lori, FamilyMed
Kalin, Michael J., FamilyMed
Kalina, Maciej, FamilyMed
Kamel, Hany M., FamilyMed
Kanadjian, Maral N., FamilyMed(EM)
Kanber, Yonca
Karanofsky, Mark, FamilyMed
Karayan, Lina, FamilyMed
Karazivan, Philippe, FamilyMed
Katz, Edward
Kavan, Petr
Kayal, Dounia
Kayssi, Hassan
Kerner, Sarah N., FamilyMed
Kettouche, Louiza
Keu, Nita, FamilyMed
Keyston, Rebecca, FamilyMed
Khadilkar, Madhusudan C.
Khadir, Saideh
Khaled, Abdelmoula
Khan, Ayesha
Khattabi, Mona, FamilyMed
Kieu, Khanh-Giao
Kieu, Vi-Thuy
Kirk, John C., FamilyMed
Klein, Benjamin D.
Klubien, Kristine E.
Kobayashi, Eliane
Kocur, Ivana
Koenig, Martial
Koniouchine, Vladimir, FamilyMed
Korany, A. Leyla, FamilyMed
Korin-Skamene, Tamara
Koss, Erica
Kounde-Tognide, Elisabeth
Koutroularas, Ekaterine
Kovacina, Nebojsa, FamilyMed
Kowalski, Odile
Kremer, Bernardo, FamilyMed
Kumka, Gillian L., FamilyMed(EM)
Kuperberg, Karol
Kuyumjian, Jirair
Kwiatkowska, Caroline
Kwong, Patrick, FamilyMed
L'Abbe, Daniel
L'Heureux, Daniele
La, Dong-Ky
La, Thuy Phuong, FamilyMed
Labadie, Caroline
Labarias-Romeo, Jose
Labateya, Nabil
Labelle, Celine
Labelle, Marie-Esther
Labelle, Martin J.

Labelle, Martine, FamilyMed(EM)
Laberge, Claude
Labrecque, Denis
Labrecque, Michele A., FamilyMed(EM)
Labrousse, Jean-Marie
Lachance, Claude
Lachance, Martin, FamilyMed
Lachance, Raymond
Lacombe, Paméla
Lacoursiere, Josiane
Lacouture Quintero, Astrid P., FamilyMed
Lacroix, Chantal
Lacroix, Vincent J., FamilyMed
Ladouceur, Roger, FamilyMed
Laferriere, Sophie
Laflamme, Marie-Pierre
Lagodich, Marina
Lajeunesse, Julie, FamilyMed
Lajeunesse, Yvette
Lajeunesse Viens, Guylaine, FamilyMed
Lalande, Johanne
Lalande, Raymond, FamilyMed
Lalla, Leonora, FamilyMed
Lalonde, Catherine
Lalonde, Eric, FamilyMed(EM)
Lalonde, Suzanne
Lam, Man-Hoa, FamilyMed
Lam, Ngoc Nga
Lam, Quoc Hung
Lam, Quoc Tru
Lam, Tai-Thuong
Lam, Vo-Hoa, FamilyMed
Lambert, Gilles
Lambert, Nicole
Lambrinos, Dimitrios J.
Lamer, Danielle
Lamothe, Marcel
Lamothe-Guay, Monique C.
Lamoureux, Manon, FamilyMed
Lamoureux, Michelle
Lanctot, Robert
Landry, Charles
Landry, Claude, FamilyMed
Landry, Gabrielle
Landry, Monique
Landry, Yves
Lanfranchi, Paola A.
Languedoc, Francine
Lanoue, Danielle
Lantagne, Christiane
Lapaige, Veronique
Laperriere, Helene, FamilyMed
Lapeyraque, Anne-Laure
Lapierre, Benoit, FamilyMed
Lapierre, Claude
Laplante, Francois
Laplante, Lucie
Laplante, Severine, FamilyMed
Lapointe, Bernard
Lapointe, Elise S., FamilyMed
Lapointe, Jacques, FamilyMed
Lapointe, Lucie
Laporte, Jean-Luc B.
Laroche, Claude
Larocque, Isabelle
Larose, Dominic
Larose, Michel
Larouche, Michel
Larouche, Nicole
Larouche, Richard
Larue, Nicole
Lasry, David A., FamilyMed(EM)
Lattermann, Ralph B.
Laurans, Muriel, FamilyMed
Laurendeau, Catherine
Laurens, Jean-Pierre
Laurier, Danielle
Laurin, Suzanne, FamilyMed
Lauriston, Christian
Lauzier, Nathalie
Lauzon, Marguerite
Lauzon, Michel
Lauzon, Pierre
Lavallee, Pierre
Lavigueur, Denis
Lavoie, Christiane-Elise
Lavoie, Stephane
Lawlor, Krista A., FamilyMed

PHYSICIANS BY PROVINCE

Lawson, Thomas
Lazarus, Michael
Le, Han
Le, Huu Phuong
Le, Melissa, FamilyMed
Le, Minh Tien
Le, Ngoc Quan
Le, Pham D T., FamilyMed(EM)
Le, Phu-Tao
Le, Phuoc Hoang
Le, Thanh-Minh
Le, Thi Qui
Le, Thien Nhan
Le, Vanessa H., FamilyMed
Le Bire, Francois
Le Deist, Francoise
Le Guerrier, Paul, FamilyMed
Le Thi, Minh-Tri
Le Van, Mai Anh, FamilyMed(EM)
Leblanc, Danielle
Leblanc, Isabelle, FamilyMed
Leblanc, Marie-Claude, FamilyMed
Lebouche, Bertrand P.
Lecavalier, Danielle
Leclerc, Jean
Leclerc, Suzanne
Leclerc, Sylvie
Lecoq, Henri
Lecours, Isabelle, FamilyMed
Leduc, Genevieve
Lefebvre, Anika, FamilyMed(EM)
Lefebvre, Helene, FamilyMed
Lefebvre, Marie-Claude, FamilyMed
Lefevre, Alain
Legault, Danielle, FamilyMed
Legault, Marie-Jose, FamilyMed
Leger, Caroline
Leger, Francine
Leibovici, Dalila
Leibovici, Theodore
Lemarquand, Janique, FamilyMed
Lemiere, Catherine
Lemieux, Bruno
Lemieux, Daniele
Lemieux, Lucie
Lemieux, Nathalie, FamilyMed
Lepage, Christiane
Lequoc, Stephane, FamilyMed(EM)
Lessard, Bernard, FamilyMed
Lessard, Louise
Lessard, Lyne
Lessard, Marthe
Letellier, Monique
Letourneau, Justin
Levan, Chau
Levejac, Chantal
Levental, Mark, FamilyMed
Levesque, Chantale, FamilyMed
Levesque, Jean
Levesque, Paul
Levi, Dahlia
Levi, Yves
Levin, Richard
Levine, Zachary A., FamilyMed(EM)
Levros, Louis-Charles
Levy, David
Lewis, John R., FamilyMed(EM)
Li, Nan
Liebich, Anne-Marie
Limoges, Michel
Lin, Roberto, FamilyMed
Lindor, Marie-Helene
Lipes, Peter M.
Lisanu, Mesfin G.
Liu Chen Kiow, Lee Ha, FamilyMed
Lizotte, Pierre
Locas, Francois
Lodygensky, Gregory A.
Loiselle, Andre
Loiselle, Maurice
Lonergan, Guy
Longpre, Daniele
Longpre, Denis
Lopes, Paulo
Lopez-Valle, Hilda R.
Lorber, Estelle, FamilyMed
Lord, Jacinthe
Lortie Forgues, Aude, FamilyMed
Loubert, Francois
Lounsbury, Catherine
Lovasco, Salvatore
Luca, Anne-Marie, FamilyMed
Luca, Virgil A.
Lucey, Michele D., FamilyMed(EM)
Luong, Diep T.
Lussier-Montplaisir, M.
Luu, Huu Ni, FamilyMed
Luu, Kiet-Quan
Luu, Thanh-Phi
Mac, Thien Hung, FamilyMed
Mac Van, Tin
MacAulay, Ann C., FamilyMed
MacDonnell, B. Jean, FamilyMed
MacKay, Charles
Magnan, Anne
Magnoux, Eric
Mah, Rick H., FamilyMed(EM)
Mahdavian, Fereydoun
Maheux, Brigitte
Mahood, Robert F., FamilyMed
Mainville, Pierre
Maiolo, Giuseppe C.
Major, Nathalie, FamilyMed(EM)
Malaise, Jacques
Malouf, Benoit
Malus, Michael, FamilyMed
Manafy, Chirina
Mandel, Romain
Mandeville, Helene
Manganas, Athena, FamilyMed
Manganas, Therese
Manoli, Sabrine, FamilyMed
Mansour, Michael
Mansour, Samer
Mantha, Jean
Maranda, Sophie, FamilyMed
Marceau, Nicole
Marchand, Ingrid, FamilyMed
Marchand, Jacques
Marchand, Michele
Marcil, Dominique
Marion, Chantal
Marmor, Goldie, FamilyMed
Marques, Sylvia
Marsan, Stephanie M., FamilyMed
Martel, Julien, FamilyMed(EM)
Martin, Jacques
Martin, Kelly M.
Martinez Marin, Jose Luis
Marzouki, Monia S.
Massey, Ephraim G.
Mathers, Paul G., FamilyMed(EM)
Mathieu, Bernard
Mathurin, Jean
Matte, Anouk
Matte, Marie-Claude, FamilyMed
Mavromichalis, Helen, FamilyMed
May, Richard
Mayer, Chantal
Mayer, Kailash K.
Mayer, Sudesh
Mayer, Sunita, FamilyMed
Mayman, Barbara, FamilyMed
Mazza, Guiseppe
Mazzella-Maiolo, Loraine
McClaran, Jacqueline
McLauchlin, Lynn R., FamilyMed
Mecarbane, Elie G.
Mehareb Redjah, Nadia
Melanson, Claude
Melnychuk, David A N.
Melnyk, Lydia C., FamilyMed
Mercier, Francois
Merouani, Aicha
Mesbahi, Karim
Messier, Alexandre, FamilyMed(EM)
Messier, Michele
Meunier, Michel
Michaels, George, FamilyMed
Michaud, Danielle
Mihic, Niko, FamilyMed
Milette, Isabelle
Miller, Wilson
Millette, Pierre
Milne, C. Michelle
Milot, Diane
Miron, Michel
Miseri, Frederic J S.
Mitnick, Howard J., FamilyMed
Mocanu, Maria
Mohamed, Ibrahim
Monahan, Barbara J., FamilyMed
Monette, Diane
Montpetit, Pierre
Montplaisir, Isabelle, FamilyMed(EM)
Moreau, Julie, FamilyMed
Moreau, Mathieu, FamilyMed
Moreau, Michele
Morel, Rene
Morel, Stephanie, FamilyMed
Moriconi, Claudette, FamilyMed
Morin, Gilbert, FamilyMed
Morin, Madeleine
Morin, Marie-Eve, FamilyMed
Morin, Michel
Morin-Bienvenu, Louise
Morissette, Nancy, FamilyMed
Morris, Lawrence
Morris, Randi E., FamilyMed
Morris, Sandra, FamilyMed
Mortezai, Berenice
Moser, Thomas P.
Motard, Alexandre, FamilyMed
Mottron, Laurent
Moukhtar, Clara F., FamilyMed
Mourey, Sophie
Moussaoui, Chloe, FamilyMed(EM)
Munoz, Gabriel
Munoz, Marie
Myara, Max N.
Myles, Virginia J., FamilyMed
Mysore, Navya M., FamilyMed
Nached, Adnan
Nadeau, Jacques E.
Nadeau, Michel
Nagy, Francine
Nally, Veronique
Naman, Nazem, FamilyMed
Nantel, A J. Albert
Naranjo, Jose
Narasiah, Lavanya
Narbonne, Sabrina, FamilyMed(EM)
Nattel, Celia A., FamilyMed
Nedelec, Joelle
Nelisse, Nicolas
Nemeth, Joe, FamilyMed(EM)
Neron, Roxane
Neveu, Alain
Neveu, Francoise
Neylon, Norah
Ng Cheong, Caroline, FamilyMed
Ngo, Thanh-Phuong
Nguyen, Andre T H.
Nguyen, Ba-Long
Nguyen, Cam-Hanh
Nguyen, Cong-Nghiem, FamilyMed
Nguyen, Daniel T.
Nguyen, Dinh Nam
Nguyen, Duy
Nguyen, Duy Toan
Nguyen, Gia-Khanh, FamilyMed
Nguyen, H. Tuong Quan
Nguyen, Hiep Huu
Nguyen, Hoang Ngoc T.
Nguyen, Hung Vuong
Nguyen, Huu Vi
Nguyen, Kim Anh, FamilyMed
Nguyen, Kim Anh
Nguyen, Kimberly, FamilyMed
Nguyen, Long Phan, FamilyMed
Nguyen, Manhluu
Nguyen, Minh Hanh
Nguyen, Minh-Duc
Nguyen, My Chau, FamilyMed
Nguyen, My Lang
Nguyen, My-Tien, FamilyMed
Nguyen, Ngoc Thien
Nguyen, Ngoc Toan
Nguyen, Ngoc-Lang
Nguyen, Olivia K., FamilyMed
Nguyen, Phu-Cuong
Nguyen, Quang Hung
Nguyen, Quang Thanh
Nguyen, Quynh Nga
Nguyen, T. Thanh Tra, FamilyMed
Nguyen, Tan-Ngoc
Nguyen, Thai Tong
Nguyen, Thanh Can, FamilyMed
Nguyen, Thi Hong
Nguyen, Thi Phuong A.
Nguyen, Thituong N.
Nguyen, Tuan Khoat.
Nguyen, Tuong Minh, FamilyMed
Nguyen, Van Dong
Nguyen, Van Thanh
Nguyen, Van-Phuc
Nguyen, Van-Tri
Nguyen, Van-Tri
Nguyen, Viet Huan
Nguyen, Vinh-Kim
Nguyen Gia, Le Thi
Nguyen-Ngoc, Bao
Nguyen-Ong, Thi Khanh Van
Nica-Danes, Doina
Nicolescu-Zinca, Alexandru, FamilyMed
Noel, Caroline, FamilyMed
Normandin, Luc
Normandin, Lucie
Notebaert, Eric
Nseir, Anas, FamilyMed
O'Brien, Robert P., FamilyMed
O'Driscoll, John K., FamilyMed(EM)
O'Shaughnessy, Gael, FamilyMed
Oberman, Saul S., FamilyMed
Ohayon-Gabbay, Huguette
Ojanguren, Andrea A.
Okan, Denis, FamilyMed
Olivie, Damien A R.
Olivier, Jeremie
Omeroglu, Gulbeyaz
Onyekwelu, Onyema A., FamilyMed
Oommen, Ashok, FamilyMed(EM)
Orlup, Gerard, FamilyMed
Orzeszyna, Magdalena M., FamilyMed
Ospina, Luis H.
Ott-Braschi, Sylvie
Ouellet, Joanie
Ouellet, Martin
Ouellet, Sylvie
Ouellet, Sylvie
Ouimet, Marie-Jo
Oulianine, Karen, FamilyMed(EM)
Ovetchkine, Philippe
Pamphile, Louis G.
Panikian, Jean-Claude
Pantel, Mitchell S., FamilyMed
Papillon, Elise, FamilyMed
Paquet, Benoit, FamilyMed(EM)
Paquette, Daniel, FamilyMed
Paquette, Pierre
Paquette-L'Ecuyer, Lucie
Paquin, Claude
Paradis, Isabelle
Paraskevopoulos, Chryssi I.
Pare, Renee
Parent, Andree-Anne
Parent, Claude
Parent, Daniel E.
Parent, Yves
Parniani, Sara
Patel, Prakash B R.
Patey, Nathalie G.
Patterson, David W., FamilyMed
Pavilanis, Alan V., FamilyMed
Payne, Allen
Payot, Antoine
Payot, Isabelle
Pearson, Eleena A., FamilyMed
Pedro, Maria E.
Pelland, Marie-France, FamilyMed
Pelletier, Bruno
Pelletier, Christine
Pelletier, Garry
Pelletier, Helene
Pelletier, Jean, FamilyMed
Pelletier, Jean
Pelletier, Marie-Chantal, FamilyMed
Pelletier, Michele
Pelletier, Paul
Pelletier, Renee
Pepin, Jean
Perez-Martinez, Jordi
Perreault, Danielle
Perron, Andre
Perrone, Maria, FamilyMed
Perrotta, Rosalba, FamilyMed
Perry, J. Christopher
Persson, Megan A., FamilyMed(EM)
Petraglia, Teresa, FamilyMed
Pham, Phuong-Vy
Pham, Thi Thanh D., FamilyMed
Pham, Van Dong H.
Pham Nhut, Huong
Phan, T H I. Dang, FamilyMed
Phan, Tuan X.
Phan, Van Thanh.
Phan, Xuan Truong
Phaneuf, Jean-Luc
Phenix, Pierre
Picard, Georges
Piche, Annie, FamilyMed
Piche, Robert
Pilarski, Robert, FamilyMed
Pilon, Dominique, FamilyMed
Pilon, Liette
Pilon, Pierre A.
Pineau, Gilles
Pinto, Antonio
Placide, Joseph E.
Plamondon, Gilles
Plante, Michel
Pless, Charles E., FamilyMed
Pluye, Pierre
Poirier, Denis
Poirier, Gerald
Poirier, Manon
Poitras, Lucie
Ponnet, Natalie
Popescu-Crainic, Sanda, FamilyMed
Pordan, Eva
Potter, Martin, FamilyMed
Potvin, Daniel
Potvin, Richard
Pou, Vitiya, FamilyMed
Pou-Youthoan, Kimlay
Poulin De Courval, Louise S., FamilyMed
Poupart, Helene
Powell, Thomas
Praseuth, Billee, FamilyMed
Pratt, J. Graham
Prefontaine, Genevieve
Prescott, Robert C.
Prevost, Francois-Yves
Prevost, Louis
Primavesi, Robert, FamilyMed(EM)
Prosper, J P. Lionel
Prossin, Albert, FamilyMed
Provencher, Robert
Provencher, Yves
Provost, Sylvie
Ptito, Linda
Pushie, Heather J., FamilyMed
Quao, Nii T.
Querleu, Denis
Quintin, Normand
Rabasa-Lhoret, Remi
Raboisson, Marie-Josee
Racine, Daniel
Racine, Daniele
Rainville, Josee, FamilyMed
Rajakesari, Meenalosany
Rajotte, Claude, FamilyMed
Ramsay, Jacques
Raphael, Frantz
Rappaport, Jerrold L.
Rappaport, Maureen E., FamilyMed
Ratte, Sonia, FamilyMed
Rauch, Frank T.
Raymond, Marie-Claude, FamilyMed
Razavi, Aram
Reid, Andrew G., FamilyMed(EM)
Remer, Zev, FamilyMed
Renaud, Sylvie
Renoult, Edith A.
Rezaeifar, Parand, FamilyMed
Rezaie, Raymond, FamilyMed
Rezende, Flavio
Rheaume, Sylvie
Ricard, Nadege
Richard, Christiane
Richard-Chesnay, Johanne
Richer, Jean-Claude
Richer, Marc
Richer, Suzanne
Richter, Anne-Katrin, FamilyMed
Riendeau, Guy
Rif, Maria, FamilyMed(EM)
Rigault, Aude
Rioux, Guylaine
Rivard, Louise-Isabelle, FamilyMed
Rivest, Jean
Rivest, Paul
Rizzuto, Anthony, FamilyMed

Robbins, Steven E.
Roberge, Claude
Roberge, Yolande
Robert, Guillaume
Robert, Marie-Michelle, FamilyMed(EM)
Robert, Yves
Robichaud-Gauvin, Nadia
Robillard, Andree, FamilyMed
Robinson, Jacques
Rodier, Irwin J.
Rodriguez Moya, Maria del Rosario
Roederer, Ghislaine
Roger-Achim, Diane, FamilyMed
Rohan, Ivan, FamilyMed
Rohan, Peter
Rohe, Philippe, FamilyMed
Roland, Pierre B.
Roman, Sandra, FamilyMed
Rompre, Anne
Rona, Mary J., FamilyMed
Rondeau, Pierre
Rosenberg, Ellen E., FamilyMed
Rosengren, A. Orin, FamilyMed
Rosenthal, Gary F.
Rossignol, Serge
Rothman, Ann, FamilyMed
Rouleau, Pierre
Roulier, Stephan, FamilyMed(EM)
Rousseau, Helene, FamilyMed
Rowen, John P., FamilyMed(EM)
Roy, Alain
Roy, Christiane
Roy, Diane
Roy, Madeleine
Roy, Marie-Andree, FamilyMed(EM)
Roy, Michelle
Rozen, Jamie, FamilyMed
Rozencwaig, Roman R.
Rubenstein, Heather, FamilyMed
Rubin, Alexandra S., FamilyMed
Rubin, Gordon, FamilyMed
Rubino, Michael, FamilyMed
Rudkin, Teresa, FamilyMed
Ruest, Richard
Russillo, Balbina, FamilyMed
Rustom, Nour
Saba, Samir E.
Sabin, Norman, FamilyMed(EM)
Sabourin, Alain
Sadani, Gaelle
Sader, John
Sahi, Nidhi, FamilyMed
Saine, Marie-Josee
Saine, Michel
Saint-Martin, Christine
Saksena, Rajni, FamilyMed
Salami, Gorgin
Sall, Gurjinder P.
Saluja, Sanjeet S., FamilyMed(EM)
Sam, Renida, FamilyMed
Samuel, Charles
Sanchez-Baracaldo, Lilia M.
Sandhu, Sangeeta
Sandhurst, Judith, FamilyMed
Santagata, Pietro
Santerre, Carole
Sarrazin-Vincelette, Lucie
Sary, Gamil
Sasseville, Elise, FamilyMed
Sauve, Agathe
Sauve, Louise, FamilyMed
Sauve, Nicolas
Sava, Renata, FamilyMed
Savage, Rachel
Savoie, Josee
Savoie, Line
Savoie, Louise
Savoie, Luc
Scarborough, Francois, FamilyMed(EM)
Schellenberg, Duncan A.
Schiff, Benjamin Z., FamilyMed
Schipper, Mitchell J., FamilyMed
Schricker, Thomas P S.
Schwarcz, Deborah, FamilyMed(EM)
Schwenter, Frank
Sebastiani, Giada
Sebbag, Sarah E., FamilyMed(EM)
Seck, Mamadou S.
Senechal, Nicole
Serero, Charles
Serero, Didier M., FamilyMed(EM)
Serfaty, Samuel
Serra, Lydia
Serrar, Jamal
Shabah, Abdo, FamilyMed
Shalom-Paz, Einat
Shapiro, Adam J.
Shenker, Hannah R., FamilyMed
Shiff, Dori, FamilyMed
Shir, Yoram
Shrier, Ian
Shuldiner, Samuel
Si-Ahmed, Fatma
Sidani, Karine, FamilyMed
Silvano, Sonia, FamilyMed
Simard, Andree-Anne
Simard, Louis-Marie
Simard, Steeve
Simion, Sonia
Simons, D. Irene, FamilyMed
Simons, Jonathan M., FamilyMed(EM)
Singer, Tamara, FamilyMed
Singerman, Jonathan, FamilyMed(EM)
Sinha, Avinash K.
Sinnreich, Michael
Siviero, Giovanni
Skinner, Natalie, FamilyMed(EM)
Slaoui, Tarik
Sleiman, Hassan
Smith, Craig A., FamilyMed(EM)
Smith, Sarah J., FamilyMed
Sohi, Julia, FamilyMed
Soldevila, Emmanuel
Soos-Kapusy, Eva D., FamilyMed
Soowamber, Mohunlall
Soucy, Eric
Sproule, Donald A., FamilyMed
Srinivasan, Anjana, FamilyMed
St-Amour, Dominic
St-Arnaud, Karine, FamilyMed(EM)
St-Arnaud, Philippe, FamilyMed(EM)
St-Aubin, Jean-Jacques
St-Hilaire, Fritz
St-Jean, Pierre
St-Laurent, Judith
St-Pierre, Guy
Stanciu, Adela E., FamilyMed
Stankova, Jitka
Stasiak, Ewa M.
Steben, Marc, FamilyMed
Steg, Doris
Steinman, Robert J.
Steinmetz, Peter O.
Stendel, Mitchell H., FamilyMed(EM)
Stern, Meira, FamilyMed
Still, Susan M., FamilyMed
Stolovitz, Cynthia, FamilyMed(EM)
Strobach, Helene G.
Stuart, Howard R., FamilyMed(EM)
Sturmer, Marcio L.
Su, Jean, FamilyMed(EM)
Sultan, Daria A.
Sun, Kathryn A., FamilyMed
Sun, Siwen, FamilyMed
Sykiniotis, John, FamilyMed
Sylvestre, Pierre A.
Szabo, Jason T., FamilyMed
Sziklas, Tibor J.
Szpilberg, Michael
Ta, Tuyet Phi
Tabakian, Ohan
Takano, Tomoko
Talaat, Mohamed S.
Talbot, Jacques R.
Tamanaha, Loree M L., FamilyMed
Tan, Rita
Tanciu, Nicolae
Tandareanu, Luminita, FamilyMed
Tang, Quoc Kiet
Tang, Thanh Q., FamilyMed
Tanguay, Daniel
Tanguay, Nicole
Tannous, Waguih N., FamilyMed
Tanoubi, Issam
Taranu, Corina
Tardif, Isabelle, FamilyMed
Tardif, Louise
Tardy, Solange
Tari, Stephane
Taussky, Daniel M.
Tehfe, Moustapha
Teira, Pierre
Tellier, Pierre-Paul, FamilyMed
Teolis, Jean-Pierre
Terrault, Daniel
Tesfaye, Yoseph
Tessier, Dominique, FamilyMed
Tessier, Lorraine
Tetreault-Deslandes, Marieve, FamilyMed
Tewfik, Yvette-Nelly, FamilyMed
Thai, Dine C K.
Thai, Quynh-Nhu, FamilyMed
Theodule, Jean-Claude
Theriault, Anne
Theriault, Nicole
Theroux, Marie-Claude
Thibault, Marie-Frederique
Thibault, Maurice
Thibault, Sonia
Thibodeau, Jacinthe
Thibodeau, Pierre G.
Thiel, Alexander
Thivierge, Claude-Yves
Thomas, Rejean
Thomas Fils-Aime, Claudette
Thomas-Guy, Catherine
Thomassin, Bruce G.
Thomassin, Michael G., FamilyMed
Thuaudet, Danielle
Tinawi, Paul, FamilyMed
Toma, Nicola
Ton-That, Quoc-Huy, FamilyMed(EM)
Ton-That, Trac
Tondreau, Genevieve, FamilyMed
Tonnu, Lienchi
Tordjman, Philippe, FamilyMed(EM)
Torres-Pardo, Carlos I.
Tourian, Leon
Tournoux, Francis B M.
Touyz, Rhian M.
Tozzi, Daniel P.
Trahan, Sabine
Tran, Cao Thang
Tran, Mong Lam
Tran, Quang Hieu
Tran, Thi Bich T.
Tran, Thi-My-Linh
Tran, Thu-Hang, FamilyMed(EM)
Tran, Van Cuong
Tran, Van-Dung
Tran, Xia Tiang, FamilyMed
Tran, Xia-Hoe
Tran Nguyen, Quoc Viet
Tran Nguyen, Thi Thu
Tremblay, Eric
Tremblay, Florence, FamilyMed
Tremblay, Francois
Tremblay, Frederic, FamilyMed(EM)
Tremblay, Marjorie
Tremblay, Michele
Trempe, Dominique
Trempe, Jocelyne
Trempe, Laurent
Trepanier, Louise, FamilyMed
Trinh Tan, Frederick, FamilyMed
Trister, Neil L.
Trottier, Benoit
Trottier, Mylene
Truchon, Valery, FamilyMed
Trudeau, Dorothee
Trudeau, Jean-Bernard
Trudeau, Vincent
Truong, Minh-Dung
Truteau, Michel
Tse, Chun Wing, FamilyMed
Tsiodras, Athanasios, FamilyMed
Tsoulos, Panagiotis, FamilyMed
Tu, My-Linh
Tugault, Julie
Tulandi, Tati
Tulin, Caroline
Turcot, Josee
Turcotte, Chantal
Turcotte, Robin
Turgeon, Pierre-Victor
Turmel, Bruno
Tétreault, Laurie, FamilyMed
Ung, Muoy
Vachon, Michel
Vaillancourt, Claude
Vaitekunas, Susan
Vaktor, Peter
Valade, Andre
Valdivia, Olga E., FamilyMed
Vallieres-Pilon, Julia, FamilyMed
Van, Quang
Van Den Eynde, Frederique
Van Duyse, Stan G.
Van Dyke, Christiane
Vandal, Johanne
Vandelli, Stefania, FamilyMed
Vandenbroucke-Menu, Franck
Vangurp, J. Gerald
Vanhuysen, Marie
Vanier, Mylene
Vanier, Stephane, FamilyMed
Vanka, Thomas
Vargas Dreyer, Maria G.
Varin, Sylvain
Vartanian, Astghik
Vartazarmian, Garabed
Varvarikos, Mariette, FamilyMed(EM)
Vary, Ana R.
Vary, Christiane, FamilyMed
Vasilikaki-Baker, Helen, FamilyMed
Vaucher, Michel P.
Vedel, Isabelle
Veillette, Rejean
Venne, Anne-Marie
Venne, Suzanne
Venne, Sylvie
Verdonck, Olivier
Vernacchia, Carlo
Vernec, Alan R.
Verret-Daigneault, Genevieve, FamilyMed
Verrette, Sylvie
Vetere, Phyllis-Marie
Vezina, Andre
Vezina, Jacques W.
Vezina, Sylvie
Vigano, Antonio A L.
Vigneault, Annie, FamilyMed(EM)
Viladevall, Hugo, FamilyMed(EM)
Villalpando Berumen, Juan M.
Villeneuve, Diane
Villeneuve, Jean-Benoit
Vincent, Martin, FamilyMed(EM)
Vo, Tai Thuan
Vo Van, Tuyen
Vrahas, Voula, FamilyMed
Vu, Dung
Vu, Ngoc Dien
Vu, The-Hung
Vu, Thi Khanh H.
Vu, Thi Thuong T.
Vu, Thien Tai T., FamilyMed
Vu-Nguyen, Caroline X L.
Waldman, Lyle H.
Ware, Mark A.
Warkus, Thomas
Wartelle-Bladou, Claire F S.
Wasfi, Atef M.
Wasser, Pnina C., FamilyMed
Wassmann, Sven
Watt, Douglas G D.
Watts, Sylvie
Wavrant, Sandrine
Weber, Marie E., FamilyMed
Weber-Bayar, Audrey
Wesson, Trevor
Whiteman, Avram D., FamilyMed
Wilson, Nagwa
Wintermark, Pia
Withington, Davinia E.
Wojcik, Joseph, FamilyMed
Wrezel, Olga A., FamilyMed(EM)
Xenos, John B.
Yaffe, Mark J., FamilyMed
Yahia Chérif, Dallel
Yao, Yu-Ju, FamilyMed
Yazdanian, Shirin O., FamilyMed
Yiannakis, Georgia
Younes, Layla, FamilyMed
Yung, Francoise
Zador, Nicolas M.
Zagury, Gaby, FamilyMed
Zaklos, Mayer M., FamilyMed
Zampini, Marisa A., FamilyMed
Zan, Nathalie, FamilyMed
Zaphiratos, Thomas A.
Zerguini, Amina A.
Zhang, Xiaosi, FamilyMed
Zigby, Jean A., FamilyMed
Zigman, Michael
Zingg, Hans H.
Zlotnik, Gregorio
Znojkiewicz, Kathia
Zoghby, Magdy
Zummo, Michel
Zwecker, Philip, FamilyMed
Zylbergold, Arnold

MONTREAL-EST

Brouillette, France
Graham, Steve
Leroux, Pierre H.
Perreault, Louis-Georges

MONTREAL-NORD

Adolphe, Sarah
Allard, Jean B.
Amsellem, Maurice
Beaulieu, Jean-Yves
Belanger, Pierre
Bherer, Serge
Binette, Nathalie, FamilyMed
Bonneau, Francois, FamilyMed
Brodeur, Jules
Campeau, Rejean
Cyr, Josiane, FamilyMed
Dang, Phu An
Dermarkar, Julie E.
Dessureault, Louise, FamilyMed
Dhaiti, Magalie
Duguay, Johanne
Fleury, Benoit
Francois, Jean
Gauthier, Carole
Gouache, Alain
Hamel, Emilie
Herard, Genevieve, FamilyMed
Hoang, Duc Hieu N.
Hoang, Tuan-Khai
Jovic, Jelena, FamilyMed
Karas, Maria, FamilyMed
Laliberte, Ariane
Laporte, Sophie
Le, Thi Xuan Mai
Lee, Ik Ju
Legros, Marie-Florence, FamilyMed
Mercier, Isabelle
Millette, Rebecca
Nadeau, Marc
Nguyen, Mau Hoang
Sayoud, Fadila
Simoncelli, Luc
Tlili, Messaoud, FamilyMed
Tran, Van-Kim
Truong, Thi Kim N.
Viau, Melanie

MONTREAL-OUEST

Yaremko-Dolan, Marie, FamilyMed

MORIN-HEIGHTS

Cadieux, Pierre

MURDOCHVILLE

Dallaire, Michel H.
Harton, Jacques
Roy, Michel R.

NANTES

Lazure, Rene

NAPIERVILLE

Gauthier, Karine, FamilyMed
Lajoie, Marc
Miron, Diane
Paradis, Denise
Pham, Huy
Robert, Diane H.

NEMISCAU

Paquet, Guy

NEUVILLE

Grenon, Jean-Francois
Simetin, Josee
Viens, Pierre

NEW RICHMOND

Levasseur, Louis

NICOLET

Bechard, Fannie, FamilyMed
Blondin, Jean
Brochu, Jean-Guy
Gamelin, Sylvain D.
Garcia, Javier
Gauthier, Guylaine
Leclerc, Roselyn, FamilyMed
Livernoche, Marie
Pelletier, Francis
Quevillon, Mylene
Tardif, Dominique
Thibault, Julie
Tremblay, Nathalie
Valois, Marie-Michelle

NOMININGUE

Dube, Paul

NORMANDIN

Rouleau, Daniel
Savard, Marie-Andree, FamilyMed
Simard, Real

NORTH HATLEY

Rock, Rejean

NOTRE DAME DE L'ILE PERROT

Laferriere, J R. Gilles A.
Moalli, Linda
Trottier, Richard

NOTRE DAME DES PRAIRIES

Bernier, Michel, FamilyMed
Bernier, Yvan, FamilyMed
Cote, Benoit
Desjardins, Lyne
Forget, Josee
Tremblay, Robert

NOTRE DAME DU LAC

Banet, Joan
Cambron, Helene
Caron, Catherine, FamilyMed
De Brouwer, Marie-Claude
Deris, Behado
Deschênes-Lapointe, Anne-Claire, FamilyMed
Dionne, Mireille, FamilyMed
Hanna, Nader
Landry, Linda
Pedneault, Janie
Poulin-Trepanier, Evelyne, FamilyMed
Rioux, Caroline
Roy, Johanne, FamilyMed

ORMSTOWN

Alipour Milajerdi, Shahryar, FamilyMed(EM)
Blonde, J. Vince, FamilyMed
Daouid, Fouad
Geukjian, S K. Gregory
Kadoch, Harry, FamilyMed
Khlil, Abderrahim, FamilyMed
Krotecki, Lech, FamilyMed
Lussier, Timothy, FamilyMed
Malec, Elizabeth A., FamilyMed
Raymond, Michel, FamilyMed
St-Amour, Annie
Vandor, Thomas A.

OTTER LAKE

Cote, Luc

OTTERBURN PARK

Boutet, Annie
Chouinard, Jean-Philippe, FamilyMed
Lafond, Michel
Lessard, Jean
Michaud, Odile

OUTREMONT

Aboussouan, Francis
Esterez, Philippe
Lamarre, Leo-Yves
Saint-Martin, Suzanne

PANET

Duhaime, Nancy

PAPINEAUVILLE

La Barre, Marc

PASPEBIAC

Basque, Marie-Helene
Bernard, Julie
Bouazra, Ahlem
Bourque, Isabelle
Dicaire, Stephanie
Galarneau-Girardin, Justine, FamilyMed
Levesque, Jean-Louis
Morissette, Pierre
Pelletier, Jacques, FamilyMed
Racine, Marie-Claude
Rycabel, Anna
Thibaudeau, Sylvie
Tremblay, Emilie, FamilyMed

PERCE

Rehel, Luc
Roberge, Andre

PIERREFONDS

Atiyabi, Haleh, FamilyMed
Boretsky, Linda, FamilyMed
Cote, Suzanne
Dadabhai, Ambreen, FamilyMed
Drapeau, Nicole
Duval, Jean-Felix
Dykhuis, Sandra, FamilyMed(EM)
Dzineku, Jean L.
Fiset, Dany
Fruth, Irmgard, FamilyMed
Gordon, Benjamin, FamilyMed
Groleau, Jean-Paul
Hermon, Orly, FamilyMed
Kayal, Magdi D.
Mathieu, Josee
Nayar, M. Jane
Neamt, Elena, FamilyMed
Poland, George
Prupas, David R.
Sandouk, Alain J S., FamilyMed
Smeja, Helen
Soulieres, Christine
Stiharu, Simona, FamilyMed
Sylvestre, Chantal
Wassef, Magdy W.
Zarruk, Ricardo

PIERREVILLE

Beauchemin, Dany, FamilyMed
Beauchemin, David, FamilyMed
Jauvin, Daniel
Shooner, Karl

PINCOURT

Bsata-Parent, Aida
Dospinescu Luliana, Simona, FamilyMed
Faucher, Marc
Gavlas, Shirley J.
Lalonde, Serge R.
Van Sterthem, Marie-Josee

PINTENDRE

Boutet, Bernard
Cusson, Diane F.
Thibeault, Marie-Helene

PLAISANCE

Villemure, Louise

PLESSISVILLE

Bedard, Daniel
Belle-Isle, Pierre
Breton, Jeannot
Dumont, Marcel
Fortier, Katie, FamilyMed
Gervais, Jean-Guy
Labonte, Genevieve, FamilyMed
Langlois, Claude
Levesque, Charles
Martel, Marie-Josee
Piche, Karine, FamilyMed
Racine, Real
Rondeau, Frederique
Samson, Vicky

POHENEGAMOOK

Bouchard, Josee
Brault, Jacques-Christian
Deschenes, Jean-Marie
Desgreniers, Guy
Gravel, Serge
Raymond, Stephane, FamilyMed
Sirois, Marco

POINTE AUX TREMBLES

Bastien, Francine
Blais, Manon
Brideau, Diane
Chirito, Edward
Comeau, Louise M.
Courteau, Jose
Do, Duy-An
Feghali, Marc
Fortin, Richard
Gourde, Marjolaine, FamilyMed
Hamelin, Christine
Hoduc, Viviane, FamilyMed
Lassonde, Pierre
Lavigne, Gisele
Lavoie, Marcel
Levenberg, Melissa, FamilyMed
Malo, Celine
Menard, Daniel
Nguyen, Huy Thang.
Normandin-Noel, Ginette
Osman, Samir
Rutkowska-Rokosz, Anna
Sanchini, Edouard R G.
Shebib, Pierre Y.
Trinh, Emilie B K., FamilyMed

POINTE CLAIRE

Abedpour Dardashti, Marzieh, FamilyMed
Bergeron, Richard
Berman, Isaac, FamilyMed
Birch, Christopher, FamilyMed
Bodor, Cristina
Bouchard, Sylvie, FamilyMed
Bounatiro, Ibrahim
Breger, Laurie T., FamilyMed
Breton, Chantal, FamilyMed
Campbell, Ian H., FamilyMed
Cosulich, Elizabeth M., FamilyMed
Dahan, Aime
Daignault, Peter G.
Darwich, Chadi
Delle Donne, Nadia, FamilyMed(EM)
Dionne, Michele
Dollois, Anne-Marie, FamilyMed
Dowell, Anthony H., FamilyMed
Dubois, Manon, FamilyMed
Duchesne, Dominique
Fasie-Neagoe, C F. Cristina, FamilyMed
Fortier, Liliane, FamilyMed
Fuchs, Aaron
Fuoco, Angelo, FamilyMed
Garber, Cheryl
Garg, Naveen, FamilyMed
Germain, Richard D.
Goldstein, Martin E.
Golgoon, Michael S.
Goulet-Page, Suzanne
Haskins, Catherine A., FamilyMed
Helou, Hussam A., FamilyMed
Hoang, Antoine
Hogenbirk, Barbara F., FamilyMed
Ionescu, Adriana, FamilyMed
Janzen, Jeannette L., FamilyMed
Kaufman, Tomas, FamilyMed
Kyle, Beverley, FamilyMed
Legault, Maurice
Loertscher, Rolf
Look, Didier S., FamilyMed
Luckow, David, FamilyMed
MacMahon, Kristian P., FamilyMed(EM)
Mamalingas, Zoe, FamilyMed
Mandeville, Dominique
Mazoff, Eric D., FamilyMed
McCarty, Tara A., FamilyMed
Mitrica, Mirela, FamilyMed
Moreau, Louise, FamilyMed
Munzar, Michael R.
Musgrave, Laurie, FamilyMed
Nghiem, Dung P.
Ogilvy, Caroline G.
Pantazopoulos, Efrosini, FamilyMed
Papic, Ognjen, FamilyMed(EM)
Pasquini, Filoteo, FamilyMed
Peters-Mainville, Dagmar, FamilyMed
Pirlog, Tiberiu, FamilyMed
Popovici, Radu G., FamilyMed
Rattray, Bruce
Reed, Katherine M.
Rus-Serban, Lenuta
Sawoniak, Robert I., FamilyMed(EM)
Soucy, Michele
Tabah, Meryl A., FamilyMed(EM)
Tagemouati, Mohammed
Tarcak, Norbert
Thibodeau, Renee
Tozer, Nancy M., FamilyMed
Trattner, Raquel, FamilyMed
Tremblay, Louise J., FamilyMed
Truong, Tuyet Lan
Vas, David W., FamilyMed(EM)
Vonniessen, Michael, FamilyMed(EM)
Weinman, Robert D., FamilyMed
Williams, Howell T.
Wilson Thomas Sorial, Mona
Yang, Una M C., FamilyMed
Zaharia, Mihai-Cristian, FamilyMed

PONT-ROUGE

Drolet, Francois
Dumont, Guy
Fortin, Celine, FamilyMed
Laverdiere, Francois M.
Sauvageau, Jocelyne

PORT-CARTIER

Bois, Christine
Clerget, Lionel
Gaudreault, Claire, FamilyMed
Gosselin, Pierre, FamilyMed
Lachapelle, Anne
Mawn, Steve
St-Gelais, Donald

POVUNGNITUK

Auclair, Genevieve, FamilyMed
Bohémier Bernard, Mathieu, FamilyMed
Boivin, Genevieve, FamilyMed
Chouinard, Gabriel, FamilyMed
Desjardins Tessier, Amelie, FamilyMed
Forget, Marc
Luna, Alberto, FamilyMed
Morin, Dominique, FamilyMed

PRINCEVILLE

Doucet, Anne-Marie
Elias-Lopez, Esmeralda
Frechette, Marie-Christine
Theriault, Lyne

QUEBEC

Abadie, Simon, FamilyMed(EM)
Abdul-Hadi, Ibada
Alary, Michel
Albert, Gabriella
Allard, Francine
Allard, Manon, FamilyMed(EM)
Allard, Marc
Allard, Melanie, FamilyMed
Allard, Suzanne
Allard-Wasajja, Kathleen A.
Amar, Maxime
Amin Hashem, Mohamed
April, Claude
April, Guy
Archambault, Maryse, FamilyMed
Archibald, Lise
Asselin, Leandre
Atamna, Chahinez
Aubin, Francois
Aubin, Michele, FamilyMed
Aubin, Sylvie
Audet, Daniel
Audet, Denis
Audet, Helene
Audet, Marie-Claude

PHYSICIANS BY PROVINCE

Auger, Claire E.
Auger, Francois
Auger, Jean-Marie
Azzaria, Samir, FamilyMed
Babakifard, Katayoun, FamilyMed
Babin, Antoine
Bagur, Rodrigo H.
Baillargeon, Lucie
Banville, Marie-Claire
Baril, Josee
Barter Leyva, Maria T., FamilyMed
Beauchemin, Christiane
Beauchemin, Pierre
Beaudet, Louis-Edmond
Beaudet, Marie-France, FamilyMed
Beaudoin, Anne
Beaudoin, Richard
Beaudry, Florent
Beaulieu, Denis
Beaulieu, Helene
Beaulieu, Lucie
Beaulieu, Nathalie
Beaulieu, Richard
Beaulieu, Samuel, FamilyMed(EM)
Beaulieu, Sophie
Beaumier, Alain
Beaupre, Richard
Becotte, Genevieve, FamilyMed(EM)
Bedard, Alain
Bedard, Caroline, FamilyMed
Bedard, Denis
Bedard, Diane, FamilyMed
Bedard, Yves
Begin, Eloise, FamilyMed
Begin, Lorraine
Begin, Marie
Begin, Thierry, FamilyMed
Beland, Guy C., FamilyMed
Belanger, Chantal
Belanger, Danielle
Belanger, Liliane
Belanger, Marc
Belanger, Norma, FamilyMed
Belle-Isle, Jasmin
Belzile, Mireille
Bensaidane, Soufiane, FamilyMed
Bergeron, Gerald, FamilyMed
Bergeron, Jean B.
Bergeron, Karine
Bergeron, Nicole
Bergeron, Rénald, FamilyMed
Bernard, Andre
Bernard, Charles
Bernard, Pascale
Bernard, Sylvie
Bernier, Daniel, FamilyMed(EM)
Bernier, David, FamilyMed
Bernier, Denyse
Bernier, Helene
Bernier, Patrick, FamilyMed
Bernier, Richard
Bernier, Suzanne
Bernier, Sylvie
Berthelot, Jacques
Bertrand, Olivier
Bertrand, Real
Berube, Nathalie
Bherer, Jean-Yves
Bherer, Luc
Biertho, Laurent
Bilodeau, Yvonne
Biron, Dominique
Bissonnette, Alain
Blais, Bernard
Blais, Helene-Gabrielle
Blais, Johanne, FamilyMed
Blanchet, Richard
Blanchet, Sylvain, FamilyMed
Blondeau, Fernand, FamilyMed
Blondeau, Helene
Blouin, Denys
Blouin, Louis
Blouin, Mario
Blouin, Patrick
Bocquier, Arnaud A F., FamilyMed
Bois, Alain
Boisclair, Philippe, FamilyMed(EM)
Boisselle, Diane
Boisvert, Paule, FamilyMed
Bolduc, Guy
Bolduc, Yves
Bordeleau, Serge
Borduas, Francine
Bouchard, Andre
Bouchard, Christiane
Bouchard, Claire
Bouchard, Claude M.
Bouchard, Jean-Claude
Bouchard, Laurent
Bouchard, Yves
Boucher, Claude
Boucher, Louis P.
Boucher, Luce
Boucher, Martin, FamilyMed(EM)
Boucher, Martine
Boucher, Rejean
Boudreau, Bernard, FamilyMed
Boudreau, Ghislain, FamilyMed
Boudreau, Ghyslain
Boudreau, Marie
Boudreau, Marie-Helene, FamilyMed
Boudreault, Nathalie
Bouffard, Jean
Bouffard-Dumais, Catherine, FamilyMed
Boulanger, Dany
Boulianne, Louise
Bourget, Danny
Boutin, Marie, FamilyMed
Boutin, Mario, FamilyMed
Bouvier, Anne-Marie, FamilyMed
Brassard, Michel P.
Breton, Claude
Breton, Lyne
Breton, Pierre
Breton, Sophie, FamilyMed(EM)
Brisson, Jacques
Brisson, Melanie, FamilyMed
Brisson, Michel
Brochu, Annie, FamilyMed
Brouillette, Bernard
Brouillette, Charles, FamilyMed
Brouw, Maryleen
Brouw, Stefan, FamilyMed
Brun, Dominique
Bruneau, Rachel, FamilyMed(EM)
Bruniau, Jean-Theo
Busque, Nadia
Caouette, Christine
Carbonneau, Diane
Cardinal, Alain
Cardinal, Bernard
Carignan, Lucie
Caron, Louise
Caron, Marjolaine
Caron, Sophie
Carpentier, Daniel
Carpentier, Louis, FamilyMed
Castel, Josette, FamilyMed
Cauchon, Michel, FamilyMed
Cayer, Suzanne
Cencig, Agnes
Chabot, Celine
Chabot, Julie V., FamilyMed
Champagne, Pierre
Charbonneau, Myriam
Charest, Jerome, FamilyMed
Charette-Martineau, Amelie
Charlton, Marco
Charron, Louise
Chartier, Jean-Claude
Chartier, Lucas
Chateauvert, Sylvie
Chenevert, Alain
Chenevert, Robert J., FamilyMed
Chetaille, Philippe
Chetaille Nezondet, Anne-Laure
Chevarie, Karine
Chevrette, Marie-Christine
Chiquette, Jocelyne
Cholette, Pascale
Chotard, Isabelle
Chouinard, Claude
Chouinard, Guy
Chouinard, Lyne
Chouinard-Chretien, Marie P., FamilyMed
Chouinard-Rousseau, Helene, FamilyMed
Cimon, Line
Claude, Sophie
Clavet, Martin, FamilyMed
Clement, Martin, FamilyMed
Cliche, Louis
Cloutier, Diane
Cloutier, Fernand
Collin, Isabelle, FamilyMed
Collin, Marie-Eve
Collin, Pierre
Collins, Evelyn
Conti, Massimo
Cooper, E. Alexander, FamilyMed
Cordeau, Karyne
Corriveau, Louis-Philippe, FamilyMed(EM)
Corriveau, Remi
Corriveau, Robert A.
Cossette, Elise
Cote, Christiane
Cote, Elizabeth, FamilyMed
Cote, Genevieve
Cote, Guy
Cote, Jean-Francois
Cote, Louise, FamilyMed
Cote, Marie-Pascale, FamilyMed
Cote, Micheline
Cote, Nicole
Cote, Remy R.
Cote, Stephane, FamilyMed
Cote, Stephanie, FamilyMed
Coulombe, Charles
Couture, Clement
Couture, Jacques A.
Crchova, Melissa
Crete, Pauline, FamilyMed
Croteau, Agathe
Cusan, Leonello
Cyr, Carole
Cyr, Dominik, FamilyMed
Cyr, Nathalie
D'Amours, Denis, FamilyMed
D'Amours, Josee, FamilyMed
Daigle, Suzanne
Dalens, Bernard J.
Dallaire, Annie, FamilyMed
Dallaire, Michel
Dansereau, L. Alexandra
De Blois, Marc, FamilyMed(EM)
De Grace, Marianne
De Serres, Gaston
Del Degan, Sandra, FamilyMed
Delafield, Mary
Delage, Martin E.
Delamarre, Samuel, FamilyMed(EM)
Delisle, Sylvie
Delmonte, Guillermo A.
Demers, Julie
Demers, Marie-Josee
Demers, Michel C.
Denis, Bruno, FamilyMed
Denis, Jocelyne
Deroy, Roma
Dery, Catherine
Desbiens, Genevieve, FamilyMed
Deschenes, Dominique, FamilyMed
Deshaies, Lucie
Deshaies, Pierre
Desilets, Odette
Desmeules, Julie
Desrochers, Diane D.
Desroches, Annie
Desroches, Olivier, FamilyMed(EM)
Deviller, Genevieve
Dewailly, Eric
Diamond, Pierre, FamilyMed
Dion, Pierre
Dionne, Langis
Dionne, Suzanne
Do, Kim-Anh
Dodin, Sylvie
Dompierre, Gervais
Dore, Jean, FamilyMed
Dorion, Julie
Dorion, Nicole
Dostaler, Louis-Pierre
Dostie, Louise
Doucet, Annie
Douville, Veronique, FamilyMed(EM)
Dow, Jamie
Drouin, Denis
Drouin, Jean
Drouin, Jean
Dube, Ghislain
Dube, Nathalie
Dube, Serge, FamilyMed
Dubois, Nadine, FamilyMed
Dubuc, Benoit
Dubuc, Jean
Ducharme, Andree
Dufour, Anne
Dufour, Marie-Helene, FamilyMed
Dufour, Marie-Josee
Dugas, Christine
Dumas, Marie-Pierre, FamilyMed
Dumas, Serge
Dumas, Sylvie
Dumont, Jacques
Dupont, Anik
Dupont, France
Dupont, Jacinthe
Dupont, Michel
Dupont, Michel, FamilyMed(EM)
Dupuis, Martine
Durand, Etienne, FamilyMed
Egedy, Maud M P.
Elysee, Jacques S.
Emond, Nathalie
Emond, Sylvie
Faber, Anne
Fallu, Bernard
Farrier, Alain
Faucher, Roland
Fecteau, David, FamilyMed
Ferron, Michele
Filion, Marie-Josee
Fiset, Caroline, FamilyMed
Fiset, Serge
Fitzback, Guy
Flambert, Florence
Fleury, Michel
Fleury, Nadine
Flynn, Anne-Josee, FamilyMed
Fortin, Christian
Fortin, Dominique, FamilyMed(EM)
Fortin, Guy
Fortin, Jean
Fortin, Josee-Melanie, FamilyMed
Fortin, Yves
Fournier, Denis
Fournier, Pierre
Fradet, Amelie, FamilyMed
Frechette, Andre
Frenette, Jacques, FamilyMed
Frigon, Michel
Gagne, Christine
Gagne, Claude
Gagne, Guy
Gagne, Helene
Gagne, Monique
Gagnon, Bruno
Gagnon, Catherine, FamilyMed
Gagnon, Fabien, FamilyMed
Gagnon, Francois
Gagnon, Genevieve
Gagnon, Louis-Simon
Gagnon, Marie-Therese
Gagnon, Rene
Gagnon, Suzanne
Gagnon, Suzanne, FamilyMed
Gamache, Suzanne
Garant, Philippe
Garon, Andre
Gaudreau, Jules
Gaudreault, Nancy
Gaulin, Colette
Gauthier, Ariane, FamilyMed
Gauthier, Claude
Gauthier, Danielle
Gauthier, Gilles
Gauthier, Remi
Gauvreau, Michel
Gelinas, Pierre
Gemme, Nathalie, FamilyMed
Gendron, Jean-Paul
Genest, Rene
Germain, Judith, FamilyMed
Germain, Violaine
Gervais, Andre
Gervais, Marie
Giguere, Genevieve, FamilyMed
Gilca, Rodica
Gill, Francis, FamilyMed(EM)
Gingras, Anne-Isabelle, FamilyMed(EM)
Girard, Benoit
Girard, Marie
Giroux, Anne-Marie
Giroux, Marc
Glenn, Joan
Gobeil, Nicole
Godin, Christian
Godin, Paul-Emile
Gomez, Jose-Luis
Gosselin, Pierre
Gourdeau, Pierre
Gourdeau, Sophie, FamilyMed
Granger-Juneau, Eugenie
Gravel, Denis
Gravel, Robert
Gregoire, Louise
Grenier, Paule
Grenon, Marie
Grimard, Marlene
Groleau, Isabelle, FamilyMed
Groleau, Nathalie
Grondin, Renee J.
Groslouis, Lise
Guay, Bernard
Guerin, Linda
Guilbault, Paul
Guilbert, Edith
Guillemette, Jeanne
Guillemot, Yolande
Guilmette, Constance
Guimond, Mauril
Guite, Christian
Hache, Nathalie
Hamelin, Lucie, FamilyMed
Harnois, Carmen
Hebert, Christian-Rene, FamilyMed
Hebert, Diane
Hebert, Michel
Hendriks, Rene
Henry, Louise
Hivon, Jacinthe
Ho Ngoc Hap, Annie
Houde, Jacques
Houde, Lucien
Houde, Madeleine
Houde, Robert
Houle, Raymond
Houle, Yves E.
Hudon, Andre
Iglesias, Juan R.
Imbeault, Carrol
Jacob, Helene
Jacob, Renee
Jacques, Denis
Jacques, Martine, FamilyMed
Jacques, Michel
Jacques, Rene
Jacques, Valerie
Jahjah, Laila
Jalbert, Yves
Jaseliunas, Odetas
Jean, Andrea
Jean, Bernard
Jeanmart, Cecile, FamilyMed
Jinchereau, Pierre, FamilyMed
Johnson, Yves
Joyal, Maryse
Julien, Rene
Keable, Andre
Kearns, Finnualla
Kirouac, Isabelle
L'Anglais, Marie-Eve, FamilyMed
L'Ecuyer, Charles
L'Esperance, Helene
L'Italien, Helene
La Rue, Suzanne
Laberge, Caroline, FamilyMed
Laberge, Janick
Laberge, Melanie
Laberge, Renee
Labrecque, Michel, FamilyMed
Labrecque, Nancy
Labrie, Claude
Lachance, Benoit
Lachance, Carole
Lachance, Lucie
Lachance, Paul
Lachance, Pierre
Lachance, Suzelle
Lacroix, Marc, FamilyMed
Lacroix, Mylene H., FamilyMed

Laflamme, Ann
Lafleur, Pierre
Lafrance, Gilles
Lafrance, Serge
Lafranchise, Karine
Lafreniere, Michel
Lajoie, Christine
Laliberte, Diane
Laliberte, Marie, FamilyMed(EM)
Laliberte, Pierre
Lalinec-Michaud, Martin
Lalonde, Christine
Lamarche, Jean
Lamarre, Martin
Lambert, Jacinthe
Lambert, Louise
Lamontagne, Claude, FamilyMed
Lamontagne, Daniel
Lamontagne, Dominique
Landry, Daniel
Landry, Danielle
Landry, France
Landry, Johanne
Landry, Josee
Landry, Martine
Landry, Michel P.
Langevin, Gilles
Langlais, Marc, FamilyMed
Langlois, Nadine
Laperriere, Daniel
Laplante, Gerald
Laroche, Liny, FamilyMed
Larochelle, Gerard
Larose, Sebastien, FamilyMed(EM)
Larouche, Darie
Lassonde, Anick
Latouche, Marie-Josee, FamilyMed
Latulippe, Dany, FamilyMed
Latulippe, Denise
Laurion, Monique
Lauze, Michelle
Lavallee, Jean
Laverdiere, Maryse
Lavertu, Caroline
Lavoie, Danielle
Lavoie, Fabien
Lavoie, Maurice
Lavoie, Michele, FamilyMed
Lavoie-Ferland, Helene
Le Moine, Lindsay
Le Roy, Marie-Claire
Le Tien Ho Thi, Kim H.
Lebel, Maude
Leblanc, Josee
Leblanc, Martin, FamilyMed(EM)
Leblanc, Renee M.
Leclair, Jean
Leclerc, Andre
Leclerc, Anne
Leclerc, Celine, FamilyMed
Leclerc, Jacinthe
Leclerc, Marie-Josee
Leclerc, Sylvie
Leclerc-Soubrier, Annie, FamilyMed
Leduc, Christian
Leduc, Julie, FamilyMed(EM)
Leduc, Yvan, FamilyMed
Lefaivre, Dominique
Lefebvre, Denis
Lefebvre, Francine
Lefebvre, Martine
Lefrancois, Katleen
Lefrancois, Nil
Legare, France, FamilyMed
Legrand, Jacques
Lehoux, Martine
Lehoux, Suzie
Lejeune, Dominique
Lemay, Marie-Claire, FamilyMed
Lemelin, Richard
Lemieux, Alain-Philippe
Lemieux, Barbara
Lemieux, Jean
Lepage, Caroline
Lepage, Robert
Lesieur, Rene
Lessard, Lucie
Lessard, Pascal
Letarte, Helene
Letourneau, Jean-Marie
Levasseur, Isabelle
Levesque, Anny
Levesque, France
Levesque, Philippe, FamilyMed
Lizotte, Michel
Loczy, Katrin
Loisel, Suzanne
Lortie, Jocelyne
Madore, Stephanie
Maheux, Claude
Mailhot, Melissa
Mailloux, Marie-Josee
Maleza, Gerard
Maltais, Catherine, FamilyMed
Manhes, Gilles
Manrique Bello, Hermes M., FamilyMed
Manseau, Serge
Marc Series, Isabelle
Marceau, Annie
Marchand, Francoise
Marcotte, Jean, FamilyMed(EM)
Marcoux, Hubert, FamilyMed
Marois, Julie, FamilyMed
Martin, Louise
Martineau, Marie E.
Maurice, Stephane
Maziade, Jean, FamilyMed
Mazur-Gekas, Severine
McGee, Michel
McKinnon, Danny
McNicoll, Johanne
Menard, Yves
Menzies, Didier P.
Mercier, Gilles
Mercier, Marie-Lise, FamilyMed(EM)
Metivier, Yves
Michaud, Patricia
Michaud, Pierrette
Michaud-Mcgee, Louise
Michel, Normand
Michou, Laetitia N F.
Montreuil, Ann, FamilyMed
Moranville, Guy
Morasse, Charles, FamilyMed
Moraud, Edouard
Morcos, Mohib
Moreau, Anne, FamilyMed
Morel, Marie-Lou, FamilyMed
Morency, Chantale
Morency, Elizabeth
Morency, Pierre
Morin, Alain
Morin, Annie
Morin, Bernard
Morin, Claude, FamilyMed(EM)
Morin, Cybele
Morin, Diane
Morin, Jean
Morin, Louise
Morin, Nadine, FamilyMed
Morin, Renee
Morin, Serge
Morin, Yan, FamilyMed
Morissette, Alain
Morneau, Jean
Motheron, Christine, FamilyMed
Moulin, Jacinthe, FamilyMed
Mourad, Nathalie
Murphy-Laverdiere, Valerie, FamilyMed(EM)
Naccache, Maya, FamilyMed(EM)
Nadeau, Denise
Nadeau, Gaetan
Nadeau, Simon
Naud, Alain, FamilyMed
Nazair, Pierre
Nguyen, Nadia, FamilyMed
Nicol, Odette
Nicole, Sophie, FamilyMed
Nolin, Clement
Nourissat, Ghislain
O'Farrell, Lisa, FamilyMed
Olivier, Marlene
Olivier, Nathalie
Oudar, Valerie
Ouellet, Caroline
Ouellet, Eric
Ouellet, Jean, FamilyMed
Ouellet, Vianney, FamilyMed
Ouellet-Pelletier, Julie
Packwood, Nadine
Painchaud, Genevieve
Painchaud, Guillaume, FamilyMed
Paloux, Jean-Philippe, FamilyMed(EM)
Paquet, Jean-Rene
Paquet, Marie, FamilyMed
Paquette, Anne, FamilyMed
Paquin, France
Paquin, Sebastien, FamilyMed(EM)
Paradis, Andre, FamilyMed
Paradis, Chantal
Paradis, France
Paradis, Joanne
Paradis, Pierre
Paradis, Rodrigue
Parent, Alain, FamilyMed
Parent, Marie-Josee
Parent, Roger
Parent, Veronique, FamilyMed(EM)
Parrot, Benoit, FamilyMed
Pasian, Sergio G.
Pasquasy, Veronique
Patry, Claude
Pelchat, Suzanne
Pelet, Stephane
Pelletier, Pierre
Peloquin, Lucie, FamilyMed
Perreault, Jacqueline
Perreault, Josee
Phaneuf, Stella
Picard, Christian, FamilyMed
Picard, Maria-Elisa
Pigeon, Marie-Andree
Pinault, France
Pineau, Raymonde
Pineau, Rene
Piuze, Francois, FamilyMed
Piuze, Genevieve
Plaisance, Yves
Plamondon, Lise
Plante, Bernard
Plante, Vicky, FamilyMed
Plourde, Simon, FamilyMed
Poitevin, Anne-Marie, FamilyMed
Poitras, Anick, FamilyMed
Potvin, Michel, FamilyMed
Poulin, Monic
Pronovost Normand, Marie-Catherine, FamilyMed
Proulx, Jean
Proulx, Jean-Francois
Proulx, Simon-Pierre
Provencher, Joanne, FamilyMed(EM)
Puymirat, Jack
Radoux, Claude
Rancourt, Cynthia
Randoin, Michele-Anne
Raymond, Denis
Raymond, Vincent
Renaud, Pascal, FamilyMed(EM)
Renzo, Alain
Rheault, Christian
Rheault, Elise
Rheaume, Caroline
Rheaume, Caroline, FamilyMed
Rheaume, Marie-Claude
Richard, Annie
Ringuet, Jean
Ringuet, Serge
Rioux, Denis
Rioux, Stephane
Rizk, Mounir
Rizzo, Daniel, FamilyMed(EM)
Roberge, Daniel
Roberge, Genevieve
Roberge, Guy
Roberge, Louise
Robert, Diane, FamilyMed
Robert, Louis
Robidoux, Nathalie, FamilyMed
Robin, Roger
Robitaille, Julie, FamilyMed
Robitaille, Michel
Robitaille, Rejean
Rochefort, Lucie, FamilyMed
Rochette, Andre
Rochette, Pascal
Rochon, Daniele
Rodes Cabau, Joseph
Rodrigue, Jean
Rodrigue, Jean-Marie
Ross, Jean
Ross, Julie, FamilyMed
Rouifed, Nora, FamilyMed
Rousseau, Lise
Roussel, Robin
Routhier, Marie-Claude
Roy, Andre
Roy, Andre
Roy, Elyse
Roy, Helene
Roy, Isabelle, FamilyMed
Roy, Jean
Roy, Julie
Roy, Louis
Roy, Lucie E.
Roy, Marie, FamilyMed
Roy, Marie-Pierre
Roy, Roger
Roy, Yvon
Royer, Helene, FamilyMed
Salman-Godin, Ariane
Samson, Christine
Samson, Isabelle, FamilyMed
Samson, Marc
Samson, Stephanie
Saucier, Danielle, FamilyMed
Sauve, Louise
Savard, Anne
Savard, Martin, FamilyMed
Savard, Sylvie
Savoie, Jean-Pierre
Schreiber, Julie, FamilyMed
Scott, Hugh A., FamilyMed(EM)
Senechal, Sylvie
Series, Frederic
Sicotte, Claude
Simard, Dominique
Simard, Frederic, FamilyMed(EM)
Simard, Marc
Sirois, Carolyne
Sirois, Marthe
Smith, Sarah
Soucy-Hirtle, Fernande
Springuel, Andre
St-Aubin, Diane, FamilyMed
St-Hilaire, Karine, FamilyMed
St-Onge, Nicole
St-Pierre, Andre J.
St-Pierre, Caroline
St-Pierre, Denis
St-Pierre, Melanie
St-Pierre, Monique
Sylvain, Sonia, FamilyMed
Tailleur, Luc
Tardif, Alain
Tardif, Johanne
Tessier, Elisabeth
Tessier, Paule
Theoret, Johanne, FamilyMed
Theriault, J. Germain-Michel
Theriault, Julie F., FamilyMed
Theriault, Julie J., FamilyMed
Theriault, Lise
Therrien, Rene
Thibault, Suzanne
Thivierge, Caroll
Thivierge, Jean-Claude
Thivierge, Maryse, FamilyMed
Tiguert, Rabi
Tissot, Jean-Marie
Tolszczuk, Michelle
Tremblay, Bruno
Tremblay, Caroline
Tremblay, Helene
Tremblay, Helene
Tremblay, Jean-Guy
Tremblay, Johanne
Tremblay, Marjolaine
Tremblay, Micheline, FamilyMed
Tremblay, Myriam
Tremblay, Nicolas, FamilyMed
Tremblay, Roger, FamilyMed
Tremblay, Sylvie
Trempe-Gourdeau, Suzanne
Trottier, Daniel
Trudeau, Gisele
Turcot, Roger
Turcotte, Alain F.
Turcotte, Jacques
Turcotte, Michel
Turgeon, Michel
Turgeon, Renee
Vachon, Andree
Vaillancourt, Catherine
Vaillancourt, Lucie
Vallee, Michele
Vallieres, Camil
Vallieres, Gerald
Vanasse, Francois
Vandal, Lyne
Vanderschuren, Abel
Veilleux, Marie-Christine
Veilleux, Martine
Veilleux, Sarto
Veilleux-Leclerc, Sylvie
Verreault, Rene, FamilyMed
Verrette, Pierre
Vezina, Andree
Vezina, Diane
Vezina, Francine
Vezina, Francine
Vezina, Lise
Vien, Helene
Vigeant, Huguette
Villeneuve, Alain-Fernand
Villeneuve, Carol
Villeneuve, Isabelle
Villeneuve, Jasmin
Villeneuve, Marie
Villeneuve, Simon
Villiard, Marie-France
Warren, Louis, FamilyMed
Wellman, Eleanor, FamilyMed
Yaccarini, Olivier, FamilyMed(EM)
Yergeau, Andree

QUYON

Gomez-Castano, Nathali, FamilyMed
Vander Stelt, Ruth E., FamilyMed

RADISSON

Goulet, Constance

RAWDON

Boudrias, Louis-David, FamilyMed
Juteau, Eric
Mondor, Thomas
Pigeon, Serge
Sylvestre, Jacques
Tremblay, Marino

REPENTIGNY

Beauchemin, Annie, FamilyMed
Bertrand, Michel
Brabant, Michel
Bugeaud, Ronald
Chaput, Andre
Chaput, Guylaine
Cossette, Helene
De Lachevrotiere, Hugues, FamilyMed
Delorme, Martine
Desjardins, Marc
Di Lallo, Kate, FamilyMed
Dube, Michel
Dumas, Jean F.
Filteau, Rene
Galipeau, Daniel
Giguere, Anick
Gravel, Jean
Gravel, Julie
Harvey, Claude
Ibrahim, Edgar
Jette-Yanire, Sylvie
Lafreniere, Marie
Lamy, Mario
Lapointe, Stephanie, FamilyMed
Le, Anh-Thu
Lefebvre, Claudette
Legault, Catherine
Marineau, Gilles
Marsan, Gilbert
Menard, Andre
Narbonne, Claude
Pigeon, Francois

Pilon, Richard
Poirier, Jacques
Prochette, Harry
Rachiele, Andre, FamilyMed
Riopel, Jocelyn
Robitaille, Chantal
Saint-Dizier, Chantal
Sarrazin, Jolaine
Schettini Vaval, Florence A M M.
So, Vay Chi
St-Laurent, Claude-Andre, FamilyMed
St-Onge, Sylvain
Thai, Nga, FamilyMed
Thibodeau, Alain
Trinh, Thao Trang, FamilyMed
Turgeon, Manon
Veilleux, Caroline, FamilyMed
Villeneuve, Jean

RICHELAIN

Dauphin, A. Marc
Fiset, Caroll
Leclerc, Clement
Morin, Heather A., FamilyMed
Tremblay, Roger J P R., FamilyMed

RICHELIEU

Barrette, Marie
Bouchard, Pierre
Cerat, Suzanne
Cournoyer-Roy, Audrey, FamilyMed
Gilbert, Christine
Hameon, Brigitte
Laliberte, Matthieu, FamilyMed
Lanoue, Linda
Lemieux, Marie-France
Moreau, Judith
Niajko, Anna
Vigneault, Diane

RICHMOND

Belanger, Louise
Cormier, Charles, FamilyMed
Cusson, Anne-Marie
Ethier, Serge
Jutras, Marie
Vincent, Natacha

RIGAUD

Ackaoui, Alexandre
Berube, Marie-Claude
Levan, Cathy-Mai, FamilyMed
Noory, Caroline, FamilyMed
Proulx, M C. Manon, FamilyMed
Rozon-Rivest, Monique

RIMOUSKI

Albert, Diane, FamilyMed
Archambault, Nicole
Azzari, Fabian A.
Beausoleil, Sebastien
Begin, Catherine
Bellavance, Louise
Benard, Sylvette
Berube, Jocelyn
Bettahar, Redouane
Blais-Morin, Pascale
Bouchard, Claude R.
Bouchard, Sylvain
Bourassa, Dominique
Brazeau, Daniel, FamilyMed
Briere, Raymond
Brisson, Kathleen
Brouillet, Mathieu
Castonguay, Benoit
Comeau, Diane
Cote, Gilles
Cote, Josee
Croteau, Myriam
Cyr, Marc
D'Amours, Melanie
Daigle, Alain
De Arantes Frota Tavares, Ana C.
De Repentigny, Gaetan
Dorval, Jean-Francois
Drapeau, Genevieve
Drapeau, Jean-Claude
Dube, Nancy
Ducharme, Pascal
Duchesne, Marie-Claude, FamilyMed
Duchesne, Marjorie, FamilyMed
Dufour, Yves
Dumais, Carol
Dumont, Isabelle, FamilyMed
Fortin, Julie, FamilyMed
Foucher, Martin
Gagne, Colombe
Gagne, Jacques
Gagne, Sandrine, FamilyMed
Gagnon, Yves-David
Gauthier, Claude P.
Girard, Alain, FamilyMed
Gonthier, Pierre
Goudreau-Michel, Joanie
Groulx, Olivier, FamilyMed
Houle, Stephanie
Jean-Louis, Carlo, FamilyMed
Lachapelle, Lucie
Landry, Isabelle, FamilyMed
Lanthier-Veilleux, Marie-Soleil
Lehoux, Virginie, FamilyMed
Lessard, Julie
Levesque, Denise
Levesque, Genevieve, FamilyMed
Levesque, Normand
Louahlia, Said
Marquis, Chantal, FamilyMed
Michaud, Ginette
Michaud, Nicole
Mill, Elizabeth
Morin, Jocelyn
Nadeau, Daniel
Nicolas, Marjolaine
Ouellet, Rodrigue
Payeur, Marie-Josee
Pouliot, Martine
Raby, France, FamilyMed
Rouleau, Richard, FamilyMed
Roy, Jean-Philippe
Roy, Mathieu
Selmani, Sabrina
Soucy, Cathya
Tessier, Jean-Francois
Tremblay, Jocelyn
Veillette, Julie, FamilyMed
Villemure, Real

RIPON

Beauregard, Michel

RIVIERE-BLEUE

Auger, Marc
Gagnon, Catherine

RIVIERE-DU-LOUP

Bastien, Nancy
Belzile, Marie-France
Beniar, Matityahu
Boudreau, Christine
Caron, Jacques
Carreras, Francisco J.
Chergui, Assia
Deschenes, Annie
Drolet, Marianne
El-Rassi, Roula
Gagnon-Ouellet, Caroline, FamilyMed
Gougoux, Fanny
Hamelin, Bernard
Herard, Jean-Francois
Khefif, Ghania
La Fontaine, Louise
Lajoie, Carole
Leblanc, Marie-Helene, FamilyMed
Lemay-Roy, Claudia
Maltais, Lucie
Maranda, Jacques
Moorjani, Anoo
Nadeau, Aubert
Nadeau, Michel
Noel, Luc
Paradis, Eric
Perrier, Caroline
Plourde, Isabelle
Poulin, Jose
Raymond, Yves
Rossignol, Guy
Salman, Raed
Savard, Gilles
Simoneau, Noella
Soucy, Genevieve
Tardif, Marc
Tourangeau-Lariviere, Marie-Eve, FamilyMed
Villemure, Jacques

RIVIERE-OUELLE

Caron, Vincent

RIVIERE-ROUGE

Aumond, Ginette
Bisaillon, Norbert
Bohamed, Annie
Debert, F. Amelina
Laflamme, Caroline, FamilyMed
Leblond, Caroline
Leclerc, Denise
Mathieu, Nicolas
Michalkova, Jana
Sigouin, Daniel

ROBERVAL

Audet, Sylvie
Bedard, Andre
Bonin-Carignan, Andreanne, FamilyMed
Bonneau, Gaston
Bouchard, Yvon
Brisson, Mario
Choquet, Benoit
Claveau, Michael E.
Cote, Julie
Dufour, Alexandre
Fortin, Robin
Gagne, Suzanne
Girard, Kevin
Guay, Joanie, FamilyMed
Guay, Serge
Guillemette, Gilles
Hevey, Simon
Larocque, Marc
Lord, Christine
Marchand, Isabelle
Raymond-Robichaud, Jean-Michel, FamilyMed
Rioux, Martin
Tremblay-Reinhardt, Nicolas-Olivier
Vien, Jeanne

ROLLET

Brouillard, Michel

ROSEMERE

Bonnaud, Jeanne
Caron, Jean-Francois
Grant, Martin, FamilyMed
Lavoie, Normand
Petit, Michel

ROUGEMONT

Bouchard, Ginette

ROUYN-NORANDA

Aad, Imad
Akil, Philippe
Arguin, Denis A.
Baz, Bechara
Beaulieu, Joelle
Benoit, Michele
Blackburn, Regine
Blagdon, Michelle
Bonin, Frederic
Bouchard, Nicole
Brisson, Nancy, FamilyMed
Bureau, Benoit
Camirand, Louis
Cayer, Alexandra, FamilyMed
Chaize, Eric
Chantal, Louise
Choquette, Julie, FamilyMed
Coulombe, François, FamilyMed
Desroches, Julie, FamilyMed
Dragoi-David, Otilia-Elena, FamilyMed
Dufresne-Beauchamp, Marie-Helene, FamilyMed
Duhaime, Francine
El Rami, Hares
Falardeau, Catherine, FamilyMed
Falardeau, Genevieve, FamilyMed
Fortin Truchon, Marie-Lea, FamilyMed
Fosso Siewe, Jean
Fournier, Yolaine
Gagnon, Christine
Gauvreau, Lyette
Germain, Estelle
Hernandez-Sanchez, Olivia
Houde, Jean
Jacques, Romeo
L'Ecuyer, Vincent, FamilyMed
Lacombe, Real
Lapointe, Richard
Latour, Sonia
Lavigne, Marie-Aimee
Lefebvre, Jocelyn
Leger, Annie
Lemieux, Marie-Pier, FamilyMed
Marchand-Drolet, Vincent, FamilyMed(EM)
Marleau, Daniel J., FamilyMed
Mayrand, Luc, FamilyMed
Molloy, Francine
Morier, Marie-Josee
Paiement-Lamothe, Anie, FamilyMed
Paquin, Marie-Josee
Parayre, Michel, FamilyMed
Parenteau, Judith, FamilyMed
Pinho, Genevieve
Plourde, Simon
Pomerleau, Anne, FamilyMed
Popa, Clara
Ricard, Jean-Guy, FamilyMed
Richer, Julie
Robitaille, Marc
Sarrouge, Tania
Taktak, Assaad
Torres-Ballen, Myriam
Turgeon, Michel
Vaillancourt, Francois
Viau, Alexandre
Vignola, Elise C.

ROXBORO

Chehade, Remi E., FamilyMed
Cohen, Steven D., FamilyMed
Delaney, David A., FamilyMed
Gotlieb, Stephanie, FamilyMed
Gut, Roman, FamilyMed
Louis-Zaher, Amani

ROXTON POND

Corbin, Serge
Cote, Guylaine

SACRE-COEUR

Cote, Stephane

SAINT-AGAPIT

Boutin, Carmen
Grenier, Louis
Kuska, Renee
Morissette, Michel

SAINT-AMABLE

Lafreniere, Celine
Le, Thanh-Y.

SAINT-ANSELME

Laliberte, Anne
Moreau, Marcel F.

SAINT-BARTHELEMY

Payette, Luc

SAINT-BERNARD

Dextraze, Pierrette
Huppe, Rivard

SAINT-BRUNO

Benjamin, Julie
Benoit, Josiane
Bolduc, Bruno
Calva, Anne-Marie
Caron, Dominique, FamilyMed
Croteau, Celine
Drolet, Denise
Falls, Elizabeth
Gauthier, Beauregard
Gorczyca, Wojciech
Hurtubise, Michel G.
Klosowski, Izabela, FamilyMed
Lemire, Eliane
Levac, Francois
Menhem, Menhem-Jean
Nadeau, Caroline
Paquette, Celine
Payette, Mario

SAINT-CALIXTE

Gaudet, Celine

SAINT-CESAIRE

De La Haye Duponsel, Ophélie
Guay, Andree A.
Harton, Elisabeth
Masson, Isabelle
Phaneuf, Veronique
Sancho, Frederic, FamilyMed
Turner, Genevieve

SAINT-CHRYSOSTOME

Lafreniere, Renee

SAINT-CONSTANT

Brunet, Herve J.
Croteau, Louis
Ferland, Christian, FamilyMed
Gelinas, Lucie M.
Larose, Gontran
Lord, Rene
Poulin, Daniel

SAINT-CYPRIEN

Cote, Richard
Juneau, Francine

SAINT-EPIPHANE

Lang, Isabelle

SAINT-ESPRIT

Bourgault, Josee, FamilyMed
Emard, Helene
Villeneuve, Francois

SAINT-EUGENE

Toussaint, Martin

SAINT-EUSTACHE

Bastien, Marie-Claude
Beauchamp, Chantal, FamilyMed(EM)
Bergeron, Annie-Claude
Bergeron, Marc
Bernier, Sandra
Bleau-Gravel, Genevieve, FamilyMed
Bonin, Catherine
Bonneville, Nathalie
Boustani, Elie
Bovo, Christiane
Boyer, Sandra, FamilyMed
Cardin, Gabrielle, FamilyMed
Cardin, Michel
Cloutier, Sophie
Cummins, Laurence, FamilyMed
Dayer Pastore, Fabienne
Demers, Francois
Di Lenardo, David
Dion, Andreanne, FamilyMed
Dionne, Melanie
Dorais, Marc
Dorion, Marie-Christine, FamilyMed(EM)
Du Cap, Alexis
Fortier, Guylaine
Fortin, Maude, FamilyMed
Francis, Johanne
Garneau, Genevieve
Gibbons, Amber, FamilyMed
Giguere, Isabelle
Gingras, Caroline
Gravel, Marie-Pascale
Hamel, Alexandra, FamilyMed
Hiller, Stella
Hogue, Nadia
Isoard, Lionel A.
Jolibois, Andree-Ann
Julien, Pierre
Kaufman-Clain, Sanda
L'Ecuyer, Genevieve, FamilyMed
Labelle, Mathieu
Lachance, Isabelle
Lacombe, Annie
Laflamme, Nathalie, FamilyMed
Lafleur, Marie-Eve, FamilyMed
Lalancette, Julie
Laplante Paquin, Tristan
Lapointe, Annie-Pier
Lavigne, Caroline, FamilyMed
Lavigne, Melanie
Lavigueur, Denis
Leblanc, Milaine, FamilyMed
Leclerc, Jonathan, FamilyMed
Ledoux, Isabelle, FamilyMed
Legault, Dominic, FamilyMed
Lemay, Louise
Levesque, Stephane, FamilyMed
Loranger, Benoit
MacKay, F. Charles
Melancon, Marie-Lise
Nassif, Rachel, FamilyMed
Ochoa Pinzon, Juan C.
Ouellette, Josiane, FamilyMed
Ouellette, Michele
Pichette, Nathalie, FamilyMed
Quenneville, Nancy
Recher, Martin O., FamilyMed(EM)
Richard, Sophie, FamilyMed
Routhier, Valerie
Roy, Sylvie
Sirois, Marie-Claude
St-Cyr Monaco, Amélie, FamilyMed
Stegaru, Astrid E., FamilyMed
Therrien, Guy, FamilyMed
Thibodeau, Emilie, FamilyMed
Turcotte, Karine
Zaharescu, Desiree

SAINT-FABIEN

Houle, Gabriel

SAINT-FELICIEN

Boudreault, Roberto
Giguere, Brigitte
Gilbert, Bernard
Nadeau, Luc, FamilyMed

SAINT-GEORGES

Al-Rikabi, Anwar
Audet, Josee, FamilyMed
Berube, Charles
Berube, Johan
Bougie, Rejean
Bourque, Berthier
Bureau Morin, Marie-Andree, FamilyMed
Bureau-Morin, Veronique
Caron-Fauconnier, Genevieve, FamilyMed
Chouinard, Denise
Cormier, Helene
Cote, Mario
Cote, Rene
Couillard, Steve
Coulong, Eric
Cournoyer-Rodrigue, Genevieve, FamilyMed(EM)
Coutellier, Maryse
Dansereau, Danielle
Dion, Marc
Ferland, Manon
Fine, Barnet
Fortier, Isabelle
Fournier, Sylvie, FamilyMed
Gagne, Pierre
Gagnon, Rebecca
Genesse, Dany
Gilbert, Lucie, FamilyMed
Gregoire, Jean, FamilyMed
Guilmette, Pierre
Hamel, Bernard
Hamel, Jean-Francois
Hebert, Isabelle
Hebert, Nancy, FamilyMed(EM)
Heredia, Maria, FamilyMed
Ingels, Anne
Janelle, Genevieve, FamilyMed
Jolicoeur, Andre
Labrecque, Carole, FamilyMed
Lapierre, Melanie
Lefebvre, Martin
Letourneau, Sandra
Levesque, Clairmont
Morin, Clement
Morin, Raymond
Paquette, Louis, FamilyMed(EM)
Parent, Nathalie
Pomerleau, Robert, FamilyMed(EM)
Rodrigue, Andre
Roussel-Canuel, Amelie
Roy, Jacques
Roy, Sophie, FamilyMed(EM)
Savard, Germain
Tardif, Eric
Tremblay, Anik
Tremblay, Claude
Vallee, Helene
Vallieres, Martin
Veilleux, Blandine
Vincent O'Keefe, Karine
Vocelle, Josee

SAINT-HIPPOLYTE

Desormeaux, Yvon
Fanzolato, Brigitte
Gossard, Francis, FamilyMed
Jacques, Nicole
Lebeau, Johanne

SAINT-HUBERT

Ah-Lan, Khim C.
Beaudry-Nehme, Angele
Beland, Normand, FamilyMed
Bergeron, Anne
Berube, Guylaine
Bouthillier, Luc
Chalut, Lise
Chauvin, Jean C.
Chung, Gia-Yen
Comtois, J. Jean-Marc
Cote, Agnes
Deschenes, Helene, FamilyMed
Gariepy, Celine
Gosselin, Isabelle I., FamilyMed
Goyette, Raphael, FamilyMed
Kuyumjian, Raffi S., FamilyMed
Lamarre, Angele, FamilyMed
Langelier, Marlene
Laurendeau, Lyne, FamilyMed
Lavoie, Jerome
Leclerc, Gilles
MacLeod, Carol
Nadeau, Nancy, FamilyMed
Paquette, Manon
Parent, Genevieve
Peterson, George
Pham, Vinh Phuc
Polletta, Sabrina, FamilyMed
Provost, Robert
Quesnel, Louise
Rajvong, Inthysone
Roy, Dominique, FamilyMed
Ruttenberg, Jacqueline I., FamilyMed
Trudel, Andre-Jean
Vandemoortele, Sylvere
Vu, Caroline T N., FamilyMed

SAINT-HYACINTHE

Ajmo, Ian
Arpin, Yves
Beaudry, Constant
Benoit, Philippe
Bernatchez, Joelle, FamilyMed
Bertrand-Bovet, Audrey, FamilyMed
Berube, Josee
Bibeau, Marie-Josee
Blouin, Julie, FamilyMed
Boisvert, Emilie, FamilyMed
Bonin, Jocelyne, FamilyMed
Bordeleau, Christian, FamilyMed
Boucher, Suzanne
Boudreault, Annie, FamilyMed
Boudreault, Johannie
Bouvier, Gilles
Brais, Marie-France
Brien, Gilles
Brodeur, Michel
Brosseau, Martine, FamilyMed
Brunet, Jocelyn, FamilyMed
Bureau, Marie-Pierre, FamilyMed(EM)
Carbonneau, Louise, FamilyMed
Collette, Myriam
Corriveau, Louisette
Dagenais, Nathalie
Dallaire, Michelle
Darche, Marie
Darsigny, Monique
Deblonde, Myriam
Decary, Jean-Marc
Delage, Catherine, FamilyMed(EM)
Delalay, Nathalie
Demers, Marie-Eve
Denault, Nathalie
Desautels, Rosaire
Desgagne, Catherine
Deslauriers, Guy
Desranleau, Jacinthe, FamilyMed
Dion, Anne-Marie, FamilyMed
Dodaro, Jocelyn, FamilyMed
Drouin, Francois
Drouin, Simon, FamilyMed
Duranceau, Robert
Durand, Isabelle
Fay, Michel
Fontaine, Geneviève, FamilyMed
Gagnon, Julie, FamilyMed
Garneau, Genevieve, FamilyMed(EM)
Gauthier, Daniel
Gemme, Michel
Germain, Gilles
Godbout, Caroline
Godin, Pierre
Guerin, Caroline, FamilyMed(EM)
Hivon, Marilene
Hudon, Pascale, FamilyMed
Kingsley, Normand
Labelle, Robert
Lachance, Nadine
Ladouceur, Sylvain
Lahaye, Pierre-Andre
Langlois, Lyne
Lapointe, Claude
Lapointe, Mario
Lariviere, France
Larouche-Marchesseault, Line
Leclerc, Louise
Leroux-Levesque, Raphaelle, FamilyMed(EM)
Luneau, Micheline
Marchand, Marie-Josee
Marchessault, Gilles
Menard, Jacinthe
Morissette, Chantale, FamilyMed
Morneau, Joanne, FamilyMed
Nadeau, Claude
Nadon, Michel
Noiseux, Pierre
Pellerin, Julie
Peloquin, Caroline, FamilyMed
Perreault, Alain
Perron, Marie-Helene
Pineault, Daniel
Poirier, Diane
Poirier, Francine, FamilyMed
Richard, Jean-Paul
Sabourin, Thomas
Soubiran, Eric
St-Julien, Louis J.
St-Pierre, Louise
Therrien, Sylvie
Thibault, Julie, FamilyMed(EM)
Tousignant, Maude
Tran, Thien-Chuong, FamilyMed
Tremblay-Wurtele, Diane
Trudel, Louise
Valiquette, Celine
Vincent, Gilles

SAINT-ISIDORE

Bisaillon, Marc
Parent, Andre

SAINT-JACQUES

Meloche, Helene
Vigeant, Alain, FamilyMed

SAINT-JEROME

Armand, Genevieve
Auger, Gilles
Auger, Julien, FamilyMed
Beaudoin, Jean-Pierre
Beaulieu, Richard
Belanger, Lucien
Bellavance, Charles
Bergeron, Maxime
Bouchard, Yves
Bourassa, Viviane, FamilyMed(EM)
Bousquet, Jean
Brissette, Claude
Carrier, Michel
Cartier, Richard
Charest, Raymond
Chartrand, Marie-Pier, FamilyMed
Chevrette, Maurice
Ciarallo, Anhony
Cote, Claude
Cote, Pierre-Paul
Couture, Lyne, FamilyMed
Couturier, Mario
Cyr, Christian
Darveau, Michelle
De Champlain, Marilou, FamilyMed(EM)
De Montigny, Catherine
Decarie, Denise
Denis, Gilles
Desautels, Michel
Deslauriers, Virginie, FamilyMed
Dufour, Amelie, FamilyMed(EM)
El Fishawy, Rami
Emond, Gilles
Forest, Daniel
Fortin, Anne-Karine
Fournier, Yvon
Gagnon, Andree, FamilyMed
Gagnon, Josee
Gareau, Jacques Y.
Gascon, Bernard
Gaston, Isabelle
Gauthier, Nicolas
Gauthier, Sylvianne
Gauthier, Veronique, FamilyMed(EM)
Gelinas, Christian
Girard, Jean-Francois
Girard, Philippe, FamilyMed(EM)
Girardin, Joel-Roger
Gosselin-Brisson, Anne
Goudreau, Stephane
Goyette, Claude
Grenier, Jean-Luc
Higgins, Eric J.
Hoquet, France
Houde, Marie-Christine
Hurtubise, Andre
Jacob, Laurent
Janelle, Sylvie
Jolicoeur, Dominique
Juneau, Pierre
Jutras, Claire
Khoury, Zahi, FamilyMed
Laberge, Micheline
Lacasse, Louis-Andre, FamilyMed
Lacombe, Jose, FamilyMed
Lacombe, Marie-Claude
Lacroix, Sebastien, FamilyMed(EM)
Lafond, Sylvain
Lalumiere, Robert
Lambert, Diane
Laporte, Sophie
Latulippe, Maude, FamilyMed(EM)
Laurin, Pierre-Michel
Leblanc-Boucher, Nicole
Leduc, Genevieve, FamilyMed(EM)
Lefebvre, Marieve, FamilyMed
Legault, Mathieu, FamilyMed
Lemaitre-Auger, Michele
Levac, Francine
Liu, Sandra A., FamilyMed
Martinez-Bellart, Josette
McDonald, Diana, FamilyMed
Millette-Francoeur, Laura-Lou
Monette, Lydia
Morin, Jean R.
Nguyen, Martin M M., FamilyMed(EM)
Nicole, Marjory
Noel, Pierre
Nwilati, Hanad
Pepin, Nancy
Potvin, Jean-Guy
Poulin, Veronique
Rheaume, Nadia
Rioux, Celine
Rioux, Gisele
Roberge, Danielle
Rouleau, Jean-Francois
Rouse, Danielle
Rousseau, Annie, FamilyMed
Savard, Michel
Schulz, Gabriella
Slythe, Christine
Solorzano Gutierrez, Silma

Soucy, Claudette
St-Germain, Myriam, FamilyMed
St-Pierre, Brigitte
Talbot, Linda A.
Trudeau, Nicolas
Vermette, Suzie
Vincent-Gaudreault, Daphne, FamilyMed
Vinette, Stephane
Weisbord, Tim
Ziegenhorn, Andreas A.

SAINT-LAMBERT

Arsenault, Isabelle, FamilyMed
Baron, Emmanuelle, FamilyMed
Blouin, Francine
Caron, Christine
Champagne, Louise, FamilyMed
Cloutier, Annie-Catherine
Couturier, Francois, FamilyMed
Crete, Elise, FamilyMed
Derigaud, Pascale
Dufour, Andre, FamilyMed
Gibeault, Robert
Goulet, Serge
Guindo, Fatouma S.
Jagan, Sarva
Labrousse, Yanouchka
Lambert, Jacques
Langlois, Martine
Leblanc, Michel
Leduc, Marie-Claude
Leonard, Marie
Magnan, Bernard
Martin, Stephanie, FamilyMed
Martineau, Catherine, FamilyMed
Metcalfe, Francine
Mikhail, Christine, FamilyMed
Morin, Gertrude
Morval, Marie-Helene
Nguyen, Lan Chau
Paul-Hus, Franck
Pelissier-Simard, Luce, FamilyMed
Pepin, Annie
Proulx, Joanne
Quintal, Louise, FamilyMed
Rancourt, Agnes
Rivard, Marie
Simard, Andre
Turcotte, Annick, FamilyMed
Turgeon, Marie-Eve
Vallieres, Nathalie
Valois, Carol, FamilyMed
Valois, Joyce, FamilyMed

SAINT-LAURENT

Agha, Amer
Allaire, Suzanne
Amar, Charles
Assayag, Y. Raphael, FamilyMed
Averback, Paul
Baram, Rola
Barbuio, Luciana
Bardakji, Zaim
Ben Salem, Bader, FamilyMed
Benhaddad, Abdeltif, FamilyMed
Benhaim, Albert
Benmebarek, Djamila
Blain, Marie
Blauer, Evan, FamilyMed(EM)
Boudiffa, Mustapha, FamilyMed
Brock, A. Jeffrey
Cote, Manon, FamilyMed
D'Allaire, Diane
Dancose, Marc
Dang, Dong My
De Serres, Jean, FamilyMed
Desrosiers, Pauline, FamilyMed
Elfassy, Bernard
Elsolh, Bashar
Ferron, Marcel
Finkelstein, Jonathan, FamilyMed
Gutman, Jimmy
Hamdad-Vitre, Nadia, FamilyMed
Hoang, Que Chi, FamilyMed
Issid, Simon
Kalash, Joseph
Kasbo, Marie-Rose
Kassissia, Ibrahim G Y.
Kaud, Robert, FamilyMed
Labissonniere, Paul-Emile
Labrecque-Sauve, Sebastien, FamilyMed
Lafreniere, Bernard
Latreille, Isabelle, FamilyMed
Le, Quang Tien
Lemay, Odette
Lussier, Normand
Machado, John, FamilyMed
Machado Contreras, A. Ricardo, FamilyMed
Marier, Sylvie
Martinez, Ricardo L.
Matouk, Ivy
Mojica Correa, Ludy, FamilyMed
Ngo, Thi Minh H.
Nguyen, Khang Huu
Nguyen, Van Hoi, FamilyMed
Pham, H. Nhat Tan
Pham, Nhu-Ngoc
Pham, Thang
Robillard, Pierre
Roy, Jacinthe
Shemesh, Tzela, FamilyMed
Sitaru, Doina, FamilyMed
Sradj, Naila
St-Jacques, Lina
Truong Hong, Bao Son
Vu, Suzanne
Zakaria, Hanaa
Zylberszac, Bernard

SAINT-LAZARE

Boulanger, Isabelle, FamilyMed
Harrison, Stephen D.
Lepage, Patrice
Miral, Henriette

SAINT-LEONARD

Bernucci, Bruno
Berthiaume, Georges
Bourbeau, Jean-Luc
Brodersen, Anne F.
Bucci, Raffaele
Charette, Francois, FamilyMed
Ciricillo, Domenico
Danan, Anny
Dischliev, Spiro
Dube, Laurier
Farruggia, Pasquale, FamilyMed
Fawaz, Nabil
Feldman, Marcel
Fernandez, Marie-Carmel
Gagnon, Claire
Gagnon, Julie
Gauthier, Bernard
Groulx, Pierre-Claude
Hani, Antoine
Lahens, Pierre
Mahfoud, Georges
Nemtean, David R.
Nguyen, Hau
Nguyen, Thi Ngoc L., FamilyMed
Nguyen Do, Uyen Ly, FamilyMed
Ocampo, Erlinda S.
Ong, Hoang
Ouellette, Gilles
Petrella, Nick J.
Pham, Gia-Trong
Pham, Huu-Trac
Poitras, Gaetan
Rabia, Djamila, FamilyMed
Robillard, Francine
Saint-Phard, Lemercier
Sioufi, Gilbert K E.
Spiridigliozzi, Mary
Toupin, Line
Vu, Minh Thuy

SAINT-LIBOIRE

Tremblay, Pierre-Paul

SAINT-MARTIN

Gingras, Alain

SAINT-NICEPHORE

Benoit, Francois
Coudert, Daniele
Danila, Alexandru-Cristian
Frechette, Solange
Jutras, Pierre
Laflamme, Denis, FamilyMed

SAINT-NICOLAS

Boivin, P. Rock, FamilyMed
Bolduc, Monique
Bouchard, Amelie
Brown, Helene
Gauvin, Constance
Higgins, Ethel, FamilyMed
Laroche, Francois, FamilyMed
Leblond, Denis
Lemieux, Gaetan
Letourneau, Francois, FamilyMed
Pare, Guylaine
Roberge, Ghislain
Robillard, Michel
St-Pierre, Antoine
Theriault, Normand
Tremblay, Marie-Helene

SAINT-OMER

Jobin, Genevieve
Theriault, Pierre

SAINT-PAMPHILE

Bertrand, Michel
Pare, Lyne
Zinga Bolenge, Roland X.

SAINT-PASCAL

Lavoie, Jean-Jacques
Lebel, Mario
Levesque, Gaetan
Levesque, Ghislain
Roussel, Renee

SAINT-PAULIN

Savard, Lise
Theberge, Jacques, FamilyMed

SAINT-PIE

Desroches, Jacques
Milette, Pierre-D.
Poulin, Eric S.

SAINT-POLYCARPE

Allard, Andree
Bloch, Didier
Boucher, Marie-Claude, FamilyMed
Dufresne, Sylvie
Rondeau, Maryse

SAINT-PRIME

Carrier, Daniel, FamilyMed
Potvin, Julie

SAINT-RAYMOND

Beaupre, Gaetane, FamilyMed
Bedard, Marc
Bilodeau, Genevieve, FamilyMed
Boissinot, Pierre
Brunet, Francois
Cameron, Nancy
Cantin, Celine
Cormier, Julie, FamilyMed(EM)
Douillard, Helene
Drolet, Michel J.
Dussault, Andreanne, FamilyMed
Georgieff, Nancy
Hamel, Gilles
Julien, Marlene
Lacharite, Karine
Lesage, Marie-Eve
Mottard, Audrey, FamilyMed
Pelletier, Caroline
Potvin, Marie-Eve
Rahmilevich, Elena, FamilyMed
Rodrigue, Lucien
Shields, Jean
Tasse, Jacynthe, FamilyMed
Verret, Gaston

SAINT-REDEMPTEUR

Bruneau, Claude
Meilleur, Carole

SAINT-REMI

Carpentier, Veronique, FamilyMed
Cloutier, Mireille
Gagnon, Claude-Francois
Gariepy, Daniel
Labbe, Robert
Lanctot, Rosaire
Marquicio De Thomas, Maria, FamilyMed
Ste-Marie, Gaston
Trudeau, Sylvie

SAINT-ROMUALD

Barthélémy, Lucie A.
Blouin, Francois
Cameron, Cynthia, FamilyMed
Camire, Raymond D.
Collin, Emilie, FamilyMed
Demers, Annie L.
Fontaine, Isabelle-Anne, FamilyMed
Fraser, Evelyne
Gagne, Eve-Marie
Genest, Pierre
Gilbert, Valerie
Jolicoeur, Denis
Lapierre, Patricia
Laroche, Julie C.
Larochelle, Julie
Lemieux, Kathleen, FamilyMed
Levesque, Yvan
Morneau, Lucie
Nadeau, Robert
Nadeau, Serge
Picard, Jean-Marc
Rousseau, Jacinthe
Taschereau, Charles
Tremblay, Claude
Tremblay, Michel

SAINT-SAUVEUR

Boutin, Mario
Dufresne, Louise
Dumontier, Real
Lapointe, Martin
Lever, Paule
Menard, Sylvain
Singer, Robert B.
Spunt, Ronald S.
Taillefer, Michel
Tardif, Pierre
Villeneuve, Lucien

SAINT-SIMEON

Gagne, Eric

SAINT-THOMAS

Depelteau, Jean
Desrosiers, Josee

SAINT-TITE

Bedard, Valerie
Cohen Bacry, Jean-Philippe
Croteau, Maryse
Francoeur, Nicolas
Grandisson, Remi, FamilyMed
Guedes-Marchand, Cecile
Leger, Alain
Lerat, Jean-Paul
Marchand-Antonin, Benoit
Petit, Karine, FamilyMed

SAINT-VICTOR

Metivier, Denis

SAINT-WENCESLAS

Landry-Frechette, Guylaine
Saint-Cyr, Claire-Marie

SAINT-ZACHARIE

Rodrigue, Bertrand

SAINT-ZOTIQUE

Nguyen, Ngoc Chi
Poirier, Denise

SAINTE-ADELE

Bessette, Michel
Desmarais, Maryse, FamilyMed
Frain, Margaret
Gladu, Yvan
Guibert, Remi
Joubert, Carole
Ouimet, Alain
Puscas, Radu
Robitaille, Brigitte
Saint-Pierre, Andre
Therrien, Ghislaine

SAINTE-CATHERINE

Barriere, Ginette
Belanger, Guy-Alain
Dallaire, Lise
Deziel, Luc
Guay, J A. Michel
Olivier, Stephane, FamilyMed

SAINTE-CLAIRE

Berger, Michelle
Roy, Rejean
Turmel, Linda, FamilyMed

SAINTE-CROIX

Cantin, Real
Drolet, Normand
Shink, Nancy
Uhlir, Anne Marie

SAINTE-FELICITE

Lavoie, Gaetan Y., FamilyMed

SAINTE-JULIE

Benoit, Suzie
Charbonneau, Jacques
Clement, Marie-Helene, FamilyMed
Dagenais, Michel
Gaul, Martine, FamilyMed
Gelinas, Marie-Christine
Jauron, Annie, FamilyMed
Lemieux, Francois
Paquet, Nadine
Plante, Martin
Roy, Andre
Roy, Daniel
Thompson, Jean-Pierre

SAINTE-MARIE

Faucher, Daniel, FamilyMed
Fleury, Manon
Fournier, Brigitte
Fournier, Claude
Giguere, Michel
Gingras, Benoit
Keskinen, Helen
Lavoie, Yvan
Lemieux, Sylvie
Lessard, Christian
Lessard, Philippe
Mathieu, Yvan
Mercier, Gaetane
Morin, Diane
Neron, Raymond
Roux, Daniel, FamilyMed
Tessier, Barbara

SAINTE-ROSE

Duperron, Marie-Josee
Goudezeune, Lynne
Tanguay, Andre

SAINTE-SOPHIE

Rochon, Jean-Louis
Seyer, Alain

SAINTE-THECLE

Cossette-Gagnon, Melanie, FamilyMed

SAINTE-THERESE

Archambault, Genevieve
Beauregard, Louis
Bernier, Carolyne
Biagioni, Cristina, FamilyMed
Blaizel Jr., Gilbert
Boudon, Emilie
Boulianne, Marie-France
Brasseur, Marie-Helene
Cardin, Louise
Clermont, Michel
Coulombe, Nicole
Delorme, Linda
Desbiens, Denis
Desjardins, Sylvie
Filiatrault-Brosseau, Carole
Gagne, Jacques
Graham, Sandra
Laplante, Raymonde
Lavallee, Claude H., FamilyMed
Leblanc, Michel
Luneau, Mance
Magnan, Pierre-Etienne, FamilyMed
Maynard, Lucie, FamilyMed
Monday, Patrick
Nadeau, Alain
Potier, Elsa
Rheault, Sylvie
Riendeau, Claudie
Roberge, Julie
Rochette, Anne
Turgeon, Mireille
Vacri, Chantal

SALABERRY DE VALLEYFIELD

Alain, Michel
Bastien, Francois
Belleville, Denis
Ben Khedher, Najoua
Berthiaume, Claude
Bessiere, Guillaume
Biabi, Mohsen
Bibi, Diaa E.
Champoux, Genevieve
Charliers-Lazure, Ariane
De Wals, Charlotte
Desilets, Jean-Francois, FamilyMed
Dominique, Lynn
Dumaine, Marcel
Gagne, Stephen
Gagnon, Yves, FamilyMed
Gigoux, Celine
Goulet, Alain
Gregoire, Gabrielle, FamilyMed
Grenier, Marie-Andree
Guay, Caroline, FamilyMed
Hallage, Marie G.
Kawerk, Jacques
Lapointe, Claude
Lareau, Ross
Larouche, Pierre
Le, Ngoc Duy
Leblanc, Daniel
Lecompte, Michele
Leonard, Julie, FamilyMed
Leroux, Maude A.
Lessard, Audrey, FamilyMed
Lussier, Richard, FamilyMed
Lussier-Plourde, Yolande
Mageau, Andre
Marchand, Guy-Ludovic
Marineau, Luc
McSween, Charles
Merahi, Ourida
Mongrain, Karine, FamilyMed
Morin, Mireille, FamilyMed
Nadeau, Julie
Ouadi, Lydia-Amina
Parent, Sylvie
Paulin, Jocelyne
Pharand, Pierre
Raymond, Margaret
Richard, Bernard
Richard, Marie-Claude
Robichaud, Jean-Luc
Robitaille, Diane
Rondeau, Nancy M., FamilyMed(EM)
Sauve, Frederic
Sauve, Michel
Simard, Christiane
Sobreira, Elizabete M., FamilyMed
Son, Florina
Szabo, Gabriel
Tanghe-Lapointe, Karina
Therrien, Jocelyne
Thibert, Alain
Turcot, Francis
Turcotte, Elisabeth
Tuvivovich, Victoria E.
Vincent, Matthieu, FamilyMed
Yelle, Jean-Pierre

SALLUIT

Fouron, Pascale

SAYABEC

Jean, Claire

SCHEFFERVILLE

Cloutier, Pierre

SENNETERRE

Charbonneau, Katerine C., FamilyMed
Cossette, Louis, FamilyMed
Denis, Jocelyne M.
Dutoy, Jean-Luc
Lambert, Jean-Marie
Ohayon, Catherine

SEPT-ILES

Baril, Chantale, FamilyMed
Belanger, Stephane, FamilyMed
Bernatchez, Annie, FamilyMed
Brassard, Richard
Cordeau, Eve
Duval, Louis-Rene
Fournier, Emilie, FamilyMed
Gagnon-Perreault, Annabelle, FamilyMed
Gagnon-Trottier, Ariane, FamilyMed
Harvey, Pierre-Claude
Herma, Messaoud
Labelle, Jean-Francois
Lalande, Bruno
Laplante, Bernard
Laporte, Guy
Lavoie, Danielle
Lebel, Annie
Leger, Julie, FamilyMed
Lemieux Potvin, Frédérique, FamilyMed(EM)
Luis, Christine, FamilyMed
Masson, Claude
Meunier, Louise
Ouellet, Sandie, FamilyMed
Plante, Denis
Poirier, Eric, FamilyMed
Popescu-Dumbrava, Laila, FamilyMed
Porlier, Caroline, FamilyMed
Ringuette, Francois, FamilyMed
Robichaud, Helene, FamilyMed
Romain, Yveline
Ross, Gilles
St-Onge, Nathalie
Turbis, Carole

SHANNON

Lafortune, Valerie, FamilyMed

SHAWINIGAN

Barabe, Pierre-Luc, FamilyMed(EM)
Boisjoli, Jacques
Boissonneault, Mario
Bonner, Marie
Bordeleau, Normand J.
Boudreau, Julie, FamilyMed
Burelle, Sebastien
Carbery, Michael
Delagrave, Jacques
Dessureault, Lucie
Grenier, Gilles
Lacombe, Louise
Laforme, Lucie
Lagace, Jean
Lavertu, Real
Lebrun, Philippe, FamilyMed
Legare, Louise
Paquin, Yvon
Philibert, Jean-Claude
Pronovost, Martine
Rousseau, Claude
Thibault, Pierre-Marc
Trahan, Gilles
Vachon, Francine

SHAWINIGAN-SUD

Barabe, Serge
Baril, Serge
Begin, Gaetan
Bernier, Julie
Blain, Samuel, FamilyMed
Brui, Nathalie, FamilyMed
Chamberland, Guy
Champagne, Anne-Marie, FamilyMed
Cloutier, Linda
Duval, Cristian
Fortier, Martin, FamilyMed(EM)
Galarneau, France
Guertin, Catherine, FamilyMed
Hassein Bey, Leila
Houle, Cynthia, FamilyMed
Huot, Denis
Jacob, Andre M.
Kachtan, Mohammed
Laferte, Noemie, FamilyMed
Lafond, Michel, FamilyMed
Lamy, Marie-Eve, FamilyMed
Lauziere, Maurice
Lavoie, Marie-Eve, FamilyMed
Lemay, Jean-Francois, FamilyMed
Leveille, Marie-Eve
Parent, Marie-Eve, FamilyMed
Pelletier, J F. Alain
Perron, Stephanie, FamilyMed
Picotte, Frederic, FamilyMed
Poudrier, Samiha
Raymond, Mario, FamilyMed
Rehel, Benoit
Renaud, Alain, FamilyMed
Rouleau, Isabelle
Savard, Martine M.
Sirois, Dany
St-Yves, Marie
Thomas, Yves
Tremblay, Diane
Trudel, Claudine, FamilyMed
Trudel, Melissa, FamilyMed
Voltz, Jean-Marc

SHAWVILLE

Cop, Milorad
Courchesne, Donna, FamilyMed
Croteau, Pascal
Homayounfar, Freydoun
Lamarche, Maurice
Lemyre, Karine, FamilyMed
MacLellan, Keith A.
O'Neill, Thomas, FamilyMed
Rivero Pinelo, Luis, FamilyMed
Roustaian, Kaveh
Smith, Genevieve A., FamilyMed
Soultan, Majed, FamilyMed
Sperduto, Michel N.
Talko, Peter
Wootton, John C S.
Zaroukian, Sevag, FamilyMed

SHEFFORD

Falardeau, Rejean

SHERBROOKE

Adjaoud, Amelie
Allard, Jacques, FamilyMed
Allard, Stephanie, FamilyMed
Arcand, Marcel, FamilyMed
Ayala Paredes, Felix A.
Bachand, Gilles
Bachand, Jacques
Badra Verdu, Mariano
Baril, Louise M C.
Bastarache, Patrice, FamilyMed(EM)
Beaudet, Lynn
Beaudet-Pleszczynska, C. Chantal
Beaulac, Emilie, FamilyMed
Beaulieu, Lysanne
Beaulieu, Marie-Claude, FamilyMed
Beaulieu, Yves
Beausejour, Denise
Bedard, Chantal
Belanger, Marie-Eve, FamilyMed(EM)
Beliveau, Melanie, FamilyMed
Benjamin, Eric, FamilyMed(EM)
Bernier, Carolle, FamilyMed
Bernier, Elise
Bertelle, Valerie
Berube, Alain
Bezeau, Marc, FamilyMed
Bigonnesse, Jean-Marc, FamilyMed
Bissonnette, Martine
Blanchard, Julie, FamilyMed
Blanchet, Chantal
Blancquaert, Ingeborg
Boilard, Yvon, FamilyMed
Boire-Lavigne, Anne-Marie, FamilyMed
Boismenu, Celine
Bordeleau, Gabriel
Bouchard, Jasmin, FamilyMed(EM)
Bouchard, Remi, FamilyMed(EM)
Bouchereau, Yves
Boudreau, Robert
Boulanger, Yves
Boule, Richard, FamilyMed
Branch, Frederic, FamilyMed(EM)
Brizard, Michele
Brochu, Caroline
Brouillet, Michel
Bruns, Alessandra
Cabana, Louise, FamilyMed
Caille, Francois-Xavier
Caouette, Benoit
Carignan, Benoit
Caron, Renee
Castonguay, Claude
Catelin, Celine
Chababi Atallah, Myrna
Champagne, Myriam, FamilyMed
Champoux, Richard J.
Chartier, Catherine, FamilyMed
Chauvette, Angele
Cherniak, Donna A G., FamilyMed
Choker, Ghassan N.
Cieuta-Walti, Cecile
Cinq-Mars, Gaetane, FamilyMed
Clavet, Diane, FamilyMed
Clement, Nathalie
Codere, Francine
Coicou, Yves
Colimon, Leslie
Collinge, Marie-Laure
Comamala Torres, Marina, FamilyMed
Comtois, Luc
Corbeil, Catherine
Corbeil, Robert P.
Corbin, Jean-Francois
Cormier, Charline
Counil, Francois-Pierre
Courteau, Jean-Marc
Courtemanche, Marie
Couture, Daniel
Daigle, Steve
Dandurand, Caroline, FamilyMed(EM)
Daniels, Lise
Delisle, Donald
Delisle, Lucie
Delli Colli, Nadia
Demers, Alain
Desgagnes, Julie
Deshaies, Jean-Francois, FamilyMed(EM)
Desrochers, Agnes, FamilyMed
Desrochers, Amelie
Desruisseaux, Benoit
Diamond, Patrick
Dionne, Jean-Francois
Doyon, Chantal
Doyon Olivier, Joelle, FamilyMed(EM)
Drapeau, Monique, FamilyMed
Dubuc, Mario, FamilyMed
Dugre, Bernard
Dumas, Jacinthe
Dussault, Marylene
Dzineku, Marie-Dominique, FamilyMed
Elazhary, Nicolas, FamilyMed(EM)
Ellyson, Josee
Farmer, Marie
Farrar, David
Faucher, Jocelyne, FamilyMed

PHYSICIANS BY PROVINCE

Ferenczi, Zoltan T.
Fluet, Bruno
Fonseca Falcao, Marcele
Fortier, Robert
Franchomme-Fosse, Violaine, FamilyMed
Frazer, Robert
Fregeau, Johanne, FamilyMed
Frenette, Louise
Gagneur, Arnaud
Gagnon, Marie-Anne, FamilyMed(EM)
Gallagher, Karen
Gaudet, Cynthia
Gaulin, Christian
Gauthier, Jacques
Geha, Sameh
Gendron, Francoise
Gendron, Jean-Sebastien
Germain, Isabelle, FamilyMed
Girard, Ginette
Girard, Ronald
Giroux, Marie, FamilyMed
Gosselin, Sophie, FamilyMed
Gosselin, Suzanne, FamilyMed
Granger, Perrine
Gregoire, Elyse
Grignon, Sylvain
Grimard, Nicole
Guay, Alain
Guerette, Pierre-Jean
Guitard, Sylvianne, FamilyMed(EM)
Harel, Simon-Pierre
Harnois, Dominic, FamilyMed(EM)
Hayes, Marie, FamilyMed
Hebert, Annie, FamilyMed(EM)
Hemond, Claude, FamilyMed
Hotte, Marie-Josee, FamilyMed
Houle, Andreane
Jacques, Andre
Jobin, Monique
Kerwin, Larkin
Labbe, Sylvie
Labrecque, Susan, FamilyMed
Lacaille, Jacques
Lachance, Eric, FamilyMed
Lafontaine-Godbout, Matthieu, FamilyMed
Lalonde, Lise, FamilyMed
Lambert, Michel
Lamontagne, Philippe
Lamothe, Sylvie, FamilyMed(EM)
Langlais, Albert
Langlois, Julie, FamilyMed(EM)
Langlois, Line, FamilyMed
Lapierre, Michel
Laplante, Patrice, FamilyMed
Lecomte, Caroline, FamilyMed(EM)
Leduc, Ghyslain, FamilyMed(EM)
Leger, Daniel
Lemay, Catherine
Lemay, Yvan
Longval, Michael, FamilyMed
Lord, Francois
Lupien, Luc
Lupien-St Pierre, Mariline, FamilyMed
Marchand, Pierre
Marquis, Isabelle
Marquis, Josee
Martel, Gilles, FamilyMed
Martial, Jocelyne
Martin, Julie, FamilyMed
Martineau, Bernard, FamilyMed
Marussi, Daphne R.
Masetto, Ariel R.
Massicotte, Caroline, FamilyMed
Masson, Judith, FamilyMed
Mathieu, Andre
Mathieu, Guy
Mathieu, Marie
McSween, Anne
Menard, Suzanne
Merat, Yves M.
Mercier, Dominique
Mercier, Helene
Meziat-Burdin, Anne
Moisan, Andree-Anne, FamilyMed
Monast, Julie
Mongeau, Laurent, FamilyMed
Morin, Martine, FamilyMed
Morin, Pierre
Munger, Andre
Nedelec, Laurence, FamilyMed
Noel, Daniel, FamilyMed
Olivier, Genevieve
Olsen, Ingrid, FamilyMed
Ouellet, Isabelle, FamilyMed(EM)
Ouellette, Marc
Ouzilleau, Christian
Pageau, Alain
Paquet, Martin
Paquet, Nathalie
Paradis, Francois, FamilyMed(EM)
Pasquier, Jean-Charles
Perreault, Sylvie
Perusse, Richard, FamilyMed
Pinard, Louis G., FamilyMed(EM)
Plante, Diane
Plante, Ludovic
Plourde, Suzie
Poirier, Eve-Marie, FamilyMed(EM)
Poulin, Claude
Proulx, Reno
Pruneau, Marc, FamilyMed
Queenton, Marie-Josee
Rateb, George
Remillard, Francine
Rinfret, Joanie, FamilyMed
Roberge, Annie
Roberge, Claude
Ross, Francis
Rottembourg, Diane
Roy, Aline
Roy, Amelia, FamilyMed
Roy, Francois, FamilyMed
Roy, Johanne
Roy, Melodie
Roy, Pierre-Michel, FamilyMed
Ruest, Pierre
Saint-Louis, Jean-Francois
Sainton, Gilles, FamilyMed
Samson, Line M I.
Schmutz, Gerard
Semaan, William
Shahidi, Mazda
Sheehy, Diane, FamilyMed
Souliere, Louise
Spacek, Jan
St-Pierre, Claude
Talbot, Marie-Claude
Tanguay-Bernard, Marie-Michèle, FamilyMed
Temmar, Rabia
Theberge, Lise
Tremblay, Genevieve, FamilyMed
Tremblay, Nathalie
Tsanaclis, Alexandre
Tsanaclis, Ana-Maria C.
Turcotte, Francois
Turcotte, Genevieve, FamilyMed
Turcotte, Jean T.
Turcotte, Suzanne
Turmel, Yves
Tzouannis, Nicholas, FamilyMed
Vaillancourt, Isabelle
Vaillancourt, Raymonde, FamilyMed
Vanasse, Alain, FamilyMed
Vanasse, Catherine
Verrier-Frechette, Veronique, FamilyMed(EM)
Vidal, Louise, FamilyMed
Viens, Christian
Vigeant, Julie
Villemure, Marie-Pier, FamilyMed
Vinette, Gaetan, FamilyMed
Voyer, Gilles
Walti, Herve
Wang, Chang Shu
Xhignesse, Marianne C.

SHIPSHAW

Stumpf, Elisabeth M.

SOREL-TRACY

Arsenault, Marie-Josee, FamilyMed
Bannour, Leila
Bernatchez, Michel
Bessaih, Nawal
Boily, Emilie, FamilyMed
Boissonneault, Josee
Boot-Neirynck, Delphine
Botros, Ussama A.
Bou Farah, Charles
Bouchal, Hachemi
Boucher, Suzanne
Castro-Contreras, Nestor E.
Charbonneau-Blouin, Renee
Chavez Guerra, Juan
Chevalier, Natalie
Cinq-Mars, Michelle
Clavel, Mathias
Colin, Francois P A.
Collin, Marianne, FamilyMed(EM)
Cote, Mylene, FamilyMed
Craciunescu, Diana, FamilyMed
Damyanova, Anastasiya, FamilyMed(EM)
Desmarais, Richard
Desrochers, Jean
Deziel, Annie, FamilyMed
Dubois, Marie-Eve, FamilyMed
Fontaine, Louis
Gilet, Danielle
Gill, Sylvie
Godbout, Francois, FamilyMed
Guillemette, Gaetan
Hamel, Caroline, FamilyMed
Hamelin, Claude
Hebert, France, FamilyMed
Jacques, Aline
Kefi, Sameh
Lacroix, Patrick, FamilyMed
Lavergne, Louis J.
Letourneau, Anne
Mallette, Yvon
Masse, Michel
McGraw, Elizabeth A.
Mena, Chantal
Menard, Claude
Morin, Claude
Mostefai, Ahmed Y.
Nakhle, Elias
Paris, Catherine, FamilyMed
Rioux, Germain
Said, Carla
Sauvageau, Eric
Senecal, Ginette
Smolla, Robert
Soroko, Oleg
Soucy, J R L. Michel
Soumis, Anne
Wauquaire, Catherine

ST-ADOLPHE D'HOWARD

Filion, Annie
Valois, Chantal

ST ALEXIS DES MONTS

Leroyer, Valerie
St-Germain, Isabelle

ST ALPHONSE RODRIGUEZ

Aubin, Alain
Legault, Jean-Pierre

ST AMBROISE DE KILDARE

Jaeger, Dominique
Landry, Suzanne

ST ANDRE ARGENTEUIL

Leclerc, Jacques

ST-ANDRE-AVELLIN

Amsellem-Abecassis, Lydie
Buchanan, G. Stuart
Charbonneau, Sylvie, FamilyMed
Daniele, Pasquale
Godin, Marie-Eve
Hanna, Jean T.
Joyeux, Nathalie
Laverdiere, Ines
Ng-Cheng-Hin, G. Tommy
Proulx, Pierrette
Taillefer, Simon

ST ANNE DE BEAUPRE

Turmel, Yvan

ST-APOLLINAIRE

Cauvier, Andree-Anne

ST AUGUSTIN DE DESMAURES

Audet, Nathalie
Boulanger, Caroline
Boutet, Sylvain
Gagnon, Elaine
Grenier, Benoit
Lachance, Sylvain
Lawless, John
Leblanc, Jacques-F.
Piche, Daniele
Robitaille, Andre
Robitaille, Julie
Rodier, Lucie
Sirois, Michel
St-Pierre, Denys
Tetu, Marie A.
Thibault, Nicole

ST BASILE LE GRAND

Cocle, Didier J.
Frechette, Jean-Rene
Laferriere, Edith
Lamoureux, Pierre
Perrier, Jean
Walker, Angela J., FamilyMed

ST-BENOIT-LABRE

Binet, Danielle

ST BONIFACE DE SHAWINIGAN

Thibeault-Caron, Helene

ST BRUNO LAC SAINT JEAN

Lalonde, Alain-Paul, FamilyMed
Larouche, Renee
Maltais, Gerard

ST-CASIMIR

Doucet, Gaetan

ST CHARLES BORROMEE

Abbas, Fadwa
Allard, Nathalie
Amand, Herve
Amyot, Marc-Andre
Apullan, Francisco J.
Asselin, Johanne
Belanger, Lucie
Belisle, Roselyne, FamilyMed
Belkadi, Ahmed Z.
Bellemare, Sylvain, FamilyMed
Bellerose-Dumontier, Marilyn, FamilyMed
Bérard, Marianik, FamilyMed(EM)
Bertrand, Josee
Bessette, Isabelle, FamilyMed
Boisse-Rheault, Emmanuelle
Boisvert, Karine E., FamilyMed
Boucher, Jean-Pierre
Bouchez, Stephane M.
Brizard, Frederic
Brouillet, Serge
Carrier, Annie
Cassan, Philippe
Champagne, Amelie
Charette, Mireille
Charlot, Lunel
Daigle, Sylvie, FamilyMed(EM)
Deschambeault, Julie
Desroches, Louise A.
Drolet, Manon
Ducharme, Jean-Luc
Dufresne, Lucille J.
Figueredo Hurtado, Sara M.
Forest, Genevieve, FamilyMed(EM)
Fortier-Riberdy, Annie
Galley, Anik
Gaudreau, Jean-Marc
Ghais, Ahmad
Godin, Johanne
Gratton, Madeleine
Hebert, Pierre A.
Hudicourt, Martine, FamilyMed
Jette, Johanie, FamilyMed
Khabazeh, Youssef
Laganiere, Marie-Josee, FamilyMed
Laporte, Helene
Leblanc, Michel
Leblanc, Valerie, FamilyMed
Leclair, Sabrina
Lefebvre, Marie-Pierre
Legare, Louise
Leroux, Elise
Levasseur, Jean
Loontjens, Bernadette
Maheu, Benoit, FamilyMed
Mayers, Alexandre
Meagher, Luc
Mebrek, Nachida
Mejri, Abdelwaheb
Miron-Pichet, Roseline, FamilyMed
Ng Ming Hing, Jackson
Paquette, Jean-Sebastien, FamilyMed
Parent, Sylvie
Pelletier, Mathieu, FamilyMed
Peloquin, Michel-Andre
Perreault, Eric
Picard-Turcot, Anae, FamilyMed
Pigeon, Amelie, FamilyMed
Plante, Virginie, FamilyMed
Pointer, Rohan, FamilyMed
Proulx, Cindy, FamilyMed
Provencher, Claude A., FamilyMed
Redburn, Alexandra, FamilyMed
Reggad, Bouchra, FamilyMed(EM)
Samson, Carine, FamilyMed(EM)
Schaefer-Zieleniak, Bozena
Simard, Jennifer M., FamilyMed
Tessier, Sylvie, FamilyMed
Thibodeau, Raymond, FamilyMed
Tremblay, Emilie
Turgeon, Sebastien, FamilyMed
Villeneuve, Etienne, FamilyMed
Zieleniak, Adam M.

ST CHARLES DE BELLECHASSE

Falardeau, Jean
Letourneau, Marc

ST-CUTHBERT

Senecal-Quevillon, Micheline

PHYSICIANS BY PROVINCE

ST CYRILLE DE WENDOVER

Fontaine, Isabelle

ST-DAMASE

Gosselin, Patrice
Lavoie, Jean-Denis

ST DENIS DE BROMPTON

Bertrand, Robert G.

ST DENIS SUR RICHELIEU

Dionne, Marie-Claude, FamilyMed
Laroche, Annie, FamilyMed

ST DONAT DE MONTCALM

Fortier, Anne
Hebert, Jean-Marc
Laflamme, Marie
Majeau, Luc
Martel, Colette

ST ETIENNE DE LAUZON

Brochu, Chantal
Gagnon, Fabienne
Gourgues, Alain
Grenon, Lisa
Laferriere, Luc
Laflamme, Paule
Marchand, Luce
Rouillier, Jean
Thomas, Eddie
Voyer, Jean

ST ETIENNE DES GRES

Boulanger, Marianne, FamilyMed
Delorme, Jacques
Dube, Marie-Helene
Dubois, David
Gelinas, Daniel
Houle, Patrick
Lefebvre, Marie-Eve
Lemieux, Jacinthe C.
Milette, David, FamilyMed
Parent, Josiane, FamilyMed

ST-EUSTACHE

Aubin, Linda, FamilyMed
Bellemare, France
Bissonnette, Jacques
Blais, Bruno
Briere, Michel
Caza, Genevieve, FamilyMed
Chartrand, Rachel
D'Annunzio, Mario
Ducharme, Martine
Gariepy, Gaetan
Goyer, Normand
Goyer, Ronald
Joron, Chantal
Kingsbury, Claude
Legare, Jean-Jacques
Monarque, Nathalie
Pannetier, Marie-France
Paquet, Roger
Paquin, Claude-Elene
Parent, Dominique
Pelletier, Daniele
Perreault, Jean
Perry, Diane
Phung, Thinh-Vinh
Plante, Jean-Francois
Restrepo, Alfonso
Robert, Martin
Robillard, Josee
Thebault, Marguerite
Thisdale, Jean

ST-FELIX-DE-VALOIS

Allard, Gaston
Allard, Jacinthe
Allard, Myriam, FamilyMed
Allard, Paul
Dulude, Michel
Mayrand, Martin
Moody, Helene
Payette, Clement

ST FERREOL LES NEIGES

Larouche, Alain

ST FRANCOIS MONTMAGNY

Morin, Simon

ST GABRIEL DE BRANDON

De Grandpre, Michel
De Serres, Marthe
Desbiens, Marie-Therese
Gagnon, Jean
Leduc, Michel
Pelland, Marcel
Truffy, Gilles

ST GEDEON DE BEAUCE

Blais, Jacques
Caron, Patricia, FamilyMed

ST GEORGES CACOUNA

Goudreau, Daniel

ST GERMAIN DE GRANTHAM

De Montigny, Rene

ST HENRI DE LEVIS

Beaudoin, Richard
Bourget, Nathalie, FamilyMed
Cote, Michel C.
Dufour, Julie
Levasseur, Jacques

ST HUBERT RIVIERE DU LAC

Harvey, Marianne

ST JEAN CHRYSOSTOME

Beaumont, Cyril
Boucher, Denis
Canuel, Jean-Pierre
Couture, Julie
Genest, Marie-Josee
Halle, Suzanne
Hetu, Marc A.
Lajoie, Danielle
Lambert, Diane
Prevost, Gilles
Renaud, Isabelle

ST JACQUES DE LEEDS

Langlois, Michel

ST JEAN PORT JOLI

Baker, Denis, FamilyMed
Blouin, Elizabeth
Coulombe, Anne-Marie
Coulombe, Paul
Gagnon, Violaine
Labrecque, Gilles F.
Lachance, Jacques R.
Paquin, Stephanie, FamilyMed
Pelchat, Veronique
Rivest, Jacques

ST JEAN DES PILES

Pepin, Sylvie
Vermette, Johanne

ST JEAN SUR RICHELIEU

Allard, Mariannick, FamilyMed(EM)
Alonzo-Proulx, Isabel
Asnong, Veronique, FamilyMed
Aubin, Stephane
Bastien, Sylvie
Begnoche, Evelyne
Belisle, Julie, FamilyMed
Benny, Frederic, FamilyMed
Bergevin, Alain A., FamilyMed
Bessette, Lucie
Binet, Jacques
Blais, Jocelyne
Boisvert, Rejean
Bouchard, Anne-Sylvie
Bouchard, Remi
Boudreau-Poissant, Karele, FamilyMed
Brais, Nathalie
Brault, Serge
Brien, Chantal
Brosseau, Jacques
Brown, Bernard H.
Brunet, Francois
Brunet, Matthieu
Carrier, Pierre
Cerat, Jean-Michel
Charlebois, Pierre
Clement, Sylvie
Crepin, Marylene
Dallaire, Genevieve, FamilyMed(EM)
Dandavino, Andre-Hector
Dang, Francois
D'Argy, Marie-Claude
De Grace, Luce, FamilyMed
Demers, Stephanie
Deneault, Luc
Desormeau, Jean
Duchesneau, Marie-Claude, FamilyMed(EM)
Dufresne, Jacques J.
Dumouchel, Richard
Faucher, Yves J L.
Fournier, Anne-Marie
Fournier, Claude
Fournier, Jean-Marie
Frenette, Jacques
Gagnon, Elyse
Gagnon, Isabelle
Gagnon, Melanie, FamilyMed
Gaucher, Christine
Gauthier, Dominic, FamilyMed
Gelinas, Jean-Pierre
Gemme, Emilie
Germain, Jean-Francois, FamilyMed
Gervais, Annie
Giguere, Marie-Chantal
Girard, Andre
Grand'Maison, Nicole
Grenier, Gilles
Grogan, Johanne
Guay, Sebastien, FamilyMed
Guillette, Lyne, FamilyMed
Hebert, Benedict, FamilyMed
Huet, Madeleine
Huot, Helene
Huot, Michele
Jutras, Serge
Kannab-Ayda, George
Kassab, Francois
Kenscoff, Jean-Michel
Khour, Hamid
Kramer, John, FamilyMed
Labrecque, Paul
Laganiere, Yves
Langlois, Yves P.
Laplante, Joanne
Lavoie, Daniel
Leclerc, Claude E.
Leger, Francine
Letovanec, Sylvie
Levesque, Isabelle
Levreault, Marie-Pier D., FamilyMed
Lortie, Marie-Noelle, FamilyMed
Marin, Louis
Martel, Rodrigue
Masson-Roy, Marie-Helene
Matouk, Zehra
Menard, Marie-Chantal
Merizzi, Marc
Messier, Nadine
Michaud, Julie-Christine, FamilyMed
Miclette Menard, Philippe-Antoine
Monette, Virginie
Mongeon, Anne
More, Philippe, FamilyMed(EM)
Moretti, Eric, FamilyMed
Moser, Josef E.
Nadeau, Chantal
Nault, Serge
Normandin, Pierre
Ouimet, Luc J.
Papineau, Cynthia, FamilyMed(EM)
Paquet, Ghislain
Paquette, Elaine
Pelletier, Stephanie
Peloquin, Sonia
Perreault, Caroline
Philibert, Bruno
Pothier, Daniel
Potvin, Helene
Prevost, Guillaume, FamilyMed
Prevost, Michel
Proulx, Francois
Quirion, Melisa, FamilyMed
Raymond, Francois
Rivard, Andre
Rivas, Jose A.
Roberge, Katerie
Roy, Suzanne, FamilyMed
Savaria, Frederick G.
Senikas, Andre
Simard, Valery
St-Germain, Pierre
Toussaint, Sebastien
Trepanier, Josee
Turenne, Yves
Turner, Michel
Vachon, Caroline
Zaidi, Houria

ST-JÉRÔME

Boisvert, Caroline

ST JOSEPH DE BEAUCE

Champagne, Pierre
Cliche, Bernard
Guay, Ghislaine
Samson, Nelson
Theberge, Helene

ST JOSEPH DU LAC

Anctil, Audrey, FamilyMed
Boyczum, Julie
Gaudet, Louise
Loiselle, Pierre
Peloquin, Jacques
Roy, Alain
Savard-Cote, Melanie, FamilyMed

ST LAMBERT DE LAUZON

Bilodeau, Elizabeth
Lambert, Roch

ST LEONARD D'ASTON

Bastin, Gauthier
Dumas, Guy
Gagnon, Mylene
Lanoue, Martin, FamilyMed
Pepin, Paul-Andre
Proulx, Richard

ST LIN LAURENTIDES

Coulombe, Martine
Dauphinais, Luc
Ducharme, Andre
Lemire, Caroline, FamilyMed
Levac, Caroline
Renaud, Andre
Roberge, Justine, FamilyMed

ST MARC DES CARRIERES

Filteau, Pierre
Frenette, Jean, FamilyMed
Grenon, Louise
Guimond, Gaston
Savoie, Louis

ST MATHIEU BELOEIL

Barbant, Andre D.
Frenette, Guy

ST-MAURICE

Trahan, Andre G.

ST-MICH-D-STS

Le Goueff, Real J.

ST MICHEL DE BELLECHASSE

Poulin, Maude, FamilyMed

ST NAZAIRE DE LAC ST JEAN

Bouchard, Myriam
Cote, Robin
Pedneault, Lisa

ST PATRICE DE BEAURIVAGE

Duquette, Louis
Nantel, Claire

ST PIERRE L'ILE D'ORLEANS

Blouin, Brigitte
Bonenfant, Paul

ST PROSPER DE DORCHESTER

Kishka, Paul
Lantagne, Louise
Lantagne, Marie-Josee

ST RAPHAEL DE BEAUCE

Bernier, Pascal
Roy, Gilles

ST-REDEMPTEUR

Bouffard, Gerald, FamilyMed

ST ROCH DE L'ACHIGAN

Belisle, Pierre
Dubois, Chantal, FamilyMed

ST SEBASTIEN DE FRONT

Laflamme, Paule

ST STANISLAS DE CHAMPLAIN

Gelinas, Louise
Martel, Jacques
Roberge, Claude
Tessier, Levis

ST-UBALD

Berlinguet, Helene

STANSTEAD

Bouchard, Gilles R.
Brazeau, Nathalie, FamilyMed
Surprenant, Anne
Tousignant, Sylvie

STE AGATHE DES MONTS

Aumont, Marie-France
Banos, Manuel
Beauchemin, Kim
Bedard, Rejean
Belanger, Josee, FamilyMed(EM)
Belanger, Pierre
Bissonnette, Bertrand
Boily, Nathalie
Boucher, Isabelle, FamilyMed
Caouette, Marie-Josee, FamilyMed
Chalifoux, Marie-Pierre, FamilyMed
Crouzier-Roux, Emmanuelle, FamilyMed
Deraspe, Emmanuel, FamilyMed
Deslauriers, Louis-Jean
Despots, Marilyne
Desrochers, Jean-Paul
Dionne, Benoit
Ethier, Lucien
Fournier, Gino
Frenette, Michel
Gagne, Eveline
Gagnon, Andree-Anne, FamilyMed
Gareau, Marilyn, FamilyMed
Gelinas, Renee-Claude
Glorion, Antoine
Gosselin, Francois
Gosselin, Marc, FamilyMed(EM)
Grenier, Valerie, FamilyMed
Guenette, Claudine
Houeto, Sohoueto
Lachaine, Colette
Lagace, Louis-Marie
Landry, Simon-Pierre, FamilyMed(EM)
Lapointe, Andre
Laroche, Jean-Pierre
Larocque, Robert
Larose, Marie
Leduc-Arbour, Nathael
Leroux, Eric
Marcoux, Francois
Martel, Laurent
Masse, Hugo
Maunders, John G., FamilyMed
Menard, Nathalie
Montini, Alexandre
Palfreeman, Mark H., FamilyMed(EM)
Paquin, Marc
Poulin, Stephane
Precourt, Julie
Prud'Homme, Veronique
Rattue, Melissa, FamilyMed
Saint-Cyr, Mathieu
Theriault, Stephane
Touchette, Jean-Sebastien
Tousignant, Maryse
Tremblay, Marie-Eve, FamilyMed
Trempe-Masson, Catherine
Trepanier, Madeleine, FamilyMed(EM)
Vallee, Sophie-Lisa

STE ANNE DE BEAUPRE

Girard, Philippe

STE ANNE DE BELLEVUE

Batalion, Hyman
Beluska, Dora-Lina, FamilyMed
Chapdelaine, Pierre
Dion, Rejean
Gingras, Serge
Joly, Dominique E.
Lillie, Eric
Nguyen, Hai Thong
Pepelea, Ancuta
Perreault, Francois
Polson, George A.
Provencal, Paul T.
Thivierge, Robert

STE ANNE DE LA PÉRADE

Boily, Pierre
Leclerc, Julie, FamilyMed
Ruel, Rejean

STE ANNE DES MONTS

Aram, Omid
Blais, Claudia T.
Bouchard-Rochette, Marie-Eve, FamilyMed
Charest, Anne-Marie, FamilyMed
Dompierre, Jean-Maurice
Dumont, Andre
Gagnon, Emilie C., FamilyMed
Garcia, Michel
Gauvreau, Alain
Hardy, Guillaume, FamilyMed
Kravchenko, Viktor
Lacoste, Daniel, FamilyMed
Lavigueur, Rene
Padron Castillo, Oswaldo E., FamilyMed
Pelletier, Alain, FamilyMed
Remy, Joseph
Simard, Michel-Xavier
Tasse, Eliane
Tremblay, Pierre-Paul
Ubeda, Ivan, FamilyMed

STE ANNE DES PLAINES

Grenier, Louise
Levesque, Robin
Prefontaine, Patrick

STE ANNE DU SAULT

Ouellette, Helene

STE BRIGITTE DE LAVAL

Bordeleau, Denis
Desy, Jean

STE CATHERINE DE LA JACQUES CARTIER

Banville, Christine
Huot, Pierre

STE CECILE DE MASHAM

Minde, Thomas, FamilyMed

STE GENEVIEVE DE BATISCAN

Cloutier, Michele
Germain, Elizabeth
Grenier, Julie
Jacques, Christine, FamilyMed
Pinard, Marie-Claude

STE-JULIENNE

Boudrias, Alain
Daneault, Michel

STE MARGUERITE ESTEREL

Gaudet, Olivier P.
Roy, Yves

STE MARTHE SUR LE LAC

Normandin, Diane M.

STE MARTINE

Ste-Marie, Pierre

STOKE

Arsenault, Pierre, FamilyMed

STONEHAM

Bergeron, Antoine
Julien, Jean-Francois

SUTTON

Balthazard, Carole
Camirand, Michel
Dion, Marie-Pierre
Fournier, Carole
Lesieur, Denis

TEMISCAMING

Brock, Gordon I., FamilyMed
Figueredo Alvarez, Roasana
Gurekas, Vydas
Raad, Samar, FamilyMed
Zivkovic Bursac, Slavica

TERREBONNE

Adams, Marc, FamilyMed
Amyot, Marie-Claudel, FamilyMed
Andre, Barnave, FamilyMed
Archambault, Julie
Aubut, Luc
Baril, Pierre
Bassal, Christine
Beauchamp, Andre
Beaudoin, Daniel
Beliveau, Vanessa
Bennett, Jean-Yves
Bergeron, Alain
Bernard, David, FamilyMed
Boisvert, Philippe, FamilyMed
Boulanger, Pascal
Boyer, Marc
Brabant, Francois
Carbonneau Girouard, Maxime, FamilyMed
Castor, Schiller, FamilyMed
Cataford, Jean
Chaabane, Sonia
Chabot, Danielle
Champagne, Myriam, FamilyMed(EM)
Charest, Francois
Chateauvert, Marie-Rose
Chevrette, Karine
Cimon, Michel
Coderre, Amélie, FamilyMed(EM)
Coll, Xavier P L.
Conseil, Jean P.
Cossette, Joanne
Cousineau, Daniel F.
Coutu, Elizabeth, FamilyMed
Couture, Marie-Claude
Darques, Loïc, FamilyMed
Delage, Eric
Desrosiers, Catherine, FamilyMed
Dion, Nathalie
Dorval, Jacqueline
Doyon, Michel
Dube, Yolande, FamilyMed
Duguay, Christine, FamilyMed
Duguay, Lyne
Dulong, Anick, FamilyMed
Duong, Giang Nghiep, FamilyMed
Dupont, Nathalie
Durand, Brigitte
Emery, France
Filion, Lucie
Fioriti, Steven
Florent, Danielle
Fontaine, Marie-Josee, FamilyMed
Fortier, Simon, FamilyMed
Frappier Chalifoux, Hamie
Gauthier, Claudie, FamilyMed(EM)
Guay-Pelletier, Louise
Heppell, Josee, FamilyMed
Houle, Noemi, FamilyMed
Kechaou, Wassim
Kerba, Jean-Paul, FamilyMed
Lacasse, Marie-Eve, FamilyMed
Ladouceur, Robert
Laflamme, Chantal
Laflamme, Jean-Claude
Lamontagne, Hugo
Lanthier, Nathalie
Laporte, Diane
Laroche, Esther
Lasalle, Luc
Lauzon, France
Lavergne, Genevieve, FamilyMed
Lavigne, Jean-Pierre, FamilyMed
Lebel, Jean-Philippe, FamilyMed
Leblanc, Martin, FamilyMed
Leveille, Daniel
Lewis, Anna M., FamilyMed
Lim, Julie, FamilyMed
Manny, Emmanuelle
Marceau, Marie-Josee
Mercier, Nicolas, FamilyMed
Methot, Renee
Nguyen, Mau Huan
Nguyen, Thanh
Oliva, Rossella
Olivier, Marc-Andre P.
Ouellet, Eve-Marie
Pagliarulo, Giovanni, FamilyMed
Payeur, Jean-Martin, FamilyMed
Potvin, Frederic
Pouliot, Claude
Racine, Stephanie, FamilyMed
Rivest, Annie
Rivest, Martin, FamilyMed(EM)
Robert, Benoit
Robert, Genevieve, FamilyMed
Robert, Melanie, FamilyMed
Rodrigue, Vincent, FamilyMed
Rodriguez, Pacita
Rousseau-Lortie, Andree
Ruffet-Bourdon, Sophie
Sanche, Stephanie
Sarrazin, Gerald
Simard, Michel
St-Jacques, Caroline, FamilyMed
Sylvestre, Nicolas, FamilyMed
Tanferna, Rosaria, FamilyMed
Thibaudeau, Johanne
Thibault, Anne
Thibault, Veronic, FamilyMed
Trottier, Cloe, FamilyMed
Turenne, Hubert
Vallee, Sophie
Wecowski, Eveline

THETFORD MINES

Arata, Martin
Bedard, Luc
Bouchard, Cindy
Breton, Steve, FamilyMed
Brossard, Michel
Cabot, Julie
Caron, Gilles J.
Chabot, Marie-Christine, FamilyMed
Champagne, Lucie
Chiquette-Pomar, Annie, FamilyMed
Cloutier-Camire, France
Cote, Pierre
Gaudreau, Eric

Giguere, Sylvie
Gilbert, Marie-Eve
Girard, Guylaine
Gourdes, Denis
Grenier, Hugo
Huet, Marc-Andre
Joubert, Pierre
Lachance, Maggie
Lafranchise, Luc
Lavigne, Philippe, FamilyMed
Lemieux, Maryse C.
Lemieux, Pierre
Lizotte, Jessica, FamilyMed(EM)
Mercier, Isabelle
Ouellet, Alain
Piuze, Jacques
Roy Talbot, Vincent, FamilyMed
Samson, Gilles
Trepanier, Line
Vallieres, Francois
Veilleux, Richard
Villeneuve, Nicole

THURSO

Boucher, Jean
Duré, Marjorie, FamilyMed

TRING-JONCTION

Nadeau, Jean-Claude
Roy, Pierre

TROIS-PISTOLES

Beaulieu, Denis
Bordeleau, Celine, FamilyMed
Bordeleau, Jacinthe
Boulianne, Annie
Cadrin, Danielle
Charbonneau, Annie
Delisle, Simon
Lavallee, Emilie
Lavoie, Eric, FamilyMed
Lemay, Isabelle, FamilyMed
Manzini, Nicolas
Ouellet, Lucie
Robillard, Claude
Streiff, Raphael

TROIS-RIVIERES

Abi Raad, Camille
Alain, Isabelle
Alarie, Hughette
Alarie, Marie-Claude, FamilyMed
Alarie, Rejean
Allard-Pigeon, Marjorie, FamilyMed
Amrani, Laila
Amstutz, Nancy
Anctil, Marylene
Archambault, Pierre
Arsenault, Sylvain, FamilyMed
Asselin, Fannie
Audet, Helene
Ayotte, Nancy
Baril, Rejean
Baron, Mireille, FamilyMed
Barrero Garcia, Miguel A.
Bastarache, Annie
Beaucage, France
Beauchemin, Denise
Beaudoin, Catherine
Beaudry, Jacques
Beland, Pierre
Belzile, Gilles
Bergeron, Anne-Catherine, FamilyMed(EM)
Bergeron, Emile
Bergeron, Jean-Pierre
Bernard, Diane, FamilyMed(EM)
Bernard, Richard, FamilyMed
Bernatchez, Marilou, FamilyMed
Berthiaume, Renee
Bessette, Maral A.
Blais, Jean-Philippe, FamilyMed
Blanchette, Agathe
Blaquiere, Martine
Boisvert, Annie, FamilyMed
Bolduc, Sebastien
Boucher, Anne-Louise
Boucher-Pilon, Amélie, FamilyMed
Bouillon, Karine
Bussieres-Labrecque, Audrey
Cadorette, Martin
Cadotte, Lucie
Caron, Andrew
Carre Desrosiers, M. Genevieve N.
Caya, Valerie
Chapuis, Frederic
Chou, Jean
Claveau, David
Clavel, Christian
Cote, Andree
Couetoux Du Tertre, Anne
Croisetiere, Guy
Cyr, Daniel R.
Dalcourt, Jean-Pierre
Dauth, Eric, FamilyMed
Daze, Pierre-Luc
Demers, Yves
Desaulniers, Jean, FamilyMed
Deschesnes, Judy
Desjardins, Marco
Deziel, Marcel
Diaz, Ariel H.
Dicaire, Caroline
Donaldson, Daniele
Donati, Johanne
Dostie, Caroline
Doyon, Yvon
Dubois, Richard
Dumas, Louise
Duplain, Rejean, FamilyMed
Dupont, Alain
Ferland, Louise
Fortier, Elise, FamilyMed
Fortin, Andre
Frechette, Julie
Gagnon, Annie, FamilyMed
Garceau, Audrey
Garneau, Jessica, FamilyMed
Garneau, Valerie
Gauthier, Celine
Gauthier, Johanne
Gauthier, Michel
Gauthier, Raphaelle, FamilyMed(EM)
Gauvin, Nathalie, FamilyMed
Gelinas, Paul R.
Gerin-Lajoie, Annie
Giguere, Dominic, FamilyMed
Gingras, Pascale
Godbout, Yves-Laurent
Gouin, Emilie, FamilyMed
Grenier, Gilles W.
Hamel, Lysianne, FamilyMed(EM)
Hassan, Youssef
Houde, Rene
Houle, Pierre-Alain
Hurtubise, Suzanne
Janelle, Christian, FamilyMed
Jeannot, Sandra, FamilyMed
Jiona, Andree
Juneau, Valerie, FamilyMed(EM)
Kauzman, George
L'Etoile, Michel, FamilyMed
Labbe, Janel, FamilyMed
Labbe, Jean C.
Labrie, Eric
Lacoursiere, Sylvie
Laflamme, Nadia
Lahaie, Pascale
Lamirande, Maxime, FamilyMed
Lamirande, Yves
Lampron, Sebastien
Landry, J. Sylvain
Lapointe, Claude
Lavallée, Philippe
Laverdiere, Annie, FamilyMed(EM)
Lavoie, Joel, FamilyMed
Lavoie-Levesque, Josiane
Leblanc, Nicole, FamilyMed
Leblanc, Steve
Leclair, Normand
Lecoeur, Daniel
Leite Vieira Costa, Ricardo
Lemay, Line
Lemieux, Marie-Eve
Lemire, Pierre-Luc, FamilyMed
Leveille, Alain
Marchand, Patricia
Martel, Louis, FamilyMed
Martin, Pierre
Matton, Jean-Francois
Mercier, Karine
Michaud, Renee
Milot, Yvon
Mirza, Asma S.
Moutier, Antoine M.
Noel, Audrey
Ouellet, Henri
Paille, Fernand
Papillon, Evelyne, FamilyMed(EM)
Parent, Francois, FamilyMed(EM)
Picotte, Rene-Paul
Pothier, Philippe
Poulin, Guy
Proulx, Nicolas
Ramalho, Denis C.
Renard, Pierre
Rioux, Samuel, FamilyMed
Roucaut, Francois-Xavier
Roy, Olivier, FamilyMed(EM)
Roy, Suzanne
Roy, Veronique-Elisabeth
Samson, Daniele
Santerre, Regine
Sigmen, Jacques
St-Onge, Benoit
Talbot, Karine
Therrien, Joelle
Thibault, Marcel
Thibault, Marie-Eve, FamilyMed
Thibault, Sebastien
Turcotte, Anna-Marie
Vallieres, Marcel
Vaugeois, Alain, FamilyMed
Veilleux, Alain
Villalobos Narvaez, Ethel H., FamilyMed
Vincent, Gilles
Vincent, Pierre R.
Youmbissi Tchetagni, Joseph

UPTON

Ouradou, Jean-Luc

VAL-MORIN

Lapointe, Pierre

VAL-D'OR

Adam, Fhameeda, FamilyMed
Authier, Alain
Bellazzi, Myriam
Bilodeau-Dubé, Anne-Michèle, FamilyMed
Blanchette, Marie-Eve
Bouchard, Catherine, FamilyMed
Chretien, Lizane
Conde, Jean-Joseph
Corriveau, Jean-Paul
Dube, Charlotte
El Koussa, Lamis
Ghattas, Aiman Y.
Gilbert, Marie-Odile
Goudreau, Veronique, FamilyMed(EM)
Kaloul, Ismail
Lapointe, Yves J.
Lee, Marc F., FamilyMed
Mailly, Christian, FamilyMed
Malenfant, Claude
Martin, Jacques
Masse, Julie, FamilyMed
McGee, Nancy, FamilyMed
Nakhostine, Nabil, FamilyMed
Nguyen, Lan-Anh, FamilyMed
Perron, Denis
Pham, Tuong-Vi, FamilyMed
Picard, Elizabeth
Salame, Charbel
Sanfacon, Lorraine, FamilyMed
Sennett, Edward S., FamilyMed(EM)
Skuherska, Romana
Souissi, Kamel
St-Amant, Lincey, FamilyMed
Sventek, Pavol, FamilyMed
Ta, Diana, FamilyMed
Tran-Le, Hong Phuc, FamilyMed
Tremblay, Chantal
Villeneuve, Regis
Wajszilber, Marcelo A.

VAL-DES-MONTS

Dube, Anne

VALCOURT

Cusson, Jacinthe
Lussier, Yvan
St-Antoine, Josee
Timmons, Amelie
Turcotte, Jean, FamilyMed

VALLEE-JONCTION

Gosselin, Johanne
Poulin, Rejean

VARENNES

Bilodeau, Francois
Cadet, Sylvie
Chagnon, Annie
Dauphinais, Lucie
Descombes, Andre
Doyon, Jean-Claude
Girard, Louise, FamilyMed
Labelle, Sylvie
Landry, Audrey
Lanouette, Pierre
Lapointe, Gerald
Lemelin, Jean-Luc
Levesque, Anne
Meunier, Pierre
Monarque, Guy
Morin, France
Nguyen, Dinh Duc
Picard, Jolene
Potvin, Nathalie
Rambaldi, Antonio
Thibault, Suzanne
Tremblay, Dominique
Trottier, Julie
Trottier, Marielle

VAUDREUIL-DORION

Anctil, Chantal, FamilyMed
Begin, M H. Julie
Bessette, Paule
Bray, Veronique
Cardin St-Antoine, Annie, FamilyMed
Caron, Jerome
Daoust, Helene, FamilyMed
Desilets-Couture, Claudette
Downs, Jean-Pierre
Drolet, Gaetan
Dufresne, Sylvain
Essaadi, Aziza
Germain, Mitchel, FamilyMed
Grenon, Denis
Iancu, Andreea, FamilyMed
Kelly, Richard
Kuganathan, Girudiha
Lam, Doan Trang, FamilyMed
Leduc, Christian
Leduc, Manon
Leduc, Michel
Padan, Callie, FamilyMed
Parent, Mariloue
Pedneault, Josee, FamilyMed
Piche, Marie-Chantal, FamilyMed
Pop, Aida M., FamilyMed
Puri-Alanoly, Lizy
Rousseau, Danielle
Saunier, Jeremy G., FamilyMed
Savard, Julie
Sharabyani, Feryal, FamilyMed
St-Amant-Cardin, Dolores

VERCHERES

Kiss, Andre L.
Roman, Jean-Pierre

VERDUN

Armand, Jean-Claude
Assaf, Christian, FamilyMed
Aubin, Richard
Awad, Stephanie, FamilyMed
Barriault, Jocelyn
Barrs, Gary B.
Beaudoin, Jacques
Beaudry, Nicole
Bedkowska, Alicja
Bedkowska, Anna
Belley, Marc, FamilyMed
Bisson, Denis
Blackburn Mailloux, Geneviève, FamilyMed
Blais, Robert
Boivin, Diane
Bouchard, Marc
Brown, Kenneth E., FamilyMed
Canaan, Julie, FamilyMed
Cernica, Maria
Chachamovich, Eduardo
Champagne, Martin
Chauvette, Michel
Choquet, Julie, FamilyMed
Choquette, Lise
Cohen, Jackie
Coutu, Louis
Côté, Nancy, FamilyMed
Damaso, Humbertino
Dauphin, Lise
Dechene, Genevieve
Demers, Christine, FamilyMed
Desforges, Johanne
Diec, Q. Diana
Drouin, Michel
Ducasse, Chantal, FamilyMed
Dunn, David
Dupont, Julie
Emond, Daniel
Ferdais, Genevieve, FamilyMed
Fourestie, Emmanuelle
Gagne, Helene
Gagne, Marc
Gervais, Daniel
Ghaderi, Bahareh
Giroux, Josee
Gregoire, Julie, FamilyMed
Guillon, Simone, FamilyMed
Handanos, Daphne, FamilyMed
Hebert, Michel, FamilyMed
Hebert-Croteau, Nicole
Henry, Caroline, FamilyMed
Hudon, Eveline, FamilyMed
Hurtubise, Severine
Iskandar, Hani
Jackson, John
Jenkins, Mark R., FamilyMed
Jollant, Fabrice B.
Joly, Caroline, FamilyMed
Joober, Ridha
Joyal, Marie
Joyal, Marie-Suzanne, FamilyMed
Lafond, Daniel
Lafortune, Jacques, FamilyMed
Lageix, Philippe
Lahlou, Hala, FamilyMed
Langevin, Dominique
Laperriere-Nguyen, Eric V.
Lapointe, Luc, FamilyMed
Larocque, Amelie, FamilyMed
Lasalle, Leo
Lehmann, Francois, FamilyMed
Marchand, Robert, FamilyMed
Mathieu, Jean-Francois
Menard, Sophie
Mereniuk, Bohdan
Moini, John, FamilyMed
Morin, Caroline, FamilyMed
Murphy, Daniel B., FamilyMed
Murray, Ariane, FamilyMed
Nasri, Nabil
Nguyen, Myvan
Paquette, Claudie, FamilyMed

Paquette, Marc
Pascual, Pierre-Gilbert
Pauyo, Eric
Phan, Amelie, FamilyMed
Picard, Lyne
Pinto, Nicholas, FamilyMed
Polak, Patrick
Proulx, Chantal
Proulx, Stephane
Pruneau, Elaine
Robert, Michel P.
Rokni, Farin, FamilyMed
Roy, Martine
Rozefort, Willine R., FamilyMed
Rusu, Gabriela, FamilyMed
Savard, Claude
Sayegh, Renee
Seguin, Eric
Sheftel, Raisa
Somera, Saundra-Lisa
St-Francois, Bernard
St-Marseille, Melanie, FamilyMed
Talbot, Genevieve
Thavundayil, Joseph X.
Thibault, Annie, FamilyMed
Tremblay, Jacques
Trudel-Brun, Amelie
Turcotte, Jean
Turecki, Gustavo X.
Vallee, Pierre
Valois, Maxime, FamilyMed(EM)
Villeneuve, Jean-Pierre
Virmani, Achla R.
Vo, Thi Minh T.

VICTORIAVILLE

Archambault, Claudine
Auger, Louis
Bedard, Michele
Belanger, Andre
Bellavance, Ethel
Bergeron, Anthony, FamilyMed
Bergeron, Pierre
Betit, Eve
Betit, Jean-Luc
Blanchette, Danielle
Champagne, Claude
Chaput, Brigitte, FamilyMed(EM)
Cotte, Celine
Couture, Dominique, FamilyMed
Croteau, Bernard, FamilyMed
Fortier, Karine
Garand, Marie-Josee, FamilyMed
Gelinas, Catherine
Girard, Jean-Marc
Grenier, Solene
Harvey, Berthold
Henri, Manon
Hould, Nathalie, FamilyMed(EM)
Huneault, Pierre
Huppe, Alain
Joly, Melissa
Labbe, Sylvain, FamilyMed
Labelle, Andre
Lamonde-Boulet, Guillaume
Lamoureux, Christian
Lemay, Marianne
Lemay, Marjorie
Leroux, Helene
Lessard, Ariane, FamilyMed
Lessard, Daniel
Lessard, Nathalie R.
Malenfant, Dominic
Menard, Carole
Nadeau, Andre
Nazair, Odette
Nitka, Monique
Parenteau, Hugues
Picard, Robert
Poirier, David
Poisson, Marco
Richard, Elise
Tardif, Chantal
Theriault, Guy
Turner, Francois

VILLE-MARIE

Aumond Beaupré, Tommy
Beauregard-Lepage, Francis
Bureau, Yanick
Dominguez Avalos, Jose A.
Lalonde, Jean
Lefebvre, Diane
Legault, Claude
Martel, France, FamilyMed
Martin, Monique
Portelance-Huot, Marjolaine
Rivet, Real J F.
Scaffidi, Carmen P., FamilyMed
Tanis, Emile J.
Theriault, Marie-Noel
Zavaleta Justiniano, Jannet

VIMONT

Bianki, Sylvain
Corbeil, Diane
Desrosiers, Line, FamilyMed
Fortier, Ginette
Grou, Fabienne, FamilyMed
Lavoie, Pauline
Lavoie, Yannick, FamilyMed
Leblanc, Claude J.
Rodrigues, Isabel, FamilyMed
Sanche, Gilbert, FamilyMed
St-Pierre, Florence

WAKEFIELD

Anya Mengue, Pierre
Cardy, Vanessa L., FamilyMed
Del Bianco, Sylvie, FamilyMed
Fellus, Youcef
Folkerson, Curtis S., FamilyMed
Gold, David I., FamilyMed
Goulet, Marie-Helene, FamilyMed
Joannisse, Valerie, FamilyMed(EM)
Lajzerowicz, Michelle, FamilyMed
Lemay, Diane
Lemelin, Tania, FamilyMed
Ngodjoum Nitcheu, Louis R.
Odell, Margaret R.
Patocka, Catherine
Satenstein, Gary H., FamilyMed
Saul, Mark E., FamilyMed
St-Amour, Pascale, FamilyMed

WARWICK

Blanchard, Pierre-Hugues
Boutin, Isabelle, FamilyMed
Chamberland, Manon
Deshaies, Pierre
Peloquin, Patrice, FamilyMed
Pichette, Monique

WASKAGANISH

Berlie, Marie C., FamilyMed
Kovitch, Ingrid

WATERLOO

Chagnon, Normand
Larkin-Chagnon, Anne
Marineau, Yves
Moore, Nathalie
Nolze, Christine
St-Onge, Robert, FamilyMed

WATERVILLE

Chia, Edison W.

WEEDON

Carne, Nicole A P.
Cloutier, Claude
Gailloux, Pierre
Kibos Talabur, Elena
Leblanc, Louise
Mathieu, Henri-Pierre
St-Pierre, Yves

WEMINDJI

Bellido Oviedo, Roxana, FamilyMed

WENDAKE

Sioui, Christian

WESTMOUNT

Backler, John H., FamilyMed
Blicher, Brian M., FamilyMed
Brzezinski, Wanda T.
Comeau, Margery
Coopersmith, Henry G., FamilyMed
Goldenberg, Barry S.
Goldsman, F. Barry
Haiek, Laura N., FamilyMed
Heisler, Stanley H., FamilyMed
Hew, Eleanor, FamilyMed
Hughes, John B.
Jednak, Irene
Josephson, Deborah
Katsounakis, John, FamilyMed
Lapointe, Michel A., FamilyMed
Larocque, Maurice
Ludman, Ronald B., FamilyMed
Lysy, Paul, FamilyMed
Martin, Stephen C., FamilyMed
Rivard, Marc
Roper, Mark, FamilyMed
Slapcoff, Barry, FamilyMed
Sunenblick, Robert E.
Tong, Christina, FamilyMed
Weigens, David, FamilyMed
White, Debrah L.
Wilson, Janet H., FamilyMed
Yajnik, Dushyant K.

WINDSOR

Ares, Francois
Belleau-Nantel, Jean F.
Bernier, Chantal
Bibeau, Marielle
Desjardins, France
Fradette, Virginie
Labrie, Christiane
Lamontagne, Suzanne
Paquet, Carine
Pontbriand, Eric
Prud'Homme, Marie L P.
Thibault, Emilie

SASKATCHEWAN

ARCOLA

Lesola, Dasual S.
Morin, Marie-Lise

ASSINIBOIA

Carulei, Victor A.
Glaeske, Daniel M.
Guirguis, Wael
Pradhan, Abhay M.

BATTLEFORD

Engelbrecht, Frederik H S., FamilyMed
Moolla, Hasan M., FamilyMed
Rodriguez Naranjo, Aristides

BEECHY

Cooper, Johan C.
Hamilton, Anthony C.

BIGGAR

Close, Alison M., FamilyMed
Crane, Neville
Laxdal, Muriel L.
Lethole, Gabriel M.
McKee, Alison M.
Muller, Anton M., FamilyMed

BLACK LAKE

Ayub, Nasir
Habib, Khawaja, FamilyMed
Urton, Jack I M.

BROADVIEW

Adam, Suleman V.
Mazamisa, Vusumzi M.

BUSHELL PARK

Padua, Raymond R., FamilyMed

CABRI

De Nysschen, Stefanus F.

CANORA

Davies, Anthony
Egbagbe, Augustine
Hari Singh, Manjeet
Newstead, Freya J.
Poon, Kea-Keu

CARLYLE

Meyer, Catharina J., FamilyMed

CARONPORT

Bell, Susan D., FamilyMed
Loper, Raymond H.

CARROT RIVER

Herbert, John W.

CHRISTOPHER LAKE

Cross, James W.

CLIMAX

Louwrens, Pierre J.

CUT KNIFE

Steenkamp, Jakobus W.

DAVIDSON

Lang Bayona, Francisco

EASTEND

Davis, Anne L., FamilyMed

EDAM

Mbaogu, Michael N., FamilyMed

EMERALD PARK

Haidash, Serhii

ESTERHAZY

Jansen Van Rensburg, Petrus
Louw, Adriaan P.
Nel, Johann W.
Nel, Mandi
Viljoen, Mighael I.

ESTEVAN

Akinsete, Folajimi
Christie, Allison
Grobler, Andre, FamilyMed
Omosigho, Osamudiamen C.
Ovueni, Efe M.
Pehlivan, Hakan
Sheikh, Khalid M.
Tsoi, Edward Y K., FamilyMed
Yekinni, Idris O.

ESTON

Holmes, Stewart E.

FILLMORE

Bell, Leslie W.
Gibbons, Patrick J.

FOAM LAKE

Bia, F. Hussain F.

FORT QU'APPELLE

Lombard, Jan H.
Saunders, Peter T R.
Tuwor, George, FamilyMed

GOODSOIL

Graham-Rowe, Sydney G.

GRAVELBOURG

Couture, Daniel C.
Pillay, Intheran P.
Ramlakhan, Larita D.

GRENFELL

Pebane, Bright D.

GULL LAKE

Kozroski, Clare J., FamilyMed

HERBERT

Kassett, Suresh P.

HUDSON BAY

Gelhorn, Donald G., FamilyMed
Maree, Pieter J., FamilyMed
Masekoameng, Ramatsiele

HUMBOLDT

Bourgeois, Jacqueline J., FamilyMed
Davids, Terence
Graf, Rose, FamilyMed
Hamman, Wessel
Huber, Warren N.
Kirchgesner, Daniel, FamilyMed
Levick-Brown, Carrie A., FamilyMed
Moola, Ashraf
Moosa, Naseeba
Ockbazghi, Russom, FamilyMed
Saul-Duke, Beverley, FamilyMed
Zwane, Mishack P.

ILE-A-LA-CROSSE

Barnett, Michael G., FamilyMed
Britton, Stephen E A., FamilyMed
Faasen, Johannes
Hanson, Jacelyn, FamilyMed
McGonigle, Darcie, FamilyMed
McGonigle, Reid M., FamilyMed(EM)
Raath, Annemie
Silva, Diana, FamilyMed
Smith, Marlene W.
Turner, Katherine A., FamilyMed

IMPERIAL

Rysbergen, Jacobus

INDIAN HEAD

Pebane, Donald M.
Zimmermann, Bruce R.

KAMSACK

Bibby, Jodi D.
Bishop, Michael B.
Davies, Murray W.
Dudley, Alistair
Ogali, Emmanuel
Rezansoff, Walter E.

KELVINGTON

Mpisi, Bulelwa

KERROBERT

Wentzel, Johann D.

KINDERSLEY

Jimenez-Guerra, Idalberto
Johnson, Daniel A., FamilyMed
Keaveney, Lynda, FamilyMed
Kleinhans, Nerine
Oberleitner, Barry H.

KINISTINO

Moe, Jan F.

KIPLING

Steyn, Johan W.

LA LOCHE

Djan, Deborah
Lefebvre, Guy R B.
Nicholls, Vaughan
Tcherenkova, Inaa A., FamilyMed
Walshe, Kevin J.

LA RONGE

Bayda, Michael C., FamilyMed
Coetzee, Direse, FamilyMed
Covenden, Kanthan L.
Delport, Christo, FamilyMed
Friesen, Lisa C., FamilyMed
Groves, Sean, FamilyMed
Jansen, Nolan P.
Khaketla, Moliehi
Kleingeld, Johannes A.
Marshall, Laura, FamilyMed
Neethling, Bertram L.
Spooner, Betty A., FamilyMed
Stoll, David L., FamilyMed
Tonn, Debra J., FamilyMed

LAFLECHE

Coneys, T. David

LAIRD

Wirth, Sandra S.

LANGENBURG

Van Eeden, Donavan C.

LANIGAN

Saxena, Onkar N.

LEADER

Fanipour, Majid
Hoque, Mohd E.
Palangi, Monga-N'Dimo
Tshabalala, Augustine K.

LLOYDMINSTER

Ajegbo, Obiora N.
Almond, Christopher J., FamilyMed(EM)
Asgari, Nilfoofar
Ashraf, Muhammad
Aslam, Muhammad R.
Bindeman, Annalene F.
Burger, Jeinien
Cassim, Mohamed R H.
Combrinck, Nantes
Dry, Marissa
Du Toit, Lionel
Ekwueme, Henry
Farhat, Najwa F.
Govender, Tinesha
Gusztak, Leo W.
Ilagan-Nyame, Matilde
Jansen Van Vuuren, Cornelius
Kamyar, Mandana
Kloppers, Allan A.
Landsberg, Hester C.
Lowton, Shamira
Mahdavifar, Alireza
Moodley, Deshinee
Mousavinejad, Kiarash
Ogunlewe, Obafemi A.
Pather, Jhodipraghasen
Pellissier, Janse V.
Sayeed, M A. Raffath
Shinyanbola, Olafimihan O.
Uddin, Iftikhar
Van Der Merwe, John S.

LOON LAKE

Bekker, Leon R.

LUMSDEN

Knaus, Russell P.
MacDonald, Susan J.

MAIDSTONE

Roman, Sherwyn
Spangenberg, David F.
Stander, Isabella C.
Stephen Gnanaraj, Leo P., FamilyMed

MAPLE CREEK

Amu-Darko, Kofi, FamilyMed
Govender, Rajan
Mudingayi, Kabuya
Naidoo, Neelandran

MARTENSVILLE

Karam-Dad, Choudhary K.

MEADOW LAKE

Babkis, Andrey Y.
Funk, Sandi, FamilyMed
Johnson, Mervin L., FamilyMed
Kalala, Tshimanga W.
Labrador Febles, Jose
Letkeman, Jacob A.
Loden, Stephen A., FamilyMed
Loots, Leani
Samuel, John P.
Seguin, Aimee M., FamilyMed
Titus, Jolene J.
Van de Venter, Gavin E.
Viljoen, Annette
Vogt, Victoria L., FamilyMed

MELFORT

Begin, Jennifer L., FamilyMed
Hanekom, Pierre
Ige, Olabode A., FamilyMed
Khan, Mohammad A.
Lavoie, Lionel A., FamilyMed
Levendall, Tamzyn D T.
Renouf, John J.
Steffen, Robert M., FamilyMed
Stoll, Michael B., FamilyMed
Strydom, Eben A.
Van Der Ross, Richard R.
Wingate, Jordan T., FamilyMed

MELVILLE

Beny, Majak T., FamilyMed
Eshawesh, Abdulhamid F., FamilyMed
Kolesky, Hendrey C., FamilyMed
Van Zyl, Johan L.

MOOSE JAW

Afolabi, Oyewale A.
Akpan, Udeme E.
Al-Begamy, Youssef S., FamilyMed
Alberts, Martin J A., FamilyMed
Awad-El-Kariem, Sawsan M.
Braun, David F., FamilyMed
Brown, Mark T.
Cruchley, Jane I.
Dautremont, Kevin J.
De Jager, Nico
De Leon, Ernesto L.
Du Toit, Abraham
Fynn, Joanne P C.
Ganesan, Arun
Geyer, Willem J.
Hassan, Ziauddin
Hetherington, Kerri, FamilyMed
Hugo, Pierre M.
Ishwarlall, Sujay
Jacobson, Roger S.
Jansen Van Rensburg, Leon
Louw, Alexander F.
Luhning, Allan H.
Magnaye, Arturo D.
Magnaye, Joyce M.
Majid, Falah S.
Maree, Narinda
Marx, Yolanda
Niaz, Majid
Oyenubi, Abimbola
Ramadan, Fawzi B.
Retief, Leon W.
Rininsland, H. Volker, FamilyMed
Sanderson, Brian J G.
Sanderson, Kirsty J.
Singh, Varsha
Soyege, Adeloye O.
Stushnoff, James J.
Thorpe, R. Brandon
Truter, Rene
Tysdal, Margaret A.
Van Der Merwe, Schalk W.
Van Heerden, Aletta J.
Van Heerden, Gert B.
Van Wyk, Gerritt C B.
Vermaak, Jan A.
Vertue, Peter J.
Vooght, Mark T R.
Wigmore, C. Frederick
Yusuf, Nureni T.

MOOSOMIN

Crouse, Ettiene J., FamilyMed
Kerkhoff, Ross V., FamilyMed
Plewes, Michael E., FamilyMed
Roets, Louisa F.
Roets, Pieter G W.
Van Jaarsveld, Iris M.

NIPAWIN

Albertyn, Albert R.
Baard, Johann
Balakrishnan, Kanapathi P., FamilyMed
Carroll, Bronwyn N.
Chernesky, Patricia A.
Fillis, Melissa R.
Francis, Eleanor
Peffer, Dale V F.
Reddy, Nelini
Smith, Corne S.
Van Der Merwe, Neville D.
Van Heerden, Hendrik G.
Van Heerden, Martha M.

NOKOMIS

Anderson, Adarine
Lim, Bee K.

NORTH BATTLEFORD

Ahmad, Shahabuddin
Anees, Muhammad
Bairagi, Niranjan
Bairagi, Ranjana
Bedi, Vishal
Bezuidenhout, Kenneth
Botha, Mattheus J.
Cholin, Brenda L., FamilyMed
Craib, Gordon G W.
Du Plessis, Aldine
Duncan, David A.
Dunhin, Anna
Fadare, Kayode
Fernandes, Geraldo A J.
Hesselson, Jeffrey P., FamilyMed
Holtzhausen, Peter J., FamilyMed
Ibarreta, Nelson Y.
Johnson, James C., FamilyMed
Khurana, Mahesh C.
La Cock, Mari C.
Lipsett, William G C.
Marcelo-Macalino, Magdalena
Mehboob, Mohammad, FamilyMed
Morton, David N.
Nwachukwu, Kingsley
Obikoya, Olubankole
Oyewole, Olusegun
Pentz, Daniel S S.
Prystupa, Aaron J., FamilyMed
Ramachandran, Kizhake V.
Ramachandran, Nirmala
Selhi, Brahm D., FamilyMed
Tootoosis, Janet J., FamilyMed
Van Der Merwe, Wynand A.
Van Vuuren, Hermanus
Viviers, Willem F.

OUTLOOK

Mtshali, Raphael T.
Mynhardt, Heinrich D., FamilyMed

OXBOW

Botha, Nicolaas C.
Hyman, David I., FamilyMed

PARADISE HILL

Warburton, Malcolm A.

PONTEIX

Barretto, Ignacio J M.

PORCUPINE PLAIN

Pieterse, Gert C S.
Scharfstein, S. Briane, FamilyMed

PREECEVILLE

Kabongo, Tshipita, FamilyMed

PRINCE ALBERT

Adamus, Allison T K., FamilyMed
Ahmad, Afzaal
Alheit, Berthold
Ardell, Dale M R., FamilyMed
Ardell, Robert A., FamilyMed
Asefa, Victor K K.
Barker, Horace R M A.
Basson, Nico
Bischoff, Jan C., FamilyMed
Botha, Lachelle G.
Brits, Annalie W.
Brown, James R., FamilyMed
Bruntrup-Taylor, Jennifer
Cantin, Craig P., FamilyMed
Chaudhry, Zubaida A.
Chokani, Khami
Chrusch, Maurice G.
Coertze, Louis J., FamilyMed
Cornelissen, Rohan
Davis, Breanna, FamilyMed
De Beer, Lodewyk N.
De Padua, Felix B.
De Villiers, Christie
Egbeyemi, Olanrewaju Y., FamilyMed
Elmer, Craig D.

Eshaghian, Reza L., FamilyMed
Furstenberg, Josias
Gallins, Colin, FamilyMed
Halyk, Mark A.
Hammond, Cecil M.
Harris, James M.
Holton, Peggy J.
Hookenson, Brenda J.
James, Michelle
Janse Van Rensberg, Annelie, FamilyMed
Kapp, Sanet
Kemp, Cornelius J.
Khan, Tariq S.
Kriel, Johannes N., FamilyMed
Lal, Sushma
Lanoie, Leo O., FamilyMed
Le Roux, Noelene
Lombard, Schalk J., FamilyMed
Lotz, Christo
Mabadeje, Oladapo
Maciel, Estanislao
Maier, Fred
Malhotra, Lalita
Marten, Dion M., FamilyMed
Martin, Allison S.
Maya, Nomtandazo P T.
Moodley, Santhiran
Moodliar, Romashnee
Mwana, N'siabar J.
Narothum, Paresh S.
Obienu, Emeka
Obrigavitch, Gregory R., FamilyMed
Oleksinski, W. Stanley, FamilyMed
Oriee, Mandhira I.
Painter, Nigel A.
Parekh, Vipul Z., FamilyMed
Pillay, Yagan
Rashid, M D. Mizanur
Rossouw, Francois P., FamilyMed(EM)
Rye, John G., FamilyMed
Sabaratnam, Rathi M.
Schemenauer, Chelsea M., FamilyMed
Silveira, Benzil M P.
Smit, Ferdie
Smith-Windsor, Thomas B., FamilyMed
Sriram, Priya N., FamilyMed
Stevens, David J.
Steyn, Jacobus A.
Sukkhu, Visham
Surkan, Donald G.
Swamy, Gandhaparimala N A.
Taj, Anita A.
Thangavelu, Dheshnie
Unsworth, Roderick J.
Van Der Merwe, Jacobus J J.
Veith, Martin
Veith, Sylvia H.
Wessels, Johann B.

RADISSON

Stalder, Lisa J., FamilyMed

RADVILLE

Helms, Nelly W.
Oberholzer, Werner, FamilyMed

REDVERS

Kgobisa, Lettie

REGINA

Abraham, J. Mathew
Achyuthan, Geeta
Adams, Mohamed N Z.
Adedipe, Olusola A.
Ahlijah, William K.
Airir, Abdelhafid
Akinloye, Olayiwola O.
Akot, Mawien M.
Al-Hayki, Maryam M A.
Ali, Amjad
Alibhai, Malyha, FamilyMed
Alibhai, Nasimbanu S.
Amjad, Asim
Anstead, Keith S.
Arndt, Susanne E., FamilyMed
Arnold, Angela J., FamilyMed(EM)
Arnold, Pamela J., FamilyMed
Arthur, Jane
Aspe Lucero, Carlos
Baldwin, Joan F D., FamilyMed
Barnard, Werner J.
Berriman, Katherine A.
Bester, Stephen C., FamilyMed
Bhagaloo, Lanishen
Bhuiyan, Salah U.
Blignaut, Lourens P G.
Boan, Jarol L.
Bodani, Jayalakshmi P.
Bouwer, Hester A.
Bowen, Francis A., FamilyMed(EM)
Bradel, Theresa M., FamilyMed
Brown, J. Donovan, FamilyMed
Brown, Tanya
Brown, Theodorah N.
Caburao, Isaac C.
Cameron, Elizabeth A.
Cameron, Mark H., FamilyMed
Casey, Maitias D.
Chalchal, Haji I.
Chandrakanth, Soornahalli
Chang, Peter S., FamilyMed
Chapple, Ruhiya B.
Cheshenchuk, Svitlana, FamilyMed
Chikukwa, Tineyi
Chin, Gordon M.
Coomaran, Vasuki
Coruzzi, James A., FamilyMed(EM)
Cowan, Ian M.
Cowley, Jennifer S., FamilyMed
Cutts, Danielle D., FamilyMed
Danielson, Jerry D.
Das, Jyoti N.
Datta, Samir, FamilyMed
De Lange, Hendrik
De Witt, Jacobus
Deb, Bakul
Deptuch, John M.
Dickson, Michael J.
Diener, Tania
Dolata, Wojciech
Draper, C. Lewis W., FamilyMed
Egware, Oluwatomi, FamilyMed
Eisa, Mohamed
Emokpare, Bernard D.
Emslie, Linda M.
Endsin, Arnold, FamilyMed
Ene, Mokelu
Ferguson, Kathleen J., FamilyMed(EM)
Fourie, Jan, FamilyMed
Ganshorn, Keren D., FamilyMed
Geddes, Carol A., FamilyMed
Gerbrands, Bea, FamilyMed
Golubovic, Dragan
Govender, Krishnasamy
Goyal, Seema, FamilyMed
Gruschenko, Pavlo
Gruszczynski, Adam, FamilyMed
Hamilton, Joan, FamilyMed
Hansia, Mohammed R.
Hanson, Johnathon, FamilyMed(EM)
Haq, M. Mansoor
Harris, Paul M., FamilyMed
Hennink, Maurice H J.
Heroux, Martin, FamilyMed(EM)
Hochban, Ty J.
Horner, Robert, FamilyMed(EM)
Hughes, Robin J., FamilyMed(EM)
Humayun, Kiran, FamilyMed
Ijaz, Mohammad S.
Islam, Mohammad Z.
Jacobsz, Nicolette
Javid, Sabiha, FamilyMed
Johnson, Carmen L., FamilyMed
Jones, Denis
Jones, Sylvie A., FamilyMed
Joseph, Jacqueline J.
Joseph, Javed
Juggernath, Nivas
Kaban, Glenda D., FamilyMed(EM)
Kamrul, Rejina, FamilyMed
Katz, Ronald
Kavulu, Anne L., FamilyMed
Kazmi, Najma
Khaladkar, Sunil V., FamilyMed
Khalifa, Amer J., FamilyMed
Khan, M. Ibrahim
Khan, Mohammad M.
Khan, Mujtaba A., FamilyMed
Kilmury, Alana J., FamilyMed
Kimball, Lauren E., FamilyMed
Kondrashov, Maxim V., FamilyMed
Konstantynowicz, Barbara R., FamilyMed
Kontsiotis, Akatereny, FamilyMed
Korley, Ebenezer K.
Kothare, Dnyanada L.
Kriek, Gileam J.
Kruger, Garth
Kumar, Patel R V.
Kuzmicz, Jennifer E., FamilyMed
Labuschagne, Barend C J.
Lai, Raymond P C.
Laursen, Brian W.
Lavelle, Nancy L.
Lawrence, Kathrine J., FamilyMed
Le Roux, Eric W.
Le Roux, Marion A.
Leibel, Sharon M.
Leung, Eric, FamilyMed
Lionel, Jesuraj
Liskowich, Sarah, FamilyMed
Llewelyn-Williams, Warwick
Logan, Dolores A F., FamilyMed
Lok, Winston A.
Lotz, Albertus B.
Lotz, Heloise
Lukubisa, Alexander
Luther, John K.
Lyster, Kish E., FamilyMed(EM)
Mahmood, Shazia T.
Mahmud, M. Hayat
Mahood, Sara S C., FamilyMed
Makiwane, Unati
Markovski, Milena, FamilyMed
Maroof, Razawa F., FamilyMed
Matand, Tshilay
Matthews, Jill A.
Mbanza, Denis B.
McLeod, Joanne M., FamilyMed
McMaster, Robin D M., FamilyMed
McMeekin-Down, Nadine R., FamilyMed
McMillan, J. Stewart, FamilyMed
Mettle, Valerie, FamilyMed
Meyer, Abraham P., FamilyMed(EM)
Michel, Joseph G., FamilyMed
Miller, Allan J., FamilyMed
Miller, Owen S., FamilyMed
Ming-Fok, Terence L.
Minnaar, Petrus A.
Montbriand, Michael W., FamilyMed
Moolla, Mohamed
Moorosi, Setsoana L.
Mordasiewicz, Merunka A., FamilyMed
Morris, John C B.
Mugerwa, Abimanyi S J.
Muhammad, Iffat A.
Muller, Pieter E.
Naidoo, Therusha
Nair, Ratheesh S., FamilyMed
Ndeke, Issa A.
Nesbitt, Raenelle E., FamilyMed
Nicholls, Michael J., FamilyMed
Nilson, Linda Lee
O'Byrne, Gregory K.
O'Carroll, Tiann F A., FamilyMed(EM)
Odenigbo, Chukwuemeka
Offiah, Francis O., FamilyMed
Oluma, Elias T.
Ooi, Teik Im
Otitoju, Chinyere
Overli-Domes, Carmel L K., FamilyMed
Parvez, Naeem
Parwez, Naumana A.
Patel, Dinubhai G.
Patel, Indravadan M.
Patel, Kalpana R.
Patel, Rajnikant L.
Paul, Ashis K.
Paul, Shefali
Pervaiz, Khalid, FamilyMed
Peti, Charles A.
Pham, Van Duc
Pillay, Kumaravel K., FamilyMed(EM)
Pillay, Nalini
Pillay, Poogendren
Pillay, Vinesh
Pineda, Maria D., FamilyMed
Pole, Meena
Potgieter, Lucas-Martin, FamilyMed
Potgieter, Tania
Rahaman, Sheriff
Rasmussen, Ole S.
Rathgeber, Lane A., FamilyMed(EM)
Rocha Michaels, Clara E.
Rose, Alwyn L E.
Ross, Terrance A., FamilyMed(EM)
Rossouw, Jacobus P.
Rossouw, Linell
Rudovica, Jelena
Rudovics, Aivars
Saczek, Krzysztof
Sadikov, Evgeny A.
Salgado De Leon, Luis A.
Salim, Muhammad
Scariah, Swapna A C.
Schonken, Willem P.
Schussler, Otto
Scott, Verna D., FamilyMed
Segu, Michael K B.
Shamsuzzaman, Mohammed, FamilyMed
Shareef, Mohammad
Sharman, Madan G.
Sheikh, Ahmad S.
Singh, Kulrajmohinder
Slabbert, Jacobus A.
Smith, Sheila M., FamilyMed(EM)
Soko, Phinda D.
Sood, Narinder
Srinivasagam, Vuthamy M R.
Sundar, Ishaan P., FamilyMed
Suri, Pravesh K.
Surtie, Faizel R.
Swart, Petrus J.
Talukdar, Sneha P.
Taylor, Ronald P., FamilyMed(EM)
Thackeray, Victor T., FamilyMed
Thomas, Biju K.
Timol, Farzana
Torri, Vamsee
Ugwumba, Rukevwe, FamilyMed
Ukabam, Sylvester O.
Ur Rahman, Asad
Van Der Merwe, Henrik
Van Der Merwe, Jan G.
Van Der Watt, Leon
Van Heerden, Jacobus J.
Van Rooyen, Hugo M., FamilyMed
Van Rooyen, Peter J.
Van Staden, Johannes J.
Vantomme, Sylvia B., FamilyMed
Vennam, Ramesh B.
Vermeulen, Abraham P M., FamilyMed
Vorster, Beukes J.
Warden, David H., FamilyMed
White, Gill N., FamilyMed
Whittick, John D R., FamilyMed
Wildenboer, Wilhelmina H., FamilyMed
Williams, Fouche, FamilyMed
Zagozeski, Cheryl A., FamilyMed
Zaidi, Syed A A., FamilyMed
Zarkovic, Mirjana

ROSETOWN

Ernst, Alfred H., FamilyMed
Igbekoyi, Olawale F.
Ledding, James D.
Ledding, M. David
Olubajo, Olabisi A., FamilyMed

ROSTHERN

Baker, Linda M.
Gandham, Prem
MacMillan, James, FamilyMed
Melle, Jesse R., FamilyMed

SASKATOON

Abbas, Tahir
Abdelmallek, Irini A A.
Abdelsayed, Nagy S I.
Abdul Hadi, Reem S O., FamilyMed
Adelugba, Olajide O.
Ahmad, Nazir
Ahmed, Osama S E.
Al-Katib, Fatih M W.
Amin, Devendra H.
Anderson, Barbara A.
Andres, Deirdre E., FamilyMed
Andres, Salvador J.
Ansell, Chantal D., FamilyMed
Anyanwu, Leonard U.
Archer, David D., FamilyMed
Arendse, Regan E.
Arnold, Florence P.
Asfour, Nabil
Baillod, Alanna B.
Balasingam, Sivadevi
Balaton, Joseph M., FamilyMed
Balaton, Julianna E K., FamilyMed
Barnardo, Georgina C., FamilyMed
Basker, Ivor G W.
Batool, Muqadas, FamilyMed
Bayly, Kenneth E.
Behl, Vernon, FamilyMed(EM)
Belak, Zenon D.
Bell, Clifford D., FamilyMed
Berger, Aimo, FamilyMed
Bettin, Leane N., FamilyMed
Billington, Robert G., FamilyMed
Blaser, Jill A., FamilyMed
Boan, Derek H., FamilyMed
Boechler, Mark D.
Bofoya, Boyale J.
Bowman, Collin P.
Brilz, Anthony P., FamilyMed(EM)
Bristol, Roger, FamilyMed(EM)
Brodie, Deborah J., FamilyMed
Bucko, Jacqueline E., FamilyMed
Butt, Peter R., FamilyMed(EM)
Buttinger, Chris S., FamilyMed
Cameron, Donna M., FamilyMed
Caspar-Bell, Gudrun M.
Chad, Jennifer M., FamilyMed
Chamarti, Venkata R.
Chan, Christopher W J.
Changela, Jayantilal J., FamilyMed
Chao, Roger W.
Chawane-Bekwayo, Nomhle N.
Chernenkoff, William, FamilyMed
Chernoff, D. Roy, FamilyMed
Chin, Joe Y J.
Clapson, J. Brian, FamilyMed
Clark, Keith M., FamilyMed
Classen, Shawn C., FamilyMed
Coates, Beverley A.
Colwell, Robin L.
Conacher, Heather J., FamilyMed
Courtney, Rosemary F., FamilyMed
Cribb, Alina, FamilyMed
Cronje, Rynier
Daguio, Glenn
Dahl, Eileen R., FamilyMed
Daniels, Gavin R.
Danilkewich, Alanna D., FamilyMed
Das, Indranil, FamilyMed
Datta, Jyotirmoy
Dattani, Indravadan D., FamilyMed
Demkiw-Bartel, Coby, FamilyMed
Deutscher, Myles, FamilyMed
Dick, Barry J M.
Doig, Anne F., FamilyMed
Dosman, John, FamilyMed
Drummond, Robbie N., FamilyMed(EM)
du Rand, Jean
du Rand, Mia
du Toit, Elmarie
Dyck, Kelly, FamilyMed
El-Gayed, Ali Abdel Halim Hussein.
El-Sayed, Assem S M.
Elemary, Mohamed

Enweani, Cyprian C., FamilyMed
Erraguntla, Vasudha
Fenton, Shanna L., FamilyMed
Ferguson, Joanne L., FamilyMed
Fern, Brian J.
Fitzpatrick, Philip, FamilyMed(EM)
Fournier Marshall, Colette S., FamilyMed(EM)
Friggstad, Aaron K., FamilyMed
Froh, John S., FamilyMed(EM)
Gabruch, Thomas K., FamilyMed
Gaertner, Paul H., FamilyMed(EM)
Gafoor, Farah, FamilyMed
Gafoor, Tasnim
Gagne, Louise E M.
Geller, Brian E., FamilyMed
Gericke, Werner
Getz, Corina, FamilyMed
Gibson, Leila
Gimon, Eglee, FamilyMed
Goluboff, Steven S., FamilyMed
Gooding, Vivian J., FamilyMed
Goojha, Devdass
Goubran Messiha, Hadi
Guselle, Tracey L., FamilyMed
Haider, Kamal-Uddin
Hailu, Tadesse
Halldorson, Heather G., FamilyMed
Hamilton, Erin, FamilyMed
Harrington, Andrew J.
Hattingh, H. Suzanne
Haug, Delmer O., FamilyMed
Haver, William J.
Helfrich, Leanne C., FamilyMed
Helliar, Stephen G.
Hey, Jonathan D., FamilyMed
Hislop, Lois
Holinaty, Carla, FamilyMed
Holmes, Vicki R.
Honish, Colin, FamilyMed
Hosain, Jason, FamilyMed
Howlett, Evan J.
Huang, Anne A., FamilyMed
Hudspith, Elizabeth
Humnicka-Szott, Malgorzata, FamilyMed
Hussain, Syed S., FamilyMed
Ibrahim, Narmin, FamilyMed
Insley, Kristyn J., FamilyMed
Iqbal, Nayyer
Ismail, Waleed S.
Ivanans, Nicholas C., FamilyMed(EM)
Iverson, Lance M., FamilyMed(EM)
Jamil, Najma
Johnson, Andrea L., FamilyMed
Johnson, Terrence R.
Johnstone, Jennifer L., FamilyMed
Jooravan, Sujeeth J.
Joubert, Hendrina J.
Jubin, Donna L., FamilyMed
Judd, Andrew S.
Jutras, Michel N., FamilyMed
Karras, Beverley E., FamilyMed
Kasmaiefar, Farzin
Kaur, Manjit
Kennedy, Shayla L.
Khan, Rukhshanda J., FamilyMed
Khanna, Charu, FamilyMed
Khayyam, Naiyar
Klassen, Ernest H.
Klym, Carol M.
Kohll, David E.
Kostyniuk, Ronald W.
Kozakavich, Ronald N.
Kriegler, Johann C.
Kundapur, Vijayananda
Kwok, Leung Sun
Labelle, Paul D., FamilyMed
Lacny, Andrew M.
Ladham, Shaun A.
Lanigan, Dennis T.
Lapetsky, Angela M., FamilyMed
Large, Barbara J.
Larson, Berwyn L., FamilyMed
Laubscher, Tessa A., FamilyMed
Le Roux, Carl J.
Leakos, Richard J., FamilyMed
Ledding, Edward C.
Ledray, Lynda L., FamilyMed
Lees, Mark, FamilyMed
Ling, Patrick M C., FamilyMed(EM)
Lubiantoro, Elsa, FamilyMed
Magee, James F.
Makinde, Oluyele A.
Malan, Catharina M.
Malan, Johann H.
Maltman, Shirley A.
Manonyane, Jacob M.
Manzini, Prince C.
Mark, M. Kit, FamilyMed
Markentin, Morris, FamilyMed
Martens, Brian R.
Marushak, Karen L.
McAllister, G. Rae
McBride, George A.
McDonald, Clint A.
McFadden, Laura L., FamilyMed
McIsaac, Matthew C., FamilyMed
McKague, Meredith, FamilyMed
McKee, Nora D., FamilyMed
McKee, W. Hugh, FamilyMed
McKinney, Veronica R., FamilyMed
McLaughlin, Sarah G., FamilyMed
McMahon, Margaret A., FamilyMed
McMahon, Selma, FamilyMed
Meier, Courtney C L., FamilyMed
Meili, Ryan D., FamilyMed
Mensah, Cynthia, FamilyMed
Merryweather, Leslie E., FamilyMed
Mettle, Armstrong N A.
Mia, Shabir M.
Miakhil, Mohsen
Misfeldt, Marlys
Mitchell, Thomas, FamilyMed
Mohamed, Adel
Mohamed, Mohamed F.
Mohr, Karen L., FamilyMed(EM)
Muller, Andries J., FamilyMed
Naidu, Diananeethie
Nataraj, Jonathon S Y., FamilyMed
Nataraj, Yellepeddy
Naugler, R. Gary
Nave, Cynthia J., FamilyMed
Nayar, Arun, FamilyMed
Nickel, Lucy C., FamilyMed
Nykiforuk, Edward M.
O'Neill, Ryan D., FamilyMed(EM)
Obayan, Aderonke O.
Ogieglo, Adam, FamilyMed
Old, C. Lee, FamilyMed
Ollegasagrem, Nirmaladevi, FamilyMed
Olszynski, Ewa P., FamilyMed
Olszynski, Paul A., FamilyMed(EM)
Opdahl, Murray D., FamilyMed
Opondo, Johnmark O.
Otani, Christine M L., FamilyMed
Owen, John S.
Padayachee, Vinogaran T.
Paley, Paula M., FamilyMed
Papenfus, William J., FamilyMed(EM)
Parker, Robert D.
Paruk, Sameer
Patenaude, Jana R., FamilyMed
Pawluck, Larissa A., FamilyMed
Pearson, W. Dallas N., FamilyMed(EM)
Pesenti, John G., FamilyMed
Pierce, Dawne E J., FamilyMed
Pilot, Lorne R.
Popick, Dallas
Poulin, David N., FamilyMed(EM)
Powalinsky, Agnes C C., FamilyMed
Prisciak, Jared S., FamilyMed
Rabin, Michael
Rajpal, Anupma, FamilyMed
Rattan, Ukesha
Rebalkin, Garry N.
Reiniger, Rhonda M., FamilyMed
Reitz, Francois
Rieder, Barry W.
Robinson, Arthur, FamilyMed
Roelens, Kurt R E.
Rubab, Shehla
Russell, Robert S.
Saad, Ali G.
Sabbagh, Zohreh
Sader, Naeem
Saleh, Dlair
Sami, Amer
Sander, Ryan A., FamilyMed
Sasbrink-Harkema, Ashley, FamilyMed(EM)
Saxena, Mitra, FamilyMed
Schubert, Roderick A., FamilyMed
Schwann, Paula G., FamilyMed
Seibel, Deborah A., FamilyMed
Shaw, John M.
Shaw, Karen
Shenouda, Amir Z.
Shukla, Karunakar
Shukla, Sushama
Singh, Madhuri
Slavik, Dalibor E., FamilyMed
Slobodzian, Donna M., FamilyMed
Smit, Shawn
Smith, Colum J J.
Smith, Joanna D., FamilyMed(EM)
Smith, Patricia R., FamilyMed
Sperling, Bradley D., FamilyMed
Stakiw, Kenneth J., FamilyMed
Stalker, Penelope E., FamilyMed
Stefiuk, Donald L.
Stempien, James E., FamilyMed(EM)
Steplewski, Jacek D.
Stewart, Lois M.
Strydom, Heinre
Suryavanshi, Sudhir K.
Syed, Badruddin
Symon, Andrea L., FamilyMed
Taillon, Paul A., FamilyMed
Tandon, Ramesh K.
Tanski, Jennifer A.
Taratibu, Mozwa B.
Tellez-Zenteno, Jose F.
Teofilov, Ivan K.
Terepa, Mary I., FamilyMed
Thompson, Katherine M E., FamilyMed
Tshiyombo, Tshala
Tymchak, Zane A.
Ullah, Ismat
Uzoho, Festus O., FamilyMed
Vachhrajani, Hareshkumar V.
Van De Kamp, Schaana M., FamilyMed(EM)
Van Der Merwe, Adam B.
Van Der Merwe, Vanessa
Van Zanten, Audrey
Van Zyl, Stephanus F., FamilyMed
Vaska, Solomon R.
Vassos, Laurie J.
Veikle, Conrad J., FamilyMed
Viden, Lonny H., FamilyMed
Viger, Marc D., FamilyMed
Vos, Andre J., FamilyMed
Wagner, Susan G., FamilyMed
Wahba, Mark Y., FamilyMed(EM)
Walker, Grace V., FamilyMed
Walton, Lloyd T.
Wanson, Laurent P.
Wardell, Florence E B.
Weetman, Sara B., FamilyMed(EM)
Wegner, Sandra L.
Werbicki, James E., FamilyMed(EM)
Whitehead, Stephen M.
Williams, Sarah L., FamilyMed
Witt, Jonathan A., FamilyMed(EM)
Wright, Heather D L., FamilyMed
Wu, Yan, FamilyMed
Wu, Yue
Yadav, Sunil K.
Yatsina, Alexandre N.
Yatsina, Oksana Y., FamilyMed
Yelland, Joel C.
Zlipko, Terrance S.

SHELLBROOK

Ajogwu, Chamberlain
Ibrahim, Imran, FamilyMed
Nguegno, Anatole

SPIRITWOOD

Person, Terri A., FamilyMed
Senzani, Farai D.
Wall, Ronald B.

SWIFT CURRENT

Addai, Stephen A.
Adwedaa, Ebenezer O.
Ahmodu, Olorunfemi S.
Ashtekar, Vijaykumar V.
Banks, Malcolm R.
Bartsch, Margaret, FamilyMed
Byker, Leonard
Claassen, Andre N.
de Klerk, Hein S.
Du Toit, Stefanus E.
Fakhir, Shamsuddin
Gatzke, Jason B., FamilyMed(EM)
Ghori, Aqeel
Gill, Jasdildar, FamilyMed
Gordon, Terrance M.
Harrison, Sarah D., FamilyMed
Ibrahim, Rizqi N.
Jagga, Michele
Johnston, David A.
Kielly, G. Andrew, FamilyMed
Lee, Tara S., FamilyMed
Moola, Dawood
Mulla, Amith A.
Muwanguzi, Michael M.
Ojo, Alaba
Radevski, Ivelin, FamilyMed
Sabri, Ali
Savoy, Effie, FamilyMed
Serwadda, Rosemary C M.
Shah, Syed M H.
Steenberg, Lourens J.
Steenberg, Melane
Tumbach, Janna L., FamilyMed
Valtchanova, Zdravka P., FamilyMed
Van Breda, Alta
Van Der Berg, Nicolaas M.
Wakefield, Tara S., FamilyMed

TISDALE

Orhadje, Charles
Richardson, Rosemarie T.
Shewchuk, John J., FamilyMed
Smith, Aleka
Sommer, Linda E.
Van Jaarsveld, Juliana B.

TURTLEFORD

Dandugula, Raghu M., FamilyMed
Ghauri, Imran K., FamilyMed
Tshatshela, Mzikayise

UNITY

Bloem, Linda
Streng-Coetzee, Ilana
Williams, Lyle K.

WADENA

Kiapway, Mosenza

WAKAW

Gholamabbas Javan, Asef
Gwiazda, Zbigniew
Lekota, Phuma J.

WARMAN

Franko, Evan P., FamilyMed(EM)
Neumann, Timothy, FamilyMed
Smit, Marcel M.

Zerajic, Sinisa, FamilyMed

WATROUS

Akhtar, Hammad, FamilyMed
Latakgomo, Lehlohonolo
Mouton, Abraham J.
Smit, Maria J.

WEYBURN

Bierman, Petrus J L.
Bigland, Karen W W.
Erhaze, Irhuo
Fong, Allan C.
Fong, Kathleen C.
Fong Wai Chin, Philip A.
Lenferna de la Motte, P. Alain
McCollam, Mary P., FamilyMed
Nyunheign, Omer
Paszkiewicz, Mariusz T.
Roy, Kamalesh C.
Shwe, Kyaw, FamilyMed
Stewart, Boyd E M.
Warren, Jessi K., FamilyMed

WHITEWOOD

Joomun, M K. Rashid

WILKIE

Kemp, David R.

WOLSELEY

Bella-Lufu, Mbuyamba

WYNYARD

Litwin, Crystal D., FamilyMed
Salter, Martin R., FamilyMed

YORKTON

Akinnawonu, Anthony
Boroto, Kahimano
de Gooijer, Lisa, FamilyMed
Eybers, Von
Fourie, Phillip J.
Groenewald, Petrus J., FamilyMed
Hahn, Johann A.
Jayasinghe, Hettiarachchige
Jokhan, Rikash
Kasim, Yusuf M.
Koudsi, Nasir M.
Kowe, Olajide O.
Lawale, Dag L., FamilyMed
Lee, Frank R.
Manyande, Tekesai T P.
Meiring, Gert J.
Nsungu, Mandiangu
O'Neill, Roger R.
Oduntan, Oluwole O.
Ogunbiyi, Ajibola
Oloko, Saliu
Onyegbule, Henry O.
Oosthuizen, Annelie
Otukoya, Folorunsho
Roodt, Johann
Salib, Michel G.
Schoeman, Corne S.
Swan, Nadine T.
Van Heerden, Andries C.
Vorster, Johannes J.
Vorster, Rene

YUKON TERRITORY

DAWSON

Devenish, Joanne M.
Parsons, J W. Gerard, FamilyMed
Scheer, Aedes N., FamilyMed
Sherrard, Adam W G., FamilyMed

MAYO

Bakri, A. Majid

WATSON LAKE

Secerbegovic, Said
Secerbegovic, Tanis R., FamilyMed
Vostretsov, Stepan

WHITEHORSE

Abraham, Jacob, FamilyMed
Ahmed, Rahel, FamilyMed(EM)
Alton, Susan H., FamilyMed
Anderson, Peter J.
Avery, Bradley C., FamilyMed
Bamford, J D. Russell, FamilyMed
Blaker, Jessica, FamilyMed
Boothroyd, Wendy M.
Breitkreutz, Cindy E., FamilyMed
Brown, Kathryn, FamilyMed
Buchanan, Stephanie, FamilyMed
Carew, Daniel A., FamilyMed
Crawford, Marjorie C.
de La Mare, Eric A.
Densmore, Lis
Gagnon, Isabelle
Gudapati, Sumathi
Hanley, Brendan E., FamilyMed(EM)
Heredia, Armando
Himmelsbach, Sherillynne, FamilyMed
Ikeji, Ngozi
Jamieson, Robin N., FamilyMed(EM)
Kanachowski, Danusia A.
Koltun, Ronald N., FamilyMed(EM)
Lazeo, Sharon R.
Macdonald, Sara E.
Mayes, Adrienne A., FamilyMed
Phillips, Ross E., FamilyMed
Pronovost, Marc E., FamilyMed(EM)
Quong, James K., FamilyMed
Reddoch, Allon
Rhein, Anke, FamilyMed
Saleheh Shoshtari, Peyman, FamilyMed
Seal, Iain D.
Starks, Stephanie A., FamilyMed
Stuart, Lucille, FamilyMed
Syed, Shahid
Tadepalli, Srinivasa R.
Tirschmann, Gunnar, FamilyMed
Todd, Bruce L S.
Williams, Anne C., FamilyMed
Zhang, Siui-Mei

SECTION 3 — CERTIFIED SPECIALISTS LISTED GEOGRAPHICALLY ACCORDING TO SPECIALTY

SPECIALTIES

Anatomical Pathology

ALBERTA

CALGARY
Abi Daoud, Marie
Alanen, Kenneth W.
Auer-Grzesiak, Iwona A.
Barber, Duane F.
Benediktsson, Hallgrimur
Bromley, Amy B.
Bruecks, Andrea K.
Bures, Nicole F.
Chebib, Ivan A.
Demetrick, Douglas
Di Francesco, Lisa M.
Duggan, Maire
Eidus, Leslie B.
Falck, Vincent G.
Fontaine, Daniel G.
George, David H.
Gorecki, Margaret A.
Gorombey, Steve J.
Gough, James
Guggisberg, Kelly A.
Hunter, Charlene A.
Jadusingh, Inderman H.
Jiang, Xiu Yan
Kelly, Margaret M.
Khalil, Moosa N G.
Kulaga, Andrzej
Larsen, Erik T.
Lee, Sandra L.
Leung, Miriam M L.
Luedtke, Chad C.
Magliocco, Anthony M.
Matshes, Evan V W.
Medlicott, Shaun A C.
Meier, Lucja U.
Morava-Protzner, Izabella
Mourad, Walid A A.
Ogilvie, R. Travis
Oryschak, Allan F.
Paslawski, Doreen E.
Pinto-Rojas, Alfredo
Schell, Andrew J.
Shabani-Rad, Meer-Taher
Sienko, Anna E.
Smith, Dean F.
Trevenen, Cynthia L.
Trotter, Martin J.
Trpkov, Kiril
Urbanski, Stefan J.
Waghray, Ranjit K.
Yang, Hua
Yilmaz, Asli
Yu, Weiming

COALDALE
Boras, Valerie F.

EDMONTON
Alakija, Pauline
Anwar, Syed S.
Bacani, Julinor T.
Balachandra, Brinda
Bano, Ather
Berendt, Richard C.
Bigras, Gilbert
Chaba, Todd P.
Chan, Suzanne
Charrois, Gregory J R.
Chiu, Brian K Y.
Deschenes, Jean L.
Dong, Wei-Feng
Dowling, Graeme P.
Ewanowich, Carol A.
Garady, Cherif Issa
Gritter, Hilda L.
Higa, Thomas E.
Hugh, Judith C.
Hwang, June H K.
Jacques, John
Lee, Mark W.
McLean, D. Ross
Moreno, Juan C.
Puttagunta, Lakshmi
Rayani, Nargis A.
Rayner, David C.
Reid, Andre
Russell, Laurie J M.
Salarieh, Afshin
Sauvageau, Anny
Sihra, Sona K.
Silverman, Svetlana
Sim, Adrian B T.
Sis, Banu
Slatnik, Jacek
Solez, Kim
Thiesen, Aducio L.
West, John R.
Wood, George O.

LETHBRIDGE
Greeff, Michael P.
Groenenboom Jankunis, Marion B.
Hegedus, Csaba
Lyon, David C.
Popma, Barbara H.

MEDICINE HAT
Chow, Wai-Kwan
Moreno Merlo, Fernando D.
O'Connor, Michael E.
Silva Martinez, Julio C.

RED DEER
Elomami, Abdulghani
Fauth, Clarissa T.
Horne, Garnet J.
Jo, Woo Je
Parai, Mira R.
Parai, Sushil K.
Sileikiene, Danguole
Thompson, Angela D.

BRITISH COLUMBIA

ABBOTSFORD
Parker, Robin L.

BOWEN ISLAND
Boone, Sharon A.

COMOX
Bellamy, Christopher D.
Donn, Wayne B.

FORT ST. JOHN
Heydarzadeh-Azar, Kamran

KAMLOOPS
Maung, Raymond T A.
McNeely, T. Bruce D.
Molgat, Gilles F.
Stephen, James W M.

KELOWNA
Bainbridge, Terry C.
Li, Qiuyan
Naghibi Torbati, Bibi A.

NANAIMO
Esakia, Elvira
Kontozoglou, Theodosios
Loken, Steven D.

NEW WESTMINSTER
Charlesworth, J. David
Cooney, Thomas P.
Cornell, I. Scott
Grabiec, Joseph T.
Law, Anthony C H.
Shiau, Carolyn J.
Straathof, Danny
Vice, Frances B.

NORTH VANCOUVER
Akbari, Majid
Chercover, David
Vaziri, Mojgan
Vischer, Gisela H.
Wolber, Robert A.

PRINCE GEORGE
Tsang, Katherine

SURREY
Berean, Kenneth W.
Darbyshire, James M.
Grant, Dennis R.
O'Connell, John X.
Shin, Doo Ho

VANCOUVER
Al-Dandan, Sadeq W A.
Allard, Michael F.
Ball, Nigel J.
Banerjee, Diponkar
Ceballos, Katherine M.
Clement, Philip B V.
Coupland, Robert W.
Crawford, Richard I.
Dorovini-Zis, Catherine
English, John C.
Filipenko, J. Douglas
Flint, Julia D A.
Gilks, C. Blake
Hayes, Malcolm M M.
Hendson, Glenda
Hiruki, Tadaaki
Holden, Janet K.
Huwait, Hassan
Ionescu, Diana
Jones, Edward C.
Klein-Parker, Helga
Lee, Carol K.
Lee, Cheng-Han
Magil, Alexander B.
Maguire, John A C.
Makretsov, Nikita A.
Martinka, Magdalena
McFadden, Deborah E.
McManus, Bruce M.
Nielsen, Torsten
O'Connor, Robert
Owen, David A.
Popescu, Oana-Eugenia
Rasmussen, Steven L.
Schaeffer, David F.
Senger, Christof
Skinnider, Brian F.
Sorensen, Paul H B.
Suen, Kenneth C H.
Tha, Susan P L.
Turbin, Dmitry
Van Niekerk, Dirk J T.
Walker, Blair A M.
Webber, Douglas L.
White, Valerie A.
Wright, Joanne L.
Wroblewski, Julius A.
Zhou, Chen Qian

VERNON
Allen Bradshaw, Barbra Y.

VICTORIA
Berry, Brian R.
Irving, Julie A.
Kelly, James K.
Martens, Mildred B.
Martin, Justin M E.
Power, Robert F.
Sawyer, Douglas M.
Tanhuanco-Kho, Grace Y.
Van Der Westhuizen, Nick G.
Watson, Peter H.
Wright, Cheryl L.

WHITE ROCK
Coret, Stephen D.

MANITOBA

BRANDON
Abidullah, Mohammad
Shapan, Mustafa F.

WINNIPEG
Aljada, Ibrahim S.
Baker, Patricia M.
Balachandra, Thambirajah
Battistuzzi, Susan C.
Bicamumpaka, Cyrille
Buksak, Raena D.
Curtis, Michael
Dupre, Marc P J.
Fischer, Gabor
Gartner, John G.
Gheorghe, Rodica C.
Gomez, Jose-Daniel
Hamza, Sate
Klein, Julianne R H.
Lategan, Belinda
Littman, Charles D.
Ludwick, Catherine L.
Mysore, Suresh M.
Phillips, Susan M.
Qing, Gefei
Qiu, Hongming
Ravinsky, Esther
Rivera, Raymond F.
Safneck, Janice R.
Santos, Cynthia B.
Wawryko, Paul M.
Wightman, Daniela M T.
Wightman, H. Robert
Willard, Martha J.
Williams, Gaynor J.
Younes, John K.

NEW BRUNSWICK

BATHURST
Sivarajah, Kalawathy
Ubaidat, Manaf

CAMPBELLTON
Lyew, Warren J.
Mills, Catherine A.

FREDERICTON
Ahmed, Itrat
Elmontaser, Ghazi I A.
Koller, Katalin E.
Ly, Thai Yen
Pugh, E. Denise
Smith, Muriel F.
Yan, Sen Rong

MIRAMICHI
Strzelczak, Dariusz

MONCTON
Colwell, Sarah J.
Husain, Almas S.
Jones, E. Shani
Maicas, Emmanuel
Mojtahedzadeh, Aghdas
Quirion, Marie-Andree A.
Shinder, Rowen
Snowdon, Jaime F.

SAINT JOHN
Godlewski, Marek
Hussein, Mahmoud R.
Obenson, Ken
Protzner, Kalman

NEWFOUNDLAND AND LABRADOR

CORNER BROOK
Karn, Eric B.

GANDER
Gallagher, Finbar P G.
Somers, Sangeeta R.

ST ANTHONY
Dankwa, Essandoh K.

ST. JOHN'S
Avis, Simon P.
Bonert, Michael
Carter, Beverley A.
Denic, Nebojsa
Gai, Luis
Hamodat, Mowafak
Pushpanathan, Chitra
Taher, Altaf
Wadden, Patricia M.

NOVA SCOTIA

ANTIGONISH
Desormeau, Leon M.
Muthu, Sarasa

BRIDGEWATER
Foyle, Annette
MacIntosh, Rebecca F.

DARTMOUTH
Bowes, Matthew J.
Murphy, Joanne S.

HALIFAX
Ahmad, Asma R.
Barnes, Penny J.
Bullock, Martin J.
Castonguay, Mathieu C.
Dakin Hache, Kelly A.
Fraser, Robert B.
Geldenhuys, Laurette
Gupta, Rekha
Heathcote, J. Godfrey
Huang, Weei-Yuarn
Magee, James Fergall.
Merrimen, Jennifer L.
Murray, Shawn K.
Offman, Saul L.
Pasternak, Sylvia
Sapp, Heidi L C.
Walsh, Noreen M G.
Werner, Dietrich
Wood, Marnie J.
Xu, Zhaolin

KENTVILLE
Tatlidil, Cuneyt
Uren, Kelly J.

SYDNEY
Cragg, Frank J.

TRURO
Boutilier, Robert G.
Jollimore, Jason V.

ONTARIO

AJAX
El-Sahrigy, Dina
Gaid, Nahed
Moussa, Bassem G F.

BARRIE
Ellison, Erin
MacNeill, Karen N.

BELLEVILLE
Gaber, Mohamed I.
Goetz, Catherine J.

BRAMPTON
Alexander, Kunniparampil N.
Curcin, Nikolina
Gardiner, Geoffrey W.
Jong, Roland C K.
Lajoie, Ginette
Medline, Paul B.
Sapp, M. Michelle

BRANTFORD
Tinguria, Mukund B.
Todd, Stanley D L.

BROCKVILLE
Yassa, Naguib H.

BURLINGTON
Hart, Julian G.
Jiang, Chaozhe

CAMBRIDGE
Bourgeois, Jacqueline M.
Brooks, Brenda
Cyr, Pamela V.
Shuhaibar, Hafez S.
Vasudev, Pooja

CHATHAM
Awad, Saadeldin M A.
Mohamed, Sarah H.

CORNWALL
Catzavelos, G. Charles
Reid, Barbara A.

ETOBICOKE
Jambrosic, Jadranka A.
Pastolero, Gemma C.
Tkachuk, Douglas C.
Torlakovic, Goran

GUELPH
Pandit, Rajani V.
Tadross, Latif A A S.

HAMILTON
Abdel-Mesih, Amal
Alexopoulou, Iakovina
Alowami, Salem O S.
Ara, Shamim
Arredondo, Jorge L.
Boutross-Tadross, Odette
Bulakhtina, Elena A.
Cutz, Jean-Claude
Daya, Dean
Deb, Pratima
Edwards, Lori M.
El-Shinnawy, Ihab H.
Elavathil, Leelamma J.
Faraji, Hamidreza
Gohla, Gabriela
Kaur, Harkiran
Lach, Boleslaw
Lytwyn, Alice
Marinescu, Mihaela
Nair, Vidhya
Ramsay, Jennifer A.
Rosati, Domenic
Ross, Catherine A.
Salama, Samih S S.
Sur, Monalisa
Tang, Shangguo
Terry, Jefferson
Toor, Jaspreet K.
Vincic, Lydia M.
Vukmirovic-Popovic, Snezana

KENORA
MacDonald, J. Kelly M.
MacDonald, James K.

KINGSTON
Abu-Abed, Suzan
Boag, Alexander H.
Chen, Chien-Hung J.
Childs, Timothy J.
Farmer, James
Farmer, Patricia L.
Hurlbut, David J.
Le Brun, David P.
Tron, Victor A.
Varma, Sonal
Young, Iain D.

KITCHENER
Batten, Adrian P.
Bhavsar, Pravin A.
Bishara, Mona
Cummings, Brian E.
Juneja, Namrata V.
Ling, Franklin C K.
Maksymov, Volodymyr I.
Melega, Douglas E.
Sawka, Barry W.

LONDON
Armstrong, Christopher
Chakrabarti, Subrata
Chan, Nancy G.
Driman, David K.
Ettler, Helen C.
Gabril, Manal Y.
Garcia, Bertha
Gomez Lemus, Jose A.
Haig, Aaron R.
Howlett, Christopher J.
McLachlin, Catherine M.
McLean, Carolyn A.
Moussa, Madeleine
Parfitt, Jeremy R.
Rizkalla, Kamilia S.
Shepherd, Jessica G.
Shibani, Areej A.
Shkrum, Michael J.
Tuck, Alan B.
Tugaleva, Elena
Tweedie, Edward J.
Walsh, Joanna C.
Wehrli, Bret M.
Weir, Michele M.

MARKHAM
Iakovleva, Gaiane K.
Lau, Michael C K.
Lee, T. Joseph
Li, Yunru
Shokry, Phoebe E.

MISSISSAUGA
Coire, Claire I.
Deodhare, Sanjeev
Dhamanaskar, Prashant K.
George, Rosamma
Hasan, Fauzia
Hu, Weimin
Iyengar, Pratibha
Kamel, Mona K.
Kapusta, Linda R.
Liaghati Nasseri, Navid
Manowski, Zbigniew J.
Nazerali, Latifa A.
Plotkin, Anna
Soares, Mark A.
Srigley, John R.
Truong, Francoise

NEPEAN
Burns, Karen L M.
Gannon, Brian

NEWMARKET
Adamiak, Anna
Chan, Susanne M.
Kanhere, Rujuta A.
Kazimi, Syed N.
Rinn, Richard W.
Rodriguez, Jennifer M.

NIAGARA FALLS
Chawla, Satish K.

NORTH BAY
Steele, Alexander A.

NORTH YORK
Barnard, Maja
Brennan, Michael
Kulkarni, Savita S.
Lee, King Siu
Leung, Chung-Shan
Macdonald, Denis F.
Miladinovic, Mirko
Niakosari, Firouzeh
Rubenchik, Illana A.
Sirkin, Wilma L.
Viero, Sandra

OAKVILLE
Edmondson, Nadeen
Liu, Jimin
Shaw, Danielle R S.
Ursani, Nafisa Ali A.

ORILLIA
Behjati, Mohammad R.
Fadavi, Ziba
Rieckenberg, R. Markus

OSHAWA
Ali-Ridha, Nihad H.
Fahim, Lisa
Fiser, Jarmila E.
Jakubovic, Henry R.

OTTAWA
Acharya, Virbala C.
Ayroud, Yasmine
Belanger, Eric C.
Burns, Bruce F.
Carlier, Maureen T.
Commons, Amiya S.
De Guzman, Ruby L.
de Nanassy, Joseph A.
Dionne, Michel
Djordjevic, Bojana
El Demellawy, Dina M S.
Gravel, Denis H.
Grynspan, David
Halwani, Fawaz
Islam, Shahidul
Jabi, Maha
Jamison, Bruce M.
Kepron, Charis A.
Lai, Chi Kien
Le Saux, Nicole M A.
Mai-Trung, Kien
Marginean, Esmeralda C.
Michaud, Jean
Milroy, Christopher M.
Moyana, Terence N.
Olberg, Bernhard J.
Padmore, Ruth F.
Parai, Jacqueline L.
Prokopetz, Robert D.
Purgina, Bibianna M.
Robertson, Susan J.
Roustan Delatour, Nicolas L D.
Senterman, Mary K.
Teo, Iris Y H.
Thomas, Mary-Janet
Veinot, John P.
Wang, Don
Wiatrowska, Beata A.
Wolfsohn, Allan L.

OWEN SOUND
Deliallisi, Ardit
Rudrick, Brian F J.
Shogan, Ahmad T K.

PARRY SOUND
Kassim, Olayiwola A.

PEMBROKE
Silva, Enrique

PETERBOROUGH
Laurence, Kelly H.
Melville, Karen A.
Moshkin, Olga M.
Radhi, Jasim M.
Sornarajah, Thangarajah

RICHMOND HILL
Lentz, John S.
Lubelsky, Sari M.
Sue-Chue-Lam, Andrew K.

SARNIA
Acharya, Chhaya V.
Kurian, Annie
Lubynski, Rosemary A.
Misir, Anil J.

SCARBOROUGH
Abdulkarim, Soran S.
Abedi, Syed T H.
Ansari, Saira
Boutros, Hedy N.
Haile Meskel, Helena
Hunt, Allan J A.
Misztal, Margaret
Noria, Dhun F.
Ren, Jian Z.
Sheikh, Tasnim K.
Sirbovan, Jane E.
Weigensberg, Corey N.
Zubovits, Judit T.

SIMCOE
Eshghabadi, Mashalah

ST CATHARINES
DeNardi, Franco
Joshi, Suhas B.
Koutsogiannis, Dimitri
Zebrowska, Grazyna A.

ST THOMAS
Battaglia, Donna
Craig, Ian D.

STRATFORD
Rouse, Tyler B.
Rowe Mahon, P. Elaine
Smith, Sharyn J.
Troster, Myron
Vetters, John M.
Walton, John C.

STRATHROY
Shah, Pravin C.

SUDBURY
Alguacil-Garcia, Antonio
Chen, Teh-Chuen
Dancea, Silvia L C.
Gaytan-Graham, Silvia R M.
Ngae, Min Yi
Patterson, Bruce J.
Queen, Martin
Rutherford, Michael N.
Tomczak-Bojarski, Anna B.
Widjanarko, Lianti

THUNDER BAY
Afshar-Ghotli, Zohreh
Arwini, Ahmed A S.
Jani, Prashant A.
Kennedy, Meagan T.

TORONTO
Adeyi, Oyedele A.
Al Habeeb, Ayman S.
Al-Haddad, Sahar F H.
Al-Maghraby, Hatim Q I.
Almohammedi, Faisal
Asa, Sylvia L.
Assaad, Dalal M.
Bailey, Denis J.
Bell, Cecil D.
Bethune, Gillian C.
Boerner, Scott
Boucher, Liza
Butany, Jagdish
Campbell, Donald M.
Cesari, Matthew
Chang, Martin C.
Chapman, William B.
Cheung, Carol
Chiasson, David A.
Chung, Catherine T.
Clarke, Blaise A.
Colgan, Terence J.
Craddock, Kenneth J.
Croul, Sidney
Cunningham, Kristopher S.
Cutz, Ernest
Cybulsky, Myron I.
Done, Susan J.
Dube, Valerie
Dubinski, William
El-Zimaity, Hala M T.
Evans, Andrew J.
Fernandes, Bernard J J.
From, Lynn
Gagne, Isabelle
Geddie, William R.
Ghaffar, Hasan
Ghazarian, Danny M D.
Goldberg, Franklin
Gotlieb, Avrum I.
Grin, Andrea
Hafezi Bakhtiari, Sara
Han, Guangming
Hanna, Wedad M.
Hegele, Richard G.
Henry, Pauline C L.
Herath, Jayantha
Howarth, David J C.
Hsieh, Eugene T K.
Hung, Lick San
Hwang, David M.
Iakovlev, Vladimir V.
Ismiil, Nadia D.
Jamali, Mina
Jothy, Serge P.
Kahn, Harriette J.
Kandel, Rita A.
Karavattathayyil, Sebastian
Keating, Sarah J.
Khalifa, Mahmoud A.
Kirsch, Richard
Kovacs, Kalman T.
Latta, Eleanor K.
Li Chang, Hector H.
Lu, Fang-I
MacMillan, Christina M.
Miller, Naomi A.
Mullen, J. Brendan M.
Musani, Rumina
Nabavi, Mitra
Naqvi, Asghar H.
Ngan, Bo-Yee
O'Malley, Frances P.
Ostrowski, Marian A.
Perez-Ordonez, Bayardo J.
Pickup, Michael J.
Pollanen, Michael S.
Pollett, Aaron F.
Pritzker, Kenneth P H.
Prud'Homme, Gerald J.
Rajagopalan, Ashwyn
Raphael, Simon J.
Rasty, Golnar
Riddell, Robert H.
Rose, Toby H.
Rouzbahman, Marjan
Rowsell, Corwyn H.
Sade, Shachar
Santos, Gilda D.
Shannon, Patrick T.
Shaw, Patricia A.
Sherman, Christopher G.
Sidiropoulos, Michael
Smart, Sydney E H.
Streutker, Catherine J.
Sugar, Linda M.
Sweet, Joan M.
Sy, Keiyan
Szentgyorgyi, Eva M.
Tanguay, Jeffrey J.
Taylor, Glenn P.
Thorner, Paul S.
Tomes, Ladislav
Tsao, Ming-Sound
Vago, Agnes
Vajpeyi, Rajkumar
Vozis, Eva E.
Walley, Virginia M.
Weinreb, Ilan
Wilson, Gregory J.
Winer, Daniel A.
Wong, John W.
Youngson, Bruce J.
Yousef, George M.
Zbieranowski, Ingrid J.

WATERLOO
Amdemichael, Esiahas

WINDSOR
Allevato, Pat A.
Alomari, Mohammad G.
El Keilani, Akram M I.
Hakim, M. Omar
Nguyen, Xong Thi.
Ra, Paul M U.
Saad, Reda S M.
Shukoor, Sajid
Shum, David T.
Smith, Pamela M.

WOODSTOCK
Engbers, Peter B.
Tauqir Naqvi, Syeda N.

YORK
Schall, W. Albrecht
Timonera, Elizabeth R.

PRINCE EDWARD ISLAND

CHARLOTTETOWN
Bowler, Lynne
Khanam, Humaira
Kim, Dae Tong
Sellers, A. Ruth

QUÉBEC

ALMA
Caron, Carole

AMOS
De Bujanda, Marilena

CHATEAUGUAY
Gosselin, Claire
Houde, Dominique

CHICOUTIMI
Gagnon, Yves
Lessard, Michel
Raymond, Catherine

DRUMMONDVILLE
Leveille, Francois

GATINEAU
Dionne, Paul G.
Logan, Cecile A M.
Perron, Nancy C.

GRANBY
Al Sabeh, Nayla
Nicholson, Robert M.

GREENFIELD PARK
Lamarre, Louis P.
Lussier, Catherine
Matte, Claire
Meunier, Caroline C.
Sauriol, Josee

LACHINE
Bouchard, Louis M.

LAVAL
Bonneau, Richard
Gutu, Liana E.
Lebeau, Annie
Marion, Alain
Masse, Janick
Nobert-Gagne, Suzanne
Peloquin, Anne
Stanasel, Cristina-Alexandra
Theoret, Gilles
Zhang, Zhi Ping

LEVIS
Bisson, Jocelyne
Lavoie, Mona
Proulx, Danielle

LONGUEUIL
Lamoureux, Diane
Milette, Francois
Piche, Jean

MONTMAGNY
Guilbault, Francois

MONTREAL
Alameldin, Mona
Albrecht, Steffen
Allaire, Guy
Amre, Ramila D.
Arseneau, Jocelyne
Auger, Manon
Bakdounes, Mhd Khldoun
Begin, Louis R.
Belisle, Annie
Bernard, Chantal
Berthelet, France
Blumenkrantz, Miriam
Bouffard, Danielle
Bourgault, Andre
Brimo, Fadi
Case, Bruce W.
Chen, Moy Fong
Cousineau, Sylvain
Croitoru, Zenovia
Daze, Yann
Desy, Delphine
Dion, Daniel
Doyon, Josee
Duarte De Almeida Brandao, Guilerme
Ellezam, Benjamin
Ferreira, Jose
Florea, Anca V.
Fraser, Richard S.
Fu, Lili
Gaboury, Louis
Gao, Zu-Hua
Gariepy, Gilles
Gologan, Olguta-Ecaterina
Guiot, Marie-Christine
Hadj Kacem, Chiraz
Hadjeres, Rachid
Haegert, David
Houde, Michelle
Jilaveanu Pelmus, Manuela
Kokta, Victor
Larose, Annie
Latour, Mathieu
Leduc, Louis-Joseph
Lussier, Christian
Maietta, Antonio
Marcus, Alexander T.
Marcus, Victoria A.
Michel, Rene P.
Nahal, Ayoub
Nguyen, Bich-Ngoc
Nguyen, Van-Hung
Omeroglu, Attila-Orhan
Onerheim, Ronald M.
Ouallouche, Karim
Pilavdzic, Dragana
Rahimi, Kurosh
Raptis, Stavros
Richardson, John B.
Rochon, Louise M A.
Romeo, Philippe
Roy, Indrojit
Royal, Virginie
Sartelet, Herve
Schurch, Walter
Sklar, Marsha C.
Soucy, Genevieve
Spatz, Alan
St-Cyr, Julie
Tanguay, Caroline
Tran-Thanh, Danh
Watters, A. Kevin

POINTE-CLAIRE
Hussain, Sajida S.
Nguyen, Jimmy
Viloria, Juan B.

QUEBEC
Beauchemin, Michel
Bergeron, Pierre
Bernier, Vincent
Boucher, Daniel A.
Caron, Chantal
Chenevert, Jacinthe
Choquette, Anne
Couture, Christian-Yves
Delage, Claude
Deschenes, Majorie
Dube, Robert
Fouquette, Bertrand G.
Gagne, Eric J.
Gould, Peter V.
Grondin, Katherine
Harvey, Isabelle
Jacob, Simon
Laberge, Sophie
Labonte, Sebastien
Latulippe, Eva
Lefebvre, Veronique
Lemay, Martin
Morency, Renald
Naud, Francoise
Nolet, Louise
Odashiro, Alexandre
Page, Sylvain
Perigny, Martine
Popa, Ion
Riopel, Julie
Roussel-Jobin, Aude
Saikali, Stephan
Tetu, Bernard
Theriault, Catherine
Trahan, Sylvain
Vaillancourt, Luc
Veilleux, Chantal

RIMOUSKI
Dermine, Jean-Francois
Gagnon, Luc
Giroux, Louise-Marie
Lagace, Real
Mailhot, Sylvain
Roman, Hassem A W.

RIVIERE-DU-LOUP
Cantin, Rejean
Gagnon, Sylvie

ROBERVAL
Bergeron, Sophie

ROUYN-NORANDA
Boucher, Danny

ROXBORO
Dupuis, Celine

SAINT-GEORGES
Nadeau, Michel

SAINT-HYACINTHE
Gervais, Daniel
Laurin, Michel A.

SAINT-JEROME
Gauthier, Jean
Lefebvre, Sebastien
Marcotte, Marie-Louise C.
Noel, Bernard

SALABERRY DE VALLEYFIELD
Chouinard, Valerie
Huttner, Istvan

SHAWINIGAN-SUD
Lanneville, Pascale
Larocque, Celine

SHERBROOKE
Doueik, Alexandre A.
Laplante, Claude
Mongeau, C. Jacques
Rizcallah, Edmond
Sawan, Bassem

SOREL-TRACY
Lussier, Sebastien

ST CHARLES BORROMEE
Allaire, Andre
Comeau, Lise
Pilon, Line

ST JEAN SUR RICHELIEU
Magown, John D.
Paquin, Francois J.
Turgeon, Pierre-Paul

TERREBONNE
Dongo Jiménez, Claudia M.
Issa-Chergui, Badia

TROIS-RIVIERES
Doucet, Caroline
Duplessis, Marc
Duval, Marie-Andree
Fortin, Simon
Gosselin, Jean
Perron, Robert

VAL-D'OR
Chatelain, Pierre C.
Vo, Tan Tai

VERDUN
Charbonneau, Sylvie G.
Huynh, Khanh-Cong
Riel, Sylvie

VICTORIAVILLE
Boudreau, Suzanne
Latendresse, Helene

SASKATCHEWAN

MOOSE JAW
Carretero, Antonio P.
Etches, R. Ian

REGINA
Al-Agha, Osama M.
Angeles, Ronald M.
Cabigon, Enrico F.
Duffy, Patrick J.
Grammatico, Dino J.
Jones, Edward A.
Khalifa, Amer J.
Seno, Hermenegildo-Rommel R.
Wooff, Jill C.

SASKATOON
Benoit, Janine L.
Brits, Nico
Chorneyko, Katherine
Diudea, Dana M.
Ezzat, Wendelin M.
Ganugapati, Usharani
Godsalve, Valerie M.
Kanthan, Rani
Meliti, Abdelrazak
Michalski, Roman T.
Quenneville, Louise A M.
Rees, Henrike
Saxena, Anurag

Anesthesia

ALBERTA

BELLEVUE
Dodd, E. Wendy

CALGARY
Ablett, David P J.
Archer, David P.
Arraf, John
Azmayesh-Fard, Arash
Baghirzada, Leyla B.
Balaton, John L.
Bands, Colin J.
Bart, Bevin B.
Berchuk, Miriam
Beriault, Michael T.
Bharwani, Fayaz
Brown, Nathan J D.
Cassidy, Michael R.
Caveno, Jordan W J.
Chan, Tommy W.
Cherry, Tadd Q.
Cheung, Kenneth S.
Chong, Michael P.
Chow, Lorraine
Chu, Alan
Chun, Rosaleen
Comm, D. Glenn
Connors, M. Ruth
Cox, Robin G.
Cuk, Aleksandar S.
Darcus, Karl L.
Davies, Jan M.
Diserens, Monique M.
Dobberthien, Marion T.
Dobson, Gary
Dodd, Colin
Donais, Phillip
Donnelly Warner, Niamh I.
Downie, Joseph A.
Drader, Keith S.
Dusevic, Myrna M E.
Duttchen, Kaylene M.
Eschun, Gerald M.
Ewen, Alastair
Farran, Rex P.
Fermor, David
Fox, Joel M.
Fraser, Louis
Froelich, Jennifer E.
Gale, Mark C.
Ghazar, Nancy J.
Gregory, Alexander J.
Guglielmin, Darryl R.
Ha, Duc Vinh
Haber, Julia A.
Hall, Gwendolen C E.
Halpenny, David G.
Hamming, Jeremy A D.
Hardy, C. David
Hawboldt, Geoffrey S.
Hiew, Moo-Khon
Hokanson, Michelle R M.
Hopper, Gordon H I.
Illing, Leigh H G.
Illing, V. Kim
Jacyna, Stephan M.
Janzen, James A.
Jordan, Dean H.
Jungen, David R A.
Kent, David A.
Korzeniewski, Peter A.
Kostash, Mark A.
Kozody, Raymond
Kruger, Marelise
Kuwahara, Brian S.
Latour, John A.
Lee, Alan Y.
Lee, Brenda C.
Letal, Michael D.
Liepert, David J.
Ligier, Bruno
Lim, Beatriz T.
MacAdams, Charles L.
Maher, Neal P.
McAllister, Debbie L.
McIntyre, Brian G.
McTaggart Cowan, Robert A.
Mensink, Fred J.
Nanji, Gulammohamed G V.
Neil, Stuart G.
Organowski, Slawomir
Parkinson, Bronwyn L.
Partridge, Bretta J.
Pash, Joel S.
Pash, Michael P.
Patterson, Steven J.
Phillips, Stephen V.
Pitter, Curt A.
Priddy, Richard E.
Prusinkiewicz, Christopher
Pysyk, Christopher L.
Pytka, Saul
Rasic, Nivez F.
Reddy, Neville
Rubin, Yair
Sachedina, Gulzar P.
Samuels, Peter L.
Sandhu, Manjot S.
Sandhu, Sabrina
Santosham, Kristi L.
Scanlon, Martin N.
Schultz, Rodney D.
Seal, Douglas D.
Shah, Misbah A.
Shing, Molly
Shinkaruk, Kelly S.
Shysh, Alexander J.
Simon, Karl D A.
Sims, Christopher H.
Smith, Marian H.
Soska, Marc A.
Spencer, Adam O.
Stacey, Shean F.
Stephan, Jarad S.
Stewart, Terry J.
Stilling, Lee S.
Sully Letal, Jillian C.
Swedlo, Dean C.
Sweet, Blythe A.
Tang, Timothy K K.
Teoh, Desiree A.
Thomas, John A.
Thompson, Robert J.
Tiessen, Alan C.
Torsher, Kevin J.
Towns, Dale K K.
Tsai, Hua-Lin
Verma, Manhar L B N.
Waechter, Jason E.
Wahba, Raouf S.
Wang, Bing
Wasserman, Paula R.
Wassill, Diane B.
Watson, Neil C.
Watterson, James G.
Willsie, W. Robert
Wilson, Joshua S M.
Wong, Vanessa P.
Wood, Daniel R.
Yang, Theresa L.
Yemen, D. Jill
Yont, Karrie R.

EDMONTON

Achen, Blaine M.
Alshankiti, Osamah H K.
Armstrong, J. Neil G.
Auld, Michael E.
Barker, Andrew P.
Barker, Michael I.
Baron, Leonard B.
Bateman, Kendall H.
Behmanesh, Saeid
Belzil, Jeanne M.
Bergstrom, Richard G.
Bhachu, Santokh
Bishop, Edward C.
Brar, Sukhpal S.
Breitling, Magnus K.
Broemling, Sunita R.
Brown, Alexander B.
Bucyk, Brent J.
Buss, Michael I.
Calvert, Robert A.
Carle, Henri L.
Cave, Cathy L.
Cave, Dominic A.
Chan, Douglas S.
Charlton, Jeff R.
Chen, Danny S.
Cheng, Alan H.
Cheng, Ronald T K.
Chiarella, Angelo B.
Chin, James
Cohen, Matthew R.
Coquet, Sean C.
Csanyi-Fritz, Yvonne
Cubitt, David
Delbecq, Bernard
Devitt, James H.
DuVal, Douglas B.
Eagle, Christopher
Eliasson, Theresa
Entwistle, Lucy M.
Ewanchuk, Mark A.
Fielding, Ariane E.
Finegan, Barry
Finucane, Brendan T.
Fitzmaurice, M. Aingeal
Flexer, William
Ford, Victor
Freed, Adam C.
Fuger, Jason J.
Godlewski, Bartosz
Godlewski, Wojciech
Gragasin, Ferrante S.
Gray, Dan P.
Gregoret-Quinn, Michael G.
Guenther, Craig R.
Gupta, Sunil N.
Hardy, Dorothy A.
Haugen, Richard D.
Hopkins, Ian A.
Hrazdil, Jiri
Hudson, Robert J.
Hui, Carolyn M W.
Jacka, Michael J.
Jensen, Valerie M.
Johnston, Richard G R.
Jolly, Donald T.
Joly Nickolet, Sarah
Kearney, Ramona A.
Kembhavie, Nikhil D.
Kindzierski, Robert
Klassen, Neil B.
Klinck, Jennifer R.
Knezevich, Mark P.
Knight, Brian
Koller, John P.
Kranjcevic, Joseph
Kropelin, Bruce W.
Kulkarni, Pradeep R.
Kwon, Elena
Lalonde, Megan M.
Lazar, Edward R.
Leighton-Lane, Dayna R.
Leung, Tanya M.
Lilley, John T.
Lin, Leslie P S.
MacDonald, A. Ian
MacNicol, Brent J.
Man, Emmeline L.
Marchak, Barbara E.
Martin, Marina
Matthey, Peter W.
Mercereau, Donald A.
Murphy, Michael F.
Muzyka, David L.
Nadeau, Louis
Nadwidny, Laurie A.
Ng, Ambrose C.
Noble, Colin J G.
Noonan, Liza M.
O'Leary, Thomas A.
Olson, Stanley A.
Paetsch, Paul R.
Paterson, Scott J G.
Patil, Deepali S.
Perez, G. Alejandro
Petriw, Boris Z.
Popoff, Jeffrey J.
Quinn, Michael G.
Rabuka, Shannon L.
Ramsey, N. Bruce
Rashiq, Saifudin
Reid, Susan J.
Rimmer, Tara J.
Rodyniuk, Andriy Y.
Saleh, Zainab A.
Sandhu, Harminder B S.
Scheelar, Leslie R.
Schneider, Oliver J.
Seal, Robert F.
Sidhu, Surita
Simmonds, Mark K.
Simmonds, Matthew R.
Smith, Graeme O.
Snider, Douglas D.
Sobolev, Igor
Soong, John H.
Steel, Graham J.
Stetsko, Samuel D.
Taam, Jason E W D.
Taggesell, Richard J.
Tang, Cathy
Terblanche, Ockert C.
Ting, Y Z. Heather
Torok-Both, Clinton J.
Tsui, Ban C.
Unger, Byron P.
Wachowski, Ireneusz
Wensveen, Quentin J.
Wiebe, Diana H.
Wildgrube, Peter D.
Yeh, Timothy W.
Yukawa, Masaru R.

FORT MCMURRAY

Wiebe, Henry

GRANDE PRAIRIE

Boldt, Charles I.
Lafontaine, Alika
McGowan, Liam
Peter, Chantelle A.

LETHBRIDGE

Bettger, Harald J.
Booth, Richard A.
Chong, Michael B.
Endersby, Ryan
Ho, Esther C Y.
Manjanatha, Channagiri P.
Nalder, Byron K.
Pounder, David R.
Setiawan, Melissa
Stewart, Barbara A.
Watson, Bryn A.
Wollach, Barry A.
Yanover, H. Clifford

MEDICINE HAT

Alhujairi, Mohammed
Cheesman, Mark E.
Goertzen, Peter J.
Hollingworth, Sean
Johnson, Thomas A.
Soklofske, Barry A.
Wardell, Gaylord C.

RED DEER

Barnard, Eduard
Christ, Albert J L.
Curtis, Robin
Goranson, Blair D.
Kapitoulski, Boris
Maragh, Vashti R.
Rudge, Trevor D.
Self, Dalton D.
Sysak, Daniel G.

ST. ALBERT

Brown, Russell J.

STONY PLAIN

Osmond, Colette

BRITISH COLUMBIA

ABBOTSFORD

Campbell, Derek W.
Forrest, Paul R.
Padda, Jagdish S.
Palmer, Christopher R T.
Smecher, Curtis A.
Underell, J. Roderick

BURNABY

Baker, Laura L.
Chuah, Elizabeth W T.
D'Arcy, Thomas M C.
Dickie-Clark, Johanna I L.
Friesen, Marvin J.
Gracias, Gavin
Krestow, Martin
Krestow, Michael
Lau, Bertrand P.
Pienaar, Petrus J.
Runzer, Timothy D.
Yu, Andrew H.

CAMPBELL RIVER

Gelinas, Jean

CHEMAINUS

Pettapiece, Kenneth G.

CHILLIWACK

Breden, Michael A.
Hellman, David

COMOX

Cook, Andrew C.
Gornall, Wayne R.
Holmes, Thomas S.
Watson, Jonathan M.

COURTENAY

Jackson, Louise M.

CRANBROOK

Nieman, Thomas E.

DAWSON CREEK

Neveling, Christoffel H.

DELTA

Cheng, Marshall A.
Hornstein, Stanley J.
Jones, Dean R.

DUNCAN

Campbell, Derek S.
Kraus, Steven L.
Ritter, Kurt A.
Robertson, William D.

KAMLOOPS

Cameron, Roderick J.
Cosman, Marvin S.
Diehl, Eberhard H.
Farren, S. Blake
Gully, Robert M.
Guy, John
Jadavji, Nadeem
Kowbel, Michael A M.
Maher, Daniel L.
Mans, Pierre L G.
Maurice, Rachel
McLaren, Drew H.
Morrow, Farrah L.
Saayman, Marius J I.
Silva, Rachel M.
Takeuchi, Lawrence
Whitehead, Michael J.

KELOWNA

Badner, Neal
Chayka, John
Collins, Ronald M.
De Souza, Duncan G.
Dickieson, Andrew
Du Toit, Corne
East, William
Eger, Robert P.
Fawcett, Wesley C.
Graham, Alistair D.
Jefferys, Stephen G.
Kuzak, Nicholai D.
Lund, Charles R.
Lutsch, Albrecht P.
Majka, Marek
Masterson, Mark F.
Nel, Stephan F.
Penner, Monica A.
Rocca, Bruno A.
Sanan, Anita
Yudin, Mark
Zimmermann, Donald L.
Zimmermann, Gordon A.

LANGLEY

Abraham, Alan
Caldwell, Chalmers W.
Goundrey, Shirley J.
Lo, Dennis L.
Michaluk, Harvey D.
Mountain, Mark A.
Sinclair, Colin M.
Storey, David G W.
Wu, Stephen C K.

LIONS BAY

Klas, Matthew J.

MAPLE RIDGE

Dmitriev, Dmitriy
Iyer, Mahalaxmi V.
Macpherson, Nicola
Wong, Joseph P C.

NANAIMO

Babst, Hans Van N.
Berkman, Alan C.
Capstick, James
Castner, Ronald P.
Coursley, Judith F.
Hall, Sarah C.
Hirst, Georgia C.
Lee, Jason K C.
McCormack, Francis W.
Neilson, R. Scott
Rieger, John
Seltenrich, Michael E.
Van Oostrom, Trevor M.

NEW WESTMINSTER

Baker, Paul F.
Banno, Dean
Bergman, Grace E.
Boisvenu, Joseph A G.
Burrill, Dean E.
Bylsma-Howell, Margaret I.
Carrie, Douglas W.
Duggan, Laura
Foulkes, Ellen F.
Gardiner, Richard R.
Ho, Cedric D S W.
Hodgson, Alyssa L.
Hoskin, Robert W.
Johnson, Patricia L.
Kahlon, Navraj
Law, Michael W.
Lipson, Adrienne
MacLennan, David J.
MacLeod, Wendy
Merchant, Richard N.
Meyler, Paula E.
Mohamedali, Feisal A H.
Morton, Roy H.
Nanaya, Neil P.
Nickel, Krista H.
Orfaly, Roland
Phu, Tommy C.
Roos, Martin R.
Scoates, Peter J.
Sharpe, Robert J.
Sun, Keith L.
Sveinbjornson, Timothy P.
Tweedle, Shelley D.
Valimohamed, Farah
Vo Nguyen, Lan
Warnick, Brady M.

NORTH VANCOUVER

Ahmadi, Hazhir
Arundell, Geoffrey W.
Fingland, Robert
Gajecki, Peter
Hewgill, Randolph T.
Kim, James K.
Kublik, Harry E.
Lipowska, Magdalena M.
Mayo, Warren G.
McAlpine, John C.
McCarter, Bryon
McDiarmid, Adam P.
Morrison, Clare
Pantel, Richard J.
Ping, Francis C.
Rajan, Yasmin A.
Rhee, Augustine Y.
Ripley, Teresa M.
Stasiuk, Russell B P.
Thobani, Shafik U F.
Veall, John W.
Vrana, Andrea P.
Walker, Jamie M.

PENTICTON

Crepeau, Brigitte A.
Crowther, John E.
Hamilton, Anderw A D.
Otruba, Zdenek
Reddekopp, Frieda J.
Weirich, Martin K.

PORT ALBERNI

Holland, Anthony J C.

PRINCE GEORGE

Ascah, John G.
Bardhan, Ashit
Schmid, Josie
Terblanche, L. Marthinus W T.

PRINCE RUPERT

Smit, Jacques-Henri

RICHMOND

Dong, Glenn L.
Huber, Christopher J.
Lister, David R A.
Navsarikar, Anup
Tang, Samuel L T.

SAANICHTON

Chana, Karam

SURREY

Bennett, Kathryn E.
Carruthers, Robert G.
Danelice, Michele
Dickson, Timothy
Findlay-Shirras, Nigel J.
Karwa, Laila
Ketabi, Salma
Kindopp, A. Shawn
Lau, Brenda W.
Lee, K. Dick
MacInnes, Aaron I.
McNeely, Patrick D.
Modi, Eesh
Mudie, Reidunn A.
Peter, Elizabeth A.
Twist, David L.

TERRACE

Gunter, Heinz J.

TRAIL

Grant, Ian R.
McCaskill, Kenneth R.
Reid, Iain C.

VANCOUVER

Abbott, William E.
Ansley, David M.
Applegarth, Oliver
Atherstone, Juliet A.

Au, Calvin L.
Bach, Paul S.
Bailey, Katherine M.
Baycroft, Sur J.
Bell, Scott C.
Berezowskyj, Jennifer
Bitter-Suermann, Bjorn F.
Blachut, Jan P.
Blackman, Lee T.
Bosma, Tymen L.
Boulton, Anthony J.
Bowering, John B.
Bright, Susan E.
Broemling, Natasha V.
Bruce, Simon
Chan, Terence C K.
Choi, Peter T.
Chow, Frances L.
Chubra-Smith, Normandie
Cole, Colm P.
Coley, Matthew A.
Demarty, Jennifer M.
Dhaliwal, Baljinder
Dolman, John F.
Douglas, M. Joanne
Doyle, Aeron
Dumitru, Ioana
Finlayson, Gordon N.
Fitzmaurice, Brett G.
Froehlich, Kevin F.
Froese, Norbert R.
Giffin, D. Mitch
Godley, Mark B.
Goresky, Gerald V.
Grant, Raymer P.
Gunka, Vit B.
Harper, Jon A.
Head, Stephen J.
Helliwell, James A.
Henderson, Cynthia L.
Herd, Stuart W.
Hudson, Jacqueline T.
Hughes, Bevan G.
Huttunen, K T. Henrik
Isac, George D.
Jee, Robert M.
Kahwaji, Raymond N.
Kamani, Allaudin A S.
Kapnoudhis, Paul C.
Khalfan, Aniz
Kilpatrick, Nevin
Kim, Alice D.
Klein, Rael
Kliffer, A. Paul
Klimek, Alexander T.
Kronitz, Naomi S.
Lampa, Martin J.
Lau, Tain Ming.
Lauder, Gillian R.
Lea, David E.
Lee, Bobby S.
Lee, Richard J.
Lennox, Pamela H.
Lo, Charles Y.
Lohser, Jens
Malherbe, David S.
Malm, David N.
Martin, Isabella L.
Massey, Simon R.
Mayson, Kelly V.
Mayson, Thomas A.
McDonald, Kenneth O.
McDonald, William N.
McEwen, Jonathan
McGinn, Peter B.
Meikle, Andrew T J.
Money, Phyllis M F.
Montemurro, Trina C.
Montgomery, Carolyne J.
Moore, Randell L.
Moult, Michael D.
Muirhead, Brian D.
Negraeff, Michael D.
O'Connor, J. Patrick
Osborn, Jill A.
Osborne, Penelope J.
Page, Michael S.
Parsons, David G.
Petrar, Steven D.
Phillips, William G B.
Prabhakar, Christopher P K.
Prasloski, P. Bruce
Prentice, James S.
Preston, Roanne L.
Price, James W.
Purdy, F. Robert
Rae, Randall J.
Randall, Thomas E.
Reichert, Clayton C.
Reimer, Eleanor J.
Ries, Craig R.
Rondi, Kevin
Ryan, Kenneth F.
Samer, Kurt K J.
Sawka, Andrew N.
Scheepers, Louis D V.
Schwarz, Stephan K W.
Setton, Deborah M.
Sirounis, Demetrios A.
Skippen, Peter W.
Stephenson, Catherine A.
Sung, Henry M H.
Swart, Petrus A.
Swenerton, Jean E.
Tang, Raymond K.
Traynor, Michael D.
Tsang, John Y C.
Umedaly, Hamed S.
Vaghadia, Himat
Villar, Giselle C P.
Vretenar, Doris F.
Vu, Mark P.
Warriner, C. Brian
Waters, Terrence S.
Weideman, Theodor
Werry, Barbara K.
White, Samuel A.
Wong, Clinton L.
Wong, David H W.
Wong, Michael
Woodhouse, I. Dorothy
Yarnold, Cynthia
Yu, Patrick Y H.

VERNON
Green, Jennifer A.
Honeywood, Kallie
Lemay, Erik
Marks, Richard
Morris, Derrick G.
Smith, Andre H D P.
Smith, Kevin F.
Viskari, Danny A.
Vvedenskyy, Oleksandr
Wong, Colin J.

VICTORIA
Atherstone, Michael J.
Bosenberg, Craig H.
Brennan, Alison T.
Caton, Brent W.
Chan, Peter A.
Coneys, Marcus C D.
Courtice, Ian D.
Davis, William
Duncan, Peter G.
Effa, Evan
Enright, Angela C.
Fancourt-Smith, Peter F.
Fenje, Nicholas
Ferreira, Susan
Herrmann, Trevor J H.
Kahn, Larry
Keane, Eimear J.
Kinahan, Michael J.
King, Wei-Shuen
Leacock, Susan L.
Leipoldt, Carl C P.
Meakes, R. Alan
Moll, Gillian
Murphy, Terence P.
Murray, Maureen E.
Pattee, Carol L.
Popova, Kalina
Porayko, Lorne D.
Quon, Leo
Ruta, Thomas S.
Sapsford, Gavin R.
Serowka, Pawel A.
Shandro, John T A.
Shaw, Lorne A W.
Shennan, Carmel F W.
Svorkdal, Nelson J.
Sweeney, Desmond H M.
Sylwestrowicz, Anna M.
Van Der Wal, Michael
Vuksic, Stanko
Wakely, Laura J.
Webster, J. Anne
Wollach, Jeffrey A.
Wood, Gordon G.

WEST VANCOUVER
Ramsden, John E.
Roston, Christina E B.

WHITE ROCK
Bachler, Markus A.
Cant, Jennifer A.
Clark, Fred J S.
Hemming, Anthony R.
Redmond, Michael P.
Robertson, Barbara J.
Rose, Sean R.

MANITOBA

BRANDON
De Wit, Simon L.
McKiernan, Bernard
Moller, Philip R.
Turner, David R.
White, K. Bruce
Wong, Clint S.

THOMPSON
Sulaiman, Ibrahim H H.

WINNIPEG
Amadeo, Ryan J J.
Aragola, Sanjay
Bagry, Hema S.
Baker, Chandran J.
Ballen, Jenifer L.
Barc, Jennine M.
Baron, Cynthia M.
Baron, Kenneth I.
Beckstead, James E.
Bell, Dean D.
Benoit, Archie G.
Booth, Steven A.
Bradley, Barry D.
Brown, Robert A.
Brownell, Laurence G.
Cameron, Murray R.
Cannon, John E.
Cappellani, Ronald B.
Christodoulou, Chris C.
Dabrowski, Piotr T.
Daya, Jayesh
De Brouwere, Roland G.
Deutscher, Raymond
Dhaliwal, Jamit S.
Dionne, Claire L.
Doak, Gregory
Docking, Leanne M.
Doerr, Jeffrey J.
Duke, Peter C.
Enns, James P I.
Esmail, Amirali M.
Ewert, Frank J.
Fedorow, Christine
Forgach, Linda G.
Freedman, Jeffrey I.
Funk, Duane J.
Gard, Sherry L.
Girard, John V J.
Govender, Prakashen
Graham, M. Ruth
Grocott, Hilary P T.
Gulati, Harleena
Haberman, Craig J.
Harms, Stefan
Harvie, Christopher J.
Hawaleshka, Adrian
Intrater, Howard M.
Jacobsohn, Eric
Kowalski, Stephen E.
Kuo, Brian Y.
Lambert, David A.
Lee, Trevor W R.
Lefevre, Gerald R.
Lemon, Peter W.
Levy, Shauna B.
Lieberman, Diane K.
Littleford, Judith A.
Loiselle, Joel A.
Lucy, Simon J.
MacKenzie, G. Scott
Maguire, Douglas S.
Mansfield, John F.
Mathieson, Angela L.
McDonald, Heather D.
McIntyre, Ian W.
McNeill, Ann M.
Miller, Michal
Miller, Tamara L.
Mutch, W. Alan C.
Mutter, Thomas C.
Mykytiuk, Patricia A.
Nugent, Linda M.
Ong, Bill Y.
Paetkau, Don J M.
Patel, Leena R.
Patel, Pravin C.
Pauls, Ryan J.
Pickering, Bryan G.
Pope, William D B.
Pretorius, Alexander P.
Putnins, Charles L.
Raghavendran, Sreekrishna
Rajamohan, Chinniampalayam
Reimer, Heinz
Ringaert, Kenneth R A.
Rohald, Pamela
Saadia, Vivien
Sabapathi, Karthik
Sareen, Sanjay
Scatliff, John E.
Segstro, Ronald J.
Sethi, Subash
Siddiqui, Faisal S.
Singh, Renate G.
Singh, Ricky D.
Stanko, Lorraine K.
Strumpher, Johann W.
Sutherland, Eric N.
Sutton, Ian R.
Swartz, Jo S.
Tenenbein, Marshall S.
Thomson, Ian R.
Tsang, Mae T.
Tulloch, Heather V.
Tweed, W. Arnold
Ullyot, Suzanne C.
Van Den Heever, Jesaja W.
Williamson, Kelvin W.
Wolfe, Scott A D.
Wong, Harley
Young, Robert S.

NEW BRUNSWICK

BATHURST
Boisvert, Catherine
Jankowska, Agnes

CAMPBELLTON
Laevski, Hristo L.

CARDIGAN
Buckenham, Sandra W.

FREDERICTON
Chisholm, Richard
Hamilton, Brian T.
Leach, James D.
McLean, Robert H.
Petrie, Edward A.
Price, Brian T.
Retallick, Ricky D.
Thompson, Geoffrey B.

MONCTON
Alturkistani, Majed
Aucoin, Sylvie
Cohen, David R.
Coimbra, Claudia
Crompton, John M.
De Grace, Raymonde F.
Dodge, David
Doiron, Paul L.
Duguay, Kirk J.
Dumais, Richard G.
Greschner, Michael
Hawkes, Christopher A.
Laplante, Renaud
Leblanc, Sophie
Pelletier, Jocelyn
Penfold, Jamie L.
Philippe, Pascal
Porter, Kenneth L.
Rafiq, Arif
Robidas, Francis
Savoie, Janie
Wilson, Peter S.
Xiang, Jianxin

NORTH TETAGOUCHE
Banville, Nathalie

QUISPAMSIS
Venkatarangam, George J M.

SAINT JOHN
Chedore, Todd R.
Chisholm, John S.
Clark, Andrew G.
Cloutier, Jennifer A.
Davies, E. Colin
Hughes, David R.
Kahn, Michael K.
Lee, Susan
Mir, Josef
Mireau, John R.
Nice, Charles A.
O'Brien, Ashley
Seidmann, Tamara

NEWFOUNDLAND AND LABRADOR

CARBONEAR
Openshaw, David J.

CORNER BROOK
Galgay, Susan M.
Sridhar, Kollipara

GANDER
Verniquet, Andrew J W.

GRAND FALLS WINDSOR
Cole, Jeffrey S.

ST. JOHN'S
Barrett, J. Alison
Bautista, Michael J.
Bishop, Robert W.
Casey, Ann P.
Chu, Christopher C.
Clarke, Barry A.
Cowan, Gail D.
Crummey, Stephen
Daly, Mary M.
Flynn, James
Forward, Robert G.
Gammal, Amir S.
Harris, Jennifer M I.
Howells, Steven R.
Jamieson, John W.
Johnston, Lesley M.
Kamra, Chander P.
King, Francis G.
Lacey, David E.
Ledez, Kenneth M.
Major, Andrew E.
Noel, Francis D.
O'Brien, Gregory M.
O'Leary, Susan D.
O'Regan, Noel B.
Pridham, Jeremy N.
Redmond, Edwin B.
Ridi, Angela
Roob, Otto V.
Samarasena, L. D. Asoka
Sampson, Sonia D.
Suppiah, Nagappan

Sweeney, Trevor A.
Thiessen, Barton P.
Williams, John T L.
Zbitnew, Geoff L.

NOVA SCOTIA

AMHERST
Hernandez, Maria D R.

BRIDGEWATER
Furey, William
Taylor, Hilary J C.

DARTMOUTH
Aylmer, Anne P.
Bent, Kevin P.
Bond, David M.
Finlayson, Alexander
Logan, Vance H.
Norman, Brian P.
Paterson, Robert A.

HALIFAX
Adamson, Henry
Allen, Christopher T B.
Audain, Colin V.
Beauprie, Ian G.
Beed, Stephen D.
Berger, Christopher W.
Bernard, Andre M.
Bird, Sally J.
Bradley, Shannon
Chisholm, Janice D.
Chisholm, Kenneth C.
Clark, Alexander J M.
Coonan, Thomas J.
Covert, Caroline R.
Delbridge, Catherine L.
Di Quinzio, Claudio
Dobson, Gregory R.
Doucet, Robyn T.
Drapeau, Dennis
Finley, G. Allen
Gallacher, William
George, Ron
Glenn, John J.
Godkin, Timothy
Gray, Allison J.
Hackmann, Thomas
Hall, Richard I.
Henderson, Jane M.
Hendy, Ayman
Henzler, Dietrich
Hinkewich, Christopher
Hirsch, Kristine J.
Hung, Orlando
Kanellakos, George W.
Kent, Blaine A.
Kolysher, Paula L.
Launcelott, Gordon O.
Law, John A.
Lehmann, Christian
Litz, D. Sharon
Livingston, Patricia L.
MacAulay, Bruce D.
MacDougall, Peter C.
MacLellan, Rochelle
MacManus, Brian J.
MacQuarrie, Kirk J.
Mariotti, Carlo U A.
McIntyre, Allan J.
McKeen, Dolores M.
McKinnon, Genevieve M.
Milne, Andrew D.
Milne, David G.
Morris, Ian R.
Muir, John G.
Mullen, Timothy J.
Ngan, Johnson C S.
Nunn, Robert T.
Roper, Fiona M.
Schelew, Benjamin L.
Schmidt, Michael
Shukla, Romesh C.
Simms, Matthew G.
Sjaus, Ana
Smith, James B.
Soder, Christian M.
Sodhi, Parvinder K.
Stevens, Sarah C.
Szerb, Jennifer J.
Vakharia, Narendra R.
Wawrzyszyn, Benigna B.
Whatley, Gordon S.
Williams, Julie M.
Wright, Alistair
Yazer, Harold

KENTVILLE
Bishop, Allen J.
Cain, Richard S.
Doyle, Robert
Hillis, Michael T.
Lloyd, R. Grayson
McArthur, Alastair
Peck, Marcus J.
Tucker, John H.

NEW GLASGOW
MacDonald, Jon K.

NORTH SYDNEY
Pollett, Harry F L.

PORT WILLIAMS
Lazaric, Daniel M.

SYDNEY
MacNeill, Robert B.
Morrison, Earl G.

TRURO
Aylmer, David A.
Smith, David Y.
Wybenga, Milton P.

WINDSOR
Kelland, Alison A.

ONTARIO

AJAX
Cooper, Christopher G.
Gaid, Magdi M A.
Huang, Harvey Y.
Kim, Linda
Liang, Lily S.
Mehta, Yatin B.
Patel, Kirit M.
Smith, Kevin J.
Yacoub, Amgad K I.

ALLISTON
Heier, Krista J.

ANCASTER
McChesney, James

BARRIE
Brasher, Jane E M.
Brooks, Christopher P.
Campbell, Rebecca M.
Chan, Emily H.
Crawford, Charles D.
Duvall, Donald E.
Gilchrist, Andrew D.
Lee, Andrew W Y.
Lewis, Mark P.
Louis, Ihab K.
Murphy, David A.
Murray, Yvonne A A.
Northcott, Michael G.
Onayemi, Adebusola O.
Poplak, Terence
Quach, Thomas
Ray, Erin K.
Rissanen, John T.
Simon, James K.
Taylor, William H.
Thiele-Kuntz, Amy M.
Webber, Paul F.
Whitty, Tina M.
Yee, Irvan

BELLEVILLE
Brown, Mitchell S.
Gibson, J. Malcolm S.
Iordanov, Kolio
McGugan, John A.
Morrison, Scott P.
Vanspall, Gordon D.
Williams, Edward A.

BOWMANVILLE
Breward, Arthur
Saad, Samy M S.

BRAMPTON
Bertlik, Maria
Bhardwaj, Arun
Bloom, Michael S.
Brown, Stephen D.
Chelico, Liza
Cooper, Andrew B.
D'Costa, Abelina S.
Dugas, Geoffrey R.
Gislason, Rachel T P.
Gold, Ileana-Maria
Ho, Kenneth S W.
Karimi Zandi, Shahram
Khalil, Raghad
Najarali, Shamim G.
Petrasek, John S.
Saccomanno, Pamela M.
Shenderey, Alexander I.
Singh, Ashley M.
Syslak, Paul H.

BRANTFORD
Chettle, Crystal A.
Dunsmuir, James T M.
Galinski, Saramin E.
Kanani, Kunal P.
Lombard, Theodore P.
Mather, Mahomed S.
Namazie, Ali M.
Reeve, Brenda K.
Scholes, Lawrence C.
Suciu, Cristina-Delia
Taylor, Roger M.

BROCKVILLE
Lipan, Carla B.
MacGillis, Murray J.
Youssef, Magdy B.

BURLINGTON
Baier, Paul A.
Barrese, Carol A.
Chavoshi, Samieh
Deshpande, Maneesh
Eidlitz, Carey J.
Harrigan, Gordon R.
Lane, Jeremy J.
Patel, Santhya
Punnen, Chinnamma
Purdell-Lewis, J. Geoffrey
Sandler, Alan N.

CAMBRIDGE
Biswas, Iqbal H.
El Alfy, Ahmed
El Ghamudi, Abdulhakim A A.
Klahsen, Andrew J.
Leone, Karen L.
Ling, Alison K W.
Nicholas, Paul R.
Shehata, Ramez S H.
Westacott, Paul C.

CHATHAM
Angeles, M. Carmen
Kapasi, Tahera Y.
Masood, Amna
Nethirasigamani, Dinesh

CONESTOGO
Grinberg, Ralph

CORNWALL
Mroz, Krzysztof S M.
Riddell, C. David

DEEP RIVER
Gow, Janet S.

DUNNVILLE
Baillie, Nigel M.

DWIGHT
McKenzie, Robert N.

EAST YORK
Tibbet, Juliana S.
Toptchieva, Anna A.
Weisbrod, Mitchell J.

ETOBICOKE
Carmichael, Frederick J.
Dhanidina, Mohammad
Hafez, Shahira O.
Hegazy, Nasr A E.
Kassam, Zarina K.
Lok, Henry T C.
Loke, Julian C P.
Makowiecka, Maria I.
Sheolal, Ravitha
Simms, Kathryn A.
Syed, Ali A.
Tam, Dorothy
Tam, Vincent S.
Van Gulik, Michael G F.
Yamka, Edward M.

FERGUS
Mercer, Nicola J.

GRAND BEND
Lampe, K. Mary

GUELPH
Al-Qadhi, Firas A L N.
Borden, Andrew T.
Burnett, Judith
Chovanec, Milan
Maykut, Andrew W.
McCormack, Noel C.
Mohammadzadeh Yaghchi, Behrooz H.
Northey, Angela J.
Refat Zaki, Maged S.
Rofaeel, Ayman S H.

HAMILTON
Ali, Madi M M.
Baxter, Frederick J.
Bell, Roger R.
Bengizi, Adel A A.
Benko, Randy R.
Bhola, Nereja
Blain, Allison M.
Blew, Philip G.
Bolis, Rafik S.
Bruce, Tracey L.
Buckley, D. Norman
Cappello, Emma M.
Chan, Philip S L.
Darby, Peter J.
Darrat, Mahmoud A.
Dauphin, Alezandre
De Graft-Johnson, Ama
De Guzman, Cecilia R.
Dingle, Jonathan A.
Fargas-Babjak, Angelica M.
Farrell, Janet C.
Gibson, Kara J.
Gourlay, Douglas L.
Hamstra, Joel M.
Hankinson, James J.
Havers, Melanie
Hollidge, Melanie G.
Isac, Michelle M.
Jackson, Paul A.
Khong, Binh K.
Kolesar, Richard E.
Korz, Linda T C.
Lajoie, Julie J M.
Lesiuk, Lawrence S.
Ligori, Tania
Ling, Elizabeth
Lubanska-Hubert, Elzbieta G.
McLean, Richard F.
Moisiuk, Peter D.
Mulcaster, Julian T.
O'Hare, Turlough J.
Olivieri, Loretta S.
Onorato, Linda
Parascandalo, Richard J.
Park, Joseph
Parlee, Katherine E.
Parrish, Michael B.
Paul, James E.
Pikaluk, D. Ryan
Pine, William E.
Puchalski, Stephen A.
Raymer, Karen E.
Reddy, Desigen
Rhydderch, Gareth M.
Ricci, Christopher J.
Rieber, Joanna C.
Rosenblood, Geoffrey S.
Rozenberg, Anna
Sawchuk, Corey W T.
Sharma, Saroo
Sirko, Peter M.
Skala, Richard A.
Skrinskas, Alena M.
Stover, Laura L.
Syed, Summer
Thomas, Tara J.
Tse, Kenneth K Y.
Turpie, Fiona H I.
Tuszynska, Hanna M.
Van Helder, Tomas
Vraets, Adrienne C.
Whyte, Robert A.
Wong, Anne K.
Woo, Joseph C H.
Zieba, Iwona E.

KEMPTVILLE
De La Salle, Gilles

KINGSTON
Ali, Samia H A.
Allard, Rene V.
Ashbury, Edwin L.
Burjorjee, Jessica E.
Cain, John P.
Cummings, Michael B.
Duggan, Scott S.
Engen, Dale A.
Erb, Jason W.
Fleming, Melinda C S.
Froese, Alison B.
Gilron, Ian
Goldstein, David
Haley, Susan L.
Henderson, Tamara A.
Henry, Richard
Jaeger, Melanie T.
Mark, David A.
McMullen, Michael C.
Meunier, Bethann D.
Milne, Brian
Murdoch, John A C.
Murphy, Gregory N.
Parlow, Joel L.
Patterson, Lindsey J.
Pietak, Stanley P.
Reimer, Cara L.
Ridi, Stacy
Rooney, Rachel A D.
Saha, Tarit K.
Seegobin, Ronald D.
Seib, Rachael K.
Shelley, Eric S.
Shyam, Vidur
Simchison, Brian L.
Sydor, Devin T.
Tanzola, Robert C.
Turner, Kim E.
Van Vlymen, Janet M.
Wang, Louie T S.
Zamora, Jorge E.

KITCHENER
Alsefaou, Abdualla O A.
Aye, Tim M.
Billing, Kulbir S.
Castano Herrera, Elkin D.
Cruchley, Patricia M A.
Drone, Troy C.
El-Brakey, Mary R R.
Fallon, Katherine
Goossen, Christine
Hanada, Philip M.
Hutfluss, Richard M.
Latchford, Kevin J.
MacKinnon, Frederick N.
Martin, Edward S G.
Mazurka, Robert A.
Morgan, Magid
Nguyen, Quoc Minh
Reinders, Francis X.

Schneider, Margaret E.
Silcox, Lisa C.
Solylo, G. Michael A.
Spenler, Valerie S M S.
Torbicki, Edward A.
Wyatt, Judith L.

LINDSAY
Badcock, Beverley S.
Don, Joan

LONDON
Ahmad, Mohamad
Al-Areibi, Arif R A.
Anderson, Ian A.
Antoniou, Andreas
Arango, Miguel F.
Arellano, Luis-Ramiro J.
Armstrong, Kevin P J.
Armstrong, Paidrig M J.
Bainbridge, Daniel T.
Banner, Robert
Batohi, Pravin
Bellingham, Geoff A.
Bernadska, Ewa
Bhandari, Rakesh
Borger, Jonathan R.
Bruni, Ida
Butler, Ronald J.
Cave, Anita L.
Champion, Lois K.
Cheng, Davy C H.
Cherry, Richard A.
Church, Brian
Clarke, Collin F M.
Coveney, Marian L.
Craen, Rosemary A P.
Cuillerier, Daniel J.
Currin, Michael R.
Dain, Steven
Dhir, Achal K.
Dobkowski, Wojciech B.
Dubois, David
Fantillo, Vanessa
Ganapathy, Sugantha
Gordon, Neil
Granton, Jeffrey T.
Griffin, Ann P.
Gros, Michelle L.
Gverzdys, Sharunas A.
Harle, Christopher
Herrick, Ian A.
Hoogstra, Jason A.
Iglesias, Ivan R.
Jones, Philip M G.
Katsiris, Sandra E.
Kutt, Judith L.
Lindsay, Peter A.
Lobb, Trevor R.
Mack, Peter H.
Marmai, Kristine L.
McCabe, Gregory P.
McConachie, Ian W.
McNamara, Jeffrey J.
Mezon, Bernard R J.
Millman, William L.
Miron, Cristiana-Octavia
Morley-Forster, Patricia K.
Morrell, Bobbi J.
Murkin, John M.
Newton, Peter T.
Nicolaou, Georghios
Ower, Katherine M.
Parkin, John A.
Rachinsky, Maxim
Railton, Craig J.
Schulz, Valerie M N.
Sharpe, Michael D.
Simon, Gary S.
Singh, Sudha I.
Sischek, William J.
Smith, David H.
St-Amand, Marc A.
Taneja, Ravi
Teague, Kevin R.
Turkstra, Timothy P.
Vannelli, Anthony M.
Watson, James T.
Wexler, Howard R.

MARKDALE
Bobik-Orchard, Francis J.

MARKHAM
Butt, Shehbaz
Harfa, Leah
Hussein, Elhadi F.
Lokoff, Paul C.
Makan, Gopal
Nandal, Vijay
Rajasingham, Menaka
Tang, Kenneth

MISSISSAUGA
Assaad, Ihab G R.
Athayde, Jitendra I.
Baig, M. Naseer
Banks, Mark D G.
Bartosik, Lidia M.
Bohay, Jordan A W.
Brovender, Andrea L.
Bruin, Gerard
Cacic, Ivan
Chhina, Tejinder S.
Chow, Chong J.
Cooke, Michael J.
Cramb, Robert J.
Cruise, Charles J E.
Curran, Sean P.
Davidson, Anna
Donnelly, Thomas
Dyke, George W.
El-Beheiry, Hossam
Flynn, Christopher A.
Ford, Meredith K.
Friedland, Michael J.
Fuchs, Marnie R.
Green, Andrew F D.
Grewal, Jasvir K.
Hirano, Gail M.
Huang, Eileen Y.
Hudes, Elliot T.
Hultzer, Michele V.
Irish, Craig L.
Kanani, Nisha
Kapala, Miroslava A.
Kathirgamanathan, Sarathadev
Kumar, Rohit
Kwan, Siu Ling
Looi-Lyons, C. Lian
Luk, Kenneth D.
MacNeil, John P.
Nishimura, Brian K.
Pollett, J. Anne W.
Roche, Mark J.
Shine, Kevin S.
Sikka, Sujata S.
Srebrnjak, Margaret J.
Sze, Augustine Y S.
Wardle, Andrew P B D.
Wong, Bill I.
Zulys, Vytas J.

NEPEAN
Chamberlain, Wayne W W.
Fong, S. Ken
Hale, Nicole
Hogan, W. Patrick D.
Kelly, C. Patrick
Kirk, Brian C T.
McCaffrey, Donald C.
Navaneelan, G. Christy
Ozard, Ian D.
Reid, Craig W.
Reid, Gordon N.

NEWMARKET
Colmenares Otero, Maria E.
Coutinho, Christopher J.
Cruickshanks, Giles F.
De Waal, Tonya R.
Hanna, Glen R.
Hatzidiakos, Peter
Heinrich, Lee E.
Hutchinson, Lisa G.
Kadiri, Yahaya Z.
Kim, Catherine Y.
Kim, Daniel H.
Mark, Trisha M.
Mawhinney, Shawn W.
Michailidis, Michael
Min, Frank
Perna, Philip
Railton, Karl T.
Scott, Julia D.
Segal, Steven H.
Shumka, David J.
Singh, Davindra
Skala, William N.
Smyth, Robert J.
Sullivan, Michael E.
Thompson, W. Kevin
Yee, May-Sann
Yue, Paul K.
Yue, Randy S.

NIAGARA FALLS
Bellinaso, John L.
Gallagher, Michael C J.
Halliday, Frederick
McCormick, Charles C K.
Phala, Everard M.
Truong, Patrick D C.

NORTH BAY
Bodley, Steven C.
Chirico, James C A.
Davies, Andrew O.
Fettes, Lisa F.
Fung, Donald E M Y.
Gagne, Kevin R.
Prychitko, Jonathan T P.
Sharifi, Shannon E.
Travers, Sean A.
Wong, Rajalaximi

NORTH YORK
Aleksandrova, Iryna G.
Balkissoon, Eric J.
Bassoon, Felix
Bernstein, Steven J.
Bloom, Ira M.
Bowry, Richard
Brose, Sylva A.
Calhoun, Todd C R.
Chan, Andrew Y.
Davidson, John R.
Dlacic, Aleksandra
Dunne, Nancy M.
Elia, Steven T.
Friedlander, Mark
Gale, George D.
Goldberg, Pamela R.
Gronas, Rolf
Hakes, John A A.
Hew, Ernest M.
Ip, Gregory J C.
Irwin, Darryl J.
Joo, Daisy T.
Kalicharran, Ubendranauth
Kashin, Brian A.
Katz, Ian L.
Kim, Joseph C.
Knapp, Charles D.
Lee, Kwok Ching
Li, Qiyu A.
Lie, Lie Ming
Martin, Bosco C F.
Mauer, Martin B.
Maxted, Grant R.
McKeown, Kevin J.
Minhas, Kuldip S.
Mustard, Janice E.
Palmgren, Elisabeth
Paterson, James G.
Powell, V. Lynette
Punja, Alim M.
Quint, Avidor
Ragos, Glenn A.
Rolbin, Stephen H.
Rothbart, Peter
Ryans, Katharine A.
Sakotic, George
Samuel, Daniella J.
Siddiqui, Tahira
Sloan, I A. Jeremy
Tang, Alexander W L.
Vosu, Helen A.
Weiss, Israel D.
Yung, Manuel M.
Zadik, Robert A.

OAKVILLE
Akinbolue, Oladele S.
Bhardwaj, Divya
Clark, James M.
Kapur, Kusum
Kay, Joseph
Lafreniere, Lynn M.
Loo, Karen M K.
Nocent, Gregory L.
Persaud, Baneshwar
Tintscheff, Mary M.
White, Gerald A.

ORANGEVILLE
Baker, Robert S.

ORILLIA
Donald, Shirley F.
Robinson, Clifford L.

OSHAWA
Bubela, Constantine B.
Doran, Richard J.
Hannouche, Fadi
Hayward, Diana
Herath, Subarathna M.
Katyal, Parul
Kriz, Robert P.
Maybee, John D.
Mitchell-Gill, Michael
Mohl, Robert W.
Simantirakis, Pantelis
Slavchenko, Paul T.
Spurrell, David W.
Tzerovska, Rayka I.
Whiting, Wilma G.

OTTAWA
Acharya, Sanjay V.
Barrows, Tammy L.
Bartosik, Lukasz P.
Basran, S K. Cindy
Baxter, Alan D.
Beauregard, Liette
Blais, Conrad
Blier, Jean
Bourke, Michael E.
Bragg, Paul R G.
Bryson, Gregory L.
Byford, Larry J.
Cattran, Charles B.
Cawadias, Alexander C.
Chaput, Alan J.
Charapov, Ilia A.
Chartrand, M L. Roxane
Chiu, Michelle
Chow, Jennifer A.
Clavel, Natalie
Connelly, Paul J J.
Conway, James B.
Corvo, Antonietta
Costache, Ioana
Crooks, Simone L.
Crosby, Edward T.
Cunningham, David G.
Curran, Michael J.
Custeau, Ingrid
Dashti, Abdullah
Di Renna, Tania
Dickie, Sean J.
Dickson, James
Doyle, Leilani
Duffy, Peter J.
Dupuis, Jean-Yves
Elliott, Robert D.
Evans, George
Evans, Holly C.
Ewing, David A.
Farrell, Mark R.
Fayad, Ashraf
Filteau, Lucie C.
Fraser, Amy B.
Frost, Ian M.
Gagne, Sylvain
Gallant, Catherine A.
Garnett, Robert L.
Gauthier, Louise F.
Ghatalia, Samir
Goddard, Yvette N.
Goheen, Mary Susan L B.
Gould, H. Marion F.
Goure, Camille A J.
Green, Ruth-Ann F.
Gupta, Sanjiv
Hall, Leslie E.
Hendy, Ramez H M.
Hladkowicz, Richard B.
Hogan, Angela
Hooper, Jonathan G V.
Hudson, Christopher C C.
Hudson, Jordan K.
Hynes, Mark S.
Johnston, Robert S.
Kim, Jarmila
Kitts, John B.
Kruger, Phil
Lambert, Andre-Stephane
Lamontagne, Christine
Landry, V L. Joseph
Lane, Alan T.
Langlois, Patrice
Lewis, Geraint W.
Lui, Anne C P.
MacDonald, John C.
MacNeil, Robert B.
McCrea, Kristin E.
McDonald, Bernard J.
McKenna, Jocelyne
Mervitz, Deborah L.
Microys, Sherissa L.
Miller, Donald R.
Moffett, Stephane
Mossdorf, Philipp
Murphy, Patti E.
Murto, Kimmo T T.
Naik, Viren
Nair, Shona
Naraine, Nadira D.
Nathan, Howard J.
Neilipovitz, David T.
Nicholson, Donna J.
Nolan, Kevin J M.
Oneschuk, Gail P.
Parent, Christine M P.
Penning, John P.
Persaud, Desiree A.
Plamondon, Marie-Jo
Po, Joseph L.
Polis, Tomasz
Power, Daniel J.
Prud'Homme, Jane M.
Ramsey, Gillian D.
Rastogi, Nikhil K.
Reid, Dennis
Robinson, Linda A.
Roeske, Amy E.
Rosen, H. David
Rostas, Aaron G.
Roze des Ordons, Amanda
Ryan, Gail L.
Schwartz, Robert A.
Shadrina, Anna G.
Silver, Lesley C A.
Skene, David S.
Skidmore, Gary B.
Smyth, Catherine E.
Sohmer, Benjamin
Splinter, William M.
Sullivan, Patrick J.
Sweet, Daniel C.
Szeto, Michael
Tallmadge, Caroline
Thompson, Calvin P.
Thompson, Ellen N.
Tran, Diem Thu T.
Walton, Kimberly J.
Watson, John B.
Wherrett, Christopher G.
Wilkes, Peter R H.
Wilson, Donald M.
Wong, Patrick B Y.
Wyand, Anna E H.
Wynne, Linda A.
Yang, Homer Y H.
Yegappan, Chidambaram
Youssef, Hany M R.
Zunder, Ian H L.

OWEN SOUND
Bell, David D.
Blight, Katherine
Brown, Eric E.
Coombes, Robin D.
Hatcher, David S.
Lalande, Phillip D N.
Nair, Vinod K.
Nairn, Travis K.
Olsen, Monica M.
Severs, S. Robert F.

PARIS
Whittier, Michael J.

PEMBROKE
Gerus, Lorraine R.
Pan, Wen-Mei
Renehan, Elizabeth M.

PERTH
Middleton, James C.

PETERBOROUGH
Bengough, Michael N.
Bonn, James R.
Edington, Robert
Geloso, Corrado G.
Goldberg, Laurie D.
Hall, David F.
Heid, Robert D.
Lewis, Jlee
Maini, Bharat
Malan, Maurice D.
Mann, R. Renwick
Pinto, Sebastian R.
Taylor, James M.
Windrim, Sean G.
Wynd, Kimberly P.
Wynd, Peter B.

PORT PERRY
Dower, Andrea M.

RICHMOND HILL
Ali, Mohamed J.
Bean, Warren A.
Butler, William J.
Chuang, Ian
Datoo, Abdulsultan A.
Gollant, Jerod
Herman, Stanley L.
Ng, Anthony T H.
Ngan, May T.
Novoshinov, Sergey
Roze, Gundars E.
Ta, Hien Minh
Yao, Zhenhai
Yeung, Raymond Y M.
Yung, Wingko W.

SARNIA
Abdulrahman, Abdulqadir M.
Al-Sadkhan, Haydar K M.
Beauchamp, Robert J.
Bertram, Barbara O B.
Lena, Anthony I.
Peregoudov, Serguei
Sherwin, Gregory D.
Singleton, Barry C.
Yarde, Muriel V.

SAULT STE MARIE
Hadley, Linda D.
Harwood, Robin
Ley, David A.
Norris, Desmond
Northan, Allan A.
O'Brien, Heather V.

SCARBOROUGH
Chan, Kenneth
Cheung, Jasmine S.
Esufali, Zakir H.
Feierabend, Martina M.
Glube, Mark L.
Hartley, Elizabeth J.
Harwood, Roger A E.
Hew, Jeremy O.
Hew-Wing, Philip
Ho-Tai, Lily M.
Hooshangi, Hedieh
Hsu, Vivienne
Huang, Louis
Jamensky, Neil T.
Kurrek, Matthias M.
Lamont, Robert W.
Lau, Lawrence C Y.
Lim, Teddy A.
Ling, Hubert H F.
Lu, Grant S T.
Malik, Nariman
Mandell, Howard B.
Markus, Jurgita R.
Panos, Larry L.
Powell-Francis, Kathryn A.
Roebuck, Marvin J.
Sharma, Vijay
Sivaganesanathan, Arumugam
Sivaji, Nirmala
Stringer, David G.
Tai-Pow, J. Malcolm
Tallmeister, Alan H.
Tsai, Olivia C.
Varty, Christopher B.
Wong, Winston Y C.
Yu, Jian Z.

ST CATHARINES
Austrup, Mona L.
Boright, William R.
Bosey, Gregory J.
Ciganovic, Olivera
Lagrotteria, David M.
Lam, Sheung L L.
Malcolm, W. Neil
Maximous, Emad F.
Shetty, Geeta R.
Smith, Philip L.
Szpejda, Witold J.

ST THOMAS
Campbell, Nicole
Marwaha, Gulshan

STRATFORD
Branson, Richard L.
Mota, Jorge A R.
Simmons, Collan J T.
Tinits, Peter

STRATHROY
Kieraszewicz, Halina
Molotiu, Nicolae
Tilsworth, Richard H.

SUDBURY
Anderson, Robert J.
Boyle, David L.
Button, Cheryl L.
Cote, Sylvain J.
Dumais, Robert
Dupuis, Natalie
Hey, Norman T P.
Hick, Anthony
Hickman, Robert S.
Kennedy, Brent A.
Lambert, A. Wayne
Lambert, Waide T.
Madden, Joanne I.
Manchuk, Derek R.
Marti, Julien A.
Mathur, Sanjiv
McKechnie, Kyle S.
Nalla, Bhanu P.
Sharan, Sumit
Sloan, Jeffrey P E.
Stewart, Jeremie R.
Wong, Kim T S.
Zalan, Peter G.

THORNHILL
Aum, Eull N.
Butler, Olivia M.
Lucas, Jan P.

THUNDER BAY
Bonneville, K. Scott
Charles, Julia C.
Dobson, Ian
Doig, George
French, Susan E.
Gareau, Rejean
Jin, Fengling
Scott, Michael A J.
Sikorski, Robert
Stallwood, Mark I.
Whittingham, Jennifer M.

TORONTO
Abbass, Syed Akbar
Abbass, Syed Ashgar
Abrahamson, Simon D.
Agellon, John D.
Ahmed, Sana A.
Ahn, Richard A.
Alakkad, Husni A O.
Angle, Pamela J.
Ararat, Alpay T.
Au-Yeung, Elizabeth J.
Avila Insambergth, Arsenio J.
Bahrey, Lisa A L.
Baird, Douglas A.
Baker, Andrew J.
Baker, James E.
Barclay, Alasdair L.
Barlow, Joseph R.
Beattie, William
Belo, Susan E.
Bender, Jennifer S.
Benedict, Christina M.
Bercovici, Mark C.
Berdock, Steven E.
Bertram, Susan G.
Bhatia, Anuj
Block, Gary
Braden, Harold P.
Bradwell, Peter J.
Braude, Bernard M.
Bremang, Joseph A.
Brown, Stephen C.
Brull, Richard T.
Byrick, Robert J.
Carstoniu, Jan K.
Carvalho, Jose C A.
Cassar-Demajo, Wilfred A.
Chan, Bok Man
Chan, Herman
Chan, Vincent W S.
Chandra, Devendr B.
Chang, Alvin
Chang, David H.
Chang, Lily
Chaudhry, Sajjad A.
Chen, Robert J B.
Chin, Ki Jinn
Chochinov, Erin M.
Choi, Mabel
Choi, Stephen
Chuang, Monica M.
Chung, Frances F T.
Cirone, Robert
Clarke, Hance A.
Constantinescu, Corina
Cooke, Mary E.
Cooper, Richard M.
Cox, Peter N.
Crago, Ronald R.
Crawford, Mark W.
Cybulskie, Karen Ann
Darrah, William C.
Dattilo, Kathleen M.
Davallou, Mojgan
Davies, Mary P.
Davies, Sharon R.
De Lacy, John L.
De Ruiter, Joost M.
Der, Tara-Diana
Devito, Isabella
Dickson, Jeffrey R.
Djaiani, George N.
Djordjevic, M. Dragan
Dodgson, Bruce G.
Edmonds, John F.
Eisen, Leonard B.
Eskandar, Sherif N F.
Evans, David
Faclier, Gil
Fan-Lun, Melissa A.
Fedorko, Ludwik M.
Fischer, Howard L.
Fisher, Joseph A.
Fleming, Ivor M.
Foster Jr., Harry L.
Fourie, Ockert J.
Fox, Gordon S.
Fried, Ben-Ari
Gates, C. Bronwen
Goldenson, Gordon L.
Goldszmidt, Eric
Govindarajulu, Arun P.
Graham, Marianne D.
Grant, Carol M R.
Griffin, Griselda K.
Grise, Ann D.
Guest, Cameron B.
Halpern, Stephen H.
Hamdy, Ahmed
Hanlon, John G.
Hare, Gregory M T.
Hawling, Christopher A.
Hayes, Jason A.
Hayter, Megan
Hegarty, C. Colette
Heggie, Jane E.
Hiscox, Michael
Ho, Alexander S.
Ho, Peter H T.
Hockmann, Edgar R.
Holt, David J.
Holtby, Helen M K.
Hong, Aaron P.
Houston, Patricia L.
Hrdina, Josef
Huang, Jane
Hussain, Kamal S.
Idestrup, Christopher
Ip, Terence K Y.
Isaac, Lisa A.
Jariani, Marjan
Jelenich, Sandra E.
John, Elizabeth
Jokhio, Raza M.
Joo, Hwan Suk
Joshi, Mital
Kamble, Vaibhav A.
Kapoor, Sunil
Karkouti, Keyvan
Karski, Jacek M.
Karsli, Cengiz H.
Kashania, Behnam
Kataoka, Mark T.
Katz, Abraham S.
Katznelson, Rita
Kavanagh, Brian P W.
Kealey, Alayne
Kelkar, Kumar V.
Kemp, Sheelagh M.
Kettles, M. Jane
Khanduja, Purva K.
Kim, H. Kenneth
Kirkham, Kyle R.
Ko, Raynauld
Kolton, Michael
Kong, Anna W S.
Kong, Audley L.
Kong, Yat Ming
Konieczny, Stanislaw J.
Kronberg, Jean E.
Kulchyk, James S.
Laflamme, Claude
Lai, Jacob K T.
Lam, Desmond K.
Lee, Henderson
Lee, Stephen L.
Leung, Peter T.
Leung, Rico P N.
Levene, Richard G.
Levine, Mark F.
Levis, Michael D.
Lilker, Suzanne J.
Lin, Ken C.
Lo, Nicholas T K L.
Loffelmann, Carol M.
Luksun, Warren J.
Lyn, Sheldon A.
Ma, Martin T.
MacArthur, Alison J.
MacPherson, Bruce A.
Mai, Ryan W.
Mallon, Joseph S.
Manninen, Pirjo H.
Marinov, Anton
Mark, Patrick W S.
Marseu, Katherin L.
Martin, Rachel S C.
Mazer, C. David
McCarthy, Vicky W K.
McCartney, Colin J L.
McCluskey, Stuart A.
McGhee, Irene D.
McGregor, Alexander P.
McGuire, Glenn P.
McHardy, Paul G.
McKnight, David J.
McLean, John S.
McLeod, M. Elizabeth
McLoone, Mary B E.
McNama, Patricia M.
McNaught, Andrew F.
McRae, Karen M.
McVicar, Jason A J.
Menikefs, Peter N.
Meschino, Alfio
Meyer, Rachel A.
Michel, Ernest R.
Middleton, Claire
Middleton, William J.
Moga, Rebecca A.
Moran, Nancy I.
Morgan, Anwar V K.
Morgan, Pamela J.
Morningstar, Beverly A.
Morton, William D.
Mosher, Emily R.
Moulton, Dagmar T.
Murphy, Patricia M.
Naser Al-Mobarak, Basem I.
Ng, Elaine K Y.
Niazi, Ahtsham U.
O'Driscoll, Martha A.
O'Leary, Gerald M.
Ondhia, Manharlal V.
Orser, Beverley A.
Oyston, John P.
Peliowski, Arie
Peng, Philip W.
Perlas Fontana, Anahi
Peterson, Carly E.
Pollard, Brian A.
Prabhu, Atul J.
Predescu, Oana
Pronovost, P. Antoine
Pyper, Elizabeth A H.
Rao, Anita U.
Riazi, Sheila
Riegert, Daniel G.
Roberts, Lisa M.
Roberts, Martyn J.
Robertson, James M.
Robison, Gordon E A.
Rose, D. Keith
Roy, W M. Lawrence
Rucker, Joshua C S.
Safa, Behnam
Salama, Said S S.
Salman, Aliya
Samahin, A. Noel
Sarmah, Anita
Sastry, Sunita G.
Shulman, Leslie S.
Silverman, Gregory L.
Sinclair, Lesley A.
Slinger, Peter D.
Smith, Terry S.
Snyman, Adam J.
Solaric, Bojana
Soliman, Ahmed O M.
Soneji, Neilesh
Spadafora, Salvatore M.
Srinivasan, Coimbatore V.
Srinivasan, Ilavajady
Steel, Andrew C.
Suess, Andrew M.
Swadi, Omar Q M.
Szabo, Elod Z.
Tamir, Diana
Tan, Chong-Jet
Tanaka, Steven H.
Tanner, Keith L.
Tarshis, Jordan C.
Tenenbein, Paul K.
Teresi, James E.
Tharmaratnam, Uma M.
Tourangeau, June A D.
Tousignant, Claude P J.
Trang, Amy J.
Tumber, P. Paul S.
Un, C C. Victor
Urbankiewicz, Lester R.
Van Der Vyver, Marthinus J.
Van Rensburg, Adriaan E.
Vegas, Annette L.
Venkat Raghavan, Lakshmi
Wasserman, Jeffrey J.
Weekes, Darlene A.
Welke, Timothy M.
Whang, Paul
Wijeysundera, Duminda N.

SPECIALISTS BY PROVINCE

Wong, Catherine K.
Wong, David T W.
Wong, Jean
Wong, Marcus G.
Wong, Sophia S F.
Wourms, Vincent P.
Yaseen, Muhammad
Yee, Doreen A.
You-Ten, Fung Voon K.

UNION
Soderman, Robert M.

WATERLOO
Loy, Frank Y.
Mahaffey, Murray E.
Rosenblum, Jerry H.

WELLAND
Gonzalez-Porras, Maria C.
Gopinathan, Asha
Hamed Abdelazim, Hala M F.
Thiyagarajan, Senthil K.

WINCHESTER
Farah, Christian
O'Connor, Timothy M.

WINDSOR
Alsaden, Mohamed-Rida A.
Banwell, Brian R.
Chopra, Ashna
Chripko, Daniel
Da Silva, Sidney J.
Desjardins, Bruce
Doerksen, David C.
Ewing, Kevin L.
Ghate, Hemant B.
Gnanendran, Kandiah P.
Hsia, Ivan K.
Laschuk, Maria J.
Lin, Mary M L.
Liolli, Americo
Manson, Henry J.
Maxwell, Timothy J.
Nanaya, Ponnettira K.
Odrcich, Mark J J.
Patel, Hasmukh G.
Roberts, A. Edwin
Salem, Eman G.
Smith, Julia A.
Taylor, William J.
Vergel De Dios, Oscar M.
Yousuf, Kashif A H.

WOODSTOCK
Lee, Susan M.
Marley, Wayne F.
Procter, Andrea M P.

YORK
Habibi, Mehri
Straka, Pavel F.
Young, James W.

PRINCE EDWARD ISLAND

CHARLOTTETOWN
Dubois, Jean-Yves
Farmer, Stephen R.
Fitzpatrick, Timothy
Kozma, David J.
Midgley, Janet E.
Moore, Anne K.
Nuechterlein, Barry

SUMMERSIDE
Vaishnav, Vandana

QUÉBEC

ALMA
Bouchard, Nadine
Moreau-Bussiere, Francois
Potvin, Pierre
Ricard, Christian

AMOS
Anctil, Pierre-Yves
Bouchard, Nadine
Cinq-Mars, Suzanne
Goyette, Anne-Marie
Martin, Daniel
Racicot, Jean-Mathieu
Vermette, Audrey

BAIE-COMEAU
Lemay, Gabriel
Tremblay, Maryse

BAIE-SAINT-PAUL
Fafard, Michel
Roberge, Rene R.

BOUCHERVILLE
Beaudoin, C. Gabriel

CAP-AUX-MEULES
Beaulieu, Pierre
Gagnon, Caroline

CHANDLER
Chretien, Angelo
Gauvin, Michel

CHATEAUGUAY
Chenier, France
Cournoyer, Alex
Gaudreau, Annie
Guay Langevin, Vincent

CHICOUTIMI
Bergeron, Jacquelin
Blackburn, Jean-Frederic
Briand, Alain
Claveau, Bernard
Dolbec, Luc
Essiembre, Christiane
Fallu, Stephane
Fortin, Marc
Gilbert, Martin
Gobeil, Gerald
Laprise-Demers, Audrey
Lelievre, Rejean
Masse, Edith
Vaillancourt, Martin

CLORIDORME
Gleeton, Dave

COWANSVILLE
Caron, Paul
Huni, Gerard E.
Jourdain, Sylvain
Saint-Laurent, Guylaine

DOLBEAU-MISTASSINI
Paul, Myriam

DRUMMONDVILLE
Cormier, Rachel M.
Durocher, Jean-Guy
Labrosse, Carl
Laplante, Francine
Pelletier, Stephan
Robert, Bruno

GASPE
Chouinard, Raynald
Hamel, Jean-Rene
Petry, Thierry

GATINEAU
Amberg, Stephane J.
De Bellefeuille, Luc
Fortin, Veronique
Giffard, Eric
Groulx, Daniel
Hamilton, Philip P.
Hennessey, Trevor
Jolin, Steeve
Katz, Joel M.
Khy, Virachit
Le Truong, Hong Hanh
Naud, Jerome
Neron-Veilleux, Sebastien
Nordstrom, Scott
Oliver, Enrique
Roy, Melanie
Sauve, Jean-Marc
Solomon, Peter H.
Sylvestre, Marie-Claude

GRANBY
Gaumond, Sylvie
Gauthier, Jean-Elzear
Martineau, Olivier
Robichaud, Remi
Trang, The Vinh

GREENFIELD PARK
Authier, Louis
Baillargeon, Robert
Desrosiers, Marie-Luce
Ferland, Lucie
Girard, Brigitte
Jodoin, Christian
Lavallee, Catherine
Lecours, Brigitte
Legrand, Jean-Claude
Menard, Lucie L.
Ng Man Sun, Joanna
Roy, Denis

JOLIETTE
Dumais, Huguette

JONQUIERE
Gagnon, Linda
St-Hilaire, Denis

LA MALBAIE
Martin, Pierre
St-Jean, Bernard

LA POCATIERE
Gingras, Rene
Proulx, Yvan D.

LA TUQUE
Errouissi, Nizar
Fafard, Andre

LACHINE
Grillas, Haralambos B.

LACHUTE
Belloncik, Yvan
Magin, Daniel

LASALLE
Aragon, Jose V.
Badawy, Mohamed
Courval, Jean-Francois
Homsy, Alfred A.
Jamali, Zainab
Jecen, Nikole
Laraya, Jose F G.
Latortue, Nicole
Woodruff, Christopher

LAVAL
Archambault, M H. Louise
Bouchard, Francois
Desormeau, Isabelle
Dubuc, Myriam
Huot, Marie-Pierre
Isabel, Liette
Mondor, Marie-Eve
Perron, Marie-Eve
Pothier, Sylvie
Raymond, Jacques
Robitaille, Olivier
Roy, Jean-Sebastien
Roy, Sebastien
Samson, Julie
Su, Antonio J.
Vezina, Daniel
Youssef, Marie D.

LEVIS
Bechard, Philippe
Bedard, O'Donnell
Charest, Eve
Cote, Marie-Chantal
Dumas-Laverdiere, Martin
Fortin, Marilyn
Fortin, Richard
Gendron, Gilles
Germain, Julie
Girard, Mario
Lacroix, Melanie
Larochelle, Denis
Laverdiere, Melanie
Leblanc, Jean-Paul R.
Masse Martel, Felix
Perron, Gino
Roy, Andre G.
Tousignant, Benoit
Tousignant, Sebastien

LONGUEUIL
Anderson, Reynald
Aubin, Christian
Bergeron, Lyne
Brouillette, Genevieve
Desnoyers, Jean-Pierre
Girard, Gilles
Gobeil, Francois
Houde, Bryan
Lemieux, Francine
Lortie, Elise
Masse, Michele-Elaine
McCaughry-Cardigos, David
Morin, Lise
Roussel, Eric
Servant, Mylene
Tremblay, Normand A G.
Tremblay-Coutu, Eleonore

MATANE
Samson, Jacques P.

MONT-LAURIER
Ricard, Pauline

MONT-ROYAL
Gilbert, Serge W.
Martel, Andre
Trottier, Anne-Marie

MONTMAGNY
Dumont, Louis
Lachance, Philippe
Letourneau, Malorie
Malenfant, Julie
Paul-Hus, Myriam
St-Pierre, Frederic

MONTREAL
Allard, Jacques
Alsenosy, Nafa
Amir, Igal M.
An, Tianyou
Angle, Michael R.
Arcand, Genevieve
Archambault, Andre
Asenjo, Juan F.
Audy, Daniel
Ayoub, Christian
Backman, Steven B.
Baldry, Craig D.
Bandi, Edith
Barry, Frances J.
Beaubien, Guy
Beaudet, Veronique
Beique, Francois A.
Bekhor, Samia
Belisle, Sylvain J.
Besner, Guy
Blain, Robert
Blaise, Gilbert A.
Bolduc, Renee
Bondy, Richard J.
Boudreault, Daniel
Boulanger, Aline
Boure, Benoit
Bozzer, Cristine
Bracco, David
Brossard, Yves
Brown, Karen A.
Brulotte, Veronique
Buu, Natalie T.
Carli, Francesco
Caron, Charles
Carrier, Francois-Martin
Carvalho, George F.
Charbonneau, Sonia
Charest, Jean
Charghi, Roshanak
Chartrand, Daniel
Chevalier, Andree
Chicha-Dzineku, Madeleine
Choiniere, Jean-Luc
Cogan-Collet, M. Jennifer
Collard, S. Vincent
Collins, Sophie
Cong, Huong
Costachescu, Tudor D.
Cote, Annie V.
Cote, Genevieve
Couture, Jacques
Couture, Pierre
Craig, Douglas B.
Crochetiere, Chantal
Crowe, Marie-Josee
Cyr, Jason
Cyrenne, Louise
DaDoun-Mchugh, Molly
Daloze, Thierry
Dekoven, Kathryn
Delabays, Eugene
Denault, Andre-Yvan
Deschamps, Alain
Desparmet, Joelle
Dickner, Martin
Donatelli, Francesco
Donati, Francois
Drolet, Pierre-A
Dumas, Diane
Dupont, Elise
Dwivedi, Shivendra
English, Michael J.
Fabrizi, Anna
Finlayson, Roderick J.
Fiset, Pierre
Fisher, Rachel
Fortier, Joanne D.
Fortier, Louis-Philippe
Fortin, Josee-Anne
Frigon, Chantal
Fuda, Giuseppe
Fugere, Francois
Furue, Koto
Garneau, Sebastien
Gauthier, Alain
Gauthier, Marlene
Georgescu, Leonida-Mihai
Germain, Hughes
Germain, R. Michel
Girard, Dominique
Girard, Francois
Girard, Marie-Andree
Girard, Martin
Girard, Michel
Girouard, Gilles R.
Gordon, Aida R.
Goyer, Caroline
Grenier, Yvan
Guay, Joanne M.
Guzzo, Angelina
Haig, Margaret J.
Hamawy, Nabil N.
Hardy, Jean-Francois
Hatzakorzian, Roupen
Hemmerling, Thomas M.
Henri, Richard
Heroux, Micheline
Heylbroeck, Christophe
Hickey, Chantal
Hickey, Donald R.
Hoffman, Shawn
Jean, Dominique
Jobin, Johanne
Joffe, Denise
Johnson, Claude
Joly, Nikola
Kaprelian, Suzan
Kardash, Kenneth J.
Kaufman, Ian
Khairy, Ramez C.
Kleiman, Simcha
Kovarik, Garrett G.
Kudish, Vitaly
Kumar, Pavan
Lagace, Annie
Lakheeram, Indrani
Lallo, Alexandre
Landry, Nicole
Laniel, Chantal
Lannes, Marcelo
Lash, Vynka C.
Lavoie, Anne
Lavoie, Claire
Lavoie, Josee
Lavoie, Nicole

Le, Anh-Tai
Lebon, Jean-Sebastien
Lenis, Serge G.
Lepage, Caroline
Lepage, Marie-Aline
Lesage, Sandra
Lessard, Nicole
Levesque, Jean-Charles
Levesque, Josette
Li Pi Shan, William
Limoges, Patrick
Loubert, Christian
Malenfant, Paul-Andre
Massicotte, Luc
Massicotte, Nathalie
Mathews, Sylvain
Maucotel, Jocelyne
Mayrand, Dominic
McKenty, Sylvie
McMillan, Patricia M.
Migneault, Brigitte
Mistry, Bergez F.
Moellenhoff, Michael E.
Moore, Albert R.
Mvilongo, Eding S.
Nguyen, Dinh Tam
Nguyen, Huu Tram Anh
Nguyen, Micheline
Nolet, Mireille
Olivier, Jean-Francois
Ouellet, Caroline
Ouellet, Pascale
Owen, Andrew J.
Paquet, Catherine
Pelland, Yves
Pelletier, Danielle
Perreault, Claude
Petit, Bruno
Pfeiffer, Uta E.
Plante, Francois
Plourde, R. Gilles
Pohl, Andrea
Popovec, Bobbi J.
Qizilbash, Baqir A.
Quance, Daniel R.
Ramadori, Francesco
Richer, Pierre
Robinson, Richard J S.
Robitaille, Arnaud
Rochon, Antoine
Rochon, Francois
Rousseau, Pierre
Roy, Jean-Denis
Roy, Louise
Ruest, Pierre
Sahab, Philippe G.
Saindon, Sophie
Salevsky, Frederick C.
Sangoul, Firooz
Slater, Marie-Eve
Sloan, James M.
St-Germain, Jean-Francois
St-Pierre, Jacques
Taillefer, Jean
Talbot, Martin
Tessler, Michael J.
Thobie, Gisele
Toledano, Karine
Tran, Quang Hieu D.
Tremblay, Isabelle
Triolet, William O.
Tsang, Janius
Valois Gomez, Teresa A.
Veillette, Yves
Villeneuve, Edith M B.
Villeneuve, Valerie
Vischoff, Daniel
Waters, Philip D.
Weeks, Sally K.
Wieczorek, Paul M.
Williams, Stephan
Zaharia, Francoise
Zaphiratos, Vasiliki V.

NOTRE-DAME-DU-LAC
St-Hilaire, Gerard

POINTE-CLAIRE
Balaban, Mihai
Doan, Julian
Hasel, Raymond
Odeh, Shaker Y H.
Zalmaev, Evgueni B.
Zuker-Fuchs, Joyce

QUEBEC
Albert, Natalie
Aucoin, Maryse
Baribault, Jean-P.
Beaubien, Jean
Beauvais, Michel
Bedard, Julie
Bergeron, Christine
Bertrand, Nadia
Bilodeau, Ruth
Blackburn, Steve
Brassard, Jean
Breton, Esther
Brochu, Jacques
Brousseau, Claude
Bussieres, Jean S.
Camire, Eric
Cantin, Isabelle
Caron, Francois
Chabot, Jacques
Chiniara, Gilles
Cote, Dany
Cote, Jacques J.
Cote, Joseph G J.
Cote, Maxime
Cote, Pierre R.
Croft, Dary
Denault, Pierre
Desgagne, Luc
Dion, Nicolas
Drolet, Guillaume
Drolet, Pierre
Duperrey, Daniel
Fournier, Louis
Gagnon, Serge
Gagnon, Sophie
Godbout, Bruno
Gourdeau, Martin
Grenier, Andre
Grenier, Lucie
Huot, Denyse
Joncas, Henri
Labrecque, Alain
Labrecque, Pascal
Lacerte, Louise
Lacroix, Gilles
Laflamme, Pierre
Laliberte, Pierre
Langevin, Jacques
Langevin, Stephan
Langlois, Denis
Lapointe, Daniel
Lavigne, Dominique
Le Bel, Lucie
Lecours, Mylene
Legendre, Luc
Lemieux, Jerome
Lessard, Martin
Letourneau, Dany-Roch
Levesque, Simon
Loisel, France
Lupien, Jacques
Marcotte, Jean
Martineau, Andre
Milot-Roy, Valerie
Montreuil, Jean P.
Morency, Jean-Pierre
Morin, Jean-Pierre
Moyen, Eric J.
Nadeau, Marie-Josee
Nadeau, Sophie M.
Nicole, Pierre
Ouellet, Jean-Marc
Ouellet, Mark
Paquet, Marie-Claude
Parent, Francois
Parent, Jean
Pellerin, Helene
Pelletier, Jacques
Pinard, Anne-Marie
Poulin, Brigitte
Rancourt, Valerie
Rheault, Michel
Rouillard, Jean-Francois
Rousseau, Annie
Savard, Jean-Francois
Somma, Jacques
St-Onge, Sophie
St-Pierre, Andre
Thiboutot, Francois
Tremblay, Denis
Tremblay, Marie-Helene
Tremblay, Pierre
Trepanier, Claude
Truchon, Rene
Turgeon-Fournier, Alexis
Veilleux, Raymond
Vezina, Marie-Claude
Vigneault, Louise
Villeneuve, Jacques

RIMOUSKI
Beaulieu, Louise
Buteau, Gaston
Lafond, Jean-Robert
Paradis, Marie-Claude
Pelletier, Julie
Picard, Philippe
Ringuette, Patricia
Rouleau, J J. Clement

RIVIERE-DU-LOUP
D'Amours, Jean-Francois
Dolbec, Pierre
Leclerc, Michel
Theriault, Stephane

ROBERVAL
Begin-Larouche, Julie
Beland, Alain
Cote, Sylvain
Michaud, Alain

ROUYN-NORANDA
Blaney, Raynald
Nguyen, Dat Nhut.
Picard, Jacques
Ricard, Mario

SAINT-EUSTACHE
Ailane, Tassadit
Beaudry, Marie-Eve
Charest, Isabelle
Lemieux, Sebastien
Monfrais, Jean-Luc
Trudel, Eric
Villeneuve, Audrey

SAINT-GEORGES
Lavoie, Marie-Josee
Mathieu, Virginie
Olivier, Stephane
Poulin, Martine
Poulin, Veronique
Tessier, Johanne

SAINT-HYACINTHE
Desgagnes, Marie-Christine
Duchesneau, Kathleen
Garneau, Sebastien
Guay, Marcel
Laberge, Stephane
Nadeau, Marie-Josee
Turcotte, Carole

SAINT-JEROME
Belliveau, Marc
Caron, Marie-Josee
Chouinard, Dany
Daigneault, Maurice
Daneau, Suzie
Demers-Pelletier, Julie
Desroches, Jean
Dingemans, Emmanuel
Dion, Marilyn
Lamontagne, Alain
Landry, Michel
Mac, Thien Bich
McSween, Audrey
Melancon, Karine
Pinsonneault, Celine
Roux, Michel

SAINT-PASCAL
Litalien, Albert

SALABERRY DE VALLEYFIELD
Bissonnette, Jean
Dagenais, Caroline
Dumais, Lynne
Fortier, Ghyslain
Martel, Brent R.
Pek, Bonavent
Rezonzew, Rebeca

SEPT-ILES
Lefebvre, Daniel L.
Page, Simon Y.
Sanfacon, Valerie

SHAWINIGAN-SUD
Cardinal, Valerie
Choquette, Jean-Francois
Leveille, Josianne
Provost, Valerie

SHERBROOKE
Beaudry, Mathieu
Berard, Dominique
Bourdua, Isabelle
Carrier, Johanne
Clairoux, Michel
Cloutier, Jean-Marc
Colas, Marie-Jose
Cormier, Francois
Cote, Daniel J.
Coutu, Stephane
D'Aragon, Frederick
De Medicis, Etienne
Doyon, Elisabeth
Drolet, Sophie
Echave, Pablo
Frigon, Veronick
Gagnon, Daniel
Lacroix, Anne
Larochelle-Girard, Marie-Noelle
Loignon, Marie-Josee
Martin, Rene
Mior, Frederic
Moliner, Peter H R.
Nadeau, Caroline
Parent, Michel
Parent, Pierre
Perrault, Michel-Antoine
Pirlet, Martine J.
Sansoucy, Yanick
Seguin, Guylaine
Theoret, Mylene
Veilleux, Leon-Jean

SOREL-TRACY
Roy, Roland

ST CHARLES BORROMEE
Arel, Luc
Bolduc, Louis
Boucher, Carl
Brault, Sophie
Deslippe, Helene
Dube, Andre
Larabee, Sonia
Nepveu, Marie-Eve

ST-EUSTACHE
Auger, Eric
Pharand, Annie

ST JEAN SUR RICHELIEU
Daher Matta, Giselle
Delorme, Mireille
Font Del Pino, Sonia
Gagne, Marcel C.
Jacques, Yvan D.
Liu Chen Kiow, Gilbert T S.
Paul, Stephane

STE AGATHE DES MONTS
Martin, Guy
Paquin, Pierre

STE ANNE DES MONTS
Duquette, Sebastien
Labart, Christian G.

TERREBONNE
Barchechat, Claude
Cousineau, Sylvie
Dionne, Sylvie
Gendron, Guy
Melnik, Howard
Richard, Anouk
Robitaille, Jean-Philippe
Thomas, David
Vaillancourt, Guy

THETFORD MINES
Bernard, Claire
Frechette, Marc
Mercier, Rheo
Roy, France

TROIS-RIVIERES
Albert, Jean-Francois
Asselin, Anne-Marie
Aubin, Patrice
Charpentier, Pascal
Cormier, Daniel
Cossette, Judith
Dansereau, Dominique
Gaulin, Francois
Gingras, France
Hakim, David
Joyal, Patricia
Lacasse, Marie-Andree
Laperriere, Gilles
Latulippe, Sebastien M.
Lemieux, Andree
Lessard, Sylvain
Monfette, Claude D.
Pellerin, Charles
Pellerin, Stephane
Tousignant, Jean

VAL-DAVID
Preville, Guy

VAL-D'OR
Guzman Bustamante, Juan

VERDUN
Bois, Sylvie
Choiniere, Andre
Curnew, George R.
Demers, Jacques
Desbiens, Paul
Gravel, Normand
Istvan, Jurai
Pepin, Paul
Roman, Ramon

VICTORIAVILLE
Becotte, Annick
Chabot, Francois
Croteau, Jacques
Fugere, Daniel
Seguin, Anick
Vasil, Dany

SASKATCHEWAN

CASA RIO
Cowie, Neil W.

PRINCE ALBERT
Arsiradam, Neethia M.
Chao, Erwin D.
Hasanni, Sameer A H.
Sriram, Konya R V.

REGINA
Akin, Suzan S.
Betcher, Jeffrey G.
Bowler, Kathleen J.
Chan-Tai-Kong, A. Joseph
Cherry, Mark S.
Crichlow, Allison
Dobson, Joy A R.
Gbinigie, Nosakhare I.
Giesinger, Carolyn L A.
Gorman, Kyle
Keeping, Brenda
Lang, Michael L.
Le Roux, Theodorus
Lett, Ryan C.
Mang, Annabelle L.
Maslany, Jurgen G.
McAllister, October E.
McAlpine, Douglas G.
McBain, Joelle H E.

McLaren, Tyler L.
Mehmood, Rashid
Mollison, Heather L.
Rosser, Timothy D.
Suri, Shashi
Zwack, Rhonda M.

SASKATOON
Banton, Keith J.
Brownbridge, Brian R.
Burris, David M.
Campbell, David C.
Chakravarti, Anita
Chaya, Malone
Clunie, Michelle L.
Dangor, Ayoub
Dease, Murray E.
Derdall, Kirstin
Gamble, Jonathan
Gore-Hickman, Wendy L.
Ha, Hang Chu.
Hodgson, Darlene
Jacobson, Perry D.
James, Mark L.
Jorgensen, Ian T.
Kawchuk, Joann M.
Lamb, Jonathan D.
Larson, Jacelyn M.
Laskowski, Kevin B.
Lim, Y C. Ben
Lougheed, Brenda L.
MacAskill, Leslie
MacDougall, Peter L R.
Malan, Albert J.
Maurer, Deborah A.
McDonald, Marguerite
McKay, William P S.
Meister, Ashley
Morris, Gary F.
Ong, Dennis D.
Pask, Barbara E.
Perverseff, Robert A.
Raazi, Mateen
Riben, Celina M.
Rooney, Michael E.
San Vicente, Monica K.
Schubert, Edward P.
Shannon, Janet L.
Shaw, Susan A.
Sheppard, Shane D.
Sirounis, H. Heather E.
Stirling, Alena M.
Surtie, Elmo A.
Szkup, Beata E.
Taylor, Brian G.
Todd, Andrea M.
Urmson, Kristine I.
Weiler, Robert L.
Wiens, Sharon A.
Wong, Kevin K.
Yip, Raymond W.

SWIFT CURRENT
Paintsil, James E.
Swica, Leszek J.

YUKON TERRITORY

WHITEHORSE
Dalinghaus, Kathleen

Cardiac Surgery

ALBERTA

CALGARY
Appoo, Jehangir J.
Borsato, Garry W.
Fedak, Paul W M.
Karolak, Wojtek

EDMONTON
Aboelnazar, Saber A.
Ghorpade, Nitin
Khani-Hanjani, Abbas
MacArthur, Roderick G G.
Meyer, Steven R.
Nagendran, Jayan
Schulze, Costas J.
Singh, Gurmeet
Wang, Shao-Hua

BRITISH COLUMBIA

KELOWNA
Peachell, John L.
Poostizadeh, Ahmad
Wan, Calvin K N.

NEW WESTMINSTER
Gunning, Derek J R.
Karim, Shahzad S.
Latham, Timothy B.
Wong, Daniel R.

VANCOUVER
Bashir, Jamil G.
Bui, Paul
Campbell, Andrew I M.
Cheung, Anson W C.
Cook, Richard C.
Danter, Matthew
Gandhi, Sanjiv
Laing, Bryce J.
Shayan, Hossein
Skarsgard, Peter L.
Ye, Jian
Yee, John

VICTORIA
Bozinovski, Jovan
Fedoruk, Lynn M.

MANITOBA

WINNIPEG
Arora, Rakesh C.
Freed, Darren H.
Lee, John J Y.
Manji, Rizwan A S.
Moon, Michael C.
Raabe, Michael A.
Singal, Rohit K.

NEW BRUNSWICK

SAINT JOHN
Hassan, Ansar
Pelletier, Marc P.

NEWFOUNDLAND AND LABRADOR

ST. JOHN'S
Lodge, Daniel J.

NOVA SCOTIA

HALIFAX
Baskett, Roger J F.
Hancock Friesen, Camille L.
Legare, Jean-Francois
O'Blenes, Stacy B.

ONTARIO

HAMILTON
Altaf, Fawaz M N S.
Chu, F. Victor
Dyub, Adel M A.
Semelhago, Lloyd C.
Singh, Steve K.
Whitlock, Richard P.

KINGSTON
Payne, Darrin

KITCHENER
Ashe, Kassem A.
Ibrahim, Moheb S.

LONDON
Chu, Michael W A.
Kiaii, Bob B.
Nagpal, Atul D.

MISSISSAUGA
Ahmed, Shafqat M.
Elghobary, Tamer
Noora, Joseph

NEWMARKET
Lee, Alexander L.
Pozeg, Zlatko I.
Teng, Carolyn J.

OTTAWA
Boodhwani, Munir
Chan, Vincent
Lam, Buu-Khanh
Lapierre, Harry
Maharajh, Gyaandeo S.
Mesana, Thierry G.
Price, Joel E.
Ruel, Marc
Saito, Simon
Shanmugam, Ganesh

SARNIA
Haddad, Michel

SUDBURY
Atoui, Rony
Bittira, Bindu
MacDonald, Derek J.

TORONTO
Ahsan, Muhammad R.
Caldarone, Christopher A.
Cohen-Nehemia, Gideon
Hill, Samantha
Huq, M. Momenul
Moussa, Fuad
Nazer, Rakan
Peterson, Mark D.
Rao, Vivek
Trop, Sebastien
Van Arsdell, Glen S.
Verma, Subodh
Yau, Terrence M.

QUÉBEC

CHICOUTIMI
Farinas, Jean-Marc
Laurendeau, Steve

MONTREAL
Bernier, Pierre-Luc
Bouchard, Denis
Chaput, Miguel
Demers, Philippe
Do, Quoc-Bao
El-Hamamsy, Ismail
Helou, Joe
Jeanmart, Hugues
Lamarche, Yoan
Ma, Felix
Noiseux, Nicolas
Poirier, Nancy C.
Samoukovic, Gordon
Stevens, Louis-Mathieu

QUEBEC
Charbonneau, Eric Y.
Dagenais, Francois
Dumont, Eric
Jacques, Frederic
Mathieu, Patrick
Mohammadi, Siamak
Perron, Jean
Voisine, Pierre

SHERBROOKE
Coutu, Marianne
Greentree, David M.
Teijeira, F. Javier

SASKATCHEWAN

REGINA
Korkola, Stephen J.
Moustapha, Ahmad
Suri, Rakesh M R.
Tsang, John C.

SASKATOON
Dalshaug, Gregory B.

Cardiology

ALBERTA

CALGARY
Aggarwal, Sandeep G.
Al-Hejily, Wesam A S.
Al-Qoofi, Faisal T Y.
Alvarez, A. Nanette
Anderson, Todd J.
Banijamali, Hamid S.
Basic, Doris
Belenkie, Israel
Bloomberg, Gary B.
Boyne, Timothy S.
Champagne, Patrick
Charbonneau, Francois
Clegg, Robin L.
Cohen, James M.
Curtis, Michael J.
Dicke, Franciscus
Duff, Henry
Exner, Derek V.
Filipchuk, Neil G.
Fruitman, Deborah S.
Giannoccaro, John P.
Gillis, Anne M.
Giuffre, R. Michael
Goodhart, David M.
Grant, Andrew D M.
Greenway, Steven
Hansen, James L.
Har, Bryan J N.
Howarth, Andrew G.
Howlett, Jonathan
Hutchison, Stuart J.
Isaac, Debra L.
Kanani, Ronak S.
Kapoor, Anmol S.
Kavanagh, Katherine
Kazmi, Mustapha H.
Kealey, Angela J.
Knudtson, Merril L.
Kryski, Albert
Kuriachan, Vikas P.
Lesoway, Robert N.
Ma, Patrick
Mason, Cindy A.
McMeekin, James D.
Meldrum, Donald
Mitchell, L. Brent
Myers, Kimberley A.
Mylonas, Ilias
O'Brien, Edward R M.
Patton, David J.
Peters, Grant L.
Prieur, Timothy G.
Schnell, Gregory B.
Sharma, Nakul C.
Sheldon, Robert S.
Slawnych, Michael P.
Spence, Frank P.
Stone, James A.
Sumner, Glen L.
Traboulsi, Mouhieddin
Veenhuyzen, George D.
Warnica, J. Wayne
Weeks, Sarah G.
Welikovitch, Lisa
White, Alan V M.
Wilton, Stephen B.
Wong, Jorge A S.
Wyse, D. George

EDMONTON
Adatia, Ian T K.
Al-Ghamdi, Hamed S A.
Alhulaimi, Naji M A.
Armstrong, Paul W.
Atallah, Joseph
Bainey, Kevin R.
Brass, Neil S.
Burton, Jeffrey R.
Butler, Craig R.
Chan, Michael C Y.
Cheung, Po Kee.
Choy, Jonathan B.
Coe, James Y.
Cujec, Bibiana
Downar, Eugene
Dyck, John D.
Ezekowitz, Justin A.
Fenske, Theodore K.
Graham, Michelle M.
Gulamhusein, Sajadhussein S.
Hruczkowski, Tomasz W.
Hui, William K.
Johnstone, David E.
Jones, Alan P.
Kantoch, Michal
Kasza, Leslie A.
Khandekar, Sayra A.
Kim, Daniel H J.
Kimber, Shane K M.
Lakhani, Zaheerali
Lalonde, Lucille D.
Leung, Raymond C M.
Lockwood, Evan E.
Mackie, Andrew S.
McMurtry, Michael S.
Miller, Donald D.
Muzyka, Timothy G.
Nsair, Ali
O'Neill, Blair J.
O'Reilly, Kenneth V.
Oudit, Gavin Y.
Pagano, Joseph J P.
Paterson, David I.
Ryerson, Lindsay M.
Senaratne, Manohara P J.
Shanks, Miriam
Sharma, Sanjay K.
Sharma, Sudheer
Sivakumaran, Sooriyakumaran T.
Smallhorn, Jeffrey F.
Sonnenberg, Brian H.
Taher, Taha H.
Taylor, Dylan A.
Toleva, Olga I.
Tymchak, Wayne J.
Tyrrell, Benjamin
Van Diepen, Sean F P.
Vonder Muhll, Isabelle F.
Wahab, Nazneem N.
Welsh, Robert C.
Williams, Randall G.
Wong, J. Szeman
Woo, Kenny S.

RED DEER
Alharbi, Abdulrahman M F.

ST. ALBERT
Khadour, Fadi

BRITISH COLUMBIA

ABBOTSFORD
Sayeh, Naser S.

BURNABY
Lee, Wilson
Wong, Lawrence H S.

COQUITLAM
Leung, Benjamin Y.

KELOWNA
Baker, Sandra E.
Fort, Stephen
Halperin, Frank A.
Hodge, Steven A.
Hooper, Richard O.
Pistawka, Kevin J.
Polasek, Petr
Townley, Richard

LANGLEY
Surkes, Jan

MAPLE RIDGE
Tsui, Winston W H.

NEW WESTMINSTER
Aminbakhsh, Amin
Barlow, Amanda J.
Blackwell, Margaret M.
Bonet, Jorge F.
Brown, Robert I G.
Chan, Albert W.
Charania, Jahangir
Dehoney, Cameron J.
Dorval, Jean-Francois
Epstein, Michael N.
Gailey, Carol B.
Kuritzky, Robin A.
Lalani, Akbar V.
Philipp, Roger K.
Rupka, Dennis W.
Simkus, Gerald J.

NORTH VANCOUVER
Doe, Sam
Imrie, John R.
Vyselaar, John R.

PRINCE GEORGE
Mousavi, Negareh

RICHMOND
Bar-Shlomo, Ben-Zion
Boroomand-Rashti, Kayoomars
Jakubowski, Andrew T.
Orenstein, Teddi L.

SURREY
Au, Stephanie Y P.
Bhagirath, Kapil M.
Bon, Richard R.
Cheung, Stephen S K.
Dong, Raymond
Hiralal, Rajesh
Manyari, Dante E.
Pearce, Stephen A.
Shariff, Salima N.
Tan, Peter K H.

VANCOUVER
Abdulla, Alnoor
Aymong, Eve D.
Bennett, Matthew T.
Boone, Robert H.
Cairns, John A.
Carere, Ronald
Chakrabarti, Santabhanu
Chan, Sammy Y.
Cowan, Simone S M.
Deyell, Marc W.
Fung, Anthony Y F.
Gin, Kenneth G.
Grewal, Jasmine
Hamburger, Jaap N.
Harris, Kevin C.
Heilbron, Brett G.
Hosking, Martin C K.
Huckell, Victor F.
Human, Derek G.
Ignaszewski, Andrew P.
Isserow, Saul H.
Jue, Johnny
Kanakos, Michael A.
Kerr, Charles R.
Kiess, Marla C.
Krahn, Andrew D.
Lee, Pui-Kee
Macdonald, Ian L.
Mancini, G B. John
Mizgala, Henry F.
Munt, Bradley I.
Nair, Parvathy
Nasmith, James B.
Rabinowitz, Alan N.
Rabkin, Simon
Ramanathan, Krishnan
Ricci, Donald R.
Sanatani, Shubhayan
Saw, Jacqueline W L.
Sedlak, Tara L.
Tang, Jonathan D.
Taylor, Carolyn M.
Thompson, Christopher R.
Todd, Jonathan K.
Toma, Mustafa
Tsang, Teresa S M.
Virani, Shahnawaz A.
Wong, Graham C.
Wood, David A.
Yang, Jiao
Yeung-Lai-Wah, A F. John

VERNON
Smylie, Paul C.

VICTORIA
Della Siega, Anthony J.
Dulay, Daisy
Fretz, Eric B.
Hilton, J. David
Kinloch, R. David
Klinke, W. Peter
Lane, Christopher J.
Leather, Richard A.
Mann, Manjeet
Mildenberger, Richard R.
Morgan, Dennis E.
Novak, Paul G.
Sinclair, Brian G.
Sochowski, Randall A.
Sterns, Laurence D.
Swiggum, Elizabeth A.
Tang, Anthony S L.
Yvorchuk, Kenneth J.

MANITOBA

WINNIPEG
Chelvanathan, Anjala
Czarnecki, Wlodzimierz
Ducas, John
Garber, Philip J.
Hussain, Farrukh
Jassal, Davinder S.
Kass, Malek
Malik, Amrit A.
Minhas, Kunal K S.
Nguyen, Thang N.
Parmar, Gurpreet
Patel, Sunil P.
Rabson, John L R.
Ravandi, Amir
Schaffer, Stephen A.
Schantz, Daryl I.
Soni, Anita
Stronger, Lyle N W.
Tam, James W L.
Tischenko, Alexander
Wolfe, Kevin B.
Zieroth, Shelley R.

NEW BRUNSWICK

DIEPPE
Baril, Jean-Francois
D'Astous, Michel
Lee, Rina
Matteau, Sylvain

MONCTON
Bourgeois, Ronald L J.
Kamel, Sherief J.
Trudeau, Chantal D.

SAINT JOHN
Barry, Colin A.
Bessoudo, Ricardo
Bewick, David J.
Corbett, Brian N.
Douglas, J. Geoffrey
Fong, Peter
Hubacek, Jaroslav
Lutchmedial, Sohrab R A.
Marr, David R.
Paddock, Vernon W.
Searles, Gregory R.
Stevenson, Robert S.
Teskey, Robert J.

NEWFOUNDLAND AND LABRADOR

ST. JOHN'S
Connors, Sean P.
Escott, Heather
Fagan, Susan M.
Furey, Michael U G.
MacCallum, G. Calvin
McPherson, Terrence P.
Paulin, Frederic L.
Pearce, Neil J.
Rose, Barry F.
Stone, Eric W.
Sussex, Bruce A.
Templeton, Christina G.
Williams, Anne E.

NOVA SCOTIA

BRIDGEWATER
Hatheway, Ronald J.

DARTMOUTH
Mears, Paul A.
Yung, Jason D K.

HALIFAX
Bata, Iqbal R.
Beydoun, Hussein K.
Clarke, Brian A.
Cox, Jafna L.
Crofts, Peter A.
Crowell, Richard H.
Curran, Helen
Gardner, Martin J.
Giacomantonio, Nicholas B.
Gray, Christopher
Horne, S. Gabrielle
Jackson, Simon D.
Josephson, E. Bruce
Kells, Catherine M.
Koilpillai, Christiansen J.
Lee, Tony C L.
Parkash, Ratika
Rajda, Miroslaw
Ramer, Sarah A.
Sapp, John
Sheridan, William J.
Stewart, Robert L.
Styles, Janet K.
Title, Lawrence M.
Warren, Andrew E.
Wong, Kenny K.

KENTVILLE
Clarke, Adam C.
Wightman, Howard A.
Woo, Daniel C.

SYDNEY
Buzaid, Amin M.
De, Sabe K.
MacDonald, Paul J.

SYDNEY RIVER
McClelland, Bruce

YARMOUTH
Merrick, Evan P.

ONTARIO

ALEXANDRIA
Sia, Ying Tung

BARRIE
Burke, Bruce R.
Dibble, Bradley J.

BELLEVILLE
Campbell, Joseph A L J.
Grant, F. Curry
Hollett, Peter M.
Kafka, Henryk P.

BRACEBRIDGE
Williams, W. Shane

BRAMPTON
Ahmad, Mayraj
Allard, Marc L.
Amlani, Shoaib
Borts, David
Gupta, Milan
Hill, Laurie L.
Jeejeebhoy, Farida M.
Joza, Paul
Jurt, Ursula
Kong, Waitak
Menon, Anilkumar S.
Raco, Dominic L F.
Singh, Narendra
Thavendiranathan, Paaladinesh
Tjandrawidjaja, Michael C.
Tsang, Wendy W C.
Turner-Gomes, Sophronia O.

BROCKVILLE
Hynd, Jamie W H.

BURLINGTON
Beaudry, Philippe R.
Carling-Chambers, Lucille B.
Darcel, Ian C.
Merali, Fatima S M.
Mody, Anita
Simmons, William W.
Stevens, Brett J D.

CAMBRIDGE
Pandey, A. Shekhar
Stinson, J. Michelle
Vizel, Saul

COLLINGWOOD
Goode, J. Eric

EAST YORK
Lefkowitz, A. Charles J.
Ovchinnikov, Vladislav L.
Pinto, Sarah R.

ETOBICOKE
Bhesania, Teosar
Drzymala, Lukasz
Fisher, Mark A.
Geranmayegan, Amir A.
Kalaparambath, Tef
Kannampuzha, Paul T.
Kirigin, Mladen J.
To, Toan Bao
Wong, Peter D.

GUELPH
Chan, Norman G.
Misterski, Jacek E.
Schwarz-Michorowski, Bogdan L.

HAMILTON
Ainsworth, Craig D.
Al Khdair, Darar A.
Belley-Cote, Emilie-Prudence
Connolly, Stuart J.
Curnew, Gregory P.
Demers, Catherine
Devereaux, Philip
Dillenburg, Rejane F.
Dokainish, Hisham
Finkelstein, Lorne
Gordon, Elaine
Ha, Andrew
Hastings, Deborah M.
Healey, Jeffrey S.
Holder, Douglas A.
Jolly, Sanjit S.
Kitching, Allan D.
Lonn, Eva M.
McKelvie, Robert S.
Mehta, Shamir
Mondal, Tapas
Moniz, Faustino P.
Montgomery, Alison G.
Mulji, Amin S.
Natarajan, Madhu K.
Rao, Rajeev V.
Rokoss, Michael J.
Salehian, Omid
Schwalm, Jon-David R.
Sheth, Tej N.
Spencer, Frederick A.
Stallwood, George R.
Stanton, Eric B.
Stimac, John M.
Sullivan, Brian J M.
Sullivan, Hugh P C.
Sullivan, Michael J J.
Tandon, Vikas
Teo, Koon Kang
Tihal, Hirawan
Valettas, Nicholas
Van Spall, Harriette G C.
Velianou, James L.
Yusuf, Salim

KINGSTON
Abdollah, Hoshiar
Adams, Gerald S.
Baird, Michael G.
Brennan, F. James
Burggraf, Gary W.
Johri, Amer M.
La Haye, Stephen A.
Matangi, Murray F.
McCans, John L.
McLellan, Catherine S.
O'Reilly, Michael G.
Pal, Raveen S.
Parfrey, Brendan P.
Redfearn, Damian P.
Sanfilippo, Anthony J.
Simpson, Christopher S.
Smythe, John F.
Thakrar, Amar

KITCHENER
Babapulle, Mohan N.
Desai, Dushyant
Kim, Hahn Hoe
Leddy, Danielle S.
McNamara, Brian T.
Pearce, Murray E.
Renner, Suzanne M.
Rinne, Claus H E.
Smith, Stuart J.
Theal, Michael D.

LONDON
Andrew, Philip J.
Bergin, M. Lynn
Brown, James E.
Chow, Lawrence H.
Diamantouros, Pantelis
Dias, Bryan F.
Finnie, Keith
Gula, Lorne J.
Hanninen, Mikael V W.
Humen, Dennis P.
Jablonsky, George
Khan, Razi
Klein, George J.
Leong-Sit, Peter
Massel, David R.
Pickering, J. Geoffrey
Rosenberg, Eli
Rosenberg, Herschel
Shoemaker, Gerard J.
Siu, Samuel C B.
Skanes, Allan C.
Sridhar, Krishnakumar
Suskin, Neville G.
Syed, Jaffer A.
Teefy, Patrick J.
Weingert, Michael E.
White, James A.
Wisenberg, Gerald
Yee, Raymond

MAPLE
Chua, Grace L.

MARKHAM
Hacker, Paul M.
Minkowitz, Joseph
Motlagh, Bahareh
Musewe, Norman N.
Newman, David M.
Simons, Derek B.

MILTON
Alter, David A.

MISSISSAUGA
Adleman, Neil L.
Bayliss, Michael
Bhatia, Rajan S.
Choudhry, Ashwani
Cyriac, Jason P.
Druck, Maurice N.
Grover, Arvinder
Gupta, Anil
Harrison, David A.
Jovanovic, John E.
Kremer, Sidney G J.
Lazzam, Charles
Le Feuvre, Catherine A.
Maingi, Manish
Nagi, Kirandeep S.
Nikhilanandhan, Janarthan Y.
Platonov, Michael
Puley, Geoffrey S.
Rebane, Thomas M.
Singh, Inderbir
Sluzar, Vladimir S.
Strauss, Hans D.
Tishler, Steven J.
Vakani, M. Tariq
Watson, K. Randal

NEPEAN
Grewal, Rasveg S.
McKibbin, Timothy G.
Miller, Fraser A.
Salcedo, Juan R.

NEWMARKET
Cantor, Warren
Chun, Robert
Fell, David A.
Goldman, Lorne E.
Habot, Juda
Hess, Allan R.
Khaykin, Yaariv
Miner, Steven E S.
Plante, Sylvain
Prabhakar, Manu
Symmes, John C.
Thangaroopan, Arulnmozhy
Tsang, Bernice
Wulffhart, Zaev A.
Zadra, Remo

NIAGARA FALLS
Poblete, Roel C.
Tannous, Rosemonde E.

NORTH YORK
Burke, Emory
Chan, Raymond H M.
Drobac, Milutin
Egri, Zoltan J.
Kagal, Darren R.
Kimball, Brian P.
Kotowycz, Mark A.
Lubelsky, Bruce J.
Mortazavi, Amir A.
Myron, Philip M B.
Rocca, Antonio S.
Rose, Randi K.
Sibbald, Matthew G.
Strauss, Martin H.
Teitelbaum, Earl J.

OAKVILLE
Chiamvimonvat, Varaporn
Feneck, Mary M.
Heffernan, Michael L.
Jedrzkiewicz, Sean J.
Mao, C. Russell
McConachie, David R.
Orfi, Jan N E.
Peat, Donald G S.

ORANGEVILLE
Wiley, Scott

OSHAWA
Alessandrini, Renato S.
Bakbak, Asaad I.
Bhargava, Rakesh K.
Rahim, Sherali A.
Tahiliani, Manoj
Tahiliani, Ravi

OTTAWA
Alanazi, Haitham A S.
Almutairi, Fawaz Q R.
Ascah, Kathryn J.
Beanlands, Rob S B.
Beauchesne, Luc M.
Burwash, Ian G.
Catching, John D.
Chamoun, Chamoun
Chan, Kwan-Leung
Chen, Shin-Yee
Chow, Benjamin J W.
Davies, Ross
Davis, Darryl R.
Dawdy, John A.
Dick, Alexander
Duchesne, Lloyd
Farag, Ashraf
Froeschl, Michael P V.
Fulop, John C.
Gardin, Letizia L.
Gauthier, Nadine
Glover, Christopher A.
Gow, Robert M.
Green, Martin S.
Haddad, Haissam A.
Hafez, Mohammed N.
Hessian, Renee C.
Higginson, Lyall A J.
Johnson, Christopher B.
Labinaz, Marino
Lai, Lillian S.
Laramee, Louise A.
Law, Angeline
Le May, J. Michel R.
Leach, Alan J.
Lee, Suzie
Lemery, Robert
Liu, Peter P.
Lougheed, Jane
Maranda, Robert C.
Marquis, Jean-Francois
Mielniczuk, Lisa M.
Moran, P. Bruce
Nair, Girish M.
Niznick, Joel M.
Quevillon, J A. Jean
Quinn, Brendan P.
Robertson, Jeffery H.
Ruddy, Terrence D.
Sabbagh, Roland
Sadek, Mouhannad M.
Seshadri, Angela
Sharma, Kamal
So, Derek Y.
Stadnick, Ellamae
Stewart, Duncan J.
Tsimiklis, Georgios
Turek, Michele A.
Wielgosz, Andreas T J.
Williams, William L.
Wong, Derek T H.
Yung, Derek

OWEN SOUND
Shelig, Khaled S.

PETERBOROUGH
Ball, Warren T.
Hartleib, Michael C.
Hughes, William G.
MacKenzie, Brian M.
Mahim, Ardavan
McLaughlin, Peter R.
Nguyen-Ho, Phong
Reesor, John N.
Shufelt, Kathryn A.

RICHMOND HILL
Chong, Paul W C.
Gangbar, Eric W.
Jevremovic, Alexandra
Raghavan, Ramya
Srivamadevan, Maheswaran
Wu, Gilbert K P.
Zeman, Peter R.

SAULT STE MARIE
Amhalhal, Ismeil M A.
Gupta, Inder P.
Mathew, M. Thomas

SCARBOROUGH
Arrazaghi, Abdelwahab A.
Beaulieu, Roland G.
Burstein, Jason M.
Cherry, James M.
D'Mello, Nisha A.
Davies, Edward G.
Dhingra, Sanjay K.
Galiwango, Paul J.
Gladstone, Peter S J.
Ho Ping Kong, Wayne
Janmohamed, Amirali K.
Kassam, Saleem A.
Kwok, Keith
Li, Christopher W H.
Ling, Michael C.
Makanjee, Bhavanesh
Mukherjee, Ashok
Naqvi, Arif
Nitkin, Robert S.
Rambihar, Vivian S.
Ricci, Joseph A.
Rosenbloom, Andrea
Ryzhak, Oleh M.
Vaughan-Neil, Edward F.
Vertes, George E.
Vijayaraghavan, Ram
Yan, Raymond T.
Yared, Kibar

SIMCOE
Naas, Abdulbasitt M.
Weeks, Andrew S.

ST CATHARINES
Abonowara, Abdulgani A M.
Chiew, S K. Sean
Hameed, Adnan K.
Kim, H. Hyung
Kotrec, Marian
MacKett, Robert L.
Pallie, Sven
Spurek, Monika J.

SUDBURY
Baigrie, Ronald S.
Charron, Thierry
Ghosh, Nina
Hourtovenko, Clyde D.
Juma, Zulfikar A H.
Labonte, Roger E.
Michaud, Josee
Nawaz, Shah
Ravi, Grama D.
Shukla, Dinkar K.
Syan, Gurcharan S.
Wong, Brian Y L.

THORNHILL
Freedman, David M.
Gomperts, Natalie R.
Langer, Galina
Nussbaum, Earl B.

THUNDER BAY
Billingsley, Ian
Henderson, Mark
Lai, Christopher C.
MacDougall, Andrea
Nigro, Frank

TORONTO
Abramson, Beth L.
Ahmad, Kamran
Ahmed, Shaheeda M.
Al Lawati, Hatim A A H.
Al-Hesayen, Abdurrahman O S.
Alghamdi, Mohammed
Ali, Naheed S.
Allan, Rebecca J.
Amad, Hani
Angaran, Paul A.
Anselm, Anjali H.
Bagai, Akshay
Barolet, Alan W.
Bauer, Robert
Beamish, Judith M.
Benson, Leland N.
Billia, Filio
Buller, Christopher E H.
Cameron, Douglas A.
Chauhan, Vijay S.
Cheema, Asim N.
Chisholm, Robert J.
Choi, Richard F Y.
Chow, Chi-Ming
Cohen, Eric A.
Colman, Jack M.
Conway, Jennifer
Courtney, Brian K.
Crystal, Eugene
Czarnecki, Andrew
D'Alessandro, Lisa C A.
Daly, Paul A.
Daniel, Lorretta B.
De Villa, Maria A.
Dighe, Kushal J.
Dipchand, Anne I.
Dorian, Paul
Dubbin, James
Dzavik, Vladimir
Edwards, Jeremy
Elmanfud, Omran R.
Elmayergi, Nader
Fam, Neil P.
Fitchett, David H.
Floh, Alejandro A.
Floras, John
Fountas, Panayiotis N.
Freeman, Michael R.
Gilbert, Brian W.
Gold, Jewel
Golding, Ian F.
Goodman, Shaun G.
Graham, Anthony F.
Gupta, Anup K.
Ha, Andrew C T.
Hamilton, Robert M.
Han, Ra Kyung
Hansen, Mark S.
Harris, Louise
Heilbut, Michele D.
Horlick, Eric M.
Howard, Robert J.
Husain, Mansoor
Iwanochko, Robert M.
Janevski, John
Joyner, Campbell D.
Kantor, Paul F.
Kilany, Ali K A A.
Kirsh, Joel A.
Ko, Dennis T.
Kobulnik, Jeremy
Korley, Victoria J.
Krimly, Ahmed M S.
Lai, Emily J.
Laksman, Zachary W.
Langer, Anatoly I.
Lau, Ching
Lee, Douglas S Y.
Leong-Poi, Howard M.
Levinson, Ari D.
Li, Qin
Logsetty, Giridhar
Madan, Minakshi
Mak, Susanna S S.
Mangat, Iqwal S.
McCrindle, Brian W.
McDonald, Michael A.
McEwan, M M. Patricia
Melvin, Kenneth R.
Mendelson, Michael
Miller, Saul
Mitoff, Peter
Moe, Gordon W.
Monge, Juan C.
Morgan, Christopher D.
Myers, Robert B H.
Naidu, Rajgopaul
Nanthakumar, Kumaraswamy
Nesbitt, Gillian C.
Newton, Gary E.
Ng, Douglas S.
Nield, Lynne E.
Oechslin, Erwin N.
Osten, Mark D.
Overgaard, Christopher B.
Pang, Jeffrey T W.
Parker, D. John
Parker, Thomas G.
Peterson, John C.
Piran, Sanaz
Poon, Stephanie C.
Prsa, Milan
Radhakrishnan, Shyam
Rakowski, Harry
Rambihar, Sherryn P.
Reial, Juri
Rewa, George
Roifman, Idan
Ross, Heather J.
Roth, Sherryn N.
Russell, Jennifer L.
Sasson, Zion S.
Schwartz, Steven M.
Silversides, Candice K.
Singh, Sheldon M S.
Sivaciyan, Vahe
Sivarajan, Venkatesan B.
Sole, Michael J.
Spears, Danna A.
Sternberg, Leonard
Strauss, Bradley H.
Szmitko, Paul E.
Thomas, Sunu S.
Udell, Jacob A.
Wald, Rachel M.
Wald, Robert W.
Wan, Andrea W.
Warren, Heather M.
Wijeysundera, Harindra C.
Wolfe, Robert E.
Woo, Anna
Yan, Andrew T.
Yu, Eric H C.
Zia, Mohammad I.

VAUGHAN
Bonafede, Nicoletta
Pourdowlat, Afsaneh

WINDSOR
Chetty, Rajendra M.
Glanz, Anthony E.
Huq, Nisarul M.
Lewis, Sheldon D.
Mikhail, Roland G.
Morsi, A. Ahmed
Rosenhek, I. Shoel

WOODBRIDGE
Daba, Ledjalem A.
Josan, Kiranbir

YORK
Klug, Andrew P.
Tiong, Irving Y H.
Vozoris, Socrates A.
Yao, Louis C H.

PRINCE EDWARD ISLAND

CHARLOTTETOWN
McMillan, Colin J.

QUÉBEC

CHATEAUGUAY
Nguyen, Quy Don
Ouellet, Gilles

CHICOUTIMI
Barabas, Julianna-Melinda
Belisle Jr., Pierre

Breton, Robert
Roy, Nathalie A M.
Tremblay, Gerald

COWANSVILLE
Lavallee, Jean-Pierre

GATINEAU
Collin, Remi
D'Amours, Georges
Ghavami, Ali
Haghighat Talab, Amir Tinouch.
Levesque, Claude
Nguyen, Tang-Thong
Vachon, Louis

GREENFIELD PARK
Benzazon, Michael
Chehayeb, Raja
Duong, Dinh Huy
Gaudreault, Gertie
Hyppolite, Renaud
Leonard, Sophie
Nguyen, Dang Khoa
Quan, Eric
Timothee, Jean-Robert

KIRKLAND
Mayer, J O. Jean-Pierre
Palaic, Mladen
Sandrin, Franco

LACHINE
Garg, Sunil
Sabe-Affaki, Georges

LASALLE
Boucher, Roger
Guimond, Claude

LAVAL
Boutros, Gebran E.
Choquet, Yves
Comtois, Hubert
Descarries, Laurence
Essiambre, Richard E.
Frenette, Marc
Gendreau, Raymond
Mayrand, Helene
Montigny, Martine
Murphy, Colm J.
Noel, Louis-Philippe
Pham, Luc Anh D.
Pohu, Andre
Ringuette, Gaetan
Roy, Annie

LEVIS
Auger, Pierre
Brulotte, Steeve
Crete, Martin
DeGrace, Michel F.
Delage, Francois
Giroux, Renald
Grondin, Francois R.
Lemieux, Ariane
Michaud, Nicolas
Poirier, Claude
Saulnier, Denis

LONGUEUIL
Charbonneau, Marcel
Colizza, Franco
Deslongchamps, Francois J.
Jarry, Michel
Lavoie, Jean-Pierre
Leduc, Francois A.
Legault, Christian
Maillette, Sylvie
Nowakowska, Dominika
Ouellet, C. Anne
Rivard, Andre
Sabbah, Eric
St-Maurice, Francois

MONT-ROYAL
Cote, Gilles
De Guise, Michele
Deschamps, Jean-Pierre
Stubington, David

MONTREAL
Addetia, Karima
Adelson, Edward I.
Afilalo, Jonathan
Amyot, Robert
Andelfinger, Gregor U.
Andrade, Jason
Argentin, Stefania
Asgar, Anita W.
Auger, Dominique
Ayas, Raouf R.
Basmadjian, Arsene J.
Beaudry, J. Pierre
Beaudry, Yves
Beaulieu, Yanick
Beland, Marie Josee
Benisty, Jacques I.
Benoualid, Henry A.
Benzaquen, Bruno
Bernier, Martin L D.
Berube, Lyne
Bigras, Jean-Luc
Bilodeau, Luc
Bogaty, Peter M.
Boileau, Laurianne
Bois, Marc-A.
Bonan, Raoul I L.
Bottega, Natalie A.
Boutin, Christine
Brassard, Myriam
Brophy, James M.
Brunet, Fabrice
Buithieu, Jean
Burelle, Denis
Cantor, Kenneth Z.
Castan, Rafael E.
Cavalle-Garrido, Maria T.
Charbonneau, Fernand
Charland, Raymond P.
Constance, Christian M.
Costi, Paolo
Coutu, Benoit
Crelinsten, Gordon L.
Crepeau, Jacques M.
Cyr, Veronique
Dahdah, Nagib S.
Dancea, Adrian B.
Dandona, Kshitij
David, Marc
De Guise, Pierre
Di Lorenzo, Maria
Diodati, Jean G.
Dore, Annie
Dorval, Jean-Francois
Doucet, Michel
Doucet, Serge
Dragatakis, Leonidas N.
Dubuc, Marc
Ducharme, Anique
Dupuis, Jocelyn
Dyrda, Katia
Eisenberg, Mark J.
El Rayess, Malak
Elstein, Eleanor
Essebag, Vidal
Fadlallah, Hussein
Fournier, Anne
Fournier, Marcel R.
Fouron, Jean-Claude
Friedrich, Matthias G W.
Gagne, Pierre
Gagnon, Roger
Gallo, Richard
Garceau, Patrick
Gelinas, Michel
Genereux, Philippe
Genest Jr., Jacques J G.
Giannetti, Nadia S.
Gobeil, Francois
Godin, Maurice
Gosselin, Gilbert
Goulet, Gilles
Gregoire, Jean
Greiss, Isabelle
Guerra, Peter G.
Hadjis, Tomy A.
Haichin, Richard N.
Hayami, Douglas A.
Honos, George N.
Huot, Roger
Husa, Regina
Huynh Thanh, Thao
Ibrahim, Reda
Jain, Deepak B.
Jolicoeur, Marc
Joyal, Dominique
Joyal, Michel
Juneau, Martin M D.
Jutras, Luc C.
Kahwati, Abed G.
Khairy, Paul
Kokis, Andre
Kornbluth, Murray
Kostiuk, David P.
Kus, Teresa K.
Lalonde, Guy
Lam-Yuk-Tseung, Jules C C.
Langleben, David
Lapierre, Andre J.
Lapointe, Jacques
Laramee, Pierre
Laverdiere, Michel
Lavoie, Vincent
Lavoie-L'Allier, Philippe
Le, Van Hoai V.
Le, Vy-Van
Lebeau, Real
Leclerc, Guy
Legault, Sylvie
Lemieux, Raymond J.
Lemire, Francois
Liszkowski, Mark
Ly, Quoc Hung
Macle, Laurent
Magder, Sheldon A.
Malcolm, Ian D.
Mansour, Fadi
Marcotte, Emile
Marcotte, Francois
Mardigyan, Vartan
Marelli, Ariane J.
Martucci, Giuseppe
Masson, Jean-Bernard
Mercier, Lise-Andree
Michel, Caroline M.
Miro, Joaquim A.
Mongeon, Francois-Pierre
Nadeau, Reginald A.
Nattel, Stanley
Nguyen, Ngoc-Huu
Nguyen, Viviane T Q.
Nguyen-Tuong, Phong
Nigam, Anil
Noel, Clement
O'Meara, Eileen
Oiknine, Albert
Ozen, Nilay
Palardy, Maryse
Palisaitis, Donald
Parent, Marie-Claude
Pelletier, Guy B.
Pelletier, Jean-Philippe
Petropoulos, Vivian
Piazza, Nicolo
Pilon, Claude
Potter, Brian J.
Potvin, Jeannot
Poulin, Frederic
Pranno, Nicolas
Primeau, Robert E.
Quan, Vu Hung
Quenneville, Stephane P.
Racine, Normand
Rahal, Deric P.
Raymond, Jean-Marc
Reeves, Francois
Reisler, Hyman
Rivard, Alain
Rivard, Lena I C.
Roberge, Guy
Rohlicek, Charles V.
Rose, Colin P.
Rouleau, Jean-Lucien
Roy, Denis
Rudski, Lawrence G.
Ruel, Monique A.
Saint-Phard, Wouter
Salem, Reda
Sami, Magdi H.
Santagata, Patrizia
Sauve, Claude
Schampaert, Erick
Schlesinger, Robert D.
Sebag, Igal A.
Serri, Karim
Sestier, Francois
Shames, Sofia
Sheppard, Richard J.
Smilovitch, Mark
Sniderman, Allan D.
Souliere, Vicky
Stewart, James A.
Talajic, Mario
Tanguay, Jean-Francois
Tardif, Jean-Claude
Terriault, Paul
Tessier, Pierre
Thanassoulis, George
Theroux, Pierre
Therrien, Judith
Thibault, Bernard
Tremblay, Annie
Tremblay, Jean-Francois
Van Doesburg, Nicolaas H.
Verma, Atul
Walker, Mathieu A D.
Walling, Ann D.
White, Michel

ORMSTOWN
Hortop, John

PIERREFONDS
Lee, Candace Y W.
Morissette, Martin M.

POINTE-CLAIRE
Chaniotis, Lambros N.
Kachra, Beheram S.
Schram, Gernot

QUEBEC
Alain, Pierre
Arsenault, Marie
Audelin, Marie-Chantal
Audet, Jean
Augustin, Charles E.
Barbeau, Gerald
Beaudoin, Jacques
Beaudoin, Jonathan
Bedard, Elisabeth
Beliveau, Patrick
Bergeron, Sebastien
Bernier, Mathieu
Blier, Louis
Boudreault, Jean-Roch
Bourgault, Christine
Cantin, Bernard
Champagne, Jean
Cote, Jean-Marc
Cote, Leonard
Cote, Marc-Andre
Coulombe, Denis A.
Couture, Jacques
D'Amours, Daniel
Dagenais, Gilles
De Blois, Jonathan
De Larochelliere, Robert
Delisle, Georges
Demeule, Eric
Dery, Jean-Pierre
Desrochers, Denis P.
Drolet, Christian
Dumesnil, Jean G.
Fillion, Nancy
Gallagher, Pierre
Gaudreault, Valerie
Gilbert, Marcel
Gilbert, Philippe
Gleeton, Onil
Houde, Christine
Houde, Gaetan
Langlais, Mario
Larose, Eric
Le Bouthillier, Pierre
Leblanc, Marie-Helene
Lemieux, Annie
Levesque, Pierre
Marchand, Francois
Molin, Franck
Morin, Annie
Morin, Josee
Nault, Isabelle
Nguyen, Can Manh
Noel, Bernard
O'Connor, Kim
O'Hara, Gilles E.
Pelletier, Marie-Josee
Philippon, Francois
Poirier, Paul
Potvin, Jean-Michel
Poulin, Jean-Francois
Proulx, Guy
Rinfret, Stephane
Robitaille, Nancy-Michelle
Rouleau, Jacques
Roy, Louis
Samson, Michel
Sarrazin, Jean-Francois
Senechal, Mario
Simard, Laval
Talbot Jr., Paul
Tessier, Yves
Theriault, Claudine
Tremblay, Benoit P.
Tremblay, J L. Guy
Turcotte, Jean
Vandal, Marie-Claude
Vinet, Elise

RIMOUSKI
Boucher, Guy
Carvalho, Jean-Christopher
Dionne, Nathalie
Hamel, Jean
Rioux, Leon

ROXBORO
Schiff, Renee L.

SAINT-GEORGES
Dion, Danielle
St-Hilaire, Richard

SAINT-HYACINTHE
Blackburn, Karl
Grandmont, Dominique
Kieu, Cong Van
Paulin, Mathieu

SAINT-JEROME
Bouchard, M. Josee
Gautier, Jean-Joseph
McNicoll, Serge
Ouimet, Dominique
Pelletier, Marie-Eve
Poupart, Robert
Rabbath, Patrick

SAINT-LAMBERT
Fortin, J B. Christian

SAINT-LAURENT
Stavrinidis, Sophie

SAINT-LEONARD
Gagnon, Andre

SEPT-ILES
Chartrand, Louis-Andre

SHERBROOKE
Bellavance, Marc
Berube, Simon
Brochu, Marie-Claude
Cote, Sarto R.
Crepeau, Jacques
Dalery, Karl
Dallaire, Frederic
Daneault, Benoit
Do, Doan Hoa
Farand, Paul
Fradet, Anne
Gagnon, Sylvie
Gervais, Andre
Harvey, Richard
Laflamme, David
Lepage, Serge
Mampuya, Warner M.
Nguyen, Michel
Paulin, Chantal
Roux, Jean-Francois

SOREL-TRACY
Godin, Daniel
Larin, Pierre
Picard, Jean-Pierre

ST AUGUSTIN DE DESMAURES
Guay, J. Michel

ST CHARLES BORROMEE
Blain, Marie-Helene
Dussureault, Martine
Kouz, Simon
Ouimet, Helene
Ton-Nu, Thanh-Thao

ST JEAN SUR RICHELIEU
Gossard, Denis
Karam, Jacques
Savard, Daniel
Simion, Oana-Maria

TERREBONNE
Desjardins, Valerie A.
Phaneuf, Denis C.

TROIS-RIVIERES
Beaudry, Pierre
Gagne, Carl E.
Garand, Mark
Gervais, Pierre B.
Gisbert, Ramon
Lainesse, Andre
Lemay, Catherine
Raymond, Alain
Rheault, Alain

VAL-D'OR
Pouliot, Joel

VERDUN
Bonny, Shawn
Gagnon, Jacques-Eric
Solignac, Alain L.
Winter, Elric D.

WESTMOUNT
Benjamin, Pierre
Maranda, Claude R.
Marpole, Derek G F.
Pasternac, Andre
Rabinovitch, Mark A.

SASKATCHEWAN

MOOSE JAW
Tarhuni, Wadea M.

REGINA
Aboguddah, Ayman A.
Booker, Jeffrey D.
Dehghani, Payam
Garbe, George J.
Gargoum, Hassan A M.
Lavoie, Andrea J.
Murthy, Dakshina
Sultan, Omar
Zimmermann, Rodney H.

SASKATOON
Akhtar, Jawed
Basran, Rashpal S.
Bree, Teresa L.
Coverett, Kelly O.
De Villiers, Jacobus
Dewa, Dalisizwe M K.
Kakadekar, Ashok P.
Nosib, Shravankumar S.
Orvold, Jason N.
PausJenssen, Erik L.
Pearce, Colin B.
Pharis, C. Scott
Rajakumar, Alphonsus R J.
Sayed, Ahmed
Stuglin, Carlo
Wells, Calvin R.

Cardiothoracic Surgery

ALBERTA

CALGARY
Ali, Imtiaz S.

BRITISH COLUMBIA

VANCOUVER
Dewar, Leith

VICTORIA
Ofiesh, John G.
Perchinsky, Michael J.

NEWFOUNDLAND AND LABRADOR

ST. JOHN'S
Mong, Kam W.

NOVA SCOTIA

HALIFAX
Hirsch, Gregory M.

ONTARIO

HAMILTON
Lamy, Andre

KINGSTON
Hamilton, G. Andrew
Petsikas, Dimitri J.

KITCHENER
Salasidis, Gary C.
Talwar, Manoj K.

LONDON
Quantz, Mackenzie A.

MISSISSAUGA
Bhatnagar, Gopal
Cutrara, Charles A.

OTTAWA
Rubens, Fraser D.

SUDBURY
Garg, Avinash

TORONTO
Keshavjee, Shaf
Ralph-Edwards, Anthony C.

WOODBRIDGE
Del Rizzo, Dario F.

QUÉBEC

MONTREAL
Cecere, Renzo
Ergina, Patrick L.
Lachapelle, Kevin J.
Shum-Tim, Dominique

Cardiovascular & Thoracic Surgery

ALBERTA

CALGARY
Burgess, John J.
Kidd, William T.
Kieser, Teresa M.
Maitland, Andrew
Prystai, Gregory D.
Rothschild, John M.

EDMONTON
Koshal, Arvind
Modry, Dennis L.
Mullen, John C.
Rebeyka, Ivan M.
Ross, David B.

BRITISH COLUMBIA

KELOWNA
Fradet, Guy

NEW WESTMINSTER
Hayden, Robert I.
Toppin, Dennis I.
Vrabec, George

VANCOUVER
Abel, James G.
Gudas, Virginia M.
Jamieson, W R. Eric
Janusz, Michael T.
Leblanc, Jacques G.
Lichtenstein, Samuel V.
Ling, Hilton
Miyagishima, Robert T.
Munro, A. Ian

MANITOBA

WINNIPEG
Menkis, Alan H.
Warrian, R. Keith

NEW BRUNSWICK

SAINT JOHN
Brown, Craig
Forgie, W. Rand

NEWFOUNDLAND AND LABRADOR

ST. JOHN'S
Melvin, Kevin N.

NOVA SCOTIA

HALIFAX
Ali, Idris M.
Stewart, Keir M.
Sullivan, John A P.
Wood, Jeremy R.

ONTARIO

BARRIE
McDonald, Sandy I R.

HAMILTON
Cybulsky, Irene J.
Lamy, Andre
Mosakoski, Joan

KINGSTON
Petsikas, Dimitri J.

KITCHENER
Leclerc, Yves

LONDON
Goldbach, Martin M.
Goodman, Robert L.
Guiraudon, Gerard M.
Guo, Lin Rui.
McKenzie, F. Neil
Myers, M. Lee
Novick, Richard

MISSISSAUGA
Ahmed, Shafqat M.

NEWMARKET
Bauset, Richard
Moon, Byung-Choo
Peniston, Charles M.
Teoh, Kevin H T.

NIAGARA FALLS
Doobay, Budhendranauth S.

OAKVILLE
Gafoor, Mohamed M.

OTTAWA
Goldstein, William
Hendry, Paul J.
Masters, Roy G.
Redmond, Mary L.
Shamji, Farid M.

SARNIA
Rosenblum, Stan

SUDBURY
Aul, Sewa S.

TORONTO
Bonneau, Daniel
Brister, Stephanie J.
Christakis, George T.
Coles, John G.
Conn, Robert D.
Cusimano, Robert J.
David, Tirone
De La Rocha, Claudio
Errett, Lee E.
Feindel, Christopher M S.
Fremes, Stephen E.
Latter, David A.
Ropchan, Glorianne V.
Scully, Hugh E.
Weisel, Richard D.

WINDSOR
Pearce, Craig R.

QUÉBEC

CHICOUTIMI
Farinas, Jean-Marc
Mathieu, John F.

CLARENCEVILLE
Jones, C. William

MONTREAL
Abdulnour, Elias M.
Basile, Fadi
Bouchard, Denis
Carrier, Michel
Cartier, Raymond
Cecere, Renzo
Choiniere, Louise
Chughtai, M. Saeed
De Varennes, Benoit
Dontigny, Leon
Ergina, Patrick L.
Ghosn, Pierre B.
Hebert, Yves
Joassin, Alfred M.
Lachapelle, Kevin J.
Lafontaine, Edwin R.
Langlois, Yves
Ma, Felix
Morin, Jean-Francois
Mulder, David S.
Normandin, Louis
Page, Pierre
Pellerin, Michel
Perrault, Louis P.
Poirier, Nancy C.
Prieto, Ignacio
Sheiner, Nathan M.
Shum-Tim, Dominique
Tchervenkov, Christo I.
Verdant, Alain G.
Vobecky, J. Suzanne

QUEBEC
Baillot, Richard
Dagenais, Francois
Desaulniers, Denis
Deslauriers, Jean
Doyle, Daniel
Gregoire, Jocelyn
Lemieux, Michel D.
Mathieu, Patrick
Metras, Jacques
Perron, Jean
Vaillancourt, Rosaire

SAINT-LAMBERT
Beaulieu, R. Claude

SHERBROOKE
Greentree, David M.
Normandin, Denyse
Teijeira, F. Javier

VERDUN
Richard, Philippe F A.

SASKATCHEWAN

SASKATOON
Mycyk, Taras R.
Thomson, Dorothy J.

Clinical Immunology & Allergy

ALBERTA

CALGARY
Cheuk, Stephen T.
Cross, David
Doctor, Joel
Kavadas, Fotini D.
Serushago, Bazir A.
Sorg, Michael K.

EDMONTON
Carr, Stuart N.
Lidman, Per G L.
Lin, Michael C.
Osundwa, Vincent M.
Russell, Anthony S.
Vander Leek, Timothy K.

BRITISH COLUMBIA

BURNABY
Chang, Ross E.
Kim, Seung

KELOWNA
Appelt, Gregory

RICHMOND
Luciuk, George H.
Wong, Chet G.

VANCOUVER
Bergman, James N.
Chan, Edmond S.
Dean, John M.
Kanani, Amin S.
Kaviani, Mandana
Schellenberg, R. Robert
Stark, Donald F.
Turvey, Stuart E.
Wong, H C. George
Yeung, Joanne P.
Yu, Joyce W.

VICTORIA
Cameron, Scott B.
Gendreau-Reid, M F. Liliane
Lee, Ching Sang
Lee, Kingsley R.

MANITOBA

WINNIPEG
Becker, Allan B.
Cisneros, Nestor F.
Drewniak, Anna
Gerstner, Thomas V.
James, J. Marion E.
Kalicinsky, Chrystyna M.
Pitt, Tracy J.
Pun, Teresa W C.
Roberts, Janet R.
Warrington, Richard J.

NOVA SCOTIA

HALIFAX
Connors, Lori A.
Kapur, Sandeep
Lacuesta, Gina A.
Rex, Gregory A.
Watson, Wade T A.

ONTARIO

AJAX
Buttoo, Kenneth

BARRIE
Clark, Jessica M.
Fischer, David A.
Haaland, Derek A.

BURLINGTON
Cyr, Michael M.
MacK, Douglas P.
Messieh, Mary L.

CORNWALL
Copeland, David

EAST YORK
Ali, Yaser M A.
Miller, Charlotte D.
Papadopoulos, Anastasios S.

ETOBICOKE
Bulley, Sean R.
McLauchlin, Michelle S.

HAMILTON
Abdurrahman, Zainab B.
Greenbaum, Joseph
Keith, Paul K.
Lebert, Phyllis A.
Ohayon, Jason A.
Waserman, Susan

KANATA
Frankish, Charles W.
Lee, Peter K O.

KINGSTON
Borici-Mazi, Rozita
Ellis, Anne K.
Tsai, Ellie L.

KITCHENER
Kim, Harold L.
Lima Filho, Jose H C.
White, Frederick A.

LONDON
Hildebrand, Kyla J.
Kloth, Debra M.
Moote, D. William
Payton, Keith B.

MISSISSAUGA
Cheema, Amarjit S.
Patel, Piyush R.
Wong, Albert G.

NEPEAN
Algom, David

NIAGARA FALLS
Alexander, Michael

NORTH YORK
Donsky, Judith E.
Herman-Kideckel, Sari M.
Hummel, David B.
Kagan, Rhoda S.
Segal, Audrey O.
Weber, Elizabeth A.
Wong, Benjamin B L.

OAKVILLE
Chung, Arthur G.
Leith, Eric S.
Marrin, Andrea K.

OSHAWA
Lemon-Mule, Heather F.
Tepper, Jamie L.

OTTAWA
Ham Pong, Antony J.
Kerr, Pauline E.

RICHMOND HILL
Yeung, Albert

SCARBOROUGH
Ching, Joyce C Y.
Mace, Sean R.

TORONTO
Al Maini, Mustafa H A.
Atkinson, Adelle R.
Betschel, Stephen D.
Binkley, Karen E.
Kim, Vy Hong-Diep N.
Lavine, Elana S.
Lee, Jason K.
Leznoff, Arthur
MacFadden, Douglas K.
Mohammed, Reem W A.
Stein, Raymond D.
Sussman, Gordon L.
Upton, Julia E M.
Vadas, Peter

UNIONVILLE
Wai, Yvonne

WATERLOO
Terpstra, Collin R.
Yip, Lisa Y.

WINDSOR
Khan, Farah I.
Liem, Joel J.
Zanganeh, Shahin

WOODBRIDGE
Liew, Kenneth Y K.
Triassi Asper, Maria

QUÉBEC

BELOEIL
Charbonneau, Yves

COTE SAINT-LUC
Segal, Lauren M.
Shahin, Edmond B N.

GATINEAU
Chad, Zave H.
Hotte, Simon L.
Pucar, Frederic

GREENFIELD PARK
Dube, Normand
Francoeur, Marie-Josee
Moore, Andrew D.

LAVAL
Caron, Andre B.
Nguyen Luu, Nha-Uyen
Weisnagel, John

MONTREAL
Alizadehfar, Reza
Banerjee, Devi
Begin, Philippe
Blaquiere, Martin
Blumer, Herbert M.
Chapdelaine, Hugo
Clarke, Ann E.
Cloutier-Marchand, Francine
Del Carpio, Jaime
Delespesse, Guy J.
Des Roches, Anne
Desjardins, Maryline
Fuks, Abraham
Gold, Phil
Haddad, Elie
Hassaine, Assia
Lejtenyi, M. Christine
Masse, Marie-Soleil
Mazer, Bruce D.
McCusker, Christine T.
Nashi, Emil
Noya, Francisco J D.
Paradis, Jean
Picard, Matthieu
Primeau, Marie-Noel
Schonfeld, Irving B.
Schulz, Jan I.
Sigman, Karen G.
Silviu-Dan, Fanny
Skamene, Emil
Small, Peter
St-Pierre, Jean-Paul
Thomson, David M P.
Watts, Craig S.

QUEBEC
Bedard, Pierre-Michel
Boursiquot, Jean-Nicolas
Drolet, Jean-Philippe
Drouin, Michel A.
Dugal, Michele
Gagnon, Remi
Hebert, Jacques R.
Lavoie, Aubert
Umemoto, Lorne N.
Verreault, Nina

REPENTIGNY
Laramée, Benoit

SAINT-HYACINTHE
Dorval, Guerin

SAINT-LAMBERT
Nguyen, Melanie M L.

SHERBROOKE
Lemire, Chantal
Lemire, Martine
Rola-Pleszczynski, Marek

ST-EUSTACHE
Paradis, Louis

VAL-D'OR
Kukhta, Allison

WESTMOUNT
Calles, Jose
Medoff, Elaine J.
Tannenbaum, Hyman

SASKATCHEWAN

SASKATOON
Persaud, Mitra M P.

Community Medicine

ALBERTA

CALGARY
Friesen, Brent T.
Fryatt, Kenneth D.
Garcia-Rodriguez, Juan A.
MacDonald, Judy
McDougall, Laura
McIntyre, L. Lynn
McLeod, Laura J.
Musto, Richard J.
Russell, Margaret L.
Sackman, Paul G.
Sarin, Christopher
Stoffel, Sandra S.
Strong, David G.
Swann, David R.
Thiara, Parminder K.
Yang, Huiming
Zimmer, Rudolf A G.

CAMROSE
Hinshaw, Deena L.

EDMONTON
Cherry, Nicola M.
Corriveau, André E.
Francescutti, Louis
Johnson, Marcia M.
Keays, Gloria E.
Koliaska, Kathryn M.
Lavoie, Martin
Predy, Gerald N.
Sikora, Christopher A.
Virani, Hakique N.
Yacoub, Wadieh R.

RED DEER
Horne, J. Digby

SHERWOOD PARK
Cheng, Jim I.

SIKSIKA
Clearsky, Lorne S.

BRITISH COLUMBIA

ABBOTSFORD
Lem, Marcus E.

BURNABY
Willaeys, Veerle R P.

COURTENAY
Enns, Charmaine L.

GIBSONS
Martiquet, Paul A.

HAZELTON
Hougesen, Bent

KELOWNA
Corneil, Trevor A.
Larder, Andrew P.
Parker, Robert A.
Pollock, Susan L.

MAPLE RIDGE
Arsenault, Gillian R.

NANAIMO
Hasselback, Paul D.

PRINCE GEORGE
Chapman, Ronald D.

RICHMOND
Lalji, Ronil S.

SALMON ARM
Barss, Peter G.

SURREY
Brodkin, Elizabeth J.
Guasparini, Roland
Swinkels, Helena M.

VANCOUVER
Barrios, Rolando A.
Bigham, J. Mark
Buxton, Jane A.
Carsley, John K.
Clair, Veronic
Daly, Patricia C.
Dawar, Meenakshi
Elliott, Catherine T.
Elwood, J. Mark
Forbes, Ian S.
Galanis, Eleni
Gilbert, Mark P J.
Gustafson, Reka Z.
Henry, Bonnie J F.
Hertzman, Clyde
Kosatsky, Thomas B.
Lee, Victoria E H.
Marion, Stephen A.
McLean, Mark E.
Moore, David M.
Scott, Ian M.
Skowronski, Danuta M.
Srour, Leila F.
Wardman, A E. Dennis
Waters, Shannon
Yassi, Annalee

VICTORIA
Fyfe, Murray W.
Kendall, Perry R W.
Rutherford, Beverly E.
Stanwick, Richard S.
Young, Eric R.

MANITOBA

BEAUSEJOUR
Robinson, Karen G.

SOUTHPORT
Buchan, Shelley M.

STONEWALL
Hilderman, Timothy E.

WINNIPEG
Butler-Jones, David A.
Demeter Jr., Sandor
Elliott, Lawrence J.
Fatoye, Olubunmi
Harlos, Sandra C.
Kettner, Joel D.
Koh, Denise M.
Kurbis, Carol A.
Libich, William G.
MacDonald, Sharon M.
Mahmud, Salaheddin M.
Poffenroth, Linda A.
Postl, Brian
Redekop, Theodore D.
Richards, Lisa K M.
Roberecki, Susan A.
Routledge, W. Michael
Wright, Brock J.

NEW BRUNSWICK

FREDERICTON
Muecke, Cristin

MONCTON
Allard, Denis G.
Donovan, Marie-Denise
Leger, Yves A.

NEWFOUNDLAND AND LABRADOR

MOUNT PEARL
Allison, David J.

ST. JOHN'S
Seviour, Rosann E.

NOVA SCOTIA

DARTMOUTH
Watson-Creed, Gaynor B.

HALIFAX
Poulin, Christiane C.
Strang, Robert A.

SYDNEY
Dutt, Monika

WOLFVILLE
Gould, John R.

ONTARIO

BARRIE
Gardner, Charles
Lee, Colin Q T.

BRAMPTON
Wallington, Tamara A.

BROCKVILLE
Stewart, Paula J.

CAMPBELLFORD
Schabas, Richard E.

DELTA
Climie, Robert C.

ETOBICOKE
Chase, Robert M.
Gibson, Brian L.

GLOUCESTER
Ellis, Edward

HAMILTON
Chong, John P.
Emili, Julie-Anne
Haines, A. Theodore S.
Jenicek, Milos
MacKie, Christopher A O.
Richardson, Elizabeth A.
Tran, Ninh Ngoc

KINGSTON
Gemmill, H. Ian M.

LONDON
Warshawsky, Bryna F.

MARKHAM
Kapoor, Vimal S.
Rottensten, Kirsten L.

MISSISSAUGA
De Villa, Eileen P.
Gindi, Medhat F.
Mowat, David L.
Ward, B. Megan

NEPEAN
Etches, Vera G.
Levy, Isra G.

NEWMARKET
Kurji, Karimmohamed H.
Moloughney, Brent W P.
Weir, Erica
Yuan, Lilian

NORTH YORK
Chan, Eng-Soon
Liss, Gary M.
Mai, Verna M.
Marchant, Rosemary E.
Pakes, Barry N.
Reynolds, Donna L.
Shapiro, Marla

OAKVILLE
Nosal, Robert M.
Taha, Monir

ORANGEVILLE
Cole, Peter N.

OTTAWA
Allard, Pierre
Archibald, Christopher
Callary, Eva
Cappon, Paul S.
Carew, Maureen T.
Cushman Jr, Robert A.
Dunkley, Geoffrey C.
Gervais, Robert-Paul
Gordon, Mary E.
Lewis, Rosamund F.
Manuel, Douglas G.
McCourt, Catherine M.
Muldoon, Laura K.
Njoo, Howard T H.
Panaro, Linda K.
Paradis, Rejean
Pelletier, Louise
Pim, Carolyn P.
Rodin, Rachel L.
Salisbury, David A.
Stieb, David M.
Taylor, Gregory W.
Tepper, Martin L.
Werker, Denise H.
Whitehead, Jeffrey J.

PETERBOROUGH
Pellizzari, Rosana

PORT HOPE
Noseworthy, A. Lynn

PORT PERRY
Hoey, John R.

SARNIA
Greensmith, Christopher T.

SCARBOROUGH
Beattie, Joan K.

STRATFORD
Tamblyn, Susan E.

SUDBURY
Lamptey, Na-Koshie
Sutcliffe, Penelope A.

THORNHILL
Kassam, Hanif
Wittes, Robert C.

THOROLD
Hopkins, Jessica P.

THUNDER BAY
Williams, David C.

TIMMINS
Ramsingh, Rosemarie

TORONTO
Armstrong, Irene E.
Berger, Lisa
Chris, Allison E.
Cole, Donald C.
DeKoven, Joel
Deeks, Shelley L.
Dubey, Vinita
Finkelstein, Michael S.
Fralick, Richard A.
Glasgow, Kevin
Goel, Vivek
Grossman, David W.
Harvey, Bartholomew J.
Hodge, Matthew J.
Holowaty, Eric J.
Hoskins, Eric W.
Johnson, Ian L.
Jones, Karen E.
Kahan, Meldon M.
Kiefer, Lori A.
King, Arlene S.
Kwong, Jeffrey C Y.
McKeown, David J.
Millson, Margaret E.
Narod, Steven A.
Nutt, Samantha J.
Pasut, George
Patel, Zeenat R.
Rachlis, Michael M.
Rea, Elizabeth H.
Sachdeva, Herveen K.
Scott, Elizabeth A F.
Shahin, Rita M.
Shapiro, Howard S.
Sider, Douglas M.
Stirling, Robert G.
Svoboda, Tomislav
Tyler, Ingrid V L.
Upshur, Ross E G.
Wilson, Sarah E.
Wong, Roland C K.
Yaffe, Barbara A.
Young, Theron K.

TWEED
Mustard, J. Charles

WATERLOO
Nolan, Liana
Wang, Hsiu-Li

WHITBY
Kyle, Robert J.

WINDSOR
Miller, Barry A.

WOODBRIDGE
Bilotta, Rosetta

QUÉBEC

CHICOUTIMI
Desmeules, Paul

GASPE
Courville, Ariane
Deck, Wilber

GATINEAU
Courteau, Jean-Pierre
Kafka, Marcella
Kom Mogto, Christelle A D.
Mohanna, Samy S M.
Paquette, Camille

GREENFIELD PARK
Blackburn, Manon

JOLIETTE
Lesage, Michel
Quirion, Sylvie
Robillard, Pierre
Trepanier, Jean-Pierre

KUUJJUAQ
Bouchard, Francoise

LAVAL
Damestoy, Nicole
Gagnon, Fabien
Irace-Cima, Alejandra
Lajoie, Mireille
Osterman, John W.
Paquette, Daniel
Poupart, Gilles
Prevost, Claude
Stefan, Mark A.

LONGUEUIL
Cambron-Goulet, Evelyne
Dufort, Julie
Guay, Maryse
Hudson, Patricia
Kadaoui, Nabila
L'Heureux, Jean
Lacroix, Christine
Lajoie, Elisabeth
Loslier, Julie
Messier, Alain
Milord, Francois
Moisan, Serge
Sauve, Jocelyne
St-Amour, Marie

MONTREAL
Adrien, Alix
Allard, Robert
Andermann, Anne
Auger, Nathalie
Battista, Renaldo N.
Bergeron, Pierre
Boivin, Jean-François
Brassard, Paul
Buckeridge, David L.
Colin, Christine
Cote, Brigitte V.
Cote, Jacques R.
Cox Jr., J. Joseph
Daneault, Serge
De Blois, Suzanne
Demers, Huguette
Denis, Geoffroy
Dery, Veronique
Deutsch-Andermann, Eva
Dougherty, Geoffrey E.
Drouin, Louis
Drouin, Mylene
Dumont, Yves G.
Duplessis, Pierre
Duval, Michel E.
Galarneau, Louise
Goulet, Lise
Goupil, Jean-Noel
Infante-Rivard, Claire
Jacques, Louis
Jen, Yun
Kossowski, Alexandra
Lague, Johanne
Lebel, Paule T.
Lessard, Richard
Levesque, Jean-Frederic
Litvak, Eric
Masse, Richard
Mercure, Claude
Morency, Patrick
Morissette, Carole
Palmieri, Sandra
Paradis, Gilles
Perron, Stephane
Pineault, Raynald
Pinsonneault, Linda
Raynault, Marie-France
Richer, Faisca
Robinson, Elizabeth
Rochon, Jean
Rossignol, Michel
Roy, Maxime
Seguin, Pierre
Sicard, Nadine
Soto, Julio C.
Stock, Susan R.
Tannenbaum, Terry-Nan
Theriault, Gilles
Thibeault, Lynda
Tousignant, Pierre
Tremblay, Michele
Valiquette, Louise
White-Guay, Brian

POINTE-A-LA-CROIX
Langlois, Richard

QUEBEC
April, Nicole
Arruda, Horacio
Aube, Denise
Bairati, Isabelle
Beaucage, Clement
Berlinguet, Marc
Cardinal, Lise
De Wals, Phillippe
Desbiens, Francois
Dionne, Marc
Dontigny, Andre
Douville-Fradet, Monique
Durand, Pierre J.
Fortin, Jean-Paul
Gagne, Denise
Girard, Jacques E.
Goupil-Sormany, Isabelle
Huot, Caroline
Hyppolite, Shirley-Rose
Lajoie, Pierre
Laliberte, Denis
Lavoie, Michel
Levallois, Patrick J.
Levesque, Benoit
Maurice, Pierre
Messely, Marie-Claude
Moreault, Louise
Morin, Real
Ouellet, Francine
Perron, Linda
Poirier, Alain
Racine, Simon
Rhainds, Marc G.
Ringuet, Jacques
Rochette, Emilien
Rochette, Marie
Roy, Denis
Roy, Guy
Sauvageau, Chantal
Theriault, A. Nathanaelle
Tourigny, Andre
Tremblay, Genevieve
Veilleux, Julien R.
Vezina, Michel
Wallot, Hubert A.

RIMOUSKI
Guyon, Akingabe
Leduc, Sylvain
Maguire, Robert

RIVIERE-DU-LOUP
Boudreau, Richard
Pouliot, Bernard

ROUYN-NORANDA
Lampron-Goulet, Eric
Letourneau, Gerald

SAINT-JEROME
Allard, Andre
Belanger-Bonneau, Helene
Goyer, Eric
Piquet-Gauthier, Blandine
Robert, Jean

SAINTE-MARIE
Bonnier-Viger, Yves
Deshaies, Pierre
Drolet, Marie-Josee
Laflamme, Patrice
Laplante, Odette
Pare, Louise
Veillette, Rene

SHERBROOKE
Baron, Genevieve
Boisvert, Richard
Clapperton, Irma
Genereux, Mélissa
Petit, Genevieve
Pronovost, Robert
Rochon, Alain
Samson, Isabelle
Simard, Robert

ST CHARLES BORROMEE
Badlissi, Dalal
Marcoux, Laurent

TROIS-RIVIERES
Grenier, Anne-Marie
Milette, Linda
Toupin, Manon

VERDUN
Cadieux, Roger
Lecours, Serge

SASKATCHEWAN

LA RONGE
Irvine, James D.

REGINA
Shahab, Saqib

SASKATOON
Findlater, A. Ross
Neudorf, Cordell O.
Reeder, Bruce A.

WEYBURN
Hudson, Shauna G.

Dermatology

ALBERTA

CALGARY
Adams, Stewart P A.
Alanen, Kenneth W.
Arlette, John P.
Barber, Kirk A.
Behm, Allan R.
Campbell, Janis P.
Cohen, Howard B.
Devani, Alim R.
Gili, Adrian F.
Haber, Richard M.
Hackett, Sharon L.
Kellner, Barbara L.
Mah-Poy, George L.
Metelitsa, Andrei
Mydlarski, P. Regine
Parsons, Laurie M.
Poelman, Susan M.
Redding, Keith G.
Remington, B. Kent
Robertson, Lynne H.
Storwick, Gregory S.
Ting, Patricia
Woo, Thomas Y.
Woolner, Derek B.
Zip, Catherine M.

CANMORE
Lubitz, Paul A.

EDMONTON
Brassard, Alain
Cheung-Lee, Melody
Chow, Eunice Y.
Dytoc, Marlene T.
El-Sawaf, Amro
Elliott, John F.
Fiorillo, Loretta
Grewal, Parbeer
Groot, Donald W.
Kalisiak, Michal S.
Keeling, Christopher P.
Liao, Janice Y.
Lin, Andrew N.
Lycka, Barry A S.
Man, Jeremy R.
Nakatsui, Thomas C.
Rao, Jaggi
Rogers, M. Bryson
Salopek, Thomas G.
Sapijaszko, Mariusz J A.
Schloss, Eric H.
Searles, Gordon E.
Taher, Muba S.
Wasel, Norman R.

GRANDE PRAIRIE
Malcolm, Christine E.

LETHBRIDGE
Low, Ronald R.

MEDICINE HAT
Taylor, William P.

BRITISH COLUMBIA

BURNABY
Dodd, William A H.
Tullis, Gary D.
Withers, Michelle C.

COQUITLAM
Prihoda, Marie B.
Tuyp, Evert J.

COURTENAY
Jenkins, Donald

KELOWNA
Anderson, Carmel R.

LANGLEY
Peter, Kevin K.

NANAIMO
Weichert, Gabriele E.

NEW WESTMINSTER
Chan, Eugene J.
Han, Christina E.
Ulmer, Marcie J.
Wong, S M. Simon

NORTH VANCOUVER
Shokravi, Mohammad B.
Yu, John T.

PENTICTON
Harris, Russell B.

PRINCE GEORGE
Martindale, Michael E.

RICHMOND
Conklin, Robert J.
Nguyen, Nhiem
Tsang, David T S.

SURREY
Albrecht, Lorne E.
Hong, Hilary C.
Jovanovic, Mile
Rahim, Zulficar K.

VANCOUVER
Akrigg, Marian R.
Au, Sheila
Bergman, James N.
Carruthers, J. Alastair
Crawford, Richard I.
Davis, Kathleen A.
De Gannes, Gillian C.
Dutz, Jan P.
Gray, Robin S.
Gregory, Brian W.
Ho, Vincent C Y.
Humphrey, Shannon D.
Jang, Frances L.
Kalia, Sunil
Kitson, C. Neil
Kunimoto, Brian T.
Lui, Harvey
McLean, David I.
McLeod, W. Alastair
Morton, Charles E.
Prendiville, Juliette S M.
Rivers, Jason K.
Shapiro, Jerry
Sigal, Cecil
Thomas, D. Richard R.
Warshawski, Laurence M.
Zhou, Youwen F.
Zloty, David M.

VICTORIA
Amiss, John D.
Hancock, Julian A.
Kenny, Patrick
Lupin, Mark H.
Rossi, Sikina F.
Telford, Gordon O.

WEST VANCOUVER
Day, Joanna
Sereda, Danya A.

MANITOBA

WINNIPEG
Afifi, Tarek J.
Collin, Marian B.
Haydey, Richard P.
Hurst, Lorne D C.
Keddy-Grant, Jill A.
Kellen, Philippa E.
Minuk, Earl S.
Sheps, Michael D.
Silver, Shane G.
Taraska, Victoria K.
Toole, John W P.
Van De Velde, Rochelle S.
Wiseman, Marni C.

NEW BRUNSWICK

BATHURST
Lepage, France

FREDERICTON
Hanson, Dana W.
Turchin, Irina

MONCTON
Bolduc, Alain
Bourcier, Marc
Hayes, Evelyn A.
Lepage, Anik

QUISPAMSIS
Keeling, Douglas N.

ROTHESAY
Hayes, Robert C.

SAINT JOHN
Baxter, Kathy L.

SHEDIAC
Chiasson, Chantal

NEWFOUNDLAND AND LABRADOR

CORNER BROOK
Sladden, Christopher S.

GRAND FALLS WINDSOR
Anandakrishnan, Canagasund
Coffey, James

ST. JOHN'S
Brown-Maher, Tracey D.
Clarke, Gillian I.
Coffey, Joseph F.
Gulliver, Wayne P.
Landells, Ian D R.
Ohson, Kamal K S.
Tomi, Zohair S.

NOVA SCOTIA

DARTMOUTH
Baxter, Mary L S.
Gallant, Christopher J.

HALIFAX
Finlayson, Laura
Green, Peter
Kelly, Colleen M.
Langley, Richard G B.
Miller, Robert A W.
Murray, Scott J.
Purdy, Kerri S.
Reardon, P. Michael
Tremaine, Robert D L.

KENTVILLE
Shaffelburg, Michael D.

SYDNEY
D'Intino, Yolanda M.
Northgrave, Stacey A.

ONTARIO

AJAX
Adam, David N.
Waitzer, Sloane M.

ANCASTER
O'Malley, Maureen P.
Wismer, Judy E M.

BARRIE
Kunynetz, Rodion A W.
Schemmer, Robert J.
Shayesteh Alam, Maryam

BELLEVILLE
Horan, P. Frank

BRAMPTON
Chang, Daniel K M.

BRANTFORD
Skolnick, Marvin

BURLINGTON
Jiaravuthisan, Michael
Muhn, Channy Y.
Rosen, Nathan A.

CAMBRIDGE
Jain, Hem C.

DUNDAS
Edstrom, Karen D.

ETOBICOKE
Alexis, Mercy E.
Fisher, Marnie E.
Jambrosic, Jadranka A.
Poulos, Elena
Redlick, Fara P.
Rosenberg, Frank W.
Saksun, Jana M B.
Simone, Andrew A.
Wasserman, Gary A.

GUELPH
Howell, Brandon G.
Tsoulis, Christopher J.
Willoughby, Joanne S.

HAMILTON
Murphy, Frank R.
Rosenthal, Donald
Saveriano, Nellina
Shukla, Rahul
Vender, Ronald B.
Vignjevic, Peter M.

HAWKESBURY
Williams, AnnaMary J.

KINGSTON
MacSween, Ruth M.

KITCHENER
Kobayashi, Kenneth A.
Lima Filho, Jose H C.

LONDON
Dilworth, Geoffrey R.
Guenther, Lyn C C.
Gupta, Aditya K.
Horgan-Bell, Caroline B.
Loo, Wei Jing
Wexler, Denise M M A.

MARKHAM
Kraft, John N.
Lynde, Charles W.
Wyse, Carl W.

MILTON
Birkett, Barbara M.

MISSISSAUGA
Alavi, Afsaneh
Eisenberg, Eric L.
Harris, Howard M.
Hinek, Anna
Lomaga, Mark
Mistry, Nisha
O'Neill, Karen A.
Panzini, Henriette A.
Sibbald, R. Gary
Webster, Christine E.

NEPEAN
Robern, Michael
Shukle, Jacqueline M C.

NEWMARKET
Katz, Arnon M.
Turner, John J.

NIAGARA FALLS
Smith, Kevin C.

NIAGARA ON THE LAKE
Hall, Susan E H.

NORTH BAY
Rosoph, Leslie A.

NORTH YORK
Amin, Smita
Barankin, Benjamin
Davis, Michael G.
Freiman, Anatoli
Ho, Nhung T C.
Leneck, Charles M.
Levy, Michelle
McKenzie, Mary A.
Monson, Rochelle L.
Natsheh, Adam
Niakosari, Firouzeh
Rajan, Poonam
Reicher, Agnes E.
Richards, Robert N.
Shapero, Jonathan
Ung, Chantelle Y W.
Weksberg, Alfred
Wine, Stanley J.
Winnicki, Monika
Wong, Maxine Y W.

OAKVILLE
Belovic, Branislav
Haider, Aamir
Hogan, Megan R.
Sapra, Sheetal
Taylor, E. Kent

ORLEANS
Brisson, Paul

OSHAWA
Cammisuli, Salvatore
Jakubovic, Henry R.
Tuppal, Raj K.
Turner, Cory C.

OTTAWA
Adam, John E.
Beecker, Jennifer R.
DesGroseilliers, Jean-Pierre
Dossetor, Clare B.
Fahim, Simone S I.
Finkelstein, Harvey
Goodall, John C.
Heughan, Caroline E.
Jackson, Robert
Kanigsberg, Nordau D.
LaBerge, Lauren E.
Laughlin, Sharyn A.
Lipson, Jennifer E.
MacDonald, Jillian A.
Mikhael, Dalia
Moses, Kathleen
Pierscianowski, Tadeusz A.
Pratt, Melanie
Prokopetz, Robert D.
Quintal, M C. Diane
Ringwald, Pierre
Roy-Boulos, Anne-Marie
Ruddy, Catherine

Swiggum, Susan M M.
Walker, James D.
Weatherhead, Louis E P.

OWEN SOUND
Cote, Stephanie J.

PETERBOROUGH
Gooderham, Melinda J.

RICHMOND HILL
Lee, Simon K W.
MacPherson, Margaret A.
Raman, Mani

SARNIA
Jose, Aurea S.

SCARBOROUGH
Abadir, Wadid W K.
Gupta, Samir
Hessami-Booshehri, Morvarid
Hofstader, Sophie L R.
Lee Choi, Kenneth

ST CATHARINES
Sloan, Kevin P.

STONEY CREEK
Lozinski, Ala Z.

THORNHILL
Bargman, Howard B.
Landolt, Sandra J.
Shapiro, Lori E.
Sharma, Shakti
Spier, Stanley

THUNDER BAY
Mahler, Ronald H.

TORONTO
Adam, Paul
Al Harithy, Ru'aa S K A.
Alhusayen, Ra'ed O S.
Almohammedi, Faisal
Assaad, Dalal M.
Baibergenova, Akerke T.
Carroll, Julia M.
Chan, An Wen
Chan, Patrick S P.
Cohen, Paul D.
Cook, Sonya M.
Curtis, M. Anne
DeKoven, Joel
Donovan, Jeffrey
Dutil, Maha Theresa
Fiala, Katarina
Florence, Ralph
From, Lynn
Gidon, Martie S.
Goldhar, John N H.
Goldstein, Eric
Haberman, Herbert F.
Ho Ping Kong, Barbara S.
Hradsky, Nadine S.
Jarvis, Ingrid M.
Joseph, Marissa O.
Kellett, Lisa M.
King, Aaron D.
Krafchik, Bernice R.
Lansang, Perla
Linzon, Charlene D.
Long, Barry H.
Medline, Norton M.
Medwidsky, Wolodymyr
Monthrope, Yvette
Murray, Christian A.
Nasseri, Eiman
Paquin, Colette
Pollack, Sheldon V.
Pon, Kucy
Rosen, Cheryl F.
Ryan, Siobhan M.
Salsberg, Jennifer M.
Schachter, G. Daniel
Shapero, Harvey G.
Shaw, James C.
Shear, Neil H.
Shiffman, Norman J.
Siddha, Sanjay K.
Singh, Davindra
Skotnicki-Grant, Sandra M.
Solish, Nowell J.
Solomon, Robert S.
Taradash, Jay B.
Unger, Walter P.
Vincent, Franklynne K.
Walsh, Scott R A.
Walter, Anthony J.
Weinstein, Miriam G.
Wilson, Maithili K.
Yeung, Jensen M.

WATERLOO
Amdemichael, Esiahas
MacEachern, William N.
Papp, Kim A.

WELLAND
Garnis-Jones, Sylvia G.

WINDSOR
Novice, Fred M.
Radin, Daniel A.
Tan, Jerry K L.
Toth, Darryl P.

WOODBRIDGE
Bertucci, Vince
Nield, Gail L.

PRINCE EDWARD ISLAND

CHARLOTTETOWN
Klein, Jean-Marc Y.

QUÉBEC

ALMA
Bouchard, Francois

BOISBRIAND
Savard, Pascal

BOUCHERVILLE
Truong, Thuy-Tien

CHICOUTIMI
Dupere, Audrey
Leclerc, Georgette
Patry, Gilles

DOLLARD DES ORMEAUX
O'Brien, Elizabeth A.

GASPE
Jacques, Pierre

GATINEAU
Alain, Guylaine
Charbonneau, Jacques
Coulibaly, Eva
Giard, Francoise
Girouard, Michele
Toscano, Marie

GRANBY
Heroux, Josee
Tanguay, Jacques

GREENFIELD PARK
Tetrault, Claire

JOLIETTE
Vera Suarez, Caridad

LASALLE
Cote, Benoit
Martel, Julie

LAVAL
Barolet, Daniel
Larocque, Annie
Mamode, Chemir
Menard, Andre
Molinari, Raynald

LEVIS
Barbeau, Francine
Dion, Pierre-Luc
Theriault, Mimi

LONGUEUIL
Baril, Joelle
Dore, Normand
Gaudreau, Pierre J.
Lefebvre, Christian
Ouellet, Alain C.
Pelletier, Jocelyne
Pham, Cuong Duc
Shaffer, Natalie

LORRAINE
Richard, Marie

MIRABEL
Cote, Jean R.

MONT-ROYAL
Demirjian, Ari
Martineau, Louise
Veilleux, Bertrand

MONTREAL
Arsenault, Theodore
Asai, Yuka
Balbul, Alfred
Bellefeuille, Jacques-P.
Benohanian, Antranik N.
Bernier-Buzzanga, Jeannine
Bernstein, Steven C.
Billick, Robin C.
Bissonnette, Robert
Bolduc, Chantal
Cameron, Judith M.
Cardinal, Francine
Chartier, Suzanne
Cohen, Dina
Collins, Micheline
Dubuc, Richard
Dumais, J R. Gaston
Durocher, Louis-Philippe
El Helou, Therese
Elie, John D.
Fish, Rowan
Fortier-Riberdy, Genevieve
Fournier-Blake, Odette
Francoeur, Marie-Alix
Friedmann, Dominique
Funaro, Deana
Gabay, Betty
Geoffrion, Genevieve
Gerstein, William
Girard, Claude
Gravel, Anne-Marie
Hacker, Peter
Hatami, Afshin
Journet, Michel
Khanna, Manish
Kohn, Thomas
Krasny, Mark J.
Lafaille, Philippe
Lanctot, Claude
Law, Teresa H L.
Lebel, Monique
Lovett, Audrey
Maari, Catherine
Marcil, Isabelle
Marcoux, Danielle
Marinier, Pascale
Mathieu-Serra, Andree
McCuaig, Catherine C.
Moreau, Linda
Moroz, Brenda E.
Nguyen, Khue Huu
Nigen, Simon R J.
Panaccio, Francois
Perras, Michel
Potoker, Steven D.
Powell, Julie C.
Provost, Nathalie
Roshdy, Osama
Rubinstein-Schipper, Rachel
Sasseville, Denis
Sissons, Wendy R.
Sonea, Michael J.
St-Jacques, Marie
Tran, Diane
Tremblay, Jean-Francois
Wang, Beatrice
Yanofsky, Howard

PIERREFONDS
Collins, Jean-Pierre
Hakim, Miriam
Raymond, Giles P.

POINTE-CLAIRE
Hebert, Denis L.
Irwin, D. June
Singer, Michael I.
Smoley, Lester B.

POINTE AUX TREMBLES
Paquette, Nicole

QUEBEC
Alain, Jimmy
Aubut, Nicolas
Auger, Isabelle
Bedard, Marie-Sophie
Bernard, Jean
Boulanger, Jean
Brulotte-Lapointe, Lise
Caron, Francine
Claveau, Joel
Cloutier, M A. Richard
Cossette, Michele
Cote, Danielle
Delisle, Bernard R.
Dessureault, Josee
Gilbert, Martin
Grenier, Raynald
Houle, Marie-Claude
Huard, Joseph
Joncas, Valerie
Mongrain, Eric
Morneau, Micheline
Poulin, Yves P.
Provencher, J J. Denis
Rochette, Linda
Rodrigue, Bertrand
Soucy, Jacques
Therien, Genevieve
Thibeault, Marie-Marthe
Veillette, Helene

REPENTIGNY
Dansereau, Alain
Garceau, Sylvie
Rozenfarb, Eva

RIMOUSKI
Lavoie, Gilles
Levesque, Marie-Helene

RIVIERE-DU-LOUP
Drouin, Christian A.

SAINT-BRUNO
Pronovost, Lyne

SAINT-EUSTACHE
Saint-Jacques, Robert R.

SAINT-GEORGES
Caron, Marilyn

SAINT-HUBERT
Normandin, Jean-Junior

SAINT-HYACINTHE
Delorme, Isabelle
Faucher, Lise
Tousignant, Jacqueline

SAINT-JEROME
Desgagnes, Jean-Francois

SAINT-LAMBERT
Roy, Marie-Christine

SAINT-LAURENT
Nault, Paul
Ohayon, Michele
Sylvestre, Guy

SAINT-SAUVEUR
Laplante, Pierre

SAINTE-THERESE
Wang, Emily J.

SEPT-ILES
Thibault, Marie-Josee

SHERBROOKE
Beauregard, Solange
Bertrand, Janie
Hanna, Dominique
Jean, Sara-Elizabeth
Loranger, Louise
Minier, Daniel

ST CHARLES BORROMEE
Meunier, Nicole

ST JEAN SUR RICHELIEU
Nguyen, Hai Hac
Trudeau-Martel, Adele

TERREBONNE
Chenier, Elisabeth
Chenier, Veronique
Girard, Liliane
Guay, Elizabeth
Lagace, Catherine

TROIS-RIVIERES
Beaudet, Louis-D.
Gagnon, Jean
Lafontaine, Nancy

VICTORIAVILLE
Schanne, Roswitha E.

VIMONT
Gagnon, Madeleine
Gagnon, Suzanne

WESTMOUNT
Carey, Wayne D.
Pehr, Kevin L.

SASKATCHEWAN

REGINA
Holfeld, Karen I.
McKay, Roberta M.

SASKATOON
Hull, Peter R.
Lichtenwald, Duane J.

Diagnostic Radiology

ALBERTA

CALGARY
Allen, Jennifer M.
Anca, Nicoleta I.
Bergen, Daryl C.
Bhagat, Kaushik K B.
Bhayana, Deepak
Boag, Graham S.
Boridy, Illya C.
Borsato, Garry W.
Brandschwei, Frank H.
Bristowe, J R. Bruce
Brunet, W. Grant
Burrowes, Paul W.
Campbell, Graham M C.
Caughlin, Cori E.
Chan, Denise
Chan, Ida H T.
Chen, Philip E.
Chlebek, Sebastian J.
Chrusch, Catherine M.
Cook, Miles C.
Davies, Robert G.
Diamond, Robert T.

Dickhoff, Peter J.
Docktor, Bobbie-Jo L.
Donnelly, Sarah
Dyke, Corinne H.
Elliot, Tracy L A.
Elliott, P. Davis
Fagnou, John M.
Fedorowicz, Andrew
Flemming, Jeffery P.
Fong, Tse Chen
Frizzell, J. Bevan
Frohlich, Dean E C.
Garry, Steven C.
Gaul, H. Penney
Godenir, Victor J B.
Goyal, Mayank
Grant, Peter A.
Gray, Robin R.
Gupta, Sanjay K.
Hall, Aaron
Hassard, Mary K.
Hochman, Mitchel I.
Hu, William Y.
Hudon, Mark E.
Hui, Gladwin C W.
Irwin, Marsha L A.
Jackson, John R.
Jones, Colin D.
Joshi, Manish D.
Katz, Nili R.
Kaura, Deepak R.
Kawamura, Nao
Kelly, Sarah A.
Kim, H L. Nancy
Kloiber, Reinhard
Koles, Sarah L.
Kolodinsky, Steve D.
Kruger, Brian M.
Kudel, Robert M.
Lalani, Amin
Larrigan, John R C.
Lautner, David
Lawrimore, Tara M.
Lee, Andrew G.
Lee, Jeffrey W.
Liew, Javier
Lipinski, J. Kenneth
Lou, Lawrence
Lydell, Carmen P.
Lyons, David J.
Lysack, John T.
MacGregor, John H M.
Mahallati, Houman
Matzinger, Dorothy J.
Medellin-Kowalewski, G. Alexandra
Menard, Shaunna L.
Merchant, Naeem
Molnar, Christine P.
Morrish, William F.
Ng, Danny G H.
Numerow, Leonard M.
Park, Roy Y.
Patel, Bijal
Patel, Shamir
Paterson, Kimiko
Pattison, Philip E.
Peppin, Andrew K.
Pham, C. Anh Ngoc
Poplawski, Stephen R.
Prevost, Jason D.
Quan, Jason K.
Raber, Earl L.
Reid, David F.
Risk, Paul J.
Romano, Clare C.
Sato, Kenneth K.
Scott, Douglas V.
Scott, James N.
Seal, Paula S.
Sevick, Robert J.
Smith, Dean F.
So, C. Benny
Spaner, Shelley J.
Steed, Barrie L.
Suchak, Amar A.
Switzer, Neil T.
Thom, Cheryl M.
Wada, Ryan
Walker, Richard E A.
Wallace, Carla J.
Watt, Donald W C.
Welsh, Michael M.
Willson, Morgan C.
Wilson, Stephanie R.
Wong, Jason K.
Yacyshyn, Brian J.
Yemen, Gary W.
Yeung, Grace W.
Zelazo, Jay A.

CAMROSE
Halls, Steven B.

CANMORE
Peachell, Milenija B.
Shaw, Paul S.

CARDSTON
Goth, Gary L.

DEVON
Conrad, Anne R.

EDMONTON
Abele, Jonathan T.
Ackerman, Thomas E.
Alexander, Timothy W.
Anderson, William W.
Andrew, George C.
Appavoo, Shushiela
Ashforth, Robert A.
Askew, Gordon R.
Baron, Jeffrey J.
Barrie, James R.
Bhalla, Sanjiv K.
Bhargava, Ravi
Birchall, Iain W J.
Bistritz, Aalo
Black, Timothy S.
Bruce, Dean E.
Campbell, Barbara E.
Carscadden, John A.
Chan, Raymond H K.
Cheng, Ah-Ling
Cheung, King
Cochrane, Nicholas W L.
Copeland, Catherine M.
Elias, Cynthia G.
Emery, Derek J.
English, Jordan H.
Fingard, Jordan E.
Foster, David A.
Friedland, Rodney
Gregoire, Scott A.
Guspie, Brian D.
Halliday, April
Hennig, Ronald C.
Hillier, Tracey L B.
Hnatiuk, Bradley
Holub, Roger V.
Horwitz, Trevor A.
Hudson, Emmanuel W.
Hung, Ryan W Y.
Hutson, Maureen L.
Hyde, J. Patrick
Ibach, Deborah M.
Jamieson, Lucy H.
Janoski, Michele M.
Jaremko, Jacob L.
Jen, Ho
Johnson, Mary A.
Kanigan, Arlene M.
Keenan, William G.
Kitay, Stanley
Korzan, Jeffrey R.
Kowand, Linda M M.
Koziarz, Peter
Kumar, Anu
Lambert, Robert G W.
Lauf, George R.
Lee, Kelvin H Y.
Ling, Bernice C.
Lummer, Charles R.
Lywood, Colin J.
MacEwan, Robert N.
Mah, Marian
Manji, Salim A.
Maslo, Nestor E.
McEwen, R. Ross
McKerlie, Ifeyinwa U.
Naik, Sandeep S.
Ng, Kai-Ling
Ngan, Elizabeth M.
Noga, Michelle L.
O'Keeffe, Margaret M.
Olson, David C.
Pandher, Darshan S.
Parker, William R.
Paskar, Lee S.
Pawluk, Randolph S.
Pereira, Raoul S.
Preville, Eric J.
Puznak, Kimbal N.
Raja, Asim J.
Rawat, Brijendra K.
Raymond, Gregory S.
Receveur, Darryn S.
Reich, M. David
Rempel, Jeremy L.
Ritchie, William L.
Rouget, Adrien C.
Samji, Rahim
Scott, Malcolm D S.
Shamchuk, David A.
Shein, Howard
Shergill, Navi
Sherlock, Richard A G.
Sidhu, Hameil S.
Sin, Margaret T W.
Singh, Anil K.
Smerdely, Marie S.
Spiers, Patrick A.
Spiers, Thomas C.
Sterling, George D.
Stoski, Douglas M.
Sugars, William P.
Sunner, Parveen K.
Swersky, Joanne F.
Tang, Allan S.
Taylor, William J B.
Terry, Timothy J.
Torbiak, Carl W.
Trepanier, Gerald P.
Turner, J. Garth E.
Turner, Richard J.
Vickar, David B.
Ward, Barbara J.
Warshawski, Robert S.
Wiebe, Edward
Winter, Christopher K.
Winters, Sean D.
Yeo, Thomas A.
Zavodni, Anna E H.

FORT MCMURRAY
Mahfud, Ahmed S.
Reid, Miles E.
Van Wyngaarden, Case B.

GRANDE PRAIRIE
Coughlin, James R.
Hydri, Muneeb S.
Jim, Gung Kyn
Lemay, Keith D.
McCabe, Richard D.

HINTON
Coppola, Joanne
Hacking, Susan M.
Helou, Tarek M.

LETHBRIDGE
Aucoin, Richard J.
Brewerton, Lee J.
Lane, Michael D.
Lee, Edward
Livingstone, Arthur G.
Martin, Rodney B.
Quon, Dick
Steed, Michael W.
Wilkins, Michael A.

MEDICINE HAT
Blair, Kenneth
Daniels, James E.
Lewall, Mark D.

OKOTOKS
Loe, Brian R.

RED DEER
Bateman, Gail E.
Bilo, John M.
Capusten, Bernice M.
Duke, Gavin G.
Harris, Thomas R.
Holmes, Donald H.
Malfair, David M.
Mamo, Andrew P T.
Mangin, James E.
Poole, Alan J.
Roth, Daniel E.
Simice, Peter
Siwak, Christopher D.
Taylor, Colin L.
Wiemer, Chad C.

SHERWOOD PARK
Hofmann, Karen H.
Loewy, John A.

ST. ALBERT
Ahamed, Karim S.
Bhutani, Sandra
Gardiner, Ian C.
Mueller, Dagmar L.
Ng, Jean S C.
Watt, James H.

WETASKIWIN
Kudel, Timothy A.

BRITISH COLUMBIA

ABBOTSFORD
Allen, Christine G.
Bajwa, Amarjit K.
Bartlett, Lewis J.
Bayat, Muhammad R H.
Chooi, Weng K.
Dion, Francoise M.
Goo, Sharon
Gupta, Shivani
Islam, Muhammad U.
Kalkman, Peter H.
Khalid, Tahir R.
Khan, Asra S.
Ko, Chung Chun
Kreml, Marian J.
Lee, Mark J.
Pon, Caroline

BURNABY
Graham, Nancy J.

CAMPBELL RIVER
Corr, Peter D.
Garber, Stanley I.
Krysl, Joseph
Reid, Ruth E.

COMOX
Astrope, Valerie J.
Chilton, Anthony P.
Kriegler, Stefan G.
Larsen, Grant A.
McKeown, Dave K.
O'Reilly, Michael L.
Thompson, William M.

COQUITLAM
Ahuja, Amit R.
Hodges, David C.
Kidney, Maria R.

CRANBROOK
Irish, Kevin E.
Maisonneuve, Daryn T.
Nicol, Julie A.
Zacharias, Abe
Zhu, Kang-Min

DAWSON CREEK
Erickson, Leroy M.

DELTA
Manning, A. Eric
Rao, Sheshagiri A S.

DUNCAN
Hagen, Paul
McCormack, Paul A.
Wilson, Robert A.
Wolfe, Brian K.

FORT ST. JOHN
Gojmerac, Frederic

KAMLOOPS
Bilbey, James H.
Clare, Michael E.
Colistro, Robert
Downey, Donal
Fache, J. Stephen
Fernandes, Dellano
Vedd, Vipal
Walter, Robert E.

KELOWNA
Anderson, David A.
D'Ovidio, Robert G.
Farnquist, Brenda
Kindrachuk, Gary W.
Kurkjian, Paul S.
Kwong, J. Stephen
Noble, John J R.
Partrick, Michael E.
Staples, Catherine A.
Tonogai, Wayne T.
Wall, David T.

LANGLEY
Campbell, Ronald M.
Lai, John T W.
Lee, Emil J Y.
Matheson, John A.
Ravindran, Aravindhan
Wong, Jerome C Y.
Wong, Xing

MAPLE RIDGE
Butchart, Michael K.
Cocquyt, Stuart R.
Mason, Andrew C.
Wong, Bobby C H.

NANAIMO
Barberie, John E.
Bissonnette, Robert T.
Carson, Brent J W.
Coupland, David B.
Johnson, Robert D A.
Kotwall, Zenobia A.
Matsuo, Kelly S A.
O'Keeffe, David
Saliken, John C.
Trepanier, Paul J.

NARAMATA
Terriff, Blake A.

NELSON
Silverthorn, Kelly G.

NEW WESTMINSTER
Ammann, Walter
Best, Andrew K.
Blake, Theodore
Chang, Debra C S.
Chen, Fred S.
Dolden, Jennifer M.
Halkier, Bradley K.
Li, Jian
MacNaughton, Heather P.
McEachern, Anita M.
Miller, Carol E.
Pirani, Aminmohamed A.
Rigby, Mark E.
Sidhu, Gary
Siu, William W Y.
Van Wiltenburg, Robert T.
Wong, Kenneth

NORTH VANCOUVER
Bicknell, Simon G.
Chan, Ian L.
Coldwell, Bobbi-Jo
Llewellyn, Patrick A.
Phillips, Catherine J.
Rowan, Kevin R.
Spielmann, Audrey L.
Spouge, David J.
Su, Jenny C.
Thompson, Andrew L.
Yoshida, Sean H.

SPECIALISTS BY PROVINCE

PARKSVILLE
Blom, Rita J M.

PENTICTON
McMillan, Victor C S.
McNicholas, Peter G.
Piche, Stacey L.
Wilkie, John A C.

PORT ALBERNI
Winn, Edward P.

PRINCE GEORGE
Breckon, Sidney L W.
Chui, Shyr Lin
Dufton, John A.
Elshazly, Shehab
Lamb, M. Nicholas
Leighton, Alasdair I M.
Lim, Chong Won
Seland, Karen L.
Shand, J. Gregory E.
Sharma, Kristina S.

PRINCE RUPERT
Stevenson, Giles W.

QUESNEL
Coffey, Charles G.

RICHMOND
Bining, Harjinder J S.
Collins, William J.
Ferrier, Donald J.
Guijon, Juan-Carlos
Huey, Henry H L.
Jenkins, Martin F.
Kai, Brian M.
Keogh, Ciaran F.
Lail, Vanindar J.
Martin, Nancy M T.
Middelkamp, Janel E.
Tanton, Elizabeth L.
Thurber, Lynette A.
White, Jeremy H.
Williamson, William D.
Wong, Ian K Y.

SALMON ARM
Beckner, Kevin
Wickert, John C.

SALT SPRING ISLAND
Shea, Donald L.

SECHELT
Dolden, Daniel A.

SQUAMISH
Schramm, William D.

SURREY
Coish, Donald L.
Eriksen, Guy R.
Janzen, Dennis L.
Lee, Dennis Y L.
Meister, Mark G.
Neyestani, Amir H.
Sisler, W. John
Timko, Livius
Tregobov, L. Earl

TERRACE
Behm, Ernest P.

TRAIL
Babensee, Susan E.
Steenkamp, Elsabe

VANCOUVER
Andrews, Gordon T.
Ashkar, Laila K.
Attariwala, Rajpaul
Becker, Annalisa K.
Bhimji, Shamim D.
Bilawich, Ana-Maria
Bray, Heather J.
Brown, Jacqueline A.
Brown, Maura J.
Buckley, Anne R.
Buckley, Miriam R E.
Cairns, Robyn A.
Chang, Silvia D.
Cheong, Yvette Y W.
Chew, Jason B.
Chipperfield, Patricia M.
Clement, Jason J.
Cresswell, Mark E.
Culham, J A. Gordon
Ellis, Jennifer D.
Fenton, David M.
Flak, Borys
Flemming, Anne K.
Forster, A. Bruce B.
Gordon, Paula B.
Graeb, Douglas A.
Hague, Cameron J.
Harris, Alison C.
Harrison, Dorothy A.
Harrison, Philip B.
Hassell, Patricia R.
Heran, Manraj K S.
Ho, Stephen G F.
Hunter, Natalie
Jamieson, Douglas H.
Jessup, Jennifer L.
Kalke, Robyn J.
Kary, Salah S M.
Kellow, Zina S.
Lapinsky, Nicola-Ann
Lee, Richard
Legiehn, Gerald M.
Leipsic, Jonathon A.
Li, David K B.
Louis, Luck J.
Lui, Yuk Ming
Machan, Lindsay S.
Manders, David C.
Mar, Colin R.
Martin, Michael L.
Martin, Montgomery A.
Mawson, John B.
Mayo, John R.
Morgan-Parkes, Jacqueline H.
Morris, Daniel C.
Muller, Nestor L.
Munk, Peter L.
Myo-Lwin, Tony Ong.
Nadel, Helen R.
Nguyen, Giang Thuy
Nicolaou, Savvakis
O'Dwyer, Helena M.
Ouellette, Hugue A.
Padilla-Thornton, Amie E.
Peramaki, Edwin R.
Poskitt, Kenneth J.
Pugash, Denise S.
Rankin, Aileen R.
Robinson, Ashley J.
Rowley, Victor A.
Rubin, David H.
Sargent, Michael A.
Shewchuk, Jason R.
Siu, Connie M.
Stilwell, Moira E.
Switzer, Philip J.
Tonseth, Rolf P.
Vertinsky, Alexandra T.
Vos, Patrick M.
Walls, Jessica
Warren, Linda J.
Wilson, Christine M.
Wong, Anthony D.
Yee, William C.
Yewchuk, Lila K.
Yong Hing, Charlotte J.
Zwirewich, Charles V.

VERNON
Bentley, Kenneth D M.
Marsh, J. Ian
Middelkamp, Graeme
Scheske, Glenn A.
Stewart, Rebekah A L.
Stuart, Thomas
Thurgur, Claire H.

VICTORIA
Anderson, Terry D.
Andrew, John
Chu, Derek D M.
Connell, Douglas G.
Eddy, Richard J.
Forkheim, Kevin E.
Greek, L. Shane
Hodgins, G. Walter
Huk, Michael
King, Christopher R.
Koopmans, Robert A.
Lawrence, D'Arcy D.
Lee, Brent R.
Mathieson, John R.
Proctor, Nicola J.
Silver, Stuart F.
Smith, Frederick J R.
Sobkin, Paul R.
Van Raalte, Vanessa A.
Warren, Melina D.
Weir, Ian H.
Wrinch, John H.
Yakemchuk, George H.
Zacks, David J.

WHITE ROCK
Clark, Eleanor J.
Hagel, Jeffrey A.
Lister, William S.

MANITOBA

BRANDON
Avila Flores, Francisco
Burnette, David M.
Fung, Harold M Y.
Harrison, Wayne D.
Kindle, Geoffrey F.
Lysack, David A.

DAUPHIN
Malik, R. Neesh

PORTAGE LA PRAIRIE
Brooker, Gary M.

SELKIRK
Brinkman, Shauna E.
Lindsay, Daniel J.
Soni, Sushane

THE PAS
Mabin, Deborah

WINKLER
Jacob, Mary V.
Lloyd, Robert L.
MacNair, Tracy L.
McGregor, Robert D.

WINNIPEG
Bay, Trevor A.
Bock, Gerhard W.
Boult, Ian F.
Bunge, Martin K.
Cassano-Bailey, Alessandra
Chapman, Leagh T.
Dashefsky, Sidney M.
Davidson, J. Michael
Eaglesham, Hugh H.
Goubran, Ashraf W H.
Greenberg, Howard M.
Greenberg, I. David
Hardy, Brian W.
Henderson, Blair T.
Higgins, Richard J.
Holt, Susan C.
Kaprowy, Richard R.
Kippen, James D.
Kirkpatrick, Iain D C.
Koenig, James K.
Kreml, Renee
Krongold, Israel J.
Kulbisky, Gordon P.
Lam, Wilson L T.
Lautatzis, Miltiade
Lawrence, Patrick H.
Levi, Clifford S.
Lindquist, Larry V.
Lyons, Edward A.
Major, Paul A.
Marantz, Jeffrey E.
Martens, M. Dawn
Maycher, Bruce W.
McClarty, Blake M.
McGinn, Gregory J.
McPhee, Lisa C.
Memauri, Brett F.
Meyers, Michael P.
Millo, Noam Z.
Moffatt, Hayley W M.
Mottola, Jeffrey C.
Nashed, Maged S.
Paquin, R. Wayne
Peterdy, Anne E.
Pierce, Garvin W.
Preachuk, Christopher T J.
Radulovic, Dejana
Reed, Martin H.
Reynolds, Jody
Rusnak, Barry W.
Shatsky, Morley A.
Stoski, Roxann M.
Strzelczyk, Jacek J.
Sutherland, I. Scott
Tsuyuki, Sean H.
Van Amstel, Leanne L.
Vivian, Mark A.
Wadhwa, Vikram S.
Wilson, Murray E.
Wrogemann, Jens J W.
Yeo, Linda I.

NEW BRUNSWICK

BATHURST
Cyr, Jean-Louis

CAMPBELLTON
McGowan, Allister J.

DIEPPE
Toupin, Michael E.

EDMUNDSTON
Leclerc, Olga

FREDERICTON
Arnason, Stephen K.
Brennan, Terrance E.
Efford, Erin
Paterson, Craig J S.
Scott, Ian R.
Teed, D. Lionel
Theriault, Cynthia H.

MIRAMICHI
Kilcup, Michael C.
MacMillan, J. Stewart
Miller, David

MONCTON
Champagne, Paul R.
Daly, J. Michael
Doiron, Anne
Finnegan, Martin M.
Fowlie, Frank E.
Francoeur, Luc
Juravsky, Louis I.
Kydd, David W.
Martel, Jean-Pierre A.
Mowat, Jeffrey J.
Pilote, Nicholas
Prasad, Vikash
Punna, Satish K.
Richard, Mario
Savoie, Isabelle
Savoie, Remi
Tingley, David R.

QUISPAMSIS
Archer, Brian

ROTHESAY
England, Michael B A.

SAINT JOHN
Allan, John C.
Anderson, Ian H.
Barry, Michael H.
Clarke, Gillian L.
Ferguson, Darren B.
Iles, David L.
King, Heidi
MacSween, J. Mark
Martin, Jennifer L.
Simms, J. David
Swan, John

SUSSEX
Leger, John

NEWFOUNDLAND AND LABRADOR

CARBONEAR
Jarvis, Tanya J.
O'Dea, Daneile F.

CORNER BROOK
Casey, William E.
Cook, Robert D.
Lombard, Jennifer J.
Mercer, Edwin E.
Pilgrim, S. Brent

GANDER
Dalton, Shelley
Kennedy, Paula M.
Skanes, Melissa D.

GRAND FALLS WINDSOR
Crocker, Kenneth
Jewer, Craig M.

ST. JOHN'S
Bartlett, Peter J.
Battcock, Stephen G.
Bhatia, Rajdeep S.
Chan, Wesley C.
Colbert, Diane A.
Collingwood, Peter W.
Cramer, Benvon
Hache, M K. Nanette D.
Hapgood, Conamara A.
Harris, Scott R.
Heale, V. Robert
Higgins, Geoffrey C.
Hogan, Maureen
Hopkins, John G.
Hoque, Asadul
Jackman, Stephanie S.
Jefford, Cheryl L.
Jenkins, Sarah J.
Jeon, Paul M.
Maguire, Conor G J.
Major, Adrian C.
O'Keefe, John B.
Pickles, Angela M.
Pike, Eric J.
Pochini, Craig M.
Rendell, M. Jane
Wadden, Nancy A T.
Walsh, Elizabeth A.

NOVA SCOTIA

AMHERST
Brady, Jolene N.
Thompson, Susan E.

ANTIGONISH
Klavina, Ieva
MacDuff, Blair A.
Nicholson, Brian M.
Silver, Michael E.

BRIDGEWATER
Church, Christopher L.
Marshall, Arthur D.
Meng, Chen
Spracklin, Ann E.

DARTMOUTH
Barton, William F.
Cheverie, Donald J.
Colter, Kimberley A.
Delaney, Susan M.
Ingham, Andrew B.
Joy, Graham A.
Oxner, James H.
Pittman, Carla E.

DIGBY
Brown, Basil S.

GLACE BAY
Kooka, Dara M.
Walker, Harmannus C G.

HALIFAX
Abraham, Robert J.
Barkova, Eva
Barnes, David C.
Berry, Robert F.
Borgaonkar, Joy N.
Boyd, Gordon J.
Brydie, Alan D.
Burrell, Steven C.
Butt, Robinette D.
Caines, Judy S W.
Clarke, James R.
Clarke, Sharon E.
Curtis, Heather
Dobson, Rebecca L.
Flemming, Bruce K.
Fraser, James D.
Gundogan, Munire
Heelan, John A.
Iles, Sian E.
Johnson, Alphonse J.
Jones, Gordon R M.
Keough, Valerie J.
Lebrun, G. Paul
Lightfoot, Christopher B.
Lo, Charles D.
Maloney, William J.
Manos, Daria K C.
Mason, William F.
McDonald, Lori J.
Miller, Robert M.
Mitchell, Michael J.
Normore, Wayne J.
O'Brien, M. Kathleen
Pringle, Christopher
Psooy, Brian J.
Ross, Andrew A.
Rowe, Judy A.
Schmidt, Matthias H.
Thompson, Deborah L.
Vandorpe, Robert A.

KENTVILLE
Acton, David C.
Bromley, Peter J.
Butler, Gregory J.
Covert, Sabrina K.
Dunn, Michael V T.
Harris, Colin J.
MacDougall, Ryan
Madigan, Maureen A.
Salat, Peter

LOWER SACKVILLE
Burke, John W.
McPhee, Michael
Murphy, George F.
Yeadon, Derek E.

NEW GLASGOW
Biernacka, Magdalena T.
Hoffman, Daniel B.
MacEachern, Ronald T.
Petrie, Daniel W.

SYDNEY
Abbasian, Ali
Hussain, Khalid M.
Latour, Anne H.
Murad, Moazzam
Naseem, Iram
Quinn, Bryan B.
Schaller, Gerald H.

TRURO
Do, Skyz
Gordon, J. David
McNeil, Nancy L.
Versnick, Eric J A.

WINDSOR
Turner, Charles G W.

YARMOUTH
Cunningham, Ian R.
Paulick, William C.
Surette, Joel Y.
Woods, Eric R.

ONTARIO

AJAX
Dan, Ratna
Gazzola, Steve
Goodman, Daniel N F.
Korwan, Claudia A.

ALLISTON
Bruno, Giovanni F.

AURORA
Graham, Robert T.

BARRIE
Baerlocher, Mark
Ball, Ian C.
Good, H. Scott
Grover, Raj Pal S.
Guest, Christopher L.
Lougheed, George E.
Mason, Robert B.
Morrison, Catherine E.
Nadeau, John G.
Paul, T. Gordon
Schemmer, Drew C.
Voorheis, Paul M.

BELLEVILLE
Biederman, Jessica L M.
Downey, Mathew T.
Gambarotta, Nicola
Gammal, Nadia T.
Holland, Sharon A.
James, Susan H.
Kadoch, Laurence
Polanski, Annette C.
Robinson, Emma
Scheffler, Rolf F.
Sutherland, Kenneth B.

BOLTON
Cameron, Glenna G.

BRACEBRIDGE
McCann, William G.

BRAMPTON
Al-Douri, Faten M.
Bloom, Carl M.
Carvalho, Preston M M A.
Chan, Bob C C.
Fairbrother, Joseph
Fitzgerald, M. Patricia
Ganguli, Satyajit N.
Giddings, C. Raymond
Haroun, Gamal W.
Kelton, David
Kurtz, Robert
Kwan, Bartholomew P.
Layton, Zeinab A.
Lee, Betty
Loucks-Gray, Teresa E.
Majesky, Ivan F.
Sheehan, Hilarie L.
Shiff, Daniel A.
Sookdeo, Sunel
Vanderburgh, Leslie C.

BRANTFORD
Fleming, Angela D.
Hendrie, Douglas S.
Jain, Vikas K.
Khan, Azra
Kunashko, Peter G.
Lighter, Mark D.
Miller, D. Lewis G.
Nicholson, R. Lawrence

BROCKVILLE
Arzoumanian, Yervant
Grant, Doris J.
Quigley, John D.
Went, John H.

BURLINGTON
Calzonetti, Elizabeth A.
Girard, Stephanie M.
Isaac, Errol B.
Lok, San-Yu
Louisy, Coventry L.
Pirani, Mohamedraza J K.
Rawlinson, John
St Louis, Eugene L.
Ting, K H. George
Torbiak, Raymond P.

CAMBRIDGE
Abrams, Mitchell W.
Jan, Edgar
Lee, Winnie
Miropolsky, Vladislav
Popuri, Ramu

CHATHAM
Musyoki, Francis
Tomney, Patricia A.
Varma, P. Victor
Yee, Main Chiong

COBOURG
Marrocco, Francis S.
Marrocco, Paul A D.
Parravano, Joseph G.

COLLINGWOOD
Leung, Mark D.
Matheson, Grant M.
O'Brien, Clare E.

CORNWALL
Assaly, Thomas R.
Bishop, David R.
Boubalos, Anastasios
Galley, Daniel J.

COURTICE
Helson, Kenneth G.

DUNDAS
Ford, Jacqueline

DUNNVILLE
Hynes, David M.

EAST YORK
Shin, Vincent H.
Spiegel, Sanford M.
Tooth, Kerry J.
Vourlas, Anastasios

ETOBICOKE
Awerbuck, Bernard
Burns, Margaret J.
Cheng, Deborah W H.
Goldenberg, Jay C.
Hayeems, Eran B Z.
Lem, Selina L.
Liu, Weldon
Lo, Patrick C C.
Mamelak, Joshua D.
Miller, Murray H.
Ornstein, David H.
Ossip, Marc G.
Patel, Nirav
Singer-Jordan, Jonathan R.
Tomashpolskaya, Janny
Tripodi, Anthony L J.
Woo, Glenn M.
Zander, Dennis R.
Zitsow, Bernard S.

FERGUS
Shewchun, James

GRIMSBY
Lindsay, George E.
Sabine, Margaret

GUELPH
Banerjee, P. Joy
Caco, Christopher C.
Foster, Michelle C.
Ghookal, Dharmendra M.
McKinstry, John E.
Mittal, Richa
Patel, Mohan C.
Patel, Samir
Plaskos, Nicholas
Wilk, Jerry P.

HAMILTON
Birchenough, Brian R.
Chiavaras, Mary M.
Chou, Sheila
Choudur, Hema N.
Coblentz, Craig L.
Colapinto, Michael N.
Dhamanaskar, Kavita P.
Di Ianni, Michael
Dobranowski, Julian
Doris, C. Ian
Elder, Janice L.
Ellins, Mary L.
Feaver, Bruce D.
Ferri, Melanie
Finlay, Karen
Franchetto, Arlene A.
Golev, Dmitry S.
Grant, Mary M.
Haider, Ehsan A H.
Harish, Srinivasan
Jurriaans, Erik
Khan, Vajid A.
Koff, David A.
Kwok-Liu, Josephine P Y.
Landry, David J.
Lee, Richard D.
Maizlin, Zeev V.
Malhotra, Rohin T.
Mensinkai, Arun
Mernagh, John R P.
Midia, Mehran
Minuk, Terry G.
Muhn, Narry Y.
Nagarajan, Naveen P.
Patlas, Michael
Rebello, Ryan P.
Ribeiro, Luciana T.
Richard, Katayoun
Schiff, David P E.
Singh, Nina R T R.
So, Genhee
Somers, Sat
Stewart, Brian G.
Stewart, Lori K.
Thomson, Andrea L.
Thomson, James G.
Tsai, Scott S W.
Vora, Parag K.
Voss, Maurice D.
Vu, Manh Huu
Walker, Michelle L.
Wang, Xi
Wat, S Y. Josephine
Wong-Pack, William K.
Woods, David M.
Yakemchuk, Valerie N.
Yemen, Brian L.
Yip, Gordon
Young, Jennifer L.

HAWKESBURY
Pagacz, Alexis A.

KANATA
Purchase, Janet E.
Whelan, Edward P.

KINGSTON
Abraham, Christopher I.
Cheeseman, Frank D.
Fenton, Paul V.
Flood, Justin R.
Grahovac, Stephen Z.
Islam, Omar S.
Jabs, Doris K.
McCallum, Annette H.
Menard, Alexandre S.
Mussari, Benedetto
Nolan, Robert L.
O'Brien, Paul G.
Pearse, Bryan F.
Ricketts, John D.
Salahudeen, Shafeequr R.
Sauerbrei, Eric E.
Scott, Charles F.
Silver, Ian M F.
Soboleski, Donald A A.
Walker, Douglas R.

KITCHENER
Doran, Dale R.
Fienberg, Samantha
Gawman, William G.
Ho-Tai, Paul
Lavallee, Chad M.
Mnyusiwalla, Yusuf A.
Moola, Cassim
Qureshi, A. Majid
Raja, Faisal S.
Stronell, Roger D.
Suleman, Mohamed R.
Venkatesh, Vikram
Wallace-Kimmel, Eda J.
Wycoco, Danilo A.
Yim, Annabella C.
Yousef, Osama A E.

LEAMINGTON
Hooper, Elizabeth D.
Leadman, Martha L.

LONDON
Amann, Justin H.
Bach, David B.
Bennett, John D.
Butler, Robert J.
Dawson, William
Elliott, James A.
Etemad-Rezai, Roya
Garvin, Gregory J.
Goela, Aashish
Gulka, Irene B.
Haddad, Richard G.
Ho, Derek C.
Hobbs, Barry B.
Hutton, Linda C.
Islam, Ali
Kornecki, Anat
Kozak, Roman I.
Kribs, Stewart W.
Landis, Mark S.
Lee, Donald H.
Leung, Andrew E.
Lum, P. Andrea
Mandel, Jonathan I.
McKillop, Scott D.
Mercado, Ashley J.
Mujoomdar, Amol
Muscedere, Giulio
O'Riordan, Ailbhe E.
Osman, Said
Pavlosky, William F.
Peck, David J M.
Pelz, David M.
Potoczny, Stefan
Rankin, Richard N.
Rogers, John M.
Romagnoli, Cesare
Romano, Walter M.
Ross, Ian G.
Shaikh, A. Allison
Shastry, Anil K.
Spouge, Alison R I.
Taves, Donald H.
Tay, Keng Y.
Vezina, William C.
Wiseman, Daniele P.
Zaleski, Witold M.

MARKHAM
Choi, Perry
Chung, Terry T H.
De Sequeira, Carlos M G.
Kan, Julio W H.
Mann, Clifford I.
McLennan, Michael K.
Mehta, Mitesh
Meindok, James R.
Sharif, Anoosh
Steirman, Michael
Stephen, Christopher M.

MISSISSAUGA
Ahmad, Afzal
Archer, Derek C.
Barsky, Michael F.
Bartucz, John P.
Bau, Alan L.
Chan, Jean-Wen
Cheung, Gordon
Florence, Stephen H.
Foga, Myrosia M.
Guram, Karmdeep
Hejjaji, Hanna E.
Ho, Yvonne
Jain, Mukesh K.
Kirsh, Joel C.
Lawrence, Janet A.

MacPhadyen, Norris B.
Magnuson, William H.
Marriott, Anne E.
Mehta, Sunil L.
Munshi, Muhammad
Pordeli, Peyvand
Quigley, Mark J R.
Raha, Ronjon
Rajput, Anshu
Rodrigues, Paulo R D.
Rodriguez-Marin, Emilio
Rosso, Dominic
Sheth, Tarang N.
Slezic, Ivo
Tran Ngoc, Cuong
Vickar, Darby K.
Ward, Susan E.
Widman, David S.
Wise, Daniel J.
Wong, Kelly D.
Zaretsky, Karolyn R.

NEPEAN
Becker, Lisa M.
Centazzo, Sophie I.
Clarke, John C.
Elliott, Alari K.
Formoso, Alfredo F.
Gandilo, Sargon B.
Gionet, Larry R.
Gitterman, Allan
Holden, Dean A.
Karamanos, Stavroula V.
Kelly, Sheila M.
Prud'Homme, Pierre T.
Raphy, Pascale
Truong, Dang-Toan

NEWMARKET
Buckler, Philip M.
Doran, James A.
Isaacson, Steven
Just, Norman W M.
Patel, Harshadrai M.
Silmberg, Erik O.
Siow, Yin-Hui

NIAGARA FALLS
Campbell, Joan P.
Chu, David K.
Legare, Lyne
Li, Thomas C H.
Perng, Richard J.

NORTH BAY
Ball, Daniel G.
Hodge, William R.
Hunter, Cameron M.
Krzeczunowicz, Dominic E J.

NORTH YORK
Armstrong, Susan A.
Baitz, Brian
Bechai, Nabil R.
Bozorgzadeh, Minoo
Cadogan, George I.
Causer, Petrina A.
Chang, Margaret K.
Chen, Julian C C.
Chow, Gilbert
Chui, Mario C.
Chung, Dae-Gyun
Cooke, Gabriel M.
Cranstoun, Kelly R.
Czosniak, Isadore J.
Deif, Hassan
Denton, P H. Omotayo
Friedman, Lawrence
Friedman, Talia
Gildiner, Michael
Ginzburg, Brian M.
Goldberg, Ronn E A.
Gonsalves, Charles G.
Grinblat, Leonard
Hausen, Doris M.
Huang, Madeline W C.
Hung, C. Francis
Isaac, Neil R A.
Jacobs, Irving G.
Kyone, Soe L.
La Mere, Elizabeth A.
Lai, Enoch K Y.
Leung, Edmond Y H.
MacAdam, Christine M.
Mak, Kelvin
Margau, Ryan
Nash, Stephen H.
O'Hayon, Bonnie B E.
Pham, Dieu Huu
Polson, Ronald
Por-Somfai, Agnes
Shumak, Rene S.
Slipacoff, Daniel
Stoneman, H. Richard
Strasberg, Zeno
Tam, Michael C C.
Tsui, Kwan-Cheung
Weisbrod, Lawrence H.
Wortsman, A. Jay
Yates, Thomas H.
Yee, Allan C N.
Yurman, Edward D.

OAKVILLE
Citren, Robert M.
Durrant, Timothy J.
Engmann, Eric C.
Feberwee, Jillian A.
Knapp, Thomas R.
Kravis, Marc M J.
Kyes, John H.
Lobo, Kevin A.
Marotta, Robert W.
Mongiardi, Christopher N.
Tlusty, Eva
Valadka, Saulius M.
Yu, Jinwoo R.

ORANGEVILLE
Dolbear, Betty E.
Kotecha, Suhas A.
Moore, April E.
Mozeg, Dan
Stefanos, Michael G F.

ORILLIA
Adkins, L. John
Kohno, Yume
Legge, A. Murray
Little, D'Arcy L.
McCloskey, Deborah A.
Swanson, Mark A.

ORLEANS
Mills, William G.

OSHAWA
Asch, Murray R.
Barton, Guy J.
Boparai, Dennis
Cnoop Koopmans, W. Michael
Donsky, Geoffrey
Dotsikas, Gus
Fong, Peter F K.
Isaac, Nicole S.
Jones, R. Stephen W.
Khan, Mustafa Z.
Lacey, Glen W.
Levine, Richard J.
Maguire, Gerard H.
Massaad, Viviane
Moore, Lori A.
Myers, Andrew B.
Nelson, James W.
Patt, Norman L.
Rastogi, Aroop
Wu, Louis

OTTAWA
Aina, Rima
Al-Rujaib, Mashael K K.
Aquino Jr, Jose
Avruch, Leonard I.
Baxter, Daniel J G.
Binkhamis, Shagran
Blair, Donald C.
Choi, Abram
Collin, Gerard A.
Curuvija, Srdjan
Dabirzadeh, Hamidreza
Dennie, Carole J.
Di Primio, Luigia G A.
Doherty, Geoffrey P.
Dube, Magalie
Duigenan, Shauna
Dunlap, Hal J.
Fraser, Margaret A.
French, Gordon J.
Glikstein, Rafael S.
Hadziomerovic, Adnan
Hammond, D. Ian
Hibbert, Rebecca
Highmore, Kerri A.
Hurteau, Julie M.
Kielar, Ania Z.
Kingstone, Michael S.
Kontolemos, Mario
Lau, Jacqueline C O.
Lee, Frank S.
Lewandowski, Bernard J.
Lobo, A L. Charlotte
Lum, Cheemun
Lyle, Terrance C.
MacDonald, D. Blair
Martin, Lucie C.
Matzinger, Mary Ann E.
Mendell, Lawrence M.
Michaud, Claudine
Miller, William D.
Nguyen, Thanh Binh
O'Kelly, Kevin F.
O'Sullivan, Joseph P.
Olivier, Andre D.
Papadatos, Demetrios
Peddle, Susan E.
Peterson, Rebecca
Putnins, Rita E.
Rakhra, Kawanpreet S.
Rasuli, Pasteur
Rhodes, Ian N.
Ritchie, R. Gordon
Ryan, John G.
Ryan, Stephen E.
Schieda, Nicola
Schweitzer, Mark E.
Seely, Jean M.
Seppala, Richard E.
Shenouda, Nazih F.
Shulakewych, Markian O.
Simantirakis, Emmanuel
Sly, Lloyd E.
Smyth, Karl R.
Taucer, Fabiano A S.
Tenaschuk, Danny S.
Udjus Teitelbaum, Kristin
Walsh, Cynthia B.
Yu, John C.

OWEN SOUND
Ador-Dionisio, Jorge B.
Baldauf, Christian G.
Drover, Shauna
Greaves, Francis W.
Hawkes, Robert P.
Howlett, Laura A.
McIver, Colin H.
Rosta, Neil I N.
Saab, George
Thomson, Scott M.

PEMBROKE
Matzinger, Frederick R.
Menzies, John E.
Van Gentevoort, Marlene A.

PERTH
Franic, Slobodan E.
Laws, Margaret-Anne
Parikh, Nimish U.

PETERBOROUGH
Aldis, Hugh W.
Bourgeois, Daniel J.
Brown, Thomas C.
Durant, Dean
Franczyk, Juliet A E.
Fung, Michael E.
Garneys, Glenn G.
Harvie, Sarah
King, Kebby F G.
Millitz, Kip
Millward, Steven
Myint, Wunna A.
O'Sullivan, Peter D.
Rafail, Ehab A.
Shalay, Katherine M.
Sobiera, Ruthanne M.
Swales, David W.
Voros, Mario
Wilson, Paul J.

RENFREW
Cunningham, Colin D B.

RICHMOND HILL
Cameron, Roderick H.
Hany, Richard W.
Hochman, Gary P.
Lan, Frederick P.
Law, Peter
McKee, John D.
Orfi, Ezel F.
Partap, Vince A.
Shorter, Anne Marie
Stroz, Peter M.
Winning, J. Barry
Yeung, Brian K P.
Zia, Peter K Y.

SARNIA
Almalki, Youssef
Cooper, Scott A.
Duggal, Rishi
Garland, Paul A.
Marcinkowski, Richard A.
Piekos, Lucyna M.
Potts, Leslie A.

SAULT STE MARIE
Jenkin, Jeffrey K.
McNair, David J.
Nguyen, Trung Khanh
Tait, Margaret V.
Tjong, Joshua K.
Yau, Jaron A.

SCARBOROUGH
Aziza, Jonathan
Bean, Sharon H.
Bell, Stuart D.
Benjamin, Matthew S.
Bruce, Robert D.
Budisin, Branko
Chait, Peter G.
Chin, Joseph M.
Clark, John A.
Clemens, Richard S.
Garces, Patricio B.
Gilloteaux, Laurent C.
Goh, Raymond H T.
Grosman, Harvey
Hodby, Elizabeth D.
Kim, Godfrey J H.
Lazarou, Lazaros P.
Levitin, Bryna S.
Liu, Yuen Chi
Mah, Michael B C.
Mehta, Mahendra H.
Murphy, John P.
Nazareno, Janice J Y.
Pecorari, Adriana I.
Prieditis, Markus P.
Rabinovitch, Samuel M.
Shuckett, Bruce M.
Verbeeten, Bernard C.
Woo, James K H.
Yeung, Eugene Y C.
Yuen, Michael L F.

SIMCOE
Chow, Sie-Chin

SIOUX LOOKOUT
McLoughlin, Diarmuid P.

ST CATHARINES
Arvinte, Andrei A.
Cheng, Gordon W.
Cook, Gregory C F.
Dyck, Christopher J.
Fan, Lily Z.
Filice, Raffaele
McGinley, Michael D.
Mehta, Amit L.
Mehta, Labhshanker S.
Nazar, Dennis M.
Prysiazny, Brian K.
Reddy, E. Rajaram
Snodgrass, Graham P.
Vilk, Jeffery K.

ST THOMAS
Harding, Kevin P.
Levin, Morris F.

STRATFORD
Erenberg, Yale A.
Harker, Lynda A.
Mnyusiwalla, Anisa
Mott, Daniel D.
Sparrow, Robert K.

SUDBURY
Ashley, Jason B.
Greco, Robert A.
Grynspan, Jonathan
Illman, Jeffery E.
Milner, Curtis A.
Neufeld, Keith T.
Nizzero, Alberto
Roberts, Evan W D.
Sloan, Richard S.
Struk, Daniel W.

TECUMSEH
Southcott, John D.

THORNHILL
Brattman, David P.
Griesman, Jordan A.
Hartman, Alexander
Jazrawy, Helen
Lee, Rose
Liu, Peter C F.
Rendak, Ian
Rideout, David F.

THUNDER BAY
Bitar, Richard
Granberg, Karl-Erik
Henderson, Donald R.
Jaward, M A. Abdul
Kim, Jae K.
O'Brien, John A.
Panu, Neety

TIMMINS
Vezina, Claude T J.

TORONTO
Adamo, Ciro A.
Agid, Ronit F.
Ainsworth, Kelly E.
Al-Humayyd, Saad S.
Alharbi, Fawaz S D.
Arenson, Anna M.
Armstrong, Derek C.
Ash, Judith M.
Atri, Mostafa
Au, W. Frederick
Aviv, Richard I.
Azzumeea, Fahad M I.
Bablad, Guru S.
Bajno, Lydia M.
Ballyk, Peter D.
Beecroft, J. Robert D.
Beresford, Meaghen J.
Betel, Cara B.
Bharatha, Aditya
Blaser, Susan I.
Bleakney, Robert R.
Blend, Ralph
Blumer, Russell D.
Bret, Patrice M.
Bukhanov, Karina
Cairns, Patricia D.
Chae, Anita S.
Chatha, Prabhdeep S.
Chawla, Punita T.
Chen, Morie
Cheran, Sendhil K.
Chiu, John H C.
Christakis, Monique S.
Chuang, Sylvester H S.
Chung, Tae Bong.
Clow, David J.
Colak, Errol
Common, Andrew A.
Connolly, Bairbre L.
Cooper, Perry W.
Curpen, Belinda N.
Daghistani, Razan
Daneman, Alan

David, Elizabeth N.
De Perrot, Marc
Deitel, Wayne L.
Donovan, Andrea
Dowdell, Timothy R.
Dua, Hemi
Eddeb, Abdurrahman A.
Ehrlich, Lisa E.
Eisen, Ari B.
Farb, Richard I.
Filakovic, Zdenko
Fleming, Rachel
Fong, Katherine W.
Fox, Allan J.
Fraser, Lorna E.
Freeman, Marc
Fruitman, Mark A.
Furey, Beth
Gardner, Douglas
Gershater, Elize
Ghandehari, Hournaz
Gilday, David L.
Glanc, Phyllis
Glickman, Aaron
Goldberg, Deborah R.
Goldberg, Franklin
Goldfinger, Morris
Gray, Bruce G.
Greyson, N. David
Hack, Kalesha
Haider, Masoom A.
Hamilton, Paul A.
Hanbidge, Anthony E.
Hendler, Aaron L.
Herman, Stephen J.
Ho, Angela L H.
Ho, Chia-Sing
Ho, Hon-Fai
Howard, Peter R S.
Ismail, Alnashir
Jacobs, Steve R.
Jaffer, Nasir M.
Jaskolka, Jeffrey D.
John, Philip R.
Jong, Roberta A.
Kachura, John R.
Karam, Rana
Kassel, Edward E.
Khalili, Korosh
Kim, Tae K.
King, Gregory P.
Kirpalani, Anish
Kleiman, J. Harry
Korb, Edwin J.
Krings, Timo
Kucharczyk, Walter
Kundu, Sanjoy
Lapin, Jonathan L.
Lata, Andrew C.
Laughlin, Suzanne
Lax, Matthew J.
Lazinski, Dorothy
Lee, Sai-Ping
Leekam, Roger N.
Leonhardt, Charlene M.
Linda, Dorota
Loreto, Michael P.
Luong, Angela
Lychacz, Bohdan I.
MacDonald, Catherine E.
MacNab, Timothy I.
Mahajan, Ashish
Mak, Walter H H.
Mandelcorn, Jeffrey N.
Mandell, Daniel M.
Mann, Erika H.
Manson, David E S.
Marcuzzi, Danny W.
Margolis, Myles
Markus, Newton
Marotta, Thomas R.
Martinovic, Elaine C.
Mascia, Anthony T.
McGregor, Caitlin T.
Mikulis, David J.
Miller, Andrea E J.
Miller, Stephen F.
Minnis, Shantel M.
Minuk, Cheryl F.
Miskin, Murray
Mohan, Ravi M.
Moktassi, Aiden
Montanera, Walter J.
Moody, Alan R.
Muradali, Derek
Murphy, Kieran P.
Nathanson, Martin M.
Newman, Harold J.
Nguyen, T. Elsie
Nitsch, Barbara A.
Noel De Tilly, Lyne
O'Malley, Martin E.
Ou Hingwan, Gilbert
Pang, Susan M W.
Pantazi, Sophia
Paul, Narinder S.
Pearce, Dawn H.
Perng, Jane
Probyn, Linda J.
Pugash, Robyn A.
Rahmani, M. Rose
Raikhlin, Anton
Rajan, Dheeraj K.
Ramprashad, Claudius A.
Ranson, Marilyn D E.
Rawal, Sapna
Raybaud, Charles A D.
Revah, Giselle
Richmond, Lara D.
Roberts, Heidi C.
Rosen, Irving E.
Rothberg, Randy D.
Rubenstein, Joel D.
Salem, Shia
Salonen, David C.
Salsberg, Barry B.
Samu, Peter C.
Sangster, Robert N.
Sarrazin, Josee
Settecase, Fabio
Shankar, Lalitha
Shaul, C. Harvey
Shin, Sharon L.
Shlomovitz, Eran
Shroff, Manohar M.
Shulman, Harry S.
Simons, Martin E.
Singer, Steven B.
Skarpathiotakis, Maria
Sniderman, Kenneth W.
Soochan, Diana C.
Sreeharsha, Boraiah
Stimec, Jennifer
Stoll, Stephen
Sussman, Sidney
Symons, Sean P.
Tan, Kong Teng
Tarulli, Giuseppe P.
Taylor, Hallie A.
Temple, Michael J.
Ter Brugge, Karel G.
Thipphavong, Seng
Thomas, Karen E.
Thurston, Wendy A.
Toi, Ants
Tomlin, Heather A.
Traubici, Jeffrey
Valikangas, Eija M.
Verbeeten, Karen M.
Walji, Moez B.
Wall, Jane M.
Wei Wei, Corie
Weisbrod, Gordon L.
Weiser, William J.
White, Lawrence M.
Williams, Tara M.
Willinsky, Robert A.
Wong, Edward Y C.
Wright, Barbara E.
Yeung, Robert
Yoo, Shi-Joon
Young, Stephanie L.
Yu, S. Eugene
Zalev, Arthur H.
Zelovitzky, Jerahmie L.

VAUGHAN

Chan, Raymond P.
Grebenyuk, Julia
Langhorne, Noel B.
Rooney, Michael S.
Thain, Lisa M F.

WELLAND

Aggarwal, Rakesh M.
Campbell, Bryan G.
Habdank-Kossowski, Krzysztof
Mittal, Charu
Tracy, Gary E.

WHITBY

Osuszek, Andrew R.

WINDSOR

Adey, Christopher K.
Ala, Brigitte D.
Beaudet, Anne-Marie
Brisson, Louis J.
Cervini, Patrick
Denath, Fareed M.
Gaisinsky, Igor
Gill, Davinder S.
Kanungo, Nachiketa M.
Lim, Meng Chee
Mitri, Ragheed K.
Mitton, Gregory D.
Newell, Paul R.
Ramsewak, Winston S.
Smith, Robert M.
Speirs, John W D.
Tabib, Mohamed A.
Tadros, Peter
Tam, Wing-Hei

WOODBRIDGE

O'Herlihy, Patrick J B.
Schneider, Kalman M.
Tsin, Thomas T Y.

WOODSTOCK

Sanders, Lawrence D.
Vinson, Robert S.

YORK

Jacobs, David A.
Walker, James D.

PRINCE EDWARD ISLAND

CHARLOTTETOWN

Foley, Colin F.
Goodwin, John L.
Hender, Kimberley J.
MacKay, Alward M.
McQuaid, Melanie A.
Neilson, Douglas J.
White, Mary E.

QUÉBEC

ALMA

Caya, Joanne
Gagne, Marie
Pineault, Claude

AMOS

Daoust, Lucie
Guay, Louise

AMQUI

Keighan, Leslie

BAIE-COMEAU

Grondin, Pierre
Jocov, Drago
Tabah, Nicolas

BOUCHERVILLE

Gelinas, Claude

BROSSARD

Duchesne, Nathalie
Dumas, Jean-Marc
Khazoom, Stephane
Vadeboncoeur, Marielle

CHANDLER

Blouin, Gilles
Simard, P. Line

CHATEAUGUAY

Brassard, Roland
Desmarais, Eric
Douziech, Maxime
Lessard, Anne-Marie
Rouleau, Yves

CHICOUTIMI

Berube, Michel
Bordeleau, Edith
Bourassa, Anne-Marie
Courcy, Claude
Daoud, Nicolas
Jobin, Philippe
Lord, Veronique
Rousseau, Isabelle

DOLBEAU-MISTASSINI

Langevin, Benoit

DRUMMONDVILLE

Bernard, Annie
Corriveau, Dominic
Drouin, Yves
Grandmont, Brigitte
Laporte, Julie
Roy, Sylvain

GASPE

Brochu, Bernard
Letourneau, Louis

GATINEAU

Abdeen, Nishard
Belair, Louis
Belley, Guy
Chang, Na Young
Chbeir, Walif
Clouatre, Andre
Damphousse, Andreanne
Deslauriers, Gilbert E.
Didomenicantonio, Gabriel
Laferriere, A. Real
Lecompte, Martin
Lemieux, Jacques
Lepage, Martin
Mercier, Jean-Francois
Place, Christopher R.
Tongue, Antonio G.

GRANBY

Asselin, Anne
Audet, Patrice
Blain Pare, Etienne
Dansereau, Yves
Dupont, Robert
Grand, Laurence
Grevillot, Marie-Helene
Robichaud, Simon
Tropper, Martin

GREENFIELD PARK

Boisvert, Genevieve
Bonin, Sylvie
Brien, Julie
Depelteau, Helene
Do, Xuan Vien
Falardeau, Julie-Anne
Francoeur, Martin
Godbout, Richard
Groleau, Sylvie
Lafontaine, Lucie
Lesage, Jacques
Pham, Thi Tam.
Rahmouni, Dalia
Roumy, Gustave
Sabourin, Thierry
Seguin, Caroline
Van Campenhout, Isabelle

JONQUIERE

Levesque, Rejean-Yves
Marceau, Jean-Charles

LA BAIE

Nadeau, Diane

LA MALBAIE

Carrier, Guy

LA POCATIERE

Demers, Jacques F.

LA SARRE

Chenier, Stephanie

LAC-MEGANTIC

Marmen, Yves

LACHUTE

Jamaty, Georges F.

LASALLE

Dallaire, Marie-Josee
Nobert, Leo
Ramani, Mathangi
Roumy, Michele B.

LAVAL

Belliveau, Kevin
Benabu, Yves
Boisjoly, Andre
Cengarle-Samak, Alexandre
Charlebois, Normand S.
Dao, Tien Trong
Dube, Louis-Jacques
Fiset, Denis
Gosselin, Gino
Hudon, Francois
Krief, Olivier
Leblanc, Marc
Lortie, Marcel
Magnan, Francine
Marcil, Pierre
Marton, Dominique
Morin, Bruno
Morin, Francois R.
Nguyen, Thi Van Anh
Ouellet, Robert
Pen, Visal
Sagredo, Sonya
Slatkoff, Robert L.
Trudel, Robert

LEVIS

Bolduc, Jean-Philippe
Boucher, Jean-Louis
Cossette-Poirier, Nicole
Cote, Jean-Francois
Dufour, Marie
Fortin, Vincent
Gagnon, Louis
Godbout, Marie-Josee
Gravel, Alain
Labourdette, Annie
Lacoursiere, Luc
Lainesse, Michel
Mathurin, Johanne
Renaud, Andre
Scherrer, Jacques
Sergerie, Franck
Tremblay, Claude

LONGUEUIL

Bellemare, Remi
Bergeron, Pierre
Bovo, Michel
Corbeil, Vincent
Desautels, Annie
Desjardins, Frederic
Fulop, Katalin
Lemieux, Marie-Josee
Ouellet, Jean-Yves
Provost, Ninon M M.
Robillard, Antoine
Tremblay, Maxime
Vu Ngoc, Quynh-Phuong
Zara, Nicolas

MARIA

Duguay, Bernard E.
Roy, Richard
Theriault, Marie-Claude

MATANE

Rioux, Michel

MONT-JOLI

Reader, Norman

MONT-ROYAL
Cardinal, Patrice-Etienne
Couture, Sophie
Ethier, Romeo
Gianfelice, David C.
Laplante, Sophie

MONTMAGNY
Bertrand, Denys

MONTREAL
Aldis, Ann E.
Andrenyi, Veronica
Assaf, Adel A.
Aubin, Benoit
Audet, Pascale
Baillargeon, Jean-Martin
Bambonye, Miriam E.
Bard, Celine
Barrette, Gaetan
Beauchamp, Daniel
Bedard, Danielle
Belair, Manon
Belley, Genevieve
Berthiaume, Marie-Josee
Bier, Rino
Bilinski, Anna
Billiard, Jean-Sebastien
Blais, Jocelyn
Boily, Mathieu
Boston, Francis M.
Bouchard, Louis
Boucher, Louis-Martin
Boulianne, Pierre A.
Bourgie, Jacques R.
Bourgouin, Pierre
Breton, Guy
Browman, Morris W.
Bureau, Nathalie J.
Camlioglu, Errol B.
Carignan, Stephane
Carpineta, Lucia
Cartier, Yannick
Cassoff, Joseph
Casullo, Joseph
Caty, Veronique
Chagnon, David-Olivier
Chalaoui, Jean
Chandonnet, Martin
Chankowsky, Jeffrey N.
Charlebois, Simon
Chartrand-Lefebvre, Carl
Chin, Anne S L.
Constantin, Andre
Cordeau, Marie-Pierre
Damphousse, Amelie
Danet, Ioana M.
David, Julie
De Albuquerque, Pedro A B.
Decarie, Jean Claude
del Carpio, Raquel
Derbekyan, Vilma A.
Dery, Julie
Dery, Renee
Deslandes, Melanie
Discepola, Federico
Drouin, Michele
Drouin, Suzanne E.
Dube, Michel
Dubois, Josee
Dufresne, Michel P.
Dugas, Alexandre
Edde, Donald J.
Ehramdjian, Vagharchag
El Jalbout, Ramy
El Khoury, Mona
Ethier, Serge
Fafard, Therese
Faingold, Ricardo
Filiatrault, Denis
Filion, Robert B.
Fontaine, Suzanne
Forghani, Reza
Frechette, France
Freire, Veronique
Garel, Laurent
Ghostine, Jimmy
Gilbert, Danielle
Gilbert, Patrick
Girard, Marc
Giroux, Marie-France
Glay, Jack D.
Gorgos, Andrei-Bogdan
Gougeon, Nicole
Grignon, Andree
Guilbeault, Helene
Guilbert, Francois
Habbab, Fadi
Hannouche, Nabil
Hanson, Robert E.
Hidvegi, Robert I S.
Hoang, Diem-Quan
Ibrahim, Nathalie
Kao, Ellen
Keller, Rhona J.
Khan, Nazir A.
Khoury, Viviane
Kintzen, George M.
Kiss, Sabrina
Kosiuk, John P.
Labelle, Maude
Lafontaine, Marc
Lafrance, Julie
Lalonde, Lucie
Lamarre, Alexandre
Lamarre, Elisabeth
Laperriere, Jean
Lapierre, Chantale
Lavallee, Gilles
Le, Binh Quoc Huy
Le, Thi Som Mai
Lepanto, Luigi
Lesperance, Jacques
Letourneau-Guillon, Laurent
Levental, Mark
Lisbona, Andre
Lisbona, Robert
Loeb, Robert S.
Lussier-Lazaroff, Jeannette
Mandalenakis, Andreas
Martin, Anne
Martin, Marie-Helene
Mathis, Christel C.
Melancon, Denis
Messier-Nepveu, Nicole
Mesurolle, Benoit
Mindel, Michael J.
Miro, Santiago M P.
Miron, Marie-Claude
Morin, Christian
Murphy-Lavallee, Jessica
Nathens, Marvin S.
Nguyen, Marie-Therese H N.
Nguyen, Thuy-Khanh
Nicolet, Viviane
Novales Diaz, Javier
O'Gorman, Augustin M.
Oei, Tjong-Leng
Oliva, Vincent
Palayew, Max J.
Papas, Konstantin
Peloquin, Laurence
Pelsser, Vincent
Perreault, Pierre
Petitclerc, Sophie
Philie, Michel
Pinsky, Merrille F.
Pistono, Andree-Anne
Pistono, Louis-Xavier
Prenovault, Julie N.
Pressacco, Josephine G.
Prosmanne, Odile
Provost, Yves L.
Rafat Zand, Khashayar
Raymond, Jean
Raymond-Tremblay, Danielle
Rehany, Mordechai
Reinhold, Caroline
Remy, M E. Huguette
Robillard, Pierre
Rosenbloom, Lorne
Rosenbloom, Marvin B.
Rosenthall, Leonard
Roy, Anne
Roy, Daniel
Roy, Marie-Christine
Rypens, Francoise
Saint-Georges, Guy
Samson, Caroline
Samson, Louise M.
Satin, Richard
Semionov, Alexandre
Soulez, Gilles
Stein, Lawrence A.
Stern, Jerry
Sygal, Vitaly
Tampieri, Donatella
Tang, Q T. An
Tarakdjian, Noushig
Taylor, Jana L.
Therasse, Eric
Theriault, Melanie
Thibodeau, Micheline
Toth, Joseph
Trop, Isabelle
Tsatoumas, Maria
Ugolini, Patricia
Valenti, David A.
Veksler, Anna L.
Wee, Christine M.
Weill, Alain F.
Wiebe, Sheldon P.
Yeghiayan, Edouard

MONTREAL-NORD
Boisvert, Jacques

ORMSTOWN
Boisvert, Guy

OUTREMONT
Cliche, Jean

POINTE-CLAIRE
Aris, Fadi
Armanious, Shadia
Sanchez-Arroyo, Emilio
Soliman, Henry
Tsipuras, Dennis J.

QUEBEC
Audet, Marie-Eve
Auger, Renee
Bedard, Fernand
Bedard, Francine
Belleville, Martin
Bergeron, Vincent
Berthelot, Christian
Berube, Anne
Bilodeau, Sylvie
Blouin, Valerie
Bouchard, Gilles
Bourget, Catherine
Brabant, Jean
Brisson, Melanie
Brochu, Marie-Claude
Brousseau, Ghislain
Camire, Myriam
Cantin, Luce
Caron, Denis F.
Chau, Luc
Chevrette, Eric
Claude-Desroches, Mederic
Cloutier, Sonia
Cote, Chantal
Cote, Francois
Cote, Gary
Dionne, Gilles
Dionne, Guy
Dorion, Anita
Dufresne, Marie-Claude
Dumas, Christiane
Duret, Jean-Sebastien
Ferguson, Natasha
Ferland, Sylvie
Fortin, Andre
Fortin, Dominique
Fougeres, Annie
Gariepy, Jean-Luc
Garneau, Guillaume
Giguere, Caroline
Gingras, Michel
Giroux, Dominique
Grenon, Hugues
Hebert, Mario
Houle, Virginie
Jodoin, Steve
Lalonde, Catherine
Lamarre, Andre
Langis, Louis
Langis, Paul-Andre
Lapointe, Marie-Noel
Laroche, Francois
Larochelle, Olivier
Levesque, Jacques
Loisel, Yves
Mailloux, Cynthia
Marceau, Julie
Morcos, Leila
Morin, Stanislas
Morissette, Jean J.
Morissette, Lucie
Noel, Patricia
Petitclerc, Michel
Plamondon, Nicole
Riederer, Barbara
Rochette, Antoine
Rodrigue, Jean
Scherrer, Louis-Philippe
St-Onge, Odette
Tesolin-Lavoie, Maude
Toutant, Robert
Trottier, Francois
Truchon, Sophie
Turcotte, Jean-Marc
Turcotte, Roc
Vignault, Francois
White, Jane

RIMOUSKI
Beauchesne, Pierre
Cote, Pierre-Luc
Levesque, Samuel
Minville, Luc
Morin, Louis-Philippe

RIVIERE-DU-LOUP
Boisclair, Chantal
Buteau, Genevieve
Dumais, Dany
Harvey, Sylvie
Morin, Francois D.
Ouellet, Annie

ROBERVAL
Bouchard, Reynald
Glaude, Yvon
Sanou, Racine

ROUYN-NORANDA
Faribault, Guy
Ouimet, Denise

ROXBORO
Pleszewski, Bartolomiej
Yip, Melissa

SAINT-ROMUALD
Laliberte, Laura

SAINT-EUSTACHE
Bissonnette, Catherine
Cote, Elisabeth
Deshaies, Claudine
Guerin, Ronald
Marchand, France
Napolitano, Giuseppe
Tehranipour, Neda

SAINT-GEORGES
Bourdeau, Guillaume
Gagnon, Alexandre
Mailhot, Vincent
Montplaisir-Gaumont, Antoine

SAINT-HYACINTHE
Journet, Charles
Nicolas, Eric
Weidner, Marie-France

SAINT-JEROME
Desjardins, Jean-Francois
Lamarre, Paul
Leroux, Patrick
Lupien, Christine A.
Remillard-Lamarre, Denise
Rene, Philippe
Sam, Karl

SAINT-LAMBERT
Hudon, J J. Gilles

SAINT-LEONARD
Trinh, Ba-Chinh

SAINT-SAUVEUR
Savoie, Pierre

SAINTE-THERESE
Rouleau, Jean-Francois

SALABERRY DE VALLEYFIELD
Carrier, Marie-Eve
Giroux, Michel
Leger, Claude

SEPT-ILES
Botton, Edouard
Crepeau, Andre
Gervais, Robert

SHAWINIGAN-SUD
Leveille, Pierre
Levesque, Jean-Daniel
Paquin, Francine
Racicot, Jean

SHAWVILLE
Lareau, Christian

SHERBROOKE
Baril, Helene
Bedard, Justine
Belzile, Francois
Benko, Andrew J.
Bergeron, Denis
Blais, Christian
Brazeau-Lamontagne, Lucie
Bui, The-Bao
Chenard, Jean
Contre, Bernard
Fisch, Christiane
Fortier, Yves
Fradet, Robert
Gahide, Gerald
Gauthier, Normand
Giguere, Caroline S.
Hamel, Erick
Langlois, Andre
Lecours, Junie
Patenaude, Yves G.
Perras, Maurice B.
Plante, Francois R.
Ste-Marie, Raymond
Voyer, Nathalie

SOREL-TRACY
Charland, Pierre
Duong, Huu Hoang
Durocher, Lorraine

ST CHARLES BORROMEE
Bourgeault, Jacques
Cadrin-Chenevert, Alexandre
Chevrette, Yves
Gauthier, Steve
Ledoux, Elisabeth
Morency, Gilles
Ouellet, Jean-Yves
Ringuette, Julie

ST-EUSTACHE
Boudrias, Claude
Ouellet, Bertrand

ST JEAN SUR RICHELIEU
Boisvert, Glenn
Djerbib, Kenza
Laflamme, Louis
Ly, Thien-Hong
Mercky, Nicolas
Poulin, Anne
Trudel, Jean-Sebastien
Vinet, Jean-Charles

STE AGATHE DES MONTS
Racette, Richard

STE ANNE DES MONTS
Aparicio, Carlos
Lacasse, Jacques E.

TERREBONNE
Aube, Francois
Belanger, Lucie

Boucher, Paule
Coulombe-Legault, Micheline
Dube, Chantal
Labrosse, Julie M.
Lacaille-Belanger, Pierre
Mainville, Karine
Ouellet, Marie-Caroline
Perreault, Lyette
Picard, Josee
Racine, Gilbert
Rochon, Michel
Sinsky, Anna B.

THETFORD MINES
Blouin, Odette
Normand, Jean-Pierre

TROIS-RIVIERES
Arseneau, Christian
Bernier, Andre
Courcy, Marie-Josee
Couture, Denis
Dion, Chantal
Gelinas, Marcien
Grondin, Luc
Halle, Amelie
Lafontaine, J A. Guy
Lavoie, Sylvain
Nolet-Levesque, Philippe
Rousseau, Daniel
Servant, Stephan
Tessier, Gilbert

VAL-D'OR
Do, Tai Hung
Stasiak, Dorota

VERDUN
Cadotte, Richard N.
Duckett, Genevieve
Germain, Veronique
Gervais, Jean-Dominique
Marinier, Helene
McAuley, David J.
Merette, Guy
Seguin, Nathalie

VICTORIAVILLE
Belanger, Gerald
Fekir, Sami
Fleurent, Dominique
Gagnon, Michel B.
Laberge, Jean
Morissette, Sebastien
Quevillon, Mathieu

WESTMOUNT
Ayala-Bustamante, Everick N.
Azouz, E. Michel
Doyon, Marie-Lucie

SASKATCHEWAN

LLOYDMINSTER
Young, Casey

MELFORT
Marais, Andre

MOOSE JAW
Tangjerd, Norvin E.

NORTH BATTLEFORD
Stevens, James D.

PRINCE ALBERT
Buglass, Tiffany D.
Chavarria, Cesar A.
Wells, Holly D.

REGINA
Adams Jr., Winston E.
Butcher, Matthew S.
Chaturvedi, Patanjali
Clarke, W. Wayne
Devitt, Neil
Farooq, Ahmed U.
Farooq, Saqba
Gourgaris, Adriana
Goyal, Kunal
Hillis, Joanne
Jeon, Albert
Kraushaar, Greg C.
Lala, Shantilal M.
Le, Brian V.
Lembke, Edward C.
Lim, Chong-Ha
Patel, Rajesh
Phillipson, Ryan T.
Rice, James H.
Schulte, Paul A.
Shaheen, Uzma
Silberberg, Phillip J.
Suchet, Ian B.
Verma, Ashok K.

SASKATOON
Babyn, Paul S.
Beck, Maxine E.
Berscheid, Bruce B.
Burbridge, Brent E.
Chappell, Brent W.
Chow, Vance
Dhir, Anita
Dixon, Brian L.
Ellchuk, Tasha
Fladeland, Derek A.
Flegg, Carolyn
Fraser, Donald K.
Gordon, Heather
Hartridge, Allan D.
Hendel, Mary-Jane
Irving, Hugh D.
Kenny, Anne
Leswick, David A.
Mack, Tyson L.
Marshall, Geoffrey B.
McIntosh, Donald B.
Norval, Ivan L.
Obaid, Haron R.
Otani, Robert K.
Rashidi, Farid
Rodriguez, Carl P.
Ross, Todd K.
Shenouda, Mark A.
Shepel, Michael L.
Stoneham, Grant W.
Szkup, Leszek P.
Tan, Kiat T.
Theoret, Christina M.
Tremeer, Cory B.
Tynan, Jennifer R.
Verrall, John R.
Waddell, Ian C.
Wall, Christopher J.
Wasif, Evet A.
Waslen, Thomas A.
White, Christopher W.

Electroencephalography(P.Q.)

ONTARIO

HAMILTON
Hollenberg, Robert D.

OTTAWA
Guzman, D. Antonio

TORONTO
Sinuff, Tasnim
Sourkes, Myra
Wennberg, Richard A.

QUÉBEC

CHICOUTIMI
Beaudry, Michel G.
Boily, Camil

DOLLARD DES ORMEAUX
Muresan, Letitia V.

GATINEAU
Therrien, Marc

GREENFIELD PARK
Duplessis, Michel
Filiatrault, Robert
Grand'Maison, Francois
Ninkovic, Svetlana
Trottier, Antonio G.

LAVAL
Archambault, Luc L P.
Lalumiere, Eric
Veilleux, Francine

LEVIS
Bergeron, Marc-Andre
Grammond, Pierre
Petitclerc, Marc
Rivest, Donald
Tremblay, Sandra

LONGUEUIL
Bui, Linh-Khue
Ducharme, Mario
Phan, Xuan Khoa.
Roy, Stephane
Thibault, Louis

MONT-ROYAL
Morcos, Rami

MONTREAL
Aube, Michel
Bekhor, Sabah
Bernier, Gilles P.
Blanchet, Pierre
Carmant, Lionel
Chayer, Celine
Copti, Michel
Cossette, Patrick
D'Amour, Monique L.
Deutsch-Andermann, Eva
Dubeau, Francois
Duchastel, Yves J.
Gendron, Daniel
Girard, J. Marc
Lachapelle, Jacques
Lebrun, Louise-Helene
Lemay, Robert
Lortie, Anne
Masson, Helene
Montplaisir, Jacques Y.
Perez-De-Leon, Adolfo J.
Poulin, Chantal
Remillard, Guy M.
Robillard, Alain A.
Rosenblatt, Bernard
Rousseau, M. Suzanne R.
Roy, Louis-Edouard
Soland, Valerie L.
Souchon, Frederique
Talbot, Jeannine
Vanasse, Michel
Veilleux, Martin
Villota, Maurilio
Wein, Howard P.
Woods, John F.

QUEBEC
Bouchard, Remi W.
Daigle, Emilien
De Lean, Jacques
Desbiens, Richard
Lafleur, Jean
Langevin, Pierre L.
Naud, Pierre G.
Radouco-Thomas, Monelly
Sylvain, Michel
Thibault, Manon
Verret, Simon

RIMOUSKI
Delisle, Francois

SHERBROOKE
Bernier, Jean-Pierre
Evoy, Francois
Frenette, Eric
Gosselin, Sylvie
Jarjoura, Samir C.
Kantardjieff, Spiridon
Lamontagne, G. Albert
Lebel, Michel L.
Rivest, Jean

ST-AMBROISE-D-KILD
Lamoureux, Louise

ST CHARLES BORROMEE
Dubreuil, Martin
Sarrazin, Anne-Marie

TROIS-RIVIERES
Arbour, Jean-Francois
Charest, Stephane
Gagnon, Andre F.
Guite, Charles

WESTMOUNT
Zifkin, Benjamin G.

Emergency Medicine

ALBERTA

BANFF
Holmen, Carol D.
Shuster, Michael

CALGARY
Abbi, Arun K.
Andruchow, James E.
Anton, Andrew R.
Berthelot, Simon
Betzner, Michael J.
Boone, Andrea
Bradley, Jeffrey A.
Bromley, Mark A.
Brulotte, Cory A.
BurTon-Macleod, Rebecca L.
Campfens, Lisa C.
Choi, Hyun D.
Curry, Donald G.
Deedo, Ryan J.
Dorrington, Catherine L.
Dowling, Shawn
Downey, Pamela M.
Erskine, Matthew
Fox, James
Francis, Marc N.
Gamble, Mardelle H.
Gant, Peter T.
Gastonguay, Johanne I.
Gaudet, Jonathan E C.
Geddes, Michael
Grant, Jeffry M.
Hall, Christopher
Hall, Robert E.
Halpenny, David G.
Harari, Maya V.
Head, Pauline W.
Huffman, James L.
Innes, Grant D.
Johnston, Robert V.
Keats, Karen L.
Lang, Eddy S.
Langhan, Trevor S.
Lazarenko, Gerald C.
Lendrum, David A.
Lord, Jason A.
Mabon, Lorraine M.
MacLeod, D. Bruce
McNeil, Gordon
McPherson, Sarah
McRae, Andrew D.
Michalchuk, Andre S.
Morris, Alyssa
Moussadji, Yael
Nesdoly, Dennis R.
Ness, Rhonda
Neufeld, John D G.
Oster, Adam
Pandya, Sudhir D.
Patterson, Heather L.
Powell, D. Gregory
Rigby, Ian J.
Robinson, Andrew J.
Schiebel, Nicola E E.
Stewart, Brian D.
Storck, Aric J.
Sztukowski, Izabela
Tourigny, Paul D.
Turner, Stuart G.
Ukrainetz, Philip J.
Vicas, Ingrid M O.
Wishart, Ian M.
Yarema, Mark C.
Young, Bryan C.
Zalmanowitz, Leo I.

EDMONTON
Barker, Andrew P.
Boulanger Jr., Michel J.
Brown, Jim J.
Bullard, Michael
Burkart, Layton D.
Chang, Eddie C.
Chen, Matthew M.
Cherniwchan, Marc A.
Dance, Erica A.
Davidow, Jonathan
Djogovic, Dennis
Dong, Kathyrn A.
Dong, Sandy
Ha, David J.
Haager, Moritz B.
Hansen, Ruben G.
Hanson, Amanda E.
Haponiuk, Adrienne D.
Holroyd, Brian R.
Jain, Praveen
Kabaroff, Alison M.
Keyes, Robert E.
Kjelland, Colleen B.
Lam, Kenneth H M.
Lam, Ni T.
Lee, Karr-Hong
Lefebvre, Dennis C.
MacDonald, Shavaun I.
MacGougan, Cameron K.
MacLachlan, Shona M.
McLelland, Kirstie
Murphy, Michael F.
Norum, Joanne N.
Pritchard, Jennifer E.
Rabuka, Curtis E.
Reitsma, Jeffrey J.
Rosenblum, Rebeccah M.
Scheirer, Richard N.
Sevcik, William E.
Shih, Elizabeth M.
Shragge, David L.
Sibley, Aaron K.
Soibelman, Felix
Sookram, Sunil M.
Taylor, John C.
Thirsk, Warren S.
Williams, Jennifer A.

GRANDE PRAIRIE
Best, Anthony H S.
Rickards, Michael R.

MEDICINE HAT
Parks, Paul

RED DEER
Junck, Randall

BRITISH COLUMBIA

ABBOTSFORD
Payrastre, Julien A O.

BURNABY
Chou, Alan F.
McGowan, Brian J.
Saunders, Robert C.

KAMLOOPS
Bilbey, James H.
Mitchell, Ian V.

KELOWNA
Clark, Kevin
Cleve, Paul D.
Eppler, Jeffrey D.

SPECIALISTS BY PROVINCE

Kuzak, Nicholai D.
Kwan, Anthony L.
McInnes, J. Gordon
Rhine, David J.
Sanz, Geoffrey
Spelliscy, Shawn D.
Tercier, John A.
Williams, David J.

LANGLEY
Anthony, Robert G.
Carthy, J. Michael
Rosenczweig, Carolyn C.

NANAIMO
Hayley, John H.

NEW WESTMINSTER
Achiam, Cimi
Ahmad, Omar
Balcar, Petr
Cheng, Amy
Choi, Christine
Davison, Aaron
Deady, Brian L.
Exner, Jason
Glazer, Sheldon
Green, Thomas J.
Ip, Joseph K H.
Janes, Shawn P.
Kelly-Smith, Carolyn H.
Khan, Idan
Lund, Adam
MacNab, Jessica M.
Mostrenko, Michael S.
Noseworthy, Robert F.
Oldring, Brian W.
Street, Robert M.
Taylor, Anthony S.
Thordarson, Ian T.
Tyson, Caroline B.
Vertesi, Leslie
Wormsbecker, Sean C.

NORTH VANCOUVER
Davidson, Adam
Kung, James H.
Severy, Philip R.
Stewart, Mark A H.

OLIVER
Lang-Hodge, Brian J.

PENTICTON
Fort, Diana K.
Plant, Jeffery R.

PORT MOODY
Grunfeld, Anton F.

RICHMOND
Huber, Alan G.

SMITHERS
Flannigan, Kelly P.

SURREY
Clarke, Anne I.
Saincher, Anurag Q.

VANCOUVER
Abu-Laban, Riyad B.
Bijlsma, Jan Jaap
Brubacher, Jeffrey R.
Cadieu, Travis M.
Campbell, Andrew S.
Chahal, Anthony M.
Cheung, Ka Wai
Christenson, James
Chung, Brian J.
DeWitt, Christopher
Dettman, Michael S.
Filiatrault, Lyne
Fleming, Bruce
Gill, Ginjeet K.
Grafstein, Eric J.
Graham, Lois E.
Harrison, David W.
Henderson, William R.
Ho, Kendall
Hohl, Corinne M.
Holmes, Allan E.
Huang, Paul B T.
Hunt, David G.
Kanji, Hussein D.
Kassen, David M.
Kestler, Andrew M.
Khazei, Afshin
Kim, Daniel J.
Lang, William J.
Lee, Donna S H.
Lee, Thomas F.
Leung, Cosmas W M.
Markel, Kenneth N.
McEwen, Jillene I.
McIntyre, Caroline M.
McKnight, R. Douglas
Morrison, A. Bruce
Moser, Meite S.
Nemethy, Kevin M.
O'Donnell, Shannon
Passi, William B.
Pickett, Tracy A.
Pledger, David J.
Pursell, Roy
Ricketson, Ian M.
Rose, Nicholas
Shirzad, Shahin
Sweet, David D.
Tallon, John M.
Teal, Philip A.
Theoret, Jonathan
Tober, Alfred E.
Trojanowski, Jan A.
Vu, Erik N.
Wanger, Karen
Yeung, Titus C.
Zahn, Karen A.

VICTORIA
Beliveau, Peter I.
Buchanan, Kenneth D.
Campana, Bruce
Cordon, Ian W.
Goshko, Victor G.
Hall, Christine A.
Hooker, Ross W.
McElgunn, Dennis M.
McFadyen, Roderick L.
Moran, Jane M.
Penner, Robert J.
Ricketson, Charles W.
Ross, Helen M.
Stewart, Samuel J.
Sun, Charles Y.
Thompson, James
Wong, Bruce M.
Wood, Victor M.
Youngash, Ronald W.

WHISTLER
Gareau, Annie

MANITOBA

WINNIPEG
Chan, Patrick B.
Chochinov, Alecs H.
Easton, David W.
Eyolfson, Douglas A.
Ffrench, Cheryl
Geurts, Jill M.
Grierson, Robert A.
Klassen, Jeffrey M.
La Riviere, Christian G.
Lefevre, Gerald R.
Ludwig, Louis W.
Minish, Travis M.
Mutz, Shane D.
Palatnick, Wesley B.
Pham, Chau
Piggott, Zoe S.
Ratanaseangsuang, Paul N.
Robertson, Adrian F.
Schindle, Rebecca L.
Snider, Carolyn E.
Steigerwald, Ronald G.
Sustrik, Ryan A.
Swirsky, S. Neil
Tetreault, Michel F.
Weldon, Erin R.
Zubert, Shelly A.

NEW BRUNSWICK

SAINT JOHN
Talbot, Jo-Ann

NEWFOUNDLAND AND LABRADOR

ST. JOHN'S
Baggs, Douglas K.
Mengual, Rose
Seviour, Catherine M.

NOVA SCOTIA

DARTMOUTH
Travers, Andrew H.

HALIFAX
Beatty, Dorothy L.
Bullock, Graham L.
Carter, Alexandra J E.
Fieldus, Warren
Green, Robert S.
Hurley, Katrina F.
Kovacs, George J.
MacIntyre, Janet K.
Magee, Kirk D.
McVey, Jennifer J.
Morris, Ian R.
Petrie, David A.
Petrie, Neil M.
Ross, John A.

KENTVILLE
McLeod, R. Bruce

ONTARIO

ALMONTE
Dolan, Michael C.

BARRIE
Armstrong, Kathryn G W.
Austgarden, Douglas A.
Eisen, Jeffrey S.
Martin, Christopher D.
Usher, Darren J.

BRAMPTON
Fan, Jerome
Karbi, Oscar A.

BRANTFORD
Komaranski, Norman

BROCKVILLE
Beveridge, Robert C.

BURLINGTON
Greenway, Keith T.
Sharma, Sangita

CAMBRIDGE
Crosby, John W.

COLLINGWOOD
Chisholm, James

CORNWALL
Burga Alvarado, Alfonso
Heeley-Ray, Timothy

ELORA
Robson, Robert J.

ETOBICOKE
McKinley, Goldwin E.
McMillan, Ronald V.
Prieditis, J. George P.
Rosenberg, Paul J.

GUELPH
Morrow, David
Squires, James S.
Tang, Patrick H.

HAMILTON
Ackerman, Margaret J.
Baw, Bandar A I.
Crossley, John G.
Eby, Roberta J.
Frank, J. Peter
Greenwald, Joseph A.
Ha, Michael
Hawley, Kristopher S.
Hayward, Melissa L.
Healey, Andrew J.
Hersi, Ali I.
Howarth, Paul A.
Jalayer, Massoud
Mallin, A. Rebecca
Marshall, Thomas D.
Martin, Douglas D.
Massarella, Carys R.
Miller, Paul Q.
Pardhan, Alim
Price, Ira M.
Richards, Douglas L.
Schiff, Karen C.
Sellens, Catherine S.
Sherbino, Jonathan D.
Upadhye, Suneel
Valani, Rahim A.
Welsford, Michelle

HUNTSVILLE
Hastie, Ian G.

KINGSTON
Ball, Ian M.
Blouin, Danielle
Bornstein, Jason
Brison, Robert J.
Brooks, Steven C.
Bruder, Eric A.
Carpenter, Jennifer L.
Caudle, Jaelyn M.
Crawford, Frances M.
Dagnone, Jeffrey
Dagnone, L. Eugene
Dungey, Paul E.
Edwards, Raymond K F.
Farnell, Barbara A.
Howes, Daniel W.
Jones, Gordon R.
Landine, James K.
McGraw, Robert C.
Messenger, David W.
Montalvo, Max
Murray, Heather E.
O'Brien, Terrence O.
O'Connor, H. Michael
Poley, Rachel
Rang, Louise C F.
Reed, Andrew D.
Sivilotti, Marco L A.
Spotswood, Wayne J.
Taylor, Murray F.

KITCHENER
Green, Jason P.
Hosek, Paul
McKinnon, Kent D L.

LONDON
Anderson, Scott B.
Armstrong, Sarah A.
Arntfield, Robert T.
Bauld Giffin, Dawn
Church, Karalyn
Cram, Gordon D.
Dagnone, R. Vico
Donovan, Keith D.
Dreyer, Jonathan
Dukelow, Adam M.
Edmonds, Marcia
Eisenhauer, Mary A.
Fuss, Jeffrey W.
Gibson, R. John
Gilkinson, Trevor L.
Hames, Heather
Innes, Marilyn E.
Jones, Andrew E.
Kalidindi, Shiva K R.
Lewell, Michael P.
Maxwell, H. Brent
McCauley, William A.
Meiwald, Allison
Millard, Wanda
Mosdossy, Gregory J.
Murphy, David G.
Ouellette, David W.
Phillips, Randall N.
Price, Laura A.
Pringle, Derrick J.
Richards, Crispen G.
Sedran, Robert J.
Shepherd, Lisa G.
Skoretz, Terry G.
Taylor, David C.
Thompson, Andrew C.

MARKHAM
Austin, David E.
Claybo, Ross A.
Moran, Philip A.

MISSISSAUGA
Allen, Timothy V.
Channan, Peter K.
Chu, Jacqueline
Ducharme, James
Everson, Edward A.
Grenier, M M. Catherine
Letovsky, Eric E.
Louis Bayliss, Amy G.
MacDonald, Russell D.
McClennan, Sarah K.
Tenn-Lyn, Nicole A.

NAPANEE
Yake, Marvin A.

NEPEAN
Godsoe, Suzanne
Makropoulos, Dimitri

NEWMARKET
Peera, Mohamed A.
Williams, David R.

NORTH YORK
Blicker, Jamie Z.
King, John W R.

OAKVILLE
Preyra, Ian J R.

ORLEANS
Ahuja, Jan
Smith, Norman A.

OSHAWA
Freeman, Kenneth C.
Vandersluis, Rudolf

OTTAWA
Al Raisi, Marwan S D.
Al Shamsi, Mohamed S M.
Alrajhi, Abdulaziz A M.
Calder, Lisa A.
Cardamore, Robin
Choi, Stephen B.
Clark, Eric A.
Corrin, Raymond G.
Cwinn, A. Adam
Davoudi, Soraya
Elder, Brian R.
Farion, Kenneth J.
Frank, Jason R.
Gee, Andrew S.
Greenberg, Gary H.
Hebert, Guy J.
Hobden, Elisabeth J.
Johns, Peter D.
Kwok, Edmund S H.
Lockman, Denis
Maloney, Justin P.
Montgomery, George D.
Montoya, David R.
Moore, Sean W.
Murnaghan, Marion A.
Nimigan, Wayne R.
Ogilvie, Kelly
Plantive, Richard
Pozgay, Anita M.
Reardon, Mark L.
Sampsel, Kari L.
Stiell, Ian G.

Terrett, Luke A.
Vaillancourt, Christian
Wallace, Gordon J.
Weitzman, Brian N.
Wiesenfeld, Lorne M.
Worthington, James R.

OWEN SOUND
Williams, Michael D.

PERTH
Del Grande, Robert W.

PETERBOROUGH
Ashbourne, John F.

PORT HOPE
Dersnah, Douglas F.

RICHMOND HILL
Jessa, Karim K.

SAULT STE MARIE
Ghosh, Rishi K.

SCARBOROUGH
Adler, Adam J.
Clasky, Howard J.

ST CATHARINES
Hatcher, Michael C E.

STRATFORD
Mann, Miriam E S.

SUDBURY
Bota, Gary
Socransky, Steven J.

THUNDER BAY
Brown, Bryce K.
MacDonald, Damian A.
McKee, David C.
Tebbenham, Troy E.

TORONTO
Atzema, Clare L.
Au, Bryan L.
Bandiera, Glen W.
Bellissimo, Agostino M.
Brzozowski, Michael S.
Caspari, David A.
Cass, Daniel E.
Cheng, Ivy S.
Chenkin, Jordan S.
Chopra, Anil
Chu, Jennifer
Cleghorn, Graham E.
Farooki, Nadia
Feldman, Michael
Freedman, Mark
Fulton, Lynne A.
Gerace, Rocco V.
Gray, Sara H.
Greenspan, Lorne
Hicks, Christopher
Horak, Martin J.
Josephson, Timothy B.
Kaul, Thomas
Kester-Greene, Nicole
Khan, Yasmin
Kovacs, Colin M.
Lampard, Robert B.
Lee, Jacques S.
Lim, Dawn Y.
Maskalyk, Milton J.
Mazurik, Laurel A.
Mazza, Christopher F.
McCallum, Andrew L.
McDonald, Andrew C.
McDonnell, Michael B.
McLellan, Barry A.
Meshkat, Nazanin
Morrison, Laurie J.
Nowacki, Anna K.
Peerbaye, Yousouf A.
Puchalski Ritchie, Lisa M.
Riley, Jennifer F.
Robles, Luis C.
Ryan, Dale T.
Sabbah, Osama R S.
Schull, Michael J.
Sinclair, Douglas E.
Slomovic, Brant M.
Smith-Gorvie, Telisha J.
Spence, Julia M.
Stefan, Raluca A.
Steinhart, Brian D.
Stone, Angela M.
Teixeira, Fernando J.
Thompson, Margaret A.
Thurgur, Lisa D.
Toma, Alina
Tyberg, Jeffrey P.
Venugopal, Raghu
Verbeek, P. Richard
Verma, Aikta
Wasserman, Jeffrey J.
Watson, Leah D.
Wolpert, Natalie
Woolfrey, Karen G H.
Wortzman, David J.
Yaphe, Joel S.
Yu, Richard S O.

UNIONVILLE
Lindzon, Ronald D.

WATERLOO
Jeffery, Deborah L.
Vernon, James D.

WINDSOR
Alsadoon, Abdulaziz A Y.
Hasan, Anwar A A.
Issley, Steven B.
MacDonald, Jay R.

PRINCE EDWARD ISLAND

CHARLOTTETOWN
Colohan, Desmond P.

SUMMERSIDE
Dickman, John H.

QUÉBEC

CHARNY
Frechette, Pierre

CHICOUTIMI
Gagnon, Louis
Hamel, Bruno
Noel, Bernard C.
Pelletier, Sylvie

GATINEAU
Assad, P. Paul
Low, Thomas D P.

GREENFIELD PARK
Baril, Bruno
Dufresne, Francois
Lamarre, Marie-Lise
Montminy, Alphonse
Ranger, Melissa

LAVAL
Gaumont, J R. Francois
Lachance, Paul-Andre
Ouellet, Jacques
Vachon, Guylaine

LEVIS
Archambault, Patrick
Beaupre, Pierre
Berger-Pelletier, Elyse
Lapointe, Jean
Lortie, Gilles
Maire, Sebastien
O'Grady, John P.
Paquet, Francois
Pigeon, Dany
Poitras, Julien
Shields, Jean-Francois
Tremblay, Stephane D.

LONGUEUIL
Beaucage, Gilles
Boucher, Marcel M.
Lefrancois, Daniel P.
Morin, Johanne
Vincent, Matthieu

MERCIER
Einagel Jr., Victor

MISTISSINI
Adjemian, Raffi A.

MONTREAL
Afilalo, Marc
Beique, Marc A.
Bernardin, Bruno
Bertrand, C. Francois
Boucher, Gilbert
Boulet, Marc
Bourque, Daniel
Carvalho, Anna-Maria
Cermignani, Monica S.
Charneux, Marco
Chauny, Jean-Marc
Collette, Francois
Coombs, Heather
Cooperman, Jonathan J.
Dankoff, Jerrald
Daoust, Raoul
De Champlain, Francois
Delaney, J. Scott
Delev, Gligor
Desaulniers, Pierre
Doyle, Kenneth R.
Dumas, Catherine
Dupre, Marguerite
Fortin, Jerome
Foxford, Robert J.
Garneau, Francois X.
Garner, Michel
Giard, Annie
Gosselin, Sophie
Grad, Willis B.
Guttman, Alex
Guy, John R.
Haggar, Carine
Homier, Valerie
Krull, Andreas
Laliberte, Martin
Larocque, Alexandre
Lee, Gary L.
Levesque, Georges
Liesegang, Nadine
Melanson, Patrick R P.
Meyers, Christine M.
Mills, Anne
Morris, Judy
Papacotsia, Jean
Pearson, Eleena A.
Piette, Claude
Piette, Eric
Poirier, Vincent
Pregent, Ernest
Rosenthal, Stephen E.
Ryder, Arthur C.
Segal, Eli
Shulman, H. Mitchell
Sigman, Eric H.
Sivaraman, Sujith K.
Stasiak, Jerome
Stern, Errol
Stewart, Jessica N.
Tratch, Alexandre
Troquet, Jean-Marc
Turner, Joel P.
Unger, Bernard
Vadeboncoeur, Alain-Michel
Welch, James C.

POINTE-CLAIRE
Gilbert, Francois
Mannard, Allan C.

QUEBEC
Baril, Pierre
Belhumeur, Marc
Bertrand, Isabelle
Blais, Rene
Bourassa, Amelie
Brochu, Pierre
Brouillard, Daniel
Cote, Remi
Couture, Marie-Maud
Deblois, Jacques
Deschenes, Michel
Dion, Jean
Dufresne, Georges
Emond, Marcel
Eramian, Douglas
Genest, Isabelle
Hamel, Pierre
Lachance, Andre
Lauzon, Robert
Le Sage, Natalie
Parent, Marc C.
Plourde, Miville
Prevost, Jean-Francois
Savard, Pierre
Tardif, Yves
Topping, Claude
Villeneuve, Jean

SAINT-EUSTACHE
Pelletier, Louis-Philippe

SAINT-JEROME
Jamaty, Chloe
Sanogo, Karine

SHAWINIGAN-SUD
Dion, Janique

SHERBROOKE
Beaudoin, Rene
Bellavance, Colette
Boisvert, Richard
Gagnon, Nathalie
Guerette, Pierre
Langlois, J L. Jean
Ouellet, Jean-Pascal
Smith, Wayne J.

SOREL-TRACY
Royal, Pierre

ST CHARLES BORROMEE
Arroyo, Jacky

SASKATCHEWAN

SASKATOON
Betz, Martin
Cload, Bruce W A.
Lalani, Nadim J.
Woods, Robert A.

Endocrinology

ALBERTA

CALGARY
Pacaud, Daniele

ONTARIO

LONDON
Dupre, John

NORTH BAY
Bowker, Blair M.

OTTAWA
Chretien, Michel
McPherson, P. Ruth
Walker, Peter

TORONTO
Kelly, Catherine M K.
Zinman, Bernard

QUÉBEC

COTE SAINT-LUC
Jukier, Lilian

DRUMMONDVILLE
Perreault, Isabelle

GATINEAU
Babin, Sandra
Lanoie, Genevieve

GRAND-MERE
Mailhot, Jean

GREENFIELD PARK
Beauchef, Jean-P
Benard, Bernard

KIRKLAND
Gilbert, François

LASALLE
Herrera-Correa, Jose R.

LAVAL
Bahsali, Georges I.
Belanger, Andre
Dumas, Richard
Long, Helene
Palardy, Jean

LEVIS
Renald, Pierre

MONT-ROYAL
Lavoie, Helene B.

MONTREAL
Assimakopoulos, Peter
Barnes, Robert D.
Beauregard, Hugues
Belanger, Raphael
Boucher, Andree
Bourdeau, Isabelle
Boutin, Jean-Marie
Breton, Donald
Brossard, Jean-Hugues
Caron, Daniel C.
Clamen, Marvin
Comtois, Ronald
D'Amour, Pierre
Duda, Barbara
Ekoe, Jean-Marie
Faure, Nacia
Garrel, Dominique
Grunbaum, David
Halle, Jean-Pierre
Hamet, Pavel
How, Jacques S.
Karaplis, Andy C.
Krishnamoorthy, Preetha
Kudo-Kyei-Aboagye, Catherine
Lacroix, Andre
Launay, Marc P.
Letendre, Michel
Mackler, Richard J.
Marcovitz, Sorana
Meissner, Les A.
Meltzer, Sara J.
Michon, Nicole
Mircescu, Hortensia S.
Mitchell, John J.
Monier, Danielle
Morris, David
Neveu, Nathalie A.
Pison, Cesar
Poirier, Lysane
Polychronakos, Constantin
Rakel, Agnes
Rasio, Eugenio A.
Rizzo, Arturo J.
Rodd, Celia J.
Schiffrin, Alicia
Schweitzer, Morris
Serri, Omar
Somma, Maurice
Ste-Marie, Louis-Georges
Tsoukas, Georges
Van Vliet, Guy
Yale, Jean-Francois

POINTE-CLAIRE
Skamene, Alexander

QUEBEC
Allen, Christyne
Coulombe, Raymond
Denis, Marie-Claire

Duclos, Pierre
Eugene, Dardye
Garrido-Russo, Maria
Lemay, Andre
Simard, Sylvain
Tremblay, Roland R.
Weisnagel, S. John
Whittom, Serge

RIMOUSKI
Boisselle, Andree

SAINT-HYACINTHE
St-Jean, Edith

SAINT-LAMBERT
Havrankova, Jana B.

SAINT-LAURENT
Saliba, Nouhad

SAINT-LEONARD
Bertrand, Sylvie

SHERBROOKE
Baillargeon, Jean-Patrice
Carpentier, Andre
Khoury, Khalil
Langlois, Marie-France
Maheux, Pierre
Perron, Patrice

ST JEAN SUR RICHELIEU
Noiseux, Daniel

TROIS-RIVIERES
Rioux, Dany

WESTMOUNT
Posner, Barry I.
Varga-Solymoss, Susan M.

Endocrinology & Metabolism

ALBERTA

CALGARY
Bassyouni, Hanan A.
Bhayana, Shelly
Butalia, Sonia
Dawrant, Jonathan M.
Donovan, Lois E.
Edwards, Alun
Grundy, Peter D.
Ho, Josephine
Huang, Carol T L.
Khosla, Munish
Kinnear, Susan E.
Kline, Gregory A.
McIlhargey, Trina L.
McKeen, Julie A.
Pacaud, Daniele
Parkins, Vicky M.
Pedersen, Susie D.
Rabi, Doreen M.
Sigal, Ronald J.
Symonds, Christopher J.

EDMONTON
Chapados, Isabelle
Chik, Constance L.
Ghosh, Mahua
Haqq, Andrea M.
Jacquier, Jennifer E.
Jetha, Mary M.
Kondi, Joma
Kwong, Sarah L.
Lewanczuk, Richard Z.
Li, Stephanie K.
Mereu, Laurie E.
Mitchell, Rebecca S.
Nelson, Jill D.
Opgenorth, Andrea A.
Pertman, Shea
Romney, Jacques S.
Ryan, Edmond A.
Siminoski, Kerry G.
Toth, Ellen L.

LETHBRIDGE
Drever, Erin
MacKay, Alison R.

BRITISH COLUMBIA

CHILLIWACK
Grills, Gordon R.

KELOWNA
Jones, Charlotte A.

NEW WESTMINSTER
Barts, Agnieszka D.
Clayton, Dale B.
Klinke, Jennifer A.
Lee, Julie
Priestman, Barbara A.
Shu, David H P.
Wallace, Clarissa

NORTH VANCOUVER
Haigh, Susan E.
Lee, D. Dae-Won
Stock, Suzanne L.

SURREY
Kang, Parmjit S.
Khurana, Reena
Schroeder, Benjamin D.
Severin, Naomi E.
Stafford, Sara G.
Watanabe, Hiroko
Yelle, Carole-Anne L.

VANCOUVER
Amed, Shazhan
Bebb, Richard A.
Dahl, Marshall A.
Dawson, Keith Granger
Elliott, Thomas G.
Francis, Gordon A.
Fung, Michelle A.
Gill, Sabrina
Johnson, Michelle D.
Kendler, David L.
Khatchadourian, Karine
Kong, Jason M.
MacKenzie-Feder, Jessica M.
Mase, Robert M.
Metzger, Daniel L.
Panagiotopoulos, Constadina
Paty, Breay W.
Sirrs, Sandra M.
Stewart, Laura L.
White, Adam S.

VICTORIA
Capes, Sarah E.
Manjoo, Prija S.
Materek, Lukasz A.
Miller, David B.
Moldoveanu, Andrei I.
Phillips, Richard A.
Tevaarwerk, Gerald J M.

MANITOBA

WINNIPEG
Hurd, Carmen A.
Katz, Pamela
Ludwig, Sora M.
Marks, Seth D.
Richardson, Cindy Jo.
Roe, E. Bruce
Salamon, Elizabeth A.
Sellers, Elizabeth A C.
Silha, Josef
Taback, Shayne P.
Wicklow, Brandy A.
Woo, Vincent C.

NEW BRUNSWICK

FREDERICTON
McGibbon, Angela M.

MONCTON
Gallant, Tania M.

SAINT JOHN
Dornan, John M.
Sanderson, Susan R.

WATERVILLE CARLETON
Pelkey, Michael C.

NEWFOUNDLAND AND LABRADOR

BURIN
Mathew, Baboo M.

ST. JOHN'S
Bridger, Tracey L.
Chandurkar, Vikram
Galway, A. Brenda
Healey, Ara A.
Joyce, Carol J.
Kovacs, Christopher S.
Murray, Cathy M.

NOVA SCOTIA

HALIFAX
Cummings, Elizabeth A.
Gee, Shirl A D.
Imran, Syed A.
Kaiser, Stephanie M.
Mokashi, Arati S.
Pinto, Teresa
Ransom, Thomas
Tugwell, Barna D.

SYDNEY
Zwicker, Deborah A.

ONTARIO

BRAMPTON
Dharmalingam, Sudharshan
Friefeld, Joanne
Kong, Yuan
May, Donna L.
Shorey, Sanam S.
Zamel, Rola

CAMBRIDGE
Bishara, Phoebe R Y.

CHATHAM
Sinnaeve, Linda J E.

CORNWALL
De Young, J. Paul
Levac, Marie-France

EAST YORK
Fine, Rebecca J.
Fung, Raymond C.
Sandler, Samantha D.
Telner, Adam H.

ETOBICOKE
Khandwala, Hasnain
Nguyen, Kinh-Tung T.
Parikh, Amish
Vaz, Camila M.
Wong, Min Min C.

GRANTON
McLean, Nicola K.

GUELPH
Purdon, Cameron J A.

HAMILTON
Bassilious, Ereny
Gerstein, Hertzel
Harper, William L.
Luthra, Meera
McAssey, Karen L.
Meyerson, Jeffrey
Morrison, Katherine M.
Prebtani, Ally K P H.
Punthakee, Zubin
Vandermeulen, John A.
Yakubovich, Natalia

KINGSTON
Houlden, Robyn L.
Kovacs, Katherine Ann.

KITCHENER
Parlea, Luciana

LONDON
Edmonds, Merrill W.
Fraser, Lisa-Ann
Haddara, Wael M.
Hegele, Robert A.
Hramiak, O M. Irene
Joy, Tisha R.
Liu, Selina L.
McDonald, Charlotte G.
McManus, Ruth M.
Morrison, Deric J.
Paul, Partha
Paul, Terri L.
Rodger, N. Wilson
Spaic, Tamara
Stein, Robert I.
Van Uum, Stanislaus H M.

MARKHAM
Bishara, Laila D.
Kogan, Eva
Sivakumar, Tharsan

MISSISSAUGA
Cheng, Alice Y.
Gottesman, Irving S.
Langlois, W. John
Lee, Elmer C C.
Milosevic, Vladimir
Piersanti, Monique
Rosenthall, Wendy
Simone, Angelo M.
Suk, Andy G.

NEWMARKET
Juta, Sunil
Wang, Henry

NORTH BAY
Bowker, Blair M.

NORTH YORK
Bain, Jerald
Kim, Rak Hay
Knight, Burton W.
Lee, Hank C.
Mojab, Hamid

OAKVILLE
Huang, Qingli L.

OSHAWA
Chong, Rachel Y V.
Willamowicz, Anna S.

OTTAWA
Abujrad, Hussein A.
Ahmet, Alexandra H.
Arnaout, Amel
Braaten, Jan T.
Chretien, Michel
Doyle, Mary-Anne
Goldbloom, Ellen B.
Hadjiyannakis, Anastasia
Keely, Erin J.
Lawrence, Sarah E.
Lawson, Margaret L.
Liu, Dora M.
Lochnan, Heather A.
Malcolm, Janine C.
McPherson, P. Ruth
Meggison, Hillary E.
O'Leary, Timothy J.
Saleh, David S.
Silverman, Mark S.
Sorisky, Alexander M.
Tailor, Chetna
Ward, Leanne M.

OWEN SOUND
Becks, Gregory

RICHMOND HILL
Kirsch, Susan E.
Leung, Nathalie M C.
Mojdami, Fatemeh

SAULT STE MARIE
Farah, Sameh S.

SCARBOROUGH
Boutros, Farid S A.
Neculau, Madalina
Sigalas, John
Tsui, Elaine Y L.
Turner, Marci R.
Zahedi, Afshan

STONEY CREEK
Babic, Bojana

SUDBURY
Varghese, Boji

THORNHILL
Daitchman, Julie F.
Goldenberg, Ronald M.
Rambaldini, Gloria M.
Schlosser, Robert J.
Singer, Debrah G C.
Wine, Nina H.

THUNDER BAY
Abu-Bakare, Asiru

TORONTO
Alguwaihes, Abdullah M A.
Arab-O'Brien, Donna M.
Aronson, Ronnie
Bayley, T. Arnold
Becker, Taryn
Booth, Gillian L.
Boright, Andrew
Briones-Urbina, Rosario
Chan, Betty L.
Curtis, Jacqueline R.
Daneman, Denis
Dawson, Ainsley E.
Donat, Diane J.
Ezzat, Shereen Z.
Fantus, Ivan G.
Feig, Denice S.
Fettes, Ivy M.
Gilbert, Jeremy D.
Gilbert, Richard E.
Goguen, Jeannette M.
Groenewoud, Yolanda A.
Grossman, Loren D.
Hamilton, Jill K.
Hanna, Amir K.
Holland, F. John
Jamal, Abida S.
James, Jacqueline
Josse, Robert G.
Khan, Shagufta U.
Kim, Sandra A.
Laredo, E. Sheila
Lega, Iliana C.
Leiter, Lawrence A.
Lipscombe, Lorraine L.
Luk, Cynthia T.
Mah-Poy, Kimberly
Mahmud, Farid H.
Millar, Adam C.
Ng, Dominic S K.
Nicholas, R. Everton S.
Perkins, Bruce J L A.
Qureshy, Kamran
Retnakaran, Ravi
Ridout, Rowena
Rothman, Laura G.
Sawka, Annie M.
Segal, Phillip H B.
Shah, Baiju R.

Shulman, Rayzel M.
Silver, Robert D.
Silverberg, Jay D H.
Sochett, Etienne B.
Stone, Elaine
Sujana Kumar, Shoba
Urbach, Stacey L.
Werb, Marsha R.
Wherrett, Diane K.
Wolfs, Maria E.
Wong, Rene
Woo, Minna N.
Yu, Catherine H.
Zeman, Robert
Zuijdwijk, Caroline S.

WATERLOO
Husein, Nadira

WINDSOR
Abouhassan, Tyceer
Cheung, M C. Raphael
Shaban, Joseph A.
Wilson, Robert J.

QUÉBEC

CHICOUTIMI
Duranceau, Caroline
Villeneuve, Helene

COTE SAINT-LUC
Schwartz, Thomas

DRUMMONDVILLE
Perreault, Isabelle

GATINEAU
Babin, Sandra
Garon, Jean
Lanoie, Genevieve

GREENFIELD PARK
Langlois, Fabienne

LAVAL
Ahlan, Jennifer C M.
Bahsali, Georges I.
Couture, Nathalie
Dumas, Richard
Long, Helene
Palardy, Jean

MONT-ROYAL
Lavoie, Helene B.

MONTREAL
Aris-Jilwan, Nahla M.
Assimakopoulos, Peter
Barnes, Robert D.
Beauregard, Catherine
Benoit, Robert
Boucher, Andree
Bourdeau, Isabelle
Breton, Donald
Brossard, Jean-Hugues
Bui, Helen
Chiasson, Jean L.
Christopoulos, Stavroula
Deal, Cheri L.
Delorme, Sophie
Duda, Barbara
Eappen, Roy
Fillion, Marc
Fournier, Helene
Garfield, Natasha
Godbout, Ariane
Grothe, Anne-Marie
Henderson, M. Melanie
How, Jacques S.
Hu, Xiao W.
Huot, Celine H.
Kader, Tina
Karaplis, Andy C.
Krishnamoorthy, Preetha
Leboeuf, Rebecca
Legault, Laurent
Leong, Aaron
Majdan, Agnieszka A.
Massicotte, Marie-Helene
Meissner, Les A.
Millette, Maude
Mircescu, Hortensia S.
Mitchell, John J.
Morin, Emilie
Nakhla, Meranda M.
Neveu, Nathalie A.
Olivier, Patricia
Poirier, Lysane
Primeau, Vanessa
Rakel, Agnes
Richards, John B.
Rivera, Juan A.
Rodd, Celia J.
Rondeau, Genevieve
Sbrocchi, Anne M.
Scott, Rachel R.
Sherman, Mark H.
Sladek, Robert G.
Tamilia, Michael
Truong, Ngoc-Uyen T T.
Vallette, Sophie
Vautour, Line M.
Wing, Simon S.
Yale, Jean-Francois
Yu, Oriana H Y.

POINTE-CLAIRE
Laib-Barama, Dalila
Wang, Ting-Yu

QUEBEC
Allen, Christyne
Baillargeon, Michel
Brassard, Maryse
D'Amours, Martin
Denis, Marie-Claire
Dupuis, Philippe
Eugene, Dardye
Forget, Genevieve
Gagne, Julie
Gagnon, Claudia
Weisnagel, S. John

RIMOUSKI
Montminy, Marie-Eve
Pelletier, Lysanne

SAINT-HYACINTHE
Sabourin, Alexis
St-Jean, Edith

SAINT-LAURENT
Yared, Zeina

SAINT-LEONARD
Bertrand, Sylvie

SHERBROOKE
Ardilouze, Jean-Luc
Baillargeon, Jean-Patrice
Bernier, Frederic
Carpentier, Andre
Gagne, Nancy
Godin, Chantal
Hivert, Marie-France
Houde, Ghislaine
Langlois, Marie-France
Maheux, Pierre
Perron, Patrice
Pesant, Marie-Helene
Simoneau-Roy, Judith
St-Pierre, Bruno
Van Rossum, Nicole

ST JEAN SUR RICHELIEU
Corbeil, Marie-Andree
Kong, Wei Lin
Noiseux, Daniel

TROIS-RIVIERES
Labrecque, Catherine
Parenteau, Chantal
Rioux, Dany

SASKATCHEWAN

REGINA
Fitzgerald, Jeremy
Mohammed, El-Fellani A.

SASKATOON
Arnason, Terra G.
Best, Thomas B.
Dala, Gideon

Gastroenterology

ALBERTA

CALGARY
Adams, Fatin M H.
Andrews, Christopher N.
Asfaha, Samuel
Aspinall, Alexander I.
Bailey, Jennifer L.
Bass, Sydney
Beck, Paul L.
Belletrutti, Paul J.
Boctor, Dana L.
Bridges, Ronald J.
Burak, Kelly W.
Buresi, Michelle
Chalmers-Nixon, Tara S.
Cheng, Edwin J.
Chopra, Angeli
Coderre, Sylvain P.
Coffin, Carla S.
Cole, Martin J.
Congly, Stephen E.
Curley, Michael A.
DeBruyn, Jennifer C C.
Devlin, Shane
Dube, Jeanne C.
Ghosh, Subrata
Gupta, Milli
Haussmann, Jessica
Heitman, Steven J.
Hilsden, Robert J.
James, Paul D.
Jayakumar, Saumya
Jijon, Humberto B.
Kaplan, Gilaad
Khaliq-Kareemi, Munaa
Kothandaraman, Maitreyi
Kumar, Puja R.
Leung, Yvette P Y.
Love, Jonathan R.
Ma, Michael Z.
McKenzie, Leanna S.
Misra, Tarun
Mohamed, Rachid
Novak, Kerri L.
Panaccione, Remo
Price, Lawrence M.
Rezaie, Ali
Rioux, Kevin P.
Rostom, Alaa M K A.
Shaffer, Eldon A.
Sherman, Thomas A.
Stapleton, Melanie P.
Stinton, Laura M.
Sutherland, Lloyd R.
Swain, Mark G.
Thompson, Robert G.
Waterhouse, Christopher C M.
Williams, Jennifer J.
Wrobel, Iwona T.
Yeung, Alfred K.

EDMONTON
AlAmeel, Turki A S.
Bain, Vincent G.
Bala, Anand
Bistritz, Lana M.
Cherry, Raeleen D.
Demeria, Denny
Fedorak, Richard N.
Ferguson, James P.
Gramlich, Leah M.
Gutfreund, Klaus S.
Halloran, Brendan P.
Johnson, Melissa A.
Kao, Dina H.
Karvellas, Constantine J.
Kroeker, Karen I.
Lazarescu, Adriana
Lim, Allen W K.
Liu, Julia J.
Lutzak, Gregory D.
Ma, Mang-Ming
Matic, Kata
McDermid, Jill C.
McKaigney, John P.
Millan, Mario S.
Morse, Amy L.
Pinchbeck, Melanie L.
Robbins, Sarah J.
Sadowski, Daniel C.
Sandha, Gurpal S.
Selvarajah, Vijeyakumar
Semlacher, Eric A.
Siffledeen, J. Shaalan
Soo, Isaac
Stead, Lori M.
Sultanian, Richard A.
Switzer, Connie M.
Syed, Atyab A N.
Tandon, Puneeta
Teshima, Christopher W.
Thomson, Alan B R.
Todoruk, Dennis N.
Van Zanten, Sander J.
Walters, Brennan M A.
Wong, Clarence K W.
Wong, Karen
Wong, Winnie W S.
Zeman, Marilyn V.

FORT MCMURRAY
Sauve, Michel D.

RED DEER
Alqahtani, Saleh A.
Simmonds, S. Douglas
Ward, Gregory J.

BRITISH COLUMBIA

BURNABY
Monkewich, Gregory J.

COMOX
Nel, Pierre R.

FERNIE
Burnett, Patricia J.

KAMLOOPS
Burgmann, Twila
Picton, Taralyn D.
Stabler, Christopher D.

KELOWNA
Agnew, Shane R.
Bak, Adrian W.
Michieletti, Pina
Nash, Carla L.
Penner, Robert M.
Perini, Rafael F.
Render, K. Craig

NEW WESTMINSTER
Atkinson, Kenneth A.
Cheung, Justin
Chung, Henry V.
Krygier, Darin S.
Lin, Cassie W.
Yik, Kwok Yeong

NORTH VANCOUVER
Hahn, Michael E J.
Haniak, William A.
Ho, Jin K.
Riley, Mark R.
Zohrab, W. John

PENTICTON
Papay, Karen D.
Wiesinger, Holly A R.

PRINCE GEORGE
Keyvani, Leila
Yacyshyn, Bruce R.

RICHMOND
Fishman, Martin J.
Wong, Victor K.

SAANICHTON
Koziol, Kathie A.

SURREY
Donaldson, Bruce W.
Karim, Zamil
Prest, Marcia E H.
Singham, Janakie
Wong, Henry D.

VANCOUVER
Amar, Jack N.
Avinashi, Vishal
Barker, Collin C.
Bressler, Brian L.
Byrne, Michael F.
Chang, Albert
Chatur, Nazira
Enns, Robert A.
Freeman, Hugh J.
Gray, James R.
Guttman, Orlee R.
Halparin, Lawrence S.
Jacobson, Kevan
Kim, Edward
Ko, Hin Hin
Kwan, Peter
Lam, Eric C S.
Law, Joanna K Y.
Ramji, Alnoor
Salh, Baljinder S.
Steinbrecher, Urs P.
Tai, Isabella T W.
Telford, Jennifer J.
Weiss, Alan A.
Whittaker, J. Scott
Yoshida, Eric M.

VICTORIA
Buckley, Alan B.
Daly, Donald S.
Holland, Stephen G.
Papp, Jamie D.
Pearson, David C.
Petrunia, Denis M.
Piercey, James R A.
Shah, Justin A.
Singh, Ranjit A.
Zandieh, Iman

MANITOBA

BRANDON
MacKalski, Barbara A M.

WINNIPEG
Bernstein, Charles N.
Cantor, Michael J.
Duerksen, Donald R.
Kippen, Robert N.
Krongold, Penina H.
Lau, Chung-Yan
Lloyd, David A.
Micflikier, Allan B.
Moffatt, Dana C H.
Peretz, David
Singh, Harminder
Targownik, Laura E.
Walli, J. Eric

NEW BRUNSWICK

BATHURST
Memiche, Nejat
Memiche, Reshat

FREDERICTON
Koller, Oscar L.
MacMillan, Mark

MONCTON
Al-Karain, Mohammad Y M.
Berger, Robert K.
Mikael, Gaby G.
Schweiger, Franzjosef
Silva, Fidelia A.
Turbide, Christian

SAINT JOHN
Cockeram, Alan W.
Gillis, Cory F.
McKnight, Lisa C.
Williams, Chadwick

NEWFOUNDLAND AND LABRADOR

CORNER BROOK
Tavenor, Anthony J.

ST ANTHONY
Al Beshir, Mohammad S A.

ST. JOHN'S
Borgaonkar, Mark R.
Bursey, R. Ford
Church, Peter C.
Critch, Jeffrey N.
Fallows, Glen A.
Fardy, John M.
Leonard, Jennifer R.
McGrath, Jerry S.
Reddy, S. Bharati

NOVA SCOTIA

ANTIGONISH
Abdelgadir, Ibrahim M.

BRIDGEWATER
Fraser, Hughie

DARTMOUTH
Sheppard, Duane G.

FALL RIVER
Fox, Roy

HALIFAX
Epstein, Ian L.
Farina, Dana M.
Gruchy, Steven E.
Laryea, Marie A.
Leddin, Desmond J.
MacIntosh, Donald G.
Patel, Sunil T.
Peltekian, Kevork M.
Turnbull, Geoffrey K.
Williams, S. Geoffrey
Williams, Stacey P.
Winsor, Wendy A.

KENTVILLE
Musgrave, Bruce L.

NEW GLASGOW
Murray, Harold S.

ONTARIO

AJAX
Shawesh, Malek H E.
Wang, James C Y.

BARRIE
Hemphill, Douglas J.
Lalor, Eoin A G.

BELLEVILLE
Pritchett, Sean B.

BRAMPTON
Bellini, Andrew B.
Chandok, Natasha
El-Takli, Issam K.
Kutty, P. Karunakaran
Puri, Vinod
Sachedina, Bashirudin
Tan, Patrick B.
Ying, Luis T J.

BRANTFORD
Jones, Mark B.
Wang, Charlie S K.

BURLINGTON
Ching, Emily K Y.
Comay, Daniel C.
Kumaranayake, A. Prasanna P.
Lad, Rameeta J.
Makhija, Sapna
Marwaha, Avantika

CAMBRIDGE
Lee, Mark J.
Nguyen, Augustin

EAST YORK
Chen, Dean L H.

ETOBICOKE
Gould, Michael I.
Greenbloom, Susan L.
Sethi, Rajiv

GUELPH
Bovell, Keith T.
Chiba, Naoki
Hewak, James C.
Kottachchi, Dan

HAMILTON
Armstrong, David
Brill, Herbert
Ganguli, Subhas C.
Greenwald, Eric R.
Khan, Khurram J.
Lumb, Barry J.
Marshall, John K.
Moayyedi, Paul
Puglia, Marco A.
Ratcliffe, Elyanne M.
Rossman, Richard L.
Sherlock, Mary E.
Spaziani, Robert
Tse, Frances W M.
Tsoi, Keith S K.
Xenodemetropoulos, Theodore T.
Zachos, Marianthi

HUNTSVILLE
Murat, Brian W.

KINGSTON
Da Costa, Laurington
Hookey, Lawrence C.
Justinich, Christopher J.
Louw, Jacob A.
Lowe, Catherine E.
Noble, Angela
Paterson, William G.
Ropeleski, Mark J.
Vanner, Stephen J.

KITCHENER
Bissonnette, Lyle V.
Ergaiey, Houda A.
Golubov, Jordan
Ismaili, Arif M A.
Meghji, M. Mohamed
Sharma, Vinod K.
Wu, Harry K C.

LINDSAY
Chan, Gabriel W L.

LONDON
Alqutub, Adel N H.
Barnett, William H.
Beaton, Melanie
Chande, Nilesh
Gregor, James C.
Howard, John M.
Hussain, Nadeem A.
Khanna, Nitin V.
Khanna, Reena
Marotta, Paul J.
McIntosh, Keith S.
Ponich, Terry
Qumosani, Karim M Y.
Rahman, Adam N.
Reynolds, Richard
Sey, Michael S L.
Sultan, Khaleel H S H.
Yan, Brian

MARKHAM
Fu, Anna
Lau, Agatha
Selucky, Michal

MISSISSAUGA
Anand, Navin
Clark, Robert N.
Correia, Adriano J.
El-Ashry, Dalia
Hollingworth, Roger W.
Joshi, Supriya
McMullen, William R.
Menon, Krishna
Nelles, Sandra E.
Newman, Jamie R.
Organ Shin, Jennifer L.
Ostro, Michael J.
Rasul, Imran A.
Sim, Keng Howe
So, Jeffrey S.

NEPEAN
Bray, Frederick T.
Inouye, Phillip K.

NEWMARKET
Faris, Andrea E.
Lin, Frank Y.
Rabie, Rania N.
Schep, Gerald N.
Stotland, Brian R.
Tripathi, Davender K.

NIAGARA FALLS
Housley, Richard J.

NORTH BAY
Shulman, Scott M.

NORTH YORK
Abdalian, Rupert S.
Al Qarshoubi, Issa S M.
Al-Harbi, Othman R A.
Desai, Milind G.
Kaila, Brinderjit K.
Khatchatourian, Marina
Medad, Ilan E.
Moskovitz, David N.
Patel, Vishal
Sam, Justina J.
Shapira, Stacey C.
Theal, Jeremy J T.
Weiner-Baron, David L.

OAKVILLE
Arya, Naveen
Bair, F. Douglas
Lau, Helena L W.
Pandya, Sudhir P.
Patel, Jayesh
Pham, Joe
Profiti, Raffaela
Wu, Arthur

ORILLIA
Anand, Nitasha

OSHAWA
Green, Daniel M.
Missiha, Sharif B.
Oravec, Michael
Pavone, Elio
Zaidi, Hasan A.

OTTAWA
Abaskharoun, Ramy R D.
Barkey, Janice L.
Benchimol, Eric I.
Boland, Margaret P.
Bolano Del Vecchio, Silvana M.
Champion, Malcolm C.
Chatterjee, Avijit
Deneault, Jocelyn J.
Dhaliwal, Harinder
Farazli, Christiane
Fournier, Marc
Hassard, Philip V.
Jolicoeur, Emilie
Kichian, Krikor
Lee, Ralph F.
Massicotte, Claude J.
Oliveira, Liliana M.
Rochon, Luc J W.
Sabbagh, Charles N J.
Saloojee, Navaaz A.
Scully, Linda J.
Sekar, Arni S C.
Shaw-Stiffel, Thomas A W.
Sy, Richmond G.
Tambay, Robert
Webster, Randall J W.
Xuan, Andrew Y.

PETERBOROUGH
Brien, Steven R.
Chan, Andrew C S.
Lee, Victor K G.
Li, Marilyn M.
Melicharkova, Andrea

PICKERING
Malhotra, Kenneth S.

RICHMOND HILL
Chan, Karen B Y.
Culnan, James G.
Fingerote, Robert J.
Nijhawan, Pardeep K.
Sarin, Nitin
Sinclair, Stephen B.

SAULT STE MARIE
Bignell, Douglas C.

SCARBOROUGH
Bierbrier, Gordon S.
Black, David R T.
Chan, Gerald C B.
Chen, Grant I.
Hurowitz, Eric E.
Lin, Edward D H.
Madala, Kiran
Nazareno, Jose V C.
Patel, Harshna
Roth, Lee S.
Shapero, Theodore F.
Thien, Vincent V S.
Tran, S. Stanley
Wong, Keith H.
Wright, John R.
Yeung, Elaine T.
Yeung, Latifa T F.

ST CATHARINES
Chan, Ronnie S.
Ibrahim, Khaled M O.
Miller, D. Alexander
Romatowski, Walter W.

THUNDER BAY
Ahmed, Nadeem A.
Alallam, A. Aboubaker
Raman, Kalyanapuram R.

TORONTO
Abadir, Amir
Allard, Johane
Appell, William A.
Baath, Kulrajbir
Baker, Jeffrey P.
Bernstein, Michael N.
Bookman, Ian
Cooper, Mary Anne
Croitoru, Kenneth
Cruz Pereira, Oscar O.
Devlin, Timothy
Elkashab, Magdy A M H.
Feld, Jordan
Friedlander, Sam A.
Fung, Scott
Gaisano, Herbert Y.
Gopinath, Nanda
Greenberg, Gordon R.
Grover, Samir C.
Habal, Flavio
Heathcote, E. Jane L.
Huang, Vivian W.
Kandel, Gabor P.
Kim, Young-In
Kortan, Paul P.
Lee Ng, Vicky
Leong, Eric W H.
Leung, Wesley D C Y.
Levy, Gary A.
Lilly, Leslie B.
Liu, Louis W C.
Margulies, Niculina M.
May, Gary R.
Murthy, Sanjay
Newman, Alvin
Nguyen, Geoffrey C.
Rabeneck, Linda
Ravindran, Nikila C.
Renner, Eberhard L.
Roberts, Eve A.
Rossos, Peter G.
Saibil, Fredric G.
Shah, Hemant A.
Silverberg, Mark S.
Springer, Jonathon E.
Stafford, Susan E.
Stal, Jeffrey M.
Steinhart, A. Hillary
Tartaro, Piero
Tinmouth, Jill M.
Tsien, Cynthia
Valentino, Pamela
Vijayaratnam, Visvalingam
Walsh, Catharine M.
Weizman, Adam
Win, Lay Lay
Wolman, Stephen L.
Wong, Florence S H.
Yogeswaran, Kumaresan
Yong, Elaine
Yu, Derek

UNIONVILLE
Murray, Iain C.

VANIER
Gregoire, Sylvie

VAUGHAN
Bilbily, Ghassan F Y.
Ford, David

WHITBY
Ho, Benjamin G M.

WINDSOR
Bacchus, Rahman
Farjalla, Salaheddin G.
Fituri, Rasem L.
Khalil, M. Arshad

WOODBRIDGE
Axler, Jeffrey L.

PRINCE EDWARD ISLAND

CHARLOTTETOWN
Beck, Jeremy N.
Clark, Donald L.

QUÉBEC

CHAMBLY
Tulin, Michel

CHATEAUGUAY
Dussault, Pierre
McNabb-Baltar, Julia
Tourigny, Marc E.

COTE SAINT-LUC
Grzywacz, Kelly

GATINEAU
Bernier, Jean-Pierre
Clement, Pierre
Dao, Catherine T.
Doumit, Maya
Lefebvre, Sonia
Sutcliffe, Ian T.

GREENFIELD PARK
Bendana, Franklin
Desilets, Etienne
Dufresne, Julie
Tran, Hanh-Khiem

JOLIETTE
Marquez Azalgara, Vladimir

LASALLE
Bastedo, Clare
Gelly, Andre L.
Godet, Patrick
Nepveu, Marie-Helene

LAVAL
Choueri, Georges N.
Doucet, Isabelle
Farber, David F.
Giroux, Yvon
Joly, Lucie
Meunier, Pierre
Nadeau, Etienne
Nudo, Carmine G.
Sabbah, Sandrine
Saheb, Nathalie

LEVIS
Bourdages, Raymond
Hache, Chantal
L'Esperance, Guy
Lavoie, Remi
Morrissette, Hugo
Robichaud, Pascal
Thivierge, Isabelle
Whittom, Steve

LONGUEUIL
Belanger, Melanie
Dommar, Gilbert
Martin, Luc P.
Nguyen, Van Vu
Plourde, Victor
Thai, Hoang Lan

MAGOG
Rousseau, Bernard

MONTREAL
Afif, Waqqas
Arakelian, Jean
Aumais, Guy L.
Barkun, Alan N G.
Beaudoin, Marc
Benhamron, Jaimes-S.
Bernard, Edmond-Jean
Bernier, Claude
Bessissow, Talat
Bilodeau, Marc
Bitton, Alain
Blum, Seymour J.
Boivin, Michel
Bouchard, Simon
Caussignac, Yves
Cleland, David P.
Clermont, Richard J.
Cohen, Albert
Cote, Simon J J.
D'Aoust, Louise
Davies, Campbell D.
Deschenes, Marc
Desir, Barbara
Deslandres, Erik
Dirks, Martha H.
Dorais, Judy
Drouin, Eric
Durivage, Gidej
Emond, Michel
Fallone, Carlo A.
Faulques, Bernard
Faure, Christophe
Fenyves, Daphna
Forget, Sylviane
Friedman, Gad
Gagnon, Michel
Ghali, Maged
Ghattas, Georges
Gratton, Jacques
Halac, Ugur
Hamel, Joanne
Herba, Karl
Hilzenrat, Nir
Huard, Genevieve
Jobin, Gilles
Katz, Saul S.
Lachance, Jean-Rene
Lahaie, Raymond
Leduc, Raymond
Lemoyne, Michel M.
Levesque, Dominique
Luterman, Leonard
Marchand, Valerie
Marleau, Denis
Matouk, Karen
Mayrand, Serge
Messekher, Ferial-Lilya
Michaud, Gilles
Morinville, Veronique D.
Mousseau, Roger
Nguyen, Thanh-Binh
Orlicka, Katarzyna
Ostiguy, Richard
Paquin, Sarto
Parent, Josee
Poitras, Pierre
Pomier Layrargues, Gilles
Ratner, Jack T.
Rioux, Louis C.
Roy, Claude C.
Sabbah, Sidney
Sahai, Anand V.
Sant'Anna, Ana M G D.
Soulellis, Constantine A.
Ste-Marie, Micheline T.
Szego, Peter L.
Szilagyi, Andrew
Tamaz, Raja
Tessier, Genevieve
Villeneuve, Jean-Pierre
Vincent, Catherine
Waschke, Kevin A.
Wild, Gary E.
Wong, Philip
Wyse, Jonathan M.

PIERREFONDS
Loutfi, Joseph

POINTE-CLAIRE
Kenick, Scott

QUEBEC
Beaudet, Isabelle-Pascale
Bergeron, Viviane
Bradette, Marc
Caouette, Pascale
Castilloux, Julie
Cayer, Sylvie
Chouinard, Pascale
Comeau, Eve-Lyne
Dallaire, Chrystian
Dube, Rejean
Dussault, Catherine
Gagnon, Pierre
Genereux, Alexandre
Gougeon, Alexandre
Gregoire, Philippe
Halle, Pierre
Lacerte, Marcel
Lavoie, Sylvain
Lemelin, Valery
Pare, Pierre
Parent, Claude
Routhier, Gaetane
St-Georges, Fernand
Sutton, Ann
Trelles, Francisco
Tremblay, Rene M.
Wieckowska, Anna

RIMOUSKI
Larose, Andre
Robillard, Jean

SAINT-EUSTACHE
Maisonneuve, Denis

SAINT-HYACINTHE
Brodeur, Guillaume
Gaboury, Jean
Robitaille, Manon

SAINT-JEROME
Laliberte, Lyne
Laurier, Louis
Stewart, Marie-Diane

SAINT-LAURENT
Farley, Alain Y A.

SHERBROOKE
Babakissa, Corentin
Bachand, Marie-Pier
Baillargeon, Jean-Daniel
Beaudoin, Annie
Carrier, Julie
Faust, Gilles
Grbic, Dusanka
Haddad, Henry
Langelier, Diane
Langevin, Serge
Lemay, Frederic
Lussier, Veronique
Menard, Charles
Menard, Daniel B.
Plamondon, Sophie
Ruel, Joannie
Watier, Alain

ST CHARLES BORROMEE
Beaulieu, Celina
Gagne, Marc-Andre
Grypinich, Michel
Kamau, Allan G.
Laflamme, Pierre
Renaud, Genevieve

ST-EUSTACHE
Nassiri, Shirin

ST JEAN SUR RICHELIEU
Lafond, Guillaume
Larocque, Martin
Remillard, Stephanie
Rousseau, Annie
Thanh, Lan Quang

TERREBONNE
Amra, Suleman
Blain, Julie
Ouellet, Vincent
Paquet, Stephanie
Plouffe, Elyse
Reid, Genevieve

TROIS-RIVIERES
Briere, Claude
Gariepy, Linda
Larouche, Jacynthe
Morin, Guy

VAL-D'OR
Binette, Alain
Lavoie, Line
Lefort, Pierre

VERDUN
Comanita, Petru
Lamoureux, Louis
Poliquin, Marc

WESTMOUNT
Mishkin, Seymour
Morelli, Gaetano

SASKATCHEWAN

REGINA
Ali, Massud A A.
Chami, George
Lewis, William F.
McHattie, James D.
Nel, Johann D L R.

SASKATOON
Bedi, Anil
Fowler, Sharyle
Jones, Jennifer L.
Larkai, Edwin N L.
Porostocky, Peter
Worobetz, Lawrence J.

General Pathology

ALBERTA

BANFF
Huhn, Otto H.

BONNYVILLE
Davey, Robert S.
Puttaswamy, Shekar

CALGARY
Abdullah, Amid K.
Larsen, Erik T.
Naugler, Christopher T.
Smith, Dean F.

EDMONTON
Bannach, Bernard G.
Berendt, Heather
Berendt, Richard C.
Brown, Stuart Z.
Chaudhry, Imran S.
Chow, Stephen W.
Danyluk, John M.
Girgis, Safwat A M.
Hodkinson, Roger G.
Johnson, Edward S.
Johnson, Gordon H.
Lai, Raymond K C.
Macyk-Davey, Andrea
McCann, Vernal L.
McLean, D. Ross
Neuman, Glen D.
Nigam, Srishti P.
O'Hara, Carolyn D.
Ramsey, Wayne R.
Rayani, Nargis A.
Saddik, Maruf S.
Satkunam, Niranjala
Sauvageau, Anny
Schloss, Eric H.
Sigurdson, Grant T.
Sin, Ignatius C F.
Tung, Dean J.
West, John R.
Wong, Kathleen S W.
Wood, George O.

LETHBRIDGE
Lyon, David C.
Wendelboe, Michael W.

MEDICINE HAT
Chow, Wai-Kwan

RED DEER
Dawson, David T P.
Morris, S. Anthony

BRITISH COLUMBIA

ABBOTSFORD
Coulter, Louise
Gates, Allan B.
Lehuquet, John B.
Nakonechny, Quentin B.

BURNABY
Earle, Elizabeth M.
Gianoulis, Mary E.
Gillen, Rael T.
Ho, Clinton
Kirby, Shane D.
Reddy, Suseela

CAMPBELL RIVER
Leia, Allan P.
Tabarsi, Aref

COMOX
Bellamy, Christopher D.
Donn, Wayne B.

CRANBROOK
Malone, Richard F.
Robertson, A. Rocke

KAMLOOPS
James, Gerald K.
McNeely, T. Bruce D.
Stefanelli, John D.
Stephen, James W M.

KELOWNA
Argatoff, Larry H.
Innes, Duncan M.
Lesack, David W.
Savard, Murray L.
Wanklyn, Beverly Jill.
Wenzel, Dwayne M.

NANAIMO
Wessler, Andreas N.

NEW WESTMINSTER
Cupples, James B.
Grabiec, Joseph T.
Hrynchak, Monica
Lau, William W L.
Litwin, Craig M E S.
Olekshy, John A.
Reich, Kurt D.
Yeung, Karen J.
Zetler, Peter J.

NORTH VANCOUVER
Chercover, David
Scholey, Janis K.
Vischer, Gisela H.
Vogrincic, Gerard S.

PENTICTON
Currie, William R.
Tebbutt-Speirs, Susan M R.
Zolein, Mohammad M.

PRINCE GEORGE
Dumont, Randall
Roden, W. Grant
Van Iderstine, Edward V.

RICHMOND
Lindsay, Leigh J.
Teng, Billy B.
Thiyagaratnam, Pathmini
Ung, Karen

SURREY
Chhanabhai, Mukesh
Darbyshire, James M.
Grant, Dennis R.
Herar, Daljit S.
Lee, Benita S M.
Lehuquet, Leslie A.
Louie, Richard A.
Shin, Doo Ho
Shokeir, M. Omar
Yu, Richard K W.

TERRACE
Laroye, Guy Jean.

TRAIL
Loyola, Vicente

VANCOUVER
Chong Kit, Renison
Crawford, Richard I.
Dalal, Bakul I.
Davis, Jennifer E.
Edwards, Enid A.
Filipenko, J. Douglas
Ford, Jason C.
Hardwick, David F.
Horsman, Douglas E.
Huntsman, David G.
Masoudi, Hamid
Matisic, Jasenka P.
Meneghetti, Victor A.
Nanthakumar, S. Selvi
Nimmo, Michael C.
Ostry, Avrum J.
Poulin, Michael P.
Slack, Graham W.
Suen, Kenneth C H.
Thomson, Thomas A.
Webber, Douglas L.
White, Valerie A.
Wroblewski, Julius A.

VERNON
Brierley, Yann
Doyle, Jason S G.
Hardy, Douglas A.

VICTORIA
Hoag, Gordon N.
Pringle, Kerry B.
Tanhuanco-Kho, Grace Y.

WHITE ROCK
Coret, Stephen D.

MANITOBA

WINNIPEG
Huzel, Leah N.
Kirkpatrick, Marilyn H.
Klein, Julianne R H.
Lucman, Lydia L.
Morales, Carmen M.
Stefanovici, Camelia
Von Kuster, Kenneth R B.

NEW BRUNSWICK

FREDERICTON
Morris, John E.
Smith, Muriel F.

SAINT JOHN
Hossain, Mohammad M.

NEWFOUNDLAND AND LABRADOR

ST. JOHN'S
Avis, Simon P.
Cook, Donald M.
Elms, Ford J.
Morris-Larkin, Carolyn
Wadden, Patricia M.

NOVA SCOTIA

BRIDGEWATER
Albiston, Brigit J.

DARTMOUTH
Thoni, Andrea J.

HALIFAX
Gaskin, David A.
Shawwa, Allam A K.
Wanless, Ian R.

KENTVILLE
Jollymore, Brian D.

NEW GLASGOW
Ashfaq, Sirajuddin

ONTARIO

BARRIE
Price, Russell G.
Salathiel, Ian P.
Wozniak, Ewa A.

BELLEVILLE
Khare, Suneeta D.
Twemlow, Gregory D.

BOWMANVILLE
Treloar, Murray E.

BRAMPTON
Olsen, Brian W.
Rabinovich, Solomon
Rajani, Shabnam S.
Ruijs, Theodora C G.
Samani, Amir A.
Swaine, Frederick B.

BRANTFORD
Hall, Ann Mary
Wentworth, Paul

BROCKVILLE
Yassa, Naguib H.

BURLINGTON
Chan, Konrad K.
Haworth, Angela C.

CAMBRIDGE
Morris, Anna G.

ETOBICOKE
Hanley, S. Anne
Scarff, Michael A.
Thomson, Bruce W.

GUELPH
Berzowski, Anna M.
Ling, Eng T.
Nguyen, Duc Truong
Tadross, Latif A A S.

HAMILTON
Aziz, Tariq
Elavathil, Leelamma J.
Fernandes, John R.
Rao, Chitra

KENORA
MacDonald, James K.

KING CITY
Mull, John D.

KINGSTON
Sengupta, Sandip K.

KITCHENER
Batten, Adrian P.
Chan, Winnie W Y.
Divaris, Dimitrios
Kumalo, Thandanani G Q.
Ling, Franklin C K.
Sawka, Barry W.

LINDSAY
Giang, Hudson K H.
Ho, Shen-Pang E.

LONDON
Ettler, Helen C.
Joseph, Mariamma G.
Kwan, Keith F.

MARKHAM
Lau, Michael C K.
Sturman, Dubravka
Villanueva Arquint, Monique

MISSISSAUGA
Coire, Claire I.
Fekete, John F.
Feltis, J. Timothy
Fox, Anthony D.
Naidoo, Jayabalan A.
Nazerali, Latifa A.
Zeng, Janice J.

NEPEAN
Frenkel, Vivien J.
Halil, Alexander
Perkins, D. Garth

NEWMARKET
Handy, Shaheda
Schatzdorfer, Julie E.
Ye, Charles C.

NIAGARA FALLS
Joshi, Sangeeta S.
Patel, Subhash K.

NORTH BAY
Courtice, Richard W.
Kerrigan, Scott A.
Ready, W. Kirkby

NORTH YORK
Brennan, Michael
Medline, Alan
Qizilbash, Ali H.
Vo, Tuyet Bach

OAKVILLE
Artinian, Berdj
Hussain, Nusrat
Walsh, Jennifer

ORILLIA
Rieckenberg, R. Markus

OSHAWA
Quantz, Marie C.

OTTAWA
Kyrollos, Maggy G H.
Lamba, Manisha
Nizalik, C L. Elizabeth
Richardson, George M J.
Robertson, Susan J.
Szumski, Roman G.

OWEN SOUND
Newell, Kenneth J.

PETERBOROUGH
Collins, Allison A P.
Horwood, John C.
Talati, Hetal H.

RICHMOND HILL
Barsoum, Nabila J.
Clerk, Nilam A.

SARNIA
Gidwani, Ram

SAULT STE MARIE
D'Agostino, Michael S.
Mozarowski, Paul T.
O'Hara, Kathleen E.

SCARBOROUGH
Fornasier, Victor
Hunt, Allan J A.

ST CATHARINES
Brennan, Michael C.
Zheng, Zuoyu

ST THOMAS
Wasty, S. Fasahat H.

STRATFORD
Carlson, Malcolm L.
Troster, Myron

STRATHROY
Shah, Pravin C.

SUDBURY
Bonin, Denis M.
Bonin, Michel L.

THUNDER BAY
Escott, Nicholas G.
Welbourne, David R.

TIMMINS
Verbeek, Johannes H.

TORONTO
Alexander, Cherupushpam
Aziz, Zared A.
Cullen, James B.
Medline, Norton M.
Moid, Farah
Turnbull, D. Ian
Van Der Kwast, Theodorus H.
Wang, Cheng T.

VIRGIL
Frendo, Marion

WELLAND
Guzowski, Ann V.
Segura, Jose

WINDSOR
Allevato, Pat A.
Helde, Michael
Yee, George E.

WOODSTOCK
Engbers, Peter B.

PRINCE EDWARD ISLAND

CHARLOTTETOWN
Fesser, Jennifer
Henderson, Rosemary
Sellers, A. Ruth
Tesch, Marvin R.

QUÉBEC

CHICOUTIMI
Prive, Myriam

DRUMMONDVILLE
Masson, Suzanne

GREENFIELD PARK
Arcand, Robert

LAVAL
Lebeau, Annie

LONGUEUIL
Lariviere, Luc

MONTREAL
Alcindor, J. Antony
Alpert, Lesley C.
Berthelet, France
Brochu, Pierre
Cadotte, Marcel
Ferenczy, Alex S.
Haliotis, Photini
Lauzon, Andre
Leung, Tack Ki.
Oligny, Luc L.
Painson, Bossuet
Pelletier, Micheline
Robitaille, Yves
Roy, Jean-Denis
Srolovitz, Herbert D.

POINTE-CLAIRE
Hussain, Sajida S.
Zaklama, Nora

QUEBEC
Paquin, Johanne
Veilleux, Chantal

ROUYN-NORANDA
Boucher, Danny

SAINT-GEORGES
Proulx, Jacques

SAINT-HYACINTHE
Gervais, Daniel
Laurin, Michel A.

SAINT-JEROME
Noel, Bernard

SALABERRY DE VALLEYFIELD
Simoneau, Jocelyne

SHAWINIGAN-SUD
Parisien, Gladys

SOREL-TRACY
Leclerc, Jean-Louis

STE ANNE DE BELLEVUE
Seemayer, Thomas A.

SASKATCHEWAN

NORTH BATTLEFORD
Murray, Robert B.

PRINCE ALBERT
Milner, Thomas G.

REGINA
Alport, Edward C.
Duffy, Patrick J.
Kirby, Angus D.
Korol, Debra A.

SASKATOON
Angel, Steven F.
Banerjee, Tamalina S.
Chibbar, Rajni
Chorneyko, Katherine
Wilde, Brent K.

General Surgery

ALBERTA

CALGARY
Abraham, Jessica
Ali, Imtiaz S.
Anderson, Ian B.
Armstrong, C. Paul
Austen, Daran L.
Ball, Chad G.
Bathe, Oliver F.
Beaudry, P. Paul
Borsato, Garry W.
Brar, Mantaj S.
Brindle, Mary E.
Buie, W. Donald
Burgess, John J.
Church, Neal G.
Datta, Indraneel
Debru, Estifanos O.
Dixon, Elijah
Drolet, Sebastien
Dunham, Michael B.
Eccles, Robin C.
Gelfand, Gary A J.
Goebel, Pamela J.
Graham, Andrew J.
Graham, John S.
Grondin, Sean C.
Hagerman, R. Neil
Harvey, Adrian M.
Heine, John A.
Hollaar, Gwendolyn L.
Jenken, Daryl A.
Johnson, Douglas R E.
Kanashiro, Jeanie
Kidd, William T.
Kieser, Teresa M.
Kirkpatrick, Andrew W.
Kortbeek, John B.
Lafreniere, Rene
Lall, Rohan N.
Lopushinsky, Steven R.
Lui, Robert C.
MacK, Lloyd A.
MacLean, Anthony R.
Maitland, Andrew
Martin, Steven A.
McConnell, Yarrow J.
McFadden, Sean D P.
McKinnon, J. Gregory
Mew, Daphne J Y.
Mitchell, Philip C.
Moore, Randy D.
Mulloy, Robert H.
Nixon, James A.
Nutley, Mark T.
Pasieka, Janice L.
Petrasek, Paul F.
Prystai, Gregory D.
Quan, May Lynn
Reddy, Esphiran
Reso, Artan M.
Rosen, Wayne S.

Rothwell, Bruce C.
Rubin, Steven Z.
Samis, Gregory A.
Selman, W. Gary
Sigalet, David L.
Sutherland, Francis R.
Taqi, Esmaeel
Temple, Walley J.
Topstad, Dawnelle R.
Vajcner, Glen A.
Way, Jeffrey C E.
Wong, Andrew L.
Wong, Joyce

CAMROSE
Fletcher, John N.
Leoni, Franco E.

CANMORE
Pagenkopf, Cort W.

CARDSTON
Hollingsworth, W. John

COLD LAKE
Parameswaran, Sandrasekeram

DRUMHELLER
Jordan, Rex W.

EDMONTON
Adams, David O.
Alibhai, Karim N.
Atwal, Sanita
Bayne, Jason P.
Bedard, Eric L.
Berg, Dale F.
Bigam, David L.
Birch, Daniel W.
Borowiec, Anna M.
Bratu, Ioana
Brisebois, Ronald J.
Cader, Sonia
Callahan, David J.
Chatenay, Michael P.
Chyczij, Harold R.
Ciona, Curtis J.
Cox, Heather L.
Dabbs, Kelly
Davey, P. Douglas
De Gara, Christopher
Dicken, Bryan J.
Engels, Paul
Evans, Mark
Fathimani, Kamran
Haase, Erika
Hadi, Ghassan M.
Hamilton, Stewart M.
Heisler, Owen R.
Jirsch, Dennis W.
Johnson, Scott T.
Karmali, Shahzeer
Kennedy, Jacqueline M.
Khadaroo, Rachel
Kneteman, Norman M.
Koshal, Arvind
Lees, Gordon
Matheson, J. Douglas
McMullen, Todd P.
Meier, Michael A.
Modry, Dennis L.
Mullen, John C.
Olson, David W.
Paton-Gay, John D.
Pelletier, Jean-Sebastien
Plewes, E. Arthur
Rebeyka, Ivan M.
Ross, David B.
Sample, Clifford B.
Sarkhosh, Kourosh
Schiller, Daniel E.
Shapiro, A M. James
Sobey, Alan V F.
Stephens, Mary H.
Stewart, James K.
Stewart, Kenneth C.
Struck, Wolfgang M.
Sutherland, John D.
Theman, Trevor W.
Turnbull, Robert G.
Valji, Azim M.
Vu, Lan Huu
Wang, Haili
White, Jonathan S.
Widder, Sandy L.
Williams, David C.
Winkelaar, Gerrit B.
Winton, Timothy L.
Yakimets, Walter J.

FORT MCMURRAY
Swenia, Mohamed M M.
Zuk, Lorne M.

FORT SASKATCHEWAN
Boora, Parveen S.
Juta, Ramesh N.
Robson, Alexander J.
Sabir, Mohamed

GRANDE PRAIRIE
Beekman, Richard A.
Ibbotson, Geoffrey C.
Miles, Peter J.
Mok, Dereck C.
Shaw, Marcus D.
St Germaine, Ronald L.

HIGH RIVER
Gougeon, Francois W.

HINTON
Pulis, Randy P.

LEDUC
MacEachern, Neil H.

LETHBRIDGE
Gomes, Anthony J.
Hebert, Richard J.
Kilam, Surendar K.
McColl, Ryan J.
Melling, Michael T.
Mortimer, Shane T.
Roxin, Gyorgy
Trautman, Allen F.

LLOYDMINSTER
Naidoo, Karunagaran

MEDICINE HAT
Bharwani, Nooral H.
Brzezinski, Wojciech S.
Elkassem, Samer
Erickson, Grant B.
Khan, Zarin P.
Nohr, Carl W.
Witzke, Ronald W.

RED DEER
Farries, Lawrence R.
Gregg, Sean M T.
Hamilton, Donald J.
Hardy, Paul E.
McFadyen, Lorraine A.
Muirhead, Robert M.
Panayides, Panayiotis
Roy, Peter D.
Warburton, Rebecca

SHERWOOD PARK
Wiens, Ernest

ST. ALBERT
Andruchow, Jennifer L.
Bennett, Athena R.
Cadili, Abdul Mujib A K M.
Jadick, Carmen H C.
Norris, Sean A.
Prakash, Anil
Wasey, Naureen

WETASKIWIN
Oad, Lachman D.

BRITISH COLUMBIA

ABBOTSFORD
Byrne, Damien F.
Dyck, Coreen
Jangra, Dalbhir
Jeffery, James W.
Lewis, Gregory M.
Schopf, Bernie W.

BURNABY
Cooke, Donald A.
Cuddington, Gary D.
Dickeson, Mark R C.
Goel, Devendra P.
Hsu, Katherine
Mahy, Jean-Noel
Okamura, James Y.

CAMPBELL RIVER
James, David N H.
Juszkiewicz, Piotr
Minnaar, Roy J.
Ring, Roger D.
Wood, Leanne J.

CHILLIWACK
Causton, Norman D.
McDonald, Susan E.
Schwarz, Richard J.
Wiggins, M. Christo

COMOX
Kimberley, Nicholas A.
Lanuke, Kathryn M.
Moise, Roger C.
T'len, Willis L.

CRANBROOK
Aleem, Abdul
Chong, Peter C.
Simons, Gertjan

DELTA
Lai, Kai-Fai
Robibo, Daniel A.
Segal, Jean M.
Woodhead, Robin V.

DUNCAN
Barton, Rachel K.
Duta, Daniel
Leckie, Peter A.

FERNIE
Nally, Colm

FORT ST. JOHN
Coetzer, Francois W.
Klompje, Jan

GOLDEN
Descoteaux, Jean-Gaston

KAMLOOPS
Azad, Aristotle
Barton, Anise C.
Baughan, James G.
Hanks, David G.
Hansen, Maxim T T.
Just, Jon D.
Leia-Stephen, Maureen
May, Douglas C.
Wallace, Thomas M.

KELOWNA
Baliski, Christopher R.
Ellett, Robert W.
Fradet, Guy
Humer, Michael F.
Jugnauth, Anand
Kluftinger, Andreas M.
Lawlor, D. Kirk
Luoma, Andrew A.
MacLeod, Michael D.
Mostowy, Stephan C.
Nelems, Bill
Pasenau, Jeffrey E H.
Poostizadeh, Ahmad
Solano, Edward B.
Sullivan, Barry J.
Wilson, Heather C.

KITIMAT
Lombard, Willem S J.

LANGLEY
Cowie, Scott E.
Fry, Peter D.
Ginting, Nadra
Ross, J. Benjamin
Shete, Charudutt D.
Shirley, Donald A.
Smith, R. Matthew M.

MAPLE RIDGE
Heed, Marni R.
Kotylak, Gregory S.
Spittel, Devin M.

NANAIMO
Carr, John A.
Frew, Euan M S.
Kingston, Gary W.
Leung, Sher-Ping
McLauchlan, Gordon
Rudston-Brown, Blair C D.
Schneidereit, Nathan P.

NEW WESTMINSTER
Blair, N. Peter
Bojm, Morris A.
Goecke, Michelle E.
Granger, Robert
Hayden, Robert I.
Kamitakahara, Alan T.
Karim, Shahzad S.
Kazemi, Kamyar
Konkin, David E.
Robb, George M M.
Toppin, Dennis I.
Turner, Laurence J.
Udwadia, Rushad T.
Van Heest, Rardi D.
Vikis, Elena A T.
Vrabec, George
Weitemeyer, Rudolf A.

NORTH VANCOUVER
Chang, George
Creedon, Kerry
Hunter, James M.
Lewis, Richard H.
Queh, Peter
Smith, Jenni

PENTICTON
Essery, Cameron R.
Marschall, Jeffery G.
McIver, D. Keith
Sawatzky, Mark E C.
Tighe, Bryan F.

PORT ALBERNI
Ferguson, James M.
Hankins, Jennifer E.
Vanderputten, Marilyn R.
Wijayanayagam, Akushla I.

POWELL RIVER
Makarewicz, Pawel A.

PRINCE GEORGE
Appleby, James P.
Babcock, Courtney A.
Caron, Nadine
Dubois, Brian J.
Lokanathan, Ramesh
Palerme, Louis-Philippe
Simpson, William T.
Sutter, F. Michelle
Wankling, Gilbert J.

PRINCE RUPERT
Nel, Philip N.

QUESNEL
Katalinic, Z. Branislav

RICHMOND
Allardyce, D. Bruce
Chuah, Teong K.
Frimer, Michael L.
Holmvang, Annette M.
Houston, Gordon T M.
Nguyen, Nam Hoang
Sampath, Sharadh

SALMON ARM
Britto, Santosh A.
Hiscock, Stephen M.
Journeau, Janice
Schneider, Johannes S J.
Wilson, Scott W J.

SECHELT
Goddard, Christopher M.

SIDNEY
Truter, Andre

SQUAMISH
Gawley, William F.

SURREY
Ashrafi, Ahmad S.
Bond, R. James
Chang, Edward N.
Doris, Peter J.
Forbes, Jason K.
Francoeur, Jason R.
Hwang, John M.
Janzen, Rhonda M.
Lauzon, Jean G.
Lee, Kathy K.
Nagra, M. Saleem
Ong, Sharon Rose Y.
Sharif, Mohammad S.
Todd, John D.
Tse, Geoffrey N W.
Wong, Andrew H K.
Yong, Yu-Sen

TERRACE
Dunfield, James I.
Evans, Warwick L.

TRAIL
Cameron, Ronald J.
Lawe, Andrew D.
Owatz, Todd S.
Schumacher, Paul A.

VANCOUVER
Abel, James G.
Baxter, Keith A.
Blair, Geoffrey K.
Brown, Carl J.
Brown, D. Ross G.
Brumwell, Mary L.
Buczkowski, Andrzej K.
Bugis, Samuel P.
Butterworth, Sonia A.
Cheifetz, Rona E.
Chen, Jerry C L.
Chung, Stephen W.
Cleator, Iain G M.
Dang, Yen
Davis, Noelle L.
Dewar, Leith
Dingee, Carol K.
Evans, David
Evans, Kenneth G.
Faulds, Jason
Finley, Richard J.
Gagnon, Joel
Gandhi, Sanjiv
Garraway, Naisan
Gentis, Edward F H.
Goodwin, Michael
Gudas, Virginia M.
Hameed, S. Morad
Hsiang, York N H.
Jamieson, W R. Eric
Janusz, Michael T.
Jones, Kirsten E.
Karimuddin, Ahmer A.
Kopac, Daniel S.
Kuusk, Urve
Lett, Ronald R.
Lichtenstein, Samuel V.
Lord, Sarah E.
MacDonald, Peter S.
McBeth, Paul B.
McFadden, Andrew W J.
McGregor, Gregor I.
McKevitt, Elaine C.
Melck, Adrienne L.
Meloche, R. Mark
Meneghetti, Adam T.
Mills, Jessica L A.
Ming-Lum, Corey
Miyagishima, Robert T.
Murphy, James J.
Nagy, Alexander G.
Panton, Ormond
Pao, Jin-Si
Pezim, Michael E.
Phang, Paul T.

Polyakov, Gregory M.
Raval, Manojkumar J.
Rebbeck, Patricia M.
Reid, John D S.
Roger, Judith A.
Salvian, Anthony J G.
Scott, Tracy M.
Scudamore, Charles H.
Shayan, Hossein
Sidhu, Ravindar S.
Sidhu, Sue P.
Simard, Laurie
Simons, Richard K.
Skarsgard, Erik D.
Skarsgard, Peter L.
Stoller, Julius L.
Taylor, David C.
Taylor, Robert H.
Tsang, Victor T L.
Warnock, Garth L.
Webber, Eric M.
Wiseman, Sam M.
Woo, Emile C.
Yee, John

VERNON
Ainslie, Scott A.
Crowley, John S.
Demetrick, Jeffrey S.
Hwang, Hamish S.
Hwang, Theng G.
Taves, Abram
Wiseman, Kevin W.

VICTORIA
Amson, Bradley J.
Biberdorf, Darren J.
Cunningham, Johann
Dewar, Gary J.
Dooner, James
Golonka, Naomi R.
Hayashi, Allen H.
Kuechler, Peter M.
Lee, Shung
Malik, Samaad M.
Mihailovic, Alexandra
Ofiesh, John G.
Orrom, William J.
Porter, George R.
Robinson, Matthew J.
Ross, Alison C.
Samphire, John
Tang, Bao Quy
Tomlinson, Corey L.

WEST VANCOUVER
Casses, Fernando

WHISTLER
Shackleton, Christopher R.

WILLIAMS LAKE
Brosseuk, Daniel T.
Oosthuizen, Jean F M.
Robbins, Nicole

MANITOBA

BRANDON
Carpenter, Noah H.
Davloor, Ramakrishna
Dhalla, Sonny
Goossen, Marvin J H.
Mohamed, Muftah A.

DAUPHIN
Lysack, Allan M.

FLIN FLON
Hoyeck, Antoine

PORTAGE LA PRAIRIE
Manuel, Paul L.
Ross, James F.

SELKIRK
Governo, Nelson J.
Kinsley, David C.

SOURIS
Myers, William E.

STEINBACH
Galessiere, Paul F.
Garba, Sule

THOMPSON
Haiart, Dominique C.

WINKLER
Abujazia, Abdurrezagh F.
Jacob, V. Chandy

WINNIPEG
Anderson, Brent R.
Andrew, Christopher G.
Assuras, George N.
Barber, Lorne E.
Bartlett, Lloyd C.
Boyd, April J.
Bracken, John H.
Cheung, Lai-Keung
Cowan, Daniel J.
Fong, Handrick
Fraser, Virginia H.
Ghazali, Susan M N.
Gillespie, Jamie L.
Gillman, Lawrence
Gray, Perry R.
Guzman, Randolph P.
Hancock, Betty
Harding, Gregory E J.
Hardy, Krista
Hebbard, Pamela
Hochman, David J.
Hutfluss, George J.
Inglis, Duncan L.
Kassum, Diamond A.
Kettner, Joel D.
Khan, Ali H.
Khan, T. Ali
Koulack, Joshua
Lee, John J Y.
Lee, Trevor J.
Lipschitz, Jeremy
Logsetty, Sarvesh
Lum Min, Suyin A.
MacEachern, Norman A.
MacIntosh, Ethel L.
Matsubara, Timothy K.
Mayba, Ihor I.
McCarthy, Brendan G.
McKay, M. Andrew
Milbrandt, Kristopher G.
Momoh, John T.
Morris, Melanie I.
Nason, Richard W.
Onotera, Rodney T.
Oppenheimer, Luis
Parham, Shelley M.
Park, Jason
Pathak, Kumar A.
Pintin-Quezada, Julio
Reimer, David J.
Robinson, James F.
Silverman, Richard E.
Srinathan, Sadeesh K.
Stimpson, Ross E J.
Tan, A. Lawrence
Taylor, Hugh R.
Thorlakson, Robert H.
Unruh, Helmut W.
Vergis, Ashley S.
Violago, Francisco C.
Warrian, R. Keith
Wirtzfeld, Deborah A.
Wiseman, Nathan E.
Woo, Nobby D.
Yaffe, Clifford S.
Yip, Benson
Zabolotny, Brent P.
Zaki, Magdy F.

NEW BRUNSWICK

BATHURST
Bartlett, Wayne C.
Houle, Francois
Savoie, Marc E.
Semerjian, Yves
Walker, Janet A.

CAMPBELLTON
Lagace, Marc
Master, Surya
Rozental-Klinger, Emmanuel

DIEPPE
Beausoleil, Sylvain
Bourgoin, Michel
Comeau, Tina
Deslauriers, Robert
Do, Lan Vinh
Hebert, Jocelyne
Skanes, Susan E.

EDMUNDSTON
Aucoin, Andre
Belanger, Jean-Francois
Cloutier, Paul

FREDERICTON
Boisvert, Rene
Bryden, Patricia L.
Franklin, John D.
Goodyear, Christopher P.
Gowan, Russell T.
Peters, Thomas H.
Redstone, Heather
Schaus, Claus P.

GRAND SAULT/ GRAND FALLS
Chowdhry, Rajendra K.

MIRAMICHI
Edward, Rex H.

MONCTON
Brown, D. Stephen
Burnett, Ralph H.
Dubois, Paul M.
Goobie, Paul W A.
Mujoomdar, Aneil A.
Murphy, John L.
Murphy, Ross W.
Nassif, Mohammed
Renfrew, Paul D.
Roberge, Roger M J.
Shakerinia, Tooraj
Tait, Heather M.
Wiebe, Shannon N.

PERTH-ANDOVER
Morales, Jose J.

ROTHESAY
McCartney, Eric D.

SAINT JOHN
Attard, Jo-Anne P.
Forgie, W. Rand
Johnston, Brian R.
Martin, Marcel
Mowatt, James I.
Mowatt, John A.
Ondiveeran, Hari K.
Scarth, Hugh M C.

ST STEPHEN
Goulding, Thomas H.

SUSSEX
Phillips, Brian C M.

NEWFOUNDLAND AND LABRADOR

CARBONEAR
Bottomley, Michael G.
Farrell, Robert T C.
Tuttle, Peggy F.

CLARENVILLE
Barnhill, John A.

CORNER BROOK
French, Gavin D.
Jefford, Valerie J.
MacKenzie, D. Scott

GANDER
Najfi, Syed M.

GRAND FALLS WINDSOR
Blackwood, Peter J.
Cheah, Huey
Clarkson, Colin A.
O'Driscoll, Mark F.
Willmore, Wendy S.

HAPPY VALLEY GOOSE BAY
Pradhan, Gautam N.

MARYSTOWN
Anjilvel, George M.

ST ANTHONY
Beveridge, J. Massey B.
Fitzgerald, G. William N.

ST. JOHN'S
Akhtar, Javed
Bohacek, Linda
Boone, Darrell C.
Browne, Gregory N.
Cox, Christopher R.
Felix, William A.
Gardiner, J. Paul
Guy, John R F.
Harrington, David M.
Heneghan, Paul D.
Hodder, Andre
Hogan, Michael P.
Mann, Catherine L.
Mathieson, Alexander
Melvin, Kevin N.
Mong, Kam W.
Pace, David E.
Pollett, William G.
Price, David I.
Smith, Christopher G.
Thavanathan, Mylvaganam J M.
Wells, Mary K.

NORTHWEST TERRITORIES

YELLOWKNIFE
Buchler, Brian
Merg, Anders R.

NOVA SCOTIA

AMHERST
MacDonald, Allan S.
Nader, Nabil
Van Boxel, Paul J.

ANTIGONISH
MacGillivray, B. Jean
Sers, Robert N.

BRIDGEWATER
Hassan, Abdalla A.
Johnson, Kevin W.
Proctor, I. Joan
Stoddart, Todd A.

CANSO
Sullivan, John H.

DARTMOUTH
Mitchell, Alexander D.
Murdoch, John L.
Nuth, Laura L.
Shih, Warren W J.

GLACE BAY
Butler, Clay K.
Chaturvedi, Prabhat K.

HALIFAX
Ali, Idris M.
Allen, Philippe
Bethune, Drew C G.
Brisseau, Guy F.
Buduhan, Gordon P.
Calverley, Virginia C.
Casey, Patrick J.
Ellsmere, James C D.
Giacomantonio, Carman A.
Giacomantonio, J. Michael
Hancock Friesen, Camille L.
Helyer, Lucy K.
Henteleff, Harry J A.
Hoogerboord, C. Marius
Jamieson, Christopher G.
Johnson, Paul M.
Klassen, Dennis R.
Lee, Min Sun
MacKean, Gerald L.
Midgley, Peter I.
Minor, Samuel F.
Plourde, Madelaine
Porter, Geoffrey A.
Stewart, Keir M.
Topp, Trevor J.
Vair, Donald B.
Walsh, Mark J.
Williams, Lara J.
Wood, Jeremy R.
Yanchar, Natalie L.

INVERNESS
Belen, Jaime O.

KENTVILLE
Clark, Frank D.
Davidson, Dion
Gallant, Paula M.
Heisler, Benjamin E.
O'Malley, Vincent P.

MIRA ROAD
Jhirad, Ronen H.

NEW GLASGOW
Alvarez, Carlos A.
Cole, Basilon C.
Sebastian, Maleakal S.
Spread, Carole-Yvonne

SYDNEY
Archibald, Alison L.
Dunn, Rex S.
Gillis, Amy E.
MacMullin, Elwood C.
McGory, Rodney W.
Naqvi, Mahmood A.
Smith, Philip M.

SYDNEY MINES
Ignacio, Bayani S.

TRURO
Dzierzanowski, Martin
Fayez, Raad M.
Jeffrey, Cam A.
McGibney, Kieron D.
McKenney, Roderick N.

WINDSOR
Crawley, Frances J M.

YARMOUTH
Janke, Edwin M.
Lefel, Oleg
Murphy, Christopher A.

NUNAVUT

IQALUIT
Canil, Katherine A.

ONTARIO

AJAX
Aleyaseen, Maryam
Goussev, Igor
Hayashida, Peter J K.
Kendall, Hugh E A.
Konn, George
Ricer, Michael W.
Siddique, Saquib M.
Umar-Khitab, Asher A.
Xeroulis, George J.

ALLISTON
Keshoofy, Mohammad

BARRIE
Anderson, Michael
Dauphinee, Peter A.
Gowing, Robert N.
Guirguis, Emad M.
Hanrahan, Renee
Kruzyk, G. Jurii K.
Maharajh, Kamla
McDonald, Sandy I R.
Powell, Scott A.
Stefanison, Henry J.
Ward, Colin J.

BELLEVILLE
Bardell, Trevor
Barnabi, Francesco
Cleminson, Douglas
Davies, Nina E.
McIlreath, Sean A.
Rizvi, Shahbano H.

BOLTON
Willard, Garry L.

BOWMANVILLE
Hamour, Faisal A.
Ibrahim, Amir A.
Lane, Robert A.
Rashid, Zaihan

BRACEBRIDGE
Gupta, Rohit
Iannantuono, Biagio
Reid, Jessica E.

BRAMPTON
Ali, Farzan
Chiasson, Paul J.
Chopra, Priya
Davison, Alan J.
Goel, Sadan K.
Gregory, Wayne D.
Hosein, Alana N.
Irshad, Kashif
Louis, Donald K.
Malik, Azhar M.
McAlister, Edward D.
Pandya, Anand H.
Park, Myung I.
Pham, Quynh N.
Smith, Ian F.

BRANTFORD
Downie, David C.
Kessaram, Robert A.
Liaconis, Haralambos
Maddison, G. David
Pawliwec, Walter J.
Rooney, Michael A.
Schnider, Denise L.

BROCKVILLE
Davison, Patrick J.
Hobden, Susan D.
Redmond, William C.
Somani, Karim
Tilley, Alison E.

BURLINGTON
Bacopulos, Sarah A.
Barnett, Carmen E.
Correia, Jason D.
Kancherla, Yasodhara
Kim, Cei-Whan
Prodger, James D.
Rogers, James D.
Ryley, Alan D C.

CAMBRIDGE
Chan, Edward
Flamand, Francois J.
Geddes, Scott A.
Green, Lawrence
Kolyn, Donna M.

CARRYING PLACE
Sue-Chue-Lam, Jerry

CHATHAM
De Pass, Ian E.
Haddad, Elizabeth M.
Mahoney, Daniel J.
Morrison, John A.
Trinh, Tram K.

COCHRANE
Brown, E J. Peter

COLLINGWOOD
Akinyele, Adegboyega A.
Lisi, Michael P.

CONCORD
Byrne, Paul G.

CORNWALL
Antunes, Rui L.
Faizer, Mohamed B H.
Menon, Rajashree K.
Moussa, Wasseem M I.
Naoum, Serge

DRYDEN
Rabbat, George R.

DUNNVILLE
Baker, Darrell K.

EAST YORK
Cyriac, Jamie S.
Eskicioglu, Cagla
Gilas, Thomas
Sawires, Hany F S.
Zeldin, Robert A.

ELLIOT LAKE
Stirling, Michael J.

ERIN
Rawling, Edward G.

ETOBICOKE
Anderson, Alvin J.
Bahasadri, Mohammad
Bury, Katherine D.
Daudi, Faiz
Hariri, Farzad
Heisler, Ryan L.
Hill, Norman S.
Jackson, Zane S.
Kahn, Frederick
King, W I. Nelson
Sandler, Jack T.
Wen, Joseph Y M.
Wooster, Douglas L.

FERGUS
Enver, Khalid
Williams, Tina W.

FORT FRANCES
Anderson, Barry J.
Shahi, Bahram
Spencer, J. Alan

GEORGETOWN
Barron, Lesley K.
Iskander, John W.

GODERICH
Anand, Parvesh

GRIMSBY
Zettel, Lenore A.

GUELPH
Bhojani, Faizal D.
Bishop, Leigh R.
Hobson, John W.
Jahromi, Afshin
Nasser, Hamid A.
Pereira-Hong, Natasha L.
Phillips, Ian G.
Reed, J. Kenneth
Ward, Mylene

HAMILTON
Al Abdulmohsin, Mohammed A H.
Al-Harbi, Khalid E A.
Ali, Abdullah
Amin, Nalin K.
Anvari, Mehran
Archibald, Stuart D.
Bailey, Karen A.
Baillie, Frank G H.
Bowser, R. Daniel
Cadeddu, Margherita O.
Cameron, Brian H.
Cybulsky, Irene J.
Dath, Deepak P.
Faidi, Samir A.
Finley, Christian
Fitzgerald, Peter G.
Flageole, Helene
Forbes, Shawn
Gagic, Nenad
Gmora, Scott B.
Gregor, Paul
Grover, Harpreet S.
Harlock, John A.
Heller, Barbara S.
Hodgson, Nicole C.
Hong, Dennis
Iyer, Vikram S.
Kahnamoui, Kamyar
Lamy, Andre
Lovrics, Peter J.
Marcaccio, Michael J.
McDonald, Charles R J.
Menon, Gopinath T.
Miller, John D.
Mosakoski, Joan
Pampaloni, Federico
Rapanos, Theodore
Reid, Susan E.
Rice, Leah L.
Ruo, Leyo
Sanders, Kenneth C.
Schieman, Colin
Semelhago, Lloyd C.
Shawyer, Anna C.
Simunovic, Marko R I.
Sne, Niv
Stephen, Wesley J.
Szalay, David A.
Tandan, Ved R.
Tittley, Jacques G.
Vander Beek, Laura E.
Walton, J. Mark
Wasserman, Lukas J.
Young, J. Edward M.

HANOVER
Duque-Rendon, Hector A.

HAWKESBURY
Friesen, Byron P P.
Wackett, Charles J L.

HEARST
McGillivray, James W.

HUNTSVILLE
Kirkpatrick, H. Roy
MacMillan, Jennifer C.
Roldan, Hector A.

KAPUSKASING
Ayeni, R. Oluwafemi

KENORA
Hristov, Hristo N.
Spielman, John M.

KINCARDINE
Gora, Michael

KINGSTON
Belliveau, Paul
Brown, Peter M.
Drover, John W.
Engel, C. Jay
Hamilton, G. Andrew
Harle, Ingrid A.
Henson, John
Jalink, Diederick W.
MacDonald, P. Hugh
Mercer, C. Dale
Nanji, Sulaiman
Petsikas, Dimitri J.
Reid, Kenneth R.
Reznick, Richard K.
Robertson, David I.
Samis, Andrew J W.
Walker, G. Ross
Winthrop, Andrea L.
Zelt, David T.

KIRKLAND LAKE
Rumball, W. James
Visbal Moreno, A. Luis

KITCHENER
Ashe, Kassem A.
Hamilton, Ronald W.
Husien, Mohamed E M.
Judges, David P.
Kilmurry, Matthew R.
Maurice, Michael J.
McKinley, Craig A.
Pace, Ronald F.
Paun, Bogdan C.
Rao, Venkat B.
Reimer, Mark W.
Saunders, Michael G.
Sharkey, Paul J.
Talwar, Manoj K.

LEAMINGTON
Ghumman, Ejaz A.

LINDSAY
Baeta, Basil R.
Matz, Alexander
McNabb, Jamie A H M.
Sherwani, Aamir S.

LONDON
Ali, Syed T.
Brackstone, Muriel
Brown, James K.
Butter, Andreana M.
Colquhoun, Patrick H D.
Croome, Kristopher P.
Davies, Edward
De Rose, Gaetano
Duff, John H.
Forbes, Thomas
Fortin, Dalilah
Gillman, Ross G.
Goodman, Robert L.
Gray, Daryl K.
Harris, Jeremy R.
Harris, Kenneth
Holliday, Ronald L.
Inculet, Richard
Jones, Sarah A.
Kiaii, Bob B.
Latosinsky, Steven
Leeper, William R.
Leslie, Kenneth A.
Malthaner, Richard A.
Manax, Stanley J.
McAlister, Vivian C.
Mele, Tina S.
Merritt, Neil
Myers, M. Lee
Novick, Richard
Ott, Michael C.
Palmer, Robert W.
Parry, Neil G.
Power, Adam H.
Quan, Douglas
Rajgopal, Chellappa
Ruz Del Pino, Ricardo
Saettler, Elizabeth B.
Sales, Jack L.
Schlachta, Christopher M.
Scott, Leslie A.
Shah, Zafar A.
Shum, Jeffrey B.
Taylor, Brian M.
Torres, Monica M.
Vig, Kartar S.
Vinden, Christopher M.
Vogt, Kelly
Wall, William J.

MALTON
Sira, Surjeet S.

MANSFIELD
Pearson, F. Griffith

MARKHAM
Cheang, Timothy S.
Frost, Peter G.
Ing, Alan F M.
Laishram, Haladhra P S.
Pallister, Crystal
Vivona, Angelo A.
Whelan, Patrick J.

MIDLAND
Tavernier, Joseph

MILTON
Aziz, Dalal A.
Kolbasnik, Jeffrey G.
Makar, Hossam S H.

MISSISSAUGA
Barnes, Patrick T.
Behzadi, Abdollah
Bhatnagar, Gopal
Black, Karen M.
Braganza, Joseph S R.
Burns, Andrew R.
Cobourn, Christopher S.
Coughlan, Donald W S.
Cutrara, Charles A.
Degani, Cassim T.
Dunin-Bell, Ola H.
Garzon, Philippe M.
Johnson, William S.
Jones, Donald P.
Kapala, Marianna M.
Kumar, Deepa
McFadyen, Craig A.
Moffat, Grant S.
Mohammed, Adam H.
Mumford, David A.
Munnings, Donald B.
Musselman, Laura J.
Niaz, Ayyan
O'Connor, Richard J A.
Orr, James F.
Padonou, Michael K.
Pariag, John K.
Pope, Marc
Rai, Sundeep
Richardson, Jeannie L.
Saleh-Elgredly, Mona
Smith, Michael A P.
Tawadros, Patrick
Tin, Lancelot K.
Uddin, Sameena
Vale, John W.
Vucemilo, Ivica
Walmsley, Michael J.
Woolfson, Neil B.
Zacharias, S. Ramesh K.

MOOSE FACTORY
Kraulis, John E.

MORRISBURG
Chande, Suryakant

NAPANEE
Hota, Venkata S V B.
Rahn, Raymond J.

NEPEAN
Bhattacharyya, Asok K.
Bigelow, Eric
Mirsky, Douglas J.
Neidert, Eric J.

NEW LISKEARD
Alsharif, Jamal A H.
Jeffery, Hartley F.

NEWMARKET
Bauset, Richard
Campbell, J. Daniel
Chia, Shea Tzi
Choi, Tat Hung J.
Delialisi, Enkelejda
Eng, Frankie
Gupta, Deepak
Moon, Byung-Choo
Peniston, Charles M.
Privitera, Salvatore
Qureshi, Alia P.
Rahimi-Darabad, Mehdi

Soutter, D. Ian
Teoh, Kevin H T.
Toth, Julius L R.

NIAGARA FALLS
Ainslie, William H.
Doobay, Budhendranauth S.
Harpur, George E.
Rajagopaul, Kreasan
Rammohan, Surianarayanan
Reddy, Kundavaram N.
Subramanian, Anantasivan

NORTH BAY
Dougall, Allan M.
Hegge, Susan G.
Lamont, D. David
Moffat, Robert C.
Paul, Margaret
Singh, Ravinder

NORTH YORK
Aminazadeh, Nasser
Anand, Sundaram
Beder, Aaron L.
Botros, Yasser
Cardella, Jonathan A.
Cina, Claudio S.
Colapinto, Nicholas D.
Corpus, Rolando T.
Down, Nancy K.
Feinberg, Stanley M.
Forrest, Ian
Goldberg, Michael R.
Hagen, John A.
Hazrati, Ali
Huynh, Quoc Hung P.
Iskander, Alexander W.
Iu, Simon C M.
Jain, Neelesh K.
Kassirian, Shima
Klein, Lazar V.
Maragh, Haridath
McRitchie, Donna I.
Osman, Fahima A.
Parekh, Jaintheelal M.
Pinchuk, Brian M.
Sohi, Herpreet S.
Stotland, Peter K.
Tan, Jensen C C.
Taylor, William H.
Whiteacre, Laura L.
Wolinska, Justyna M.

OAKVILLE
Byrne, Alan J.
Callan, Nicole
Gafoor, Mohamed M.
Kealey, Miles S.
Khan, Qasim S.
Rozario, Duncan R.
Sayal, Manoj K.
Valiulis, Algis P J.

ORANGEVILLE
Bergen, Harry J.
Lane-Smith, D. Mark
Salih, Raafat B.
Wang, Grace T.

ORILLIA
Bauman, Nicholaus L L.
Campbell, James A.
Harrison, Lloyd W.
Makar, Magdy S I.
Riordon, Michele A.
Saettler, Erik R J.

OSHAWA
Amurawaiye, Emmanuel O.
Chin, Ian D.
Coutu, Pierre A.
Dickie, A. John
Jones, Julia J.
Marcus, Herbert I.
Moozar, Kouros
Sengar, Pankaj S.
Trainor, Shannon E.
Wherrett, Laurie J.
Woolfson, Ian K.

OTTAWA
Alobaid, Abdulhakeem M S.
Arnaout, Angel
Arnold, Ian M F.
Auer, Rebecca A C.
Balaa, Fady K.
Barron, Philip T.
Bass, Juan A.
Beaulieu, Chantal
Bodurtha, Audley J.
Boushey, Robin P.
Brandys, Timothy M.
Brar, Balpreet S.
Cagiannos, Catherine
Chadwick, Chris D J.
Chou, Shirley H Y.
Cowan, Kyle N.
Dervish, Greta A.
Dervish, H. Zihni
Desai, Dennis
Dion, Louise
Fairfull-Smith, Robert J.
Forse, Raymond A.
Freeman, Joel B.
Friedlich, Martin S.
Garber, Bryan
Gauthier, Jean-Claude
Gay, Brian C.
Gay, Raymond B.
Gilbert, Sebastien
Goldstein, William
Guilbert, Jacques
Gutauskas, Andrea
Gutauskas, Jose
Hajjar, Georges E.
Hendry, Paul J.
Hill, Andrew B.
Jarmuske, Mario B.
Jayaram, Srinidhi K.
Jetty, Prasad
Kaminsky, Victor M.
Kendal, Wayne S.
Kubelik, Dalibor
Lampron, Jacinthe
Legrand Westfall, Lorraine
Lewis, Ronald T.
Lokhat, M. Hossen
Lorimer, John W.
Mamazza, Joseph
Martel, Guillaume V D.
Masters, Roy G.
Maziak, Donna E.
Methot, Mireille
Mimeault, Richard E.
Moloo, Husein
Monaghan, Ronald A.
Moonje, Vijay B.
Nagpal, Sudhir K.
Nasr, Ahmed L.
Pagliarello, Giuseppe
Pires, Jose M.
Pitt, Dennis F.
Porte, Alexis N.
Poulin, Eric C.
Raiche, Isabelle M M.
Redmond, Mary L.
Redwan, Hani A S.
Rubens, Fraser D.
Saito, Simon
Saleh, Wasfy S.
Seely, Andrew J E.
Shamji, Farid M.
St-Jean, Benoit
Stedman Jr., Alfred S.
Sundaresan, R. Sudhir
Syme, Roderick G.
Tadros, Shaheer
Taylor, R. Dale
Todd, Thomas R J.
Trottier, Daniel C J.
Villeneuve, Patrick J.
Watters, James M.
Weaver, Joel G R.
Weekes, Andrew N.
Winckel, Christopher P.
Yang, Ilun
Yelle, J P. Jean-Denis
Zolfaghari, Shahram

OWEN SOUND
Caulfeild, Jonathan D.
Lamont, R. Neil
Lozon, Alan M.
Milencoff, G. Scott
Nechala, Patrik

PARRY SOUND
Decker, Christopher
Foster, Kenneth D.
Hunt, George D.

PEMBROKE
El Fitori, Adel
Graham, Christopher S.
Haney, Colleen M.

PENETANGUISHENE
Pigeon, Michel B J.
Sacks, Eileen
Walc, Leslie C.

PERTH
Morell, Thomas P.

PETERBOROUGH
Ebisuzaki, Lawrence K.
Gibb, Graham K.
Mikula, Lynn A.
Minor, Adrian A.
Nie, Robert G.
Petrasek, Anthony J.
Rowsom, John T.
Scott, Jaime M.
Thompson, Alan A.

PICKERING
Salmon, Ernest A T.

PORT HOPE
Al-Ali, Kaes A S.
Basmajian, Haig
Stratford, Andrew F C.

PORT PERRY
Dobbin, Karolyn M.
Evans, John
Stewart, Martin C.
Stryde, Trevor S.

RENFREW
Krajewski, Susan A.
Miller, J. Lance

RICHMOND HILL
Bhargava, Reena
Bhat, K. Rama
Bui, Luke L Q.
Fiture, Ali O.
Klevan, Ariel E.
Lee, Justin T.
Lee, Mark H.
Ortega, Sarah J.
Tassis, Andreas

SARNIA
Balachandra, Vasthare K.
Cuccarolo, Glenna
Gray, W. Alexander
Kareemi, Raza K.
Muhunthan, Arumairajah
Pratt, Kathleen J.
Ross, Joan E.
Suryavanshi, Rajeev K.
Taylor, John P T F.
Taylor, Mark C.

SAULT STE MARIE
Abdurahman, Adel
Allen, Stephen M.
Fratesi, Sante J.
Mossing, Morley S.
Reich, Joseph A.
Taylor, Kerri-Ann S.

SCARBOROUGH
Anderson, Thomas H.
Asano, Tracey K.
Au, How Hoong
Azoubel, Gustavo A P.
Chan, Joseph E.
Chan, Michael C K.
Chiu, Arthur K K.
Hodgkiss, David R.
Huhlewych, Roman
Jackson, Steven J.
Kawun, Ulana B.
Law, Lorraine T.
Leung, Winnie W C.
Maaz, Umar
Mandelbaum, Saul H.
Moffat, John G.
Mohan, Naresh
Nallapaneni, Sailaja P.
Nanda, Arvind
Norman, Nadine I E.
Pennington, Jason J.
Rosenthal, Gary A.
Stitt, Robert B.
Tabari, Mohammad
Walkovich, Peter
Wong, Jason H P.
Wong, Kevin H.
Yasser, Zaid J.
Yau, Patrick W N.
You, John M S.

SIMCOE
Al-Aqeel, Aqeel I M.
Al-Kassem, Anas
Mattar, Nabih
Olsson, Larry S M.
Soenen, Gary M.

SIOUX LOOKOUT
Chaudhuri, Monica M.
Touzin, Eric S.

ST CATHARINES
Azabi, Tareq O.
Blewett, Christopher J.
Cranford, Jeffrey W H.
Kobylecky, Anna A.
MacMillan, James I.
Phillips, Stephanie E.
Sawula, Donald A.

ST THOMAS
Black, Robert T.
Collins, Paul J.
McLachlin, Hugh A.
Sostaric, John V.

STRATFORD
Gonser, Randal J.
Hardwick, James M.
Lefebvre, Kevin L.
Maciver, Angus G.
McCune, Marcie L.
O'Neill, Craig D.
Sorsdahl, A. Kent

STRATHROY
Elgamal, Akram S.
Jain, Vipan K.

SUDBURY
Aul, Sewa S.
Benedict, Richard R.
Bhatia, Pankaj
Brule, Michele F M.
Caycedo, Antonio J.
Fenton, John A.
Garg, Avinash
Gay, Raymond J.
Hendel, Raymond
Kealy, Ciaran L.
Luison, Fabio
Muir, Craig F.
Paradis, Rachelle L.
Pudupakkam, Santosh R.
Smith, Robert A.
Smith, Shona E.
Snider, John M.
Willoughby, Rodney P N.
Wright, Frederick F.

THORNHILL
Affifi, Rasheed A E.
Alexander, Michael A J.
Burul, Claude J.
Chan, Chin K.
Melamedov, Daniel
Singal, Ram K.

THUNDER BAY
Armstrong, Barry D.
Davenport, Eric
Gehman, Kenneth E.
Gooding, John T.
Harris, William A.
Holmes, Matthew C.
Kirk, Allan A G.
MacLeod, Heather C.
Mapeso, Gabriel V.
Remus, John L.
Telang, Harshad
Thibert, Mark R.
Wyant, John D.

TILLSONBURG
Colaco, Carmo D D.
Crosby, Jacqueline A.

TIMMINS
Beres, Alana
Kelly, Daniel M.
Labelle, Eric R.
Squires, William E.
Swidinsky, Teddi L D.
Voogjarv, Harry M.

TORONTO
Aarts, Mary-Anne W.
Abawi, Walid
Abraham, T. Easo
Ahmed, Najma A.
Al Sawafi, Yaqoub A R.
Al Shaibi, Maha A N.
Al Shareef, Basem H M.
Ali, Jameel
Ashamalla, Shady
Atherton, William
Azzie, Georges R.
Basian, Herbert
Bawazeer, Mohammed A.
Baxter, Nancy N.
Beckett, Andrew N.
Bendzsak, Anna M.
Bernick, Paul E.
Blitz, Maurice
Bohnen, John M A.
Boutros, John
Brar, Savtaj S.
Brenneman, Frederick D.
Brister, Stephanie J.
Burke, Bonnie A.
Burnstein, Marcus J.
Cassie, Scott G.
Cattral, Mark S.
Chiu, Priscilla P L.
Christakis, George T.
Cil, Tulin D.
Cleary, Sean P.
Coburn, Natalie S G.
Cohen, Zane
Compeau, Christopher G.
Cordeiro, Erin D.
Craddock, Graham N.
Cusimano, Robert J.
Daar, Abdallah S.
Darling, Gail
Davies, Dafydd A.
De La Rocha, Claudio
De Montbrun, Sandra L.
Devon, Karen M.
Doyle, Jeffrey D.
Dueck, Andrew D.
Easson, Alexandra M.
Errett, Lee E.
Escallon, Jaime M.
Fecteau, Annie H.
Feindel, Christopher M S.
Fenech, Darlene
Finn, William P.
Fischer, Gerhardt E.
Fremes, Stephen E.
Fung, F. Siu-Yue
Gallinger, Steven
George, Ralph L.
Gerstle Jr, Justin T.
Ghanekar, Anand
Gladdy, Rebecca A.
Govindarajan, Anand
Grant, David R.
Greig, Paul D.
Gryfe, Robert
Hamilton, J. Douglas
Hanna, Sherif S.
Harmantas, Athanasios
Hart, Richard S.
Hassan, Saima
Hendrick-Hallet, Julie

Himal, Harry S.
Himidan, Sharifa A.
Holloway, Claire M B.
Huseynov, Khumar
Jackson, Timothy D.
Jayaraman, Shiva
Johnston, K. Wayne
Kapila, Varun
Karanicolas, Paul J.
Kennedy, Erin D.
Keshavjee, Shaf
Kim, Peter T W.
King, William
Ko, Michael A.
Koo, Jarley
Kucey, Daryl S.
Langer, Jacob C.
Latter, David A.
Lau, Tak Sang
Law, Calvin H L.
Lawless, Bernard W.
Leong, Wey-Liang
Lickley, H. Lavina A.
Lindsay, David R.
Lindsay, Thomas F.
Look Hong, Nicole J.
MacLellan, Steven J.
MacRae, Helen M.
Mackenzie, Robert L.
Maggisano, Robert
Marshall, John C.
McCart, Judith A.
McCready, David R.
McGilvray, Ian D.
McKenna, Joseph P.
McLeod, Robin S.
Minna, Roberta
Mueller, Carmen L.
Mustard, Robert A.
Nathens, Avery B.
Nenshi, Rahima N.
Nessim, Carolyn
Noria, Sabrena
O'Brien, Catherine
Okrainec, Allan E P P.
Oreopoulos, George D.
Papia, Giuseppe
Penner, Todd P.
Pierre, Andrew F.
Piper, Hannah G.
Quereshy, Fayez A.
Ralph-Edwards, Anthony C.
Reedijk, Michael J.
Rizoli, Sandro B.
Ropchan, Glorianne V.
Rosen, Irving B.
Ross, Theodore M.
Rotstein, Lorne E.
Rotstein, Ori D.
Rudd, William Warren H.
Safieddine, Najib N.
Saleh, Fady
Schaal, Peter G H.
Scheer, Adena S.
Scully, Hugh E.
Segedi, Maja
Shahrokhi Ebrahimipour, Shahriar
Simpson, Jory S.
Singh, Arun K.
Smith, Andrew J.
Smith, David E.
Smith, Lloyd C.
Spence, William J E.
Spencer Netto, Fernando A C.
Starr, David M.
Sullivan, Paul A.
Swallow, Carol J.
Tanner, Wayne R.
Taylor, Bryce R.
Tien, Homer C.
Tremblay, Lorraine N.
Tse, Leonard W H.
Urbach, David R.
Waddell, Thomas K.
Wales, Paul W.
Walker, Paul M.
Wei, Alice C C.
Weizel, Harold A E.
Williams, Eldon S V.
Wright, Frances C.
Yau, Terrence M.
Zakrison, Tanya L.
Zlotta, Alexandre R.

UNIONVILLE
Pendergast, Patrick J F.

VAUGHAN
Kundhal, Prabhsharan S.
Weizman, David A.

VINELAND
Hyatt, H. John

WALKERTON
Graham, Duncan C M.

WALLACEBURG
Vaughan, George E R.

WELLAND
Abdel-Malik Ghali, Rafik R.
Kapijimpanga, Lowesha B.
Khan, Iqbal A.
Koziarz, Piotr
Railton, Richard H.
Willard, Peter T.

WINCHESTER
Blakslee, James M.
Davey, Michelle A L.
Oberoi, Malika

WINDSOR
Ben-Ibrahim, Mohamed A.
Coughlin, Michael P.
Elalem, Abdusalam
Gyetvai, Kristen M.
Heartwell, Barbara J E.
Kanji, Amirali
Khokhotva, Vladislav
Laschuk, Bohdan S.
Liebman, Shael M.
McKay, A. Robert
McKinnon, John R.
Mehta, Sowmil K.
Moodley, Mathaven
Parashar, Rakesh K.
Petrakos, Andrew
Ravid-Einy, Anat
Ristic, Miodrag A.
Singh, Minesh
Sion, David M.
Takahashi Monroy, Takeshi

WOODBRIDGE
Del Rizzo, Dario F.
Harrison, Alan W.

WOODSTOCK
El-Salviti, Gamal I.
Humphrey, Robert J.
MacLeod, Malcolm K.
Oung, Christopher M.

YORK
Boszko, Andres
Gebrechristos, Ephrem

PRINCE EDWARD ISLAND

CHARLOTTETOWN
Ashby, David
Cottreau, G. Thomas
Craswell, Jeffrey D.
Fleming, D A. Barry
Gulati, Brahm B.

SUMMERSIDE
Dawes, Peter
Schaefer, J. Paul
Walker, William L.

QUÉBEC

ALMA
Gagnon, Marie-Claude
Harnois, Yves
Pettersen, Carl
Poulin, Renald M.

AMOS
Bosse, Charles
Dupras, Eric
Gaillard, Felix
Le Regent, Linda

AMQUI
Hasan, Omar N.

BAIE-COMEAU
Brie, Michele
Gitlan, Dan Liviu
Nadeau, Richard

BAIE-SAINT-PAUL
Carrier, Jude
Potvin, Martin
Tourville, Yves V.

BOUCHERVILLE
Gauthier, Louise

BROSSARD
Arbour, Rejean

CAP-AUX-MEULES
Arsenault, Lorne J A.
Bourque, Marjolaine
Duguay, R. Lester

CHANDLER
Bedard, Christine

CHATEAUGUAY
Doyon, Caroline
Gyopar, Andrew F.
Hogue, Dominique
Lamarre, Claudine
Levesque, Christian
Mazerolle, Richard

CHIBOUGAMAU
Beaudoin, Gaetan
Gelinas, Denis

CHICOUTIMI
Blackburn, Michel
Carignan, Sebastien
Dery, Marie-Claude
Farinas, Jean-Marc
Ferland, Olivier
Houde, Jean-Luc
Lafortune-Payette, Annie
Larochelle, Guillaume
Mathieu, John F.
Michaud, Pierre
Pilotte, Marie-Natacha
Tousignant, Julie
Trudeau, Patrick

CLARENCEVILLE
Jones, C. William

COWANSVILLE
Demers, Philippe
LaRue, Nathalie
O'Sullivan, Katherine
Robitaille, Josee
Stevens Lebel, Miriane

DOLBEAU-MISTASSINI
Menard, Christian
Tremblay-Allan, Fannie

DORVAL
Polson, Herbert A.

DRUMMONDVILLE
Chapdelaine, Joyaube
Labreche, Jacques
Lalancette, Mathieu
Laplante, Richard
Miller, Steven

ENTRELACS
Galarneau, Pierre

GASPE
De Bie, Jacques
Gaul, Karine
Leclerc, Pierre J A.
Soucy, Genevieve

GATINEAU
Begin, Eric V.
Bothwell, Jody N.
Cote, Frederic
Cournoyer, Julie
Duchesne, Annie
Germain, Louis-Philippe
Lessard, Caryne
Malak, M. Nabil
Mathew, Jane M.
Nadkarni, Gauri
Nault, Patrice
Perodin, Farah
Roy, Nancy
Salib, Samir
Tavassoli, Massoud

GRANBY
Bellemare, Benoit
Gharib, Rami
Jacquemin, Jean-Pierre
Richard, Michel
Saint-Jean, Claude

GREENFIELD PARK
Bergeron, Eric
Clas, David
Coutu, Diane E.
Gauvreau, Frederic
Larose, Pierre
Laurin, Gilles
Le Guillan, Marie-Pierre
Loriot, Marie-Helene
Pichette, Maude
Ratte, Sebastien
Robinson, Patrick N.

JOLIETTE
Berlinguet, Jean-Claude
Villiard, Roselyne
Windisch, Louis

JONQUIERE
Al-Chaddad, Elias

LA MALBAIE
Letourneau, Serge
Smith, Jacques

LA POCATIERE
Couture, Gilles
Nadeau, Patrick

LA SARRE
El-Haddad, Issam

LA TUQUE
Djaknoun, Djaoeida

LAC-MEGANTIC
Breton, Denys
Paradis, Paul E.
Sfeir, Antoine

LACHINE
Kass, Theodore
Nguyen, Ngoc-Van
Woo, Debbie

LACHUTE
Gingras, Marc
Mutch, David O.

LASALLE
Badro, Emile
Meunier, Mathieu

LAVAL
Belhumeur, Jacinthe S V.
Bilodeau, Lucie
Bouchard, Patrick
Coulloudon, Alain
Couture, J G R. Guy
Danylewick, Richard
Flanagan, Guy
Forgues, Richard P.
Gravel, Denis
Houle, Jean-Rene
Lamoureux, Patrice
Laurion, Marcel
Legault, Serge
Montpetit, Patrick
Provencher, Josee
Thibault, Elise

LEVIS
Bertrand, Annie
Couture, Jean
Desaulniers, Rene C.
Dubreuil, Daniel
Imbeau, Eric
Laliberte, Jean
Sasseville, Nicole D.

LONGUEUIL
Chagnon, Francois
Chouinard, Christian
Cloutier, Alexis-Simon
Des Groseilliers, Sylvain
Deshaies, Gaetan
Deslauriers, Nancy
Diec, Hung Long
Gosselin, Michel
Jette, Pierre
Letellier, Francois
Roy, Mathieu
Simon, Renee
Vo, Thanh Truc

MAGOG
Petraki, Nabil
Sauve, Marie

MARIA
Allard, Valere
Gagne, Thierry
Larue, Marie

MATANE
Dufour, Claude
Ouellet, Daniel

MONT-LAURIER
Celestin-Noel, S. Marie
Loungnarath, Vilaysoun
Ouellet, Kim

MONT-ROYAL
Atlas, Henri
Denis, Ronald
Garneau, Pierre Y.
Le Guillan, Soazig
Panic, Stephane
Synnott, Dominique

MONTMAGNY
Laprise, Christine
Lavigne, Alexandre
Leveille, Germaine

MONTREAL
Abdulnour, Elias M.
Abraham, Cherrie Z.
Alshaikhi, Abdullah Y.
Anderson, Dawn L.
Arena, Orazio
Aspirot, Ann
Baird, Robert
Barama, Azemi A.
Barkun, Jeffrey S T.
Basik, Mark
Basile, Fadi
Beauchamp, Gilles
Beaudoin, Nathalie
Beaunoyer, Mona
Beaupre, Andre
Bejerman, Mario
Bellemare, Jean-Francois
Bendavid, Yves
Bergman, Simon
Bernard, Denis
Blair, Jean-Francois
Boileau, Jean-Francois
Bouchard, Sarah
Brabant, Gordon V.
Breton, Gail
Brown, Rea A.
Bruneau, Luc
Caron, Josee
Carrier, Michel
Cartier, Raymond
Cecere, Renzo
Chagnon, Michel
Chan, Gabriel
Chaput, Veronique
Charlebois, Patrick
Chaudhury, Prosanto K.
Choiniere, Louise

Chughtai, M. Saeed
Chughtai, Talat S.
Corriveau, Marc M.
Court, Olivier
Dagenais, Michel H.
Daloze, Pierre M.
De Broux, Eric
De Varennes, Benoit
Deckelbaum, Dan L E.
Dejoie, Carl Louis A.
Demyttenaere, Sebastian V.
Derossis, Anna M.
Dionisopoulos, Tassos
Dube, Pierre
Dube, Serge
Duranceau, Andre C H.
Elkouri, Stephane
Emil, Sherif G S.
Emond, Carl P.
Ergina, Patrick L.
Faria, Julio
Fata, Paola M.
Feghali, Joseph
Feldman, Liane S.
Fenster, Roger F.
Ferraro, Pasquale
Ferri, Lorenzo E.
Fleiszer, David M.
Fraser, Shannon A.
Freedman, Arthur N.
Fried, Gerald M.
Gagner, Michel
Garzon, Jacob
Genest, Jocelyne
Ghali, Rafik
Ghitulescu, Gabriela
Ghosn, Pierre B.
Gordon, Philip H.
Granger, Beatrice
Hardy, Mark
Hassanain, Mazen
Hebert, Yves
Henri, Margaret
Heyen, Francoise
Ho, Quang Nhan
Huynh, Phuoc Hai
Keyserlingk, R.. John R.
Khoury, Nagib
Khwaja, Kosar A.
Kordich, Miroslav
Laberge, Jean-Martin
Lachapelle, Kevin J.
Lacharite, Sophie
Lafontaine, Edwin R.
Lallier, Michel
Lamontagne, Yvan
Langlois, Yves
Lapointe, Real
Latulippe, Jean-Francois
Lauzon, Gilles
Leblanc, Guy
Leclerc, Yves E.
Letourneau, Richard
Liberman, A. Moishe
Liberman, Alexander S.
Loungnarath, Rasmy
Loutfi, Antoine
MacKenzie, Kent S.
Marcoux, Raymond
Margolese, Richard G.
Martin, Ginette
Martin, Jocelyne
Meguerditchian, Ari N.
Meterissian, Sarkis H.
Metrakos, P. Peter
Milne, Catherine A.
Mitmaker, Benjamin
Mitmaker, Elliot
Montreuil, Bernard
Moralejo, Richard V.
Morgan, Stephen R.
Morin, Jean-Francois
Morin, Michel
Morin, Nancy A.
Mulder, David S.
Nassif, Edgard
Nassif, Raymond
Neville, Amy A.
Normandin, Louis
Nouh, Thamer A.
Obrand, Daniel
Otaky, Naim F.
Ouellette, M A. Denise
Ouimet, Alain A.
Page, Pierre
Papenburg, Robert R.
Paraskevas, Steven
Patocskai, Erica J.
Pearl, Gerald J.
Pellerin, Michel
Perrault, Louis P.
Plasse, Marylene
Poenaru, Dan
Poirier, Madeleine
Poljicak, Mate
Puligandla, Pramod S.
Rakovich, George
Ratelle, Richard
Razek, Tarek S A.
Richard, Carole S.
Rivilis, Jeffrey
Robidoux, Andre
Rodriguez, Joseph
Rosenberg, Lawrence
Roy, Andre F.
Rusnov, Mladen V.
Safa, Nagi
Saint-Vil, Dickens
Salasidis, Robert
Salem, Nabil
Sebajang, Herawaty
Shanfield, Isidore
Shaw, Kenneth S.
Shibata, Henry R.
Shum-Tim, Dominique
Sideris, Lucas
Sigman, Harvey H.
Sirois, Cateline
Sirois, Christian
Spicer, Jonathan
Stein, Barry L.
Steinmetz, Oren K.
Stern, Hartley S.
Tabah, Roger J.
Tardif, Caroline
Tataryn, Donna N.
Tavassoli, Mohammed
Tchervenkov, Christo I.
Tchervenkov, Jean I.
Than Trong, An
Tremblay, Francine
Tremblay, Yves
Ubani, Nelson C.
Vanounou, Tsafrir
Vasilevsky, Carol-Ann
Vassiliou, Melina
Verdant, Alain G.
Vo, Kim
Vobecky, J. Suzanne
Vollant, Stanley
Wassef, Ramses
Weissglas, Issie S.
Wexler, Marvin J.
Yeretsian, Sarkis
Younan, Rami J.
Youssef, Sami A.
Zaharia, Florin
Zogopoulos, George

MONTREAL-NORD
Legros, Guy

NOTRE-DAME-DU-LAC
Hanna, Hala

ORMSTOWN
Aikin, Kenneth A.
Dupras, Genevieve
Zalai, Christian V.

POINTE-CLAIRE
Benchetrit, Arie
Bourdon, Gilles
Dalrymple, Sharon A.
Lamarre, Pascal
McLeod, Robert A H.
Polyhronopoulos, Gerry
Znajda, Tamara L.

QUEBEC
Auger-Dufour, Etienne
Baillot, Richard
Belanger, Mathieu
Biron, Simon
Blair, Duane
Bouchard, Alexandre
Bouchard, Philippe
Brochu, Gaetan
Chhiv, Mony
Clement, Julien
Croft, Dary
Dagenais, Francois
Daigle, Carl
Desbiens, Christine
Deshaies, Isabelle
Deslauriers, Jean
Dion, Yves-Marie
Douville, Yvan
Doyle, Daniel
Dussault, Jean
Frechette, Eric
Gagne, Jean-Pierre
Gagnon, Josee
Garneau, Pierre
Gilbert, Alain
Gilbert, Nathalie
Gregoire, Jocelyn
Gregoire, Roger C.
Guimond, Marie-France
Hareth, Rezkallah
Hould, Frederic S.
Kibrite, Antoine
Labbe, Raymond
Lebel, Stefane
Leclerc, Suzanne G.
Lemieux, Michel D.
Lemire, Luc
Lescelleur, Odette
Marceau, Picard
Marceau, Simon
Marois, Denis
Morin, Jacques
Moustarah, Fady
Noel, Henri-Paul
Ouellet, Jean-Francois
Ouellet, Jean-Francois
Pap, Genevieve
Peloquin, Jean
Perron, Jean
Poirier, Brigitte
Poirier, Eric
Prasil, Pascale
Provencher, Louise
Rainville, J C. Bruno
Rheaume, Pascal
Rouleau, Claude A.
Roy, Guy
St-Germain, Pascal
Thauvette, Daniel
Thibault, Claude
Trottier, Vincent
Vaillancourt, Rosaire
Vallee, Nicole

REPENTIGNY
Benoit, Yvon

RIMOUSKI
Bilodeau, Josee
Brisson, Vincent
Chouinard, Jerome
Cousineau, Martin
Demalsy, Jean-Claude
Gagne, Richard
St-Georges, Regent

RIVIERE-DU-LOUP
Arsenault, Jean-Pierre
Blanchet, Richard
Gaudreault, Judith
Gervais, Normand
Lapointe, Louis
St-Onge, Gerard R.

ROBERVAL
Dubois, Pierre
Noel, Guylaine
Trudeau, Alain

ROUYN-NORANDA
Saint-Marseille, Sophie

SAINT-EUSTACHE
Guindon, Karine
Malhotra, Vikram K.
Marceau, Pierre
Ouellet, Frederic
Savard, Philippe

SAINT-GEORGES
Drouin, Simon
Faucher, Dorothee
Lavoie, Perrine
Pazira, Hassibollah
Pomerleau, Serge

SAINT-HYACINTHE
Boily, Helene
Caron, Patricia-Anne
Charbonneau, Maxime
Levesque, Sonia

SAINT-JEROME
Allard, Michel
Chapleau, Denis
Gaffiero, Patricia
Gaudreault, Nicolas
Genest, Sylvain
Gravel, Stephane
Huynh Bao, Giang Thanh
Larouche, Alain L.
Luu, Thanh Phi Y.
Martel, Karine
Minville, Nathalie
Tardif, Eric
Vafiadis, Petros

SAINT-LAMBERT
Beaulieu, R. Claude

SAINT-LAURENT
Christou, Nicolas V.

SAINT-ROMUALD
Gosselin, Claire

SALABERRY DE VALLEYFIELD
Barrette, Pierre
Cartier, Benoit
Chamberland, Pierre
Guyot, Catherine
Lemieux, Francois
Martin, Michel
Provencal, Annie
Simard, Stephanie
Surowaniec, Tadeusz
Talbot, Michel N.

SEPT-ILES
L'Esperance, Marion
Michaud, Nathalie
Nantais, Michel
Perrin, Nadege

SHAWINIGAN-SUD
Abel, Sylvain
Cyr, Jonathan
Lavoie, Frederic
Marchand, Valerie
Poissant, Jean-Francois

SHAWVILLE
Potvin, Earl G.

SHERBROOKE
Bedard, Valerie
Begin, Andre
Blouin, Yvan
Comeau, Emilie
Despatis, Marc-Antoine
Devroede, Ghislain J.
Forget, Andre
Gonzalez-Amaya, Gonzalo
Greentree, David M.
Hamel, Jean-Yves
Hellou, Gisele
Hetu, Jessika
Lapie, Veronique
Leblanc, Valerie
Mayer, Sandeep K.
McFadden, Nathalie
Mosimann, Francois
Normandin, Denyse
Paris, Catherine
Sirois, Chantal
Sirois, Marco
Viens, Mario

SOREL-TRACY
Belanger, Julie
Comtois, Andre
Martin, Pierre
Perron, Thierry
Royal, Pierre

ST CHARLES BORROMEE
Aubree, Nicolas
Beaulieu, Gaston
Dunberry, Michel
Eloy, Laurence
Fleury, Alain
Klopfenstein, Jean-Jacques
Koch, Patricia
Legault, Michel
Lemieux, Patrice
Martel, Elise
Morency, Isabelle
Racicot, Caroline

ST-EUSTACHE
Pigeon, Pierre D.

ST JEAN SUR RICHELIEU
Boulais, Genevieve
Lapostolle, Annie-Claude
Legare, Genevieve
Levesque, Jean-Luc
Perreault, Yves
Poisson, Jacques
Poliquin, Denis

STE AGATHE DES MONTS
Camire, Jean-Sebastien
Dugas, Renee
Emond, Benoit
Giard, Alain
Richer, Bernard
Sabourin, Francois

STE ANNE DES MONTS
Nadeau, Marie-Eve

TERREBONNE
Benitez, Bella
Bouchereau-Eyegue, Mila-Denise
Bourbonnais, David
Chevalier, Christine
Despres, Cathy
Giroux, Manon
Legare, Alain
Nguyen Buu, Paul
Viger, Pierre

THETFORD MINES
Bilodeau, Audrey
Magnan, Michel
Pidgeon, Jean-Francois
Roy, Anthony

TROIS-RIVIERES
Blouet, Sylvie
Bourgouin, Daniel
Boyer, Rene
Brosseau, Isabelle
Contant, Chantal
Doyon, Annabelle
Dufresne, Jose
Dumont, Yannick
Girouard, Marie-Helene
Jutras, Jean-Francois
Lamy, Martin
Rheault, Michel

VAL-D'OR
Booth, Janet M.
Brouillette, Denis
Mijangos-Pelaez, Jose L.

VERDUN
Azzi, Melhem
Beauregard, Gilles N.
Ferland, Marc-Andre
Hermans, Pierre
Karam, Boutros
Nguyen, Phuoc Ngoc Diem
Richard, Philippe F A.

VICTORIAVILLE
Baril, Claude
Laganiere, Michel

Levesque, Yves
Rouillard, Martin
Toure, Lossany E.

VILLE-MARIE
Vien, Daniel

WESTMOUNT
Adle, Mansour
Zadeh, Teanoosh

SASKATCHEWAN

MELFORT
Laosebikan, Adeyemi O.

MOOSE JAW
Cadili, Ali
Cheddie, Nishaan
Miller, George B.

NORTH BATTLEFORD
Du Plessis, Hendrik
Gieni, Melissa E.
Retief, Malcolm W.

PRINCE ALBERT
Friesen, Randall W.
Lumb, Kathleen J.
Nel, Joshka A.
O'Carroll, Ruth F.
Olsen, Valerie P.
Royeppen, Edmund C.

REGINA
Baird, Jennifer E.
Butler, Matthew S.
Cameron, Robert D A.
Carter, James W.
Cuddington, Gordon W.
Gorman, Peter R.
Jacob, Sanjay M.
Kaban, Gordie K.
Kopriva, David
Kurtz, Ingrid L.
McCarville, Donald J.
Meiers, Suzanne L.
Moustapha, Ahmad
Pooler, Stephen D.
Rao, Jagadish
Sood, Om Prakash
Suri, Rakesh M R.
Tcherni, Marly B L.
Tin, Wendy W T.

SASKATOON
Awan, Saeed-Ur-Rehman
Beck, Gavin
Bharadwaj, Steven C.
Bigsby, Richard J.
Casson, Alan G.
Chandrakanthan, Selliah
Christian, Francis T.
Dalshaug, Gregory B.
Duval, Bruce J.
Gaboury, Jeffrey P.
Groot, Gary
Harington, Michael B.
Hayes, Paul R.
Hayton, Susan
Keith, Roger G.
Kenyon, Christopher R.
Kvinlaug, Kylie E.
Luo, Yigang
Meiers, Pamela J.
Miller, Grant G.
Moser, Michael A J.
Mycyk, Taras R.
Oleniuk, Fredrick H.
Oucharek, Jennifer J.
Pfeifer, Joseph J T.
Seshadri, Pieter A.
Spelay, Jodi L.
Stevenson, Kevin W.
Ulmer, Brian G.

SWIFT CURRENT
Vasquez, Virgilio B.

YORKTON
Wanis, Nashat S.

YUKON TERRITORY

WHITEHORSE
Huang, Felicia
Poole, Alexander J.
Samuelson, Samantha L.
Storey, David L.

Geriatric Medicine

ALBERTA

CALGARY
Burback, Darren C.
Cohen, Adrienne F.
Fruetel, Karen
Hogan, David B.
Kwok, Jimmy C W.
Rodgers, Lynne K.
Schmaltz, Heidi N.
Silvius, James L.

EDMONTON
Alagiakrishnan, Kannayiram
Lawson, Fiona M E.
Lechelt, Katherine
McCracken, Peter
Robertson, Duncan
Rolfson, Darryl B.
Rucker, Diana

LETHBRIDGE
Ikuta, Roland M.

BRITISH COLUMBIA

CAMPBELL RIVER
Man-Son-Hing, Malcolm G.

NANAIMO
King, Kim W.

NEW WESTMINSTER
Chase, Jocelyn M.
Chin, Ying Wai
Jain, Leena
Mian, Mamta
O'Connor, M. Peter
Petrossian, Caroline

PORT ALBERNI
Williams, Dorothy L.

RICHMOND
Barnett, Kim E.
Forbes, Anastasia F.

SURREY
Liao, Joy
Pillay, Shunmoogam W.
Vohra, Sanjeev

VANCOUVER
Alimoradi, Ima
Beattie, B. Lynn
Bell, Kathryn A.
Chung, A. Maria
Cook, Wendy L.
Dian, Larry
Hill, Amanda J.
Kushner Kow, Janet V.
Lee, Philip E.
Lo, Lawrence S.
Madden, Kenneth M.
Meneilly, Graydon S.
Menezes, Janice A.
Ranchod, Hetesh A.
Rauscher, Christopher J.
Sztramko, Richard W K.
Villanyi, Diane
Wong, Roger Y M.

VICTORIA
Bater, Marilyn G.
Jenkins, Catherine A.
Malone, Marilyn L.
Montgomery, Patrick R.
Pai, Rajeev N.

WEST VANCOUVER
Comeau, Scott M.
Maher, Deviani

WHITE ROCK
Gayton, David C.
Thornton, Pamela J.

MANITOBA

WINNIPEG
Boustcha, Elizabeth M.
St John, Philip D.
Strang, David G.
Thille, Suzanne M L.
Van Ineveld, Cornelia H M.
Watson, A. Elizabeth W.

NEW BRUNSWICK

FREDERICTON
Feltmate, Patrick J G.

MONCTON
Chiasson, Guylaine

SAINT JOHN
Hobbs, Cynthia A.
Jarrett, Pamela G.
MacDonald, Elizabeth A.
MacNeil, Donna M.
Rhynold, Elizabeth S.

NOVA SCOTIA

GLACE BAY
Creighton, Paula A.

HALIFAX
Andrew, Melissa K.
Carver, Daniel J.
Freter, Susan H.
Ginther, D. Glen
Gordon, Janet E.
Koller, Katalin E.
MacKnight, Christopher R.
Mallery, Laurie H.
Moorhouse, Paige A.
Rockwood, Kenneth J.

ONTARIO

BARRIE
McKenzie, Kim R.

BRAMPTON
Baath, Jasbir S.
Baker, Andrew D.
Hussain, Fatima M.
Nesdoly, Christine H.

BRANTFORD
Braun, E. Anne

BURLINGTON
Nisker, William A.

CAMBRIDGE
Yang, John C.

ETOBICOKE
Joshipura, Mini G.

GUELPH
Noor, Amra

HAMILTON
Cowan, David D.
Gagnon, Micheline D M.
Keen, Sabina L C.
Marr, Sharon A.
McLeod, Heather C.
Misiaszek, Brian
Papaioannou, Alexandra
Patterson, Christopher J.
Peat, Mary I.
St-Onge, Joye A.
Turpie, Irene D.
Woo, Tricia K W.

KINGSTON
Armour, Christine M.
Garcia-Ameijeiras, Maria A.
Gill, Sudeep S.
Puxty, John A H.

KITCHENER
Didyk, Nicole E.
Heckman, George A W.
Sarkaria, Gagandeep S.

LONDON
Al-Aama, Tareef Y A.
Borrie, Michael
Brymer, Christopher D.
Dasgupta, Monidipa
Diachun, Laura L.
Kane, Sheri-Lynn
Montero Odasso, Manuel M.
Wells, Jennie L.

MISSISSAUGA
Chandrakumar, Sandrasegaram
Cheung, Catherine Z.
Clive, Barbara A.
Devaraj, Chikkahanumaiah
Grant, Margaret H.
Ott, Carol L B.
Page, Vesna

NEPEAN
Miller, Fraser A.

NIAGARA FALLS
Puvendran, Samuel N.

NORTH YORK
Gordon, Michael
Gotesman, Galina
Krajewski, Adam
Marotta, Giovanni C.
Petrut, Bianca
Varlese, Fabio
Veinish, Shelley L.
Yeung, Kam-Tong
Yogaparan, Thirumagal

OAKVILLE
Abid, Simona
Khan, Aliya A.

ORILLIA
Byles, Nancy I A.
Young, Kevin J.

OSHAWA
Nicula, Mihaela

OTTAWA
Afshari-Azad, Nahid
Byszewski, Anna M.
Cranney, Blanid A.
Ellen, Ruth L B.
Fitt, Nicole S.
Huang, Allen R.
Khoury, Lara
Molnar, Frank J.
Power, Barbara E.

PETERBOROUGH
Doell, Donald
Ingram, K. Jennifer
Tainsh, Susan M M.

RICHMOND HILL
Dighe, Krupa H.

SCARBOROUGH
Chan, Gabriel F P.
Lessard, Janice E.
Peto, John J.

ST CATHARINES
Safranyos, Richard G A.

SUDBURY
Clarke, Jo-Anne M.
McElhaney, Janet E.

THUNDER BAY
Bon, Trevor J.

TORONTO
Adler, Reva N.
Alibhai, Shabbir M H.
Bierman, Arlene S.
Cheng, Calvin K Y.
D'Silva, Karen
Gandell, Dov
Gilley, Heather J.
Goldenberg, Leslie
Goldlist, Barry J.
Ho, Joanne M.
Katz, Paul R.
Kirshen, Albert J.
Kormendi, Ferenc
Liu, Barbara A.
Malik, Kartika
Mehta, Rajin
Naglie, I. Gary
Ng, Karen
Norris, Mireille A.
Rochon, Paula A.
Ruth, Jonathan
Sinha, Samir K.
Straus, Sharon E.
Tal, David T.
Tsui, Vincent T.
Varga, Marica
Wong, Camilla L.
Zorzitto, Maria L.

WINDSOR
Sclater, Anne L.
Torrible, Susan J.
Yap, Hanle O.

QUÉBEC

BAIE-COMEAU
Pare, Chantal

CHICOUTIMI
Gagnon, Elisabeth

GATINEAU
Brousseau-Tremblay, Isabelle

GREENFIELD PARK
Bisson, Sebastien

LAVAL
Becker, Rubin M.

LEVIS
Thivierge, Isabelle

MONTREAL
Bacher, Yves
Bailey, Robert F.
Bergman, Howard
Bonnycastle, Michael J.
Boucher, Lucie
Brodeur, Catherine
Chiu, Wendy S W.
Dupras, Annik
Filion, Josee
Friedman, Ruby
Fung, Shek Hong
Gaba Idiamey, Francine
Gold, Susan L.
Inglis, Gary
Kergoat, Marie-Jeanne
Kissel, Catherine
Kravitz, Elliot
Lafleur, Martine
Larente, Nadine
Latour, M P. Judith
Lussier, David
Massoud, Fadi A.
Mondou, Melanie
Monette, Johanne

Morais, Jose A.
Ratner, Jack T.
Saint-Martin, Monique
Tannenbaum, Cara B.
Thibodeau, Marie-Pierre
Verdon, Josee
Vu, Thien-Tuong M.
Wan Chow Wah, Doreen Y L.

QUEBEC
Beauchemin, Jean-Pierre
Caron, Stephanie
Chevalier, Manon
Couture, Julie
Dionne, Christine
Dugas, Michel
Durand, Pierre J.
Fontaine, Jean-Guy
Fortin, Marie-Pierre
Hains, Melanie
Marchand, Eric
Morin, Jacques
Morin, Michele
Plante, Valerie
St-Laurent, Maurice

SHAWINIGAN-SUD
Savard, Pierre-Alexandre

SHERBROOKE
Baron, Michel
Brazeau, Serge
Fulop, Tamas
Hebert, Rejean
Lacombe, Guy
Lapierre, Julie
Peloquin, Marie M.
Ricard, Genevieve
Tessier, Daniel

TROIS-RIVIERES
Lavoie, Lucie

VICTORIAVILLE
Monaghan, Deborah

SASKATCHEWAN

SASKATOON
Basran, Jenny F S.

Hematological Pathology

ALBERTA

CALGARY
Fourie, Thomas M.

EDMONTON
Clarke, Gwendolyn M.
Hannon, Judith L.
Nahirniak, Susan N.
Onell, Rodrigo I.
Shier, Luke R.
Szkotak, Artur J.
Wong, Kathleen S W.

BRITISH COLUMBIA

ABBOTSFORD
Yeung, Wilson T.

BURNABY
Daw, Zohra M A.
Ho, Clinton

NEW WESTMINSTER
Haley, Lawrence P.
Morrison, Douglas M.

SURREY
Ferguson, David J.
Krikler, Samuel H.
Wong, Michelle P.

VANCOUVER
Au, Nicholas H.
Bested, Alison C.
Chipperfield, Katherine M.
Coupland, Robert W.
Dmitrienko, Svetlana
Gascoyne, Randall D.
Griswold, Deborah J.
Hudoba De Badyn, Monika
Karsan, Aly
Pi, David W.
Ramadan, Khaled M A.
Roland, Kristine J.
Smith, Tyler W.
Vercauteren, Suzanne M.
Wadsworth, Louis D.

VICTORIA
Berry, Brian R.
Cuthbert, Donna A.
Manna, Jonaki
Xu, Qiwei
Zayed, Ekram

MANITOBA

WINNIPEG
Lane, Debra
Moltzan, Catherine J.
Musuka, Charles
Sun, Ping

NEW BRUNSWICK

MONCTON
Cameron, Bruce D.
Erfaei, Afaf A E.

NOVA SCOTIA

HALIFAX
Cheng, Calvino K.
Liwski, Robert S.
Pambrun, Chantale A.
Sadek, Irene

ONTARIO

CAMBRIDGE
Saeed, Niloufer

ETOBICOKE
Adesanya, Arinola O.
Wozniak, Miranda L.

KINGSTON
Good, David J.
Matthews, John H.
Rapson, Dilys A.
Rauh, Michael J.
Shepherd, Lois E.

MISSISSAUGA
Ninos, Adam G.

NORTH YORK
Macdonald, Denis F.

OTTAWA
Giulivi, Antonio
Leung, Elaine W Y.
McBride, Eileen R A.
Padmore, Ruth F.
Sher, Graham D.
Xu, Zhaodong

SUDBURY
Gill, Kulwant S.

TORONTO
Abdelhaleem, Mohamed M M S.
Barth, David
Brien, William F.
Chang, Hong
Fernandes, Bernard J J.
Gordon, Philip
Lau, Wendy W.
Reis, Marciano D.
Sheridan, Brian L.
Wang, Chen

QUÉBEC

CHATEAUGUAY
Belanger, Robert

GRANBY
Clement, Serge

MONTREAL
Ayoub, Joseph I.
Beaulieu, Raymond
Belanger, Carl
Biron, Guy L.
Boileau, Jacques
Bonny, A M. Yvette
David, Michele
Gyger, Martin
Haliotis, Photini
Lapointe, Yves
Le May, Jacques P.
Leclerc, Jean-Marie
Neemeh, Jean A.
Perreault, Claude
Trempe, Germain L.

QUEBEC
Dumas, Olivier

SAINT-HYACINTHE
Cuirot, Gilles

ST CHARLES BORROMEE
Comtois, Robert
Ghobril, Victor P.

TERREBONNE
Maheu, Michel
Noel, Daniel R.

VERDUN
Arjane, Georges

SASKATCHEWAN

REGINA
Alseraye, Faisal M.
Deverajalu, Ramachandran
Ledingham, Donna L.

SASKATOON
Dallas, Karen
De Coteau, John F.

Hematology

ALBERTA

CALGARY
Al-Hashmi, Hani
Blahey, Walter B.
Bosch, Mark J.
Brown, Christopher B.
Daly, Andrew
Duggan, Peter R.
Geddes, Michelle N.
Goodyear, M. Dawn
Grossman, Jennifer K.
Guilcher, Gregory M T.
Jenkins, Deirdre A.
Jones, David M.
Le, Doan Thuy
Leaker, Michael T.
Lee, Adrienne
Owen, Carolyn J.
Poon, Man-Chiu
Rydz, Natalia
Savoie, Mary-Lynn
Sayani, Farzana A.
Shafey, Mona N.
Steele, J. MacGregor
Street, Lesley E.
Thaell, John F.
Valentine, Karen A.
Wong, Michael D.
Wu, John W Y.

EDMONTON
Belch, Andrew R.
Bodnar, Melanie R.
Bolster, Lauren D.
Dower, Nancy A.
Fontaine, Amelie
Hamilton, Marlene A.
Larratt, Loree M.
Mant, Michael J.
Patterson, Jeffery M.
Peters, Anthea C.
Ritchie, D. Bruce C.
Saini, Lalit K.
Sandhu, Irwindeep
Shier, Luke R.
Turner, A. Robert
Venner, Christopher P.
Wu, Cynthia M J.
Zhu, Nancy Y.

LETHBRIDGE
Benke, Stanley M.
Brigden, Malcolm L.

BRITISH COLUMBIA

ABBOTSFORD
Galbraith, Paul F.
Hebb, Jonathan P O.

BURNABY
Lam, Wendy Y H.
Mangal, Anil
Telio, David

KELOWNA
Delorme, Michael A.
Jones, Allan R.
Khoo, Kong E.
Sutherland, Judith A.

NEW WESTMINSTER
Chan, Vicky W K.
Constantine, Maggie M.
Noble, R. Michael C.

RICHMOND
Lim, Gloria

SURREY
Gill, Karamjit K.
Shustik, Jesse D.

VANCOUVER
Ambler, Kimberley L S.
Ballem, Penny J D.
Barnett, Michael J.
Benny, W. Barrett
Boldt, Camilla L.
Carter, Cedric J.
Chen, Luke Y C.
Chipperfield, Katherine M.
Conway, Edward M.
Denegri, Jorge F.
Dix, David B.
Ezzat, Hatoon M.
Foltz, Lynda M.
Forrest, Donna L.
Hogge, Donna E.
Jackson, Shannon C.
Lee, Agnes Y Y.
Leger, Chantal S.
Leitch, Heather A.
Li, Charles H.
Nantel, Stephen
Nevill, Thomas J.
Petraszko, Tanya R.
Rodrigo, Judith A.
Shepherd, John D.
Skalska, Ursula
Song, Kevin W.
Sreenivasan, Gayatri M.
Sutherland, Heather
Toze, Cynthia L.
Tsang, Peter W K.
Ward, John H.
Wu, John K M.
Yenson, Paul R.
Zypchen, Leslie N.

VICTORIA
Browman, George P.
Cuthbert, Donna A.
Hart, Jason J.
Sparling, Terence G.
Wass, Hilary
Yee, Adrian S Y.

MANITOBA

WINNIPEG
Banerji, Versha
Bow, Eric J.
Cham, Bonnie P.
Dao, Vi Vinh B.
Doyle, John
Grimes, Ruth B.
Harris, Patricia E.
Houston, Donald S.
Israels, Sara J.
Kumar, Rajat
Lezack, Jack D.
McCusker, Patricia J.
Moltzan, Catherine J.
Ponnampalam, Arjuna
Rimmer, Emily K.
Rubinger, Morel
Seftel, Matthew D.
Skrabek, Pamela J.
Stoffman, Jayson M.
Szwajcer, David
Zarychanski, Ryan L.

NEW BRUNSWICK

MONCTON
Finn, Nicholas G.
Rubin, Sheldon H.
St-Hilaire, Eve
Whitlock, Pierre

SAINT JOHN
Comeau, Terrance B W.

NEWFOUNDLAND AND LABRADOR

ST. JOHN'S
Bergstrom, Debra J.
Grewal, Kuljit S.
Hickey, Joanne
Scully, Mary-Frances
Tompkins, Kirsty A.
Whitman, Lucinda A.

NOVA SCOTIA

DARTMOUTH
Keating, Mary-Margaret

HALIFAX
Anderson, David R.
Bernstein, Mark L.
Couban, Stephen
Fernandez, Louis A V.
Hasegawa, Wanda
Kew, Andrea K.

MacDonald, David A.
Robinson, K. Sue
Shivakumar, Sudeep P.
White, Darrell J.

ONTARIO

ANCASTER
Webert, Kathryn E.

BRAMPTON
Hammouda, M. Wahbi
Kim, Christie Y.

BRANTFORD
Kagoma, Peter K.

BURLINGTON
Christjanson, Lisa J.
Gee, Sydney R.

ETOBICOKE
Damji, Nazim F.
Lau, Robert C.

GEORGETOWN
Browning, Craig J.

HAMILTON
Arnold, Donald M.
Bacchus, Farzana R.
Bates, Shannon M.
Benger, Ann M.
Bhagirath, Vinai C.
Blajchman, Morris A.
Chan, Anthony K C.
Chan, Howard H W.
Crowther, Mark A.
Denburg, Judah
Foley, Stephen R.
Fraser, Graeme
Ghanny, Shari
Ginsberg, Jeffrey
Grand'Maison, Anne
Hayward, Catherine P M.
Kelton, John G.
Klein, Cheryl A.
Kouroukis, Chrisostomos
Leber, Brian F.
Leonard, Blair J N.
Lepic, Kylie L.
Levine, Mark N.
Lim, Wendy P W.
Marcellus, Deborah C.
Pai, Menaka
Portwine, Carol Ann.
Powers, Peter J.
Takach Lapner, Sarah L D.
Trus, Michola R.
Verhovsek, Madeleine M.
Walker, Irwin R.
Warkentin, Theodore E.
Wasi, Parveen
Weitz, Jeffrey I.

KINGSTON
Dudebout, Jill J.
Duffin, Jacalyn M.
Eisenhauer, Elizabeth A.
James, Paula D.
Lee, David H.
Lillicrap, David P.
Meyer, Ralph M.
Smith, Anne M.

KITCHENER
MacEachern, Janet A.
McCarron, Bonnie I.
Stevens, Robert L.
Tam, Amy S.

LONDON
Chin-Yee, Ian
Dingle, Brian
Gob, Alan
Hsia, Cyrus C.
Kocha, Walter H.
Lohmann, Reinhard C.
Mangel, Joy E.
Minuk, Leonard
Xenocostas, Anargyros
Zeller, Michelle P.

MISSISSAUGA
Ernst, Blair D.
Kwan, Terry
Lee, Christina D.
Zaretsky, Yael S.

NEPEAN
Morrin, Sharon M L.

NEWMARKET
Anglin, Peter J.
Luk, Cynthia S Y.
Rahim, Yasmin H.
Villeneuve, Pierre

NORTH YORK
Berger, Sam
Ingber, Sarah A.
Roitman, Daryl S.
Silverman, Jeffrey A.

OAKVILLE
Lee, Andrea
McPhaden, John

OSHAWA
Chiu, Hak M.
Naassan, Anthony E.
Paramsothy, Koushalya
Schattner, Ariah J.
Woods, Anthony C.

OTTAWA
Allan, David
Alwasaidi, Turki A M.
Bence-Bruckler, Isabelle A.
Bormanis, Janis
Carrier, Marc
Conrad, David
Duffett, Lisa D M.
Faught, Carolyn R.
Forgie, Melissa A.
Goldman, Mindy R.
Gonsalves, Carol
Hamadah, Abdulaziz A.
Ho, Jenny M.
Huebsch, Lothar B.
Jacques, Cindi N.
Khamisa, Karima
Klaassen, Robert J.
Lacroix, Linda A M.
Mandel, Karen M.
McBride, Eileen R A.
Padmos, M. Andrew
Rodger, Marc A.
Saidenberg, Elianna
Scarvelis, Dimitrios
Sheppard, Dawn C.
Sullivan, Arthur K.
Tay, Jason
Taylor, J. Robert M.
Tinmouth, Alan T.
Toupin, Melissa
Van Der Jagt, Richard H C.
Wells, Philip S.
Wu, Grace C Y.
Young, Vincent P J.

PETERBOROUGH
Swain, Gordon J.

RICHMOND HILL
Grossman, Lawrence
Muir, Erin E A.
Tweeddale, Mary E.

SAULT STE MARIE
Hill, Danny G.

SCARBOROUGH
Colwill, Richard W.
Krieger, Henry

ST CATHARINES
Samosh, Martin L.

SUDBURY
Gill, Kulwant S.
Herst, Jordan A.
Lopez, Pedro G.

THUNDER BAY
Kahlon, Amrit
Kotchetkov, Rouslan I.
Laferriere, Nicole B.
Vergidis, Dimitrios

TORONTO
Al-Tarshi, Muna T A.
Amato, Dominick J.
Andreou, Efrosini R.
Baker, Michael A.
Barth, David
Blanchette, Victor S.
Boyd, Norman F.
Brandwein, Joseph
Buckstein, Rena
Callum, Jeannie L.
Carcao, Manuel
Castonguay, Vincent
Chen, Christine I.
Cheng, Susanna Y.
Cheung, Matthew C T.
Chodirker, Lisa
Crump, Michael R.
Cserti-Gazdewich, Christine M.
Disperati, Patricia
Dror, Yigal
Guirguis, Hany R Y.
Hannach, Barbara R.
Hicks, Lisa K.
Hitzler, Johann K.
Hogg, David H.
Hsiao, Janey S C.
Imrie, Kevin R.
Jay, Richard M.
Kahr, Walter H A.
Keating, Armand
Kukaswadia, Sadiya S.
Kukreti, Vishal
Kuo, Kevin H.
Kuruvilla, John G.
Liew, Elena
Lin, Yulia
McLeod, Anne G.
Meharchand, Jacinta M.
Naessens, Veronique
Olivieri, Nancy F.
Pavenski, Katerina
Pearson, Derek S.
Pendergrast, Jacob M.
Piliotis, Eugenia
Poldre, Peeter A.
Prica, Anca
Sawka, Carol A.
Schimmer, Aaron D.
Schuh, Andre C.
Seidenfeld, Allan M.
Selby, Rita
Shehata, Nadine
Shepherd, Frances A.
Sholzberg, Michelle
Sung, Lillian
Teitel, Jerome M.
Trinkaus, Martina A.
Trudel, Suzanne M.
Wang, Jean C Y.
Wells, Richard A.
Williams, Brent A.
Wilson, Jonathan J.
Yee, Karen W L.
Yeo, Erik L.

WINDSOR
Abu-Zahra, Hakam T.
Kanjeekal, Sindu M.

YORK
Rudinskas, Leona C.

PRINCE EDWARD ISLAND

CHARLOTTETOWN
Dryer, Dagny E.

QUÉBEC

CHATEAUGUAY
Belanger, Robert

CHICOUTIMI
Rousseau, Come
Simard, Herve
Simard, Raynald

COWANSVILLE
Koopmann, Peter
Sirhan, Shireen M.

GATINEAU
Abou-Nassar, Karim E.
Azzouzi, Khalid
Gaudet, Sylvie

GREENFIELD PARK
Boisjoly, Josie-Anne
Desjardins, Pierre
Devaux, Celine
Fox, Susan B.
Latreille, Jean
Nguyen, Trung Nghia
Samson, Benoit
Sperlich, Catherine

LACHINE
Brox, Alan G.

LAVAL
Aucoin, Nathalie
Boursier, Manon
Comeau, Reginald
Lapointe, Carole
Lavoie, Catherine
Raymond, Nicolas
Talbot, Danielle
Tremblay, Christine

LEVIS
Belanger, Mario
Lavoie, Andre

LONGUEUIL
Ferland, Emery
Poupart, Charles

MONT-LAURIER
Peloquin, Robert

MONTREAL
Abish, Sharon B.
Alcindor, Jean J T.
Assouline, Sarit
Aubin, Francine
Ayoub, Joseph I.
Bachand, Andre
Balicki, Danuta M.
Bambace, Nadia
Beaudet, Julie
Beaulieu, Raymond
Belanger, Carl
Belanger, Daniel
Bergeron, Julie
Bernard, Lea
Bestawros, Alain
Biron, Guy L.
Blais, Normand
Blake, Geoffrey P.
Blostein, Mark D.
Boileau, Jacques
Bonny, A M. Yvette
Busque, Lambert
Caplan, Stephen N.
Cassis, Chantal
Cellot, Sonia
Chamakhi, Ines
Champagne, Josette
Charpentier, Danielle
Cohen, Sandra R A.
Cournoyer, Denis
Dalfen, Richard
David, Michele
Delisle, Jean-Sebastien
Diaconescu, Razvan
Dionne, Jean-Luc
Doucet, Stephane
Duval, Michel
Fish, Douglas
Fleury, Isabelle
Gaudet, Guylaine P.
Girouard, Caroline
Guevin, Raymond
Gyger, Martin
Hebert, Josee
Hings, Ingrid M.
Hirsh, Vera
How, Jonathan
Hume, Heather
Jamal, Rahima
Johnson, Nathalie
Kassis, Jeannine
Khakee, Shamshuddin G.
Kiss, Thomas L.
Lachance, Sylvie
Laneuville, Pierre J.
Langleben, Adrian
Laplante, Jacques
Lavallee, Vincent P.
Laverdiere, Caroline
Le May, Jacques P.
Leblanc, Richard
Leclerc, Jean-Marie
Lemieux, Bernard
Lemieux-Blanchard, Emilie
Lesperance, Bernard
Letendre, Francois
Mitchell, David A.
Mollica, Luigina
Moquin, Jean-Pierre
Mouaikel, Elie
Neemeh, Jean A.
Olney, Harold J.
Patenaude, J J. Francois
Pelletier, Patricia
Perreault, Claude
Pichette, Roxanne
Popradi, Gizelle A.
Prchal, Jaroslav F.
Rajan, Raghu D.
Rioux-Massé, Benjamin
Rivard, Georges E.
Robitaille, Danielle
Robitaille, Nancy
Rosenberg, Arthur
Rousseau, Julie
Routy, Jean-Pierre G.
Roy, Denis-Claude
Roy, Jean
Roy, Josee-Anne
Samson, Yvan
Sauvageau, Guy J L.
Sebag, Michael
Seguin, Chantal
Shamy, April A.
Shustik, Chaim
Solymoss, Susan
Soulieres, Denis
Spurll, Gwendoline M.
St-Louis, Jean
Stern, Donna
Storring, John M.
Tosikyan, Axel
Trempe, Germain L.
Vincent, Anne-Marie
Warner, Margaret N.
Whittemore, N. Blair
Whittom, Renaud
Winikoff, Rochelle
Yelle, Louise
Zidulka, Joan R.

POINTE-CLAIRE
Katz, Max G.

QUEBEC
Auger, Pierre L.
Barabe, Frederic
Bergeron, Marc
Cantin, Guy
Cloutier, Stephanie
Cote-Brisson, Linda
Couture, Felix
Delage, Robert
Demers, Christine
Doyle, A I. Catherine
Drolet, Yvan
Filion, Alain
Gallagher, Genevieve
Lalancette, Marc
Laroche, Vincent

Larouche, Jean-Francois
Larouche, Valerie
Lavoie, Marianne
Leblond, Pierre F.
Lemieux, Julie
Levesque, Eric
Lyonnais, Jean
Marceau, Daniele
Martel, Nadine
Michon, Bruno
Ouellet, Pierre
Petitclerc, Claude
Shields, Claude
Tessier, Claude
Villeneuve, Bertrand

RIMOUSKI
Allard, Joffre C.
Blais, Andre
Gagnon, Gabrielle
Lepine, Jean
Letourneau, Yves
Levesque, Georges
Marquis, Katerine

SAINT-EUSTACHE
Jao, Kevin

SAINT-HYACINTHE
Cuirot, Gilles
Girard-Desbiens, Catherine
Perreault, Francois

SAINT-JEROME
Charron, Maryse
Cournoyer, Ghislain
De Bellefeuille, Claude
Desy, Madeleine
Lessard, Marie-Claude
Montminy-Metivier, Stephane

SAINT-LAURENT
Lebrun, Andre

SAINT-LEONARD
Derghazarian, Chahe B.

SALABERRY DE VALLEYFIELD
Buck, Michael

SHERBROOKE
Beauregard, Patrice
Brossard, Josee
Castilloux, Jean-Francois
Delisle, Line
Dufresne, Jean
Knecht, Hans
Le Blanc, Richard
Lepine-Martin, Mariette

SOREL-TRACY
St-Germain, Paul

ST CHARLES BORROMEE
Comtois, Robert
Santikyan, Sarkis

ST JEAN SUR RICHELIEU
Dubreuil-Moisan, Nathalie
Foley, Marie-Claude
Lacroix, Annie
Nouh, Elias

TERREBONNE
Ah-Lan, Christopher
Archambault-Grenier, Marie-Anne
Jamali, Hossein
Noel, Daniel R.

TROIS-RIVIERES
Aucoin, Jean-Sebastien
Blanchette, Pierre J.
Caron, Johanne
Carrier, Christian
Chapdelaine, Sylvie
Mignault, Chantal
Peters, Claire
Tremblay, Anouk

VERDUN
Arjane, Georges
Barrette, Stephane
Champagne, Martin A.
Moghrabi, Albert

SASKATCHEWAN

SASKATOON
Brose, Kelsey M J.
Card, Robert T.
Harding, Sheila M R.
MacKay, Rebecca E.
Moodley, U. Otto
Sheridan, David P.
Stakiw, Julie

YUKON TERRITORY

WHITEHORSE
Kaegi, Andrew

Infectious Diseases

ALBERTA

CALGARY
Chaubey, Vikas P.
Chawla, Rupesh
Chu, Angel K M.
Church, Deirdre L.
Conly, John M.
Culman, Kate N.
Gill, M. John
Gregson, Daniel B.
Ho, Tze May
Holton, Donna L.
Horne, Duff D.
Jadavji, Tajdin P.
Janvier, Jack A.
Johnson, Andrew S.
Kellner, James D.
Kim, Joseph
Kuhn, Susan M.
Larios, Oscar
Laupland, Kevin B.
Lemay, Mireille D.
Louie, Marie
MacPhail, Gisela L P.
Meatherall, Bonnie L.
Megran, David W.
Parkins, Michael D.
Pattullo, Andrew L S.
Rabin, Harvey R.
Read, Ronald R.
Vanderkooi, Otto G.
Vaughan, Stephen D.
Vayalumkal, Joseph

EDMONTON
Ahmed, Rabia A.
Akai, Peter S.
Bowman, Michael E.
Boychuk, Lesia R.
Chiu, Isabelle
Cooper, Ryan D.
Doucette, Karen E.
Forgie, Sarah
Harrison, Robyn A.
Hoang, Holly
Houston, Stanley C.
Humar, Atul
Joffe, A. Mark
Joffe, Ari
Kanji, Jamil
Kumar, Deepali
Lee, Bonita E.
Robinson, Joan
Rosser, Stuart J.
Saxinger, Lynora M.
Shafran, Stephen D.
Singh, Ameeta E.
Sligl, Wendy I.
Smith, Stephanie W.
Taylor, Geoffrey D.
Tse-Chang, Alena W.
Vaudry, Wendy L A.

ST. ALBERT
Hussein, Ahmed

BRITISH COLUMBIA

DUNCAN
MacKenzie, Louisa K.

KELOWNA
Blondel-Hill, Edith M.
Ferris, Dwight A N.

NANAIMO
Forrest, David M.

NEW WESTMINSTER
Malhotra, Sangita
Reynolds, Steven C.

PRINCE GEORGE
Abelson, William H.
Hamour, Abuobeida

RICHMOND
Vortel, Jerry J.

SURREY
Chapman, Michael G.
Henwick, Scott
Leblanc, Louiselle
MacK, Benjamin J.
Mirzanejad, Yazdan

VANCOUVER
Brunham, Robert C.
Cunningham, Jane A.
Deans, Gregory
Dinh, Quynh-Dao
Finlay, Jane D C.
Grant, Jennifer M.
Hajek, Jan J.
Hull, Mark
Krajden, Mel
Lester, Richard
Leung, Victor
Montessori, Valentina C.
Murray, Melanie C M.
Patrick, David M.
Peters, Laurenna D.
Phillips, Peter
Plewes, Katherine A.
Press, Natasha M.
Reynolds, Robert P.
Roberts, Ashley D.
Sauve, Laura J.
Stefanovic, Aleksandra
Yang, Tung C.

VICTORIA
Galbraith, John C T.
Ghesquiere, Wayne
Hammond, Karsten M.
Partlow, Eric S.

MANITOBA

WINNIPEG
Becker, Marissa
Bovell, Frank M.
Bow, Eric J.
Bullard, Jared M P.
Crockett, Maryanne E.
Embil, John
Embree, Joanne
Fanella, Sergio T.
Hammond, Gregory W.
Kabani, Amin M.
Kasper, Kenneth D.
Lo, Evelyn
Nicolle, Lindsay E.
Orr, Pamela H.
Plourde, J J. Pierre
Smith, Catherine A.
Thottingal, Paul A.
Walkty, Andrew J.

NEW BRUNSWICK

FREDERICTON
Doroshenko, Alexander

MONCTON
Dow, Gordon C K.
Girouard, Gabriel
Smyth, Daniel J.

SAINT JOHN
Salmon, Joanne

NEWFOUNDLAND AND LABRADOR

ST. JOHN'S
Bridger, Natalie A.
Daley, Peter

NOVA SCOTIA

DARTMOUTH
Hermann, Laura L.

HALIFAX
Davis, Ian R C.
Forward, Kevin R.
Haase, David A.
Hatchette, Todd F.
Johnston, B. Lynn
Langley, Joanne M.
MacDonald, Nora Noni E.
Mailman, Timothy L.
Marrie, Thomas J J.
McNeil, Shelly A.
Top, Karina A M.

KENTVILLE
DiQuinzio, Melanie L.

ONTARIO

AJAX
Kitai, Ian C.
Silverman, Michael S.

BARRIE
Khosrovaneh, Amir K.

BELLEVILLE
Zoutman, Dick E.

BRAMPTON
Borgia, Sergio M.
Richardson, David C.

BRANTFORD
Pennie, Ross A.
Szakacs, Thomas A.

BURLINGTON
Jeans, E. Rose

CAMBRIDGE
Glavin, Verne J.

ETOBICOKE
Al Mohri, Huda A G.
Allen, Vanessa G.
Baqi, S. Mahin

HAMILTON
Bader, Mazen
Goldfarb, David M.
Haider, Shariq
Johnstone, Jennie
Lee, Christine H C.
Leto, Daniela L.
Loeb, Mark B.
Main, Cheryl L.
O'Shea, Timothy M.
Pernica, Jeffrey M.
Singhal, Nishma
Smaill, Fiona M.
Smieja, Marek J.
Woodward, Kevin S.
Yamamura, Deborah L R.

KINGSTON
Evans, Gerald A.
Onyett, Heather A.
Wobeser, Wendy L.

KITCHENER
Ciccotelli, William A.
Liu, Theresa T.

LONDON
Elsayed, Sameer
Salvadori, Marina I.
Thompson, Guy W S.
Zahariadis, George

MARKHAM
Lingley, Michael D.
Sales, Valerie

MISSISSAUGA
Chakrabarti, Sumontra
Graham, Christopher
Ostrowska, Krystyna I.
Sarabia, Alicia
Small, Lorne N.

NEPEAN
Law, Barbara J.

NIAGARA FALLS
Elkout, Lotfia

NORTH YORK
Baghdadlian, Hovsep
Lee, Vivian T P.
Minnema, Brian J.
Yip, Clarwyn

OAKVILLE
Rau, Neil V.
Warren, Thomas A.

OSHAWA
Chkrebtii, Natalia O.
Ricciuto, Daniel R.

OTTAWA
Angel, Jonathan B.
Brooks, James I.
Brophy, Jason C.
Cooper, Curtis L.
Costiniuk, Cecilia T.
Garber, Gary E.
Hui, Charles P S.
Jessamine, Peter G.
Le Saux, Nicole M A.
Lee, B. Craig
MacPherson, Paul A.
Majewski, Jakub
McCarthy, Anne E.
Pham-Huy, Anne
Rose, Gregory W.
Roth, Virginia R.
Samson, Lindy M.
Schreiber, Yoko S.
Slinger, Robert W.
Suh, Kathryn N.
Tam, W S. Theresa
Touchie, Claire E.
Toye, Baldwin W.
Varghese, Sunil A.

RICHMOND HILL
Chen, Danny K.

SAULT STE MARIE
Barrett, Lisa

SCARBOROUGH
John, Susan
Lovinsky, Reena
Ricci, Joseph A.

SUDBURY
Sandre, Roger M.

THUNDER BAY
Gamble, D. Gregory

TORONTO
Al-Maani, Amal S S.
Allen, Upton D.
Banerji, Anna
Bitnun, Sean A.
Bogoch, Isaac I.
Bunce, Paul E.
Chan, Adrienne K.
Christian, Michael D.
Daneman, Nick
Desai, Shalini
Downing, Mark
Gardam, Michael A.
Gold, Wayne L.
Gough, Kevin A.
Grennan, J. Troy
Hota, Susy S.
Katz, Kevin C.
Kaul, Rupert
Khan, Kamran M.
Liles, W. Conrad
Loutfy, Mona R.
Low, Donald E.
MacDonald, Kelly S.
Matlow, Anne G.
Matukas, Larissa M.
Mazzulli, Tonino
McCready, Janine
McGeer, Allison J.
Mishra, Sharmistha
Morris, Andrew M.
Morris, Shaun K.
Mubareka, Samira
Muller, Matthew P.
Murthy, Srinivas
Nadarajah, Jeya T.
Ostrowski, Marian A.
Ota, Kaede
Page, Andrea V.
Poutanen, Susan M.
Powis, Jeff E.
Rachlis, Anita R.
Richardson, Susan E.
Rosenthal, Alana J.
Science, Michelle E I.
Sharkawy, Abdul Q A.
Simor, Andrew E.
Song, Howard H.
Srigley, Jocelyn A.
Sung, Lillian
Taggart, Linda R.
Tan, Darrell H S.
Thampi, Nisha
Tran, D. Jeffrey
Vellend, Hillar
Wadhwa, Anupma
Walmsley, Sharon L.
Waters, Valerie J.

WINDSOR
Quan, Corinna M.

QUÉBEC

COWANSVILLE
Michaud, Sophie

GATINEAU
Baptiste-Desruisseau, Dinah

GREENFIELD PARK
Mak, Anton
Yared, Nada

LACHINE
Teltscher, Marty S.

LAVAL
Bergevin, Marco

LONGUEUIL
Blouin, Valerie
Cohen, Linda

MONTREAL
Autmizguine, Julie
Barriga, Peter C.
Beauchamp, Elizabeth
Behr, Marcellus A.
Bourgault, Anne-Marie
Buteau, Chantal
Coutlee, Francois
Dascal, Andre
Demers, Anne-Marie
Di Iorio, Daniela
Frenette, Charles H.
Girouard, Yves
Greenaway, Christina A.
Horn, Ruth
Kakkar, Fatima
Karatzios, Christos
Kelly, Mirabelle
Klein, Marina B.
Knowles, Kathleen F.
Labbe, Annie-Claude
Labrecque, Louise-Genevieve
Laferriere, Celine
Lalonde, Richard G J.
Lamarre, Valerie
Laroche, Marc C.
Lavallee, Christian
Laverdiere, Michel
Lebel, Marc
Lee, Todd C.
Lemieux, Claude
Libman, Michael D.
Loo, Vivian G.
Luong, Me-Linh
McDonald, Jane C.
Mendelson, Jack
Moore, Dorothy L.
Oughton, Matthew T.
Papenburg, Jesse
Plamondon, Mireille
Quach-Thanh, Caroline
Qureshi, Salman T.
Renaud, Christian
Rouleau, Danielle
Rubin, Earl E.
Saint-Jean, Maude
Semret, Makeda
Sheppard, Donald
Su, Shih-Hann
Trifiro, Silvana G.
Turner, Stephen A.
Vinh, Donald C.
Yansouni, Cedric
Zaharatos, Gerasimos J.

POINTE-CLAIRE
Arrieta, Maria-Jesus
Billick, Kendall

QUEBEC
Cote, M E G. Louise
Gourdeau, Marie
Ruest, Annie
Senay, Helene
Soucy, Genevieve
Thibeault, Roseline

RIMOUSKI
Jutras, Philippe A.

SAINT-EUSTACHE
Lamothe, Francois

SAINT-HYACINTHE
Eymard, Daniel

SAINT-JEROME
Bailey, Luc

SALABERRY DE VALLEYFIELD
Allan, James P.
Vigeant, Patrice

SHERBROOKE
Allard, Catherine
Bergeron, Cybele
Sinave, Christian P.
Valiquette, Louis

ST JEAN SUR RICHELIEU
Lauzon, Dominique

VERDUN
Yechouron, Ariane

SASKATCHEWAN

REGINA
Wong, Alexander

SASKATOON
McClean, Karen L.
McConnell, Athena
Robichaud, Sophie
Sanche, Stephen E.
Skinner, Stuart J.
Takaya, Sachiko
Tan, Ben J K.
Williams, Kurt E.
Wong, Alice H M.

Internal Medicine

ALBERTA

BONNYVILLE
Ndovi, Edwards D.

CALGARY
Abu-Hakima, Maysan
Adamiak, Eugene J.
Adams, Fatin M H.
Aggarwal, Sandeep G.
Ahmed, Sofia B.
Al-Hashmi, Hani
Al-Hejily, Wesam A S.
Al-Qoofi, Faisal T Y.
Ali, Khan
Altabbaa, Ghazwan
Alvarez, A. Nanette
Alvarez, George F.
Anderson, Todd J.
Andrews, Christopher N.
Asfaha, Samuel
Aspinall, Alexander I.
Atkinson, Martin H.
Au, Selena S.
Bacchus, Catherine M.
Bailey, Jennifer L.
Banijamali, Hamid S.
Barber, Claire
Barnabe, Cheryl C M.
Barr, Susan G.
Basic, Doris
Bass, Adam
Bass, Sydney
Bassyouni, Hanan A.
Baylis, Barry W.
Bebb, Dafydd G.
Beck, Paul L.
Belenkie, Israel
Belletrutti, Paul J.
Berthiaume, Luc R.
Bharwani, Aleem M.
Bhayana, Shelly
Blahey, Walter B.
Bloomberg, Gary B.
Blustein, Philip K.
Boiteau, Paul J E.
Boscan, Alejandra
Bosch, Mark J.
Boucher, Paul E.
Boyne, Timothy S.
Bramwell-Wesley, Vivien H C.
Bridges, Ronald J.
Brown, Christopher B.
Burak, Kelly W.
Burback, Darren C.
Buresi, Michelle
Burgess, Ellen D.
Burns, Michele A.
Burs, Simona C.
Butalia, Sonia
Campbell, Norman R.
Card, Cynthia M.
Castillo, Eliana
Chalmers-Nixon, Tara S.
Champagne, Patrick
Chan, John S.
Charbonneau, Francois
Chaubey, Vikas P.
Chee, C M. Alex
Cheng, Edwin J.
Cheng, Ting
Chopra, Angeli
Chou, Julie P.
Chou, Sophia H.
Chrusch, Carla A.
Chu, Angel K M.
Chu, Yuen Mei
Church, Deirdre L.
Cleary, Cynthia E.
Coderre, Sylvain P.
Coffin, Carla S.
Cohen, Adrienne F.
Cohen, James M.
Cole, Martin J.
Congly, Stephen E.
Conly, John M.
Conradie, Johan A.
Cook, D. Roy
Cook, Donald R.
Corenblum, Bernard
Crawford, Anne-Marie
Cross, David
Curley, Michael A.
Curtis, Michael J.
Daly, Andrew
Datta, Partha
Dave, Amritlal
Davidson, Warren
Davis, John
Dear, Richard A R.
Deol, Sandeep
Desreux, Michelle R.
Devlin, Shane
Doctor, Joel
Doig, Christopher
Donovan, Lois E.
Dowden, Scott D.
Dube, Jeanne C.
Duggan, Peter R.
Duncan, Stephen C.
Dunne, Fiona M.
Easaw, Jacob C.
Easton, Paul A.
Edwards, Alun
Edworthy, Steven
Exner, Derek V.
Fabreau, Gabriel
Fell, Charlene D.
Feng, Xiumei
Ferland, Andre
Field, Stephen K.
Fifi-Mah, Aurore
Filipchuk, Neil G.
Fisher, Dina A.
Fisher, Michael J.
Fitzgerald, Avril
Flemons, W. Ward
Ford, Gordon
Fraser, Kristin L.
Fripp, Amber G.
Fritzler, Marvin J.
Fruetel, Karen
Geddes, Michelle N.
Gelberg, Jacob
Ghali, William A.
Giannoccaro, John P.
Gibson, Paul S.
Gill, M. John
Gilmour, Janet G.
Girard, Louis-Phillipe
Godinez-Luna, Tomas
Goodhart, David M.
Goodyear, M. Dawn
Grant, Andrew D M.
Gregson, Daniel B.
Grinman, Susana E Z.
Grisdale, William R.
Groshaus, Horacio
Grossman, Jennifer K.
Groves, Terence
Grundy, Peter D.
Gupta, Milli
Hames, Linda
Hamilton, Douglas R.
Hanley, David A.
Hanly, Patrick J.
Hansen, James L.
Har, Bryan J N.
Haussmann, Jessica
Haw For Chin, Oliver R.
Hawkins, Ralph G.
Hawkins, T. Lee-Ann
Hazlewood, Glen S.
Heitman, Steven J.
Helmersen, Douglas S.
Hemmelgarn, Brenda
Heng, Daniel Y C.
Henning, Jan-Willem
Herman, Robert J.
Hershfield, Noel B.
Hill, Michael
Hilsden, Robert J.
Hirani, Naushad
Ho, Tze May
Hogan, David B.
Holroyd-Leduc, Jayna M.
Holton, Donna L.
Hons, Ronald B.
Horne, Duff D.
Howarth, Andrew G.
Howlett, Jonathan
Hoyte, Keith M.
Huan, Susan D.
Hull, Russell D.
Hulme, W. Terrance
Hutchison, Stuart J.
Isaac, Debra L.
James, Matthew T.
James, Paul D.
Janovcik, Juraj E.
Janvier, Jack A.
Jarand, Julie M.
Jayakumar, Saumya
Jenkins, Deirdre A.
Jhandir, Muhammad F M.
Jibb, Norma E.
Jijon, Humberto B.
Johannson, Kerri A M.
Johnson, Andrew S.
Jones, David M.
Jordan, Michaela R V.
Jung, Marek A.
Kaminska, Elzbieta A.
Kanani, Ronak S.
Kaplan, Gilaad
Kapoor, Anmol S.
Kavanagh, Katherine
Kazmi, Mustapha H.
Kealey, Angela J.
Kennedy, Richard J.
Khaliq-Kareemi, Munaa
Khosla, Munish
Kim, Joseph
Kinnear, Susan E.
Kirby, Ann S.
Klassen, John
Kline, Gregory A.
Knudtson, Merril L.
Kothandaraman, Maitreyi
Kramer, Andreas H.
Krause, Vanessa S.
Kryski, Albert
Kumar, Puja R.
Kuriachan, Vikas P.
Kwok, Jimmy C W.
Lam, Calvin
Landry, Jennifer M.
Larios, Oscar
Lau, David C W.
Laupland, Kevin B.
Lautner, David
Le Clercq, Sharon
Leblanc, Paul E.
Lee, Adrienne
Lee, Samuel S.
Leigh, Richard
Lemaire, Jane B.
Lesoway, Robert N.
Leung, Alexander A.
Leung, Yvette P Y.
Lewkonia, Raymond M.
Li, Pin
Lim, Thomas W P.
Loewen, Andrea H S.
Lohmann, Tara E.
Louie, Marie
Louie, Thomas J.
Love, Jonathan R.

SPECIALISTS BY PROVINCE

Lupichuk, Sasha M.
Lutterodt, Alfred
Ma, Irene W Y.
Ma, Ling Ling
Ma, Michael Z.
Ma, Patrick
MacEachern, Paul
MacKay, Elizabeth A.
MacPhail, Gisela L P.
MacRae, Jennifer M.
Manns, Braden J.
Martin, William O.
Mason, Cindy A.
McIlhargey, Trina L.
McKeen, Julie A.
Meatherall, Bonnie L.
Meddings, Jonathan
Megran, David W.
Meldrum, Donald
Mellor, Jeffrey
Minty, Evan
Mintz, Marcy J.
Misra, Tarun
Mitchell, L. Brent
Mody, Christopher H.
Mohamed, Rachid
Monzon, Jose G.
Morris, Donald G.
Morris, Gary L.
Mortis, Garth P.
Mosher, Dianne P.
Muruve, Daniel A.
Mustata, Stefan
Myers, Robert P.
Mylonas, Ilias
Nanji, Alykhan
Niven, Daniel J.
Noseworthy, Thomas W.
Novak, Kerri L.
O'Brien, Edward R M.
Owen, Carolyn J.
Panaccione, Remo
Parekh, Praful K.
Parhar, Kuljit S.
Parkins, Michael D.
Parkins, Vicky M.
Patry, David G.
Pattullo, Andrew L S.
Pedersen, Susie D.
Pederson, D. Troy
Pendharkar, Sachin R.
Penney, Christopher J.
Penz, Erika D.
Peters, Grant L.
Pollak, P. Timothy
Poon, Man-Chiu
Povitz, Marcus
Price, Lawrence M.
Prieur, Timothy G.
Purdy, Anna C.
Quinn, Robert R.
Rabi, Doreen M.
Rabin, Harvey R.
Read, Ronald R.
Rezaie, Ali
Rimmer, Karen P.
Rioux, Kevin P.
Robertson, Lynne H.
Rodgers, Lynne K.
Roman, Michael A.
Rorstad, Otto P.
Ross, Stuart A.
Rostom, Alaa M K A.
Roy, Andre L.
Ruether, Joseph D.
Ryan, John P.
Rydz, Natalia
Sabur, Natasha F.
Sam, David X.
Sargious, Peter
Sarna, Magdalena A.
Savoie, Mary-Lynn
Sayani, Farzana A.
Schaefer, Jeffrey P.
Schmaltz, Heidi N.
Schnell, Gregory B.
Schoenroth, Leeanne J.
Schorr, Samuel
Scott, Ian M.
Scott-Douglas, Nairne W.
Sepandj, Farshad
Shafey, Mona N.
Shaffer, Eldon A.
Sharma, Nakul C.
Sheldon, Robert S.
Sherman, Thomas A.
Sigal, Ronald J.
Silvius, James L.
Simon, Jessica E.
Singh, Gurpreet
Singh, Ram R.
Slawnych, Michael P.
Smith, Eldon R.
Sood, Nidhi
Spence, Frank P.
Sporina, Jan
Stajkovic, Svetlana
Stapleton, Melanie P.
Stather, David R.
Stelfox, Henry T.
Stewart, Douglas A.
Stinton, Laura M.
Stone, James A.
Street, Lesley E.
Sumner, Glen L.
Sutherland, Lloyd R.
Swain, Mark G.
Symonds, Christopher J.
Tam, Vincent C.
Tang, Karen
Tang, Patricia A.
Taub, Kenneth J.
Ter Keurs, Hendrik
Thaell, John F.
Thakrar, Mitesh V.
Thomas, Chandra M.
Thompson, Robert G.
Tibbles, Lee Anne
Tilley, Stephen E.
Tourin, Olga
Traboulsi, Mouhieddin
Tremblay, Alain
Tsai, Willis H.
Tsang, Roger
Valentine, Karen A.
Van Olm, T M. Matthew J.
Varma, Sonya
Vaughan, Stephen D.
Veenhuyzen, George D.
Vickers, Michael M.
Viner, Sidney M.
Vitale, George D.
Walker, Brandie L.
Walley, Barbara A.
Walsh, John M.
Wang, Wenjie
Wang, Xiangyu
Warnica, J. Wayne
Warshawski, Frank J.
Watanabe, Mamoru
Webster, Marc A.
Weeks, Sarah G.
Welikovitch, Lisa
White, Alan V M.
Williams, Jennifer J.
Wilton, Stephen B.
Winston, Brent W.
Wong, Jorge A S.
Wong, Michael D.
Wong, Norman C W.
Wu, Caren M.
Wyse, D. George
Yacyshyn, Vincent J.
Yau, Jonathan C.
Yipp, Bryan G.
Zarnke, Kelly B.
Zaw-Tun, Ni Ni S.
Ziouzina, Olga
Zuege, Danny J.

EDMONTON

Aaron, Stephen L.
Abdulsamad, Atef A M.
Ahmed, Rabia A.
Akai, Peter S.
Akbar, Shafiq F.
Al-Ghamdi, Hamed S A.
AlAmeel, Turki A S.
Alagiakrishnan, Kannayiram
Alherbish, Aws J A.
Alhulaimi, Naji M A.
Almutawa, Mohammad
Alsehli, Riyadh N M.
Archibald, James S.
Au, Dick
Au, Heather-Jane
Bagshaw, Sean M.
Bailey, Robert J.
Bain, Vincent G.
Bainey, Kevin R.
Bala, Anand
Ballermann, Barbara J.
Bartha, David J.
Basappa, Naveen S.
Baur, Martin
Belch, Andrew R.
Bhutani, Mohit
Bibeau, Marc D.
Bistritz, Lana M.
Black, William R.
Bodnar, Melanie R.
Bolster, Lauren D.
Borgersen, Kaj
Bowering, C. Keith
Boychuk, Lesia R.
Boyington, Curtiss R.
Bradley, John
Brass, Neil S.
Bridgland, Lindsay J.
Brindley, Peter G.
Brisebois, Amanda J.
Bryan, Tracey L.
Buckle, Patricia M.
Butler, Craig R.
Butts, Charles A.
Caldwell, Steven S.
Campbell, Duncan A.
Campbell, Patricia M.
Carney, Dominic P.
Cernohorsky, Karel
Chaba, Todd P.
Chan, Kris H K.
Chan, Michael C Y.
Chea, Rith
Cherry, Raeleen D.
Cheung, Lawrence A.
Cheung, Po Kee.
Chiam, Benjamin T H.
Chichak, Vernon R.
Chik, Constance L.
Chin, Wu Dat N.
Chiu, Isabelle
Chiu, Peter L S L.
Choy, Jonathan B.
Chu, Siu-Chung
Chua, Neil S.
Chui, Betty K.
Cockfield, Sandra M.
Colbourne, S. Ann
Cooper, Ryan D.
Courtney, Mark J.
Craig, Kelly L.
Cujec, Bibiana
Damant, Ronald W.
Daniels, Vijay J.
Dasgupta, Mrinal
Davis, Paul
Davison, Sara
Demeria, Denny
Deved, Vinay
Dhawan, Vivek
Dickout, William J.
Dimitry, John R.
Doucette, Karen E.
Duggan, Shelley
El-Sawaf, Amro
Enenajor, Aweriarue G.
Ezekowitz, Justin A.
Fedorak, Richard N.
Fenske, Theodore K.
Ferguson, James P.
Feroe, Raquel L.
Ferrari, Robert
Fields, Anthony L A.
Fisher, Bruce W.
Fontaine, Amelie
Fulton, Dorcas S.
Ghani, Afshan Y.
Ghosh, Mahua
Gilchrist, Dawna M.
Gillson, Ashley
Goldstein, Cheryl E.
Goodhart, Joseph M.
Gourishankar, Sita
Graham, Michelle M.
Gramlich, Leah M.
Grynoch, A. Robert
Grynoch, J. Richard
Gulamhusein, Sajadhussein S.
Guo, Peter Y.
Gutfreund, Klaus S.
Halloran, Brendan P.
Halloran, Kieran
Halloran, Philip F.
Hamilton, Marlene A.
Hamilton, Peter G.
Hammer, Debra M.
Haraphongse, Mant
Hardin, Philip A.
Harley, Charles H.
Harrison, Robyn A.
Hayward, Robert S A.
Henry, Monica M.
Heule, Mark K.
Ho, Maria Y.
Hoang, Holly
Homik, Joanne E.
Hosein, Rasheed A.
Houston, Stanley C.
Hrimiuc, Ramona
Hruczkowski, Tomasz W.
Hrynchyshyn, Gregory J.
Hudson, Darren A.
Hui, William K.
Humar, Atul
Hwang, Peter M.
Ip, Shannon
Jacquier, Jennifer E.
Jindal, Kailash K.
Joffe, A. Mark
Johnson, Melissa A.
Johnston, Curtis W.
Johnstone, David E.
Jones, Alan P.
Jones, H. Niall
Kachope, J. Twinomujuni
Kaila, Kendeep S.
Kalenga, Jean-Claude M.
Kanji, Jamil
Kao, Dina H.
Kapasi, Ali M.
Karolak, Michael M.
Karvellas, Constantine J.
Kassam, Narmin
Kasza, Leslie A.
Katz, Steven J.
Keeling, Stephanie O.
Khandekar, Sayra A.
Khurana, Rshmi
Kim, Daniel H J.
Kimber, Shane K M.
King, Karen M.
Klarenbach, Scott
Kohansal Vajargah, Ali R.
Kondi, Joma
Koski, Sheryl L.
Kretzul, Eugene M.
Kroeker, Karen I.
Kumar, Deepali
Kunimoto, Dennis Y.
Kutsogiannis, Demetrios J.
Kwong, Sarah L.
Lakhani, Zaheerali
Lam, Paul H S.
Larratt, Loree M.
Lauzon, Matthew A.
Lawson, Fiona M E.
Lazarescu, Adriana
Lechelt, Katherine
Lee, Mao-Cheng
Lee, Suk-Kun
Lee, Tzu-Kuang
Leung, Raymond C M.
Leung, Winnie M W.
Lewanczuk, Richard Z.
Li, Stephanie K.
Lien, Dale C.
Lim, Allen W K.
Lim, Lawrence
Liu, Allen T L.
Liu, Julia J.
Lockwood, Evan E.
Long, G. Richard
Lutzak, Gregory D.
Lyons, Kristin J.
Ma, Mang-Ming
MacDonald, Colin F.
Mackey, John R.
Majumdar, Sumit R.
Maksymowych, Wolodymyr P.
Malowany, Leo E R.
Man, Godfrey C W.
Mant, Michael J.
Marcushamer, Samuel L.
Marion, Dennis A.
Markland, Darren M.
Matheson, J. Douglas
Matic, Kata
Mayers, Irvin
McAlister, Finlay A.
McCracken, Peter
McDermid, Jill C.
McDermid, Robert C.
McKaigney, John P.
McMahon, Alan W.
McMurtry, Michael S.
McNab, Brian D.
Melenka, Lyle S.
Mereu, Laurie E.
Michalska, Magdalena A.
Miedzinski, Lilly J.
Millan, Mario S.
Miller, Donald D.
Mitchell, Rebecca S.
Morales, Fraulein
Morrish, Donald W.
Morse, Amy L.
Mulchey, Kimberley D.
Mulder, Karen E.
Murray, Allan G.
Muzyka, Timothy G.
Nelson, Jill D.
Nerenberg, Kara A.
Nicholson, Joanne M.
Nijjar, Tirath S.
North, Scott A.
Nsair, Ali
Nutting, Michael G.
O'Neill, Blair J.
O'Reilly, Kenneth V.
Opgenorth, Andrea A.
Osman, Maisoon A.
Oswald, Anna E.
Oudit, Gavin Y.
Padwal, Rajdeep S.
Pannu, Neesh I.
Paterson, David I.
Patterson, Jeffery M.
Pauly, Robert P.
Pedersen, John E.
Pertman, Shea
Peters, Anthea C.
Pinchbeck, Melanie L.
Pisani, Amin
Preiksaitis, Jutta K.
Price Hiller, Julie A.
Qarni, Muhammad U.
Raff, Errol
Ramesh, Warren P.
Ramsay, Gillian I.
Reddy, Suresh P.
Richman-Eisenstat, Janice B Y.
Ringrose, Jennifer S.
Ritchie, D. Bruce C.
Robbins, Sarah J.
Roberts, R. Neil
Robertson, Duncan
Rockx, Marie A J.
Rokosh, Elizabeth T.
Rolfson, Darryl B.
Romanovsky, Adam S.
Romanowski, Barbara
Romney, Jacques S.
Rosser, Stuart J.
Rouget, Julia E.
Rucker, Diana
Ryan, Edmond A.
Sadowski, Daniel C.
Saini, Lalit K.
Salman, Sadik
Sandha, Gurpal S.
Sandhu, Irwindeep
Sangha, Randeep
Sasmal, Pulin B.
Sawyer, Michael B.
Saxinger, Lynora M.
Scarfe, Andrew G.
Searles, Gordon E.
Sebastian, Justin C.
Sehgal, Tarun
Selvarajah, Vijeyakumar
Semlacher, Eric A.
Senaratne, Manohara P J.
Senaratne, Savitri C.
Shafran, Stephen D.
Shanks, Miriam
Sharma, Sanjay K.
Sharma, Sudheer
Sherbaniuk, Richard W.
Shier, Luke R.

Sholter, Dalton E.
Shurraw, Sabin C N.
Shustack, Allan
Sia, Winnie W K.
Siffledeen, J. Shaalan
Siminoski, Kerry G.
Simpson, Christine L.
Singh, Ameeta E.
Sivakumaran, Sooriyakumaran T.
Skeith, Kenneth J.
Slabu, Dan L.
Sligl, Wendy I.
Smith, Stephanie W.
Smylie, Michael G B.
Sonnenberg, Brian H.
Soo, Isaac
Spratlin, Jennifer L.
Stead, Lori M.
Stollery, Daniel E.
Sugars, Benjamin J A.
Sultanian, Richard A.
Switzer, Connie M.
Syed, Atyab A N.
Szudek, Jacek
Taher, Taha H.
Takats, Laszlo N.
Tandon, Puneeta
Tapardel, Anca F.
Taylor, Dylan A.
Taylor, Geoffrey D.
Teo, Michele M.
Teshima, Christopher W.
Thompson, Stephanie E.
Thomson, Alan B R.
Todoruk, Dennis N.
Toleva, Olga I.
Tonelli, Marcello A.
Tonkin, Katia S.
Toth, Ellen L.
Turner, A. Robert
Tymchak, Wayne J.
Tyrrell, Benjamin
Tyrrell, D. Lorne J.
Ullah, Saif
Van Diepen, Sean F P.
Van Zanten, Sander J.
Venner, Christopher P.
Venner, Peter M.
Verma, Geetika E.
Vethanayagam, Dilini P.
Vijay, Sheela M.
Villeneuve, Pierre-Marc
Vonder Muhll, Isabelle F.
Voth, Arnold J.
Wahab, Nazneem N.
Walters, Brennan M A.
Watanabe, Sharon M.
Wei, Peter Y.
Weinkauf, Justin G.
Weisz, Samuel I.
Welsh, Robert C.
Williams, C. Noel
Williams, Randall G.
Wirzba, Brian J.
Wong, Clarence K W.
Wong, Eric Y L.
Wong, J. Szeman
Wong, Karen
Wong, Winnie W S.
Woo, Kenny S.
Wu, Cynthia M J.
Yacyshyn, Elaine A.
Yan, Alexander
Yehya Aladin, Jaled W.
Yeung, Albert A C L.
Zeman, Marilyn V.
Zhu, Nancy Y.
Zia, Shahzad
Zibdawi, M. Mohamad
Zygun, David A.

FORT MCMURRAY
Al-Ghamdi, Khalid H S.
Khinda, Surinder S.
Sauve, Michel D.

GRANDE PRAIRIE
Bertozzi, Hugo A R.
Best, Anthony H S.
Burris, Robert J.
Moreau, Marie A.
Nikoleychuk, Gerald
Strehlke, Claudia T.
Westra, Yolande N.

LEDUC
Bhargava, Keshav
Sprague, John H.

LETHBRIDGE
Au, Chi-Cheong
Benke, Stanley M.
Brigden, Malcolm L.
Drever, Erin
Forestell, Clair F.
Holland, David R.
Hunt, Gordon S.
Ikuta, Roland M.
Janzen, Ernest P.
Koegler, David P.
Low, Richard A.
MacKay, Alison R.
Oviatt, Patrick L.
Schuld, Richard L.
Villar, Erwin
Wilde, Eric R.
Wong, Morley P.

LLOYDMINSTER
Kostic, Zlatko
Rogers, Raymond M.

MEDICINE HAT
Azam, Adeel
Jahandardoost, Mohammad R.
Javier, Joseph J.
Soo, Tony Y.
Trudeau, Marc
Weigel, Michael A.

RED DEER
Alharbi, Abdulrahman M F.
Alqahtani, Saleh A.
Bailey, Gordon R.
Donnelly, Regina
Glady, Christine A.
Hart, Meryl E.
Heathcote, Karen
Heinrichs, Irvin H.
Jenkins, Huw
Jim, Kym Lee
Lim, Leonard
Pimm, Jeff R.
Simmonds, S. Douglas
Singh, Jitendra
Sokolowski, Colleen A.
Tarukandirwa, Callisto
Ward, Gregory J.

SHERWOOD PARK
Skjodt, Neil M.

SPRUCE GROVE
Allen, Joel
Cesarz, John A.

ST ALBERT
Bharmal, Azim A.
Gibson, Neil E.
Hoque, Mohamed N.
Hussein, Ahmed
Khadour, Fadi
Te, Luis D.
Zucker, Tal

STONY PLAIN
Chihrin, Stephen

WETASKIWIN
Au, Anita G.
Crocket, Jennifer A.
York, Ernest L.

BRITISH COLUMBIA

ABBOTSFORD
Burke, Donald G.
Chang, Peter C.
Chum, Elliott S.
Cooper, Susan E.
Costantino, Anthony D.
Friesen, Marlyce
Galbraith, Paul F.
Habib, Naiyer
Hebb, Jonathan P O.
Keith, Bruce D.
Keshmiri, Mehdi
Kucerak, Martin
Markanday, Anurag
Maung, Tun Zan
McIntyre, Grant
Min, Simon T.
Pluta, Henryk
Sayeh, Naser S.
Uhlman, Dorothy L.
Williams, Dave J.
Winston, Robert D.
Wong, Henry C H.
Yao, Shaoyee
Zulfiqar, Muhammad

BURNABY
Anderson, Heather D.
Brunt, Margaret E.
Carpenito, Gerardo
Chang, Ross E.
Chisholm, Sherrie-Anne
Dong, Sunny R.
Ghatak, Sasanka S.
Hiller, Bruce
Horne, Bruce D.
Jain, Sajal
Kang, Anna
Kim, Seung
Kwan, Susan Y L.
Lam, Wendy Y H.
Lau, Chuen-Ping
Lee, Mervin M F.
Lee, Wilson
Luongo, Rolfe M.
Monkewich, Gregory J.
Pimstone, Simon N.
Qureshi, Ehsan U.
Saberi, Farzad
Shahparaki, Aram
Sing, George
Stuart, David S.
Telio, David
Wong, Lawrence H S.
Yu, Simon
Zaidel, Patrick A.

CAMPBELL RIVER
Grace, Jennifer E.
Heath, John W.
Lee, Randolph
Mahoney, Charles J.
Man-Son-Hing, Malcolm G.

CHILLIWACK
Grills, Gordon R.
MacFadyen, Donald R.
Son, Wai Kon
Vivian, Anthony C H.
Wilson, Jennifer M.

COMOX
Camacho Maldonado, Pedro
Dang, Bao Pham N.
Engman, Richard T.
Humphreys, Karen M.
Mahmudi-Azer, Salahaddin
Nel, Pierre R.
Simice, Jaroslav J.
Thomas, Trace S.

COQUITLAM
Leung, Benjamin Y.
Sadowski, Henry A.

COURTENAY
Jenkins, Donald

CRANBROOK
Baverstock, Marcus B.
Browne, Kevin P.
Janbey, Ehsan M.
Newsome, William E.
Sawatsky, Errin L.
Wik, Lori M.

DELTA
Dhillon, Avtar S.
Jaffer, Shahin
Shaw, Robert Y.
Shin, Amanda L.
Shin, T W. Thomas

DUNCAN
O'Malley, Brendan D.
O'Shea, A. Mary
Pewarchuk, Willie J.

FERNIE
Burnett, Patricia J.

FOREST GROVE
Hughes, Ariana

KAMLOOPS
Avanessian, Ardashes
Beall, Franklin R.
Blumenauer, Barbara T.
Burgmann, Twila
Hudson, Nancy
Michaud, Marie T.
Navratil, Jan J.
Picton, Taralyn D.
Prasad, Shailendra
Proctor, Bradley R.
Schmidt, Timothy
Stabler, Christopher D.
Teichrob, Deanna M.
Tynan, Iain E T.
Wijeyesinghe, E. Cornel R.

KELOWNA
Agnew, Shane R.
Bak, Adrian W.
Baker, Sandra E.
Blondel-Hill, Edith M.
Borthistle, Bruce K.
Czerkawski, Barbara A.
Davies, Janine
Delorme, Michael A.
Dueck, Gregory
Ellard, Susan L.
Ferris, Dwight A N.
Finch, Daygen
Fort, Stephen
Foster, Ryan
Fox, Lorne M.
Godin, Anick
Halperin, Frank A.
Hodge, Steven A.
Holmes Boulton, Cheryl L.
Hooper, Richard O.
Jones, Allan R.
Jones, Charlotte A.
Kates, David M.
Khoo, Kong E.
McCauley, Graeme
McLeod, B. Daniel
Michieletti, Pina
Nash, Carla L.
Penner, Robert M.
Perini, Rafael F.
Pistawka, Kevin J.
Polasek, Petr
Rao, Sanjay C.
Render, K. Craig
Rolf, J. Douglass
Sarbit, Jay L.
Sauciuc, Nicoleta D.
Seigel, Stuart N.
Stewart, Alan R.
Sutherland, Judith A.
Taylor, Marianne J.
Taylor, Sara K.
Topic, Delilah L.
Townley, Richard
Victor, Gary H.
Welsh, Edward V.

LANGLEY
Chandler, David E.
Hollands, Laurence S.
Korosi, Judit
McDermid, Kevin P.
O'Brien, Michael M.
Surkes, Jan
Wittmann, Rita

MAPLE RIDGE
Auersperg, Edward V.
Ervin, Francis L C.
George, Deepu J.
Hughes, Barbara L.
Stanger, Hilda A D.
Tsui, Winston W H.
Wallach, Jean-Philippe

NANAIMO
Baillie, Hector M.
Baur, Nicole
Booth, Anthony D.
Carson, Rachel C C.
Croome, Alison J G.
Forrest, David M.
Glick, Naomi H G.
King, Kim W.
Kydd, Alison S.
Lai, Kevin
Lang, Michael P.
McHugh, Sean M.
McLaren, Andrew A.
McLean, Laura E.
Mitenko, Paul A.
Park, Kirily
Rasaiah, Suvi B.
Ronald, John A.
Schwarz, Niels E.
Sheriff, Maqbool K.
Silva, Vincent E.
Trajan, Marc
Winkler, Lawrence H.

NELSON
Malpass, Phillip B.
Tuvel, Brandon R.

NEW WESTMINSTER
Aminbakhsh, Amin
Arikan, Yasemin
Atkinson, Kenneth A.
Barts, Agnieszka D.
Bernard, Matthew D.
Blackie, Stephen P.
Blackwell, Margaret M.
Blake, Erin A.
Brown, Melanie L.
Brown, Robert I G.
Chan, Albert W.
Chan, Edward Y.
Chan, Vicky W K.
Chan, Victor R.
Charania, Jahangir
Chase, Jocelyn M.
Cheung, Justin
Chin, Ying Wai
Chung, Henry V.
Chung, Randy D.
Clayton, Dale B.
Constantine, Maggie M.
Da Roza, Gerald
Dehoney, Cameron J.
Dorval, Jean-Francois
Epstein, Michael N.
Fava, Craig S.
Fenton, Stanley F.
Flanagan, Cathy
Gabana, Cori-Ann
Gailey, Carol B.
Glezos, James D.
Jain, Leena
Kerrie, Jeffrey P.
Klinke, Jennifer A.
Krygier, Darin S.
Kuritzky, Robin A.
Lai, Emily J.
Lalani, Akbar V.
Lam, Sui-Sang
Lee, Julie
Li, Anson H Y.
Lin, Cassie W.
MacCarthy, John A J.
Malhotra, Samir
Malhotra, Sangita
Matossian, Sebouh M.
Mian, Mamta
Nazerali-Sunderji, M. Muni
Noble, R. Michael C.
O'Connor, M. Peter
Petrossian, Caroline
Philipp, Roger K.
Priestman, Barbara A.
Ramsden, Michael F.
Reynolds, Steven C.
Ross, Jeffrey S.
Rothwell, Robert S.
Rupka, Dennis W.
Schaffrin, Roger M.
Schwartz, Daniel

Shu, David H P.
Simkus, Gerald J.
Starko, Robert J.
Stolar, Marguerite A.
Torng, Shirley
Wallace, Clarissa
Webster, Sheila B.
Wong, Christopher K.
Yik, Kwok Yeong

NORTH VANCOUVER

Bains, Puneet
Boldt, Michael J.
Bourchier, Takashi D.
Brunham, Liam R.
Cunningham, Kenneth F.
Dewar, Catharine
Doe, Sam
Graff, Peter
Hahn, Michael E J.
Haigh, Susan E.
Haniak, William A.
Hariton, Nicolas C.
Ho, Jin K.
Imrie, John R.
Lee, D. Dae-Won
Mahmoudi, Nasim
Mainra, Rajesh R.
Mayo, Warren G.
McLeod, Kevin I.
Molavi, Massood
Rafi-Zadeh, Ebrahim
Sandhu, Naveen S.
Smiljanic, Sasha R.
Vyselaar, John R.

PENTICTON

Ashton, Thomas H.
Broder, Sarah L.
Casilla, Vanbric R.
Cleveland, David R.
Clouatre, Yves J J.
Dyck, Chadwyn L.
Forzley, Brian R.
Hochman, Jay
Kincade, David D.
Papay, Karen D.
Schneider-MacRae, Margaret L N.
Stewart, Jacqueline C.
Walker, Shannon L.
Wiesinger, Holly A R.

PORT ALBERNI

O'Dwyer, Robert L.
Taylor, Susan A.
Williams, Dorothy L.

POWELL RIVER

Hoffert, Blake M.
Takhar, Sneeta K.

PRINCE GEORGE

Bashir, Khalid
Bishop, Winston T.
Buchanan, Michael L.
Din, Fareen
Hamour, Abuobeida
Hennessy, Colleen
Hirji, Alim
Iqbal, Zafar
Katakkar, Suresh B.
Keyvani, Leila
Khalid, Muhammad R.
Lowry, Robin P.
MacRitchie, Donald M.
Mansour, Firas
Mousavi, Negareh
Olsen, Sharla-Rae J.
Smith, John T.
Winwood, Paul J.
Yacyshyn, Bruce R.

QUESNEL

Aziz, Ahmed T.

RICHMOND

Ahmed, Iqbal H.
Bar-Shlomo, Ben-Zion
Barnett, Kim E.
Boroomand-Rashti, Kayoomars
Caswell, Sherri L.
Choi, Hyon K.
Cibere, Jolanda
Dirnfeld, Victor
Fam, Ezz
Fishman, Martin J.
Forbes, Anastasia F.
Gabra, Genevieve
Haljan, Gregory
Ho, Jeremy J.
Hoeschen, Lawrence
Jakubowski, Andrew T.
Kherani, Raheem B.
Koehler, Barry E.
Lacaille, Diane V.
Lau, Edgar S T.
Lee-Son, Llewellyn
Lim, Gloria
Martinka, Grzegorz P.
Minhas, Avinder S.
Orenstein, Teddi L.
Perlman, Shelley D.
Sahiholnasab, S. Vahid
Vortel, Jerry J.
Wong, Chet G.
Wong, Steven
Wong, Victor K.
Yeung, Margaret M W.
You, Yong Dong
Yun, John W S.

SAANICHTON

Koziol, Kathie A.

SALMON ARM

Main, Christopher D.
McKee, Scott D.

SALT SPRING ISLAND

Morse, John W I.

SECHELT

Morantz, Jesse
Wadge, Sara M.

SIDNEY

Seigo, Raymond L.

SURREY

Abrahams, Zuheir
Al-Tourah, Abdulwahab J.
Ali, M. Iqbal
Au, Stephanie Y P.
Bhagirath, Kapil M.
Bon, Richard R.
Bourque, Sylvie A.
Cass, Aaron I.
Chan, Theresa W.
Chapman, Michael G.
Cheung, Stephen S K.
Constantine, Charles T.
Davidson, James A.
Do, Thuan Hieu
Donaldson, Bruce W.
Dong, Raymond
Feige, Richard R R.
Gill, Karamjit K.
Giustino, Giuseppe
Hiralal, Rajesh
Ho, Hip Wah
Hong, Harry H L.
Janda, Surinder P.
Johal, Balvindar S.
Kang, Parmjit S.
Karim, Mohamud A.
Karim, Zamil
Khan, A M. Safiqul I.
Khurana, Reena
Kornder, Jan M.
Kwan, Winkle B.
Lawson, Edward J.
Le, Lyly H.
Leblanc, Louiselle
Lee, Christopher W K.
Lee, Ursula J Y M.
Leonard, Russell K.
Liao, Joy
MacK, Benjamin J.
Mahony, Christopher J.
Martin, Lee Ann
Martin, Perry M.
McCormack, Grant S.
Mirzanejad, Yazdan
Nagaria, Neelam
Oja, Conrad D.
Pansegrau, Gary K.
Pearce, Stephen A.
Perlman, Michael J.
Pillay, Shunmoogam W.
Prakash, Suma
Prest, Marcia E H.
Rudnik, James E.
Sawhney, Ravinder P S.
Schachter, Michael E.
Schroeder, Benjamin D.
Severin, Naomi E.
Shariff, Salima N.
Shustik, Jesse D.
Singham, Janakie
Smith, John S.
Stafford, Sara G.
Tan, Peter K H.
Turner, Mark O.
Vohra, Sanjeev
Watanabe, Hiroko
Wong, Henry D.
Yelle, Carole-Anne L.
Yerman, Todd J.
Yorke, Alan J.

TERRACE

Kenyon, Michael R.
Lim, Jean-Paul
Phillips, Barrie L.

TRAIL

Ghosh, Surajit
Ksiazek, Danuta
Mountain, Scott A.
Scotland, Newborne
Zhang, Chi

VANCOUVER

Abdulla, Alnoor
Abou Mourad, Yasser
Alenezi, Osamah H S S.
Alimoradi, Ima
Amar, Jack N.
Ambler, Kimberley L S.
Arseneau, Richard R.
Ayas, Najib
Aymong, Eve D.
Badii, Maziar
Bains, Perminder S.
Barbour, Sean J.
Barnett, Michael J.
Beattie, B. Lynn
Beaulieu, Monica C.
Bebb, Richard A.
Beckman, Jeffrey H.
Bell, Kathryn A.
Bennett, Matthew T.
Bernstein, Victoria
Birmingham, C. Laird
Blocka, Kenneth L N.
Boldt, Camilla L.
Boone, Robert H.
Boyd, John
Bressler, Brian L.
Brunham, Robert C.
Bryce, Cicely J.
Bryce, Elizabeth A.
Busser, James R.
Byrne, Michael F.
Cairns, John A.
Carere, Ronald
Carlsten, Christopher R.
Carter, Cedric J.
Chalmers, Andrew
Chan, Alex C H.
Chan, Angela S A.
Chan, Sammy Y.
Chan, Wee Shian
Chan-Yan, Clifford
Chang, Albert
Chatur, Nazira
Chaun, Hugh
Chen, Luke Y C.
Cheung, Winson Y T.
Chi, Kim Nguyen
Chia, Stephen K L.
Chipperfield, Katherine M.
Chittock, Dean R.
Chiu, Anthony S Y.
Choi, Heywood S.
Choi, Mark
Chong, Carolyn C.
Chow, Katherine S.
Chung, A. Maria
Collins, David R.
Connors, Joseph M.
Conway, Brian
Conway, Edward M.
Cook, Victoria J.
Cook, Wendy L.
Copland, Michael A.
Cowan, Simone S M.
Craig, Katherine G.
Cummins, Nora R.
Cuncic, Cary F.
Cunningham, Jane A.
Dahl, Marshall A.
Das, Sharmistha
Dawson, Keith Granger
De Luca, Linda G.
DeWitt Talbot, Dawn
Deans, Gregory
Deyell, Marc W.
Dhingra, Vinay K.
Dian, Larry
Dinh, Quynh-Dao
Dodek, Peter M.
Dorscheid, Delbert R.
Duncan, John
Dunne, James V.
Dutz, Jan P.
Eaves, Allen
Ebtia, Mahasti
Eigl, Bernhard
Elliott, Thomas G.
Elwood, Richard K.
Enns, Robert A.
Ensworth, Stephanie
Erb, Siegfried R.
Ezzat, Hatoon M.
Farah, Myriam
Farley, John D.
Fera, Tharwat A E.
Firoz, Tabassum
FitzGerald, J. Mark
Fleetham, John A.
Fok, Mark
Foltz, Lynda M.
Fordyce, Christopher B.
Forrest, Donna L.
Francis, Gordon A.
Freeman, Hugh J.
Fung, Anthony Y F.
Fung, Michelle A.
Gelmon, Karen A.
Gill, Jagbir
Gill, John S.
Gill, Sabrina
Gill, Sharlene
Gillies, Jean H.
Gin, Kenneth G.
Grant, Jennifer M.
Gray, James R.
Grewal, Jasmine
Growe, Gershon H.
Hajek, Jan J.
Halparin, Lawrence S.
Harris, David
Hatala, Rosemarie A.
Hawley, Philippa H.
Hayden, Michael R.
Heilbron, Brett G.
Henning, Hartmut
Hill, Amanda J.
Ho, Cheryl C.
Hogge, Donna E.
Hoskins, Paul J.
Hsu, Tina Y.
Huang, Simon H K.
Huckell, Victor F.
Hui, Philip L Y.
Hull, Mark
Ignaszewski, Andrew P.
Ioannou, K. Panagiotis
Isserow, Saul H.
Jackson, Shannon C.
Jacobson, Kevan
Jamal, Abeed
Jamal, Shahin
Jastrzebski, Jacek P.
Johnson, Michelle D.
Johnston, James C.
Jue, Johnny
Jung, Beverly
Kanakos, Michael A.
Kanani, Amin S.
Kassen, Barry O.
Kaviani, Mandana
Keebler, Conrad G.
Kelsall, John T.
Kendler, David L.
Kennecke, Hagen F.
Kennedy, James R.
Keown, Paul A.
Kerr, Charles R.
Khalil, Nasreen
Khan, Nadia A.
Kiaii, Mercedeh
Kim, Edward
Kimel, Gilad
Klasa, Richard J.
Klinkhoff, Alice V.
Knowling, Margaret A.
Ko, Hin Hin
Kohen, Samuel A.
Kollmannsberger, Christian
Kong, Jason M.
Krahn, Andrew D.
Krajden, Mel
Kreisman, Stuart H.
Kumar, Aalok
Kur, Jason K.
Kushner Kow, Janet V.
Kwan, Peter
Kyskan, Robert
Lam, Eric C S.
Lam, Stephen C T.
Landsberg, David N.
Laskin, Janessa J.
Law, Joanna K Y.
Lee, Agnes Y Y.
Lee, Philip E.
Lee, Pui-Kee
Leger, Chantal S.
Leitch, Heather A.
Lester, Richard
Leung, Janice M.
Leung, Victor
Levin, Adeera
Levy, Robert D.
Li, Charles H.
Lim, Howard J.
Lo, Lawrence S.
Lohrisch, Caroline A.
Lysyshyn, Mark A.
MacKenzie-Feder, Jessica M.
MacLeod, Stuart M.
MacRedmond, Ruth E.
Macdonald, Ian L.
Mackie, Iain D F.
Madden, Kenneth M.
Magee, Laura A.
Man, S F. Paul
Mancini, G B. John
Mandl, Michael A J.
Mase, Robert M.
McCormick, Iain A.
McDonald, William N.
McKay, Rhonda J.
McKinney, James
McKnight, R. Douglas
Melosky, Barbara L.
Meneilly, Graydon S.
Menezes, Janice A.
Metcalf, Corey M.
Mizgala, Henry F.
Montaner, Julio S G.
Montessori, Valentina C.
Morton, Charles E.
Moss, Robert R.
Munt, Bradley I.
Murray, Melanie C M.
Murray, Robert C N.
Nagi, Harpinder S.
Nair, Parvathy
Nakielna, Edina M.
Nantel, Stephen
Nasmith, James B.
Nayar, Shalini
Neufeld, Peter R.
Nevill, Thomas J.
Nijjar, Aman P.
Noble, Michael A.
Nolan, Sheila M.
O'Reilly, Susan E.
Ong-Lam, May C.
Onrot, John M.
Ostrow, David N.
Palepu, Anita
Pare, Peter D.

Parmar, Naaz
Patrick, David M.
Paty, Breay W.
Peets, Adam D.
Perry, Thomas L.
Peters, Laurenna D.
Petraszko, Tanya R.
Petrovic, Vanja
Phillips, Peter
Pick, Neora
Plewes, Katherine A.
Powe, John E.
Prchal, David
Press, Natasha M.
Purkiss, Susan E.
Quon, Bradley S.
Rabinowitz, Alan N.
Rabkin, Simon
Ragaz, Joseph
Rahmani Gorji, Anna P.
Rajala, Jennifer L.
Ramanathan, Krishnan
Ramji, Alnoor
Ranchod, Hetesh A.
Rauscher, Christopher J.
Reid, Callum G.
Reid, Graham D.
Reiner, Neil E.
Rekart, Michael L.
Renouf, Daniel J.
Reynolds, Jennifer L.
Reynolds, Robert P.
Ricci, Donald R.
Road, Jeremy D.
Roberts, James M.
Rodrigo, Judith A.
Ronco, Juan J.
Rosenbaum, Debbie A.
Rosenfeld, Gregory A.
Russell, James A.
Ryan, C. Frank P.
Ryerson, Christopher J.
Salh, Baljinder S.
Savage, Kerry J.
Saw, Jacqueline W L.
Schellenberg, R. Robert
Sedlak, Tara L.
Sehn, Laurie H.
Shah, Amil M.
Shaipanich, Tawimas
Shanks, David J.
Shapiro, R. Jean
Shenkier, Tamara N.
Shepherd, John D.
Shojania, Kamran
Shuckett, Rhonda
Simmons, Christine E.
Sin, Donald D H.
Singh, Gurdayal
Singh, R. Suneet
Sirrs, Sandra M.
Skalska, Ursula
Smith, Alan D.
Song, Kevin W.
Sreenivasan, Gayatri M.
Stark, Donald F.
Stefanovic, Aleksandra
Steinbrecher, Urs P.
Steiner, Theodore S.
Stiver, H. Grant
Strijak, Bradford J.
Sun, Sophie
Sutcliffe, Steven D I.
Sutherland, Heather
Sutton, Roger A L.
Swiston, John R.
Sztramko, Richard W K.
Tai, Charles C F.
Tai, Isabella T W.
Tam, Edward
Tam, Penny K.
Tang, Jonathan D.
Taylor, Carolyn M.
Taylor, Paul A.
Telford, Jennifer J.
Thompson, David M.
Tildesley, Hugh D.
Tinker, Anna
Todd, Jonathan K.
Toma, Mustafa
Tothill, Andrea E.
Toze, Cynthia L.
Trutsov, Zdravko B.
Tsang, Ian K.
Tsang, Peter W K.
Tsang, Teresa S M.
Tung, K K. Stanley
Uh, Mitchell
Ur, Ehud
Van Eeden, Stephanus F.
Vandegriend, Richarad A.
Verdejo-Aguilar, N. Alfonso
Villa Restrepo, Diego
Villanyi, Diane
Virani, Shahnawaz A.
Voyer, Stephane M.
Vyas, Mukul N.
Wade, John P D.
Wade, N. Kevin
Wakefield, Robert G.
Walley, Keith R.
Ward, John H.
Watterson, John R.
Weerasinghe, Chandana P.
Weiss, Alan A.
Werb, Ronald
White, Adam S.
Whittaker, J. Scott
Wilcox, Pearce G.
Wilk, Lucie A.
Wojtowska, Ewa
Wong, Graham C.
Wong, H C. George
Wong, Roger Y M.
Wood, David A.
Wood, Evan G R.
Wright, James M.
Yang, Jiao
Yang, Tung C.
Yenson, Paul R.
Yeung, Choi Kit
Yeung-Lai-Wah, A F. John
Yoshida, Eric M.
Yu, Jen Zhen
Zalunardo, Nadia Y.
Zypchen, Leslie N.

VERNON

Armanious, Finley
Chai, Brian C.
Hardy, Edward L G.
Humphreys, Michael R.
Naude, David F.
Smylie, Paul C.
Vaz, Glenn F.
Yacyshyn, Harold P.

VICTORIA

Allan, Sharon J.
Anderson, Helen L.
Antonsen, John E.
Attwell, Andrew J.
Baker, Milton F.
Bater, Marilyn G.
Bernstein, Vanessa
Browman, George P.
Buckley, Alan B.
Capes, Sarah E.
Clark, Heather E.
Connolly, Thomas P.
Coppin, Christopher M L.
Cuthbert, Donna A.
Daly, Donald S.
De Champlain, J. Paul
Della Siega, Anthony J.
Dulay, Daisy
Eddy, Richard J.
Farrell, Laura
Fenton, David W.
Fitzgerald, Catherine A.
Fretz, Eric B.
Galbraith, John C T.
Ganz, Gregory M F.
Ghesquiere, Wayne
Gillett, Dennis G.
Gough, Ellen R.
Hammond, Karsten M.
Hargrove, Gaylene M.
Hart, Jason J.
Holland, Stephen G.
Horgan, Kevin P.
Jenkins, Catherine A.
Jones, Christopher M.
Kinloch, R. David
Klinke, W. Peter
Ksienski, Doran S.
Lane, Christopher J.
Law, Genevieve
Leather, Richard A.
Lee, Ching Sang
Lee, Kingsley R.
Lundy, Stephen E.
MacPherson, Nicol A.
Malone, Marilyn L.
Manjoo, Prija S.
Mann, Manjeet
Marshall, Harvey P.
Martins, Heidi
Materek, Lukasz A.
McDonald, David I.
McGhie, John P.
Meakes, R. Alan
Mildenberger, Richard R.
Miller, David B.
Moldoveanu, Andrei I.
Montgomery, Patrick R.
Morgan, Dennis E.
Myers, Danny M.
Northcott, Kimberly A.
Novak, Paul G.
Ovakim, Daniel H.
Pai, Rajeev N.
Papp, Jamie D.
Partlow, Eric S.
Paul, Terrance W.
Pearson, David C.
Petrunia, Denis M.
Pewarchuk, Jesse A.
Phillips, Richard A.
Piercey, James R A.
Polson, Alasdair L.
Reynolds, Clayton
Sanders, Bruce R.
Shah, Justin A.
Sherk, Peter A.
Singh, Ranjit A.
Skinnider, Douglas J.
Sochowski, Randall A.
Souliere, Sheila F.
Sparling, Terence G.
Spence, James W.
Sterns, Laurence D.
Stigant, Caroline E.
Swiggum, Elizabeth A.
Tang, Anthony S L.
Telford, Gordon O.
Tevaarwerk, Gerald J M.
Von Westarp, Christian H A.
Wass, Hilary
Waters, C. Ian
Weinerman, Brian H.
Weir, Rene V.
Williams, Malcolm B.
Wilson, Kenneth S.
Yee, Adrian S Y.
Young, Aaron M.
Yvorchuk, Kenneth J.
Zandieh, Iman

WEST VANCOUVER

Comeau, Scott M.
Day, Heather M.
Maher, Deviani
Zentner, Alissa S.

WESTBANK

Shojania, Nima

WHISTLER

Shackleton, Christopher R.

WHITE ROCK

Butt, Mohammad I.
Gayton, David C.
Offer, Robert C.
Thornton, Pamela J.

MANITOBA

BRANDON

Bookatz, Brian J.
Cartagena, Ricardo A.
Dunsmore, Sara E.
MacKalski, Barbara A M.
Mshiu, Merlyn E.
Penner, Charles G.
Riche, Barry R.
Turabian, B. Michael

DAUPHIN

Hrabarchuk, Blair E.

THE PAS

Kostyk, Richard J.

THOMPSON

Ramadan, Abdul-Nasser J.

WINNIPEG

Ahmadi Torshizi, Ali
Ainslie, Martha D.
Allan, Donald R.
Anastasiades, Lefkos
Anderson DeCoteau, Marcia
Aoki, Fred Y.
Armstrong, Sean W.
Baillie, Cory S.
Banerji, Shantanu
Banerji, Versha
Barac, Snezana
Battad, Anthony B.
Becker, Marissa
Bellas, Jonathon S.
Bernstein, Charles N.
Bernstein, Keevin N.
Blakeley, Ellen D.
Bohm, Clara J.
Bourque, Christopher N.
Boustcha, Elizabeth M.
Bovell, Frank M.
Bow, Eric J.
Brandes, Lorne J.
Brar, Adarshdip
Bshouty, Zoheir
Bueti, Giuseppe A.
Cantor, Michael J.
Chelvanathan, Anjala
Cleghorn, Scott A.
Cohen, Barry A.
Cooke, Andrew
Corne, Stephen I.
Cumming, Gordon R.
Czarnecki, Wlodzimierz
Czaykowski, Piotr M.
Daeninck, Paul J.
Dao, Vi Vinh B.
Dhindsa, Navjot
Drobot, Glen R.
Ducas, John
Duerksen, Donald R.
Duffy, Gerard
Eggertson, Douglas E.
El-Gabalawy, Hani S.
Embil, John
Eschun, Gregg M.
Fournier, Marc R.
Gabor, Jonathan
Garber, Philip J.
Giannouli, Eleni
Gingerich, Joel R.
Goldenberg, David J.
Gordon, Vallerie L.
Goulet, Stephen C.
Grenier, Debjani
Griffin, Patrick M G.
Hajidiacos, Nicholas P.
Hameed, Kazi A.
Hammond, Gregory W.
Handford, Robert G.
Harding, Gary A J.
Harris, Patricia E.
Hechtenthal, Norman
Henry, Stephen F.
Hershfield, Earl S.
Hiebert, Tim
Hitchon, Carol A.
Ho, Juliet
Homik, Lawrence A.
Horton, Jillian J.
Houston, Donald S.
Hurd, Carmen A.
Hussain, Farrukh
Hutchison, Trevor
Ilnyckyj, Alexandra
Ilse, Werner K.
Jackson, Alan C.
Jacob, Thomas K.
Jassal, Davinder S.
Johnson, Bijai
Johnston, James B.
Jolly, Kanwaljit S.
Junaid, Asad I.
Kahanovitch, I I. David
Kaita, Kelly D E.
Kalicinsky, Chrystyna M.
Karpinski, Martin E.
Kasper, Kenneth D.
Kass, Malek
Katz, Pamela
Kaufman, Ruebin
Kepron, M. Wayne
Kippen, Robert N.
Komenda, Paul V J.
Krahn, Marianne J.
Kramer, Matthias P A.
Kraut, Allen G.
Kroeker, L. Robert
Krongold, Penina H.
Kumar, Anand
Lam, Herman P Y.
Lamba, Kiraninder S.
Lau, Chung-Yan
Lee, Harvey B.
Lerner, Neal Z.
Leslie, William D.
Lezack, Jack D.
Light, Robert B.
Lloyd, David A.
Lo, Evelyn
Lucman, Tahir S.
Ludwig, Sora M.
MacDiarmid, Andrew L.
MacDougall, Brendan K.
Maksymiuk, Andrew W.
Malik, Amrit A.
Manishen, Wayne J.
Marantz, Susan G.
Mathew, George
Matthews, Nicola E.
Maxwell, Ian
McCarthy, Timothy G.
McCusker, Patricia J.
Meyrowitz, David M.
Micflikier, Allan B.
Miller, Anthony
Miller, Lisa M.
Minhas, Kunal K S.
Minuk, Earl S.
Minuk, Gerald Y.
Moffatt, Dana C H.
Moltzan, Catherine J.
Muthiah, Karuppan
Myers, Renelle L.
Naimark, Arnold
Navaratnam, Srisaladevi
Nguyen, Thang N.
Nickerson, Peter W.
Nicolle, Lindsay E.
Nkosi, Joel E.
Olafson, Kendiss P.
Orr, Pamela H.
Padua, Rodolfo N.
Parmar, Gurpreet
Patel, Sunil P.
Paunovic, Bojan N.
Penner, S. Brian
Peretz, David
Peschken, Christine A.
Pilkey, Jana L.
Pitz, Marshall W.
Plourde, J J. Pierre
Ponnampalam, Arjuna
Poon, Wayne W C.
Porhownik, Nancy R.
Pun, Teresa W C.
Ramsey, Clare D.
Ravandi, Amir
Reslerova, Martina
Richardson, Cindy Jo.
Rigatto, Claudio
Rimmer, Emily K.
Roberts, Daniel
Robinson, David B.
Roe, E. Bruce
Ronald, Allan R.
Rowe, Richard C.
Rubinger, Morel
Rush, David N.
Salamon, Elizabeth A.
Salih, Bashar
Sandham, J. Dean
Sathianathan, Christie
Schacter, Brent A.

Schaffer, Stephen A.
Seftel, Matthew D.
Selaman, Mustafa H.
Semus, Michael J.
Sharma, Satyendra
Shepertycky, Martha R.
Silha, Josef
Simonsen, J. Neil
Singh, Harminder
Singh, Ramandip
Sinha, Sachchida N.
Skrabek, Pamela J.
Smith, Catherine A.
Smith, Hugh W E.
Sochocki, Michael P.
Soni, Anita
Sood, Manish M.
St John, Philip D.
Storsley, Leroy J.
Strang, David G.
Stronger, Lyle N W.
Szwajcer, David
Tam, James W L.
Tangri, Navdeep
Taraska, Vincent A.
Targownik, Laura E.
Thille, Suzanne M L.
Thomson, Glen T D.
Thottingal, Paul A.
Tischenko, Alexander
Van Ameyde, Kenneth J L.
Van Ineveld, Cornelia H M.
Venkatesan, Nithya
Verrelli, Mauro
Walkty, Andrew J.
Walli, J. Eric
Walters, Justin J.
Wanono, Revital
Warrington, Richard J.
Watson, A. Elizabeth W.
Wiebe, Kim L.
Wiseman, David G H.
Wolfe, Kevin B.
Wong, Jonathan K.
Wong, Justin K F.
Wong, Ralph P W.
Wong, Stephen G.
Wong, Turnly
Woo, Vincent C.
Yeung, Clement S L.
Zacharias, James M.
Zarychanski, Ryan L.
Zieroth, Shelley R.

NEW BRUNSWICK

BATHURST
Al Zain, Khalid A H.
Hickey, Dean
Memiche, Reshat
Robichaud, Sylvie
Satyanarayana, Bellura S.
Violette, Claude P.

CAMPBELLTON
Whalen, Mark G.

DIEPPE
Baril, Jean-Francois
D'Astous, Michel
Lee, Rina
Matteau, Sylvain

EDMUNDSTON
Clavette, Paul F.
Lang, Anik
Malenfant, Laurie
Paillard, Christian
Soucie, Jean-Joseph
Violette, Chantal L.

FREDERICTON
Anan, Ghadeer
Ecker, George A.
Feltmate, Patrick J G.
Harvey, Richard D.
Koller, Oscar L.
MacMillan, Mark
McGibbon, Angela M.
McMullen, David H.
Moore, D. Jeffrey H.
Solven, Frederick G.

MIRAMICHI
Khan, Niaz A.
Rigley, Joseph

MONCTON
Al-Karain, Mohammad Y M.
Alqdah, Maen A A.
Baer, Carolyn E H.
Balfour, Shana C.
Berger, Robert K.
Bourgeois, Ronald L J.
Brideau, Eric
Chiasson, Guylaine
Cohen, David R.
D'Astous, Julien R.
Docherty, Peter S.
Dorval, Marc
Dow, Gordon C K.
Ferguson, Kathy
Finn, Nicholas G.
Gallant, Tania M.
Gallien, Annelise
Gaudet, Matthieu
Girouard, Gabriel
Kamel, Sherief J.
Kemp, Kristina M.
LeBlanc, Remi
Lightfoot, Peter D.
MacSween, Mary C.
Mallet, Marcel
McAvinue, Thomas
Mikael, Gaby G.
Ouellette, Sylvie A.
Picard, Leo
Roux, Veronique
Rubin, Sheldon H.
Schweiger, Franzjosef
Silva, Fidelia A.
Smyth, Daniel J.
St-Hilaire, Eve
Thibeault, Yves
Trudeau, Chantal D.
Turbide, Christian
Whitlock, Pierre
Williston, Maryse

SAINT JOHN
Barry, Colin A.
Bessoudo, Ricardo
Bewick, David J.
Bishop, Graham W.
Burnell, Margot J.
Cockeram, Alan W.
Comeau, Terrance B W.
Costain, Gary A.
Dolan, Sean P.
Dornan, John M.
Douglas, J. Geoffrey
Fong, Peter
Gillis, Cory F.
Gogan, Nessa R.
Grant, Eric N.
Gray, Samantha
Hobbs, Cynthia A.
Hubacek, Jaroslav
Jarrett, Pamela G.
Joshi, Prakash C.
Lutchmedial, Sohrab R A.
MacDonald, Elizabeth A.
MacKinnon, Martin G.
MacNeil, Donna M.
Marr, David R.
McKnight, Lisa C.
Paddock, Vernon W.
Pippy, Christine C.
Raju, Mahesh K.
Reiman, Anthony J.
Rhynold, Elizabeth S.
Sadowska, Ewa
Salmon, Joanne
Searles, Gregory R.
Sohi, Paul S.
Stevenson, Robert S.
Sullivan, Glendon E.
Teskey, Robert J.
Webster, Duncan V.
West, Peter H F.
Williams, Chadwick

WATERVILLE CARLETON
Pelkey, Michael C.

WOODSTOCK
Milton, John R.

NEWFOUNDLAND AND LABRADOR

BURIN
Mathew, Baboo M.

CORNER BROOK
Graham, Jamie
Krishnan, Venkataraman S G.
Murphy, Stephen T.
Sharif, Ismail A A.
Tavenor, Anthony J.

GRAND FALLS WINDSOR
King, Amy C.
Lush, Richard B.
Sheridan, James J.
Wadhwa, Kanwar J S.

ST ANTHONY
Al Beshir, Mohammad S A.

ST. JOHN'S
Adams, Grenfell B.
Ahmad, Chaudhary E.
Anees, Iram
Anwar, Muhammad A Q.
Bandrauk, Natalie A.
Barrett, Brendan J.
Bergstrom, Debra J.
Bhalla, Sunil
Borgaonkar, Mark R.
Borgaonkar, Ram D.
Bowmer, Michael I.
Bursey, R. Ford
Chandra Sekhar, Harnahalli B.
Chandurkar, Vikram
Clarke, Gillian I.
Connors, Sean P.
Curtis, Bryan M.
Daley, Peter
Duguid, Nigel J D.
Fagan, Susan M.
Fallows, Glen A.
Fardy, John M.
Farrell, Jamie
Fox, George A.
Furey, Michael U G.
Furlong, Michael B.
Galway, A. Brenda
Genge, Stephanie I.
Grewal, Kuljit S.
Hamilton, Sean F.
Hannaford, Maureen C.
Hickey, Joanne
Hiscock, Jeffery G.
Ingram, David W.
Iqbal, Muhammad
Iqbal, Sahar J.
Joshi, Pradip J.
Joyce, Carol J.
Khraishi, Majed M.
Kovacs, Christopher S.
Laing, Kara E T.
Leonard, Jennifer R.
Lockyer, Joseph M.
MacCallum, G. Calvin
McCarthy, Joy S.
McGrath, Jerry S.
McPherson, Terrence P.
Murphy, Sean W.
Murray, Cathy M.
O'Brien, Mary H.
Parfrey, Patrick S.
Paul, Michael D.
Paulin, Frederic L.
Pearce, Neil J.
Peters, Sharon D.
Pike, Pamela A.
Powell, Erin D.
Rahman, Al-Amin M P.
Reddy, S. Bharati
Rorke, Stewart
Rose, Barry F.
Seal, Melanie D.
Shik, John W C.
Siddiqui, Jehan Z.
Stefanelli, Mark G.
Stone, Eric W.
Sussex, Bruce A.
Taylor, Douglas S.
Tompkins, Kirsty A.
Tong, Amy Y M.
Trahey, Julia C.
Williams, Anne E.
Young, Robert W.

STEPHENVILLE
Qureshi, Amer S H.

NOVA SCOTIA

AMHERST
Bowen, A. Scott L.
Szczesny, Krystian M.

ANTIGONISH
Abdelgadir, Ibrahim M.
Boyd, Matthew
Miles, Graham C.
Pereira, Leo V.

BRIDGEWATER
Atkinson, Anthony R.
Fraser, Hughie
Hatheway, Ronald J.
Nestel, Anthony W.
Nestel, Magdalena D.
Ratushny, Jeffrey V.
Shirley, Margaret A.

DARTMOUTH
Al Harbi, Mousa A R.
Duke, Stephen M.
Hermann, Laura L.
Ing, Vincent W.
Keating, Mary-Margaret
Knight, Deborah C.
Lindensmith, Jorin M.
McCarville, Clifford
Mears, Paul A.
Rappard, Scott C.
Shaw, Emily J.
Sheppard, Duane G.
Smith, Peter K L.
Theriault, M Y. Diane
Yung, Jason D K.
Zaman, Khawar-Uz

GLACE BAY
Creighton, Paula A.
McNeil, Kevin S.
Rebelo, Raul A.

HALIFAX
Acres, John C.
Anderson, David R.
Andrew, Melissa K.
Badley, Bernard W D.
Bakowsky, Volodko S.
Bata, Iqbal R.
Beydoun, Hussein K.
Carver, Daniel J.
Charlebois, Paul B.
Chiasson, Meredith D.
Clarke, Brian A.
Colwell, Bruce D O.
Connors, Lori A.
Cookey, Benedict J.
Couban, Stephen
Cox, Jafna L.
Crofts, Peter A.
Crowell, Richard H.
Curran, Helen
Davis, Ian R C.
Dipchand, Christine S.
Dorreen, Mark S.
Drucker, Arnold M.
Dupere, David
Epstein, Ian L.
Farina, Dana M.
Fernandez, Louis A V.
Finkle, Simon N.
Forward, Kevin R.
Freter, Susan H.
Gee, Shirl A D.
Giacomantonio, Nicholas B.
Ginther, D. Glen
Gordon, Janet E.
Gray, Christopher
Green, Peter
Gruchy, Steven E.
Haase, David A.
Hancock, Jennifer
Hanly, John G.
Hasegawa, Wanda
Hatchette, Todd F.
Hernandez, Paul
Hirsch, David J.
Horne, S. Gabrielle
Imran, Syed A.
Jackson, Simon D.
Jeyakumar, Alwin
Johnston, B. Lynn
Josephson, E. Bruce
Kaiser, Stephanie M.
Kells, Catherine M.
Keough-Ryan, Tammy M.
Kew, Andrea K.
Kiberd, Bryce A.
Klaus, E. Markus
Koilpillai, Christiansen J.
Koller, Katalin E.
Krueger-Naug, Anne M.
Lacuesta, Gina A.
Laryea, Marie A.
Leddin, Desmond J.
Lee, Tony C L.
Little, Cameron D.
Lodge, Richard
MacDonald, David A.
MacDonald, Nancy L.
MacIntosh, Donald G.
MacKnight, Christopher R.
MacNeil, Mary V.
Macfarlane, Robyn
Mallery, Laurie H.
Mann, Elizabeth
Manning, J. David
Marrie, Thomas J J.
McKiggan, John J.
McMullen, Sarah M.
McNeil, Shelly A.
McParland, Columba
Michael, Roger T.
Moorhouse, Paige A.
Morrison, Debra L.
Morrison, Nancy J.
Morzycki, Wojciech
Panek, Romuald
Parkash, Rajender
Parkash, Ratika
Patel, Sunil T.
Patrick, Ward D.
Peltekian, Kevork M.
Poyah, Penelope
Purdy, Kerri S.
Rajda, Miroslaw
Ramer, Sarah A.
Ransom, Thomas
Rayson, Daniel
Rebello, Rosario
Rheaume, Dorianne E.
Robinson, K. Sue
Rocker, Graeme
Rockwood, Kenneth J.
Sapp, John
Schlech III, Walter F.
Shatshat, Souad M.
Sheridan, William J.
Shivakumar, Sudeep P.
Simpson, C. David
Snow, Stephanie L.
Soroka, Steven D.
Stewart, John W.
Stewart, Robert L.
Styles, Janet K.
Sutton, Evelyn D.
Taylor, Trudy A.
Title, Lawrence M.
Tugwell, Barna D.
Turnbull, Geoffrey K.
West, Kenneth A.
West, L. Michael

White, Darrell J.
Williams, S. Geoffrey
Williams, Stacey P.
Winsor, Wendy A.
Wong, Jill M.
Wood, Lori A.
Workman, Stephen R.

KENTVILLE
Burch, Karen A.
Clarke, Adam C.
DiQuinzio, Melanie L.
Gordon, Ann
Harrigan, Lynne A.
Merryweather, Rachel J.
Musgrave, Bruce L.
Wightman, Howard A.
Woo, Daniel C.

LIVERPOOL
Crawford, Kim R.

LUNENBURG
Wilson, Diane B.

NEW GLASGOW
Ashfaq, Sirajuddin
El-Zubeidi, Wassim
Hack, M. Imran
Roy, A. Michael
Shaarbaf, Raid

NORTH SYDNEY
Igoe, Michael P.

PORT WILLIAMS
Hadlaw, Violetta A.
Marsters Jr., David W.
Mindrum, Michael
Stern, Richard B.

SYDNEY
Bedard, Richard J.
Brake, David J.
Buzaid, Amin M.
De, Sabe K.
Hewlett, Thomas J C.
Jensen, John L.
MacCormick, Ronald E.
MacDonald, Paul J.
Shaaban, Hani
Thanamayooran, Siva
Wong, Dave
Yeung, Gordon K.
Zwicker, Deborah A.

SYDNEY RIVER
McClelland, Bruce

TRURO
Perk, Masis
Singh, Jagmohan K.

WINDSOR
Kasina, Rafal A.
Machel, Teresa M.

YARMOUTH
Merrick, Evan P.
Moses, Brian G.
Prabhu, Umesh H.
Tarakji, Ahmad R.

ONTARIO

AJAX
Blumer, Ian R.
Buttoo, Kenneth
Campbell, Peter J.
Clements-Baker, Marie I.
Elfirjani, Ali Salem B.
Jeyalingam, Kanapathipillai
Leader, Rolland M.
Philteos, George S R.
Price, Carman S.
Pushpapalan, Jegathesan
Shawesh, Malek H E.
Sheikh, Gul Nawaz
Silverman, Michael S.
Wang, James C Y.
Wei, Charles C Y.

ALEXANDRIA
Sia, Ying Tung

AMHERSTVIEW
Macdonald, Colin A W.

ANCASTER
Pavlova, Viktoria V.
Webert, Kathryn E.

ARNPRIOR
Greenough, M. Catherine

AYTON
Clarke, Peter V.

BALA
Jacyk, William R.

BARRIE
Abdel Salam, Suzan Y.
Aitken, A. Stewart
Amba, Sudhir
Benjamin, Derek S.
Burke, Bruce R.
Campbell, Rebecca M.
Di Diodato, Giulio
Dibble, Bradley J.
El-Maraghi, Robert H.
Fischer, David A.
Haaland, Derek A.
Hemphill, Douglas J.
Khosrovaneh, Amir K.
Krishnan, Mukta M.
Krishnan, Murali
Krishnan, Usha
Kutcher, R. Walter W.
Lalor, Eoin A G.
Li, Isabel
McKenzie, Kim R.
Nay, Derek W.
Ng, Dawn M.
Petroniene, Rima
Pressnail, Bryn L.
Rask, Sara J.
Rassouli-Rashti, Mohammad
Tailor, Adarsh
Tebbutt, L. Christopher
Visentin, Diana E.
Yuen, Kenneth W H.
Zatelny, Diane L.

BELLEVILLE
Berezny, Gary M.
Campbell, Joseph A L J.
Courtland, Michael R.
Grant, F. Curry
Grieve-Eglin, Leandra H.
Heffernan, Paul
Hollett, Peter M.
Kafka, Henryk P.
Leong, Roger
Levesque, Roger
Link, Catherine A.
Marcotte, Laura S.
Masood, Mujaddid
Milne, Laura A.
Pritchett, Sean B.
Theodorou, Maria E.
Yee, Ernest
Zoutman, Dick E.

BOWMANVILLE
Islam, Ashiqul
Shickh, Ali M.
Shrives, David M.
Sridhar, Srilata K.

BRACEBRIDGE
Caughey, William G.
Deketele, Anthony G.
Moran, Keith W V.
Williams, W. Shane

BRAMPTON
Ahluwalia, Vandana
Ahmad, Mayraj
Allard, Marc L.
Amin, Reham
Amlani, Shoaib
Baath, Jasbir S.
Bajaj, Sangeeta
Baker, Andrew D.
Balcewicz, Malgorzata
Bellini, Andrew B.
Borgia, Sergio M.
Borts, David
Chandok, Natasha
Chaudhry, Love R.
Chaudhry, Muhammad S.
Ciric, Ioana E.
Dharmalingam, Sudharshan
Donnelly, M. Sandra
El-Takli, Issam K.
Friefeld, Joanne
Gill, Paramjit
Gupta, Milan
Hammouda, M. Wahbi
Hayani, Omar
Hill, Laurie L.
Hussain, Fatima M.
Jeejeebhoy, Farida M.
Joshi, V. Raman
Joza, Paul
Jurt, Ursula
Kajbaf, Sahar
Kim, Christie Y.
Kohn, Magdie L.
Kong, Waitak
Kong, Yuan
Kuruvilla, Philip G.
Kutty, P. Karunakaran
Lim, Ki Dong
Luk, Tracy C C.
May, Donna L.
Mehta, Hitesh
Moltyaner, Yuri
Murray, Shirley Y.
Naraine, Virjanand
Nesdoly, Christine H.
Omer, Saeed A.
Papneja, Tripti
Pinto, Michael A.
Powell, Elizabeth
Puri, Vinod
Qureshi, Tariq M.
Raco, Dominic L F.
Ravindran, Vikram C.
Reen, Bajinder S.
Reingold, Stephen M.
Richardson, David C.
Sachdeva, Jasdip S.
Sachedina, Bashirudin
Sadak, Yuksel
Sehdev, Sandeep R.
Shan, Xi
Shorey, Sanam S.
Singh, Jagdeep
Singh, Narendra
Soicher, Avrum A.
Suneja, Sumeet K.
Tan, Patrick B.
Thavendiranathan, Paaladinesh
Tjandrawidjaja, Michael C.
Tsang, Wendy W C.
Varadarasa, Arulanandam
Walele, Abdul A.
Ying, Luis T J.
Zamel, Rola

BRANTFORD
Ajayi, Abayomi
Braun, E. Anne
Carlton, Timothy J.
Cordell, Bruce A.
Dabreo, Derek E J.
Jones, Mark B.
Kagoma, Peter K.
Kathrada, Yacoob A H.
Koubaesh, Yousery Y R.
Lee, Bryan C W.
Nikore, Vinay
Pastuszewska, Natalia M.
Rusthoven, James J.
Sarkar, Ujjaini
Somerton, Stephen C.
Szakacs, Thomas A.
Wang, Charlie S K.

BROCKVILLE
Beveridge, Robert C.
Bhatt, Jayant S.
Brook-Williams, Penelope
Hebert Croteau, Nicolas
Hynd, Jamie W H.
Iqbal, Tariq
Steyn, Jacobus J.

BURLINGTON
Beaudry, Philippe R.
Berlingieri, Joseph C.
Carling-Chambers, Lucille B.
Cheung, Lily S K.
Ching, Emily K Y.
Chow, Mabel Y T.
Christjanson, Lisa J.
Comay, Daniel C.
Cyr, Michael M.
Darcel, Ian C.
Dixit, Sanjay
Gee, Sydney R.
Haddon, Roger W T.
Jaroszynska, Anna M.
Jeans, E. Rose
Killorn, W. Patrick
Kumaranayake, A. Prasanna P.
Lad, Rameeta J.
Ladha, Al-Karim
Lang, Jefferey D.
Lipsit, Sharon E.
Makhija, Sapna
Martin, David H.
Marwaha, Avantika
Merali, Fatima S M.
Messieh, Mary L.
Mody, Anita
Mulgund, Manisha M.
Nisker, William A.
Pandith, Vikas
Phillips, Callista M.
Robbins, Stephanie J.
Saxena, Akash D.
Simmons, William W.
Stevens, Brett J D.
Todd, David C.
Wilkinson, Sharon I.
Youssef, George M Y.

CAMBRIDGE
Bishara, Phoebe R Y.
Chouinard, Edmond E.
Famorca, Leilani Casilda de Leon
Hanna, Brian D.
Kumar, Ragbir S.
Lee, Mark J.
Liutkus, Joanne F.
Macie, Christine M G.
Martin, Glenn E.
Mathai, George
Nguyen, Augustin
Pandey, A. Shekhar
Sivakumaran, Thevaki
Stinson, J. Michelle
Vizel, Saul
Yang, John C.

CAMPBELLFORD
Schabas, Richard E.

CAYUGA
Sethi, Jagmeet

CHATHAM
Bain-Atoe, Gemma H.
Ben Issa, Entisar M.
Brisbin, Donald P.
Iyer, R. Padmanabhan
Khalifa, Nagib M A.
Letarte, Pierre
Rajabale, Mahmud A.
Sinnaeve, Linda J E.
Tran, Quoc Hung.
Xue, Shuwen

CHELTENHAM
MacPherson, Douglas W.

CLAREMONT
Steyn, Antony W.

CLINTON
Flowers, Raymond W.

COBOURG
Beck, John R.
Krishnan, Rajesh
Moorsom, David M.

COLLINGWOOD
Goode, J. Eric
MacFarlane, J. Grant

CONCORD
Kagal, Allan D.

CORNWALL
Al-Saadon, Khalid
Baitz, Thomas
Copeland, David
Dandurand, Ronald
De Young, J. Paul
Ghaly, Ezzat G.
Levac, Marie-France
Soodan, Baldev S.

DUNDAS
Booth, John D.

EAST YORK
Ali, Yaser M A.
Bin, James
Chen, Dean L H.
Dunn, Anita Y.
Fine, Rebecca J.
Fung, Raymond C.
Lefkowitz, A. Charles J.
Ovchinnikov, Vladislav L.
Pinto, Sarah R.
Sandler, Samantha D.
Shao, Richard H.
Singer, William
Telner, Adam H.
Tran, Kham Quang.
Vasiliou, Denise M.

ETOBICOKE
Adesanya, Arinola O.
Al Mohri, Huda A G.
Allen, Vanessa G.
Amin, Leena
Arif, Saroosh
Baqi, S. Mahin
Barchan, Olexander
Bhesania, Teosar
Birkin, Brenda L.
Bulley, Sean R.
Chu, Joseph Y C.
Clements, L E. Gotham
Cuthbert, Anthony L.
Damji, Nazim F.
Drzymala, Lukasz
Fisher, Mark A.
Florica, Brandusa
Foster, Sandra
Geranmayegan, Amir A.
Goldstein, Sheldon H.
Gould, Michael I.
Greenbloom, Susan L.
Huang, Max
Jancelewicz, Zygmunt
Joshipura, Mini G.
Kalaparambath, Tef
Kannampuzha, Paul T.
Karani, Yasir
Karasik, Arthur E.
Khandwala, Hasnain
Killinger, Donald W.
Kirigin, Mladen J.
Lam, Peter J.
Likar, Ivan
Lumb, Kevin A.
Miletin, Michael S.
Mukherjee, Sanjib K.
Nedilski, Morris
Nelson, Sarah L.
Newbigging, Peter D.
Ngai, Benjamin Y C.
Nguyen, Kinh-Tung T.
Oh, Clifford
Parikh, Amish
Perl, Avishay
Rajkotwala, Victor A.
Rosenberg, Joseph I.
Sameshima, Takaki
Seth-Sharma, Anila
Sethi, Rajiv
Sevitt, Brian M.
Silverberg, Samuel

Sklar, Lawrence S.
Taher, Fakhruddin
To, Toan Bao
Varkul, Mark D.
Warren, William P.
Wilansky, Douglas L.
Wong, Min Min C.

FORT ERIE
Tayab, Syed M A.

GEORGETOWN
Browning, Craig J.

GODERICH
Fiaani, Majed M S.

GRANTON
McLean, Nicola K.

GRIMSBY
Ginsburg, Jonathan C.
Lam, Andy S C.
Peller, Joseph A.

GUELPH
Agarwal, Anil
Bovell, Keith T.
Chan, Norman G.
Chapman, Larry S.
Chiba, Naoki
Friedman, Oded
Grebenyuk, Liliya
Hewak, James C.
Hollinger, C. Gerald
Kottachchi, Dan
Landis, Stephan J.
Misterski, Jacek E.
Morris, Catherine A W.
Nemni, Jacqueline C.
Noor, Amra
Purdon, Cameron J A.
Raso, Dean A.
Schwarz-Michorowski, Bogdan L.
Shende, Vasanti N.
Sirek, Ann Maria T.
Somerville, Peter J.

HAGERSVILLE
Chiu, Sylvester S.

HAMILTON
Achong, Michael R.
Adachi, Jonathan D R.
Ainsworth, Craig D.
Al Khdair, Darar A.
Al-Saleh, Ayman M O.
Al-Shamsi, Humaid O.
Ali, Asma
Alshehhi, Maryam H A D.
Amaratunga, Kanchana R.
Amer, Rebecca K.
Amlani, Salima
Anand, Sonia S.
Anjum, Mahraz
Arlen, Dianne J.
Armstrong, David
Arnold, Andrew M.
Arnold, Donald M.
Azharuddin, Mohammed
Bacchus, Farzana R.
Bader, Mazen
Bajaj, Girish
Barr, Ronald D.
Bates, Shannon M.
Batool, Tahira
Belley-Cote, Emilie-Prudence
Benger, Ann M.
Bensen, William G.
Bhagirath, Vinai C.
Bianchi, Fernando A.
Blajchman, Morris A.
Bobba, Raja
Bojcevski, Alexandra T.
Bordeleau, Louise J.
Boulos, Pauline
Bradley, Christine A.
Brandt Vegas, Daniel
Brimble, K Scott.
Carlisle, Euan
Carmona, Rajendra
Chakroborty, Amitabha
Chan, Howard H W.
Chelvanathan, Anushya
Chung, Han-Oh
Cividino, Alfred A.
Clark, David A.
Clase, Catherine M.
Cohen, Jeremy I.
Collins, Stephen M.
Cook, Deborah J.
Cowan, David D.
Crabbe, Lindsay A.
Crowther, Mark A.
Cunnington, John P W.
Curnew, Gregory P.
Davis, Clive
Dawe, David
Demers, Catherine
Denburg, Judah
Derby, Ian R G.
Devereaux, Philip
Dhesy-Thind, Sukhbinder
Dokainish, Hisham
Dominguez, Ada L.
Dorasamy, Punginathn
Douketis, James D.
Dragomir, Alina R.
Drost, Nicole Z A.
Eikelboom, John
El-Helou, Philippe P.
Ellis, Peter
Evans, William
Figueredo, Alvaro
Foley, Stephen R.
Fox-Robichaud, Alison E.
Fraser, Graeme
Freitag, Andreas P.
Fuller, Hugh D.
Gagnon, Micheline D M.
Gangji, Azim
Ganguli, Subhas C.
Gerstein, Hertzel
Ghanny, Shari
Gibson, James
Ginsberg, Jeffrey
Goffin, John
Goodwin, Jodi L.
Goodwin, Susan E B.
Gordon, Elaine
Gottschalk, Raymond
Grand'Maison, Anne
Greenbaum, Joseph
Greenwald, Eric R.
Gross, Peter L.
Gulenchyn, Karen Y.
Guyatt, Gordon H.
Guzman Orduz, Juan
Ha, Andrew
Haider, Shariq
Hamielec, Cindy M.
Hanmiah, Rajendar
Harper, William L.
Hart, Lawrence
Hastings, Deborah M.
Haynes, R. Brian
Hayward, Catherine P M.
Healey, Jeffrey S.
Hess, Talvi M.
Higgins, David A.
Hirsh, Jack
Hirte, Holger
Holbrook, Anne M.
Holder, Douglas A.
Hotte, Sebastien J.
Hunt, Dereck L.
Hunt, Richard H.
Husain, Saima F.
Ingram, Alistair J.
Iorio, Alfonso
Ip, W. William
Jaeschke, Roman Z.
Jalali, Subash
Johanson, Curtis R.
Johnstone, Jennie
Jolly, Sanjit S.
Jones, Graham L.
Joseph, Geena
Kaki, Reham M S.
Karachi, Timothy A.
Kean, Walter F.
Kearon, M. Clive
Keen, Sabina L C.
Keith, Paul K.
Kelton, John G.
Khalid, Zahira
Khalidi, Nader A.
Khan, Khurram J.
Killian, Kieran J.
Kitching, Allan D.
Klein, Cheryl A.
Kouroukis, Chrisostomos
Kraeker, Christian B.
Kraus, Peter A.
Krepinsky, Joan C.
Kruisselbrink, Rebecca J.
Lau, Arthur
Leber, Brian F.
Lebert, Phyllis A.
Lee, Christine H C.
Legassie, Jenny M.
Legault, Kimberly J.
Leonard, Blair J N.
Lepic, Kylie L.
Lester, Frances T.
Leto, Daniela L.
Lim, Wendy P W.
Lo, Raymond C T.
Loeb, Mark B.
Lonn, Eva M.
Ludwin, David
Lumb, Barry J.
Luthra, Meera
Mahabir, Vishwanath K.
Main, Cheryl L.
Major, Pierre P.
Mann, Nooreen
Marcellus, Deborah C.
Margetts, Peter J.
Marr, Sharon A.
Marshall, John K.
Mathivanan, Meena
Matsos, Mark
McIvor, R. Andrew
McKelvie, Robert S.
McLellan, Allan P.
McLeod, Heather C.
McMullin, Joseph P.
McWhirter, Elaine
Meade, Maureen O.
Medina, Damien R.
Mehta, Shamir
Menzies, Fiona V.
Merali, Abbas M.
Meyers, Brandon M.
Meyerson, Jeffrey
Miller, Matthew C.
Misiaszek, Brian
Mizera, Ryszard
Moayyedi, Paul
Mohammed, Naufal
Moniz, Faustino P.
Montgomery, Alison G.
Morgan, David
Mukherjee, Som D.
Mukherji, Atreyi
Mulji, Amin S.
Natarajan, Madhu K.
Neary, John D D.
Neville, Alan J.
Noroozi, Nastaran
O'Byrne, Paul M.
O'Shea, Timothy M.
Pai, Menaka
Paikin, Jeremy
Panju, Akbar A.
Panju, Mohamed
Papaioannou, Alexandra
Patel, Alex
Patel, M. Ameen
Patriquin, Christopher J.
Patterson, Christopher J.
Peat, Mary I.
Perez, Gavino R D.
Perri, Danny
Pillai, Geetha
Potts, Jayson M.
Powers, Peter J.
Powles, A C. Peter
Prebtani, Ally K P H.
Puglia, Marco A.
Pugsley, Stewart O.
Puksa, Serge
Punthakee, Zubin
Rabbat, Christian G.
Radwi, Ghazala R H K.
Raghavan, Natya
Ramsdale, E. Helen
Rao, Rajeev V.
Ribic, Christine M.
Rokoss, Michael J.
Rudkowski, Jill C.
Russell, J. David
Ryan, Thomas J.
Salehian, Omid
Salena, Bruno J.
Savelli, Gordina E.
Schuenemann, Holger J.
Schulman, Sam
Schwalm, Jon-David R.
Scocchia, Tulio G.
Sealey, Brian J.
Seaton, Trevor L C.
Sebaldt, Rolf J.
Sheth, Tej N.
Sindi, Anees A S.
Singh, Jessica
Singhal, Nishma
Smaill, Fiona M.
Smieja, Marek J.
Sohal, Avtar S.
Soth, Mark D.
Spaziani, Robert
St-Onge, Joye A.
Stallwood, George R.
Stimac, John M.
Subramanian, Ganesh K.
Sullivan, Brian J M.
Sullivan, Hugh P C.
Sullivan, Michael J J.
Suryanarayan, Deepa
Takach Lapner, Sarah L D.
Talman, Marianne R.
Tandon, Vikas
Tiboni, Maria-Elena
Tihal, Hirawan
To, Karen C.
Tomlinson, Charles W.
Tougas, Manon
Tozer, Richard G.
Treleaven, Darin J.
Trus, Michola R.
Tsang, Michael B.
Tse, Frances W M.
Tsega, Edemariam
Tsoi, Keith S K.
Tunks, Marcel G.
Turnbull, John D.
Turpie, Alexander G G.
Turpie, Fiona H I.
Turpie, Irene D.
Valettas, Nicholas
Van Spall, Harriette G C.
Vander Meer, Rachel L.
Velianou, James L.
Verhovsek, Madeleine M.
Visram, Farzin M.
Walker, Irwin R.
Walsh, Michael W.
Warkentin, Theodore E.
Waserman, Susan
Wasi, Parveen
Wharton, Sean N.
Whelan, Timothy J.
Whitehead, Lori N.
Whittingham, Heather A.
Witt-Sullivan, Helga B.
Woo, Tricia K W.
Woodward, Kevin S.
Wright, Douglas S.
Xenodemetropoulos, Theodore T.
Yakubovich, Natalia
Yamamura, Deborah L R.
Yang, Robert C.
You, John J.
Yuan, George
Yudin, Jovana
Zbuk, Kevin M.

HAWKESBURY
Hay, W. John
Thibodeau, Michel E.

HUNTSVILLE
Jindal, Sanjay K.
Johnstone, David W.
Murat, Brian W.
Wilson, Malcolm A G.

INGERSOLL
Hanoman, Marguerite B C.
Sharma, Maheshwar D.

KANATA
Choudhri, Omer H.
Frankish, Charles W.
Smith, Bryan V.

KAPUSKASING
Boucher, Daniel A.

KINGSTON
Adams, Gerald S.
Aggarwal, Aaron N.
Aloudat, Sarah I M.
Anastassiades, Tassos P.
Archer, Stephen
Baetz, Tara D.
Bechara, Robert
Beyak, Michael J.
Biagi, James J.
Booth, Christopher M.
Borici-Mazi, Rozita
Boseovski, James
Brouillard, Daniel D.
Brunet, Donald G.
Cain, John P.
D'Arsigny, Christine L.
Da Costa, Laurington
Dancey, Janet E.
Depew, William T.
Diamant, Nicholas E.
Dudebout, Jill J.
Dudgeon, Deborah J.
Duffin, Jacalyn M.
Eisenhauer, Elizabeth A.
Ellis, Anne K.
Evans, Gerald A.
Fanaras, Effie
Ferguson, Michelle J.
Fitzpatrick, Michael F.
Garcia-Ameijeiras, Maria A.
Garland, Jocelyn S.
Ghazan-Shahi, Sassan
Gill, Sudeep S.
Gregg, Richard W.
Harrison, Mariam N.
Heyland, Daren K.
Hibbert, Nadira D.
Holden, Rachel M.
Holland, David C.
Hookey, Lawrence C.
Houlden, Robyn L.
Hudson, Robert W.
Iliescu, Eduard A.
James, Paula D.
Johri, Amer M.
Joneja, Mala
Kovacs, Katherine Ann.
Kumar, Vikaash N C.
Kunanithy, Vitharani
La Haye, Stephen A.
Lee, David H.
Lillicrap, David P.
Lougheed, M. Diane
Lowe, Catherine E.
Madarnas, Yolanda
Martinez Cajas, Jorge L.
Matangi, Murray F.
Mates, Mihaela
McLellan, Catherine S.
Meyer, Ralph M.
Mocanu, Brindusa I.
Moffatt, Susan L.
Moran-Mendoza, A. Onofre
Morton, A. Ross
Murphy, Johanna M.
Muscedere, John G.
O'Donnell, Denis E M.
O'Reilly, Michael G.
Pal, Raveen S.
Parfrey, Brendan P.
Parker, Christopher M.
Parulekar, Wendy R.
Paterson, William G.
Patton, Daniel M.
Puxty, John A H.
Ramjeesingh, Ravi A.
Redfearn, Damian P.
Riolo, Giovanna

Riopelle, Richard J.
Ropeleski, Mark J.
Sanfilippo, Anthony J.
Shamsseddin, Mohammad K.
Simon, Jerome B.
Simpson, Christopher S.
Singer, Michael A.
Smith, Christopher A.
Stalker, M. John B.
Thakrar, Amar
Toffelmire, Edwin B.
Tomiak, Anna T.
Towheed, Tanveer E.
Tsai, Ellie L.
Vanner, Stephen J.
Walker, David M C.
Wasserman, David W.
Wattam, David P.
Waymouth, Heather E.
White, Christine A.
Wigle, Ronald D.
Wobeser, Wendy L.
Yeates, Karen E.
Yendt, Edmund R.

KIRKLAND LAKE

Isenberg, Joel H.

KITCHENER

Babapulle, Mohan N.
Bahl, Mala
Bahrgard Nikoo, Mohammad J.
Benaroia, Mark
Bissonnette, Lyle V.
Bouttell, Elaine S.
Brickell, Sandra E.
Califaretti, Nadia B.
Campbell, Carolyn N J.
Champagne, Caro Line.
Chaudhry, M. Usman L.
Chernish, Robert N.
Ciccotelli, William A.
Desai, Dushyant
Didyk, Nicole E.
Ergaiey, Houda A.
Faraawi, Rafat Y.
Fowlis, Ronald A F.
Golubov, Jordan
Gregor, Laura H.
Gulan, Mirjana
Heckman, George A W.
Hentschel, Eric P.
Ho, Victoria Y W.
Hubay, Stacey A.
Ismaili, Arif M A.
Jackson, Mary E.
Jolly, Shivinder S.
Kim, Hahn Hoe
Kim, Harold L.
Knight, Gregory J.
Langridge, Jonathon M D.
Leddy, Danielle S.
Liu, Theresa T.
Liu, Tom T T.
MacEachern, Janet A.
McCarron, Bonnie I.
McNamara, Brian T.
Meghji, M. Mohamed
Molckovsky, Andrea
Nagpal, Anil K.
Needham-Nethercott, Natalie
Parlea, Luciana
Pearce, Murray E.
Plaxton, William R.
Prasad, Sadhana
Puley, Ronald J.
Racz, Heather N.
Renner, Suzanne M.
Rinne, Claus H E.
Rosenstein, Gerald A.
Sarkaria, Gagandeep S.
Saxena, Shiv K.
Sharieff, Saleem
Sharma, Vinod K.
Singer, Lorne
Smith, Stuart J.
Spanglet, Offir
Stevens, Robert L.
Strban, Martin
Suhail, Tariq
Tam, Amy S.
Theal, Michael D.
Van Walraven, Adrianus A.
Vitou, Louise Y.
White, Frederick A.
Wu, Harry K C.

LEAMINGTON

El Tawil, Basel A.
Guerra, Enrique C.
Leung, Wai Ming.
Naom, Nashwan A I.

LINDSAY

Chan, Gabriel W L.
Jones, Jeremy C.
Kazhila, David G.
Krishnan, Narayanan
Miletskaia, Galina N.
Syed, Abu A.
Zavery, Oanali T.

LISTOWEL

Brow, James R.

LONDON

Adams, Paul C.
Ahmad, Dildar
Al Jawad, Mohammed S.
Al Katheeri, Ali M A.
Al-Aama, Tareef Y A.
Alhozali, Hanadi
Allen, Susan J.
Alqutub, Adel N H.
Andrew, Philip J.
Arnold, J. Malcolm O.
Aswald, Jorg M.
Austin, Thomas W.
Barnett, William H.
Barra, Lillian
Bashir, Abdelnasir
Beaton, Melanie
Bergin, M. Lynn
Blake, Peter
Bodak, Ann-Marie
Borrie, Michael
Bosma, Karen
Boughner, Derek R.
Brownscombe, Larry
Brymer, Christopher D.
Butchey, Joseph R K.
Chande, Nilesh
Chehadi, Waleed
Chin-Yee, Ian
Chopra, Nikhil
Chow, Lawrence H.
Clark, William F.
Clemens, Kristin K.
Crilly, Richard G.
Dasgupta, Monidipa
Davey, Ryan A.
Diachun, Laura L.
Diamantouros, Pantelis
Dias, Bryan F.
Dingle, Brian
Dresser, George K.
Driedger, Albert
Dupre, John
Eberhard, R. Stuart
Edmonds, Merrill W.
Elsayed, Sameer
Ernst, D. Scott
Farag, George
Farquhar, Donald R E.
Feagan, Brian
Feldman, Ross D.
Finnie, Keith
Fraser, Lisa-Ann
Garg, Amit
George, Charles F P.
Gilbert, Kenneth
Gob, Alan
Goddard, Michele D.
Goldszmidt, Mark
Gregor, James C.
Gula, Lorne J.
Hackam, Daniel G.
Haddara, Wael M.
Hahn, Karin M E.
Haig, Sara L.
Hanninen, Mikael V W.
Harth, Manfred M.
Hegele, Robert A.
Hildebrand, Ainslie M.
Hinkkala, Kaarlo S.
Hodsman, Anthony B.
Hollomby, David J.
House, Andrew A.
Howard, John M.
Howson-Jan, Kang
Hramiak, O M. Irene
Hsia, Cyrus C.
Huang, Shih-Han S.
Huda, Noureen
Humen, Dennis P.
Hurwitz, Joel S.
Jain, Arsh K.
Jevnikar, Anthony M.
Johnson, John F.
Joy, Tisha R.
Kane, Sheri-Lynn
Kao, Raymond L C.
Kashgari, Alia Y A.
Kashgary, Abdullah Y A.
Kathirgamanathan, Kalaimakal
Kay, John D.
Kertesz, Andrew
Khan, Airudin S.
Khan, Razi
Khanna, Nitin V.
Khanna, Reena
Kim, Richard B.
Klein, George J.
Koo, Karen
Kortas, Claude
Kostuk, William J.
Kuruvilla, Mridula S.
Lam, Ngan
Lam, Selay
Lannigan, Robert
Larocque, Brian J.
Le Riche, Nicole G H.
Leasa, David J.
Leong-Sit, Peter
Levstik, Mark A.
Lewis, James F.
Licskai, Christopher J.
Lindsay, Robert M.
Liu, Selina L.
Logan, Diane M.
Lohmann, Reinhard C.
MacKenzie, Mary J F.
Mahon, Jeffrey L.
Mangel, Joy E.
Marotta, Paul J.
Martell, Rafael
Martin, Claudio M.
Massel, David R.
Mazza, Jorge A.
McCormack, David G.
McDonald, Charlotte G.
McDonald, John W D.
McFadden, Robin G.
McGillen, Joseph E M.
McIntosh, Keith S.
McKeown, Emily J.
McManus, Ruth M.
Mehta, Sanjay
Minuk, Leonard
Moist, Louise M.
Montero Odasso, Manuel M.
Moore, P. Mary
Moote, D. William
Morrison, Deric J.
Mrkobrada, Marko
Muinuddin, Ahmad
Muirhead, Norman
Myers, Kathryn A.
Patel, Paulum U.
Patrick, Lawrence
Paul, Partha
Paul, Terri L.
Payton, Keith B.
Pflugfelder, Peter W.
Pickering, J. Geoffrey
Ponich, Terry
Pope, Janet E.
Potvin, Kylea
Qumosani, Karim M Y.
Rahman, Adam N.
Ralph, Edward D.
Rehman, Faisal
Reynolds, Richard
Rodger, N. Wilson
Rohekar, Gina
Rohekar, Sherry
Romsa, G. Jonathan
Rosenberg, Eli
Rydz, Frederick
Sanatani, Irina
Sanatani, Michael S.
Sears, Gerald A.
Sen, Mithu
Sey, Michael S L.
Shah, Sachin J.
Shoemaker, Gerard J.
Siu, Samuel C B.
Skanes, Allan C.
Smaggus, Andrew C.
Spaic, Tamara
Spence, J. David
Sridhar, Krishnakumar
Stiller, Calvin R.
Strauss, Matthew S.
Sultan, Khaleel H S H.
Sultan, Nabil M.
Sun, Dongmei
Syed, Jaffer A.
Taabazui, Mary-Margaret
Taabazuing, Mary-Margaret
Tangri, Vikram
Teefy, Patrick J.
Thibert, Robert F.
Thompson, Andrew E.
Thompson, Guy W S.
Thomson, Benjamin K A.
Tsai, Gina Y.
Turkistani, Yosra A A.
Van Uum, Stanislaus H M.
Vandenberg, Theodore A.
Veldhuis, Keimpe
Vincent, Mark D.
Weingert, Michael E.
Weir, Matthew A.
Welch, Stephen A.
Wells, Jennie L.
White, James A.
Wilson, Aze S A.
Wilson, Janet L.
Winquist, Eric W.
Wisenberg, Gerald
Wojcik, John P.
Wong, Dennis S.
Wyllie, Blair F.
Xenocostas, Anargyros
Yadegari, Andrew B.
Yamashita, Cory M.
Yan, Brian
Yik, David K H.
Younus, Jawaid
Zabani, Najla A H I.
Zafar, Saira
Zahariadis, George
Zeller, Michelle P.
Zhao, Ying Ying

MANOTICK

Nishikawa, James A.

MAPLE

Chua, Grace L.

MARKHAM

Bansal, Atul
Bishara, Laila D.
Cook, Timothy J.
Dancey, David R.
Doobay, Anand V.
Forse, Monique I S.
Fu, Anna
Gnanapandithen, Kumudini
Goodman, Rusty C J.
Hacker, Paul M.
Hajra, Leena
Kogan, Eva
Lau, Agatha
Le, Khoa-Anh
Lewtas, Joanne L.
Lingley, Michael D.
Mak, Vincent C W.
Minkowitz, Joseph
Motlagh, Bahareh
Newman, David M.
Nimchonok, Punam M.
Oyenubi, Ademilola N.
Selucky, Michal
Simons, Derek B.
Sivakumar, Tharsan
Solow, Henry L.
Sultana, Shahida
Thirugnanam, Subarna
Trinkaus, Mateya E.
Tupchong, Michele A.
Van Wert, Ryan J F.
Wan, John C.
Yee, Allan J.

MEAFORD

McCall, Joann C.

MIDLAND

Dolezel, Josef
Fahy, James F A.

MILTON

Alter, David A.
Beshara, Hani M N.
Hui, Gavin
Sawhney, Gulshan

MISSISSAUGA

Al Sawi, Mohamed A M.
Al-Sabbagh, Ahmad
Alled, Jalal A.
Amer, Emad E.
Anand, Navin
Antman, Neil S.
Bahrami-Esferjani, Azar
Barboza, Milan K.
Bayliss, Michael
Bhatia, Rajan S.
Boll, Philip R.
Chakrabarti, Sumontra
Chan, Edwin S L.
Chandi, Rajpal S.
Chandrakumar, Sandrasegaram
Cheema, Amarjit S.
Cheng, Alice Y.
Cheung, Catherine Z.
Choi, Young S.
Choudhry, Ashwani
Chow, Andrew
Clark, Robert N.
Clive, Barbara A.
Correia, Adriano J.
Cyriac, Jason P.
Danial, Bahauddin H.
Devaraj, Chikkahanumaiah
Dhillon, Gagandeep S.
Di Prizito, Claudio D.
Digges, Deborah D.
Druck, Maurice N.
El-Ashry, Dalia
Enright, Katherine A.
Ernst, Blair D.
Fine, Sheldon
Flood, Diane A.
Gapski, John A P.
Ginzburg, Amir
Gottesman, Irving S.
Graham, Christopher
Grant, Margaret H.
Green, Kevin W.
Grossman, Ronald F.
Grover, Arvinder
Gupta, Anil
Harrison, David A.
Higgins, Brian P.
High, Sasha M.
Hollingworth, Roger W.
Huang, Eileen Y.
Hung, Anthony R T.
Hussain, Mohammad A.
Inouye, Tetsuo
Joshi, Supriya
Jovanovic, John E.
Kaizer, Leonard
Khan, Imtiaz M S.
Khanna, Parul
Khera, Vikas
Ki, Vincent
Kim, Donald D.
King, Michael H.
Kremer, Sidney G J.
Kumar, Sameer
Kundhal, Kiran K.
Kwan, Terry
Lange-Mechlen, Ilse
Langlois, W. John
Lazzam, Charles
Le Feuvre, Catherine A.
Lee, Christina D.
Lee, Elmer C C.
Levy, Harold L.
Lipscombe, Jennifer B.

Lipson, Frank
Liu, Yan
Maham, Nava
Maingi, Manish
McColl, Christopher
McMullen, William R.
Mehdi, Nadya B.
Menon, Krishna
Milosevic, Lawrence M.
Milosevic, Vladimir
Mody, Ami N.
Mohammed, Michelle J.
Montgomery, Angela B.
Murthy, Anant N.
Myers, Jeffrey A.
Myers, Robert E.
Nagi, Kirandeep S.
Nelles, Sandra E.
Newman, Jamie R.
Nguyen, Dang Minh.
Nikhilanandhan, Janarthan Y.
O'Connor, Thomas C.
Organ Shin, Jennifer L.
Ostro, Michael J.
Ostrowska, Krystyna I.
Ott, Carol L B.
Page, Vesna
Pataki, Janos J.
Patel, Milan V.
Pereira, W. Malathi D.
Perkins, David N.
Piersanti, Monique
Platonov, Michael
Price, Charles M.
Puley, Geoffrey S.
Quinton-Gladstone, Cindy
Rajagopal, Sudhashree
Rasul, Imran A.
Rebane, Thomas M.
Ritacca, Frank V.
Rosenthall, Wendy
Rother, Mark J.
Sarabia, Alicia
Schwarz, Rosemarie R.
Sharman, Asheer
Sibbald, R. Gary
Silva Gomez, Cecilia V.
Sim, Keng Howe
Singh, Inderbir
Sluzar, Vladimir S.
Small, Lorne N.
So, Jeffrey S.
Soghrati, Kamyar
Soh, Joo-Meng
Soucy, Elaine
Spring, Melanie J.
Strauss, Hans D.
Strevel, Elizabeth L.
Sud, Sachin
Suk, Andy G.
Temple, Bryan K.
Thompson, Kerry
Tishler, Steven J.
Tucker, A. George
Vakani, M. Tariq
Wadgymar, J. Arturo
Walz, Barbara A E.
Watson, K. Randal
Wolski, Winicjusz M.
Wong, Albert G.
Wong, Gordon K T.
Wong, Robert A.
Wu, George G.
Yip, T C. Kathy
Zaretsky, Yael S.

MORRISBURG
Schnurr, Lawrence P.

MOUNT ALBERT
Wojcicki, Andre T.

NAPANEE
Chen, Benjamin H.

NEPEAN
Beanlands, Donald S.
Bray, Frederick T.
Chawla, Jasmeet S.
Chawla, Ramandeep K.
Cohn, Adam Y.
Grewal, Rasveg S.
Harczy, Martha
Inouye, Phillip K.
Kapur, Suneil
Keses, Natalie
Kyrollos, Adel G H.
Liu, Bin
McKibbin, Timothy G.
Miller, Fraser A.
Morassut, Patricia A.
Morrin, Sharon M L.
Raju, Dharmapaul L.
Robern, Michael
Salcedo, Juan R.
Shukle, Pravin J.
Suri, Permjit S.
Whetter, Christine R.

NEW LISKEARD
Leger-Nolet, Celine N.

NEWMARKET
Anglin, Peter J.
Atwal, Gulshandeep S.
Aubrey, Michael E.
Bida, Adriana
Cantor, Warren
Chun, Robert
Evans, Kirby J.
Faris, Andrea E.
Fell, David A.
Goldman, Lorne E.
Habot, Juda
Hess, Allan R.
Hutchinson, Lisa G.
Juta, Sunil
Kachoei, Babak A.
Kassam, Farrah
Khaykin, Yaariv
Kouchakan, Mohsen
Lin, Frank Y.
Luk, Cynthia S Y.
Metawee, Mohamed L M.
Miner, Steven E S.
Nathanson, Barry N.
Ng Tung Hing, Edward K K.
Nikon, Yaghoub
Patel, Harshadrai M.
Persyko, Lucien
Plante, Sylvain
Prabhakar, Manu
Qureshi, Shahzad
Rabie, Rania N.
Rahim, Yasmin H.
Ramakrishnan, Srikanth
Roberts, D. Kenneth
Samadi, Nooshin
Schep, Gerald N.
Shafai-Sarshar, Roshan S.
Stotland, Brian R.
Symmes, John C.
Thangaroopan, Arulnmozhy
Thorne, J. Carter
Towns, Kathryn A.
Tripathi, Davender K.
Tsang, Bernice
Villeneuve, Pierre
Wang, Henry
Weingarten, Murray D.
Wulffhart, Zaev A.
Zadra, Remo
Zafar, Moiz M.
Zibdawi, Labib A A.

NIAGARA FALLS
Alexander, Michael
Chan, Terence
Chan, Yun Kai.
Dhillon, Rajwinder S.
El Zuway, Rabeh M A.
Gill, Gurpreet S.
Goodarzi, Masoud
Housley, Richard J.
Mulaisho, Chilango
Poblete, Roel C.
Puvendran, Samuel N.
Tannous, Rosemonde E.
Werhun, Robert S.
Zimakas, George W.

NIAGARA ON THE LAKE
Kischuk, Robert P.
Nolan, John

NORTH BAY
Andrews, John E.
Bowker, Blair M.
Finnis, William
Lavoie, Roberto
Saunders, Darren D.
Shulman, Scott M.
Shulman, Tanya S.

NORTH YORK
Abbott, Michael M.
Abdalian, Rupert S.
Abramson, Harry
Al Qarshoubi, Issa S M.
Al-Harbi, Othman R A.
Al-Hellawi, Ali Z D.
Alegado, Eli
Amin, Smita
Arhanchiague, Eneko R.
Bader, Russell T.
Baghdadlian, Hovsep
Bain, Jerald
Bassoon-Zaltzman, Caroline
Bastien, Pascal
Bell, Benjamin R.
Berger, Sam
Bergman, Arik
Borenstein, Harold B.
Braude, Andrew
Carr, Sean A.
Chaiton, Abraham
Chan, Frank S M.
Chan, Raymond H M.
Chen, Jia-De
Cheng, Anthony
Chidambaram, Malathi
Davidson, Derek A.
De Veber, George A.
Desai, Milind G.
Devenyi, Paul
Dostrovsky, Nathaniel
Drobac, Milutin
Dunne, Shelly M.
Edwards, Lawrence A J.
Egri, Zoltan J.
Elia, Steven T.
Esmail, Sherali G.
Etlin, David D.
Fishbein, David L S.
Fishman, Paula N.
Gayle, Barrington A.
Ghafouri, Seyed M.
Glazer, Stephen A.
Glenns, Vivian P.
Gordon, Michael
Gotesman, Galina
Graham, Caroline H.
Gray, Gary W.
Gutzin, Sheryl J.
Handelsman, Sam
Herman-Kideckel, Sari M.
Ingber, Sarah A.
Jacob, Moire S.
James, Richard G G.
Jeyaranjan, A. Richard
Kagal, Darren R.
Kaila, Brinderjit K.
Kaminker, Arthur
Kanawaty, David S.
Kanji, Dilshad A.
Katchan, Brian M.
Khatchatourian, Marina
Kim, Rak Hay
Kimball, Brian P.
Klein, Stuart W.
Knight, Burton W.
Koren, Sharon
Kotowycz, Mark A.
Krajewski, Adam
Kreaden, David A.
Kreidstein, Sharon H.
Kruczynski, Krystyna H.
Lee, Hank C.
Lee, Vivian T P.
Lekas, Poli
Liang, Dana Y.
Lubelsky, Bruce J.
Malkin, Aaron
Marotta, Giovanni C.
McKenzie, Mary A.
Medad, Ilan E.
Mederski, Barbara D.
Minnema, Brian J.
Mojab, Hamid
Monson, Rochelle L.
Morgenthau, David R.
Mortazavi, Amir A.
Moskovitz, David N.
Myron, Philip M B.
Patel, Vishal
Petrut, Bianca
Potashner, Wayne J.
Prabhakar, Maneesh K.
Ptak, Theadore W.
Rahimi Darabad, Parisa
Robson, Daniel
Rocca, Antonio S.
Roitman, Daryl S.
Rose, Randi K.
Roussev, Rossen
Rush, Perry J.
Sam, Justina J.
Sanders, Kevin M.
Shapira, Stacey C.
Sherkin, Marc D.
Shin, Phillip C.
Sibbald, Matthew G.
Silverman, Jeffrey A.
Singh, Arjune B.
Skrinskas, Gailius J.
Spiegelman, Jamie
Strauss, Martin H.
Teitelbaum, Earl J.
Theal, Jeremy J T.
Varlese, Fabio
Veinish, Shelley L.
Weber, Elizabeth A.
Weiner-Baron, David L.
Wong, Benjamin B L.
Yeung, Kam-Tong
Yip, Clarwyn
Yogaparan, Thirumagal
Zupnik, Joseph

OAKVILLE
Abid, Simona
Arya, Naveen
Bair, F. Douglas
Ball, Adrianne M M.
Bhandhal, Sharn
Chau, Laurence K L.
Chiamvimonvat, Varaporn
Chung, Arthur G.
Feneck, Mary M.
Goldstein, Jeffrey L.
Hameed, Nageen
Heffernan, Michael L.
Huang, Qingli L.
Jedrzkiewicz, Sean J.
Khan, Aliya A.
Kim, Christina K.
Kirby, John G.
Kohli, Sandeep S S.
Lau, Helena L W.
Lee, Andrea
Leith, Eric S.
MacKenzie, B. Ross
Mao, C. Russell
McConachie, David R.
McPhaden, John
Meindok, Harry
Orfi, Jan N E.
Pandeya, Sanjaya
Pandya, Sudhir P.
Patel, Jayesh
Patodia, Shaila
Peat, Donald G S.
Pham, Joe
Profiti, Raffaela
Rau, Neil V.
Rehsia, Sachdeep S.
Salazar, Charlene L.
Sapir, Daniel
Twum-Barima, David Y.
Warren, Thomas A.
Wu, Arthur
Zawadowski, Andrew G A.

ORANGEVILLE
Apps, Robert C.
Arunasalam, Kiritharan
Joshi, Atul
Martin-Smith, Paul
Mauro, Marina
McKinnon, Jeffrey L.
Mohsin, Afshan
Wiley, Scott
Willans, Gordon W.

ORILLIA
Alexander, David J.
Anand, Nitasha
Bailey, Mark N.
Byles, Nancy I A.
Collins, David S.
Crewe, Shawn G.
Jefferies, John W.
Lam, Leo T Y.
MacFadyen, John C.
Poulopoulos, Vassilios
Sriharsha, Hindupuram V.
Tascona, Daniel J.
Young, Kevin J.

ORLEANS
Tan, Kim-Weng

OSHAWA
Alessandrini, Renato S.
Bakbak, Asaad I.
Barrese, Nancy
Bhargava, Rakesh K.
Birbrager, Donna R.
Bridge, Suzanne K.
Buldo, George P.
Cha, James Y M.
Chang, Jose
Chiang, Mae S M.
Chiu, Hak M.
Chiu, Leo
Chkrebtii, Natalia O.
Chong, Angeline Y W.
Chong, Christopher A K.
Chong, Rachel Y V.
Crisp, David T.
Eisenstat, L. Jonathan
El-Keeb, Rabea A H.
Fisher, Myles G.
Forbes, Leta M.
Freedman, Orit C.
Green, Daniel M.
Huzel, Lisa L.
Jeyabalan, Neera
Koneru, Rama D.
Kwan, Michael W H.
Lenga, Ilan
Lisnevskaia, Larissa A.
Lo, Gregory K.
Long, Edward G S.
Missiha, Sharif B.
Monchesky, Theodore C.
Morra, Pasqualino
Naassan, Anthony E.
Nicula, Mihaela
Oravec, Michael
Paramsothy, Koushalya
Pavone, Elio
Rahim, Sherali A.
Ricciuto, Daniel R.
Ross, David J.
Rothenstein, Jeffrey
Sandhu, Manindar K.
Sangaralingham, Sinnadurai
Schattner, Ariah J.
Sharma, Arunabh B.
Shim, Katharine J.
Silecky, Walter B.
Soliman, Karim A F.
Steele, Andrew W.
Tahiliani, Manoj
Tahiliani, Ravi
Tepper, Jamie L.
Tuppal, Raj K.
Wax, Randy S.
Wierzbicki, Rafal F.
Willamowicz, Anna S.
Woods, Anthony C.
Zaidi, Hasan A.
Zalewski, Pawel G.

OTTAWA
Aaron, Shawn D.
Abaskharoun, Ramy R D.
Abujrad, Hussein A.

Abunassar, Joseph G.
Abunassar, Ramzi Y.
Afshari-Azad, Nahid
Akbari, Ayub
Al-Turbak, Haytham
Alanazi, Haitham A S.
Alikhan, Qasim R.
Allan, David
Almutairi, Fawaz Q R.
Alnajjar, Abdulsalam
Alqahtani, Abdulrahman
Alshahrani, Ali M G.
Alvarez, Gonzalo G.
Alwasaidi, Turki A M.
Amaratunga, Ruwan T.
Amjadi, Kayvan
Angel, Jonathan B.
Antar, Ramy
Argent, Nicholas B.
Arnaout, Amel
Ascah, Kathryn J.
Asmis, Timothy R.
Atkins, Harold L.
Auclair, Francois
Baldo, Allain
Banihashemi, Sayed-Benham
Beanlands, Rob S B.
Beauchesne, Luc M.
Begin, Micheline
Bell, Robert C.
Bence-Bruckler, Isabelle A.
Bencze, Istvan T.
Bishop, Douglas R.
Block, Jennifer K.
Boate, Brian W.
Boivin, Daniel
Bolano Del Vecchio, Silvana M.
Boyle, Loree L.
Braaten, Jan T.
Brooks, James I.
Bugeja, Ann L.
Bukowskyj, Maria
Burns, Kevin D.
Burwash, Ian G.
Byszewski, Anna M.
Cameron, D. William
Canil, Christina M B.
Cardinal, Pierre
Carrier, Marc
Castellucci, Lana A.
Catching, John D.
Chamoun, Chamoun
Champion, Malcolm C.
Chan, James W T.
Chan, Kwan-Leung
Chander, Sanjeev
Chandy, George P.
Chatha, Neel-Kamal K.
Chatterjee, Avijit
Chauret, Denis
Chen, Shin-Yee
Chow, Benjamin J W.
Clark, Edward G.
Clark, Heather D.
Code, Catherine C.
Conrad, David
Cooper, Curtis L.
Costiniuk, Cecilia T.
Cranney, Blanid A.
Cripps, M. Christine
D'Egidio, Gianni
Dahche, Khaled M.
Dahche, Tarek
Dales, Robert E.
Davies, Ross
Davis, Darryl R.
Davis, Janet L.
Davis, Kathleen A.
Dawdy, John A.
De Boer, Aglaia K.
Dehejia, Harsha V.
Deneault, Jocelyn J.
Dent, Robert R M.
Dent, Susan F.
Dhaliwal, Harinder
Di Valentin, Tanya
Dick, Alexander
Doyle, Mary-Anne
Duchesne, Lloyd
Duff, Susie
Duffett, Lisa D M.
Dugan, Alison K.
Ede, Megeri
Edwards, Cedric A W.
Eliosoff, Ronald V.
Ellen, Ruth L B.
English, Shane
Fairhead, Todd R.
Farag, Ashraf
Farazli, Christiane
Faught, Carolyn R.
Fitt, Nicole S.
Forgie, Melissa A.
Forster, Alan
Fournier, Marc
Froeschl, Michael P V.
Froeschl, Sandra
Garber, Gary E.
Gauthier, Nadine
Geiger, Glen W.
Gertler, Stanley Z.
Glover, Christopher A.
Goel, Rakesh
Goldman, Mindy R.
Gollob, Michael H.
Gonsalves, Carol
Goodall, John C.
Goodwin, Rachel
Goss, Glenwood D.
Gray, Catherine
Green, Martin S.
Haddad, Haissam A.
Hafez, Mohammed N.
Halman, Samantha
Hamadah, Abdulaziz A.
Haq, Anwar U.
Hartwick, Karl
Hasimja Saraqini, Delvina
Hassard, Philip V.
Hazra, Samir K.
Hebert, Guy J.
Hebert, Paul C.
Heshka, Jodi
Hessian, Renee C.
Hierlihy, Phyllis J.
Higginson, Lyall A J.
Ho, Jenny M.
Ho, W Steve.
Hoar, Stephanie E.
Hossenbux, Farook
Huang, Allen R.
Huang, Shirley C.
Huebsch, Lothar B.
Humphrey, Susan M.
Ismaeil, Nabeel H A.
Iyengar, Akshai M.
Jacques, Cindi N.
Jamison, Bruce M.
Jessamine, Peter G.
Jiwa, Nizarali H.
Johnson, Christopher B.
Jolicoeur, Emilie
Jones, Gwynne
Jonker, Derek J.
Jovaisas, Algis V.
Karovitch, Alan J.
Karpinski, Jolanta A M.
Karsh, Jacob
Keays, Tara N.
Keely, Erin J.
Keller, Oliver R.
Kelly, Erin M.
Khamisa, Karima
Khan, M. Gabriel
Khan, Shajia
Khoury, Lara
Kichian, Krikor
Kim, John
Knoll, Gregory A.
Kraag, Gunnar R.
Kravcik, Stephen
Kronick, Stanley H.
Kuriakose, Binny C.
Kyeremanteng, Kwadwo S.
Labinaz, Marino
Lacroix, Linda A M.
Laramee, Louise A.
Laurie, Scott A.
Lavoie, Susan D.
Law, Angeline
Le May, J. Michel R.
Le Saux, Nicole M A.
Lee, B. Craig
Lee, Ralph F.
Leech, Judith A.
Lemay, Genevieve
Lemery, Robert
Liu, Dora M.
Lochnan, Heather A.
Lui, Clementine J P M.
MacIntyre, Erika J.
MacMillan, Suzanne M.
MacPherson, Paul A.
Magner, Peter O.
Majewski, Jakub
Makar, Sherif S M.
Malakieh, Nadia
Malcolm, Janine C.
Maranda, Robert C.
Maroun, Jean A.
Marovac, M. Misha
Marquis, Jean-Francois
Massicotte, Claude J.
McCarthy, Anne E.
McCormick, Brendan B.
McIntyre, Lauralyn A.
McKendry, Robert J R.
McKim, Douglas A.
McPherson, P. Ruth
Meggison, Hillary E.
Mielniczuk, Lisa M.
Mierins, Egils
Millington, Scott J.
Milman, Nataliya
Moghadam, Soraya
Molnar, Frank J.
Moran, P. Bruce
Moudgil, Rohit
Mulligan, Matthew D.
Mulpuru, Sunita S.
Mustafa, Hassan A.
Nadler, Steven P.
Nair, Girish M.
Nicholas, Garth A.
Nichols, Robert B.
Nixon, Judith P.
Niznick, Joel M.
O'Keefe, Deborah L.
O'Leary, Timothy J.
Oliveira, Liliana M.
Ooi, Teik Chye
Padmos, M. Andrew
Pakhale, Smita S.
Patel, Rakesh V.
Peticca, Patricia
Pierscianowski, Tadeusz A.
Power, Barbara E.
Psarras, Thomas E.
Pugh, Debra
Quevillon, J A. Jean
Quinn, Brendan P.
Reaume, M. Neil
Reimche, Leanne D.
Rhodes, Ian N.
Rivington, Robert N.
Roberts, Robert
Robertson, Jeffery H.
Rochon, Luc J W.
Rodger, Marc A.
Rose, Gregory W.
Rosenberg, Erin A.
Roth, Virginia R.
Rousseau, Melissa
Roy, Mononita
Ruddy, Terrence D.
Russell, Kent R.
Ruzicka, Marcel
Sabbagh, Charles N J.
Sabbagh, Roland
Sabloff, Mitchell
Sadek, Mouhannad M.
Saginur, Raphael
Saidenberg, Elianna
Saloojee, Navaaz A.
Sandoz, Jacqueline S.
Sant, Nadia P.
Sarti, Aimee J.
Scarvelis, Dimitrios
Schneiderman, David A.
Schreiber, Yoko S.
Scott, Kenneth C.
Scully, Linda J.
Segal, Roanne J.
Sekar, Arni S C.
Shamess, Charles J.
Sharma, Kamal
Sharma, Krishna B.
Shaver, Charles S.
Shaw-Stiffel, Thomas A W.
Sheppard, Dawn C.
Shiau, Judy Y.
Silverman, Mark S.
Simos, Demetrios
Sitwell, Lucian D.
Skinner, Christopher R R.
Smith, C. Douglas
Smith, Mark A.
So, Derek Y.
Song, Xinni
Sorisky, Alexander M.
Spitale, Naomi S.
Srour, Nadim
Stadnick, Ellamae
Stewart, David J.
Stewart, Duncan J.
Sud, Shelly
Suh, Kathryn N.
Sulpher, Jeffrey A.
Sy, Richmond G.
Tailor, Chetna
Tambay, Robert
Tay, Jason
Taylor, J. Robert M.
Tharson, Carolyn C.
Thomson, John G.
Tinmouth, Alan T.
Tomiak, Eva M.
Touchie, Claire E.
Toupin, Melissa
Toye, Baldwin W.
Troppmann, Leticia A.
Tsimiklis, Georgios
Tsvetkov, Elena V.
Tugwell, Peter S L.
Turek, Michele A.
Turnbull, Jeffrey M.
Turner, Lary J.
Tyndall, Mark W.
Van Der Jagt, Richard H C.
Van Walraven, Carl G.
Varghese, Sunil A.
Verma, Shailendra
Vimalendran, Suthaharan
Visram, Hasina
Voduc, Nha
Walker, Peter
Watanabe Duffy, Karen N.
Webster, Randall J W.
Weinberg, Anthony L.
Wells, Philip S.
Wielgosz, Andreas T J.
Williams, William L.
Willis, Kenneth R.
Wilson, Kumanan R.
Wong, Thomas
Wooller, Krista R.
Wu, Grace C Y.
Xuan, Andrew Y.
Yang, William H.
Yung, Derek
Zanke, Brent W.
Zimmerman, Deborah L.

OWEN SOUND

Becks, Gregory
Johnson, Suni J.
Kaal, Nuri I M B.
Newton, F. Marcus
Ostrander, John J.
Shelig, Khaled S.

PARRY SOUND

Fargher, Terence J.
Jakubowski, Marek J.
Mills, Karen C.

PEMBROKE

Kify, Omar H.
Li, Kong Ching
Mgbemena, Benjamin E.

PERTH

Del Grande, Robert W.

PETERBOROUGH

Ball, Warren T.
Beaubien, Eliot R.
Bishop, Gregory M.
Boyle, David A.
Brien, Steven R.
Brown, Jamie C.
Butan, Radu
Chan, Andrew C S.
Cheung, Vincent S J.
Doell, Donald
Doell, Donald V.
Doris, J. Frederick
Hanson, Garth J.
Hartleib, Michael C.
Hughes, William G.
Ingram, K. Jennifer
Kammila, Srinu
Lee, Victor K G.
Li, Marilyn M.
MacKenzie, Brian M.
Mahim, Ardavan
McLaughlin, Peter R.
McMillan, David R.
Melicharkova, Andrea
Nguyen-Ho, Phong
Ninan, Vadakethu T.
Pike, Malcolm J.
Purvis, Jane
Rajendran, Bakirathan
Reesor, John N.
Shufelt, Kathryn A.
Stelzer, Hans J.
Sudbury, M. Susan F.
Swain, Gordon J.
Tainsh, Susan M M.
Vlasschaert, John J.
Wilkins, Warren T.

PICKERING

Basser, Wilma V.
Lee, Martin M S.
Malhotra, Kenneth S.

PORT PERRY

Hoey, John R.
Nasser-Sharif, Farah J.

RENFREW

Collins, Sharon C.
Delbrouck, Nicole F L.
Musawir, Amtul
Nemani, Shantiprakash S.

RICHMOND HILL

Aujla, Prince S S.
Bensoussan, Karen
Blakely, John A.
Chan, Karen B Y.
Chan, Victoria M Y.
Charest, Andre
Chen, Danny K.
Chong, Paul W C.
Chu, Eric K.
Culnan, James G.
Dighe, Krupa H.
Dwosh, Hy Avi
Fabian, Jacqueline
Fingerote, Robert J.
Fong, Edwin M Y C.
Gangbar, Eric W.
Gladman, Aviv S.
Grossman, Lawrence
Hart, R. Allan
Illamperuma, Chamani
Lai, Joe H.
Lam, Tukien M.
Lee, Kar Cheong
Leung, Nathalie M C.
Liu, L. Felix
Manuel, Mogamat A.
Maslove, David M.
Mojdami, Fatemeh
Muir, Erin E A.
Nathoo, Bharat C.
Ng, Matilda W.
Nijhawan, Pardeep K.
Pandes, Michael S.
Passaperuma, Kavitha
Plenk, Katharina
Raghavan, Ramya

Razian, Ali
Redstone, Carol S.
Richmond, Martin I.
Sarin, Nitin
Shin, Anne Y.
Sinclair, Stephen B.
Sirca, Florica C.
Srivamadevan, Maheswaran
Sugai, Michael K.
Syed, Nazia
Szaky, Esther A.
Thayaparan, Jeyasakthy J.
Turner, Penny A.
Tweeddale, Mary E.
Wu, Gilbert K P.
Yahyavi, Pooneh
Zeman, Peter R.

SARNIA

Ali, S. Nasir
Cornila, Angelica M.
Davies, Brian J.
Dhar, Jag Mohan
Jose, Aurea S.
Khan, M A. Rauf
Naidu, Renuka S.
Sahay, Bal Makund.
Shetty, Panduranga Y.
Soparkar, Gautam R.
Syan, Rajinder S.
Willans, Martin J.
Yoshida, Kenneth M.

SAULT STE MARIE

Amhalhal, Ismeil M A.
Barrett, Lisa
Berg, Gregory M A.
Berry, William A D.
Bignell, Douglas C.
Ciaschini, Patricia M.
Farah, Sameh S.
Gupta, Inder P.
Hill, Danny G.
Jenkins, Charles O.
Maharaj, Neil
Mathew, M. Thomas
Robertson, John W.
Shafiee, Mir
Spadafora, Silvana
Walde, Paul L D.

SCARBOROUGH

Acker, John J.
Al-Khayyat, Shadi S M.
Almakki, Nazar E M.
Anthony, John S.
Arnott, James H.
Arrazaghi, Abdelwahab A.
Baer, Philip A.
Bay, Ariel M.
Bierbrier, Gordon S.
Birman, Harry
Black, David R T.
Bongard, Howard B.
Boutros, Farid S A.
Burstein, Jason M.
Chan, Gabriel F P.
Chan, Gerald C B.
Chan, Patricia C K.
Chee, Jung Hoon
Chen, Grant I.
Cherry, James M.
Chiarotto, James A.
Chien, S M. Joseph
Clasky, Howard J.
Colwill, Richard W.
D'Mello, Nisha A.
Davies, Edward G.
Dhingra, Sanjay K.
Finkelstein, Sandy
Fung, Jason
Galiwango, Paul J.
Georgevich, Lila L.
Gladstone, Peter S J.
Ho Ping Kong, Wayne
Hurowitz, Eric E.
Iyer, L. Priya
Janmohamed, Amirali K.
Jethalal, Hirendrarai D.
John, Susan
Kassam, Saleem A.
Khan, Farrukh A.
Kong, Kester
Krieger, Henry
Kumar, Ganraj
Kwok, Eva
Kwok, Keith
Lazongas, Chris
Le, Brian B.
Lee, Julietta C T.
Lee, Ronita S M.
Lee Choi, Kenneth
Lefebvre, Jeanne M J.
Lessard, Janice E.
Leung, Felix K Y.
Li, Christopher W H.
Lin, Edward D H.
Ling, Michael C.
Lorraine, Joanne
Lovinsky, Reena
Low, George A.
Mace, Sean R.
Madala, Kiran
Majl, Lance B.
Makanjee, Bhavanesh
Mandell, Lionel
Manogaran, Mansula
Marqus, Sami S.
McMillan, Alexandra E.
Moosavian, Mona
Mukherjee, Ashok
Nadon, J W. Grant
Nagai, Gordon R.
Naqvi, Arif
Nazareno, Jose V C.
Neculau, Madalina
Ng, Paul S Y.
Nitkin, Robert S.
Patel, Harshna
Peress, Leonard
Peto, John J.
Pflug, Michael
Price, Howard L.
Punjani, Yasmeen A B.
Rambihar, Vivian S.
Rana, Afshan N.
Ricci, Joseph A.
Robes, Reynaldo P.
Roscoe, Janet M.
Rose, David B.
Rosen, Fred
Rosenbloom, Andrea
Roth, Lee S.
Ryzhak, Oleh M.
Sadiq, Shehla
Shahriaree, Pegah
Shainhouse, J. Zevi
Shapero, Theodore F.
Sigalas, John
Sikaneta, Tabo G.
Simmons, Pamela A.
Sivaji, Ponnuthurai
Stein, Jacob L.
Sundaralingam, Theepa
Swan, James H.
Syed, Uzma
Syed, Zareen
Tadiboyina, Venu T.
Tam, Denise H.
Tam, Paul Y W.
Tepperman, Arnold D.
Thien, Vincent V S.
Ting, Robert H.
Tobe, Lauren E.
Tran, S. Stanley
Tsui, Elaine Y L.
Tsui, Simon Y T.
Turner, Marci R.
Tyndel, Felix J.
Vador, Gunjan M.
Vaughan-Neil, Edward F.
Vertes, George E.
Vijayaraghavan, Ram
Wan, Peter S K.
Wong, Daniel M T.
Wong, Harvey H.
Wong, Keith H.
Wright, John R.
Yan, Raymond T.
Yared, Kibar
Yassa, Teraiza S S.
Yeung, Elaine T.
Zahedi, Afshan

SIMCOE

Bard, Timothy D.
Kennedy, David R.
Naas, Abdulbasitt M.
Nia, Ali
Weeks, Andrew S.

SMITHS FALLS

Moore, Stephen B.

ST CATHARINES

Abonowara, Abdulgani A M.
Agarwala, Ravi
Beshay, Alfi M.
Broski, Anthony P.
Chan, Ronnie S.
Chiew, S K. Sean
D'Sa, Ryan A.
De Souza, Henry R.
Delrue, Andrea N J.
Dickson, John R.
Ditor, Allan S.
Fernandez, Peter G.
Findlay, Brian P.
Giesbrecht, Janice L.
Griffiths, Gregory B.
Gruber, Wayne M.
Hameed, Adnan K.
Hazra, Sachin K.
Hughes, Philip F D.
Ibrahim, Khaled M O.
Jany, Mark J.
Kim, H. Hyung
Kim, Simon Y.
Kotrec, Marian
Lagrotteria, Danny D.
Lee, Linda M.
Levesque, Michael A.
Lowe, Gregory J J T.
MacKett, Robert L.
Marshall, Cheryl P.
Miller, D. Alexander
Minkarious, Edmon F W.
Nagai, Ryuta
Nolan, Thomas J.
Pallie, Sven
Rabin, Elijah Z.
Raimondo, F. Emilio
Rempel, Brenda M.
Romatowski, Walter W.
Sadikali, Fakhruddin
Safranyos, Richard G A.
Samosh, Martin L.
Shaikh, Saeed A.
Soliman, Gamal M L.
Spurek, Monika J.
Stoltz, Katherine J.
Velasquez Malvehy, Juan M.
Yelamanchili, Radhika

ST THOMAS

Burns, Timothy
Donahue, Paula C.
Ferguson, Kathleen
Hawken, Katherine A S.
Leaf, Suzanne C.
Nimir, Asim B.
Soliman, Samy

STRATFORD

Caines, Angela E.
Feltham, Matthew D.
Gillett, Michael K.
Haffner, Thomas D.
MacNaughton, Janis A.
Narayan, Shanil V.
Nicholson, Janis L.
Tamblyn, C. David

STRATHROY

Gomes, David R.
Sanders, David B.

STURGEON FALLS

Wadhwa, Atma S.

SUDBURY

Brabant, Angele Y.
Cameron, Sandra J.
Cano, Pablo O.
Cavanagh, Matthew N.
Charron, Thierry
Clarke, Jo-Anne M.
Fay, William P.
Ghosh, Nina
Gill, Kulwant S.
Goluch, Richard J.
Herst, Jordan A.
Hourtovenko, Clyde D.
Juma, Zulfikar A H.
Kalu, Uduma O.
Kerr, Mary
Kivinen, Gary W.
Labonte, Roger E.
Lopez, Pedro G.
MacDonald, Ian A G.
McElhaney, Janet E.
McKibbon, Christopher D.
Mehta, Navdeep K.
Michaud, Josee
Nawaz, Shah
Nistico, Amy R.
Noble, Jonathan C S.
Oliphant, Lawrie D.
Puranam, Padma
Ravi, Grama D.
Reddy, G. Jagan Mohan.
Robinson, Andrew G.
Roy, Denis
Sandre, Roger M.
Shivakumar, Ranganayaky
Shukla, Dinkar K.
Syan, Gurcharan S.
Theriault, Josee
Tilbe, Kim S.
Varghese, Boji
Wong, Brian Y L.
Young, Scott D.

THORNHILL

Bishinsky, Jonathan
Daitchman, Julie F.
Freedman, David M.
Goldenberg, Ronald M.
Gomperts, Natalie R.
Landolt, Sandra J.
Langer, Galina
Nussbaum, Earl B.
Rambaldini, Gloria M.
Schlosser, Robert J.
Shapiro, Lori E.
Singer, Debrah G C.
Warner, Leonard C.
Wine, Nina H.

THUNDER BAY

Abu-Bakare, Asiru
Ahmed, Nadeem A.
Ahmed, Syed Z.
Alallam, A. Aboubaker
Anderson, William D.
Ashater, Elsharif M M.
Billingsley, Ian
Biman, Birubi R.
Boake, Armour I.
Bon, Trevor J.
Chan, Adrien M T.
Chessex, Noemie
Czolpinski, Thaddeus R.
Dueck, Dorie-Anna C.
Fidler, Wesley
Gamble, D. Gregory
George, Philip
Gooding, Geoffrey T.
Holtby, Stuart G.
Joanes, Joseph F.
Kahlon, Amrit
Kellett, John G.
Kolobov, Anton
Kotchetkov, Rouslan I.
Laferriere, Nicole B.
Lai, Christopher C.
Latella, Jennifer
MacDougall, Andrea
Malik, Saleem T.
Masood, Khaja M.
McCready, William G.
Melton, Ellen
Mitchell, Catherine J.
Morrison, George H.
Nigro, Frank
O'Hara, William J.
Rafilovich, Seda S.
Raman, Kalyanapuram R.
Roussos, Marios
Shahbazi, Nasim
Sicheri, Dolores A.
Smith, H. James
Vergidis, Dimitrios
Watson, Paul A.
Wong, Mark A.

TILLSONBURG

Liwanpo, Paul T F.

TIMMINS

Adesanya, Augustine T.
Kalra, Savita
Parmar, Malvinder S.

TORONTO

Abadir, Amir
Abdel-Qadir, Husam-Eldin M.
Abdullah, Nadine
Aberman, Arnold
Abosh, Dory B.
Abrahamson, John L A.
Abrams, Howard B.
Abramson, Beth L.
Abufayyah, Mohammed
Abuzeid, Wael
Adam, Paul
Adams, Jeremy
Adhikari, Neill
Adler, Reva N.
Ahmad, Ghias
Ahmad, Kamran
Ahmad, S. Zareen
Ahmed, Shaheeda M.
Al Awamy, Mohammed B H.
Al Ghanim, Nayef S A.
Al Hussein, Mosaad A.
Al Lawati, Hatim A A H.
Al Maini, Mustafa H A.
Al-Busaidi, Mujahid
Al-Hesayen, Abdurrahman O S.
Al-Tarshi, Muna T A.
Albert, Lori J.
Albert, Shelley E.
Alguwaihes, Abdullah M A.
Ali, Naheed S.
Alibhai, Shabbir M H.
Allan, Rebecca J.
Allard, Johane
Allegro, Sabrina
Almogbel, Osama A.
Alnaqbi, Khalid
Alsarraf, Adel
Amad, Hani
Anand, Anju
Andreou, Efrosini R.
Andres, Mario R.
Angaran, Paul A.
Angel, Aubie
Anselm, Anjali H.
Appell, William A.
Arab-O'Brien, Donna M.
Aronson, Ronnie
Aslahi, Ramona
Atin, Mark D.
Avendano Alvarez, Monica
Baath, Kulrajbir
Bagai, Akshay
Bagovich, Maria A.
Bain, Douglas J G.
Baker, Jeffrey P.
Baker, Michael A.
Balter, Meyer S.
Bargman, Joanne M.
Barolet, Alan W.
Barth, David
Batt, Jane A E.
Bauer, Robert
Bayley, T. Arnold
Bayoumi, Ahmed M M.
Beamish, Judith M.
Becker, Taryn
Bedard, Philippe L.
Bekier, Estera
Bell, Charles M.
Bell, Mary J.
Ben Musa, Sirajeddin A A.
Berall, Murray J.
Berbece, Adriana N.
Berinstein, Neil L.

SPECIALISTS BY PROVINCE

Berlyne, Graham S.
Berman, Hershl
Bernstein, Michael N.
Berry, Henry
Berry, Scott R.
Betschel, Stephen D.
Bezjak, Andrea
Bhan, Vineet
Bhella, Sita D.
Bierman, Arlene S.
Billia, Filio
Binkley, Karen E.
Binnie, P. Alexandra
Binnie, William M H.
Bjarnason, Georg A.
Blackmore, Michael G.
Blackstein, Martin
Blondal, John A.
Blundell, Ross S.
Bogoch, Isaac I.
Bombardier, Claire
Bonta, Mark J.
Bookman, Arthur A M.
Bookman, Ian
Booth, Gillian L.
Boright, Andrew
Born, Abraham
Borowoy, Alan M.
Boyd, Norman F.
Bradley, T. Douglas
Brandwein, Joseph
Brezden-Masley, Christine
Briggs, Alice E.
Briones-Urbina, Rosario
Brode, Sarah K.
Bruni, Joseph
Buckstein, Rena
Buller, Christopher E H.
Bunce, Paul E.
Burkes, Ronald
Burns, Karen E A.
Burrell, Althea A.
Bykerk, Vivian
Callum, Jeannie L.
Cameron, Douglas A.
Campbell, Doreen J.
Cardella, Carl J.
Cardew, Savannah S C R.
Carette, Simon
Casella, Luigi
Casey, Deborah K.
Cass, William
Cassar-Demajo, Wilfred A.
Castelli, Mario F.
Castonguay, Vincent
Catton, Charles N.
Cattran, Daniel C.
Cavalcanti, Rodrigo B.
Cescon, David W.
Chaklader, Mohsina
Chan, Adrienne K.
Chan, Betty L.
Chan, Charles K N.
Chan, Chris C W.
Chan, Christopher T M.
Chan, Kelvin K.
Chandy, Mark J K.
Chapman, Kenneth R.
Chau, Vicky
Chauhan, Vijay S.
Cheema, Asim N.
Cheema, Harpaul S.
Cheema, Parneet K.
Chen, Christine I.
Chen, Xueyu
Cheng, Calvin K Y.
Cheng, Susanna Y.
Cheng, Wing K.
Chepesiuk, Martin A.
Cherney, David Z I.
Chessex, Caroline
Cheung, Angela C.
Cheung, Angela M.
Cheung, C Y. Mark
Cheung, Matthew C T.
Chien, Vincent
Chisholm, Robert J.
Cho, Brian J H.
Chodirker, Lisa
Choi, Richard F Y.
Chow, Chi-Ming
Chow, Chung Wai
Chow, Shirley
Chow, Stephen S.
Choy, Gregory W.
Christian, Michael D.
Chun, Soohun
Chung, Carmen W H.
Ciofani, Amelia
Cohen, Eric A.
Cohen, Lawrence B.
Coke, William J.
Cole, Edward H.
Colman, Jack M.
Colman, Rebecca E.
Cooligan, Terrance
Cooper, Mary Anne
Courtney, Brian K.
Croitoru, Kenneth
Crump, Michael R.
Cruz Pereira, Oscar O.
Cserti-Gazdewich, Christine M.
Curtis, M. Anne
Czarnecki, Andrew
D'Silva, Karen
Da Costa, Rhiannon
Daneman, Nick
Daniel, Lorretta B.
Davidson, Murray
Dawson, Ainsley E.
Day, Anna
De Villa, Maria A.
Del Campo, J C. Martin
Delaney, Jesse W.
Detsky, Allan S.
Dev, Shelly P.
Devine, Luke
Devlin, Timothy
Dhalla, Irfan A N.
Dhani, Neesha
Dicum, Francis D.
Dighe, Kushal J.
Disperati, Patricia
Docheva, Diyana S.
Donat, Diane J.
Dorian, Paul
Dotten, Dale A.
Dounaevskaia, Vera
Downar, James A.
Downey, James F.
Downing, Mark
Drucker, Daniel J.
Dubbin, James
Dwosh, Isaac
Dzavik, Vladimir
Earle, Craig C.
Economopoulos, Peter A.
Edwards, Jeremy
Eisen, Andrea
Elimova, Elena
Elkashab, Magdy A M H.
Elmanfud, Omran R.
Elmayergi, Nader
Elsobky, Reem
Elzawi, Abdul F M.
Epstein, Stanley W.
Esquivel, Manuel N.
Etchells, Edward
Ezzat, Shereen Z.
Fam, Neil P.
Fan, Eddy
Fantus, Ivan G.
Farkouh, Michael
Faughnan, Marie E.
Feig, Denice S.
Feinman, Saya V.
Feld, Jordan
Feld, Ronald
Ferguson, Niall D.
Ferreira, Ivone M.
Fettes, Ivy M.
Fieghen, Heather E.
Filate, Woganne
Fisher, Jolene H.
Fisher, Joseph A.
Fisher, Murray M.
Fisher, Rory H G.
Fisman, David N.
Fletcher, David M.
Fong, Ignatius W.
Fountas, Panayiotis N.
Fowler, Robert A.
Fraser, Ian
Freedman, Stephen M.
Freeman, Michael R.
Friedlander, Sam A.
Friedrich, Jan Oliver.
Frost, David
Fung, Scott
Gaisano, Herbert Y.
Gakhal, Natasha K.
Gandell, Dov
Gandhi, Shital
Gandhi, Sonal
Gardam, Michael A.
Garvey, M. Bernadette
Geerts, William H.
Geisler, William O.
George, Susan R.
Gerard, Lauren M.
Gershon, Andrea S.
Gershon, Sydney L.
Gilbert, Jeremy D.
Gilbert, Richard E.
Gilley, Heather J.
Ginsburg, Shiphra R.
Gladman, Dafna D.
Goddard, Shannon L.
Goguen, Jeannette M.
Golan, Eyal
Gold, Jewel
Gold, Wayne L.
Goldenberg, Leslie
Goldlist, Barry J.
Goldstein, Marc B.
Goldstein, Roger S.
Goligher, Ewan C.
Goluboff, Lanny
Goodman, Shaun G.
Goodwin, Pamela J.
Gopinath, Nanda
Gospodarowicz, Maria K.
Gough, Kevin A.
Graczyk, Joanna
Granton, John T.
Greenberg, Gordon R.
Grennan, J. Troy
Grigoriadis, Elizabeth
Grinman, Michelle
Groenewoud, Yolanda A.
Grossman, Loren D.
Grover, Samir C.
Gudgeon, Patrick
Guirguis, Hany R Y.
Gupta, Anup K.
Gupta, Rajesh
Gupta, Samir
Ha, Andrew C T.
Habal, Flavio
Hall, David A.
Hamilton, M. Lynn
Hanna, Amir K.
Hannach, Barbara R.
Hansen, Mark S.
Haq, Rashida
Harel, Ziv
Hawker, Gillian
Hawryluck, Laura A.
Hayes, Christopher W.
Heathcote, E. Jane L.
Heffer, Matthew
Hendler, Aaron L.
Hercz, Gavril
Herridge, M. Margaret S.
Hicks, Lisa K.
Hillmer, Melinda
Hingwala, Jay P.
Hladunewich, Michelle A.
Ho, Joanne M.
Hochman, Jacqueline R.
Hogg, David H.
Horlick, Eric M.
Hota, Susy S.
Howard, Robert J.
Hsiao, Janey S C.
Huang, David J T.
Huang, Vivian W.
Hurwitz, Gilbert A.
Husain, Mansoor
Hutcheon, Michael A.
Hutchinson-Jaffe, Adam B.
Hwang, Stephen W.
Hyland, Robert H.
Hyman, Andrew R.
Imrie, Kevin R.
Ing, Douglas J.
Inman, Robert D.
Irvine, Elizabeth Jan.
Iscoe, Neill A.
Iwanochko, Robert M.
Izukawa, Terumi A.
Jamal, Abida S.
James, Jacqueline
Jamieson, William T.
Janevski, John
Jang, Raymond W.
Jassal, S. Vanita
Jay, Richard M.
Jeejeebhoy, Khursheed N.
Jerome, Dana C.
Johnson, Sindhu R.
Josse, Robert G.
Joyner, Campbell D.
Juurlink, David N.
Juvet, Stephen C.
Kahr, Walter H A.
Kamel, Kamel S.
Kandel, Gabor P.
Kang, Amrit K.
Kapral, Moira K.
Karanicolas, Stavros
Kargel, Marcus J.
Katz, Kevin C.
Katz, Miriam
Kaul, Rupert
Keating, Armand
Keefe, Peter H.
Keesal, Nancy B.
Kelly, Catherine M K.
Kempston, John D.
Kenny, Lisa P.
Kenshole, Anne B.
Kevork, Raymond B.
Keystone, Edward C.
Keystone, Jay
Khamsi, Firouz
Khan, A H. Mahmood
Khan, Kamran M.
Khan, Shagufta U.
Kilany, Ali K A A.
Kim, Raymond H.
Kim, S. Joseph
Kim, Sandra A.
Kim, Young-In
Kirshen, Albert J.
Kitchell, Latiff A.
Kitchens, James M.
Klein, David J.
Knight, Allan
Knox, Jennifer J.
Ko, Dennis T.
Ko, Yoo Joung
Kobulnik, Jeremy
Kopplin, Peter A.
Korley, Victoria J.
Kormendi, Ferenc
Kortan, Paul P.
Kovacs, Julie A J.
Krahn, Murray D.
Krajden, Sigmund
Krajny, Milos J.
Krimly, Ahmed M S.
Krzyzanowska, Monika K.
Kukaswadia, Sadiya S.
Kukreti, Vishal
Kung, Tabitha N.
Kuo, Kevin H.
Kuper, Ayelet
Kuriya, Bindee
Kuruvilla, John G.
Kutryk, Michael J B.
La Delfa, Ignazio
Lai, Emily J.
Lakhani, Aly
Laksman, Zachary W.
Laluck, Bohdan
Landolt-Marticorena, C. Maria
Landy, Joshua S.
Lang, Anthony E T.
Langer, Anatoly I.
Lapinsky, Stephen E.
Laranjeiro, Joao M V.
Laredo, E. Sheila
Laskin, Carl A.
Lau, Ambrose K.
Lau, Ching
Laupacis, Andreas
Lazar, Neil M.
Lee, Christie M.
Lee, Cindy H Y.
Lee, Douglas S Y.
Lee, Jason K.
Lee, Kut Yau
Lee, Mary C Y.
Lee, Peter
Lee, Warren L.
Lee, Yuna
Lega, Iliana C.
Lehnert, Dominic C.
Leighl, Natasha B.
Leis, Jerome A.
Leiter, Lawrence A.
Leong, Eric W H.
Leong-Poi, Howard M.
Leung, Frances Y K.
Leung, Richard S T.
Leung, Wesley D C Y.
Levene, Richard G.
Levin, Leslie
Levinson, Ari D.
Levinson, Wendy
Levy, Gary A.
Lewis, Gary F.
Leznoff, Arthur
Li, Christopher K.
Li, Dorothy Y Y.
Li, Jing
Li, Qin
Liberman, Dan
Liew, Elena
Liles, W. Conrad
Lilker, Emmanuel S.
Lilly, Leslie B.
Lin, Yulia
Lingas, Rania I.
Lipscombe, Lorraine L.
Lipton, Jeffrey H.
Liu, Barbara A.
Liu, Fei-Fei
Liu, Geoffrey
Liu, Louis W C.
Livingstone, Donald J.
Lo, Dorothy S.
Locke, Kenneth A.
Logan, Alexander G.
Logsetty, Giridhar
Lok, Charmaine E.
Long, Barry H.
Loutfy, Mona R.
Low, Donald E.
Luk, Adriana C.
Luk, Cynthia T.
Ly, Joseph P H.
MacDonald, Kelly S.
MacFadden, Douglas K.
MacKenzie, Robert G.
MacMillan, Leslie G.
Madan, Minakshi
Mah-Poy, Kimberly
Mahendira, Dharini
Mak, Susanna S S.
Maldonado, Juan E.
Maleki-Yazdi, Mohammad R.
Malik, Kartika
Man, Hon-Sum J.
Mangat, Iqwal S.
Maniate, Jerry M.
Manocha, Sanjay
Marcon, Norman E.
Margulies, Niculina M.
Marras, Theodore K.
Marwaha, Seema
Maser, Joel E.
Mason, Warren P.
Matlow, Anne G.
Matukas, Larissa M.
May, Gary R.
Mazzulli, Tonino
McCready, Janine
McCredie, Victoria A.
McDonald, Michael A.
McDonald Blumer, M. Heather
McEwan, M M. Patricia
McFarlane, Philip A.
McGeer, Allison J.

SPECIALISTS BY PROVINCE

McIntyre, Kieran P D.
McKenna, Anne M.
McLeod, Anne G.
McNeely, David J.
Meharchand, Jacinta M.
Mehta, Rajin
Mehta, Sangeeta
Melvin, Kenneth R.
Mendelssohn, David C.
Messner, Hans A.
Mewa, Amirudin A M.
Meyer, L. Joanne
Millar, Adam C.
Miller, Judith A.
Miller, Saul
Minden, Mark D.
Mintz, Sheldon
Minuk, Howard L.
Mishra, Sharmistha
Mitoff, Peter
Mittoo, Shikha
Moe, Gordon W.
Moffatt, Josiah B.
Monge, Juan C.
Moore, Malcolm J.
Moore, Terrence L.
Morgan, Christopher D.
Morgan, Matthew W.
Moric, Jakov
Morra, Dante J.
Morris, Andrew M.
Mosko, Jeffrey D.
Mourad, Ophyr
Mubareka, Samira
Mukerji, Geetha
Muller, Matthew P.
Munshi, Laveena
Murthy, Sanjay
Myers, Martin G.
Myers, Robert B H.
Nadarajah, Jeya T.
Nadeau-Fredette, Annie C.
Nadjafi, Maral
Naeem, Nauman
Naessens, Veronique
Naglie, I. Gary
Naidu, Rajgopaul
Naimark, David M J.
Najeeb, Umberin
Nanthakumar, Kumaraswamy
Naylor, C. David
Nesbitt, Gillian C.
Nesrallah, Gihad E.
Newton, Gary E.
Ng, Dominic S K.
Ng, Douglas S.
Ng, Karen
Nguyen, Geoffrey C.
Nicholas, R. Everton S.
Niroumand-Sarvestani, Mitra
Noronha, Luis C E.
Norris, Erin B.
Norris, Mireille A.
O'Brien, Tara E.
Oechslin, Erwin N.
Ogilvie, Richard I.
Oh, Paul I T.
Okrainec, Karen
Oliver, Matthew J.
Olivieri, Nancy F.
Osten, Mark D.
Ostrowski, Marian A.
Otremba, Mirek
Ottaway, Clifford
Overgaard, Christopher B.
Oza, Amit M.
Paco, Charles A.
Page, Andrea V.
Pain, Tarun K.
Pang, Jeffrey T W.
Panisko, Daniel M.
Parker, D. John
Parker, Thomas G.
Patel, Yashesh
Pavenski, Katerina
Payne, David G.
Pearson, Derek S.
Pedvis, Stacey R.
Pei, York P C.
Pendergrast, Jacob M.
Perkins, Bruce J L A.
Perl, Jeffrey
Perlin, Louise R B.
Peterson, John C.
Petrella, Teresa M.
Phillipson, Eliot A.
Pierratos, Andreas
Piliotis, Eugenia
Piquette, Dominique
Piran, Sanaz
Poldre, Peeter A.
Poon, Stephanie C.
Popovic, Stanislav
Poutanen, Susan M.
Powis, Jeff E.
Prasad, G V. Ramesh
Prica, Anca
Pritchard, Kathleen I.
Pruzanski, Waldemar
Puchyr, Martina
Quaggin, Susan E.
Quansah, Joseph S T.
Qureshy, Kamran
Ra, Greta S.
Rabeneck, Linda
Rachlis, Anita R.
Radhakrishnan, Shyam
Rambihar, Sherryn P.
Rana, Amira
Rana, Punam
Ranganathan, Narasimhan
Rao, Myurathy
Rauchwerger, Martin
Ravindran, Nikila C.
Ray, Joel G.
Rebick, Gabriel
Redelmeier, Donald A.
Reece, Donna E.
Reial, Juri
Reich, Heather N.
Reiss, Dina
Retnakaran, Ravi
Rewa, George
Rewa, Oleksa G.
Richardson, Beverley J.
Richardson, Lisa A.
Richardson, Robert M A.
Richardson, Susan E.
Richter, Suzanne C.
Ridout, Rowena
Roberts, Eve A.
Rocha, Roland C.
Rochon, Paula A.
Rodriguez, Carlos H.
Rogovein, Ted S.
Roifman, Idan
Ross, Heather J.
Rossos, Peter G.
Roth, Sherryn N.
Rothman, Laura G.
Rotstein, Coleman M F.
Rottapel, Robert K.
Rowat, Bruce M T.
Rozenberg, Dmitry
Ruth, Jonathan
Ryan, Clodagh-Mai
Ryan, Douglas R.
Safinia, Layla
Sagman, Uri
Sahebjam, Solmaz
Sahni, Puja K.
Saibil, Fredric G.
Salit, Irving E.
Salmasi, Ghazal
Saltzman, Abraham J.
Sands, Alex
Santos, Claudia
Sapir-Pichhadze, Ruth
Sargeant, Robert J.
Sarin, Michael K.
Sasal, Joanna T.
Sasson, Zion S.
Sawka, Annie M.
Sawka, Carol A.
Scales, Damon C.
Schiff, Jeffrey
Schimmer, Aaron D.
Schipper, Harvey
Scholey, James W.
Schreiber, Martin
Schuh, Andre C.
Schwartz, Leonard
Segal, Phillip H B.
Seidelin, Peter H.
Seidenfeld, Allan M.
Selby, Deborah M.
Selby, Rita
Seyed Akhavan, Pooneh
Shadowitz, Steven B.
Shafiee Nyestanak, Mohammad A.
Shah, Baiju R.
Shah, Hemant A.
Shalby, Moustafa A M M.
Shapera, Shane M.
Sharkawy, Abdul Q A.
Sharma, Malika
Shaw, Tammy Y.
Shear, Neil H.
Shehata, Nadine
Shepherd, Frances A.
Sherman, Morris
Sholzberg, Michelle
Shumak, Steven L.
Shupak, Rachel
Siddiqi, Ferhan S.
Siddiqui, Nausheen F.
Silver, Robert D.
Silver, Samuel A.
Silverberg, Jay D H.
Silverberg, Mark S.
Silverman, Melvin
Silversides, Candice K.
Siminovitch, Katherine A.
Simor, Andrew E.
Singal, Sewa R.
Singer, Lianne G.
Singer, Peter A.
Singh, Jeffrey M.
Singh, Sheldon M S.
Singh, Simron
Singh, Sunita K S.
Singhal, Rajni
Sinha, Samir K.
Sinuff, Tasnim
Siu, Lillian L Y.
Sivaciyan, Vahe
Sivjee, Khalil Y.
Skrastins, Roland
Slaughter, Graham R D.
Slegr, Marie N.
Smith, Christopher N C.
Smith, Terry S.
Snihura, Robert
Sohi, Davedeep S.
Sokoluk, Craig A.
Song, Howard H.
Sourkes, Myra
Sovran, Steven A.
Spaner, David E.
Spears, Danna A.
Spears, John C.
Springer, Jonathon E.
Sridhar, Srikala S.
Srigley, Jocelyn A.
Srikanthan, Amirrtha
St George-Hyslop, Peter H.
Stafford, Susan E.
Stal, Jeffrey M.
Stanbrook, Matthew J B.
Stanley, Katherine S.
Staples, John A.
Steiman, Amanda J.
Stein, Jonathan D.
Stein, Raymond D.
Steiner, George
Steinhart, A. Hillary
Stephenson, Anne L.
Sternberg, Leonard
Stewart, Thomas E.
Stone, Elaine
Straus, Sharon E.
Strauss, Bradley H.
Stroud, Lynfa F.
Sue-A-Quan, Gregory T.
Sugar, Linda M.
Sujana Kumar, Shoba
Sussman, Gordon L.
Szmitko, Paul E.
Taggart, Linda R.
Tal, David T.
Tan, Darrell H S.
Tandon, Anu
Tanna, Gemini V.
Tannock, Ian F.
Tarlo, Susan M.
Tartaro, Piero
Teitel, Jerome M.
Tenenbaum, Jerry
Tennankore, Karthik K.
Thapar, Natasha
Thenganatt, John
Thomas, Peter
Thomas, Sunu S.
Thongthai, Kanyabhorn
Tile, Lianne E.
Tinckam, Kathryn J.
Tinmouth, Jill M.
Tobe, Sheldon W.
Toma, Alina
Tram, Carolyn Q N.
Tram, Khai Minh
Tran, Maithy N.
Trinh, K Y. Denny
Trinkaus, Martina A.
Trivieri, Maria G.
Trudeau, Maureen E.
Trudel, Suzanne M.
Tsang, Jennifer L.
Tsang, Richard W C.
Tse, Yvonne Y W.
Tsien, Cynthia
Tsui, Vincent T.
Tu, Jack V.
Tullis, D. Elizabeth
Tzanetos, Katina
Uddin, A H M. Jamal
Udell, Jacob A.
Upton, Julia E M.
Urback, Percy G.
Urowitz, Murray B.
Vadas, Peter
Valois, Maria
Van Den Berg, Lucretia
Vanek, Arthur W.
Varga, Marica
Varshney, Nishi K.
Vellend, Hillar
Verma, Sunil
Volpini, Brie V.
Voorneveld, Colin R.
Vozoris, Nicholas T.
Wadhwa, Gagan D D.
Wald, Ron
Walfish, Paul G.
Walmsley, Sharon L.
Walsh, Christopher J.
Wang, Jean C Y.
Warner, Ellen
Warner, Michael B.
Warr, David G.
Warren, Heather M.
Waxman, Menashe B.
Webster, Peter M.
Weinstein, Jordan J.
Weizman, Adam
Wells, Richard A.
Wells, Woodrow A.
Werb, Marsha R.
Whiteside, Catharine I.
Wijeysundera, Harindra C.
Wilcox, M. Elizabeth
Wilson, Jonathan J.
Win, Lay Lay
Wither, Joan E.
Wolfe, Robert E.
Wolfs, Maria E.
Wolman, Stephen L.
Wong, Brian M.
Wong, Camilla L.
Wong, David K H.
Wong, David T W.
Wong, Florence S H.
Wong, Natalie
Wong, Rene
Woo, Anna
Woo, Minna N.
Wu, Robert C.
Yan, Andrew T.
Yazdani, Arash
Yeboah, Ophelia
Yee, Karen W L.
Yeo, Erik L.
Yogeswaran, Kumaresan
Yong, Elaine
Yu, Catherine H.
Yu, Derek
Yu, Eric H C.
Yu, Joanne L.
Yuan, Jane
Yuen, Darren A.
Zahirieh, Alireza
Zaltzman, Jeffrey S.
Zeman, Robert
Zia, Mohammad I.
Zimmermann, Camilla C U.
Zinman, Bernard
Zorzitto, Maria L.
Zownir, Jerry R.
Zurawska, Joanna H.
Zurawska, Urszula

TRENTON

Hilton, Jack G.
Koshy, Varghese C.

UNIONVILLE

Murray, Iain C.
Wai, Yvonne

VANIER

Gregoire, Sylvie

VAUGHAN

Bilbily, Ghassan F Y.
Bonafede, Nicoletta
Cohen, Dana R.
Ford, David
Pourdowlat, Afsaneh

WATERLOO

Husein, Nadira
Sharad, Sunil
Steingart, Christopher R.
Terpstra, Collin R.
Yip, Lisa Y.

WELLAND

Abraham, E. George
Gallab, Nagy F A E.
Habdank-Kossowski, Katherine
Khandelwal, Mukesh Kumar N.
Sobkowski, Wojciech W.

WHITBY

Heslop, Winston L.
Ho, Benjamin G M.
Kumar, Naresh
Man, Kwok-Chu
McAlister, Neil H.
Singh, Jitendra K.

WINCHESTER

Gupta, Kaveri
Irobi, Clara C.
MacLean, Mary J.

WINDSOR

Abdelgader, Abdelgalel
Abouhassan, Tyceer
Aboulisayen, Abdullah M.
Abu-Zahra, Hakam T.
Ahmed, Abdelaziz A E.
Alam, Zeenat Y.
Bacchus, Rahman
Bagga, Amit
Bautista, Alberto
Callaghan, Wayne D.
Chahine-Malus, Natalie
Chan, Vanessa P S.
Chao, Stephen
Chaudhry, Sukarno N.
Chetty, Rajendra M.
Cheung, M C. Raphael
Dhar, Anil
Farjalla, Salaheddin G.
Fituri, Rasem L.
Glanz, Anthony E.
Hamm, Caroline M.
Hellyer, Deborah J.
Huq, Nisarul M.
Hussaini, Syed M.
Jacobs, Lawrence
Jeun, Bing W.
Jina, Abdul F.
Kadri, Albert
Kanjeekal, Sindu M.

Khalil, M. Arshad
Kidd, Arthur D F.
Kooner, Sukhdev S.
Kulkarni, Swati
Lewis, Sheldon D.
Liem, Tiang-Ham
Malus, Eli
Mandal, Amal B.
Mathews, John
McFarlane, Martin H.
Mikhail, Roland G.
Morsi, A. Ahmed
Nwadiaro, Nduka
Peer, Ismail G H.
Quan, Corinna M.
Rajkumar, Winston D.
Rodrigues, Jude F N.
Rosenhek, I. Shoel
Saad, Wassim
Sclater, Anne L.
Shaban, Joseph A.
Shanfield, Simon E.
Sieniawski, Rafal
Simeunovic, Branko
Tan, Jerry K L.
Tan, Lee Puan
Tan, Richard Y.
Tarabain, Osman A.
Torrible, Susan J.
Treki, Ibrahim M.
Upneja, Harpreet K.
Wasserman, Avi
Wilson, Robert J.
Wong, George K K.
Yap, Hanle O.
Yoshida, Sam S.
Zanganeh, Shahin

WINGHAM
Flowers, Michele A.

WOODBRIDGE
Aggarwal, Ram K.
Axler, Jeffrey L.
Bertucci, Vince
Daba, Ledjalem A.
Josan, Kiranbir
Listgarten, Charles

WOODSTOCK
Al-Mane, Faisal M.
Fullerton, Gary M.

YORK
Balsys, Aras J.
Cheung, Ming-Tat
Klug, Andrew P.
Rudinskas, Leona C.
Slaughter, David N.
Tiong, Irving Y H.
Varadi, Robert G.
Vozoris, Socrates A.

PRINCE EDWARD ISLAND

CHARLOTTETOWN
Adams, Lenley S.
Beck, Jeremy N.
Bergin, Patrick C.
Champion, Philip E.
Clark, Donald L.
Deziel, Francois
Dryer, Dagny E.
Harris-Eze, Ayodeji
Hunt, Barry H.
McCarthy, Kenneth G A.
McMillan, Colin J.
Seviour, J. Paul
Shetty, Karunakara N.

SUMMERSIDE
Carmody, Douglas E.
Hoare, Constance D.
Irvine, Michael A.

QUÉBEC

ALMA
Couture-Villeneuve, Francois
Gagnon, Michel P.

AMOS
Boyer, Liette
Govig, Bert A.
Javaheri, Sepehr
Roy, Pierre-Olivier
Theriault, Benoit
Warren, Paule

BAIE-COMEAU
Bonin, Patricia
Girard, Yves
Lapointe, Veronique
Pare, Chantal

BELOEIL
Charbonneau, Yves

CAP-AUX-MEULES
Berube, Michel J A.
Dansereau, Luc
Hanel, Robert

CHANDLER
Bechard, David
Bonenfant, Francis
Ferland, Mario
Hebert, Isabelle
Walker, Caroline

CHATEAUGUAY
Alwin, David M.
Bourrellis, Sonia
Chenier, France
Dussault, Pierre
Fortin, Charles
Gamache, Ghislaine
Garceau, Nicole
Granger, Nathalie
McCabe, Pierre
McNabb-Baltar, Julia
Nguyen, Cong Du
Ouellet, Pierre-Luc
Skaburskis, Martin W.

CHICOUTIMI
Allard, Christian
Begin, Paul
Belisle, Damien
Belisle Jr., Pierre
Bilodeau, Jean-Sebastien
Bouchard, Hugues
Breton, Robert
Breton-Thibodeau, Marianne
Cote, Fanny
Duranceau, Caroline
Gagnon, Elisabeth
Grondin Beaudoin, Brian
Houle, Marie-Andree
Joncas, Sebastien X.
Labbe, Patrick
Laverdiere, David
Leblanc, Jean-Pierre
Massy, Caroline
Paradis, Eric
Roy, Nathalie A M.
Simard, Raynald
Villeneuve, Helene

COTE SAINT-LUC
Baltzan, Marcel A.
Jukier, Lilian
Rotaple, Michael J.

COURCELETTE
Drolet, Patrice

COWANSVILLE
Gottke, Markus U.
Koopmann, Peter
Macek, Daniel B.
Michaud, Sophie
Nguyen, Jennifer
Sirhan, Shireen M.

DOLBEAU-MISTASSINI
Bouchard, Elise
Lachance, Nathalie
Lizotte, Marie-Eve

DRUMMONDVILLE
Allard, Yves
Carrier, Daniel J.
Falardeau, Simon
Gallant, Marco
Larose, Andre
Noel, Alain
Paquette, Odile
Perreault, Isabelle
Roux, Rene
Sanfacon, Martin
St-Georges, Catherine
Viens, Daniel L.

GASPE
Bourget, Philippe
Couture, Caroline
Laverdiere, Patrick

GATINEAU
Abou-Nassar, Karim E.
Babin, Sandra
Bernier, Jean-Pierre
Berris, Kenneth
Boisvert, Denis
Boufassa, Meriem
Brousseau-Tremblay, Isabelle
Clement, Pierre
Cote, Gilles E.
D'Amours, Georges
Dallaire, Mario
Dao, Catherine T.
Doumit, Maya
Engfield, Marc
Forget, Eric J.
Frechette, Dominique
Garon, Jean
Gaudet, Sylvie
Halle, Denis
Jolicoeur, Gilbert
Julien, Natalie A.
Lalonde, Andrea E S.
Lanoie, Genevieve
Lefebvre, Sonia
Levesque, Claude
MacDonald, Sara E.
Moleski, Luc
Nguyen, Khiem Ngoc
Nguyen, Tang-Thong
Proulx, Normand L.
Pucar, Frederic
Starra, Ronald F.
Sutcliffe, Ian T.
Tatu, Dan-Marius
Valcourt, Dieudonné
Zadorozny, Oleg G.

GRANBY
Bourgeois, Stephanie
Clement, Serge
Germain, Caroline
Morisset, Anne
Rivard, Marc-Antoine
Robert, Caroline
Robichaud, Philippe

GREENFIELD PARK
Angle, James D.
Beauchef, Jean-P
Beauchemin, Julie
Begin, Violaine
Benard, Bernard
Benzazon, Michael
Bisson, Patrick
Bisson, Sebastien
Boisjoly, Josie-Anne
Chasse, Marc L.
Cournoyer, Serge
Cusson, Jean
Dery, Lorraine
Desilets, Etienne
Desjardins, Pierre
Devaux, Celine
Diec, Olivier H Q.
Dube, Normand
Dufresne, Julie
Duong, Dinh Huy
Faucher, Jacques-Philippe
Fox, Susan B.
Gaudreault, Gertie
Guillet, Mario A.
Kanji, Mohammed I.
Langlois, Fabienne
Latreille, Jean
Lavigne, Annie
Lebovich, Irith
Leonard, Sophie
Mak, Anton
Moore, Andrew D.
Morissette, Nathalie
Nguyen, Dang Khoa
Nguyen, Trung Nghia
Passerini, Louise
Pietrangelo, Maria G.
Poirier, Germain
Quan, Eric
Rivet, Roxanne
Rodier, Francois
Samson, Benoit
Savoie, Lisa
Soltys, George I M.
Sperlich, Catherine
Tran, Hanh-Khiem
Vallee, Chantal
Yared, Nada

JOLIETTE
Duchesne, Line
Dussault, Charles
Marquez Azalgara, Vladimir
Morisset, Julie
Riahi, Mounir
Roberge, Guillaume
Sabbagh, Ramsey
Thivierge, Marie-France
Yergeau, Stephanie

JONQUIERE
Carrier, Stephane
Plourde, Patrice

KIRKLAND
Gilbert, François
Mayer, J O. Jean-Pierre
Palaic, Mladen
Sandrin, Franco

LA POCATIERE
Racine, Marie-Claude

LAC-MEGANTIC
Pusca, Adrian
Saad, Wadih-Pierre

LACHINE
Brox, Alan G.
Edwards, Michelle
Farooki, M. Sarwar
Garg, Sunil
Sairam, Charith
Teltscher, Marty S.
Toledano, Thierry E.

LACHUTE
Exantus, Marjorie
Liu Chen Kiow, Khim Sew H.

LASALLE
Bastedo, Clare
Bellon, Marie-Michelle
Brossoit, Real
Gelly, Andre L.
Gilman, Sean A.
Godet, Patrick
Lahoud, Nadine J.
Langlais, Francois
Lapin, Henry D.
Nepveu, Marie-Helene
Van Vo, Thi Hai

LAVAL
Ahlan, Jennifer C M.
Aucoin, Nathalie
Bahsali, Georges I.
Becker, Rubin M.
Belanger, Andre
Bergeron, Marie-France
Bergevin, Marco
Boutros, Gebran E.
Caron, Andre B.
Charbonneau, Marc
Chronopoulos, Alexandra
Ciolofan, Oana C.
Comeau, Reginald
Comtois, Hubert
Couture, Nathalie
Descarries, Laurence
Desjardins, Marie-Helene
Doucet, Isabelle
Dumas, Richard
Essiambre, Richard E.
Farber, David F.
Gelston, Arthur L.
Gendreau, Raymond
Giroux, Yvon
Haddad, Henri K.
Hadjoudj, Hachemi
Hamel, Melanie
Hazeltine, Mark
Joly, Lucie
Langlais, Rebecca
Lapointe, Carole
Long, Helene
Marcotte, Jean
Mayrand, Helene
Monette, Marie-Jose
Murphy, Colm J.
Nadeau, Etienne
Nguyen, Anh Tu
Nguyen Thanh, Hien-Tu
Nudo, Carmine G.
Osseni, Fadel
Palardy, Jean
Paradis, Bruno
Pham, Luc Anh D.
Prud'Homme, Louis
Raymond, Martine
Raymond, Nicolas
Ringuette, Gaetan
Roy, Annie
Saheb, Nathalie
Talbot, Danielle
Tremblay, Christine
Tremblay, Richard
Verschelden, Paul
Vezina, Danielle

LEVIS
Auger, Pierre
Belanger, Mario
Blier, Claude
Bourdages, Raymond
Brulotte, Steeve
Crete, Martin
DeGrace, Michel F.
Deschenes, Dominique
Drouin, Christine
Dupuis, Marie-Josee
Giguere, Richard
Gonthier, Genevieve
Grondin, Francois R.
Hache, Chantal
Landry, Stephanie
Lavoie, Remi
Lemieux, Ariane
Marchand, Helene
Michaud, Nicolas
Morrissette, Hugo
Pelletier, Clarence
Plante, Julie
Robichaud, Pascal
Roy, Nathalie
Saulnier, Denis
Sirois, Isabelle
Thivierge, Isabelle
Trudeau, Judith
Vincent, Andre
Whittom, Steve

LONGUEUIL
Belanger, Melanie
Blouin, Valerie
Braidy, Joseph F.
Cohen, Linda
Colizza, Franco
Deschenes, Julie
Deslongchamps, Francois J.
Desmarais, Sylvie
Doummar, Gilbert
Elstein, Jack
Ferland, Emery
Gauthier, Sylvie
Germain, David

Haraoui, Louis-Patrick
Huynh, Huu Hung
Laberge, Marc Andre
Lavoie, Jean-Pierre
Leduc, Francois A.
Legault, Christian
Maillette, Sylvie
Mathieu, Genevieve
Nguyen, Duy Quynh H.
Nguyen, Van Vu
Nowakowska, Dominika
Pinsonneault, Monique
Poulin, Eric
Poupart, Charles
Rivard, Andre
Sabbah, Eric
Speranza, Giovanna
St-Maurice, Francois
Thai, Hoang Lan
Tran, Paul C D.

MAGOG

Gauthier, Christine
Rousseau, Bernard

MANIWAKI

Haidar, Rafid

MARIA

Audet, Richard
Carignan, Pierre
Girard, Claude
Laliberte, Alain L.

MIRABEL

Cote, Jean R.

MONT-LAURIER

Clermont, Genevieve
Garcia, Sebasian

MONT-ROYAL

Cote, Gilles
De Guise, Michele
Deschamps, Jean-Pierre
Lavoie, Helene B.
Stubington, David

MONTMAGNY

Carrier, Alexis
Carrier, Jerome
Denault, Isabelle

MONTREAL

Addetia, Karima
Adelson, Edward I.
Afif, Waqqas
Afilalo, Jonathan
Agulnik, Jason S.
Ahern, Stephane P.
Ahlgren, Paul D.
Ahmad Khan, Faiz
Alam, Ahsan
Albert, Martin
Amyot, Robert
Anderson, Kim
Andrade, Jason
Angle, Michael R.
Argentin, Stefania
Aris-Jilwan, Nahla M.
Asgar, Anita W.
Aslanian, Pierre
Assayag, Deborah
Assimakopoulos, Peter
Assouline, Sarit
Aubin, Francine
Auger, Dominique
Ayoub, Jean-Pierre M.
Azar, Rani M.
Azarbar, Sayena
Azuelos, Ilan
Bacher, Yves
Badir, Badir Francis
Bailey, Robert F.
Balicki, Danuta M.
Bambace, Nadia
Banerjee, Devi
Baran, Dana
Barkun, Alan N G.
Baron, Murray
Barre, Paul E.
Barriga, Peter C.
Basmadjian, Arsene J.
Batist, Gerald
Beaucage, Francois
Beauchamp, Elizabeth
Beaudet, Francois
Beaudet, Julie
Beaudoin, Andre
Beaudoin, Marc
Beaudry, J. Pierre
Beaudry, Yves
Beaulieu, Yanick
Beauregard, Catherine
Beauregard, Hugues
Begin, Philippe
Begin, Rejean
Behr, Marcellus A.
Belanger, Daniel
Belanger, Raphael
Bellemare, Patrick
Benaroya, Samuel H.
Benhamron, Jaimes-S.
Benisty, Jacques I.
Benzaquen, Bruno
Bercovitch, David D.
Bergeron, Celine
Bergeron, Julie
Berkson, Laeora
Bernard, Edmond-Jean
Bernard, Francis
Bernard, Lea
Bernardin, Sandra R.
Bernatsky, Sasha R.
Bernier, Martin L D.
Bertrand, Carole
Bertrand, Michel
Berube, Lyne
Bessissow, Talat
Bestawros, Alain
Bettache, Nazila
Bichet, Daniel
Bielinski, Michael
Bilefsky, Ralph
Billick, Robin C.
Bilodeau, Luc
Bilodeau, Marc
Birnbaum, Leora
Bissonnette, Bernard F.
Bissonnette, Julien
Bitton, Alain
Blair, Louis
Blais, Normand
Blake, Geoffrey P.
Blaquiere, Martin
Blondin, Claude
Bloom, Walter S.
Blostein, Mark D.
Blumer, Herbert M.
Bogaty, Peter M.
Boileau, Laurianne
Bonnardeaux, Alain
Bonnycastle, Michael J.
Bottega, Natalie A.
Boubez, Walid I.
Bouchard, Josee
Bouchard, Simon
Boucher, Andree
Boucher, Anne
Boucher, Lucie
Boudreau, J. Donald
Bouganim, Nathaniel
Bourbeau, Jean
Bourdeau, Isabelle
Bourgault, Anne-Marie
Bourgouin, Paul-A.
Bourre Tessier, Josiane
Bourrelle, Dominique
Boutet, Kim
Brachemi, Soumeya
Breton, Donald
Briedis, Dalius J.
Brodeur, Catherine
Brossard, Jean-Hugues
Brunette, Veronique
Buithieu, Jean
Bunea, Ruxandra
Burelle, Denis
Busque, Lambert
Cailhier, Jean-Francois
Campbell, Bruce A.
Cantor, Kenneth Z.
Cardinal, Heloise
Cardoso, Manuel R.
Cassis, Chantal
Caussignac, Yves
Chagnon, Isabelle
Chagnon, Karine
Chagnon, Pierre-Marc
Chamakhi, Ines
Chang, Harvey Y.
Chapdelaine, Hugo
Chapdelaine, Isabelle
Charpentier, Danielle
Chatillon, Annick M.
Chiu, Wendy S W.
Christopoulos, Stavroula
Chrysler, Bernard
Churchill-Smith, Michael J.
Ciubotariu, Elena
Clamen, Marvin
Clarke, Ann E.
Cleland, David P.
Clermont, Richard J.
Cohen, Albert
Cohen, Sandra R A.
Cohen, Victor
Coiteux, Isabelle
Collette, Suzon
Colman, Neil C.
Constance, Christian M.
Corsilli, Daniel
Costa, Jean-Pascal
Costi, Paolo
Cote, Isabelle
Cote, Simon J J.
Cournoyer, Denis
Coutu, Benoit
Crelinsten, Gordon L.
Cummings, Beth-Ann M.
Cumyn, Annabelle L.
Cybulsky, Andrey V E.
Cyr, Veronique
D'Amico, Patrick
D'Aoust, Louise
Dagenais, Pierre
Dalfen, Richard
Dandona, Kshitij
Darsaklis, Konstadina
Dascal, Andre
Dasgupta, Kaberi
Davidman, Michael
Davies, Campbell D.
Davignon, Jean
Dawson, David J.
Dayan, Natalie
De Bortoli, Bruno J.
De Guise, Pierre
De Marchie, Michel
Debay, Badri
Del Carpio, Jaime
Delgado, Alfonso
Deligne, Benoit
Delisle, Jean-Sebastien
Delorme, Sophie
Denault, Andre-Yvan
Deschenes, Marc
Desir, Barbara
Desjardins, Alain
Deslandres, Erik
Di Iorio, Daniela
Di Lorenzo, Maria
Diaconescu, Razvan
Dial, M. Sandra
Diodati, Jean G.
Dionne, Jean-Luc
Dominguez, J. Manuel
Dorais, Judy
Dore, Annie
Doucet, Michel
Doucet, Serge
Doucet, Stephane
Dube, Suzanne
Dubois, Marc-Jacques
Dubuc, Marc
Duceppe, Emmanuelle
Ducharme, Anique
Duda, Barbara
Dugas, Mario
Dupras, Annik
Dupuis, Jocelyn
Durand, Madeleine
Durivage, Gidej
Dylewski, Irving M.
Dylewski, Joe S.
Dyrda, Katia
Eappen, Roy
Eidelman, David H.
Eisenberg, Mark J.
El Rayess, Malak
Elizov, Michelle
Elstein, Eleanor
Emond, Michel
Ernst, Pierre-Paul
Essebag, Vidal
Ethier, Jean
Ezer, Nicole
Fafard, Josee
Fallavollita, Sabrina
Fallone, Carlo A.
Falutz, Julian M.
Fares, Leila
Favreau, Marc B.
Fenyves, Daphna
Ferron, Jean-Paul
Filion, Josee
Fish, Douglas
Flegel, Kenneth M.
Fleury, Isabelle
Florescu, Marie
Foldes, Eva
Fortin, Louise
Fortin, Marie-Chantal
Fournier, Helene
Fournier, Marcel R.
Frenette, Charles H.
Friedman, Gad
Frisch, Gershon D.
Froment, Daniel
Fung, Shek Hong
Gaba Idiamey, Francine
Gagnon, Michel
Gagnon, Raymonde F.
Gallo, Richard
Garceau, Patrick
Garfield, Natasha
Garneau, Pascale
Gascon, Michel
Gaudet, Guylaine P.
Gauthier, Andreanne
Genereux, Philippe
Genest Jr., Jacques J G.
Genge, Angela L.
Germain, Guy
Gervais, Andre J G.
Ghali, Maged
Ghattas, Georges
Giannetti, Nadia S.
Giasson, Marc
Gilbert, Philippe
Girard, Marc-A
Girardin, Catherine
Girouard, Caroline
Gobeil, Francois
Godbout, Ariane
Godin, Maurice
Goh, Chor
Gold, Phil
Goldberg, Peter
Goldman, Gail
Goltzman, David
Gomberg, Charles L.
Gonzalez, Anne V.
Gougoux, Andre
Goulet, Gilles
Goulet, Michelle
Granger Vallee, Alexandre
Gratton, Jacques
Green, Laurence D.
Greenaway, Christina A.
Gregoire, Genevieve
Gregoire, Jean
Gregoire, Pierre
Gregory, Walter
Greiss, Isabelle
Grenier, Louis-Pierre
Grodzicky, Tamara C.
Grothe, Anne-Marie
Grover, Steven A.
Gruber, James M.
Grunbaum, David
Guerra, Peter G.
Guevin, Raymond
Guimond, Jean-Gilles
Gursahaney, Ashvini H.
Gyger, Genevieve
Hadjis, Tomy A.
Haichin, Richard N.
Halle, Jean-Pierre
Hamel, Joanne
Haraoui, Boulos
Hayami, Douglas A.
Hazel, Elizabeth
Hebert, Josee
Hebert, Marie-Josee
Heilpern, Paul L.
Helou, Maggy
Herba, Karl
Hercz, Amos R.
Hings, Ingrid M.
Hirsch, Andrew M.
Hoffer, L. John
Honos, George N.
Horn, Ruth
Hornstein, David
How, Jonathan
Hu, Xiao W.
Huard, Genevieve
Hudson, Marie
Husa, Regina
Hutchinson, Tom A.
Huynh Thanh, Thao
Ibrahim, Ragui A B.
Ibrahim, Reda
Inglis, Gary
Iqbal, Sameena Z.
Jain, Deepak B.
Jamal, Rahima
Jayaraman, Dev
Jeanneret-Grosjean, Alphonse
Jobin, Vincent
Johnson, Nathalie
Jolicoeur, Marc
Joyal, Dominique
Joyal, France
Joza, Jacqueline
Kader, Tina
Kahn, Susan R.
Kaminska, Marta
Kang, Harbhajan S.
Kapusta, Morton A.
Karaplis, Andy C.
Kassis, Jeannine
Katz, Saul S.
Kelly, Mirabelle
Khairy, Paul
Kimoff, R. John
Kiss, Thomas L.
Kissel, Catherine
Klein, Marina B.
Kokis, Andre
Kopel, Tal
Kornbluth, Murray
Kostiuk, David P.
Kravitz, Elliot
Kristof, Arnold S.
Kus, Teresa K.
Labrecque, Louise-Genevieve
Labrecque, Manon
Lachance, Sylvie
Lafleur, Martine
Lafond, Chantal
Laforest-Renald, Alexandra
Lafrance, Dominique
Lafrance, Jean-Philippe
Lagrenade-Verdant, Colin
Lahaie, Raymond
Lalonde, Guy
Lalonde, Richard G J.
Lam-Yuk-Tseung, Jules C C.
Lamarre-Cliche, Maxime
Landry, Jennifer S.
Laneuville, Pierre J.
Langleben, Adrian
Langleben, David
Langlois, Robert P.
Lapierre, Louis
Laplante, Jacques
Lapointe, Jacques
Laporta, Donald P.
Laramee, Pierre
Larente, Nadine
Laroche, Marc C.
Larochelle, Pierre
Latour, M P. Judith
Laufer, Brian

Launay, Marc P.
Laurier, Michel
Lavallee, Vincent P.
Laverdiere, Michel
Lavoie, Annick
Lavoie, Marc-Andre
Lavoie-L'Allier, Philippe
Le, Philippe
Le, Van Hoai V.
Le, Vy-Van
Le Lorier, Jacques
Le Van Long, Maurice
Le-Ngoc, A. Anne
LeBlanc, Roger P.
Leblanc, Martine
Leblanc, Richard
Leboeuf, Rebecca
Leclerc, Guy
Lecours, Rene
Leduc, Raymond
Lee, Todd C.
Legare, Martin
Legault, Louis
Legault, Sylvie
Legler, Christine M.
Lemay, Serge
Lemieux, Bernard
Lemieux-Blanchard, Emilie
Leong, Aaron
Lesperance, Bernard
Lessard, Myriam
Letendre, Francois
Letendre, Michel
Leveille, Michel P.
Levesque, Marianne
Levesque, Renee
Levy, Mortimer
Liberge, Johanne
Libman, Michael D.
Ligier, Sophie
Lipes, Jed
Lipman, Mark L.
Lipnowski, Martin
Liszkowski, Mark
Lize, Jean-Francois
Loo, Vivian G.
Lord, Helene
Ludwig, Mara S.
Luong, Me-Linh
Lussier, David
Lussier, Marielle
Luterman, Leonard
Ly, Quoc Hung
Ly, T. Nhu-Khue
M'Seffar, Abdelmajid
MacLean, Alan J.
Mackler, Richard J.
Macle, Laurent
Madore, Francois
Magder, Sheldon A.
Mahone, Michele
Maida, Reem
Majdan, Agnieszka A.
Malcolm, Ian D.
Manganas, Helene
Mangel, Roman
Maniatis, Thomas
Mannix, Sharyn E.
Mansour, Anne-Marie
Mansour, Fadi
Marchand, Richard
Marcotte, Emile
Marcotte, Francois
Marcovitz, Sorana
Mardigyan, Vartan
Mardini, Louay
Marelli, Ariane J.
Marleau, Denis
Marliss, Errol B.
Marquis, Francois
Marsolais, Pierre
Martucci, Giuseppe
Masse, Marie-Soleil
Massicotte, Frederic
Massicotte, Marie-Helene
Masson, Jean-Bernard
Massoud, Fadi A.
Matouk, Elias
Matouk, Karen
Mayer, Pierre
Mayrand, Serge
McConnell, Todd A.
McMillan, Patricia M.
Meagher, Timothy W.
Meissner, Les A.
Meltzer, Sara J.
Menzies, Richard I.
Mercille, Suzanne
Messekher, Ferial-Lilya
Meunier, Rosalie-Selene
Michel, Caroline M.
Michon, Nicole
Mihalcioiu, Catalin L D.
Mindru, Cristina S.
Mircescu, Hortensia S.
Miron, Marie-Jose F.
Mollica, Luigina
Mondou, Melanie
Monette, Johanne
Mongeon, Francois-Pierre
Moquin, Jean-Pierre
Morais, Jose A.
Morency, Nathalie
Morin, Emilie
Morin, Francine N.
Morin, Suzanne N.
Morin, Suzanne T.
Moroz, Leonard A.
Nadeau, Reginald A.
Nadler, Norman J.
Naiman, Lada
Nanci, Vanessa
Narine, Nyan K.
Nashi, Emil
Nattel, Stanley
Neiman, Gregory
Nessim, Sharon J.
Neveu, Nathalie A.
Ng Cheong, Nathalie
Nguyen, Chinh Nhan
Nguyen, Dao
Nguyen, Diem-Quyen
Nguyen, Doan-Trang
Nguyen, Duy Don
Nguyen, Ngoc Bich
Nguyen, Ngoc-Huu
Nguyen, Thanh-Thao
Nguyen, Viviane T Q.
Nguyen Van Nguyen, Paul
Nguyen-Tuong, Phong
Nigam, Anil
Numainville, Louise
O'Meara, Eileen
Olivenstein, Ronald
Olney, Harold J.
Opatrny, Lucie
Orlicka, Katarzyna
Ostiguy, Gaston L.
Ouellet, Georges
Oughton, Matthew T.
Owen, Scott
Ozen, Nilay
Palardy, Maryse
Palayew, Mark D.
Palisaitis, Donald
Palumbo, Michel
Pamidi, Sushmita
Panasci, Lawrence
Panopalis, Pantelis
Panzini, Benoit-Pierre
Paquet, Michel R.
Paquin, Sarto
Paradis, Jean
Parent, Josee
Parent, Marie-Claude
Parent, Roch
Parenteau, Simon
Patenaude, J J. Francois
Patenaude, Jean-Victor
Paulin, Claude
Pelletier, Guy B.
Pelletier, Jean-Philippe
Pelletier, Jean-Pierre
Pelletier, Patricia
Pepe, Carmela
Pepin, Marie-Noelle
Perraton-Brillon, Melanie
Perrault, Jean L.
Petrof, Basil J.
Petropoulos, Vivian
Piazza, Nicolo
Picard, Matthieu
Pichette, Vincent
Pickering, Joyce L.
Pierre-Louis, Schiller
Pilon, Claude
Pilote, Louise
Pineau, Christian A.
Plamondon, Mireille
Podymow, Tiina L.
Poirier, Charles D.
Poirier, Claude
Poirier, Lysane
Pollak, Michael N.
Popradi, Gizelle A.
Potter, Brian J.
Potvin, Jeannot
Poulin, Frederic
Pranno, Nicolas
Primeau, Robert E.
Primeau, Vanessa
Prud'Homme, Michel
Quan, Vu Hung
Quenneville, Stephane P.
Querin, Serge
Qureshi, Salman T.
Rabinovitch, Barry
Racine, Normand
Raffoul, Joseph I.
Rahal, Deric P.
Rajan, Raghu D.
Rakel, Agnes
Ratner, Jack T.
Raymond, Jean-Marc
Raymond-Carrier, Stephanie
Raynauld, Jean-Pierre
Reeves, Francois
Reisler, Hyman
Remillard, Marie-Anais
Rene, Pierre
Renzi, Gildo
Renzi, Paolo
Rey, Evelyne
Rheaume, Maxime
Rich, Eric
Richards, John B.
Rico, Philippe
Rioux, Jean-Philippe
Rioux, Louis C.
Rioux-Massé, Benjamin
Rivard, Alain
Rizzo, Arturo J.
Roberge, Guy
Robson, Hugh G.
Rola, Philippe
Rondeau, Genevieve
Rosenberg, Arthur
Rouleau, Jean-Lucien
Rousseau, Julie
Roussin, Andre
Routhier, Nathalie
Roy, Denis-Claude
Roy, Jean
Roy, Josee-Anne
Roy, Louise
Rudski, Lawrence G.
Rudwal, Christopher T.
Ruel, Monique A.
Saad, Nathalie
Sabbah, Sidney
Sahai, Anand V.
Saint-Martin, Monique
Saint-Phard, Wouter
Sakr, Lama
Salem, Reda
Sami, Magdi H.
Santagata, Patrizia
Saumart-Dufour, Nicolas
Sauvageau, Guy J L.
Sauve, Claude
Schampaert, Erick
Schiffrin, Ernesto L.
Schlesinger, Robert D.
Schulz, Jan I.
Schwartz, Blair C.
Schwartzman, Kevin J.
Schweitzer, Morris
Seah, Stanley K K.
Sebag, Igal A.
Sebag, Michael
Segal, Jeffrey S.
Seguin, Chantal
Semret, Makeda
Senecal, Jean-Luc
Senecal, Lynne
Sergerie, Mathieu
Serri, Karim
Shahin, Jason
Shamekh, Farzaneh
Shames, Sofia
Shamy, April A.
Sheppard, Donald
Sheppard, Richard J.
Sherman, Mark H.
Shustik, Chaim
Sidorowicz, Ewa
Silvestri, Isabelle
Silviet-Carricart, Maite
Silviu-Dan, Fanny
Sirdar, Emmanuel
Sirdar, Marie-Eve
Skrobik, Yoanna K.
Sladek, Robert G.
Small, David I.
Smilovitch, Mark
Smith, Benjamin M.
Snell, Linda S.
Sniderman, Allan D.
Solymoss, Susan
Somma, Maurice
Soulellis, Constantine A.
Souliere, Vicky
St-Louis, Gilles
St-Louis, Jean
St-Pierre, Anne
Stein, Michael A.
Stewart, James A.
Storring, John M.
Sturgeon, Jeremy F G.
Sun, Ning-Zi
Suri, Rita
Szego, Peter L.
Szilagyi, Andrew
Tagalakis, Vasiliki V.
Talajic, Mario
Tamaz, Raja
Tamilia, Michael
Tanguay, Jean-Francois
Tannenbaum, Cara B.
Tardif, Jean-Claude
Tellier, Claudia
Terriault, Paul
Tessier, Genevieve
Tessier, Pierre
Thanassoulis, George
Therrien, Judith
Thibault, Bernard
Thibodeau, Marie-Pierre
Thirlwell, Michael P.
Thomson, David M P.
Tosikyan, Axel
Tousignant, Pierre
Tran, Duy
Tremblay, Annie
Tremblay, Francois
Tremblay, Jean-Francois
Trifiro, Mark A.
Trifiro, Silvana G.
Troyanov, Stephan
Troyanov, Yves
Trudeau, Luc
Truong, Ngoc-Uyen T T.
Tsoukas, Alexander
Tsoukas, Christos M.
Tsoukas, Georges
Tsoukas, Michael
Turner, Howard M.
Turner, Stephen A.
Unikowsky, Bernie
Vallee, Michel
Vanasse, Madeleine
Vandemoortele, Thomas
Vasilevsky, Murray L.
Vat, Sopharat
Vautour, Line M.
Veillette, Andre
Verdon, Josee
Verma, Atul
Villeneuve, Edith
Vincent, Catherine
Vinet, Evelyne
Vinh, Donald C.
Vu, Thien-Tuong M.
Vuong, Te
Wahhab, Ramzy
Walker, Mathieu A D.
Walling, Ann D.
Wan Chow Wah, Doreen Y L.
Ward, Brian J.
Warner, Margaret N.
Warshawsky, Paul J.
Waschke, Kevin A.
Watts, Craig S.
Weber, Florence A.
White, Michel
Whittemore, N. Blair
Whittom, Renaud
Wild, Gary E.
Willemot, Patrick
Willems, Bernard E.
Wilson, Thomas R.
Wing, Simon S.
Winikoff, Rochelle
Wiseman, Jeffrey G.
Wistaff, Robert
Wong, Philip
Wyse, Jonathan M.
Yansouni, Cedric
Yeadon, Carol A M.
Yelle, Louise
Yiannopoulos, Anna
Young, Barbara M.
Yu, Oriana H Y.
Yuen, Sai Yan
Zackon, Harold M.
Zaharatos, Gerasimos J.
Zanelli, Patrizia A C.
Zidulka, Arnold
Zummer, Michel

NOTRE-DAME-DU-LAC

Gagne, Nathalie

OUTREMONT

Couture, Francois

PIERREFONDS

Lee, Candace Y W.

POINTE-CLAIRE

Arrieta, Maria-Jesus
Biem, H. Jay
Billick, Kendall
Cohen, Martin A.
Dascalu, Petronela
Dumont, Charles H.
Fox, Joel M.
Katz, Max G.
Kenick, Scott
Labuda, Marcin
Laryea, Horace D.
Morris, Leo C.
Muhtadie, Lina
Schram, Gernot
Siddiqui, Anita K.
Skamene, Alexander
Smoley, Lester B.
Starr, Michael R.
Thibert, Gilberte
Wang, Ting-Yu
Weber, Catherine L C.
Yee, Daphne P.

QUEBEC

Adams, Karen
Agharazii, Mohsen
Albert, Alexandra
Allen, Christyne
Arsenault, Marie
Babin, Guillaume
Baillargeon, Michel
Barabe, Frederic
Barbeau, Gerald
Bastien, Marie-Helene
Beaudet, Isabelle-Pascale
Beaudoin, Jonathan
Beaudry, Jean-Marc
Bedard, Elisabeth
Bedard, Marie-Eve
Bedard, Pierre-Michel
Beliveau, Patrick
Bellemare, Jean-Francois
Bergeron, Julie
Bergeron, Michel
Bergeron, Sebastien
Bergeron, Vincent

Bergeron, Viviane
Bernier, Mathieu
Bessette, Louis
Bibeau, Virginie
Bilodeau, Lara
Blackburn, Robert
Blier, Louis
Bourgault, Christine
Bourgeois, Jacques
Boursiquot, Jean-Nicolas
Boutin, Isabelle
Bradette, Marc
Brassard, Maryse
Cadrin, Camille
Cantin, Bernard
Caouette, Pascale
Caron, Stephanie
Champagne, Jean
Charbonneau, Robert
Chasse, Michael
Chevalier, Manon
Chouinard, Pascale
Chouinard, Sylvain R.
Claveau, Suzanne
Cloutier, Stephanie
Comeau, Eve-Lyne
Cote, Fabien
Cote, Isabelle
Cote, Johanne
Cote, Marc-Andre
Cote, Marie-Noelle
Cote, Stephane
Couture, Felix
Couture, Ghislaine
Couture, Julie
Couture, Louis P.
Couture, Patrick
D'Amours, Martin
D'Amours, Pierre
Dallaire, Chrystian
De Blois, Jonathan
De Larochelliere, Robert
De Serres, Sacha
Delage, Antoine
Delage, Robert
Demers, Christine
Demeule, Eric
Denis, Marie-Claire
Dery, Jean-Pierre
Desmeules, Marc
Desmeules, Simon
Dion, Genevieve
Dionne, Christine
Doyle, A I. Catherine
Drouin, Michel A.
Dube, Francois
Dube, Rejean
Dubrule, Charles-Etienne
Duclos, Pierre
Dufresne, Louis R.
Dugal, Michele
Dugas, Michel
Dumas, Olivier
Dupuis, Philippe
Dussault, Catherine
Emond, Danielle
Fekete, Ferenc
Filion, Alain
Fillion, Nancy
Fontaine, Jean-Guy
Forget, Genevieve
Fortin, Marie-Pierre
Fortin, Paul
Gagne, Dominique
Gagnon, Claudia
Gagnon, Nathalie
Gagnon, Pierre
Gagnon, Remi
Gallagher, Genevieve
Garceau, Claude
Garceau, Daniel
Garrido-Russo, Maria
Gaudreau, Vincent
Gaudreault, Valerie
Genereux, Alexandre
Gilbert, Philippe
Gleeton, Onil
Gorman, Todd E.
Gougeon, Alexandre
Gregoire, Philippe
Grondin, Charlotte
Hains, Melanie
Halle, Pierre
Houde, Isabelle
Isenring, Paul
Kirouac, Isabelle
Labbe, Michel
Laberge, Francis
Labonte, Isabelle
Labrie, Michel
Lacasse, Yves
Lacerte, Marcel
Lachance, Carl-Hugo
Lacourciere, Yves
Lafleur, Alexandra
Lalancette, Marc
Lampron, Noel
Langelier, Michel
Langlais, Mario
Langlois, Serge
Lapointe, Isabelle
Laroche, Vincent
Larochelle, Bernard
Larose, Eric
Larouche, Jean-Francois
Laterreur, Marie-Eve
Laughrea, John B.
Lauzier, Francois
Lavoie, Aubert
Lavoie, Marianne
Le Bouthillier, Pierre
Leblanc, Francois
Leblond, Martin
Leclerc, Renee
Leclerc, Valerie
Lefebvre, Jean-Claude
Lemaire, Jean-Rene
Lemay, Julie
Lemelin, Valery
Lemieux, Annie
Lemieux, Julie
Levesque, Eric
Mac-Way, Fabrice
Maltais, Francois
Marceau, Daniele
Marchand, Eric
Marchand, Francois
Marcoux, Claude
Martel, Alain Y.
Martel, Nadine
Martel, Simon
Michaud, Isabelle
Milot, Alain
Milot, Julie
Minville, Caroline
Montambault, Louis
Morin, Annie
Morin, Jacques
Morin, Josee
Morin, Jovette
Morin, Michele
Morissette, Nadesh
Nault, Isabelle
Nguyen, Can Manh
Noel, Bernard
Noel, Real
Normand, Michel
O'Connor, Kim
O'Hara, Gilles E.
Ong, Geraldine
Pare, Pierre
Parent, Claude
Pelletier, Marie-Josee
Pelletier, Marie-Josee
Philibert, David
Philippon, Francois
Plamondon, Isabelle
Plante, Valerie
Poirier, Alain
Poirier, Paul
Pothier, Jacques
Potvin, Jean-Michel
Poulin, Jean-Francois
Poulin, Louis-Denis
Poulin, Marie-Claude
Poulin, Sonya
Pouliot, Rene
Provencher, Steeve
Raby, Bruno
Raby, Kathleen
Rene De Cotret, Paul
Rinfret, Stephane
Riopel, Caroline
Rousseau, Mario
Roy, Andre
Ruest, Annie
Samson, Michel
Sarrazin, Jean-Francois
Savard, Sebastien
Senay, Helene
Senechal, Mario
Shields, Claude
Simard, Helene
Simon, Mathieu
St-Georges, Fernand
St-Laurent, Maurice
Theriault, Claudine
Trelles, Francisco
Tremblay, Benoit P.
Tremblay, Lise
Tremblay, Samuel L.
Tremblay Laroche, Dave
Turcotte, Angele
Vallieres, Michel
Vandal, Marie-Claude
Villeneuve, Josee
Vinet, Elise
Weisnagel, S. John
Whittom, Serge

REPENTIGNY

Laramée, Benoit

RIMOUSKI

Allard, Joffre C.
Bergeron, Claudie
Bernier, Maude
Blais, Andre
Boucher, Guy
Boulanger-Dorval, Jean-Philippe
Carvalho, Jean-Christopher
Dion, Marie-Josee
Dionne, Nathalie
Fortin, Isabelle
Gafsi, Aicha
Gagnon, Gabrielle
Goulet, Steeve
Hamel, Jean
Jutras, Philippe A.
Lebreux, Elie
Lepine, Jean
Marquis, Katerine
Montminy, Marie-Eve
Mony, Marc F.
Pelletier, Lysanne
Rioux, Leon
Robillard, Jean
Touzel, Christine

RIVIERE-DU-LOUP

Brunet, Daniel
Carignan, Suzanne
Czech, Eric
Gagnon, Francois
Landry, Jean-Francois
Lefebvre, Martin
Raymond, Daniel
Verret, Benoit

ROBERVAL

Boily, Yves
Hebert, Odette

ROUYN-NORANDA

Delorme, Hugo
Heroux, Julie
Meunier, Philippe
Voglimacci-Stephanopoli, P.

ROXBORO

Schiff, Renee L.
Zarruk, Alexandro R L.

SAINT-CONSTANT

St-Louis, Jean

SAINT-EUSTACHE

Birri, Lino
Cote-Page, Veronique
Dessain, Mathieu
Jao, Kevin
Lacelle, Marie-Josee
Maisonneuve, Denis
Racette, Francois
Serban, Alexandrina
Tremblay, Vanessa

SAINT-GEORGES

Beliveau, Samuel
Delisle, Marie-Noelle
Dion, Danielle
Doyon, Julie
Francoeur, Helene
Giroux, Sylvie
Karzazi, Meryem

SAINT-HYACINTHE

Blackburn, Karl
Brodeur, Guillaume
Brunet, Sylvain
Courteau, Maryse
Dansereau, Jean-Yves
Diallo, Soraya V.
Eymard, Daniel
Gaboury, Jean
Gaudreau, Andre
Girard-Desbiens, Catherine
Grandmont, Dominique
Kieu, Cong Van
Lemoine, Bernard
Oster, Eric
Paulin, Mathieu
Perreault, Francois
Robitaille, Manon
Sabourin, Alexis
St-Jean, Edith

SAINT-JEROME

Amyot, Sylvain L.
Arsenault, Isabelle
Bastien, Yves
Bienvenue, Veronique
Bouchard, M. Josee
Carrier, Jean-Sebastien
Cartier, Pierre
Chalifour, Jean-Francois
Charron, Maryse
Chevalier, Pierre
Clement Major, Sebastien
Cournoyer, Ghislain
De Bellefeuille, Claude
Deslauriers, Guy
Gosselin, Eve
Hofmann, Adam
Jolivet, Jacques
Joly, Jean-Gil
Laliberte, Lyne
Laurier, Louis
Lessard, Marie-Claude
Levesque Rouleau, Maude
Mongeau, Frederic
Montminy-Metivier, Stephane
Ouimet, Dominique
Pelletier, Marie-Eve
Perpignan, Frantz
Pesant, Yves
Rabbath, Patrick
Stewart, Marie-Diane

SAINT-LAMBERT

Havrankova, Jana B.
Nguyen, Melanie M L.

SAINT-LAURENT

Champagne, Kateri
Farley, Alain Y A.
Saliba, Nouhad
Stavrinidis, Sophie
Yared, Zeina

SAINT-LEONARD

Bertrand, Sylvie
Derghazarian, Chahe B.
Gagnon, Andre

SAINTE-GENEVIEVE

Gabbay, Moshe

SALABERRY DE VALLEYFIELD

Baggio, Daniel
Beaulieu-Boire, Genevieve
Buck, Michael
Gilbert, Elise
Kempf, Christina
Kennedy, Richard
Lam, Thuc Bao.
Plourde, Pierre
Tahan, Majd
Tran, T S. Paul
Vigeant, Patrice
Wong Wong Keet, Annick

SEPT-ILES

Bedard, Jinny
Chartrand, Louis-Andre
Forget, Anne-Marie
Gionet, Dominique
Hogan, Marie-Pier
Imbeault, Bruno
Lafortune, Pascale

SHAWINIGAN-SUD

Beaule, Caroline
Courtoy, Gregory
Gervais, Jocelyn
Kerkerian, Eric J.
Lafreniere, Anne-Marie
Perron, Sebastien
Robert, Bruno
Savard, Pierre-Alexandre
Sultanem, Ibrahim A.

SHAWVILLE

Karabatsos, Athanassios

SHERBROOKE

Abel, Julie
Arsenault, Guylaine
Bachand, Marie-Pier
Baillargeon, Jean-Daniel
Baillargeon, Jean-Patrice
Baron, Michel
Beaudoin, Annie
Beauregard, Patrice
Bedard, Jacques
Begin, Raymond O.
Ben Yedder, Naim
Bernier, Frederic
Berube, Simon
Bilodeau, Jean-Francois
Boileau, Robert
Boire, Gilles
Bouchard, Nicole
Boulais, Isabelle
Brazeau, Serge
Brochu, Marie-Claude
Bromwich, Carl R.
Caron, Nadia
Carpentier, Andre
Carrier, Julie
Castilloux, Jean-Francois
Chamberland, Martine S.
Charron, Pierre
Coll, Bernard
Cormier, Luc
Cossette, Pierre
Cote, Anne-Marie
Crepeau, Jacques
Dalery, Karl
Daneault, Benoit
Deland, Eric
Delisle, Line
Dion, Louise
Do, Doan Hoa
Dufresne, Jean
Duperval, Raymond
Echenberg, Donald
Ethier, Jean-Francois
Farand, Paul
Faust, Gilles
Fradet, Anne
Fulop, Tamas
Gagne, Eve-Reine
Gagnon, Melanie
Gagnon, Sylvie
Gaudette, Emilie
Godin, Chantal
Grbic, Dusanka
Haddad, Henry
Hivert, Marie-France
Houde, Ghislaine
Lacombe, Guy
Laflamme, David
Lajoie, Jean-Francois
Lamontagne, Francois
Langelier, Diane
Langevin, Serge

Langlois, Marie-France
Langlois, Nathalie
Lanthier, Luc
Lapierre, Julie
Larivee, Pierre
Le Blanc, Richard
Le Templier, Genevieve
Leclair, Marc-Andre
Lemay, Frederic
Lemire, Martine
Lepage, Serge
Lepine-Martin, Mariette
Lessard, Andre
Liang, Patrick
Lussier, Veronique
Maheux, Pierre
Mampuya, Warner M.
Masse, Melanie
Mayette, Michael
Menard, Charles
Montambault, Paul A.
Nawar, Tewfik W.
Nguyen, Michel
Paulin, Chantal
Peloquin, Marie M.
Pepin, Jacques
Pepin Dubois, Yanek
Perron, Patrice
Pesant, Marie-Helene
Pilon, Danielle
Plamondon, Sophie
Poulin, Yannick
Ricard, Genevieve
Robb, John A.
Roux, Jean-Francois
Ruel, Joannie
Sauve, Nadine
Setrakian, Jean C.
Sinave, Christian P.
St-Arnaud, Charles
St-Pierre, Bruno
St-Pierre, Catherine
Tessier, Daniel
Touchette, Matthieu
Valiquette, Louis
Van Rossum, Nicole
Vezina, Yves

SOREL-TRACY
Can, T. Bich Dao.
Godin, Daniel
Guirguis, Hesham S R.
Tincoca, Lorenzo P.

ST CHARLES BORROMEE
Beaulieu, Celina
Blain, Marie-Helene
Boule, Marie-Eve
Cayouette, Maryse
Dussureault, Martine
Gagne, Marc-Andre
Grypinich, Michel
Lachance, Richard
Laflamme, Pierre
Landry, Pierre
Langlais, Nathalie
Letourneau, Isabelle
Levallois-Gignac, Jasmin
Pek, Bonavuth
Renaud, Genevieve
Ton-Nu, Thanh-Thao

ST-EUSTACHE
Gagne, Michel
Nassiri, Shirin
Paradis, Louis

ST JEAN SUR RICHELIEU
Babin, Jacinthe
Corbeil, Marie-Andree
De Smet, Eric
Deschenes, Isabelle
Filion, Serge
Foley, Marie-Claude
Fournier, Sylvie
Kong, Wei Lin
Lacroix, Annie
Lafond, Guillaume
Larocque, Martin
Laroussi, Leila
Noiseux, Daniel
Preville, Marie-Josee
Remillard, Stephanie
Rousseau, Annie
Simion, Oana-Maria
Umapathy, Dhiviya

STE AGATHE DES MONTS
Bernard, Maude
Cloutier, Jonathan

STE ANNE DES MONTS
Deschenes, Jean-Pierre
Emond, Julie
Leblond, Richard

TERREBONNE
Ah-Lan, Christopher
Amra, Suleman
Archambault-Grenier, Marie-Anne
Blain, Julie
Chayer, Sebastien
Cottenoir, Nattacha
Coutu, Amelie
Desjardins, Valerie A.
Duong, Hoang
Jamali, Hossein
Lamargese, Isabella
Maheu, Michel
Ouellet, Vincent
Paquet, Isabelle
Paquet, Stephanie
Petrucci, Martin
Plouffe, Elyse
Reid, Genevieve
Robitaille, Yves
Woods, Philippe

THETFORD MINES
Audet, Maryse
Boulianne, Marc
Campeau, Jean
Dupuis, Robert
Lauzon, Claude
Pruneau, Guylaine
Senay, Bobby
Taillon, Joseph E A C.

TROIS-RIVIERES
Absi, Farid
Arcand-Bosse, Jean-Francois
Aucoin, Jean-Sebastien
Beriault, Marie-Josee
Bourque, Solange
Briere, Claude
Caron, Johanne
Carrier, Christian
Chapdelaine, Sylvie
Corbeil, Francois
Dessureault, M. Michele
Drapeau, Christine
Drouin, Julie
Dube, Jean-Nicolas
Garand, Mark
Gariepy, Linda
Gauthier, Patrice
Goulet-Dion, Sophie
Labrecque, Catherine
Lapointe, Michel
Larouche, Jacynthe
Lavoie, Lucie
Lemay, Catherine
Lessard, Clode
Mignault, Chantal
Moreau, Vincent
Morin, Frederic
Naud, Jean-Francois D.
Parenteau, Chantal
Peters, Claire
Raymond, Alain
Rioux, Dany
Tousignant, Karine
Tremblay, Anouk
Tremblay, Jean-Luc
Turcot, Richard

VAL-D'OR
Germain-Lacroix, Nicolas
Lauzon, Ghyslain
Lavoie, Line
Pouliot, Joel
Tremblay, Charles

VERDUN
Ahad, Victor A.
Ayoub, Paul
Bazin, Anne-Marie
Bonny, Shawn
Canzani, Genevieve
Champagne, Martin A.
Comanita, Petru
Cossette, Pierre-Yves
Dubois, Pascale
Gagnon, Jacques-Eric
Ghannoum, Marc
Giard, Marie-Claude
Guerin, Lucie C.
Lachance, Yves
Moghrabi, Albert
Poliquin, Marc
Smith, Terry A.
Winter, Elric D.
Yechouron, Ariane

VICTORIAVILLE
Beaurivage, Charles
Chagnon, Patrick
Desrochers, Georges W.
Lamothe, Marc
Lecours, Simon
Mercier, Maryse
Monaghan, Deborah
Proulx, Pierre-Yvon
Quintin, Isabel
Richard, Claude
Robert, Ghislain
Tousignant, Eric

WESTMOUNT
Knight, Lawrence
Maranda, Claude R.
Marpole, Derek G F.
Mishkin, Seymour
Morelli, Gaetano
Petrovich, Milenko
Posner, Barry I.
Rabinovitch, Mark A.
Shannon, David J.
Tannenbaum, Hyman
Varga-Solymoss, Susan M.

SASKATCHEWAN

LLOYDMINSTER
Abdulla, Agiela M K.

MOOSE JAW
Amies, David R.
Rodwan, Omar M A.
Tarhuni, Wadea M.

PRINCE ALBERT
Ali, Syed A.
Ben Saleh, Adel Hassen
Ilie-Haynes, Radu T.

REGINA
Abdulhadi, Mohamed H.
Abdulla, Ramzan H.
Aboguddah, Ayman A.
Ali, Massud A A.
Belak, Zenon A.
Bohn, Mary C.
Booker, Jeffrey D.
Chami, George
Dehghani, Payam
Duffy, Patrick J.
Ellwood, Amanda D.
Fahlman, Nicole M.
Fitzgerald, Jeremy
Garbe, George J.
Gargoum, Hassan A M.
Gebhardt, Vernon A.
Hopkins, Howard
Jancewicz, Miroslav T.
Karunakaran, Kumudhini
Karunakaran, Siva
Lavoie, Andrea J.
Lewis, William F.
Lwanga, Steven K.
Mann, Suba S.
McDougall, Robert S.
McHattie, James D.
Milne, Ardyth A.
Mohammed, El-Fellani A.
Momenkhan, Ibrahim M M.
Muftah, Abdalla G.
Muftah, Anwar S A.
Murthy, Dakshina
Nel, Johann D L R.
Patel, Prakash C.
Rayson, Sandra
Rehman, Habib
Richardson, Bonnie R.
Sridhar, Guruswamy
Sultan, Omar
Tikkisetty, Bhanu P.
Wilson, Cameron B.
Wojcik, Wladyslaw
Wong, Alexander
Zacharias, Sherma R.
Zimmermann, Rodney H.

SASKATOON
Ahmed, Ayesha A.
Ahmed, Shahid
Akhtar, Jawed
Arnason, Terra G.
Baldelli, Angela M.
Baltzan, Richard B.
Barton, James W.
Basi, Raviqubal S.
Basran, Jenny F S.
Basran, Rashpal S.
Bedi, Anil
Bhalerao, Uddhav K.
Bose, Sabyasachi
Bree, Teresa L.
Brose, Kelsey M J.
Card, Robert T.
Card, Sharon E.
Cockcroft, Donald W.
Cotton, David J.
Coverett, Kelly O.
Dala, Gideon
De Coteau, W. Earle
De Villiers, Jacobus
Degenhart, Nathan
Dewa, Dalisizwe M K.
Dosman, James A H.
Dyck, Roland F.
Fenton, Mark
Fenton, W. James
Fowler, Sharyle
Ghoorah, Sanyukta K.
Gjevre Jr., John A.
Gowda, Kempe
Hafezi, Rodmehr
Harding, Sheila M R.
Hassan, Abubaker M M.
Hergott, Christopher A.
Hoeppner, Vernon H.
Joanis, Norman D J.
Jones, Jennifer L.
Kappel, Joanne E.
Klassen, Judith T.
Kundapur, Rekha
Laframboise, Karen F.
Larkai, Edwin N L.
Lopez, Jose F.
Lubiantoro, Elsa
MacKay, Rebecca E.
Mainra, Rahul R.
Mamchur, Lori L.
Marciniuk, Darcy D.
Markland, Janet J.
McClean, Karen L.
Moodley, U. Otto
Naik, Latha D.
Nair, Bindu V.
Newstead-Angel, Jill C.
Nosib, Shravankumar S.
Nuri, Humayun
Olszynski, Wojciech P.
Orvold, Jason N.
PausJenssen, Erik L.
Pausjenssen, Anne Marie
Pausjenssen, Elizabeth S.
Pearce, Colin B.
Pierce, Cameron W.
Pollock, A. Patrice
Porostocky, Peter
Pylypchuk, George B.
Rajakumar, Alphonsus R J.
Reid, John K.
Sanche, Stephen E.
Sayed, Ahmed
Sharma, Nawal K.
Sheridan, David P.
Shoker, Ahmed S A H.
Skinner, Stuart J.
Skomro, Robert
Stakiw, Julie
Stein, Jeffrey C.
Stewart, Kristofor B.
Stryker, Rodrick K.
Stuglin, Carlo
Sylwestrowicz, Thomas A.
Szabo, Eileen M.
Tai, Davina J.
Takaya, Sachiko
Taylor Gjevre, Regina M.
Truchan, Margaret B.
Ubhi, Mandeep S.
Wall, Alastair R.
Ward, Heather A.
Wells, Calvin R.
Williams, Kurt E.
Wilson, Thomas W.
Wong, Alice H M.
Worobetz, Lawrence J.
Zawadowski, Michael A J.

SWIFT CURRENT
Khonje, Tadeyo T.
Tagboto, Senyo K.

YORKTON
Wickert, Wayne A.

YUKON TERRITORY

WHITEHORSE
Kaegi, Andrew

Medical Biochemistry

ALBERTA

CALGARY
Ferreira, Patrick

EDMONTON
Bamforth, Fiona

BRITISH COLUMBIA

BURNABY
Moss, Michael A.

NEW WESTMINSTER
Garg, Arun K.

SURREY
Cleve, Richard H.
Heathcote, John C.

VANCOUVER
Bondy, Gregory P.
Frohlich, Jiri
Fung, Vincent W H.
Halstead, A. Catherine
Holmes, Daniel T.
Mattman, Andre
Seccombe, David W.
Vallance, Hilary D.

NEW BRUNSWICK

MONCTON
Cartier, Louis-Jacques

NOVA SCOTIA

HALIFAX
Nanji, Amin A.
Nassar, Bassam A.

ONTARIO

BRAMPTON
Mickle, Donald A G.

ETOBICOKE
Gandhi, Shruti

HAMILTON
Chetty, Vasudhevan
Don-Wauchope, Andrew
McQueen, Matthew J.
Pare, Guillaume
Potter, Murray A.

LONDON
Ainsworth, Peter
Prabhakaran, Varagur M.

MISSISSAUGA
Abdelshaheed, Nabegh N.

OTTAWA
Chakraborty, Pranesh K.
Gertler, Stanley Z.
Ooi, Daylily
Sorisky, Alexander M.

ST THOMAS
Ho, Darius M S.

TORONTO
Bromberg, Irwin L.
Cheung, C Y. Mark
Cole, David E C.
Karambolova, Kristi K.

QUÉBEC

BAIE-COMEAU
Robitaille, Daniel

CHICOUTIMI
Cote-Richer, Melanie
Miron, Michel

GATINEAU
Alain, Jean
Champagne, Marie-Rose

GREENFIELD PARK
Carrier, Gaëtan
Tang, Jianqing

LAVAL
Kanj, Nada
Madarnas, Alexandre
Pu, Qian

LEVIS
Deslauriers, Daniel
Lachance, Pierre

MONTREAL
Aleyassine, Hassan
Baass, Alexis
Blank, David W.
Eintracht, Shaun L.
Gilfix, Brian M.
Kadri, Nadine
Kremer, Richard B.
Lariviere, Francois
Lessard, Francois Y.
Letendre, Elaine
MacNamara, Elizabeth M.
Parente, Fabienne
Petitclerc, Claude
Radwan, Farouk
Shuster, Joseph
St-Cyr, Julie
Wesolowska, Ewa B.

QUEBEC
Belanger, Luc
Bergeron, Jean
Douville, Pierre
Forest, Jean-Claude
Fruteau-De-Laclos, Bernard
Gervais, Philippe
Giguere, Yves
Girouard, Joel
Lavoie, Robert
Leclerc, Pierre
Lemay, Andre
Masse, Jacques
Mourabit Amari, Karim
Nadeau, Linda
Rousseau, Francois
Talbot, Jean
Turcotte, Gilles

RIMOUSKI
Medane, Nadia

SAINT-JEROME
Joly, Jean-Gil

SALABERRY DE VALLEYFIELD
Bachand, Isabelle

SHERBROOKE
Chevrier, Pierre
Chouiali, Ahlem
Corbin, Francois
Dube, Jean
Grant, Andrew M.
Kelly, Anthea G.
Lehouillier, Philippe

ST CHARLES BORROMEE
Westerlund, John A R.

TERREBONNE
Lesiege, Daniel

TROIS-RIVIERES
Pelletier, Pascal

SASKATCHEWAN

REGINA
Mali, Bahera

SASKATOON
Kalra, Jawahar

Medical Genetics

ALBERTA

CALGARY
Bernier, Francois P.
Ferreira, Patrick
Gerritsen, Jennifer A.
Innes, A. Micheil
Johnson, Carey L.
Lauzon, Julie L.
Lowry, R. Brian
McLeod, D. Ross
Perrier, Renee L.
Sparkes, Rebecca L.
Thomas, Mary Ann
Yee, Harris A.

EDMONTON
Bamforth, J. Stephen G.
Caluseriu, Oana
Jain, Shailly
Leonard, Norma J.

BRITISH COLUMBIA

PORT ALBERNI
Hughes, Rhiannon M.

VANCOUVER
Armstrong, Linlea
Boerkoel, Cornelius F.
Dias, Angela C.
Friedman, Jan
Gibson, William T.
Goldberg, Yigal P.
Lehman, Anna M.
Lopez, Elena
McGillivray, Barbara C.
Patel, Millan S.
Van Allen, Margot I.

VICTORIA
Aubertin, Gudrun
MacLeod, Patrick M J.
Steinraths, Michelle R.

MANITOBA

WINNIPEG
Chodirker, Bernard N.
Chudley, Albert E.
Marles, Sandra L.
Mhanni, Aizeddin A M.
Rockman-Greenberg, Cheryl

NEWFOUNDLAND AND LABRADOR

ST. JOHN'S
Fernandez, Bridget

NOVA SCOTIA

HALIFAX
Gillis, L. Jane
Penney, Lynette S.

ONTARIO

HAMILTON
Kozenko, Mariya A.
Li, Chumei

KINGSTON
MacKenzie, Jennifer J.
Walia, Jagdeep S.

LONDON
Goobie, Sharan L.

MISSISSAUGA
Farrell, Sandra A.
Goh, Elaine S.

NORTH YORK
Aul, B. Ritu
Nezarati, Marjan

OSHAWA
Blumenthal, Andrea
So, Joyce

OTTAWA
Boycott, Kym
Dyment, David A.
Graham, Gail E.
Hunter, Alasdair G W.
Nikkel, Sarah M.
Richer, Julie
Sawyer, Sarah L.

TORONTO
Carter, Melissa T.
Chitayat, David A.
Cole, David E C.
Faghfoury, Hannaneh
Lefebvre, Maude
Lines, Matthew A.
Morel, Chantal F J.
Yoon, Grace

QUÉBEC

MONTREAL
Al-hertani, Walla
Ben Amor, Ibtihel M.
Brunel-Guitton, Catherine
Buhas, Daniela C.
De Bie, Isabelle
Desilets, Valerie
Deutsch-Andermann, Eva
El Haffaf, Ahmed Z A.
Foulkes, William
Karalis, Aspasia
Laberge, Anne-Marie
Lambert, Marie
Lemyre, Emmanuelle
Melancon, Serge B.
Michaud, Jacques
Mitchell, Grant A.
Rosenblatt, David S.
Rouleau, Guy A.
Russell, Laura
Soucy, Jean-Francois

QUEBEC
Gagne, Richard
Laframboise, Rachel

SHERBROOKE
Chenier, Sebastien
Drouin, Regen
Levesque, Sebastien
Maranda, Bruno

SASKATCHEWAN

SASKATOON
Lemire, Edmond G.

Medical Microbiology

ALBERTA

CALGARY
Carson, Julie-Ann
Chan, Wilson W.
Gregson, Daniel B.
Johnson, Andrew S.
Larios, Oscar
Louie, Marie
Pillai, Dylan R.
Tellier, Raymond J M.
Vanderkooi, Otto G.

EDMONTON
Ahmed-Bentley, Jasmine
Chandran, A. Uma
Kanji, Jamil
Kowalewska-Grochowska, Kinga
Kulkarni, Shobhana P.
Lee, Mao-Cheng
Nigrin, Jana
Solomon, Natalia
Talbot, James A.
Verity, Robert A.

BRITISH COLUMBIA

BURNABY
Imperial, Miguel
Reyes, Romina C.

KELOWNA
Blondel-Hill, Edith M.
Wang, Bing

NEW WESTMINSTER
Purych, Dale B.
Tomblin, Joan L.

SURREY
Henwick, Scott
Leblanc, Louiselle
MacK, Benjamin J.

VANCOUVER
Al Rawahi, Ghada N.
Bryce, Elizabeth A.
Champagne, Sylvie
Cimolai, Nevio
Doyle, Patrick W.
Grant, Jennifer M.
Isaac-Renton, Judith L.
Krajden, Mel
Leung, Victor
Noble, Michael A.
Romney, Marc G.
Roscoe, Diane L.
Sherlock, Christopher H.
Stefanovic, Aleksandra
Tan, Rusung
Tang, Patrick K C.
Thomas, Elizabeth
Thomas, Eva E.
Tilley, Peter A G.
Wong, Titus T T.
Yang, Tung C.

VICTORIA
Galbraith, John C T.
Hutchinson, James M.
Kibsey, Pamela C.
Martinez, Luis A.
Tan, Kennard E K.

MANITOBA

WINNIPEG
Bullard, Jared M P.
Hammond, Gregory W.
Kabani, Amin M.
Lagace-Wiens, Philippe R.
Ronald, Allan R.
Van Caeseele, Paul G.
Walkty, Andrew J.

NEW BRUNSWICK

MONCTON
Bourque, Christine
Garceau, Richard
Girouard, Gabriel
Kuhn, Magdalena
Thibault, Louise

SAINT JOHN
Webster, Duncan V.

NEWFOUNDLAND AND LABRADOR

ST. JOHN'S
Daley, Peter

NOVA SCOTIA

HALIFAX
Davis, Ian R C.
Forward, Kevin R.

Haldane, David J M.
Hatchette, Todd F.
Mailman, Timothy L.

WOLFVILLE
Gould, John R.

ONTARIO

BELLEVILLE
Zoutman, Dick E.

BRAMPTON
Richardson, David C.

BURLINGTON
Jeans, E. Rose

CHELTENHAM
MacPherson, Douglas W.

ETOBICOKE
Al Mohri, Huda A G.
Allen, Vanessa G.

HAMILTON
Goldfarb, David M.
Lee, Christine H C.
Leto, Daniela L.
Loeb, Mark B.
Main, Cheryl L.
O'Shea, Timothy M.
Smaill, Fiona M.
Smieja, Marek J.
Yamamura, Deborah L R.

KITCHENER
Ciccotelli, William A.

LONDON
Colby, W. David
Elsayed, Sameer
Hammerberg, Ole
John, Michael A.
Lannigan, Robert
Zahariadis, George

MISSISSAUGA
Couroux, Peter R.
Ostrowska, Krystyna I.
Sarabia, Alicia

NORTH YORK
Baghdadlian, Hovsep
Gerson, Marvin
Stuart, Philip F.

OAKVILLE
Rau, Neil V.
Warren, Thomas A.

OTTAWA
Chacon, Danelia D.
Jessamine, Peter G.
Saginur, Raphael
Slinger, Robert W.
Touchie, Claire E.
Toye, Baldwin W.

SCARBOROUGH
Belhaj, Abdelbaset
Choi, Edwin D.
Mucklow, Michael G.

SUDBURY
Diaz-Mitoma, Francisco

TORONTO
Boggild, Andrea K.
Devlin, H. Roslyn
Diamandis, Eleftherios P.
Downey, James F.
Fearon, Margaret A.
Grennan, J. Troy
Gubbay, Jonathan B.
Hii, John
Jamieson, Frances
Kain, Kevin C.
Karmali, Mohamed A.
Katz, Kevin C.
Krajden, Sigmund
Low, Donald E.
MacDonald, Kelly S.
MacMillan, Leslie G.
Matlow, Anne G.
Matukas, Larissa M.
Mazzulli, Tonino
Mubareka, Samira
Nadarajah, Jeya T.
Ota, Kaede
Poutanen, Susan M.
Richardson, Susan E.
Simor, Andrew E.
Srigley, Jocelyn A.
Vearncombe, Mary E.
Walmsley, Sharon L.
Walter, Anthony J.
Yau, Yvonne C W.

PRINCE EDWARD ISLAND

CHARLOTTETOWN
German, Gregory

QUÉBEC

CHATEAUGUAY
Sanchez, Miguelle

CHICOUTIMI
Grimard, Doria
Lavoie, Myriam
Paradis, Jean-Francois
Savard, Roger

COWANSVILLE
Michaud, Sophie

GATINEAU
Baptiste-Desruisseau, Dinah
Bonin, Richard A.

GRANBY
Joly, Jean R.

GREENFIELD PARK
Delorme, Laurent
Le Corre, Isabelle
Lussier, Nathalie
Mak, Anton
Yared, Nada

LACHINE
Elie, Kathryn D.
Teltscher, Marty S.

LAVAL
Bergevin, Marco
Carrier, Marc
Castonguay, Stephanie
Haeck, Olivier
Nguyen, Thi Thanh T.
Rivest, Natalie
Simoneau, Esther

LEVIS
Marcoux, Diane
Roy, Marie-Hélène
Vincent, Andre

LONGUEUIL
Cohen, Linda
Haraoui, Louis-Patrick
Pelletier, Lorraine

MONTREAL
Albert, Guy
Auger, Pierre
Barriga, Peter C.
Bayardelle, Paul
Beauchamp, Elizabeth
Behr, Marcellus A.
Beliveau, Claire
Bourgault, Anne-Marie
Charbonneau, Louise
Coutlee, Francois
Demers, Anne-Marie
Di Iorio, Daniela
Doss, Arulraj F.
Dufresne, Simon
Dylewski, Joe S.
Fortin, Claude
Frenette, Charles H.
Gaudreau, Christiane
Girouard, Yves
Greenaway, Christina A.
Horn, Ruth
Kelly, Mirabelle
Knowles, Kathleen F.
Labbe, Annie-Claude
Labrecque, Louise-Genevieve
Laferriere, Celine
Laflamme, Pierre J.
Laroche, Marc C.
Lavallee, Christian
Laverdiere, Michel
Lavergne, Valery
Lebel, Pierre
Lemieux, Claude
Libman, Michael D.
Loo, Vivian G.
Luong, Me-Linh
Marchand, Richard
McDonald, Jane C.
Mendelson, Jack
Montplaisir, Serge
Morisset, Richard
Noel, Gregoire E.
Oughton, Matthew T.
Papenburg, Jesse
Phaneuf, Denis
Pichette, Gilbert
Plamondon, Mireille
Poirier, Louise
Poisson, Michel
Portnoy, David
Portnoy, Joseph
Quach-Thanh, Caroline
Renaud, Christian
Rene, Pierre
Robson, Hugh G.
Roger, Michel
Rouleau, Danielle
Rousseau, Celine
Rubin, Earl E.
Saint-Jean, Maude
Savard, Patrice
Semret, Makeda
Sheppard, Donald
St-Antoine, Pierre
St-Jean, Lise A.
Su, Shih-Hann
Thivierge, Benoit E.
Toma, Emil
Tremblay, Cecile
Trifiro, Silvana G.
Tsimiklis, Catherine
Turner, Stephen A.
Vincelette, Jean
Vinh, Donald C.
Ward, Brian J.
Weiss, Karl A.
Yansouni, Cedric
Zaharatos, Gerasimos J.

POINTE-CLAIRE
Arrieta, Maria-Jesus

QUEBEC
Auger, Francois
Bergeron, Michel
Bestman-Smith, Julie
Boivin, Guy
Boudreault, Alexandre
Claveau, Suzanne
Cote, M E G. Louise
Deschenes, Louise
Desjardins, Anne
Germain, Marc
Gourdeau, Marie
Hivon, Pierre
Longtin, J D N. Yves
Longtin, Jean
Loungnarath, Vilayvong
Martel, Alain Y.
Paradis, Alain
Pelletier, Gilles
Pelletier, Rene
Picard, Anne-Claude
Roy, Marie-Claude
Ruest, Annie
Senay, Helene
Soucy, Genevieve
Tetrault, Isabelle
Tremblay, Claude A.
Trottier, Sylvie
Turgeon, Nathalie
Vachon, Marie-Louise C.

RIMOUSKI
Bernatchez, Harold
Dolce, Patrick
Jutras, Philippe A.
Tourangeau, Francine

RIVIERE-DU-LOUP
Harvey, Pierre
Moisan, Danielle

SAINT-EUSTACHE
Lalancette, Linda
Lamothe, Francois

SAINT-HYACINTHE
Beaulieu, Andree-Anne
Eymard, Daniel
Vibien, Anne

SAINT-JEROME
Bailey, Luc
Lapointe, Veronique
Levreault, Jean-Guy
Riberdy-St Pierre, Catherine
Robert, Jean
Tremblay, Julie

SAINT-LAURENT
Delage, Gilles

SALABERRY DE VALLEYFIELD
Allan, James P.
Vigeant, Patrice

SEPT-ILES
Laberge, Pierre-R.

SHERBROOKE
Alarie, Isabelle
Allard, Catherine
Bergeron, Cybele
Carignan, Alex
Dion, Louise
Piche, Alain
Sinave, Christian P.
Valiquette, Louis

SOREL-TRACY
Carrier, Marie-Andree
Turgeon, Pierre L.

ST CHARLES BORROMEE
Boisvert, Jean-Francois
Boukhoudmi, Soraya
Cayouette, Maryse
Lauzon-Laurin, Anais
Lavergne, Martine

ST JEAN SUR RICHELIEU
Baril, Melanie
Lauzon, Dominique
Morissette, Isabelle
Thuot, Amelie

TERREBONNE
Charbonneau, Alain
Fafard, Judith
Khadir, Amir A H.
Maziade, Pierre-Jean
Murray, Gilles

TROIS-RIVIERES
Bouchard, Jean
Galarneau, Lise-Andree
Goyette, Monique
Houle, Claudia
Poirier, André
Tremblay, Carole

VERDUN
Ishak, Maged
Jolivet, Marie
Yechouron, Ariane

WESTMOUNT
Ahronheim, Gerald A.

SASKATCHEWAN

REGINA
Horsman, Gregory B.
Minion, Jessica L.

SASKATOON
Robichaud, Sophie
Sanche, Stephen E.

Medical Oncology

ALBERTA

CALGARY
Al-Hashmi, Hani
Bebb, Dafydd G.
Card, Cynthia M.
Cheng, Ting
Dowden, Scott D.
Easaw, Jacob C.
Heng, Daniel Y C.
Henning, Jan-Willem
Huan, Susan D.
Krause, Vanessa S.
Lupichuk, Sasha M.
Monzon, Jose G.
Morris, Donald G.
Ruether, Joseph D.
Stewart, Douglas A.
Tam, Vincent C.
Tang, Patricia A.
Tsang, Roger
Vickers, Michael M.
Walley, Barbara A.
Webster, Marc A.
Yau, Jonathan C.

EDMONTON
Au, Heather-Jane
Basappa, Naveen S.
Butts, Charles A.
Chu, Siu-Chung
Chua, Neil S.
Fields, Anthony L A.
Hamilton, Marlene A.
Ho, Maria Y.
King, Karen M.
Koski, Sheryl L.
Mackey, John R.
Mulder, Karen E.
Nijjar, Tirath S.
North, Scott A.
Price Hiller, Julie A.
Ritchie, D. Bruce C.
Sangha, Randeep
Sawyer, Michael B.
Scarfe, Andrew G.
Smylie, Michael G B.
Spratlin, Jennifer L.
Tonkin, Katia S.
Turner, A. Robert
Venner, Peter M.
Watanabe, Sharon M.

LETHBRIDGE
Holland, David R.

MEDICINE HAT
Trudeau, Marc

BRITISH COLUMBIA

ABBOTSFORD
Keith, Bruce D.
Winston, Robert D.
Zulfiqar, Muhammad

BURNABY
Stuart, David S.
Telio, David
Yu, Simon

KAMLOOPS
Proctor, Bradley R.

KELOWNA
Davies, Janine
Dueck, Gregory
Ellard, Susan L.
Finch, Daygen
Jones, Allan R.
Khoo, Kong E.
Rao, Sanjay C.
Sauciuc, Nicoleta D.
Sutherland, Judith A.
Taylor, Marianne J.
Taylor, Sara K.
Topic, Delilah L.

NORTH VANCOUVER
Bains, Puneet
Smiljanic, Sasha R.

RICHMOND
Ho, Jeremy J.
Yun, John W S.

SURREY
Al-Tourah, Abdulwahab J.
Bourque, Sylvie A.
Chan, Theresa W.
Davidson, James A.
Do, Thuan Hieu
Gill, Karamjit K.
Johal, Balvindar S.
Le, Lyly H.
Lee, Christopher W K.
Lee, Ursula J Y M.
Martin, Lee Ann
Oja, Conrad D.
Pansegrau, Gary K.
Sawhney, Ravinder P S.
Shustik, Jesse D.

VANCOUVER
Bryce, Cicely J.
Chan, Angela S A.
Cheung, Winson Y T.
Chi, Kim Nguyen
Chia, Stephen K L.
Eigl, Bernhard
Gelmon, Karen A.
Gill, Sharlene
Ho, Cheryl C.
Hoskins, Paul J.
Hsu, Tina Y.
Kennecke, Hagen F.
Klasa, Richard J.
Kollmannsberger, Christian
Laskin, Janessa J.
Lim, Howard J.
Lohrisch, Caroline A.
Melosky, Barbara L.
Renouf, Daniel J.
Savage, Kerry J.
Sehn, Laurie H.
Shenkier, Tamara N.
Simmons, Christine E.
Smith, Alan D.
Sun, Sophie
Tinker, Anna
Villa Restrepo, Diego

VERNON
Hardy, Edward L G.
Humphreys, Michael R.

VICTORIA
Allan, Sharon J.
Attwell, Andrew J.
Bernstein, Vanessa
Coppin, Christopher M L.
Cuthbert, Donna A.
Fenton, David W.
Fitzgerald, Catherine A.
Hart, Jason J.
Ksienski, Doran S.
MacPherson, Nicol A.
Martins, Heidi
McGhie, John P.
Souliere, Sheila F.
Wilson, Kenneth S.

MANITOBA

WINNIPEG
Banerji, Shantanu
Czaykowski, Piotr M.
Gingerich, Joel R.
Gordon, Vallerie L.
Grenier, Debjani
Harding, Gary A J.
Krahn, Marianne J.
Maksymiuk, Andrew W.
Pitz, Marshall W.
Rubinger, Morel
Wong, Ralph P W.

NEW BRUNSWICK

FREDERICTON
Anan, Ghadeer

MONCTON
Whitlock, Pierre

SAINT JOHN
Burnell, Margot J.
Gray, Samantha
Reiman, Anthony J.

NEWFOUNDLAND AND LABRADOR

ST. JOHN'S
Ahmad, Chaudhary E.
Laing, Kara E T.
McCarthy, Joy S.
Powell, Erin D.
Rorke, Stewart
Seal, Melanie D.
Siddiqui, Jehan Z.

NOVA SCOTIA

HALIFAX
Bernstein, Mark L.
Colwell, Bruce D O.
Dorreen, Mark S.
Drucker, Arnold M.
Jeyakumar, Alwin
Little, Cameron D.
MacNeil, Mary V.
Macfarlane, Robyn
Morzycki, Wojciech
Rayson, Daniel
Snow, Stephanie L.
Wood, Lori A.

KENTVILLE
Merryweather, Rachel J.

SYDNEY
Jensen, John L.
MacCormick, Ronald E.

ONTARIO

BARRIE
El-Maraghi, Robert H.
Li, Isabel
Nay, Derek W.
Ng, Dawn M.
Rask, Sara J.
Rassouli-Rashti, Mohammad

BELLEVILLE
Levesque, Roger

BRAMPTON
Kuruvilla, Philip G.
Reingold, Stephen M.
Sehdev, Sandeep R.

BRANTFORD
Lee, Bryan C W.
Rusthoven, James J.

BURLINGTON
Phillips, Callista M.

CAMBRIDGE
Chouinard, Edmond E.

EAST YORK
Bin, James
Shao, Richard H.

HAMILTON
Al-Shamsi, Humaid O.
Ali, Asma
Bordeleau, Louise J.
Dawe, David
Dhesy-Thind, Sukhbinder
Evans, William
Goffin, John
Hirte, Holger
Hotte, Sebastien J.
Levine, Mark N.
Major, Pierre P.
McWhirter, Elaine
Meyers, Brandon M.
Mukherjee, Som D.
Neville, Alan J.
Tozer, Richard G.
Vander Meer, Rachel L.
Zbuk, Kevin M.

KINGSTON
Baetz, Tara D.
Biagi, James J.
Booth, Christopher M.
Dancey, Janet E.
Dudgeon, Deborah J.
Gregg, Richard W.
Kumar, Vikaash N C.
Madarnas, Yolanda
Parulekar, Wendy R.
Smith, Anne M.
Tomiak, Anna T.

KITCHENER
Bahl, Mala
Bouttell, Elaine S.
Califaretti, Nadia B.
Campbell, Carolyn N J.
Hubay, Stacey A.
Knight, Gregory J.
Molckovsky, Andrea

LONDON
Ernst, D. Scott
Hahn, Karin M E.
Kuruvilla, Mridula S.
Logan, Diane M.
MacKenzie, Mary J F.
Potvin, Kylea
Sanatani, Michael S.
Vandenberg, Theodore A.
Vincent, Mark D.
Welch, Stephen A.
Winquist, Eric W.
Younus, Jawaid

MARKHAM
Hajra, Leena
Trinkaus, Mateya E.

MISSISSAUGA
Enright, Katherine A.
Higgins, Brian P.
Kaizer, Leonard
Myers, Jeffrey A.
Quinton-Gladstone, Cindy
Rajagopal, Sudhashree
Rother, Mark J.
Strevel, Elizabeth L.

NEPEAN
Harczy, Martha

NEWMARKET
Anglin, Peter J.
Kassam, Farrah
Luk, Cynthia S Y.
Rahim, Yasmin H.
Towns, Kathryn A.
Zibdawi, Labib A A.

NORTH YORK
Fishman, Paula N.
Glenns, Vivian P.
Robson, Daniel
Roitman, Daryl S.

OSHAWA
Chang, Jose
Chiu, Hak M.
Forbes, Leta M.
Freedman, Orit C.
Jeyabalan, Neera
Koneru, Rama D.
Lo, Gregory K.
Rothenstein, Jeffrey
Shim, Katharine J.
Wierzbicki, Rafal F.
Zalewski, Pawel G.

OTTAWA
Asmis, Timothy R.
Canil, Christina M B.
Clemons, Mark J.
Dent, Susan F.
Di Valentin, Tanya
Gertler, Stanley Z.
Goel, Rakesh
Goodwin, Rachel
Goss, Glenwood D.
Jonker, Derek J.
Keller, Oliver R.
Laurie, Scott A.
Maroun, Jean A.
Nicholas, Garth A.
Reaume, M. Neil
Segal, Roanne J.
Simos, Demetrios
Song, Xinni
Stewart, David J.
Tomiak, Eva M.
Verma, Shailendra
Zanke, Brent W.

RICHMOND HILL
Passaperuma, Kavitha

SARNIA
Yoshida, Kenneth M.

SAULT STE MARIE
Spadafora, Silvana
Walde, Paul L D.

SCARBOROUGH
Al-Khayyat, Shadi S M.
Chiarotto, James A.
Lee, Ronita S M.
Rana, Afshan N.
Sundaralingam, Theepa

ST CATHARINES
Findlay, Brian P.
Giesbrecht, Janice L.
Lee, Linda M.
Levesque, Michael A.
Yelamanchili, Radhika

SUDBURY
Lopez, Pedro G.
Noble, Jonathan C S.
Robinson, Andrew G.
Young, Scott D.

THUNDER BAY
Chan, Adrien M T.
Dueck, Dorie-Anna C.
Malik, Saleem T.
Sicheri, Dolores A.

TORONTO
Allegro, Sabrina
Baruchel, Sylvain
Bedard, Philippe L.
Berinstein, Neil L.
Berry, Scott R.
Bjarnason, Georg A.
Blondal, John A.
Brezden-Masley, Christine
Castonguay, Vincent
Cescon, David W.
Chan, Kelvin K.
Cheema, Parneet K.
Chen, Xueyu
Cheng, Susanna Y.
Dhani, Neesha
Earle, Craig C.
Eisen, Andrea
Gandhi, Sonal
Goodwin, Pamela J.
Haq, Rashida
Iscoe, Neill A.
Jang, Raymond W.
Knox, Jennifer J.
Krzyzanowska, Monika K.
Leighl, Natasha B.
Li, Jing
Lingas, Rania I.
Lipton, Jeffrey H.
Lo, Dorothy S.
Moore, Malcolm J.
Petrella, Teresa M.
Pritchard, Kathleen I.
Puchyr, Martina
Rana, Amira
Rana, Punam
Richter, Suzanne C.
Sahebjam, Solmaz
Sawka, Carol A.
Singh, Simron
Siu, Lillian L Y.
Sridhar, Srikala S.
Trudeau, Maureen E.
Verma, Sunil
Wadhwa, Gagan D D.
Warner, Ellen
Warr, David G.
Wilson, Jonathan J.

WINDSOR
Hamm, Caroline M.
Kanjeekal, Sindu M.
Kulkarni, Swati
Mathews, John

YORK
Rudinskas, Leona C.

PRINCE EDWARD ISLAND

CHARLOTTETOWN
Champion, Philip E.

QUÉBEC

AMOS
Boyer, Liette
Osili, Maed

CHICOUTIMI
Rousseau, Come
Simard, Herve
Simard, Raynald

COWANSVILLE
Sirhan, Shireen M.

GATINEAU
Azzouzi, Khalid
Brisson, Sonia L.
Frechette, Dominique
Gaudet, Sylvie

GRANBY
Clement, Serge

GREENFIELD PARK
Boisjoly, Josie-Anne
Devaux, Celine
Latreille, Jean
Nguyen, Trung Nghia
Samson, Benoit

LAVAL
Aucoin, Nathalie
Comeau, Reginald

Lapointe, Carole
Lavoie, Catherine
Raymond, Nicolas
Talbot, Danielle
Tremblay, Christine

LEVIS
Belanger, Mario
Couture, Jean
Lavoie, Andre

LONGUEUIL
Ferland, Emery
Speranza, Giovanna

MONT-LAURIER
Peloquin, Robert

MONTREAL
Abdulkarim, Bassam S.
Abish, Sharon B.
Ahlgren, Paul D.
Alcindor, Jean J T.
Aubin, Francine
Ayoub, Jean-Pierre M.
Ayoub, Joseph I.
Bachand, Andre
Balicki, Danuta M.
Batist, Gerald
Beaudet, Julie
Beaulieu, Raymond
Belanger, Carl
Belanger, Daniel
Bergeron, Julie
Bestawros, Alain
Blais, Normand
Blostein, Mark D.
Bouganim, Nathaniel
Chamakhi, Ines
Champagne, Josette
Charpentier, Danielle
Cohen, Victor
Dalfen, Richard
Daoud, Aida
David, Michele
Dionne, Jean-Luc
Doucet, Stephane
Fleury, Isabelle
Florescu, Marie
Gaudet, Guylaine P.
Girouard, Caroline
Guevin, Raymond
Hings, Ingrid M.
Hirsh, Vera
Hume, Heather
Jamal, Rahima
Langleben, Adrian
Laplante, Jacques
Le May, Jacques P.
Leblanc, Richard
Leclerc, Jean-Marie
Legler, Christine M.
Lemieux, Bernard
Lemieux-Blanchard, Emilie
Lesperance, Bernard
Letendre, Francois
Mihalcioiu, Catalin L D.
Mollica, Luigina
Moquin, Jean-Pierre
Mouaikel, Elie
Neemeh, Jean A.
Olney, Harold J.
Owen, Scott
Panasci, Lawrence
Patenaude, J J. Francois
Pichette, Roxanne
Pollak, Michael N.
Prchal, Jaroslav F.
Rajan, Raghu D.
Rivard, Georges E.
Rousseau, Julie
Samson, Yvan
Seguin, Chantal
Shustik, Chaim
Soulieres, Denis
St-Louis, Jean
Stern, Donna
Sturgeon, Jeremy F G.
Thirlwell, Michael P.
Tosikyan, Axel
Trempe, Germain L.
Veillette, Andre
Vuong, Te
Whittom, Renaud
Yelle, Louise
Zidulka, Joan R.

POINTE-CLAIRE
Katz, Max G.
Laryea, Horace D.

QUEBEC
Bergeron, Marc
Cantin, Guy
Cote-Brisson, Linda
Couture, Felix
Doyle, A I. Catherine
Drolet, Yvan
Dumas, Olivier
Filion, Alain
Lalancette, Marc
Larouche, Jean-Francois
Lavoie, Marianne
Lemieux, Julie
Levesque, Eric
Marceau, Daniele
Martel, Nadine
Ouellet, Pierre
Tessier, Claude

RIMOUSKI
Allard, Joffre C.
Blais, Andre
Gagnon, Gabrielle
Lepine, Jean
Letourneau, Yves
Levesque, Georges
Marquis, Katerine

SAINT-HYACINTHE
Cuirot, Gilles

SAINT-JEROME
Charron, Maryse
Cournoyer, Ghislain
Desy, Madeleine
Jolivet, Jacques
Lessard, Marie-Claude
Montminy-Metivier, Stephane

SAINT-LAURENT
Lebrun, Andre

SALABERRY DE VALLEYFIELD
Wong Wong Keet, Annick

SHERBROOKE
Castilloux, Jean-Francois
Delisle, Line
Lepine-Martin, Mariette

SOREL-TRACY
St-Germain, Paul

ST CHARLES BORROMEE
Comtois, Robert
Ghobril, Victor P.
Santikyan, Sarkis

ST JEAN SUR RICHELIEU
Lacroix, Annie
Nouh, Elias

TERREBONNE
Ah-Lan, Christopher
Archambault-Grenier, Marie-Anne
Jamali, Hossein
Maheu, Michel
Noel, Daniel R.

TROIS-RIVIERES
Aucoin, Jean-Sebastien
Blanchette, Pierre J.
Caron, Johanne
Carrier, Christian
Chapdelaine, Sylvie
Mignault, Chantal
Tremblay, Anouk

VERDUN
Arjane, Georges
Champagne, Martin A.
Moghrabi, Albert

SASKATCHEWAN

SASKATOON
Ahmed, Shahid

Medical Scientist

ALBERTA

EDMONTON
Dursun, Serdar M.
Jugdutt, Bodh I.

BRITISH COLUMBIA

BURNABY
Kelly, Michael T.

VANCOUVER
Bruchovsky, Nicholas
Churg, Andrew M.
McGeer, Patrick L.
Schechter, Martin T.

MANITOBA

WINNIPEG
Anthonisen, Nicholas R.
Cowden, Elizabeth Anne M.

ONTARIO

AURORA
Sweeney, George D.

HAMILTON
Hirsh, Jack

LONDON
Dupre, John

NORTH YORK
Levine, David Z.

OTTAWA
Chretien, Michel
Leenen, Frans H H.
Radziuk, Jerry M.
Renaud, Leo P.

TORONTO
Bruce, W. Robert
Diamandis, Eleftherios P.
Hryniuk, William M.
Jenkins, David J A.
Koren, Gideon
Roifman, Chaim M.
Zamel, Noe

QUÉBEC

MONTREAL
Chang, Thomas M S.
Hamet, Pavel
Petitclerc, Claude
Rosenblatt, David S.
Shuster, Joseph

QUEBEC
Forest, Jean-Claude
Tremblay, Roland R.

SASKATCHEWAN

SASKATOON
Prasad, Kailash

Nephrology

ALBERTA

CALGARY
Ahmed, Sofia B.
Altabbaa, Ghazwan
Bass, Adam
Burgess, Ellen D.
Chou, Sophia H.
Girard, Louis-Phillipe
Hamiwka, Lorraine A.
Haw For Chin, Oliver R.
Hawkins, Ralph G.
Hemmelgarn, Brenda
James, Matthew T.
Ma, Irene W Y.
MacRae, Jennifer M.
Manns, Braden J.
Mortis, Garth P.
Muruve, Daniel A.
Mustata, Stefan
Quinn, Robert R.
Samuel, Susan M.
Sarna, Magdalena A.
Scott-Douglas, Nairne W.
Sepandj, Farshad
Taub, Kenneth J.
Tee, James B.
Thomas, Chandra M.
Tibbles, Lee Anne
Vitale, George D.
Wang, Wenjie
Wang, Xiangyu

EDMONTON
Alabbas, Abdullah E.
Alexander, Robert
Alsehli, Riyadh N M.
Bradley, John
Caldwell, Steven S.
Campbell, Patricia M.
Chui, Betty K.
Cockfield, Sandra M.
Courtney, Mark J.
Craig, Kelly L.
Davison, Sara
Deved, Vinay
Duggan, Shelley
Gourishankar, Sita
Gowrishankar, Manjula
Guo, Peter Y.
Harley, Frances L.
Jindal, Kailash K.
Johnston, Curtis W.
Kalenga, Jean-Claude M.
Klarenbach, Scott
Markland, Darren M.
McMahon, Alan W.
Michalska, Magdalena A.
Morgan, Catherine J.
Murray, Allan G.
Osman, Maisoon A.
Pannu, Neesh I.
Pauly, Robert P.
Pinsk, Maury N.
Pisani, Amin
Qarni, Muhammad U.
Reddy, Suresh P.
Rockx, Marie A J.
Romanovsky, Adam S.
Shurraw, Sabin C N.
Thompson, Stephanie E.
Tonelli, Marcello A.
Yiu, Verna W Y.

LETHBRIDGE
Wong, Morley P.

RED DEER
Jim, Kym Lee

ST. ALBERT
Bharmal, Azim A.

BRITISH COLUMBIA

ABBOTSFORD
Chum, Elliott S.
Cooper, Susan E.
Wong, Henry C H.
Yao, Shaoyee

BURNABY
Carpenito, Gerardo

KAMLOOPS
Michaud, Marie T.
Wijeyesinghe, E. Cornel R.

KELOWNA
Jugnauth, Eleonora M.
Kates, David M.
Welsh, Edward V.

NANAIMO
Booth, Anthony D.
Carson, Rachel C C.
Croome, Alison J G.
Glick, Naomi H G.
Rasaiah, Suvi B.

NEW WESTMINSTER
Brown, Melanie L.
Chan, Victor R.
Da Roza, Gerald
Lam, Sui-Sang
Schwartz, Daniel
Starko, Robert J.
Torng, Shirley

PENTICTON
Casilla, Vanbric R.
Clouatre, Yves J J.
Forzley, Brian R.
Hochman, Jay

PRINCE GEORGE
Bashir, Khalid
Din, Fareen
Lowry, Robin P.

SURREY
Cass, Aaron I.
Constantine, Charles T.
Humphreys, Robert A.
Karim, Mohamud A.
Prakash, Suma
Schachter, Michael E.

TRAIL
Zhang, Chi

VANCOUVER
Barbour, Sean J.
Beaulieu, Monica C.
Chiu, Anthony S Y.
Copland, Michael A.
De Luca, Linda G.
Dionne, Janis
Duncan, John
Farah, Myriam
Gill, Jagbir
Gill, John S.
Jamal, Abeed
Jastrzebski, Jacek P.
Jung, Beverly
Kiaii, Mercedeh
Landsberg, David N.
Lee-Son, Kathy K Y.
Levin, Adeera
Mammen, Cherry
Matsell, Douglas G.
Matsuda-Abedini, Mina
Neufeld, Peter R.
Prchal, David
Rosenbaum, Debbie A.
Singh, R. Suneet
Strijak, Bradford J.
Taylor, Paul A.
White, Colin T.
Yeung, Choi Kit
Zalunardo, Nadia Y.

VICTORIA
Antonsen, John E.
Ganz, Gregory M F.
Hargrove, Gaylene M.
Horgan, Kevin P.
Jones, Christopher M.
Stigant, Caroline E.

WHISTLER
Shackleton, Christopher R.

MANITOBA

BRANDON
Dunsmore, Sara E.
Riche, Barry R.

WINNIPEG
Allan, Donald R.
Armstrong, Sean W.
Birk, Patricia E.
Bohm, Clara J.
Bueti, Giuseppe A.
Cohen, Barry A.
Dart, Allison B.
Goldberg, Aviva M.
Henry, Stephen F.
Ho, Juliet
Karpinski, Martin E.
Komenda, Paul V J.
Lam, Herman P Y.
Miller, Lisa M.
Pederson, Kristen L.
Reslerova, Martina
Rigatto, Claudio
Sathianathan, Christie
Sood, Manish M.
Storsley, Leroy J.
Tangri, Navdeep
Verrelli, Mauro
Walters, Justin J.
Zacharias, James M.

NEW BRUNSWICK

BATHURST
Hickey, Dean
Robichaud, Sylvie

MONCTON
Balfour, Shana C.
Dorval, Marc
Ferguson, Kathy
Roux, Veronique
Thibeault, Yves

SAINT JOHN
Gogan, Nessa R.
MacKinnon, Martin G.
Pippy, Christine C.
Sohi, Paul S.

NEWFOUNDLAND AND LABRADOR

CORNER BROOK
Murphy, Stephen T.

ST. JOHN'S
Anees, Iram
Barrett, Brendan J.
Bhalla, Sunil
Curtis, Bryan M.
Murphy, Sean W.
Paul, Michael D.
Pike, Pamela A.
Shik, John W C.

NOVA SCOTIA

HALIFAX
Dipchand, Christine S.
Finkle, Simon N.
Hirsch, David J.
Keough-Ryan, Tammy M.
Kiberd, Bryce A.
McLaughlin, Robyn A.
Panek, Romuald
Poyah, Penelope
Soroka, Steven D.
West, Kenneth A.
West, L. Michael

SYDNEY
Hewlett, Thomas J C.
Thanamayooran, Siva
Yeung, Gordon K.

TRURO
Wornell, Philip A.

YARMOUTH
Tarakji, Ahmad R.

ONTARIO

AJAX
Elfirjani, Ali Salem B.
Wei, Charles C Y.

BARRIE
Benjamin, Derek S.

BRAMPTON
Donnelly, M. Sandra
Kajbaf, Sahar
Mehta, Hitesh
Pearl, Rachel J.
Sachdeva, Jasdip S.
Shan, Xi
Suneja, Sumeet K.
Walele, Abdul A.

BURLINGTON
Youssef, George M Y.

EAST YORK
Dunn, Anita Y.

GUELPH
Friedman, Oded
Somerville, Peter J.

HAMILTON
Arlen, Dianne J.
Arora, Steven K.
Brimble, K Scott.
Carlisle, Euan
Clase, Catherine M.
D'Souza, Sudhir J A.
Gangji, Azim
Ingram, Alistair J.
Joseph, Geena
Krepinsky, Joan C.
Lau, Keith K H.
Ludwin, David
Margetts, Peter J.
Rabbat, Christian G.
Ribic, Christine M.
Russell, J. David
Sohal, Avtar S.
To, Karen C.
Treleaven, Darin J.
Walsh, Michael W.
Yang, Robert C.

KENORA
Blydt-Hansen, Tom D.

KINGSTON
Aloudat, Sarah I M.
Garland, Jocelyn S.
Holden, Rachel M.
Holland, David C.
Iliescu, Eduard A.
Morton, A. Ross
Shamseddin, Mohammad K.
White, Christine A.
Yeates, Karen E.

KITCHENER
Benaroia, Mark
Gregor, Laura H.
Jolly, Shivinder S.
Rosenstein, Gerald A.
Vitou, Louise Y.

LONDON
Al Katheeri, Ali M A.
Alhozali, Hanadi
Blake, Peter
Garg, Amit
Grimmer, Joanne
Hildebrand, Ainslie M.
Hollomby, David J.
House, Andrew A.
Huang, Shih-Han S.
Jain, Arsh K.
Johnson, John F.
Kortas, Claude
Lam, Ngan
Moist, Louise M.
Rehman, Faisal
Sultan, Nabil M.
Thomson, Benjamin K A.
Weir, Matthew A.
Wyllie, Blair F.
Zabani, Najla A H I.

MISSISSAUGA
Al Sawi, Mohamed A M.
Boll, Philip R.
Ki, Vincent
Kim, Donald D.
Kundhal, Kiran K.
Lipscombe, Jennifer B.
Perkins, David N.
Silva Gomez, Cecilia V.
Teskey, Lindsay S.
Wadgymar, J. Arturo
Wong, Gordon K T.
Wu, George G.

NEPEAN
Chawla, Jasmeet S.
Cohn, Adam Y.
Raju, Dharmapaul L.

NORTH BAY
Saunders, Darren D.
Shulman, Tanya S.

NORTH YORK
Bergman, Arik
Borenstein, Harold B.
Chidambaram, Malathi
Davidson, Derek A.
Lekas, Poli
Levine, David Z.

OAKVILLE
Ball, Adrianne M M.
Bhandhal, Sharn
Goldstein, Jeffrey L.
Kim, Christina K.
Pandeya, Sanjaya
Sapir, Daniel

ORILLIA
Lam, Leo T Y.
Poulopoulos, Vassilios
Tascona, Daniel J.

OSHAWA
Barrese, Nancy
Birbrager, Donna R.
Buldo, George P.
Lenga, Ilan
Steele, Andrew W.

OTTAWA
Ahmed, Maheen
Akbari, Ayub
Argent, Nicholas B.
Bell, Robert C.
Bugeja, Ann L.
Burns, Kevin D.
Clark, Edward G.
Davis, Janet L.
Edwards, Cedric A W.
Fairhead, Todd R.
Hoar, Stephanie E.
Karpinski, Jolanta A M.
Knoll, Gregory A.
Magner, Peter O.
McCormick, Brendan B.
Moghadam, Soraya
Mustafa, Hassan A.
Nadler, Steven P.
Ruzicka, Marcel
Tsampalieros, Anne K.
Vethamuthu, Jennifer M.
Vimalendran, Suthaharan
Weiler, Gabrielle S.
Zimmerman, Deborah L.

PETERBOROUGH
Beaubien, Eliot R.
Butan, Radu
Cheung, Vincent S J.
Hanson, Garth J.
Kammila, Srinu

RENFREW
Delbrouck, Nicole F L.

RICHMOND HILL
Aujla, Prince S S.
Charest, Andre
Fong, Edwin M Y C.
Nathoo, Bharat C.
Pandes, Michael S.
Roushdi, Amani E.
Szaky, Esther A.
Turner, Penny A.

SAULT STE MARIE
Berry, William A D.
Shafiee, Mir

SCARBOROUGH
Fung, Jason
Manogaran, Mansula
Roscoe, Janet M.
Sikaneta, Tabo G.
Tam, Denise H.
Ting, Robert H.
Tsui, Simon Y T.
Wong, Hubert M C.
Yassa, Teraiza S S.

ST CATHARINES
Broski, Anthony P.
Lagrotteria, Danny D.
Minkarious, Edmon F W.
Nagai, Ryuta
Soliman, Gamal M L.

SUDBURY
Goluch, Richard J.
MacDonald, Ian A G.
Mehta, Navdeep K.
Nistico, Amy R.
Roy, Denis

THORNHILL
Warner, Leonard C.

THUNDER BAY
Boake, Armour I.
Shahbazi, Nasim
Watson, Paul A.
Wong, Mark A.

TIMMINS
Parmar, Malvinder S.

TORONTO
Albert, Shelley E.
Aslahi, Ramona
Berall, Murray J.
Berbece, Adriana N.
Cattran, Daniel C.
Chan, Christopher T M.
Cherney, David Z I.
Chow, Stephen S.
Cole, Edward H.
Cummings, Marion
Harel, Ziv
Hercz, Gavril
Hladunewich, Michelle A.
Hyman, Andrew R.
Kamel, Kamel S.
Kang, Amrit K.
Kim, S. Joseph
Langlois, Valerie
Licht, Christoph P B.
Lok, Charmaine E.
Ly, Joseph P H.
McFarlane, Philip A.
Mendelssohn, David C.
Miller, Judith A.
Nadeau-Fredette, Annie C.
Naimark, David M J.
Nesrallah, Gihad E.
Oliver, Matthew J.
Parekh, Rulan S.
Pei, York P C.
Perl, Jeffrey
Pierratos, Andreas
Prasad, G V. Ramesh
Quaggin, Susan E.
Radhakrishnan, Seetha
Rao, Myurathy
Reich, Heather N.
Sands, Alex
Sapir-Pichhadze, Ruth
Sasal, Joanna T.
Schiff, Jeffrey
Scholey, James W.
Schreiber, Martin
Siddiqui, Nausheen F.
Singh, Sunita K S.
Singhal, Rajni
Tanna, Gemini V.
Tennankore, Karthik K.
Tinckam, Kathryn J.
Tobe, Sheldon W.
Wald, Ron
Weinstein, Jordan J.
Whiteside, Catharine I.
Yuen, Darren A.
Zahirieh, Alireza
Zaltzman, Jeffrey S.

WINDSOR
Bagga, Amit
Callaghan, Wayne D.
Kadri, Albert

YORK
Slaughter, David N.

QUÉBEC

CHICOUTIMI
Belisle, Damien
Berthiaume, Pierre
Bouchard, Hugues
Breton-Thibodeau, Marianne
Filiatrault, Jacques

GATINEAU
Boisvert, Denis
Farah, Antoine
Julien, Natalie A.
MacDonald, Sara E.
Proulx, Normand L.

GREENFIELD PARK
Begin, Violaine
Cournoyer, Serge
Diec, Olivier H Q.
Giroux, Charlotte
Lebovich, Irith
Savoie, Lisa
Soltys, George I M.

JOLIETTE
Sabbagh, Ramsey

LASALLE
Van Vo, Thi Hai

LACHINE
Farooki, M. Sarwar

LAVAL
Corneille, Louise
Desjardins, Marie-Helene
Faucher, Claire
Hamel, Melanie
Marcotte, Jean
Prud'Homme, Louis

Raymond, Martine
Tremblay, Richard
Vezina, Danielle

MONTREAL
Alam, Ahsan
Barre, Paul E.
Bell, Lorraine E.
Benoit, Genevieve
Bercovitch, David D.
Bichet, Daniel
Bilefsky, Ralph
Bonnardeaux, Alain
Bouchard, Josee
Boucher, Anne
Bourgouin, Paul-A.
Brachemi, Soumeya
Cailhier, Jean-Francois
Cantarovich, Marcelo
Cardinal, Heloise
Chapdelaine, Isabelle
Clermont, Marie-Jose
Collette, Suzon
Cybulsky, Andrey V E.
Dandavino, Raymond
Davidman, Michael
De Bortoli, Bruno J.
Deziel, Clement
Douyon, Frantz
Eid, Jouhaina
Ethier, Jean
Falardeau, Pierre
Fortin, Marie-Chantal
Foster, Bethany J.
Frisch, Gershon D.
Froment, Daniel
Gagnon, Raymonde F.
Gascon, Michel
Gervais, Marc H.
Girardin, Catherine
Goh, Chor
Goodyer, Paul R.
Gougoux, Andre
Granger Vallee, Alexandre
Gupta, Indra R.
Hebert, Marie-Josee
Houde, Marc
Hutchinson, Tom A.
Iqbal, Sameena Z.
Kopel, Tal
Laforest-Renald, Alexandra
Lafrance, Jean-Philippe
Langlois, Robert P.
Leblanc, Martine
Legault, Louis
Lemay, Serge
Lessard, Myriam
Leveille, Michel P.
Levesque, Renee
Levy, Mortimer
Liberge, Johanne
Lipman, Mark L.
Lord, Helene
Madore, Francois
Mangel, Roman
Mucsi, Istvan
Nessim, Sharon J.
Ng Cheong, Nathalie
Nolin, Linda
Ouellet, Georges
Ouimet, Denis
Paquet, Michel R.
Pepin, Marie-Noelle
Phan, Veronique
Pichette, Vincent
Podymow, Tiina L.
Prud'Homme, Michel
Querin, Serge
Raymond-Carrier, Stephanie
Rioux, Jean-Philippe
Robitaille, Pierre O.
Roy, Louise
Rudwal, Christopher T.
Senecal, Lynne
Sharma, Atul K.
St-Louis, Gilles
Suri, Rita
Tran, Duy
Troyanov, Stephan
Unikowsky, Bernie
Vallee, Michel
Vasilevsky, Murray L.
Vinay, Patrick
Zappitelli, Michael

POINTE-CLAIRE
Muhtadie, Lina
Weber, Catherine L C.

QUEBEC
Agharazii, Mohsen
Brown, Michael S.
Charbonneau, Robert
Cote, Isabelle
De Serres, Sacha
Desmeules, Simon
Dufresne, Louis R.
Emond, Danielle
Garceau, Daniel
Houde, Isabelle
Isenring, Paul
Lachance, Jean-Guy
Langlois, Serge
Lapointe, Isabelle
Mac-Way, Fabrice
Noel, Real
Philibert, David
Plamondon, Isabelle
Poulin, Louis-Denis
Poulin, Sonya
Pouliot, Rene
Rene De Cotret, Paul
Roy, Marie-Claude
Savard, Sebastien

RIMOUSKI
Dion, Marie-Josee
Gafsi, Aicha

SAINT-HYACINTHE
Brunet, Sylvain
Courteau, Maryse
Diallo, Soraya V.

SAINT-JEROME
Bienvenue, Veronique
Cartier, Pierre
Levesque Rouleau, Maude
Mongeau, Frederic

SHERBROOKE
Bilodeau, Jean-Francois
Cote, Anne-Marie
Gagne, Eve-Reine
Langlois, Nathalie
Masse, Melanie
Montambault, Paul A.
Nawar, Tewfik W.
Wolff, Jean-Luc

ST CHARLES BORROMEE
Boule, Marie-Eve
Gascon, Georges
Landry, Pierre
Letourneau, Isabelle
Levallois-Gignac, Jasmin
Proulx, Jean

ST JEAN SUR RICHELIEU
Babin, Jacinthe
De Smet, Eric
Fournier, Sylvie
Pichette, Carole
Preville, Marie-Josee

TROIS-RIVIERES
Arcand-Bosse, Jean-Francois
Bourque, Solange
Lambert, France
Moreau, Vincent
Tousignant, Karine
Turcot, Richard

VERDUN
Ahad, Victor A.
Ayoub, Paul
Cossette, Pierre-Yves
Ghannoum, Marc
Jobin, Jacques R.

SASKATCHEWAN

REGINA
Abdulhadi, Mohamed H.
Ellwood, Amanda D.
Essalah, Abdulhafid A.
Karunakaran, Siva
Richardson, Bonnie R.
Tikkisetty, Bhanu P.

SASKATOON
Ahmed, Ayesha A.
Barton, James W.
Dyck, Roland F.
Erickson, Robin
Hassan, Abubaker M M.
Kappel, Joanne E.
Klassen, Judith T.
Mainra, Rahul R.
Shoker, Ahmed S A H.
Stryker, Rodrick K.
Tai, Davina J.

SWIFT CURRENT
Tagboto, Senyo K.

Neurology

ALBERTA

CALGARY
Agha Khani, Yahya
Almekhlafi, Mohammed A G.
Amoozegar, Farnaz
Barber, Philip A.
Becker, Werner J.
Bell, Robert B.
Brownell, A. Keith W.
Burton, Jodie M.
Busche, Kevin D.
Chhibber, Sameer
Cooke, Lara J.
Costello, Fiona E.
Couillard, Philippe L.
Coutts, Shelagh B.
Davenport, William J.
Demchuk, Andrew M.
Desai, Jamsheed
Esser, Michael
Feasby, Thomas E.
Federico, Paolo
Fletcher, William
Furtado, J C. Sarah
Hagen, Neil A.
Hanson, Alexandra J.
Hill, Michael
Ho, Alice W.
Hoyte, Keith M.
Jarvis, Scott E.
Jette, Nathalie
Kirton, Christopher A.
Klassen, Brian D.
Klein, Gary M.
Kohli, Jagdeep
Korngut, Lawrence W.
Kraft, Scott W.
Mah, Jean K.
Metz, Luanne M.
Mineyko, Aleksandra
Moore, Alison J.
Murphy, William F.
Patry, David G.
Pillay, Neelan
Pringsheim, Tamara M.
Ranawaya, Ranjit N.
Sarna, Justyna R.
Sarnat, Harvey B.
Sereda, Andrew W.
Shamy, Michel C F.
Smith, Eric E.
Smyth, Kimberley A.
Stys, Peter K.
Subramaniam, Suresh
Toth, Cory C.
Watson, Timothy W J.
White, Christopher M.
Wiebe-Velazquez, Samuel
Wilson, Scott F.
Wiltshire, Katie M.
Yeung, Michael M C.
Zochodne, Douglas W.

EDMONTON
Ahmed, S. Nizamuddin
Billinghurst, Lori L.
Blevins, Gregg
Bolduc, Francois
Boyle, Carol A J.
Brooke, Michael
Buck, Brian H.
Bussiere, Miguel E.
Butcher, Kenneth S.
Camicioli, Josepeh R M.
Edguer, Beste
Elleker, M. George
Fulton, Dorcas S.
Gross, Donald W.
Jacob, Francois-Dominique J R.
Jassal, Rajive
Jeerakathil, Thomas J.
Jhamandas, Jack H.
Jirsch, Jeffrey D.
Johnston, Wendy S W.
Kalra, Sanjay
Kashmere, Jodi
Khan, Khurshid A.
Knash, Michael E.
Kolski, Hanna
Makus, Kenneth G.
Martin, W R. Wayne
Marynowski, Bohdan
McCombe, Jennifer A.
McDermott, John
Muayqil, Taim A.
Obaid, Mona
Pokroy, Robert
Power, Christopher N.
Richer, Lawrence
Roberts, R. Neil
Roberts, Theodore E.
Saqqur, Maher
Schellenberg, Kerri L.
Scozzafava, Giuseppe J.
Shuaib, Ashfaq
Siddiqui, Muzaffar M.
Sim, Valerie L.
Sinclair, D. Barry
Smyth, Penelope S.
Starreveld, Elout
Stenerson, Paul E.
Stewart, Bradley J.
Suchowersky, Oksana
Sudharshan, Namratha
Tai, Chao
Tang-Wai, Richard F.
Warren, Kenneth G.
Witt, Norbert J.

LETHBRIDGE
Winder, Anthony R.

MEDICINE HAT
Salih, Emad A A S.

RED DEER
Bakker, Jacqueline I.
Bestard, Jennifer A.
Heinrichs, Irvin H.

BRITISH COLUMBIA

ABBOTSFORD
Botha, Stephanus S.
Costantino, Anthony D.
Punambolam, Ryan J.
Tanha, Farzad

BURNABY
Bozek, Christopher B.
Rees, Peter M.
Van den Elzen, Marketa
Vorobeychik, Galina

COQUITLAM
Sadowski, Henry A.

DUNCAN
Moll, Alexander S G.

KAMLOOPS
Collier, Todd G.
Mosewich, Russell K.
Oyler, Jeffrey R.
Takahashi, Jennifer L.

KELOWNA
Adams, Dermot A A.
Craig, David R.
Donat, Jeffrey R.
Falconer, John B.
Meckling, Scott K.
Seland, T. Peter

NANAIMO
Waterman, Kimberley R.

NELSON
Berry, Marian E.

NEW WESTMINSTER
Chahal, Chaman P S.
Ho, Kennely J.
Lee, Julian S.
Medvedev, Gueorgui A.
Tessler, Bernard B.

NORTH VANCOUVER
Cameron, Donald A.
Cheung, Christina S.
Devonshire, Virginia
Purves, Sherrill J.
Stewart, John D.

PENTICTON
Davidson, Niall J.
Novak, David J.

PRINCE GEORGE
Daly, Lyle F.
Ilyas, Amir
Pettersen, Jacqueline A.

RICHMOND
MacKie, Gordon F.
Varelas, Michael A N.

SAANICHTON
Shtybel, Wayne W.
Wambera, Katherine M.

SURREY
Diggle, John L.
Hinnell, Claire J.
Singh, Gurwant
Smyth, Allan J.
Sutton-Brown, Martin A.

VANCOUVER
Anzarut, Andre R.
Asdaghi, Negar
Barton, Jason J S.
Beckman, Jeffrey H.
Benavente, Oscar R.
Bjornson, Bruce H.
Briemberg, Hannah R.
Cashman, Neil R.
Chapman, Kristine M.
Chau, Vann
Clarke, Stephen D.
Connolly, Mary B C.
Demos, Michelle K.
Dilli, Esma
Feldman, Howard
Foti, Dean J.
Gibson, Gillian M.
Grosch, Richard D.
Hashimoto, Stanley A.
Hill, Alan
Hooge, John P.
Hrazdil, Chantelle T.
Hsiung, G Y. Robin
Huh, Linda L.
Hukin, Juliette
Hurwitz, Trevor A.
Javidan, Manouchehr
Johnston, Dean C C.
Kastrukoff, Lorne F.
Keyes, Robert D.

SPECIALISTS BY PROVINCE

Krieger, Charles
Leavitt, Blair R.
McKeown, Martin J.
Mezei, Michelle M.
Miller, Steven P.
Moore, G R. Wayne
Murphy, Colleen B.
Oger, Joel J.
Panenka, William J.
Pfeffer, Gerald
Prout, Alister J E.
Raymond, Lynn A.
Robinson, R. Gordon
Roland, Elke H.
Sayao, Ana Luiza
Schrader, Dewi V.
Selby, Kathryn A.
Spacey, Sian D.
Stockler-Ipsiroglu, Gerda S.
Stoessl, A. Jonathan
Stowe, Robert M.
Tai, Charles C F.
Teal, Philip A.
Thiessen, Brian A.
Townsend, Tiffany N.
Traboulsee, Anthony L.
Tsui, Joseph K.
Wada, Juhn A.
Wong, Milton J.
Wong, Peter K H.
Woolfenden, Andrew R.
Yip, Samuel

VICTORIA
Attwell, Kristen A.
Boulton, Peter G.
Hostetler, John C.
Hrebicek, Olinka K.
Kemble, Frank
Parton, David E.
Pathak, Parbeen K.
Penn, Andrew M W.
Saly, Viera
Scott, James L.

WEST VANCOUVER
Makin, G J. Vance

MANITOBA

BRANDON
Tang-Wai, Robert

WINNIPEG
Al-Kaabi, Atheer
Anderson, Brian A.
Barnes, Jeffrey G.
Borys, Andrew E.
Chan-Lui, W Y. Winifred
Cossoy, Michael B.
Dominique, Francis
Eggertson, Douglas E.
Fast, Mallory D.
Gomori, Andrew J.
Hobson, Douglas
Ilse, Werner K.
Jackson, Alan C.
Johnston, Janine L.
Leung, Edward C W.
Marriott, James J.
Nijjar, Satnam S.
Pacin, Stefan
Schmidt, Brian J.
Shelton, Paul A.
Vosoughi, Reza
Yankovsky, Alexei E.
Young, Mark R.

NEW BRUNSWICK

MONCTON
Harper, Byrne D J.
MacEachern, Michael H.
Weston, Lyle E.

ROTHESAY
Stewart, Wendy A.

SAINT JOHN
Al-Amri, Ahmed S A.
MacLean, Gregg L.

NEWFOUNDLAND AND LABRADOR

GANDER
Hussey, Danielle M.

ST. JOHN'S
Alam, Muhammad F.
Buckley, David J.
Eustace, Marsha L.
Goodridge, Alan E.
House, A. Maxwell
Jacob, Jacob C.
Ogunyemi, Abayomi O.
Pryse-Phillips, William E.
Squarey, Kyna J.
Stefanelli, Mark G.

NOVA SCOTIA

BEDFORD
Leckey, Richard N.

DARTMOUTH
McKelvey, J. Roger
Moeller, Jeremy J.

HALIFAX
Benstead, Timothy J.
Bhan, Virender
Brna, Paula M.
Camfield, Peter R.
Darvesh, Sultan
Gordon, Kevin E.
Grant, Ian
Gubitz, Gordon J.
King, David B.
Kirby, Sarah
MacDougall, Alexander D.
Maxner, Charles E.
Mohamed, Ismail S.
Phillips, Stephen J.
Purdy, R. Allan
Sadler, R. Mark
Schoffer, Kerrie L.
Weaver, Donald F.
Wood, Ellen P.

SYDNEY
Maharaj, Mandat
Shimon, Laith D.

ONTARIO

AJAX
Gupta, Aparna

ALMONTE
Atack, David M.

BARRIE
Arts, Rudolf J.
Maher, John

BRACEBRIDGE
Ursell, Melanie R M.

BRAMPTON
Angel, Michael J.
Best, Brian R.
Koponen, Glynis M.
Tullio, Gerald C.
Zaitlen, Marshall S.

BURLINGTON
Ganesan, Ramakrishnan
Lad, Tara L.

CAMBRIDGE
Giles, Kathryn A.
Stewart, Dwight J.

CORNWALL
Suranyi, Leslie

EAST YORK
Stefurak, Taresa L.

ETOBICOKE
Chu, Joseph Y C.
Watson, Christoper P N.
Yufe, Robert S.

GUELPH
Jichici, Draga
Singh, Ranjit

HAMILTON
Brown, William F E.
Callen, David J A.
De Rubeis, Debra A.
Derby, Ian R G.
Giammarco, Rosella
Goodwin, Susan E B.
Kronby, Michael H.
Lo, Raymond C T.
Mazurek, Michael F.
Meaney, Brandon F.
Mesterman, Ronit
Morillo, Luis E.
Oczkowski, Wieslaw J.
Paulseth, John E.
Picard, Pierre
Ramachandran, N. Rajesh
Rathbone, Michel P.
Ronen, Gabriel M.
Sahlas, Demetrios D J.
Savelli, Gordina E.
Shapiro, Michelle J.
Silva, Jaime E.
Turnbull, John D.
Upton, Adrian R M.
Yegappan, Chidambaram M.

HUNTSVILLE
Foell, R. Blaine T.

KINGSTON
Abdollah, Azad
Baranchuk, Adrian M.
Bolton, Charles F.
Bonni, Azad
Boyd, John G.
Brunet, Donald G.
Dinsdale, Henry
Jin, Albert Y.
Melanson, Michel
Pari, Giovanna
Reid, Stuart E.
Riopelle, Richard J.
Spiller, Allison E.
Taylor, Sean W.

KITCHENER
Mandalfino, Patricia
Sloka, Jeffery S.
Steckley, Jamie L.

LONDON
Alavian Ghavanini, Ahmad
Blume, Warren T.
Campbell, Craig G N.
Cooper, Paul E.
Diosy, David C.
Fraser, John A.
Ganapathy, Gobi R.
Hachinski, Vladimir
Hahn, Angelika F G.
Hyson, H. Christopher
Jack, Kristin L.
Jenkins, Mary E.
Jog, Mandar S.
Jones, Michelle-Lee
Kay, John D.
Kaye, Kathy L.
Kertesz, Andrew
Kimpinski, Kurt
Kremenchutzky, C. Marcelo M.
MacDonald, Maria J.
MacDonald, Penny A.
Macdonald, David R.
McLachlan, Richard S.
Mirsattari, Seyed M.
Morrow, Sarah A.
Moulin, Dwight E.
Nicolle, Michael W.
Pasternak, Stephen H.
Prasad, Asuri
Salmon, Andrea K.
Shoesmith, Christen L.
Spence, J. David
Strong, Michael J.
Van Adel, Brian A.
Venance, Shannon L.
Watling, Christopher J.
Young, G. Bryan

MAPLE
Markson, Lisa A.

MARKHAM
Adams, John R.
Geenen, Caroline L.
Guttman, Mark
Kim, David H.
Robinson, Dale K.

MILTON
Marchetti, Paul J.

MISSISSAUGA
Blair, R D. Gordon
Dhanani, Al-Noor
Douen, Andre
Friedman, Yael
Israelian, Gaspar
John, Verity J.
Margaliot, Adit
McKenzie, Stephen W.
Mehdiratta, Manu
Perez, Yael
Sawa, Gordon M J.
Temple, Bryan K.
Tsiaprailis, Alexandros

NEPEAN
Briscoe, Natalie K.
Christie, Suzanne N.
Dhalla, Zahir A K.
Giaccone, Roberto A.
Rabinovitch, Hyman E.

NEWMARKET
Baryshnik, Devra B.
Baryshnik, Sheldon M.

NIAGARA FALLS
Chew, Donald L.

NORTH YORK
Baskind, Roy D.
Bryer, Mark A.
Cohen, Sharon
Esmail, Sherali G.
Freedman, Morris
Gladstone, Jonathan P.
Henri-Bhargava, Alexandre R.
Kasravi, Neema
Koo, Betty K K.
Levitan, Maurice D.
Morgenthau, David R.
Mossanen, Ayoob
Munn, Robert I.
Roussev, Rossen
Schiffer, Laura J.
Serebrin, Raold G.
Wong, Daniel C.
Yahmad, Nagib Y R.

OAKVILLE
Gazala, Khalid
Stirling, Denise S.
Trott, Jeffrey N.

OSHAWA
Crisp, David T.
Guppy, Barry R.
Jiaravuthisan, Somchai

OTTAWA
Beaulieu, J. Marc-Andre
Blacquiere, Dylan P V.
Bourque, Pierre R.
De Meulemeester, Christine
Doja, M. Asifud
Dowlatshahi, Dariush
Frank, Andrew
Freedman, Mark S.
Grimes, David A.
Guberman, Alan
Guzman, D. Antonio
Hakim, Antoine M.
Hogan, Matthew J.
Humphreys, Peter
Keene, Daniel L.
Krelina, Michael
MacLean, Heather J.
McIlraith, Duncan M.
McMillan, Hugh J.
Mendis, Tilak
Nelson, Robert F.
Nguyen, The-Minh
Ponesse, Jonathan S.
Pringle, C. Elizabeth
Schlossmacher, Michael G.
Sharma, Mukul
Sitwell, Lucian D.
Skinner, Christopher R R.
Stotts, Grant J.
Venkateswaran, Sunita
Warman Chardon, Jodi P.
Whiting, Sharon E.
Zwicker, Jocelyn C.

PARIS
Dost, Rehan

PETERBOROUGH
Lan, John S F.
Semmler, Robert T.

RICHMOND HILL
Fu, Ping
Goldstein, Warren C.
Licorish, Paulette M.
Santhiramohan, Ratha

SARNIA
Muhunthan, Jothimalar

SAULT STE MARIE
Nolan, William T.

SCARBOROUGH
Castagna, Avril E.
Chakrabarti, Gobinda L.
Dindar, Farouk
Gardner-Maher, Bertha
Georgevich, Lila L.
Jensen, Paul
Kong, Kester
Lim, Chern W.
Majl, Lance B.
Parekh, Neal A.
Ramanathan, Usha
Rana, Abdul Q.
Tyndel, Felix J.
Wilson, Ronald H.

ST CATHARINES
Klimek, Edwin H.
Stoltz, Katherine J.
Tokar, Judith L.

SUDBURY
Gupta, Salil Kumar
Mathew, Cizy

THORNHILL
Langburt, Wayne

THUNDER BAY
Howse, David C N.
Sweet, Margaret E.

TORONTO
Abunaji, Mohamed A.
Alkhater, Reem A A.
Anagnostou, Evdokia
Ashby, Peter
Askalan, Rand A.
Banwell, Brenda L.
Basile, Vincenzo S.
Berry, Henry
Birnbaum, Alexander
Black, Sandra E.
Bondar, Roberta L.
Borrett, Donald S.
Boulos, Mark I.
Breiner, Ariel

Bril, Vera
Bruni, Joseph
Bui, Esther
Carlen, Peter L.
Casaubon, Leanne K.
Chan, David K W.
Chen, Robert E W.
Chepesiuk, Martin A.
Connolly, Barbara S.
Consky, Earl S.
Crookshank, Emily
DeVeber, Gabrielle A.
Del Campo, J C. Martin
Dimitrakoudis, Dimitrios P.
Dodig, Dubravka
Donner, Elizabeth J.
Ellis, Paul D.
Fornazzari, Luis R.
Gawel, Marek J.
Gladstone, David J.
Gladstone, Richard M.
Goldman, Marvin B.
Gordon, Allan S.
Grek, Adrian
Hahn, Cecil D A.
Hohol, Maria J.
Hopyan, Julia J.
Hung, Ryan M T.
Huot, Philippe
Hwang, Paul A L S.
Jaigobin, Cheryl S.
Katzberg, Hans
Kleiner-Fisman, Galit
Lam, Benjamin
Lang, Anthony E T.
Lay, Christine L.
Lazarou, Jason
Lee, Liesly
Lena, Tanya S.
Lim, Andrew S.
Lin, Liping
Lindsay, Shanna L.
Logan, William J.
MacGregor, Daune L.
Makhani, Naila
Marras, Laurie C.
Masellis, Mario
Mason, Warren P.
Meloff, Keith L.
Midroni, Gyl
Minassian, Berge A.
Miyasaki, Janis M.
Moddel, Garry
Murray, Brian J.
Narayansingh, Marc J.
Nulman, Irena
O'Connor, Paul W.
Oh, Jiwon
Ong, Alan P Y.
Payne, Eric
Perry, James
Picard, Larry M.
Ranalli, Paul J.
Safinia, Layla
Saposnik, Gustavo
Sawa, Michael T.
Schneiderman, Jacob H.
Selchen, Daniel H.
Shandling, Maureen R.
Sharpe, James A.
Silver, Frank L.
Singerman, Jennifer D.
Slegr, Marie N.
Snead III, Orlando C.
Sourkes, Myra
St George-Hyslop, Peter H.
Steeves, Thomas D L.
Stewart, Bruce M.
Strafella, Antonio P.
Sundaram, Arun N E.
Supala-Berger, Agnes Z.
Swartz, Richard H.
Tai, Peter C.
Tam, Emily W Y.
Tang-Wai, David F.
Turley, Judith J E.
Vajsar, Jiri
Veidlinger, Otto F.
Weiss, Shelly K.
Wennberg, Richard A.
Wherrett, John R.
Zahn, Catherine A.
Zinman, Lorne H.

WATERLOO
Carleton, Susan A.

WINDSOR
Desai, Hiren B.
Moodley, Logan G.
Mustafa, Abdalhakim I.
Winger, Michael J.

PRINCE EDWARD ISLAND

CHARLOTTETOWN
Hutchings, Reginald S.
Silverberg, David C.

QUÉBEC

AMOS
Roux, Louise

CHATEAUGUAY
Dahan, Benjamin

CHICOUTIMI
Beaudry, Michel G.
Boily, Camil
Mathieu, Jean
Theodore, Sylvie

DOLLARD DES ORMEAUX
Muresan, Letitia V.

GATINEAU
Gagnon, Alexis
Gagnon, Sophie
Hadj Tahar, Abdallah
Halle, Denis
Jacques, Francois H.
Therrien, Marc

GREENFIELD PARK
Berger, Leo R.
Boulanger, Jean-Martin
Clement, Jean-Francois
Cloutier, Martin
Duplessis, Michel
Filiatrault, Robert
Grand'Maison, Francois
Larue, Sandrine
Nasreddine, Ziad
Ninkovic, Svetlana
Pinard-D'Amour, Catherine A.
Trottier, Antonio G.

KAHNAWAKE
Vanast, Walter J.

LASALLE
Rosa Neto, Pedro

LAVAL
Archambault, Luc L P.
Lalumiere, Eric
Ledoux, Stephane
Monette, Marie-Jose
Nadeau, Amelie
Rabinovitch, Daniel E.
Veilleux, Francine

LEVIS
Bergeron, Marc-Andre
Bouchard, Manon
Gagnon, Marie-Eve
Grammond, Pierre
Letourneau, Karine
Petitclerc, Marc
Rivest, Donald
Tremblay, Sandra

LONGUEUIL
Bui, Linh-Khue
Ducharme, Mario
Jutras, Marie-France
Phan, Xuan Khoa.
Roy, Stephane
Thibault, Louis

MAGOG
Vaucher, Robert-Yves

MASCOUCHE
Pepin, E. Paul

MONT-ROYAL
Morcos, Rami

MONTREAL
Al Hashmi, Amal
Altman, Robert D.
Antel, Jack P.
Arnold, Douglas L.
Aube, Michel
Ayotte, Charles
Bar-Or, Amit
Barkas, William J.
Bekhor, Sabah
Bernard, Genevieve
Bernier, Gilles P.
Berube, Arline
Blanchet, Pierre
Boghen, R. Dan
Boileau, Jean
Botez, Stephan
Bourgeau, Pierre
Brais, Bernard
Carlton, Joseph A.
Carmant, Lionel
Chalk, Colin H.
Charron, Louise F.
Chayer, Celine
Chertkow, Howard M.
Chouinard, Sylvain
Copti, Michel
Cossette, Patrick
Cote, Robert
D'Amour, Monique L.
D'Anjou, Guy
Dagher, Alain
Daneault, Nicole
De Villers-Sidani, Etienne
Desautels, Alex
Deschaintre, Yan
Diadori, Paola
Dilenge, Marie-Emmanuelle
Dion, Marie-Helene
Diorio, Diane L.
Dubeau, Francois
Duchastel, Yves J.
Duquette, Antoine
Durcan, Liam V.
Durocher, Andre
Ehrensperger, Eric
Ender, Peter
Fellows, Lesley K.
Fon, Edward A.
Gagnon, Stephan
Gendron, Daniel
Genge, Angela L.
Giacomini, Paul S.
Girard, J. Marc
Goudreau, Guy
Gupta, Meera
Houde, Sylvie
Jobin, Celine M.
Jodoin, Nicolas
Keezer, Mark R.
Khairallah, Nicole
Labrecque, Raymonde
Lachapelle, Jacques
Lafontaine, Anne-Louise
Lanthier, Sylvain
Lapierre, Yves L.
Laplante, Pierre
Larbrisseau, Albert
Larochelle, Catherine
Lauzier, Sylvie
Lebrun, Louise-Helene
Lemay, Robert
Leroux, Elizabeth
Lortie, Anne
Lubarsky, Stuart E.
Major, Philippe
Marchand, Luc
Massie, Rami
Masson, Helene
Matte, Genevieve
Melmed, Calvin A.
Minuk, Jeffrey
Moore, Fraser G A.
Moussette, Normand
Nguyen, Dang Khoa.
O'Ferrall, Erin K.
Odier, Celine
Oskoui, Maryam
Panisset, Michel
Parpal, Helene
Perez-De-Leon, Adolfo J.
Poppe, Alexandre Y.
Postuma, Ronald B.
Poulin, Chantal
Prat, Alexandre
Rasminsky, Michael
Rasmussen, Lisa A.
Remillard, Guy M.
Robillard, Alain A.
Rosenblatt, Bernard
Rossignol, Elsa
Rouleau, Guy A.
Rousseau, M. Suzanne R.
Roy, Jean-Pierre
Roy, Louis-Edouard
Schipper, Hyman M.
Schondorf, Ronald
Shevell, Michael I.
Sidel, Michael
Soland, Valerie L.
Souchon, Frederique
Srour, Myriam
Stumpf, Erika
Talbot, Jeannine
Teitelbaum, Jeanne S.
Vanasse, Michel
Veilleux, Martin
Villota, Maurilio
Wein, Howard P.
Wein, Theodore H.
Woods, John F.
Ziller, Matthias G.

POINTE-CLAIRE
Roberts, Richard D.
Vieira, Lucy M.

QUEBEC
Bouchard, Jean-Pierre L.
Bouchard, Remi W.
Boucher, Renee-Myriam
Brunet, Denis
Camden, Marie-Christine
Daigle, Emilien
De Lean, Jacques
Desbiens, Richard
Desbiens, Serge
Dionne, Annie
Dupre, Nicolas
Emond, Francois
Guillemette, Annie
Lafleur, Jean
Laforce, Robert
Langevin, Pierre L.
Langlois, Melanie
MacKey, Ariane
Naud, Pierre G.
Parent, Carole
Pourcher, Emmanuelle
Quirion, Annie
Savard, Martin
Sylvain, Michel
Thibault, Manon
Thibeault-Eybalin, Marie-Pierre
Verreault, Steve
Verret, Louis
Verret, Simon

RIMOUSKI
Delisle, Francois
Gonzalez Herrera, Luis A.

RIVIERE-DU-LOUP
Attig, Ezzedine

ROUYN-NORANDA
Cote-Mantha, Evelyne
Jacques, Stephanie
Nadeau, Yannick
Neveu, Marc

SAINT-HYACINTHE
Berube-Desrosiers, Maxime
Kovitz-Lensch, Jessica M.

SAINT-JEROME
Girard, Marie-Eve
Langlois, Marie-Josee
McGuire, Claudie
Pham-An, Minh-Thy
Prevost, Julie
Ricard, Genevieve
Sirois-Bergeron, Elise

SAINT-LEONARD
Prelevic, Stanislav

SHERBROOKE
Bernier, Jean-Pierre
Bocti, Christian
Deacon, Charles M A.
Evoy, Francois
Frenette, Eric
Gosselin, Sylvie
Jarjoura, Samir C.
Kantardjieff, Spiridon
Lamontagne, G. Albert
Lebel, Michel L.
Moreau, Francois P.
Pannetier, Evelyne
Riou, Emilie
Rioux, Marie-France
Rivest, Jean
Sebire, Guillaume

ST-AMBROISE-D-KILD
Lamoureux, Louise

ST CHARLES BORROMEE
Dubreuil, Martin
Guevremont, Mylene
Sarrazin, Anne-Marie

ST JEAN SUR RICHELIEU
Tudorescu, Aurel

TERREBONNE
Rosu, Liliana
Varga, Caroline

TROIS-RIVIERES
Arbour, Jean-Francois
Arsenault, Marie-Eve
Charest, Stephane
Delisle, Richard R.
Durand-Martel, Pascali
Gagnon, Andre F.
Guite, Charles
Lapalme, Sophie

VERDUN
Dvorkin, Gary S.
Gauthier, Serge G.
Prescott, Lise
Saltiel, Philippe
Wu, Ying

WESTMOUNT
Lechter, Mortimer
Zifkin, Benjamin G.

SASKATCHEWAN

REGINA
Raghig, Abdulhakim M.
Rehman, Ziaur
Shawush, Melad F R.
Veloso, Felix M.

SASKATOON
Atkins, Edward J.
Block, Haley J.
Datta, Anita
Fitzpatrick, Wendi
Hunter, Gary R W.
Huntsman, Richard J.
Kirk, Andrew
Lowry, Noel J.
Masiowski, A. Paul

Moien Afshari, Farzad
Rajput, Alexander H.
Rajput, Ali H.
Savedia-Cayabyab, Sheila M.
Voll, Christopher L.

Neuropathology

ALBERTA

CALGARY
Chan, Jennifer A.
Resch, Lothar

EDMONTON
Johnson, Edward S.
Lacson, Atilano G.
Lu, Jian-Qiang

BRITISH COLUMBIA

VANCOUVER
Al-Dandan, Sadeq W A.
Dunham, Christopher P.
MacKenzie, Ian R A.
Maguire, John A C.
Moore, G R. Wayne
Neumann, Etela
Yip, Stephen T.

MANITOBA

WINNIPEG
Del Bigio, Marc R.

NEW BRUNSWICK

MONCTON
Kydd, David W.

NEWFOUNDLAND AND LABRADOR

ST. JOHN'S
Barron, Jane R.

NOVA SCOTIA

HALIFAX
Easton, Alexander
MacAulay, Robert J B.

ONTARIO

HAMILTON
Lach, Boleslaw
Provias, John P.

KINGSTON
Rossiter, John P.

LONDON
Ang, Lee-Cyn
Hammond, Robert R.
Ramsay, David A.

OTTAWA
Jansen, Gerard H.
Woulfe, John M J.

ST CATHARINES
Davidson, George

SUDBURY
Gaytan-Graham, Silvia R M.

TORONTO
Babiak, Taras
Bilbao, Juan M.
Croul, Sidney
Hawkins, Cynthia E.
Hazrati, Lili-Naz
Jay, Venita
Keith, Julia L.
Munoz, David G.
Shannon, Patrick T.
Yucel, Yeni H.

QUÉBEC

MONTREAL
Albrecht, Steffen
Auer, Roland N.
Richardson, John B.

SASKATCHEWAN

SASKATOON
Robinson, Christopher A.

Neurosurgery

ALBERTA

CALGARY
Ajani, Olufemi A.
Alant, Jacob D V.
Casha, Steven
Gallagher, Clare N.
Hader, Walter J.
Hamilton, Mark G.
Hurlbert, R. John
Jacobs, W. Bradley
Kelly, John J P.
Khuong, Helene T.
Kiss, Zelma H T.
Leblanc, Francis E.
Louw, Deon F.
Midha, Rajiv
Mitha, Alim
Myles, S. Terence
Serrano Almeida, Cesar A.
Starreveld, Yves P.
Sutherland, Garnette R.
Wong, John H Y.

EDMONTON
Alflouse, Atya
Aronyk, Keith E.
Benour, Mahmoud A.
Broad, Robert W.
Chan, Patrick D S.
Chow, Michael M C.
Darsaut, Timothee E.
Findlay, J. Max
Fox, Richard J.
McKean, John D S.
Mehta, Vivek
Nataraj, Andrew
O'Kelly, Cian
Petruk, Kenneth C.
Pugh, Jeffrey A.
Quateen, Ahmed S.
Ryan, Robert W J.
Sankar, Tejas
Shandro, Gerald L.
Souster, Jenny D.
Steinke, David E.
Weir, Bryce K A.
Wheatley, B. Matthew

BRITISH COLUMBIA

BURNABY
Hudoba De Badyn, Peter

KAMLOOPS
Brownlee, Richard D.
Chevalier, Jean-Francois
Faridi, Majid
Nikolakis, Michael A.
Omahen, David A.

KELOWNA
Goplen, Gary B.
Govender, Preneshlin V.
Lefevre, Kim M.

NEW WESTMINSTER
Chan, Richard C.
Gittens, Winston O.
Heran, Navraj S.
Lee, Andrew S Y.
Matishak, Mark Z.

NORTH VANCOUVER
Gul, Shahid M.
Hunt, Brian M.
Janicki, Ryan R.
Mutat, Abdurrazag M.
Padilla, Julio R.
Sahjpaul, Ramesh L.

VANCOUVER
Akagami, Ryojo
Boyd, Michael C.
Cochrane, D. Douglas
Dea, Nicolas
Griesdale, Donald E.
Haw, Charles S.
Honey, Christopher R.
Kestle, John R W.
Paquette, Scott J.
Redekop, Gary J.
Singhal, Ashutosh
Steinbok, Paul
Toyota, Brian D.
Turnbull, Ian M.
Zwimpfer, Thomas J.

VICTORIA
Cameron, G. Stuart
Fleetwood, Ian
Frangou, Evan M.
Hentschel, Stephen J.
Joaquin, Andrew J.
Matwijecky, Cornelius
Reid, Richard A S.
Sun, John C L.
Warren, Daniel T.

MANITOBA

WINNIPEG
Beiko, Jason
Fewer, H. Derek
Kaufmann, Anthony M.
Krcek, Jerry P.
McDonald, Patrick J.
Silvaggio, Joseph A.
West, Michael
Williams, Owen R T.

NEW BRUNSWICK

MONCTON
Adams, Robert
Charest, Dhany T.
Fawaz, Charbel S.
Gorman, Peter B C.
Kenny, Brendan G.
Quartey, Gilbert R C.

SAINT JOHN
Al-Shayji, Ayman F.
Attabib, Najmedden A.
Kolyvas, George
Wheelock, W. Brian

NEWFOUNDLAND AND LABRADOR

ST. JOHN'S
Avery, Roger A.
Maroun, Falah B.
Murray, Gerald P.

NOVA SCOTIA

HALIFAX
Brownstone, Robert M.
Christie, Sean D.
Clarke, David B.
Lwu, Shelly H.
McNeely, P. Daniel
Mendez, Ivar M.
Pickett, Gwynedd E.
Walling, Simon A.

SYDNEY
Malik, Hatim G.

ONTARIO

HAMILTON
Algird, Almunder R R.
Cenic, Aleksa
Hollenberg, Robert D.
Kachur, Edward
Reddy, Kesava K V.
Singh, Sheila K.
Wells, John D.

KINGSTON
Ellis, Peter M.
Levy, Ron
Pokrupa, Ronald P.
Saunders, Fraser W.
Wallace, M. Christopher

LONDON
Al-Otibi, Merdas H F.
Boulton, Melfort R.
Duggal, Neil
Dyer, Erin
Hebb, Matthew O.
Lownie, Stephen P M.
MacDougall, Keith
Megyesi, Joseph F.
Ng, Wai-Pui
Parrent, Andrew
Ranger, Adrianna
Siddiqi, Fawaz
Steven, David A.

MISSISSAUGA
Duncan, Eric G.
Izukawa, Dennis M S.
Kis, Mihaly
Li, Hui
Marmor, Eric
Smyth, Harley S.

OTTAWA
Agbi, Charles B.
Alkherayf, Fahad A E.
Benoit, Brien G.
Da Silva, Vasco F.
Kassam, Amin
Labib, Mohamed A M.
Lesiuk, Howard J.
Moulton, Richard J.
Richard, Michael T.
Sinclair, John
Tsai, Eve C.
Vassilyadi, Michael
Ventureyra, Enrique C G.

SUDBURY
Adegbite, Andrew B O.
De Marchi, Ryan
Mantle, Ross E.
Ogundimu, Fadegbola
Schneider, Elizabeth A.

THUNDER BAY
Haq, Iftikhar U.
Marchuk, Graeme G.
McCluskey, Stephen D.

TORONTO
Barry, Sean P.
Bernstein, Mark
Cusimano, Michael D.
Dirks, Peter
Drake, James
Elashaal, Abdurrahim A.
Fazl, Mahmood
Fehlings, Michael
Gentili, Fred
Ginsberg, Howard J.
Hodaie, Mojgan
Jha, Neilank K.
Johnston, Karen M.
Kalia, Suneil K.
Kim, Betty Y S.
Kongkham, Paul N.
Kulkarni, Abhaya V.
Lo, Benjamin W Y.
Lozano, Andres M.
Macdonald, Robert Loch.
Mainprize, Todd G.
Massicotte, Eric M.
Mohammadzadeh, Gelareh
Muller, Paul J.
Perrin, Richard G.
Phan Cong, Nicolas
247Pirouzmand, Farhad
Rowed, David W.
Rutka, James T.
Schacter, Irving B.
Schwartz, Michael L.
Shamji, Mohammed F.
Spears, Julian
Tasker, Ronald R.
Tator, Charles H.
Taylor, Michael D.
Tucker, William S.
Tymianski, Michael
Valiante, Taufik A.
Yang, Victor X D.

WINDSOR
Dang, Tommy
Jhawar, Balraj
Morassutti, Dante J.
Shamisa, Abdalla R M.

QUÉBEC

BROSSARD
Gariepy, Jacques

CHICOUTIMI
McLelland, Hans

GATINEAU
Brien, Susan E.
Khalaf, Khalil
Lieu, Hung-Ba

GREENFIELD PARK
Demers, Jacques
Gauthier, Nathalie
Malak, Ramez
Michaud, Yzabel
Roux, Alain

LAVAL
Giroux, Marc F.
Khoueir, Jihad P.

MONTREAL
Atkinson, Jeffrey D.
Bojanowski, Wieslaw M.
Bouthillier, Alain
Chaalala, Chiraz
Chatillon, Claude E.
Couillard, Philippe L.
Crevier, Louis
Del Maestro, Rolando
Dimaio, Salvatore
Farmer, Jean-Pierre
Fournier-Gosselin, Marie
Giguere, Jean-Francois

Golan, Jeff D.
Goulet, Benoit
Hall, Jeffery A.
Hardy, Jules J.
Hebert-Blouin, Marie-Noelle
Jacques, Line
L'Esperance, Georges
Laroche, Mathieu
Leblanc, Richard
Li, Maria S.
Maleki, Mohammad
Marcoux, Judith
Mercier, Claude
Mohr, Gerard
Molina-Negro, Pedro
Montes, Jose
Moumdjian, Robert A.
Olivier, Andre
Petrecca, Kevin
Sadikot, Abbas F.
Shedid, Daniel
Sinclair, David S.
Sirhan, Denis

POINTE-CLAIRE
Balasingam, Vijayabalan

QUEBEC
Cantin, Leo
Francoeur, Jacques
Lapointe, Genevieve
Lavoie, Pascale
Mercier, David
Michaud, Karine
Milot, Genevieve
Paquet, Jerome
Picard, Claude
Prud'Homme, Michel
Thomas, Tina E.
Turcotte, Jean-Francois
Turmel, Andre

SAINT-ROMUALD
Laliberte, Laura

SAINT-BRUNO
Potvin, Jacques A.

SAINT-EUSTACHE
Ladouceur, Denis

SHERBROOKE
Blanchard, Jocelyn
Cloutier, Christian
Fortin, David
Luneau, Colette P.
Mathieu, David
Seguin, Mario

TROIS-RIVIERES
Bilocq, Alain
Gendron, Cathy
Pelletier, Mario
Truffer, Eric

SASKATCHEWAN

REGINA
Al Hayek, Ali I K.
Buwembo, Joseph E.
Ekong, Chris E U.
Kumar, Anil
Kumar, Krishna
Zwai, Akram M.

SASKATOON
Fourney, Daryl R.
Kelly, Michael E.
Meguro, Kotoo
Sadanand, Venkatraman
Vitali, Aleksander M.
Wu, Adam S G.

Nuclear Medicine

ALBERTA

CALGARY
Chan, Denise
Chan, Ida H T.
Fedorowicz, Andrew
Flemming, Jeffery P.
Frohlich, Dean E C.
Kloiber, Reinhard
Lou, Lawrence
Matzinger, Dorothy J.
Molnar, Christine P.
Numerow, Leonard M.
Scott, Douglas V.

EDMONTON
Abele, Jonathan T.
Buteau, Francois-Alexandre
Chan, Raymond H K.
Hoskinson, Michael E.
Hudson, Emmanuel W.
Jen, Ho
Ling, Bernice C.
MacEwan, Robert N.
McEwan, Alexander J B.
Scott, Malcolm D S.
Singh, Anil K.
Warshawski, Robert S.
Winter, Christopher K.

LETHBRIDGE
Aucoin, Richard J.
Lee, Edward

BRITISH COLUMBIA

ABBOTSFORD
Maharaj, Damien D.

COMOX
Thompson, William M.

KELOWNA
Kindrachuk, Gary W.
Kwong, J. Stephen

NANAIMO
Coupland, David B.
Johnson, Robert D A.

NEW WESTMINSTER
Ammann, Walter
Joshi, Urvi
Ross, Jeffrey S.

NORTH VANCOUVER
Cohen, Philip F.
Tarzwell, Robert R.

RICHMOND
Guijon, Juan-Carlos

SURREY
Dowey, Michael T J.

TRAIL
Babensee, Susan E.

VANCOUVER
Attariwala, Rajpaul
Belzberg, Allan S.
Benard, Francois
Nadel, Helen R.
Powe, John E.
Sexsmith, George P.
Stilwell, Moira E.
Tonseth, Rolf P.
Wilson, Donald C.
Worsley, Daniel F.

VERNON
Mohamed, Curtis R.

VICTORIA
Andrew, John
Chu, Derek D M.
Forkheim, Kevin E.
Yakemchuk, George H.

MANITOBA

BRANDON
Makis, Viliam

WINNIPEG
Demeter Jr., Sandor
Dupont, Jacqueline O.
Greenberg, I. David
Leslie, William D.
Levin, Daniel P.
Peterdy, Anne E.
Stern, Sheryl

NEW BRUNSWICK

BATHURST
Leblanc, John L.

MONCTON
Savoie, Isabelle

SAINT JOHN
Martin, Jennifer L.

NEWFOUNDLAND AND LABRADOR

GANDER
Kennedy, Paula M.

ST. JOHN'S
Hollett, Peter D.
Jefford, Cheryl L.
Maguire, Conor G J.

NOVA SCOTIA

HALIFAX
Barnes, David C.
Boyd, Gordon J.
Burrell, Steven C.
Clarke, James R.
Iles, Sian E.
Ross, Andrew A.

ONTARIO

BARRIE
Paul, T. Gordon

BELLEVILLE
Barette, Rene
Nguyen, Thien Huong

BRAMPTON
Boxen, Izzie
Ganguli, Satyajit N.
Murray, Shirley Y.

BRANTFORD
Nicholson, R. Lawrence
O'Brien, Christopher J M.
Urbain, Jean-Luc C P.

BURLINGTON
Louisy, Coventry L.

CAMBRIDGE
Coates, Geoffrey

CHATHAM
Mattar, Adel G.

ETOBICOKE
Bienenstock, Eli A.
Wilansky, Douglas L.
Willems, Cara L M.

HAMILTON
Gulenchyn, Karen Y.
Marriott, Christopher J C.
Singnurkar, Amit
Wong-Pack, William K.
Yakemchuk, Valerie N.

KINGSTON
Cheeseman, Frank D.
Dutchak, Peter A.

KITCHENER
Champagne, Caro Line.
Dubeau, Richard A.

LONDON
Akincioglu, Cigdem
Driedger, Albert
Mandel, Jonathan I.
Pavlosky, William F.
Rachinsky, Irina V.
Reid, Robert H.
Romsa, G. Jonathan
Shastry, Anil K.
Vezina, William C.
Warrington, James C.
Yuoness, Salem A H.

MARKHAM
Sharif, Anoosh

MISSISSAUGA
Foga, Myrosia M.
Kirsh, Joel C.
Yip, T C. Kathy

NEWMARKET
Siow, Yin-Hui

NORTH BAY
Hunter, Cameron M.

NORTH YORK
Cranstoun, Kelly R.
Grinblat, Leonard
Hausen, Doris M.

OAKVILLE
Kyes, John H.
Meindok, Harry

OSHAWA
Hershkop, Marlon S.
Kwan, Michael W H.
Lee, Norman K K.

OTTAWA
Bazarjani, Sadrollah S.
Dinh, Laurent
Leung, Eugene Y C.
Pham, Xuan H.
Raymond, Francois
Taucer, Fabiano A S.
Zeng, Wanzhen
Zuckier, Lionel S.

RICHMOND HILL
Yeung, Brian K P.

SCARBOROUGH
Nagai, Gordon R.
Nazareno, Janice J Y.
Vaughan-Neil, Edward F.

ST CATHARINES
McGinley, Michael D.

SUDBURY
Carr, Thomas J.
Webster, David L.

THORNHILL
Griesman, Jordan A.
Rendak, Ian

THUNDER BAY
Boekhoud, Jonathan J W.
Masood, Khaja M.

TORONTO
Ash, Judith M.
Bayley, T. Arnold
Charron, Martin
Cliche, Jean-Pierre
Ehrlich, Lisa E.
Eisen, Ari B.
Freeman, Marc
Gilday, David L.
Gray, Bruce G.
Greyson, N. David
Hendler, Aaron L.
Houle, Sylvain
Hurwitz, Gilbert A.
Mandelcorn, Jeffrey N.
Shammas, Amer
Verbeeten, Karen M.
Zeman, Robert

WINDSOR
Chang, Edward Y.
Ghali, Samia S K.
O'Donoghue, J. Paul
Tracey, Kevin P.

WOODBRIDGE
Tsin, Thomas T Y.

QUÉBEC

BAIE-COMEAU
Marquis, Michel

CHICOUTIMI
Brassard, Anne
Claveau, Rosaire
Leblond, Richard

DRUMMONDVILLE
Djeredjian, Sarkis

GATINEAU
Lalonde, Daniel

GRANBY
Blais, Gregoire

GREENFIELD PARK
Jeannotte, Simon
McNamara, Daniel
Recoskie, Mary Jo

LAVAL
Bouchard, Guillaume
Graveline, Ronald
Morais, Jacques

LEVIS
Lefebvre, Bernard

LONGUEUIL
Caron, Michelle
Carrier, Lucie

MONTREAL
Abikhzer, Gad S.
Arsenault, Andre M.
Beaulieu, Sylvain
Boucher, Luc
Chartrand, Raymonde
Cohade, Christian
Derbekyan, Vilma A.
Eybalin, Marie-Claire
Gregoire, Jean
Harel, Francois
Hickeson, Marc P.
Laflamme, Louis
Lambert, Raymond
Lamoureux, Francois
Laufer, Jerome R.
Leblond, Antoine
Lemieux, Raymond J.
Lepanto, Luigi
Lette, Jean L.
Levasseur, Andre
Levert, Valerie
Lisbona, Robert
Lord, Martin
Menard, Stephanie
Novales Diaz, Javier

Picard, Michel A.
Pison, Cesar
Probst, Stephan
Rosenthall, Leonard
Roy, Felix-Nicolas
Rush, Christopher L.
Soucy, Jean-Paul
Stern, Jerry
Turpin, Sophie M B.
Veilleux, Martin J P L.

POINTE-CLAIRE
Charest, Mathieu

QUEBEC
Beauregard, Jean-Mathieu
Cote, Christian
Dumont, Marcel
Friede, Juan
Guimond, Jean C.
Lacourciere, Yves
Lebrun, Josee
Morin, Francis
Tessier, Michel
Trottier, Mikael
Villemaire, Jean-Marc

REPENTIGNY
Labonte, Chantal

RIMOUSKI
Boucher, Yvan
Dionne, Daniel
Gravel, Maxime
Poisson, Frederic

SAINT-GEORGES
Guay, Christian

SAINT-HYACINTHE
Perrault, Roger

SAINT-JEROME
Dupras, Georges
Larocque, Jean-Francois
Mehrabian, Ali
Picard, Daniel

SAINTE-MARIE
Bisson, Guy

SALABERRY DE VALLEYFIELD
Ton-That, Quoc-Tuan

SEPT-ILES
Deslauriers, Patrice

SHERBROOKE
Keu, Khun Visith
Lamoureux, Guy
Leclerc, Yves
Paquet, Nancy
Prevost, Sylvain
Turcotte, Eric
Verreault, Jean

SOREL-TRACY
Leveille, Jean

ST CHARLES BORROMEE
Cerino, Michel
Lebel, Lisa

ST-JEAN-RICHELIEU
Taillefer, Raymond

TERREBONNE
Bernier, Helene
Lamargese, Isabella

THETFORD MINES
Huot, Denys

TROIS-RIVIERES
Bruneau, Virginie
Desroches, Joel
Gagne, Pierre
Laurin, Norman R.
Leblanc, Michel
Tremblay, Dominic
Vallieres, Bertrand J.

VAL-D'OR
Hebert, Jean

VERDUN
Kerouac, Marcel

VICTORIAVILLE
Drapeau, Gervais
Leveillee, Felix

SASKATCHEWAN

REGINA
Ollenberger, Glenn P.
Trivedi, Vijay K.

SASKATOON
Almgrahi, Abdulaziz
Dudzic, Edyta M.
Nijjar, Sundeep S.
Wesolowski, Carl A.

Obstetrics & Gynecology

ALBERTA

AIRDRIE
Currie, James

CALGARY
Albrecht, Kelly D.
Allan, Bruce B.
Ball, Allison L.
Baranowski, Susan L.
Belland, Liane M.
Birch, Colin
Brain, Philippa H.
Brar, Simrit K.
Brennand, Erin A.
Cenaiko, David F.
Chadha, Rati
Chang, Viviana
Chow, Clinton J.
Chu, Pamela
Connors, Gregory
Cooper, Stephanie L.
Cusano, Ronald E.
Docksteader, Brian
Donnelly, Jocelyn
Dwinnell, Shannon
Edwards, Heather E.
Ekwalanga, Pauline R.
Fahey, Meriah S.
Foong, Shu Ching.
Galan, Neville E.
Ghatage, Prafull
Gibbons, Sherri
Glaze, Sarah J.
Graham, James A.
Grant, Heather A.
Greene, Calvin A.
Hauck, Brian A.
Igras-Kulach, Dorothy
Iwanicki, Stanislaw M.
Jarrell, John F.
Johnson, Jo-Ann M.
Jones, Donna V.
Lam, Gail
Lamb, Kendra M.
Lange, Ian R.
Le Jour, Caroline
Leung, Wynne I.
Li, Andrew W.
Lyndon, Charlene A.
Mahalingham, Aisling M.
Martyn, Paul L.
Mattatall, Fiona M.
Min, Jason K.
Moscovitz, Walter
Motta, James A T.
Murphy, Magnus
Nation, Jill G.
Nelson, Gregg S.
O'Keane, Joseph A.
Pollard, Jeffrey K.
Robert, Magali
Roggensack, Anne
Rosengarten, Albert M.
Sabourin, Jeanelle N.
Schachar, Jaime D.
Scott, Selma G.
Shumsky, Anne G.
Simrose, Rebecca L.
Somerset, David A.
Steed, Joel D.
Suri, Michelle D.
Thompson, Elu M.
Tran, Quynh Mong
Wagner, Elisabeth M.
Wallace-Chau, Dhea
Watson, Sheila D.
Wilson, R. Douglas
Wong, Benjamin C.
Wood, Stephen L.

CAMROSE
Hugo, Wouter L.

COCHRANE
Adanlawo, Adewumi M.

CONSORT
Usher, Ann K.

DRUMHELLER
Smith, Laurel L.

EDMONTON
Aiken, Amanda M.
Bader, Erin L.
Baker, Philip N.
Ballermann, Charlotte A.
Barnes, Charlene A.
Baydock, Sandra A.
Black, Gail L.
Black, Robert C.
Bow, Michael R.
Brassard, Graeme M.
Brown, Alexander M.
Brown, Ronald J.
Burnett, Charles E.
Caddy, Sheila C.
Capstick, Valerie A.
Chandra, Sujata
Chari, Radha S.
Chua, Robert C M.
Corbett, Thomas F X.
Cumming, David C.
Danial, Hajira F.
Demianczuk, Nestor N.
Dolhaniuk, Christina
Evenson, Leonard G.
Flood, Catherine G.
Fraser, Derek
Genuis, Stephen J.
Gleason, Thomas P.
Griffiths, Jill C.
Gupta, Neelam K.
Halleran, Sarah
Hodges, Daniel J.
Hoskins, Christopher F.
Jain, Venu
Jiwa, Gulnaz B.
Kim, Amanda L.
Langton, Stephen R.
Larose, Dwaine L.
Lee, Agnes S.
Lieberman, Murray
Long, Ann Marie E.
Mah, May Sue
Mayo, Jorge P.
McCubbin, Jacqueline M.
Motan, Tarek
Neilson, Andrea M.
Robinson, Heather E.
Romanovsky, Amanda J.
Roy, Martine N.
Sabourin, J. Georges
Sacks, Juliette Y.
Sagle, Margaret A.
Schepansky, Alexandra
Schulz, Jane A.
Schuurmans, S. Nanette
Skorenki, Andrea H.
Steed, Helen L W.
Tankel, Jonathan
Tataryn, Ivanna V.
Tauh, Mangi N.
Tsui, Floria P L.
Turnell, Roger W.
Uretsky, Aubrey D.
Uretsky, H. Richard
Verma, Pramod K.
Wang, Jingwei
Wells, Tiffany H.
Wittner-Smith, Carlissa R.
Wong, Billy R.
Young, Carmen B.

FORT MCMURRAY
Wong, Keet Peng

GRANDE PRAIRIE
Barreth, Drew
De La Cruz, Christa Lynn.
Muir, Brian P.

HIGH RIVER
Bailey, Karen J.
Lukwinski, Angelina T.
Mueller, Harry D.

LETHBRIDGE
Adolph, Allyson J.
Browne, Philip M.
Davey, Stanley J.
Khan, Karla E.
Malach, Jaye A.
Stanzl, Valerie I.

LLOYDMINSTER
Abouhamra, Musbah M.
Elghdewi, Turia A.

MEDICINE HAT
Jeffery, John
McCubbin, Duncan

RED DEER
Apantaku, Olubukola J.
Awad, S. Michael
Cassis, Irene M.
Marais, Nico F.
Whitford, Amber L L.
Wiebe, Kevin M A.
Young, William R.

ST. ALBERT
Coe, Michael J O.
De Doming, Eva N.
Fernandez de Lara Nieto, Jose
Linton, Carol A V.
Tam, Florence M S.
Unger, D. Terrance

WETASKIWIN
Badawi, Mohammad

BRITISH COLUMBIA

ABBOTSFORD
Ahman, Frank W.
Goswami, Duna D.
Kenyon, Jennifer A.
Poon, Jason S Y.
Shone, Neal A.
Tregoning, Shaun K.
Tuffnell, Clayton E E.

BURNABY
Anand, Sarah-Jane
Coll, Oisin P.
Havelock, Jon C.
Lalani, Salim
Muir, Jennifer C.
Roberts, Jeffrey E.
Roy, Robert P A.
Seethram, Kenneth
Waterman, Elizabeth J.
Wong, Carrie K.

CAMPBELL RIVER
Duckitt, Kirsten

CHILLIWACK
Deacon, Sean D S.
Robertson, John G M.
Smith, Jan D W.

COMOX
Bagdan, Barry M.
Hartman, Dennis L.
Rodgers, Tracy L.
Wilson, Donald G.

CRANBROOK
Hugo, Daniel
Huyser, Charles A.
Post, William D.
Rode, Paul B.

DUNCAN
Beaudet, Luc
Fleige-Zahradka, Bettina G.
Liston, Fiona A.

KAMLOOPS
Adams, Erin R M.
Baikie, Hilary A.
Human, Anthony P.
Lott, Paula M.
Sproule, Pamela
Treissman, Mark J B Y E.
Wroz, Thom W.

KELOWNA
Benoit, A. Glenn
La Berge, Shelley-Ann A.
Leon, Roberto
McGregor, Sumathi
Meathrel, Karen A.
Valnicek, Stanislav
Wilson, Peter S.
Wise, Katherine E.
Yakimov, Margaret C.
Yoshida, Owen I.

LANGLEY
Abrahams, Ruth S.
Busletta, Angela V.
Mah, Elaine
Mohtashami-Gozellou, Fariba
Phelps, Erica L.
Taneda, Barbara L.

MAPLE RIDGE
Lampen, Ockert
Obioha, Godwin E.
Yeung, William H W.

NANAIMO
Arbelaez Correa, Luz J.
Hamilton, Janet
Hunt, Alan P.
Lajoie, Jennifer M.
Mitchell, Patrick J.
Renner, Regina-Maria A K.
Somerville, Jeffrey A.

NELSON
Alger, Sheryl
Moola, Shiraz

NEW WESTMINSTER
Altas, Melanie J.
Beauchamp, Aude
Beresford, Peter
Farquharson, Duncan F.
Nakatsuka, Nao
Neapole, Laurie A.
Pedersen, Sara A.
Ubhi, Jagdeep S.
Waterman, Douglas H.

NORTH VANCOUVER
Donnelly, Carolyn P.
Dy, Colleen
Goojha, Ciaran
Hoyer, Emelie M L.
Kaye, Stephen H.
Lipp, Michele M.
Sadeghi Tehrani, Susan
Scali, Vincent C.
Schouls, Jacquelynn J.
Sharpe, Kimberley A.

PENTICTON
Dela Cruz, M C. Armellie
Goncalves, Jose L.
Rublee, Catherine H.

PORT ALBERNI
Fouad, Magdy A M.

POWELL RIVER
Du Plessis, Pierre

PRINCE GEORGE
Galliford, Brian W.
Kingston, William G R.
Odulio, Maria J.
Tsang, Henry H K.

PRINCE RUPERT
Pienaar, Marius P.

RICHMOND
Arkuran, Cigdem
Heslip, Laura A M.
Kowalczyk, Jill C.
Mackoff, Harley P.
Monahan, Sarah K.
Mueller, Caroline P.
O'Connell, Jacqueline M.
Robson, Helen J.
Wagner, Brenda L M.

SECHELT
Kellett, Russell H.

SURREY
Abrahams, Ismail
Bakhet, Maged M S.
Bleszynski, Maria E.
Burrows, Jason B.
Gustafson, Kerstin D.
Ho, Peter S C.
Huckell, Caitlin L.
Price, Duncan A.
Still, Douglas K.
Tam, Winston T L.
Tkatch, Shelin
Yeung, Peter K.

TERRACE
Almas, Leilani T.
Janse Van Rensburg, Dawid A.

TRAIL
Dobson, Ann E.
Hale, Kathryn B.

VANCOUVER
Abdessamad, Hasan
Allaire, Catherine
Anderson, Robert B.
Belanger, Michelle A.
Bloomenthal, Dena F.
Brunner, Monica
Butler, Blair W E.
Carey, Mark S.
Chen, Innie
Cheung, Anthony P Y.
Christilaw, Jan E.
Dahlgren, Leanne S.
Delisle, Marie-France
Doersam, Gerald B.
Ehlen, Thomas G.
Ezzat, Hanna
Finlayson, Sarah J.
Fisher, Stephanie A.
Fitzsimmons, Brian P.
Fluker, Margo R.
Gagnon, Alain
Garrey, Matthew M.
Geoffrion, Roxana
Ghahremani, Mandana
Giesbrecht, Ellen M.
Gogela-Spehar, Marketa
Gomel, Victor
Grabowska, Kirsten M.
Guijon, Fernando B.
Gupta, Madhu
Heywood, Mark
Hitkari, Jason A.
Hyakutake, Momoe T.
Joa, Elisabet A E.
Johnson, Stephanie
Kalyanpur, Yamuna
Kanke, Lorena J.
Kashyap, Sonya
Kent, Nancy E.
Kim, Susan
Kinney, Gary E J.
Kuret, Verena
Kwon, Janice S.
Lalji, Sayrin S.
Lazare, Darren M.
Lee, Marette H.
Lee, Mary
Lee, Patrick
Lim, Kenneth I.
Liston, Robert M.
Marquette, Gerald
Massey, Andrea
Mayer, Chantal M H.
McAlpine, Jessica
McComb, Peter F.
Mehra, Neeraj
Millar, Debra M.
Miller, Dianne M.
Mitenko, Nancy L.
Money, Deborah M.
Moukhortova-Von Lipinski, Olga
Oakes, Jennifer
Pressey, Tracy L.
Pride, Sheila M.
Purcell, Jacqueline L.
Racette, Nicole
Reimer, Shirley A.
Rhone, Stephanie A.
Rivera, Loida R.
Robertson, Julie E.
Romalis, Garson
Rosengarten, Mark I.
Rowe, Timothy C.
Rychel, Valerie C.
Sadownik, Leslie A.
Salvador, Shannon C.
Sanders, Barry H.
Selke, Petra A.
Shaw, Dorothy
Simpson, M. Lynn
Skoll, M. Amanda L.
Steele, Dale R.
Stuart, Gavin C E.
Taylor, Elizabeth L.
Tessier, Francine
Thomson, Sydney L.
Unger, Waldemar G.
Van Schalkwyk, Julianne E.
Von Dadelszen, Peter
Whitehill, Kellie J.
Wilkie, David H L.
Williams, Christina
Woo, Henry L.
Yong, Paul J.
Yue, Jenise J W.
Yuen, Chui Kin
Yuzpe, A. Albert

VERNON
Daniel, Kimberly B.
Golosinski, Agata A.
Half, Nicholas P.
Hatfield, M. Christine
Jordan, Laurance T.
Mobbs, Christopher J.
Upton, Kenneth J.

VICTORIA
Bos, Hayley B.
Bourgeois-Law, Gisele
Cohen, Trevor
Cooper, John K.
Cox, Michael J.
Dansereau, Jerome
Dennie, Joelle
Hancock, Sherri R M.
Hudson, Stephen P.
Hunt, Harold G.
Ingram, Diana R.
McMurtrie, Elissa J.
Quinlan, David J.

WHITE ROCK
Jackson, Gary C.
Jackson, Roy P.

WILLIAMS LAKE
Gill, Glenn H.
Johnson, Robin L.
Raffard, Skye

MANITOBA

BRANDON
Akintola, Olalekan M.
Helms, Johan B.
Lee-Kwen, Johnson
Sutter, Joan A.

SELKIRK
Stearns, Eric L.

THE PAS
Jackson, Andora T K.

THOMPSON
Azzam, Hussam M.
Azzam, Lina
Mustafa, Arjowan

WINNIPEG
Al-Rujaib, Turky
Altman, Alon
Ambrose, Devon J.
Anttila, Lisa K.
Arneja, Jagmit
Avery, Lisa S.
Awadalla, Alaa
Bernier, Mark J.
Black, Denise R A.
Boroditsky, Michael L.
Burnett, Margaret A.
Burym, Craig J.
Corbett, Caroline A.
Dean, Erin C.
Debnath, Pranab K.
Diamond, Heather D.
Dubyna, Dale S.
Dzikowski, Dana
Elliott, Jason E.
Gertenstein, Robyn J.
Gupta, Anjali
Gupta, Chander K.
Helewa, Michael E.
Hooper, Wendy M.
Hunt, Jennifer
Katz, Guido A.
Kredentser, Jeremy V.
Lee, Francis F W.
Lee, Vivian K.
Logan, Alison C.
Lotocki, Robert J.
Maslow, Kenny D.
Masoud, Ibtisam A R.
McCarthy, Gerard F.
McNaught, Jennifer L.
McTavish, William G B.
Menticoglou, Savas M.
Morris, Margaret L.
Naugler, Sharon M M.
Palatnick, Carrie S.
Paterson, Corinne R S.
Popowich, Shaundra L.
Pymar, Helen C.
Reid, Gregory J.
Ring, Heather L.
Robinson, Debbie J.
Rogozinska, Ludwika
Ruddock, Deanne L.
Sabeski, Lynne M.
Schneider, Carol E.
Seager, Mary-Jane
Sett, Sikhor N.
Sinha, Meera
Srichandra, Withaya
Taylor, Susan N.
Yamamoto, Kenneth K.

NEW BRUNSWICK

BATHURST
Lebouthillier, Anne

CAMPBELLTON
Habaz, Yehuda

DIEPPE
McLaughlin, Nathalie
Nadeau, Sylvie

FREDERICTON
Adam, Christian
Butler, Kimberly A.
Butt, Kimberly D.
Christie, Garth B.
Collins, Samantha M.
Frecker, Erica
Holloway, Erica
Landau, Petr
Mills, Martha L.
Mullaly, Christa L.
Murdock, H. Ward
Samson, Sheri-Lee

MONCTON
Bernardin, Jeanne
Brodie, Glen
Caddick, Robert
Desrosiers, Karen
Gaudet, Laura
Gillespie, Kenneth E.
Kogon, David P.
Lamoureux, Marie-Catherine
Leblanc, Carole
Murphy-Kaulbeck, Lynn
Roberts, Carla D.
Robichaud, Alfred
Savoie, Rejean
Smallwood, Katharine R.
Williams, Carole

ROTHESAY
Lord, H. Leavinson

SAINT JOHN
Andrews, James S.
Colford, Donald F.
Leyenaar, Laurina K.
Ojuawo, Akinlolu B.
Patterson, Leslie S.
Reardon, Edward P.
Sanderson, Francis L.
Satya, Suma
Trites, Kimberly L.
Walsh, Jennifer D.

NEWFOUNDLAND AND LABRADOR

CORNER BROOK
Caines, Nadean M.
Carpenter, Jillian A.
Healey, Christopher J.
Hema, Karumpuzha

GANDER
Muise, Suzanne L.
Torraville, Douglas A.

GRAND FALLS WINDSOR
Mercer, Jennifer L.
Parsons, Steven M.

LABRADOR CITY
Sheppard, Kerry J.

ST. JOHN'S
Bajzak, Krisztina I.
Bartellas, Elias I.
Brown, Krista D.
Crane, Joan M G.
Dawson, Lesa
Delaney, Martina
Farrell-Cook, Colleen L.
Fowler, Erika
Gill, Atamjit
Healey, Sarah
Kennedy, Robert C.
Kravitz, Heidi
Kum, Franklin N.
Martin, Vickie J.
Murphy, Deanna M.
O'Grady, Teresa
Pike, Cherry J.
Popadiuk, Catherine M.
Power, R. Patricia
Strand, Timothy C O.
White, Joanne E.

NORTHWEST TERRITORIES

YELLOWKNIFE
Guthrie, Bing D.
Krushel, Robert F.

NOVA SCOTIA

AMHERST
MacQuarrie, Robyn M.
Sandland, Helen

ANTIGONISH
Hegarty, Raymond
MacLean-Fraser, Erin E.
Wescott, Donald D.

BRIDGEWATER
Jorgensen, Sally H.
Nicholson, Jennifer
Owen, Stephen M.
Pugh, Cheryl

DARTMOUTH
Craig, Catherine M.
Delisle, Isabelle M G.
Lee, Winifred
Mawdsley, Scott D.
Zilbert, Arthur W.

HALIFAX
Abu Rafea, Basim F A.
Allen, Victoria M.
Amirkhalkhali, Baharak
Armson, B. Anthony
Bentley, James R.
Bouzayen, Renda
Brock, Jo-Ann K.
Clermont, Marie-Eve
Coolen, Jillian D.
Corkum, Thomas P.
Dempster, Jeffrey J.
Farrell, Scott A.
Gilmour, Donna T.
Graves, Gillian R.
Grimshaw, Robert
Hamilton, Linda D.
Khalil, Hisham A.
Kieser, Katharina E.
McCarthy, Leanne S.
McLeod, N. Lynne
Murphy, Sean F.
Parish, Barbara M.
Pierce, Marianne
Rittenberg, David A.
Rittenberg, Paula V C.
Scott, Heather M.
Van Den Hof, Michiel C.
Van Eyk, Nancy A.
Wenning, Joan B.
Young, David C.

KENTVILLE
Hamm, Charles
Nette, Farrell
Rudd, Michael W.
Singh, Jaspal
Tynski, Gregory F.
Watts, Peter W S.

MIRA ROAD
Dolhanty, Dorothy A.

NEW GLASGOW
Jony, Louai
Joshi, Changulanda M.

SYDNEY
Conrod, Cheryl K.
Gardner, Angus J.

TRURO
Bent, Alfred E.
Clague, Nicholas P.
Folinsbee, Catherine D.
Houck, Leslie V H.

YARMOUTH
Agboola, Olaniyi B.
Madhvani, Ashwin K.

ONTARIO

AJAX
Eltayeb, Suha
Gordillo, Andres E.
Odueke, Adebayo W.

ALLISTON
Barrett, Alison P.
Narine, Andy J.
Simms, Richard J.

ALMONTE
Prevost, Michel R.
Stillman, Karen L.

BARRIE
Bologna, John T.
Browning, Andrew D.
Causey, Shannon E.
Kilani, Mehrak M.
Moreau, Jan P.
Reyes, Enrique G.
Scheeres, Jan J.
Wu, Vincent M Y.

BELLEVILLE
Ademidun, Aderotimi O.
Adu-Poku, Yaw
Chanda, Melanie N.
Clarke, Donald H.
Gwizdal, Mary
Kovacs, David P R.
O'Brien, David M.

BOLTON
Michael, Essam S N.

BOWMANVILLE
Singh, Padamjit M.

BRAMPTON
Abou-Seido, Maher K M.
Alexander, Kimberly A.
Ayodele, Kayode I.
Ben Omran, Karima
Braithwaite, Nicholas D J.
Caloia, David V.
Chandran, Indira
Cheng, Henry J C K.
ElSugy, Ramadan E.
Girvitz, Sheldon C.
Gronau, Karen A.
Jaffer, Kassamali M F.
Khan, Nayla M.
Le, Quynh M T.
Persad, Vidia L.
Sahi, Kiranjit
Soliman, Samuel R H.
Suleman, Shiraz
Vaidyanathan, Sankar

BRANTFORD
Azzam, Joseph E.
Bates, K. Stephen
Cowan, Christopher J.
Docrat, Zohra
Langlois, David A.
Powell, Anne C.
Rooney, Rebecca A.
Roye, Charmaine A.
Sorge, Cindy R.

BROCKVILLE
Froats, Timothy R.
Hafazalla, Basem K.
LeRiche, Tammy G.
Ng-Cheng-Hin, Raymond

BURLINGTON
Amin, Shilpa
Baillie, Jane I.
Beliveau, Caroline A.
De Jong, Christine
Faghih, Mehrnoosh
Hughes, Edward G.
Hunter, J. Barry
Karnis, Megan M F.
Komer, Lawrence D.
Mangaloglu, Leyla F.
Psarakis, Stella
Wu, Paul T K.

CAMBRIDGE
Butler, Deborah J.
Chan, Clifford C.
Cvetic, Valentina
Green, Jeremy A.
Strauss, Paul L.
Znamirowski, Anna I M.

CHATHAM
Nasello, Constance M.
Singh, Baljit

CLIFFORD
Tyson, John E A.

COLLINGWOOD
O'Toole, Susan A.
Yeates, Gillian R.

CORNWALL
Dehinbo, Olugbenga O.
Udoeyop, Emmanuel U J.
Ywakim, Fikry M.

COURTICE
Tauseef, Nazia

EAST YORK
MacLeod, Tara Lee.
Shore, Eliane M.

ETOBICOKE
Addison, Anthony M.
Ayoade, Gbade A.
Bhangu, Dalip K.
Caetano, Melanie G.
Cherry, Nicole A.
Chun, Kooyeon
Claessens, E. Anne
Colman, Laurence D.
Del Valle Rebeil, Alfonso P.
Friedman, Esti
Gringorten, Natalie A.
Grygowski, Beata K.
Johnston, Brenda A.
Judah, Sybil
Melchior, Maria F.
Rosset, Michael A.
Ryan, Edward A J.
Shinoff, Susan
Sutandar, Marilyn
Vaidyanathan, Prema

FERGUS
Reilly, Daniel R.

GEORGETOWN
Fiel, Naiema M.
Gunaratnam, Selvaratnam

GLOUCESTER
Dawood, Dawood G.

GODERICH
Moore, Julie B.

GRIMSBY
Gai, Tina D.
Nwebube, Nwachukwu I.

GUELPH
Ayanbadejo, Benjamin O.
Elliott, Elizabeth A.
Fraser, Gordon A D.
Huband, Donald M.
Jadi, Mohamed S.
Mueller, Valerie M L.
Namis, Nabil N.
Perron, Roger J W.
Strode, Kelly K.

HAMILTON
Akinsooto, Victor S.
Berndl, Anne M L.
Best, Carolyn
Brennan, Barbara G.
Cepeda, Rolando
Chamberlain, Jean E.
Chen, Ann Marie C.
Chomej, Anna K.
Cowan, William D.
Cullimore, Amie J.
De France, Bryon F.
Donnery, Cara-Anne
Dube, Marie-Josee
Dzaja, Nancy
Elit, Lorraine
Ellis, Susan M O.
Fedorkow, Donna M.
Fernandes, John R.
Gangam, Nirupama
Hamoudi, Aseel
Hoang, T. Boi-Ngoc
Hutchison, Robert J.
Lamont, John A.
Leyland, Nicholas A.
Lightheart, Margaret R.
Loosley-Millman, Margot E.
Mazurka, John
McDonagh, Roderick J.
McDonald, Sarah D.
Moens, Francois O P.
Mohide, Patrick T.
Morais, Michelle L.
Murji, Ally
Persadie, Richard J.
Ramanna, Raj
Roth, Paula
Sayed Ahmed, Raid M S H.
Sciarra, Carmela
Sibley, Caroline A.
Small, David R J.
Smith, Lauren
Smith, Patricia A.
Sobel, Mara L.
Stopps, Richard G.
Torrance, Shona M.
Winsor, Stephanie H M.

KANATA
Anderson, Lucyna J.

KINGSTON
Bryson, S C. Peter
Chamberlain, Susan M.
Costescu, Dustin J W.
Davies, Gregory
Francis, Julie-Ann R.
Harvey, Marie-Andree
Hillen, James
Huber, Jonathan D.
Jamieson, Mary Anne
Jeffrey, John F.
Johnston, Edward E.
Johnston, Shawna L.
McGrath, Michael M J.
Nitsch, Romy
O'Neill, J. Peter
Reid, Robert L.
Smith, Graeme N.
Tessier, Julie L.
Thomas, Richard P.
Waddington, Ashley

KITCHENER
Anstett, Robert J.
Campanaro, Judith M.
Carruthers, Danny E.
Halmo, Stephen D.
McCuaig, Wendy S.
Oliver, Gillian D.
Potts, Peter G G.
Raby, Patricia M.
Ross, Dana I.
Schnarr, Jennifer J.
Shannon, Michael A.
Tsandelis, Nickoli
Wakim, Emma G.

LEAMINGTON
Campeau, Denise L.
Carroll, Bryan W.
Chan, Angelina G J.
Gruneir, Richard K.

LINDSAY
Adelasoye, Oluremi F.
Bhatia, Gargi

LONDON
Akhtar, Saima S.
Arntfield, Shannon L.
Bertrand, Monique
Brown, Stanley E.
Chou, Queena
Crumley, Tracey L.
Di Cecco, Robert
Eastabrook, Genevieve D M.
Fellows, G. Fraser
Feyles, Valter
Frank, Cathy S.
Gratton, Robert
Hollett-Caines, Jackie R.
Kirby, Joanne N.
Lopes, Laudelino M.
MacMillan, J. Barry
Marks, Jennifer
Martin, James S B.
Maruncic, Michael A.
McGee, Jacob D.
McNaught, John J.
Milne, John K.
Natale, Renato
Nisker, Jeffrey
Oraif, Ayman M K.
Penava, Deborah A.
Power, Stephen G A.
Prefontaine, J E J. Michel
Rebel, Margaretha
Richardson, Bryan S.
Robins, Ronald N.
Schmidt, Jordan P.
Sugimoto, Akira K.
Tew, William L.
Vilos, Angelos G C.
Vilos, George A.
White, Andrea A.

MARKHAM
Arnold, George M.
Chang, Neil G.
Chouinard, Renee R.
Garcia-Erdeljan, Meivys
Gilmour, Jeffrey L.
Hall, Robert O M.
Lackman, Felice D.
Linkenheil, Edith
Peters, Christyne J.
Pyselman, Colette R.
Ranken, Kersti A.
Singh, Gita
Virro, Michael R.

MIDLAND
O'Halloran, Patrick J.

MILTON
Hunter, Glen A.
Karah, Munia M A.
Nadkarni, Dipti A.
Rajasingham, Melodye
Wilkinson, Jane E.

MISSISSAUGA
Attuah, Kwame
Bonde, Veena
Chu, Kelly S.
Corbey, Leigh A.
Cowal, Catherine A.
Daya, Salim H.
De Petrillo, A. Dennis
Doyle, Patricia M.
Duemler, Marianne R.
Ewaschuk, Ernest J.
Goodrow, Gwendolyn J.
Greisman, Bernard
Gurland, Paul R.
Gysler, Mathias
Hakim, Ronnie
Jong, Winston M.
Kanee, Allan S.
Lee, Joseph Y.
Leone-Tomaschoff, Sylvie L.
Liao, Patrick M.
Mark, Siobhan E V.
Myckan, Kerry A.
Nahas, Samar H A.
Newell, Kendra N.
Rogers, Kimberly A M.
Scheufler, Peter W.
Smith, John R.
Stein, Richard A M.
Thurairajah, Rajeswary
Tigert, Scott S.
Wade, Carol L.
Woolford, Lorraine

NEPEAN
Beshara, Nasser R.
Cargill, Yvonne M.
Cochen, Douglas A.
Gagne, Helene M.
Honey, Liisa L.
Huard, Pierre J.
Lamensa, John W E.
Ling, Constance M.
Pascali, Dante U.
Schachter, Joyce
Straszak-Suri, Marina A.
Tawagi, F. Georges
Treehuba, Kathryn E.

NEWMARKET
Atack, D. Barry
Chang, Genevieve
Dervaitis, Kristina L.
Fortier, Anne M.
Joutsi, Pentti A.
Mantay, Erica M E.
Rouselle, David A.
Svystonyuk, Oleksandr I.
Walsh, Anne J.
Watt, Peter D.

NIAGARA FALLS
Cheema, Gurnam S.
Jackiewicz, Allan W.
Olufowobi, Olufemi O.
Yegappan, Muthulakshmi

NORTH BAY
Agboola, Julius A.
Kulkarni, Ramesh
Waja, Lukmaan
Wong, Tsing San
Zeman, George J.

NORTH YORK
Brown, Adrian R H.
Cha, Lily S L.
Chan, Dora
Chu, K C. Dennis
D'Souza, Mirabelle
Dixon, Marjorie
Gans, Maja G.
Grynspan-Sredhi, Shlomo
Hew, Lincoln R.
Ho, Man Fan
Kang, Angela M.
Kosalka, Tadeusz
Kreichman, Daniel
Lackie, Elyse G.
Lee, Clive C M.
Lee, Joseph S K.
Lee, Sabrina K.
Leung, Peter C S.
Mariampillai, Grace I.
Nadel, Mendel R.
Nevin Lam, Alexandra C.
Nicholson, R. Derek
Pairaudeau, Nicholas V J.
Pettle, Alvin
Ray, Dalia
Revah, Ayala
Rosenthal, David M.
Sam, Francis B.
Sarraf, Morad K.
Shilletto, D.W. Nicholas
Shuen, Paul K.
Smith, Kirsten L.
Stirk, Linda J.
Tai, R W. Melissa
The, B L. Linda
Tse, Man Buen
Tunde-Byass, Modupe O J.
Weisberg, Fay G.
Wong, George P L.
Zolis, Lynne R.

OAKVILLE
Andrighetti, Santina
Cockwell, Heather A.

SPECIALISTS BY PROVINCE

Elford, Kimberly
Feroze, Sleem
Liske, Sabine I.
Morrow, Robert J.
Prouse, Kristy A.
Sharma, Sandeep K.
Tam, David W.

ORANGEVILLE
Chatterjee, Sukhamay
Murad, Khulood J.
Umeh, Jude I.

ORILLIA
Abdel-Razek, Khaled H.
Ingles, Julia
Johnston, Richard U.
Olupona, Samuel M.
Rheault, Katherine M.
Will, Stephen B.

ORLEANS
Aubin, Fanny
Begin, Nicolas A.
Faucher, Catherine
Lussier, Robert
Marleau, Alain
Moreau, Daniel
Palerme, Stephanie
Valcourt, Edith E.

OSHAWA
Beatty, Myles F.
Crawford-Bourke, Denise
Hepburn, Douglas S.
Jana, Elizabeth V.
Pancham, Paul I.
Rowe, Charles D.
Sun, Christina H Y.
Tremblay, Pamela M.

OTTAWA
Amankwah, Yaa Obesebea
Attie, Catherine
Aubin, M. Susan L.
Aubry, Joan
Aziz, S. Yasmin
Baker, Kevin R.
Bell, E. Douglas
Berger, Pamela S.
Black, Amanda Y.
Black, Douglas M.
Blanchet, Genevieve
Bonin, Brigitte
Buckley, M. Joyce B R.
Campbell, Craig E.
Caughey, Sharon C.
Claman, Paul
Cohen, Elliott S.
Corbett, Shannon
Dome, Valerie
Dudley, Denis K L.
Dumont, Tania
Dy, Jessica G.
Edwards, Lesley C.
Farrell, Christopher J.
Faught, J. Wylam
Feigel, Roman
Fleming, Nathalie
Fung Kee Fung, Karen M C.
Fung Kee Fung, Michael
Gofton, Emma N.
Goulet, Marie
Gravelle, Catherine
Gruslin, Andree M R.
Haebe, James R.
Haebe, Jeffrey J.
Harrison, Warren E.
Hopkins, M. Laura
Jackson, Aaron L.
Jolly, Elaine E.
Jones, Griffith D.
Kotarba, Delani D.
Lal, Sunita T.
Lapointe-Milot, Korine
Laroche, Andre M.
Le, Tien Dung
Leader, Arthur
Legault, Paul J W.
Leroux, Andre-Marie
Lortie, Karine J.
McCoubrey, David R.
McFaul, Susan M.
Nakajima, Amy K.
Newton, Arnold
Onochie, Lawrence M.
Oppenheimer, Lawrence W.
Posner, Glenn D.
Rousseau, Genevieve D.
Roy-Lacroix, Marie-Eve
Ruparelia, Bhagwanji C.
Senikas, Vyta M.
Senterman, Mary K.
Shabib, Gihad M H.
Shenassa, Hassan
Shepherd, Lynn J.
Shmorgun, Doron
Singh, S. Sony
Sylvain, Jacques P E.
Vassiliou, Demetra
Vause, Tannys D R.
Visser, Karen A L.
Walker, Mark C.
Warraich, Gunwant
Weberpals, Johanne I.
Wolfish, Karen R.
de la Ronde, Sandra K.

OWEN SOUND
Berezowski, Riva E.
Caulley, Emmanuel N N.
Comette, Melissa J.
Ekong, Enobong
El-Hajj, May I.
Moore, Britt
Savasi, Ingrid

PEMBROKE
Mukherjee, Siddhartha
Yacoub, Ashraf K I.

PETERBOROUGH
Bos, Carlo
Harrington, Brian D.
Kramer, Barry N.
Maskens, Peter D.
Pakenham, Susan E.
Sobowale, Oluyomi A.
Zahradnik, Joseph

PICKERING
McConville, Fiona C.
Ruggles, Janice L.

POINT EDWARD
Ferreira, Bernard E.
Ghazarian, Boulos A.

PORT HOPE
Green, Michael

RICHMOND HILL
Amankwah, Kofi S.
Laseinde, Olufunto O.
Ng, Esther
Nicholas, Cynthia S.
Ou, Che-Wei R.

SARNIA
Blunt, Marie E.
Elkelani, Saad M A.
Pressey, David B.
Rutledge, Sharon M.
Saraf, Rajni

SAULT STE MARIE
Amimi, Myriam N.
Awwad, Bahaa E D H.
Fam, Alice P N.
Gupta, Hemi
Hergott, Paul A.
Kelly, Michael J A.
Lingurar, Maxine A.
Willett, Janice A.
Zehr, Patricia A.

SCARBOROUGH
Abdelrazek, Nermean M.
Barnwell, Donna M.
Blankier, Joseph
Cheng, Mary M L.
Chu, Katherine H C.
Cooke, Carolyn J.
Costa, Stacy L.
Cramer, Joseph H.
Damla, Garo
Davis, Victoria J.
Easton, William A.
Ekeh, Norbert I.
Forman, Rachel A.
Freedman, Dayna M.
Fruitman, Sheldon
Harikumar, Usha
Hew, Karen E.
Huh, Caroline C.
Jegatheeswaran, Rajadurai
Jibodh, Rawle M.
Kalaichandran, Sivasamboo
Kirupananthan, Coomarasamy
Ko, Jevan
Ko, Samuel
Kurup, Asha
Logaridis, Terry E.
Ma, Joanne L C.
Mahmoud, Haidar A.
Mo, Anita B.
O'Brien, Sharon R.
Owen, Catherine M.
Padmore, Lloyd G.
Peng, Carol Y M.
Roth, Nathan L.
Rutherford, Colette M.
Samra, David
Silver, Michael
Tam, Larissa E.
Turner, Marci R.
Venkatarangam, Nina E N.
Wilcock, Georgina E M.
Williams, Tanya-Gay M.
Wong, Jeremy C.

SMITHS FALLS
Kerner, Cecilia M.
Wang, Yan

ST CATHARINES
Bedkowski, Wojciech A.
Chan, Anthony K H.
Dobosiewicz, Andrzej
Nowicki, Robert D.
Okon, Marquis M A.
Shetty, Rathnakar B.
Viljoen, Johan

ST THOMAS
O'Brien, Meagan R.
Reddy, Natalie Y M.
Roe, Michael

STRATFORD
Bloch, Christine L.
Hancock, Gregg W.
Hillyer, Cheryl
Nascu, Camelia P.
Neilsen, Philip D.
Szirmay-Kalos, Tibor Z.
Whitmore, Nancy A.

SUDBURY
Dufour, Marc E.
Franklin, R. Bernard
Garisa, Padma L.
Huneault, David R.
Provatopoulos, John
Righi, Roxanna V.
Splinter, Karen L N.
Vijayakanthan, Kandiah
Wallace, Sarah G.

THORNHILL
Benzaquen, Susan
Grossman, Stacey

THUNDER BAY
Baunemann, Heiko
Dudar, Amber
Fairley, Henry S.
Knowles, Louise M B.
Novak, Rudolf
Pokrant, Colleen M.
Potestio, Frank A.
Siren, Andrew J E.

TIMMINS
Munnoch, Katherine M.
Pond, Donald G.
Raveendran, Arulpiragasam

TORONTO
Abrol, Kaajal
Aggarwal, Anjali
Akoury, Hani A G.
Alanjari, Abdulmohsen K A A.
Allen, Lisa M.
Aneja, Ambika
Ang, Miriam
Arthur, Rebecca H.
Auyeung, Anthony
Badmos, Oluleke S.
Bambao, M. Clarissa
Baratz, Ari Y.
Barkin, Marshall P.
Barrett, Jon F R.
Batarseh, Samir J.
Bernardini, Marcus
Bernstein, Abraham
Bernstein, E. Paul
Bocking, Alan D.
Bodley, Janet
Boutet, Marianne
Brill, Yoav
Cadesky, Kenneth I.
Casper, Robert F J.
Chang, Paul T.
Cohen, Howard R.
Covens, Allan L.
Cram, Jennifer A.
Cruickshank, Barbara
Cruickshank, Beth
Curtis, Nickola J.
Czikk, Marie J.
Daly, Lanval J.
Daniel, Ariadne
Dawood, Ashraf M.
Derzko, Christine M.
Di Pierdomenico, Anthony P.
Drutz, Harold P.
Durand, Nancy E.
Eiriksson, Lua
El-Chaar, Darine
Engle, Fredric M.
Evaniuk, Debra A.
Farine, Dan
Farrugia, M. Michele
Ferguson, Sarah E.
Freire-Lizama, Tatiana
Gare, Douglas J.
Gerber, David
Gerulath, Alan H.
Giannoulias, Dimitrios
Gien, Lilian T.
Glass, Karen B.
Graham, Janice S.
Greenblatt, Ellen M.
Gunn, Beth M.
Hannam, Thomas G.
Hawrylyshyn, Peter A.
Herer, Elaine R.
Hewlett, Patrick T.
Ho, Harmony A.
Ho, Helen H Y.
Hui, Dini
Im, Stephen S.
Jones, Claire A.
Khambhla, Arvind D.
Kingdom, John C P.
Kirkham, Yolanda A.
Kives, Sari L.
Kroach, Murray N.
Kroft, Jamie
Kumar, C L. Prasanna
Kung, Rose C.
Kupets, Rachel S.
Ladhani, Noor N N.
Laframboise, Stephane
Laskin, Matthew D.
Lausman, Andrea Y.
Lee, Patricia E.
Lefebvre, Guylaine G.
Leong, Yvonne W.
Levinsky, Elyse S.
Librach, Clifford L.
Librach, Samuel
Lickrish, Gordon M.
Lie, Kay I.
Liu, Grace
Liu, Kimberly E.
Livingstone, Ronald A.
Lo, Katherine A.
Lovatsis, Danny
Lyons, Elliott R.
MacKenzie, Roberta C F.
Malinowski, Ann
Martoglio, Adelmo E.
Maxwell, Cynthia V.
McDermott, Colleen
Meffe, Filomena M.
Mocarski, Eva J M.
Morency, Anne-Maude
Morton, Matthew L.
Murphy, K. Joan
Murphy, Kellie E.
Okun, Nanette B.
Ornstein, Melanie P.
Osborne, Raymond J.
Paek, Wusun
Page, Andrea E.
Park, Esther M.
Pham, Alice Trang
Phillips, Perry
Pittini, Richard J.
Qaadri, Mussarrat K.
Raymond, Elin L.
Reade, Clare J M.
Redmond, Carol A.
Ritchie, J W. Knox
Robertson, Deborah G.
Rosen, Barry P.
Ryan, Greg
Satkunaratnam, Abheha
Seaward, P. Gareth R.
Selk, Amanda
Sermer, Mathew
Shah, Rajiv R.
Shapiro, Heather M.
Shapiro, Jodi L.
Sharma, Kalpana S.
Sharma, Kawal J.
Shier, R. Michael P.
Shime, Jerry
Sierra, Sony
Sims, Richard H.
Sinasac, Sarah
Sohn, Brenda
Soroka, Dana J.
Spitzer, Rachel F.
Steele, Donna M.
Steinberg, Wilfred M.
Sved, Michael H.
Ternamian, Artin M.
Tessler, Karen M.
Thomas, Bruce
Thomas, Jacqueline A.
Tremblay, Catherine
Windrim, Rory C.
Wolfman, Wendy L.
Wong, Herbert M.
Wong, Suzanne T.
Woo, George H K.
Woods, Brenda T.
Yudin, Mark H.
Yung, Yick Shing
Zaltz, Arthur P.

TRENTON
Omaboe, Narh

VAUGHAN
Badi, Entisar M.
Belej-Rak, Timea
Rosman, David E.

WATERLOO
Frank, Sheldon M.
Macdonald, Alison H.
Stewart, Andrew E F.

WELLAND
Beyani-Mulaisho, Nambizi
Chaudhry, Naheed M.
Sternadel, Jerzy

WESTON
Caccia, Nicolette C.

WHITBY
Abdel Hadi, Farid M.
Akingbola, Olurotimi A.
Athaide, Gregory O.
Chirayilkalam, Shereen B.
McIntyre, R. Alan
Rubabaza, Jean-Placide

WINCHESTER
Adetola, Ejibunmi
Deeb, Shamsa
St-Cyr, Dominique

WINDSOR
Bourke, Richard A.
Brkovich, Andrea
Glowacki, Adam R.
Handscomb, Arthur
Hasen, Gregory A.
Jasey, Bradley
Jasey, Gordon M.
Mundle, William R.
Patel, Shobhana J.
Pattinson, Howard A.
Polsky, Joshua N.
Rawlins, Jenna R.
Suga Rak, Michelle S.
Tomc, John E.
Victory, Rahi

WOODBRIDGE
Cash, Rebecca L.
Fried, Eve L M.
Osak, Roberta
Sisca, Lyana I.

WOODSTOCK
Antolinez-Uribe, Edgar
Smith, Christopher J.
Snider, D. David

PRINCE EDWARD ISLAND

CHARLOTTETOWN
Bethune, Peter N.
Cassell, Krista
Connors, Shelagh
Coolen, Anna L.
Ferguson, Shaun
Knickle, David A.
MacDonald, Francis

STRATFORD
Brodie, Beverly L.

SUMMERSIDE
Barbrick-Crozier, Elizabeth
Farag, Hani

QUÉBEC

ALMA
Fortin, Denis
Gagne, Alexandra
Langevin, Anny
Rouleau, Lucie

AMOS
Allen, Diane
Gaudet, Pascale

BAIE-COMEAU
Lebel, Marie-Claude
Millaire, Melanie
Roberge, Suzanne
Thalabot, Marie-Claude

BROSSARD
Ah-Sue, Michael J.

CAP-AUX-MEULES
Lajeunesse, Simon

CHANDLER
Giroux, Cynthia
Poirier, Annick
Soucy, Renee

CHATEAUGUAY
Fernandez, Roberto
Hebert, Josee
Latraverse, Frederique
Loiselle, Francois

CHICOUTIMI
Bouchard, Laurier
Carre, Valerie
Dubois, Suzy
Dumont, Julie
Fisch, Patricia A.
Gagnon, Sylvain
Guimond, Richard
Mareschal, Veronique
Simard, Catherine
Simard, Fabien

COWANSVILLE
Cadrin, Christine
De Saint-Victor, Jean R.
Fadin, Anne
Lemay, Michel

DRUMMONDVILLE
Brassard, Liliane
Doucet, Paul R.
Lincourt, Isabelle
Philibert, Marie-Claude
Raymond, Chantal
St-Onge, Anick

GASPE
Blain, Marie-Yanouk
Bureau, Marc
Guilbeault, Nathalie

GATINEAU
Blais, Francine
Chartrand, Lisa-Marie
Gamache, Nathalie
Garcia, Elio D.
Le Goff, Gilbert
Nadeau, Karine
Poungui Moungondo, Lionel A.
Roumain, Marie H C.
Vollinoti, Carlos A.

GRANBY
Bouchard-Richard, Marie-Claude
Labelle, Genevieve
Larouche, Lucie
Lemonnier, Marie-Chantal
Saad, Antoine

GREENFIELD PARK
Chan, Kenneth L.
Mansour, Nabil

JOLIETTE
Gascon, Chantal
Gervais, Hugues

JONQUIERE
Bolduc, Serge
Larochelle, Andre

KIRKLAND
Shalaby, Karam

LA PRAIRIE
Paquet, Jean-Claude

LASALLE
Arsenault, Marc-Yvon
Dontigny, Lorraine
Douyon, Sylvie
Engel, Francis
Filion, Rosalie
Fortin, Anne
Fortin, Claude A.
Goyet, Martine
Lafortune, Chantal
Lalande, Johanne
Lamb, Fanny
Laporte, Nathalie

LAVAL
Arbour-Levert, Melanie
Bertrand, Genevieve
Carette, Marie-Eve
Charles, Yolande
Choquette, Pierre
Desjardins, Caroline
Dubois, Chantal
Dupont-Chalaoui, Katrie
Durocher, France
Lacerte, Maxime
Lamontagne, Annie
Lanctot, Jean-Francois
Peloquin, Anne
Piche, Yves
Theriault, Dominique
Tremblay, Dominique

LEMOYNE
Lebrun, Manon

LEVIS
Berube, Laurie
Chamberland, Henri
Farley, Julie
Fortin, Suzette
Gennaoui, Jean-Pierre
Morency, Jacques
Renald, Marie-Helene
Tellier, Lyne
Verret, Nadine

LONGUEUIL
Beauregard, Melanie
Cerat, Yves
Couturier, Bernard L.
Desautels, Pascale
Fortier, Andre J.
Jodoin, Marcel R.
Ladouceur, Diane
Larochelle, Annick
Paradis, Desmond
Paradis, Eric
Tanguay, Marie-Claude
Venne, Sophie

MERCIER
Cabana, Diane T.

MONT-LAURIER
Bastien, Pierre

MONT-ROYAL
Beaudoin, Francois
Bielinski, Stanislaw
Bourque, Jacques
Dubuc, Elise
Duperron, Louise
Francoeur, Diane
Gascon, Suzy
Kattygnarath, Tiao
St-Michel, Pierre

MONTREAL
Abenhaim, Haim A.
Antaki, Roland
Asselin, Guylaine
Audet-Lapointe, Pierre
Beauchamp, Coralie
Beaumont, Louis
Bedard, Marie-Josee
Behamdouni, Mounir E.
Belisle, Serge
Benjamin, Alice
Benoit, Joanne
Bernard, Martine
Bissonnette, Francois
Bodmer, A. Barbara
Boucher, Marc
Brochu, Ian
Buzaglo, Karen
Cassar, Nagib L.
Chemaly, Rene
Climan, Allan B.
Cohen, Deborah R.
Colantoni, Guido
Cormier, Beatrice
Dahan, Michael H.
De Koos, Edmond B.
Desaulniers, Gilles
Desilets, Valerie
Desjardins, Celine
Desjardins, Jocelyne
Di Zazzo, Anne
Drouin, Pierre
Dube, Johanne
Dupuis, Marie-Josee
Dzineku, Frederick
El Fakir, Abdelghani
El-Messidi, Amira
Farag, Reda A.
Faruqi, Faez
Faucher, Guy L.
Feochari, Konstantin
Fortin, Suzanne
Fournier, Paul J R.
Fraser, William D.
Frydman, Rita B.
Fugere, Pierre
Gagnon, Robert
Gagnon, Sonia I.
Gauthier, Philippe
Gauthier, Robert J.
Geumei, Ahmed
Gilbert, Lucy
Gillett, Peter G.
Girard, Isabelle
Girard, Yvan M.
Goldsmith, William J.
Goorah, Berenice
Gotlieb, Walter H.
Granger, Louis R.
Grigoriu, Ariadna
Guimond, Julie
Haber, George D.
Hall, Melinda H.
Hallak, Jean J.
Hamilton, Emily F.
Hemmings, Robert
Himaya, Eric
Hudon, Lynda
Hum, Hing-Sang
Iglesias, Marie-Helene
Jamal, Wael H.
Jammal, Wael H.
Jasmin, Yvon
Jean, Catherine
Johansson, Dawn A.
Johnson, Carolyne
Johnson, Louise M.
Kamga-Ngande, Carole N.
Khalife, Samir
Khoday, Shanta S.
Kiely, Daniel J.
Klam, Stephanie
Koby, Robert D.
Korcaz, Yves A.
Lachapelle, Marie-France
Lambert, Bernard
Landry, Daniel
Lapensee, Louise
Lau, Susie K S.
Lavoie-St-Gelais, Genevieve
Leduc, Line
Lemieux, Marie-Claude
Leroux, Nathalie
Lord, Julien
Luskey, Gary W.
MacFarlane, Sonia T.
Mahutte, Neal G.
Mallouh, George E.
Mallozzi, Angelina
Mansour, Fady W.
Marcon, Loretta
Marcoux, Violaine
Martin, Markus C.
Masse, Andre
Mayrand, Marie-Helene
Menard, Sylvain
Merovitz, Lisa
Michaud, Raymonde
Michon, Bertrand
Miner, Louise
Mok, Andrew K C.
Monnier, Patricia
Monton, Luis R.
Morin, Lucie
Moutquin, Jean-Marie
Nguyen, Ngoc Thuy
Noel, Ann
Ouellet, Stephane
Ouhilal, Sophia A.
Pilorge, Robert P.
Ponette, Vincent B.
Press, Joshua Z.
Provencher, Diane M.
Quiros-Calinoiu, Elsa S.
Racicot, Marie-Helene
Reichetzer, Barbara
Reinblatt, Shauna L.
Rivard, Chantal
Rizos, Nick
Robillard, Andre
Roy, Genevieve
Sabbah, Robert
Sabin, I. Morris
Sansregret, Andree
Saumet Chilito, Julio
Seropian, Lilliane
Shams, Sherif A A.
Shatz, Richard M.
Shear, Roberta M.
Shinder, Janet
Shine, Joseph F.
Sidani, Paul M.
Sim, Wee-Lim
Simard-Emond, Laurence
Stanimir, Gerald W.
Sylvestre, Camille V.
Taillefer, Catherine
Tan, Seang Lin
Tchervenkov, Sophia B.
Truchon, Josee
Tucker, Elrie C.
Tulandi, Togas
Wagner, Marie-Soleil
Walter, Jens-Erik
Wo, Bi Lan
Wolde-Giorghis, Rahel
Zeng, Xing
Ziegler, Cleve

OUTREMONT
Rousseau, Serge

PIERREFONDS
Vilain, Luc S.

PINTENDRE
Lemieux, Rejean

POINTE-CLAIRE
Bakare, Stephanee O.
Biem, Sandra R D.
Bray, John C.
Krackovitch, Stephanie
Mercier, Gilles G.
Saxon, Daniel J A.
Simon, Jeannine G M.
Vasilie, Yvonne B.

QUEBEC
Bastide, Adrien
Bazin, Sylvie
Belhumeur, Francois
Bellemare, Guy
Bergeron, Jacques
Bergeron, Marie-Eve
Blackburn, Line
Blanchet, Jean J.
Blanchet, Pierre
Bouchard, Celine
Brassard, Normand
Brien, Marie-Chantal
Bujold, Emmanuel
Camire, Bruno
Carrier, Simon
Cyr, Elphege
Daris, Marleen
Fontaine, Jean-Yves
Fortier, Michel
Gagnon, Genevieve
Gauthier, Cajetan M.
Gekas, Jean
Girard, Karine
Gouin, Katy
Gregoire, Jean
Guillemette, Julie
Huot, Celine
Hurtubise, Johann
Jean, Christian
Laberge, Philippe-Yves
Leboeuf, Mathieu
Legare, Denis
Lemyre, Madeleine
Levesque, Isabelle
Mailloux, Jacques
Morin, Valerie
Noel, Suzanne
Paris, Gaetan
Pinault, Jean-Jacques
Renaud, Marie-Claude
Rheaume, Caroline I.
Rousseau, Julie-Anne

Roy, Marie-Christine
Roy, Michel
Sebastianelli, Alexandra
Thomas, Nancy
Verreault, Jean-Pierre
Villeneuve, Marc

REPENTIGNY
Gagnon, Martine
Girard, Guy
Langlois, Daniel
Topakian, Arman

RIMOUSKI
Beaudet, Christine
Bouchard, Roger
Chenard, Elaine
Faucher, Elise
Levesque, Stephanie
Poirier, Isabelle
Premont, Pierre

RIVIERE-DU-LOUP
Blair, Tony
Lambert, Marie-France
Nadeau, Yves
Plourde, Diane

ROUYN-NORANDA
Beaumont, Marie-Claude
Bouthiette, Pierre
Charlebois, Manon
East, Nathalie
Guimond, Joanne

ROXBORO
Hassan, Durreshahwar

SAINT-CONSTANT
Petit, Francine

SAINT-EUSTACHE
Bertrand, Marie
Dostie, Sarah
Gendron, Claudie
Mercky, Jocelyn
Piche, Jacqueline

SAINT-GEORGES
Bedard, Natacha
Belair, Jacques D.
Berube, Andree-Anne
Caron, Michelle
Pomerleau, Claude V.

SAINT-HUBERT
Rabbani, Shahida N.

SAINT-HYACINTHE
Arpin, Marie-Helene
Aube, Marie-Helene
Mathieu, Jean-Luc
Poirier, Caroline

SAINT-JEROME
Allard, Marie-Eve
Bourque, Manon
Dubois, Emmanuelle
Girard, Anne-Marie
Hamel, Annick
Laroche, Caroline
Rivet, Caroline
Vezina, Louise
Vezina, Yannik

SAINT-LAURENT
Koufogianis, Vayia
Maraghi, Kamal E.
Welt, Michel

SAINT-LEONARD
Gemayel, Kange P.
Girgis, Emile F.
Ketchian, Leon V.

SAINT-ROMUALD
Dansereau, Benoit

SALABERRY DE VALLEYFIELD
Bedrossian, Roupen
Lalonde, Carole
Paquin, Michel

SEPT-ILES
Bosse, Isabelle
Martel, Michelle
Simard, Martine

SHAWINIGAN
Ayotte, Normand J.
Roy-Matton, Naome

SHAWINIGAN-SUD
Cantin, Jerome
Gervais, Carolyne

SHERBROOKE
AinMelk, Youssef
Bertholet-Anku, Catherine L.
Bessette, Paul
Blouin, Daniel J.
Bureau, Yves-Andre
Caron, Marcel
Carranza Mamane, Belina
Constantineau, Louise
Cote, Michel J.
Desindes, Sophie
Girard, Isabelle
Lajoie, Francois
Ouellet, Annie
Pinsonneault, Odette
Raiche, Evelyne
Thibodeau, Daniel
Waddell, Guy

SOREL-TRACY
Claveau, Jacques

ST CHARLES BORROMEE
Brosseau-Roberge, Anais
Grenier, Julie
Hetu, Valerie
Seguin, Marc
St-Jacques, Frederic

ST-EUSTACHE
Boily, Karine
Ouellet, Nathalie

ST JEAN SUR RICHELIEU
Albert, Emilie
Aubin, Dominique
Bernier, Danielle A.
Cyr, Nathalie
Landry, Gerard
Larente, Amelie
Perreault, Gilles

STE AGATHE DES MONTS
Chouinard, Marie-Josee
Dery, Jean-Paul
Lague, Nadine

STE ANNE DES MONTS
Levesque, Francine

TERREBONNE
Beaudry, Genevieve
Beauregard, Pascale
Lemay, Nadia
Lepine, Sylviane
Major, Brigitte
Michaluk, Audrey
Miron, Pierre

THETFORD MINES
Dorval, Gaston
Gagnon, Serge R.

TROIS-RIVIERES
Babineau, Veronique
Belanger, Estelle
Bellemare, Marc
Boucher, Julie
Bouvet, Sylvie
Bussiere, Veronique
Dion, Jean-Paul
Malenfant, Sylvain
Malmedy, Natacha
Patry, Michel
Theriault, Nancy

VAL-DAVID
Aubin, Yvan

VAL-D'OR
Parent, Josee
Rojas Orozco, Ledy
Turbide, Manon

VERDUN
Gagne, Guy-Paul
Lefebvre, Josee
Samaan, Magdy K.

VICTORIAVILLE
Aubry, Martine
Charest, Nicole
Leclercq, Corinne
Long, Jack A.
St-Pierre, Luc

WESTMOUNT
Boyd, Mark E.
Guralnick, Melvin S.

SASKATCHEWAN

NORTH BATTLEFORD
Prollius, Almereau

PRINCE ALBERT
Clark, C. Eric
Mircea, Carmen
Moodliar, Santhosian
Sivertson, Joanne D.
Tennent, Alison C.
Udayasankar, Vijayalakshmi

REGINA
Abed, Mohammed M.
Akinbiyi, Amos A.
Bastian, James S.
Bhargava, Rashmi
Briggs, Martha M.
Brydon, Lizabeth A.
Cardoso, Reynaldo
Carson, George D.
Hilton, Jennifer
Jabs, Corrine F I.
Kamencic, Huse
Lett, Christine D.
Onasanya, Olanrewaju
Poole, Angela M.
Rattray, Darrien D.
Shepherd, Debra-Jo
Stryker, Trina D.
Thiel, John A.

SASKATOON
Agrawal, Anita
Case, Allison M.
Chizen, Donna R.
Davidson, Marilyn J.
Epp, Annette M.
Ezzat, Ahmed M.
Gamelin, Adrian
Giede, K. Christopher
Gilliland, G. Barry
Harding, Anita
Mainprize, Thomas C.
Martel, Marie-Jocelyne
Mirosh, Melissa D.
Mytopher, Kristine D.
Olatunbosun, Olufemi A.
Payton, Natasha A.
Podilsky, Natalia M.
Ravichander, Ann Meera
Regush, Lexy C.
Schubert, Matthew
Sheridan, Mark A.
Simpson, Charles W.
Smith, Thirza E.
Stewart, Sabrina
Tyson, Nerissa A.
Yeboah, Emmanuel K.

SWIFT CURRENT
Malleck, Naseem

YORKTON
Spies, Cornelius A.

YUKON TERRITORY

WHITEHORSE
Bendall, Michael G.
MacNicol, Wayne M.

Occupational Medicine

ALBERTA

CALGARY
Corbet, Kenneth J.
Cowell, John W F.
Razavi, Jalees M S.

EDMONTON
Abbasi Dezfouly, Nader
Beach, Jeremy R.
Hoffman, Harold E.
Karpluk, Philip F.
Lappi, Vernon G.
Lauzon, Matthew A.
Liu-Shum, Alice T.
Rani, Ritu
Sperka, Paul J.

FORT MCMURRAY
Lawley, Thomas M.

SHERWOOD PARK
Cheng, Jim I.

BRITISH COLUMBIA

VANCOUVER
Carlsten, Christopher R.
Kaboli, Fariba
Yamanaka, Michael W.
Yassi, Annalee

VICTORIA
Addo, Sylvia M.
Youakim, Sami

MANITOBA

WINNIPEG
Kraut, Allen G.

ONTARIO

BELLEVILLE
Wills, Michael C.

BRAMPTON
Markus, Yaacov M.

BURLINGTON
Cheung, Lily S K.

ETOBICOKE
Isles, Katherine K.
Sax, Solly E.

HAMILTON
Haines, A. Theodore S.

LONDON
Siu, Sidney K.

NORTH YORK
Liss, Gary M.
Marchant, Rosemary E.
Roy, Marie L.

OSHAWA
Dykeman, Ronald

OTTAWA
Arnold, Ian M F.
Tsekrekos, Stephen N.

TORONTO
Cole, Donald C.
Genesove, Leon J.
Holness, D. Linn
House, Ronald A.
McGoveran, Bruce M.
Qureshi, Roohi Y.
Saary, M. Joan
Schweigert, Michael K.
Smith, Carol A.
Thompson, Aaron M S.
Wong, Lillian

VAUGHAN
Sandhu, Charanjit S.

QUÉBEC

LAVAL
Levesque, Christian
Osterman, John W.

MONTREAL
Baillargeon, Martine
Isler, Monique
Jacques, Louis
Patry, Louis
Rossignol, Michel
Stock, Susan R.

QUEBEC
Auger, Pierre L.
Lambert, Nicole

SAINTE-MARIE
Turcot, Alice

TROIS-RIVIERES
Poulin, Maurice

SASKATCHEWAN

SASKATOON
Koehncke, Niels K.

Ophthalmology

ALBERTA

CALGARY
Adatia, Feisal A.
Al-Ghoul, Ahmed R.
Anand, Jagdish R.
Anderson Penno, Ellen E.
Ashenhurst, Michael E.
Astle, William F.
Ball, Arlene E.
Bhamra, Jamie
Chow, Bill P C.
Cooper, Linda L.
Crichton, Andrew
Culver, Ronald L.
Demong, Thaddeus
Douglas, Gordon R.
Dyer, Alan M.
Ells, Anna L.
Fielden, Michael P.
Ford, Bryce A.
Gibson, Peter F.
Gimbel, Howard V.
Goel, Nand K.
Gohill, Jitendra
Gordon, Robert
Hammamji, Karim
Hill, Vivian E.

Huang, John T.
Huang, Peter T S.
Kassab, Jacinthe
Kherani, Amin
Kirk, Angus H.
Krebes, Andrew J.
Lakra, Arun
Lang, Robert M.
Leger, Richard
McWhae, John A.
Mitchell, Patrick C.
Mitchell, Robert J.
Punja, Karim G H.
Romanchuk, Kenneth G.
Savage, Paul R G.
Shah, Chirag R.
Skov, Carolyn M B.
Smith, Stanley S.
Van Westenbrugge, John A.
Verstraten, Karin L.
Warrian, Kevin J.
Williams, R. Geoffrey
Wong, Jonathan Y.
Wyse, J. Patrick H.
Yau, Ryan J H.

EDMONTON
Baker, Chad F.
Buski, Z. John
Carle, Michelle V.
Chan, Stanley M.
Climenhaga, David B.
Climenhaga, Harold W.
Cote, David S.
Damji, Karim F.
Denton, Paul D.
Dorey, Michael W.
Dotchin, Stephanie A.
Drummond, Garry T.
Edwards, Marianne C.
Filaferro, Danny L.
Foy, James J.
Greve, Mark D J.
Hennig, Kevin R.
Heston, Jonathan P A.
Hinz, Bradley J.
Hodges, Ernest J.
Johnson, Michael C.
Johnson, Royce L C.
Kassiri, Kamrouz
Kaye, Geoffrey B.
King, Joseph W.
Kutzner, Morley R.
Leong-Sit, Fook Lin
Leong-Sit, Joseph P T.
Lewis, James R.
MacDonald, Ian M.
Macdonald, E. Anne
Mah, Dean
McCabe, James B.
Morgan, Roderick A.
Pearce, William G.
Rawlings, Nigel G.
Rudnisky, Christopher J.
Rudnisky, Eugene J.
Shutt, Harold K R.
Somani, Rizwan
Tennant, Matthew T S.
Ting, Andrew Y C.
Uniat, Linda M.
Weis, Ezekiel

FORT MCMURRAY
Sutton, Hugh F S.

GRANDE PRAIRIE
Roberts, Steve A I.

LETHBRIDGE
Heyns, Daniel B.
Kwan, Eddie
Leishman, Robert G.
Novak, John J.

MEDICINE HAT
Carlsson, Anthony M.
Chaudhary, Ripan
Rinaldi, Brent D.

RED DEER
Bozdech, Miloslav B.
Lythgoe, Elizabeth S.
Okada, William T.
Skochylas, Edwin P.

ST. ALBERT
Chornell, J. Gary

BRITISH COLUMBIA

ABBOTSFORD
Blaylock, John F.
Chu, Gabriel K.
Nisbett, Samuel
Tadrous, Zakaria L T.
Walker, Randy A.

BURNABY
Aroichane, Maryam
Boyd, Michael J.
Butler, Michael T W.
Dhaliwal, Harjinder S.
Finlay, Kelvin R.
Hwang, Norman H.
Kherani, Femida
Matheson, Donald C.
Pratt, Arthur W.
Saunders, Patrick P R.
Yu, Y W. Edward

CAMPBELL RIVER
Moosbrugger, Karen A.

CHILLIWACK
De Bruin, Walter
Heinrichs, David A.

COMOX
Cornock, Elizabeth
Hoar, Glen G.

COQUITLAM
Parkinson, Kevin M.

COURTENAY
Claasen, J. Pieter
Shaver, Steven W.

CRANBROOK
Ho Yuen, Vernon

DELTA
Bayne, John M.
Giligson, Ari

DUNCAN
Hoar, Karen
MacGregor, Donald G.
MacLeod, John N.
Polack, Stanley S G.
Ramstead, Cory L.
Wakelin, David L.

KAMLOOPS
Brown, Dennis B.
Hopp, Peter M.
Jelfimow, Peter V.

KELOWNA
Baldassare, Ronald D.
Chambers, Jeffrey D.
Hoonjan, Malvinder S.
Ramsey, Kevin M.
Ruthnum, Manorgaren
Theriault, J. Francois A.
Yap, Keith D.

LANGLEY
Anderson, Carolyn K.
Clarke, Margo S.
Gottner, Michael J.
Ma, Steven S.
McFadden, D. Murray
Zakrzewski, Peter A.

MAPLE RIDGE
Bright, Michael A.

NANAIMO
Bowen, Richard A.
Hay, Elizabeth J.
Johnston, William H.
Jones, Carl V.
O'Donnell, Michael
Piemontesi, Roberto L G.
Spencer, Martin H.
Yearsley, George C.

NELSON
Maytom, Peter A N.

NEW WESTMINSTER
Cottle, Robin W.
D'Souza, Annette M.
Dhanda, Dharminder S.
Lam, Simon R.
Miller, James R.
Neima, David R S.
Nelson, David E.
Parsons, Hugh M.
Townsend, Anthony L.
Wallace, Susan M A.
Wittenberg, Leah A.

NORTH VANCOUVER
Chen, Lydia M.
Diep, Tung M.
Forooghian, Farzin
Godinho, Derek V.
Goldberg, Aron
Maerov, Perry H.
Mohaseb, Kamyar
Tischler, Aron M.

PENTICTON
Peters, Carl W.
Post, Joel
Semeniuk, Robert M.

PORT COQUITLAM
Hay, Gregory J.

PRINCE GEORGE
Konkal, P. John
Lukaris, Andrew D.
Roesch, Marian T.
Veselinovic, Aleksandra

RICHMOND
Cherry, Jason
Lee, Shui Hing
Thomas, Roger H.

SALMON ARM
Seth, Aditya
Tjaden, Janice M.

SECHELT
Woodburn, Bruce D.

SIDNEY
Green, Larry T.
Quinlan, Michael F.

SURREY
Cline, Roy A.
Kennedy, Ross A.
Napier, Lee B.
Paul, Tania
Tong, Melissa G Y.
Tsuyuki, Kurt T.
Zack, Barend N.

TERRACE
Nagy, Thomas

TRAIL
Morency, Rene-Louis

VANCOUVER
Akkor, Sueda
Albiani, David A.
Anderson, Duncan P.
Blicker, Jeffrey A.
Broome, Samuel J.
Buffam, Frank V.
Butler, David M.
Carruthers, Jean D A.
Chen, Sylvia H.
Chew, Jesse
Chui, Lica
Chuo, Jean Y.
Demco, Thomas
Dobrogowski, Michael J J.
Dolman, Peter J.
Dubord, Paul
Faber, Pierre
Gardiner, Jane A.
Gill, Harpreet
Gregory-Evans, Kevin
Hass, Ian
Holland, Simon P.
Kirker, Andrew W.
Kirzner, Steven L.
Law, Francis C H.
Lee, Peter
Lin, David T.
Lindley, Janette I.
Lyons, Christopher J.
Ma, Patrick E.
Maberley, Alan L.
Maberley, David A L.
MacIntosh, Jocelyn M.
Mallek, Noa K.
McCarthy, J. Martin
Merkur, Andrew B.
Mikelberg, Frederick S.
Moloney, Gregory T.
Orton, Tanya D.
Paton, Katherine E.
Pollock, Christopher S.
Rees, Megan G.
Richards, John S F.
Rollins, David F.
Rootman, Jack
Ross, William H.
Rossman, David W.
Sanmugasunderam, Suren
Schertzer, Robert M.
Scott, Krista S.
Sexton, K. Briar
Smith, Stuart W.
Sullivan, Kathleen M C.
Wade, N. Kevin
Walker, Diane
Warner, Simon J.
Wong, Vincent A.
Yeung, Sonia N.

VERNON
Fellenz, Mathias O.
Hollands, Hussein
Ingram, Wessel J.

VICTORIA
Baker, Stephen M.
Behn, Darren
Bell, Raymond A.
Brierley, Lawrence A.
Burnett, Andrew J.
Dam, Olivia
Dragicevich, John T.
Erasmus, Murray J.
Jackson, Mary L.
Jones, Michele L.
Khan, Hamza N.
Kilshaw, Margaret W.
Lowden, Bruce A.
Matvenko, Jack
Nelson, Colvin
Orr, W. Malcolm
Pegado, Victor D.
Shortt, Stanley G.
Taylor, James D N.
Young, David W.

WEST VANCOUVER
Chubb, P. David
Isbister, Carolyn M.
MacKenzie, Paul J.

WHITE ROCK
Berman, Michael
Tam, Mae Yit M.

MANITOBA

BRANDON
Rocha, Guillermo

WINNIPEG
Beldavs, Robert A.
Bellan, Lorne D.
Bracken, John
Brodovsky, Stephen C.
Chin, Daniel D Y.
Clark, Ian H.
Dookeran, Ravi I.
Ekins, Marilyn B C.
Gdih, Gdih Abulgasem M.
Gillespie, Brian G.
Gooi, Teong Lam
Gould, Lisa F.
Gupta, Daya K.
Kadambi, Desikan R.
Kellen, Rodney I.
Kogan, Sylvia
Lee-Wing, Matthew
Leicht, Richard T.
Macrodimitris, Angelo G.
Manusow, David N.
Mathen, K. Mathen
Mis, Andrew A.
Nigam, Rashmi
Rahman, Jennifer W.
Rehsia, Davinder
Sanders, Robert W.
Shuckett, E. Paul
Wiens, James J.

NEW BRUNSWICK

BATHURST
Javidi, Robert R.
Roy, Melanie

CAMPBELLTON
Cortin, Paul M.

DIEPPE
Cormier, Daniel
Cormier, Gilles J.
Sekhavat, Houfar

EDMUNDSTON
Guinard, Francois

FREDERICTON
Harrison, R. Joseph
Noftall, Lachelle V.
Roberts, Kenneth F.
Seymour, Robert G.

MIRAMICHI
Sharma, Vijay K.

MONCTON
Aucoin Savoie, Isabelle
Eid, Clovis
Leblanc, Guy D.
Taylor, Vicki L.

ROTHESAY
Steeves, Jeffrey H.

SAINT JOHN
Farrell, Donald H.
Goodfellow, A. Frank
Polya, Daniel G.
Smrz, Iva
Symonds, J. Christopher

WATERVILLE CARLETON
Goodine, C. William

NEWFOUNDLAND AND LABRADOR

CORNER BROOK
French, Justin
Wijayanayagam, Yoganathan

GANDER
Collins, Edmund W.

ST. JOHN'S
Bautista, Dorothy V.
Bense, Michael H J.
Bramwell, Lori A.
Conway, Valentine H.
Dunphy, Derek J.
Jackman, Christopher S.
LaPierre, Paul D.

McEachren, Todd M.
McNicholas, P. John
Murphy, Bradley D.
O'Leary, Sean W.
Whelan, James H A.
Williams, Kenneth B.

STEPHENVILLE
Abdeen, Aboosaly Z.

NORTHWEST TERRITORIES

YELLOWKNIFE
Smith, Leonard F G.

NOVA SCOTIA

ANTIGONISH
Hamilton, John R.
Mohandas, Rajender N.
Silver, M. Margaret

BRIDGEWATER
De Saint Sardos, Alexandre
Falvey, Denis M.
Himmelman, Donald W.
Mann, Colin G.

BROOKFIELD
Carpenter, Frederick J.
Rogers, Jamie B.

CHESTER
Sapp, George A.

DARTMOUTH
Humayun, Muhammad

HALIFAX
Alotaibi, Noor H A.
Andrews, David M H.
Archibald, Curtis W.
Belliveau, Daniel J.
Cruess, Alan F.
Dahrab, Mishari M.
Dayal-Gosine, Lystra
Dickinson, John D.
George, Stanley P.
Hoskin-Mott, Ann E D.
Kozousek, Vladimir
Lakosha, Hesham M M A.
Laroche, G. Robert
MacNeill, James R.
Maleki, Babak
Mishra, Aditya V.
Nicolela, Marcelo T.
O'Brien, Daniel M.
Orr, Andrew C.
Rafuse, Paul E.
Ramsey, Michael S.
Read, Robert M.
Ritenour, Rusty J.
Robitaille, Johane M.
Samad, Arif
Seamone, Christopher D.
Shuba, Lesya M.
Tan, Alexander Y.

NEW GLASGOW
Archibald, J. David
Hammel, Kenneth H.

NEW MINAS
Schaffner, John P.
Scott, Robert C.
Taiani, Edward J.

SYDNEY
Al Karmi, Rani N I.
Mayer, Kristine L.
Sivakumar, Saraswati
Snow, William M F.

YARMOUTH
Cheevers, Paul M.
Shetty, Banakesari N.

ONTARIO

BARRIE
Emon, Steven J.
Letwin, Kenneth M.
Macrae, William G.
Nixon, Donald R.

BELLEVILLE
Davies, Andrew
Sakamoto, Terence K.

BRAMPTON
Alizadeh-Ebadi, Mahmoud
Braithwaite, Desmond L.
Chen, Roy Y.
Dickson, David H.
Hammoudi, Dena
Khan, Yasser A.
Klein, Thomas B.
Radford, Charles
Somani, Sohel
Tam, Eric S L.
Yuen, Darana W.

BRANTFORD
Skrypuch, Orest W I.
Thomsen, J. Eric
Zanetti, Fabio G.

BROCKVILLE
Lindsay, Ardis B.
Stevens, Samuel D.

BURLINGTON
McGillivray, Daniel L.
Singer, Robert H.

CAMBRIDGE
Anderson, David M.
Desai, Nimesh
Wilkinson, John W.

CHATHAM
Anjema, Christopher
Fraser, Grant R I.
McMahon, Robert G.

CORNWALL
Guindon, Benoit
Suess, Christine J.

DUNDAS
Mann, Keith D.

EAST YORK
Morrow, Gary L.
Morton, Philip L.
Rutherford, Susan M.

ETOBICOKE
Abel, Selwyn L.
Breslin, Calvin W.
Derzko-Dzulynsky, Larissa A.
Flora, Pietro G.
Kaplan, Henry D.
Kravetz, Arnold I.
Kraw, Nicholas M.
Mandell, Mark A.
McDonald, Donald J.
Mednick, Edward B.
Smythe, Donna E.
Spencer, John A.

FORT ERIE
Teal, Patricia K.

GLOUCESTER
Chevrier, Robert L A.
Harding, Peter W.
Morgan, Robert B.
Murphy, M. Madeleine H.

GRAVENHURST
Cripps, John R.
Nia, Keon M.

GUELPH
Johnson, Robert E.
Neufeld, Mark V.
Rodriguez, Sylvia L.
Thompson, Marian P.

HAMILTON
Ahuja, Nina
Arora, Vineet I.
Beattie, Anne M.
Chaudhary, Varun
Harvey, John T.
Hasanee, Khalid
Kobetz, Lawrence E.
Liszauer, Allan D.
Martin, James A.
Mihic, Annette M C.
Nash, Wesley A.
O'Brien, Dermot B.
Rifkind, Aaron W.
Sharda, Rajeshvar K.
Sogbesan, Enitan A.
Vayalumkal, Antony J.

HAWKESBURY
Mihalovits, Helena

KINGSTON
Arthur, Brian W.
Baxter, Stephanie A.
Bona, Mark D.
Camoriano Nolasco, Gerardo
Campbell, Robert
Cheung, John P.
Farmer, James
Gale, Jeffrey S.
Jinapriya, Delan
Kratky, Vladimir
Schweitzer, Kelly D.
Sharma, Sanjay
Smallman, Donald S.
Strube, Y N. Johanna
Ten Hove, Martin W.
Urton, Todd E.

KIRKLAND LAKE
Sales, Karl H.

KITCHENER
Chan, Toby Y B.
Jellie, Hugh G.
Kiskis, Anthony A.
McCuaig, Bradley M.
Pocrnich, Dante M.
Weinstein, Richard D.
Yepes Restrepo, Natasha
Zafar, Aftab

LINDSAY
Cooper, T. James
Lane, David P P.

LONDON
Allen, Larry H.
Bains, Rick A B S.
Gonder, John R.
Hodge, William G.
Hooper, Philip L.
Hutnik, Cindy M.
Mailer, Colin M.
Mather, Rookaya
McIlraith, Ian P.
Merchea, M. Mohan
Motolko, Michael A.
Nichols, Bruce
Nicolle, David A.
Orton, Robert B.
Proulx, Alain A.
Sheidow, Thomas G.
Siebert, Lee F.
Tingey, David P.
Tokarewicz, Alexander C.

MARKHAM
Hussein, Naushad
MacDonald, Alan L.
Martow, Jeffrey
Weinstock, V. Moss

MIDLAND
Scanlan, Daniel T.

MISSISSAUGA
Ahmed, Iqbal K.
Ali, Fareed A.
Allin, Warren D.
Armogan, Narendra
Budning, Andrew S.
Daily, Robert F.
Davidson, Joseph K.
De Angelis, Dan
Fakhry, Yousef M S.
Gooi, Patrick C H.
Kelly, Robert G M.
Kent, Jerrod S.
Kent, Shefalee
Kosaric, Alan
Markowitz, Samuel N.
Mathew, Benjamin
Miller, Michael
Mills, Michael D.
Roy, Mili
Seetner, A. Ashley
Smith, Dean A.
Varma, Devesh K.
Vettese, Antonio

NEPEAN
Bastianelli, Francesco E.
Britton, J. Robert
Engel, Bruce E.
MacInnis, Brent J.
Marshall, David H.
Munro, Shane M.
Myles, W. Michael
Zabel, Ralph W.

NEWMARKET
Landecker, Leslie S.
Liu, Eugene S.
Walker, Robin M C.

NIAGARA FALLS
Merritt, Richard D.
Sheikh, Amber Z.
Smith, Nancy I.
Taylor, Andrew W.

NORTH BAY
Bullen Kesty, Cynthia L.
Kesty, Kenneth R.
Spencer, Jon R L.

NORTH YORK
Arshinoff, Steve
Brent, Henry P.
Cao, Y. Kathy
Dorfman, Jason K.
Elder, John R.
Eplett, Catherine J.
Erlich, Christine M.
Goldlist, Gerald I.
Grader, Joseph
Gray, Dale E H.
Hinton, Patricia V.
Kamel, Ibrahim D.
Kranemann, Christoph F.
Lu, Ying
Lutchman, Carla N R.
Ma, Joseph J K.
McGowan, Hugh D.
Pashby, Robert C.
Rabinovitch, Theodore
Rathee, Rajinder S.
Samis, William D.
Shin, John H.
Sigesmund, Dayle A.
Silvera, Dwight A.
Simpson, E. Rand
Squires, W. Gordon D.
Tanzer, Herbert
Velos, Pamela
Waisberg, Jon W.
Weisbrod, Lawrence
Yoganathan, Pradeepa

OAKVILLE
Amy, Robert J P M.
Bindlish, Rajiv
Eino, Dalia M.
Hakim, Omar
Kates, W. Bradley

ORANGEVILLE
Seto, Raymond J.

ORILLIA
Hillson, Tim R.

OSHAWA
Baziuk, Natalie
Korzinstone, Clifford A.
Misra, Manjula
Nijhawan, Navdeep
Ro, Athanasius S K.
Yassein, Hossam

OTTAWA
Agapitos, Peter J.
Al Kandari, Salem
Al-Breiki, Danah H M S.
Baig, Kashif M.
Bhargava, Anuj
Bonn, Gary E.
Britton Jr, William A A.
Brownstein, Seymour
Buhrmann, Ralf R.
Cameron, James A.
Delpero, Walter
Desroches, Gilles
Edmison, David R.
Entwistle, Catherine M A.
Fournier, Annick V.
Gilberg, Steven M.
Gottlieb, Chloe
Hurley, Bernard R.
Jackson, W. Bruce
Jordan, David R.
Konzuk, Peter J.
Lapointe, Marie-Louise
Lee, Thomas K M.
Leonard, Brian C.
McCunn, P. Donald
McDonald, Hector
Miller, Garfield L A.
Mintsioulis, George
Patel, Vivek R.
Pirbhai, Adnan K.
Poleski, Steven A.
Sabourin, Marcel J L.
Smith, Kevin D.
Tuli, Raman
Weston, Bonnie C.
Zackon, David H.
Ziai, Setareh

OWEN SOUND
Lewis, David C.
Mainville, Norman P.
Orr, Richard J.
Sherif, Hesham

PEMBROKE
Canniff, Wayne W.
Shoughary, Ali T.

PETERBOROUGH
Cheung, Cindy H.
Drysdale, Ian O.
McDonald, J. Christopher
McReelis, Kylen D.
Rogers, William L.
Yeung, Jacky Y.

POINT EDWARD
Ibrahim, Fahim K F.

PORT COLBORNE
Ventresca, Mario R.

RICHMOND HILL
Karas, Yair
Liang, Edmund K K.
Woo, Elaine K J.

SARNIA
Patodia, Murari L.

SAULT STE MARIE
Bariciak, Mark D.
Giroux, Jason P.
Golesic, George F.
Mitchell, Brian J.
Sharp, Daniel C.
Stevenson, Robert F.

SCARBOROUGH
Assaad, David M.
Cheskes, Jordan W.
Goldberg, Chaim J.
Goldhar, Sheldon W.

Henen, Raafat
Liao, H. Robert
Noble, Jason
Rabinovitch, Jed
Znajda, James P.

SIMCOE
Thorpe, John B.

ST CATHARINES
Aedy, Lawrence J.
Beiko, George H H.
Cabrera, Anthony E.
Rhemtulla, El-Karim F J.
Scaife, Gerald D.

ST THOMAS
Brydon, Kyle W.

STRATFORD
Walker, J. Roberts

STRATHROY
Rogelstad, Michael L.

SUDBURY
Kosar, Stephen E.
Lee, Kevin K.
Sayuchchiyadevan, Ganeshan
Schonberger, Lawrence S.
Sorgini, Curtis J.

THORNHILL
Chung, Thomas
Feldman, Fredrick
Hershenfeld, Seymour
Kazdan, Jerome J.

THUNDER BAY
Czarnecki, Jan S C.
Dhurjon, Leland M.
Francis, Christopher J.
Gupta, Sanjoy
Schoales, Blair R.

TIMMINS
Oliver Fernandez, Alejandro

TORONTO
Adam, Robert S.
Ali, Asim
Altomare, Filiberto
Azadeh, Minoo
Bakshi, Nupura K.
Berger, Alan R.
Birt, Catherine M.
Boyd, Shelley R.
Braga-Mele, Rosa M.
Braude, Laurence
Brazel, Sheila M.
Brent, Michael H.
Bujak, Matthew C.
Buncic, J. Raymond
Buys, Yvonne M.
Chan, Clara C.
Chan, Wing Chow.
Cherry, Paul M H.
Cheskes, Albert
Chew, Hall F.
Chin Fook, Trevor J.
Choudhry, Netan
Chow, David R.
Christakis, John T.
Cohen, Mark J.
Cooper, Marvin
Dekany, Eva C.
Devenyi, Robert G.
Dixon, William S.
Easterbrook, W. Michael
El-Defrawy, Sherif
Eng, Kenneth
Epstein, Nancy E.
Fearon, S. Blair
Gallie, Brenda L.
Gasser, Joseph
Giavedoni, Louis R.
Gill, Harmeet
Girschek, Peter K.
Gorfinkel, John A.
Gupta, Neeru
Harvey, Patricia T.
Henry, Michael M.
Heon, Elise
Herzig, Sheldon
Hurwitz, Jeffrey J.
Iizuka, Megumi
Ing, Edsel B.
Kertes, Peter J.
Kohly, Radha P.
Kraft, Stephen P.
Lam, Wai-Ching
Leung, Christina C W.
Lichter, Myrna
Lloyd, John C.
MacDonald, Angus L.
Machat, Jeffrey J J.
Mandelcorn, Efrem D.
Mandelcorn, Mark S.
Margolin, Edward
Muni, Rajeev H.
Najm-Tehrani, Nasrin
Navajas, Eduardo V.
Nazemi, Fariba
Nianiaris, Nicholas
Oestreicher, James H.
Parker, John A.
Pavlin, Charles J.
Reginald, Arunun Y.
Rootman, David S.
Rosenstock, Ted
Sanghera, Gurinder P.
Schwartz, Carol E.
Singal, Neera
Singer, Shaun
Sit, Marisa
Skouras, Nicholas
Slomovic, Allan R.
Smith, David R.
Sniderman, Barry P.
Somerville, Glasier M.
Stein, Harold A.
Stein, Raymond M.
Tadros, Monir L.
Trope, Graham E.
Tucker, Nancy A.
Vanek, Irene J.
Wagman, Robert D.
Wedge, Charlotte I.
Weinstock, David J.
Weinstock, S. Joseph
Weiser, Brent A.
Wolpert, Maureen
Wong, David T W.
Wong, M F. Agnes
Yan, David B.
Yin, Vivian

TRENTON
Lachapelle, Kevin R.
Rao, Krishna B G.
Whiteman, Donald W.

VANIER
Rock, William J.
Ross, Ella A.

VAUGHAN
Dorrepaal, Stephen
Fava, Mark A.
Khan, Baseer U.
McGuire, Kwesi C.
Salyani, M. Asif
Weisbrod, Daniel J.

WATERLOO
Waind, Peter B.

WELLAND
Hassard, Frank A.
Vahdat, Jamie H.

WINDSOR
Chiu, Ann M.
Colev, Gheorghe
Curran, Brian M.
Deans, Robin M.
Emara, Barry
Ing, Tom G E.
Tayfour, Fouad

WOODSTOCK
Johnson, David W.
Lui, Derek P K.
Szasz, John

PRINCE EDWARD ISLAND

CHARLOTTETOWN
Boswall, Guy J.
Drysdale, Anne
O'Hanley, Gerald P.
Sefau, Suleiman O A.

CORNWALL
Price, Paul A.

QUÉBEC

ALMA
Carriere, Marc

AMOS
Dube, Pascale

BAIE-COMEAU
Dreige, Danny

BELOEIL
Ta, To-Quyen

BOISBRIAND
Lalonde, Laurent
Lepage, Robert
Racine, Suzanne

BROSSARD
Nasr, Kamil

CAP-AUX-MEULES
Delorme, Chantal

CHATEAUGUAY
Landry, Hubert

CHICOUTIMI
Beaulieu, Sophie
Chevrette, David
Gaudreault, Gilles
Lapointe, Andre
Trottier, Pierre

CHISASIBI
Sirois, Claude

COWANSVILLE
Gosselin, Michel P.
Simard-Lebrun, Adele
Weldon, Charles J.

DORVAL
Silver, Barry L.

DRUMMONDVILLE
Esper, Philip
Gagnon, Pauline R.
Saurel, Patrick

GATINEAU
Behki, Rama R.
Blair, Jason D.
Do, Minh-Thu
Gagnon, Marjolaine M.
Menard, Claude
Patenaude, Brian L.
Teboul, Nathalie

GRANBY
Dupont, Stephane
Fortin, Come
Guertin, Benoit-Jean
Labbe, Sebastien

GREENFIELD PARK
Menassa, Johanne

JOLIETTE
Yu, B W. Daniel

LACHINE
Laflamme, Michel-Yves
Lim, Khian-Kok
Mechaly-Chokron, Jeannine
Perrier, Manuel
Youhnovska, Pavlina

LASALLE
Segal-Ardman, Laura

LAVAL
Boileau, Martin
Duchesne, Raymond
Ferremi, Christian
Laflamme, Pierre
Le Francois, Michel
Marquis, Helene
Roberge, Francois
Uleckas, Jurate K.

LEVIS
Byrns, Katherine
Chmielewska, Karolina
Des Roches, Renee
Guay, Francine
Leblanc-Simard, Virginie
Marquis, Catherine
Samson, Jacques

LONGUEUIL
Assalian, Alfred
Cayer, Marie-Michelle
Deslauriers, Francine
Devaux, Angele
Duranceau, Alfred M.
Giroux, Louise
Robidas, Lorraine
Tassot, Pierre-Marie

MARIA
Morrissette, Roger

MONT-ROYAL
Balazsi, A. Gordon
Discepola, Marino J.
Mullie, Marc A.

MONTMAGNY
Asselin, Yves
Morin, Stephane P.

MONTREAL
Agoumi, Younes
Albert, Darren L.
Arbour, Jean-Daniel
Ares, Chantal
Arthurs, Bryan P.
Aubin, Marie-Josee
Bashour, Mounir
Basmadjian, Girair
Belair, Marie-Lyne
Belanger, Caroline
Bergeron, Richard F.
Boisjoly, Helene
Boucher, Marie Carole
Brais, Pierre M.
Brochu, Jocelyne
Brunette, Isabelle
Callejo, Sonia A.
Carignan, Renee
Chaput, Gilles R.
Charbonneau, Louise
Cheema, Devinder P.
Choremis, Johanna
Codere, Francois
Coffey, Alan J H.
Cohen, Shawn L.
Connolly, W. Edward S.
Corriveau, Christine
Corriveau, Louis
Demers, Jean-P
Demers, Pierre
Deschenes, Jean
Desjardins, Daniel C J.
Duperre, Jean A.
Edelstein, Chaim Z I.
Edelstein, Eugene
El-Achkar, Ghassan G.
El-Saheb, Hady
Fallaha, Nicole
Fichman, Stephen H.
Fortin, Eric
Gagne, Sebastien
Gans, Mark S.
Gariepy, Elizabeth L.
Gauthier, Danny
Gomolin, Julius E S.
Goodyear, Emilie
Gravel, Michel
Hafez, Ali
Hamel, Patrick
Harasymowycz, Paul J.
Hardy, Isabelle
Harissi Dagher, Mona
Heredia, Cesar
Hladky, Eugene N.
Jaworski, Laurence
Kapusta, Michael A.
Kasner, Oscar P.
Kattleman, Barry S.
Kavalec, Conrad
Koenekoop, Robert K.
Labelle, Pierre F.
Lahoud, Salim
Lederer, David
Leduc, Sophie M.
Lesk, Mark R.
Levin, Leonard A.
Li, Gisele
Lindley, Susan K.
Little, John M.
Lord, Frederic
Luneau, Katie
Mabon, Michele
Marcil, J E. Gilles
Mathieu-Millaire, Francine
Meere, Stephane B.
Montas, Lys B.
Mydlarski, Marc B.
Nguyen, Cong L.
Nguyen, Thi Bich T.
Nguyen, Tuan Quynh T.
Oliver, Karin
Olivier, Sebastien
Orquin, Jacqueline
Panisset, Alain
Papanagnu, Paraskevi-Eleni
Paquin, Michel
Pelletier, Conrad R.
Pop, Mihai
Quevillon, Andree
Quigley, Michael G.
Racine, Louis
Rheaume, Marc-Andre
Robillard, Nicole
Rosen, Joel
Rouleau, Jacinthe
Saheb, Nabil E.
Salem, Jacques
Sebag, Mikael
Silver, David A.
Solomon, Leon D.
Superstein, Rosanne
Svarc, Emile D.
Tardif, Denis
Thompson, Paul
Toffoli, Daniela
Wallerstein, Avi
Wein, Francine B.
Wong, Jamie
Zaharia, Marian-Ananda

NOTRE DAME DES PRAIRIES
Deschenes, Christian
Jeanson, Pierre

POINTE-CLAIRE
Archambault, Patrice
Chartrand, Jean-Pierre
Hasegawa, Naomi A.
Kraus, Danielle
Nguyen, Tuong-Nam

QUEBEC
Achim, Catherine
Anctil, Jean-Louis
Bazin, Richard
Bergeron, Dan
Black, Daniel O.
Blanchette, Francois
Boudreault, Ghislain A.
Boulanger, Claude
Boutin, Yannick
Caissie, Mathieu
Carignan, Jacqueline
Caron, Louis
Cinq-Mars, Benoit
Clement, Jean-Rene
Couture, Simon

SPECIALISTS BY PROVINCE

Des Marchais, Beatrice
Dinh, Rene N.
Dube, Paule
Dube, Yolande
Duguay, Pierre
Duquette, Claude
Foster, William
Fredette, Marie-Josee
Garand, Lise J.
Gelinas, Guy
Gourdeau, Alain
Goyette, Annie
Gravel, Jean-Pierre
Hoffman, Bertrand
Labrecque, Nathalie
Lachance, Guy
Lafond, Gilles-Philippe
Lajoie, Caroline
Laliberte, Isabelle
Lalonde, Gilles
Laughrea, Patricia A.
Legare, Marie-Eve
Letartre, Laurence
Malenfant, Mario
Marcoux, Louis-Etienne
Mathieu, Anne-Marie
Meyer, Dominique H.
Molgat, Yvonne M.
Morency, Johanne
Rodrigue, Denis
Schmit, Isabelle
Tardif, Yvon-Maurice
Toren, Andrew J.
Tourigny, Richard
Tourville, Eric
Turcotte, Pierre
Vaillancourt, Luc

RIMOUSKI
Duguay, Claude
Dumas, Bruno
Laplante, Alain
Leblanc, Jean-Paul M.
Mercille, Genevieve
Saab, Marc
Simard, Raymond
Smith, Gaetan M.

RIVIERE-DU-LOUP
Gravel, Celine
Grenier, Rejean

ROBERVAL
Laroche, Maxime
Mathieu, R. Brian
Plante, Denis

SAINT-GEORGES
Belanger, Paul
Lachance, Alain
St-Gelais, Philippe

SAINT-HYACINTHE
Bergeron, Elise
Ghali, Zineb
Jodoin, Caroline
Julien, Pierre G.
Leclerc, Michele
Silvestri, Alexandre

SAINT-JEROME
Montplaisir, Sylvie

SAINT-LAURENT
Amyot, Marcel A.
Fanous, Sameh
Khouri, Lucie M.
Khoury, Elie G.

SAINT-NICEPHORE
Gauthier, Daniel

SAINTE-THERESE
Desgroseilliers, Anik
Tremblay, Marie-Claude

SALABERRY DE VALLEYFIELD
Hammami, Hachmi
Swieca, Richard O.
Teboul, Barbara K.

SEPT-ILES
Cote, Gilles M.
Turbide, Pascale

SHAWINIGAN-SUD
Le Bel, Stephane
Sultan, Mazen

SHERBROOKE
Blondeau, Pierre
Boulos, Patrick R.
Carbonneau, Marjorie
Doyon, Guy
Faucher, Anne
Giunta, Michel
Gregoire, Alain D.
Gregoire, Jacques C.
Grenier, Benoit
Mazerolle, Eric
Olivier, Patrick
Roberge, Jean-Francois

SOREL-TRACY
Blouin, Marie-Claude
Demay, Francois L.
Lamoureux, Alain

ST CHARLES BORROMEE
Lor, Huy Sroy
Mayer, Jean

ST JEAN SUR RICHELIEU
Betournay, Nicole
Boucher, Serge
Joyal, Helene
Legris, Celine
Staudenmaier, Christa

STE AGATHE DES MONTS
Guilbault, Normand

TERREBONNE
Chehade, Nicolas
Mwilambwe wa Mwilambwe, Annick
Perreault, Christian

TROIS-RIVIERES
Bazin, Genevieve
Charbonneau, Alain
De Groot, Jean-Andre
Letourneau, Steeve
Maamar-Samet, Maamar
Roberge, Marcel
Roy, Francis F.
St-Arnaud, Claude

VAL-D'OR
Barrette-Delorme, Michelle
Daniel, Shannon M.

VERDUN
Louis, Melissa A.
Noel, Francoise
Podtetenev, Michel

VICTORIAVILLE
Corriveau, Marie-Noel
Denhez, Paul
Grondin, Valerie
Martel, Sophie

WESTMOUNT
Alotaibi, Majed
Chen, John C C.
Chevrette, Line
Flanders, Michael E.
Galic, John I.
Polomeno, Robert C.
Waldron, James B.
Wise, Jack S.

SASKATCHEWAN

BATTLEFORD
O'Keeffe, Patrick D.

MOOSE JAW
Botha, Jan-Beyers

PRINCE ALBERT
Buglass, Todd D.
Wandzura, Michael J.

REGINA
Avram, Darrell R.
Coupal, Dustin J.
Courtney, Anthony O.
Eidsness, Ryan
Garcia-Salinas, Raul
Judelson, Jeffrey
Mervitz, Michael D.
Ong-Tone, Lindsay
Varma, Renatta

SASKATOON
Blackwell, Thomas E R.
Colleaux, Kevin M.
Conlon, M. Ronan
Hamilton, W. Keith
Murphy, Paul H.
Nrusimhadevara, Ravikrishna
Pekush, Robert D.
Riyaz, Rehan R.
Sharma, Vikas
Van Der Zweep, John B.

YORKTON
Smith, Harold M B.

Orthopedic Surgery

ALBERTA

BANFF
Buchko, Gregory M L.
Heard, S. Mark A.
Hiemstra, Laurie A.
O'Brien, Catherine L.

BELLEVUE
Hurdle, Ian B.

CALGARY
Abelseth, Gregory A.
Bauman, John
Bois, Aaron J.
Boorman, Richard S.
Bouchard, J. Jacques A.
Bowen, C. Vaughan A.
Brauer, Carmen A.
Bray, Robert C.
Buckley, Richard E.
Burkart, Brian C.
Cho, Roger K N.
Clark, Marcia L.
Cundal, Cory S.
De Souza, Francis K.
Dhaliwal, Gurpreet S.
Donaghy, John J.
Dougall, Hugh R.
Duffy, Paul J.
England, Ronald M.
Frank, Cyril B.
Goldstein, Simon G.
Hamdi, Amre
Harder, James A.
Hildebrand, Kevin A.
Hollinshead, Robert M.
Hu, Richard W.
Huang, Eric M.
Hunt, Stephen B.
Hutchison, Carolyn
Johnston, Kelly D.
Joughin, V. Elaine
Keetbaas, Shayne D.
Kiefer, Gerhard N.
Korley, Robert
Kuchinad, Raul A.
Le, Ian L D.
Lewkonia, Peter D.
Lo, Ian K Y.
Longino, Peter D.
MacKenzie, James R.
Miller, Stephen D.
Mohtadi, Nicholas G H.
Monument, Michael J.
Mrkonjic, Linda A.
O'Brien, Maureen D.
Parsons, David L.
Penner, Darrell A.
Powell, James N.
Puloski, Shannon K T.
Rendall, Edward O.
Russell, Iain S.
Salo, Paul T.
Schachar, Norman S.
Shihata, Shadi S A.
Spiess, Michael P.
Stewart, James I.
Swamy, Ganesh
Thomas, Kenneth C.
Timmermann, Scott A.
Van Zuiden, Lowell J.
Werle, Jason R.
White, Neil J.

CAMROSE
Kumar, Sunail

EDMONTON
Arnett, Gordon D.
Balyk, Robert A.
Bergman, Joseph W.
Bouliane, Martin J.
Bury, Jeffrey H.
Cinats, John G.
Cole, William G.
Dick, Donald
Dulai, Sukhdeep K.
Durand, D'Arcy C.
Ekert, Lee
Esmail, Salim M A.
Glasgow, Donald L M.
Glasgow, Robert M.
Glasgow, Robert R M.
Goplen, Gordon R.
Greenhill, Brian J.
Greidanus, Thomas H.
Hedden, Douglas M.
Henderson, Ronald L.
Hui, Catherine M T.
Hunka, Larry E.
Jiang, Hongxing
Johnston, D. William C.
Jomha, Nadr M.
Kortbeek, Frank B.
Lalani, Aleem
Lavoie, Guy J.
Lavoie, Michel V M.
Leung, Paul M K.
Mahood, James K.
Masson, Edward C O.
McIvor, John B.
McKenzie, Alvin H.
McMillan, James F.
Menon, Matthew R G.
Moreau, Marc J.
O'Connor, Gregory J.
Otto, David D.
Panaro, Carlo D A.
Paul, Paulose J.
Pedersen, M. Elizabeth
Pisesky, Wayne A.
Reid, David C.
Rigal, Wynne M.
Russell, G. Gordon Q.
Scharfenberger, Angela V.
Sheps, David M.
Stiegelmar, Robert E.
Tadros, Cherif
Weber, Donald W.
Wiens, Scott W.

FORT MCMURRAY
Qureshi, Irfan T.

GRANDE PRAIRIE
Akinbiyi, Oluwatosin A.
Al-Ghamdi, Mohammed

LETHBRIDGE
Anderson, S. Lance
Chang, Malcolm E.
Chaudhary, Reyhan A.
Costello, Bernard G.
Fernhout, Mark J.
Kwan, Stephen F.
Storey, Benjamin L.
Vincent, Nancy E.

LLOYDMINSTER
Kowalczyk, Earl S.

MEDICINE HAT
Bering, Michael P.
Jena, Debakanta
Martin, Robert P.

RED DEER
Batuyong, Eldridge D.
Beuerlein, Murray J.
Bredo, Lance K.
Henderson, Winston B.
Korbyl, Robert E.
Maragh, Krishna K.
Pearce, Timothy J.
Perlau, Robert J R.
Reikie, W. Roddick
Wolstenholme, Keith R.

ST. ALBERT
Chan, Robert K W.
Narang, Rajendra

BRITISH COLUMBIA

ABBOTSFORD
Lee, David C.
Mehin, Ramin
Rose, James C.
Sovio, Olli M.
Wickham, David

BURNABY
Belle, Ralph M.
Dunwoody, James M.
Goel, Danny P.
Hill, Kenneth C.
Kokan, Peter A.
Kostamo, Timothy
Popovic, Dina
Tarazi, Fadi

CAMPBELL RIVER
Botsford, Deke J.
Crosby, Andrew J R.
Leete, Stanley F.
Sohmer, Stephen

CHILLIWACK
Grover, Deepak
Kousaie, Kenneth N.
Locht, Randall C.

COMOX
Bell, Timothy H.
Sundby, Kirk A.
Van Sittert, Jacobus J.
Woods, Thomas C H.

CRANBROOK
Buckley, Charles K R.
Chan, Alex D M.
Chaney, Jonathan W.
Driedger, Bernhard E.

DUNCAN
Anderson, A. Robert
Austin, Thomas M.
Lake, David M.
Velazquez, Ricardo J.

KAMLOOPS
Ackermann, Carel W.
Beaton, William N.
Langevin, Jean
McLeod, Richard A.
Outerbridge, A. Ross
Plausinis, Derek J A.
Porter, Andrew D.
Toreson, Jeffrey A.
Zeznik, Laura A.

KELOWNA
Boyce, David W.
Bridge, Michael A.
Krywulak, Steven
Malish, Dean G.
Moreau, Paul G.
Myden, Curtis A.
O'Connor, Gary D.
O'Farrell, Terrance A.
Oliver, John H W.

KITIMAT
Van Der Merwe, Ignatius

LANGLEY
Chan, K H. Albert
Chiu, Mark H N.
Elkoussy, Moustafa A.
Favero, Kenneth J.
Grypma, Martin P.
Hicks, Tracy E.
Syal, Abeer

MAPLE RIDGE
Bhachu, Davinder S.
Chancey, Ann B.
Kim, Won Oh
Patel, Surendra K.

NANAIMO
Birchard, John G.
Cameron, Christopher D.
Ellis, David R.
Gutmanis, Peter
Malone, William C.
Markland, Brenda A.
Smith, Erasmus J.
Woodruff, Brian G.

NEW WESTMINSTER
Apostle, Kelly L.
Boyer, Dory
Dacambra, Mark
Dommisse, Iain G.
Hansen, Gregory
Loomer, Richard L.
Lopez, Carlos A.
McCormack, Robert G.
Moola, Farhad O.
Pate, Graham C.
Perey, Bertrand H.
Piper, Michael S.
Pirani, Shafique P.
Stone, Trevor B.
Viskontas, Darius G.

NORTH VANCOUVER
Baggoo, Alan K.
Boyle, Marc R.
Jando, Victor T.
Panagiotopoulos, Konstantino P.
Preto, Antonio F.
Sabiston, Colin P.
Samler, Shannon R.
Sidky, Adam O.
Thompson, J. Paul
Vaisler, Barry J.
Zarkadas, Peter C.

PENTICTON
Naude, Roelof J T.
Pinsonneault, Troy G.
Tatebe, Rodney Y.
Taylor, Cameron R.

PRINCE GEORGE
Costa, Anthony J.
Dreyer, Hendrik A.
MacKey, Denise A.
Moran, Michael M.
Nelson, David R.
Purnell, Roger A.
Van Zyl, Johannes P.

RICHMOND
Arthur, John S.
Calvert, Erik
Fenton, Jonathan A S.
Hughes, Kenneth F.
Kendall, Richard W.
Leung, Fay
Lu, Thomas S.
Lui, Spenser M Y.
McConkey, Mark O.
Smith, Derek B.

ROSSLAND
McVicar, Stephen F.

SQUAMISH
McConkey, John P.

SURREY
Aitken, George S.
Brown, David S.
Bubbar, Vikrant K.
Froh, Robert G.
Jackson, Colin M.
Lescheid, Jonathan M.
Maloon, Stephen
Matthew, James R.
Rickards, Robin C.
Sabir, M. Munawar
Sabo, Marlis T.
Schweigel, Robert C.
Shahid, Riad M A.
Telfer, Charles D.
Yao, Peter Y O.

TRAIL
Bitting, Seth S.
Hjelkrem, Michel
Laverty, Lee-Anne
Sproul, Cathryn D.

VANCOUVER
Alvarez, Christine M.
Beauchamp, Richard D.
Blachut, Piotr A.
Broekhuyse, Henry M.
Brown, Kenneth L B.
Chin, Y K. Patrick
Clarkson, Paul W.
Day, Brian
Douglas, James
Duncan, Clive
Dvorak, Marcel F S.
Fisher, Charles G.
Forsythe, Caroline M.
Garbuz, Donald S.
Gatha, Mark
Gilbart, Michael K.
Goetz, Thomas J.
Greidanus, Nelson V.
Gropper, Peter T.
Guy, Pierre
Hawkins, Robert H.
Hepburn, Andrew
Horlick, Simon G D.
Kelly, Adrienne M.
Kolla, Lee A.
Kwon, Brian K.
Lefaivre, Kelly A.
Leith, Jordan M.
Masri, Bassam A.
McCormick, William D.
McGraw, Robert W.
McKenzie, Gerard M.
McPherson, G. Duncan
Miyanji, Firoz
Nadeau, Melissa M T A.
O'Brien, Peter J.
Penner, Murray J.
Pike, Jeffrey M.
Pinney, Stephen J.
Regan, William D.
Reilly, Christopher W.
Smith, Donna
Stothers, Keith A.
Umran, Tamim
Van Der Merwe, Johannes M.
Werry, Donald G.
Wing, Kevin J.
Wing, Peter C.
Younger, Alastair S E.
Yu, William Y.

VERNON
Ball, Mary Kate
Christian, Keith M W.
O'Brien, R. Jason
Parfitt, Christopher J.
Richardson, Alan J.
Secretan, Charles C.
Splawinski, Jan B.

VICTORIA
Burnett, R. Stephen J.
Cloutier, Frederic-Charles
Dryden, Peter J.
Jacks, Duncan A.
Landells, Colin D.
Lapp, Ralph A.
Lundine, Kristopher M.
Mathes, Sonja K.
McAllister, Patrick J.
Nelson, Charles A.
O'Neill, Michael O.
Penny, J. Norgrove
Stanger, Michael A.
Stone, James E.
Torstensen, Eric T.
Wahl, Adalbert E.
White, James P.
Yoneda, Bruce T.
Zarzour, Zane D S.

WHISTLER
Brooks-Hill, Alexandra L.

WHITE ROCK
Kwee, Jeffrey K.
Kwee, Kai Liang
Smit, Bernardus H W G M.

MANITOBA

BRANDON
Klippenstein, Norman L.

WINKLER
Engel, Jeff S.
Mazek, Fawzi R E.

WINNIPEG
Adduri, V. Rao
Arnot, James B.
Balageorge, Dimitrios
Baria, Kaikhushroo
Barron, Laurie W.
Barske, Heather L.
Birt, Douglas F.
Black, G. Brian
Bohm, Eric R.
Burnell, Colin D.
Clark, Tod A.
Crosby, Jason A.
De Korompay, Victor L L.
Dillon, John
Dubberley, James
Elkurbo, Mohamed
Foerster, David R.
Froese, Warren G.
Goytan, Michael J.
Graham, Christopher
Hammond, Allan
Hedden, David
Huebert, David M.
Huebert, Helmut T.
Irving, James E.
Jellicoe, Paul A.
Johnson, Michael G.
Kayler, Douglas E.
Longstaffe, Albert E.
MacDonald, Peter B.
Mayba, Ihor I.
McPherson, John A M.
Monson, Ronald C.
Muller Delgado, Hellmuth A.
Nasser-Sharif, Susan B.
Old, Jason A.
Pilkey, Bradley D.
Sharif, Manoutch N.
Shariff, Fariduddin K.
Stranges, Gregory A.
Tufescu, Tudor V.
Tung, Taranjit S.
Turgeon, Thomas R.
Wiens, John L.

NEW BRUNSWICK

BATHURST
Bosse, Marilyn
Branch, Neil
Caron, Michel

BERESFORD
Frenette, Remi J.

DALHOUSIE JUNCTION
Verret, Gilles W.

DIEPPE
Bourque, Luc
David, Herve
Le Breton, Michel A.

EDMUNDSTON
Paillard, Jean-Francois

FREDERICTON
Barnhill, Thomas A.
Berkshire, Andrew J.
Bowden, Scott H.
Burton, Philip J.
De Vries, Gwyneth
Touchie, Harold W.

MIRAMICHI
Norris, Philip L.

MONCTON
Allanach, William W.
Clark, Andrew E.
Comstock, Sean A.
Daigle, Jean-Pierre
Forsythe, Michael E.
Forsythe, Michael G.
Massoeurs, Steven J.

ROTHESAY
Acker, John C.

SAINT JOHN
Abraham, Edward P.
Connolly, Stephen H.
Fletcher, Jennifer A.
Grant, John A.
Kerr, Darren
Manson, Neil A.
Steeves, John M.
Wagg, James P.

SHEDIAC
de Yturralde, Daniel

NEWFOUNDLAND AND LABRADOR

CORNER BROOK
Lewis, Brendan D.
Wentzell, Tracey M.

GANDER
Kennedy, Carl J.
Russell, Robert S.
Tumilty, Joseph A.
Woolridge, Bryan S.

ST. JOHN'S
Au, Keegan P.
Deane, Robert H.
Jackman, Heather R.
Martin, Roderick D.
Moores, Carl D.
Noftall, Francis E.
O'Dea, Francis J.
Rockwood, Peter R.
Sahajpal, Viki
Squire, Daniel S.
Stone, Norman C.

NORTHWEST TERRITORIES

YELLOWKNIFE
Corkal, James F.
Younge, Derek A.

NOVA SCOTIA

DARTMOUTH
Anderson, K. Eric
LeGay, Douglas A.
O'Brien, David A L.
Venugopal, Vikram

HALIFAX
Alexander, David I.
Amirault, J. David
Biddulph, Michael P.
Coady, Catherine M.
Coles, Chad P.
Dunbar, Michael
El-Hawary, Rany
Gauthier, Luke E.
Glazebrook, Mark A.
Gross, Michael
Howard, Jason J.
Hyndman, John C.
Johnston, David G.
Lefrancois, Tina I.
Leighton, Ross K.
Orlik, Benjamin C.
Oxner, William M.
Reardon, Gerald
Richardson, C. Glen
Stanish, William D.
Taylor, J E. Scott
Thibaudeau, Pascale
Trenholm, J. Andrew
Zhang, Lu

KENTVILLE
Beveridge, William K.
Clarke, Gregory V.
Hewins, Edward A.
Howatt, Eric B.
Murphy, Nadia L.
Veljkovic, Andrea N.

MIRA ROAD
Brien, Donald M.
Orrell, Kevin G S.

NEW GLASGOW
Boudreau, D. Todd
Lincoln, Maximillian C.
Sequeira, Stanislaus P.

SYDNEY
Collicutt, James A.
Dodd, Faith
O'Neill, Michelle E.

ONTARIO

AJAX
Abuzgaya, Fathi H.
Benfayed, Hamdi H.
Gallay, Stephen H.
Lobo, Joel J A.

ANCASTER
Ogilvie, Rick A.

BARRIE
Casses, Alberto
Crawford, Gordon A.
Delaney, James
Ikejiani, Charles E.
Korkola, Michael L.
McKenzie, J. Scott
O'Sullivan, John J.
Vennettilli, Marco C.

BELLEVILLE
Birchard, James D.
Deans, James R A.
Kawam, Michael P.
Langer, Joseph
Ling, Herbert S C.
Pickle, Andrew R.
Steinitz, Daniel K.

BRAMPTON
Alexander, Pradeep J.
Benmoftah, Osama S A.

Hanna, Samer K F.
Harrington, John P.
Hockmann, Guido I.
Karabatsos, Charalabos B.
Newall, John R.
Paitich, C. Bruce
Sekyi-Otu, Ato
Tavazzani, Franco G.

BRANTFORD

Dill, James R.
Pugh, David M W.
Rabinovich, Alexander
Rerri, Bernard
Richie, Steven J.
Whately, Christopher G.
Woolfrey, Michael R.

BROCKVILLE

Beg-Mirza, Athar
Gambrel, Jason
Shim, Paul S.

BURLINGTON

Armstrong, R. Douglas
Carbin, Robert J.
Jaroszynski, Grzegorz C.
Manjoo, Ajay
Pyper, J. Alexander
Smith, Benjamin M.
Smith, Frank C.
Wong, Ivan H.

CAMBRIDGE

Daly, Joyce L.
Haddad, Dimitri E.
Leone, James M.
Mathew, Paul K.
Stapleton, John K.

CHATHAM

Kukkadi, Zaheer
Stone, Jonathan F.
Turnbull, John R.

COLLINGWOOD

Cheng, Y Y. Olivia
Koo, Henry

CORNWALL

Chang, Chih-Peng
Corrigan, Michael J.
Tombler, Richard D.

EAST YORK

Catre, Melanio G.
Wong, Paul K C.

ETOBICOKE

Angelini, Mark P.
Bhargava, Manoj
Cartan, Stephen J.
Gordon, Robert G.
Gyomorey, Sandor
McGonigal, Donald J.
Quinn, Andrew P.
Roscoe, Martin W A.
Sadoughi, Mehdi
Townley, John B.

GEORGETOWN

Lu, Christopher M.

GUELPH

Armstrong, Donald R.
Fung, Wayne A.
Hoey, Steven A.
McKenzie, Kenneth A.
Stamp, Gary W.
White, Ernest J.

HAMILTON

Adili, Anthony
Alshakman, Khalad
Alshaya, Osama S I.
Avram, Victoria R A.
Ayeni, Olufemi R.
Badawi, Abdelrahman K.
Bednar, Drew A.
Bhandari, Mohit
Burrow, Sarah R.
De Beer, Justin
Deheshi, Benjamin
Denkers, Matthew R.
Drew, Brian M.
Dunlop, R H. Brett
Gandhi, Harjeet S.
Ghert, Michelle A.
Hetaimish, Bandar
Kwok, Desmond C.
Lachowski, Richard J.
Mah, Jung Y.
Missiuna, Paul
Moro, Jaydeep K.
Peterson, Devin C.
Petrisor, Bradley A.
Porte, Arthur M.
Punthakee, Dinshaw K.
Rajaratnam, Krishan
Ristevski, Bill
Robles, Harold I.
Sadler, John T S.
Scriven, Edward A K.
Williams, Dale
Winemaker, Mitchell J.
Wismer, David I A.
Zabtia, Nazar R.

INGLEWOOD

Prior, Donald F.

KINGSTON

Bardana, Davide D.
Bicknell, Ryan T.
Borschneck, Daniel P.
Bow, Jennifer K.
Campbell, Aaron
Cooke, T. Derek V.
Davidson, Lindsay K.
Harrison, Mark M.
Hiscox, Christina M.
Lau, Rick L.
Pichora, David R.
Rudan, John F.
Sawan, Hasan M S.
Wood, Gavin C A.
Yach, Jeff D.
Yen, David

KITCHENER

Grosso, Paul M.
Hupel, Thomas M.
Moammer, Gemah M A.
Schuringa, Peter C R.
Snider, Matthew G.
Stevenson, Peter

LINDSAY

Al-Beer, Ali
Noronha, Charles A.

LONDON

Alomar, Abdulaziz Z M.
Apostol, Tony A.
Athwal, George G S.
Bailey, Christopher
Bailey, Stewart
Bartley, Debra
Carey, Timothy
Cashin, Megan S.
Chant, Chris B.
Chess, David G.
Copithorne, Peter G.
Drosdowech, Darren S.
Faber, Kenneth J.
Fowler, Peter J.
Gammon, Braden
Giffin, J. Robert
Grewal, Ruby
Gurr, Kevin R.
Howard, James L.
King, Graham J W.
Lanting, Brent A.
Lapner, Michael A C.
Lawendy, Abdel-Rahman
Lebel, Marie-Eve
Lee, W J. Kenny
Litchfield, Robert B.
MacDonald, Steven J M.
MacLeod, Mark D.
McAuley, James P.
McCalden, Richard W.
Naudie, Douglas D R.
Rorabeck, Cecil H.
Sanders, David W.
Sharma, Rajrishi
Taylor, David C.
Vasarhelyi, Edward M.
Willits, Kevin R.

MAITLAND

Mussett, Steven A.

MARKDALE

Hall, Hamilton

MARKHAM

Alpert, Brian
Haider, Syed Y A.
McMahon, J. Stephen
Shirali, Hemant R.
Smith, Crystal A.

MILTON

Bischoff, Markus

MISSISSAUGA

Boynton, Erin L.
Cheah, Henry K.
Clements, Nigel D.
Di Pasquale, Dennis J.
French, Geoffrey R.
Gelinas, Jill M J.
Getahun, Tajedin Y.
Jinnah, Rashid A.
Levesque, Jerome
Manolopoulos, Vaselios
McBroom, Robert J.
McGoey, Brian V.
Nguyen, Can Dinh
Rosenfeld, Steven A.
Saplys, Ramunas F J.
Sennik, Vir Bhushan.
Skipper, R. James
Soriano, Samuel
Stewart, John A.
Taromi, Bejzad
Turchin, Diana C.
Weisleder, Louis M.
Wilson, Dana F.

NEPEAN

Oliver, Steven W.
Young, Darryl K.

NEWMARKET

Bertoia, J. Thomas D.
Devlin, S. Rueben
Gamble, Patrick
Lee, Moo-Hyung
Lindsay, Christopher S.
Randle, John A.
Rogakou, Cleo C.
Tuli, Vikas

NIAGARA FALLS

Flores, Luis A.
Le Roux, Bartholomeus J M.
Offierski, Chris M.
Ostrowski, John D.

NORTH BAY

Holmes, John E.
Khodabandehloo, Mohammed R.
Lewis, Timothy E.
Van Vliet, Aaron J.
Wallace, Thomas H.
Yadav, Mahesh P.

NORTH YORK

Ali, Pervez
Alvi, Mansour I.
Barrington, Thomas W.
Bent, Maurice A.
Brock, Robert M.
Cayen, Barry
Chan, Gladys K Y.
Chan, Henry
Chan, Tommy K C.
Charendoff, Morris D.
Dantzer, Dale
Efala, Khal Mabru
Faulkner, John R.
Grant, Kevin
Halman, Stephen I.
Harrington, Ian
Heller, Martin
Indech, Michael
Kwok, M K. Joseph
Mehdian, Hossein
Peskun, Christopher J.
Reed, Stephen C.
Rodriguez-Elizalde, Sebastian
Rumble, Edward J.
Seligman, James V.
Smith-Auguste, Jacqueline A.
Tansey, Patrick A H.
Tountas, Apostolos A.
West, Michael
Yee, Gilbert Y M.

OAKVILLE

Brien, Heather
Deakon, R. Timothy
Ginty, Mark R.
Naumetz, Victor A.
Thompson, Stephen R.
Weening, Bradley S.
Zalzal, Paul K.

ORILLIA

Hickey, Michael

OSHAWA

Chhabra, Samir R.
Dessouki, Esmat A.
Fern, Ken T C.
Gharsaa, Osama
Ibrahim, Abdulmajid S.
Martin, Michael
Osinga, Christopher J.

OTTAWA

Agarwala, Vinod K.
Baxter, Maureen
Beaule, Paul E.
Bessette, Benoit J.
Bienkowski, Peter
Brown, Christopher W.
Brunet, Jacques A.
Charles, Mark N.
Chauhan, Rameshchandra P.
Chow, Donald
Dervin, Geoff
Desjardins, JP. Jean-Pierre
Di Silvestro, Matthew
Feibel, Robert J.
Fleuriau-Chateau, Philip B.
Forget, Robert J.
Gartke, Kathleen
Giachino, A. Alan
Gittens, Rudolph
Gofton, Wade T.
Gordon, John A.
Goulding, Krista A.
Hradecky, Cyril M.
Illical, Emmanuel M.
Jarvis, James G.
Johnson, Donald H.
Johnson, Garth E.
Khanna, Vickas
Kim, Paul R.
Kingwell, Stephen P.
Kontio, Ken K.
Lafleche, Jean-Pierre
Lalonde, Karl-Andre R.
Lapner, Peter L C.
Lawton, Louis J.
Liew, Allan S L.
Marshall, Andrew G.
Moreau, Guy
Moroz, Paul J.
O'Neil, D. Joseph
O'Neill, Brendan D.
Papp, Steven R.
Parai, Milton S.
Phan, Philippe T N.
Pollock, J. Whitcomb
Portner, Oliver T.
Prihar, Rajiv K.
Randall, James P.
Raynor, Christopher F.
Ritter, Douglas J.
Sharma, Sanjeev P.
Simon, David A.
Steeves, Mark A.
Thurston, Peter R.
Wai, Eugene K.
Werier, Joel M.
Wilkinson, Ross S.
Willis Jr., R. Baxter

OWEN SOUND

Adlington, Jay B.
Haider, Esam M S.
Henning, Jan L.
Manwell, Stuart E E.

PARRY SOUND

Smyth, William-Lee R.

PERTH

Anderson, P. Paul A.
Roberts, Mark S.

PETERBOROUGH

Blastorah, Bernard J.
Dobson, J. Crawford
Lever, James P.
Parker, Stuart M.
Veri, John-Paul

PICKERING

Thompson, Charles V.

RICHMOND HILL

Camazzola, Daniele
Marchie, Anthony
Nourhosseini, Seyed H.
Soon-Shiong, Gregory
Wang, Robert Y.
Watson, Christopher H C.

SARNIA

Garach, Anil
MacKinlay, Duncan C.
March, Gerard M J.
Southcott, W. Peter
Wong, George A.

SAULT STE MARIE

Burrell, John
Cheong, Y. Michele
Costain, Darren J.
Elder, Graham M.
Fraser, Brian P.
Jacqmin, Marc L.
McAllister, Terrance B.
Slagel, Bradley E.
Tait, John H.

SCARBOROUGH

Abughaduma, Read M A.
Bushuk, Michael B.
Chapman, Michael T.
Deonarain, Sue
Ghazavi, Mohammed T.
Guerra Paez, Jose G.
Hahn, Miah
Hummel, Jonathan S.
Kaminker, Richard S.
Latham, Warren C W.
Luba, Robert M A.
Maistrelli, Gianni
Rathbun, James B.
Sattarian, Javad
Siller, Theodore N.
Smith, Jason C.
Sue-A-Quan, Errol A.
Tabloie, Farshid
Tran, Franklin T V.
Urovitz, Edwin P.
Vandersluis, Ronald
Woolford, Bernard J.
Young, M. Christine

ST CATHARINES

Blackman, Eric R.
Josefchak, Robert G.
Kalchman, Marc J.
Martin, David C.
Masnyk, Robert D.
Robert, Christopher E.
Robert, Paul F.

ST THOMAS

Cervinka, Anthony G.
Van Houwelingen, Andrew P.

STRATFORD

Guy, K. James
Pototschnik, Ralph

STRATHROY
Blokker, Catherine P.
Rajgopal, Vaishnav

SUDBURY
Allison, Patrick J.
Cisa Bergos, Jordi C.
Healey, David C.
Robinson, Eric J.
Saidi, Kevan
Tubin, Stanislaw
Vokey, Susan E.

THORNHILL
Dakin, Edward B.

THUNDER BAY
Clark, Russell P.
Cullinan, Claude A.
Droll, Kurt P.
French, Stephen J.
Hoffman, David V.
McCormick, Myra J C.
Payandeh, Jubin B.
Porter, Gordon A.
Porter, John
Puskas, David A.
Remus, John L.
Wilson, Tracy L.

TIMMINS
Al-Sahan, Mohammad
Harding, David M.
Lafontaine, Robert E.

TORONTO
Abbas, Harith A.
Abdelbary, Hesham A M M.
Abouali, Jihad A K.
Ahn, Henry
Al Saied, Mohamed
Alman, Benjamin A.
Axelrod, Terry S.
Backstein, David J.
Bell, Robert S.
Bogoch, Earl R.
Bouchard, Maryse L.
Cameron, Hugh U.
Cameron, John C.
Chahal, Jaskarndip S.
Chakravertty, Rajesh
Conn, Garson S.
Daniels, Timothy R.
Davey, J. Roderick
De Demeter, Dorrit A.
Dodwell, Emily
Elmaraghy, Amr W.
English, Edward
Ferguson, Peter C.
Fielden, Robert H N.
Finkelstein, Joel A.
Ford, Michael H G.
Gallimore, Christopher H.
Gandhi, Rajiv
Garbedian, Shawn
Goldstein, Christina
Gollish, Jeffrey D.
Graham, Brent A.
Gross, Allan E.
Gupta, Sumit
Hall, Jeremy A.
Hamam, Al-Walid
Hayward, Andrew C.
Heng, Marilyn M.
Holtby, Richard M.
Hopyan, Sevan
Howard, Andrew W.
Hunter, Gordon A.
Jenkinson, Richard J.
Kliman, Michael E.
Kraemer, William J.
Kreder, Hans J.
Kumar, Ashesh
Kuzyk, Paul R T.
Langer, Frederick
Lansang, Edward P.
Lau, Johnny T.
Leitch, K. Kellie
Lewis, Stephen J.
Lexier, Reuven R.
Lloyd, Geoffrey J.
Mahmoudi, Ali
Mahomed, Nizar N.
Malcolm, Barry
Marks, Paul H.
Marshall, K. Wayne
Mastrogiacomo, Frank F.
Mayich, D. Joshua
McKee, Michael D.
Murnaghan, John J.
Murnaghan, Michael L.
Nam, Diane
Narayanan, Gopalakrishnan
Nauth, Aaron
Nguyen, Duong H.
Nousiainen, Markku T.
Oda, Ninos M.
Ogilvie-Harris, Darrell J.
Okusanya, Olanrewaju O.
Qamirani, Erion
Rampersaud, Yoga R.
Richards, Robin R.
Riedel, Kelly D.
Safir, Oleg A.
Schatzker, Joseph
Schemitsch, Emil H.
Sernik, Julian B.
Sharma, Om Prakash
Silverstein, Ezra A.
Singer, Syndie B.
Slobogean, Myron G P.
Stephen, David J G.
Syed, Khalid A.
Theodoropoulos, John S.
Tile, Marvin
Tom-Pack, Maurice
Truong, Walter
Veillette, Christian J H.
Vincent, George M F.
Von Schroeder, Herbert P.
Waddell, James P.
Wadey, Veronica M R.
Walton, Christine C.
Wasserstein, David N.
Wedge, John H.
Weiler, Peter J.
Whelan, Daniel B.
Wiley, Alan M.
Wood, Michael R.
Wright, C. Stewart
Wright, James G.
Wright, Thomas A.
Wunder, Jay S.
Yardley, Nicholas J.
Yee, Albert J M.
Zarnett, Mark E R.
Zeller, Reinhard D.

WATERLOO
Chris, Anthony D.
Stevens, David G.

WELLAND
Rakem, Jamal A M H.
Rittenhouse, Bryan R.
Song, John Y.

WHITBY
Ali, Abdulhafid O.

WINDSOR
Annisette, Garth K M.
Bartol, Stephen W.
Elashaal, Abdelrahman A B.
Fleming, Dana A.
Jasey, Gregory S.
Koppert, George J.
Lopez, Christopher J.
McCaffrey, Michael C.
Pepin, John W.
Yousif, Thair H.
Yovanovich, Robert M.

WOODSTOCK
Ahmer, Abubaker A.
Bigham, Aaron T.
Kruger, Gordon D.
Reid, Robert L.
Xenoyannis, George L.

PRINCE EDWARD ISLAND

CHARLOTTETOWN
Campbell, Gordon S.
Campbell, John
Miller, Stephen
Profitt, Allen W.
Wotherspoon, Scott D M.

QUÉBEC

ALMA
Cantin, Simon
Gimael, Jean-Francois
Harvey, Guy
Laprise, Benoit
Tremblay, Marc-Andre

AMOS
Adam, Robert A.
Aubin, Mario
Beauregard, Edith
Bellemare, Louis

BOIS-DES-FILION
Rizkallah, Rizkallah

BROSSARD
Lambert, David C.

CHANDLER
Larocque, Martine

CHATEAUGUAY
Bissonnette, Guillaume
Browman, Catherine
Levesque, Jean-Marc
Moise, Paul

CHICOUTIMI
Allard, Jean-Pascale
Belanger, Louis R.
Boivin, Eric
Lefebvre, Francois
Lemieux, Remy
Seguin, Bernard

COWANSVILLE
Bruneau, Nathalie
Duval, Pierre
Leclerc, Etienne

DOLLARD DES ORMEAUX
Coughlin, Larry P.

DRUMMONDVILLE
Camire, Michel
Dorion, Martin
Sinclair, Karine
Turgeon, Jean-Martin

GASPE
Jean, Gabriel

GATINEAU
Carter, Christopher J.
Gaspard, Henry S.
Matar, Wadih Y.
Morin, Andre J.
Papadopoulos, Platon V K.
Richards, Corey J.
Therriault, Natalie
Varin, Jean R.

GRANBY
Arsenault, Francois
Rodrigue, Luc
Younes, Chahine

GREENFIELD PARK
Germain, Michel M.
Loranger, Christian

KIRKLAND
Jones, Pamela L.
Ortaaslan, Sevan G.

LAVAL
Bah, Chaikou
Baillargeon, David
Bertrand, Pierre
Dahan, Philippe
Guimond-Simard, Sebastien
Hamel, Nathalie
Kouncar, Nathalie
Lemieux, Real
Masri, Khalil
Quiniou, Alain-Andre
Renaud, Eric G.
Roy, Louis
Thiffault, Gilbert
Toueg, Jacques

LEMOYNE
Desautels, Charles
Desloges, Danielle
Desnoyers, Jacques
Ferron, Serge
Fournier, Karl
Gravel, Charles A.
Mac, Thien Vu
Nguyen, Hai

LEVIS
Angers, Yves
Begin, Jean-Francois
Ferland, Yves
Giguere, Michel
Lacoursiere, Jean-Pierre
Laflamme, Denis
Lapointe, Pierre
Lessard, Pierre
Mercier, Denis

LONGUEUIL
Bamdadian, Farshid
Chafai, Parviz
Co, Thanh Ngoc C.
Fraser, Myriam
Megarbane, Farid
Sutton, John R.
Valeriote, Josee

MANIWAKI
Perron, Odette

MARIA
Leblond, Christian
Mercier, Simon
Rouleau, Claude

MATANE
Nault, Theodore

MONTMAGNY
Belanger, Jean-Philippe
Garneau, Daniel
Potvin, Jean

MONTREAL
Amiot, Louis-Philippe
Antoniou, John
Beauchamp, Marc
Beaumont, Pierre
Benaroch, Thierry E.
Benoit, Benoit
Bergeron, Stephane
Berry, Gregory K.
Besner, Louis
Blanchette, David
Boubez, Ghassan
Brooks, Caleb E.
Burman, Mark L.
Cantin, Marie-Andree
Chaytor, E. Ruth
Dehnade, Faramarze
Des Marchais, Jacques E.
Dimentberg, Ronald A.
Duhaime, Maurice
Dupuis, Pierre R.
Duquette, Maurice
Fallaha, Michel
Fassier, Francois
Fernandes, Julio C.
Fisher, William D.
Gagnon, Sylvain
Gaudelli, Cinzia A.
Gdalevitch, Marie
Glavas, Panagiotis
Godbout, Veronique
Godin, Claude
Goulet, Marc
Grimard, Guy
Grondin, Philippe P.
Hamdy, Reggie C A.
Han, Yung
Harvey, Edward J.
Heron, Timothy A.
Huk, Olga L.
Isler, Marc H.
Jacques, Ulrick
Janelle, Chantal
Jarzem, Peter F.
Jodoin, Alain
Johansson, Joyce E.
Labelle, Hubert B.
Laflamme, George-Yves
Laflamme, Georges
Lavigne, Martin
Lavigne, Patrick
Lavoie, Frederic
Leduc, Stephane
Lenczner, Eric M.
Levesque, Martine
Lichtblau, Ethan
Lincoln, Lawrence
Mac-Thiong, Jean-Marc
Major, Pierre
Malo, Michel
Marcoux, Luc
Marien, Robert J.
Martineau, Paul A.
Masse, Vincent
Maurais, Gilles
Morelli, Moreno
Mottard, Sophie
Newman, Nicholas M.
Nguyen, Tuan Khoan
Ouellet, Jean-Albert
Parent, Stefan
Perreault, Andre
Pilon, Luc
Poitras, Benoit P.
Racine, Luc
Ranger, Pierre
Reindl, Rudolf
Rivard, Charles H.
Rosen, Leonard
Rouleau, Dominique
Roy, Alain
Sabouret, Pierre J J.
Saidi, Kaveh
Saran, Neil
Sepehr-Arae, Arash
Sioufi, Georges
Stanciu, Constantin
Stephenson, Paul K.
Sullivan, James D.
Talbot, Maxime
Tanzer, Michael
Tetreault, Patrice
Tremblay, Gilles R.
Turcotte, Robert
Vendittoli, Pascal-Andre
Volesky, Monika
Weber, Michael H.
Zukor, David J.

POINTE-CLAIRE
Girard, Pierrette
Knight, Richard S.
Rhodes, Michael E.
Wiltshire, David G.

QUEBEC
Angers, Michele
Arteau, Annie
Bedard, Anne-Marie
Bedard, Luc
Bedard, Martin
Belzile, Etienne
Belzile, Sylvain
Blanchet, Michel
Blanchette, Michel-Henri
Boivin, Jules
Bouchard, Henri-Louis
Bouchard, Marc
Cloutier, Rejean
Denault, Alexandre
Dion, Norbert

Du Tremblay, Pierre
Dufour, Marcel
Fradet, Jean-Francois
Gallien, Roger
Garneau, Jacques
Kinnard, Patrick R G.
Lacasse, Bernard
Laflamme, Melissa
Laliberte, Bernard
Lamontagne, Jean
Latour, Marc-Andre
Lavallee, Pierre
Leclerc, Alexandre
Lemire, Luc
Lepine, Jean-Marc
Lesieur, Martin
Lirette, Richard
Marquis, Francois
Mercier, Pierre
Montminy, Patrice
Morin, Francois
Nadeau, Paul O.
Paradis, Gaston R.
Petitclerc, Luc
Roger, Marie-Eve
Roy, Jean-Francois
St-Cyr, Yvan

RIMOUSKI
Asselin, Clement
Bachand, Stephane
Bouchard, Ludovic
Dugas, Luc-Antoine
Gendron, Tina-Louise
Genest, Mathieu
Hudon, Claude
Masse, Nicholas

RIVIERE-DU-LOUP
Cojocaru, Andre N.
Cournoyer, Jean C J.
Dudon, Emmanuelle M J.
Perreault, Rene

ROBERVAL
Abinader, Naji
De La Huerta, Francois

SAINT-EUSTACHE
Greenfield, Garry
Jacob-Goudreau, Philippe
Vezina, Pascale

SAINT-GEORGES
Arsenault, Sarto
Beaudoin, Simon
Durand, Sebastien
Gagnon, Serge
Rodrigue, Jean-Philippe
Vachon, Pierre

SAINT-HYACINTHE
Daigle, Michel
Dionne, Julien
Pouliot, Catherine
Roy, Louis J.

SAINT-JEROME
Alami, Ghassan
Carrier, Mathieu
Farmer, Carl
Makinen, Patrice
Tasse, Michel
Tasse, Pierre
Toriz, Luis
Tran-Van, Bernard
Turcotte, Antoine
Wang, Zhi

SAINT-LEONARD
Rosman, Michael A.

SALABERRY DE VALLEYFIELD
Gaspard, Antoine

SEPT-ILES
Griffiths, Nancy
Guay, Stephane
Porlier, Jean-Paul

SHAWINIGAN
Groarke, Marie-Therese
Navarre, Pierre
Rodrigue-Vinet, Ani-Raphaelle

SHAWINIGAN-SUD
Rodrigue-Vinet, Marie-Lou

SHERBROOKE
Angers, Magalie
Balg, Frederic
Cabana, Francois
Decarie, Paul R.
Deshaies, Annie
Dumais, Rejean
Dumont, Alain
Joncas, Jean-Francois
Lamoureux, Gilles
Langlois, Gaetan
Larue, Bernard
Magalhaes-Grave, Marc-Andre
Morcos, Roger
Patenaude, Nicolas
Ricard, Stephane
St-Pierre, Michel
Theoret, Chantal
Vezina, Francois

ST CHARLES BORROMEE
Bogusz, Sharlene
Bonin, Richard
Le Bouthillier, Guy
Rousseau, Jean

ST-EUSTACHE
Clermont, Pierre-Andre

ST JEAN SUR RICHELIEU
Blanchet, Florent
Corriveau, Mario
Jodoin-Fontaine, Xavier
Lachance, Nadia
Leclerc, Georges-Edouard
Leroux, Michel
Michaud, Guillaume
Morazain, Louis
Raymond, Louis-David
Viens, Hugo

TERREBONNE
Desjardins, Andre L.
Duchesne, Robert
Girard, Bruno
Grenier, Stefanie
Simion, Teodor
Tanguay, Frederic

THETFORD MINES
Dorval, Nicolas
Dumont, Luc
Miville-Deschenes, Marc

TROIS-RIVIERES
Antoniades, Marc
Beaulieu, Marie-Pier
Bureau, Etienne
Dafniotis, Olga
Gelinas Chaine, Karine
Giroux, Mario
Horth, Caroline
La Haye, Bruno
Milot, Martin
Page, Alain
Rheault, Louis-Serge

VERDUN
Cirkovic, Alain
Coriaty, Paul
Kornacki, Joseph B.
Massie, Dani H.
Tohme, Serge

VICTORIAVILLE
Cote, Jean-Paul
Fleury, Dominique
Fournier-Gosselin, Simon
Hould, Raymond
Lamontagne, Janie M F.
Larochelle, Pascale

VIMONT
Duval, Nicolas

WESTMOUNT
Fournier, Guy

SASKATCHEWAN

PRINCE ALBERT
Brijlall, Shashi
Martins, Sandrew

REGINA
Ailsby, Ronald L.
Alshrif, Moustfha A.
Beggs, Alan J.
De Jager, Jacobus F.
Fraser, James M.
Jones, Alan W R.
Mahmood, Tahir
Patel, Satyam R.
Reed, Jeremy G R.
Rodwan, Khaled S O.
Shawush, Mohamed F.
Silver, William A.
Sivasundaram, Ramanan

SASKATOON
Allen, Lauren A.
Beavis, R. Coleson
Dust, William N.
Dzus, Anne K.
Ernst, Mark A.
Hussain, Tousief
Johnston, Geoffrey H F.
Kim, David E.
King, Anthony E.
Loback, Dwight R.
Loback, Trevor J.
McIvor, Graeme W D.
McKerrell, Jeffrey G.
Pally, Elliott M.
Rees, Huw G.
Sauder, David J.
Shannon, Robert
Taillon, Mario R.
Thiessen, Trent E.
Urmson, Andrew T.
Woo, Allan K H.
Yong-Hing, Ken Yow

Otolaryngology

ALBERTA

CALGARY
Bosch, J. Douglas
Brookes, James T.
Burke, Robert C.
Chandarana, Shamir
Chau, Justin K C.
Cho, John J W.
Dort, Joseph C.
Drummond, Derek S.
Gillis, Thomas M.
Hoshowsky, Borys O.
Huang, Ian T.
Hui, Anita K W.
Lange, Elizabeth J.
Marck, Paul A.
Matthews, T. Wayne
Mechor, Bradford D.
Park, Phillip S.
Rudmik, Lucas R.
Shandro, W G. Bud
Wagner, Garth A L.
Warshawski, S. Joseph
Yunker, Warren
Zakhary, Kristina

EDMONTON
Adamis, Jon M.
Allegretto, Michael W.
Almarzouki, Hani Z M.
Alrajhi, Yaser A M.
Ansari, Khalid
Carter, Clifford S.
Chowdhury, Ryan H.
Cote, David W J.
Di Toppa, John C.
Eksteen, Eduard C.
Harris, Jeffrey R.
Keohane, John D.
Khetani, Justin D.
Kudryk, William H.
Liu, Richard
MacNeil, S. Danielle
Morrissey, Andrew T.
O'Connell, Daniel A.
Richardson, Keith
Seemann, Robert P.
Seikaly, Hadi R.
Szudek, Jacek
Uwiera, Trina C.
Will, David R A.
Wright, Erin D.

GRANDE PRAIRIE
De La Cruz, Romelito
Wong, Kevin K M.

LETHBRIDGE
Balderston, Janet I.
Monaghan, Anthony J T.

MEDICINE HAT
Harris, Neil S.

RED DEER
Monaghan, Patrick N.
Pabbies, Arone

RED DEER COUNTY
Hjertaas, Richard J.

BRITISH COLUMBIA

ABBOTSFORD
Miller, Mark J.
Tsai, Vance C.

BURNABY
Manarey, Casey R A.
Samad, Imran

CAMPBELL RIVER
Van Rooy, Charles H.

CHILLIWACK
Steinberg, Johannes L.

COQUITLAM
Mah, Stanley M.
Smyth, Richard R J.

CRANBROOK
Cain, Ryan A.
Jewett, Lawrence C.

KAMLOOPS
Cleland, W. John D.
Kramer, David

KELOWNA
Achtem, Benjamin
Bakala, Cameron D.
Kramer, Timothy A.
Povah, W. Bruce

LANGLEY
Gill, Curtis R.
Maharaj, Mitra G.

NANAIMO
Bartlett, Clark G.
Dumper, Jamie W.

NEW WESTMINSTER
Harriman, Maureen M A.
Tsaparas, Panagiotis F.

NORTH VANCOUVER
Buonassisi, Thomas J.
David, Eytan
Diamond, Ronald C.
Smith, J. Michael H.

PENTICTON
Moshaver, Ali
Prabhu, Vilas S.
Stevens, Holly E.

PRINCE GEORGE
Filatov, Sergei

RICHMOND
Bartlett, J. Andrew
Nabi, Shahin
Wong, David L H.
Wong, Lillian

SURREY
Dickson, John M.
Kwak, John J.
Mickelson, Jon-Ivar
Mori, Tyler Y H.
Morzaria, Sanjay
Strecker, Harvey D.
Vargas, Danilo R.

TERRACE
Gheriani, Heitham A A.

TRAIL
Cook, David B.

VANCOUVER
Alandejani, Talal
Anderson, Donald W.
Blokmanis, Andris
Denton, Andrew B.
Dickson, Robert I.
Dubeta, Kenneth R.
Durham, James S.
Gillanders, David A.
Irvine, Robert A.
Janjua, Arif S.
Javer, Amin R.
Kibblewhite, Douglas J.
Kozak, Frederick K.
Lau, B. Chung
Lea, Jane
Lee, Patricia
Longridge, Neil S.
Ludemann, Jeffrey P.
Maloney, Amanda P.
Man, S S. Christopher
Mick, Paul
Mintz, Donald R.
Morrison, Murray D.
Moxham, John P.
Nunez, Desmond A.
Thong, Chee Nyok
Ummat, Sunil K.
Westerberg, Brian D.
Woodham, Jeremy D.
Younger, Ritchie A L.

VERNON
Massa, Noah

VICTORIA
Cheung, Roy L H.
Clarke, Kevin D.
Mostachfi, Omid
Noel, Fraser L.
Pathak, Irvin K.
Pieprzak, Patricia S.
Wong, Frank S H.

MANITOBA

WINNIPEG
Barker, Mark F.
Blakley, Brian W.
Chan, Laura H.
Chau, Jason K.
Duval, Lindsay A.
Fishman, Lawrence
Frohlich, Arnold M.
Gall, Richard M.
Garber, Lesley Z.
Gooi, Adrian C C.
Hochman, Jordan
Jones, Jodi L P.
Kerr, Paul D.
Leitao, Darren J.

Levin, Brenda L.
Levin, Heather A.
Meen, Eric K.
Mina, Mina M F.
Osler, Flordeliz G.
Qureshy, Kaiser A.
Sutherland, Donna E.
Varma, Amrit B.
Viallet, Norbert R J.

NEW BRUNSWICK

BATHURST
Stephenson, Marie-France
Tremblay, Guy-Luc
Yousuf, Mohammad

DIEPPE
Allard, Marie-Josee
Lemaire, David
Robichaud, Ronald

FREDERICTON
Hoyt, Benjamin J A.
Thompson, Gregory

MONCTON
Giberson, Warren G.
MacCallum, Patricia L.

SAINT JOHN
Garland, Andrea D.
Rae, Robert E.
Tees, David A.

NEWFOUNDLAND AND LABRADOR

CARBONEAR
Fowler, Robert D.

ST. JOHN'S
Batten, Tony F.
Burrage, Kenneth J.
Drover, Chris
Kirby, Simon D.
Lee, Boyd S.
Redmond, Wayne M.
Savoury, Loran W.
Smith, Thomas J.
Tibbo, Jamie J.
Tjan, Eng-Tjie

NORTHWEST TERRITORIES

YELLOWKNIFE
McArthur, Peter D.

NOVA SCOTIA

AMHERST
MacDonald, J. Gerard
Wallace, Timothy D J.

DARTMOUTH
Amoodi, Hosam A M.
Dempsey, Ian
Leblanc, Robin B.
McGrail, J. Simon
Smith, Andrew N.

HALIFAX
Aron, Margaret
Bance, Manohar L.
Brown, Timothy F E.
Corsten, P. Gerard
Hart, Robert D.
Hong, Paul
Johnson, Liane B.
Kirkpatrick, David A.
Massoud, Emad
Nasser, Joseph G.
Taylor, S. Mark
Trites, Jonathan R B.

KENTVILLE
Maltby, C. Christine
Ruddy, James

LAKESIDE
Cron, Charles C.

LOWER SACKVILLE
Balys, Richard
Walling, Keith E.

SYDNEY
Chokshi, Rashmikant G.
Curry, Philip L.
Hafidh, Maky

ONTARIO

AJAX
Huang, Henry Y.

BARRIE
Ballagh, Robert H.
Hekkenberg, Robert J.
Leung, Randy M H.
Quadri, Syed M A.
Thornley, Glenn D.

BELLEVILLE
Braig, Florian G A.
Stone, Peter C A.

BRAMPTON
Belchetz, Gregory J.
Chow, Kan-Yan
Dickson, Thomas G.
Korman, Mark J.
McClure, Douglas L.
North, Robert H.
Stewart, Craig L.

BRANTFORD
Lam, Allen K L.
Wiesenthal, Alain A.

BROCKVILLE
Robertson, Kerri D.

BURLINGTON
Batchra, Nandita
Korkis, Joseph A.
MacRae, John D C.

CAMBRIDGE
Ward, Kenneth M.

CHATHAM
Da Samy, Santhi P P.

DUNDAS
Lemckert, Ronald

EAST YORK
Chiodo, Albino

ETOBICOKE
Hacker, David C.
Sky, Kenneth
Toth, Adam A.

GUELPH
Diwan, Murtaza A.
Lin, Denny
Wellman, Mark B.

HAMILTON
Archibald, Jason D.
Grabec, Jaroslav
Gupta, Michael
Jackson, Bernard S.
Jeney, Elizabeth V M.
Korman, S. Bruce
MacLean, Jonathan A.
Menkarios, Gamil N.
Reid, Diane E.
Robertson, Donald D.
Sommer, Doron D.
Zhang, Irene

KANATA
Love, Robert B.

KINGSTON
Franklin, Jason
Hall, Stephen F.
Hollins, Russell J.
Jones, Edmund F.
MacNaughton, Donald M.
Vukovic, Ljubomir

KITCHENER
Banerjee, Avik U.
Bharadwaj, Vinod K.
Bindlish, Vinita
Cameron, Billie-Rose H.

LONDON
Agrawal, Sumit K.
Belzile, Mathieu
Fung, Irving C.
Fung, Kevin
Husein, Murad
LeBoldus, Gordon M.
MacRae, Duncan L.
MacRae, Emerson E.
Moore, Corey C.
Nichols, Anthony
Parnes, Lorne
Rotenberg, Brian W.
Roth, Kathryn E.
Ruby, Ralph R F.
Sowerby, Leigh J.
Sukerman, Sydney
Yoo, John H J.

MARKHAM
Halik, Jerry J.
Lui, Bosco T M.
Maxwell, E. Linda
Ng, Raymond H W.
Werger, Jeffrey P.

MISSISSAUGA
Beard, D. Glenn
Brandt, Michael G.
Chan, Yvonne
De Souza, Fructuoso M.
Mendelsohn, Jeffrey D.
Nazarali, Karim B.
Segall, Lorne E.
Vojvodich, Sandra M.
Wong, Joseph K.

NAPANEE
Tan, K W. Andre

NEPEAN
Matyas, Miklos

NEWMARKET
Davids, Taryn
Finkelstein, David M.
Lee, Annesse Y.
Naiberg, Jerry B.
Rival, Richard A.

NIAGARA FALLS
Caetano, Helen M.
Makerewich, Leonard A.

NORTH BAY
Prinja, Navin
Tremblay, Valerie M C.

NORTH YORK
Bonaparte, James
Chaban, Roman J.
Elahi, Mohammed
Ellis, David A F.
Goldfarb, David R.
Gooden, Everton A.
Miller, Robert B.
Morrow, Nathan J.
Ogilvie, Robert V.
Seaberg, Raewyn M.
Shah, Manish D.
Smitheringale, Alma J.

OAKVILLE
Debreceni, Andrew E.
Kolenda, Jacek
Lai, Philip
Mabini, Aimee J V.

ORILLIA
Ngo, Kenny Q P.
Price-Jones, R. Greg

OSHAWA
Ho, Ru-Chie
Kassel, Robert N.
Siomra, Stephen W.

OTTAWA
Antoniak, Gregory P.
Bromwich, Matthew A.
Brownrigg, Peter J.
Corsten, Martin J.
Gerin-Lajoie, Jean
Girard, Lynne
Guay, Benoit
Henry, Eric L.
Kherani, Safeena
Kilty, Shaun J.
Lamothe, J P. Andre
MacCormick, Johnna A.
Macdonald, Kristian I.
Marsan, Joseph G.
McLean, Laurie E.
Murphy, Patrick G.
Odell, Michael J.
Odell, Paul F.
Planet, Jean-Francois
Scherer, Nita
Schramm, David R.
Shahnavaz, Shahryar-Ali
Souaid, Jean-Pierre
Vaccani, Jean-Philippe
Young, John G.

OWEN SOUND
Akyurekli, Deniz
Marsh, Alexander S.
McKenna, Joseph M.

PEMBROKE
Jones, Jeffery B.

PETERBOROUGH
Conlin, Anne
Fagan, John
Fuoco, Gabriel G C.
Hamilton, Scott
Minet, Wyatt W.
Rumball, William G.
Sewchand, Kenneth

PICKERING
Asgarali, Saied

RICHMOND HILL
Kaul, William H.
Lee, Ambrose W M.

SARNIA
Hynes, Brian P.

SAULT STE MARIE
Micomonaco, Damian C.

SCARBOROUGH
Anand, Sumeet M.
Brown, Deron J.
Chang, Michael B.
Crotin, Abraham M.
Kou, Brenda S H M.
Marcarian, Berge
Minz, Lorna B H.
Mounsey, Robert A.
Naiberg, David
Shahin, Jack
Tatham, Robert B.

ST CATHARINES
Amin, Sushma
Lo, Shirley M H.
Robichaud, Jeffrey M.

ST THOMAS
Fetterly, Alexander C.
Hanson, Wayne G.

STRATFORD
Hughes, Brian D.
Scott, F G. Ellis

STRATHROY
Raymond, Marc R.

SUDBURY
Filippone, Daniela G S.
Ishak, Fadel A.
Robinson, Marie-Brigitte
Szeto, Christopher C.

THORNHILL
Guirgis, Hany
Kane, Nolan P.
Solomon, Philip R.

THUNDER BAY
Abdel-Hamid, M. Nabile
Turner, Andrew J.

TIMMINS
Ethier, Jean-Luc

TORONTO
Adamson, Peter A.
Al-Saffar, Hussain A A.
Anderson, Jennifer A.
Asaria, Jamil
Atlas, Jason T.
Brown, Dale H.
Campisi, Paolo
Castillo, Guillermo I.
Chapnik, Jerry S.
Chen, Joseph M.
Conrad, Krzysztof
Cushing, Sharon
Davidson, M. Jean
El Masri, William S.
Enepekides, Danny J.
Fenton, Ronald S.
Forte, Vito
Fox, Rick
Freeman, Jeremy L.
Friedberg, Jacob
Gantous, Andres
Gevorgyan, Artur
Gilbert, Ralph W.
Goldstein, David P.
Gullane, Patrick J.
Haight, James S J.
Hands, Brian W.
Hawke, W. Michael
Hay, Marshall A.
Higgins, Kevin
Holler, Theresa A M.
Irish, Jonathan C.
Johnson-Obaseki, Stephanie E.
Josephson, Robert L.
Katyal, Anil
Lee, John
Lin, Vincent Y.
MacNab, Timothy I.
McIntosh, Frederick E A.
Michell, Marcus J.
Middleton, William G.
Morong, Sharon E.
Nedzelski, Julian M.
Noyek, Arnold M.
Papsin, Blake C.
Propst, Evan J.
Punthakee, Xerxes D.
Rutka, John A.
Smith, Oakley D.
Tarshis, Lorne M.
Torgerson, Cory S.
Vescan, Allan D.
Wade, Phillip S.
Witterick, Ian J.
Zirkle, Molly S.

TRENTON
Lee, John Y H.

VAUGHAN
Chauhan, Nitin

WATERLOO
Prudencio, Jose A.

SPECIALISTS BY PROVINCE

WELLAND
Nussbaum, Marvin A.
Tang, Alan C.

WHITBY
Bravo, Francisco

WINDSOR
Abdallah, Omar E M.
Brisson, Dennis A T.
Dwyer, Joseph G.
Elbreki, Mustafa M.
Hilal, Ali Abbas M.
Lan, Robert H M.
Ling, Francis T K.
Tietze, Linda

WOODBRIDGE
Oh, Alfred Y G.

WOODSTOCK
Jeremic, Goran

YORK
Toran, Victor A.

PRINCE EDWARD ISLAND

CHARLOTTETOWN
Fong, Michael W M.

SUMMERSIDE
Campos, Alfredo

QUÉBEC

AMOS
Levesque, Daniel

BAIE-COMEAU
El Gandli, Daw Saad

CHATEAUGUAY
Larose, Pierre-Philippe

CHICOUTIMI
Harvey, Michel
Lavoie, Janie
Lavoie, Raynald
Moisescu, Razvan

COTE SAINT-LUC
Shapiro, Robert S.

COWANSVILLE
Abourjaili, Radwan

DRUMMONDVILLE
Bathalon, Sebastien
Darveau, Simon
Drolet, Richard
Nappert, Catherine

GASPE
Savage, Marie-Claude

GATINEAU
Boucher, Carl
Caouette, Richard
Dionne, Renee
Doepner, Michael
Lalonde, Michel
Monette, Luc

GRANBY
Horth, Marie-Christine
Larivee, Yanick

GREENFIELD PARK
Charbonneau, Nicolas

LACHINE
Abboud, Samir

LAVAL
Belanger, Claude
Bilodeau, Eric
Boutin, Guy R.
Landry, Ivan
Morin, Christian G.
Trinh, Ba-Truc
Yoskovitch, Adi

LEVIS
Drolet, Isabelle
Labbe, Caroline
Langis, Denis
Sevigny, Bernard
Sfriso, Anna

LONGUEUIL
Bissada, Eric
Charlin, Bernard D.
Deschamps, Nicole
Dupuis, Paule
Guertin, Louis
Haikal, Youssef
Laferriere, Jacques
Larochelle, Daniel
Spenard, Jean-Raymond
Tropper, J R. Guy

MARIA
Dagher, Chady

MONT-ROYAL
Lavigne, Francois G.
Samaha, Mark
Ste-Marie, Pierre

MONTMAGNY
Caouette, Helene
Gregoire, Danielle

MONTREAL
Abboud, Olivier
Abela, Anthony
Abou Chacra, Zahi
Arcand, Pierre H.
Ayad, Tareck
Bertrand, Robert A.
Black, Martin J.
Chagnon, Francoise
Christopoulos, Apostolos
Daniel, Sam J.
Desnoyers, Lyne
Desrosiers, Martin
Dufour, Jean-Jacques
Finesilver, Allan M.
Forest, Veronique I.
Forget, Guy
Fradette, Clermont
Frenkiel, Saul
Gaudreault, Lynn
Gauze, Joseph
Giguere, Chantal M.
Hier, Michael
Ho, Suzanne
Katsarkas, Athanasios
Keyserlingk, R.. John R.
Korban, Nadim
Kost, Karen M.
Lacroix, Yolene
Lapointe, Annie
Lessard, M. Lucie
Manoukian, John J V.
Marceau, Michel
Mlynarek, Marcin A.
Nagi, Mohamed M.
Ngo, Hieu-Hanh
Nguyen, C L. Remy
Nguyen, Ha-Nam P.
Novick, William H.
Payne, Richard J.
Peloquin, Louis
Pham-Dang, Huong
Poulin, Mark D.
Quintal, Marie-Claude
Rappaport, Jamie M.
Rothstein, Jack
Saliba, Issam
Schloss, Melvin D.
Sejean, Georges
Sicard, Fernand
Sidani, Zouhair
Sierra-Dupont, Sergio
Sweet Jr, Robert C G.
Tabet, Jean-Claude
Tarantino, Leopold
Tewfik, Marc A.
Tewfik, Tewfik L.
Trinh, Nathalie
Vo-Doan, Kim-Loan
Vu, Thien Tuong V.
Young, Jonathan
Zeitouni, Anthony G.

MONTREAL-NORD
Ahmarani, Christian
Clairoux, Marc I.
Olivier, Marie-Jo
Rahal, Akram

NOTRE DAME DU PORTAGE
Roussel, Guy

POINTE-CLAIRE
Belisle, Gilles-Michel
Lafleur, J. Richard
Le Bel, Roger E.

QUEBEC
Audet, Nathalie
Beaudoin, Danielle
Boisvert, Pierre
Bussieres, Richard
Camire, Marcel
Corriveau, Marie-Noelle
Cote, Mathieu
Demers, Georges
Ferland, Renald
Ferron, Pierre
Fournier, Jacques
Fradet, Gaetan
Gagnon, Simon
Giguere, Paul
Harbour, Jacques
Lachance, Sophie
Leclerc, Jacques-Ernest
Marin, Patrick
Nadeau, Sylvie
Parent, Francois
Philippon, Daniel
Pouliot, Denis
Rouillard, Roger
Savard, Patrick
St-Pierre, Sylvain
Thuot, Francois J L.
Vezina, Jean-Philippe

RIMOUSKI
Desjardins, Gilles
Gauthier, Marie-Sophie
Marion, Andre

RIVIERE-DU-LOUP
Cote, Andre

ROBERVAL
Bouchard, Caroline
Dufresne, Diane
Morin, Pascal

ROUYN-NORANDA
Moukheiber, Alain

SAINT-CONSTANT
Durr, Dory G.

SAINT-GEORGES
Carrier, Isabelle
Lachance, Marianne
Lemelin, Michel J R.

SAINT-HYACINTHE
Brown, Erik D.
Conti, Sylvain
Cormier, Chantale
Kim, Julie
Wurtele, Paul

SAINT-JEROME
Allaire, Denis
Dorion, Michel
Granger, Jean
Helie, Frederic
Lanoie, Marie-Claude
Roberge, Stephane
Tardif, Jacques

SAINT-LAURENT
Alami, Ziad

SAINT-LEONARD
Lemire, Anouc

SALABERRY DE VALLEYFIELD
Guilbeault, Julie
Kiwan, Emile

SEPT-ILES
Guevremont, Pierre

SHAWINIGAN
Arteau-Gauthier, Isabelle

SHAWINIGAN-SUD
Dufour, Georges
Fortin, Michel R.
Tremblay, Sylvie S.

SHERBROOKE
Dorion, Dominique
Fortier, Pierre-Hugues
Gervais, Mireille
Grenier, Jean-Paul
Paradis, Serge J.
Rouleau, Michel O.
Savage, Julian
Tardif, Sylvie
Tremblay, Chantal

SOREL-TRACY
St-Pierre, Raymond

ST CHARLES BORROMEE
Bilodeau, Gilles
Desrochers, Pascal
Desrosiers, Sophie
Gauthier, Pierre
Lemlin, Pierre

ST-EUSTACHE
Amar, Yannick G.

ST JEAN SUR RICHELIEU
Cataphard, Isabelle
Fournier, Andre
Hilareguy, Natacha
Leroux, Jean-Francois

TERREBONNE
Cerat, Jean
Martinez, Jose A.
Sarrazin, Janik G.

THETFORD MINES
Carignan, Marisol
Chabot, Magda
Nguyen, N. Vinh-Thuy

TROIS-RIVIERES
Kirouac, Jacques
Larouche, Andre
Nadeau, Claude

VAL-D'OR
Sarrazin, Janik G.

VERDUN
Cloutier, Jean-Francois
Iordanescu, Vlad
Picard, Lyne

VICTORIAVILLE
Bernier, Linda
Brousseau, Valerie J.
Ouellet, Yves
Rouillard, Gervais

WESTMOUNT
Fanous, Nabil E.

SASKATCHEWAN

LLOYDMINSTER
Mohamed, Mohamed A.

REGINA
Fritz, James R.
Ogrady, Mark J.

SASKATOON
Franke, Gordon
Gore-Hickman, Patrick O.
Mia, Mahomed
Shoman, Nael M.
Spafford, Peter D.
Wright, W D. Grant

Pediatric Cardiology

ALBERTA

CALGARY
Harder, Joyce A R.

BRITISH COLUMBIA

VANCOUVER
Duncan, Walter
Sandor, George G S.
Tipple, Marion A.

MANITOBA

WINNIPEG
Soni, Nandini R.

NEWFOUNDLAND AND LABRADOR

ST. JOHN'S
Shah, Suryakant K.

NOVA SCOTIA

HALIFAX
Chen, Robert P.
Finley, John P.

ONTARIO

TORONTO
Gross, Gil
Lee, Kyong-Jin

QUÉBEC

MONTREAL
Van Doesburg, Nicolaas H.

Pediatric General Surgery

ALBERTA

CALGARY
Beaudry, P. Paul
Brindle, Mary E.
Eccles, Robin C.
Rubin, Steven Z.

Sigalet, David L.
Taqi, Esmaeel
Wong, Andrew L.

EDMONTON
Bratu, Ioana
Dicken, Bryan J.
Evans, Mark
Lees, Gordon

BRITISH COLUMBIA

VANCOUVER
Blair, Geoffrey K.
Butterworth, Sonia A.
Mills, Jessica L A.
Skarsgard, Erik D.
Webber, Eric M.

VICTORIA
Golonka, Naomi R.
Hayashi, Allen H.

MANITOBA

WINNIPEG
Hancock, Betty
Lum Min, Suyin A.
Milbrandt, Kristopher G.
Morris, Melanie I.
Wiseman, Nathan E.

NEWFOUNDLAND AND LABRADOR

ST. JOHN'S
Akhtar, Javed
Hodder, Andre
Price, David I.

NOVA SCOTIA

HALIFAX
Brisseau, Guy F.
Giacomantonio, J. Michael
Yanchar, Natalie L.

ONTARIO

HAMILTON
Al-Harbi, Khalid E A.
Bailey, Karen A.
Cameron, Brian H.
Fitzgerald, Peter G.
Flageole, Helene
Walton, J. Mark

KINGSTON
Winthrop, Andrea L.

LONDON
Butter, Andreana M.
Jones, Sarah A.
Merritt, Neil
Scott, Leslie A.

NORTH YORK
Taylor, William H.

OTTAWA
Bass, Juan A.
Chou, Shirley H Y.
Cowan, Kyle N.
Nasr, Ahmed L.

TORONTO
Azzie, Georges R.
Chiu, Priscilla P L.
Fecteau, Annie H.
Himidan, Sharifa A.
Langer, Jacob C.
Wales, Paul W.

QUÉBEC

DRUMMONDVILLE
Chapdelaine, Joyaube

MONTREAL
Aspirot, Ann
Baird, Robert
Beaunoyer, Mona
Bouchard, Sarah
Emil, Sherif G S.
Laberge, Jean-Martin
Lallier, Michel
Poenaru, Dan
Puligandla, Pramod S.
Saint-Vil, Dickens
Shaw, Kenneth S.
Youssef, Sami A.

QUEBEC
Leclerc, Suzanne G.
Prasil, Pascale

SHERBROOKE
Mayer, Sandeep K.
Paris, Catherine

SASKATCHEWAN

SASKATOON
Awan, Saeed-Ur-Rehman
Miller, Grant G.

Pediatrics

ALBERTA

CALGARY
Aitken, Susan E.
Akierman, Albert R.
Al Wassia, Haydi
Al-Ghaithi, Ibrahim S M.
Al-Shaibani, Wifaq
Amin, Harish J.
Anderson, Ronald A.
Andrews, Christopher W.
Angeles, Hilda A N.
Anselmo, Mark A.
Arasu, Mala
Bailey, Michelle J A.
Bannister, Susan L.
Barnard, Chantelle B.
Belanger, Francois P H.
Bendiak, Glenda N.
Bjornson, Candice L.
Bjornson, Michele E.
Blackwood, Jaime S.
Boctor, Dana L.
Bond, Rachel L.
Boulton, Jill E.
Bowen, Thomas J.
Brenner, Jennifer L.
Burgess, Gavin
Burkholder, Shauna C.
Butzner, J. Decker
Cardwell, Starr E M.
Chan, Nathaniel I.
Chaulk, David C.
Chawla, Rupesh
Cheng, Adam M.
Cheuk, Stephen T.
Chow, Gary C H.
Chung, Seen Taek
Clark, Deborah J.
Clarke, Margaret E.
Clegg, Robin L.
Cooke, Suzette R.
Cooper, Neil D J.
Culman, Kate N.
D'Mello, Jennifer
Davies, Laura M.
Dawrant, Jonathan M.
DeBruyn, Jennifer C C.
Dei-Baning, Alfred
Dibartolo-King, Marielena L.
Dicke, Franciscus
Donsky, Allan
Drews, Tanya
Elliott, April S.
Eustace, Dominique M.
Evans, Amanda
Evashuk, Kristin
Farrelly, Geraldine A.
Ferreira, Patrick
Fisher, Julie
Forbes, Natalie K.
Fras, Mary
Freedman, Stephen
Fruitman, Deborah S.
Galbraith, Roger
Gerschman, Tommy D.
Gibbard, W. Benton
Gilfoyle, Elaine
Gilman, Cara E.
Giuffre, R. Michael
Goldade, Roxanne M.
Graham, Heather R.
Grant, Estee C.
Grant, Vincent J.
Greenway, Steven
Gross, Melissa L.
Guilcher, Gregory M T.
Guilfoyle, F. Jonathan
Hadi, Hani
Hall, Sarah A.
Hamiwka, Lorraine A.
Harabor, Andrei
Harder, Joyce A R.
Hasan, Shabih U.
Heard, Janice
Hegde, Hardally R.
Ho, Della S W.
Ho, Josephine
Howlett, Alexandra A.
Huang, Carol T L.
Jackman, Michelle L.
Jackson, Renee N M.
Jadavji, Tajdin P.
Johnson, Carey L.
Johnson, Kristen M.
Johnson, Nicole A.
Jorgenson, Keith F.
Kalny, Michele T.
Kam, Karen J.
Kao, Cham-Pion
Kardal, Lori J.
Karthikeyan, Suba
Kavadas, Fotini D.
Kellner, James D.
Kelly, Brian R.
Kendrick, Victoria L.
Kennedy, Christine D.
Khan, Aneal A.
Kirk, Valerie G.
Kodeeswaran, Tanuja
Kuhn, Susan M.
Lam, Quyen Kim.
Lam, Russell A.
Landry, Kerri L.
Landry, Marc-Antoine
Le, Doan Thuy
Leaker, Michael T.
Lemay, Jean-Francois
Lemay, Mireille D.
Lemieux, Lisa B.
Les, Jacob E.
Leung, Alexander K C.
Lever, Christopher G.
Levere, Kevin C.
Long, Lindsay C.
Loovere, Linda A.
Lowry, R. Brian
MacKenzie, Roderick M.
MacNeil, Catherine M.
MacPherson, Jennifer R.
Machida, Helen M.
Mah, Jean K.
Mahoney, Meagan E.
Markowsky, Donald G.
Martin, Steven R.
McKenzie, Leanna S.
McLeod, D. Ross
Miettunen, Paivi M H.
Mihalicz, Patrick A.
Mikrogianakis, Angelo
Millar, Kelly R.
Mitchell, Ian
Mitchell, Kathleen S.
Montgomery, Mark D.
Myers, Kimberley A.
Nelson, Danielle L.
Ng, Jane W Y.
Nieman, Peter
Nijssen-Jordan, Cheri L D.
Noseworthy, Mary E.
O'Byrne, Mary L.
Olliver, Steven B.
Pacaud, Daniele
Palmer, Darrell J.
Parsons, Simon J.
Patton, David J.
Pinzon, Jorge L.
Prieur, Beverley J.
Prince, Theodore A.
Rabi, Yacov
Racher, Laine
Rastogi, Swati
Roberts, R. Avalon
Robertson, Marli A.
Robinson, Elizabeth L.
Robson, W. Lane M.
Ross, B. Catherine
Ross, Daniel A.
Sabir, Aaliya P.
Samuel, Susan M.
Sandhu, Amonpreet K.
Sandhu, Naminder
Sarpal, Amrita
Saunders, Anne-Corinne
Schroter, Heidemarie
Scott, R. Brent
Serushago, Bazir A.
Shyleyko, Elizabeth M.
Singhal, Nalini
Smart, Katharine L.
Smith, Derrick M.
Soraisham, Amuchou S.
Sorg, Michael K.
Spicer, Sharron L.
Stang, Antonia S.
Stanzeleit, Cheri A.
Steele, J. MacGregor
Stephure, David K.
Stoian, Cristina A.
Stone, Pamela J.
Sztukowski, Izabela
Taylor, Tracy L.
Tee, James B.
Thakore, Siddharth
Thompson, Graham C.
Thomson, Margaret B.
Tierney, Anne J.
Tobler, Kathleen R.
Truong, Tony H.
Truscott, David H R.
Unwala, Hussein A.
Vanderkooi, Otto G.
Vayalumkal, Joseph
Veale, Pamela M.
Vila, J. Michael
Vomiero, Gemma F.
Vyver, Ellie E.
Wade, Andrew W.
Wainer, Stephen
Walker, Lori L.
Waterhouse, Christopher C M.
Winston, Karin Y.
Wong, Byron E.
Wright, Monique D M.
Wright, Nicola A M.
Wrobel, Iwona T.
Wu, John W Y.
Wu, Theresa F.
Yee, Wendy H.
Yeung, Alfred K.
Yeung, Douglas E.
Yow, Desiree S.

CAMROSE
Saini, Neel

CANMORE
Cooke, Kathryn J.
Redel, Lioba
Robertson, Dale F.

EDMONTON
Ackland-Snow, Julia C.
Adatia, Ian T K.
Alabbas, Abdullah E.
Alexander, Robert
Ali, Samina
Allain, Dominic
Anand, Vijay
Andersen, John C.
Anderson, Kelly B.
Andrew, Gail H.
Andrews, Debra
Angelski, Carla L.
Anton, Natalie R.
Apostol, Georgeta
Atallah, Joseph
Aziz, Khalid
Baxter, Cecilia I.
Baydala, Lola T.
Belletrutti, Mark J.
Berry, David A.
Bhambhani, Mahesh N.
Billinghurst, Lori L.
Bolster, Edwin L.
Bowman, Michael E.
Brar, Jagdeep
Bruce, Aisha A K.
Buka, Irena S.
Byrne, Paul J.
Carr, Stuart N.
Chan, Alicia K J.
Chapados, Isabelle
Chatur, Rehana
Cheung, Po-Yin
Chibuk, Thea K.
Clark, Brenda G.
Conradi, Alf G.
Couch, Robert M.
Craig, William
Curtis, Sarah J.
Danielson, Dawn A.
Dansereau, Angela
Davidson, Mark R.
Davies, Dawn
De Caen, Allan R B.
Desai, Sunil
Dhunnoo, Indra M C.
Dibden, Lionel
Dixon, Andrew C.
Dosman, Cara F.
Doughty, Paul
Dower, Nancy A.
Doyle-Chan, Wai-Kuen
Duff, Jonathan P.
Dyck, John D.
Ellsworth, Janet
Enarson, Mark
Estey, Andrea
Evered, Lisa
Fiedrich, Elsa C.
Fiorillo, Loretta
Forbes, Karen
Forgie, Sarah
Galante, Samy
Gilmour, Susan
Gonzalez, Hernan
Goulden, Keith J.
Gowrishankar, Manjula
Grewal, Simran
Grundy, Paul E.
Haqq, Andrea M.
Harley, Frances L.
Harris, Evan W.
Hartfield, Dawn
Harvey-Blankenship, Michele
Hendson, Leonora
Hornberger, Lisa
Hutchings, Robyn J.
Huynh, Hien
Islam, Bonnieca F.
Janicka, Alicja W.
Jetha, Mary M.
Joffe, Ari
Jou, Hsing
Joynt, Chloe A.
Kantoch, Michal
Kyriakides, Christine P.
Ladha, Tehseen S.
Lang, Mia E.
Lappa, Scot V.
Lee, Bonita E.

SPECIALISTS BY PROVINCE

Lee, Jacqueline A.
Lee, Kan Chee
Lee, Sze Lap.
Lemke, Robert P.
Leonard, Heather E.
Lequier, Laurance
Lewis, Melanie A.
Lidman, Per G L.
Lin, Michael C.
Lopatka, Joan E.
MacLean, Joanna E.
Mackie, Andrew S.
Majaesic, Carina M.
Malanowska, Anna J.
Malik, Anita C.
Malinowski, Ben A.
Mandhane, Piushkumar J.
Massicotte, Mary P.
Masterson, Tami
McConnell, Donald W.
McCook, Breanne T.
McGonigle, Lyle F.
McKillop, Sarah
Mian, A. Nadeem
Montgomery, Matthew R.
Morgan, Catherine J.
Moriartey, Robert R.
Obaid, Laila
Ortega, Gustavo A.
Osundwa, Vincent M.
Pabst, Henry F.
Pagano, Joseph J P.
Peliowski, Abraham
Persad, Rabindranath
Persson, Erika B.
Phillipos, Ernest Z.
Pierse, Patrick M.
Pinsk, Maury N.
Pon, Darlene C.
Qureshi, Mosarrat J.
Rabinovitch, Edward M.
Radisic, Djordje G.
Rahman, Amaly
Rajani, Hasmukhlal R.
Ramlall, A. Kumar
Reichert, Amber E.
Robertson, Charlene M T.
Robinson, Joan
Roseman, David
Rutledge, Jennifer M.
Ryerson, Lindsay M.
Salter, Elizabeth
Sim, Lois
Siu, Victoria W M.
Smith, Lesley J.
Sonnenberg, Lyn K.
Spavor, Maria L.
Stevens, Jonathan P.
Stevens, Kelly A J.
Stobart, Kent
Sukhrani, Geeta
Szymanski, Waldemar A.
Talwar, K K. Joan
Teoh, Johnny C.
Thebaud, Bernard C F.
Thomas, Daina
Toye, Jennifer M.
Tse-Chang, Alena W.
Turner, Troy W S.
Tyebkhan, Juzer M.
Van Manen, Michael A.
Vander Leek, Timothy K.
Vaudry, Wendy L A.
Vohra, Sunita
Walton, Jennifer M.
Warmington, Lise M.
Waters, Kellie L.
Watt, Man-Joe
West, Lori J.
Wilson, Beverly A.
Wincott, J. Leigh
Wong, Kan Shick
Wong, Sam Ken
Wright, Robert B.
Yager, Jerome Y.
Yiu, Verna W Y.
Zhang, Mona M.
Zuberbuhler, Peter C.
Zubi, Kalfalla M.
Zwaigenbaum, Lonnie

FORT MCMURRAY
James, Thresiamma

GRANDE PRAIRIE
Libsekal, Kebreab
Odaibo, Felix S.

LETHBRIDGE
Chan, Kerry K.
Harilal, Mayadevi
Holland, John E.

MEDICINE HAT
Foulston, Charlotte
Hak, Hendrik C.
Vaz, Gerald A.

OKOTOKS
Friesen, Frank R.
Klym, Kelleigh K A.
Redgate, Lauren M.

RED DEER
Driedger, G. Emmi
Mahood, J. Mark
McKenzie, Kyle C.
Molberg, Carey R.

SHERWOOD PARK
Ramji, Munira M.
Witmans, Manisha B.

ST. ALBERT
Abu-Sa'da, Omar S D.
Murdock, Alan I.
Paton, Thomas J.

BRITISH COLUMBIA

ABBOTSFORD
Anquist, K. Warren
Cohen, Jasmine S.
Hewes, Deborah K M.
Sorial, Mark Z.
Traverse, Lionel D B.

BURNABY
Baldwin, Gregory A.
Guralnick, Marla S.
How, Angela R.
Kee, I. Heather
Kim Sing, Malcolm
Lloyd-Jones, Philip M.
Lotocka-Reysner, Hanna
Winters, Michael J.

CAMPBELL RIVER
Lund, Mark A.
Russell, Brian F.

CHILLIWACK
Harries, Vladimira D.

COMOX
Aird, Natalie J.
Theron, Jan J H.

COQUITLAM
Kesavan, Vinod
O'Toole, John D.

DELTA
Ghufran, Shazia

DUNCAN
MacKenzie, Louisa K.

GOLDEN
Wilson, Robert W.

KAMLOOPS
Chapple, Denise L.
Davey, Allyson L.
Okano, Kyle S K.
Smith, Trent J.
Van Leeve, Karenza

KELOWNA
Appelt, Gregory
Baba, Carolyn M.
Burrows, Kim J.
Cronin, Catherine
Duncan, Mark A.
Jugnauth, Eleonora M.
Ranchod, Neelesh
Rosolowsky, Elizabeth
Slater, Jonathan D.
Storoz, Linda L.
Szombathy, Stanley P.
Warshawski, Thomas J.
Wires, Shannon M.

LANGLEY
Bamber, Karen E.
Horvath, Zoltan
Jia, Xiaoyan
Poynter, Aven J.
Tandan, Tara C A.
Ward, Glen K.

MAPLE RIDGE
Archer, John W.
Iyer, Sriram N.
Korada, Srinivasa M.

MILL BAY
Brienz, Deborah D.
Zinkiew, Kristi

NANAIMO
Arruda, Wilma G.
Bartleman, Betty P.
Cox, Kelly A K.
Francis, Michelle C.
MacDougall, Peter E.
Menard, Keith M.
Pegg, S. Jane

NELSON
Fitzsimons, Carrie L.

NEW WESTMINSTER
Al-Mudaffer, Mudaffer A.
Barlow, Amanda J.
Cieslak, Zenon
Duggan, Laura
Kalaher, Susan G.
Ou Tim, David Ou.
Sorokan, S. Todd

NORTH VANCOUVER
Critchley, David D.
Ebbeson, Regan L.
Ladki, Alena
Riley, Mark R.
Robertson, Glenn
Stock, Suzanne L.
Toma, Warda S.

PENTICTON
Gross, Katherine R.
Lannon, Karen P.

PORT ALBERNI
Hughes, Rhiannon M.
McCollister, Christopher D.

PRINCE GEORGE
Abelson, William H.
Arockiasamy, Vincent S.
Chaudhry, Tahir S.
Earl, Simon F.
Hay, Marie D.
Miller, Kirsten K.

PRINCE RUPERT
Simons, Jeffrey A.

RICHMOND
Atkinson, Victoria E.
Behrmann, Bernard A.
Gill, Balbinder S.
Louie, Heather M.
Luciuk, George H.
Luu, Kelly
Neufeld, Kelsey M.
Swartz, Erik N.

SAANICHTON
Wambera, Katherine M.

SMITHERS
Moisey, Clarence G.

SURREY
Alisharan, Robert M.
Bhui, Paramjit S.
Bhurji, Pargat S.
Chan, Ruby W Y.
Chou, Jenny W.
Greenstone, Gerrard C.
Henwick, Scott
Hirsh, Denton
Humphreys, Robert A.
Kwee, Yee-Nga Yong.
Laswick, Alison J.
Moodley, Anithadevi
Ng, Kathryn W.
Poole, Colleen E.
Prevost, Derek
Ramdhani, Hemendra B.
Ramesh, Kuppuchipalayam K.
Ruthnum, L. Poovendren
Singh, Sunira
Stritzke, Amelie I.
Tan-Dy, Cherrie R.
Van Aerde, John E E.
Venkatesh, Vugranam C.
White, Robert W.
Yousfie, Samer
Zajaczkowska-Kielska, Anna

TERRACE
Adlam, Anita

TRAIL
Ukpeh, Henry A.

VANCOUVER
Abu Aish, Mohammed
Adderley, Robert J.
Albersheim, Susan G.
Allaire, Jasmine
Amed, Shazhan
Anson, Shelagh
Antrim, Anne A.
Anzarut, Andre R.
Au, Sheila
Avinashi, Vishal
Bansal, Nina-Karen
Barker, Collin C.
Barr, Ronald G.
Baumgard, Godfrey M.
Beimers, Mary Ann
Bennett, Mary M.
Bergman, James N.
Bhanji, Nazmudin M F.
Bigg, Cristina M.
Binnie, Rosemary C.
Bjornson, Bruce H.
Bond, Mason C.
Cabral, David A.
Carroll, Allison B.
Casey, Linda M.
Chakrabarti, Santabhanu
Champagne, Sylvie
Chan, Edmond S.
Chan, Mercedes O.
Cheng, James W K.
Choi, Margaret S.
Clarke, Lorne A.
Clarke, Michelle S.
Coates, Edward G.
Cogswell, Arthur F.
Colbourne, Margaret L.
Davidson, A. George
Davies, Carolyn
De Levie, Melvin I.
Dean, John M.
Dehghani, Navid
Demos, Michelle K.
Denny, Sarah K.
Dewan, Tammie J.
Deyell, Rebecca J.
Dionne, Janis
Dix, David B.
Dmytryshyn, Amie
Doan, Quynh Huong
Dobson, Simon R M.
Druker, Jennifer
Duncan, Walter
Ebbert, Kirsten V J.
Eddy, Allison A.
Enarson, Paul J.
Erendzhinova, Ekaterina P.
Escudero, Carolina A.
Everett, Robert J.
Feng, Ann Qian
Finlay, Jane D C.
Fitzgerald, Barbara E.
Fryer, Christopher J H.
George, Shawn S.
Gilmer, Deborah
Glodjo, Armansa
Goldman, Ran D.
Graham, Jennifer M.
Grant, Elizabeth R L.
Guttman, Orlee R.
Hadad, Keyvan
Hailey, Jane
Harris, Kevin C.
Hassall, Eric
Haughton, David A.
Hedrei, Philip
Hill, Alan
Hlady, Lois J.
Horvath, Gabriela A.
Hosking, Martin C K.
Hoube, Jill S.
Huh, Linda L.
Hukin, Juliette
Human, Derek G.
Hung, Geoffrey R.
Israel, David M.
Jain, Nita
Jamal, Shelina M.
Jan, James E.
Jetha, Nasir
Junker, Anne K.
Kaikov, Yigal
Khangura, Simi
Khatchadourian, Karine
Kissoon, Niranjan
Kitson, Hilary F.
Korn, Paul M A.
Kovacs, Mark A.
Lam, Joseph M.
Langlois, Sylvie
Lavoie, Pascal
Leatherbarrow, Zoe A.
Lee-Son, Kathy K Y.
Leung, Vicki W K.
Liang, Howard S H.
Lillquist, Yolanda P.
Lipson, Alisa B.
Loock, Christine A.
Louie, Peter
Lupton, Brian A.
MacNab, Andrew J.
Mammen, Cherry
Manhas, Deepak
Marriage, Keith J.
Matsell, Douglas G.
Matsuba, Carey A.
Matsuda-Abedini, Mina
McGillivray, Barbara C.
Mendoza, Patricia M.
Metzger, Daniel L.
Mickelson, Elizabeth C R.
Miller, Anton R.
Moodley, Shreya
Morishita, Kimberley A.
Mutch, Cheryl L.
O'Donnell, Maureen E.
Oberlander, Timothy F A.
Odendal, Lisa T.
Ogborn, Malcolm R.
Osiovich, Horacio C.
Panagiotopoulos, Constadina
Parsons, Howard G.
Perreault, Christine M.
Petty, Ross E.
Phang, Min Sen
Phillips, Bruce A.
Pitfield, Alexander F.
Prisman, Larraine D.
Pritchard, Sheila L.
Radziminski, Nicole A.
Rassekh, Shahrad R.
Retallack, Jennifer E.
Roberts, Ashley D.
Rogers, Paul C J.
Roopani, Seemi H.
Rotecka, Joanna M.
Rozmus, Jacob
Rutkunas, Zita M.

SPECIALISTS BY PROVINCE

Ruzic, Svjetlana
Salvarinova-Zivkovic, Meni R.
Sanatani, Shubhayan
Sandor, George G S.
Sauve, Laura J.
Scheifele, David W.
Schreiber, Richard A.
Seear, Michael D.
Selby, Kathryn A.
Shepherd, Margaret A.
Sheps, Samuel B.
Sherlock, Rebecca L.
Siden, Harold B.
Singal, Mona
Singh, Avash J.
Smith, David F.
Smyth, John A.
Solimano, Alfonso J.
Speert, David P.
Spier, Sheldon
Stewart, Laura L.
Straatman, Lynn P.
Synnes, Anne R.
Tang, Clementine
Thiessen, Paul N.
Tiah, Ai Lin
Tipple, Marion A.
Tremblay, Sophie
Trudel, Karen
Turvey, Stuart E.
Van Den Brekel, Antoinette M.
Van Rensburg, Esias R.
Virji, Mumtaz A.
Wellington, Stephen R.
Wensley, David F.
White, Colin T.
Whitehouse, Sandra R.
Whitfield, Michael F.
Wingerin, Ruth C.
Wishart, Robert L.
Wolfe, Judith S.
Wong, Peggy P C.
Wu, John K M.
Yang, Connie L.
Yeung, Joanne P.
Yong, Collin K K.
Yong, Sharon H.
Yong, Siu-Li
Yu, Grace W.
Yu, Joyce W.
Zwicker, Kelly A.

VERNON

Cooke, Michael D.
Gingras, Michele S.
Harris, Lia C.
Snook, Jody E R.
Waida, Eiko

VICTORIA

Arbour, Laura T.
Balfour, Jennifer
Barclay, Amanda D.
Beck, Raphael
Bishop, Jeffrey M S.
Bolaria, Roxana K.
Breikss, Karlina A.
Cameron, Scott B.
Casiro, Oscar G.
Condello, Adriana S.
Gendreau-Reid, M F. Liliane
Harrison, Adele M.
Kang, Maria
Kent, Steven N.
Lunaczek-Motyka, Ewa M.
MacLeod, Patrick M J.
Manthorne, Janice L A.
Pelligra, Gustavo
Pillay, Thevanisha
Rose, Spencer G.
Sinclair, Brian G.
Stanwick, Richard S.
Taylor, Richard S.
Tulsiani, Suresh R K.
Zuin, Claudia C.

WEST VANCOUVER

Bucke, Rodney J.

MANITOBA

BRANDON

Elves, Emmett J.

SELKIRK

Smith, Robert G J.

THOMPSON

Bowes, R. Carla
Hamson, Andrew C.

WINNIPEG

Ali, Abdalla M.
Alsomali, Faisal M.
Alto, Lauri E C.
Anyadike, Ignatius O.
Baier, R. John
Becker, Allan B.
Beer, Darcy L.
Benoit, Teresa C.
Bermack, Barry A.
Birk, Patricia E.
Blampy, Janice
Booth, Frances A.
Bowman, M. Nancy
Brennan, Gerald D G.
Bullard, Jared M P.
Burzynski, Jeffrey H.
Caces, Rebecca F.
Caplan, Aubrey H.
Carson, James B.
Cham, Bonnie P.
Chan, Ming-Ka
Chan-Lui, W Y. Winifred
Chiu, Aaron
Chodirker, Bernard N.
Chudley, Albert E.
Cisneros, Nestor F.
Collison, Linda M.
Collison, Susan L.
Connor, David D.
Coombs, Jennifer M L.
Cranston, Meghan E.
Crockett, Maryanne E.
Cuvelier, Geoffrey
Dakshinamurti, Shyamala L.
Dart, Allison B.
David, Mirla F.
Deally, Carole M R.
Dean, Heather J.
Deonarine, Linda A.
Doyle, Elisabete R.
Doyle, John
Drewniak, Anna
Embree, Joanne
Fanella, Sergio T.
Feierstein, Michele E.
Ferguson, Charles A.
Fischer, Annette D.
Fleming, Fiona L.
Gerrard, Jonathan M.
Gerstner, Thomas V.
Giles, Brenda-Louise
Goldberg, Aviva M.
Goldberg, Norman A.
Goldner, Sarah
Grabowski, Janet L.
Griffin, Jennifer A.
Grimes, Ruth B.
Hamilton, Joanne M.
Hamilton, Kristin
Hanlon-Dearman, Ana C.
Hanna, Marni K.
Haresha, Abdullatif
Hildes-Ripstein, G. Elizabeth E.
Hohl, Christopher M.
Hyman, Jeffrey R.
Israels, Sara J.
Istasy, Victor F.
James, J. Marion E.
Jebamani, Samuel
Kabani, Amin M.
Kerr, Lorraine M R.
Kesselman, Murray S.
Klassen, Terry P.
Kovnats, Sylvia F.
Kumar, Aparna
Lane, Margo A.
Lazar, Matthew H.
Leung, Edward C W.
Lindsay, Deborah A.
Lipnowski, Stan
Longstaffe, Sally E A.
MacDougall, Eleanor R E.
MacDougall, Grant L.
MacKenzie, Shelagh K.
Madison, Adena M.
Magwood, Bryan D.
Margolis, Neil
Marks, Seth D.
Marles, Sandra L.
Martinez, Eddsel R.
McLeod, Jaret K.
Miller, David L.
Moddemann, Diane M.
Moffatt, Michael E K.
Moisiuk, Sharon E.
Muruve, Gabriel N.
Mustapha, Shareef F.
Narvey, Michael R.
Oen, Kiem G.
Pasterkamp, Hans
Pederson, Kristen L.
Pitt, Tracy J.
Pollock, Bradley J.
Postl, Brian
Raizen, Marilyn
Rajani, Kantilal R.
Rempel, Regina R.
Ridley, Tracy S.
Roberts, Janet R.
Robinson, Wesley K.
Rockman-Greenberg, Cheryl
Ruth, Chelsea A.
Sawyer, Scott K.
Schantz, Daryl I.
Schroeder, Maria-Louise
Schur, Natalie K.
Sellers, Elizabeth A C.
Silver, Norman A.
Silvester, Jocelyn A.
Simons, Frances E R.
Soni, Nandini R.
Stoffman, Jayson M.
Strong, James E.
Taback, Shayne P.
Tapper, Jason
Tenenbein, Milton
Teskey, Jennifer F.
Verma, Mradula R.
Veroukis, Stasa
Warda, Lynne J.
Webb, Susan M.
Wicklow, Brandy A.
Wiebe, Tannis H.
Wilkie Gilmore, Andrea
Yamsuan, Marlen C.
Yanofsky, Rochelle A.
Yung, Grant S Y.
Zetaruk, Merrilee N.

NEW BRUNSWICK

BATHURST

Ashur, Mohamed S A.
Memiche, Nejat

DIEPPE

Bernatchez, Josee
Hebert, Natacha
Leblanc, Genevieve
Leblanc, Nicole

FREDERICTON

Bulleid, Barbara A.
Doroshenko, Alexander
Kennedy, Tara J T.
Krishnaswamy, Ramaiyer
Messenger, Mark D.
Ouellette, Rachel E.

MEMRAMCOOK

Deschenes, Elaine

MIRAMICHI

Dickinson, Michael T.
Perry, Stephanie L.

MONCTON

Canning, G. Anne
Canning, Roderick O.
Carlson-Reid, Heidi M.
Leger, Gabriel R.

ROTHESAY

Alexander, Wendy J.
Schollenberg, Edmund G A.
Stewart, Wendy A.

SAINT JOHN

Gander, Sarah L G.
Lambert, Todd B.
McKenna, Marianne M.
Meek, David C.
Murphy, Anne M.
Nicholson, Marc D.
Ojah, Cecil R.
Paras, Emilyos
Sanderson, Susan R.

NEWFOUNDLAND AND LABRADOR

CORNER BROOK

Chrappa, Jarmila
Feener, Tricia A.

GANDER

Kemp, Ilse

GRAND FALLS WINDSOR

Cheriyan, Mammen

MOUNT PEARL

Muram, Bhanu P.

ST ANTHONY

Guntamukkala, Padmavathy

ST. JOHN'S

Akhtar, Yasmeen J.
Andrews, Wayne L.
Barter, Ola J.
Beck, Allon
Bowes, B. Lynette
Bridger, Natalie A.
Bridger, Tracey L.
Church, Peter C.
Cooper, Austin R.
Critch, Jeffrey N.
Crosbie, Victoria
Curtis, Joseph A.
Dancey, Paul
Doherty, Delores S.
Dominic, Anna
Downton, Geoffrey F.
Doyle, G. Tyna
Emberley, Julie
Escott, Heather
Goodyear, Lisa
Hall, Michael S.
Healey, Ara A.
Henderson, Kenneth J.
Hickey, Denise M.
Hobeika, Chaker A.
Kamra, Palinder
Kelly, C. Maeve
Kwa, Poh Gin
Martin, John H.
Morris, Robert F.
Newhook, Leigh A.
O'Brien, Colleen M.
O'Dea, Jennifer
Reid, Debbie H R.
Ryan Drover, Anne E.
Sathya, Pushpa
Scully, Mary-Frances
Shah, Suryakant K.
Smith, Mary J.
Templeton, Christina G.
Turner, Lesley A.
Vardy, Cathy L.
Vivian, Laura D.
Waheed, Shahzad B.

NORTHWEST TERRITORIES

YELLOWKNIFE

Scott, Darcy J S.

NOVA SCOTIA

ANTIGONISH

Amit, Minoli N.
Maloney, Paul A.
Ortiz-Alvarez, Oliva

DARTMOUTH

McCulloch, Donna M.
Torok, Maria T.
Webster, Susan D.

HALIFAX

Acott, Philip D.
Allen, Alexander C.
Berman, Jason N.
Bernstein, Mark L.
Black, Karen J L.
Blackie, Barbara J.
Blake, Kim
Bortolussi, Robert A.
Brna, Paula M.
Burns, Emma
Camfield, Carol S.
Camfield, Peter R.
Chen, Robert P.
Chobotuk, Tara
Crocker, John F S.
Cummings, Elizabeth A.
Dooley, Joseph M.
Dyack, Sarah
Fernandez, Conrad V.
Fraboni, Theresa
Frager, Gerri
Gatien, John G.
Goldbloom, Richard B.
Gregoire, Marie-Claude
Halperin, Scott
Hawkins, Ann E.
Holland, Joanna
Huber, Adam M.
Hughes, Daniel M.
Issekutz, Andrew C.
Issekutz, Thomas B.
Jangaard, Krista A L.
Kapur, Sandeep
Kawchuk, Janet
Lang, Bianca A.
Langley, Joanne M.
Larson, Alfhild J.
LeBlanc, John C.
MacDonald, Nora Noni E.
MacPhee, Shannon P.
Mailman, Timothy L.
Manos, Sarah H.
McLaughlin, Robyn A.
McMillan, Douglas D.
McRobert, Elizabeth A.
McTimoney, C A. Michelle
Mokashi, Arati S.
Morley, Charlotte M.
Ornstein, Amy E.
Otley, Anthony R.
Parkash, Sandhya
Pinto, Teresa
Ramsey, Suzanne E.
Rashid, Mohsin
Rex, Gregory A.
Schwartz, Stacey A.
Scott, Jeffrey W.
Shea, Sarah E.
Simpson, Charles D A.
Skidmore, David L.
Smith, Deborah J.
Soder, Christian M.
Stinson, Dora A.
Stringer, Elizabeth
Szudek, Ewa A.
Taylor, Brett W.
Top, Karina A M.
Vincer, Michael J.
Vitale, William R.

Warren, Andrew E.
Watson, Wade T A.
Whyte, Robin K.
Wong, Kenny K.
Wood, Ellen P.
Wren, Patricia L.
Yhap, Margaret C.
Young, Michael J.

KENTVILLE
Bolivar, Patricia E.
Brown, Charles A.
Davis, Heather S.
Hilliard, Jennifer
MacLeod, Alison D.
Nash, Michael B.

LUNENBURG
Yamada, Drew C.

MAHONE BAY
McNeill, Laurie K.

MUSQUODBT HBR
Rose, Heather P.

SYDNEY
Abenheimer, Martin S M.
Bird, Roderick A.
Budden, Heidi L.
Lynk, Andrew D.
Sasani, Najat

TRURO
Cox, Katharine S.
MacPherson, Marilyn P.
White, Michael L.
Williams, Tracey L.
Wornell, Philip A.

YARMOUTH
Couture, J. Dominique

ONTARIO

AJAX
Abdurrahman, Murtala B.
Aref, Karim G.
Kitai, Ian C.
Lewis, Valerie S.
Meinert, Paul C.
Odhiambo, Raphael L S.
Umamaheswaran-Maharaj, Meera
Veale, John L.

ANCASTER
Pinto, Barbara B.

BARRIE
Bartlett, Leah D.
Chen, Chee Pyn
Clark, Jessica M.
Davidson, Cara E.
Hansen, Miriam
Hazlett, Melinda M.
Hiram-Karasmanis, Rania
Ho, Vincent W G.
Kazmi, Asif A.
Kuzik, Brian A.
Osswald, Ivana G.
Sauro, Victor S.
Simms, R. Gregory
Surry, Susan A M.

BELLEVILLE
Dempsey, G. Paul
Gosse, Gordon D.
Gregoire, Keith R.
Morrison, Kristin R.
Nguyen, Tuyet Thi
Shipman, Richard R.
Vanier, Kelly L.

BOLTON
Kanwal, Tejpreet K.

BRAMPTON
Bikangaga, Peter M.
Brown, Mijin
Dwight, Prabo J.
Feanny, Stephen J.
Ghaffar, Abdul
Gill, Kulvinder K.
Gupta, Rajeev
Kao, Shawn S K.
Kawai, Susan H.
Leet, Carol A.
Luthra, Sanjeev S.
Margolis, Ivor J.
Mehra, Sunil
Mehrmanesh, Flora Z.
Menon, Anilkumar S.
Pearl, Rachel J.
Rayar, Umesh
Saund, Gagandeep K.
Selliah, Prasanna S.
Sur, Smeeksha S.
Turner-Gomes, Sophronia O.
Vaz, Simone S.
Zakhary, Gamel S.

BRANTFORD
Dost, Ismat Z.
McIntyre, Martin T J.
Padamadan, Philsamma G.
Pearson, Brooke E.
Pennie, Ross A.
Salim, Asim

BROCKVILLE
Chawla, Harmeet K.
Chawla, Harvinder K.

BURLINGTON
Cadman, David T.
Carson, Sharon K.
Federici, Guiliana M.
Ford-Jones, Anthony E A.
Gerber, Laura K.
Hughes, Frances J.
MacK, Douglas P.
Malik, Arinder K.
Murthy, Trisha R.
Neame, Peter Dion
Shalan Al-Gazi, Mohanad J.
Walker, Roxanne E.
Weisz, Janet I.

CAMBRIDGE
Glavin, Verne J.
Hua, Johnson T S.
Mantynen, Philip R.
Moyo, Margaret S.
Paikatt, Santosh C.
Rajguru, Manjulata

CHATHAM
Clowater, Julie L.
Edwards, Wendy E.
Johnston, Ian G.
Tithecott, Gary A.

CORNWALL
Kirtsman, Irina
Nchama, M. Dokiso
Roumeliotis, Paul
Wickramasinghe, Senani D.

DELAWARE
Poonai, Naveen P C.

DELHI
Norton, Seamus

DUNDAS
Calvert, Chrystella K.
Seigel, Sandra A.
Steele, Brian T.

EAST YORK
De Veber, Hilary R H.
Hanley, William B.
Miller, Charlotte D.
Papadopoulos, Anastasios S.

ETOBICOKE
Al-Hashmi, Ibrahim M M.
Bishay, Azhar
Calpin, Carolyn
Chattergoon, Dhurbassa S.
Contreras, Carlos E.
Dorey, J. Michael
Fung, Kee-Wai
George, Sabine R.
Ginzberg, Hedy H.
Grad, Elliott
Harrington, Leah D.
Ho, Philip C.
Lau, Robert C.
Manson, Peter
McLauchlin, Michelle S.
Miller, Annette F.
Moodie, Rosemary G.
Smiltnieks, Barbara M A.
Vaz, Camila M.
Wong, Peter D.
Zakhary, Liliane H.

FENWICK
Rau, Sabnavis M.

FORT ERIE
Makken, Hilda A.

GRIMSBY
Nwebube, Anne O.

GUELPH
Afadapa-Ipaye, Morenike A.
Hoegler, Kathy A.
Laszlo, Theodore A.
Loy Son, Glenn
Naidoo, Balakrishna P.
Promnitz, Michael
Shethwala, Nahid K.

HAMILTON
Abdurrahman, Zainab B.
Arora, Steven K.
Athale, Uma H.
Ayad, Misaa M S.
Baird, J. Burke
Bassilious, Ereny
Breakey, Vicky
Brill, Herbert
Canisius, Elisabeth M.
Carter, Teresa A.
Cellucci, Tanya
Chan, Anthony K C.
Cheung, Wendy H.
Chitayat, Samara G.
Choong, Karen
Conner, William T.
Crocco, Anthony G.
Cupido, Cynthia
D'Souza, Sudhir J A.
Dent, Peter
Doyle, Marijane
Dutta, Sourabh
Ernst, Caroline
Findlay, Sheri
Fitzpatrick, Kelly P.
Fusch, Christoph
Gambarotto, Kathryn R.
Giglia, Lucia G.
Gilleland, Jonathan C.
Goldfarb, David M.
Grant, Christina
Harman, Karen E.
Horwood, Sargent P.
Hotz, Harry
Hunter, Andrea J.
Issenman, Robert
Johnson, Kassia J.
Johnson, Natasha I.
Kam, April J.
Kraus De Camargo, Olaf
Ladhani, Moyez
Latchman, Andrew R.
Lim, Audrey Y.
Lloyd, Robert J.
MacNay, Ramsay G.
Mahoney, William J.
Malcolmson, Charles H.
Marrin, Michael L.
Marshall, Daniel R.
McAssey, Karen L.
Meaney, Brandon F.
Mesterman, Ronit
Modi, Anjana
Mondal, Tapas
Morrison, Katherine M.
Ngo, Quang
Niec, Anne
Nolan, Kathleen J.
Nowaczyk, Malgorzata J M.
O'Toole, Francis J.
Ohayon, Jason A.
Paes, Bosco A.
Parker, Melissa J.
Pedder, Linda
Peer, Joseph
Pernica, Jeffrey M.
Portwine, Carol Ann.
Punthakee, Narsys
Purcell, Laura K.
Ramachandran, N. Rajesh
Ramji, Taheera
Ratcliffe, Elyanne M.
Rosenbaum, Peter L.
Roy, Madan M.
Saigal, Saroj
Shah, Jay K.
Shahid, Shaneela
Shbash, Iman A M.
Sherlock, Mary E.
Solh, Ziad
Somani, Arif
Sulowski, Christopher A.
Thomas, Sumesh P.
Thompson, Penelope J.
Twiss, Jennifer E.
Vandermeulen, John A.
Wahi, Gita
Wahi, Shobha
Williams, Constance L.
Xu, Y. Sophia
Zachos, Marianthi

KANATA
Chan, Kevin C Y.
Joly, Jacqueline L.
Lee, Peter K O.

KENORA
Blydt-Hansen, Tom D.

KINGSTON
Acker, Amy E.
Clarke, Maxine C W.
Connelly, Robert J.
Dow, Kimberly E.
Flavin, Michael P.
Hefferon, Michael D.
Johannes, Christine J.
Justinich, Christopher J.
Kiruluta, Sheila M.
MacDonald, E. Athen
MacKenzie, Jennifer J.
Mehlomakulu, Mtimkulu
Moore, Andrea M L.
Moorehead, Paul C.
Noble, Angela
Onyett, Heather A.
Richardson, Donald W.
Samdup, Dawa Z.
Silva, Mariana
Smith, R. Garth
Smythe, John F.
Stidham, Gregory L.
Storr, Michael
Van Wylick, Richard C.
Wherrett, Brian A.

KITCHENER
Backway, Karen L.
Cresswell, David A.
Davey, Cecile D.
Di Gravio, Bruno
Hutzal, Carolyn E.
Pineau, Linda A.
Rosner, Jodi L S.
Sichilima, Tangu
Smith, David P.
Walia, Manjit S.
Wilson, Ian M.

LONDON
Al-Selahi, Eiman M S A.
Atkinson, David I.
Atkison, Paul R.
Belda, Antonio A.
Berard, Roberta A.
Cairney, A. Elizabeth
Campbell, Craig G N.
Cheng, Anita K.
Clarson, Cheril L.
Coughlin, Kevin W.
Da Silva, Orlando P.
Filler, Guido
Forward, Karen
Foster, Jennifer R.
Fraser, Douglas D.
Frewen, Timothy C.
Frid, Pamela
Gammon, Jessica
Gibson, Paul J.
Gloor, Jane
Gorodzinsky, Fabian P.
Grimmer, Joanne
Hammerberg, Ole
Han, Victor
Helleman, Krista
Hildebrand, Kyla J.
Hussain, Asmaa S.
Jardine, Lawrence F.
Jenner, Morris
Johnston, Maureen R.
Joubert, Gary I E.
Jung, Jack H.
Kalidindi, Shiva K R.
Kenyon, Cynthia F.
Kilgar, Jennifer L.
Killorn, Erin E.
Kloth, Debra M.
Kornecki, Aleksander
Lee, David S C.
Levin, Simon
Li, Mok-Dock
Lim, Rodrick K.
Loubani, Eman M.
Lubell, Richard F.
Lynch, Timothy P.
Lyttle, Brian D B.
Manchanda, Meera
Matsui, Doreen M.
McLean, Jennifer L.
McNeely, Michael P.
McNeill, Michelle M.
Mehrotra, Shruti
Misir, Amita T R.
Mitchell, Clare E.
Mohammed, Afzal
Nanda, Sunit K.
Nasreen, Ruksana
Norozi, Kambiz
Pavri, Daisy R.
Ponti-Sgargi, Michelle G.
Prasad, Asuri
Prasad, Chitra
Price, April K.
Radhakrishnan, Dhenuka K.
Ralyea, Evan P.
Ramadan, Said
Rieder, Michael J.
Rosenberg, Herschel
Roukema, Henry W.
Rovis, Katarina
Salvadori, Marina I.
Sangha, Gurinder S.
Shaheed, Wagih K A.
Sharma, Ajay
Singh, Ram N.
Sottosanti, Maria
Stare, Liga
Stein, Robert I.
Stoffman, John M.
Van Hooren, Tamara A.
Walker, C. Robin
Warren, David W.
Wellington, Nancy E F.
Yuen, Doris E.
Zelcer, Shayna M.

MAPLE
Cellupica, Umberto
Merchant, Saba M.

MARKHAM
Cole, Mara
Ehrlich, Robert M.
Fazal, Haydarally H.
Grewal, Deepa
Haney, Isabel M M.
Khan, Shahida R.
Lee, Kevin A.
Levin, Leo
Musewe, Norman N.
Pancer, Larry B.

Sales, Valerie
Singh, Munesh C S.
Telch, Joseph
Tobin, Cathryn E.
Turlapati, Padmini N.
Wong, Helen H L.
Wong, Richard L.
Yoon, Yeung-Seu

MILTON
Khalefih, Tarek A.

MISSISSAUGA
Abdullah, Rukhsana A.
Abraham, Marilyn
Adleman, Neil L.
Ahmed, Uzma
Allen, Tara
Bai, Helen H K.
Bayliss, Patricia A.
Binnington, Melanie E.
Blanchette, Nicholas S.
Chandra, Ranjit K.
Chiavaro, Hector L.
Chlebus, Andrew
Coates, Pamela J K.
Davidson, William
Egger, Gian
Erez, Hanna J.
Farrell, Sandra A.
Folman, Raphael R.
Goldenberg, Donna A.
Gwiazda, Katarzyna M.
Hafiz, Shujauddin F.
Hamed, Azza A W M.
Healey, Jane
Hogan, Gillian M M.
Horsham, Patricia A M.
Kim, M. Marie
Lester, Michael L.
Ma, Tze Y.
MacKinnon, James A.
Makhene, Edward
Mandoff, Nedka
Mansour, Yasser M A.
Morra, Antonella
Nadarajah, Sumathi
Narikuzhy, Anna
Oman-Ganes, A. Loraine
Pachai, Indira
Patel, Kirit B.
Patel, Piyush R.
Rojnica, Lillian M.
Simone, Angelo M.
Strachan, Peter G.
Szymonowicz, Wanda M.
Taylor, Catherine Y.
Terespolsky, Deborah
Teskey, Lindsay S.
Weaver, Lana M.
Yim, Conrad C Y.
Zaazou, Mostafa A F T I.
Zajdman, Michael L.

NEPEAN
Assemi, Manutchehr
Bialik, Mark J.
Grodinsky, Stephen H.
Kardash, Sidney
Law, Barbara J.
Liddle, Jane E.
McConville, James M.
Morawska-Jablonska, Joanna
Pasquet, Eric A.
Sadana, Sumeet
Sisto, Alfred
Van Stralen, Judy P M.

NEWMARKET
Balogh, Louis
Chang, Lawrence J A.
Doherty, Colleen
Lee, Sai-Kui
Liquornik, Karen N.
Mulera, Muniini K.
Rajan, Aziza A.
Van Schaik, Charmaine S.

NIAGARA FALLS
Bhagirath, Chander P.
Donkor, Kwame L.
Elkout, Lotfia
Jackiewicz, Grazyna
Snyder, Donna A.

NORTH BAY
Ahmed, Shakeela R.
Clayton, Cheryl A.
Fazzari, Frank
Grise, Mary E.
Madden, Joseph K.
Mutch, Linsey S.

NORTH YORK
Al-Dabbagh, Muroog
Ardeshiri, Farnaz
Baine, Sherri D.
Baker, Stephen R.
Barron, Alexander C.
Bedford, H. Melanie
Berall, Glenn
Carr, Jordan P.
Cheng, Malcolm H F.
Cohen, Susan B.
Comay, Stephen A.
Dave, Malini G.
Dhillon, Jasvinder
Doctor, Shaheen S.
Donsky, Judith E.
Fazeli Chaghoshi, Leila
Feldman, Kayla S.
Filderman, Ronald B.
Fishman-Shapiro, Leona
Gallant, Lee Ann
Geft, Colin H.
Givelas, Danny
Goldfarb, Cynthia E.
Gordner, Stuart
Govan, Jairaj J.
Granovsky, Shawna
Greenwald, Mark
Grosser, Elana
Gruber, Dinah C.
Ho, Nhung T C.
Hsuen, John S C.
Hummel, David B.
Hung, Richard H.
Hutchinson, Clare M.
Jin, Edward G J.
Kagan, Rhoda S.
Kanani, Ronik
Kosoy, Martin H.
Kupfert, Beverly
Lakdawalla, Nadira F.
Lee, John Y C.
Levichek, Zinaida
Lo, Louis Y C.
Meschino, Wendy S.
Mills-Tettey, Diana B.
Milne, Janette A.
Moss, Steven M.
Munn, Robert I.
Murray, John D M.
Newman, Jack
Pape, Karen E.
Parent, Jocelyne
Patel, Neeta
Porepa, Michelle E.
Porepa, S. Joseph
Pucholt, Vladimir
Rajchgot, Percy
Sacks, Diane P G.
Schelberg, Kenneth
Segal, Audrey O.
Shu, Y W. Maggie
Siemiatycki, Deborah G.
Singh, Narendra C.
Tolkin, Jonathan B.
Velsher, Lea S.
Weizman, Samuel I.
Wise, Sheldon A.

OAKVILLE
Ansari, Zeba I.
Balakrishnan, Sadhana L.
Culbert, Erin L.
Dekna, Maisa M A.
Fathollahzadeh, Afsoon
Fox, Michael J.
Galanter, Elizabeth
Hierlihy, Lynn E.
Kathuria, Sangeet
MacDonald, Richard J.
MacGregor, Todd M.
Marrin, Andrea K.
Mistry, Silloo B.
Parameswaran, Krishanthan
Sam, Jonathan C M.

ORANGEVILLE
Murphy, Ronald G.

ORILLIA
Barker, Sarah
Colpitts, Melanie H.
Gordon, Michelle
Hudak, Alan P.
Jones-Stokreef, Nicola J.
Meeder, Robert J J.
Smith, W. Gary

ORLEANS
Bhargava, Someshwar
Joseph, Mathew B.
Tirado, Rossana M.
Wong, Eddy K K.

OSHAWA
Almadani, Mahmud H M.
Cammisuli, Salvatore
Hunt, Carolyn P.
Lai Fatt, Peter H.
Lemon-Mule, Heather F.
MacDonald, Mary R A.
Montgomery, Christopher W.
Rajah, Rashid

OTTAWA
Adams, Barrett R.
Adegbite, A. Manna
Ahmed, Ahmed A A.
Ahmed, Maheen
Ahmet, Alexandra H.
Al-Bakkal, Sahar
AlQurashi, Waleed D A.
Alnaji, Fuad S.
Amid, Ali
Audcent, Tobey A M.
Baldwin, Katherine L.
Bariciak, Erika D.
Barkey, Janice L.
Batra, Gurumukh D.
Belder, Diana
Bellemare, Steven J Y R.
Ben Fadel, Nadya M.
Benchimol, Eric I.
Bennett, Susan
Bergh, Rodney M.
Boland, Margaret P.
Bomela, Hlwelekazi N.
Bowie, Paul R.
Brill-Edwards, Michele
Brophy, Jason C.
Chacon, Danelia D.
Chadha, Uday
Chakraborty, Pranesh K.
Cook, Nathalie
Cornet, Anne M J.
Creery, W. David
Dabee, Vassant
Daboval, Thierry
Davis, Deborah J.
Dehejia, Sudha H.
Doyle, David A.
Duffy, Ciaran
Dust, Nicholas
Engel, Andre
Farhadi, Elham
Feber, Janusz
Fraser-Roberts, D. Leigh
Gardin, Letizia L.
Gerein, Richard B.
Gfeller, Kenneth F.
Ghobrial, Mahassen M.
Gillies, Anne M W.
Goldbloom, Ellen B.
Gravelle, M R. Joan
Grondin, Danielle
Gunz, Anna C.
Hadjiyannakis, Anastasia
Halton, Jacqueline M L.
Ham Pong, Antony J.
Harman, Stuart
Harrison, Megan E.
Harrold, JoAnn E.
Hillier, Linda G.
Hollinger, Shawn M.
Huang, Pein-Pein
Hui, Charles P S.
Hunter, Alasdair G W.
Issa, Kheirie
Jabbour, Mona L.
Jain, Raagini
James, William
Jaworski, Martine A.
Jetty, Radha
Jocelyn, Leslie J.
Johnston, Donna L.
Karwowska, Anna
Katz, Sherri L.
Keely, Kathryn L.
Keene, Daniel L.
Kerr, Pauline E.
King, W. James B.
Klaassen, Robert J.
Kotarba, Jan A.
Kovesi, Thomas A.
LaBerge, Robert C.
Lai, Lillian S.
Langevin, Melissa K.
Lapner, Manfred
Lau, Anita S.
Lawrence, Sarah E.
Lawrence, Sarah L.
Lawson, Margaret L.
Lee, Suzie
Leifso, Kirk R.
Lemyre, Brigitte
Lena, Sujatha M.
Leung, Elaine W Y.
Lobos, Anna-Theresa
Losier, Andrea M.
Lougheed, Jane
Luke, Koon-Hung
MacDonnell, Heather M M.
MacKenzie, Alexander E.
MacLusky, Ian B.
Mack, David R.
Macklin, G. Elizabeth
Mandel, Karen M.
McBride, Eileen R A.
McCormick, Anna M.
McGregor-Shaw, Alyson M.
McMillan, Hugh J.
McNally, James D.
Menon, Kusum
Merchant, Pradeep
Milanska, Janina
Moineau, Genevieve
Moore, Gregory P.
Morgan, Susan G M.
Murray, C. Louise
Nair, Asha
Nault, Julie R.
Nayar-Kingwell, Sunita M.
Neto, Gina M P.
Nguyen, The-Minh
Norris, Mark L.
Noseworthy, Stephen
O'Kelly, Fionnuala
Osmond, Martin H.
Palayew, Karen S.
Parker, Kristy A.
Patel, Serina V.
Pham-Huy, Anne
Pierse, Michael P.
Pitters, Carrol A.
Plint, Amy C.
Pothos, Mary
Pound, Catherine M.
Rajakumar, Derek D.
Reid, Sarah M.
Reisman, John J.
Richler, Michael E.
Ristoski, Nikolce
Saginur, Michael D.
Saleh, David S.
Sambasivan, Aarathi S.
Samiee Zafarghandy, Samira
Samson, Lindy M.
Seshadri, Angela
Shariff, Aftab M.
Shefrin, Allan E.
Simpson, Ewurabena A.
Slinger, Robert W.
Stockwell, Margaret J.
Suk, Jean C.
Tam, Ronald K H.
Tam, W S. Theresa
Tjahjadi, Anindita
Tsai, Ellen
Tsampalieros, Anne K.
Tse, Sandra T.
Tucker, Tara L.
Turner, D. Christopher
Udupa, Sharmila
Vadeboncoeur, Christina M.
Vaidyanathan, Chandraprabha
Venkateswaran, Sunita
Vethamuthu, Jennifer M.
Ward, Leanne M.
Ward, Michelle G K.
Weiler, Gabrielle S.
Whiting, Sharon E.
Williams, Robin L.
Wong, Derek T H.
Writer, Hilary K.
Zemek, Roger L.
Zucker, Marc E.

OWEN SOUND
Cato, Shani A.
Dick, Paul
Ham, Trevor J.
Porter, Ewan A.

PETERBOROUGH
Boyer, Michael E.
Comerford, Thomas A.
Hardy-Brown, Karolyn W.
Hughes, Peter L.
Jamieson, Iain C.
Loukras, Lucinda
Moradhassel, Fariedeh P.
Thain, Mary E.
White, Richard A.

PICKERING
Schwartz, Clive J.

POINT EDWARD
Rashed, Nashed

RICHMOND HILL
Andre, J. Kurt
Blustein, Norman S.
Fabbro, Julie F.
Grouhi, Masoud
Gryn, David M.
Gunawardena, S. Yamuna
Ho, Gerald C L.
Iu, Alvin C L.
Jethwa, Anita
Jevremovic, Alexandra
Kirsch, Susan E.
Levin, Martin R.
Mak, Wang-Cheong
Man, Gregory C K.
Roushdi, Amani E.
Singer, Michael O.
Smith, Eileen M.
Weisbrot, Jeffrey J.
Yamashiro, Hirotaka
Yeung, Albert

SARNIA
Lacroix, Thomas B.
Singh, Kunwar K.

SAULT STE MARIE
Burrows, David R.
Keuhl, Jonathan R.
Leung, Kevin S N.
Stevenson, Sandra J.
Zufelt, Kirk W.

SCARBOROUGH
Amarasekera, Sukeshini
Azzopardi, Peter
Beaulieu, Roland G.
Bezu, Kesete T.
Castagna, Luigi A.
Chang, Karen D.
Cherian, Alice T.
Chin, Vincent V.
Ching, Joyce C Y.
D'Cunha Rebello, Chrysal D E.
Dar, Shahnaz
Durno, Carol A.

Gamulka, Beth D.
Gan-Gaisano, Margaret C.
Gurwitz, E. Dennis
Hsieh, Tauyee
Jagdeo, Dayanand G.
Lee, Cinda B S.
Lieberman, Lani D.
Lowe, Aviva H.
Madikiza, Aggrey P.
Mo, Lup-Ho
Morzaria, Rasik N.
Neumann, Peter Z.
Noticewala, Neelam N.
Petrou, Constantine S.
Raghubir, Kushal V.
Saxena, Rahul
Shaikh, Wajid A.
Shawn, David H.
Shu, Raymond M.
Simon, Sonia H.
Solomon, Jill K.
Tattum, Leah E.
Vermaat, Jentien H.
Weinberg, Eitan
Wong, Hubert M C.
Yeung, Latifa T F.

ST CATHARINES
Brar, Parminder S.
Burger, Michael
Crysler, John G.
Dorah, Nicholas H.
McMain, Peter B.
Nash, Leslie A X.
Ogunkeye, Alarape
Pirbhai, Kalimuddin H.
Shakhatreh, Hala D S.
Szpejda, Monika A.
Zapata, Myrna B.

ST THOMAS
Ahmed, Syed T.
Bertoldi, Margaret E.
Kerr, Paul A.
Ndur, Joshua D.

STONEY CREEK
Babic, Bojana
Hallett, Kristen M.
Orovec, Natalie M.

STOUFFVILLE
Cooper, Pamela J.

STRATFORD
Blaine, Kirsten Ann.
Mitchell, Nadine C.
Montiveros, Carolina
Squires, Philip J R.
Tejpar, Shamim J.

SUDBURY
Baron, Tara
Blacklock, Elaine G.
Blayney, Marc P.
Corbeil, Chantal P.
Kumar, Gautam
Kumar, Vijay
Murray, Sean R.
Odulana-Ogundimu, Adebola O.
Pluta, Catherine J.

THORNHILL
Berzen, Alan
Freedman, John S.
Friedman, Gerald
Greenberg, Manuel S.
Kamalia, Fatima R.
Langburt, Wayne
Lavi, Sasson
Levy, Maurice
Maze, Aubrey H.
Miller, Gilbert
Sturm, Heshy
Widrich, Guy V.

THUNDER BAY
Baboolal, Ranjit T.
Bruni, Teresa
De, Nibhas
De Sa, Vincent
Derbyshire, George
Jagger, Justin
Minnes, Shir
Warkentin, Joel D.

TIMMINS
Bhatia, Sanjay
Verbeek, Johannes H.
Verbeek, Willem C.

TORONTO
Abbott, Lesleigh S.
Abu Kuwaik, Ghassan Z K.
Al Saleh, Hani Q A M.
Al-Maani, Amal S S.
Alghamdi, Mohammed
Ali, Khaled
Allen, Upton D.
Asztalos, Elizabeth D V.
Atkinson, Adelle R.
Atkinson, Celia N.
Au, Hosanna C M.
Avdic, Sanja
Baker, Jillian M.
Banerji, Anna
Banwell, Brenda L.
Barnor, Nah-Amakuma
Barozzino, Antonio
Batthish, Michelle
Bayer, Nessa A.
Beck, Carolyn E.
Belik, Jaques
Benjamin, Candice N.
Beno, Suzanne M.
Benson, Leland N.
Berger, Elizabeth D.
Bernhard, Nirit
Bernstein, Stacey E.
Bhattacharjee, Rakesh
Biggar, W. Douglas
Birken, Catherine S.
Bismilla, Zia
Bitnun, Sean A.
Blanchette, Victor S.
Bonifacio, Herbert J.
Bouffet, Eric
Boutis, Kathy
Cada, Michaela
Cameron, Bonnie J.
Campbell, Douglas M.
Carcao, Manuel
Chan, Helen S L.
Chan, Kevin J.
Cheng, Sylvia S.
Chisamore, Brian C.
Chong, Karen L.
Clarke, Joseph T R.
Coates, Allan L.
Coffey, Maitreya S.
Cohen, Eyal
Colangelo, Patricia C.
Conway, Jennifer
Coombs, Susan
Cory, Emma J.
Cummings, Marion
Curtis, Jacqueline R.
D'Alessandro, Lisa C A.
Danayan, Karoon C.
Daneman, Denis
Davy, Till
Dell, Sharon D M.
Denburg, Avram
Desai, Shalini
Desjardins, Marie-Pier
Diambomba, Yenge
Dipchand, Anne I.
Do, Anh Phuong
Donsky, Gordon
Dorenbaum, David
Driver, Katy F.
Dror, Yigal
Duic, Andrew D.
Duke, Anthony S R.
Dunn, Michael
Durie, Peter R.
El Gouhary, Enas El Gouhary
Ens, Andrea R D.
Epstein, Norman
Farber, Robert
Farine, Michelle
Feerasta, Sharmeen H.
Fehlings, Darcy
Feigenbaum, Annette S J.
Feldman, Brian M.
Feldman, Mark E.
Flanagan, Janine
Flanders, Daniel I.
Flanders, Tamar Y.
Floh, Alejandro A.
Ford-Jones, Elizabeth L.
Foster, Heather P M.
Freedman, Melvin H.
Freeman, Sloane J.
Fregonas, Claudio G.
French, Amy E.
Friedman, Jeremy N.
Gans, Marvin H.
Garfield, Hartley
Geary, Denis F.
Gelman, Tara D.
Giesinger, Regan E.
Goldbach, Morton
Goldberg, Eudice
Golding, Ian F.
Goodis, Leslie
Grant, Ronald M.
Greenberg, Mark L.
Greenberg, Saul
Griffiths, Anne-Marie
Gross, Gil
Guerguerian, Anne-Marie
Gupta, Abha A.
Gupta, Sumit
Guttmann, Astrid
Haasz, Maya
Haka-Ikse, Katerina K.
Hamilton, Jill K.
Hamilton, Robert M.
Han, Ra Kyung
Handley-Derry, Mark H.
Harvey, Elizabeth A.
Hasan, Fyeza
Haynes, Alison
Hebert, Diane
Heilbut, Michele D.
Hellmann, Jonathan
Hick, Katherine M.
Hilliard, Robert I.
Hilton, James D.
Hitzler, Johann K.
Ho, Tommy K L.
Holland, F. John
Huang, Annie A.
Huber, Joelene F H.
Hui, Anthony Y T.
Hung, Ryan M T.
Inch, Nicole G.
Ipp, Moshe M.
Irwin, Meredith S.
Islur, Jaya M.
Ito, Shinya
Jacobson, Sheila J.
Jaeggi, Edgar T.
Jagiello, Lukasz W.
Jain, Preeti
Jain, Shauna A.
James, Andrew G.
James, J. Walter
Jean-St-Michel, Emilie M.
Jefferies, Ann Louise
Jimenez, Elizabeth
Johnstone, Julie C.
Jones, Nicola L.
Joseph, Marissa O.
Kadar, Paul-Lewis
Kantor, Paul F.
Kassam, Alisha
Katzman, Debra K.
Kaufman, Miriam E.
Kawamura, Anne
Kelly, Edmond N.
Kempinska, Anna
Keogh, Kelly A.
Kim, Vy Hong-Diep N.
Kirby, Melanie-Ann
Kirsh, Joel A.
Kobayashi, Jeffrey S.
Koelink, Eric A.
Komar, Luba N V.
Korah, Nadine
Korczak, Daphne J.
Kotsakis, Afrothite
Kovacs, Susan V B.
Kronick, Jonathan B.
Kulik, Dina M.
Kwan, Charisse W.
Lalani, Amina P.
Lamenza, Cecilia
Langer, Howard M.
Langlois, Valerie
Lau, Eddy C H.
Lavine, Elana S.
Laxer, Ronald M.
Le, Hoang Yen
Lee, Kyong-Jin
Lee, Kyong-Soon
Lee, Shoo Kim
Lee Ng, Vicky
Leslie, Karen M.
Levy, Deborah M.
Levy, Lance D.
Licht, Christoph P B.
Liebman, Mira F.
Linders, Patricia M.
Lindzon, Aaron J.
Loh, Alvin W H.
Luca, Nadia J C.
MacGregor, Daune L.
Magder, Ilana
Maguire, Jonathon L.
Mah, Catherine L.
Mahant, Sanjay
Mahmud, Farid H.
Malkin, David D.
Manji, Arif
Marcon, Margaret A.
Maresky, David C.
Massam, Joanna L.
McAdam, Laura
McCrindle, Brian W.
Mehta, Dilipkumar H.
Mehta, Sanjay V.
Meloff, Keith L.
Mema, Briseida
Mendelson, Michael
Mendes, John M.
Mennie, Mary K.
Milo-Manson, Golda
Minhas, Ripudaman S.
Minnes, Bruce G.
Mistry, Niraj K.
Mizzi, Trent D.
Mohammed, Javed
Mohammed, Reem W A.
Moore, Aideen M A.
Moore, Charlotte
Moraes, Theo J.
Morinis, Julia B S.
Morris, Shaun K.
Mounstephen, William J.
Muise, Aleixo M.
Mukerji, Amit
Munk, Paul
Murthy, Srinivas
Nag, Shudeshna
Nathan, Paul C.
Naymark, Sharon I.
Neelands, Patricia J.
Newman, Christine J.
Ng, Eugene H L.
Nguyen, Tram T.
Nield, Lynne E.
Noriega, Eleazar H.
O'Beirne, Carole P.
O'Brien, Karel K E.
Orsino, Angelina
Ota, Kaede
Papadouris, Evangelia
Parekh, Rulan S.
Parkin, Patricia C.
Parvez, Boriana
Peebles, Erin R.
Peer, Michael
Pencharz, Paul B.
Penner, Melanie J.
Perlman, Kusiel
Perlmutar, Marty
Philpott, John F.
Pirie, Jonathan R.
Piscione, Tino D.
Pope, Elena
Popovic, Jelena
Prasad, Aduvala V.
Principi, Tania
Prsa, Milan
Pugh, James E V.
Punnett, Angela S.
Rachlis, Alisa C.
Radhakrishnan, Seetha
Randhawa, Harkamal
Rapoport, Adam L.
Ratjen, Felix
Ratnapalan, Savithiri
Rayar, Meera S.
Read, Stanley E.
Richards, H. Anne
Roberts, S. Gwendoline
Robinson, Lisa A.
Rosenblum, Norman D.
Rosenfield, Jay D.
Rosenstein, Karen A.
Rosenthal, Alana J.
Rossi, Miriam F..
Roth, Daniel E.
Roth, Leah H.
Rumney, Peter G.
Russell, Jennifer L.
Sabapathy, Christine A.
Samanta, Tania
Sanchez, Arturo
Saunders, Natasha R.
Saunderson, Janet L.
Savlov, Deena J.
Schneeweiss, Suzan
Schneider, Rayfel
Schuh, Suzanne
Schulze, Andreas
Schwartz, Kevin
Schwartz, Sarah B.
Schwartz, Steven M.
Science, Michelle E I.
Scolnik, Dennis
Sgro, Michael D.
Shah, Chandrakant P.
Shah, Prakeshkumar S.
Shah, Vibhuti S.
Shaikh, Furqan K S.
Shalish, Wissam
Shamsah, Abdullah A.
Shennan, Andrew T.
Sherman, Philip M.
Shouldice, Michelle K.
Shulman, Rayzel M.
Sickinger, Tina M.
Silver, Shawna E.
Silverman, Earl D.
Simmons, Brian S.
Sivarajan, Venkatesan B.
Skidmore, Martin B.
Sochett, Etienne B.
Solomon, Melinda P.
Soon, Gordon S.
Spiegel, Lynn R.
Star, Janet A.
Subbarao, Padmaja
Sung, Lillian
Superina-Bell, Diann J.
Sutton, Robert E.
Sweezey, Neil B.
Talarico, Susanna
Talbot, Yves R.
Tamayo Estrada, Catalina M.
Tanswell, A. Keith
Taylor, Carolyn V.
Tein, Ingrid
Thakur, Varsha
Thampi, Nisha
Tijssen, Janice A.
Toulany, Alene A.
Tran, D. Jeffrey
Tran, Kim A T.
Tran, Thai Hoa
Tse, Shirley M L.
Unger, Sharon L.
Urbach, Stacey L.
Valentino, Pamela
Vaughan, Joanne
Vijayaratnam, Visvalingam
Villani, Anita
Wadhwa, Anupma
Wald, Rachel M.
Walsh, Catharine M.
Wan, Andrea W.
Waters, Valerie J.
Weingarten, Kevin A.

Weinstein, Michael J.
Weinstein, Miriam G.
Weiss, Shelly K.
Weisz, Dany
Weitzman, Sheila S.
Weksberg, Rosanna
Wherrett, Diane K.
Whyte, Hilary E A.
Wilejto, Marta
Williams, Brent A.
Williams, Suzan A.
Wise, Talya C.
Wormsbecker, Anne E.
Yang, Heather C.
Yeh, Eluen A.
Yeung, Rae S M.
Ying, Ethel
Young, Elizabeth Y F.
Young Tai, Kin Fan W.
Zlotkin, Stanley H.
Zuijdwijk, Caroline S.

UNIONVILLE
Lau, Ho-Yin
Tsui, I L. Helen

UXBRIDGE
Kirkpatrick, Sybil M L.
Mohile, Sonali A.

VANIER
Huot, David J.

WATERLOO
Graham, John W.
Polevoy, Terry A.

WELLAND
Al-Darazi, Youness
Bhetasi, Fatima
Bonsu, Peter O.
Visbal Amador, Fernando A.

WHITBY
Campbell, Susan M C.
Dockrill, Karen G.
Godfrey, Sean E.
Khattak, M. Sohail
Mitchell, Marianna K.
Styles, Scott G.

WINDSOR
Adie, Mohammad A.
Armour, Edouard F H.
Awuku, Mark A.
Bacheyie, Godfrey S.
Burey, Sharon T A.
Chow, Sing W.
Deshpande, Ashish
Galiwango, Joseph
Hahn-Lee, June H.
Kazmie, Huma
Khan, Farah I.
Liem, Joel J.
Morgan, Lenna M.
Nwaesei, Chukwuma G.
Rahman, Riffat Ur
Ross, Donald C.
Zaher, Amjad N.

WOODBRIDGE
Cannitelli, Alberto
Hamat, Richard B.
Liew, Kenneth Y K.
Rosenberg, Jacob J.
Sit, Shirley M.
Triassi Asper, Maria

YORK
Feldman, Jacob

PRINCE EDWARD ISLAND

CHARLOTTETOWN
Bethune, Margaret D.
Bigsby, Kathryn M.
Morrison, Kathryn S.
Noonan, Peter G.
Sweet, Lamont E.
Vitullo, Bennedetto B.
Zelman, Mitchell I.

SUMMERSIDE
Gandy, Alan C.
Wong, David T W.

QUÉBEC

ALMA
Carriere, Brigitte
Harvey, Dany
Rouillard-Lafond, Joelle
Rousseau, Claudyne

AMOS
Mamet, Francoise G.
Paul, Adrien
Savoie, Liette

BAIE-D'URFE
Westwood, Michael

BOISBRIAND
Savard, Pascal

BROSSARD
Beaulieu, Lucie
Deschamps, Lyne
Dionne, Anne
Landry, Martine
Rabin, Irving
St-Onge, Gisele

CHATEAUGUAY
Giraldo, Hernan
Marc, Maya
Rossy, Paul E.

CHICOUTIMI
Bouchard, Jean-Benoit
Grenier Cliche, Catherine
Harvey, Johanne
Milot, Marcel
Morin, Charles
Parizeault, Guy
St-Pierre, Julie

COTE SAINT-LUC
Burko, Benjamin
Champagne, Elaine M C.
Cummings, Carl
Grzywacz, Kelly
Schwartz, Thomas
Segal, Lauren M.
Shahin, Edmond B N.

DOLBEAU-MISTASSINI
Fortin, Danielle

DOLLARD DES ORMEAUX
Graves, Nana
Ngassam, Philippe

DRUMMONDVILLE
Foucault, Nathalie

GASPE
Lebeau, Marie-Claude

GATINEAU
Bedard, Sonia
Belanger, Eve-Marie
Bergeron, Sophie
Boisvert, Mariette
Chad, Zave H.
Charette, Luc
Clement, Karine
Couture, Yohann
Fortin, Henriete
Gagne, Chantal
Grenier, Danielle
Hebert, Louis P.
Hotte, Simon L.
King, Dionne V.
Lafrance, Elise
Landreville, Marie-Helene
Lemonde, Jean
Marchand, Celine
Waterston, Sarah E.

GRANBY
Guay, Patrice
Khalil, Riad A.

GREENFIELD PARK
Calabrese, Julie
Doray, Jean-Luc
Doray, Jean-Pierre
Francoeur, Marie-Josee
Ninkovic, Svetlana
St-Denis-Demers, Monique

JOLIETTE
Legault, Luc
Martin, Charles

KIRKLAND
Metrakos, Stephanie

LA SARRE
Cardinal, Godefroy A.

LACHINE
Mandich, George H.

LACHUTE
Comte, Pierre

LASALLE
Archambault, Lisa M J.
Ardila-Romero, Jesus A.
Jeanneau, Robert
Scholten, Vicki
Urbanski, R. Pierre

LAVAL
Alloul, Sophie
Bailon-Poujol, Julie
Blanchette, Donald E.
Blanchette, Suzanne
Chevalier, Claudia
Gradinger, Charles
Gradinger, Harvey
Hamel, Pascale
Hausser, Christian
Lajoie, Mireille
Langlois, Michel
Le Siege, Michele
Michaud, Guy A.
Nguyen Luu, Nha-Uyen
Phan, Quynh Giao
Piche, Louise
Poitras, Pierre
Riopel, M. Eve
Rouette, Justine
Roussy, Jacques
Seddiki, Fatiha
Simard, Fernand
Simard, Jacques
Therrien, Elyse
Tourigny, Daniel
Weisnagel, John

LEVIS
Beaudry, Caroline
Belanger, Celine
Belanger, Lise
Cote, Jean
Labbe, Valerie
Mondor, Claire
Plante, Jessica
Rheault, Mylene
Rousseau, Andre

LONGUEUIL
Belley, Jacques
Boucher, Chantale
Bouhairie, Torik
De Belle, Ross C.
Dunn, Carolyn M.
Filiatrault, Michele
Frechette-Pelletier, Emilie
Hebert, Nathalie
Latraverse, Veronique
Lehuu, Phung
Pedneault, Caroline
Raymond, Francois
Roy, Marie-Josee
Villeneuve, Nadia

MARIA
Dumas, Francois
Martin, Elise J.
Robineault, Antoine

MONT-ROYAL
Lawandi, Philip

MONTREAL
Abish, Sharon B.
Ageranioti-Belanger, Stacey
Agostino, Holly
Ahmed, Najma N.
Ali, Nabeel
Alizadehfar, Reza
Allard-Dansereau, Claire
Amyot, Isabelle
Arsenault, Michael A.
Auger, Louise T.
Autmizguine, Julie
Bailey, Benoit
Bank, Ilana M.
Bardin, Claudette L.
Barnes, Robert D.
Barrington, Keith J.
Bartholomew, Julie-Anne
Beaudry, Claude
Beaumier, Louis
Beland, Marie
Beland, Marie Josee
Belhumeur, Celine
Bell, Lorraine E.
Benoit, Genevieve
Bergeron, Sylvie
Bernard-Bonnin, Anne-Claude
Berry, Margaret A.
Berube, Denis
Bhanji, Farhan
Bhatt, Maala
Bigras, Jean-Luc
Bimbi-Kovacs, Agnes E.
Blaise, Fritz
Bonny, A M. Yvette
Bouthillier, Renee
Boutin, Christine
Boutin, Manon
Brassard, Myriam
Bretholz, Adam
Brody, Daniel
Brousseau, Yves F.
Brunet, Suzanne M.
Bui, Helen
Buithieu, Maria
Buteau, Chantal
Buu, C. Dung Anh
Campillo, Sarah
Canakis, Anne-Marie
Carceller, Ana M.
Carriere, Benoit
Cavalle-Garrido, Maria T.
Cellot, Sonia
Chabot, Gilles
Chalut, Dominic
Champagne, Josette
Chartrand, Caroline
Chauvin-Kimoff, Laurel A.
Chemtob, Sylvain
Chessex, Philippe
Chevalier, Isabelle M.
Chicoine, Jean-Francois
Clermont, Marie-Jose
Colombini, Linda M.
Constantin, Evelyn J T.
Costom, Bruce H.
Cote, Aurore
Cousineau, Dominique
Couture, Elise
CuMmins-Mcmanus, Barbara J.
D'Angelo, Antonio F.
Dancea, Adrian B.
Dandavino, Mylene
Daoud, Aida
Dassa, Justine
Deal, Cheri L.
Debs, Negib
Decaluwe, Hélène
Decell, Mary K.
Del Valle-Pison, Maria
Demers, Anne-Marie
Des Roches, Anne
Desjardins, Maryline
Deslandres, Colette
Desmarchais, Louise
Di Genova, Tanya
Di Liddo, Lydia
Diksic, Dubravka A.
Dirks, Martha H.
Dobrescu, Otilia-M.
Dore-Bergeron, Marie-Joelle
Dorval, Veronique G.
Dougherty, Geoffrey E.
Douyon, Frantz
Doyon-Trottier, Evelyne
Drouin, Eric
Dube, Robert
Dubrovsky, Alexander
Ducharme, Francine M.
Eisman, Harley N.
Farrell, Catherine A.
Faucher, Daniel J.
Faucher, Frederic
Ferdinand, Jae-Marie
Ficara, Giuseppe
Fillion, Marc
Fleming, Adam J.
Forbes, Patricia A.
Forget, Sylviane
Foster, Bethany J.
Fournier, Anne
Fouron, Jean-Claude
Frappier, Jean-Yves
Friedman, Jack
Gafoor, Tamara A.
Gagnon, Christiane
Gaucher, Nathalie
Gaudreault, Pierre
Gauthier-Chouinard, Marie
Gauvin, France
Geoffroy, Louis
Gervais, Marc H.
Girodias, Jean-Bernard
Gorgos, Andreea-Bogdana
Gosselin, Richard
Gosselin-Hunter, Anne-Marie
Gottesman, Ronald D.
Gouin, Serge
Goyette, Anne-Marie
Gravel, Caroline
Gravel, Jocelyn
Greenstone, Ilana R.
Gref, Pauline
Guay, Joanne M.
Gupta, Indra R.
Haley, Nancy
Hamaoui, Charles
Hardy, Pierre
Harrington, Karen P.
Hassaine, Assia
Hazan, Joelle
Henderson, M. Melanie
Henin, Catherine Y.
Hervouet-Zeiber, Catherine
Hume, Heather
Huot, Celine H.
Hussain, Samiruddin S.
Jacob, Sheila V.
Jamoulle, Olivier
Janvier, Annie F.
Joyal, Jean-Sebastien
Julien, Gilles
Jutras, Luc C.
Kakkar, Fatima
Karatzios, Christos
Key, Fiona M.
Khairy, May
Khakee, Shamshuddin G.
Khalil, Elene O.
Khediguian, Varoujan
Khoury, Samir
Kleiber, Niina M.
Koclas, Louise
Kovacs, Lajos B.
Krishnamoorthy, Preetha
Laberge, Sophie
Laberge-Malo, Marie E.
Lachance, Christian
Lachapelle, Jean
Lacroix, Jacques
Laferriere, Celine
Lamarre, Valerie
Lambert, Marie
Lands, Larry C.

SPECIALISTS BY PROVINCE

Lapierre, Jean-Guy
Lapointe, Anie
Lapointe, Normand
Larbrisseau, Albert
Larose, Guylaine
Laverdiere, Caroline
Lazaro-Lopez, Francisco J.
Le, Tuyet-Diem
Lebel, Marc
Leblanc, Claire
Leblond, Helene
Lefebvre, Francine
Legault, Laurent
Lejtenyi, M. Christine
Lemyre, Emmanuelle
Leroux, Jacques-Rene
Levesque, Dominique
Levy, Arielle R.
Li, Patricia T.
Liben, Stephen B.
Litalien, Catherine
Liu, Joanne
Longtin, Pierre
Lortie, Anne
Lucas, Nathalie
Luong, Tinh-Nhan
Lupu, G. Harvey
Lussier, Anne
Luu, Thuy Mai
MacDonald, Suzanne F.
MacDonald, Wendy A.
MacLellan, Anne-Marie
Mandel, Ruth J.
Marchand, Valerie
Marcotte, Jacques-Edouard
Marin, Pierre
Markus, Arthur J.
Martens, David J.
Mattimoe, Claire A.
Mazer, Bruce D.
McCusker, Christine T.
McDonald, Jane C.
McKinney, Martha L.
Melancon, Serge B.
Melcuk, Ekaterina
Meloche, Judith
Menard, Marc
Mercure, Claude
Michaud, Jacques
Millar, Catherine
Millette, Maude
Miro, Joaquim A.
Mitchell, David A.
Mitchell, Grant A.
Mitchell, John J.
Moore, Dorothy L.
Morantz-Ornstein, Gillian
Morel, Johanne
Morin, Marie-Paule
Morinville, Veronique D.
Morrison, Jessica A.
Mouaikel, Elie
Moussa, Ahmed
Nakhla, Meranda M.
Nguyen, Bich-Hong
Nguyen, The Thanh D.
Nguyen, Uyen-Phuong
Noel, Melanie
Nogarede, Annick
Noya, Francisco J D.
Nuyt, Anne M.
Olivier, Patricia
Ortenberg, June
Ouellet, Caroline
Paice, Naomi
Panet-Raymond, Dominique
Papageorgiou, Apostolos
Papenburg, Jesse
Patel, Hema
Pekeles, Gary S.
Pelausa, Ermelinda O.
Pelletier, Veronique A.
Pepin, Michelle
Perreault, Therese
Perron, Jean-Marc
Pettersen, Geraldine
Phan, Veronique
Phi, Chi-Minh
Plotnick, Laurie H.
Pluviose, William
Polychronakos, Constantin
Pomerleau, Damien
Pomerleau, Genevieve
Powell, Julie C.
Primeau, Marie-Noel
Proulx, Francois
Quach-Thanh, Caroline
Quansah, Samuel B.
Rabin, David
Rabinovitch, Eric A.
Rajabieh Shayan, Yasaman
Rashed, Selim
Rasquin-Weber, Andree
Razack, Saleem I.
Reiter, Stephanie L.
Rich, Harold A.
Riley, Sheilagh P.
Rivard, Georges E.
Roberge, Claude A.
Robert, Monique
Robitaille, Nancy
Rodd, Celia J.
Rohlicek, Charles V.
Rosenblatt, David S.
Rossignol, Elsa
Rousseau, Celine
Rousseau-Harsany, Elisabeth
Roy, Claude C.
Roy, Michel
Roy-Fleising, Celine
Rubin, Earl E.
Saint-Cyr, Claire H.
Saint-Jean, Maude
Saintonge, Jacques P A.
Samotis-Tchervenkov, Linda
Samson, Yvan
Sanchez, Marisol
Sant'Anna, Guilherme M.
Saylor, Kent D.
Sbrocchi, Anne M.
Scarinci, Christine
Schonfeld, Irving B.
Scott, Rachel R.
Scuccimarri, Rosie
Seidman, Ernest G.
Setton, Nora S.
Sharma, Atul K.
Shemie, Sammy D.
Sigman, Karen G.
Sigman, Terry E.
Sioufi, Guy
Sirard, Alain
Soulieres, Denis
Spigelblatt, Linda S.
St-Laurent-Gagnon, M H L. Therese
Ste-Marie, Micheline T.
Sterescu, Anca E.
Stewart, Jessica N.
Stojanovic, Sanja
Taddeo, Danielle
Tapiero, Bruce
Teasdale, Francois
Thivierge, Robert L.
Toledano, Baruch J.
Toussi, Tahmouresse
Tucci, Marisa A.
Turgeon, Jean
Turnbull, Jennifer E S.
Vaillancourt, Suzanne M.
Van Doesburg, Nicolaas H.
Vartian, Michele
Veilleux, Annie
Vekemans, Gaelle
Verdy, Isabelle
Vezina, Catherine
Villeneuve, Andreanne
Vincent, Anne-Marie
Vincent, Melanie A.
Vo, Thuy Tien
Wilkins, Jean
Zappitelli, Michael
Zavalkoff, Samara
Zielinski, Dawid K.
Znojkiewicz, Maria H.
Zylbergold-Schonfeld, Betty

ORMSTOWN

Hortop, John

PIERREFONDS

Erdstein, Julius
Ismail, Laila
Kugelmass, Robin
Loyer, Deborah M.
Magnani, Lucia B.
Ouellette, Nathalie
Shiller, Mitchell B.
Waxman, David H.

POINTE-CLAIRE

Lubkiewicz, Krzysztof
Ricot, Pierre-Jacques
Wiseman, Fred

QUEBEC

Bailey Vera, Dennis
Bairam, Aida
Bedard, Veronique
Belanger, Richard
Belanger, Sylvie
Beliveau, Sylvie
Bernard, Brigitte
Bernier, Nadia
Blanchard, Pierre W.
Blanchet, Jacques
Bouchard, Isabelle
Bouchard, Maurice
Boucher, Francois
Boucher, Marie-Danielle R.
Bourdages, Macha
Bourgault, Francois
Brodeur, Anne
Brousseau, Marie-Claude
Brown, Michael S.
Caouette, Georges
Castilloux, Julie
Catellier, Priscilla
Cayer, Sylvie
Cote, Jean-Marc
Cote-Brisson, Linda
Couet, Hugues
Daigneault, Patrick
Delisle, Georges
Dery, Pierre
Deschenes, Marianne
Donlan, Matthew
Drolet, Christian
Drolet, Christine
Drolet, Jean-Philippe
Drolet, Yvan
Dubois, Danielle
Dugas, Marc-Andre N.
Duquette, Marie-Camille
Duval, Renee-Claude
Falardeau, Guy
Fecteau, David
Ferland, Louise M.
Frenette, Marie G L.
Gagne, Julie
Gagnon, Josee A.
Gaumont, Yves A.
Gervais, Pascale
Giroux, Roger
Goulet, Richard
Houde, Christine
Hudon, Claire
Jobin, Catherine
Labbe, Jean
Laflamme, Julie
Langevin, Pierre L.
Larouche, Valerie
Lessard, Julie
Marcotte, Marie-Eve
Masson, Michel
Mercier, Jean-Claude
Michon, Bruno
Naccache, Lamia
Nadeau, Sophie
Pelletier, Luc
Pichette, Jeanne L.
Piedboeuf, Bruno
Piuze, Genevieve-Helene
Plante, Monique
Rousseau, Anne
Roy, Genevieve
Roy, Helene
Roy, Marie-Claude
Saikali, Emilie
Samson, Marie-Eve
St-Laurent Lemerle, Catherine
Thibeault, Roseline
Tremblay, Pierre
Umemoto, Lorne N.
Veilleux-Lemieux, Maude
Verreault, Nina
Verret, Simon
Weiss, Matthew J.
Wieckowska, Anna

REPENTIGNY

Antaki, Aline
Bonin, Diane
Chouinard, Josee
Lacaille, Luc
Lafond, Lucie
Rock, Nathalie

RIMOUSKI

Belanger, Yvan
Boucher, Jacques A.
Boutin, Caroline
Gamache, Sylvie
Kimpton, Susan
Riberdy, Jocelyne
St-Pierre, Yohann
Synnott, Jocelyne

RIVIERE-DU-LOUP

Caissie, Romeo
Charest, Veronie
Desrosiers, Lucie
Deziel, Francois
Ouellet, Linda
Sauvageau, Jean-Paul

ROBERVAL

Blanchette, Christine

ROUYN-NORANDA

Leclerc, Roland
Perreault, Louise
Vincelette, Pierre

ROXBORO

Goldman, Hyman

SAINT-BRUNO

Pelletier, Suzanne

SAINT-EUSTACHE

Janssen, Lyne

SAINT-GEORGES

Dery, Catherine
Lemieux-Roy, Marie-Josee
Poulin, Pierre-Claude

SAINT-HUBERT

Albert, Gilles R.
Desgranges, Marie-Francoise
Nehme, Edgard W.

SAINT-HYACINTHE

Barnabe, Gerard
Binet, Marie-Eve
Boulay, Remi
Charette, Christiane
Duchesne, Sylvane
Lavigne, Jocelyn
Lemoine, Marie-Helene
Morin, Julie
Pepin, Marie-Pascale
Renaud, Jacques
Turcotte, Jean-Jacques

SAINT-JEROME

Audet, Catherine
De Villers, France
Desmarais, Dominique
Filiatrault, Danielle C.
Germain, Sophie
Haccoun, Charles
Khayat, Kamal
Poupart, Robert
Racette, Julie-Maude
Robidas, Isabelle
Roy, Lucie E.

SAINT-LAURENT

Attye, Aly
Chidiac, Abdallah
Delifer, Jean-Claude

SAINT-LAZARE

Jarjour, Allan M.

SAINT-LEONARD

Chaer, Sanae

SAINTE-THERESE

Anctil, Suzanne
Aubin, Genevieve
Girouard, France
Lemay, Nathalie
Nguyen, Thi Ngoc Diep
Roy, Valerie

SALABERRY DE VALLEYFIELD

Bellemare, Johanne
Lanctot, Guy

SEPT-ILES

Belanger, Pierre
Gauthier, Pierre
Sirois, Nathalie

SHAWINIGAN

Trudel, Judith

SHAWINIGAN-SUD

Chretien, Francois

SHERBROOKE

Beaulieu, Genevieve
Bellavance, Marc
Bergeron, Cybele
Brossard, Josee
Cote, Sylvie
Cote-Boileau, Therese
Cyr, Claude
Dallaire, Frederic
Demers, Charlotte
Fortin-Pellerin, Etienne
Gagne, Nancy
Girardin, Colette
Graillon, Ann
Harpin, Chantal
Jarjoura, Samir C.
Khoury, Khalil
L'Allier, Johanne
Laflamme, Sophie
Lafrenaye, Sylvie
Langlais, Caroline
Lavoie, Eric
Lemire, Chantal
Lessard, Sophie
Lippe, Julie
Loignon, Julie
Masse, Edith
Maurice, Pascale
Pare, Gilles
Pesant, Caroline
Pigeon, Nicole
Quesnel, Josee
Rivard, Lyne
Robinette, Mylene
Rola-Pleszczynski, Marek
Roulier, Sebastien
Roy, Marie-Claude
Santschi, Miriam
Simoneau-Roy, Judith
Soucy, Marc
Therien, Serge
Toulouse, Krystel
Tremblay, Stephane
Vlachos, Helen

SOREL-TRACY

Daoud, Maha
Haddad, Georges
Leveille, Jean
Robitaille, J. Michel J P.

ST AUGUSTIN DE DESMAURES

Guay, J. Michel

ST JEAN SUR RICHELIEU

Dubreuil-Moisan, Nathalie
Grondin, Anne
Guay, Michel A.
Guillemette-Grignet, Helene
Lefebvre, Denis
Letellier, Manon
Provost, Francine

STE AGATHE DES MONTS
Barron, Teresa
Roy, Ann-Veronique

STE ANNE DE BELLEVUE
Haber, L. Richard

TERREBONNE
Guilbault, Nathalie
Montulet, Evelyne C.
Pepin, Karine

THETFORD MINES
Gagne, Louise

TROIS-RIVIERES
Caumartin, Marie-Celine
Fecteau, Claude
Garneau, Suzanne
Guillemette, Fernand
Lacerte, Caroline
Marchand, Line
Nadeau, Marie-Claude
Perrault, Raymond
Valois, M S. Nadine

VAL-D'OR
Kukhta, Allison
Malaab, Suzanne
Medou-Ntyame, Leopold
Petit, Normand
Woods, Sandra G B.

VERDUN
Barrette, Stephane

VICTORIAVILLE
Cantin, Jean-Claude
Caya, Nathalie
De Serres, Sonia

WESTMOUNT
Ahronheim, Gerald A.
Allard, Manon
Baltzer, Franziska
Blaichman, Shirley
Di Meglio, Giuseppina
Francoeur, T. Emmett
Kimia, Dyan
Lalonde, Richard A.
Leduc, Denis G.
Medoff, Elaine J.
Moneta, Ilaria
Munz, Diane L.
Stein, Naomi B.
Treherne, Stephen E.
Tse, Olivia Q.
Yaremko, John F.
Zeliger, Agnes M.

SASKATCHEWAN

LLOYDMINSTER
Kowalczyk, Amie J.

PRINCE ALBERT
Bulat, Duane C.
Du Russel, Michelle
Lambos, Peggy
Malhotra, Tilak R.
Ramji, Ayaaz

REGINA
Datta, Biswa R.
Essalah, Abdulhafid A.
Flavelle, Shauna C.
Hobeika, Sharon L.
Holmes, S. Bruce
Lodhi, Abid M D.
Murthy, Poornima S.
Petryk, Susan C.
Soper, Juliet
Sotomi, Omopelola O.
Talukdar, Chiranjib

SASKATOON
Adamko, Darryl J.
Albritton, William L.
Ali, S. Kaiser
Baerg, Krista L.
Bedard, Vanessa
Best, Thomas B.
Bingham, William T.
Blakley, Patricia M.
Bruce, Garth A.
Brusky, Janna D.
Erickson, Robin
Gamble, Carmen
Gamer, Meghan
Givelichian, Laurentiu M.
Hewitt, Morgan
Hodgson-Viden, Heather
Holt, Tanya
Huntsman, Richard J.
Jones, Angela M.
Kakadekar, Ashok P.
Krochak, Carla A M.
Kurji, Ayisha
Leis, Karen S.
Lothian, James B.
Lowry, Noel J.
Martin, Susanna M.
Mater, Ahmed M A.
McConnell, Athena
Mehtar, Maryam
Mpofu, Christopher
Neufeld, Ruth E.
Ninan, Abraham
Paquin, Raphael
Persaud, Mitra M P.
Pharis, C. Scott
Robichaud, Sophie
Rosenberg, Alan M.
Sankaran, Koravangattu
Shiff, Natalie J.
Siemens, Ronald K.
Sinha, Roona
Streilein, Karen F.
Tan, Ben J K.
Wiens, Sharon A.
Wonko, Neil A.
Woods, Erin L.
Yee, Edgar H.

YUKON TERRITORY

WHITEHORSE
Grueger, Barbara

Physical Medicine & Rehabilitation

ALBERTA

CALGARY
Apel, Maryana
Barton, Pamela M.
Burkholder, Lee M.
Debert, Chantel T.
Dukelow, Sean P.
Flaschner, David M.
Gabriel, Vincent
Giantomaso, Tony
Gupta, Arun T.
Hill, Denise C.
Lam, K S. Kenneth
Latter, John E.
Li Pi Shan, Rodney
McGovern, Christine H.
McGowan, M. Daniel
McNeil, Stephen M.
Plamondon, Stephanie A.
Simonett, Gillian R.
Ubhi, Perminder S.
Virani, Noorshina S.

EDMONTON
Acharya, Hernish J.
Ashworth, Nigel L.
Chan, Kam Ming.
Currie, Angela S.
Dafoe, William
Di Persio, Mario B.
Gonzales, Sean
Guthrie, John B.
Hebert, Jacqueline S.
Hlushak, Curtis R.
Irvine, Jamie J.
Kulkarni, Sharmila N.
Lesiuk, Thomas P.
Naidu, Dhiren J.
Paleksic, Sanja
Pappachan, Michael J.
Prowse, Matthew T.
Rambaransingh, Brian S.
Sampson, Evan E.
Satkunam, Lalith E.
Thiara, Rajpal S.
Townsend, Judy A.
Tuchak, Carmen C.
Watt, Man-Joe
Yablon, Stuart
Yen, Tien
Zaki, Sami F.

LACOMBE
Burnham, Robert S.
McLean, Deirdre E.

LETHBRIDGE
Gumbs, Darren G.
LeBlond, Daniel

PONOKA
Gray, D. Shaun

SHERWOOD PARK
Amirjani, Nasim

SPRUCE GROVE
Al-Feeli, Aziz K.
El Maadawy, Sherif S.

BRITISH COLUMBIA

BURNABY
Watson, J. David

DELTA
Caillier, Lisa A.

KAMLOOPS
Calder, C. Jill
Raghavan, Prathapakumar T.

KELOWNA
McCann, Shawn C.
Nowak, Jozef E.
Vallentyne, Stephen W.
Yu, Jaime C.

LANGLEY
Chu, Ansel L.

MAPLE RIDGE
Hughes, Barbara L.

NANAIMO
Deutscher, Timothy R.
Hawkeswood, Jonathan P.
Willmott, Andrew D.

NEW WESTMINSTER
Reebye, Nittin K.

NORTH VANCOUVER
Craig, William H.
Le Nobel, John C.

PORT MOODY
Dawson, Andrew S.

SIDNEY
Graboski, Corrie L.

SURREY
Jaworski, Jerzy S.

VANCOUVER
Acob, Constante A.
Adrian, Mark D.
Anton, Hubert A.
Bohorquez, Anibal F.
Crossman, Mark W.
Deforge, Daniel A.
Dhawan, Pankaj M.
Fan, H I. Anita
Feldman, Rubin M.
Finlayson, Heather C.
Guzman, Jaime
Helper, Steven R M.
Hershler, Cecil
Hirsch, Gabriel H.
Koo, David W K.
Krassioukov, Andrei
Lau, Herman H M.
Mills, Patricia B.
Murray, Andrew I S.
Nguyen, Viem Chung
O'Connor, Russell J.
Paramonoff, Catherine E.
Purtzki, Jacqueline S.
Reebye, Rajiv N.
Stewart, Rosemary N.
Sudol, Malgorzata M.
Townson, Andrea F.
Travlos, Andrew
Ummat, Samira
Underwood, Heather
Van Rijn, Theo A.
Vondette, Michael J.
Weeks, Claire Ann O.
Weiss, Elliott P.
Willms, Rhonda L.
Yao, Jennifer K.
Yasin, Nasif I.

VERNON
Inkpen, Peter C.

VICTORIA
Bass, Alan L.
Chapman, Paul D.
Filbey, James A.
Killian, Fionnuala M.
Lafreniere, Ronald T J.
MacKean, Lynne C.
Quartly, Caroline A.
Rocheleau, Michael G.
Winston, Paul J.
Yip, Todd R.

WEST KELOWNA
Laidlow, Duncan M.

WESTBANK
Coghlan, John K.

MANITOBA

WINNIPEG
Arneja, Amarjit S.
Casey, Alan R.
Daniels, Valsa
Engel, Christopher V W.
Ethans, Karen D.
Galimova, Lena
Hooper, Davyd R.
Hoy, Conrad S G.
Johnson, Charles N.
Perry, Daryl
Pooyania, Sepideh
Priestley, Douglas W.
Salter, Jennifer E.
Skrabek, Ryan Q.
Sommer, Hillel M.
Stitz, Marshall Y.

NEW BRUNSWICK

FREDERICTON
Leckey, J. Robert
Milczarek, John J.
O'Connell, Colleen M.
Poole, Bruce J.
Taillon, A. Monique
Worley, Scott W.

MONCTON
Giroux, Patrick
Pike, Jeffrey H.

ROTHESAY
Forgeron, M. Patricia
Reid, Philip H.

NEWFOUNDLAND AND LABRADOR

BAY L'ARGENT
Acharya, Meenaxi S.

CORNER BROOK
Woolfrey, Paul G W.

NOVA SCOTIA

HALIFAX
Hanada, Edwin Y.
Joyce, Brenda M.
Kirby, R. Lee
Koshi, Edvin
Loane, Thomas D.
Mahar, Robert K.
Majaess, George G.
McVeigh, Sonja A.
Mountain, Anita D.
Saric, Amra
Short, Christine A.

SYDNEY MINES
Watt, Douglas A.

ONTARIO

AJAX
Katz, Dan G.
Singh, Jogindra

BARRIE
Wilkins, Kathryn R.

BELLEVILLE
McInnes, Craig M.

BRAMPTON
Armitage, Kathleen J.

BRANTFORD
Ballyk, Catherine J.
Varey, Peter A.

BURLINGTON
Bowler, Kenneth A.
Clark, Benjamin B.
Garner, Scott H.
Henriques, Tania R.
Muhlstock, Joshua P.

CAMBRIDGE
Ballard, Tonya G.

CORNWALL
Reen, Mehar S.

DUNDAS
Trotter, Judy E.

ETOBICOKE
Chizen, Lawrence S.
Czok, Anna A.
Dziedzic, Margaret

GRIMSBY
Samways, Michelle L.

GUELPH
Galvin, Patti A.
MacCallum, Johnstone S.

HAMILTON
Baker, Steven K.
Bentley, Todd C.
Chari, Vinjamuri R.
Chmiel, Agnes E.
Darracott, John
Farrauto, Leonardo A.
Ghouse, Ali T.
Grad, Sharon

Gwardjan, Andrzej J.
Harvey, David T.
Kumbhare, Dinesh A.
Letcher, Kevin V.
Mathoo, Julian
Muniz Rodriguez, Flor M.
Nesathurai, Shanker
Tarnopolsky, Mark A.
Williams, Ryan A.

HUNTSVILLE
Lapp, Timothy J.

KINGSTON
Bagg, Stephen D.
Delaney, Gail
Faris, Matthew W.
Ruggles, David J M.
Shanks, Gavin L.
Smith, Karen M.
Wee, Joy Y M.

KITCHENER
Heitzner, John D.

LONDON
Bhardwaj, Asha
Clifford, John C.
Death, A. Barry
Doherty, Timothy
Lacerte, Michel
Loh, Eldon
Miller, Thomas
Payne, Michael W C.
Potter, Patrick J.
Sequeira, Keith A J.
Teasell, Robert W.

MARKHAM
Ko, Gordon D.

MISSISSAUGA
Lipson, Frank
Smith, Ruth E.
Stolee, Karen A.

NEPEAN
Lentini, Anthony C.
Sitaram, Kadambi P.

NEWMARKET
Tam, Emily J S.
Wong, Samuel

NORTH BAY
Mitchell, W. Murray

NORTH YORK
Ameis, Arthur
Feigelson, Lori
Gyenes, Tal Ora
Han, Thomas M K.
Khoury, Shahira S.
Kirwin, Pierre J.
Kleinman, Max
Patcai, John T.
Prutis-Misterska, Krystyna
Rado, George
Sreenivasan, Barathi R.
Wong, Joseph Y S.

OAKVILLE
Labuda, Anna
Lang, J. Michael
Waseem, Zeeshan

ORILLIA
Ray, George M.

OSHAWA
John, Thomas
Park, Y. James
Tseng, Leo

OTTAWA
Besemann, Markus
Blackmer, Jeffrey E.
Buenger, Usha R.
Dojeiji, Suzan
Dudek, Nancy L.
El-Sawy, Reda M.
Finestone, Hillel M.
MacGregor, Lynne S.
Marks, Meridith B.
Marshall, Shawn C.
McCormick, Anna M.
McKee, Alexander C.
Quon, Deanna L.
Racine, Francois R J.
Sreenivasan, Vidya A.
St-Pierre, Taunya A.
Trudel, Guy
Wiebe, Scott C.
Wolff, Gerald K.
Yang, Christine P.

OWEN SOUND
Meikle, Ben G.
O'Doherty, Brian M J.

PEMBROKE
Timpson, Deborah J.

PERTH
Stolee, Kathrine J.

PETERBOROUGH
Krete, Derek M.

RICHMOND HILL
Chen, Yen-Fu
Ko, Yong-Kyong

SCARBOROUGH
Cheng, Albert S.
Kachooie, Alireza
Liao, Sunu M.
Nguyen, Melody H H.
Wong, Joseph S.

ST CATHARINES
Fulton, Gerald A.
Khan, Omar D M.
McMillan, Richard W.

SUDBURY
Graham, Anthony D.

THORNHILL
Somogyi, Daniel M.
Tepperman, Perry S.

THUNDER BAY
Hargadon, John M.
Rao, Pramila

TORONTO
Amani, Hossein
Awan, Raza A.
Bayley, Mark T.
Becker, Lisa
Berbrayer, David
Bhangu, Sukhinder K.
Bharatwal, Nirmala
Boulias, Christos
Bruno, Tania R.
Campbell, Doreen J.
Chow, Raphael K T.
Cohodarevic, Tea
Craven, B. Catharine
De Haan, Melanie N.
Devlin, H T. Michael
Flannery, John F.
Geisler, William O.
Godfrey, Charles M.
Ismail, Farooq F.
Kekosz, Veronica N H.
Lo, Alexander J.
Lo, Julian K.
MacNeill, Heather L.
Mailis, Angela H.
Masanic, Cheryl A.
McGillivray, Colleen F.
Muir, Sylvia K.
Rabinovitch, Deborah L.
Richardson, Denyse L.
Sangha, Harpreet S.
Sharma, Satyendra
Somerville, Josephine H.
Soric, Rajka
Tardif, Gaetan
Unarket, Milan
Vaidyanath, Chantal G.
Yap, Audrey P G.

WINDSOR
Burke, Bradley D.
Charron, Patrick M.
Liem, Nathania R.

WOODSTOCK
Tugalev, Oleg

YORK
Cullen, Nora K.
Dilkas, Steven M.
Rambihar, Nadira

PRINCE EDWARD ISLAND

CHARLOTTETOWN
Harrison, Edmund R.

QUÉBEC

BROMONT
Duranceau, Jacques A.

CHANDLER
St-Pierre, Michel

COWANSVILLE
Perreault, Nathalie

GATINEAU
Dehoux, Eric
Lanoie, Nathalie

GREENFIELD PARK
Blier, Francois

LAVAL
Bazinet, Brigitte
Imbeault, Sarto

LEVIS
D'Anjou, Jean-Maurice
Levasseur, Marie-Eve

LONGUEUIL
Dube, Julie
Fournier, Christine

MONT-JOLI
Guimond, Nathalie

MONT-ROYAL
Roy, Andre

MONTREAL
Beaudoin, Nicole
Benhaim, Patrick
Bergeron, Yves M.
Bouthillier, Claude
Dahan, Valerie
Denis, Isabelle
Duranleau, Denis
Filiatrault, Marc
Fleury, Jean
Fortin, Luc
Gupta, Gaurav
Habra, Natalie
Harissi Dagher, Jehan
Haziza, Muriel
Houde, Sylvie
Jacquemin, Geraldine
Laberge-Malo, Marie E.
Lamarre, Celine
Lambert, Richard
Lamontagne, Martin
Leclaire, Richard
Leduc, Bernard E.
Ling, Elisabeth
Luong, Dien Hung
Marois, Pierre
Michaud, Johan
Nguyen, Bich Han
Nguyen, Oanh Thi
Pelletier, Michel
Plante, Pierre
Radhakrishna, Mohan
Raymond, Denis
Remillard, Jean
Spacek, Elena
Susset, Veronique
Talbot, J H. Bernard
Tinawi, Simon
Trojan, Daria A.
Vadeboncoeur, Roger

QUEBEC
Baribeault, Alain
Beliveau, Pierre
Boulet, Daniel
Boulet, Melanie
Brault, Yves
Cote, Isabelle M H.
Fecteau, Serge
Lacroix, Remi
Lavoie, Suzanne
Morand, Claudine
Parent, Rene
Saucier, Danie
Sirois, Genevieve

SAINT-EUSTACHE
Korkmaz, Paul

SAINT-HUBERT
Filion, Gaetan
Lussier, Sylvain
Rivet, Ghislain

SAINT-HYACINTHE
Desbiens, Isabelle

SAINTE-ADELE
Lacoste, Pierre

SALABERRY DE VALLEYFIELD
Latreille, Jean-Marie

SHERBROOKE
Harvey, Anne
St-Pierre, Michel

TROIS-RIVIERES
Cote, Isabelle
Fortier, Josee

SASKATCHEWAN

REGINA
Chrusch, Wendy M.
Fink, Milo P.
Kraushaar, Jacqueline

SASKATOON
Bernacki, Barry A.
Hader, Walter
Knox, Katherine B.
Linassi, A. Gary
Rudachyk, Lila M.
Sankaran, Rajini
Selk, Bradley A.
Wang, Sherry X.

Plastic Surgery

ALBERTA

BANFF
Hall-Findlay, Elizabeth J.

CALGARY
Beveridge, John A.
Birdsell, Dale C.
Campbell, Earl A D.
Dawes, Jeffrey
De Haas, William
Dilay, Jocelyn E.
Frank, Ryan C.
Fraulin, Frankie
Hamilton, George D.
Harrop, A. Robertson
Haugrud, Mark J.
Humphreys, Douglas B.
Kennedy, James M C.
Lee, Jonathan P.
Lin, Alan N.
Lindsay, Robert L.
Magi, Enzio
McPhalen, Donald F.
Nickerson, Duncan A.
Perron, Wayne R.
Schrag, Christian H.
Sutton, Frank R.
Temple-Oberle, Claire F.
Waslen, Gregory D.
Whidden, Paul G R.
Whidden, Peter G.
Yau, Farrah M.

CAMROSE
Wong, Diana

CANMORE
Sinclair, Thomas M.

EDMONTON
Campbell, David D.
Chong, Tze-Feng
Edwards, David C.
Giuffre, Martin J.
Lobay, Gerald L W.
Louie, Gorman
Mehling, Blair M.
Morhart, Michael J.
Murabit, Amera
Olson, Jaret L.
Riegel, Timothy M.
Schembri, Paul J.
Toy, Jonathan W M.
Tredget, Edward E.
Wilkes, Gordon H.
Wolfli, James N.

LETHBRIDGE
Grover, Ramon S.
Hasell, John S.
Hein, Kent S.

MEDICINE HAT
Cassar, Stephen L.

RED DEER
Furness, Robert A H.
McDonald, David S.
Westberg, Kirsten I.

SYLVAN LAKE
Carter, Robert B.

BRITISH COLUMBIA

ABBOTSFORD
Brown, Aaron D.
Musto, David J.
Tung, Andrew S.

BURNABY
Horton, Ross C.
Peers, Robert R.

CAMPBELL RIVER
Evans, Robin J.
Fowler, Peter S.
Loiselle, Frederick B.
Olesen, Peter R.

CUMBERLAND
Classen, Dale A.

DUNCAN
Anzarut, Alexander D.

KAMLOOPS
Jacoby, Michael E.
Meredith, Steven R.
Sunderland, Mark P.

KELOWNA
Allazzam, Abdulmohsen
Miller, Brian J.
Peterson, Brian D.
Valnicek, Stanley M.
Williamson, David G.
Williamson, J. Scott

LANGLEY
Mosher, Mathew C.

NANAIMO
Barnsley, G. Philip
Cheng, Jenny S.
Christensen, L. Blair
Robinson, Richard G.
Tang, Lawrence L.

NEW WESTMINSTER
MacDonald, Patricia J.
Nelson, Rebecca A.
Pugash, Eric S.
Rai, D. Kimit

NORTH VANCOUVER
Chew, Roderick T.
Osberg, Peter E.

PORT MOODY
Nguyen, Dao Q T.
Ukani, Hanif

PRINCE GEORGE
Kurz, Christine J.
Malpass, Kristian G.

RICHMOND
Brady, Stephen C.
Brown, W. Lorne
Reid, Owen G.
Watts, Robyn J.

SURREY
French, Rodney J.
Guichon, Donald M P.
Lee, Adrian T.
Mian, Rizwan A.
Oxley, Paul J.
Prince, Jennifer M.
Ward, David K.

VANCOUVER
Arneja, Jugpal S.
Bowman, Cameron C.
Boyle, James C.
Bristol, Sean G.
Brown, Erin E.
Bush, Kevin L.
Carr, Nicholas J.
Courtemanche, Douglas J.
Cowan, Bryce J.
Cundiff, Geoffrey W.
Demianczuk, Arkadiy
Gdalevitch, Perry
Gelfant, Benjamin M.
Hill, Mark K.
Joughin, Karen E.
Lennox, Peter A.
MacAdam, Sheina A.
Papp, Anthony A.
Seal, Alexander N.
Son-Hing, Quintin R.
Sproul, M. Jane
Thompson, Robert P.
Van Laeken, Nancy Y.
Verchere, Cynthia G.
Warren, Richard J.
Wells, Neil J.

VICTORIA
Djurickovic, Slobodan
Gray, Jason H.
Hollis, Harlow R.
Morley, Rebecca E.
Naysmith, J. David
Robinson, Jennifer W.
Smith, Kenneth A.
Taylor, Christopher D.

WEST VANCOUVER
Morris, Rolf D T.

MANITOBA

WINNIPEG
Ali, M. Ben
Dolynchuk, Kenneth
Giuffre, Jennifer L.
Hayakawa, Thomas E J.
Islur, Avinash
Lockwood, Anthony P F.
Murray, Kenneth A.
Rosenfeld, Iris
Ross, Lonny L.
Sigurdson, Leif J.
Singh, Gurbalbir
Turner, Robert B.
Ziesmann, Manfred

NEW BRUNSWICK

BATHURST
Gomez-Jimenez, Alfonso
Sirois, Michel

DIEPPE
Dool, Jayson
Husain, Ali M A.
Skanes, Susan E.

FREDERICTON
Haswell, W. Timothy F.
Ismail, Abdel-Raouf
Menesi, Wisam A.
Oja, Mihkel A.

MONCTON
Howley, D. Brent
Inglis, Douglas S.

SAINT JOHN
Cook, Geoffrey S.
Lalonde, Donald H.
O'Brien, James P.

NEWFOUNDLAND AND LABRADOR

ST. JOHN'S
Anderson, Kenneth
Cluett, M. Joy
Fitzpatrick, Donald G.
Jewer, David D.
Rideout, Arthur A.
Seal, Shane K F.

NOVA SCOTIA

ANTIGONISH
Brennan, Michael B.

BRIDGEWATER
Hayden, David S.

HALIFAX
Bendor-Samuel, Richard L.
Bezuhly, Michael
LeBlanc, Martin R.
Morris, Steven
Paletz, Justin L.
Stein, John D.
Tang, David T T.
Williams, Jason G.
Wilson, Kenneth L.

NEW WATERFORD
Atiyah, Abdulrazzak O.

ONTARIO

AJAX
Eckhaus, Allan A.
Hayashida, Peter J K.

BARRIE
Dickie, Kenneth E.
Hassa, Agnieszka
Tumi, Kamaleddin H.

BRAMPTON
Haywood, Catherine T.
Kim, Sharon
Krajden, Selig
Sleightholm, Robert L.

BRANTFORD
Drakos, Demetrios A.
Nguyen, The Lac

BURLINGTON
Assad, Christopher J.
Grace, Douglas E.
Harris, Leonard
Weiglein, Otto

CAMBRIDGE
Sproat, Janet E.

CONCORD
Madronich, J. Robert

CORNWALL
Harris, Robert W.

EAST YORK
Dvali, Linda

ETOBICOKE
Baum, Joseph B.
Goldberg, Cory S.
Kasrai, Leila
Levine, Ronald H.
Panchapakesan, Vivek
Rebot, Morris T M.
Roach, Muriel P.
Tang, Christine L.
Wanzel, Kyle R.

HAMILTON
Avram, Ronen
Bain, James R.
Campbell-Moscrop, Alan J.
Collins, Jessica
Cooper, Michael J.
Dal Cin, Arianna
Hynes, Nicolas M.
Levis, Carolyn M.
Martin, Stuart
Patterson, Robert S.
Strumas, Nick
Thoma, Achilleas

KANATA
Lacey, James D.

KINGSTON
Davidson, John S D.
McKay, Douglas R.
Meathrel, Kimberley E.
Watkins, J. Frederick
Watters, Conrad W L.

KITCHENER
Chahal, Vickramjit S.
De Lorenzi, Claudio
Evans, Peter D.
Law, Warren C.

LONDON
Colcleugh, Robert
Evans, H. Brian
Gan, Bing Siang
Marignani, Marilena
Matic, Damir
Richards, Robert S.
Ross, Douglas C.
Scilley, Christopher G.
Yazdani, Arjang

MARKHAM
Kao, John T S.
Wallman, Ronald A.

MISSISSAUGA
Ahmad, Jamil
Inman, Richard J.
Lista, Francesco R.
Margaliot, Zvi
McLean, Hugh A.
Turley, Conor B.
Weinberg, Michael J.

NEPEAN
Callaghan, W. Bryan

NEWMARKET
Andrade, William N.
Ayeni, Olubimpe
Beatty, Steven E.
Knight, Casey T.
Van Vliet, Deborah

NIAGARA FALLS
Huq, Nasimul S.

NORTH YORK
Backstein, Robert S.
El-Sheikh, Yasser S.
Elahi, Mohammed
Golger, Alexander
Hong, Collin
Mahoney, Mary-Helen
Martin, Daniel C.
McCain, W. Gregory
Motakis, Dimitrios
Neu, Bernd R.
Rice, Sean B.
Samuel, Steve E S.
Schiller, Petra P.
Schlosser, Holli-Ellen
Starr, Joseph A.

OAKVILLE
Brown, Stephen C.
De Kleer, Nancy M A.
Khanna, Julie J.
Knowlton, Robert J.
Shortt, Rodger A D.

ORANGEVILLE
Taylor, John R.

ORILLIA
Seki, John T.
Toye, John W.

OSHAWA
Narini, Philip P.
Ruszkowski, Alexandra D.
Simmons, Elizabeth L.

OTTAWA
Allen, Murray W.
Benoit, Paul R.
Boyd, Kirsty U.
Chitte, Sachin A.
Duncan, Mary Jean
Ferron, Charles
Gallant, Michel
Gross, Ian G.
Guay, Nicolas A.
James, M. Ray
Jarmuske, Mario B.
Labow, Stanley S.
Nodwell, S A. Trefor
Peters, Daniel A.
Rockwell, Gloria M.
Silverman, Howard J.
Van Wyck, Lloyd G.
White, Colin P.
Ying, Yvonne

PETERBOROUGH
Mok, Lawrence M S.
Nimigan, Andre S.
Van Brenk, Bert

POINT EDWARD
Kaila, Sanjeev

PORT HOPE
Hutchinson, Neil T.

SAULT STE MARIE
Best, Timothy J.
Woolner, Douglas S.

SCARBOROUGH
Bendago, Mansour M.
Carlsen, Lloyd N.
Nandagopal, Narayanan
Shammas, Nouri I.
Sproule, Timothy R.
Voice, Sandra D.
Wong, Sarah H M.
Wong, Vanessa H.
Zorn, Marietta L T.

ST CATHARINES
Bush, Keith J.
Cohen, Richard S.
Young, Peter G J.

STRATFORD
Hasegawa, Brian J.

SUDBURY
Barr, Scott K M.
Fortin, Amanda J.
Hendel, Raymond
Kettle, Charles A.

THUNDER BAY
Thibert, Mark R.

TORONTO
Adibfar, Ali
Afolabi, Oluwatola
AlKudmani, Amer S B.
Anastakis, Dimitrios J.
Antonyshyn, Oleh M.
Beber, Brett
Bell, Thomas A B.
Binhammer, Paul A.
Born, Trevor M.
Bray, Peter W.
Brown, Mitchell H.
Carman, Wayne W.
Cartotto, Robert C.
Chesney, Amy L.
Chivers, Quinton
Clarke, Howard
DuPere, Marc
Edelstein, Jerome
Fialkov, Jeffrey
Fish, Joel
Fisher, David
Ford, Derek
Forrest, Christopher R.
Hofer, Stefan O P.
Hynes, Sally L.
Jeschke, Marc
Jugenburg, Martin
Kattan, Abdullah E.
Kreidstein, Michael L.
Lipa, Joan
Mahoney, James L.
Martou, Glykerie
McCabe, Steven J.
McKee, Nancy H.
Mrad, Mohamed A A M.
Musgrave, Melinda A.
Peters, Walter J.
Phillips, John H.
Pirani, Asif
Pritchard, Sandy J.
Salter, Margaret J.
Sandor, George K B.
Semple, John L.
Sliwin, Sammy J.
Snell, Laura J.
Stubbs, Robert H.
Tate, Laura J.
Tong, Lawrence
Wong, Karen W.
Zhong, Toni
Zuker, Ronald M.

VAUGHAN
O'Grady, Kevin

WATERLOO
Elmaraghy, Mohamed
Shenker, Robert L.

WELLAND
Bengezi, Omar

WHITBY
Kara, Mahmud

WINDSOR
Adams, Howard F.
Chow, Isabel J S.
Niessen, Marcus P.
Sion, David M.
Snowdon, Bruce A.

PRINCE EDWARD ISLAND

CHARLOTTETOWN
Kontor, Jurgen A.

STRATFORD
McLean, Gary D.

QUÉBEC

AMOS
Jodoin, Richard R.

BOUCHERVILLE
Daigle, Jean-Pierre

CHATEAUGUAY
Durand, Daniel L.

CHICOUTIMI
Dufresne, Marc L G.
Lopez-Valle, Carlos A.

GATINEAU
Berbari, Patricia
Dubois, Robert
Germain, Louis-Philippe
St-Amand, Hugo
Thompson, Tracey A.
Toupin, Yves

GREENFIELD PARK
Bourget, Amelie
Mok, David
Sauvageau, J. Johanne

KIRKLAND
Cunningham, David M.

LAVAL
Bernier, Mario F.
Brodeur, Andre
Charbonneau, Roland
Delorme, Roger P.
Dolmajian, Jennifer
Duranceau, Paul
Pellemans, Wilhelm B.

LEVIS
Arsenault, Frederic
Boa, Olivier
Leveille, Andre
Leveille, Claude

LONGUEUIL
Cote, Serge

MONT-ROYAL
Proulx, Claude
Zelt, Ronald G.

MONTREAL
Alshaikhi, Abdullah Y.
Baillargeon, Martine
Belanger, Maud
Bensimon, Eric
Bergeron, Leonard
Bernier, Christina
Borsuk, Daniel E.
Borsuk, Ronnie M.
Bortoluzzi, Patricia
Bou-Merhi, Joseph
Brassard, Pierre J.
Brutus, Jean-Paul
Caouette-Laberge, Louise
Chollet, Andre
Cianciulli, Rino
Cohen, Jack
Cordoba, J. Carlos
Crepeau, Rene
Dionisopoulos, Tassos
Duclos, Lucie
Duranceau, Louise A.
Egerszegi, E. Patricia
Frenette, Gilles A.
Gagnon, Alain
Gaudreau, Genevieve
Gilardino, Miroslav
Guberman, Daniel S.
Guertin, Charles
Harris, Patrick G.
Hashim, Ezat
Hyacinthe, Jean M F.
Lapointe, Richard H.
Lauzon, Gilles
Leblanc, Benoit
Lee, Chen
Lessard, M. Lucie
Lin, Jenny C.
Luc, Mario
Mercier, Jean-Francois
Moufarrege, Richard
Nicolaidis, Stephen C.
Nikolis, Andreas
Pelletier, Johanne
Perreault, Isabelle
Schwarz, Gaston
Schwarz, Karl A.
St-Laurent, Jean-Yves
Tardif, Michele
Tremblay, Dominique M.

POINTE-CLAIRE
Benchetrit, Arie
Pavlin, Jeanette E.
Tawile, Carolyne

QUEBEC
Chabot, Denys
Cloutier, Daniel
Dumas, Amelie
Gagnon, Isabelle
Genest, Herve
Houle, Normand
Lavertu, Denis J R.
Lecours, Catherine
Mailhot, Emilie
Montalin, Livia
Nguyen, Sebastien
Roberge, Celine
Roy, Alphonse
Roy, Michel A.
Tetu, Felix-Andre

REPENTIGNY
Cange, Sylvie

RIMOUSKI
Theriault, Claude

SAINT-HYACINTHE
Bussieres, Claude
Charbonneau, Ivan
Duguay, Pierre
Dupere, Sophie
Lampron, Carmen

SAINT-JEROME
Badran, Haitham
Borsanyi, Jean-Pierre
Loizides, Photis
Picard, Martine

SAINT-LAMBERT
Nonnenman, David K.

SAINT-LEONARD
Ciaburro, Hugo E.

SHERBROOKE
Cardin-Langlois, Etienne
Croteau, Frederic
El-Haddad, Jacques
Haddad, Jacques
Nootens, Jean V.
Olivier, Stephanie
Orfali, Charles G.

SOREL-TRACY
Dubois, Claude

TROIS-RIVIERES
Haddad, Jacob P.
Salib, George E.

VERDUN
Beaudoin, Jean-Louis
Beauregard, Gilles N.
Bouchard, Jacques

WESTMOUNT
McGill, Sandra N.
Papanastasiou, Vasilios W.
Schwarz, Jorge A.
Swift, Arthur
Zadeh, Teanoosh

SASKATCHEWAN

REGINA
Chandran, Geethan J.
Chang, Peter S.
Ghremida, Shukri A M.
Ledding, Kristopher M W.
Souf, Shawki A.

SASKATOON
Burwell, M. Shayne
Card, Annika M.
Clapson, J. Brian
Duval, Carolyn R.
Sunderland, Ian R P.
Thomson, Christopher J.
Tokaryk, Robert A M.
Zondervan, James H.

Psychiatry

ALBERTA

CALGARY
Abdel-Keriem, Mohamed A.
Adams, Beverly L.
Addington, Donald E.
Adrian, Carl H D.
Amadala, Stephen L.
Anderson, Kent S.
Angus, Donald R.
Appavoo, Lalitha L.
Atkinson, Carla M.
Ayas, Timmy
Baird, Kevin J.
Barnes, Daphne
Bawa, Hussam-Ul H.
Baxter, Cynthia L.
Beck, Cynthia A.
Benjamin, Joshua
Besant, Joan E.
Bhanji, Nadeem H.
Binder, Sara K.
Birkett, Leanne D.
Bodenstein, Christel E.
Boucher, Stephen A.
Brager, Nancy P D.
Brownell, Susan M.
Caldwell, Lyle H.
Carpenter, Susan P C.
Cassity, Sheri-Lynn E.
Chang, Christine H Y.
Chang, Samuel Y Y.
Chetner, Cynthia S.
Chohan, Inderjit S.
Cohen, Jordan S.
Coll, Patrick G.
Costello, Kathleen A.
Crockford, David N.
Culver, Timothy D.
Czechowsky, Diana
Dang, Chi Bao
Darlington, Paul
Dawson, David
De Groot, Janet M.
De Vries, Johannes D.
Dickson, Ruth
Donsky, Allan
Duffy, Anne C.
Duska, George P.
El-Guebaly, Nady A.
Elliott, John F.
Esche, Irena
Farnalls, Raymond B.
Fauvel, C. Terry
Fawcett, Arlie
Filyk, Maria
Fischer, Thomas I.
Fisher, Jennifer
Fitch, Kathryn
Fitzgerald, Cristin A.
Fraser, Suzanne M.
Gabriel, Adel A R.
Gagnon, Lisa M.
Gibbs, David J.
Haalboom, Erijka W.
Hamid, Salim
Harpur, Lisa L.
Hart, Claire
Hashman, Kenneth
Hibbard, Jennifer
Hirst, Clinton G.
Hnatowich, Rachel
Hogg, Lori M.
Hussain, Seema
Ihsan, Novin
Ismail, Zahinoor
Jalali, Fereshteh
Jericho, Monique C.
Kirova, Juliana S.
Kozman, Mervat N.
Kroll, Ian T.
Lakusta, Cherelyn M.
Lam, Peter C Y.
Lo, Tony H.
Lucido, Barbara M.
Lyons, Jessica E.
MacGougan, Donald D.
MacQueen, Glenda M.
Mackie, Aaron P.
Madan, Suparna
Malhotra, Sonya
Mann, A. Douglas
Manning, Pamella A M.
Marcus, Lawrence A.
Mason, Christine R.
Mason, Stephanie A.
Maybaum, Lloyd E M.
Mayer, Katalin E.
McCrank, Ernest W T.
McIlwrick, Joann G.
McKercher, Catherine D.
McLennan, John
McMullen, David M.
Mew, Jenny S.
Miyauchi, David K.
Mohamed, Zahra
Montgomery, Gregory P J.
Morin, M T. Caroline
Morrison, Dennis
Muir, Darcy G.
Naylor, John D.
Norbash, Adrian A.
Okoro, Daniel C.
Olaosun, Oluremi T.
Oluboka, Oloruntoba J.
Oluwadairo, Samuel A.
Onugha, Edward C.
Oosman, Jodie J.
Pandya, Rupang
Patten, Scott B.
Perpick-Breton, Marion L.
Petrov, Elena
Pierson, Kathleen E.
Pirlot, Tyler S.
Plowman, Brian K.
Postnikoff, Ian M.
Prior, Trevor I.
Quickfall, Jeremy P.
Rahman, Abdul
Ramasubbu, Rajamannar
Reinhardt, Paul H.
Rickhi, Badri G.
Ritchie, Blair D.
Roberts, R. Avalon
Rodway, Megan R.
Ryan, John P.
Sanders, Stuart B.
Sargeant, John K.
Schulz, Monika
Scott, Heather E.
Sellmer, Rory C.
Sgouromitis, Efthimios T.
Simpson, John S A.
Singh, Nandini J.
Smart, Marlene A.
Smith, Reilly G.
Solty, Heidi L.
Sowa, Bernard
Spivak, Mitchel H.
Stach, Misty J.
Stokes, Philip M A.
Stubbs, Michael D.
Taggart, Jason J.
Tang-Wai, Raymond M.
Tanguay, Karen E.
Tano, David S.
Toews, John A.
Tomm, Karl M.
Trew, Michael E.
Turner, Roy
Tuttle, John R.
Urquhart, Robert J.
Waheed, Waqar
Wallace, Elizabeth M.
Watson, G. Douglas
White, William D.
Wilkes, Thomas C R.
Yacoub, Maged F S.
Yates, Timothy T.
Yeung, Helen P.
Zanussi, Lauren W.
Zanussi, Ursula

CAMROSE
Edstrom, John P.

CANMORE
Perkins, C. Suzanne

CLARESHOLM
Cohen, Herbert L.
McCruden, Jane E.

COLD LAKE
Rees, Sylvia M.

EDMONTON
Adams, Leyland M.
Al Faraj, Noura J B.
Al-Ghamdi, Mohammad S.
Al-Sibani, Nasser K M.
Alghamdi, Mohammad S.
Alikouzehgaran, Maryam
Astorga, Maria Fe V.
Bailey, Darrin L.
Balachandra, Bhamini
Balachandra, Krishna
Banasch, Jan L.
Bhatia, Niti
Blackman, Adam S.
Blackman, Maurice
Bland, Roger C.
Blashko, Carl A.
Block, David N H.
Boffa, Ernest J.
Bondurant, Helen M.
Bottas, Alexandra
Bowman, Sylvia A.
Brooks, J. Hamilton
Brown, Roger T A.
Buchholz, Craig J.
Buchinski, Michael B.
Burback, Lisa M.
Caffaro, Leslie E.
Carr, Jane C.
Carr, Padraic E.
Carroll, Alan M.
Carter, Christine M.
Ceresney, Maureen N.
Chimich, William T.
Chokka, Pratap R.
Choy, Alberto L.
Chrenek, Carson
Chu, Jack Y L.
Chue, Pierre
Cojocaru, Alice
Collinson, Kathleen M.
Cooney, John A E.
Cummins, Mary G.
Czarnecki, Cory
Demaries, Sandra
Demas, Michael L.
Dewart, John M.
Din, Omar Shuja U.
Dobrofsky, Shirley
Drebit, Robert H.
Ede, Anizor
Flor-Henry, Pierre
Florence, Peter

Fogarty, Finola M.
Folescu, Simona
Frank, Sandi C.
Freed, Jennene L M.
Friend, William C.
Froelich, Christine K.
Gendemann, Klaus D.
Gibson, Keith K.
Gillese, J. Timothy
Ginter, Douglas
Girvin, Theresa C.
Gollapudi, Shreyasi R.
Gordon, Alan
Granger, Robert D C.
Guinhawa, Dante R.
Gurke, Richard A.
Hapchyn, Carole A.
Hesse, Stephen R.
Hetherington, Gabrielle S E.
Hibbard, Kate
Hibbard, Richard E.
Hugie, Tammy R.
Hunting, Erika A.
Jahandar, Parveen F.
Jegadesh, Beula S.
Joffe, Kenneth M.
John, Nicholas D.
Johnston, Jean F.
Kagan, Leon J.
Kasamali, Naureen N.
Kelly, Gordon J.
Khaliq, Anisa L.
Khullar, Atul
Kirdeikis, Katherine L.
Ko, Benjamin
Kostynuk, Carol D.
Kovithavongs, Carl S.
Kumpula, Iris M.
LaFrance, Rena S.
Lawless, Kevin
Lefebvre, Genevieve
Lefko-Singh, Karen J.
Leicht, Krista K.
Leiper, Thomas R.
Leung, Alice C.
Li, Daniel M.
Litwinson, Laurie
Long, Jason A.
Lorrain, Brandene L.
Lundeen, Richard C.
MacSween, Margaret J.
Mahil, Neelam
Maitra, Rajat
Malmberg, James L.
Marsh-Joyal, Melanie A.
Matthews, Sarah
McCahill, John A.
McCay, William A.
McKaigney, Eimear P.
McManus, David J.
McPherson, Alexandra M C.
Meakins, Diana M.
Meakins, Douglas W.
Mills, Philip
Mirtle, Brian R.
Mitchell, Andrea R.
Mitchell, Nicholas D.
Moreau, Chantal M M.
Morhaliek, Cameron S.
Morin, Kevin W.
Nadon, Philippe C.
Nahirney, David B.
Nair, Bina V.
O'Kelly, John G.
Osinchuk, James W.
Ostolosky, Lara J.
Oswald, Ronald E.
Parsons, Mitchel B.
Pawluk, Lawrence K.
Perez-Parada, Jorge E.
Phillips, Catherine L.
Piktel, Henry M.
Polak-Furigay, Yvetta M.
Rabeeh, Richard H.
Rajwani, Talib
Read, Daniel L.
Rodd, Peter M.
Rosie, John S.
Rourke, Margaret
Salsali, Mahnaz
Sanderman, Blaine S.
Scott, J. Rowan
Segal, Perry M.
Shapiro, Yakov
Shih, David
Silverstone, Peter H.
Simonds, Patricia E.
Singh, Vijay P.
Smit, Louwrens E.
Soper, Paul
Spaner, Douglas L.
Spence, David C.
Stich, Beverley R.
Stonehocker, Brian K.
Stovel, Laura E.
Studer, Lea H.
Swainson, Jennifer N.
Swanson, Murray C J.
Talsky, Mark A.
Taubner, Eric P.
Tomy, Nadia N.
Ustina, Judith K.
Vallabh, Pravesh K.
Walker, Candace M.
Warneke, Lorne B.
White, Wendy L.
Wilkes, Heidi R.
Woods, Curtis J.
Wright, Janet L.
Yaltho, C. Mathew
Youssef, Nagy A G.
Zedkova, Lenka

LETHBRIDGE
D'Agnone, John J.
Edwards, Wayne J.
Kotkas, Lawrence J.
Owen, Michael L S.
Rampling, Roger C.
Smart, Wallace D.
Sugars, John G.

MEDICINE HAT
Nandy, Saibal
Patel, Aditi J.

PONOKA
Danyluk, Dale E.
Hicken, W. Blair
Mott-Trille, Helen R.
Urness, Douglas

RAYMOND
Kennedy, John S.

RED DEER
Abelseth, David P.
D'Costa, Joseph A.
Dua, Manjula
Hansen, Frederick M.
Leung, Henry H Y.
Todd, Susan E.

SHERWOOD PARK
Elwell, Leo B.
Vozar, Jiri G.

ST ALBERT
Eades, Barnett R.
Lysak, Pauline S.
Petryk, Justin
Rogan, Ernest
Simpson, Patricia L.

BRITISH COLUMBIA

ABBOTSFORD
Arojojoye, Oyebode
Barbieri, Norma
Grasswick, Linda
Healey, Linda M.
Lamba, Rakesh K.
Saini, Mandeep S.
Sidhu, Parmjit K.
Strauss, Pieter
Uppal, Sonia
Zaghloul, Emad

AHOUSAT
Kamil, Rifaat

BURNABY
Agbayewa, M. Oluwafemi
Bostinariu, Anca Ioana.
Burns, Kyle D.
Chee, Hwa Kim
Friedlander, Robin I.
Gubanov, Alexander
Gutteridge, Ursula
Holland, Roy V.
Hyrman, Vaclav
Kang, Nirmal S.
Lee, Jerome B.
Murphy, Emlene M.
Napier, Robert L.
Paredes, Jaime P.
Rana, Babra M.
Ronsley, John C.
Sienicki, Marcin
Stefanelli, Michael N.
Thakur, Aruna K.
Thompson, Darren J.
Waraich, Paul S.
Wu, Johnny J.
Yuen, Sze-Ming

CAMPBELL RIVER
Bredenkamp, Barend J.

CHILLIWACK
Antony, Saju
Hope, Kim
Lilla, Mogamad N.
Tewfik Moussa, Laila

COMOX
Coxon, Carol E.
Frolic, Natasha K.
Lupton, P. Lauren
Schovanek, Stefan P J.
Tapper, C. Mark
Whetter, Kevin M.

COQUITLAM
Brink, Johann H.
De Freitas, Brian A.
Iskander, Sam
Meldrum, Lee Anne H.
Oduwole, Olusegun
Widajewicz, Witold J.

COURTENAY
Barber, Jeffrey L.

CRANBROOK
Van Der Lugt, Hubertus

DAWSON CREEK
Cilliers, Denise
Garbett, Sally E.
Kotze, Dirk A.

DELTA
Faris, Glenn D.
Gandhi, Amita
Kope, Teresa M.

DUNCAN
Derocher, Christopher S.
Pachal, Richard G.
Routledge, Robin
Saunders, Jane N.
Watler, Crosbie L.

FERNIE
Cote Beck, Martin E J.

FORT ST. JOHN
Jones, Carolyn S S.

GALIANO
Parfitt, Kathleen P.
Sousa-Poza, Joaquin F.

HERIOT BAY
McIntosh, Mary G.

KAMLOOPS
Baril, Marie-Claire
Buller, Kurt W.
Dagg, Paul
Hosenbocus, Sheik N.
Kusler, Janet L.
MacBeath, Lyn S.
Molgat, Carmen V.
Nwachukwu, Ikechukwu C.
Prystawa, Barbara M.
Pusztai, Edit Esther
Thibeault, Amy B.
Ward, Carol L.
Wiehahn, George J.

KELOWNA
Chin, James E.
De Luca, Marina
Derry, Heather
Diaz-Bobadilla, Julio F.
Hanon, Neil H.
Jones, Valerie A.
Latimer, Paul R.
Lok, Jennifer S.
McFayden, Ryan W C.
Ocana, Michael A.
Pipher, Bruce E.
Schuster, Lidia M.
Smith, Grant D.
Stevens, Annette C.
Wasti, Zahid
Wisniewska, Anna B.

LAKE COUNTRY
Coulter, David

LANGLEY
Hayden, Huguette S.
Hoffman, Joanne M.
Mistry, Prabhudas N.
Mohamed, Shiraz N.
Nair, Gangadharan N.
Seminiano, Pascualito A.
Shete, Shilpa C.

MAPLE RIDGE
Achong, Eamon H.
Benning, Tony B.
Bright, Britt
Daszkiewicz-Recizac, Maria
Dmitrieva, Victoria
Gopinath, Hirekatur V.
Killick, Lyn M.
Mathew, Biju
Nanda, Atul K.

MISSION
Frew, Patricia A.

NANAIMO
Ballance, D. Lee-Ann
Bowering, M. Rex
Goodhue, Angelique
Likwornik, Victor
McHugh, Sean M.
McPherson, Kathleen E.
Myronuk, Lonn D S.
O'Breasail, Aindrias M.
Okereke, Sunday O.
Rusak, Anysia M.
Smith, Sarah C.
Vincent, Merville A.
Walker, Joseph
Wiggers, Joris A J.

NELSON
Brownstein, Michael P.
Magee, Richard E L.

NEW WESTMINSTER
Anwar, Muhammad M.
Babbage, Christopher A.
Bowering, Tricia A.
Buttle, Jeffrey W.
Casey, Janel B.
Cheng, Ambrose C S.
Guan, Brian
Irani, Kaizad S.
Isomura, M. Theresa K.
Joshi, Hemlata S.
Khan, Mohammad A.
Koo, Anson
Lari, Harris
Lax, Stuart A.
Nazif, A. Aziz
Phaterpekar, Hem M.
Robertson, Christopher M.
Rogers, Jenny S.
Scarth, Brian A.
Wang, Eugene

NORTH VANCOUVER
Abdel-Fattah, Mohamed M.
Abdoulraman, Hamed
Barnett, Thomas W.
Basson, Denise I.
Booth, Christopher A.
Burgmann, Allan J F.
Freedman, Glen L.
Holdsworth, Rosalynd E.
Hunter, Christopher D.
Kang, Arvind
Laroche, Catherine
Lim, Meng Eng
Lim, Peter S H.
Severy, Philip R.
Shane, H. Frederick
Tang, Betty W.
Tarzwell, Robert R.
Termansen, Paul E.

PARKSVILLE
Juralowicz, Pawel
Whelton, Charles L M.

PENTICTON
Drew-Scott, Ryan N.
McIntyre, Alexander W.
Nichols, Melinda
Sheoran, Rajeev

PORT COQUITLAM
McKibbin, R. Douglas
Parfitt, Hugh L.
Ramsundhar, Rohan
Sharan, Richa

PORT MOODY
Turner, Julia A.

POWELL RIVER
Howard, Robert S.
Ramirez Moreno, Saby E M.

PRINCE GEORGE
Boulding, Rachel A.
Frye, June C O.
Giede, Johannes A.
Grant-Oyeye, Lind
Jani, Aarti
Kane, Barbara J.
Khan, Isfandyar
Kolisang, Mohau P.

REVELSTOKE
Brooks-Hill, Robin

RICHMOND
Adam, Trudy J.
Au, Raymond
Bhopal, Jaswant S.
Brandt, E. Lorne
Choo, Caroline W H.
Cohen, David J.
Costin, Avrum
Fung, Jonathan
Fung, Kathryn C.
Gibson, Peter
Harris, James G.
Karlinsky, Harry J.
Katta, Balaraju B.
Minhas, Avinder S.
Moorthy, Ramachandra N.
Rabin, David G.
Shabbits, Michael S.
Steinberg, Carolyn R.
To, Agnes S.
Ye, Zhongbo J.
Zipursky, Sheldon

SALMON ARM
Britto, Ericka L.

SALT SPRING ISLAND
Montalbetti, David J.
Sladen-Dew, Nicholas S.

SECHELT
Altman, Siemion
Barale, Anthony E.
White, Norman F.

SIDNEY
Lohrasbe, Shabehram S.
Nixon, G. William H.
Prowse, Arthur W H.

SOOKE
Ney, Philip G F.

SURREY
Catona, Tamara
Devlin, Paul G.
Dowey, Michael T J.
Ellis, G. Graham
Eswar, Shruthi
French, Kelly M.
Griffin, Desmond J.
Harrad, Upninderjit S.
Heilbrunn, David L.
Jassal, Kuldip
Kostolowski-Kondysar, Malgorzata H.
Mallavarapu, Harinath
Miremadi, Saman
Narang, Satinder P S.
Pole, Chak L.
Proulx, Francois
Riley, Mark P.
Saffy, Samantha C.
Sandhu, Jatinder S.
Selvaraj, Madhavan
Sidhu, Rajreet S S.
Thillainadarajah, Pandaram
Van Den Berg, Marietta
Wand, Reginald R.
Zielonka, Lucjan J.

TRAIL
Naicker, Sharman M.
Okonkwo, Cletus C.

VANCOUVER
Adams, Leona
Ainsworth, Geoffrey
Allen, Judith M.
Anderson, Cameron M.
Anderson, Stephen D.
Andrews, Lorraine D.
Axler, Auby H.
Baer, Susan
Baerg Hall, Elizabeth A.
Berzen, Leon
Black, Tyler R.
Blank, Myles K.
Bond, David J.
Borowska, Anna M.
Braunstein, Ronald E.
Broster, Brett S.
Cabalo, Eve C.
Caldis, Efstratios V.
Cameron, Kristjana G.
Campbell, D. Paula
Carter, Diana M G.
Chan, Peter K Y.
Chan, Ryan
Chapman, Andrea J M.
Chaudhary, Muzumel A.
Chauhan, Harpreet
Chen, Chi Nan
Chernick, Grant M P.
Cho, Caroline E.
Chodkiewicz, Adam C.
Chow, Matthew C.
Claman, Jeffrey M.
Cockhill, Leslie A.
Comey, Robert
Constance, Peter D A.
Cook, Michael I.
Corral, Maria D R.
Coupland, Jason E.
Cunningham, Linda D.
D'Oyley, Heather M.
Davidson, Jana-Lea
Davis, Lindsay E.
Debbane, Elie G.
Dilli, Melih
Dimov, Marius
Doherty, Mary P.
Donaldson, Heather J.
Donnelly, Martha L.
Drance, Elisabeth
Driscoll, Miriam A.
Dryer, Donna A.
Drysdale, Elaine R.
Dua, Vikram
Duke, Margaret H.
Dunn, Patrice M.
Fahy, Mellisa J.
Falconer, Clark W.
Fan, Nancy C.
Fast, Diane
Fitzpatrick, Stephen J.
Fleming, Jonathan A E.
Flynn, Sean W.
Forbes, Ian S.
Frankland, Allan G.
Fredrikson, Diane H.
Freeman, Roger D.
Friesen, Wesley H.
Froese, Colleen L.
Fullagar, Ernest W.
Fung, David A.
Gambetti, Andrea
Ganesan, Soma
Garland, E. Jane
Geizer, Marie
Genge, Margot M.
Gibson, Ronald E.
Golden, Susan J.
Goldner, Elliot M.
Gorman, Christopher
Gosselin, Caroline
Goumeniouk, Alexander D.
Grabovac, Andrea D.
Greenaway, Masa'il
Gregson, Alison N.
Gruson, Valerie J.
Hadjipavlou, George A.
Hardin, Earl D.
Hay, William L.
Hewko, Robert A.
Honer, William G.
Howard, Andrew K.
Hui, Jacqueline C W.
Hunter, Julia D.
Hurwitz, Trevor A.
Hutnyk, David J.
Ilcewicz-Klimek, Magdalena I.
Illing, Martin A J.
Irwin, David A J.
Janke, Paul G.
Jiwa, Abdulkarim M.
Jokhani, Krishna
Jones, Russet L.
Kalda, Riho
Kalenchuk, Anna L.
Kang, G. Shimi
Kasapi, Marina S.
Kelleher, Samantha M A.
Kennedy, Andrea L.
Kerr, Clifford G.
Khanbhai, Irfan A.
Kline, Stephen A.
Koczapski, Andrzej B A.
Koritar, Endre L.
Korkuczanska, Svetlana
Krausz, R. Michael
Kroeker, Garth D.
Kulpas, Leila
Kunkel, Lucinda C.
Kwan, Man Wai
Kwok, Winnie W.
Lafleur, Daniel L.
Lam, Raymond W.
Lament, Richard
Lazar, Gary A.
Lazar, Susan F.
Lee, Tih-Shih W.
Leech-Porter, J. Colin G.
Leong, Judith M.
Levin, Alexander L.
Levy, J. Mark
Liang, Raymond A.
Lin, Daniel C.
Lisiak, Elena
Livesley, W. John
Locke, Jake J.
Loh, Diana P Y.
Lomax, Susan M.
Louie, Donald F.
Lu, Shao-Hua
MacFadden, Megan E.
Madhani, Kurban J.
Mador, Joseph A.
Marcus, Harvey V.
Marriage, Keith J.
Mathias, Steven M.
Matrick, Lawrence E.
Maurice, William L.
McAleer, Dominic J.
McGarvey, Kathleen A.
McIntosh, Diane M.
McLachlan, Siobhan C.
McMillan, M. Janette
McWatters, Dorothy L.
Melck, Cyril I.
Mendoza, Valentina I.
Miki, Nancy P H.
Mildenberger, Sheila J.
Millar, Grant A.
Miller, Ashley P.
Miller, Debra S.
Minnes, Yoram
Mirmiran, S. Jamaluddin
Misri, Shaila
Mittler, Gerald R.
Mok, Hiram L H.
Moniwa, Emiko
More, Susan G.
Mulvey, Michael R.
Murray, Christopher B.
Musacchio, Mafalda S.
Nazif, Anna S K.
Neelakant, Harish K.
Ngan, Elton T C.
Nolan, Sean P.
Nolan, Sheila M.
Noone, Joseph A.
Northcott, Colleen J.
O'Kane, Janine M.
O'Shaughnessy, Roy J.
Ong, Larry S.
Panenka, William J.
Parker, Anne M.
Passey, D. Greg
Passmore, Michael J.
Patrick, Lancelot L C.
Patterson, Bruce D.
Pattison, Mark A.
Patton, Sheila W.
Penfold, P. Susan
Perry, Katherine F.
Persaud, Rainer
Perzow, Sidney M.
Pezzot, Donald E.
Price, William E H.
Pullmer, Lewis Z.
Quan, James L.
Raina, Raj Binder S.
Randhawa, Ramandeep S.
Raudzus, Julia A.
Raycraft, Stephen W.
Reebye, Pratibha N.
Remick, Ronald A.
Riar, Kulwant S.
Richford, Carole M.
Risling, Eva M.
Rivera, Karen A.
Roberts, Megan
Robertson, Heather
Rosenauer, Helen L.
Rosin, Richard A.
Rothschild, Carl J.
Rungta, Kamal N.
Russel, Jennifer M.
Ryan, Deirdre M A.
Saari, Carol-Ann
Sadrehashemi, Ladan
Sanders, Andrew P.
Saran, Kalwinder S.
Scamvougeras, Anton
Scarfe, Sarah E.
Schaffer, Nathan
Schenk, Christian H.
Schertzer, Stephen J.
Schwartz, Deborah C.
Schwartz, Patricia L T.
Segal, Barry M.
Sehon, Anthony A P.
Shaw, Nur Deniz.
Sheldon, Leslie J.
Sherwood, Megan E.
Shetty, Maithili R.
Shick, Roger D.
Shoja, Sheila
Shore, Resa S.
Shulman, Barbara
Sidhu, Jesse A.
Sidky, Abdallah Y.
Singh, Kulbir I.
Smith, Derryck H.
Smith, Jeanette E.
Solomons, Kevin
Solyom, Ildiko E.
Stein, Paul B.
Steinberg, Paul I.
Sternthal, David S.
Stevenson, Ronald W D.
Stewart, S. Evelyn
Stikarovska, Irena
Straszak, Irena M.
Sucharov, Maxwell S.
Tam, Edwin M.
Taylor, Christine G.
Telio, Summer L.
Tesler-Mabe, Carlos
Tham, C W. Joseph
Tidmarsh, Mary E L.
Tomita, Todd M.
Tremblay, Madeleine D.
Tsang, Nicole
Uppal, Loveleen
Vallance, Maelor
Vassar, Elizabeth V.
Vik, Astrid L.
Vila-Rodriguez, Fidel
Vogt, Lori A.
Voutsilakos, Emorphea
Waddell, Charlotte A.
Wanis, Wahan
Ward, David G H.
Weiss, Margaret D.
Whelan, John M.
White, Randall F.
Wicholas, Bertrand L.
Wicholas, Leslie
Wide, Jennifer K.
Wiebe, Carl H B.
Wiese, Bonnie S.
Wilkins-Ho, Michael
Wilt, Frances R.
Wiseman, Stephen R.
Wong, Allan P G.
Wong, Angela S W.
Wong, Monique L.
Wrixon, Katherine J.
Wulff, Tanya A.
Yatham, Lakshmi N.
Yeh, Jennifer N.
Young, Allan H.
Young, Kay
Yuswack, Timothy J.
Zhang, Dajiang
Zis, Athanasios P.
Zoffmann, Elisabeth
Zuberbier, Oonagh A.

VERNON
Abdel-Kader, Mahmoud A K.
Acton, Gillian R.
Eaman, Stanley G.
McGregor, F. Fiona K.
Smith, David H.
Stevenson, Kevin W.
Tomm, Bill G.
Williams, Russell G.

VICTORIA
Argouarch, Sylvie J.
Atkins, Mark H.
Bardell, Andrea
Blashko, Christopher D.
Bosley, Laurence A.
Bouffard, Rachelle E.
Breitman, Deanne R.
Burrell, Erin C.
Campbell, Helen
Chamitoff, Shayna E.
Chapman, Laura M.
Cheek, Joanna P.
Collins, Nelson C.
Connolly, Mary C C.
Cooper, Michael C.
Copen, Brenda Y K.
Copen, John V W.
Crouse, Wanda J.
Culo, Sandi
Dalsin, Judith
Drabkin, Rodney
Edward-Chandran, Therese S.
Emes, Craig E.
Firstbrook, Peggy J.
Gillespie, Ian A.
Gould, Brent
Gunn, Adam M.
Halischuk, Grant F.
Holden, Timothy J.
Immelman, Lynleigh J.
Ingram, Diana R.
Johnson, F. Gordon
Knudson, Gail A.
Korn, Miriam
Kowalchuk, Shauna L.
Leishman, David J.
Lilley, Kenneth
Lohrasbe, Harpreet
Lydon, Patrick
Malaviarachchi, Pushpa K.
Megahed Gheis, Mohamed A.
Mestelman, Bryan P.
Miller, Marian R.
Miller, Robert E W.
Milliken, A. Donald
Musgrave, S. Ian
Nerenberg, Lucila
Nixon, Mary K.
O'Neill, Kevin B.
Palmer, Karen A.
Pawliuk, George K.
Preuss, Jeannette
Ramstead, Margaret J.
Robinow, R. Oliver
Roth, Victoria E.
Rudnick, Abraham
Sacamano, James T.
Schieldrop, Peter
Semrau, Stanley R.
Sheinbaum, Deborah
Shrikhande, Satish
Sigurdson, Wilfred F.
Simms, Kiri J M.
Sinai, Joanne
Song, Wei-Yi
Stern, Richard J.
Stovel, Duncan C.
Strueby, Brian J D.
Swan, David M A.
Tuka, Andrea
Watt, John A.
Whitaker, Katherine J.
Williams, Richard
Witt, Alvera
Wood, Clare M P F.
Wooder, E. Jeffrey
Yaxley, David T.

WEST VANCOUVER
Azim, Hassan F A.
Bawden, Carole A.
Blunderfield, G. Mark
Buchanan, R. Alan
Chesko, Jennifer C.
Fabian, James E.
Kiraly, Stephen J.
Kirkpatrick, David
Kjernisted, Kevin D.
Pankratz, Werner J.
Paragas, Pedro G.
Reddy, Dorothy
Warrian, W. Garnet
Weiss, Jacqueline R.

WHITE ROCK
Baksh, Arlene D.
Bergen, Dorothea
Bondar, Jay S.
Kennedy, Lindsay C.
Kyne, Peter T.
MacEwan, Gordon W.
Maskall, Douglas D.
Paquet, Karine
Zaitzow, Michael D.

WILLIAMS LAKE
Priest, Vona G.

MANITOBA

BRANDON
Jenkins, Keith A.
Lee, Gilbert Q.
Lint, Donald W.
McIntyre, Ian L.
Tavares, Alexandre G.
Varley, Kevin R.
Vasconcelos, Jose A.
Vipulananthan, Manohary
Vipulananthan, Velluppillai

DAUPHIN
Sandhu, Sukhbir S.

OAKBANK
Steinbart, Murray R.

SELKIRK
Barchet, Paul M.
Graham, Roger C.
Kremer, Steven
MacKay, Maralyn J.
Malchy, Brian A.
Teillet, Marc E.
Walji, Mohammediqbal F H.
Wilkie, W. Clarke

THE PAS
Medd, Thomas M.

THOMPSON
Pandey, Anil K.

WINKLER
Dyck, Michael
Funk, Kathryn M.
Ivey, Jeffrey A.
Klassen, Larry J.
Miller, William W J.
Wiebe, Hazel L J.

WINNIPEG
Altman, Gary N.
Anderson, Donna M.
Anderson, Erin
Anderson, Ryan A.
Anderson, Shelley D.
Andrew, Hugh G.
Armstrong, Brent J.
Ballegeer, Trevor
Barakat, Samia M.
Bolton, David R.
Bolton, James M S.
Boman, Jonathan C.
Bristow, Kristin M.
Buchik, Glenda M.
Calhoun, Laura L.
Campbell, Barry I.
Casiano, Hygiea
Chochinov, Harvey M.
De Rocquigny, Andre J.
Downs, Allan C.
Ducas, Diane A.
Edye, Frances
Eghtedari-Namin, Fariba
El-Gaaly, Sherief
Eleff, Michael K.
Enns, Murray W.
Enyingi, Juliette A.
Etkin, Mark S.
Fast, Henry V.
Fleisher, William
Fotti, Sarah A.
Gallagher, Katherine L.
Gill, Eunice C.
Globerman, Daniel J.
Gonzalez-Pino, Fernando
Goossen, Randolph B.
Gordon, Jeremy
Gregoryanz, Tatiana
Hall, Andrew
Harrington, Michael
Hawe, Richard
Hershberg, Dane M.
Hildahl, V. Keith
Hosain, Shahid
Hynes, Adrian F M.
Ingimundson, Janice C.
Ingram, Peter F.
Jagdeo, Amit
Karvelas, Lisa M.
Katz, Laurence Y.
Katz, Philip
Kettler, Jack J.
Kettner, Adrian S.
Kirshner, Alla
Klaponski, Stanka
Koltek, Mark M.
Koodoo, Stanley R.
Kowalchuk, Ivan J.
Kreviazuk, Jessica L.
Kroft, Cara D L.
Kuzenko, Nina J L.
Lambert, Kerri L.
Lander, Debra A.
Lander, S. Mark
Lavitt, Gail B.
Lebedin, Walter W.
Levin, Giovanna V D A.
Li, Xin-Min
Ludwig, Louis W.
McCartney, Dawn M.
McPhee, James S.
Moody, Jane K.
Morier, Gisele S L.
Mowchun, Leon
Mowchun, Neil
Mysore, Munithanamma J.
Newman, Francis
O'Keeffe, Kieran M.
Omelan, Craig K.
Partap, Nadine A.
Penner, Layna R.
Perlov, Jack
Phillips, Michael L.
Polimeni, Joseph O.
Prasad, Benjamin A A.
Prober, Mark A.
Rolls, Rodney E.
Rosenthal, Peter
Sala, Tanya N.
Sam, Diana L.
Sareen, Jitender
Savage, Bonita H.
Sawyer, Jeremy A.
Schachter, Murray A.
Schaub, J. Christian
Schwartz, Leonard D.
Seifer, Roman
Shane, Marvin D.
Sharkey, Rowan D.
Shelton, Lynne J.
Sigurdson, Eric S.
Simm, James F.
Skakum, Kurt K.
Skinner, James T.
Sloan, Gary W.
Steinberg, Robert J G.
Sutherland, Karen E.
Szelazek, Joanna T.
Thompson, Thomas R.
Trepel, Simon P.
Vanderwert, Ruwani T.
Vattheuer, Frank B.
Vickar, Eric L.
Wakeman, M. Stewart A.
Waldman, Jeffrey C.
Wightman, Nancy A.
Wightman, Patricia A.
Willows, James R.
Winogrodzki, Arthur
Wirch, M. Faye
Woods, Anna K.
Yaren, Stanley
Zimmer, Kenneth W.
Zloty, Richard B.

NEW BRUNSWICK

BATHURST
Bordeaux, Patrick
Dru, Gilbert
Godin, Stephane
Hache, Mireille C.

CAMPBELLTON
Binette, Marcel
Laevski, Aleksandar L.

DIEPPE
Marquis, Etienne
Theriault, Louis F J.

FREDERICTON
Addleman, David
Doucet, John R.
Hoyt, Linda C.
Jayaram, Kadamby P.
Poder, Kulli
Scholten, Monique C.
Tran, Simone M P.

MIRAMICHI
Mahfoudi, Redha

MONCTON
Akinmokun, Adebusola
Alatishe, Moses A.
Aucoin, Colette
Bhalla, Dinesh
Chianetta, Jean-Marc
Dandenault, Brigitte L M.
Doucet, Jerome
Levesque, Andree
Liashko, Vitaly A.
Mahmud, Syed
Marcotte, Patrick
Poirier, Mylene
Ross, Barbara M.
Tahir, Laeeq A.
Trudeau, Terrence R.
Vautour, Marc

SAINT JOHN
Aicher, Joseph
Bryniak, Christopher S.
Forsythe, Pamela
John, Omana E.
Joshi, Vinod S.
Kubacki, Andrzej
Maxan, Emily E.
Morehouse, Rachel L.
Onuora, Abraham N.
Potter, Laurie A.
Rowe, Helen S.
Satyanarayana, Satyendra
Thompson, Sarah J.
Yuzda, Edward S.

NEWFOUNDLAND AND LABRADOR

CARBONEAR
Porter, M. Anne
Vokey, Keith A.

CORNER BROOK
Power, Y. Mark E.

GRAND FALLS WINDSOR
Luscombe, Kristopher D.
Manhas, Surender S.

HAPPY VALLEY GOOSE BAY
Walsh, Gilbert D.

ST. JOHN'S
Adey, Tanis L.
Bonnell, Weldon
Brace, Alec W.
Broaders, Marguerite A.
Callanan, Terrence S.
Caravan, Christine L.
Collins, David J.
Dalton, Susan M.
Dolezalek, Jan A.
Gill, Jasbir
Hancock, E. Jolene
Hearn, Taryn L.
Hickey, Catherine
Hofner, Anne Marie
Hogan, Kevin P.
Jat, Khalid M.
Kennedy, Norman R.
Ladha, Nizar B.
Latus, Andrew M.
Ledrew, Kellie K.
Lynch, Sheila M P.
MacLaughlin, Deirdre A.
Maddigan, Barbara A.
Martins, Isabel M.
McWilliam, Tina M.
Noble, Sarah E.
Noseworthy, Gordon W.
O'Keefe, Erin L.
Penney, Angela M.
Pratt, Douglas R.
Reid, Chantelle A.
Slade, Cynthia S.
Snelgrove, Christine
St John, Kimberly A.
Walsh, Anthony D.
Walsh, Coleen P.
Weiner, Marta A.
Wheeler, Leslie
White, Hubert P.

NORTHWEST TERRITORIES

YELLOWKNIFE
Clemmey, W. Robert L.
Laureijs, Pauweliena P M.

NOVA SCOTIA

AMHERST
Lock, Elizabeth A.
MacNeill, Kara E.
Moss, Philippa A.

ANTIGONISH
Rideout, Carolyn M.
Slayter, Ian M.

BEDFORD
Birnie, William A.
Curtis, John C.
Gosse, G. Craig
Ring, Melanie S.
Wawer, Ursula B.

BRIDGEWATER
Brooks, Simon A L.
Casey, J. Stephanie
Milliken, Jacqueline H J.
Morgan, Neal A.
Wood Jr., William C.

CANNING
Garvey, Brian M.

DARTMOUTH
Bergin, Siobhan M.
Black, Katharine A.
Brunet, Aileen S.
Flynn, Michael S.
Fraser, Ronald I.
Gordon, Edward G.
Hazelton, Lara D K.
Hipwell, Alexander E.
Kronfli, Risk
Mills, Philip J.
Muir, Ava J F.
Muthu, M. Saravana
Neilson, Grainne E.
Peters, Curt S.
Pottle, Robert A.
Rubens, Mark J.
Sadek, Joseph A.
Theriault, P. Scott
Tomlinson, H. Mary M.
Walentynowicz, Magdalena A.

HALIFAX
Abbass, Allan A.
Abidi, Sabina
Alda, Martin
Bagnell, Alexa L.
Bilski-Piotrowski, Miroslaw
Borst, Sjoerd A.
Bosma, Mark A.
Brake, Jonathan A.
Calkin, Cynthia V.
Carrey, Normand J.
Cassidy, Keri-Leigh
Chehil, Sonia
Chengapa, Vinnie
Chisholm, Blanche T.
Cooper, Kenneth J.
Davis, Joann E.
Delva, Nicholas
Freer, Janya M.
Gray, Gerald
Harris, Andrew S.
Howard, Richard J.
Hudec, Mary-Ann
Jha, Umesh C.
Junek, R. Wade
Keshen, Aaron R.
Kutcher, Stanley P.
Lovas, David A.
Lynch, Mary E.
MacDonald, Dianne D.
MacDonald, Joanne L.
MacDonald, Shannon L.
MacKay, Thomas J.
Marval Ospino, Heizer Jose
Maynes, Douglas F.
Milliken, Heather I.
Morrison, Jason M.
Murphy, Cheryl L.
O'Donovan, M. Claire
O'Neill, Marie-Therese A.
Orlik, Herbert
Parker, Deborah J R.
Pearce, Patricia A.
Pellow, Tanya R.
Rajda, Malgorzata
Rosenberg, Edwin M.
Ross, Dawn L.
Ruzickova, Martina
Sokolenko, Marina
Stokes, Aidan
Tait, Glendon R.
Teehan, Michael D.
Thurgood, Ann M.
Tibbo, Philip G.
Tulipan, Tanya M.
Ursuliak, Zenovia B J.
Watt, Garth B.
White, Kimberley D.
Wilson, Adriana E.
Zinck, Mary S.

HUBBARDS
Jellema, Dick

KENTVILLE
George, Puthenkalathil P.
Johnston, J. Mark
Mulhall, David R.
Thompson, Karen M.

LOWER SACKVILLE
Bhaskara, Sreenivasa M.
James, Sherry L.
McCormick, William O.
Morgan, Matthew

NEW GLASGOW
Basecqz, Guy M.
Vienneau, Theresa L.

SYDNEY
Akinsola, Oluwatosin A.
Aldridge, David J.
Ali, Javed E.
Christians, Neil J.
Curwin, Julie M.
Foley, Brian M.
Libbus, Yvonne E.
Milligan, Scott R.
Munshi, Autar K.
Rogers, John C.
Udolu, Owhoede J.

TRURO
Curley, William F.
De Boer, Cornelis
Ginnish, Amanda
Hofner, Grazyna W.
Maguire, Hugh P.
Penn, Jeffrey R.
Pogosyan, Maryna
Warren, Jo-Ann L.

WINDSOR
Burke, Brian J.
Lazier, Lorraine L.
Warren, Katherine J.

WOLFVILLE
Cassidy, Beverley-Dawn

YARMOUTH
Banjo, Olufemi
Chandler, James D.

ONTARIO

AJAX
Devi, Bijayalaxmi
Drandic, Marijana
Lachmann, Mark H.
Omoruyi, Enosakhare B.
Thangaroopan, Arulanantham

ANCASTER
Epelbaum, Mikhail
Morgan, Jane A.

AURORA
Madden-Fitzsimons, Therese
Waese, Adam S.

BALA
Wright, David C.

BARRIE
Ali, Liaqat
Benjamin, Marcia D.
Bilkey, Timothy S.
Hakim, Hassan R.
Hector, R. Ian
Horsey, Mary E.
Khan, Sher B.
Kraus, Peter J.
Luczak, L. Alexander
Menuck, Morton N.
Mulder, Eric M.
Rajkhowa, Sudhir
Reichmann, Jaak T.
Seevaratnam, David M.

BARRYS BAY
McKay, Suzanne J.

BELLEVILLE
Al-Nakhli, Mohammed
Arboleda-Florez, Julio E.
Ash, Leslie C.
El Saidi, Mohammed
Fahy, Maeve P.
King, Robert J.
MacPherson, Colin J.
Singh, Amarendra N.

BORDEN
Ewing, David G.
Labonte, Anne

BOWMANVILLE
Ledger, Gabrielle H.

BRACEBRIDGE
Wilson, G. Andrew C.

BRAMPTON
Acharyya, Partha
Asayesh, Khalil
Bakht, M. Murad
Bami, Harmeet K.
Banik, Tapan K.
Cryer, Elizabeth J.
Dhaliwal, Jagtaran S.
El-Kholi, Vivian M.
Faux, Peter J.
Gyimah, Albert
Koczerginski, David
Kruger, Kenneth
Mansour, Ahmed M.
Mech, Zdzislaw R.
Nagpurkar, Ranjana
Noorani, Naushad A.
Nyhus, Nadine J.
Ohene-Darkoh, Charles
Sayeed, Muhammad R U.
Soliman, Wassim G F.

BRANTFORD
Book, Ronald W.
Briskin, Jonathan K.
Clarke, Theresa-Ann
Luthra, Atul
Olejarova, Emilia
Prayaga, Rama S R.
Ratnayake, Quintine
Sharma, Poonam
Sharma, Shreekant

BROCKVILLE
Ahmed, Adekunle G.
Bradford, John M W.
Brook-Williams, Penelope
Calleia, Sarah G E.
Cameron, Colin J.
Deshauer, Dorian
Feltham, Ian
Jackson, R. Jeffrey D.
James, Elizabeth D F.
Malone, Robert D.
Messina, Sarina
Sim, Franklin H.
Smith, Robert G.
Watson, Diane B.

BURLINGTON
Amaladoss, Noel R.
Aziz, Mariam
Bishop, W. Mary E.
Colonne, D D. Prasannajith
Dermer, Stanley W.
Dziurdzy, Stanley A.
Freebury, David R.
Lam, David B W.
Purohit, Nimishchandra N.
Skladman, Irina
Taynen, Howard D.
Turner, Peter G.

CAMBRIDGE
Dawson, David F L.
Matti, Edward T.
Power, A. Martina H.
Senior, Susan E.

CAMPBELLFORD
Schabas, Patti A.

CARLETON PLACE
Rae, Christopher J.

CHATHAM
Barral, Myrlinda V.
Chandrasena, Ranjith D.
Devarajan, Sivakumaran
Fairbairn, Robert F.
Swaminath, Sam

COBOURG
Brooks, Kathleen M.
Carlyle, Robert W.

COLLINGWOOD
Josiukas, Anne N N E.

CONESTOGO
Ligate, Loys J.

CORNWALL
Hanna, Magda W.
Khan, A. Ghaffar
Wassef, Kawsar K.

DRAYTON
Polak, Vivian A.

DRYDEN
Hampe, Kyle

DUNDAS
Buie, Robert
King, Caroline A.
Ryerse, Cynthia L.

EAST YORK
Armstrong, Harvey A.
Smith, George E D.
Tamakloe, Barnaby E A.

ETOBICOKE
Armstrong, Taylor C.
Bismonte, Maria Dulce B.
Cho, Brian
Clarke, June M.
Clarke, Michelle B.
Jokay, Eva M.
Kantor, A. David
Khan, Naeem A H.
Kodsi, Maged S.
Kulesha, Denis
Kulkarni, Chetana A.
Lodenquai, Gregory M.
Morris, Paul S.
O'Brien, Elizabeth P.
Panjwani, Dilkhush D.
Rzadki, Edward J J.
Sandor, Zsuzsanna S.
Shafro, Ariel
Sood, Balbhadar D.
Srinivasan, Vasundhara
Swierczek, Janusz S.

FERGUS
Thurling, M. Lynne

FLINTON
Connell, Stephen L.

GODERICH
Al Darwish, Mahdi E A.
Conlon, Patrick S J.
Hudson, Craig J.
MacLeod, Valerie A.
McAuley, Thomas J.

GUELPH
Alvarez- Higuera, Andrea D.
Badoe, Kwame E.
Balakrishnan, Pradeep
Braida, Raymond L.
Clements, Karen H.
Coulter, H. Joan
Fareau-Weyl, Joelle M T.
Furlong, Brian G.
Glumac, George
Johnston, Anita G C.
Kukreja, Kanwal
Lalonde, Carlos D.
Litch, Stanley W.
Long, Briar A.
McColl, Linda C P.
Moorthy, Sathasivam W.
Mulder, Erik W.
Papadopoulos, Yousef G.
Pittman, C. Dianne
Reade, Elizabeth A.
Savage, Martha H B.
Teferi, Amde M.
Velamoor, Varadaraj R.
Zarins, Eric D.

HAMILTON
Adam, Christina M.
Agrawal, Sacha
Akintan, Olabode O.
Alatishe, Yuri
Anglin, Rebecca E S.
Archie, Suzanne M.
Arciszewska, Halszka T.
Auron, Samuel
Bartolucci, Giampiero
Bennett, Teresa Ann
Bibr, Henry J.
Bienenstock, Audrie M.
Bigelow, Gayle S.
Boylan, Khrista R A.
Brasch, Jennifer S.
Brotea, Alina R.
Carr, Anthony C.
Cebrian, Clara
Chaimowitz, Gary A.
Cheng, Tracy T.
Clinton, Jean M.
Collins, Stephen
Cook, Peter E.
Corey, Jo Ann M.
Cornfield, Mark J I.
Cote, Isabelle
Couturier, Jennifer L.
Czernikiewicz, Wojciech
Davine, Jonathan
Deadman, John
Dudley, John
Duff, Sharon
Edwards, Carla
Ennis, Jeffrey
Eppel, Alan B.
Ferencz, Joseph C.
Gaind, Gagan S.
Garside, Sarah L.
George, Lindsey J.
Gilani, Sadia
Goldberg, Jeremy
Gunasekera, Shiny D.
Guscott, Richard G.
Harms, Sheila C.
Hasey, Gary M.
Hategan, Ana
Johnston, David G.
Kates, Nicholas S.
Kiang, Michael W J.
Kolawole, Olubukola F.
Kondra, Peter M.
Korzekwa, Marilyn I.
Krasnik, Catherine E.
Levinson, Anthony J.
Lewis, Jennifer E.
Lipman, Ellen L.
List, Stephen J.
Lough, Rodney D.
MacCrimmon, Duncan J.
MacLeod, Roderick J.
Mancini, Catherine L.
Martin, Lawrence S.
Masterson, Julia A.
McFarlane, Allan H.
Menes, Catharine E.
Menezes, Natasja M.
Monti, Liliana L.
Munn, Catharine J.
Murphy, Patricia M.
Nagy, Joan C.
Nichols, Dorin
Ofosu, Kofi E A.
Padgett, Richard W W.
Parthasarathi, Usha D.
Patelis-Siotis, Irene
Patterson, Janet A.
Puddu, Silvana
Pytka, Pauline S.
Rosebush, Patricia I.
Rotstein, Edward A.
Rutherford, Patricia A.
Saperson, Karen
Savenkov, Oleg A.
Siegel, Belle M B.
Siekierski, Michal M.
Soares, Claudio D N.
Spinner, Miriam R.
Steiner, Meir
Swinson, Richard P.
Szatmari, Peter
Tam, William Y.
Taylor, Lorraine
Tunks, Eldon R.
Van Ameringen, Michael A.
Van Lieshout, Ryan J.
Van Reekum, Robert
Veltman, Albina
Waldenberg, Stuart S A.
Warsi, Mohammed A.
Watling, Mark A.
Webb, Stephen P.
Weerasekera, Priyanthy
Wesley, Steven J.
Zamora, Emil N.
Zipursky, Robert B.

HANOVER
Macdonald, D. James

HAWKESBURY
Ferguson, Pierre A.
L'Heureux, Francine
Morissette, Diane
Ouellette, Jean
Rocheleau, France D.

KANATA
Bedford, Robert M.
Gaudet, Michael E.
Koritnik, Angela R.

KENORA
Bains, Ravinder
Zahlan, Usama

KESWICK
Brennagh, Michael C.

KINGSTON
Andrew, Melissa H.
Boyd, Michele
Carlile, John B.
Chan, Michael P.
Conacher, G. Neil
Du Toit, Regina M.
Elliott, Deborah
Finch, Susan J.
Fitzpatrick, Catherine M R.
Flynn, Leslie V.
Furst, Katherine A.
Goff, Valerie M.
Hampel, Elizabeth
Hanna, Samia
Hillen, James
Hucker, Stephen J C.
Hussain, Maria
Iftene, Felicia
Ilkov-Moor, Snezana S.
Jadot, Sabina
Jarrett, Francis J.
Jokic, Ruzica
Jones-Hiscock, Cherie L.
Le Clair, J. Kenneth
Leverette, John S.
Linn Iii, George F.
MacDonald, Brian K.
Mazhar, Mir Nadeem
McCulloch, Janet R.
McNevin, Stephen H.
Milev, Roumen
Millson, Richard C.
Monaghan, Michael J.
Nashed, Yousery H.
O'Brien, Simon J.
Oliver, Dijana
Parenteau, Pierre R.
Pearson, Heather J.
Potopsingh, Desmond M.
Prabhu, Vijayalaxmi
Prost, Eric W.
Roberts, Nasreen
Scott, Duncan A.
Seitz, Dallas P.
Stevenson, Cameron M.
Szymczak, Peter S.
Teitelbaum, Louise E.
Weaver, Gerald B.
Woogh, Carolyn M.

KITCHENER
Al-Battran, Mazin H M.
Botros, Wagdy
Coppolino, Andrew G.
Dennis, Jane D.
Easo, Hyacinth S E.
Gangolli, Vinod K.
Ghuman, Harleen K.
Heath, David S.
Heintzman, John D.
Helmi, Sanaa T H A.
Juneja, Ravneet S.
Kelly, Michael J.
Khan, Arshad
Kumar, Hullur V.
Lang, Peter J.
Mabifa, Olasunkanmi L.
O'Doherty, James J.
Parveen, Nighat
Patel, Sujay
Popoola, Abraham J.
Saleem, Mohammad
Santoro, Dino
Sethi, Berjinder J.
Singh, Manbir
Singleton, Paul J W.
Surapaneni, Ramakrishna R.
Tadross, Emmanuel H.
Vanderkooy, John D.

KOMOKA
Lockhart, Robert J M.

LAMBTON SHORES
Galbraith, Donald A.

LEAMINGTON
Burdett, Rachel L.

LONDON
Ahluwalia, Simran
Allen, Susan J.
Alzaben, Faten
Barr, Jennifer
Blichowski, Teresa D.
Bogue, Lisa A.
Brownstone, Desi Y.
Burdan, Lyudmila N.
Bush, Haydn
Butchey, Janki
Campbell, D. Robert
Carew, Marjorie C.
Chamberlaine, Charles H.
Chandarana, Prafulchandra C.
Craven, John L.
Crozier, Robert S.
Doering, Michele M.
Dourova, Nevena
Dua, Varinder
Dubois, John R.
Duggal, Vikas
Duncan, Jacqueline
Eastwood, Diane E.
Egan, Raymond R.
Fisman, Michael Z.
Fisman, Sandra N.
Ganjavi, Hooman
Garcia, Carla S.
Goldberg, Benjamin
Gupta, Madhulika A.
Haensel, Heidi M.
Hall, Patricia
Harricharan, Rajendra
Harris, David J.
Hartford, James A J.
Haslam, David R S.
Hertzman-Chalouh, Daniel
Hocke, Volker S.
Isaac, Isaac F.
Ismail, Aden A.
Isserlin, Leanna E.
Jain, Subhash C.
Jerome, Laurence
Kaye, Valerie N.
Kerfoot, Karin E.
King, Rebecca R.
Kligman, David H.
Kumar, M M. Sujana
Lanius, Ruth A.
Laporte, Noel P.
Lefcoe, Daniel H.
Links, Paul S.
Loveday, Benjamin D.
Malhotra, Birinder
Manchanda, Rahul
McCarthy, Gregory
McCready, John R.
McKinney, Katherine A.
Mehta, Viraj
Mejia, Jose H.
Merskey, Harold
Milo, Michael E.
Mirza, Rida K.
Molnar, Laura A.
Mount, John H.
Ngo, Michelle A.
Nicolson, Robert J.
Ninan, Ajit T.
Noce, Emilia
Northcott, Sandra J.
Nowicki, Aleksandra
O'Donnell, David A.
O'Reilly, Richard
Oates, Jennifer
Osuch, Elizabeth A.
Park, Hae-Ryun
Pelz, Margaret A.
Phegan, Warren D.
Plowright, Linda R.
Przysiezny, Janine M.
Ralyea, Evan P.
Rao, Jayasimha M.
Reid, Brian S.
Reiss, Jeffrey P.
Repo-Hendsbee, S. Michele
Richard, Julie C.
Richardson, J. Donald
Ritchie, Hendrica
Rizvi, Syed N A.
Ross, James W M.
Rybak, Iouri E.
Sadek-Botros, Gamal E.
Saleem, Azra K.
Sanjeev, Doraiswamy
Sharma, Verinder
Sidhu, Gurpreet S.
Silcox, Jo Ann T.
Singh, Abhay K.
Steele, Margaret M.
Surti, Bhadreshchandra V.
Swamy, Guruswamy N.
Takhar, Jatinder
Templeman, F. David
Thorpe, Marilyn B.
Tidd, Christopher M.
Truant, Gregory S.
Turner, Timothy J.
Van Bussel, Elisabeth M.
Varapravan, Sreelatha P.
Venkatesan, Bogeswari
Veresezan, Alexa P.
Wadden, Paul C.
Weijer, Charles E.
Williamson, Peter C.
Wojakowski, Krystyna H.
Zilli, Cheryl A.

MANOTICK
Biggar, Ruth A.

MARKHAM
Berber, Mark J.
Chan, Angeline W L.
Garbharran, Hari N.
Kakar, Ravi
Karapareddy, Venugopal R.
Oyewumi, L. Kola
Persad, Emmanuel
Qian Lee, Ivy H.
Sethna, Rustom H.
Snyder, Brian L.
Ticoll, Brian
Wallani, Zulfikarali A.

METCALFE
Kerr, PJK. Peter J.

MIDLAND
Barker, Elliott T.

MILLGROVE
Marriott, John A S.

MILTON
Ahmed, Abul B M.
Ben-Aron, Mark H.
Busse, Erhard W.
Mangar, Mohini

MISSISSAUGA
Aleksiejuk, Zofia K.
Banoub, Tahany D.
Battigelli, Marino
Butler, Anna L.
D'Iorio, A M. Michele
Davison, Kristina
Dayal, Naveen R.
Dimanno, Domenic
Doyle, Christopher S.
Eusebio-Torres, Engracia D.
Flynn, Colleen S.
Gallant, Stephen E.
Head, Donald R.
Johnson, Manamohan
Johnson, Sunny V.
Lalani, Sartajali G.
Laurencic, Djurdjica
Legault, M. Suzanne E.
Lezon-Giacomelli, Dianne
Maindonald, Kevin L.
Manohar, Prethima
Manohar, Savalai V.
Moran, Peter I M.
Muhammad, Amin A.
Naidoo, Suryakumari
O'Riordan, John
O'Riordan, John W.
Orchard, Basil C L.
Peltz, Lou
Pendharkar, Raveendra B.
Pendharkar, Sushama R.
Petruccelli, Karen
Philips, Nabil A.
Porter, Jean E.
Ram, Katherine
Rehman, Mujeeb U.
Sandhu, Ravinder V.
Senthelal, Sashikala
Staab, Randolf A.
Sumner, Michael G.
Syed, Arif M.
Tirovolas, Konstantinos
Virey, Maselle G.
Wadhwa, Uttam J K.

NEPEAN
Batth, Sue K.
Brown, Mary M.
Browne, Michael
Deangelis, Matthew A.
Dhesi, Ravinderjit K.
Dimock, John L.
Firth, S. Terry
Hamilton, David M P.
Kassam, Azaad
Kovacs, Katalin
Kraitberg, Neil J.
Pande, Suniti
Stavrakaki, Chrissoula S.

NEWMARKET
Boachie, Ahmed
Brill, Francine
Cruickshanks, Sonia M.
Felcenbuch-Dachis, Harry L.
Garcia, Cesar P.
Grigoreva, Diana
Joseph, Llewellyn W.
Katz, Mark R.
Look Hong, William A.
Memarpour, Mahdi
Paramsothy, Rasiah
Stokl, Stephen B.
Ulic, Liliana

NIAGARA FALLS
Ahmed, Syed A.
Danial, Sarah B.
Gopidasan, Balaji
Mitchell, Wallace M M.
Naqvi, Imran H.
Santher, Kathiraveloo
Yu-Siao, Barbara A.

NORTH BAY
Achiume, Patricia M.
Adams, Susan
Beddage, Victorine
Boss, Kenneth
Cochrane, David K.
Crawford, Barbara
Denson, John R.
Fretz, Norman
Hackett, R. Andrew
Henry, Rachel
Hlusek, Emilia
Holtby, Joanne L.
Howard, Jane M.
Jacques, Ian R.
Johnston, Susan A.
O'Toole, Eamon A.
Renwick, Robert B.
Sanhueza Luco, Pablo E R F.
Slataroff, Youssef A.
Talarico, Brian N.

NORTH YORK
Appleton, Darryl E.
Arbitman, Ruben
Arfai, Esmail K.
Baker, Brian
Baker, Gordon A.
Barankin, Tatyana
Ben-Arie, Oved
Berger, Joseph
Berkal, Allen B.
Bogo, Norman H.
Bordbar, Kamran
Borsook, Cathi
Caplan, Joseph
Cohen, Sherry T.
Conn, David K.
Cooper, Jerry J I.
Edward, Raouf K A.
Emelianova, Svetlana
Erdman, Florence A.
Eryavec, Goran M.
Feder, Victor M.
Fraser, David
Fung, W L. Alan
Furlong, F. Wayne
Gallay, Henry M.
Gelber, Stephen G.
Gertsman, Cynthia M.
GhaemMaghami, Toghra
Girgis, Mona M.
Goldstein, Sol J.
Grant, Peter
Grief, Cindy J.
Guimond, Marie-Claude
Hanson, Mark D.
Hill, Mariana G.
Hoffman, Brian F.
Joglekar, Anvita S.
Jones, Arthur L.
Jones, Victoria J.
Kamel, Sahar S F.
Kim, Hae Ryong
Kugelmass, Michael I.
Lee, Francis K.
Lee, Michael S W.
Levitsky, Neil S.
Lin, Judy
Lowe, Alan D.
MacRitchie, Kenneth J.
Maerov, Phillip J.
Mallia, Salvatore
Mamelak, Mortimer
Mandelman, Krystyna
Marks, Saul I.
Martens-Kmiotek, Ewa L.
McLean, Mary K.
Moscovitch, Adam
Myran, David D.
Naidu, Mary
Nathanson, Jay A.
Nkansah, John
Notkin, Robert M.
Oguntoyinbo, Funmi A.
Ozersky, Sam
Pakes, Eddy H.
Pakes, Judith B.
Patel, Jayanti B.
Paupst, Millie M M.
Posner, Paul L.
Prasad, Lakshman
Prince, Garry E.
Propst, Lara G.
Raghuraman, Anusha
Raghuraman, Varadarajan
Rapp, Morton S.
Ratnanather, Kingsley V J.
Rehaluk, Robert M.
Robillard, Matthew T.
Roldan Lozano, Luis O.
Rosenberg, Marsha H.
Salama, Gamal M S.
Sarid, Esther
Schofield, Sally A.
Schwartz, Kenneth M.
Shapiro, Joel A.
Singh, Lakha
Sklar, Donald
Solomon, Leigh
Stein, Adam M.
Stein, Bernard A.
Sussman, Jillian
Tewfik, Sherif
Tucker, Joan M.
Ungar, Thomas E.
Vania, Mariam
Verhoeff, Nicolaas P L G.
Waisman, Zohar
Weinroth, Ian S.
Weinstein, Robert P.
Wong, Franklin T.
Wright, Leslie C.
Yeung, Michael K.
Yousef, Jakline M Y.
Zalan, Robert M.
Zare-Parsi, Mojgan

OAKVILLE
Awad, Awad I.
Barakat, Sammy W.
Bhattacharya, Ashok
Bradley, Carl A.
Brown, Alan D.
Butler, Brian T.
Crosby, Janet E.
De Souza, Darina
Gilbert, Jane C.
Girgla, Satpal S.
Handelman, Kenneth L.
Hastings, Thomas J E K.
Holub, Darren J.
Kis, Joanna K.
Layne, Elizabeth C.
Mace, Frank J.
Mollot, Kimberley D.
Muhamedagic, Tatjana
O'Sullivan, S. Karl C B.
Parlow, Carol M.
Seli Uzelac, Antonia
Treyvaud, Stephane N.
Voruganti, Lakshmi N P.

OHSWEKEN
MacDonald, Kathryn J.

ORANGEVILLE
Daniel, Geoffrey B.
De Marco, Vincent P.

ORILLIA
Chawla, Anjana
Desjardins, Nina
Guirguis, Ezzat F.
Guller, Dmitry
Rodway-Norman, Mark T.

ORLEANS
Augustin, Jean
Cattan, Edward F E.
Dion, Maryse
Malik, Vinod
West, Dixy Lee

OSHAWA
Betlen, Cerasela E.
Gnaneswaran, Aiyathurai
Keesari, Manohar
Kwamie, Yosef K.
Majeed, Arshad
Malamed, Phillip J.
Massabki, R. Albert Y.
Mistry, Dalpatbhai B.
Ojiegbe, Chinyere C.
Racicovshi, Daria S.
Sagi, Eliyhoo A.
Sorial, Ihab Z N.
Udaya Shankar, Sachidanandam
Zakaria, Muhammed

OTTAWA
Ad-Dab'bagh, Yasser
Allidina, Diamond A.
Amjad, Afsari B.
Anderson, Keith H.
Antochi, Ruxandra M.
Arora, Sunder S.
Attwood, David G.
Baines, Alexandra S.
Bajramovic, Hifzija H.
Bakish, David
Baksh, Anton D.
Bali, Neena
Balmaceda, Rufino B.
Barlow, Jane M.
Beck, Gail M.
Ben Cheikh, Imen
Bhatla, Rajiv
Bismil, Ramprasad
Bissada, Hany E.
Boafo, Addo
Boisvert, Denis E.
Boodoosingh, Lal A.
Booth, Bradley D.
Boucher, Catherine
Bourget, Dominique
Bourgon, Luc N.

Boyles, Peter
Bradwejn, Jacques
Braidek, Catherine M.
Brathwaite, Shirley N.
Brault, Jennifer
Brown, C. Donald
Brzezinska-Pytlak, Hanna G.
Cadotte, Helene
Campbell, Carolyne A.
Campbell, Martin
Carrier, Louise
Charbonneau, Sylvia M.
Charbonneau, Yoland R.
Chasse, Hughes
Cheifetz, Philip N.
Clement, Pierre
Cosico-De Jesus, Corazon
Courtney, Darren B.
Czechowicz, Dominika
Davidson, Simon I.
De Guzman, Ruby L.
Dickson, Christine
Doiron, Daniel
Dollin, Barry
Douglass, Alan B.
Druss, Elizabeth C.
Ducharme, Rene
Eapen, Tamina
Eaton, Christopher J.
Erak, Drago
Eshleman, Paul
Esmond, Elizabeth M.
Evans, Jane B.
Faucher, Lucien L.
Featherston, Carlos R.
Fedoroff, J. Paul
Flament, Martine
Fleury, Gilles
Fogl, Tomas
Freeland, Alison D.
Galipeau, Anne V.
Gandhi, Jasmine
Gandy, Hazen M.
Garnham, Jennifer A.
Gautam, Mamta
Gawlik, Janusz D.
Gerin-Lajoie, Caroline M A.
Gervais, Carole
Gillis, Katharine A.
Gobessi, Linda
Gray, Clare E.
Gray, Jonathan D.
Green, Douglas S.
Grof, Paul
Grondin, Fernande M H.
Habib, Rami
Halliday, Sarah M F.
Hamilton, Matthew J.
Hatcher, Simon
Heber, Alexandra S.
Hennessy, Anne D M.
Hoe, Walter
Howell, Kathleen
Hrycko, Sophia
Huehn, Linda L.
Huntington, Katrina D.
Husband, Carol A.
Ilivitsky, Vadim B.
Jardine, Julie A.
Jayasuriya, D. Sushila
Jetly, Rakesh
Jocelyn, Leslie J.
Jones, A. Frank
Jones, Barbara A.
Kaluzienski, Mark H.
Kay, Gary P.
Kealey, N. Lynn S.
Khan, Asifjehan
Khan, Badarunisa
Klein, Jack
Kolodziej, Alexander W.
Krane, Sam D.
Krelina, Michael
Krishnaprasad, Degala V.
Krul, L. Edward
Kua, Jimmy
Kunjukrishnan, Reghuvaran
Labelle, Alain
Lantos, Veronica M.
Lau, Timothy E.
Lee, Elliott K.
Lena, Boneventure
Lenz, Radomila
Lepadatu, Silvia I.
Lessard, Serge
Levine, Norman B.
Levine, Richard H.
Levine, Sharon S.
Lodha, Vinay
Lougheed, Donna C.
MacNeill, Susan J.
Mai, Francois M M.
Mann, Catherine D.
Martin, Mary M.
Masliyah, Tamara N.
Mathias, Michelle D.
Mauguin, Marc L P.
McBride, David R.
McCarthy, Veronica J.
McLean, David A.
McMurray, Lisa A.
Meitin, Joan M.
Melanson, Gilles G J.
Mendis, Tilak
Mercer, Deanna M.
Milin, Robert P.
Mirzaei, Ameneh
Miura, Carlos
Moise, John P.
Morse, Linda A.
Morton, Grazyna
Motayne, Gregory G.
Mouldey, R. Gordon
Mullin, James G.
Mylvaganam, Rock R X.
Nadeau, Johane M.
Nadon, Dominique J.
Navarro, Joaquin X R.
Navarro, Margaret E.
Nigam, Tara
Norman, David W.
Norris, Sandhaya
Northey, Robert A W.
O'Brien, Brian P.
Palframan, David S.
Patel, Surendra R.
Paterniti, Sabrina
Pentland, Neomi
Petit, Lyndal C.
Polis, Ilona C.
Potoczny, Walter M.
Powell, Garry W.
Powell, Gerald W.
Puddester, Derek G.
Pulman, Jonathan R.
Quan, F. Wayne
Rabheru, Kiran
Ribeyre, Jean-Marie
Richard, Hugues J.
Ripley, Carl D.
Robaey, Philippe
Robertson, Sharman J.
Rogers, Tabitha M C.
Roscoe, Clare L.
Roy, Paul D.
Royle, Mary-Clare H.
Rusalovska, Svitlana
Sachdeva, Rajeev
Saul, Daniel I.
Sedge, Paul A.
Shea, Catherine L.
Simon, Jonathan R.
Smith, Susan C.
Sokolowska, Anna M.
Solomon, M A. Andrew
Soucy, Louis J.
Spees, Richard C.
Spettigue, Wendy J.
Spindler, Eric E.
Stewart, Andrea K.
Suddaby, Kenneth W G.
Suh, Matthew C K.
Sullivan, Arthur K.
Swenson, J. Robert
Tahirkheli, Surriya J.
Talbot, Jeanne D.
Taylor, Ruth L.
Tempier, Raymond P L.
Temple, Michelle T.
Tessier, J L. Pierre F.
Thatte, Smita V.
Thomas, Gordon R.
Tighe, Spencer A.
Tourigny-Rivard, Marie F.
Tremblay, Michele M.
Trudel, Jean-René
Vervaeke, Robert J.
Vollrath, Thilo E.
Walsh-Bergin, Paula
Ward, Helen C.
Whelan, Chantal I.
Wiatrowska, Beata A.
Wiebe, Patricia K.
Wiens, Andrew S.
Wilkins, Douglas F.
Wilson, Bonnie L.
Woods, Si-Ann H L.
Yack, Mary E.
Zeglinski, Joie A.
Zolpis, Edward C A.

OWEN SOUND
Gormandy, Winston D.
Morrison, David E.

PARRY SOUND
Golombek, Harvey

PEMBROKE
Ferri, R. Michael
Vijay, Nishka R.

PENETANGUISHENE
Bergstrome, Brant E.
Bishop, Joan E H.
Cameron, Glenn G.
Dickey, Robert L.
Fleming, Russel
Gasewicz, Wilson R J.
Hossie, Helen L.
Jones, Ann D.
Kolchak, Andriy
Livermore, Craig A.
Lorberg, Gunter W.
Pigeon, Michel B J.
Van Impe, Jeffrey J H.
Wagg, L. Allison

PERTH
Goldstein, Stanley E.

PETAWAWA
Magar, Janice D.
Meakin, Carmen R.
Quinn, Joan M.
Tompalski, Sherry L.

PETERBOROUGH
Adel, Anoushirvan
Chawla, Bharat B.
Dancel, Mary Lou.
Dayot-Venida, Madeline
Ghatavi, Kayhan R.
Maher, John T.
McNestry, Fergus G.
Momi, Rajinder S.
Nugent, Kevin B.
Ravindran, Girija
Smith, Karen A.
Thornton, Mary D.
Wynd, Henriette D.

RENFREW
Simson, Stanley E.

RICHMOND HILL
Abaya-Comendador, Albina
Barabtarlo, Jack
Chan, John
Eisen, Joel N.
Grossman, Harold A.
Krishnalingam, Chinniah
Kurup, Lekha M G.
Leung, Albert S H.
Mottaghian, Mojgan
Perez-Youssoufian, Steven A.
Risman, Jared P.
Seif-Zadeh, Atih
Urson, Shoshana
Vardy, Rhonda M.
Zelina, Peter I.

SARNIA
Aguilar Rivera, Omar D J.
Hussey, Linda S.
Jegede, R. Olukayode
LaForte, Anne R.
Lubczanski, Aron
Naidu, Kumar
Robinson, David J.
Scholz, John F.

SAULT STE MARIE
Barrett, Elizabeth A.
Hopgood, Derek C.
Marshall, Emmalee V.
Pistor, Lino A.
Rogers, Anna E.
Stejar, Dana C.
Wallenius, Samantha C.

SCARBOROUGH
Barron, Stanley P.
Barsky, Stephen
Birdi, Girish
Chakrabarti, Gobinda L.
Choy, Thomas W.
Cruz, Caridad M.
Ferguson, Anne L.
Ferguson, Ian
Fishman, Steven
Gagarin, Ruben
Gelber, Herman
Gokcen, M. Ilhami
Gorguy, Verkeen S.
Gratzer, David
Guest, William A.
Hanna Dief, Sarwat K.
Isenberg, Meyer L.
Jamal, Parviz A.
John, Verghese
Lau, Man Pang.
Liu, Regina C Y.
Lo, Hung-Tat
Lowe, David W W.
Mantro, Kiran B.
Ng, David
O'Dea, Dominic A.
Okyere, Ebenezer
Pinto, Tanya R.
Rajendra, Jegapathy
Ramshaw, Peter J.
Sahyoun, Hani N I.
Sai, Obodai
Shin, Karen H.
Siu, Kien G J.
Sooriabalan, Thuraisamy
Sy, William Y.
Sze, Jacqueline Y M.
Vukovic, Milorad

SHARBOT LAKE
Burley, H. Joseph

SHARON
Mandryk, Eugene W.

SIMCOE
Robertson Moore, Rohan K.

SMITHS FALLS
Goodwin, Beverly J.
MacEwan, Elspeth

ST CATHARINES
Asti, Melina
Hunter, Kathryn L.
Johnston, Ronald E.
Perez, Edgardo L.
Porter, P. Michael
Shukla, Avanish K.
Van Kampen, Janice Y.
Wheeler, Maxwell
Zebrowski, Andrzej

ST THOMAS
Arun-Prakash, M. Venugopal
Chaya, Jihad Y.
Chiu, Simon S.
Ellis, Jack M.
Goldman, David
Jarmain, Sarah H.
Keshav, Dattatri L.
Komer, William J.
Norris, Phillip D.
Nowicki, Iwona M.
Roopchand-Mohammed, Rupa R.
Srivastava, Amresh K.

STRATFORD
Bucur, Mirela S M.
Cleto, Luis F.
Johnston, William H.
Marshall, Marilyn C.
Neilsen, Philip D.
Salo, Rosaline
Verny, Thomas R.

SUDBURY
Bhagavatula, Subramanya
Boylan, Declan P.
Gagnon, Jean-Guy R.
Joseph, Anil P.
Koka, Hanumantha R.
Kumar, Rajender
Lavallee, Carol L.
MacLeod, Eric C.
Marr, Douglas F.
Mathew, Beena
Okoronkwo, Elendu
Pearsall, Donald F.
Sanchez, Angelita R.
Shivakumar, Kuppuswami
Sutherland, Kristiina A.
Veluri, Ramamohan

THORNHILL
Azadian, Abbas G.
Jablonowski, Karin
Roher, Luna S.
Saffer, Linda S.
Saffer, Mark D.
Wohlgelernter, Joseph I O.

THOROLD
Boyd, Kerry E.

THUNDER BAY
Allain, Suzanne M.
Braunberger, Peter
Chakrabarti, Anita
Cheng, Chiachen
Corcoran, Edan P.
Czolpinska, Elizabeth
Fogolin, Jane
Gyomorey, Katalin
Haggarty, John M.
Heapes, Mary B.
Husni, Mariwan H.
Hutchinson, Lois J.
Johnson, Pamela J.
Lapointe, Carole S M.
Lepage, Patricia A.
Mulzer, Paul G G.
Sacevich, Tegan F.
Schubert, Peter J.
Sheppard, Robert R B.
Stewart, R. Jay
Vandenberg, Ingrid L.
Whitney, Diane K.
Wilberforce, Kevin C.

TILLSONBURG
Hussain, Farida K.

TIMMINS
Raveendran, Manoranjitham R.
Tuhan Mirza Baranowski, Izolda L.

TORONTO
Abadi, Babak
Abbey, Susan E.
Abi-Jaoude, Elia
Abouelnasr, Wahid A.
Abraham, Gebrehiwot
Abrams, Karen M.
Adams, Martha E.
Addae, Gina A O.
Agarwal, Parul
Al Mosyab, Nemer
Albuquerque, Joy M.
Aleem, Nadia
Ali, Faizal H.
Allodi, Federico A.
Almagor, Doron
Alsuwaidan, Mohammad
Alter, Howard M.
Ameis, Stephanie

Andermann, Lisa F S.
Arnold, Paul D.
Awad, Awad G.
Babiak, Taras
Bagheri, Aghdas
Baici, Wayne C V.
Bail, Monte H.
Bakshi, Shameet N.
Balaban, Kayli
Balchand, Kamlesh
Balderson, Kenneth E.
Ballon, Bruce C.
Ballon, Lawrence L.
Baluyut, Crystal A.
Barbera, Joseph
Barlas, Joanna
Barrenechea, Ana-Maria
Barrie, Gordon
Baruch, Ruth
Bassarath, Lindley E.
Bassett, Anne
Beaver, Susan A.
Behar, Beatriz M R.
Behesnilian, Katyg
Beitchman, Joseph H.
Beitel, Allan
Bender, Ash D.
Benes, Catherine
Benoit, Diane
Berdichevsky, Raul
Berg, Joseph M.
Berntson, Andrea M.
Bhalerao, Shree U.
Bhide, Devayanee M.
Blank, Diana S.
Bloom, Hyman
Blumberger, Daniel M.
Bogomolny, Howard H E.
Book, Howard E.
Borins, Elaine
Borsch, Roman N.
Boulos, Carolyn M.
Bourdeau, Danielle
Bowins, Brad E.
Bradley, Elspeth A.
Brandes, Jack S.
Brar, Simuran K.
Braverman, Jennifer R.
Brenken, Ernst G.
Brodziak, Helene E.
Brook, Shelley C.
Brotman, Michael C.
Brown, Edward
Brown, Gregory
Bruno, Deanna M E.
Bruun-Meyer, Sturla E.
Buckingham, Robert A.
Buckley, Leslie L.
Bukhari, Rukhsana N.
Burhan, Amer M A.
Burra, Tara A R.
Burrows, Gary T.
Butany, Vidya J.
Byers, David S.
Byrne, Miriam R.
Campbell, Wayne H.
Canella, Louis F.
Cardish, Robert J.
Carlier, Michelle A.
Carlisle, Corine E.
Caro, Jonathan
Carr, Melanie L.
Carter, Erin
Cashman, Frank E.
Casola, Paul G.
Castel, Saulo
Cavanagh, Patricia D.
Chad, Lawrence L.
Chagoya, Leopoldo
Chandler, Gregory M.
Chang, Peter P.
Charach, Alice E.
Charach, Ronald H.
Charlton, Katharine
Chatterjee, Sumeeta
Cheok, Andy S.
Cheung, Amy H Y.
Chisvin, Martin J.
Choi, Julianna
Chopra, Kevin K.
Chopra, Sabeena B.
Chow, Eva W C.
Chua, Boon-Chye
Cliche-Fontaine, Marie-Michele
Cochrane-Brink, Katherine A.
Cohen, Carole A.
Cohen, Miles A.
Cohen, Steven N.
Cohn, Tony A.
Cole, Howard J.
Colleton, Michael J.
Collins, Evan J.
Collins, Peter I.
Colton, Patricia A.
Cook, Katherine A.
Cooke, Robert G.
Cooper, James P.
Craigen, Gerrard P.
Crawford, Allison M J.
Crocker, Thomas C.
Cvejic, Elizabeth
D'Alessandro, Enzo
Dalfen, Ariel K.
Dang, Kien Trung
Danielson, Kimberly J.
Darani, Shaheen
Darby, Padraig L.
Daskalakis, Zafiris
Davies, William M.
De Bosset, Farideh
De Roche, Peter L.
De Souza, Claire
Dean, Margaret S.
Debow, Stanley L.
Dembo, Justine S.
Desai, Devanshu
Deutsch, James
Diaz-Hermosillo, Pablo
Digiacomo, Danny A.
Distin, Kiloran E.
Dixon, David J.
Doan, Richard J.
Doidge, Norman
Dorenbaum, David
Downar, Jonathan
Driver, Kelly L.
Druckman, Paul B.
Dubo, Elyse D.
Duchen, Suzanne
Duckworth, Geoffrey S.
Duff, Virginia A.
Dukszta, Janusz R.
Dundas, Susan D.
Dy Pac, Emily T.
Dyer, Cinda R.
Eayrs, Gertrude E.
Elliott, Mary E.
Ellis, Janet W M.
Enchin, Adam M.
Ennis, Jonathan D.
Epstein, Irvin
Erlich, Murray
Farcnik, Karl D.
Farewell, John C.
Farid Araki, Keyghobad
Fefergrad, Mark D.
Feinstein, Anthony
Feldmann, Joseph
Fenner, Danuta Z.
Filipczuk, Mark J.
Finkel, Richard M.
Finkelberg, Fred
Finnegan, A. Paul J.
Fischer, Corinne E.
Fishell, Alicja D.
Fishman, S. Brian
Flak, Edred A.
Fleming, Jan E.
Flett, Heather L.
Flint, Alastair J.
Fornazzari, Ximena
Foussias, Agoritsa T.
Foussias, Athanassios
Foussias, George
Frantseva, Marina
Freedman, M. Lee
Fridman, Ida
Friedman, Jerry A.
Friedman, Robert N.
Fulgosi, Zoran D.
Fung, Kenneth P L.
Futerman, David H.
Gabel, Kevin D.
Gafni, Inbal
Gage, Laura E.
Gaind, Karandeep S.
Galler, Shelly
Gangbar, Randy A.
Ganguli, Rohan
Garfinkel, Paul
Geagea, Justin
Geist, Rose
George, Tony P.
Gerber, Lionel
Gerretsen, Philip M.
Ghabbour, Nagi N R.
Ghaffar, Omar
Giacobbe, Peter
Gilbert, Barry L R.
Ginsberg, Leonard S.
Gisladottir, Kristin
Gitev, Margarita
Glancy, Graham D.
Gnam, William H.
Gocker, Marianne
Gofine, Timothy
Gojer, Julian A C.
Goldberg, Mark A.
Goldbloom, David S.
Golden, Ross S.
Goldenberg, Lesley P.
Goldhamer, Paul M.
Goldstein, Benjamin I.
Goldstein, Mara S.
Golts, Marianna
Goodwin, Grainne M.
Gorman, Daniel A.
Gorman, Howard E.
Gorman, Richard F.
Gotlib, David A.
Gotowiec, Andrew P.
Graham, Ian Davidson
Greben, Daniel H.
Grek, Adrian
Grewal, Seena
Grigoriadis, Sophie
Grujich, Nikola
Guimond, Timothy H.
Gulens, Voldemars
Gupta, Malati
Hahn, Margaret K.
Hales, Sarah
Halman, Mark H.
Halpern, Janice R.
Hamer, Edward S.
Hamidi, Jinous
Hand, Karen M.
Hanick, Adrian N.
Hanson, Mary K.
Harman, Jeremy J.
Hassan, Sameh A.
Hawa, Raed J.
Hazan, Sandra J.
Heasman, Kaaren Z.
Henderson, Julie L.
Hercig, Dragan
Herrmann, Nathan
Hersch, Edwin L.
Herschman, Peter L.
Hershkop, Susan K.
Hershler, Abby
Hidvegi, Sylvia
Higgins, Darren S.
Hill, Robert W.
Hodges, Brian D.
Hoffer, Mayer
Hood, Eric
Horodezky, L. Sandford
Horowitz, Glenda A.
Howlett, Andrew L.
Hunter, Jonathan J.
Huntley, Margaret E.
Hurdalek, Jiri T.
Hurtig, Avery I.
Iaboni, Andrea
Ickowicz, Abel
Iosif, Alina R.
Iscove, Melvyn L.
Israel, Aliza T.
Izenberg, O. Samuel
Jamal, Laila T.
Jaunkalns, Robert
Jeavons, Michael M.
Jeeva, Imraan
Jeffries, J. Joel
Joannou, Jason A J.
Johnston, Carolina
Kahn, Alan S.
Kanji, Diamond M.
Kaplan, Allan S.
Kaplansky-Gold, Cathy S.
Katzman, Martin A.
Kay, L. Rex K.
Keefe, Peter H.
Kennedy, James L.
Kennedy, Sidney H.
Keren, Ron
Keyhan, Nicola T.
Khan, Yasir
Khorasani, Kasra
Kim, Donna M.
Kimmons, Gerard M J.
Kingstone, Eddie
Kiraly, Leslie T.
Kirkpatrick, Xenia R.
Kirsh, Brian S.
Kirsh, Shari G.
Kirshner, Caroline M.
Kleinman, Irwin
Kljenak, Diana
Klukach, John J.
Koczorowska, Maria T.
Kohl, Jack H M.
Kolla, Nathan J.
Koochesfahani, Kasra M.
Korczak, Daphne J.
Korenberg, Lela C.
Korenblum, Marshall S.
Korostil, Michele C.
Koutsoukos, Georgios
Kozerawski, G. Margaret
Kreindler, David
Kreindler, Simon
Krisman, Avery A.
Krstich, Desanka
Kumar, Sameer
Kurdyak, Paul A.
Kussin, Dennis J.
La Croix, Eileen L.
Lamba, Wiplove R.
Lamon, Richard D.
Langley, John H.
Law, Samuel F.
Lazenby, Anne L.
LeBlanc, Serge R.
Lee, Victoria
Lefebvre, Arlette M L.
Leibow, Deborah F.
Leibow, Stephen R.
Leith, Mark G.
Lemke, Krista K.
Leon, Chloe M.
Leon, Paola
Leszcz, Molyn
Levinson, Andrea J.
Levitan, Robert D.
Levitt, Anthony J.
Lewis, Ralph B.
Li, Madeline T.
Lieff, Susan J.
Lilley, Mary M.
Little, Sian C C.
Lofchy, Jodi S.
Logan, Vance M.
Lorefice, Sylvia E.
Loszak, Karl G.
Lukaszewska-Andziak, Bozenna
Lulic-Hrvojic, Ana
Lustig, Andrew J M.
Maal-Bared, Haya
MacDonald, Ophelia L.
MacKenzie, Susan E.
MacLachlan, Donna J.
MacLean, George W A.
Madan, Robert I.
Magder, David M.
Maggi, Julie D.
Mah, K. Bill
Mah, Linda
Malat, Jan
Malcolm, Jacqueline I.
Manassis, Katharina M.
Mansfield, Joanna K.
Marcilio, Milton P.
Margittai, Katalin J.
Margolese, Ellen A.
Margulies, Alfred I.
Marshall, Michelle T.
Marta, Janet A.
Martin, Barry A.
Martin, Freda E.
Marzouk, Sherief E M.
Masri, Sam
Masson, Jacqueline E.
Maunder, Robert G.
McCallum, Nancy L.
McCormick, John W.
McCullagh, Scott R.
McCurley, Robert
McDonald, D. Angus
McDonough, Erin T.
McEvilly, Rebecca
McIntosh, Christopher A.
McIntyre, Roger S.
McMaster, Jeffry J.
Meen, Richard
Meier, H M. Rosemary
Melnyk, Tatiana C.
Menchions, C W. Bruce
Mesaros, J. Helen
Meschino, Diane D.
Meyer, Jeffrey H.
Mian, Irfan A.
Michell, Marcus J.
Milenkovic, Svetlana
Miller, Kimberley L.
Moldofsky, Harvey
Molleken, Lynda L.
Moller, Henry J.
Monga, Suneeta
Moore, Wendy A L.
Morgan, Andrew W.
Moss, Jay J H.
Mulsant, Benoit H.
Munshi, Alpna
Necas, Lucille M.
Nguyen, Jennifer
Nguyen, San Duy
Nkungu, B. Mandisa
Novick, Jon S.
Nynkowski, Peter A.
O'Brien, Thomas H B.
O'Hanlon, Jacinta S M.
O'Mahony, Michael
Offman, Hilary J.
Olive, Christopher M.
Owens, Mary C.
Pain, Clare M.
Pallandi, Derek V.
Papatheodorou, George
Parikh, Sagar V.
Parker, Vivien M.
Pasricha, Suvercha
Patel, Mitesh
Payne, Donald E.
Pearce, Mark A.
Pearce, Michelle M.
Peck, Jared R.
Peterkin, Allan D.
Philipp, Diane A.
Pignatiello, Antonio
Pinhas, Leora
Pollock, Bruce G.
Posel, Clifford H.
Postl, Lara A.
Poynter, Brittany A.
Prendergast, Peter J.
Preston, Helen A.
Proulx, Genevieve C.
Pytyck, Jennifer M.
Quastel, Adam G.
Quesnel, Susan D.
R Riopel, Marie Eve
Rabinovitch, Gerald I.
Rajabi-Asl, Akbar
Rajji, Tarek K.
Raju, Priyadarshani
Rakoff, David
Rakoff, Vivian M.
Ralley, Len
Ramsay, J. Douglas
Ramshaw, Lisa A L.
Rapoport, Mark J.
Raskin, Joel
Ravindran, Arumuga V.

Ravindran, Lakshmi N.
Ravindran, Nisha I.
Ravitz, Paula J.
Rawkins, Sian R.
Razmy, Ajmal
Reddick, D. Susan
Redman, Linda M.
Reiter, Sharon R.
Remington, Gary J.
Renecker, Glenn T.
Reznek, Lawrence R.
Richter, Margaret A.
Roberge, Johanne N.
Robertson, Carolyn J.
Robertson, David W.
Robinson, G. Gail E.
Robinson, William E.
Rochwerger, Felisa L.
Rodin, Gary M.
Rogers, Joseph E.
Rootenberg, Jonathan H.
Rosenblat, Henry
Rosenbluth, Allan B.
Rosenbluth, Michael B.
Rosenthal, Greta
Ross, Michael S.
Rowe, Cheryl J.
Rumm, Ellen B H.
Ruskin, Ronald
Sadavoy, Joel
Sagman, Doron
Sakinofsky, Isaac
Salim, Syeeda S S.
Salter, Nancy E.
Salvendy, John T.
Sanchez, Adolfo
Sandor, Paul
Saruk, Cynthia M.
Scalco, Andreia Z.
Scalco, Monica Z.
Schachar, Russell J.
Schachter, Debbie C.
Schaffer, Ayal
Schamberger-Keren, Beatrice M.
Scharf, Nathan D.
Schneider, Kathleen C.
Schneiderman, Gerald
Schogt, Barbara
Schonbach, Karen M.
Schuller, Deborah R.
Scroggie, David G.
Seeman, Mary V.
Selchen, Steven K.
Seyone, Chanthirasekaram
Shapir Kahan, Marcia H.
Shapiro, Colin M.
Shapiro, Sergey
Shapiro, Solomon M.
Shepherd, Anne L.
Sherret, David
Shoichet, Roy P.
Shomair, Garry Y.
Shugar, Gerald
Shulman, Kenneth I.
Shulman, Richard W.
Sibalis, Stephen J.
Silveira, Jose M A D.
Silver, Ivan L.
Silverstein, Paul V.
Simpson, Richard B.
Sinha, Smit S.
Sinyor, Mark J.
Sirota, Marcia
Siu, Maurice K.
Sivasubramanian, Velan
Skorzewska, Anna K.
Sloan, Eileen P.
Sloane, John A.
Sloman, Leon
Slonim, Rodney O N.
Small, Fern E.
Snaiderman, Abraham
Snelgrove, W. John
Sockalingam, Sanjeev
Sokolov, Stephen T H.
Sommers, Frank G.
Soni, Jorge
Soulios, Christos
Spivak, Harold I.
Spring, Paul
Srinivasan, Janaki
Stall, Richard J.
Stein, Debra G.
Stein, Marvin D.
Steingart, Allan B.
Stergiopoulos, Victoria
Stewart, Donna E.
Stewart, Mary F M.
Stewart, Pamela A.
Stone, Karina A.
Strauss, John S.
Styra, Rima G.
Sullovey, Amanda J.
Sunderji, Nadiya A.
Sutandar, Kalam
Sutton, Bruce M.
Svartberg, Martin
Svihra, Martin W.
Swayze, Allan G.
Swayze, Ian G.
Swoboda, Ewa
Szmuilowicz, Julio
Szmuilowicz, Sharon
Taerk, Gary S.
Tafler, Gitta E.
Tan, Adrienne O.
Tao, Tina Maria M L.
Taylor, Christine M.
Taylor, Valerie H.
Tennen, Gayla B.
Teplitsky, Mark
Teshima, John S.
Theohar, Carl
Thirlwell, Celeste J.
Thomas, Danielle A.
Thornton, John F R.
Thurairajah, Indranee
Thurley, Jane
Tisdall, Gordon W.
Tozman, Seymour
Tran, P P. Peter
Traub-Werner, Daniel Z.
Trossman, Bernard
Truong, Hau Van
Tseng, Michael
Tugg, Lorne A.
Turner, Tyrone S.
Tuters, Kaspars B.
Ulic, Bogdan-Christian I.
Vallabhaneni, M. Rao
Van Zyl, Louis T.
Vasdev, Shawn
Veisman, Aneta
Vidal Peralta, Bertha C R B.
Vigod, Simone N.
Vohra, Anita
Voineskos, Aristotle N.
Voineskos, George
Voore, Peter M.
Voysey, Mark A.
Wachsmuth, J. Rodney
Waddell, Andrea E.
Walsh, Kilian B.
Walsh, Mary G A.
Wanono, Oshrit
Warme, Gordon
Warsh, Jerry J.
Waserman, Jack
Wasserman, Lori B.
Wasylenki, Donald A.
Watson, Priya N.
Wehrspann, William H.
Weir, Douglas C.
Weir, Heather N.
Weisberg, Lori M.
Weissglas, Juma J M.
Werry, Elizabeth A.
Wesson, Virginia A.
Westkirk, Russell C.
Westlind, Paul E.
Westreich, Neal M.
Whitfield, Margaret D.
Whitton, Joel L.
Wiebe, Carmen E.
Wieman, Cornelia G.
Wiener, John S.
Wiesenfeld, Lesley A.
Wiesenthal, Stephanie R.
Wilansky, Hannah
Wilkie, Treena D.
Wilkins, Judy A.
Willer, Christopher C.
Wilson, David A K.
Wittenberg, Jean-Victor P.
Wolf, M. Uri
Wolkoff, Irvin I.
Wong, Albert H C.
Woo, Vincent L.
Woodside, D. Blake
Woodside, Scott M.
Wright, Martha E.
Wright, Mary A.
Yanchyshyn, Gordon W.
Yiu, Wendy W S.
Young, Beverly
Young, L. Trevor
Youssoufian de Perez, Never
Zaheer, Juveria S.
Zarb, Marie-Therese A.
Zaretsky, Ari E.
Zbuk, Randall S.
Zemans, Marcia S.
Zener, Shery H K.
Zielinsky, N. Ariel
Zurowski, Mateusz-Jerzy

TOWNSEND
Taylor, Charlene

TRENTON
Zimmerman, Paul R.

VANIER
Aggarwal, Dhiraj
Buteau, Jacques
Cheng, Michael K S.
Menard-Buteau, Carole
Monpremier, Pierre
Morel, Richard F.
Page, Francine M G.
Pierre-Louis, Faudry
Robb, Marjorie E.
Simeon, Jovan G.
Spenser, Helen R.

VAUGHAN
Costa, A. Daniel

WATERLOO
Appavoo, Siva
Galarraga-Carrero, C. Willy
Panjwani, Gulshan D.
Wolkoff, David A.

WELLAND
Abraham, Thoppil M.
Kumaran, Raghunath
Pallen, Alphie
Unoh, Emma S.

WHITBY
Byers, Jean E F.
Coleman, Elizabeth J.
Dawe, Ian
De Freitas, Karen D.
Fadel, Marc
Fischler, Ilan
Hasan, Sadiq
Hlousek, Daniela B.
Kevorkian, Agavni
Klassen, Philip E.
Kounine, Michael
Kriegel Perez, Graciela Ruth R.
Leung, Debbie W S.
McCormack, Brian C.
Olsen, Jeanine
Payne, Kira L.
Pham, Hoa Cong
Shammi, Chekkera M.
Shiffman, Kevin
Sohail, Mohammad K.
Sonbol, Soliman M.
Srivastava, Anil
Sundaralingam, Nirmala
Tam, Christopher H.
Usha, Sama P.
Waxman, Robyn E.

WINDSOR
Ahmad, Saima W.
Akinlosotu, Adewale A.
Bhangu, Raminder K.
Bordoff, Benjamin
Burke, Brian R.
Cassidy, Walter J.
Cortese, Leonardo
Doey, Tamison
Fernando, F. Priyalal
Finkelstein, Sheldon C.
Jwely, Ahmed M.
Malempati, N. Rao
Mape, Avelino M.
Miller, Barry A.
Mirza, Yousha K.
Nassr, Donald G.
Ndubisi, Ihuoma U.
Omoseni, Olusegun B.
Rai, Prem K K.
Rajan, Idumban A.
Roberge, Jean-Guy R.
Ross, Donald C.
Shenava, Ravishankar T.
Velehorschi, Corina M.
Villella, Giovanni
Warsi, Mustafa K.

WOODBRIDGE
Patmanidis, Stefanos

WOODSTOCK
Fernando, M. Lakshman
Tahlan, Pramil

YORK
Dudek, Malgorzata
Edwards, D. Virginia
McNichol, Kim L.
Morris, Monica K.
Packer, Samuel
Rasasingham, Rajeevan
Rudky, Rina
Simon, Barry J.
Sirman, Mehmet R.
Stefaniu, Rodica
Stenn, Peter G.
Styrsky, Eva M.

PRINCE EDWARD ISLAND

CHARLOTTETOWN
Amanullah, Shabbir
Beck, Angus W.
Cronin, Terence J.
Dada, Nadeem
Jay, Robert L.
Keizer, Heather E.
Moore, Douglas R.
Stewart, Susan E.

SUMMERSIDE
Singh, Arvind G.
Stewart, Christopher C.

QUÉBEC

ALMA
Cossette, Luc
Delisle, Gilles
Imbeault, Stephanie

ANJOU
Lesage, Jacques

BAIE-COMEAU
Cote, Serge
Mainguy, Nicole
Plante, Marie
Thibeault, Laurent

BAIE-SAINT-PAUL
Camirand, Yannick
Dussault, Martin

BEAUPRE
Cousineau, Pierre E.

BROSSARD
Martial, Johanne

CAP-AUX-MEULES
Finn, Celine
Poirier, Hugues

CHAMBLY
Langevin, Catherine

CHANDLER
Rivard, Paul
Segura, Jose A C.

CHARLEMAGNE
Des Rosiers, Joel
Ferland-Lavigne, Katia
Forget, Sylvie
Jomphe, Julie
Paquette, Suzanne

CHATEAUGUAY
Cote, Philippe
Dao, Thu-Van
Gagnon, Pierre
Malec, Tadeusz S.
Milovan, Eduard
Saleh, Fatehia
Veljanova Peeva, Elizabeth

CHIBOUGAMAU
Vachon, Natalie

CHICOUTIMI
Bernier, Annick
Bouchard, Marcel
Brassard, Nathalie
Chouinard, Catherine
Croteau, Benoit
Gravel, Christine
Grenier, Mathieu
Lavallee, Yvon-Jacques
Lavoie, Lise
Lessard, Rupert
Morin, Catherine
Ouimet, Luc
Rochette, Denis
Simard, Normand
Voisine, Claude
Voisine, Jean-Francois

COURCELETTE
Bernier, Joelle
Bilodeau, Mathieu
Blanchette, Tania
Samson, Esther
Turgeon, Josee-Anne
Vanier, Lyne

DOLLARD DES ORMEAUX
Belec, Daniel

DRUMMONDVILLE
Belanger, Philippe
Cyr, Jean-Francois
Deslandes, Carole
Dragon, Normand
Gilbert, Luc
Laprise, Genevieve
Lessard, Melanie
Martel, Julie
Morin, Andre
Parent, Marie-Claude
Vaillancourt, Jean-Philippe

GASPE
Boisvert, Rene
Chiniara, Gisele
Denis, Francois
Thouin, Dominique

GATINEAU
Attia-Galand, Samia
Basque, Andre-Denis
Beaudry, Louise F.
Bergeron, Richard
Bernard, Claude
Bertrand, Danyelle
Blais, Isabelle
Boily, Marcel
Bunea, Mioara
Cealicu Toma, Florina
Cote, Paul L.
Darwich, Walid
Gagnon, Andre
Goulard, Ginette
Gouriou, Louis

SPECIALISTS BY PROVINCE

Joly, Sylvain
Labonte, Roger A.
MacCordick, Alexander
Menard, Claude E.
Michaud, Dominick A.
Ngo-Minh, Tin
O'Donnell, James P.
Pierre-Louis, Marie-Laurette
Quintal, Marie
Seguin, Joseph J Y.
Tremblay, Alain
Triffault, Olivier

GRANBY

Bedard, Nancy
Bourassa, Marie-Claude
Bourget, Yves
Breton, Genevieve
Delorme, Andre
Huppe, Diane
Petitpas, Anick
Pinard, Julie
Therien, Manon
Trudeau, Marie-Helene

GREENFIELD PARK

Aiello, Marie-Jose
Beauchemin, Nathalie
Bedard, Mylene
Benoit, Frederic
Bienvenu, Jean-Pierre
Borduas Page, Stephanie
Bouchard, Denyse
Breault, Annie
Delisle, Marc
Des Parois, Lucie
Deschamps, Benoit
Dussault, Louis-Martin
Gougeon, Nathalie
Grenier, Claude
Jalbert, Maya
La Haye, Andre
Leblond, Martin
Lemire, Myriam
Noel, Caroline P.
Ouimet, Stephane
Pelland, Camille
Peloquin, Jean
Ponton, Anne-Marie
Poulin, Pierre
Proulx, Alexandre
Ricard, Jean-Francois
Rioux, Johanne
Roberge, Anne-Marie
Robitaille, Georges
Soulard, Isabelle
St-Germain, Marc-Andre
Theriault-Viger, Nicolas
Thibault-Chabot, Isabelle
Thomassin-Girard, Caroline

JOLIETTE

Olivier, Jerome

L'ASSOMPTION

Dao, Ba Anh L.

LA TUQUE

Norris, Stanley
Tessier, Jocelyne

LACHINE

Germain, Louis

LACHUTE

Gendron, Louise

LASALLE

Brebion, Carol M J.
Etienne, Pierre E G.
Steger, Katherine A.
Vachon, Jean-Francois

LAVAL

Boucher-Arseneau, Yannick
Bugeaud, Eric
Chaloult, Louis
Denis, Jean-Francois
Denis, Sylvain
Filiatrault, Liliane
Frare, Paola
Gamache, Claire
Gauthier, Serge
Goulet, Jean
Hayes, Claire L.
Lamoureux, Daniel
Lavoie, Ginette
Lopez, Isabelle
Parratte, Jean
Prevost, Alexandra
Proulx, Andree-Anne
Robitaille, Erik
Roy, Ivan
Sarrasin, Francois
Vezina, Martin
Viau, Lucie

LES CEDRES

Waszczuk, Madeleine

LEVIS

Beaudoin, Melanie
Bedard, Alain
Bond, Lorraine
Brouillette, Johanne
Caron, Suzanne
Chiasson, Myriam
Delage, Marie
Desmarais, Paul-Andre
Gagnon, Caroline
Girard, Claude
Lajeunesse, Charles
Laliberte, Richard
McNicoll, Julie
Mercier, Claude
Noiseux, Robert
Painchaud, Magalie
Plante, Isabelle
Poirier, Francois
Primeau, Francois J.
Riverin, Sylvie
Roussel, Stephane
Roy, Genevieve
Tanguay, Stephane
Tosti, Roberto
Toupin, Genevieve
Turcotte, Claudine
Turgeon, Marie-Helene
Wapler, Michel F.

LONGUEUIL

Anctil, Mylene
Beaudin, Jean-Hugues
Bouayed, Rita
Bouchard, Jacques
Brisson, Henri R J.
Chouinard, Marie-Josee
Fortin, Marie-Eve
Garnier, Marie-Lise
Houde-Sauve, Mathieu
Labrie, Christian
Lefebvre, Julie
Mailhot, Marie-Pierre
Marquette, Claude
Masson, Pascale
Michaud, Isabelle
Nguyen, Phan Nha T.
Paradis, Serge
Picard, Marie-Eve
Richer, Claude
Robitaille, David
Scherer, Gilles
Tetreault, Pierre L J.
Trahan, Linda

LOUISEVILLE

Mailloux, Pierre

MAGOG

Lemieux, Raymond G.
Poirier, Roger M.

MALARTIC

Gendron, Sebastien

MANIWAKI

Payeur, Richard

MARIA

Breton, Serge
Cote, Gilles A.
Ernest-Bizet, Florence
Laroche, Julie

MONT-LAURIER

Rosner, Sophie

MONT-ROYAL

Beliveau, Lionel

MONT-SAINT-HILAIRE

Des Roches, Benoit P.

MONTMAGNY

Auger-Dufour, Alexis
Daudelin, Ghislaine
L'Heureux, Caroline
Morin, Audree
Morin, Jacques
Robert, Nicole
Robitaille, Manon

MONTREAL

Abdel-Baki, Amal
Adams, Mark P.
Amar, Simon
Amirali, Evangelia-Lila
Amyot, Arthur
Andres, Cedric
Arjane, Mylene
Artaud, Laurence
Assalian, Pierre
Aubut, Jocelyn
Baillargeon, Joanne
Banon, Elisabeth
Barabe, Patrick
Barbezieux, Maurice-C.
Bazinet, Andree
Beauclair, Linda
Beaudry, Melanie
Beck, Philip R.
Bedard-Charette, Kim
Bedwani, Nagy C.
Belanger, Jean-Francois
Belanger, Michele
Belisle, Marie-Claude
Belkheir, Kamel
Belotte, Danielle
Belzile, Gabriel
Benierakis, Constantin E.
Benoit, Suzanne
Berard, Louis J.
Bergeron, Nicolas
Bernazzani, Odette
Bernier, Jacques
Bertelli, Christiane
Bertrand, Jean-Claude
Berube, Felix-Antoine
Bexton, Brian G.
Biard, Wanda
Billon, Eric
Biskin, Robert S.
Blanchet, Luc
Blanchet, Raymond
Bleau, Pierre
Blondeau, Claude
Blouin, Guy A.
Boileau, Bernard
Boivin, Johanne
Boivin, Marie-Christine
Bond, Michael
Borgeat, Francois
Bouchard, Anne-Marie
Bouchard, Chantale
Boucher, Lorraine
Boudreau, Anne
Bouthillier, Genevieve
Bouvier, Helene
Brahm, Evan J.
Brault, Jocelyne
Breton, J. Jacques
Brochu, Lise
Brouillette, Marie-Josee
Brown, Ronald D.
Bruneau, Marie-Andree
Brunelle, Sarah
Brunet, Andre
Bucci, Clotilde
Bureau, Nathalie
Campbell, Laurence
Canfield, Joyce
Caron, Chantal
Carriere, Nicole
Cartier, Georges-Etienne
Casacalenda, Nicola
Cervantes, Pablo
Chamard-Bergeron, Thomas
Chamberland, Gilles
Chamelian, Laury
Chan, Paul P.
Chanut, Florence
Charney, Dara A.
Charron, Maryse
Chicoine, Michel
Chouinard, Guy
Claveau, Denis
Clerc, Doris
Cloutier, Richard
Cole, Martin G.
Collette, Sebastien
Constantinides, Prometheas
Cote, Louis
Cote, Marie-Claude
Cotton, Marie-Eve
Cournoyer, Jocelyne
Couture, Claudine
Couture-Trudel, Pierre-Marc
Crombez, Jean-Charles
Cyr, Joanne
Czarlinska, Alina
Daigneault, Andree
Dao, T. Trang
Dassylva, Benoit
David, Pierre
Davis, M. Eric
De Benedictis, Luigi
De Plaen, Sylvaine
Delisle, Marie-Claude
Des Rosiers, Pascale
Desautels, Sophie
Desjardins, Monique
Desmarais, Julie
Deumie, Louis
Di Nicola, Vincenzo
Drouin, Jacques
Dubreucq, Jean-Luc
Ducharme, Simon
Dufour, Georges E.
Dufour, Natasha
Dufresne, Roger A.
Dumais, Alexandre
Dumont, Daniel
Dumont, Michelle
Dumoulin, Lyne
Durivage, Antoine
Elie, Andreanne
Elie, Louis-Michel
Ellman, Jon P.
Emond, Anne
Emond, Mutsuko
Errunza, Jennifer
Fabian, Jose L.
Faridi, Kia
Farmer, Olivier R.
Fedorowicz, Valerie
Fielding, Allan G.
Forget, Yvon A.
Fortin, Helene
Fournier, Gilbert
Franck, Robert E.
Frank, Daniel E.
Friedland, Jess N.
Fugere, Renee
Fulicea, Laurentiu
Gagne, Guylaine
Gagne, Serge
Gagnier, Stephane
Gagnon, Jacques R.
Galbaud Du Fort, Guillaume
Gamache, Andre
Garel, Patricia
Gascon, Louis
Gaudet, Adrienne
Gauthier, Bernard G A.
Gauthier, Jacques
Gauthier, Martin G.
Geagea, Khalil
Geloso, Angela
Gervais, Maryse
Ghadirian, A. Missagh
Gignac, Martin
Girard, Sylvie
Glass, Judy E.
Gobbi, Gabriella
Gobeil, Marie-Helene
Goddard, Karin G.
Goineau, Jacques
Goldhaar, Haviva
Granger, Beatrice
Granich, Annette
Greenfield, Brian J.
Gregoire, Ginette
Gregoire, Michel F.
Gregoire, Pascale
Groenewege, Donald R.
Grondin, Gaetan
Guay, Louise
Gupta, Mona
Guzder, Jaswant K B.
Haddad, Georges
Heyman, Marsha R.
Hoffman, Lawrence H.
Hoffman, Norman
Hudon, Marcel
Ianni, Floriana
Igartua, Karine J.
Imbeault, Jean
Jarvis, G. Eric
Jutras-Aswad, Didier
Kapuscinska, Maria M.
Keller, Robert
Kemp, Isabelle
Key, Fiona M.
Kirmayer, Laurence J.
Kolivakis, Theodore T.
Kolivakis, Thomas N.
Kraus, Daniel J.
Kunicki, Stephane
Kuyumjian, Rita
L'Esperance, Paul
Laberge, Pierre
Lacerte, Jean-F.
Lacroix, Yvon
Lafleur, Paul-Andre
Lafontaine, Sylvain-Louis
Laliberte, Marc-Andre
Lalonde, Pierre
Lamarre, Hans
Lamarre, Suzanne
Lamontagne, Yves
Lamoureux, Pierre
Landry, Pierre
Laniel, Sylvain
Lapierre, Odile
Laporta, Marc
Laramee, Michel
Larose, Michele
Larouche, Leon-Maurice
Larrivee, Marie-Pier
Laurendeau, Denis
Laverdure, Julie
Lavigne, Louise
Lavoie, Michel
Lebel, Alain
Leblanc, Guy
Leblanc, Helene
Leblanc, Jean
Leclair, Suzanne E.
Legault, Louis
Legault, Lucie
Legendre, Andree
Leger, Caroline
Lelievre, Andre
Lemay, Michel
Leouffre, Pierre J.
Lepine, Suzanne
Leroux, J. Robert
Lesage, Alain D.
Lesperance, Francois
Letourneau, Genevieve
Leveille, J E. Guy
Levesque, Alain
Levesque, Sylvie
Lipp, Olivier R.
Lizondo, Enrique E.
Lonergan, Marc
Looper, Karl J.
Lortie, Sylvie
Low, Graeme L.
Low, Nancy
Luyet, Joseph-Andre
Maranda, Francois
Margolese, Howard C.
Marier, Jean-Jacques
Marullo, Carolle
Massac, Charles-Henri
Masse, Andre P M.

Mauffette, Andre A.
Measham, Toby J.
Melancon, Geoffroy
Melun, Jean-Pierre G.
Messier, Rejean L.
Meterissian, Gregory B.
Millaud, Frederic
Milroy, Thomas M.
Minde, Klaus K.
Miresco, Marc J.
Monday, Jacques
Montagne, Gerard
Monti De Flores, Silvia
Montoro, Richard
Montplaisir, Jacques Y.
Morin, Francine P.
Morissette, Louis
Morissette, Raymond
Mottard, Jean-Pierre
Muanza, Thierry M.
Murphy, Carole
Myhr, Gail A.
Myron, Kathleen S.
Nadeau, Lucie
Nadeau, Nicole
Nadeau, Pierre-Olivier
Nantel, Andre P.
Navidzadeh, Adel
Navidzadeh, Niassa
Negrete, Juan C.
Ngo, Thanh-Lan
Nguyen, Bich Ngoc
Nicole, Luc
Noel, Francois
Nowakowski, Christophe
O'Neil, John A.
Oskoui, Ahmad
Ouellet, Robin
Ouellet-Plamondon, Clairelaine
Ouimet, Marie-Andree
Paiement, Isabelle
Palacios-Boix, Jorge A.
Palardy, Sylvain
Papamarkakis, Crystalia
Paquette, Isabelle
Paradis, Michel
Pare, Maryse
Paris, Joel F.
Payne, Jennifer R.
Pelletier, Gilles
Pelletier, Yvan
Pepin, Jean-Pierre
Perreault, J J. Daniel
Perreault, Line
Perreault, Robert
Perrin, Clifford
Peters, Lynne S.
Pichette, Francois
Pierre-Louis, Gerard
Pilon, Jean-Claude
Pinard, Georges-F.
Pinard, Louis
Plante, Gilles C.
Plante, Marie-Carmen
Poirier, Helene
Portnoy, Aron
Poulin, Sacha
Prelevic, Zorana
Presser, Baldomero
Propst, Arthur
Proulx, France
Proulx, Stephane
Provencher, Anne-Marie
Punti, Rosita
Quenneville, Yves
Rabinovitch, Eric A.
Racicot, Pierre
Ramsay, R. Alec
Reid-Perreault, Micheline
Richard, Johanne
Richter, Kenneth
Ritchie, Janet
Rivest, Jacynthe
Rochette, Pierre
Rochon, Denise T.
Rochon, Michelle
Rodriguez, Jean-Pierre
Rousseau, Anne-Marie
Rousseau, Cecile
Rousseau, Louise
Roy, Carmella A.
Roy, Mario
Roy, Renee
Russell, Ruth C.
Safadi, Gabriel
Said, Tewfik
Saint-Aubin, Catherine
Saint-Jean, Pierre
Saint-Laurent, Daniel
Saint-Laurent, Marie
Sanchez, Marie-Alice
Sansfacon, Chantal
Sasseville, J A. Marc
Saucier, Jean-Francois
Sauriol, Diane
Savard, Pierre
Schwartz, Hannah
Segal, Marilyn
Semeniuk, Trent T.
Serrano, Manuel
Shamlian, Nathalie
Sheiner, Richard H.
Sieu, Nida
Simard, Hugues
Singh, Santokh
Solomon, Martin L.
Soulieres, Annie
St-Andre, Elise
St-Andre, Martin
St-Denis, Pierre
St-Hilaire, Sophie
St-Jacques, Helene M.
Steiner, Warren
Sterlin, Carlo
Stern, Lara
Stip, Emmanuel
Sultan, Soraya G S.
Szkrumelak, Nadia
Talbot, Jacques
Tellier, Genevieve
Tessier, Louis
Thibault, A. Alfred
Thibodeau, Martin
Thuot, Evelyne
Todorov, Christo
Tourjman, Smadar V.
Tran, Trong Quang
Tranulis, Constantin
Tremblay, Martin
Tremblay, Nancy
Tremblay, Pierre H.
Tremblay-Jolicoeur, Claudine
Trudeau, Sonia
Turcot, France
Turcotte, Jean-Robert
Turcotte, Julie
Vadnais, Marjorie
Vanier, Claude
Vasil, Nancy
Verrier, Pierre
Vida, Stephen
Villeneuve, Claude
Villeneuve, Marie
Vogel, Judith A.
Watts, Joel C.
Wazana, Ashley D.
Wilner, Asher P.
Wisebord, Susan R.
Wiviott, Gerald S.
Wolde-Giorghis, Rahel
Zack, Deborah E.
Zahirney, Georgina M.
Zarrelli, Marianna
Zicherman, Viviane
Zigman, Daniel
Zikos, Eugenia

NOTRE DAME DES PRAIRIES
Desjardins, J. Jacques

OUTREMONT
De Montigny, Claude
Doucet, Pierre L.
Fortier, Claude
Patoine, Claude
Reid, Wilfrid
Scarfone, Dominique

POINTE-CLAIRE
Ait Bentaleb, Lahcen
Cattan, Candice
De Ciccio, Maria A.
Korpassy, Andras
Lalla, Fiore R.
Pilon, Normand
Rivest, Jean-Francois
Rodier, Mitchell
Rzepecki, Isabela
Solonyna, Daniel

QUEBEC
Archambault, Line
Audet, Marie-Josee
Auger, Edouard
Baruch, Philippe
Beauchemin, Marie-Josee
Bedard, Mathieu
Belanger, Helene
Bergeron, Danielle
Bernatchez, Jean-Pierre
Bertrand, Estelle
Binette-Gagnon, Marylyn
Bolduc, Michel
Bouchard, Guylain
Bouchard, Roch H.
Bouffard, Anne-Pierre
Bourget, Martine
Brassard, Catherine
Brien, Louis
Brochu, Michel
Brochu-Blain, Annie
Bussieres, Helene
Cardinal, Andree
Caron, Lucie
Carrier, Marie-France
Carriere, Jacques
Charland, Frederic
Chenard, Marise
Cimon, Marie-Juie
Cloutier, Annie
Cote, Isabelle J.
Cote, Jean-Francois
De Bonville, Marianne
Dion, Alain
Dionne, Suzanne
Dorion, Julie
Dorion, Pierre
Doucet, Rene
Douville, Lucie
Dube, Valerie
Faucher, Sylvain
Fillion, Mylene
Filteau, Marie-Josee
Fleury, Catherine
Fournier, Christiane
Fournier, Jean-Pierre
Gagnon, Fabien
Gagnon, Nadine
Gagnon, Pierre R.
Gagnon, Stephanie
Garneau, Yvon
Gaudet, Lyne
Gauthier, Benoit
Gauthier, Yvan
Gingras, Nathalie
Gourgue, Martin
Hebert, Julien
Houde, Michele
Huppe, Rene
Jacques, Paul
Jobidon, Denis
Keller, Evelyn-Elizabeth
L'Heureux, Sophie
Labonte, Edith
Labrecque, Judith
Lajoie, Genevieve C.
Lanctot, Guy R.
Laplante, Bruno T.
Laroche Savard, Amelie
Larose, Michel
Lavoie, Claude A.
Leblanc, Diane
Leblanc, Gerard A.
Legris, Genevieve
Lemay, Andree
Lemieux, Maude
Levesque, Suzie L.
Lord, Marie-Josee
Maziade, Michel
Michea, Rodrigo
Montgrain, Noel-H.
Montreuil, Jean-Francois
Ouellet, Francine
Ouellet, Paul G.
Ouellet, Pierre A.
Ouellet, Ronald
Panneton, Isabelle
Patry, Simon
Pelletier, Julien
Picard, Sylvie
Pires, Arthur E.
Plamondon, Jacques
Poirier, Simon
Pomerleau, Guy
Potvin, Anne
Potvin-Girard, Marie-Claude
Poulin, Marie-Josee
Poulin, Stephane
Pouliot, Claudie
Proteau, Guylaine
Proulx, Sebastien
Quintal, Marie-Luce
Radermaker, Steve
Radouco-Thomas, Monelly
Ratte, Carole M R.
Robichaud, Renee
Rouillard, Pierre
Rousseau, Francois
Rousseau, Louis
Roy, Jean-Yves
Roy, Marc-Andre
Saindon, Jacinthe
Shriqui, Christian L.
Simard, Michele
Sirois, Alain
Sirois, Francois
Skalli, Leila
St-Hilaire, Gilles
St-Hilaire, Michel
Thibodeau, Nicole
Thiffeault, Line
Touchette, Catherine
Tremblay, Annie
Tremblay, Guy
Tremblay, Julie
Tremblay, Lambert
Tremblay, Philippe
Tremblay, Pierre G.
Trottier-Hebert, Valerie
Trudeau, Nadine
Turmel, France
Villeneuve, Evens
Vincent, Pierre M.
Wallot, Hubert A.

REPENTIGNY
Gil, Michel R.
Ilies, Drigissa A.
Lemire, Isabelle

RICHELAIN
Tremblay, Monique

RIMOUSKI
Bastien-Chretien, Christine
Begin, Simon
Charneau, Manon
Cote, Serge
Dallard, Laurence-Raphaelle
Lamarre, Marc
Landry, Sarah
Lebel, Catherine
Poulin, Yves
Turmel, Roger

RIVIERE-DU-LOUP
Binet, Stephanie
Bosse, Genevieve
Breault, Jacques
Cormier, Julie
De La Sablonniere, Jean F.
De Vriendt, Xavier
Gougoux, David
Marquis, Elisabeth
Melen, Veronique C.
St-Onge, Gerard R.

RIVIERE-ROUGE
Barbarosie, Michaela
Fabbro, Franck

ROBERVAL
Monette, Yvan
Senechal, Alain
Zwiebel, Pierre

ROUYN-NORANDA
Barbes-Morin, Guillaume
Cloutier, Guylene
Dube, Christian
Lamontagne, Renee

SAINT-BRUNO
Giguere, Eric

SAINT-CONSTANT
Lessard, Stephanie

SAINT-EUSTACHE
Belair, Patricia
Calouche, Sonia
Dumaraix, Nathalie
Fliesen, Willy E J.
Rosca Stredie, Gianina
Suhani, N. Gabriel

SAINT-GEORGES
Cliche, Denis
Doyon, Martin
Lapierre, Yves
Leduc, Martin
Nobecourt, Philippe

SAINT-HUBERT
Coupal, Gerald

SAINT-HYACINTHE
Adam, Germain
Arpin, Jacinthe
Brochu, Stephanie
Croteau, Dominique
Filiatreault, Manon
Lavigueur, Catherine
Nguyen, Ngoc-Tram
Paille, Catherine
Payeur, B. Jacques
Phaneuf, Julie
Pineault, Jacinthe
Prayal-Pratte, Marie-Eve
Valiquette-Lavigne, Mylene

SAINT-JEROME
Bego, Anne
Caron, Edith
Caron, Marie C.
Comtois, Pierre
Dallal, Abdallah
Delbarre, Marthe
Labine, Robert
Lafreniere, Marie-France
Maheu, Marie-Lise
Ng, Albert
Sarrat-Vezina, Mijouk-Ariane
Teboul, Eric A.

SAINT-LAMBERT
Garant, Jacques

SAINT-LEONARD
Benoit, Elise
Cormier, Hugues
Poirier, Diane
Wolfe, Marcel
Wolwertz, John

SAINT-SAUVEUR
Dworetz, Arthur

SAINTE-THERESE
Aragones, Rafael
Ayala Arevalo, M. Angelica
Fortin, Lucie

SALABERRY DE VALLEYFIELD
Bedrossian, Taline
Biard, Christian
Bilodeau, Denis
Monette, Andre

SEPT-ILES
Beaudry, Veronique
Charbonneau, Manon
Dumont, Guillaume
Gingras, Isabelle
Marchand, Julie
Michaud, Sylvie Y.

SHAWINIGAN
Allard, Marie-Frederique A.
Beauchemin, Lyne
Bell, Caroline
Bois, Marie-Lou
Cossette, Jean-Rene
Gervais, Michel
Goulet, Karine
Laverdiere, Marianne
Olivier, David
Swenor, Rachel

SHAWINIGAN-SUD
Brady, Annick M.
Lamarre, Monique

SHERBROOKE
Allary, Catherine
Arbour, Claude
Beauregard, Carmen
Beausejour, Pierre
Bergeron, Claude
Berube, Martine
Bilodeau, Marie-Claude
Carle, Roger
Chagnon, Gilles
Chiasson, Eric
Cook, Allan M.
Djahanbakhsh Asli, Khashayar
Dumoulin, Joanne
Durand, Myriam
Fallu, Angelo
Forget, Karine
Fortier, Anne-Marie
Gagne, Pierre
Gagnon, Stephane
Gaudreault, Lynn
Godbout, Sylvie
Goulet, Ronald
Guimaraes, Daniel B S.
Hassoun, Joelle
Hottin, Paule
Lajoie, Yves
Lapierre, Patrick
Legare, Marie-Christine
Lepage, Denis J B.
Mailloux, Stephanie
Matte, Gilbert
Matte, Raymond
Michel, Julie
Morin, Luc
Mury, Muriel
Perrier, Marie-Pascale
Pinero-Medina, Francisco
Renaud, Sylvain
Saint-Pierre, Jean-Yves
Tittley, Matthieu
Trudel, Jean-Francois

SOREL-TRACY
Boulet, Daniel
Dion, Yves
Habib, Adel F.
Mohamed Abdou, Mohamed S.
Morin, Johanne

ST AUGUSTIN DE DESMAURES
Vincent, Annick

ST CHARLES BORROMEE
Albert, Jean-Marie
Allard, Magali
Cournoyer, Gerard
Lefebvre, Marc
Lemire, Magali
Major, Bertrand
Mireault, Gilles
Morin, Nive
Nguyen, Hai-Nam
Simard, Lyne

ST-EUSTACHE
Gilbert, Linda
Patenaude, Nathalie

ST JEAN SUR RICHELIEU
Agnaou, Hocine
Beaulieu, Lucie
Cerat, Nathalie
Chaput, Yves
Choquette, Marie
Cusson, Sylvie
Dreyfuss, Valerie
Fortin, Raymond-Yves
Guay, Pierre
Hamdani, Aziza
Moss, Genevieve
Ouasti, Abdessebar
Prevost, Catherine
Savereux, Michael
Tran, M A. Marie
Wagner, Marie-Helene
Yale, Pierre-Paul

STE AGATHE DES MONTS
Dumitrescu, Luiza A A.
Pouliot, Michele
Quenneville, Robert

STE ANNE DE BELLEVUE
Ouellette, Robert A.
White, Michel B.

STE ANNE DES MONTS
Beltrami, Edouard
Lew, Viviane A.

STE ANNE DES PLAINES
Hebert, Jean
Roy, Michelle

TERREBONNE
Beauchemin, Marie-Andree
Blanchet, Chantale N.
Boudreau, Dany
Curras, Pablo
Doree, Jean-Pierre
Forest, Isabelle
Fouquette, Yves
Grandmont, Julie
Hobden, Alexandra
Laroche, Steve
Lassonde, Sophie
Le Mevel-Moreira, Francoise
Scheid, Frederic J.

THETFORD MINES
Belanger, Carole
Lesperance, Jean

TROIS-RIVIERES
Boucher, Henri
Pelletier, Fabrice
Veilleux, Johanne

VAL-D'OR
Badescu, Felicia
Chassé, Claudel
Lapointe, Nicole
Theberge, Josee

VAUDREUIL-DORION
Benoit, Chantale
Costisella, Marie-Agnes
Couillard, Fernand
Filotto, Jean-Francois

VERDUN
Beaudry, Paul
Beaulieu, Serge
Belair, Jean-Francois
Belisle, Dominique
Bloom, David
Boisvert, Marianne
Bourque, Jean-Marc
Brunet, Robert
Casimir-Tordjman, Euphrosyne
Cauchois, Emmanuel
Cvejic, Helen
Debruille, J. Bruno
Desautels, Rene
Di Tomasso, Maria
Dongier, Maurice H J.
Dongier, Suzanne
Farquhar, James A.
Giguere, Catherine
Grizenko, Natalie
Guerin, Marc
Guile, Jean M.
Harvey, Janique
Israel, Mimi
Jolicoeur, Claude
Joly, Johanne
Karama, Sherif
Lake-Richards, Ruby B V.
Lalinec, Martine
Laperriere, Rene
Levy, Emmanuelle
Malla, Ashok K.
Messier, Michel J.
Nair, N P. Vasavan
Nakhost, Arash
Rabinovitch, Mark H.
Renaud, Johanne
Renaud, Suzane M.
Simoneau, Roger
Suranyi-Cadotte, Barbara E.
Wolf, Marc A.

VICTORIAVILLE
Ares, Isabelle
Brethes, Jean-Ianic
Doyon, Julie
Frechette, Guillaume
Hoang, Ngoc Bich
Morency, Mario B.
Parenteau, Rosaire
Perreault, Gerard A.

VILLE-MARIE
Lapointe, Marc-Henry

WAKEFIELD
Koch, Marion D.

WATERLOO
Beaudry-Remillard, Janine

WESTMOUNT
Fombonne, Eric
Grignon, Michel
Hagen, Arlene D.
Hechtman, Lily T.
Levinson, Edward D.
Magill, Chandra A.
McPherson, David E.
Olders, Henry G.
Pecknold, John C.
Reyburn, Thomas H.
Riven, Linda
Roper, Peter D L.
Zoccolillo, Mark

SASKATCHEWAN

CARLYLE
MacRae, Donald K.

MOOSE JAW
Adewumi, Adegboyega A.

NORTH BATTLEFORD
Mahmood, Yasin

PRINCE ALBERT
Cooper, Lilanie H.
Cruickshank, Lindsay
Husain, S. Baqir
Hussain, M. Zulfiquar

REGINA
Damodharan, Senthil
Falkenberg, Kornelia
Gbinigie, Victoria A.
Haque, M. Samiul
Harold, S. Brent
Jayaprakash, Makam S.
Messer, Charles J.
Mirchandani, Mukesh G.
Natarajan, Dhanapal
Papish, Andriyka L M.
Reddi, Krishnavellie
Verma, Kamla R.

SASKATOON
Adams, Gheorghita C.
Adams, Stephen G.
Aftab, Huma
Baetz, Marilyn D A.
Baziany, Azaad A.
Bennett, Vernon L.
Blackshaw, Stella L.
Bowen, Rudradeo C.
Brennan, Stefan D.
Cherland, Esther E.
Clark, Malin K.
Conacher, Heather J.
Davidson, Marla
De Souza, Dawn P.
Felstrom, Anna
Ferguson, Gisele M C.
Gillies, Pamela M.
Hendrickson, Donna V.
Holt, Alana
Hooper, Monika
Karuthedath, Rajesh
Keegan, David L.
Kok, Kevin D.
Kukha-Mohamad, Shirwan
Lau, Bienca
Lawson, Dennis M.
Lizon, Marina J.
Lowry, Helen A.
Marcoux, Eugene S.
Mela, Mansfield A.
Okunola, Olubusola A.
Peluola, Akinlolu O.
Pham, Vu Hoang
Qayyum, Saba
Quinn, Declan M P.
Rahmani, Mohammad F.
Reisner, Debra M.
Renuka-Prasad, Mysore S.
Thorpe, Lilian U.
Wanson, Annabelle S.
Zimmer, Rachelle C.

WEYBURN
Oyebode, Omoniyi O.
Suberu, Ganiyu B.

YORKTON
Adefolarin, Oluremi A.
Kotin, Svetlana N.
Lombard, Hermanus E.

Public Health

NOVA SCOTIA

TRURO
Taylor, Robin S L.

QUÉBEC

JOLIETTE
Robillard, Pierre

LONGUEUIL
L'Heureux, Jean

MONTREAL
Infante-Rivard, Claire

Public Health & Preventive Medicine

ALBERTA

CALGARY
McIntyre, L. Lynn
Russell, Margaret L.
Zimmer, Rudolf A G.

EDMONTON
Keays, Gloria E.
Sikora, Christopher A.
Williams, David C.
Yacoub, Wadieh R.

SHERWOOD PARK
Cheng, Jim I.

BRITISH COLUMBIA

COURTENAY
Enns, Charmaine L.

HAZELTON
Hougesen, Bent

KELOWNA
Larder, Andrew P.

NORTH VANCOUVER
Skuridina, Nataliya

RICHMOND
Lalji, Ronil S.

SURREY
Swinkels, Helena M.

VANCOUVER
Campbell, Audrey C.
Carsley, John K.
Daly, Patricia C.
Dawar, Meenakshi
Elwood, J. Mark
McLean, Mark E.
Mu, Lisa J.
Naus, Monika
Scott, Ian M.
Skowronski, Danuta M.

VICTORIA
Johnson, Roger J.
Stanwick, Richard S.

MANITOBA

BRANDON
Allison, Sandra J.

SOUTHPORT
Buchan, Shelley M.

WINNIPEG
Fatoye, Olubunmi
Roussin, Brent C.

NEW BRUNSWICK

BATHURST
Paquet, Mariane

MONCTON
Allard, Denis G.

NEWFOUNDLAND AND LABRADOR

MOUNT PEARL
Allison, David J.

NOVA SCOTIA

BRIDGEWATER
Earle, Lynda M M.

HALIFAX
Strang, Robert A.

TRURO
Taylor, Robin S L.

ONTARIO

BRAMPTON
Loh, Lawrence C.

HAMILTON
Chong, John P.
Kouyoumdjian, Fiona
Singh, Sheila K.

KINGSTON
Moore, Kieran M.

MARKHAM
Ge, Hong
Kapoor, Vimal S.

MISSISSAUGA
De Villa, Eileen P.
Hau, Monica
Mowat, David L.
Ward, B. Megan

NEWMARKET
Kurji, Karimmohamed H.
Weir, Erica

NORTH YORK
Pakes, Barry N.
Shapiro, Marla

OTTAWA
Allard, Pierre
McCourt, Catherine M.
Panaro, Linda K.
Paradis, Rejean
Pim, Carolyn P.
Tanuseputro, Peter
Werker, Denise H.

PETERBOROUGH
Pellizzari, Rosana

SCARBOROUGH
Nnorom, Onyenyechukwu

SUDBURY
Sutcliffe, Penelope A.

THORNHILL
Wittes, Robert C.

THOROLD
Hopkins, Jessica P.

THUNDER BAY
De Mille, Janet K.
Williams, David C.

TORONTO
Deeks, Shelley L.
Grossman, David W.
Jones, Karen E.
Kiefer, Lori A.
Meghani, Hamidah K.
Murti, Michelle
Patel, Zeenat R.
Pinto, Andrew
Rachlis, Michael M.
Rea, Elizabeth H.
Tyler, Ingrid V L.
Yaffe, Barbara A.

WOODBRIDGE
Bilotta, Rosetta

QUÉBEC

BAIE-COMEAU
Trepanier, Stephane

GASPE
Courville, Ariane

GATINEAU
Courteau, Jean-Pierre
Kom Mogto, Christelle A D.
Paquette, Camille

JOLIETTE
Lesage, Michel

LAVAL
Osterman, John W.
Prevost, Claude
Stefan, Mark A.

LONGUEUIL
Dufort, Julie
Guay, Maryse
Kadaoui, Nabila
St-Amour, Marie

MONTREAL
Andermann, Anne
Bergeron, Pierre
Cote, Brigitte V.
Cox Jr., J. Joseph
Dehghani, Kianoush
Denis, Geoffroy
Dery, Veronique
Drouin, Mylene
Duplessis, Pierre
Levesque, Jean-Frederic
Palmieri, Sandra
Paradis, Gilles
Roy, Maxime
Tannenbaum, Terry-Nan
White-Guay, Brian

QUEBEC
Arruda, Horacio
Berlinguet, Marc
Desbiens, Francois
Dionne, Marc
Fortin, Jean-Paul
Huot, Caroline
Lajoie, Pierre
Levallois, Patrick J.
Levesque, Benoit
Messely, Marie-Claude
Moreault, Louise
Racine, Simon
Rochette, Marie
Theriault, A. Nathanaelle
Tourigny, Andre
Tremblay, Genevieve
Wallot, Hubert A.

RIMOUSKI
Aube-Maurice, Joanne

RIVIERE-DU-LOUP
Pouliot, Bernard

ROUYN-NORANDA
Lampron-Goulet, Eric
Letourneau, Gerald

SAINT-JEROME
Allard, Andre
Goyer, Eric
Perreault, Genevieve

SAINTE-MARIE
Pare, Louise

SHERBROOKE
Boisvert, Richard
Clapperton, Irma
Pronovost, Robert
Simard, Robert

ST CHARLES BORROMEE
Badlissi, Dalal
Marcoux, Laurent

TROIS-RIVIERES
Brousseau, Nicholas

SASKATCHEWAN

LA RONGE
Irvine, James D.

SASKATOON
Kryzanowski, Julie A.
Reeder, Bruce A.

Radiation Oncology

ALBERTA

CALGARY
Angyalfi, Steve J.
Balogh, Alexander G.
Brunet, Bryan L.
Chan, Alexander K P.
Corbett, Peter J.
Craighead, Peter S.
Doll, Corinne M.
Husain, Siraj M.
Kurien, Elizabeth C.
Lau, Harold Y H.
Lim, Gerald W K.
Liu, Hongwei
MacKinnon, John A.
Nordal, Robert A.
Phan, Tien Thi
Sia, Michael A.
Sinha, Siddhartha R.
Skarsgard, David P.
Trotter, Theresa
Voroney, Jon-Paul J.
Wu, Jackson S Y.

EDMONTON
Amanie, John O.
Capelle, Lisa R.
Chafe, Susan M J.
Chu, Karen P.
Cuartero, Julie
Danielson, Brita L.
Fairchild, Alysa M.
Gabos, Zsolt
Huang, Fleur
Jha, Naresh
Joseph, Kurian J T.
Krause, Barbara E.
Murtha, Albert D.
Nijjar, Tirath S.
Parliament, Matthew B.
Patel, Samir I.
Pearcey, Robert G.
Pedersen, John E.
Pervez, Nadeem
Roa, Wilson H Y.
Scrimger, Rufus A.
Severin, Diane M.
Tankel, Keith
Urtasun, Raul C.
Usmani, Nawaid H.
Wiebe, Ericka M.
Yee, Don

LETHBRIDGE
Ghose, Abhijit
Wilson, Jane

BRITISH COLUMBIA

ABBOTSFORD
Ahmed, Sheikh N.
Bahl, Gaurav S.
Hsu, Fred H C.
Lester, Beverley H.
Panjwani, Dilip D.

KELOWNA
Bachand, Francois
Chowdhury, Rezwan H.
Crook, Juanita M.
Germain, Francois
Halperin, Ross M.
Hoegler, David
Kim, David
Leco, Pamela A.
Manji, Mohamed
Mohamed, Islam G.
Petrik, David W.
Reed, Melanie J.

PRINCE GEORGE
Miller, Stacy

SURREY
Agranovich, Alexander L.
Balkwill, Susan L.
Cheung, Arthur
Ingledew, Paris-Ann
Karvat, Anand
Kostashuk, Edmund C.
Kwan, Winkle B.
Leong, Carson
Lund, Chad R.
Po, Milton C.
Schellenberg, Devin D.
Wong, Frances L W.

VANCOUVER
Aquino-Parsons, Christina
Berthelet, Eric
Cao, Jeffrey Q.
Carolan, Hannah
Chan, Elisa K Y.
Duncan, Graeme G.
Fryer, Christopher J H.
Goddard, Karen J.
Hay, John H.
Keyes, Mira
Kim Sing, Charmaine
Lim, Peter
Liu, Mitchell C C.
Ma, Roy M K.
McKenzie, Michael R.
Morris, William J.
Nichol, Alan M.
Olson, Robert A.
Owen, Dawn
Pickles, Thomas A.
Tyldesley, Scott K.
Voduc, Kim D.
Voss, Nicholas J S.
Weir, Lorna M.
Wilson, Donald C.
Wu, Jonn S.

VICTORIA
Alexander, Abraham S.
Berrang, Tanya S.
Blood, Paul A.
Canavan, Joycelin
Goulart, Jennifer M.
Holloway, Caroline L.
Joe, Howard A.
Kader, Hosam E H A.
Larsson, Stephan N.
Lim, Jan T W.
Ludgate, Charles M.
Olivotto, Ivo A.
Pai, Howard H.
Smith, Sally L.
Truong, Pauline T.
Wai, Elaine S S.

MANITOBA

BRANDON
Bashir, Bashir M.

WINNIPEG
Ahmed, Naseer
Ahmed, Shahida
Akra, Mohamed A M.
Butler, James B.
Cooke, Andrew
Liu, Junliang
Loewen, Shaun K.
Lyn, Basil E.
Nashed, Maged S.
Ong, Aldrich D T.
Quon, Harvey C.
Schroeder, Garry C B.

NEW BRUNSWICK

MONCTON
Filice, Santo
LeBlanc, Linda M.
Lirette, Andree
Rojas-Lievano, Fernando

SAINT JOHN
Campbell, Holly A.
Carson, John H.

NEWFOUNDLAND AND LABRADOR

ST. JOHN'S
Greenland, Jonathan
Kamran, Asim
Norman, Alia W.
Sathya, Jinka R.
Stuckless, Teri L.
Thoms, John W.
Tompkins, Brent W.
Verma, Mukesh K.

NOVA SCOTIA

DIGBY
Brown, Basil S.

HALIFAX
Ago, C. Tetteh
Bowes, David M C.
Cwajna, Wladyslawa
Hollenhorst, Helmut
Joseph, Paul K.
Mulroy, Liam A.
Nolan, Maureen C.
Rajaraman, Murali M.
Rheaume, Dorianne E.
Rutledge, Robert D H.
Wilke, Derek R.

SYDNEY
Wajstaub, Sandra

ONTARIO

BARRIE
Kamra, Juhu
Stevens, Christiaan S M.
Yoon, Frederick H.

HAMILTON
Chang, Lynn
Corbett, Thomas B.
Dayes, Ian S.
Greenspoon, Jeffrey N.
Hodson, D. Ian
Johanson, Curtis R.
Kim, Do-Hoon
Kong, Iwa
Lukka, Himanshu R.
McMillan, William G.
Okawara, Gordon S.
Patel, Maltibehn P.
Reiter, Harold I.
Sagar, Stephen M.
Sharieff, Waseem
Strang, Barbara K.
Sur, Ranjan K.
Sussman, Jonathan
Swaminath, Anand
Tsakiridis, Theodoros
Voruganti, Sachi M.
Whelan, Timothy J.
Whitton, Anthony C.
Wright, James R.

INVERARY
Froud, Peter J.

KINGSTON
Brundage, Michael D.
Duplan, Danny
Falkson, Conrad
Kalyvas, Maria
MacKillop, William J.
Mahmud, Aamer
Owen, Timothy E.
Rose, James N.
Shenfield, Carey B.
Thain, Sou K.
Zaza, Khaled O A.
de Metz, Catherine E.

KITCHENER
Basrur, Vasanth R.
Fortin, Pierre
Gopaul, Darindra D.
Kobeleva, Sofya
Kuk, Joda
Rachakonda, Ramanamurthy V.
Shahi, Sundeep

LONDON
Ahmad, Belal
Ashworth, Allison B.
Bauman, Glenn S.
Bush, Haydn
D'Souza, David
Dar, A. Rashid
Fisher, Barbara J.
Gilchrist, James A.
Hammond, J. Alex
Lock, Michael I.
Palma, David A.
Perera, Francisco E.
Read, Nancy E.
Rodrigues, George B.
Sexton, Tracy L.
Venkatesan, Varagur M.
Vujovic, Olga
Yaremko, Brian P.
Yu, Edward W T.

MISSISSAUGA
Finlay, Marisa H D.
Hayter, Charles
Jones, Glenn W.
Lian, Jidong
McGowan, Thomas S.
Radwan, John S.
Rauth, Sarah J.
Senthelal, Senthe S.
Tsao, Jonathan R.
Wang, Yongjin
Yuen, Jasper S Y.

NEWMARKET
Cho, Charles Y.
Fenkell, Louis L.
Kassam, Fatma-Zahra
Taremi, Mojgan

OSHAWA
Banihashemi, Sayed B.
Dixon, Peter F.
El-Mallah, Medhat W.
Iqbal, Fawaad O.
Koll, Wayne A L.
Li, Audrey M W.
Maguire, Gerard H.
Mui, Jimmy K Y.
Youssef, Youssef M R.

OTTAWA
Agboola, Olusegun O.
Caudrelier, Jean-Michel
Cross, Peter W.
Dennis, Kristopher
E, C. Choan
Eapen, Libni J.
El-Sayed, Samy M.
Esche, Bernd A.
Genest, Jacques A P R.
Grimard, Laval J.
Kendal, Wayne S.
Lochrin, Catherine A.
Lupe, Krystine K.
MacRae, Robert M.
Malone, Shawn C.
Meng, Joanne
Morgan, Scott C.
Pantarotto, Jason R.
Perry, Gad A.
Samant, Rajiv S.

SUDBURY
Andronowski, Adam K.
Bissett, Randall J.
Bowen, Julie L.
Pearce, Andrew G.
Prichard, Hugh L.
Shehata, Sarwat W M.
Want, David A.

THUNDER BAY
Anthes, Margaret L.
Gulavita, Sunil
Kotalik, Jaroslav F.
Ramchandar, Kevin

TORONTO
Ackerman, Ida
Balogh, Judith M.
Barbera, Lisa C.
Barnes, Elizabeth A.
Bayley, Andrew J S.
Bezjak, Andrea
Brade, Anthony M.
Brierley, James D.
Bristow, Robert G.
Carlson, Ryan G.
Catton, Charles N.
Catton, Pamela A.
Charpentier, Anne-Marie
Cheung, Patrick C F.
Cho, B C. John
Chow, Edward L W.
Chu, William
Chung, Caroline
Chung, Hans T K.
Chung, Peter W.
Cummings, Bernard J.
Czarnota, Gregory Jan.
Danjoux, Cyril J E.
Davey, Phillip
Dawson, Laura A.
Dinniwell, Robert
Doherty, Mary A.
Elantholi Parameswaran, Saibishkumar
Fyles, Anthony W.
Gospodarowicz, Maria K.
Hodgson, David C.
Hope, Andrew
Ishkanian, Adrian S.
Kim, J. John
Koch, Christine A.
Laperriere, J. Normand
Lee, Justin W.
Levin, Wilfred
Liu, Fei-Fei
Liu, Stanley K.
Loblaw, Douglas A B.
MacKenzie, Robert G.
Manchul, Lee A.
Marchand, Eve-Lyne
McLean, Michael
Menard, Cynthia M M.
Millar, Barabara-Ann M.
Milosevic, Michael F.
Morton, Gerard C.
O'Sullivan, Brian
Paszat, Lawrence F.
Payne, David G.
Pignol, Jean-Philippe
Poon, Ian D T.
Rakovitch, Eileen
Ringash, Jolie G.
Sahgal, Arjun
Soliman, Hany
Spayne, Jacqueline A.
Sun, Alexander Y.
Szumacher, Ewa F.
Thibault, Isabelle
Thomas, Gillian M.
Tsang, Richard W C.
Tsao, May N.
Ung, Yee C.
Vesprini, Daniel J.
Waldron, John N.
Warde, Padraig R D.
Wells, Woodrow A.
Wojcicka, Anna M.
Wong, Chong Shun
Wong, K S. Rebecca

WINDSOR
Hirmiz, Khalid J.
Leighton, Christopher C.
Pan, Ming
Schneider, Kenneth M.
Springer, Colvin D.
Yousuf, Junaid A H.

PRINCE EDWARD ISLAND

CHARLOTTETOWN
Laukkanen, Ethan
Pan, Larry

QUÉBEC

CHICOUTIMI
Brassard, Marc-Andre
Brochet, Nicolas
Vass, Sylvie
Villeneuve, Hugo

GATINEAU
Archambault, Robert
Ferland, Stephanie
Gaudet, Marc
Haddad, Alain
Laferriere, A. Real
Martens, Chandra G R.

GREENFIELD PARK
Ballivy, Olivier
Derashodian, Talar
Jean Mary, Evelyne
Jolicoeur, Marjory
Mhiri, Selma
Racine, Marie Lynn

LAVAL
Clavel, Sebastien
Fortin, Marie-Andree
Gauthier-Pare, Anne-Sophie
Houle, Annie
Igidbashian, Levon

LONGUEUIL
Wakil, Georges

MONT-ROYAL
Ethier, Romeo

MONTREAL
Alfieri, Joanne
Bahary, Jean-Paul
Bahoric, Boris
Barkati, Maroie
Beauchemin, Marie-Claude
Bernard, Maryse
Bou Karam, Christian E.
Bujold, Alexis
Campeau, Marie-Pierre
Carbonneau, Annie
Chabot, Pierre
Coulombe, Genevieve
David, Marc
Del Vecchio, Pierre
Delouya, Guila
Donath, David J.
Duclos, Marie
Faria, Sergio L.
Filion, Edith
Fortin, Bernard
Freeman, Carolyn R.
Guay, Jean-Pierre
Hijal, Tarek
Khaouam, Nader
Kopek, Neil J.
Laliberte, Benoit
Lambert, Carole
Lambert, Christine
Lambert, Louise
Lavertu, Sophie
Lefebvre, Pierre D.
Lemaire, Celine
Lessard, Monique
Masucci, Giuseppina L.
Menkarios, Cathy
Methot, Francis
Muanza, Thierry M.
Nguyen, David H A.
Nguyen-Huynh, Thu-Van
Nguyen-Tan, Felix Phuc.
Niazi, Mohammad T.
Palayew, Max J.
Panet-Raymond, Valerie
Portelance, Lorraine
Porter, Arthur
Roberge, David
Rosenthall, Leonard
Rousseau, Pierre
Roux, Audrey
Roy, Isabelle
Shenouda, George
Souhami, Luis
Sultanem, Khalil
Sylvestre, Alma D.
Vavassis, Peter
Vu, Thi-Trinh T.
Vuong, Te
Wan, Jonathan F H.
Yassa, Mariam
Yassa, Michael

QUEBEC
Archambault, Jean
Blondeau, Lucie
Dagnault, Anne
Diaz de Bedoya, Luis Victor
Fortin, Andre
Foster, William
Froment, Marie-Anne
Germain, Isabelle
Larochelle-Beland, Marie
Lavoie, Caroline
Lessard, Nathalie J.
Martin, Andre-Guy
Theberge, Valerie
Vallieres, Isabelle
Vigneault, Eric

RIMOUSKI
Gionet, Melanie
Raymond, Paul-Emile

ROUYN-NORANDA
Ouimet, Denise

SHERBROOKE
Bouchard, Myriam
Bujold, Rachel
Ebacher, Annie
Gauthier, Isabelle
Masson-Cote, Laurence
Nabid, Abdenour
Provencher, Sawyna

TROIS-RIVIERES
Dahmane, Rafika
Harvey, Julie
Lebrun, Benoit
Sicard, Marie-Eve
Vincent, Francois
Vincent, Linda S.

SASKATCHEWAN

REGINA
Behl, Monica A A.
Dubey, Arbind A.
Kakumanu, Ankineedu S.
Koul, Rashmi
Tai, T H. Patricia

SASKATOON
Gardiner, Donald B.
Le, Duc M.
Wright, Philip H.

Respirology

ALBERTA

CALGARY
Anselmo, Mark A.
Bendiak, Glenda N.
Berthiaume, Luc R.
Bjornson, Candice L.
Boiteau, Paul J E.
Chan, John S.
Chee, C M. Alex
Chou, Julie P.
Chrusch, Carla A.
Davidson, Warren
Dibartolo-King, Marielena L.
Easton, Paul A.
Fell, Charlene D.
Field, Stephen K.
Fisher, Dina A.
Flemons, W. Ward
Fras, Mary
Fraser, Kristin L.
Gelberg, Jacob
Hanly, Patrick J.
Helmersen, Douglas S.
Hirani, Naushad
Hulme, W. Terrance
Janovcik, Juraj E.
Jarand, Julie M.
Johannson, Kerri A M.
Kam, Karen J.
Kennedy, Richard J.
Kirk, Valerie G.
Lim, Thomas W P.
Loewen, Andrea H S.
Lohmann, Tara E.
MacEachern, Paul
Mody, Christopher H.
Montgomery, Mark D.
Noseworthy, Mary E.
Pendharkar, Sachin R.
Penz, Erika D.
Povitz, Marcus
Rimmer, Karen P.
Roman, Michael A.
Sabur, Natasha F.
Stather, David R.
Thakrar, Mitesh V.
Tourin, Olga
Tremblay, Alain
Tsai, Willis H.
Van Olm, T M. Matthew J.
Viner, Sidney M.
Walker, Brandie L.
Warshawski, Frank J.
Winston, Brent W.
Zuege, Danny J.

CANMORE
Robertson, Dale F.

EDMONTON
Bhutani, Mohit
Bibeau, Marc D.
Brown, Neil E.
Bryan, Tracey L.
Carney, Dominic P.
Cheung, Lawrence A.
Chiam, Benjamin T H.
Chin, Wu Dat N.
Damant, Ronald W.
Deutscher, Clive O.
Dhawan, Vivek
Dickout, William J.
Gibney, R T. Noel
Gillson, Ashley
Halloran, Kieran
Kapasi, Ali M.
Leung, Winnie M W.
Lien, Dale C.
Liu, Allen T L.
MacLean, Joanna E.
Majaesic, Carina M.
Man, Godfrey C W.
Mandhane, Piushkumar J.
Marcushamer, Samuel L.
Mayers, Irvin

McDermid, Robert C.
McNab, Brian D.
Melenka, Lyle S.
Mulchey, Kimberley D.
Ramesh, Warren P.
Ramlall, A. Kumar
Shustack, Allan
Stollery, Daniel E.
Ullah, Saif
Verma, Geetika E.
Vethanayagam, Dilini P.
Wei, Peter Y.
Weinkauf, Justin G.
Wong, Eric Y L.
Yehya Aladin, Jaled W.

LETHBRIDGE
Oviatt, Patrick L.
Wilde, Eric R.

RED DEER
Glady, Christine A.
Heathcote, Karen

SHERWOOD PARK
Skjodt, Neil M.
Witmans, Manisha B.

WETASKIWIN
Crocket, Jennifer A.
York, Ernest L.

BRITISH COLUMBIA

ABBOTSFORD
Williams, Dave J.

BURNABY
Dong, Sunny R.
Kwan, Susan Y L.
Saberi, Farzad

CHILLIWACK
Wilson, Jennifer M.

COMOX
Dang, Bao Pham N.

KELOWNA
Fox, Lorne M.
McCauley, Graeme
Rolf, J. Douglass
Sarbit, Jay L.

LANGLEY
Wittmann, Rita

MAPLE RIDGE
Ervin, Francis L C.

NANAIMO
McLean, Laura E.
Park, Kirily
Ronald, John A.
Trajan, Marc

NEW WESTMINSTER
Blackie, Stephen P.
Chung, Randy D.
Fava, Craig S.
Glezos, James D.
MacCarthy, John A J.
Malhotra, Samir
Webster, Sheila B.

NORTH VANCOUVER
Mainra, Rajesh R.

PENTICTON
Broder, Sarah L.
Schneider-MacRae, Margaret L N.
Walker, Shannon L.

PRINCE GEORGE
Hirji, Alim
Olsen, Sharla-Rae J.
Smith, John T.

RICHMOND
Ahmed, Iqbal H.
Lau, Edgar S T.

SURREY
Feige, Richard R R.
Giustino, Giuseppe
Hong, Harry H L.
Janda, Surinder P.
Lawson, Edward J.
McCormack, Grant S.
Turner, Mark O.

VANCOUVER
Ayas, Najib
Boyd, John
Carlsten, Christopher R.
Chittock, Dean R.
Cook, Victoria J.
Dodek, Peter M.
Elwood, Richard K.
Fera, Tharwat A E.
FitzGerald, J. Mark
Fleetham, John A.
Johnston, James C.
Khalil, Nasreen
Lam, Stephen C T.
Leung, Janice M.
Levy, Robert D.
Man, S F. Paul
Nayar, Shalini
Pare, Peter D.
Quon, Bradley S.
Road, Jeremy D.
Ryan, C. Frank P.
Ryerson, Christopher J.
Shaipanich, Tawimas
Sin, Donald D H.
Spier, Sheldon
Swiston, John R.
Tothill, Andrea E.
Wensley, David F.
Wilcox, Pearce G.
Yang, Connie L.

VICTORIA
Beck, Raphael
Clark, Heather E.
Connolly, Thomas P.
Gough, Ellen R.
Paul, Terrance W.
Polson, Alasdair L.
Sanders, Bruce R.
Sherk, Peter A.
Waters, C. Ian
Young, Aaron M.

MANITOBA

BRANDON
Penner, Charles G.

WINNIPEG
Ainslie, Martha D.
Bshouty, Zoheir
Corne, Stephen I.
Eschun, Gregg M.
Giannouli, Eleni
Homik, Lawrence A.
Myers, Renelle L.
Porhownik, Nancy R.
Ramsey, Clare D.
Sandham, J. Dean
Sharma, Satyendra
Shepertycky, Martha R.
Wanono, Revital

NEW BRUNSWICK

MONCTON
Alqdah, Maen A A.
Beaudry, Daniel
Brideau, Eric
Gaudet, Matthieu
Kemp, Kristina M.
Mallet, Marcel
Williston, Maryse

SAINT JOHN
Bishop, Graham W.
Joshi, Prakash C.

NEWFOUNDLAND AND LABRADOR

ST. JOHN'S
Duguid, Nigel J D.
Farrell, Jamie
Fox, George A.
Lockyer, Joseph M.

NOVA SCOTIA

ANTIGONISH
Boyd, Matthew

DARTMOUTH
Rappard, Scott C.

HALIFAX
Acres, John C.
Chiasson, Meredith D.
Hernandez, Paul
McParland, Columba
Morrison, Debra L.
Morrison, Nancy J.

KENTVILLE
Gordon, Ann

ONTARIO

AJAX
Philteos, George S R.

BARRIE
Tailor, Adarsh

BELLEVILLE
Heffernan, Paul

BRAMPTON
Bikangaga, Peter M.
Ciric, Ioana E.
Kohn, Magdie L.
Moltyaner, Yuri
Naraine, Virjanand
Powell, Elizabeth
Ravindran, Vikram C.
Soicher, Avrum A.

BRANTFORD
Carlton, Timothy J.

BURLINGTON
Killorn, W. Patrick
Martin, David H.
Todd, David C.

CAMBRIDGE
Macie, Christine M G.

CORNWALL
Dandurand, Ronald

EAST YORK
Tran, Kham Quang.

ETOBICOKE
Huang, Max
Lumb, Kevin A.
Miletin, Michael S.
Nelson, Sarah L.
Perl, Avishay
Rosenberg, Joseph I.
Varkul, Mark D.

GRIMSBY
Lam, Andy S C.

GUELPH
Nemni, Jacqueline C.
Shende, Vasanti N.

HAMILTON
Allen, Christopher J.
Amer, Rebecca K.
Amlani, Salima
Bradley, Christine A.
Chelvanathan, Anushya
Drost, Nicole Z A.
Gottschalk, Raymond
Hamielec, Cindy M.
Higgins, David A.
Jones, Graham L.
Kearon, M. Clive
Killian, Kieran J.
McIvor, R. Andrew
McLellan, Allan P.
Nair, Parameswaran K.
O'Byrne, Paul M.
Puksa, Serge
Raghavan, Natya
Ramsdale, E. Helen
Rudkowski, Jill C.
Sears, Malcolm R.
Sindi, Anees A S.
Soth, Mark D.
Subramanian, Ganesh K.
Tunks, Marcel G.
Visram, Farzin M.
Whitehead, Lori N.

KINGSTON
Aggarwal, Aaron N.
D'Arsigny, Christine L.
Fanaras, Effie
Fitzpatrick, Michael F.
Forkert, Lutz
Harrison, Mariam N.
Lougheed, M. Diane
Moffatt, Susan L.
Moran-Mendoza, A. Onofre
Muscedere, John G.
O'Donnell, Denis E M.
Parker, Christopher M.

KITCHENER
Chernish, Robert N.
Hentschel, Eric P.
Ho, Victoria Y W.
Jackson, Mary E.
Langridge, Jonathon M D.
Nagpal, Anil K.
Racz, Heather N.
Strban, Martin

LONDON
Bosma, Karen
Farquhar, Donald R E.
George, Charles F P.
Kashgari, Alia Y A.
Leasa, David J.
Lewis, James F.
Licskai, Christopher J.
Lyttle, Brian D B.
McCormack, David G.
McFadden, Robin G.
Mehta, Sanjay
Price, April K.
Radhakrishnan, Dhenuka K.
Sen, Mithu
Yamashita, Cory M.

MARKHAM
Dancey, David R.
Forse, Monique I S.
Nimchonok, Punam M.

MISSISSAUGA
Allen, Tara
Antman, Neil S.
Flood, Diane A.
Green, Kevin W.
Inouye, Tetsuo
Maham, Nava
O'Connor, Thomas C.
Patel, Milan V.
Price, Charles M.
Ritacca, Frank V.
Soghrati, Kamyar
Wolski, Winicjusz M.

NEWMARKET
Ramakrishnan, Srikanth
Roberts, D. Kenneth
Zafar, Moiz M.

NIAGARA FALLS
Werhun, Robert S.

NORTH YORK
Braude, Andrew
Carr, Sean A.
Fishbein, David L S.
Kanawaty, David S.
Rahimi Darabad, Parisa
Sanders, Kevin M.
Sherkin, Marc D.
Singh, Arjune B.

OAKVILLE
Chau, Laurence K L.
Kirby, John G.
Salazar, Charlene L.

ORILLIA
Alexander, David J.

OSHAWA
El-Keeb, Rabea A H.
Huzel, Lisa L.
Ross, David J.
Sharma, Arunabh B.

OTTAWA
Aaron, Shawn D.
Alikhan, Qasim R.
Alvarez, Gonzalo G.
Amjadi, Kayvan
Block, Jennifer K.
Bukowskyj, Maria
Cardinal, Pierre
Chandy, George P.
Chatha, Neel-Kamal K.
Dales, Robert E.
Katz, Sherri L.
Keays, Tara N.
Kovesi, Thomas A.
Leech, Judith A.
MacLusky, Ian B.
Marovac, M. Misha
McKim, Douglas A.
Mulpuru, Sunita S.
Pakhale, Smita S.
Reisman, John J.
Rivington, Robert N.
Sandoz, Jacqueline S.
Schneiderman, David A.
Sharma, Krishna B.
Smith, Mark A.
Spitale, Naomi S.
Srour, Nadim
Voduc, Nha
Willis, Kenneth R.

OWEN SOUND
Newton, F. Marcus

PEMBROKE
Kify, Omar H.

PETERBOROUGH
Stelzer, Hans J.
Vlasschaert, John J.

RICHMOND HILL
Chan, Victoria M Y.
Chu, Eric K.
Liu, L. Felix

SAULT STE MARIE
Berg, Gregory M A.
Maharaj, Neil

SCARBOROUGH
Bongard, Howard B.
Chee, Jung Hoon
Chien, S M. Joseph
Hsieh, Tauyee
Iyer, L. Priya
Kwok, Eva
Wong, Harvey H.

ST CATHARINES
Jany, Mark J.
Nolan, Thomas J.

ST THOMAS
Ferguson, Kathleen

SUDBURY
Cameron, Sandra J.
Kivinen, Gary W.
Oliphant, Lawrie D.

THUNDER BAY
Anderson, William D.
Biman, Birubi R.
Holtby, Stuart G.

TORONTO
Adhikari, Neill
Anand, Anju
Bain, Douglas J G.
Balter, Meyer S.
Batt, Jane A E.
Bhattacharjee, Rakesh
Binnie, William M H.
Bradley, T. Douglas
Brode, Sarah K.
Burns, Karen E A.
Casey, Deborah K.
Chan, Charles K N.
Chapman, Kenneth R.
Cheng, Wing K.
Chow, Chung Wai
Coates, Allan L.
Cooligan, Terrance
Day, Anna
Dell, Sharon D M.
Faughnan, Marie E.
Ferguson, Niall D.
Ferreira, Ivone M.
Fraser, Ian
Geerts, William H.
Gershon, Andrea S.
Ginsburg, Shiphra R.
Goldstein, Roger S.
Granton, John T.
Gupta, Samir
Hall, David A.
Heffer, Matthew
Herridge, M. Margaret S.
Hoffstein, Victor
Hutcheon, Michael A.
Hyland, Robert H.
Juvet, Stephen C.
Kargel, Marcus J.
Lau, Ambrose K.
Lazar, Neil M.
Lee, Christie M.
Lee, Cindy H Y.
Lee, Warren L.
Leung, Richard S T.
Li, Christopher K.
Maleki-Yazdi, Mohammad R.
Man, Hon-Sum J.
Manocha, Sanjay
Marras, Theodore K.
Massam, Joanna L.
Mate, Eva S.
McIntyre, Kieran P D.
Mehta, Sangeeta
Moraes, Theo J.
Moric, Jakov
Niroumand-Sarvestani, Mitra
Rodriguez, Carlos H.
Sahni, Puja K.
Samanta, Tania
Shapera, Shane M.
Singer, Lianne G.
Sinuff, Tasnim
Sivjee, Khalil Y.
Skrastins, Roland
Solomon, Melinda P.
Stanbrook, Matthew J B.
Stephenson, Anne L.
Subbarao, Padmaja
Sweezey, Neil B.
Tandon, Anu
Tarlo, Susan M.
Thenganatt, John
Tullis, D. Elizabeth
Vanek, Arthur W.
Vozoris, Nicholas T.
Yuan, Jane

WELLAND
Habdank-Kossowski, Katherine

WINDSOR
Chahine-Malus, Natalie
Chao, Stephen
Denys, Allen P.
Dhar, Anil
Hellyer, Deborah J.
Malus, Eli
Rajkumar, Winston D.
Tan, Richard Y.

YORK
Varadi, Robert G.

PRINCE EDWARD ISLAND

CHARLOTTETOWN
Hunt, Barry H.

QUÉBEC

ALMA
Gagnon, Michel P.

CHATEAUGUAY
Skaburskis, Martin W.

CHICOUTIMI
Allard, Christian
Begin, Paul
Houle, Marie-Andree
Laforte, Mario
Leblanc, Jean-Pierre
Massy, Caroline

COTE SAINT-LUC
Baltzan, Marcel A.
Dabrusin, Richard A.
Rotaple, Michael J.

COWANSVILLE
Jodoin, Gilles

GATINEAU
Cote, Gilles E.
Forget, Eric J.

GREENFIELD PARK
Chasse, Marc L.
Corbeil, Claude
Matar, Nadim
Passerini, Louise
Rodier, Francois

LASALLE
Gilman, Sean A.

LAVAL
Bergeron, Marie-France
Charbonneau, Marc
Daigle, Micheline
Dehaut, Pierre
Langlais, Rebecca
Nguyen, Anh Tu
Paradis, Bruno
Verschelden, Paul

LEVIS
Deschenes, Dominique
Drouin, Christine
Lecours, Richard
Pelletier, Clarence
Plante, Julie
Sirois, Isabelle

LONGUEUIL
Braidy, Joseph F.
Deschenes, Julie
Germain, David
Le Duc, Tam
Pinsonneault, Monique
Simard, Marc
Tran, Paul C D.

MONTREAL
Agulnik, Jason S.
Ahmad Khan, Faiz
Amyot, Robert
Assayag, Deborah
Azuelos, Ilan
Beaucage, Francois
Beaupre, Alain
Bellemare, Patrick
Bergeron, Celine
Berthiaume, Yves
Berube, Denis
Bolduc, Philippe
Boudreau, J. Donald
Bourbeau, Jean
Boutet, Kim
Canakis, Anne-Marie
Cartier, Andre
Chagnon, Karine
Chatillon, Annick M.
Chrysler, Bernard
Colman, Neil C.
Colombini, Linda M.
Cote, Aurore
Cote, Isabelle
Desjardins, Alain
Dial, M. Sandra
Dugas, Mario
Eidelman, David H.
Ernst, Pierre-Paul
Ezer, Nicole
Gauthier, Andreanne
Gauthier, Richard
Gervais, Andre J G.
Goldberg, Peter
Gonzalez, Anne V.
Gottfried, Stewart B.
Gregoire, Pierre
Gruber, James M.
Gursahaney, Ashvini H.
Hirsch, Andrew M.
Jacob, Sheila V.
Jeanneret-Grosjean, Alphonse
Jobin, Vincent
Julien, Marcel
Kaminska, Marta
Kimoff, R. John
Kristof, Arnold S.
Laberge, Sophie
Labrecque, Manon
Lafond, Chantal
Landry, Jennifer S.
Lands, Larry C.
Lapierre, Jean-Guy
Laporta, Donald P.
Lavoie, Annick
Leblanc, Pierre-P.
Legare, Martin
Levesque, Marianne
Lize, Jean-Francois
Ludwig, Mara S.
Malo, Jacques
Malo, Jean-Luc
Manganas, Helene
Mannix, Sharyn E.
Marcotte, Jacques-Edouard
Martin, James G.
Matouk, Elias
Mayer, Pierre
McKinney, Martha L.
Menzies, Richard I.
Nepveu, Francois
Nguyen, Dao
Nguyen, Ngoc Bich
Nguyen, The Thanh D.
Olivenstein, Ronald
Ostiguy, Gaston L.
Palayew, Mark D.
Pamidi, Sushmita
Parenteau, Simon
Pepe, Carmela
Perraton-Brillon, Melanie
Perrault, Jean L.
Petrof, Basil J.
Poirier, Charles D.
Poirier, Claude
Qureshi, Salman T.
Rabinovitch, Barry
Renzi, Gildo
Renzi, Paolo
Rizzi, Mario C.
Saad, Nathalie
Sakr, Lama
Schwartzman, Kevin J.
Shahin, Jason
Silvestri, Isabelle
Silviet-Carricart, Maite
Small, David I.
Smith, Benjamin M.
Tremblay, Francois
Tremblay, Jacques
Vandemoortele, Thomas
Vat, Sopharat
Warshawsky, Paul J.
Wilson, Thomas R.
Wolkove, Norman
Yiannopoulos, Anna
Zackon, Harold M.
Zidulka, Arnold
Zielinski, Dawid K.

POINTE-CLAIRE
Fox, Joel M.
Yee, Daphne P.

QUEBEC
Bedard, Marie-Eve
Bilodeau, Lara
Boucher, Serge S B.
Boulet, Louis-Philippe
Boutin, Isabelle
Catellier, Priscilla
Cormier, Yvon F.
Cote, Fabien
Cote, Johanne
D'Amours, Pierre
Daigneault, Patrick
Delage, Antoine
Desmeules, Marc
Dion, Genevieve
Gagne, Dominique
Gaudreau, Vincent
Jobin, Catherine
Laberge, Francis
Labrie, Michel
Lacasse, Yves
Laforge, Jacques M.
Lampron, Noel
Laughrea, John B.
Laviolette, Michel
Leblanc, Pierre
Lemay, Julie
Maltais, Francois
Martel, Simon
Milot, Julie
Minville, Caroline
Parent, Jean-Guy
Provencher, Steeve
Raby, Bruno
Rouleau, Michel
Simon, Mathieu
Tremblay, Lise

RIMOUSKI
Goulet, Steeve
Lebreux, Elie

ROUYN-NORANDA
Farah, Majdeline

SAINT-EUSTACHE
Serban, Alexandrina

SAINT-HYACINTHE
Lemoine, Bernard

SAINT-JEROME
Arsenault, Isabelle
Carrier, Jean-Sebastien
Chalifour, Jean-Francois
Cournoyer, Guy
Deslauriers, Guy
Ouimet, Gilles

SAINT-LAURENT
Champagne, Kateri

SEPT-ILES
Hogan, Marie-Pier
Imbeault, Bruno

SHERBROOKE
Begin, Raymond O.
Boileau, Robert
Bouchard, Nicole
Cantin, Andre M.
Coll, Bernard
Dumas, Mario E.
Gaudette, Emilie
Larivee, Pierre
Lesur, Olivier J.
Poulin, Yannick
Praud, Jean-Paul
Vezina, Yves
Vlachos, Helen

SOREL-TRACY
Can, T. Bich Dao.
Godin, Jacques

ST CHARLES BORROMEE
Eid, Soheil E.
Lachance, Richard
Pek, Bonavuth

ST JEAN SUR RICHELIEU
Filion, Serge
Umapathy, Dhiviya

TERREBONNE
Paquet, Isabelle
Tremblay, Candide

TROIS-RIVIERES
Corbeil, Francois
Drapeau, Christine
Gauthier, Patrice
Goulet-Dion, Sophie
Lapointe, Michel
Noorolahi, Babak

VAL-D'OR
Germain-Lacroix, Nicolas
Lauzon, Ghyslain
Tremblay, Charles

VERDUN
Jacquemin, Paul J.
Lachance, Yves
Plante, Francois J.
Smith, Terry A.

WESTMOUNT
Knight, Lawrence

SASKATCHEWAN

REGINA
Abdulla, Ramzan H.
Belak, Zenon A.
Muftah, Abdalla G.
Sridhar, Guruswamy

SASKATOON
Adamko, Darryl J.
Fenton, Mark
Gjevre Jr., John A.
Hafezi, Rodmehr
Hergott, Christopher A.
Hoeppner, Vernon H.
Laframboise, Karen F.
Lothian, James B.
Marciniuk, Darcy D.
Pausjenssen, Elizabeth S.
Pierce, Cameron W.
Reid, John K.
Skomro, Robert
Ubhi, Mandeep S.
Ward, Heather A.

Rheumatology

ALBERTA

CALGARY
Atkinson, Martin H.
Barber, Claire
Barnabe, Cheryl C M.
Barr, Susan G.
Crawford, Anne-Marie
Edworthy, Steven
Fifi-Mah, Aurore
Fitzgerald, Avril
Fritzler, Marvin J.
Gerschman, Tommy D.
Hazlewood, Glen S.

Jibb, Norma E.
Johnson, Nicole A.
Kaminska, Elzbieta A.
Le Clercq, Sharon
Lewkonia, Raymond M.
Martin, William O.
Miettunen, Paivi M H.
Morris, Gary L.
Mosher, Dianne P.
Penney, Christopher J.
Ryan, John P.
Schoenroth, Leeanne J.
Ziouzina, Olga

EDMONTON
Aaron, Stephen L.
Akbar, Shafiq F.
Chiu, Peter L S L.
Davis, Paul
Homik, Joanne E.
Jones, H. Niall
Katz, Steven J.
Keeling, Stephanie O.
Maksymowych, Wolodymyr P.
Oswald, Anna E.
Senaratne, Savitri C.
Sholter, Dalton E.
Skeith, Kenneth J.
Teo, Michele M.
Yacyshyn, Elaine A.
Yan, Alexander

BRITISH COLUMBIA

BURNABY
How, Angela R.
Luongo, Rolfe M.

KAMLOOPS
Blumenauer, Barbara T.
Hudson, Nancy
Navratil, Jan J.

KELOWNA
Godin, Anick
McLeod, B. Daniel
Seigel, Stuart N.

NANAIMO
Baur, Nicole
Kydd, Alison S.
Sheriff, Maqbool K.

NEW WESTMINSTER
Fenton, Stanley F.
Flanagan, Cathy
Ramsden, Michael F.
Rothwell, Robert S.
Stolar, Marguerite A.

NORTH VANCOUVER
Dewar, Catharine

PENTICTON
Gross, Katherine R.
Stewart, Jacqueline C.

RICHMOND
Choi, Hyon K.
Cibere, Jolanda
Kherani, Raheem B.
Koehler, Barry E.
Lacaille, Diane V.

VANCOUVER
Badii, Maziar
Blocka, Kenneth L N.
Chalmers, Andrew
Chan, Mercedes O.
Collins, David R.
Dutz, Jan P.
Ensworth, Stephanie
Gillies, Jean H.
Jamal, Shahin
Kelsall, John T.
Klinkhoff, Alice V.
Kur, Jason K.
Morishita, Kimberley A.
Petty, Ross E.
Reid, Graham D.
Reynolds, Jennifer L.
Shojania, Kamran
Shuckett, Rhonda
Tsang, Ian K.
Verdejo-Aguilar, N. Alfonso
Wade, John P D.
Watterson, John R.
Wilk, Lucie A.

VICTORIA
Bolaria, Roxana K.
De Champlain, J. Paul
Law, Genevieve
Northcott, Kimberly A.

WESTBANK
Shojania, Nima

MANITOBA

WINNIPEG
Baillie, Cory S.
Brar, Adarshdip
Dhindsa, Navjot
El-Gabalawy, Hani S.
Hitchon, Carol A.
Jacob, Thomas K.
McCarthy, Timothy G.
Peschken, Christine A.
Robinson, David B.
Singh, Ramandip
Thomson, Glen T D.

NEW BRUNSWICK

FREDERICTON
Ecker, George A.
Henderson, James M.

MONCTON
Docherty, Peter S.
Ouellette, Sylvie A.
Picard, Leo

SAINT JOHN
Grant, Eric N.
Sadowska, Ewa

NEWFOUNDLAND AND LABRADOR

ST. JOHN'S
Dancey, Paul
Hamilton, Sean F.
Khraishi, Majed M.
Rahman, Al-Amin M P.

NOVA SCOTIA

DARTMOUTH
Shaw, Emily J.
Theriault, M Y. Diane

HALIFAX
Bakowsky, Volodko S.
Hanly, John G.
Huber, Adam M.
Lang, Bianca A.
Ramsey, Suzanne E.
Shatshat, Souad M.
Stringer, Elizabeth
Sutton, Evelyn D.
Taylor, Trudy A.
Wong, Jill M.

LUNENBURG
Wilson, Diane B.

ONTARIO

AJAX
Clements-Baker, Marie I.

ANCASTER
Pavlova, Viktoria V.

BARRIE
Haaland, Derek A.
Yuen, Kenneth W H.

BOWMANVILLE
Shickh, Ali M.

BRAMPTON
Ahluwalia, Vandana
Bajaj, Sangeeta
Joshi, V. Raman
Papneja, Tripti
Pinto, Michael A.

BROCKVILLE
Iqbal, Tariq

BURLINGTON
Dixit, Sanjay
Jaroszynska, Anna M.
Mulgund, Manisha M.
Pandith, Vikas
Wilkinson, Sharon I.

CAMBRIDGE
Famorca, Leilani Casilda de Leon

CONCORD
Kagal, Allan D.

EAST YORK
Ali, Yaser M A.

ETOBICOKE
Florica, Brandusa
Karasik, Arthur E.

GUELPH
Alderdice, Catherine A.

HAMILTON
Adachi, Jonathan D R.
Bensen, William G.
Bobba, Raja
Boulos, Pauline
Carmona, Rajendra
Cellucci, Tanya
Cividino, Alfred A.
Khalidi, Nader A.
Legault, Kimberly J.
Matsos, Mark
Scocchia, Tulio G.
Sebaldt, Rolf J.

KINGSTON
Brouillard, Daniel D.
Joneja, Mala
Towheed, Tanveer E.

KITCHENER
Faraawi, Rafat Y.

LONDON
Barra, Lillian
Berard, Roberta A.
Chopra, Nikhil
Haig, Sara L.
Le Riche, Nicole G H.
McKeown, Emily J.
Pope, Janet E.
Rohekar, Gina
Rohekar, Sherry
Thompson, Andrew E.

MARKHAM
Goodman, Rusty C J.
Lewtas, Joanne L.
Mak, Vincent C W.
Tupchong, Michele A.

MISSISSAUGA
Bahrami-Esferjani, Azar
Blanchette, Nicholas S.
Chan, Edwin S L.
Chow, Andrew
Khan, Imtiaz M S.
Liu, Yan
Mody, Ami N.
Montgomery, Angela B.
Soucy, Elaine
Walz, Barbara A E.

NEPEAN
Kapur, Suneil
Liu, Bin
Morassut, Patricia A.

NEWMARKET
Aubrey, Michael E.
Ng Tung Hing, Edward K K.
Thorne, J. Carter

NIAGARA FALLS
Dhillon, Rajwinder S.

NORTH YORK
Dostrovsky, Nathaniel
Dunne, Shelly M.
Greenwald, Mark
Handelsman, Sam
Hutchinson, Clare M.
Kanji, Dilshad A.
Koren, Sharon
Kreidstein, Sharon H.
Potashner, Wayne J.
Rush, Perry J.

OAKVILLE
Patodia, Shaila

ORILLIA
Collins, David S.

OSHAWA
Silecky, Walter B.

OTTAWA
Boate, Brian W.
Cranney, Blanid A.
Davis, Kathleen A.
Duff, Susie
Duffy, Ciaran
Humphrey, Susan M.
Jovaisas, Algis V.
Karsh, Jacob
Kraag, Gunnar R.
MacMillan, Suzanne M.
McKendry, Robert J R.
Milman, Nataliya
O'Keefe, Deborah L.
Shamess, Charles J.
Smith, C. Douglas
Thomson, John G.

PETERBOROUGH
Doris, J. Frederick
Purvis, Jane
Sudbury, M. Susan F.

PICKERING
Lee, Martin M S.

RICHMOND HILL
Sugai, Michael K.

SCARBOROUGH
Acker, John J.
Baer, Philip A.
Lee, Julietta C T.
Leung, Felix K Y.

ST CATHARINES
Dickson, John R.
Griffiths, Gregory B.
Shaikh, Saeed A.

ST THOMAS
Leaf, Suzanne C.

SUDBURY
Cano, Pablo O.

THUNDER BAY
Ashater, Elsharif M M.
Fidler, Wesley

TORONTO
Abrahamson, John L A.
Abufayyah, Mohammed
Ahmad, S. Zareen
Al Ghanim, Nayef S A.
Al Maini, Mustafa H A.
Albert, Lori J.
Alnaqbi, Khalid
Batthish, Michelle
Bell, Mary J.
Blackmore, Michael G.
Bombardier, Claire
Bookman, Arthur A M.
Bykerk, Vivian
Cameron, Bonnie J.
Campbell, Doreen J.
Carette, Simon
Chow, Shirley
Choy, Gregory W.
Danayan, Karoon C.
Feldman, Brian M.
Gakhal, Natasha K.
Gladman, Dafna D.
Grigoriadis, Elizabeth
Hamilton, M. Lynn
Hawker, Gillian
Hochman, Jacqueline R.
Inman, Robert D.
Jerome, Dana C.
Johnson, Sindhu R.
Keesal, Nancy B.
Keystone, Edward C.
Kovacs, Julie A J.
Kung, Tabitha N.
Kuriya, Bindee
Landolt-Marticorena, C. Maria
Laskin, Carl A.
Laxer, Ronald M.
Lee, Mary C Y.
Lee, Peter
Leung, Frances Y K.
Luca, Nadia J C.
Mahendira, Dharini
McDonald Blumer, M. Heather
Mewa, Amirudin A M.
Mittoo, Shikha
Norris, Erin B.
Pedvis, Stacey R.
Perlin, Louise R B.
Seyed Akhavan, Pooneh
Shupak, Rachel
Silverman, Earl D.
Siminovitch, Katherine A.
Sokoluk, Craig A.
Soon, Gordon S.
Steiman, Amanda J.
Stein, Jonathan D.
Tenenbaum, Jerry
Tse, Shirley M L.
Voorneveld, Colin R.
Wither, Joan E.

VAUGHAN
Cohen, Dana R.

WINDSOR
Abdelgader, Abdelgalel
Rodrigues, Jude F N.

QUÉBEC

GATINEAU
Zadorozny, Oleg G.

GREENFIELD PARK
Angle, James D.
Beauchemin, Julie
Kanji, Mohammed I.

JOLIETTE
Duchesne, Line

LAVAL
Ciolofan, Oana C.
Hazeltine, Mark

LEVIS
Blier, Claude
Roy, Nathalie
Trudeau, Judith

MONTREAL
Baron, Murray
Beaudet, Francois
Berjat, Michel E.
Berkson, Laeora
Bernatsky, Sasha R.
Bertrand, Carole
Bissonnette, Bernard F.
Blondin, Claude
Bourre Tessier, Josiane

Bourrelle, Dominique
Campillo, Sarah
Choquette, Denis
Ciubotariu, Elena
Dagenais, Pierre
Fallavollita, Sabrina
Favreau, Marc B.
Fitzcharles, Mary-Ann
Garfield, Bruce
Germain, Guy
Grodzicky, Tamara C.
Gyger, Genevieve
Haraoui, Boulos
Hazel, Elizabeth
Hudson, Marie
Kang, Harbhajan S.
Kapusta, Morton A.
Krasny, Jiri L.
Leblanc, Claire
Ligier, Sophie
M'Seffar, Abdelmajid
Massicotte, Frederic
Mathieu, Jean-Pierre
Menard, Henri A.
Mercille, Suzanne
Morency, Nathalie
Morin, Marie-Paule
Moroz, Leonard A.
Naiman, Lada
Nashi, Emil
Numainville, Louise
Panopalis, Pantelis
Pelletier, Jean-Pierre
Pineau, Christian A.
Radoux, Victor
Raynauld, Jean-Pierre
Remillard, Marie-Anais
Rich, Eric
Scuccimarri, Rosie
Senecal, Jean-Luc
St-Pierre, Anne
Stein, Michael A.
Troyanov, Yves
Villeneuve, Edith
Vinet, Evelyne
Watts, Craig S.
Yeadon, Carol A M.
Yuen, Sai Yan
Zummer, Michel

OUTREMONT
Couture, Francois

POINTE-CLAIRE
Cohen, Martin A.
Starr, Michael R.

QUEBEC
Adams, Karen
Albert, Alexandra
Beaulieu, Andre
Bessette, Louis
Brown, Jacques
Fortin, Paul
Grondin, Charlotte
Leclerc, Valerie
Marcoux, Claude
Poubelle, Patrice E E.
Turcotte, Angele

RIMOUSKI
Bergeron, Claudie
Fortin, Isabelle

SAINT-HYACINTHE
Dansereau, Jean-Yves
Gaudreau, Andre

SAINT-LEONARD
Attie, Nabil

SHERBROOKE
Arsenault, Guylaine
Boire, Gilles
Camerlain, Monique
Fernandes, Artur J D B.
Liang, Patrick

ST CHARLES BORROMEE
Langlais, Nathalie

ST-EUSTACHE
Gagne, Michel

ST JEAN SUR RICHELIEU
Deschenes, Isabelle

TROIS-RIVIERES
Dessureault, M. Michele
Drouin, Julie
Lessard, Clode
Morin, Frederic
Rouleau, Louise
Tremblay, Jean-Luc

VERDUN
Giard, Marie-Claude

WESTMOUNT
Tannenbaum, Hyman

SASKATCHEWAN

REGINA
Fahlman, Nicole M.
McDougall, Robert S.
Milne, Ardyth A.

SASKATOON
Nair, Bindu V.
Rosenberg, Alan M.
Shiff, Natalie J.
Taylor Gjevre, Regina M.

Thoracic Surgery

ALBERTA

CALGARY
Gelfand, Gary A J.
Graham, Andrew J.
Grondin, Sean C.
McFadden, Sean D P.

EDMONTON
Bedard, Eric L.
Johnson, Scott T.
Stewart, Kenneth C.
Valji, Azim M.
Winton, Timothy L.

BRITISH COLUMBIA

KELOWNA
Humer, Michael F.
Jugnauth, Anand
Luoma, Andrew A.
Nelems, Bill

NEW WESTMINSTER
Hayden, Robert I.

PENTICTON
Essery, Cameron R.

SURREY
Ashrafi, Ahmad S.
Bond, R. James
Ong, Sharon Rose Y.

VANCOUVER
Brumwell, Mary L.
Evans, Kenneth G.
Finley, Richard J.
Laing, Bryce J.
Yee, John

VICTORIA
Dewar, Gary J.
Samphire, John

MANITOBA

BRANDON
Mohamed, Muftah A.

WINNIPEG
Parham, Shelley M.
Srinathan, Sadeesh K.
Tan, A. Lawrence
Unruh, Helmut W.

NEW BRUNSWICK

FREDERICTON
Gowan, Russell T.
Peters, Thomas H.

MONCTON
Burnett, Ralph H.
Dubois, Paul M.
Mujoomdar, Aneil A.

NEWFOUNDLAND AND LABRADOR

ST. JOHN'S
Gardiner, J. Paul
Guy, John R F.
Mann, Catherine L.

NOVA SCOTIA

HALIFAX
Bethune, Drew C G.
Buduhan, Gordon P.
Henteleff, Harry J A.
Johnston, Michael R.
Plourde, Madelaine

SYDNEY
McGory, Rodney W.

ONTARIO

BRAMPTON
Chiasson, Paul J.
Irshad, Kashif

EAST YORK
Zeldin, Robert A.

HAMILTON
Altaf, Fawaz M N S.
Finley, Christian
Miller, John D.
Schieman, Colin
Shargall, Yaron

KINGSTON
Reid, Kenneth R.

KITCHENER
Kilmurry, Matthew R.
Talwar, Manoj K.

LONDON
Fortin, Dalilah
Inculet, Richard
Malthaner, Richard A.

MISSISSAUGA
Behzadi, Abdollah
Jones, Donald P.
Mohammed, Adam H.
Uddin, Sameena

NEWMARKET
Lee, Alexander L.
Privitera, Salvatore
Toth, Julius L R.

OSHAWA
Dickie, A. John
Marcus, Herbert I.
Trainor, Shannon E.

OTTAWA
Gilbert, Sebastien
Maziak, Donna E.
Seely, Andrew J E.
Sundaresan, R. Sudhir
Todd, Thomas R J.
Villeneuve, Patrick J.

OWEN SOUND
Nechala, Patrik

RICHMOND HILL
Lee, Mark H.

SCARBOROUGH
Anderson, Thomas H.
Chan, Michael C K.

ST THOMAS
McLachlin, Hugh A.

SUDBURY
Ewing-Bui, T. David
Luison, Fabio
Smith, Shona E.

THUNDER BAY
Gehman, Kenneth E.

TORONTO
Blitz, Maurice
Compeau, Christopher G.
Darling, Gail
Ko, Michael A.
Pierre, Andrew F.
Safieddine, Najib N.
Simone, Carmine
Waddell, Thomas K.

WINDSOR
Coughlin, Michael P.
Elalem, Abdusalam

QUÉBEC

CHICOUTIMI
Michaud, Pierre

LEVIS
Dubreuil, Daniel

MONTREAL
Beauchamp, Gilles
Choiniere, Louise
Ferraro, Pasquale
Ferri, Lorenzo E.
Liberman, A. Moishe
Martin, Jocelyne
Ouellette, M A. Denise
Rakovich, George
Rusnov, Mladen V.
Sheiner, Nathan M.
Sirois, Cateline
Sirois, Christian

QUEBEC
Frechette, Eric

SHERBROOKE
Sirois, Chantal

SASKATCHEWAN

SASKATOON
Bharadwaj, Steven C.
Bigsby, Richard J.
Casson, Alan G.
Kennedy, Renee S.

Urology

ALBERTA

CALGARY
Barr, Richard E.
Baverstock, Richard J.
Carlson, Kevin V.
Cook, Anthony J.
Donnelly, Bryan
Duffy, Martin
Dushinski, John W.
Gotto, Geoffrey T.
Hyndman, C. William
Hyndman, Matthew E.
Kawakami, Jun
Kozak, Gregory N.
Lee, Jay C H.
Leong, James P.
Metcalfe, Donald
Weber, Bryce A.
Wilkin, Richard P.

EDMONTON
Bochinski, Dariuz
Chetner, Michael P.
Estey, Eric P.
Evans, Howard
Gray, Gary J.
Hobart, Michael G.
Jacobsen, Niels-Erik B.
Kiddoo, Darcie A.
Mador, David R.
Metcalfe, Peter D.
Moore, Ronald B.
Rourke, Keith F.
Schuler, Trevor D.
St Martin, Blair A.
Todd, Gerald T.
Weisler, Marvin N.
Wollin, Timothy A.

GRANDE PRAIRIE
Torbey, Camille

LEDUC
Foda, Mohamed M R.
McCallum, Theresa J.

LETHBRIDGE
Lavens, Nathan T.
Shields, William R.
Taylor, Jonathan S.

MEDICINE HAT
Alphin, Mohamed T.

RED DEER
San Vicente, Juan J.
Thomas, Robert G.
Walz, Norman C H.

BRITISH COLUMBIA

ABBOTSFORD
Evani, Subbarao
Neville, Christopher S.
Vrabec, George J.

BURNABY
Truong, Vu Ngoc
Warner, John A.
Woo, Young-Chi

CHILLIWACK
Goodman, Saul H.

COQUITLAM
Este, Francis A.

COURTENAY
Beristain, Guillermo R.
Chartrand, James G H.
Clark, Aaron T D.
Tinmouth, William W.

CRANBROOK
Schieman, Steven M.

DUNCAN
Nielsen, William R.

KAMLOOPS
Faddegon, Stephen P.
Jonat, Lee M.
Ottem, Derek P.
Treissman, Simon P I D.

KELOWNA
Carter, Michael D.
Jaklis, Ziad
Kinahan, Thomas J.
Prestage, Keith T.
Wiesenthal, Joshua D.

LANGLEY
Cripps, Stephanie M.
Perks, Alexandra E.
Stogryn, Russell D.

MAPLE RIDGE
Harrington, Gregory D R.

NANAIMO
Carlson, William H.
Morrison, Kevin B.
Palmer, Geoffrey M.

NEW WESTMINSTER
Hershfield, Melvyn
Paulus, Edmund M.
Yang, Brian P T.

NORTH VANCOUVER
Chow, Victor D W.
Crofts, Paul G.
Hoag, Christopher C.
Poon, Christina I.

PENTICTON
Crofts, Neil G.

PORT ALBERNI
Mohamedali, Zeid

PRINCE GEORGE
Cassidy, Darby J.
Hampole, Rahul K.
Jamieson, Clark B.
Paterson, Guy S.

RICHMOND
Hennessey, Katherine K.
Krahn, Corrie G.
Mickelson, Jennifer J.
Poon, Kenneth S.
Rapoport, Daniel

SIDNEY
Grace, Donald A.

SURREY
Andreou, Charalambos
Kwan, Herman C.
Nazif, Omar A.
Skepasts, Peter K.
Yong, Yu-Sen

TERRACE
Osei-Tutu, Francis K.

TRAIL
Livingstone, Roy R.

VANCOUVER
Afshar, Kourosh
Black, Peter C V.
Chew, Ben H.
Eng, Michael K.
Fenster, Howard N.
Gleave, Martin E.
Goldenberg, S. Larry
Gourlay, William A.
Leone, Ercole F.
MacNeily, Andrew E.
Masterson, John S T.
McDougall, Elspeth M.
McLoughlin, Martin G.
Nguan, Christopher Y.
Nigro, Mark K.
Paterson, Ryan
Perler, Zelick
Phillips, Elliott J.
Piszel, Lloyd M.
So, Alan I.
Stothers, Mary-Ann L.
Taylor, William N.
Teichman, Joel M H.
Toren, Paul J.
Wright, Jamie E.

VERNON
Houle, Gregory A.
Lavoie, Denis J.
Schultz, Troy D.

VICTORIA
Kinahan, John F J D.
McAuley, Iain W.
McCracken, Jeffrey M.
Pommerville, P. John
Steinhoff, Gary E J.

MANITOBA

BRANDON
Kassier, Karl E.

WINNIPEG
Al Essawi, Turki H M.
Bard, Robert J.
Cho, Patrick A.
Dharamsi, Nafisa
Drachenberg, Darrel E.
Hildebrand, Brenda
Hosking, Denis H.
Jason, Marlowe A.
Jensen, Christopher W B.
Karvelas, John P.
MacMahon, Ross G.
McGregor, Thomas B.
Milner, John F.
Paquin, R. Wayne
Peters, Brian G T.
Psooy, Karen J.
Ritchie, Brian
Saranchuk, Jeffery W.
Wong, Simon W C.

NEW BRUNSWICK

BATHURST
Daigle, Sebastien
Ngo, Duc Sieu

DIEPPE
Breault, Guy

FREDERICTON
Feero, Peter G.
Hickey, Liam
McLellan, Rowen A.
Patrick, Allan B.

MONCTON
Anthony, Francis R.
Boudreau, Luc
Dwyer, Neil
LeBlanc, Guy
Savoie, Marc
Sitland, Troy D.

RIVERSIDE-ALBERT
Garston, Ronald G.

SAINT JOHN
Ashfield, James E.
Bryniak, Steven
Morse, Michael J.
Whelan, Thomas F.

NEWFOUNDLAND AND LABRADOR

GRAND FALLS WINDSOR
Sutherland, David J.

ST. JOHN'S
Best, Leoncio M.
Drover, Douglas N.
Duffy, Gavin R.
French, Christopher G.
Hewitt, Richard J.
Johnston, Paul H.
Pike, John G.

NOVA SCOTIA

DARTMOUTH
Chun, Samuel S S.
T'ien, Wallace

HALIFAX
Anderson, Peter A M.
Bagnell, P. Scott
Bailly, Gregory G.
Bell, David G.
Gajewski, Jerzy
Grantmyre, John E.
Lawen, Joseph G.
MacLellan, Dawn L.
Rendon, Ricardo A.
Schwarz, Robert D.

KENTVILLE
Butler, Trevor J.
McCarthy, John-Paul
Palmer, Bruce W.

SYDNEY
Miller, Mervyn D.

TRURO
Padmore, Dave E.
Puthenparumpil, Jacob J.

UPPER TANTALLON
Norman, Richard W.

ONTARIO

AJAX
Grabowski, Arthur
Smith, Steven I.

BARRIE
Hartsburg, Cory J.
Iocca, Angelo J.
Ray, A. Andrew
Zadra, Joseph A.

BELLEVILLE
Campbell, Thomas A.
Guan, Meng
Leal, Gregory R J.
Woods, Edward F A.

BRACEBRIDGE
Drohomyrecky, Anthony

BRAMPTON
Beheshti, Mojtaba N.
Chatterjee, Suman
Farivar-Mohseni, Hesam
Giddens, Jonathan L.
Ibrahim, Mohammed A.
Tisdale, Britton E.

BRANTFORD
Beasley, Kenneth A.
Dickson, Dann W.
Leung, Wilson W S.

BROCKVILLE
Earle, John M.
Noss, Mark B.

BURLINGTON
Jansz, G. Kenneth
Love, William
Sowery, Richard S D.

CAMBRIDGE
Kim, Dennis
Roth, Kirk M.

CHATHAM
Pakulis, Valdis
Williams, Charles A.

CONCORD
Kogon, Michael D.

CORNWALL
Weinberg, Garry B.
Yassa, Samir A R.

EAST YORK
Vlaovic, Peter D.

ETOBICOKE
Dagnone, A. Joel
Gupta, Rajiv
Harry, Gervais A.
Morrell, John D.
Skeldon, Simon C.
Tsihlias, John

GUELPH
Hirshberg, Eric D.
Morris, Thomas J.
Wesley-James, Timothy

HAMILTON
Davies, Timothy O.
De Maria, Jorge
Fischer, Marc
Greenspan, Michael
Kapoor, Anil
Matsumoto, Edward D.
Orovan, William L.
Piercey, Kevin R.
Rehsia, Sabeer S.
Shayegan, Bobby
Tsai, Shian-Yih
Whelan, John P J.
Winter, A. Leo
Zikman, Jerrold M.

KINGSTON
Beiko, Darren T.
Leveridge, Michael J.
Morales, Alvaro
Nickel, J. Curtis
Siemens, D. Robert
Steele, Stephen S.
Touma, Naji J.
Wilson, James W L.

KITCHENER
Borth, Christopher S.
Cybulski, Peter A.
Egerdie, Russell B.
Hamilton, Ronald W.
McFarlane, Nicholas A.
Rangaswamy, Satish

LONDON
Brock, Gerald B.
Chin, L K. Joseph
Denstedt, John
Fahmy, Nader
Izawa, Jonathan I.
Luke, Patrick P W.
Pautler, Stephen E.
Power, Nicholas E.
Razvi, Hassan A S.
Rowe, Ernest N.
Sales, Jack L.
Sener, Alp
Welk, Blayne K.

MARKHAM
Boudakian, Avidis H.
Di Costanzo, Giovanni A.

MILTON
Kwan, Kevin

MISSISSAUGA
Carnat, Toby A.
Desai, Rashmikant J.
Feifer, Andrew H.
Jamal, Munir A.
McIsaac, Gary P.
Papanikolaou, Frank F.
Short, Thomas W D.

NEPEAN
Girvan, Andrew
Pierre, Sean A.
Power, Kevin V.
Proudlove, Steven G.
Sahajpal, Riki

NEWMARKET
Green, Jerome A.
Klinghoffer, Zachary D.
Liquornik, Morrie S.
Preiner, John L.
Woo, Stanley K C.

NIAGARA FALLS
Brown, Ian R.
Mattar, Kamal
Reddy, Kundavaram N.

NORTH BAY
Goldfarb, Bernard
Sogbein, S. Kolawole

NORTH YORK
Barkin, Jack
Buckley, Roger
Charendoff, Jeffrey S.
Comisarow, Richard H.
Defreitas, Gina
Durier, Jean-Louis M.
Fazio, Luke M.
Flax, Stanley
Hajek, David M.
Juriansz, Allan R.
Kong, Y S. Peter
Noakes, Jeffrey E.
Punnen, Punnamkuzhil C.
Radzinski, Charles A.
Sharir, Sharon
Spevack, Leslie M.

OAKVILLE
Casey, Richard W.
Incze, Peter F.
Prince, W. Ross

ORILLIA
Lee, Livia K Y.
Minich, Peter J.
Okafo, Benjamin A.
Sing, Roland I.

OSHAWA
Chang, C. Michael
Gibson, Sean
Mathur, Arun K.
Morton, Thomas J.
Sachdeva, Krishan K.

OTTAWA
Bella, Anthony J.
Blew, Brian D M.
Bourdeau, Gilles
Breau, Rodney H.
Cagiannos, Ilias
De Jesus Jr., Filemon
Gerridzen, Ronald
Kamal, Fadi A B.
Leonard, Michael P G.
Mahoney, John E.
Morash, Christopher G L.
Oake, J. Stuart
Roberts, Matthew T.
Saleh, Wasfy S.
Saltel, Marc E J.
Tessier, Jocelyne
Tran, Viet Tan
Warren, Jeffrey
Watterson, James D.
Wong, James W.

OWEN SOUND
Middlebrook, Paul F.
Webster, Todd M.
Wignall, Geoffrey R.

PEMBROKE
Murray, J. Scott

PETERBOROUGH
El Harram, Mohamed A.
Meade, William M.
Weir, Michael J.

POINT EDWARD
Singh, Rajiva R.

RICHMOND HILL
Abara, O. Emmanuel
Mak, Victor
Samsoondar, Wayne R.

SARNIA
Ramirez, Alvaro

SAULT STE MARIE
Aziz, Anis
Haidar, Nadim
Mathur, Vinod K.
Mohamed, John K.

SCARBOROUGH
Abramovitch, Allan
Baldwin, William E.
Buzon, Antonio A.
Chan, Jonathan E K.
Erdeljan, Petar
Logarakis, Nick F.
Singer, Henry N.
Soon, Shawn J.
Spodek, Jeffrey M.
Toguri, Allan G.
Trottier, Gregory T.

SMITHS FALLS
Roney, Peter D.

ST CATHARINES
Casselman, Ronald C.
Heritz, Dianne M.
Lee, James L.

ST THOMAS
Cheng, Michael J C.
McKenzie, John A.

STRATFORD
Bukala, Bernard P.
Hussey, Andrew A.

STRATHROY
Ferguson, Ian K.

SUDBURY
Abourbih, Jacques
Bilgasem, Solieman A.
Bora, Bishwajit
D'Aloisio, Joseph F.
Moskalyk, Tara M.
Pianezza, Michael L.

THUNDER BAY
Abdel-Malak, Mamdouh Z.
Prowse, Owen A.
Skehan, Anthony M.

TIMMINS
Hares, Mark

TORONTO
Bagli, Darius J.
Barsoum, Milad K.
Blumenfeld, Aaron J.
Carr, Lesley K.
Chawla, Ashis K.
Cox, Ashley R.
Farhat, Walid A.
Finelli, Antonio
Fleshner, Neil E.
Grober, Ethan
Groll, Ryan J.
Hassouna, Magdy
Herschorn, Sender
Honey, R. John D'A.
Jain, Umesh
Jarvi, Keith A.
Jewett, Michael A S.
Juda, Tibor
Kell, John S.
Kim, Steve Y.
Klotz, Laurence H.
Kodama, Ronald T.
Koyle, Martin A.
Kulkarni, Girish S.
Kwok, Harold K Y.
Lantz, Andrea G.
Lee, Jason Y.
Lo, Kirk C L.
Lorenzo, Armando J.
Marcuzzi, Alfonso
McLean, Anthony R.
Nadeau, Genevieve
Nam, Robert
Ordon, Michael
Pace, Kenneth T.
Pippi-Salle, Joao L P.
Radomski, Sidney B.
Robinette, Michael A.
Shaikh, Bashiruddin N.
Singal, Rajiv K.
Stewart, Robert J.
Tam, Stephanie
Trachtenberg, John
Wehbi, Elias
Yap, Stanley A.
Zlotta, Alexandre R.

VAUGHAN
Shahani, Rohan

WELLAND
Mazmanian, Hagop K.
Shoebridge, Jeffrey J.
Song, Tom T Y.

WINDSOR
Al-Farra, Bassel
Deklaj, Tom
Elsdon, Thomas C.
Goel, Raj K.
Khalaff-Abourawai, Hussein
Sherghin, Ahmed S O.
Sorensen, Ronald B.

WOODSTOCK
Voegelin, Richard E.

PRINCE EDWARD ISLAND

CHARLOTTETOWN
Mulligan, John M.
Mundle, R. Murray
Reid, R. Ian

QUÉBEC

ALMA
Robert, Jean G.

BAIE-SAINT-PAUL
Simard, Jacques

CHATEAUGUAY
Antebi, Elie
Sioufi, Richard

CHICOUTIMI
Barrette, Louis-Rene
Blackburn, Frederic
Paradis, Jean-Benoit

COURCELETTE
Gosselin, Gabriel

COWANSVILLE
Deblois, Michel

DRUMMONDVILLE
Debs, Chaouki
Godbout, Manon

GATINEAU
Bouchard, Claude
Duclos, Benoit
Faddoul, Said F.
Quirouet, Adrienne
Saliba, Nasri

GRANBY
Dagenais, Louis J.
Ouellette, Paul

GREENFIELD PARK
Aaron, Lorne E.
Arjane, Philippe
Desbiens, Rene
Gilchrist, Lawrence I.
Nachabe, Mahmoud

KIRKLAND
Kurgansky, Vladimir

LAVAL
Bettez, Mathieu
Cossette, Jean
Duval, Louis
Guertin, Benoit
Hage, Bechir
Hanna, Samer
Jammal, Marie-Paule
Lapointe, Steven P.
Laurent, Guy
Simard, Jean
Trudel, Claude

LEVIS
Bazinet, Jocelyn
Emond, Jean-Paul
Gagnon, Louis-Olivier
Lemelin, François
Paradis, Gaetan
Patry, Genevieve

LONGUEUIL
Marois, Carlos
Steinberg, Andrew P.

MONTREAL
Andonian, Sero
Aprikian, Armen-Garo
Aronson, Samuel A.
Barrieras, Diego
Belair, Guy
Benard, Francois
Benayoun, Serge
Bertrand, Pierre E.
Brzezinski, Alex E.
Capolicchio, Gianpaolo
Carrier, Serge
Chan, Peter T K.
Charghi, Ali
Chiricosta, Albert A.
Cianciulli, Bruno
Corcos, Jacques
Desbiens, Genevieve
Drouin, Guy
Duclos, Alain J.
El-Sherbiny, Mohamed T.
Elhilali, Mostafa M.
Firszt, Jose
Franc-Guimond, Julie
Girard, Guy
Houle, Anne-Marie
Jacobson, Stephen A.
Jednak, Roman
Jolivet-Tremblay, Martine
Jolly, Patrick
Karakiewicz, Pierre
Kassouf, Wassim
Lapointe, Steven
Lattouf, Jean-Baptiste
Lebeau, Thierry
Leboeuf, Line
Letendre, Julien
Matthews, Keith L.
McCormack, Michael
Morehouse, Douglas D.
Morris, Brian M.
Paquin, Jean-Marie
Peloquin, Francois A.
Perreault, Jean-Paul
Perrotte, Paul
Pharand, Daniel
Racine, Pierre Y.
Saad, Fred
Schick, Erik
Shaigetz, Daniel
Taguchi, Yoshinori
Tanguay, Simon
Trinh, Quoc-Dien
Tukaram, Khoday T.
Valiquette, Luc
Widmer, Hugues
Zini, Armand S.
Zorn, Kevin C.

POINTE-CLAIRE
Eiley, David
El-Hakim, Assaad
Jacobson, Avrum I.

QUEBEC
Audet, Jean-Francois
Bolduc, Stephane
Caumartin, Yves
Dujardin, Thiery
Fradet, Vincent
Fradet, Yves
Gregoire, Mireille
Imbeault, Annie
Lacombe, Louis
Laroche, Bruno
Moore, Katherine
Naud, Alain
Pouliot, Frederic
Roy, Rejean
Soucy, Frederic

REPENTIGNY
Bellavance, Gilles B.

RIMOUSKI
Boutin, Helene
Daignault, Robert
Desjardins, Richard
Lebel, Michel H.
Vary, John R C M.

RIVIERE-DU-LOUP
Boisvert, Isabelle
Gagnon, Nathalie

ROBERVAL
Adamo, George
Delisle, Rejean

ROUYN-NORANDA
Liandier, Frederic

SAINT-HYACINTHE
Baillargeon-Gagne, Sara
Gagnon, Bernard
Lessard, Annie
Matte, Hugues

SAINT-JEROME
Alcaidinho, Duarte
Allard, Denis
Cantin, Aline
Leblanc, Bruno
Lewinshtein, Daniel J.

SAINT-LAURENT
Libman, Jamie

SAINT-LEONARD
Papazian, Apkar

SALABERRY DE VALLEYFIELD
Al Mandil, Majid
Boman, Jason M.
Itovitch, Joseph J.

SHERBROOKE
Carmel, Michel
Khoury, Elie-Philippe
Martel, Arold M.
Ponsot, Yves
Sabbagh, Robert
Tu, Le Mai

SOREL-TRACY
Hejeily, Antoine

ST CHARLES BORROMEE
Crevier, Jean
Sajous, Franck J A.

ST JEAN SUR RICHELIEU
Dessureault, Jean
Drouin, Johanne
Walsh, Philippe

THETFORD MINES
Girard, Jean-Guy

TROIS-RIVIERES
Duchesnay, Gaetan
Fortier, Serge
Fournier-Cloutier, Vincent
Lapierre, Sylvain
Maillette, Alain
Marchand, Luc
Morisset, Julie

VAL-D'OR
Tremblay, Thierry

VANIER
Le May, Claude

VERDUN
Bourque, Jean-Louis

VICTORIAVILLE
Auger, Michel
Lemieux, Marguerite

SASKATCHEWAN

REGINA
Abuhjar, Abdussalam K.
Crichlow, Michael W.
Tse, Edward T W.

SASKATOON
Domes, Trustin
Gonor, Saul E.
Jana, Kunal K.
Lau, Peter C K.
McKinny, Shari-Lee C.
Taranger, Lawrence A.
Visvanathan, Kishore
Weckworth, Paul F.

SWIFT CURRENT
Arwini, Mohamed A S.

Vascular Surgery

ALBERTA

CALGARY
Moore, Randy D.
Nutley, Mark T.
Petrasek, Paul F.
Samis, Gregory A.
Wong, Joyce

EDMONTON
Alibhai, Karim N.
Bayne, Jason P.
Chyczij, Harold R.
Cox, Heather L.
Davey, P. Douglas
Turnbull, Robert G.
Winkelaar, Gerrit B.

RED DEER
Hamilton, Donald J.

BRITISH COLUMBIA

ABBOTSFORD
Lewis, Gregory M.

KAMLOOPS
Azad, Aristotle

KELOWNA
Ellett, Robert W.
Lawlor, D. Kirk
Mostowy, Stephan C.
Pasenau, Jeffrey E H.

LANGLEY
Fry, Peter D.
Ginting, Nadra
Smith, R. Matthew M.

NEW WESTMINSTER
Kazemi, Kamyar

NORTH VANCOUVER
Hunter, James M.

PRINCE GEORGE
Lokanathan, Ramesh
Palerme, Louis-Philippe

RICHMOND
Holmvang, Annette M.
Houston, Gordon T M.

SURREY
Sharif, Mohammad S.

VANCOUVER
Baxter, Keith A.
Chen, Jerry C L.
Gagnon, Joel
Hsiang, York N H.
MacDonald, Peter S.
Reid, John D S.
Salvian, Anthony J G.
Sidhu, Ravindar S.
Taylor, David C.

VICTORIA
Dooner, James
Kuechler, Peter M.
Lee, Shung
Robinson, Matthew J.

MANITOBA

WINNIPEG
Boyd, April J.
Fong, Handrick
Guzman, Randolph P.
Harding, Gregory E J.
Koulack, Joshua
Violago, Francisco C.

NEW BRUNSWICK

DIEPPE
Bourgoin, Michel

EDMUNDSTON
Cloutier, Paul

FREDERICTON
Schaus, Claus P.

MONCTON
Brown, D. Stephen
Burnett, Ralph H.
Murphy, John L.

NEWFOUNDLAND AND LABRADOR

ST. JOHN'S
Browne, Gregory N.
Harrington, David M.
Heneghan, Paul D.

NOVA SCOTIA

HALIFAX
Casey, Patrick J.
Lee, Min Sun
MacKean, Gerald L.
Midgley, Peter I.

KENTVILLE
Davidson, Dion
Heisler, Benjamin E.

MIRA ROAD
Jhirad, Ronen H.

SYDNEY
Dunn, Rex S.
Naqvi, Mahmood A.

ONTARIO

BARRIE
Gowing, Robert N.

BRAMPTON
Louis, Donald K.

BRANTFORD
Maddison, G. David

ETOBICOKE
Wooster, Douglas L.

GUELPH
Hobson, John W.
Jahromi, Afshin
Nasser, Hamid A.

HAMILTON
Harlock, John A.
Iyer, Vikram S.
Rapanos, Theodore
Szalay, David A.
Tittley, Jacques G.

KINGSTON
Brown, Peter M.
Petsikas, Dimitri J.
Zelt, David T.

KITCHENER
Ashe, Kassem A.

LONDON
De Rose, Gaetano
Forbes, Thomas
Harris, Jeremy R.
Harris, Kenneth
Power, Adam H.

MISSISSAUGA
Johnson, William S.
O'Connor, Richard J A.
Orr, James F.
Pope, Marc
Vucemilo, Ivica

NEWMARKET
Campbell, J. Daniel
Gupta, Deepak
Lossing, Alan G.

NIAGARA FALLS
Rammohan, Surianarayanan

NORTH BAY
Moffat, Robert C.

NORTH YORK
Beder, Aaron L.
Cardella, Jonathan A.
Cina, Claudio S.
Forrest, Ian
Goldberg, Michael R.

OSHAWA
Coutu, Pierre A.

OTTAWA
Brandys, Timothy M.
Cagiannos, Catherine
Dervish, Greta A.
Hajjar, Georges E.
Hill, Andrew B.
Jayaram, Srinidhi K.
Jetty, Prasad
Kubelik, Dalibor
Lewis, Ronald T.
Lorimer, John W.
Nagpal, Sudhir K.
Syme, Roderick G.

PETERBOROUGH
Nie, Robert G.
Thompson, Alan A.

RICHMOND HILL
Fiture, Ali O.

SAULT STE MARIE
Fratesi, Sante J.

SCARBOROUGH
Au, How Hoong
Azoubel, Gustavo A P.
Huhlewych, Roman
You, John M S.

STRATFORD
Gonser, Randal J.

SUDBURY
Fenton, John A.
Pudupakkam, Santosh R.
Willoughby, Rodney P N.

THORNHILL
Kalman, Peter G.

TORONTO
Ameli, F. Michael
Atherton, William
Campbell, Vern
Dueck, Andrew D.
Huseynov, Khumar
Johnston, K. Wayne
King, William
Kucey, Daryl S.
Lindsay, Thomas F.
Maggisano, Robert
Oreopoulos, George D.
Papia, Giuseppe
Rubin, Barry B.
Tanner, Wayne R.
Tse, Leonard W H.
Walker, Paul M.

WINDSOR
Iannicello, Carman M.
Mehta, Sowmil K.
Ristic, Miodrag A.

QUÉBEC

CHICOUTIMI
Michaud, Pierre

GATINEAU
Nault, Patrice

GREENFIELD PARK
Larose, Pierre
Le Guillan, Marie-Pierre

JOLIETTE
Berlinguet, Jean-Claude

LAVAL
Couture, J G R. Guy
Danylewick, Richard
Houle, Jean-Rene
Thibault, Elise

LONGUEUIL
Vo, Thanh Truc

MONTREAL
Abraham, Cherrie Z.
Beaudoin, Nathalie
Blair, Jean-Francois
Cartier, Raymond
Chaput, Miguel
Corriveau, Marc M.
Elkouri, Stephane
Emond, Carl P.
Ghali, Rafik
Ghosn, Pierre B.
MacKenzie, Kent S.
Montreuil, Bernard
Morin, Jean-Francois
Obrand, Daniel
Steinmetz, Oren K.

QUEBEC
Douville, Yvan
Gilbert, Nathalie
Guimond, Marie-France
Labbe, Raymond
Marois, Denis
Rheaume, Pascal

SAINT-JEROME
Chapleau, Denis
Gaffiero, Patricia
Luu, Thanh Phi Y.

SAINT-ROMUALD
Gosselin, Claire

SHERBROOKE
Despatis, Marc-Antoine
Lapie, Veronique

TROIS-RIVIERES
Bourgouin, Daniel
Dufresne, Jose

VERDUN
Karam, Boutros

SASKATCHEWAN

REGINA
Jacob, Sanjay M.
Kopriva, David
McCarville, Donald J.

SASKATOON
Duval, Bruce J.
Kvinlaug, Kylie E.
Spelay, Jodi L.
Ulmer, Brian G.

SECTION 4 — HOSPITALS & HEALTH CENTRES IN CANADA

HOSPITALS & HEALTH CENTRES IN CANADA

If you know the hospital name but not its province or city, refer to the Index of Hospitals immediately following this section. The Index lists all Canadian hospitals alphabetically by name. The numbers in the Index refer you back to page numbers in the Hospitals in Canada section.

ALBERTA

ATHABASCA

ATHABASCA COMMUNITY HEALTH SERVICES
3401 48 Ave
Athabasca AB T9S 1M7
Tel. 780 675-2231
Fax 780 675-3111
www.albertahealthservices.ca

ATHABASCA HEALTHCARE CENTRE
3100 48 Ave
Athabasca AB T9S 1M9
Tel. 780 675-6000
Fax 780 675-7050
www.albertahealthservices.ca

ATIKAMEG

ATIKAMEG HEALTH CENTRE
GD
Atikameg AB T0G 0C0
Tel. 780 767-3941
Fax 780 767-3900
www.informalberta.ca

BANFF

COVENANT HEALTH - BANFF MINERAL SPRINGS HOSPITAL
301 Lynx St
PO BOX 1050 Stn Main
Banff AB T1L 1H7
Tel. 403 762-2222
Fax 403 762-4193
banffmineralspringshospital.ca

BARRHEAD

BARRHEAD COMMUNITY CANCER CENTRE
4815 51st Ave
Barrhead AB T7N 1M1
Tel. 780 305-3304
Fax 780 305-3326
www.albertacancer.ca

BARRHEAD COMMUNITY HEALTH SERVICES
6203 49 St
Barrhead AB T7N 1A1
Tel. 780 674-3408
Fax 780 674-3941

BARRHEAD CONTINUING CARE CENTRE
5336 59 Ave
PO Box 1330
Barrhead AB T7N 1L2
Tel. 780 674-4506
Fax 780 674-3003

BARRHEAD HEALTHCARE CENTRE
4815 51 Ave
Barrhead AB T7N 1M1
Tel. 780 674-2221
Fax 403 674-3541
www.albertahealthservices.ca

BASHAW

BASHAW CARE CENTRE
5308 53rd St
PO Box 449
Bashaw AB T0B 0H0
Tel. 780 372-3731
Fax 780 372-4050
www.albertahealthservices.ca

BASSANO

BASSANO HEALTH CENTRE
608 5th Ave
PO Box 120
Bassano AB T0J 0B0
Tel. 403 641-6100
Fax 403 641-2157
www.albertahealthservices.ca

BEAVERLODGE

BEAVERLODGE MUNICIPAL HOSPITAL
422 10A St
PO Box 480
Beaverlodge AB T0H 0C0
Tel. 780 354-2136
Fax 780 354-8355
www.albertahealthservices.ca

BENTLEY

BENTLEY CARE CENTRE
4834 52nd Ave
PO Box 30
Bentley AB T0C 0J0
Tel. 403 748-4115
Fax 403 748-2727
www.albertahealthservices.ca

BLACK DIAMOND

EDEN VALLEY WELLNESS CENTRE
PO Box 178
Black Diamond AB T0L 0H0
Tel. 403 558-3656
Fax 403 558-2145

OILFIELDS GENERAL HOSPITAL
717 Government Rd
PO Box 1
Black Diamond AB T0L 0H0
Tel. 403 933-2222
Fax 403 933-2031
www.albertahealthservices.ca

BLAIRMORE

CROWSNEST PASS HEALTH CENTRE
2001 107 St
PO Box 510
Blairmore AB T0K 0E0
Tel. 403 562-5011
Fax 403 562-8992
www.albertahealthservices.ca

BONNYVILLE

BONNYVILLE COMMUNITY HEALTH SERVICES
4904 50 Ave
Bonnyville AB T9N 2G4
Tel. 780 826-3381
Fax 780 826-6470

BONNYVILLE HEALTHCARE CENTRE
5001 Lakeshore Dr
PO Box 1008 Stn Main
Bonnyville AB T9N 2J7
Tel. 780 826-3311
Fax 780 826-6526
www.covenanthealth.ca

KEHEWIN HEALTH CENTRE
PO Box 7550
Bonnyville AB T9N 2H8
Tel. 780 826-2913
Fax 780 826-1915
www.informalberta.ca

BOW ISLAND

BOW ISLAND HEALTH CENTRE
938 Centre St
PO Box 3990
Bow Island AB T0K 0G0
Tel. 403 545-3200
Fax 403 545-2281
www.albertahealthservices.ca

BOYLE

BOYLE HEALTHCARE CENTRE
5004 Lake View Rd
PO Box 330
Boyle AB T0A 0M0
Tel. 780 689-3731
Fax 780 689-3951
www.albertahealthservices.ca

BRETON

BRETON HEALTH CARE CENTRE
4919 49 Ave
PO Box 340
Breton AB T0C 0P0
Tel. 780 696-4713
Fax 780 696-4747
www.albertahealthservices.ca

BROOKS

BROOKS HEALTH CENTRE
440 3rd St E
PO Box 300 Stn Main
Brooks AB T1R 1B3
Tel. 403 501-3232
Fax 403 362-6039
www.albertahealthservices.ca

CALGARY

ALBERTA CHILDREN'S HOSPITAL
2888 Shaganappi Trail NW
Calgary AB T3B 6A8
Tel. 403 955-7211
Fax 403 955-7214
www.albertahealthservices.ca

THE ALEX COMMUNITY HEALTH CENTRE
101-1318 Centre St N
Calgary AB T2E 2R7
Tel. 403 266-2622
Fax 403 266-2692
www.thealex.ca

THE ALEX SENIORS HEALTH CENTRE
630 9 Ave SE
Calgary AB T2G 4V9
Tel. 403 920-0011
Fax 403 920-0014
www.thealex.ca

THE ALEX YOUTH HEALTH CENTRE
101-1318 Centre St N
Calgary AB T2E 2R7
Tel. 403 520-6270
Fax 403 266-2692
www.thealex.ca

BETHANY CARE CENTRE
916 18A St NW
Calgary AB T2N 1C6
Tel. 403 284-6000
Fax 403 284-6085
www.bethanycare.com

BONNYVILLE COMMUNITY HEALTH SERVICES MENTAL HEALTH
5201 44 St
Calgary AB T2N 2H3
Tel. 780 826-2404
Fax 780 826-6114
www.albertahealthservices.ca

CAREWEST GLENMORE PARK
6909 14 St SW
Calgary AB T2V 1P8
Tel. 403 258-7650
Fax 403 258-7676
www.albertahealthservices.ca

CAREWEST SARCEE HOSPICE
3504 Sarcee Rd SW
Calgary AB T3E 2L3
Tel. 403 685-6460
Fax 403 685-6465
www.carewest.ca

DR VERNON FANNING EXTENDED CARE CENTRE
722 16 Ave NE
Calgary AB T2E 6V7
Tel. 403 230-6900
Fax 403 230-6902
www.carewest.ca

EAST CALGARY HEALTH CENTRE
4715 8 Ave SE
Calgary AB T2A 3N4
Tel. 403 955-1000
Fax 403 955-1011
www.albertahealthservices.ca

FOOTHILLS MEDICAL CENTRE
1403 29 St NW
Calgary AB T2N 2T9
Tel. 403 944-1110
Fax 403 944-2400
www.calgaryhealthservices.ca

PETER LOUGHEED CENTRE
3500 26th Ave NE
Calgary AB T1Y 6J4
Tel. 403 943-4555
Fax 403 252-8575
www.albertahealthservices.ca

ROCKYVIEW GENERAL HOSPITAL
7007 14 St SW
Calgary AB T2V 1P9
Tel. 403 943-3000
Fax 403 212-1242
www.albertahealthservices.ca

THE SALVATION ARMY AGAPE HOSPICE
1302 8 Ave NW
Calgary AB T2N 1B8
Tel. 403 282-6588
Fax 403 284-1778
www.agapehospice.ca

TOM BAKER CANCER CENTRE
1331 29 St NW
Calgary AB T2N 4N2
Tel. 403 521-3723
Fax 403 521-3723
www.albertacancer.ca

TSUU T'INA HEALTH CENTRE
3700 Anderson Rd SW
Calgary AB T2W 3C4
Tel. 403 251-7575
Fax 403 251-1627

CAMROSE

CAMROSE COMMUNITY CANCER CENTRE
4607 53 St
c/o St Mary's Hospital
Camrose AB T4V 1Y5
Tel. 780 679-2822
Fax 780 679-2821
www.albertacancer.ca

COVENANT HEALTH - ST MARY'S HOSPITAL
4607 53 St
Camrose AB T4V 1Y5
Tel. 780 679-6100
Fax 780 679-6196
www.stmayscamrose.com

CANMORE

BOW VALLEY COMMUNITY CANCER CENTRE
1100 Hospital Place
Canmore AB T1W 1N2
Tel. 403 678-7226
www.albertacancer.ca

CANMORE GENERAL HOSPITAL
1100 Hospital Pl
Canmore AB T1W 1N2
Tel. 403 678-5536
Fax 403 678-9874
www.albertahealthservices.ca

CARDSTON

CARDSTON HOSPITAL
144 Second St W
PO Box 1440
Cardston AB T0K 0K0
Tel. 403 653-4411
Fax 403 653-4399
www.albertahealthservices.ca

CASTOR

CASTOR COMMUNITY HEALTH CENTRE
4909 50 Ave
Box 49
Castor AB T0C 0X0
Tel. 403 882-3404
Fax 403 882-2387
www.albertahealthservices.ca

COVENANT HEALTH - OUR LADY OF THE ROSARY HOSPITAL
5402 67 St
PO Box 329
Castor AB T0C 0X0
Tel. 403 882-3434
Fax 403 882-2751
www.covenanthealth.ca

CHARD

JANVIER HEALTH CENTRE
Gen Delivery
Chard AB T0P 1G0
Tel. 780 559-2375
Fax 780 559-2050
www.albertahealthservices.ca

CHATEH

HAY LAKES NURSING STATION
PO Box 90
Chateh AB T0H 0S0
Tel. 780 321-3971
Fax 780 321-3520

CLARESHOLM

CALGARY ZONE CLARESHOLM PUBLIC HEALTH
5221 2 St W
Box 1391
Claresholm AB T0L 0T0
Tel. 403 625-4061
Fax 403 625-4062

CLARESHOLM CENTRE FOR MENTAL HEALTH AND ADDICTIONS
139 43 Ave W
PO Box 490
Claresholm AB T0L 0T0
Tel. 403 682-3500
Fax 403 625-4318
www.claresholmcentre.com

CLARESHOLM GENERAL HOSPITAL
221 43 Ave W
PO Box 610
Claresholm AB T0L 0T0
Tel. 403 682-3700
Fax 403 682-3789
www.albertahealthservices.ca

WILLOW CREEK CONTINUING CARE CENTRE
4221 8 St W
PO Box 700
Claresholm AB T0L 0T0
Tel. 403 625-3361
Fax 403 625-3822
www.albertahealthservices.ca

COALDALE

COALDALE HEALTH CENTRE
2100 11 St
Coaldale AB T1M 1L2
Tel. 403 345-3075
Fax 403 345-2681
www.albertahealthservices.ca

COLD LAKE

COLD LAKE COMMUNITY HEALTH SERVICES
4720 55 St
Cold Lake AB T9M 1V8
Tel. 780 594-4404
Fax 780 594-2404

COLD LAKE COMMUNITY HEALTH SERVICES MENTAL HEALTH
208-314 25 St
Cold Lake AB T9M 1G6
Tel. 780 639-4922
Fax 780 639-4990

COLD LAKE FIRST NATION HEALTH CENTRE
PO Box 8100
Cold Lake AB T9M 1N1
Tel. 780 594-2473
Fax 780 594-0084

COLD LAKE HEALTHCARE CENTRE
314 25 St
Cold Lake AB T9M 1G6
Tel. 780 639-3322
Fax 780 639-2255
www.albertahealthservices.ca

CONSORT

CONSORT COMMUNITY HEALTH CENTRE
5410 52nd Ave
Consort AB T0C 1B0
Tel. 403 577-3770
Fax 403 577-2235
www.albertahealthservices.ca

CONSORT HOSPITAL AND CARE CENTRE
5402 52nd Ave
PO Box 310
Consort AB T0C 1B0
Tel. 403 577-3555
Fax 403 577-3950
www.albertahealthservices.ca

CORONATION

CORONATION COMMUNITY HEALTH CENTRE
4909 Royal St
Coronation AB T0C 1C0
Tel. 403 578-3200
Fax 403 578-2702
www.albertahealthservices.ca

CORONATION HOSPITAL & CARE CENTRE
PO Box 500
Coronation AB T0C 1C0
Tel. 403 578-3803
Fax 403 578-3918
www.albertahealthservices.ca

DAYSLAND

DAYSLAND HEALTH CENTRE
5920 51 Ave
PO Box 27
Daysland AB T0B 1A0
Tel. 780 374-3746
Fax 780 374-2111
www.albertahealthservices.ca

DEVON

DEVON GENERAL HOSPITAL
101 Erie St S
Devon AB T9G 1A6
Tel. 780 342-7000
Fax 780 342-7125
www.albertahealthservices.ca

DIDSBURY

DIDSBURY DISTRICT HEALTH SERVICES
1210 20th Ave
PO Box 130
Didsbury AB T0M 0W0
Tel. 403 335-9393
Fax 403 335-4816
www.albertahealthservices.ca

DRAYTON VALLEY

CENTRAL ZONE DRAYTON VALLEY COMMUNITY HEALTH CENTRE
4110 50 Ave
Drayton Valley AB T7A 0B3
Tel. 780 542-4415
Fax 780 621-4998
www.albertahealthservices.ca

DRAYTON VALLEY HOSPITAL & CARE CENTRE
4550 Madsen Ave
Drayton Valley AB T7A 1N8
Tel. 780 542-5321
Fax 780 621-4966
www.albertahealthservices.ca

DRAYTON VALLEY MENTAL HEALTH CENTRE
4110 50 Ave
Drayton Valley AB T7A 0B3
Tel. 780 542-3140
Fax 780 542-4461
www.albertahealthservices.ca

DRIFTPILE

DRIFTPILE HEALTH CENTRE
PO Box 120
Driftpile AB T0G 0V0
Tel. 780 355-3931
Fax 780 355-2055
www.driftpilecreenation.com

DRUMHELLER

DRUMHELLER COMMUNITY CANCER CENTRE
351 9 St NW
SS 1 Drumheller Health Centre
Drumheller AB T0J 0Y1
Tel. 403 823-6500
Fax 403 820-7234
www.albertacancer.ca

DRUMHELLER HEALTH CENTRE
351 9 St NW
Drumheller AB T0J 0Y1
Tel. 403 823-6500
Fax 403 823-5076
www.albertahealthservices.ca

ECKVILLE

ECKVILLE COMMUNITY HEALTH CENTRE
5120 51st Ave W
PO Box 150
Eckville AB T0M 0X0
Tel. 403 746-2201
Fax 403 746-2185
www.albertahealthservices.ca

EDMONTON

ALBERTA HOSPITAL EDMONTON
17480 Fort Rd
PO Box 307 Stn Main
Edmonton AB T5J 2J7
Tel. 780 472-5555
Fax 780 472-5508
www.albertahealthservices.ca

ALLEN GRAY CONTINUING CARE CENTRE
5005 28 Ave NW
Edmonton AB T6L 7G1
Tel. 780 469-2371
Fax 780 465-2073
www.allengray.ab.ca

BOYLE MCCAULEY HEALTH CENTRE
10628 96 St NW
Edmonton AB T5H 2J2
Tel. 780 422-7333
Fax 780 422-7343
www.albertahealthservices.ca/

CAPITAL CARE - DICKINSFIELD
14225 94 St NW
Edmonton AB T5E 6C6
Tel. 780 371-6500
Fax 780 371-6583
www.capitalcare.net

CAPITAL CARE - GRANDVIEW
6215 124 St NW
Edmonton AB T6H 3V1
Tel. 780 496-7100
Fax 780 496-7150
www.capitalcare.net

CAPITAL CARE - LYNWOOD
8740 165th St NW
Edmonton AB T5R 2R8
Tel. 780 341-2300
Fax 780 341-2363
www.capitalcare.net

CAPITAL CARE - NORWOOD
10410 111 Ave NW
Edmonton AB T5G 3A2
Tel. 780 496-3200
Fax 780 474-9806
www.capitalcare.net

COMMUNITY NURSING STATION
10014 105A Ave
Edmonton AB T5H 0M6
Tel. 780 423-3434
Fax 780 423-3436
www.bmhc.net

COVENANT HEALTH - EDMONTON GENERAL CONTINUING CARE CENTRE
11111 Jasper Ave NW
Edmonton AB T5K 0L4
Tel. 780 342-8000
Fax 780 342-8477
www.covenanthealth.ca

COVENANT HEALTH - GREY NUNS COMMUNITY HOSPITAL
1100 Youville Drive West NW
Edmonton AB T6L 5X8
Tel. 780 735-7000
Fax 780 735-7368
www.albertahealthservices.ca

COVENANT HEALTH - MISERICORDIA COMMUNITY HOSPITAL
16940 87 Ave NW
Edmonton AB T5R 4H5
Tel. 780 735-2000
Fax 780 735-2774
www.covenanthealth.ca

COVENANT HEALTH - ST. JOSEPH'S AUXILLIARY HOSPITAL
10707 29 Ave NW
Edmonton AB T6J 6W1
Tel. 780 430-9110
Fax 780 430-9777
www.stjosephs.ab.ca

CROSS CANCER INSTITUTE
11560 University Ave NW
Edmonton AB T6G 1Z2
Tel. 780 432-8771
Fax 780 432-8411
www.albertacancer.ca

GLENROSE REHABILITATION HOSPITAL
10230 111 Ave NW
Edmonton AB T5G 0B7
Tel. 780 735-7999
Fax 780 735-7976
www.albertahealthservices.ca

THE GOOD SAMARITAN SOCIETY
8861 75 St NW
Edmonton AB T6C 4G8
Tel. 780 431-3600
Fax 780 431-3699
www.gss.org

LOIS HOLE HOSPITAL FOR WOMEN
10240 Kingsway NW
Edmonton AB T5H 3V9
Tel. 780 735-4111
www.albertahealthservices.ca

MAZANKOWSKI ALBERTA HEART INSTITUTE
8440 112 St
Edmonton AB T6G 2B7
Tel. 780 407-8583
Fax 780 407-7418
www.albertaheartinstitute.ca

MOTHER ROSALIE HEALTH SERVICES CENTRE
16930 87 Ave
Edmonton AB T5R 4H5
Tel. 780 735-2000
Fax 780 735-2774
www.albertahealthservices.ca

NORTHEAST COMMUNITY HEALTH CENTRE
14007 50 St
Edmonton AB T5A 5E4
Tel. 780 342-4000
Fax 780 472-5188
www.albertahealthservices.ca

ROYAL ALEXANDRA HOSPITAL
10240 Kingsway NW
Edmonton AB T5H 3V9
Tel. 780 491-5116
Fax 780 735-4777
www.albertahealthservices.ca

ST. MARGUERITE'S HEALTH SERVICES CENTRE
1090 Youville Dr NW
Edmonton AB T6L 5X8
Tel. 780 735-7268
www.albertahealthservices.ca

STOLLERY CHILDREN'S HOSPITAL
8440 112 St NW
Edmonton AB T6G 2B7
Tel. 780 407-8822
Fax 780 407-3301
www.capitalhealth.ca

UNIVERSITY OF ALBERTA HOSPITAL
8440 112 St NW
Edmonton AB T6G 2B7
Tel. 780 407-8822
Fax 780 407-7418
www.albertahealthservices.ca

WOMEN'S CENTRE FOR HEALTH
9611 101A Ave
Edmonton AB T5H 0C8
Tel. 780 423-4209
Fax 780 423-4421
www.albertahealthservices.ca

EDSON

EDSON COMMUNITY HEALTH SERVICES
5028 3rd Ave
Edson AB T7E 1X4
Tel. 780 723-4421
Fax 780 723-6299

EDSON COMMUNITY HEALTH SERVICES MENTAL HEALTH
111 54 St
Edson AB T7E 1T2
Tel. 780 723-8294
Fax 780 723-8297
www.albertahealthservices.ca

EDSON HEALTHCARE CENTRE
4716 5 Ave SS 3
Edson AB T7E 1S8
Tel. 780 723-3331
Fax 403 723-2135
www.albertahealthservices.ca

ELK POINT

ELK POINT HEALTHCARE CENTRE
5310 50 Ave
PO Box 3
Elk Point AB T0A 1A0
Tel. 780 724-3847
Fax 780 724-3085
www.albertahealthservices.ca

ELNORA

ELNORA COMMUNITY HEALTH CENTRE
PO BOX 659
Elnora AB T0M 0Y0
Tel. 403 773-3636
Fax 403 773-3949
www.albertahealthservices.ca

ENILDA

SUCKER CREEK HEALTH CENTRE
PO Box 65
Enilda AB T0G 0W0
Tel. 780 523-4390
Fax 780 523-5934
www.informalberta.ca

FAIRVIEW

FAIRVIEW HEALTH COMPLEX
10628 110 St
PO Box 2201
Fairview AB T0H 1L0
Tel. 780 835-6100
Fax 780 835-5789
www.albertahealthservices.ca

FORT CHIPEWYAN

NUNEE HEALTH BOARD SOCIETY
PO Box 476
Fort Chipewyan AB T0P 1B0
Tel. 780 697-3875
Fax 780 697-3031
www.nunee.org

FORT MACKAY

FORT MACKAY HEALTH CENTRE
Gen Del
Fort MacKay AB T0P 1C0
Tel. 780 828-4229
Fax 780 828-4132

FORT MACLEOD

FORT MACLEOD HEALTH CENTRE
744 26th St
PO Box 520
Fort Macleod AB T0L 0Z0
Tel. 403 553-5311
Fax 403 553-4567
www.albertahealthservices.ca

FORT MCMURRAY

NORTH ZONE FORT MCMURRAY PUBLIC HEALTH CENTRE
113 Thickwood Blvd
Fort McMurray AB T9H 5E5
Tel. 780 793-7353
www.albertahealthservices.ca

NORTHERN LIGHTS REGIONAL HEALTH CENTRE
7 Hospital St
Fort McMurray AB T9H 1P2
Tel. 780 791-6161
Fax 780 791-6019
www.albertahealthservices.ca

FORT SASKATCHEWAN

FORT SASKATCHEWAN HEALTH CENTRE
9430 95 St
Fort Saskatchewan AB T8L 1R8
Tel. 780 998-2256
Fax 780 992-1532
www.albertahealthservices.ca

FORT VERMILION

NORTH TALLCREE HEALTH CENTRE
PO Box 100
Fort Vermilion AB T0H 1N0
Tel. 780 927-3956
Fax 780 927-4312

ST THERESA GENERAL HOSPITAL
4506 46 Ave
PO Box 128
Fort Vermilion AB T0H 1N0
Tel. 780 927-3761
Fax 780 927-4271
www.albertahealthservices.ca

SOUTH TALLCREE HEALTH CENTRE
PO Box 100
Fort Vermilion AB T0H 1N0
Tel. 780 927-4605
Fax 780 927-2391

FOX CREEK

FOX CREEK HEALTH CARE CENTRE
600 3rd St
PO Box 990
Fox Creek AB T0H 1P0
Tel. 780 622-3545
Fax 780 622-3474
www.albertahealthservices.ca

FOX LAKE

FOX LAKE NURSING STATION
GD
PO Box 330
Fox Lake AB T0H 1R0
Tel. 780 659-3730
Fax 780 659-3960
www.albertahealthservices.ca

FROG LAKE

MORNING SKY HEALTH & WELLNESS SOCIETY
Gen Del
Frog Lake AB T0A 1M0
Tel. 780 943-3777
Fax 780 943-2193

GALAHAD

GALAHAD CARE CENTRE
102 Lady Helen Ave
PO Box 88
Galahad AB T0B 1R0
Tel. 780 583-3788
Fax 780 583-2105
www.albertahealthservices.ca

GLENDON

GLENDON COMMUNITY HEALTH CLINIC
Railway Ave-2nd St E
PO Box 570
Glendon AB T0A 1P0
Tel. 780 635-3861
Fax 780 635-4213
www.albertahealthservices.ca

GLENEVIS

ALEXIS HEALTH CENTRE
PO Box 39
Glenevis AB T0E 0X0
Tel. 780 967-1091
Fax 780 967-1097
www.informalberta.ca

GOODFISH LAKE

GOODFISH LAKE HEALTH CENTRE
PO Box 272
Goodfish Lake AB T0A 1R0
Tel. 780 636-3638
Fax 780 636-3457
www.informalberta.ca

GRANDE CACHE

GRANDE CACHE COMMUNITY HEALTH COMPLEX
10200 Shand Ave
PO Box 629
Grande Cache AB T0E 0Y0
Tel. 780 827-3701
Fax 780 827-2859
www.albertahealthservices.ca

GRANDE PRAIRIE

GRANDE PRAIRIE CANCER CENTRE - QUEEN ELIZABETH II HOSPITAL
10409 98 St
Grande Prairie AB T8V 2E8
Tel. 780 538-7588
Fax 780 532-9120
www.albertacancer.ca

QUEEN ELIZABETH II HOSPITAL
10409 98 St
Grande Prairie AB T8V 2E8
Tel. 780 538-7100
Fax 780 538-7500
www.albertahealthservices.ca

GRIMSHAW

GRIMSHAW/BERWYN AND DISTRICT COMMUNITY HEALTH CENTRE
5621 Wilcox Rd
PO Box 648
Grimshaw AB T0H 1W0
Tel. 780 332-6500
Fax 780 332-1177
www.albertahealthservices.ca

GROUARD

KAPAWE'NO HEALTH CENTRE
Box 10
Grouard AB T0G 1C0
Tel. 780 751-2284
Fax 780 751-2363
www.informalberta.ca

HANNA

HANNA HEALTH CENTRE
904 Centre St N
PO Box 730
Hanna AB T0J 1P0
Tel. 403 854-3331
Fax 403 854-3253
www.albertahealthservices.ca

HARDISTY

HARDISTY HEALTH CENTRE
4531 47 Ave
PO Box 269
Hardisty AB T0B 1V0
Tel. 780 888-3742
Fax 780 888-2427
www.albertahealthservices.ca

HIGH LEVEL

BEAVER FIRST NATION HEALTH CENTRE
Bag 270
High Level AB T0H 1Z0
Tel. 780 927-4059
Fax 780 927-4064

GARDEN RIVER HEALTH CENTRE
PO Bag 5000
Fort Vermillion AB T0H 1Z0
Tel. 780 659-3636
Fax 780 659-2171
www.informalberta.ca

JEAN D'OR PRAIRIE HEALTH CENTRE
PO Box 1100
High Level AB T0H 1Z0
Tel. 780 759-3872
Fax 780 759-3770
www.informalberta.ca

MEANDER RIVER HEALTH STATION
PO Box 1889
High Level AB T0H 1Z0
Tel. 780 535-2272
Fax 780 535-6641
www.informalberta.ca

NORTHWEST HEALTH CENTRE
11202 100 Ave
High Level AB T0H 1Z0
Tel. 780 841-3200
Fax 780 926-7373
www.albertahealthservices.ca

HIGH PRAIRIE

HIGH PRAIRIE HEALTH COMPLEX
4620 53rd Ave
PO Box 1
High Prairie AB T0G 1E0
Tel. 780 523-6440
Fax 780 523-6442
www.albertahealthservices.ca

HIGH RIVER

HEADWATERS COMMUNITY CANCER CENTRE
560 9 Ave SW
High River AB T1V 1B3
Tel. 403 652-0139
Fax 403 652-0165
www.calgaryhealthregion.ca

HIGH RIVER GENERAL HOSPITAL
560 9 Ave SW
High River AB T1V 1B3
Tel. 403 652-2200
Fax 403 652-0199
www.albertahealthservices.ca

HINTON

GOOD SAMARITAN MOUNTAIN VIEW CENTRE
1280A Switzer Dr
Hinton AB T7V 1T5
Tel. 780 865-4926
Fax 780 865-4098
www.albertahealthservices.ca

HINTON COMMUNITY CANCER CENTRE
General Delivery
Hinton AB T7V 1V2
Tel. 780 865-3333
Fax 780 817-5034
www.albertacancer.ca

HINTON HEALTHCARE CENTRE
1280 Switzer Dr
Hinton AB T7V 1V2
Tel. 780 865-3333
Fax 780 865-1099
www.albertahealthservices.ca

HOBBEMA

HOBBEMA HEALTH CENTRE
Box 189
Hobbema AB T0C 1N0
Tel. 780 585-3982
Fax 780 585-2203
www.informalberta.ca

INNISFAIL

INNISFAIL HEALTH CENTRE
5023 42 St
Innisfail AB T4G 1A9
Tel. 403 227-7800
Fax 403 227-7801
www.albertahealthservices.ca

ISLAY

ISLAY ASSISTED LIVING
5016 53rd St
PO Box 55
Islay AB T0B 2J0
Tel. 780 744-3795
Fax 780 744-3922
www.albertahealthservices.ca

JASPER

JASPER COMMUNITY HEALTH SERVICES
300 Miette Ave
PO Box 1740
Jasper AB T0E 1E0
Tel. 780 852-4759
Fax 780 852-4752
www.albertahealthservices.ca

SETON JASPER HEALTHCARE CENTRE
518 Robson St
PO Box 310
Jasper AB T0E 1E0
Tel. 780 852-3344
Fax 780 852-3413
www.albertahealthservices.ca

KILLAM

COVENANT HEALTH - KILLAM HEALTH CENTRE
5203 49 Ave
PO Box 40
Killam AB T0B 2L0
Tel. 780 385-3741
Fax 780 385-3901
www.covenanthealth.ca

KINUSO

SWAN RIVER HEALTH STATION
PO Box 71
Kinuso AB T0G 1K0
Tel. 780 775-3544
Fax 780 775-2002
www.informalberta.ca

LAC LA BICHE

BEAVER LAKE HEALTH CENTRE
PO Box 1950
Lac La Biche AB T0A 2C0
Tel. 780 623-4276
Fax 780 623-4569
www.informalberta.ca

HEART LAKE HEALTH CENTRE
PO Box 447
Lac La Biche AB T0A 2C0
Tel. 780 623-7477
Fax 780 623-8155

LAC LA BICHE COMMUNITY HEALTH SERVICES
9503 Beaverhill Rd
PO Box 869
Lac La Biche AB T0A 2C0
Tel. 780 623-4471
Fax 780 623-2615
www.albertahealthservices.ca

LAC LA BICHE HEALTHCARE CENTRE - WILLIAM J. CADZOW BUILDING
9100 93 St
PO Box 507
Lac La Biche AB T0A 2C0
Tel. 780 623-4404
Fax 780 623-5904
www.albertahealthservices.ca

LACOMBE

LACOMBE COMMUNITY HEALTH CENTRE
5010 51 St
Lacombe AB T4L 1W2
Tel. 403 782-3218
Fax 403 782-2866
www.albertahealthservices.ca

LACOMBE HOSPITAL & CARE CENTRE
5430 47 Ave
Lacombe AB T4L 1G8
Tel. 403 782-3336
Fax 403 782-2818
www.albertahealthservices.ca

LACOMBE MENTAL HEALTH CENTRE
5033 52 St
Suite 12
Lacombe AB T4L 2A6
Tel. 403 782-3413
Fax 403 782-2866
www.albertahealthservices.ca

LAMONT

LAMONT HEALTH CARE CENTRE
5216 53rd St
PO Box 10
Lamont AB T0B 2R0
Tel. 780 895-2211
Fax 780 895-7305
lamonthealthcarecentre.com

LEDUC

LEDUC COMMUNITY HOSPITAL
4210 48 St
Leduc AB T9E 5Z3
Tel. 780 986-7711
Fax 780 980-4490
www.albertahealthservices.ca

LETHBRIDGE

CHINOOK REGIONAL HOSPITAL
960 19th St S
Lethbridge AB T1J 1W5
Tel. 403 388-6111
Fax 403 388-6011
www.albertahealthservices.ca

COVENANT HEALTH - ST MICHAEL'S HEALTH CENTRE
1400 9 Ave S
Lethbridge AB T1J 4V5
Tel. 403 382-6400
Fax 403 382-6413
www.covenanthealth.ca

JACK ADY CANCER CENTRE
960 19 St S
Lethbridge AB T1J 1W5
Tel. 403 329-0633
www.albertacancer.ca

LETHBRIDGE CANCER CENTRE
960 19 St S
Lethbridge AB T1J 1W5
Tel. 403 329-0633
Fax 403 320-0508
www.insite.cancerboard.ab.ca

LLOYDMINSTER

DR COOKE EXTENDED CARE CENTRE
3915 56 Ave
Lloydminster AB T9V 1N9
Tel. 780 871-7900
Fax 780 875-3505
www.albertahealthservices.ca

MAGRATH

MAGRATH COMMUNITY HEALTH
37 East 2nd Ave N
PO Box 550
Magrath AB T0K 1J0
Tel. 403 758-4422
Fax 403 388-3332
www.albertahealthservices.ca

MANNING

MANNING COMMUNITY HEALTH CENTRE
600 2nd St NE
PO Box 1260
Manning AB T0H 2M0
Tel. 780 836-3391
Fax 780 836-7352
www.albertahealthservices.ca

MANNVILLE

MANNVILLE CARE CENTRE
5007 46 St
PO Box 1000
Mannville AB T0B 2W0
Tel. 780 763-3621
Fax 780 763-3678
www.albertahealthservices.ca

MAYERTHORPE

MAYERTHORPE HEALTH CARE CENTRE
4706 54th Street
Mayerthorpe AB T0E 1N0
Tel. 780 786-2261
Fax 780 786-2023
www.albertahealthservices.ca

MCLENNAN

SACRED HEART COMMUNITY HEALTH CENTRE
350 3rd Ave NW
PO BOX 2000
McLennan AB T0H 2L0
Tel. 780 324-3730
Fax 780 324-2267
www.albertahealthservices.ca

MEDICINE HAT

MARGERY E. YUILL CANCER CENTRE
666 5 St SW
Medicine Hat AB T1A 4H6
Tel. 403 529-8817
Fax 403 529-8007
www.albertahealthservices.ca

MEDICINE HAT REGIONAL HOSPITAL
666 5 St SW
Medicine Hat AB T1A 4H6
Tel. 403 529-8000
Fax 403 529-8950
www.albertahealthservices.ca

MILK RIVER

MILK RIVER HEALTH CENTRE
517 Centre Ave E
PO Box 90
Milk River AB T0K 1M0
Tel. 403 647-2337
Fax 403 647-2197
www.albertahealthservices.ca

MORINVILLE

ALEXANDER HEALTH CENTRE
PO Box 3570
Morinville AB T8R 1S3
Tel. 780 939-4787
Fax 780 939-2951
www.informalberta.ca

MUNDARE

COVENANT HEALTH - MARY IMMACULATE HOSPITAL
165018-534 Twp Rd
Mundare AB T0B 3H0
Tel. 780 764-3730
Fax 780 764-3039
www.covenanthealth.ca

NANTON

CALGARY ZONE NANTON COMMUNITY HEALTH CENTRE
2218 20th St
PO Box 940
Nanton AB T0L 1R0
Tel. 403 646-2218
Fax 403 646-3046

NORDEGG

BIGHORN HEALTH CENTRE
Box 1617
Nordegg AB T0M 2H0
Tel. 403 721-2264
Fax 403 721-2170
www.informalberta.ca

OLDS

OLDS COMMUNITY HEALTH CENTRE
103-5030 50 St
Olds AB T4H 1S1
Tel. 403 556-8441
Fax 403 556-6842
www.albertahealthservices.ca

OLDS HOSPITAL & CARE CENTRE
3901 57th Ave
Olds AB T4H 1T4
Tel. 403 556-3381
Fax 403 556-2199
www.albertahealthservices.ca

OLDS MENTAL HEALTH CENTRE
5025 50 St
Olds AB T4H 1R9
Tel. 403 507-8174
Fax 403 556-1584
www.albertahealthservices.ca

ONOWAY

ONOWAY COMMUNITY HEALTH SERVICES
4919 Lac Ste Anne Trail
Onoway AB T0E 1V0
Tel. 780 967-4440
Fax 780 967-4433
www9.albertahealthservices.ca

ONOWAY COMMUNITY HEALTH SERVICES MENTAL HEALTH
5115 Lac Ste Anne Trail
Onoway AB T0E 1V0
Tel. 780 967-9117
Fax 780 967-3547
www9.albertahealthservices.ca

OYEN

BIG COUNTRY HOSPITAL
312 3rd Ave E
PO Box 150
Oyen AB T0J 2J0
Tel. 403 664-4300
Fax 403 664-4325
www.albertahealthservices.ca

PEACE RIVER

PEACE RIVER COMMUNITY HEALTH CENTRE
10101 68 St
PO Box 400 Stn Main
Peace River AB T8S 1T6
Tel. 780 624-7500
Fax 780 618-3472
www.albertahealthservices.ca

PEERLESS LAKE

PEERLESS LAKE COMMUNITY HEALTH SERVICES
PO Box 90
Peerless Lake AB T0G 2W0
Tel. 780 869-3930
Fax 780 869-2053
www.albertahealthservices.ca

PICTURE BUTTE

PIYAMI HEALTH CENTRE
301A Cowan Ave
PO Box 430
Picture Butte AB T0K 1V0
Tel. 403 388-6751
Fax 403 732-5062
www.albertahealthservices.ca

PINCHER CREEK

PINCHER CREEK HEALTH CENTRE
1222 Bev McLaughlin Dr
PO Box 968
Pincher Creek AB T0K 1W0
Tel. 403 627-1234
Fax 403 627-5275
www.albertahealthservices.ca

PONOKA

CENTENNIAL CENTRE FOR MENTAL HEALTH & BRAIN INJURY
53 2 Km at Hwy S
PO Box 1000 Stn Main
Ponoka AB T4J 1R8
Tel. 403 783-7600
Fax 403 783-7774
www.albertahealthservices.ca

PONOKA COMMUNITY HEALTH CENTRE
5900 Hwy 2A
Ponoka AB T4J 1P5
Tel. 403 783-4491
Fax 403 783-3825
www.albertahealthservices.ca

PONOKA HOSPITAL & CARE CENTRE
5800 57 Ave
Ponoka AB T4J 1P1
Tel. 403 783-3341
Fax 403 783-6907
www.albertahealthservices.ca

PONOKA MENTAL HEALTH CENTRE
223-5110 49 Ave
Ponoka AB T4J 1R6
Tel. 403 783-7903
Fax 403 783-7926
www.albertahealthservices.ca

PROVOST

PROVOST HEALTH CENTRE
5002 54 Ave
PO Box 270
Provost AB T0B 3S0
Tel. 780 753-2291
Fax 780 753-6132
www.albertahealthservices.ca

RADWAY

RADWAY CONTINUING CARE CENTRE
5002 52nd St
PO Box 70
Radway AB T0A 2V0
Tel. 780 736-3740
Fax 780 736-2353
www.albertahealthservices.ca

RAYMOND

RAYMOND HEALTH CENTRE
150N 4th St E
PO Box 599
Raymond AB T0K 2S0
Tel. 403 752-4561
Fax 403 752-3554
www.albertahealthservices.ca

SENIORS MENTAL HEALTH
328 Broadway S
PO Box 260
Raymond AB T0K 2S0
Tel. 403 752-3316 Ext. 301
Fax 403 752-3933
www.albertahealthservices.ca

RED DEER

CENTRAL ALBERTA CANCER CENTRE
3942 50A Ave
PO Box 5030 Stn Postal
Red Deer AB T4N 6R2
Tel. 403 343-4526
Fax 403 346-1160
www.albertacancer.ca

RED DEER 49TH ST. COMMUNITY HEALTH CENTRE
4755 49th St
Red Deer AB T4N 1T6
Tel. 403 314-5225
Fax 403 314-5230
www.albertahealthservices.ca

RED DEER BREMNER AVE COMMUNITY HEALTH CENTRE
2845 Bremner Ave
Red Deer AB T4R 1S2
Tel. 403 341-2100
Fax 403 346-2610
www.albertahealthservices.ca

RED DEER JOHNSTONE CROSSING COMMUNITY HEALTH CENTRE
300 Jordan Parkway
Red Deer AB T4P 0G8
Tel. 403 356-6300
Fax 403 356-6440
www.albertahealthservices.ca

RED DEER REGIONAL HOSPITAL CENTRE
3942 50A Ave
Red Deer AB T4N 4E7
Tel. 403 343-4422
Fax 403 343-4866
www.albertahealthservices.ca

RED DEER COUNTY

SYLVAN LAKE COMMUNITY HEALTH CENTRE
4602 49 Ave
Sylvan Lake AB T4S 1M7
Tel. 403 887-2241
Fax 403 887-2610
www.albertahealthservices.ca

RED EARTH CREEK

LOON RIVER FIRST NATION HEALTH CENTRE
Box 329
Red Earth Creek AB T0G 1X0
Tel. 780 649-3490
Fax 780 649-2214
www.loonriver.net

RED EARTH CREEK COMMUNITY HEALTH SERVICES
PO Box 109
Red Earth Creek AB T0G 1X0
Tel. 780 649-2242
Fax 780 649-2029
www.albertahealthservices.ca

REDWATER

REDWATER HEALTH CENTRE
4812 58 Street
PO Box 39
Redwater AB T0A 2W0
Tel. 780 942-3932
Fax 780 942-2373
www.albertahealthservices.ca

RIMBEY

RIMBEY COMMUNITY HEALTH CENTRE
4709 51 Ave
Rimbey AB T0C 2J0
Tel. 403 843-2288
Fax 403 843-3050
www.albertahealthservices.ca

RIMBEY HOSPITAL & CARE CENTRE
5228 50th Ave
PO Box 440
Rimbey AB T0C 2J0
Tel. 403 843-2271
Fax 403 843-2506
www.albertahealthservices.ca

ROCKY MOUNTAIN HOUSE

O'CHIESE HEALTH CENTRE
PO Box 2348
Rocky-Mtn-House AB T4T 1B7
Tel. 403 989-3900
Fax 403 989-3905
www.informalberta.ca

ROCKY MOUNTAIN HOUSE HEALTH CENTRE
5016 52 Ave
Rocky-Mtn-Hse AB T4T 1T2
Tel. 403 845-3347
Fax 403 845-7030
www.albertahealthservices.ca

SADDLE LAKE

SADDLE LAKE HEALTH AND WELLNESS CENTRE
5051 11th Ave
PO Box 160
Saddle Lake AB T0A 3T0
Tel. 780 726-3930
Fax 780 726-2776
www.saddlelakehealth.com

ST. ALBERT

STURGEON COMMUNITY HOSPITAL
201 Boudreau Rd
St. Albert AB T8N 6C4
Tel. 780 418-8200
Fax 780 418-8262
www.albertahealthservices.ca

ST. PAUL

ST. PAUL COMMUNITY HEALTH SERVICES
5610 50 Ave
St Paul AB T0A 3A1
Tel. 780 645-3396
Fax 780 645-6609
www.albertahealthservices.ca

ST. PAUL (ST. THERESE) HEALTHCARE CENTRE
4713 48th Ave
St Paul AB T0A 3A3
Tel. 780 645-3331
Fax 780 645-1702
www.albertahealthservices.ca

SHERWOOD PARK

CAPITAL CARE - STRATHCONA
12 Brower Dr
Sherwood Park AB T8H 1V3
Tel. 780 467-3366
Fax 780 467-4095
www.capitalcare.net

HEALTH FIRST STRATHCONA
140-80 Chippewa Rd
Athabasca Professional Ctre
Sherwood Park AB T8A 4W6
Tel. 780 449-5380
Fax 403 467-9829
www.albertahealthservices.ca

SLAVE LAKE

SLAVE LAKE HEALTH CARE CENTRE
309 6th St NE
SS 2
Slave Lake AB T0G 2A2
Tel. 780 805-3500
Fax 780 805-3574
www.albertahealthservices.ca

SMOKY LAKE

GEORGE MCDOUGALL - SMOKY LAKE HEALTHCARE CENTRE
4212 55 Ave
PO Box 340
Smoky Lake AB T0A 3C0
Tel. 780 656-3034
Fax 780 656-5010
www.albertahealthservices.ca

SMOKY LAKE COMMUNITY HEALTH SERVICES
4212 55 Ave
PO Box 127
Smoky Lake AB T0A 3C0
Tel. 780 656-3595
Fax 780 656-2242
www.albertahealthservices.ca

SPIRIT RIVER

CENTRAL PEACE HEALTH COMPLEX
5010 45 Ave
PO Box 339
Spirit River AB T0H 3G0
Tel. 780 864-3993
Fax 780 864-3495
www.albertahealthservices.ca

SPRUCE GROVE

ENOCH HEALTH CENTRE
PO Box 60
Enoch AB T7X 3Y3
Tel. 780 470-5440
Fax 780 470-0683
ww.enochecdev.ca

STAND OFF

LEVERN HEALTH STATION
PO Box 148
Stand Off AB T0L 1Y0
Tel. 403 737-3933
Fax 403 737-2377

STETTLER

STETTLER COMMUNITY HEALTH CENTRE
5911 50 Ave
Box 550
Stettler AB T0C 2L0
Tel. 403 742-3326
Fax 403 742-1353
www.albertahealthservices.ca

STETTLER HOSPITAL AND CARE CENTRE
5912 47 Ave
PO Box 500
Stettler AB T0C 2L0
Tel. 403 742-7400
Fax 403 742-1244
www.albertahealthservices.ca

STONY PLAIN

WESTVIEW HEALTH CENTRE
4405 South Park Dr
Stony Plain AB T7Z 2M7
Tel. 780 968-3600
Fax 780 963-7192
www.albertahealthservices.ca

STRATHMORE

STRATHMORE DISTRICT HEALTH SERVICES
200 Brent Blvd
Strathmore AB T1P 1J9
Tel. 403 361-7000
Fax 403 361-7048
www.albertahealthservices.ca

SUNDRE

SUNDRE COMMUNITY HEALTH CENTRE
212-6 Ave NE
Box 101
Sundre AB T0M 1X0
Tel. 403 638-4063
Fax 403 638-4460
www.albertahealthservices.ca

SUNDRE HOSPITAL & CARE CENTRE
709 1st St NE
PO Box 3
Sundre AB T0M 1X0
Tel. 403 638-3033
Fax 403 638-4971
www.albertahealthservices.ca

SWAN HILLS

SWAN HILLS HEALTHCARE CENTRE
29 Freeman Dr
PO Box 266
Swan Hills AB T0G 2C0
Tel. 780 333-7000
Fax 780 333-7009
www.albertahealthservices.ca

TABER

TABER HEALTH CENTRE
4326 50 Ave
Taber AB T1G 1N9
Tel. 403 223-7211
Fax 403 223-1703
www.albertahealthservices.ca

THORHILD

THORHILD COMMUNITY HEALTH SERVICES
302 2nd Ave
PO Box 366
Thorhild AB T0A 3J0
Tel. 780 398-3879
Fax 780 398-2671
www.albertahealthservices.ca

THREE HILLS

THREE HILLS HEALTH CENTRE
1504 2nd St N
PO Box 340
Three Hills AB T0M 2A0
Tel. 403 443-2444
Fax 403 443-5565
www.albertahealthservices.ca

THREE HILLS MENTAL HEALTH CENTRE
160-3 Ave S
Box 1717
Three Hills AB T0M 2A0
Tel. 403 443-8532
Fax 403 443-8541
www.albertahealthservices.ca

TOFIELD

TOFIELD HEALTH CENTRE
5543 44 St
PO BOX 1200
Tofield AB T0B 4J0
Tel. 780 662-3263
Fax 780 662-3835
www.albertahealthservices.ca

TROCHU

COVENANT HEALTH - ST. MARY'S HEALTH CARE CENTRE
451 DeChauney Ave
Trochu AB T0M 2C0
Tel. 403 442-3955
Fax 403 442-3945
www.covenanthealth.ca

TWO HILLS

TWO HILLS HEALTH CENTRE
4401 53rd Ave
PO Box 160
Two Hills AB T0B 4K0
Tel. 780 657-3344
Fax 780 657-2508
www.albertahealthservices.ca

VALLEYVIEW

STURGEON LAKE HEALTH CENTRE - VALLEYVIEW
Box 757
Valleyview AB T0H 3N0
Tel. 780 524-5520
Fax 780 524-2903

VALLEYVIEW HEALTH CENTRE
4802 Hwy St
PO Box 358
Valleyview AB T0H 3N0
Tel. 780 524-3356
Fax 780 524-2107
www.albertahealthservices.ca

VEGREVILLE

COVENANT HEALTH - ST JOSEPH'S GENERAL HOSPITAL
5241 43 St
PO Box 490 Stn Main
Vegreville AB T9C 1R5
Tel. 780 632-2811
Fax 780 603-4401
www.covenanthealth.ca

VEGREVILLE CARE CENTRE
4525 50 St
Vegreville AB T9C 1A0
Tel. 780 632-2871
Fax 780 632-6680
www.albertahealthservices.ca

VERMILION

VERMILION HEALTH CENTRE
5720 50 Ave
Vermilion AB T9X 1K7
Tel. 780 853-5305
Fax 780 853-4786
www.albertahealthservices.ca

VIKING

EXTENDICARE VIKING
5020 57th Ave
PO Box 430
Viking AB T0B 4N0
Tel. 780 336-4790
Fax 780 336-4004
www.albertahealthservices.ca

VIKING HEALTH CENTRE
5110 57 Ave
PO Box 60
Viking AB T0B 4N0
Tel. 780 336-4786
Fax 780 336-4983
www.albertahealthservices.ca

VULCAN

VULCAN COMMUNITY HEALTH CENTRE
610 Elizabeth St S
PO Box 299
Vulcan AB T0L 2B0
Tel. 403 485-3333
Fax 403 485-2336
www.albertahealthservices.ca

WABASCA

BIGSTONE HEALTH CENTRE
PO Box 1020
Wabasca AB T0G 2K0
Tel. 780 891-2000
Fax 780 891-2623
www.informalberta.ca

WABASCA / DESMARAIS HEALTHCARE CENTRE
813 Hwy
PO Box 450
Wabasca AB T0G 2K0
Tel. 780 891-3007
Fax 780 891-3784
www.albertahealthservices.ca

WAINWRIGHT

WAINWRIGHT HEALTH CENTRE
530 6 Ave
Wainwright AB T9W 1R6
Tel. 780 842-3324
Fax 780 842-4290
www.albertahealthservices.ca

WESTLOCK

WESTLOCK HEALTHCARE CENTRE
10220 93 St
Westlock AB T7P 2G4
Tel. 780 349-3301
Fax 780 349-6973
www.albertahealthservices.ca

WETASKIWIN

WETASKIWIN COMMUNITY HEALTH CENTRE
5610 40 Ave
Wetaskiwin AB T9A 3E4
Tel. 780 361-4333
Fax 780 361-4335
www.albertahealthservices.ca

WETASKIWIN HOSPITAL & CARE CENTRE
6910 47 St
Wetaskiwin AB T9A 3N3
Tel. 780 361-7100
Fax 780 361-4107
www.albertahealthservices.ca

WETASKIWIN MENTAL HEALTH CENTRE
5201 50 Ave
Wetaskiwin AB T9A 0S7
Tel. 780 361-1245
Fax 780 361-1387
www.albertahealthservices.ca

WHITECOURT

WHITECOURT HEALTHCARE CENTRE
20 Sunset Blvd
Whitecourt AB T7S 1M8
Tel. 780 778-2285
Fax 780 778-5161
www.albertahealthservices.ca

WILLINGDON

WILLINGDON COMMUNITY HEALTH CENTRE
5303 49 St
Box 120
Willingdon AB T0B 4R0
Tel. 780 367-2374
Fax 780 367-2379
www.albertahealthservices.ca

WINFIELD

WINFIELD COMMUNITY HEALTH CENTRE
10 2 Ave
PO Box 114
Winfield AB T0C 2X0
Tel. 780 682-4755
Fax 780 682-4750
www.albertahealthservices.ca

BRITISH COLUMBIA

100 MILE HOUSE

100 MILE HOUSE DISTRICT GENERAL HOSPITAL
555 Cedar Ave
PO Box 399
100 Mile House BC V0K 2E0
Tel. 250 395-7600
Fax 250 395-7607
www.interiorhealth.ca

ABBOTSFORD

ABBOTSFORD REGIONAL HOSPITAL & CANCER CENTRE
14-32900 Marshall Rd
Abbotsford BC V2S 0C2
Tel. 604 851-4700
Fax 604 851-4891
www.fraserhealth.ca

BC CANCER AGENCY ABBOTSFORD CENTRE
32900 Marshall Rd
Abbotsford BC V2S 0C2
Tel. 604 851-4710
www.bccancer.bc.ca

MENNO EXTENDED CARE HOSPITAL
32945 Marshall Rd
Abbotsford BC V2S 1K1
Tel. 604 859-7631
Fax 604 859-6931
www.mennoplace.ca

REGIONAL TREATMENT CENTRE & PACIFIC INSTITUTION
33344 King Rd
PO Box 3000 Stn Del Ctr
Abbotsford BC V2S 4P4
Tel. 604 870-7700
Fax 604 870-7746
www.csc-scc.gc.ca

AGASSIZ

HEALTH AND FAMILY SERVICES
4690 Salish Way
Agassiz BC V0M 1A1
Tel. 604 796-2116
Fax 604 796-3946
www.stsailes.com

SEABIRD HEALTH CENTRE
Box 765
Agassiz BC V0M 1A0
Tel. 604 796-2177
Fax 604 796-1124

ALERT BAY

CORMORANT ISLAND HEALTH CENTRE
49 School Rd
PO Box 223
Alert Bay BC V0N 1A0
Tel. 250 974-5585
Fax 250 974-5422
www.viha.ca

NAMGIS HEALTH CENTRE
Box 49
Alert Bay BC V0N 1A0
Tel. 250 974-5522
Fax 250 974-5952
www.namgis.bc.ca

ALEXIS CREEK

ALEXIS CREEK HEALTH CENTRE
2591 Morton Rd
PO Box 39
Alexis Creek BC V0L 1A0
Tel. 250 394-4313
Fax 250 394-5179
www.interiorhealth.ca

ANAHIM LAKE

ANAHIM LAKE NURSING STATION
PO Box 207
Anahim Lake BC V0L 1C0
Tel. 250 742-3305
Fax 250 742-3336
www.interiorhealth.ca

ANGLEMONT

BARRIERE MENTAL HEALTH
537-4521 Barrierre Town Rd
Anglemont BC V0E 1A0
Tel. 250 672-9731
www.interiorhealth.ca

ASHCROFT

ASHCROFT & DISTRICT HOSPITAL AND COMMUNITY HEALTH CENTRE
700 Ash-Cache Creek Hwy
PO Box 488
Ashcroft BC V0K 1A0
Tel. 250 453-2211
Fax 250 453-1926
www.interiorhealth.ca

ATLIN

ATLIN HEALTH CENTRE
164 3rd St
PO Box 330
Atlin BC V0W 1A0
Tel. 250 651-7677
Fax 250 651-7687
www.northernhealth.ca

BAMFIELD

BAMFIELD HEALTH CENTRE
353 Bamfield Rd
PO Box 40
Bamfield BC V0R 1B0
Tel. 250 728-3312
Fax 250 728-3054
www.viha.ca

BARRIERE

BARRIERE HEALTH CENTRE
4537 Barriere Town Rd
Barriere BC V0E 1E0
Tel. 250 672-9731
Fax 250 672-5144
www.interiorhealth.ca

SIMPCW HEALTH CENTRE
500 Dunn Lake Rd
PO Box 220
Barriere BC V0E 1E0
Tel. 250 672-9995
Fax 250 672-5500
www.interiorhealth.ca

BELLA COOLA

BELLA COOLA GENERAL HOSPITAL
1025 Elcho St
PO Box 220
Bella Coola BC V0T 1C0
Tel. 250 799-5311
Fax 250 799-5635
www.vch.ca

BELLA COOLA HEALTH CENTRE
PO Box 93
Bella Coola BC V0T 1C0
Tel. 250 799-5311
Fax 250 799-5635
www.vch.ca

BLUE RIVER

BLUE RIVER HEALTH CENTRE
858 Main St
PO Box 18
Blue River BC V0E 1J0
Tel. 250 673-8311
Fax 250 673-2380
www.interiorhealth.ca

BURNABY

BURNABY HOSPITAL
3935 Kincaid St
Burnaby BC V5G 2X6
Tel. 604 434-4211
Fax 604 412-6170
www.fraserhealth.ca

FELLBURN CARE CENTRE
6050 East Hastings St
Burnaby BC V5B 1R6
Tel. 604 412-6513
Fax 604 299-1015
www.fraserhealth.ca

MAPLES ADOLESCENT TREATMENT CENTRE
3405 Willingdon Ave
Burnaby BC V5G 3H4
Tel. 604 660-5800
Fax 604 660-5814
www.mcf.gov.bc.ca

ST MICHAEL'S CENTRE
7451 Sussex Ave
Burnaby BC V5J 5C2
Tel. 604 434-1323
Fax 604 434-6469
www.stmichaels.bc.ca

WILLINGDON PARK HOSPITAL
4435 Grange St
Burnaby BC V5H 1P4
Tel. 604 433-2455
Fax 604 433-5804
www.fraserhealth.ca

BURNS LAKE

CARRIER SEKANI FAMILY SERVICES
102 2nd Ave
Burns Lake BC V0J 1E2
Tel. 250 692-2387
Fax 250 592-2389
www.csfs.org

LAKES DISTRICT HOSPITAL & HEALTH CENTRE
741 Centre St
PO Box 7500
Burns Lake BC V0J 1E0
Tel. 250 692-2400
Fax 250 692-2403
www.northernhealth.ca

SOUTHSIDE HEALTH & WELLNESS CENTRE
27920 Wellness Way
Burns Lake BC V0J 1E4
Tel. 250 694-3270
Fax 250 694-3290
www.southsidewellness.ca

CAMPBELL RIVER

CAMPBELL RIVER & DISTRICT GENERAL HOSPITAL
375 2nd Ave
Campbell River BC V9W 3V1
Tel. 250 850-2141
Fax 250 286-9675
www.viha.ca

CASTLEGAR

CASTLEGAR & DISTRICT COMMUNITY HEALTH CENTRE
709 10th St
Castlegar BC V1N 2H7
Tel. 250 365-7711
Fax 250 304-1234
www.interiorhealth.ca

CHASE

ADAMS LAKE HEALTH STATION
PO Box 1009
Chase BC V0E 1M0
Tel. 250 679-7726
Fax 250 679-7731

CHASE HEALTH CENTRE
825 Thompson Ave
PO Box 1099
Chase BC V0E 1M0
Tel. 250 679-3312
Fax 250 679-5329
www.interiorhealth.ca

CHEMAINUS

CHEMAINUS HEALTH CARE CENTRE
9909 Esplanade St
PO Box 499
Chemainus BC V0R 1K1
Tel. 250 739-2040
Fax 250 737-2059
www.viha.ca

CHETWYND

CHETWYND GENERAL HOSPITAL
5500 Hospital Rd
PO Box 507
Chetwynd BC V0C 1J0
Tel. 250 788-2236
Fax 250 788-7547
www.northernhealth.ca

CHILLIWACK

CHILLIWACK GENERAL HOSPITAL
45600 Menholm Rd
Chilliwack BC V2P 1P7
Tel. 604 702-2885
Fax 604 702-2882
www.fraserhealth.ca

SKWAH FIRST NATION HEALTH CENTRE
619 Wellington St
Chilliwack BC V2P 6H7
Tel. 604 792-9204
Fax 604 792-3419

CLEARWATER

CLEARWATER COMMUNITY HEALTH
640 Park Dr
Clearwater BC V0E 1N0
Tel. 250 674-3141
www.interiorhealth.ca

DR HELMCKEN MEMORIAL HOSPITAL
640 Park Dr
RR 1
Clearwater BC V0E 1N0
Tel. 250 674-2244
Fax 250 674-2477
www.interiorhealth.ca

CLINTON

CLINTON HEALTH & WELLNESS CENTRE
834 Thompson Ave
Clinton BC V0K 1K0
Tel. 250 459-2080
www.interiorhealth.ca

COMOX

ST JOSEPH'S GENERAL HOSPITAL
2137 Comox Ave
Comox BC V9M 1P2
Tel. 250 339-2242
Fax 250 339-1432
www.sjghcomox.ca

CRANBROOK

CRANBROOK HEALTH CENTRE
20 23rd Ave S
Cranbrook BC V1C 5V1
Tel. 250 420-2207
Fax 250 420-2201
www.interiorhealth.ca

EAST KOOTENAY REGIONAL HOSPITAL
13 24th Ave N
Cranbrook BC V1C 3H9
Tel. 250 426-5281
Fax 250 426-5285
www.vch.ca

CRAWFORD BAY

EAST SHORE COMMUNITY HEALTH CENTRE
15985 Hwy 3A
PO Box 161
Crawford Bay BC V0B 1E0
Tel. 250 227-9006
www.interiorhealth.ca

CRESTON

CRESTON VALLEY HOSPITAL & HEALTH CENTRE
312 15th Ave N
Bag 3000
Creston BC V0B 1G0
Tel. 250 428-2286
Fax 250 428-4860
www.interiorhealth.ca

CUMBERLAND

CUMBERLAND HEALTH CENTRE
2696 Windermere Ave
PO Box 400
Cumberland BC V0R 1S0
Tel. 250 331-8505
Fax 250 336-2100
www.viha.ca

DAWSON CREEK

DAWSON CREEK & DISTRICT HOSPITAL
11100 13 St
Dawson Creek BC V1G 3W8
Tel. 250 782-8501
Fax 250 784-7301
www.northernhealth.ca

DEASE LAKE

STIKINE HEALTH CENTRE
7171 Hwy 37
Box 386
Dease Lake BC V0C 1L0
Tel. 250 771-4444
Fax 250 771-3911
www.northernhealth.ca

DELTA

DELTA HOSPITAL
5800 Mountain View Blvd
Delta BC V4K 3V6
Tel. 604 946-1121
Fax 604 946-3086
www.fraserhealth.ca

DENNY ISLAND

BELLA BELLA HEALTH CENTRE
PO Box 819
Denny Island BC V0T 1Z0
Tel. 250 957-2308
Fax 250 957-2311
www.vch.ca

R W LARGE MEMORIAL HOSPITAL
88 Waglisla St
Bella Bella BC V0T 1Z0
Tel. 250 957-2314
Fax 250 957-2612
rwlargememorialhospital.com

DOG CREEK

DOG CREEK HEALTH STATION
Gen Del
Dog Creek BC V0L 1J0
Tel. 250 440-5822
Fax 250 440-5866
www.cha-bc.org

DUNCAN

COWICHAN DISTRICT HOSPITAL
3045 Gibbins Rd
Duncan BC V9L 1E5
Tel. 250 737-3000
Fax 250 746-4247
www.viha.ca

COWICHAN HEALTH CENTRE
5768 Allenby Rd
Duncan BC V9L 5J1
Tel. 250 746-6184
Fax 250 748-8815

ECHO BAY

GILFORD ISLAND HEALTH STATION
Gilford Village
Echo Bay BC V0P 1S0
Tel. 250 974-8099

EDGEWOOD

EDGEWOOD HEALTH CENTRE
322 Monashee Ave
PO Box 5
Edgewood BC V0G 1J0
Tel. 250 269-7313
Fax 250 269-7520
www.interiorhealth.ca

ELKFORD

ELKFORD HEALTHCARE CENTRE
212 Alpine Way
PO Box 640
Elkford BC V0B 1H0
Tel. 250 865-2247
Fax 250 865-2797
www.interiorhealth.ca

ENDERBY

ENDERBY COMMUNITY HEALTH CENTRE
707 3rd Ave
Enderby BC V0E 1V0
Tel. 250 838-2450
www.interiorhealth.ca

SPALLUMCHEEN HEALTH STATION
PO Box 460
Enderby BC V0E 1V0
Tel. 250 838-9538
Fax 250 838-9548

FERNIE

ELK VALLEY HOSPITAL
1501 5th Ave
PO Box 670
Fernie BC V0B 1M0
Tel. 250 423-4453
Fax 250 423-3732
www.interiorhealth.ca

FERNIE HEALTH CENTRE
1501 5th Ave
Fernie BC V0B 1M0
Tel. 250 423-8288
www.interiorhealth.ca

FORT NELSON

FORT NELSON GENERAL HOSPITAL
5315 Liard St
Bag 1000
Fort Nelson BC V0C 1R0
Tel. 250 774-8100
Fax 250 774-8110
www.northernhealth.ca

FORT ST. JAMES

BINCHI HEALTH STATION
Box 670
Fort St James BC V0J 1P0
Tel. 250 648-3673
Fax 250 648-3685

NESCOLIE HEALTH CENTRE
Box 1238
Fort St James BC V0J 1P0
Tel. 250 996-7400
Fax 250 996-2262

STUART LAKE HOSPITAL
600 Stuart Dr E
PO BOX 1060
Fort St. James BC V0J 1P0
Tel. 250 996-8201
Fax 250 996-8777
www.northernhealth.ca

FORT ST. JOHN

FORT ST JOHN HOSPITAL & HEALTH CENTRE
8704 112 Ave
Fort St. John BC V1J 0J5
Tel. 250 262-5200
Fax 250 262-5294
www.northernhealth.ca

FRASER LAKE

FRASER LAKE COMMUNITY HEALTH CENTRE
130 Chowsunket Rd
PO Box 98
Fraser Lake BC V0J 1S0
Tel. 250 699-7742
Fax 250 699-6987
www.northernhealth.ca

GALIANO

GALIANO ISLAND HEALTH CARE CENTRE
908 Burrill Rd
Galiano BC V0N 1P0
Tel. 250 539-3230
www.galianohealth.org

GOLD RIVER

GOLD RIVER HEALTH CENTRE
601 Trumpeter Dr
PO Box 580
Gold River BC V0P 1G0
Tel. 250 283-2626
Fax 250 283-7561
www.viha.ca

GOLDEN

GOLDEN & DISTRICT GENERAL HOSPITAL
835 9th Ave S
PO Box 1260
Golden BC V0A 1H0
Tel. 250 344-5271
Fax 250 344-2511
www.interiorhealth.ca

GOLDEN HEALTH CENTRE
835 9th Ave S
Golden BC V0A 1H0
Tel. 250 344-3001
www.interiorhealth.ca

GOOD HOPE LAKE

GOOD HOPE LAKE HEALTH CLINIC
37 Hwy
PO Box 79
Good Hope Lake BC V0C 2Z0
Tel. 250 239-3000
Fax 250 239-3003
www.find.healthlinkbc.ca

GRAND FORKS

BOUNDARY COMMUNITY HEALTH CENTRE
7649 22nd St
Grand Forks BC V0H 1H2
www.interiorhealth.ca

BOUNDARY HOSPITAL
7649 22nd St
PO Box 2647
Grand Forks BC V0H 1H0
Tel. 250 443-2100
Fax 250 442-8331
www.interiorhealth.ca

GRANISLE

GRANISLE COMMUNITY HEALTH CENTRE
1 Hagen St
PO Box 209
Granisle BC V0J 1W0
Tel. 250 697-2251
Fax 250 697-6221
www.northernhealth.ca

HAISLA

HAISLA HEALTH CENTRE
351 Haisla Ave
PO Box 1041
Haisla BC V0T 2B0
Tel. 250 639-9361
Fax 250 632-3686
www.haisla.ca

HARTLEY BAY

HARTLEY BAY NURSING STATION
341 Wee Xaa Ave
Hartley Bay BC V0V 1A0
Tel. 250 841-2556
Fax 250 841-2554
www.cha-bc.org

HAZELTON

GITANMAAX HEALTH STATION
PO Box 223
Hazelton BC V0J 1Y0
Tel. 250 842-6320
Fax 250 842-6399
www.gitxsanhealth.com

GLEN VOWELL HEALTH STATION
c/o Gitxsan Health Society
Hazelton BC V0J 1Y0
Tel. 250 842-6876
Fax 250 842-5925
www.northernhealth.ca

HAZELTON COMMUNITY HEALTH
2510 Hwy 62
Bag 999
Hazelton BC V0J 1Y0
Tel. 250 842-4640
Fax 250 842-4642
www.northernhealth.ca

HAZELTON MENTAL HEALTH AND ADDICTIONS
70-2510 Hwy 62
Hazelton BC V0J 1Y0
Tel. 250 842-5144
Fax 250 842-2179
www.northernhealth.ca

KISPIOX HEALTH CENTRE
2215 Mary Blackwater Ave
Hazelton BC V0J 1Y0
Tel. 250 842-6320
Fax 250 842-5319
www.gitxsanhealth.com

WRINCH MEMORIAL HOSPITAL
2510 Hwy 62
PO Bag 999
Hazelton BC V0J 1Y0
Tel. 250 842-5211
Fax 250 842-5865
www.northernhealth.ca

HOPE

FRASER CANYON HOSPITAL
1275 7th Ave
RR 4
Hope BC V0X 1L4
Tel. 604 869-5656
Fax 604 860-7732
www.fraserhealth.ca

HOUSTON

HOUSTON HEALTH CENTRE
3202 14th St
PO Box 538
Houston BC V0J 1Z0
Tel. 250 845-2294
Fax 250 845-2259
www.northernhealth.ca

HUDSON'S HOPE

HUDSON'S HOPE GETHING DIAGNOSTIC & TREATMENT CENTRE
10309 Kyllo St
PO Box 599
Hudson's Hope BC V0C 1V0
Tel. 250 783-9991
Fax 250 783-9125
www.northernhealth.ca

INVERMERE

INVERMERE & DISTRICT HOSPITAL
850 10th Ave
PO Box 5001
Invermere BC V0A 1K0
Tel. 250 342-9201
Fax 250 342-6303
www.interiorhealth.ca

ISKUT

ISKUT VALLEY NURSING STATION
PO Box 90
Iskut BC V0J 1K0
Tel. 250 234-3511
Fax 250 234-3516

KAMLOOPS

OVERLANDER RESIDENTIAL CARE
953 Southill St
Kamloops BC V2B 7Z9
Tel. 250 554-2323
Fax 250 554-5557
www.interiorhealth.ca

ROYAL INLAND HOSPITAL
311 Columbia St
Kamloops BC V2C 2T1
Tel. 250 374-5111
Fax 250 314-2333
www.interiorhealth.ca

KASLO

VICTORIAN COMMUNITY HEALTH CENTRE OF KASLO
PO Box 607
Kaslo BC V0G 1M0
Tel. 250 353-2211
Fax 250 353-2747
www.interiorhealth.ca

KELOWNA

BC CANCER AGENCY SINDI AHLUWALIA HAWKINS CENTRE FOR THE SOUTHERN INTERIOR
399 Royal Ave
Kelowna BC V1Y 5L3
Tel. 250 712-3900
Fax 250 712-3911
www.bccancer.bc.ca

KELOWNA GENERAL HOSPITAL
2268 Pandosy St
Kelowna BC V1Y 1T2
Tel. 250 862-4000
Fax 250 862-4058
www.interiorhealth.ca

KEREMEOS

SOUTH SIMILKAMEEN HEALTH CENTRE
700 3rd St
Keremeos BC V0X 1N3
Tel. 250 499-3000
Fax 250 499-3026
www.rccbc.ca

KIMBERLEY

KIMBERLEY HEALTH CENTRE & HOME SUPPORT
260 4th Ave
Kimberley BC V1A 2R6
Tel. 250 427-2215
Fax 250 427-7389
www.interiorhealth.ca

KINCOLITH

KINCOLITH HEALTH CENTRE
General Delivery
Kincolith BC V0V 1B0
Tel. 250 326-4251
Fax 250 326-4276

KITIMAT

KITIMAT HOSPITAL & HEALTH CENTRE
920 Lahakas Blvd S
Kitimat BC V8C 2S3
Tel. 250 632-2121
Fax 250 632-8726
www.northernhealth.ca

KITKATLA

KITKATLA NURSING STATION
PO Box 149
Kitkatla BC V0V 1C0
Tel. 250 848-2254
Fax 250 848-2263

KITWANGA

GITANYOW HUMAN SERVICES
PO Box 130
Kitwanga BC V0J 2A0
Tel. 250 849-5572
Fax 250 849-5267
www.health.gitanyow.com

GITWANGAK HEALTH CENTRE
149 Bridge St
PO Box 550
Kitwanga BC V0J 2A0
Tel. 250 849-5555
Fax 250 849-5531
www.find.healthlinkbc.ca

KLEMTU

KLEMTU NURSING STATION
General Delivery
Klemtu BC V0T 1L0
Tel. 250 839-1221
Fax 250 839-1184

KYUQUOT

KYUQUOT HEALTH CENTRE
100 Okime Island
Kyuquot BC V0P 1J0
Tel. 250 332-5289
Fax 250 332-5215
www.viha.ca

VANCOUVER ISLAND HEALTH AUTHOFITY HEALTH CENTRE
100 Okime Island
GD
Kyuquot BC V0P 1J0
Tel. 250 332-5289
Fax 250 332-5215
www.viha.ca

LADYSMITH

LADYSMITH COMMUNITY HEALTH CENTRE
1111 4th Ave
PO Box 10 Stn Main
Ladysmith BC V9G 1A1
Tel. 250 739-5777
Fax 250 740-2689
www.ladysmith.ca

LANGLEY

LANGLEY MEMORIAL HOSPITAL
22051 Fraser Hwy
Langley BC V3A 4H4
Tel. 604 534-4121
Fax 604 534-8283
www.fraserhealth.ca

LILLOOET

LILLOOET DISTRICT HOSPITAL
951 Murray St
PO Box 300
Lillooet BC V0K 1V0
Tel. 250 256-4233
Fax 250 256-1336
www.interiorhealth.ca

LOGAN LAKE

LOGAN LAKE PRIMARY HEALTH CENTRE
5 Beryl Ave
PO Box 1089
Logan Lake BC V0K 1W0
Tel. 250 523-9414
Fax 250 523-6869
www.interiorhealth.ca

LYTTON

ST BARTHOLOMEW'S HEALTH CENTRE
531 Main St
Lytton BC V0K 1Z0
Tel. 250 455-2221
Fax 250 455-6621
www.interiorhealth.ca

MACKENZIE

MACKENZIE & DISTRICT HOSPITAL & HEALTH CENTRE
45 Centennial Dr
PO Box 249
Mackenzie BC V0J 2C0
Tel. 250 997-3263
Fax 250 997-3940
www.northernhealth.ca

MAPLE RIDGE

RIDGE MEADOWS HOSPITAL & HEALTH CARE CENTRE
11666 Laity St
Maple Ridge BC V2X 7G5
Tel. 604 463-4111
Fax 604 463-1888
www.fraserhealth.ca

MASSET

HAIDA HEALTH CENTRE
347 Eagle Ave
PO Box 176
Masset BC V0T 1M0
Tel. 250 626-3911
Fax 250 626-3357
www.northernhealth.ca

MASSET COMMUNITY HEALTH
2520 Harrison Ave
PO Box 215
Masset BC V0T 1M0
Tel. 250 626-4727
Fax 250 626-5279
www.northernhealth.ca

NORTHERN HAIDA GWAII HOSPITAL AND HEALTH CENTRE
2520 Harrison Ave
PO Box 319
Masset BC V0T 1M0
Tel. 250 626-4700
Fax 250 626-4709
www.northernhealth.ca

MAYNE ISLAND

MAYNE ISLAND HEALTH CARE CENTRE
526 Felix Jack Rd
PO Box 120
Mayne Island BC V0N 2J0
Tel. 250 539-2312
Fax 250 539-3215
www.mayneisland.com

MCBRIDE

MCBRIDE & DISTRICT HOSPITAL
1136 5th Ave
McBride BC V0J 2E0
Tel. 250 569-2251 Ext. 202
Fax 250 569-2313
www.northernhealth.ca

MERRITT

NICOLA VALLEY HEALTH CENTRE
3451 Voght St
Merritt BC V1K 1C6
Tel. 250 378-2242
Fax 250 378-3287
www.interiorhealth.ca

MISSION

MISSION MEMORIAL HOSPITAL
7324 Hurd St
Mission BC V2V 3H5
Tel. 604 826-6261
Fax 604 826-9513
www.fraserhealth.ca

MOUNT CURRIE

PQUSNALHCW HEALTH CENTRE
PO Box 161
Mount Currie BC V0N 2K0
Tel. 604 894-6656
Fax 604 894-6643
www.vch.ca

NAKUSP

ARROW LAKES HOSPITAL
97 1st Ave NE
PO Box 87
Nakusp BC V0G 1R0
Tel. 250 265-3622
Fax 250 265-4435
www.interiorhealth.ca

NANAIMO

ADULT FORENSIC PSYCHIATRIC COMMUNITY SERVICES
101-190 Wallace St
Nanaimo BC V9R 5B1
Tel. 250 739-5000
Fax 250 739-5001
www.bcmhas.ca

NANAIMO REGIONAL GENERAL HOSPITAL
1200 Dufferin Cres
Nanaimo BC V9S 2B7
Tel. 250 755-7691
Fax 250 755-7633
www.viha.ca

NELSON

KOOTENAY LAKE GENERAL HOSPITAL
3 View St
Nelson BC V1L 2V1
Tel. 250 352-3111
Fax 250 354-2320
www.interiorhealth.ca

MCKIM COTTAGE
916 11th St
Nelson BC V1L 7A6
Tel. 250 352-2022
Fax 250 352-2023
www.interiorhealth.ca

MOUNT ST FRANCIS HOSPITAL
1300 Gordon Rd
Nelson BC V1L 3M5
Tel. 250 352-3531
Fax 250 352-6942
www.interiorhealth.ca

NEMAIAH VALLEY

ENIYUD HEALTH CENTRE
Box 51
Nemaiah Valley BC V0L 1X0
Tel. 250 394-7020
Fax 250 394-7028

NEW DENVER

SLOCAN COMMUNITY HEALTH CENTRE
401 Galena Ave
PO Box 129
New Denver BC V0G 1S0
Tel. 250 358-7911
Fax 250 358-7117
www.interiorhealth.ca

NEW HAZELTON

HAGWILGET HEALTH STATION
PO Box 460
New Hazelton BC V0J 2J0
Tel. 250 842-5272
Fax 250 842-6792
www.northernhealth.ca

NEW WESTMINSTER

EAGLE RIDGE HOSPITAL & HEALTH CARE CENTRE
475 Guildford Way
Port Moody BC V3H 3W9
Tel. 604 461-2022
Fax 604 461-9972
www.fraserhealth.ca

FORENSIC PSYCHIATRIC HOSPITAL
70 Colony Farm Rd
Coquitlam BC V3C 5X9
Tel. 604 524-7700
Fax 604 524-7775
www.bcmhas.ca

ROYAL COLUMBIAN HOSPITAL
330 Columbia St E
New Westminster BC V3L 3W7
Tel. 604 520-4253
Fax 604 520-4327
www.rchfoundation.com

NORTH VANCOUVER

CENTRAL COMMUNITY HEALTH CENTRE
132 W Esplanade
North Vancouver BC V7M 1A2
Tel. 604 983-6700
Fax 604 983-6839
www.vch.ca

LIONS GATE HOSPITAL
231 15th St E
North Vancouver BC V7L 2L7
Tel. 604 988-3131
Fax 604 984-5838
www.vch.ca

OLIVER

SOUTH OKANAGAN GENERAL HOSPITAL
911 McKinney Rd
Oliver BC V0H 1T0
Tel. 250 498-5000
Fax 250 498-5004
www.interiorhealth.ca

PARKSVILLE

TRILLIUM LODGE EXTENDED CARE HOSPITAL
401 Mailliet St
PO Box 940 Stn Main
Parksville BC V9P 2G9
Tel. 250 248-8230
www.viha.ca

PEMBERTON

PEMBERTON HEALTH CENTRE
1403 Portage Rd
PO Box 310
Pemberton BC V0N 2L0
Tel. 604 894-6939
Fax 604 894-6918
www.vch.ca

PENDER ISLAND

PENDER ISLANDS HEALTH CENTRE
5715 Canal Rd
Pender Island BC V0N 2M1
Tel. 250 629-3326
www.penderislandhealth.ca

PENTICTON

PENTICTON HEALTH CENTRE
740 Carmi Ave
Penticton BC V2A 8P9
Tel. 250 770-3434
Fax 250 770-3410
www.interiorhealth.ca

PENTICTON REGIONAL HOSPITAL
550 Carmi Ave
Penticton BC V2A 3G6
Tel. 250 492-4000
Fax 250 492-9068
www.vch.ca

PORT ALBERNI

WEST COAST GENERAL HOSPITAL
3949 Port Alberni Hwy
Port Alberni BC V9Y 4S1
Tel. 250 731-1370
Fax 250 724-8805
www.viha.ca

PORT ALICE

PORT ALICE HEALTH CENTRE
1090 Marine Dr
PO Box 69
Port Alice BC V0N 2N0
Tel. 250 284-3555
Fax 250 284-6163
www.viha.ca

PORT COQUITLAM

BC MENTAL HEALTH & ADDICTION SERVICE
2601 Lougheed Hwy
Coquitlam BC V3C 4J2
Tel. 604 524-7000
Fax 604 524-7016
www.bcmhas.ca

PORT HARDY

PORT HARDY HOSPITAL
9120 Granville St
PO Box 790
Port Hardy BC V0N 2P0
Tel. 250 902-6011
Fax 250 949-7000
www.viha.ca

PORT MCNEILL

PORT MCNEILL & DISTRICT HOSPITAL
2750 Kingcome Place
PO Box 790
Port McNeill BC V0N 2R0
Tel. 250 956-4461
Fax 250 956-4823
www.viha.ca

PORT SIMPSON

PORT SIMPSON NURSING STATION
206 Shashaak St
Port Simpson BC V0V 1H0
Tel. 250 625-3331
Fax 250 625-3488
www.northernhealth.ca

POUCE COUPE

POUCE COUPE CARE HOME
5216 50 Ave
Pouce Coupe BC V0C 2C0
Tel. 250 786-6116
Fax 250 786-0197
www.northernhealth.ca

POWELL RIVER

POWELL RIVER GENERAL HOSPITAL
5000 Joyce Ave
Powell River BC V8A 5R3
Tel. 604 485-3211
Fax 604 485-3243
www.vch.ca

PRINCE GEORGE

BC CANCER AGENCY CENTRE FOR THE NORTH
1215 Lethbridge St
Prince George BC V2M 7E9
Tel. 250 645-7300
www.bccancer.bc.ca

CARRIER SEKANI FAMILY SERVICES
987 4th Ave
Prince George BC V2L 3H7
Tel. 250 562-3591
Fax 250 562-2272
www.csfs.org

CARRIER SEKANI FAMILY SERVICES
1010 4th Ave
Prince George BC V2L 3H9
Tel. 250 561-1271
Fax 250 561-1871
www.csfs.org

CARRIER SEKANI FAMILY SERVICES
301-1705 3rd Ave
Prince George BC V2L 3G7
Tel. 250 564-4079
Fax 250 564-7097
www.csfs.org

NORTHERN HEALTH CENTRE FOR HEALTHY LIVING
1788 Diefenbaker Dr
Prince George BC V2N 4V7
Tel. 250 649-7011
www.northernhealth.ca

UNIVERSITY HOSPITAL OF NORTHERN BRITISH COLUMBIA
1475 Edmonton St
Prince George BC V2M 1S2
Tel. 250 565-2000
Fax 250 565-2343
www.northernhealth.ca

PRINCE RUPERT

PRINCE RUPERT COMMUNITY HEALTH
300 3rd Ave W
Prince Rupert BC V8J 1L4
Tel. 250 622-6380
Fax 250 622-6391
www.northernhealth.ca

PRINCE RUPERT REGIONAL HOSPITAL
1305 Summit Ave
Prince Rupert BC V8J 2A6
Tel. 250 624-2171
Fax 250 622-2195
www.northernhealth.ca

PRINCETON

PRINCETON GENERAL HOSPITAL
98 Ridgewood
PO Box 610
Princeton BC V0X 1W0
Tel. 250 295-3233
Fax 250 295-3344
www.interiorhealth.ca

QUEEN CHARLOTTE

QUEEN CHARLOTTE CITY HEALTH CENTRE
302 Second Ave
Queen Charlotte BC V0T 1S0
Tel. 250 559-8765
Fax 250 559-8765
www.northernhealth.ca

QUEEN CHARLOTTE ISLANDS COMMUNITY HEALTH
3211 3rd Ave
Queen Charlotte BC V0T 1S0
Tel. 250 559-2350
www.northernhealth.ca

QUEEN CHARLOTTE ISLANDS GENERAL HOSPITAL - QUEEN CHARLOTTE SITE
3209 Oceanview Dr
Queen Charlotte BC V0T 1S0
Tel. 250 559-4300
Fax 250 559-4312
www.qcihealth.com

SKIDEGATE HEALTH CENTRE
156 2nd Ave
PO Box 1348
Queen Charlotte BC V0T 1S1
Tel. 250 559-4610
Fax 250 559-4619
www.northernhealth.ca

QUESNEL

G R BAKER MEMORIAL HOSPITAL
543 Front St
PO Box 4000
Quesnel BC V2J 2K7
Tel. 250 985-5600
Fax 250 992-5652
www.northernhealth.ca

REVELSTOKE

QUEEN VICTORIA HOSPITAL
1200 Newlands Rd
PO Bag 5000
Revelstoke BC V0E 2S0
Tel. 250 837-2131
Fax 250 814-2285
www.interiorhealth.ca

RICHMOND

RICHMOND HOSPITAL
7000 Westminster Hwy
Richmond BC V6X 1A2
Tel. 604 278-9711
Fax 604 244-5552
www.richmondhealth.ca

ROSE PRAIRIE

DOIG HEALTH STATION
Rose Prairie
PO Box 56
Rose Prairie BC V0C 2H0
Tel. 250 827-3776
Fax 250 827-3778

SAANICHTON

SAANICH PENINSULA HOSPITAL
2166 Mount Newton Cross Rd
Saanichton BC V8M 2B2
Tel. 250 544-7676
Fax 250 652-3553
www.viha.ca

SALMON ARM

SHUSWAP LAKE GENERAL HOSPITAL
601 10th St NE
PO Box 520 Stn Main
Salmon Arm BC V1E 4N6
Tel. 250 833-3600
Fax 250 833-3609
www.interiorhealth.ca

SALT SPRING ISLAND

LADY MINTO GULF ISLANDS HOSPITAL
135 Crofton Rd
Salt Spring Island BC V8K 1T1
Tel. 250 538-4800
Fax 250 538-4870
www.viha.ca

SECHELT

ST MARY'S HOSPITAL
5544 Sunshine Coast Hwy
PO Box 7777
Sechelt BC V0N 3A0
Tel. 604 885-2224
Fax 604 885-8628
www.vch.ca

SETON PORTAGE

ROSE CASPER HEALING CENTRE
Module 2, Site 4
Box 5
Seton Portage BC V0N 3B0
Tel. 250 259-8232
Fax 250 259-8167

SMITHERS

BULKLEY VALLEY DISTRICT HOSPITAL
3950 8th Ave
PO Box 370
Smithers BC V0J 2N0
Tel. 250 847-2611
Fax 250 847-2446
www.northernhealth.ca

SMITHERS COMMUNITY HEALTH
3793 Alfred Ave
PO Bag 5000
Smithers BC V0J 2N0
Tel. 250 847-6400
Fax 250 847-5908
www.northernhealth.ca

SOUTH HAZELTON

GITSEGUKLA HEALTH PROGRAMS & SERVICES
Seymour Ave
RR #1
South Hazelton BC V0J 2R0
Tel. 250 849-5231
Fax 250 849-5235

SPARWOOD

SPARWOOD HEALTHCARE CENTRE
570 Pine Ave
PO Box 9
Sparwood BC V0B 2G0
Tel. 250 425-6212
Fax 250 425-2313
www.interiorhealth.ca

SPENCES BRIDGE

HESKW'EN'SCUTXE HEALTH SERVICES
3691 Deer Lane
Box 188
Spences Bridge BC V0K 2L0
Tel. 250 458-2212
Fax 250 458-2213
www.interiorhealth.ca

SQUAMISH

SQUAMISH GENERAL HOSPITAL / HILLTOP HOUSE
38140 Behrner Dr
P O Box 6000
Squamish BC V8B 0J3
Tel. 604 892-5211
Fax 604 892-9417
www.vch.ca

STEWART

STEWART HEALTH CENTRE
904 Brightwell St
PO Box 8
Stewart BC V0T 1W0
Tel. 250 636-2221
Fax 250 636-2715
www.northernhealth.ca

SUMMERLAND

SUMMERLAND MEMORIAL HEALTH CENTRE
12815 Atkinson Rd
PO Box 869
Summerland BC V0H 1Z0
Tel. 250 404-8000
Fax 250 404-8005
www.interiorhealth.ca

SURREY

ADULT FORENSIC PSYCHIATRIC COMMUNITY SERVICES
10022 King Geoge Hwy
Surrey BC V3T 2W4
Tel. 604 529-3300
Fax 604 529-3333
www.bcmhas.ca

BC CANCER AGENCY FRASER VALLEY CENTRE
13750 96 Ave
Surrey BC V3V 1Z2
Tel. 604 930-4055
Fax 604 930-4049
www.bccancer.bc.ca

SURREY MEMORIAL HOSPITAL
13750 96 Ave
Surrey BC V3V 1Z2
Tel. 604 581-2211
Fax 604 588-3320
www.fraserhealth.ca

TAHSIS

TAHSIS HEALTH CENTRE
1085 S Maquinna Dr
PO Box 399
Tahsis BC V0P 1X0
Tel. 250 934-6322
Fax 250 934-6404
www.viha.ca

TAKLA LANDING

TAKLA NURSING STATION
GD
Takla Landing BC V0J 2T0
Tel. 250 564-9334
Fax 250 564-9334

TATLA LAKE

WEST CHILCOTIN HEALTH CENTRE
16452 Hwy 20
Box 48
Tatla Lake BC V0L 1V0
Tel. 250 476-1114
Fax 250 476-1266
www.interiorhealth.ca

TELEGRAPH CREEK

TELEGRAPH CREEK NURSING STATION
PO Box 112
Telegraph Creek BC V0J 2W0
Tel. 250 235-3211
Fax 250 235-3213
www.northernhealth.ca

TERRACE

KITSUMKALUM HEALTH STATION
3531 West Kalum Rd
PO Box 544
Terrace BC V8G 4B5
Tel. 250 635-6172
Fax 250 635-6182
www.northernhealth.ca

MILLS MEMORIAL HOSPITAL
4720 Haugland Ave
Terrace BC V8G 2W7
Tel. 250 635-2211
Fax 250 638-4017
www.northernhealth.ca

TERRACE COMMUNITY MENTAL HEALTH SERVICES
34-3412 Kalum St
Terrace BC V8G 4T2
Tel. 250 631-4202
Fax 250 631-4282
www.northernhealth.ca

TOFINO

TOFINO GENERAL HOSPITAL
261 Neill St
PO Box 190
Tofino BC V0R 2Z0
Tel. 250 725-4010
Fax 250 725-3324
www.viha.ca

TRAIL

KOOTENAY BOUNDARY REGIONAL HOSPITAL
1200 Hospital Bench
Trail BC V1R 4M1
Tel. 250 368-3311
Fax 250 364-3422
www.kbrh.ca

TUMBLER RIDGE

TUMBLER RIDGE COMMUNITY HEALTH CENTRE
220 Front St
PO Box 80
Tumbler Ridge BC V0C 2W0
Tel. 250 242-5271
Fax 250 242-3889
www.northernhealth.ca

TUMBLER RIDGE MENTAL HEALTH AND ADDICTIONS
1205 Front St
Tumbler Ridge BC V0C 2W0
Tel. 250 242-5505
Fax 250 242-3595
www.northernhealth.ca

VALEMOUNT

VALEMOUNT COMMUNITY HEALTH CENTRE
1445 5th Ave
PO Box 697
Valemount BC V0E 2Z0
Tel. 250 566-9138
Fax 250 566-4319
www.northernhealth.ca

VANCOUVER

AMHERST PRIVATE HOSPITAL
375 W 59 Ave
Vancouver BC V5X 1X3
Tel. 604 321-6777
Fax 604 322-0123
www.vch.ca

BC CANCER AGENCY VANCOUVER CENTRE
600 10th Ave W
Vancouver BC V5Z 4E6
Tel. 604 877-6000
Fax 604 877-4596
www.bccancer.bc.ca

BC CHILDREN'S HOSPITAL
4480 Oak St
Vancouver BC V6H 3V4
Tel. 604 875-2345
Fax 604 875-3448
www.bcchildrens.ca

BC WOMEN'S HOSPITAL & HEALTH CENTRE
4500 Oak St
Vancouver BC V6H 3N1
Tel. 604 875-2424
Fax 604 875-3582
www.bcwomens.ca

EVERGREEN COMMUNITY HEALTH CENTRE
3425 Crowley Dr
Vancouver BC V5R 6G3
Tel. 604 872-2511
www.vch.ca

G F STRONG REHABILITATION CENTRE
4255 Laurel St
Vancouver BC V5Z 2G9
Tel. 604 734-1313
Fax 604 737-6359
www.gfstrong.com

GEORGE PEARSON CENTRE
700 57th Ave W
Vancouver BC V6P 1S1
Tel. 604 321-3231
Fax 604 321-7833
www.vch.ca

GORDON & LESLIE DIAMOND HEALTH CARE CENTRE
2775 Laurel St
Vancouver BC V5Z 1M9
Tel. 604 875-4111
Fax 604 875-5701

LOUIS BRIER HOME & HOSPITAL
1055 41st Ave W
Vancouver BC V6M 1W9
Tel. 604 261-9376 Ext. 4000
Fax 604 266-8712
www.louisbrier.com

MARY PACK ARTHRITIS PROGRAM
895 10th Ave W
Vancouver BC V5Z 1L7
Tel. 604 875-4111 Ext. 68853
Fax 604 875-4321
www.vch.ca

PROVIDENCE HEALTH CARE - HOLY FAMILY HOSPITAL
7801 Argyle St
Vancouver BC V5P 3L6
Tel. 604 321-2661
Fax 604 321-6886
www.providencehealthcare.org

PROVIDENCE HEALTH CARE - MOUNT SAINT JOSEPH HOSPITAL
3080 Prince Edward St
Vancouver BC V5T 3N4
Tel. 604 874-1141
Fax 604 877-8733
www.providencehealthcare.org

PROVIDENCE HEALTH CARE - ST PAUL'S HOSPITAL
1081 Burrard St
Vancouver BC V6Z 1Y6
Tel. 604 682-2344
Fax 604 806-8811
www.providencehealthcare.org

PROVIDENCE HEALTH CARE - ST VINCENT'S HOSPITAL-BROCK FAHRNI SITE
4650 Oak St
Vancouver BC V6H 4J4
Tel. 604 806-9710
Fax 604 806-9706
www.providencehealthcare.org

PROVIDENCE HEALTH CARE - ST VINCENT'S HOSPITAL-LANGARA SITE
255 West 62nd Ave
Vancouver BC V5X 4V4
Tel. 604 325-4116
Fax 604 806-9756
www.providencehealthcare.org

PROVIDENCE HEALTH CARE -YOUVILLE RESIDENCE
4950 Heather St
Vancouver BC V5Z 3L9
Tel. 604 261-9371
Fax 604 261-9047
www.providencehealthcare.org

SUNNY HILL HEALTH CENTRE FOR CHILDREN
3644 Slocan St
Vancouver BC V5M 3E8
Tel. 604 453-8300
Fax 604 453-8301
www.bcchildrens.ca

UBC HOSPITAL - DETWILLER PAVILION
2255 Wesbrook Mall
Vancouver BC V6T 2A1
Tel. 604 822-7118
Fax 604 822-7653
www.vch.ca

UBC HOSPITAL - KOERNER PAVILLION
2211 Wesbrook Mall
Vancouver BC V6T 2B5
Tel. 604 822-7121
Fax 604 822-7186
www.brain.ubc.ca

UBC HOSPITAL - PURDY PAVILLION
2221 Wesbrook Mall
Vancouver BC V6T 1Z9
Tel. 604 822-7131
www.vch.ca

VANCOUVER GENERAL HOSPITAL - CENTENNIAL PAVILLION
855 12th Ave W
Vancouver BC V5Z 1M9
Tel. 604 875-4111
Fax 604 875-4686
www.vch.ca

VANDERHOOF

CARRIER SEKANI FAMILY SERVICES
240 W Stewart St
PO BOX 1219
Vanderhoof BC V0J 3A0
Tel. 250 567-2900
Fax 250 567-2975
www.csfs.org

ST JOHN HOSPITAL
3255 Hospital Rd
Vanderhoof BC V0J 3A2
Tel. 250 567-2211
Fax 250 567-9713
www.northernhealth.ca

VERNON

OKANAGAN INDIAN HEALTH DEPARTMENT
12420 Westside Rd
Vernon BC V1H 2A9
Tel. 250 542-4328
Fax 250 542-4990
www.okib.ca

VERNON JUBILEE HOSPITAL
2101 32 St
Vernon BC V1T 5L2
Tel. 250 545-2211
Fax 250 545-5602
www.interiorhealth.ca

VICTORIA

ABERDEEN HOSPITAL
1450 Hillside Ave
Victoria BC V8T 2B7
Tel. 250 370-5626
Fax 250 370-5610
www.viha.ca

ADULT FORENSIC PSYCHIATRIC COMMUNITY SERVICES
2840 Nanaimo St
Victoria BC V8T 4W9
Tel. 250 213-4500
Fax 250 213-4532
www.bcmhas.ca

BC CANCER AGENCY VANCOUVER ISLAND CENTRE
2410 Lee Ave
Victoria BC V8R 6V5
Tel. 250 519-5500
Fax 250 519-2002
www.bccancer.bc.ca

CANADIAN FORCES HEALTH SERVICES - PACIFIC CENTRE
1200 Colville Rd
PO Box 17000 Stn Forces
Victoria BC V9A 4P7
Tel. 250 363-4112
Fax 250 363-4119

COOL AID COMMUNITY HEALTH CENTRE
713 Johnson St
Victoria BC V8W 1M8
Tel. 250 385-1466
Fax 250 383-1327

GLENGARRY HOSPITAL
1780 Fairfield Rd
Victoria BC V8S 1G7
Tel. 250 370-5626
Fax 250 370-5727
www.viha.ca

GORGE ROAD HOSPITAL
63 Gorge Rd E
Victoria BC V9A 1L2
Tel. 250 519-3500
Fax 250 995-4759
www.viha.ca

MOUNT ST MARY HOSPITAL
861 Fairfield Rd
Victoria BC V8V 5A9
Tel. 250 480-3100
Fax 250 480-3110
www.mtstmary.victoria.bc.ca

MOUNT TOLMIE HOSPITAL
3690 Richmond Rd
Victoria BC V8P 4R6
Tel. 250 370-5626
Fax 250 370-5755
www.viha.ca

PRIORY HOSPITAL
567 Goldstream Ave
Victoria BC V9B 2W4
Tel. 250 370-5626
Fax 250 370-5779
www.viha.ca

QUEEN ALEXANDRA CENTRE FOR CHILDREN'S HEALTH
2400 Arbutus Rd
Victoria BC V8N 1V7
Tel. 250 519-5390
Fax 250 721-6837
www.viha.ca

ROYAL JUBILEE HOSPITAL
1952 Bay St
Victoria BC V8R 1J8
Tel. 250 370-8000
Fax 250 370-8750
www.viha.ca

SANDRINGHAM CARE CENTRE
1650 Fort St
Victoria BC V8R 1H9
Tel. 250 595-2313
Fax 250 595-4137

VICTORIA GENERAL HOSPITAL
1 Hospital Way
Victoria BC V8Z 6R5
Tel. 250 727-4212
Fax 250 727-4106
www.viha.ca

VICTORIA HOSPICE - PALLIATIVE CARE
1952 Bay St
Victoria BC V8R 1J8
Tel. 250 370-8715
Fax 250 370-8625
www.victoriahospice.org

VICTORIA YOUTH FORENSIC PSYCHIATRIC SERVICES
1515 Quadra St
Victoria BC V8V 3P3
Tel. 250 387-2830
Fax 250 387-3217
www.mcf.gov.bc.ca

WHISTLER

WHISTLER HEALTH CARE CENTRE
201-4380 Lorimer Rd
RR 4
Whistler BC V0N 1B4
Tel. 604 932-3977
Fax 604 932-0660

WHITE ROCK

PEACE ARCH HOSPITAL
15521 Russell Ave
White Rock BC V4B 2R4
Tel. 604 531-5512
Fax 604 541-5862
www.peacearchhospital.com

WILLIAMS LAKE

CARIBOO HEALTH UNIT
3F-540 Borland St
Williams Lake BC V2G 1R8
Tel. 250 302-5000
www.interiorhealth.ca

CARIBOO MEMORIAL HOSPITAL AND HEALTH CENTRE
517 Sixth Ave N
Williams Lake BC V2G 2G8
Tel. 250 392-4411
Fax 250 392-2157
www.interiorhealth.ca

MENTAL HEALTH ADDICTION SERVICES - WILLIAMS LAKE
487 Borland St
Williams Lake BC V2G 1R9
Tel. 250 392-1483
Fax 250 398-4484
www.interiorhealth.ca

THREE CORNERS HEALTH SERVICES SOCIETY
PO Box 4728
Williams Lake BC V2G 1Y8
Tel. 250 398-9814
Fax 250 398-9824

WINDERMERE

COLUMBIA LAKE HEALTH STATION
3048 Hwy 93/95
Windermere BC V0B 2L2
Tel. 250 342-6379
Fax 250 342-6279

ZEBALLOS

ZEBALLOS HEALTH CENTRE
500 Pkwy Dr
Zeballos BC V0P 2A0
Tel. 250 761-4274
Fax 250 761-4027
www.viha.ca

MANITOBA

ALTONA

ALTONA COMMUNITY MEMORIAL HEALTH CENTRE/EASTVIEW PLACE
240 5th Ave NE
PO Box 660
Altona MB R0G 0B0
Tel. 204 324-2280
Fax 204 324-1299
www.rha-central.mb.ca

AMARANTH

BIRDTAIL SIOUX HEALTH OFFICE
PO Box 190
Beulah MB R0H 0B0
Tel. 204 568-4545
Fax 204 568-4615

ARBORG

ARBORG & DISTRICT HEALTH CENTRE
234 Gislason St
PO Box 10
Arborg MB R0C 0A0
Tel. 204 376-5247
Fax 204 376-5669
www.irha.mb.ca

ASHERN

LAKESHORE HEALTH CENTRE
1 Steenson Dr
PO Box 110
Ashern MB R0C 0E0
Tel. 204 768-2461
Fax 204 768-2337
www.irha.mb.ca

BALDUR

BALDUR HEALTH CENTRE
531 Elizabeth Ave E
PO Box 128
Baldur MB R0K 0B0
Tel. 204 535-2373
Fax 204 535-2116
www.assiniboine-rha.ca

BEAUSÉJOUR

BEAUSEJOUR DISTRICT HOSPITAL
151 1st St S
PO Box 550
Beausejour MB R0E 0C0
Tel. 204 268-1076
Fax 204 268-1207
www.neha.mb.ca

BENITO

BENITO HEALTH CENTRE
200 1st Ave
PO Box 490
Benito MB R0L 0C0
Tel. 204 539-2815
Fax 204 539-2482
www.prha.mb.ca

BERENS RIVER

BERENS RIVER NURSING STATION
PO Box 131
Berens River MB R0B 0A0
Tel. 204 382-2265
Fax 204 382-2005
www.First Nations & Inuit Hlth

BINSCARTH

GAMBLER HEALTH OFFICE
Box 250
Binscarth MB R0J 0G0
Tel. 204 532-2192
Fax 204 532-2359
www.prdp1.ctt.gov.mb.ca

BIRCH RIVER

INDIAN BIRCH HEALTH OFFICE (WUSKWI SIPIKH)
Gen Del
Box 188
Birch River MB R0L 0E0
Tel. 204 236-4894
Fax 204 236-4836

BIRTLE

BIRTLE HEALTH CENTRE
843 Gertrude St
PO Box 2000
Birtle MB R0M 0C0
Tel. 204 842-3317
Fax 204 842-3375
www.assiniboine-rha.ca

BLOODVEIN

BLOODVEIN NURSING STATION
GD
Bloodvein MB R0C 0J0
Tel. 204 395-2161
Fax 204 395-2087

BOISSEVAIN

BOISSEVAIN HEALTH CENTRE
305 Mill Rd
PO Box 899
Boissevain MB R0K 0E0
Tel. 204 534-2451
Fax 204 534-6487
www.assiniboine-rha.ca

BRANDON

BRANDON REGIONAL HEALTH CENTRE
150 McTavish Ave E
Brandon MB R7A 2B3
Tel. 204 578-4000
Fax 204 578-4969
www.brandonrha.mb.ca

BROCHET

BROCHET NURSING STATION
General Delivery
Brochet MB R0B 0B0
Tel. 204 323-2120
Fax 204 323-2650

CAMPERVILLE

PINE CREEK HEALTH CENTRE
PO Box 70
Camperville MB R0L 0J0
Tel. 204 524-2422
Fax 204 524-2801

CARBERRY

CARBERRY PLAINS HEALTH CENTRE
220 1st Ave
PO Box 2000
Carberry MB R0K 0H0
Tel. 204 834-2144
Fax 204 834-3333
www.assiniboine-rha.ca

CARMAN

CARMAN MEMORIAL HOSPITAL
350 4th St SW
PO Box 610
Carman MB R0G 0J0
Tel. 204 745-2021
Fax 204 745-2756
www.rha-central.mb.ca

CARTWRIGHT

DAVIDSON MEMORIAL HEALTH CENTRE
345 Division St
Box 118
Cartwright MB R0K 0L0
Tel. 204 529-2483
Fax 204 529-2562
www.assiniboine-rha.ca

CHURCHILL

CHURCHILL HEALTH CENTRE
PO Box 2500
Churchill MB R0B 0E0
Tel. 204 675-8318
Fax 204 675-2243

CORMORANT

CORMORANT HEALTH CENTRE
Box 42
Cormorant MB R0B 0G0
Tel. 204 357-2161
Fax 204 357-2259

CRANBERRY PORTAGE

CRANBERRY PORTAGE WELLNESS CENTRE
PO Box 186
Cranberry Portage MB R0B 0H0
Tel. 204 472-3338
Fax 204 472-3389
www.norman-rha.mb.ca

CRANE RIVER

O-CHI-CHAK-KO-SIPI HEALTH CENTRE
Gen Del
Crane River MB R0L 0M0
Tel. 204 732-2076
Fax 204 732-2422

CROSS LAKE

CROSS LAKE NURSING STATION
PO Box 160
Cross Lake MB R0B 0J0
Tel. 204 676-2011
Fax 204 676-2055

CRYSTAL CITY

ROCK LAKE HEALTH DISTRICT HOSPITAL
135 Machray Ave
PO Box 130
Crystal City MB R0K 0N0
Tel. 204 873-2132
Fax 204 873-2185
www.rocklakehealthdistrict.ca

DAKOTA TIPI

DAKOTA TIPI HEALTH CENTRE
1090 Dakota Dr
Dakota Tipi MB R1N 3X6
Tel. 204 857-9715
Fax 204 856-0279

DALLAS

KINONJEOSHTEGON HEALTH CENTRE (JACKHEAD)
PO Box 30
Dallas MB R0C 0S0
Tel. 204 394-2220
Fax 204 394-2194

DAUPHIN

DAUPHIN REGIONAL HEALTH CENTRE
625 3rd St SW
Dauphin MB R7N 1R7
Tel. 204 638-3010
Fax 204 638-4471
www.prha.mb.ca

DELORAINE

DELORAINE HEALTH CENTRE
109 Kellett St
PO Box 447
Deloraine MB R0M 0M0
Tel. 204 747-2745
Fax 204 747-2160
www.assiniboine-rha.ca

EDWIN

DAKOTA PLAINS HEALTH CENTRE
PO Box 9
Edwin MB R0H 0G0
Tel. 204 252-2830
Fax 204 252-2111

ELPHINSTONE

KEESEEKOWENIN HEALTH CENTRE
PO Box 130
Elphinstone MB R0J 0N0
Tel. 204 625-2043
Fax 204 625-2171

EMERSON

EMERSON HEALTH CENTRE
26 Main St
PO Box 428
Emerson MB R0A 0L0
Tel. 204 373-2109
Fax 204 373-2748
www.rha-central.mb.ca

ERICKSON

ERICKSON HEALTH CENTRE
60 Queen Elizabeth St
PO Box 25
Erickson MB R0J 0P0
Tel. 204 636-7777
Fax 204 636-2471
www.assiniboine-rha.ca

ROLLING RIVER HEALTH OFFICE
PO Box 246
Erickson MB R0J 0P0
Tel. 204 636-2989
Fax 204 636-2307
www.prdp1.ctt.gov.mb.ca

ERIKSDALE

ELIZABETH M CROWE MEMORIAL HOSPITAL
40 Railway Ave
PO Box 130
Eriksdale MB R0C 0W0
Tel. 204 739-2611
Fax 204 739-2065
www.ierha.ca

FAIRFORD

PINAYMOOTANG HEALTH CENTRE
Gen Del
Fairfords First Nations Hlth
Fairford MB R0C 0X0
Tel. 204 659-5786
Fax 204 659-5841

FLIN FLON

FLIN FLON GENERAL HOSPITAL INC
50 Church St
PO Box 340 Stn Main
Flin Flon MB R8A 1N2
Tel. 204 687-7591
Fax 204 687-8494
www.norman-rha.mb.ca

GILBERT PLAINS

GILBERT PLAINS COMMUNITY HEALTH CENTRE
100 Cutforth St North
PO Box 368
Gilbert Plains MB R0L 0X0
Tel. 204 638-2118
Fax 204 548-2516
www.prha.mb.ca

GILLAM

FOX LAKE HEALTH OFFICE
PO Box 369
Gillam MB R0B 0L0
Tel. 204 652-2954
Fax 204 652-6519

GILLAM HOSPITAL
115 Gillam Dr
PO Box 2000
Gillam MB R0B 0L0
Tel. 204 652-2600
Fax 204 652-2536
www.brha.mb.ca

GIMLI

GIMLI COMMUNITY HEALTH CENTRE (JOHNSON MEMORIAL HOSPITAL)
120 Sixth Ave
PO Box 250
Gimli MB R0C 1B0
Tel. 204 642-5116
Fax 204 642-5860
www.irha.mb.ca

GINEW

ROSEAU RIVER HEALTH CENTRE
PO Box 90
Ginew MB R0A 2R0
Tel. 204 427-2384
Fax 204 427-2484
www.prdp1.ctt.gov.mb.ca

GLADSTONE

SEVEN REGIONS HEALTH CENTRE
24 Mills St
PO Box 1000
Gladstone MB R0J 0T0
Tel. 204 385-2968
Fax 204 385-3053
www.rha-central.mb.ca

GLENBORO

GLENBORO HEALTH DISTRICT HOSPITAL
219 Murray St
PO Box 310
Glenboro MB R0K 0X0
Tel. 204 827-2438
Fax 204 827-2199
www.assiniboine-rha.ca

GOD'S LAKE NARROWS

GOD'S LAKE NARROWS NURSING STATION
GD
Gods Lake Narrows
MB R0B 0M0
Tel. 204 335-2557
Fax 204 335-2043
www.prdp1.ctt.gov.mb.ca

GODS RIVER

GOD'S RIVER NURSING STATION
Gen Del
Gods River MB R0B 0N0
Tel. 204 366-2355
Fax 204 366-2474
www.prdp1.ctt.gov.mb.ca

GRAND RAPIDS

GRAND RAPIDS HEALTH CENTRE
Box 351
Grand Rapids MB R0C 1E0
Tel. 204 639-2417
Fax 204 639-2332

GRANDVIEW

GRANDVIEW DISTRICT HOSPITAL
644 Mill St
PO Box 339
Grandview MB R0L 0Y0
Tel. 204 546-2425
Fax 204 546-3269
www.prha.mb.ca

GYPSUMVILLE

DAUPHIN RIVER HEALTH CENTRE
PO Box 129
Gypsumville MB R0C 1J0
Tel. 204 659-5370
Fax 204 659-2109
www.prdp1.ctt.gov.mb.ca

HAMIOTA

HAMIOTA DISTRICT HEALTH CENTRE
177 Birch Ave
Hamiota MB R0M 0T0
Tel. 204 764-2412
Fax 204 764-2049
www.assiniboine-rha.ca

HARTNEY

HARTNEY HEALTH CENTRE
PO Box 280
Hartney MB R0M 0X0
Tel. 204 858-2054
Fax 204 858-2303
www.assiniboine-rha.ca

HODGSON

PERCY E MOORE HOSPITAL
PO Box 190
Hodgson MB R0C 1N0
Tel. 204 372-8444
Fax 204 372-6991

ILFORD

ILFORD COMMUNITY HEALTH CENTRE
Gen Delivery
Ilford MB R0B 0S0
Tel. 204 288-4315
Fax 204 288-4371

ISLAND LAKE

GARDEN HILL NURSING STATION
General Delivery
Island Lake MB R0B 0T0
Tel. 204 456-2343
Fax 204 456-2866
www.prdp1.ctt.gov.mb.ca

KILLARNEY

TRI-LAKE HEALTH CENTRE
86 Ellise Dr
PO Box 5000
Killarney MB R0K 1G0
Tel. 204 523-4661
Fax 204 523-8948
www.assiniboine-rha.ca

KOOSTATAK

FISHER RIVER HEALTH CENTRE
Box 362
Koostatak MB R0C 1S0
Tel. 204 645-2689
Fax 204 645-2461
www.prdp1.ctt.gov.mb.ca

LAC BROCHET

LAC BROCHET NURSING STATION
General Delivery
Lac Brochet MB R0B 2E0
Tel. 204 337-2161
Fax 204 337-2143

LAC DU BONNET

LAC DU BONNET DISTRICT HEALTH CENTRE
89 McIntosh St
Lac du Bonnet MB R0E 1A0
Tel. 204 345-8647
Fax 204 345-8609
www.ierha.ca

LEAF RAPIDS

LEAF RAPIDS PRIMARY HEALTH CENTRE
PO Box 370
Leaf Rapids MB R0B 1W0
Tel. 204 473-2441
Fax 204 473-8273
www.brha.mb.ca

LITTLE-GRAND-RAPIDS

LITTLE GRAND RAPIDS NURSING STATION
General Delivery
Ltle-Grnd-Rap MB R0B 0V0
Tel. 204 397-2115
Fax 204 397-2016

PAUINGASSI NURSING STATION
PO Box 32
Paungassi MB R0B 0V0
Tel. 204 397-2395
Fax 204 397-2104
www.prdp1.ctt.gov.mb.ca

LYNN LAKE

LYNN LAKE HOSPITAL
PO Box 2030
Lynn Lake MB R0B 0W0
Tel. 204 356-2474
Fax 204 356-8023
www.brha.mb.ca

MACGREGOR

MACGREGOR & DISTRICT HEALTH CENTRE
87 Grafton St S
PO Box 250
MacGregor MB R0H 0R0
Tel. 204 685-2850
Fax 204 685-2529
www.rha-central.mb.ca

MANITOU

PEMBINA-MANITOU HEALTH CENTRE
232 Carrie St
PO Box 129
Manitou MB R0G 1G0
Tel. 204 242-2744
Fax 204 242-3062
www.rha-central.mb.ca

MARIUS

SANDY BAY HEALTH CENTRE - MARIUS
Box 110
Marius MB R0H 0T0
Tel. 204 843-2304
Fax 204 843-3088
www.prdp1.ctt.gov.mb.ca

MCCREARY

MCCREARY / ALONSA HEALTH CENTRE
613 Government Rd
PO Box 250
McCreary MB R0J 1B0
Tel. 204 835-2482
Fax 204 835-2713
www.prha.mb.ca

MELITA

MELITA HEALTH CENTRE
147 Summit St
PO Box 459
Melita MB R0M 1L0
Tel. 204 522-3403
Fax 204 522-3161
www.assiniboine-rha.ca

MINNEDOSA

MINNEDOSA HEALTH CENTRE
334 1st St SW
PO Box 960
Minnedosa MB R0J 1E0
Tel. 204 867-2701
Fax 204 867-2239
www.assiniboine-rha.ca

MORRIS

MORRIS GENERAL HOSPITAL
215 Railroad Ave E
PO Box 519
Morris MB R0G 1K0
Tel. 204 746-2301
Fax 204 746-2197
www.rha-central.mb.ca

NEEPAWA

NEEPAWA DISTRICT MEMORIAL HOSPITAL
500 Hospital St
PO Box 1240
Neepawa MB R0J 1H0
Tel. 204 476-2394
Fax 204 476-5007
www.assiniboine-rha.ca

NEGGINAN

POPLAR RIVER NURSING STATION
GD
Negginan MB R0B 0Z0
Tel. 204 244-2102
Fax 204 244-2001
www.prdp1.ctt.gov.mb.ca

NORWAY HOUSE

NORWAY HOUSE INDIAN HOSPITAL
PO Box 730
Norway House MB R0B 1B0
Tel. 204 359-6731
Fax 204 359-6599
www.prdp1.ctt.gov.mb.ca

NOTRE DAME DE LOURDES

NOTRE DAME HOSPITAL
283 Notre Dame Ave W
PO Box 130
Notre-Dame-Lourdes
MB R0G 1M0
Tel. 204 248-2112
Fax 204 248-2499
www.rha-central.mb.ca

OAKBANK

KIN PLACE PRIMARY HEALTH CARE CENTRE
689 Main St
Box 28
Oakbank MB R0E 1J0
Tel. 204 444-2227
Fax 204 444-7851
www.ierha.ca

O'HANLY

BLACK RIVER HEALTH CENTRE
Gen Delivery
O'Hanly MB R0E 1K0
Tel. 204 367-8089
Fax 204 367-4188
www.prdp1.ctt.gov.mb.ca

OXFORD HOUSE

OXFORD HOUSE NURSING STATION
Gen Del
Oxford House MB R0B 1C0
Tel. 204 538-2347
Fax 204 538-2445
www.prdp1.ctt.gov.mb.ca

THE PAS

CREE NATION TRIBAL HEALTH CENTRE
PO Box 2760
The Pas MB R9A 1M5
Tel. 204 627-1500
Fax 204 623-7809

THE PAS (OTINEKA) HEALTH CENTRE
PO Box 509
The Pas MB R9A 1K6
Tel. 204 627-7025
Fax 204 623-5496
www.prdp1.ctt.gov.mb.ca

ST. ANTHONY GENERAL HOSPITAL
67 1st St W
PO Box 240
The Pas MB R9A 1K4
Tel. 204 623-6431
Fax 204 623-9263
www.norman-rha.mb.ca

PEGUIS

PEGUIS HEALTH CENTRE
PO Box 690
Peguis MB R0C 3J0
Tel. 204 645-2869
Fax 204 645-2874
www.rdp1.ctt.gov.mb.ca

PELICAN RAPIDS

SAPOTAWEYAK CREE NATION HEALTH CENTRE
PO Box 149
Pelican Rapids MB R0L 1L0
Tel. 204 587-2058
Fax 204 587-2072
www.scnha.com

PINAWA

PINAWA HOSPITAL
30 Vanier Dr
PO Box 220
Pinawa MB R0E 1L0
Tel. 204 753-2334
Fax 204 753-2219
www.ierha.ca

PINE FALLS

FORT ALEXANDER HEALTH CENTRE
PO Box 70
Pine Falls MB R0E 1M0
Tel. 204 367-2208
Fax 204 367-4587
www.ierha.ca

PINE FALLS HEALTH COMPLEX
37 Maple St
PO Box 2000
Pine Falls MB R0E 1M0
Tel. 204 367-4441
Fax 204 367-8981
www.ierha.ca

PIPESTONE

CANUPAWAKPA HEALTH OFFICE
Old Lake Sioux
PO Box 11
Pipestone MB R0M 1T0
Tel. 204 854-2990
Fax 204 854-2221

PORTAGE LA PRAIRIE

LONG PLAINS HEALTH CENTRE
PO Box 580
Portage la Prairie MB R1N 3B9
Tel. 204 252-2369
Fax 204 252-2898
www.prdp1.ctt.gov.mb.ca

MANITOBA DEVELOPMENTAL CENTRE
840 3rd St NE
PO Box 1190 Stn Main
Portage La Prairie MB R1N 3C6
Tel. 204 856-4200
Fax 204 856-4258

PORTAGE DISTRICT GENERAL HOSPITAL
524 5th St SE
Portage La Prairie MB R1N 3A8
Tel. 204 239-2211
Fax 204 239-1941
www.rha-central.mb.ca

PUKATAWAGAN

NIKAWAY HEALTH CENTRE
Missisippi River
GD
Pukatawagan MB R0B 1G0
Tel. 204 553-2271
Fax 204 553-2241

PUKATAWAGAN NURSING STATION
GD
Pukatawagan MB R0B 1G0
Tel. 204 553-2271
Fax 204 553-2241

RED SUCKER LAKE

RED SUCKER LAKE NURSING STATION
General Delivery
Red Sucker Lake MB R0B 1H0
Tel. 204 469-5351
Fax 204 469-5769
www.prdp1.ctt.gov.mb.ca

RESTON

RESTON COMMUNITY HEALTH CENTRE
1st St N
PO Box 250
Reston MB R0M 1X0
Tel. 204 877-3925
Fax 204 877-3998
www.assiniboine-rha.ca

RIVERS

RIVERDALE HEALTH CENTRE
512 Quebec Street
PO Box 428
Rivers MB R0K 1X0
Tel. 204 328-5321
Fax 204 328-7130
www.assiniboine-rha.ca

ROBLIN

ROBLIN & DISTRICT HEALTH CENTRE
15 Hospital St
PO Box 940
Roblin MB R0L 1P0
Tel. 204 937-2142
Fax 204 937-8892
www.prha.mb.ca

ROSSBURN

ROSSBURN HEALTH CENTRE
116 Parkview Dr
PO Box 40
Rossburn MB R0J 1V0
Tel. 204 859-2413
Fax 204 859-2526
www.assiniboine-rha.ca

RUSSELL

RUSSELL HEALTH CENTRE
426 Alexandria Ave
PO Box 2
Russell MB R0J 1W0
Tel. 204 773-2125
Fax 204 773-2142
www.assiniboine-rha.ca

STE. ANNE

STE ANNE HOSPITAL
52 Gerard St
Ste Anne MB R5H 1C4
Tel. 204 422-8837
Fax 204 422-9929
www.sehealth.mb.ca

ST. CLAUDE

ST CLAUDE HEALTH CENTRE
33 Roy St
St Claude MB R0G 1Z0
Tel. 204 379-2585
Fax 204 379-2655
www.rha-central.mb.ca

ST. MARTIN

LITTLE SASKATCHEWAN HEALTH OFFICE
Gen Del
St. Martin MB R0C 2T0
Tel. 204 659-5278
Fax 204 659-5782

ST. PIERRE JOLYS

DESALABERRY DISTRICT HEALTH CENTRE
354 Prefontaine Ave
St Pierre Jolys MB R0A 1V0
Tel. 204 433-7611
Fax 204 433-7455
www.sehealth.mb.ca

STE. ROSE DU LAC

STE ROSE GENERAL HOSPITAL
480 Third Ave SE
PO Box 60
Ste Rose du Lac MB R0L 1S0
Tel. 204 447-2131
Fax 204 447-2250
www.prha.mb.ca

ST. THERESA POINT

ST THERESA POINT NURSING STATION
GD
St Theresa Point MB R0B 1J0
Tel. 204 462-2693
Fax 204 462-2642
www.prdp1.ctt.gov.mb.ca

SCANTERBURY

BROKENHEAD HEALTH CENTRE
PO Box 88
Scanterbury MB R0E 1W0
Tel. 204 766-2740
Fax 204 766-2634
www.prdp1.ctt.gov.mb.ca

SELKIRK

SELKIRK & DISTRICT GENERAL HOSPITAL
100 Easton Dr
PO Box 5000 Stn Main
Selkirk MB R1A 2M2
Tel. 204 482-5800
Fax 204 785-9113
www.ierha.ca

SELKIRK MENTAL HEALTH CENTRE
825 Manitoba Ave
PO Box 9600 Stn Main
Selkirk MB R1A 2B5
Tel. 204 482-3810
Fax 204 785-8936
www.gov.mb.ca

SHAMATTAWA

SHAMATTAWA NURSING STATION
General Delivery
Shamattawa MB R0B 1K0
Tel. 204 565-2370
Fax 204 565-2519
www.prdp1.ctt.gov.mb.ca

SHERRIDON

SHERRIDON HEALTH CENTRE
Gen Del
Sherridon MB R0B 1L0
Tel. 204 468-2012
Fax 204 468-2167

SHOAL LAKE

SHOAL LAKE/STRATHCLAIR HEALTH CENTRE
524 Mary St
PO Box 490
Shoal Lake MB R0J 1Z0
Tel. 204 759-2336
Fax 204 759-2230
www.assiniboine-rha.ca

SNOW LAKE

SNOW LAKE HEALTH CENTRE
PO Box 453
Snow Lake MB R0B 1M0
Tel. 204 358-2287
Fax 204 358-7310
www.norman-rha.mb.ca/

SOURIS

SOURIS HEALTH CENTRE
155 Brindle St
PO Box 10
Souris MB R0K 2C0
Tel. 204 483-2121
Fax 204 483-2310
www.assiniboine-rha.ca

SOUTH INDIAN LAKE

SOUTH INDIAN LAKE NURSING STATION
PO Box 22
South Indian Lake MB R0B 1N0
Tel. 204 374-2013
Fax 204 374-2039
www.prdp1.ctt.gov.mb.ca

SPLIT LAKE

SPLIT LAKE NURSING STATION
GD
Split Lake MB R0B 1P0
Tel. 204 342-2033
Fax 204 342-2319
www.prdp1.ctt.gov.mb.ca

STEINBACH

BETHESDA HOSPITAL STEINBACH
316 Henry St
Steinbach MB R5G 0P9
Tel. 204 326-6411
Fax 204 326-6931
www.sehealth.mb.ca

STONEWALL

STONEWALL & DISTRICT HEALTH CENTRE
601 3rd Ave S
Stonewall MB R0C 2Z0
Tel. 204 467-5514
Fax 204 467-4431
www.ierha.ca

SWAN LAKE

LORNE MEMORIAL HOSPITAL
9 2nd St N
PO Box 40
Swan Lake MB R0G 2S0
Tel. 204 836-2132
Fax 204 836-2044
www.rha-central.mb.ca

SWAN LAKE HEALTH CENTRE
9 2nd St N
Swan Lake MB R0G 2S0
Tel. 204 836-2132
Fax 204 836-2044
www.rha-central.mb.ca

SWAN RIVER

SWAN RIVER VALLEY HOSPITAL
1011 Main St
PO Box 1450
Swan River MB R0L 1Z0
Tel. 204 734-3441
Fax 204 734-9081
www.prha.mb.ca

TADOULE LAKE

TADOULE LAKE NURSING STATION
Gen Del
Tadoule Lake MB R0B 2C0
Tel. 204 684-2031
Fax 204 684-2049

TEULON

TEULON/HUNTER MEMORIAL HOSPITAL
PO Box 89
Teulon MB R0C 3B0
Tel. 204 886-2433
Fax 204 886-2653
www.ierha.ca

THOMPSON

THOMPSON GENERAL HOSPITAL
871 Thompson Dr
Thompson MB R8N 0C8
Tel. 204 677-2381
Fax 204 778-1508
www.brha.mb.ca

TREHERNE

TIGER HILLS HEALTH DISTRICT
64 Clark St
PO Box 130
Treherne MB R0G 2V0
Tel. 204 723-2133
Fax 204 723-2869
www.assiniboine-rha.ca

VIRDEN

VIRDEN HEALTH CENTRE
480 King St E
PO Box 400
Virden MB R0M 2C0
Tel. 204 748-1230
Fax 204 748-2053
www.assiniboine-rha.ca

VITA

VITA & DISTRICT HEALTH CENTRE
217 First Ave W
PO Box 160
Vita MB R0A 2K0
Tel. 204 425-3804
Fax 204 425-3545
www.sehealth.mb.ca

WAASAGOMACH

WASAGAMACK NURSING STATION
GD
Waasagomach MB R0B 1Z0
Tel. 204 457-2024
Fax 204 457-2348
www.prdp1.ctt.gov.mb.ca

WANIPIGOW

ADAM HARDISTY (HOLLOW WATER)
PO Box 2567
Wanipigow MB R0E 2E0
Tel. 204 363-7364
Fax 204 363-7201
www.prdp1.ctt.gov.mb.ca

WAWANESA

WAWANESA & DISTRICT MEMORIAL HEALTH CENTRE
506 George St
PO Box 309
Wawanesa MB R0K 2G0
Tel. 204 824-2335
Fax 204 824-2148
www.assiniboine-rha.ca

WAYWAYSEECAPPO

WAYWAYSEECAPPO HEALTH CENTRE
PO Box 129
Waywayseecappo MB R0J 1S0
Tel. 204 859-2311
Fax 204 859-2998
www.prdp1.ctt.gov.mb.ca

WHITEMOUTH

WHITEMOUTH DISTRICT HEALTH CENTRE
75 Hospital St
PO Box 160
Whitemouth MB R0E 2G0
Tel. 204 348-7191
Fax 204 348-7911
www.ierha.ca

WINKLER

BOUNDARY TRAILS HEALTH CENTRE
PO Box 2000 Stn Main
Winkler MB R6W 1H8
Tel. 204 331-8820
Fax 204 331-8801
www.rha-central.mb.ca

EDEN HEALTH CARE SERVICES
309 Main St
PO Box 129
Winkler MB R6W 4A4
Tel. 204 325-5355
Fax 204 325-8742
www.edenhealth.mb.ca

EDEN MENTAL HEALTH CENTRE
1500 Pembina Ave
Winkler MB R6W 1T4
Tel. 204 325-4325
Fax 204 325-8429
www.edenhealth.mb.ca

PATHWAYS COMMUNITY MENTAL HEALTH SERVICES
351 Main St
PO Box 1840 Stn Main
Winkler MB R6W 4B6
Tel. 204 325-0946
Fax 204 325-0834
www.edenhealth.mb.ca

WINNIPEG

CONCORDIA GENERAL HOSPITAL
1095 Concordia Ave
Winnipeg MB R2K 3S8
Tel. 204 667-1560
Fax 204 667-1049
www.concordiahospital.mb.ca

HEALTH ACTION CENTRE - HEALTH SCIENCES CENTRE
425 Elgin Ave
Winnipeg MB R3A 1P2
Tel. 204 947-1626
Fax 204 942-7828
www.hsc.mb.ca

HEALTH SCIENCES CENTRE
820 Sherbrook St
Winnipeg MB R3A 1R9
Tel. 204 774-8511
Fax 204 787-3912
www.hsc.mb.ca

HOPE CENTRE HEALTH CARE INC
240 Powers St
Winnipeg MB R2W 5L1
Tel. 204 589-8354
Fax 204 586-4260

KLINIC COMMUNITY HEALTH CENTRE
870 Portage Ave
Winnipeg MB R3G 0P1
Tel. 204 784-4090
Fax 204 772-7998
www.klinic.mb.ca

MANITOBA ADOLESCENT TREATMENT CENTRE
120 Tecumseh St
Winnipeg MB R3E 2A9
Tel. 204 477-6391
Fax 204 783-8948
www.matc.ca

MISERICORDIA HEALTH CENTRE
99 Cornish Ave
Winnipeg MB R3C 1A2
Tel. 204 774-6581
Fax 204 783-6052
www.misericordia.mb.ca

NINE CIRCLES COMMUNITY HEALTH CENTRE
705 Broadway
Winnipeg MB R3G 0X2
Tel. 204 940-6000
Fax 204 940-6003
www.ninecircles.ca

NOR'WEST COOPERATIVE HEALTH & SOCIAL SERVICE CENTRE INC.
103-61 Tyndall Ave
Winnipeg MB R2X 2T4
Tel. 204 940-2020
Fax 204 632-4666
www.norwesthealth.ca

REHABILITATION CENTRE FOR CHILDREN
633 Wellington Cres
Winnipeg MB R3M 0A8
Tel. 204 452-4311
Fax 204 477-5547
www.rccinc.ca

RIVERVIEW HEALTH CENTRE
1 Morley Ave
Winnipeg MB R3L 2P4
Tel. 204 478-6203
Fax 204 478-6261
www.riverviewhealthcentre.com

ST BONIFACE GENERAL HOSPITAL
409 Tache Ave
Winnipeg MB R2H 2A6
Tel. 204 233-8563
Fax 204 231-0640
www.sbgh.mb.ca

THE SALVATION ARMY GRACE HOSPITAL
300 Booth Dr
Winnipeg MB R3J 3M7
Tel. 204 837-0391
Fax 204 831-0029
www.gracehospital.ca

SEVEN OAKS GENERAL HOSPITAL
2300 McPhillips St
Winnipeg MB R2V 3M3
Tel. 204 632-7133
Fax 204 697-2106
www.sogh.mb.ca

VICTORIA GENERAL HOSPITAL
2340 Pembina Hwy
Winnipeg MB R3T 2E8
Tel. 204 269-3570
Fax 204 261-0223
www.vgh.mb.ca

WRHA - DEER LODGE CENTRE
2109 Portage Ave
Winnipeg MB R3J 0L3
Tel. 204 837-1301
Fax 204 889-0430
www.deerlodge.mb.ca

WINNIPEGOSIS

WINNIPEGOSIS & DISTRICT HEALTH CENTRE
230 Bridge St
PO Box 280
Winnipegosis MB R0L 2G0
Tel. 204 656-4881
Fax 204 656-4402
www.prha.mb.ca

YORK LANDING

YORK LANDING NURSING STATION
Gen Del
York Landing MB R0B 2B0
Tel. 204 341-2325
Fax 204 341-2179
www.prdp1.ctt.gov.mb.ca

NEW BRUNSWICK

BATHURST

HOPITAL REGIONAL CHALEUR
1750 Sunset Dr
Bathurst NB E2A 4L7
Tel. 506 544-3000
Fax 506 544-2440
www.santevitalitehealth.ca

BELLEDUNE

JACQUET RIVER HEALTH CENTRE
41 Mack St
Belledune NB E8G 2R3
Tel. 506 237-3222
Fax 506 237-3224
www.santevitalitehealth.ca

BLACKS HARBOUR

FUNDY HEALTH CENTRE
34 Hospital St
Blacks Harbour NB E5H 1K2
Tel. 506 456-4200
Fax 506 456-4259
www.horizonnb.ca

BOIESTOWN

BOIESTOWN HEALTH CENTRE
2-6154 Route 8
Boiestown NB E6A 1M4
Tel. 506 369-2700
Fax 506 369-2702
www.horizonnb.ca

CAMPBELLTON

CENTRE HOSPITALIER RESTIGOUCHE
65 Gallant Dr
PO Box 10 Stn Main
Campbellton NB E3N 3G2
Tel. 506 789-7000
Fax 506 789-7065
www.santerestigouchehealth.com

HÔPITAL RÉGIONAL CAMPBELLTON
189 Lily Lake Rd
PO Box 880
Campbellton NB E3N 3H3
Tel. 506 789-5000
Fax 506 789-5025
www.santevitalitehealth.ca

CARAQUET

HÔPITAL DE L'ENFANT-JÉSUS RHSJ
1 boul St-Pierre O
Caraquet NB E1W 1B6
Tel. 506 726-2166
Fax 506 726-2188
www.santevitalitehealth.ca

CHIPMAN

CHIPMAN HEALTH CENTRE
9 Civic Crt
Chipman NB E4A 2H8
Tel. 506 339-7650
Fax 506 339-7652
www.horizonnb.ca

DALHOUSIE

CENTRE DE SANTÉ COMMUNITAIRE - ST-JOSEPH
1-280 Victoria St
Dalhousie NB E8C 2R6
Tel. 506 684-7000
Fax 506 684-4751
www.santevitalitehealth.ca

DEER ISLAND

DEER ISLAND HEALTH CENTRE
999 Route 772
Fairhaven NB E5V 1P2
Tel. 506 747-4150
Fax 506 747-4151
www.horizonnb.ca

DOAKTOWN

CENTRAL MIRAMICHI COMMUNITY HEALTH CENTRE
11 Prospect St
Doaktown NB E9C 1C3
Tel. 506 365-6100
Fax 506 365-6104
www.horizonnb.ca

EDMUNDSTON

HÔPITAL REGIONAL D'EDMUNDSTON
275 Hebert Blvd
Edmundston NB E3V 4E4
Tel. 506 739-2200
Fax 506 739-2248
www.santevitalitehealth.ca

FREDERICTON

DR EVERETT CHALMERS REGIONAL HOSPITAL
700 Priestman St
PO Box 9000 Stn A
Fredericton NB E3B 5N5
Tel. 506 452-5400
Fax 506 452-5500
www.horizonnb.ca

FREDERICTON ADDICTION SERVICES
65 Brunswick St
Fredericton NB E3B 1G5
Tel. 506 452-5558
Fax 506 452-5533
www.horizonnb.ca

STAN CASSIDY CENTRE FOR REHABILITATION
800 Priestman St
Fredericton NB E3B 0C7
Tel. 506 452-5225
Fax 506 443-2169
www.horizonnb.ca

FREDERICTON JUNCTION

FREDERICTON JUNCTION HEALTH CENTRE
233 Sunbury Dr
Fredericton-Jntn NB E5L 1S1
Tel. 506 368-6501
Fax 506 368-6502
www.horizonnb.ca

GRAND FALLS

HÔPITAL GÉNÉRAL DE GRAND-FALLS
625 boul Évérard H Daigle
PO Box 7061
Grand Falls NB E3Z 1J5
Tel. 506 473-7555
Fax 506 473-7530
www.santevitalitehealth.ca

GRAND MANAN ISLAND

GRAND MANAN ADDICTION AND MENTAL HEALTH SERVICES
3-130 Route 776
Grand Manan Island
NB E5G 1A3
Tel. 506 662-7023
Fax 506 662-7029
www.horizonnb.ca

GRAND MANAN HOSPITAL
196 Route 776
Grand Manan NB E5G 1A3
Tel. 506 662-4060
Fax 506 662-4050
www.horizonnb.ca

HARVEY

HARVEY HEALTH CENTRE
2019 Route 3
Harvey Station NB E6K 3E9
Tel. 506 366-6400
Fax 506 366-6403
www.horizonnb.ca

LAMÈQUE

HÔPITAL DE CSC DE LAMÈQUE
29 rue de L'Hopital
Lameque NB E8T 1C5
Tel. 506 344-2261
Fax 506 344-3403
www.santevitalitehealth.ca

MCADAM

MCADAM HEALTH CENTRE
15 Saunders Rd
PO Box 311
McAdam NB E6J 1K9
Tel. 506 784-6300
Fax 506 784-6306
www.horizonnb.ca

MINTO

QUEENS NORTH COMMUNITY HEALTH CENTRE
1100 Pleasant Dr
PO Box 1004
Minto NB E4B 3Y6
Tel. 506 327-7800
Fax 506 327-7899
www.horizonnb.ca

MIRAMICHI

MIRAMICHI HEALTH CENTRE
679 King George Hwy
Miramichi NB E1V 1N9
Tel. 506 627-7511
Fax 506 627-7515
www.horizonnb.ca

MIRAMICHI REGIONAL HOSPITAL
500 Water St
Miramichi NB E1V 3G5
Tel. 506 623-3000
Fax 506 623-3465
www.horizonnb.ca

MONCTON

DR GEORGES-L-DUMONT UNIVERSITY HOSPITAL CENTRE
330 av Universite
Moncton NB E1C 2Z3
Tel. 506 862-4000
Fax 506 862-4256
www.santevitalitehealth.ca

THE MONCTON HOSPITAL
135 MacBeath Ave
Moncton NB E1C 6Z8
Tel. 506 857-5111
Fax 506 857-5545
www.horizonnb.ca

NACKAWIC

NACKAWIC HEALTH CENTRE
201-135 Otis Dr
Nackawic NB E6G 1H1
Tel. 506 575-6600
Fax 506 575-6603
www.horizonnb.ca

NEGUAC

NEGUAC HEALTH CENTRE
38 Otho St
Neguac NB E9G 4H3
Tel. 506 776-3876
Fax 506 776-3877
www.horizonnb.ca

OROMOCTO

OROMOCTO PUBLIC HOSPITAL
103 Winnebago St
Oromocto NB E2V 1C6
Tel. 506 357-4710
Fax 506 357-4735
www.horizonnb.ca

PERTH-ANDOVER

HÔTEL-DIEU OF ST JOSEPH HOSPITAL
10 Woodland Hill
Perth-Andover NB E7H 5H5
Tel. 506 273-7100
Fax 506 273-7200
www.horizonnb.ca

PETITCODIAC

PETICODIAC HEALTH CENTRE
32 Railway Ave
Petitcodiac NB E4Z 6H4
Tel. 506 756-3400
Fax 506 756-3406
www.horizonnb.ca

PLASTER ROCK

TOBIQUE VALLEY COMMUNITY HEALTH CENTRE
120 Main St
Plaster Rock NB E7G 2E5
Tel. 506 356-6600
Fax 506 356-6618
www.horizonnb.ca

PORT ELGIN

PORT ELGIN AND REGION HEALTH CENTRE
33 Moore Rd
PO Box 1557
Port Elgin NB E4M 2E6
Tel. 506 538-2140
Fax 506 538-2142
www.horizonnb.ca

RIVERSIDE-ALBERT

ALBERT COUNTY HEALTH AND WELLNESS CENTRE
8 Forestdale Rd
Riverside-Albert NB E4H 3Y7
Tel. 506 882-3100
Fax 506 882-3101
www.horizonnb.ca

SACKVILLE

SACKVILLE MEMORIAL HOSPITAL
8 Main St
Sackville NB E4L 4A3
Tel. 506 364-4100
Fax 506 536-1983
www.horizonnb.ca

SAINTE-ANNE-DE-KENT

HÔPITAL STELLA-MARIS-DE-KENT
7714 Route 134
Sainte-Anne-de-Kent
NB E4S 1H5
Tel. 506 743-7800
Fax 506 743-7813
www.santevitalitehealth.ca

SAINT JOHN

CENTRACARE
414 Bay St
PO Box 3220 Stn B
Saint John NB E2M 7L4
Tel. 506 649-2550
Fax 506 649-2520
www.horizonnb.ca

MEDISANTE SAINT JEAN
67 Ragged Point Rd
Saint John NB E2K 5C3
Tel. 506 648-8020
Fax 506 648-8028
www.horizonnb.ca

RIDGEWOOD ADDICTION SERVICES TREATMENT CENTRE
416 Bay street
Saint John NB E2M 7L4
Tel. 506 674-4300
Fax 506 674-4374
www.horizonnb.ca

RIDGEWOOD VETERANS WING
422 Bay St
PO Box 2100
Saint John NB E2L 4L2
Tel. 506 635-2420
Fax 506 635-2425
www.horizonnb.ca

SAINT JOHN REGIONAL HOSPITAL
400 University Ave
PO Box 5200
Saint John NB E2L 4L2
Tel. 506 648-6000
Fax 506 648-6060
www.horizonnb.ca

ST JOSEPH'S HOSPITAL
130 Bayard Dr
Saint John NB E2L 3L6
Tel. 506 632-5555
Fax 506 632-5551
www.horizonnb.ca

WORKSAFE NB REHABILITATION CENTRE
1 Portland St
PO Box 160
Saint John NB E2L 3X9
Tel. 506 738-8411
Fax 506 738-3470
www.worksafenb.ca

SAINT-QUENTIN

HÔTEL-DIEU ST-JOSEPH DE SAINT-QUENTIN
9 Canada St
Saint-Quentin NB E8A 1J2
Tel. 506 235-2300
Fax 506 235-7202
www.santevitalitehealth.ca

ST. STEPHEN

CHARLOTTE COUNTY ADDICTION & MENTAL HEALTH SERVICES
41 King St
St Stephen NB E3L 2C1
Tel. 506 466-7380
Fax 506 466-7501
www.horizonnb.ca

CHARLOTTE COUNTY HOSPITAL
4 Garden St
St Stephen NB E3L 2L9
Tel. 506 465-4444
Fax 506 465-4418
www.horizonnb.ca

STANLEY

STANLEY HEALTH CENTRE
PO Box 340
Stanley NB E6B 2K5
Tel. 506 367-7730
Fax 506 367-7738
www.rivervalleyhealth.nb.ca

SUSSEX

SUSSEX HEALTH CENTRE
75 Leonard Dr
Sussex NB E4E 2P7
Tel. 506 432-3100
Fax 506 432-3106
www.horizonnb.ca

TRACADIE-SHEILA

HÔPITAL DE TRACADIE-SHEILA
400 rue des Hospitalieres
CP 3180 Stn Main
Tracadie-Sheila NB E1X 1G5
Tel. 506 394-3000
Fax 506 394-3034
www.santevitalitehealth.ca

WATERVILLE

UPPER RIVER VALLEY HOSPITAL - WATERVILLE
11300 Rte 130
Watervil-Carleton NB E7P 0A4
Tel. 506 375-3740
Fax 506 375-2681
www.horizonnb.ca

WELSHPOOL

CAMPOBELLO ISLAND HEALTH CENTRE
1-640 Route 774
Welshpool NB E5E 1A5
Tel. 506 752-4100
Fax 506 752-4101
www.horizonnb.ca

NEWFOUNDLAND AND LABRADOR

BAIE VERTE

BAIE VERTE PENINSULA HEALTH CENTRE
1 Columbus Dr
Baie Verte NL A0K 1B0
Tel. 709 532-4281
Fax 709 532-4939
www.centralhealth.nl.ca

BELL ISLAND

DR WALTER TEMPLEMAN HEALTH CENTRE
PO Box 580
Bell Island NL A0A 4H0
Tel. 709 488-2821
Fax 709 488-2600
www.easternhealth.ca

BLACK TICKLE

BLACK TICKLE NURSING STATION
GD
Black Tickle NL A0K 1N0
Tel. 709 471-8872
Fax 709 471-8893
www.lghealth.ca

BONAVISTA

BONAVISTA PENINSULA HEALTH CENTRE
123 Confederation Dr
PO Box 1510
Bonavista NL A0C 1B0
Tel. 709 468-7881
Fax 709 468-7690
www.easternhealth.ca

BROOKFIELD

BROOKFIELD BONNEWS HEALTH CARE CENTRE
PO Box 349
Brookfield NL A0G 1J0
Tel. 709 536-2405
Fax 709 536-2433
www.centralhealth.nl.ca

BUCHANS

A M GUY MEMORIAL HEALTH CENTRE
15 Water St
PO Box 10
Buchans NL A0H 1G0
Tel. 709 672-3304
Fax 709 672-3390
www.centralhealth.nl.ca

BURIN

BURIN PENINSULA HEALTH CARE CENTRE
51-85 Main St
PO Box 340
Burin NL A0E 1E0
Tel. 709 891-1040
Fax 709 891-3375
www.easternhealth.ca

CARBONEAR

CARBONEAR GENERAL HOSPITAL
86 Highroad S
Carbonear NL A1Y 1A4
Tel. 709 945-5111
Fax 709 945-5158
www.easternhealth.ca

CHANNEL-PORT-AUX -BASQUES

DR CHARLES L LEGROW HEALTH CENTRE
1 Grand Bay Rd
PO Box 250
Channel-Pab NL A0M 1C0
Tel. 709 695-2175 Ext. 546
Fax 709 695-3118
www.westernhealth.nl.ca

CHARLOTTETOWN (LABRADOR)

CHARLOTTETOWN NURSING STATION
GD
Charlottetown Lab NL A0K 5Y0
Tel. 709 949-0259
Fax 709 949-0317
www.lghealth.ca

CHURCHILL FALLS

CHURCHILL FALLS HEALTH CENTRE
1 Ossak St
PO Box 100 Stn Main
Churchill Falls NL A0R 1A0
Tel. 709 925-3381
Fax 709 925-3246
www.lghealth.ca

CLARENVILLE

THE DR G B CROSS MEMORIAL HOSPITAL
67 Manitoba Dr
Clarenville NL A5A 1K3
Tel. 709 466-3411
Fax 709 466-3300
www.easternhealth.ca

CORNER BROOK

WESTERN MEMORIAL REGIONAL HOSPITAL
1 Brookfield Ave
PO Box 2005 Stn Main
Corner Brook NL A2H 6J7
Tel. 709 637-5000
Fax 709 634-2649
www.westernhealth.nl.ca

FLOWER'S COVE

STRAIT OF BELLE ISLE HEALTH CENTRE
PO Box 59
Flowers Cove NL A0K 2N0
Tel. 709 456-2401
Fax 709 456-2562
www.lghealth.ca

FOGO

FOGO ISLAND HEALTH CENTRE
5-7 North Shore Rd
PO Box 9
Fogo NL A0G 2B0
Tel. 709 266-2221
Fax 709 266-2409
www.centralhealth.nl.ca

FORTEAU

LABRADOR SOUTH HEALTH CENTRE
1 Main St
PO Box 70
Forteau NL A0K 2P0
Tel. 709 931-2450
Fax 709 931-2000
www.lghealth.ca

GANDER

JAMES PATON MEMORIAL HOSPITAL
125 Trans Canada Hwy
Gander NL A1V 1P7
Tel. 709 256-2500
Fax 709 256-7800
www.centralhealth.nl.ca

GRAND BANK

GRAND BANK HEALTH CENTRE
3 Grandview Blvd
PO Box 310
Grand Bank NL A0E 1W0
Tel. 709 832-2500
Fax 709 832-1164
www.easternhealth.ca

GRAND FALLS-WINDSOR

CENTRAL NEWFOUNDLAND REGIONAL HEALTH CENTRE
50 Union St
Grnd-Falls-Wi NL A2A 2E1
Tel. 709 292-2500
Fax 709 292-2249
www.centralhealth.nl.ca

HAPPY VALLEY - GOOSE BAY

LABRADOR HEALTH CENTRE
227 Hamilton River Rd
PO Box 7000 Stn C
Happy-Valley-Goose
NL A0P 1C0
Tel. 709 897-2000
Fax 709 896-4032
www.lghealth.ca

HARBOUR BRETON

CONNAIGRE PENINSULA COMMUNITY HEALTH CENTRE
Alexander Ave
PO Box 70
Harbour Breton NL A0H 1P0
Tel. 709 885-2359
Fax 709 885-2358
www.centralhealth.nl.ca

HOPEDALE

HOPEDALE COMMUNITY CLINIC
General Delivery
Hopedale NL A0P 1G0
Tel. 709 933-3857
Fax 709 933-3744
www.lghealth.ca

LABRADOR CITY

CAPTAIN WILLIAM JACKMAN MEMORIAL HOSPITAL
410-410 Booth St
Labrador City NL A2V 2K1
Tel. 709 944-2632
Fax 709 944-6045
www.lghealth.ca

MAKKOVIK

MAKKOVIK NURSING STATION
GD
Box 58
Makkovik NL A0P 1J0
Tel. 709 923-2229
Fax 709 923-2428
www.lghealth.ca

MARY'S HARBOUR

MARY'S HARBOUR NURSING STATION
GD
Marys Harbour NL A0K 3P0
Tel. 709 921-6228
Fax 709 921-6975
www.lghealth.ca

NAIN

NAIN COMMUNITY HEALTH CENTRE
General Delivery
Nain NL A0P 1L0
Tel. 709 922-2912
Fax 709 922-2103
www.lghealth.ca

NORRIS POINT

BONNE BAY HEALTH CENTRE
131-13 Main St
PO Box 70
Norris Point NL A0K 3V0
Tel. 709 458-2201
Fax 709 458-3069
www.westernhealth.nl.ca

NORTH WEST RIVER

NORTH WEST RIVER MANI ASHINI HEALTH CENTRE
North West River NL A0P 1M0
Tel. 709 497-8202
Fax 709 497-8521
www.lghealth.ca

OLD PERLICAN

DR A A WILKINSON MEMORIAL HEALTH CENTRE
428-438 Station Dr
PO Box 70
Old Perlican NL A0A 3G0
Tel. 709 587-2200
Fax 709 587-2338
www.easternhealth.ca

PLACENTIA

PLACENTIA HEALTH CENTRE
PO Box 480
Placentia NL A0B 2Y0
Tel. 709 227-2061
Fax 709 227-5476
www.easternhealth.ca

PORT HOPE SIMPSON

PORT HOPE SIMPSON NURSING STATION
GD
Port Hope Simpson
NL A0K 4E0
Tel. 709 960-0271
Fax 709 960-0461
www.lghealth.ca

PORT SAUNDERS

RUFUS GUINCHARD HEALTH CENTRE
PO Box 40
Port Saunders NL A0K 4H0
Tel. 709 861-3533
Fax 709 861-3772
www.westernhealth.nl.ca

POSTVILLE

POSTVILLE NURSING STATION
GD
Postville NL A0P 1N0
Tel. 709 479-9851
Fax 709 479-9715
www.lghealth.ca

RIGOLET

RIGOLET NURSING STATION
General Delivery
Rigolet NL A0P 1P0
Tel. 709 947-3386
Fax 709 947-3401
www.lghealth.ca

RODDICKTON

WHITE BAY CENTRAL HEALTH CENTRE
PO Box 70
Roddickton NL A0K 4P0
Tel. 709 457-2215
Fax 709 457-2076
www.lghealth.ca

ST. ANTHONY

CHARLES S CURTIS MEMORIAL HOSPITAL
178-200 West St
St Anthony NL A0K 4S0
Tel. 709 454-3333
Fax 709 454-2052
www.lghealth.ca

ST. JOHN'S

DR H BLISS MURPHY CANCER CENTRE
300 Prince Phillip Dr
St. John's NL A1B 3V6
Tel. 709 752-6715
www.easternhealth.ca

DR LEONARD A MILLER CENTRE
100 Forest Rd
St. John's NL A1A 1E5
Tel. 709 777-6555
Fax 709 777-6969

HEALTH SCIENCES CENTRE
300 Prince Philip Dr
St. John's NL A1B 3V6
Tel. 709 737-6300
Fax 709 737-6400
www.easternhealth.ca

JANEWAY CHILDREN'S HEALTH & REHABILITATION CENTRE
300 Prince Phillip Dr
St John's NL A1B 3V6
Tel. 709 777-6300
Fax 709 778-4333
www.easternhealth.ca

ST CLARE'S MERCY HOSPITAL
154 Lemarchant Rd
St. John's NL A1C 5B8
Tel. 709 777-5000
Fax 709 777-5883
www.easternhealth.ca

WATERFORD HOSPITAL
306 Waterford Bridge Rd
St. John's NL A1E 4J8
Tel. 709 777-3300
Fax 709 777-1302
www.easternhealth.ca

ST. LAWRENCE

US MEMORIAL HEALTH CENTRE
1 Memorial Dr
PO Box 398
St Lawrence NL A0E 2V0
Tel. 709 873-2330
Fax 709 873-2299
www.easternhealth.ca

ST. LEWIS

ST LEWIS NURSING STATION
General Delivery
St Lewis NL A0K 4W0
Tel. 709 939-2230
Fax 709 939-2342

SPRINGDALE

GREEN BAY COMMUNITY HEALTH CENTRE
292 Main St
PO Box 280
Springdale NL A0J 1T0
Tel. 709 673-3911
Fax 709 673-3186
www.centralhealth.nl.ca

STEPHENVILLE

SIR THOMAS RODDICK HOSPITAL
142 Minnesota Dr
PO Box 5000 Stn Main
Stephenville NL A2N 2V6
Tel. 709 643-5111
Fax 709 643-2700
www.westernhealth.nl.ca

TWILLINGATE

NOTRE DAME BAY MEMORIAL HEALTH CENTRE
Hospital Lane
Twillingate NL A0G 4M0
Tel. 709 884-2131
Fax 709 884-2586
www.centralhealth.ca

NORTHWEST TERRITORIES

AKLAVIK

SUSY HUSKEY HEALTH CENTRE
PO Box 114
Aklavik NT X0E 0A0
Tel. 867 978-2516
Fax 867 978-2160

DÉLINE

DELINE HEALTH CENTRE
PO Box 199
Deline NT X0E 0G0
Tel. 867 589-3111
Fax 867 589-5570

FORT GOOD HOPE

FORT GOOD HOPE HEALTH CENTRE
GD
PO Box 9
Fort Good Hope NT X0E 0H0
Tel. 867 598-2211
Fax 867 598-2605

FORT LIARD

FORT LIARD HEALTH CENTRE
GD
Fort Liard NT X0G 0A0
Tel. 867 770-4301
Fax 867 770-3235

FORT MCPHERSON

FORT MCPHERSON - WILLIAM FIRTH HEALTH CENTRE
PO Box 56
Fort Mcpherson NT X0E 0J0
Tel. 867 952-2586
Fax 867 952-2620
www.bdhssa.nt.ca

FORT PROVIDENCE

FORT PROVIDENCE HEALTH CENTRE
GD
PO Box 260
Fort Providence NT X0E 0L0
Tel. 867 669-4311
Fax 867 699-3811
www.hlthss.gov.nt.ca

FORT RESOLUTION

FORT RESOLUTION HEALTH CENTRE
PO Box 1997
Fort Resolution NT X0E 0M0
Tel. 867 394-4511
Fax 867 394-3117
www.hlthss.gov.nt.ca

FORT SIMPSON

FORT SIMPSON HEALTH CENTRE
10101 100th Ave
PO Box 246
Fort Simpson NT X0E 0N0
Tel. 867 695-7000
Fax 867 695-7017

FORT SMITH

FORT SMITH HEALTH CENTRE
PO Box 1080
Fort Smith NT X0E 0P0
Tel. 867 872-6200
Fax 867 872-6299
www.hlthss.gov.nt.ca

HAY RIVER

H H WILLIAMS MEMORIAL HOSPITAL
3 Gaetz Dr
Hay River NT X0E 0R8
Fax 867 874-7118
www.hss.gov.nt.ca

INUVIK

INUVIK REGIONAL HOSPITAL
285 MacKenzie Rd
PO Box 2
Inuvik NT X0E 0T0
Tel. 867 777-8000
Fax 867 777-8054
http://bdhssa.nt.ca

LUTSELK'E

LUTSEL K'E HEALTH CENTRE
PO Box 56
Lutsel K'E NT X0E 1A0
Tel. 867 370-3111
Fax 867 370-3022
www.hlthss.gov.nt.ca

NORMAN WELLS

NORMAN WELLS HEALTH CENTRE
Box 8
Norman Wells NT X0E 0V0
Tel. 867 587-2250
Fax 867 587-2934

PAULATUK

PAULATUK HEALTH CENTRE
PO Box 114
Paulatuk NT X0E 1N0
Tel. 867 580-3231
Fax 867 580-3300

SACHS HARBOUR

SACHS HARBOUR HEALTH CENTRE
PO Box 14
Sachs Harbour NT X0E 0Z0
Tel. 867 690-4181
Fax 867 690-3802
www.bdhssa.nt.ca

TSIIGEHTCHIC

TSIIGEHTCHIC HEALTH CENTRE
General Delivery
Tsiigehtchic NT X0E 0B0
Tel. 867 953-3361
Fax 867 953-3408
www.bdhssa.nt.ca

TUKTOYAKTUK

TUKTOYAKTUK HEALTH CENTRE
PO Box 1000
Tuktoyaktuk NT X0E 1C0
Tel. 867 977-2321
Fax 867 977-2535

TULITA

TULITA HEALTH CENTRE
GD
Tulita NT X0E 0K0
Tel. 867 588-4251
Fax 867 588-3000
www.hlthss.gov.nt.ca

ULUKHAKTOK

HOLMAN HEALTH & SOCIAL SERVICES CENTRE
PO Box 160
Ulukhaktok NT X0E 0S0
Tel. 867 396-3111
Fax 867 396-3221

WHA TI

WHATI HEALTH CENTRE
GD
Whati NT X0E 1P0
Tel. 867 573-3261
Fax 867 573-3701

YELLOWKNIFE

STANTON TERRITORIAL HEALTH AUTHORITY
550 Byrne Rd
PO Box 10 Stn Main
Yellowknife NT X1A 2N1
Tel. 867 669-4111
Fax 867 669-4361
www.stha.ca

NOVA SCOTIA

ADVOCATE HARBOUR

BAYVIEW MEMORIAL HEALTH CENTRE
3375 Hwy 209
PO Box 61
Advocate Harbour NS B0M 1A0
Tel. 902 392-2859
Fax 902 392-2625
www.cha.nshealth.ca

AMHERST

CUMBERLAND REGIONAL HEALTH CARE CENTER
19428 Highway 2
Amherst NS B4H 1N6
Tel. 902 667-3361
Fax 902 667-6306
www.cha.nshealth.ca

ANNAPOLIS ROYAL

ANNAPOLIS COMMUNITY HEALTH CENTRE
821 St George St
PO Box 426
Annapolis Royal NS B0S 1A0
Tel. 902 532-2381
Fax 902 532-2113
www.avdha.nshealth.ca/

ANTIGONISH

ST MARTHA'S REGIONAL HOSPITAL
25 Bay St
Antigonish NS B2G 2G5
Tel. 902 863-4500
Fax 902 867-1059
www.gasha.nshealth.ca

BADDECK

VICTORIA COUNTY MEMORIAL HOSPITAL
30 Old Margaree Rd
PO Box 220
Baddeck NS B0E 1B0
Tel. 902 295-2122
Fax 902 295-3432
www.cbdha.nshealth.ca

BERWICK

WESTERN KINGS MEMORIAL HEALTH CENTRE
121 Orchard St
PO Box 490
Berwick NS B0P 1E0
Tel. 902 538-3111
Fax 902 538-0770
www.avdha.nshealth.ca

BRIDGEWATER

SOUTH SHORE REGIONAL HOSPITAL
90 Glen Allan Dr
Bridgewater NS B4V 3S6
Tel. 902 543-4603
Fax 902 543-4719
www.ssdha.nshealth.ca

CANSO

EASTERN MEMORIAL HOSPITAL
1746 Union St
PO Box 10
Canso NS B0H 1H0
Tel. 902 366-2794
Fax 902 366-2740
www.gasha.nshealth.ca

CHETICAMP

SACRED HEART HOSPITAL
15102 Cabot Trail
PO Box 129
Cheticamp NS B0E 1H0
Tel. 902 224-1500
Fax 902 224-2903
www.cbdha.nshealth.ca

CLEVELAND

STRAIT RICHMOND HOSPITAL
138 Hospital Rd
RR 1
Cleveland NS B0E 1J0
Tel. 902 625-3100
Fax 902 625-3804
www.gasha.nshealth.ca

DARTMOUTH

DARTMOUTH GENERAL HOSPITAL
325 Pleasant St
Dartmouth NS B2Y 4G8
Tel. 902 465-8300
Fax 902 465-8537
www.cdha.nshealth.ca

THE EAST COAST FORENSIC PSYCHIATRY HOSPITAL
88 Gloria McCluskey Ave
Burnside Industrial Park
Dartmouth NS B3B 2B8
Tel. 902 460-7300
Fax 902 460-7337
www.cdha.nshealth.ca

THE NOVA SCOTIA HOSPITAL
300 Pleasant St
PO Box 1004 Stn Main
Dartmouth NS B2Y 3Z9
Tel. 902 464-3111
Fax 902 464-3460
www.cdha.nshealth.ca

DIGBY

DIGBY GENERAL HOSPITAL
75 Warwick St
PO Box 820
Digby NS B0V 1A0
Tel. 902 245-2502
Fax 902 245-2803
www.swndha.nshealth.ca

ELMSDALE

LLOYD E. MATHESON CENTRE
150-50 Commerce Crt
Elmsdale NS B2S 3K5
Tel. 902 883-8444
Fax 902 883-3400
www.cehha.nshealth.ca

GLACE BAY

GLACE BAY HEALTHCARE FACILITY
300 South St
Glace Bay NS B1A 1W5
Tel. 902 849-5511
Fax 902 849-9775
www.cbdha.nshealth.ca

GUYSBOROUGH

GUYSBOROUGH MEMORIAL HOSPITAL
10560 Hwy 16
PO Box 170
Guysborough NS B0H 1N0
Tel. 902 533-3702
Fax 902 533-4066
www.gasha.nshealth.ca

HALIFAX

CANADIAN FORCES HEALTH SERVICES CENTRE (ATLANTIC)
PO Box 99000 Stn Forces
Halifax NS B3K 5X5
Tel. 902 427-8700
Fax 902 427-8866

CAPITAL HEALTH/QEII CANCER CARE PROGRAM
5820 University Ave
Halifax NS B3H 1V7
Tel. 902 473-6441
Fax 902 473-4224
www.cdha.nshealth.ca

COBEQUID COMMUNITY HEALTH CENTRE
5788 University Ave
Halifax NS B3H 1V8
Tel. 902 869-6130
Fax 902 865-4816
www.cdha.ns health .ca

IWK HEALTH CENTRE
5850-5980 University Ave
PO Box 9700 RPO CSC
Halifax NS B3K 6R8
Tel. 902 470-8888
Fax 902 428-8826
www.iwk.nshealth.ca

NOVA SCOTIA REHABILITATION CENTRE
1341 Summer St
Halifax NS B3H 4K4
Tel. 902 473-5757
Fax 902 473-3581
www.cdha.nshealth.ca

QUEEN ELIZABETH II HEALTH SCIENCES CENTRE - HALIFAX INFIRMARY SITE
1796 Summer St
Halifax NS B3H 3A7
Tel. 902 473-2700
Fax 902 496-2719
www.cdha.ns.ca

QUEEN ELIZABETH II HEALTH SCIENCES CENTRE - VICTORIA GENERAL SITE
1276 South Park St
Halifax NS B3H 2Y9
Tel. 902 473-2700
Fax 902 473-3317
www.cdha.ns.ca

INVERNESS

INVERNESS CONSOLIDATED MEMORIAL HOSPITAL
39 James St
PO Box 610
Inverness NS B0E 1N0
Tel. 902 258-2100
Fax 902 258-3025
www.cbdha.nshealth.ca

KENTVILLE

ANNAPOLIS VALLEY HEALTH ADULT MENTAL HEALTH PROGRAM
15 Chipman Dr
Kentville NS B4N 3V7
Tel. 902 364-1701
Fax 902 678-4917
www.avdha.nshealth.ca

VALLEY REGIONAL HOSPITAL
150 Exhibition St
Kentville NS B4N 5E3
Tel. 902 678-7381
Fax 902 679-1904
www.avdha.nshealth.ca

LIVERPOOL

QUEENS GENERAL HOSPITAL
175 School St
PO Box 370
Liverpool NS B0T 1K0
Tel. 902 354-3436
Fax 902 354-4614
www.ssdha.nshealth.ca

LOWER SACKVILLE

COBEQUID COMMUNITY HEALTH CENTRE
40 Freer Lane
Lower Sackville NS B4C 0A2
Tel. 902 869-6100
Fax 902 865-4816
www.cdha.nshealth.ca

LUNENBURG

FISHERMEN'S MEMORIAL HOSPITAL
14 High St
PO Box 1180
Lunenburg NS B0J 2C0
Tel. 902 634-8801
Fax 902 634-3668
www.southshorehealth.ca

MIDDLE MUSQUODOBOIT

MUSQUODOBOIT VALLEY MEMORIAL HOSPITAL
492 Archibald Brook Rd
Mid Musquodoboit NS B0N 1X0
Tel. 902 384-2220
Fax 902 384-3310
www.cdha.nshealth.ca

MIDDLETON

SOLDIERS MEMORIAL HOSPITAL
462 Main St
PO Box 730
Middleton NS B0S 1P0
Tel. 902 825-3411
Fax 902 825-0599
www.avdha.nshealth.ca

MUSQUODOBOIT HARBOUR

TWIN OAKS MEMORIAL HOSPITAL
7704 7 Highway
RR1
Musquodbt Hbr NS B0J 2L0
Tel. 902 889-2200
Fax 902 889-2470
www.cdha.nshealth.ca

NEILS HARBOUR

BUCHANAN MEMORIAL HOSPITAL
32610 Cabot Trail
Neil's Harbour NS B0C 1N0
Tel. 902 336-2200
Fax 902 336-2399
www.cbdha.nshealth.ca

NEW GLASGOW

ABERDEEN HOSPITAL
835 East River Rd
New Glasgow NS B2H 3S6
Tel. 902 752-7600 Ext. 3875
Fax 902 752-2356
www.pcha.nshealth.ca

NEW WATERFORD

NEW WATERFORD CONSOLIDATED HOSPITAL
716 King St
New Waterford NS B1H 3Z5
Tel. 902 862-6411
Fax 902 862-8277
www.cbdha.nshealth.ca

NORTH SYDNEY

NORTHSIDE GENERAL HOSPITAL
PO BOX 399 St n Main
North Sydney NS B2A 3M4
Tel. 902 794-8521
Fax 902 794-3355
www.cbdha.nshealth.ca

PARRSBORO

SOUTH CUMBERLAND COMMUNITY CARE CENTRE
50 Jenks Ave
Parrsboro NS B0M 1S0
Tel. 902 254-2540
Fax 902 254-2504
www.cha.nshealth.ca

PICTOU

SUTHERLAND-HARRIS MEMORIAL HOSPITAL
222 Haliburton Rd
PO Box 1059
Pictou NS B0K 1H0
Tel. 902 485-4324
Fax 902 485-8835
www.pcha.nshealth.ca

PUGWASH

NORTH CUMBERLAND MEMORIAL HOSPITAL
260 Church St
PO Box 242
Pugwash NS B0K 1L0
Tel. 902 243-2521
Fax 902 243-2941
www.cha.nshealth.ca

SHEET HARBOUR

EASTERN SHORE MEMORIAL HOSPITAL
22637 Rte 7
Sheet Harbour NS B0J 3B0
Tel. 902 885-2554
Fax 902 885-3200
www.cdha.nshealth.ca

SHELBURNE

ROSEWAY HOSPITAL
1606 Sandy Point Rd
PO Box 610
Shelburne NS B0T 1W0
Tel. 902 875-3011
Fax 902 875-1580
www.swndha.nshealth.ca

SHERBROOKE

ST MARY'S MEMORIAL HOSPITAL
91 Hospital Rd
PO Box 299
Sherbrooke NS B0J 3C0
Tel. 902 522-2882
Fax 902 522-2556
www.gasha.nshealth.ca

SPRINGHILL

ALL SAINTS SPRINGHILL HOSPITAL
10 Princess St
PO Box 700
Springhill NS B0M 1X0
Tel. 902 597-3773
Fax 902 597-3440
www.cha.nshealth.ca

SYDNEY

CAPE BRETON HEALTHCARE COMPLEX
1482 George St
Sydney NS B1P 1P3
Tel. 902 567-8000
Fax 902 567-7921
www.cbdha.nshealth.ca

SYDNEY MINES

HARBOURVIEW HOSPITAL
22 Richard St
Sydney Mines NS B1V 2H7
Tel. 902 736-2831
www.cbdha.nshealth.ca

TATAMAGOUCHE

LILLIAN FRASER MEMORIAL HOSPITAL / PRIMARY HEALTH CARE CENTRE
110 Blair Ave
PO Box 40
Tatamagouche NS B0K 1V0
Tel. 902 657-2382
Fax 902 657-3745
www.cehha.nshealth.ca

TRURO

COLCHESTER EAST HANTS HEALTH CENTRE IS
600 Abenaki Rd
Truro NS B2N 5A1
Tel. 902 893-5554
Fax 902 893-5559
www.cehha.nshealth.ca

WATERVILLE

KINGS REGIONAL REHABILITATION CENTRE
1349 County Home Rd
PO Box 128
Waterville NS B0P 1V0
Tel. 902 538-3103
Fax 902 538-7022
www.krrc.nsnet.org

WINDSOR

HANTS COMMUNITY HOSPITAL
89 Payzant Dr
Windsor NS B0N 2T0
Tel. 902 792-2000
www.cdha.nshealth.ca

WOLFVILLE

EASTERN KINGS MEMORIAL HEALTH CENTRE
23 Earnscliffe Ave
Wolfville NS B4P 1X4
Tel. 902 542-2266
Fax 902 542-4619

YARMOUTH

YARMOUTH REGIONAL HOSPITAL
60 Vancouver St
Yarmouth NS B5A 2P5
Tel. 902 742-3541
Fax 902 742-0369
www.swndha.nshealth.ca

NUNAVUT

ARCTIC BAY

ARCTIC BAY HEALTH CENTRE
PO Box 60
Arctic Bay NU X0A 0A0
Tel. 867 439-8816
Fax 867 439-8315

ARVIAT

ARVIAT HEALTH CENTRE
Bag 510
Arviat NU X0C 0E0
Tel. 867 857-3100
Fax 867 857-3149
www.irespectmyself.ca

CAMBRIDGE BAY

CAMBRIDGE BAY HEALTH & SOCIAL SERVICES CENTRE
PO Box 53
Cambridge Bay NU X0B 0C0
Tel. 867 983-4500
Fax 867 983-4509
www.irespectmyself.ca

KITIKMEOT HEALTH CENTRE
PO Box 53
Cambridge Bay NU X0B 0C0
Tel. 867 983-4500
Fax 867 983-4509
www.irespectmyself.ca

CAPE DORSET

CAPE DORSET HEALTH CENTRE
PO Box 180
Cape Dorset NU X0A 0C0
Tel. 867 897-8820
Fax 867 897-8194
www.irespectmyself.ca

CHESTERFIELD INLET

CHESTERFIELD INLET HEALTH CENTRE
PO Box 9
Chesterfield NU X0C 0B0
Tel. 867 898-9968
Fax 867 898-9122
www.irespectmyself.ca

CLYDE RIVER

CLYDE RIVER HEALTH CENTRE
PO Box 40
Clyde River NU X0A 0E0
Tel. 867 924-6377
Fax 867 924-6244
www.irespectmyself.ca

CORAL HARBOUR

CORAL HARBOUR HEALTH CENTRE
PO Box 120
Coral Harbour NU X0C 0C0
Tel. 867 925-9916
Fax 867 925-8380

GJOA HAVEN

KATIVIK HEALTH & SOCIAL SERVICES CENTRE
General Delivery
Gjoa Haven NU X0B 1J0
Tel. 867 360-7441
Fax 867 360-6110
www.irespectmyself.ca

GRISE FIORD

GRISE FIORD HEALTH CENTRE
PO Box 81
Grise Fiord NU X0A 0J0
Tel. 867 980-9923
Fax 867 980-9067
www.irespectmyself.ca

HALL BEACH

HALL BEACH HEALTH CENTRE
General Delivery
Hall Beach NU X0A 0K0
Tel. 867 928-8827
Fax 867 928-8847
www.irespectmyself.ca

IGLOOLIK

IGLOOLIK HEALTH CENTRE
PO Box 260
Igloolik NU X0A 0L0
Tel. 867 934-2100
Fax 867 934-2149
www.irespectmyself.ca

IQALUIT

BAFFIN REGIONAL HOSPITAL
PO Box 1000 Stn 1040
Iqaluit NU X0A 0H0
Tel. 867 979-7300
Fax 867 979-7328

QIKIGTANI GENERAL HOSPITAL
PO Box 1000
Station 1040
Iqaluit NU X0A 0H0
Tel. 867 975-8600
Fax 867 979-2032

KIMMIRUT

KIMMIRUT HEALTH CENTRE
PO Box 30
Kimmirut NU X0A 0N0
Tel. 867 939-2217
Fax 867 939-2068
www.irespectmyself.ca

KUGAARUK

PELLY BAY HEALTH CENTRE
General Delivery
Kugaaruk NU X0B 1K0
Tel. 867 769-6441
Fax 867 769-6059

KUGLUKTUK

KUGLUKTUK HEALTH CENTRE
General Delivery
Box No 288
Kugluktuk NU X0B 0E0
Tel. 867 982-4531
Fax 867 982-3115

PANGNIRTUNG

PANGNIRTUNG HEALTH CENTRE
PO Box 454
Pangnirtung NU X0A 0R0
Tel. 867 473-8977
Fax 867 473-8519
www.irespectmyself.ca

POND INLET

POND INLET HEALTH CENTRE
PO Box 216
Pond Inlet NU X0A 0S0
Tel. 867 899-7500
Fax 867 899-7538

QIKIQTARJUAQ

QIKIQTARJUAQ HEALTH CENTRE
PO Box 911
Qikiqtarjuaq NU X0A 0B0
Tel. 867 927-8916
Fax 867 927-8217
www.irespectmyself.ca

RANKIN INLET

KIVALLIQ HEALTH CENTRE
PO Box 008
Rankin Inlet NU X0C 0G0
Tel. 867 645-8300
Fax 867 645-8324

RANKIN INLET HEALTH CENTRE
PO Box 871
Ranklin Inlet NU X0C 0G0
Tel. 867 645-8070
Fax 867 645-8079

REPULSE BAY

REPULSE BAY HEALTH CENTRE
GD
Repulse Bay NU X0C 0H0
Tel. 867 462-9916
Fax 867 462-4212

RESOLUTE

RESOLUTE BAY HEALTH CENTRE
PO Box 180
Resolute Bay NU X0A 0V0
Tel. 867 252-3844
Fax 867 252-3601
www.irespectmyself.ca

SANIKILUAQ

SANIKILUAQ HEALTH CENTRE
General Delivery
Sanikiluaq NU X0A 0W0
Tel. 867 266-8965
Fax 867 266-8802

TALOYOAK

TALOYOAK BAY HEALTH CENTRE
GD
Taloyoak NU X0B 1B0
Tel. 867 561-5111
Fax 867 561-6906

WHALE COVE

WHALE COVE HEALTH CENTRE
PO Box 30
Whale Cove NU X0C 0J0
Tel. 867 896-9916
Fax 867 896-9115

ONTARIO

AJAX

ROUGE VALLEY HEALTH SYSTEM - AJAX & PICKERING HEALTH CENTRE SITE
580 Harwood Ave S
Ajax ON L1S 2J4
Tel. 905 683-2320
Fax 905 683-2618
www.rougevalley.ca

ALEXANDRIA

GLENGARRY MEMORIAL HOSPITAL
20260 County Rd 43
PO Box 910
Alexandria ON K0C 1A0
Tel. 613 525-2222
Fax 613 525-4515
www.hgmh.on.ca

ALLISTON

STEVENSON MEMORIAL HOSPITAL
200 Fletcher Cres
PO Box 4000 Stn Main
Alliston ON L9R 1W7
Tel. 705 435-6281
Fax 705 434-5138
www.smhosp.on.ca

ALMONTE

ALMONTE GENERAL HOSPITAL
75 Spring St
Almonte ON K0A 1A0
Tel. 613 256-2500 Ext. 2220
Fax 613 256-4889
www.almontegeneral.com

ARMSTRONG STATION

NORWEST COMMUNITY HEALTH CENTRE - ARMSTRONG
PO Box 104
Armstrong Station ON P0T 1A0
Tel. 807 583-1145
Fax 807 583-1147
www.norwestchc.org

WHITESANDS HEALTH OFFICE
PO Box 68
Armstrong Station ON P0T 1A0
Tel. 807 583-2177
Fax 807 583-2858
www.firstnation.ca

ARNPRIOR

ARNPRIOR & DISTRICT MEMORIAL HOSPITAL
350 John St N
Arnprior ON K7S 2P6
Tel. 613 623-3166
Fax 613 623-4844
www.arnpriorhospital.com

ATIKOKAN

ATIKOKAN GENERAL HOSPITAL
120 Dorothy St
Atikokan ON P0T 1C0
Tel. 807 597-4215
Fax 807 597-4305
www.aghospital.on.ca

ATTAWAPISKAT

ATTAWAPISKAT HEALTH CENTRE
PO Box 248
Attawapiskat ON P0L 1A0
Tel. 705 997-2166
Fax 705 997-2116
www.firstnation.ca

JAMES BAY GENERAL HOSPITAL - ATTAWAPISKAT
General Delivery
Attawapiskat ON P0L 1A0
Tel. 705 997-2150
Fax 705 997-2121
www.jbgh.org

AURORA

BLUE HILLS CHILD AND FAMILY CENTRE
402 Bloomington Rd
Aurora ON L4G 0A9
Tel. 905 773-4323
Fax 905 773-8133
www.bluehillschildandfamily.ca

THE SOUTHDOWN INSTITUTE
1335 St John's Sideroad
RR 2 Stn Main
Aurora ON L4G 3G8
Tel. 905 727-4214
Fax 905 727-4214
www.southdown.on.ca

BALA

WAHTA NURSING STATION
2664 Muskoka Rd 38
Box 260
Bala ON P0C 1A0
Tel. 705 762-2354 Ext. 243
Fax 705 762-4809
www.wahtamohawks.ca

BANCROFT

QHC NORTH HASTINGS
1H Manor Lane
PO Box 157
Bancroft ON K0L 1C0
Tel. 613 332-2825
Fax 613 332-3847
www.qhc.on.ca

BARRIE

BARRIE COMMUNITY HEALTH CENTRE
56 Bayfield St
Barrie ON L4M 3A5
Tel. 705 734-9690
www.bchc.ca

ROYAL VICTORIA HOSPITAL OF BARRIE'S COMMUNITY CARE CENTRE FOR SUBSTANCE ABUSE
70 Wellington St W
Barrie ON L4N 1K4
Tel. 705 728-4226
Fax 705 728-7308
www.rvh.on.ca

ROYAL VICTORIA REGIONAL HEALTH CENTRE
201 Georgian Dr
Barrie ON L4M 6M2
Tel. 705 728-9802
Fax 705 726-0822
www.rvh.on.ca

BARRY'S BAY

ST FRANCIS MEMORIAL HOSPITAL
7 St Francis Memorial Dr
PO Box 129
Barrys Bay ON K0J 1B0
Tel. 613 756-3044
Fax 613 756-0106
www.sfmhosp.com

BEACHBURG

LANARK HEALTH & COMMUNITY SERVICES (BEACHBURG)
20 Robertson Dr
RR#1
Beachburg ON K0J 1C0
Tel. 613 582-3685
www.ontariochc.ca

BEAR ISLAND

DOREEN POTTS HEALTH CENTRE
Bear Island PO
Bear Island ON P0H 1C0
Tel. 705 237-8900
Fax 705 237-8959
www.temagamifirstnation.ca

BEARSKIN LAKE

BEARSKIN LAKE NURSING STATION
GD
Bearskin Lake ON P0V 1E0
Tel. 807 363-2582
Fax 807 363-1021
www.firstnation.ca

BEAVERTON

BROCK COMMUNITY HEALTH CENTRE
720 Simcoe St
Beaverton ON L0K 1A0
Tel. 705 432-3322
Fax 705 426-4215
www.brockchc.ca

BROCK COMMUNITY HEALTH CENTRE - GERIATRIC ASSESSMENT
720 Simcoe St
Beaverton ON L0K 1A0
Tel. 705 426-2175
Fax 705 426-4215
www.brockchc.ca

BELLEVILLE

BELLEVILLE AND QUINTE WEST COMMUNITY HEALTH CENTRE
161 Bridge St W
Belleville ON K8P 1K2
Tel. 613 962-0000
www.bqwchc.com

QHC BELLEVILLE GENERAL
265 Dundas St E
Belleville ON K8N 5A9
Tel. 613 969-7400
Fax 613 968-8234
www.qhc.on.ca

BIG TROUT LAKE

BIG TROUT LAKE NURSING STATION
PO Box 327
Big Trout Lake ON P0V 1G0
Tel. 807 537-2262
Fax 807 537-2587
www.firstnation.ca

BLIND RIVER

BLIND RIVER DISTRICT HEALTH CENTRE
525 Causley St
PO Box 970
Blind River ON P0R 1B0
Tel. 705 356-2265
Fax 705 356-1220
www.brdhc.on.ca

BOWMANVILLE

LAKERIDGE HEALTH - BOWMANVILLE SITE
47 Liberty St S
Bowmanville ON L1C 2N4
Tel. 905 623-3331
Fax 905 697-4685
www.lakeridgehealth.on.ca

BRACEBRIDGE

SOUTH MUSKOKA MEMORIAL HOSPITAL - MUSKOKA ALGONQUIN HEALTHCARE
75 Ann St
Bracebridge ON P1L 2E4
Tel. 705 645-4404 Ext. 102
Fax 705 645-4594
www.mahc.ca

BRAMPTON

BRAMALEA COMMUNITY HEALTH CENTRE
40 Finchgate Blvd
Brampton ON L6T 3J1
Tel. 905 451-6951
Fax 905 451-5217
www.bramaleachc.ca

WILLIAM OSLER HEALTH SYSTEM - BRAMPTON CIVIC HOSPITAL
2100 Bovaird Dr E
Brampton ON L6R 3J7
Tel. 905 494-2120
Fax 905 796-4289
www.williamoslerhc.on.ca

BRANTFORD

THE BRANT COMMUNITY HEALTHCARE SYSTEM -BRANTFORD GENERAL HOSPITAL SITE
200 Terrace Hill St
Brantford ON N3R 1G9
Tel. 519 752-7871
Fax 519 752-0098
www.bchsys.org

DE DWA DA DEHS NYE'S ABORIGINAL HEALTH ACCESS CENTRE (BRANTFORD)
36 King St
Brantford ON N3T 3C5
Tel. 519 752-4340
Fax 519 752-6096
www.aboriginalhealthcentre.com

GRAND RIVER COMMUNITY HEALTH CENTRE -BRANTFORD
347 Colborn St
Brantford ON N3S 3N2
Tel. 519 754-0777
Fax 519 754-0727
www.grandriverchc.ca

LANSDOWNE CHILDREN'S CENTRE
39 Mount Pleasant St
Brantford ON N3T 1S7
Tel. 519 753-3153
Fax 519 753-5927
www.lansdownecentre.ca

BROCKVILLE

BROCKVILLE GENERAL HOSPITAL - CHARLES STREET
75 Charles St
Brockville ON K6V 1S8
Tel. 613 345-5649
Fax 613 345-8336
www.bgh-on.ca

BROCKVILLE GENERAL HOSPITAL - GARDEN STREET
42 Garden St
Brockville ON K6V 2C3
Tel. 613 345-2522
Fax 613 345-4111
www.bgh-on.ca

ACUTE CARE MENTAL HEALTH SERVICES - ELMGROVE SITE
PO Box 1050 Stn Main
Brockville ON K6V 5W7
Tel. 613 345-5645
Fax 613 345-7431
www.bgh-on.ca

BURK'S FALLS

BURK'S FALLS & DISTRICT HEALTH CENTRE - MUSKOKA ALGONQUIN HEALTHCARE
150 Hudson St
PO Box 520
Burks Falls ON P0A 1C0
Tel. 705 382-2900
Fax 705 382-3131
www.mahc.ca

BURLINGTON

JOSEPH BRANT MEMORIAL HOSPITAL
1230 North Shore Blvd E
Burlington ON L7S 1W7
Tel. 905 632-3737
Fax 905 336-6480
www.jbmh.com

CAMBRIDGE

CAMBRIDGE MEMORIAL HOSPITAL
700 Coronation Blvd
Cambridge ON N1R 3G2
Tel. 519 621-2333
Fax 519 621-4938
www.cmh.org

KIDSABILITY CENTRE FOR CHILD DEVELOPMENT - CAMBRIDGE
250 Hespler Rd
Cambridge ON N1R 3H3
Tel. 519 886-7292
Fax 519 886-7292
www.kidsability.ca

CAMPBELLFORD

CAMPBELLFORD MEMORIAL HOSPITAL
146 Oliver Rd
PO Box 1027
Campbellford ON K0L 1L0
Tel. 705 653-1140
Fax 705 653-4371
www.cmh.ca

CANNINGTON

BROCK COMMUNITY HEALTH CENTRE - DIABETES EDUCATION PROGRAM
20 Cameron St W
Cannington ON L0E 1E0
Tel. 705 432-2446
Fax 705 426-3039
www.brockchc.ca

CARLETON PLACE

CARLETON PLACE & DISTRICT MEMORIAL HOSPITAL
211 Lake Ave E
Carleton Place ON K7C 1J4
Tel. 613 257-2200
Fax 613 257-3026
www.carletonplacehospital.ca

CAT LAKE

CAT LAKE NURSING STATION
Gd
Cat Lake ON P0V 1J0
Tel. 807 347-2110
Fax 807 347-2140
www.firstnation.ca

CHAPLEAU

BRUNSWICK HOUSE HEALTH OFFICE
PO Box 1178
Chapleau ON P0M 1K0
Tel. 705 864-0174
Fax 705 864-1960
www.firstnation.ca

CHAPLEAU CREE HEALTH CLINIC
Fox Lake Reserve
PO Box 400
Chapleau ON P0M 1K0
Tel. 705 864-0200
Fax 705 864-1760

CHAPLEAU GENERAL HOSPITAL - DIVISION OF SERVICES DE SANTÉ DE CHAPLEAU HEALTH SERVICES
6 Broomhead Rd
PO Box 757
Chapleau ON P0M 1K0
Tel. 705 864-1520
Fax 705 864-0449
www.sschs.ca

CHATHAM

CHATHAM/KENT COMMUNITY HEALTH CENTRE
150 Richmond St
Chatham ON N7M 1N9
Tel. 519 397-5455
www.ckchc.ca

CHATHAM-KENT HEALTH ALLIANCE
80 Grand Ave W
PO Box 2030 Stn Main
Chatham ON N7M 5L9
Tel. 519 352-6400
Fax 519 352-2536
www.ckha.on.ca

CHILDREN'S TREATMENT CENTRE OF CHATHAM-KENT
355 Lark St
Chatham ON N7L 5B2
Tel. 519 354-0520
Fax 519 354-7355
www.childrenstreatment-ck.com

CHESLEY

SOUTH BRUCE GREY HEALTH SERVICES - CHESLEY SITE
39 2nd St SE
PO Box 40
Chesley ON N0G 1L0
Tel. 519 363-2340
Fax 519 363-9871
www.sbghc.on.ca

CLINTON

CLINTON PUBLIC HOSPITAL - HURON PERTH HEALTHCARE ALLIANCE
98 Shipley St
Clinton ON N0M 1L0
Tel. 519 482-3440
Fax 519 482-8762
www.hpha.ca

COBOURG

NORTHUMBERLAND HILLS HOSPITAL
1000 DePalma Dr
Cobourg ON K9A 5W6
Tel. 905 372-6811
Fax 905 372-4243
www.nhh.ca

COCHRANE

LADY MINTO HOSPITAL COCHRANE
241 8th St
PO Box 4000
Cochrane ON P0L 1C0
Tel. 705 272-7200
Fax 705 258-2624
www.micsgroup.com

NEW POST HEALTH CENTRE
RR 2
PO Box 3310
Cochrane ON P0L 1C0
Tel. 705 272-5685
Fax 705 272-6352
www.communities.knet.ca

COLLINGWOOD

COLLINGWOOD GENERAL & MARINE HOSPITAL
459 Hume St
Collingwood ON L9Y 1W9
Tel. 705 445-2550
Fax 705 444-2679
www.cgmh.on.ca

COLLINGWOOD HEALTH CENTRE
186 Erie St
Collingwood ON L9Y 4T3
Tel. 705 444-2268
Fax 705 444-2809

CORNWALL

CORNWALL COMMUNITY HOSPITAL
840 McConnell Ave
Cornwall ON K6H 5S5
Tel. 613 938-4240
Fax 613 930-4502
www.cornwallhospital.ca

CORNWALL COMMUNITY HOSPITAL - SECOND STREET SITE
510 Second St E
Cornwall ON K6H 1Z6
Tel. 613 932-3300
Fax 613 936-4610
www.cornwallhospital.ca

OTTAWA CHILDREN'S TREATMENT CENTRE - CORNWALL SITE OF SERVICE
100-600 Campbell St
Cornwall ON K6H 6C9
Tel. 613 932-2327
Fax 613 932-5688
www.octc.ca

ST JOSEPH'S CONTINUING CARE CENTRE - CORNWALL
14 York St
Cornwall ON K6J 5T2
Tel. 613 938-6040
Fax 613 933-0163
www.sjccc.ca

SEAWAY VALLEY COMMUNITY HEALTH CENTRE
353 Pitt St
Cornwall ON K6J 3R1
Tel. 613 936-0306
www.seawayvalleychc.ca

CURVE LAKE

CURVE LAKE HEALTH CENTRE
Gen Del
Curve Lake ON K0L 1R0
Tel. 705 657-2557
Fax 705 657-2095
www.communities.knet.ca

CUTLER

KENABUTCH HEALTH CENTRE
40 Ball Park Rd
Cutler ON P0P 1B0
Tel. 705 844-2152
Fax 705 844-2414

N'MNINOEYAA COMMUNITY HEALTH ACCESS CENTRE
473B Hwy #17W
Cutler ON P0P 1B0
Tel. 705 844-2021
www.ontariochc.ca

DEEP RIVER

DEEP RIVER & DISTRICT HOSPITAL
117 Banting Dr
Deep River ON K0J 1P0
Tel. 613 584-3333
Fax 613 584-4920
www.drdh.org

DEER LAKE

JEANNETTE OSCAR LINDOKKEN NURSING STATION
PO Box 10
Deer Lake ON P0V 1N0
Tel. 807 775-2054
Fax 807 775-2309
www.deerlakehealth.ca

DESERONTO

THAYENDANEGA HEALTH CENTRE
50 York Rd
Deseronto ON K0K 1X0
Tel. 613 967-3603
Fax 613 962-4010

DEVLIN

NAICATCHEWENIN HEALTH STATION
RR 1
PO Box 56
Devlin ON P0W 1C0
Tel. 807 486-3560
Fax 807 486-3704

DRYDEN

DRYDEN REGIONAL HEALTH CENTRE
58 Goodall St
PO Box 3003 Stn Main
Dryden ON P8N 2Z6
Tel. 807 223-8201
Fax 807 223-2370
www.dh.dryden.on.ca

FIREFLY
75 C Van Horne Ave
Dryden ON P8N 2B2
Tel. 807 223-8550
Fax 807 223-2791
www.fireflynw.ca

DUNNVILLE

HALDIMAND WAR MEMORIAL HOSPITAL
206 John St
Dunnville ON N1A 2P7
Tel. 905 774-7431 Ext. 211
Fax 905 774-6776
www.hwmh.on.ca

DURHAM

SOUTH BRUCE GREY HEALTH CENTRE - DURHAM SITE
320 College St
PO Box 638
Durham ON N0G 1R0
Tel. 519 369-2340
Fax 519 369-6180
www.sbghc.on.ca

EABAMET LAKE

EABAMETOONG HEALTH SERVICES
PO Box 179
Eabamet Lake ON P0T 1L0
Tel. 807 242-1484
www.firstnation.ca

FORT HOPE NURSING STATION
PO Box 70
Eabamet Lake ON P0T 1L0
Tel. 807 242-7221
Fax 807 242-1440
www.firstnation.ca

EAR FALLS

EAR FALLS COMMUNITY HEALTH CENTRE/FAMILY HEALTH TEAM
25 Spruce St
PO Box 520
Ear Falls ON P0V 1T0
Tel. 807 222-3728
Fax 807 222-2053
www.ear-falls.com

ELLIOT LAKE

ST JOSEPH'S GENERAL HOSPITAL ELLIOT LAKE
70 Spine Rd
Elliot Lake ON P5A 1X2
Tel. 705 848-7181
Fax 705 848-6239
www.sjgh.ca

EMO

EMO HEALTH CENTRE -RIVERSIDE HEALTH CARE FACILITY
170 Front St
Emo ON P0W 1E0
Tel. 807 482-2881
Fax 807 482-3089
www.riversidehealthcare.ca

MANITOU RAPIDS ISAAC BARKMAN HEALTH STATION
PO Box 450
Emo ON P0W 1E0
Tel. 807 482-2021
Fax 807 482-2603
www.firstnation.ca

ENGLEHART

ENGLEHART & DISTRICT HOSPITAL INC
61 5th St
PO Box 69
Englehart ON P0J 1H0
Tel. 705 544-2301
Fax 705 544-5222
www.edhospital.on.ca

ESPANOLA

ESPANOLA REGIONAL HOSPITAL AND HEALTH CENTRE
825 McKinnon Dr
Espanola ON P5E 1R4
Tel. 705 869-1420
Fax 705 869-2608
www.esphosp.on.ca

ETOBICOKE

REXDALE COMMUNITY HEALTH CENTRE - HEAD OFFICE
8 Taber Rd
Etobicoke ON M9W 3A4
Tel. 416 744-0066
Fax 416 744-1881
www.rexdalechc.com

REXDALE COMMUNITY HEALTH CENTRE - SATELLITE OFFICE
1071 Martingrove Rd
Etobicoke ON M9V 4N4
Tel. 647 288-0281
Fax 647 288-0284
www.rexdalechc.ca

STONEGATE COMMUNITY HEALTH CENTRE
150 Berry Rd
Etobicoke ON M8Y 1W3
Tel. 416 231-7070
Fax 416 231-2663
www.stonegatechc.org

TRILLIUM HEALTH CENTRE - WEST TORONTO
150 Sherway Dr
Etobicoke ON M9C 1A5
Tel. 416 259-6671
Fax 416 521-4000
www.trilliumhealthcentre.org

WILLIAM OSLER HEALTH SYSTEM - ETOBICOKE GENERAL HOSPITAL
101 Humber College Blvd
Etobicoke ON M9V 1R8
Tel. 416 494-2120
Fax 416 747-8608
www.williamoslerhc.on.ca

EXETER

SOUTH HURON HOSPITAL ASSOCIATION
24 Huron St W
Exeter ON N0M 1S2
Tel. 519 235-2700
Fax 519 235-3405
www.shha.on.ca

FERGUS

GROVES MEMORIAL COMMUNITY HOSPITAL
235 Union St E
Fergus ON N1M 1W3
Tel. 519 843-2010
Fax 519 843-7288
www.gmch.ca

KIDSABILITY CENTRE FOR CHILD DEVELOPMENT - FERGUS
160 St David St S
Fergus ON N1M 2L3
Fax 519 843-7597
www.kidsability.ca

TRELLIS MENTAL HEALTH AND DEVELOPMENTAL SERVICES - FERGUS
234 St Patrick St E
Fergus ON N1M 1M6
Tel. 519 843-6191
Fax 519 843-7608
www.trellis.on.ca

FOREST

KETTLE & STONY POINT HEALTH CENTRE
6247 Indian Lane RR 2
PO Box 670
Forest ON N0N 1J0
Tel. 519 786-5647
Fax 519 786-4541
www.kettlepoint.org/healthservices

NORTH LAMBTON COMMUNITY HEALTH CENTRE - FOREST SITE
3-59 King St W
Forest ON N0N 1J0
Tel. 519 786-4545
Fax 519 786-6318
www.nlchc.com

NORTH LAMBTON COMMUNITY HEALTH CENTRE - KETTLE POINT SITE
6275 Indian Lane
Forest ON N0N 1J0
Tel. 519 786-2770
Fax 519 786-4992
www.nlchc.com

FORT ALBANY

FORT ALBANY HEALTH CENTRE
Gen Del
Fort Albany ON P0L 1H0
Tel. 705 278-3333
Fax 705 278-1069

JAMES BAY GENERAL HOSPITAL - FORT ALBANY HOSPITAL WING
5 Airport Rd
Fort Albany ON P0L 1H0
Tel. 705 278-3330
Fax 705 278-1121
www.weeneebaykohealth.ca

FORT ERIE

BRIDGES COMMUNITY HEALTH CENTRE - FORT ERIE
1485 Garrison Rd
Fort Erie ON L2A 1P8
Tel. 905 871-7621
www.bridgeschc.ca

NIAGARA HEALTH SYSTEM - DOUGLAS MEMORIAL HOSPITAL SITE
230 Bertie St
Fort Erie ON L2A 1Z2
Tel. 905 378-4647
Fax 905 871-7765
www.niagarahealth.on.ca

FORT FRANCES

COUCHICHING (BAND) HEALTH OFFICE
RMB 2027
RR 2
Fort Frances ON P9A 3M3
Tel. 807 274-3228
Fax 807 274-6199
www.firstnation.ca

FORT FRANCES HEALTH CENTRE
PO Box 626
Fort Frances ON P9A 3M9
Tel. 807 274-7771
Fax 807 274-4285

LA VERENDRYE HOSPITAL -RIVERSIDE HEALTH CARE FACILITY
110 Victoria Ave
Fort Frances ON P9A 2B7
Tel. 807 274-3266
Fax 807 274-2898
www.riversidehealthcare.ca

RAINY RIVER HEALTH CENTRE -RIVERSIDE HEALTH CARE FACILITY
115 Fourth St
Rainy River ON P0W 1L0
Tel. 807 852-3261 x 6560
www.riversidehealthcare.ca

STANJIKOMING HEALTH OFFICE
PO Box 609
Fort Frances ON P9A 3M4
Tel. 807 274-2188
Fax 807 274-4774
www.firstnation.ca

FORT SEVERN

FORT SEVERN NURSING STATION
GD
Fort Severn ON P0V 1W0
Tel. 807 478-2575
Fax 807 478-2541

GEORGETOWN

HALTON HEALTHCARE SERVICES CORPORATION - GEORGETOWN HOSPITAL
1 Princess Anne Dr
Georgetown ON L7G 2B8
Tel. 905 873-0111
Fax 905 873-4574
www.haltonhealthcare.com

GERALDTON

GERALDTON DISTRICT HOSPITAL
500 Hogarth Ave W
Geraldton ON P0T 1M0
Tel. 807 854-1862
Fax 807 854-1568
www.geraldtondh.com

GODERICH

ALEXANDRA MARINE & GENERAL HOSPITAL
120 Napier St
Goderich ON N7A 1W5
Tel. 519 524-8689 Ext. 5271
Fax 519 524-5579
www.amgh.ca

GRAND BEND

GRAND BEND COMMUNITY HEALTH CENTRE - GRAND BEND
69 Main St E
Grand Bend ON N0M 1T0
Tel. 519 238-2362
Fax 519 238-6478
www.gbachc.ca

GRIMSBY

WEST LINCOLN MEMORIAL HOSPITAL
169 Main St E
Grimsby ON L3M 1P3
Tel. 905 945-2253
Fax 905 945-0504
www.wlmh.on.ca

GUELPH

GUELPH COMMUNITY HEALTH CENTRE
176 Wyndham St N
Guelph ON N1H 8N9
Tel. 519 821-6638
Fax 519 821-6148
www.guelphchc.ca

GUELPH COMMUNITY HEALTH CENTRE - SHELLDALE
20 Shelldale Cres
Guelph ON N1H 1C8
Tel. 519 821-6638
Fax 519 821-2080
www.guelphchc.ca

GUELPH GENERAL HOSPITAL
115 Delhi St
Guelph ON N1E 4J4
Tel. 519 837-6440
Fax 519 822-2170
www.gghorg.ca

HOMEWOOD HEALTH CENTRE
150 Delhi St
Guelph ON N1E 6K9
Tel. 519 824-1010
Fax 519 824-8751
www.homewood.org

KIDSABILITY CENTRE FOR CHILD DEVELOPMENT - GUELPH (IMPERIAL RD SITE)
21 Imperial Rd S
Guelph ON N1K 1X3
Fax 519 780-0470
www.kidsability.ca

KIDSABILITY CENTRE FOR CHILD DEVELOPMENT - GUELPH (WOODLAWN RD SITE)
18 & 19-340 Woodlawn Rd W
Guelph ON N1H 7K6
Tel. 519 780-0186
Fax 519 886-7292
www.kidsability.ca

ST JOSEPH'S HEALTH CENTRE
100 Westmount Rd
Guelph ON N1H 5H8
Tel. 519 824-2620
Fax 519 763-0264
www.sjhh.guelph.on.ca

TRELLIS MENTAL HEALTH AND DEVELOPMENTAL SERVICES - DELHI ST
147 Delhi St
Guelph ON N1E 4J3
Tel. 519 821-2060
Fax 519 821-6139
www.trellis.on.ca

TRELLIS MENTAL HEALTH AND DEVELOPMENTAL SERVICES - SILVERCREEK
1-485 Silvercreek Pkwy N
Guelph ON N1H 7K5
Tel. 519 836-4991
Fax 519 836-7459
www.trellis.on.ca

TRELLIS MENTAL HEALTH CLINIC
1-485 Rivercreek Pkwy N
Guelph ON N1H 7K5
Tel. 519 824-5544
Fax 519 824-0178
www.cmhcgwd.on.ca

GULL BAY

GULL BAY HEALTH STATION
Gull Bay PO
via Armstrong
Gull Bay ON P0T 1P0
Tel. 807 982-2104
Fax 807 982-2232

HAGERSVILLE

WEST HALDIMAND GENERAL HOSPITAL
75 Parkview Rd
Hagersville ON N0A 1H0
Tel. 905 768-3311
Fax 905 768-1820
www.whgh.ca

HALIBURTON

HALIBURTON HIGHLANDS HEALTH SERVICES - HALIBURTON SITE
7199 Gelert Rd
PO Box 115
Haliburton ON K0M 1S0
Tel. 705 457-1392
Fax 705 457-2398
www.hhhs.on.ca

HAMILTON

DE DWA DA DEHS NYE'S ABORIGINAL HEALTH ACCESS CENTRE
678 Main St E
Hamilton ON L8M 1K2
Tel. 905 544-4320
Fax 905 544-4247
www.aboriginalhealthcentre.com

HAMILTON COMMUNITY HEALTH CENTRE
M6-414 Victoria Ave N
Hamilton ON L8L 5G8
Tel. 905 525-5656
Fax 905 525-4242

HAMILTON HEALTH SCIENCES CENTRE - CHEDOKE HOSPITAL
559 Sanatorium Rd
Hamilton ON L9C 7W8
Tel. 905 521-2100
Fax 905 521-5067
www.hamiltonhealthsciences.ca

HAMILTON HEALTH SCIENCES CENTRE - HAMILTON GENERAL HOSPITAL
237 Barton St E
Hamilton ON L8L 2X2
Tel. 905 527-4322
Fax 905 527-1941
www.hamiltonhealthsciences.ca

HAMILTON HEALTH SCIENCES CENTRE - JURAVINSKI CANCER CENTRE
699 Concession St
Hamilton ON L8V 5C2
Tel. 905 387-9495
Fax 905 575-6323
www.hrcc.on.ca

HAMILTON HEALTH SCIENCES CENTRE -JURAVINSKI SITE
711 Concession St
Hamilton ON L8V 1C3
Tel. 905 521-2100
Fax 905 521-5067
www.hamiltonhealthsciences.ca

HAMILTON HEALTH SCIENCES CENTRE - MCMASTER CHILDREN'S HOSPITAL
1200 Main St W
PO Box 2000 Stn Lcd 1
Hamilton ON L8N 3Z5
Tel. 905 521-2100
Fax 905 521-5090
mcmasterchildrenshospital.ca

HAMILTON HEALTH SCIENCES CENTRE - MCMASTER UNIVERSITY MEDICAL CENTRE
1200 Main St W
PO Box 2000 Stn Lcd 1
Hamilton ON L8N 3Z5
Tel. 905 521-2100 Ext. 5387
Fax 905 521-5092
www.hamiltonhealthsciences.ca

HAMILTON HEALTH SCIENCES CENTRE - ST PETER'S HOSPITAL
88 Maplewood Ave
Hamilton ON L8M 1W9
Tel. 905 777-3837
Fax 905 545-0822
www.stpetes.ca

HAMILTON URBAN CARE COMMUNITY HEALTH CENTRE
71 Rebecca St
Hamilton ON L8R 1B6
Tel. 905 522-3233
Fax 905 522-3433
www.hucchc.com

NORTH HAMILTON COMMUNITY HEALTH CENTRE
438 Hughson St N
Hamilton ON L8L 4N5
Tel. 905 523-6611 Ext. 300
Fax 905 523-5173
www.nhchc.ca

NORTH HAMILTON COMMUNITY HEALTH CENTRE - WENTWORTH
460 Wentworth St N
Hamilton ON L8L 5W8
Tel. 905 521-8295
www.nhchc.ca

ST JOSEPH'S HEALTHCARE - CHARLTON CAMPUS
50 Charlton Ave E
Hamilton ON L8N 4A6
Tel. 905 522-4941
Fax 905 521-6140
www.stjoes.ca

ST JOSEPH'S HEALTHCARE HAMILTON - KING CAMPUS
2757 King St E
Hamilton ON L8G 5E4
Tel. 905 573-7777
Fax 905 573-4828
www.stjoes.ca

ST JOSEPH'S HEALTHCARE HAMILTON - WEST 5TH CAMPUS
100 West 5th St
PO Box 585 Stn Lcd 1
Hamilton ON L8N 3K7
Tel. 905 388-2511
Fax 905 575-6038
www.stjoes.ca

WELLWOOD RESOURCE CENTRE - COMMUNITY SITE
501 Sanatorium Rd
Hamilton ON L9C 0C3
Tel. 905 667-8870
www.wellwood.on.ca

WELLWOOD RESOURCE CENTRE - HOSPITAL SITE
711 Concession St
Hamilton ON L8V 1C3
Tel. 905 389-5884
www.wellwood.on.ca

HANOVER

HANOVER & DISTRICT HOSPITAL
90 7th Ave
Hanover ON N4N 1N1
Tel. 519 364-2340
Fax 519 364-6602
www.hanoverhospital.on.ca

HAWKESBURY

HAWKESBURY & DISTRICT GENERAL HOSPITAL
1111 Ghislain St
Hawkesbury ON K6A 3G5
Tel. 613 632-1111
Fax 613 636-6161
www.hgh.ca

HEARST

HÔPITAL NOTRE DAME HOSPITAL - HEARST
1405 Edward St
PO BOX 8000
Hearst ON P0L 1N0
Tel. 705 362-4291
Fax 705 372-2923
www.ndh.on.ca

HENSALL

GRAND BEND COMMUNITY HEALTH CENTRE - HENSALL SITE
122 King St
PO Box 159
Hensall ON N0M 1X0
Tel. 519 238-2362
Fax 519 238-2448
www.gbachc.ca

HERON BAY

PICK RIVER HEALTH CENTRE
Gen Del
Heron Bay ON P0T 1R0
Tel. 807 229-1836
Fax 807 229-3367

HORNEPAYNE

HORNEPAYNE COMMUNITY HOSPITAL
278 Front St
PO Box 190
Hornepayne ON P0M 1Z0
Tel. 807 868-2442
Fax 807 868-2697
www.hornepayne.com

HUNTSVILLE

HUNTSVILLE DISTRICT MEMORIAL HOSPITAL - MUSKOKA ALGONQUIN HEALTHCARE
100 Frank Miller Dr
Huntsville ON P1H 1H7
Tel. 705 789-2311
Fax 705 789-0557
www.mahc.ca

IGNACE

MARY BERGLUND COMMUNITY HEALTH CENTRE
Hwy 7 & 599
Ignace ON P0T 1T0
Tel. 807 934-6719
www.ontariochc.ca

INGERSOLL

ALEXANDRA HOSPITAL
29 Noxon St
Ingersoll ON N5C 1B8
Tel. 519 485-1700
Fax 519 485-9606
www.alexandrahospital.on.ca

INNISFIL

BARRIE COMMUNITY HEALTH CENTRE - NORTH INNISFIL
902 Lockhart Rd
Innisfil ON L9S 4V2
www.bchc.ca

IROQUOIS FALLS

ANSON GENERAL HOSPITAL
58 Anson Dr
Iroquois Falls ON P0K 1E0
Tel. 705 258-3911
Fax 705 258-2618
www.micsgroup.com

KAPUSKASING

SENSENBRENNER HOSPITAL
101 Progress Cres
Kapuskasing ON P5N 3H5
Tel. 705 337-6111
Fax 705 337-4021
www.senhosp.ca

KASABONIKA

EMILY ANDERSON MEMORIAL NURSING STATION
Kasabonia Lake
via Pickle Lake
Kasabonika ON P0V 1Y0
Tel. 807 535-1189
Fax 807 535-1192

KASHECHEWAN

KASHECHEWAN NURSING STATION
PO Box 243
Kashechewan ON P0L 1S0
Tel. 705 275-4444
Fax 705 275-1010

KEEWATIN

WASHAGAMIS HEALTH STATION
PO Box 571
Keewatin ON P0X 1C0
Tel. 807 543-2532
Fax 807 543-2964

KEEWAYWIN

KEEWAYWIN HEALTH OFFICE
PO Box 59
Keewaywin ON P0V 3G0
Tel. 807 771-1210
Fax 807 771-1053
www.keewaywin.firstnation.ca

KEJICK

SHOAL LAKE #39 HEALTH STATION
Gen Del
Kejick ON P0X 1E0
Tel. 807 733-3318
Fax 807 733-2871

KEMPTVILLE

KEMPTVILLE DISTRICT HOSPITAL
2675 Concession Rd
PO Box 2007
Kemptville ON K0G 1J0
Tel. 613 258-6133
Fax 613 258-4997
www.kdh.on.ca

KENORA

KENORA HEALTH CARE CENTRE
100 Park St
Federal Bldg
Kenora ON P9N 1Y6
Tel. 807 468-8961
Fax 807 468-6257

LAKE OF THE WOODS DISTRICT HOSPITAL
21 Sylvan St
Kenora ON P9N 3W7
Tel. 807 468-9861 Ext. 230
Fax 807 468-3939
www.lwdh.on.ca

RAT PORTAGE HEALTH STATION
PO Box 1850
Kenora ON P9N 3X1
Tel. 807 548-6340
Fax 807 548-4877
www.firstnation.ca

KILLALOE

LANARK HEALTH & COMMUNITY SERVICES (RAINBOW VALLEY)
49 Mill St
Killaloe ON K0J 2A0
Tel. 613 757-0004
www.ontariochc.ca

KINCARDINE

SOUTH BRUCE GREY HEALTH CENTRE - KINCARDINE SITE
43 Queen St
Kincardine ON N2Z 2Z2
Tel. 519 396-3331
Fax 519 881-0452
www.sbghc.on.ca

KINGSTON

CANCER CENTRE OF SOUTHEASTERN ONTARIO
25 King St W
Kingston ON K7L 5P9
Tel. 613 544-2630 Ext. 6830
Fax 613 544-9708
www.krcc.on.ca

HOTEL-DIEU HOSPITAL
166 Brock St
Kingston ON K7L 5G2
Tel. 613 544-3310
Fax 613 544-9897
www.hoteldieu.com

KINGSTON COMMUNITY HEALTH CENTRE
400 Elliott Ave
Kingston ON K7K 6M9
Tel. 613 542-2949
Fax 613 542-3872
www.kchc.ca

KINGSTON COMMUNITY HEALTH CENTRE - BETTER BEGINNINGS FOR KINGSTON CHILDREN
900 Monteal St
Kingston ON K7K 3J9
Tel. 613 542-2835
Fax 613 542-3861
www.kchc.ca

KINGSTON COMMUNITY HEALTH CENTRE - KINGSTON IMMIGRATION PARTNERSHIP
500-837 Princess St
Kingston ON K7L 1G8
Tel. 613 544-4661
Fax 613 544-2916
www.khc.ca

KINGSTON COMMUNITY HEALTH CENTRE - NAPANEE
6 Dundas St E
Kingston ON K7K 6M9
Tel. 613 354-8937
Fax 613 354-8940
www.kchc.ca

KINGSTON COMMUNITY HEALTH CENTRE - STREET HEALTH CENTRE
235 Wellington St
Kingston ON K7K 0B5
Tel. 613 549-1440
Fax 613 549-7986
www.kchc.ca

KINGSTON GENERAL HOSPITAL
76 Stuart St
Kingston ON K7L 2V7
Tel. 613 549-6666 Ext. 3232
www.kgh.on.ca

KINGSTON REGIONAL TREATMENT CENTRE
560 King St W
PO Box 22 Stn Main
Kingston ON K7L 4V7
Tel. 613 536-6901
Fax 613 536-4115
www.csc-scc.gc.ca

ONGWANADA RESOURCE CENTRE
191 Portsmouth Ave
Kingston ON K7M 8A6
Tel. 613 548-4417
Fax 613 548-8135
www.ongwanda.com

PROVIDENCE CARE - MENTAL HEALTH SERVICES
752 King St W
PO BOX 603 Stn Main
Kingston ON K7L 4X3
Tel. 613 546-1101
Fax 613 548-5588
www.providencecare.ca

PROVIDENCE CARE - ST MARY'S OF THE LAKE HOSPITAL SITE
340 Union St
PO BOX 3600 Stn Main
Kingston ON K7L 5A2
Tel. 613 544-5220
Fax 613 544-8558
www.providencecare.ca

KIRKLAND LAKE

KIRKLAND & DISTRICT HOSPITAL
145 Government Rd E
PO BOX 3000 Stn Main
Kirkland Lake ON P2N 3P4
Tel. 705 567-5251
Fax 705 568-2102
www.kdhospital.com

KITCHENER

GRAND RIVER HOSPITAL - FREEPORT SITE
3570 King St E
PO Box 9056
Kitchener ON N2A 2W1
Tel. 519 749-4300
Fax 519 749-4208
www.grhosp.on.ca

GRAND RIVER HOSPITAL - KITCHENER/WATERLOO HEALTH CENTRE
835 King St W
PO Box 9056 Stn C
Kitchener ON N2G 1G3
Tel. 519 749-4300
Fax 519 749-4208
www.grhosp.on.ca

GRAND RIVER REGIONAL CANCER CENTRE
835 King St W
PO Box 9056
Kitchener ON N2G 1G3
Tel. 519 749-4370
Fax 519 749-4274
www.grhosp.on.ca

KIDSABILITY CENTRE FOR CHILD DEVELOPMENT - KITCHENER
65 Hanson AVe
Kitchener ON N2C 2H6
Tel. 519 886-8886
Fax 519 886-7292
www.kidsability.ca

KITCHENER DOWNTOWN COMMUNITY HEALTH CENTRE
44 Francis St S
Kitchener ON N2G 2A2
Tel. 519 745-4404
Fax 519 745-3709
www.kdchc.org

ST MARY'S GENERAL HOSPITAL
911 Queens Blvd
Kitchener ON N2M 1B2
Tel. 519 744-3311
Fax 519 749-6426
www.smgh.ca

TRELLIS MENTAL HEALTH AND DEVELOPMENTAL SERVICES - KITCHENER
202-130 Weber St W
Kitchener ON N2H 4A2
Tel. 519 576-2333
Fax 519 576-8980
www.trellis.on.ca

LANARK

LANARK HEALTH & COMMUNITY SERVICES
207 Robertson Dr
Lanark ON K0G 1K0
Tel. 613 259-2372
www.lanarkhealth.on.c

LANSDOWNE HOUSE

LANSDOWNE HOUSE NURSING STATION
GD
via Pickle Lake
Lansdowne House ON P0T 1Z0
Tel. 807 479-2533
Fax 807 479-2588

LEAMINGTON

LEAMINGTON DISTRICT MEMORIAL HOSPITAL
194 Talbot St W
Leamington ON N8H 1N9
Tel. 519 326-2373
Fax 519 322-5584
www.leamingtonhospital.com

LINDSAY

COMMUNITY CARE CITY OF KAWARTHA LAKES
34 Cambridge St S
Lindsay ON K9V 3B8
Tel. 705 321-7323
www.community-care.on.ca

ROSS MEMORIAL HOSPITAL
10 Angeline St N
Lindsay ON K9V 4M8
Tel. 705 324-6111
Fax 705 328-2817
www.rmh.org

LIONS HEAD

GREY BRUCE HEALTH SERVICES - LION'S HEAD
22 Moore St
PO Box 220
Lions Head ON N0H 1W0
Tel. 519 793-3424
Fax 519 534-4407
www.gbhs.on.ca

LISTOWEL

LISTOWEL MEMORIAL HOSPITAL - LISTOWEL WINGHAM HOSPITALS ALLIANCE
255 Elizabeth St E
Listowel ON N4W 2P5
Tel. 519 291-3120
Fax 519 291-5440
www.lwha.ca

LITTLE CURRENT

MANITOULIN HEALTH CENTRE - LITTLE CURRENT
11 Meredith St
PO Box 640
Little Current ON P0P 1K0
Tel. 705 368-2300
Fax 705 368-3566
manitoulinhealthcentre.com

NAANDWEGAMIK HEALTH CENTRE
PO Box 21
Little Current ON P0P 1K0
Tel. 705 368-3171
Fax 705 368-0293
www.aundeckomnikaningfn.com

NOOJMOWIN TEG HEALTH CENTRE
48 Hillside Rd
Hwy 540; Postal Bag 2002
Little Current ON P0P 1K0
Tel. 705 368-2182
Fax 705 368-2229
www.ontariochc.ca

LONDON

CHILD & PARENT RESOURCE INSTITUTE
600 Sanatorium Rd
London ON N6H 3W7
Tel. 519 858-2774
Fax 519 858-3913
www.cpri.ca

LONDON HEALTH SCIENCES CENTRE - CHILDREN'S HOSPITAL
800 Commissioners Rd E
PO Box 5010
London ON N6A 4G5
Tel. 519 685-8500
Fax 519 685-8127
www.childrenshospitallhsc.ca

LONDON HEALTH SCIENCES CENTRE - LONDON REGIONAL CANCER CENTRE
790 Commissioners Rd E
London ON N6A 4L6
Tel. 519 685-8600
Fax 519 685-8614
www.lhsc.on.ca

LONDON HEALTH SCIENCES CENTRE - SOUTH STREET
375 South St
London ON N6A 4G5
Tel. 519 685-8500
Fax 519 667-6628
www.lhsc.on.ca

LONDON HEALTH SCIENCES CENTRE - UNIVERSITY HOSPITAL
339 Windermere Rd
PO Box 5339 Stn B
London ON N6A 5A5
Tel. 519 685-8500
www.lhsc.on.ca

LONDON HEALTH SCIENCES CENTRE - VICTORIA CAMPUS
800 Commissioners Rd E
PO Box 5010 Stn B
London ON N6A 5W9
Tel. 519 685-8500
www.lhsc.on.ca

LONDON INTERCOMMUNITY HEALTH CENTRE - DUNDAS STREET
659 Dundas St
London ON N5W 2Z1
Tel. 519 660-0874
Fax 519 642-1532
www.lihc.on.ca

LONDON INTERCOMMUNITY HEALTH CENTRE - HURON STREET
7-1355 Huron St
London ON N5V 1R9
Tel. 519 659-6399
Fax 519 659-9930
www.lihc.on.ca

PARKWOOD HOSPITAL - ST JOSEPH'S HEALTH CARE
801 Commissioners Rd E
London ON N6C 5J1
Tel. 519 685-4000
Fax 519 685-4052
www.sjhc.london.on.ca

REGIONAL MENTAL HEALTH CARE-ST JOSEPH'S HEALTH CARE
850 Highbury Ave
PO Box 5532 Stn B
London ON N6A 4H1
Tel. 519 455-5110
Fax 519 455-9986
www.sjhc.london.on.ca

ST JOSEPH'S HOSPITAL - ST JOSEPH'S HEALTH CARE
268 Grosvenor St
PO Box 5777 Stn B
London ON N6A 4V2
Tel. 519 646-6000
Fax 519 646-6054
www.sjhc.london.on.ca

ST MARY'S HOSPITAL - ST JOSEPH'S HEALTH CARE LONDON
21 Grosvenor St
London ON N6A 1Y6
Tel. 519 646-6000
Fax 519 646-6148
www.sjhc.london.on.ca

THAMES VALLEY CHILDREN'S CENTRE
779 Base Line Rd
London ON N6C 5Y6
Tel. 519 685-8700
Fax 519 685-8699
www.tvcc.on.ca

LONGLAC

GINOOGAMING HEALTH STATION
PO Box 89
Longlac ON P0T 2A0
Tel. 807 876-2732
Fax 807 876-1614

LONGLAC #58 FIRST NATIONS HEALTH STATION
PO Box 817
Longlac ON P0T 2A0
Tel. 807 876-4553
Fax 807 876-1615

NORWEST COMMUNITY HEALTH CENTRE - LONGLAC
99 Skinner Ave
PO Box 910
Longlac ON P0T 2A0
Tel. 807 876-2271
Fax 807 876-2473
www.norwestchc.org

MACDIARMID

ROCKY BAY HEALTH STATION
Gen Del
Macdiarmid ON P0T 2B0
Tel. 807 885-3204
Fax 807 885-3206

MANITOUWADGE

MANITOUWADGE GENERAL HOSPITAL
1 Healthcare Cres
Manitouwadge ON P0T 2C0
Tel. 807 826-3251
Fax 807 826-4216
www.mh.on.ca

MARATHON

WILSON MEMORIAL GENERAL HOSPITAL
26 Peninsula Rd
PO Bag W
Marathon ON P0T 2E0
Tel. 807 229-1740
Fax 807 229-1721
www.wmgh.net

MARKDALE

GREY BRUCE HEALTH SERVICES - MARKDALE
55 Isla St
PO Box 406
Markdale ON N0C 1H0
Tel. 519 986-3040
Fax 519 986-4562
www.gbhs.on.ca

MARKHAM

MARKHAM STOUFFVILLE HOSPITAL
381 Church St
PO Box 1800 Stn Main
Markham ON L3P 7P3
Tel. 905 472-7000
Fax 905 472-7086
www.msh.on.ca

MASSEY

SAGAMOK HEALTH CENTRE
4005 Espaniel St
PO Box 610
Massey ON P0P 1P0
Tel. 705 865-2171
Fax 705 865-3131
www.sagamok.ca

MATHESON

BINGHAM MEMORIAL HOSPITAL
507 8th Ave
PO Box 70 Stn Main
Matheson ON P0K 1N0
Tel. 705 273-2424
Fax 705 273-2515
www.micsgroup.com

WAHGOSHIG HEALTH STATION
PO Box 722
Matheson ON P0K 1N0
Tel. 705 268-9066
Fax 705 268-8554

MATTAWA

MATTAWA HOSPITAL
217 Turcotte Park Rd
PO Box 70 Stn Main
Mattawa ON P0H 1V0
Tel. 705 744-5511
Fax 705 744-6020
www.mattawahospital.ca

M'CHIGEENG

M'CHIGEENG HEALTH CENTRE
689 Hwy 551
Po Box 308
M'Chigeeng ON P0P 1G0
Tel. 705 377-5347
Fax 705 377-5090
www.mchigeeng.ca

MEAFORD

GREY BRUCE HEALTH SERVICES - MEAFORD SITE
229 Nelson St W
Meaford ON N4L 1A3
Tel. 519 538-1311
Fax 519 538-5500
www.gbhs.on.ca

MERRICKVILLE

RIDEAU COMMUNITY HEALTH SERVICES - MERRICKVILLE DISTRICT COMMUNITY HEALTH CENTRE
354 Read St
PO Box 550
Merrickville ON K0G 1N0
Tel. 613 269-3400
Fax 613 269-4958
www.rvds.ca

MIDLAND

GEORGIAN BAY GENERAL HOSPITAL - MIDLAND
1112 St Andrew's Dr
PO BOX 760 Stn Main
Midland ON L4R 4P4
Tel. 705 526-3751
Fax 705 526-2007
www.gbgh.on.ca

MIGISI SAHGAIGAN

EAGLE LAKE HEALTH OFFICE
122 Aspen Road
PO Box 1001
Migisi Sahgaigan ON P0V 3H0
Tel. 807 755-1157
Fax 807 755-1161
www.eaglelakefirstnation.ca

MILTON

HALTON HEALTHCARE SERVICES CORPORATION - MILTON DISTRICT HOSPITAL
7030 Derry Rd
Milton ON L9T 7H6
Tel. 905 878-2383
Fax 905 878-7047
www.haltonhealthcare.com

MINDEMOYA

MANITOULIN HEALTH CENTRE - MINDEMOYA SITE
2120A-Hwy 551
PO Box 170
Mindemoya ON P0P 1S0
Tel. 705 377-5311
Fax 705 368-5799

MINDEN

HALIBURTON HIGHLANDS HEALTH SERVICES - MIDEN SITE
6 McPherson St
PO Box 30
Minden ON K0M 2K0
Tel. 705 286-2140
Fax 705 286-6384
www.hhhs.on.ca

MINE CENTRE

SEINE RIVER HEALTH STATION
Gen Del
Mine Centre ON P0W 1H0
Tel. 807 599-2224
Fax 807 599-2865

MISSISSAUGA

THE CREDIT VALLEY HOSPITAL
2200 Eglinton Ave W
Mississauga ON L5M 2N1
Tel. 905 813-2200
Fax 905 813-4444
www.cvh.on.ca

ERINOAK KIDS CENTRE FOR TREATMENT AND DEVELOPMENT
120-2695 North Sheridan Way
Mississauga ON L5K 2N6
Tel. 905 855-2690
Fax 905 855-9404
www.erinoakkids.ca

TRILLIUM HEALTH CENTRE - MISSISSAUGA
100 Queensway W
Mississauga ON L5B 1B8
Tel. 905 848-7100
Fax 905 848-7356
www.trilliumhealthcentre.org

MOBERT

PIC MOBERT HEALTH STATION
Gen Delivery
Mobert ON P0M 2J0
Tel. 807 822-2625
Fax 807 822-2975

MONETVILLE

DOKIS HEALTH STATION
Gen Del
Monetville ON P0M 2K0
Tel. 705 763-2112
Fax 705 763-2663

MOOSE FACTORY

MOOSE FACTORY HEALTH CENTRE
22 Jonathan Cheechoo Dr
PO Box 190
Moose Factory ON P0L 1W0
Tel. 705 658-4619
Fax 705 658-4734
www.firstnation.ca

WEENEEBAYKO GENERAL HOSPITAL
19 Hospital Dr
PO Box 34
Moose Factory ON P0L 1W0
Tel. 705 658-4544
Fax 705 658-4917
www.weeneebaykohealth.ca

MOOSONEE

JAMES BAY GENERAL HOSPITAL - MOOSONEE, FORT ALBANY, AND ATTAWAPISKAT
4 Ferguson Rd N
PO Box 370
Moosonee ON P0L 1Y0
Tel. 705 336-2947
Fax 705 336-2637
www.jbgh.org

MOOSONEE HEALTH CENTRE
PO Box 370
Moosonee ON P0L 1Y0
Tel. 705 336-2341
Fax 705 336-2066
www.moosecree.com

MORSON

BIG ISLAND HEALTH OFFICE
GD
Morson ON P0W 1J0
Tel. 807 488-5602
Fax 807 488-5942

MOUNT BRYDGES

SOUTHWEST MIDDLESEX HEALTH CENTRE
22262 Mill Rd at Hwy 81
RR 5
Mount Brydges ON N0L 1W0
Tel. 519 264-2800
Fax 519 264-2742
www.smhc.net

MOUNT FOREST

COMMUNITY MENTAL HEALTH CLINIC - MOUNT FOREST
392 Main St
Suite 1
Mount Forest ON N0G 2L2
Tel. 519 323-4004
Fax 519 323-3771
www.trellis.on.ca

NORTH WELLINGTON HEALTH CARE - LOUISE MARSHALL HOSPITAL
630 Dublin St
Mount Forest ON N0G 2L3
Tel. 519 323-2210
Fax 519 323-3741
www.nwhealthcare.ca

TRELLIS MENTAL HEALTH AND DEVELOPMENTAL SERVICES - MOUNT FOREST
1-392 Main St N
Mount Forest ON N0G 2L2
Tel. 519 323-4004
Fax 519 323-3771
www.trellis.on.ca

MUNCEY

CHIPPEWAS OF THE THAMES HEALTH SERVICES
322 Chippewas Rd
RR #1
Muncey ON N0L 1Y0
Tel. 519 289-5641
www.firstnation.ca

MUNCEY HEALTH CENTRE
PO Box 426
RR 1
Muncey ON N0L 1Y0
Tel. 519 289-2220
Fax 519 289-5121

MUSKRAT DAM

MUSKRAT DAM HEALTH STATION
Muskrat Dam
via Pickle Lake
Muskrat Dam ON P0V 3B0
Tel. 807 471-2573
Fax 807 537-2699
www.ifna.ca

NAKINA

OGOKI HEALTH STAION
Gen Del via Nakina
Nakina ON P0T 2H0
Tel. 807 349-2510
Fax 807 349-2688

NAPANEE

LENNOX & ADDINGTON COUNTY GENERAL HOSPITAL
8 Richmond Park Dr
Napanee ON K7R 2Z4
Tel. 613 354-3301 Ext. 202
Fax 613 354-7157
www.lacgh.com

NAUGHTON

SHAWENEKEZHIK HEALTH CENTRE WHITEFISH LAKE FIRST NATION
25 Reserve Rd
Naughton ON P0M 2M0
Tel. 705 692-3674
Fax 705 692-7255

NESTOR FALLS

ONEGAMING HEALTH STATION
PO Box 160
Nestor Falls ON P0X 1K0
Tel. 807 484-2339
Fax 807 484-2789

NEW LISKEARD

TEMISKAMING HOSPITAL
421 Shepherdson Rd
New Liskeard ON P0J 1P0
Tel. 705 647-8121
Fax 705 647-5800
www.temiskaming-hospital.com

NEWBURY

FOUR COUNTIES HEALTH SERVICES - MIDDLESEX HOSPITAL ALLIANCE
1824 Concession Dr
RR 3
Newbury ON N0L 1Z0
Tel. 519 693-4441
Fax 519 693-7084
www.mhalliance.on.ca

NEWMARKET

SOUTHLAKE REGIONAL HEALTH CENTRE
596 Davis Dr
Newmarket ON L3Y 2P9
Tel. 905 895-4521
Fax 905 830-5972
www.southlakeregional.org

NIAGARA FALLS

NIAGARA FALLS COMMUNITY HEALTH CENTRE
4481 Queen St
Niagara Falls ON L2E 2L4
Tel. 905 356-4222
Fax 905 356-5676
www.nfchc.ca

NIAGARA HEALTH SYSTEM - GREATER NIAGARA GENERAL SITE
5546 Portage Rd
Niagara Falls ON L2E 6X2
Tel. 905 378-4647
Fax 905 358-8435
www.niagarahealth.on.ca

NIAGARA-ON-THE-LAKE

NIAGARA HEALTH SYSTEM - NIAGARA-ON-THE-LAKE HOSPITAL SITE
176 Wellington St
PO Box 1270
Niagara-on-the-Lke ON L0S 1J0
Tel. 905 378-4647
Fax 905 468-7690
www.niagarahealth.on.ca

NIPIGON

LAKE HELEN HEALTH OFFICE
PO Box 1030
Nipigon ON P0T 2J0
Tel. 807 887-2510
Fax 807 887-0063

NIPIGON DISTRICT MEMORIAL HOSPITAL
125 Hogan Rd
PO Box 37
Nipigon ON P0T 2J0
Tel. 807 887-3026
Fax 807 887-2800
www.ndmh.ca

NORTH BAY

NORTH BAY REGIONAL HEALTH CENTRE - REGIONAL MENTAL HEALTH
50 College Dr
PO Box 2500
North Bay ON P1B 5A4
Tel. 705 474-7525
Fax 705 495-7896
www.nbrhc.on.ca

ONE KIDS PLACE/LA PLACE DES ENFANTS
400 400 Mckeown Ave
North Bay ON P1B 0B2
Tel. 705 476-5437
Fax 705 474-0127
www.onekidsplace.ca

NORTH SPIRIT LAKE

NORTH SPIRIT LAKE HEALTH STATION
Gen Del
North Spirit Lake ON P0V 2G0
Tel. 807 776-0019
Fax 807 776-0063
www.firstnation.ca

NORTH YORK

BLACK CREEK COMMUNITY HEALTH CENTER
5-2202 Jane St
North York ON M3M 1A4
Tel. 416 249-8000
Fax 416 249-4594
www.bcchc.com

BLACK CREEK COMMUNITY HEALTH CENTER YORKGATE
1 York Gate Blvd
North York ON M3N 3A1
Tel. 416 246-2388
Fax 416 650-0971
www.bcchc.com

CHILD DEVELOPMENT INSTITUTE
197 Euclid Ave
Toronto ON M3H 6A7
Tel. 416 603-1827
Fax 416 603-6655
www.childdevelop.ca

DONWAY HOSPITAL
800-12 Concorde Place
North York ON M3C 4J2
Tel. 416 442-5600
Fax 416 510-5128

FLEMINGDON COMMUNITY HEALTH CENTRE
10 Gateway Blvd
North York ON M3C 3A1
Tel. 416 429-4991
Fax 416 422-3573
www.fhc-chc.com

FLEMINGDON COMMUNITY HEALTH CENTRE - FAIRVIEW COMMUNITY HEALTH
5 Fairview Mall Dr
North York ON M2J 2Z1
Tel. 416 640-5298
www.fhc-chc.com

THE HINCKS-DELLCREST CENTRE - SHEPPARD
1645 Sheppard Ave W
North York ON M3M 2X4
Tel. 416 633-0515
Fax 416 633-7141
www.hincksdellcrest.org

HUMBER RIVER REGIONAL HOSPITAL - FINCH AVENUE SITE
2111 Finch Ave W
North York ON M3N 1N1
Tel. 416 744-2500
Fax 416 747-3882
www.hrrh.on.ca

HUMBER RIVER REGIONAL HOSPITAL - KEELE STREET SITE
2175 Keele St
Toronto ON M6M 3Z4
Tel. 416 249-8111
Fax 416 243-4547
www.hrrh.on.ca

NORTH YORK GENERAL HOSPITAL
4001 Leslie St
North York ON M2K 1E1
Tel. 416 756-6000
Fax 416 756-6384
www.nygh.on.ca

NORTH YORK GENERAL HOSPITAL - BRANSON DIVISION
555 Finch Ave W
North York ON M2R 1N5
Tel. 416 633-9420
Fax 416 635-2537
www.nygh.on.ca

ST JOHN'S REHABILITATION HOSPITAL
285 Cummer Ave
Toronto ON M2M 2G1
Tel. 416 226-6780
Fax 416 226-6265
www.stjohnsrehab.com

ST JOSEPH'S INFIRMARY
2 O'Connor Dr
North York ON M2K 2K1
Tel. 416 467-3080
Fax 416 467-8939

UNISON HEALTH AND COMMUNITY SERVICES - BATHURST-FINCH
104-5987 Bathurst St
North York ON M2R 1Z3
Tel. 647 436-0385
Fax 647 436-0215
www.unisonhcs.org

UNISON HEALTH AND COMMUNITY SERVICES - JANE-TRETHEWAY
1541 Jane St
North York ON M9N 2R3
Tel. 416 645-7575
Fax 416 645-7570
www.unisonhcs.org

UNISON HEALTH AND COMMUNITY SERVICES - LAWRENCE HEIGHTS
12 Flemington Rd
Toronto ON M6A 2N4
Tel. 416 787-1661
Fax 416 787-3761

OAKVILLE

CENTRAL WEST SPECIALIZED DEVELOPMENTAL SERVICES
53 Bond St
Oakville ON L6K 1L8
Tel. 905 844-7864
Fax 905 844-3545
www.cwsds.ca

HALTON HEALTHCARE SERVICES CORPORATION - OAKVILLE SITE
327 Reynolds St
Oakville ON L6J 3L7
Tel. 905 845-2571
Fax 905 338-4457
www.haltonhealthcare.com

OHSWEKEN

GANE YOHS COMMUNITY HEALTH CENTRE
PO Box 220
Ohsweken ON N0A 1M0
Tel. 519 445-2672
Fax 519 445-4525

ORANGEVILLE

HEADWATERS HEALTH CARE CENTRE - ORANGEVILLE SITE
100 Rolling Hills Dr
Orangeville ON L9W 4X9
Tel. 519 941-2410
Fax 519 942-0483
www.headwatershealth.ca

TRELLIS MENTAL HEALTH AND DEVELOPMENTAL SERVICES - ORANGVILLE
15 Brenda Blvd
Orangeville ON L9W 3Y5
Tel. 519 941-0465
Fax 519 941-0580
www.trellis.on.ca

ORILLIA

HURONIA REGIONAL CENTRE
700 Memorial Ave
PO Box 1000 Stn Main
Orillia ON L3V 6L2
Tel. 705 326-7361 Ext. 2315
Fax 705 326-2606
www.mcss.gov.on.ca

ORILLIA SOLDIERS' MEMORIAL HOSPITAL
170 Colborne St W
Orillia ON L3V 2Z3
Tel. 705 325-2201
Fax 705 325-7953
www.osmh.on.ca

OSHAWA

GRANDVIEW CHILDREN'S CENTRE MAIN SITE
600 Townline Rd S
Oshawa ON L1H 7K6
Tel. 905 728-1673
Fax 905 728-2961
www.grtc.ca

LAKERIDGE HEALTH - OSHAWA SITE
1 Hospital Crt
Oshawa ON L1G 2B9
Tel. 905 576-8711
Fax 905 721-7798
www.lakeridgehealth.on.ca

OSNABURGH HOUSE

MISHKEEGOGAMANG NURSING STATION
1 First Nation St
Osnaburgh House ON P0V 2H0
Tel. 807 928-2414
Fax 807 928-2077
www.mishkeegogamang.ca

OTTAWA

BRUYÈRE CONTINUING CARE - ELISABETH BRUYERE HOSPITAL
75 Bruyere St
Ottawa ON K1N 5C8
Tel. 613 562-6262
Fax 613 241-1971
www.bruyere.org

BRUYÈRE CONTINUING CARE - SAINT-VINCENT HOSPITAL
60 Cambridge St N
Ottawa ON K1R 7A5
Tel. 613 233-4041
Fax 613 782-2785
www.bruyere.org

CANADIAN FORCES HEALTH SERVICES CENTRE
1745 Alta Vista Dr
Ottawa ON K1A 0K6
Tel. 613 945-6600
Fax 613 991-1543

CARLINGTON COMMUNITY HEALTH CENTRE
900 Merivale Rd
Ottawa ON K1Z 5Z8
Tel. 613 722-4000
Fax 613 761-1805
www.carlington.ochc.org

CENTRETOWN COMMUNITY HEALTH CENTRE
420 Cooper St
Ottawa ON K2P 2N6
Tel. 613 233-4443
Fax 613 233-3987
www.centretownchc.org

CHILDREN'S HOSPITAL OF EASTERN ONTARIO (CHEO)
401 Smyth Rd
Ottawa ON K1H 8L1
Tel. 613 737-7600
Fax 613 738-3216
www.cheo.on.ca

HERRIDGE COMMUNITY HEALTH
59 Herridge St
Ottawa ON K1S 0G8
Tel. 613 236-7609

MONTFORT HOSPITAL
713 Montreal Rd
Ottawa ON K1K 0T2
Tel. 613 746-4621 Ext. 2006
Fax 613 748-4914
www.hopitalmontfort.com

OTTAWA CHILDREN'S TREATMENT CENTRE - CENTRAL LOCATION #1
395 Smyth Rd
Ottawa ON K1H 8L2
Tel. 613 737-0871
Fax 613 523-5167
www.octc.ca

OTTAWA CHILDREN'S TREATMENT CENTRE - CENTRAL LOCATION #2
401 Smyth Rd
2nd Fl
Ottawa ON K1H 8L1
Tel. 613 737-0871
Fax 613 738-4230
www.octc.ca

OTTAWA CHILDREN'S TREATMENT CENTRE - THURSTON RD SITE OF SERVICE
2211 Thurston Dr
Ottawa ON K1G 6C9
Tel. 613 688-2126
Fax 613 688-2142
www.octc.ca

OTTAWA CHILDREN'S TREATMENT CENTRE - WESTERN OTTAWA-KANATA SITE OF SERVICE
2 MacNeil Court
Ottawa ON K2L 4H7
Tel. 613 831-5098
Fax 613 831-9098
www.octc.ca

OTTAWA HOSPITAL CANCER CENTRE - CANCER CARE ONTARIO
501 Smyth Rd
Ottawa ON K1H 8L6
Tel. 613 737-7700 Ext. 6880
Fax 613 247-3503
www.cancercare.on.ca

THE OTTAWA HOSPITAL - CIVIC CAMPUS
1053 Carling Ave
Ottawa ON K1Y 4E9
Tel. 613 722-7000
Fax 613 761-4600
www.ottawahospital.on.ca

THE OTTAWA HOSPITAL - GENERAL CAMPUS
501 Smyth Rd
Ottawa ON K1H 8L6
Tel. 613 722-7000
Fax 613 737-8470
www.ottawahospital.on.ca

THE OTTAWA HOSPITAL REHABILITATION CENTRE
505 Smyth Rd
Ottawa ON K1H 8M2
Tel. 613 737-7350
Fax 613 737-9638
www.ottawahospital.on.ca/rehabcentre

THE OTTAWA HOSPITAL - RIVERSIDE CAMPUS
1967 Riverside Dr
Ottawa ON K1H 7W9
Tel. 613 722-7000
Fax 613 737-8526
www.ottawahospital.on.ca

THE PERLEY & RIDEAU VETERANS' HEALTH CENTRE
1750 Russell Rd
Ottawa ON K1G 5Z6
Tel. 613 526-7170
Fax 613 526-7172
www.prvhc.com

PINECREST-QUEENSWAY COMMUNITY HEALTH CENTRE
1365 Richmond Rd
2nd Floor
Ottawa ON K2B 6R7
Tel. 613 820-4922
Fax 613 288-3407
www.pqchc.com

QUEENSWAY CARLETON HOSPITAL
3045 Baseline Rd
Nepean ON K2H 8P4
Tel. 613 721-2000
Fax 613 721-4770
www.qch.on.ca

ROYAL OTTAWA MENTAL HEALTH CENTRE - ROYAL OTTAWA HEALTH CARE GROUP
1145 Carling Ave
Ottawa ON K1Z 7K4
Tel. 613 722-6521
Fax 613 722-7686
www.theroyal.ca

SANDY HILL COMMUNITY HEALTH CENTRE
221 Nelson St
Ottawa ON K1N 1C7
Tel. 613 789-8458
Fax 613 789-8710
www.sandyhillchc.ca

SCO HEALTH SERVICE - ÉLISABETH BRUYÈRE HOSPITAL
43 Bruyère St
Ottawa ON K1N 5C8
Tel. 613 562-6262
Fax 613 562-6367
www.bruyere.org

SOMERSET WEST COMMUNITY HEALTH CENTRE
55 Eccles St
Ottawa ON K1R 6S3
Tel. 613 238-8210
Fax 613 235-7595
www.swchc.on.ca

SOUTH-EAST OTTAWA COMMUNITY HEALTH CENTRE
1355 Bank St
Ottawa ON K1H 8K7
Tel. 613 737-5115
Fax 613 739-8199
www.seochc.on.ca

SOUTH-EAST OTTAWA COMMUNITY HEALTH CENTRE - BETTER BEGINNINGS BETTER FUTURES PROGRAM
22-1485 ch Heatherington Rd
Ottawa ON K1V 8Z4
Tel. 613 523-2223
Fax 613 523-2360
www.betterbeginnings.ca

UNIVERSITY OF OTTAWA HEART INSTITUTE
40 Ruskin St
Ottawa ON K1Y 4W7
Tel. 613 761-5000
Fax 613 761-5323
www.ottawaheart.ca

OWEN SOUND

GREY BRUCE HEALTH SERVICES - OWEN SOUND
1800 8th St E
PO Box 1800 Stn M
Owen Sound ON N4K 6M9
Tel. 519 376-2121
Fax 519 376-1846
www.gbhs.on.ca

PALMERSTON

NORTH WELLINGTON HEALTH CARE - PALMERSTON & DISTRICT HOSPITAL
500 White's Rd
Palmerston ON N0G 2P0
Tel. 519 343-2030
Fax 519 343-3821
www.nwhealthcare.ca

PALMERSTON & DISTRICT HOSPITAL
500 White Road
Palmerston ON N0G 2P0
Tel. 519 343-2030
Fax 519 343-3821
www.nwhealthcare.ca

PARIS

THE BRANT COMMUNITY HEALTHCARE SYSTEM - WILLETT HOSPITAL SITE
238 Grand River St N
Paris ON N3L 2N7
Tel. 519 442-2251
Fax 519 442-1641
www.bchsys.org

PARRY SOUND

PARRY SOUND HEALTH CENTRE
74 James St
PO Box 89
Parry Sound ON P2A 2X2
Tel. 705 746-5807
Fax 705 746-1421

WASAUKSING HEALTH CENTRE
PO Box 253
Parry Sound ON P2A 2X4
Tel. 705 746-2531 Ext. 2249
Fax 705 746-5984
www.wasauksing.ca

WEST PARRY SOUND HEALTH CENTRE
6 Albert St
Parry Sound ON P2A 2L8
Tel. 705 746-9321
Fax 705 746-7364
www.wpshc.com

PEAWANUCK

PEAWANUCK NURSING STATION
Gen Del
Peawanuck ON P0L 2H0
Tel. 705 473-2554
Fax 705 473-2588
www.firstnation.ca

PEMBROKE

PEMBROKE REGIONAL HOSPITAL INC
705 Mackay St
Pembroke ON K8A 1G8
Tel. 613 732-2811
Fax 613 732-9986
www.pemreghos.org

PENETANGUISHENE

BEAUSOLEIL FAMILY HEALTH CENTRE
156 Mkade Kegwin Miikan
Christian Island ON L9M 0A9
Tel. 705 247-2035
Fax 705 247-2006
www.bfhc.ca

GEORGIAN BAY GENERAL HOSPITAL - PENETANGUISHENE
25 Jeffery St
PO Box 670
Penetanguishene ON L9M 1K5
Tel. 705 549-7431
Fax 705 549-4031
www.gbgh.on.ca

HÔPITAL PRIVÉ BEECHWOOD PRIVATE HOSPITAL
58 Church St
Penetanguishene ON L9M 1B3
Tel. 705 549-7473
Fax 705 549-7194

WAYPOINT CENTRE FOR MENTAL HEALTH CARE
500 Church St
Penetanguishene ON L9M 1G3
Tel. 705 549-3181 Ext. 2214
Fax 705 549-3446
www.waypointcentre.ca

PERTH

PERTH & SMITHS FALLS DISTRICT HOSPITAL - PERTH SITE (GREAT WAR MEMORIAL SITE)
33 Drummond St W
Perth ON K7H 2K1
Tel. 613 267-1500
Fax 613 264-0365
www.psfdh.on.ca

PETERBOROUGH

FIVE COUNTIES CHILDREN'S CENTRE
872 Dutton Rd
Peterborough ON K9H 7G1
Tel. 705 748-2221
Fax 705 748-3526
www.fivecounties.on.ca

PETERBOROUGH REGIONAL HEALTH CENTRE - HOSPITAL DRIVE
1 Hospital Dr
Peterborough ON K9J 7C6
Tel. 705 743-2121
Fax 705 876-5120
www.prhc.on.ca

PETERBOROUGH REGIONAL HEALTH CENTRE - ROGERS ST SITE
384 Rogers St
Peterborough ON K9H 7B6
Tel. 705 743-4251
Fax 705 740-8005
www.prhc.on.ca

PETROLIA

BLUEWATER HEALTH -CHARLOTTE ELEANOR ENGLEHART HOSPITAL
450 Blanche St
Petrolia ON N0N 1R0
Tel. 519 882-4325
Fax 519 882-3711
www.bluewaterhealth.ca

PICTON

QHC PRINCE EDWARD COUNTY MEMORIAL
403 Main St E
Box 1900
Picton ON K0K 2T0
Tel. 613 476-1008
Fax 613 476-8600
www.qhc.on.ca

PIKANGIKUM

PIKANGIKUM NURSING STATION
GD
Pikangikum ON P0V 2L0
Tel. 807 773-5550
Fax 807 773-5923
www.gov.on.ca

POPLAR HILL

POPLAR HILL HEALTH STATION
PO Box 78
Poplar Hill ON P0V 3E0
Tel. 807 735-1381 Ext. 1369
Fax 807 772-8869
www.communities.knet.ca

PORT COLBORNE

BRIDGES COMMUNITY HEALTH CENTRE - PORT COLBORNE/WAINFLEET
177 King St
Port Colborne ON L3K 4G5
Tel. 289 479-5017
www.bridgeschc.ca

NIAGARA HEALTH SYSTEM - PORT COLBORNE GENERAL SITE
260 Sugarloaf St
Port Colborne ON L3K 2N7
Tel. 905 378-4647
Fax 905 834-0404
www.niagarahealth.on.ca

PORT HOPE

PORT HOPE COMMUNITY HEALTH CENTRE
99 Toronto Rd
Port Hope ON L1A 3S5
Tel. 905 885-2626 Ext. 212
Fax 905 885-2646
www.porthopechc.ca

PORT HOPE MEDICAL CENTRE
249 Ontario St
Port Hope ON L1A 3Y9
Tel. 905 885-0611
www.porthope.ca

PORT PERRY

LAKERIDGE HEALTH - PORT PERRY SITE
451 Paxton St
PO Box 960 Stn Main
Port Perry ON L9L 1A8
Tel. 905 985-7321
Fax 905 721-5829
www.lakeridgehealth.on.ca

MISSISSAUGA OF SCUGOG ISLAND HEALTH & RESOURCE CENTRE
22600 Island Rd
Port Perry ON L9L 1B6
Tel. 905 985-1826
Fax 905 985-7958
www.scugogfirstnation.com

PORTLAND

COUNTRY ROADS COMMUNITY HEALTH CENTRE
4319 Cove Road at Hwy 15
PO Box 58
Portland ON K0G 1V0
Tel. 613 272-3302
Fax 613 272-3463
www.crchc.on.ca

RAMA

CHIPPEWAS OF RAMA
200-5884 Rama Rd
Rama ON L3V 6H6
Tel. 705 325-3611
Fax 705 329-0879
www.mnjikaning.ca

RED LAKE

RED LAKE MARGARET COCHENOUR MEMORIAL HOSPITAL
51 Hwy 105
PO Box 5005
Red Lake ON P0V 2M0
Tel. 807 727-2066
Fax 807 727-2923
www.redlakehospital.ca

RENFREW

OTTAWA CHILDREN'S TREATMENT CENTRE - RENFREW
499 Raglan St N
Renfrew ON K7V 1P6
Tel. 613 433-8239
Fax 613 433-8265
www.octc.ca

RENFREW VICTORIA HOSPITAL
499 Raglan St N
Renfrew ON K7V 1P6
Tel. 613 432-4851
Fax 613 432-8649
www.renfrewhosp.com

RICHARDS LANDING

SAULT AREA HOSPITAL - MATTHEWS MEMORIAL HOSPITAL
1180 Richard St
PO Box 188
Richards Landing ON P0R 1J0
Tel. 705 246-2570
Fax 705 246-2569
www.sah.on.ca

RICHMOND HILL

EAST MISSISSAUGA COMMUNITY HEALTH CENTRE - SATELLITE OF LAMP CHC
7-2555 Dixie Rd
Mississauga ON L4C 4C4
Tel. 905 602-4082
Fax 905 602-5432
www.eastmississaugachc.org

MACKENZIE RICHMOND HILL HOSPITAL
10 Trench St
Richmond Hill ON L4C 4Z3
Tel. 905 883-1212
Fax 905 883-2455
www.yorkcentral.on.ca

ROSENEATH

ALDERVILLE HEALTH STATION
8467 Country Rd 45
PO Box 46
Roseneath ON K0K 2X0
Tel. 905 352-2140
Fax 905 352-3824
www.aldervillefirstnation.ca

SACHIGO LAKE

SACHIGO LAKE NURSING STATION
General Delivery
Sachigo Lake ON P0V 2P0
Tel. 807 595-2527
Fax 807 595-1119
www.firstnation.ca

ST. CATHARINES

HÔTEL DIEU SHAVER HEALTH & REHABILITATION CENTRE
541 Glenridge Ave
St Catharines ON L2T 4C2
Tel. 905 685-1381
Fax 905 687-4871
www.hoteldieushaver.org

NIAGARA HEALTH SYSTEM - ONTARIO STREET SITE
155 Ontario St
St Catharines ON L2R 5K3
Tel. 905 378-4647
Fax 905 682-5533
www.niagarahealth.on.ca

NIAGARA HEALTH SYSTEM - ST CATHARINES GENERAL SITE
142 Queenston St
St Catharines ON L2R 7C6
Tel. 905 378-4647
Fax 905 684-1468
www.niagarahealth.on.ca

NIAGARA PENINSULA CHILDREN'S CENTRE
567 Glenridge Ave
St Catharines ON L2T 4C2
Tel. 905 688-3550
Fax 905 688-1055
www.npcc.on.ca

QUEST COMMUNITY HEALTH CENTRE
100-145 Queenston St
St Catharines ON L2R 2Z9
Tel. 905 688-2558
Fax 905 688-4678
www.questchc.ca

ST. JACOBS

WOOLWICH COMMUNITY HEALTH CENTRE - WOOLWICH SITE
10 Parkside Dr
St Jacobs ON N0B 2N0
Tel. 519 664-3794
Fax 519 664-2184
www.wchc.on.ca

ST. MARYS

ST MARYS MEMORIAL HOSPITAL - HURON PERTH HEALTHCARE ALLIANCE
267 Queen St
PO Box 940 Stn Main
St Marys ON N4X 1B6
Tel. 519 284-1330
Fax 519 284-8324
www.hpha.ca

ST. THOMAS

CENTRAL COMMUNITY HEALTH CENTRE
359 Talbot St
St Thomas ON N5P 1B7
Tel. 519 633-7989
Fax 519 633-8467
www.centralchc.com

REGIONAL MENTAL HEALTH CARE-ST JOSEPH'S HEALTH CARE
467 Sunset Dr
PO Box 2004 Stn Main
St Thomas ON N5P 3V9
Tel. 519 631-8510
Fax 519 633-0852
www.sjhc.london.on.ca

ST THOMAS ELGIN GENERAL HOSPITAL
189 Elm St
St Thomas ON N5R 5C4
Tel. 519 631-2020
Fax 519 631-1825
www.stegh.on.ca

SANDY LAKE

SANDY LAKE NURSING STATION
Via Favourable Lake
General Delivery
Sandy Lake ON P0V 1V0
Tel. 807 774-3461
Fax 807 774-1585

SARNIA

BLUEWATER HEALTH - MITTON SITE
220 Mitton St N
Sarnia ON N7T 6H6
Tel. 519 464-4400
Fax 519 336-8780
www.bluewaterhealth.ca

BLUEWATER HEALTH - NORMAN SITE
89 Norman St
Sarnia ON N7T 6S3
Tel. 519 464-4400
Fax 519 464-4407
www.bluewaterhealth.ca

CHIPPAWAS OF SARNIA HEALTH CENTRE
978 Tashmoo Ave
Sarnia ON N7T 7H5
Tel. 519 336-6770
Fax 519 336-0382
www.aamjiwnaang.ca

NORTH LAMBTON COMMUNITY HEALTH CENTRE - WEST LAMBTON SITE
100-429 Exmouth St
Sarnia ON N7T 5P1
Tel. 519 344-3017
Fax 519 344-7535
www.nlchc.com

PATHWAYS HEALTH CENTRE FOR CHILDREN
1240 Murphy Rd
Sarnia ON N7S 2Y6
Tel. 519 542-3471
Fax 519 542-4115
www.pathwayscentre.org

SAULT STE. MARIE

BATCHEWANA HEALTH CENTRE
210 Gran St
SS 2
Sault Ste Marie ON P6A 5K9
Tel. 705 252-7827
Fax 705 759-8716
www.batchewana.ca

CHILDREN'S REHABILITATION CENTRE - ALGOMA
74 Johnson Ave
Sault Ste Marie ON P6C 2V5
Tel. 705 759-1131
Fax 705 759-0783
www.crcalgoma.ca

GARDEN RIVER WELLNESS CENTRE
23 Shingwauk St
Sault Ste Marie ON P6A 7B2
Tel. 705 946-5710
Fax 705 946-5702
www.gardenriver.org

SAULT AREA HOSPITAL - SAULT STE MARIE
750 Great Northern Rd
Sault Ste. Marie ON P6B 0A8
Tel. 705 759-3434
Fax 705 759-3640
www.sah.on.ca

SAVANT LAKE

WABIGOON LAKE OJIBWAY NATION NURSING STATION
GD
Savant Lake ON P0V 2S0
Tel. 807 928-2351
Fax 807 735-3392
www.communities.knet.ca

SCARBOROUGH

BELLWOOD HEALTH SERVICES
1020 McNicoll Ave
Scarborough ON M1W 2J6
Tel. 416 495-0926
Fax 416 495-7943
www.bellwood.ca

PROVIDENCE HEALTHCARE
3276 St Clair Ave E
Scarborough ON M1L 1W1
Tel. 416 285-3666
Fax 416 285-3758
www.providence.on.ca

ROUGE VALLEY HEALTH SYSTEM - CENTENARY HEALTH CENTRE SITE
2867 Ellesmere Rd
Scarborough ON M1E 4B9
Tel. 416 284-8131
Fax 416 281-7323
www.rougevalley.ca

SCARBOROUGH CENTRE FOR HEALTHY COMMUNITIES
3545 Kingston Rd
Scarborough ON M1M 1R6
Tel. 416 642-9445
Fax 416 284-1964
www.schcontario.ca

SCARBOROUGH CENTRE FOR HEALTHY COMMUNITIES - SATELLITE OFFICE
4002 Sheppard Ave E
Scarborough ON M1S 4R5
Tel. 416 642-9445
Fax 416 284-1964
www.schcontario.ca

THE SCARBOROUGH HOSPITAL - BIRCHMOUNT CAMPUS
3030 Birchmount Rd
Scarborough ON M1W 3W3
Tel. 416 495-2400
Fax 416 495-2631
www.tsh.to

THE SCARBOROUGH HOSPITAL - GENERAL CAMPUS
3050 Lawrence Ave E
Scarborough ON M1P 2V5
Tel. 416 431-8200
Fax 416 431-8204
www.tsh.to

TAIBU COMMUNITY HEALTH CENTRE
1-27 Tapscott
Scarborough ON M1B 4Y7
Tel. 416 644-3539
Fax 416 644-3542
www.taibuchc.ca

SEAFORTH

SEAFORTH COMMUNITY HOSPITAL - HURON PERTH HEALTHCARE ALLIANCE
24 Centennial Dr
PO Box 99
Seaforth ON N0K 1W0
Tel. 519 527-1650
Fax 519 527-2665
www.hpha.ca

SHELBURNE

HEADWATERS HEALTH CARE CENTRE - SHELBURNE SITE
301 First Ave E
PO Box 190
Shelburne ON L0N 1S2
Tel. 519 925-3340
Fax 519 925-2130
www.headwatershealth.ca

SHESHEGWANING

SHESHEGWANING HEALTH STATION
Gen Del
Sheshegwaning ON P0P 1X0
Tel. 705 283-3030
Fax 705 283-3642

SIMCOE

NORFOLK GENERAL HOSPITAL
365 West St
Simcoe ON N3Y 1T7
Tel. 519 426-0750
Fax 519 429-6998
www.ngh.on.ca

SIOUX LOOKOUT

SIOUX LOOKOUT MENO-YA-WIN HEALTH CENTRE
1 Meno Ya Win Way
PO Box 909
Sioux Lookout ON P8T 1B4
Tel. 807 737-3030
Fax 807 737-5127
www.slmhc.on.ca

WAWAKAPEWIN HEALTH STATION
PO Box 449
Sioux Lookout ON P8T 1A5
Tel. 807 442-2567
Fax 807 442-1162
www.firstnation.ca

SIOUX NARROWS

NORTHWEST #37 HEALTH STATION
PO Box 267
Windigo Island & Regina Bay
Sioux Narrows ON P0X 1N0
Tel. 807 226-5353
Fax 807 226-1164
www.communities.knet.ca

WHITEFISH BAY HEALTH STATION
Gen Del
Sioux Narrows ON P0X 1N0
Tel. 807 226-5383
Fax 807 226-5752

SMITHS FALLS

PERTH & SMITHS FALLS DISTRICT HOSPITAL - SMITHS FALLS SITE
60 Cornelia St W
Smiths Falls ON K7A 2H9
Tel. 613 283-2330
Fax 613 283-8990
www.psfdh.on.ca

RIDEAU COMMUNITY HEALTH SERVICES - SMITHS FALLS
2 Gould St
Smiths Falls ON K7A 2S5
Tel. 613 283-1952
Fax 613 283-6322
www.rvds.ca

SMOOTH ROCK FALLS

SMOOTH ROCK FALLS HOSPITAL
107 Kelly Rd
PO Box 219
Smooth Rock Falls ON P0L 2B0
Tel. 705 338-2781
Fax 705 338-4410
www.srfhosp.ca

SOUTHAMPTON

GREY BRUCE HEALTH SERVICES - SOUTHAMPTON SITE
340 High St
Southampton ON N0H 2L0
Tel. 519 797-3230
Fax 519 797-2442
www.gbhs.on.ca

MINO BIMAADSAWIN HEALTH CENTRE
57 Mason Dr
RR 1
Southampton ON N0H 2L0
Tel. 519 797-3336
Fax 519 797-5275
www.firstnation.ca

SOUTHWOLD

ONEIDA NATION OF THE THAMES HEALTH CENTRE
RR 2
Southwold ON N0L 2G0
Tel. 519 652-0500
Fax 519 652-9287

STRATFORD

STRATFORD GENERAL HOSPITAL - HURON PERTH HEALTHCARE ALLIANCE
46 General Hospital Dr
Stratford ON N5A 2Y6
Tel. 519 271-8120
Fax 519 272-8198
www.hpha.ca

STRATHROY

STRATHROY MIDDLESEX GENERAL HOSPITAL - MIDDLESEX HOSPITAL ALLIANCE
395 Carrie St
Strathroy ON N7G 3J4
Tel. 519 245-5295
Fax 519 245-0366
www.mhalliance.on.ca

STURGEON FALLS

LAWRENCE COMMANDA HEALTH CENTRE
58 Semo Rd
RR 1 Garden Village
Sturgeon Falls ON P2B 3K2
Tel. 705 753-3312
Fax 705 753-5087
www.nfn.ca

WEST NIPISSING GENERAL HOSPITAL
725 Coursol Rd
Sturgeon Falls ON P2B 2Y6
Tel. 705 753-3110
Fax 705 753-0210
www.wngh.ca

SUDBURY

HEALTH SCIENCES NORTH -CARDIAC/PULMONARY REHABILITATION CENTRE
140 Durham St
Sudbury ON P3E 3M7
Tel. 705 688-7310
www.hsnsudbury.ca

HEALTH SCIENCES NORTH -KIRKWOOD SITE
680 Kirkwood Dr
Sudbury ON P3E 1X3
Tel. 705 675-5900
www.hsnsudbury.ca

HEALTH SCIENCES NORTH -LAURENTIAN SITE
41 Ramsey Lake Rd
Sudbury ON P3E 5J1
Tel. 705 522-7100
Fax 705 523-7112
www.hsnsudbury.ca

HEALTH SCIENCES NORTH - MEMORIAL SITE
865 Regent St
Sudbury ON P3E 3Y9
Tel. 705 523-7100
Fax 705 523-7116
www.hsnsudbury.ca

HEALTH SCIENCES NORTH -ST JOSEPH'S HEALTH CENTRE
700 Paris St
Sudbury ON P3E 3B5
Tel. 705 523-7100
Fax 705 523-7116
www.hsnsudbury.ca

HEALTH SCIENCES NORTH -SUDBURY CHILDREN'S TREATMENT CENTRE
41 Ramsey Lake Rd
Sudbury ON P3E 5J1
Tel. 705 523-7337
Fax 705 560-4273
www.hsnsudbury.ca

HEALTH SCIENCES NORTH -SUDBURY MENTAL HEALTH & ADDICTIONS CENTRE
127 Cedar St
Sudbury ON P3E 1B1
Tel. 705 523-4988
www.hsnsudbury.ca

NORTH BAY REGIONAL HEALTH CENTRE - KIRKWOOD
680 Kirkwood Dr
Sudbury ON P3E 1X3
Tel. 705 675-9193
Fax 705 675-6817
www.nbrhc.on.ca

SHKAGAMIK-KWE HEALTH CENTRE
161 Applegrove St
Sudbury ON P3C 1N2
Tel. 705 675-5430 Ext. 256
www.skhc.ca

SHKAGAMIK-KWE HEALTH CENTRE - SATELLITE OFFICE
202-109 Elm St
Sudbury ON P3C 1T4
Tel. 705 675-5430 Ext. 256
www.skhc.ca

SUDBURY HEALTH CENTRE
282-40 Elm St
Sudbury ON P3C 1S8
Tel. 705 671-0608
Fax 705 671-4112
www.hsnsudbury.ca

SUMMER BEAVER

SUMMER BEAVER (NIBINAMIK) NURSING STATION
Gen Del
Summer Beaver ON P0T 3B0
Tel. 807 593-2211
Fax 807 593-2253

SUTTON WEST

GEORGINA ISLAND HEALTH CENTRE
RR 2
Sutton West ON L0E 1R0
Tel. 705 437-4242
Fax 705 437-2071

TERRACE BAY

THE MCCAUSLAND HOSPITAL
20B Cartier Dr
Terrace Bay ON P0T 2W0
Tel. 807 825-3273
Fax 807 825-9623
www.mccauslandhospital.com

THAMESVILLE

DELAWARE NATION HEALTH CENTRE
14737 School House Line
RR 3
Thamesville ON N0P 2K0
Tel. 519 692-3969
Fax 519 692-3182
www.firstnation.ca

THESSALON

SAULT AREA HOSPITAL - THESSALON DIVISION
135 Dawson St
PO Box 60
Thessalon ON P0R 1L0
Tel. 705 842-2014
Fax 705 842-3214
www.sah.on.ca

THESSALON FIRST NATION HEALTH CENTRE
35 Sugarbush Rd
Thessalon ON P0R 1L0
Tel. 705 842-2323
Fax 705 842-2332
www.firstnation.ca

THORNHILL

SHOULDICE HOSPITAL
7750 Bayview Ave
Thornhill ON L3T 4A3
Tel. 905 889-1125
Fax 905 889-4216
www.shouldice.com

THUNDER BAY

FORT WILLIAM FIRST NATION HEALTH CENTRE
200-90 Anekki Dr
Thunder Bay ON P7J 1L3
Tel. 807 623-9543
Fax 807 623-5190
www.fwfn.com

GEORGE JEFFREY CHILDREN'S CENTRE
2nd E Brock St
Thunder Bay ON P7E 0A2
Tel. 807 623-4381
Fax 807 623-6626
www.georgejeffrey.com

LAKE SUPERIOR HEALTH CENTRE
33 South Court St
Thunder Bay ON P7B 2W6
Tel. 807 345-1443
Fax 807 343-9196

LAKEHEAD PSYCHIATRIC HOSPITAL - ST. JOSEPH'S CARE GROUP
580 Algoma St N
PO Box 2930 Stn P
Thunder Bay ON P7B 5G4
Tel. 807 343-4300
Fax 807 343-4373
www.sjcg.net

NORTHWESTERN ONTARIO REGIONAL CANCER CENTRE - CANCER CARE ONTARIO
980 Oliver Road
Thunder Bay ON P7B 6V4
Tel. 807 684-7200
Fax 807 684-5800
www.nw-rcp.on.ca

NORWEST COMMUNITY HEALTH CENTRE - THUNDER BAY
525 Simpson St
Thunder Bay ON P7C 3J6
Tel. 807 622-8235
Fax 807 622-7637
www.norwestchc.org

ST JOSEPH'S CARE GROUP - BALMORAL CENTRE -WITHDRAWAL MANAGEMENT PROGRAMS
667 Sibley Dr
Thunder Bay ON P7B 6Z8
Tel. 807 623-6515
Fax 807 623-4988
www.sjcg.net

ST JOSEPH'S CARE GROUP -BEHAVIOURAL SCIENCES CENTRE
300 Lillie St N
Thunder Bay ON P7C 4Y7
Tel. 807 623-7677
Fax 807 623-7697
www.sjcg.net

ST JOSEPH'S CARE GROUP - DIABETES HEALTH THUNDER BAY
285 A Montreal Ave
Thunder Bay ON P7B 6H4
Tel. 807 344-3422
Fax 807 346-8006
www.sjcg.net

ST JOSEPH'S CARE GROUP - SISTER MARGARET SMITH CENTRE
301 Lillie St N
Thunder Bay ON P7C 0A6
Tel. 807 684-5100
Fax 807 622-1779
www.sjcg.net

ST JOSEPH'S CARE GROUP - ST JOSEPH'S HEALTH CENTRE
710 Victoria Ave E
Thunder Bay ON P7C 5P7
Tel. 807 624-3400
Fax 807 624-3522
www.sjcg.net

ST JOSEPH'S CARE GROUP - ST JOSEPH'S HOSPITAL
35 Algoma St N
PO Box 3251 Stn P
Thunder Bay ON P7B 5G7
Tel. 807 343-2431
Fax 807 343-0144
www.sjcg.net

THUNDER BAY REGIONAL HEALTH SCIENCES CENTRE PORT-ARTHUR
460 Court St N
Thunder Bay ON P7A 4X6
Tel. 807 343-6621
Fax 807 343-7165

THUNDER BAY REGIONAL HEALTH SCIENCES CENTRE
980 Oliver Rd
Thunder Bay ON P7B 6V4
Tel. 807 684-6000
Fax 807 343-3122
www.tbrhsc.net

TILLSONBURG

TILLSONBURG DISTRICT MEMORIAL HOSPITAL
167 Rolph St
Tillsonburg ON N4G 3Y9
Tel. 519 842-3611
Fax 519 842-6733
www.tillsonburghospital.on.ca

WOODSTOCK AND AREA COMMUNITY HEALTH CENTRE - TILLSONBURG
96 Tillson Ave
Tillsonburg ON N4G 3A1
Tel. 519 539-1111
Fax 519 539-9111
www.wachc.ca

TIMMINS

COCHRANE TEMISKAMING CHILDREN'S TREATMENT CENTRE
733 Ross Ave E
Timmins ON P4N 8S8
Tel. 705 264-4700
Fax 705 268-3585
www.ctctc.org

MISIWAY MILOPEMAHTESEWIN COMMUNITY HEALTH CENTRE
130 Wilson Ave
Timmins ON P4N 2S9
Tel. 705 264-2200
Fax 705 267-2243
www.misiway.ca

TIMMINS & DISTRICT HOSPITAL
700 Ross Ave E
Timmins ON P4N 8P2
Tel. 705 267-2131
Fax 705 267-6311
www.tadh.com

WABUN TRIBAL COUNCIL HEALTH UNIT
313 Railway St
Timmins ON P4N 2P4
Tel. 705 268-9066
Fax 705 268-8554
www.wabun.on.ca

TORONTO

ACCESS ALLIANCE MULTICULTURAL HEALTH AND COMMUNITY SERVICES
500-340 College St
Toronto ON M5T 3A9
Tel. 416 324-8677
Fax 416 324-9074
www.accessalliance.ca

ANISHNAWBE HEALTH TORONTO
225 Queen St E
Toronto ON M5A 1S4
Tel. 416 360-0486
Fax 416 365-1086
www.ontariochc.ca

ANNE JOHNSTON HEALTH STATION
2398 Yonge St
Toronto ON M4P 2H4
Tel. 416 486-8666
Fax 416 486-8660
www.ajhs.ca

BAYCREST CENTRE FOR GERIATRIC CARE
3560 Bathurst St
Toronto ON M6A 2E1
Tel. 416 785-2500
Fax 416 785-2378
www.baycrest.org

BRIDGEPOINT HEALTH CENTRE
14 St Matthews Rd
Toronto ON M4M 2B5
Tel. 416 461-8252
Fax 416 461-5696
www.bridgepointhealth.ca

CANCER CARE ONTARIO - PROVINCIAL OFFICE
1500-620 University Ave
Toronto ON M5G 2L7
Tel. 416 971-9800
Fax 416 971-6888
www.cancercare.on.ca

CENTRAL TORONTO COMMUNITY HEALTH CENTRES
168 Bathurst St
Toronto ON M5V 2R4
Tel. 416 703-8482
Fax 416 703-6190
www.ctchc.com

CENTRE FOR ADDICTION & MENTAL HEALTH (CAMH) - BRENTCLIFFE RD SITE
175 Brentcliffe Rd
Toronto ON M4G 3Z1
Tel. 416 425-8501
Fax 416 425-7896
www.camh.net

CENTRE FOR ADDICTION & MENTAL HEALTH (CAMH) - COLLEGE STREET SITE
250 College St
Toronto ON M5T 1R8
Tel. 416 535-8501
Fax 416 583-4316
www.camh.net

CENTRE FOR ADDICTION & MENTAL HEALTH (CAMH) - QUEEN SITE
1001 Queen St W
Toronto ON M6J 1H4
Tel. 416 535-8501
Fax 416 595-6881
www.camh.net

CENTRE FOR ADDICTION & MENTAL HEALTH (CAMH) - RUSSELL STREET SITE
33 Russell St
Toronto ON M5S 2S1
Tel. 416 595-6878
Fax 416 595-6881
www.camh.net

DAVENPORT-PERTH NEIGHBOURHOOD & COMMUNITY HEALTH CENTRE
1900 Davenport Rd
Toronto ON M6N 1B7
Tel. 416 656-8025
Fax 416 656-1264
www.dpnchc.ca

EAST END COMMUNITY HEALTH CENTRE
1619 Queen St E
Toronto ON M4L 1G4
Tel. 416 778-5858
Fax 416 778-5855
www.eastendchc.ca

FOUR VILLAGES COMMUNITY HEALTH CENTRE
1700 Bloor St W
Toronto ON M6P 4C3
Tel. 416 604-3361
www.4villageschc.ca

FOUR VILLAGES COMMUNITY HEALTH CENTRE - DUNDAS
3446 Dundas St W
Toronto ON M6S 2S1
Tel. 416 604-0640
www.4villageschc.ca

HINCKS-DELLCREST CENTRE -GAIL APPEL INSTITUTE
114 Maitland St
Toronto ON M4Y 1E1
Tel. 416 924-1164
Fax 416 924-8208
www.hincksdellcrest.org

THE HINCKS-DELLCREST CENTRE - TORONTO
440 Jarvis St
Toronto ON M4Y 2H4
Tel. 416 924-1164
Fax 416 924-8208
www.hincksdellcrest.org

HOLLAND BLOORVIEW KIDS REHABILITATION HOSPITAL
150 Kilgour Rd
Toronto ON M4G 1R8
Tel. 416 425-6220
Fax 416 425-6591
www.hollandbloorview.ca

THE HOSPITAL FOR SICK CHILDREN
555 University Ave
Toronto ON M5G 1X8
Tel. 416 813-1500
www.sickkids.ca

HUMBER RIVER REGIONAL HOSPITAL - CHURCH STREET SITE
200 Church St
Toronto ON M9N 1N8
Tel. 416 249-8111
Fax 416 243-4547
www.hrrh.on.ca

MOUNT SINAI HOSPITAL
600 University Ave
Toronto ON M5G 1X5
Tel. 416 596-4200
Fax 416 586-8899
www.mountsinai.on.ca

PARKDALE COMMUNITY HEALTH CENTRE
1229 Queen St W
Toronto ON M6K 1L2
Tel. 416 537-2455
Fax 416 537-5133
www.pchc.on.ca

HOSPITALS & HEALTH CENTRES

PRINCESS MARGARET HOSPITAL - UNIVERSITY HEALTH NETWORK
610 University Ave
Toronto ON M5G 2M9
Tel. 416 946-2000
Fax 416 946-6563
www.theprincessmargaret.ca

QUEEN WEST COMMUNITY HEALTH CENTRE
168 Bathurst St
Toronto ON M5V 2R4
Tel. 416 703-8480
Fax 416 703-8479
www.ctchc.com

REGENT PARK COMMUNITY HEALTH CENTRE
465 Dundas St E
Toronto ON M5A 2B2
Tel. 416 364-2261
Fax 416 364-0822
www.regentparkchc.ca

REGENT PARK COMMUNITY HEALTH CENTRE - PARENTS FOR BETTER BEGINNINGS
38 Regent St
Upper Level
Toronto ON M5A 3N7
Tel. 416 362-0805 Ext. 228
Fax 416 362-5899
www.regentparkchc.org

RUNNYMEDE HEALTHCARE CENTRE
625 Runnymede Rd
Toronto ON M6S 3A3
Tel. 416 762-7316 Ext. 201
Fax 416 762-3836
www.runnymedehc.ca

ST JOSEPH'S HEALTH CENTRE
30 The Queensway
Toronto ON M6R 1B5
Tel. 416 530-6000
Fax 416 530-6078
www.stjoe.on.ca

ST MICHAEL'S HOSPITAL
30 Bond St
Toronto ON M5B 1W8
Tel. 416 360-4000
Fax 416 864-5937
www.stmichaelshospital.com

THE SALVATION ARMY TORONTO GRACE HEALTH CENTRE
650 Church St
Toronto ON M4Y 2G5
Tel. 416 925-2251
Fax 416 926-3211
www.torontograce.org

SHERBOURNE HEALTH CENTRE
333 Sherbourne St
Toronto ON M5A 2S5
Tel. 416 324-4180
Fax 416 324-4188
www.sherbourne.on.ca

SOUTH RIVERDALE COMMUNITY HEALTH CENTRE
955 Queen St E
Toronto ON M4M 3P3
Tel. 416 461-1925
www.srchc.ca

SUNNYBROOK HEALTH SCIENCES CENTRE
2075 Bayview Ave
Toronto ON M4N 3M5
Tel. 416 480-6100
Fax 416 480-6033
www.sunnybrook.ca

SUNNYBROOK HEALTH SCIENCES CENTRE - EDMOND ODETTE CANCER CENTRE
2075 Bayview Ave
Toronto ON M4N 3M5
Tel. 416 480-6100
Fax 416 480-6002
www.sunnybrook.ca

SUNNYBROOK HEALTH SCIENCES CENTRE - HOLLAND ORTHOPAEDIC & ARTHRITIC CENTRE
43 Wellesley St E
Toronto ON M4Y 1H1
Tel. 416 967-8500
Fax 416 967-8521
www.sunnybrook.ca

THISTLETOWN REGIONAL CENTRE FOR CHILDREN & ADOLESCENTS
51 Panorama Crt
Rexdale ON M9V 4L8
Tel. 416 326-0600
Fax 416 326-9078
www.children.gov.on.ca

TORONTO EAST GENERAL HOSPITAL INC
825 Coxwell Ave
Toronto ON M4C 3E7
Tel. 416 461-8272
Fax 416 469-6106
www.tegh.on.ca

TORONTO GENERAL HOSPITAL - UHN
200 Elizabeth St
Toronto ON M5G 2C4
Tel. 416 340-3111
www.uhn.ca

TORONTO REHABILITATION INSTITUTE - E W BICKLE CENTRE FOR COMPLEX CONTINUING CARE
130 Dunn Ave
Toronto ON M6K 2R7
Tel. 416 597-3422 Ext. 2000
Fax 416 530-2470
www.torontorehab.com

TORONTO REHABILITATION INSTITUTE - LYNDHURST CENTRE
520 Sutherland Dr
Toronto ON M4G 3V9
Tel. 416 597-3422 Ext. 6000
Fax 416 422-5216
www.torontorehab.com

TORONTO REHABILITATION INSTITUTE - RUMSEY CENTRE
345 Rumsey Rd
Toronto ON M4G 1R7
Tel. 416 597-3422 Ext. 5200
Fax 416 597-7160
www.torontorehab.com

TORONTO REHABILITATION INSTITUTE - UNIVERSITY CENTRE
550 University Ave
Toronto ON M5G 2A2
Tel. 416 597-3422 Ext. 3000
Fax 416 597-1977
www.torontorehab.com

TORONTO WESTERN HOSPITAL - UNIVERSITY HEALTH NETWORK
399 Bathurst St
Toronto ON M5T 2S8
Tel. 416 603-2581
Fax 416 603-5553
www.uhn.ca

WOMEN'S COLLEGE HOSPITAL
76 Grenville St
Toronto ON M5S 1B2
Tel. 416 323-6400
Fax 416 323-7314
www.womenscollegehospital.ca

TRENTON

QHC TRENTON MEMORIAL
242 King St
PO Box 1600 Stn Main
Trenton ON K8V 5S6
Tel. 613 392-2540
Fax 613 392-3749
www.qhc.on.ca

TWEED

GATEWAY COMMUNITY HEALTH CENTRE
41 McClellan St
Bag Service 99
Tweed ON K0K 3J0
Tel. 613 478-1211
Fax 613 478-6692
www.gatewaychc.or

UXBRIDGE

MARKHAM STOUFFVILLE HOSPITAL - UXBRIDGE SITE
4 Campbell Dr
PO Box 5003 Stn Main
Uxbridge ON L9P 1S4
Tel. 905 852-9771
Fax 905 852-2642
www.msh.on.c

VAUGHAN

VAUGHAN COMMUNITY HEALTH CENTRE
9401 Jane St
Vaughan ON L6A 4H7
Tel. 905 303-8490
Fax 905 303-4227
vaughanhealthcarechc.com

WALKERTON

SOUTH BRUCE GREY HEALTH CENTRE - WALKERTON SITE
21 McGivern St
PO Box 1300
Walkerton ON N0G 2V0
Tel. 519 881-1220
Fax 519 881-0452
www.sbghc.on.ca

WALLACEBURG

CHATHAM/KENT COMMUNITY HEALTH CENTRE - WALLACEBURG SATELLITE
800 Dufferin Ave
Wallaceburg ON N8A 2V4
Tel. 519 397-5455
www.ckchc.ca

CHATHAM/KENT COMMUNITY HEALTH CENTRE - WALPOLE SITE
2-785 Tecumseh Rd
Wallaceburg ON N8A 4K9
Tel. 519 397-5455
www.ckchc.ca

CHATHAM-KENT HEALTH ALLIANCE - SYDENHAM HOSPITAL CAMPUS
325 Margaret Ave
Wallaceburg ON N8A 2A7
Tel. 519 627-1461
Fax 519 628-8121
www.ckha.on.ca

WALPOLE ISLAND HEALTH CENTRE
RR 3
Wallaceburg ON N8A 4K9
Tel. 519 627-0765
Fax 519 627-0440

WASAGA BEACH

SOUTH GEORGIAN BAY COMMUNITY HEALTH CENTRE
14 Ramblewood Dr
Wasaga Beach ON L9Z 0C4
Tel. 705 422-0900
www.ontariochc.ca

WATERLOO

KIDSABILITY CENTRE FOR CHILD DEVELOPMENT - WATERLOO
500 Hallmark Dr
Waterloo ON N2L 3G1
Tel. 519 886-8886
Fax 519 886-7292
www.kidsability.ca

WATFORD

NORTH LAMBTON COMMUNITY HEALTH CENTRE - EAST LAMBTON SITE
536 Simcoe St
Watford ON N0M 2S0
Tel. 519 333-2747
Fax 519 333-6447
www.nlchc.com

WAWA

LADY DUNN HEALTH CENTRE
17 Government Rd
PO Box 179
Wawa ON P0S 1K0
Tel. 705 856-2335
Fax 705 856-7533
www.ldhc.com

MICHIPICOTEN HEALTH OFFICE
Box 1 Site 8
RR 1
Wawa ON P0S 1K0
Tel. 705 856-1993
Fax 705 856-1642
www.michipicoten.com

WEBEQUIE

WEBIQUE NURSING STATION
PO Box 90
Webequie ON P0T 3A0
Tel. 807 353-7241
Fax 807 353-1551

WELLAND

NIAGARA HEALTH SYSTEM - WELLAND HOSPITAL SITE
65 Third St
Welland ON L3B 4W6
Tel. 905 738-4647
Fax 905 732-3268
www.niagarahealth.on.ca

WELLESLEY

WOOLWICH COMMUNITY HEALTH CENTRE - WELLESLEY SITE
1180 Queens Bush Rd
Wellesley ON N0B 2T0
Tel. 519 656-9025
Fax 519 656-9027
www.wchc.on.ca

WEST LORNE

WEST ELGIN COMMUNITY HEALTH CENTRE
153 Main St
PO Box 761
West Lorne ON N0L 2P0
Tel. 519 768-1715
Fax 519 768-2548
www.wechc.on.ca

WHITBY

LAKERIDGE HEALTH - WHITBY SITE
300 Gordon St
Whitby ON L1N 5T2
Tel. 905 668-6831
Fax 905 665-2406
www.lakeridgehealth.on.ca

ONTARIO SHORES CENTRE FOR MENTAL HEALTH SCIENCES
700 Gordon St
Whitby ON L1N 5S9
Tel. 905 430-4055
Fax 905 430-4032
www.ontarioshores.ca

WIARTON

CHIPPAWAS OF NAWASH HEALTH CENTRE
RR 5
Wiarton ON N0H 2T0
Tel. 519 534-0373
Fax 519 534-0964
www.firstnation.ca

GREY BRUCE HEALTH SERVICES - WIARTON SITE
369 Mary St
Wiarton ON N0H 2T0
Tel. 519 534-1260
Fax 519 534-4450
www.gbhs.on.ca

WIKWEMIKONG

WIKWEMIKONG HEALTH CENTRE
16A Complex Dr
PO Box 101
Wikwemikong ON P0P 2J0
Tel. 705 859-3164
Fax 705 859-3300
www.wikyhealth.ca

WINCHESTER

WINCHESTER DISTRICT MEMORIAL HOSPITAL
566 Louise St
Winchester ON K0C 2K0
Tel. 613 774-2420
Fax 613 774-0453
www.wdmh.on.ca

WINDSOR

DIABETES WELLNESS
107-2885 Lauzon Pkwy
Windsor ON N8T 3H5
Fax 519 945-7864
www.ontariochc.ca

HÔTEL-DIEU GRACE HOSPITAL
1030 Ouellette Ave
Windsor ON N9A 1E1
Tel. 519 973-4411
Fax 519 977-0018
www.hdgh.org

JOHN MCGIVNEY CHILDREN'S CENTRE
3945 Matchette Road
Windsor ON N9C 4C2
Tel. 519 252-7281 Ext. 227
Fax 519 252-5873
www.jmccentre.ca

TEEN COMMUNITY HEALTH CENTRE
1585 Ouellette Ave
Windsor ON N8X 1K5
Tel. 519 253-8481

WINDSOR ESSEX COMMUNITY HEALTH CENTRE
1585 Ouellette Ave
Windsor ON N8X 1K5
Tel. 519 253-8481
www.wechc.org

WINDSOR REGIONAL HOSPITAL - METROPOLITAN SITE
1995 Lens Ave
Windsor ON N8W 1L9
Tel. 519 254-5577
Fax 519 254-3150
www.wrh.on.ca

WINDSOR REGIONAL HOSPITAL - REGIONAL CHILDREN'S CENTRE
3901 Connaught Ave
Windsor ON N9C 4H4
Tel. 519 257-5215
Fax 519 257-5212
www.wrh.on.ca

WINDSOR REGIONAL HOSPITAL - TAYFOUR SITE
1453 Prince Rd
Windsor ON N9C 3Z4
Tel. 519 254-5577
Fax 519 254-2469
www.wrh.on.ca

WINDSOR REGIONAL HOSPITAL - WINDSOR REGIONAL CANCER CENTRE
2220 Kildare Rd
Windsor ON N8W 2X3
Tel. 519 253-5253
Fax 519 255-8670
www.wrh.on.ca

WINGHAM

WINGHAM & DISTRICT HOSPITAL - LISTOWEL WINGHAM HOSPITALS ALLIANCE
270 Carling Terrace
Wingham ON N0G 2W0
Tel. 519 357-3210
Fax 519 357-2931
www.lwha.ca

WOODBRIDGE

COSMETIC SURGERY HOSPITAL
4650 Highway 7
Woodbridge ON L4L 1S7
Tel. 905 851-7701
Fax 905 856-4406
www.cosmeticsurgeryhospital.com

WOODSTOCK

WOODSTOCK AND AREA COMMUNITY HEALTH CENTRE - WOODSTOCK
400 Dundas St
Woodstock ON N4S 1B9
Tel. 519 539-1111
Fax 519 539-9111
www.wachc.ca

WOODSTOCK GENERAL HOSPITAL
310 Juliana Dr
Woodstock ON N4V 0A4
Tel. 519 421-4211
Fax 519 537-5142
www.wgh.on.ca

WOODSTOCK PRIVATE HOSPITAL
369 Huron St
Woodstock ON N4S 7A5
Tel. 519 537-8162
Fax 519 537-7204
www.thehealthline.ca

WUNNUMMIN LAKE

WUNNUMMIN LAKE NURSING STATION
PO Box 101
Wunnummin Lake ON P0V 2Z0
Tel. 807 442-2573
Fax 807 442-2532

YORK

UNISON HEALTH AND COMMUNITY SERVICES - KEELE-ROGERS
1651 Keele St
York ON M6M 3W2
Tel. 416 653-5400
Fax 416 653-1696
www.unisonhcs.org

WEST PARK HEALTHCARE CENTRE
82 Buttonwood Ave
Toronto ON M6M 2J5
Tel. 416 243-3600
Fax 416 243-8947
www.westpark.org

PRINCE EDWARD ISLAND

ALBERTON

WESTERN HOSPITAL - HEALTH PEI
148 Poplar St
PO Box 10
Alberton PE C0B 1B0
Tel. 902 853-8650
Fax 902 853-8651

CHARLOTTETOWN

FOUR NEIGHBOURHOODS MEDICAL CENTRE
152 St. Peters Rd
Charlottetown PE C1A 5P8
Tel. 902 569-7772
Fax 902 368-6936
www.healthpei.ca

HILLSBOROUGH HOSPITAL & SPECIAL CARE CENTRE
115 Murchison Lane
PO Box 1929 Stn Central
Charlottetown PE C1A 7N5
Tel. 902 368-5400
Fax 902 368-5467

QUEEN ELIZABETH HOSPITAL
60 Riverside Dr
PO Box 6600 Stn Ctrl
Charlottetown PE C1A 8T5
Tel. 902 894-2111
Fax 902 894-2416

HUNTER RIVER

CENTRAL QUEENS HEALTH CENTRE
4276 Hopedale Rd
Hunter River PE C0A 1N0
Tel. 902 621-3050
Fax 902 621-3069
www.healthpei.ca

LENNOX ISLAND

TYNE VALLEY HEALTH CENTRE
6905 Route 12
PO Box 145
Lennox Island PE C0B 1P0
Tel. 902 831-5800
Fax 902 831-5828
www.healthpei.ca

MONTAGUE

KINGS COUNTY MEMORIAL HOSPITAL
409 McIntyre Ave
PO Box 490
Montague PE C0A 1R0
Tel. 902 838-0736
Fax 902 838-0777
www.healthpei.ca

MONTAGUE HEALTH CENTRE
407 MacIntyre Ave
Montague PE C0A 1R0
Tel. 902 838-0830
Fax 902 838-0834
www.healthpei.ca

NORTH RUSTICO

GULF SHORE HEALTH CENTRE
7379 Cavendish Rd
North Rustico PE C0A 1X0
Tel. 902 963-7835
Fax 902 963-7836
www.healthpei.ca

O'LEARY

COMMUNITY HOSPITAL INC
14 MacKinnon Dr
PO Box 160
O'Leary PE C0B 1V0
Tel. 902 859-8700
Fax 902 859-8774

O'LEARY HEALTH CENTRE
15 MacKinnon Dr
PO Box 550
O'Leary PE C0B 1V0
Tel. 902 859-3929
Fax 902 859-3922
www.healthpei.ca

SOURIS

EASTERN KINGS HEALTH CENTRE
7 Green St
PO Box 640
Souris PE C0A 2B0
Tel. 902 687-7033
Fax 902 687-7166
www.healthpei.ca

SOURIS HOSPITAL INC
17 Knights Ave
PO Box 640
Souris PE C0A 2B0
Tel. 902 687-7150
Fax 902 687-7175

SUMMERSIDE

HARBOURSIDE HEALTH CENTRE
243 Harbour Dr
Summerside PE C1N 5R1
Tel. 902 432-2600
Fax 902 432-2610
www.healthpei.ca

PRINCE COUNTY HOSPITAL
65 Roy Boates Ave
PO Box 3000 Stn Main
Summerside PE C1N 2A9
Tel. 902 438-4200
Fax 902 438-4381
www.gov.pe.ca

TYNE VALLEY

STEWART MEMORIAL HOSPITAL
6926 Route #12
PO Box 10
Tyne Valley PE C0B 2C0
Tel. 902 831-7900
Fax 902 831-7901

WELLINGTON STATION

EVANGELINE COMMUNITY HEALTH CENTRE
60 Sunset Dr
PO Box 119
Wellington PE C0B 2E0
Tel. 902 854-7259
Fax 902 854-7270

QUÉBEC

ALMA

CSSS DE LAC-SAINT JEAN-EST
300 boul Champlain S
CP 1300 Succ Bureau-Chef
Alma QC G8B 5W3
Tel. 418 669-2000 Ext. 6655
Fax 418 668-9695
www.santealma.ca

AMOS

CH HÔTEL-DIEU D'AMOS
622 4e rue O
Amos QC J9T 2S2
Tel. 819 732-3341 Ext. 2175
Fax 819 732-7054
www.sante-abitibi-temiscamingue.gouv.qc.ca

AMQUI

CSSS DE LA MATAPEDIA
135 rue de l'Hopital
Amqui QC G5J 2K5
Tel. 418 629-2211
Fax 418 629-4498
www.santeautravail.net

ASBESTOS

CSSS DES SOURCES D'ASBESTOS
475 3e av
Asbestos QC J1T 1X6
Tel. 819 879-7151
Fax 819 879-0075
www.santeestrie.qc.ca

BAIE-COMEAU

CENTRE HOSPITALIER RÉGIONAL BAIE-COMEAU
635 boul Jolliet
Baie-Comeau QC G5C 1P1
Tel. 418 589-3701 Ext. 2601
Fax 418 589-9654
www.csssmanicouagan.qc.ca

BAIE-DU-POSTE

MISTISSINI COMMUNITY CLINIC
203 Mistissini Blvd
PO Box 1016
Baie-du-Poste QC G0W 1C0
Tel. 418 923-3376
Fax 418 923-3240

BEAUCEVILLE

CENTRE D'HÉBERGEMENT DE BEAUCEVILLE
253 Route 108
Beauceville QC G5X 2Z3
Tel. 418 774-3304
Fax 418 774-5517
www.csssbeauce.qc.ca

BEAUPRÉ

HÔPITAL SAINTE ANNE DE BEAUPRÉ
11000 rue des Montagnards
Beaupré QC G0A 1E0
Tel. 418 827-3726
Fax 418 827-8452
www.rrsss03.gouv.qc.ca

BEDFORD

CHSLD ET CLSC DE BEDFORD
34 rue St-Joseph
CP 1140
Bedford QC J0J 1A0
Tel. 450 248-4304
Fax 450 248-4676

BELOEIL

CENTRE HOSPITALIER CHAMPLAIN-BELOEIL
221 rue Brunelle
Beloeil QC J3G 2M9
Tel. 514 467-3356
Fax 514 467-3357

BERTHIERVILLE

CHSLD LE CHATEAU
1231 rue Dr Olivier-M.-Gendron
Berthierville QC J0K 1A0
Tel. 450 836-6241
Fax 450 836-4013
www.wpp01.msss.gouv.qc.ca

CAP-AUX-MEULES

HÔPITAL DE L'ARCHIPEL
430 ch Principal
Cap-aux-Meules QC G4T 1R9
Tel. 418 986-2121 Ext. 8310
Fax 418 986-6845
www.csssdesiles.qc.ca

CHANDLER

CENTRE HOSPITALIER DE CHANDLER
451 rue Monseigneur Ross E
CP 3300
Chandler QC G0C 1K0
Tel. 418 689-2261 Ext. 2144
Fax 418 689-5049
www.csssrocherperce.com

CHÂTEAUGUAY

HÔPITAL ANNA-LABERGE
200 boul Brisebois
Chateauguay QC J6K 4W8
Tel. 450 699-2425
www.santemonteregie.qc.ca

CHIBOUGAMAU

CENTRE DE SANTE DE CHIBOUGAMU
312 3e Rue
Chibougamau QC G8P 1N5
Tel. 418 748-3575 Ext. 2473
Fax 418 748-7123
www.crsssbaiejames.gouv.qc.ca

CRSSS DE LA BAIE-JAMES
51 3e rue
Chibougamau QC G8P 1N1
Tel. 418 748-2676
Fax 418 748-3662
www.crsssbaiejames.gouv.qc.ca

CHICOUTIMI

COMPLEXE HOSPITALIER DE LA SAGAMIE
305 rue Saint-Vallier
CP 5006
Chicoutimi QC G7H 5H6
Tel. 418 541-1000
Fax 418 541-1144
www.csss-chicoutimi.qc.ca

CHISASIBI

CREE BOARD OF HEALTH & SOCIAL SERVICES JAMES BAY
PO Box 250
Chisasibi QC J0M 1E0
Tel. 819 855-2744
Fax 819 855-2098
www.creehealth.org

WEMINDJI COMMUNITY CLINIC
PO Box 9
Wemindji QC J0M 1E0
Tel. 819 978-0225
Fax 819 978-0280

WHAPMAGOOSTUI COMMUNITY CLINIC
PO Box 180
Chisasibi QC J0M 1E0
Tel. 819 929-3307
Fax 819 929-3526

COATICOOK

CENTRE HOSPITALIER DE COATICOOK
138 rue Jeanne-Mance
Coaticook QC J1A 1W3
Tel. 819 849-9102
Fax 819 849-6735
www.cssscoaticook.ca

COWANSVILLE

HÔPITAL BROME -MISSISQUOI-PERKINS
950 rue Principale
Cowansville QC J2K 1K3
Tel. 450 266-4342 Ext. 5508
Fax 450 263-8669
www.santemonteregie.qc.ca

DOLBEAU-MISTASSINI

CENTRE MARIA -CHAPDELAINE -CH DE DOLBEAU-MISTASSINI
2000 boul du Sacre-Coeur
Dolbeau-Mistassini
QC G8L 2R5
Tel. 418 276-1234
Fax 418 276-4355
www.csssmariachapdelaine.com

DONNACONA

CSSS DE PORTNEUF
250 boul Gaudreau
Donnacona QC G3M 1L7
Tel. 418 285-3025
Fax 418 285-3656
www.csssdeportneuf.qc.ca

DRUMMONDVILLE

CHSLD COEUR-DU-QUÉBEC
75 rue Saint-Georges
Drummondville QC J2C 4G6
Tel. 819 477-0544
Fax 819 477-3888
www.csssdrummond.qc.ca

HÔPITAL SAINTE-CROIX
570 rue Heriot
Drummondville QC J2B 1C1
Tel. 819 478-6464
Fax 819 478-6410
www.csssdrummond.qc.ca

EASTMAIN

EASTMAIN COMMUNITY CLINIC
PO Box 149
Eastmain QC J0M 1W0
Tel. 819 977-0241
Fax 819 977-0342

FERMONT

CLSC DE L'HÉMATITE
1 rue Aguilon
CP 550
Fermont QC G0G 1J0
Tel. 418 287-5461 Ext. 262
Fax 418 287-5281
www.wpp01.msss.gouv.qc.ca

FORT-COULONGE

CSSS DU PONTIAC
160 chemin de la Chute
CP 340
Mansfld-et-Ponterf QC J0X 1V0
Tel. 819 683-3000
Fax 819 647-2409
www.santepontiac.qc.ca

GASPÉ

CENTRE HOSPITALIER DE GASPE
215 boul de York O
Gaspé QC G4X 2W2
Tel. 418 368-3301 Ext. 3153
Fax 418 368-6850
www.csssctedegaspe.ca

INSTALLATION CLSC GASPE
154 boul Renard E
Gaspé QC G4X 5R5
Tel. 418 269-2572
Fax 418 269-5294

GATINEAU

CH-CHSLD DE PAPINEAU - PAVILLON DU CENTRE D'ACCUEIL
111 rue Lucerne
Buckingham QC J8L 3C9
Tel. 819 986-1043
Fax 819 986-9602

CH-CHSLD DE PAPINEAU - PAVILLON DU CENTRE HOSPITALIER
500 rue Belanger
Gatineau QC J8L 2M4
Tel. 819 986-3341
Fax 819 986-4000
www.cssspapineau.qc.ca

CSSS DE GATINEAU
777 boul de la Gappe
Gatineau QC J8T 8R2
Tel. 819 966-6560
Fax 819 966-6565
www.csssgatineau.qc.ca

CENTRE D'HÉBERGEMENT - LA PIETÀ
273 rue Laurier
Gatineau QC J8X 3W8
Tel. 819 771-7362
Fax 819 771-3710

CENTRE HOSPITALIER PIERRE-JANET
20 rue Pharand
Gatineau QC J9A 1K7
Tel. 819 771-7761
Fax 819 771-2908
www.pierre-janet.qc.ca

HÔPITAL DE GATINEAU
909 boul de la Verendrye O
Gatineau QC J8P 7H2
Tel. 819 966-6100
Fax 819 566-6333
www.csssgatineau.qc.ca

HÔPITAL DE PAPINEAU
155 rue MacLaren Est
Gatineau QC J8L 0C2
Tel. 819 986-3341
Fax 819 986-4000
www.cssspapineau.qc.ca

HULL HOSPITAL
116 boul Lionel-Emond
Gatineau QC J8Y 1W7
Tel. 819 595-6000
Fax 819 595-6306
www.csssgatineau.qc.ca

GRANBY

CENTRE HOSPITALIER DE GRANBY
205 boul Leclerc O
Granby QC J2G 1T7
Tel. 450 375-8000 Ext. 2156
Fax 450 375-8032
www.chgranby.qc.ca

GRAND-MÈRE

CENTRE LAFLECHE GRAND-MERE
1650 6e av
Grand'Mere QC G9T 2K4
Tel. 819 533-2500
Fax 819 538-7640
www.agencesss04.qc.ca

HAVRE-SAINT-PIERRE

CSSS DE LA MINGANIE
1035 prom des Anciens
CP 190
Havre-Saint-Pierre QC G0G 1P0
Tel. 418 538-2212 Ext. 401
Fax 418 538-3066
www.csssminganie.com

HUNTINGDON

HUNTINGDON COUNTY HOSPITAL CENTRE
PO Box 370
Huntingdon QC J0S 1H0
Tel. 450 264-6111
Fax 450 264-4932

JOLIETTE

CENTRE HOSPITALIER RÉGIONAL DE LANAUDIÈRE
RC D27-1000 Sainte-Anne Blvd
Joliette QC J6E 6J2
Tel. 450 759-8222 Ext. 2501
Fax 450 759-7969
www.csssnl.qc.ca

JONQUIÈRE

CENTRE HOSPITALIER JONQUIERE
2230 rue de l'Hopital
Jonquière QC G7X 4H6
Tel. 418 695-7700
Fax 418 695-7729
www.jonquiere.qc.ca

KAHNAWAKE

KAHNAWAKE YOUTH CENTRE
PO Box 1440
Kahnawake QC J0L 1B0
Tel. 450 632-6601
Fax 450 632-5943
kahnawakeyouthcenter.com

KATERI MEMORIAL HOSPITAL CENTRE
PO Box 10
Kahnawake QC J0L 1B0
Tel. 450 638-3930
Fax 450 638-4634
www.kmhc.ca

KAWAWACHIKAMACH

CLSC NASKAPI
9 Naskapi Rd
PO Box 5154
Kawawachikamach
QC G0G 2Z0
Tel. 418 585-2897
Fax 418 585-3126

KUUJJUAQ

CENTRE DE SANTE TULATTAVIK DE L'UNGAVA
CP 149
Kuujjuaq QC J0M 1C0
Tel. 819 964-2905
Fax 819 964-6353

LA BAIE

CHSLD-CLSC CLEOPHAS -CLAVEAU
1000 rue du Dr Desgagné
CP 38 succ La Baie
La Baie QC G7B 3P9
Tel. 418 544-3381
Fax 418 544-6012
www.santesaglac.gouv.qc.ca

LA MALBAIE

CSSS DE CHARLEVOIX
535 boul de Comporté
La Malbaie QC G5A 1S8
Tel. 418 665-1700 Ext. 2101
Fax 418 665-7297
www.chdc.charlevoix.net

HÔPITAL DE LA MALBAIE
303 rue St-Etienne
CP 340 Succ Bureau-Chef
La Malbaie QC G5A 1T8
Tel. 418 665-1711
Fax 418 665-1706

LA POCATIÈRE

HÔPITAL NOTRE-DAME-DE -FATIMA
1201 6e av
La Pocatière QC G0R 1Z0
Tel. 415 856-7000
Fax 418 856-4737

LA PRAIRIE

CSSS JARDINS-ROUSSILLON
87B boul Marie-Victorin
La Prairie QC J5R 1C3
Tel. 450 659-7661 Ext. 251
Fax 450 699-2425
www.santemontérégie.qc.ca

LA SARRE

CENTRE HOSPITALIER LA SARRE
679 2e Rue E
CP 6000
La Sarre QC J9Z 2X7
Tel. 819 333-2311
Fax 819 333-4316
www.csssab.qc.ca

LA TUQUE

CENTRE HOSPITALIER SAINT -JOSEPH DE LA TURQUE
885 boul Ducharme
La Tuque QC G9X 3C1
Tel. 819 523-4581
Fax 819 523-6176
www.cssshsm.qc.ca

LAC-ETCHEMIN

CSSS DES ETCHEMINS
331 rue du Sanatorium
Lac-Etchemin QC G0R 1S0
Tel. 418 625-3101
Fax 418 625-2038
www.csssetchemins.qc.ca

LAC-MÉGANTIC

CARREFOUR SANTE GRANIT
3569 rue Laval
Lac-Megantic QC G6B 1A5
Tel. 819 583-0330
Fax 819 583-5664
www.wpp01.msss.gouv.qc.ca

LACHINE

CHSLD BUSSEY INC
2069 boul Saint-Joseph
Lachine QC H8S 4B7
Tel. 514 637-1127
Fax 514 637-1129
www.chsldbussey.com

CSSS DE DORVAL -LACHINE-LASALLE
1900 rue Notre-Dame
Lachine QC H8S 2G2
Tel. 514 637-8634
Fax 514 637-1632
www.csssdll.qc.ca

CENTRE HOSPITALIER DE LACHINE
650 16th Ave
Lachine QC H8S 3N5
Tel. 514 637-2351
Fax 514 637-5270
www.cusm.ca

LACHUTE

CENTRE HOSPITALIER D'ARGENTEUIL
145 av de la Providence
Lachute QC J8H 4C7
Tel. 450 562-3761
Fax 450 566-3316
www.csssargenteuil.qc.ca

LASALLE

CENTRE D'HÉBERGEMENT CHAMPLAIN
1325 rue Crawford
Verdun QC H4H 2N6
Tel. 514 766-8513 Ext. 8501
Fax 514 769-6552
www.champlain-manoir.org

CENTRE HOSPITALIER DE LASALLE
8585 Terrasse Champlain
Lasalle QC H8P 1C1
Tel. 514 362-8000
Fax 514 367-8634
www.csssdll.qc.ca

CENTRE HOSPITALIER DE VERDUN
4000 boul Lasalle
Verdun QC H4G 2A3
Tel. 514 362-1000
Fax 514 765-7306
www.ch-verdun.fr

DOUGLAS MENTAL HEALTH UNIVERSITY INSTITUTE
6875 boul LaSalle
Verdun QC H4H 1R3
Tel. 514 761-6131
Fax 514 888-4067
www.douglas.qc.ca

LAVAL

CHSLD ST-JUDE-DE-LAVAL LTÉE
4410 boul Saint-Martin O
Laval QC H7T 1C3
Tel. 450 687-7714
Fax 450 682-0330
www.age-3.com

HOPITAL DE LA CITE DE LA SANTÉ
1755 boul René-Laennec
Laval QC H7M 3L9
Tel. 450 668-1010
Fax 450 975-5545
www.csssl.qc.ca

JEWISH REHABILITATION HOSPITAL
3205 Place Alton-Goldbloom
Laval QC H7V 1R2
Tel. 450 688-9550
Fax 450 688-3673
www.hjr-jrh.qc.ca

LEBEL-SUR-QUÉVILLON

CENTRE DE SANTÉ LEBEL
950 boul Quevillon N
CP 5000
Lebel-s-Quevillon QC J0Y 1X0
Tel. 819 755-4881
Fax 819 755-3581

LES ESCOUMINS

CENTRE DE SANTÉ DES CÔTÉ-NORD
4 rue de l'Hopital
CP 1000
Les Escoumins QC G0T 1K0
Tel. 418 233-2931 Ext. 2214
Fax 418 233-2608
www.agencesante09.gouv.qc.ca

LÉVIS

CSSS DU GRAND LITTORAL
975 rue de la Concorde
Saint-Romuald QC G6W 8A7
Tel. 418 883-3359
Fax 418 883-4204
www.csssgrandlittoral.qc.ca

CENTRE HOSPITALIER PAUL-GILBERT
9330 du Centre-Hospitalier
Charny QC G6X 1L6
Tel. 418 380-2050
Fax 418 832-9041
www.cspg.qc.ca

HÔTEL-DIEU DE LÉVIS
143 rue Wolfe
Levis QC G6V 3Z1
Tel. 418 835-7121
Fax 418 835-7143
www.hdl.qc.ca

LONGUEUIL

CHSLD DE LA MRC DE CHAMPLAIN-CENTRE SAINT-LAMBERT
831 av Notre-Dame
Saint-Lambert QC J4R 1S1
Tel. 450 672-3320
Fax 450 672-3370
www.lesresidences.com

CHSLD VIGI MONTÉRÉGIE
2042 boul Marie
Saint-Hubert QC J4T 2B4
Tel. 450 671-5596
Fax 450 671-5079
www.vigisante.com

CSSS CHAMPLAIN
5928 boul Cousineau
bureau 200
Longueuil QC J3Y 7R9
Tel. 450 445-4452 Ext. 2543
Fax 450 678-7586
www.santemonteregie.qc.ca

CENTRE D'HEBERGEMENT CHAMPLAIN RIVE-SUD
5300 ch de Chambly
Longueuil QC J3Y 3N7
Tel. 450 445-0123
Fax 450 445-1175
www.reseau411.ca

CENTRE HOSPITALIER PIERRE BOUCHER
1333 boul Jacques-Cartier E
Longueuil QC J4M 2A5
Tel. 450 468-8111 Ext. 2555
Fax 450 468-8188
www.santemonteregie.qc.ca

HOPITAL CHARLES LEMOYNE
3120 boul Taschereau
Greenfield Park QC J4V 2H1
Tel. 450 466-5000
Fax 450 466-8887
www.hclm.qc.ca

LOUISEVILLE

CSSS DE MASKINONGÉ
450 2e rue
Louiseville QC J5V 1V3
Tel. 819 228-2731
Fax 819 228-2973
www.csssm.qc.ca

LOURDES-DU-BLANC -SABLON

CSSS DE LA BASSE CÔTÉ-NORD
1070 boul Dr Camille Marcou
CP 130
Lourdes-D-Bl-Sabl
QC G0G 1W0
Tel. 418 461-2144 Ext. 400
Fax 418 461-2731
www.csssbcn.gouv.qc.ca

MACAMIC

CENTRE HOSPITALIER ST-JEAN
169 7e av E
Macamic QC J0Z 2S0
Tel. 819 782-4661
Fax 819 782-2400

MAGOG

CENTRE HOSPITALIER ET CLSC DE MEMPHREMAGOG
50 rue Saint-Patrice E
Magog QC J1X 3X3
Tel. 819 843-3381
Fax 819 843-8262
csssm.santeestrie.qc.ca

MALARTIC

HÔPITAL PSYCHIATRIQUE DE MALARTIC
1141 rue Royale
CP 800
Malartic QC J0Y 1Z0
Tel. 819 825-5858
Fax 819 757-4330
www.csssvo.qc.ca

MANIWAKI

CSSS DE LA VALLÉE DE LA GATINEAU
309 boul Desjardins
Maniwaki QC J9E 2E7
Tel. 819 449-2300
Fax 819 449-6137
www.csssvg.qc.ca

MARIA

CSSS DE LA BAIE-DES-CHALEURS
419 boul Pérron
RR 2
Maria QC G0C 1Y0
Tel. 418 759-3443 Ext. 2193
Fax 418 759-5063
www.csssbc.ca

MATAGAMI

CENTRE DE SANTE ISLE-DIEU MATAGAMI
130 boul Matagami
CP 790
Matagami QC J0Y 2A0
Tel. 819 739-2515
Fax 819 739-4777
www.crsssbaiejames.gouv.qc.ca

MATANE

CENTRE HOSPITALIER DE MATANE
333 rue Thibault
Matane QC G4W 2W5
Tel. 418 562-3135
Fax 418 562-9374
www.santeautravail.net/

MÉTABETCHOUAN-LAC -À-LA-CROIX

HÔPITAL DE MÉTABETCHOUAN
1895 Hwy 169
Métabetchouan QC G0W 2A0
Tel. 418 349-2861

MONT-JOLI

CSSS DE LA MITIS
800 av du Sanatorium
Mont-Joli QC G5H 3L6
Tel. 418 775-7261
Fax 418 775-1989
www.centremitissien.net

MONT-LAURIER

CSSS D'ANTOINE-LABELLE
757 rue de la Madone
Mont-Laurier QC J9L 1T3
Tel. 819 623-6127 Ext. 6345
Fax 819 623-9451
www.csssal.org

MONTMAGNY

CSSS DE MONTMAGNY -L'ISLET
350 boul Tache O
Montmagny QC G5V 3R8
Tel. 418 248-0630 Ext. 223
Fax 418 248-6838
www.csssml.qc.ca

MONTRÉAL

CHSLD BOURGET INC
11570 rue Notre-Dame E
Pte-aux-Trembles QC H1B 2X4
Tel. 514 645-1673
Fax 514 645-8451
www.chsldbourget.com

CHSLD CARDINAL INC
12900 rue Notre-Dame E
Pte-aux-Trembles QC H1A 1R9
Tel. 514 645-2766
Fax 514 640-6267
www.reseau411.ca

CHSLD CENTRE-VILLE DE MONTRÉAL
66 boul Rene-Levesque E
Montreal QC H2X 1N3
Tel. 514 861-9331
Fax 514 861-8385
www.santemontreal.qc.ca

CHSLD LUCILLE-TEASDALE
3095 rue Sherbrooke E
Montreal QC H1W 1B2
Tel. 514 523-1173 Ext. 316
Fax 514 528-2711
www.santemontreal.qc.ca

CHSLD PAUL-GOUIN
5900 rue de Saint-Vallier
Montréal QC H2S 2P3
Tel. 514 848-0707
Fax 514 273-1099
www.arrondissement.com

CLSC CÔTE SAINT-PAUL - VILLE EMARD
6161 rue Laurendeau
Montréal QC H4E 3X6
Tel. 514 766-0546
Fax 514 732-5128
www.sov.qc.ca

CSSS D'AHUNTSIC ET MONTRÉAL-NORD
1725 boul Gouin E
Montréal QC H2C 3H6
Tel. 514 384-2000
Fax 514 384-4245
www.csssamn.ca

CSSS DU COEUR DE L'ISLE HÔPITAL JEAN-TALON
1385 rue Jean-Talon E
Montreal QC H2E 1S6
Tel. 514 495-6754
Fax 514 495-6734
www.santemontreal.qc.ca

CSSS JEANNE MANCE
155 boul. Saint-Joseph E
Montréal QC H2T 1H4
Tel. 514 525-1900 Ext. 6388
Fax 514 380-5152
www.msss.gouv.qc.ca

CSSS DE LA MONTAGNE
314-5700 ch Côte des Neiges
Montreal QC H3T 2A8
Tel. 514 731-1386 Ext. 2331
Fax 514 731-9600
www.msss.gouv.qc.ca

CSSS DE LA POINTE DE ÎLE
9503 rue Sherbrooke Est
Montréal QC H1L 6P2
Tel. 514 356-2572
Fax 514 356-2571
www.santemontreal.qc.ca

CSSS SAINT-LEONARD ET SAINT-MICHEL
3130 Jarry est
Montréal QC H1Z 4N8
Tel. 514 722-3000
Fax 514 593-7400
csss-stleonardstmichel.qc.ca

CSSS DU SUD-OUEST VERDUN
6161 rue Laurendeau
Montreal QC H4E 3X6
Tel. 514 762-2777
Fax 514 762-4139
www.sov.qc.ca

CATHERINE BOOTH HOSPITAL
4375 av Montclair
Montreal QC H4B 2J5
Tel. 514 481-0431
Fax 514 481-0029
www.santemontreal.qc.ca

CENTRE DE RÉADAPTATION MARIE ENFANT DU CHU SAINTE-JUSTINE
5200 rue Belanger
Montreal QC H1T 1C9
Tel. 514 374-1710
Fax 514 374-7944
www.chu-sainte-justine.org

CENTRE DE SOINS PROLONGÉS GRACE DART
5155 rue Sainte-Catherine Est
Montréal QC H1V 2A5
Tel. 514 255-2833
Fax 514 255-0650
www.gracedart.ca

CENTRE D'HÉBERGEMENT ST-GEORGES
3550 rue St Urbain
Montréal QC H2X 4C5
Tel. 514 849-1357
Fax 514 849-8465

CENTRE HOSPITALIER JACQUES VIGER
1051 rue Saint-Hubert
Montréal QC H2L 3Y5
Tel. 514 842-7181
Fax 514 842-7689

CENTRE HOSPITALIER L'UNIVERSITÉ DE MONTRÉAL (CHUM) - HÔPITAL NOTRE-DAME
1560 rue Sherbrooke E
Montréal QC H2L 4M1
Tel. 514 890-8000
Fax 514 842-7689
www.chumtl.qc.ca

CENTRE HOSPITALIER L'UNIVERSITÉ DE MONTRÉAL (CHUM) - HÔPITAL SAINT-LUC
1058 rue Saint-Denis
Montreal QC H2X 3J4
Tel. 514 890-8000
Fax 514 412-7382
www.chumtl.qc.ca

CENTRE HOSPITALIER L'UNIVERSITÉ DE MONTRÉAL (CHUM) - HÔTEL-DIEU
3840 rue Saint-Urbain
Montréal QC H2W 1T8
Tel. 514 890-8000
Fax 514 412-7224
www.chumtl.qc.ca

CENTRE METROPOLITAN DE CHIRURGIE PLASTIQUE
999 rue de Salaberry
Montreal QC H3L 1L2
Tel. 514 332-7091
Fax 514 332-7095
www.weightlosssurgery.ca

DONALD BERMAN MAIMONIDES GERIATRIC CENTRE
5795 av Caldwell
Cote Saint-Luc QC H4W 1W3
Tel. 514 483-2121
Fax 514 483-1086
donaldbermanmaimonides.net

GRACE DART EXTENDED CARE CENTRE
5155 rue Sainte-Catherine E
Montreal QC H1V 2A5
Tel. 514 255-2833
Fax 514 255-0650
www.gracedart.ca

GRACE DART PAVILLION
6085 Sherbrooke St E
Montréal QC H1N 1C2
Tel. 514 256-9021
Fax 514 251-2391
www.gracedart.com

HÔPITAL CHINOIS DE MONTRÉAL
189 av Viger E
Montreal QC H2X 3Y9
Tel. 514 871-0961
Fax 514 871-0966

HÔPITAL DE RÉADAPTATION VILLA MEDICA
225 rue Sherbrooke E
Montreal QC H2X 1C9
Tel. 514 288-8201
Fax 514 288-6370
www.villamedica.ca

HÔPITAL DU SACRE-COEUR DE MONTRÉAL
5400 boul Gouin O
Montreal QC H4J 1C5
Tel. 514 338-2222
Fax 514 338-2384
www.hscm.ca

HOPITAL LOUIS-H LAFONTAINE
7401 rue Hochelaga
Montréal QC H1N 3M5
Tel. 514 251-4000
Fax 514 251-0856
www.hlhl.qc.ca

HOPITAL MAISONNEUVE -ROSEMONT
5415 boul de l'Assomption
Montreal QC H1T 2M4
Tel. 514 252-3400
Fax 514 252-3506
maisonneuve-rosemont.org

HÔPITAL RIVIERE DES PRAIRIES
7070 boul Perras
Montreal QC H1E 1A4
Tel. 514 323-7260
Fax 514 323-8622
www.hrdp.qc.ca

HÔPITAL SANTA CABRINI OSPEDALE
5655 rue Saint-Zotique E
Montreal QC H1T 1P7
Tel. 514 252-6000
Fax 514 252-6453
www.santacabrini.qc.ca

HÔPITAL STE-JUSTINE
3175 ch Côte-Sainte-Catherine
Montréal QC H3T 1C5
Tel. 514 345-4931
Fax 514 345-4800
www.chu-sainte-justine.org

INSTITUT DE CARDIOLOGIE DE MONTRÉAL
5000 rue Belanger
Montreal QC H1T 1C8
Tel. 514 376-3330
Fax 514 593-2540
www.icm-mhi.org

INSTITUT DE RÉADAPTATION GINGRAS-LINDSAY DE MONTRÉAL
6300 av de Darlington
Montreal QC H3S 2J4
Tel. 514 340-2085
Fax 514 340-2091
www.irglm.qc.ca

INSTITUT PHILIPPE-PINEL DE MONTREAL
10905 boul Henri-Bourassa E
Montreal QC H1C 1H1
Tel. 514 648-8461
Fax 514 494-4406
www.pinel.qc.ca

INSTITUT UNIVERSITAIRE DE GÉRIATRIE DE MONTRÉAL
4565 ch Queen-Mary
Montreal QC H3W 1W5
Tel. 514 340-2800
Fax 514 340-3525
www.iugm.qc.ca

JEWISH ELDERCARE CENTRE - CHSLD JUIF DE MONTRÉAL
5725 av Victoria
Montreal QC H3W 3H6
Tel. 514 738-4500
Fax 514 738-2611
www.jewisheldercare.ca

MCGILL UNIVERSITY HEALTH CENTRE - MONTREAL CHEST INSTITUTE
3650 rue Saint-Urbain
Montreal QC H2X 2P4
Tel. 514 934-5201
Fax 514 843-2088
www.muhc.ca

MCGILL UNIVERSITY HEALTH CENTRE - MONTREAL CHILDREN'S HOSPITAL
2300 rue Tupper
Montreal QC H3H 1P3
Tel. 514 412-4400
Fax 514 412-4477
www.thechildrens.com

MCGILL UNIVERSITY HEALTH CENTRE - MONTREAL GENERAL CAMPUS
1650 av Cedar
Montreal QC H3G 1A4
Tel. 514 934-1934
Fax 514 934-8200
www.muhc.ca

MCGILL UNIVERSITY HEALTH CENTRE - MONTREAL NEUROLOGICAL HOSPITAL
3801 rue University
Montreal QC H3A 2B4
Tel. 514 398-6644
Fax 514 398-8540
www.muhc.ca

MCGILL UNIVERSITY HEALTH CENTRE - ROYAL VICTORIA HOSPITAL
687 av des Pins O
Montreal QC H3A 1A1
Tel. 514 934-1934
www.mcgill.ca

MOUNT SINAI HOSPITAL CENTER
5690 boul Cavendish
Cote Saint-Luc QC H4W 1S7
Tel. 514 369-2222
Fax 514 369-2225
www.sinaimontreal.ca

PAVILLON NOTRE-DAME DE LA MERCI
555 boul Gouin O
Montreal QC H3L 1K5
Tel. 514 331-3020 Ext. 209
Fax 514 331-3358
www.csssbcstl.qc.ca

PAVILLON ST-JOSEPH DE LA PROVIDENCE
11844 av du Bois-de-Boulogne
Montreal QC H3M 2X7
Tel. 514 334-3120
Fax 514 334-5881

PROVIDENCE NOTRE-DAME -DE-LOURDES INC
1870 boul Pie-IX
Montréal QC H1V 2C6
Tel. 514 527-4595
Fax 514 527-4475

RICHARDSON HOSPITAL CENTRE
5425 av Bessborough
Montreal QC H4V 2S7
Tel. 514 484-7878
Fax 514 483-4596
www.cssscavendish.qc.ca

ST MARY'S HOSPITAL CENTRE
3830 av Lacombe
Montreal QC H3T 1M5
Tel. 514 345-3511
Fax 514 734-2636
www.smhc.qc.ca

SHRINERS HOSPITALS FOR CHILDREN - CANADA
1529 av Cedar
Montreal QC H3G 1A6
Tel. 514 842-4464
Fax 514 842-7553
www.shrinershq.org

SIR MORTIMER B DAVIS JEWISH GENERAL
3755 ch Côte-Sainte-Catherine
Montréal QC H3T 1E2
Tel. 514 340-8222
Fax 514 340-7510
www.jgh.ca

MONTRÉAL-NORD

CHSLD MARIE CLARET
3345 boul Henri-Bourassa E
Montréal-Nord QC H1H 1H6
Tel. 514 322-4380
Fax 514 326-8811
www.vigisante.com

CHSLD STE-ELISABETH
11720 av desy
Montreal-Nord QC H1G 4C3
Tel. 514 788-2085
Fax 514 788-2905

HOPITAL MARIE CLARAC
3530 boul Gouin E
Montréal-Nord QC H1H 1B7
Tel. 514 321-8800
Fax 514 321-9626
www.hopitalmarie-clarac.qc.ca

MUTTON BAY

CLSC MUTTON BAY (POINT DE SERVICE)
Direction Gen
Mutton Bay QC G0G 2C0
Tel. 418 773-2212
Fax 418 773-2635

NEMISCAU

NAMASKA COMMUNITY CLINIC
Nemiscau QC J0Y 3B0
Tel. 819 673-2511
Fax 819 673-2554

NICOLET

HÔPITAL DE CHRIST-ROI
675 rue Saint-Jean-Baptiste
Nicolet QC J3T 1S4
Tel. 819 293-2071 Ext. 2280
Fax 819 293-6160
www.csssbny.qc.ca

NOTRE-DAME-DU-LAC

CENTRE HOSPITALIER NOTRE-DAME-DU-LAC
58 rue de l'Eglise
CP 310
Notre-Dame-du-Lac
QC G0L 1X0
Tel. 418 899-6751
Fax 418 899-2809
www.cssstemiscouata.com

OKA

KANESATAKE HEALTH CENTRE
12 Joseph Swan Rd
Kanehsatake QC J0N 1E0
Tel. 450 479-6000
Fax 450 479-8313
www.kanesatakehealthcentre.ca

ORMSTOWN

BARRIE MEMORIAL HOSPITAL
28 Gale St
CP 2000
Ormstown QC J0S 1K0
Tel. 450 829-2321
Fax 450 829-3582
www.santemonteregie.qc.ca

OUJÉ-BOUGOUMOU

OUJE-BOUGOUMOU - PLACE WHERE PEOPLE GATHER
203 Opemiska Meskino
Oujé-Bougoumou QC G0W 3C0
Tel. 418 745-3901
Fax 418 745-3043
www.ouje.ca

PLESSISVILLE

CLSC DE L'ERABLE
1331 rue Saint-Calixte
Plessisville QC G6L 1P4
Tel. 819 362-6301
Fax 819 362-6300

POHÉNÉGAMOOK

CLSC DE POHÉNÉGAMOK
1922 rue St-Vallier
CP 70
Saint-Éleuthère QC G0L 2T0
Tel. 418 859-2450
Fax 418 859-3484

POINTE-CLAIRE

CHSLD BAYVIEW INC
27 ch du Bord-du-Lac
Pointe-Claire QC H9S 4H1
Tel. 514 695-9384 Ext. 222
Fax 514 695-5723
www.chsldbayview.com

LAKESHORE GENERAL HOSPITAL - POINTE CLAIRE
160 av Stillview
Pointe-Claire QC H9R 2Y2
Tel. 514 630-2225 Ext. 5253
Fax 514 630-3302

PORT-CARTIER

CLSC-CSSS DE PORT-CARTIER
3 rue de Shelter Bay
Port-Cartier QC G5B 2W9
Tel. 418 766-2572
Fax 418 766-5229

POVUNGNITUQ

INUULITSIVIK HEALTH CENTRE
General Delivery
Puvirnituq QC J0M 1P0
Tel. 819 988-2957
Fax 819 988-2796
www.inuulitsivik.ca

QUÉBEC

CH NOTRE-DAME DU CHEMIN
510 ch Sainte-Foy
Quebec QC G1S 2J5
Tel. 418 681-7882
Fax 418 681-5387

CH ST-FRANCOIS INC
1604 1e av
Quebec QC G1L 3L6
Tel. 514 524-6033
Fax 514 524-9542

CH ST-SACREMENT LTEE
1165 ch Sainte-Foy
Quebec QC G1S 2M8
Tel. 418 527-4836
Fax 418 527-1743

CSSS DE LA VIEILLE-CAPITALE
1 av du Sacré-Coeur
Québec QC G1N 2W1
Tel. 418 529-4777 Ext. 366
Fax 418 691-0711
www.csssvc.qc.ca

CSSS DE QUEBEC NORD
2915 av Bourg-Royal
Québec QC G1C 3S2
Tel. 418 661-5666
Fax 418 780-8726
www.csssqn.qc.ca

CSSS DE QUEBEC-SUD
300 boul Wilfrid-Hamel
Vanier QC G1M 2R9
Tel. 418 682-1711
Fax 418 682-1773
www.ramq.gouv.qc.ca

CENTRE D'HEBERGEMENT SAINT-AUGUSTIN
2135 rue de Terrasse-Cadieux
Beauport QC G1C 1Z2
Tel. 418 667-3910
Fax 418 667-4094
www.rrsss03.gouv.qc.ca

CENTRE HOSPITALIER AFFILIÉ UNIVERSITAIRE DE QUÉBEC-HÔPITAL DE L'ENFANT JÉSUS
1401 rue 18E
Québec QC G1J 1Z4
Tel. 418 649-0252
Fax 418 649-5557
www.cha.quebec.qc.ca

CENTRE HOSPITALIER AFFILIÉ UNIVERSITAIRE DE QUÉBEC - HÔPITAL DU ST-SACREMENT
1050 ch Sainte-Foy
Quebec QC G1S 4L8
Tel. 418 682-7511
Fax 418 682-7977
www.cha.quebec.qc.ca

CENTRE HOSPITALIER CHAUVEAU
29 rue de L'Hôpital
Quebec QC G2A 2T7
Tel. 418 842-3651
Fax 418 842-8931

CENTRE HOSPITALIER UNIVERSITAIRE DE QUÉBEC-CHUL
2705 boul Laurier
Quebec QC G1V 4G2
Tel. 418 656-4444
Fax 418 654-2247
www.chuq.qc.ca

CENTRE HOSPITALIER UNIVERSITAIRE DE QUÉBEC (CHUQ) - SIEGE SOCIAL
11 Cote du Palais
Quebec QC G1R 2J6
Tel. 418 525-4444
Fax 418 691-5331
www.chuq.qc.ca

CENTRE HOSPITALIER UNIVERSITAIRE DE QUÉBEC - PAVILLON DE ST-FRANÇOIS-D'ASSISE
10 rue de l'Espinay
Quebec QC G1L 3L5
Tel. 418 525-4444
Fax 418 525-6338
http://www.crchuq.ulaval.ca

HÔPITAL GÉNÉRAL DE QUÉBEC - CHSLD
260 boul Langelier
Quebec QC G1K 5N1
Tel. 418 529-0931
Fax 418 529-5801

HÔPITAL LAVAL
2725 ch Sainte-Foy
Québec QC G1V 4G5
Tel. 418 656-8711
Fax 418 656-4829
www.hopitallaval.qc.ca

HOPITAL STE-MONIQUE INC
4805 boul Wilfrid-Hamel
Quebec QC G1P 2J7
Tel. 418 871-8701
Fax 418 871-0105
www.rrsss03.gouv.qc.ca

HOTEL-DIEU DU SACRE -COEUR DE JESUS DE QUEBEC
1 av du Sacre-Coeur
Quebec QC G1N 2W1
Tel. 418 529-6851
Fax 418 529-2971

INSTITUT UNIVERSITAIRE SANTE
2601 ch de la Canardiere
Québec QC G1J 2G3
Tel. 418 663-5126
Fax 418 663-9774
www.institutsmq.qc.ca

JEFFERY HALE HOSPITAL -SAINT BRIGID'S
1250 ch Sainte-Foy
Quebec QC G1S 2M6
Tel. 418 684-5333
Fax 418 527-6862
www.chuq.qc.ca

MAISON MICHEL SARRAZIN
2101 ch Saint-Louis
Quebec QC G1T 1P5
Tel. 418 688-0878
Fax 418 681-8636
www.michel-sarrazin.ca

RAWDON

MANOIR HEATHER LODGE
3462 3rd av
Rawdon QC J0K 1S0
Tel. 450 834-2512
Fax 450 834-5805
www.manoirheather.com

RESTIGOUCHE

CENTRE DE SANTÉ LISTUGUJ
6 Pacific Dr
CP 338
Restigouche QC G0C 2R0
Tel. 418 788-2155
Fax 418 788-3155

RIMOUSKI

HÔPITAL REGIONAL RIMOUSKI
150 av Rouleau
CP 3150 succ Bureau Chef
Rimouski QC G5L 5T1
Tel. 418 724-8441
Fax 418 724-8632
www.chrr.qc.ca

RIVIÈRE-DU-LOUP

CENTRE HOSPITALIER REGIONAL DU GRAND-PORTAGE
75 rue Saint-Henri
Riviere-Du-Loup QC G5R 2A4
Tel. 418 868-1010
Fax 418 868-1035
www.csssrivieredulop.qc.ca

RIVIÈRE-ROUGE

CENTRE DE L'ANNONCIATION
1525 rue l'Annonciation N
Rivière-Rouge QC J0T 1T0
Tel. 819 275-2118
Fax 819 275-2464
www.csssal.org

ROBERVAL

CENTRE RÉADAPTATION EN DÉFICIENCE INTELLECTUALLE DU SAGUENAY-LAC-ST-JEAN
835 rue Roland
Roberval QC G8H 3J5
Tel. 418 275-1360
Fax 418 275-6595
www.santesaglac.gouv.qc.ca

HOTEL-DIEU DE ROBERVAL
450 rue Brassard
Roberval QC G8H 1B9
Tel. 418 275-0110 Ext. 2226
Fax 418 275-8087
www.cmdp-roberval.com

ROUYN-NORANDA

CENTRE HOSPITALIER ROUYN-NORANDA
4 9e rue
Rouyn-Noranda QC J9X 2B2
Tel. 819 764-5131 Ext. 45159
Fax 819 764-2900
www.csssrn.qc.ca

SAINTE-ADÈLE

CSSS DES PAYS D'EN HAUT
707 boul de Sainte-Adèle
Sainte-Adèle QC J8B 2N1
Tel. 450 229-6601
Fax 450 229-8513
www.cssspdh.net

SAINTE-AGATHE-DES-MONTS

CENTRE HOSPITALIER LAURENTIEN
234 rue Saint-Vincent
Ste-Agathe-des-Mts
QC J8C 2B8
Tel. 819 324-4000
Fax 819 324-4010
www.csss-sommets.com

SAINT-AMABLE

QUAQTAQ HEALTH SERVICES
539 rue Principale
Saint-Amable QC J0L 1N0
Tel. 450 468-5250
Fax 450 922-5251

SAINT-ANDRÉ

CLSC LES ABOITEAUX - SAINT-ANDRÉ
122 rue Principale
Saint-André QC G0L 2H0
Tel. 418 856-7000
Fax 418 493-2142
www.wpp01.msss.gouv.qc.ca

SAINTE-ANNE-DE-BELLEVUE

HOPITAL STE-ANNE
305 boul des Anciens-Combattants
Ste-Anne-de-Bellev
QC H9X 1Y9
Tel. 514 457-3440
Fax 514 457-5741
www.veterans.gc.ca

SAINTE-ANNE-DES-MONTS

CENTRE HOSPITALIER DES MONTS
50 rue du Belvedere
Ste-Anne-des-Monts
QC G4V 1X4
Tel. 418 763-2261
Fax 418 763-1221
www.hautegaspesie.com

SAINT-EUSTACHE

HÔPITAL DE SAINT-EUSTACHE
520 boul Arthur-Sauvé
Saint-Eustache QC J7R 5B1
Tel. 450 473-6811 Ext. 2000
Fax 450 473-6966
www.moncsss.com

SAINT-FERDINAND

CENTRE D'HEBERGEMENT DE SACRE-COEUR
230 rue Principale
Saint-Ferdinand QC G0N 1N0
Tel. 418 428-3266
www.csssae.qc.ca

SAINT-GEORGES

CHSLD DE L'ASSOMPTION
16750 boul Lacroix
Saint-Georges QC G5Y 2G4
Tel. 418 228-2041
Fax 418 228-9366
www.groupechamplain.qc.ca

CENTRE HOSPITALIER BEAUCE-ETCHEMIN
1515 17e rue
Saint-Georges QC G5Y 4T8
Tel. 418 774-3304 Ext. 3304
Fax 418 227-3825
www.csssbeauce.qc.ca

SAINT-HYACINTHE

CENTRE D HEBERGEMENT DE L HÔTEL-DIEU DE SAINT-HYACINTHE
1800 rue dessaulles
Saint-Hyacinthe QC J2S 2T2
Tel. 450 774-3333
Fax 450 774-9900

CENTRE HOSPITALIER HONORE-MERCIER
2750 boul Laframboise
Saint-Hyacinthe QC J2S 4Y8
Tel. 450 771-3333 Ext. 4972
Fax 450 771-3246
www.rsry.qc.ca

SAINT-JEAN-PORT-JOLI

CSSS DE MONTMAGNY -L'ISLET
430 rue Jean-Leclerc
RR 1
St-Jean-Port-Joli QC G0R 3G0
Tel. 418 598-3355
Fax 418 598-9800

SAINT-JEAN-SUR-RICHELIEU

HÔPITAL DU HAUT-RICHELIEU
920 du Seminaire Blvd N
St-Jean-sur-Richel QC J3A 1B7
Tel. 450 359-5000
Fax 450 359-5251
www.santemonteregie.qc.ca

SAINT-JÉRÔME

HÔTEL-DIEU DE SAINT-JÉRÔME
290 rue de Montigny
Saint-Jérôme QC J7Z 5T3
Tel. 450 431-8200 Ext. 2551
Fax 450 431-8244
www.cdsj.org

SAINT-MICHEL-DE -BELLECHASSE

CHSLD VIGI OUR LADY OF LOURDES
80 rue Principale
CP 10
St-Michel-De-Bell QC G0R 3S0
Tel. 418 884-2811
Fax 418 884-3714
www.vigisante.com

SAINT-PACÔME

RESEAU SANTE KAMOURASKA-HÔPITAL D'ANJOU INC
127 rue Galarneau
St-Pacome QC G0L 3X0
Tel. 418 852-2281
Fax 418 852-3230

SAINT-PASCAL

CSSS DE KAMOURASKA
575 av Martin
Saint-Pascal QC G0L 3Y0
Tel. 418 856-7000 Ext. 3229
Fax 418 492-5742

SAINT-RAYMOND

CENTRE HOSPITALIER PORTNEUF
700 rue Saint-Cyrille
Saint-Raymond QC G3L 1W1
Tel. 418 337-4611
Fax 418 337-4808
www.csssdeportneuf.qc.ca

SAINTE-THÉRÈSE -DE-BLAINVILLE

CSSS DE THÉRÈSE DE BLAINVILLE
125 rue Duquet
Sainte-Thérèse QC J7E 0A5
Tel. 450 430-4553 Ext. 5106
Fax 450 430-0140
cssstheresedeblainville.qc.ca

SAINT-TITE

CSSS DE LA VALLÉE DE LA BATISCAN
750 rue du Couvent
CP 430
Saint-Tite QC G0X 3H0
Tel. 418 365-7556
Fax 418 365-6009
www.csssvalleebatiscan.qc.ca

SALABERRY -DE-VALLEYFIELD

CENTRE HOSPITALIER RÉGIONAL DU SUROÎT
150 rue Saint-Thomas
Salaber-de-Valleyf QC J6T 6C1
Tel. 450 371-9920 Ext. 2000
Fax 450 377-1372
www.rocler.qc.ca

SENNETERRE

CENTRE DE SANTE VALLEE-DE-L'OR
961 rue de la Clinique
CP 4000
Senneterre QC J0Y 2M0
Tel. 819737-5858
Fax 819 737-3122
www.csssvo.qc.ca

SEPT-ÎLES

CENTRE HOSPITALIER REGIONAL DE SEPT-ILES
45 rue du Pere-Divet
Sept-Îles QC G4R 3N7
Tel. 418 962-9761 Ext. 2402
Fax 418 962-2701
www.cssssi.qc.ca

SHAWINIGAN

CENTRE HOSPITALIER DU CENTRE LA MAURICIE
50 119e rue
Shawinigan QC G9P 5K7
Tel. 819 536-7500
Fax 819 536-7658
www.chcm.qc.ca

CH DU CENTRE-DE-LA -MAURICIE (STE-THÉRÈSE DE SHAWINIGAN)
1705 av Georges
Shawinigan QC G9N 2N1
Tel. 819 537-9351
Fax 819 537-4737

SHAWVILLE

PONTIAC HOSPITAL CENTRE
200 rue Argue
Shawville QC J0X 2Y0
Tel. 819 647-2211
Fax 819 647-2409
www.santepontiac.qc.ca

SHERBROOKE

CSSS INSTITUT UNIVERSITAIRE DE GÉRIATRIE DE SHERBROOKE
1036 rue Belvedere S
Sherbrooke QC J1H 4C4
Tel. 819 821-1150
Fax 819 829-7149
www.csss-iugs.ca

CENTRE HOSPITALIER UNIVERSITAIRE DE SHERBROOKE-HOPITAL FLEURIMONT
3001 12e av N
Sherbrooke QC J1H 5N4
Tel. 819 346-1110
Fax 819 820-6417
www.usherbrooke.ca

CENTRE HOSPITALIER UNIVERSITAIRE DE SHERBROOKE-HÔPITAL HÔTEL-DIEU
580 rue Bowen S
Sherbrooke QC J1G 2E8
Tel. 819 346-1110
Fax 819 822-6766
www.chus.qc.ca

CENTRE HOSPITALIER UNIVERSITAIRE DE SHERBROOKE-MURRAY BUILDING
500 Murray St
Sherbrooke QC J1G 2K6
Tel. 819 346-1100
Fax 866 638-2601
www.chus.qc.ca

INSTITUT UNIVERSITAIRE DE GERIATRIE DE SHERBROOKE-PAVILLON ARGYLL
375 rue Argyll
Sherbrooke QC J1J 3H5
Tel. 819 821-1150
Fax 819 829-7146

SOREL-TRACY

CHSLD DU BAS-RICHELIEU
151 rue George
Sorel-Tracy QC J3P 1C8
Tel. 450 746-5555
Fax 450 746-4897
www.soreltracyregion.net

HÔPITAL RICHELIEU
30 rue Ferland
CP 590
Sorel-Tracy QC J3P 3C7
Tel. 450 743-5569
Fax 450 743-1803

HÔTEL-DIEU DE SOREL
400 av de l'Hôtel-Dieu
Sorel-Tracy QC J3P 1N5
Tel. 450 746-6062
Fax 450 746-6063
www.santemonteregie.qc.ca

TASIUJAQ

TASIUJAQ HEALTH SERVICES
Gen Del
Tasiujaq QC J0M 1T0
Tel. 819 633-9977
Fax 819 633-5098

TÉMISCAMING

CENTRE DE SANTÉ DE TÉMISCAMING
180 rue Anvik
CP 760
Temiscaming QC J0Z 3R0
Tel. 819 627-3385
Fax 819 627-9497
www.cssstr.ca

TERREBONNE

CENTRE HOSPITALIER PIERRE LE GARDEUR
911 montée des Pionniers
Terrebonne QC J6V 2H2
Tel. 450 654-7525 Ext. 42148
Fax 450 582-4439
www.csss.sudlanaudiere.ca

TÊTE-À-LA-BALEINE

CLSC DE TÊTE-À-LA-BALEINE (POINT DE SERVICE)
Tête-à-la-Baleine QC G0G 2W0
Tel. 418 242-2112
Fax 418 242-2133

THETFORD MINES

HOPITAL DU CSS DE LA REGION DE THETFORD
1717 rue Notre-Dame E
Thetford Mines QC G6G 2V4
Tel. 418 338-7777
Fax 418 338-7616
www.centresantethetford.ca

TROIS-PISTOLES

CENTRE HOSPITALIER TROIS-PISTOLES
550 rue Notre-Dame E
Trois-Pistoles QC G0L 4K0
Tel. 418 851-1111
Fax 418 851-2934
csssbasques@ssss.gouv.qc.ca

TROIS-RIVIÈRES

CHSLD LE TRIFLUVIEN
3450 rue Sainte-Marguerite
Trois-Rivieres QC G8Z 1X3
Tel. 819 375-7713
Fax 819 375-5659
www.indexsante.ca

CSSS DE TROIS-RIVIÈRES
731 rue Sainte-Julie
Trois-Rivières QC G9A 1Y1
Tel. 819 697-3333
Fax 819 372-3581
www.msss.gouv.qc.ca

CENTRE DE SANTÉ CLOUTIER-DU-RIVAGE
155 rue Toupin
Trois-Rivières QC G8T 3Z8
Tel. 819 370-2100
Fax 819 379-9644
www.cssstr.qc.ca

CENTRE HOSPITALIER REGIONAL DE TROIS-RIVIERES
731 rue Sainte-Julie
Trois-Rivieres QC G9A 1Y1
Tel. 819 697-3333
Fax 819 372-3581
www.allerplusloin.ca

VAL-D'OR

CENTRE HOSPITALIER DE VAL D'OR
725 6e rue
Val-d'Or QC J9P 3Y1
Tel. 819 825-6711 Ext. 2220
Fax 819 825-7909
www.csssvo.qc.ca

VAUDREUIL-DORION

CSSS DE VAUDREUIL -SOULANGES
490 boul Harwood
Vaudreuil-Dorion QC J7V 7H4
Tel. 450 445-6171 Ext. 134
Fax 450 455-9086
www.cldvs.com

VICTORIAVILLE

HOTEL-DIEU D'ARTHABASKA
5 rue des Hospitalieres
Victoriaville QC G6P 6N2
Tel. 819 357-2030
Fax 819 357-7406
www.csssae.qc.ca

VILLE-MARIE

CSSS DU TÉMISCAMINGUE
22 rue Notre-Dame N
Ville-Marie QC J9V 1W8
Tel. 819 629-2773
Fax 819 629-3257
www.cssst.qc.ca

WAKEFIELD

CENTRE HOSPITALIER GATINEAU MÉMORIAL
101 ch Burnside
PO Box 160
Wakefield QC J0X 3G0
Tel. 819 459-1112
Fax 819 459-3947
www.santedescollines.qc.ca

WASKAGANISH

WASKAGANISH COMMUNITY CLINIC
PO Box 493
Waskaganish QC J0M 1R0
Tel. 819 895-8833
Fax 819 895-8871

WASWANIPI

WASWANIPI COMMUNITY CLINIC
1 Chief Louis R. Gull St
Waswanipi QC J0Y 3C0
Tel. 819 753-2587
Fax 819 753-2555
www.waswanipi.com

WATERLOO

CHSLD HORACE-BOIVIN -CENTRE WATERLOO
5300 av Courville
CP 1230
Waterloo QC J0E 2N0
Tel. 514 539-5512
Fax 514 539-1830

WEEDON

CSSS DU HAUT -SAINT-FRANÇOIS
460 2E Avenue
Weedon QC J0B 3J0
Tel. 819 877-3434
Fax 819 877-3714
www.wpp01.msss.gouv.qc.ca

WINDSOR

CSSS DU VAL -SAINT-FRANÇOIS
79 rue Allen
Windsor QC J1S 2P8
Tel. 819 542-2777
Fax 819 845-5521
www.csssvsf.com

SASKATCHEWAN

ARBORFIELD

ARBORFIELD & DISTRICT HEALTH CARE CENTRE
5th Ave
Box 160
Arborfield SK S0E 0A0
Tel. 306 769-8757
Fax 306 769-8759
www.kelseytrailhealth.ca

ARCOLA

ARCOLA HEALTH CENTRE
607 Prairie Ave
PO Box 419
Arcola SK S0C 0G0
Tel. 306 455-2771
Fax 306 455-2397
www.suncountry.sk.ca

RADVILLE MARIAN HEALTH CENTRE
217 Warren St
Box 310
Arcola SK S0C 0G0
Tel. 306 869-2224
Fax 306 869-2653
www.suncountry.sk.ca

ASSINIBOIA

ASSINIBOIA UNION HOSPITAL
509 6th Ave E
PO Box 1120
Assiniboia SK S0H 0B0
Tel. 306 642-3351
Fax 306 642-3804
www.fhhr.ca

BALCARRES

BALCARRES INTEGRATED CARE CENTRE
100 South Elgin
PO Box 340
Balcarres SK S0G 0C0
Tel. 306 334-6260
Fax 306 334-2674
www.rqhealth.ca

STAR BLANKET HEALTH CENTRE
Box 456
Balcarres SK S0G 0C0
Tel. 306 334-2206
Fax 306 334-2606

BEAUVAL

BEAUVAL HEALTH CENTRE
PO Box 68
Beauval SK S0M 0G0
Tel. 306 288-4800
Fax 306 288-2225
www.ehealth-north.sk.ca

BEECHY

BEECHY HEALTH CENTRE
226 1st Ave N
Beechy SK S0L 0C0
Tel. 306 859-2118
Fax 306 859-2206
www.hrha.sk.ca

BENGOUGH

BENGOUGH HEALTH CENTRE
PO Box 429
Bengough SK S0C 0K0
Tel. 306 268-2840
Fax 306 268-4339
www.suncountry.sk.ca

BIG RIVER

ANGELIQUE CANADA HEALTH CENTRE
PO Box 380
Pelican Narrows SK S0J 0E0
Tel. 306 632-2046
Fax 306 632-4502
www.ehealth-north.sk.ca

BIG RIVER HEALTH CENTRE
220 1st Ave N
PO Box 100
Big River SK S0J 0E0
Tel. 306 469-2220
Fax 306 469-2193
www.ehealth-north.sk.ca

BIGGAR

BIGGAR HOSPITAL
501 1st Ave W
PO Box 130
Biggar SK S0K 0M0
Tel. 306 948-3323
Fax 306 948-2011
www.hrha.sk.ca

BIRCH HILLS

BIRCH HILLS HEALTH CENTRE
3 Wilson St
Birch Hills SK S0J 0G0
Tel. 306 749-3331
Fax 306 749-2440
www.paphr.sk.ca

BLACK LAKE

ATHABASCA HEALTH FACILITY
224 Chicken Indian Reserve
PO Box 124
Black Lake SK S0J 0H0
Tel. 306 439-2200
Fax 306 439-2211
www.ehealth-north.sk.ca

BLACK LAKE NURSING STATION
Gen Del
PO Box 135
Black Lake SK S0J 0H0
Tel. 306 284-2020
Fax 306 284-2090
www.athabascahealth.ca

BROADVIEW

BROADVIEW UNION HOSPITAL
901 Nina St
Box 100
Broadview SK S0G 0K0
Tel. 306 696-2441
Fax 306 696-2611
www.rqhealth.ca

KAHKEWISTAHAW HEALTH CENTRE
PO Box 850
Broadview SK S0G 0K0
Tel. 306 696-2660
Fax 306 696-3154

BUFFALO NARROWS

BUFFALO NARROWS HEALTH CENTRE
PO Box 40
Buffalo Narrows SK S0M 0J0
Tel. 306 235-5800
Fax 306 235-4500
www.kyrha.ca

CABRI

PRAIRIE HEALTH CARE CENTRE
517 1st St N
PO Box 79
Cabri SK S0N 0J0
Tel. 306 587-2623
Fax 306 587-2751
www.cypresshealth.ca

CANOE NARROWS

CANOE LAKE HEALTH CENTRE
PO Box 229
Canoe Narrows SK S0M 0K0
Tel. 306 829-2140
Fax 306 829-4312
www.ehealth-north.sk.ca

CANORA

CANORA HOSPITAL
1219 Main St
PO Box 749
Canora SK S0A 0L0
Tel. 306 563-5621
Fax 306 563-1257
www.sunrisehealthregion.sk.ca

CARLYLE

CARLYLE COMMUNITY HEALTH CENTRE
206 Railway Ave E
Carlyle SK S0C 0R0
Tel. 306 453-6131
Fax 306 453-6799
www.suncountry.sk.ca

WHITE BEAR HEALTH CENTRE
PO Box 700
c/o Band Office
Carlyle SK S0C 0R0
Tel. 306 577-4482
Fax 306 577-4888

CARROT RIVER

CARROT RIVER HEALTH CENTRE
4101 1st Ave W
PO Box 250
Carrot River SK S0E 0L0
Tel. 306 768-3100
Fax 306 768-3233
www.kelseytrailhealth.ca

CENTRAL BUTTE

CENTRAL BUTTE REGENCY HOSPITAL
601 Canada St
PO Box 40
Central Butte SK S0H 0T0
Tel. 306 796-2190
Fax 306 796-4610
www.fhhr.ca

CHRISTOPHER LAKE

LITTLE RED RIVER HEALTH CENTRE
PO Box 330
Christopher Lake SK S0J 0N0
Tel. 306 982-4294
Fax 306 982-3672
www.ehealth-north.sk.ca

CLEARWATER RIVER

CLEARWATER HEALTH CENTRE
PO Box 5040
Clearwater River SK S0M 3H0
Tel. 306 822-2378
Fax 306 822-2297

CLIMAX

BORDER HEALTH CENTRE
301 1st St W
PO Box 60
Climax SK S0N 0N0
Tel. 306 293-2222
Fax 306 293-2860
www.cypresshealth.ca

CORONACH

CORONACH HEALTH CENTRE
240 South Ave E
PO Box 150
Coronach SK S0H 0Z0
Tel. 306 267-2022
Fax 306 267-2324
www.suncountry.sk.ca

COWESSESS

COWESSESS HEALTH CENTRE
PO Box 100
Cowessess SK S0G 5L0
Tel. 306 696-2263
Fax 306 696-2374

CRAIK

CRAIK & DISTRICT HEALTH CENTRE
620 Mary St
PO Box 208
Craik SK S0G 0V0
Tel. 306 734-2288
Fax 306 734-2248
www.fhhr.ca

CREIGHTON

CREIGHTON HEALTH CENTRE
298 1st St E of Creighton
PO Box 219
Creighton SK S0P 0A0
Tel. 306 688-8620
Fax 306 688-8629
www.mcrrha.sk.ca

HOSPITALS & HEALTH CENTRES

CUMBERLAND HOUSE

CUMBERLAND HOUSE HEALTH CENTRE
2nd Ave
PO Box 8
Cumberland House SK S0E 0S0
Tel. 306 888-2244
Fax 306 884-2269
www.kelseytrailhealth.ca

CUPAR

CUPAR HEALTH CENTRE
PO BOX 100
Cupar SK S0G 0Y0
Tel. 306 723-4300
Fax 306 723-4416
www.rqhealth.ca

CUT KNIFE

CUT KNIFE HEALTH COMPLEX
102 Dion Ave
PO Box 220
Cut Knife SK S0M 0N0
Tel. 306 398-4718
Fax 306 398-2206
www.pnrha.ca

DAVIDSON

DAVIDSON HEALTH CENTRE
900 Government Rd
PO Box 758
Davidson SK S0G 1A0
Tel. 306 567-2801
Fax 306 567-2073
www.hrha.sk.ca

DEBDEN

BIG RIVER HEALTH CENTRE DEBDEN
PO Box 160
Debden SK S0J 0S0
Tel. 306 724-4664
Fax 306 724-4555

DELISLE

DELISLE PRIMARY HEALTH CENTRE
305 First St W
PO Box 119
Delisle SK S0L 0P0
Tel. 306 493-2810
Fax 306 493-2812
www.saskatoonhealthregion.ca

DESCHAMBAULT LAKE

DESCHAMBAULT LAKE NURSING STATION
Gen Del
Deschambault Lake
SK S0P 0C0
Tel. 306 632-2106
Fax 306 632-4555
www.mcrrha.sk.ca

DILLON

BUFFALO RIVER FIRST HEALTH CENTRE
Gen Del
Dillon SK S0M 0S0
Tel. 306 282-2011
Fax 360 282-2132
www.kyrha.ca

DINSMORE

DINSMORE HEALTH CARE CENTRE
207 1st St E
PO Box 219
Dinsmore SK S0L 0T0
Tel. 306 846-2222
Fax 306 846-2225
www.hrha.sk.ca

DUCK LAKE

BEARDY'S & OKEMASIS HEALTH CENTRE
PO Box 96
Duck Lake SK S0K 1J0
Tel. 306 467-4402
Fax 306 467-4404
www.beardysband.net

EASTEND

WOLF WILLOW HEALTH CENTRE
555 Red Coat D
PO Box 490
Eastend SK S0N 0T0
Tel. 306 295-3534
www.cypresshealth.ca

EATONIA

EATONIA HEALTH CARE CENTRE INC.
205 2nd Ave W
PO Box 400
Eatonia SK S0L 0Y0
Tel. 306 967-2591
Fax 306 967-2373

EDAM

LADY MINTO HEALTH CARE CENTER
1513 1st Ave S
PO BOX 330
Edam SK S0M 0V0
Tel. 306 397-5560
Fax 306 397-2225
www.pnrha.ca

ELROSE

ELROSE HEALTH CENTRE
505 Main St
Box 100
Elrose SK S0L 0Z0
Tel. 306 378-2882
Fax 306 378-2812
www.hrha.sk.ca

ESTERHAZY

ST ANTHONY'S HOSPITAL
216 Ancona St
PO Box 280
Esterhazy SK S0A 0X0
Tel. 306 745-3973
Fax 306 745-3245
www.sunrisehealthregion.sk.ca

ESTEVAN

ST JOSEPH'S HOSPITAL
1174 Nicholson Rd
PO Box 5000
Estevan SK S4A 2V6
Tel. 306 637-2400
Fax 306 637-2490
www.stjosephsestevan.ca

ESTON

ESTON HEALTH CENTRE
822 Main St
PO Box 667
Eston SK S0L 1A0
Tel. 306 962-3215
Fax 306 962-3900
www.hrha.sk.ca

FILLMORE

FILLMORE UNION HEALTH CENTRE
100 Main St
PO Box 246
Fillmore SK S0G 1N0
Tel. 306 722-3331
Fax 306 722-3877
www.suncountry.sk.ca

FOAM LAKE

FOAM LAKE HEALTH CENTRE
715 Saskatchewan Ave E
PO Box 190
Foam Lake SK S0A 1A0
Tel. 306 272-3325
Fax 306 272-4449
www.sunrisehealthregion.sk.ca

FOND DU LAC

FOND DU LAC DENESULINE HEALTH CENTRE/NURSING STATION
PO Box 213
Fond du Lac SK S0J 0W0
Tel. 306 686-2003
Fax 306 686-2114
www.ehealth-north.sk.ca

FORT QU'APPELLE

ALL NATIONS HEALING HOSPITAL
450 Eight St
PO Box 300
Fort Qu'Appelle SK S0G 1S0
Tel. 306 332-5611
Fax 306 332-5033
www.fortquappelle.com

FORT QU'APPELLE COMMUNITY HEALTH SERVICES CENTRE
178 Boundary Ave N
Fort Qu'Appelle SK S0G 1S0
Tel. 306 332-3300
www.rqhealth.ca

MUSCOWPETUNG HEALTH CENTRE
Box 1310
Fort Qu'Appelle SK S0G 1S0
Tel. 306 723-4747
Fax 306 723-4509

PASQUA HEALTH CENTRE
PO Box 50
Fort Qu'Appelle SK S0G 5M0
Tel. 306 332-3763
Fax 306 332-3766

STANDING BUFFALO HEALTH CENTRE
PO Box 818
Fort Qu'Appelle SK S0G 1S0
Tel. 306 332-4681
Fax 306 332-4945

GAINSBOROUGH

GAINSBOROUGH & AREA HEALTH CENTRE
312 Stephens St
PO Box 420
Gainsborough SK S0C 0Z0
Tel. 306 685-2277
Fax 306 685-4636
www.suncountry.sk.ca

GOODSOIL

L GERVAIS MEMORIAL HEALTH CENTRE
First Ave N
PO Box 100
Goodsoil SK S0M 1A0
Tel. 306 238-2100
Fax 306 238-4449
www.pnrha.ca

GRASSWOOD

STUDENT HEALTH SERVICES
1 Campus Dr
4th Fl Place Riel Student Ctre
Grasswood SK S7N 5A3
Tel. 306 966-5768
Fax 306 966-5786

GRAVELBOURG

ST JOSEPH'S HOSPITAL /FOYER D'YOUVILLE
Box 810
Gravelbourg SK S0H 1X0
Tel. 306 648-3185
Fax 306 648-3440
www.stjosephsgbourg.com.

GREEN LAKE

GREEN LAKE HEALTH CENTRE
PO Box 29
Green Lake SK S0M 1B0
Tel. 306 832-6257
www.ehealth-north.sk.ca

GRENFELL

GRENFELL HEALTH CENTRE
721 Stella St
PO Box 243
Grenfell SK S0G 2B0
Tel. 306 697-2853
Fax 306 697-3459
www.rqhealth.ca

SAKIMAY HEALTH CENTRE
PO Box 339
Grenfell SK S0G 2B0
Tel. 306 697-2970
Fax 306 697-3461

GULL LAKE

GULL LAKE SPECIAL CARE CENTRE
751 Grey St
Gull Lake SK S0N 1A0
Tel. 306 672-4700
www.cypresshealth.ca

HAFFORD

HAFFORD HOSPITAL & SPECIAL CARE CENTRE
213 South Ave E
PO Box 130
Hafford SK S0J 1A0
Tel. 306 549-2108
Fax 306 549-4660
www.paphr.sk.ca

HERBERT

HERBERT AND DISTRICT INTEGRATED HEALTH FACILITY
405 Herbert Ave
PO Box 520
Herbert SK S0H 2A0
Tel. 306 784-2466
Fax 306 784-2449
www.cypresshealth.ca

HODGEVILLE

HODGEVILLE HEALTH CENTRE
105 Main St
Box 332
Hodgeville SK S0H 2B0
Tel. 306 677-2292
Fax 306 677-2584
www.cypresshealth.ca

HOSPITALS & HEALTH CENTRES

HUDSON BAY

HUDSON BAY HEALTH CARE FACILITY
614 Prince St
PO Box 940
Hudson Bay SK S0E 0Y0
Tel. 306 865-2219
Fax 306 865-2429
www.kelseytrailhealth.ca

HUMBOLDT

HUMBOLDT DISTRICT HOSPITAL
515 14th Ave
PO Box 10
Humboldt SK S0K 2A0
Tel. 306 682-2603
Fax 306 682-4046
www.saskatoonhealthregion.ca

ÎLE-À-LA-CROSSE

ST JOSEPH'S HOSPITAL
PO Bag 500
Ile-A-La-Crosse SK S0M 1C0
Tel. 306 833-2016
Fax 306 833-2556
www.kyrha.ca

IMPERIAL

LONG LAKE VALLEY INTEGRATED FACILITY
125 Prince St
PO Box 180
Imperial SK S0G 2J0
Tel. 306 963-2210
Fax 306 963-2518
www.rqhealth.ca

INDIAN HEAD

INDIAN HEAD HOSPITAL
300 Hospital St
PO Box 340
Indian Head SK S0G 2K0
Tel. 306 695-2272
Fax 306 695-2525
www.rqhealth.ca

INVERMAY

INVERMAY HEALTH CENTRE
303 Fourth Ave N
PO Box 160
Invermay SK S0A 1M0
Tel. 306 593-2133
Fax 306 593-4566
www.sunrisehealthregion.sk.ca

ISLAND LAKE

MINISTIKWAN HEALTH CENTRE
PO Box 162
Island Lake SK S0M 3G0
Tel. 306 837-2265
Fax 306 837-4480

ITUNA

ITUNA PIONEER HEALTH CARE CENTRE
320 Fifth Ave NE
Ituna SK S0A 1N0
Tel. 306 795-2471
Fax 306 795-3592
www.sunrisehealthregion.sk.ca

KAMSACK

COTE HEALTH CENTRE
PO Box 1776
Kamsack SK S0A 1S0
Tel. 306 542-4074
Fax 306 542-3532

KAMSACK HOSPITAL & NURSING HOME
341 Stewart St
PO Box 429
Kamsack SK S0A 1S0
Tel. 306 542-2635
Fax 306 542-4360
www.sunrisehealthregion.sk.ca

KELVINGTON

KELVINGTON HOSPITAL
512 1st Ave S
PO Box 70
Kelvington SK S0A 1W0
Tel. 306 327-4711
Fax 306 327-5115
www.kelseytrailhealth.ca

KERROBERT

KERROBERT HEALTH CENTRE
635 Alberta Ave
PO Box 320
Kerrobert SK S0L 1R0
Tel. 306 834-2646
Fax 306 834-1007
www.hrha.sk.ca

KINCAID

KINCAID WELLNESS CENTRE
PO Box 179
Kincaid SK S0H 2J0
Tel. 306 264-3233
Fax 306 264-3878
www.fhhr.ca

KINDERSLEY

KINDERSLEY & DISTRICT HEALTH CENTRE
1003 1st St W
Kindersley SK S0L 1S2
Tel. 306 463-2611
Fax 306 463-4577
www.hrha.sk.ca

KINISTINO

JAMES SMITH HEALTH CENTRE
Box 506
Kinistino SK S0J 1H0
Tel. 306 864-2454
Fax 306 864-2536
www.ehealth-north.sk.ca

KINISTINO JUBILEE LODGE
401 Myers Ave
PO Box 370
Kinistino SK S0J 1H0
Tel. 306 864-2851
Fax 306 864-2440

KIPLING

KIPLING COMMUNITY HEALTH CENTRE
602 Main St
PO Box 480
Kipling SK S0G 2S0
Tel. 306 736-2522
Fax 306 736-2300
www.suncountry.sk.ca

KIPLING MEMORIAL HEALTH CENTRE
803 First St
PO Box 420
Kipling SK S0G 2S0
Tel. 306 736-2553
Fax 306 736-8407
www.suncountry.sk.ca

KISBEY

PHEASANT RUMP HEALTH CENTRE
PO Box 158
Kisbey SK S0C 1L0
Tel. 306 462-4808
Fax 306 462-2003

KYLE

KYLE AND DISTRICT HEALTH CENTRE
208 3rd Ave E
PO Box 70
Kyle SK S0L 1T0
Tel. 306 375-2251
Fax 306 375-2422

KYLEMORE

FISHING LAKE HEALTH CENTRE
Box 9
Kylemore SK S0A 1Z0
Tel. 306 338-2680
Fax 306 338-3988

LA LOCHE

LA LOCHE HEALTH CENTRE AND HOSPITAL
Bag Service 1
La Loche SK S0M 1G0
Tel. 306 822-2221
Fax 306 822-2112
www.kyrha.ca

LA RONGE

LA RONGE HEALTH CENTRE
227 Backlund St
PO Box 6000
La Ronge SK S0J 1L0
Tel. 306 425-2422
Fax 306 425-3298
www.mcrrha.sk.ca

LAC LA RONGE HEALTH SERVICES
PO Box 1770
La Ronge SK S0J 1L0
Tel. 306 425-3600
Fax 306 425-5520

NEMEIBAN RIVER HEALTH CENTRE
PO Box 1770
La Ronge SK S0J 1L0
Tel. 306 425-5590
Fax 306 425-3153

LAFLECHE

LAFLECHE & DISTRICT HEALTH CENTRE
315 Main St
PO Box 159
Lafleche SK S0H 2K0
Tel. 306 472-5230
Fax 306 472-5405
www.fhhr.ca

LAMPMAN

LAMPMAN COMMUNITY HEALTH CENTRE
309 Second Ave E
PO Box 100
Lampman SK S0C 1N0
Tel. 306 487-2561
Fax 306 487-3103
lampman.sasktelwebsite.net

LANGENBURG

LANGENBURG HEALTH CARE COMPLEX
200 Heritage Dr
PO Box 370
Langenburg SK S0A 2A0
Tel. 306 743-2661
Fax 306 743-5025
www.sunrisehealthregion.sk.ca

LANIGAN

LANIGAN HOSPITAL
36 Downing St E
PO Box 609
Lanigan SK S0K 2M0
Tel. 306 365-1400
Fax 306 365-3354
www.saskatoonhealthregion.ca

LEADER

LEADER HOSPITAL
423 Main St E
PO Box 129
Leader SK S0N 1H0
Tel. 306 628-3845
Fax 306 628-4413
www.cypresshealth.ca

LEASK

MISTAWASIS HEALTH CENTRE
PO Box 148
Leask SK S0J 1M0
Tel. 306 466-4507
Fax 306 466-2220
www.ehealth-north.sk.ca

LEOVILLE

EVERGREEN HEALTH CENTRE
238 Second St
PO Box 160
Leoville SK S0J 1N0
Tel. 306 984-2136
Fax 306 984-2046
www.ehealth-north.sk.ca

PELICAN LAKE (CHITEK) HEALTH CENTRE
GD
PO Box 361
Leoville SK S0J 1N0
Tel. 306 984-4716
Fax 306 984-4728
www.ehealth-north.sk.ca

LEROY

LEROY COMMUNITY HEALTH & SOCIAL CENTRE
211 1st Ave N E
Leroy SK S0K 2P0
Tel. 306 286-3347
Fax 306 286-3888
www.saskatoonhealthregion.ca

LESTOCK

MUSKOWEKWAN HEALTH CENTRE
PO Box 59
Lestock SK S0A 2G0
Tel. 306 274-4640
Fax 306 274-2644

ST JOSEPH'S INTEGRATED CARE CENTRE
508 Westmoore St
PO Box 280
Lestock SK S0A 2G0
Tel. 306 274-2215
Fax 306 274-2045
www.rqhealth.ca

LLOYDMINSTER

LLOYDMINSTER & DISTRICT COMMUNITY HEALTH CENTRE
4806 50th St
PO Box 530
Lloydminster SK S9V 0M8
Tel. 306 825-4427
Fax 306 825-2028
www.pnrha.ca

LLOYDMINSTER HOSPITAL
3820 43 Ave
Lloydminster SK S9V 1Y5
Tel. 306 820-6000
Fax 306 825-6516
www.pnrha.ca

LOON LAKE

LOON LAKE HOSPITAL & SPECIAL CARE HOME
510 2nd Ave
PO Box 69
Loon Lake SK S0M 1L0
Tel. 306 837-2114
Fax 306 837-2268
www.pnrha.ca

MAKWA SAHGAIEHCAN FIRST NATION HEALTH CENTRE
PO Box 559
Loon Lake SK S0M 1L0
Tel. 306 837-2208
Fax 306 837-4469
www.ehealth-north.sk.ca

LUCKY LAKE

LUCKY LAKE HEALTH CENTRE
1st Ave
Box 250
Lucky Lake SK S0L 1Z0
Tel. 306 858-2133
Fax 306 858-2312
www.hrha.sk.ca

MACKLIN

ST JOSEPH'S HEALTH CENTRE
Hwy 31 N
PO Box 190
Macklin SK S0L 2C0
Tel. 306 753-2115
Fax 306 753-2181
www.hrha.sk.ca

MAIDSTONE

MAIDSTONE HEALTH COMPLEX
214 Fifth Ave E
PO Box 160
Maidstone SK S0M 1M0
Tel. 306 893-2622
Fax 306 893-2922
www.pnrha.ca

MANKOTA

PRAIRIE VIEW HEALTH CENTRE
241 1st Ave
PO Box 390
Mankota SK S0H 2W0
Tel. 306 478-2200
Fax 306 478-2462
www.cypresshealth.ca

MAPLE CREEK

MAPLE CREEK HOSPITAL
575 Hwy 21 S
PO Box 1330
Maple Creek SK S0N 1N0
Tel. 306 662-2611
Fax 306 662-2307
www.cypresshealth.ca

MARCELIN

MUSKEG LAKE HEALTH STATION
PO Box 224
Marcelin SK S0J 1R0
Tel. 306 466-4914
Fax 306 466-4919
www.ehealth-north.sk.ca

MARYFIELD

MARYFIELD HEALTH CENTRE
PO Box 164
Maryfield SK S0G 3K0
Tel. 306 646-2133
Fax 306 646-2088
www.suncountry.sk.ca

MCMAHON

NEKANEET HEALTH STATION
PO Box 1252
McMahon SK S0N 1M0
Tel. 306 662-5022
Fax 306 662-5088

MEADOW LAKE

FLYING DUST FIRST NATION HEALTH CENTRE
8001 Flying Dust Reserve
Meadow Lake SK S9X 1T8
Tel. 306 236-8670
Fax 306 236-2835
www.ehealth-north.sk.ca

MEADOW LAKE HOSPITAL
7-711 Centre St
Meadow Lake SK S9X 1E6
Tel. 306 236-1500
Fax 306 236-3215
www.pnrha.ca

MELFORT

MELFORT HOSPITAL
510 Broadway Ave N
PO Box 1480
Melfort SK S0E 1A0
Tel. 306 752-8700
Fax 306 752-8711
www.kelseytrailhealth.ca

MELVILLE

ST PETER'S HOSPITAL
200 Heritage Dr
PO Box 1810
Melville SK S0A 2P0
Tel. 306 728-5407
Fax 306 728-4870
www.sunrisehealthregion.sk.ca

MONTMARTRE

MONTMARTRE HEALTH CENTRE
237 2nd Ave E
Box 206
Monmartre SK S0G 3M0
Tel. 306 424-2222
Fax 306 424-2227
www.rqhealth.ca

MONTREAL LAKE

MONTREAL LAKE HEALTH CENTRE
Gen Del
Montreal Lake SK S0J 1Y0
Tel. 306 663-5995
Fax 306 663-5986

MOOSE JAW

MOOSE JAW UNION HOSPITAL
455 Fairford St E
Moose Jaw SK S6H 1H3
Tel. 306 694-0200
Fax 306 692-5596
www.fhhr.ca

MOOSOMIN

SOUTHEAST INTEGRATED CARE CENTRE - MOOSOMIN
601 Wright Rd
PO Box 1
Moosomin SK S0G 3N0
Tel. 306 435-3303
Fax 306 435-3211
www.rqhealth.ca

MOSSBANK

MOSSBANK HEALTH CENTRE
Box 322
Mossbank SK S0H 3G0
Tel. 306 354-2300
Fax 306 354-2819
www.fhhr.ca

NEILBURG

MANITOU HEALTH CENTRE
105 2nd Ave W
PO Box 190
Neilburg SK S0M 2C0
Tel. 306 823-4262
Fax 306 823-4590
www.pnrha.ca

NIPAWIN

NIPAWIN HOSPITAL
800 6th St E
PO Box 389
Nipawin SK S0E 1E0
Tel. 306 862-4643
Fax 306 862-9310
www.kelseytrailhealth.ca

NIPAWIN PUBLIC HEALTH OFFICE
210 2nd St W
Nipawin SK S0E 1E0
Tel. 306 862-0761
Fax 306 862-0763
www.ehealth-north.sk.ca

NORQUAY

KEY HEALTH CENTRE
PO Box 368
Norquay SK S0A 2V0
Tel. 306 594-2291
Fax 306 594-2168

NORQUAY HEALTH CENTRE
355 East Rd Allowance
PO Box 190
Norquay SK S0A 2V0
Tel. 306 594-2133
Fax 306 594-2488
www.sunrisehealthregion.sk.ca

NORTH BATTLEFORD

BATTLEFORDS UNION HOSPITAL
1092 107th St
North Battleford SK S9A 1Z1
Tel. 306 446-6600
Fax 306 937-2258
www.pnrha.ca

BTC INDIAN HEALTH SERVICES
1192 101St St
North Battleford SK S9A 0Z6
Tel. 306 937-6700
Fax 306 445-8355
www.firstnation.ca

SASKATCHEWAN HOSPITAL - NORTH BATTLEFORD
1 Jersey St
PO Box 39 Stn Main
North Battleford SK S9A 2X8
Tel. 306 446-6800
Fax 306 445-5392
www.pnrha.ca

SWEETGRASS HEALTH CENTRE
PO Box 1658
North Battleford SK S9A 3W2
Tel. 306 937-6770
Fax 306 937-3630

ONION LAKE

ONION LAKE HEALTH CENTRE
PO Box 70
Onion Lake SK S0M 2E0
Tel. 306 344-2330
Fax 306 344-4762
www.pnrha.ca

OUTLOOK

OUTLOOK HEALTH CENTRE
500 Semple St
PO Box 369
Outlook SK S0L 2N0
Tel. 306 867-8676
Fax 306 867-9449
www.hrha.sk.ca

OXBOW

GALLOWAY HEALTH CENTRE
917 Tupper St
PO Box 268
Oxbow SK S0C 2B0
Tel. 306 483-2956
Fax 306 483-5178
www.suncountry.sk.ca

PAKWAW LAKE

SHOAL LAKE HEALTH CENTRE
PO Box 55
Pakwaw Lake SK S0E 1G0
Tel. 306 768-3457
Fax 306 768-2950
www.kelseytrailhealth. Ca

PANGMAN

PANGMAN HEALTH CENTRE
211 Keeler St
PO Box 90
Pangman SK S0C 2C0
Tel. 306 442-2044
Fax 306 442-4227
www.suncountry.sk.ca

PARADISE HILL

PARADISE HILL HEALTH CENTRE
1st Ave
PO Box 179
Paradise Hill SK S0M 2G0
Tel. 306 344-2255
Fax 306 344-2277
www.pnrha.ca

PATUANAK

ENGLISH RIVER HEALTH CENTRE
Gen Del
PO Box 60
Patuanak SK S0M 2H0
Tel. 306 396-2072
Fax 306 396-2177
www.ehealth-north.sk.ca

PIERCELAND

BIG ISLAND CREE NATION HEALTH CENTRE
PO Box 508
Pierceland SK S0M 2K0
Tel. 306 839-2330
Fax 306 839-4556
www.ehealth-north.sk.ca

PINEHOUSE LAKE

PINEHOUSE HEALTH CENTRE
PO Box 70
Pinehouse Lake SK S0J 2B0
Tel. 306 884-5670
Fax 306 884-5699
www.mcrrha.sk.ca

PONTEIX

PONTEIX HEALTH CENTRE
428 2nd Ave
PO Box 600
Ponteix SK S0N 1Z0
Tel. 306 625-3382
Fax 306 625-3764

PORCUPINE PLAIN

PORCUPINE CARRAGANA HOSPITAL
Windsor Ave
PO Box 70
Porcupine Plain SK S0E 1H0
Tel. 306 278-2211
Fax 306 278-3088
www.kelseytrailhealth.ca

PREECEVILLE

PREECEVILLE & DISTRICT HEALTH CENTRE
712 7th St NE
PO Box 469
Preeceville SK S0A 3B0
Tel. 306 547-2102
Fax 306 547-2223
www.sunrisehealthregion.sk.ca

PRINCE ALBERT

MENTAL HEALTH SERVICES
2345 10th Ave
PO Box 3003
Prince Albert SK S6V 6G1
Tel. 306 765-6055
Fax 306 765-6349
www.ehealth-north.sk.ca

PRINCE ALBERT CO -OPERATIVE HEALTH CENTRE
110 8th St E
Prince Albert SK S6V 0V7
Tel. 306 763-6464
Fax 306 763-2101
www.coophealth.com

VICTORIA HOSPITAL
1200 24th St W
PO Box 3000 Stn Main
Prince Albert SK S6V 5T4
Tel. 306 765-6000
Fax 306 763-2871
www.paphr.sk.ca

WAHPETON HEALTH CENTRE
PO Box 128
Prince Albert SK S6V 5R4
Tel. 306 922-6772
Fax 306 922-6774
www.ehealth-north.sk.ca

PUNNICHY

DAY STAR HEALTH CENTRE
PO Box 277
Punnichy SK S0A 3C0
Tel. 306 835-2883
Fax 306 835-2724

GORDON HEALTH CENTRE
PO Box 416
Punnichy SK S0A 3C0
Tel. 306 835-2020
Fax 306 835-2142

QUILL LAKE

QUILL LAKE COMMUNITY HEALTH & SOCIAL CENTRE
PO Box 126
Quill Lake SK S0A 3E0
Tel. 306 383-2266
Fax 306 383-2255
www.saskatoonhealthregion.ca

RAYMORE

KAWACATOOSE HEALTH CENTRE
PO Box 384
Raymore SK S0A 3J0
Tel. 306 835-2720
Fax 306 835-2630

RAYMORE COMMUNITY HEALTH & SOCIAL CENTRE
806 2nd Ave
Box 134
Raymore SK S0A 3J0
Tel. 306 746-2231
Fax 306 746-4639
www.rqhealth.ca

RED EARTH

RED EARTH HEALTH CENTRE
PO Box 106
Red Earth SK S0E 1K0
Tel. 306 768-3617
Fax 306 768-3440
www.kelseytrailhealth.ca

REDVERS

REDVERS HEALTH CENTRE
18 Eichorst St
PO Box 30
Redvers SK S0C 2H0
Tel. 306 452-3553
Fax 306 452-3556
www.suncountry.sk.ca

REGINA

AL RITCHIE HEALTH ACTION CENTRE
325 Victoria Ave
Regina SK S4N 0P5
Tel. 306 766-7660
www.rqhealth.ca

FOUR DIRECTIONS COMMUNITY HEALTH CENTRE
3510 5th Aves4
Regina SK S4T 0M2
www.rqhealth.ca

PASQUA HOSPITAL
4101 Dewdney Ave
Regina SK S4T 1A5
Tel. 306 766-2222
www.rqhealth.ca

REGINA GENERAL HOSPITAL
1440 14th Ave
Regina SK S4P 0W5
Tel. 306 766-4444
Fax 306 766-5414
www.rqhealth.ca

SASKATCHEWAN CANCER AGENCY
400-2631 28th Ave
Regina SK S4S 6X3
Tel. 306 585-1831
Fax 306 584-2733
www.saskcancer.ca

WASCANA REHABILITATION CENTRE
2180 23rd Ave
Regina SK S4S 0A5
Tel. 306 766-5100
www.rqhealth.ca

ROCKGLEN

GRASSLANDS HEALTH CENTRE
Gen Del
Rockglen SK S0H 3R0
Tel. 306 476-2030
www.fhhr.ca

ROSE VALLEY

ROSE VALLEY & DISTRICT HEALTH CENTRE
119 McCallum St
PO Box 310
Rose Valley SK S0E 1M0
Tel. 306 322-2115
Fax 306 322-2037
www.kelseytrailhealth.ca

ROSETOWN

ROSETOWN & DISTRICT HEALTH CENTRE
409 Hwy 4 North
PO Box 850
Rosetown SK S0L 2V0
Tel. 306 882-2672
Fax 306 882-3335
www.hrha.sk.ca

ROSTHERN

ROSTHERN HOSPITAL
2016 2nd St
PO Box 309
Rosthern SK S0K 3R0
Tel. 306 232-4811
Fax 306 232-4887
www.saskatoonhealthregion.ca

ST. ISIDORE DE BELLEVUE

ONE ARROW HEALTH CENTRE
PO Box 147
St-Isidore-Bllevue SK S0K 3Y0
Tel. 306 423-5493
Fax 306 423-5441

ST WALBURG

ST WALBURG HEALTH COMPLEX
410 3rd Ave W
Box 339
St Walburg SK S0M 2T0
Tel. 306 248-6719
Fax 306 248-3413
www.pnrha.ca

SANDY BAY

SANDY BAY HEALTH CENTRE
PO Box 210
Sandy Bay SK S0P 0G0
Tel. 306 754-5400
Fax 306 754-5429
www.mcrrha.sk.ca

SASKATOON

NUTANA COLLEGIATE HEALTH CENTRE
411 11th St E
Saskatoon SK S7N 0E9
Tel. 306 655-4565
Fax 306 655-3951
www.saskatoonhealthregion.ca

PRIMARY HEALTH CENTRE SOUTH EAST
100-2501 Louise St
Scott-Forget Towers
Saskatoon SK S7J 3M1
Tel. 306 655-4552
Fax 306 655-4555
www.saskatoonhealthregion.ca

REGIONAL PSYCHIATRIC CENTRE - PRAIRIES
2520 Central Ave N
PO Box 9243 Stn Main
Saskatoon SK S7K 3X5
Tel. 306 975-5400
Fax 306 975-6024

ROYAL UNIVERSITY HOSPITAL
103 Hospital Dr
Saskatoon SK S7N 0W8
Tel. 306 655-1000
Fax 306 655-1037
www.saskatoonhealthregion.ca

ST PAUL'S HOSPITAL (GREY NUNS) OF SASKATOON
1702 20th St W
Saskatoon SK S7M 0Z9
Tel. 306 655-5000
Fax 306 664-5555
www.saskatoonhealthregion.ca

SASKATOON CANCER CENTRE
20 Campus Dr
Saskatoon SK S7N 4H4
Tel. 306 655-2662
Fax 306 655-0935
www.saskcancer.ca

SASKATOON CITY HOSPITAL
701 Queen St
Saskatoon SK S7K 0M7
Tel. 306 655-8000
Fax 306 655-8269
www.saskatoonhealthregion.ca

WESTSIDE COMMUNITY CLINIC
1528 20th St W
Saskatoon SK S7M 0Z6
Tel. 306 644-4310
Fax 306 934-2506
saskatooncommunityclinic.ca

WHITECAP HEALTH CENTRE
182 Chief Whiltecap Trail
Saskatoon SK S7K 2L2
Tel. 306 477-0908
Fax 306 343-8855
www.saskatoonhealthregion.ca

SHAUNAVON

SHAUNAVON HOSPITAL & CARE CENTRE
660 4th St E
PO Box 789
Shaunavon SK S0N 2M0
Tel. 306 297-2644
Fax 306 297-2502
www.cypresshealth.ca

SHELLBROOK

SHELLBROOK HOSPITAL
211 Second Ave W
PO Box 70
Shellbrook SK S0J 2E0
Tel. 306 747-2603
Fax 306 747-3004
www.paphr.sk.ca

STURGEON LAKE HEALTH CENTRE
726 Education Rd
Site 12, RR1
Sturgeon Lake SK S0J 2E1
Tel. 306 764-9352
Fax 306 763-0767
www.ehealth-north.sk.ca

SINTALUTA

CARRY THE KETTLE HEALTH CENTRE
PO Box 180
Sintaluta SK S0G 4N0
Tel. 306 727-2101
Fax 306 727-2052

SMEATON

SMEATON & DISTRICT HEALTH CENTRE
2nd Ave N
PO Box 158
Smeaton SK S0J 2J0
Tel. 306 426-2051
Fax 306 426-2229
www.kelseytrailhealth.ca

SOUTHEND

ARTHUR MORIN MEMORIAL HEALTH CENTER (SOUTHEND)
PO Box 40
Southend SK S0J 2L0
Tel. 306 758-2063
Fax 306 758-2052
www.ehealth-north.sk.ca

SOUTHEY

SOUTHEY HEALTH ACTION CENTRE
280 Burns Ave
PO Box 519
Southey SK S0G 4P0
Tel. 306 726-2239
Fax 306 726-4472
www.rqhealth.ca

SPALDING

SPALDING COMMUNITY HEALTH CENTRE
12-318 2nd St S
PO Box 220
Spalding SK S0K 4C0
Tel. 306 872-2011
Fax 306 872-2186
www.saskatoonhealthregion.ca

SPIRITWOOD

SPIRITWOOD & DISTRICT HEALTH COMPLEX
400 First St E
PO Box 69
Spiritwood SK S0J 2M0
Tel. 306 883-2133
Fax 306 883-4440
www.ehealth-north.sk.ca

WITCHEKAN LAKE HEALTH CENTRE
PO Box 359
Spiritwood SK S0J 2M0
Tel. 306 883-2552
Fax 306 883-2578
www.ehealth-north.sk.ca

STANLEY MISSION

STANLEY MISSION HEALTH CENTRE
PO Box 310
Stanley Mission SK S0J 2P0
Tel. 306 635-2090
Fax 306 635-2189
www.stanleymission.com

STOUGHTON

OCEAN MAN HEALTH CENTRE
PO Box 157
Stoughton SK S0G 4T0
Tel. 306 457-4160
Fax 306 457-4163

STRASBOURG

STRASBOURG AND DISTRICT HEALTH CENTRE
303 Edward St
Box 217
Strasbourg SK S0G 4V0
Tel. 306 725-3220
Fax 306 725-4060
www.saskatoonhealthregion.ca

STURGEON LANDING

STURGEON LANDING HEALTH CENTRE
Box 2451
Sturgeon Landing SK S0P 0H0
Tel. 306 688-4510
Fax 306 688-2148
www.mcrrha.sk.ca

SWIFT CURRENT

COMMUNITY HEALTH SERVICES
350 Cheadle St W
Swift Current SK S9H 4G3
Tel. 306 778-5280
www.cypresshealth.ca

CYPRESS REGIONAL HOSPITAL
499 4th Ave NE
Swift Current SK S9H 2J9
Tel. 306 778-9400
Fax 306 778-9431
www.cypresshealth.ca

SWIFT CURRENT CARE CENTRE
700 Aberdeen St SE
Swift Current SK S9H 3E3
Tel. 306 773-9371
www.cypresshealth.ca

THEODORE

THEODORE HEALTH CENTRE
615 Anderson Av
Box 70
Theodore SK S0A 4C0
Tel. 306 647-2115
Fax 306 647-2238
www.sunrisehealthregion.sk.ca

TISDALE

TISDALE HOSPITAL
2010 10th Ave W
PO Box 1630
Tisdale SK S0E 1T0
Tel. 306 873-2621
Fax 306 873-5994
www.kelseytrailhealth.ca

TURNOR LAKE

BIRCH NARROWS FIRST NATION HEALTH CENTRE
Gen Del
PO Box 149
Turnor Lake SK S0M 3E0
Tel. 306 894-2112
Fax 306 894-2201
www.mltc.ca

TURTLEFORD

RIVERSIDE HEALTH COMPLEX
First Street South
PO Box 10
Turtleford SK S0M 2Y0
Tel. 306 845-2195
Fax 306 845-2772
www.pnrha.ca

UNITY

UNITY & DISTRICT HEALTH CENTRE
PO Box 741
Unity SK S0K 4L0
Tel. 306 228-2666
Fax 306 228-2292
www.hrha.sk.ca

URANIUM CITY

URANIUM CITY HEALTH CENTRE
PO Box 360
Uranium City SK S0J 2W0
Tel. 306 498-2412
Fax 306 498-2577
www.athabascahealth.com

VANGUARD

VANGUARD HEALTH CENTRE
PO Box 190
Vanguard SK S0N 2V0
Tel. 306 582-2044
Fax 306 582-4833
www.cypresshealth.ca

WADENA

WADENA HOSPITAL
533 5th St NE
PO Box 10
Wadena SK S0A 4J0
Tel. 306 338-2515
Fax 306 338-2720
www.saskatoonhealthregion.ca

WAKAW

WAKAW HOSPITAL
300 1st St N
PO Box 309
Wakaw SK S0K 4P0
Tel. 306 233-4611
Fax 306 233-5990
www.saskatoonhealthregion.ca

WATERHEN LAKE

WATERHEN LAKE HEALTH CENTRE
PO Box 16
Waterhen Lake SK S0M 3B0
Tel. 306 236-3151
Fax 306 236-6377

WATROUS

WATROUS HOSPITAL & HEALTH CENTRE
702 4th St E
PO Box 130
Watrous SK S0K 4T0
Tel. 306 946-1200
Fax 306 946-2369
www.saskatoonhealthregion.ca

WAWOTA

WAWOTA MEMORIAL HEALTH CENTRE
201 Wilfred St
PO Box 60
Wawota SK S0G 5A0
Tel. 306 739-2244
Fax 306 739-2802
www.suncountry.sk.ca

WEYAKWIN

WEYAKWIN HEALTH CENTRE
General Delivery
Weyakwin SK S0J 1W0
Tel. 306 663-6100
Fax 306 663-6165
www.mcrrha.sk.ca

WEYBURN

WEYBURN COMMUNITY HEALTH SERVICES (MENTAL HEALTH)
PO Box 2003 Stn Main
Weyburn SK S4H 2Z9
Tel. 306 842-8665
Fax 306 842-8690
www.suncountry.sk.ca

WEYBURN GENERAL HOSPITAL
201 1st Ave NE
Weyburn SK S4H 0N1
Tel. 306 842-8400
Fax 306 842-8374
www.suncountry.sk.ca

WHITEWOOD

OCHAPOWACE HEALTH CENTRE
Box 550
c/o Band Office
Whitewood SK S0G 5C0
Tel. 306 696-3557
Fax 306 696-3446

WHITEWOOD COMMUNITY HEALTH CENTRE
921 Gambetta St
PO Box 699
Whitewood SK S0G 5C0
Tel. 306 735-2688
Fax 306 735-2512
www.rqhealth.ca

WILKIE

WILKIE HEALTH CENTRE
304 7th Ave E
PO Box 459
Wilkie SK S0K 4W0
Tel. 306 843-2644
Fax 306 843-3222
www.hrha.sk.ca

WILLOW BUNCH

WILLOW BUNCH HEALTH CENTRE
Box 6
Willow Bunch SK S0H 4K0
Tel. 306 473-2310
Fax 306 473-2677
www.fhhr.ca

WOLLASTON LAKE

HATCHET LAKE HEALTH CENTRE
GD
Wollaston Lake SK S0J 3C0
Tel. 306 633-2167
Fax 306 633-2080
www.mcrrha.sk.ca

WOLSELEY

WOLSELEY MEMORIAL HOSPITAL
801 Quimet St
PO Box 458
Wolseley SK S0G 5H0
Tel. 306 698-2213
Fax 306 698-2988
www.rqhealth.ca

WYNYARD

WYNYARD COMMUNITY HEALTH CENTRE
315 Bosworth St
PO Box 1359
Wynyard SK S0A 4T0
Tel. 306 554-3363
Fax 306 554-2994
www.saskatoonhealthregion.ca

WYNYARD HOSPITAL
300 10th St E
PO Box 670
Wynyard SK S0A 4T0
Tel. 306 554-2586
Fax 306 554-2765
www.saskatoonhealthregion.ca

YORKTON

YORKTON MENTAL HEALTH & ADDICTION CENTRE
270 Bradbrooke Dr
Yorkton SK S3N 2K6
Tel. 306 786-0558
Fax 306 786-0556
www.sunrisehealthregion.sk.ca

YORKTON REGIONAL HEALTH CENTRE
270 Bradbrooke Dr
Yorkton SK S3N 2K6
Tel. 306 782-2401
Fax 306 786-6295
www.sunrisehealthregion.sk.ca

ZEHNER

PIOPOT HEALTH CENTRE
Gen Del
Zehner SK S0G 5K0
Tel. 306 781-4833
Fax 306 781-7063

YUKON TERRITORY

DAWSON

DAWSON CITY NURSING STATION
PO Box 10
Dawson YT Y0B 1G0
Tel. 867 993-4444
Fax 867 993-5811

FARO

FARO HEALTH CENTER
PO Box 99
Faro YT Y0B 1K0
Tel. 867 994-4444
Fax 867 994-3457

HAINES JUNCTION

HAINES JUNCTION HEALTH CENTRE
131 Bates St
PO Box 5369
Haines Junction YT Y0B 1L0
Tel. 867 634-4444
Fax 867 634-2733
www.ykhealthguide.org

MAYO

MAYO HEALTH CENTRE
PO Box 98
Mayo YT Y0B 1M0
Tel. 867 996-4444
Fax 867 996-2018

OLD CROW

OLD CROW NURSING STATION
PO Box 92
Old Crow YT Y0B 1N0
Tel. 867 966-4444
Fax 867 966-3614
www.ykhealthguide.org

PELLY CROSSING

PELLY CROSSING HEALTH CENTRE
Box 20
Pelly Crossing YT Y0B 1P0
Tel. 867 537-4444
Fax 867 537-3611
www.ykhealthguide.org

ROSS RIVER

ROSS RIVER HEALTH CENTRE
GD
Ross River YT Y0B 1S0
Tel. 867 969-4444
Fax 867 969-2014
www.ykhealthguide.org

TESLIN

TESLIN HEALTH CENTRE
PO Box 70
Teslin YT Y0A 1B0
Tel. 867 390-4444
Fax 867 390-2217
www.ykhealthguide.org

WATSON LAKE

WATSON LAKE HEALTH CENTRE
PO Box 500
Watson Lake YT Y0A 1C0
Tel. 867 536-7483
Fax 867 536-7011
www.hss.gov.yk.ca

WATSON LAKE HOSPITAL
PO Box 866
Watson Lake YT Y0A 1C0
Tel. 867 536-4444
Fax 867 536-7302
www.yukonhospitals.ca

WHITEHORSE

KWANLIN DUN HEALTH CENTRE
35 McIntyre Dr
Whitehorse YT Y1A 5A5
Tel. 867 633-7800
Fax 867 668-5057
www.kwanlindun.com

WHITEHORSE GENERAL HOSPITAL
5 Hospital Rd
Whitehorse YT Y1A 3H7
Tel. 867 393-8700
Fax 867 393-8771
www.yukonhospitals.ca

WHITEHORSE HEALTH CENTRE
9010 Quartz Rd
Whitehorse YT Y1A 2Z5
Tel. 867 667-8864
Fax 867 393-6407
www.hss.gov.yk.ca

INDEX OF HOSPITALS & HEALTH CENTRES IN CANADA

1

A

B

C

D

E

F

G

H

I

J

K

L

M

HOSPITALS & HEALTH CENTRES

N

O

P

Q

R

S

T

U

V

W

Y

Z

SECTION 5 — RESOURCE SECTION

THE ROYAL COLLEGE OF PHYSICIANS AND SURGEONS OF CANADA

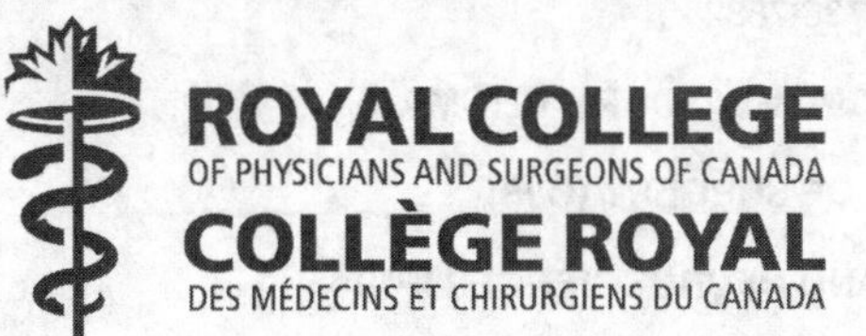

774 Echo Drive, Ottawa, ON, Canada K1S 5N8
Tel: 1-800-668-3740/(613) 730-8177
Fax: (613) 730-8830
E-mail: info@royalcollege.ca
Web site: www.royalcollege.ca

MEMBERS OF COUNCIL

President, Dr. Cecil Rorabeck, FRCSC, London, ON
Past President Elect, Dr. Louis Francescutti, FRCPC, Sherwood Park, AB

DIVISION OF MEDICINE
Dr. Máire Duggan, FRCPC, Calgary, AB
Dr. Robin Cox, MBBS, MRCP, FRCA, Calgary, AB
Dr. Bill Pope, FRCPC, Winnipeg, MB
Dr. Elizabeth Cowden, FRCPC, Winipeg, MB
Dr. Kevin Imrie, FRCPC, Toronto, ON
Dr. Katherine Gills, FRCPC, Ottawa, ON
Dr. Christopher O'Brien, FRCPC, Brantford, ON
Dr. Donald Palisaitis, Senneville, QC
Dr Louise Côté, Sainte-Foy, QC
Dr. Marie-Hélène LeBlanc, FRCPC, Sainte Foy, QC
Dr. Minoli Amit, FRCPC, Antigonish, NS

DIVISION OF SURGERY
Dr. Peter Anderson, FRCSC, Halifax, NS
Dr. Céline Bouchard, FRCSC, Québec, QC
Dr. Geoffrey Johnston, FRCSC, Saskatoon, SK
Dr. Roger Turnell, FRCSC, Edmonton, AB
Dr. Francoise Chagnon, FRCSC, Montreal, QC
Dr. Robert Sabbagh, FRCSC, Sherbrooke, QC
Dr. Amy Nakajima, Nepean, ON
Dr. James O'Brien, Saint John, NB
Dr. Jim Wilson, FRCSC, Kingston, ON
Dr. Vivian McAlister, FRCSC, London, ON

Appointed Members:
Dr. John Hamm, Stellarton, Public Member
Mrs. Louise Simard, Regina, Public member
Dr. Glenn Brimacombe, Public Member
Dr. David Smithson, Resident Member
Dr. Richard Reznick, FRCSC, Fellow-at-Large

Directors/Staff:

Chief Executive OFficer,
M. Andrew Padmos, MD, FRCPC 613-730-6205
Director, Office of Health Policy,
Danielle Fréchette, MPA 613-730-6269
Director, Office of Education,
Kenneth A. Harris, MD, FRCSC 613-730-6283
Associate Director, Specialty Standards, Policy and Development,
Jason Frank, MD, MA(Ed), FRCSC . . . . 613-730-8177 x: 170
Associate Director, Assessment,
Tim Allen, MD, MA(Ed), MCFP, FRCPC. 613-730-8177
Assistant Director, Accreditation and Liaison,
Margaret Kennedy, MA 613-730-6202

Director, Office of Professional Affairs,
Craig Campbell, FRCPC. 613-730-6243
Associate Director, Professional Affairs,
Susan Brien, MD, FRCSC . . . . 613-730-8177 x: 177
Chief Financial Officer,
Tim Julien, CA, CAE 613-730-6227
Chief People Officer/Director,
Bonnie Seidman, CHRP 613-730-6221
CIO and Director eSolutions,
David Perfetti . . . . 613-730-8177 x: 183

The Royal College of Physicians and Surgeons of Canada is the national, not-for-profit organization that oversees the medical education in 61 specialties and subspecialties in Canada by setting high standards for postgraduate medical education and continuing professional development. In collaboration with health organizations and government agencies, the Royal College also plays a role in developing sound health policy in Canada. The Royal College is committed to working together for excellence in specialty medicine for healthy Canadians.

CANADIAN MEDICAL ASSOCIATION

1867 Alta Vista Dr., Ottawa, ON K1G 5W8
Tel: 1-800-267-9703/(613) 731-9331
Fax: (613) 736-7882

CANADIAN MEDICAL ASSOCIATION JOURNAL (CMAJ)

CANADIAN JOURNAL OF SURGERY (CJS)

JOURNAL OF PSYCHIATRY AND NEUROSCIENCE (JPN)

OFFICERS

Chair, Board of Directors, Dr. M. Golbey, Kelowna, BC
President, Dr. Anna Reid, Yellowknife, NT
Honorary Treasurer, Dr. Brian Brodie, Chilliwack, BC
President-Elect, Dr. Louis Francescutti, Sherwood Park, AB
Past President, Dr. John Haggie, Gander, NL

SECRETARIAT

Secretary General & CEO, Mr. Paul-Émile Cloutier
Vice President, Health Policy & Research, Mr. O. Adams
Vice President, Advocacy & Public Affairs, Mr. J. Lefebvre
Vice President, Community Building, Dr. M. Vogel
Vice President, Professional Services & Leadership (PSL), Mr. T. Smith

CMAJ

Editor-In-Chief, Dr. J. Fletcher, Ottawa, ON

CJS

Coeditors, Dr. E.J. Harvey, Montré, QC and
Major V.C. McAlister, London, ON

JPN

Editor-In-Chief, P. Boska, PhD, Montréal, QC
and R. Joober, MD, PhD, Montréal, QC

PROVINCIAL/TERRITORIAL MEDICAL ASSOCIATIONS EXECUTIVE DIRECTORS

ALBERTA - Mr. Michael Gormley, Executive Director
12230 106 Ave. N.W., Edmonton, AB T5N 3Z1
Tel: (780) 482-2626 Fax: (780) 482-5445
Email: amamail@albertadoctors.org Web: www.albertadoctors.org

BRITISH COLUMBIA - Mr. Allan Seckel, CEO
115-1665 Broadway W, Vancouver, BC V6J 5A4
Tel: (604) 736-5551 Fax: (604) 638-2919
Web: www.bcma.org

MANITOBA - Mr. Robert (Bobby) Cram, CEO
20 Desjardins Dr, Winnipeg, MB R3X 0E8
Tel: (204) 985-5888 Fax: (204) 985-5844
Web: www.docsmb.org

NEW BRUNSWICK - Mr. Anthony Knight, Executive Director
176 York St., Fredericton, NB E3B 3N7
Tel: (506) 458-8860 Fax: (506) 458-9853
Email: nbms@nbnet.nb.ca Web: nbms.nb.ca

NEWFOUNDLAND AND LABRADOR
- Mr. Robert Ritter, Executive Director
164 MacDonald Dr., St. John's, NL A1A 4B3
Tel: (709) 726-7424 Fax: (709) 726-7525
Email: nfma@nlma.nl.ca
Web: www.nlma.nl.ca

NORTHWEST TERRITORIES - Dr. Peter McArthur, President/CEO
P.O. Box 1732, Stn. Main, Yellowknife, NT X1A 2P3
Tel: (867) 920-4575 Fax: (867) 920-4578
Email: nwtmedassoc@ssimicro.com Web: www.mwtma.ca

NOVA SCOTIA - Ms. Nancy MacCready-Williams, CEO
25 Spectacle Lake Dr., Dartmouth, NS B3B 1X7
Tel: (902) 468-1866 Fax: (902) 468-6578
Web: doctorsNS.com

ONTARIO - Mr. Ron Sapsford, CEO
900-150 Bloor St W., Toronto, ON M5S 3C1
Tel: (416) 599-2580 Fax: (416) 599-9309
Email: info@oma.org Web: www.oma.org

PRINCE EDWARD ISLAND
- Mr. Alexander (Sandy) Irwin, Executive Director
2 Myrtle St., Stratford, PE C1B 2W2
Tel: (902) 368-7303 Fax: (902) 566-3934
Email: mspei@mspei.org Web: www.mspei.org

QUÉBEC - Normand Laberge, Executive Director
3200-380, rue Saint-Antoine Ouest, Montréal, QC H2Y 3X7
Tel: (514) 866-0660 Fax: (514) 866-0670
Email: admin@amq.ca Web: www.amq.ca

SASKATCHEWAN - Dr. Vino Padayachee, Executive Director
402-321A 21st St. E, Saskatoon, SK S7K 0C1
Tel: (306) 244-2196 Fax: (306) 653-1631
Email: sma@sma.sk.ca Web: www.sma.sk.ca

YUKON - Dr. Rao Tadepalli, President/CEO
5 Hospital Road, Whitehorse, YT Y1A 3H7
Tel: (867) 393-8749 Fax: (867) 393-6601
Email: yma@yukondoctors.ca Web: www.yukondoctors.ca

THE MEDICAL COUNCIL OF CANADA

The Medical Council of Canada was established in 1912 by the *Canada Medical Act* to examine candidates for medical registration on behalf of the provincial medical licensing authorities.

Dan Small
Rose Carter
Gwen Haliburton
Nancy MacBeth

MEDICAL REGULATORY AUTHORITIES' APPOINTEES

Alberta — Dr. Trevor Theman; Dr. Karen Mazurek
British Columbia — Dr. Jack Burak; Dr. Heidi Oetter
Manitoba — Dr. William Pope; Dr. Robert Menzies
New Brunswick — Dr. Edmund G. A. Schollenberg; Dr. John C. McCrea
Newfoundland and Labrador — Dr. Robert Young; Dr. William Moulton
Northwest Territories — Dr. Theresa Farrell; Dr. Bing Guthrie
Nova Scotia — Dr. Douglas Grant; Dr. William Lowe
Ontario — Dr. Rocco Gerace; Dr. James Watters
Prince Edward Island — Dr. Cyril A. Moyse; Dr. Geraldine Johnson
Quebec — Dr. Anne-Marie McLellan; Dr. Markus C. Martin
Saskatchewan — Dr. Edward Tsoi; Dr. Karen Shaw
Yukon Territory — Dr. Bruce Beaton
Nunavut — Dr. William MacDonald; Dr. Patricia DeMaio

UNIVERSITY APPOINTEES

Alberta — Dr. Kent Stobart
British Columbia — Dr. Oscar Casiro
Calgary — Dr. Bruce Wright
Dalhousie — Dr. Simon Field
Laval — Dr. Joan Glenn
Manitoba — Dr. Bruce Martin
McGill — Dr. Joyce Pickering
McMaster — Dr. Michael L. Marrin
Memorial — Dr. Cathy Vardy
Montreal — Dr. Christian Bourdy
Northern Ontario — Dr. Lisa Graves
Ottawa — Dr. Melissa Forgie
Queen's — Dr. Anthony Sanfilippo
Saskatchewan — Dr. Grant Stoneham
Sherbrooke — Dr. Daniel Côté
Toronto — Dr. Jay Rosenfield
Western Ontario — Dr. Chris Waitling

STUDENT AND RESIDENT APPOINTEES

Student, — Safia Chatur/Laurence Bernard
Resident, — Meggie Raymond/Dipinder Keer

RESOURCE SECTION

PROVINCIAL REGISTRARS

Dr. Trevor Theman, Registrar
College of Physicians & Surgeons of Alberta
2700 - 10020 100 Street NW, Edmonton, AB T5J 0N3
Tel. (780)423-4764. Fax: (780)420-0651.
E-mail: info@cpsa.ab.ca
Web: www.cpsa.ab.ca

Dr. Heidi M. Oetter, Registrar
College of Physicians & Surgeons of British Columbia
300-669 Howe St, Vancouver, BC V6C 0B4
Tel. (604)733-7758. Fax: (604)733-3503
Web: www.cpsbc.ca

Dr. William D.B. Pope, MD LL.B FRCPC, Registrar/CEO
The College of Physicians & Surgeons of Manitoba
1000 - 1661 Portage Avenue, Winnipeg, MB R3J 3T7
Tel. (204)774-4344. Fax: (204)774-0750.
E-mail: bpope@cpsm.mb.ca

Dr. Ed Schollenberg, MD LLB FRCPC, Registrar
College of Physicians & Surgeons of New Brunswick
1 Hampton Rd., Suite 300, Rothesay, NB E2E 5K8
Tel. (506)849-5050. Fax: (506)849-5069
E-mail: info@cpsnb.org
Web: www.cpsnb.org

Dr. Robert W. Young, MD, FRCPC, Registrar
College of Physicians & Surgeons of Newfoundland & Labrador
120 Torbay Road, Suite W100, St. John's, NL A1A 2G8
Tel. (709)726-8546. Fax: (709)726-4725
E-mail: cpsnl@cpsnl.ca
Web: www.cpsnl.ca

Ms. Samantha Van Genne, Registrar
Medical Profession, Dept. of Health & Social Services
Government of the Northwest Territories
P.O. Box 1320, Yellowknife, NT X1A 2L9
Tel. (867)920-8058. Fax: (867)873-0484

Dr. D.A. (Gus) Grant, Registrar & CEO
College of Physicians & Surgeons of Nova Scotia
Suite 5005, 7071 Bayers Road, Halifax, NS B3L 2C2
Tel. (902)422-5823. Fax: (902)422-5035.
E-mail: dagrant@cpsns.ns.ca
Web: www.cpsns.ns.ca

Dr. Rocco Gerace, Registrar
The College of Physicians & Surgeons of Ontario
80 College St, Toronto, ON M5G 2E2
Tel. (416)967-2600 Ext. 400
Toll Free: (800) 268-7096 Ext. 400
Fax: (416)967-2618
Web: www.cpso.on.ca

Dr. C.A. Moyse, Registrar
The College of Physicians & Surgeons of Prince Edward Island
14 Paramount Dr, Charlottetown, PE C1A 0C7
Tel. (902)566-3861. Fax: (902)566-3986
E-mail: mmacdonald@cpspei.ca
Web: www.cpspei.ca

D' Yves Robert, Secretary
Collège des médecins du Québec
2170 boul. René-Lévesque Ouest, Montréal, QC H3H 2T8
Tel. (514)933-4441. Fax: (514)933-3112
E-mail: info@cmq.org
Web: www.cmq.org

Dr. Karen Shaw, Registrar
College of Physicians & Surgeons of Saskatchewan
500, 321A - 21st Street East, Saskatoon, SK S7K 0C1
Tel. (306)244-7355. Fax: (306)244-2600
E-mail: karen.shaw@cps.sk.ca
Web: www.cps.sk.ca

Fiona Charbonneau, Registrar of Medical Practitioners
Yukon Medical Council
Box 2703 (C-18), Whitehorse, YT Y1A 2C6
Tel. (867)667-3774. Fax: (867)393-6483
E-mail: ymc@gov.yk.ca
Web: www.yukonmedicalcouncil.ca

COLLEGE OF FAMILY PHYSICIANS OF CANADA

2630 Skymark Ave., Mississauga, ON L4W 5A4
Tel. (905) 629-0900
Fax: (905) 629-0893
Web: www.cfpc.ca

EXECUTIVE COMMITTEE MEMBERS (2012-2013)

President, Dr. Marie-Dominique Beaulieu
Past President, Dr. Sandy Buchman
President-Elect and Chair of the Board, Dr. Kathy Lawrence
Honorary Secretary-Treasurer, Dr. Gary Mazowita
Member-at-Large (1 year term), Dr. Jennifer Hall
Member-at-Large (3 year term), Dr. Claudette Chase
Executive Director & CEO, Dr. Francine Lemire
Communications Manager, Jayne Johnston

COLLEGE OF FAMILY PHYSICIANS OF CANADA - PROVINCIAL OFFICES

BC College of Family Physicians
V. Jim Thorsteinson, Executive Director
350-1665 W Broadway
Vancouver BC, V6J 1X1
Tel. (604) 736-1877 Fax: (604) 736-4675

Alberta College of Family Physicians
Terri Potter, Executive Director
Suite 370 10403-172 St, Centre 170
Edmonton AB, T5S 1K9
Tel. (780) 488-2395 Fax: (780) 488-2396

Saskatchewan College of Family Physicians
Lois Hislop, Administrator
P.O. Box 7111
Saskatoon SK, S7K 4J1
Tel. (306) 665-7714 Fax: (306) 665-7714

Manitoba College of Family Physicians
Susan Patek, Administrator
240 - 1695 Henderson Highway
Winnipeg MB, R2G 1P1
Tel. (204) 668-3667 Fax: (204) 668-3663

Ontario College of Family Physicians
Janet Kasperski, Executive Director & CEO
340 Richmond St, W. (Richmond & John)
Toronto ON, M5V 1X2
Tel. (416) 867-9646 Fax: (416) 867-9990

Collège Québécois des médecins de famille
Nicole Cloutier, Directrice générale
3210 avenue Jacques, Bureau 202
Laval QC, H7P 0A9
Tel. (450) 973-2228 Fax: (450) 973-4329

New Brunswick College of Family Physicians
950 Picot Ave, Bathurst NB, E2A 4Z9
Tel. (506) 548-4707 Fax: (506) 548-4761

Nova Scotia College of Family Physicians
Cathie W. Carroll, Executive Director
Suite 207, Mill Cove Plaza, 967 Bedford Hwy
Bedford NS, B4A 1A9
Tel. (902) 499-0303 Fax: (902) 457-2584

P.E.I. College of Family Physicians
Rosemary Burke-Perry, Administrator
14 Royalty Road, Charlottetown, PE C1E 1T8
Tel. (902) 894-2605 Fax: (902) 894-3975

NL/LAB College of Family Physicians
Debbie Rideout, Administrator
c/o The Discipline of Family Medicine
Room 2422 Health Sciences Centre
300 Prince Phillip Drive
St John's NL, A1B 3V6
Tel. (709)782-4343 Fax: (709) 782-4363

THE DECLARATION OF GENEVA

Adopted by the 18th General Assembly of the World Medical Association, Helsinki, Finland, June 1964
and amended by the 29th World Medical Association General Assembly, Tokyo, Japan, October 1975
35th World Medical Association General Assembly, Venice, Italy, October 1983
41st WMA General Assembly, Hong Kong, September 1989
46th WMA General Assembly, Stockholm, Sweden, September 1994
48th WMA General Assembly, Somerset West, Republic of South Africa, October 1996
52nd WMA General Assembly, Edinburgh, Scotland, October 2000
53rd General Assembly of WMA, Washington, DC, USA, October 2002
54th General Assembly of the WMA, Helsinki, Finland, September 2003
55th General Assembly of the WMA, Tokyo, Japan, October 2004
56th General Assembly of the WMA, Latin America, October 2005
57th General Assembly of the WMA, Pilanesburg, South Africa, October 2006
58th General Assembly of the WMA, Coopenhagen, Denmark, October 2007
59th General Assembly of the WMA, Seoul, Korea, October 2008
General Assembly of the WMA, New Delhi, India, October 2009
General Assembly of the WMA, Vancouver, Canada, October 2010
General Assembly of the WMA, Montevideo, Uruguay, October 2011
General Assembly of the WMA, Bangkok, Thailand, October 2012
Council Meetings of WMA, Bali, Indonesia, April 2013.

AT THE TIME OF BEING ADMITTED AS A MEMBER OF THE MEDICAL PROFESSION:

I SOLEMNLY PLEDGE myself to consecrate my life to the service of humanity;
I WILL GIVE to my teachers the respect and gratitude which is their due;
I WILL PRACTICE my profession with conscience and dignity;
THE HEALTH OF MY PATIENT will be my first consideration;
I WILL RESPECT the secrets which are confided in me, even after the patient has died;
I WILL MAINTAIN by all the means in my power, the honour and the noble traditions of the medical profession;
MY COLLEAGUES will be my sisters and brothers;
I WILL NOT PERMIT considerations of age, disease or disability, creed, ethnic origin, gender, nationality, political affiliation, race, sexual orientation, or social standing to intervene between my duty and my patient;
I WILL MAINTAIN the utmost respect for human life;
I WILL NOT USE my medical knowledge to violate human rights and civic liberties, even under threat;
I MAKE THESE PROMISES solemnly, freely, and upon my honour.

HEALTH CANADA
Ottawa

Brooke Claxton Bldg, Tunney's Pasture, A.L. 0906C, Ottawa, ON K1A 0K9
Gen. Inquiries: (613) 957-2991, TDD (T.Free): 1-800-267-1245; Fax: (613) 941-5366; E-mail: info@hc-sc.gc.ca; Web: www.hc-sc.gc.ca

Health Canada is responsible for matters related to the promotion and preservation of the health of the people of Canada over which the Parliament of Canada has jurisdiction. Major examples of these responsibilities include administration of legislation relating to the health of the people of Canada; investigation and research into public health; information services relating to health conditions and practices; health services for Indian and Inuit people, federal government employees, immigrants and civil aviation personnel; public health matters affecting Canada's boundary with the United States; cooperation and coordination with provincial governments on matters of health, and collection, publication and distribution of information relating to health.

Minister of National Health, The Honourable Leona Aglukkaq

Chief of Staff, Mr. Leah Canning
Deputy Minister, Ms. Glenda Yeates
Associate Deputy Minister, Paul Rochon
Scheduling Assistant, Ms. Isabelle Beaudry
Departmental Liaison, Ellen Birnbaum

CORPORATE SERVICES BRANCH Tel: (613) 946-3200

Assistant Deputy Minister, Sony Perron

Executive Assistant, Kateri Beauregard
CIO & Director General, Information Management Services, Guylaine Montplaisir
Director General. Real Property & Security Directorate, Gary Lacey
Administrative Officer, Planning Integration & Management, Véeronique Armit
Director General, Human Resources Services, Stephen Black
Chief Financial Officer, Melissa Gautier

FIRST NATIONS AND INUIT HEALTH BRANCH Tel: (613) 957-7701

Senior Assistant Deputy Minister, Michel Roy

Senior Dir General, Internal Client Services & Transition, Debbie L. Reid
Director General, Interprofessional Advisory & Program Support, Anthony Sangster
Director, Health Funding Arrangements, Catherine Jones
Director, Health Infrastructure Division, France Dauphin
A/Director General, Strategic Policy Planning & Information, Aruna Sadana
Senior Policy Analyst, Health Services Integration, Kaila-Lea Clarke
Director General, Insured Benefits, Sandra Bruce

STRATEGIC POLICY BRANCH Tel: (613) 946-1791

Assistant Deputy Minister, Abby Hoffman
Manager, Executive Services, Paula Crupi
Manager, Adinistrative Services & Finance, Shehmina Shamsi

Dir General, Health Care Programs & Policy Directorate, Robert Shearer
Dir General, Policy Coordinator & Planning Directorate, Cheryl Grant
Exec Dir, Office of Nursing Policy, Ms Sandra MacDonald-Rencz
Director, Health Acts Division, Gigi Mandy
Director Gen, Applied Research and Analysis Directorate, Sylvain Paradis
Executive Dir, Pharmaceutical Management Strategies, Jean Pruneau
Senior Policy Analyst, Policy Priorities & Analysis Division, Kelly Connor

PUBLIC HEALTH AGENCY OF CANADA AND REGIONAL OFFICES (613) 957-3507

CHIEF PUBLIC HEALTH OFFICER, Dr. David Butler-Jones
HEALTH CANADA
19th Floor - PL 1919A5 Jean Mance Building, Tunney's Pasture, Ottawa, ON K1A 1B4

Atlantic Region
Regional Director, Beth Sherwood
1525-1505 Barrington St, Halifax, NS B3J 3Y6
Tel: (902) 426-2700 Fax: (902) 426-9689

Quebec Region
Regional Director, Danielle Gagnon
Guy-Favreau Complexe, East Tower,
200 René Levesque Blvd West
Montreal, QC H2Z 1X4
Tel: (514) 283-2858 Fax: (514) 496-7012

Ontario/ Nunavut Region
Regional Director, Mauricette Howlett
180 Queen St W, 11th Fl,
Toronto, ON M5V 3L7
Tel: (416) 973-0003 Fax: (416) 954-8211

Manitoba/ Saskatchewan
Regional Dir, Larry Flynn
7th Fl, 275 Portage Ave, Winnipeg, MB R3B 2B3
Mailing Address: 1015, Arlington St,
Winnipeg, MB R3E 3R2
Tel: (204) 789-2000 Fax: (204) 789-7878

Alberta/ Northwest Territories
A/Regional Dir, Rashmi Joshee
815-9700 Jasper Ave
Edmonton, AB T5J 4C3
Tel: (780) 495-2754 Fax: (780) 495-7842

British Columbia/ Yukon Region
A/Regional Dir, Christine Burgess
Suite 405, Winch Bldg, 757 West Hastings St
Vancouver, BC V6C 1A1
Tel: (604) 666-2083 Fax: (604) 666-2258

HEALTH PRODUCTS AND FOOD BRANCH Tel: (613) 957-1806

Assistant Deputy Minister, Paul Glover

Associate Assistant Deputy Minister, N. Lamar

Therapeutic Products Directorate, Dir Gen, Barbara Sabourin
Biologics and Genetic Therapies, Dir Gen, Robert Cushman
Natural Health Products Directorate, Dir Gen, Scott Sawler
Inspectorate, Dir Gen, Diana Dowthwaite
Marketed Health Products Directorate, Dir Gen, Cindy Ezamus
Policy, Planning & International Affairs Directorate, Dir Gen, Kendal Weber

REGIONAL OFFICES & LABORATORIES

Atlantic
Health Canada
1505, Barrington St, Maritime Centre
Health Products and Food Branch
Suite 1625, 16th Floor,
Halifax, NS B3J 3Y6
Health Canada
1st Floor, Government of Canada Building
10 Highfield St, Moncton NB E1C 9V5

Québec
Santé Canada
Direction générale des produits de santé et des aliments
1001, rue St-Laurent ouest, 3e étage
Longueuil QC J4K 1C7

Saskatchewan
Health Canada
103-1855, Smith Street
Regina SK S4P 2N5
Health Canada
Federal Building
101-22nd St E, Room 412
Saskatoon SK S7K 0E1

Manitoba
Health Canada
510 Lagimodière Blvd, 1st Floor
Winnipeg, MB R2J 3Y1

Ontario
Health Canada
2301 Midland Avenue,
Toronto, ON M1P 4R7

British Columbia
Office: Health Canada
Health Products and Food Branch
#400-4595 Canada Way,
Burnaby, BC V5G 1J9
Lab: Health Canada
Health Products and Food Branch
Western Regional Lab
3155 Wellingdon Green,
Burnaby, BC V5G 4P2

Assistant Deputy Minister, Samuel Godefroy

DISTRICT OFFICES

St. John's	Sir Humphrey Gilbert Bldg, 165 Duckworth St, St. John's, NL A1C 1G4
Saint John	New Customs Bldg, Rm. 517, 189 Prince William St, Saint John, NB E2L 2B9
Charlottetown	Kelly Bldg, 3 Harbour Side, Ste 101, Charlottetown, PE C1A 8R4
Halifax	1625-1505, 16th Fl, Barrington St, Halifax, NS B3J 3Y6
Quebec	901 Cap Diamant St, Maritime Champlain Station, Ste 267, Quebec, QC G1K 4K1
Sherbrooke	50 Place de la Cité, Ste 319, PO Box 1120, Sherbrooke, QC J1H 5L5
Trois-Rivières	25, rue des Forges, Trois-Rivières, QC G9A 6AJ
Hamilton	150 Main St W, Rm 530, Hamilton, ON L8P 1H8
London	Federal Bldg, 451 Talbot St, Rm 201, London, ON N6A 5C9
Thunder Bay	Public Bldg, 33 Court St S, Rm 313, Thunder Bay, ON P7B 2W6
Ottawa	SBI Bldg, 2323 Riverside Dr, 11th Fl, Ottawa, ON K1A 0L2
Winnipeg	510 Lagimodière Blvd, Winnipeg, MB R2J 3Y1
Regina	103-1855 Smith St, Regina, SK S4P 2N5
Saskatoon	Federal Bldg, 101-22nd St E, Rm 412, Saskatoon, SK S7K 0E1
Edmonton	Suite 710, Canada Place, 9700 Jasper Ave, Edmonton, AB T5K 1C5
Calgary	220-4th Ave SE, Rm 282, Calgary, AB T2P 3C3
Victoria	Customs Bldg, 816 Government St, Rm 231, Victoria, BC V8W 1W9
Burnaby	3155 Willingdon Green, Burnaby, BC V5G 4P2
Vancouver	757 West Hastings St, Vancouver, BC V6C 1A1

Hazardous Materials Information Review Commission, 427 Laurier Ave West, 7th Floor, Ottawa, ON K1A 1M3
Corporate Service Officer: Karen Berndt E-mail: hmirc-ccrmd@hc-sc.gc.ca Tel: (613) 993-4331 Fax: (613) 993-4686
Patented Medicine Prices Review Board, PO Box L40, Standard Life Centre, 333 Laurier Ave W, Ste 1400, Ottawa, ON K1P 1C1
Dir of Board Secretariat & Communications: Sylvie Dupont
Tel: (613) 954-8299
Fax: (613) 952-7626
E-mail: pmprb@pmprb-cepmb.gc.ca

THE CONTROLLED DRUGS AND SUBSTANCES ACT

The Controlled Drugs and Substances Act (CDSA) came into force in 1997 and fulfils Canada's obligations under the 1961 Single Convention on Narcotic Drugs, the 1971 Convention on Psychotropic Substances, and the 1988 United Nations Convention against Illicit Traffic in Narcotic Drugs and Psychotropic Substances.

The CDSA, which is administered by the Controlled Substances and Tobacco Directorate within Health Canada, includes six Schedules identifying the controlled substances, e.g., narcotics, anabolic steroids, benzodiazepines, etc., and precursor chemicals regulated under the Act.

The legislative framework is completed by a series of regulations including the *Narcotic Control Regulations, Part G of the Food and Drug Regulations, Part J of the Food and Drug Regulations, the Benzodiazepines and Other Targeted Substances Regulations, the Marihuana Medical Access Regulations, the Precursor Control Regulations, the New Classes of Practitioners Regulations and the Industrial Hemp Regulations.* These regulations set out the circumstances under which activities with controlled substances and precursor chemicals are permitted. If an activity is not permitted by the regulations or other provisions in the Act, it is an offence and subject to potential prosecution.

A copy of the CDSA and its associated regulations can be obtained by writing to the Canada Communications Group - Publishing, Ottawa, Canada, K1A 0S9 or online via the LAWS page on the Department of Justice Website at: http://laws.justice.gc.ca.

PROVINCIAL & TERRITORIAL DIRECTORS OF SEXUALLY TRANSMITTED INFECTION (STI) CONTROL

Each province has its own Sexually Transmitted Infection prevention act and regulations. In British Columbia, Ontario and Saskatchewan, physicians are required to report cases directly to the local medical officer of health. In the other provinces, reporting is directly to the provincial department of health - either to the physician employed as S.T.I. Control Director or as provincial epidemiologist. Notification forms are available from these sources as shown below:

NEWFOUNDLAND

Dr. Faith Stratton, Chief Medical Officer of Health
Public Health, Department of Health and Community Services
P.O. Box 8700
St. John's, NL A1B 4J6
Tel. (709) 729-3430; Fax: (709) 729-0730

PRINCE EDWARD ISLAND

Chief Public Health Officer, Dr. Heather Morrison
Deputy Chief Public Health Officer, Dr. Lamont Sweet
Tel. (902) 368-4996; Fax: (902) 620-3354
Department of Health & Wellness
16 Fitzroy St, PO Box 2000
Charlottetown, PE C1A 7N8

NOVA SCOTIA

Chief Medical Officer of Health, Dr. Robert Strang
Department of Health and Wellness
1894 Barrington St.,
3rd Floor, Barrington Tower
P.O. Box 488
Halifax, NS B3J 2R8
Tel. (902) 424-2358; Fax: (902) 424-4716

NEW BRUNSWICK

Chief Medical Officer of Health, Dr. Eilish Cleary
Department of Health
PO Box 5100, Carleton Place
Fredericton, NB E3B 5G8
Tel. (506) 444-2112; Fax: (506) 453-8702
Email: eilish.cleary@gnb.ca

QUEBEC

Dr. Monique Douville-Fradet, MD, MHSc, FRCP(C)
Institut National de santé publique du Québec
2400, rue d'Estimauville, 3e etage
Québec, Province de Québec, Canada, G1S 7G9
Tel. (418) 666-7000 Ext.313; Fax: (418) 666-2776
Email: monique.fradet@inspq.qc.ca

ONTARIO

Dr. Eileen de Villa, Associate Medical Officer of Health, Region of Peel
7120 Hurontario St, PO Box 630 Mississauga, ON L5M 2C5
Tel.(905) 791-7800 ; Fax: (905) 564-2683

MANITOBA

Chief Provincial Public Health Officer, Dr. Michael Routledge
Manitoba Health
4003-300 Carlton St
Winnipeg, MB R3B 3M9
Tel. (204) 788-6636; Fax: (204) 948-2204

SASKATCHEWAN

Chief Medical Health Officer, Dr. Saquib Shahab,
Population Health Branch
Saskatchewan Health
3475 Albert St
Regina, SK S4S 6X6
Tel. (306) 787-3235; Fax: (306) 787-3237;
Email: mmckinnon@health.gov.sk.ca

ALBERTA

Chief Medical Officer of Health, Dr. James Talbot
Alberta Health and Wellness
24th Fl, Telus Plaza North Tower, 10025 Jasper Ave
Edmonton, AB T5J 1S6
Tel. (780) 427-5263; Fax: (780) 427-7683

BRITISH COLUMBIA

Medical Director, Dr. Gina Ogilvie
STI/HIV Prevention and Control
BC Centre for Disease Control
655 W 12th Ave
Vancouver, BC V5Z 4R4
Tel. (604) 707-2422; Fax: (604) 707-5604

NORTHWEST TERRITORIES

Chief Public Health Officer, Dr André Corriveau, MD, MBA, FRCPC
Deputy Chief Public Health Officer, Dr.Kami Kandola, MD, MPH, CCFP, DTM&H, ABPM
Department of Health and Social Services
Government of the Northwest Territories
PO Box 1320
Yellowknife, NT X1A 2L9
Tel. (867) 920-3286; Fax: (867) 873-0442

NUNAVUT

Chief Medical Health Officer, Dr. Maureen Baikie
Department of Health and Social Services
Fl 3, Sivummut Bldg
PO Box 1000
Iqaluit, NU X0A 0H0
Tel. (867) 975-5774; Fax: (867) 975-5755

YUKON TERRITORY

Chief Medical Officer of Health, Dr. Brendan Hanley
Manager, Lori Tudwick
Yukon Communicable Disease Control
Department of Health and Social Services
#4 Hospital Road
Whitehorse, Yukon Y1A 3H8
Tel. (867) 667-8323; Fax: (867) 667-8349

Dr. Tom Wong
Director, Professional Guidelines & Public Health Practice Division
Public Health Agency of Canada - AL:0602C
Room 2391-C
100 Eglantine Driveway
Tunney's Pasture AL: 0602C
Ottawa, ON K1A 0K9
Tel. (613) 946-5700 Fax: (613) 941-9813
E-mail: tom.wong@phac-aspc.gc.ca

RESOURCE SECTION

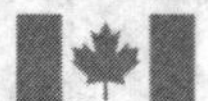
Health Canada Santé Canada

Canada Vigilance Adverse Reaction Reporting Form

Report of suspected adverse reactions to marketed health products in Canada

See instructions and information on adverse reaction reporting and confidentiality on Page 2.

Complete all mandatory items, marked by a *, and provide as much information as possible for the remaining items. PROTECTED WHEN COMPLETED – B**

A. Patient Information

1. Identifier

2. Age ☐ Years ☐ Months | 3. Sex* ☐ Male ☐ Female | 4. Height cm feet | 5. Weight kg lbs

B. Adverse Reaction

1. Outcome attributed to adverse reaction (Select all that apply)

- ☐ Death: (yyyy-mm-dd)
- ☐ Life-threatening
- ☐ Hospitalization
- ☐ Hospitalization – prolonged
- ☐ Disability
- ☐ Congenital malformation
- ☐ Required intervention to prevent damage/impairment
- ☐ Other:

2. Reaction date (yyyy-mm-dd) | 3. Report date (yyyy-mm-dd)

4. Describe reaction or problem*

5. Relevant tests/laboratory data (including dates (yyyy-mm-dd))

6. Relevant history and pre-existing medical conditions (e.g. allergies, pregnancy, smoking/alcohol use, hepatic/renal dysfunction)

C. Suspected Health Product(s)

1. Name*, strength and manufacturer (if known)

#1

#2

2. Dose, frequency and route used

#1 | #2

3. Therapy dates (or duration)

#1 From (yyyy-mm-dd) - To (yyyy-mm-dd) | #2 From (yyyy-mm-dd) - To (yyyy-mm-dd)

4. Indication for use

#1 | #2

5. Reaction abated after use stopped or dose reduced

#1 ☐ Yes ☐ No ☐ Does not apply | #2 ☐ Yes ☐ No ☐ Does not apply

6. Lot #

#1

#2

7. Expiration

#1 (yyyy-mm-dd)

#2 (yyyy-mm-dd)

8. Reaction reappeared after reintroduction

#1 ☐ Yes ☐ No ☐ Does not apply | #2 ☐ Yes ☐ No ☐ Does not apply

9. Concomitant health products, excluding treatment of reaction (name, dose, frequency, route used and therapy dates (yyyy-mm-dd))

10. Treatment of reaction, including dates (yyyy-mm-dd)

D. Reporter Information

1. Name*, occupation, address, telephone number*

2. Health professional? ☐ Yes ☐ No

3. Reported to manufacturer? ☐ Yes ☐ No

** As per the Treasury Board of Canada Secretariat Government Security Policy.

A program of MedEffect™ Canada

HC Pub.: 100251 (September 2012)

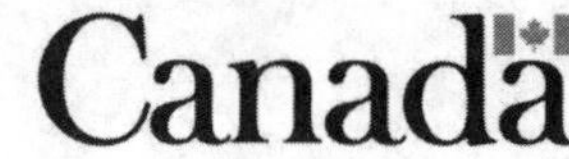

Instructions to Complete the Canada Vigilance Adverse Reaction Reporting Form

- Use this form only to report adverse reactions to Canadian marketed health products, including prescription and non-prescription medications; natural health products; biologically derived products; cells, tissues and organs; radiopharmaceuticals; and disinfectants and sanitizers with disinfectant claims.
- All sections of the form should be filled in as completely as possible. Use a separate form for each patient. Up to two suspected health products for a particular adverse reaction may be reported on one form. Attach an additional form if there are more than two suspected health products for the adverse reaction being reported. Additional pages may be attached if more space is required.
- For the "Identifier" box, provide some type of identifier that will allow you, the reporter, to readily locate the case if you are contacted for more information; do not use the patient's name. See the Confidentiality disclaimer at the bottom of this page.
- Any follow-up information for an adverse reaction that has already been reported can be submitted using a new form, indicating that it consists of follow-up information, including, if known, the date of the original report and the Adverse Reaction Number provided in the acknowledgement letter.
- **Reports can be faxed** to 1-866-678-6789 (toll-free) **or mailed** to: Canada Vigilance Program, Marketed Health Products Directorate, Health Canada, Postal Locator 0701E, Ottawa, Ontario K1A 0K9. Postage paid labels are available at www.health.gc.ca/medeffect or by calling 1-866-234-2345 (toll-free). Do not send reports by e-mail.

Information on Adverse Reaction Reporting

What is an adverse reaction?

An adverse reaction is a harmful and unintended response to a health product. This includes any undesirable patient effect suspected to be associated with health product use. Unintended effect, health product abuse, overdose, interaction (including drug-drug and drug-food interactions) and unusual lack of therapeutic efficacy are all considered to be reportable adverse reactions.

A serious adverse reaction is one that requires in-patient hospitalization or prolongation of existing hospitalization, causes congenital malformation, results in persistent or significant disability or incapacity, is life-threatening or results in death. Adverse reactions that require significant medical intervention to prevent one of these listed outcomes are also considered to be serious.

Which adverse reactions should be reported?

All suspected adverse reactions should be reported, especially those that are:

- *unexpected*, regardless of their severity, i.e., not consistent with product information or labelling; or
- *serious*, whether expected or not; or
- reactions to *recently marketed health products* (on the market for less than five years), regardless of their nature or severity.

Alternative ways to report

You can also report side effects to health products to the Canada Vigilance Program:

- By calling 1-866-234-2345 (toll-free)
- Online: www.health.gc.ca/medeffect

The Canada Vigilance Adverse Reaction Reporting Form is also available online at www.health.gc.ca/medeffect or at the back of the *Compendium of Pharmaceuticals and Specialties* (CPS).

Other Information

- Submission of a report does not constitute an admission that medical personnel or the product caused or contributed to the adverse reaction.
- Adverse reaction reports are, for the most part, only suspected associations. A temporal or possible association is sufficient for a report to be made. Reporting of an adverse reaction does not imply a definitive causal link.
- Health professionals and consumers may also report adverse reactions to the market authorization holder (MAH). Indicate on your adverse reaction report sent to Health Canada if a case was also reported to the product's MAH.
- To report an Adverse Event Following an Immunization (AEFI) for a vaccine used in the prevention of infectious disease, health professionals should complete a copy of the AEFI reporting form that is available online at http://www.phac-aspc.gc.ca/im/aefi-form-eng.php These forms also exist as customized provincial/territorial adverse event forms which can be obtained either from local public health departments or from the provincial/territorial health authorities.

For additional information, contact a Canada Vigilance Regional Office by telephone at 1-866-234-2345 (toll-free) or:

Canada Vigilance Regional Office – British Columbia and Yukon
400-4595 Canada Way, Burnaby, BC V5G 1J9
CanadaVigilance_BC@hc-sc.gc.ca

Canada Vigilance Regional Office – Alberta and Northwest Territories
Suite 730, 9700 Jasper Ave, Edmonton, AB T5J 4C3
CanadaVigilance_AB@hc-sc.gc.ca

Canada Vigilance Regional Office – Saskatchewan
Room 412 – 101 22nd Street East, Saskatoon, SK S7K 0E1
CanadaVigilance_SK@hc-sc.gc.ca

Canada Vigilance Regional Office – Manitoba
510 Lagimodière Blvd, Winnipeg, MB R2J 3Y1
CanadaVigilance_MB@hc-sc.gc.ca

Canada Vigilance Regional Office – Ontario and Nunavut
2301 Midland Ave, Toronto, ON M1P 4R7
CanadaVigilance_ON@hc-sc.gc.ca

Canada Vigilance Regional Office – Québec
Suite 202-40, East Tower
200 René-Lévesque Blvd. West, Montréal, QC H2Z 1X4
CanadaVigilance_QC@hc-sc.gc.ca

For New Brunswick, Nova Scotia, Prince Edward Island, Newfoundland and Labrador:

Canada Vigilance Regional Office – Atlantic
Suite 1625, 1505 Barrington St., Halifax, NS B3J 3Y6
CanadaVigilance_ATL@hc-sc.gc.ca

Confidentiality

Personal information collected, used or disclosed under the Canada Vigilance Program is confidential and protected. For the purposes of the Canada Vigilance Program, information related to the identity of a patient and/or reporter of the adverse reaction will be protected as personal information under the *Privacy Act*, and under the *Access to Information Act*, in the case of an access to information request. Provision of the information requested on this form is voluntary. Information from adverse reaction reports is maintained in a computerized database and used for the monitoring of marketed health products, which may contribute to the detection of potential product-related safety issues, as well as to the benefit-risk assessments of these products. For details about personal information collected under this program, visit the Government of Canada web site on Institution-Specific Personal Information Banks under Health Canada, Health Products and Food Branch, Branch Incident Reporting System, PIB # ppu 088 at: http://infosource.gc.ca/inst/shc/fed07-eng.asp (Health Products and Food Branch, Branch Incident Reporting System).

Page 2 of 2

RESOURCE SECTION

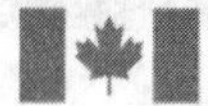

Santé Canada Health Canada

Formulaire de déclaration des effets indésirables de Canada Vigilance

Déclaration d'effets indésirables présumés dus à des produits de santé commercialisés au Canada

Voir les directives ainsi que l'information sur la déclaration d'effets indésirables et la confidentialité en page 2.
Compléter tous les items obligatoires, indiqués par un *, et fournir autant d'information que possible pour les autres items.

PROTÉGÉ LORSQUE COMPLÉTÉ – B**

A. Information reliée au patient

1. Identification

2. Age	3. Sexe*	4. Taille	5. Poids
☐ Ans ☐ Mois	☐ Homme ☐ Femme	___ cm ___ pi	___ kg ___ lb

B. Effet indésirable

1. Suite de l'effet indésirable (sélectionner ceux qui s'appliquent)

- ☐ Décès : (aaaa-mm-jj)
- ☐ Met la vie en danger
- ☐ Hospitalisation
- ☐ Hospitalisation – prolongée
- ☐ Incapacité
- ☐ Malformation congénitale
- ☐ Besoin d'intervention pour prévenir lésion/invalidité
- ☐ Autre :

2. Date de l'effet (aaaa-mm-jj)

3. Date de déclaration (aaaa-mm-jj)

4. Décrire l'effet ou le problème*

5. Tests/données de laboratoire pertinents (incluant les dates (aaaa-mm-jj))

6. Historique pertinente et conditions médicales préexistantes (p. ex. allergies, grossesse, consommation de tabac/d'alcool, dysfonctionnement hépatique/rénal)

C. Produit(s) de santé soupçonné(s)

1. Nom*, teneur et fabricant (si connu)

N°1

N°2

2. Dose, fréquence et voie d'administration

N°1 N°2

3. Date du traitement (ou durée)

N°1 Du (aaaa-mm-jj) - au (aaaa-mm-jj) | N°2 Du (aaaa-mm-jj) - au (aaaa-mm-jj)

4. Indication pour l'utilisation

N°1 N°2

5. Effet disparu après arrêt d'utilisation ou réduction de dose

N°1 ☐ Oui ☐ Non ☐ Ne s'applique pas | N°2 ☐ Oui ☐ Non ☐ Ne s'applique pas

6. N° de lot	7. Expiration
N°1	N°1 (aaaa-mm-jj)
N°2	N°2 (aaaa-mm-jj)

8. Effet réapparu après réadministration

N°1 ☐ Oui ☐ Non ☐ Ne s'applique pas | N°2 ☐ Oui ☐ Non ☐ Ne s'applique pas

9. Produits de santé concomitants, excluant le traitement de l'effet (nom, dose, fréquence, voie d'administration et date du traitement (aaaa-mm-jj))

10. Traitement de l'effet, incluant les dates (aaaa-mm-jj)

D. Information reliée au déclarant

1. Nom*, profession, adresse, numéro de téléphone*

2. Professionnel(le) de la santé? ☐ Oui ☐ Non

3. Déclaré au fabricant? ☐ Oui ☐ Non

** Selon la Politique du gouvernement du Canada émise par le Secrétariat du Conseil du Trésor du Canada.

Un programme de **MedEffet**[MC] **Canada**

SC Pub. : 100252 (septembre 2012)

Page 1 de 2

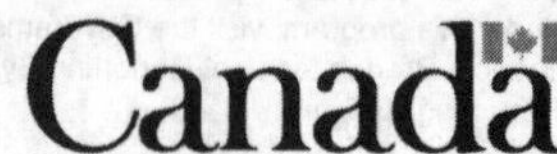

Directives pour compléter le Formulaire de déclaration des effets indésirables Canada Vigilance

- Utilisez ce formulaire seulement pour déclarer les effets indésirables dus aux médicaments d'ordonnance ou en vente libre; les produits de santé naturels; les produits d'origine biologique; les cellules, les tissus et les organes; les produits radiopharmaceutiques; les désinfectants et les produits d'hygiène comportant des allégations de propriétés de désinfection.
- Complétez le présent formulaire en fournissant autant de détails que possible et en utilisant un formulaire distinct pour chaque patient. On peut déclarer jusqu'à deux produits de santé soupçonnés sur un même formulaire. S'il y a plus de deux produits soupçonnés d'être responsables de l'effet indésirable, il faut joindre un autre formulaire. Des pages supplémentaires peuvent être jointes au formulaire au besoin.
- Pour la case « Identification », indiquez un code d'identification quelconque qui vous permettra, à vous le déclarant, de trouver le cas facilement si l'on communique avec vous pour davantage de renseignements; n'employez pas le nom du patient. Voir l'énoncé de confidentialité au bas de cette page.
- Tout renseignement concernant le suivi d'un effet indésirable qui a déjà été déclaré peut être communiqué sur un autre formulaire, signalant qu'il s'agit d'un suivi, incluant, si connus, la date de la déclaration initiale et le numéro d'effet indésirable fournis dans l'accusé de réception.
- **Les déclarations peuvent être envoyées par télécopieur** au 1-866-678-6789 (sans frais) **ou par courrier** à : Santé Canada, Direction des produits de santé commercialisés, Programme Canada Vigilance, Indice postal 0701E, Ottawa (Ontario) K1A 0K9. Des étiquettes d'adresse préaffranchies sont offertes à www.sante.gc.ca/medeffet ou en appelant au 1-866-234-2345 (sans frais). Ne pas soumettre une déclaration par courriel.

Information au sujet de la déclaration d'effets indésirables

Qu'est-ce qu'un effet indésirable?

Un effet indésirable est une réponse nuisible et non voulu à un produit de santé. Ceci inclut tout effet indésirable présumé d'être associé au produit de santé utilisé. L'abus de médicament, la surdose de médicament, les interactions médicamenteuses et les interactions entre les médicaments et les aliments et l'absence inhabituelle d'efficacité sont considérés comme étant des effets indésirables pouvant être déclarés.

Un effet indésirable grave est une réaction qui nécessite/prolonge l'hospitalisation, une malformation congénitale ou une invalidité/incapacité persistante ou importante, met la vie en danger ou entraîne la mort. Les effets indésirables qui nécessitent une intervention médicale importante pour éviter l'un des autres effets énumérés plus haut sont aussi jugés graves.

Quels effets indésirables devrait-on déclarer?

Tous les effets indésirables présumés doivent être déclarés, surtout s'ils sont :

- *imprévus*, peu importe leur gravité (compte tenu des renseignements sur le produit ou de l'étiquetage);
- *graves*, qu'ils soient prévus ou non;
- liés à des *produits récemment mis sur le marché* (commercialisés depuis moins de 5 ans), peu importe leur nature ou leur gravité.

Autres façons de déclarer

Vous pouvez déclarer les effets secondaires des produits de santé au Programme Canada Vigilance :

- par téléphone : 1-866-234-2345 (sans frais)
- en ligne : www.sante.gc.ca/medeffet

Le Formulaire de déclaration des effets indésirables de Canada Vigilance est également disponible en ligne à www.sante.gc.ca/medeffet ou à la fin du *Compendium des produits et spécialités pharmaceutiques* (CPS).

Renseignements supplémentaires

- Une déclaration n'équivaut pas à reconnaître que le personnel médical ou le produit a causé ou contribué à causer l'effet indésirable.
- Les déclarations sont, dans la plupart des cas, des associations soupçonnées. Une association temporelle ou possible peut justifier une déclaration, laquelle n'implique pas un lien causal définitif.
- Les professionnels de la santé et les consommateurs peuvent déclarer les effets indésirables au détenteur d'une autorisation de mise en marché. Indiquez, dans votre déclaration faite à Santé Canada, si le cas a été déclaré au détenteur d'une autorisation de mise en marché pour le produit.
- Pour déclarer un effet secondaire suivant l'immunisation (ESSI) de vaccins administrés pour prévenir des maladies infectieuses, les professionnels de la santé doivent remplir Le formulaire de rapport des effets secondaires suivant l'immunisation, disponible en ligne à http://www.phac-aspc.gc.ca/ im/aefi-form-fra.php Il existe aussi des formulaires propres aux provinces/territoires qu'on peut se procurer auprès des services de santé publique locaux ou des autorités sanitaires des provinces ou territoires.

Pour plus d'information, contactez un bureau régional de Canada Vigilance par téléphone au 1-866-234-2345 (sans frais) ou :

Bureau régional de Canada Vigilance – Colombie-Britannique et Yukon
400-4595, Canada Way, Burnaby (CB) V5G 1J9
CanadaVigilance_BC@hc-sc.gc.ca

Bureau régional de Canada Vigilance – Alberta et Territoires du Nord-Ouest
730-9700, avenue Jasper, Edmonton (AB) T5J 4C3
CanadaVigilance_AB@hc-sc.gc.ca

Bureau régional de Canada Vigilance – Saskatchewan
Bureau 412 – 101, 22e rue E., Saskatoon (SK) S7K 0E1
CanadaVigilance_SK@hc-sc.gc.ca

Bureau régional de Canada Vigilance – Manitoba
510, boul. Lagimodière, Winnipeg (MB) R2J 3Y1
CanadaVigilance_MB@hc-sc.gc.ca

Bureau régional de Canada Vigilance – Ontario et Nunavut
2301, avenue Midland, Toronto (ON) M1P 4R7
CanadaVigilance_ON@hc-sc.gc.ca

Bureau régional de Canada Vigilance – Québec
Bureau 202-40, Tour Est
200, boulevard René-Lévesque Ouest, Montréal (QC) H2Z 1X4
CanadaVigilance_QC@hc-sc.gc.ca

Pour Nouveau-Brunswick, Nouvelle-Écosse, Île-du-Prince-Édouard, Terre-Neuve et Labrador :

Bureau régional de Canada Vigilance – Atlantique
1625-1505, rue Barrington, Halifax (NS) B3J 3Y6
CanadaVigilance_ATL@hc-sc.gc.ca

Confidentialité

Les renseignements personnels recueillis, utilisés ou diffusés dans le cadre du Programme Canada Vigilance sont confidentiels et protégés. De la même manière, les renseignements sur l'identité des patients ou des personnes ayant déclaré les effets secondaires, recueillis par l'entremise du Programme Canada Vigilance, sont protégés comme renseignements personnels en vertu de la *Loi sur la protection des renseignements personnels* et, dans les cas de demande d'accès à l'information, en vertu de la *Loi sur l'accès à l'information*. La présentation des renseignements demandés sur ce formulaire estfacultative. Les renseignements tirés des déclarations d'effets indésirables sont maintenus dans une base de données informatisée et sont utiliséesdans le cadre de l'évaluation des produits de santé commercialisés, ce qui peut contribuer à la détection de problèmes potentiels en matière d'innocuitéainsi qu'à l'évaluation de leurs bienfaits et de leurs risques. Pour en connaître davantage sur les renseignements recueillis dans le cadre de ce programme, veuillez consulter la section « Système de déclaration des incidents » (Direction générale des produits de santé et des aliments) (numéro du fichier : Scan PPU 088) de la page « Fichiers de renseignements personnels spécifiques aux institutions » (http://infosource.gc.ca/inst/shc/fed07-fra.asp).

Page 2 de 2

RESOURCE SECTION

PROVINCIAL WORKERS' COMPENSATION BOARDS

THE WORKERS' COMPENSATION HEALTH AND SAFETY BOARD - YUKON

401 Strickland St, WHITEHORSE, YT Y1A 5N8
Tel. (867) 667-5645 Fax: (867) 393-6279 Web: wcb.yk.ca

President & CEO, Joy Waters
Vice President of Operations & CFO, Jim Stephens
Director of Claimant Services, Karen Branigan
Medical Consultant, Dr. Allon Reddoch
Medical Administrative Assistant, Donna Chambers

THE WORKERS' SAFETY AND COMPENSATION COMMISSION - NORTHWEST TERRITORIES AND NUNAVUT

5022 49th St, 5th Floor, Centre Square Tower PO Box 8888, YELLOWKNIFE, NT X1A 2R3
Tel. (867) 920-3888 Fax: (867) 873-4596 Toll Free Tel: 1-800-661-0792 Toll Free Fax: 1-866-277-3677

Box 669, Qamutiq Building, 2nd Floor, IQALUIT, NU X0A 0H0
Tel: (867) 979-8500 Fax: (867) 979-8501 Toll Free Tel: 1-877-404-4407 Toll Free Fax: 1-866-979-8501

151 Mackenzie Rd, 3rd Floor Mack Travel Bldg, Box 1188, INUVIK, NT X0E 0T0
Tel. (867) 678-2301 Fax: (867) 678-2302

Chair, William (Bill) Aho
President & CEO, Dave Grundy
VP, Prevention Services, Cara Benoit
VP, Corporate Services, Harmeet Jagpal
Senior Advisor/Corporate Secretary, Melanie Walters
Occupation Health & Safety Nurses, Angela Fraser & LeeAnna Carson
VP, Executive Services , Edith Johnston-Ryder
VP, Skateholder Services, Kim Collins Riffel
VP, Financial Services, Len MacDonald
Associate VP, Susan Abernethy
General Counsel, Shirley Walsh

WORKSAFEBC

6951 Westminster Hwy, RICHMOND, BC V7C 1C8
or PO Box 5350 Stn. Terminal, VANCOUVER, BC V6B 5L5
Tel. (604) 273-2266 Fax: (604) 276-3191 Web: www.worksafebc.com

Chair, Public Interest, George Morfitt
President & Chief Executive Officer, David Anderson
Senior Vice-President, Human Resources & Corporate Affairs, Roberta Ellis
Senior Vice-President, Operations, Diana Miles
Vice-President, Industry Services & Sustainability, Donna Wilson
General Counsel & Secretary to WorkSafeBC, Ed Bates
Health Care & Rehabilitation Representative, Henry Harder
Employer Representative, Joe Lindgren
Vice Chair, Public Interest Representative, Rick Roger
Public Interest Representative, Tazeem Nathoo
Actuarist, Alan Cooke
Director of Governance, John Panusa

WORKERS' COMPENSATION BOARD - ALBERTA

9925-107 St, PO Box 2415, EDMONTON, AB T5J 2S5
Tel. (780) 498-4000 Fax: (780) 498-7878

President & Chief Executive Officer, Guy Kerr
Vice-President, Information & Disability Management, Wendy King
Chief Financial Officer, Ron Helmhold
Secretary & General Counsel, Douglas R. Mah
Vice-President, Employee & Corporate Services, Roxy Shulha-Mckay
Vice-President, Customer Service & Risk Management, Dieter Brunsch

APPEALS COMMISSION FOR ALBERTA WORKERS' COMPENSATION

Edmonton Office
Energy Square Building
901, 10109 - 106 St, Edmonton, AB T5J 3L7
Tel. (780) 412-8700 Fax: (780) 412-8701 Web: www.appealscommission.ab.ca

Calgary Office
Braithwaite Boyle Building
206, 1701 Centre Street North, Calgary, AB T2E 7Y2
Tel. (403) 508-8800 Fax: (403) 508-8822 Web: www.appealscommission.ab.ca

Chairman & Chief Appeals Commissioner, Mr. Douglass M. Tadman

THE WORKERS' COMPENSATION BOARD - SASKATCHEWAN

200-1881 Scarth St, REGINA, SK S4P 4L1
Tel. (306) 787-4370 Fax: (306) 787-0213 1-800-667-7590 Web: www.wcbsask.com

Chair, David Eberle
Board Member, Karen Smith
Board Member, Walter Eberle
Chief Executive Officer, Peter D. Federko
Vice-President, Operations, Graham Topp
Vice-President, Prevention & Employer Services, Phil Germain
Vice-President, Administration, Mick Williams
Chief Financial Officer, Ann Schultz
Vice-President, Human Resources & Communications, Donna Kane

THE WORKERS COMPENSATION BOARD OF MANITOBA

333 Broadway, WINNIPEG, MB R3C 4W3
Tel. (204) 954-4922 Fax. (204) 954-4999 Email: wcb@wcb.mb.ca Web: wcb.mb.ca

Chairperson, Michael Werier
President & Chief Executive Officer, Winston Maharaj
Chief Financial Officer, Finance & Administrative Services, Lorena Trann
Vice-President, Compensation Services, Darren Oryniak
Vice-President, People, Technology & Innovation Services, David Scott
Vice-President, Strategy & Assessment Services, Alice Sayant
Chief Appeal Commissioner, Alan Scramstad

WORKPLACE, SAFETY & INSURANCE BOARD - ONTARIO

200 Front St W, TORONTO, ON M5V 3J1
Tel. (416) 344-4433 Fax. (416) 344-4366 Web: www.wsib.on.ca

Chair, Elizabeth Witmer
President and CEO, I. David Marshall
General Counsel, VP Compliance Services & Corporate Secretary, Brenda Abrams
Acting Chief Corporate Services Officer and Vice-President, Prevention, Steve Jackson
Chief Operating Officer, John Slinger
Chief Financial Officer, Lawrence Davis
Acting Vice-President, Human Resources & Executive Director, Strategic Transformation Branch, Rod Cook
Vice-President & Chief Information Officer, Business Technology Services, John Hill
Chief Investment Officer, John Denham
Vice-President, Health Services Division, Donna Bain
Vice-President & Chief Actuary, Actuarial Services, Don Blue
Vice-President, Work Reintegration Program & Provider Effectiveness, Linda Kelly
Vice-President, Communications and Public Affairs Division, Catherine Allman
Director, Serious Injury Services, Sal Cavaricci
Director, Health Services Program & Provider Effectiveness, Richard Morrison
Director, Occupational Disease & Survivor Benefits Program, Irene Dias

COMMISSION DE LA SANTÉ ET DE LA SÉCURITÉ DU TRAVAIL DU QUÉBEC (CSST)

1199, rue de Bleury, C.P. 6056, Succursale Centre-Ville, MONTRÉAL, QC H3C 4E1 Tél. (514) 906-3503 Fax: (514) 906-3781
524, rue Bourdages, C.P. 1200, Terminus Postal, QUÉBEC, QC G1K 7E2 Tél. (418) 266-4414 Fax: (418) 266-4369 Web: www.csst.qc.ca

Chairman of the Board and Chief Executive Officer, Michel Després
Vice President, Administration, Communications & Public Relations, Carole Théberge
Vice President, Finance, André Beauchemin
Vice President, Operations, Gaétan Theriault
Vice President, Partnership & Expert Consulting, Claude Sicard
Vice President, Information System, Michel Dumas
Director of Corporate Affairs and Secretary General, Paul Gendron
Director, Communications, Josée Delisle
Director, Crime Victims Compensation, Suzanne Mailhot
Director, Legal Services (Québec), Pierre Vigneault
Assistant Director, Legal Services (Montréal), Carole Bergeron
Assistant Director, Legal Services (Québec), Nancy Thibodeau
Director, Medical Services, Sylvie Verrette
Director, Administrative Review, Jeannine Dubé (Interim)

THE WORKERS COMPENSATION BOARD - PRINCE EDWARD ISLAND

PO Box 757, CHARLOTTETOWN, PE C1A 7L7
Tel. (902) 368-5680 Fax: (902) 368-5705 Web: www.wcb.pe.ca

Chairperson, Nancy Guptill
Chief Executive Officer, Sharon Cameron
Medical Advisor, Dr. Steve O'Brien
Director of Client Services, Wendy McIsaac
Director of Corporate Services, Tammy Turner
Director of Corporate Development, Bonnie Blakney
Director of Occupational Health & Safety, Bill Reid

RESOURCE SECTION

WORKSAFENB

1 Portland St, PO Box 160, SAINT JOHN, NB E2L 3X9
Tel. (506) 632-2200 Fax: (506) 632-4999 Web: www.worksafenb.ca

Chairperson of the Board of Directors, Sharon Tucker
Chairperson, Appeals Tribunal, Ronald Gaffney
President & CEO, Gerald M Adams
Executive Assistant to the President & CEO and Chariperson, Diane Green
Corporate Secretary & General Counsel, Christine Fagan
Vice-President, WorkSafe Services, Shelly Dauphinee
Vice-President, Corporate Services, Peter Murphy
Chief Medical Officer, Dr. Douglas Margison
Director, Program Development & Evaluation, Barbara Keir

THE WORKERS' COMPENSATION BOARD - NOVA SCOTIA

Halifax Office

5668 South St, PO Box 1150, HALIFAX, NS B3J 2Y2
Tel. (902) 491-8999 Fax: (902) 491-8002 Email: info@wcb.gov.ns.ca Web: www.worksafeforlife.ca

Chief Executive Officer, Stuart MacLean . . . . (902) 491-8304
Chief Financial Officer, Leo McKenna . . . . (902) 491-8402
Executive Corporate Secretary, Brad Fraser. . . . . . . (902) 491-8303
VP, Prevention & Service Delivery, Shelley Rowan . . . . (902) 491-8901
VP, People & Planning, Wendy Griffin . . . . (902) 491-8323
Chair, Board of Directors, Elaine Sibson. . . . . (902) 491-8380
Deputy Chair, Board of Directors, Chris Power . . . . (902) 491-8380
Financial Analyst, Kim Garnier . . . . (902) 491-8401
Director, Finance, Maureen Boyd . . . . (902) 491-8406
Director, Partnerships, Mary Kingston . . . . (902) 491-8101
Director, Communications, Steve McDonald. . . . . . (902) 491-8105
Director, Human Resources, Carla Hurley . . . . (902) 491-8508
Director, Business Transformation, Dennita Fitzpatrick. (902) 491-8351
Director, Workplace Services, Erin Flannery. . . . . . . (902) 491-8375
Director, Information Technology Services, George Crowdis . . . . (902) 491-8722
Director, Service Delivery Large Workplace, Andrea Vardy . . . . (902) 491-8828
Director, Central Services, John Banks . . . . (902) 491-8068
Director, Business Intelligence, Sandra Keefe . . . . . (902) 491-8405
Director, Cape Breton Service Unit, Rob MacDonald . . (902) 563-2083

WORKPLACE HEALTH, SAFETY AND COMPENSATION COMMISSION - NEWFOUNDLAND & LABRADOR

St. John's

146-148 Forest Road, PO Box 9000, St. John's, NL A1A 3B8
Tel. (709) 778-1000 Fax: (709) 738-1714
Toll Free: 1-800-563-9000
general.inquiries@whscc.nl.ca
Web: www.whscc.nl.ca

Grand Falls-Windsor

26 High Street, PO Box 850, Grand Falls-Windsor, NL A2A 2P7
Tel. (709) 489-1600 Fax: (709) 489-1616
Toll Free: 1-800-563-3448
general.inquiries@whscc.nl.ca

Corner Brook

Suite 201B Millbrook Mall 2 Herald Ave, PO Box 474, Corner Brook, NL A2H 6E6
Tel. (709) 637-2700 Fax: (709) 639-1018
Toll Free: 1-800-563-2772
general.inquiries@whscc.nl.ca

Chief Executive Officer, Leslie Galway
Executive Director, Worker Services, Tom Mahoney
Executive Director, Employer Services, Brenda Greenslade
Executive Director, Corporate Services, Eric Bartlett
Executive Director, Chief Financial/Information Officer, Paul Kavanagh
General Counsel and Corporate Secretary, Ann Martin
Director, Assessment Services, Lena Griffis
Director, Information Technology Services, Joan McCarthy-Wiseman
Director, Worker Services-Occupational Disease, Fabian Philpott
Director, Compensation Services, Craig Noseworthy
Director, Prevention Services, Charlie Coady
Director, Health Care Services, Dr. Carrie Comerford
Director, Regional Office, Grand Falls-Windsor, Brenda Hayter
Director, Regional Office, Corner Brook, Derek Murphy
Director, Communications, Chris Flanagan
Director, Human Resources & Facilities Management, Glenda Peet
Director, Corporate Governance and Planning, Anna Tapper
Director, Internal Audit, Kevin Lannigan
Sr. Health Care Services Assistant, Leah Atkinson

DEPARTMENT OF HEALTH & COMMUNITY SERVICES NEWFOUNDLAND & LABRADOR

1st Floor, West Block, Confederation Bldg, PO Box 8700, St. John's, NL A1B 4J6
Tel.: (709) 729-4984 Fax: (709) 729-0121 Email: healthinfo@gov.nl.ca Web: www.health.gov.nl.ca/health

MINISTER'S OFFICE

Minister, The Honourable Susan Sullivan . . . . (709) 729-3124
Administrative Assistant, Colleen Power . . . . (709) 729-3124
Executive Assistant, Lisa Lindall . . . . (709) 729-5980
Parliamentary Secretary, Sandy Collins . . . . (709) 729-1390

DEPUTY MINISTER'S OFFICE

Deputy Minister, Bruce Cooper . . . . (709) 729-3125
Administrative Assistant, Pam Bennett. . . . . (709) 729-3125
Program Coordinator, Rhonda Fleming . . . . (709) 729-6162
Director of Communications, Jennifer Tulk . . . . (709) 729-1377
Administrative Assistant, Geri Young . . . . (709) 729-2667
Marketing Consultant, Gillian Hussey . . . . (709) 729-6986
Communications Manager, Blair Medd. . . . . (709) 729-1399

MEDICAL CARE PLAN

Regional Director, Glenn Budgell . . . . (709)292-4009
Assistant Executive Director, Tony Maher. . . . . (709)758-1599
Manager, Medical Affairs, Dr. Blair Fleming . . . . (709)292-4003

MEDICAL SERVICES BRANCH

Associate Deputy Minister, Dr. Cathi Bradbury . . . . . (709) 729-1574
Director, Pharmaceutical Services, Keith Sheppard . . . . . (709) 729-6507
Assistant Deputy Minister (Acting), Population Health Branch, Colleen Stockley . . . . . (709) 729-1716
Director, Physician Services, Dr Larry Alteen . . . . . (709) 729-3508

REGIONAL HEALTH OPERATIONS (709) 729-3105

Assistant Deputy Minister (Acting), Beverly Griffiths . . (709) 729-3103
Administrative Assistant, Mary Crotty, ... (709) 729-5265
Director, Board Services, Debbie Morris . . . . (709)729-0717
Secretary, Connie Fry. (709)729-3105

POLICY & PLANNING BRANCH

Assistant Deputy Minister, Tracy King . . . . (709) 729-3103
Administrative Assistant, Elaine Power. . . . . (709) 729-3103
Director, Policy Development, Wanda Legge . . . . (709) 729-3421
Legislative Analyst, Suzanne Osborne . . . . (709) 729-2472

CORPORATE SERVICES BRANCH

Assistant Deputy Minister, Denise Tubrett . . . . (709) 729-0620
Administrative Assistant, Denise French . . . . (709) 729-0620

PUBLIC HEALTH BRANCH

Chief Medical Officer, Dr. Faith Stratton . . . . (709) 729-3430
Administrative Assistant, Juanita Follett . . . . (709) 729-3430

NOTIFICATION TO MEDICAL EXAMINERS (Newfoundland and Labrador)

Dr. Simon P. Avis, Chief Medical Examiner
Province of Newfoundland and Labrador
300 Prince Philip Dr
St. John's, NL A1B 3V6
(709) 777-6402 Fax: (709) 777-6975
E-mail: ocme@gov.nl.ca

Attention is directed to the following sections in the Act Respecting the Investigation of Fatalities, 1995, Chapter F-6.1:

5. A person having knowledge of or reason to believe that a person has died under one of the following circumstances shall immediately notify a medical examiner or an investigator:
(a) as a result of violence, accident or suicide;
(b) unexpectedly when the person was in good health;
(c) where the person was not under the care of a physician;
(d) where the cause of death is undetermined; or
(e) as a result of improper or suspected negligent treatment by a person.

6. (1) Where a person dies while in a health care facility, or another place where patients are received for treatment or care and there is reason to believe that,
(a) the death occurred as a result of violence, attempted suicide or accident, no matter how long the patient had been hospitalized:
(b) the death occurred as a result of suspected misadventure, negligence or accident on the part of the attending physician or staff;
(c) the cause of death is undetermined;
(d) the death occurred during or following pregnancy in circumstances that might reasonably be related to pregnancy;
(e) a stillbirth or a neonatal death has occurred where maternal injury has occurred or is suspected, either prior to admission or during delivery; or
(f) the death occurred within 10 days of an operative procedure or the patient is under initial induction, under anaesthesia or during the recovery from anaesthesia.

the person responsible for that facility shall immediately notify a medical examiner or an investigator.

(2) Where a person is declared dead on arrival or dies in the emergency department of a health care facility as a result of a condition referred to in section 5, the person responsible for that facility shall immediately notify a medical examiner or an investigator.

7. Where a person dies
(a) while detained in a correctional institution, such as a jail, penitentiary, guard room, remand centre, detention centre, youth facility, lock-up or any other place where a person is in custody;
(b) while an inmate or patient in treatment facilities or parts, or psychiatric divisions of treatment facilities or parts, or classes of treatment facilities designated under the Mental Health Act;
(c) while in the custody of the Director of Child Welfare: or
(d) while in the custody of a peace officer.

the person in charge of that institution or the person having the custody of that person shall immediately notify a medical examiner or an investigator.

8. Where a person dies as a result of
(a) a disease or ill-health;
(b) an injury sustained by the person; or
(c) a toxic substance introduced into the person,

probably caused by the person's employment or occupation or in the course of one or more of his or her former employments or occupations, the person attending the person shall immediately notify a medical examiner or an investigator.

RESOURCE SECTION

DEPARTMENT OF HEALTH PRINCE EDWARD ISLAND

95-105 Rochford Street, PO Box 2000, Charlottetown, PEI, C1A 7N8
Gen Enquiries:Tel. (902) 368-6414 Fax. (902) 368-4121 Web: www.gov.pe.ca/health

MINISTER'S OFFICE

Minister, Honourable Doug Currie (902) 368-5250

Deputy Minister, Dr. Michael Mayne . . . . . . (902) 368-5290
. . . . . . Fax: (902) 368-4121

Chief Public Health Officer, Dr. Heather Morrison . . . . (902) 368-4996
. . . . . . Fax: (902) 620-3354

Director, Finance & Corporate Management,
Kevin Barnes . . . . . . (902) 894-0399
. . . . . . Fax: (902) 368-4224

Manager, Recruitment & Retention Secretariat,
Marney MacRae . . . . . . (902) 620-3874
. . . . . . Fax: (902) 620-3875

Director, Sport Recreation & Healthy Living,
John Morrison . . . . . . (902) 620-3875
. . . . . . Fax: (902) 368-4224

A/Director of Health Policy & Planning,
Kevin Barnes . . . . . . (902) 894-0399
. . . . . . Fax: (902) 368-4224

HEALTH PEI

A/CEO, Dr. Richard Wedge (902) 368-4935

Board Chair, Leo Steven (902) 368-5810

Executive Director, Corporate Development & Innovation,
Pamela Trainor . . . . . . (902) 368-5804
. . . . . . Fax: (902) 368-4969

Executive Director, Community Hospitals & Primary Health Care,
Deborah Bradley . . . . . . (902) 368-6157
. . . . . . Fax: (902) 569-0579

Executive Director, Financial Services,
Denise Lewis Fleming . . . . . . (902) 368-6125
. . . . . . Fax: (902) 368-6136

Executive Director, Home-Based & Long-Term Care,
Cecil Villard . . . . . . (902) 894-0337
. . . . . . Fax: (902) 368-6136

Executive Director, Medical Affairs, Dr. Richard Wedge (902) 368-6261
. . . . . . Fax: (902) 620-3072

Executive Director, Health Information Management,
Liam Whitty . . . . . . (902) 368-3165
. . . . . . Fax: (902) 368-6136

Executive Director, Prince County Hospital,
Arlene Gallant-Bernard . . . . . . (902) 438-4514
. . . . . . Fax: (902) 438-4381

Executive Director, Queen Elizabeth Hospital,
Rick Adams . . . . . . (902) 894-2351
. . . . . . Fax: (902) 894-2416

Executive Director, Provincial Clinical Services,
Jamie MacDonald . . . . . . (902) 569-7768
. . . . . . Fax: (902) 368-6136

NOTIFICATION TO CORONERS (Prince Edward Island)

Dr. Charles St. Clair Trainor
Chief Coroner
Chief Coroner's Office
2 Myrtle St
Stratford, PE C1B 2W2
Tel. (902) 628-6974 Fax: (902) 566-3934 Web: www.gov.pe.ca/oag/

5. (1) Where a death has occurred in the province, or as a result of events that occurred in the province, every person shall immediately report the death to a coroner or a police officer, if the person has reason to believe that the death

(a) occurred as a result of violence, accident, suicide, or other cause other than disease, sickness or old age;

(b) occurred as a result of negligence or misconduct or malpractice;

(c) occurred suddenly or unexpectedly when the deceased had been in apparent good health;

(d) occurred under circumstances in which the body is not available because the body or part of the body

(i) has been destroyed
(i) is in a place from which it cannot be recovered, or
(i) cannot be located

(e) occurred within 10 days after a surgical procedure or while the deceased was under or recovering from anaesthesia;

(f) occurred as a direct or immediate consequence of the deceased being engaged in employment, an occupation or a business;

(g) was a stillbirth that occurred without the presence of a duly qualified medical practitioner;

(h) occurred while the deceased was detained or in custody involuntarily pursuant to law in a jail, lock-up, correctional facility, medical facility or other institution;

(i) occurred while the deceased was detained by or in the custody of a police officer

(j) occurred while the deceased was under the care, custody or supervision of the Director of Child Welfare; or

(k) occurred in circumstances that require investigstion,

the Coroner, whether the cause of death arose within his jurisdiction or not, shall, as soon as practicable, issue his warrant to take possession of the body and shall view the body and make such further investigation as may be required to enable him to determine whether or not an inquest is necessary.

DEPARTMENT OF HEALTH AND WELLNESS

Joseph Howe Building, 1690 Hollis St, PO Box 488, Halifax, N.S. B3J 2R8
Tel. (902) 424-5818 Toll Free 1-800-387-6665 Departmental TTY 1-800-670-8888 Fax (902) 424-0730
E-mail: dohweb@gov.ns.ca Web: www.gov.ns.ca/heal

MINISTER'S OFFICE

Fax (902) 424-0559

Minister, Hon. David A. Wilson . . . . . (902) 424-3377
Sr Policy Advisor, Jen Smith . . . . . (902) 424-1691
Executive Secretary, Wendy Anderson . . . . . (902) 424-3377
Executive Assistant, Jenny Benson . . . . . (902) 424-7952

DEPUTY MINISTER'S OFFICE

Fax (902)424-4570

Deputy Minister, Kevin McNamara . . . . . (902) 424-7570
Executive Secretary, Joanne Bolger . . . . . (902) 424-7570
Legal Counsel, Sara Gorelick . . . . . (902) 424-3585
Director, Human Resources, Colette Curran . . . . . (902) 424-2049

PUBLIC HEALTH BRANCH

Fax (902) 424-4716

Chief Public Health Officer, Dr. Robert Strang . . . . . (902) 424-2358
Administrative Assistant, Kelly Dean . . . . . (902) 424-2358

FINANCIAL SERVICES BRANCH

Fax (902) 424-0615

Chief Financial Officer, Linda Penny . . . . . (902) 424-5948
Executive Assistant, Irene Dockendorff . . . . . (902) 424-5948

OFFICE OF THE CHIEF OF PROGRAM DELIVERY

Fax (902) 424-4570

Chief of Program Delivery, Paula English . . . . . Tel.(902) 424-3730
Administrative Assistant, Sandra Bennett . . . . . Tel.(902) 424-3730

CHIEF INFORMATION OFFICER

Fax (902) 424-0763

Chief Information Officer, Sandra Cascadden . . . Tel: (902) 424-4838
Administrative Assistant, Jane Whittaker . . . . . Tel: (902) 424-4514

MENTAL HEALTH, CHILD HEALTH & ADDICTION TREATMENT SERVICES

Fax (902) 424-0647

Executive Director, Lynn Cheek . . . . . (902) 424-7895
Administrative Assistant, Colleen Hartling . . . . . (902) 424-7895

ACUTE & TERTIARY CARE

Fax (902) 424-0605

Executive Director, Sandra Christie . . . . . (902) 424-4489
Administrative Assistant, Donna Mattie . . . . . (902) 424-4489

CONTINUING CARE

Fax (902) 424-0558

Executive Director, Ruby Knowles, ... (902) 424-3221
Administrative Assistant, Heather Miller, ... (902) 424-7233

NOTIFICATION TO MEDICAL EXAMINERS (Nova Scotia)

Dr. Mathew J. Bowes, MD, FRCPC
Chief Medical Examiner for Nova Scotia
51 Garland Ave
Dartmouth, NS B3B 0J2
(902) 424-0607 Fax: (902) 424-8349

When the medical cause of death is unknown (unexplained) or of unnatural origin (violence; injury/poisoning) a medical examiner must be informed. The medical examiner will investigate (together with police and others as required) and usually complete the medical certificate of death. Examples include vehicular, industrial, self-inflicted and homicidal injuries, or where the medical cause albeit apparently natural, is not reasonably explained. An attending doctor should not sign the certificate of death in these cases but rather notify the medical examiner's office or local municipal police/RCMP.

Note: The Chief Medical Examiner's Office is an independent agency affiliated with the Department of Justice.

DEPARTMENT OF HEALTH NEW BRUNSWICK

HSBC Place, PO Box 5100, Fredericton, NB, E3B 5G8 General Inquiries (506) 453-2536 Fax: (506) 444-4697
Web: www.gnb.ca

Minister of Health, Hugh J Flemming, QC

Policy Advisor, Peter Josselyn
Executive Assistant, Cal Cipolla
Deputy Minister, Health, Marc Léger
Associate Deputy Minister of Health , Lyne St-Pierre Ellis
Assistant Deputy Minister, Addictions and Mental Health Services Division, Ken Ross
Director, Governance Transition Office, Lise Daigle

Assistant Deputy Minister, Corporate Services, Tom Maston
Director, Communication Branch, Tracey Burkhardt
Chief Ex Officers, NB Cancer Network, Dr. S. Eshwar Kumar & Dr Réjean Savoie
Assistant Deputy Minister, Planning, Sustainability and E-Health, Kelli Simmonds
Human Resources Director, Joanne Stone

PUBLIC HEALTH AND MEDICAL SERVICES DIVISION

Chief Medical Health Officer, Dr. Eilish Cleary
Executive Director, Health Protection, Scott MacLean

Deputy Chief Medical Officer of Health, Dennis Allard
Executive Director, Operations, Luc Sirois

Medical Officers of Health

Saint John	Dr. Scott Giffin 55 Union St, Saint John, NB
Fredericton	Dr. Cristin Muecke 300 St Mary's St, Fredericton, NB
Edmundston	Dr. Yves Leger 121 Church St, Edmundston, NB
Bathurst	Dr. Yves Leger 165 St. Andrew St, Bathurst, NB
Campbellton	Dr. Yves Leger 6 Arran St, Campbellton, NB
Fredericton	Dr. Alexander Doroshenko 520 King St, Fredericton, NB

Director, Communicable Disease Control, Cheryl Yates
Director, Public Health & Population Health, Claudette Landry
Director, Healthy Environments, Karen White

INSTITUTION SERVICES

Senior Consultant, Institutional Services, John McGarry
Director, Hospital Operations, Kathy Perrin

Director, Hospital Clinical Services, Francine Bordage

ADDICTION, MENTAL HEALTH AND PRIMARY HEALTH CARE SERVICES

Director, Addictions & Mental Health, Barb Whitenect
Director, Quality Management & Executive Support, John Esley
Director, Child & Adolescent Services, Yvette Doiron-Brun

Director, Primary Care, Bronwyn Davies
Director, Adult Services, Sylvie Martin
Director, Extra Mural Program, Jean Bustard

CORPORATE SERVICES

Director, IT Services, Dawn O' Donnell
Director, Contact Management & Corporate Support Services, Mark Thompson
Executive Director, Financial Services, Renée La Forest
Director, Accontability and Health Information Management, John Boyne

Director, Federal-Provincial Relations, Tom Fetter
Director, Health Emergency Management Services, Joanne Rosevear
Executive Director, Health, Business & Technology Solutions, Cheryl Hansen

OFFICE OF THE ASSOCIATE DEPUTY MINISTER

Associate Deputy Minister and Acting Assistant Deputy Minister, Institutional Services, Lyne St-Pierre Ellis
Nursing Resources Advisor, Mary Okeefe-Robak
Health Human Resource Advisor, Michèle Roussel
Physician Resources Advisor, Eric Levesque

Medicare-Insured Services & Physician Remuneration, Michel Léger
Acting Director, Salaried Physician Services, Nada Sarkis
Director, Medicare, Eligibility & Claims, Carole Sharpe
Director, Health Human Resources Information, James Ayles

PLANNING, PHARMACEUTICAL SERVICES AND PRIVACY

Assistant Deputy Minister, Kelly Simmonds

Director, Pharmaceutical Services, Leanne Jardine
Privacy Officer, Sara Smallwood

NOTIFICATION TO CORONERS (New Brunswick)

Gregory Forestell, Chief Coroner
Department of Public Safety
364 Argyle, 3rd Floor, PO Box 6000
Frederiction, NB E3B 5H1
(506) 453-3604 Fax: (506) 453-7124
E-mail: greg.forestell@gnb.ca

Attention is drawn to 31 (1) of the Vital Statistics Act:

Section 31 (1) If there is reason to believe that a person has died under any of the circumstances set out in section 4 of the Coroners Act, no acknowledgement of registration of death and no burial permit shall be issued unless

- (a) the body has been examined by a coroner or the coroner has made inquiry into the circumstances of the death or held an inquest as provided by the Coroners Act,
- (b) the coroner has signed the medical certificate of cause of death portion of the death registration form, and
- (c) the other provisions of this Act regarding the registration of the death have been complied with.

Coroner's Act:

Section 4 Every person who has reason to believe that a person died

- (a) as a result of
  - (i) violence
  - (ii) misadventure
  - (iii) negligence
  - (iv) misconduct, or
  - (v) malpractice,
  - (a.1) during pregnancy or following pregnancy in circumstances that might reasonably be attributable to the pregnancy;
  - (a.2) suddenly and unexpectedly;
  - (a.3) from disease or sickness for which there was no treatment given by a medical practitioner;
- (b) from any cause other than disease or natural causes; or
- (c) under such circumstances as may require investigation;

shall, unless he knows that a coroner has already been notified, immediately notify a coroner of the facts and circumstances relating to the death. R.S., c.41; s.4, 1971, c.20, s.3; 1999, c.11, s.2.

RESOURCE SECTION

MINISTÈRE DE LA SANTÉ ET DES SERVICES SOCIAUX

1075, chemin Sainte-Foy, Québec G1S 2M1
Renseignements généraux: Québec: (418) 266-8900 Renseignements: 1-800-707-3380
Courrier: info@msss.gouv.qc.ca Adresse internet: www.msss.gouv.qc.ca

CABINET DES MINISTRES

Télécopieur: (418) 266-7197

Ministre de la Santé et des Services sociaux et ministre responsable des ainés, Dr. Réjean Hébert
Directrice de cabinet, France Amyot . . . . (418) 266-7171
Ministre déleguée aux Services sociaux et à la Protection de la jeunesse,, Dominique Hivon
Directeur de cabinet, Monique Richard. . . . . (418) 266-7181

DIRECTION SUPÉRIEURE

Sous-ministre, Jacques Cotton . . . . (418) 266-8989
Secrétariat général, André Giguère . . . . (418) 266-8989
Secrétariat administratif, Anne-Marie Tremblay . . . (418) 266-7140
Service de l'accès à l'information et de la propriété intellectuelle, Claude Lamarre . . . . (418) 266-7005
Direction des affaires juridiques, Jean-Paul Dupré. . . . (418) 266-8950
Direction des communications, Michèle St-Jean . . . . (418) 266-8905
Direction des relations ministérielles et de la vérification interne, Dominique Breton. . . . . (418) 266-8989
Direction québécoise de cancérologie, Jean Rodrigue . (418)266-6940

PLANIFICATION, PERFORMANCE ET QUALITÉ

Sous-ministre adjoint, Luc Castonguay . . . . (418) 266-5990
Direction générale adjointe de la performance, Éric Fournier . . . . (418) 266-7025
Direction des l'évaluation, Harold Côté . . . . (418) 266-7025
Direction des études et des analyses, Éric Fournier . . . . (418) 266-7025
Direction de la qualité, Sylvie Bernier. . . . . (418) 266-7505
Direction des affaires intergouvernementales et de la coopération internationale, Anne Marcoux . . . (418) 266-8740
Direction des affaires pharmaceutiques et du médicament, Hélène Beaulieu . . . . (418) 266-8810
Direction de la planification et des orientations stratégiques, Lynda Fortin . . . . (418) 266-7088
Direction de la recherche de l'innovation et du transfert des connaissances, Manon St-Pierre . . . . (418) 266-7056

SANTÉ PUBLIQUE

Sous-ministre adjoint, Horacio Arruda . . . . (418) 266-6700
Direction de la protection de la santé publique, Danielle Auger . . . . (514) 873-1587
Direction du développement des individus et de l'environnement social, André Dontigny . . . . . . (418) 266-6714
Direction de la planification, de l'évaluation et du développement en santé publique, Lyne Jobin. . . . (418) 266-6780
Direction de la surveillance de l'état de santé, Lyne Jobin (par interim) . . . . (418) 266-6778
Direction de la prévention des maladies chroniques et des traumatismes, Marie Rochette . . . . (418) 266-6750

SERVICES DE SANTÉ ET MÉDECINE UNIVERSITAIRE

Sous-ministre adjointe, Jean Rodrigue. . . . . (418) 266-6930
Direction de la main-d'oeuvre médicale, Isabelle Savard . . . . (418) 266-6975
Direction des soins infirmiers, Danielle Fleury . . . . (418) 266-8485
Direction de la santé mentale, André Delorme . . . . . (418) 266-6835
Direction nationale des urgences, des services de traumatologie et des services préhospitaliers d'urgence, François Scarborough (par interim) . . . . (418) 266-6948
Direction des services hospitaliers et des affaires universitaires, Louis Dufresne . . . . (418) 266-7500
Direction des services généraux, Jeannine Auger . . . (418) 266-5827
Direction de l'accès, des technologiques et de la biologie médicale, Yves Jalbert . . . . (418) 266-6946
Direction de l'organisation des services de première ligne intégres, Antoine Groulx . . . . . . (418) 266-6976

PERSONNEL RÉSEAU ET MINISTÉRIEL

Sous-ministre adjointe, Édith Lapointe . . . . (418) 266-8400
Direction des ressources humaines, ministérielles, Claude Tremblay . . . . (418) 266-8710
Direction génerale adjointe des relations de travail et professionnelles, Alexandre Hubert. . . . . (418) 266-8408
Direction du personnel syndiqué, Alexandre Hubert (par interim). . . . . (418) 266-8408
Direction du personnel de la santé et du personnel d'encadrement, Yves Lapointe . . . . (418) 266-8420
Direction du personnel hors-établissement et de la classification réseau, Luc Bouchard . . . . (418) 266-8410
Direction des relations professionnelles avec les fédérations médicales, Marco Thibault . . . . (418) 266-8430
Direction de la planification de la main-d'oeuvre et du soutien au changement, Gilles Le Beau . . . . . . (418) 266-8835
Direction de l'analyse et du soutien informationnel, Marie-Pierre Legault . . . . (418) 266-8450

TECHNOLOGIES DE L'INFORMATION

Sous-ministre associée, Lisé Verreault . . . . (418) 266-8770
Direction génerale adjointe des projets (DSQ), Gilles Simard (par intérim) . . . . (514) 597-2066
Direction des relations d'affaires avec les clienteles, Clermont Saucier . . . . (418) 266-6935
Direction des relations avec les partenaires et les mandataires, Clermont Saucier (par intérim) . . . . (418) 266-6935
Direction de la sécurité des technologies de l'information, Sonia Ray . . . . (418) 266-6935
Direction des services financiers et administratifs, Philippe Moss . . . . (418) 266-7118
Direction du soutien ministériel et des infrastructures communes, Michel Rochette . . . . (418) 266-2287

SERVICES SOCIAUX

Sous-ministre associé, Sylvain Gagnon . . . . (418) 266-6800
Secrétariat à l'adoption internationale, Luce de Bellefeuille . . . . (514) 873-4747
Direction des dépendances et de l'itinérance, Lynne Duguay . . . . (418) 266-6830
Direction des personnes ayant une déficience, Josette Chouinard . . . . (418) 266-6874
Direction des services sociaux généraux, et des activités communautaires, Mario Fréchette . . . . (418) 266-6863
Direction des services jeunes et des familles, Natalie Rosebush (par intérim) . . . . (418) 266-6840
Direction générale adjointe des des services aux aînés , Chantal Maltais . . . . (418) 266-7072
Direction du soutien à domicile , Chantal Maltais (par intérim) . . . . (418) 266-6818
Direction de projet pour la mise en oeuvre de la Loi sur la représentation de RI-RTF, Chantal Maltais (par intérim) . (418) 266-6818

COORDINATION, FINANCEMENT, IMMOBILISATIONS ET BUDGET

Direction générale adjointe du budget et des politiques de financement, François Dion . . . . (418) 266-5965
Direction de la gestion budgétaire et comptable ministérielle, André Bolduc . . . . (418) 266-5986
Direction de la gestion financière - réseau, Guylaine Lajoie . . . . (418) 266-5920
Direction des ressources matérielles, Marie-Claude Beauchamp . . . . (418) 266-8760
Direction des générale adjointe des investissements, Sylvain Périgny . . . . (418) 266-5830
Direction des investissements et du financement, Marlène Sinclair . . . . (418) 266-5850
Direction de l'expertise et de la normalisation, Pierre Gauthier . . . . (418) 266-5956
Direction de la logistique sociosanitaire, Caroline Imbeau . . . . (418) 266-5835
Direction générale adjointe à la coordination et aux ententes de gestion, Pierre Lafleur . . . . (418) 266-5812
Direction de la gestion intégree de l'information, Alain Saucier . . . . (418) 266-8399
Secrétariat à l'accès aux services en langue anglaise et aux communautés culturelles, Ronald McNeil . . . . (514) 873-2292
Direction des affaires autochtones, ethnoculturelles et régions nordiques, Louise Rondeau . . . . (418) 266-7128
Direction des ententes de gestion et de l'imputabilité, Yves Villieneuve . . . . (418) 266-6822
Direction de l'inspection, Jean-François Therrien . . . (418) 643-6084
Direction des relations institutionnelles, Martin Simard (418) 266-5800

SECRÉTARIAT AUX AÎNÉS

Sous-ministre adjointe, Catherine Ferembach . . . . . (418) 643-7811
Direction du développement stratégique et des innovations aînés, Élise Paquette . . . . (418) 643-0837
Direction du développement des programmes et des partenariats, Marie-Josée Poulin . . . . (418) 646-2859

ORGANISMES RELEVANT DU MINISTRE

COMMISSAIRE À LA SANTÉ ET AU BIEN-ÊTRE

Robert Salois . . . . (418) 643-3040

RÉGIE DE L'ASSURANCE-MALADIE DU QUÉBEC

Marc Giroux . . . . (418) 682-5162

OFFICE DES PERSONNES HANDICAPÉES DU QUÉBEC

Céline Giroux . . . . (819) 475-8530

HÉMA QUÉBEC

Jean De Serres . . . . (514) 832-5000

BUREAU DES PROJETS CHUM, CUSM ET CHU SAINTE-JUSTINE

Clermont Gignac . . . . (514) 873-9289

INSTITUT NATIONAL D'EXCELLENCE EN SANTÉ ET EN SERVICES SOCIAUX

Juan Roberto Iglesias . . . . (514) 873-2563

INSTITUTE NATIONAL DE SANTÉ PUBLIQUE DU QUÉBEC

Luc Boileau . . . . (418) 650-5155

URGENCES SANTÉ

Nicola Stephan D'Ulisse . . . . (514) 723-5601

CURATEUR PUBLIC

Diane Lavallée . . . . (514) 873-4898

RESOURCE SECTION

NOTIFICATION TO CORONERS (Québec)

Docteure Louise Nolet, Chief Coroner
Édifice Le Delta 2, bur. 390
2875, boul. Laurier
Québec, QC G1V 5B1
(418) 643-1845, ext. 20231 Fax: (418) 644-4157

Obligation of physicians

34. Every physician who certifies a death for which he is unable to establish the probable causes or which appears to him to have occurred**as a result of negligence** or in obscure or violent circumstances shall immediately notify a coroner or peace officer.
1983, c. 41, s. 34; 2011, c27, s.35.

Death

35. Where a death occurs in a facility maintained by an institution operating a hospital centre, the director of professional services of the institution or a person under his authority may take measures to have the probable causes of death established by a physician.

Coroner's authorization

However, in the case of a death contemplated in section 36, the director of professional services or a person under his authority shall obtain the coroner's authorization before taking measures to have the probable causes of death established.
1983, c. 41, s. 35; 1992, c. 21, s. 281.

Obscure circumstances

36. Unless he has reasonable cause to believe that a coroner, a physician or a peace officer has already been informed, every person having knowledge of a death must immediately notify a coroner or a peace officer where it appears that the death has occurred**as a result of negligence** or in obscure or violent circumstances or where the identity of the deceased person is unknown to him.
(1) 1983, c. 41, s. 36; 2011, c.27, s.36.

Notification to coroner

37. The director of, or, in his absence, the person in authority in an institution contemplated in this section shall immediately notify a coroner or peace officer where a death occurs
(1) in a reception centre classified as a rehabilitation centre within the meaning of the Act respecting health services and social services for Cree Native persons(chapter S-5) and the regulations made thereunder;
(1.1) in a facility maintained by an institution within the meaning of the Act respecting health services and social services (chapter S-4.2) which operates a rehabilitation centre;
(2) in an adapted enterprise within the meaning of the Act to secure handicapped persons in the exercise of their rights with a view to achieving social, school and workplace integration (chapter E-20.1);
(3) in a facility maintained by a health and social services institution, where the person in whose respect death occurred was under confinement.
1983, c. 41, s. 37; 1991, c. 44, s. 1; 1992, c. 21, s. 282, s.375; 1994, c23, s. 23; 1997, c. 75, s. 48; 2004, c. 31, s.71, s. 72.

Notification to coroner

38. The director of, or, in his absence, the person in authority in an establishment contemplated in this section shall immediately notify a coroner where a death occurs
(1) in a house of detention within the meaning of the Act respecting correctional services (chapter S-4.01);
(2) in a penitentiary within the meaning of the Penitentiary Act (Revised Statutes of Canada, 1985, chapter P-5);
(3) in a security unit within the meaning of the Youth Protection Act (chapter P-34.1);
(4) in a police station.
1983, c. 41, s. 38; 1991, c. 43, s. 22.

Death of a child

39. Where a child dies while he is in the custody of the holder of a permit issued by the Minister of Child and Family Welfare, the permit holder, or in his absence, the person in authority at the place where the child is in custody shall immediately notify a coroner or a peace officer.
1983, c. 41, s. 39; 1997, c. 58, s. 144.

Death in a foster family

40 Where a person dies while in the care of a foster family within the meaning of the Act respecting health services and social services for Cree Native persons (chapter S-5) or by a family-type resource within the meaning of the Act respecting health services and social services (chapter S-4.2), the person in authority in the family shall immediately notify a coroner or a peace officer.
1983, c. 41, s. 40; 1992, c.21, s. 283; 1994, c. 23, s. 23.

(Repealed)

41. 1983, c. 41, s. 41; 1985, c. 29, s. 38.

Death during an event.

42. Where a death occurs during an event to which the Civil Protection Act (chapter S-2.3) applies, the person in charge of response operations shall immediately inform a coroner.
1983, c. 41, s. 42; 2001, c. 76, s. 149.

Notice to the coroner

43. The person who is required to transport into Québec the body of a person who died outside Québec shall first notify the coroner of the place where the body is to be buried or cremated if the death occurred**as a result of negligence** or in obscure or violent circumstances, the identity of the deceased person is unknown or the probable causes of death could not be established.

Transport outside Québec

Every person who is required to transport out of Québec the body of a person who died in Québec shall first notify the coroner of the place where the body was found.
1983, c. 41, s. 43; 1991, c. 44, s. 2; 2011, c.27, s.37.

Duty of the coroner

44. Every coroner or peace officer who is notified or informed in accordance with sections 34 to 42 shall immediately notify the coroner having jurisdiction in the place where the dead body was found or the place where the dead body is presumed to be.
1983, c. 41, s. 44.

Repealed.

44.1. 1985, c. 29, s. 39; 1991, c. 44, s. 3.

ONTARIO MINISTRY OF HEALTH AND LONG TERM CARE

Hepburn Block, 80 Grosvenor St, Toronto, Ontario M7A 2C4
Tel. (416) 327-4327 Toll Free: 1-866-532-3161 TTY: 1-800-387-5559 Fax: (416) 314-8721
E-mail: infoweb@moh.gov.on.ca Web: www.health.gov.on.ca

MINISTER'S OFFICE

General Enquiries: (416) 327-4300 Fax: (416) 326-1571 Email: ccu.moh@ontario.ca

Minister of Health, Hon. Deb Matthews

Chief of Staff, Chris Carson . . . . (416) 326-3985
Director of Communications, Sheamus Murphy . . . . . (416) 327-4388
Senior Policy Advisor, Michael Coe . . . . (416) 212-1140

DEPUTY MINISTER'S OFFICE

General Inquiries: (416) 327-4496 Fax: (416) 326-1570

Deputy Minister, Saäd Rafi . . . . (416) 327-4496
Deputy Minister Support Coordinator, Lisa Benvenuto . . (416) 327-4294

ASSOCIATE DEPUTY MINISTER'S OFFICE

General Inquiries: (416) 327-2600

Associate Deputy Minister, David Hallett. . . . . (416) 327-2605
Executive Support Coordinator, Cathy Shoup . . . . . (416) 327-2600

HEALTH SYSTEM MANAGEMENT

COMMUNICATIONS,
Kevin Finnerty, Assistant Deputy Minister . . . . (416) 327-4352

DIRECT SERVICES,
Patricia Li, Assistant Deputy Minister . . . . (416) 327-4490

CORPORATE SERVICES, Ruth Hawkins, Assistant Deputy Minister & Chief Administrative Officer . . . . . (416) 327-4387

HEALTH HUMAN RESOURCS STRATEGY DIVISION,
Suzanne McGurn, Assistant Deputy Minister . . . . . (416) 212-7688

HEALTH SERVICES CLUSTER, I&IT,
Lorelle Taylor, Chief Information Officer . . . . (416) 314-1279

HEALTH SYSTEM ACCOUNTABILITY & PERFORMANCE DIVISION,
Ken Deane, Assistant Deputy Minister. . . . . (416) 212-1134

HEALTH SYSTEM INFORMATION MANAGEMENT AND INVESTMENT,
Don Young, Assistant Deputy Minister . . . . (416) 327-8854

HEALTH SYSTEM STRATEGY & POLICY DIVISION,
Dr. Vasanthi Srinivasan, Assistant Deputy Minister . . . (416) 327-7261

NEGOTIATIONS & ACCOUNTABILITY MANAGEMENT,
Susan Fitzpatrick, Assistant Deputy Minister . . . . . (416) 212-7012

LEGAL SERVICES, Janice Crawford, Director . . . . (416) 327-8565

MEDICAL ADVISORY SECRETARIAT,
Dr. Leslie Levin, Head Sr. Medical Advisor . . . . . . (416) 314-0249

ONTARIO PUBLIC DRUG PROGRAMS, Diane McArthur, Assistant Deputy Minister & Executive Officer. . . . . (416) 327-0902

PUBLIC HEALTH,
Dr. Arlene King, Chief Medical Officer of Health
Debra Bournes, Provincial Chief Nursing Officer
Dr. Robin Williams, Associate Chief Medical Officer of Health, Infrastructure & System (Transition). . . . . (416) 327-7513

TRANSITION, Debbie Fischer, Assistant Deputy Minister . (416) 325-1432

STAKEHOLDERS

Ontario Hospital Association

200 Front St. W, Ste 2800, Toronto, ON M5V 3L1
Tel: (416) 205-1300 Fax: (416) 205-1301
Email: info@oha.com Website: www.oha.com

Ontario Medical Association

150 Bloor St West, Ste 900, Toronto, ON M58 3C1
Tel: (416) 599-2580 Fax: (416) 340-2944 Email: info@oma.org
Website: www.oma.org

Ontario Nurses Association

85 Grenville St, Suite 400, Toronto, ON, M5S 3A2
Tel: (416) 964-8833 Fax: (416) 964-8864
Email: onamail@ona.org Website: www.ona.org

Registered Nurses Association of Ontario

158 Pearl St, Toronto, ON M5H 1L3
Tel: (416) 599-1925 Fax: (416) 599-1926
Website: www.rnao.org

Registered Practical Nurses Association of Ontario

5025 Orbitor Dr, Bldg. 4, Suite 200, Mississauga, ON L4W 4Y5
Tel: (905) 602-4664 Fax: (905) 602-4666
Email: info@rpnao.org Website: www.rpnao.org

Ontario Association of Non-Profit Homes and Services for Seniors

7050 Weston Road Suite 700, Woodbridge, ON L4L 8G7
Tel: (905) 851-8821 Fax: (905) 851-0744
Website: www.oanhss.org

Association of Local Public Health Agencies

2 Carlton Street, Ste 1306, Toronto, ON M5B 1J3
Tel: (416) 595-0060 Fax: (416) 595-0030
Email: info@alphaweb.org Website: www.alphaweb.org

Ontario Long-Term Care Association

345 Renfrew Drive 3rd Flr, Markham, Ontario L3R 9S9
Tel: (905) 470-8995 Fax: (905) 470-9595
Email: info@oltca.com Website: www.oltca.com

Ontario Pharmacists' Association

375 University Ave. Suite 800, Toronto ON M5G 2J5
Tel: (416) 441-0788 Fax: (416) 441-0791
Email: mail@opatoday.com Website: www.opatoday.com

Ontario Home Care Association

PO Box 68018, Hamilton, ON L8M 3M7
Tel: (905) 543-9474 Fax: (905) 545-1568
Email: info@homecareontario.com
Website: www.homecareontario.com

Ontario Association of Community Care Access Centres

200-130 Bloor St W, Toronto, ON M5S 1N5
Tel: (416) 750-1720 Email: frontdeskservices@ccac-ont.ca
Website: www.ccac-ont.ca

LOCAL HEALTH INTEGRATION NETWORK (LHIN)

CENTRAL

60 Renfrew Dr, Markham, L3R 0E1
Tel: (905) 948-1872 Fax: (905) 948-8011
Email: central@lhins.on.ca
Website: www.centrallhin.on.ca
Communications Manager, Sandra Upeslacis . (416) 327-4352 ext:214

CENTRAL EAST

314 Harwood Ave S, Suite 204A, Ajax L1S 2J1
Tel: (905) 427-5497 Fax: (905) 427-9659
Email: centraleast@lhins.on.ca
Website: www.centraleastlhin.on.ca
Chief Executive Officer, Ms Deborah Hammons

CENTRAL WEST

8 Nelson St W, Suite 300, Brampton L6X 4J2
Tel: (905) 455-1281 Fax: (905) 455-0427
Email: centralwest@lhins.on.ca
Website: www.centralwestlhin.on.ca
Senior Director of Planning, Mr. David Colgan

CHAMPLAIN

1900 City Park Dr, Suite 204, Ottawa K1J 1A3
Tel: (613) 747-6784 Fax: (613) 747-6519
Email: chaplain@lhins.on.ca
Website: www.chaplainlhin.on.ca
Communications Coordinator, Ms. Elaine Medline

ERIE ST. CLAIR

180 Riverview Dr, Chatham ON N7M 5Z8
Tel: (519) 351-5677 Fax: (519) 351-9672
Email: eriestclair@lhins.on.ca
Website: www.eriestclairlhin.on.ca
Communications Coordinator, Ms. Elaine Medline

HAMILTON NIAGARA HALDIMAND BRANT

264 Main St E, Units 1-6, Grimsby L3M 1P8
Tel: (905) 945-4930 Fax: (905) 945-1992
Email: hamiltonniagarahaldimandbrant@lhins.on.ca
Website: www.hnhblhin.on.ca
Communications Advisor, Ms. Laura Bruccoleri

MISSISSAUGA HALTON

700 Dorval Dr, Suite 500, Oakville L6K 3V3
Tel: (905) 337-7131 Fax: (905) 337-8330
Email: mississaugahalton@lhins.on.ca
Website: www.mississaugahaltonlhin.on.ca
Chief Executive Officer, Mr. Bill MacLeod

NORTH SIMCOE MUSKOKA

210 Memorial Ave, Suite 127-130, Orillia L3V 7V1
Tel: (705) 326-7750 Fax: (705) 326-1392
Email: northsimcoemuskoka@lhins.on.ca
Website: www.nsmlhin.on.ca
Senior Manager, Planning & Development, Ms Cheryl Faber

NORTH EAST

555 Oak St E. 3rd Flr, North Bay P1B 8E3
Tel: (705) 840-2872 Fax: (705) 840-0142
Email: northeast@lhins.on.ca
Website: www.nelhin.on.ca
Senior Corporate Advisor, Communications & Community Engagement, Ms. Cynthia Stables

NORTH WEST

975 Alloy Dr, Suite 201, Thunder Bay P7B 5Z8
Tel: (807) 684-9425 Fax: (807) 684-9533
Email: northwest@lhins.on.ca
Website: www.northwestlhin.on.ca
Senior Director, Health System Performance, Mr. Brian Ktytor

SOUTH EAST

71 Adam St., Belleville K8P 5K3
Tel: (613) 967-0196 Fax: (613) 967-1341
Email: southeast@lhins.on.ca
Website: www.southeastlhin.on.ca
Communications & Community Engagement, Mr. Michael Alexander

SOUTH WEST

201 Queens Ave, Suite 700, London N6A 1J1
Tel: (519) 672-0445 Fax: (519) 672-6562
Email: southwest@lhins.on.ca
Website: www.southwestlhin.on.ca
Senior Dir, Planning, Integration and Community Engagement, Ms. Kelly Gillis

TORONTO CENTRAL

425 Bloor St E., Suite 201, Toronto M4W 3R4
Tel: (416) 921-7453 Fax: (416) 921-0117
Email: torontocentral@lhins.on.ca
Website: www.torontocentrallhin.on.ca
Senior Director, Performance Management, Mr William B. Manson

WATERLOO WELLINGTON

50 Sportsworld Crossing Rd, East Bldg, Suite 200, Kitchener N2P 0A4
Tel: (519) 650-4472 Fax: (519) 650-3155
Email: waterloowellington@lhins.on.ca
Website: www.waterloowellingtonlhin.on.ca
Senior Manager, Communications and Public Affairs, Ms Toni Adey

NOTIFICATION TO CORONERS (Ontario)

Dr. A. McCallum
Chief Coroner
c/o Ms. Cathy Craig, Chief Administrative Officer,
Province of Ontario
26 Grenville St
Toronto, ON M7A 2G9
(416) 314-4000 Fax: (416) 314-4030

Duty to give information

10. (1) Every person who has reason to believe that a deceased person died,
   (a) as a result of,
      (i) violence,
      (ii) misadventure,
      (iii) negligence,
      (iv) misconduct, or
      (v) malpractice;
   (b) by unfair means;
   (c) during pregnancy or following pregnancy in circumstances that might reasonably be attributable thereto;
   (d) suddenly and unexpectedly;
   (e) from disease or sickness for which he or she was not treated by a legally qualified medical practitioner;
   (f) from any cause other than disease; or
   (g) under such circumstances as may require investigation,
shall immediately notify a coroner or a police officer of the facts and circumstances relating to the death, and where a police officer is notified he or she shall in turn immediately notify the coroner of such facts and circumstances. R.S.O. 1990, c. C.37, s. 10 (1).

Deaths to be reported

(2) Where a person dies while resident or an in-patient in,
   (a) . . .Repealed: 2007, c. 8, s. 201 (1).
   (b) a children's residence under Part IX (Licensing) of the Child and Family Services Act, 1984 or premises approved under subsection 9 (1) of Part I (Flexible Services) of that Act;
   (c) . . .Repealed: 1994, C. 27, s. 136(1)
   (d) a supported group living residence or an intensive support residence under the Services and Supports to Promote the Social Inclusion of Persons with Developmental Disabilities Act, 2008;
   (e) a psychiatric facility designated under the Mental Health act;
   (f) . . .Repealed: 2009, c. 33, Sched. 18, s. 6.
   (g) . . .Repealed: 1994, c. 27, s. 136 (1).
   (h) a public or private hospital to which the person was transferred from a facility, institution or home referred to in clauses (a) to (g),
the person in charge of the hospital, facility, institution, residence or home shall immediately give notice of the death to a coroner, and the coroner shall investigate the circumstances of the death and, if as a result of the investigation he or she is of the opinion that an inquest ought to be held, the coroner shall hold an inquest upon the body. R.S.O. 1990, c. C.37, s. 10 (2); 1994, c. 27, s. 136 (1); 2001, c. 13, s. 10; 2007, c. 8, s. 201 (1); 2008, c. 14, s. 50; 2009, c. 15, s. 6 (1); 2009, c. 33, Sched. 8, s. 11; 2009, c. 33, Sched. 18, s. 6.

Deaths in nursing homes and homes for the aged.

(2.1) Where a person dies while resident in a long-term care home to which the *Long-Term Home Act, 2007* applies, the person in charge of the home shall immediately give notice of the death to a coroner and, if the coroner is of the opinion that the death ought to be investigated, he or she shall investigate the circumstances of the death and if, as a result of the investigation, he or she is of the opinion that an inquest ought to be held, the coroner shall hold an inquest upon the body. 2007, c. 8, s. 201 (2); 2009, c. 15, s. 6 (3).

Deaths off premises of psychytric facilities, correctional institutions, Youth custody facilities

(3) Where a person dies while,
   (a) a patient of a psychiatric facility;
   (b) committed to a correctional institution;
   (c) committed to a place of temporary detention under the Youth Criminal Justice Act (Canada); or
   (d) committed to secure or open custody under section 24.1 of the Young Offenders Act (Canada), whether in accordance with section 88 of the Youth Crimincal Justice Act (Canada) or otherwise,
but while not on the premises or in actual custody of the facility, institution or place, as the case may be, subsection (2) applies as if the person were a resident of an institution named in subsection (2). 2009, c. 15, s. 6 (4).

Death on premises of detention facility or lock-up

(4) Where a person dies while detained in and on the premises of a detention facility established under section 16.1 of the Police Services Act or a lock-up, the officer in charge of the facility or lock-up shall immediately give notice of the death to a coroner and the coroner shall hold an inquest upon the body. 2009, c. 15, s. 6 (4).

Death on premises of place of temporary detention

(4.1) Where a person dies while committed to and on the premises of a place of temporary detention under the Youth Criminal Justice Act (Canada), the officer in charge of the place shall immediately give notice of the death to a coroner and the coroner shall hold an inquest upon the body. 2009, c. 15, s. 6 (4).

Death on premises of place of secure custody

(4.2) Where a person dies while committed to and on the premises of a place or facility designated as a place of secure custody under section 24.1 of the Young Offenders Act (Canada), whether in accordance with section 88 of the Youth Criminal Justice Act (Canada) or otherwise, the officer in charge of the place or facility shall immediately give notice of the death to a coroner and the coroner shall hold an inquest upon the body. 2009, c. 15, s. 6 (4).

Death on premises of correctional institution

(4.3) Where a person dies while committed to and on the premises of a correctional institution, the officer in charge of the institution shall immediately give notice of the death to a coroner and the coroner shall investigate the circumstances of the death and shall hold an inquest upon the body if as a result of the investigation he or she is of the opinion that the person may not have died of natural causes. 2009, c. 15, s. 6 (4).

Non-application of subs. (4.3)

(4.4) If a person dies in circumstances referred to in subsection (4), (4.1) or (4.2) on the premises of a lock-up, place of temporary detention or place or facility designated as a place of secure custody that is located in a correctional institution, subsection (4.3) does not apply. 2009, c. 15, s. 6 (4).

Death in custody off premises of correctional institution

(4.5) Where a person dies while committed to a correctional institution, while off the premises of the institution and while in the actual custody of a person employed at the institution, the officer in charge of the institution shall immediately give notice of the death to a coroner and the coroner shall investigate the circumstances of the death and shall hold an inquest upon the body if as a result of the investigation he or she is of the opinion that the person may not have died of natural causes. 2009, c. 15, s. 6 (4).

Other deaths in custody

(4.6) If a person dies while detained by or in the actual custody of a peace officer and subsections (4), (4.1), (4.2), (4.3) and (4.5) do not apply, the peace officer shall immediately give notice of the death to a coroner and the coroner shall hold an inquest upon the body. 2009, c. 15, s. 6 (4).

Death while restrained on premises of psychiatric facility, etc.

(4.7) Where a person dies while being restrained and while detained in and on the premises of a psychiatric facility within the meaning of the Mental Health Act or a hospital within the meaning of Part XX.1 (Mental Disorder) of the Criminal Code (Canada), the officer in charge of the psychiatric facility or the person in charge of the hospital, as the case may be, shall immediately give notice of the death to a coroner and the coroner shall hold an inquest upon the body. 2009, c. 15, s. 6 (4).

Death while restrained in secure treatment program

(4.8) Where a person dies while being restrained and while committed or admitted to a secure treatment program within the meaning of Part VI of the Child and Family Services Act, the person in charge of the program shall immediately give notice of the death to a coroner and the coroner shall hold an inquest upon the body. 2009, c. 15, s. 6 (4).

Notice of death resulting from accident at or in construction project, mining plant or mine

(5) Where a worker dies as a result of an accident occurring in the course of the worker's employment at or in a construction project, mining plant or mine, including a pit or quarry, the person in charge of such project, mining plant or mine shall immediately give notice of the death to a coroner and the coroner shall hold an inquest upon the body. R.S.O. 1990, c. C.37, s. 10 (5); 2009, c. 15, s. 6 (5).

Certificate as evidcence

(6) A statement as to the notification or non-notification of a coroner under this section, purporting to be certified by the coroner is without proof of the appointment or signature of the coroner, receivable in evidence as proof, in the absence of evidence to the contrary of the facts stated therein for all purposes in any action, proceeding or prosecution. R.S.O. 1990, c. C.37, s. 10 (6).

Interference with body

11. No person who has reason to believe that a person died in any of the circumstances mentioned in section 10 shall interfere with or alter the body or its condition in any way until the coroner so directs by a warrant. R.S.O. 1990, c. C.37, s. 11.

If there is any doubt about the interpretation of Section 10 of the Coroners Act it would be advisable for the person reporting the death to contact the local Coroner for advice.

RESOURCE SECTION

PROVINCE OF MANITOBA DEPARTMENT OF HEALTH

300 Carlton St, Winnipeg, MB R3B 3M9 Tel. (204) 786-7101 Fax: (204) 783-2171 Web: www.gov.mb.ca/health

MINISTER OF HEALTH

Rm 302, The Legislative Building of Manitoba
450 Broadway, MB R3C 0V8

Minister, Honourable Theresa Oswald (204) 945-3731 Fax: (204) 945-0441
Email: minhlt@leg.gov.mb.ca

Project Manager, Keir Johnson (204) 945-3731

Secretary to Minister, Linda Freed . . . . (204) 945-3749

MANITOBA HEALTH APPEAL BOARD

Rm 102 (Main Floor), 500 Portage Ave, Winnipeg, MB R3C 3X1
Tel: (204) 788-5408 Fax: (204) 948-2024 Email: appeals@gov.mb.ca

Administrator to Board, Marcia Ewatski . . . . (204) 788-5408

Administrative Assistant, Gosia Parada . . . . (204) 945-5806

MINISTER OF HEALTHY LIVING, SENIORS & CONSUMER AFFAIRS MENTAL HEALTH & SPIRITUAL HEALTH CARE

300 Carlton St, Winnipeg, MB R3B 3M9
Tel: (204) 786-7101

Minister Honourable, Jim Rondeau. . . . . (204) 945-1373

Scheduling Assistant to the Minister, Marina Portz . . . (204) 945-2221

ADDICTIONS FOUNDATION OF MANITOBA

Chief Executive Officer, John Borody . . . . (204) 944-6237

MANITOBA SENIORS AND HEALTHY AGING SECRETARIAT

1610-155 Carlton St, Winnipeg, MB R3C 3H8 Tel. (204) 945-2127 Email: seniors@gov.mb.ca

Director, Policy Development, Patti Chiapetta . . . . . . (204) 945-1825

Deputy Minister, Jan Sanderson . . . . (204) 945-3771

DEPUTY MINISTER OF HEALTH OFFICE - Milton Sussman

Rm 327, The Legislative Building of Manitoba
450 Broadway, MB R3C 0V8
Tel: (204) 945-3771 Fax: (204) 945-4564

Assistant Deputy Minister Cross Department Coordination Initiatives, Marcia Thompson . . . . (204) 945-4895

Administrative Officer to the Deputy Minister, Janice Kereluk . . . . (204) 945-0869

Dir, Emergency Preparedness & Response, Gerry Delorme . . . . (204) 945-6382

Health Communications, Kelly Keith . . (204) 945-8525/(204) 945-0750

Chief Provincial Public Health Officer, Michael Routledge . . . . (204) 788-6636

Special Policy Director, Ulrich Wendt . . . . (204) 788-6611

Executive Director, Provincial Policy Support Unit, Joanna Platter . . . . (204) 788-7347

ADMINISTRATION, FINANCE AND ACCOUNTABILITY

300 Carlton Street

Chief Financial Officer & Assistant Deputy Minister, Karen Herd . . . . (204) 788-2525

Executive Director, Finance, Nardia Maharaj . . . . . . (204) 786-7138

Executive Director, Health Information Management, Deborah Malazdrewicz . . . . (204) 786-7149

Consultant, Accountability Support Branch, Nettle Pentland . . . . (204) 788-6747

Comptroller, Finance, Tony Messner . . . . (204) 786-7135

Senior Policy Analyst, Residential Charges Unit , Peter Senychych . . . . (204) 786-7173

CORPORATE AND PROVINCIAL PROGRAM SUPPORT

300 Carlton St, Winnipeg, MB R3B 3M9

Assistant Deputy Minister, Bernadette Preun . . . . (204)786-6439

Coordinator, French Language Services, Richard Loiselle . . . . (204) 788-6698

PROVINCIAL DRUG PROGRAMS - PROFESSIONAL SERVICES

Director, Provincial Drug Programs Drug Management Policy Unit, Olaf Koester. . . . . (204) 788-6670

A/Director, Gail Keeley . . . . (204) 786-7396

PROVINCIAL BLOOD PROGRAMS OFFICE

Director, Carol Renner . . . . . . (204) 786-7395
A/Director, Information Systems Branch, Ken Browne . (204) 788-2521

PUBLIC HEALTH

Chief Provincial Public Health Officer, Michael Routledge . (204) 788-6636
Executive Director, Public Health, Lorraine Adam . . . . . . (204) 788-6781
Director, Provincial Blood Program Office, Carol Renner. . . . . . (204) 786-7395
Medical Director Cadham Provincial Laboratory, Dr. Paul Van Caessele . . . . . . (204) 945-6456

REGIONAL PROGRAMS & SERVICES

300 Carlton St, Winnipeg, MB R3B 3M9

Assistant Deputy Minister, Jean Cox. . . . . . (204) 786-7301
Director, Office of Emergency Medical Services, Brenda Gregory . . . . . . (204) 945-5613
Administrative Officer, Wait Time Task Force , Brie DeMone . . . . . . (204) 786-7137
Administrative Officer, Primary Health Care & Public Health, Donalda Walker . . . . . . (204) 788-6657

REGIONAL SUPPORT SERVICES

Executive Director, Teresa Mrozek . . . . . . (204) 786-7358

PRIMARY HEALTH CARE BRANCH

1090-300 Carlton St, Winnipeg, MB R3B 3M9
Tel: (204) 786-6732 Fax: (204) 943-5305 Email: phc@gov.mb.ca

Associate Deputy Minister, Marie Perchotte . . . . . . (204) 788-6656
Minister, Aboriginal & Northern Health, Hon. Eric Robinson . . . . . . (204) 788-6649
Director, Healthy Living and Populations, Mark Robertson . . . . . . (204) 788-6654
Provincial Coordinator, Healthy Together Now, Betty Kozac. . . . . . (204) 788-6746
Executive Director, Health Systems Innovation, Barb Wasilewski . . . . . . (204) 786-7176
Executive Director, Mental Health, Addictions & Spiritual Care, Fran Schellenberg. . . . (204) 786-7281
Director, Northern Provincial Nursing Stations, Kim Hutcherson . . . . . . (204) 788-6642
Chief Provincial Psychiatrist, Dr. Hugh Andrew . . . . . (204) 788-6677
Executive Director, Public Health Planning, Debbie Nelson . . . . . . (204) 786-7336

HEALTH WORKFORCE

1038-300 Carlton St, Winnipeg, MB R3B 3M9

Asst Deputy Minister, Terry Goertzen. . . . . . (204) 788-6674
Administrative Assistant, Medical Labour Relations, Candace Butler . . . . . . (204) 945-8065
Director, Physician Resource Coordination Office, Michele Mathae-Hunter . . . . . . (204) 788-6405
Executive Director, Workforce Strategies, Brenna Shearer. . . . . . (204) 786-7316
Senior Advisor, Medical Labour Relations, Rick Boyd (204) 786-7282
Director, Insured Benefits, Jackie Sul . . . . . . (204) 783-8482
Manager, Complex Claims Insured Benefits, Debbi Guay. . . . . . (204) 788-2554
Manager, Medical Claims Program, Insured Benefits, Linda Ladabruk-Lahn . . . . . . (204) 786-7394
Manager, Registration/Client Services Insured Benefits, Yves Vandal. . . . . . (204) 788-6462
Director, Medical Labour Relations, Sean Brygidyr . . (204) 786-6767
Labour Relations Officer/Medical Labour Relations, Gayle Martens . . . . . . (204) 788-6623
Committee Coordinator Medical Review/Patient Utilization Committee, Betty Melvin Harder . . . . . (204) 786-7341
Medical Consultant, Medical Consulting Group, Dr. Ali Khan. . . . . . (204) 786-7198

DEPARTMENTAL AGENCIES

HEARING AID BOARD

302-258 Portage Ave, Winnipeg, MB R3C 0B6

Chair, James Ryan . . . . . . (204) 945-3800
Secretary, Nancy Anderson. . . . . . (204) 945-3457

CANCERCARE MANITOBA

675 McDermot Ave, Winnipeg, MB R3E 0V9

President & CEO, Dr. Dhali Dhaliwal . . . . . . (204) 787-2241
Chairman, Lorne F. Daejaeger. . . . . . (204) 787-2241

MANITOBA HEALTH RESEARCH COUNCIL

205-445 Ellice Ave, Winnipeg MB R3B 3P5

Executive Director, Christina Weise. . . . . . (204) 772-1072

MANITOBA LUNG ASSOCIATION/SANATORIUM BOARD OF MANITOBA

629 McDermot Ave, Winnipeg, MB R3A 1P6

Executive Director, Margaret Bernhardt-Lowdon (204) 774-5501 x 225

NOTIFICATION TO MEDICAL EXAMINERS (Manitoba)

Dr. A. Thambirajah Balachandra
Chief Medical Examiner
Manitoba Justice
210 - 1 Wesley Avenue
Winnipeg, MB R3C 4C6
(204) 945-2088 Fax: (204) 945-2442

Manitoba's Fatality Inquiries Act reads:

Reporting Deaths

6(1) A person who is a witness to or has knowledge of a death to which clause 7(9)(a), (b), (c), or (d) applies shall immediately report the death to a medical examiner, an investigator or to the police.

Deaths to which subsection 5 applies

7(9) Subsection (5) applies to a death where

(a) the deceased person died

(i) as a result of an accident,

(ii) by an act of suicide, negligence or homicide,

(iii) in an unexpected or unexplained manner,

(iv) as a result of poisoning,

(v) as a result of contracting a contagious disease that is a threat to public health,

(vi) suddenly of unknown cause,

(vii) during a pregnancy or during recovery from a pregnancy,

(viii) while under anesthesia or while recovering from an anesthesia or within 10 days of a surgical operation performed upon by the person,

(ix) while in the custody of a peace officer,

(x) as a result of

(A) contracting a disease or condition,

(B) sustaining an injury, or

(C) ingesting a toxic substance, at the place of employment or former employment of the person,

(xi) within 24 hours of admission of the person to a hospital,

(xii) in a place, institution of facility that is prescribed or is of a class of place, institution or facility that is prescribed, or

(b) at the time of death, the deceased person

(i) was not under the care of a duly qualified medical practitioner for the condition that brought on the death, or

(ii) was a resident of an institution or care facility that is licensed, or is required by an Act of the Legislature to be licensed, to operate as a residential institution or care facility:

(c) the deceased person died while a resident in a correctional institution, jail, prison or military guardroom, in a psychiatric facility as defined in The Mental Health Act or in a developmental centre as defined in The Vulnerable Persons Living with a Mental Disability Act; or

(d) the deceased person is a child.

MINISTRY OF HEALTH SASKATCHEWAN

3475 Albert St, Regina, Sask. S4S 6X6 Web: www.health.gov.sk.ca

MINISTER'S OFFICE

Minister of Health, Honourable Duncan Dustin, ... (306) 787-7345
Room 204, Legislative Building

Minister Responsible for Rural & Remote Health, Randy Weekes, ... (306) 798-9014
Room 208, Legislative Building

Chief of Staff, Brenda Barootes . . . . . (306) 787-9091

DEPUTY MINISTER'S OFFICE

Deputy Minister, Dan Florizone . . . . . (306) 787-3041

Assistant to the Deputy Minister, Michelle Schmalenberg . . . . . (306) 787-3444

Assistant Deputy Minister, Max Hendricks . . . . . (306) 787-4695

Assistant Deputy Minister, Lauren Donnelly . . . . . (306) 787-0513

Special Advisor to the Deputy Minister, Duncan Fisher . . (306) 787-3147

COMMUNICATIONS BRANCH

Executive Director, Kimberley Kratzig. . . . . (306) 787-8433

PUBLIC HEALTH BRANCH

Chief Medical Officer of Health, Dr. Saquib Shahab (306) 787-3220

STRATEGIC PLANNING, QUALITY & PROCESS IMPROVEMENTS BRANCH

Executive Director, Pauline Rousseau . . . . . (306) 787-3951

MEDICAL SERVICES BRANCH

Executive Director, Shaylene Salazar. . . . . (306) 787-3423

DRUG PLAN & EXTENDED BENEFITS BRANCH

Executive Director, Kevin Wilson . . . . . (306) 787-3301

SASKATCHEWAN DISEASE CONTROL LABORATORY

Executive Director, Patrick O'Bryne. . . . . (306) 787-3129

eHEALTH SASKATCHEWAN

Chief Operating Officer, Brenda Jameson . . . . . (306) 337-0662

PRIMARY HEALTH SERVICES BRANCH

Executive Director, Ron Knaus . . . . . (306) 787-0875

ACUTE & EMERGENCY SERVICES BRANCH

Executive Director, Deb Jordan. . . . . (306) 787-3200

POPULATION HEALTH BRANCH

Executive Director, Donna Magnusson. . . . . (306) 787-5136

COMMUNITY CARE BRANCH

Executive Director, Roger Carriere . . . . . (306) 787-6092

HEALTH REGISTRATION

Director, Pat Cambridgee . . . . . (306) 787-3249

WORKFORCE PLANNING BRANCH

Executive Director, Brad Havervold. . . . . (306) 787-6672

PRINCIPAL NURSING ADVISOR

Lynn Digney-Davis . . . . . (306) 787-7195

RISK & RELATIONSHIP MANAGEMENT BRANCH

Executive Director, Lori Hutchinson Hunter . . . . . (306) 787-7954

STRATEGY AND INNOVATION BRANCH

Executive Director, Pauline Rousseau . . . . . (306) 787-3951

SASKATCHEWAN SURGICAL INITIATIVE BRANCH

Executive Director, Mark Wyatt . . . . . (306) 787-3153

NOTIFICATION TO CORONERS (Saskatchewan)

THE CORONERS ACT, 1999

R. Kent Stewart, Chief Coroner
Office of the Chief Coroner
#920, 1801 Hamilton St
Regina, SK S4P 4B4
(306) 787-5541 Fax: (306) 787-5503
Toll Free: (866) 592-7845

PART III

Duty to Notify Coroner of a Death

General duty to notify coroner

7 (1) Every person shall immediately notify a coroner or a peace officer of any death that the person knows or has reason to believe:
(a) occurred as a result of an accident or violence or was self-inflicted;
(b) occurred from a cause other than disease or sickness;
(c) occurred as a result of negligence, misconduct or malpractice on the part of others;
(d) occurred suddenly and unexpectedly when the deceased appeared to be in good health;
(e) occurred in Saskatchewan under circumstances in which the body is not available because:
(i) the body or part of the body has been destroyed;
(ii) the body is in a place from which it cannot be recovered; or
(iii) the body cannot be located;
(f) was a stillbirth that occurred without the presence of a duly qualified medical practitioner;
(g) occurred as a direct or immediate consequence of the deceased being engaged in employment, an occupation or a business; or
(h) occurred under circumstances that require investigation.

(2) Every peace officer who is notified of a death pursuant to subsection (1) shall immediately notify a coroner of the death. 1999,c.C-38.01, s.7.

Duty of institutions to notify coroner

8 (1) Where an inmate of a jail, military guardroom, remand centre, penitentiary, lock-up or place where the person is held under a warrant of a judge or a correctional facility as defined in *The Correctional Services Act* dies, the person in charge of that place shall immediately notify a coroner of the death.

(2) When a person dies while in custody facility as defined in *The Youth Justice Administration Act*, the person in charge of that facility shall immediately notify a coroner of the death.

(3) Where a minor dies while a resident of a foster home, group home or place of safety within the meaning of *The Child and Family Services Act*, the person in charge of that place shall immediately notify a coroner of the death.

(4) Where an involuntary patient admitted pursuant to section 23 or 24, or detained pursuant to section 24.1, of *The Mental Health Services Act* to an inpatient facility within the meaning of that Act dies, the person in charge of that facility shall immediately notify a coroner of the death.

(5) The duty mentioned in this section applies whether or not:
(a) the person died on the premises or in actual custody; or
(b)the person was an inmate, resident or patient at the time of death if the death was caused at that place.

(6) Where a person dies while in hospital to which the person was transferred from a place mentioned in this section, the person in charge of the hospital shall immediately notify the coroner of the death. 1999, c.C-38.01, s.8; 2004, c.65, s.7

Duty of police to notify coroner

9 Where a person dies as a result of an act or omission of a peace officer in the course of duty or while detained by or in the custody of a peace officer, the peace officer shall immediately notify a coroner of the death. 1999,c.C-38.01,s.9

Duty of social workers to notify coroner

10 While a minor dies while under the care, custody or supervision of the Minister of Community Resources and Employment, officers or employess of the Department of Community Resources and Employment or its designates or an agency that has entered into an agreement with the Minister of Community Resources and Employment pursuant to section 61 of *The Child and Family Services Act*, an officer or employee of the Department of Community Resources and Employment, its designate or the agency who has knowledge of the death shall immediately notify a coroner of the death. 1999,c.C-38.01,s.10; 2004, c.65, s.7

RESOURCE SECTION

ALBERTA HEALTH AND WELLNESS

OFFICE OF THE MINISTER

208, Legislature Bldg, 10800-97 Ave NW, Edmonton, Alberta, T5K 2B6 Fax: (780) 415-0961 Web: www.health.alberta.ca

Minister, Honourable Fred Horne . . . . (780) 427-3665
Executive Assistant, Carol Anderson . . . . (780) 427-3665
Special Advisor, Matthew Hebert . . . . (780) 427-3665

ASSOCIATE MINISTER SENIORS

227, Legislature Bldg,
10800-97 Ave NW, Edmonton, Alberta, T5K 2B6 Fax: (780) 415-0961 Web: www.health.alberta.ca

Associate Minister Senior, Hon. George VanderBurg . . (780) 415-9550
Chief of Staff, Remo Padovani . . . . (780) 638-3229

ASSOCIATE MINISTER WELLNESS

418, Legislature Bldg,
10800-97 Ave NW, Edmonton, Alberta, T5K 2B6 Fax: (780) 415-0961 Web: www.health.alberta.ca

Associate Minister, Hon. Dave Rodney . . . . (780) 415-0482
Chief of Staff, Robert Whittaker . . . . (780) 415-0482

OFFICE OF THE DEPUTY MINISTER

Fl 22, Telus Plaza N Tower,
10025 Jasper Ave, Edmonton, Alberta, T5J 2N3 Fax: (780) 427-1016

Deputy Minister, Marcia Nelson . . . . (780) 422-0747
Executive Assistant, Jill Nimmo . . . . (780) 422-0747

COMMUNICATIONS

Fl 22, Telus Plaza N Tower,
10025 Jasper Ave, Edmonton, Alberta, T5J 2N3 Fax: (780) 427-1171

Director, Carol Chawrun . . . . (780) 427-5344
A/Assistant Director, Paul Michna . . . . (780) 643-6350
A/Assistant Director, John Muir . . . . (780) 422-7951
A/Assistant Director, Micky Elabdi . . . . (780) 415-1231
Executive Assistant, Alison Reid . . . . (780) 643-1012

OFFICE OF THE CHIEF MEDICAL OFFICER

Fl 24, Telus Plaza N Tower,
10025 Jasper Ave, Edmonton, Alberta, T5J 2N3 Fax: (780) 427-7683

Chief Medical Officer of Health, Dr. James Talbot . . . (780) 415-2809
Deputy Chief Medical Officer of Health, Dr. Martin Lavoie. . . . . (780) 644-7557
Administrative Assistant, Jo-Anne Bacon . . . . (780) 415-1400

STRATEGIC SERVICES

Fl 19, Telus Plaza N Tower,
10025 Jasper Ave, Edmonton, Alberta, T5J 1S6 Fax: (780) 643-9421

Assistant Deputy Minister, Christine Couture . . . . . . (780) 643-9287
Issue Coordination, Shannon Haggarty . . . . (780) 415-0953
Executive Assistant, Brenda Johnston. . . . . (780) 427-5387

HEALTH INFORMATION TECHNOLOGY AND SYSTEMS

Fl 21, Telus Plaza N Tower,
10025 Jasper Ave, Edmonton, Alberta, T5J 1S6 Fax: (780) 422-5176

A/Assistant Deputy Minister, Mark Brisson . . . . (780) 427-1572
Executive Assistant, Leslie Majeau . . . . (780) 415-1598

FAMILY AND POPULATION HEALTH

Fl 24, Telus Plaza N Tower,
10025 Jasper Ave, Edmonton, Alberta, T5J 1S6 Fax: (780) 422-3671

A/Assistant Deputy Minister, Neil Mac Donald . . . . . (780) 415-2759
Executive Assistant, Linda McKay . . . . (780) 427-5206

HEALTH WORKFORCE

Fl 10, Telus Plaza N Tower
10025 Jasper Ave, Edmonton, Alberta, T5J 1S6 Fax: (780) 415-8455

A/Assistant Deputy Minister, Deb Kaweski . . . . (780) 415-0212 **A/Executive Assistant**, Donna Lefurgey . . . . (780) 644-3094

FINANCIAL AND CORPORATE SERVICES

Fl 16, Telus Plaza N Tower
10025 Jasper Ave, Edmonton, Alberta, T5J 1S6 Fax: (780) 422-3672

Assistant Deputy Minister, Dave Breakwell . . . . (780) 415-1599 **Executive Assistant**, Vera Krawec. . . . . (780) 644-5151

HUMAN RESOURCES

Fl 22, Telus Plaza N Tower
10025 Jasper Ave, Edmonton, Alberta, T5J 1S6 Fax: (780)422-1700

A/Executive Director, Michelle Dorval. . . . . (780) 427-1294 **Executive Assistant**, Karen Huxley . . . . (780) 427-1118

CHIEF DELIVERY

Fl 22, Telus Plaza N Tower
10025 Jasper Ave, Edmonton, Alberta, T5J 1S6

Chief Delivery Officer, Glen Monteith. . . . . (780) 415-2745 **Executive Assistant**, Deb Dorege . . . . (780) 415-4781

CHIEF STRATEGY OFFICER

Fl 18, Telus Plaza N Tower
10025 Jasper Ave, Edmonton, Alberta, T5J 1S6

Chief Strategy Officer, Susan Williams . . . . (780) 644-3086 **Executive Assistant**, Karleen Carlson. . . . . (780) 422-0788

SENIORS SERVICES AND CONTINUING CARE

Fl 6, 10405 Standard Life Centre, Edmonton, Alberta, T5J 4R7 Fax: (780) 644-7602

Assistant Deputy Minister, Chi Loo. . . . . (780) 422-3179 **Executive Assistant**, Angie Moscaluk. . . . . (780) 638-3125

HEALTH BENEFITS AND COMPLIANCE

Fl 19, Telus Plaza N Tower
10025 Jasper Ave, Edmonton, Alberta, T5J 1S6 Fax: (780) 422-3674

A/Assistant Deputy Minister, Lorraine McKay . . . . . (780) 415-1424 **A/Executive Assistant**, Amanda Nolet . . . . (780) 415-0808

PRIMARY HEALTH CARE

Fl 18, Telus Plaza N Tower
10025 Jasper Ave, Edmonton, Alberta, T5J 1S6 Fax: (780) 985-7699

A/Assistant Deputy Minister, Joan Berezanski. . . . . (780) 422-9325 **A/Executive Assistant**, Chrissy Searle . . . . (780) 422-6614

MENTAL HEALTH PATIENT ADVOCATE OFFICE

Fl 12, Centre W Bldg
10035-108 St NW, Edmonton, Alberta, T5J 3E1 Fax: (780) 422-0695

Patient Advocate, Ms Fay Orr . . . . (780) 422-1812 **Administrative Assistant**, Ronda Gauthier . . . . (780) 422-1812

NOTIFICATION TO MEDICAL EXAMINER (Alberta) FATALITY INQUIRIES ACT

Dr. Anny Sauvageau
Chief Medical Examiner
Medical Examiner's Office
7007 116 St
Edmonton, AB T6H 5R8
(780) 427-4987 Fax: (780) 422-1265

10. (1) Any person having knowledge or reason to believe that a person has died under any of the circumstances referred to in subsection (2) or section 11, 12 or 13 shall immediately notify a medical examiner or an investigator.

(2) Deaths that occur under any of the following circumstances require notification under subsection (1):

(a) deaths that occur unexplainedly;
(b) deaths that occur unexpectedly when the deceased was in apparent good health;
(c) deaths that occur as the result of violence, accident or suicide;
(d) maternal deaths that occur during or following pregnancy and that might reasonably be related to pregnancy;
(e) deaths that may have occurred as the result of improper or negligent treatment by any person;
(f) deaths that occur
  (i) during an operative procedure,
  (ii) within 10 days after an operative procedure,
  (iii) while under anesthesia, or
  (iv) any time after anesthesia and that may reasonably be attributed to the anesthesia;
(g) deaths that are the result of poisoning;
(h) deaths that occur while the deceased person was not under the care of a physician;
(i) deaths that occur while the deceased person was in the custody of a peace officer or as a result of the use of force by a peace officer while on duty;
(j) deaths that are due to
  (i) any disease or ill-health contracted or incurred by the deceased,
  (ii) any injury sustained by the deceased, or
  (iii) any toxic substance introduced into the deceased,

as a direct result of the deceased's employment or occupation or in the course of one or more of the deceased's former employments or occupations.

11. If a person dies while

(a) detained in a correctional institution as defined in the "Corrections Act" or a jail, including a military guard room, remand centre, penitentiary, secure services facility as defined in the "Child, Youth and Family Enhancement Act", facility or place designated as a place of open or secure custody pursuant to the "Youth Criminal Justice Act" (Canada), detention centre or a place where a person is held under a warrant of a judge,
(b) a formal patient in any facility as defined by the "Mental Health Act", or
(c) an inmate or patient in any institution specified in the regulations,

the person in charge of that institution, jail, facility or other place shall immediately notify a medical examiner.

12. If a person dies while

(a) committed to a correctional institution as defined in the *Corrections Act* or a jail, including a military guard room, remand centre, penitentiary, secure services facility as defined in the *Child, Youth and Family Enhancement Act*, facility or place designated as a place of open or secure custody pursuant to the *Youth Criminal Justice Act* (Canada), detention centre or a place where a person is held under a warrant of a judge,
(b) a formal patient in any facility as defined by the *Mental Health Act*, or
(c) an inmate or patient in any institution specified in the regulations,

but while not on the premises or in actual custody of that facility or institution, jail or other place, the person in charge of that facility or institution, jail or other place, shall, immediately on receiving notice of the death, notify a medical examiner.

13. A director under the *Child, Youth and Family Enhancement Act* shall immediately notify a medical examiner of the death of any child under the director's guardianship or in the director's custody.

BRITISH COLUMBIA MINISTRY OF HEALTH

MINISTER OF HEALTH

Parliament Bldgs, Room 337, PO Box 950, Victoria, BC V8V 1X4
Tel: (250) 953-3547 Fax: (250) 953-9587 E-mail: hlth.minister@gov.bc.ca Web: www.gov.bc.ca/health

Minister Of Health, Honourable Margaret MacDiarmid . . . . (250) 953-3547
Ministerial Assistant, Richard Maksymetz . . . . (250) 953-3547
Ministerial Assistant, Jennifer Wright . . . . (250) 953-3547
Executive Assistant, Mario Miniaci . . . . (250) 953-3547
Executive Assistant, John Manning . . . . (250) 953-3547

DEPUTY MINISTER OF HEALTH OFFICE

5-3, 1515 Blanshard St, Victoria, BC V8W 3C8
Tel: (250) 952-1911 Fax: (250) 952-1909 Email: hlth.dmoffice@gov.bc.ca

Deputy Minister, Graham Whitmarsh . . . . (250) 952-1911
Senior Executive Assistant, Joanne Boomer . . . . . . (250) 952-1911
Chief Operating Officer, John Bethel . . . . (250) 952-2402
Senior Executive Assistant, Linda Zilkie . . . . (250) 952-2402
Chief Administrative Officer, Elaine McKnight . . . . . (250) 952-1764
Senior Executive Assistant, Cheryl Weiss . . . . (250) 952-1764

PROVINCIAL HEALTH OFFICER

4-2, 1515 Blanshard St, Victoria, BC V8W 3C8 Tel: (250) 952-1330 Fax: (250) 952-1362

Provincial Health Officer, Dr. Perry Kendall . . . . (250) 952-1330
Executive Administrative Assistant, Sheila Kowalewsky . (250) 952-1330
Deputy Provincial Health Officer, Dr. Eric Young . . . . (250) 952-1329

HEALTHLINK BC

PO Box 9600 Stn Prov Govt, Victoria, BC V8W 9P1 Tel: (250) 952-6314 Fax: (250) 952-6509

Executive Lead, Bob Bell . . . . (250) 356-0767
Executive Administrative Assistant, Sarah Obee . . . . (250) 356-0767

NOTIFICATION TO CORONERS (British Columbia)

Chief Coroner
Metrotower II, Suite 800
4720 Kingsway
Burnaby, BC V5H 4N2
(604) 660-7745 Fax: (604) 660-7766 Email: BC.CorSer@gov.bc.ca

Part 2 - Reporting Deaths :

Deaths that must be reported by anyone

2 (1) A person must immediately report to a coroner or peace officer the facts and circumstances relating to the death of an adult or child who the person has reason to believe has died

(a) as a result of violence, accident, negligence, misconduct or malpractice,

(b) as a result of self-inflicted illness or injury,

(c) suddenly and unexpectedly, when the person was apparently in good health and not under the care of a medical practitioner,

(d) from disease, sickness or unknown cause, for which the person was not treated by a medical practitioner,

(e) during pregnancy, or following pregnancy in circumstances that might reasonably be attributable to pregnancy,

(f) if the chief coroner reasonably believes it is in the public interest that a class of deaths be reported and issues a notice in accordance with the regulations, in the circumstances set out in the notice, or

(g) in any prescribed circumstances.

2 (2) If a child died in circumstances other than those described in subsection (1), a person who, by regulation, must report child deaths, must immediately report to the chief coroner, in the form required by the chief coroner,

(a) the facts and circumstances relating to the child's death, and

(b) any other information required by the chief coroner.

Deaths that must be reported by peace officers

2 (1) If a peace officer receives a report of a death under section 2 [*deaths that must be reported by anyone*], the peace officer must immediately report to a coroner the facts and circumstances relating to the death.

2 (2) A peace officer must immediately report to a coroner the facts and circumstances relating to the death of a person who dies

(a) while detained by or in the custody, or in a custodial facility, of a peace officer, or

(b) as a result, directly or indirectly, of an act of a peace officer performed in the course of his or her duty.

Deaths that must be reported by institutional administrators.

4 The person in charge of an institution referred to in this section must immediately report to a coroner the facts and circumstances relating to the death of a person who dies

(a) while a patient of a designated facility or private mental hospital within the meaning of *Mental Health Act*, whether or not on the premises or in actual detention,

(b) while the person is committed to a correctional centre, youth custody centre or penitentiary or a police prision or lockup, whether or not on the premises or in custody, or

(c) while a patient of a hospital within the meaning of the Hospital Act, if the patient was transferred to the hospital from a place referred to in the paragraph (a) or (b).

REGIONAL CORONERS
Addresses and Phone Numbers

ISLAND REGIONAL CORONERS OFFICE
PO Box 9772, 5th Floor, 910 Govt St, Victoria, BC V8X 3W4
Phone: (250) 356-9133 . . . . Toll Free Phone: 1-877-741-3707
Fax: (250) 356-9289 . . . . Toll Free Fax: 1-866-229-2226

FRASER REGIONAL CORONERS OFFICE
Metrotower II 800 - 4720 Kingsway, Burnaby, BC V5H 4N2
Phone: (604) 775-1051 . . . . Fax: (604) 775-1049

VANCOUVER METRO REGIONAL CORONERS OFFICE
Metro Tower II, Suite 800-4720 Kingsway, Burnaby, BC V5H 4N2
Phone: (604) 660-7708 . . . . Fax: (604) 660-5290

INTERIOR REGION CORONERS OFFICE
103 - 1420 St Paul St, Kelowna, BC V1Y 2E6
Phone: (250) 861-7429 . . . . Fax: (250) 861-7515

NORTHERN REGION CORONERS OFFICE
Plaza 400 - 4th floor, Room 440 - 1011 4th Ave,
Prince George, BC V2L 3H9
Phone: (250) 565-6040 . . . . Fax: (250) 565-6606

NORTHWEST TERRITORIES DEPARTMENT OF HEALTH & SOCIAL SERVICES

Government of The Northwest Territories, PO Box 1320, Centre Square Tower, Yellowknife, N.W.T. X1A 2L9
Tel. (867) 669-2344 Fax: (867) 873-0481 Web: www.hlthss.gov.nt.ca

MINISTER OFFICE

Minister, Tom Beaulieu . . . . . (867) 669-2399
Executive Assistant, Doug Pon . . . . . (867) 669-2315
Executive Secretary, Soledad Boado . . . . . (867) 669-2399
Fax . . . . . (867) 873-0274

DIRECTORATE

Deputy Minister,
Debbie Delancey . . . . . (867) 920-6173
Executive Secretary, Tiffany Digness . . . . . (867) 920-6173
Fax . . . . . (867) 873-0266

POLICY, PLANNING & EVALUATION

Director, Lisa Cardinal . . . . . (867) 873-7906
Administrative Assistant, Marlene Keeling . . . . . (867) 920-3361
Fax . . . . . (867) 873-0484

CHILDREN & FAMILY SERVICES

Director, Andy Langford . . . . . (867) 873-7046
Program Assistant, Kimberley Galbaransingh . . . . . (867) 873-7991
A/Manager, Sara Chorotkowski . . . . . (867) 920-3109
Fax . . . . . (867) 873-7706

POPULATION HEALTH

Director, Donna Allen . . . . . (867) 873-7400
Administrative Assistant, Kim Austin . . . . . (867) 873-7715
Chief Public Health Officer, André Corriveau . . . . . (867) 920-3286
Administrative Assistant, Rachel Kirizopoulos . . . . . (867) 920-3286

NOTIFICATION TO CORONERS (Northwest Territories)

Ms. Cathy Menard, Chief Coroner
Department of Justice
Government of the Northwest Territories
Box 1320
Yellowknife, NT X1A 2L9
(867) 873-7460 Fax: (867) 873-0426

The Coroners Act of the NWT states that:

Appointment of Coroners

1. (1) The Minister may appoint one or more persons as coroners for the Territories.

Term of Office

(2) A coroner appointed under subsection (1) holds office for a term of three years. 1985 (3), c. 2, s. 4.

Chief Coroner

2. The Minister may appoint a person as the Chief Coroner for the Territories. 1985 (3), c. 2, s. 5.

Duties of Chief Coroner

3. (1) The Chief Coroner shall:
(a) administer this Act and the regulations; and
(b) supervise all coroners in the performance of their duties and the exercise of their powers.

Powers of Chief Coroner

(2) The Chief Coroner may
(a) assist coroners in obtaining medical and other experts where necessary;
(b) establish and conduct programs for the instruction of coroners;
(c) bring the findings and recommendations of coroners and juries to the attentions of appropriate persons, agencies or departments of governments;
(d) issue public reports;
(e) prepare, publish and distribute a code of ethics for coroners and guidelines on the performance of their duties and the exercise of their powers; and
(f) make recommendations to the Minister respecting the appointment and removal of coroners.

Duty to Notify

4. (1) Every person shall immediately notify a coroner or a police officer of any death of which he/she has knowledge that occurs in the Territories, or as a result of events that occur in the Territories, where the death:
(a) occurs as a result of apparent violence, accident, suicide or other apparent cause OTHER THAN disease, sickness or old age;
(b) occurs as a result of apparent negligence, misconduct or malpractice;
(c) occurs suddenly and unexpectedly when the deceased was in apparent good health;
(d) occurs within 10 days after a medical procedure or while the deceased is under or recovering from anesthesia;
(e) occurs as a result of
(i) a disease or sickness incurred or contracted by the deceased,
(ii) an injury sustained by the deceased, or
(iii) an exposure of the deceased to a toxic substance,
as a result or in the course of any employment or occupation of the deceased;
(f) is a stillbirth that occurs without the presence of a medical practitioner;
(g) occurs while the deceased is detained or in custody involuntarily pursuant to law in a jail, lock-up, correctional facility, medical facility or other institution; or
(h) occurs while the deceased is detained by or in the custody of a police officer.

NUNAVUT DEPARTMENT OF HEALTH & SOCIAL SERVICES

Fl 3, Sivummut Bldg, PO Box 1000, Stn 1000 Iqaluit NU X0A 0H0
Tel. (867) 975-5700 Fax (867) 975-5705 Web: www.gov.nu.ca/health
*Unless otherwise indicated, use above phone number.

MINISTER'S OFFICE (867) 975-5007

Minister, Hon. Keith Peterson
Executive Assistant, Nick Pashkoski

DEPUTY MINISTER'S OFFICE (867) 975-5702

Deputy Minister, Peter MA
Executive Services Coordinator, Christie Akearok
Assistant Deputy Minister, Monita O'Connor
Child & Family Services, Mark Arnold

POPULATION HEALTH

Executive Director, Gogi Greeley
Manager, External Public Health Relations, Ainiak Korgak
Chief Medical Officer, Maureen Baikie

POLICY & PLANNING

A/Director,Policy & Planning Natalie Chafe-Yuan
Policy Analyst, Lynn Matte
Policy Analyst, Natalie Strijak

CORPORATE SERVICES (867) 975-5700

A/Executive Director, Bill Neish
Director, Finance Ram Kamath
Manager, Information Technology, Martin Joy

HEALTH INSURANCE PROGRAMS (867) 645-8002

RSO Bldg, Bag 003, Rankin Inlet, X0C 0G0

Manager, Annamarie Hedley. . . . . (867) 645-8002
Registration Specialist, Zellie Nooldok . . . . (867) 645-8016
Specialist, Vital Statistics, Margaret Nokkikok . . . . (867) 645-8017

INSURED SERVICES

Health Benefits Coordinator, Kathleen Irwin . . . . (867) 645-8027
Coordinator & Supervisor, Non-Insured Health Benefits, Kathleen Irwin . . . . (867) 645-8027
Specialist, Extended Health Benefits/Non-Insurance, Suzanne Thompson . . . . (867) 645-8029
Medicare Specialist, Nellie Ussak. . . . . (867) 645-8030

NOTIFICATION TO CORONERS (Nunavut Territory)

Ms. Padma Suramala
Chief Coroner
Court Services Division
Department of Justice
Government of Nunavut Territory
Box 1000, Stn. 590
Iqaluit, NU X0A 0H0
Tel: (867) 975-7292 Fax: (867) 975-7294 E-mail: psuramalajus@gov.nu.ca

The Coroners Act of Nunavut states that:

Appointment of Coroners

1. (1) The Minister may appoint one or more persons as coroners for the Territories.

Term of Office

(2) A coroner appointed under subsection (1) holds office for a term of three years. S.N.W.T. 1995,c.11,s.12.

Chief Coroner

2. The Minister may appoint a person as the Chief Coroner for the Territories.

Duties of Chief Coroner

3. (1) The Chief Coroner shall:
(a) Administer this Act and the regulations; and
(b) Supervise all coroners in the performance of their duties and the exercise of their powers.

Powers of Chief Coroner

(2) The Chief Coroner may
(a) Assist coroners in obtaining medical and other experts where necessary;
(b) Establish and conduct programs for the instruction of coroners;
(c) Bring the findings and recommendations of coroners and juries to the attention of appropriate persons, agencies or departments of governments;
(d) Issue public reports;
(e) Prepare, publish and distribute a code of ethics for coroners and guidelines on the performance of their duties and the exercise of their powers; and
(f) Make recommendations to the Minister respecting the appointment and removal of coroners.

REPORTING OF DEATH

Duty to Notify

8. (1) Every person shall immediately notify a coroner or a police officer of any death of which he/she has knowledge that occurs in the Territories, or as a result of events that occur in the Territories, where the death:
(a) Occurs as a result of apparent violence, accident, suicide or other apparent cause OTHER THAN disease, sickness or old age;
(b) Occurs as a result of apparent negligence, misconduct or malpractice;
(c) Occurs suddenly and unexpectedly when the deceased was in apparent good health;
(d) Occurs within 10 days after a medical procedure or while the deceased is under or recovering from anesthesia;
(e) Occurs as a result of
(i) A disease or sickness incurred or contracted by the deceased,
(ii) An injury sustained by the deceased, or
(iii) An exposure of the deceased to a toxic substance, as a result or in the course of any employment or occupation of the deceased;
(f) Is a stillbirth that occurs without the presence of a medical practitioner;
(g) Occurs while the deceased is detained or in custody involuntarily pursuant to law in a jail, lock-up, correctional facility, medical facility or other institution; or
(h) Occurs while the deceased is detained by or in the custody of a police officer.

Exception

(2) Notwithstanding subsection (1), a person need not notify a coroner or a police officer of a reportable death where the person knows that a coroner or police officer is already aware of the death.

Duty of a Police Officer

(3) A police officer who has knowledge of a reportable death shall immediately notify a coroner of the death.

Special reporting arrangements

(4) The Chief Coroner may make special arrangements with medical facilities, correctional facilities, and the Royal Canadian Mounted Police for the efficient notification of reportable deaths by persons in these facilities or that organization.

DEPARTMENT OF HEALTH AND SOCIAL SERVICES YUKON TERRITORY

2071 Second Ave, PO Box 2703, Whitehorse, YT Y1A 2C6 Tel. (867) 667-5770 Web: www.hss.gov.yk.ca

MINISTER'S OFFICE

Tel.: (867) 667-5800 Fax: (867) 393-6252

Minister of Health & Social Services, Hon. Doug Graham
Executive Assistant, Jess Staffen
Administrative Assistant, Lisa McConnell

ADMINISTRATION

Deputy Minister, Health & Social Services, Paddy Meade . . . (867) 667-5770
Executive Assistant, Kelly Pollard . . . (867) 667-5770
Assistant Deputy Minister, Health, Sherri Wright . . . (867) 667-5689
Administrative & research Assistant, Karla Scott . . . (867) 667-5689
Director, Insured Health & Hearing Services, Paul Gudaitis . . . (867) 667-5202
Chief Medical Health Officer, Dr. Brendan Hanley . . . (867) 456-6136
Medical Travel Officer, Chrissy Campbell . . . (867) 667-3740
Manager, Corporate Strategic Initiatives & Priorities, Cynthia Lyslo . . . (867) 667-5092
Chronic Disease Officer, Karen Carriere

NOTE:

Hospitals - under Director, Health Insurance Programs

Health Centres - under Director of Nursing

Dental Programs, Public Health, Mental Health and Environmental Health-under Director, Health Programs

Deputy Registrar, Vital Statistics, Sylvia Kitching . . . (867) 667-5207
Assistant Deputy Minister, Continuing Care, Cathy Morton-Bielz . . . (867) 667-8922
Administrative & Research Assistant, Yvonne Clarke . . (867) 667-5945
A/Director, Community Health Programs, Cathy Stannard . . . (867) 667-8340
Director of Community Nursing, Joy Kajiwara . . . (867) 667-8324
Director, Communications & Social Marketing, Patricia Living . . . (867) 667-3673
Director, Safety & Clinical Evaluation, Nancy Kidd . . . (867) 667-8750
Manager, Health Human Resources, Tiffany Duncan . . (867) 667-3636
Senior Policy Analyst, James Smith . . . (867) 456-6728

NOTIFICATION TO CORONERS (Yukon Territory)

CORONER'S SERVICE

Ms. Kristen Macdonald
Chief Coroner
Department of Justice
Box 2703, J-10A
Whitehorse, Yukon, Y1A 2C6
(867) 667-5317 Fax: (867) 456-6826
E-mail: kristen.macdonald@gov.yk.ca

The Coroners Act, 1986, of the YT states that:

Appointment and Removal

1. (1) The Commissioner in Executive Council may appoint one or more coroners for the Yukon and may at any time remove, supersede or dispense with any or all of them and appoint others in their place.
   (2) The Commissioner in Executive Council may appoint a chief coroner who shall have jurisdiction throughout the Yukon.
   (3) The powers, duties and remuneration of the chief coroner shall be those that are from time to time defined and set forth by order of the Commissioner in Executive Council.

Duty to Notify Coroner of Death

5 A medical practitioner, undertaker, embalmer, peace officer or any person residing in the house in which the deceased resided immediately before death or any other person who has reason to believe that a deceased person died as a result of violence, misadventure or unfair means, from any cause other than disease or sickness, as a result of negligence, misconduct or malpractice on the part of others or under any other circumstances as require investigation shall immediately notify the coroner who ordinarily has jurisdiction in the locality in which the body of the deceased person is found, of the circumstances relating to the death.

PROVINCIAL HEALTH UNITS

BRITISH COLUMBIA

Provincial Health Officer, Dr Perry Kendall Tel: (250) 952-1330

FRASER HEALTH AUTHORITY CORPORATE OFFICE
400-13450 102nd Ave
Surrey BC V3T 0H1
Tel. (604) 587-4600
Fax. (604) 587-4666
Email: feedback@fraserhealth.ca
Pres/CEO Dr. Nigel Murray
Chief MOH Dr. Paul Van Buynder
Consultant, IRHA Dr. Mary E L Tidmarsh

FRASER EAST SERVICE

Abbotsford Health Protection
2776 Bourquin Cres W
Abbotsford BC V2S 6A4
Tel. (604) 870-7900
Fax. (604) 870-7901
Email: feedback@fraserhealth.ca
Admv Support Ms. Cecilene Schembri

Abbotsford Public Health Unit
104-34194 Marshall Rd
Abbotsford BC V2S 5E4
Tel. (604) 864-3400
Fax. (604) 864-3410
Email: feedback@fraserhealth.ca
Staff Hematopath Dr. Wilson T Yeung

Agassiz Public Health
7243 Pioneer Ave
PO Box 104
Agassiz BC V0M 1A0
Tel. (604) 793-7160
Fax. (604) 796-8587
Email: feedback@fraserhealth.ca
Supvr Ms. Elma Pauls

Chilliwack Public Health Unit
45470 Menholm Rd
Chilliwack BC V2P 1M2
Tel. (604) 702-4900
Fax. (604) 702-4901
Email: feedback@fraserhealth.ca

Cloverdale Health Unit
205-17700 56 Ave
Surrey BC V3S 1C7
Tel. (604) 575-5100
Fax. (604) 574-3738
feedback@fraserhealth.ca
Nurs Supvr Ms. Janice Germaine

Hope Public Health
444 Park St
PO Box 176
Hope BC V0X 1L0
Tel. (604) 860-7630
Fax. (604) 869-2332
Email: feedback@fraserhealth.ca
Pub Hlth Nurse Kim Roberts

FRASER NORTH SERVICE

Burnaby Public Health
305-4946 Canada Way
Burnaby BC V5G 4H7
Tel. (604) 918-7605
Fax. (604) 918-7630
Email: feedback@fraserhealth.ca
Mgr-Environ Serv Mr. Gordon Stewart
Regd Dent Hygienist Mrs. Jacqueline Gerry

Maple Ridge Health Unit
400-22470 Dewdney Trunk Rd
Maple Ridge BC V2X 5Z6
Tel. (604) 476-7000
Fax. (604) 476-7077
Email: feedback@fraserhealth.ca
Chair Med Advisor Dr. Laura J Kelly
Med Officer of Hlth Dr. Nadine Loewen
Env Mgr Mr. Ken Shaw

New Port Public Health
Environ Hlth Serv-Hlth Protection
300-205 Newport Dr
Port Moody BC V3H 5C9
Tel. (604) 949-7700
Fax. (604) 949-7706
Email: feedback@fraserhealth.ca
Med Officer of Hlth Dr. Nadine Loewen
Mgr-EHS Ms. Oonagh Tyson
Staff Dr. Patrick P Leung

New Westminster Health Unit
610 Sixth St
New Westminster BC V3L 3C2
Tel. (604) 777-6740
Fax. (604) 525-0878
Email: feedback@fraserhealth.ca
Coord-Waste & Env Svcs Mr. Kevin McClain

Port Coquitlam Public Health Unit
2266 Wilson Ave
Port Coquitlam BC V3C 1Z5
Tel. (604) 777-8700
Fax. (604) 941-2409
Email: feedback@fraserhealth.ca
Med Officer of Hlth Dr. Nadine Loewen

SOUTH FRASER SERVICE

Delta North Public Health Unit
11245 84 Ave
Delta BC V4C 2L9
Tel. (604) 507-5400
Fax. (604) 507-4617
Email: feedback@fraserhealth.ca

Delta South Public Health
4470 Clarence Taylor Cres
Delta BC V4K 3W3
Tel. (604) 952-3550
Fax. (604) 946-6953
Email: kathy.koop@fraserhealth.ca
Admin Ms. Kathy Koop
Office Coord Ms. Cassandra Cocar

Guilford Public Health
100-10233 153 St
Surrey BC V3R 0Z7
Tel. (604) 587-4750
Fax. (604) 587-4777
Email: feedback@fraserhealth.ca
Med Officer of Hlth Dr. Veronic Ouellette

Langley Environmental Health
22051 Fraser Hwy
Langley BC V3A 4H4
Tel. (604) 507-6121
Fax. (604) 514-6122
Email: feedback@fraserhealth.ca
Med Officer of Hlth Dr. Veronic Ouellette
Env Mgr Mr. Bill Koberstein

Langley Public Health
20389 Fraser Hwy
Langley BC V3A 7N2
Tel. (604) 539-2900
Fax. (604) 514-8036
Email: feedback@fraserhealth.ca
Med Officer of Hlth Dr. Veronic Ouellette

Mission Public Health Unit
32618 Logan Ave
Mission BC V2V 6C7
Tel. (604) 814-5500
Fax. (604) 814-5517
Email: feedback@fraserhealth.ca

Newton Public Health
200-7337 137 St
Surrey BC V3W 1A4
Tel. (604) 592-2000
Fax. (604) 501-4814
Email: feedback@fraserhealth.ca
Admv Asst Ms. Ray Badh

Surrey North Public Health
220-10362 King George Hwy
Surrey BC V3T 2W5
Tel. (604) 587-7900
Fax. (604) 582-4811
Email: feedback@fraserhealth.ca
Med Officer of Hlth Dr. Veronic Ouellette
Supvr Ms. Michelle Donaldson

White Rock Public Health
15476 Vine Ave
Berkeley Pav
White Rock BC V4B 5M2
Tel. (604) 542-4000
Fax. (604) 542-4009
Email: feedback@fraserhealth.ca
Med Officer of Hlth Dr. Veronic Ouellette
Env Mgr Mr. Bill Koberstein

INTERIOR HEALTH AUTHORITY CORPORATE OFFICE
220-1815 Kischner Rd
Kelowna BC V1Y 4N7
Tel. (250) 862-4200
Fax. (250) 862-4201
Pres/CEO Dr. Robert Halpenny
VP Med & Quality Dr Jeremy Etherington
Sr Med Hlth Officer Andrew Larder

Castlegar Public Health Office
709 10th St
Castlegar BC V1N 2H7
Tel. (250) 365-4300
Fax. (250) 365-4303
Email: kellywaage@interiorhealth.ca
Admin Ms. Heather Allen
Adm Coord Ms. Kelly Waage

Central Okanagan Kelowna Health Unit
2F-1340 Ellis St
Kelowna BC V1Y 9N1
Tel. (250) 868-7817
Fax. (250) 868-7826
Admv Asst Ms. Monica Wilson
Family Med Dr. Adriaan I Kellerman
Med Microbiol Dr. Edith M Blondel-Hill

Cranbrook Public Health Unit
20 23rd Ave S
Cranbrook BC V1C 5V1
Tel. (250) 420-2207
Fax. (250) 420-2295
Email: feedback@interiorhealth.ca
Adm Coord Ms. Glenda Montggomery

Creston Health Unit
312 15th Ave N
Creston BC V0B 1G0
Tel. (250) 428-3873
Fax. (250) 428-3649
Dir Dr. Robert C Brunham

EAST KOOTENAY

Fernie Health Unit
1501 5th Ave
Bag 100
Fernie BC V0B 1M0
Tel. (250) 423-8288
Fax. (250) 423-8280
Med Officer of Hlth Dr. Doug Kittel

Golden Mental Health Unit
907 9th St S
PO Box 369
Golden BC V0A 1H0
Tel. (250) 344-3015
Fax. (250) 344-7570
Med Officer of Hlth Dr. Doug Kittel

Invermere Health Centre
850 10th Ave
PO Box 2069
Invermere BC V0A 1K0
Tel. (250) 342-2360
Fax. (250) 342-2373
Contact Ms. Shauna Power
Pub Hlth Nurse Mr. Jeff Quinn
Pub Hlth Nurse Ms. Brenda Maroman

Kimberley Health Unit
260 4th Ave
Kimberley BC V1A 2R6
Tel. (250) 427-2215
Fax. (250) 865-2797
Med Officer of Hlth Dr. Doug Kittel

Sparwood Health Unit
570 Pine Ave
Po Box 1120
Sparwood BC V0B 2G0
Tel. (250) 425-6212
Fax. (250) 425-2378
Med Officer of Hlth Dr. Doug Kittel

KOOTENAY BOUNDARY

Castlegar Health Unit
813 10th St
Castlegar BC V1N 2H7
Tel. (250) 365-4301
Fax. (250) 365-4344
Med Officer of Hlth Dr. Doug Kittel
Staff Dr. Margaret C Yakimov

Grand Forks Health Unit
1200 Central Ave
PO Box 2647
Grand Forks BC V0H 1H0
Tel. (250) 443-3150
Fax. (250) 442-3780
Clerk Ms. Dorothy Swimarchuk

Kaslo Heath Unit
Kaslo Primary Health Service
673A Ave
PO Box 670
Kaslo BC V0G 1M0
Tel. (250) 353-2291
Fax. (250) 353-2738
Med Officer of Hlth Dr. Doug Kittel

Midway Health
Midway Health Centre
540 7th Ave
Midway BC V0H 1M0
Tel. (250) 449-2887
Med Officer of Hlth Dr. Doug Kittel

Nakusp Health Unit
611 Broadway St
Box 315
Nakusp BC V0G 1R0
Tel. (250) 265-3608
Fax. (250) 265-3104
Med Officer of Hlth Dr. Doug Kittel

Nelson Health Unit
2F-333 Victoria St
Nelson BC V1L 4K3
Tel. (250) 505-7200
Fax. (250) 505-7211
Admv Serv Supvr Ms. Barb Patterson

Trail Health Unit
2-1500 Columbia Ave
Trail BC V1R 1J9
Tel. (250) 364-6219
Fax. (250) 364-6218
Med Officer of Hlth Dr. Doug Kittel

NORTH OKANAGAN

Armstrong Health Unit
3800 Patten Dr
Armstrong BC V0E 1B0
Tel. (250) 546-4720
Fax. (250) 546-4721
Med Officer of Hlth Dr. Rob Parker
Pub Hlth Nurse Ms. Wendy Morgan
Pub Hlth Nurse Ms. Jane Macnabb

Vernon Health Unit
1440 14th Ave
Vernon BC V1B 2T1
Tel. (250) 549-5700
Fax. (250) 549-6367
Physician Sexual Hlth Dr Louise Coetzer

SOUTH OKANAGAN

Penticton Health Unit
2F-740 Carmi St
Penticton BC V2A 8P9
Tel. (250) 770-3434
Fax. (250) 770-3470
Med Officer of Hlth Dr. Rob Parker
Med Officer of Hlth Dr Paul Hasselback
Staff Dr. Rajeev Sheoran

THOMPSON CARIBOO SHUSWAP

Chase Public Health
825 Thompson Ave
Chase BC V0E 1M0
Tel. (250) 679-3312
Fax. (250) 679-5329
Email: donna.dube@interiorhealth.ca
Admin Ms. Tina Dillon
Contact Ms. Anne McDonald
Regd Nurse Ms. Donna Dube

Kamloops Health Unit
519-B Columbia St
Kamloops BC V2C 2T8
Tel. (250) 851-7300
Fax. (250) 851-7375
Med Officer of Hlth Dr. J Digby Horne
Supvr Ms. Jodi Helm

Revelstoke Health
1200 Newlands Rd
Box 5000
Revelstoke BC V0E 2S0
Tel. (250) 814-2244
Fax. (250) 814-2243

Salmon Arm Health Unit
851 16th St NE
Salmon Arm BC V1E 4N7
Tel. (250) 833-4100
Fax. (250) 832-1714
Med Officer of Hlth Dr. Digby Horne

Williams Lake Health Unit
3rd Fl 540 Borland St
Williams Lake BC V2G 1R8
Tel. (250) 302-5000
Fax. (250) 302-5002
Med Officer of Hlth Dr. Digby Horne
Office Supvr Ms. Sharon Morgan

NORTHERN HEALTH CORPORATE OFFICE
600-299 Victoria St
Prince George BC V2L 5B8
Tel. (250) 565-2649
Fax. (250) 565-2640
Email: hello@northernhealth.ca
Pres/CEO Ms. Cathy Ulrich
Chief MOH Dr. Ronald Chapman
MOH Northwest Dr. David Bowering
MOH Northeast
Dr. Charles Badenhorst
MOH Northern Interior HSDA William Osei

Chetwynd Public Health
5500 Hospital Rd
Bag 105
Chetwynd BC V0C 1J0
Tel. (250) 788-7200
Fax. (250) 788-7247
Med Officer of Hlth Dr. Charles Badenhorst
Clerk Ms. Wendy Ricketts

NORTH WEST

Hazelton Health Unit
2510 Hwy 62
Bag 999
Hazelton BC V0J 1Y0
Tel. (250) 842-4640
Fax. (250) 842-4642
Email: ruth.carle@northernhealth.ca
Admin Ms. Ruth Carle
Regd Nurse Ms. Dennis Thomsen
Regd Nurse Ms. Pauline Juhasz

Rupert Public Health Unit
300 3rd Ave W
Prince Rupert BC V8J 1L4
Tel. (250) 622-6380
Fax. (250) 622-6391
Mgr-Pub Hlth Ms. Debie Gray

NORTH EAST HEALTH SERVICE

Dawson Creek
1001 110 Ave
Dawson Creek BC V1G 4X3
Tel. (250) 719-6500
Fax. (250) 719-6513
Med Officer of Hlth Dr. Charles Badenhorst

Fort Nelson
5217 Airport Dr
Bag 1000
Fort Nelson BC V0C 1R0
Tel. (250) 774-7092
Fax. (250) 774-7096

Fort St John
10115 110 Ave
Fort St. John BC V1J 6M9
Tel. (250) 263-6000
Fax. (250) 263-6086
Med Officer of Hlth Dr. Charles Badenhorst
Mgr-Pub Hlth Nick Oliphant
Commun Dental Hygienist Susanne Doetzel

Hudson's Hope
10309 Kyllo St
PO Box 599
Hudson's Hope BC V0C 1V0
Tel. (250) 783-9991
Fax. (250) 783-9125
Med Officer of Hlth Dr. Charles Badenhorst

Tumbler Ridge
220 Front St
Box 1090
Tumbler Ridge BC V0C 2W0
Tel. (250) 242-4262
Fax. (250) 242-4009
Admiv Support Ms. Brenda Klages

NORTHERN INTERIOR HEALTH SERVICE

Burns Lake
741 Centre St
Box 7500
Burns Lake BC V0J 1E0
Tel. (250) 692-2460
Fax. (250) 692-2403
Med Officer of Hlth Dr. William Osei

Fort St James
121-250 Stuart Dr
Bag 1268
Fort St James BC V0J 1P0
Tel. (250) 996-7178
Fax. (250) 996-2216
Med Officer of Hlth Dr. William Osei

Fraser Lake
130 Chowsunket Rd
PO BOX 369
Fraser Lake BC V0J 1S0
Tel. (250) 699-7742
Fax. (250) 699-6987
Med Officer of Hlth Dr. William Osei

Mackenzie
45 Centennial Rd
PO Box 249
Mackenzie BC V0J 2C0
Tel. (250) 997-3263
Fax. (250) 997-3940
Med Officer of Hlth Dr. William Osei

Prince George
1444 Edmondson St
Prince George BC V2M 6W5
Tel. (250) 565-7311
Fax. (250) 565-6674
Med Officer of Hlth Dr. William Osei
Staff Dr. Dmitrij Zanozin

Quesnel
523 Front St
Quesnel BC V2J 2K7
Tel. (250) 991-7571
Fax. (250) 991-7577
Med Officer of Hlth Dr. William Osei
Mgr Mr. Jill Walker

Quesnel Health Service Valemount
1445 5th Ave
PO Box 697
Valemount BC V0E 2Z0
Tel. (250) 566-9138
Fax. (250) 566-4319
Admv Asst Ms. Kira Wilkinson

Quesnel Health Service Vanderhoof
3299 Hospital Rd
Vanderhoof BC V0J 3A2
Tel. (250) 567-6900
Fax. (250) 567-6170
Clerk Ms. Leslie Thiessen

McBride Public Health Unit
1126 5th Ave
PO Box 97
McBride BC V0J 2E0
Tel. (250) 569-2251 Ext.2026
Fax. (250) 569-2232
Admv Asst Ms. Heather Callaghan
Pub Hlth Nurse Ms. Cary Savarella

NORTHWEST HEALTH SERVICE

Dease Lake
7171 Hway #37
Bag 2000
Dease Lake BC V0C 1L0
Tel. (250) 771-5024
Fax. (250) 771-5026
Chief MOH Dr. David Bowering

Houston
3202 14th St
PO Box 538
Houston BC V0J 1Z0
Tel. (250) 845-2294
Fax. (250) 845-2259
Admin Ms. Pauline Watson

Kitimat
920 Lahakad Blvd South
Kitimat BC V8C 1S3
Tel. (250) 632-3181
Fax. (250) 632-7081
Admv Asst Ms. Michelle Christmas

Masset
2520 Harrison Ave
PO BOX 215
Masset BC V0T 1M0
Tel. (250) 626-4727
Fax. (250) 626-5279
Pub Hlth Admv Asst Ms. Casie Jarvis

Queen Charlotte Health
3209 Oceanview Dr
PO Box 419
Queen Charlotte BC V0T 1S0
Tel. (250) 559-4447
Chief MOH Dr. David Bowering

Smithers
3793 Alfred Ave
PO Bag 5000
Smithers BC V0J 2N0
Tel. (250) 847-6400
Fax. (250) 847-5908
Mgr Ms. Rachael Lecher

Stewart
904 Brightwell St
PO Box 8
Stewart BC V0T 1W0
Tel. (250) 636-2221
Fax. (250) 636-2715
Mgr Ms. Christie Heuston

Terrace
3412 Kalum St
Terrace BC V8G 4T2
Tel. (250) 638-4200
Fax. (250) 638-2264
Nurse Mgr Ms. Edna Mclellan
NW Dental Leader Mrs. Shirley Gray

Provincial Health Office of British Columbia
4th Floor 1515 Blanshard St
Victoria BC V8W 3C8
Tel. (250) 952-1330
Fax. (250) 952-1362
Email: perry.kendall@gov.bc.ca
Provincial Hlth Officer Dr. Perry Kendall
Provincial Hlth Officer Ms. Andrea Berkes
Dep Provincial Hlth Off Dr. Eric Young

VANCOUVER COASTAL HEALTH CORPORATE OFFICE
904-601 W Broadway
11th Floor
Vancouver BC V5Z 4C2
Tel. (604) 675-3900
Fax. (604) 731-2756
Email: feedback@vch.ca
Chief Med Officer of Hlth Dr. Patricia Daly
Med Officer of Hlth Dr. John Carsley
Asst Ms. Mavis Chu

Central Community Health Service
132 Esplanade W
North Vancouver BC V7M 1A2
Tel. (604) 983-6700
Fax. (604) 983-6839
Med Officer of Hlth Dr Brian O'Connor

Richmond Public Health
8100 Granville Ave
Richmond BC V6Y 3T6
Tel. (604) 233-3150
Fax. (604) 233-3198
Email: feedback@vch.ca
Med Officer of Hlth Dr. James Lu
Asst Ms. Karmel Tanner

VANCOUVER ISLAND HEALTH AUTHORITY CORPORATE OFFICE
1952 Bay St
Victoria BC V8R 1J8
Tel. (250) 370-8699
Fax. (250) 370-8750
Email: info@viha.ca
Chief Med Off of Hlth Dr Richard Stanwick
Corp Dir Risk Mgmt Mr. Graham Sanderson
Commun Dent Hygien Mrs. Heather Buchanan

Central Duncan Health Unit
4th Fl 238 Government St
Duncan BC V9L 1A5
Tel. (250) 737-2010
Fax. (250) 737-2008
Med Officer of Hlth Dr. Fred Rockwell

Central Duncan Public Health Unit
675 Canada Ave
Duncan BC V9L 1T9
Tel. (250) 709-3050
Fax. (250) 709-3055
Adm Supvr Jean Valleau
Pub Hlth Mgr Mr. Joy Stott

Central Parksville/Qualicum Health Unit
New Family Place Bldg 494 Bay Ave
Parksville BC V9P 1C7
Tel. (250) 947-8242
Fax. (250) 947-8241
Adm Mgr Ms. Deanna Shanley

Central Port Alberni Health Unit
4227 6th Ave
Port Alberni BC V9Y 4N1
Tel. (250) 731-1315
Fax. (250) 731-1316
Med Officer of Hlth Dr. Fred Rockwell
Adm Mgr Ms. Deanna Shanley

Esquimalt Health Unit
530 Fraser St
Victoria BC V9A 6H7
Tel. (250) 519-5311
Fax. (250) 519-5312

Health Protection & Environmental Services
6475 Metral Dr, 3rd Fl
Nanaimo BC V9T 2L9
Tel. (250) 739-6304
Fax. (250) 755-3372
Email: christal.lawson@viha.ca
Med Officer of Hlth Dr. Paul Hasselback
Admin Ms. Michelle Whyte
Admv Asst Ms. Christal Lawson

Ladysmith Public Health Unit
1111 4th Ave
Ladysmith BC V9G 1A1
Tel. (250) 755-3342
Pub Hlth Nurse Ms. Faith Thompson

Lake Cowichan Health Unit
58 Cowichan Ave W
PO Box 590
Lake Cowichan BC V0R 2G0
Tel. (250) 749-6878
Fax. (250) 709-3095
Pub Hlth Nurse Ms. Carolyn Yablonski
Pub Hlth Nurse Ms. Patricia Fothergill

Nanaimo Princess Royal Family Public Health Unit
260 Irwin St
Nanaimo BC V9R 4X5
Tel. (250) 739-5845

Nanaimo Public Health Unit
1655 Grant Ave
Nanaimo BC V9S 5K7
Tel. (250) 755-3342
Fax. (250) 755-3369
Clerical Supvr Ms. Lynn Mason

North Campbell River Health Unit
200-1100 Island Hwy
Campbell River BC V9W 8C6
Tel. (250) 850-2110
Fax. (250) 850-2454
Nurs Coord Ms. Linda Carlson

North Comox Valley Health Unit
961 England Ave
Courtenay BC V9N 2N7
Tel. (250) 338-8520
Fax. (250) 338-9985
Nurse Mgr Ms. Jan Adam

North Port Hardy Health Unit
7070 Market st
Port Hardy BC V0N 2P0
Tel. (250) 902-6071
Fax. (250) 902-6072
Med Officer of Hlth Dr. Charmaine Enns

North Port McNeil Health Unit
1775 Grenville St
Port McNeill BC V0N 2R0
Tel. (250) 956-4711
Fax. (250) 956-2031

North Saanich Health Unit
3995 Quadra St
Victoria BC V8X 1J8
Tel. (250) 519-5100
Fax. (250) 744-1042
Commun Dental Hygienist Holly McDonald

North Salt Spring Island Health Unit
1-137 Crofton Rd
Salt Spring Island BC V8K 2R8
Tel. (250) 538-4880
Fax. (250) 538-4899

North Sooke Health Unit
104-2145 Townsend Rd
Sooke BC V9Z 0H3
Tel. (250) 642-5464
Fax. (250) 642-5467

North Ucluelet Health Unit
Coastal Family Place 265 First St
PO Box 1078
Tofino BC V0R 2Z0
Tel. (250) 725-4020
Med Officer of Hlth Dr. Fred Rockwell

North Victoria Health Unit
1947 Cook St
Victoria BC V8T 3P7
Tel. (250) 388-2200
Fax. (250) 388-2249

North Westshore Health Unit
345 Wale Rd
Victoria BC V9B 6X2
Tel. (250) 519-3490
Fax. (250) 519-3491
Med Officer of Hlth Dr. Murray Fyfe

Peninsula Health Unit
2170 Mount Newton X Rd
Saanichton BC V8M 2B2
Tel. (250) 544-2400
Fax. (250) 544-2403
Med Officer of Hlth Dr. Murray Fyfe

South Gateway Village Public Health
201-771 Vernon Ave
Victoria BC V8X 5A7
Tel. (250) 519-3401
Fax. (250) 519-3402
Nurse Mgr Mr. Gary Gibson

Victoria Public Health
430-1900 Richmond Rd
Victoria BC V8R 4R2
Tel. (250) 519-3046
Fax. (250) 519-3441
Email: info@viha.ca
Med Officer of Hlth Dr. Richard Stanwick
Exec Dir-Pub Hlth Mr. Allison Cutler
Reg Mgr Ms. Ann Thomas

ALBERTA

Chief Medical Officer of Health, Dr James Talbot Tel: (780) 427-5263

ALBERTA HEALTH SERVICES CORPORATE OFFICE
7th Street Plaza 10030 107 St NW
Edmonton AB T5J 3E4
Tel. (780) 342-2000
Fax. (780) 342-2060
Email: ahsinfo@albertahealthservices.ca.
Chair Stephen Lockwood
Consultant Dr. Herbert L Cohen
Consultant Med Dr. Anthony R Winder

CALGARY ZONE

Alberta Health Services Calgary
10101 Southport Rd SW
Calgary AB T2W 3N2
Tel. (403) 943-1111
Fax. (403) 943-1138
Pres/CEO Dr. Christopher Eagle
Med Officer of Hlth Dr. Brent Friesen
Med Officer of Hlth Dr. Richard Musto
Dep Med Officer of Hlth Dr. Lorne Clearsky

Black Diamond Public Health
717 Government Rd
PO Bag 1
Black Diamond AB T0L 0H0
Tel. (403) 933-8505
Fax. (403) 933-2031

Canmore Public Health
104-800 Railway Ave
Canmore AB T1W 1P1
Tel. (403) 678-5656
Fax. (403) 678-5068
Mgr Ms. Pat Brooks

Claresholm Public Health
5221 2 St W
Box 1391
Claresholm AB T0L 0T0
Tel. (403) 625-4061
Fax. (403) 625-4062
Pub Hlth Nurse/Admin Ms. Nancy K Miller

Didsbury Public Health Unit
1210 20th Ave
Bag 130
Didsbury AB T0M 0W0
Tel. (403) 335-7292
Fax. (403) 335-7610

High River Public Health
310 MacLeod Trail
Box 5638
High River AB T1V 1M7
Tel. (403) 652-5450
Fax. (403) 652-5455
Mgr Ms. Erin MacKay

Nanton Community Health Centre
2218 20th St
PO Box 940
Nanton AB T0L 1R0
Tel. (403) 646-2218
Fax. (403) 646-3046
Physician Dr. Mohammed Shoaib Alam
Physician Dr. John Tenove
Nurse Pract Ms. Janice Giles

Strathmore Public Health Office
650 Westchester Rd
Strathmore AB T1P 1H8
Tel. (403) 361-7200
Fax. (403) 361-7244

Valleyview Public Health Centre
5112 50th Ave
Valleyview AB T0H 3N0
Tel. (780) 524-3338
Fax. (780) 524-3153
Admv Asst Ms. Rose Shaver

Vulcan Public Health
610 Elizabeth St
PO Box 214
Vulcan AB T0L 2B0
Tel. (403) 485-3333
Fax. (403) 485-2336
Admin Ms. Wendy Shearer

CENTRAL ZONE

Camrose Public Health
5510 46 Ave
Camrose AB T4V 4P8
Tel. (780) 679-2980
Fax. (780) 679-2999
Office Mgr Mr. Brent Poirier

David Thompson Health Region
602-4920 51 St
Red Deer AB T4N 6K8
Tel. (403) 341-8622
Fax. (403) 341-8632
Assoc VP Med Dr. Lawrence A Olfert
Medical Director Dr. Evan Lundall
Dir Community Med Dr. Shirley Hovan

Drayton Valley Community Health Centre
4110 50 Ave
Drayton Valley AB T7A 0B3
Tel. (780) 542-4415
Fax. (780) 621-4998
Reg Pres/CEO Dr. Christopher Eagle

Hughenden Public Health Centre
33 Mackenzie Ave
PO BOX 25
Hughenden AB T0B 2E0
Tel. (780) 753-6180
Fax. (780) 753-2064

Kitscoty Public Health
4922 49 Ave
Kitscoty AB T0B 2P0
Tel. (780) 846-2824
Fax. (780) 846-2731

Myrnam Health Centre
4802 49th Ave
PO Box 220
Myrnam AB T0B 3K0
Tel. (780) 366-3891
Fax. (780) 366-3919
Admin Ms. Shirley Kobewka

Provost Public Health
Provost Provincial Bldg 5419 44 St
PO Box 729
Provost AB T0B 3S0
Tel. (780) 753-6180
Fax. (780) 753-2064
Prog Sec Ms. Beth Breunig

Sedgewick Public Health
4822 50 St
PO Box 12
Sedgewick AB T0B 4C0
Tel. (780) 384-3652
Fax. (780) 384-3699
Prog Asst Ms. Judy Scott

Vegreville Public Health
5318 50 St
PO Box 99
Vegreville AB T9C 1R1
Tel. (780) 632-3331
Fax. (780) 632-4334

Vermilion Public Health
Vermilion Provincial Bldg 11-4701 52 St
Vermilion AB T9X 1J9
Tel. (780) 853-5270
Fax. (780) 853-7362
Site Mgr Ms. Joanne Brady

Viking Public Health
5224 50 St
Viking AB T0B 4N0
Tel. (780) 336-4782
Fax. (780) 336-4916

Wainwright Public Health
22-810 14 Ave
Wainwright AB T9W 1R2
Tel. (780) 842-4077
Fax. (780) 842-3151
Team Leader Ms. Linda Cookson

EDMONTON ZONE

Beaumont Public Health Centre
4918 50 Ave
Beaumont AB T4X 1J9
Tel. (780) 929-4822
Fax. (780) 929-4828
Mgr Ms. Lindsay Stark

Bonnie Doon Public Health Centre
8314 88 Ave NW
Edmonton AB T6C 1L1
Tel. (780) 342-1520
Fax. (780) 466-3110
Ops Mgr Ms. Lisa Sereda

Devon Health Unit
101 Erie St S
Devon AB T9G 1A6
Tel. (780) 342-7069
Fax. (780) 342-7097
Team Coord Ms. Shauna Gallaugher

East Edmonton Public Health Centre
7910 112 Ave
Edmonton AB T5B 0C2
Tel. (780) 342-4719
Fax. (780) 342-4720

Edmonton Public Health Services
8440 112 St N W
Edmonton AB T6G 2B7
Tel. (780) 735-3000
Fax. (780) 482-4194
VP Mike Conroy
Consultant Psy Dr. Atul Khullar
Sec Head Dr. Sander J Van Zanten

Fairview Public Health
10628 110 St
Bag 2201
Fairview AB T0H 1L0
Tel. (780) 835-4951
Fax. (780) 835-3879
Hlth Info Mgmt Clerk Ms. Sherri Bilous

Gibbons Health Unit
4720 50th Ave
Gibbons AB T0A 1N0
Tel. (780) 923-2660
Fax. (780) 923-3939
Operations Mgr Ms. Jeanette Rigby
Receptionist Ms. Lindsay Connolly

Leduc Public Health Centre
4219 50 St
Leduc AB T9E 8C9
Tel. (780) 980-4644
Fax. (780) 980-4666

Millwoods Public Health Centre
7525 38 Ave NW
Edmonton AB T6K 3X9
Tel. (780) 342-1660
Fax. (780) 461-2504
Oerationps Mgr Ms. Farida Etoroma
Admv Asst Kim Watt

Morinville Public Health Centre
101-10008 107 St
Morinville AB T8R 1L3
Tel. (780) 342-2600
Fax. (780) 939-7126

Sprucegrove Health Unit
505 Queen St
Spruce Grove AB T7X 2V2
Tel. (780) 342-1301
Fax. (780) 342-1328

St Albert Public Health Centre
23 Sir Winston Churchill Ave
St Albert AB T8N 2S7
Tel. (780) 459-6671
Fax. (780) 460-7062
Mgr Ms. Jeanette Rigby

Thorsby Public Health Centre
4825 Hankin St
Box 314
Thorsby AB T0C 2P0
Tel. (780) 789-4800
Fax. (780) 789-4811
Mgr Ms. Lindsay Stark

Twin Brooks Public Health Centre
201-1110 113 St NW
Edmonton AB T6J 7J4
Tel. (780) 342-1560
Fax. (780) 437-6240
Mgr Ms. Marg Loitz

Woodcroft Public Health Centre
13221 115 Ave NW
Edmonton AB T5M 4B7
Tel. (780) 342-1600
Fax. (780) 451-5886
Mgr Ms. Chery Smith-John

NORTH ZONE

Beaverlodge Public Health Centre
412 10A St
PO Box 120
Beaverlodge AB T0H 0C0
Tel. (780) 354-2647
Fax. (780) 354-8410

Fort McMurray Public Health Centre
113 Thickwood Blvd
Fort McMurray AB T9H 5E5
Tel. (780) 793-7353

Fox Creek Public Health Unit
600 3rd St
PO Box 430
Fox Creek AB T0H 1P0
Tel. (780) 622-3730
Fax. (780) 622-3474
Pub Hlth Nurse Ms. Jan Cox

Gift Lake Public Health Centre
PO Box 60
Gift Lake AB T0G 1B0
Tel. (780) 767-2101
Fax. (780) 767-2095

Grande Cache Public Health Centre
10001 Hope Ave
PO Box 478
Grande Cache AB T0E 0Y0
Tel. (780) 827-3504
Fax. (780) 827-2728
Hlth Info Clerk Ms. Crystal Goodyear

Grande Prairie Public Health Centre
Main Floor 10320 99 St
Grande Prairie AB T8V 6J4
Tel. (780) 513-7500
Fax. (780) 532-1550
Exec Dir Ms. Donna Koch
Med Dir Kevin Worry

RESOURCE SECTION

Grande Prairie Vienne Building Public Health Centre
10121 97 Ave
Grande Prairie AB T8V 0N5
Tel. (780) 532-4447
Fax. (780) 532-2477

Grimshaw Public Health
1st Fl 5612 Wilcox Rd
Box 648
Grimshaw AB T0H 1W0
Tel. (780) 332-6500
Fax. (780) 332-6504
Admv support Ms. Debbie Herman

High Prairie Public Health
PO Box 1
High Prairie AB T0G 1E0
Tel. (780) 523-6450
Fax. (780) 523-6458
Mgr Ms. Valerie Beynon

Kinuso Public Health Centre
230 Centre St
PO Box 208
Kinuso AB T0G 1K0
Tel. (780) 775-3501
Fax. (780) 775-3944
Sec Ms. Kelly Penny

Manning Public Health
600 2nd St NE
PO BOX 1260
Manning AB T0H 2M0
Tel. (780) 836-7361
Fax. (780) 836-7351
Hlth Registry Clerk Ms. Carla Bieleski

Peace River Public Health
10101 68 St
Bag 400
Peace River AB T8S 1T6
Tel. (780) 624-7260
Fax. (780) 618-3405
Sec Ms. Evan Ruel

Sacred Heart Community Public Health
PO Box 2000
McLennan AB T0H 2L0
Tel. (780) 324-3750
Fax. (780) 324-4256
Sec Ms. Sheila Seary

Spirit River Public Health Centre
5005 45 Ave
Box 187
Spirit River AB T0H 3G0
Tel. (780) 864-3063
Fax. (780) 864-4187
Mgr-Info Ms. Mary Twernichuk

West Jasper Place Public Health
9720 182 St NW
Edmonton AB T5T 3T9
Tel. (780) 342-1234
Mgr Ms. Andrea Guthrie

Westlock Public Health Services
10003 100 Ave
Westlock AB T7P 2E8
Tel. (780) 349-6079
Fax. (780) 349-7055

SASKATCHEWAN

Chief Medical Officer of Health, Dr Saqib Shahab Tel: (306) 787-4722

ATHABASCA HEALTH AUTHORITY CORPORATE OFFICE
Box 124
Black Lake SK S0J 0H0
Tel. (306) 439-2200
Fax. (306) 439-2211
Email: vrobillard@athabascahealth.ca
Chair Ms Caroline Isadore
CEO Ms Jennifer Conley
Dep Chief-MO Dr. Susan Roberecki

CYPRESS REGIONAL HEALTH AUTHORITY CORPORATE OFFICE
429 4th Ave NE
Swift Current SK S9H 2J9
Tel. (306) 778-5100
Fax. (306) 773-9513
Email: info@cypressrha.ca
Chair Mr. Tyler Bragg
CEO Ms Beth Vachon

First Nations & Inuit Health Branch Health Canada
2045 Broad St
Regina SK S4P 3T7
Tel. (306) 780-5414
Fax. (306) 780-8826
Email: ibrahim_khan@hc-sc.gc.ca
Reg Med Off of Hlth Dr. M Ibrahim Khan
Gen Admv Asst Ms. Sharon Martin

FIVE HILLS HEALTH REGION CORPORATE OFFICE
455 Fairford St E
Moose Jaw SK S6H 1H3
Tel. (306) 694-0296
Fax. (306) 694-0282
Email: inquiries@fhhr.ca
Chair Ms. Betty Collicott
CEO Ms. Cheryl Craig
Med Officer of Hlth Dr. Mark Vooght

Five Hills Health Region Assiniboia Public Health
800 1st St E
Box 489
Assiniboia SK S0H 0B0
Tel. (306) 642-2200
Fax. (306) 642-2211
Pub Hlth Nurse Dr. Leisa Vaessen

Gravelburg Public Health
216 Bettez St
PO Box 158
Gravelburg SK S0H 0X0
Tel. (306) 648-1400
Fax. (306) 648-3533

Moose Jaw Public Health
107-110 Ominica St W
Moose Jaw SK S6H 6V2
Tel. (306) 691-1500
Fax. (306) 691-1523
Email: mvoo@fhhr.ca
Med Officer of Hlth Dr. Mark Vooght
Dental Hlth Educator Ms. Jennifer Pituley

HEARTLAND HEALTH REGION CORPORATE OFFICE
110 Hwy 4 S
PO Box 2110
Rosetown SK S0L 2V0
Tel. (306) 691-4111
Fax. (306) 691-1389
Chair Mr Richard Anderson
CEO Gregory Cummings
Med Officer of Hlth Dr. David Torr

Davidson Public Health
900 Government Rd
PO Box 449
Davidson SK S0G 1A0
Tel. (306) 567-2801
Fax. (306) 567-2073

Kerrobert Public Health
635 Alberta Ave
Box 320
Kerrobert SK S0L 1R0
Tel. (306) 834-2646 Ext.251
Fax. (306) 834-1007

Kindersley Public Health
1003 1st St W
Kindersley SK S0L 1S0
Tel. (306) 463-1000 Ext.201
Fax. (306) 463-4550
Facilities Mgr Ms. Wanda Desrosiers

Outlook Public Health
500 Semple St
Outlook SK S0L 2N0
Tel. (306) 867-8676
Fax. (306) 867-2069

Rosetown Public Health
Hwy 4 N
Box 1300
Rosetown SK S0L 2V0
Tel. (306) 882-6413 Ext.3
Fax. (306) 882-6474
Lab Supvr Mrs. Barb Cowell
Clin Supvr Ms. Debby Milton

Unity Public Health
Airport Rd
PO Box 741
Unity SK S0K 4L0
Tel. (306) 228-2666
Fax. (306) 228-2292

KEEWATIN YATTHE REGIONAL HEALTH AUTHORITY
1321 Peterson Ave
PO Box 40
Buffalo Narrows SK S0M 0J0
Tel. (306) 235-2220
Fax. (306) 235-2229
Email: richard.petit@kyrha.sk.ca
Chair Ms Tina Rasmussen
CEO Mr Richard Petit
Dir-Emerg Serv Dr. Megan Koskie
Dental Hygienist Mrs. Glenda Burnouf

KELSEY TRAIL HEALTH REGION CORPORATE OFFICE
901 108 Ave
PO Box 1780
Tisdale SK S0E 1T0
Tel. (306) 873-6600
Fax. (306) 873-6605
Email: lkisil@kthr.sk.ca
Chair Rennie Harper
CEO Mr. Glen Kozak

Cumberland House Public Health Office
2nd Ave
Box 8
Cumberland House SK S0E 0S0
Tel. (306) 888-2244
Fax. (306) 888-2269
CEO Mr. Richard Petit

Hudson Bay Public Health Office
614 Prince St
Po Box 980
Hudson Bay SK S0E 0Y0
Tel. (306) 865-2634
Fax. (306) 865-3425
Pub Hlth Nurse Ms. Margaret Rudychuk

Melfort Public Health
107 Crawford Ave E
PO BOX 6500
Melfort SK S0E 1A0
Tel. (306) 752-6310
Fax. (306) 752-6353
Email: mkhan@kthr.sk.ca
CEO Glen Kozac
Med Off of Hlth Dr. Mohammad Khan

Nipawin Public Health
210 2nd St W
Box 389
Nipawin SK S0E 1E0
Tel. (306) 862-0761
Fax. (306) 862-0763
Pub Hlth Nurse Ms. Bonnie Mair

Tisdale Public Health Office
800 1st St W
Po Box 1297
Tisdale SK S0E 1T0
Tel. (306) 873-8282
Fax. (306) 873-2168

MAMAWETAN CHURCHILL RIVER HEALTH REGION CORPORATE OFFICE
Box 6000
La Ronge SK S0J 1L0
Tel. (306) 425-2422
Fax. (306) 425-5513
Email: information@mcrrha.sk.ca
CEO Mr. Andrew McLetchie
Contact Kim Vancoughnett
Staff Dr. James D Irvine

PRAIRIE NORTH HEALTH REGION
101-4910 50th St
Lloydminster SK S9V 0Y5
Tel. (306) 446-6622
Fax. (306) 446-4114
CEO Mr David Fan
Med Officer of Hlth Dr. Brenda Cholin

Maidstone Public Health Centre
8-120 1st Ave W
Box 629
Maidstone SK S0M 1M0
Tel. (306) 893-4850
Fax. (306) 893-4488
Pub Hlth Nurse Ms. Jan Mitchell

North Battleford Public Health
101-11427 Railway Ave
North Battleford SK S9A 3G6
Tel. (306) 446-6400
Fax. (306) 446-6432
Email: brenda.c@pnrha.ca
Med Officer of Hlth Dr. Brenda Cholin

PRINCE ALBERT PARKLAND HEALTH REGION CORPORATE OFFICE
1521 6th Ave W
Po Box 5700
Prince Albert SK S6V 5K1
Tel. (306) 765-6400
Fax. (306) 765-6401
Sr Med Officer of Hlth Dr. Edmund Royeppen

Big River Public Health
Big River Health Centre
220 1st Ave N
Box 100
Big River SK S0J 0E0
Tel. (306) 469-2220
Fax. (306) 469-2193
Dir-Care Ms. Helen Donald

Blaine Lake Public Health
370 Main St
Blaine Lake SK S0J 0J0
Tel. (306) 497-2494

Hafford Public Health Centre
213 South Ave E
Hafford SK S0J 1A0
Tel. (306) 549-2323

Kinistino Public Health Centre
401 Meyers Ave
Kinistino SK S0J 1H0
Tel. (306) 864-2212

Prince Albert Public Health
PO Box 5700 Stn Main
Prince Albert SK S6V 7V6
Tel. (306) 765-6500
Fax. (306) 765-6536
Admv Asst Ms. Jane Schultz

Spiritwood Public Health
401 1st St E
Spiritwood SK S0J 2M0
Tel. (306) 883-4470
Med Officer of Hlth Dr. Brenda Cholin

REGINA QU'APPELLE HEALTH REGION
2180 23rd Ave
Regina SK S4S 0A5
Tel. (306) 766-5279
Fax. (306) 766-5222
Email: publicaffairs@rqhealth.ca
CEO Mr. Dwight Nelson
Med Dir Dr. Omar Sultan
Sr Med Officer of Hlth Dr. Joy Dobson

Regina Population & Public Health Services
2110 Hamilton St
Regina SK S4P 2E3
Tel. (306) 766-7770
Fax. (306) 766-7607
Email: tania.diener@rqhealth.ca
Med Officer of Hlth Dr. Tania Diener
Dep Med Officer of Hlth Dr. Maurice Hennink
Sec Ms. Bev Pastaruk

Saskatchewan Health
3475 Albert St
Regina SK S4S 6X6
Tel. (306) 787-3235
Fax. (306) 787-3237
Email: mmckinnon@health.gov.sk.ca
Chief MOH Dr. Moira McKinnon

SASKATOON HEALTH REGION CORPORATE OFFICE
701 Queen St
Saskatoon SK S7K 0M7
Tel. (306) 655-7500
Fax. (306) 655-3394
general.inquiries@saskatoonhealthregion.ca
Pres/CEO Ms. Maura Davies
Dir-Risk Mgmt Ms. Lori Frank
Legal Counsel Mr. Evert Van Olst

Humboldt Public Health
1515 14th Ave
PO Box 1930
Humboldt SK S0K 2A0
Tel. (306) 682-2626
Fax. (306) 682-4417
Mgr Ms. Jan Berger

Lanigan & Nokomis Population & Public Health
PO Box 130
Watrous SK S0K 4T0
Tel. (306) 946-2102
Fax. (306) 946-2369
marni.hicks@saskatoonhealthregion.ca
Pub Hlth Nurse Ms. Wendy Yanoshewski
Pub Hlth Nurse Ms. Marni Hicks

Rosthern Public Health
2014 6th St
Rosthern SK S0K 3R0
Tel. (306) 232-6001
Fax. (306) 232-4269
Pub Hlth Nurse Ms. Diane Fehr

Saskatoon Public Health
101-310 Idylwyld Dr N
Saskatoon SK S7L 0Z2
Tel. (306) 655-4620
Fax. (306) 655-4414
neudorf@saskatoonhealthregion.ca
Chief MOH Dr. Cordell Neudorf
Med Officer of Hlth Dr. Johnmark O Opondo
Staff MOH Office Dr. Julie A Kryzanowski

Strasbourg Public Health
303 Edward St
PO Box 457
Strasbourg SK S0G 4V0
Tel. (306) 725-3371
Fax. (306) 725-2053
Pub Hlth Nurse Ms. Marilyn Crasswell

Wadena Public Health
533 5th St NE
PO Box 10
Wadena SK S0A 4J0
Tel. (306) 338-2538
Fax. (306) 338-2510
Admv Asst Ms. Leona Smail
Regd Nurse Ms. Connie Wagner

Wakaw Public Health
301 1st St
Wakaw SK S0K 4P0
Tel. (306) 682-2626

Watrous Public Health
704 4th St
PO Box 130
Watrous SK S0K 4T0
Tel. (306) 946-2102

Wynyard Public Health
300 10th St E
PO Box 670
Wynyard SK S0A 4T0
Tel. (306) 554-3335
Admin Tera Shewchuk

SUN COUNTRY HEALTH REGION CORPORATE OFFICE
808 Souris Valley Rd
PO Box 2003
Weyburn SK S4H 2Z9
Tel. (306) 842-8718
Fax. (306) 842-8738
Email: info@schr.sk.ca
CEO Marga Cugnet
Med Officer of Hlth Dr. Shauna Hudson

Estevan Public Health
1174 Nicholson Rd
Box 5000-201
Estevan SK S4A 2V6
Tel. (306) 637-3626
Fax. (306) 637-2496
Pub Hlth Coord R Gammack

Gravelbourg Public Health
216 Better St
Box 158
Gravelbourg SK S0H 1X0
Tel. (306) 648-1400
Fax. (306) 648-3533

SUNRISE HEALTH REGION CORPORATE OFFICE
270 Bradbrooke Dr
Yorkton SK S3N 2K6
Tel. (306) 786-0100
Fax. (306) 786-0620
CEO Ms. Suann Laurent
Dir-Pub Hlth Mr. James Wallace
Med Off of Hlth Dr. Mandiangu Nsungu
Corp Serv Coord Mr. Perry Froehlich

Canora Public Health Services
1219 Main St
PO Box 685
Canora SK S0A 0L0
Tel. (306) 563-1259
Fax. (306) 563-1257
Pub Hlth Nurse Ms. Kelly Streliof

Esterhazy Public Health Office
216 Ancona St
PO Box 849
Esterhazy SK S0A 0X0
Tel. (306) 745-3200
Fax. (306) 745-3207
Pub Hlth Nurse Ms. Michele Kuntz
Pub Hlth Nurse Ms. Melanie Nagy

Kamsack Public Health Office
359 Queen Elizabeth Blvd
PO Box 218
Kamsack SK S0A 1S0
Tel. (306) 542-4295 Ext.202
Fax. (306) 542-2995
Pub Hlth Nurse Ms. Gail Strukoff

Langenburg Public Health Office
200 Heritage Dr
PO Box 160
Langenburg SK S0A 2A0
Tel. (306) 743-2801
Fax. (306) 743-2899
Pub Hlth Nurse Ms. Shuna P

Melville Public Health Office
200 Heritage Dr
PO Box 62
Melville SK S0A 2P0
Tel. (306) 728-7310
Fax. (306) 728-4925
Sec Ms. Shauna Bassingthwaite

Norquay Public Health Office
355 East Rd Allowance S
PO Box 190
Norquay SK S0A 2V0
Tel. (306) 594-2262
Fax. (306) 594-2488

Preeceville Public Health Office
239 Hwy Ave E
PO Box 466
Preeceville SK S0A 3B0
Tel. (306) 547-2815
Fax. (306) 547-2092

Theodore Public Health Office
615 Anderson Ave
PO Box 292
Theodore SK S0A 4C0
Tel. (306) 647-2353
Fax. (306) 647-2238
Med Off of Hlth Dr. Mandiangu Nsungu

Yorkton Public Health Office
150 Independent St
Yorkton SK S3N 0S7
Tel. (306) 786-0600
Fax. (306) 786-0620
Email: james.wallace@shr.sk.ca
Dir-Pub Hlth Mr. James Wallce
Med Off of Hlth Dr. Mandiangu Nsungu

MANITOBA

Chief Provincial Health Officer, Dr Michael Routledge Tel: (204) 788-6636

INTERLAKE EASTERN REGIONAL HEALTH AUTHORITY PINAWA
24 Aberdeen Ave
PO Box 339
Pinawa MB R0E 1L0
Tel. (204) 753-2012
Fax. (204) 753-2015
Med Officer of Hlth Dr. Karen Robinson
Exec Asst Ms. Lydia Mccoi

INTERLAKE EASTERN REGIONAL HEALTH AUTHORITY SELKIRK
100 Easton Dr
Selkirk MB R1A 2M2
Tel. (204) 482-5800
Fax. (204) 785-9113

INTERLAKE EASTERN REGIONAL HEALTH AUTHORITY STONEWALL
589 3rd Ave S
Stonewall MB R0C 2Z0
Tel. (204) 467-4742
Fax. (204) 467-4750
CEO Mr. Kevin Beresford
Med Officer of Hlth Dr. Tim Hilderman
Exec Asst Ms. Donna Stevens

NORTHERN HEALTH FLIN FLON REGIONAL OFFICE
84 Church St
PO Box 130
Flin Flon MB R8A 1M7
Tel. (204) 687-1300
Fax. (204) 687-6405
Email: nrha@normanrha.mb.ca
CEO Ms. Helga Bryant
Chief Med Officer of Hlth Dr. Hussam Azzam
Mgr Ms. Beverley Hill

Flin Flon Public Health
1 North Ave
Flin Flon MB R8A 1V9
Tel. (204) 687-1340
Fax. (204) 687-8602

Gillam Public Health Unit
15 Gillam Dr
Gillam MB R0B 0L0
Tel. (204) 652-2576
Fax. (204) 652-2536
Admin Ms. Denise Macdirmid
Pub Hlth Nurse Ms. Mandy Hedman

The Pas Public Health
111 Cook Ave
The Pas MB R9A 1K4
Tel. (204) 623-9650
Fax. (204) 627-8285

NORTHERN HEALTH THE PAS REGIONAL OFFICE
67 1st St W
The Pas MB R9A 1K4
Tel. (204) 623-6431
CEO Ms. Helga Bryant
Chief MOH Dr. Hussam Azzam

NORTHERN HEALTH THOMPSON REGIONAL OFFICE
867 Thompson Dr S
Thompson MB R8N 1Z4
Tel. (204) 677-5350
Fax. (204) 340-6742
CEO Ms. Helga Bryant
Chief MOH Dr. Hussam Azzam

PRAIRIE MOUNTAIN HEALTH CORPORATE OFFICE BRANDON
150A 7th St
Brandon MB R7A 7M2
Tel. (204) 578-2301
Fax. (204) 578-2820
CEO Mr. Brian Schoonbaert
Med Officer of Hlth Dr. Elise Weiss
Exec Asst Ms. Doreen Lawrence

PRAIRIE MOUNTAIN HEALTH CORPORATE OFFICE DAUPHIN
625 3rd St SW
Dauphin MB R7N 1T7
Tel. (204) 638-2118
Fax. (204) 622-6232
Email: prha@prha.mb.ca
Med Officer of Hlth Dr Anna Johnston
Commun/Pub Aff Ms. Blaine Kraushaar

PRAIRIE MOUNTAIN HEALTH REGIONAL OFFICE SHOAL LAKE
344 Elm St
PO Box 310
Shoal Lake MB R0J 1Z0
Tel. (204) 759-3441
Fax. (204) 759-3127
CEO Penny Gibson

PRAIRIE MOUNTAIN HEALTH CORPORATE OFFICE SOURIS
Corporate Office 192 1st Ave W
PO Box 579
Souris MB R0K 2C0
Tel. (204) 483-5000
Fax. (204) 759-5005
Email: assiniboinerha@arha.ca
VP Medical Services Dr. Elise C Weiss

Brandon Public Health Services
A5-800 Rosser Ave
Brandon MB R7A 6N5
Tel. (204) 578-2500
Fax. (204) 578-2523
Dir Ms. Janice Loe

Hamiota Public Health
177 Birch Ave E
Hamiota MB R0M 0T0
Tel. (204) 764-2412
Fax. (204) 764-2049
Email: ryaremchuk@assiniboine-rha.ca
Area Mgr Ms. Roseanne Yaremchuk
Pub Hlth Nurse Ms. Susie Paddock

Melita Public Health Unit
PO Box 459
Melita MB R0M 1L0
Tel. (204) 522-3403
Fax. (204) 522-3161
Email: koberlin@arha.ca
Dir-Pub Hlth Ms. Pam Walker

SOUTHERN HEALTH/SANTÉ SUD CORPORATE OFFICE LA BROQUERIE
94 Principale St
Box 470
La Broquerie MB R0A 0W0
Tel. (204) 424-5880
Fax. (204) 424-5888
Email: corp@sehealth.mb.ca
Med Officer of Hlth Dr. Jan Roberts
Commun Coord Ms. Maria Siemens

SOUTHERN HEALTH/SANTÉ SUD CORPORATE OFFICE SOUTHPORT
180 Centennaire Dr
Southport MB R0H 1N1
Tel. (204) 428-2726
Fax. (204) 428-2774
Email: sbuchan@gov.mb.ca
Med Officer of Hlth Dr. Shelley Buchan
Admv Asst Ms. Tanis Durnin

Altona Public Health
240 5th Ave NE
Box 660
Altona MB R0G 0B0
Tel. (204) 324-2351
Fax. (204) 324-8482
Email: ecalder@rha-central.mb.ca
Dir-Health Mr. Brad Street
Pub Hlth Nurse Ms. Julie French

Boundary Trails Public Health
Po Box 2000
Stn Main
Winkler MB R6W 1H8
Tel. (204) 331-8841
Fax. (204) 331-8801
Email: lbuhr@rha-central.mb.ca
Dir-Health Ms. Linda Buhr

Carman Public Health
350 4th St SW
Box 610
Carman MB R0G 0J0
Tel. (204) 745-2426
Fax. (204) 745-2756
Email: mheard@rha-central.mb.ca
Dir-Health Ms. Mary Heard

East Borderland Primary Health
80147 Hwy 12
PO Box 11
Sprague MB R0A 1Z0
Tel. (204) 437-3015
Fax. (204) 437-2884

Elie Public Health
7 Main St E
Box 27
Elie MB R0H 0H0
Tel. (204) 353-2043
Fax. (204) 353-4077
Email: dbleakney@rha-central.mb.ca
Dir-Health Ms. Donna Bleakney
Pub Hlth Nurse Ms. Val Carignan

Gladstone Public Health
24 Mill St
PO Box 1000
Gladstone MB R0J 0T0
Tel. (204) 385-3137
Fax. (204) 385-2663
Email: jegilson@rha-central.mb.ca
Dir-Health Ms. JoAnn Eglison

MacGregor Public Health
87 Grafton St S
PO Box 250
Macgregor MB R0H 0R0
Tel. (204) 685-5705
Fax. (204) 685-2983
Email: chafletcher@rha-central.mb.ca
Pub Hlth Nurse Ms. Chancie Fletcher

Montcalm Public Health
26 Main St
PO Box 428
Emerson MB R0A 0L0
Tel. (204) 373-2109
Fax. (204) 373-2748
Email: penns@rha-central.mb.ca
Dir-Health Mr. Paul Enns

Morris Public Health
215 Railroad Ave E
Box 837
Morris MB R0G 1K0
Tel. (204) 746-7354
Fax. (204) 746-2197
Email: penns@rha-central.mb.ca
Dir-Health Mr. Paul Enns
Pub Hlth Nurse Ms. Laurie Reid-Jones

Pilot Mound Public Health
135 Machray Ave
PO Box 130
Crystal City MB R0K 0N0
Tel. (204) 825-2466
Fax. (204) 825-2185
Email: vcollins@rha-central.mb.ca
CEO/Dir-Health Ms. Ginger Collins

Portage Public Health
25 Tupper St N
Portage la Prairie MB R1N 3K1
Tel. (204) 239-2408
Fax. (204) 239-2444
Email: dbleakney@rha-central.mb.ca
Dir-Health Ms. Donna Bleakney

Rosenort Public Health
124-14 Spruce Cres
PO Box 313
Rosenort MB R0G 1W0
Tel. (204) 746-8885
Fax. (204) 746-2197
Email: penns@rha-central.mb.ca
Dir-Health Mr. Paul Enns

Sanford Public Health
215 Railroad Ave E
PO Box 519
Morris MB R0G 1K0
Tel. (204) 746-2388
Fax. (204) 746-2659
Email: penns@rha-central.mb.ca
Dir-Health Mr. Paul Enns

Somerset Public Health
40 Rogers St
PO Box 190
Notre-Dame-Lourdes MB R0G 1M0
Tel. (204) 744-2092
Fax. (204) 248-2499
kmckitrick-bazin@rha-central.mb.ca
Dir-Health Ms. Kristal McKitrick-Bazin

St. Adolphe Public Health
353 Main St
St Adolphe MB R5A 1A1
Tel. (204) 883-2243
Fax. (204) 883-2916

Steinbach Public Health
365 Reimer Ave
PO Box 2560 Stn Main
Steinbach MB R5G 0R9
Tel. (204) 346-6348
Fax. (204) 326-1046
Email: bunger@sehealth.mb.ca
Med Officer of Hlth Dr. Jan Roberts
Admv Asst Ms. Karen Richardson
Pub Hlth Prog Mgr Ms. Bev Unger

WINNIPEG REGIONAL HEALTH AUTHORITY CORPORATE OFFICE
4F-650 Main St
Winnipeg MB R3B 1E2
Tel. (204) 926-7000
Fax. (204) 926-7007
Chief/Med Officer of Hlth Dr. Brock Wright
Med Dir Dr. Michael E K Moffatt

Churchill Office
Churchill MB R0B 0E0
Tel. (204) 675-8318
Fax. (204) 675-2243
Med Officer of Hlth Dr. Randy Gesell
Pub Hlth Nurse Ms. Melanie S

Fort Garry Office
2735 Pembina Hwy
Winnipeg MB R3T 2H5
Tel. (204) 940-2015
Fax. (204) 261-0888
Commun Team Mgr Ms. Jeanette Patrick

Winnipeg Public Health Branch
4th Fl 100-300 Carlton St
Winnipeg MB R3B 3M9
Tel. (204) 788-6766
Fax. (204) 948-2204
Chief MOH Dr. Joel Kettner
Dep Chief MOH Dr. Susan Roberecki

RESOURCE SECTION

ONTARIO

Chief Medical Officer of Health, Dr Arlene King Tel: (416) 212-3831

Algoma Public Health Blind River Office
9B Lawton St
Blind River ON P0R 1B0
Tel. (705) 356-2551
Fax. (705) 356-2494
Email: anorthan@algomapublichealth.com
Med Officer of Hlth Dr. Allan Northan
Dist Dir Mr. Marshall Chow
Public Hlth Nurse Ms. Angela Schock

Algoma Public Health Elliot Lake Office
Algo Centre Mall 151 Ontario Ave
Elliot Lake ON P5A 2T2
Tel. (705) 848-2314
Fax. (705) 848-1911
Email: anorthan@algomapublichealth.com
Med Officer of Hlth Dr. Allan Northan
Pub Hlth Nurse Ms. Lucy Cywink

Algoma Public Health Sault Ste Marie
294 Willow Ave
Sault Ste. Marie ON P6B 0A9
Tel. (705) 759-5421
Fax. (705) 759-1534
Email: anorthan@algomapublichealth.com
Med Officer of Hlth Dr. Allan Northan
Exec Asst to MOH Ms. Trina Mount
Dental Hygienist Mrs. Kim Sexsmith

Algoma Public Health Wawa Office
18 Ganley St
Wawa ON P0S 1K0
Tel. (705) 856-7208
Fax. (705) 856-1752
Email: anorthan@algomapublichealth.com
Med Officer of Hlth Dr. Allan Nothan
Pub Hlth Nurse Ms. Remee Mellish

Brant County Health Unit
194 Terrace Hill St
Brantford ON N3R 1G7
Tel. (519) 753-4937 Ext.421
Fax. (519) 753-2140
Email: email@bchu.org
Exec Dir Jo Ann Tober
Med Officer of Hlth Dr. Malcolm S Lock
Admv Asst Ms. Lorraine Johnson

Chatham-Kent Public Health Unit
435 Grand Ave W
PO Box 1136
Chatham ON N7M 5L8
Tel. (519) 352-7270 Ext.2500
Fax. (519) 352-2166
Email: CKhealth@chatham-kent.ca
Med Officer of Hlth Dr. David Colby
Admv Asst Ms. Heather Bakker
Regd Dental Hyg Mrs. Leeanne Pepper

DURHAM REGIONAL HEALTH DEPARTMENT CORPORATE OFFICE
605 Rossland Rd E
PO Box 730
Whitby ON L1N 6A3
Tel. (905) 668-7711 Ext.3110
Fax. (905) 666-6214
Email: Robert.Kyle@durham.ca
Med Officer of Hlth Dr. Robert Kyle
Exec Asst Ms. Helen Cialone
Hlth Exec Coord Ms. Annette Laferriere

North Office
200-181 Perry St
Port Perry ON L9L 1B8
Tel. (905) 985-4889
Fax. (905) 982-0840
Admv Asst Ms. Marion Megesi

Oshawa Sexual Health Clinic
Office Galleria 419 King St W
Suite 180
Oshawa ON L1J 2K5
Tel. (905) 433-8901
Fax. (905) 433-8010
Prog Mgr Ms. Vicki Olmstead
Admv Asst Ms. Marion Megesi

Pickering Sexual Health Clinic
14A-1355 Kingston Rd
Pickering ON L1V 1B8
Tel. (905) 420-8781
Fax. (905) 420-9765

Whitby Office
101 Consumers Dr
Whitby ON L1N 1C4
Tel. (905) 723-3818
Fax. (905) 666-1887
Email: ken.gorman@durham.ca
Dir Mr. Ken Gorman
Med Officer of Hlth Dr. Robert Kyle

Whitby Emergency Medical Services
4040 Anderson St
Whitby ON L1R 3P6
Tel. (905) 665-6313
Fax. (905) 444-2042
Dir-Emer Med Serv Mr. Richard Armstrong

EASTERN ONTARIO HEALTH UNIT CORPORATE OFFICE
1000 Pitt St
Cornwall ON K6J 5T1
Tel. (613) 933-1375
Fax. (613) 933-7930
Email: proumeliotis@eohu.ca
Med Officer of Hlth Dr. Paul Roumeliotis
Dir-Pub Hlth Ms. Suzanne Ross
Exec Asst Ms. Nicole Desautels

Alexandria Office
2-60 Anik St
Alexandria ON K0C 1A0
Tel. (613) 525-1112
Fax. (613) 525-2603
Mgr-Hlth Info Dr. Gamil Shahein

Casselman Office
787 Principale St
Box 338
Casselman ON K0A 1M0
Tel. (613) 764-2841
Fax. (613) 764-0264
Dir-Pub Hlth Ms. Susan Ross

Hawkesbury Office
301-134 Main St E
Hawkesbury ON K6A 1A3
Tel. (613) 632-4355
Fax. (613) 632-4171
Email: ndesautels@eohu.ca
Exec Asst Ms. Nicole Desautels

Rockland Office
200-2229 Laurier St
Rockland ON K4K 0B7
Tel. (613) 446-1400
Fax. (613) 446-1454
Email: ndesautels@eohu.ca
Exec Asst Ms. Nicole Desautels
Supvr Ms. Nicole Latlante

Winchester Office
457 Main St E
PO Box 616
Winchester ON K0C 2K0
Tel. (613) 774-2739
Fax. (613) 774-4079
Email: nesautels@eohu.ca
Exec Asst Ms. Nicole Desautels
Supvr Ms. Darlene Rose

ELGIN ST THOMAS PUBLIC HEALTH CORPORATE OFFICE
99 Edward St
St Thomas ON N5P 1Y8
Tel. (519) 631-9900
Fax. (519) 633-0468
Email: estph@elginhealth.on.ca
A-Med Officer of Hlth Dr. Frank Warsh
Dir-Hlth Protection Ms. Laura Mclachlin
Exec Asst Ms. Kim Eitel

GREY BRUCE HEALTH UNIT CORPORATE OFFICE
101 17th St E
Owen Sound ON N4K 0A5
Tel. (519) 376-9420 Ext.224
Fax. (519) 376-0605
publichealth@publichealthgreybruce.on.ca
Med Officer of Hlth Dr. Hazel R Lynn
Exec Asst MHO Ms. Erin Meneray
Regd Dental Hygienist Heather Prior

Walkerton Office
30 Park St
PO Box 248
Walkerton ON N0G 2V0
Tel. (519) 881-1920
Fax. (519) 881-3920
publichealth@publichealthgreybruce.on.ca
Contact Mr. Drew Ferguson

HALDIMAND-NORFOLK HEALTH UNIT CORPORATE OFFICE
12 Gilberson Dr
PO Box 247
Simcoe ON N3Y 4L1
Tel. (519) 426-6170 Ext.3235
Fax. (519) 426-9974
Email: hnmoh@hnhu.org
A-Med Officer of Hlth Dr. Malcoln S Lock
Admv Asst Ms. Helen Hazlewood
Mgr-Pub Hlth Mr. Jill Steen

Caledonia Branch Office
282 Argyle St S
Caledonia ON N3W 1K7
Tel. (905) 318-5367
Fax. (905) 765-8905
Email: hnmoh@hnhu.org
Admv Asst Ms. Helen K Hazlewood
Office Mgr Ms. Rosanne Maracle-Ringuette

Dunville Branch Office
117 Forest St E
Dunnville ON N1A 1B9
Tel. (905) 318-6623
Fax. (905) 774-1538
Email: hnmoh@hnhu.org
Dir Ms. Karen Boughner
Admv Asst Ms. Helen K Hazlewood

Langton Branch Office
22 Albert St
PO Box 128
Langton ON N0E 1G0
Tel. (519) 875-4485
Fax. (519) 875-4789
Email: hnmoh@hnhu.org
Admv Asst Ms. Helen K Hazlewood

HALIBURTON, KAWARTHA, PINE RIDGE DISTRICT HEALTH UNIT CORPORATE OFFICE
200 Rose Glen Rd
Port Hope ON L1A 3V6
Tel. (905) 885-9100 Ext.223
Fax. (905) 885-9551
Email: rmcdonald@hkpr.on.ca
Med Officer of Hlth Dr. Lynn Noseworthy
Exec Asst Ms. Rosemary McDonald

Haliburton Office
301-191 Highland St
PO Box 570
Haliburton ON K0M 1S0
Tel. (705) 457-1391
Fax. (705) 457-1336
Email: info@hkpr.on.ca
Exec Asst Ms. Rosemary McDonald

Lindsay Office
108 Angeline St S
Lindsay ON K9V 3L5
Tel. (705) 324-3569
Fax. (705) 324-0455
Exec Asst Ms. Rosemary McDonald
Dir-Hum Res/Admn Ms. Susan Bicke

HALTON REGION HEALTH DEPARTMENT
1151 Bronte Rd
Oakville ON L6M 3L1
Tel. (905) 825-6000 Ext.7806
Fax. (905) 825-8588
Email: healthdep@halton.ca
Med Officer of Hlth Dr. Robert Nosal
Assoc Med Officer of Hlth Dr. Monir Taha
Admv Asst Ms. Brenda Christopher

Hamilton Public Health Services
4th Floor 1 Hughson St N
Hamilton ON L8R 3L5
Tel. (905) 546-2424 Ext.3501
Fax. (905) 546-4075
Email: richardson@hamilton.ca
Med Officer of Hlth Dr. Elizabeth Richardson
Assoc Med Officer of Hlth Dr. Julie Emili
Admv Asst Ms. Cindy Purnomo

HASTINGS & PRINCE EDWARD COUNTIES HEALTH UNIT CORPORATE OFFICE
179 North Park St
Belleville ON K8P 4P1
Tel. (613) 966-5500
Fax. (613) 966-9418
Email: rschabas@hpechu.on.ca
Med Officer of Hlth Dr. Richard Schabas
Admv Asst Ms. Lisa Cote
Dental Hygienist Mr. Brian Convey

Bancroft Office
2nd Floor 1 Manor Lane
PO Box 99
Bancroft ON K0L 1C0
Tel. (613) 332-4555
Fax. (613) 332-5418
Sec Ms. Patti Inwood

Madoc Office
101-108 Russell St
PO Box 740
Madoc ON K0K 2K0
Tel. (613) 473-4247
Fax. (613) 473-2320
Email: lcote@hpechu.on.ca
Exec Asst Ms. Lisa Cote

Picton Office
74A King St
PO Box 1080
Picton ON K0K 2T0
Tel. (613) 476-7471
Fax. (613) 476-2919
Exec Asst Ms. Lisa Cote

Trenton Office
499 Dundas St W
Trenton ON K8V 6C4
Tel. (613) 394-4831
Fax. (613) 965-6535
Exec Asst Ms. Lisa Cote

HURON COUNTY HEALTH UNIT CORPORATE OFFICE
77722B London Rd
RR 5
Clinton ON N0M 1L0
Tel. (519) 482-3416 Ext.2280
Fax. (519) 482-7820
Email: hchu@huroncounty.ca
Med Officer of Hlth Dr. Nancy Cameron
Exec Asst Ms. Angela Sturdy

Wingham Office
288 Josephine St
Wingham ON N0G 2W0
Tel. (519) 357-4993
Fax. (519) 357-4062
Email: hchu@huroncounty.ca
Exec Asst Ms. Angela Sturdy

KINGSTON, FRONTENAC AND LENNOX & ADDINGTON PUBLIC HEALTH CORPORATE OFFICE
221 Portsmouth Ave
Kingston ON K7M 1V5
Tel. (613) 549-1232
Fax. (613) 549-7896
Med Officer of Hlth Dr. Ian Gemmill
OHN, Train & Dev Spec Ms. Stephanie Blasko

Cloyne Public Health
14209 Hwy 41
PO Box 59
Cloyne ON K0H 1K0
Tel. (613) 336-8989
Fax. (613) 336-0522
Exec Asst Ms. Carol Kobb

Napanee Public Health
41 Dundas St W
Napanee ON K7R 1Z5
Tel. (613) 354-3357
Fax. (613) 354-6267
Exec Asst Ms. Carol Kobb

Sharbot Lake Public Health
1130 Elizabeth St
PO Box 149
Sharbot Lake ON K0H 2P0
Tel. (613) 279-2151
Fax. (613) 279-3997
Exec Asst Ms. Carol Kobb

LAMBTON COMMUNITY HEALTH SERVICES DEPARTMENT CORPORATE OFFICE
160 Exmouth St
Sarnia ON N7T 7Z6
Tel. (519) 383-8331 Ext.3500
Fax. (519) 383-7092
Email: joane.clark@county-lambton.on.ca
Med Officer of Hlth Dr. Sudit Ranade
Admv Asst Ms. Joanne Clarke
Reg'd Dental Hygienist Mrs. Leslie Lambert

Forest Office
59 King St
Forest ON N0N 1J0
Tel. (519) 786-2148
Fax. (519) 786-2149
andrew.taylor@county-lambton.on.ca
Gen Mgr Mr. Andrew Taylor

Petrolia Office
C/O Blue Water Hlth CEE
Petrolia ON N0N 1R0
Tel. (519) 882-4844
Fax. (519) 882-3853
harriet.nagle@county-lambton.on.ca
Admv Asst Ms. Harriet Nagle

Lambton Shared Services Centre
2nd Floor 150 Christina St N
Sarnia ON N7T 8H3
Tel. (519) 344-2062
Fax. (519) 344-2025
Mgr-Health Mr. Kevin Churchill

LEEDS, GRENVILLE & LANARK DISTRICT HEALTH UNIT CORPORATE OFFICE
458 Laurier Blvd
Brockville ON K6V 7A3
Tel. (613) 345-5685 Ext.2248
Fax. (613) 345-2879
Email: heather.bruce@healthunit.org
Med Officer of Hlth Dr. Paula Stewart
Exec Asst Ms. Heather Bruce
Oral Health Promoter Ms. Rebecca Shams

Gananoque Branch Office
200-375 William St S
Gananoque ON K7G 1T2
Tel. (613) 382-4231
Fax. (613) 382-7599
Dir-Corp Serv Ms. Joanne Pearce
Med Officer of Hlth Dr. Paula Stewart

Kemptville Branch Office
2-8 Assa St
PO Box 343
Kemptville ON K0G 1J0
Tel. (613) 258-5941
Fax. (613) 382-1407
Dir-Corp Serv Ms. Joanne Pearce
Med Officer of Hlth Dr. Paula Stewart

Smiths Falls Branch Office
25 Johnson St
Smiths Falls ON K7A 0A4
Tel. (613) 283-2740
Fax. (613) 283-1679
Email: joanne.pearce@healthunit.org
Dir-Corp Serv Ms. Joanne Pearce
Med Officer of Hlth Dr. Paula Stewart

MIDDLESEX-LONDON HEALTH UNIT CORPORATE OFFICE
50 King St (at Ridout)
London ON N6A 5L7
Tel. (519) 663-5317 Ext.2444
Fax. (519) 663-9581
Email: health@mlhu.on.ca
MOH/CEO Dr. Graham L Pollett
Assoc MOH Dr. Bryna Warshawsky
Exec Asst Ms. Lynn Guy

RESOURCE SECTION

London Office
201 Queens Ave
London ON N6A 1J1
Tel. (519) 663-5317
Fax. (519) 663-9276
Exec Asst Ms. Lynn Guy

Strathroy Office
Kenwick Mall 51 Front St E
Strathroy ON N7G 1Y5
Tel. (519) 245-3230
Fax. (519) 245-4772
Email: health@mlhu.on.ca
Exec Asst Ms. Lynn Guy

Mississauaga-Halton Public Health Centre
7330 Goreway Dr
Mississauga ON L4T 4J2
Tel. (905) 799-7700
Fax. (905) 848-9176
Inspector Mr. Paul Theodorlis
Lab Supvr Ms. Molly Balraju

NIAGARA REGION PUBLIC HEALTH CORPORATE OFFICE
2201 St David's Rd Campbell E
PO Box 1052 Station Main
Thorold ON L2V 0A2
Tel. (905) 688-3762
Fax. (905) 682-3901
Email: valerie.jaeger@niagararegion.ca
Med Officer of Hlth Dr. Valerie Jaeger
Exec Asst Ms. Jane Bonaldo
Regd Dental Hygienist Mrs. Karen Hemingway

Fort Erie Public Health
43 Hagey Ave
Fort Erie ON L2A 1W4
Tel. (905) 871-6513
Fax. (905) 871-3020
Exec Asst Ms. Jane Bonaldo

Niagara Falls Public Health
5710 Kitchener St
Niagara Falls ON L2G 1C1
Tel. (905) 536-1538
Fax. (905) 356-7377
Admv Asst Ms. Diane Sutherland

St Catharines Public Health
277 Welland Ave
St Catharines ON L2R 2P7
Tel. (905) 688-3817
Fax. (905) 688-6063
Exec Asst Ms. Catherine O'Leary

Welland Public Health
200 Division St
Welland ON L3B 4A2
Tel. (905) 735-5697
Fax. (905) 735-4895
Exec Asst Ms. Jane Benaldo

NORTH BAY PARRY SOUND DISTRICT HEALTH UNIT CORPORATE OFFICE
681 Commercial St
North Bay ON P1B 4E7
Tel. (705) 474-1400 Ext.2214
Fax. (705) 474-8252
Email: jim.chirico@nbdhu.on.ca
Med Officer of Hlth Dr. James C A Chirico
Admv Asst Ms. Lynn Ringler
Regd Dental Hygienist Mrs. Roxane Hopton

Burks Fall Office
17 Copeland St
Box 484
Burks Falls ON P0A 1C0
Tel. (705) 382-2018
Fax. (705) 382-2931
Email: lynn.ringler@nbpsdhu.ca
Man Admv Asst Ms. Lynn Ringler

Parry Sound Office
70 Joseph St
Parry Sound ON P2A 2G5
Tel. (705) 746-5801
Fax. (705) 746-2711
Email: lynn.ringler@nbpsdhu.ca
Man Admv Asst Ms. Lynn Ringer

NORTHWESTERN HEALTH UNIT CORPORATE OFFICE
21 Wolsley St
Kenora ON P9N 3W7
Tel. (807) 468-3147 Ext.252
Fax. (807) 468-4874
Email: jarthurs@nwhu.on.ca
CEO Mr. Mark Perrault
Med Officer of Hlth Dr. James Arthurs
Exec Asst Ms. Dorothy Strain

Atikokan
Voyageur Mall 115 Main St
PO BOX 1317
Atikokan ON P0T 1C0
Tel. (807) 597-6871
Fax. (807) 597-5217
Email: dstrain@nwhu.on.ca
Exec Asst Ms. Dorothy Strain

Dryden
75D Van Horne Ave
Dryden ON P8N 2B2
Tel. (807) 223-3301
Fax. (807) 223-5754
Email: dstrain@nwhu.on.ca
Prog Mgr Dental Health Dawn Sauve
Regd Dental Hygienist Silvana Edenburn

Ear Falls
25 Spruce St
Box 688
Ear Falls ON P0V 1T0
Tel. (807) 222-3098
Fax. (807) 222-3324
Prog Asst Ms. Glenda Wigle

Emo
76 Front St
Box 539
Emo ON P0W 1E0
Tel. (807) 482-2211
Fax. (807) 482-1678
Prog Asst Mr. Michael Dawber

Kenora Family Services Program
308 Second St S
Unit 209
Kenora ON P9N 1G4
Tel. (807) 468-3436
Fax. (807) 468-8940
Prog Asst Ms. Denise Adams

Fort Frances
396 Scott St
Fort Frances ON P9A 1G9
Tel. (807) 274-9827
Fax. (807) 274-0779
Prog Asst Ms. Kathy Jewell
Regd Dental Hygienist Miss Nicole Rogozinski

Ignace
599&17 Corner of Hwy
Box 420
Ignace ON P0T 1T0
Tel. (807) 934-2236
Fax. (807) 934-2879
Prog Asst Ms. Rosa Harrington

Pickle Lake
3 Anne St
Box 208
Pickle Lake ON P0V 3A0
Tel. (807) 928-2234
Fax. (807) 928-2584
Prog Asst Ms. Ms Denise

Rainy River
210 Atwood Ave
Box 36
Rainy River ON P0W 1L0
Tel. (807) 852-3268
Fax. (807) 852-3015
Pub Hlth Nurse Ms. Gaylene Jasper

Red Lake
234 Howie St
Box 414
Red Lake ON P0V 2M0
Tel. (807) 727-2626
Fax. (807) 727-3001
Prog Asst Ms. Brenda McDonald

Sioux Lookout
47B Front St
Box 246
Sioux Lookout ON P8T 1A3
Tel. (807) 737-2292
Fax. (807) 737-3711
Prog Asst Ms. Leeanne O'Donohue

Sioux Narrows
Hwy 71
Box 246
Sioux Narrows ON P0X 1N0
Tel. (807) 226-9626
Fax. (807) 226-9807
Hlth Educator Ms. Holly Kropelin

Vermilion Bay
84B Spruce St
PO Box 237
Vermilion Bay ON P0V 1V0
Tel. (807) 227-2088
Fax. (807) 227-2418
Chief Adv Officer Mr. Mark Perrault

Ottawa Public Health
100 Constellation Cres
Nepean ON K2G 6J8
Tel. (613) 580-6744 Ext.23681
Fax. (613) 580-9641
Email: isra.levy@ottawa.ca
Med Officer of Hlth Dr. Isra Levy
Exec Asst Ms. Bernadette Martin
Corp Librarian Ms. Mary O'Donnell

Oxford County Public Health & Emergency Services
410 Buller St
Woodstock ON N4S 4N2
Tel. (519) 539-9800
Fax. (519) 539-6206
CEO/Dir-Health Mr. Lynn Beath
A-Med Officer of Hlth Dr. Douglas Neal
Admv Asst Ms. Karen Vance

PERTH DISTRICT HEALTH UNIT CORPORATE OFFICE
653 West Gore St
Stratford ON N5A 1L4
Tel. (519) 271-7600 Ext.255
Fax. (519) 271-2195
Email: mklassen@pdhu.on.ca
Med Officer of Hlth Dr. Miriam Klassen
Admv Asst Ms. Nancy Contois
Dental Hygienist Anna Read

Listowel Public Health
570 Main St W
Listowel ON N4W 1A8
Tel. (519) 291-2812
Fax. (519) 291-6914
Email: ncontois@pdhu.on.ca
Admv Asst Ms. Nancy Contois

Stratford Public Health
Festival Square Office 10 Downie St
2nd Floor
Stratford ON N5A 7K4
Tel. (519) 271-0375
Fax. (519) 271-5368
Email: rhill@pdhu.on.ca
Commun Mgr Ms. Rebecca Hill

Peterborough County-City Health Unit
10 Hospital Drive
Peterborough ON K9J 8M1
Tel. (705) 743-1000 Ext.264
Fax. (705) 743-2897
Email: info@pcchu.ca
Med Officer of Hlth Dr. Rosana Pellizzari
Admv Asst Ms. Aida Tanna

PORCUPINE HEALTH UNIT CORPORATE OFFICE
169 Pine St S
PO BOX 2012 Stn Main
Timmins ON P4N 8B7
Tel. (705) 267-1181 Ext.310
Fax. (705) 264-3980
rosemarie.ramsingh@porcupinehu.on.ca
Med Officer of Hlth Dr. Rosemarie Ramsingh
Admv Asst Ms. Maria Cook
Mgr Infectious Diseases Ms. Lynn Leggett
Dental Hygienist Mrs. Lisa Barber

Cochrane
233 8th St
Box 550
Cochrane ON P0L 1C0
Tel. (705) 272-3394
Fax. (705) 272-4996
Email: maria.cook@porcupinehu.on.ca
Exec Asst Ms. Maria Cook

Hearst
1403 Edward St
Box 2470
Hearst ON P0L 1N0
Tel. (705) 362-4854
Fax. (705) 362-7462
Email: hrst@porcupinehu.on.ca
Med Officer of Hlth Dr Rosemarie Ramsingh
Sec Ms. France Nolet-Vaillancourt
Pub Hlth Nurse Ms. Diane Fillion

Hornepayne
200 Front St
Box 127
Hornepayne ON P0M 1Z0
Tel. (807) 868-2091
Fax. (807) 868-2225
Email: info4you@porcupinehu.on.ca
Pub Hlth Nurse Ms. Chantal Arenovich

Iroquois Falls
58A Anson Dr
Box 575
Iroquois Falls ON P0K 1G0
Tel. (705) 258-2247
Fax. (705) 258-2249
Email: info4you@porcupinehu.on.ca
Sec Ms. Helen Desormeau

Kapuskasing
4 Ash St
Kapuskasing ON P5N 2C8
Tel. (705) 335-6101
Fax. (705) 337-1895
Email: info4you@porcupinehu.on.ca
Sec Ms. Pirette Tremblay

Matheson
507 8th Ave
PO Box 490
Matheson ON P0K 1N0
Tel. (705) 273-2954
Fax. (705) 273-2522
Email: info4you@porcupinehu.on.ca
Admv Asst Ms. Margaret Anne

Moosonee
Revillion St
PO Box 57
Moosonee ON P0L 1Y0
Tel. (705) 336-2294
Fax. (705) 336-2919
Email: info4you@porcupinehu.on.ca
Exec Asst Ms. Maria Cook

Smooth Rock Falls
141 5th St
Box 388
Smooth Rock Falls ON P0L 2B0
Tel. (705) 338-2654
Fax. (705) 338-2250
Email: info4you@porcupinehu.on.ca
Sec Ms. Diane Bernier

Region of Peel Public Health
8F-7120 Hurontario St
Mississauga ON L5W 1N4
Tel. (905) 799-7700
Fax. (905) 789-1604
Med Officer of Hlth Dr. Megan Ward
Assoc MOH Dr. Eileen De Villa
Admin Ms. Cassandra Julien

REGION OF WATERLOO PUBLIC HEALTH CORPORATE OFFICE
99 Regina St S
PO Box 1633 Stn Waterloo
Waterloo ON N2J 4V3
Tel. (519) 883-2000
Fax. (519) 883-2241
Email: lnolan@region.waterloo.on.ca
Med Officer of Hlth Dr. Liana Nolan
Sr Admv Asst Ms. Melody Hurllbut
Mktg Coord Ms. Lu-Ann Procter

Cambridge Public Health
150 Main St
Cambridge ON N1R 6P9
Tel. (519) 621-6110
Fax. (519) 622-5868
Sr Admv Asst Ms. Melody Hurllbut

Regional Municipality of Peel Health Department
7120 Hurontario St
PO Box 667
Mississauga ON L5M 2C2
Tel. (905) 791-7800 Ext.2566
Fax. (905) 564-2683
Email: david.mowat@peelregion.ca
Med Officer of Hlth Dr. David Mowat
Assoc MOH Dr. Eileen De Villa
Admv Asst Ms. Dianne Wiegand

RENFREW COUNTY & DISTRICT HEALTH UNIT CORPORATE OFFICE
7 International Dr
Pembroke ON K8A 6W5
Tel. (613) 735-8650 Ext.503
Fax. (613) 735-3067
Email: nwoodtke@rcdhu.com
Med Officer of Hlth Dr. Michael R A Corriveau
Contract Admin Noreen Woodtke

Arnprior Public Health
156-346 John St N
PO Box 188
Arnprior ON K7S 3H4
Tel. (613) 623-2991
Fax. (613) 623-8939
Email: mcorriveau@rcdhu.com
Med Officer of Hlth Dr. Michael Corriveau
Office Sec Ms. Betty Dunlop

Barry's Bay Public Health
12 Dunn St
Barrys Bay ON K0J 1B0
Tel. (613) 756-2744
Fax. (613) 756-5248
Email: nwoodtke@rcdhu.com
Med Officer of Hlth Dr. Michael Corriveau
Contract Admin Ms. Noreen Woodtke
Sec Ms. Barb Yskolskie

Renfrew Public Health
106-450 O'Brien Rd
Renfrew ON K7V 4B1
Tel. (613) 432-5853
Fax. (613) 432-3382
Sec Ms. Rose Mchale

SIMCOE MUSKOKA DISTRICT HEALTH UNIT CORPORATE OFFICE
15 Sperling Dr
Barrie ON L4M 6K9
Tel. (705) 721-7520 Ext.7219
Fax. (705) 721-1495
Email: charles.gardner@smdhu.org
Med Officer of Hlth Dr. Charles Gardner
Assoc Med Officer of Hlth Dr. Jim Pfaff
Assoc MOH Dr. Susan Surry
Exec Asst Ms. Phyllis Graham-Crowe

Collingwood Office
280 Pretty River Pky N
Collingwood ON L9Y 4J5
Tel. (705) 445-0804 Ext.720
Fax. (705) 445-6498
Managing Asst Ms. Susan Munroe
Admv Asst Mr. Maxime Holmes

Gravenhurst Office
5 Pineridge Gate
Gravenhurst ON P1P 1Z3
Tel. (705) 684-9090
Fax. (705) 684-9887
Prog Asst Ms. Diane Brie

Huntsville Office
34 Chaffey St
Huntsville ON P1H 1K1
Tel. (705) 789-8813
Fax. (705) 789-7245
Prog Asst Ms. Cheryl Spalding

Midland Office
B-865 Hugel Ave
Midland ON L4R 1X8
Tel. (705) 526-9324
Fax. (705) 526-1513
Prog Asst Ms. Rose Leonard

Orillia Office
120-169 Front St S
Orillia ON L3V 4S8
Tel. (705) 325-9565
Fax. (705) 325-2091
Sec Ms. Laury Mccullough

South Simcoe Office
2-25 King St S
Cookstown ON L0L 1L0
Tel. (705) 458-1103
Fax. (705) 458-0105
Prog Asst Ms. Bobbie Fullarton

SUDBURY & DISTRICT HEALTH UNIT CORPORATE OFFICE
1300 Paris St
Sudbury ON P3E 3A3
Tel. (705) 522-9200 Ext.291
Fax. (705) 522-5182
Email: sutcliffep@sdhu.com
CEO/Med Officer of Hlth Dr. Penny Sutcliffe
Assoc Med Officer of Hlth Dr. Na-Koshie Lamptey
Exec Dir Ms. Denise Lafond

Chapleau Office
101 Pine St E
Box 485
Chapleau ON P0M 1K0
Tel. (705) 864-1610
Fax. (705) 864-0820
Admv Office Asst Ms. Susie Mccoleman

Espanola Office
Espanola Mall 100C-800 Centre St
Espanola ON P5E 1J3
Tel. (705) 222-9202
Fax. (705) 869-5583
Sec Ms. Sandy Miles

Manitoulin Island Office
6163 Hwy 542
Box 87
Mindemoya ON P0P 1S0
Tel. (705) 370-9200
Fax. (705) 377-5580

Sudbury East Office
1 King St
Box 52
St Charles ON P0M 2W0
Tel. (705) 222-9201
Fax. (705) 867-0474
Office Asst Ms. Andree Lantaigne

THUNDER BAY DISTRICT HEALTH UNIT CORPORATE OFFICE
999 Balmoral St
Thunder Bay ON P7B 6E7
Tel. (807) 625-5900
Fax. (807) 623-2369
Email: david.williams@tbdhu.com
Med Officer of Hlth Dr. David Williams
Exec Asst Ms. Barabara Moro
Regd Dental Hygienist Mrs. Ruth Currie

Espanola
100-800 Centre St
Espanola ON P5E 1J3
Tel. (705) 222-9202
Fax. (705) 869-5583
Exec Asst Ms. Rachel Quesnel

Geraldton
510 Hogarth Ave W
Box 1360
Geraldton ON P0T 1M0
Tel. (807) 854-0454
Fax. (807) 854-1871
Mgr Ms. Laurie Malendyk

Manitouwadge
1 Health Care Court
Box 385
Manitouwadge ON P0T 2C0
Tel. (807) 826-4061
Fax. (807) 826-8664
Pub Hlth Nurse Ms. Shirley Saasto-Stopvra

Marathon
Marathon Library Building
24 Peninsula Rd
PO Box 384
Marathon ON P0T 2E0
Tel. (807) 229-1820
Fax. (807) 229-3356
Exec Asst Ms. Rachel Quesnel

Nipigon
Nipigon District Memorial Hosp
125 Hogan Road
PO Box 125
Nipigon ON P0T 2J0
Tel. (807) 887-3031
Fax. (807) 887-3489
Exec Asst Ms. Rachel Quesnel

Terrace Bay
McCausland Hospital 20B Cartier Rd
PO Box 1030
Terrace Bay ON P0T 2W0
Tel. (807) 825-7770
Fax. (807) 825-7774

TIMISKAMING HEALTH UNIT CORPORATE OFFICE
421 Shepherdson Rd
New Liskeard ON P0J 1P0
Tel. (705) 647-4305 Ext.2223
Fax. (705) 647-5779
Email: marlene.spruyt@timiskaminhu.com
Med Officer of Hlth Dr. Marlene Spruyt
COO Mrs. Esther Millar
Exec Asst Ms. Rachelle Leveiller

Dymond
3-883317 Hwy 65
PO Box 1090
New Liskeard ON P0J 1P0
Tel. (705) 647-4305
Fax. (705) 647-5779

Englehart
81 Fifth St
Englehart ON P0J 1H0
Tel. (705) 544-2221
Fax. (705) 544-8698
Exec Asst Ms. Rachelle Leveille

Kirkland Lake
31 Station Rd
Kirkland Lake ON P2N 3M6
Tel. (705) 567-9335
Fax. (705) 567-5476
Exec Asst Ms. Rachelle Leveille

TORONTO PUBLIC HEALTH CORPORATE OFFICE
277 Victoria St
Toronto ON M5B 1W2
Tel. (416) 392-7820
Fax. (416) 392-0713
Email: dmckeown@toronto.ca
Med Officer of Hlth Dr. David J McKeown
Assoc MOH Dr. Rita M Shahin
Assoc MOH Dr. Elizabeth A F Scott
Admv Asst Ms. Helen Tolvaisa

EAST REGION

Markham Road
1530 Markham Rd
Scarborough ON M1B 3G4
Tel. (416) 338-7420
Fax. (416) 338-6299
Email: publichealth@toronto.ca
Admv Support Ms. Joanne Nina

Scarborough
160 Borough Dr
Scarborough ON M1P 4N8
Tel. (416) 338-7600
Fax. (416) 338-7584
Email: publichealth@toronto.ca
Admv Asst Ms. Helen Tolvaisa

Toronto Memorial Park
175 Memorial Park
East York ON M4J 4Y6
Tel. (416) 338-0900
Fax. (416) 392-0714
Email: publichealth@toronto.ca
Admv Asst Ms. Janet Melanson

NORTH REGION

North York Sheppard West
3rd Floor 2300 Sheppard Ave W
North York ON M9M 3A4
Tel. (416) 338-8650
Fax. (416) 338-8651
Email: publichealth@toronto.ca
Admv Asst Ms. Janet Melanson

North York Yonge St
5100 Yonge St
2nd Floor
North York ON M2N 5V7
Tel. (416) 338-8500
Fax. (416) 338-8550
Email: publichealth@toronto.ca
Admv Asst Ms. Janet Melanson

Toronto Duncan Mill Office
225 Duncan Mill Rd
Suite 302
Toronto ON M3B 3K9
Fax. (416) 338-8610
Email: publichealth@toronto.ca
Admv Asst Ms. Janet Melanson

SOUTH REGION

Dundas West
2340 Dundas St W
Toronto ON M6P 4A9
Tel. (416) 392-0715
Fax. (416) 392-0645
Email: publichealth@toronto.ca
Admv Asst Ms. Janet Melanson

Queen West
1115 Queen St W
Toronto ON M6J 1J1
Fax. (416) 392-0631
Email: publichealth@toronto.ca
Admv Asst Ms. Janet Melanson

St Claire Ave
55 St Clair Ave E
Toronto ON M4T 1M2
Tel. (416) 392-0962
Fax. (416) 392-0716
Email: publichealth@toronto.ca
Med Officer of Hlth Dr. David McKeon
Assoc MOH Dr. Barbara Yaffe

WEST REGION

Etobicoke
399 The West Mall
Etobicoke ON M9C 2Y2
Tel. (416) 338-1515
Fax. (416) 338-1780
Email: publichealth@toronto.ca
Admv Asst Ms. Janet Melanson
Dental Hygienist Tara Prendergast

WELLINGTON-DUFFERIN-GUELPH PUBLIC HEALTH CORPORATE OFFICE
100-474 Wellington Rd 18
RR1
Fergus ON N1M 2W3
Tel. (519) 846-2715 Ext.2500
Fax. (519) 846-0323
Email: sylvia.muir@wdgpublichealth.ca
Med Officer of Hlth Dr. Nicola J Mercer
Exec Asst Ms. Sylvia Muir

Mount Forest
311 Foster St
Mount Forest ON N0G 2L1
Tel. (519) 846-2715 Ext.2301
Fax. (519) 323-9312
Email: sylvia.muir@wdgpublichealth.ca
Med Officer of Hlth Dr. Nicola Mercer
Exec Asst Ms. Sylvia Muir

North Guelph
20 Shelldale Cres
Guelph ON N1H 1C8
Tel. (519) 846-2715 Ext.2301
Fax. (519) 824-7399
Email: sylvia.muir@wdgpublichealth.ca
Med Officer of Hlth Dr. Nicola Mercer
Exec Asst Ms. Sylvia Muir
Regd Dental Hygienist Ms. Emilyrose Burns

Orangeville Office
71 Broadway St
Orangeville ON L9W 1K1
Tel. (519) 846-2715 Ext.2301
Fax. (519) 941-1600
Email: sylvia.muir@wdgpublichealth.ca
Med Officer of Hlth Dr. Nicola Mercer
Exec Asst Ms. Syliva Muir

Shelburne Office
Mel Lloyd Ctre 167 Centre St
Entrance C
Shelburne ON L0N 1S4
Tel. (519) 846-2715 Ext.2301
Fax. (519) 925-3744
Email: sylvia.muir@wdgpublichealth.ca
Exec Asst Ms. Sylvia Muir

South Guelph
600 Southgate Dr
Guelph ON N1G 4P6
Tel. (519) 846-2175 Ext.2301
Fax. (519) 836-7215
Email: sylvia.muir@wdgpublichealth.ca
Exec Asst Ms. Sylvia Muir
Staff Dr. Mary T Wilson

WINDSOR-ESSEX COUNTY HEALTH UNIT CORPORATE OFFICE
1005 Ouellette Ave
Windsor ON N9A 4J8
Tel. (519) 258-2146 Ext.1402
Fax. (519) 258-6003
Email: aheimann@wechealthunit.org
Med Officer of Hlth Dr. Allan Heimann
Admv Asst Ms. Rosanne St. Denis
Support Services Officer D Gemmell

Essex Office
215-360 Fairview Ave W
Essex ON N8M 3G4
Tel. (519) 776-5933
Fax. (519) 776-6102
Dir-Health Dr. G Allen Heimann
Exec Asst Ms. Rosanne St. Denis

Leamington Office
215 Talbot St E
Leamington ON N8H 3X5
Tel. (519) 326-5716
Fax. (519) 326-4642
Med Officer of Hlth Dr. G Allen Heimann
Exec Asst Ms. Rosanne St. Denis

YORK REGION COMMUNITY & HEALTH SERVICES DEPARTMENT CORPORATE OFFICE
17250 Yonge St
PO Box 147 Stn Main
Newmarket ON L3Y 6Z1
Tel. (905) 895-4444 Ext.4012
Fax. (905) 895-3166
Email: karim.kurji@york.ca
Med Officer of Hlth Dr. Karim Kurji
Assoc MOH Dr. Erica Weir
Admv Asst Ms. Paula Ferreira

Newmarket
22 Prospect St
Newmarket ON L3Y 3S9
Tel. (905) 895-4512
Fax. (905) 895-7520
Email: karim.kurji@york.ca
Med Officer of Hlth Dr. Karim Kurji
Regd Dental Hygienist Ms. Jennifer McLean
Regd Dental Hygienist Mrs. Teresa Siddons

Newmarket Davis Dr
240-465 Davis Dr
Newmarket ON L3Y 2P1
Tel. (905) 895-4511
Fax. (905) 895-6602
Email: karim.kurji@york.ca
Med Officer of Hlth Dr. Karim Kurji
Admv Asst Ms. Paula Ferreira

Richmond Hill
50 High Tech Rd
2nd Floor
Richmond Hill ON L4B 4N7
Tel. (905) 762-2090
Fax. (905) 762-2091
Email: karim.kurji@york.ca
Med Officer of Hlth Dr. Karim Kurji
Admv Asst Ms. Paula Ferreira

Unionville
B6 9-4261 Highway 7
Unionville ON L3R 9W6
Tel. (905) 940-1333
Fax. (905) 940-9872
Email: karim.kurji@york.ca
Med Officer of Hlth Dr. Karim Kurji
Admv Asst Ms. Paula Ferreira

QUÉBEC

Director of Public Health, Dr Horacio Arruda Tel: (418) 266-6720

Agence de développement de réseaux locaux des services de santé et des services sociaux de l'Abitibi-Témiscamingue
1-9 e rue
3 étage, Pavillion Laramée
Rouyn-Noranda QC J9X 2A9
Tel. (819) 764-3264
Fax. (819) 797-1947
Email: lise_stamour@ssss.gouv.qc.ca
Prés/Dir gén Mr. Jacques Boissonneault
Dir-Pub Hlth Dr. Réal Lacombe

Agence de développement de réseaux locaux des services de santé et des services sociaux de la Côte-Nord
691 rue Jalbert
Baie-Comeau QC G5C 2A1
Tel. (418) 589-9845
Fax. (418) 295-8574
Email: pascal.paradis.09asss@ssss.gouv.qc.ca
Prés/Dir gén Ms. Gaetan Garon
Dir-Pub Hlth Dr. Raynald Cloutier
Staff Dr. Stephane Trepanier

Agence de développement de réseaux locaux des services de santé et des services sociaux de Lanaudière
5 è étage 245 rue du Curé-Majeau
Joliette QC J6E 8S8
Tel. (450) 759-1157
Fax. (450) 759-0023
Email: agencelanaudiere@ssss.gouv.qc.ca
Coord santé, séc, enviro Mr. Rivard Jonathan

Agence de développement de réseaux locaux des services de santé et des services sociaux du Saguenay-Lac St-Jean
930 Jacques-Cartier est
Chicoutimi QC G7H 7K9
Tel. (418) 545-4980
Fax. (418) 545-8791
Email: info@santesaglac.gouv.qc.ca
Prés/Chef dir Martine Couture
Dir-Pub Hlth Dr. Andrew Kennedy

Agence de santé et des services sociaux du Bas Saint-Laurent
288 rue Pierre-Saindon
Rimouski QC G5L 9A8
Tel. (418) 724-5231
Fax. (418) 723-1597
Prés/Dir gén Ms. Isabelle Malo

Agence de la santé et des services sociaux de la Capitale-Nationale
Direction rég de santé pub 2400 aveue D'Estimauville
Québec QC G1E 7G9
Tel. (418) 666-7000
Fax. (418) 666-2776
Email: 03_rrsss@ssss.gouv.qc.ca
Prés/Dir gén Mr. Guy Thibodeau

Agence de la santé et des services sociaux de Chaudière-Appalaches
363 route Cameron
Sainte-Marie QC G6E 3E2
Tel. (418) 386-3363
Fax. (418) 386-3361
Email: reception.rr12@ssss.gouv.qc.ca
Prés/Dir gén Marc Tanguay
Dir santé pub Phiippe Lessard
Admin Ms. Maryse Asselin

Agence de la santé et des services sociaux de l'Estrie
300-300 King St E
Sherbrooke QC J1G 1B1
Tel. (819) 566-7861
Fax. (819) 569-8894
Email: information.agence05@ssss.gouv.qc.ca
Prés/Dir gén Ms. Johanne Turgeon

RESOURCE SECTION

Agence de la santé et des services sociaux des Laurentides
1000 rue Labelle
Local 210
Saint-Jérôme QC J7Z 5N6
Tel. (450) 436-8622
Fax. (450) 432-8712
Email: infosantelaurentides@ssss.gouv.qc.ca
Prés/Dir gén Mr. Marc Fortin
Dir commun Mr. Marc Angers
Dir ress hum Mr. Luc Bergeron

Agence de la santé et des services sociaux de Laval
TA-800 boul Chomedey
Laval QC H7V 3Y4
Tel. (450) 978-2000
Fax. (450) 978-2100
Email: regie-laval@ssss.gouv.qc.ca
Dir Reg-Qual/Res/Gestion Mr. Yves St-Onge
Admin Mr. Francine Prévost

Agence de la santé et des services sociaux de la Mauricie et du Centre du-Québec
3e étage 550 rue Bonaventure
Trois-Rivières QC G9A 2B5
Tel. (819) 693-3636
Fax. (819) 373-1627
commissaires.plaintes04@ssss.gouv.qc.ca
Prés/Dir gén Mr. Gaétan Lamy

Agence de santé et des services sociaux de la Montérégie
1255 rue Beauregard
Longueuil QC J4K 2M3
Tel. (450) 928-6777 Ext.4300
Fax. (450) 679-6443
Email: agencemonteregie@ssss.gouv.qc.ca
Prés/Chef dir Claire Pagé
Dir Ms. Jocelyne Sauve
Med Consultant Dr. Lyne Judd

Agence de la santé et des services sociaux de Montréal
3725 rue Saint-Denis
Montréal QC H2X 3L9
Tel. (514) 286-6500
Fax. (514) 286-5669
Email: prenom_nom@ssss.gouv.qc.ca
Prés/Dir gén Ms. Danielle McCann

Agence de la santé et des services sociaux de l'Outaouais
104 rue Lois
Gatineau QC J8Y 3R7
Tel. (819) 770-7747
Fax. (819) 771-8632
Email: lucie_lemieux@ssss.gouv.qc.ca
Prés/Dir gén Mr. Guy Morissette

Centre régional de santé et de services sociaux de la Baie-James
312 3è rue
Chibougamau QC G8P 1N5
Tel. (418) 748-3575
Fax. (418) 748-2081
Email: info.crsssbj@ssss.gouv.qc.ca
Prés/Dir gén Ms. Nathalie Boisvert

Cree Board of Health & Social Services James Bay
PO Box 250
Chisasibi QC J0M 1E0
Tel. (819) 929-3596
Fax. (819) 929-3851
Infirm chef Ms. Ghislaine Télémaque

Direction de santé publique
205-1 York Ouest
Gaspé QC G4X 2W5
Tel. (418) 368-2443
Fax. (418) 368-1317
Email: agence11@ssss.gouv.qc.ca
Prés/Dir gén Gilles Pelletier
Dir-Pub Hlth Mr. Christian Bernier

Institut National de Santé Publique du Québec
945 av Wolfe
Québec QC G1V 5B3
Tel. (418) 650-5115 Ext.5336
Fax. (418) 646-9328
Prés/Dir gén Mr. Luc Boileau
Med Consultant Dr. Rejean Dion
Physician Epidemiol Dr. Agathe Croteau

Régie régionale de la santé et des services sociaux du Nunavik
PO Box 900
Kuujjuaq QC J0M 1C0
Tel. (819) 964-2222
Fax. (819) 964-2888
Email: information_rrsss17@ssss.gouv.qc.ca
Dir santé Serge Déry

NEW BRUNSWICK

Chief Medical Officer of Health, Dr Eilish Cleary Tel: (506) 444-2112

HORIZON HEALTH NETWORK CORPORATE OFFICE
155 Pleasant St
Miramichi NB E1V 1Y3
Tel. (506) 623-5500
Fax. (506) 623-5533
President/CEO John McGarry
VP Med Acad Affairs Dr. J A Edouard Hendriks
COO Andrea Seymour
Corp Dir of Communications Janet Hogan

Blackville Public Health
2A Shaffer Lane
Blackville NB E9B 1P4
Tel. (506) 843-2959
Fax. (506) 543-2911
Dir Ginette Pellerin
Sec Ms. Erica Robichaud

Boiestown Public Health
1-6154 Route 8
Boiestown NB E6A 1M4
Tel. (506) 453-5200
Fax. (506) 444-5108
Email: horizon@horizonnb.ca
Pub Hlth Nurse Ms. Jeane MacWilliams

Chipman Public Health
2-9 Civic Court
PO Box 280
Chipman NB E4A 2H8
Tel. (506) 453-7076
Fax. (506) 339-7181
Pub Hlth Nurse Ms. Tracy Busson

Fredericton Public Health Office
1200-300 St. Mary's St
Fredericton NB E3B 5H1
Tel. (506) 453-5200
Fax. (506) 453-5108
Med Officer of Hlth Dr. Cristin Muecke
Reg Admin Faye Skaarup

Gibson Health
700 Priestman St
PO Box 9000
Fredericton NB E3B 5N5
Tel. (506) 452-5678
Fax. (506) 452-5670
Reg Mgr Infection Ctrl Jane Stafford
Reg Mgr Lab Ms. Jennifer Sutherland
Mgr-Health Mr. Brett Fraser

Grand Manan Public Health Office
4-130 Route 776
Grand Manan NB E5G 1A3
Tel. (506) 662-7024
Fax. (506) 662-3067
Pub Hlth Nurse Ms Jackie

Miramichi-Chatham Public Health
300-1780 Water St
Miramichi NB E1N 1B6
Tel. (506) 778-6102
Fax. (506) 773-6611
Reg Dir Ms. Ginette Pellerin
Sec Ms. Marian Whitty

Neguac Public Health
60-1175 rue Principale
Neguac NB E9G 1T1
Tel. (506) 776-3824
Fax. (506) 776-3897
Dir Ginette Pellerin
Sec Ms. Erica Robichaud

Oromocto Public Health
275A Restigouche Rd
Oromocto NB E2V 2H1
Tel. (506) 453-5200
Fax. (506) 444-5108
Pub Hlth Nurse Ms. Kathy Levesque

Perth-Andover Public Health Office
35 Tribe Rd
Perth-Andover NB E7H 0A8
Tel. (506) 325-4630
Fax. (905) 325-4724
Pub Hlth Nurse Ms. Barb O'Donnell

Plaster-Rock Public Health
120 Main St
Plaster Rock NB E7G 2E5
Tel. (506) 325-4630
Fax. (506) 325-4724

St George Public Health
5 Riverview Ave
PO Box 300
St George NB E5C 3M1
Tel. (506) 755-4022
Fax. (506) 658-3067
Pub Hlth Nurse Ms. Darlene Lambert

Saint John Public Health
55 Union St
Saint John NB E2L 5B7
Tel. (506) 658-2454
Fax. (506) 658-3067
Pres/CEO Ms. Dora Nicinski
VP-Corp Aff/CFO Mr. Michael R Chisholm
Reg Dir-Enviro Mr. Roy Hess

St Stephen Public Health
41 King St
St Stephen NB E3L 2C1
Tel. (506) 466-7504
Fax. (506) 658-3067
Pub Hlth Nurse Ms. Leslie Sharkey
Staff Dr. David J M Green

Sussex Public Health
30 Moffatt Ave
Sussex NB E4E 1E8
Tel. (506) 432-2003
Fax. (506) 658-3067
Pub Hlth Nurse Marti Traston

Woodstock Public Health
145-200 King St
Woodstock NB E7M 1R8
Tel. (506) 325-4630
Fax. (506) 325-4724
Pub Hlth Nurse Ms. Marjorie Allison-Ross

VITALITE HEALTH NETWORK CORPORATE OFFICE
600-275 Main St
Bathurst NB E2A 1A9
Tel. (506) 544-2133
Fax. (506) 544-2145
Email: info@vitalitenb.ca

Bathurst Public Health
2nd Floor 165 St. Andrew St
Bathurst NB E2A 1C1
Tel. (506) 549-5550
Fax. (506) 547-7459
Email: yves.leger@gnb.ca
Med Officer of Hlth Dr. Yves Leger

Belledune Public Health Office
Jacquet River Health Centre
41B Mack St
Belledune NB E8G 2R3
Tel. (506) 237-3206
Fax. (506) 237-3209
Sec Ms. Melissa Power

Campbellton Health Protection
Regional Pub Hlth Office
15-10 Village Ave
!st Floor
Campbellton NB E3N 3S8
Tel. (506) 789-2549
Fax. (506) 759-6648
Exec Dir Mr. Yves Goudreau
Adm Support Right Hon. Toni Blanchard
Sec Ms. Melissa Power

Caraquet Public Health
295 Blvd St Pierre W
PO Box 5590
Caraquet NB E1W 1B7
Tel. (506) 726-2025
Fax. (506) 726-2493
Sec Ms. Roseline Chiasson

Edmundston Public Health Office
PO Box 5001 Stn Main
Edmundston NB E3V 3L3
Tel. (506) 737-4800
Fax. (506) 735-3142
Email: Health.Sante@gnb.ca
Med Officer of Hlth Dr. Yves Leger
Reg Admin Ms. Diane Levasseur
Sec Ms. Michele Dianchette

Grand Falls Public Health Office
Municipal Bldg 131 Pleasant St
PO Box 5001
Grand Falls NB E3Z 1G1
Tel. (506) 457-4800
Fax. (506) 475-2443
Email: Health.Sante@gnb.ca
Pub Hlth Nurse Ms. Ginette Desjardins

Kedgwick Public Health Office
D-39 Notre-Dame St
PO Box 158
Kedgwick NB E8B 1H5
Tel. (506) 284-3422
Fax. (506) 284-3447
Med Officer of Hlth Dr. Jessie Turcotte
Pub Hlth Nurse Ms. Manon Bujold

Moncton Public Health Office
81 Albert St
PO Box 5001
Moncton NB E1C 8R3
Tel. (506) 856-2401
Fax. (506) 856-2623
Dep Chief MOH Dr. Denis G Allard
Staff Dr. Yves A Leger

Plaster Rock Public Health Office
120 Main St
Plaster Rock NB E7G 2E5
Tel. (506) 325-4630
Fax. (506) 325-4724
Pub Hlth Nurse Ms. Pauline Cormier

Richibucto Public Health Office
Cartier place 153-25 Cartier boul
Richibucto NB E4W 5R5
Tel. (506) 523-7620
Fax. (506) 523-7678
Pub Hlth Mgr Murielle Wade
Pub Hlth Nurse Ms. Brenda Basgarasche

Sackville Public Health Office
B-95 Queens Rd
Sackville NB E4L 4H2
Tel. (506) 364-4080
Fax. (506) 364-4099
Pub Hlth Mgr Ms. Nicole Poirier

Shediac Public Health Office
Centre Ville Mall 160-342 Main St
Shediac NB E4P 2E7
Tel. (506) 533-3354
Fax. (506) 533-3376
Email: info@vitalitenb.ca
Med Officer of Hlth Dr. Denis Allard
Pub Hlth Mgr Ms. Murielle Wade

Shippagan Public Health
239B Blvd J D Gauthier
PO Box 5001
Shippagan NB E8S 1N2
Tel. (506) 336-3061
Fax. (506) 336-3068
Adm Sec Ms. Dina Noel

Tracadie-Sheila Public Health
Tracadie place 3520 Main St
Tracadie-Sheila NB E1X 1C9
Tel. (506) 394-3888
Fax. (506) 394-3858
Dir Ms. Violette Benhamed
Mgr Ms. Livain Doucett

NOVA SCOTIA

Chief Public Health Officer, Dr Robert Strang Tel: (902) 424-2358

ANNAPOLIS VALLEY HEALTH

Public Health Services Annapolis
Annapolis Royal Hlth Ctre
821 St George St
PO Box 426
Annapolis Royal NS B0S 1A0
Tel. (902) 532-2381
Fax. (902) 532-2113
Email: pr@avdha.nshealth.ca
Reg Med Officer of Hlth Dr. Richard Gould

Public Health Services Middleton
462 Main St
Box 730
Middleton NS B0S 1P0
Tel. (902) 825-3411
Fax. (902) 825-0599
Commun Health Nurse Ms. Stacey Ben

Public Health Services Wolfville
23 Earnscliffe Ave
Wolfville NS B4P 1X4
Tel. (902) 542-2266
Fax. (902) 542-4619
Email: jhillier@avdha-nshealth.ca
Med Officer of Hlth Dr. J Richard Gould
Sec-MOH Ms. J Hillier

CAPE BRETON DISTRICT HEALTH AUTHORITY

Public Health Baddeck
30 Old Margaree Road
PO Box 6
Baddeck NS B0E 1B0
Tel. (902) 295-2178
Fax. (902) 295-3432
Pub Hlth Nurse Ms. Cindy Gillis-McDougall

Public Health Cheticamp
15102 Cabot Trail
PO Box 111
Cheticamp NS B0E 1H0
Tel. (902) 224-2410
Fax. (902) 224-2903
Email: public.health@cbdha.nshealth.ca
Mgr Mr. Bruce Morrison

Public Health Glace Bay
Ground Floor 633 Main St
Glace Bay NS B1A 4X9
Tel. (902) 842-4050
Fax. (902) 842-4004
Admv Asst Ms. Carol Gallagher

RESOURCE SECTION

Public Health Inverness
26 Upper Railway St
PO Box 118
Inverness NS B0E 1N0
Tel. (902) 258-1920
Fax. (902) 258-2721

Public Health Neil's Harbour
Buchanan Mem'l Comm Hlth Ctre PO Box 46
Neils Harbour NS B0C 1N0
Tel. (902) 336-2295
Fax. (902) 336-2202

Public Health New Waterford
New Waterford Consolidated Hospital
716 King St
PO Box 26
New Waterford NS B1H 3Z5
Tel. (902) 862-2204
Fax. (902) 862-3155
Admv Asst Ms. Patsy Hayes
Pub Hlth Nurse Ms. Kathy MacNeil
Pub Hlth Nurse Ms. Antoinette Hillier

Public Health Sydney
235 Townsend St
2nd Floor
Sydney NS B1P 5E7
Tel. (902) 563-2214
Fax. (902) 563-0508
Dir-Community Hlth Ms. Kathy Bell
Admv Asst Ms. Julie Hawco

Public Health Sydney Mines
7 Fraser Ave
Sydney Mines NS B1V 2B8
Tel. (902) 736-6245
Fax. (902) 736-7909

CAPITAL HEALTH IWK HEALTH CENTRE

Public Health Dartmouth
5-7 Mellor Ave
Dartmouth NS B3B 0E8
Tel. (902) 481-5800
Fax. (902) 481-5803
Dir Ms. Linda Young
Med Officer of Hlth Dr. Gaynor B Watson-Creed

COLCHESTER EAST HANTS HEALTH AUTHORITY

Elmsdale Public Health Services
Lloyd E. Matheson Centre
150-15 Commerce Court
Elmsdale NS B2S 3K5
Tel. (902) 883-8444
Fax. (902) 883-3400
Dir-Pub Rel Ms. Krista Woods

Truro Public Health Office
Public Health Services 3F-201 Willow St
Truro NS B2N 4Z9
Tel. (902) 893-5820
Fax. (902) 893-5839
Med Officer of Hlth Dr. Shelley Sarwal
Admv Asst Ms. Sherry Brander

CUMBERLAND HEALTH AUTHORITY CORPORATE OFFICE

Amherst public Health
34 Prince Arthur St
Amherst NS B4H 1V6
Tel. (902) 661-1090
Fax. (902) 667-1125
Med Officer of Hlth Dr. Shelly Sarwal
Dir-Pub Affairs Ms. Ann Keddy
Mgr Ms. Darla Macpherson

GUYSBOROUGH ANTIGONISH STRAIT HEALTH AUTHORITY

Antigonish Public Health Services
23 Bay St
Antigonish NS B2G 2G7
Tel. (902) 867-4500 Ext.4800
Fax. (902) 863-5111
Donalda.Macgillivary@gasha.nshealth.ca

Arichat Public Health
14 Bay St
PO Box 224
Arichat NS B0E 1A0
Tel. (902) 226-2944
Fax. (902) 226-1594
Pub Hlth Nurse Ms. Joanne DeCouste

Canso Public Health Canso
Eastern Memorial Hospital
PO BOX 299
Canso NS B0H 1H0
Tel. (902) 366-2925
Fax. (902) 366-2900
Pub Hlth Nurse Ms. Angela Dobson

Guysborough Public Health
Guysborough Hospital
PO Box 106
Guysborough NS B0H 1N0
Tel. (902) 533-3502
Fax. (902) 533-2167

Neil's Harbour Public Health
PO Box 46
Neils Harbour NS B0C 1N0
Tel. (902) 336-2295
Fax. (902) 336-2202
Email: heather.budge@cbdha.nshealth.ca
Pub Hlth Nurse Ms. Heather Budge

Port Hawkesbury Public Health
Public Health Services 3-708 Reeves St
Port Hawkesbury NS B9A 2S1
Tel. (902) 625-1693
Fax. (902) 625-4091
sharon.spencer@publichealth.ns.ca
Mgr Ms. Donna Samson
Contact Ms. Sharon Spencer

Sherbrooke Public Health
St Mary's Hospital PO Box 275
Sherbrooke NS B0J 3C0
Tel. (902) 522-2212
Fax. (902) 522-2094

PICTOU COUNTY HEALTH AUTHORITY

Public Health Services New Glasgow
835 East River Rd
New Glasgow NS B2H 3S6
Tel. (902) 752-5151
Fax. (902) 755-7175
Med Officer of Hlth Dr. Shelly Sarwal
Dir Ms. Lubin Bourque
Mgr Mr. Patrick Mullaly

SOUTH SHORE HEALTH

Public Health Services Bridgewater
200-215 Dominion St
Health Authority
Bridgewater NS B4V 2K7
Tel. (902) 543-0850
Fax. (902) 543-8024
Reg Med Officer of Hlth Dr. Richard Gould
Dir Ms. Carol MacKinnon
Sec Ms. Amanada Nauss

Public Health Services Liverpool
175 School St
PO Box 694
Liverpool NS B0T 1K0
Tel. (902) 354-5737
Fax. (902) 354-2127
Pub Hlth Nurse Ms. Nadeen A

Public Health Services Lunenberg
14 High St
PO Box 96
Lunenburg NS B0J 2C0
Tel. (902) 634-4014
Fax. (902) 634-7330
Reg Med Officer of Hlth Dr. Richard Gould

Public Health Services New Germany
5246 Hwy 10
PO Box 106
New Germany NS B0R 1E0
Tel. (902) 644-2710
Fax. (902) 624-8650
Nurse-in-Charge Ms. Susie Wood

SOUTH WEST HEALTH

Public Health Services Barrington
Barrington Plaza 3640 Hwy 3
PO Box 68
Barrington Passage NS B0W 1G0
Tel. (902) 637-2430
Fax. (902) 637-4502
Reg Med Officer of Hlth Dr. Richard Gould

Public Health Services Digby
Digby General Hospital
67 Warwick St
PO Box 820
Digby NS B0V 1A0
Tel. (902) 245-2557
Fax. (902) 245-1302

Public Health Services Meteghan
Clare Medical Centre
PO Box 150
Meteghan Centre NS B0W 2K0
Tel. (902) 645-2325
Fax. (902) 645-3250

Public Health Services Shelburne
Roseway Hospital
1606 Sandy Pont Rd
PO Box 610
Shelburne NS B0T 1W0
Tel. (902) 875-2623
Fax. (902) 875-4502
Pub Hlth Nurse Krissy Muise

Public Health Services Yarmouth
4th Fl Yarmouth Reg Hosp
60 Vancouver St
Yarmouth NS B5A 2P5
Tel. (902) 742-7141
Fax. (902) 742-6062
Reg Med Officer of Hlth Dr. Richard Gould

PRINCE EDWARD ISLAND

Chief Public Health Officer, Dr Heather Morrison Tel: (902) 368-4996

Chief Public Health Office Prince Eward Island
16 Fitzroy St
2nd Floor; PO Box 2000
Charlottetown PE C1A 7N8
Tel. (902) 368-4996
Fax. (902) 620-3354
Chief Pub Hlth Officer Dr. Heather Morrison
Dep Chief Hlth Officer Dr. Lamont Sweet

Primary Care Services Speech & Nutrition
17 Knights Ave
PO Box 550
Souris PE C0A 2B0
Tel. (902) 687-7049
Fax. (902) 687-7048
Nurse Ms. Jean MacDonald
Regd Dietician Ms. Lynne Faubert

Public Health Nursing
205 Linden Ave
Summerside PE C1N 2K4
Tel. (902) 888-8160
Fax. (902) 888-8153
Pub Hlth Coord W Joan Savage

Queens Health Region
Sherwood Business Centre
161 St Peters Rd
PO Box 2000 Stn Central
Charlottetown PE C1A 7N8
Tel. (902) 368-4530
Fax. (902) 368-4497
Med Dir Dr. Alfred Morais
Mgr-Pub Hlth Nurse Valerie Nicholson

NEWFOUNDLAND AND LABRADOR

Chief Medical Officer of Health, Dr Faith Stratton Tel: (709) 729-3430

CENTRAL HEALTH CORPORATE OFFICE
21 Carmelight Rd
Grnd-Falls-Windsor NL A2A 2E1
Tel. (709) 292-2500
Fax. (709) 292-2249
VP Ms. Rosemarie Goodyear
Exec Sec Ms. Dale Winsor

EASTERN HEALTH CORPORATE OFFICE
Building 532
PO Box 13122
St. John's NL A1B 4A4
Tel. (709) 752-4192
Fax. (709) 752-4873
Med Officer of Hlth Dr. David J Allison
Asst Medical Officer Dr. Sandeep Mangat
Physician Emerg Dr. H Blair Drover

EASTERN HEALTH RURAL
Hawco Building 34 Salmonair Line
PO Box 70
St. John's NL A1A 2R0
Tel. (709) 229-1551
Fax. (709) 229-1591
Email: catherinedonovan@hcse.ca
Med Officer Hlth Dr. Catherine Donovan
Sec Ms. Shirley Doran

LABRADOR-GRENFELL HEALTH CORPORATE OFFICE
PO Box 7000, Station C
Happy-Valley-Goose NL A0P 1C0
Tel. (709) 897-2267
Fax. (709) 896-4032
CEO Mr. Boyd Rowe
Sec Ms. Angie Elliot

Happy-Valley-Goose Public Health
Confederation Bldg W Block
PO Box 8700
St John's NL A1B 4J6
Tel. (709) 729-0724
Reg'l Dir-Env Hlth Michele Leblanc-Havard
CDC Nurse Ms Sylvia Doody

WESTERN HEALTH
1 Brookfield Ave
PO Box 2005 Stn Main
Corner Brook NL A2H 6J7
Tel. (709) 637-5245
Fax. (709) 637-5410
CEO Ms. Susan Gillam
Med Officer of Hlth Dr. Greg Mercer

YUKON TERRITORY

Beaver Creek Health Facility
GD
PO Box 3
Beaver Creek YT Y0B 1A0
Tel. (867) 862-4444
Fax. (867) 862-7909
Nurse-in-Charge Ms. Sandra Frost

Carcross Health Centre
PO Box 27
Carcross YT Y0B 1B0
Tel. (867) 821-4444
Fax. (867) 821-3909
Nurse-in-charge Ms. Patricia Lincoln

Carmacks Health Centre
PO Box 230
Carmacks YT Y0B 1C0
Tel. (867) 863-4444
Fax. (867) 863-6612
Email: hc.caramacks@gov.yk.ca
Admin Ms. Helena Belanger
Nurse-in-charge Ms. Deb Crosby

Destruction Bay Health Centre
GD
Destruction Bay YT Y0B 1H0
Tel. (867) 841-4444
Fax. (867) 841-5274
Email: nic.destruction-bay@gov.yk.ca
Nurse-in-Charge Ms. Sharon Kerr

Faro Health Center
PO Box 99
Faro YT Y0B 1K0
Tel. (867) 994-4444
Fax. (867) 994-3457
Email: faro.hc@gov.yk.ca
Nurse Mgr Ms. Debra Edwards

Haines Junction Health Centre
131 Bates St
PO Box 5369
Haines Junction YT Y0B 1L0
Tel. (867) 634-4444
Fax. (867) 634-2733

Kwanlin Dun Health Centre
35 McIntyre Dr
Whitehorse YT Y1A 5A5
Tel. (867) 633-7800
Fax. (867) 668-5057
Email: reception@kwanlindun.com
Dir Ms. Cameron Gibbons

Mayo Health Centre
PO Box 98
Mayo YT Y0B 1M0
Tel. (867) 996-4444
Fax. (867) 996-2018
Email: hc.mayo@gov.yk.ca
Staff Dr. A Majid Bakri
RN/NIC Ms. Linda Heasley
Nurse Pract Ms. Rachalle Desharnais

Office of the Medical Health Officer
4 Hospital Rd
Whitehorse YT Y1A 3H8
Tel. (867) 667-8323
Fax. (867) 667-8349
Med Officer of Hlth Dr. Brendan Hanley

Old Crow Nursing Station
PO Box 92
Old Crow YT Y0B 1N0
Tel. (867) 966-4444
Fax. (867) 966-3614
Email: nic.old-crow@gov.yk.ca
Chief Nurse P Arey
A-Nurse-in-charge Ms. Maurice Chiasson

Pelly Crossing Health Centre
Box 20
Pelly Crossing YT Y0B 1P0
Tel. (867) 537-4444
Fax. (867) 537-3611
Nurse-in-charge Ms. Jody Saul

Ross River Health Centre
GD
Ross River YT Y0B 1S0
Tel. (867) 969-4444
Fax. (867) 969-2014
Nurse-in-Charge Ms. Lynne Harris

Teslin Health Centre
PO Box 70
Teslin YT Y0A 1B0
Tel. (867) 390-4444

Fax. (867) 390-2217
Gen Practitioner Dr. Rao Tadepali
Primary Nurse practioner Ms. Shari Comerford
Primary Health Nurse Ms. Deb Chadwick

Watson Lake Health Centre
PO Box 500
Watson Lake YT Y0A 1C0
Tel. (867) 536-7483
Fax. (867) 536-7011
Support Serv Super Ms. Laura Hauser

Watson Lake Hospital
PO Box 866
Watson Lake YT Y0A 1C0
Tel. (867) 536-4444
Fax. (867) 536-7302
Email: hosp.watson-lake@wgh.yk.ca
Facility Admin Ms. Carol Chiasson
Admv Asst Ms. Holly Brown
Support Serv Supvr Ms. Laura Hauser

Whitehorse Health Centre
9010 Quartz Rd
Whitehorse YT Y1A 2Z5
Tel. (867) 667-8864
Fax. (867) 393-6407

NORTHWEST TERRITORIES

Chief Public Health Officer, Dr Lorne Clearsky Tel: (867) 920-8646

BEAUFORT-DELTA HEALTH & SOCIAL SERVICES AUTHORITY

Inuvik Public Health Unit
106 Veteran's Way 1st Floor
Bag Service #2
Inuvik NT X0E 0T0
Tel. (867) 777-7246
Fax. (867) 777-3255
Email: jeannie_greenland@gov.nt.ca
Admv Asst Ms. Jennie Greenland
Medical Doctors Office Dr. Roohina Virk
Nurse-in-charge Ms. Barbara Lennie

DEH CHO HEALTH & SOCIAL SERVICES AUTHORITY

Fort Simpson Public Health Unit
Box 246
Fort Simpson NT X0E 0N0
Tel. (867) 695-3815
Fax. (867) 695-2920
Email: health_beat@gov.nt.ca
Mgr-Health Ms. Cindy MacDonald

FORT SMITH HEALTH & SOCIAL SERVICES AUTHORITY

Fort Smith Public Health Unit
41 Breynat St
Box 1080
Fort Smith NT X0E 0P0
Tel. (867) 872-6203
Fax. (867) 872-6251
Chair Ms. Brenda Johnson
CEO Mr. Robert Tardiff

HAY RIVER HEALTH & SOCIAL SERVICES AUTHORITY

Hay River Public Health Unit
3 Gaetz Dr
Hay River NT X0E 0R8
Tel. (867) 874-7100
Fax. (867) 874-7109
CEO Ms. Sue Cullen
Exec Asst Mrs. Erin Griffiths
Enviro. Hlth. Offr. Rhiam Harrison

Office of the Chief Public Health Officer
5022 49 St, CST-6
Box 1320
Yellowknife NT X1A 2L9
Tel. (867) 920-3231
Fax. (867) 873-0442
Email: rachel_kirizopoulos@gov.nt.ca
Chief Pub Hlth Officer Dr. Lorne Clearsky
Asst to Chief Pub Hlth Off Ms. Rachel Kirizopoulos
Dep Chief Pub Hlth Officer Dr. Kami Kandola

SATHU HEALTH & SOCIAL SERVICES AUTHORITY

Regional Public Health Norman Wells
Box 340
Norman Wells NT X0E 0V0
Tel. (867) 587-3650
Fax. (867) 587-3436
Email: mireille_gionet@gov.nt.ca
Dir-Health/Social Serv Mireille Hamlyn

Stanton Health Promotion and Protection Office
102-5204 50 Ave
Yellowknife NT X1A 1E2
Tel. (867) 669-8979
Fax. (867) 669-7517
Chief Environ Hlth Officer Duane Fleming

TICHO COMMUNITY SERVICES AGENCY

Regional Public Health Bechoko
Nishi Khon Bldg
Bag 5
Bechoko NT X0E 0Y0
Tel. (867) 392-3007
Fax. (867) 392-3001
Dir-Hlth & Social Services Ms. Anna Beals

YELLOWKNIFE HEALTH & SOCIAL SERVICES AUTHORITY

Yellowknife Public Health Unit
Jan Stirling Building
4702 Franklin Ave
Yellowknife NT X1A 2N5
Tel. (867) 920-6570
Fax. (867) 873-0158
Email: yhssa@gov.nt.ca
Mgr Ms. Laurie Parton

NUNAVUT

Chief Medical Officer of Health, Dr Geraldine Osbourne Tel: (867) 975-5755

BAFFIN REGIONAL OFFICE DEPARTMENT OF HEALTH & SOCIAL SERVICES
PO Box 437
Pangnirtung NU X0A 0R0
Tel. (867) 473-2638
Fax. (867) 473-2657
Email: rstuckless@gov.nu.ca
Chief Med Off of Hlth Geraldine Osborne
Exec Dir Roxanne Stuckless

DEPARTMENT OF HEALTH & SOCIAL SERVICES KIVALLIQ REGION
PO Box 1000
Rankin Inlet NU X0C 0G0
Tel. (867) 975-6000
Fax. (867) 645-2409
Email: info@gov.nu.ca
Exec Dir Norman Hatlevik
Exec Serv Coord Ms. Anne Noolook

Office of the Chief Medical Officer of Health
Sivummut Bldg 1107 Dept of HSS, Govt of Nunavut
PO Box 1000, Station 1000
Iqaluit NU X0A 0H0
Tel. (867) 975-5774
Fax. (867) 975-5755
Email: isobol@gov.nu.ca
Chief Med Officer Hlth Dr. Maurine Baikie

PROVINCIAL CANCER CENTRES & CLINICS

BRITISH COLUMBIA

BC Cancer Agency

Executive and Provincial Offices

600 West 10th Ave
Vancouver, BC V5Z 4E6
Tel. (604) 877-6000 Fax: (604) 877-6146 Web: www.bccancer.bc.ca
Interim President, Dr. Max Coppes

Sindi Ahluwalia Hawkins Centre for the Southern Interior
399 Royal Ave, Kelowna, BC V1Y 5L3
Tel. (250) 712-3900 Fax: (250) 712-3911

Abbotsford Centre
32900 Marshall Rd, Abbotsford, BC V2S 0C2
Tel. (604) 851-4710 Toll-free: (877) 547-3777

Fraser Valley Cancer Centre
13750-96th Ave, Surrey, BC V3V 1Z2
Tel. (604) 930-2098 Fax: (604) 930-4049

Vancouver Cancer Centre
600 W. 10th Ave, Vancouver, BC V5Z 4E6
Tel. (604) 877-6000 Fax: (604) 872-4596

Vancouver Island Cancer Centre
2410 Lee Ave, Victoria, BC V8R 6V5
Tel. (250) 519-5500 Fax: (250) 519-2002

BC Cancer Foundation
600-686 W Broadway, Vancouver, BC V5Z 1G1
Tel. (604) 877-6040 Fax: (604) 877-6161

BC Cancer Agency's Research Centre
675 W 10th Ave, Vancouver, BC V5Z 1L3
Tel. (604) 675-8000 Fax: (604) 675-8187

ALBERTA

Alberta Health Services/Cancer Care

1500, 10123 - 99 Street, Edmonton, AB T5J 3H1
Senior Vice-President & Senior Medical Director, Cancer Care,
Dr. Paul Grundy . . . . Tel. (780) 643-4387
. . . . Fax. (780) 643-4397

Administering:

NORTHERN ALBERTA:

Cross Cancer Institute
11560 Univ Ave, Edmonton, AB T6G 1Z2
Executive Director: Dr. Scott Fielding . . . . Tel. (780) 432-8543
. . . . Fax. (780) 432-8886

Responsible for:

Barrhead Community Cancer Centre
Barrhead Healthcare Centre
4815-51 Ave, Barrhead, AB T7N 1M1
Physician Contact:
Dr. Kent Barnes/Dr. Abdeldaim Tawfik
. . . . Tel. (780) 674-2447
. . . . Fax. (780) 674-6773

Bonnyville Community Cancer Centre
Bonnyville Health Centre
P.O. Bag 1008, 5001 Lakeshore Dr
Bonnyville, AB T9N 2J7
Physician Contact:
Dr. Guy Lamoureux . . . . Tel. (780) 826-3346
. . . . Fax. (780) 826-6526

Camrose Community Cancer Centre
St. Mary's Hospital
4607-53 St Camrose, AB T4V 1Y5
Physician Contact:
Dr. Dr. Willem Slabbert . . . . Tel. (780) 672-2425
. . . . Fax. (780) 608-2401

Central Alberta Cancer Centre
3942-50A Ave, P O Bag 5030, Red Deer, AB T4N 4E7
Physician Contact, Dr. Callisto Tarukandirwa . . Tel. (403) 314-6956
. . . . Fax. (403) 346-1160

Fort McMurray Community Cancer Centre
Northern Lights Regional Health Centre
7 Hospital St Fort McMurray, AB T9H 1P2
Physician Contact:
Dr. Surinder Khinda . . . . Tel. (780) 791-2268
. . . . Fax. (780) 791-0023
Dr. Josef Largoza . . . .

Drayton Valley Community Cancer Centre

Drayton Valley Hospital & Care Centre
4550 Madsen Ave, Drayton Valley, AB T7A 1N8
Physician Contact:
Dr. Antoinette Gossmann
. . . . Tel. (780) 542-3366
. . . . Fax. (780) 542-6207

Lloydminster Community Cancer Centre

Lloydminster Hospital
3820-43 Ave, Lloydminster, AB/SK S9V 1Y5
Physician Contact:
Dr. Raymond Rogers/Dr. Zlatko Kostic/Dr. Mark Chapelshi
. . . . Tel. (780) 875-4930
. . . . Fax. (780) 875-8361

Grande Prairie Cancer Centre
10409-98 St, Grande Prairie, AB T8V 2E8
Director, Dr. Marie Moreau . . . . Tel. (780) 538-7588
. . . . Fax. (780) 532-9120

Hinton Community Cancer Centre
Hinton Community Health Services, 1280 Switzer Dr, Hinton, AB T7V 1T5
Physician Contact:
Dr. Margaret (Peggy) Allan . . . . Tel. (780) 865-3333
. . . . Fax. (780) 865-1099

Peace River Community Cancer Centre
Peace River Community Health Centre, 10101-68 St, Box 400,
Peace River, AB T8S 1T6
Physician Contact:
Dr. Thomas McKeown . . . . Tel. (780) 624-2581
. . . . Fax. (780) 624-7549

SOUTHERN ALBERTA:

Tom Baker Cancer Centre
1331-29th St NW, Calgary, AB T2N 4N2
Director, Dr. Peter Craighead . . . . Tel. (403) 521-3701
. . . . Fax. (403) 521-3128

Responsible for:

Drumheller Community Cancer Centre
Drumheller District Health Services
351 - 9th St NW, Drumheller, AB T0J 0Y1
Physician Contact:
Dr. Joachim F. Neffgen . . . . Tel. (403) 823-3345
Dr. Elizabeth Racz . . . . Tel. (403) 823-3345
. . . . Fax. (403) 823-7823

Lethbridge Cancer Centre
Rm. 2H209, 960-19th St S, Lethbridge, AB T1J 1W5
Physician Contact, Dr. Brigden . . . . Tel. (403) 388-6869
. . . . Fax. (403) 327-4160

Medicine Hat Cancer Centre
666-6th St SW, Medicine Hat, AB T1A 4H6
Physician Contact: Dr. J. Foley . . . . Tel. (403) 529-8817
. . . . Fax. (403) 529-8007
Dr. Marc Trudeau, Medical Director . . . . . . Tel. (403) 529-8817
. . . . Fax. (403) 529-8007

High River Community Cancer Centre,
High River General Auxiliary Hospital
560-9th Ave W, High River, AB T1V 1B3
Physician Contact: Dr. Adam Vyse/Dr. C. Powell . Tel. (403) 652-0145
. . . . Fax. (403) 652-0198

Bow Valley Community Cancer Centre
c/o Canmore General Hospital
Hospital Place, Canmore, AB T1W 1N2
Physician Contact:
Dr. Catherine Hinds. . . . . Tel. (403) 678-5585
. . . . Fax. (403) 678-6262

SASKATCHEWAN

Saskatchewan Cancer Agency

Ste 400, 2631-28th Ave, Regina, SK S4S 6X3
Tel. (306) 585-1831 Fax: (306) 584-2733
Chief Executive Officer, Scott Livingstone

Allan Blair Cancer Centre

4101 Dewdney Ave, Regina, SK S4T 7T1
Tel. (306) 766-2213 Fax: (306) 766-2688

Saskatoon Cancer Centre

20 Campus Dr, Saskatoon, SK S7N 4H4
Tel. (306) 655-2662 Fax: (306) 655-2910

MANITOBA

CancerCare Manitoba

675 McDermot Ave, Winnipeg, MB R3E 0V9
President and CEO, Dr. H.S. Dhaliwal Tel. (204) 787-2241
Chairman, Mr. Lorne DeJaeger Tel. (204) 787-2241

M.R. MacCharles Unit (675 McDermot Ave., Winnipeg)
St. Boniface Unit ("O" Block, 409 Tache Ave., Winnipeg)

ONTARIO

Cancer Care Ontario,

Provincial Office, 620 University Ave, Toronto, M5G 2L7
President & Chief Executive Officer, Dr. Michael Sherar
Tel. (416) 971-9800 Fax. (416) 971-6888

R. S. McLaughlin Durham Regional Cancer Centre
1 Hospital Court, 2nd Floor, Supportive Care
Oshawa, ON L1G 2B9
RVP, Regional Cancer Services, Mr. Tom McHugh
Tel. (905) 576-8711 . . . . Fax: (905) 721-4741

Grand River Regional Cancer Centre
835 King St W, Kitchener, ON N2G 1G3
Acting RVP, Regional Cancer Services, Mr. Mark Berry
Tel. (519) 749-4370 . . . . Fax. (519) 749-4274

Juravinski Cancer Centre
699 Concession St, Hamilton, ON L8V 5C2
RVP, Regional Cancer Services, Dr. Bill Evans
Tel. (905) 387-9711 . . . . Fax. (905) 575-6323

Cancer Centre of Southeastern Ontario at Kingston General Hospital
25 King St W, Kingston, ON K7L 5P9
RVP, Regional Cancer Services, Ms. Brenda Carter
Tel. (613)544-2630 . . . . Fax. (613) 544-4967

London Regional Cancer Program
790 Commissioners Rd E, London, ON N6A 4L6
RVP, Regional Cancer Services, Mr. Neil Johnson
Tel.(519) 685-8466 . . . . Fax. (519) 685-8611

Sudbury Regional Hospital Regional Cancer Program
41 Ramsey Lake Rd, Sudbury, ON P3E 5J1
RVP, Regional Cancer Services, Mr Mark Hartman
Tel. (705) 522-6237 . . . . Fax. (705) 523-7328

Thunder Bay Regional Health Sciences Centre Regional Cancer Care
980 Oliver Road, Thunder Bay, ON P7B 6V4
RVP, Regional Cancer Services, Dr. Mark Henderson
Tel. (807) 684-7213 . . . . Fax. (807) 684-5800
Web: www.tbrhsc.net/nworcc

Ottawa Hospital Regional Cancer Centre
501 Smyth Rd, Ottawa, ON K1H 8L6
RVP, Regional Cancer Services, Ms. Paula Doering
Tel. (613) 737-8464 . . . . Fax. (613) 247-3503

Carlo Fidani Peel Regional Cancer Centre
2200 Eglinton Ave W, Mississauga, ON L5M 2N1
RVP, Regional Cancer Services, Dr. Craig McFadyen
Tel. (905) 313-1100 . . . . Fax. (905) 813-4024

Odette Cancer Centre
2075 Bayview Ave, Toronto, ON M4N 3M5
RVP, Cancer Services, Dr. Andy Smith
Tel. (416) 480-4825 . . . . Fax. (416) 480-6002

Windsor Regional Cancer Centre
2220 Kildare Rd, Windsor, ON N8W 2X3
RVP, Regional Cancer Services, Ms. Claudia Den Boer Grima
Tel. (519) 253-3191 x 58545 . . . . Fax. (519) 971-9922

Stronach Regional Cancer Centre, Southlake Regional Cancer Centre
596 Davis Drive, Newmarket, ON L3Y 2P9
RVP, Regional Cancer Services, Dr. Louis Balogh
Tel. (905) 895-4521 . . . . Fax. (905) 853-2220

North Simcoe Muskoka Regional Cancer Centre
201 Georgian Drive, Barrie, ON L4M 6M2
RVP, Regional Cancer Services, Ms. Lindsey Crawford
Tel. (705) 728-9090 . . . . Fax. (705) 728-2408

Princess Margaret Hospital, University Health Network
610 University Avenue, Toronto, ON M5G 2M9
RVP, Regional Cancer Services, Dr. Mary Gospodarowicz
Tel. (416) 946-4501 . . . . Fax. (416) 340-4896

QUÉBEC

The treatment of cancer by radiation in the Province of Québec is undertaken in hospitals with qualified radiation therapists.

NEW BRUNSWICK

Atlantic Health Sciences Corporation Dept. of Oncology

Saint John Regional Hospital, P O Box 2100, Saint John, NB E2L 4L2
Tel. (506) 648-6884 Fax: (506) 649-2810
Department Head, Dr. Margot Burnell, Oncology Department
Horizon Health Network

NOVA SCOTIA

Nova Scotia Cancer Centre

Queen Elizabeth II Health Sciences Centre, Nova Scotia Cancer Centre
Dickson Bldg, 5820 University Ave, Halifax, NS, B3H 1V7
Tel. (902) 473-6000 Fax: (902) 473-1273
Head Radiation Oncology, Dr. Tetteh Ago

PRINCE EDWARD ISLAND

PEI Cancer Treatment Centre, Queen Elizabeth Hospital

Box 6600
Charlottetown, PE C1A 8T5
Medical Director, Dr. Philip Champion . . . . Tel. (902) 894-2027
. . . . Fax: (902) 894-2187
Manager, Liz Dobbin

NEWFOUNDLAND & LABRADOR

Eastern Health

Chief Executive Officer/President, Ms. Vickie Kaminski

Cancer Care Program

Dr. H. Bliss Murphy Cancer Centre
300 Prince Philip Drive
St. John's, NL A1B 3V6
Tel. (709) 777-6480, Fax: (709) 753-0927
VP, Cancer Care, Ms. Katherine Chubbs
Program Director, Ms. Elaine Warren
Clinical Chief, Dr. Jehan Siddiqui

Provinces which have a specially appointed Provincial Group responsible for the treatment of cancer are as follows: British Columbia - BC Cancer Agency; Alberta - Alberta Cancer Board Alberta - Alberta Cancer Board, which also operates the: Alberta Program for the Early Detection of Breast Cancer - Edmonton & Calgary, and the Edmonton Radio Pharmaceutical Centre; Saskatchewan - Saskatchewan Cancer Agency; Manitoba - CancerCare Manitoba; Ontario - Cancer Care Ontario; New Brunswick - Atlantic Health Sciences Corporation Dept. of Oncology; Nova Scotia - Nova Scotia Cancer Centre; Prince Edward Island - PEI Cancer Treatment Centre; Newfoundland & Labrador - Cancer Care Program.

THE ASSOCIATION OF FACULTIES OF MEDICINE OF CANADA L'ASSOCIATION DES FACULTÉS DE MÉDECINE DU CANADA (AFMC)

265 Carling Avenue, Suite 800 Ottawa, Ontario K1S 2E1
Tel: (613) 730-0687 Fax: (613) 730-1196 Web: www.afmc.ca

Executive Committee 2013

Chair, Dr. Jacques Bradwejn
Dean, Faculty of Medicine
University of Ottawa
451 Smyth Road - Room 2037
Ottawa, OM K1H 8M5
Tel: (613) 562-5800 Ext.: 8113 Fax: (613) 562-5457
E-mail: jacques.bradwejn@uottawa.ca
Assistant: Martine Desaulniers (mdesauln@uottawa.ca)

Past Chair, Dr. James Rourke
Dean, Faculty of Medicine
Memorial University of Newfoundland
Health Sciences Centre
St-John's, NL A1B 3V6
Tel: (709) 777-6602 Fax: (709) 777-6746
E-mail: dean.medicine@mun.ca

Members-at-Large, Dr. Catharine I. Whiteside
Dean, Faculty of Medicine
University of Toronto
Room 2109 Medical Sciences Bldg
1 King's College Circle
Toronto, ON M5S 1A8
Tel: (416) 946-7810 Fax: (416) 978-1774
E-mail: catharine.whiteside@utoronto.ca
Assistant: Amy Lee (amy.lee@utoronto.ca)

Members-at-Large, Dr. Rénald Bergeron
Doyen, Faculté de médecine
Université Laval
Pavillon Ferdinand Vandry - Local 1219
Québec, QC G1K 7P4
Tel: (418) 656-2301 Fax: (418) 656-5062
E-mail: renald.nergeron@fmed.ulaval.ca
Assistant: Suzanne Gamache (suzanne.gamache@fmed.ulaval.ca)

Members-at-Large, Dr. Roger Strasser
Founding Dean of Medicine
Northern Ontario School of Medicine
Parker Building - Room L1124
935 Ramsey Lake Road
Sudbury ON P3E 2C6
Tel: (705) 671-3874 Fax: (705) 671-3830
E-mail: roger.strasser@nosm.ca
Assistants: Natalie Raymond-Marois & Nicole Lauzon
E-mail: natalie.raymond-marois@nosm.ca
E-mail: nicole.lauzon@nosm.ca

AFMC Staff

President & CEO, Dr. Nick Busing
E-mail: nbusing@afmc.ca

The Association of Faculties of Medicine (AFMC) represents the country's 17 faculties of medicine and is the national voice for academic medicine. AFMC was founded in 1943 and functions to support individually and collectively Canada's medical schools through promotion of medical education, research and critical care.

CANADIAN POST-M.D. EDUCATION REGISTRY SYSTÈME INFORMATISÉ SUR LES STAGIAIRES POST-M.D. EN FORMATION CLINIQUE (CAPER)

265 Carling Avenue, Suite 800, Ottawa, ON K1S 2E1
Tel: (613) 730-1204 Fax: (613) 730-1196
E-mail: caper@afmc.ca Web: www.caper.ca

V. P. Research & Analysis, CAPER/ORIS, Steve Slade

CAPER is the central repository for statistical information on postgraduate medical education in Canada. The CAPER Annual Census of Post-MD Trainees provides comprehensive data on residency training. CAPER also prepares custom research and analysis, and responds to client requests on a cost-recovery basis.

RESOURCE SECTION

CANADIAN ASSOCIATION OF INTERNES & RESIDENTS (CAIR)

412-151 Slater St, Ottawa, ON K1P 5H3
Tel: (613) 234-6448 Fax: (613) 234-5292
E-mail: cair@cair.ca Website: www.cair.ca

President, Dr. Simon Moore (2012 - 2013)

The Canadian Association of Internes & Residents (CAIR) is the national representative body of over 8,000 Resident Physicians in Canada. It delivers improvement to the lives of Residents in such areas as personal well-being, medical education quality, and professionalism.

PROVINCIAL HOUSESTAFF ORGANIZATIONS

PAR-BC
2010-401 West Georgia, Vancouver, BC V6B 5A1
Toll-Free: 1-888-877-2722
Tel: (604) 876-7636 Fax: (604) 876-7690
E-mail: par@par-bc.org

PARA
11044 82nd Ave, Suite 340 Edmonton, AB T6G 0J2
Tel: (780) 432-1749 Fax: (780) 432-1778
E-mail: para@para-ab.ca

PAIRS
P.O. Box 23, Royal University Hospital
103 Hospital Drive, Saskatoon, SK S7N 0W8
Tel & Fax: (306) 655-2134
E-mail: pairs.sk@usask.ca

PARIM
GF132 Health Sciences Centre
820 Sherbrook Ave
Winnipeg, MB R3A 1R9
Tel: (204) 787-3673 Fax: (204) 787-2692
E-mail: parim@mts.net

PAIRO
1901-400 University Ave, Toronto, ON M5G 1S5
Tel: (416) 979-1182 Toll-free: 1-877-979-1183
Fax: (416) 595-9778
E-mail: pairo@pairo.org

PARI-MP
Halifax Professional Centre
5991 Spring Garden Road, Suite 460
Halifax, NS B3H 1T6
Tel: (902) 404-3595 Fax: (902) 404-3599
Website: www.parimp.ca

PAIRN
Student Affairs Office, Room 2713
Memorial University Medical School
Health Sciences Complex
St. John's, NF A1B 3V6
Tel: (709) 777-7118 Fax: (709) 777-6968
E-mail: pairn@mun.ca

MÉDECINS FRANCOPHONES DU CANADA

8355, rue Saint-Laurent, Montréal, QC H2P 2Z6
Tel: (514) 388-2228 Fax: (514) 388-5335
E-mail: info@medecinsfrancophones.ca Web: www.medecinsfrancophones.ca

President, Dr. Louis Conrad Pelletier

Council Members

Céline Monette, CEO
Dr. Michel Carrier, président
Dr. Raymond Lalande, vice-président
Dr. Louis Conrad Pelletier, président sortant
Dr. Françis Reeves, administrateur, secrétaire-trésorier
Dr. André Roch, administrateur
Dr. Sébastien Toussaint, administrateur
Dre Francine Borduas, administratrice
Dr. Réjean Savoie, administrateur

CANADIAN MEDICAL PLACEMENT SERVICE

148 York St, London, Ontario N6A 1A7
Tel.: (519) 672-0777; Toll-Free: 1-800-991-6661; Fax: (519) 672-0830
E-mail: info@cmps.ca Web: www.cmps.ca

President & CEO: Joseph Verga, MBA, MS CHE

Canadian Medical Placement Service is dedicated to matching medical professionals with practice opportunities in Canada and international locations. They are currently being utilized by over 300 hospitals and clinics across Canada to recruit medical professionals matching both the needs of the hospital or clinic and the needs of the medical professional. Physicians seeking practices can obtain advice on availability of practices matching the physicians' criteria including quality of work life, financial potential, geographic preference and administrative support.

CANADIAN MEDICALERT FOUNDATION

2005 Sheppard Ave E, #800
Toronto, ON M2J 5B4
Toll-Free: 1-800-668-1507 (English) Mon-Fri: 9am-5pm (EST), 1-800-668-6381 (French)
Telephone: (416) 696-0267 Fax: (416) 696-0156
E-mail: medinfo@medicalert.ca Web: www.medicalert.ca/

President, Dr. Robert Ridge
Communications, Nina Doiron

As Canada's largest national member-based charity with over one million members, MedicAlert is the leading provider of medical information services linked to customized medical bracelets and necklaces

When you become a MedicAlert member, our Medical Profile Specialists will help you to create your electronic MedicAlert Emergency Health Record, detailing your medical history, a list of personal emergency contacts and physician information. You also receive a custom-engraved bracelet or necklace and International coverage with the MedicAlert® 24-hour Emergency Hotline, which gives medical responders instant access to your Personal Health Record, including family contacts and medical history. The hotline is available 24/7, worldwide, supported in more than 150 engraved languages.

MedicAlert: Recognized & Recommended,
MedicAlert is recommended by many leading health professionals, including the Canadian Association of Emergency Physicians (CAEP) and the National Emergency Nurses Association (NENA). MedicAlert also educates medical professionals and first responders to look for the MedicAlert symbol first. MedicAlert could save your life.

There are hundreds of medical conditions applicable to adults and children that should be known by health professionals in emergencies or non-critical medical situations.

Sample Medical Conditions and Diseases Prompting Membership in MedicAlert

Condition
Adrenal Insufficiency
Addison's Disease
Alzheimer's Disease
Anaphylaxis
Aneurysms
Angina
Arrhythmia
Asthma
Bleeding Disorders
Clotting Disorder
Colitis
Congenital Heart, Lung, Kidney Disease
Coronary Bypass
Crohn's Disease
Diabetes
Epilepsy
Glaucoma
Head Injury
Heart Valve Disease
Hemolytic Anemia
Hemophilia
Hypertension
Hypoglycemia
Hypopituitarism
Hypothyroidism
Laryngectomy
Leukemia
Lymphomas
Malignant Hyperthermia
Migraines
Multiple Sclerosis
Myasthenia Gravis
Myocardial Infarction
Parkinson's Disease
Porphyria
Renal Failure/Dialysis
Seizure Disorder
Sickle Cell Anemia
Situs Inversus
Sleep Apnea
Stroke

Allergies
Chemicals
Drugs
Foods
Insects
Latex

Medications
Anticoagulant
Beta Blocker
Chemotherapy
DDAVP
Epinephrine (EpiPen)
Immunosuppressant
Insulin
Lithium
MAOI & RIMA
Steroid Therapy
Streptokinase

Devices/Implants
Pacemaker
Intraocular Lenses
VP Shunt, Stents, Catheters, Metal Pins, Plates or Clips
Prostheses
Artificial heart valves, hips, knees
Lens Implants

Special Needs/Other
Clinical Studies
Contact Lenses
Developmental Challenges
Existence of advance directives or living wills
Hearing/Visual/Speech impairment
Immunosuppressant
No blood transfusions
No known medical condition
Organ Donor
Scuba Diver

CANADIAN PUBLIC HEALTH ASSOCIATION

404-1525 Carling Ave, Ottawa, ON K1Z 8R9
Tel: 613-725-3769 Fax: 613-725-9826
E-mail: info@cpha.ca
Web-site: www.cpha.ca

Chair, Dr. Lynn McIntyre
Chair-Elect, Ms Ardene Robinson Vollman

The Canadian Public Health Association (CPHA) is a national, independent, not-for-profit, voluntary association representing public health in Canada with links to the international public health community.

CPHA's mission is to constitute a special national resource in Canada that advocates for the improvement and maintenance of personal and community health according to the public health principles of disease prevention, health promotion and protection and healthy public policy.

MÉDECINS SANS FRONTIÈRES/DOCTORS WITHOUT BORDERS

National Office
402-720 Spadina Ave, Toronto, ON M5S 2T9
Toll-Free: 1-800-982-7903 Tel: (416) 964-0619 Fax: (416) 963-8707
E-mail: msfcan@msf.ca
Web-site: www.msf.ca

President, Dr. Bruce Lampard

Executive Director, Stephen Cornish
Director of Communications, Nicol Zarb
Director of Fundraising, Ms. Rebecca Davies

Médecins Sans Frontières / Doctors Without Borders is an international independent medical relief organization, in operation now for over 40 years. The Canadian office was founded in 1991, and has sent more than 2,000 doctors, nurses, specialists and support staff abroad to help victims of war, epidemics, natural disasters and poverty, irrespective of their race, religion, creed or political affiliation. The organization is a registered Canadian charity. MSF is the recipient of the 1999 Nobel Peace Prize.

CANADIAN NURSES ASSOCIATION

50 Driveway, Ottawa, ON K2P 1E2
Tel. 1-800-361-8404 / (613) 237-2133 Fax: (613) 237-3520
E-mail: reception@cna-aiic.ca Web-site: www.cna-nurses.ca

Executive Director, Rachel Bard, RN, MEd

PROVINCIAL / TERRITORIAL MEMBERS

College & Association of Registered Nurses of Alberta
11620-168 Street, Edmonton, AB T5M 4A6
Tel. (780) 451-0043 Fax: (780) 452-3276
E-mail: carna@nurses.ab.ca

College of Registered Nurses of British Columbia
2855 Arbutus Street, Vancouver, BC V6J 3Y8
Tel. (604) 736-7331 Fax: (604) 738-2272
E-mail: info@crnbc.ca

College of Registered Nurses Of Manitoba
890 Pembina Hwy, Winnipeg, MB R3M 2M8
Tel. (204) 774-3477 Fax: (204) 775-6052
E-mail: info@crnm.mb.ca

Nurses Association of New Brunswick/Association des Infirmières et Infirmiers du Nouveau-Brunswick
165 Regent Street, Fredericton, NB E3B 7B4
Tel. (506) 458-8731 Fax: (506) 459-2838
E-mail: nanb@nanb.nb.ca

Association of Registered Nurses of Newfoundland and Labrador
55 Military Road, St. John's, NL A1C 2C5
Tel. (709) 753-6040 Fax: (709) 753-4940
E-mail: info@arnnl.nf.ca

Registered Nurses Association of the Northwest Territories and Nunavut
Box 2757, Yellowknife, NT X1A 2R1
Tel. (867) 873-2745 Fax: (867) 873-2336
E-mail: admin@rnantnu.ca

College of Registered Nurses of Nova Scotia
Suite 4005-7071 Bayers Rd, Halifax, NS B3L 2C2
Tel. (902) 491-9744 Fax: (902) 491-9510
E-mail: info@crnns.ca
web-site: www.crnns.org

Registered Nurses Association of Ontario
158 Pearl St, Toronto, ON M5H 1L3
(416) 599-1925 Toll Free: 1-800-268-7199 Fax: (416) 599-1926
E-mail: info@rnao.org

Association of Registered Nurses of Prince Edward Island
53 Grafton Street, Charlottetown, PE C1A 1K8
Tel. (902) 368-3764 Fax: (902) 628-1430
E-mail: anpei@pei.aibn.com

Saskatchewan Registered Nurses Association
2066 Retallack Street, Regina SK S4T 7X5
Tel. (306) 359-4200 Toll Free: 1-800-667-9945 Fax: (306) 525-0849
E-mail: info@srna.org
Web-site: www.srna.org

Yukon Registered Nurses Association
204-4133-4th Avenue, Whitehorse, YT Y1A 1H8
Tel. (867) 667-4062 Fax: (867) 668-5123
E-mail: admin@yrna.ca

MEMORIAL UNIVERSITY OF NEWFOUNDLAND

St. John's, Newfoundland

Health Sciences Centre, St. John's, Newfoundland Postal Code A1B 3V6
Tel. (709) 777-6602 Fax. (709) 777-6746 Website: www.med.mun.ca/med

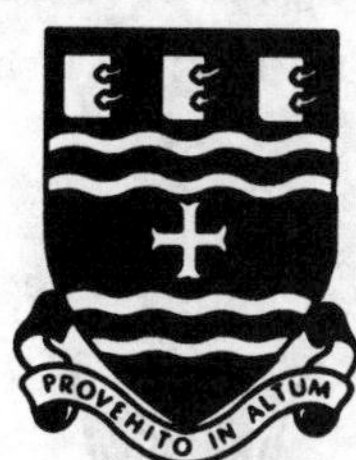

Official Visitor, His Honor the Lieutenant Governor, John C. Crosbie, P.C., O.C., Q.C., B.A (Hons) (Queen's), LLB (Dalhousie), LL.D. (Dalhousie), LL.D. (Memorial)
Chancellor, General Rick J. Hillier (Retired), CMM, MSC, CD, BSc (Memorial)
President & Vice-Chancellor, Dr. Gary Kachanoski, BSc (Hons), (Univ of Sask), MSc (Univ of Sask), PhD (Univ of California)
Provost and Vice-President (Academic), Dr David Wardlaw, BSc, PhD (Univ of Toronto)
Vice-President, Administration & Finance, Kent Decker, BComm (Hons), (Memorial), C.A. (Newfoundland)
Vice President, Research, Chris Loomis, BSc (Hons), MSc, PhD (Queen's)

Faculty of Medicine

Dean, James T.B. Rourke, MD, CCFP(EM), MClinSci(FM), FCFP, FRRMS, LLD
Vice Dean, Sharon Peters, MD, MPH, FRCP(C)
Associate Dean, (Acting), Biomedical Sciences, Gary D. Paterno, BSc., MSc (Toronto), PhD (Ottawa)
Associate Dean for Research and Graduate Studies (Medicine) Reza Tabrizchi, BSc (Hons) Sunderland, MSc, PhD, British Columbia
Associate Dean, Clinical Research, Proton Rahman, MD (Mem'l), MSc (Toronto), FRCPC
Associate Dean, Community Health and Humanities, Shree Mulay, MSc (McGill), PhD (McGill)
Assistant Dean, Admissions, Dr. Wanda Parsons, MD, Memorial, CCFP
Assistant Dean, Postgraduate Medical Studies, Dr. Asoka Samarasena, MBBS (Ceylon), FRCPC
Assistant Dean, Student Affairs, Dr. Scott Moffatt, M., BSc, Acadia, B.A. (New Brunswick), MD (Memorial), CCFP, FCFP
Assistant Dean, Continuing Medical Education, Dr. Ford Bursey, BSc, MD (Memorial) FRCPC
Assistant Dean (Acting), Graduate Studies, Dr. Diana Gustafson, B.A. McMaster, MEd, Brock, PhD. Toronto: Social Sciences and Health
Assistant Dean, Rural Clinical School Medical Education Network (RCSMEN), Dr. Mohamed Ravalia; LRCP(ED) (Zimbabwe) CCFP, ChB (Rhodesia), LRCPS, MB (Rhodesia)
Associate Dean, Undergraduate Medical Education, Dr. Don McKay, BSc, MS, PhD (Michigan State)

Chairs of Clinical Disciplines

Anesthesia, Dr. Jeremy Pridham, (Acting Clinical Chair) MD (Western Ontario), FRCPC
Family Medicine , Dr. Catherine MacLean, BSc (Dalhousie), M.Clin.Sc (UWO), MD (Dalhousie)
Genetics, Dr. Bridget Fernandez (Acting Clinical Chair); MD (Memorial), FRCPC, FCCMG
Laboratory Medicine, Dr. Simon Avis, BMedSc (Memorial), MD (Memorial), FRCPC
Medicine (Acting), Dr. Alan E. Goodridge, MD (Memorial), FRCPC
Obstetrics & Gynecology, Dr. Atamjit Gill, MBBS (India), FRCSC, FACOG
Oncology (Interim), Dr. Kara Laing, MD (Memorial), FRCPC
Pediatrics, Dr. Cathy Vardy, MD (Memorial), FRCPC
Psychiatry, Dr. Ted S. Callanan, BSc, MD (Memorial), FRCPC
Radiology, Dr. Benvon Cramer, MB, BCh, BAO(NUI), FRCPC
Surgery, Dr. Darrell Boone (Clinical Chair), DC, MD (Meorial), FRCSC

The Medical School at Memorial University came into existence in 1967, following the recommendations of the (Federal) Hall Royal Commission, a Newfoundland Royal Commission on Health Services, chaired by the late Lord Brain and a careful Feasibility Study by a team of international experts under the chairmanship of the late Dr. J.A. MacFarlane. The rapid build-up of an experienced Faculty made it possible to admit the first class of undergraduate students in September 1969 - one year ahead of the original schedule. The first class graduated in 1973. The Faculty of Medicine is located in a modern Health Sciences Centre which is shared with The Schools of Pharmacy and Nursing and Health Care Corporation of St John's

Admissions

Students are ordinarily admitted to the first year of medical studies after completing a bachelors degree. In exceptional circumstances, an application may be considered from someone who does not hold a bachelor's degree; such an applicant will have completed at least 20 one-semester courses and be a student who has work related or other experience acceptable to the Admissions Committee. The course of study must include two courses in English. All applicants must take the new MCAT (revised in 1991) prior to the application deadline.

Programs

The M.D. degree is granted at the conclusion of the fourth year of Medical Studies. Masters and Ph.D. degree programs are offered in the Divisions of Biomedical Sciences, Community Health and Humanities and Clinical Sciences to appropriately qualified candidates. Biomedical Sciences and Community Health and Humanities are non-departmentalized.

Residency Programs

Residency programs are provided in all major clinical disciplines within the Affiliated Teaching Hospitals of Memorial University.

RESOURCE SECTION

DALHOUSIE UNIVERSITY

Halifax, Nova Scotia

Faculty of Medicine

5849 University Ave, CRC Building, Halifax, Nova Scotia Postal Code B3H 4H7

Tel. (902) 494-6592 Fax. (902) 494-7119 Website: www.medicine.dal.ca/

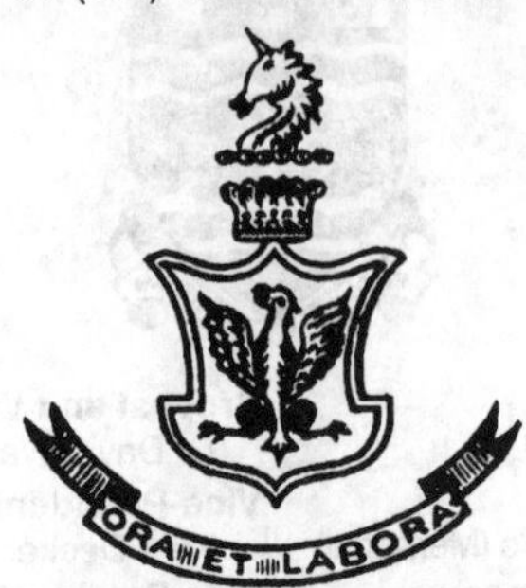

Principal Officers

President & Vice-Chancellor, T. Traves, BA, MA, PhD
Dean of Medicine, T. Marrie, MD
Vice-President, Acting Academic & Provost, C. Watters, PhD
Vice-President, Research, M. Crago, PhD
Vice-President, Finance & Administration, K. Burt
Vice-President, External, F. Dykeman
Vice-President, Student Services, B. Neuman, PhD
Assistant Vice-President, Enrolment Managment & Registrar, Asa Kachan
Senior Associate Dean, P. Smith, MD
Associate Dean, Postgraduate Medical Education, A. Warren, MD
Assistant Dean, Operations & Policy, D. Gorsky, MD
Associate Dean, Dalhousie Medicine New Brunswick, J. Steeves, MD
Associate Dean, Research, G. Johnston, PhD
Associate Dean, Undergraduate Medical Education, M. Matte, MD
Associate Dean, Continuing Medical Education, Dr Connie LeBlanc
Secretary to Faculty, B. Tait-Persaud
Assistant Dean, Operations, A. Weeden
Assistant Dean, Graduate Medical Education, New Brunswick, T. Lambert, MD (Acting)
Assistant Dean, Student Affairs, Dr. Michael Teeham
Assistant Dean, Admissions, E. Sutton, MD
Head, Division of Medical Education, B. Frank, PhD

Heads or Directors of Departments & Divisions

Anesthesia, R. Shukla, MD
Biochemistry & Molecular Biology, S. Bearne
Bioethics, C. Simpson, PhD
Bimedical Engineering, G. Mcksym, PhD
Community Health & Epidemiology, A. Levy, PhD
Emergency Medicine, D. Petrie, MD
Medicine, D. Anderson, MD
Microbiology & Immunology, J. Marshall
Obstetrics & Gynecology, A. Armson, MD
Ophthalmology & Visual Sciences, A. Cruess, MD
Pathology, G. Heathcote, MD
Pediatrics, M. Bernstein, MD
Pharmacology, C. McMaster
Physiology/Biophysics, N. Morgunov, PhD
Psychiatry, N. Delva, MD
Radiation Oncology, T. Ago, MD
Radiology, D. Barnes, MD
Surgery, D. Kirkpatrick, MD (Acting)
Urology, D. Bell, MD

The Faculty of Medicine was inaugurated in 1858 and continued until 1875. In that year, the Halifax Medical College, affiliated with Dalhousie, took over the responsibilities which it bore until 1911, when Dalhousie resumed the teaching of Medicine.

Present Course - The Faculty provides a four-year medical Training leading to the degree MD. The Faculty provides and has responsibility for specialty training in the major medical and surgical disciplines, under the approval of the Royal College of Physicians and Surgeons of Canada and is conducted in affiliated teaching hospitals in the Maritime Provinces. Dalhousie currently holds Royal College approval for specialty training programmes. The Family Medicine Resident Training Programme is approved by the College of Family Physicians of Canada. Dalhousie Continuing Medical Education takes responsibility for the continuing education of the practitioners of the three Maritime Provinces.

UNIVERSITÉ LAVAL

Québec, Québec

Faculty of Medicine

Pavillion Ferdinand-Vendry, 1050, av. de la médécine, Local 4684, Québec, Québec Postal Code G1V 0A6

Tel. (418) 656-5245 Fax: (418) 656-7706 Website: www.fmed.ulaval.ca

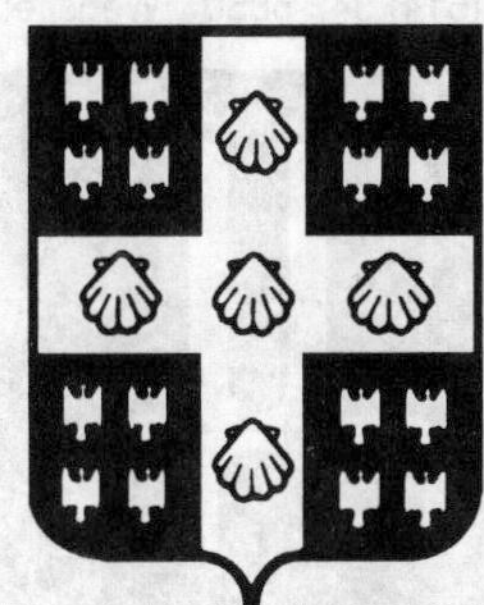

Rector, Denis Brière
Vice-Rector, Administration, Éric Bauce
Vice-Rector, Academic Affairs & Students, Bernard Gernier
Vice-Rector, Research, Sophie D'Amours
Vice-Rector, Human Resources, Michel Beauchamp
Vice-Rector, Administration & Finances, Josée Germain
Secretary-General, Monique Richer
Director of Communications, Hélène Côté
Dean, Faculty of Medicine, Rénald Bergeron
Executive Assistant to the Dean, Marielle Lapointe
Associate Dean, Research, Michel J Tremblay
Associate Dean, Clinical Affairs, Julien Poitras
Associate Dean, Teaching, Jean-Francois Montreuil
Associate Dean, Administration, Bruno Piedboeuf
Associate Dean, Pedagogy and Continued Education, Gaëtane Routhier
Secretary, Sylvie Marcoux
Executive Director, Patrice Lemay
Public Relations, Geneviève Bhérer

Department Heads

Anesthesiology, Jean Beaubien
Family Medicine and Emergency Medicine, Guy Béland
Médecine, Pierre LeBlanc
Microbiologie-Infectious Diseases & Immunology, Sylvie Trottier
Molecular Biology, Medical Biochemistry and Pathology, Pierre Leclerc
Molecular Medicine, Jean Gosselin
Obstetrics & Gynecology, Jacques Mailloux
Ophthalmology and O.R.L., Yoland Dubé
Pediatrics, Marc-André Dugas
Psychiatry and Neurosciences, Nathalie Gingras
Radiology, André Lamarre, Interim
Rehabilitation, Claude H. Côté
Social & Preventive Medicine, Yv Bonnier-Viger
Surgery, Yvan Douville

The School of Medicine was established in the Fall of 1853, less than a year after the foundation of Laval University. In 1847, a medical school had been incorporated by the city of Quebec and in 1850 twenty students were registered. In 1852 some of the teachers were invited to become the first Professors of the new Faculty, and they were officially granted the degree of Doctor of Medicine by Lord Elgin, the Governor General of Canada.

The curriculum is divided into two parts, the preclerkship phase, which is composed of courses using a variety of pedagogical methods (lectures, workshops, problem-based learning, independent study modules, etc.) and the clerkship phase, which is composed of clinical rotations. An MD degree is granted after four or five years of medical studies, because the student can elect to do the preclerkship phase in two or three years. For clinical teaching purposes, the School of Medicine has a network of partly affiliated hospitals.

RESOURCE SECTION

UNIVERSITÉ DE MONTRÉAL

Montréal, Québec

Faculty of Medicine

C.P. 6128 Succursale Centre-Ville
Montréal, Québec Postal Code H3C 3J7
Tel. (514) 343-6267 Fax: (514) 343-5850 Website: www.med.umontreal.ca

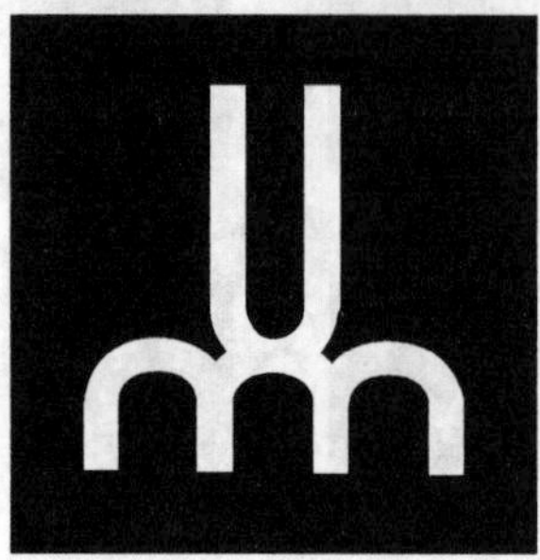

Rector, Guy Breton, MD
Vice-Rector, Academic Affairs, Raymond Lalande, MD
Vice-Rector, Finances & Infrastructure, Éric Filteau, MBA
Vice-Rector, Student Affairs & Sustainable Development, Louise Béliveau, PhD
Vice-Rector, Human Resources & Planning, Anne-Marie Boisvert, LLM
Vice-Rector, Research, Creation & Innovation, Geneviève Tanguay, PhD
Vice-Rector, International Affairs & Francophoneie, Hélène David, PhD
Vice-Rector, Student Affairs & Sustainable Development, Louise Béliveau, PhD
Vice-Rector, Major Academic Projects, Joseph Hubert, PhD
Secretary-General, Alexandre Chabot, BSc
Chief of Staff, Jean Renaud, MPA
Registrar, Marie-Claude Binette, MSc

Faculty of Medicine

Dean, Hélène Boisjoly, MD
Executive Vice-Dean & Clinical Affairs, Pierre Bourgouin, MD
Vice-Dean, Research & Innovation, Daniel Bourbonnais, PhD
Vice-Dean, Basic Sciences, & Graduate Studies, Daniel Lajeunesse, PhD
Vice-Dean, Undergraduate Studies, Christian Boudry, MD
Vice-Dean, Faculty Affairs, Pierre Belhumeur, MD
Vice-Dean, Postgraduate Studies, Josée Dubois, MD
Vice-Dean, Pedagogy & Continuing Professional Development, Andrée Boucher, MD
Assistant Vice-Dean, Student Life, Hughes Cormier, MD & Rainses Wassef, MD
Assistant Vice-Dean, Campus Maurice, Réjean Duplain, MD
Director, MD Programs, Éric Drouin, MD
Secretary of the Faculty & Assistant Vice-Dean Student Life, Josette Noël, PhD
Assistant Vice-Dean, Health Sciences, Louise Demers, PhD; Louise Getty, MA; Marielle Ledoux, PhD

Department Heads

Anesthesiology, Pierre Drolet, MD
Biochemistry, Christian Baron, PhD
Family Medicine, Jean Pelletier, MD
Health Administration, Régis Blais, PhD
Medicine, Mario Talajic, MD,
Microbiology & Immunology, Hugho Soudeyns, PhD
Nutrition, Marielle Ledoux, PhD
Obstetrics-Gynecology, Line Leduc, MD (interim)
Occupational Medicine & Environmental Health, André Dufresne, PhD
Ophthalmology, Jean-Daniel Arbour, MD
Pathology & Cellular Biology, Pierre Drapeau, PhD
Pediatrics, Jean-Yves Frappier, MD
Pharmacology, Patrick du Souich, MD, PhD
Physiology, Michèle Brochu, PhD
Psychiatry, Emmanuel Stip, MD
Radiology, Radio-Oncology & Nuclear Medicine, Gilles Soulez, MD
Social & Preventive Medicine, Louise Potvin, PhD
Surgery, Luc Valiquette, MD

Schools

Audiology & Speech Therapy, Louise Getty, MA
Rehabilitation, Louise Demers, PhD

The Faculty of Medicine of the Université de Montréal can be traced back to a school established in Montreal in 1843 under the name of "École de Médecine et de Chirurgie de Montréal". In 1891, this school merged with the Faculty of Medicine of the Montreal branch of Laval University, and, in 1920, it was granted its independence and became known as the Université de Montréal Faculty of Medicine.

The course consists of four professional years at the end of which the degree of Doctor of Medicine (M.D.) is conferred. Applicants with a CEGEP diploma must complete one premedical year.

The Faculty has residency programs in all subspecialties as well as a number of M.Sc. and Ph.D. programs. Programs in Nutrition, Physiotherapy, Occupational Therapy and in Speech Therapy and Audiology are also available.

Application for admission to the Faculty of Medicine must be made upon the regular application forms which may be obtained from the Registrar. For graduate training or for admission to residency in a specialty program, application forms may be obtained from the Secretary for the Post-graduate Medical Education.

For undergraduate studies, all documents must be submitted before March 1st, immediately preceding the session to which admittance is contemplated. For residency training, all documents must be submitted before October 1st.

McGILL UNIVERSITY

Montréal, Québec

Faculty of Medicine
McIntyre Medical Sciences Building, 3655 Promenade Sir-William-Osler, Suite 605
Montréal, Québec Postal Code H3G 1Y6

Tel. (514) 398-1768 Fax: (514) 398-3595 Website: www.med.mcgill.ca

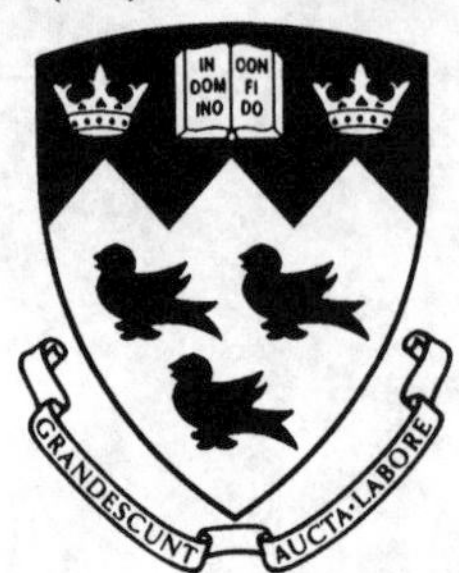

Principal & Vice-Chancellor, Heather Munroe-Blum, PhD, MSW, BA, BBW
Principal as of September 2013, Dr. Suzanne Fortier, BSc, PhD
Deputy Provost (Student Life and Learning), Morton J. Mendelson, PhD
Vice-Principal, Administration & Finance, Michael Di Grappa
Provost, Anthony C. Masi, PhD
Executive Head of Public Affairs, Vaughan Dowie
Vice-Principal, Health Affairs & Dean, David Eidelman, MDCM, FRCPC, FACP
Director of Admissions and Recruitment, Kim Bartlett, BA, MA
Registrar, Executive Director of Enrolment Services, Kathleen Massey
Associate Dean, Faculty Development, Miriam Boillat, MD
Secretary General, Stephen Strople
Associate Dean, Research, Marianna Newkirk, PhD
AVP Health Affairs & Associate Dean, Inter-Hospital Affairs, Sam Benaroya, BSc (McG), MD, CM (McG)
Associate Dean, Postgraduate Medical Education & Professional Affairs, Sarkis Meterissian, MD, MSc, FRCS(C), FACS
Associate Dean, Undergraduate Medical Education & Student Affairs, Robert Primavesi, MDCM, FCFP(EM)
Assistant Dean, Admissions (Faculty of Medicine), Saleem Razack, MD, FRCPC
Director, Centre for Medical Education, Yvonne Steinert, BA (McG), MA (Tor), PhD (Mtl)
Associate Dean, Faculty Affairs, Dr. Mara Ludwig, MD
Director, Curriculum Development & Physicianship Program, J. Donald Boudreau, BSc (Mt.Allison), MD (Dal)
Assistant Dean, Student Affairs, Namta Gupta, MD
Head of Life Sciences & Osler Library, Susan Murray

Departmental Heads

Anatomy & Cell Biology, Craig A. Mandato, BSc, PhD
Anesthesia, Steven Backman, MDCM, PhD, FRCPC
Biochemistry, David Y. Thomas, PhD (London), FRSC
Biomedical Engineering, Robert Kearney, PhD
Biomedical Ethics Unit, Eugene Bereza, MD, CM
Epidemiology, Biostatistics, & Occupational Health, Gilles Paradis, MD, MSc, FRCPC
Family Medicine, Howard Bergman, MD, FCFP, FRCPC
Human Genetics, David Rosenblatt, BSc(McG), MD(McG)
Medicine, James Martin, MD (Interim)
Microbiology & Immunology, Joaquin Madrenas, MD, PhD
Neurology & Neurosurgery, Lesley Fellows, MD, CM, DPhil (Interim)
Obstetrics & Gynecology, Denis Querleu, MD
Oncology, Eduardo Franco, MPH, DrPH
Ophthalmology, Leonard A. Levin, MD, PhD
Otolaryngology-Head & Neck Surgery, Saul Frenkiel, MD, CM(McG), FRCSC
Pathology, Zu-hua Gao, MD, PhD, FRCPC
Pediatrics, Michael Shevell, MDCM, FRCPC, FANA, FAAN
Pharmacology & Therapeutics, Gerhard Multhaup, MD, PhD.
Physiology, John Orlowski, PhD
Psychiatry, Mimi Israel, MD, FRCP

The Faculty of Medicine of McGill University was established in 1829.

Radiology (Diagnostic), Robert Lisbona, BSc(McG), MD,CM (McG)
Social Studies of Medicine, Alberto Cambrosio, MA, PhD
Surgery, Gerald M. Fried, MD
Animal Resources Centre, Jim C. Gourdon, DVM
Artificial Cells & Organs Research Centre, T.M.S. Chang, BSc, MD, CM, PhD(McG), FRCPC
Centre for Studies in Aging, Jens Pruessner, PhD
Centre for Host Resistance, Emil Skamene, MD(Charles), PhD(Czech.Acad.Sci.), FRCPC, FACP
Centre for Non Linear Dynamics, Michael Mackey, BA(Kan), PhD(Wash)
Centre for Translational Research, Gerald Batist, BS(Col.), MD, CM(McG)
Centre for Tropical Diseases, Michael Libman, MDCM
Centre for Bone and Periodontal Research, David Goltzman, MD
Experimental Medicine, , Hugh Bennett, PhD
Goodman Cancer Centre, Peter Siegel, PhD (Interim Director)
McGill A.I.D.S. Centre, Mark Wainberg, BSc(McG), PhD(Colum)
Nutrition & Food Science Centre, Errol B. Marliss, MD(Tor), FRCPC
School of Communication Sciences & Disorders, Marc Pell, PhD
Ingram School of Nursing, Helene Ezer, N, PhD
School of Physical & Occupational Therapy, Annette Majnemer OT, PhD, FCAHS
Medical Physics Unit, Jan P.F. Seuntjens, PhD, FAAPM, MCCPM

UNIVERSITÉ DE SHERBROOKE

Sherbrooke, Québec

Faculty of Medicine and Health Sciences

3001 12th Ave N, Sherbrooke, Québec Postal Code J1H 5N4

Tel. (819) 564-5200 Fax: (819) 564-5378 Website: www.usherbrooke.ca/medecine

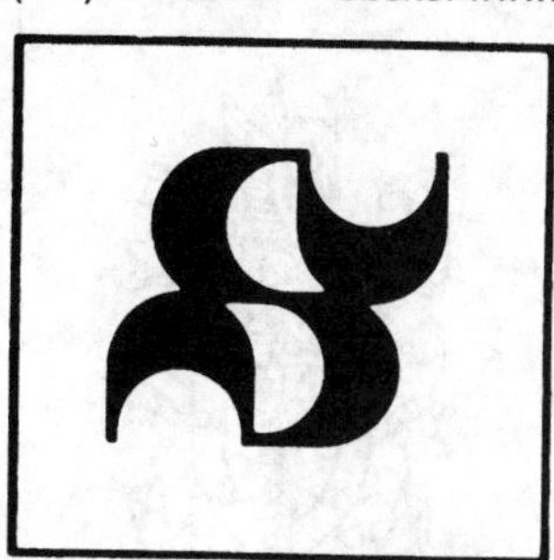

Chancellor, His Excellency Monseignor André Gaumond
Rector, Luce Samoisette, M. Fisc.
Director of Communications, Jacques Viens
Rector Graduate Studies, Denis Marceau, PhD
Vice Rector, Research, Jacques Beauvais, PhD
Vice Rector, Longueuil Campus and Information Technologies, Lyne Bouchard, PhD
Vice Rector, Human Resources and Students Life, Martin, Buteau, D.Sc
General Secretary and Vice Rector, International Relations, Jocelyne Faucher, MD
Vice Rector, Academic, Lucie Laflamme, DESS
Vice Rector, Administration, Joanne Roch, PhD
Vice Rector, Sustainable Development and Government Relations, Alain Webster, PhD

Medical School Administrative Staff

Dean, Pierre Cossette, MD
Vice-Dean, Research, Jean-Pierre Perreault, PhD
Vice-Dean, Predoctoral Medical Studies, Eve-Reine Gagne, MD
Vice-Dean, Resources and Assistant Dean, Dominique Dorion, MD
Vice-Dean, Postgraduate Medical Studies, Serge Langevin, MD
Faculty Secretary and Vice-Dean, Student Services, Sophie Laflamme, MD
Director, Centre for Continuing Education, Gilles Voyer, MD
Vice-Dean, Nursing, Luc Mathieu, DBA
Vice-Dean, Rehabilitation, Johanne Desrosiers, PhD
Director, Information Technologies and Communications Services, David Serouge
Vice-Dean, Pedagogue Development, Diane Clavet, MD
Chairperson of Admission Committee, Daniel J. Côté, MD
Administrator Director, René Gagnon, MBA
Director-Administration, Predoctoral Medical Studies, Sylvie Lamarche
Vice-Dean, Development & Partnership, Mr. Luc Paquet
Medical Librarian, Marthe Brideau

Department Heads

Anatomy & Cellular Biology, Nathalie Rivard, MSc, PhD
Anesthesia, René Martin, MD
Biochemistry, Dr. Martin Bisaillon, PhD
Community Health Sciences, Richard Côte, MD
Family Medicine, Marie Giroux, MD
Medicine, Patrice Perron, MD
Microbiology and Infectiology, Raymond Wellinger, PhD
Nuclear Medicine & Radiobiology, Benoit Paquette, PhD
Nursing, Luc Mathieu, Inf., DBA
Obstetrics & Gynecology, Guy Waddell, MD
Pathology, Dr. Edmund Rizcallah, MD
Pediatrics, Hervé Walti, MD
Pharmacology, Richard Leduc
Physiology & Biophysics, Eric Rousseau, PhD
Psychiatry, Pierre Beauséjour, MD
Radiology, The Bao Bui, MD
Rehabilitation, Johanne Desrosiers, PhD
Surgery, Gaétan Langlois, MD

General Information

The Faculty of Medicine of the Université de Sherbrooke received its first students in 1966.

The objectives of the Faculty of Medicine are to graduate practitioners of the best quality, to promote research and to raise the standards of the practice of medicine to better meet the needs of communities they serve. The four-year Medical School works in cooperation with an extensive network of affiliated health care institutions of which Sherbrooke University Hospital is the most important. Since 2001, the Faculty is a World Health Organization Collaborating Centre on, "The education and practice of health professionals responsive to health needs of communities".

UNIVERSITY OF OTTAWA

Ottawa, Ontario

Faculty of Medicine

451 Smyth Road, Ottawa, Ontario Postal Code K1H 8M5

Dean's Office - Tel. (613) 562-5800 Ext. 8117 Fax (613) 562-5457 Email: infomed@uottawa.ca Website: www.medecine.uottawa.ca

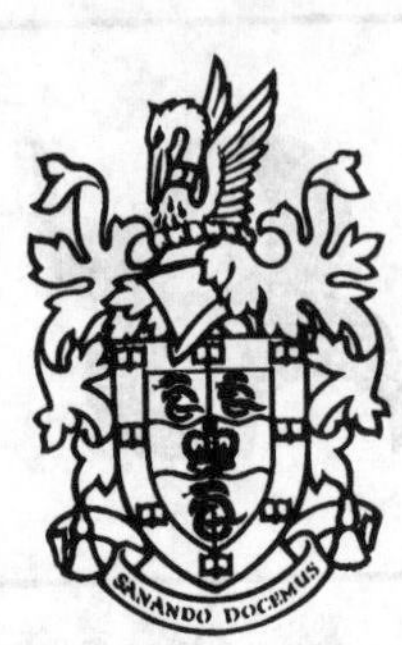

The Faculty of Medicine was established in 1945. Between 1978 and 1988, the School of Medicine was regrouped into a Faculty of Health Sciences along with the School of Nursing and the School of Human Kinetics. The Faculty of Medicine was reestblished as an entity in 1989.

Type: public

2012 Total Enrolment: 165

Clinical facilities: The Ottawa Hospital, Royal Ottawa Health Care Group, Children's Hospital of Eastern Ontario, Montfort Hospital, Queensway Carleton Hospital, Sisters of Charity of Ottawa, Winchester District Memorial, Pembroke Regional Hospital, Cornwall Community Hospital, Hawkesbury & District General Hospital (French Stream)

Medical School

Dean, Faculty of Medicine, Jacques Bradwejn, MD
Vice Dean, Research, Bernard Jasmin, PhD
Vice Dean, Professional Affairs, Rama C. Nair, PhD
Vice Dean, Postgraduate Medical Education, Paul Bragg, MD (interim)
Vice Dean, Undergraduate Medical Education, Melissa Forgie, MD
Vice Dean, Office of Francophone Affairs, Jean Roy, MD
Vice Dean, Continuing Medical Education, Paul Hendry, MD
Vice Dean, Health/Hospital Services, Sharon Whiting, MD
Assistant Dean, Academy for Innovation in Medical Education (AIME), Stanley Hamstra, PhD. (acting)
Assistant Dean, Admissions, Gary Hollingworth, MD
Assistant Dean, Student Affairs, Louise Laramée, MD
Assistant Dean, Research and Special Projects, David Park, PhD
Assistant Dean, Graduate and Postdoctoral Studies, Ruth Slack, PhD
Director, Faculty Development, Catharine Robertson, MD
Director, Faculty Wellness Program, Tara Tucker, MD
Director, Office of Equity, Diversity and Gender Issues, Catherine Tsilfidis, MD
Director, Global Health, Anne McCarthy, MD
Director, Professionalism, Homer Yang, MD
Director, Distributed Medical Education, Charles Su, MD
Director, E-curriculum, Pippa Hall, MD
Director, Alumni & Student Affairs-Aboriginal Students, Darlene Kitty, MD
Secretary of the Faculty, Vasek Mezl, PhD
Director, Animal Care Services, Marilyn Keaney, DVM
Director, Health Sciences Library, Lee-Anne Upholz
Chief Administrative Officer, Vanessa Sutton, FCIS., CMA
Operations Manager, Linda Chenard
Human Resources Manager, Heidi Baier
Director of Advancement, Sharon Cardiff
Financial Services Manager, Yudy Bengoa
Marketing & Communications Manager, Susan Maroun

University of Ottawa Faculty of Medicine: Department Chairs

Basic Sciences

Biochemistry, **Microbiology & Immunology**, Zemin Yao, PhD
Cellular and Molecular Medicine, David Lohnes, PhD
Epidemiology & Community Medicine, Julian Little, PhD.

Clinical Sciences

Anesthesia, Homer Yang, MD, FRCPC
Emergency Medicine, Ian Stiell, MD
Family Medicine, Michael Hirsh, MD (interim)
Medicine, Phil Wells, MD
Obstetrics & Gynecology, Andrée Gruslin, MD (interim)
Ophthalmology, Steven M. Gilberg, MD
Otolaryngology, Martin Corsten, MD
Pediatrics, Ciarán Duffy, MD
Pathology & Laboratory Medicine, John Veinot, MD
Psychiatry, Katharine Gillis, MD
Radiology, Mark E. Schweitzer, MD
Surgery, Sudhir Sundaresan, MD (interim)

Admission Requirements

Candidates in the following categories are eligible to apply for admission to the first year of the four-year program of undergraduate medical studies:

(a) Candidates for admission must have completed successfully three years of full-time studies in a recognized university (minimum of five full-year courses/year) in an undergraduate program leading to a bachelor degree; including four specific prerequisite courses:

- One full-year course in General Biology or Zoology including laboratory session;
- One full-year course in Humanities (ex: Literature, History, Logic, Philosophy, Psychology, Expository Writing, Sociology, Anthropology, Art History, etc. . . .)
- Two of the following full-year courses in Chemistry:

i) General Biochemistry (without laboratory session);
ii) General Chemistry (with laboratory session);
iii) Organic Chemistry (with laboratory session).
Science prerequisites should be completed before the beginning of June preceding registration.
iv) Applicants are not required to write the MCAT (Medical College Admission Test) to be eligible for admission.
v) Candidates must be Canadian citizens or permanent residents.

Equivalence to be determined by the Faculty of Medicine of the University of Ottawa.
N.B. Meeting the above requirements does not guarantee admission.

RESOURCE SECTION

QUEEN'S UNIVERSITY

Kingston, Ontario

Faculty of Health Sciences
Macklem House
18 Barrie St, Kingston, Ontario Postal Code K7L 3N6
Tel. (613) 533-2544 Fax (613) 533-6884 Website: http://meds.queensu.ca

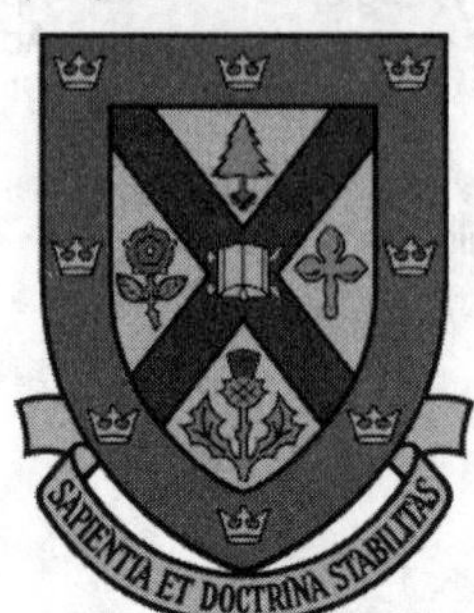

Chancellor, David Dodge
Principal & Vice-Chancellor, Daniel Woolf, PhD
Dean, Faculty of Health Sciences and Director, School of Medicine, Richard Reznick, MD, MEd, FRCSC, FACS, FRCSEd (hon), FRCSI (hon)
Executive Vice Dean, Iain Young, MD, FRCPC
Vice Dean, Research, Roger Deeley, PhD
Vice Dean, Medical Education, Leslie Flynn, MMus, MD, CCFP, FRCPC (Interim)
Associate Dean, Postgraduate Medical Education, Ross Walker, MD, FRCSC, FACS
Associate Dean, Continuing Professional Development, Karen Smith, PhD, FRCPC
Associate Dean, Undergraduate Medical Education, Anthony Sanfilippo, MD, FRCPC
Associate Dean, Graduate & Postdoctoral Education, Brian Bennett, PhD
Associate Dean, Life Sciences & Biochemistry, Michael Kawaja, PhD
Associate Dean, Finance & Administration, David Edgar, CMA, MBA, MSc
Associate Dean, Regional Education, Eugene Dagnone, MD, CCFP, FACEP, FRCPC
Vice Dean (Health Sciences) and Director, School of Nursing, Jennifer Medves, RN, PhD
Vice Dean (Health Sciences) and Director, School of Rehabilitation Therapy, Marcia Finlayson, PhD

Department Heads

Anesthesiology & Perioperative Medicine, Joel Parlow, MD, FRCPC
Biomedical & Molecular Sciences, Michael Adams, PhD
Community Health & Epidemiology, William Pickett, PhD
Diagnostic Radiology, Annette McCallum, MSc, MD
Emergency Medicine, Gord Jones, MD, FRCPC
Family Medicine, Glenn Brown, MD, CCFP(EM), FCFP, MPH
Medicine, Stephen Archer, MD, FRCPC, FAHA, FACC
Obstetrics & Gynaecology, Michael McGrath, MD, FRCSC, FSOGC
Oncology, Elizabeth Eisanhauer, MD, FRCPC
Ophthalmology, Martin ten Howe, MD, MEng, FRCSC
Otolaryngology, Russell Hollins, BScH, MD, FRCSC
Pathology & Molecular Medicine, Victor Tron, MD, FRCPC, PhD
Paediatrics, Kimberley Dow, MD, FRCPC (Acting)
Physical Medicine & Rehabilitation, Stephen Bagg, MD, FRCPC
Psychiatry, Roumen Milev, MD,, PhD, FRCPsych, FRCPC
Surgery, John Rudan, MD, FRCSC
Urology, Robert Siemens, MD, FRCSC

Queen's University owes its origin to the efforts of the Synod of the Presbyterian Church in Canada to found a college at Kingston along the lines of the Scottish National Universities. On October 16, 1841, a Royal Charter was issued and the first classes were opened at Kingston in March, 1842. The Faculty of Medicine was established in 1854. In 1866, it was reorganized as the Royal College of Physicians and Surgeons in affiliation with the University, but, in 1892, the original status was resumed. The Faculty was renamed as the Faculty of Health Sciences in 1997.

The Medical Course

There are one hundred places in the first year of a four year program leading to the degree of Doctor of Medicine. The minimum academic requirements for admission are three full years of study at university in any program and successful completion of the following prerequisite university subjects: general biology, general chemistry, general physics and organic chemistry. All candidates are required to write the revised (1991) Medical College Admission Test.

Further information concerning admission may be obtained from the Admissions Office, School of Medicine, or by Consulting the Calendar of the Faculty of Health Sciences.

Graduate and Postgraduate Training

In co-operation with the School of Graduate Studies, courses are offered leading to the degrees of Master of Science and Doctor of Philosophy. In the clinical departments, training is provided to meet the requirements for certification and fellowship of the Royal College of Physicians and Surgeons of Canada. A combined MD/PhD program is also offered.

Continuing Education

An active program of continuing medical education for physicians includes weekly lectures, special courses, and decentralized clinics.

UNIVERSITY OF TORONTO

Toronto, Ontario

Medical Sciences Building

One King's College Circle, Suite 2109, Toronto, Ontario   Postal Code M5S 1A8

Tel. (416) 978-6585   Fax: (416) 978-1774   Website: www.medicine.utoronto.ca

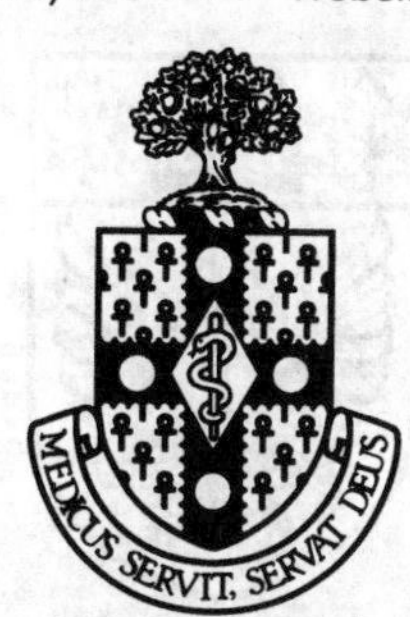

Faculty of Medicine

President, David Naylor, MD, DPhil, FRCPC
Dean, Catharine Whiteside, MD, PhD., FRCPC
Deputy Dean, Sarita Verma, LLB, MD, CCFP, FCFP
Vice-President & Provost, Cheryl Misak, PhD
Vice-Provost, Relations with Health Care Institutions, Catharine Whiteside, MD, PhD, FRCPC
Vice-Dean, Research & International Relations, Alison Buchan, PhD, FCAHS
Vice-Dean, Graduate Affairs (Interim), Avrum Gotlieb, MDCM, FRCPC
Vice-Dean, Continuing Education & Professional Development, Dimitri Anastakis
Vice-Dean, Clinical Affairs, J. Bohnen, MD, FACS
Vice-Dean, Undergraduate Medical Education, Jay Rosenfield, MD, MEd, FRCPC
Vice-Dean, Postgraduate Medical Education(PGME), Salvatore Spadofora, MD, FRCPC, MHPE
Associate Dean, Equity & Professioanalism, David McKnight, MD, FRCPC
Associate Dean, Undergraduate Medicine, Admissions & Student Finances, Mark Hanson, MEd
Senior Academic Advisor, Avrum Gotlieb, MDCM, FRCPC
Associate Dean, Health Professions Student Affairs, Prof. Leslie Nickell, MSW, MD, CCFP
Chief Administrative Officer, Tim Neff, MBA, CMA
Faculty Comptroller & CFO, Nancy Edwards, BSc, MBA, CMA

Departmental Chairs

Anesthesia, B. Kavanagh, MD, FRCPC
Biochemistry, R. Reithmeier, PhD
Biomaterials and Biomedical Engineering, P. Santerre, PhD
Family & Community Medicine, L. Wilson, MD, CCFP
Health Policy, Management and Evaluation (institute of), Adalsteinn Brown, AB, DPhill
Immunology, J.C. Zunigra-Pflücker, PhD
Laboratory Medicine and Pathobiology, R. Hegele, MD, PhD, FRCPC
Medical Imaging, A. Moody, FRCR, FRCP
Medicine, W. Levinson, MD, FRCPC
Molecular Genetics, H. Lipshitz
Medical Biophysics, P. Burns, PhD
Nutritional Sciences, M. L'Abbé, PhD
Obstetrics & Gynaecology, A. Bocking, MD, FRCSC
Occupational Sciences and Occupational Health, S. Rappolt, PhD
Ophthalmology and Vision Sciences, S. El-Defrawy, MD, PhD, FRCSC
Otolaryngology-Head & Neck Surgery, I. Witterick, MD, MSc, FRCSC
Pediatrics, D. Daneman, MD, FRCPC
Pharmacology and Toxicology, R.A. Ross, PhD
Physical Therapy, K. Berg, PhD, MSc, BSc, BPT
Physiology, S. Matthews, PhD
Psychiatry, T Young, MD, PhD, FRCPC
Public Health (Dalla Lana School of), H. Hu, MD, MPH, MS, ScD
Radiation Oncology, F.F. Liu, MD, FRCPC
Speech-Language Pathology, L. Girolametto, PhD
Surgery , J. Rukta, MD, PhD, FRCSC, FACS, FAAP

The Medical School was founded in 1843. Through the University of Toronto, the Faculty of Medicine is fully affiliated with 10 teaching hospitals and partially affiliated with a further 15 teaching healthcare sites and with the Toronto Academic Health Science Network (TAHSN).

The course consists of four professional years at the end of which the degree of Doctor of Medicine (M.D.) is conferred.

McMASTER UNIVERSITY

Hamilton, Ontario

Faculty of Medicine Health Sciences Centre,

1200 Main St W, Hamilton, Ontario Postal Code L8N 3Z5

Tel. (905) 525-9140 Fax. (905) 528-4727 Website: www.fhs.mcmaster.ca/

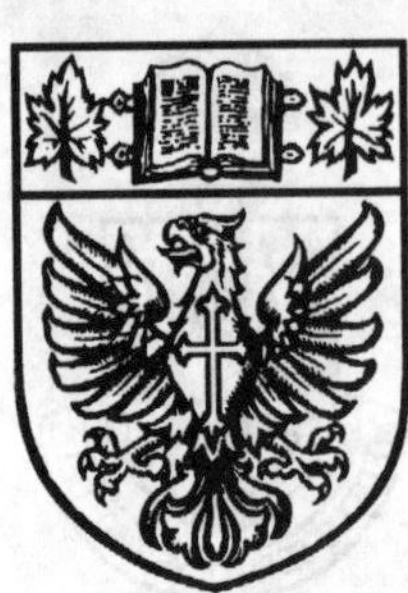

Chancellor, L. Wilson
President & Vice-Chancellor, P.Deane
Provost & Vice-President, Academic, D. Wilkinson
Vice-President, Administration, R. Couldrey
Dean and Vice-President, Health Sciences, J.G. Kelton, MD, FRCPC
Vice-President, Research & International affairs, M.A. Elbestawi, PhD, FCAE, PEng
Assistant Vice-President, Administration, D. Henne
Acting Registrar, M. Pool
Associate Vice-President, Institutional Research & Analysis, K. Menard, BA, MA, PhD
Librarian, J. Trzeciak, BS, MLS

Faculty of Health Sciences Administrative Staff

Dean and Vice-President, Health Sciences, J.G. Kelton, MD, FRCPC
Associate Dean, Academic, S. Denburg
Associate Dean, Research, S. Collins
Associate Dean, Nursing, C. Tompkins
Associate Dean, Graduate Studies, C. Hayward
Associate Dean & Director, School of Rehabilitation Sciences, P. Solomon
Health Sciences Librarian, L. Bayley
Chair, Undergraduate MD Program, R. Whyte
Chair, Postgraduate Medical Programme, H.M. Walton

Departmental Heads

Anesthesia, N. Buckley, MD
Biochemistry, E. Brown, MD
Clinical Epidemiology & Biostatistics, H. Schunemann, MD
Family Medicine, D. Price, BSc, MD, CCFP
Medicine, P. O. O'Byrne, MD
Nursing (School of), Catherine Tompkins
Obstetrics & Gynecology, N. Leyland, MD
Oncology, M. N. Levine, MD
Pathology, F. Smaill, MD
Pediatrics, L. Huang
Psychiatry, N. Kates (Acting), MD
Radiology, D. Koff, MD
Rehabilitation Science (School of), P, Solomon
Surgery, B. Orovan MD(McM), FRCSC

The MD Programme at McMaster University operates on a year-round basis with a duration of three calendar years at the end of which the degree, Doctor of Medicine, is conferred. To be eligible for consideration for admission, applicants must have completed or will have completed before registration, at least three years of undergraduate degree studies at a recognized university, with an overall second class ("B") average.

The Northwestern Ontario medical programme has been developed in cooperation with the Thunder Bay Medical Society and physicians in towns in Northwestern Ontario to provide clinical training opportunities for Medical students and Residents from all other various medical schools. Clinical training opportunities also exist in affiliated teaching hospitals adjacent to Hamilton, and experience in these settings is part of both the undergraduate and postgraduate medical programmes.

Graduate Training

Opportunities for postgraduate training for higher professional qualifications are available in university-directed programmes in accord with a regional plan to coordinate health services at the Chedoke-McMaster Hospitals; Chedoke Hospital Division, McMaster University Medical Centre Division; Hamilton Civic Hospitals; Hamilton General Hospital; Henderson General Hospital; Hamilton Psychiatric Hospital; St. Joseph's Hospital.

Physicians are offered residency training certified by the Royal College of Physicians and Surgeons of Canada and the College of Family Physicians of Canada.

RESOURCE SECTION

WESTERN UNIVERSITY

London, Ontario

The Schulich School of Medicine & Dentistry

Don Rix Clinical Skills Building, Rm 3700
London, Ontario Postal Code N6A 5C1

Tel. (519) 661-2111 Fax. (519) 850-2357 Web: www.schulich.uwo.ca

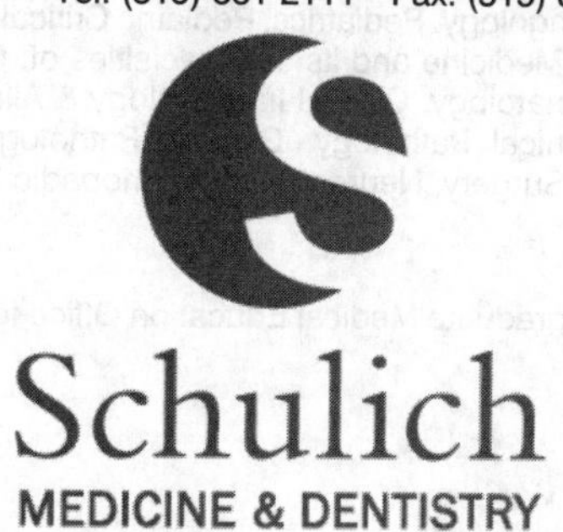

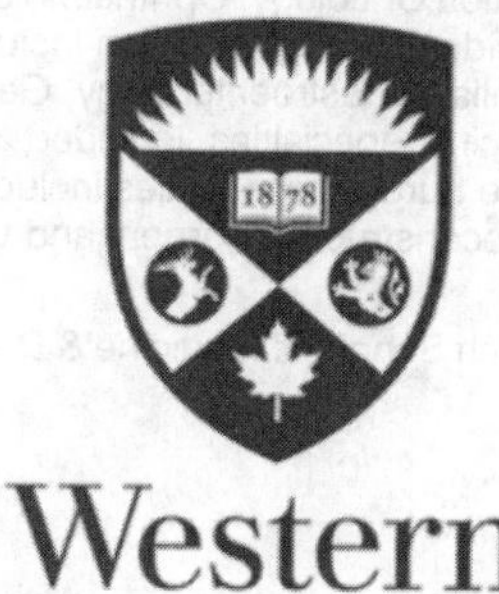

Senior Administration

President & Vice-Chancellor, Amit Chakma, PhD (UBC)
Provost & Vice-President, Academic, Janice Deakin
Vice-President (Resources & Operations), Gitta Kulczycki

The Schulich School of Medicine & Dentistry

Dean, Michael Strong, MD, FRCPC, FAAN, FCAHS
Chief Operating Officer, Dwayne Martins
Vice Dean, Education, Bertha Garcia, MD, FRCPC
Vice Dean, Hospital & Interfaculty Relations, Margaret Steele, MD, FRCPC
Vice Dean, Research & Innovations, Denise Figlewicz, PhD
Associate Dean, Admissions, Robert Hammond, MD, FRCPC
Vice Dean, Basic Medical Sciences, Doug Jones, PhD
Associate Dean, Continuing Professional Development, Jatinder Takhar, MD, FRCPC
Associate Dean, Equity and Professionalism, Terri Paul, MD, FRCPC
Associate Dean, Research (Graduate & Postdoctoral Studies), Andrew Watson, PhD
Associate Dean, Postgraduate Medical Education, Christopher J. Watling, MD, FRCPC
Associate Dean, Undergraduate Education, Gary Tithecott, MD, FRCPC
Associate Dean, Rural & Regional Medicine, Shamin Tejpar, MD, FRCPC
Associate Dean, Student Affairs, Michael Rieder, MD, FRCPC
Associate Dean, Windsor Program, Gerry Cooper, PhD
Associate Dean, Windsor Program-Faculty & Governmental Affairs, Mark Awuku, MD, FRCPC
Vice Dean, Director, Schulich Dentistry, Harinder Sandhu, DDS
Clinical Medicine Librarian, Robin Featherstone

Department Chairs

Anaesthesia & Perioperative Medicine, Davy Cheng, MD, MSc, FRCPC
Anatomy & Cell Biology, Kem Rogers, PhD, MSc
Biochemistry, David Litchfield, BSc, PhD
Clinical Neurological Sciences, Acting Chair, Paul Cooper, MD, FRCPC
Epidemiology & Biostatistics, Karen Campbell, MSc, PhD
Family Medicine, Stephen J. Wetmore, MD, CCFP
History of Medicine, Shelley McKellar
Medical Biophysics, Jerry Battista, PhD, FCCPM
Medical Imaging, Andrea Lum, MD, FRCPC
Medicine, Rob McFadden, MD, FRCPC
Microbiology & Immunology, Bhagi Singh
Obstetrics & Gynaecology, Maggie Rebel, MD, FRCSC
Oncology, Glenn Bauman, MD, FRCPC
Ophthalmology, William Hodge, MD, FRCPC, PhD
Otolaryngology-Head & Neck Surgery, John Yoo, MD, FRCSC, FACS
Pathology, Subrata Chakrabarti, MD, FRCPC, PhD
Paediatrics, Guido Filler, MD, FRCPC, PhD
Physiology & Pharmacology, Jane Rylett, PhD
Physical Medicine & Rehabilitation, Timothy Doherty, MD, FRCPC, PhD
Psychiatry, Paul Links, MD, FRCPC
Surgery, John Denstedt, MD, FRCSC
Dentistry, Harinder Sandhu, DDS (Director & Vice-Dean)
Robarts Research Institute, Michael Strong, MD, FRCPC, FAAN, FCAHS

The Schulich School of Medicine & Dentistry, Western University, provides outstanding education within a research-intensive, distributed learning environment where tomorrow's physicians, dentists, health researchers and other scholars learn to be socially responsible leaders in the advancement of human health locally, regionally and globally. There is a long-standing tradition of excellence, beginning with the founding of the medical school in 1881 and continuing with the formation of the dental school in 1964. Today, the school is a leading Canadian centre of outstanding education and research shaping health care for the next generation.

Postgraduate Training in Clinical Specialties

Schulich School of Medicine & Dentistry and its affiliated teaching sites offer about 52 postgraduate programs accredited by the College of Family Physicians of Canada or the Royal College of Physicians & Surgeons of Canada. We are committed to providing an outstanding resident experience, whether in London or in our diverse distributed sites. Our programs offer an outstanding depth and breadth of education experiences that will prepare learners for challenging and productive careers.

Some of our nationally accredited residency programs include Family Medicine and the clinical specialties of: Anesthesia, Diagnostic Radiology, Emergency Medicine, Neurology, Neuroradiology, Nuclear Medicine, Obstetrics & Gynecology, Maternal-Fetal Medicine, Reproductive Endocrinology and Infertility, Medical Oncology, Radiation Oncology, Ophthalmology, Otolaryngology, Pediatrics, Pediatric Critical Care, Neonatal-Perinatal Medicine, Psychiatry and Adult Critical Care. Residency programs also include Internal Medicine and its subspecialties of: Cardiology, Clinical Pharmacology, Dermatology, Endocrinology & Metabolism, Gastroenterology, Geriatrics, Hematology, Clinical Immunology & Allergy, Nephrology, Respirology and Rheumatology. The Laboratory Medicine specialties included are: Anatomical Pathology, General Pathology, Medical Microbiology, Medical Biochemistry, and Neuropathology. The Surgical specialties include: General Surgery, Neurosurgery, Orthopedic Surgery, Cardiac Surgery, Vascular Surgery, Thoracic Surgery, Plastic & Reconstructive Surgery and Urology.

Applicants should contact the Schulich School of Medicine & Dentistry Postgraduate Medical Education Office for information regarding application procedures.

NORTHERN ONTARIO SCHOOL OF MEDICINE

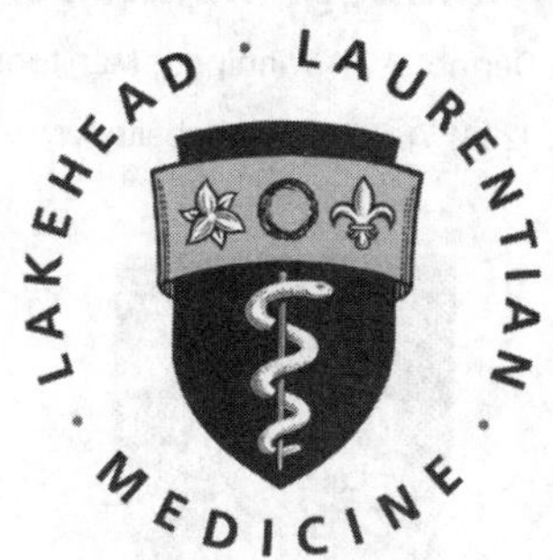

LAKEHEAD UNIVERSITY
Thunder Bay, Ontario

Northern Ontario School of Medicine

West Campus

955 Oliver Road, Thunder Bay, Ontario Postal Code P7B 5E1

Tel. (807) 766-7300 Fax. (807) 766-7370
Email: communications@nosm.ca Website: www.nosm.ca

LAURENTIAN UNIVERSITY
Sudbury, Ontario

Northern Ontario School of Medicine

East Campus

935 Ramsey Lake Road, Sudbury, Ontario Postal Code P3E 2C6

Tel. (705) 675-4883 Fax. (705) 675-4858
Email: communications@nosm.ca Website: www.nosm.ca

Faculty of Medicine Administrative Staff

Dean, CEO & Professor, Roger Strasser, MBBS, BMedSci, MClSc, DA, Dip RACOG, FRACGP, FACRRM, FRGP, AM (AU)
Associate Dean, Community Engagement, David Marsh, MD, CCSAM
Associate Dean, Faculty Affairs, William McCready, MB, BCh, MRCP(UK), FRCP
Associate Dean, Postgraduate Medical Education, Catherine Cervin, MD, FCFP
Associate Dean, Undergraduate Medical Education, Lisa Graves, MD
Associate Dean, Research, Greg Ross, PhD
Director, Learner Affairs, John Friesen
Chief Administrative Officer, Ken Adams, CMA, MHSA, CHE
Division Head, Medical Sciences , Douglas Boreham, PhD
Division Head, Human Sciences, Elizabeth Levin, PhD
Division Head, Clinical Sciences, Janice Willett, FRCSC

Postgraduate Programs

Assistant Dean, Family Medicine, Dr. Tom Crichton
Program Director, Family Practice Anaesthesia, Dr. Rob Anderson
Program Director, Public Health & Preventive Medicine, Dr. Na-Koshie Lamptey
Program Director, Emergency Medicine, Dr. Williams MacGregor
Program Director, Family Medicine, Dr. Richard Almond
Program Director, Anesthesia, Dr. Rob Anderson
Program Director, Psychiatry, Dr. Shiva Kumar
Program Director, Pediatrics, Dr. Tara Baron
Program Director, Orthopedic Surgery, Dr. David Puskas
Regional Director, Internal Medicine, Dr. Kim Tilbe
Regional Director, Obstetrics & Gynecology, East: Dr. Stephen Fairley
Regional Director, Psychiatry, Dr. Kuppuswami Shivakumar
Program Director, General Surgery, Dr. Pankaj Bhatia

About the Northern Ontario School of Medicine

A medical school for the whole of Northern Ontario, the Northern Ontario School of Medicine (NOSM) is a joint initiative of Lakehead University in Thunder Bay and Laurentian University in Sudbury. NOSM has been established by the two universities as a not-for-profit corporation which serves as the Faculty of Medicine both for Laurentian University and for Lakehead University. With main campuses in Thunder Bay and Sudbury, NOSM has multiple teaching and research sites distributed across Northern Ontario, including large and small communities. NOSM contributes to improving the health of the people of Northern Ontario.

NOSM offers a world-class four year MD Program organized around five themes: Northern and Rural Health, Personal & Professional Aspects of Medical Practice, Social and Population Health. It lays the foundations of medicine, and clinical Skills in healthcare. Classroom learning is mostly in small groups, Patient Centered Class Based Learning, complemented by Whole Group Sessions and clinical learning from the beginning of year one. Clinical placements occur in a diverse range of communities and clinical settings supported by high quality electronic communications in the Virtual Learning Environment, with a full year of Community Based Medical Education outside Sudbury and Thunder Bay in year three.

Specialty residency programs are available at the Northern Ontario School of Medicine. These include Family Medicine, Enhanced Skills in Emergency Medicine, Anesthesia, Public Health & Preventive Medicine, General Surgery, Internal Medicine, Orthopedic Surgery, Pediatrics and Psychiatry.

RESOURCE SECTION

UNIVERSITY OF MANITOBA

Winnipeg, Manitoba

260 Brodie Centre, 727 McDermot Ave, Winnipeg, Manitoba Postal Code R3E 3P5

Tel. (204) 789-3557 Fax. (204) 789-3928 Website: www.umanitoba.ca/medicine

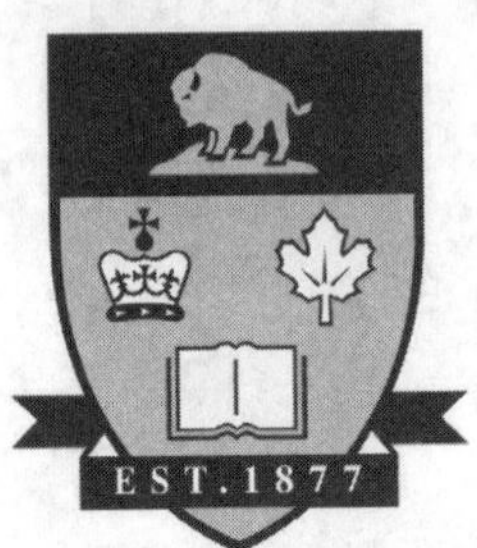

Faculty of Medicine

President, David T. Barnard, PhD

Dean, Faculty of Medicine, Brian Postl, MD

Associate Deans

Academic Terry Klassen, MD, MSc, FRCPC
Undergraduate Medical Education Ira Ripstein, MD, MSc, CCFP
Postgradate Medical Education Cliff Yaffe, MD, FRCSC, FACS
Clinical Affairs Brock Wright, BSc., MD, FRCPC, MBA
Continuing Professional Development Jose Francois, MD, CCFP, MEd
Research Peter Nickerson, BSc, MD, FRCPC
Professionalism & Diversity Samia Barakat, MD, FRCPC
Students Bruce Martin, MD, MSc, CCFP, FRCPC
First Nations, Metis & Inuit Health Catherine Cook, MD, MSc, CCFP, FCFP
Accreditation Gary Harding, MD, FRCPC

Assistant Deans

Academic Heather Dean, MD, FRCPC
Grad Studies Ed Kroeger, BSc (Biol), MSc (Physiology), PhD (Physiology)
Research Kevin Coombs, PhD

Departmental Heads

Anesthesia, E. Jacobsohn, MBChB (Capetown), FRCPC, MHPE (Illinois)
Biochemistry & Medical Genetics, L. Simard, BSc, PhD
Clinical Health Psychology, R. McIlwraith, PhD (Psych)
Community Health Sciences, Sharon Macdoanld, BSc (Med), FRCPC
Medical Education, A. MacDiarmid, MD
Family Medicine, R. James Boyd, MD, CCFP, FCFP
Human Anatomy and Cell Science, Thomas Klonisch, MD, PhD(Germany)
Immunology, Dr. Redwan Moqbel, MSc, PhD (UK)
Medical Microbiology, J.E. Embree, FRCPC, Peds, InfectDis
Medicine, D. Roberts, MD(Tor), FRCPC
Emergency Medicine, Alecs Chochinov, MD, FRCPC
Obstetrics, Gynecology & Reproductive Sciences, Margaret Morris, MD, FRCSC
Ophthalmology, L.D. Bellan, FRCSC, Ophth
Otolaryngology, P. Kerr, FRSCS
Pathology, J. Gartner, MD, CH, LMCC, FRCPC
Pediatrics & Child Health, C. Rockman-Greenberg, MD, CM, FRCPC, FCCMG
Pharmacology & Therapeutics, F. Parkinson
Physiology, J. Dodd, BSc, PhD(Tor)
Psychiatry, P. Cattini, BSc. Hons. PhD (UK)
Radiology, S. Demeter, MHSc, MSc, FRCPC
Surgery, J. McPherson, A.M., MD, FRCS(C), (Interim)

In 1883 thirteen physicians applied to the local legislature for a charter to form Manitoba Medical College, Dr. James Kerr was the Dean and Dr. James Patterson, Registrar. Dr. Kerr delivered an introductory lecture on November 15th, 1883, and the first lectures of the medical course were given in the Central Collegiate Building on November 21st. The first practical work was done in a cottage on Isabel Street. With funds entirely furnished by members of the Faculty, a building was erected on the corner of McDermot and Kate Streets, and was utilized for teaching purposes during the second session. The College from its beginning, was affiliated with the University of Manitoba and the first graduating class of six students received their degrees from the University in May, 1886.

Present Course

The present medical course at the University of Manitoba is of four years' duration and full details may be secured from the Admissions Office. Application for admission should be made before Nov. 30.

Degrees Offered

The degrees offered are Doctor of Medicine (MD), Bachelor of Science in Medicine (BScMed), Master of Science (MSc), and Doctor of Philosophy (PhD).

UNIVERSITY OF SASKATCHEWAN

Saskatoon, Saskatchewan

College of Medicine
B103 Health Sciences Building
107 Wiggins Road, Saskatoon, Saskatchewan Postal Code S7N 5E5
Tel. (306) 966-6149 Fax (306) 966-6164 Website: www.medicine.usask.ca

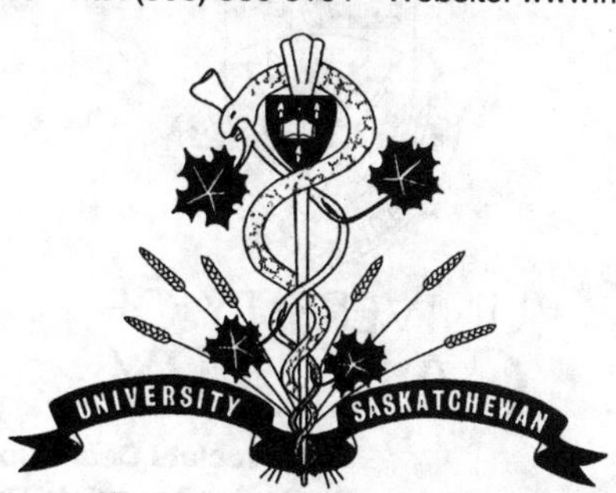

President, I. J. Busch-Vishnlac, BS/BA, MSc, PhD
Associate VP Student & Enrolment Services, D. Hannah, BEd, PhD
Registrar & Director, Academic Services & Financial Assistance, Student Enrolment Services Division, R. Isinger

College of Medicine

Dean of the Faculty of Medicine, L.F. Qualtiere (Acting)
Associate Dean, Undergraduate Medical Education, S.R. Rutledge Harding, MD, FRCPC
Associate Dean, Physical Therapy & Rehabilitation Sciences, E.L. Harrison, BPT, MSc, MCPA, PhD
Associate Dean, Biomedical Sciences, N. Ovsenok, BSc, MS, PhD
Associate Dean, Research, L. F. Qualtiere, PhD
Associate Dean, Faculty Affairs, O.A. Olatunbosun, MD, FRCSC, FACOG
Associate Dean, Saskatoon, G.S. Stoneham, MD, FRCPC
Associate Dean, Rural & Northern Medical Education, T. Smith-Windsor, BSc, MD, FCFP
Associate Dean, Postgraduate Medical Education, A. Saxena, MD, MBBS, FACA, FRCPC
Assistant Dean, Undergradute Medical Education, G. Linassi, BSc, MB, FRCPC
Assistant Dean, CME and Professional Development, A. Muller, MBChB, CFPC
Director of Admissions, B. Ziola, BSc, PhD
Chair, Global Health, L. Buhler, BSc, MSc

Departmental Heads

Anatomy and Cell Biology, B. Rosser, BSc, MSc, PhD
Anesthesiology, D. Campbell, MD, FRCPC
Biochemistry, W. Roesler, BSc, MSc, PhD
Community Health & Epidemiology, N. Muhajarine, PhD
Family Medicine, A. Danilkewich, MD, CCFP
Medicine, V. Hoeppner, MD, FRCPC
Medical Imaging, P. S. Babyn, MDCM, FRCPC
Microbiology & Immunology, P. Bretscher, PhD
Obst, Gyn & Reproductive Sciences, T. Mainprize, MD, FRCSC
Pathology & Laboratory Medicine, J. Blondeau, BSc, MSc, PhD (Acting)
Pediatrics, L. Givelichian, MD, FRCPC
Pharmacology, V. Gopal, BSc, MSc, PhD
Physical Medicine and Rehabilitation, L.M. Rudachyk, MD, CCFP, FRCPC
Physiology, M. Desautels, PhD
Psychiatry, M. Baetz, MD, FRCPC
Surgery, I. Mendez, MD, PhD, FRCSC
School of Physical Therapy, S. Milosavljevic, MMPhty, PhD

The University prepares students for entrance to and graduation in Medicine. The affiliated Royal University Hospital opened with 420 beds in January, 1955 and is the major teaching hospital. Instruction is also carried out in other hospitals affiliated with the Saskatoon and Regina Health Regions, namely Saskatoon City and St. Paul's in Saskatoon, and the Regina General in Regina.

The College of Medicine is developing a combined MD/PhD or MD/MSc degree programs for interested, qualifying students with the College of Graduate Studies.

Admission

The number of students admitted to the first year of the medical course will be 100 in 2013, 10% of which are reserved for aboriginal applicants. The selection will depend upon academic records, prerequisites/MCAT, references, interviews and general qualifications. Up to 10% of the positions may be offered to out-of-province residents.

The curriculum is four years in length.

The regulations governing admission will be found on the College of Medicine website at www.medicine.usask.ca/admissions

Registration

Orientation is August 15 and 16; August 19 is the first day of classes.

UNIVERSITY OF CALGARY

Calgary, Alberta

Faculty of Medicine

3330 Hospital Dr NW, Calgary, Alberta Postal Code T2N 4N1

Tel. (403) 220-4404 Fax. (403) 283-4740 Website: www.med.ucalgary.ca

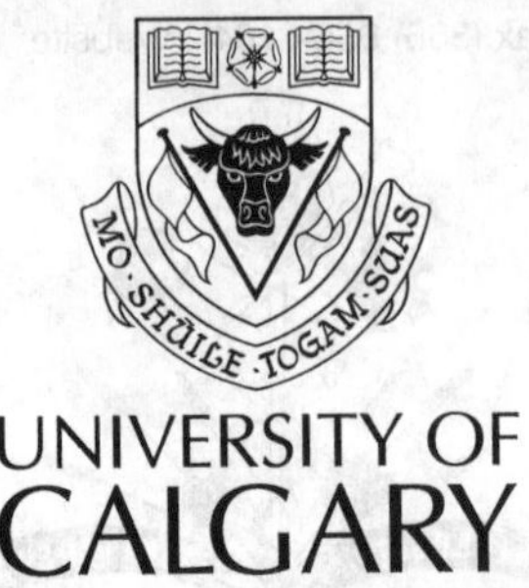

UNIVERSITY OF CALGARY

Chancellor, J. Dinning, BCom, MPA, LLD
President & Vice Chancellor, E. Cannon, PhD
Dean of the Faculty of Medicine, J. B. Meddings, MD, FRCPC
Vice Dean, G. M. MacQueen, PhD, MD, FRCPC
Associate Dean, Undergrad Medical Education, B. J. Wright, MD
Senior Associate Dean, Research, G. W. Zamponi, PhD
Associate Dean, Basic Research, J. D. Reynolds, PhD
Associate Dean, Distributed Learning & Rural Initiatives, D.L. Myhre, MD, CCFP
Associate Dean, Postgrad Medical Education, M. H. Topps, MB ChB
Senior Associate Dean, Education, J. Lockyer, PhD
Associate Dean, Faculty Assessment and Development, K. D. Patel, PhD
Associate Dean, Continuing Medical Education, L. J. Cooke, MD
Senior Associate Dean, Faculty Affairs, R. J. Bridges, MD
Associate Dean, Graduate Sciences Education, F.A. van der Hoorn, PhD
Associate Dean, Global Health and International Partnerships, J. M. Hatfield, PhD
Associate Dean, Clinical Trials, M.D. Hill, MD, FRCPC
Associate Dean, Undergraduate Science Education, A. B. Schryvers, PhD, MD
Associate Dean, Clinical Research, S. Wiebe, MD, FRCPC
Associate Dean, Equity & Professionalism, J. M. de Groot, MD, FRCPC
Executive Director, M. G. Levy, CA, CIRP

Department Heads

Anaesthesia, J.N. Armstrong, MD
Biochemistry & Molecular Biology, J. Lytton, PhD
Cardiac Sciences, T. J. Anderson, MD, FRCPC
Cell Biology & Anatomy, N.I. Syed, PhD
Clinical Neurosciences, R. Midha, MD, FRCSC
Community Health Sciences, C. J. Doig, MD, FRCPC
Critical Care Medicine, P.J.E. Boiteau, MD, FRCPC
Family Medicine, Dennis Kreptul (Interim)
Medical Genetics, F. P. Bernier, MD, FCCMG
Medicine, S. Ghosh, MD, MBBS
Microbiology & Infectious Diseases, G.D. Armstrong, PhD
Obstetrics & Gynaecology, R.D. Wilson, MD, FRCSC
Oncology, P.S. Craighead, MB ChB.
Pathology & Laboratory Medicine, J.R. Wright, Jr., PhD, MD
Paediatrics, J.D. Kellner, MD, FRCPC
Physiology & Pharmacology, W. K. MacNaughton, PhD
Psychiatry, B. L. Adams, MD, FRCPC (Acting)
Radiology, R.J. Sevick, MD, FRCPC
Surgery, J.B. Kortbeek, MD

The Faculty of Medicine at the University of Calgary was created in 1967 with the appointment of the then Dean, Dr. W.A. Cochrane. The first class of undergraduate students was accepted in September 1970 and graduated in June, 1973.

The 3-year program leads to the degree of Doctor of Medicine (MD). Each academic year consists of 11 months of instruction, and one month of unassigned vacation time. In addition, it is recommended that each student commit himself/herself to a minimum of 2 years postgraduate training.

The number of positions in the entering class is limited to 150. Students may apply for admission after completion of two years of university-level study. Most, however, will have completed a baccalaureate degree before admission to the Faculty of Medicine. The Faculty does not require that students undertake a formal pre-medical program, rather, some courses are recommended as providing the necessary background for medical studies.

The curriculum is based on systems. Each system is designated as a "course", and is complemented by parallel courses which focus on learning clinical skills and exploring human interactions relative to medicine. Each course is divided into "units". Defining all course units as clinical problems enables each course subcommittee to create a summary statement of clinical problems in which medical students need to achieve a certain level of competence. Since acquisition of skills and attitudes is as important as acquisition of knowledge, competence is defined in terms of behaviour to be developed. Clerkship objectives are defined in the same manner as the objectives in the first two years of the curriculum. Learning opportunities in the clerkship are designed to meet the stated objectives.

Postgraduate Training

At the present time a MSc and a PhD in medical sciences and a MBT (Master of Biomedical Technology) are awarded by the Faculty of Graduate Studies. Residency Programs in the major specialty areas are offered.

Research Funds

Arrangements may be made to carry on research within the Health Sciences Centre.

Continuing Medical Education

These courses are directed from the office of the Associate Dean (Continuing Medical Education.)

UNIVERSITY OF ALBERTA

Edmonton, Alberta

Faculty of Medicine & Dentistry

2J2.00 Walter C Mackenzie Health Sciences Centre, Edmonton, Alberta Postal Code T6G 2R7

Tel. (780) 492-6621 Fax: (780) 492-7303 Web. www.med.ualberta.ca/

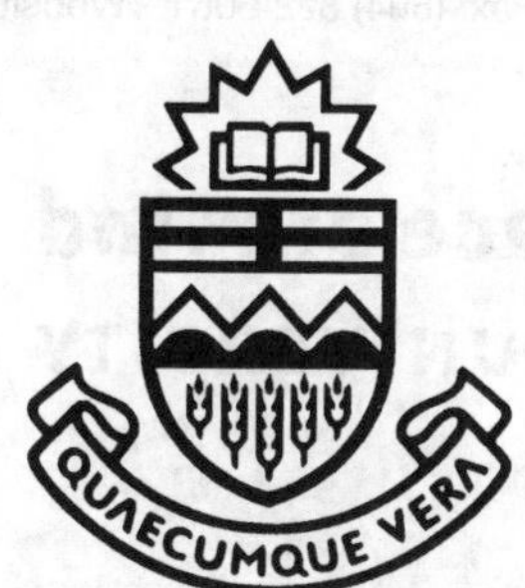

Faculty of Medicine and Dentistry

President, I. Samarasekera, PhD
Registrar, G. Kendal
Director, Financial Services, M. Coutts
Dean, Faculty of Medicine and Dentistry, D.D. Miller, MD, CM, MBA, FRCPC
Vice Dean, Faculty Affairs, D. Kunimoto, MD, FRCPC
Vice Dean, Education, F. Brenneis, MD, CCFP, FCFP
Vice Dean, Research, M. Michalak, PhD
Associate Dean, Undergraduate Medical Education, K. Stobart, MD, MSc
Chief Operating Officer, V. Wulff
Assistant Dean, Admissions, M. Moreau, MD, CCFP, FCFP
Director, Pre Clinical Education, R. Damant, MD
Associate Dean, Learner Advocacy & Wellness, M. Lewis, MD, MMedEd, FRCPC
Chair, Dentistry, P. Major, BSc, DDS, MSc
Associate Dean, Postgraduate Medical Education, R. Kearney, MD
Assistant Dean, Research, H. Ostergaard, PhD

Department Chairs

Anesthesiology & Pain Medicine, M. Murphy, MD, FRCPC (EM)
Biochemistry, C. Holmes, PhD
Biomedical Engineering, R. Burrell, PhD
Cell Biology, R. Rachubinski, PhD
Dentistry, P. Major, BSc, DDS, MSc
Emergency Medicine, B. Holroyd, MD, FACEP, FRCPC
Family Medicine, L. Green, MD, MPH
Laboratory Medicine & Pathology, M. Mengel, MD (Acting)
Medical Genetics, M. Walter, PhD
Medicine, B. Ballermann, BSc, MD
Medical Microbiology & Immunology, D. Evans, PhD
Obstetrics & Gynecology, M. Sagle, MD, MSc
Oncology, A. McEwan, MD
Ophthalmology, I. MacDonald, MD, CM
Pediatrics, S. Gilmour, MD, MSc
Pharmacology, J. Hammond, BSc, PhD
Physiology, J. Young, PhD
Psychiatry, G. Baker (Interim), PhD, DSc, FCAHS
Radiology & Diagnostic Imaging, R. Lambert, MB, BCh
Surgery, D. Hedden, MD

Division Directors

Anatomy, D. Livy, PhD
Critical Care Medicine, D. Zygun, MD, MSc, FRCPC
Health Sciences Laboratory Animal Services, N. Bosvik, DVM (Acting)
Medical Laboratory Sciences, M. Mengel (Acting), MD
Centre for Neurosciences, J. Greer, PhD
Physical Medicine and Rehabilitation, S. Gray, MD, PhD
Studies in Medical Education, B. B. Fisher, MD
Alberta Diabetes Institute, P. Light, PhD

The Faculty of Medicine and Dentistry of the University of Alberta was founded in 1913. The principal course offered leads to the MD degree. The number of candidates accepted for entrance into the first year of the program is restricted. All students who wish to enter are required to make application to the Registrar, University of Alberta by November 1st each year. The course leading to the degree of MD is a four year program following a minimum of 2 years of University work.

Other Degrees

The degrees of MSc and PhD are obtainable in certain departments of the Faculty. Candidates for these degrees are under the jurisdiction of the Faculty of Graduate Studies & Research, University of Alberta.

The Department of Dentistry offers an accredited four-year program leading to the degree of Doctor of Dental Surgery (DDS). At least two pre-dental years at University are required before admission to this program. Other programs offered by the Department include a three-year program leading to the Diploma in Dental Hygiene, a four-year program leading to a Bachelor of Science (Dental Hygiene Specialization) Degree, an MSc and PhD Degree program in Oral Health Sciences, and an MSc and PhD Degree in Orthodontics. The DDS and Dental Hygiene Programs are quota programs. All students who wish to enter are required to make application to the Registrar, University of Alberta by November 1st of the year prior to the year admission is sought. All students who wish to enter the Dental Hygiene programs are required to make application to the Registrar, University of Alberta by January 2nd each year.

A full programme of graduate training in all clinical specialties is available under the direction of a Faculty Committee on Graduate Training.

Continuous Professional Learning

An active programme in Continuous Professional Learning is conducted by the Faculty in co-operation with the College of Physicians & Surgeons of Alberta.

Allied Training

A course in Medical Laboratory Science leading to a BSc (MLS) degree is conducted under the jurisdiction of the Faculty of Medicine and Dentistry.
A programme leading to the degree of Master of Public Health Sciences (MPHS) is also offered.
As of April 1, 1996 the Faculty of Medicine has amalgamated with the Faculty of Dentistry to become the new Faculty of Medicine and Dentistry.

UNIVERSITY OF BRITISH COLUMBIA

Vancouver, British Columbia

Faculty of Medicine
Room 317-2194 Health Sciences Mall, Vancouver, British Columbia Postal Code V6T 1Z3
Tel. (604) 822-2421 Fax. (604) 822-6061 Website: www.med.ubc.ca/

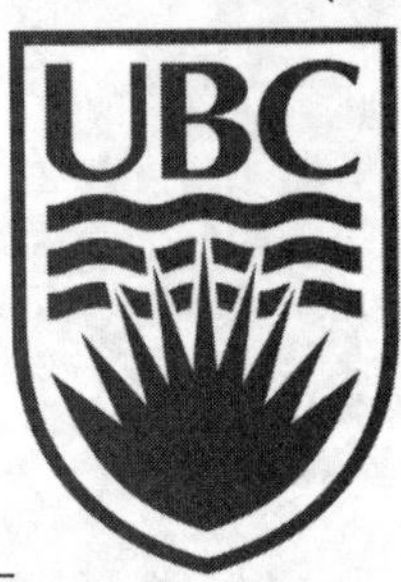

a place of mind
THE UNIVERSITY OF BRITISH COLUMBIA

Faculty of Medicine

President & Vice-Chancellor, Stephen Toope, PhD
Dean and Vice Provost, Health, Gavin C.E. Stuart, MD, FRCSC
Vice Dean, Academic Affairs, Frederick Mikelberg, MD, CM, FRCPC

Executive Associate Deans

Clinical Affairs, Robert Liston, MB ChB, FRCSC, FRCOG
Education, David Snadden, MB, ChB, MClSc, MD
Research, Howard Fieldman, MD, FRCP(C)

Regional Associate Deans

Interior, Allan Jones, MD, FRCPC
Northern BC, Paul Winwood, MB BS, DM, FRCPC
Vancouver Fraser, Dawn Dewitt, BA, MSc, MD, FACP, FRACP
Vancouver Island, Oscar Casiro, MD, FRCPC

Associate Deans

Equity & Professionalism, Gurdeep Parhar, MD
Graduate & Postdoctoral Education, Peter Leung, PhD
Admissions, Bruce Fleming, MD
MD Undergraduate Program, Student Affairs, Sharon Salloum, MD, CCFP
MD Undergraduate Education, Dawn DeWitt, BA, MSc, MD, FACP, FRACP
Postgraduate Medical Education, Roger Wong, BMSc, MD, FRCPC, FACP
Professional Development, Gisèle Bourgeois-Law, MD, MEd, FRCSC
Health Professions, William Miller, PhD, FCAOT

Associate Deans, Research

B.C. Cancer Agency, Sam Abraham, PhD
Children & Family Research Institute (CFRI), Michael O'Shaughnessy, PhD (Interim)
Providence Health Care Research Institute, Robert D. Sindelar, PhD
Vancouver Coastal Research Institute (VCHRI), Robert McMaster, PhD, DPhil

Department Heads & School Directors

Anesthesiology, Pharmacology & Therapeutics, Roanne Preston, MD, FRCPC
Biochemistry & Molecular Biology, Roger Brownsey, PhD
Cellular & Physiological Sciences, Geoffrey Hammond, PhD
Dermatology & Skin Science, Harvey Lui, MD, FRCPC
Emergency Medicine, Jim Christenson, MD, FRCPC
Family Practice, Martin Dawes, MB BS, MD, DRCOG, FRCGP
Medical Genetics, Carolyn Brown, PhD
Medicine, Graydon Meneilly, MD, FRCPC
Obstetrics & Gynecology, Geoffrey Cundiff, MD, FACOG, FACS, FRCPSC
Occupational Science and Occupational Therapy, Catherine Backman, PhD, FCAOT
Ophthalmology and Visual Sciences, David Maberley, MD
Orthopaedics, Bassam Masri, MD, FRCSC
Pathology & Laboratory Medicine, Michael Allard, BSc, MD, FRCP(C)
Pediatrics, Allison Eddy, MD
Physical Therapy, S. Jayne Garland, BSc (PT), PhD
Psychiatry, William Honer, MD, FRCPC
Radiology, Bruce Forster, MD
Surgery, John Kestle, MD, MSc, FRCSC, FACS
Urological Sciences, Larry Goldenberg, CM, OBC, MD, FRCSC, FACS, FACHS, DABU
School of Audiology & Speech Sciences, Valter Ciocca, PhD
School of Population & Public Health, David Patrick, MD, FRCPC, MHSc

Research Centre Directors

Biomedical Research Centre, John W. Schrader, BSc, MD, PhD
Brain Research Centre,
Max Cynader, CM, OBC, PhD, FRSC, FCAHS
Centre for Blood Research, Ed Conway, MD, PhD, MBA
UBC Centre for Disease Control, Robert C. Brunham, MD, FRCPC
Centre for Health Education Scholarship,
Joanna Bates, MDCM, CCFP, FCFP
Centre for Hip Health & Mobility, Heather McKay, PhD
Centre for Health Services & Policy Research,
Morris L. Barer, BSc, PhD, MBA
Centre for Molecular Medicine & Therapeutics,
Michael Hayden, MB, ChB, PhD, FRCP(C), FRSC
Child & Family Research Institute,
J. M. Friedman (Acting), MD, PhD, FAAP, FABMG, FCCMG, FRCPC
ICORD - International Collaboration on Repair Discoveries (ICORD),
Tom Oxland, P.Eng (Acting)
UBC James Hogg Research Centre,
Bruce McManus, MD, PhD, FRSC, FCAHS
Life Sciences Institute, Christian Naus, MSc, PhD
Vancouver Prostate Centre, Martin Gleave, MD, FRCSC, FACS

The UBC Faculty of Medicine Distributed Learning Model

4 University Academic Campuses
11 Clinical Academic Campuses
14 Affiliated Regional Centres
80+ Community Educational Facilities

Medical Undergraduate Program

The UBC Faculty of Medicine offers an innovative MD undergraduate program and is one of the largest in North America. It currently accepts 288 students in the first year and after the first four months students are distributed to one of our teaching sites across the province. The first two years of the undergraduate program consist of two components. The first component uses small group problem-based learning where the students learn the basic sciences of medicine in the context of clinical cases. These experiences are supplemented by lectures and laboratories. The second component consists of the longitudinal courses: the doctor-patient-society course that emphasizes societal issues, the family practice continuum which is an experience in family physicians' offices and, finally, clinical skills. Third year begins with the Rural Family Medicine Clerkship, a 4-week rotation in rural or underserved urban medicine delivered by the Department of Family Practice. The remainder of third year clerkship involves the following disciplines: Anesthesiology, Orthopaedics, Dermatology, Emergency, Medicine, Obstetrics & Gynaecology, Pediatrics, Psychiatry and Surgery. The fourth year consists of senior clinical electives and approximately five weeks of "Preparation for Medical Pracice".

Graduate and Postgraduate Programs

The UBC Faculty of Medicine hosts Masters, Doctoral and Postdoctoral programs in a wide range of health-related fields, with more than 1,200 students and 250 fellows enrolled. Our research-based programs provide oportunities for training in subjects ranging from the diversity of basic biomedical sciences to clinical and health services research at all geographical sites, including our affiliated hospitals and institutes. Graduate programs are also offered for the professions of audiology, speech-language pathology, occupational therapy, physical therapy, genetic counselling and health administration.

The clinical departments offer training towards Certification and Fellowship of the Royal College of Physicians and Surgeons of Canada and Certification of the College of Family Physicians of Canada.

Additional Programs

The UBC Faculty of Medicine also offers: Bachelor of Medical Laboratory Science, Midwifery, and Continuing Medical Education & Professional Development.

RESOURCE SECTION

2012 GRADUATES

Memorial University of Newfoundland

ACHIKE, Olisa
ATKINSON, Stephanie
BLANCHARD, Crystal
BOLAND, Paul
BUDDEN, Curtis
CALLAGHAN, Laura
CARROLL, David
CLAYTON, Jonathan
COFFEY, Jessica C.
COLBOURNE, Amy J.
COLLIER, Amanda T.
CORBETT, Jessica
CRANE, Ashley
DAIGLE-MALONE, Trisha
DUPLISEA, Jonathan
EDWARDS, Laura
FAGAN, Richard
FARRELL, James
GOUDIE, Shaina
GRAVES, Natalie
GUIGNE, Francoise
HAMILTON, Christopher
HARDING, Lacey
HERRINGTON, Katharine
HICKEY, Cindy L.
HOFFE, Sharleen N.
JOSHI, Nikhil
KIRBY, Raie L.
KOOPS, Joel
LEDREW, Robyn
LESTER, Erica
LEUNG, Jason
LI, K. Karen
MA, Karen M.
MACPHERSON, Ian
MARSHALL, Alexis G.
MERCER, Jamison
METCALFE, Shawn
MONG, Christopher C.K.
MURPHY, Laura
MYERS, Nicole
O'HAGAN, Joshua
PARSONS, Amanda
POWELL, Rebecca E.
POWER, Jennifer
POWER, Robert
PRITCHETT, Erica
QUIGLEY, Stephen
QUINTON, C. Brianne
RAJABALEE, Nadiim
REID, Stephanie
RICHARD, Pierre R.
RYAN, Matthew
SAMPLE, Megan L.
SMITH, Andrew
SMITH, Andrew L.
STENBACK, Melanie
STRATTON, Julia L.
TAYLOR, Jenelle
THOMS, Kathie
WAREHAM, Angela
WILLIAMS, Heather C.

Dalhousie University

ABIDALI, Asra'a
ALLEN, Elizabeth K.
AMOS, Elizabeth J.
ARSENAULT, Kory M.
ASHTON, Rosalind J.
BAKER, Noel T.
BEBBINGTON, Erica M.
BEGUM, Afroza
BENNETT, Sean A.
BEST, William J.
BEZANSON, Sarah S.
BLACK, Coleman R.
BLACKLAWS, Brydon D.
BLANCHARD, Mathieu M.
BLIGH, Mathew P.
CAMPBELL, Jeffrey D.
CARVER, David A.
COLLICOTT, Cherie C.
COSTAIN, Nicholas A.
COTTENDEN, Jennifer
CREASER, Jenna C.
CUNNINGHAM, Natalie P.
DATTA, Nilanjana
DAVIES, Elaine C.
DELANEY, Nicole C.
DI PENTA, Jillian C.
DICKSON, Cory M.
DOBROWOLSKI, Sarah L.
DOOLEY, Jessica D.
DORREEN, Alastair P.
DUMBARTON, Tristan C.
EMMS, Mandy D.
EMSLEY, Jason G.
FANCY, Sarah A.
FORWARD, Nicholas A.
GIBSON, Julia L.
GILLIS, Joshua A.
GOODINE, Carrie L.
GOUZOULES, Thera E.
GRAHAM, Marie-Elise R.
GREEN, Jordan A.
GREENLAW, Kristin E.
HARRIS, Adam A.
KADING, Adam R.
KALE, Shoan C.
KEITH, Melissa M.M.
KELLY, Aliya B.
LAVRANOS, Haralambos
LEE, Jeffrey A.
LEE, Le Min
LEIGHTON, Jennifer L.
LEROUX, Yves A.
MACCORMICK, Hilary K.
MACDONALD, Jeffery E.
MACDONALD, Jillian M.
MACDONALD, Lindsey D.
MACDONALD, M. Jason
MACINNES, Emily H.
MACLELLAN, Brenton J.
MACNEARNEY, Robin
MACNEIL, John R.G.
MACNEIL, Scott A.
MACSWAIN, Sarah A.
MCCARVILL, Terrence P.
MELVIN, Jennifer E.
MOHAMED ARIS, Nur Haizum
MORTON, Craig C.
MUIR, Robin M.
MUIR, Thomas F.
NEWMAN, Alana M.
O'BRIEN, Cliona M.
OULTON, Hayley
PATRIQUIN, Glenn M.
PERCY, Jennifer H.
PHILLIPS, Timothy J.
POUSHAY, Heather M.
QUACKENBUSH, Katherine E.
REYNOLDS, Luke F.
ROBERTSON, Mark W.
ROBICHAUD, Aaron S.
ROSTOM, Ahmed A.
SARTY, Ian F.
SCHLIEWINSKY, Kharim J.
SEARLE, Samuel D.
SIMPSON, Andrew M.
SKINNER, Thomas A.A.
SMITH, Daniel Y.
SMITH, Thomas D.
STEVENS, Michael S.
STEWART, Riley D.
SUTHERLAND, Kailee N.
VANINETTI, Nadine M.
VELDHUIJZEN VAN ZANTEN, Stephanie D.
VON MALTZAHN, Maia F.
VUONG, Sebastian
WILLIAMS, Mark R.
WILSON, David A.
WING, Andrew C.
WOLFE, Deanna C.
YAZID, Mohd D.F.
YEATES, Jessica L.
YOUNG, Paul D.

Université Laval

ALLEN, Myriam
ANDONIAM, Nvart
ASFOUR, Sara
AUBE-PETERKIN, Melanie
AUDETTE, Louis-David
BARBE, Joanie
BARRETTE, Penelope
BEAUDRY, Edith
BEAULIEU, Alain
BEAULIEU, Marie-Christine
BEAULIEU, Marie-Pier
BEDARD, Melanie
BELANGER, Steven
BERDUGO, Jeremie
BERGERON-DUPRAS, Thea
BERNARD-GENEST, Julie
BERNIER-OUELLET, Anick
BLAIS, Anne-Sophie
BLANCHETTE-GOBEIL, Remi
BLOUIN, Pierre-Luc
BOUCHARD, Jean-Emmanuel
BOUEILH, Sandrine
BOURDUA-ROY, Evelyne
BOURQUE, Amelie
BOURRET-MASSICOTTE, Dominique
BRASSARD, Paul-Eric
BUSSIERES, Marie-Claude
BUTEAU, James P.
CADIEUX-SIMARD, Marie-Lie
CAIRE, Josianne
CAISSIE, Marie-Claude
CALABRINO, Sabrina
CAMIRÉ, Julie
CANTIN, Alexandre
CARRIER-BOLDUC, Myriam
CHEVRETTE, Marianne
CHIBANE, Imane-Samah
CHICOINE, Marie-Eve
CHOQUETTE, Andre
CLAVEAU, Valerie
CLOUTIER, Daphne
COMEAU, Marie-Pier
COMEAU-LEVESQUE, Paul
CORBIN, Julie
CORMIER, Catherine
CORMIER, Marie-Helene
CORNEAU, Audree
CORRIVEAU, Lucie
CORRIVEAU-DUSSAULT, Amelie
COUPAL, Eve
COUTU, Myriam
COUTURE, Veronique
DAVID, Sebastien
DE LAFONTAINE, Alexandre
DE REPENTIGNY, Janie
DEMERS-GAGNON, Nicolas
DESGAGNE-HEROUX, Gabrielle
DION, Genevieve
DIONNE, Anne-Isabelle
DONATI-DAOUST, Paule
DROUIN, Stephanie
DUPUIS VAILLANCOURT, Marie-Helene
FORTIN, Joanie
FRANCOEUR, Elissa
FRIEDMANN, Daniel
GABOURY, Amelie
GAGNON, Louis-Philippe
GAGNON, Maude-Marie
GALESANU, Roxana G.
GARANT, Aurelie
GAUQUELIN, Laurence
GAUTHIER, David
GAUVIN, Valerie
GIARD, Marilou
GIONET PES, Marie-Michelle
GIRARD, Marie-Eve
GOBEIL, Marie-Pascale
GOSSELIN, Genevieve
GOSSELIN, Myriam
GRAVEL, Genevieve
GUILLEMETTE, Myriam
GUIMEZAP-TSOPMO, Jackson
HAFFAF, Redha
HO, Erick
HOUDE, Maryse
ISSA, Rami
KASEKA, Matsanga-Leyila
KHREISS, Tarek
KINNEAR, Danielle
LABRECHE, Evelyne
LABRECQUE, Marie-Noel
LABROSSE, Roxane
LACHANCE, Caroline
LACHANCE-FORTIN, Aubert
LACROIX, Genevieve
LACROIX, Stephanie
LAFLAMME, Emilie
LAFLAMME, Jonathan
LAGACE, Sonia
LAJEUNESSE, Remi
LALIBERTE, Vincent
LALIBERTE-ROY, Lawrence
LAMBERT-JULIEN, Renaud
LAMY, Claudel
LANDRY-GAGNE, Maryse
LANG, Denis P.
LANGLAIS, Eve-Lyne
LANTHIER-VEILLEUX, Mathieu
LAPOINTE, Sarah
LAROCHELLE, Pierre-Paul
LARUE, Melissa
LAURIN, Jean-Carroll
LAVOIE-GAGNON, Claudie
LEBLANC, Xavier
LEBLOND, Veronique
LECLERC, Marianne
LEFRANCOIS, Kate
LEMELIN, Annie
LEPAGE-COTE, Noemi
LESSARD, Elisabeth
LIM TI YAN, David
MANIS, Adam
MORIN, Valerie
MORIN SIMARD, Vanessa
MORIN-BRASSARD, Hugo
MUSTAPHA, Noura
NACHEF, Alexandra
NADEAU, Fannie
NADEAU, Nadia
NERON, Genevieve
NORMANDIN, Marie-Michele
NUMAINVILLE, Sarah
OCHOA BONILLA, Carlos A.
OUELLET, Camille
OUELLET, Marie-Claude
OUELLET, Myriam
OUELLET, Philippe
OUELLET, Sarah
PANA, Raluca M.
PAQUET-DE-VARENNES, Anne-Claire
PARFENOVA, Maria
PELLETIER, Maude
PEREIRA, Luciana G.
PICHARD-JOLICOEUR, Alexia
PLAISANCE, Julie
PLOURDE, Anne
POIRIER-HARVEY, Andreanne
POULIN, Alexandre
POULIN, Thomas
RACICOT, Jean-Nicolas
RACINE, Samuel
RENAUD, Marie-Pierre
RHEAUME, Maude
RIOUX, Emmanuelle
RIZK, Aida
ROBERT, Marisa
ROCHETTE, Elise
RODRIGUE, Stephanie
RONDEAU-LEGAULT, Judith
ROUSSEAU, Genevieve
ROY, France E.
SABELLA, Lisa
SCHREIBER, Ariane
ST-AMOUR, Annie
ST-LAURENT, Guillaume
ST-PIERRE, Melanie
TESSIER, Jeremie
THEBERGE, Simon
TOURIGNY, Erick
TRAN, Cong Dung
TREMBLAY, Jonathan
TREMBLAY, Melanie
TREMBLAY, Pierre-Luc
TREMBLAY-LEMAY, Rosemarie
TREPANIER, Anne
TRUDEL, Simon
TURCOTTE, Karine
TURCOTTE, Mireille
VALIQUETTE, Annie-Claude
VAUCHER, Jonathan
VERGER DEMERS, Sarah
VERMETTE, Sarah
VIENS, Francoise
VILLEMARIE-COTE, Emmanuelle
VILLENEUVE, Sarah-Christine
WAGNER-LEVEILLE, Veronique
WAHBA-MORCOS, Mina-Waheed

Université de Montréal

ANCTIL, Marie-Christine
AUGER-BELLAVANCE, Marie-Pierre
AWADA, Fahd
AZIZI, Mounsif
BAINBRIDGE-BERUBE, Claudia
BARA, Elie
BARIL, Sabrina
BASILE, Georges
BEATTIE, Hannah
BEAULIEU-DORE, Roxane
BEAULIEU-TRUCHON, Samantha
BEDARD, Virginie
BELANGER, Marie-Pier
BELANGER-DESJARDINS, Elise
BELLEFLEUR-MERCIER, Elisabeth
BERGERON, Jennifer
BERNIER, Fanny-Emmanuelle
BIDET, Gwenaelle
BLAIN-HEBERT, Andreane
BLEAU, Nathalie
BOIVIN, Marie H.
BOUCHARD-DECHENE, Vincent
BOUHABEL, Sarah
BOUKAS, Ibtissama
BOULANGER, Marie-Michele
BOULE, Marie-Pier
BOURASSA, Ariane
BOURGEOIS, Andreane
BOUTIN, Ariane
BRASSARD, Karine
BROUSSEAU-FOLEY, Magali
BURELLE, Stephanie
CAMIRAND, Viviane
CAMIRE, Julie
CARRIERE, Chantale
CATANA, Dragos
CAUDRELIER, Marie
CENTOMO, Hugo
CHABOT, Salome
CHAER, Laila
CHALFOUN, Claire
CHALIFOUX, Francisca
CHALIFOUX, Frederic
CHAN, Marie-Agnes
CHAREST-MARCOTTE, Alexis
CHARRETTE, Etienne
CHETRIT, Michael
CHEUNG, Yi Ting
CHOQUETTE-FUKS, Adam
CLAVEL, Virginie
CLERMONT-CHAMPAGNE, Cindy
COHEN, Vanessa
COLIZZA, Melissa
CORNUT, Gilbert
COTE-POIRIER, Gabrielle
COURNOYER, Alexis
COUTURIER, Charles
CROTEAU, Jerome
CYR, Caroline
DAOUST, Sarah E.
DECARY-GUIMOND, Gabrielle
DELLERBA, Maria
DELMAS-FRENETTE, Catherine
DENIS, Julie-Anne
DENISSOVA, Daria
DEROME, Pascale
DESBOIS, Melina
DESGROSEILLIERS, Liliane
DESLAURIERS, Laurence
DEVIN, Anne
DEZIEL MALOUIN, Marc O.
DIALLO, Mamadou B.
DIONNE, Francois
DIXIT, Ashwin
DU, Qin
DUFRESNE, Alix
DUFRESNE, Anne-Marie
DUMOUCHEL, Vincent
DUPONT, Magdeleine
DUPUIS, Katherine
DURR, George M.
DUTILLEUL, Aurore
ELFASSY, Hannah L.
FILION, Marianne
FOLEY, Catherine J.
FORTIN, Claudia
FOURNIER, Emilie
GAUDREAU-GOUACHE, Olivier
GAUTHIER, Christophe
GAUTHIER, Melanie
GAZDOVICH, Mathieu
GEAGEA, Anna
GENEREUX, Vincent
GHINDA, Cristina D.
GHUMMAN, Simranjit S.
GIASSON-GARIEPY, Karine
GIFUNI, Anthony
GIRARDOT, Daphne
GODIN, Anny
GOSSELIN, Gabriel
GOSSELIN -PAPADOPOULOS, Rania
GRABLY, Melissa
GRAHAM, Francois
GRAVELINE, Francis
GUILBERT-VANDAL, Gabrielle
HADDADI, Dalal
HADJ-AISSA, Nadia
HAJJAR, Albert
HAMEL-PAQUET, Catherine
HASSANALY, Salima
HEBERT-LALONDE, Maude
HEDARALY, Sabera
HELIE MARTEL, Nicolas
HENRY LEBEL, Jean-Sebastien
HINDIE, Jade
HOFF ARCAND, Lea
HUARD, Gabriel
HUEBER, Pierre-Alain
HUYNH, Minh Tung
IANNATTONE, Lisa
IMBAULT-DAGNEAU, Gabrielle
JACQUES-TURCOTTE, Lauriane
JAMALI, Redouane
JOANETTE-SAMSON, Fannie
JOH, Yung Kyu
JULIEN, Marco
KILEY, Lee
KYRILLOS, Ralph
L'HEUREUX-LEBEAU, Benedicte
LABBE, Myrlande
LAFLAMME, Jeanne
LAM SHANG LEEN, Laetitia
LAMARCHE, Caroline
LAMBERT, Isabelle
LAMBERT GAUTHIER, Kim
LANDRY, Anne-Marie
LANGLOIS-MICHAUD, Samuel
LAPLANTE, Marie-Helene
LAPOINTE, Alexis
LAPOINTE, Julie
LAROCHE, Ann-Sophie
LAUGHREA, Catherine
LAVOIE, Ghislain
LAVOIE, Marie-Eve
LE, Laurent H.
LEBEL, Marie-Lou
LEBEL, Pierre-Olivier
LECLERC, Andreanne
LECLERC, Andree-Anne
LECLERC, Genevieve
LEFEBVRE, Aizhen J.
LEFEBVRE, Tracy
LEMIRE-THERIEN, Gabrielle
LEPAGE, Melanie
LEROUX GROLEAU, Etienne
LESSARD BONAVENTURE, Paule
LEVEILLE, Cathy
LEVY, Genevieve
LI, Kevin
LIU, Kun Peng
LOIGNON, Maude
LOUIS, Kerby M.
LUU, Stefan H.
MAHER LAPORTE, Marjolaine
MAILHOT, Jean-Philippe
MALHAME, Isabelle
MARCHAND, Emilie
MARCHAND, Gabrielle
MARCHE, Melanie
MARDINI, Joelle
MCCONNELL-LEGAULT, Sarah
MENARD, Dominique
MENHEM, Elise
MOORE, Marie-Claude
MORAMARCO, Veronica
MORIN-ROY, Florence
MOTTILLO, Salvatore
NADON, Gabrielle
NAULT-COUSINEAU, Blanche
NETCHIPOROUK, Elena
NGUYEN, Lila
NGUYEN, Marie Q.C.
NORMAND, Blanche
NUTTER, Alison
O'BRIEN, Alan
OLIGNY LONGPRE, Genevieve
PAGEAU, Felix
PAQUET, Suzie
PAQUETTE, Vanessa
PARADIS, Alexandra
PARE, Xavier
PARE-PLANTE, Andree-Anne
PARENT-VACHON, Mathilde
PARISIEN, Brigitte
PARVIN, Sacha
PATENAUDE-BLAIS, Renee A.
PERRAULT, Jean-David
PERRAULT-HARVEY, Sophie
PERUSSE, Philippe
PETIT, Fannie
PHAM, Kimberly
PHAM, Le Phuong Q.
PILON, Magalie
POMERLEAU, Valerie
POPA, Ioana
POULIN-GROULX, Emilie
PROULX, Alexandra
PURCELL-LEVESQUE, Vanessa
QIABI, Mehdi
QUACH, My Van
QUESNEL, Marylene
QUINN-LAURIN, Vanessa
RAYMOND, Katherine
RAYNER-HARTLEY, Erin M.
REBEYROL, Maud
REGIMBAL-ETHIER, Maxin
RICHARD, Claudie-Anne
RIGUTTO, Pamela
RIVARD, Stephanie
ROCHON, Audrey
ROCHON, Isabelle
ROUILLARD, Elise
ROUSSEAU-SAINE, Nicolas
ROY, Jean-Philippe
ROYER-PERRON, Elise
SAMMAN, Michael G.
SANTERRE, Audrey G.
SAUTHIER, Michael
SCHWEIGER, Marie-Eve
SENOUCI, Majda I.
SIMARD, Francois
SIROIS, Jennifer
SOUISSI, Nour E.
ST-AUBIN, Thomas
ST-ONGE, Janie
TAHIRI-HASSANI, Mohamed M.
TALEB, Amir
TANASIE, Christiana
TAWIL, Youssef
TESSIER-JASMIN, Jean-Michel
TETREAULT, Catherine
TETREAULT, Simon
THIBEAULT, Marie-Eve
THURAISINGAM, Thusanth
TISSEVERASINGHE, Steven A.
TRAHAN, Emilie
TREMBLAY, Mireille
TRINH, Bao-Huy
TRUSSART, Rachel
TURCOTTE, Jessica
TURMEL, Jean-Francois
TURNBLOM, Jean-Patrick
VAN, Tuong Dieu C.
VANDAL, Mylene
VEILLET, Frederic
VERVILLE, Jean-Francois
VU, Kim-Nhien
VU, Minh-Quan
WATERS, Alexandra
WILHELMY, Mylene
WISE, Bryan
WOZNIAK, Katarzyna
XIAO, Yao
YANG, Dan Y.
YIN, Lu
ZHANG, Xi Sophie
ZHU, Ping S.
ZOU, Xue
ZUMMO-SOUCY, Mathieu

McGill University

AGUILAR, Martin
AL-MASRI, Ahmad
AMIR, Alexander
ANGELUS, Amanda
ANGHEL, Tiberiu
BAKER, Alyson
BALAYLA, Jacques
BALENDRA, Haran
BANASZEK, Daniel
BANON, David
BARBARIAN, Mher
BATTAT, Robert
BENMASSAOUD, Amine
BERGER-RICHARDSON, David
BILEK, Aaron
BLANCHARD, Ana
BOGATY, Chloe
BOON, Adrienne
BOUDIER-REVERET, Mathieu
BOUHAIRIE, Caleb A.
BOULANGER, Elise
BRAGANZA, Michael
BRAR, Seeminder
CASTELINO, Tanya
CAUDARELLA, Alexander
CHABOT, Julia
CHADI, Nicholas
CHANDA, Mohammed Y.
CHARTIER, Marie-Eve
CHEN, Yue Xi
CHENG, Hang
CHERTKOW, Elizabeth J.A.
CHETRIT, Estelle
CLERMONT, Valérie
CLERMONT DEJEAN, Nayima
CORDUKES, Colleen
COSTA-VON AESCH, Zoe F.
CURTIS, James
DESCHAMPS, Jean
DESCHAMPS, Rachel
DIWAN, Maheen
DOWNS, Allyson
DRAGER, Justin
DUCHARME-BENARD, Stephanie
DUMONT-MAURICE, Raven
DUNBAR-YAFFE, Richard J.
ESFAHANI, Khashayar
FARZIN, Houman
FERNANDEZ, Miguel
FILEWOD, Niall C.J.
FILIP, Constatin
FILIP, Iulia L.
FORTIER-MORISSETTE, Zoe
FRAGAPANE, Joseph-Donato
FREEDMAN, Laura
GANS, Nathalie
GARFINKLE, Jarred
GARFINKLE, Michael
GAROFALO, Milena
GO, Belinda
GOSSELIN-PAPADOPOULOS, Nayla M.
GOTRA, Akshat
GUILBAULT, Catherine
GUPTA, Mayuri
HAMLIN-DOUGLAS, Lauren K.
HART, Adam
HASSAN, Noura
HATHAWAY, Andrea
HERNANDEZ TORRES, Catalina
HOSSEINI, Shahine
HUANG, Kenneth H.
HULL, Margaret
HULME, Jennifer M.
HUTCHINSON, Nora
ISCHAYEK, Amanda
IULIUS, Ioana G.
JIANG, Fan
KADLUBOWSKA, Dorota
KAMINSKI, Radoslaw
KARAM, Sani
KARLS, Shawn
KATZ, Lauren E.
KONG, Ling Yuan
KORKIDAKIS, Ann K.
KOURI, Andrew J.T.
KUDRINA, Irina
LABELLE, Alexandre
LABELLE, Maxime
LAMBRINAKOS-RAYMOND, Alicia
LAVOIE, Jean-Michel
LEE, Brian
LEE, Michelle S.
LEFEBVRE, Benedicte
LEFEBVRE, Claire
LEVIN, Josh
LEVINE, Phillip
LI, Annie
LI, Yi
LIN, Yalin
MA, Lei
MACKENZIE-FEDER, Julian
MAMANE, Samuel
MARTELLO, Cristiano
MARTINEAU, Patrick J.G.
MCGRUTHERS, Lauren
MCKAY, Erin
MICIELI, Jonathan A.
MILOT, David M.
MISRA, Paraish
MOOSAVI, Mandana
MUTTALIB, Fiona
NATAROS, Alexander
NAYAN, Madhur
NEHME, Jessica
NG, Joshua S.
NGUYEN, Julie
NILES, Kirsten M.
NITCHKE, Brett
NOREAU-NGUYEN, Maxime
OBAID, Sami
PHARAND, Leigh C.
PILOZZI-EDMONDS, Laura
PIRAU, Samuel
PRAKASH, Ipshita
PROULX, Alexandre
PUT, Daryline
QUIGLEY, Philip
RADOVANOVIC, Bojana
RAMJI, Naila
RAMKUMAR, Stephanie R.
RANKIN-JARDIN, Glynn
REICHMAN, Lee E.
RICHARD ALBERT, Marc
RICHARD-ROSS, Justin
ROBERTSON, Dale
ROBINSON, Marie-Eve
ROBINSON, Matthew
ROSKIES, Michael
SALIBA, Joe
SAYEGH, Mireille
SEIDMAN, Amanda
SELF, Lauren
SOLASKI, Myrill
STEINMAN, Andrew N.
STOYNOVA, Valeria
SURESH, Himabindu
TANAKA, Yumi
THOMAS, Hana
THOMAS, Zoe
TIKASZ, Dorottya
TRAN, Shiao J.
TRUDEAU, Maeve L.
TRUDEAU-RIVEST, Raphaele
TRUONG, Catherine
VERMA, Karan
VON AESCH, Zoe F.
VULPE, Horia
WAKIL, Susan
WANG, Qian Q.
WEINSTOCK, Andrew
WHYTE POTTER-MAL, Majenta
WIVIOTT, Robin
WONG, Stephanie
WU, Yang Y.
WU, Y.Y. Jenny
XU, Liqin
YANG, Ji Wei
YIM, Yolaine
YOON, Joong C.
ZENG, Han
ZHENG, Jia
ZHENG, Jiamin
ZYSMAN-COLMAN, Zofia

Université de Sherbrooke

AKL, Elie
ARCHAMBAULT, Patrick
ARSENAULT, Karyne
ASSAYAG, Jonathan
BASILE, Karim
BEAUDOIN, Jonathan
BEGIN, Yannick
BELANGER, Valerie
BENMOHAMMED, Farah
BENNY, Alexandre
BENOIT, Charlie
BERGERON, Antoine
BERNARD, Julia
BERNIER, Valerie
BIGRAS, Antony
BOILEAU, Jean C.
BOURSIQUOT, Marie-Laure
BRASSARD, Caroline
BRISSON, Jean-Denis
BROUSSEAU, Sylvie
BROUSSEAU, Tomy
CARETTE, Marie-Christine
CARRIERE, Sophie
CHAPUT, Danelle
CHARTRAND POIRIER, Catherine
CHRETIEN, Raphaelle
CLOUTIER, Francis
CLOUTIER LAMBERT, Christophe
CORMIER, Denny L.
CORRIVEAU-DURAND, Simon
COSSETTE-LAVALLEE, Malika
COTE, Elodie
COTE, Marie-Pier
COURTEMANCHE, Karim
COUTURE, Lucie
COUTURE-COSSETTE, Antoine
COUTURIER, Jonathan
CYR, Amelie
CYR, Eric
D'EON, Charelle
DAIGLE, Jean-Sebastien L.
DAIGLE, Josee L.
DECKER, Ainsley L.
DESJARDINS, Melanie
DODIER, Veronique
DORE-VEILLETTE, Sophie
DUBE, Catherine
DUFOUR, Stephanie
DUGAS, Jean-Luc
DUMOUCHEL, Emilie
EL OUTARI, Ahmad
FAUST, Joanie
FERGUSON, Crystal
FIZAZI, Meryem
FLAMAND, Audrey
FORTIN, Elzabeth
FOURNIER, Maryse
GAGNER, Pascal
GAGNON, Catherine
GAGNON, Emily
GAGNON, Valerie-Anne
GAGNON-MCMAHON, Audrey
GALLANT, Marilyn-Renee
GARANT, Michelle
GAUDET, Veronique C.
GAUTHIER, Marianne
GAUTHIER-POULIN, Sunnie
GEMME, Isabelle
GEORGES, Samer
GIBEAULT, Catherine
GILBERT, Alexandre
GILBERT, Rachel
GOSSELIN ARCOUET, Laurent
GRENIER GAUTHIER, Pierre P.
GRONDINES, Laurent
GUEVIN, Marie-Eve
GUEZ, Manon
HAGENIMANA, Nadia
HARVEY, Janie
HUNT, Anne-Marie
ICAZA ORDONEZ, Nydia
ISEPPON, Massimiliano
JALBERT, Maxime
JEANSON, Chloe
JOLY, Simon
KIROUAC, Patricia C.
LAFRANCE, Judith
LAFRENAYE, Julie
LAGACÉ, Marie Ève
LAMARRE, Kathia
LAMONTAGNE, Christina
LAMOUREUX-AUCLAIR, Antoine
LANGLOIS, Annie
LAUZIERE, Alex
LAVIGNE, Philippe
LAVOIE, Sarah
LE BLANC, Myriam
LEBLANC, Jolene
LEBLANC, Marie-Eve
LEBLANC, Martin
LEBLANC, Mathieu
LEFEBVRE, Marco
LEMIEUX, Marie-Line
LEMIRE, Andrea
LEPAGE, Jean-Philippe
LEROUX, Pierre-Andre
LESSARD, Anne-Sophie
LEVESQUE-DANIEL, Sarah
LEVY, Albert
LUSSIER, Alexandre
LY, Hoang-Kim
MAILHOT, Laurence
MALLET, Genevieve
MALLETTE-LEBLANC, Fanny
MALO, Francois C.
MALTAIS, Sabrina
MARCHAND-SENECAL, Xavier
MARKEY, Stephanie
MARQUIS, Marc-Antoine
MAZLOUM, Noura
MELANSON, Jules
MERCIER, Christine
MERCIER-LINTEAU, Catherine
MONTREUIL, Erika
MORIN, Caroline
MORIN-BEN ABDALLAH, Sami
MORISSETTE, Erika
MORISSETTE, Jessica
MUHOZA BUTOKE, Christian
MUNGER, Michael
NADEAU, Marie-Claude
NADON, Valerie
NOEL, Marie-Christine
NORMAND LAUZIERE, Francois
OUELLET, Marie-Eve
P BECOTTE, Pierre-Luc
PARENT, Stephanie
PARMAR, Robin
PELLETIER, Marie-Eve
PERRIN, David
PHUNG, Stephen
POIRIER, Clemence
POIRIER, Matthieu B.J.
POTVIN, Catherine
POTVIN-DULUDE, Philippe
RACINE, William
RACINE CHARETTE, Elaine
RAYMOND, Isabelle
RICHARD, Nicolas
ROCHON, Marie-Eve
ROY, Mylene
SALIBA, Emile
SALVAIL, Mia
SANCHE, Joannie
SCHWARTZ, Alexandra
SIMARD, Stephanie
SIROIS, Patricia
ST-AMAND, Carl F.
ST-JACQUES, Vicky
ST-JEAN, Matthieu
ST-PIERRE, Claude
ST-PIERRE, Mathilde
SURPRENANT, Marie-Claude
TALAB, Yasmine
TASEEN, Khadijah
TCHEUMI, Guy B.
THEBEAU, Annette C.
THERRIAULT, Valerie
THERRIEN, Edith
THIBAULT, Alexis
THIBEAULT, Patrick
THIBODEAU, Caroline
TO, Vincent
TREMBLAY, Patrice
TROTTIER-TELLIER, Felix
URENA CAMPOS, Sally R.
VAIRY, Stephanie
VEILLETTE, Catherine
VENNE, Sebastien
VEZINA, Mark
VIENNEAU, Jeremie S.
WADDELL, Andreanne
WARD, Charlene
ZAKANI, Marouane

University of Ottawa

ABUNASSAR, Michael J.
AL-ATTAR, Salam
AL-DABBAGH, Raed
ANDREWS, Jessica L.
APSIMON, Megan
BAHRAMIFARID, Nasim
BAINS, Jupinder
BALLOU, Eloise
BASMAJI, Samir
BATEMAN, Katherine
BELL, William
BELLACK, Neil
BEN-EZRA, Michael
BERUBE, Marie-Eve
BLAKE, Anastasia
BOECKNER, Jennifer N.
BOGLER, C. Talia A.
BORKOVICH, Renee
BRANDIGAMPOLA, Sarah
CAMPBELL, Ryan K.
CARMICHAEL, Scott A.G.
CARONZO, Fortunato
CHANG, Nina
CHUGH, Shaan
CHUNG, Justin C.
CICALO, Michelle
CLARK, David
COHEN, Elissa
COLTER, Ashley L.
D'SYLVA, Christopher
DALY, Colleen
DE WIT, Jose
DENIS, Rachelle
DHAMKO, Helena
DICKINSON, Michelle
DRUCE, Irena S.
DURLING, Bethany
EL-ZABET, Ajda
ELDJAMA, Tarik
ESUFALI, Susmita
FARBER, Allison
FERNANDEZ, Sarah
FORTINSKY, Kyle
FRATESI, Jennifer
FRENCH, Lauren
GAGNE, Austin
GAGNE, Owen
GAJARIA, Amy
GALLAGHER, Erin
GAUVIN, Gabrielle
GAWRYLUK, Marielle
GHAZAL, Jean-Christophe
GONSALVES, Allison
GOYAL, Prateek
GRADY, Rosheen
GRAY, George
GUPTA, Madhu
HARTMAN, Jason
HAYNE, Laura
HEIMRATH, Olivier
HEIPEL, Heather
HIJAZI, Ramsey
HOCHSTADTER, Elana F.
HOGG, Ryan
HOLLA, Aimee
HUKUI, Julie N.M.
IAFOLLA, Marco
IBRAHIM, Hicham
IVORY, Catherine P.A.
KADHOM, Noha
KATZ, Noam S.
KLING, Rakel
KOUZMITCHEVA, Elizabeth
KOVAL, Dmitrii
KUCERA, Marsha
KWAN, Benjamin Y.M.
KWAPISZ, Lukasz
LAFLECHE, Catherine M.
LAJEUNESSE, Benoit
LAST, Christine J.
LAU, Christine W.
LEBLANC, Danielle
LEMIRE-ELMORE, Chloe
LEWIS, Darrell
LI, Bo
LIANG, Shuyin
LIM FAT, Mary-Jane
LOGANATHAN, Mayura
MACDONALD, Anthony G.
MACDONALD, Ashley J.
MACGREGOR, Kathleen
MALAK, Mariem I.
MARTIN, Leslie J.
MAUGER, Sophie
MCGILLIS, Eric
MCVICAR, Lisa
METHIWALLA, Adnan
MICLETTE, Alain
MILLER, Ashley
MONTPETIT, Catherine-Anne
MOORE, Emily K.
MUCCILLI, Alexandra
MURPHY, Matthew J.
MURRAY, Marie-Eve
MURZIN, Diane L.
NEHME, Jak S.
NETTING, Caleb
NGUYEN, Melanie L.
NOLAND, Marie
ORGAN, Brock
PELLAND, Amelie
PERRI, Nicholas
PIETRZYNSKA, Magdalena A.
POIRIER, Lynne D.
POMERLEAU, Francois
PUETZ, Judith
QUAYE, Victor
RAJANI VILLEGAS, Anjali M.
RAMZAN, Sarah
REINGLAS, Jason M.
REYNOLDS, Katelyn B.
ROFAIEL, James
ROY, Jessica J.
SANCI, Vito
SARDANA, Vandit
SAWA, Kathryn
SCHERLING, Nicole D.
SHAW, Jordan E.
SIMARD, Trevor
SKAFF, Elie R.
SLADE, Laura A.
SOUDI, Nima
SRIVARATHARAJAH, Kajenny
STALLWOOD, Rebecca K.
SYLVAIN, Josee E.
TAKHAR, Simran S.
TEPPERMAN, Elissa D.
TETREAULT-PAQUIN, Jean-Olivier
THERIAULT, Amelie
TOOMEY, Patricia C.
TOTH, Jason A.
TOUPIN, Philippe N.
TWEEDIE, Jessica
TWEEDLE, Jessica L.
VALE, Rachel
VAN WALRAVEN, Michelle
VIEIRA, Amanda M.
VIRANI, Sabah S.
WAITE, Melanie M.S.
WALKE, Monica
WALSH, Valerie
WASSERMAN, Jason K.
WEINSTANGEL, Hannah
WOODS, Lindsay A.
YEUNG, Alison R.
YOO, Solina S.K.
YU, Andrea
ZHANG, Hanfei
ZHANG, Jerry

Queen's University

AHUJA, Christopher S.
ALIYARZADEH, Hoda
ANSELM, Daniel D.
ATFIELD, Alexandre D.
BAKAR, Shahrukh
BATRA, Poonam
BAXTER, Jennifer
BHARATH, Vighnesh
BOOY, Jason D.
BRIJBASSI, Melissa M.
BROWN, Christopher A.
BRUNI, Silvio
CHOWDHURY, Chinmoy
COE, Emma K.
DATOO, Natasha
DEMSEY, Daniel
DINELEY, Brigid
DISIPIO, Christina
DOAN, John
DOBSON, Jessica
DOUMOURAS, Aristithes
DRANDIC, Ana
FONG, Jeremy
FUNG, Filgen
FURTADO, Louis
GAI, Nan
GARUBA, Habibat
GLICKSMAN, Amy S.
GRANT, Robin
GREENWOOD, Allen
HABEEB, Syed
HARVEY, Philip
HOOSAINNY, Waseema
HORVATH, Aaron I.
IBRAHIM, Ali Z.
JASWAL, Gurpreet
JOHN, Sanjna M.
KAMAL, Ramy
KAWAGUCHI, Sarah K.
KHAN, Zainab
KOIFMAN, Julius Y.
KONVISER, Michael
KOZIAK, Adrian M.Y.
LAMBA, Jasmine K.
LAW, Tyler J.
LEE, Paul K.P.
LESLIE, Robert J.
LEVIS, Ruth E.
LIAK, Christina Y.Y.
LOUGHEED, Taylor P.
LYTLE, Lindsey
MA, Elaine F.
MARTINOVIC, Jovana
MEDNICK, Zale D.
MILLER, Elizabeth C.
MILLMAN, Adrian A.
MIRSKY, Leah C.
MOE, Jessica
MUTTER, Eric L.
NGUYEN, Henry
NOORMOHAMED, Salma
PATAFIO, Francis M.
PHILP, Lauren A.C.
PLENER, Ian
QAZALBASH, Ali H.
RAGHAVAN, Gita
RANA, Jesleen K.
RAPHAEL, Michael J.
RAYAT, Jaspreet
REID, Robert J.E.
ROBINSON, Mark M.
RODRIGUES, Melanie
RUSH, Raphael
SALEHI, Fateme
SANDERS, Sheilagh
SARANGAPANI, Aparna
SARKAR, Medina G.
SAUNDERS, Brooke
SETTERFIELD, Jeremy
SHARMA, Varun
SHEIKH, Hasan M.
SHETH, Ujash
SHUM, Serena

SMITH, Whitney B.F.
SRIRAM, Swetha
STAROVA, Blerta
STEEDMAN, Michael J.
TARULLI, Emidio
THOMAS, Sanjna
TIERNEY, Sarah L.
TREBB, Christopher J.
VAN DOORMAAL, Curtis J.
WAIS, Marta E.
WILLINSKY, Jacqueline L.
WONG, Jellena
WONG, Jonathan
WONG, Chung-Kwun
XU, Shuo
YAZDAN-ASHOORI, Payam
YU, Huan
ZHU, Cici R.

University of Toronto

ALANGH, Avreet
ALFONSI, Jeffrey E.
ALINGARY, Nelab
ALSTON, Jillian T.
ANSARI, Shahmeer
BAIK, Sonya
BARIBEAU, Danielle A.
BARRON, Laura
BARRON, Marcus A.
BARTENS, Michelle L.
BASMA, Sarah
BENNITZ, Joshua D.
BERGER, Warren
BESWICK, Melanie
BINEPAL, Navneet K.
BOIMER, Corey
BORYS, Jacob
BOYD, Erin M.R.
BRADLEY, Carl J.
BRUCE, Erin M.
BURKE, Matthew J.M.
BURRY, Erica M.
CAPE, David L.D.
CARTER, Michael D.
CAULLEY, Lisa M.
CHAMPION, Caitlin E.
CHAN, Andrea H.W.
CHANDHOKE, Gursimran
CHANG, Jin Yop
CHAUKOS, Deanna
CHEN, Ing Je
CHIN, Jessica W.S.
CHIU, Ernest H.
CHUNG, Andrew D.
CLARKSON, Rosemary F.
CONKLIN, John M.L.
COWELL, Alison
CRAWFORD, Eric J.
CRISTIAN, Alexandra L.
CUSHNIE, Duncan W.
DELORME, Alison C.C.
DHANJANI, Dhiraj
DOBKIN, Karen J.
DOUGLAS, Stephen C.
DOWNIE, Mallory L.
DU, Lei
DUBE, Rebecca-Joy
DUGANI, Chandrasagar
DUNSTAN, Jane D.
DURBIN, Adam D.
EGLENCE, Aline
FARIA, Sarah
FERNANDES, Russell W.
FINKBEINER, Melanie
FIORELLINO, Joseph
FONG, Bryan
FOSTER, Cheryl
FRALICK, Michael P.F.
FULLER, Elisa
GALLINGER, Zane
GAO, Andrew F.
GAUTHIER, Stephen
GEURTJENS, Carla M.
GIILCK, Steve M.
GILCHRIST, Christopher
GILLIES, Alison R.
GOELA, Kapil
GOTHA, Lara K.
GREWAL, Keerat K.
GUHA, Daipayan
GUTTMAN, Ashley
HAHN, Sara C.
HAJIHA, Mohammad
HAN, Mihan
HAN, Vanessa
HANSRAJ, Priyanka
HENSHAW, Christena J.
HO, Meghan J.
HOFFMAN, Nicola A.
HOLLAND, Anna C.
HONG, Jonathan C.
HUANG, Guan
HUITEMA, Ashlay
HUYNH, Lise J.
JEIMY, Samira
JENNINGS, Angela
JUNG, J. James
KAGEDAN, Daniel J.
KALAICHANDRAN, Amitha
KALIAZINA, Margarita
KANAGALINGAM, Ambi
KANG, Han Na
KANJEE, Raageen
KASHIGAR, Aida
KATZ, David L.
KE, Calvin
KECSKES, Agoston
KEGEL, Stefan P.L.
KHAN, Sofia
KHEZRI, Navid
KIROU-MAURO, Andrea M.
KLOSTRANEC, Jesse M.
KNIGHT, Jeffrey D.
KOCULYM, Alexander G.
KOLIN, David L.
KRYSKO, Kristen M.
KUGATHASAN, Kapilan
KWOK, Yvonne
LAI, Ingrid
LAM, Andrea S.M.
LAM, H.Y. Eunice
LAM, Karen K.L.
LAWLOR, Raymond
LAZARE, Kimberly D.
LE NOBEL, Gavin J.
LEE, Hanna
LEE, Seung-Jun
LEE, Kenneth
LEONARDI, Mathew J.
LEVIN, David N.
LEVITZ, Joshua A.
LEVY, Jonathan M.S.
LI, K. Bryan
LI, K. Karen
LI, Melinda Y.
LI, Michael M.
LIAN, Kevin S.
LIM, Caesar S.H.
LIM, Terrence C.W.
LIN, Amy E.
LIONTOS, Larissa M.
LIU, Jerome J.
LO, Tiffany
LOO, C.K. Jennifer
LUNGU, Monica R.
MACKENZIE, Melissa
MAKINO, Amber
MAMMO, Zaid
MATEI, Anca
MCGIRR, Robert A.A.
MCGREGOR, Tara A.
MCLEAN, Kristopher W.
MILLER, James M.
MISCH, Michael R.
MITAR, Michael D.
MOORES, Andrew R.
MURRAY, Gerrit
NASR EL HAG ALI, Maha
NGUYEN, Tri Hoang
NIKOLIC, Ana
NIROOPAN, Gavinn R.
NOLAN, Brodie T.J.
OKUBO, Nobuhiko
ORAVA, Matthew V.
PAGE, Jessica L.
PAJAK, Carla R.
PALLAN, Smiley
PARIAG, Lee J.S.
PARKER, Colleen H.
PASIC, Ivan
PATEL, Nikita
PEERANI, Al-Raheem
PELC, Jordan R.
PETERS, Craig
PETRE, Maria A.
PHAN, Eugenie
PLATZKER, Tal
PODOLSKY, Dale J.
PRESS, Delna R.
QU, Xuan L.
QUERENGESSER, Kate M.
RAE, Rachel E.
RAGHURAM, Kamini
RAGUNATHAN, Subhani D.
RAMBIHAR, Vanessa S.
RAPHAEL, David J.
RASTOGI, Anjali
RAY, Matthew D.
RIDLEY, Jane
ROBERT, Joshua M.
ROCHMAN, Arielle
RODIN, Danielle L.
ROY, Trisha
RUSTAD, Clare A.
RYAN, Michelle
SACHEDINA, Ayaaz K.
SAITO, Gregory K.
SALTMAN, Alexandra P.
SETO, Eva
SHARMA, Tanu
SHOUCRI, Rami
SMIRNOVA, Alina
SOEYONGGO, Tony
SPANO, Vincent R.
STEIN, Corey M.
STERLING, Cara L.
STERLING, Lynn E.
SY, Jennifer
TEHRANI, Mandana
TIMMONS, Matthew J.
TOLE, Soumitra S.
TOM, Stephanie
UMASUTHAN, Nishani
VAN DEWARK, Kenneth
VANDERLAAN, Rachel D.
VOLLING, Cheryl A.
WINATA, Nathaniel
WAGNER, Laura A.
WANG, Jenny Y.
WANG, Shelly
WEGENER, Stephen P.
WHITE, Alexander N.J.
WHITE, David G.B.
WIEGELMANN, Julian R.
WILLOUGHBY, Lauren I.
WOLF, Amparo M.
WONG, Janice C.Y.
WOOLFSON, Jessica P.
WRIGHT, Julie F.K.
XIANG, Shuo
YANG, Peter S.
YEUNG, Darwin F.T.
YU, Savio K.H.
YUNG, Terence C.H.
ZARETSKY, Ashley B.
ZHAI, Jacqueline
ZHANG, Phil X.
ZHANG, Yimeng
ZHU, Sijia
ZHU, Tina R.Y.
ZOCHOWSKI, Thomas
ZROBACK, Christopher D.

McMaster University

ACTON, Christine
AGARWAL, Anshi
AL-BALDAWI, Danya
ALLARD, Charlotte
ALOLABI, Noor
ALVAREZ DE LORENZANA, John
AMBRASKA, Heather K.
ANANTHARAJAH, Rokeni
ARMANIOUS, Monica
ARORA, Sourabh
ASMER, M. Selim
ASSAL, Angela F.
ATTIA, Menat
AU, Michael
AUGUSTE, Bourne L.A.
BAKEWELL, Francis W.
BANG, Andrew
BHULLAR, Supreet
BIRK-UROVITZ, Elizabeth
BOGZA, Iulia A.
BOUGHAN, Diana
BROADHURST, Peter K.
BRONICHESKI, Alicia V.
BURNS, David M.
CAMPBELL, Clinton J.V.
CANNON, Lesley M.
CHACKERY, Rosemary C.
CHACKERY-PALMIERI, Rosemary C.
CHAN, Alice C.M.
CHAN, Brian J.
CHAN, Stephanie C.Y.
CHAN, Winnie W.
CHEN, Jerry Y.
CHORLEY, Alexander G.
CICERO, Mark
CLARK-GALLANT, Lauren V.
COMPEAU, Sarah M.
CORBO, Michael D.
CORDUKES, Mary C.
CORONEOS, Marie K.
CORRIVEAU, Nathalie
COTHROS, Nicholas
CRAWFORD, Nicola A.
DAHROUJ, Dalal M.
DALES, Laurence B.
DASON, Shawn
DAVIS, Andrew
DE SA, Darren
DE ZOYSA, Maya K.
DERIA, Mariam M.
DILAURO, Marc
DIONNE, Joanna C.
ELGEBEILY, Seifeldin
EUSTACE, Gregory J.
FABBRO, Sarah A.
FALLEN, Robyn S.
FARAJ, Zein
FISHMAN, Haley R.
FLORINDO, Tiffany M.
FLOWERS, Brendan J.S.
FOX, Andrew S.
FU, Lisa W.
GILROY, Nadin C.
GIORDANI, Christine E.
GRANT, Erin N.
GRAYBIEL, Christopher E.
GUPTA, Nandini
HEASLIP, Ashley M.
HERMAN, Michael
HESKETH, Caitlin C.
HODKINSON, Keira J.
HOLM, Nicolle
HOPPE, Tamara L.
HOWARTH, Briana S.
HOWATT, Neil M.
HUNT, Kyle D.
HUSSAIN, Mohamad A.
IBRAHIM, Christine M.S.
IQBAL, Ali
JACKSON, Ted G.
JAKOVLJEVIC, Ivana
JIANG, Y. Claire
JIANG, Ming Y.
JIANG, Yue
JOHNSON, Emily R.
JOHNSON, Richard B.
JREARZ, Ricky
KALIDINDI, Navya
KAPLAN, Alexander
KHAN, Mohammed N.
KHAN, M. Abdul-Wahab
KIM, S. Katherine
KIZUIK, Meghan T.
KLASSEN, Hilary B.
KLINE, Jordana L.
KNAPP, Gregory
LAMPTEY, Brent A.
LEE, Tiffany W.M.
LEE, Erika Y.
LEUNG, Stephanie P.
LI, Jennifer Z.
LIAO, Willa
LIEDERMAN, Zachary H.
LIU, Cindy
LUCHKIW, Crystal
LUKOVIC, Jelena
MA, Evelyn
MA, Heung K.
MACGILLIVRAY, Lindsey E.S.
MAEDLER-KRON, Chelsea
MAJEED, Habeeb
MALACH, Jessica H.
MALDENIYA, Pramudith M.
MARKOVIC, Nevena
MARTORELLI, Christina M.
MASOTTI, Mary
MATTELIANO, Andre A.
MATTHEWS, Michele
MAYRAND, Kerry E.M.
MAZUREK, Emma M.
MCCARREL, Heather E.
MCDONELL, Tyler H.
MCKAY, Katherine A.
MCLAUGHLIN, Christopher R.
MIKHAIL, Mikel
MOBO, Gerson
MOHAMED, Nourhan S.
MOITRI, Misha O.
MOLNAR, Iulia A.
MOORE, Jennifer E.M.
MULLER, Horatiu
MURDOCH, James C.
NADEL, Maya
NEWTON, Kathryn
NIGLAS, Mark R.
NOBLE, Rosemarie
O'TOOLE, Ashley
OLSEN, Julie A.
ORAAS, Kathryn L.
ORLANDO, Laura
PATEL, Ashish D.
PEEL, Alexandrea C.
PLUME, Julie T.J.
POON, Elizabeth
PRANGER, Emily R.
QUINN, Kathleen M.
QUINN, Stephany M.
RAVEENDRAN, Gayathtri
REDEKOP, Kylie J.
ROBERTS, Lauren E.
ROBSON, Gail
ROSEN, Benjamin F.
ROSTAS, Aviva Y.
RUSSO, Miguel A.
SALIB, Mary
SETIADI, Audi F.
SHACHAR, Orli M.
SHAIKH, Sameer Y.
SHEFFIELD, Holden A.
SHENOUDA, Caroline
SHETHWALA, Shazli
SHIGWADJA, Melissa A.C.
SIDAHMED, Aalla
SIEMIENIUK, Reed A.C.
SILVER, Mara J.
SIMONS, Janet E.
SINGH, Parkash K.
SITZER, Nicole B.
SMITH, Amanda M.
STEINBERG, Rosalie J.
STEINMANN, Tamra M.
TAFLER, Kathleen J.
TAM, Benjamin H.
TAN, Eva Y.
TAUQIR, Madiha
TAYLOR, Jody
TOMA, Monica
TSAO, Miriam W.S.
TSAY, Nataliya E.
TSE, Tabitha J.
VALE, Kayla
VAN MEER, Ryan D.
VARLEY, Talia L.
VIGIL, Humberto R.
WHELLAMS, Diana J.
WIGLE, Hannah J.M.
WILDGOOSE, Petra J.
WONG, Arthur D.W.
WOOD, Thomas
XU, Kunyong
YAN, Ran
YEUNG, Marco C.H.
ZAHANOVA, Stacy
ZAKERIYA, Raziya A.
ZANDI RIAHI, Shervin
ZAVALISHINA, Yelena
ZELOVITZKY, Jennifer H.

RESOURCE SECTION

Western University

AHRENS, Katlin J.P.
ALBION, Caroline
ARMSTRONG, Mitchel
AVANESSY, Aida
AVERY, Michael
BARNETT, Rebecca P.
BEHZADPOOR, Doreh
BEVAN, Rachel
BEZAIRE, Martin
BIELAS, Katarzyna
BISCH, Steven P.
BOL, Eric
BONDY, Jennifer
BROWN, Kaitlyn
BULATOVIC, Ranko
BUSATO, Gian-Marco C.
CAMPAGNA, Craig
CAO, Yang
CHEUNG, Valerie
CHIA, Justin
CHO, Dennis D.
CHOY, Stephen
CHUNG SIK YUEN, Sabrina
CONNOLLY, Michael M.
COOKSON, Christina A.
COOPER, Joel A.
COULSON, Jennifer N.
CRABBE, Rory A.
DATERS, Aaron
DI LABIO, Anthony
ERNST, Jaclyn
FALCONER, Erin
FEHR, Adam
FOK, Tommy
FREUND, Paul
FULTON, Courtney
GALL, Chris
GALL, Robert
GEERLINKS, Ashley
GORMAN, Claude
GRAY, Andrew
HAQUE, Nihal
HAYWARD, Victoria
HEALE, Liane
HEMPHILL, Andrew
HEWSON, Gillian
HO, Joyce K.
HOLMES, Meghan D.
HONTSCHARUK, Rayisa
HUANG, Julie M.
HUANG, Yi Min
HUGHES, Julie K.J.
HUTCHINSON, Marie
JEWELL, Kirsten
JOHNSON, Anna
JOHNSON, Taylor A.
JUMA, Salina
KAGOMA, Yoan K.
KALEN, Chemanthi R.
KATCHKY, Ryan N.
KEDDY, Maeghan
KHALAF, Roy
KHANDEKAR, Neha
KHIMDAS, Sarit S.
LANKTREE, Matthew B.
LASKI, Matthew
LEBNER, Adrianne C.
LEE, Ashley
LI, Allanah
LIU, Daisy M.
LUU, Kimberly
MACLELLAN, Adam C.
MACKERACHER, Kathleen
MAGGISANO, Kevin
MASCARENHAS, Jeffrey E.
MCCLURE, Adam
MCINTYRE, Kathryn S.
MCKNIGHT, Sarah K.S.
MCLAUGHLIN, Heather M.
MCPHERSON, Victor A.
MCWILLIAM, Morgan
MELOCHE, Craig A.C.
MEYER-MACAULAY, Colin
MILLER, Eli
MILLER, Lance S.
MIR, Hassan
MITCHELL, Michael A.
MITHOOWANI, Hamid
MORRISON, Leslie A.
MORTERA, Genevieve
MOSS, Matthew
MULAOSMANOVIC, Stephanie
MUSSEN, Lauren E.
MYERS, Mallory
MYSLIK, Frank E.
NJARLANGATTIL, Anna P.
PATEL, Neeraj
PEASE, Christopher A.
PEIRCE, Michael W.K.
PEREIRA, Ian J.
PRENDERGAST, Patrick
QUINN, Jason J.
RAI, Bikramjit S.
RAJAKUMAR, Chandheeb
REISMAN, William J.
RICHARDSON, Michael
RIEDER, Scott W.
ROACH, Elizabeth E.
ROCHON, Matthew D.
ROGERS, Eamonn
ROSSONI, Melissa T.
ROZANSKI, Camilla
RUBIN, Erica S.
RYCERZ, Katarzyna W.
RYU, Won
SAUNDERS, Samantha J.
SAWCHUK, Michael A.
SCHNEIDER, Kara
SCHULTZ, William J.
SCOTT, Kristen V.
SHAH, Kalpa
SHAPIRO, Cal A.J.
SHEPHARD, Lauren
SHESHGIRI, Rachit
SHETTY, Akshay
SHU, Jenny
SLOMER, Adam
SMITH, Mara
STALL, Nathan M.
STECHO, William M.
STRAUSS, Benjamin J.
SUN, Yuan
SYMONETTE, Caitlin J.
TABOUN, Fatima S.
TANCIO, Michael B.P.M.
TELLIER, Sylvie
TENBERGEN, Melissa M.
THOMPSON, Caitlin E.
THOMASSON, Kathleen E.
THOMPSON, Kimberly C.
THOMSON, Steven
TSANG, Gordon F.
VIVAS, Lucas
WARSHAFSKY, Daniel
WEISS, Edward S.
WEISZ, Karen
WEPPLER, Alison M.
WONG, Jay S.M.
XIAO, Yue V.
YAU, Joyce K.
ZHAO, Yun Wei
ZULYS, Matthew
ZWIEP, Terry M.

Northern Ontario School of Medicine

AGOSTINO, Kevin D.
ANDERSON, Kathleen
AZZOLA, Alescia
BEDUHN, John
BEVERIDGE, Julia
BODKIN, Brienne
BURKHART, Aaron R.
BUTT, Aeysha
CARIA, Laura
CARLUCCI, Courtney
CARRIER, Morgan M.
CHASE, Teena D.
COMSTOCK, Shawna M.C.
CONWAY, Jessica
COSSAR, Kathryn E.
DADGOSTAR, Neema
DITTARO, Jade
DONALESHEN, Jeniva
EDWARDS, Jacqueline
ETTIE, Suzanne
GARON, Jennifer
GERVAIS, Sophie
GRAVELLE, Sean
HEIDMAN, Jaimi T.
HEIDMAN, Scott
HERINGER, Jeffrey
HOBBS, Hailey
KUCHERAN, Jacob N.
LANDRY, Yves D.
LANTHIER, Claudine
LOCKE-ROBINSON, Kirsty C.I.A.
MATHEW, Rebecca T.
MIDDLETON, Sean C.
MILLS, Melissa M.
MONTPELLIER, Renee-Anne
MOORE, Aimee L.
MOORE, Amanda
NEEDHAM-REGAN, Leslie-Darlene
PARLETT, Brittney L.
PENFOLD, Sarah B.J.
PENHEAROW, Janie
POULIN, Josee
QUIRION, Christine
RODY, Caelen
RYS, Trisha M.
SELLICK, Megan
SPRAGUE, Celia
ST-ONGE, Natasha E.
SULLIVAN, Sean T.
SWEENEY, Allison
VALENTE, Colleen R.
VEITCH, Zachary
ZALAN, Elise J.
ZROBACK, Jesse P.

University of Manitoba

ADAMSON, Lori G.
ADELMANN, Susan J.
AGRAWAL, Veena R.
ALEXANDER, Ian S.
ALKANA, Matthew R.J.
BELL, William O.
BERGEN, Calvin J.
BERSCHEID, Amber W.
BHULLAR, Navdeep
BIGDER, Mark G.
BRAUN, Monica D.
BURKETT, Kyle C.
BZURA, Thomas J.
CHATWIN, Meghan K.
CHEN, Joel
CHEUNG, Paul*
CHIU, Sidney S.
CHOWDHURY, Farah N.
CHRISTIANSEN, David
COISH, Rebecca
CONEYS, John G.D.
CRAIG, Lisa A.
CUDMORE, Jessica A.M.
DE BLONDE, Riley T.
DOW, Nathan W.
ELIMBAN, Vinit V.
ESPINO, M. Paula M.
FENSKE, Mark A.
FORSYTH, Mark D.
FREEMAN, Lisa K.
FRIDFINNSON, Jason A.
FRIESEN, Janis E.
FURNISH, Sandra D.
GLOBA, Ashley J.
GLOVER, Sean A.I.
GOUSSEAU, Michael E.
GRAHAM, Jeffrey R.
GREEN, Susan L.
GUIRGIS, Mina
GULAVITA, Natasha K.
HALL, William P.
HAN, Zhifei
HILDAHL, Erik J.
HOLLAND, Darren R.W.
HOSSEINI, Boshra
IRVING, Heather D.
JAVELLANA, Audrey D.
JAWANDA, Gurswinder G.
JIANG, Kailun
KUUSSELKA, Christopher D.
LAKHI, Sunjay
LEE, Gloria S.Y.
LEONHART, Michael W.
LEYLEK, Melike L.
LINDSAY, Duncan C.
LIPSON, Mark E.
LOFTUS, Russell G.
LONGSTAFFE, Robert C.
LU, Peter H.
LUONG, Erica K.
MACDONALD, Karen E.
MACLEAN, Rebecca
MAHAL, Mandeep K.
MAILEY, Trevor F.
MARSHALL, Stephanie J.
MARTIN, David G.E.
MARTIN, Richard K.M.
MATHEN, Peter G.
MCLEAN, Norman
MENDOZA, Francisco
MOLLISON, Scott W.N.
MONGRU, Padma P.
MYSORE, Priyanka K.
O'NEIL, Liam J.
OOMAH, Sacha
PEITSCH, Lorraine S.
PETERS, Harold J.A.
RAMSAY, Andrea M.
RENKAS, Rebecca L.
ROCKENSTEIN, Johanna V.
ROSENFIELD, Lana A.
ROUSSEAU, Skye R.
SCOTT, Kristen M.
SERRANO, Griselda N.
SHAW, James A.
SHEPS, Daniel J.
SHIN, Amber H.
SIMMONDS, Reesa
SINNEMAKI, Lauren C.
SPOONER, Aaron
STANIFORTH, Christopher J.
STASIUK, Allison Dianne*
SURAJBALLI, Llewellyn
TUNOVIC, Edin
VAN, Royce
WANG, Neng Jack
WEIDMAN, Danielle R.
WELIHINDA, Hasitha
WENGEL, Tiffany
WETTIG, Kara B.
WINOGRODZKI, Olga
WITIW, Christopher D.
WYKES, Benjamin C.
YAWORSKI, Helen E.
ZAMAN-HAQUE, Abeyat

*(2011 MD Graduates)

University of Saskatchewan

BALATON, Breanna
BAPTISTE, Roryck
BAXTER, Julie
BEVANS, Trent
BLACKSTOCK, Kalah
BOLLINGER, Megan L.
BOURGAULT, Joanne
BRAHMANIA, Poorvi
BULL, Lauren
BUTLER, Russell
CHALOUPKA, Marketa
CURRIE, Kristopher
DE GUZMAN, Jolly
DENIS, Jason
DINSMORE, Michael
DOLMAN, Petra
DOMUSCHIEVA, Hristina
DUMANSKI, Sandra
ELLIOTT, William
ERICKSON, Bree
FAIRFIELD, Janice
FERGUSON, Heather
FITTERER, Taffeta
FORDHAM, Karen
FOWLER, Adam
FROMBACH, Aaron
GACO, Damjan
GARTNER, Kali
GILL, Jillian
GRAHAM, Alexsis
HAGEL, Kimberly
HARRIMAN, Suzanne
HOIUM, Jason
HORNE, David
HUBENIG, Lindsay
HUYNH, James
IRADUKUNDA, Diphile
JUST, Celeste
KHAN, Mohammad
KLEISINGER, Amanda
KOHLENBERG, Jennifer
KURJI, Khaliq
LAMONTAGNE, Megan
LAUGHLIN, Caitlin
LENARTOWICZ, Magdalena
LITTLE, Gregory
MAMCHUR, Joel
MCEWEN, Heather
MISSKEY, Jonathan
MITCHELL, Cheryl
MOAZENI RIZI, Afra
NG, Katherine
OLENIUK, Ashley
OLSON, Lanna
OROZ, Irina
OTTENBREIT, Rachel
OVERLI-DOMES, Taffeta
PABANI, Aliyah
PAHWA, Dave R.
PARIHAR, Rishi
PATEL, Krupal B.
PEKRUL, Christopher
POLLEY, Gina
PREMKUMAR, Kamini
REMPEL, Benjamin
REWUSKI, Nicole
RUSSELL, Jordan
SELVARAJ, Saumya
SHARMA, Ankur
SHUMILAK, Geoffrey
SIELSKI, Afton
SIEMENS, Kristen
SILBERNAGEL, Lana R.
SKLAR, Michael C.
SMITH, Alistair J.
SMITH, Kristine
STEED, McKay
STRUBLE, Jennifer
SULLIVAN, Emily
TYMCHAK, Zane
UPPAL, Sundeep
VARGO, Michael
VOLL, Alexandra
WALKER, Crystal
WALLER, Brittany A.M.
WASLAK, Robin
WEISGARBER, Danielle
WEISGERBER, Grahme
WUDEL, Beverly
XIA, Lei
XIAO, Linda
YAM, Stephen
ZHENG, James
ZIOLA, Kirsti

University of Calgary

AHMED, Khaled
AMBASTA, Anshula
ANAND, Arun
ANDERSON, Kathryn
ASCIONE, Marc
ATHWAL, Tarndeep
BALUTIS, Kelsey
BANDALI, Murad
BARSS, Leila
BELL, Alexandra
BJAZEVIC, Jennifer
BODNARCHUK, Kaylee N.
BORGSTROM, Matthew
BOX, Alan
BRAICH, Kanwar
BRAR, Sandeep
BRIN, Geoffrey
BROWN, Gordon
BURROWES, David
BYRNE, Roisin
CAMATEROS, Pierre
CASAULT, Colin
CHEE, Caroline
CHEEMA, Kim
CHENG, James J.
CHIVERS-WILSON, Kaitlin
CHRETIEN, Marc
COLL, Neasa
COLLINS, Jovian A.E.
COMMODORE, Amy L.
CORMACK, Stacy
DALEY, Tara
DAS, Debanjana
DE VERE, Stephanie
DE VETTEN, Giselle
DEBOSZ, Joanna
DESILETS, Nichelle
DI NINNO, Alexandra
DIRKSEN, Meghan
DISSANAYAKE, Tharindri
DMYTRASH, Andrea
DUNBAR, Mary
ELDOMA, Maysoon
EPP, Rebecca
ESMAIL, Kaisra
FLEXHAUG, Cody
FONG, Carmen
FOUST, Leanne
FRANZ, Colin
GANESH, Aravind
GIBSON, Katherine
GILL, Sukhdeep
GILLRIE, Mark
GIRGIS, Mina
GRANBERG, Brad
GURSKY, Lucas
GUSTAFSON, Karla
HAGEL, Carly
HAJJAR, Sarah
HANASYK, Brent
HAWS, Jolene
HEATH, Peter
HOLLAND, Megan
HONEYMAN, Graeme
HYUN, Eric
JIVRAJ, Aman
JOWHARI, Fahd
KAHLON, Maninder
KANUNGO, Anish
KENNEDY, Rebecca
KHAMBATI, Husain
KILB, Brett
KIM, Esther H.
KRAKOWSKI, Katrina
KRALL, Randall
LAFFIN, Michael
LAIL, Parabhdeep
LALONDE, Sarah
LAM, Joyce N.H.
LAU, Jenny
LEE, Joohyun
LEMMEX, Devin
LEWIS, Clinton
LIU, Che
LIVINGSTONE, Aaron
LORINCZ-PILLING, Caeley
LUONG, Micah
LUYKENAAR, Kevin
MA, Christopher
MADEJ, Ursula H.Z.
MALLET, Mark
MATTHEWS, Selena
MAXWELL, Jay P.
MCCAFFREY, Carmen M.
MCCONNELL, Allison H.
MCPHERSON, Robyn
MICHAELS, Danielle
MILLAR, Vanessa
MORRISON, Carlyn
MUMMERY, Ashley
NADERKHANI, Golnaz
NANTAIS, Jordan
NIELSEN, Christopher
O'CONNOR, Pamela
O'LEARY, Frances M.
O'LEARY, Moira
PANDYA, Anjli
PARKIN, Stephen
PERREAULT, Alexander
PERSAUD, Steven
PETERS, Tess
PETRIE MCCONNELL, Allison
POLLOCK, Cody
PREMJI, Nahbeel
PRYSTAJECKY, Michael
RAMJI, Qahir
RATANSHI, Imran
REGLIN, Paul
REICHENAUER, Jeffrey
RITTBERG, Naomi
ROBERTSON-MORE, Connal
ROLLICK, Natalie
RUBENSOHN, Hayden
RYPIEN, Candace
SARAN, Sandeep
SAWATZKY-MARTENS, Jeremy
SCHWARTZENBERGER, Edward
SETO, Anthony
SHAFRAN, Daniel M.
SHAH, Nikhil
SHAW, Jeffrey
SIDHU, Bikrampal S.
SIDHU, Robinder
SINGENDONK, Erik
SLOMP, Stefan
SMITH, Jena L.
SMITH, Miles A.
SONTAG, Daniel
STEINER, Mia I.
STOLTE, Erin
STONE, Jill
STORNESS-BLISS, Claudine
SURETTE, Sarah
SWINTON, Lindsay
SYED, Ali S.
SYED, Raheel
SZABO, Lian
TAYLOR, Regan
TEITELBAUM, Lisa
TEJA, Salina
THIESSEN, Jeshiah
THOMPSON, Jenny
TODD, Ryan A.
TRUONG, Jacky
TRUONG, Kathy
TYMCHUK, Sarah
VAN ROOYEN, Francine
VAZ, Gina
WALSH, Richelle
WALSH, Sarah K.
WANG, Ying
WARSHAWSKI, Timothy
WAUGH, Alistair
WEATHERBEE, Pamela
WOO, Albert
YANG, Stephanie P.
YARASKAVITCH, Megan
YOUNG, Courtney
YU, Andrea C.
YUAN, Su
YUEN, Gilbert
ZARETSKY, Mark

University of Alberta

ABDULWAHAB, Kamal
ABOU-GHAIDA, Maen
AGUSTO, Clarissa
AL-SABEQ, Basil
ANDERSON, Blaire
AUBREY, Christa
BACH, Tammy
BADRE, Armin
BANMANN, Aaron
BARTELL, Nicholas
BASCOM, Alexandra
BEAMISH, Leigh
BENZ, Jennifer
BIRKHOLZ, Kristina
BLACKSHAW, Lee A.
BLACKSHAW, Michael
BRENNEIS, Mikayla K.
BRISTOW, Erin
BROWN, Taryn
BURKE, Paula
BYERS, Justin
BYRNS, Simon
CAMPBELL, Lindsey
CAPTAN, Virgil
CARPENTER, Travis D.
CHAKRABARTY, Trisha
CHAMPAGNE, Chantelle
CHAN, F.W. Philip
CHAN, Timothy W.C.
CHAPMAN, Kimberley
CHAU, Johnny
CHEUNG, Serena
CHEVALIER, James
CHOW, Renfred
COOK, Victoria
COOPER, Timothy
COTTON, Darrel
COUGHLIN, Jason
CROSSMAN, Roberta
CURIAL, Marc
DEAN, Lucas
DEY, Anita
DHALLA, Muhammed
DINGELDEIN, Genelle
DIXON, Tara
DU PLESSIS, Jean
DUROCHER, Shauna
DYTE, Christopher
FANAEIAN, Joshua
FORSBERG, Daniel
FROBB, Devin
FU, David
GANTA, Ninada
GHAZNAVI, Sana
GOEKJIAN, Serge
GORDEY, Erin
GROESCHEL, Michael
GUNAWARDENA, Harshitha
HALEY, Kevin
HARRIS, Matthew
HARTFEIL, Misha
HEGAN, Kathleen
HENKELMAN, Josh
HO, Michael L.
HOFFART, Kaili
HRYCIUK, Stacey
HU, Jia
HUANG, James
HUSSEIN, Abbeir
ILNITSKY, Sara
JIANG, Di
KAHLKE, Paul
KALAICHANDRAN, Sivanesan
KAPUSTA, Michael
KHARRAT, Ashraf
KORO, Konstantin
KULAGA, Adam
KUZEL, Paul
KWAN-WONG, Terence
LEE, Maria
LEE, Rene
LEE, Sang-Oh
LEE, Victoria
LEISHMAN, Eric
LEUNG, William P.H.
LI, Mathew
LIM, Charles H.
LIM, Lillian
LIU, Hebert
LYNCH, Meredith
MACPHERSON, Peter
MADLUNG, Alison
MATEMISZ, Laura
MAWDSLEY, Stewart
MCCREA, Richard
MCFARLANE, Alexandra
MCLEOD, Scott
MEHTA, Rahul
MORRIS, Tammy
MORRISON, Laura
NABETA, David
NADEAU, Brandon R.A.
NAGJI, Alim
NANJI, Jalal
NGUYEN, Vina
NICOLL, Jessica
NIGAM, Aparna
O'DUNN-ORTO, Alexandra
OMAN, Kathleen M.
PANDYA, Shawna
PARIY, Maria
PAWA, Jasmine
PENNEY, Todd
PETERS, Amber
POPEL, Jillian
POWER, Hollie
PUI, Odell
RAJABALI, Naheed
RAO, Adarsh S.
RODYCH, Murray
ROSENBERG, Zale
SAMYCIA, Michael
SAWCHUK, Brett
SEDLAK, Robert
SHI, Jing
SIBTAIN, Alyzee
SIY, Anna-Kristen
SKLAR, Cameron
SPELLISCY, Courtney C.D.
STASIUK, Samantha M.
SUE, Kyle
TAYLOR, Andrew M.J.
TAYLOR, Ian
TEJPAR, Qassim Z.
TENNESE, Alysa
TRAN, Allen
TULIS, Roman
VALJI, Rafiaa
VERMA, Shawn
VIPULANANTHAN, Nirupan
WASILENKO, Shawn
WOLFF, Jordan
WONG, Daniel
WONG, Peter
WOZNEY, Sarah
YANG, Christina
YIP, Steven
YUAN, Linda
ZDRILL, Everett
ZHANG, Lili
ZHU, Julie

University of British Columbia

ADHAMI, Nassir
ALI, Salman
APPERLEY, Scott
ASTANEHE, Arezoo
BAKER, Sarah
BAKKER, Ashley T.
BARIBEAU, Anne-Marie
BARNES, Tavish
BEAUDRY, Jeffrey
BEAUDRY, Ruth-Ann
BENHAM, Jamie
BENTZON, Brianne
BERG, Mattias
BERKHOUT, Suze G.
BOLDT, Leah J.
BRAR, Rupinder
BRIEMON, Dayna
BROSSEAU, Ami
BUDLOVSKY, Joshua
BUNNEY, Alli
BUTLER, Myra
CAIRNS, Stephanie L.
CANNON, Tracy
CASAGRANDE, Magdalena D.
CHAMBERLAIN, Ciara
CHAN, Aaron
CHAN, Angela
CHAN, Irene
CHANG, Jack
CHANG, Brent
CHAPMAN, Chris
CHAWORTH-MUSTERS, Tessa
CHEEMA, Rajinder
CHEN, Becky
CHEN, Patrick
CHEUNG, Jessica
CHIN, Carson
CHING, K.Y. Carrie
CHNG, Laura
CHOI, Wayne
CHOI, J.W. James
CHUANG, Michael
CLEAVE, Spencer
COOPER, Matthew
CORDONIER, Genevieve
CUNNINGHAM, Cameron
DEDHAR, Alysha
DETILLIEUX, Sonia
DHARAMPAL, Navjit
DIAO, Diana
DRAHT, Lisa
DRESSEKR, Sarah
DREW-MCKINSTRY, Meg
DUKE, Carlie
DUMONT, Michael
DUPUIS, Elaine
EADIE, Brennan
EAMER, Gil
ELEFANTE, Julius
ELIASON, Scott
ENSOM, Asia
EPPINGA, Peter
EVANS, Morgan
FARAJI, Reza
FAULKNER, Launny
FELDHOFF, Lauren
FENG, Florina
FENRICH, Mark
FLYNN, Caley
FOX, Chris
FRANCIS, George
FREDRICKSEN, Brynn
FUKUNAGA, Marcia
GALLIE, Annie
GALM, Brandon
GALWAY, Shannon M.
GARDNER, James
GIANG, Karen
GILL, Amar
GILL, Hardave
GILLEY, Meghan
GLEN, Mary
GREWAL, Karan
GRIFFITHS, Tanya
GUAN, Camila
GUSTAFSON-VICKERS, Sabrina
HADDON, Craig
HADISFAR, Omeed
HAIDUK, Tasha
HALL, Grayson
HAMMOND, Judith
HARRIMAN, David
HARRIS, Claire
HEINRICHS, Ryan
HENDERSON, Christine
HERNANDEZ-LEE, Jacalynne
HETLAND, Karissa
HEWITSON, Leanne
HIEBERT, Stephanie
HILL, Megan
HILL, Shannon
HO, Karina
HOP WO, Nolan
HOPE, Maralyn
HUGET-PENNER, Sawyer
HUNG, Gabriel
JAMIESON, Blake
JANG, Wesley
JANJUA, Irvin
JANKOLA, Lauchlan J.
JANSSEN, Jesse

JARVIE, Amber T.
JIANG, Steven
JIM, Brent
JOHAL, Gurp
JOHNSON, Chad
JUN, Moses B.
KARIM, Naila A.
KENNAH, Erin
KENNEDY, Megan
KHALSA, Tejinder S.
KHORASANI, Mohammadali
KHORASANI, Sepehr
KING, Ashlee
KOLKER, Sabrina M.
KONDRA, Jennifer
KOZORIZ, Michael
KRUEGER, Joel
KUMAR, Ritu
KUO, K.H. Daniel
KWAN, Kelvin S.K.
KWOK, Evelyn
LAI, Leo
LAI, Tina
LAM, Godfrey
LAM, Morgan
LARATTA, Peter
LAU, Monica
LAW, Tamryn K.
LAWSON, Mark
LEE, Bryan
LEE, Gibong
LEE, Karen G.
LEE, Lauren
LEE, Lawrence
LEE, Stephanie G.
LERCH, Lindsey
LEUNG, David
LIAO, Pamela
LIDSTONE, Sarah C.
LIEPH, Ryan
LIN, Wendy
LITTLE, Kelly
LIU, Iris
LO, P. Andy
LOU, Cindy K.K.
LOW, Katrina
LUNG, Rita
MA, Janet
MA, Vivian
MACNAB, Magnus
MACHUK, Andrew
MADDEN, Anne-Marie
MALMBERG, Dustin D.
MANOCHA, Ranita H.
MARACLE, Kelly
MARCOTTE, Greg
MARINO, Michael
MARK, Sarah M.
MARK, Shelly T.
MARKO, Crystal A.
MATCHETT, Stephanie
MCEACHERN, Cyrus
MCINNES, Colin
MCKAY, Jeff
MCKENZIE, Karie-Jean
MCLEOD, Troy
MCPHEE, Jan
METRIE, Mary M.H.
MITRA, Anish
MITROVIC, Suzana
MOORE, Steven
MORGAN-JONKER, Cecily
MORRISON, Kathryn
MUNSHEY, Farrukh
NAJAFI LARIJANI, Omid
NATHWANI, Shahana
NELSON, Hilary
NGAI, Jacqueline
NGAI, Tyler
NGUYEN, David
NOBLE, Emma
O'CONNOR, Deirdre
OLVER, Amy
OMIDVAR, Vida
OTTO, Alexandra
PARSA, Ashkan
PATTERSON, Loni
PETZOLD, Matthew
PHILLIPS, Melanie
POURSHAHNAZARI, Persia
PRITCHARD, Julia
QUIGLEY, Nicole
QUINN, Hillary
RANDHAWA, Nikkie
RATTAN, Navi N.
RAZAGHI KASHANI, Nima
READ, Alison
ROCCAMATISI, Dawn
ROSE, Peter
ROSE, Simon
ROSTON, Kathryn
RYAN, Jane
SANDERS, Ari
SARAVANA-BAWAN, Samantha
SCALI, Elena
SCHAMUHN, Ruth-Ann M.
SCHARF, Jed
SEBASTIAN, Renee M.
SHERWOOD, Michelle
SINGLETON-POLSTER, Amy J.
SIOW, Serena
SKITCH, Steven A.
SOMA, Rahul
SOMANI, Alysalim
SPINELLI, Egidio
STEVENS, Emilie
STOKVIS, Lindsay
STREGGER, Anthony M.
SUEN, Alexander T.H.
SULEMAN, Shazeen
SWANEY, Laura
SWEENEY, Colleen
TAM, Andrea W.K.
TAM, Jennifer M.
TAM, Nicola
TANSLEY, Gavin
THONG, Nicole
TIMPERLEY BERG, Tonia Q.G.
TRUSCOTT, Sarah
TSO, David
TURA, Emanuela
TURKO, Britteny
URQUHART, David J.
VAID, Moni
VAUGHAN, Mariko
VERMA, Pamela
VIDA, Omidvar
WADHWA, Devina D.
WALKER, Caroline A.
WAN, Tony
WATSON, Elizabeth
WEINBERG, Alex
WENNER, Joshua B.
WILLMS, Elizabeth
WILSON, Julie L.
WISE, Stephanie
WITHEFORD, Miranda
WONG, Benedict
WONG, Catherine C.
WOO, Simon
WOODWARD, Elizabeth R.
WOOLNOUGH, Bonnie O.
WU, Christopher H.
YAO, Sabrina
YAU, Alan
YOKOGAWA, Tomonori A.
YOUSSEF, David
ZHENG, Q. Gina

SECTION 6 — CANADIAN HEALTH CARE ASSOCIATIONS

CANADIAN HEALTH CARE ASSOCIATIONS

ADDICTIONS

Action on Women's Addictions - Research and Education
Mailing: PO Box 86 Stn Main, Kingston ON K7L 4V6
613 545-0117; Fax: 613 545-1508
E: aware@kos.net
W: www.aware.on.ca
Languages: English

Addiction Services - Red Deer
104-4920 51 St, Red Deer AB T4N 6K8
403 340-5274; Fax: 403 340-4804
E: reddeer@albertahealthservices.ca
W: www.albertahealthservices.ca
Executive:
Mgr: Pat McNulty

Al-Anon Family Group Headquarters (Canada), Inc.
900-275 Slater St, Ottawa ON K1P 5H9
613 723-8484
Toll-free: 888 425-2666
E: wso@al-anon.org
W: www.al-anon.alateen.org
Year Founded: 1951
Criteria: *Open to any person who has been affected by someone else's drinking.*
Speakers Available
Languages: English; French; Spanish
◈Toronto:
222 Yonge St, PO Box 47007, Toronto ON M5B 2H0
416 410-3806
E: gtais.chair@gmail.com

Alberta Health Services, Adult Addiction Services - Calgary
1177 11 Ave SW, Floor 2, Calgary AB T2R 1K9
403 297-3071; Fax: 403 297-3036
Toll-free: 866 332-2322 AB only
W: www.albertahealthservices.ca
Languages: English

Alcoholic Anonymous - Regina Office
312-845 Broad St, Regina SK S4R 8G9
306 545-9300
E: a.a@sasktel.net
W: www.aaregina.com

Alcoholics Anonymous
Location: 17A St & 10 Ave S, Lethbridge AB T1J 3Y5
Mailing: PO Box 212 Stn Main
403 327-8049
W: www.alcoholicsanonymous.com
Executive:
Trusted Server: Alex Slobodian
Languages: English

Alcoholics Anonymous - Abbotsford Intergroup Committee
17-1961 Eagle St, Abbotsford BC V2S 3A7
604 850-0811
E: abbotsfordintrgrp@hotmail.com
W: www.theabbotsfordintergroup-aa.org
Executive:
A-Rep: Daniel Harder

Alcoholics Anonymous - Calgary Central Service Office
2-4015 1 St SE, Calgary AB T2G 4X7
403 777-1212; Fax: 403 287-6540
E: aaoffice@telusplanet.net
W: www.calgaryaa.org
Executive:
Office Mgr: Mathew Marshall
No of Paid Staff: 2
Speakers Available
Languages: English

Alcoholics Anonymous - District 1 & 2 Central Service Committee
Location: 3 Dundas St, Dartmouth NS B2Y 2T6
Mailing: PO Box 31338 RPO Gladstone, Halifax NS B3K 5Y5
902 461-1119
E: webmaster@aahalifax.org
W: www.aahalifax.org
Criteria: *Open to any person who has a desire to stop drinking.*
Languages: English

Alcoholics Anonymous - District 30 Quinte West-Trenton
Mailing: RR 4 Stn Main, Trenton ON K8V 5P7
Toll-free: 866 951-3711
E: secretary@quintewestaa.org
W: www.quintewestaa.org

Alcoholics Anonymous - District 35
Mailing: 3916 Ragged Ass Rd, Yellowknife NT X1A 2T4
867 444-4230
E: jstlouis44@hotmail.com
Executive:
Dist committee member: Irene Savoy

Alcoholics Anonymous - Edmonton Central Office
8-11041 105 Ave NW, Edmonton AB T5H 3Y1
780 424-5900; Fax: 780 426-1929
E: edmontonaa@hotmail.com
W: www.edmontonaa.org
Executive:
Mgr: JoAnn Oscar
Year Founded: 1945
No of Paid Staff: 1
Speakers Available
Languages: English
Membership: 5,000

Alcoholics Anonymous - Elgin County
Location: 204 First Ave, St Thomas ON N5R 6A1
Mailing: PO Box 22001, RPO Elmwood Square
519 633-0430
W: www.aa.org
Languages: English

Alcoholics Anonymous - Greater Vancouver Intergroup Office
3457 Kingsway, Vancouver BC V5R 5L5
604 434-3933; Fax: 604 434-2553
E: intrgrp@vancouveraa.ca
W: www.vancouveraa.ca
Executive:
Mgr: John McCormick
Languages: English
◈Greater Vancouver Intergroup Office:

Alcoholics Anonymous - Greater Victoria Intergroup Association
8-2020 Douglas St, Victoria BC V8T 4L1
250 383-7744; Fax: 250 383-0417
W: www.aavictoria.ca
Criteria: *Any alcoholic with a desire to stop drinking.*
No of Paid Staff: 1
Speakers Available
Languages: English

Alcoholics Anonymous - GTA Intergroup
McConnell Bldg
202-234 Eglinton Ave E, Toronto ON M4P 1K5
416 487-5591; Fax: 416 487-5855
Toll-free: 877 404-5591
E: office@aatoronto.org
W: www.aatoronto.org
Executive:
Literature Dept Mgr: Helen Gillan
Office Mgr: Gail Dobbs
Year Founded: 1935
Criteria: *The only requirement for AA membership is a desire to stop drinking.*
Budget: $250,000
No of Paid Staff: 3
Speakers Available
Library: Y *(Open to the public)*
Languages: English
Membership: 12,000

Alcoholics Anonymous - Hamilton Central Office
205-627 Main St E, Hamilton ON L8M 1J5
905 522-8399; Fax: 905 522-1946
E: info@aahamilton.com
W: www.aahamilton.com
Executive:
Office Coord: Martin Aire
Languages: English

Alcoholics Anonymous - Kawartha District Intergroup
625 Cameron St, Peterborough ON K9J 3Z9
705 745-6111
W: www.peterboroughaa.org
Executive:
Chair: Jack Delfry
Languages: English

Alcoholics Anonymous - Lakehead Intergroup Office
3-516 Victoria Ave E, Thunder Bay ON P7C 1A7
807 623-1712
E: lakeheadintergroup@tbaytel.net
W: www.aa-nwo-area85.org
Languages: English

Alcoholics Anonymous - London
137 Consortium Crt, London ON N6E 2S8
519 438-9006
E: hugh.hughes@hotmail.com
W: www.aalondon.org
Executive:
Office Mgr: Mike Dynes
Languages: English

Alcoholics Anonymous - Manitoba Central Office
208-323 Portage Ave, Winnipeg MB R3B 2C1
204 942-0126
E: aambco@mts.net
W: www.aamanitoba.org
Year Founded: 1935
Criteria: *There are no age or education requirements. Membership is open to anyone who wants to do something about his or her drinking problem.*
No of Paid Staff: 1
Languages: English

Alcoholics Anonymous - Mid-Island Intergroup Society
212-285 Prideaux St, Nanaimo BC V9R 2N2
250 753-7513; Fax: 250 753-7513
E: nanaimoaa@shaw.ca
W: www.nanaimoaa.org
Library: Y
Languages: English

HEALTHCARE ASSOCIATIONS

Alcoholics Anonymous - Montréal
3920 rue Rachel E, Montréal QC H1X 1Z3
514 350-3444; Fax: 514 374-2250
Toll-free: 888 424-2975
E: area@aa87.org
W: www.aa-quebec.org
Year Founded: 1935
Criteria: *Le désir d'arrêter de boire.*
No of Paid Staff: 2
Speakers Available
Languages: English; French
Membership: 2,000,000/150 countries

Alcoholics Anonymous - Niagara District Intergroup
Location: 125 Carlton St, St Catharines ON L2R 1R0
Mailing: PO Box 23091 RPO Carlton,
St Catharines ON L2R 7P6
905 682-2140
E: info@aaniagara.org
W: www.aaniagara.org
Languages: English

Alcoholics Anonymous - Oshawa
102-124 Wilson Rd S, Oshawa ON L1H 6C1
905 728-1020
E: aa.oshawa@live.com
W: www.aaoshawa.org
Executive:
Admn/Office Mgr: Linda Sawyer
No of Paid Staff: 1
Languages: English

Alcoholics Anonymous - Ottawa Area Intergroup Office
108-211 Bronson Ave, Ottawa ON K1R 6H5
613 237-6000
E: help@ottawaaa.org
W: www.ottawaaa.org
Languages: English

Alcoholics Anonymous - Québec
3-75 rue des Épinettes, Québec QC G1L 1N6
418 523-9993; Fax: 418 523-9997
Toll-free: 877 523-9993
E: region89@qc.aira.com
W: www.aa-quebec.org
Executive:
Sec: Joanne Gagnon
Languages: French; Bilingual(French/English)

Alcoholics Anonymous - Saskatoon Central Office
311-220 3rd Ave S, Saskatoon SK S7K 1M1
306 665-6727; Fax: 306 665-6753
E: aasaskatoon@sasktel.net
W: www.aasaskatoon.org
Languages: English

Alcoholics Anonymous - Sudbury
4-109 Elm St, Sudbury ON P3C 1T4
705 674-6217
E: sudburydistricts@gmail.com
W: www.aaneontarioarea84.org
Languages: English

CDD des GFA
101-777 rue de Bellechasse, Montréal QC H2S 1X7
514 270-3277
Languages: English; French

Canadian Addiction Counsellors Certification Federation
C-81 Bruce St, Kitchener ON N2B 1Y7
519 772-0533; Fax: 519 772-0535
Toll-free: 866 624-1911
E: info@caccf.ca
W: www.caccf.ca
Executive:
Exec Dir: Jeff Wilbee
Year Founded: 1985
Languages: English

Canadian Centre on Substance Abuse
500-75 Albert St, Ottawa ON K1P 5E7
613 235-4048; Fax: 613 235-8101
E: info@ccsa.ca
W: www.ccsa.ca
Executive:
Chairperson: Leanne Lewis
CEO: Michel Perron
Dep CEO: Rita Notarandrea
Year Founded: 1988
Budget: $7,200,000
No of Paid Staff: 45
Speakers Available
Library: Y *(Open to the public)*
Languages: English
Membership list available to the public

Chilliwack Men's Centre
4166 Eckert St, Yarrow BC V2R 5J6
604 823-0133; Fax: 604 823-0139
Toll-free: 866 866-0701
W: www.bcteenchallenge.com

Council On Drug Abuse
120-215 Spadina Ave, Toronto ON M5T 2C7
416 763-1491; Fax: 416 979-3936
E: info@drugabuse.ca
W: www.drugabuse.ca
Year Founded: 1969
Budget: $350,000
No of Paid Staff: 2
Speakers Available
Library: Y
Languages: English; French
Library:
Library Digest Package *(Open to the public)*

Défi Jeunesse Mauricie
100 ch Petite Rivière Souris,
St-Mathieu-du-Parc QC G0X 1N0
819 532-2335; Fax: 819 532-2929
W: www.defijeunessemauricie.com
Executive:
Dir/Fondateur: René Couture
Dir/Fondateur: Anne Demers Couture

Labrador Inuit Association
Mailing: GD, Rigolet NL A0P 1P0
709 947-3383; Fax: 709 947-3371
E: pmsheppard@nunatsiavut.com

Langley Intergroup Office
16-20449 Douglas Cres, Langley BC V3A 4B6
604 533-2600

Makkovik Field Office
Mailing: GD, Makkovik NL A0P 1J0
709 923-2365; Fax: 709 923-2366
E: cgear@nunatsiavut.com

Native Alcohol and Drug Abuse Counselling Association
Paqtnkek First Nation
128 Saqamaw Rd, RR 1, Afton Station NS B0H 1A0
902 386-2048; Fax: 902 386-2828
E: molly.peters@paqtnkek.ca
Executive:
Chairman: Juliana Julian
Coun: Thomas Christmas
Languages: English

Okanagan Men's Centre
4550 Glenmore Rd, Winfield BC V4V 1L7
888 575-3930; Fax: 250 766-5079
Toll-free: 877 777-7344
W: www.bcteenchallenge.com
Membership Fee: $1,000 one time fee

Responsible Gambling Council (RGC)
205-411 Richmond St E, Toronto ON M5A 3S5
416 499-9800; Fax: 416 499-8260
Toll-free: 888 391-1111
E: mail@rgco.org
W: www.responsiblegamblingcouncil.org
Executive:
Chair: Terry Finn
Sec: Michael Hunter
Year Founded: 1983
Criteria: Open
Budget: $800,000
No of Paid Staff: 12
Speakers Available
Library: Y *(Open to the public)*
Languages: English
Membership: 100
Membership Fee: $50 /year

Teen Challenge Inc.
Location: 9340 Sharon Rd, London ON N6P 1R6
Mailing: PO Box 777 Stn Lambeth
519 652-0777
Toll-free: 888 417-7777
W: www.teenchallenge.ca/tcfarm
Executive:
CEO: George Glover

◈Teen Challenge Alberta
Mailing: PO Box 1000 Stn A, Calgary AB T2H 3B7
403 931-3501; Fax: 403 931-3853
Toll-free: 800 856-8902
E: info@tcalberta.org
Executive:
Exec Dir: Juan Manigault

◈Manitoba:
Location: 260 Jean Marc Ave, Winnipeg MB R2C 2Z2
Mailing: RR 5, Site 525 Comp 55
204 949-9484; Fax: 204 949-9479
E: info@teenchallenge.tc
W: www.teenchallenge.tc
Executive:
Exec Dir: Steve Paulson
Languages: English

◈Teen Challenge Atlantic
Mailing: PO Box 911 Stn Main, Moncton NB E1C 8N8
506 758-2377; Fax: 506 758-9227
Toll-free: 800 965-7170
W: www.teenchallenge.ca/tcatlantic
Executive:
Exec Dir: Juan Manigault

◈Teen Challenge GTA Women's Centre
Mailing: PO Box 100 Stn Main, Aurora ON L4G 3H1
905 727-3913
Toll-free: 877 979-7770
W: www.teenchallenge.ca/tcgta
Executive:
Exec Dir: Garry Cox

◈Teen Challenge Ontario North
Mailing: PO Box 20012 Rpo Churchill Pl, Sault Ste. Marie ON P6A 6W3
705 942-7771; Fax: 705 942-8164
Toll-free: 800 480-3153
W: teenchallenge.ca/tcnorth
Executive:
Exec Dir: Dean Waddell

◈Teen Challenge Ottawa Valley Centre
Mailing: PO Box 61 Stn Main, Renfrew ON K7V 4A2
519 652-0777 1287
Toll-free: 888 417-7777
W: www.teenchallenge.ca/tcottawavalley

◈Thunder Bay:
Location: 545 Simpson St, Thunder Bay ON P7B 6T8
Mailing: PO Box 10443 Stn P
807 345-2873; Fax: 800 322-9230
E: thunderbay@teenchallenge.tc
W: www.teenchallengethunderbay.com
Executive:
Dir-Dev: Robby Ahuja
Year Founded: 2007
Speakers Available

◈Teen Challenge Saskatchewan
Location: 2155 Airport Dr, Bay 12, Saskatoon SK S7L 6M5
Mailing: PO Box 21111 RPO Grosvenor Prk, Saskatoon SK S7H 5N9
306 664-4673; Fax: 306 664-1982
E: info@tcsk.org
W: www.tcsk.org
Executive:
Dir: Denis Smail
Admv Asst: Rita Glass
Languages: English

CARE FACILITIES & HOMES

Alberta Continuing Care Association
Center 104
120-9405 50 ST NW, Edmonton AB T6B 2T4
780 435-0699; Fax: 780 436-9785
E: info@ab-cca.ca
W: www.ab-cca.ca
Executive:
Exec Dir: Bruce West
Dir- Member Serv/ Spec Proj: Denise MacDonald
Commun Coord: Jamie Wilson
Year Founded: 1981
Criteria: *Must be a Long Term Care Facility in Alberta.*
No of Paid Staff: 34
Speakers Available
Languages: English
Membership: 88

The Alberta Foster Parent Association
9750 35 Ave NW, Edmonton AB T6E 6J6
780 429-9923; Fax: 780 426-7151
Toll-free: 800 667-2372 within Alberta
E: info@afpaonline.com
W: www.afpaonline.com
Executive:
Pres: Norm Brownell
VP: Sylvia Thompson
Exec Dir: Katherine Jones

BC Care Providers Association
301-1338 Broadway W, Vancouver BC V6H 1H2
604 736-4233; Fax: 604 736-4266
E: info@bccare.ca
W: www.bccare.ca
Executive:
CEO: Daniel Fontaine
Languages: English

Bethany Care Society
1001 17 St NW, Calgary AB T2N 2E5
403 210-4600; Fax: 403 284-1992
Toll-free: 888 410-4679
E: info@bethanycare.com
W: www.bethanycare.com
Executive:
VP-Pastoral Serv: Jean Morris
Year Founded: 1945
Budget: $43,000,000
No of Paid Staff: 1,200
Languages: English
Membership Fee: Institutional: $100/year; Personal: $20/year

Business Information Group/BIG Magazines LP
80 Valleybrook Dr, North York ON M3B 2S9
416 442-5600; Fax: 416 442-2230
Toll-free: 800 268-7742
W: www.businessinformationgroup.ca
Executive:
Pres: Bruce Creighton
VP-Publishing: Alex Papanou
Mktg Mgr: Jennepher Hunter

Calgary Centre for Spiritual Living
103 17 Ave SE, Calgary AB T2G 1H3
403 244-8728; Fax: 403 245-3016
E: cploffice@positiveliving.org
W: www.calgary.csl.org
Executive:
Minister: Rev Carol Carnes
Languages: English

Coopérative de soutien à domicile du Pays des Vergers
276 av des Érables, Cowansville QC J2K 4C9
450 266-5484; Fax: 450 266-1919
W: www.soutienadomicile.coop
Executive:
Dir gén: Christine-Marie Gladu

Houselink Community Homes
805 Bloor St W, Toronto ON M6G 1L8
416 539-0690; Fax: 416 539-0693
E: info@houselink.on.ca
W: www.houselink.on.ca
Executive:
Pres: Luke Bowden
VP: Dana Gregoire
Exec Dir: Brian Davis
Treas: Peter Adamson
Mgr-Admin/Hum Res: Sian Ferguson
Fin Mgr: Charles Lior
Mgr-Prop Svcs: Carl Melvin

Long Term Care Association of Manitoba
103-1483 Pembina Hwy, Winnipeg MB R3T 2C6
204 477-9888; Fax: 204 477-9889
E: info@ltcam.mb.ca
W: www.ltcam.mb.ca
Year Founded: 1959
No of Paid Staff: 2
Speakers Available
Languages: English
Membership: 25

Mon Sheong Foundation
11199 Yonge St, Richmond Hill ON L4S 1L2
905 883-9288; Fax: 905 883-9855
E: msf@monsheong.org
W: www.monsheong.org
Executive:
Chair/Pres: Tim Kwan
CEO: Bernard Cheung

Ontario Association of Residences Treating Youth
210-550 Alden Rd, Markham ON L3R 6A8
905 475-5437; Fax: 905 475-5430
E: info@oarty.net
W: www.oarty.net
Executive:
Membership/Events Coord: Erin Vanderstelt
Year Founded: 1990
Criteria: *Licensed from M.C.Y.S.*
No of Paid Staff: 2
Languages: English
Membership: 80

Ontario Long Term Care Association
345 Renfrew Dr, Floor 3, Markham ON L3R 9S9
905 470-8995; Fax: 905 470-9595
E: info@oltca.com
W: www.oltca.com
Executive:
CEO: Christina Bisanz
Dir-Commun/Pub Affairs: Gilbert Heffern
Dir-Fin Policy: Brian Pollard
Dir-Health Plan: Paula Neves
Dir-Policy/Prof Dev: Nancy Cooper
Dir-Member Serv: Brian Baillie
Accnt: Greig Nishio
Budget: $3,000,000
No of Paid Staff: 15
Speakers Available
Library: Y
Languages: English
Membership: 410
Membership Fee: $260 + $29.78 per bed

Recovery Acres Calgary Society
1835 27 Ave SW, Calgary AB T2T 1H2
403 245-1196; Fax: 403 244-4019
E: info@recoveryacres.org
W: www.recoveryacres.org
Executive:
Exec Dir: John O'Reilly
Pub Rel Dir: Jim Calverley
Year Founded: 1973
Budget: $425,000
No of Paid Staff: 10
Speakers Available
Languages: English
Membership: 1,500
Membership Fee: $5/year

DISABLED

AiMHi - Prince George Association for Community Living
950 Kerry St, Prince George BC V2M 5A3
250 564-6408; Fax: 250 564-6801
E: aimhi@aimhi.ca
W: www.aimhi.ca
Executive:
Exec Dir: J (Bill) W Fildes
Exec Dir: Melinda Heidsma
Supplies Prop Coord: Lee Miners
Dir-Hum Res: Keith Dennison
Year Founded: 1951
Speakers Available
Languages: English
Membership list available to the public
Membership Fee: $10 Per Year

HEALTHCARE ASSOCIATIONS

ALSO - Assisted Living Southwestern Ontario
3141 Sandwich St, Windsor ON N9C 1A7
519 969-8188; Fax: 519 969-0390
E: info@alsogroup.org
W: www.appdgroup.org
Executive:
Pres: Katharen Hynes
Pres Elect: Ron Kerr
VP: Stan McDowell
Exec Dir: Lynn Calder
Hum Res Mgr: Leo Muzzatti
Treas: Paul Boyes

ARCH Disability Law Centre
110-425 Bloor St E, Toronto ON M4W 3R4
416 482-8255; Fax: 416 482-2981
Toll-free: 866 482-2724
Toll-free Fax: 866 881-2723
E: archlib@lao.on.ca
W: www.archdisabilitylaw.ca
Executive:
Exec Dir: Ivana Petricone
Prog/Litigation Asst: Theresa Sciberras
Languages: English

Ability New Brunswick / Capacité Nouveau-Brunswick
Park Office Centre
102-440 Wilsey Rd, Fredericton NB E3B 7G5
506 462-9555; Fax: 506 458-9134
E: info@abilitynb.ca
W: www.abilitynb.ca
Executive:
Pres: Courtney Keenan
VP: Pat Guest
Dir-Dev: Suzanne Wood
Exec Dir: Haley Flaro
Treas: Beth Corey
Sec: Chris Aalders
Year Founded: 1956
Criteria: *Open to anyone interested in the goals of the Association.*
No of Paid Staff: 5
Speakers Available
Languages: English; French
Membership Fee: $10

Ability New Brunswick / Capacité Nouveau-Brunswick - Moncton
Commerce House
20-236 St. George St, Moncton NB E1C 1W1
506 858-0311; Fax: 506 858-8290
Toll-free: 866 462-9555
E: info@abilitynb.ca
W: www.abilitynb.ca
Executive:
Rehab Counsellor: Liane Gould
No of Paid Staff: 5
Languages: English; French
Accnt: Greig Nishioeers

Ability Society of Alberta
331 41 Ave NE, Calgary AB T2E 2N4
403 262-9445; Fax: 403 262-4539
E: info@abilitysociety.org
W: www.abilitysociety.org
Executive:
Pres/CEO: Adrian Bohach
Dir-Ops: Kelly Gurtin
Year Founded: 1979
No of Paid Staff: 10
Languages: English
Library:
ACT Library

AboutFace
1003-123 Edward St, Toronto ON M5G 1E2
416 597-2229; Fax: 416 597-8494
Toll-free: 800 665-3223
E: info@aboutface.ca
W: www.aboutface.ca
Executive:
Exec Dir: Anna Pileggi
Year Founded: 1985
No of Paid Staff: 4
Speakers Available
Languages: English

Action Committee of People with Disabilities
948 View St, Victoria BC V8V 3L5
250 383-4105; Fax: 250 383-4835
E: acpd@actioncommittee.ca
W: www.actioncommittee.ca
Executive:
Pres: Jim Franklin
VP: Joanne Neubauer
Year Founded: 1975
Criteria: *Open to all.*
Budget: $96,000
No of Paid Staff: 1
Speakers Available
Library: Y *(Open to the public)*
Languages: English
Membership: 180
Membership Fee: $5 per year and up

Active Living Alliance for Canadians with a Disability
104-720 Belfast Rd, Ottawa ON K1G 0Z5
613 244-0052; Fax: 613 244-4857
Toll-free: 800 771-0663
E: ala@ala.ca
W: www.ala.ca
Executive:
Exec Dir: Jane Arkell
All abilities welcome Coord: Jason Dunkerley
Year Founded: 1988
Criteria: *Interest in active living and/or disability.*
No of Paid Staff: 10
Speakers Available
Languages: English; French
Membership: 5,000 +

Adaptation Inc.
1-3025 rue Girard, Trois-Rivières QC G8Z 2M4
819 372-0102; Fax: 819 372-0443
Executive:
Prop: Francis Giroux

Aide aux Personnes Obèses Handicapées du Québec Inc.
12716 boul Industriel, Pte-aux-Trembles QC H1A 3V2
514 254-8415; Fax: 514 256-6627
E: cdat@qc.aira.com
Executive:
Dir: André Beauchamp
Languages: English; French

Aim Croit
450-750 boul Marcel-Laurin,
Saint-Laurent QC H4M 2M4
514 744-2944; Fax: 514 744-5711
E: emploi@aimcroitqc.org
W: www.aimcroitqc.org
Executive:
Dir: May Polsky
Adj admin: Céline Turner
Speakers Available
Library: Y
Languages: English; French

Alice Saddy Association
401-111 Waterloo St, London ON N6B 2M4
519 433-2801; Fax: 519 433-1435
W: www.alicesaddy.com
Executive:
Exec Dir: Ken MacLellan
Dir-Coord Prog: Kathy Peters
Dir-Fin: Gail Lafreniere
Dir-Hum Res: Kathie Wolcott
Pub Rel Mgr/Fundraiser: Cindy Rektor
Supvr Support Serv: Barb Smith
Criteria: *Open to all.*
No of Paid Staff: 52
Languages: English

Alliance for Equality of Blind Canadians
Mailing: PO Box 20262 RPO Towne Centre,
Kelowna BC V1Y 9H2
Fax: 250 862-3966
Toll-free: 800 561-4774
E: info@blindcanadians.ca
W: www.blindcanadians.ca
Executive:
Pres: Donna Jodhan
1st VP: Lui Greco
2nd VP: Rajesh Malik
Treas: Charles Bailey
Languages: English

Amalgame Montréal Inc.
5970 rue Bannantyne, Verdun QC H4H 1H8
514 362-9551
E: rcaron@amalgamemontreal.com
W: www.amalgamemontreal.com
Executive:
Dir: Renée Caron

Les Amputés de guerre - Québec
Location: 530-606 rue Cathcart, Montréal QC H3B 1K9
Mailing: CP 11027 succ Centre Ville,
Montréal QC H3C 4W6
514 398-0759; Fax: 514 398-0699
Toll-free: 800 250-3030
Toll-free Fax: 800 219-8988
E: serviceclientele@amputesdeguerre.ca
W: www.amputesdeguerre.ca
Executive:
Dir gén: Marlène Girard
Year Founded: 1918
Criteria: *Personne amputée (âgée de moins de 19ans)*
Speakers Available
Library: Y *(Open to the public)*
Languages: French; English

Antigonish Guysborough Early Childhood Intervention Program
Martha Centre
25 Bay St, Floor 2, Antigonish NS B2G 2G5
902 863-2298; Fax: 902 867-1037
E: agecip@ns.aliantzinc.ca
W: www.nsnet.org
Executive:
Exec Dir: Brenda MacInnis
No of Paid Staff: 7
Speakers Available
Languages: English

Association de Montréal pour la déficience intellectuelle
100-633 boul Crémazie E, Montréal QC H2M 1L9
514 381-2307; Fax: 514 381-0454
E: info@amdi.info
W: www.amdi.info
Executive:
Dir gén: Nadia Bastien
Year Founded: 1935
Languages: French; English

Association de personnes handicapées physiques de Cowansville et région
Location: 495 rue du Sud, Cowansville QC J2K 3S7
Mailing: CP 307
450 266-4744; Fax: 450 266-1263
E: info@aphpcr.qc.ca
W: www.aphpcr.qc.ca
Executive:
Dir: Francine Tremblay
Adj à la dir: Ruth Potvin

Association des parents et amis du malade émotionel Centre du Québec Inc.
1090 rue Lafontaine, Drummondville QC J2B 1M9
819 478-1216; Fax: 819 478-5799
E: apamedr@cgocable.ca
W: www.apamedrummondville.org
Executive:
Prés: Diane Clavet
VP: Michel Laroche
Dir: Karine Leroux
Sec/Comptable: Guylaine Manseau
Intervenante: Céline Mondou
Year Founded: 1985
Languages: French

Association du Québec pour enfants avec problèmes auditifs
A446-3700 rue Berri, Montréal QC H2L 4G9
514 842-8706; Fax: 514 842-4006
Toll-free: 877 842-4006
E: aqepa@aqepa.org
W: www.aqepa.org
Executive:
Dir gén: Édith Keays
Resp des commun: Sarrah Osama
Year Founded: 1972
Criteria: *Lien avec la surdite.*
No of Paid Staff: 4
Speakers Available
Library: Y *(Open to the public)*
Languages: French
Membership: 600

Association for Community Living -Algoma/East Algoma Office
The Lester B. Pearson Civic Ctre
255 Hwy 108 N, Elliot Lake ON P5A 2T1
705 848-2475; Fax: 705 848-2520
Toll-free: 800 385-7235
W: www.communitylivingalgoma.org
Languages: English

Association for Community Living - Quesnel Satellite Office
611 Anderson Dr, Quesnel BC V2J 3K6
250 992-7774; Fax: 250 992-6651
Executive:
Exec Dir: Colleen Hackler
Mgr: Pat Marshall
Budget: $80,000
No of Paid Staff: 24
Speakers Available
Library: Y *(Open to the public)*
Languages: English
Membership: 30 *(Lists available to the public)*
Membership Fee: $5 per year

Association Garagona Inc.
23 ch Garagona, Frelighsburg QC J0J 1C0
450 298-5159; Fax: 450 298-5554
E: info@campgaragona.qc.ca
W: www.campgaragona.qc.ca
Executive:
Dir gén: Nicholas Brien

Association pour l'Intégration Sociale d'Ottawa
150-235 Donald St, Ottawa ON K1K 1N1
613 744-2241; Fax: 613 744-4898
E: info@aiso.org
W: www.aiso.org

Association pour l'intégration sociale - région de Québec
5225 3e Av O, Québec QC G1H 6G6
418 622-4290; Fax: 418 622-1683
E: aisq@aisq.org
W: www.aisq.org
Executive:
Prés: Jean Lafrance
Dir gén: Marie Boulanger-Lemieux
Agent d'info: Rachel Germain
Admin adj: Céline Paré
Year Founded: 1961
Budget: $175,000
No of Paid Staff: 4
Speakers Available
Library: Y *(Open to the public)*
Languages: French
Membership: 330
Membership Fee: Range $12 - $25 Per année aux membres

The BC Lions Society for Children With Disabilities
2095 Granite St, Victoria BC V8S 3G5
250 370-0518; Fax: 250 370-5098
E: info@forthekidsbc.org
W: www.lionsbc.ca
Executive:
Office Mgr: Eileen Torgeson
Year Founded: 1952
Languages: English

Banner Residence Association
624 Banner Ave, North Bay ON P1A 1X8
705 472-4844
Criteria: *Services are open to the physically disabled.*
No of Paid Staff: 16
Languages: English

Beaufort Association for the Mentally Handicapped
536A 5th St, Courtenay BC V9N 1K3
250 338-9398
E: coptions@shaw.ca
Executive:
Pres: Gil Hudgin
VP: Carol McLaughlin
Mgr: Joky Winton
Sec: Shirley McCann
No of Paid Staff: 7
Speakers Available
Languages: English

Blissymbolics Communication International
300-1370 Don Mills Rd, Toronto ON M3B 3N7
416 644-8291; Fax: 905 481-2389
E: bcic@blissymbolics.ca
W: www.blissymbolics.ca
Executive:
Dir/Teacher: Sherly Thankappan
Volunteer Consultant: Shirley McNaughton
Languages: English

The Bob Rumball Centre for the Deaf
2395 Bayview Ave, Toronto ON M2L 1A2
416 449-9651; Fax: 416 449-8881
E: info@bobrumball.org
W: www.bobrumball.org
Executive:
Chairman: Alistair Fraser
Exec Dir: Derek Rumball
Year Founded: 1979
No of Paid Staff: 18
Speakers Available
Languages: English

The Bob Rumball Foundation for the Deaf
2395 Bayview Ave, Toronto ON M2L 1A2
416 449-9651; Fax: 416 449-8881
E: joannebursa@bobrumball.org
W: bobrumball.org
Executive:
Foundation Dir: Suzanne Prosser

British Columbia Coalition of People with Disabilities
204-456 Broadway W, Vancouver BC V5Y 1R3
604 875-0188; Fax: 604 875-9227
Toll-free: 800 663-1278
E: feedback@bccpd.bc.ca
W: www.bccpd.bc.ca
Executive:
Pres: Johanna Johnson
External VP: Lucy Goncalves
Internal VP: Derek Isobe
Treas: Al Hanet
Languages: English

Brockville & District Association for Community Involvement
4-2495 Parkedale Ave, Brockville ON K6V 3H2
613 345-4092; Fax: 613 345-7469
E: bdaci@ripnet.com
W: www.bdaci.com
Executive:
Pres: Bobbi Stephen
Exec Dir: Beth French

Burnaby Association for Community Inclusion
2702 Norland Ave, Burnaby BC V5B 3A6
604 299-7851; Fax: 604 299-5921
E: reception@gobaci.com
W: www.gobaci.com
Executive:
Pres: Merrilyn Cook
VP: Troy Nikolai
VP: Susan Anthony
Exec/Dir-Serv: Richard Faucher
Exec Dir-Support Serv: Tayna Sather
Languages: English

CNIB - National Office
1929 Bayview Ave, Toronto ON M4G 3E8
416 486-2500; Fax: 416 480-7000
Toll-free: 800 563-2642
E: info@cnib.ca
W: www.cnib.ca
Executive:
Pres/CEO: John Rafferty
VP-Hum Res: Sandra Levy
IS Dir: Vicki Mains
Year Founded: 1918
Speakers Available
Library: Y *(Open to the public)*
Languages: English; French
Library:
CNIB Library for the Blind
◈ ***CNIB Western Canada:***
15 Colonel Baker Pl NE, Calgary AB T2E 4Z3
403 266-8831; Fax: 403 265-5029
Toll-free: 800 365-2642
E: alberta@cnib.ca
W: www.cnib.ca

HEALTHCARE ASSOCIATIONS

Executive:
Exec Dir: Cathy McFee
Year Founded: 1918
Languages: English; French

◇ ***Calgary District Office***
15 Colonel Baker Pl NE, Calgary AB T2E 4Z3
403 266-8831; Fax: 403 265-5029
Toll-free: 800 376-2642
E: alberta@cnib.ca
W: www.cnib.ca
Year Founded: 1918
Criteria: *Services are available to anyone experiencing vision loss that cannot be corrected with ordinary lenses.*
No of Paid Staff: 33
Speakers Available
Languages: English
Membership: 9,500 clients in Alberta

◇ ***Grande Prairie District Office:***
105-9919 99 Ave, Grande Prairie AB T8V 0R6
780 539-4719; Fax: 780 539-3331
Toll-free: 800 365-2642
E: alberta@cnib.ca
W: www.cnib.ca
Year Founded: 1918
No of Paid Staff: 1
Speakers Available
Languages: English; French

◇ ***Lethbridge District Office:***
100-410 Stafford Dr S, Lethbridge AB T1J 2L2
403 327-1044; Fax: 403 380-2672
Toll-free: 800 563-2642
E: alberta@cnib.ca
W: www.cnib.ca
Year Founded: 1918
Speakers Available
Library: Y *(Open to the public)*
Languages: English

◇ ***Medicine Hat District Office:***
102-520 2 St SE, Medicine Hat AB T1A 0C6
403 527-2211; Fax: 403 526-3548
Toll-free: 800 376-2642
E: alberta@cnib.ca
W: www.cnib.ca
Executive:
Admv Asst/Fund Dev Rep: Susan Storozuk
Client Supp Spec: Bob Short
Year Founded: 1918
Speakers Available
Library: Y *(Open to the public)*
Languages: English; French
Membership: 9,500 in AB

◇ ***Red Deer***
4-5015 48 St, Red Deer AB T4N 1S9
403 346-0037; Fax: 403 341-3925
E: alberta@cnib.ca
W: www.cnib.ca
Executive:
Chm: Donald Biberdorf
Exec Dir: Cathy McFee
Year Founded: 1918
Languages: English; French

◇ ***Yellowknife District Office:***
Location: 4-5003 48th St, Yellowknife NT X1A 2N6
Mailing: PO Box 872 Stn Main
867 873-2647; Fax: 867 873-2657
Toll-free: 800 563-2642
E: alberta@cnib.ca
W: www.cnib.ca
Executive:
Reg Mgr: Norma Jarvis
Year Founded: 1918
Speakers Available
Library: Y *(Open to the public)*
Languages: English; French

◈ ***British Columbia/Yukon:***
200-5055 Joyce St, Vancouver BC V5R 6B2
604 431-2121; Fax: 604 431-2099
E: bcy@cnib.ca
W: www.cnib.ca
Executive:
Exec Dir: John Mulka
Assoc Dir-Serv/Ops: Andrea Gronfeldt
Year Founded: 1918
Budget: $8,500,000
No of Paid Staff: 70
Speakers Available
Library: Y *(Open to the public)*
Languages: English
Membership: 18,500
Membership Fee: $150 - Lifetime; $15 - Annual

◇ ***Kamloops District Office***
145-540 Seymour St, Kamloops BC V2C 2G9
250 374-8080; Fax: 250 374-8033
Toll-free: 877 374-8080
E: les.nolin@cnib.ca
W: www.cnib.ca
Executive:
Chair: Rob Sleath
Exec Dir: John Mulka
Year Founded: 1918
No of Paid Staff: 2
Languages: English

◇ ***Prince George District Office***
100-490 Quebec St, Prince George BC V2L 5N5
250 563-1702; Fax: 250 563-1787
Toll-free: 800 563-2642
E: bcy@cnib.ca
W: www.cnib.ca
Executive:
Exec Dir: John Mulka
Year Founded: 1918
Budget: $250,000
No of Paid Staff: 4
Speakers Available
Languages: English

◇ ***Southern Interior District Office***
101-1456 St. Paul St, Kelowna BC V1Y 2E6
250 763-1191; Fax: 250 763-1129
Toll-free: 800 563-2642
E: bcy@cnib.ca
W: www.cnib.ca
Languages: English

◇ ***Vancouver Island District Office***
2340 Richmond Rd, Victoria BC V8R 4R9
250 595-1100; Fax: 250 595-1129
E: bcy@cnib.ca
W: www.cnib.ca
Year Founded: 1818
Speakers Available
Library: Y
Languages: English; French

◈ ***Manitoba:***
1080 Portage Ave, Winnipeg MB R3G 3M3
204 774-5421; Fax: 204 775-5090
Toll-free: 800 563-2642
E: manitoba@cnib.ca
W: www.cnib.ca
Executive:
Pres/CEO: Bob Brennan
Exec Dir: Delcy-Ann Selymes
Year Founded: 1918
Speakers Available
Languages: English; French

◇ ***Brandon District Office:***
354 10th St, Brandon MB R7A 4G1
204 727-0631; Fax: 204 727-1139
Toll-free: 800 563-2642
E: manitoba@cnib.ca
W: www.cnib.ca
Criteria: *Payment of membership fee.*
No of Paid Staff: 5
Speakers Available
Library: Y
Languages: English
Membership Fee: $25

◈ ***New Brunswick:***
130-77 Westmorland St, Fredericton NB E3B 6Z3
506 458-0060; Fax: 506 458-9219
Toll-free: 800 563-2642
E: newbrunswick@cnib.ca
W: www.cnib.ca
Executive:
Dir-Govt Rels: Lui Greco
Year Founded: 1918
Library: Y *(Open to the public)*
Languages: English; French

◇ ***Bathurst District Office:***
Keystone Place
270 Douglas Ave, Floor 1, Bathurst NB E2A 1M9
506 546-9922; Fax: 506 546-0179
Toll-free: 800 563-2642
E: newbrunswick@cnib.ca
W: www.cnib.ca
Executive:
Mgr: Denise Coward
Year Founded: 1918
No of Paid Staff: 2
Languages: English; French

◇ ***Moncton District Office:***
T120-22 Church St, Moncton NB E1C 0P7
506 857-4240; Fax: 506 857-3019
E: newbrunswick@cnib.ca
W: www.cnib.ca
Executive:
Pres: John M. Rafferty
No of Paid Staff: 7
Speakers Available
Languages: English; French
Membership: 800 +

◇ ***Saint John District Office:***
A150-40 Charlotte St, Saint John NB E2L 2H6
506 634-7277; Fax: 506 634-7202
Toll-free: 800 563-2642
E: newbrunswick@cnib.ca
W: www.cnib.ca
Executive:
Mgr: Ruth Edmondson
Year Founded: 1918
No of Paid Staff: 6
Languages: English; French

◈ ***Newfoundland & Labrador Division:***
70 The Boulevard, St. John's NL A1A 1K2
709 754-1180; Fax: 709 754-2018
Toll-free: 800 563-2642
E: nl@cnib.ca
W: www.cnib.ca
Year Founded: 1918
Criteria: *Open to all to be volunteers. Client status is available to individuals whose daily life is affected by vision loss.*
No of Paid Staff: 17
Speakers Available
Library: Y
Languages: English
Membership: 2,410
Membership Fee: $15

◇ ***Corner Brook District Office:***
CNIB Downtown Health Center
1F-3 Herald Ave, Corner Brook NL A2H 4B8
709 639-9167; Fax: 709 639-9290
Toll-free: 800 563-2642

E: nl@cnib.ca
W: www.cnib.ca
Year Founded: 1918
No of Paid Staff: 27
Speakers Available
Library: Y *(Open to the public)*
Languages: English
Membership: 2,210 *(Lists available to the public)*
Membership Fee: $15

◇ **Grand Falls-Windsor District Office:**
Location: 1A O'Neill Ave,
Grnd-Falls-Windsor NL A2A 2J8
Mailing: PO Box 442 Stn Main
709 489-6515; Fax: 709 489-6516
Toll-free: 800 563-2642 8366
E: nl@cnib.ca
W: www.cnib.ca
Year Founded: 1918
Library: Y *(Open to the public)*
Languages: English; French
Membership list available to the public

◈ **Nova Scotia & PEI Division:**
6136 Almon St, Halifax NS B3K 1T8
902 453-1480; Fax: 902 454-6570
Toll-free: 800 563-2642
E: nspei@cnib.ca
W: www.cnib.ca
Executive:
Mgr-Progs/Serv: Peter Parsons
Dir-Dev: Warren Spires
Exec Dir-Atlantic Cda: Pam Gow-Boyd
Commun Mgr Atlantic Cda: Catherine Kieran
Dir-Fin Eastern Zone: Rosalind Moyst
Dir-Hum Res: Colleen Fitzgerald
Exec Asst: Wendy Constable
Year Founded: 1918
Criteria: *Open to anyone experiencing vision loss that cannot be corrected with ordinary lenses.*
No of Paid Staff: 32
Speakers Available
Languages: English
Membership: 4,600 people served

◇ **Charlottetown District Office:**
201-342 Grafton St, Charlottetown PE C1A 1L8
902 566-2580; Fax: 902 628-1445
Toll-free: 800 563-2642
E: nspei@cnib.ca
W: www.cnib.ca
Executive:
Dir-Dev: Warren Spires
Registrar: Maryann Robinson
Exec Dir: Pam Gow-Boyd
Commun Mgr Atlantic Cda: Catherine Kieran
Dir-Hum Res: Colleen Fitzgerald
Year Founded: 1918
Criteria: *Anyone with a vision loss that cannot be corrected using an ordinary lense.*
No of Paid Staff: 4
Languages: English; French

◇ **Sydney District Office:**
45 Weatherbee Rd, Mira Road NS B1M 0A1
902 564-5711; Fax: 902 562-9802
Toll-free: 800 563-2642
E: nspei@cnib.ca
W: www.cnib.ca
Year Founded: 1918
No of Paid Staff: 2
Languages: English; French

◈ **Central Regional Hub:**
10-20 Anne St S, Barrie ON L4N 2C6
705 728-3352; Fax: 705 722-5305
Toll-free: 800 563-0887
E: ontario@cnib.ca
W: www.cnib.ca
No of Paid Staff: 10
Speakers Available
Languages: English

◇ **Durham Service Centre:**
D-1 Mary St N, Oshawa ON L1G 7W8
905 436-7732; Fax: 905 436-1202
Toll-free: 800 563-0887
E: ontario@cnib.ca
W: www.cnib.ca
Year Founded: 1918
No of Paid Staff: 4
Languages: English; French

◇ **Peterborough District Office:**
300-159 King St, Peterborough ON K9J 2R8
705 745-6918; Fax: 705 745-9899
E: info@cnib.ca
W: www.cnib.ca
Executive:
Reg Serv/Ops Mgr: Rosemary Kitney
Year Founded: 1918
Criteria: *Vision Problem*
No of Paid Staff: 7
Speakers Available
Library: Y
Languages: English; French
Membership list available to the public

◇ **Simcoe-Muskoka District Office:**
10-20 Anne St S, Barrie ON L4N 2C6
705 728-3352; Fax: 705 722-5305
Toll-free: 800 563-0887
E: info@cnib.ca
W: www.cnib.ca
Executive:
Man Dir-Serv/Ops Central Reg: Paul Ting
Languages: English

◈ **North Regional Hub:**
303 York St, Sudbury ON P3E 2A5
705 675-2468; Fax: 705 675-6635
Toll-free: 888 275-2468
E: ontario@cnib.ca
W: www.cnib.ca
Executive:
Mgr-Info Sys: Vaden Stoodley
Year Founded: 1918
No of Paid Staff: 20
Speakers Available
Languages: English; French

◇ **Nispissing/Parry Sound District Office:**
Location: 310-222 McIntyre St W,
North Bay ON P1B 2Y8
Mailing: 303 York St, Sudbury ON P3E 2A5
705 675-2468; Fax: 705 675-6635
E: ontario@cnib.ca
W: www.cnib.ca
Executive:
Mgr-Info Sys: Vaden Stoodley
No of Paid Staff: 4
Library: Y *(Open to the public)*
Languages: English; French
Membership: 650

◇ **Northern Ontario District Office:**
Location: 312-60 Wilson Ave, Timmins ON P4N 2S7
Mailing: 303 York St, Sudbury ON P3E 2A5
705 264-2312; Fax: 705 264-9851
Toll-free: 888 675-2468
E: ontario@cnib.ca
W: www.cnib.ca
Executive:
Mgr-Info Sys: Vaden Stoodley
Year Founded: 1918
No of Paid Staff: 6
Languages: English; French

◇ **Northwest Ontario:**
Location: 229 Camelot St, Thunder Bay ON P7A 4B2
Mailing: 303 York St, Sudbury ON P3E 2A5
807 345-3341; Fax: 807 345-0786
Toll-free: 800 411-3337
E: ontario@cnib.ca
W: www.cnib.ca
Executive:
Mgr-Info Sys: Vaden Stoodley
Year Founded: 1918
Budget: $800,000
No of Paid Staff: 9
Languages: English
Membership list available to the public
Membership Fee: $15

◇ **Sault-Algoma District Office**
Location: 205-477 Queen St E,
Sault Ste. Marie ON P6A 1Z5
Mailing: 303 York St, Sudbury ON P3E 2A5
705 949-2610 5454; Fax: 705 949-2291
Toll-free: 888 675-2468
E: ontario@cnib.ca
W: www.cnib.ca
Executive:
Rehab/Coord Client Serv: Terry Caporossi
Mgr-Info Sys: Vaden Stoodley
Languages: English

◈ **Ontario Central West Regional Hub:**
115 Parkdale Ave S, Hamilton ON L8K 6K4
905 528-8555; Fax: 905 527-9536
Toll-free: 888 275-5332
E: ontario@cnib.ca
W: www.cnib.ca
Executive:
Sec/Dir-Client Serv: Tammy McLellan
Year Founded: 1918
No of Paid Staff: 64
Languages: English; French

◇ **Brantford**
Location: 67 King St, Brantford ON N3T 3C8
Mailing: 115 Parkdale Ave S, Hamilton ON L8K 6K4
519 752-6831; Fax: 519 752-4920
Toll-free: 888 275-5332
E: ontario@cnib.ca
W: www.cnib.ca
Year Founded: 1918
Criteria: *Open to those experiencing visual difficulties in both eyes.*
No of Paid Staff: 9
Speakers Available
Library: Y
Languages: English
Library:
CNIB Library Services

◇ **Halton/Peel District**
Location: 300-50 Burnhamthorpe Rd W, Mississauga ON L5B 3C2
Mailing: 115 Parkdale Ave S, Hamilton ON L8K 6K4
905 275-5332; Fax: 905 527-9536
Toll-free: 888 275-5332
E: info@cnib.ca
W: www.cnib.ca
Year Founded: 1918
Criteria: *People with visual impairment.*
Languages: English
Membership: 3,849

◇ **Niagara District Office**
Location: Ina Grafton Gage Village, 413 Linwell Rd, St Catharines ON L2M 7Y2
Mailing: 115 Parkdale Ave S, Hamilton ON L8K 6K4
905 938-9250; Fax: 905 938-3188
E: ontario@cnib.ca
W: www.cnib.ca

Executive:
Reg Mgr: Thom Burger
Speakers Available
Library: Y
Languages: English; French

◈ ***Ontario Southwest Regional Hub:***
749 Base Line Rd E, London ON N6C 2R6
519 685-8420; Fax: 519 685-8419
Toll-free: 800 265-4127
E: sherry.malcho@cnib.ca
W: www.cnib.ca
Year Founded: 1918
Criteria: *Eye report no older than 12 mos. Can be obtained after registration.*
Budget: $1,000,000
No of Paid Staff: 25
Speakers Available
Library: Y
Languages: English

◇ ***Bruce/Dufferin/Grey***
Location: 202-908 2nd Ave E,
Owen Sound ON N4K 6H6
Mailing: 749 Base Line Rd E, London ON N6C 2R6
519 371-2721; Fax: 519 371-2741
Toll-free: 800 265-4127
E: sherry.malcho@cnib.ca
W: www.cnib.ca
Year Founded: 1918
No of Paid Staff: 5
Languages: English; French

◇ ***Essex/Kent Office***
Location: 245 Janette Ave, Floor 1,
Windsor ON N9A 4Z2
Mailing: 749 Base Line Rd E, London ON N6C 2R6
519 253-1900; Fax: 519 253-4440
E: sherry.malcho@cnib.ca
W: www.cnib.ca
Year Founded: 1918
Budget: $900,000
No of Paid Staff: 10
Speakers Available
Library: Y
Languages: English; French

◇ ***Waterloo/Wellington***
Location: 160-180 King St S, Waterloo ON N2J 1P8
Mailing: 160-749 Base Line Rd E, London ON N6C 2R6
519 742-3536; Fax: 519 742-4003
Toll-free: 800 265-4127
E: sherry.malcho@cnib.ca
W: www.cnib.ca
Year Founded: 1918
No of Paid Staff: 16
Speakers Available
Languages: English; French
Membership: 2,000

◈ ***Ottawa/Lanark Regional Hub:***
101-1355 Bank St, Ottawa ON K1H 8K7
613 563-4021; Fax: 613 563-1898
Toll-free: 866 842-9071
E: info@cnib.ca
W: www.cnib.ca
Executive:
Reg Dir: Mike Nicholson
Year Founded: 1918
Languages: English; French

◇ ***Eastern Counties***
203-4 Montreal Rd, Cornwall ON K6H 1B1
613 936-2300; Fax: 613 936-2296
Toll-free: 866 842-9071
E: info@cnib.ca
W: www.cnib.ca
Executive:
Reg Dir: Michael Nicholson
Year Founded: 1918
No of Paid Staff: 3
Speakers Available
Languages: English; French

◇ ***Hastings/Prince Edward Counties***
Belleville Shopping Plaza
8-470 Dundas St E, Belleville ON K8N 1G1
613 966-8833; Fax: 613 962-0414
Toll-free: 866 842-9071
E: info@cnib.ca
W: www.cnib.ca
Executive:
Reg Dir: Mike Nicholson
Year Founded: 1918
Languages: English; French

◇ ***Kingston***
826 Princess St, Kingston ON K7L 1G3
613 542-4975; Fax: 613 542-8639
Toll-free: 866 842-9071
E: donna.norman@cnib.ca
W: www.cnib.ca
Executive:
Mgr: Donna Norman
Receptionist: Cathy Radnor
Year Founded: 1918
Speakers Available
Languages: English; French

◈ ***Québec Division:***
3044 rue Delisle, Montréal QC H4C 1M9
514 934-4622; Fax: 514 934-2131
Toll-free: 800 465-4622
W: www.inca.ca
Executive:
Dir gén: Marie-Camille Blais
Year Founded: 1918
No of Paid Staff: 14
Speakers Available
Library: Y
Languages: English; French
Membership: 98 *(Lists available to the public)*

◈ ***Saskatchewan Division:***
2550 Broad St, Regina SK S4P 3Z4
306 525-2571; Fax: 306 565-3300
Toll-free: 800 563-2642
E: saskatchewan@cnib.ca
W: cnib.ca
Executive:
Ops Mgr: Debby Cuninghame
Year Founded: 1918
Criteria: *All members in any class of membership shall be elected by a majority vote of the Board.*
Languages: English
Membership Fee: $15

◇ ***Saskatoon District Office:***
1705 McKercher Dr, Saskatoon SK S7H 5N6
306 374-4545; Fax: 306 955-6224
Toll-free: 800 563-2642
E: saskatchewan@cnib.ca
W: www.cnib.ca
Executive:
Mgr-Client Serv: Selene Daniel-Whyte
Criteria: *Referral from Doctor/Eye Report.*
Speakers Available
Library: Y *(Open to the public)*
Languages: English

Calgary Board of Education - Service for the Deaf and Hard-of-Hearing

728 32 St NW, Calgary AB T2N 2V9
403 777-7240; Fax: 403 777-6016
W: www.cbe.ab.ca
Executive:
Principal: Norma-Jean Taylor
Languages: English

Calgary HandiBus Association

231 37 Ave NE, Calgary AB T2E 8J2
403 276-8028; Fax: 403 276-1434
W: www.calgaryhandibus.com
Executive:
Dir-Fin: Louis Jesudason
Year Founded: 1971
Criteria: *Subject to approval by Board of Directors.*
Budget: $13,000,000
No of Paid Staff: 200
Speakers Available
Languages: English
Membership: 220
Membership Fee: $10

Calgary Society for Persons with Disabilities

3410 Spruce Dr SW, Calgary AB T3C 3A4
403 246-4450; Fax: 403 246-4530
E: cspd@cspd.ab.ca
Executive:
Exec Dir: Mickey Greiner
Year Founded: 1974
Criteria: *Open to anyone except employees.*
Budget: $1,500,000
No of Paid Staff: 50
Languages: English
Membership: 50
Membership Fee: $10

Camrose Association for Community Living

4604 57 St, Camrose AB T4V 2E7
780 672-0257; Fax: 780 672-7484
W: www.cafcl.org
Executive:
Prog Dir: Lisa Kosinski
Prog Dir: Leevi Hasso
Tech Serv Mgr: Brian Stevens

Canadian Association for Community Living -National Office

York University Kinsmen Bldg
4700 Keele St, Toronto ON M3J 1P3
416 661-9611; Fax: 416 661-5701
Toll-free: 800 856-2207
E: inform@cacl.ca
W: www.cacl.ca
Executive:
Treas: Peter Chivers
Sec: Michael Bach
Year Founded: 1958
No of Paid Staff: 9
Speakers Available
Languages: English; French
Membership: 42,000

◈ ***Alberta:***
11724 Kingsway NW, Edmonton AB T5G 0X5
780 451-3055; Fax: 780 453-5779
Toll-free: 800 252-7556
E: mail@aacl.org
W: www.aacl.org
Executive:
CEO: Bruce Uditsky
Librarian: Lisa Snyder
Year Founded: 1956
No of Paid Staff: 10
Speakers Available
Library: Y *(Open to the public)*
Languages: English
Library:
Reg Peters Resource Centre *(Open to the public)*

◇ ***Calgary:***
212-4014 Macleod Trail SE, Calgary AB T2G 2R7
403 717-0361; Fax: 403 228-2132
W: www.aacl.org

Executive:
Exec Dir: Lori Adamchick
Year Founded: 1984
No of Paid Staff: 2
Speakers Available
Library: Y
Languages: English
Library:
Resource Library *(Open to the public)*

◇ ***Edmonton:***
104-18304 105 Ave NW, Edmonton AB T5S 0C6
780 454-0701; Fax: 780 454-0843
W: www.gatewayassociation.ca
Executive:
Exec Dir: Cindy de Bruijn
Office Mgr: Sarah Preston
Commun Mgr: Christine Spottiswood
Year Founded: 1975
No of Paid Staff: 18
Speakers Available
Library: Y
Languages: English
Membership: 220
Membership Fee: $20 - Family
Library:
Family Resource Room *(Open to the public)*

◇ ***Fort McMurray:***
10010 Franklin Ave, Fort McMurray AB T9H 2K6
780 791-3009; Fax: 780 791-7506
W: www.aacl.org
Executive:
Exec Dir: Tracy Condon
Year Founded: 1969
No of Paid Staff: 12
Speakers Available
Library: Y *(Open to the public)*
Languages: English

◇ ***Red Deer:***
6010 45 Ave, Red Deer AB T4N 3M4
403 347-3333; Fax: 403 342-2677
W: www.parklandclass.org
Executive:
CEO: Phil Stephan
COO: Dan Verstraete
CFO: Roxanne MacKenzie
Chief Educ Serv: Trudy Lewis
Hum Res Mgr: Joy Smith
Bus Dev Mgr: Brendon Krygsveld
No of Paid Staff: 40
Languages: English

◈ ***Lethbridge***
401 21A St N, Lethbridge AB T1H 6L6
403 329-1525; Fax: 403 329-1435
W: www.sacla.ca
Year Founded: 1980
No of Paid Staff: 150
Speakers Available

◈ ***British Columbia***
227 Sixth St, New Westminster BC V3L 3A5
604 777-9100; Fax: 604 777-9394
Toll-free: 800 618-1119
E: info@bcacl.org
W: www.bcacl.org
Executive:
Pres: Annette Delaplace
Exec Dir: Faith Bodnar
Dir-Fin/Admv: Frank Peng
Dir-Commun: Danielle Kelliher
Year Founded: 1955
Speakers Available
Languages: English
Membership: 70 *(Lists available to the public)*
Membership Fee: Varies

◈ ***Campbell River and District***
1153 Greenwood St, Campbell River BC V9W 3C5
250 286-0391; Fax: 250 286-3732
E: aclpub@conected.bc.ca
W: www.cradacl.bc.ca/
No of Paid Staff: 150
Speakers Available
Library: Y
Languages: English
Membership: 150

◈ ***Kelowna & District***
555 Fuller Ave, Kelowna BC V1Y 7W8
250 763-4837; Fax: 250 763-4837
E: cdaley@kdscl.bc.ca
W: www.kdscl.bc.ca
Executive:
Exec Dir: Charisse Daley
Year Founded: 1953
No of Paid Staff: 90
Speakers Available
Languages: English

◈ ***Langley***
23535 44 Ave, Langley BC V2Z 2V2
604 534-8611; Fax: 604 534-4763
E: main@langleyacl.com
W: www.langleyacl.com
Executive:
Exec Dir: Dan Collins
HR Mgr/Labour Rel: Corrine Barton
Qual Assur Mgr: Kim Bucholtz
Admv Asst: Gillian Sutcliffe
Year Founded: 1959
No of Paid Staff: 150
Languages: English
Membership list available to the public

◈ ***Powell River***
201-4675 Marine Ave, Powell River BC V8A 2L2
604 485-6411; Fax: 604 485-6419
E: ltipton@pracl.ca
W: www.pracl.ca
Executive:
Exec Dir: Lilla Tipton
Year Founded: 1954
Budget: $7,000,000
No of Paid Staff: 194
Speakers Available
Library: Y *(Open to the public)*
Languages: English
Membership: 75
Membership Fee: $5/year

◈ ***Prince Rupert***
Mailing: PO Box 442 CDO Prince Rupert,
Prince Rupert BC V8J 3R2
250 624-5256; Fax: 250 627-7182
E: duchsher@citytel.net
W: www.bcacl.org
Executive:
Exec Dir: Shirley Duchsherer
Languages: English

◈ ***Sunshine Coast***
Location: 105-5711 Mermaid St, Sechelt BC V0N 3A3
Mailing: PO Box 165, Sechelt BC V0N 3A0
604 885-7455; Fax: 604 885-7702
E: info@scacl.ca
W: www.scacl.ca
Executive:
Exec Dir: Glen McClughan
Ops Mgr: Xerez Haffenden
Year Founded: 1958
No of Paid Staff: 35
Speakers Available
Library: Y
Languages: English
Membership: 50 *(Lists available to the public)*
Membership Fee: $15

◈ ***Surrey***
17687 56A Ave, Surrey BC V3S 1G4
604 574-7481; Fax: 604 574-4731
E: admin@commliv.com
W: www.commliv.com
Executive:
Exec Dir: Coreen Windbiel
Year Founded: 1958
Criteria: *Interest in the work of the society.*
Budget: $3,000,000
No of Paid Staff: 100
Languages: English
Membership: 60
Membership Fee: $15

◈ ***Williams Lake***
Location: 51 Fourth Ave S, Williams Lake BC V2G 1J6
Mailing: PO Box 6001 Stn Main,
Williams Lake BC V2G 3W2
250 398-7633; Fax: 250 398-7623
E: wlacl@telus.net
W: www.wlacl.org
Executive:
Exec Dir: Ian McLaughlin
Year Founded: 1961
Budget: $2,000,000
No of Paid Staff: 54
Speakers Available
Languages: English

◈ ***Brandon***
Career Connections Inc.
710 3rd St, Brandon MB R7A 3C8
204 726-2348; Fax: 204 726-5242
W: www.aclmb.ca
Speakers Available
Library: Y *(Open to the public)*
Languages: English
Membership: 300 *(Lists available to the public)*

◈ ***Flin Flon***
76 Channing Dr, Flin Flon MB R8A 0S4
204 687-7050; Fax: 204 687-7976
E: vtc@mts.net
Executive:
Exec Dir: Michelle Cooper
Year Founded: 1961
No of Paid Staff: 6
Languages: English

◈ ***Interlake***
Mailing: PO Box 1222, Stonewall MB R0C 2Z0
204 467-9169; Fax: 204 467-2743
Executive:
Exec Dir: Tara Smith

◈ ***Manitoba:***
6-120 Maryland St, Winnipeg MB R3G 1L1
204 786-1607; Fax: 204 789-9850
E: aclmb@aclmb.ca
W: www.aclmb.ca
Executive:
Exec Dir: Rose Flag
Office Mgr: Cheryl Duffy
Year Founded: 1951
No of Paid Staff: 5
Speakers Available
Library: Y *(Open to the public)*
Languages: English

◇ ***Beauséjour:***
Location: 917 Park Ave, Beauséjour MB R0E 0C0
Mailing: PO Box 1015
204 268-1803; Fax: 204 268-2879
Toll-free: 800 268-1803
W: www.aclbb.com
Executive:
Exec Dir: Linda Gmiterek

◇ ***Brandon:***
Career Connections Inc.
710 3rd St, Brandon MB R7A 3C8
204 726-2348; Fax: 204 726-5242
W: www.aclmb.ca
Speakers Available
Library: Y *(Open to the public)*
Languages: English
Membership: 300 *(Lists available to the public)*

◇ ***Flin Flon***
76 Channing Dr, Flin Flon MB R8A 0S4
204 687-7050; Fax: 204 687-7976
E: vtc@mts.net
Executive:
Exec Dir: Michelle Cooper
Year Founded: 1961
No of Paid Staff: 6
Languages: English

◇ ***Interlake:***
Mailing: PO Box 1222, Stonewall MB R0C 2Z0
204 467-9169; Fax: 204 467-2743
Executive:
Exec Dir: Tara Smith

◇ ***Manitoba***
6-120 Maryland St, Winnipeg MB R3G 1L1
204 786-1607; Fax: 204 789-9850
E: aclmb@aclmb.ca
W: www.aclmb.ca
Executive:
Pres: Val Surbey
Exec Dir: Rose Flaig
Year Founded: 1959
No of Paid Staff: 4
Speakers Available
Languages: English
Membership: 100 *(Lists available to the public)*
Membership Fee: $10 - Family; $5 - Individual

◇ ***Portage la Prairie:***
Mailing: PO Box 773 Stn Main,
Portage la Prairie MB R1N 3C2
204 857-9242; Fax: 204 239-0878

◇ ***Red River:***
Mailing: PO Box 280, St Malo MB R0A 1T0
204 347-5418; Fax: 204 347-5378
E: rrws@mts.net

◇ ***Selkirk & District:***
306 Jemima St, Selkirk MB R1A 1X1
204 785-8484; Fax: 204 785-8161
E: arcind@mts.net
W: www.aclmb.ca

◇ ***Steinbach:***
Mailing: PO Box 730 Stn Main,
Steinbach MB R5G 1M5
204 326-7539; Fax: 204 346-3639
W: www.aclmb.ca
Executive:
Exec Dir: Ed Barkman

◇ ***Swan River:***
Mailing: PO Box 1282, Swan River MB R0L 1Z0
204 734-9114; Fax: 204 734-3704
E: aclswanriver@nvcn.mb.ca
W: www.aclmb.ca
Executive:
Pres: John Christensen
1st VP: Fran Mullin
2nd VP: Ray Lepholtz

◇ ***Virden:***
Location: 216 Bridge St, Virden MB R0M 2C0
Mailing: PO Box 1957
204 748-1444; Fax: 204 748-1737
W: www.aclmb.ca

◇ ***Surrey***
17687 56A Ave, Surrey BC V3S 1G4
604 574-7481; Fax: 604 574-4731
E: admin@commliv.com
W: www.commliv.com
Executive:
Exec Dir: Coreen Windbiel
Year Founded: 1958
Criteria: *Interest in the work of the society.*
Budget: $3,000,000
No of Paid Staff: 100
Languages: English
Membership: 60
Membership Fee: $15

◈ ***Manitoba:***
6-120 Maryland St, Winnipeg MB R3G 1L1
204 786-1607; Fax: 204 789-9850
E: aclmb@aclmb.ca
W: www.aclmb.ca
Executive:
Pres: Val Surbey
Exec Dir: Rose Flaig
Year Founded: 1959
No of Paid Staff: 4
Speakers Available
Languages: English
Membership: 100 *(Lists available to the public)*
Membership Fee: $10 - Family; $5 - Individual

◈ ***Portage la Prairie***
Mailing: PO Box 773 Stn Main, Portage la Prairie MB R1N 3C2
204 857-9242; Fax: 204 239-0878

◈ ***Red River***
Mailing: PO Box 280, St Malo MB R0A 1T0
204 347-5418; Fax: 204 347-5378
E: rrws@mts.net

◈ ***Selkirk & District***
306 Jemima St, Selkirk MB R1A 1X1
204 785-8484; Fax: 204 785-8161
E: arcind@mts.net
W: www.aclmb.ca

◈ ***Steinbach***
Mailing: PO Box 730 Stn Main, Steinbach MB R5G 1M5
204 326-7539; Fax: 204 346-3639
W: www.aclmb.ca
Executive:
Exec Dir: Ed Barkman

◈ ***Swan River***
Mailing: PO Box 1282, Swan River MB R0L 1Z0
204 734-9114; Fax: 204 734-3704
E: aclswanriver@nvcn.mb.ca
W: www.aclmb.ca
Executive:
Pres: John Christensen
1st VP: Fran Mullin
2nd VP: Ray Lepholtz

◈ ***Virden***
Location: 216 Bridge St, Virden MB R0M 2C0
Mailing: PO Box 1957
204 748-1444; Fax: 204 748-1737
W: www.aclmb.ca

◈ ***New Brunswick:***
800 Hanwell Rd, Fredericton NB E3B 2R7
506 453-4400; Fax: 506 453-4422
Toll-free: 866 622-2548
E: nbacl@nbnet.nb.ca
W: www.nbacl.nb.ca
Executive:
Pres: Joy Bacon
Exec Dir: Krista Carr
Year Founded: 1957
No of Paid Staff: 40
Speakers Available
Library: Y *(Open to the public)*
Languages: English; French
Membership: 26 *(Lists available to the public)*
Library:
Resource Library *(Open to the public)*

◇ ***Bathurst:***
Mailing: PO Box 1031 Stn Main, Bathurst NB E2A 4H8
506 548-9488
W: www.nbacl.nb.ca
Executive:
VP: Albert Lavigne
Treas: Anne Jamieson

◇ ***Campbellton:***
Location: 6 Union St, Campbellton NB E3N 3G1
Mailing: PO Box 54 Stn Main
506 759-6668; Fax: 506 759-6661
E: rra@nb.aibn.com
W: www.nbacl.nb.ca
Executive:
Pres: Romain Leclair
Languages: English; French

◇ ***Eastern Charlotte:***
401-124 Main St, St George NB E5C 3S3
506 755-3730; Fax: 506 755-8188
E: nbacl@nbnet.nb.ca
W: www.nbacl.nb.ca
Executive:
Pres: John Norman

◇ ***Edmundston:***
3631 rue Principale, Baker Brook NB E7A 1V1
516 737-6829; Fax: 506 455-3318
Executive:
Pres: Joan Levesque
Languages: English; French

◇ ***Fredericton:***
1079 York St, Fredericton NB E3B 3S4
506 458-2198; Fax: 506 458-9821
E: facl@nb.aibn.com
W: www.nbacl.nb.ca
Executive:
Pres: Wynn Everett
Exec Dir: Diane Latouche
Languages: English; French

◇ ***Grand Falls:***
475 rue Terrace, Grand Falls NB E3Z 1B3
506 475-4060; Fax: 506 473-5998
E: aicgs@nb.sympatico.ca
Executive:
Dir: Brigitte LaPointe
Year Founded: 1965
No of Paid Staff: 25
Speakers Available
Languages: French; English
Membership list available to the public

◇ ***Greater Moncton:***
Location: 112 High St, Moncton NB E1C 6B5
Mailing: PO Box 1715 Stn Main, Moncton NB E1C 9X5
506 857-8899; Fax: 506 858-7883
E: gmacl@nb.aibn.com
W: www.gmacl.no-ip.org
Executive:
Exec Dir: C Melanson-Savoy
Year Founded: 1987
No of Paid Staff: 2
Speakers Available
Library: Y *(Open to the public)*
Languages: English; French
Membership: 200
Membership Fee: $15 Adult; $5 Student; $20 Family

HEALTHCARE ASSOCIATIONS

◇ ***Kennebecasis Valley:***
Mailing: PO BOX 4616 Stn Main, Rothesay NB E2E 5X3
E: nbacl@nbnet.nb.ca
W: www.nbacl.nb.ca
Executive:
Pres: Gail Hines
Treas: Kathy Turnbull
Languages: English; French

◇ ***Memramcook:***
280 Old Shediac Rd, Memramcook NB E4K 1W3
506 758-2751; Fax: 506 758-3237
E: vleblanc71@rogers.com
Executive:
Pres: Donald Bourque

◇ ***Néguac:***
978 Route 445, Fairisle NB E9G 2X7
506 776-8848; Fax: 506 776-5687
E: beausoleil@nb.aibn.com
Executive:
Pres: Ferdinande Comeau Robichaud
Languages: English; French

◇ ***Saint John:***
Location: Hilyard Place Bldg C, 203-600 Main St, Saint John NB E2K 1J5
Mailing: PO Box 803 Stn Main, Saint John NB E2L 4B3
506 652-1544; Fax: 506 648-9687
E: n6employ@nb.aibn.com
W: www.sjacl.ca
Executive:
Pres: Cathy O'Donel
Coord: Rick Seely
Year Founded: 1955
Budget: $240,000
No of Paid Staff: 5
Speakers Available
Languages: English
Membership: 200 *(Lists available to the public)*

◇ ***Sussex:***
26 Gordon St, Sussex NB E4E 1Z4
506 432-2021
Executive:
Pres: Cindy Ross
Languages: English; French

◇ ***Woodstock:***
120 Kirkpatrick St, Woodstock NB E7M 2A8
506 328-8027
Executive:
Pres: Ken Nichols
VP: Anne Marie Gullison
Treas: Teri Dickinson
Languages: English; French

◈ ***Newfoundland/Labrador:***
Location: 31 Peet St, St. John's NL A1B 3N7
Mailing: PO Box 8414 Stn A
709 722-0790; Fax: 709 722-1325
Toll-free: 800 701-8511
E: nlacl@nf.aibn.com
W: www.nlacl.ca
Executive:
Pres: Ray McIsaac
Exec Dir: Natasha McDonald
Year Founded: 1956
Criteria: *To be involved with a local ACL*
No of Paid Staff: 3
Speakers Available
Library: Y *(Open to the public)*
Languages: English
Membership: 23

◈ ***Northwest Territories:***
Location: 4912 53rd St, Yellowknife NT X1A 2N7
Mailing: PO Box 981 Stn Main
867 920-2644; Fax: 867 920-2348
E: info@ykacl.ca
W: www.ykacl.ca
Executive:
Pres: Pamela Weeks-Beaton
Exec Dir: Lynn Elkin
Year Founded: 1962
No of Paid Staff: 24
Library: Y *(Open to the public)*
Languages: English
Membership: 20 *(Lists available to the public)*
Membership Fee: $5/year

◈ ***Nova Scotia:***
Seacoast Towers
22-24 Dundas St, Suite 100, Dartmouth NS B2Y 4L2
902 469-1174; Fax: 902 461-0196
E: nsacl@eastlink.ca
W: nsacl.wordpress.com
Executive:
Pres: Lewis Crews
Exec Dir: Jean Coleman
No of Paid Staff: 3
Library: Y *(Open to the public)*
Languages: English
Membership: 16 *(Lists available to the public)*

◇ ***Halifax:***
2557 Maynard St, Halifax NS B3K 3V6
902 463-4752; Fax: 902 463-5007
E: hacl@eastlink.ca
W: www.hacl.ca
Executive:
Exec Dir: Peggy Weaver
Year Founded: 1953
No of Paid Staff: 13
Speakers Available
Library: Y *(Open to the public)*
Languages: English

◈ ***Ajax, Pickering, Whitby***
36 Emperor St, Ajax ON L1S 1M7
905 427-3300; Fax: 905 427-3310
E: info@apwcommunityliving.org
W: www.cl-apw.org
No of Paid Staff: 130
Languages: English

◈ ***Barrys Bay***
Location: 19491 Opeongo Line, Barrys Bay ON K0J 1B0
Mailing: PO Box 1178
613 756-3817; Fax: 613 756-0616
E: info@mvacl.ca
W: www.mvacl.ca
Executive:
Pres: Bridget Gutoskie
Exec Dir: Darcy Lacombe
Languages: English

◈ ***North Halton***
917 Nipissing Rd, Milton ON L9T 5E3
905 878-2337; Fax: 905 878-5413
E: khayward@clnh.on.ca
W: www.clnh.on.ca
Executive:
Pres: Hugh Williams
Exec Dir: Greg Edmiston

◈ ***Oakville***
301 Wyecroft Rd, Oakville ON L6K 2H2
905 844-0146; Fax: 905 844-1832
W: www.oakcl.org

Executive:
Pres: Tom Crawford
Exec Dir: John Wilson
Hum Res Mgr: Shannon Coles
Fin Mgr: Nancy Steptoe

◈ ***Ontario:***
403-240 Duncan Mill Rd, Toronto ON M3B 3S6
416 447-4348; Fax: 416 447-8974
Toll-free: 800 278-8025
E: info@communitylivingontario.ca
W: www.communitylivingontario.ca
Executive:
I-Exec Dir: Alan McWhorter
Dir-Commun Dev: Kimberley Gavan
Dir-Social Policy/Gov Rel: Gordon Kyle
Dir-Membership: Keith Dee
Year Founded: 1953
Criteria: *Members of affiliated local associations are members of Community Living Ontario.*
No of Paid Staff: 12
Speakers Available
Languages: English
Membership: 12,000

◇ ***Ajax, Pickering, Whitby:***
36 Emperor St, Ajax ON L1S 1M7
905 427-3300; Fax: 905 427-3310
E: info@apwcommunityliving.org
W: www.cl-apw.org
No of Paid Staff: 130
Languages: English

◇ ***Algoma:***
99 Northern Ave E, Sault Ste. Marie ON P6B 4H5
705 253-1700; Fax: 705 253-1777
Toll-free: 800 448-8097
W: www.communitylivingalgoma.org
Executive:
Exec Dir: John Policicchio
Criteria: *Services are open to the physically disabled.*
No of Paid Staff: 40
Library: Y *(Open to the public)*
Languages: English
Membership: 175 *(Lists available to the public)*
Membership Fee: $15

◇ ***Algoma:***
Location: 26 St Marie St, Floor 2, Wawa ON P0S 1K0
Mailing: PO Box 387
705 856-2423; Fax: 705 856-1046
W: www.communitylivingalgoma.org
Executive:
Case Mgr: Joan Ruebsam
Exec Dir: John Pollicicchio
Languages: English

◇ ***Almaguin Highlands:***
Location: 78 Ontario St, Sundridge ON P0A 1Z0
Mailing: PO Box 370
705 384-5384; Fax: 705 384-7695
Toll-free: 888 293-2425
E: admin@ahcl.org
W: www.ahcl.org
Executive:
Pres: Jackie Matthews
Exec Dir: Kerry Carnevale
Year Founded: 1973
No of Paid Staff: 56

◇ ***Almonte:***
Location: 6 Mill St, Almonte ON K0A 1A0
Mailing: PO Box 443
613 256-5459; Fax: 613 256-3963
Executive:
Exec Dir: Rick Tutt
No of Paid Staff: 6
Speakers Available
Library: Y
Languages: English
Membership list available to the public

HEALTHCARE ASSOCIATIONS

◊ ***Atikokan:***
Location: 114 Gorrie St, Atikokan ON P0T 1C0
Mailing: PO Box 2054
807 597-2259; Fax: 807 597-1495
E: info@cl-atikokan.ca
W: www.cl-atikokan.ca
Executive:
Pres: Bob Wilson
Exec Dir: Jim Turner

◊ ***Barrys Bay:***
Location: 19491 Opeongo Line, Barrys Bay ON K0J 1B0
Mailing: PO Box 1178
613 756-3817; Fax: 613 756-0616
E: info@mvacl.ca
W: www.mvacl.ca
Executive:
Pres: Bridget Gutoskie
Exec Dir: Darcy Lacombe
Languages: English

◊ ***Brampton/Caledon:***
34 Church St W, Brampton ON L6X 1H3
905 453-8841; Fax: 905 453-8853
E: info@bramptoncaledoncl.ca
W: www.bramptoncaledoncl.ca
Executive:
Exec Dir: Jim Triantafilou
Hum Res Mgr: Joan McGovern
Public/Admv Liasion: Jane Cerdic
Year Founded: 1947
Languages: English

◊ ***Brant:***
366 Dalhousie St, Brantford ON N3S 3W2
519 756-2662; Fax: 519 756-7668
E: communitylivingbrant@clbrant.com
W: www.clbrant.com
Executive:
Exec Dir: Janet Reansbury
Dir: Deb Cavers
Dir: Kathryn Dubicki
Dir: Edie Mous
Year Founded: 1952
Budget: $11,000,000
No of Paid Staff: 220
Speakers Available
Library: Y
Languages: English
Membership: 150 *(Lists available to the public)*

◊ ***Bruce Peninsula:***
Location: 314 George St, Wiarton ON N0H 2T0
Mailing: PO Box 95
519 534-0553; Fax: 519 534-2739
E: bpacl@bmts.com
W: www.communitylivingbp.org
Year Founded: 1968

◊ ***Cambridge:***
160 Hespeler Rd, Cambridge ON N1R 6V7
519 623-7490; Fax: 519 740-8073
W: www.communitylivingcambridge.ca
Executive:
Exec Dir: Michael Mullen
Year Founded: 1954
No of Paid Staff: 240
Library: Y
Languages: English
Membership Fee: $10/year

◊ ***Campbellford/Brighton:***
Location: 65 Bridge St E, Campbellford ON K0L 1L0
Mailing: PO Box 1360
705 653-1821; Fax: 705 653-5738
Toll-free: 866 528-0825
E: admin@communitylivingcampbellford.com
W: www.communitylivingcampbellford.com
Executive:
Pres: Chris Park
Exec Dir: Nancy Brown

◊ ***Central Huron:***
Location: 267 Suncoast Dr E, Goderich ON N7A 4H8
Mailing: PO Box 527, Goderich ON N7A 4C7
519 524-7362; Fax: 519 524-1511
E: clch@hurontel.on.ca
W: www.clch.ca
Executive:
Exec Dir: Rosemary Foran
Budget: $266,000
No of Paid Staff: 75
Speakers Available
Library: Y
Languages: English
Membership: 12
Membership Fee: $3

◊ ***Chatham-Kent:***
Location: Riverview Ent, 2-650 Riverview Dr, Chatham ON N7M 5J5
Mailing: PO Box 967 Stn Main, Chatham ON N7M 5L3
519 352-1174; Fax: 519 352-5459
W: www.clc-k.ca
Executive:
Pres: Gordon Crompton
Exec Dir: Lu-Ann Cowell
Dir-Fin/Admn: Linda D Karnas
Year Founded: 1955
No of Paid Staff: 215
Speakers Available
Library: Y *(Open to the public)*
Languages: English; French
Membership: 150+

◊ ***Cochrane:***
Location: 18 Aurora Ave, Cochrane ON P0L 1C0
Mailing: PO Box 2330
705 272-2999; Fax: 705 272-4983
E: icccl@puc.net
W: www.communitylivingontario.ca
Executive:
Pres: Gaston Gauthier
Supvr: Jane Williams

◊ ***Chapleau:***
Mailing: PO Box 1377, Chapleau ON P0M 1K0
705 864-2932; Fax: 705 864-1720
W: www.communitylivingontario.ca
Executive:
Pres: Lise Jewett
Project Mgr: Diana Taylor

◊ ***Dryden & District:***
280 Arthur St, Dryden ON P8N 1K8
807 223-3364; Fax: 807 223-5784
W: www.communitylivingdryden.com
Executive:
Pres: Vince Kastrukoff
Exec Dir: Mike Hull
Dir-Fin: Corrine Owen
Dir-Serv: Lynda Ménard-Penner

◊ ***Dufferin:***
065371 County Road 3, Orangeville ON L9W 2Y9
519 941-8971; Fax: 519 941-9121
E: info@communitylivingdufferin.ca
W: www.communitylivingdufferin.ca
Executive:
Pres: Sylvia Cheuy
Year Founded: 1954
Languages: English

◊ ***Dundas County***
Location: 55 Allison Ave, Morrisburg ON K0C 1X0
Mailing: PO Box 678
613 543-3737; Fax: 613 543-4432
E: cldc@cldc.ca
W: www.cldc.ca
Executive:
Exec Dir: Deborah (Debbie) Boardman
Criteria: *Must be physically disabled.*
Languages: English

◊ ***Durham North:***
Location: 2-60 Vanedward Dr, Port Perry ON L9L 1G3
Mailing: PO Box 964, Port Perry ON L9L 1A8
905 985-8511; Fax: 905 985-0799
W: www.communitylivingdurhamnorth.ca
Executive:
Exec Dir: Glenn Taylor

◊ ***Espanola:***
345 Centre St, Espanola ON P5E 1E4
705 869-0442; Fax: 705 869-0446
E: info@communitylivingontario.ca
W: www.clespanola.ca/
Languages: English

◊ ***Essex County:***
372 Talbot St N, Essex ON N8M 2W4
519 776-6483; Fax: 519 776-6972
Toll-free: 800 265-5820
E: nancywallacegero@communitylivingessex.org
W: www.communitylivingessex.org
Executive:
Pres: Michael Groot
Exec Dir: Nancy Wallace-Gero
Year Founded: 1961
Budget: $10,000,000
No of Paid Staff: 300
Speakers Available
Languages: English
Membership: 200
Membership Fee: $10/year
Library:
Resource Library *(Open to the public)*

◊ ***Etobicoke/York Region:***
204-295 The West Mall, Etobicoke ON M9C 4Z4
416 236-7621; Fax: 416 236-7673
W: www.communitylivingtoronto.ca
Executive:
Reg Exec Dir: Brad Saunders
Volunteer Coord: Faruk Hossan
Dir-Pub Rel/Fundraising: Angela Bradley

◊ ***Fort Erie:***
Location: 615 Industrial Dr, Fort Erie ON L2A 5M4
Mailing: PO Box 520 Stn Main, Fort Erie ON L2A 5Y1
905 871-6770; Fax: 905 871-3339
W: www.clfe.ca
Executive:
Exec Dir: Maureen Brown
Fin Mgr: Joan Haist
Year Founded: 1957
Languages: English

◊ ***Gananoque & District:***
26 Mill St, Gananoque ON K7G 3A6
613 382-7702; Fax: 613 382-7705
W: www.gdacl.com
Executive:
Exec Dir: Colleen Kelly-Jansen
Hum Res Coord: Debbie Lameront

◊ ***Georgina:***
Location: 26943 Hwy 48, Sutton West ON L0E 1R0
Mailing: PO Box 68
905 722-8947; Fax: 905 722-9591
W: www.communitylivinggeorgina.com

◊ ***Glengarry:***
332 MacDonald Blvd, Alexandria ON K0C 1A0
613 525-4357; Fax: 613 525-4360
W: www.clglen.on.ca
Executive:
Exec Dir: Danielle Duranceau
Admn Office Mgr: Lise-Marie Papadopoulos
Mgr-Day Programs: Carol White
Mgr-Commun Serv: Laurie McKay-Levac

Year Founded: 1966
No of Paid Staff: 60
Languages: English; French

◇ ***Greater Sudbury:***
241-303 York St, Sudbury ON P3E 2A5
705 671-7181; Fax: 705 671-1238
W: www.communitylivinggreatersudbury.ca
Executive:
Pres: Rob Franceschini
Year Founded: 1967
Criteria: *Open to any person who has attended three meetings. Must be nominated by a member in good standing.*
No of Paid Staff: 120
Languages: English; French
Membership: 35
Membership Fee: $7

◇ ***Grimsby/Lincoln/West Lincoln:***
Location: 8-5041 King St, Beamsville ON L0R 1B0
Mailing: PO Box 220
905 563-4115; Fax: 905 563-8887
E: info@cl-grimsbylincoln.ca
W: www.cl-grimsbylincoln.ca
Executive:
Exec Dir: Sarina Labonte
No of Paid Staff: 170
Library: Y
Languages: English
Membership Fee: $5 per year

◇ ***Guelph-Wellington:***
8 Royal Rd, Guelph ON N1H 1G3
519 824-2480; Fax: 519 821-6174
E: admin@clgw.ca
W: www.clgw.ca
Executive:
Exec Dir: Bob Butella
Languages: English

◇ ***Haldimand:***
Location: 2256 River Rd, Cayuga ON N0A 1E0
Mailing: PO Box 396
905 772-3344; Fax: 905 772-3155
Executive:
Pres: J D Anderson
Exec Dir: Susan Wavell

◇ ***Haliburton County:***
Location: 713 Mountain St, PO Box 90, Haliburton ON K0M 1S0
Mailing: PO Box 90
705 457-2626; Fax: 705 457-9287
E: info@communitylivinghaliburtoncounty.com
W: www.communitylivinghaliburtoncounty.com
Executive:
Exec Dir: Maureen O'Hara

◇ ***Hamilton:***
191 York Blvd, Hamilton ON L8R 1Y6
905 528-0281; Fax: 905 528-5156
E: bshields@clham.com
W: www.communitylivinghamilton.com
Executive:
Exec Dir: Sherry Parsley
Criteria: *Open to all.*
Budget: $7,000,000
No of Paid Staff: 300
Library: Y *(Open to the public)*
Languages: English

◇ ***Hearst & Area:***
Location: 923 Edward St, Hearst ON P0L 1N0
Mailing: PO Box 12000
705 362-5758; Fax: 705 362-8093
E: dillonc@cscdgr.on.ca
W: www.communitylivingontario.ca
Executive:
Coord - NE Region: Cristy Webb

◇ ***Hornepayne:***
Location: 200 Front St, Hornepayne ON P0M 1Z0
Mailing: PO Box 1532
807 868-3052; Fax: 807 868-3052
W: www.communitylivingalgoma.com
Languages: English

◇ ***Huronia:***
339 Olive St, Midland ON L4R 2R4
705 526-4253; Fax: 705 526-8299
E: clhmid@clhmidland.on.ca
W: www.clhmidland.on.ca
Executive:
CEO: Tony Vipond
Dir-Fin: Mitchell Stewart
Dir-Hum Res: Angela Larmand
Year Founded: 1960
Budget: $5,500,000
No of Paid Staff: 180
Library: Y *(Open to the public)*
Languages: English
Membership: 120
Membership Fee: $5

◇ ***Iroquois Falls:***
Location: 9 Veterans Rd, Iroquois Falls ON P0K 1E0
Mailing: PO Box 310
705 258-3971; Fax: 705 258-3119
E: ifacl@onlink.net
Executive:
Pres: Jackie Irvine
Exec Dir: Carol Gauthier

◇ ***Kapuskasing & District:***
12 Kimberly Dr, Kapuskasing ON P5N 1L5
705 337-1417; Fax: 705 337-6538
E: kdacl@nt.net
W: www.communitylivingontario.ca

◇ ***Kenora:***
501 Eighth Ave S, Kenora ON P9N 3Z9
807 467-5225; Fax: 807 467-5247
E: central@kacl.ca
W: www.kacl.ca
Executive:
Pres: Coleen Neil
Exec Dir: James Retson
Criteria: *Open to all.*
Budget: $4,000,000
No of Paid Staff: 115
Speakers Available
Languages: English
Membership: 125
Membership Fee: $10

◇ ***Kingston:***
1412 Princess St, Kingston ON K7M 3E5
613 546-6613; Fax: 613 546-0436
E: amcwhorter@kdacl.on.ca
W: www.communitylivingkingston.org
Executive:
Exec Dir: Peter Sproul

◇ ***Kirkland Lake:***
Location: 51 Government Rd W, Kirkland Lake ON P2N 2E5
Mailing: PO Box 274, Kirkland Lake ON P2N 3H7
705 567-9331; Fax: 705 567-5005
E: kdadh@nt.net
Executive:
Pres: Annice Tilley
Exec Dir: Heather Topliss
Dir-Fin: Traci Fong
Pers Clerk: Cheryl Peever
Mtce Coord: Sylvie Adams
Criteria: *Open to any person who is developmentally handicapped.*
Languages: English

◇ ***Lanark County CSS Perth:***
87 Gore St E, Perth ON K7H 1J1
613 264-0876; Fax: 613 264-8433
E: cssperth@clalanark.ca
W: www.clalanark.ca
Executive:
Reg Mgr: Alice-Anne Patterson Collinge
Criteria: *Services are open to the physically disabled.*
No of Paid Staff: 5
Library: Y *(Open to the public)*
Languages: English
Membership: 30

◇ ***Lennox and Addington:***
99 Richmond Blvd, Napanee ON K7R 3S3
613 354-2184; Fax: 613 354-0815
Year Founded: 1967
Criteria: *Members must live in Lennox and Addington county.*
No of Paid Staff: 30
Library: Y *(Open to the public)*
Languages: English
Membership: 24
Membership Fee: $5

◇ ***Manitoulin:***
Location: 6062 Hwy 542, Mindemoya ON P0P 1S0
Mailing: PO Box 152
705 377-6699; Fax: 705 377-7175
E: clmhayes@eastlink.ca
W: www.clmanitoulin.ca
Executive:
Exec Dir: Marguerite Hayes
Year Founded: 1976
No of Paid Staff: 60
Languages: English

◇ ***Mississauga:***
1-6695 Millcreek Dr, Mississauga ON L5N 5R8
905 542-2694; Fax: 905 542-0987
E: info@clmiss.ca
W: www.clmiss.ca
Executive:
Exec Dir: Keith Tansley
Languages: English

◇ ***Newmarket/Aurora District:***
757 Bogart Ave, Newmarket ON L3Y 2A7
905 898-3000; Fax: 905 898-6441
E: info@clnad.com
W: www.clnad.com
Executive:
Exec Dir: Colleen Zakoor
Dir-Servs: Maureen MacFayden
Languages: English

◇ ***North Bay:***
161 Main St E, North Bay ON P1B 1A9
705 476-3288; Fax: 705 476-4788
Toll-free: 866 821-7770
E: info@communitylivingnorthbay.org
W: www.communitylivingnorthbay.org
Executive:
Exec Dir: Jennifer Valenti
Library: Y *(Open to the public)*
Languages: English

◇ ***North Bay and District:***
161 Main St E, North Bay ON P1B 1A9
705 476-3288; Fax: 705 476-4788
E: info@communitylivingnorthbay.org
W: www.communitylivingnorthbay.org
Executive:
Exec Dir: Jennifer Valenti
Year Founded: 1954
Criteria: *Services are open to the physically disabled.*
Languages: English; French

HEALTHCARE ASSOCIATIONS

◇ ***North Frontenac:***
Location: 1025 Elizabeth St, Sharbot Lake ON K0H 2P0
Mailing: PO Box 76
613 279-3731; Fax: 613 279-3732
Executive:
Pres: Phyllis Badour
Exec Dir: Donald W Nielsen

◇ ***North Halton***
917 Nipissing Rd, Milton ON L9T 5E3
905 878-2337; Fax: 905 878-5413
E: khayward@clnh.on.ca
W: www.clnh.on.ca
Executive:
Pres: Hugh Williams
Exec Dir: Greg Edmiston

◇ ***North Perth:***
Location: 820 Main St E, Listowel ON N4W 3H4
Mailing: PO Box 220 Stn Main
519 291-1350; Fax: 519 291-2747
E: clnp@shm.ca
W: www.communitylivingontario.ca
Year Founded: 1971
No of Paid Staff: 35
Languages: English
Membership: 75 *(Lists available to the public)*
Membership Fee: $100 Lifetime; $5 Per Year

◇ ***Oakville***
301 Wyecroft Rd, Oakville ON L6K 2H2
905 844-0146; Fax: 905 844-1832
W: www.oakcl.org
Executive:
Pres: Tom Crawford
Exec Dir: John Wilson
Hum Res Mgr: Shannon Coles
Fin Mgr: Nancy Steptoe

◇ ***Oshawa/Clarington:***
39 Wellington Ave E, Oshawa ON L1H 3Y1
905 576-3011; Fax: 905 576-9754
E: info@communitylivingoc.ca
W: www.communitylivingoc.ca
Executive:
Exec Dir: Steve Finlay
Dir-Ops: Terri Gray
Dir-Hum Res: Kay Corbier

◇ ***Owen Sound & Dist:***
769 4th Ave E, Owen Sound ON N4K 2N5
519 371-9251; Fax: 519 371-5168
E: info@comlivos.on.ca
W: www.communitylivingowensound.ca

◇ ***Parry Sound:***
38 Joseph St, Parry Sound ON P2A 2G5
705 746-9330; Fax: 705 746-6151
E: mail@clps.ca
W: www.clps.ca
Executive:
Exec Dir: Jo-Anne Demick
Year Founded: 1962
Criteria: *Services are open to those who are developmentally disabled.*
Library: Y
Languages: English

◇ ***Peterborough:***
223 Aylmer St N, Peterborough ON K9J 3K3
705 743-2411; Fax: 705 743-3722
E: contact@communitylivingpeterborough.ca
W: www.communitylivingpeterborough.ca
Executive:
CEO: Jack Gillan
Year Founded: 1953
Criteria: *Services are open to the physically disabled.*
Budget: $5,500,000
No of Paid Staff: 145
Speakers Available
Library: Y *(Open to the public)*
Languages: English
Membership: 123
Membership Fee: $20 individual; $50 corporate; $30 family

◇ ***Port Colborne/Wainfleet:***
100 McRae Ave, Port Colborne ON L3K 2A8
905 835-8941; Fax: 905 835-5515
W: www.portcolbornecommunityliving.com
Executive:
Exec Dir: Vickie Moreland
Criteria: *Services are open to the physically disabled.*
No of Paid Staff: 11
Library: Y *(Open to the public)*
Languages: English

◇ ***Prince Edward:***
1-67 King St, Picton ON K0K 2T0
613 476-6038; Fax: 613 476-2868
E: info@clpe.on.ca
W: www.clpe.on.ca
Executive:
Exec Dir: Brian Smith

◇ ***Quinte West:***
1 Greenleaf Crt, Belleville ON K8N 5T5
613 394-2222; Fax: 613 394-0381
E: communitylivingquintewest@clqw.ca
W: www.clqw.ca
Executive:
Pres: Michelle Earle
Exec Dir: Starr Olsen
Languages: English

◇ ***Red Lake & District:***
Location: 26 Young St, Red Lake ON P0V 2M0
Mailing: PO Box 906
807 727-2828; Fax: 807 727-1102
Executive:
Exec Dir: Margaret Kudlowsky
Cust Serv Coord: Georgie McCann

◇ ***Renfrew County South:***
Location: 326 Raglan St S, Renfrew ON K7V 1R5
Mailing: PO Box 683 Stn Main, Renfrew ON K7V 4E7
613 432-6763; Fax: 613 432-9465
E: commliving@clrcs.com
W: www.clrcs.com
Executive:
Exec Dir: Jennifer Creeden
Year Founded: 1964
Languages: English

◇ ***Sarnia/Lambton:***
202-551 Exmouth St, Box 610, Sarnia ON N7T 5P6
519 332-0560; Fax: 519 332-3446
W: www.communitylivingsarnia.org
Executive:
Pres: Earle Kilner
Exec Dir: John Hagens
Controller: Pam Atkinson
Commun Involvement Coord: Norma Hills
A-Exec Asst to Exec Dir: Tammy Langis
Year Founded: 1656
Budget: $5,100,000
No of Paid Staff: 150
Languages: English

◇ ***St. Catharines:***
437 Welland Ave, St Catharines ON L2M 5V2
905 688-5222; Fax: 905 688-9926
E: administration@clstcatharines.ca
W: www.clstcatharines.ca
Executive:
Exec Dir: Al Moreland

◇ ***St. Marys & Area:***
Location: 300 Elgin St E, St Marys ON N4X 1B9
Mailing: PO Box 1618
519 284-1400; Fax: 519 284-3120
E: info@communitylivingstmarys.ca
W: www.communitylivingstmarys.ca
Executive:
Pres: Al Slater
Exec Dir: Marg McLean

◇ ***Scarborough Region:***
1712 Ellesmere Rd, Scarborough ON M1H 2V5
416 438-6099; Fax: 416 438-6144
W: www.communitylivingtoronto.ca
Executive:
Reg Exec Dir: Sue Lynch
Membership Coord: Karla Galvez
Membership Coord: Anne-Marie Binetti
Dir-Pub Rel/Fundraising: Angela Bradley

◇ ***Sioux Lookout:***
Location: 41 King St, Sioux Lookout ON P8T 1B8
Mailing: PO Box 1258
807 737-1447; Fax: 807 737-3833
Executive:
Exec Dir: Michael Hall

◇ ***Simcoe:***
89 Culver St, Simcoe ON N3Y 2V5
519 426-0007; Fax: 519 426-9549
E: access@kwic.com
W: www.access-support.on.ca
Executive:
Pres: Jennie Chanda
Exec Dir: Patricia Morris
Dir-Fin: Vivian Fuller
Treas: Jennifer Baie
Year Founded: 1981
Library: Y
Languages: English

◇ ***South Huron:***
Location: 146 Main St, Dashwood ON N0M 1N0
Mailing: PO Box 29
519 237-3637; Fax: 519 237-3190
E: clsh@hay.net
W: clsh.ca
Executive:
Exec Dir: Bruce Shaw

◇ ***Stormont County:***
280 Ninth St W, Cornwall ON K6J 3A6
613 938-9550; Fax: 613 938-2033
E: information@clstormont.ca
W: www.communitylivingstormontcounty.ca
Executive:
Pres: Stephan Perreault
Exec Dir: Richard D'Alessio
Asst Exec Dir: Michelle Alguire
Year Founded: 1958
Criteria: *Any person aged 18 or older who supports CLSC.*
Budget: $2,500,000
No of Paid Staff: 70
Speakers Available
Library: Y *(Open to the public)*
Languages: English; French
Membership: 60 *(Lists available to the public)*
Membership Fee: $5/yr

◇ ***Stratford & Area:***
112 Frederick St, Stratford ON N5A 3V7
519 273-1000; Fax: 519 273-6277
E: info@clsa.ca
W: www.community-living.com
Year Founded: 1958
Speakers Available
Languages: English

◇ ***Superior Greenstone:***
Location: 206 Hogarth Ave W, Geraldton ON P0T 1M0
Mailing: PO Box 970, Nipigon ON P0T 2J0
807 854-0924; Fax: 807 854-1047
W: www.communitylivingontario.ca
Executive:
Exec Dir: Bob Tkaczyk
Criteria: *Services are open to developmentally disabled adults & children.*
Budget: $2,400,000
No of Paid Staff: 70
Languages: English
Membership: 20
Membership Fee: Family: $5; Single: $2

◇ ***Temiskaming South:***
Location: 513 Amwell St, Haileybury ON P0J 1K0
Mailing: PO Box 1149
705 672-2000; Fax: 705 672-2722
W: www.communitylivingontario.ca
Executive:
Pres: Mark Sargent
Exec Dir: Sherwin Knight
Admin/Supvr: Pat Lauder
Languages: English; French

◇ ***Thunder Bay:***
1501 Dease St, Thunder Bay ON P7C 5H3
807 622-1099; Fax: 807 622-8528
E: info@cltb.ca
W: www.cltb.ca
Executive:
Pres/Board Member: Gary Ferguson
I-Exec/Dir-Fin: Sandra Buosi
Dir-Hum Res: Jill Symington

◇ ***Tillsonburg & District:***
The Livingston Centre
96 Tillson Ave, Tillsonburg ON N4G 3A1
519 842-9000 226; Fax: 519 842-7628
E: communitylivingtillsonburg@ocl.net
W: www.communitylivingtillsonburg.ca
Languages: English

◇ ***Timmins:***
166A Brousseau Ave, Timmins ON P4N 5Y4
705 268-8811; Fax: 705 267-2011
E: admin@cltic.ca
W: www.communitylivingtimmins.com
Executive:
Pres: Robert Tremblay
Exec Dir: Johanne Rondeau

◇ ***Toronto:***
20 Spadina Rd, Toronto ON M5R 2S7
416 968-0650; Fax: 416 968-6463
W: www.cltoronto.ca
Executive:
Pres: Chris Stringer
CEO: Garry Pruden
CFO: Flavian Pinto
Reg Exec Dir: Francis MacNeil
Dir-Pub Rel/Fundraising: Angela Bradley
Year Founded: 1948
Budget: $45,000,000
No of Paid Staff: 1,200
Speakers Available
Languages: English
Membership: 650
Membership Fee: $30/year

◇ ***Upper Ottawa Valley:***
Location: 894 Pembroke St W, Pembroke ON K8A 5P8
Mailing: PO Box 1030 Stn Main, Pembroke ON K8A 6Y6
613 735-0659; Fax: 613 735-1373
E: info@communitylivingupperottawavalley.ca
W: www.communitylivingupperottawavalley.ca
Executive:
Exec Dir: Paul Melcher
Criteria: *Services are open to the physically disabled.*
Languages: English; French

◇ ***Walkerton & District:***
Location: 19 Durham St E, Walkerton ON N0G 2V0
Mailing: PO Box 999
519 881-3713; Fax: 519 881-0531
W: www.clwalkerton.org
Executive:
Pres: Nancy Skiba
Exec Dir: Brodie Hart
Fin/Admn Mgr: Rose Weber
Ops Mgr: Ron Spitzig
Mgr-Measures/Best Practices: Carol Patterson
Support Serv Mgr: Kathy Kieffer
Support Serv Mgr: Sheryl Marshall
Year Founded: 1956

◇ ***Wallaceburg:***
1100 Dufferin Ave, Wallaceburg ON N8A 2W1
519 627-0777; Fax: 519 627-8905
Toll-free: 800 620-4425
W: www.getintocommunityliving.com
Executive:
Exec Dir: David Katzman

◇ ***Welland-Pelham:***
535 Sutherland Ave, Welland ON L3B 5A4
905 735-0081; Fax: 905 735-9431
E: communityliving@cl-wellandpelham.ca
W: www.cl-wellandpelham.ca
Executive:
Exec Dir: Barbara Vyrostko
Dir-Ops: Saro Stranges
Admn Mgr: Theresa Terreberry
Coord-Day Prog Adult: Cindy Bradley
Supvr-Child Serv: Judy Bonsignore

◇ ***West Northumberland:***
275 Cottesmore Ave, Cobourg ON K9A 4E3
905 372-4455; Fax: 905 372-2783
E: communitylivingwn@yahoo.ca
W: www.communitylivingwn@yahoo.ca
Executive:
Exec Dir: Cathy Timlin
Year Founded: 1959
No of Paid Staff: 40
Languages: English

◇ ***Wikwemikong Anishinabe:***
11 Fox Lake Rd, Wikwemikong ON P0P 2J0
705 859-2174; Fax: 705 859-2147
W: www.communitylivingontario.ca
Executive:
Pres: Leland Bell
Prog Dir: Jeannette Assinewai

◇ ***Wingham & District:***
Location: 153 John St W, Wingham ON N0G 2W0
Mailing: PO Box 818
519 357-3562; Fax: 519 357-4283
W: www.wdcla.org
Executive:
Pres: Graeme Craig
Exec Dir: Debbie Hopper
Fin Mgr: Lois Darling

◇ ***York South:***
101 Edward Ave, Richmond Hill ON L4C 5E5
905 884-9110; Fax: 905 737-3284
W: www.communitylivingyorksouth.ca
Executive:
Exec Dir: Don Wilkinson
Dep Exec Dir: Ursula Rehdner
Dir-Fin: Steve Klein
Bus Mgr-Bright Ideas Cust Pkg: Wayne Kitto
Hum Res Coord: Dianna Thompson
Year Founded: 1954
Budget: $10,000,000
No of Paid Staff: 250
Library: Y *(Open to the public)*
Languages: English
Membership: 900
Membership Fee: Family - $35; Senior - $10; Single - $20

◇ ***York South-Markham Office:***
5-144 Main St N, Markham ON L3P 5T3
905 294-4971; Fax: 905 472-5409
W: www.communitylivingyorksouth.ca
Languages: English

◇ ***York South-Vaughan Office***
136 Winges Rd, Woodbridge ON L4L 6C3
905 264-7262; Fax: 905 264-7850
Executive:
Commun Support Coord: Cheri Evans
Commun Support Coord: Kula Kulasegaram
Commun Support Coord: Anita Leung
Commun Support Coord: Rhitu Bhasin

◈ ***Prince Edward Island:***
Location: 161 St. Peters Rd, Charlottetown PE C1A 5P6
Mailing: PO Box 280 Stn Central, Charlottetown PE C1A 7K4
902 566-4844; Fax: 902 368-8057
Toll-free: 888 360-8681
E: info@peiacl.ca
W: www.peiacl.ca
Executive:
Pres: Frank Driscoll
Exec Dir: Bridget Cairns
Year Founded: 1955
No of Paid Staff: 2
Speakers Available
Languages: English; French
Membership: 250
Membership Fee: Affiliate - $75/year; Families - $10/year
Library:
PEI Resource Library *(Open to the public)*

◈ ***Quebec:***
3958 rue Dandurand, Montréal QC H1X 1P7
514 725-7245; Fax: 514 725-2796
E: direction_generale@aqis-iqdi.qc.ca
W: www.aqis-iqdi.qc.ca
Executive:
Prés: Jacqueline Babin
Dir gén: Diane Milliard
Year Founded: 1951
No of Paid Staff: 10
Speakers Available
Library: Y *(Open to the public)*
Languages: English; French
Membership: 84
Library:
Centre de documentation *(Open to the public)*

◈ ***Saskatchewan:***
3031 Louise St, Saskatoon SK S7J 3L1
306 955-3344; Fax: 306 373-3070
E: sacl@sacl.org
W: www.sacl.org
Executive:
Pres: Gloria Mahussier
Exec Dir: Kevin McTavish
Year Founded: 1956
No of Paid Staff: 25
Speakers Available
Languages: English
Membership list available to the public
Membership Fee: $20
Library:
John Dolan Resource Centre *(Open to the public)*

◇ **Regina and District:**
2216 Smith St, Regina SK S4P 2P4
306 790-5680; Fax: 306 586-7899
E: mainrdacl@sasktel.net
W: www.rdacl.ca
Executive:
Pres: Stuart Mason
Exec Dir: Larry Deters
Year Founded: 1952
Criteria: *Open to all, however membership status may vary.*
No of Paid Staff: 3
Speakers Available
Library: Y
Languages: English

◇ **Saskatoon:**
102-135 Robin Cres, Saskatoon SK S7L 6M3
306 652-9111; Fax: 306 652-9112
E: sacl1@sasktel.net
W: www.clasaskatoon.org
Executive:
Exec Dir: Jerome Nicol
Office Admin/Bookkeeper: Donna Parkinson
Year Founded: 1955
Criteria: *Open to all.*
Budget: $450,000
No of Paid Staff: 40
Speakers Available
Languages: English
Membership: 150
Membership Fee: Family - $20

◈ **Yukon:**
Location: 40-986 Range Rd, Whitehorse YT Y1A 4V1
Mailing: PO Box 31478 RPO Main Street, Whitehorse YT Y1A 6K8
867 667-4606; Fax: 867 668-8169
E: yaclwhse@northwestel.net
Executive:
Pres: Chris Hale
Coord: Vicki Wilson
Year Founded: 1964
Criteria: *Open to persons who believe in best practices to enable community inclusion for people with intellectual disabilities.*
Budget: $150,000
No of Paid Staff: 1
Speakers Available
Library: Y *(Open to the public)*
Languages: English
Membership: 50 *(Lists available to the public)*
Membership Fee: $1 per year
Library:
YACL Resource Library *(Open to the public)*

Canadian Association of Educators of the Deaf and Hard-of-Hearing

871 Centennial St, Winnipeg MB R3N 1R6
204 918-2651; Fax: 204 945-1767
E: info@caedhh.ca
W: www.caedhh.ca
Executive:
Natl Dir: Nancy Schenkeveld
Year Founded: 1973
Languages: English
Membership Fee: $85 - Full member; $55 - Student/Retired member; $65 - Associate member

Canadian Association of the Deaf

303-251 Bank St, Ottawa ON K2P 1X3
613 565-2882; Fax: 613 565-1207
E: info@cad.ca
W: www.cad.ca
Executive:
Exec Dir: James Roots
Year Founded: 1940
No of Paid Staff: 5
Speakers Available
Languages: English; French
Membership Fee: $25

Canadian Council of the Blind - National

100-20 James St, Ottawa ON K2P 0T6
613 567-0311; Fax: 613 567-2728
Toll-free: 877 304-0968
E: ccb@ccbnational.net
W: www.ccbnational.net
Executive:
Pres: Louise Gillis
1st VP: Jim Tokes
2nd VP: Linda Sobey
3rd VP: Heather Hannett
Year Founded: 1944
No of Paid Staff: 10
Speakers Available
Languages: English
Membership: 1,600 +
Membership Fee: $10

◈ **Alberta:**
Location: 69 Grand Meadow Cres NW, Edmonton AB T6L 1A3
Mailing: PO Box 74006 RPO Pepper Tree, Edmonton AB T5K 2S7
780 462-8879
W: www.ccbnational.net
Executive:
Natl Pres: Harold Schnellert
Languages: English

◈ **Manitoba:**
Location: 305-960 Portage Ave, Winnipeg MB R3G 0R4
Mailing: PO Box 2454 Stn Main, Winnipeg MB R3C 4A7
204 942-8722
E: ccbmb.division@gmail.com
W: www.ccbmb.ca
Executive:
1st VP: Norman Lyons
Year Founded: 1950
Criteria: *Blind or visually impaired or Associate member with voice but no vote.*
Budget: $102,000
No of Paid Staff: 1
Speakers Available
Languages: English
Membership: 42 *(Lists available to the public)*
Membership Fee: $12

◈ **Saskatchewan:**
1105 Campbell St, Regina SK S4T 5P5
306 352-9458
Executive:
Board Member: Jerome Kuntz
Criteria: *Class One membership is open to visually impaired persons. Associate membership is open to friends of the CCB.*
Speakers Available
Languages: English
Membership: 158

Canadian Deafblind Association - National Office

Location: 5160 Lampman Ave, Burlington ON L7L 6K1
Mailing: 421-2000 Appleby Line, Burlington ON L7L 7H7
905 319-9243; Fax: 905 319-2027
Toll-free: 866 229-5832
E: info@cdbanational.com
W: www.cdbanational.com
Executive:
Pres: Carolyn Monaco
Exec Dir: Tom McFadden
Year Founded: 1975
Budget: $200,000
No of Paid Staff: 3
Languages: English; French
Membership: 25

◈ **Alberta Chapter:**
Mailing: PO Box 89006 MacKenzie RPO Towne, Calgary AB T2Z 3W3
780 425-9444
E: mrttrouttours@shaw.ca
W: www.deafblindalberta.ca
Executive:
Pres: Wayne Turnbull

◈ **British Columbia Chapter:**
227 Sixth Street, New Westminster BC V3L 3A5
604 528-6170; Fax: 604 528-6174
E: theresa@cdbabc.ca
W: www.cdbabc.ca
Executive:
Early Intervention Prog Dir: Sue Gawne
Family Servs Coord: Theresa Tancock
Criteria: *Open to anyone who pays the fee.*
No of Paid Staff: 3
Speakers Available
Library: Y *(Open to the public)*
Languages: English
Membership: 88

◈ **Manitoba Chapter:**
201-1100 Concordia Ave, Winnipeg MB R2K 4B8
204 949-3730; Fax: 204 949-3732
Executive:
Pres: Don Ernst
Dir-Ops: Heather Greenwood
Prog Dir: Erin Gendreau
Year Founded: 1991
Criteria: *Open to anyone who supports the mission and objectives of the CDBRA.*
No of Paid Staff: 35
Speakers Available
Languages: English
Membership: 21
Membership Fee: Associate - $15; Corporate - $30; Family - $25; Individual - $20

◈ **New Brunswick Chapter:**
408-212 Queen St, Fredericton NB E3B 1A8
506 452-1544; Fax: 506 451-8309
Toll-free: 877 452-1544
E: office@cdba-nb.ca
W: cdba-nb.ca
Executive:
Exec Dir: Kevin Symes
Dir-Intervention Reg: Gisele Gaudet
Office Mgr: Shari Holmes
Year Founded: 1982
No of Paid Staff: 40
Speakers Available
Languages: English
Membership: 100
Membership Fee: Ranges from $10 - $20

◈ **Ontario Chapter:**
54 Brant Ave, Floor 3, Brantford ON N3T 3G8
519 759-0520; Fax: 519 759-1425
Toll-free: 877 760-7439
E: info@cdbaontario.com
W: www.cdbraontario.ca
Executive:
Exec Dir: Cathy Proll
Dir-Intervention Serv: Diane Wilcock
Year Founded: 1990
Criteria: *Support the objectives of the organization.*
No of Paid Staff: 130
Speakers Available
Library: Y
Languages: English
Membership: 250
Membership Fee: $15

◈ Saskatchewan Chapter:
83 Tucker Cres, Saskatoon SK S7H 3H7
306 374-0022; Fax: 306 374-0004
E: cdba.sk@shaw.ca
W: www.cdbanational.com
Executive:
Pres: J Theo Gonari
Exec Dir: Dana Heinrichs
Year Founded: 1985
No of Paid Staff: 40
Languages: English
Membership: 15

Canadian Foundation for Physically Disabled Persons

265-6 Garamond Crt, Toronto ON M3C 1Z5
416 760-7351; Fax: 416 760-9405
E: whynot@sympatico.ca
W: www.cfpdp.com
Executive:
Chair: Vim Kochhar
Exec Dir: Dorothy Price
No of Paid Staff: 1
Languages: English

Canadian Guide Dogs for the Blind

Location: 4120 Rideau Valley Dr N, Manotick ON K4M 1B2
Mailing: PO Box 280, Manotick ON K4M 1A3
613 692-7777; Fax: 613 692-0650
E: info@guidedogs.ca
W: www.guidedogs.ca
Executive:
Co-Founder/COO: Jane E Thornton
Year Founded: 1984
Speakers Available
Library: Y
Languages: English; French

Canadian Hard of Hearing Association

1459 Brock Rd, Dundas ON L9H 5E4
905 659-7347
E: info@chha-hamilton.ca
W: www.chha-hamilton.ca
Executive:
Pres: Linda Baine

Canadian Hard of Hearing Association

205-2415 Holly Lane, Ottawa ON K1V 7P2
613 526-1584; Fax: 613 526-4718
Toll-free: 800 263-8068
E: chhanational@chha.ca
W: www.chha.ca
Executive:
Pres: Louise Normand
Exec Dir: Robert Corbeil
Year Founded: 1982
Criteria: *Anyone who supports CHHA*
No of Paid Staff: 3
Speakers Available
Library: Y
Languages: English
Membership: 2,100
Membership Fee: $25 per year - Singles; $300 - Lifetime Membership; $40 per year - Family; $70 per year - Organization

◈ Alberta

◇ Calgary Branch
63 Cornell Rd NW, Calgary AB T2L 0L4
403 284-6224; Fax: 403 276-5080
E: info@chha-calgary.ca
W: www.chha-calgary.ca
Executive:
Pres: Jade Coultman
Year Founded: 1982
Languages: English; French

◇ Edmonton Branch
10-9912 106 St NW, Edmonton AB T5K 1C5
780 428-6622; Fax: 780 420-6661
E: chha-ed@shaw.ca
W: www.chha-ed.com/CHHA-HOME.html
Executive:
Pres: Cindy Gordon
Treas: Jeffrey Resnick
Office Coord: Frances Tallon
Year Founded: 1997
No of Paid Staff: 1
Speakers Available
Library: Y *(Open to the public)*
Languages: English
Membership: 65 *(Lists available to the public)*

◇ High River/Okotoks Branch
100 Lineham Acres Grove NW, High River AB T1V 1S6
403 652-1811; Fax: 403 652-1811
E: lbetker@telus.net
Executive:
Treas: Les Betker

◇ Lethbridge Branch
1010 18A St N, Lethbridge AB T1H 3J3
403 328-2929
E: dgyorkos@telusplanet.net
Executive:
Pres: Doreen Gyorkos
Speakers Available
Languages: English; French

◈ BC Chapter
101-9300 Nowell St, Chilliwack BC V2P 4V7
604 795-9238; Fax: 604 795-9628
Toll-free: 866 888-2442 in BC
Toll-free Fax: 866 888-2443 in BC
E: info@chha-bc.org
W: www.chha-bc.org
Executive:
Pres: Nora McKellin
VP: Rodney George
Admin: Sharon Perry
No of Paid Staff: 3
Speakers Available
Library: Y
Languages: English
Membership: 425

◇ Alberni Valley Branch
4262 Michigan Rd, Port Alberni BC V9Y 5Z5
250 723-3750
Toll-free: 866 888-2442
Toll-free Fax: 866 888-2443
E: neilabe@shaw.ca
W: www.chha-bc.org
Executive:
Pres: Neil Abrahamson
Languages: English; French

◇ BC Parents' Branch
10150 Gillanders Rd, Chilliwack BC V2P 6H4
604 794-3772; Fax: 604 794-3960
E: info@chhaparents.bc.ca
W: www.chhaparents.bc.ca
Executive:
Pres: Leila Lolua
Editor: Janet Les
Languages: English; French

◇ Chilliwack Branch
101-9300 Nowell St, Chilliwack BC V2P 4V7
604 795-9238; Fax: 866 888-2443
Toll-free: 866 888-2442
E: info@chha-bc.org
W: www.chha-bc.org
Executive:
Pres: Nora McKellin
Languages: English; French

◇ Comox Valley Branch
Location: PO Box 433, Lazo BC V0R 2K0
Mailing: PO Box 433
250 339-5770
Toll-free: 866 888-2442
E: fstrotter@shaw.ca
W: www.chha-bc.org
Executive:
Pres: Sarah Trotter
Languages: English; French

◇ HEAR Branch
60-5221 Oakmount Cres, Burnaby BC V5H 4R4
604 438-2500
E: bettymac@telus.net
W: www.chha-bc.org
Executive:
Co-Chair: Hank Erickson
Co-Chair: Betty MacGillivray
Treas: Anna Bernard
Year Founded: 1982
Speakers Available
Languages: English
Membership: 25

◇ Nanaimo Branch
21 Haliburton St, Nanaimo BC V9R 4V6
250 591-6206
Toll-free: 866 888-2442 in BC
Toll-free Fax: 866 888-2443 in BC
Executive:
Br Mgr: Linda Chartrand
Languages: English; French

◇ North Shore Branch
600 Queens Rd W, North Vancouver BC V7N 2L3
604 926-5222; Fax: 604 925-2286
E: chha_nsb@telus.net
W: www.chha-nsb.com
Executive:
Pres: Mike Hocevar
Treas: Hugh Hetherington
Year Founded: 1989
Speakers Available
Languages: English
Membership: 75

◈ Manitoba

◇ Manitoba Chapter
SMD Self-help Clearinghouse
825 Sherbrook St, Winnipeg MB R3A 1M5
204 975-3037; Fax: 204 975-3027
E: mbchha@mts.net
W: www.chha-mb.ca
Year Founded: 1984
Speakers Available
Languages: English; French

◈ New Brunswick

◇ Fredericton Branch
563 Canada St, Fredericton NB E3A 4A8
613 526-1584
E: yeehaw@nbnet.nb.ca
W: chha.ca
Executive:
Pres: Louise Normand
VP: Michael Curriev
Treas: André Hurtubise
Languages: English; French

◇ Moncton Branch
809 Bernard St, Dieppe NB E1A 5Y2
506 855-3799
E: legerrh@rogers.com
Executive:
Pres: Rhéal Léger
Languages: English; French

◇ ***New Brunswick Chapter***
201-400 Douglas Ave, Saint John NB E2K 1E7
506 657-7643; Fax: 506 657-7643
E: winslow@nbnet.nb.ca
W: www.chha.ca
Executive:
Pres: Ian Hamilton
Languages: English; French

◈ ***Newfoundland***

◇ ***Exploits Valley Branch***
576 Main St, Bishops Falls NL A0H 1C0
709 258-5658
E: chha-evb@nl.rogers.com
Languages: English; French

◇ ***Gander Branch***
16 Griffin Pl, Gander NL A1V 2L3
709 651-3272
E: gordon.baker@nl.rogers.com
Languages: English; French

◇ ***Happy Valley Goose Bay Branch***
Mailing: PO Box 192 Stn C,
Happy-Valley-Goose NL A0P 1C0
709 896-5434
E: cgpeach@hotmail.com
Executive:
Pres: Cyril Peach

◇ ***Newfoundland & Labrador Chapter***
1081 Topsail Rd, Mount Pearl NL A1N 5G1
709 753-3224; Fax: 709 753-5640
Toll-free: 888 753-3224
E: chhanl@nfld.net
W: www.chha-nl.nl.ca
Executive:
Pres: Myrtle Barrett
VP: Glenn Kolonel
Exec Dir: Leon Mills
Treas: Robert Young
Sec: Mike Devine
Year Founded: 1984
Criteria: *Membership open to any interested party.*
Budget: $1,600,000
No of Paid Staff: 7
Speakers Available
Library: Y *(Open to the public)*
Languages: English
Membership: 100 *(Lists available to the public)*
Membership Fee: $15/year

◈ ***Northwest Territories Branch***

◇ ***Northwest Territories Branch***
252 Borden Dr, Yellowknife NT X1A 3R4
867 873-5446
E: billadkins@sunlife.com
Executive:
Principal: Bill Adkins
Languages: English; French

◈ ***Nova Scotia***

◇ ***Nova Scotia Chapter***
2 Homestead Rd, Fergusons Cove NS B3V 1S6
902 475-1277
E: understandingwhatsnext@gmail.com
W: www.chha.ca

◈ ***Ontario Chapter***
205-2415 Holly Lane, Ottawa ON K1V 7P2
613 526-1584; Fax: 613 526-4718
Toll-free: 800 263-8068
W: www.chha.ca
Executive:
Pres: Michel David
Criteria: *must be a member of CHHA-National and residing in Ontario*
Speakers Available
Languages: English; French
Membership: 700

◇ ***Hamilton Branch***
122-726 Upper James St, Hamilton ON L9C 2Z9
905 575-4964
E: info@chha-hamilton.ca
W: www.chha-hamilton.ca
Executive:
Pres: R Diehl
Treas: Craig Ellis
Sec: Kim Martin
Year Founded: 1985
Speakers Available
Languages: English

◇ ***Kingston Branch***
Mailing: 517-829 Norwest Rd, Kingston ON K7P 2N3
613 378-2457
E: mshenton@sympatico.ca
Executive:
Pres: Al Hiddema
Past Pres: M Shenton
Year Founded: 1980
Languages: English
Membership: 30

◇ ***London Branch***
3-1615 Churchill Ave, London ON N5W 2L1
613 526-1584
E: ossa_travis@hotmail.com

◇ ***Muskoka-Parry Sound Branch***
613 526-1584
E: chhanational@chha.ca

◇ ***National Capital Region Branch***
205-2415 Holly Lane, Ottawa ON K1V 7P2
613 526-1584; Fax: 613 526-4718
E: nicole@chhancr.com
W: chhancr.com
Executive:
Pres: Nicole Synowski

◇ ***Outaouais Branch***
205-2415 Holly Lane, Ottawa ON K1V 7P2
E: lnormand@justice.gc.ca
Executive:
Exec Dir: Louise Normand

◇ ***Sault Ste. Marie Branch***
613 526-1584; Fax: 613 526-4718
Toll-free: 800 263-8068
E: chhanational@chha.ca

◇ ***Sudbury Branch***
101-435 Notre Dame Ave, Sudbury ON P3C 5K6
705 523-5695; Fax: 705 523-8621
Toll-free: 866 300-2442
E: chha@vianet.ca
W: www.chha.ca
Executive:
Pres: Lorraine O'Brien
Languages: English; French

◇ ***Thunder Bay Branch***
5909 Mapleward Rd, Thunder Bay ON P7G 1L5
807 768-7668
E: donhalpert@gmail.com
W: www.chha.ca

◇ ***Toronto Hard of Hearing Branch***
101-55 Neptune Dr, North York ON M6A 1X2
416 781-4787
E: dc946@torfree.net
W: www.chha.ca
Executive:
Pres: Valerie Eaton
Languages: English; French

◇ ***York Branch***
147 Primeau Dr, Aurora ON L4G 6Z6
905 505-2578
E: dmac773@gmail.com
Executive:
Pres: Dan McDonnell

◈ ***Prince Edward Island***

◇ ***PEI Chapter***
RR 1, Augustine Cove, Borden-Carleton PE C0B 1X0
902 855-2382; Fax: 902 855-2382
E: annmerdon@pei.sympatico.ca
W: www.chha.ca
Executive:
Pres: Annie Lee MacDonald
Languages: English; French

◈ ***Quebec Chapter***
25 rue des Rapides, Gatineau QC J8T 5K2
613 526-1584
E: president@chha.ca
W: www.chha.ca
Executive:
Prés: Carole Willans

◈ ***Saskatchewan***

◇ ***Maple Creek Branch***
Mailing: PO Box 6, Richmound SK S0N 2E0
306 669-4212
E: abbischoff@sasktel.net
W: www.chha.ca
Executive:
Pres: Bernadette Bischoff
Treas: Doris Berreth
Languages: English; French

◇ ***Regina and District Branch Inc***
2341 Broad St, Regina SK S4P 1Y9
306 352-3323; Fax: 306 757-3252
Toll-free: 800 565-3323
E: glochha@sasktel.net
W: www.chha.ca
Executive:
Pres: Ruth McKim
Treas: George Thomas
Sec: Crystal Montoya
Year Founded: 1981
Budget: $6,500
Speakers Available
Languages: Sign Language; English
Membership: 34 *(Lists available to the public)*

◇ ***Saskatoon Branch***
267 Sylvian Way, Saskatoon SK S7H 5G1
306 665-2845
E: kelly.read@shaw.ca
Executive:
Pres: Joan Read
Languages: English; French

◈ ***Yukon Chapter***
613 526-1584
E: chhanational@chha.ca

The Canadian Hearing Society
271 Spadina Rd, Toronto ON M5R 2V3
416 928-2500; Fax: 416 928-2523
Toll-free: 877 347-3427 (Voice)
E: info@chs.ca
W: www.chs.ca
Executive:
Chair: Len Mitchell
Pres/CEO: Chris Kenopic
VP-Prog/Serv: Karen McDonald
VP-Fundraising/Strat Commun: Susan Main
COO: Katherine Hum-Antonopoulos
CFO: Stephanus Greeff
Dir-Hum Res: Donald Prong
Spec Advisor to Pres/Public Affairs: Gary Malkowski
Year Founded: 1940
Budget: $37,000,000
No of Paid Staff: 350
Speakers Available
Languages: English; American Sign Language; French
Membership: 600

Membership Fee: $250 - Lifetime; $25 per year - Regular
Library:
Phyllis Stephen Memorial Library *(Open to the public)*

◈Barrie:
1009-74 Cedar Pointe Dr, Barrie ON L4N 5R7
705 737-3190; Fax: 705 722-0381
E: abyl@chs.ca
W: www.chs.ca
Executive:
Counsellor (Hearing Care): Cathy O'Connor
Counsellor (Hearing Care): Peggy Norton-Harris
Reg Dir: Tim Maloney
No of Paid Staff: 4
Speakers Available
Languages: English

◈Belleville:
Bayview Mall
51-470 Dundas St E, Belleville ON K8N 1G1
613 966-8995; Fax: 613 966-8365
E: jvanderheyden@chs.ca
W: www.chs.ca
Executive:
Area Office Sec: Jen Vanderheyden
Prog Mgr: Anna Strati-Morrison
Speakers Available
Library: Y *(Open to the public)*
Languages: English; American Sign Language

◈Brantford:
139-225 Colborne St, Brantford ON N3T 2H2
519 753-3162; Fax: 519 753-7447
E: nmcalonen@chs.ca
W: www.chs.ca
Executive:
Prog Mgr: Natalie McAlonen

◈Brockville:
205-68 William St, Brockville ON K6V 4V5
613 498-3933; Fax: 613 498-3317
E: sbaker@chs.ca
W: www.chs.ca
Executive:
Hearing Care Couns: Dianne McConkey

◈Chatham:
75 Thames St, Floor 2, Chatham ON N7L 1S4
519 354-9347; Fax: 519 354-2083
E: gbaker@chs.ca
W: www.chs.ca
Executive:
Reg Dir: David Kerr

◈Elliot Lake
Huron Lodge
130 Queen St E, Sault Ste. Marie ON P6A 1Y5
705 848-5306
Toll-free: 855 819-9169
E: wking@chs.ca
W: www.chs.ca
Executive:
Prog Mgr: Wayne King

◈Guelph:
200-2 Quebec St, Guelph ON N1H 2T3
519 821-4242; Fax: 519 821-8846
E: info@chs.ca
W: www.chs.ca
Executive:
Reg Info Officer: Amanda Hogan
Hearing Care Counsellor: Mary Anne Melanson
Hearing Care Counsellor: Mary Young
Year Founded: 1978
Speakers Available
Languages: English; American Sign Language
Membership list available to the public

◈Hamilton:
21 Hunter St E, Floor 2, Hamilton ON L8N 1M2
905 522-0755; Fax: 905 522-1336
E: dtaylor@chs.ca
W: www.chs.ca
Executive:
Reg Dir: Monte Hardy
Reg Prog Mgr: Natalie McAlonen
Hearing Care Couns: Jill Gittings

◈Kenora
136 Main St S, Kenora ON P9N 1S9
807 468-7230; Fax: 807 468-8496
E: agriffeth@chs.ca
W: www.chs.ca
Executive:
Reg Dir: Nancy Frost
Admv Asst: Loris Letain
Hearing Care Counsellor: Dianne Griffiths

◈Kingston:
Frontenac Mall
D4-1300 Bath Rd, Kingston ON K7M 4X4
613 544-1927; Fax: 613 544-1975
E: smarigold@chs.ca
W: www.chs.ca
Executive:
Reg Dir: Brian McKenzie
Admn/Support Serv Mgr: Debbie Oakley
Year Founded: 1940

◈Kitchener:
200-120 Ottawa St N, Kitchener ON N2H 3K5
519 744-6811; Fax: 519 744-2390
Toll-free: 800 668-5815
E: info@chs.ca
W: www.chs.ca
Executive:
Reg Dir: Victoria Baby
Reg Info Officer: Amanda Hogan
Hearing Care Counsellor: Joyce Haynes
Hearing Care Counsellor: Mary Anne Melanson
Year Founded: 1978
Criteria: *Open to all. Anyone interested.*
No of Paid Staff: 20
Speakers Available
Library: Y
Languages: English; American Sign Language
Membership Fee: $25
Library:
Hickman Community Resource Centre *(Open to the public)*

◈London:
181 Wellington St, London ON N6B 2K9
519 667-3325; Fax: 519 667-9668
E: info@chs.ca
W: www.chs.ca
Executive:
Hearing Care Counsellor: Kim Paulton
Reg Dir: Marilyn Reid
Commun Spec: Dawn Vandaele

◈Mississauga:
300-2227 South Millway, Mississauga ON L5L 3R6
905 608-0271; Fax: 905 608-8241
E: info@chs.ca
W: www.chs.ca
Executive:
Reg Dir: Victoria Baby
Reg Prog Mgr: Darrin Ballard

◈North Bay:
432-101 Worthington St E, North Bay ON P1B 1G5
705 474-8090; Fax: 705 474-6075
E: nbleach@chs.ca
W: www.chs.ca
Executive:
Intervenor: Jackie Cardy
Counsellor: Robin Osborne
GSS Counsellor: Francesca Morabito
Sec/Receptionist: Nicole Bleach

◈Oshawa:
Braemor Center Plaza
7-575 Thornton Rd N, Oshawa ON L1J 8L5
905 404-8490; Fax: 905 404-2012
Toll-free: 800 213-3848
E: info@chs.ca
W: www.chs.ca
Executive:
Hearing Care Counsellor: Anna McIntosh
Office Mgr: Kim Nicholson
Reg Dir: Maggie Doherty-Gilbert

◈Ottawa:
600-2197 Riverside Dr, Ottawa ON K1H 7X3
613 521-0509; Fax: 613 521-0838
E: office@ottawa.chs.ca
W: www.chs.ca
Executive:
Hearing Care Couns: Doris Brownlee
Hearing Care Couns: Barb Christopher
Reg Dir: Philippe Ramsay

◈Peterborough:
315 Reid St, Peterborough ON K9J 3R2
705 743-1573; Fax: 705 741-0708
Toll-free: 800 213-3848
E: amulligan@chs.ca
W: www.chs.ca
Executive:
Hearing Care Counsellor: Rose Watson
Office Mgr: Kim Nicholson
Reg Dir: Maggie Doherty-Gilbert

◈Point Edward:
420 East St N, Sarnia ON N7T 6Y5
519 337-8307; Fax: 519 337-6886
Toll-free: 877 634-0178 TDD
E: jbartlett@chs.ca
W: chs.ca
Executive:
Reg Dir: Marilyn Reid
Year Founded: 1940
Speakers Available
Languages: Sign Language
Membership list available to the public

◈Sault Ste Marie:
130 Queen St E, Sault Ste. Marie ON P6A 1Y5
705 946-4320; Fax: 705 256-7231
E: tcollins@chs.ca
W: www.chs.ca
Executive:
Hearing Care Counsellor: Kerri Tuckett
Hearing Care Counsellor: Gisella Krezek
Gen Support Serv Counsellor: Anna Riseng
Connect Counsellor: Linda Schraeder
Reg Prog Mgr: Wayne King
Sign Language Interpreter: Lesley Sawchyn
Literacy Instructor: Gieselle Bourgault

◈St. Catharines
501-55 King St, St Catharines ON L2R 3H5
905 984-4412; Fax: 905 984-8298
E: dflor@chs.ca
W: www.chs.ca
Executive:
Reg Dir: Chris Kenopic
Year Founded: 1940
No of Paid Staff: 7
Speakers Available
Languages: English; American Sign Language

◈ ***Sudbury:***
1233 Paris St, Sudbury ON P3E 3B6
705 522-1020; Fax: 705 522-1060
Toll-free: 800 479-4562
E: gcosh@chs.ca
W: www.chs.ca
Executive:
Hearing Care Counsellor: Angele Chandler
Office Mgr: Kim Irving
Reg Dir: Silvy Coutu
Year Founded: 1940

◈ ***Thunder Bay:***
35-125 Syndicate Ave S, Thunder Bay ON P7E 6H8
807 623-1646; Fax: 807 623-4815
Toll-free: 866 646-0514
Toll-free Fax: 866 646-0514
E: smetzner@chs.ca
W: www.chs.ca
Executive:
Hearing Care Counsellor: Jody Carrier
Reg Dir: Nancy Frost
Criteria: *Join CHS Thunder Bay Today! Your membership allows you to vote at the CHS Annual General Meeting and you will receive a year's subscription to the 'Vibes' magazine. 1 year individual membership is $25. Other family members living at the same address who wish to obtain voting privileges must pay an additions $5 each. A lifetime membership is $250. Call (807) 623-1646 for further information.*

◈ ***Timmins:***
20 Wilcox St, Timmins ON P4N 3K6
705 268-0771; Fax: 705 268-4598
Toll-free: 877 872-0580 TTY
W: www.chs.ca
Executive:
GSS Counsellor/Emp Consultant: Amy Fleury
Deaf/Blind Intervenor: Regina St-Denis

◈ ***Windsor:***
A3-300 Giles Blvd E, Windsor ON N9A 4C4
519 253-7241; Fax: 519 253-6630
E: info@chs.ca
W: www.chs.ca
Executive:
Hearing Care Counsellor: Bonnie Petryschuk
Reg Dir: David Kerr

◈ ***Saskatchewan:***
2341 Broad St, Regina SK S4P 1Y9
306 352-3323; Fax: 306 757-3252
Toll-free: 800 565-3323
E: glochha@sasktel.net
W: www.chha.ca
Executive:
Pres: Ruth McKim
Treas: George Thomas
Sec: Crystal Montoya
Year Founded: 1981
Budget: $6,500
Speakers Available
Languages: Sign Language; English
Membership: 34 *(Lists available to the public)*

Canadian National Society of the Deaf-Blind
405-422 Willowdale Ave, North York ON M2N 5B1
416 730-9501; Fax: 416 730-1350
W: www.cnsdb.ca
Executive:
Treas: Jennifer Robbins
Languages: English; French

Canadian Paraplegic Association (Alberta)
305-11010 101 St NW, Edmonton AB T5H 4B9
780 424-6312; Fax: 780 424-6313
Toll-free: 888 654-5444
E: edmonton@cpa-ab.org
W: www.cpa-ab.org
Year Founded: 1961
No of Paid Staff: 35
Speakers Available
Library: Y *(Open to the public)*
Languages: English

◈ ***Calgary:***
5211 4 St NE, Calgary AB T2K 6J5
403 228-3001; Fax: 403 229-4271
E: calgary@cpa-ab.org
W: www.cpa-ab.org
Executive:
Mgr: Cal Schuler
Languages: English

◈ ***Fort McMurray***
Gregoire Park Centre
194 Grenfell Cres, Fort McMurray AB T9H 2M6
780 743-0307; Fax: 780 743-4563
E: fortmcmurray@cpa-ab.org
W: www.cpa-ab.org

◈ ***Lethbridge:***
300-515 7 St S, Lethbridge AB T1J 2G8
403 327-7577; Fax: 403 320-0269
E: lethbridge@cpa-ab.org
W: www.cpa-ab.org
Executive:
Client Serv Coord: Dylan Adkins
Languages: English

◈ ***Lloydminster***
Mailing: PO Box 1691 Stn Main, Lloydminster SK S9V 1K6
780 875-1046; Fax: 780 875-1046
E: lloydminster@cpa-ab.org
W: www.cpa-ab.org

◈ ***Medicine Hat:***
26-419 3 St SE, Medicine Hat AB T1A 0G9
403 504-4001; Fax: 403 504-5172
Toll-free: 888 654-5444
E: medicinehat@cpa-ab.org
W: www.cpa-ab.org
Executive:
Mgr: Sue Edwards
No of Paid Staff: 60
Speakers Available
Library: Y *(Open to the public)*
Languages: English
Membership list available to the public

◈ ***Red Deer:***
103-4719 48 Ave, Red Deer AB T4N 3T1
403 341-5060; Fax: 403 343-1630
Toll-free: 888 654-5444
E: reddeer@cpa-ab.org
W: www.cpa-ab.org
Executive:
Reg Mgr: Doug Manderville
No of Paid Staff: 4
Speakers Available
Library: Y *(Open to the public)*
Languages: English

◈ ***St. Paul***
Mailing: PO Box 653, St Paul AB T0A 3A0
780 645-5116; Fax: 780 645-5141
E: stpaul@cpa-ab.org
W: www.cpa-ab.org
Executive:
Aboriginal Serv Coord: Ken Kwiatkowski

Canadian Paraplegic Association (Manitoba) Inc.
211-825 Sherbrook St, Winnipeg MB R3A 1M5
204 786-4753; Fax: 204 786-1140
Toll-free: 800 720-4933 within manitoba only
E: winnipeg@canparaplegic.org
W: www.cpamanitoba.ca
Executive:
Exec Dir: Ron Burky
Year Founded: 1945
No of Paid Staff: 11
Speakers Available
Library: Y *(Open to the public)*
Languages: English
Membership Fee: $10/year

Canadian Paraplegic Association Newfoundland and Labrador
Location: 342 Freshwater Rd, St. John's NL A1B 1C2
Mailing: PO Box 21284, RPO MacDonald Drive, St. John's NL A1A 5G6
709 753-5901; Fax: 709 753-4224
E: cpa.stj@cpa.nfld.net
W: www.canparaplegic.org
Executive:
Exec Dir: Michael Burry
Year Founded: 1976
Budget: $1,500,000
No of Paid Staff: 40
Speakers Available
Languages: English
Membership: 9,000

◈ ***Conception Bay/Placentia Office:***
Location: PMC Prof Bldg, 25 Bareneed Rd, Bay Roberts NL A0A 1G0
Mailing: PO Box 1309
709 786-1440; Fax: 709 786-1441
E: cpabayroberts@nf.aibn.com
W: www.canparaplegic.org
Executive:
Exec Dir: Michael Burry
Languages: English

◈ ***Gander Regional Office***
Location: 304-9 Main St, Corner Brook NL A2H 1C2
Mailing: PO Box 764 Stn Main, Corner Brook NL A2H 6G7
709 634-9909; Fax: 709 634-7395
E: cornerbrook@cpa.nfld.net
Executive:
Exec Dir: Michael Burry
Dir-Client Serv: Marilyn Bonnell
Languages: English

◈ ***Labrador:***
Location: 21 Bloomfield St, Happy-Valley-Goose NL A0P 1E0
Mailing: PO Box 848
709 896-3010; Fax: 709 896-3716
E: cpalab@nf.aibn.com
W: www.canparaplegic.org
Languages: English

◈ ***Northern Regional Office:***
Mailing: PO Box 319, Port Saunders NL A0K 4H0
709 861-3244; Fax: 709 861-3248
E: portsaunders@nf.aibn.com
W: www.canparaplegic.org
Executive:
Exec Dir: Michael Burry
Languages: English

◈ ***Stephenville Regional Office:***
Mailing: PO Box 281 Stn Main, Stephenville NL A2N 2Z4
709 643-9649; Fax: 709 643-3293
E: cpa.stv@nf.aibn.com
W: www.canparaplegic.org

Executive:
Exec Dir: Michael Burry
Languages: English

◈ ***Windsor Regional Office:***
Upper Level,Town Square Mall
7 High St, Grnd-Falls-Windsor NL A2A 1C3
709 489-8410; Fax: 709 489-8460
E: gdflpa@nf.aibn.com
W: www.canparaplegic.org
Executive:
Career/Empl Dis Case Mgr: Denyse Goulding
Languages: English; French

Canadian Paraplegic Association Nova Scotia
Mumford Towers 1
317A-7001 Mumford Rd, Halifax NS B3L 2H8
902 423-1277; Fax: 902 492-1213
Toll-free: 800 889-1889 NS only
E: halifax@canparaplegic.org
W: www.thespine.ca
Executive:
Dir: Nancy Beaton
Year Founded: 1952
No of Paid Staff: 9
Speakers Available
Languages: English
Membership: 900
Membership Fee: $15 per year

Canadian Paraplegic Association of Saskatchewan
311 38th St E, Saskatoon SK S7K 0T1
306 652-9644; Fax: 306 652-2957
E: saskatoon@canparaplegic.org
W: www.canparaplegic.org
Budget: $620,000
No of Paid Staff: 10
Languages: English
Membership: 1,200

Canadian Paraplegic Association Ontario Provincial & Toronto Office
520 Sutherland Dr, Toronto ON M4G 3V9
416 422-5644; Fax: 416 422-5943
Toll-free: 877 422-1112
E: info@cpaont.org
W: www.cpaont.org
Executive:
Chair: Michael Gottlieb
Exec Dir: Bill Adair
Treas: Daniel Ross
Year Founded: 1945
Budget: $7,000,000
No of Paid Staff: 150
Speakers Available
Library: Y *(Open to the public)*
Languages: English
Membership: 2,000
Membership Fee: $25

◈ ***Barrie:***
Barrie by the Bay
111-80 Bradford St, Barrie ON L4N 6S7
705 726-4546; Fax: 705 726-5054
Toll-free: 800 870-5670
E: barrie@cpaont.org
W: www.cpaont.org
Executive:
Reg Serv Coord: Heather Hollingshead
Languages: English

◈ ***Hamilton***
Location: 300 Wellington St N, Room B1-3, Hamilton ON L8L 0A4
Mailing: 237 Barton St E, Hamilton ON L8L 2X2
905 383-0216; Fax: 905 383-5021
Toll-free: 877 262-3366
W: www.cpaont.org
Executive:
Community Dev: Chelsea Crealock

◈ ***Kearney***
Mailing: PO Box 327, Kearney ON P0A 1M0
705 636-5827; Fax: 705 636-7223
Executive:
Reg Serv Coord: Yvonne Green

◈ ***Kingston***
772 Blackburn Mews, Kingston ON K7P 2N7
613 547-1391; Fax: 613 547-1393
Toll-free: 866 220-7539
W: www.cpaont.org
Executive:
Reg Serv Coord: Michelle Smith

◈ ***London***
3-1111 Elias St, London ON N5W 5L1
519 433-2331; Fax: 519 433-3987
Toll-free: 866 433-9888
W: www.cpaont.org
Executive:
Reg Serv Coord: Elizabeth Zarnowiecki
Library: Y *(Open to the public)*
Languages: English

◈ ***North York***
306-1120 Finch Ave W, Toronto ON M3J 3H7
416 241-1433; Fax: 416 241-2466
Toll-free: 866 318-9990
E: AttendantServices@sciontario.org
W: www.sciontario.org
Executive:
Ops Mgr Attendant Serv: Vera Harris
Dir-Client Serv: Gillian Bone

◈ ***Peterborough***
Mailing: PO Box 131, Warsaw ON K0L 3A0
705 652-7496; Fax: 705 743-2508
Toll-free: 888 643-2507
W: www.cpaont.org
Executive:
Reg Serv Coord: Stephanie Bolton

◈ ***Sault Ste. Marie***
3-260 Elizabeth St, Sault Ste. Marie ON P6A 6J3
705 759-0333; Fax: 705 759-0335
Toll-free: 866 531-1513
W: www.cpaont.org
Executive:
Reg Serv Coord: Diane Morrell

◈ ***Sudbury***
ICAN Bldg
765 Brennan Rd, Sudbury ON P3C 1C4
705 671-2444; Fax: 705 671-2446
Toll-free: 877 671-2444
E: marjorie.mccann@cpaont.org
W: www.cpaont.org
Executive:
Reg Serv Coord: Marjorie McCann

◈ ***Thunder Bay***
B-1201 Jasper Dr, Thunder Bay ON P7B 6R2
807 344-3743; Fax: 807 344-9490
Toll-free: 866 344-4159
W: www.cpaont.org
Executive:
Reg Serv Coord: Darren Lillington

◈ ***Windsor***
Western Campus,Windsor Regional Hospital
1453 Prince Rd, Windsor ON N9C 3Z4
519 253-7272; Fax: 519 253-7279
Toll-free: 877 253-7279
W: www.cpaont.org
Executive:
Reg Serv Coord: Peggy Koelin

Canadian Paraplegic Association Prince Edward Island
Location: 14 Exhibition Dr, Charlottetown PE C1A 5Z5
Mailing: PO Box 2188 Stn Central, Charlottetown PE C1A 8B9
902 626-9523
E: myrtle@eventsinc.ca
W: www.canparaplegic.org
Executive:
Exec Dir: Paul Cudmore
Languages: English

Canadian Therapeutic Riding Association
11-5420 Hwy 6, RR 5, Guelph ON N1H 6J2
519 767-0700; Fax: 519 767-0435
E: ctra@golden.net
W: www.cantra.ca
Executive:
Schl Prin: Daphne Davey
Year Founded: 1980
No of Paid Staff: 2
Speakers Available
Languages: English; French
Membership: 500
Membership Fee: $30

Canadian Wheelchair Foundation Canada
Mailing: PO Box 75038 RPO White Rock, White Rock BC V4B 5L3
604 536-2022; Fax: 604 536-9831
Toll-free: 866 666-2411
E: info@cdnwheelchair.ca
W: www.cdnwheelchair.ca
Executive:
Exec Dir: Christiana Flessner
Languages: English; French

Cardston and District Association for the Handicapped
Location: 474 5th Ave W, Cardston AB T0K 0K0
Mailing: PO Box 1467
403 653-3766; Fax: 403 653-3785
Executive:
Exec Dir: Kim Flickinger
Year Founded: 1990
Criteria: *Parent, guardian, interest*
No of Paid Staff: 30
Languages: English
Membership: 50
Membership Fee: $5

Career Services of Brockville Inc.
89 Hubbell St, Brockville ON K6V 4K6
613 342-5775; Fax: 613 342-1733
E: info@careerservices.ca
W: www.careerservices.ca
Executive:
Chair: Candy Burkitt
Vice Chair: Valerie Kines
Mktg Mgr: Bill Hart
Sec-Treas: Robert Croxall
Office Mgr: Brenda Donovan
OH&S Mgr: Carol Roy

Carewest Dr. Vernon Fanning Centre
722 16 Ave NE, Calgary AB T2E 6V7
403 230-6900; Fax: 403 230-6902
W: www.carewest.ca
Executive:
Dir: Mark Ewan
Adm Sec: Lynne Johnson
Languages: English

Carrefour Jeunesse Emploi Charlevoix Côte-de-Beaupré
85 rue Saint-Jean-Baptiste, Baie-Saint-Paul QC G3Z 1M5
418 435-2503; Fax: 418 435-3739
E: appui@charlevoix.net
W: www.cje-appui.qc.ca
Executive:
Dir exéc: Martin Larouche

Centre d'intégration à la vie active (CIVA)
330-525 rue Dominion, Montréal QC H3J 2B4
514 935-1109; Fax: 514 935-8597
E: info@civa.qc.ca
W: www.civa.qc.ca
Executive:
Dir: Daniel Vézina
Coord commun: Chantale Montpetit
Budget: $250,000
No of Paid Staff: 5
Languages: French

Child & Family Services
7055 Alberni St, Powell River BC V8A 2C2
604 485-6077; Fax: 604 485-6017
E: jpcsecretary@pracl.ca
W: www.pracl.ca
Executive:
Exec Dir: Lilla Tipton
Year Founded: 1954

Christian Blind Mission International - CBM
Location: 3844 Stouffville Rd, Stouffville ON L4A 7X5
Mailing: PO Box 800 Stn Main, Stouffville ON L4A 7Z9
905 640-6464; Fax: 905 640-4332
Toll-free: 800 567-2264
E: cbm@cbmcanada.org
W: www.cbmcanada.org
Executive:
CFO: Steven Baal
Exec Dir: Ed Epp
Dir-Overseas Ops: Winston Miller
Dir-Mktg/Commun: Beth Jost-Reimer
Dir-Hum Res: Jill Bartley
Year Founded: 1908
Budget: $10,000,000
No of Paid Staff: 25
Speakers Available
Languages: English
Library:
Talking Book Library -- Manager, Mrs. Jill Bartley
(Open to the public)

Civil Rights Now!
425-1489 Marine Dr, West Vancouver BC V7T 1B8
604 928-1644
W: www.palsbc.org
Executive:
Founder/Exec Dir: Paul Caune

Coalition of Persons with Disabilities - Newfoundland & Labrador
48-15 Hamlyn Rd, St. John's NL A1E 6E2
709 722-7011; Fax: 709 722-4424
E: info@codnl.ca
W: www.codnl.ca
Executive:
Exec Dir: Kelly White
Year Founded: 1983
No of Paid Staff: 1
Library: Y
Languages: English

Colchester Residential Services
201-35 Commercial St, Box 1860, Truro NS B2N 3H9
902 893-4273; Fax: 902 895-4192
E: crss@ns.aliantzinc.ca
W: crss.info/contact-us
Executive:
Exec Dir: Shannon McLellan

Community Association for Riding for the Disabled
4777 Dufferin St, North York ON M3H 5T3
416 667-8600; Fax: 416 739-7520
E: info@card.ca
W: www.card.ca
Executive:
Exec Dir: Penny Smith
Prog Dir: Seana Waldon
Finl Coord: Vivienne Hennie
Fundraising/Spec Events: Bonnie Hartley
Year Founded: 1969
Criteria: *A voting member must be 18 years of age and must have paid $25 fee. A non-voting member is under 18 years of age and must have paid $25 fee.*
Budget: $850,000
No of Paid Staff: 11
Speakers Available
Languages: English
Membership: 175
Membership Fee: Ranges from $25 to $l000 Per Year

Community Living Association South Simcoe
125 Dufferin St S, Alliston ON L9R 1E9
705 435-4792; Fax: 705 435-2766
W: www.class.on.ca
Executive:
Exec Dir: Vito Facciolo

Community Living Burlington
3057 Mainway, Burlington ON L7M 1A1
905 336-2225; Fax: 905 335-9919
W: www.clburlington.ca
Executive:
Exec Dir: Judy Pryde
Dir-Fin: Lisa Morikawa
Hum Res Coord: Donna Clausnitzer
Sr Mgr: Donna Vandermeulen

Community Living - Fort Frances & District
Location: 340 Scott St, Fort Frances ON P9A 1G9
Mailing: PO Box 147 Stn Main,
Fort Frances ON P9A 3M5
807 274-5556; Fax: 807 274-5009
E: clffd@vianet.ca
W: www.communitylivingfortfrances.com
Executive:
Exec Dir: Alanna J Barr
Year Founded: 1965
Budget: $4,354,000
No of Paid Staff: 93
Speakers Available
Languages: English
Membership: 25

Community Living - Victoria
3861 Cedar Hill Cross Rd, Victoria BC V8P 2M7
250 477-7231; Fax: 250 477-6944
E: info@clvic.ca
W: www.clvic.ca
Executive:
Exec Dir: Ellen Tarshis
IT/Fin Mgr: Rob Turner

Community Living Windsor
7025 Enterprise Way, Windsor ON N8T 3N6
519 974-4221; Fax: 519 974-4157
E: info@clwindsor.org
W: www.clwindsor.org
Executive:
Pres: John Fairley
Exec Dir: Xavier Noordermeer
Dir-Fin: Brian Cutler
Year Founded: 1953
No of Paid Staff: 450
Library: Y
Languages: English

Connect Society Deafness Advocacy and Family Services
6240 113 St NW, Edmonton AB T6H 3L2
780 454-9581; Fax: 780 447-5820
W: www.connectsociety.org
Executive:
Exec Dir/CEO: Clare Gallant
Year Founded: 1963
Languages: English
Membership: 100

Cope Rocky Mountain House
Location: 4940 50th Ave,
Rocky-Mtn-House AB T4T 1A8
Mailing: PO Box 1120 Stn Main
403 845-4080; Fax: 403 845-6951
Executive:
Exec Dir: Laurel Ponich

Corbrook Awakening Abilities
1-931 Progress Ave, Scarborough ON M1G 3V5
416 431-9000; Fax: 416 431-4227
W: www.corbrook.com
Executive:
Exec Dir: Deepak Soni
Dir-Servs: Toni Grillo
Bus Mgr: Vahan Palamoudian
Mgr-Serv: Paulette Cross
Year Founded: 1950

Council of Canadians with Disabilities
926-294 Portage Ave, Winnipeg MB R3C 0B9
204 947-0303; Fax: 204 942-4625
E: ccd@ccdonline.ca
W: www.ccdonline.ca
Executive:
Chairperson: Tony Dolan
1st V-Chair: John Rae
2nd V-Chair: Susan Ralph
Year Founded: 1976
Criteria: *Open to all consumer controlled organizations whose primary purpose is advocacy.*
Budget: $1,600,000
No of Paid Staff: 6
Speakers Available
Library: Y
Languages: English; French
Membership: 17

Dawson Creek Society of Community Living
1334 102 Ave, Dawson Creek BC V1G 2C6
250 782-2611; Fax: 250 782-2662
E: info@dcscl.org
W: www.dcscl.org

Deaf & Hard of Hearing Society
63 Cornell Rd NW, Calgary AB T2L 0L4
403 284-6200; Fax: 403 282-7006
Toll-free: 877 711-3447
E: leslie.brachman@dhhs.ca
W: www.dhhs.ca

Executive:
Exec Dir: Christina Smith
Mgr-Strat Partnership: Lynne Nieman
Fin/Hum Res/Admn Mgr: Leslie Brachman
Tinnitus Coord: Sylvia Bird
Coord: Kathy Harrison
Interpreter Booking Coord: Jason Huddlestone
Interpreter Booking Coord: Deanna Lilley
Hard of Hearing Serv Coord: Jan Stewart
Equip Spec: Rytch Newmiller
Year Founded: 1971
No of Paid Staff: 62
Speakers Available
Languages: English; Sign Language
Membership: 150
Membership Fee: $25 per year

Deaf Children's Society of BC
200-7355 Canada Way, Burnaby BC V3N 4Z6
604 525-6056; Fax: 604 525-7307
Toll-free: 877 525-6056
E: deafbc@deafchildren.bc.ca
W: www.deafchildren.bc.ca
Executive:
Exec Dir: Janice Springford
Year Founded: 1981
Budget: $700,000
No of Paid Staff: 12
Speakers Available
Library: Y *(Open to the public)*
Languages: Sign Language; English
Membership: 200
Membership Fee: $40 - Organization; $25 - Individual/Family (non-voting)
Library:
DCS Library *(Open to the public)*

DeafBlind Ontario Services Inc.
15-17665 Leslie St, Newmarket ON L3Y 3E3
905 853-2862; Fax: 905 853-3407
Toll-free: 855 340-3267
E: execasst@deafblindontario.com
W: www.deafblindontario.com
Year Founded: 1989
No of Paid Staff: 140
Library: Y *(Open to the public)*
Languages: English
Membership list available to the public

Delta Community Living Society
1-3800 72 St, Delta BC V4K 3N2
604 946-9508; Fax: 604 940-9683
E: dcls@dcls.ca
W: www.dcls.ca
Executive:
Exec Dir: Anita Sihota
Dir-Commun/Residential Serv: Tara Asquith
Fin Mgr: Alison Betts
Year Founded: 1963
No of Paid Staff: 200
Languages: English
Membership: 120
Membership Fee: Individual: $10; Family $15; Corporate/Community $75.

Developmental Disabilities Resource Centre of Calgary
4631 Richardson Way SW, Calgary AB T3E 7B7
403 240-3111; Fax: 403 240-3230
E: info@ddrcc.com
W: www.ddrcc.com
Executive:
CEO: Helen Cowie
Dir-Hum Res: Janice Cutforth
Bus Dev Mgr: Eric Koo
Year Founded: 1952
Criteria: *Anyone 18 years of age or older.*
Budget: $10,327,608
No of Paid Staff: 394
Speakers Available
Languages: English
Membership: 108
Membership Fee: Single or Associate: $15, Family: $20

Disabled Peoples' International
874 Topsail Rd, Mount Pearl NL A1N 3J9
709 747-7600; Fax: 709 747-7603
E: info@dpi.org
W: www.dpi.org
Executive:
Fin Off: Chris Morrissey
Proj Coord: Elizabeth da Silva
Year Founded: 1981
No of Paid Staff: 4
Languages: English; French; Spanish
Membership: 134 member countries

Dog Guides Canada
152 Wilson St, Oakville ON L6K 0G6
905 842-2891; Fax: 905 842-3373
E: info@dogguides.com
W: www.dogguides.com
Executive:
Exec Dir: Sandy Turney
Controller: Don Duncan
Commun Mgr: Natalie Moncur
Year Founded: 1983
Languages: English

Easter Seals Alberta - Calgary Office
103-811 Manning Rd NE, Calgary AB T2E 7L4
403 235-5662; Fax: 403 248-1716
Toll-free: 877 832-7837
E: calgary@easterseals.ab.ca
W: www.easterseals.ab.ca
Executive:
CEO: Susan Boivin
Dir-Ops Edmonton: Jodi Zabludowski
Year Founded: 1951
Budget: $4,000,000
No of Paid Staff: 25
Speakers Available
Languages: English

◈Bragg Creek:
Mailing: PO Box 540, Bragg Creek AB T0L 0K0
403 949-3818; Fax: 403 949-3388
E: info@telusplanet.net/public/easter
Executive:
CEO: Mary Thompson

◈Edmonton:
1408-10025 106 St NW, Edmonton AB T5J 1G4

Easter Seals New Brunswick (CRCD)
65 Brunswick St, Fredericton NB E3B 1G5
506 458-8739; Fax: 506 457-2863
Toll-free: 888 280-8155
E: info@easterseals.nb.ca
W: www.easterseals.nb.ca
Executive:
Pres: Doug Bridgeman
Past Pres: Glen Hughes
Fin Mgr: Dora Buchanan
Exec Asst: Jennifer Griffin
Contact: Julie Walker
Year Founded: 1966
Budget: $1,000,000
No of Paid Staff: 12
Speakers Available
Library: Y
Languages: English; French
Membership Fee: $10

Easter Seals - Newfoundland and Labrador
Location: 206 Mount Scio Rd, St. John's NL A1B 4L5
Mailing: PO Box 23033 Churchill Sq
709 754-1399; Fax: 709 754-1398
Toll-free: 888 601-6767
W: www.easterseals.nf.ca
Executive:
Pres: Gerry Olscamp
Exec Dir: Deirdre Greene
No of Paid Staff: 7
Speakers Available
Languages: English

Easter Seals Nova Scotia
3670 Kempt Rd, Halifax NS B3K 4X8
902 453-6000; Fax: 902 454-6121
E: easterseals@easterseals.ns.ca
W: www.easterseals.ns.ca
Executive:
Pres/CEO: Thomas G Merriam
Coord-Assistive Devices/Client Info Serv: Faye Joudrey
Year Founded: 1931
No of Paid Staff: 18
Speakers Available
Languages: English
Membership: 125
Membership Fee: $10

Elmira District Community Living
118 Barnswallow Dr, Elmira ON N3B 2Y9
519 669-3205; Fax: 519 669-3444
E: elmiraacl@elmiraacl.com
W: www.elmiraacl.com
Executive:
Exec Dir: Greg Bechard
Hum Res Mgr: Laurie Thomson

Employment Solutions Society
215 Dominion St, Bridgewater NS B4V 2K7
902 543-2479; Fax: 902 543-0284
E: info@empsolutions.ca
W: www.empsolutions.ca
Executive:
Exec Dir: Margaret Matthews
Job Dev Officer: Jim Key

Employment Support Services
105-4675 Marine Ave, Powell River BC V8A 2L2
E: empsupport@pracl.ca

L'ÉTAPE, un projet de La Bourgade Inc.
527-1001 boul de Maisonneuve E, étage 5, Montréal QC H2L 4P9
514 526-0887; Fax: 514 527-1028
E: letape@letape.org
W: www.letape.org
Executive:
Dir gén: François Huard
Year Founded: 1982
No of Paid Staff: 10
Languages: French; English

◈Laval
320-1865 rue Fleetwood, Laval QC H7N 4B2
Executive:
Contact: Françoise Préfontaine

Exploits Disability Association
Location: 109 Main St, Grnd-Falls-Windsor NL A2B 1J8
Mailing: PO Box 736 Stn Main, Grnd-Falls-Windsor NL A2B 2K2
709 489-3900; Fax: 709 489-3546
E: eda@nf.aibn.com
W: www.grandfallswindsor.com

Executive:
Pres: Job Goudie
Library: Y *(Open to the public)*
Languages: English
Membership list available to the public

Fondation Mira Inc.
114-2700 rue Jean-Perrin, Québec QC G2C 1S9
418 845-6472; Fax: 418 845-1000
E: quebec@mira.ca
W: www.mira.ca
Executive:
Dir: Rachel Lunardi

Foundation Équilibre Saguenay-Lac-St-Jean
Location: 150 rue Pinel, Chicoutimi QC G7G 3N8
Mailing: CP 2250 succ Nord, Chicoutimi QC G7G 3W4
418 549-5474; Fax: 418 543-4584
E: info@fondationequilibre.com
W: www.fondationequilibre.com
Executive:
Dir gén: Francine Leblond

Foundation Fighting Blindness-Canada
890 Yonge St, Floor 12, Toronto ON M4W 3P4
416 360-4200; Fax: 416 360-0060
Toll-free: 800 461-3331
W: www.ffb.ca/
Executive:
Chair: Donna Green
Vice Chair: Ken Kirk
Pres/CEO: Sharon M Colle
Treas: Rahn Dodick
Corp Sec: Andrew Burke
Mktg/Commun Mgr: Erin George
Year Founded: 1974
No of Paid Staff: 7
Speakers Available
Languages: English; French

G.F. Strong Rehabilitation Centre - Vancouver Coastal Health Authority
4255 Laurel St, Vancouver BC V5Z 2G9
604 734-1313; Fax: 604 737-6359
W: www.gfstrong.com
Executive:
COO: Mary Ackenhusen
Dir: Annette Lange
Year Founded: 1949
No of Paid Staff: 339
Speakers Available
Library: Y
Languages: English

Garth Homer Society
813 Darwin Ave, Victoria BC V8X 2X7
250 475-2270; Fax: 250 475-2279
Executive:
MIS Mgr: Jon Lepas
Dir-QA: Mary Ann Snowden

Gateway Resources Inc.
Location: 1582 Pembina Ave, Winkler MB R6W 4B4
Mailing: PO Box 1448 Stn Main
204 325-7304; Fax: 204 325-1958
E: gradmin@gatewayresourcesinc.com
W: www.gatewayresourcesinc.com/
Executive:
CEO: Jim McNeil
Prog Dir: Kim Nelson
Dir-Woodroom/Transp: Jake Heide
Dir-Housing: Jody Nobes
Dir-Recycling/Packaging: Ron Gerbrandt
Year Founded: 1970
Budget: $4,200,000
No of Paid Staff: 105
Speakers Available
Languages: English

Greek Community of Toronto
30 Thorncliffe Park Dr, Toronto ON M4H 1H8
416 425-2485; Fax: 416 425-2954
E: info@greekcommunity.org
W: www.greekcommunity.org
Executive:
Pres: Nikona Georgakopoulos
No of Paid Staff: 7
Library: Y
Languages: English; French

Groupe Action pour l'enfant, la famille et la communauté de Prescott-Russell
210-250 Main St E, Hawkesbury ON K6A 1A5
613 632-7837; Fax: 613 632-5648
Toll-free: 866 363-3210
W: www.groupeaction.ca
Executive:
Exec Dir: Yves Séguin
Supvr Outreach: Sheila Lacroix
Supvr de fiers nos enfants: Brigitte Williams
Criteria: *Tous citoyens.*
No of Paid Staff: 34
Library: Y
Languages: English; French
Membership: 29 *(Lists available to the public)*
Membership Fee: $5

Hagi Community Services for Independence
A-1201 Jasper Dr, Thunder Bay ON P7B 6R2
807 343-0414; Fax: 807 344-6140
E: info@hagi.ca
W: www.hagi.ca
Executive:
Chief Admv Off: Allan Buchan
Year Founded: 1975
Languages: English
Membership: 180
Membership Fee: $10 - Family; $5 - Individual

Handicapped Action Group Inc.
A-1201 Jasper Dr, Thunder Bay ON P7B 6R2
807 343-0414; Fax: 807 344-6140
E: info@hagi.ca
W: www.hagi.ca
Executive:
Exec Dir: Cal Rankin
Mgr-Transport: Brenda Deck
Mgr-Commun Serv: Arlene Morris
Budget: $12
Languages: English

Hartmanns Community Centre
41 Main St E, Milton ON L9T 1N2
905 749-9246; Fax: 905 693-8800
E: maria@caattts.org
Executive:
Dir: Maria Reis
Dir: J Harry Reis

The Hearing Foundation of Canada
1801-1 Yonge St, Toronto ON M5E 1W7
416 364-4060; Fax: 416 214-2043
Toll-free: 866 432-7968
E: info@hearingfoundation.ca
W: www.hearingfoundation.ca
Executive:
Chair: John Pepperell
Chair-Finl Committee: Jason F Gorel
Pres: Dino Sophocleous
Dir: Peter Alberti
Mgr-Dev/Progr: Janice Eales
Year Founded: 1979
Budget: $1,500,000
No of Paid Staff: 7
Speakers Available
Languages: English
Membership: 21 *(Lists available to the public)*

Hutton House Association For Adults With Disability
654 Wonderland Rd N, London ON N6H 3E5
519 472-6381; Fax: 519 472-1051
E: hhservices@huttonhouse.com
W: www.huttonhouse.com
Executive:
Pres: Paul Coulter
VP: Carmen Sprovieri
Treas: Susan Mrnik
No of Paid Staff: 25
Library: Y *(Open to the public)*
Languages: English

In-Definite Arts
8038 Fairmount Dr SE, Calgary AB T2H 0Y1
403 253-3174; Fax: 403 255-2234
E: ida@indefinitearts.com
W: www.indefinitearts.com
Executive:
Exec Dir: Darlene Murphy
Year Founded: 1975
Criteria: *Open to any person supporting the mandate.*
Budget: $500,000
No of Paid Staff: 10
Speakers Available
Languages: English
Membership: 200

Independence Plus Inc.
115-66 Waterloo St, Saint John NB E2L 3P4
506 643-7004; Fax: 506 643-7009
E: independence@nb.aibn.com
W: saintjohn.cioc.ca
Executive:
Exec Dir: David Black
Languages: English

Independent Living Canada
402-214 Montreal Rd, Vanier ON K1L 8L8
613 563-2581; Fax: 613 563-3861
E: info@ilc-vac.ca
W: www.ilcanada.ca
Executive:
Natl Dir: Traci Walters
Year Founded: 1986
No of Paid Staff: 11
Speakers Available
Languages: English; French
Membership: 2000+ *(Lists available to the public)*
Membership Fee: Varies

Independent Living Services of Simcoe County and Area
1102-44 Cedar Pointe Dr, Barrie ON L4N 5R7
705 737-3263; Fax: 705 737-1874
Toll-free: 800 465-1133
E: ilssimcoe@ilssimcoe.ca
W: www.ilssimcoe.ca
Executive:
Chair: Kimberley Simpson
Treas: Albert Stein
Sec: Dan McGale
Year Founded: 1977
Criteria: *Eighteen years of age, physical disability, family or interested community member.*
Budget: $3,600,000
No of Paid Staff: 130
Speakers Available
Library: Y *(Open to the public)*
Languages: English
Membership: 70
Membership Fee: $5 Per Year

Integra for Children and Adults of Prescott-Russell

Location: 173 Old Hwy 17, Plantagenet ON K0B 1L0
Mailing: PO Box 248
613 673-5148; Fax: 613 673-4800
Toll-free: 800 675-6168
E: info@integra-pr.ca
W: www.integra-pr.ca
Executive:
Pres: Kevin McBride
VP: Raymond Parisien
Exec Dir: Raymond Lemay
Treas: Jean Dugas
Criteria: *Services are open to the physically disabled.*
Library: Y *(Open to the public)*
Languages: English; French
Membership: 90

K-W Habilitation Services

108 Sydney St S, Kitchener ON N2G 3V2
519 744-6307; Fax: 519 571-1629
E: generalinquiries@kwhab.ca
W: www.kwhab.ca
Executive:
Exec Dir: Ann Bilodeau
Dir-Fin: Lorie Datta
Dir-Hum Res: Steven Plaum
Dir-Res Serv: Chris Gefucia
Asst Dir-Res Serv: Tracy Franks
Languages: English

L'Amicale des Personnes Handicapés Physiques de L'Outaouais

405 rue Notre-Dame, Gatineau QC J8P 1L7
819 663-2999; Fax: 819 663-5124
E: info@amicale.ca
W: www.amicale.ca
Executive:
Dir gén: Jacques de Bellefeuille
Aide-compt: Jean-Paul Potvin
Coord: Julie Villeneuve
Languages: French

Lethbridge Association for Community Living

527 6 St S, Lethbridge AB T1J 2E1
403 327-2911; Fax: 403 320-7054
E: mail@lacl.ca
W: www.lacl.ca
Executive:
Exec Dir: Dave Lawson
Office Admin: Lesley Sawers
Year Founded: 1957
Criteria: *Individuals, families, guardians, interested citizens.*
Budget: $135,000
No of Paid Staff: 3
Speakers Available
Library: Y *(Open to the public)*
Languages: English
Membership: 75
Membership Fee: $20 - Family; $10 - Individual

Lions Foundation of Canada - Dog Guides

Location: 152 Wilson St, Oakville ON L6K 0G6
Mailing: PO Box 907 Stn Main, Oakville ON L6J 5E8
905 842-2891; Fax: 905 842-3373
Toll-free: 800 768-3030
E: info@dogguides.com
W: www.dogguides.com
Executive:
Chairperson: Bev Semple
Vice Chairperson/Dir QC: Daniel Poulin
Dir NB: Jan Phillips
Dir PE: Douglas Cook
Dir ON: Ralph Krueger
Sec/Dir NS: Sharon Dykeman
Treas/Dir MB/N ON/NU: Gary Hutchinson
Dir NF: Doreen Burton
Dir SK: Gordon Ziegler
Exec Member at Large/Dir BC/YT: Rosemary Small
Dir AB/NT: David Dalby
Year Founded: 1983
Languages: English

Low Vision Association of Ontario

Mailing: PO Box 156 Stn Q, Toronto ON M4T 2M1
416 486-3442; Fax: 416 486-3442
E: lvao@sympatico.ca
Executive:
Man Dir: Bill Carroll
Budget: $250,000
No of Paid Staff: 3
Languages: English

Manitoba League of Persons With Disabilities Inc.

105-500 Portage Ave, Winnipeg MB R3C 3X1
204 943-6099; Fax: 204 943-6654
Toll-free: 888 330-1932 Manitoba only
E: mlpd@shawcable.com
W: www.mlpd.mb.ca
Year Founded: 1975
Criteria: *An interest in disability issues.*
Budget: $200,000
No of Paid Staff: 2
Speakers Available
Library: Y
Languages: English
Membership: 600
Membership Fee: $2 Youth; $10 Family; $8 Couple; $5 Individuals

Medical Interpreting Services - WIDHH

2125 7th Ave W, Vancouver BC V6K 1X9
604 736-7012; Fax: 604 736-7786
Toll-free: 877 736-7012
E: mis@widhh.com
W: www.widhh.com
Executive:
Dept Head: Janice Lyons
Dispatcher: Jacky Jickels
Year Founded: 1998
No of Paid Staff: 4
Languages: English

Meta Centre for the Developmentally Disabled

Meta Centre
401 Champagne Dr, North York ON M3J 2C6
416 736-0199; Fax: 416 736-9181
W: www.metacentre.ca
Executive:
Pres: Jim Johnston
Exec Dir: Antonet Orlando
Dir-Fin: Raymond Thai
Dir-Res Serv: Frank Grosso
Sec-Treas: Adrienne Sordi
Hum Res Coord: Sandra Connors
Year Founded: 1986
No of Paid Staff: 170
Speakers Available
Languages: English; Italian

Metropolitan Montréal Deaf Community Centre

Location: 207-2200 boul Crémazie E, Montréal QC H2E 2Z8
Mailing: 203-2200 boul Crémazie E
514 279-7609; Fax: 514 279-5373
E: ccsmm.membres@videotron.ca
W: www.ccsmm.net
Executive:
Dir gén: Gilles Read
Adj au dir gén: Jeanne D'Arc Paradis
Year Founded: 1978
Criteria: *Pour tout.*
Budget: $115,000
No of Paid Staff: 1
Speakers Available
Languages: English; French
Membership: 350 *(Lists available to the public)*

Miramichi Physically Disabled and Handicapped Association

Location: 80 University Ave, Miramichi NB E1N 3W4
Mailing: PO Box 1053 Stn Chatham
506 773-9437; Fax: 506 773-9439
Executive:
Pres: Leona Isiah
VP: Delores Landry
Office Mgr: Shirley Forrest
Year Founded: 1980
No of Paid Staff: 4
Speakers Available
Languages: English
Membership: 10 *(Lists available to the public)*

Mission Association for Community Living

33345 Second Ave, Mission BC V2V 1K4
604 826-9080; Fax: 604 826-9611
E: macl@macl.bc.ca
W: macl.bc.ca
Executive:
Pres: Bob Ingram
VP: Michael Taggart
Treas: Linda Golightly
Sec: Tracy Martin
Year Founded: 1958
Budget: $6,000,000
No of Paid Staff: 130
Speakers Available
Library: Y
Languages: English
Membership: 25
Membership Fee: $5

Moelle épinière et motricité Québec

400-6020 rue Jean-Talon E, Saint-Léonard QC H1S 3B1
514 341-7272; Fax: 514 341-8884
Toll-free: 877 341-7272
E: info@moelleepiniere.com
W: www.moelleepiniere.com
Executive:
Dir gén: Walter Zelaya
Dir serv d'interv: Nathalie Michaud
Adj à la dir gén: Karine Laplante
Year Founded: 1946
No of Paid Staff: 20
Speakers Available
Languages: French
Membership: 2,100
Membership Fee: $25-$35/year

Multi-Ethnic Association for the Integration of Persons with Disabilities

6462 boul Saint-Laurent, Montréal QC H2S 3C4
514 272-0680; Fax: 514 272-8530
Toll-free: 866 318-0680
E: ameiph@ameiph.com
W: www.ameiph.com
Executive:
Dir gén: Luciana Soave
Admin: Sylvio Caddeo
Year Founded: 1981
Criteria: *Personnes handicapées/parents, amis/sympathisants/professionels, organismes, de soutien.*
Persons with disabilities, Family members, friends, professional, Organizations
Budget: $350,000
No of Paid Staff: 12
Speakers Available
Languages: English; French; Italian
Membership: 455
Membership Fee: Ranges from $5 - $25

National Educational Association of Disabled Students

Carlton University
426-1125 Colonel By Dr, Ottawa ON K1S 5B6
613 380-8065; Fax: 613 369-4391
Toll-free: 877 670-1256
E: info@neads.ca
W: www.neads.ca
Executive:
Project Mgr: Jennifer Dillon
Sr Advisor: Jennison Asuncion
Natl Coord: Frank Smith
Year Founded: 1986
No of Paid Staff: 5
Speakers Available
Library: Y *(Open to the public)*
Languages: English; French

North Hastings Community Integration Association

Location: 2 Alice St, Bancroft ON K0L 1C0
Mailing: PO Box 1508
613 332-2090; Fax: 613 332-4762
E: communityliving@nhcia.ca
W: www.communitylivingontario.ca

Nova Scotia League for Equal Opportunities

1211-5251 Duke St, Halifax NS B3J 1P3
902 455-6942; Fax: 902 454-4781
Toll-free: 866 696-7536
E: nsleo@eastlink.ca
W: www.novascotialeo.org/
Executive:
Chair: Earl Flynn
V-Chair: David Monney
Treas: Claredon Robicheau
Sec: Vera Stapleton
Prov Coord: Gail Bruhm
Year Founded: 1979
Criteria: *Cross-disability groups must be consumer controlled (at least 51% of the members of the Board of Directors must be persons with a disability) and must support the goals and objectives of the league.*
No of Paid Staff: 1
Speakers Available
Languages: English
Membership: Represent disabled consumers provincally. *(Lists available to the public)*
Membership Fee: $50/year

ORW Opportunities Through Rehabilitation and Work Society

17355 27A Ave, Surrey BC V3S 0E9
604 535-6384; Fax: 604 535-6385
E: info@orw.ca
W: www.orw.ca
Executive:
Exec Dir: Winston Leckie
Year Founded: 1965
Budget: $100,000
No of Paid Staff: 1
Speakers Available
Languages: English
Membership: 10 *(Lists available to the public)*

Ottawa-Carleton Association for Persons with Developmental Disabilities

229 Colonnade Rd, Nepean ON K2E 7K3
613 569-8993; Fax: 613 569-9865
E: ocapdd@ocapdd.on.ca
W: www.ocapdd.on.ca
Executive:
Exec Dir: David Ferguson
Prog Supvr: Ann-Marie Cousineau
Library: Y *(Open to the public)*
Languages: English

Pacific Assistance Dogs Society

9048 Stormont Ave, Burnaby BC V3N 4G6
604 527-0556; Fax: 604 527-0558
E: info@pads.ca
W: www.pads.ca
Executive:
Exec Dir: Laura Watamanuk
Dir-Canine Prog: Margaret Hicks
Dir-Client Serv: Ron Tymrick
Puppy Trng Inst-Calgary: Heather Kidd
Year Founded: 1987
Budget: $1,200,000
No of Paid Staff: 7
Speakers Available
Languages: English
Membership: 284 *(Lists available to the public)*
Membership Fee: Adult - $25; Senior - $15; Family - $50

Pacific Riding for Developing Abilities

1088 208 St, Langley BC V2Z 1T4
604 530-8717; Fax: 604 530-8617
E: mmeacher@prda.ca
W: www.prda.ca
Executive:
Exec Dir: Michelle Meacher
Year Founded: 1973
No of Paid Staff: 8
Speakers Available
Languages: English
Membership: 160
Membership Fee: $20/yr

Participation House

9 Butternut Lane, Markham ON L3P 3M1
905 294-0944; Fax: 905 294-7834
W: www.participationhouse.net
Executive:
Exec Dir: Frances DiCarlo

PEI Council of People with Disabilities

Landmark Plaza
2-5 Lower Malpeque Rd, Charlottetown PE C1E 1R4
902 892-9149; Fax: 902 566-1919
E: peicod@peicod.pe.ca
W: www.peicod.pe.ca
Executive:
Exec Dir: Marcia Carroll
Fund Dev Coord: Judith Bayliss
Year Founded: 1975
Criteria: *Individualized membership paid each year.*
No of Paid Staff: 12
Speakers Available
Languages: English
Membership: 6,000
Membership Fee: $2

Penticton & District Society for Community Living

180 Industrial Ave W, Penticton BC V2A 6X9
250 493-0312; Fax: 250 493-9113
E: tony@pdscl.org
W: www.pdscl.org
Executive:
Board Pres: Bill Baird
Year Founded: 1958
Budget: $5,000,000
No of Paid Staff: 85
Speakers Available
Languages: English
Membership: 22

Persons United for Self-Help in Northwestern Ontario Inc.

B-1201 Jasper Dr, Thunder Bay ON P7B 6R2
807 345-3400; Fax: 807 345-3533
Executive:
Pres: Donna Wiitala
Prog Coord: Amy Vaillant
Year Founded: 1989
Criteria: *People with disabilities and people and organizations interested in helping achieve goals.*
Budget: $175,000
Speakers Available
Languages: English
Membership: 30 *(Lists available to the public)*
Membership Fee: $5

Physically Handicapped Adults' Rehabilitation Association (PHARA)

280 Oakwood Ave, North Bay ON P1B 9G2
705 476-0733; Fax: 705 476-9287
E: phara@phara.org
W: www.phara.org
Executive:
Exec Dir: Alice Radley
Budget: $2,100,000
No of Paid Staff: 61
Speakers Available
Languages: English; French

Planned Lifetime Networks (Waterloo-Wellington-Oxford)

306, 5-420 Erb St W, Waterloo ON N2L 6K6
519 746-1188
E: plninfo@plannedlifetimenetworks.ca
W: www.plannedlifetimenetworks.ca
Executive:
Board Member: Arlene Smith

Queens Association for Supported Living

Location: 44 Pleasant St, Milton NS B0T 1P0
Mailing: PO Box 520
902 354-2723; Fax: 902 354-2262
E: info@qasl.ca
W: www.qasl.ca
Year Founded: 1968
Budget: $2,000,000
No of Paid Staff: 55
Speakers Available

Languages: English
Membership: 8
Membership Fee: $5

Red Deer Action Group
301-4805 48 St, Red Deer AB T4N 1S6
403 343-1198; Fax: 403 343-8945
E: rdag@telus.net
W: www.rdactiongroup.ca
Executive:
Office Coord: Sharon Freeman

Reena
927 Clark Ave W, Thornhill ON L4J 8G6
905 889-6484; Fax: 905 889-3827
W: www.reena.org
Executive:
Pres: Sandy Keshen
CFO: Sol Fleising
Dir-Fin: Mike Kligman

Regional Residential Services Society
LKD1-202 Brownlow Ave, Dartmouth NS B3B 1T5
902 465-4022; Fax: 902 465-3124
E: irina.vassitchko@rrss.ns.ca
W: www.rrss.ns.ca
Executive:
Exec Dir: Carol Ann Brennan
Sr Dir: Brenda Dixon
Controller: Irena Vassitzhko

Rehabilitation Society of Calgary
7 11 St NE, Calgary AB T2E 4Z2
403 263-8341; Fax: 403 264-4579
E: anna_rehab@shaw.ca
W: www.rehabcalgary.ca
Executive:
Prog Mgr: Anna Skalka
Team Coord: Noreen Branagh
Year Founded: 1948
Criteria: *18 years and older*
Budget: $200,000
No of Paid Staff: 2
Languages: English
Membership: 75 *(Lists available to the public)*

Rehoboth Christian Ministries
3920 49 Ave, Stony Plain AB T7Z 2J7
780 963-4044; Fax: 780 963-3075
E: stonyplain@rehoboth.ab.ca
W: www.rehoboth.ab.ca
Executive:
CEO/Exec Dir: Wally Mulder
Dir-Ops: Kelvin Van Dasselaar
Reg Dir: Janice Blake
Year Founded: 1976
Criteria: *Must state acceptance of objectives and mission statement.*
Budget: $19,000,000
No of Paid Staff: 426
Speakers Available
Languages: English
Membership: 5,046
Membership Fee: $10

Richmond Society for Community Living
170-7000 Minoru Blvd, Richmond BC V6Y 3Z5
604 279-7040; Fax: 604 279-7048
E: info@rscl.org
W: www.rscl.org
Executive:
Exec Dir: Janice Barr
Year Founded: 1982
Budget: $4,000,000
No of Paid Staff: 150
Languages: English; French

Rick Hansen Foundation
300-3820 Cessna Dr, Richmond BC V7B 0A2
604 295-8149; Fax: 604 295-8159
Toll-free: 800 213-2131
E: info@rickhansen.com
W: www.rickhansen.com
Executive:
Pres/CEO: Rick Hansen
Exec VP: Doramy Ehlinge
Mgr: Nathalie Earley
Languages: English

Robin Hood Association
141 Broadway Blvd, Sherwood Park AB T8H 2A4
780 467-7140; Fax: 780 449-2028
E: riediger@robinhoodassoc.com
W: www.robinhoodassoc.com
Executive:
CEO: Ed Riediger
Year Founded: 1963
Budget: $15,000,000
No of Paid Staff: 400
Speakers Available
Languages: English
Membership: 100

Saint John Deaf and Hard of Hearing Services, Inc.
324 Duke St W, Saint John NB E2M 1V2
506 633-0599; Fax: 506 652-3382
E: sjdhhs@nb.sympatico.ca
W: www.sjdhhs.com
Executive:
Exec Dir: Lynn LeBlanc
Admv Asst: Rosemary Blanchard
Year Founded: 1979
Budget: $150,000
No of Paid Staff: 2
Speakers Available
Library: Y *(Open to the public)*
Languages: English; French; Sign Language
Membership: 300 *(Lists available to the public)*
Membership Fee: Free
Library:
SJDHHS Video Library & Resources *(Open to the public)*

Sair Training & Employment Placement Services (STEPS)
1-201 Scott St, Winnipeg MB R3L 0L4
204 474-2303; Fax: 204 453-3959
E: sair@mts.net
W: www.steps2work.ca
Executive:
Exec Dir: Ron Fortier
Sr Prog Mgr: Scott Byiers

Saskatchewan Abilities Council Inc.
2310 Louise Ave, Saskatoon SK S7J 2C7
306 374-4448; Fax: 306 373-2665
E: provincialservices@abilitiescouncil.sk.ca
W: www.abilitiescouncil.sk.ca
Executive:
Exec Dir: Ian Wilkinson
Dir-Prov Serv: Keith Appleton
Dir-Rehab Serv: Heather Rasmussen
Exec Asst: Joan Nelson
Year Founded: 1950
Criteria: *Open to those who give an annual donation.*
Budget: $34,000,000
No of Paid Staff: 370
Languages: English
Membership: 2,800
Membership Fee: $10

Saskatchewan Voice of People with Disabilities Inc.
984 Albert St, Regina SK S4R 2P7
306 569-3111; Fax: 306 569-1889
Toll-free: 877 569-3111
E: voice@saskvoice.com
W: www.saskvoice.com
Executive:
Chairperson: Ron Bort
Exec Dir: Bev Duncan
Prog Dir: Amber-Joy Boyd
Year Founded: 1973
Criteria: *Full: open to any person with a disability, Advocate: represents a member who cannot speak for themselves, Associate: open to persons without disabilites interested in the work of the Voice.*
Budget: $250,000
No of Paid Staff: 3
Speakers Available
Languages: English
Membership: 850
Membership Fee: $10

Society for Manitobans with Disabilities Inc.
825 Sherbrook St, Winnipeg MB R3A 1M5
204 975-3010; Fax: 204 975-3073
Toll-free: 866 282-8041
E: info@smd.mb.ca
W: www.smd.mb.ca
Executive:
CEO SMD Series: Maria Marone
Admv Asst: Denise Bellesia
Year Founded: 1946
No of Paid Staff: 120
Speakers Available
Languages: English
Library:
SMD Library *(Open to the public)*

South-East Grey Support Services
Location: 24 Toronto St, Flesherton ON N0C 1E0
Mailing: PO Box 12
519 924-3339; Fax: 519 924-3575
E: segss@bmts.com
W: www.communitylivingontario.ca
Executive:
Pres: Richard Gott
Exec Dir: Maurice Voisin

South Saskatchewan Independent Living Centre Inc.
2220 Albert St, Regina SK S4P 2V2
306 757-7452; Fax: 306 757-5892
E: info@ssilcsk.ca
W: www.ssilcsk.ca
Executive:
Exec Dir: Michael Richter

Southern Alberta Society for the Handicapped
Location: 22N 1st St W, Magrath AB T0K 1J0
Mailing: PO Box 280
403 758-3334; Fax: 403 758-3644
E: sash_@telus.net
Executive:
Exec Dir: Darren Bennett
Commun Access Coord: Heather Johnston
Community Living Coord: Tami Tolley
Year Founded: 1987
Criteria: *Caring advocate for persons with developmental disabilities.*
Budget: $1,400,000
No of Paid Staff: 54
Speakers Available
Languages: English
Membership list available to the public

Spectrum Society for Community Living
3231 Kingsway, Vancouver BC V5R 5K3
604 323-1433; Fax: 604 321-4144
W: www.spectrumsociety.org
Executive:
Exec Dir: Ernest Baatz
Office Mgr: Judy Wong
Year Founded: 1987
Criteria: *Families, friends and individuals receiving service.*
No of Paid Staff: 150
Speakers Available
Library: Y
Languages: English

Spinal Cord Injury British Columbia
780 Marine Dr SW, Vancouver BC V6P 5Y7
604 324-3611; Fax: 604 326-1229
Toll-free: 800 689-2477
E: info@sci-bc.ca
W: www.bcpara.org
Executive:
Chair: Bernard Fahy
V-Chair: Scott McCloy
Pres/CEO: Anthony Ariganello
Year Founded: 1957
Library: Y *(Open to the public)*
Languages: English
Membership Fee: $25

◈Kootenays:
102-1617 Baker St, Cranbrook BC V1C 1B4
250 417-0416; Fax: 250 489-1438
Toll-free: 877 410-0416
E: vancouver@bcpara.org
W: www.bcpara.org
Languages: English

◈Okanagan South:
3-1873 Spall Rd, Kelowna BC V1Y 4R2
250 860-8700; Fax: 250 712-0977
Toll-free: 877 816-8700
E: kelowna@bcpara.org
W: www.bcpara.org
Library: Y
Languages: English

◈North Okanagan Office:
830 Seymour St, Kamloops BC V2C 2H5
250 851-0882; Fax: 250 851-0038
Toll-free: 877 851-0882
E: cfriars@bcpara.org
W: sci-bc.ca
Year Founded: 1957
Speakers Available
Languages: English

◈Northeast & Central:
777 Kinsmen Pl, Prince George BC V2M 6Y7
250 563-6942; Fax: 250 563-6992
Toll-free: 800 689-2477
E: info@sci-bc.ca
W: www.bcpara.org
Languages: English

Spinal Cord Injury Canada
230-1101 Prince of Wales Dr, Ottawa ON K2C 3W7
613 723-1913; Fax: 613 723-1060
Toll-free: 888 723-1033
E: info@canparaplegic.org
W: www.canparaplegic.org
Executive:
Pres: Myrtle Jenkins-Smith
VP/Sec: Bruce Drewett
Exec Dir: Robert (Bobby) White
Treas: Ron Swan
Reg Serv Coord: Stacey Moore
Year Founded: 1945
Criteria: *Open to any person interested in the objectives of the Association.*
Budget: $2,000,000
No of Paid Staff: 8
Speakers Available
Languages: English; French
Membership: 7,000
Membership Fee: Varies by province: $15-$25

◈NWT Council of Persons with Disabilities:
Location: B-321 Old Airport Rd, Yellowknife NT X1A 3T3
Mailing: PO Box 1387 Stn Main, Yellowknife NT X1A 2P1
867 873-8230; Fax: 867 873-4124
Toll-free: 800 491-8885 Disability Info. Line
E: disabilitynwt@yk.com
W: www.nwtability.ca
Executive:
Exec Dir: Andra Malcolm
Year Founded: 1978
Criteria: *Full Members: residents of NWT willing to further the goals & objectives of the council Associate Members: organization within or outside of NWT, or resident outside of NWT willing to further the goals & objectives of the Council.*
Budget: $500,000
No of Paid Staff: 10
Languages: English
Membership Fee: Business/organization: $20; Individual: $10
Library:
Resource Library *(Open to the public)*

Starworks Packaging & Assembly
276 Marine Dr SW, Vancouver BC V5X 2R5
604 879-8457; Fax: 604 879-7441
E: starworks@develop.bc.ca
W: www.starworks.ca
Executive:
Gen Mgr: Kirsti Inglis
Dir: Deanne Ziebart
No of Paid Staff: 40
Languages: English

Sunrise Therapeutic Riding & Learning Centre Inc.
6920 Concession 1, Puslinch ON N0B 2J0
519 837-0558; Fax: 519 837-1233
E: info@sunrise-therapeutic.ca
W: www.sunrise-therapeutic.ca
Executive:
Exec Dir: Ann Caine

Surex Community Services
311-40 Wynford Dr, Toronto ON M3C 1J5
416 469-4109; Fax: 416 469-4184
E: colin.hamilton@surexcs.com
W: www.surexcs.com
Executive:
Exec Dir: Colin Hamilton

Témabex Inc.
52 rue Perreault O, Rouyn-Noranda QC J9X 2T4
819 762-7711; Fax: 819 762-7456
Toll-free: 866 836-2239
E: temabex@temabex.qc.ca
W: www.temabex.qc.ca

Témabex Inc.
375 av Centrale, Val-D'Or QC J9P 1P4
819 825-2944; Fax: 819 759-8212
E: temabex@temabex.qc.ca
Executive:
Chef dir: Jean-Pierre Roy

Tetra Society of North America
207-3077 Granville St, Vancouver BC V6H 3J9
604 688-6464; Fax: 604 688-6463
Toll-free: 877 688-8762
E: tetra@disabilityfoundation.org
W: www.tetrasociety.org
Executive:
Exec Dir: Duane Geddes
Natl Coord: Pat Tweedie
Year Founded: 1987
Speakers Available
Languages: English

Transitions Rehab Association of St Albert
100-365 Carleton Dr, St. Albert AB T8N 7L1
780 458-7371; Fax: 780 460-7078
E: info@transitions-ab.org
W: www.transitions-ab.org
Executive:
Exec Dir: Paul Fujishige
Hum Res Coord: Hanna Gorecka

Tremploy Inc.
Location: Enman Cres, Charlottetown PE C1A 7M4
Mailing: PO Box 936 Stn Central
902 892-5338; Fax: 902 892-5334
E: swatts@tremploy.com
W: www.tremploy.com
Executive:
Bus Mgr: Shelley Watts
Exec Dir: Nick Blanchard

Under the Banyan Tree Centre for the Developmentally Disabled
106-1020 Denison St, Markham ON L3R 3W5
905 947-0036; Fax: 905 947-0052
E: info@underthebanyantree.ca
W: www.underthebanyantree.ca
Executive:
Pres: May Ip
Exec Dir: David Yung
Treas: Wilfred Luk
Sec: Veronica Lam
Year Founded: 1996
No of Paid Staff: 8
Speakers Available
Languages: English; Cantonese

Variety Place Association Inc.
Location: 600 Conquest Ave, Outlook SK S0L 2N0
Mailing: PO Box 1362
306 867-9363; Fax: 306 867-9543
E: variety.place@sasktel.net
Executive:
Pres: Randy Kangas
Exec Dir: Angela Knapik
Exec Asst: Susan Ptolemy
Prog Coord: Margaret MacLeod
Year Founded: 1983
Criteria: *Open to any mentally handicapped adults.*
Budget: $1,800,000
No of Paid Staff: 39
Languages: English
Membership: 12 *(Lists available to the public)*

Variety - The Children's Charity of Alberta
Location: 14-11625 Elbow Dr SW, Calgary AB T2W 1G8
Mailing: PO Box 83040, RPO Canyon Meadows, Calgary AB T2W 6G8
403 228-6168; Fax: 403 245-9282
E: varietyalberta@shaw.ca
W: www.varietyalberta.ca
Executive:
Exec Dir: Lesley Gomez
No of Paid Staff: 1
Speakers Available
Languages: English
Membership list available to the public

Variety, the Children's Charity of Manitoba
2-1313 Border St, Winnipeg MB R3H 0X4
204 982-1050; Fax: 204 475-3198
E: businessmanager@varietymanitoba.com
W: www.varietymanitoba.com
Executive:
Exec Dir: Wayne Rogers
Dir-Fund Develop: Janet McLeod
Admv Asst: Ashley Irwin
Spec Events/Volunteer Coord: Nancy Militano
Prog Coord: Shanlee Johnson
Year Founded: 1978
No of Paid Staff: 5
Speakers Available
Languages: English
Membership: 150
Membership Fee: $50/year

Vegreville Association for Living in Dignity
4843 49 St, Vegreville AB T9C 1K7
780 632-2418; Fax: 780 632-3882
Toll-free: 888 632-9842
E: valid@valid-assoc.org
W: www.valid-assoc.org
Executive:
Exec Dir: Jody Nicholson
Year Founded: 1992
Speakers Available
Library: Y
Languages: English
Membership: 26 *(Lists available to the public)*
Membership Fee: $5

Venture Works - Div. of Community Living Windsor
2840 Temple Dr, Windsor ON N8W 5J5
519 944-2464; Fax: 519 944-0199
E: steve@clwindsor.org
W: www.clwindsor.org
Executive:
Mgr: Steve Shearer

VOICE for Hearing Impaired Children
I.N.A. Bldg
704-161 Eglinton Ave E, Toronto ON M4P 1J5
416 487-7719; Fax: 416 487-7423
Toll-free: 866 779-5144
E: info@voicefordeafkids.com
W: www.voicefordeafkids.com
Executive:
Exec Dir: Norah-Lynn McIntyre
Fin Mgr: Jessica Chan
Library: Y
Languages: English

Western Institute for the Deaf & Hard of Hearing
2125 7th Ave W, Vancouver BC V6K 1X9
604 736-7391; Fax: 604 736-4381
Toll-free: 888 736-7391
E: info@widhh.com
W: www.widhh.ca
Executive:
Exec Dir: Susan Masters
Hd-Interpreting Serv: Janice Lyons
Hd-Employment Ser: Linda Franchi
Hd-Audiology Serv: Grace Shyng
Year Founded: 1956
No of Paid Staff: 36
Speakers Available
Languages: English; French; American Sign Language; Mandarin; Spanish
Membership: 203 *(Lists available to the public)*
Membership Fee: $15/year, $100 Lifetime

◈ *Western Institute for the Deaf & Hard of Hearing*
514-2525 Willow St, Vancouver BC V5Z 3N8
778 329-0870; Fax: 778 329-0875
E: willowinfo@widhh.com
Executive:
Mgr/Regd Audiologist: Charles Fontaine
Audiology Admv Asst: Sacha Diprose
Regd Audiologist: Praise Chow

Wetaskiwin & District Association for Community Service
5211 54 St, Wetaskiwin AB T9A 1T2
780 352-2241
E: wdacs@incenter.net
Executive:
Pres: Lavern Buchert
Exec Dir: Marilyn Conner
No of Paid Staff: 60
Speakers Available
Library: Y
Languages: English
Membership: 25
Membership Fee: $10 per year

EATING DISORDERS

Bulimia Anorexia Nervosa Association
100-1500 Ouellette Ave, Windsor ON N8X 1K7
519 969-2112; Fax: 519 969-0227
E: info@bana.ca
W: www.bana.ca
Executive:
I-Exec Dir: Luciana Rosu-Sieza
Year Founded: 1985
Criteria: *Promotes size acceptance and promotes agency's mission and vision.*
Budget: $550,000
No of Paid Staff: 8
Speakers Available
Library: Y *(Open to the public)*
Languages: English
Membership: 300 *(Lists available to the public)*
Membership Fee: $20
Library:
BANA Library *(Open to the public)*

New Realities Eating Disorders Recovery Centre
103-62 Charles St E, Toronto ON M4Y 1T1
416 921-9670; Fax: 416 921-8923
E: newrealities@rogers.com
W: www.newrealitiescan.com
Executive:
Co-Founder: Orit Morse
Co-Founder: Patricia Kelly
Year Founded: 1996
No of Paid Staff: 2
Speakers Available
Languages: English

HEALTH

Accreditation Canada
1150 Cyrville Rd, Gloucester ON K1J 7S9
613 738-3800; Fax: 800 811-7088
Toll-free: 800 814-7769
Toll-free Fax: 800 811-7088
W: www.accreditationcananda.ca
Executive:
Pres/CEO: Wendy Nicklin
VP Bus Dev/Client Engagement: Paula McColgan
CFO: Patrick Girard
CIO: Su Huynh
Dir-Prog Dev: Christine Niro
Dir-Strategist Commun: Liane Craig
Year Founded: 1958
Criteria: *Compliance with accreditation standards.*
Budget: $7,000,000
No of Paid Staff: 60
Speakers Available
Languages: English; French
Membership list available to the public
Publications
Standards for Acute Care Organizations 1995
Standards for Cancer Treatment Centres 1995
Standards for Community Health Services 1996
Standards for Home Care Organizations 1997

Action on Smoking and Health
Location: 208-17420 Stony Plain Rd NW, Edmonton AB T5S 1K6
Mailing: PO Box 4500 Stn South Cro, Edmonton AB T6E 6K2
780 426-7867; Fax: 780 488-7195
W: www.ash.ca
Executive:
Exec Dir: Les Hagen
Languages: English

The Advanced Coronary Treatment Foundation of Canada
379 Holland Ave, Ottawa ON K1Y 0Y9
613 729-3455; Fax: 613 729-5837
Toll-free: 800 465-9111
Toll-free Fax: 888 697-7747
E: act@actfoundation.ca
W: www.actfoundation.ca
Year Founded: 1985
Languages: English

Alberta Centre for Active Living
11759 Groat Rd NW, Edmonton AB T5M 3K6
780 427-6949; Fax: 780 427-2677
Toll-free: 800 661-4551 Alberta
E: active.living@ualberta.ca
W: www.centre4activeliving.ca
Executive:
Dir: Judith Down
Year Founded: 1989
Library: Y
Languages: English

Alive Publishing Group - Live Magazine
100-12751 Vulcan Way, Richmond BC V6V 3C8
604 295-9333; Fax: 604 295-9101
Toll-free: 800 663-6580
Toll-free Fax: 800 663-6597
E: sales@alive.com
W: www.alive.com
Executive:
Pres: Ryan Benn
VP/Assoc Pub: Rick Kroetsch
Publications
Canadian Journal of Health and Nutrition

Association des Cadres Supérieurs de la Santé et des Services Sociaux
Place du Commerce
160-8 rue de la Place-du-Commerce,
Brossard QC J4W 3H2
450 465-0360; Fax: 450 465-0444
E: cadres.superieurs@acssss.qc.ca
W: www.acssss.qc.ca

HEALTHCARE ASSOCIATIONS

Executive:
Prés: Lise Giroux
Dir admin: Chantal Beaulieu
Criteria: *Être cadres supérieurs oeuvrant dans les établissements de santé et de services sociaux du Québec.*
No of Paid Staff: 6
Languages: French

Association des Établissements Privés Conventionnés-Santé Services Sociaux
200-204 rue Notre-Dame O, Montréal QC H2Y 1T3
514 499-3630 224; Fax: 514 873-7063
E: info@aepc.qc.ca
W: www.aepc.qc.ca
Executive:
Dir gén: Jean Hébert
Dir gest fin: Richard Désy
Year Founded: 1979
Criteria: *Détenir un permis d'opération d'établissment privées conventionnés.*
No of Paid Staff: 9
Languages: French
Membership: 67 *(Lists available to the public)*

Association des gestionnaires des établissements de santé et de service sociaux (AGESSS)
101-601 rue Adoncour, Longueuil QC J4G 2M6
450 651-6000; Fax: 450 651-9750
Toll-free: 800 361-6526
E: direction@agesss.qc.ca
W: www.agesss.qc.ca
Executive:
Prés/Prop: François Jean
Year Founded: 1970
Speakers Available
Membership: 8,200

Association Manger Santé Bio
Mailing: CP 325 Succ C, Montréal QC H2L 4K3
514 332-1005
E: info@mangersantebio.org
W: www.mangersantebio.org
Executive:
Prés: Renée Frappier
Trés: Bernard Lalonde

Association of Local Public Health Agencies
1306-2 Carlton St, Toronto ON M5B 1J3
416 595-0006; Fax: 416 595-0030
E: info@alphaweb.org
W: www.alphaweb.org
Executive:
Exec Dir: Linda Stewart
Mgr/Public Health Issues: Gordon Fleming
Mgr Admin/Assoc Serv: Susan Lee
Year Founded: 1986
No of Paid Staff: 4
Languages: English
Membership: 36

Association of Ontario Health Centres
500-970 Lawrence Ave W, Toronto ON M6A 3B6
416 236-2539; Fax: 416 236-0431
E: mail@aohc.org
W: www.aohc.org
Executive:
Pres: Jocelyne Maxwell
VP: Cate Melito
CIO: Rodney Burns
Exec Dir: Adrianna Tetley
Dir-Corp Serv: Hugh Hassan
Sec: Janet Bowes
Office Mgr: Sandra Wong
Treas: Peter Szota
Year Founded: 1926
No of Paid Staff: 12
Speakers Available
Library: Y *(Open to the public)*
Languages: English; French
Membership: 125

Association of Sexologists of Quebec
709-1100 boul Crémazie E, Montréal QC H2P 2X2
514 270-9289; Fax: 514 270-6351
E: info@associationdessexologues.com
W: www.associationdessexologues.com
Executive:
Prés: Alain Gariépy
Resp compte: Dan Li
Criteria: *Must have a Master's degree in clinical sexology or equivalent.*
Budget: $75,000
No of Paid Staff: 1
Speakers Available
Library: Y
Languages: English; French
Membership list available to the public

Association pour la santé publique du Québec
200-4126 rue Saint-Denis, Montréal QC H2W 2M5
514 528-5811; Fax: 514 528-5590
E: info@aspq.org
W: www.aspq.org
Year Founded: 1943
No of Paid Staff: 9
Languages: French

COTA Health Inc.
2901 Dufferin St, North York ON M6B 3S7
416 785-9230; Fax: 416 785-9358
Toll-free: 888 785-9358
E: info@cotahealth.ca
W: www.cotahealth.ca
Executive:
Exec Dir: Paul Bruce
Dir-Corp Serv: Apolone Gentles
Technology Mgr: Graham Taylor

Calgary Health Trust
Executive Tower
800-11012 MacLeod Trail SE, Calgary AB T2J 6A5
403 943-0615; Fax: 403 943-0628
E: fundraising@calgaryhealthtrust.ca
W: www.thetrust.ca
Executive:
CEO: Sally Flintoft
I-CFO/COO: Jill Olynyk
Year Founded: 1996
No of Paid Staff: 30
Speakers Available
Languages: English

Canadian Association of Specialized Kinesiology
Mailing: PO Box 45071 RPO Dunbar, Vancouver BC V6S 2M8
604 669-8481
E: office@canask.org
W: www.canask.org
Executive:
Exec Dir: Denise Cambiotti

Canadian Blood Services
2540 Lancaster Rd, Ottawa ON K1B 4S5
613 560-7440
E: feedback@blood.ca
W: www.blood.ca
Executive:
CIO: Kerry Cairnes
Hum Res Mgr: William Eagan

◈ Ottawa
1800 Alta Vista Dr, Ottawa ON K1G 4J5
613 739-2300; Fax: 613 731-1411
E: feedback@blood.ca
W: www.blood.ca
Executive:
CEO: Dr Graham Sher
Languages: English; French

Canadian Blood Services - Winnipeg
777 William Ave, Winnipeg MB R3E 3R4
204 789-1000; Fax: 204 775-9215
Toll-free: 888 236-6283
E: winnipegfb@bloodservices.ca
Languages: English; French

Canadian College of Health Leaders
292 Somerset St W, Ottawa ON K2P 0J6
613 235-7218; Fax: 613 235-5451
Toll-free: 800 363-9056
E: info@cchl-ccls.ca
W: www.cchl-ccls.ca
Executive:
Pres/CEO: Ray Racette
VP-Membership/Corp Serv: Jaime Cleroux
Year Founded: 1970
Budget: $2,000,000
No of Paid Staff: 15
Speakers Available
Languages: English; French
Membership: 3,000
Membership Fee: $40-$385

Canadian Council for Tobacco Control (CCTC)
192 Bank St, Ottawa ON K2P 1W8
613 567-3050; Fax: 613 567-2730
Toll-free: 800 267-5234
E: info-services@cctc.ca
W: www.cctc.ca
Executive:
Exec Dir: Robert Walsh
Ops Mgr: Jocelyne Koepke
Year Founded: 1974
No of Paid Staff: 10
Speakers Available
Library: Y
Languages: English; French

Canadian Health Coalition
105-2841 Riverside Dr, Ottawa ON K1V 8X7
613 277-6295
E: info@medicare.ca
W: www.medicare.ca
Executive:
Coord: Michael McBane
Languages: English

Canadian Healthcare Engineering Society
310-4 Cataraqui St, Kingston ON K7K 1Z7
613 531-2661; Fax: 613 531-0626
E: ches@eventsmgt.com
W: www.ches.org
Executive:
Exec Dir: Donna Dennison
Year Founded: 1980
Criteria: *Annual - calendar year renewal.*
Languages: English
Membership: 573
Membership Fee: $105 + GST

Canadian Hospice Palliative Care Association
Location: 41 Empress Ave, Ottawa ON K1R 7E9
Mailing: Annex D, 60 Cambridge St N,
Ottawa ON K1R 7A5
613 241-3663; Fax: 613 241-3986
Toll-free: 800 668-2785
E: info@chpca.net
W: www.chpca.net
Executive:
Exec Dir: Sharon Baxter
No of Paid Staff: 4
Languages: English; French
Membership: 3,500
Membership Fee: $20

Canadian Institute for Health Information
600-495 Richmond Rd, Ottawa ON K2A 4H6
613 241-7860; Fax: 613 241-8120
E: communications@cihi.ca
W: www.cihi.ca
Executive:
Pres/CEO: John Wright
Mgr-Infrastructure Tech: Ross Stewart
IT Coord: Karen Schlesiger
Year Founded: 1994
No of Paid Staff: 450
Languages: English; French
Membership: 600

◈CIHI Victoria:
600-880 Douglas St, Victoria BC V8W 2B7
250 220-4100; Fax: 250 220-7090
W: www.cihi.ca
Executive:
Exec Dir: Anne McFarlane

◈St. John's
701-140 Water St, St. John's NL A1C 6H6
709 576-7006; Fax: 709 576-0952

◈CIHI Toronto;
300-4110 Yonge St, Toronto ON M2P 2B7
416 481-2002; Fax: 416 481-2950
W: www.cihi.ca
Executive:
Hum Res Admin: Kathy Harris
Team Leader-IT: Satish Nair

Canadian Institute of Public Health Inspectors - National Office
720-999 Broadway W, Vancouver BC V5Z 1K5
604 543-0935; Fax: 604 738-4080
Toll-free: 888 245-8180
E: exec@ciphi.ca
W: www.ciphi.ca
Executive:
Pres: Keir Cordner
Year Founded: 1934
Criteria: *See website - www.ciphi.ca/memtypes.htm*
Languages: English
Membership: 1,000
Membership Fee: See website - www.ciphi.ca/memforms.htm

◈British Columbia:
Vancouver Coastal Health
132 Esplanade W, Floor 6,
North Vancouver BC V7M 1A2
604 675-3810; Fax: 604 736-8651
E: president@ciphi.bc.ca
Executive:
Pres: Jasmina Egeler

◈Winnipeg
Location: 208 Provencher Blvd,
Winnipeg MB R2H 3B4
Mailing: PO Box 171 CSP St Boniface
204 667-1655
W: www.ciphi.mb.ca
Executive:
Pres: Darcy Chrisp

◈Clarenville
Location: 8 Myers Ave, Clarenville NL A5A 1T5
Mailing: PO Box 243
709 466-4065; Fax: 709 466-5674
W: www.ciphi.nl.ca
Executive:
Pres: Chris Hart
Past Pres: Darryl Johnson
VP: Terry Battcock
Sec-Treas: Karen Hann
Rep Western: Nita MacLean
Rep Eastern: Sharon Williams
Rep Central: Sara Timpa
Year Founded: 1913
Speakers Available
Languages: English
Membership: 25

◈London
Ministry of Environment
3232 White Oak Rd, London ON N6E 1L8
519 873-5090; Fax: 519 873-5096
W: www.ciphi.on.ca
Executive:
Pres: Adam Grant
Languages: English

Canadian MedicAlert Foundation
800-2005 Sheppard Ave E, Toronto ON M2J 5B4
416 696-0142; Fax: 416 696-0156
Toll-free: 800 668-1507 English
Toll-free Fax: 800 338-1507
E: medinfo@medicalert.ca
W: www.medicalert.ca
Executive:
Pres/CEO: Robert Ridge
VP-Mktg: Camille Krupa
Year Founded: 1961
Criteria: *Anyone with a medical condition, special need, allergies and organ donors.*
No of Paid Staff: 60
Speakers Available
Languages: English; French
Membership: 1000000 +
Membership Fee: $39 or $49 annually

Canadian Public Health Association
300-1565 Carling Ave, Ottawa ON K1Z 8R1
613 725-3769; Fax: 613 725-9826
E: info@cpha.ca
W: www.cpha.ca
Executive:
Chair: Erica Diruggiero
CEO: Debra Lynkowski
A-Reg Dir/Office Mgr: Shawn Bostick
Year Founded: 1910
No of Paid Staff: 45
Languages: English
Membership: 1,400

Canadian Red Cross - Atlantic Zone
Mailing: Burnside Business Park
133 Troop Ave, Dartmouth NS B3B 2A7
902 423-3680; Fax: 902 422-6247
No of Paid Staff: 120
Languages: English

◈Moncton
246 Lutz St, Moncton NB E1C 5G3
506 863-2650 0; Fax: 506 863-2662
No of Paid Staff: 14
Speakers Available
Languages: English; French
Membership list available to the public

◈Atlantic Zone:
300-170 Metcalfe St, Ottawa ON K2P 2P2
613 740-1900; Fax: 613 740-1911
Toll-free: 877 280-9673
E: feedback@redcross.ca
W: www.redcross.ca
Executive:
Sec Gen/CEO: Conrad Sauvé
Natl Dir-Info Serv: Almin Surani
Natl Dir-Hum Res Volunteer Serv: Ann Clancy
Year Founded: 1909
No of Paid Staff: 5,900
Languages: English

◈Atholville
3 Savoie Ave, Atholville NB E3N 4A8
506 759-8521; Fax: 506 753-2487
Toll-free: 800 588-4881
W: www.redcross.ca
Languages: English

Canadian Society for Exercise Physiology
370-18 Louisa St, Ottawa ON K1R 6Y6
613 234-3755; Fax: 613 234-3565
Toll-free: 877 651-3755
E: info@csep.ca
W: www.csep.ca
Executive:
Mgr-Exercise in Medicine Cda: Susan Yungblut
Mgr: Mary Duggan
Health/Fitness Prog Dir: Bridget Lett
Year Founded: 1967
Criteria: *Graduate degree or above. Complete application form and return with fee.*
Budget: $900,000
No of Paid Staff: 2
Languages: English; French
Membership: 5,000
Membership Fee: $125 + GST/HST

Canadian Society for International Health
1105-1 Nicholas St, Ottawa ON K1N 7B7
613 241-5785; Fax: 613 241-3845
E: csih@csih.org
W: www.csih.org
Executive:
Co-Chair: Dr Karan Ranotar
Co-Chair: Sam Lanfranco
Exec Dir: Janet Hatcher Roberts
Dir-Fin: Bob Abma
Year Founded: 1977
Criteria: *Open to all*
No of Paid Staff: 20
Library: Y
Languages: English

Canadian Society of Nutrition Management
300-1370 Don Mills Rd, North York ON M3B 3N7
416 441-9622; Fax: 416 441-0591
Toll-free: 866 355-2766
E: csnm@csnm.ca
W: www.csnm.ca
Executive:
Office Admin: Debbie Cullen
No of Paid Staff: 3
Languages: English

Cardiac Fitness Association
1010 Hopewell Creek Rd, RR 2, Breslau ON N0B 1M0
519 648-2252; Fax: 519 648-3686
W: www.cfaheart.com
Executive:
Med Dir: Dr John Schaman
Year Founded: 1980
Criteria: *Rehabilitation program for cardiac patients.*
Languages: English

HEALTHCARE ASSOCIATIONS

Catholic Health Association of Saskatchewan
1702 20th St W, Saskatoon SK S7M 0Z9
306 655-5330; Fax: 306 655-5333
E: cath.health@sasktel.net
W: www.chassk.ca
Executive:
Exec Dir: Sandra Kary
Year Founded: 1943
Criteria: *Persons or organized groups who are interested in Catholic health care and wish to show their support for the work of the Association.*
Budget: $250,000
No of Paid Staff: 3
Speakers Available
Library: Y
Languages: English
Membership: 550
Membership Fee: $25 Personal; $250 Affiliate; $75 Associate
Library:
CHAS Library *(Open to the public)*

Catholic Health Corporation of Ontario
Location: 712 College Ave W, Guelph ON N1G 1V1
Mailing: PO Box 1879 Stn Main, Guelph ON N1H 7A1
519 767-5600; Fax: 519 767-5602
E: chco@chco.ca
W: www.chco.ca
Executive:
Pres: Don McDermott
Year Founded: 1997
No of Paid Staff: 1
Languages: English

Centre de Santé Communautaire Hamilton/Niagara
460 Main St E, 2nd Floor, Hamilton ON L8N 1K4
905 528-0163; Fax: 905 528-9196
E: cschwn@iaw.on.ca
W: www.cschn.ca
Executive:
Gen Mgr: Marcel Castonguay
No of Paid Staff: 25
Languages: English

Christian Health Association of Alberta
Location: 132 Warwick Rd NW, Edmonton AB T5X 4P8
Mailing: PO Box 4173 Stn South Cro, Edmonton AB T6E 4T2
780 488-8074; Fax: 780 475-7968
E: chaaa@compusmart.ab.ca
W: www.chaaa.ab.ca
Executive:
Admin: Glyn Smith
Year Founded: 1943
Budget: $85,000
Languages: English
Membership: 200

COACH: Canada's Health Informatics Association
301-250 Consumers Rd, Toronto ON M2J 4V6
416 494-9324; Fax: 416 495-8723
Toll-free: 888 253-8554
E: info@coachorg.com
W: www.coachorg.com
Executive:
CEO: Don Newsham
Exec Dir CTF: John Schinbein
Exec Dir Ops: Shannon Bott
Exec Dir CHIEF: Linda Miller
Prog Dir: Alison Gardner
Year Founded: 1975
No of Paid Staff: 5
Speakers Available
Languages: English
Membership: 1,500
Membership Fee: $165

Common Ground Publishing Corp.
204-4381 Fraser St, Vancouver BC V5V 4G4
604 733-2215; Fax: 604 733-4415
Toll-free: 800 365-8897
E: admin@commonground.ca
W: www.commonground.ca
Executive:
Pub: Joseph Roberts
Publications
Common Ground

Community Health Services Association (Regina) Ltd.
1106 Winnipeg St, Regina SK S4R 1J6
306 543-7880; Fax: 306 543-5545
E: admin@reginacommunityclinic.ca
W: www.reginacommunityclinic.ca
Executive:
Exec Dir: Lorna Knudson
Medical Coord: Dr Robin McMaster
Year Founded: 1962
No of Paid Staff: 50
Speakers Available
Library: Y *(Open to the public)*
Languages: English
Membership: 12,382
Membership Fee: $5
◈Regina
20A Sangster Blvd, Regina SK S4R 7B4

Consumer Health Organization of Canada
1901-355 St Clair Ave W, Toronto ON M5P 1N5
416 924-9800; Fax: 416 924-6404
Toll-free: 877 389-0996
W: www.consumerhealth.org
Executive:
Pres: Libby Gardon
Dir: Helen McLellan
Year Founded: 1975
No of Paid Staff: 1
Library: Y
Languages: English

Corporation l'Espoir
55 av Dupras, LaSalle QC H8R 4A8
514 367-3757; Fax: 514 367-0444
E: info@corporationespoir.org
W: www.corporationespoir.org
Executive:
Dir: Caroline Langevin
Year Founded: 1976
Criteria: *Adhésion*
No of Paid Staff: 10
Languages: French
Membership: 450 families
Membership Fee: $15/ans

Croissance Travail
215 rue Caron, Québec QC G1K 5V6
418 522-1244; Fax: 418 524-5809
E: serealiser@croissancetravail.qc.ca
W: www.croissancetravail.com
Executive:
Resp de l'atelier: Hélène Plamondon
Year Founded: 1992
No of Paid Staff: 20
Languages: French

Croix Rouge Canadienne
325 rue de la Croix-Rouge, Quebec QC G1K 2L4
418 648-9066; Fax: 418 648-1320
W: www.croixrouge.ca
Executive:
Dir fin: Pascal Mathieu
Dir-servs d'intervention: Claudie Laberge

Dietitians of Canada - Canadian Journal of Dietetic Practice & Research
604-480 University Ave, Toronto ON M5G 1V2
416 596-0857; Fax: 416 596-0603
E: centralinfo@dietitians.ca
W: www.dietitians.ca
Executive:
CEO: Marsha Sharp
Editor: Dawna Royall
Cust Serv Rep: Helena Asfaw
Year Founded: 1958
Criteria: *Qualifying membership available*
Budget: $2,500,000
No of Paid Staff: 20
Languages: English; French
Membership list available to the public
Publications
Canadian Journal of Dietetic Practice and Research (English, Quarterly)

Fédération Québécois des Laryngectomisés
5565 rue Sherbrooke E, Montréal QC H1N 1A2
514 259-5113; Fax: 514 259-8946
E: fqlar@fqlar.qc.ca
W: www.fqlar.qc.ca
Executive:
Prés: Michel Lafortune
Year Founded: 1979
No of Paid Staff: 1
Languages: French
Membership: 900

Fondation Des Sourds Du Quebec
3348 boul Monseigneur-Gauthier, Québec QC G1E 2W2
418 660-6800; Fax: 418 666-0123
W: www.fondationdessourds.net
Executive:
Adj exéc: Patricia Nemeth

Fung Loy Kok Institute of Taoism
2029 North Park St, Halifax NS B3K 4B2
902 422-8142; Fax: 902 422-1998
E: halifax@taoist.org
W: www.taoist.org
Year Founded: 1980
No of Paid Staff: 1
Speakers Available
Languages: English; French

Health & Safety Conference Society Of Alberta
Mailing: PO Box 38009 Rpo Country Hills, Calgary AB T3K 5G9
403 236-2225; Fax: 403 206-7099
E: info@hsconference.com
W: www.hsconference.com
Executive:
Pres: Guy Clyne
VP: Arlene Ledi-Thom

Health Action Network Society
202-5262 Rumble St, Burnaby BC V5J 2B6
604 435-0512
E: hans@hans.org
W: www.hans.org
Executive:
Co-Founder/Dir: Lorna J Hancock
Year Founded: 1984
Budget: $200,000
No of Paid Staff: 4
Speakers Available
Library: Y

Languages: English
Membership: 3,000
Membership Fee: $35 Individual; $180 Business; $50 Family
Library:
HANS Library

Health Association Nova Scotia
2 Dartmouth Rd, Bedford NS B4A 2K7
902 832-8500; Fax: 902 832-8505
E: contactus@healthassociation.ns.ca
W: www.healthassociation.ns.ca
Executive:
Pres/CEO: Mary Lee
Year Founded: 1960
No of Paid Staff: 83
Speakers Available
Library: Y *(Open to the public)*
Languages: English
Membership: 118

Health Association of Prince Edward Island Inc.
10 Pownal St, Charlottetown PE C1A 3V6
902 368-3901; Fax: 902 368-3231
Executive:
Exec Dir: Ken Ezeard
Exec Sec: Earlene Holmes
No of Paid Staff: 3
Languages: English
Membership: 1

Health Employers Association of British Columbia
200-1333 Broadway St W, Vancouver BC V6H 4C6
604 736-5909; Fax: 604 736-2715
E: contact@heabc.bc.ca
W: www.heabc.bc.ca
Executive:
Chair: Betsy Gibbons
Year Founded: 1993
No of Paid Staff: 80
Library: Y
Languages: English

Health Professions Regulatory Advisory Council
56 Wellesley St W, Floor 12, Toronto ON M5S 2S3
416 326-1550; Fax: 416 326-1549
Toll-free: 888 377-7746
E: hpracwebmaster@ontario.ca
W: www.hprac.org
Executive:
Pol Analyst: Susana Tam
Exec Coord: Laura Niles
Speakers Available
Languages: English

Health Quality Council
Atrium Bldg Innovation Pl
241-111 Research Dr, Saskatoon SK S7N 3R2
306 668-8810; Fax: 306 668-8820
E: info@hqc.sk.ca
W: www.hqc.sk.ca
Executive:
CEO: Bonnie Brossart
Year Founded: 2003

Health Sciences Association of Alberta
10212 112 St NW, Edmonton AB T5K 1M4
780 488-0168; Fax: 780 488-0534
Toll-free: 800 252-7904
E: mail@hsaa.ca
W: www.hsaa.ca
Executive:
Pres: Elisabeth Ballermann
Dir-Labor Rel: Lynette McAvoy
Languages: English
Membership list available to the public

◈ Calgary
204-200 Country Hills Landing NW, Calgary AB T3K 5P3
403 250-8999; Fax: 403 250-8576
W: www.hsaa.ca
Executive:
Dir: Lynette McAvoy
Admv Asst: Correna Phillips
No of Paid Staff: 5
Languages: English

Health Sciences Association of British Columbia
300-5118 Joyce St, Vancouver BC V5R 4H1
604 439-0994; Fax: 604 439-0976
Toll-free: 800 663-2017
E: webmaster@hsabc.org
W: www.hsabc.org
Executive:
Pres: Reid Johnson
Exec Dir-Labour Rels/Legal Serv: Jeanne Meyers
Dir-Ops: Rebecca Maurer
Dir-Commun: Miriam Sobrino
Year Founded: 1971
Criteria: *Unionized paramedical professional employees.*
No of Paid Staff: 50
Speakers Available
Library: Y
Languages: English
Membership: 14,000
Membership Fee: Varies as per union constitution.

Health Sciences Centre Foundation
MS107-820 Sherbrook St, Winnipeg MB R3A 1R9
204 787-2022; Fax: 204 787-2804
Toll-free: 800 679-8493
E: hsc_foundation@hsc.mb.ca
W: www.hscfoundation.mb.ca
Executive:
VP/COO: Dawne Smithson
Dir-Mktg/Commun: Tammy Wood
Dir-Sponsorships/Partnerships: Seri Blatt
Year Founded: 1981
Budget: $14,000,000
No of Paid Staff: 15
Speakers Available
Languages: English

Hospice Toronto
400-2221 Yonge St, Toronto ON M4S 2B4
416 364-1666; Fax: 416 364-2231
E: info@hospicetoronto.ca
W: www.hospicetoronto.ca
Executive:
Pres: Brian T Glasspoole
Exec Dir: Dena Maule
Dir Clinical Serv: Belinda Marchese
Mgr Volunteer Svcs: Sally Blainey
Treas: Sheena Kotecha
Office Coor: Janice Nyarko-Mensah

Institut de réadaptation Gingras Lindsay de Montréal
6300 av de Darlington, Montréal QC H3S 2J4
514 340-2085; Fax: 514 340-2091
W: www.irglm.qc.ca
Executive:
Dir gén: Jean-Philippe Cotton
Dir ress hum: Marie-Ève Lemieux
Adj admin: Janet Campbell
Year Founded: 1949
Budget: $25,000,000
No of Paid Staff: 400
Library: Y *(Open to the public)*
Languages: French

Institute for Clinical Evaluative Sciences
G-106-2075 Bayview Ave, Toronto ON M4N 3M5
416 480-4055; Fax: 416 480-6048
E: info@ices.on.ca
W: www.ices.on.ca
Executive:
Pres/CEO: Dr David Henry
Dep CEO/Sr Scientist: Michael Schull
Sr Dir-Corp Serv: Cathy Hazell
Sr Dir-Data,Tech & Sec: Leslie Howard
Dir-Commun: Susan Shiller
Dir-Fin: Pauline Yick
Facilities/Admn Mgr: Jim Park
Hum Res Mgr: Christopher Tan
Technology Mgr: Felix Zhang
Languages: English

International Health Collaboration (C.S.I.)
1001 ch de la Canardière, Québec QC G1J 5G5
418 522-6065; Fax: 418 522-5530
E: csi@csiquebec.org
W: www.csiquebec.org
Year Founded: 1975
Budget: $1,000,000
No of Paid Staff: 10
Languages: French
Membership: 3,000

Joint Centre For Bioethics
University Of Toronto
754-155 College St, Toronto ON M5T 1P8
416 978-2709; Fax: 416 978-1911
E: jcb.info@utoronto.ca
W: www.jointcentreforbioethics.ca/
Executive:
Dir-Admn/Ops: Brenda Knowles
Exec Asst: Rhonda Martin

KinVillage Association West Court
5410 10 Ave, Delta BC V4M 3X8
604 943-0155; Fax: 604 943-1542
W: www.kinvillage.org
Executive:
CEO: Donna Ellis
Dir-Fin/Admn: Mike Skelly
Dir-Rec Serv/Volunteers: John Lusted
Dir Hlth Serv: Cynthia Langenberg

Life Science Association of Manitoba
1000 Waverley St, Winnipeg MB R3T 0P3
204 272-5095; Fax: 204 272-2961
E: info@lsam.ca
W: www.lsam.ca
Executive:
Pres: Tracey Maconachie
Board Member: Philip Unger
Year Founded: 1990
Criteria: *Manufacturer/Research & Development, Life Sciences*
Budget: $200,000
No of Paid Staff: 4
Speakers Available
Library: Y *(Open to the public)*
Languages: English
Membership: 100 *(Lists available to the public)*

Manitoba Tobacco Reduction Alliance Inc.

192B Goulet St, Winnipeg MB R2H 0R8
204 784-7030; Fax: 204 784-7039
E: admin@mantrainc.ca
W: www.mantrainc.ca
Executive:
Chair: Dr Beverley Temple
Exec Dir: Murray Gibson

Manufacturers' Health and Safety Association

225 Parsons Rd SW, Edmonton AB T6X 0W6
780 428-1006; Fax: 780 487-4529
W: www.mhsa.ab.ca
Executive:
Exec Dir: Lorne Kleppe
Budget: $500,000
No of Paid Staff: 8
Speakers Available
Library: Y
Languages: English

Nature's Way North Publishers Inc - Vitality Magazine

356 Dupont St, Toronto ON M5R 1V9
416 964-0528
E: info@vitalitymagazine.com
W: www.vitalitymagazine.com
Executive:
Editor: Julia Woodford

Newfoundland and Labrador Health Boards Association

Beothuck Bldg
20 Crosbie Pl, Floor 2, St. John's NL A1B 3Y8
709 364-7701; Fax: 709 364-6460
W: www.nlhba.nl.ca
Executive:
Exec Dir: Dr Patricia Conrad
Year Founded: 1962
No of Paid Staff: 12
Languages: English
Membership: 14 *(Lists available to the public)*
Membership Fee: Based on portion of Provincial Health Budget

Non-Smokers' Rights Association

221-720 Spadina Ave, Toronto ON M5S 2T9
416 928-2900; Fax: 416 928-1860
E: toronto@nsra-adnf.ca
W: www.nsra-adnf.ca
Executive:
Exec Dir: Lorraine Fry
Office Mgr: Elsa Sykes
Membership Svcs: Peter Holt
Year Founded: 1975
No of Paid Staff: 9
Speakers Available
Languages: English; French

North Eastman Health Association

24 Aberdeen Ave, PO Box 339, Pinawa MB R0E 1L0
204 753-2012; Fax: 204 753-2015
Toll-free: 877 753-2012
E: neha@neha.mb.ca
W: www.neha.mb.ca
Executive:
CEO: Jim Hayes
Exec Asst: G Wilson
No of Paid Staff: 800
Speakers Available
Languages: English

OPDQ - Ordre professionnel des diététistes du Québec

1220-2155 rue Guy, Montréal QC H3H 2R9
514 393-3733; Fax: 514 393-3582
Toll-free: 888 393-8528
E: opdq@opdq.org
W: www.opdq.org
Executive:
Prés: Anné Gagné
Dir gén: Annie Chapados
Year Founded: 1956
No of Paid Staff: 10
Speakers Available
Languages: French
Membership: 2,300 *(Lists available to the public)*

Occupational Hygiene Association of Ontario

6519B Mississauga Rd, Mississauga ON L5N 1A6
905 567-7196; Fax: 905 567-7191
E: office@ohao.org
W: www.ohao.org
Executive:
Pres: Paul Bozek
Pres Elect: Nancy Wilk
Dir: Negin Ghanvatian
Dir: Bernardino Grande
Dir: Tim Kelsall
Dir: Don K Webb
Dir: John J Prince
Dir: John Petherick
Exec Mgr: Jason Boyer
Sec-Treas: Altaire Hildebrand
Year Founded: 1964
Criteria: *Full Membership: must have a total of 6 years combined post-secondary education and work experience in occupational hygiene.*
Associate Membership: a combined post-secondary education and work experience of 6 years, but the work experience consists of continuing practice of occupational hygiene for less than the majority but more than one quarter of the applicant's time, or, less than 6 years combined post-secondary education and work experience, but the work experience consists of the continuing practice of occupational hygiene for the majority of the applicant's time.
Student Membership: open to any person who has an interest in occupational hygiene and is registered full-time in an occupational hygiene, environmental, health or safety related program at a post secondary institution in Canada.
Speakers Available
Languages: English
Membership: 300 *(Lists available to the public)*
Membership Fee: $80 per year

Ontario Fitness Council

496 Taylor Cres, Burlington ON L7L 6G2
800 671-4632; Fax: 905 738-7797
W: ontariofitnesscouncil.com
Executive:
Man Dir: Jeff Angus
Year Founded: 1986
Criteria: *Certification*
No of Paid Staff: 1
Speakers Available
Languages: English; French; Italian
Membership: 700
Membership Fee: $125 for 2 years

Ontario Home Care Association

Mailing: PO Box 68018 RPO Blakely, Hamilton ON L8M 3M7
905 543-9474; Fax: 905 545-1568
E: suevan@homecareontario.ca
W: www.homecareontario.ca
Executive:
Exec Dir: Sue VanderBent
Languages: English

Ontario Public Health Association (OPHA)

1850-439 University Ave, Toronto ON M5G 1Y8
416 367-3313 238; Fax: 416 367-2844
Toll-free: 800 267-6817 Ontario only
E: info@opha.on.ca
W: www.opha.on.ca
Executive:
Pres: Sue Makin
VP: Larry Stinson
Treas: Monica Mitchell
Sec: Marty Mako
Year Founded: 1949
Criteria: *Interest in public and community health.*
Languages: English
Membership: 850 +
Membership Fee: $70

Ontario Tobacco Research Unit

33 Russell St, Toronto ON M5S 2S1
416 595-6888; Fax: 416 595-6068
E: info@otru.org
W: www.otru.org
Year Founded: 1993
Criteria: *Academic/Public Health Affiliation*
No of Paid Staff: 40
Speakers Available
Library: Y
Languages: English
Membership: 130 *(Lists available to the public)*
Library:
Resource Centre

Pathways Health Promotion

3040 Bradburn Rd, Main Floor, Blackstock ON L0B 1B0
Toll-free: 866 921-9355
E: info@pathwayshealthpromotion.com
W: www.PathwaysHealthPromotion.com
Executive:
Coach: Rae-Anne Jammer

Physical and Health Education Canada

301-2197 Riverside Dr, Ottawa ON K1H 7X3
613 523-1348; Fax: 613 523-1206
Toll-free: 800 663-8708
E: info@phecanada.ca
W: www.phecanada.ca
Executive:
CEO: Chris Jones
COO: Bryan Merrett
Bus Dev/Memb Mgr: Jordan Burwash
Year Founded: 1933

Physicians for a Smoke-Free Canada

1226 Wellington St W, Ottawa ON K1Y 3A1
613 233-4878; Fax: 613 233-7797
Toll-free: 800 540-5418
E: psc@smoke-free.ca
W: www.smoke-free.ca
Executive:
Pres: Dr Atul Kapur
Dir-Research: Neil Collishaw
Budget: $180,000
No of Paid Staff: 2
Speakers Available
Languages: English

Les Promotions Rodel Inc.

1350 rue Marie-Victorin, Saint-Bruno QC J3V 6B9
450 653-1337; Fax: 450 653-9924
Toll-free: 800 463-4961
E: reception@rodel.ca
W: www.promotionsrodel.com
Executive:
Prés: Alain Delorme

Quebec Council on Tobacco and Health
302-4126 rue Saint-Denis, Montréal QC H2W 2M5
514 948-5317; Fax: 514 948-4582
E: info@cqts.qc.ca
W: www.cqts.qc.ca
Executive:
Prés: Dr André-H Dandabino
Dir gén: Mario Bujold
Year Founded: 1976
No of Paid Staff: 14
Languages: French; English
Membership: 25

St. John Ambulance - National Headquarters
400-1900 City Park Dr, Ottawa ON K1J 1A3
613 236-7461; Fax: 613 236-2425
Toll-free: 800 268-7581
E: info@nhq.sja.ca
W: www.sja.ca
Executive:
COO: Dawn Roach
No of Paid Staff: 260
Speakers Available
Languages: English; French
Membership: 25,000

◈Alberta
12304 118 Ave NW, Edmonton AB T5L 5G8
780 452-6565; Fax: 780 453-1632
Toll-free: 800 665-7114
E: edmonton@stjohn.ab.ca
W: www.sja.ca/ab
Executive:
Pres/CEO: David J Hook
VP-Fin/Corp Serv: Rick Stewart
VP-Training/Commun Serv: Beverly Lafortune
Dir-Reg Dev N-AB: Barbara Walters
Dir-Reg Dev S-AB: Kim Laing
Year Founded: 1897
Budget: $8,000,000
No of Paid Staff: 80
Speakers Available
Languages: English
Membership: 3,000

◇Red Deer:
6519 67 St, Red Deer AB T4P 1A3
403 342-7744; Fax: 403 342-0222
E: rdeer@stjohn.ab.ca
W: www.sja.ca/Alberta
Executive:
Admv Coord: Sherry McMullen

◈St. John Society (British Columbia and Yukon)
201-6111 Cambie St, Vancouver BC V5Z 3B2
604 321-2652; Fax: 604 321-5316
Toll-free: 866 321-2651
E: info@bc.sja.ca
W: www.sja.ca/bc
Executive:
Dir-Mktg: Rene Bernstein
Hum Res Coord: May Foggo
Year Founded: 1898
Criteria: *Various categories*
Budget: $7,000,000
No of Paid Staff: 65
Speakers Available
Library: Y *(Open to the public)*
Languages: English

◇Fort St John
Location: 10066 Tundra St, Fort St. John BC V1J 4M6
Mailing: RR 1 Stn Main
250 785-7233; Fax: 250 785-6127
E: ftstjohn@bc.sja.ca
W: www.sja.ca

◇Vancouver:
6111 Cambie St, Vancouver BC V5Z 3B2
604 321-2651; Fax: 604 321-2650
E: register@bc.sja.ca
W: www.sja.ca/bc
Executive:
Cust Serv Coord: John Serrano
Languages: English

◈Manitoba
1 St. John Ambulance Way, Winnipeg MB R3G 3H5
204 784-7000; Fax: 204 786-2295
Toll-free: 800 471-7771
E: info@mb.sja.ca
W: www.sja.ca/mb
Executive:
CEO: Steven D Gaetz
Reg Ops Mgr: Brent Fowler
Dir-Fin/Corp Serv: Marilee Eldridge
Dir-Commun Serv: Christine Armstrong
Year Founded: 1911
No of Paid Staff: 15
Speakers Available
Languages: English
Membership: 500

◈New Brunswick
Location: 200 Miles St, Fredericton NB E3A 3J7
Mailing: PO Box 3599 Stn B, Fredericton NB E3A 5J8
506 458-9129; Fax: 506 452-8699
Toll-free: 800 563-9998
E: stjohnnb@nbnet.nb.ca
W: www.sja.ca/
Executive:
CEO: Larry Broad
Year Founded: 1896
No of Paid Staff: 18
Languages: English; French
Membership: 500

◈Newfoundland and Labrador
8 Thomas Byrne Dr, Mount Pearl NL A1N 0E1
709 726-4200; Fax: 709 726-4117
Toll-free: 800 801-0181 outside St. John's and surrounding area
E: sja@nl.sja.ca
W: www.sja.ca/nl
No of Paid Staff: 9
Languages: English

◈Sydney
479 George St, Sydney NS B1P 1K5
902 564-4189; Fax: 902 539-2730
Toll-free: 800 565-5056
E: info@ns.sja.ca
W: www.sja.ca/ns
Executive:
CEO: Paul Millen
No of Paid Staff: 20
Languages: English

◈Cambridge
56 Jaffray St, Cambridge ON N1R 3H9
519 740-8895; Fax: 519 740-8642
E: cambridge@on.sja.ca
W: www.sja.ca
Executive:
Br Mgr: Myra Klaassen

◈Federal District Council
Ottawa Carleton Region
5 Corvus Crt, Nepean ON K2E 7Z4
613 722-2002; Fax: 613 722-7024
E: fd@fdgd.sja.ca
W: www.sja.ca/ottawa
Executive:
CEO: Les Johnson
Year Founded: 1931
Criteria: *Recruiting criteria for adults & cadets.*
Budget: $1,500,000
No of Paid Staff: 12
Speakers Available
Languages: English; French
Membership: 250 *(Lists available to the public)*

◈Hamilton
65 Nebo Rd, Hamilton ON L8W 2C9
905 387-1880; Fax: 905 387-1444
E: hamilton@on.sja.ca
W: www.sja.ca
Executive:
Mgr: Kevin Keith
Year Founded: 1912
No of Paid Staff: 3
Speakers Available
Languages: English
Membership: 150

◈Lindsay
210 Kent St W, Lindsay ON K9V 2Y8
705 324-9894; Fax: 705 324-1833
E: info@sja.ca
W: www.sja.ca
Executive:
Mgr: Judy Hartin

◈Ontario
15 Toronto St, Floor 8, Toronto ON M5C 2E3
416 923-8411; Fax: 416 923-4856
Toll-free: 800 268-7581
E: info@on.sja.ca
W: www.sja.ca
Executive:
Exec Dir: Terry Wardrop
Languages: English

◇Hamilton:
65 Nebo Rd, Hamilton ON L8W 2C9
905 387-1880; Fax: 905 387-1444
E: hamilton@on.sja.ca
W: www.sja.ca
Executive:
Mgr: Kevin Keith
Year Founded: 1912
No of Paid Staff: 3
Speakers Available
Languages: English
Membership: 150

◇Lindsay
210 Kent St W, Lindsay ON K9V 2Y8
705 324-9894; Fax: 705 324-1833
E: info@sja.ca
W: www.sja.ca
Executive:
Mgr: Judy Hartin

◇Owen Sound
Location: 1580 20th St E, Owen Sound ON N4K 5P5
Mailing: PO Box 632 Stn Main,
Owen Sound ON N4K 5R4
519 376-4813; Fax: 519 376-4981
E: owen.sound@on.sja.ca
W: www.sja.ca
Year Founded: 1912
Criteria: *Desire to help your community.*
No of Paid Staff: 2
Speakers Available
Library: Y *(Open to the public)*
Languages: English
Membership: 40

◇Thunder Bay
518 Fort William Rd, Thunder Bay ON P7B 2Z8
807 345-1712; Fax: 807 343-0295
W: www.sja.ca
Executive:
Exec Dir: Diana Sustawenko
Year Founded: 1923
No of Paid Staff: 10
Languages: English
Membership list available to the public

◈ **Québec**
400-529 rue Jarry E, Montréal QC H2P 1V4
514 842-4801; Fax: 514 842-4807
Toll-free: 877 272-7607
Toll-free Fax: 866 856-4728
E: info@qc.sja.ca
W: www.sja.qc.ca
Executive:
Prés: Jacques Carrier
Contrôleuse: Aline Patenaude
Year Founded: 1918
No of Paid Staff: 30
Speakers Available
Languages: English; French
Membership: 4,000

◈ **North Battleford**
1225C 100th St, North Battleford SK S9A 0V6
306 445-3472; Fax: 306 445-3796
E: north.battleford@sk.sja.ca
W: www.sja.ca
Executive:
Mgr: Shirley Blyan
Criteria: *Open to all.*
Languages: English

◈ **Saskatchewan**
2625 3rd Ave, Regina SK S4T 0C8
306 522-7226; Fax: 306 525-4177
Toll-free: 888 273-0003
E: inquiries@sk.sja.ca
W: www.sja.ca
Executive:
CEO: Kevin Moore
Languages: English

◇ **North Battleford:**
1225C 100th St, North Battleford SK S9A 0V6
306 445-3472; Fax: 306 445-3796
E: north.battleford@sk.sja.ca
W: www.sja.ca
Executive:
Mgr: Shirley Blyan
Criteria: *Open to all.*
Languages: English

St. Joseph's Home Care
201-1550 Upper James St, Hamilton ON L9B 2L6
905 522-6887; Fax: 905 522-5579
Toll-free: 800 463-6612
E: admin@stjhc.ca
W: www.stjoeshomecare.on.ca
Executive:
Pres: Kim Ciavarella
Dir-CSS: Glenys Currie
Dir-Nursing: Fran Sullivan
Hum Res Coord: Lisa Vincelli
Year Founded: 1921
No of Paid Staff: 300
Languages: English

Saskatchewan Association of Health Organizations
800-2002 Victoria Ave, Regina SK S4P 0R7
306 347-5500; Fax: 306 525-1960
E: info@saho.org
W: www.saho.org
Executive:
Pres/CEO: Susan Antosh
Admv Asst/Member Rel: Cindy Robison
Exec Coord: Janet Steinhubl
Year Founded: 1993
Criteria: *Must be a health organization.*
Budget: $5,000,000
No of Paid Staff: 100
Speakers Available
Languages: English
Membership: 140
Membership Fee: Varies

Saskatchewan Coalition for Tobacco Reduction (SCTR)
Mailing: 1080 Winnipeg St, Regina SK S4R 8P8
306 766-6327; Fax: 306 766-6945
E: sctr@rqhealth.ca
W: www.sctr.ca
Executive:
Pres: Lynn Greaves
VP/Treas: Bill Bray
Sec: Crystal Storey
Year Founded: 1972
Criteria: *Organizations and individuals interested in reducing tobacco use.*
Languages: English
Membership: 20 *(Lists available to the public)*

Saskatchewan Prevention Institute
1319 Colony St, Saskatoon SK S7N 2Z1
306 655-2512; Fax: 306 655-2511
E: info@preventioninstitute.sk.ca
W: www.preventioninstitute.sk.ca
Executive:
Exec Dir: Noreen Agrey
Sec: Donna Anderson
Year Founded: 1980
Criteria: *Board of Directors*
No of Paid Staff: 20
Speakers Available
Languages: English
Membership: 18

Smoke-Free Nova Scotia
Mailing: PO Box 822, Lower Sackville NS B4C 3V3
902 864-9633; Fax: 902 864-6946
E: carivanlingen@smokefreens.ca
W: www.smokefreens.ca
Executive:
Pres: Krista McMullen

Smoking and Health Action Foundation
221-720 Spadina Ave, Toronto ON M5S 2T9
416 928-2900; Fax: 416 928-1860
E: toronto@nsra-adnf.ca
W: www.nsra-adnf.ca
Executive:
Exec Dir: Lorraine Fry
Office Mgr: Elsa Sykes
Membership Svcs Coor: Peter Holt
Languages: English

Unity Centre of Northeast Edmonton
101-14530 72 St NW, Edmonton AB T5C 0R7
780 478-6521; Fax: 780 473-4548
E: lindaunity@shaw.ca
W: www.unitycentreofedmonton.ca
Executive:
Exec Dir: Linda Armstrong
Year Founded: 1970
Criteria: *Open to anyone who accesses the Centre's programs or services.*
Budget: $250,000
No of Paid Staff: 8
Languages: English
Membership: 150

HEALTH CARE

Alberta Public Health Association
ACICR 4075 RTF
8308 114 St NW, Edmonton AB T6G 2E1
780 492-6014
E: info@apha.ab.ca
W: www.apha.ab.ca
Executive:
Pres: Dr P K Doyle-Baker

BCS Communications Ltd.
803-255 Duncan Mill Rd, Toronto ON M3B 3H9
416 421-7944 302; Fax: 416 421-8418
Toll-free: 800 798-6282
E: dostal@bcsgroup.com
W: www.bcsgroup.com
Executive:
Pres: Helmut H Dostal
Dir-Mktg: Caroline Tapp-McDougall

Blue Heron Support Service Association - Keir Building
Location: 4925 51st Ave, Barrhead AB T7N 1A2
Mailing: PO Box 4238
780 674-4944; Fax: 780 674-2837
E: admin@bhssa.com
W: www.bhssa.com
Executive:
Hum Res Supvr: Marilyn Badduik
Admin Supvr: Peggy Swanson

The Canadian Association of Chain Drug Stores
301-45 Sheppard Ave E, North York ON M2N 5W9
416 226-9100; Fax: 416 226-9185
E: cacds@cacds.com
W: www.cacds.com
Executive:
Dir - Membership & Trade Issues: Heather Tyrrell
Year Founded: 1995
No of Paid Staff: 10
Languages: English
Membership: 180 Associate members; 22 Traditional Drug Store Chains

The Canadian Chiropractic Association
600-30 Saint Patrick St, Toronto ON M5T 3A3
416 585-7902; Fax: 416 585-2970
Toll-free: 877 222-9303
W: www.chiropracticcanada.ca
Executive:
CEO: Alison Dantas
Dir-Ops: Marlene Paulin
Year Founded: 1953
Criteria: *Must be a chiropractor.*
Budget: $2,000,000
No of Paid Staff: 9
Speakers Available
Languages: English; French
Membership: 5,590

◈ **College of Chiropractors of Alberta**
11203 70 St NW, Edmonton AB T5B 1T1
780 420-0932; Fax: 780 425-6583
E: office@albertachiro.com
W: www.albertachiro.com
Executive:
CEO: Deb Manz
Registrar: Brian Gushaty
No of Paid Staff: 11
Speakers Available
Library: Y
Languages: English
Membership: 888

◈ **Manitoba Chiropractors' Assn**
610-1445 Portage Ave, Winnipeg MB R3G 3P4
204 942-3000; Fax: 204 942-3010
W: www.mbchiro.org
Executive:
Exec Dir: Taras Luchak
Languages: English

◈ **New Brunswick Chiropractors' Association**
206-944 Prospect St, Fredericton NB E3B 9M6
506 455-6800; Fax: 506 455-4430
W: www.nbchiropractic.ca

Executive:
Exec Dir: Mohamed El Bayoumi
Year Founded: 1958
Criteria: *Legislated by the New Brunswick Chiropractors' Act 1958 & 1997.*
No of Paid Staff: 1
Speakers Available
Languages: English; French; Arabic
Membership: 52 *(Lists available to the public)*

◈ *Ontario Chiropractic Association*
200-20 Victoria St, Toronto ON M5C 2N8
416 860-0070; Fax: 416 860-0857
Toll-free: 877 327-2273
E: oca@chiropractic.on.ca
W: www.chiropractic.on.ca
Executive:
Pres: Dr Natalia Lishchyna
VP: Dr Kristina Peterson
Media Rel/Adv: M Pacheo
Exec Dir: Dr Robert Haig
Sec-Treas: Dr Ayla Azad
Year Founded: 1929
Criteria: *Open to any person licensed by the College of Chiropractors of Ontario.*
Budget: $2,000,000
No of Paid Staff: 12
Speakers Available
Languages: English
Membership: 2,500

◈ *Association des Chiropraticiens du Québec*
7960 boul Métropolitain E, Anjou QC H1K 1A1
514 355-0557; Fax: 514 355-0070
Toll-free: 866 292-4476
E: acq@chiropratique.com
W: www.chiropratique.com
Executive:
Prés: Richard Giguère
VP: Richard Valade
Dir gén: Sylvie Des Ruisseaux
Year Founded: 1966

◈ *Québec*
7950 boul Métropolitain E, Anjou QC H1K 1A1
514 355-8540; Fax: 514 355-2290
Toll-free: 888 655-8540
E: info@ordredeschiropraticiens.qc.ca
W: www.ordredeschiropraticiens.qc.ca
Executive:
Prés: Dr Georges Lepage
Year Founded: 1974
Languages: French

◈ *Chiropractors' Association of Saskatchewan*
3420A Hill Ave, Regina SK S4S 0W9
306 585-1411; Fax: 306 585-0685
W: www.saskchiropractic.ca
Executive:
Exec Dir: Jim Stewart
Sec: Sandra England
Languages: English; French

Canadian Chiropractic Examining Board
230-1209 59 Ave SE, Calgary AB T2H 2P6
403 230-5997; Fax: 403 230-3321
E: exams@cceb.ca
W: www.cceb.ca
Executive:
CEO: Pat Frank
Year Founded: 1962
No of Paid Staff: 8
Speakers Available
Languages: English; French

Canadian Healthcare Association
100-17 York St, Ottawa ON K1N 9J6
613 241-8005; Fax: 613 241-5055
Toll-free: 855 236-0213
E: info@cha.ca
W: www.cha.ca
Executive:
I-Pres/CEO: Phil Dresch
Dir-CHA Lrng: Dale Shierbeck
Commun Spec: Teresa Neuman
Year Founded: 1931
Criteria: *Membership composed of provincial and territorial hospitals and healthcare organizations.*
No of Paid Staff: 19
Speakers Available
Languages: English
Publications
Guide to Canadian Healthcare Facilities (English, Annual)

Canadian Healthcare Technology
207-1118 Centre St, Thornhill ON L4J 7R9
905 709-2330; Fax: 905 709-2258
E: info2@canhealth.com
W: www.canhealth.com
Executive:
Pub/Editor: Jerry Zeidenberg
Office Mgr: Neil Zeidenberg

Canadian Institute for Health Information
600-495 Richmond Road, Ottawa ON K2A 4H6
613 241-7860 6432
W: www.cihi.ca
Executive:
Dir-Strategy & Operations: Francine Anne Roy

Classic Lifecare
1550-1200 73rd Ave W, Vancouver BC V6P 6G5
604 263-3621; Fax: 604 263-4139
E: info@classiclifecare.com
W: www.classiclifecare.com
Executive:
Pres: John Sherwood
Year Founded: 1974
Languages: English

College of Massage Therapists of British Columbia & License Board
Business Building
304-1212 Broadway W, Vancouver BC V6H 3V1
604 736-3404; Fax: 604 736-6500
Toll-free: 877 321-3404
E: office@cmtbc.bc.ca
W: www.cmtbc.bc.ca
Executive:
Registrar: Susan Addario
Dep Registrar: Annette Ruitenbeek
Year Founded: 1994
Criteria: *By examination.*
No of Paid Staff: 4
Languages: English
Membership: 2400+
Membership Fee: $330

DT Publishing Group Inc.
2276 Rosedene Rd, RR 1, St Anns ON L0R 1Y0
905 957-6016; Fax: 877 385-6418
E: admin@activelivingmagazine.com
W: www.play2podium.com
Executive:
Pub: Jeff Tiessen
Publications
Active Living Magazine

Healthcare Information Management & Communications Canada
12-9196 Tronson Rd, Vernon BC V1H 1E8
780 489-4521; Fax: 780 489-3290
E: healthcare@shaw.ca
W: www.healthcareimc.com
Executive:
Pub/Editor: Elaine Huesing

Healthcare Materials Management Service
188 Stronach Cres, London ON N5V 3A1
519 453-7888; Fax: 519 455-4495
W: www.hmms.on.ca
Executive:
Gen Mgr: Toby O'Hara
Controller: Pat Klein
Coord Bus Solutions: Karen Sessions

Institute for Quality Management in Healthcare (IQMH)
1500-393 University Ave, Toronto ON M5G 1E6
416 323-9540; Fax: 416 323-9324
E: info@iqmh.org
W: iqmh.org
Executive:
CEO: Greg Flynn
Proj Coord: Gertrude Welsh

Medec
1515A-740 rue Notre-Dame O, Montréal QC H3C 3X6
514 871-8096; Fax: 514 398-0902
Toll-free: 866 586-3332
E: medec@medec.org
W: www.medec.org
Executive:
VP: Diane Côte
Dir-princ commun/projets spéc: Claudia Ouellet
Year Founded: 1897
No of Paid Staff: 5
Languages: French; English

Medical Device Development Centre
Mailing: 1099 8th Ave W, Vancouver BC V6H 1C3
604 742-3808
E: info@mddc.org
W: www.mddc.org/mainpage.htm
Executive:
Chm: Geoffrey Auchinleck
Ops Mgr: Graham Wickham
Languages: English

National Eating Disorder Information Centre
Doctors Bldg
200 Elizabeth St, ES 7-421, Toronto ON M5G 2C4
416 340-4156; Fax: 416 340-4736
Toll-free: 866 633-4220
E: nedic@uhn.ca
W: www.nedic.ca
Executive:
Dir: Merryl Bear
Prog Coord: Suzanne Phillips
Year Founded: 1985
Speakers Available
Languages: English

Ontario Hospital Association
2800-200 Front St W, Toronto ON M5V 3L1
416 205-1300; Fax: 416 205-1301
Toll-free: 800 598-8002
E: info@oha.com
W: www.oha.com

HEALTHCARE ASSOCIATIONS

Executive:
Pres/CEO: Patricia Campbell
VP-Educ Servs/COO: Warren DiClemente
CFO: Douglas Miller
Chief Hum Res Officer/VP Health Hum Res Leadership: Julie Giraldi
VP-Policy/Pub Affairs: Anthony Dale
Media Mgr: A Clark
Year Founded: 1924
Budget: $25,000,000
No of Paid Staff: 84
Speakers Available
Languages: English
Membership: Assoc/Affil - 200; Full - 160
Membership Fee: Ranges from $1,000 - $3,000

Pacific Health & Development Sciences
Mailing: PO Box 44125 RPO Gorge, Victoria BC V9A 7K1
250 380-1538
E: pacificsci@shaw.ca
W: www.pacificsci.org
Executive:
Pres: Franklin White
VP: Debra Nanan
Year Founded: 2003
No of Paid Staff: 2
Speakers Available
Library: Y
Membership: 2

Psychologist Registration Committee
Mailing: Dept-Health & Social Serv
PO Box 1320 Stn Main, Yellowknife NT X1A 2L9
Fax: 867 873-0484
E: professional_licensing@gov.nt.ca
Executive:
Registrar: Samantha Van Genne

Public Health Association of British Columbia
219-2187 Oak Bay Ave, Victoria BC V8R 1G1
250 595-8422; Fax: 250 595-8622
E: admin@phabc.org
W: www.phabc.org
Executive:
Exec Dir: Michael Barnes

Pulsus Group Inc.
2902 South Sheridan Way, Floor 3, Oakville ON L6J 7L6
905 829-4770; Fax: 905 829-4799
Toll-free: 866 829-4770
E: pulsus@pulsus.com
W: www.pulsus.com
Executive:
Pub: Robert Kalina
VP: Ann Leblanc
Man Editor: Brian Vukusic
Dir-Adv Sls: Lisa Robb
Publications
Canadian Journal of Cardiology
Pain Research & Management
The Canadian Journal of Clinical Pharmacology
Canadian Respiratory Journal
The Canadian Journal of Infectious Diseases
The Canadian Journal of Plastic Surgery
The Canadian Journal of Gastroenterology

Société de Gestion Informatique SOGIQUE Inc.
150-3000 av Saint-Jean-Baptiste, Québec QC G2E 6J5
418 527-5211; Fax: 418 527-2773
W: www.sogique.qc.ca
Executive:
Dir gén adj: Paul Moreau

VON Canada - Ontario Branch - Brantford Site
204-446 Grey St, Brantford ON N3S 7L6
519 759-7750; Fax: 519 759-3924
E: aberdeen@aberdeenhealth.ca
W: www.aberdeenhealth.ca
Executive:
Dir-Clinical Serv: Deb Cockerill
Year Founded: 1907
Budget: $7,000,000
No of Paid Staff: 220
Languages: English
Membership: 350

◈Alzheimer's Respite Service
87 Culver St, Simcoe ON N3Y 2V5
519 426-8111; Fax: 519 426-2474
E: aberdeen@aberdeenhealth.ca
W: www.aberdeenhealth.ca
Executive:
Dir Clinical Srv: Deb Cockerill

◈Home Support Services
87 Culver St, Simcoe ON N3Y 2V5
519 426-8111; Fax: 519 426-2474
W: www.von.ca
Executive:
Dist Exec Dir: Irene Pasel
Year Founded: 1907
No of Paid Staff: 200

Valley Integration to Active Living Society
156D Government St, Duncan BC V9L 1A2
250 748-5899; Fax: 250 748-5877
W: www.vitals.ca
Executive:
Asst Exec Dir: Angela Milligan
Year Founded: 1991
No of Paid Staff: 55

Vancouver Coastal Health - Home Care Services
Location: 5630 Inlet Ave, Sechelt BC V0N 3A0
Mailing: PO Box 2420
604 741-0726; Fax: 604 741-0728
W: www.vch.ca
Speakers Available
Languages: English

HOLISTIC HEALTH

Acupuncture Foundation of Canada Institute
204-2131 Lawrence Ave E, Scarborough ON M1R 5G4
416 752-3988; Fax: 416 752-4398
E: afciweb@afcinstitute.com
W: www.afcinstitute.com
Executive:
Pres: Mac Mierzejewski
Dir: Marjorie Hammond
Year Founded: 1995
Criteria: *Physicians, dentists, physiotherapists, chiropractors, baccalaureate RNs, naturopaths, licensed acupuncturists*
No of Paid Staff: 2
Languages: English
Membership: 1,400
Membership Fee: $195 + taxes

British Columbia Chiropractic Association
125-3751 Shell Rd, Richmond BC V6X 2W2
604 270-1332; Fax: 604 278-0093
E: dnixdorf@allstream.net
W: www.bcchiro.com
Executive:
Exec Dir: Dr Don Nixdorf
Speakers Available
Membership: 900 *(Lists available to the public)*

British Columbia Naturopathic Association
2238 Pine St, Vancouver BC V6J 5G4
604 736-6646; Fax: 604 736-6048
E: bcna@bcna.ca
W: www.bcna.ca
Executive:
Exec Dir: Glenn Cassie
No of Paid Staff: 2
Speakers Available
Languages: English
Membership list available to the public
Membership Fee: $25/yr

Canadian Academy of Homeopathy Inc.
1173 boul Mont-Royal, Outremont QC H2V 2H6
514 279-6629; Fax: 514 279-0111
E: cah@videotron.ca
W: www.homeopathy.ca
Executive:
Doyen/Docteur de Homéopathique: Dr André Saine
Chef bur: Francine Gauthier
Languages: English

Canadian Federation of Aromatherapists
110 Thorndale Pl, Waterloo ON N2L 5Y8
519 746-1594; Fax: 519 746-9493
E: manager@cfacanada.com
W: www.cfacanada.com
Executive:
Pres: Tricia Eagle
Office Mgr: Patricia Dimeck
Year Founded: 1993
No of Paid Staff: 1
Languages: English
Membership: 325 *(Lists available to the public)*

Canadian Memorial Chiropractic College
6100 Leslie St, Toronto ON M2H 3J1
416 482-2340; Fax: 416 646-1114
Toll-free: 800 463-2923
E: communications@cmcc.ca
W: www.cmcc.ca
Executive:
Pres: Dr Jean Moss
Year Founded: 1945
Languages: English

Canadian Reiki Association
Location: 7155 Kingsway, Burnaby BC V5E 4J6
Mailing: PO Box 54570 RPO Highgate
604 669-9049; Fax: 866 734-4540
Toll-free: 866 835-7525
E: reiki@reiki.ca
W: www.reiki.ca
Executive:
Pres: Bonnie Smith
VP: Barb Weston
Dir: Carell Mehl
A-Dir: Virginia Smith
Dir: Louise Vigneault
Year Founded: 1996
Speakers Available
Languages: English; French
Membership: 650 *(Lists available to the public)*

The Chi Kung Association of Canada
545 St Clair Ave W, Toronto ON M6C 1A3
416 653-4105; Fax: 416 653-4105
Executive:
Pres: Dr Chu Chow
Languages: English

The Chinese Medicine and Acupuncture Association of Canada
154 Wellington St, London ON N6B 2K8
519 642-1970; Fax: 519 642-2932
E: cmaac@execulink.com
W: www.cmaac.ca
Executive:
Mgr: Hsi Ping Lin
Year Founded: 1983
Languages: English

Homeopathic Medical Council of Canada
Mailing: PO Box 605 Stn Adelaide, Toronto ON M5C 2J8
416 788-4622
E: ontario@hmcc.ca
W: www.hmcc.ca
Languages: English

International Academy of Natural Health Sciences
380 Forest St, Ottawa ON K2B 8E6
613 820-0318; Fax: 613 820-7478
Toll-free: 800 267-8732
E: info@intlacademy.com
W: www.intlacademy.com
Executive:
Prog Coord: Gregory Scott
Exec Dir: Dorothy Marshall
Year Founded: 1980
Languages: English

Iridologists' Association of Canada
Mailing: PO Box 421 Stn D, Etobicoke ON M9A 4X4
416 233-9837; Fax: 905 824-0063
W: www.professionaliridology.com
Executive:
Chm: Agota Csekey
Year Founded: 1994
Speakers Available
Languages: English

Nova Scotia College of Chiropractors
Location: 700-6009 Quinpool Rd, Halifax NS B3K 5J7
Mailing: PO Box 9410 Stn A, Halifax NS B3K 5S3
902 407-4255; Fax: 902 425-2441
E: inquiries@chiropractors.ns.ca
W: www.chiropractors.ns.ca
Executive:
V-Chair: Dr Janis Noseworthy
Pres: Dr Ward MacDonald
VP: Dr Lisa VanZoost
Exec Dir: John K Sutherland
Treas: Dr Brad Lohrenz
Languages: English; French

Ontario Association of Naturopathic Doctors
603-789 Don Mills Rd, North York ON M3C 1T5
416 233-2001; Fax: 416 233-2924
Toll-free: 877 628-7284
E: info@oand.org
W: www.oand.org
Executive:
I-CEO/Dir-Policy: Michael Heitshu
Dir-Mktg: Ronda Parkes
Year Founded: 1950
Criteria: *Licensed naturopathic doctors practising in Ontario.*
Budget: $750,000
No of Paid Staff: 8
Speakers Available
Languages: English
Membership: 425

Ontario Herbalists' Association (OHA)
Mailing: PO Box 123 Stn D, Etobicoke ON M9A 4X1
416 236-0090
Toll-free: 877 642-4372
E: info@herbalists.on.ca
W: www.herbalists.on.ca
Executive:
Pres: Diane Kent
VP: Rick De Sylva
Sec-Treas/Office Mgr: Joanne Watson
Media Contact: Kathleen Leeson
Year Founded: 1982
Languages: English

Ontario Kinesiology Association (OKA)
6519B Mississauga Rd, Mississauga ON L5N 1A6
905 567-7194; Fax: 905 567-7191
E: info@oka.on.ca
W: www.oka.on.ca
Executive:
Pres: Sabrina Francescut
Pres Elect: Jennifer Chapman
Dir-Mktg/Pub Rel: Scott Tate
Dir-Educ: Paul Schuster
Exec Dir: Stuart Moulton
Dir Gov Rel: Janice Ray
Dir Fundraising/SponsorshipSpec Proj: Karen Quan
Sec-Treas: Andrew Zbyrko
Office Mgr: Leslie Wright
Criteria: *Certified members are bound by Professional Standards and Ethics policies and accountable to Professional Disciplinary Hearings and Appeals proceedings. Continuing professional development and education is encouraged with a mandatory Continuing Education Standards Program.*
No of Paid Staff: 2
Speakers Available
Languages: English
Membership: 1,500
Membership Fee: $225

World Natural Medicine Foundation
9904 106 St NW, Edmonton AB T5K 1C4
780 424-2231; Fax: 780 424-8520
Toll-free: 800 815-1116
E: draung@aung.com
W: www.aung.com
Executive:
Pres: Dr Steven Aung
Year Founded: 1994
No of Paid Staff: 10
Speakers Available
Languages: English

LEARNING DISABILITIES

Cosmopolitan Industries Ltd.
28 34th St E, Saskatoon SK S7K 3Y2
306 664-3158; Fax: 306 244-5509
E: info@cosmoindustries.com
W: www.cosmoindustries.com
Executive:
Exec Dir: Peter Gerrard
Year Founded: 1971
No of Paid Staff: 130

Learning Disabilities Association of British Columbia - Fraser South Chapter
201-13766 72 Ave, Surrey BC V3W 2P4
604 591-5156; Fax: 604 591-1669
E: info@ldafs.org
W: www.ldafs.org
Executive:
Pres: Steven Sapinsky
Resource Coord: Tania Wittal
Commun Initiatives: Vicki Nelson
Year Founded: 1977
Criteria: *Open to anyone who would benefit from membership.*
No of Paid Staff: 3
Speakers Available
Languages: English
Membership: 150 *(Lists available to the public)*
Membership Fee: $30

Learning Disabilities Association of Canada
616-250 City Centre Ave, Ottawa ON K1R 6K7
613 238-5721; Fax: 613 235-5391
Toll-free: 877 238-5332 National office only
E: info@ldac-acta.ca
W: www.ldac-acta.ca
Executive:
CEO: Judy Kerr
Dir-Public Policy/Prog: Claudette Larocque
Year Founded: 1963
No of Paid Staff: 3
Languages: English; French
Membership: 8,500 to 10,000
Membership Fee: Varies

◈Alberta:
Mailing: PO Box 29011 RPO Lendrum, Edmonton AB T6H 5Z6
780 462-9497
E: info@ldalberta.ca
W: www.ldalberta.ca
Executive:
Exec Dir: Kathryn Burke
Commun Dir: Dina Hendzel
Languages: English

◇Edmonton Chapter:
St. Gabriel's School
5540 106 Ave NW, Edmonton AB T6A 1G3
780 466-1011; Fax: 780 466-1095
E: ldaec@nucleus.com
W: www.ldaa.ca
Year Founded: 1967
Membership: 120

◇Calgary Chapter:
340-105 12 Ave SE, Calgary AB T2G 1A1
403 283-6606; Fax: 403 270-4043
Toll-free: 866 408-5322
E: info@ldaa.net
W: www.ldaa.net
Executive:
Prog Coord: Colleen Wall
Exec Dir: Marty Hornstein
Year Founded: 1974
Criteria: *Adults 18 years of age or over and Families, schools.*
Budget: $800,000
No of Paid Staff: 5
Speakers Available
Library: Y *(Open to the public)*
Languages: English
Membership: 300 *(Lists available to the public)*
Membership Fee: Individual - $35 per year; Corporate - $120; Schools - $75; Students - $20

◇Red Deer Chapter:
Lower Level
3757 43 Ave, Red Deer AB T4N 3B7
403 340-3885; Fax: 403 340-3884
E: execdir@ldreddeer.ca
W: www.ldreddeer.ca
Executive:
Pres/Chair: Janet de Laforest
Budget: $250,000
No of Paid Staff: 7

Speakers Available
Library: Y *(Open to the public)*
Languages: English
Membership: 45

◈ Vancouver Chapter:
3292 Broadway E, Vancouver BC V5M 1Z8
604 873-8139; Fax: 604 873-8140
E: info@ldav.ca
W: www.ldav.ca
Executive:
Exec Dir: Susan Keyes
Info/Support Coord: Nicole Makortoff
Program Coord: Victoria Walters
Comm Invest/Commun Coord: Diana Squires
Year Founded: 1970
Budget: $223,000
No of Paid Staff: 4
Speakers Available
Library: Y
Languages: English
Membership: 200
Membership Fee: $35/year

◇ Vancouver Chapter
1562 Fort St, Victoria BC V8S 5J2
250 370-9513; Fax: 250 370-9421
E: info@ldasvi.bc.ca
W: www.ldasvi.bc.ca
Year Founded: 1981
No of Paid Staff: 2
Speakers Available
Library: Y *(Open to the public)*
Languages: English
Membership: 165
Membership Fee: $40/year

◈ Manitoba:
617 Erin St, Winnipeg MB R3G 2W1
204 774-1821; Fax: 204 788-4090
E: ldamb@mts.net
W: www.ldamanitoba.org
Executive:
Exec Dir: Marilyn Mackinnon
Year Founded: 1966
Budget: $100,000
No of Paid Staff: 3
Speakers Available
Library: Y
Languages: English
Membership: 250
Membership Fee: $15-$25
Library:
Learning Disabilities Association of Manitoba *(Open to the public)*

◇ Brandon & District Office
Location: 129B 12th St, Brandon MB R7A 4L8
Mailing: PO Box 22146 RPO Downtown, Brandon MB R7A 6Y9
204 727-4669
E: ldambdn@mts.net
W: www.ldambrandon.org
Executive:
Pres: Michelle Poole
V-Prin: Peggy Fortier
Admv Off: Edy Clayton

◈ New Brunswick:
203-403 Regent St, Fredericton NB E3B 3X6
506 459-7852; Fax: 506 455-9300
Toll-free: 877 544-7852 within NB
E: ldanb_taanb@nb.aibn.com
W: www.ldanb-taanb.ca
Executive:
Pres: Mary Jones
VP-Admn: Fabienne McKay
Exec Dir: André Deschênes
Treas: Sylvianne Caron
Sec: Kailha Winter
Admin: Nila Christensen
VP-Funding: Shelley Clayton
VP-Programs: Rhonda Rubin
Year Founded: 1970
Budget: $180,000
No of Paid Staff: 1
Speakers Available
Library: Y
Languages: English; French
Membership list available to the public
Membership Fee: $25/year
Library:
Resource Centre

◈ Newfoundland and Labrador:
301-66 Kenmount Rd, St. John's NL A1B 3V7
709 753-1445; Fax: 709 753-4747
E: info@ldanl.org
W: www.nald.ca/ldanl/
Year Founded: 2001
No of Paid Staff: 3
Speakers Available
Library: Y
Languages: English
Membership Fee: $25

◈ Northwest Territories:
Mailing: PO Box 242 Stn Main, Yellowknife NT X1A 2N2
867 873-6378; Fax: 867 873-6378
W: www.ldac-acta.ca
Year Founded: 1981
Criteria: *People 16 years of age or older.*
Languages: English
Membership: 25
Membership Fee: $20

◈ Nova Scotia:
2 Dartmouth Rd, Floor 3, Bedford NS B4A 2K7
902 423-2850; Fax: 902 423-2834
Toll-free: 877 238-5322
E: info@ldans.ca
W: www.ldans.ca
Executive:
Exec Dir: Marilyn O'Neil
Year Founded: 1989
Budget: $70,000
No of Paid Staff: 4
Speakers Available
Library: Y *(Open to the public)*
Languages: English
Membership: 500
Membership Fee: Ranges from $25 - $45/year

◈ Ontario:
202-365 Evans Ave, Toronto ON M8Z 1K2
416 929-4311; Fax: 416 929-3905
W: www.ldao.ca
Executive:
Pres/CEO: Lawrence Barns
Sr Mgr-Pub Policy/Educ: Diane Wagner
Year Founded: 1963
No of Paid Staff: 10
Speakers Available
Library: Y *(Open to the public)*
Languages: English
Membership: 3,000
Membership Fee: $50
Library:
LDAO Library *(Open to the public)*

◇ Kitchener-Waterloo Chapter:
Location: 171 Frederick St, Kitchener ON N2H 2M6
Mailing: PO Box 23002 RPO Frederick, Kitchener ON N2B 3V1
519 743-9091; Fax: 519 743-9027
E: ldakw@golden.net
W: www.ldakw.on.ca
Executive:
Exec Dir: Annette Zegers
Year Founded: 1966
No of Paid Staff: 1
Library: Y *(Open to the public)*
Languages: English
Membership: 50
Membership Fee: $50 per year

◇ LDA of Toronto - Resource Centre
203-121 Willowdale Ave, Toronto ON M2N 6A3
416 229-1680; Fax: 416 229-1681
W: www.ldatd.on.ca
Executive:
Exec Dir: Mimi Hoffman
Languages: English; French

◇ London Region:
101-333 Horton St E, London ON N6B 1L5
519 438-6213; Fax: 519 438-0368
E: ldainfo@ldalondon.ca
W: www.ldalondon.ca
Executive:
Resource Cons: Jennifer Paterson
Year Founded: 1967
Criteria: *Open to all.*
No of Paid Staff: 4
Speakers Available
Library: Y *(Open to the public)*
Languages: English
Membership: 50
Membership Fee: $50

◇ Mississauga:
800-165 Dundas St W, Mississauga ON L5B 2N6
905 272-4100; Fax: 905 272-4863
E: lda1@bellnet.ca
W: www.ldanp.ca
Executive:
Exec Dir: Carla Warwick
Year Founded: 1986
No of Paid Staff: 5
Speakers Available
Library: Y
Languages: English
Membership: 193
Membership Fee: $50
Library:
Charles Fournier *(Open to the public)*

◇ Ottawa-Carleton Resource Centre Library
160 Percy St, Room 2, Ottawa ON K1R 6E5
613 567-5864
E: resources@ldaottawa.com
W: www.ldaottawa.com

◈ Prince Edward Island:
Location: 40 Enman Cres, Charlottetown PE C1E 1E6
Mailing: PO Box 400 Stn Central, Charlottetown PE C1A 7K7
902 894-5032
E: info@ldapei.ca
W: www.ldapei.ca/
Executive:
Exec Dir: Nills Ling
Languages: English

◈ Yukon:
107 Main St, Whitehorse YT Y1A 2A7
867 668-5167; Fax: 867 668-6504
E: ldayoffice@northwestel.net
W: www.ldayukon.com

Executive:
Exec Dir: Stephanie Hammond
Year Founded: 1973
Speakers Available
Library: Y *(Open to the public)*
Languages: English
Membership: 140
Membership Fee: $10
Library:
Laurie Briggs Library *(Open to the public)*

Learning Disabilities Association of North Peel - Div. of Learning Disabilities Association of Ontario
150 Central Park Dr, Suite 104, Brampton ON L6T 2T9
905 791-4100; Fax: 905 791-5189
E: info@ldanp.ca
W: www.ldanp.ca
Executive:
Exec Dir: Carla Warwick
Languages: English; French

Learning Disabilities Association of York Region
221-11181 Yonge St, Richmond Hill ON L4S 1L2
905 884-7933; Fax: 905 770-9377
E: info@ldayr.org
W: www.ldayr.org

Society for the Education of Children with Specific Learning Disabilities
420 Seymour River Pl, North Vancouver BC V7H 1S8
604 985-5224; Fax: 604 985-4562
E: kgsprincipal@shaw.ca
W: www.kgms.ca
Executive:
Principal: John Wilson
V-Prin: Rosita Tam
Year Founded: 1973
Budget: $1,400,000
No of Paid Staff: 33
Speakers Available
Library: Y
Languages: English
Membership: 85 Families; 33 Staff

MEDICAL & HEALTH (1) —Education & Research

AMREF - African Medical & Research Foundation
407-489 College St, Toronto ON M6G 1A5
416 961-6981; Fax: 416 961-6984
Toll-free: 888 318-4442
E: info@amrefcanada.org
W: www.amrefcanada.org
Executive:
Dir-Programmes: Todd Carmichael
Dir-Fundraising/Mktg: Rachel Lancaster
Exec Dir: Anne-Marie Kamanye
Dir-Commun: Jennifer Foulds
Year Founded: 1973
No of Paid Staff: 6
Speakers Available
Languages: English; French
Membership list available to the public

Alberta Diabetes Foundation
University of Alberta
1-020 Li Ka Shing Centre, Edmonton AB T6G 2E1
780 492-6537; Fax: 780 492-6046
Toll-free: 800 563-2450
E: info@afdr.ab.ca
W: www.afdr.ab.ca
Year Founded: 1988
No of Paid Staff: 3
Languages: English

Alberta Innovates Health Solutions
1500-10104 103 Ave NW, Edmonton AB T5J 4A7
780 423-5727; Fax: 780 429-3509
E: health@albertainnovates.ca
W: www.albertainnovates.ca
Executive:
Pres: Jacques Magnan
CEO: Dr Cyril Frank
COO: Pamela Valentine
VP-Corp Aff: Joseph Gebran
Research Lib: Liza Chan
Advisor: Ivan Pylypow
Dir-Commun: Kathleen Thurber
Year Founded: 1980
Budget: $5,000,000
No of Paid Staff: 35
Speakers Available
Library: Y
Languages: English
Library:
Research Library

The Association of Faculties of Medicine of Canada
800-265 Carling Ave, Ottawa ON K1S 2E1
613 730-0687; Fax: 613 730-1196
E: nbusing@afmc.ca
W: www.afmc.ca
Executive:
Pres/CEO: Dr Nick Busing
Year Founded: 1943
Criteria: *Open to accredited Canadian Faculties of Medicine*
No of Paid Staff: 23
Languages: English; French
Membership: 17 *(Lists available to the public)*
Membership Fee: Fixed fee and a capitation fee based on first time enrollment.

The Banting Research Foundation
Banting Institute
10-6 Queen's Park Cres W, Toronto ON M5S 3H2
416 595-9046
E: banting.foundation@utoronto.ca
W: www.utoronto.ca/bantresf
Executive:
Chair/Brd of Trustees: Dr John Floras
Year Founded: 1925
Languages: English

British Columbia Surgical Society
115-1665 Broadway W, Vancouver BC V6J 5A4
604 638-2843; Fax: 604 638-2938
E: dwong@bcma.bc.ca
W: www.bcss.ca
Executive:
Coord: Diane Wong
Criteria: *Open to all certified surgeons of the Royal College of Physicians and Surgeons of Canada or Diplomats of the American Board of Surgery.*
Languages: English
Membership: 200

Canadian Academy of Sport and Exercise Medicine
1400-180 Elgin St, Ottawa ON K2P 2K3
613 748-5851; Fax: 613 231-3739
Toll-free: 877 585-2394
E: admin@casem-acmse.org
W: www.casem-acmse.org
Executive:
Exec Dir: Dawn Haworth
Year Founded: 1970
Criteria: *Must be either a medical doctor, post-graduate medical trainee or medical student.*
No of Paid Staff: 2
Languages: English; French
Membership: 700

Canadian Advanced Medical Service International
4531 Emily Carr Dr, Victoria BC V8X 2N5
250 881-3622; Fax: 250 479-3569
E: info@camsi.org
W: www.camsi.org
Executive:
Exec Dir: Steve Kenny
Year Founded: 1995
Speakers Available
Languages: English

Canadian Association for the Study of the Liver
307-10328 81 Ave NW, Edmonton AB T6E 1X2
780 436-0983 233; Fax: 780 437-5984
E: casl@hepatology.ca
W: www.hepatology.ca
Executive:
Pres: Dr Marc Deschênes
Sec-Treas: Dr Kevork Peltekian
Languages: English; French

Canadian Association of Gastroenterology
224-1540 Cornwall Rd, Oakville ON L6J 7W5
905 829-2504; Fax: 905 829-0242
Toll-free: 888 780-0007
E: general@cag-acg.org
W: www.cag-acg.org
Executive:
Sr Mgr: Sandra Daniels
Exec Dir: Paul Sinclair
Office Admin: Palma Colacino
Year Founded: 1962
Languages: English

Canadian Association of Nuclear Medicine
774 Echo Dr, Ottawa ON K1S 5N8
613 730-6254; Fax: 613 730-1116
E: canm@royalcollege.ca
W: www.canm-acmn.ca
Executive:
Pres: Dr Norman Laurin
Exec Dir: Hélène Samson
Year Founded: 1977
No of Paid Staff: 2
Speakers Available
Languages: English; French
Membership: 100

Canadian Cardiovascular Society
1403-222 Queen St, Ottawa ON K1P 5V9
613 569-3407; Fax: 613 569-6574
Toll-free: 877 569-3407
E: info@ccs.ca
W: www.ccs.ca

HEALTHCARE ASSOCIATIONS

Executive:
CEO: Anne E Ferguson
Dir-Ext Rel: Nick Neuheimer
Dir Knowledge Trans: Susan Oliver
Dir-Membership Serv: Linda Palmer
Year Founded: 1947
No of Paid Staff: 18
Speakers Available
Library: Y
Languages: English; French
Membership: 1,700

Canadian Fertility and Andrology Society
1107-1255 rue University, Montréal QC H3B 3W7
514 524-9009; Fax: 514 524-2163
E: info@cfas.ca
W: www.cfas.ca
Executive:
Dir exéc par intérim: Christian Orfali
Year Founded: 1954
Criteria: *Cotisation annuelle et approbation du C.A.*
Budget: $500,000
No of Paid Staff: 2
Speakers Available
Languages: French; English
Membership: 550
Membership Fee: $100

Canadian Fitness and Lifestyle Research Institute
201-185 Somerset St W, Ottawa ON K2P 0J2
613 233-5528; Fax: 613 233-5536
E: info@cflri.ca
W: www.cflri.ca
Year Founded: 1980
Budget: $500,000
No of Paid Staff: 8
Speakers Available
Languages: English
Membership list available to the public

Canadian Foundation for AIDS Research
710-165 University Ave, Toronto ON M5H 3B8
416 361-6281; Fax: 416 361-5736
Toll-free: 800 563-2873
W: www.canfar.com/
Executive:
Pres: Christopher Bunting
Office Mgr: Lynne Butler
Year Founded: 1988
Budget: $2,000,000
No of Paid Staff: 7
Speakers Available
Languages: English

Canadian Foundation for Healthcare Improvement
700-1565 Carling Ave, Ottawa ON K1Z 8R1
613 728-2238; Fax: 613 728-3527
E: beth.everson@chsrf.ca
W: www.chsrf.ca
Executive:
Commun Coord: Véronique Leduc
Year Founded: 1997
Criteria: *Eligibility Criteria: i) individuals who make significant contributions to the endowment. ii) organizations (represented by their leaders) which have either made significant contributions to the endowment or which are associated with significant contributions to the endowment. iii) organizations (represented by their leaders) which have made a contractual commitment for at least ten years of significant contributions to the costs of ongoing Foundation programs.*
Budget: $9,110,000
No of Paid Staff: 20
Languages: English; French

Canadian Foundation for the Study of Infant Deaths
403-60 James St, St Catharines ON L2R 7E7
905 688-8884; Fax: 905 688-3300
Toll-free: 800 363-7437
E: sidsinfo@sidscanada.org
W: www.sidscanada.org
Executive:
Exec Dir: Jamie King
Year Founded: 1973
No of Paid Staff: 2

Canadian Foundation for Trauma Research & Education, Inc.
207-346 Lawrence Ave, Kelowna BC V1Y 6L4
250 860-8860; Fax: 604 694-0086
Toll-free: 888 960-8860
E: info@cftre.com
W: www.cftre.com
Executive:
Clinical Psychologist: Dr Lynne Zettl
Languages: English

Canadian Institute for the Relief of Pain and Disability
204-916 Broadway W, Vancouver BC V5Z 1K7
604 684-4148; Fax: 604 684-6247
Toll-free: 800 872-3105
E: admin@cirpd.org
W: www.cirpd.org
Executive:
Exec Dir: Dr Marc White
Prog Mgr: Tonya Hide
Year Founded: 1985
No of Paid Staff: 2
Speakers Available
Library: Y *(Open to the public)*
Languages: English
Membership: 350

Canadian Network of Toxicology Centres
Location: Bovey Bldg 80, Gordon St, Floor 2, Guelph ON N1G 2W1
Mailing: 50 Stone Rd E, University of Guelph
519 824-4120 58918
E: lritter@uoguelph.ca
W: www.uoguelph.ca/cntc/
Executive:
Exec Dir: Dr Len Ritter
Languages: English

Canadian Neurological Sciences Federation
709-7015 MacLeod Trail SW, Calgary AB T2H 2K6
403 229-9544; Fax: 403 229-1661
E: info@cnsfederation.org
W: www.cnsfederation.org
Executive:
Pres: Derek Fewer
CEO: Dan Morin
Membership Fee Required: Y
No of Paid Staff: 7
Languages: English
Membership: 4 Societies - total membership 1,100
Membership Fee: Varies

Canadian Post-M.D. Education Registry - The Caper Annual Census of Post-M.D. Trainees
800-265 Carling Ave, Ottawa ON K1S 2E1
613 730-1204; Fax: 613 730-1196
W: www.caper.ca
Executive:
Dir: Steve Slade
Year Founded: 1986
No of Paid Staff: 3
Speakers Available
Languages: English
Publications
Caper Annual Census of post-M.D. Trainees (English, Annual)

Canadian Society for Clinical Investigation
114 Cheyenne Way, Ottawa ON K2J 0E9
877 968-9449; Fax: 613 491-0073
E: info@csci-scrc.ca
W: www.csci-scrc.ca
Executive:
Pres: Dr Brent W Winston
Sec-Treas: Dr Bing Siang Gan
Year Founded: 1951
Criteria: *General Membership: The application should indicate clearly that the applicant is making a significant contribution to research. Authorship of at least 3 publications in a journal with an editorial review process is the usual evidence required. The applicant should clearly indicate what his/her specific contribution has been to work reported in these publications. Other critieria which may be considered in the evaluation will be the award of an operating grant, the award of a career development grant, and the authority to supervise graduate students. Associate Membership: Any person who holds a doctoral level degree (M.D., Ph.D.) and is still in training is eligible. Applicants for this category will normally be pursuing careers in medical research. The application for membership in this category must be supported in writing by a regular member of the CSCI.*
Speakers Available
Languages: English; French
Membership: 440
Membership Fee: $5,000 - Corporate; Ranges from $45 - $145 - Individual

Canadian Society for Transfusion Medicine
774 Echo Dr, Ottawa ON K1S 5N8
613 260-6198; Fax: 613 730-1116
Toll-free: 800 668-3740
E: cstm@royalcollege.ca
W: www.transfusion.ca
Executive:
Pres: Debbie Lauzon
VP: Gwen Clark
Eastern Dir: Anne Marie Robinson
Central Dir: Ann Wilson
Western Dir: Julia Hendry
Mgr: Christiane Dowsing
Sec-Treas: Wendy Owens
Year Founded: 1978
Criteria: *Membership should be individual. There shall be no limit to the number of individual members. However, an institution may be considered for membership. Anyone professionallly involved in Transfusion Medicine may submit a completed application form to the Treasurer. The Board of Directors shall, if necessary, make decisions on individual cases, and these decisions shall be final. The Treasurer shall inform the applicant whether the application has been accepted or rejected. It is the privilege of any individual member to recommend to the Board of Directors persons who have rendered distinguished service to the Society or in Transfusion Medicine for Honourary Membership. This must be done at least sixty (60) days before the next meeting of the Board of Directors. To be successful, such nominations shall require the unanimous approval of the Board of Directors.*
Languages: English; French
Membership: approx 500
Membership Fee: International Individual: US$60; International: US$300; Institutional Membership Application: CDN$300; Individual Canadian Resident: CDN$90

The Canadian Society of Allergy and Clinical Immunology (CSACI)
Mailing: PO Box RPO Bilberry Villge, Orleans ON K1E 3W4
613 986-5869; Fax: 613 839-7501
E: info@csaci.ca
W: www.csaci.ca
Executive:
Pres: Dr Paul Keith
VP: Dr Sandy Kapur
Exec Dir: Louise Tremblay
Sec-Treas: Dr David Fischer
Year Founded: 1945
Criteria: *See website*
Membership Fee Required: Y
No of Paid Staff: 2
Languages: English; French
Membership: 450
Membership Fee: $100

Canadian Society of Endocrinology and Metabolism
774 Echo Dr, Ottawa ON K1S 5N8
613 730-6224; Fax: 613 730-1116
E: csem@royalcollege.ca
W: www.endo-metab.ca
Executive:
Pres Elect: Dr Stephanie Kaiser
Pres: Dr Lawrence Leiter
Past Pres: Dr Cherri Deal
Assoc Mgr: Christiane Dowsing
Sec-Treas: Dr Jean-Patrice Baillargeon
Languages: English
Membership: 300

Canadian Spinal Research Organization
2-120 Newkirk Rd, Richmond Hill ON L4C 9S7
905 508-4000; Fax: 905 508-4002
Toll-free: 800 361-4004
E: info@csro.com
W: www.csro.com
Executive:
Chairman: Barry Munro
Year Founded: 1984
No of Paid Staff: 7
Speakers Available
Languages: English

Canadian Thoracic Society
c/o Lung Association,National Office
300-1750 Courtwood Cres, Ottawa ON K2C 2B5
613 569-6411 270; Fax: 613 569-8860
E: ctsinfo@lung.ca
W: www.lung.ca/cts
Executive:
Pres: Dr Robin McFadden
Pres Elect: Dr Mark FitzGerald
Dir: Janet Sutherland
Mgr-Commun/Membership: Suzanne Desmarais
Treas: Dr Jean Bourbeau
Sec: Dr Diane Lougheed
Admn Coord: Chantal Bégin-Ghanem
Year Founded: 1958
Criteria: *Specialists in respiratory diseases as well as other physicians, surgeons, medical practitioners and scientists.*
No of Paid Staff: 3
Languages: English; French
Membership: 526
Membership Fee: $50

Cancer Research Society
402-625 av du Président-Kennedy, Montréal QC H3A 3S5
514 861-9227; Fax: 514 861-9220
Toll-free: 866 343-2262
E: info@src-crs.ca
W: www.CancerResearchSociety.ca
Executive:
Prés: Domenic Pilla
Dir exéc: Andy Chabot
Dir exéc adj: Nathalie Giroux
Dir admin/fin: Alain Laurendeau
Dir rég Ottawa: Trista Lynch-Black
Year Founded: 1945
Budget: $17,000,000
No of Paid Staff: 22
Speakers Available
Languages: French

College and Association of Respiratory Therapists of Alberta (CARTA)
370-6715 8 St NE, Calgary AB T2E 7H7
403 274-1828; Fax: 403 274-9703
Toll-free: 800 205-2778
W: www.carta.ca
Executive:
Exec Dir: Bryan Buell
Languages: English

Community and Hospital Infection Control Association Canada
Location: Membership Services Office, Winnipeg MB R3R 3S3
Mailing: PO Box 46125 RPO Westdale
204 897-5990; Fax: 204 895-9595
Toll-free: 866 999-7111
E: chicacanada@mts.net
W: www.chica.org
Executive:
Admin: Gerry Hansen
Year Founded: 1976
Criteria: *Open to any person occupationally interested in infection prevention and control in health care settings.*
No of Paid Staff: 2
Speakers Available
Languages: English; French
Membership: 1,700
Membership Fee: $100

Fondation BMP
950 rue Principale, Cowansville QC J2K 1K3
450 266-5548; Fax: 450 266-5040
E: info@fondationbmp.ca
W: www.fondationbmp.ca
Executive:
Trés: Mario Lagimonière

Foundation of Stars
317-300 rue de la Berge-du-Canal, Lachine QC H8R 1H3
514 595-5730; Fax: 514 595-5745
Toll-free: 800 665-2358
E: info@fondationdesetoiles.ca
W: www.fondationdesetoiles.ca
Executive:
PDG: Josée Saint-Pierre
Year Founded: 1977
Budget: $5,500,000
No of Paid Staff: 14
Languages: French
Membership: 5,000

Fragile X Research Foundation of Canada
167 Queen St W, Brampton ON L6Y 1M5
905 453-9366; Fax: 905 453-0095
E: info@fragilexcanada.ca
W: www.fragilexcanada.ca
Executive:
Pres/Med Dir: Dr Carlo Paribello
VP-Mktg: Lori Beesley
Treas: Lawrence Spero
Languages: English

Genesis Research Foundation
92 College St, Toronto ON M5G 1L4
416 978-2667; Fax: 416 978-8350
E: info@genesisresearch.org
W: www.genesisresearch.org
Executive:
Chair: Dr Alan Bocking
Vice Chair: Dr Jennifer Blake
Med Dir Research: Dr Stephen Lye
Year Founded: 1983
No of Paid Staff: 2
Speakers Available
Languages: English

JDRF Canada
800-2550 Victoria Park Ave, North York ON M2J 5A9
647 789-2000; Fax: 416 491-2111
Toll-free: 877 287-3533
E: general@jdrf.ca
W: www.jdrf.ca
Executive:
Pres/CEO: Andrew McKee
Exec Admin to Pres: Ruby Archer
Year Founded: 1974
Speakers Available
Languages: English; French

◈ Northern Alberta Region:
First Edmonton Place
17321 108 Ave NW, Edmonton AB T5S 1G2
780 428-0343; Fax: 780 428-0348
E: edmonton@jdrf.ca
W: www.jdrf.ca/chapters/edmonton
Executive:
Reg Mgr-N Central/NWT: Barbara J Armstrong
Fundraising Coord: Karen Zabinski
Year Founded: 1984
No of Paid Staff: 2
Languages: English
Membership: 600

◈ Vancouver:
150-6450 Roberts St, Burnaby BC V5G 4E1
604 320-1937; Fax: 604 320-1938
E: vancouver@jdrf.ca
W: www.jdrf.ca
Executive:
Reg Mgr: Chris Lowe
Year Founded: 1974
No of Paid Staff: 7
Speakers Available
Languages: English

◈ The Prairies:
1101-191 Lombard Ave, Winnipeg MB R3B 0X1
204 953-4477; Fax: 204 953-4470
E: winnipeg@jdrf.ca
W: www.jdrf.ca
Executive:
Reg Mgr Prairie Reg: Dorothy Ross
Year Founded: 1974
No of Paid Staff: 3
Speakers Available
Languages: English; French
Membership: 500

◈ ***Halifax***
Bedford Place Mall
2055-1658 Bedford Hwy, Bedford NS B4A 2X9
902 453-1009; Fax: 902 453-2528
Toll-free: 888 439-5373
E: halifax@jdrf.ca

◈ ***Kitchener***
103-684 Belmont Ave W, Kitchener ON N2M 1N6
519 745-2426; Fax: 519 745-2626
E: waterloo@jdrf.ca
W: www.jdrf.ca
Executive:
Dev Coor: Lisa Milligan

◈ ***Nepean:***
206-1600 Merivale Rd, Nepean ON K2G 5J8
613 244-4818; Fax: 613 244-4822
Toll-free: 866 796-5373
E: ncr@jdrf.ca
W: www.jdrf.ca
Executive:
Mgr NE Ontario: Kerry Winnemore
No of Paid Staff: 3
Speakers Available
Languages: English

◈ ***Quebec Region:***
330-615 boul René-Lévesque O, Montréal QC H3B 1P5
514 744-5537; Fax: 514 744-0516
Toll-free: 877 634-2238
E: montreal@jdrf.ca
W: www.jdrf.ca
Executive:
Dir rég: Agathe Grinberg
Adj admin: Rocio Valencia
Year Founded: 1974
No of Paid Staff: 10
Speakers Available
Languages: French

◈ ***Saskatoon:***
Location: 1624 33rd St W, Saskatoon SK S7L 7M6
Mailing: PO Box 30055 RPO 32
306 314-9533; Fax: 306 955-2140
E: saskatoon@jdrf.ca
W: www.jdrf.ca
Executive:
Fundraising Coord: Lori Farkas
Speakers Available
Languages: English

◈ ***South Saskatchewan Chapter:***
Mailing: PO Box 3924 Stn Main, Regina SK S4P 3R8
306 789-8474; Fax: 306 543-5451
E: regina@jdrf.ca
W: www.jdrf.ca
Languages: English

JDRF - Southern Alberta
204-1608 17 Ave SW, Calgary AB T2T 0E3
403 255-7100; Fax: 403 253-6683
Toll-free: 877 287-3533
E: calgary@jdrf.ca
W: www.jdrf.ca
Executive:
Reg Mgr South AB: Myles D Rusak
Speakers Available
Languages: English

The M.S.I. Foundation
12230 106 Ave NW, Edmonton AB T5N 3Z1
780 421-7532; Fax: 780 425-4467
E: info@msifoundation.ca
W: www.msifoundation.ca
Executive:
Chairman: Dr Doug Wilson
Sec: Jennifer McCombe
Year Founded: 1971
Budget: $350,000
No of Paid Staff: 2
Speakers Available
Languages: English

Manitoba Medical Service Foundation Inc.
Location: 499 Empress St, Winnipeg MB R3G 3P3
Mailing: MB Blue Cross, PO Box 1046 Stn Main, Winnipeg MB R3C 2X7
204 788-6801; Fax: 204 774-1761
E: info@mmsf.ca
W: www.mmsf.ca
Executive:
Chair: Allen Rouse
V-Chair: Dr Lindsay DuVal
Exec Dir: Greg Hammond
Asst Exec Dir: Dr John Wade
Year Founded: 1971
Languages: English
Membership: 30

Partners In Research (PIR)
700 York St, London ON N5W 2S8
519 433-7866; Fax: 519 645-8899
E: info@pirweb.org
W: www.pirweb.org
Executive:
Exec Dir: Kevin Cougler
VROC Natl Project Mgr: Nicole Tate-Hill
Commun Mgr: Jesse Cressman-Dickinson
Dir-Spec Projects: Brent Peltola
Year Founded: 1986
Criteria: *Interest in educating about Health Research in Canada.*
Budget: $150,000
No of Paid Staff: 4
Speakers Available
Languages: English; French
Membership: 50

Public Health Association of Nova Scotia
Mailing: PO Box 33074 Rpo Quinpool Ctr, Halifax NS B3L 4T6
902 477-2960; Fax: 902 477-4584
W: www.phans.ca
Executive:
Pres: Marie McCully Collier

St. Boniface Hospital Foundation
C1026-409 Tache Ave, Winnipeg MB R2H 2A6
204 237-2067; Fax: 204 231-0041
W: www.saintboniface.ca
Executive:
CEO: Charles La Fleche

Society of Toxicology of Canada
Mailing: CP 55094 CSP MacKay, Montréal QC H3G 2W5
514 697-9219; Fax: 514 697-9309
W: www.stcweb.ca
Executive:
Prés: Louise Winn

Toronto West Society for Vascular Surgery
1202-1243 Islington Ave, Toronto ON M8X 1Y9
416 516-4399; Fax: 416 516-1704
E: drdwooster@bellnet.ca
Executive:
Owner: Dr Douglas Wooster
Languages: English

University of Waterloo - Propel Centre for Population Health Impact
Propel Centre LHN
200 University Ave W, Waterloo ON N2L 3G1
519 888-4567; Fax: 519 886-6424
W: www.uwaterloo.ca/
Executive:
Exec Officer: Katherine Marshall
Languages: English

MEDICAL & HEALTH (2) —General

Alberta College of Pharmacists
1100-8215 112 St NW, Edmonton AB T6G 2C8
780 990-0321; Fax: 780 990-0328
Toll-free: 877 227-3838
W: www.pharmacists.ab.ca
Executive:
Registrar: Greg Eberhart
Dep Registrar: Dale Cooney
Bus Mgr: Lynn Paulitsch
Cust Serv Admin: Janet Bradshaw
Languages: English

Associated Medical Services, Inc.
228-162 Cumberland St, Toronto ON M5R 3N5
416 924-3368; Fax: 416 323-3338
W: www.ams-inc.on.ca
Executive:
Chm/Pres: Dorothy Pringle
Dir-Ops/Corp Sec: Sheila McDougall
Year Founded: 1937
No of Paid Staff: 2
Library: Y
Languages: English
Membership: 9 directors

BC Medical Journal
115-1665 Broadway W, Vancouver BC V6J 5A4
604 638-2815; Fax: 604 638-2917
Toll-free: 800 665-2262
E: journal@bcma.bc.ca
W: www.bcmj.org
Executive:
Man Editor: Jay Draper
Ed in Chief: Dr David Richardson
Sr Editorial/Prod Coord: Kashmira Suraliwalla

College of Medical Laboratory Technologists of Ontario
950-36 Toronto St, Toronto ON M5C 2C5
416 861-9605; Fax: 416 861-0934
Toll-free: 800 323-9672
E: mail@cmlto.com
W: www.cmlto.com
Executive:
Registrar/Exec Officer: Kathy Wilkie

Filter - NOW AN ONLINE NEWS BRIEF
Location: 101-233 Colborne St, Brantford ON N3T 2H4
Mailing: PO Box 1054 Stn Main, Brantford ON N3T 5S7
519 753-6037; Fax: 519 753-6408
Toll-free: 800 387-4674
W: www.oamrs.org
Executive:
Dep CEO/Mgr-Prof Serv: Greg Toffner
Year Founded: 1935

International Society For Evolutionary Protistology
University of BC,Botany Dept
3529-6270 University Blvd, Vancouver BC V6T 1Z4
604 822-4906; Fax: 604 822-6089
W: www.isepsociety.com
Executive:
Pres: Ken Ishida
Office Mgr: Dr Patrick Keeling

MEDEC Canada Medical Technology Company
900-405 The West Mall, Toronto ON M9C 5J1
416 620-1915; Fax: 416 620-1595
E: medec@medec.org
W: www.medec.org
Executive:
Pres/CEO: Stephen Dibert
VP: Lawrence Fereacki

Medical Devices Canada
900-405 The West Mall, Etobicoke ON M9C 5J1
416 620-1915; Fax: 416 620-1595
Toll-free: 866 586-3338
E: medec@medec.org
W: www.medec.org
Executive:
Pres/CEO: Brian Lewis
Year Founded: 1973
Criteria: *Open to any company which has a Canadian business address and is involved in the medical devices industry.*
Budget: $850,000
No of Paid Staff: 8
Languages: English

ACOUSTIC NEUROMA

Acoustic Neuroma Association of Canada
Mailing: PO Box 144, Dunnville ON N1A 2X1
416 546-6426; Fax: 905 701-0970
Toll-free: 800 561-2622
E: info@anac.ca
W: www.anac.ca
Executive:
Pres: Dr Carol-Anne Sullivan
Natl Coord: Yvonne Bottcher
Year Founded: 1983
No of Paid Staff: 1
Languages: English
Membership: 483
Membership Fee: $32

AIDS

Bruce House
402-251 Bank St, Ottawa ON K2P 1X3
613 729-0911; Fax: 613 729-0959
E: admin@brucehouse.org
W: www.brucehouse.org
Executive:
Office/Prog Admin: Jennifer Bruce
Year Founded: 1988
Languages: English
Membership Fee: $10

CATIE (Canadian AIDS Treatment Information Exchange), Canada's Source for HIV and Hepatitis C Information
505-555 Richmond St W, Toronto ON M5V 3B1
416 203-7122; Fax: 416 203-8284
Toll-free: 800 263-1638
E: info@catie.ca
W: www.catie.ca
Executive:
Exec Dir: Laurie Edmiston
Dir-Commun/Social Mktg: Jim Pollock
Year Founded: 1991
Budget: $2,500,000
No of Paid Staff: 40
Speakers Available
Library: Y
Languages: English; French
Membership: 1,500 *(Lists available to the public)*
Library:
National HIV/AIDS Reference Library

CIHR Canadian HIV Trials Network
588-1081 Burrard St, Vancouver BC V6Z 1Y6
604 806-8327; Fax: 604 806-8005
Toll-free: 800 661-4664
E: ctninfo@hivnet.ubc.ca
W: www.hivnet.ubc.ca
Executive:
CAO: David Cox
Dir: Martin T Schechter
Mgr- Commun: Kevin Pendergraft
Chief Science Off: Jim Pankovich
Year Founded: 1991
Speakers Available
Languages: English; French
Membership list available to the public

Canadian AIDS Society
100-190 O'Connor St, Ottawa ON K2P 2R3
613 230-3580; Fax: 613 563-4998
Toll-free: 800 499-1985
E: casinfo@cdnaids.ca
W: www.cdnaids.ca
Executive:
CEO: Monique Doolittle-Romas
Prog Dir: Kim Thomas
Year Founded: 1986
Criteria: *Canadian Community-based AIDS service organizations and non-profit organizations working in the field of AIDS only.*
No of Paid Staff: 8
Speakers Available
Languages: English; French
Membership: Approx. 125 community-based AIDS organizations. *(Lists available to the public)*

◈Alberta:

◇Aids Jasper:
Location: 622 Connaught Dr, Upper Floor, Jasper AB T0E 1E0
Mailing: PO Box 2427
780 852-5274; Fax: 780 852-5273
Toll-free: 877 291-8811
E: director@hivwestyellowhead.com
W: www.hivwestyellowhead.com
Executive:
Exec Dir: Andrea Watson
Year Founded: 1988
Criteria: *Open to any interested member of the public.*
Budget: $58,000
No of Paid Staff: 2
Speakers Available
Languages: English; French
Membership list available to the public

◇Bow Valley
Location: 302 Buffalo St, Banff AB T1L 1C8
Mailing: PO Box 3160
403 762-0690; Fax: 403 762-0694
E: programs@aidsbowvalley.com
W: www.aidsbowvalley.com
Executive:
Chairperson: Dr Priscilla Wilson
Treas: Alison Eason
Year Founded: 1988
No of Paid Staff: 1
Speakers Available
Languages: English

◇Calgary
110-1603 10 Ave SW, Calgary AB T3C 0J7
403 508-2500; Fax: 403 263-7358
E: info@aidscalgary.org
W: www.aidscalgary.org
Executive:
Exec Dir: Susan Cress
Year Founded: 1983
Criteria: *A member supports the philosophy and work of the Association, endeavours to enhance the successful achievement of goals by the Association, endeavours to remain informed of the issues relevant to HIV/AIDS, registers annually with the Association, pays the annual membership fee, if any, as required.*
No of Paid Staff: 18
Speakers Available
Library: Y *(Open to the public)*
Languages: English
Membership: 100 approx.
Membership Fee: $10

◇Edmonton:
9702 111 Ave NW, Edmonton AB T5G 0B1
780 488-5742; Fax: 780 488-3735
E: contact@hivedmonton.com
W: www.hivedmonton.com
Executive:
Chair: James Mabey
Dir-Res Dev/Pub Engagement: Laura Keegan
Exec Dir: Shelley Williams
Ops Coord: John Gee
Year Founded: 1986
No of Paid Staff: 10
Speakers Available
Languages: English
Membership: 60
Membership Fee: $25

◇Grande Prairie:
303-9804 100 Ave, Grande Prairie AB T8V 0T8
780 538-3388; Fax: 780 538-3368
E: info@hivnorth.org
W: www.hivnorth.org
Executive:
Pres: Shannon Dunfield
Exec Dir: Brenda Yamkowy
Year Founded: 1987
No of Paid Staff: 5
Speakers Available
Library: Y *(Open to the public)*
Languages: English

◇Lethbridge:
1206 6 Ave S, Lethbridge AB T1J 1A4
403 328-8186; Fax: 403 328-8564
E: lethhiv@telusplanet.net
W: lethbridgehiv.com
Executive:
Admv Asst: Pat DeBoer
Year Founded: 1988
Criteria: *To qualify for membership an individual must be in agreement with the vision, mission and mandate of the organization.*
No of Paid Staff: 3
Speakers Available
Languages: English
Membership: 200
Membership Fee: $10

◇Red Deer:
4611 50 Ave, Red Deer AB T4N 3Z9
403 346-8858; Fax: 403 346-2352
Toll-free: 877 346-8858
E: info@caans.org
W: www.caans.org
Executive:
Exec Dir: Jennifer Vanderschaeghe
Admin/NightReach Prog Mgr: Ashley Fleming
Year Founded: 1988
Criteria: *none*
No of Paid Staff: 12
Speakers Available

Languages: English
Membership list available to the public
Membership Fee: $10

◇ ***The SHARP Foundation:***
2-3012 17 Ave SE, Box 172, Calgary AB T2A 0P9
403 272-2912; Fax: 403 272-9792
E: info@thesharpfoundation.com
W: www.thesharpfoundation.com
Executive:
Pres: Gerald Hart
Exec Dir: Floyd Visser
Case Mgr: Patricia Hinds
Mgr-Health: Caitlin Palmer
Year Founded: 1990
Budget: $900,000
No of Paid Staff: 13
Speakers Available
Languages: English
Membership: 150
Membership Fee: $25

◈ ***British Columbia:***
Languages: English

◇ ***AIDS and Disability Action Program***
204-456 Broadway W, Vancouver BC V5Y 1R3
604 875-0188; Fax: 604 875-9227
E: feedback@bccpd.bc.ca
W: www.bccpd.bc.ca
Executive:
Prog Dir: Shelley Hourston
Exec Dir: Jane Dyson
Year Founded: 1977
No of Paid Staff: 25
Library: Y
Languages: English
Library:
WDI/ADAP Resource Centre *(Open to the public)*

◇ ***AIDS Network, Outreach & Support Society***
205 14th Ave N, Cranbrook BC V1C 3W3
250 426-3383; Fax: 250 426-3221
Toll-free: 800 421-2437
E: info@ankors.bc.ca
W: www.ankors.bc.ca
Executive:
Exec Dir: Cheryl Dowden
Harm Red/Needle Exch: Alex Sherstibitoff
Community Care Team: Gary Dalton
Year Founded: 1992
Budget: $243,000
No of Paid Staff: 2
Speakers Available
Library: Y
Languages: English

◇ ***Kamloops:***
433 Tranquille Rd, Kamloops BC V2B 3G9
250 376-7558; Fax: 250 376-7530
Toll-free: 800 661-7541 Area Code 250 only
E: info@askwellness.ca
W: askwellness.ca
Executive:
Exec Dir: Bob Hughes
Year Founded: 1992
No of Paid Staff: 13
Speakers Available
Library: Y *(Open to the public)*
Languages: English
Membership: 48 *(Lists available to the public)*
Membership Fee: $1
Library:
Resource & Education Centre *(Open to the public)*

◇ ***Okanagan and Region:***
168 Asher Rd, Kelowna BC V1X 3H6
778 753-5830; Fax: 778 753-5832
E: info@lprc.ca
W: www.lprc.ca
Executive:
Exec Dir: Clare MacDonald
Year Founded: 1992
Budget: $730,000
No of Paid Staff: 7
Speakers Available
Library: Y *(Open to the public)*
Languages: English
Membership: 63
Membership Fee: $12
Library:
LPRC Library *(Open to the public)*

◇ ***Persons with AIDS Society of British Columbia***
1107 Seymour St, Floor 2, Vancouver BC V6B 5S8
604 893-2200; Fax: 604 893-2251
Toll-free: 800 994-2437
E: info@positivelivingbc.org
W: www.positivelivingbc.org
Executive:
Chair: John Bishop
Exec Dir: Ross Harvey
Criteria: *Persons with an HIV+ status.*
No of Paid Staff: 25
Speakers Available
Languages: English
Membership: 4,900 *(Lists available to the public)*
Library:
Pacific AIDS Resource Centre *(Open to the public)*

◇ ***Positive Living North Society - Prince George***
1-1563 2nd Ave, Prince George BC V2L 3B8
250 562-1172; Fax: 250 562-3317
Toll-free: 888 438-2437
E: info@positivelivingnorth.ca
W: positivelivingnorth.ca
Executive:
Admv Serv Mgr: Gail Brawn
Co-Exec Dir: Carmen Nutter
Co-Exec Dir: Vanessa West
Year Founded: 1990
Criteria: *Volunteers must be members, clients are automatically members (fee waived).*
No of Paid Staff: 16
Speakers Available
Library: Y *(Open to the public)*
Languages: English
Membership: 50
Membership Fee: $5

◇ ***Positive Women's Network:***
614-1033 Davie St, Vancouver BC V6E 1M7
604 692-3000; Fax: 604 684-3126
Toll-free: 866 692-3001 in BC only
E: pwn@pwn.bc.ca
W: www.pwn.bc.ca
Executive:
Exec Dir: Marcie Summers
Commun Coord: Janet Madsen
Year Founded: 1989
Criteria: *HIV positive status*
Budget: $750,000
No of Paid Staff: 7
Library: Y *(Open to the public)*
Languages: English
Membership: 600
Membership Fee: Free to HIV positive women

◇ ***Vancouver:***
1107 Seymour St, Vancouver BC V6B 5S8
604 893-2201; Fax: 604 893-2205
E: contact@aidsvancouver.org
W: www.aidsvancouver.org
Executive:
Exec Dir: Dr Brian Chittock
Year Founded: 1983
Budget: $2,100,000
No of Paid Staff: 33
Speakers Available
Languages: English
Membership: 350
Membership Fee: Free to volunteers or those who have AIDS; $25
Library:
Pacific AIDS Resource Centre Library *(Open to the public)*

◇ ***Vancouver Island:***
Access Health Centre
713 Johnson St, Floor 3, Victoria BC V8W 1M8
250 384-2366; Fax: 250 380-9411
Toll-free: 800 665-2437 Island Wide Infoline
E: info@avi.org
W: www.avi.org
Executive:
Mgr-Fund Dev: James Boxshall
Exec Dir: Katrina Jensen
Dir-Fin: Bryson Hawkins
Year Founded: 1986
Criteria: *Any person, organization of persons or corporation subscribing to the aims, purposes and by-laws of the society may apply for membership.*
Budget: $1,800,000
No of Paid Staff: 32
Speakers Available
Languages: English
Membership: 120
Membership Fee: $1 - People with HIV/AIDS; $15
Library:
AVL Resource Centre *(Open to the public)*

◇ ***Victoria AIDS Respite Care Society:***
1284F Gladstone Ave, Victoria BC V8T 1G6
250 388-6220; Fax: 250 388-7011
E: info@varcs.org
W: www.varcs.org
Executive:
Pres: Art Holbrook
Exec Dir: Karen Dennis
Year Founded: 1991
Criteria: *Open to all.*
Budget: $99,000
No of Paid Staff: 3
Speakers Available
Library: Y *(Open to the public)*
Languages: English
Membership: 113
Membership Fee: Others - $15; Free to HIV + people registered with VARCS

◇ ***Victoria Persons with AIDS Society:***
101-1139 Yates St, Victoria BC V8V 3N2
250 382-7927; Fax: 250 382-3232
Toll-free: 877 382-7927
E: support@vpwas.com
W: www.vpwas.org
Executive:
Office Mgr: Richard Mallory
Year Founded: 1992
Criteria: *Be HIV positive and live on Vancouver Island or Gulf Islands.*
No of Paid Staff: 1
Speakers Available
Library: Y *(Open to the public)*
Languages: English
Membership: 530

◇ ***Wings Housing Society***
12-1041 Comox St, Vancouver BC V6E 1K1
604 899-5405; Fax: 604 899-5410
E: wingsinfo@shaw.ca
W: www.wingshousing.bc.ca
Executive:
Exec Dir: Dallas Kolomay
Year Founded: 1991
Criteria: *Persons who are HIV positive.*
No of Paid Staff: 1
Speakers Available

Languages: English
Membership: 215

◈ **Manitoba:**
Languages: English

◇ **Nine Circles Community Health Centre**
705 Broadway, Winnipeg MB R3G 0X2
204 940-6000; Fax: 204 940-6006
Toll-free: 888 305-8647
E: ninecircles@ninecircles.ca
W: www.ninecircles.ca
Languages: English

◈ **New Brunswick:**
Languages: English

◇ **Fredericton:**
Victoria Health Centre
65 Brunswick St, Fredericton NB E3B 1G5
506 459-7518; Fax: 506 459-5782
Toll-free: 800 561-4009 NB only
E: info@aidsnb.com
W: www.aidsnb.com
Executive:
Exec Dir: Nick Scott
Year Founded: 1986
Budget: $125,000
No of Paid Staff: 5
Speakers Available
Library: Y *(Open to the public)*
Languages: English; French
Membership: 200
Membership Fee: $15

◇ **Saint John:**
205-115 Hazen St, Saint John NB E2L 3L3
506 652-2437; Fax: 506 652-2438
E: aidssj@mb.aibn.com
W: www.aidssaintjohn.com
Executive:
Pres: Dr Leslie Jeffrey
VP: Patricia Scott
Treas: SarahRose Werner
Sec: Mike Gravel
Budget: $110,000
No of Paid Staff: 4
Speakers Available
Library: Y *(Open to the public)*
Languages: English
Membership: 50 *(Lists available to the public)*

◈ **Newfoundland & Labrador:**
Languages: English

◇ **AIDS Committee of Newfoundland and Labrador**
47 Janeway Pl, St. John's NL A1A 1R7
709 579-8656; Fax: 709 579-0559
Toll-free: 800 563-1575 (in Newfoundland)
E: info@acnl.net
W: www.acnl.net
Executive:
Exec Dir: Gerrard Yetman
Harm Reduction Outreach/SWAP Wkr: Julie Crouse
Languages: English

◈ **Nova Scotia:**
Languages: English

◇ **AIDS Coalition of Cape Breton**
Location: 150 Bentinck St, Sydney NS B1P 6G1
Mailing: PO Box 177 Stn A, Sydney NS B1P 6H1
902 567-1766; Fax: 902 567-1766
Toll-free: 877 597-9255
W: www.accb.ns.ca
Executive:
Exec Dir: Christine Porter
PHA Prog Coord: Jo-Anne Rolls
Year Founded: 1992
Budget: $65,000
No of Paid Staff: 1
Speakers Available
Languages: English

◇ **AIDS Coalition of NS - Halifax**
401-1668 Barrington St, Halifax NS B3J 2A2
902 425-4882; Fax: 902 422-6200
Toll-free: 800 566-2437 within Nova Scotia
E: acns@acns.ns.ca
W: www.acns.ns.ca
Year Founded: 1995
No of Paid Staff: 6
Speakers Available
Library: Y *(Open to the public)*
Languages: English

◇ **Mainline Needle Exchange**
Location: 5511 Cornwallis St, Halifax NS B3K 3B4
Mailing: 2158 Gottingen St
902 423-9991; Fax: 902 423-1619
Toll-free: 877 904-4555
E: mainline2@eastlink.ca
W: www.mainlineneedleexchange.ca
Executive:
Prog Dir: Diane Bailey
Year Founded: 1992
No of Paid Staff: 8
Speakers Available
Languages: English

◇ **Picton County AIDS Coalition**
Location: 35 Riverside St, New Glasgow NS B2H 5K7
Mailing: PO Box 964 Stn Main
902 752-6218; Fax: 902 752-2233
E: picaids@north.nsis.com

◈ **Ontario:**
201-468 Queen St E, Toronto ON M5A 1T7
416 364-4555; Fax: 416 364-1250
Toll-free: 800 839-0369
E: info@ontarioaidsnetwork.on.ca
W: www.ontarioaidsnetwork.on.ca
Executive:
Exec Dir: Rick Kennedy
Year Founded: 1986
No of Paid Staff: 5
Speakers Available
Languages: English
Membership: 49

◇ **Africans in Partnership Against AIDS**
101-314 Jarvis St, Toronto ON M5B 2C5
416 924-5256; Fax: 416 924-6575
E: info@apaa.ca
W: www.apaa.ca
Executive:
Exec Dir: Fanta Ongoiba
Year Founded: 1993
Budget: $60,000
No of Paid Staff: 6
Languages: English
Membership: 100

◇ **Alliance for South Asian AIDS Prevention**
315-120 Carlton St, Toronto ON M5A 4K2
416 599-2727; Fax: 416 599-6011
E: info@asaap.ca
W: www.asaap.ca
Executive:
Exec Dir: Vijaya Chikermane
Year Founded: 1989
Criteria: *South Asians committed to the mission of the agency.*
Budget: $200,000
No of Paid Staff: 5
Library: Y
Languages: Tamil
Membership list available to the public
Library:
Resource Centre *(Open to the public)*

◇ **Asian Community AIDS Services**
410-260 Spadina Ave, Toronto ON M5T 2E4
416 963-4300; Fax: 416 963-4371
Toll-free: 877 630-2227
E: info@acas.org
W: www.acas.org
Executive:
Exec Dir: Noulmook Sutdhibhasilip
Youth Prog Coord: Wilson Ho
Support Prog Coord: Patrick Truong
Year Founded: 1994
Criteria: *Program client and volunteering experience*
Languages: English

◇ **Black Coalition for AIDS Prevention**
20 Victoria St, Floor 4, Toronto ON M5C 2N8
416 977-9955; Fax: 416 977-7664
E: info@black-cap.com
W: www.black-cap.com
Executive:
Chair: Angela Robertson
Co-Chair: Trevor Gray
Treas: Michael Went
Sec: Aakilah Ade
No of Paid Staff: 5
Languages: English

◇ **Cambridge, Kitchener, Waterloo & Area**
2B-625 King St E, Kitchener ON N2G 4V4
519 570-3687; Fax: 519 570-4034
Toll-free: 877 770-3687
E: volunteer@acckwa.com
W: www.acckwa.com
Executive:
Dir-Ops: Lynn Cashubec
Year Founded: 1987
Criteria: *Membership is limited to persons 18 years of age and over.*
Budget: $420,000
No of Paid Staff: 5
Speakers Available
Library: Y *(Open to the public)*
Languages: English
Membership: 29 *(Lists available to the public)*
Library:
ACCKWA Resource Library *(Open to the public)*

◇ **Fife House Foundation**
490 Sherbourne St, Floor 2, Toronto ON M4X 1K9
416 205-9888; Fax: 416 205-9919
E: info@fifehouse.org
W: www.fifehouse.org
Executive:
Pres: Bruce Mayhew
Dir-Dev/Commun: David Currah
Exec Dir: Keith Hambly
Sec-Treas: Linda Stewart
Dir-Fin/Admv: Annette Williams
Languages: English

◇ **Guelph & Wellington County**
115-89 Dawson Rd, Guelph ON N1H 1B1
519 763-2255; Fax: 519 763-8125
Toll-free: 800 282-4505
E: director@aidsguelph.org
W: www.aidsguelph.org
Executive:
Exec Dir: Tom Hammond
Year Founded: 1989
Criteria: *Must support the aims and objectives of ACGWC.*
Budget: $900,000
No of Paid Staff: 12
Speakers Available
Languages: English
Membership: 32
Membership Fee: $20

HEALTHCARE ASSOCIATIONS

◇ ***Hamilton***
101-140 King St E, Hamilton ON L8N 1B2
905 528-0854; Fax: 905 528-6311
Toll-free: 866 563-0563
E: info@aidsnetwork.ca
W: www.aidsnetwork.ca
Executive:
Exec Dir: Ruthann Tucker
Year Founded: 1986
No of Paid Staff: 9
Speakers Available
Library: Y *(Open to the public)*
Languages: English
Membership: 40
Membership Fee: $10

◇ ***London***
30-186 King St, London ON N6A 1C7
519 434-1601; Fax: 519 434-1843
Toll-free: 866 920-1601
E: info@aidslondon.com
W: info@hivaidsconnection.ca
Executive:
Exec Dir: Brian Lester
Year Founded: 1985
Criteria: *Support the mission and services of the agency.*
Budget: $750,000
No of Paid Staff: 12
Speakers Available
Library: Y
Languages: English; French
Membership: 100
Library:
Resource Centre *(Open to the public)*

◇ ***London Regional Aids Hospice***
596 Pall Mall St, London ON N5Y 2Z9
519 433-3951; Fax: 519 433-1314
E: johngordonhome@lrah.ca
W: www.johngordonhome.ca
Executive:
Exec Dir: Bruce Rankin
Coord-Residence-Care: Yvonne Rimbult
Year Founded: 1991
No of Paid Staff: 12
Library: Y *(Open to the public)*
Languages: English
Membership Fee: $10

◇ ***Niagara***
120 Queenston St, St Catharines ON L2R 2Z3
905 984-8684; Fax: 905 988-1921
Toll-free: 800 773-9843
E: info@aidsniagara.com
W: www.aidsniagara.com
Executive:
Exec Dir: Steve Byers
Year Founded: 1989
No of Paid Staff: 23
Speakers Available
Library: Y *(Open to the public)*
Languages: English
Membership: 80 *(Lists available to the public)*

◇ ***North Bay & Area***
201-269 Main St W, North Bay ON P1B 2T8
705 497-3560; Fax: 705 497-7850
Toll-free: 800 387-3701
E: acnba@efni.com
W: www.aidsnorthbay.com
Executive:
Exec Dir: Dr Stacey Mayhall
Year Founded: 1992
Criteria: *Support of mission.*
Budget: $350,000
No of Paid Staff: 7
Speakers Available
Library: Y *(Open to the public)*
Languages: English; French
Membership: 60 *(Lists available to the public)*
Membership Fee: $10/year

◇ ***Ottawa***
700-251 Bank St, Ottawa ON K2P 1X3
613 238-5014; Fax: 613 238-3425
Toll-free: 800 461-2182
W: www.aco-cso.ca
Executive:
A-Exec Dir: Khaled Salam
Mgr-Educ/Prev: Heather Money
No of Paid Staff: 12
Speakers Available
Library: Y *(Open to the public)*
Languages: English; French
Membership: 160

◇ ***Peel Region***
1-160 Traders Blvd E, Mississauga ON L4Z 3K7
905 361-0523; Fax: 905 361-1004
Toll-free: 866 896-8700
E: info@phan.ca
W: www.phan.ca
Executive:
Co-Chair: Tania Fernandes
Co-Chair: Rob Gearing
Exec Dir: Keith Wong
Dir: Ted Koosterman
Dir: Rose Colacci
Treas: Dorothy Binkley
Sec: Sanya Khan
Coord-Admv/Fin: Skha Mpofu
Year Founded: 1991
No of Paid Staff: 6
Languages: English
Membership: 29
Membership Fee: $10

◇ ***Peterborough***
302-159 King St, Peterborough ON K9J 2R8
705 749-9110; Fax: 705 749-6310
Toll-free: 800 361-2895
E: getinformed@parn.ca
W: www.parn.ca
Executive:
Exec Dir: Kim Dolan
Office Admin: Peg Town
Year Founded: 1990
No of Paid Staff: 6
Speakers Available
Library: Y *(Open to the public)*
Languages: English
Membership: 350
Membership Fee: Organization - $25 per year; Individual - $10 per year
Library:
PARN Resource Centre *(Open to the public)*

◇ ***Regional Services***
844A Princess St, Kingston ON K7L 1G5
613 545-3698; Fax: 613 545-9809
Toll-free: 800 565-2209 (613 exchange only)
E: hars@kingston.net
W: www.hars.ca
Executive:
Exec Dir: John MacTavish
Year Founded: 1988
Criteria: *Agreement with mission*
No of Paid Staff: 6
Speakers Available
Library: Y *(Open to the public)*
Languages: English
Membership Fee: $5 - $15 for others; Free to people who are HIV +

◇ ***Simcoe County***
Location: Barrie by the Bay, 337-80 Bradford St, Barrie ON L4N 6S7
Mailing: PO Box 744 Stn Main, Barrie ON L4M 4Y5
705 722-6778; Fax: 705 722-6560
Toll-free: 800 372-2272
E: acscexecutivedirector@rogers.com
W: www.acsc.ca
Executive:
Exec Dir: Gerry Croteau
Health Consultant: Edith Reyes
Year Founded: 1995
No of Paid Staff: 2
Speakers Available
Library: Y *(Open to the public)*
Languages: English; French
Membership Fee: $20

◇ ***The Teresa Group***
300-124 Merton St, Toronto ON M4S 2Z2
416 596-7703; Fax: 416 596-7910
E: theteresagroup@on.aibn.com
W: www.teresagroup.ca
Executive:
Exec Dir: Karen Vance-Wallace
Year Founded: 1990
Criteria: *Open to any person who gives a donation in money, goods or services.*
Budget: $469,000
No of Paid Staff: 6
Speakers Available
Languages: English
Membership list available to the public

◇ ***Thunder Bay***
574 Memorial Ave, Thunder Bay ON P7B 3Z2
807 345-1516; Fax: 807 345-2505
Toll-free: 800 488-5840
E: info@aidsthunderbay.org
W: www.aidsthunderbay.org
Executive:
Exec Dir: Lawrence Korhonen
Educ Commun Coord: Bob Manson
Year Founded: 1985
No of Paid Staff: 13
Speakers Available
Library: Y *(Open to the public)*
Languages: English; French
Membership Fee: $10

◇ ***Toronto***
399 Church St, Floor 4, Toronto ON M5B 2J6
416 340-2437; Fax: 416 340-8224
E: ask@actoronto.org
W: www.actoronto.org
Executive:
Serv Coord: Peter Stevenson
Exec Asst - Mgmt Team: Doreen Davies
Year Founded: 1983
Criteria: *Agreement with ACT's mission and values statement.*
Budget: $2,100,000
No of Paid Staff: 35
Library: Y
Languages: English; French
Library:
AIDS Committee Toronto - Library *(Open to the public)*

◇ ***Toronto People with AIDS***
200 Gerrard St E, Floor 2, Toronto ON M5A 2E6
416 506-1400; Fax: 416 506-1404
E: info@pwatoronto.org
W: www.pwatoronto.org
Executive:
Prog/Dir-Servs: Suzanne Paddock
Exec Dir: Murray Josi
Year Founded: 1987
Criteria: *Open to any Toronto resident.*

Budget: $1,500,000
No of Paid Staff: 17
Speakers Available
Languages: English
Membership: 5,600
Membership Fee: $10

◇ ***Voices of Positive Women***
104-66 Isabella St, Toronto ON M4Y 1N3
E: voices@vopw.org
W: www.vopw.org
Executive:
Exec Dir: Wendy Pinder
Board Member: Khatundi Masinde
Budget: $400,000
No of Paid Staff: 6
Speakers Available
Library: Y *(Open to the public)*
Languages: English

◇ ***Windsor***
511 Pelissier St, Windsor ON N9A 4L2
519 973-0222; Fax: 519 973-7389
Toll-free: 800 265-4858 Kent & Lambton
E: admin@aidswindsor.org
W: www.aidswindsor.org
Year Founded: 1985
Budget: $900,000
No of Paid Staff: 16
Speakers Available
Library: Y
Languages: English; French
Library:
AIDS Committee of Windsor Resource Library *(Open to the public)*

◈ ***Prince Edward Island:***
Languages: English

◇ ***AIDS Prince Edward Island***
2-375 University Ave, Charlottetown PE C1A 4N4
902 566-2437; Fax: 902 626-3400
Toll-free: 800 314-2437 (PEI, NS only)
E: info@aidspei.com
W: www.aidspei.com
Executive:
Exec Dir: Alana Leard
Year Founded: 1991
Budget: $110,000
No of Paid Staff: 2
Speakers Available
Library: Y *(Open to the public)*
Languages: English; French
Membership: 50 *(Lists available to the public)*
Membership Fee: $10

◈ ***Québec:***
Languages: English

◇ ***AIDS Community Care Montreal***
2075 rue Plessis, Montréal QC H2L 2Y4
514 527-0928; Fax: 514 527-0701
E: info@accmontreal.org
W: www.accmontreal.org
Executive:
Dir gén: Mark Hapanowicz
Criteria: *Open to all.*
Budget: $230,000
No of Paid Staff: 6
Speakers Available
Languages: English; French
Membership: 700
Membership Fee: $1

◇ ***Centre des ROSÉS de l'Abitibi-Témiscamingue***
380 av Richard, bureau 220, Rouyn-Noranda QC J9X 4L3
819 764-9111; Fax: 819 762-9697
Toll-free: 800 783-9002 Ligne régionale sans frais
E: centre-r.o.s.e.s@cablevision.qc.ca
Executive:
VP: René-Pierre LaFrenière
Dir: Ginette Guay
Year Founded: 1993
Criteria: *Avoir à coeur la cause du sida.*
No of Paid Staff: 4
Speakers Available
Library: Y
Languages: French
Membership: 46 *(Lists available to the public)*
Membership Fee: $10 année

◇ ***Centre SIDA amitié***
527 rue Saint-Georges, Saint-Jérôme QC J7Z 5B6
450 431-7432; Fax: 450 431-6536
Toll-free: 888 431-7432
Executive:
Dir: Hugo Bissonnet
Year Founded: 1954
Criteria: *Conseil d'ecole d'une école francophone cathdrique ou pubizue*
No of Paid Staff: 2
Speakers Available
Languages: French
Membership: 328
Membership Fee: $5 per année

◇ ***Coalition SIDA des Sourds du Québec***
320-2075 rue Plessis, Montréal QC H2L 2Y4
877 535-5556; Fax: 514 521-1137
Toll-free: 800 855-0511 Service relais pour Sourds
E: info@cssq.org
Executive:
Dir gén: Michel Turgeon
Adj admin: Nicky Blouin
Year Founded: 1992
No of Paid Staff: 3
Speakers Available
Languages: Sign Language; English; French
Membership: 100
Membership Fee: $10-$100

◇ ***Équipe Multidisciplinaire d'Intervention en Santé Sexuelle***
101-1005 boul Curé-Poirier O, Longueuil QC J4K 2E2
450 651-9229; Fax: 450 651-3420
W: www.emiss-ere.ca
Executive:
Dir gén: Sylvain Gauthier
Languages: French

◇ ***Gatineau***
410-109 rue Wright, Gatineau QC J8X 2G7
819 568-9986; Fax: 819 568-1582
E: info@trocao.org
W: www.trocao.org
Executive:
Prés: Fabienne Lachapelle
Dir gén: Isabelle Boespflug
Year Founded: 1991
Budget: $100,000
No of Paid Staff: 2
Speakers Available
Library: Y
Languages: English; French
Membership: 130 *(Lists available to the public)*
Membership Fee: $5/yr

◇ ***Intervention régionale et information sur le SIDA en estrie***
505 rue Wellington S, Sherbrooke QC J1H 5E2
819 823-6704; Fax: 819 823-5537
E: iris.estrie@videotron.ca
W: www.iris-estrie.com
Executive:
Dir: Susan Garand
Year Founded: 1988
No of Paid Staff: 4
Speakers Available
Library: Y *(Open to the public)*
Languages: English; French
Membership: 50

◇ ***Séro Zéro***
Location: 207-2075 rue Plessis, Montréal QC H2L 2Y4
Mailing: CP 246 succ C, Montréal QC H2L 4K1
514 521-7778; Fax: 514 521-7665
E: info@rezosante.org
W: www.rezosante.org
Executive:
Dir gén: Robert Rousseau
Year Founded: 1994
No of Paid Staff: 17
Languages: French

◇ ***SIDAction Inc.***
Location: 515 rue Sainte-Cécile, Trois-Rivières QC G9A 1K9
Mailing: CP 1142 PDF 1, Trois-Rivières QC G9A 5K8
819 374-5740; Fax: 819 374-5932
Toll-free: 866 433-7432
E: information@sidactionmauricie.ca
W: www.sidactionmauricie.ca
Executive:
Coord: Faye Héroux
Agent d'info: Christine Boisvert
Criteria: *Les personnes intéress à promouvoir les objectifs de la corporation.*
Library: Y
Languages: French
Library:
Centre de documentation

◇ ***Victoriaville***
116-59 rue Monfette, Victoriaville QC G6P 1J8
819 758-2662; Fax: 819 758-8270
E: blits@cdcbf.qc.ca
W: www.blits.ca
Executive:
Prés: Gabrielle Bergeron
VP: Jacques Gélinas
Trés: Denis Hébert
Year Founded: 1989
No of Paid Staff: 6
Speakers Available
Library: Y *(Open to the public)*
Languages: French
Membership Fee: $5 per year

◈ ***Saskatchewan***

◇ ***Persons Living With AIDS Network of Saskatchewan***
Location: 127C Avenue D N, Saskatoon SK S7L 1M5
Mailing: PO Box 7123 Stn Main, Saskatoon SK S7K 4J1
306 373-7766; Fax: 306 374-7746
Toll-free: 800 226-0944 Saskatchewan only
E: plwa@sasktel.net
Executive:
Pres: Lorraine Stewart
Exec Coord: Laurie Schuette
Year Founded: 1987
Criteria: *HIV/AIDS suffers, their family and/or partners.*
Budget: $125,000
No of Paid Staff: 3
Speakers Available
Library: Y *(Open to the public)*
Languages: English
Membership: 146 *(Lists available to the public)*

◇ ***Saskatoon:***
Location: 1143 Ave F N, Saskatoon SK S7L 1X1
Mailing: PO Box 4062 Stn Main, Saskatoon SK S7K 4E3
306 242-5005; Fax: 306 665-9976
Toll-free: 800 667-6876 Western Canada Only

E: admin@aidssaskatoon.ca
W: www.aidssaskatoon.ca
Executive:
Exec Coord: Nicole White
Year Founded: 1987
Criteria: *Anyone who agrees with the goals of AIDS Saskatoon and abides by AIDS Saskatoon's by-laws.*
No of Paid Staff: 8
Speakers Available
Library: Y *(Open to the public)*
Languages: English
Membership list available to the public
Membership Fee: $10

◇ **South Saskatchewan:**
2911 5th Ave, Regina SK S4T 0L4
306 924-8420; Fax: 306 525-0904
E: aidsprograms@sasktel.net
W: www.aidsprogramssouthsask.com
Executive:
Exec Dir: Sope Ogunrinde
Admn Coord: Cindy O'Connor
Educ/Outreach Coord: Alicia Slywka
Empowerment Life Skills Coord: Doreen Lloyd
Needle Exchange Facilitator: Laurie Pellerin
Support Serv Coord: Morag Hurn
Year Founded: 1986
Criteria: *None*
Budget: $300,000
No of Paid Staff: 6
Speakers Available
Library: Y *(Open to the public)*
Languages: English
Membership: 35 *(Lists available to the public)*
Membership Fee: $75 Year-Organizations; $10 Year-Individuals
Library:
HIV/AIDS Resource Centre *(Open to the public)*

◈ **Yukon:**
Languages: English

◇ **Yukon:**
307 Strickland St, Whitehorse YT Y1A 2J9
867 633-2437; Fax: 867 633-2447
Toll-free: 877 333-2437
E: bloodties@klondiker.com
W: www.bloodties.ca
Executive:
HIV/HCV Counsellor: Leigh Ayton
Exec Dir: Patricia Bacon
Health Promo Worker: Amelia Merhar
Year Founded: 1993
No of Paid Staff: 6
Library: Y *(Open to the public)*
Languages: English
Membership: 30 *(Lists available to the public)*
Membership Fee: Individual - $10; Family - $15; Corporate - $25

Interagency Coalition on AIDS and Development
726-1 Nicholas St, Ottawa ON K1N 7B7
613 233-7440; Fax: 613 233-8361
E: info@icad-cisd.com
W: www.icad-cisd.com
Executive:
Pres: Daniel Townsend
VP: Marnie Davidson
Exec Dir: Nicci Stein
Treas: Anne Garder
Sec: Tricia Smith
Admv Off: Kate Alexander
Sr Prog Officer: Shayna Buhler
Year Founded: 1990
Criteria: *All Canadian voluntary sector organizations, including international development NGOs, AIDS service organizations, universities, research institutes, and individuals that support the mission of ICAD are eligible to join.*
Budget: $800,000
No of Paid Staff: 4
Speakers Available
Library: Y *(Open to the public)*
Languages: English; French
Membership: 100+ *(Lists available to the public)*
Membership Fee: Ranges from $25 - $300 per year

ALLERGIES

Allergy/Asthma Information Association
118-295 The West Mall, Toronto ON M9C 4Z4
416 621-4571; Fax: 416 621-5034
Toll-free: 800 611-7011
E: national@aaia.ca
W: www.aaia.ca
Executive:
Exec Dir: Mary Allen
Sls/Membership Admin: Fauzia Adamally
Year Founded: 1964
Speakers Available
Languages: French
Membership: 3,000

◈ **Prairies/Northwest Territories:**
16531 114 St NW, Edmonton AB T5X 3V6
780 456-6651; Fax: 780 456-6651
Toll-free: 866 456-6651
E: prairies@aaia.ca
W: www.aaia.ca
Year Founded: 1964
Languages: English

◈ **British Columbia/Yukon:**
4730 Redridge Rd, Kelowna BC V1W 3A6
250 764-7507; Fax: 250 764-7587
Toll-free: 877 500-2242
E: bc@aaia.ca
W: www.aaia.ca
Executive:
Reg Coord: Yvonne Rousseau
Year Founded: 1964
Criteria: *Open to all.*
No of Paid Staff: 1
Speakers Available
Languages: English; French
Membership Fee: $35

◈ **Bedford NS**
70 Snowy Owl Dr, Bedford NS B4A 3L3
Toll-free: 800 611-7011
E: atlantic@aaia.ca
W: www.aaia.ca
Executive:
Reg Coord: Ruth Roberts

◈ **Collingwood**
30 Patten St, Collingwood ON L9Y 0E4
705 444-0477; Fax: 705 444-5705
Toll-free: 888 250-2298
E: ontario@aaia.ca
W: www.aaia.ca

ALZHEIMER'S

Alzheimer Society London and Middlesex
435 Windermere Rd, London ON N5X 2T1
519 680-2404; Fax: 519 680-2864
Toll-free: 888 495-5855
E: info@alzheimerlondon.ca
W: www.alzheimerlondon.ca
Executive:
CEO: Betsy Little
Commun Mgr: Bruce Wray
Intake Coord: Betty Rutledge
First Link Prog Coord: Nancy O'Regan
Pub Educ Coor/Hum Res Advisor: Susan Oster
Fund Dev Coord: Leslie Rand
Social Worker: Rick Bunt
Social Worker: Brooke Hurley
Social Worker: Carolyn Underwood
Spec Event Coord: Brenda Miedema
Acct Coord/Ops Coord: Rose Brochu
Hlthy Community Proj/Volunteer Serv Coord: Rae Belcourt
Year Founded: 1982
Criteria: *Open to all.*
Budget: $1,000,000
No of Paid Staff: 15
Speakers Available
Library: Y *(Open to the public)*
Languages: English
Membership: 230 *(Lists available to the public)*
Membership Fee: $15
Library:
Resource Centre *(Open to the public)*

Alzheimer Society of Belleville-Hastings-Quinte
Belleville Shopping Plaza
470 Dundas St E, Belleville ON K8N 1G1
613 962-0892; Fax: 613 962-1225
Toll-free: 800 361-8036
E: info@alzheimersocietyofbhq.com
W: www.alzheimersocietyofbhq.com
Year Founded: 1987
Budget: $159,000
No of Paid Staff: 4
Speakers Available
Library: Y *(Open to the public)*
Languages: English
Membership: 100
Membership Fee: $10-$15/year
Library:
Alzheimer Society Resource Centre *(Open to the public)*

Alzheimer Society of Calgary
201-222 58 Ave SW, Calgary AB T2H 2S3
403 290-0110; Fax: 403 269-8836
Toll-free: 877 569-4357
E: info@alzheimercalgary.com
W: www.alzheimercalgary.com
Executive:
Exec Dir: Barbara Ferguson
Year Founded: 1981
Languages: English

Alzheimer Society of Cambridge
1145 Concession Rd, Cambridge ON N3H 4L5
519 650-1628; Fax: 519 650-1629
E: admin@alzheimercambridge.on.ca
W: www.alzheimercambridge.on.ca
Executive:
Exec Dir: Dr Jennifer Gillies
Year Founded: 1991
Budget: $200,000
No of Paid Staff: 4
Speakers Available
Library: Y *(Open to the public)*
Languages: English
Membership: 80
Membership Fee: $10-$15/year

Alzheimer Society of Canada
1600-20 Eglinton Ave W, Toronto ON M4R 1K8
416 967-5900; Fax: 416 967-3826
Toll-free: 800 879-4226 only in Canada
E: staff@alzheimeront.org
W: www.alzheimer.ca
Year Founded: 1978
Budget: $4,006,087
No of Paid Staff: 24
Library: Y
Languages: English; French

◈ ***Alberta:***
10531 Kingsway NW, Edmonton AB T5H 4K1
780 488-2266; Fax: 780 488-3055
Toll-free: 866 950-5465 Alberta only
E: info@alzheimer.ab.ca
W: www.alzheimer.ab.ca
Executive:
Mgr-Client Serv/Prog: Arlene Huhn
Year Founded: 1988
Criteria: *Support group or regional office of the society.*
Budget: $1,500,000
No of Paid Staff: 25
Speakers Available
Library: Y *(Open to the public)*
Languages: English
Membership list available to the public

◇ ***Grande Prairie:***
10531 Kingsway NW, Edmonton AB T5H 4K1
780 488-2266; Fax: 780 488-3055
Toll-free: 866 950-5465
E: info@alzheimer.ab.ca
W: www.alzheimer.ab.ca
Executive:
CEO: B Gaudette

◇ ***Lethbridge and Area:***
402-740 4 Ave S, Lethbridge AB T1J 0N9
403 329-3766; Fax: 403 327-3711
Toll-free: 888 329-3766
W: www.alzheimer.ab.ca
Executive:
Mgr: Brenda Hill
Year Founded: 1983
No of Paid Staff: 2
Speakers Available
Library: Y *(Open to the public)*
Languages: English
Membership: 35
Membership Fee: $15/Year
Library:
Lending Library *(Open to the public)*

◇ ***Palliser:***
401D 3 St SE, Medicine Hat AB T1A 0G8
403 528-2700; Fax: 403 526-4994
E: palliser1@alzheimer.ab.ca
W: www.alzheimer.ab.ca
Executive:
Community Rel Coord: Alariss Schmid
Client Serv Coord: Brenda Lorencz

◇ ***Red Deer and Central Alberta:***
101-4805 48 Ave, Red Deer AB T4N 3T2
403 346-2540; Fax: 403 342-0448
E: reddeer@alzheimer.ab.ca
W: www.alzheimer.ab.ca
Executive:
Reg Mgr: Donna Durand
Dir-Commun: Tash Taylor

◇ ***Wood Buffalo:***
Mailing: Redpoll Centre, 207-10010 Franklin Ave, Fort McMurray AB T9H 2K6
780 743-6175; Fax: 780 791-0088
Toll-free Fax: 866 950-5465

◇ ***Yellowknife:***
1-5710 50 Ave, Yellowknife NT X1A 1G1
867 669-9390; Fax: 403 250-8251

◈ ***British Columbia:***
300-828 8th Ave W, Vancouver BC V5Z 1E2
604 681-6530; Fax: 604 669-6907
Toll-free: 800 667-3742
E: info@alzheimerbc.org
W: www.alzheimerbc.org
Executive:
Pres: Bob Hastings
Past Pres: Nicole Bertrand
CEO: Jean Blake
VP: Jeff Woodburn
Sr Mgr-Reg Serv: Kathy Kennedy
Year Founded: 1981
Speakers Available
Library: Y *(Open to the public)*
Languages: English

◇ ***Kelowna***
865 Bernard Ave, Kelowna BC V1Y 6P6
250 860-0305; Fax: 250 860-0418
Toll-free: 800 634-3399
W: www.alzheimerbc.org
Executive:
First Link Coord: Lila Sofonoff
Coord-Minds in Motion: Melanie Wasylyshen
No of Paid Staff: 3
Speakers Available
Library: Y *(Open to the public)*
Languages: English

◈ ***Manitoba:***
10-120 Donald St, Winnipeg MB R3C 4G2
204 943-6622; Fax: 204 942-5408
Toll-free: 800 378-6699
E: alzmb@alzheimer.mb.ca
W: www.alzheimer.mb.ca
Executive:
CEO: Sylvia Rothney
Prog Dir: Norma Kirkby
Dir-Fin/Admn: Sarbjit Bal
Commun/Event Mgr: Kimberly Mardero
No of Paid Staff: 15
Speakers Available
Library: Y *(Open to the public)*
Languages: English

◈ ***New Brunswick:***
Location: 100-320 Maple St, Fredericton NB E3A 3R4
Mailing: PO Box 1553 Stn A, Fredericton NB E3B 5G2
506 459-4280; Fax: 506 452-0313
Toll-free: 800 664-8411
E: info@alzheimernb.ca
W: www.alzheimernb.ca
Year Founded: 1987
Budget: $240,000
No of Paid Staff: 3
Speakers Available
Library: Y
Languages: English; French
Membership list available to the public
Library:
Resource Library *(Open to the public)*

◇ ***Miramichi***
Location: 222 Wellington St, Miramichi NB E1N 1N1
Mailing: PO Box 205 Stn Chatham, Miramichi NB E1N 3A6
506 773-7093; Fax: 506 773-7093
Toll-free: 800 664-8411
E: alzmir@nb.aibn.com
Executive:
Pres: Kathy Campbell
Year Founded: 1993
No of Paid Staff: 1
Speakers Available
Library: Y *(Open to the public)*
Languages: English; French
Library:
Alzheimer Society Lending Library *(Open to the public)*

◈ ***Newfoundland and Labrador:***
Location: 685 Water St, St. John's NL A1E 1C2
Mailing: PO Box 37013 Rpo Water St West, St. John's NL A1E 5Y2
709 576-0608; Fax: 709 576-0798
Toll-free: 877 776-0608
E: alzheimersociety@nf.aibn.com
W: www.alzheimernl.org
No of Paid Staff: 5
Speakers Available
Library: Y *(Open to the public)*
Languages: English

◈ ***Nova Scotia:***
112-2717 Gladstone St, Halifax NS B3K 0A4
902 422-7961; Fax: 902 422-7971
Toll-free: 800 611-6345
W: www.alzheimer.ca/ns
Executive:
Pres: John Mullowney
VP: Chris Wilson
Exec Dir: Lloyd Brown
Prog/Dir-Servs: Linda Bird
Dir-Fin/Admin: Carla Dolomont
Mgr-Comm/Media Rels: Michele Charlton
Mgr-Fund Dev: Sarah Lyon
Year Founded: 1982
No of Paid Staff: 12
Speakers Available
Library: Y
Languages: English
Membership Fee: $15 Per Year

◈ ***Prince Edward Island:***
166 Fitzroy St, Charlottetown PE C1A 1S1
902 628-2257; Fax: 902 368-2715
Toll-free: 866 628-2257
E: society@alzpei.ca
W: www.alzheimer.ca/pei
Executive:
CEO: C Hendricken-Eldershaw
Year Founded: 1991
Budget: $150,000
No of Paid Staff: 8
Speakers Available
Library: Y *(Open to the public)*
Languages: English

◈ ***Quebec:***
Immeuble Commercial
211-5165 rue Sherbrooke O, Montréal QC H4A 1T6
514 369-7891; Fax: 514 369-7900
Toll-free: 888 636-6473
E: info@alzheimerquebec.ca
W: www.alzheimerquebec.ca
Executive:
Dir gén: Diane Roch
Year Founded: 1986
No of Paid Staff: 4
Languages: French; English

◇ ***Bas-Saint-Laurent***
114 av Saint-Jérôme, Matane QC G4W 3A2
418 562-2144; Fax: 418 562-7449
Toll-free: 877 446-2144
E: info@alzheimer-bsl.com
W: www.alzheimer-bsl.com
Executive:
Prés: Céline Lefrançois
Dir gén: Josée Lefrançois
Intervenante/animatrice/formatrice: Anne Tremblay
Year Founded: 1995
No of Paid Staff: 20

HEALTHCARE ASSOCIATIONS

Library: Y
Languages: French
Membership: 98
Membership Fee: $10
Library:
Centre de documentation *(Open to the public)*

◇ ***Centre du Québec***
880 rue Côté, St-Charles-de-Drum QC J2C 4Z7
819 474-3666; Fax: 819 474-3133
E: glamoureux@alzheimer-centre-du-quebec.org
W: www.alzheimer-centre-du-quebec.org
Executive:
Dir gén: Ghislaine Lamoureux
Languages: French

◇ ***Chaudière-Appalaches***
Location: 440 boul Vachon S, Sainte-Marie QC G6E 1X9
Mailing: CP 1 Succ Bureau-Chef, Sainte-Marie QC G6E 3B4
418 387-1230; Fax: 418 387-1360
Toll-free: 888 387-1230
E: sachap@globetrotter.net
W: www.alzheimerchap.qc.ca
Executive:
Dir gén: Sonia Nadeau
Year Founded: 1997
No of Paid Staff: 9
Speakers Available
Library: Y *(Open to the public)*
Languages: French; English
Membership: 150

◇ ***Chibougamau-Chapais***
Location: 32 3e Ave, Chapais QC G0W 1H0
Mailing: CP 1300
418 745-2591 247; Fax: 418 745-3038
Executive:
Dir gén: Nathalie Boisvert
Adj admin: Linda Boisvert

◇ ***Cote-Nord:***
373 av Jolliet, Sept-Îles QC G4R 2B1
418 968-4673; Fax: 418 962-4161
Toll-free: 866 366-4673
E: coord.sacn@globetrotter.net

◇ ***Domaine-du-Roy et Maria Chapdelaine:***
Location: CLSC des Prés-Blues, 1228 boul du Sacré-Coeur, Saint-Félicien QC G8K 2R2
Mailing: 1209 boul du Sacré-Coeur, CP 10 Succ Bureau-Chef, Saint-Félicien QC G8K 2P8
418 679-5270 8412; Fax: 418 275-7118
Toll-free: 877 668-0161
E: melfort@live.ca
W: www.alzheimersagamie.com
Executive:
Conseillière: Mélissa Fortin
Dir gén: Josée Pearson

◇ ***Estrie***
Édifice Norton
0625-375 rue Argyll, Sherbrooke QC J1J 3H5
819 821-5127; Fax: 819 820-8649
E: info@alzheimerestrie.com
W: www.alzheimerestrie.com
Executive:
Conseillière auprès des familles: Danielle Yergeau
Dir gén: Caroline Giguère
Agente commun/dév: Geneviève Lapointe
Year Founded: 1985
No of Paid Staff: 15
Speakers Available
Languages: French; English
Membership: 250

◇ ***Gaspésie Les Îles***
114C av Grand-Pré, Bonaventure QC G0C 1E0
418 534-1313; Fax: 418 534-1312
Toll-free: 866 380-4959
E: bernard.sagim@navigue.com
W: www.alzheimerquebec.ca
Languages: French
Membership: 185

◇ ***Granby et Région***
201-66 rue Court, Granby QC J2G 4Y5
450 777-3363; Fax: 450 777-8677
E: sagrinfo@videotron.ca
W: alzheimergranby.ca
Executive:
Dir gén: Julie Desgranges
Dir/Coord: Diane Laliberté
No of Paid Staff: 2
Languages: French

◇ ***Haut-Richelieu***
Location: 2-125 rue Jacques-Cartier N, St-Jean-sur-Richel QC J3B 8C9
Mailing: CP 485 succ Bureau-Chef, St-Jean-sur-Richel QC J3B 6Z8
450 347-5500; Fax: 450 347-7370
Toll-free: 514 990-8262
E: info@sahr.ca
W: www.sahr.ca
Executive:
Dir gén: Lise Marcoux

◇ ***L'Outaouais***
380 boul Saint-Raymond, Gatineau QC J9A 1V9
819 777-4232; Fax: 819 777-0728
Toll-free: 877 777-0888
E: saoq@saoq.org
W: www.saoq.org
Executive:
Dir gén: Hubert Grégoire
Coord: Marisol Pizarro
Budget: $1,100,000
No of Paid Staff: 31
Speakers Available
Library: Y *(Open to the public)*
Languages: French
Membership: 140 *(Lists available to the public)*

◇ ***La Baie-Bas-Saguenay***
Foyer Bagotville
562 rue Victoria, La Baie QC G7B 3M6
418 544-4964; Fax: 418 668-2639
W: www.alzheimerquebec.ca
Executive:
Conseiller: René Tremblay

◇ ***Labal***
2525 boul René-Laennec, Laval QC H7K 0B2
450 975-0966 230; Fax: 450 975-0517
E: info@alzheimerlaval.org
W: www.alzheimerlaval.org
Executive:
Dir gén: Lise Lalande
Year Founded: 1995
No of Paid Staff: 27
Library: Y *(Open to the public)*
Languages: French
Membership: 200

◇ ***Lanaudière***
190 rue Montcalm, Joliette QC J6E 5G4
450 759-3057; Fax: 450 760-2633
Toll-free: 877 759-3077
E: sadl@videotron.ca
Executive:
Prés: Jean-François Denault
Dir gén: Janie Duval

◇ ***Laurentides***
Location: 37 rue Principale E, étage 2, Ste-Agathe-des-Mts QC J8C 1J5
Mailing: CP 276, Ste-Agathe-des-Mts QC J8C 3A3
819 326-7136; Fax: 819 326-9664
Toll-free: 800 978-7881
E: salaurentides@bellnet.ca
W: www.alzheimerlaurentides.com
Executive:
Dir gén: Catherine Vaudry
Year Founded: 1983
Languages: English; French

◇ ***Maison J. Arthur Desjardins***
11 av d'Amours, Matane QC G4W 2X3
418 562-2110; Fax: 418 562-7449
W: www.alzheimerquebec.ca

◇ ***Maskoutains-Vallée des Patriotes***
1955 av Pratte, Saint-Hyacinthe QC J2S 7W5
450 771-4536 6218; Fax: 450 771-5499
E: caroline.croteau@rrsss16.gouv.qc.ca
Executive:
Coord: Caroline Croteau
Languages: French

◇ ***Mauricie - Maison CARPE DIEM***
1765 boul Saint-Louis, Trois-Rivières QC G8Z 2N7
819 376-7063; Fax: 819 376-3538
W: www.alzheimercarpediem.com
Executive:
Prés: Jean Poliquin
VP: Denyse Bellemare
Dir: Nicole Poirier
Trés: Caroline Gélinas
Sec: Marguerite Paquet
Coord: Marie-Claude Savard
Adj: Marianne Vaveluy

◇ ***Montreal:***
410-5165 rue Sherbrooke O, Montréal QC H4A 1T6
514 369-0800; Fax: 514 369-4103
E: info@alzheimermontreal.ca
W: www.alzheimermontreal.ca
Executive:
Dir gén: Gérald Hubert
Year Founded: 1981
Budget: $1,600,000
No of Paid Staff: 40
Speakers Available
Library: Y *(Open to the public)*
Languages: English; French
Membership: 500
Membership Fee: $20 Family; $20 'Friend'

◇ ***Québec***
312-1040 av Belvédère, Québec QC G1S 3G3
418 527-4294; Fax: 418 527-9966
Toll-free: 866 350-4294
E: hthibault@societealzheimerdequebec.com
W: www.societealzheimerdequebec.com
Executive:
Dir gén: Hélène Thibault

◇ ***Rive-Sud***
1160 boul Nobert, Longueuil QC J4K 2P1
450 442-3333; Fax: 450 442-9271
E: info@alzheimerrivesud.ca
W: www.alzheimerrivesud.ca
Executive:
Dir gén: Geneviève Grégoire
Languages: French

◇ ***Rouyn-Noranda***
Location: 58 rue Monseigneur-Tessier E, Rouyn-Noranda QC J9X 3B9
Mailing: CP 336 succ Bureau-Chef, Rouyn-Noranda QC J9X 5C3
819 764-3554; Fax: 819 764-3534
E: sam@cablevision.qc.ca
Executive:
Consultante: Ginette Blouin
Coord: Guillaume Parent

◇ ***Sagamie-Saguenay - Lac St-Jean***
1657 av du Pont N, Alma QC G8B 5G2
418 668-0161; Fax: 418 668-2639
Toll-free: 877 668-0161
E: alzheimersag@bellnet.ca
W: www.alzheimersagamie.com
Executive:
Dir gén: Josée Pearson

◇ ***Suroît***
101-340 boul du Havre, Salaber-de-Valleyf QC J6S 1S6
450 373-0303; Fax: 450 373-0388
Toll-free: 877 773-0303
E: lsauve@alzheimersuroit.com
W: www.alzheimersuroit.com
Executive:
Dir gén: Lorraine Sauvé
Year Founded: 1998
No of Paid Staff: 12
Library: Y *(Open to the public)*
Languages: French; English

◇ ***Vallée de l'Or***
734 4E Av, Val-d'Or QC J9P 1J2
819 825-7444; Fax: 819 825-7448
E: sco.alz.valdor@tlb.sympatico.ca
Executive:
Coord: Danielle Lapointe
No of Paid Staff: 1
Languages: French

◈ ***Saskatchewan:***
301-2550 12th Ave, Regina SK S4P 3X1
306 949-4141; Fax: 306 949-3069
Toll-free: 800 263-3367
E: info@alzheimer.sk.ca
W: www.alzheimer.sk.ca
Executive:
CEO: Joanne Bracken
Fin/Admn Mgr: Kathleen Defoe
Fund Dev/Commun Mgr: Kristina Gebhard
Prog Serv Mgr: Joanne Michael
Year Founded: 1982
Criteria: *Payment of fees.*
Budget: $1,000,000
No of Paid Staff: 12
Speakers Available
Library: Y *(Open to the public)*
Languages: English
Membership: 250
Membership Fee: $15/year

Alzheimer Society of Greater Simcoe County
Location: 103-12 Fairview Rd, Barrie ON L4N 4P3
Mailing: PO Box 1414 Stn Main, Barrie ON L4M 5R4
705 722-1066; Fax: 705 722-9392
Toll-free: 800 265-5391
E: alzgsc@alzheimersociety.ca
W: www.alzheimer.ca/gsc
Executive:
Educ Coord: Laura-Lynn Bourassa
Support Counsellor: Melissa Martinson
Support Counsellor: Heidi Haupt
Exec Dir: Debbie Islam
Support Serv Coord: Leslie Nemisz
Coord-Volunteers: Marguerite Glanfield
Fund Dev Coord: Erika Rice
Social Worker Behavioural Support Mobile Team: Donna Gordon
Social Worker Behavioural Support Mobile Team: Stephanie Saunders
Occup Ther Behavioural Support Mobile Team: Jennifer Keresztesi
Year Founded: 1985
Criteria: *Open to all persons upon receipt of application and payment of dues.*
No of Paid Staff: 12
Speakers Available
Library: Y *(Open to the public)*
Languages: English
Membership: 136
Library:
Resource Centre *(Open to the public)*

Alzheimer Society of Guelph-Wellington
111 MacDonell St, Guelph ON N1H 2Z7
519 836-7672; Fax: 519 836-1041
E: office@alzheimer.guelph.org
W: www.alzheimer.guelph.org
Executive:
Exec Dir: Paul Visschedyk
Public Educ Coord: Robin Smart
Family Supp Cord: Kayla Belanger
Office Admin/Fundraiser: Rachel Hopf
Year Founded: 1987
Budget: $200,000
No of Paid Staff: 5
Speakers Available
Library: Y *(Open to the public)*
Languages: English
Membership: 135
Membership Fee: $15

Alzheimer Society of North East Simcoe County
Location: Trillium Manor, 169 Front St S, Orillia ON L3V 4S8
Mailing: PO Box 486 Stn Main, Orillia ON L3V 6K2
705 329-0909; Fax: 705 329-2378
E: info@alzheimerorillia.com
W: www.alzheimerorillia.com
Executive:
Exec Dir: Leila Sherriff
Counsellor: Susan Nagy
Year Founded: 1986
Criteria: *Open to all.*
No of Paid Staff: 1
Library: Y *(Open to the public)*
Languages: English

Alzheimer Society Peel
60 Briarwood Ave, Mississauga ON L5G 3N6
905 278-3667; Fax: 905 278-3964
W: www.alzheimerpeel.com
Executive:
CEO: Christopher Rawn-Kane
Year Founded: 1984
No of Paid Staff: 100

AMYOTROPHIC LATERAL SCLEROSIS

ALS Ontario
402-3100 Steeles Ave E, Markham ON L3R 8T3
905 248-2101; Fax: 905 248-5620
Toll-free: 866 611-8545
E: info@alsont.ca
W: www.alsont.ca
Executive:
Pres/CEO: Maureen Sheahan
Exec Asst/Office Mgr: Frida Mazarello

Amyotrophic Lateral Sclerosis Society of Canada
200-3000 Steeles Ave E, Markham ON L3R 4T9
905 248-2052; Fax: 905 248-2019
Toll-free: 800 267-4257
E: info@als.ca
W: www.als.ca
Executive:
Pres: Mike Gardner
Dir-Dev: Eno Raponi
Dir-Fin: Karen Hunter
Dir-Research: David Taylor
Year Founded: 1988
Criteria: *Open to any person with an interest in the objects of the society and who pays a membership fee.*
No of Paid Staff: 11
Speakers Available
Languages: English; French
Membership: 500
Membership Fee: $25

◈ ***Alberta:***
250-4723 1 St SW, Calgary AB T2G 4Y8
403 228-3857; Fax: 403 228-7752
Toll-free: 888 309-1111
E: info@alsab.ca
W: www.alsab.ca
Executive:
Chm: Cathy Martin
Exec Dir: Karen Caughey
Mgr-Resource Dev/Commun: Rahael Chester
Year Founded: 1986
No of Paid Staff: 9
Speakers Available
Library: Y *(Open to the public)*
Languages: English
Membership: 150
Membership Fee: $10; Free to those with ALS

◈ ***Manitoba:***
493 Madison St, Winnipeg MB R3J 1J2
204 831-1510; Fax: 204 837-9023
Toll-free: 866 718-1642
E: HOPE@alsmb.ca
W: www.alsmb.ca
Executive:
Pres: Lorna McLeod
Exec Dir/Client Serv Coord: Diana Rasmussen
Treas: George Pastera
Office Mgr: Sharon Carter
Year Founded: 1986
No of Paid Staff: 4
Speakers Available
Library: Y *(Open to the public)*
Languages: English
Membership list available to the public

◈ ***New Brunswick***
Mailing: PO Box 295 Stn Main, Moncton NB E1C 8K9
506 532-5786; Fax: 506 388-7466
Toll-free: 866 722-7700
E: info@alsnb.ca
W: www.alsnb.ca
Executive:
Exec Dir: Carol Cottrill
Library: Y
Languages: English; French
Membership: 50

◈ ***Newfoundland:***
Location: Downtown Health Centre, 3 Herald Ave, Corner Brook NL A2H 4B8
Mailing: PO Box 844 Stn Main, Corner Brook NL A2H 6H6
709 634-9499
Toll-free: 888 364-9499
E: alssocietyofnfld@nf.aibn.com
W: www.envision.ca/webs/alsnl
Executive:
Pres: Peter Puddester
Year Founded: 1988
No of Paid Staff: 1
Speakers Available
Library: Y *(Open to the public)*
Languages: English
Membership: 100
Membership Fee: Others - $25; Patients/Families - Free

HEALTHCARE ASSOCIATIONS

◈ ***Ottawa***
204A-1150 Morrison Dr, Ottawa ON K2H 8S9
613 820-2267; Fax: 613 820-2255
Toll-free: 866 858-4226
W: www.alsont.ca
Executive:
Reg Dir: Tracey Martin
Reg Dir: Lianne Johnston

◈ ***Nova Scotia***
Location: 7071 Bayers Rd, Halifax NS B3L 4T7
Mailing: PO Box 22112 RPO Bayers Road
902 454-3636; Fax: 902 453-3646
Toll-free: 866 625-7257
E: info@alsns.ca
W: www.alsns.ca
Executive:
Pres/CEO: Kimberly Carter
Languages: English

Amyotrophic Lateral Sclerosis Society -Victoria Chapter
Location: 3335 Oak St, Victoria BC V8X 3G2
Mailing: PO Box 43054 RPO Victoria N
250 598-4172; Fax: 604 278-4257
Executive:
Pres (Victoria Chapter): George Stewardson
Treas (Victoria Chapter): Merle Stewardson

ARTHRITIS

The Arthritis Society - National Office
1700-393 University Ave, Toronto ON M5G 1E6
416 979-7228; Fax: 416 979-8366
E: info@arthritis.ca
W: www.arthritis.ca
Executive:
Chair: Ken Ready
Pres/CEO: Janet Yale
Sr Dir-Info Tech: Nigel Carpenter
No of Paid Staff: 50
Languages: English
Membership: 600
Membership Fee: $15 -$20

◈ ***Alberta and Northwest Territories:***
300-1301 8 St SW, Calgary AB T2R 1B7
403 228-2571; Fax: 403 229-4232
Toll-free: 800 321-1433
E: info@ab.arthritis.ca
W: www.arthritis.ca
Executive:
I-Exec Dir: Shirley Philips
Year Founded: 1948
Criteria: *Membership fees*
Budget: $2,900,000
No of Paid Staff: 11
Speakers Available
Library: Y
Languages: English
Membership: 500
Membership Fee: $30

◇ ***Northern Region:A***
307-10109 106 St NW, Edmonton AB T5J 3L7
780 424-1740; Fax: 780 428-6198
Toll-free: 800 321-1433
E: info@ab.arthritis.ca
W: www.arthritis.ca/alberta
Executive:
Exec Dir: Shirley Philips
Speakers Available
Library: Y *(Open to the public)*
Languages: English

◈ ***British Columbia and Yukon Region:***
101-1645 7th Ave W, Vancouver BC V6J 1S4
604 714-5550; Fax: 604 714-5555
Toll-free: 866 414-7766
E: info@bc.arthritis.ca
W: www.arthritis.ca
Year Founded: 1948
Speakers Available
Library: Y *(Open to the public)*
Languages: English

◇ ***Fraser Regional Centre:***
Fraser Arthritis Centre
101-5501 204 St, Langley BC V3A 5N8
604 514-9902; Fax: 604 514-0401
Toll-free: 800 321-1433 Arthritis Answers Line
E: info@arthritis.ca
W: www.arthritis.ca
Year Founded: 1948
Speakers Available
Library: Y *(Open to the public)*
Languages: English; French

◇ ***Kelowna:***
150A-1855 Kirschner Rd, Kelowna BC V1Y 4N7
250 868-8643; Fax: 250 868-0779
W: www.arthritis.ca

◇ ***Vancouver:***
895 10th Ave W, Main Floor, Vancouver BC V5Z 1L7
604 875-5051; Fax: 604 875-5048
Toll-free: 800 321-1433
E: info@bc.arthritis.ca
W: www.arthritis.ca/bc

◇ ***Victoria:***
2680 Richmond Rd, Victoria BC V8R 4S9
250 519-4000; Fax: 250 598-1901
Toll-free: 800 321-1433
E: info@bc.arthritis.ca
W: www.arthritis.ca
Year Founded: 1948
Speakers Available
Library: Y *(Open to the public)*
Membership: 450

◈ ***Manitoba:***
105-386 Broadway, Winnipeg MB R3C 3R6
204 942-4892; Fax: 204 942-4894
Toll-free: 800 321-1433
E: info@mb.arthritis.ca
W: www.arthritis.ca
Executive:
Exec Dir: Carol Hiscock
Admv Asst: Sheliza Wheatland
No of Paid Staff: 8
Speakers Available
Library: Y *(Open to the public)*
Languages: English

◈ ***New Brunswick:***
107-146 Main St, Fredericton NB E3A 1C8
506 452-7191; Fax: 506 459-3925
Toll-free: 800 321-1433
E: info@nb.arthritis.ca
W: www.arthritis.ca
Executive:
Exec Dir: Susan Tilley-Russell
Commun Educ Coord: Krista Phillips
Year Founded: 1950
No of Paid Staff: 5
Speakers Available
Languages: English; French
Membership: 1,000
Membership Fee: $5

◈ ***Newfoundland and Labrador:***
78 O'Leary Ave, St. John's NL A1B 2C7
709 579-8190; Fax: 709 579-8191
Toll-free: 800 321-1433
E: info@nl.arthritis.ca
W: www.arthritis.ca/nl
Executive:
Exec Dir Atlantic Reg: S Tilley-Russell
Dir-Dev Atlantic Reg: Jone Mitchell
Year Founded: 1973
Criteria: *Persons with arthritis or having an interest in arthritis.*
Budget: $600,000
No of Paid Staff: 3
Speakers Available
Library: Y *(Open to the public)*
Languages: English
Membership: 750
Library:
Arthritis Lending Library *(Open to the public)*

◈ ***Nova Scotia :***
210-3770 Kempt Rd, Halifax NS B3K 4X8
902 429-7025; Fax: 902 423-6479
Toll-free: 800 321-1433
E: info@ns.arthritis.ca
W: www.arthritis.ca/novascotia
Executive:
Exec Dir Atlantic Reg: Susan Tilley-Russell
Dir-Dev Atlantic Reg: Jone Mitchell
Accntg Coord: Sue Keenan
Year Founded: 1948
Budget: $900,000
No of Paid Staff: 7
Speakers Available
Library: Y *(Open to the public)*
Languages: English; French
Membership: 7,000 +

◈ ***Algoma, Temiskaming and Districst:***
316 Wellington St W, Sault Ste. Marie ON P6A 1J1
705 253-7750; Fax: 705 253-7900
Toll-free: 888 253-7752
W: www.arthritis.ca
Executive:
Physiotherapist: Mary Ellen Marcon

◈ ***Grey - Bruce:***
210B-1717 2nd Ave E, Owen Sound ON N4K 6V4
519 372-0060; Fax: 519 372-0056
E: info@on.arthritis.ca
W: www.arthritis.ca

◈ ***Halton & Peel Region:***
214-40 Finchgate Blvd, Brampton ON L6T 3J1
905 455-6273; Fax: 905 455-6989
Toll-free: 888 434-0009
W: www.arthritis.ca
Executive:
Mgr: Lorna Catranbone
Admin: Kim Rainford
Year Founded: 1948
No of Paid Staff: 2
Languages: English

◈ ***Hamilton & Halton Region:***
Upper Canada Place
11-460 Brant St, Burlington ON L7R 4B6
905 632-9390; Fax: 905 632-6801
Toll-free: 866 273-2229
E: info@on.arthritis.ca
W: www.arthritis.ca
Executive:
Coord-Community Engagement: Heather Pickles
Specialist-Community Engagement: Lorna Anstruther
Speakers Available

◈ ***Hamilton & Niagara:***
218-245 Pelham Rd, St Catharines ON L2S 1X8
905 646-7284; Fax: 905 646-0513
E: info@on.arthritis.ca
W: www.arthritis.ca
Executive:
Specialist-Community Engagement: Lorna Anstruther

◈ ***Kenora & Rainy River Districts:***
35 Wolsley St, Kenora ON P9N 0H8
807 468-2298; Fax: 807 468-1284
W: www.arthritis.ca

◈ ***Kingston Region:***
The Kidd House
100 Stuart St, Room 114, Kingston ON K7L 2V6
613 546-2546; Fax: 613 546-3819
Toll-free: 800 410-4033
W: www.arthritis.ca
Executive:
Dir-Eastern ON: Phil Ambury
Fundraising Mgr Reg Dev: Nancy Lawlor

◈ ***London, Middelsex County:***
204-400 York St, London ON N6B 3N2
519 433-2191; Fax: 519 433-7035
Toll-free: 866 466-0501
E: info@on.arthritis.ca
W: www.arthritis.ca
Executive:
Dir-Reg/Volunteer Dev: Margaret Wills
Rsch/Dev Mgr: Shelly White

◈ ***Muskoka & Parry Sound Districts:***
110-95 Manitoba St, Bracebridge ON P1L 2B3
705 645-8548; Fax: 705 645-8548

◈ ***Ottawa:***
20-2269 Riverside Dr, Ottawa ON K1H 8K2
613 723-1083; Fax: 613 723-1172
Toll-free: 800 410-4033
E: info@on.arthritis.ca
W: www.arthritis.ca
Executive:
Specialist-Community
Engagement: Melissa Courmier
Commun Engagement Mgr: Jason Hussak

◈ ***Sudbury***
202-10 Elm St, Sudbury ON P3C 5N3
705 673-4641; Fax: 705 673-2337
Toll-free: 800 224-0296
E: mhussak@on.arthritis.ca
W: www.arthritis.ca
Executive:
Mgr-Reg Development: Jana Schilkie
Year Founded: 1948

◈ ***Toronto & Central East Ontario:***

◇ ***Peterborough:***
20B-159 King St, Peterborough ON K9J 2R8
705 742-7191; Fax: 705 742-3560
Executive:
Dir-Client Serv: Susan Ross
Commty Engmnt Spec: Karen Thomson
Occup Ther/Physiotherapist: Osk Jenkins
Year Founded: 1948
Speakers Available
Languages: English

◇ ***Muskoka and Parry Sound Districts:***
110-95 Manitoba St, Bracebridge ON P1L 2B3
705 645-8548; Fax: 705 645-8548

◈ ***Toronto, York Region & Simcoe County:***
1700-393 University Ave, Toronto ON M5G 1E6
416 979-7228; Fax: 416 979-8366
Toll-free: 800 321-1433
E: info@on.arthritis.ca
W: www.arthritis.ca
Executive:
Dir: Susan Ross
Year Founded: 1948

◈ ***Waterloo Region & Wellington County***
9-41 River Rd E, Kitchener ON N2B 2G3
519 743-2820; Fax: 519 743-4142
Toll-free: 800 854-6445
W: www.arthritis.ca
Executive:
Dir-Prog/Serv: Lynne Tintse
Fundraising Mgr Reg Dev: Shirley Mitchell

◈ ***PEI:***
Liesure World Building
95 Capital Dr, Charlottetown PE C1E 1E8
902 628-2288; Fax: 902 628-6035
Toll-free: 800 321-1433
E: info@pe.arthritis.ca
W: www.arthritis.ca/pei
Executive:
Exec Dir Atl Region: Susan Tilley-Russell
Budget: $65,000
No of Paid Staff: 2
Speakers Available
Library: Y *(Open to the public)*
Languages: English
Membership: 85
Membership Fee: $25 per year

◈ ***Québec:***
3280-380 rue Saint-Antoine O, Montréal QC H2Y 3X7
514 846-8840; Fax: 514 846-8999
Toll-free: 800 321-1433
E: info@qc.arthrite.ca
W: www.arthrite.ca/quebec
Executive:
Dir gén: Mark Bordeleau
Agente support serv éduc: Nicole Rochette
Year Founded: 1948
Budget: $1,500,000
No of Paid Staff: 21
Languages: French

◇ ***Québec***
400-845 boul René-Lévesque O, Québec QC G1S 1T5
418 692-0220; Fax: 418 692-0110
W: www.arthrite.ca/qc
Executive:
Dir rég: Yves Genest
Coord: Manon Cloutier
Coord: Violaine Mailloux
Adj admin: Martine Pouliot
Year Founded: 1948
Speakers Available
Languages: French

◇ ***Sherbrooke:***
564 rue King E, Sherbrooke QC J1G 1B5
819 562-5551; Fax: 819 562-2917
E: info@qc.arthrite.ca
W: www.arthritis.ca/quebec
Executive:
Resp dév/revenus: Marie-Eve D'Aoust

◈ ***Saskatchewan:***
110-2550 12th Ave, Regina SK S4P 3X1
306 352-3312; Fax: 306 565-8731
Toll-free: 800 321-1433
E: info@sk.arthritis.ca
W: www.arthritis.ca
Executive:
Exec Dir: Carol Hiscock
Coord Arthritis Educ Prog: Sheila Fahlman
Dev Officer: Erin Marchuk
Speakers Available
Library: Y *(Open to the public)*
Languages: English
Membership list available to the public

◇ ***Saskatoon:***
1851D Lorne Ave, Saskatoon SK S7H 1Y5
306 244-9922; Fax: 306 244-9903
W: www.arthritis.ca
Executive:
Commun Dev: Sondra Livingston
Joints in Motion Coord: Tracey Shewciw
Year Founded: 1948
No of Paid Staff: 2
Speakers Available
Library: Y *(Open to the public)*
Languages: English
Membership Fee: $25/year

The Arthritis Society - Thunder Bay District
5-895 Tungsten St, Thunder Bay ON P7B 6H2
807 345-9535; Fax: 807 344-1915
Toll-free: 800 268-9535
W: www.arthritis.ca
Executive:
Mgr Comm Engagement: Linda Urry
Languages: English

ASTHMA

Asthma Society of Canada
401-124 Merton St, Toronto ON M4S 2Z2
416 787-4050; Fax: 416 787-5807
Toll-free: 866 787-4050
E: info@asthma.ca
W: www.asthma.ca
Executive:
Pres/CEO: Dr Robert Oliphant
Dir-Commun: Noah Farber
Year Founded: 1974
Budget: $750,000
No of Paid Staff: 3
Languages: English; French
Membership: 500 + members *(Lists available to the public)*

Canadian Network for Respiratory Care
16851 Mount Wolfe Rd, Caledon ON L7E 3P6
905 880-1092; Fax: 905 880-9733
E: cconnors@cnrchome.net
W: cnrchome.net
Executive:
Exec Dir: Cheryl Connors
Year Founded: 1994
No of Paid Staff: 2
Speakers Available
Languages: English
Membership: 25 *(Lists available to the public)*

ATAXIA

Canadian Association for Familial Ataxias - Claude St-Jean Foundation
110-3800 rue Radisson, Montréal QC H1M 1X6
514 321-8684
Toll-free: 855 321-8684
E: ataxie@lacaf.org
W: www.lacaf.org
Executive:
Admin: Jean Phenix
Year Founded: 1972
Criteria: *Ataxique-symphatisant-association, organisation*
No of Paid Staff: 1
Languages: English; French
Membership: 250

AUTISM

AATEDEQ
Location: 111-125 boul René-Lepage E, Rimouski QC G5L 1N9
Mailing: CP 44 succ A, Rimouski QC G5L 7B7
418 725-2575; Fax: 418 725-2638
Toll-free: 877 725-2575
E: info@aatedeq.com
W: www.aatedeq.com

HEALTHCARE ASSOCIATIONS

Executive:
Prés: Martine Martin
Coord: Mélanie Lavoie

Autism Society Canada

Location: 1670 Heron Rd, Ottawa ON K1V 0C2
Mailing: PO Box 22017 RPO Heron Gate, Ottawa ON K1V 0W2
613 789-8943; Fax: 613 789-8943
Toll-free: 866 476-8440
E: info@atismsocietycanada.ca
W: www.autismsocietycanada.ca/
Executive:
Exec Dir: Kathleen Provost
Languages: English; French

◈Alberta:
101-11720 Kingsway NW, Edmonton AB T5G 0X5
780 453-3971; Fax: 780 447-4948
E: autism@autismedmonton.org
W: www.autismedmonton.org
Executive:
Exec Dir: Freda Badry
Dir-Comm Awareness/Dev: Deborah Barrett

◈Calgary
174-3359 27 St NE, Calgary AB T1Y 5E4
403 250-5033; Fax: 403 250-2625
E: info@autismcalgary.com
W: www.autismcalgary.com
Executive:
Chair: Daria Skibington
Vice Chair: Rod Onoferychuck
Exec Dir: Lyndon Parakin
Treas: Dan Tran
Sec: Allen Schultz

◈Burnaby
303-3701 Hastings St, Burnaby BC V5C 2H6
604 434-0880; Fax: 604 434-0801
Toll-free: 888 437-0880
E: administrator@autismbc.ca
W: www.autismbc.ca
Executive:
Pres: Michael Lewis
Info Worker: Lindy Chau
Year Founded: 1974
Criteria: *Families, Individuals, Professionals, Students*
Budget: $660,000
No of Paid Staff: 5
Library: Y
Languages: English; Mandarin; Cantonese
Membership: 300
Membership Fee: $25/yr
Library:
Autism Society of British Columbia - Library

◇Prince George
n/a Home Based, Prince George BC V2M 3S3
250 961-7620; Fax: 604 434-0801
Toll-free: 888 437-0880
E: info@autismbc.ca
W: http://www.autismbc.ca/the-society/branches/prince-george-branch/
Executive:
Br Coord: Corey Walker

◇Nanaimo
Mailing: PO Box 180 Stn A, Nanaimo BC V9R 5K9
250 714-0801; Fax: 250 714-0802
Toll-free: 888 437-0880
E: info@autismbc.ca
W: www.autismbc.ca/nanaimo.php
Executive:
Br Coord: Alexandria Stuart
Year Founded: 1970
Speakers Available
Library: Y
Languages: English; French

◈Manitoba:
825 Sherbrook St, Winnipeg MB R3A 1M5
204 783-9563; Fax: 204 975-3027
Toll-free: 888 444-9563
E: info@autismmanitoba.com
W: www.autismmanitoba.com/
Executive:
Pres: Kim Campbell
Languages: English

◈Fredericton
Mailing: PO Box 1493 Stn A, Fredericton NB E3B 5G2
Toll-free: 866 773-1916
E: autism_nb@yahoo.com
W: www.autismnb.org
Executive:
Pres: Tamara Downey

◈Newfoundland & Labrador:
Location: 70 Clinch Cres, St. John's NL A1B 4G8
Mailing: PO Box 14078 Stn A
709 722-2803; Fax: 709 722-4926
E: info@autism.nf.net
W: www.autism.nf.net
Executive:
Exec Dir: Wendy Skinner
Languages: English; French

◈Yellowknife
4904 Matonabee St, Yellowknife NT X1A 1X8
867 920-4206; Fax: 867 873-0235
E: lynnelkin@hotmail.com
W: autism@hotmail.com
Executive:
Pres: Lynn Elkin

◈Halifax
1456 Brenton St, Halifax NS B3J 2K7
902 429-5529; Fax: 902 446-4997
Toll-free: 877 544-4495
E: info@provincialautismcentre.ca
W: www.provincialautismcentre.ca
Executive:
Pres: Nancy Walker
Exec Dir: Vicki Harvey

◈Ottawa:
210-211 Bronson Ave, Ottawa ON K1R 6H5
613 230-6305; Fax: 613 288-1423
E: ottawa@autismontario.com
W: www.autismontario.com/ottawa
Criteria: *Open to all.*
Speakers Available
Library: Y *(Open to the public)*
Languages: English
Membership: 140

◈St Catharines:
401-36 Page St, St Catharines ON L2R 4A7
905 682-2776; Fax: 905 682-5609
E: chaptermgr.niagara@autismontario.com
W: www.autismontario.com/niagara
Year Founded: 1983
No of Paid Staff: 5
Speakers Available
Library: Y *(Open to the public)*
Membership: 200

◈Toronto
004-1179 King St W, Toronto ON M6K 3C5
416 246-9592 232; Fax: 416 246-9417
E: mail@autismontario.com
W: www.autismontario.com
Executive:
Pres: Tanya Stephenson
Exec Dir: Margaret Spoelstra
Mgr: Ethel Berry
Treas: Deborah Woodland
Sec: Wendie Vieselmeyer
Year Founded: 1973

Criteria: *Open to all 18 years and over. Membership form on website.*
No of Paid Staff: 15
Languages: English; French
Membership: 1,900
Membership Fee: Ranges from $10 - $50

◈Charlottetown
Location: Sherwood Business Centre, 161 St Peters Rd, Charlottetown PE C1A 5P6
Mailing: 135 Kent St, PO Box 3243 Stn Central, Charlottetown PE C1A 8W5
902 566-4844; Fax: 902 368-8057
Toll-free: 888 360-8681
E: Nathalie@autismsociety.pe.ca
W: www.autismsociety.pe.ca
Executive:
Exec Dir: Nathalie Walsh

◈Chicoutimi
415 rue Racine E, Chicoutimi QC G7H 1S8
418 543-7088
Toll-free: 888 543-7088
E: sarsaglac@autisme02.com
W: www.autisme02.com
Executive:
Adj admin: Isabelle Simard
Speakers Available
Languages: French
Membership: 110

◈Montreal:
Location: 104-65 rue de Castelnau O, Montréal QC H2R 2W3
Mailing: 200-7675 boul Saint-Laurent, Montréal QC H2R 1W9
514 270-7386; Fax: 514 270-9261
E: info@autisme.qc.ca
W: www.autisme.qc.ca
Executive:
Prés: Ginette Côté
Dir gén: Jo-Ann Lauzon
Year Founded: 1976
Criteria: *Les organismes qui offrent des services notamment aux personnes autistes.*
No of Paid Staff: 3
Languages: English; French
Membership: 80
Library:
Centre de documentation *(Open to the public)*

◈Quebec:
1055 boul des Chutes, Québec QC G1E 2E9
418 624-7432; Fax: 418 624-7444
E: info@autismequebec.org
Executive:
Dir gén: Lili Plourde
Year Founded: 1977
Library: Y *(Open to the public)*
Languages: French

◈Saskatoon:
609 25th St E, Saskatoon SK S7K 0L7
306 665-7013; Fax: 306 665-7011
E: admin@autismservices.ca
W: www.autismservices.ca
Executive:
Chair: David Ambrose
Exec Dir: Shannon Zook
Admv Asst: Bonita Harman
Admv Asst: Pat Kuechle
Year Founded: 1979
Criteria: *Membership open to everyone.*
No of Paid Staff: 30
Speakers Available
Library: Y *(Open to the public)*
Languages: English
Membership: 300
Membership Fee: $20

◈Tisdale
Mailing: PO Box 2150, Tisdale SK S0E 1T0
306 862-4768; Fax: 306 862-3899
E: saskfeat@hotmail.com
W: www.saskfeat.com
Executive:
Pres: Tim Verklan

◈Whitehorse
503B Steele St, Whitehorse YT Y1A 2E1
867 667-6406; Fax: 867 667-6408
E: asca@rdcsc.ca
W: www.autismyukon.org
Executive:
Exec Dir: Leah Davy Ryckman

Autism Treatment Services (Ontario) Inc.
113 Gardiner Shore Rd, Carleton Place ON K7C 0C4
613 762-7752; Fax: 613 257-2209
Toll-free: 800 257-7618 728
E: tekirkp@sympatico.ca
W: www.autism.ca
Executive:
Chair: Terry Kirkpatrick
VP: Heather Ballinger
Year Founded: 1989
Criteria: *Professional interest in Autism.*
Budget: $1,000
Speakers Available
Languages: English
Membership list available to the public

Autisme et troubles envahissants du développement Montréal
320-4450 rue Saint-Hubert, Montréal QC H2J 2W9
514 524-6114; Fax: 514 524-6420
E: atedm@autisme-montreal.com
W: www.autisme-montreal.com
Executive:
Prés: Carmen Lahaie
Dir gén: Julie Champagne
Year Founded: 1991
No of Paid Staff: 8
Library: Y *(Open to the public)*
Languages: French; English
Membership: 530

Gateway Society
4807 Georgia St, Delta BC V4K 2T1
604 946-0401
W: www.gatewaysociety.org
Executive:
Hum Res Mgr: Jan Armstrong

Geneva Centre for Autism
112 Merton St, Toronto ON M4S 2Z8
416 322-7877; Fax: 416 322-5894
Toll-free: 800 436-3829
E: info@autism.net
W: www.autism.net
Executive:
Pres: Abe Evreniadis
CEO: Dr Lindy Zaretsky
COO Prog/Serv: Debbie Irish
CFO: Jim Gilmour
VP: Bob Langlois
Dir-Dev: Debbie Drewett
Sec-Treas: Christian Gingras
Hum Res Mgr: Claudia Kugelmass

Reading & Writing Consultants Inc.
Malcolm Tweddle School
10-2340 Millbourne Road West NW, Edmonton AB T6K 1Y9
780 439-8120; Fax: 780 439-8125
E: reading@telus.net
W: www.readingandwriting.ab.ca
Executive:
Pres: Peggy Kickham
Treas: Judy Pool
Sec: Debbie Sniderman
Year Founded: 1994
No of Paid Staff: 6
Speakers Available
Library: Y

Société d'autisme et TED de Laval
34 boul Bellerose E, Laval QC H7K 1S4
450 663-5551; Fax: 450 663-0694
E: lechatbotte@videotron.ca
W: www.autismelaval.org
Executive:
Dir gén: Germain Lafrenière

Société de l'autisme et des autres troubles envahissants du developpement de l'Abitibi-Témiscamingue
101-19 rue Gamble O, Rouyn-Noranda QC J9X 2R3
819 762-2700
E: satedat@hotmail.com
W: www.satedat.wordpress.com/
Executive:
Dir gén: Enrik Cliche
Year Founded: 1985
No of Paid Staff: 3
Speakers Available
Library: Y *(Open to the public)*
Languages: French
Membership: 50

Société de l'autisme région Lanaudière
200 rue de Salaberry, Joliette QC J6E 4G1
450 759-9788; Fax: 450 759-8749
Toll-free: 866 759-9788
E: autisme.lanaudiere@cepap.ca
W: autisme-lanaudiere.org
Executive:
Coord: Manon Champigny
Library: Y *(Open to the public)*
Membership: 200

Sociétés de l'autisme S.A.R. Laurentides
474 rue Laviolette, Saint-Jérôme QC J7Y 2T7
450 569-1794; Fax: 450 569-6022
E: info@autismelaurentides.org
W: www.autismelaurentides.org
Executive:
Prés: Chantal Thériault
VP: Sylvie Lejeune
Dir gén: Jean-Pierre Leboeuf
Trés: Hélène Giard

Society for Treatment of Autism - Alberta
404 94 Ave SE, Calgary AB T2J 0E8
403 253-2291; Fax: 403 253-6974
E: atsc@autism.ca
W: www.autism.ca
Executive:
Board Pres: Peter Johnson
Exec Dir: David Mikkelsen
Languages: English

Society for Treatment of Autism - Nova Scotia
Location: 541 Charlotte St, Sydney NS B1P 1E6
Mailing: PO Box 392 Stn A, Sydney NS B1P 6H2
902 567-6441; Fax: 902 567-0425
E: autism@ns.sympatico.ca
W: www3.ns.sympatico.ca/autism
Executive:
Exec Dir: Denise Whalen
Year Founded: 1988
No of Paid Staff: 98
Speakers Available
Languages: English

Trait d'Union Outaouais Inc.
004-109 rue Wright, Gatineau QC J8X 2G7
819 595-1290; Fax: 819 595-7099
Toll-free: 866 355-8864
E: admintuoi@bellnet.ca
W: www.traitdunionoutaouais.com
Executive:
Dir gén: Jocelyne Sylvestre
Agente d'admin: Monique Fortier
Languages: French; English

BRAIN INJURY

Alan Stewart Homes Limited
349 Reid St, Peterborough ON K9H 4G3
705 743-8043; Fax: 705 743-5736
E: info@stewart-homes.com
W: www.stewart-homes.com
Executive:
Owner/Dir: Alan Stewart
Dir-Hum Res: Kim Erskin
Prog Mgr: Pegi Hanley

Association for the Rehabilitation of the Brain Injured
3412 Spruce Dr SW, Calgary AB T3C 3A4
403 242-7116; Fax: 403 242-7478
E: info@arbi.ca
W: www.arbi.ca
Executive:
Prog Dir: Mary Anne Ostapovitch
Exec Dir: Judy Stawnychko
Year Founded: 1978
No of Paid Staff: 31
Speakers Available
Library: Y *(Open to the public)*
Languages: English
Membership list available to the public

Brain Injury Association of Alberta
4916 50 St, Red Deer AB T4N 1X7
403 309-0866; Fax: 403 342-3880
Toll-free: 888 533-5355 Alberta & NWT
E: admin@biaa.ca
W: www.biaa.ca
Year Founded: 1988
No of Paid Staff: 1
Speakers Available
Library: Y *(Open to the public)*
Languages: English

Brain Injury Association of Canada
200-440 Laurier Ave W, Ottawa ON K1R 7X6
Fax: 613 782-2228
Toll-free: 866 977-2492
E: info@biac-aclc.ca
W: www.biac-aclc.ca
Executive:
Exec Dir: Harry Zarins

◈Maple Ridge:
11948 207 St, Box 143, Maple Ridge BC V2X 1X7
604 465-1783; Fax: 888 429-0656
Toll-free: 877 858-1788 outside Vancouver
E: info@bcbraininjuryassociation.com
W: www.bcbraininjuryassociation.com
Year Founded: 1983
Budget: $85,000
No of Paid Staff: 1
Speakers Available
Membership: 100 +

◈***Manitoba:***
204-825 Sherbrook St, Winnipeg MB R3A 1M5
204 975-3280; Fax: 204 975-3027
E: mbia@mymts.net
W: www.mbia.ca

◈***Newfoundland and Labrador:***
Location: Miller Centre Southcott Hall, 21 Merrymeeting Rd, St. John's NL A1C 5T9
Mailing: PO Box 21063 Rpo MacDonald Drive, St. John's NL A1A 5B2
709 579-3070; Fax: 709 579-3109
Toll-free: 877 525-6242
W: www.nlbia.ca
Executive:
Pres: Tom Lush
VP: Brad Wicks
No of Paid Staff: 1
Speakers Available
Library: Y *(Open to the public)*
Languages: English

◈***Nova Scotia:***
Location: Victoria Building, Room 13-009/010 Floor 13, Halifax NS B3H 2Y9
Mailing: PO Box 8804 RPO CSC, Halifax NS B3K 5M4
902 473-7301; Fax: 902 473-7302
E: bians1@ns.sympatico.ca
W: www3.ns.sympatico.ca/bians1

◈***Eastern Ontario:***

◇***Oshawa:***
24-850 King St W, Oshawa ON L1J 8N5
850 723-2732; Fax: 905 723-4936
Toll-free: 866 354-4464
E: information@biad.ca
W: www.biad.ca

◇***Ottawa Valley:***
300-211 Bronson Ave, Ottawa ON K1R 6H5
613 233-8303; Fax: 613 233-8422
E: braininjuryottawavalley@bellnet.ca
W: biaov.org
Executive:
Pres/Chairperson: Wendy Charbonneau
Library: Y *(Open to the public)*
Languages: English; French

◇***Peterborough:***
158 Charlotte St, Peterborough ON K9J 2T8
705 741-1172
Toll-free: 800 854-9738
E: fcbia@nexicom.net
Executive:
Exec Dir: Cheryl Ann Hassan

◈***Northern Ontario:***

◇***North Bay and Area:***
280 Oakwood Ave, North Bay ON P1B 9G2
705 840-8882
E: contact@bianba.ca
W: www.bianba.ca
Executive:
Chairperson: Beth Ward

◇***Sault Ste. Marie:***
127-31 Old Garden River Rd, Sault Ste. Marie ON P6B 5Y7
705 946-0172; Fax: 705 946-0594
Toll-free: 888 772-5701
E: biassmd@shaw.ca
W: www.braininjuryssm.ca
Executive:
Pres: Debbie Scarfone
Year Founded: 1990
Speakers Available
Library: Y *(Open to the public)*
Languages: English
Membership: 60

◈***Ontario:***
Mailing: PO Box 2338 Stn Main, St Catharines ON L2R 7R9
905 641-8877; Fax: 905 641-0323
Toll-free: 800 263-5404
E: obia@obia.on.ca
W: www.obia.ca

◈***Sarnia-Lambton:***
1032-1705 London Line, Sarnia ON N7W 1B2
519 337-5657
E: braininjuryassoc@cogeco.net
Executive:
Pres: Ken McRae
Year Founded: 1990
Criteria: *Membership open to any interested person, except for brain injury survivors' meetings.*
No of Paid Staff: 1
Library: Y
Languages: English
Library:
Head Injury Lending Library *(Open to the public)*

◈***Southcentral Ontario:***

◇***Belleville:***
281 Front St, Belleville ON K8N 2Z6
613 967-2756; Fax: 613 967-1108
Toll-free: 866 894-8884
E: biaqd@bellnet.ca
W: www.biaqd.ca
Executive:
Office Admin: Pam Ferrill

◇***Mississauga:***
204-2155 Leanne Blvd, Mississauga ON L5K 2K8
905 823-2221; Fax: 905 823-9960
Toll-free: 800 565-8594
W: www.biaph.com
Executive:
Exec Dir: Jorun Rucels

◈***Southwestern Ontario:***

◇***Chatham-Kent/New Beginnings Club:***
9 Maple Leaf Dr, Chatham ON N7M 6H2
519 351-0297; Fax: 519 351-7600
E: biack@biack.com
W: www.newbeginning-cksl.com
Executive:
Pres: Jerry O'Brien
VP: Greg Davenport
Exec Dir: Michelle Chernets
Year Founded: 1996
Membership Fee Required: Y
Speakers Available
Library: Y *(Open to the public)*
Languages: English; French
Membership Fee: Individual - $10; Corporate - $50; Family - $20

◇***Grey-Bruce:***
Mailing: PO Box 481 Stn Main, Owen Sound ON N4K 5P7
519 373-8555
W: www.biagb.com

◇***Waterloo Region:***
5A-607 King St W, Kitchener ON N2G 1C7
519 579-5300
E: biaww@bellnet.ca
W: www.biaww.com
Executive:
Exec Dir: Patti Lehman

◇***Windsor & Essex County:***
201-200 West Grand Blvd, Windsor ON N9E 3W7
519 981-1329; Fax: 519 250-7124
Toll-free: 800 263-5404
E: info@biawe.com
W: www.biawe.com

Executive:
Exec Dir: Laura Kay

◈***Prince Edward Island:***
81 Prince St, Charlottetown PE C1A 4R3
902 314-4228
E: info@biapei.com
W: www.biapei.com
Executive:
Pres: Kenneth Murnaghan

◈***Quebec:***
106-911 rue Jean-Talon E, Montréal QC H2R 1V5
514 274-7447; Fax: 514 274-1717
E: aqtc@aqtc.ca
W: www.aqtc.ca
Executive:
Dir gén: Pierre Mitchell
Languages: French

◈***Saskatchewan:***
PO Box 3843 Stn Main, Regina SK S4P 3R8
306 373-1555; Fax: 306 373-5655
W: www.sbia.ca

Brain Injury Association of Niagara
4-36 Page St, St Catharines ON L2R 4A7
905 984-5058; Fax: 905 984-5354

Brain Injury Relearning Services - Div. of Redi Enterprise
856 Allowance Ave SE, Medicine Hat AB T1A 7S6
403 528-2661; Fax: 403 528-2647
E: birs@redi.ca
W: www.redi.ca
Executive:
Mgr: Donna Stein
No of Paid Staff: 10
Speakers Available
Library: Y *(Open to the public)*
Languages: English

Buckley Valley Brain Injury Association
3862B Broadway Ave, Box 634, Smithers BC V0J 2N0
250 877-7723; Fax: 250 877-7724
E: executive_director@bvbia.ca
W: www.bvbia.ca

Cheshire Homes Society of British Columbia
202-625 Fifth Ave, New Westminster BC V3M 1X4
604 540-0686; Fax: 604 540-0684
E: john@cheshirehomes.ca
W: www.cheshirehomes.ca
Executive:
Exec Dir: John Millard
Year Founded: 1973
No of Paid Staff: 70
Library: Y *(Open to the public)*
Languages: English

Northern Alberta Brain Injury Society
229-10106 111 Ave NW, Edmonton AB T5G 0B4
780 477-7575; Fax: 780 474-4415
Toll-free: 800 425-5552
E: shamim@braincarecentre.com
W: www.braincarecentre.com
Executive:
Pres: Stephanie Boldt
CFO: Kaitlin Cluff
Treas/VP: Ryan Barry
Ops Mgr: Louise Jensen
Exec Dir: Dr Garnet Cummings
Office Coor: Shamim Khanbhai
Prog Mgr Client Serv: Michael Ryan
Year Founded: 1983
No of Paid Staff: 13
Speakers Available
Library: Y *(Open to the public)*

Languages: English
Membership: 200 *(Lists available to the public)*
Membership Fee: $30/Year
Library:
Mathewson LIbrary on Brain Injury *(Open to the public)*

◈***Edson Office:***
Location: 4916 50 St, Red Deer AB T4N 1X7
Mailing: PO Box 30105 RPO Tag West, Edson AB T7E 1Y2
780 712-7560; Fax: 780 712-7567
Toll-free: 866 712-7560
E: tannis@braincarecentre.com
W: www.braincarecentre.com
Executive:
Svc/Support Coor: Tannis Arsenault
Serv Coord: Laura See
Languages: English

Northern Brain Injury Association
Location: 1273 4th Ave, Prince George BC V2L 3J5
Mailing: PO Box 951 Stn A, Prince George BC V2L 4V1
250 562-4673
Toll-free: 866 979-4673
E: info@nbia.ca

Southern Alberta Brain Injury Society
102-2116 27 Ave NE, Calgary AB T2E 7A6
403 521-5212; Fax: 403 283-5867
E: natasha@sabis.ab.ca
W: www.sabis.ab.ca
Executive:
Exec Dir: Dr Denis J Cooney
Prog Mgr: Joe Schreiber
Fund Dev Coor: Natasha Bodei
Year Founded: 1985
Criteria: *Survivor of brain injury, family member or caregiver.*
Budget: $420,000
No of Paid Staff: 8
Library: Y
Languages: English
Membership: 200

Victoria Brain Injury Society
D-E-830 Pembroke St, Victoria BC V8T 1H9
250 598-9339; Fax: 250 598-9363
Toll-free: 877 598-9399
E: admin@vbis.ca
W: www.vbis.ca
Executive:
Admn Mgr: Anna McLauchlan
Dir-Client Serv: Helen Lang
Year Founded: 1983
No of Paid Staff: 5
Speakers Available
Library: Y
Languages: English

CANCER

Alberta Cancer Foundation
Cross Cancer Institute
11560 University Ave NW, Edmonton AB T6G 1Z2
780 432-8500; Fax: 780 432-8357
Toll-free: 866 412-4222
W: www.albertacancerfoundation.ca
Executive:
CEO: Myka Osinchuk
Sr Dev Officer: Jane Weller

Alberta Cancer Foundation
710-10123 99 St NW, Edmonton AB T5J 3H1
780 643-4400; Fax: 780 643-4398
W: www.albertacancer.ca
Executive:
CEO: Myka Osinchuk
Year Founded: 1984
No of Paid Staff: 40
Speakers Available
Languages: English

Brain Tumour Foundation of Canada
301-620 Colborne St, London ON N6B 3R9
519 642-7755; Fax: 519 642-7192
Toll-free: 800 265-5106
E: braintumour@braintumour.ca
W: www.braintumour.ca
Executive:
Chair: Dr Joseph Megyesi
Vice Chair: Sean Taggart
Exec Dir: Susan Marshall
Sec: Sarah Keels
Mgr-Mktg/Pub Affairs: Megan Winkler
Fin/Office Mgr: Jeff Howard
Community Rels Officer: A Paul Mitchell
Natl Spec Event Mgr: Sharon Whiteside
Year Founded: 1982
Budget: $1,500,000
No of Paid Staff: 13
Speakers Available
Library: Y *(Open to the public)*
Languages: English
Membership: 10 *(Lists available to the public)*
Membership Fee: $5

Breast Cancer Action
301-1390 Prince of Wales Dr, Ottawa ON K2C 3N6
613 736-5921; Fax: 613 736-8422
E: info@bcaott.ca
W: www.bcaott.ca
Executive:
Pres-Board of Dir: Julia Ringma
Exec Dir: Karen Graszat

Breast Cancer Action Montreal
201-5890 av Monkland, Montréal QC H4A 1G2
514 483-1846; Fax: 514 483-9221
E: info@bcam.qc.ca
W: www.bcam.qc.ca
Year Founded: 1991
Criteria: *Membership open to everyone.*
Library: Y *(Open to the public)*
Languages: French

Breast Cancer Society Of Canada
420 East St N, Sarnia ON N7T 6Y5
519 336-0746; Fax: 519 336-5725
Toll-free: 800 567-8767
E: bcsc@bcsc.ca
W: www.bcsc.ca
Executive:
Exec Dir: Marsha Davidson

Canadian Breast Cancer Foundation
375 University Ave, Floor 6, Toronto ON M5G 2J5
416 596-6773; Fax: 416 596-7857
Toll-free: 800 387-9816
E: info@cbcf.org
W: www.cbcf.org
Executive:
CEO: Colleen Fleming
Languages: English

Canadian Breast Cancer Network (CBCN)
602-331 Cooper St, Ottawa ON K2P 0G5
613 230-3044; Fax: 613 230-4424
Toll-free: 800 685-8820
E: cbcn@cbcn.ca
W: www.cbcn.ca
Executive:
Pres: Cathy Ammendolea
VP: Sharon Young
Year Founded: 1994
Criteria: *$25 yearly*
Budget: $700,000
No of Paid Staff: 8
Speakers Available
Languages: English; French
Membership: 300 *(Lists available to the public)*

Canadian Cancer Society - BC/Yukon
565 10th Ave W, Vancouver BC V5Z 4J4
604 872-4400; Fax: 604 879-9267
Toll-free: 800 663-2524
E: cancerinfo@bc.cancer.ca
W: www.cancer.ca
Executive:
CEO: Barbara Kaminsky
Year Founded: 1938
No of Paid Staff: 165
Languages: English

◈***Fraser Valley - Surrey & Delta:***
202-20434 64 Ave, Langley BC V2Y 1N4
604 533-1668; Fax: 604 533-8511
Toll-free: 888 222-2240
E: fraservalley@bc.cancer.ca
Executive:
Mgr: Mike Glass
Languages: English

◈***Greater Vancouver:***
230-3689 1st Ave E, Vancouver BC V5M 1C2
604 253-8470; Fax: 604 253-8403
Toll-free: 888 229-8288
E: greatervan@bc.cancer.ca
W: www.cancer.ca
Executive:
Pres: Justin Stephenson
Reg Mgr: Brad Beattie
Languages: English

◈***Kootenays:***
19 9th Ave S, Cranbrook BC V1C 2L9
250 426-8916; Fax: 250 426-3947
Toll-free: 800 656-6426
E: kootenay@bc.cancer.ca
W: www.bc.cancer.ca
Executive:
Reg Dir: Sally Ginter
Languages: English

◈***Northern BC:***
300-500 Victoria St, Prince George BC V2L 2J9
250 564-0885; Fax: 250 563-0385
Toll-free: 800 811-5666
E: north@bc.cancer.ca
W: www.bc.cancer.ca
Executive:
Reg Mgr: Margaret Jones-Bricker
Languages: English

◈***Vancouver Island:***
101-1537 Hillside Ave, Victoria BC V8T 4Y2
250 592-2244; Fax: 250 382-8130
Toll-free: 800 663-7892
E: vanisland@bc.cancer.ca
W: www.bc.cancer.ca
Executive:
Reg Dir: Kathy Ilott
Languages: English

◈***Yukon Territory:***
2-211 Wood St, Whitehorse YT Y1A 2E4
867 668-6440; Fax: 867 668-6442
E: yukon@bc.cancer.ca
W: www.bc.cancer.ca
Languages: English

HEALTHCARE ASSOCIATIONS

Canadian Cancer Society - Eastern Region
329 George St, Sydney NS B1P 1J7
902 564-8263; Fax: 902 539-2526
Toll-free: 800 639-0222
E: sydney@ns.cancer.ca
W: www.cancer.ca

Canadian Cancer Society - Manitoba Division
193 Sherbrook St, Winnipeg MB R3C 2B7
204 774-7483; Fax: 204 774-7500
Toll-free: 888 532-6982
E: info@mb.cancer.ca
W: www.cancer.ca
No of Paid Staff: 20
Languages: English

Canadian Cancer Society - National Office
300-55 St Clair Ave W, Toronto ON M4V 2Y7
416 961-7223; Fax: 416 961-4189
Toll-free: 800 268-8874
E: ccs@cancer.ca
W: www.cancer.ca
Executive:
CEO-Ont Div: Martin Kabat
Year Founded: 1938
No of Paid Staff: 75
Languages: English
Membership: All donors

◈***Alberta:***
200-325 Manning Rd NE, Calgary AB T2E 2P5
403 205-3966; Fax: 403 205-3979
Toll-free: 800 661-2262
E: info@cancer.ab.ca
W: www.cancer.ca
Executive:
Exec Dir: Dan Holinda
No of Paid Staff: 95
Speakers Available
Library: Y
Languages: English

◇***Edmonton & District:***
201-9452 51 Ave NW, Edmonton AB T6E 5A6
780 455-7181; Fax: 780 455-0277
E: katyt@cancer.ab.ca
W: www.cancer.ca
Executive:
Admin: Katy Tsang
Year Founded: 1938
No of Paid Staff: 20
Speakers Available
Languages: English

◇***Fort McMurray & District:***
150 MacDonald Cres, Fort McMurray AB T9H 4B2
780 791-0174; Fax: 780 791-3178
E: fortmcMurray.relayforlife@cancer.ab.ca
Executive:
Coord: Jon Tupper
Criteria: *Anyone who donates is a member.*
No of Paid Staff: 2
Speakers Available
Library: Y
Languages: English
Library:
Esther Robbies Lending Library *(Open to the public)*

◇***Grande Prairie:***
103-9805 97 St, Grande Prairie AB T8V 8B9
780 538-8205; Fax: 780 538-2707
Toll-free: 888 939-3333
E: theresec@cancer.ab.ca
W: www.cancer.ca
Executive:
Commun Serv Coord: Thérèse Chauvin
Year Founded: 1936
No of Paid Staff: 4
Speakers Available
Languages: English; French

◇***Lethbridge & District:***
Lethbridge & District Unit
317 10 St S, Lethbridge AB T1J 2M7
403 327-5452; Fax: 403 327-5883
E: kelly.archibald@cancer.ab.ca
W: www.cancer.ab.ca
Executive:
Reg Office Admin Asst: Kelly Archibald
No of Paid Staff: 4
Speakers Available
Languages: English

◇***Medicine Hat:***
102-1865 Dunmore Rd SE, Medicine Hat AB T1A 1Z8
403 528-2125; Fax: 403 528-2235
E: info@cis.cancer.ca
W: www.cancer.ca
Executive:
Admv Asst: Janice Montgomery
No of Paid Staff: 3
Speakers Available
Languages: English

◇***Red Deer:***
101-6751 52 Ave, Red Deer AB T4N 4K8
403 347-3662; Fax: 403 347-9690
E: reddeer.office@cancer.ab.ca
W: www.cancer.ab.ca
Executive:
Admv Asst: Dhwani Parikh
No of Paid Staff: 3
Speakers Available
Languages: English

◇***Northwest Territories:***
Location: Bowling Green Bldg, 207-4817 49 St, Yellowknife NT X1A 2P5
Mailing: PO Box 2007 Stn Main
867 920-4428; Fax: 867 920-4162
W: www.cancer.ca
Executive:
Voulunteer Resources Coord: Lorna Deveau
No of Paid Staff: 1
Speakers Available
Library: Y *(Open to the public)*
Languages: English; French
Membership: 2

◈***Central Toronto:***
500-55 St Clair Ave W, Toronto ON M4V 2Y7
416 480-7901; Fax: 416 480-7902
E: toronto@ontario.cancer.ca
W: www.cancer.ca
Executive:
CEO: Martin Kabat
Languages: English

◇***London:***
123 St George St, London ON N6A 3A1
519 432-1137; Fax: 519 432-1900
Toll-free: 800 465-4838
E: elginmiddlesex@ontario.cancer.ca
W: www.cancer.ca
No of Paid Staff: 15
Library: Y *(Open to the public)*
Languages: French

◇***North Bay:***
101-147 McIntyre St W, North Bay ON P1B 2Y5
705 472-9072; Fax: 705 472-9084
Toll-free: 888 208-2125
E: northbay@ontario.cancer.ca
W: www.cancer.ca
Executive:
Unit Mgr: Andrew Layne
Criteria: *Open to all.*
No of Paid Staff: 2
Library: Y *(Open to the public)*
Languages: English

◇***Cornwall:***
1-837 Pitt St, Cornwall ON K6J 3S4
613 932-1283; Fax: 613 932-1284
Toll-free: 800 669-4181
E: sdgprescott@ontario.cancer.ca
W: www.cancer.ca
No of Paid Staff: 3
Speakers Available
Library: Y *(Open to the public)*
Languages: English; French

◇***Markham:***
100-30 East Beaver Creek Rd, Richmond Hill ON L4B 1J2
905 709-4978; Fax: 905 709-1240
Toll-free: 866 889-2345
E: southyorkregionunit@ontario.cancer.ca
W: www.cancer.ca

◇***Mississauga:***
The Southcom Bldg
202-2227 South Millway, Mississauga ON L5L 3R6
905 608-8411; Fax: 905 608-2266
E: mississauga@ontario.cancer.ca
W: www.cancer.ca
Executive:
Unit Mgr: Barry Edington
Unit Mgr: Niambi Martin'John
Year Founded: 1938
No of Paid Staff: 7
Speakers Available
Library: Y
Languages: English

◈***National Public Issues Office - Ottawa:***
1010-116 Albert St, Ottawa ON K1P 5G3
613 565-2522; Fax: 613 565-2278
E: ccs@ottawa.cancer.ca
W: www.cancer.ca
Executive:
Dir-Public Issues: Dan Demers

◈***Frontenac-Lennox & Addington:***
496 Days Rd, Kingston ON K7M 5R4
613 384-2361; Fax: 613 384-9783
Toll-free: 866 877-0309
E: frontenac@ontario.cancer.ca
W: www.cancer.ca
Executive:
Unit Mgr: Craig Faucette
Year Founded: 1945
Criteria: *Open to all.*
No of Paid Staff: 3
Speakers Available
Languages: English
Membership: 1,500

◈***Guelph:***
4-214 Speedvale Ave W, Guelph ON N1H 1C4
519 824-4261; Fax: 519 824-8923
W: www.cancer.ca
Executive:
Mgr: Lorraine Skarratt
Office Coord: Robyn St. Jules
No of Paid Staff: 2
Speakers Available
Library: Y *(Open to the public)*
Languages: English; French
Membership list available to the public

◈***Oshawa:***
3-12 Stanley Crt, Whitby ON L1N 8P9
905 430-5770; Fax: 905 430-9971
Toll-free: 800 668-7830
E: durham@ontario.cancer.ca
W: www.cancer.ca
Criteria: *Open to all.*
No of Paid Staff: 6
Languages: English

◈Ottawa:
1745 Woodward Dr, Ottawa ON K2C 0P9
613 723-1744; Fax: 613 723-8967
Toll-free: 800 268-8874
E: ottawa@ontario.cancer.ca
W: www.cancer.ca
Executive:
Reg Dir ON East: Mary Hobbs
Unit Mgr: Dawn Cooper
Year Founded: 1938
Criteria: *None*
Speakers Available
Library: Y *(Open to the public)*
Languages: English; French

Canadian Cancer Society - New Brunswick Division

Location: 201-133 Prince William St, Saint John NB E2L 2B5
Mailing: PO Box 2089 Stn Main, Saint John NB E2L 3T5
506 634-6272; Fax: 506 634-3808
Toll-free: 800 455-9090
E: ccsnb@nb.cancer.ca
W: www.cancer.ca
Executive:
Exec Dir: Anne McTiernan-Gamble
Languages: English

Canadian Cancer Society -Newfoundland/Labrador Division

Location: Daffodil Place, 70 Ropewalk Lane, St. John's NL A1B 3R9
Mailing: PO Box 8921 Stn A
709 753-6520; Fax: 709 753-9314
Toll-free: 888 753-6520
E: ccs@nl.cancer.ca
W: www.cancer.ca
Library: Y *(Open to the public)*
Languages: English

◈Central Regional Office:
10 Pinsent Dr, Grnd-Falls-Windsor NL A2A 2R6
709 489-5822; Fax: 709 489-2795
Toll-free: 866 545-9534
E: centralregion@nl.cancer.ca
W: www.cancer.ca
Speakers Available
Languages: English
Membership: 30 *(Lists available to the public)*

◈Western Regional Office:
CIBC Building
304-9 Main St, Corner Brook NL A2H 1C2
709 634-6542; Fax: 709 634-6030
Toll-free: 866 545-9533
E: westernregion@nl.cancer.ca
W: www.cancer.ca
Executive:
Community Resource Coord: Heidi Kirby
Community Services Coord: Cara-Leigh Wyllie
No of Paid Staff: 2
Speakers Available
Library: Y *(Open to the public)*
Languages: English

Canadian Cancer Society - Nova Scotia Division

5826 South St, Halifax NS B3H 1S6
902 423-6183; Fax: 902 429-6563
Toll-free: 800 639-0222
E: ccs.ns@ns.cancer.ca
W: www.cancer.ca
Executive:
CEO: Maureen Summers
Hum Res Mgr: Kendra Morton
Exec Asst to CEO: Kelly Boyce
Year Founded: 1948
Criteria: *Open to any person who donates $1 or more and who holds a valid receipt.*
Budget: $6,200,000
No of Paid Staff: 52
Speakers Available
Languages: English
Membership Fee: $1

Canadian Cancer Society - PEI Division

1-1 Rochford St, Charlottetown PE C1A 9L2
902 566-4007; Fax: 902 628-8281
Toll-free: 866 566-4007
E: info@pei.cancer.ca
W: www.cancer.ca
Year Founded: 1958
Criteria: *Open to anyone who has made a donation and received a receipt in the current year.*
No of Paid Staff: 13
Languages: English

Canadian Cancer Society - Saskatchewan Division

1910 McIntyre St, Regina SK S4P 2R3
306 790-5822; Fax: 306 569-2133
Toll-free: 877 977-4673
E: ccssk@sk.cancer.ca
W: www.cancer.ca
Executive:
Exec Dir: Keith Karasin
Criteria: *Open to any donor to the CCS.*
Budget: $5,000,000
Speakers Available
Languages: English; French
Membership: 13,000

◈Lloydminster:
Location: 105-4910 50 St, Lloydminster SK S9V 0Y5
Mailing: PO Box 2071 Stn Main, Lloydminster SK S9V 1R5
306 825-7722; Fax: 306 825-6822
Toll-free: 888 939-3333
E: lloyd.ccssk@sk.cancer.ca
W: www.cancer.ca
Executive:
Unit Mgr: Linda Ferguson
Office Asst: Karen Dela Rosa
Year Founded: 1984
Criteria: *All members who make a donation in the past year can vote.*
Budget: $25,795
No of Paid Staff: 2
Library: Y *(Open to the public)*
Languages: English
Membership: 15 Board members *(Lists available to the public)*

◈Moose Jaw:
61B Ross St W, Moose Jaw SK S6H 2M2
306 692-2333; Fax: 306 692-6125
Toll-free: 888 939-3333
E: mj.ccssk@sk.cancer.ca
W: www.cancer.ca/saskatchewan
Executive:
Mgr: Gaye Stewart
Criteria: *Open to all.*
Budget: $175,000
No of Paid Staff: 1
Speakers Available
Library: Y *(Open to the public)*
Languages: English

◈North Battleford:
Location: 1141 101th St, North Battleford SK S9A 0Z5
Mailing: PO Box 112 Stn Main, North Battleford SK S9A 2X6
306 445-3339; Fax: 306 446-6200
E: nb.ccssk@sk.cancer.ca
W: www.cancer.ca
Executive:
Mgr: Janice Foley
No of Paid Staff: 1
Speakers Available
Library: Y *(Open to the public)*
Languages: English

◈Prince Albert:
54 11th St E, Prince Albert SK S6V 0Z9
306 764-4808; Fax: 306 764-4065
Toll-free: 888 939-3333
W: www.cancer.ca
Year Founded: 1938
Criteria: *Open to all.*
Budget: $25,000
No of Paid Staff: 1
Speakers Available
Library: Y *(Open to the public)*
Languages: English
Membership: 20 *(Lists available to the public)*

◈Saskatoon:
101-440 2nd Ave N, Saskatoon SK S7K 2C3
306 244-4389; Fax: 306 244-5657
E: sktn.ccssk@sk.cancer.ca
W: www.cancer.ca
Executive:
Mgr: Dean Butcher
Languages: English

◈Swift Current:
43 1st Ave NE, Swift Current SK S9H 2A9
306 773-6422; Fax: 306 773-5130
E: sw.ccssk@sk.cancer.ca
W: www.cancer.ca
Executive:
Mgr-Southwest Unit: Roxana Fryklund
Event Coord: Verena Marsden
No of Paid Staff: 2
Speakers Available
Library: Y *(Open to the public)*
Languages: English
Membership Fee: donation

CancerCare Manitoba Foundation Inc.

675 McDermot Ave, Room ON1160, Winnipeg MB R3E 0V9
204 787-4143; Fax: 204 786-0627
Toll-free: 877 407-2223
E: donate@cancercare.mb.ca
W: www.cancercare.mb.ca
Year Founded: 1930
Criteria: *Appointed by Lieutenant Governor in Council.*
Budget: $47,000,000
No of Paid Staff: 547
Speakers Available
Library: Y
Languages: English; French
Membership: 22 *(Lists available to the public)*
Library:
CancerCare Manitoba Library

Childhood Cancer Canada Foundation

801-21 St Clair Ave E, Toronto ON M4T 1L9
416 489-6440; Fax: 416 489-9812
Toll-free: 800 363-1062
E: info@childhoodcancer.ca
W: www.childhoodcancer.ca
Executive:
Pres/CEO: Megan Davidson
Dir-Mktg/Commun Prog: Dana Stanescu
Year Founded: 1987
No of Paid Staff: 5
Library: Y *(Open to the public)*
Languages: English
Membership: 11

Kids Cancer Care Foundation of Alberta
302-609 14 St NW, Calgary AB T2N 2A1
403 216-9210; Fax: 403 216-9215
Toll-free: 888 554-2267
E: staff@kidscancercare.ab.ca
W: www.kidscancercare.ab.ca
Executive:
CEO: Christine Wandzura
Dir-Fund Dev/Comm: Trish Matheson
Dir-Camp/Outreach: Mike Mackay
Commun Mgr: Gail Anne Corbett
Year Founded: 1991
No of Paid Staff: 16
Speakers Available
Languages: English

Montreal Cancer Institute
1560 rue Sherbrooke E, Montréal QC H2L 4M1
514 890-8213; Fax: 514 412-7591
E: anne-marie.mes-masson@umontreal.ca
W: www.icm.qc.ca
Executive:
Dir gén: Maral Tersakian
Dir scientif: Anne-Marie Mes-Masson

Société canadienne du cancer - Division Québec
5151 boul de l'Assomption, Montréal QC H1T 4A9
514 255-5151; Fax: 514 255-2808
Toll-free: 888 939-3333
E: info@sic.cancer.ca
W: www.cancer.ca
Executive:
Dir gén: Suzanne Dubois
Dir gén adj: Jean-Pierre Laurin
Dir aff pub: Jean-Daniel Hamelin
Admin réseau: Michel Ducharme
Year Founded: 1938
Criteria: *bénévolat*
Budget: $8,500,000
No of Paid Staff: 86
Speakers Available
Languages: English; French

◊Chicoutimi:
Immeuble Commercial
B210-930 rue Jacques-Cartier E,
Chicoutimi QC G7H 7K9
418 543-2222; Fax: 418 543-5912
E: rgirard@quebec.cancer.ca
W: www.quebec.cancer.ca
Executive:
Coord rég: Raymond Girard
Criteria: *Open to all.*
No of Paid Staff: 5
Languages: French

◊Drummondville:
209 rue Dorion, Drummondville QC J2C 1T8
819 478-3261; Fax: 819 478-0479
E: ssevigny@quebec.cancer.ca
W: www.cancer.ca
Executive:
Coord rég: Diane Grondin
No of Paid Staff: 1
Languages: French

◊Gatineau:
105-15 rue Buteau, Gatineau QC J8Z 1V4
819 777-4428; Fax: 819 777-7164
Toll-free: 888 939-3333 Cancer Info
W: www.quebec.cancer.ca
Executive:
Coord rég: Martin Lessard
No of Paid Staff: 4
Languages: French

◊Laval:
1419 rue Michelin, Laval QC H7L 4S2
450 668-1013; Fax: 450 668-1092
Toll-free: 888 668-1013
W: www.cancer.ca
Executive:
Dir gén: Suzanne Dubois
Dir opér: Alain Deschamps
Ress hum: Nada Horth
Languages: French

◊Longueuil:
110-550 ch de Chambly, Longueuil QC J4H 3L8
450 442-9430; Fax: 450 442-0592
W: www.cancer.ca
Executive:
Agente: Gisèle Richard
Coord: Suzanne Barnabé
No of Paid Staff: 6
Languages: French

Trillium Childhood Cancer Support Centre
940 Queensdale Ave E, Hamilton ON L8V 1N4
905 527-1992; Fax: 905 527-5314
Toll-free: 888 999-2267
W: www.camptrillium.com
Executive:
Exec Dir: Marci Shea-Perry
Acct Mgr: Pat Garbett
Admin: Cheryl Rogerson
Year Founded: 1984
Criteria: *Open to any child or parent of a child who has cancer.*
Budget: $1,800,000
No of Paid Staff: 15
Library: Y *(Open to the public)*
Languages: English; French

CELIAC DISEASE

Canadian Celiac Association
Bldg 1
400-5025 Orbitor Dr, Mississauga ON L4W 4Y5
905 507-6208; Fax: 905 507-4673
Toll-free: 800 363-7296
E: info@celiac.ca
W: www.celiac.ca
Year Founded: 1973
Criteria: *Open to all.*
No of Paid Staff: 2
Library: Y *(Open to the public)*
Languages: English

Canadian Celiac Association - Edmonton Chapter
212-5004E 98 Ave NW, Edmonton AB T6A 0A1
780 485-2949; Fax: 780 485-2940
E: info@celiacedmonton.ca
W: www.celiac.edmonton.ab.ca
Executive:
Pres: Don Briggs
VP: Dan Wiebe
Treas: Trish Wayne
Sec: Sherri Tirschmann
Year Founded: 1982
No of Paid Staff: 1
Speakers Available
Languages: English
Membership: 700

CEREBRAL PALSY

BC Centre For Ability
2805 Kingsway, Vancouver BC V5R 5H9
604 451-5511; Fax: 604 451-5651
W: www.centreforability.bc.ca
Executive:
Exec Dir: Angela Kwok
Dir-Info Tech: Wade Fung
Commun Mgr: Audrey Kwan
Library: Y *(Open to the public)*
Languages: English

Cerebral Palsy Association in Alberta
12001 44 St SE, Calgary AB T2Z 4G9
403 543-1161; Fax: 403 543-1168
Toll-free: 800 363-2807
E: admin@cpalberta.com
W: www.cpalberta.com
Executive:
Exec Dir: Janice Bushfield
Year Founded: 1976
Criteria: *Family with child with CP or individual (18 yrs. or older) with CP.*
Budget: $1,200,000
No of Paid Staff: 15
Library: Y *(Open to the public)*
Languages: English
Membership: 2,100
Library:
Community Resource Centre *(Open to the public)*

◊Edmonton:
17231 105 Ave NW, Edmonton AB T5S 1H2
780 477-8030; Fax: 780 471-0855
Toll-free: 800 363-2807
E: info@cpalberta.com
W: www.cpalberta.com
Executive:
Exec Dir: Janice Bushfield
Office Mgr: Elizabeth Kaleta
Year Founded: 1976
Criteria: *Individuals affected by cerebral palsy.*
Budget: $600,000
No of Paid Staff: 10
Speakers Available
Library: Y
Languages: English
Membership: 1,600
Library:
Cerebral Palsy Resource Centre *(Open to the public)*

Cerebral Palsy Association of British Columbia
801-409 Granville St, Vancouver BC V6C 1T2
604 408-9484; Fax: 604 408-9489
Toll-free: 800 663-0004
E: info@bccerebralpalsy.com
W: www.bccerebralpalsy.com
Executive:
Pres: Craig Langston
VP: Trish McKay
Dir-Prog/Admin: Feri Dehdar
Treas: Andy Yu
Year Founded: 1954
Criteria: *Payment of membership fees.*
Budget: $200,000
No of Paid Staff: 3
Speakers Available
Library: Y *(Open to the public)*
Languages: English
Membership: 900 *(Lists available to the public)*
Membership Fee: $20
Library:
Cerebral Palsy Association Lending Library *(Open to the public)*

Cerebral Palsy Association of Manitoba
Colony Square
105-500 Portage Ave, Winnipeg MB R3C 3X1
204 982-4842; Fax: 204 982-4844
Toll-free: 800 416-6166 (Manitoba only)
E: office@cerebralpalsy.mb.ca
W: www.cerebralpalsy.mb.ca
Executive:
Membership/Prog Dir: David Kron
Year Founded: 1974
Criteria: *Open to all*
Budget: $100,000
No of Paid Staff: 1
Speakers Available
Library: Y
Languages: English
Membership: 350
Membership Fee: $10, $25 Corporate/Orginization

Cerebral Palsy Association of P.E.I.
Location: 13 Linden Ave, Charlottetown PE C1A 5Y5
Mailing: PO Box 22034, RPO Ch'Twn Parkdale, Charlottetown PE C1A 9J2
902 892-9694; Fax: 902 628-8751
E: info@peicpa.com
W: www.peicpa.com
Year Founded: 1953
Speakers Available
Languages: English

Child Development Centre of Prince George and District Association
1687 Strathcona Ave, Prince George BC V2L 4E7
250 563-7168; Fax: 250 563-8039
W: www.cdcpg.org
Executive:
Exec Dir: Darrell Roze
Year Founded: 1968
Criteria: *Receiving support service from CPA.*
Budget: $3,200,000
No of Paid Staff: 65
Speakers Available
Library: Y *(Open to the public)*
Languages: English
Membership: 600

Halifax Regional Cerebral Palsy Association
Mailing: PO Box 33075, RPO Quinpool Centre, Halifax NS B3L 4T6
902 479-0963; Fax: 902 479-0963
E: cerebral.palsy@ns.sympatico.ca
W: www.hrcpa.ca
Languages: English

Newfoundland Cerebral Palsy Association Inc.
Mailing: PO Box 23059 RPO Churchill Sq, St. John's NL A1B 4J9
709 753-9922; Fax: 709 753-9922
E: cerebralpalsy@nf.aibn.com
W: www.cpnl.ca
Executive:
Pres: Darren Martin
VP: Marvin Chaulk
Sec: Cindy Bishop
Budget: $20,000
Speakers Available
Library: Y *(Open to the public)*
Languages: English

Ontario Federation for Cerebral Palsy
104-1630 Lawrence Ave W, Toronto ON M6L 1C5
416 244-9686; Fax: 416 244-6543
Toll-free: 877 244-9686
W: www.ofcp.on.ca
Executive:
Sr Mgr: Steve Chandler
Exec Dir: Clarence Meyers
Year Founded: 1947
Speakers Available
Library: Y *(Open to the public)*
Languages: English

Saskatchewan Cerebral Palsy Association
2310 Louise Ave, Saskatoon SK S7J 2C7
306 955-7272; Fax: 306 373-2665
Toll-free: 800 925-4524
E: saskcpa@shaw.ca
Executive:
Pres: Holly Flett
Admin/Receptionist: Heather Frehlick
Languages: English
Membership Fee: $15 Family; $10 Individual

Voice of the Cerebral Palsied of Greater Vancouver
103-577 8th Ave E, Vancouver BC V5T 1S9
604 874-1741; Fax: 604 874-1746
E: vcpgv@vcn.bc.ca
W: www.vcpgv.org
Executive:
Exec Dir: Yoshinori Tanabe
Year Founded: 1977
No of Paid Staff: 3
Library: Y
Languages: English

CHRONIC PAIN

Chronic Pain Association of Canada - CPAC
Location: 7-10329 61 Ave NW, Edmonton AB T6H 1K9
Mailing: PO Box 66017 RPO Heritage, Edmonton AB T6J 6T4
780 482-6727; Fax: 780 435-8758
E: cpac@chronicpaincanada.com
W: www.chronicpaincanada.com
Executive:
Pres: Heather Divine
Exec Dir: Barry Ulmer
Criteria: *Open to any person interested in joining.*
Languages: English

CROHN'S AND COLITIS

Cancer Advocacy Coalition of Canada
204-60 St Clair Ave E, Toronto ON M4T 1N5
416 538-4874; Fax: 416 538-7319
Toll-free: 877 472-3436
E: cacc@canceradvocacy.ca
W: www.canceradvocacy.ca
Executive:
Chm: Dr Dauna Crooks
Vice Chm: Larry Broadfield
Vice Chm: David Saltman
Sec-Treas: Elizabeth Whamond

Crohn's and Colitis Foundation of Canada - National Office
600-60 St Clair Ave E, Toronto ON M4T 1N5
416 920-5035; Fax: 416 929-0364
Toll-free: 800 387-1479
E: ccfc@ccfc.ca
W: www.ccfc.ca
Executive:
Natl Pres: Marty Cutler
Natl Treas: Byron Sonberg
Natl Sec: Paul McCarten
Year Founded: 1974
No of Paid Staff: 35
Languages: English; French
Membership: 50,000

◈Alberta/NWT/Nunavut:
3100-246 Stewart Green SW, Calgary AB T3H 3C8
403 569-8477; Fax: 403 569-1552
Toll-free: 888 884-2232
E: alberta@ccfc.ca
W: www.ccfc.ca
Executive:
Reg Dir: Carolle Anderson
Languages: English; French

◈British Columbia/Yukon:
Location: 11108 84 Ave, Delta BC V4C 2L7
Mailing: PO Box 33060 Rpo Nordel, Delta BC V4C 8E6
604 596-2305; Fax: 604 596-3187
Toll-free: 800 513-8202
E: aobrecht@ccfc.ca
W: www.ccfc.ca
Executive:
Reg Dir-BC & Yukon: Shona Brown
Chapter Dev Coord: Alison Obrecht
Year Founded: 1938
Speakers Available
Languages: English

◈Manitoba/Saskatchewan:
Location: 3310 Portage Ave, Winnipeg MB R3K 2E5
Mailing: PO Box 20009 RPO Westwood
204 231-2115; Fax: 204 237-8214
Toll-free: 866 856-8551
W: www.ccfc.ca
Executive:
Reg Dir: Shari Haydaman
No of Paid Staff: 2
Speakers Available
Languages: English

◈Newfoundland/Labrador:
Mailing: PO Box 39093 RPO Topsail Rd, St. John's NL A1E 5Y7
709 579-3700; Fax: 709 579-3744
Toll-free: 800 563-4843
W: www.ccfc.ca
Executive:
Reg Dir: Julie Bowering
Year Founded: 1974
No of Paid Staff: 1
Speakers Available
Languages: English
Membership: 100

◈Maritimes:
5816 St Margarets Bay Rd, Hd St Margts NS B3Z 2E4
902 422-8137; Fax: 902 422-6552
Toll-free: 800 265-1101
W: www.ccfc.ca
Executive:
Reg Dir: Tracy Durkee Jones
Chapter Dev Coord: Tradina Meadows-Forgeron
Languages: English

◈Ontario:
600-60 St Clair Ave E, Toronto ON M4T 1N5
416 920-5035; Fax: 416 929-0364
Toll-free: 800 387-1479
E: ccfc@ccfc.ca
W: www.ccfc.ca
Executive:
Reg Dir Ontario: Rea Ganesh
Languages: English
Membership: 3,391

◇East District Office:
Mailing: PO Box 141, Dunrobin ON KOA 1T0
613 832-9344; Fax: 613 832-7231
Toll-free: 877 338-7426
W: www.ccfc.ca
Executive:
Chapter Dev Coord: Sherry Pang

◈ ***Québec:***
223-3767 boul Thimens, Saint-Laurent QC H4R 1W4
514 342-0666; Fax: 514 342-1011
Toll-free: 800 461-4683
E: info@ccfc.ca
W: www.fcmii.ca
Executive:
Adj admin: Daniela Santinelli
No of Paid Staff: 2
Languages: English; French
Membership Fee: $30

CYSTIC FIBROSIS

Cystic Fibrosis Canada
Location: 1300 Garth St, Hamilton ON L9C 4L7
Mailing: PO Box 79005 RPO Garth, Hamilton ON L9C 7N6
519 717-8898
Toll-free: 800 378-2233
E: kgcf@sympatico.ca
W: www.cysticfibrosishamilton.com
Executive:
Pres: Karen Gliddon
Languages: English

Cystic Fibrosis Canada - National Office
601-2221 Yonge St, Toronto ON M4S 2B4
416 485-9149; Fax: 416 485-0960
Toll-free: 800 378-2233 Canada-Wide
E: info@cysticfibrosis.ca
W: www.cysticfibrosis.ca
Executive:
Pres/CEO: Maureen Adamson
Year Founded: 1960
Criteria: *Open to any person interested in cystic fibrosis.*
No of Paid Staff: 24
Speakers Available
Languages: English; French
Membership: 60,000
Membership Fee: N/A

◈ ***Prairies:***

◇ ***Calgary & Southern Alberta Chapter:***
403 266-5295; Fax: 403 262-7556
E: ccffcal@telus.net
Executive:
Admin: Debbie Matthews

◇ ***Central Alberta Chapter:***
403 347-5075; Fax: 403 347-5075
E: jmeulenbelt@shaw.ca
Executive:
Pres: Joanne Meulenbelt

◇ ***Edmonton & Northern Alberta Chapter:***
St. James Catholic School
7814 83 St, Edmonton AB T6C 2Y8
780 466-2265; Fax: 780 437-7655
E: ecfs@telusplanet.net

◇ ***North Saskatchewan Chapter:***
Mailing: PO Box 3088 Stn Main, Saskatoon SK S7K 3S9
306 979-8688
E: bjlid@shaw.ca
Executive:
Pres: Joan Lidington
Languages: English

◇ ***South Saskatchewan Chapter:***
Mailing: PO Box 721 Stn Main, Regina SK S4P 3A8
306 949-1515
E: info@southsaskcf.ca
W: www.southsaskcf.ca/
Executive:
Co-Pres: Mike Weger
Co-Pres: Cara Weger
Speakers Available
Languages: English

◇ ***Winnipeg Chapter:***
157 Lake Ridge Rd, Winnipeg MB R2Y 1K3
204 663-1037
E: info@cysticfibrosis.ca
W: www.cysticfibrosis.ca
Languages: English

◈ ***Vancouver & Interior BC:***

◇ ***Kamloops Chapter:***
250 314-1606
E: catchnrelease@shaw.ca
Executive:
Pres: John Bowers

◇ ***Prince George Chapter:***
Mailing: PO Box 1402 Stn A, Prince George BC V2L 4V4
250 330-4494; Fax: 250 330-4494
E: kkellett@netbistro.com
Executive:
Pres: Lesley Girard
Languages: English

◇ ***Vancouver/Lower Mainland Chapter:***
119-1600 6th Ave W, Vancouver BC V6J 1R3
604 436-1158; Fax: 604 436-1154
W: www.cfvancouver.ca
Languages: English

◈ ***Vancouver Island:***

◇ ***Campbell River Chapter:***
573 Nature Park Dr, Campbell River BC V9W 7Z9
250 923-4992; Fax: 250 286-3679
W: www.crcf.ca
Executive:
Pres: Jo-Ann Wallis
Languages: English

◇ ***Nanaimo***
140 Tait Rd, Nanaimo BC V9X 1C2
250 753-1597
Executive:
Pres: Debra Tuck
Languages: English

◇ ***Powell River Satellite:***
604 485-9337; Fax: 604 485-2120
E: lorvilla@shaw.ca
Executive:
Pres: Lorne Villani

◈ ***Atlantic Provinces:***

◇ ***Moncton Chapter:***
Location: 57 Colonial Dr, Moncton NB E1G 2J1
Mailing: 164 Collishaw St, Moncton NB E1C 9R3
506 852-9341; Fax: 506 382-2571
E: smithviv@nb.sympatico.ca
W: www.cysticfibrosis.ca
Executive:
Principal: Vivian Smith
Languages: English

◇ ***Prince Edward Island Chapter:***
902 672-1624
E: roberta_d_clark@hotmail.com
Executive:
Pres: Roberta Clark

◇ ***Scotia Chapter:***
902 425-2462; Fax: 902 422-2956
E: jennifer@cfnovascotia.ca
Executive:
Pres: Bruce Thompson
Dev Coord: Jennifer Gillis

◇ ***West Coast Nfld/Labrador Satellite:***
709 944-3359; Fax: 709 944-5798
E: pfurlong@crrstv.net
Executive:
Principal: Erica Furlong

◈ ***Central Ontario:***

◇ ***Durham Region Chapter:***
905 725-9524
E: j_thow23@hotmail.com
Executive:
Pres: Jo-Ann Thow
Executive:
Pres: Frank Aucoin
Mgr/Fundraising Coord: Dolores Adams
Year Founded: 1976
No of Paid Staff: 1
Languages: English

◇ ***Niagara Chapter:***
7051 Dolphin St, Niagara Falls ON L2E 6Y3
289 296-7941
E: mscotney2@cogeco.ca
W: www.cysticfibrosis.ca
Executive:
Pres: Mary-Ellen Scotney
Criteria: *Open to all.*
Library: Y *(Open to the public)*
Languages: English

◇ ***Peel & District Chapter:***
227 Wilkinson Rd, Brampton ON L6T 4M2
905 450-1882; Fax: 905 450-1908
E: admin@ccffpeel.org
W: www.ccffpeel.org

◇ ***Toronto & District Chapter:***
817-2 Carlton St, Toronto ON M5B 1J3
416 932-3900; Fax: 416 932-3010
Toll-free: 888 289-7923
E: toronto@cysticfibrosis.ca
W: www.ccfftoronto.ca
Executive:
Exec Dir: Jackie Bloom
Fundraising/Acct Coord: Laura Ferguson
Event Mgr: Shannon Carkner
Year Founded: 1960
Criteria: *An interest in supporting the Foundations' cause.*
No of Paid Staff: 3
Speakers Available
Languages: English
Membership: 350

◈ ***Eastern Ontario:***

◇ ***Cornwall***
Mailing: PO Box 1385 Stn Main, Cornwall ON K6H 5V4
613 933-5851
E: bairdjk@cogeco.ca
W: www.cysticfibrosis.ca
Executive:
Pres: Kim Baird
Languages: English

◇ ***Kingston Chapter:***
613 549-3240; Fax: 613 634-9090
E: jeff.q@bellnet.ca
Executive:
Pres: Jeff Quanz

◇ ***Ottawa Chapter:***
120 Amberwood Cres, Nepean ON K2E 7H8
613 230-6643; Fax: 613 230-3628
Toll-free: 800 378-2233
E: amberkandy@rogers.com
Executive:
Pres: André Chartrand
VP Fundraising: Karen Chartrand
Year Founded: 1961
Budget: $500,000
Speakers Available
Languages: English; French
Membership: All volunteers

◇ ***Peterborough Chapter:***
705 657-7119
Toll-free: 800 378-2233
E: peterboroughbreathe_cf@hotmail.com
W: www.cysticfibrosis.ca
Executive:
Pres: Erin Stewart
Languages: English

◈ ***Northern Ontario:***

◇ ***North Bay Chapter:***
705 474-7487
E: microkin@sympatico.ca
Executive:
Pres: Mike Croghan

◇ ***Sault Ste. Marie Chapter:***
705 942-0273
E: brasonking@shaw.ca
Executive:
Pres: Marilyn King

◇ ***Sudbury Chapter:***
4650 Robert Dr, Val Therese ON P3P 1S4
705 969-5520
E: cysticfibrosissudbury@hotmail.com
Languages: English

◇ ***Thunder Bay Chapter:***
807 344-6824
E: glowar@tbaytel.net
Executive:
Pres: Gloria Houghton

◈ ***Western Ontario:***

◇ ***Huron-Oxford-Perth:***
519 291-5837
E: head2toe@sympatico.ca
Executive:
Pres: Donna Mitchell

◇ ***Kitchener/Waterloo District:***
Location: 69 Sydney St S, Kitchener ON N2G 3V1
Mailing: PO Box 2151 Stn C, Kitchener ON N2H 6M1
519 772-2300; Fax: 519 772-2301
E: kwdcfc@golden.net
W: www.kwdcfc.ca
Languages: English

◇ ***London Chapter:***
Location: 154 Inverary Cres, London ON N6G 3L8
Mailing: PO Box 1131 Stn B, London ON N6A 5K2
519 615-1355; Fax: 519 471-4131
Toll-free: 800 378-2233
E: info@cysticfibrosislondon.ca
W: www.cysticfibrosislondon.ca
Executive:
Chapter Admin: Carol Cooper
Library: Y *(Open to the public)*
Languages: English

◇ ***Sarnia-Lambton Chapter:***
519 337-0560
E: info@cysticfibrosissarnia.com
Executive:
Pres: Paul Croft

◇ ***Windsor Chapter:***
Mailing: PO Box 21001 RPO University Mall, Windsor ON N9B 3T4
519 252-2850
E: windsorcysticfibrosis@cogeco.ca
W: www.ccffwindsor.ca
Executive:
Dev Coord: Chantelle Foreman
Languages: English

◈ ***Eastern & Western Quebec:***
505-625 av du Président-Kennedy, Montréal QC H3A 1K2
514 877-6161; Fax: 514 877-6116
Toll-free: 800 363-7711
E: info@fibrosekystiquequebec.ca
W: www.fibrosekystiquequebec.ca
Executive:
Prés: Julie Saucier
Dir gén: Benoit Vigneau
Sec exéc: Bettina Ehlers
Year Founded: 1981
Criteria: *Parents, amis, partenaires corporatifs*
Budget: $3,000,000
No of Paid Staff: 10
Speakers Available
Languages: French; English
Membership: 600 à 700
Membership Fee: $15

◇ ***Bas Saint-Laurent/Gaspésie:***
418 723-9291; Fax: 418 725-5442
E: gilbert.berube@globetrotter.net
Executive:
Prés: Gilbert Bérubé

◇ ***Centre du Québec:***
819 379-7272
E: drtrahan@drtrahan.com
Executive:
Prés: Dr André Trahan

◇ ***Charlevoix-Ouest:***
418 435-6308
E: hdall@sympatico.ca
Executive:
Prés: Henriette Dallaire

◇ ***Côte-Nord:***
1049 rue Henri, Baie-Comeau QC G5C 2K6
418 589-6428
E: sofaca@globetrotter.net
Executive:
Prés: Sophie Girard
Languages: English; French

◇ ***Estrie:***
819 569-4924
E: rene.lacasse@sympatico.ca
Executive:
Prés: Michel Roy

◇ ***Montréal:***
514 238-7088
E: sectionmontreal@aqfk.qc.ca
Executive:
Prés: Julie Saucier

◇ ***Outaouais:***
48A rue Saint-Antoine, Gatineau QC J8T 3L6
819 243-8619; Fax: 819 561-7907
E: lyne.r.lacroix@aexp.com
W: www.fibrosekystique.ca
Executive:
Prés: Lyne Lacroix
VP: Daniel Raymond
Speakers Available
Languages: French; English

◇ ***Québec:***
Centre Plaza Laval
227-2750 ch Sainte-Foy, Québec QC G1V 1V6
418 653-2086; Fax: 418 653-1152
Toll-free: 877 653-2086
E: mgamache@fibrosekystiquequebec.ca
W: www.fibrosekystiquequebec.ca
Executive:
Prés: Guy Pagé
Coord: Marielle Gamache
No of Paid Staff: 1
Languages: French

◇ ***Sept-Îles Satellite:***
418 961-2247
Executive:
Principal: Ronald Lévesque

DIABETES

Canadian Diabetes Association - National Office

National Life Bldg
1400-522 University Ave, Toronto ON M5G 2R5
416 363-3373; Fax: 416 408-7117
Toll-free: 800 226-8464
E: info@diabetes.ca
W: www.diabetes.ca
Executive:
Exec Dir HR: Heather Angel
Year Founded: 1953
Membership Fee Required: Y
Speakers Available
Library: Y *(Open to the public)*
Languages: English
Membership Fee: Senior - $18; Individual - $28

◈ ***Northern Alberta & NWT Regional Leadership Centre:***
100-12220 Stony Plain Rd NW, Edmonton AB T5N 3Y4
780 423-1232; Fax: 780 423-3322
Toll-free: 800 226-8464
E: abinfo@diabetes.ca
W: www.diabetes.ca
No of Paid Staff: 30
Speakers Available
Library: Y *(Open to the public)*
Languages: English

◇ ***Foothills:***
Holy Cross Centre
101-138 18 Ave SE, Calgary AB T2G 5P9
403 283-1500; Fax: 403 283-1527
W: www.diabetes-foothills.org
Executive:
Exec Dir: Marjorie Snaith
Year Founded: 1993
No of Paid Staff: 4
Speakers Available
Languages: English
Membership: 2,200

◇ ***Grande Prairie & District:***
Mailing: 1010-10117 Jasper Ave NW, Edmonton AB T5J 1W8
Toll-free: 800 563-0032
E: freda.badry@diabetes.ca
Executive:
Reg Dir: Freda Badry

◇ ***NWT, Wood Buffalo & District:***
Mailing: 10117 Jasper Ave NW, Edmonton AB T5J 1W8
Toll-free: 800 563-0032 AB only
E: freda.badry@diabetes.ca
Executive:
Reg Dir: Freda Badry

◈ ***Southern Alberta Regional Leadership Centre:***
204-2323 32 Ave NE, Calgary AB T2E 6Z3
403 266-0620; Fax: 403 269-8927
Toll-free: 403 440-3717
W: www.diabetes.ca
Executive:
PPS/Br Cood Red Deer: Helen Robertson
PPS/Br Cood Medicine Hat: Karen Rodgers
Reg Dir: Laura Kempi
Speakers Available
Library: Y *(Open to the public)*
Languages: English
Membership Fee: $18 Seniors; $28 Regular

◇ ***Business Operations***
7A-2835 19 St NE, Calgary AB T2E 7A2
403 509-0070; Fax: 403 509-0072

Executive:
Ops Mgr: Carolyn Farago
Area Dir Western Cda: Danny Nykolaychuk

◈Pacific Area:

◇Greater Vancouver & District:
360-1385 8th Ave W, Vancouver BC V6H 3V9
604 732-1331; Fax: 604 732-8444
Toll-free: 800 665-6526
E: infobc@diabetes.ca
W: www.diabetes.ca
Executive:
Exec Dir Pacific Area: Connie Abram
Br Coord: Franca Lattanzio
Year Founded: 1953
No of Paid Staff: 25
Speakers Available
Library: Y *(Open to the public)*
Languages: English; Mandarin
Membership Fee: $18 Seniors; $28 Regular
Library:
Diabetes Information & Support Centre

◇Kelowna:
1589 Sutherland Ave, Kelowna BC V1Y 5Y7
250 762-9447; Fax: 250 717-3199
Toll-free: 888 628-9494
W: www.diabetes.ca
Year Founded: 1953
Speakers Available
Library: Y *(Open to the public)*
Languages: English; French; Chinese; Punjabi
Membership: 321
Membership Fee: $18-$28
Library:
Diabetes Information and Support Centre

◇Nanaimo & District:
255-2000 Island Hwy N, Nanaimo BC V9S 5W3
250 729-3824; Fax: 250 729-3825
Toll-free: 800 665-6526 Vancouver
W: www.diabetes.ca
Library: Y *(Open to the public)*
Languages: English

◇Penticton & District:
Location: 1589 Sutherland Ave, Kelowna BC V1Y 5Y7
Mailing: PO Box 24008 RPO Government St, Penticton BC V2A 8L9
250 862-9447; Fax: 250 492-2865
E: pentictoncda@img.net
Languages: English

◇Prince George & District:
103-490 Quebec St, Prince George BC V2L 5N5
250 561-9284; Fax: 250 561-0009
E: boyanne.young@diabetes.ca
W: www.diabetes.ca
Executive:
Northern Br Coord: Boyanne Young
No of Paid Staff: 4
Speakers Available
Library: Y *(Open to the public)*
Languages: English
Membership: 200 *(Lists available to the public)*
Membership Fee: Senior - $18; Regular - $28
Library:
Diabetes Resource Centre

◇Vernon & District:
Location: 1589 Sutherland Ave, Kelowna BC V1Y 5Y7
Mailing: PO Box 1301 Stn Main, Vernon BC V1T 6N6
250 549-5002
E: cdn_diabetes_vernon@telus.net
Languages: English

◇Williams Lake & District:
1589 Sutherland Ave, Kelowna BC V1Y 5Y7
250 392-1129; Fax: 250 392-4776
Toll-free: 800 665-6526
E: cdawilliamslake@uniserve.com
Year Founded: 1984
Budget: $6,000
Speakers Available
Library: Y *(Open to the public)*
Languages: English
Membership: 40

◈Winnipeg Regional Leadership Centre:
200-310 Broadway, Winnipeg MB R3C 0S6
204 925-3800; Fax: 204 949-0266
Toll-free: 800 226-8464
Languages: English

◇Westman Branch & District:
727B 10th St, Brandon MB R7A 4G7
204 728-2382; Fax: 204 726-1603
Toll-free: 800 226-8464
E: laura.neely-carter@diabetes.ca
W: www.diabetes.ca
Languages: English

◈New Brunswick:
2-61 Carleton St, Fredericton NB E3B 3T2
506 452-9009; Fax: 506 455-4728
Toll-free: 800 884-4232
E: nbinfo@diabetes.ca
W: www.diabetes.ca
Executive:
Reg Dir: Jake Reid
Membership Fee Required: Y
No of Paid Staff: 4
Speakers Available
Library: Y *(Open to the public)*
Languages: English; French
Membership: 1,500
Membership Fee: $18 Senior; $28 Regular

◈Newfoundland & Labrador:
2007-29 31 Pippy Pl, St. John's NL A1B 3X2
709 754-0953; Fax: 709 754-0734
W: www.diabetes.ca
Executive:
Reg Dir: Carol Ann Smith
Year Founded: 1953
No of Paid Staff: 22
Languages: English

◈Nova Scotia Branch:
101-137 Chain Lake Dr, Halifax NS B3S 1B3
902 453-4232; Fax: 902 453-4440
Toll-free: 800 326-7712
W: www.diabetes.ca
Executive:
Exec Dir-Cmmty Engmnt: Jim Casey
Reg Dir Maritimes: Lisa Matte
Exec Asst: Tracy Clarke
Speakers Available
Library: Y *(Open to the public)*
Languages: English

◇Sydney Branch:
42 Coxheath Rd, Sydney NS B1R 1R3
902 564-6461; Fax: 902 564-5354
E: arlene.parsons@diabetes.ca
Executive:
Br Coord: Arlene Parsons
Languages: English

◈Ontario:

◇Brantford:
99 Wayne Gretzky Pky, Floor 5, Brantford ON N3S 6T6
519 756-9131; Fax: 519 756-4262
W: www.diabetes.ca
Executive:
Exec Dir: Kerry Bruder
Br Coord: Lorraine Hagan
Year Founded: 1953
No of Paid Staff: 1
Speakers Available
Library: Y *(Open to the public)*
Languages: English
Membership Fee: $18 Senior; $28 Individual

◇Chatham & District:
Location: 180 McNaughton Ave W, Chatham ON N7L 4Z7
Mailing: PO Box 724 Stn Main, Chatham ON N7M 5L1
519 351-6020; Fax: 519 351-5167
Toll-free: 800 226-8464
W: www.diabetes.ca
Executive:
Br Coord: Peter Jones
Languages: English

◇Cornwall & District:
119 Sydney St, Cornwall ON K6H 3H1
613 938-7497; Fax: 613 938-9782
Toll-free: 800 226-8464
W: www.diabetes.ca
Executive:
Br Coord: Linda Rodgers
Languages: English

◇Durham Region:
1400-522 University Ave, Toronto ON M5G 2R5
416 408-7087; Fax: 416 363-7465
Toll-free: 800 226-8464 7144
E: info@diabetes.ca
W: www.diabetes.ca
Executive:
Reg Dir: Kerry Bruder
Languages: English

◇Elmira & District:
1-14 Irvin St, Kitchener ON N2H 1K8
519 742-1481; Fax: 519 742-1282
E: kitchener.office@diabetes.ca
W: www.diabetes.ca
Executive:
Reg Dir: Kerry Bruder
No of Paid Staff: 4
Languages: English

◇Hamilton & District:
17-1685 Main St W, Hamilton ON L8S 1G5
905 528-3111; Fax: 905 528-1263
W: www.diabetes.ca
Executive:
Pub Prog/Serv Coord: Lucy Florio
Reg Dir: Kerry Bruder
Year Founded: 1953
No of Paid Staff: 9
Speakers Available
Library: Y *(Open to the public)*
Languages: English
Membership: 2,500
Membership Fee: $18 Senior; $28 Regular

◇Hastings & Prince Edward Branch
49 Millennium Pky, Belleville ON K8N 4Z5
613 962-6520; Fax: 613 962-1624
W: www.diabetes.ca
Executive:
Reg Dir: Terry Cavanaugh
Languages: English

◇Kawarthas:
102-294 Rink St, Peterborough ON K9J 2K2
705 742-2733; Fax: 705 742-1185
E: kawarthas@diabetes.ca
W: www.diabetes.ca
Executive:
Reg Chairperson: Michael Brierley
Reg Serv Coord: Elaine Petreman
Year Founded: 1953
Criteria: *Open to all.*
No of Paid Staff: 1
Speakers Available
Library: Y *(Open to the public)*
Languages: English
Membership: 800 Kawarthas Branch
Membership Fee: $20 Seniors; $28 Regular

◊ ***Lindsay & District:***
189 Kent St W, Lindsay ON K9V 5G6
705 878-0131; Fax: 705 786-2277
Toll-free: 800 226-8464
E: cda19@nexicom.net
W: www.diabetes.ca
Year Founded: 1969
Speakers Available
Library: Y
Languages: English
Membership: 462
Membership Fee: $18 Seniors; $28 Regular
Library:
Resource Centre *(Open to the public)*

◊ ***London***
1150 Frances St, London ON N5W 5N5
519 858-3443; Fax: 519 858-9133
Toll-free: 800 505-5525
W: www.diabetes.ca
Executive:
Ops Mgr: Jeb Aarts
Reg Mgr: Sylvia Krampelj
Criteria: *Open to all.*
Library: Y *(Open to the public)*
Languages: English

◊ ***Midland-Penetanguishene:***
25 Jeffery St, Penetanguishene ON L9M 1K6
705 549-0881; Fax: 705 549-0745
Toll-free: 800 226-8464
W: www.diabetes.ca
Executive:
Chairperson: Fran Moreau
Criteria: *Open to all.*
Library: Y *(Open to the public)*
Languages: English; French

◊ ***Niagara & District:***
Mailing: Rear Unit
PO Box 20158 RPO Grantham, St. Catharines ON L2M 7W7
Fax: 905 646-1130
Toll-free: 800 226-8464
E: terri.young@diabetes.ca
W: www.diabetes.ca
Executive:
Public Prog/Serv Coord: Terri Young
Year Founded: 1953
No of Paid Staff: 2
Speakers Available
Library: Y
Languages: English
Membership: 1,200
Membership Fee: $18 Senior; $28 Family
Library:
Reference Centre *(Open to the public)*

◊ ***Ottawa & District:***
45 Montreal Rd, Vanier ON K1L 6E8
613 521-1902; Fax: 613 521-3667
W: www.diabetes.ca
Executive:
Reg Dir: Terry Cavanaugh
Criteria: *None*
No of Paid Staff: 13
Speakers Available
Library: Y *(Open to the public)*
Languages: English; French
Membership: 2,300
Membership Fee: $20

◊ ***Peel Region:***
1400-522 University Ave, Toronto ON M5G 2R5
416 408-7087; Fax: 416 363-7465
W: www.diabetes.ca
Executive:
Reg Dir: Kerry Bruder

◊ ***Pembroke & District:***
103-227 Lake St, Pembroke ON K8A 5M2
613 735-1605; Fax: 613 735-1205
Toll-free: 800 226-8464
E: laura.murphy@diabetes.ca
W: www.diabetes.ca
Executive:
Mgr: Laura Murphy
Criteria: *Open to all.*
Library: Y *(Open to the public)*
Languages: English; French

◊ ***Sault Ste. Marie & District:***
134 Northern Ave E, Sault Ste. Marie ON P6B 4H4
705 759-1233; Fax: 705 759-3985
Toll-free: 800 226-8464
W: www.diabetes.ca
Executive:
Br Coord: Janie Bringleson
Languages: English

◊ ***Simcoe County/Muskokas/Parry Sound:***
4-556 Bryne Dr, Barrie ON L4N 9P6
705 737-3611; Fax: 705 737-4912
Toll-free: 800 224-8464
E: centraleastontario@diabetes.ca
W: www.diabetes.ca
Executive:
Br Coord: JoAnn Warren
Reg Dir: Kerry Bruder
Speakers Available
Library: Y *(Open to the public)*
Languages: English

◊ ***South East Ontario Regional Leadership Centre***
10-541 Days Rd, Kingston ON K7M 3R8
613 384-9374; Fax: 613 384-1079
E: terry.cavanaugh@diabetes.ca
W: www.diabetes.ca
Executive:
Reg Dir SE ON: Terry Cavanaugh
Languages: English

◊ ***South West Ontario Regional Leadership Centre:***
442 Adelaide St N, London ON N6B 3H8
519 673-1630; Fax: 519 660-8992
Toll-free: 800 226-8464
W: www.diabetes.ca
Executive:
Reg Dir: Sue Taylor
Criteria: *Open to all.*
No of Paid Staff: 8
Speakers Available
Library: Y *(Open to the public)*
Languages: English
Membership: 9
Membership Fee: $18 Seniors; $28 Regular

◊ ***Sudbury & District:***
F-2141 Lasalle Blvd, Sudbury ON P3A 2A3
705 670-1993; Fax: 705 670-1995
E: kirsikka.corradi@diabetes.ca
W: www.diabetes.ca
Executive:
Reg Dir: Jennifer MacKinnon
Languages: English

◊ ***Timmins & District:***
206-670 Airport Rd, Timmins ON P4P 1J2
705 267-1191; Fax: 705 267-1151
E: julie.st-onge@diabetes.ca
W: www.diabetes.ca
Executive:
Mgr: Bonnie Swietek
Coord: Julie St-Onge
Speakers Available
Library: Y *(Open to the public)*
Languages: English

◊ ***Toronto:***
1400-522 University Ave, Toronto ON M5G 2R5
416 408-7087; Fax: 416 363-7465
E: info@diabetes.ca
W: www.diabetes.ca
Executive:
Reg Dir: Kerry Bruder
Criteria: *Open to all.*
No of Paid Staff: 4
Languages: English

◊ ***Tri-County Branch***
Location: 42 George St, Brockville ON K6V 6N4
Mailing: PO Box 1911 Stn Main
613 345-0992; Fax: 613 345-6545
Toll-free: 877 240-2224
E: tricounty.office@diabetes.ca
W: www.diabetes.ca
Year Founded: 1968
Criteria: *Open to everyone.*
Speakers Available
Library: Y
Languages: English
Membership: 300
Membership Fee: $18 Senior; $28 Regular

◊ ***Thunder Bay & District:***
501-200 Syndicate Ave S, Thunder Bay ON P7E 1C9
807 577-4232; Fax: 807 623-0851
Toll-free: 800 226-8464
W: www.diabetes.ca
Executive:
Reg Dir: Terry Cavanaugh
Commun Engagement Coord: Danica Logan
Public Prog/Serv Coord: Richard Boon
Year Founded: 1953
No of Paid Staff: 3
Speakers Available
Library: Y *(Open to the public)*
Languages: English
Membership: 400 +
Membership Fee: Seniors - $18; Household - $28

◊ ***Windsor & District:***
3-2605 Howard Ave, Windsor ON N8X 3W7
519 253-1797; Fax: 519 253-6305
Toll-free: 800 226-8464
W: www.diabetes.ca
Executive:
Reg Dir SW Ont: Sue Taylor
Languages: English

◈ ***Prince Edward Island Branch:***
161 St. Peters Rd, Charlottetown PE C1A 5P7
902 894-3195; Fax: 902 368-1928
E: sandra.leblanc@diabetes.ca
W: www.diabetes.ca
Year Founded: 1953
No of Paid Staff: 3
Languages: English

◈ ***Montreal:***
630-6020 rue Jean-Talon E,
Saint-Léonard QC H1S 3B1
514 274-9461; Fax: 514 256-6907
E: artmars@securenet.net

◈ ***Québec:***
300-8550 boul Pie-IX, Montréal QC H1Z 4G2
514 259-3422; Fax: 514 259-9286
Toll-free: 800 361-3504
E: info@diabete.qc.ca
W: www.diabete.qc.ca

Executive:
Prés/Dir gén: Serge Langlois
Chef des ops/Dir Dev: Sylvie Lauzon
Dir rel assoc: Georges Quellos
Dir fin/admin: Marcelle Paquette
Dir commun: Marc Aras
Dir aff pub: Édouard Kilanowski
Dir serv enseignement: Louise Tremblay
Year Founded: 1954
Criteria: *Adhesion annuelle*
No of Paid Staff: 16
Speakers Available
Languages: French; English
Membership: 30,000
Membership Fee: $16
Library:
Diabète Québec - Bibliothèque *(Open to the public)*

◇ ***Abitibi-Ouest:***
23 av Leclerc, La Sarre QC J9Z 3A4
819 333-4493; Fax: 819 333-9056
E: ghislaine_mayer@tlb.sympatico.ca
Executive:
Prés: Claire Lemoyne
Sec: Ghislaine Mayer
Languages: English

◇ ***Bas St-Laurent:***
Location: 380 av de la Cathédrale, porte 8, Rimouski QC G5L 7C5
Mailing: CP 622 succ A
418 722-4746; Fax: 418 725-4780
Toll-free: 866 722-4746
E: diabetebsl@globetrotter.net
W: www.diabetebsl.com
Executive:
Coord: Lise Fortin
Year Founded: 1987
Budget: $14,000
No of Paid Staff: 1
Languages: French
Membership: 450

◇ ***Bas St-Laurent - KRTB:***
Location: 28 rue Joly, Rivière-du-Loup QC G5R 4M1
Mailing: CP 1463 Succ Bureau-Chef
418 862-7428; Fax: 418 862-7428
E: da-krtb@bellnet.ca
Executive:
Prés: Noël Thériault
Languages: French

◇ ***Beauce-Etchemin:***
101-999 17e Rue, Saint-Georges QC G5Y 4W1
418 227-1608; Fax: 418 227-1608
E: diabetebce@hotmail.com
W: www.diabetebce.com
Executive:
Prés: Jacqueline Poulin
Languages: French

◇ ***Bois-Francs:***
213-59 rue Monfette, Victoriaville QC G6P 1J8
819 795-3360; Fax: 819 795-3300
E: diabete.boisfrancs@cdbcf.qc.ca
Executive:
Prés: Michèle Côté
Coord: Ghislaine H Landry
Speakers Available
Library: Y
Languages: French
Membership: 535

◇ ***Châteauguay:***
176 boul Rameau, Châteauguay QC J6K 4P8
450 844-3627; Fax: 450 844-3657
Toll-free: 855 299-3627 227
E: diabetesoleilroussillon@gmail.com
W: www.diabete.qc.ca
Executive:
Dir fin: Marcelle Paquette
Comptable: Annie Maiyer

◇ ***Côte-Nord - Baie-Comeau:***
25 av Laurier, Baie-Comeau QC G4Z 1N9
418 296-2959
E: levesque.jean@globetrotter.net
Executive:
Prés: Jean Levesque
Languages: French; English

◇ ***Côte-Nord - Haute Côte-Nord:***
11 rue de la Réserve, Les Escoumins QC G0T 1K0
418 233-2541
E: carolinebruno@msn.com
Executive:
Prés: Caroline Ross
Languages: French; English

◇ ***Côte-Nord - Sept-Îles:***
652 av de Quen, Sept-Îles QC G4R 2R5
418 961-2424
E: jeannette.canuel@cgocable.ca
Executive:
Prés: Jeannette Canuel
Languages: French; English

◇ ***Côté-Sud:***
Mailing: CP 432 Succ Bureau-Chef, Montmagny QC G5V 3S7
418 248-5784
E: diabetecotesud@hotmail.com
W: www.diabete.qc.ca
Executive:
Prés: Roland Pouliot

◇ ***Drummondville***
206 rue Saint-Marcel, Drummondville QC J2B 2E2
819 478-4630; Fax: 819 472-1783
E: info@diabetedrummond.com
Executive:
Prés: Joel Lavoie
Dir gén: Marie Préfontaine
Languages: French

◇ ***Estrie:***
100-600 rue Woodward, Sherbrooke QC J1G 1W3
819 823-8558; Fax: 819 823-1445
E: info@diabete-estrie.ca
W: www.diabete-estrie.ca
Executive:
Prés: Renaud Labbé
Dir: Josée Delage
Year Founded: 1972
Library: Y *(Open to the public)*
Languages: French
Membership: 1,200

◇ ***Gaspésie-îles-de-la-Madeleine - la Baie des Chaleurs:***
181 Perron E, Caplan QC G0C 1H0
418 388-2832
E: wilson.grant@globetrotter.net
Executive:
Prés: Michel Hughes

◇ ***Gaspésie-îles-de-la-Madeleine - Îles-de-la-Madeleine:***
7B-315 ch Principal, Cap-aux-Meules QC G4T 0L7
418 969-2705
E: langford@lino.com
Executive:
Prés: Sylvie Arsenault
Languages: French; English

◇ ***Haut St-Laurent:***
Hôpital Barrie Memorial
28 rue Gale, Ormstown QC J0S 1K0
450 829-2321 3225; Fax: 450 829-4329
E: danielle.thibert@rrsss16.gouv.qc.ca
Executive:
Prés: François Verner
Languages: French

◇ ***Haute-Yamaska:***
Mailing: CP 117 Succ Bureau-Chef, Granby QC J2G 8E2
450 372-1151
Executive:
Prés: Andrée Lamarche
Languages: French

◇ ***Lanaudière Inc.***
SB-F 341-1000 boul Sainte-Anne, St-Charles-Brromée QC J6E 6J2
450 759-8222 2231; Fax: 450 752-5233
E: diabetlanau@citenet.net
W: www.diabetiquesdelanaudiere.org
Executive:
Prés: Henri Chapdelaine
Languages: French

◇ ***Laval:***
905-3030 boul Le Carrefour, Laval QC H7T 2P5
450 686-0330; Fax: 450 686-1159
E: info@diabetelaval.qc.ca
W: www.diabetelaval.qc.ca
Executive:
Prés: Jean-Louis Chenail
Coord: Jocelyne St-Amour
Languages: French

◇ ***Lotbinière:***
104 rang 2E E, St-Janvier-Joly QC G0S 1M0
418 380-2439
E: diabete.lotbiniere@gmail.com
Executive:
Prés: Jean Beaupré
Languages: French

◇ ***Mauricie - Trois-Rivières:***
1-575 rue du Père-Daniel, Trois-Rivières QC G9A 5Z7
819 373-8931; Fax: 819 693-0056
W: www.diabete.qc.ca
Executive:
Prés: Marc Lamoureux
Languages: French

◇ ***Mont-Laurier:***
Mailing: CP 114 stn Bureau-Chef, Mont-Laurier QC J9L 3G9
819 585-3085
E: diabetemontlaurier@hotmail.ca
W: diabete.qc.ca
Executive:
Prés: Denis Cloutier

◇ ***Mont-Laurier:***
929 rue Labelle, Mont-Tremblant QC J8E 2W5
819 425-3873; Fax: 819 587-2741
Executive:
Prés: Lise Fecteau
Languages: French

◇ ***Montréal:***
Location: 44 Saint-Alphonse St S, Thetford Mines QC G6G 3T7
Mailing: CP 222 succ Bureau-Chef, Thetford Mines QC G6H 5R9
418 423-5377
E: diabeteamiante@hotmail.com
Executive:
Prés: Monique Boulé Nadeau
Languages: French

◇ ***Montréal - l'Hôpital Notre-Dame/Maisonneuve-Rosemont:***
2065 rue Alexandre-DeSève, étage 9 - Z-5358, Montréal QC H2L 2W5
514 890-8000 25358
E: amicale.diabetique.chum@ssss.gouv.qc.ca
W: www.amicaledesdiabetiques.com

Executive:
Prés: Pierre Boileau
Dir gén: Francine Léveillé
Year Founded: 1989
No of Paid Staff: 2
Languages: French; English

◇ ***Montréal - NDG:***
2525 boul Cavendish, Montréal QC H4B 2Y4
514 484-7878 3102; Fax: 514 485-6406
E: judith.shapiro@ssss.gouv.qc.ca
Executive:
Prés: Elinor Alleyne
Languages: French; English

◇ ***Montréal Nord***
Hôpital Sacré-Coeur
5400 boul Gouin O, Montréal QC H4J 1C5
438 828-3565
E: diabetenordmtl@yahoo.ca
W: www.diabete.qc.ca
Executive:
Prés: Lise Giguère

◇ ***Outaouais:***
111-331 boul de la Cité-des-Jeunes, Gatineau QC J8Y 6T3
819 770-0442; Fax: 819 770-5919
E: diabetiquesoutaouais@gmail.com
Executive:
Prés-cons admin: Lise Boudreault
Prés: Roland Blondin
Languages: French

◇ ***Pabos:***
531 boul Pabos, Pabos QC G0C 2H0
418 689-4100
E: majuki@globetrotter.net
Executive:
Prés: Jules Monfette

◇ ***Québec City:***
12-3175 ch des Quatre-Bourgeois,
Québec QC G1W 2K7
418 656-6241 2; Fax: 418 656-6323
E: info@diabec.com
W: www.lesdiabetiquesdequebec.com
Executive:
Prés: Ève Vanelslande
Dir gén: Hélène House
Year Founded: 1986
Languages: French

◇ ***Québec City - Charlevoix:***
Centre Communautaire
324-367 rue Saint-Étienne, La Malbaie QC G5A 1M3
418 665-7755
E: diabetecharlevoix@bellnet.ca
Executive:
Prés: Georges Levasseur
Languages: French

◇ ***Rive Nord:***
12 Place de Beaujeu, Repentigny QC J6A 3S9
450 654-7561
E: velocontrediabete@hotmail.com
W: www.diabeterivenord.org
Executive:
Prés: Jacques Dupuis
Languages: English

◇ ***Rive-Sud:***
210-150 rue Grant, Longueuil QC J4H 3H6
450 928-3422; Fax: 450 748-0925
E: diabeterivesud@videotron.ca
Executive:
Prés: Monique P Jacob
Languages: French

◇ ***Rouyn-Noranda***
220 8e Rue, Rouyn-Noranda QC J9X 2A8
819 797-0905
E: gillesnaud@hotmail.com
Executive:
Prés: Gilles Naud
Languages: French

◇ ***Saguenay - Lac-St-Jean:***
150 rue Pinel, Chicoutimi QC G7G 3N8
418 549-8136; Fax: 418 549-8349
E: diabetesaguenay@gmail.com
Executive:
Prés: René Durocher
Languages: French
Membership: 800

◇ ***Saguenay-Lac-St-Jean:***
Mailing: CP 62 succ Bureau-Chef,
Roberval QC G8H 2N4
418 275-5298; Fax: 418 275-7991
Toll-free: 877 775-5298
E: legermar@qc.aira.com
W: www.diabete.qc.ca
Executive:
Prés: Marielle Lavoie
Languages: French

◇ ***Sorel-Tracy:***
111-71 rue de Ramezay, Sorel-Tracy QC J3P 3Z1
450 743-7461
E: diabetest@bellnet.ca
Executive:
Prés: Ghislaine Cournoyer

◇ ***Val d'Or***
Mailing: CP 444 succ Bureau-Chef, Val-d'Or QC J9P 4P4
819 825-0633
E: diabetevaldor@hotmail.com
Executive:
Prés: Georges Michaud
Prés: Philippe Tremblay

◇ ***Valleyfield:***
16-521 boul du Hâvre, Salaber-de-Valleyf QC J6S 4Z5
450 371-6444 303; Fax: 450 371-5315
E: diabete.suroit@bellnet.ca
W: diabetesuroit.com
Executive:
Prés: Germain Daoust
Coord: Annie Boilard

◇ ***Victoriaville:***
2 rue Adhémar Cusson, Bedford QC J0J 1A0
450 248-2224; Fax: 450 248-2224
E: dbm@bellnet.ca
W: fdbmhr.org/DBMHR.htm
Executive:
Prés: Robert Fontaine
Languages: French

◈ ***Northern Regional Leadership Centre:***
104-2301 Avenue C N, Saskatoon SK S7L 5Z5
306 933-1238; Fax: 306 244-2012
Toll-free: 800 996-4446
W: www.diabetes.ca
Languages: English

◈ ***South Regional Leadership Centre:***
917A Albert St, Regina SK S4R 2P6
306 584-8445; Fax: 306 586-9704
Toll-free: 800 297-7488
E: reginainfo@diabetes.ca
W: www.diabetes.ca
No of Paid Staff: 5
Speakers Available
Library: Y *(Open to the public)*
Languages: English
Membership Fee: Senior - $18; Individual/Family - $28

Diabète Saint-Hyacinthe inc.
1955 av Pratte, Saint-Hyacinthe QC J2S 7W5
450 778-2572 6331; Fax: 450 799-1176
E: chiplagace@cgocable.ca
Executive:
Prés: Pierrette Chicoine
Languages: French

Diabète Senneterre
49 rue des Pins, Senneterre QC J0Y 2M0
418 737-4409
E: solange51@hotmail.fr
Executive:
Prés: Lise Gignac
Languages: French

DOWN SYNDROME

Canadian Down Syndrome Society
283-5005 Dalhousie Dr NW, Calgary AB T3A 5R8
403 270-8500; Fax: 403 270-8291
Toll-free: 800 883-5608
E: info@cdss.ca
W: www.cdss.ca
Executive:
Exec Dir: Kirk Crowther
Year Founded: 1987
Criteria: *Interest in Down Syndrome*
No of Paid Staff: 10
Speakers Available
Languages: English
Membership: 1,400
Membership Fee: Company - $40; Family/Individual - $20

Ups and Downs - Calgary Down Syndrome Association
Location: 1940 6 Ave NW, Calgary AB T2N 0W3
Mailing: PO Box 61180 RPO Kensington,
Calgary AB T2N 4S6
403 289-4394; Fax: 403 289-1015
Toll-free: 866 230-0979
E: info@upsdowns.org
W: www.upsdowns.org
Executive:
Office Mgr: Amber Boyd
Year Founded: 1984
Criteria: *Payment of dues.*
No of Paid Staff: 1
Speakers Available
Library: Y
Languages: English
Library:
Ups & Downs Lending Library *(Open to the public)*

EPILEPSY

Edmonton Epilepsy Association
11007 124 St NW, Edmonton AB T5M 0J5
780 488-9600; Fax: 780 447-5486
Toll-free: 866 374-5377
E: info@edmontonepilepsy.org
W: www.edmontonepilepsy.org
Executive:
Exec Dir: Gary Sampley
Volunteer Coord: Cameron Reid
Social Worker: Sunny Kim
Prog Mgr: Sharon Otto
Year Founded: 1960
Criteria: *Membership is open to anyone.*
Budget: $230,000
No of Paid Staff: 4
Speakers Available
Library: Y
Languages: English
Membership: 300
Membership Fee: $10 Per Year

HEALTHCARE ASSOCIATIONS

Epilepsy and Seizure Association of Manitoba
4-1805 Main St, Winnipeg MB R2V 2A2
204 783-0466; Fax: 204 784-9689
Toll-free: 866 374-5377
E: epilepsy.seizures.mb@mts.net
W: www.manitobaepilepsy.org
Executive:
Pres: Jim Cook
VP: Chris Vander Aa
Year Founded: 1975
Criteria: *Must have epilepsy or be affected by epilepsy or have a genuine interest in improving the quality of life for people with epilepsy.*
No of Paid Staff: 1
Speakers Available
Languages: English
Membership: 100
Membership Fee: $10

Epilepsy and Seizure Disorder Resource Centre for Eastern Ontario
100 Stuart St, Kingston ON K7L 2V6
613 542-6222; Fax: 613 548-4162
E: ed@epilepsyresource.org
W: www.epilepsyresource.org
Executive:
Exec Dir: Kimberly Neill
Client Serv Coord: Angie Smith
Outreach Coord: Paula Muir
Criteria: *Open to all.*
No of Paid Staff: 5
Speakers Available
Library: Y *(Open to the public)*
Languages: English
Membership: 150
Membership Fee: $10/yr

◈Brockville Outreach Office
42 George St, Brockville ON K6V 3V5
613 498-3288
Toll-free: 866 374-5377
E: paula@epilepsyresource.org
W: www.epilepsyresource.org/
Executive:
Exec Dir: Kim Neill
Educ/Client Serv Coord: Paula Muir

Epilepsy Association of Calgary
4112 4 St NW, Calgary AB T2K 1A2
403 230-2764; Fax: 403 230-5766
Toll-free: 866 374-5379 (1-866 EPILEPSY)
W: www.epilepsycalgary.com
Executive:
Pres: Donna Bernreuther
VP: Paul Kelly
Exec Dir: Kathy Fyfe
Year Founded: 1955
Budget: $235,000
No of Paid Staff: 5
Speakers Available
Library: Y *(Open to the public)*
Languages: English
Membership: 150
Membership Fee: Life - $200; Annual - $20

◈Calgary
4811 48 St, Red Deer AB T4N 1S6
403 358-3358
Toll-free: 866 374-5379

The Epilepsy Association of Nova Scotia -Member of Canadian Epilepsy Alliance
306-5880 Spring Garden Rd, Halifax NS B3H 1Y1
902 429-2633; Fax: 902 425-0821
Toll-free: 866 374-5377
E: info@epilepsyns.com
W: www.epilepsyns.com
Executive:
Pres: Deirdre Floyd
VP: Suzanne Robichaud
Year Founded: 1980
Criteria: *Open to anyone*
No of Paid Staff:
Speakers Available
Library: Y *(Open to the public)*
Languages: English
Membership: approx. 600
Membership Fee: $15

Epilepsy Canada - National Office
Location: 308-1 A Promenade Cir, Thornhill ON L4J 4P8
Mailing: 336-2255B Queen St E, Toronto ON M4E 1G3
905 764-9991; Fax: 905 764-1231
Toll-free: 877 734-0873
E: epilepsy@epilepsy.ca
W: www.epilepsy.ca
Executive:
Epilepsy Ontario Volunteer: Dianna Findlay
Year Founded: 1966
Criteria: *Individual, Association, Corporations*
Budget: $200,000
Languages: English; French
Membership: 150
Membership Fee: Associations/Corporations - $50; Individual - $30

◈British Columbia:
2500-900 8th Ave W, Vancouver BC V5Z 1E5
604 875-6704; Fax: 604 875-0617
E: info@bcepilepsy.com
W: www.bcepilepsy.com
Executive:
Exec Dir: Shawn Laari
Prog/Commun Coord: Elvira Balakshin
Year Founded: 1959
Budget: $200,000
No of Paid Staff: 2
Speakers Available
Library: Y *(Open to the public)*
Languages: English
Membership: 2,000
Membership Fee: $25
Library:
Dr. Aukland Resource Centre

◈Halifax:
306-5880 Spring Garden Rd, Halifax NS B3H 1Y1
902 429-2633; Fax: 902 425-0821
Toll-free: 866 374-5377
E: info@epilepsyns.com
W: www.epilepsyns.com

◈Ontario:
803-3100 Steeles Ave E, Markham ON L3R 8T3
905 474-9696; Fax: 905 474-3663
Toll-free: 800 463-1119
E: info@epilepsyontario.org
W: epilepsyontario.org
Executive:
Exec Dir: Rozalyn Werner-Arcé
Year Founded: 1956
No of Paid Staff: 4
Languages: English; French

◇Durham Region:
20-850 King St W, Oshawa ON L1J 8N5
905 571-2099; Fax: 905 571-0995
E: support@epilepsydurham.com
W: www.epilepsydurham.com
Executive:
Exec Dir: Dianne McKenzie
Year Founded: 1987
Languages: English

◇Huron-Perth-Bruce:
Location: 52 Main St S, Floor 2, Seaforth ON N0K 1W0
Mailing: PO Box 1111
519 527-0033; Fax: 519 527-2533
E: epilepsy@tcc.on.ca
W: www.epilepsyontario.org
Executive:
Pres: Lorraine Devereaux
Exec Dir: Lynne Armstrong
Year Founded: 1960
No of Paid Staff: 3
Speakers Available
Library: Y *(Open to the public)*
Languages: English
Membership list available to the public

◇London
234 Riverside Dr, London ON N6H 1E6
519 433-4073; Fax: 519 433-4079
E: support@epilepsysupport.ca
W: www.epilepsysupport.com

◇Mississauga
4-2160 Dunwin Dr, Mississauga ON L5L 5M8
905 450-1900
Toll-free: 855 734-2111
E: info@epilepsyhaltonpeel.org
W: www.epilepsyhaltonpeel.org

◇Niagara:
5017 Victoria Ave, Niagara Falls ON L2E 4C9
905 353-1096; Fax: 905 353-0758
E: info@epilepsyniagara.org
W: www.epilepsyniagara.org
Executive:
Exec Co-Dir: Kristin Welton
Exec Co-Dir/Support Serv Coord: Dawn Giroux
Year Founded: 2003
No of Paid Staff: 2
Speakers Available
Library: Y *(Open to the public)*
Languages: English
Membership: 100

◇Ottawa Carleton:
207-211 Bronson Ave, Ottawa ON K1R 6H5
613 594-9255; Fax: 613 594-4971
Toll-free: 866 374-7377
E: info@epilepsyottawa.ca
W: www.epilepsyottawa.ca
Executive:
Dev Officer: Lynn Andrews
Library: Y *(Open to the public)*

◇Peterborough & Area:
Location: Charlotte Mews, 4-203 Simcoe St, Peterborough ON K9J 7Y8
Mailing: PO Box 2453 Stn Main
705 876-0311; Fax: 705 876-0109
Toll-free: 800 463-1119
E: epilepsyptbo@yahoo.ca
W: www.epilepsyontario.org
Executive:
Exec Dir: Tom Appleby
Languages: English

◇Seizure and Brain Injury Centre Timmins:
733 Ross Ave E, Timmins ON P4N 8S8
705 264-2933; Fax: 705 264-0350
Toll-free: 866 374-5377
E: sabicrl@ntl.sympatico.ca
W: www.seizurebraininjurycentre.com
Executive:
Exec Dir: Rhonda Latendresse
Year Founded: 1988
Budget: $100,000
No of Paid Staff: 2
Library: Y *(Open to the public)*
Languages: English; French
Membership: 100+

◇ ***Sudbury Manitoulin:***
Waterview Apartments
409-1290A Bancroft Dr, Sudbury ON P3B 4C8
705 688-0188; Fax: 705 688-1685
E: epilepsysudbury@yahoo.ca
W: www.epilepsyontario.org
Year Founded: 1986
Library: Y *(Open to the public)*
Languages: English
Membership list available to the public

◇ ***Waterloo-Wellington:***
5-165 Hollinger Cres, Kitchener ON N2K 2Z2
519 745-2112; Fax: 519 745-2435
E: epilepsy@epilepsyww.com
W: www.epilepsyww.com
Executive:
Exec Dir: Karen Reeves
Year Founded: 1982
No of Paid Staff: 2
Speakers Available
Library: Y *(Open to the public)*
Languages: English
Membership: 100 *(Lists available to the public)*

◇ ***York Region:***
11181 Yonge St, Floor 2, Richmond Hill ON L4S 1L2
905 508-5404; Fax: 905 508-0920
Toll-free: 866 374-5377
E: info@epilepsyyork.org
W: www.epilepsyyork.org
Executive:
Bus Mgr: David Harper
Exec Dir: Paul Raymond
Year Founded: 1988
Criteria: *Open to all.*
No of Paid Staff: 1
Speakers Available
Library: Y
Languages: English
Membership: 100
Membership Fee: $20
Library:
Epilepsy Family Resource Centre *(Open to the public)*

◈ ***Prince Edward Island:***
RR 1, Richmond PE C0B 1Y0
902 854-2063
E: epilepsy_pei@yahoo.ca
Executive:
Commun/Publicity: Dorothy Farish
Languages: English

◈ ***Quebec:***
204-1650 boul de Maisonneuve O,
Montréal QC H3H 2P3
514 875-5595; Fax: 514 875-6734
E: aqe@cooptel.qc.ca
W: www.associationquebecoiseepilepsie.com
Executive:
Dir gén: France Picard
Budget: $1,500,000
No of Paid Staff: 3
Speakers Available
Languages: English; French
Membership: 3,000
Membership Fee: $5

◇ ***Abitibi-Témiscamingue:***
Mailing: CP 1392 Succ Bureau-Chef, Rouyn-Noranda QC J9X 6P1
819 279-7992
E: epilepsieat@yahoo.fr
W: www.associationepilepsieat.com
Executive:
Coord: Jacques Bouffard
Languages: French; English

◇ ***Côte-Nord:***
652 av de Quen, Sept-Îles QC G4R 2R5
418 968-2507; Fax: 418 962-5982
Toll-free: 866 968-2507
E: adm@epilepsiecn.org
Executive:
Coord: Sonya De Rosby
Year Founded: 1985
No of Paid Staff: 1
Speakers Available
Languages: French
Membership: 43

◇ ***Gaspésie-Sud:***
Location: 176 boul Gérard-D-Lévesque O,
Paspébiac QC G0C 2K0
Mailing: PO Box 337
418 752-6819; Fax: 418 752-5959
E: info@epilepsiegaspesiesud.com
W: www.epilepsiegaspesiesud.com
Executive:
VP: Yvan Blais
Coord: Diane Horth
Languages: French; English

◇ ***Granby & Région:***
207-17 boul Mountain, Granby QC J2G 9M5
450 378-8876
Toll-free: 866 374-5377
E: info@epilepsiegranby.com
W: www.epilepsiegranby.com
Executive:
Coord: Giselle Paquette
Coord: Anie Roy
No of Paid Staff: 4
Library: Y *(Open to the public)*
Languages: French
Membership list available to the public

◇ ***Outaouais:***
111-115 boul Sacré-Coeur, Gatineau QC J8X 1C5
819 595-3331; Fax: 819 771-3286
E: info@epilepsieoutaouais.org
W: www.epilepsieoutaouais.org
Executive:
Dir gén: Roger Hébert
Serv sociale: Suzanne Guérin
Coord: Sylvie Deschambault

◇ ***Québec:***
1411 boul Père-Lelièvre, Québec QC G1M 1N7
418 524-8752; Fax: 418 524-5882
E: epilepsiequebec@megaquebec.net
W: www.epilepsiequebec.com
Executive:
Dir: Nicole Bélanger

◇ ***Région 02:***
218-371 rue Racine E, Chicoutimi QC G7H 1S8
418 549-9888; Fax: 418 549-3547
E: arpe@bellnet.ca
Executive:
Dir: Nicole Bouchard
Languages: French; English

Epilepsy Canada - Simcoe County
Victoria Village
6-72 Ross St, Barrie ON L4N 1G3
705 737-3132; Fax: 705 737-5045
E: epilepsysimcoecounty@rogers.com
W: www.epilepsyontario.org/simcoe
Executive:
Pres: Heather Allen
Exec Dir: Elizabeth Thomas
Year Founded: 1978
Criteria: *Open to anyone who wants to join.*
No of Paid Staff: 1
Speakers Available
Library: Y
Languages: English
Membership: 65 *(Lists available to the public)*
Membership Fee: $20/yr
Library:
Resource Library *(Open to the public)*

Epilepsy Newfoundland & Labrador - Member of Canadian Epilepsy Alliance
351 Kenmount Rd, St. John's NL A1B 3P9
709 722-0502; Fax: 709 722-0999
E: info@epilepsynl.com
W: www.epilepsynl.com
Executive:
Exec Dir: Gail Dempsey
No of Paid Staff: 20
Speakers Available
Library: Y *(Open to the public)*
Languages: English

Epilepsy Toronto
210-468 Queen St E, Toronto ON M5A 1T7
416 964-9095
Toll-free: 866 374-5377
E: info@epilepsytoronto.org
W: epilepsytoronto.org
Executive:
Exec Dir: Geoff Bobb
Year Founded: 1999
Languages: English; French

Focus On Epilepsy
11007 124 St NW, Edmonton AB T5M 0J5
780 488-9600; Fax: 780 447-5486
Toll-free: 866 374-5377
E: info@edmontonepilepsy.org
W: www.edmontonepilepsy.org
Executive:
Exec Dir/COO: Gary Sampley
Admn Mgr: Wendy Sauve
Prog Mgr: Sharon Otto
Volunteer Coord: Cameron Reid
Social Worker: Sunny Kim

HEAD INJURY

Association Québécoise des Traumatisés Crâniens
220 av du parc, Laval QC H7N 3X4
514 274-7447; Fax: 450 629-8807
E: aqtc@aqtc.ca
W: www.aqtc.ca
Executive:
Dir gén: Pierre Mitchell
Year Founded: 1987
Budget: $500,000
No of Paid Staff: 10
Library: Y
Languages: French; English
Membership: 380
Library:
Centre de documentation *(Open to the public)*

Head Injury Association of Fort Erie
649 Niagara Blvd, Fort Erie ON L2A 3H7
905 871-7789; Fax: 905 871-7832
E: hiafeadmin@bellnet.ca
Executive:
Pres: Julie Anthony
Prog Dir: Donna Summerville
Year Founded: 1987
Criteria: *Individuals who have sustained a brain injury and their extended families.*
Budget: $100,000
No of Paid Staff: 2

Speakers Available
Library: Y *(Open to the public)*
Languages: English
Membership: 250
Membership Fee: $15

HEART & STROKE

Heart and Stroke Foundation of Canada
1402-222 Queen St, Ottawa ON K1P 5V9
613 569-4361; Fax: 613 569-3278
Toll-free: 888 473-4636
E: itstaff@hsf.ca
W: www.heartandstroke.ca
Executive:
CEO/Exec Dir: Bobbe Wood
Speakers Available
Library: Y
Languages: English; French
Membership list available to the public

◈ ***Alberta/Northwest Territories/Nunavut:***
100-119 14 St NW, Calgary AB T2N 1Z6
403 264-5549; Fax: 403 237-0803
Toll-free: 888 473-4636
W: www.heartandstroke.ab.ca
Executive:
CEO: Donna Hastings
Coord-Rsrch: Dan Leffelaar
Exec Asst: Sharon Meikle
Speakers Available
Library: Y
Languages: English

◇ ***Lethbridge:***
Mailing: PO Box 2211 Stn Main, Lethbridge AB T1J 4K7
403 327-3239; Fax: 403 327-9928
W: www.heartandstroke.ca
Executive:
Area Mgr: Valerie Fraser
No of Paid Staff: 2
Speakers Available
Library: Y *(Open to the public)*
Languages: English

◇ ***Medicine Hat:***
124-430 6 Ave SE, Medicine Hat AB T1A 2S8
403 527-0028; Fax: 403 526-9655
W: www.heartandstroke.ca
Executive:
Area Mgr: Valerie Fraser
Languages: English

◇ ***Northwest Territories and Nunavut***
10985 124 St NW, Edmonton AB T5M 0H9
780 451-4545; Fax: 780 454-1593
W: www.heartandstroke.ab.ca
No of Paid Staff: 10
Speakers Available
Languages: English

◇ ***Red Deer:***
202-5913 50 Ave, Red Deer AB T4N 4C4
403 342-4435; Fax: 403 342-7088
W: www.heartandstroke.ca
Year Founded: 1957
No of Paid Staff: 4
Speakers Available
Library: Y *(Open to the public)*
Languages: English

◈ ***British Columbia and Yukon:***
200-1212 Broadway W, Vancouver BC V6H 3V2
604 736-4404; Fax: 604 736-8732
E: info@hsf.bc.ca
W: www.heartandstroke.bc.ca
Executive:
Pres/CEO: Bobbe Wood
Year Founded: 1955
Speakers Available
Languages: English

◈ ***Manitoba:***
Heart and Stroke Bldg
200-6 Donald St, Winnipeg MB R3L 0K6
204 949-2000; Fax: 204 957-1365
Toll-free: 888 473-4636
W: www.heartandstroke.mb.ca
Executive:
Pres/CEO: Debbie Brown
VP-Admn/Fin: Randy Dueck
VP-Fund Dev: Susan Punter
VP-Philanthropy: Marc Desrosiers
VP-Hlth Promo: Jackie Zalnasky
VP-Commun: Katherine Gador
No of Paid Staff: 40
Library: Y *(Open to the public)*
Languages: English

◈ ***New Brunswick:***
Harbour Bldg
133 Prince William St, Floor 5, Saint John NB E2L 2B5
506 634-1620; Fax: 506 648-0098
Toll-free: 800 663-3600
E: heart.stroke@hsf.nb.ca
W: www.heartandstroke.ca
Executive:
CEO: Daniel Connolly
Dir-Revenue Dev: Kurtis Sisk
Fin Admin: Cathy Densmore
Commun Mgr: Darcy LeBlanc
Health Promo Dir: Moira Gagnon
Year Founded: 1965
Budget: $2,600,000
No of Paid Staff: 15
Speakers Available
Library: Y *(Open to the public)*
Languages: English; French
Membership list available to the public

◈ ***Corner Brook:***
9 Main St, Corner Brook NL A2H 1C2
709 639-8507; Fax: 709 639-8122
W: www.heartandstroke.ca
Executive:
Mgr: Rita Calahan
No of Paid Staff: 1
Speakers Available
Library: Y *(Open to the public)*
Languages: English

◈ ***Newfoundland and Labrador:***
Location: 1037 Topsail Rd, Mount Pearl NL A1N 5E9
Mailing: PO Box 670 RPO Centennial S, Mount Pearl NL A1N 2X1
709 753-8521; Fax: 709 753-3117
Toll-free: 888 473-4636
E: info@hsf.nl.ca
W: www.heartandstroke.ca
Executive:
CEO: Mary Ann Butt
No of Paid Staff: 5
Speakers Available
Library: Y *(Open to the public)*
Languages: English
Membership: 100 *(Lists available to the public)*

◈ ***Nova Scotia:***
Park Lane Mall - Level 3
5657 Spring Garden Rd, Box 245, Halifax NS B3J 3R4
902 423-7530; Fax: 902 492-1464
Toll-free: 800 423-4432
E: contactus@heartandstroke.ns.ca
W: www.heartandstroke.ns.ca
Executive:
Program Coord: Brenda Gallagher
Year Founded: 1958
No of Paid Staff: 32
Speakers Available
Languages: English
Membership: 5,000 + volunteers

◈ ***Ontario:***
Location: Yonge-Eglinton Centre, 1300-2300 Yonge St, Toronto ON M4P 1E4
Mailing: PO Box 2414
416 489-7111; Fax: 416 489-6885
Toll-free: 888 473-4636
E: heartandstroke@hsf.on.ca
W: www.heartandstroke.on.ca
Executive:
CEO: David Sculthorpe
VP-Hum Res: Cindy Dunn
Dir-Pub Rel: Teresa Roncon
VP/Chief Philanthropy Officer: Shannon Von Kaldenberg
Mgr-Network/Infrastructure: Christopher Snell
Year Founded: 1952
No of Paid Staff: 200
Speakers Available
Languages: English

◇ ***Barrie Office:***
1-112 Commerce Park Dr, Barrie ON L4N 8W8
705 737-1020; Fax: 705 737-0902
E: vholland@hsf.on.ca
W: www.heartandstroke.ca
Languages: English

◇ ***Belleville Office:***
106A-121 Dundas St E, Belleville ON K8N 1C3
613 962-2502; Fax: 613 962-6080
Toll-free: 888 473-4636
E: hhedley@hsf.on.ca
W: www.heartandstroke.ca
Speakers Available
Languages: English

◇ ***Brampton Office - Peel Region:***
306-201 County Court Blvd, Brampton ON L6W 4L2
905 451-0021; Fax: 905 452-0503
W: www.heartandstroke.ca
Year Founded: 1952
No of Paid Staff: 4
Speakers Available
Languages: English

◇ ***Brantford Office:***
A-442 Grey St, Brantford ON N3S 7N3
519 752-1301; Fax: 519 752-5554
Toll-free: 888 246-9040
E: mail@hsf.on.ca
W: www.heartandstroke.ca
Year Founded: 1952
No of Paid Staff: 4
Library: Y
Languages: English

◇ ***Brockville Office:***
310-51 King St E, Brockville ON K6V 1A8
613 345-6183; Fax: 613 345-3037
W: www.heartandstroke.ca
Year Founded: 1952
No of Paid Staff: 2
Speakers Available
Languages: English

◇ ***Burlington Office - Halton Region:***
7-4391 Harvester Rd, Burlington ON L7L 4X1
905 634-7732; Fax: 905 634-1353
W: www.heartandstroke.ca
Executive:
Area Mgr: Michelle Fox
Area Admin: Vicki Roy
No of Paid Staff: 2
Speakers Available
Library: Y *(Open to the public)*
Languages: English

◇ **Chatham Office:**
214 Queen St, Chatham ON N7M 2H1
519 354-6232; Fax: 519 354-6351
W: www.heartandstroke.ca
Languages: English

◇ **Cornwall Office:**
36 Second St E, Cornwall ON K6H 1Y3
613 938-8933; Fax: 613 938-0655
W: www.heartandstroke.ca
Languages: English

◇ **Guelph Office:**
204-21 Surrey St W, Guelph ON N1H 3R3
519 837-4858; Fax: 519 837-9209
W: www.heartandstroke.ca
Executive:
Area Mgr: Sara Felske
Area Admin: Beth Kerr
Year Founded: 1952
No of Paid Staff: 4
Speakers Available
Library: Y *(Open to the public)*
Languages: English

◇ **Hamilton Office:**
7-1439 Upper Ottawa St, Hamilton ON L8W 3J6
905 574-4105; Fax: 905 574-4380
Toll-free: 888 476-4636
E: mcollura@hsf.on.ca
W: www.heartandstroke.ca
Executive:
Area Mgr: Gloria Picanco
Area Admin: Marianna Collura
Criteria: *Open to all.*
No of Paid Staff: 5
Speakers Available
Languages: English
Membership: 5

◇ **Kingston Office:**
720 Progress Ave, Kingston ON K7M 4W9
613 384-2871; Fax: 613 384-2899
W: www.heartandstroke.com
Languages: English

◇ **Kitchener Office:**
2A-1373 Victoria St N, Kitchener ON N2B 3R6
519 571-9600; Fax: 519 571-9832
Toll-free: 888 473-4636
W: www.heartandstroke.ca
Executive:
Area Mgr: Bernie Westfall
Year Founded: 1852
Criteria: *Potential volunteers are screened to see if they meet with the Heart and Stroke Foundation's mission statement.*
No of Paid Staff: 5
Speakers Available
Library: Y *(Open to the public)*
Languages: English
Membership: 2,000

◇ **London Area**
150-633 Colborne St, London ON N6B 2V3
519 679-0641; Fax: 519 679-6898
W: www.heartandstroke.ca
Year Founded: 1951
No of Paid Staff: 6
Speakers Available
Languages: English
Membership list available to the public

◇ **Newmarket Office:**
29-17665 Leslie St, Newmarket ON L3Y 3E3
905 853-6355; Fax: 905 853-7961
W: www.heartandstroke.on.ca
Year Founded: 1952
No of Paid Staff: 5
Speakers Available
Languages: English

◇ **Ottawa Office**
100-1101 Prince of Wales Dr, Ottawa ON K2C 3W7
613 727-5060; Fax: 613 727-1895
Toll-free: 888 473-4636
W: www.heartandstroke.ca
Languages: English; French

◇ **Owen Sound Office:**
795 1st Ave E, Owen Sound ON N4K 2C6
519 371-0083; Fax: 519 371-8164
W: www.heartandstroke.on.ca
No of Paid Staff: 5
Speakers Available
Languages: English

◇ **Peterborough Office**
3-824 Clonsilla Ave, Peterborough ON K9J 5Y3
705 749-1044; Fax: 705 749-1470
W: www.heartandstroke.ca
Executive:
Area Admin: Victoria Thompson
Year Founded: 1952
Criteria: *Open to all.*
Speakers Available
Library: Y *(Open to the public)*
Languages: English

◇ **Richmond Hill - York Region South Office**
204-9251 Yonge St, Richmond Hill ON L4C 9T3
905 709-4899; Fax: 905 709-0883
E: hsfoyork@hsf.on.ca
W: www.heartandstroke.ca
Languages: English

◇ **Sarnia Office**
774 London Rd, Sarnia ON N7T 4Y1
519 332-1415; Fax: 519 332-3139
W: www.heartandstroke.ca
Executive:
Area Mgr: Kim Vanhooft
Area Admin: Sue McKinlay
No of Paid Staff: 2
Speakers Available
Languages: English

◇ **Sault Ste. Marie Office:**
59 Great Northern Rd, Sault Ste. Marie ON P6B 4Y7
705 253-3775; Fax: 705 946-5760
No of Paid Staff: 2
Speakers Available
Languages: English

◇ **Stratford Office:**
556 Huron St, Stratford ON N5A 5T9
519 273-5212; Fax: 519 273-7024
Toll-free: 888 287-7775
W: www.heartandstroke.ca
Year Founded: 1957
No of Paid Staff: 5
Languages: English

◇ **Sudbury Office**
130-43 Elm St, Sudbury ON P3C 1S4
705 673-2228; Fax: 705 673-7406
Toll-free: 888 473-4636
W: www.heartandstroke.ca
Year Founded: 1952
Languages: English
Membership list available to the public

◇ **Thunder Bay Office:**
104-979 Alloy Dr, Thunder Bay ON P7B 5Z8
807 623-1118; Fax: 807 622-9914
W: www.heartandstroke.ca
Languages: English

◇ **Timmins Office:**
301-60 Wilson Ave, Timmins ON P4N 2S7
705 267-4645; Fax: 705 268-6721
W: www.heartandstroke.ca
Languages: English

◇ **Windsor Office:**
350-4570 Rhodes Dr, Windsor ON N8W 5C2
519 254-4345; Fax: 519 254-4215
W: www.heartandstroke.ca
Executive:
Area Mgr: Bambi Blondin
Area Coord: Diane DeMarco
Year Founded: 1957
Languages: English

◈ **Prince Edward Island:**
Location: 180 Kent St, Charlottetown PE C1A 1N9
Mailing: PO Box 279 Stn Central, Charlottetown PE C1A 7K4
902 892-7441; Fax: 902 368-7068
Toll-free: 888 473-4636
E: info@hsfpei.ca
W: www.heartandstroke.pe.ca
Executive:
Chair: Jason Roberts
Budget: $250,000
No of Paid Staff: 8
Speakers Available
Library: Y
Languages: English

◈ **Québec:**
500-1434 rue Sainte-Catherine O, Montréal QC H3G 1R4
514 871-1551; Fax: 514 871-9385
Toll-free: 888 473-4636
W: www.fmcoeur.qc.ca
Executive:
Chef dir: Edmée Métivier
Adj admin: Marie-Eve Lefebvre
Dir-mktg/commun: Serge Breton
Year Founded: 1955
No of Paid Staff: 49
Speakers Available
Languages: English; French
Membership: 20,000 *(Lists available to the public)*

◇ **Chicoutimi**
251-152 rue Racine E, Chicoutimi QC G7H 1R8
418 543-8959; Fax: 418 543-5872
Executive:
Dir rég: Manon Bissonnette

◇ **Dorval**
18-795 av Carson, Dorval QC H9S 1L7
514 636-4599; Fax: 514 636-8576
Executive:
Dir rég: Dalia Sodo

◇ **Eastern Townships:**
100-2630 rue King O, Sherbrooke QC J1J 2H1
819 562-7942; Fax: 819 564-0690
W: www.heartandstroke.qc.ca
Executive:
Dir rég: François Demarais
Coord porte à porte: Anne-Marie Leclerc
Adj admin: Katy Côté
No of Paid Staff: 6
Languages: French

◇ **Gatineau:**
007-109 rue Wright, Gatineau QC J8X 2G7
819 771-8595; Fax: 819 771-7070
Toll-free: 888 473-4636
E: christiane.matte@fmcoeur.qc.ca
W: www.fmcoeur.qc.ca
Executive:
Dir rég: Christiane Matte
Coord: Véronique Sicennes
Year Founded: 1955
Languages: French

◇ **Laval:**
Place Val Des Arbres
410-1600A boul Saint-Martin E, Laval QC H7G 4R8
450 669-6909; Fax: 450 669-8987
Toll-free: 888 473-4636
W: www.fmcoeur.qc.ca
Executive:
Dir gén: Nathalie Goyer
Year Founded: 1955
Languages: French

◇ **Longueuil:**
200-1194 ch de Chambly, Longueuil QC J4J 3W6
450 442-6387; Fax: 450 442-3329
Toll-free: 888 473-4636
W: www.fmcoeur.qc.ca
Executive:
Prés/Chef de la dir: Jean Noël
Dir rég: Hélène Gagné
Coord porte-à-porte: Marie-Eve Lacombe
Coord d'activités: Karoline Theriault
Adj admin: Claudine Piché
Year Founded: 0004
No of Paid Staff: 1,955
Languages: French

◇ **Québec City:**
261-4715 av des Replats, Québec QC G2J 1B8
418 682-6387; Fax: 418 682-8214
E: josee.giguere@fmcoeur.qc.ca
W: www.fmcoeur.qc.ca
Executive:
Dir dév commun Quebec E: Josée Giguère
Languages: French

◇ **Rimouski**
204-125 rue de l'Évéché O, Rimouski QC G5L 4H4
514 723-7270; Fax: 418 722-8556
Executive:
Dir rég: Louisella Bérubé

◇ **Trois Rivieres**
137 rue Radisson, Trois-Rivières QC G9A 2C5
819 375-9565; Fax: 819 375-0233
Toll-free: 888 473-4636
W: www.heartandstroke.ca
Executive:
Dir rég: Lysette Boivin
Year Founded: 1955
Languages: French

◈ **Saskatoon:**
279 3rd Ave N, Saskatoon SK S7K 2H8
306 244-2124; Fax: 306 664-4016
Toll-free: 888 473-4636 (in Sask.)
E: heart.stroke@hsf.sk.ca
W: www.heartandstroke.sk.ca
Executive:
Dir-Fund Dev: Lorie Langenfurth
Dir-Missions: Graham Addley
Dir-Fin/Admn: Cloude Hounjet
Dir-Commun: Rhae Ann Bromley
Year Founded: 1956
Criteria: *Interest in heart disease, stroke and healthy lifestyles.*
No of Paid Staff: 7
Speakers Available
Library: Y *(Open to the public)*
Languages: English

Stroke Recovery Association - Hamilton Wentworth
5-65 Nebo Rd, Hamilton ON L8W 2C9
905 385-1639; Fax: 905 385-9257
W: www.strokerecovery.org
Executive:
Pres: Patricia Kopita
Year Founded: 1978
Criteria: *Open to any person who has had a stroke, and their families.*
Budget: $25,000
No of Paid Staff: 1
Speakers Available
Library: Y *(Open to the public)*
Languages: English
Membership: 82
Membership Fee: $10

Stroke Recovery Association of British Columbia
Business Bldg
301-1212 Broadway W, Vancouver BC V6H 3V1
604 688-3603; Fax: 604 688-3660
Toll-free: 888 313-3377
E: office@strokerecoverybc.ca
W: www.strokerecoverybc.ca
Executive:
Pres: Dan Kennedy
Exec Dir: Tim Readman
Dir-Fin: Ali Mahdiyar
Year Founded: 1976
Criteria: *Be a stroke survivor or a caregiver/family member of a stroke survivor.*
Budget: $250,000
No of Paid Staff: 4
Speakers Available
Languages: English
Membership: 1,500
Membership Fee: $12

Stroke Recovery Association of London & District Chapter
Mailing: 2033 Vanneck Rd, RR 3, Komoka ON N0L 1R0
519 457-6715
Executive:
Pres: Jean Blackwell
Treas: Nola Doherty
Year Founded: 1978
Criteria: *Open to all.*
Budget: $60,000
Languages: English

Stroke Recovery Association of Manitoba Inc.
B-247 Provencher Blvd, Winnipeg MB R2H 0G6
204 942-2880; Fax: 204 944-1982
E: info@strokerecovery.ca
W: www.strokerecovery.ca
Executive:
Admin: Russ Down
Year Founded: 1973
Criteria: *Stroke survivors and others interested in supporting the welfare of stroke survivors.*
No of Paid Staff: 3
Speakers Available
Languages: English
Membership: 250 *(Lists available to the public)*
Membership Fee: $25/yr

◈ **Winnipeg:**
404-56 Sparks St, Ottawa ON K1P 5A9
613 236-7041; Fax: 613 236-3087
Toll-free: 800 267-8221
E: info@unitedway.ca
W: www.unitedway.ca
Executive:
Pres/CEO: Dr Jacline Abray-Nyman
VP-Dev Resource: Bonnie Morris
Sr VP: Eva Kmiecic
Year Founded: 1933
Budget: $8,400,000
No of Paid Staff: 27
Languages: English; French
Membership: 124 *(Lists available to the public)*

HEMOCHROMATOSIS

Canadian Hemochromatosis Society
285-7000 Minoru Blvd, Richmond BC V6Y 3Z5
604 279-7135
Toll-free: 877 233-4766
E: office@toomuchiron.ca
W: www.toomuchiron.ca
Executive:
Pres/Chair: Patrick Haney
Exec Dir/CEO: Robert (Bob) Rogers
Year Founded: 1982
Criteria: *Payment of fee.*
Budget: $150,000
No of Paid Staff: 5
Speakers Available
Library: Y *(Open to the public)*
Languages: English
Membership: 1,200
Membership Fee: $25

HEMOPHILIA

Canadian Hemophilia Society
400-1255 rue University, Montréal QC H3B 3B6
514 848-0503; Fax: 514 848-9661
Toll-free: 800 668-2686
E: chs@hemophilia.ca
W: www.hemophilia.ca
Executive:
Dir gén natl: David Page
Dir-ress hum/Rélation sect: Hélène Bourgaize
Responsable commun natl: Chantal Raymond
Year Founded: 1953
No of Paid Staff: 8
Speakers Available
Languages: English; French

◈ **Toronto**
501-65 Wellesley St E, Toronto ON M4Y 1G7
416 972-0641; Fax: 888 958-0307
Toll-free: 888 838-8846
E: tcor@hemophilia.on.ca
Executive:
Exec Dir: Terri Lee Higgins
Exec Asst: Susan Turner

Canadian Hemophilia Society - New Brunswick Chapter
43 Parkin St, Salisbury NB E4J 2N3
506 962-1477
E: president@chsnb.com
W: www.chsnb.com
Executive:
Pres: Bucky Buchanan
VP: Tara Curwin

Canadian Hemophilia Society of Ontario - Alberta Chapter
Mailing: PO Box 44171 RPO Garside, Edmonton AB T5V 1N6
780 421-9851; Fax: 780 459-2548
Toll-free: 866 425-9851
E: albertachapter@hemophilia.ca

Canadian Hemophilia Society of Ontario -British Columbia Chapter
Mailing: PO Box 21161 RPO Square, Maple Ridge BC V2X 1P7
778 230-9661
E: chsbc@shaw.ca

Canadian Hemophilia Society of Ontario -Manitoba Chapter
944 Portage Ave, Winnipeg MB R3G 0R1
204 775-8625; Fax: 204 772-0399
E: chsmb@hemophilia.mb.ca

Canadian Hemophilia Society of Ontario -Newfoundland and Labrador Chapter
38 Larkhall St, St. John's NL A1B 4C7
709 754-4879
E: chsnlcc@nf.sympatico.ca

Canadian Hemophilia Society of Ontario -Nova Scotia Chapter
Location: 988 J. Jordan Rd, Canning NS B0P 1H0
Mailing: PO Box 494
902 403-2208
E: nshemophiliasociety@hotmail.com

Canadian Hemophilia Society of Ontario -Prince Edward Island Chapter
Mailing: PO Box 2951 Stn Central, Charlottetown PE C1A 8C5
E: craigjoann@eastlink.ca

Canadian Hemophilia Society of Ontario -Saskatchewan
213-2366 Avenue C N, Saskatoon SK S7L 5X5
306 653-4366; Fax: 306 653-4368
Toll-free: 866 953-4366
E: hemosask@hemophilia.ca

Canadian Hemophilia Society - Ontario
501-65 Wellesley St E, Toronto ON M4Y 1G7
416 972-0641; Fax: 888 958-0307
Toll-free: 888 838-8846
E: info@hemophilia.on.ca
W: www.hemophilia.on.ca
Executive:
Exec Dir: Terri Higgins
Year Founded: 1956
Speakers Available

◈ ***Central West Ontario:***
19-10 George St, Floor 4, Hamilton ON L8P 1C8
905 522-2545; Fax: 905 522-0976
Toll-free: 800 267-8563
E: cwor@hemophilia.on.ca

◈ ***Ontario:***
501-65 Wellesley St E, Toronto ON M4Y 1G7
416 972-0641; Fax: 888 958-0307
Toll-free: 888 838-8846
W: www.hemophilia.on.ca
Executive:
Exec Dir: Terri Lee Higgins
Exec Asst: Susan Turner

◈ ***South Western Ontario:***
30-186 King St, London ON N6A 1C7
519 432-2365
Toll-free Fax: 888 958-0307
E: swor@hemophilia.on.ca
W: www.hemophilia.on.ca
Executive:
Reg Serv Coord: Matthew Maynard

Hemophilia Ontario
501-65 Wellesley St E, Toronto ON M4Y 1G7
416 972-0641; Fax: 888 958-0307
Toll-free: 888 838-8846
E: info@hemophilia.on.ca
W: www.hemophilia.ca
Executive:
Exec Dir: Terri-Lee Higgins
Finl Asst/Admv Asst: Susan Turner
Year Founded: 1957
No of Paid Staff: 9
Speakers Available
Library: Y *(Open to the public)*
Languages: English; French
Membership: 2,000
Membership Fee: $15

Hemophilia Ontario - Ottawa and Eastern Ontario Region
B151-2445D St. Laurent Blvd, Ottawa ON K1G 6C3
613 739-3845; Fax: 613 739-3820
Toll-free: 888 838-8846
E: cpatterson@hemophilia.on.ca
W: www.hemophilia.on.ca
Executive:
Reg Serv Coord: Colin Patterson
Year Founded: 1955
No of Paid Staff: 1
Library: Y *(Open to the public)*
Languages: English

World Federation of Hemophilia
1010-1425 boul René-Lévesque O, Montréal QC H3G 1T7
514 875-7944; Fax: 514 875-8916
E: wfh@wfh.org
W: www.wfh.org
Executive:
Prés: Alain Weill
Chef dir: John Bournas
Year Founded: 1963
No of Paid Staff: 27
Speakers Available
Library: Y
Languages: Spanish; English; French
Membership Fee: 50 US$

HEREDITARY HEMMORHAGIC TELANGIECTASIA

Hereditary Hemorrhagic Telangiectasia Foundation International Inc. (HHT)
8651 Tulsy Cres, Surrey BC V3W 6C5
604 596-3418
E: hhtinfo@hht.org
W: www.hht.org
Executive:
Cdn Rep: Trish Linke
Languages: English

HEREDITARY METABOLIC DISEASES

Canadian Association of Centres for the Management of Hereditary Metabolic Diseases
Dept of Genetics,Children's Hospital of Eastern Ontario
401 Smyth Rd, Ottawa ON K1H 8L1
613 737-7600 3427; Fax: 613 738-4822
E: pchakraborty@cheo.on.ca
W: www.garrod.ca
Executive:
Sec-Treas: Dr Pranesh Chakraborty
Criteria: *All interested professionals*
Speakers Available
Languages: English
Membership: 150
Membership Fee: $10

HUNTINGTON'S DISEASE

Huntington Society of Canada
400-151 Frederick St, Kitchener ON N2H 2M2
519 749-7063; Fax: 519 749-8965
Toll-free: 800 998-7398
E: info@huntingtonsociety.ca
W: www.huntingtonsociety.ca
Executive:
Chair: Anne Brace
CEO/Exec Dir: Bev Heim-Myers
Dir-Fin: Ean Robertson
Dir-Dev/Mktg: Cindy Moffat
Office Admin: Shirley Barnes
Treas: Glenda Rowein
Sec: Sean Dewart
Commun Coord: Christina Steinmann
Year Founded: 1973
Criteria: *Payment of annual membership donation or lifetime membership.*
Budget: $1,600,000
No of Paid Staff: 33
Speakers Available
Languages: English

INFERTILITY

Infertility Network
160 Pickering St, Toronto ON M4E 3J7
Fax: 416 690-8015
E: info@infertilitynetwork.org
W: www.infertilitynetwork.org
Executive:
Exec Dir: Diane Allen
Year Founded: 1990
Criteria: *Open to all.*
Budget: $30,000
No of Paid Staff: 2
Languages: English
Membership: 10,000 *(Lists available to the public)*
Membership Fee: $10

KABUKI SYNDROME

Kabuki Syndrome Network
8060 Struthers Cres, Regina SK S4Y 1J3
306 543-8715
E: margot@kabukisyndrome.com
W: www.kabukisyndrome.com
Executive:
Dir: Margot Schmiedge
Dir: Dean Schmiedge
Dir: Jen Morton
Dir: Lois Ross
Year Founded: 1997
Speakers Available
Languages: English; Spanish
Membership: 250+
Membership Fee: $15

KIDNEY DISEASE

Fondation Canadienne du Rein - Division Québec
2300 boul René-Lévesque O, Montréal QC H3H 2R5
514 938-4515; Fax: 514 938-4757
W: www.rein.ca
Executive:
Adj: Jocelyne Renaud

Kidney Foundation of Canada
208-29 Gervais Dr, North York ON M3C 1Y9
416 446-1620; Fax: 416 446-7884
Toll-free: 800 414-3484
W: www.kidney.on.ca
Executive:
Ops Mgr: Angela Solozano

The Kidney Foundation of Canada
300-5165 rue Sherbrooke O, Montréal QC H4A 1T6
514 369-4806; Fax: 514 369-2472
Toll-free: 800 361-7494
E: info@kidney.ca
W: www.rein.ca
Executive:
Dir gén ntl: Paul Shay
Year Founded: 1964
Criteria: *Paiement du droit d'inscription et particpation aux activités de la succursale.*
Budget: $2,000,000
No of Paid Staff: 8
Languages: English; French
Membership: 200
Membership Fee: $10/an

The Kidney Foundation of Canada
Location: 102-10 Pippy Pl, St. John's NL A1B 3X3
Mailing: PO Box 8032 stn A, St John's NL A1B 3M7
709 753-8999; Fax: 709 753-5708
Toll-free: 800 563-0626 Newfoundland only
W: www.kidney.ca
No of Paid Staff: 3
Speakers Available
Languages: English

The Kidney Foundation of Canada - BC Branch
200-4940 Canada Way, Burnaby BC V5G 4K6
604 736-9775; Fax: 604 736-9703
Toll-free: 800 567-8112 B.C. only
E: info@kidney.bc.ca
W: www.kidney.bc.ca
Executive:
Exec Dir: Karen Philp
Admv Asst: Claudine Fernandes
Year Founded: 1964
No of Paid Staff: 11
Speakers Available
Library: Y *(Open to the public)*
Languages: English
Membership Fee: $10 per year

The Kidney Foundation of Canada - Kingston Chapter
100 Stuart St, Kingston ON K7L 2V6
613 542-2121; Fax: 613 542-7258
E: alabrash@kidney.on.ca
W: www.kidney.on.ca
Executive:
Chapter Coord: Ann LaBrash
Year Founded: 1981
Criteria: *Open to all.*
No of Paid Staff: 2
Speakers Available
Languages: English
Membership: 18

The Kidney Foundation of Canada - Manitoba Branch
1-452 Dovercourt Dr, Winnipeg MB R3Y 1G4
204 989-0800; Fax: 204 989-0815
Toll-free: 800 729-7176
E: info@kidney.mb.ca
W: www.kidney.ca
Executive:
Exec Dir: Val Dunphy
Languages: English

The Kidney Foundation of Canada - National Office
300-5165 rue Sherbrooke O, Montréal QC H4A 1T6
514 369-4806; Fax: 514 369-2472
Toll-free: 800 361-7494
E: info@kidney.ca
W: www.kidney.ca
Executive:
Dir opér: Silvana Anania
Dir dév: Susan McKenzie
Dir exéc: Paul Shay
Dir ress hum: Teresa Havill
Dir recherche prog: Wim Wolfs
Dir natle programmes/politique d'ordre public: Nadine Valk
Year Founded: 1964
Languages: English; French

The Kidney Foundation of Canada - Northern Alberta & The Territories Branch
202-11227 Jasper Ave NW, Edmonton AB T5K 0L5
780 451-6900; Fax: 780 451-7592
Toll-free: 800 461-9063 Within Alberta & Territories only
E: info@kidney.ab.ca
W: www.kidney.ab.ca
Languages: English

The Kidney Foundation of Canada - Ontario Branch
201-1599 Hurontario St, Mississauga ON L5G 4S1
905 278-3003; Fax: 905 271-4990
Toll-free: 800 387-4474
E: kidney@kidney.on.ca
W: www.kidney.ca/ontario
Executive:
Dir-Mktg/Commun: Wendy Kudeba
Exec Dir: Jim O'Brien
Dir-Commun Serv: Tony Tirone
Year Founded: 1967
Criteria: *Interest in volunteering to improve health or quality of life of people living with kidney disease.*
No of Paid Staff: 10
Speakers Available
Languages: English
Membership: 10,000

◊ ***London Chapter:***
119-379 Dundas St, London ON N6B 1V5
519 850-5362; Fax: 519 850-5360
E: rramzanali@kidney.on.ca
W: www.kidney.ca
Executive:
Sr Dev Mgr: Michael Brennan
Dev Officer: Rizwana Ramzanali
Languages: English

◊ ***Windsor Chapter:***
310-1368 Ouellette Ave, Windsor ON N8X 1J9
519 977-9211; Fax: 519 977-9768
E: kidney@mnsi.net
W: www.kidney.ca
Executive:
Sr Mgr-Dev Western ON: Mike Brennan

The Kidney Foundation of Canada Regina & District Chapter
1545C McAra St, Regina SK S4N 6H4
306 347-0711
W: www.kidney.ca
Executive:
Reg Mgr: Iris Lord

The Kidney Foundation of Canada, Sarnia-Lambton Chapter
546 Christina St N, Main Floor, Sarnia ON N7T 5W6
519 344-3462; Fax: 519 344-4038
E: ehayter@kidney.on.ca
W: www.kidney.ca
Executive:
Pres: Phil Litrenta
Sr Dev Mgr: Elaine Hayter
No of Paid Staff: 2
Speakers Available
Library: Y *(Open to the public)*
Languages: English
Membership: 50 *(Lists available to the public)*

The Kidney Foundation of Canada - Saskatchewan Branch
1-2217 Hanselman Crt, Saskatoon SK S7L 6A8
306 664-8588; Fax: 306 653-4883
Toll-free: 888 664-8588
E: info@kidney.sk.ca
W: www.kidney.ca/saskatchewan
Executive:
Exec Dir: Joyce Van Deurzen
Office Mgr: Peggy Mausch
Year Founded: 1982
Membership Fee Required: Y
No of Paid Staff: 5
Speakers Available
Languages: English
Membership: 200
Membership Fee: $10

The Kidney Foundation of Canada - Sault Ste. Marie & District Unit
1-514 Queen St E, Floor 2, Sault Ste. Marie ON P6A 2A1
705 949-0400; Fax: 705 949-0030
E: ssmkidney@shaw.ca
W: www.kidney.on.ca
Executive:
Campaign Coord: Penny Marquis
No of Paid Staff: 1
Speakers Available
Library: Y *(Open to the public)*
Languages: English
Membership Fee: $10

The Kidney Foundation of Canada - Southern Alberta Branch
6007 1A St SW, Calgary AB T2H 0G5
403 255-6108; Fax: 403 255-9590
Toll-free: 800 268-1177
E: info@kidneyfoundation.ab.ca
W: www.kidney.ca
Executive:
Exec Dir: Joyce Van Deurzen
Year Founded: 1964
Criteria: *Open to any Canadian resident who pays the $10 fee and who agrees to the aims and objects of the Kidney Foundation.*
Budget: $2,000,000
No of Paid Staff: 10
Speakers Available
Languages: English
Membership Fee: $10

LEPROSY

The Leprosy Mission Canada
200-90 Allstate Pky, Markham ON L3R 6H3
905 886-2885; Fax: 905 886-2887
Toll-free: 888 537-7679
E: info@leprosy.ca
W: www.leprosy.ca

Executive:
Dir-Ops: Harin Watson
Mgr Donor Serv: Wayne Chung
Dir-Dev: Glenn Waterman
Exec Dir: Peter Derrick
Year Founded: 1892

Le Secours aux Lepreux Canada - Leprosy Relief Canada
305-1805 rue Sauvé O, Montréal QC H4N 3H4
514 744-3199; Fax: 514 744-9095
Toll-free: 866 744-3199
E: info@slc-lr.ca
W: www.slc-lr.ca
Executive:
Prés: Paul E Legault
VP: Jacques Chapleau
Dir exéc: Maryse Legault
Trés: Christiane Beauvais
Year Founded: 1961
Budget: $1,550,555
No of Paid Staff: 3
Languages: French; English
Membership: 10 *(Lists available to the public)*
Membership Fee: $10/an

LEUKEMIA

The Leukemia & Lymphoma Society of Canada
804-2 Lansing Sq, Toronto ON M2J 4P8
416 661-9541; Fax: 416 661-7799
Toll-free: 877 668-8326
W: www.lls.org/canada
Executive:
Pres: Nancy Allen
Year Founded: 1955
Criteria: *Open to all.*
No of Paid Staff: 39
Speakers Available
Languages: English; French
Membership: 4,000 +

Van der Jagt Medical Prof Corporation
Dept of Medicine,Ottawa Hosp General Campus
501 Smyth Rd, Ottawa ON K1H 8L6
613 737-8804; Fax: 613 739-6227
E: rvanderjagt@toh.on.ca
Executive:
Chair: Richard H C van der Jagt
Studies Coord: Judith Koolwine
Speakers Available
Library: Y
Languages: English

LIVER DISEASE

Canadian Liver Foundation - National Office & Toronto/GTA Chapter
801-3100 Steeles Ave E, Markham ON L3R 8T3
416 491-3353; Fax: 905 752-1540
Toll-free: 800 563-5483
E: clf@liver.ca
W: www.liver.ca
Executive:
Pres: Gary A Fagan
VP-Commun: Melanie Kearns
Natl Dir Health Promo/Patient Servs: Billie Potkonjak
Year Founded: 1969
No of Paid Staff: 25
Speakers Available
Library: Y *(Open to the public)*
Languages: English; French; Chinese

◈***CLF - Alberta/Northwest Territories:***
309-1010 1Ave NE, Calgary AB T2E 7W7
780 444-1547; Fax: 780 481-7781
Toll-free: 888 557-5516
E: thebert@liver.ca
W: www.liver.ca
Executive:
Prov Dir-AB: Todd Hebert
Year Founded: 1969
Budget: $500,000
No of Paid Staff: 2
Speakers Available
Library: Y *(Open to the public)*
Languages: English
Membership: 300
Membership Fee: $30/yr

◈***CLF - Calgary/Southern Alberta Regional Office***
309-1010 1 Ave NE, Calgary AB T2E 7W7
403 276-3390; Fax: 403 276-3423
Toll-free: 888 557-5516
E: thebert@liver.ca
W: www.liver.ca
Executive:
Reg Dir: Todd Hebert
Languages: English

◇***CLF - Edmonton Office:***
309-1010 1Ave NE, Calgary AB T2E 7W7
780 444-1547; Fax: 780 481-7781
Toll-free: 888 557-5516
E: thebert@liver.ca
W: www.liver.ca
Executive:
Prov Dir-AB: Todd Hebert
Year Founded: 1969
Budget: $500,000
No of Paid Staff: 2
Speakers Available
Library: Y *(Open to the public)*
Languages: English
Membership: 300
Membership Fee: $30/yr

◈***CLF - British Columbia/Yukon:***
109-828 8th Ave W, Vancouver BC V5Z 1E2
604 707-6430; Fax: 604 681-6067
Toll-free: 800 856-7266
E: emurgoci@liver.ca
W: www.liver.ca
Executive:
Reg Dir: Elena Murgoci
Speakers Available
Library: Y
Languages: English
Library:
Information Resource Centre (by appointment only) *(Open to the public)*

◈***CLF - Manitoba:***
210-375 York Ave, Winnipeg MB R3C 3J3
204 831-6231; Fax: 204 786-6292
E: rmagnuson@liver.ca
W: www.liver.ca
Executive:
Reg Mgr: Ruth Magnuson
Year Founded: 1988
No of Paid Staff: 1
Speakers Available
Languages: English
Membership: 125

◈***CLF - Newfoundland/Labrador:***
346 Newfoundland Dr, St. John's NL A1A 4A2
709 753-9989; Fax: 709 753-9989
E: clfst.johnchapter@nf.aibn.com
Executive:
Pres: Leonard Stacey
Languages: English

◈***CLF - Atlantic Canada Regional Office:***
103-287 Lacewood Dr, Halifax NS B3M 3Y7
902 423-8538; Fax: 902 423-8811
Toll-free: 866 423-8538
E: atlantic@liver.ca
W: www.liver.ca
Executive:
Exec Dir: Shayla Steeves
Languages: English; French
Membership: 15

◈***CLF - Central Ontario Regional Office:***

◈***CLF - Southwestern Ontario:***
519 659-0951; Fax: 519 659-4232

◇***CLF - Chatham/Kent Office***
Mailing: PO Box 23 Stn Main, Chatham ON N7M 5K1
519 682-9805; Fax: 519 682-2184
E: clfchatham@liver.ca
W: www.liver.ca
Executive:
Dev Mgr: Sheila Hughes
Year Founded: 2001
No of Paid Staff: 1

◇***CLF - London Chapter***
Royal Bank Bldg
1206-383 Richmond St, London ON N6A 3C4
519 659-0951; Fax: 519 659-4232
W: www.liver.ca
Executive:
Fund Dev Mgr: Christine McKinlay
Year Founded: 1969
Speakers Available
Languages: English

◇***CLF - Sarnia/Lambton Chapter***
Mailing: PO Box 1011 Stn Main, Sarnia ON N7T 7K2
519 336-5223
E: shughes@liver.ca
W: www.liver.ca
Executive:
Exec Dir: Sheila Hughes
No of Paid Staff: 1

◈***Kapuskasing:***
56 Radisson Cres, Kapuskasing ON P5N 3C3
705 335-5665
Executive:
A-Chapter Pres: Lise Genier

LUNG DISEASE

Canadian Lung Association - National Office
300-1750 Courtwood Cres, Ottawa ON K2C 2B5
613 569-6411; Fax: 613 569-8860
Toll-free: 888 566-5864
E: info@lung.ca
W: www.lung.ca
Executive:
A-Pres/CEO: Mary-Pat Shaw
VP-Fin: Debbie Smith
Dir-Mktg/Commun: Janis Hass
Year Founded: 1900
Budget: $1,500,000
No of Paid Staff: 25
Speakers Available
Languages: English; French
Membership: 2 Health professional groups; 10 Provincial lung associations

◈***Alberta/NWT***
Location: 208-17420 Stony Plain Rd NW, Edmonton AB T5S 1K6
Mailing: PO Box 4500 Stn South CRO, Edmonton AB T6E 6K2
780 488-6819; Fax: 780 488-7195

HEALTHCARE ASSOCIATIONS

Toll-free: 888 566-5864
E: info@ab.lung.ca
W: www.ab.lung.ca
Executive:
Pres/CEO: Leigh Allard
Year Founded: 1939
Budget: $4,000,000
No of Paid Staff: 20
Speakers Available
Library: Y
Languages: English
Membership Fee: $20 Year

◈British Columbia Lung Association
2675 Oak St, Vancouver BC V6H 2K2
604 731-5864; Fax: 604 731-5810
Toll-free: 800 665-5864
E: info@bc.lung.ca
W: www.bc.lung.ca
Executive:
Exec Dir: Scott McDonald
Year Founded: 1900
Budget: $4,000,000
No of Paid Staff: 20
Speakers Available
Languages: English

◈Manitoba Lung Association
629 McDermot Ave, Floor 2, Winnipeg MB R3A 1P6
204 774-5501; Fax: 204 772-5083
Toll-free: 888 566-5864
E: info@mb.lung.ca
W: www.mb.lung.ca
Executive:
Chair: Neil Johnston
V-Chair: Andrew Halayko
Treas: Gail Sigurdson
Year Founded: 1904
No of Paid Staff: 12
Speakers Available
Languages: English

◇Brandon:
940 Princess Ave, Brandon MB R7A 0P6
204 725-4230; Fax: 204 726-5800
Toll-free: 888 262-5864
E: westman@mb.lung.ca
W: www.mb.lung.ca
Executive:
Dir-Tobacco Red Init: Jo-anne Douglas
Year Founded: 1974
No of Paid Staff: 2
Speakers Available
Library: Y *(Open to the public)*
Languages: English

◈New Brunswick Lung Association
65 Brunswick St, Fredericton NB E3B 1G5
506 455-8961 101; Fax: 506 462-0939
Toll-free: 800 565-5864
E: info@nb.lung.ca
W: www.nb.lung.ca
Executive:
Pres/CEO: Dr Barbara MacKinnon
No of Paid Staff: 6
Speakers Available
Library: Y *(Open to the public)*
Languages: English; French
Membership: 35,000

◈Newfoundland and Labrador:
Location: Carnell Bldg, 15 Pippy Pl, Floor 2, St. John's NL A1B 3X2
Mailing: PO Box 13457 Stn A, St. John's NL A1B 4B8
709 726-4664; Fax: 709 726-2550
Toll-free: 888 566-5864
E: info@nf.lung.ca
W: www.nf.lung.ca
Executive:
Pres: John Hodder
VP/Treas: Peter Collens
Year Founded: 1944
No of Paid Staff: 7
Speakers Available
Languages: English

◈Lung Association of Nova Scotia
17 Alma Cres, Halifax NS B3N 2C4
902 443-8141; Fax: 902 445-2573
Toll-free: 888 566-5864 (LUNG)
E: info@ns.lung.ca
W: www.ns.lung.ca
Executive:
Pres/CEO: Louis Brill
Commun Mgr: Rose Poirier
Mgr-Fin/Spec Events: Nick McBride
Year Founded: 1905
Budget: $750,000
No of Paid Staff: 10
Languages: English

◈Ontario Lung Association
401-18 Wynford Dr, Toronto ON M3C 0K8
416 864-9911; Fax: 416 864-9916
Toll-free: 800 972-2636 General Information
E: olalung@on.lung.ca
W: www.on.lung.ca
Executive:
Chair: Hélène Michaud
Chair Elect: John Granton
Treas: Eric Bentzen
Coord: Stephanie Lear
Year Founded: 1945
Budget: $15,000,000
No of Paid Staff: 100
Languages: English

◇Algoma Area:
Cornwall Bldg
99-503 Queen St E, Sault Ste Marie ON P6A 2A2
705 256-2335; Fax: 705 256-1210
E: algoma@on.lung.ca
Executive:
Area Mgr: Rosalie Graham

◇Brant:
104-233 Colborne St, Brantford ON N3T 2H4
519 753-4682; Fax: 519 753-4667
E: brant@on.lung.ca
Executive:
Area Mgr: Vicky Spadoni

◇Bluewater-Thames Valley:
480 Egerton St, London ON N5W 3Z6
519 453-9086; Fax: 519 453-9184
W: www.on.lung.ca
Executive:
Reg Mgr: Lori Pallen
Year Founded: 1990
Criteria: *Open to all.*
No of Paid Staff: 3
Speakers Available
Languages: English

◇Hastings-Prince Edward:
Century Place Building
107-199 Front St, Belleville ON K8N 5H5
613 969-0323; Fax: 613 969-0359
Toll-free: 888 344-5864
W: www.on.lung.ca
Executive:
Volunteer/Fund Dev Coord: Debby Nolan
No of Paid Staff: 2
Speakers Available
Library: Y *(Open to the public)*
Languages: English
Membership list available to the public

◇Hamilton:
4-1447 Upper Ottawa St, Hamilton ON L8W 3J6
905 383-1616; Fax: 905 383-1213
Toll-free: 800 790-5527
E: hamilton@on.lung.ca
W: www.on.lung.ca
Executive:
Area Mgr: Jean Foster
Volunteer/Fund Raising Dev Coord: Sandy Lee
Criteria: *Open to all.*
No of Paid Staff: 3
Languages: English

◇Huron-Perth:
Jenny Trout Centre
121-342 Erie St, Stratford ON N5A 2N4
519 271-7500; Fax: 519 271-7503
E: huronperth@on.lung.ca
Executive:
Area Mgr: Deedee Herman

◇Kingston and The 1000 Islands Area:
The Woolen Mill
301-4 Cataraqui St, Kingston ON K7K 1Z7
613 545-3462; Fax: 613 545-1007
E: kingston@on.lung.ca
W: www.on.lung.ca
Executive:
Mgr: Jody Forman
Year Founded: 1900
Criteria: *Open to all.*
No of Paid Staff: 2
Speakers Available
Languages: English

◇Ottawa, Renfrew County, Cornwall & Area:
500-2319 St. Laurent Blvd, Ottawa ON K1G 4J8
613 230-4200; Fax: 613 230-5210
E: melanie@on.lung.ca
W: www.on.lung.ca
Executive:
Corp/Community Dev Officer: Melanie Estable-Porter
Res Therapist: Rosario Holmes
Year Founded: 1947
Languages: English; French

◈Ontario Lung Association - Ottawa
500-2319 St. Laurent Blvd, Ottawa ON K1G 4J8
613 230-4200; Fax: 613 230-5210
E: melanie@on.lung.ca
W: www.on.lung.ca
Executive:
Corp/Community Dev Officer: Melanie Estable-Porter
Res Therapist: Rosario Holmes
Year Founded: 1947
Languages: English; French

◈L'Association pulmonaire du Quebec
5790 av Pierre-de Coubertin, Montréal QC H1N 1R4
514 287-7400; Fax: 514 287-1978
Toll-free: 888 768-6669
E: info@pq.poumon.ca
W: www.pq.poumon.ca
Executive:
Dir gén: Dominique Massie
Dir fin: Raymond Jabbour
Dir d'évènement: Carole Bouchard
Year Founded: 1938
Budget: $1,600,000
No of Paid Staff: 12
Languages: English; French
Membership: 600

◈Lung Association of Saskatchewan Inc.
1231 8th St E, Saskatoon SK S7H 0S5
306 343-9511; Fax: 306 343-7007
E: info@sk.lung.ca
W: www.sk.lung.ca

Executive:
Pres/CEO: Dr Brian L Graham
VP-Fin/Ops: Leah Sullivan
VP-Dev: Sharon Kremeniuk
VP Health Promo: Jennifer Miller
VP Prof Educ: Jan Neumann
Year Founded: 2002
No of Paid Staff: 16
Speakers Available
Library: Y
Languages: English
Membership: 133 *(Lists available to the public)*
Membership Fee: $25

Ontario Lung Association - Windsor-Essex, Chatham-Kent
104-647 Ouellette Ave, Windsor ON N9A 4J4
519 256-3433; Fax: 519 256-8179
Toll-free: 888 566-5864
W: www.on.lung.ca
Executive:
Coord: Michelle Gellatly
No of Paid Staff: 1
Languages: English
Membership list available to the public

LUPUS

Lupus Canada
3-3555 14th Ave, Markham ON L3R 0H5
905 513-0004; Fax: 905 513-9516
Toll-free: 800 661-1468
E: info@lupuscanada.org
W: www.lupuscanada.org
Executive:
Pres: Kendra MacDonald
Mgr - Ntl Ops: Leanne Mielczarek
Speakers Available
Library: Y *(Open to the public)*
Languages: English
Membership: 375 *(Lists available to the public)*

◈Alberta:
200-1301 8 St SW, Calgary AB T2R 1B7
403 228-7956; Fax: 403 228-7853
Toll-free: 888 242-9182
E: lupuslsa@shaw.ca
W: www.lupus.ab.ca
Executive:
Past Pres: Norma Jaenen
VP: Muriel Kaun
Exec Dir: Rosemary Church
Year Founded: 1973
Budget: $150,000
No of Paid Staff: 2
Speakers Available
Library: Y *(Open to the public)*
Languages: English
Membership: 369 *(Lists available to the public)*
Membership Fee: $20

◈British Columbia:
329-720 Sixth St, New Westminster BC V3L 3C5
604 714-5564
Toll-free: 866 585-8787
E: info@bclupus.org
W: www.bclupus.org
Executive:
Pres: Josie Bradley
Adm Coord: Val Bishop
Year Founded: 1977
No of Paid Staff: 1
Speakers Available
Library: Y *(Open to the public)*
Languages: English
Membership: 500
Membership Fee: $20 per year

◈Manitoba:
105-386 Broadway, Winnipeg MB R3C 3R6
204 942-6825; Fax: 204 942-4894
Toll-free: 888 942-6825 Manitoba only
E: lupus@mts.net
W: www.lupusmanitoba.com
Year Founded: 1991
Criteria: *Affected by lupus.*
Speakers Available
Library: Y *(Open to the public)*
Languages: English
Membership: 190

◈New Brunswick:
17-55 Grant St, Moncton NB E1A 3R3
506 384-6227; Fax: 506 384-6227
Toll-free: 877 303-8080
E: lupins@rogers.com
W: lupusnb.ca
Executive:
Pres: Nancy Votour
Languages: English

◈Nova Scotia:
Mailing: PO Box 38038 Stn Burnside, Dartmouth NS B3B 1X2
902 425-0358; Fax: 902 789-0772
Toll-free: 800 394-0125 Nova Scotia only
E: info@lupusns.org
W: www.lupuscanada.org/novascotia/
Year Founded: 1981
Speakers Available
Languages: English

◈Ontario:
301-2900 John St, Markham ON L3R 5G3
905 415-1099; Fax: 905 415-9874
Toll-free: 877 240-1099
E: info@lupusontario.org
W: www.lupusontario.org
Executive:
Office Coord: Karen Furlotte
Support Serv/Prov Support Group Liaison: Juanita Butler
Coord-Fundraising/Events: Nicole Wright
Year Founded: 1999
Budget: $250,000
No of Paid Staff: 2
Speakers Available
Languages: English
Membership: 1,000
Membership Fee: $25

Lupus Foundation of Ontario
Location: 294 Ridge Rd N, Ridgeway ON L0S 1N0
Mailing: PO Box 687
905 894-4611; Fax: 905 894-4616
Toll-free: 800 368-8377
E: lupusont@vaxxine.com
W: www.vaxxine.com/lupus
Executive:
Pres: Patricia Leece
Past Pres: Patricia Aikenhead
Dir: Wally Kroeke
Treas: Michelle Leece
Office Mgr: Kathy Crowhurst
Year Founded: 1977
Criteria: *Open to all.*
No of Paid Staff: 1
Speakers Available
Library: Y *(Open to the public)*
Languages: English
Membership: 375 *(Lists available to the public)*
Membership Fee: $15

MALIGNANT HYPERTHERMIA

University Health Network - Malignant Hyperthermia Investigation Unit
ES3 323-200 Elizabeth St, Toronto ON M5G 2C4
416 340-3128; Fax: 416 340-4960
Executive:
Med Dir: Dr Sheila Riazi
Sec: Anna Atkinson
Year Founded: 1979
No of Paid Staff: 1
Languages: English

MARFAN

Canadian Marfan Association
Location: 128 Queen St S, Mississauga ON L5M 1K8
Mailing: PO Box 42257 RPO Centre Plaza, Mississauga ON L5M 4Z4
905 826-3223; Fax: 905 826-2125
Toll-free: 866 722-1722
E: info@marfan.ca
W: www.marfan.ca
Executive:
Exec Dir: Sharmin Jamal
Admn Mgr: Eva Theofilopoulos
Year Founded: 1986
Budget: $200,000
No of Paid Staff: 1
Speakers Available
Library: Y
Languages: English; French; Greek
Membership: 300

MUCOPOLYSACCHARIDE

Canadian Society for Mucopolysaccharide & Related Diseases Inc.
Location: 202-173 Forester St, North Vancouver BC V7H 0A6
Mailing: PO Box 30034 RPO Parkgate Vlg, North Vancouver BC V7H 2Y8
604 924-5130; Fax: 604 924-5131
Toll-free: 800 667-1846
W: www.mpssociety.ca
Executive:
Exec Dir: Kirsten Harkins
Year Founded: 1984
Criteria: *Open to all.*
Budget: $350,000
No of Paid Staff: 12
Speakers Available
Languages: English
Membership: 200

MULTIPLE SCLEROSIS

Multiple Sclerosis Society of Canada
North Tower
700-175 Bloor St E, Toronto ON M4W 3R8
416 922-6065; Fax: 416 922-7538
Toll-free: 800 268-7582
E: info@mssociety.ca
W: www.mssociety.ca
Executive:
Pres/CEO: Yves Savoie
Year Founded: 1948
Criteria: *Interest in MS*
Membership Fee Required: Y
Budget: $24,500,000
No of Paid Staff: 200
Speakers Available
Library: Y

Languages: English; French
Membership: 30,000
Membership Fee: $10-$12
Library:
MS Information Resource Centre *(Open to the public)*

◈Edmonton
150-9405 50 St NW, Edmonton AB T6B 2T4
780 463-1190; Fax: 780 463-7298
Toll-free: 800 268-7582
E: info.edmonton@mssociety.ca
W: www.mssociety.ca/alberta
Executive:
Pres Alberta Div: Neil Pierce
VP Edmonton Chapter: Garry Wheeler
Exec Asst: Dorothy Marshall
Year Founded: 1980
Budget: $2,100,000
No of Paid Staff: 14
Speakers Available
Languages: English
Membership: 2,400
Membership Fee: Family: $15; Single: $10

◇Calgary:
150-110 Quarry Park Blvd SE, Calgary AB T2C 3G3
403 250-7090; Fax: 403 250-8937
E: info@mscalgary.org
W: www.mscalgary.org
Executive:
Exec Dir: Mark Wolff
Year Founded: 1959
Criteria: *Members must reside within the Chapter boundaries.*
Budget: $2,500,000
No of Paid Staff: 15
Speakers Available
Library: Y *(Open to the public)*
Languages: English
Membership: 500 *(Lists available to the public)*
Membership Fee: $10 per year

◇Edmonton:
150-9405 50 St NW, Edmonton AB T6B 2T4
780 471-3034; Fax: 780 463-7298
W: www.mssociety.ca
Executive:
Exec Dir: Neil Pierce
Year Founded: 1948
Criteria: *Open to anyone.*
Budget: $750,000
No of Paid Staff: 8
Speakers Available
Languages: English
Membership list available to the public
Library:
Edmonton Chapter Library

◇Southeastern Alberta:
101-1201A Kingsway Ave SE,
Medicine Hat AB T1A 2Y2
403 529-6797; Fax: 403 504-1385
E: info.sealberta@mssociety.ca
W: www.mssociety.ca
Executive:
Chapter Mgr: Cheryl Cowling
Client Serv Coord: Terri Sailer
Year Founded: 1979
No of Paid Staff: 2
Speakers Available
Library: Y *(Open to the public)*
Languages: English
Membership: 150 *(Lists available to the public)*
Membership Fee: $15 Family; $10 Individual

◈Burnaby
1501-4330 Kingsway, Burnaby BC V5H 4H9
604 689-3144; Fax: 604 689-0377
Toll-free: 800 268-7582
E: info.bc@mssociety.ca
W: www.mssociety.ca
Executive:
Pres: Janet Palm
Commun Mgr: Suzanne Jay
Dir-Client Serv: Sharon Farrish
Year Founded: 1975
Budget: $3,600,000
No of Paid Staff: 40
Speakers Available
Library: Y *(Open to the public)*
Languages: English
Membership: 6,000
Membership Fee: $10
Library:
MS Library *(Open to the public)*

◈Brandon
5B-457 9th St, Brandon MB R7A 1K2
204 571-5671; Fax: 204 571-5678
E: melissa.rothwell@mssociety.ca
W: www.mssociety.ca
Year Founded: 1979
No of Paid Staff: 2
Speakers Available
Library: Y *(Open to the public)*
Languages: English
Membership: 200
Membership Fee: $10/year

◈Winnipeg
100-1465 Buffalo Pl, Winnipeg MB R3T 1L8
204 943-9595; Fax: 204 988-0915
Toll-free: 800 268-7582
E: info.manitoba@mssociety.ca
W: www.mssociety.ca
Year Founded: 1948
Library: Y *(Open to the public)*
Languages: English

◇Brandon:
5B-457 9th St, Brandon MB R7A 1K2
204 571-5671; Fax: 204 571-5678
E: melissa.rothwell@mssociety.ca
W: www.mssociety.ca
Year Founded: 1979
No of Paid Staff: 2
Speakers Available
Library: Y *(Open to the public)*
Languages: English
Membership: 200
Membership Fee: $10/year

◇Morden Office:
101-400 Stephen St, Morden MB R6M 1W3
204 822-1397; Fax: 204 822-6944

◇Parkland Chapter:
B1-101 1st Ave NW, Dauphin MB R7N 1G8
204 622-2940; Fax: 204 622-2949

◇South Central Chapter:
306 Saskatchewan Ave E,
Portage la Prairie MB R1N 0K8
204 239-1308; Fax: 204 239-4012
Toll-free: 800 268-7582
W: www.mssociety.ca/manitoba
Executive:
Office Admin/Event Coord: Cindy Hope
Client Serv Coord: Nadine Konyk
Criteria: *Open to all.*
Languages: English; French
Membership Fee: $10/yr

◇South East Chapter:
Steinbach 55 Plus
10 Chrysler Gate, Steinbach MB R5G 2E6
204 471-0402; Fax: 204 326-1434

◇Swan River Branch Office:
516 Main St, Swan River MB R0L 1Z0
204 734-6343; Fax: 204 734-6344

◈Dartmouth
1-109 Ilsley Ave, Dartmouth NS B3B 1S8
902 468-8230; Fax: 902 468-5328
Toll-free: 800 268-7582
E: info.atlantic@mssociety.ca
W: www.mssociety.ca
Executive:
Commun/Public Affairs: Jessesar Mitchell
Year Founded: 1974
Budget: $1,900,000
No of Paid Staff: 14
Speakers Available
Library: Y *(Open to the public)*
Languages: English
Membership: 1,433
Membership Fee: $10 to non-MS clients; Complimentary to MS clients

◈Ottawa
1826 Woodward Dr, Ottawa ON K2C 0P7
613 728-1583; Fax: 613 728-0342
E: info.ottawa@mssociety.ca
W: www.mssociety.ca/ottawa
Executive:
Exec Dir: Laurel Mackenzie
Year Founded: 1950
Budget: $1,000,000
No of Paid Staff: 9
Languages: English
Membership: 1,100
Membership Fee: $15-$25

◇Frontenac, Lennox and Addington:
3-637 Norris Crt, Kingston ON K7P 2R9
613 384-8500; Fax: 613 384-8706
E: msking@kingston.net
W: www.mssociety.ca/chapters/kingston
Executive:
Chair: Kelly Fraser
VP: K Fraser
Treas: Dona Riddell
Office Mgr: Linda Marks
Year Founded: 1952
Criteria: *Open to all.*
Budget: $105,000
No of Paid Staff: 1
Speakers Available
Library: Y *(Open to the public)*
Languages: English
Membership: 180 *(Lists available to the public)*
Membership Fee: $18 2 yrs; $10 1 yr

◈Montreal
Tour E
1010-550 rue Sherbrooke O, Montréal QC H3A 1B9
514 849-7591; Fax: 514 849-8914
Toll-free: 800 268-7582 Québec
E: info.qc@scleroseenplaques.ca
W: www.scleroseenplaques.ca
Executive:
Dir gén: Louis Adam
Year Founded: 1967
Budget: $4,175,000
No of Paid Staff: 35
Speakers Available
Languages: English; French
Membership: 8,300

◇Joliette:
200 rue de Salaberry, Joliette QC J6E 4G1
450 753-5545; Fax: 450 759-8749
E: asepl@intermonde.net
W: www.asepl.org
Executive:
Coord: Monique Boissy

Year Founded: 1986
No of Paid Staff: 1
Speakers Available
Library: Y
Languages: French; English

◊ **Laval:**
210A-387 boul des Prairies, Laval QC H7N 2W4
450 663-4911; Fax: 450 663-4584
E: scsp-sectionlaval@videotron.ca
W: www.scleroseenplaques.ca/laval
Executive:
Prés: Suzanne Chartrand
VP: Dina Lachapelle
Gest section: Sophie Marcil
Coord: Dina Tazi
Coord servs: Lina Atallah
Year Founded: 1974
No of Paid Staff: 3

◈ **Regina:**
150 Albert St, Regina SK S4R 2N2
306 522-5600; Fax: 306 565-0477
Toll-free: 800 268-7582
E: laurie.murphy@mssociety.ca
W: www.mssociety.ca/sask
Executive:
Sec: Melanie Oberg
Speakers Available
Languages: English
Membership: 2,000
Membership Fee: $5

MUSCULAR DYSTROPHY

Muscular Dystrophy Canada (MDC)
900-2345 Yonge St, Toronto ON M4P 2E5
416 488-0030; Fax: 416 488-7523
Toll-free: 866 687-2538
E: info@muscle.ca
W: www.muscle.ca
Executive:
CEO: Catherine Sherrard
CFO: Melanie Towell
Mktg/Commun Coord: Tori Laird
Year Founded: 1954
Budget: $8,300,000
No of Paid Staff: 60
Speakers Available
Languages: English; French
Membership: 2,000
Membership Fee: $10 Family; $5 Individual

◈ **Edmonton:**
200-8944 182 St NW, Edmonton AB T5T 2E3
780 489-6322; Fax: 780 486-1948
Toll-free: 800 661-9312
E: infoedmonton@muscle.ca
W: www.muscle.ca
Executive:
Reg Mgr Prairies/NWT: Jo-Ann Burton
Year Founded: 1954
Criteria: *Registered clients must be diagnosed with one of the over 40 neuromuscular disorders under the umbrella of MDAC. Chapter members must pay $5 annual membership fee.*
Budget: $9,117,166
No of Paid Staff: 4
Speakers Available
Languages: English
Membership: 1,200 + *(Lists available to the public)*
Library:
MOAC Resource Library *(Open to the public)*

◈ **Western Canada Region:**
1401 Broadway W, Floor 7, Vancouver BC V6H 1H6
604 732-8799; Fax: 604 731-6127
Toll-free: 800 366-8166
E: infowest@muscle.ca
W: www.muscle.ca
Year Founded: 1954
No of Paid Staff: 9
Speakers Available
Library: Y *(Open to the public)*
Languages: English

◈ **Fredericton:**
203-56 Avonlea Crt, Fredericton NB E3C 1N8
506 450-6322; Fax: 506 458-2205
Toll-free: 888 647-6322
E: infoatlantic@muscle.ca
W: www.muscle.ca
Executive:
Dir-Servs Atlantic: Tracy Ryan

◈ **Saint John:**
13 Minstrel Drive, Quispamsis NB E2E 1S5
506 849-8459
E: infosaintjohn@muscle.ca
W: www.muscle.ca
Languages: English; French

◈ **London:**
915-383 Richmond St, London ON N6A 3C4
519 850-8700; Fax: 519 850-8701
Toll-free: 877 850-8720
E: infoontario@muscle.ca
W: www.muscle.ca

◈ **Ontario:**
215-150 Isabella St, Ottawa ON K1S 1V7
613 232-7334; Fax: 613 567-2288
Toll-free: 866 337-3365
E: info.ottawa@muscle.ca
W: www.muscle.ca
Year Founded: 1954
Budget: $10,000,000
No of Paid Staff: 54
Languages: English; French

◈ **Jonquiere:**
Location: 7.37-2230 rue de l'Hôpital, Jonquière QC G7X 7X2
Mailing: CP 15
418 695-7760; Fax: 418 695-7761
Toll-free: 877 295-7911
E: infovillesaguenay@muscle.ca
W: www.muscle.ca
Languages: French

◈ **Quebec:**
506-1425 boul René-Lévesque O, Montréal QC H3G 1T7
514 393-3522; Fax: 514 393-8113
Toll-free: 800 567-2236
E: infoquebec@muscle.ca
W: www.muscle.ca
Executive:
Dir gén: Dominique Richard
Adj admin: Maryse Lapensée
Year Founded: 1954
Budget: $1,450,000
No of Paid Staff: 11
Languages: French

Society for Muscular Dystrophy Information International
Mailing: PO Box 479 Stn Main, Bridgewater NS B4V 2X6
902 685-3961; Fax: 902 685-3962
E: smdi@auracom.com
W: www.nsnet.org/smdi
Year Founded: 1983
Criteria: *People interested in Muscular Dystrophy or allied disorders.*
Languages: English
Membership: 260 organizations and individuals

MYALGIC ENCEPHALOMYELITIS

National ME / FM Action Network
512-33 Banner Rd, Nepean ON K2H 8V7
613 829-6667; Fax: 613 829-8518
E: mefminfo@mefmaction.com
W: www.mefmaction.net
Executive:
Pres: Margaret Parlor
CEO: Lydia E Neilson
VP: Lynda Cregan
Year Founded: 1993
Budget: $24,000
No of Paid Staff: 1
Speakers Available
Languages: English; French

NEUROFIBROMATOSIS

Association de la Fibromyalgie - Montréal
105-1140 rue Jean-Talon E, Montréal QC H2R 1V9
514 259-7306; Fax: 438 381-9376
E: afim_mtl@yahoo.ca
W: www.afim.qc.ca
Executive:
Prés: Renée Marleau
Languages: French; English

The British Columbia Neurofibromatosis Foundation
Mailing: PO Box 5339 Stn B, Victoria BC V8R 6S4
250 743-2678; Fax: 250 743-2027
Toll-free: 250 743-2678
E: info@bcnf.bc.ca
W: www.bcnf.bc.ca
Executive:
Exec Dir: Desiree Sher
Prog Coord: Susan Wood
Year Founded: 1984
Budget: $200,000
No of Paid Staff: 3
Speakers Available
Library: Y *(Open to the public)*
Languages: English
Membership: 300
Membership Fee: Family - $50; Single - $35

OSTEOPOROSIS

Centre Ostéopathique du Québec
103-2210 boul Henri-Bourassa E, Montréal QC H2B 1T3
514 384-1271; Fax: 514 384-2725
E: info@coq.org
W: www.coq.org
Executive:
Dir: Andrée Aubin
Languages: French

Osteoporosis Canada - National Office
301-1090 Don Mills Rd, Toronto ON M3C 3R6
416 696-2663; Fax: 416 696-2673
Toll-free: 800 463-6842 English
E: info@osteoporosis.ca
W: www.osteoporosis.ca
Executive:
Pres/CEO: Dr Famida Jiwa
Year Founded: 1982
Budget: $7,500,000
No of Paid Staff: 160
Speakers Available
Languages: English; French; Chinese; Punjabi
Membership: 3,000

Membership Fee: $20
Library:
Lindy Fraser Library *(Open to the public)*

◈Alberta Chapter
Currie Barracks Bldg B8
104-2526 Battleford Ave SW, Calgary AB T3E 7J4
403 237-7022; Fax: 403 220-1727
E: alberta@osteoporosis.ca
W: www.osteoporosis.ca
Executive:
Admin: Val Freeman

◈British Columbia Chapters:

◇North Shore Chapter
1691 Davenport Pl, North Vancouver BC V7J 1N4
604 985-5430
E: NorthShore@osteoporosis.ca
W: www.osteoporosis.ca
Executive:
Chairperson: Mary Hamm

◇Surrey/White Rock Chapter
13845 18 Ave, Surrey BC V4A 1W6
604 541-1942
E: surrey-whiterock@osteoporosis.ca
W: www.osteoporosis.ca
Executive:
Chair: Rycarda Smith

◈Manitoba Chapter:
123 St Anne's Rd, Winnipeg MB R2M 2Z1
204 772-3498; Fax: 204 772-4200
E: manitoba@osteoporosis.ca
W: www.osteoporosis.ca
Executive:
Chair: Cherylle Unryn
Exec Dir: Janet Choboter
Prog Asst: Sheila McBeath
Year Founded: 1982
No of Paid Staff: 3
Speakers Available
Languages: English; French
Membership list available to the public

◈New Brunswick Chapter:
195-527 Dundonald St, Fredericton NB E3B 1X5
506 459-4901; Fax: 506 488-1995
E: newbrunswick@osteoporosis.ca
W: www.osteoporosis.ca

◈Nova Scotia Chapter:
90 Drillio Cres, Halifax NS B3N 3K7
902 445-2448; Fax: 902 445-5257
Toll-free: 800 463-6824 405
E: novascotia@osteoporosis.ca
W: www.osteoporosis.ca

◈Niagara Chapter:
406-36 Page St, St Catharines ON L2R 4A7
905 227-9646
E: niagara@osteoporosis.ca
W: www.osteoporosis.ca
Executive:
Chair: Judy Cline

◈Ontario Chapters:

◇Hamilton-Burlington:
2-10 George St, Floor 4, Hamilton ON L8P 1C8
905 525-5398; Fax: 905 577-0396
E: hamilton@osteoporosis.ca
W: www.osteoporosis.ca

◇Niagara Chapter:
406-36 Page St, St Catharines ON L2R 4A7
905 227-9646
E: niagara@osteoporosis.ca
W: www.osteoporosis.ca
Executive:
Chair: Judy Cline

◇Ottawa
301-1090 Don Mills Rd, North York ON M3C 3R6
416 696-2663
Toll-free: 800 463-6842 411
W: www.osteoporosis.ca
Executive:
Ottawa Area Mgr, ON Osteo Strat: Marq Nelson
No of Paid Staff: 1
Speakers Available
Languages: English; French

◇Peterborough:
3-360 George St N, Peterborough ON K9H 7E7
705 740-2776; Fax: 705 740-2107
Toll-free: 866 376-2776
E: peterborough@osteoporosis.ca
W: www.osteoporosis.ca

◈Quebec Chapters:

◇Québec
100-1200 av de Germain-des-Prés,
Québec QC G1V 3M7
418 651-8661; Fax: 418 650-2916
Toll-free: 800 977-1778
E: sectiondequebec@osteoporosecanada.ca
W: www.osteoporosis.ca
Executive:
Coord-section QC: Elizabeth Shaver
Year Founded: 2004
No of Paid Staff: 1
Speakers Available
Languages: French; English

◈Saskatchewan Chapters:

◇Regina
90C Cavendish St, Regina SK S4N 5G7
306 757-2663; Fax: 306 789-2663
E: osteoporosis.regina@sasktel.net
W: www.osteoporosis.ca
Executive:
Chair: Sylvia Fiske
Pub Rel Mgr: Alice Gaveronski
Fundraiser: R Kapoor
Year Founded: 2002
Budget: $30,000
No of Paid Staff: 1
Speakers Available
Library: Y *(Open to the public)*
Languages: Chinese; Punjabi
Membership list available to the public

◇Saskatoon
1926 St George Ave, Saskatoon SK S7M 0K5
306 931-2663; Fax: 306 249-9065
E: saskatoon@osteoporosis.ca
W: www.osteoporosis.ca
Executive:
Chair: Carole Young
Off administrator: Joanne Harbottle
No of Paid Staff: 1
Speakers Available

OSTOMY

Association Iléostomie & Colostomie de Montréal
5151 boul de l'Assomption, Montréal QC H1T 4A9
514 255-3041; Fax: 514 645-5464
E: jean-pierre.lapointe@sympatico.ca
W: www.aicm-montreal.org
Executive:
VP: Jean-Pierre Lapointe
Year Founded: 1958
Speakers Available
Languages: French; English

United Ostomy Association of Canada Inc.-Head Office
501-344 Bloor St W, Toronto ON M5S 3A7
416 595-5452; Fax: 416 595-9924
Toll-free: 888 969-9698
W: www.ostomycanada.ca
Executive:
Pres: Les Kehoe
Treas: Eugene Zapf
Sec: Ferne Oliver
Office Coord: Marion Whate
No of Paid Staff: 1
Speakers Available
Library: Y *(Open to the public)*
Languages: English
Membership: 4,000

◈Ontario

◇Brantford Chapter
Mailing: 56 Banbury Rd, Brantford ON N3P 1C3
519 752-5037
E: poohbear17@sympatico.ca
Executive:
Pres: Marie Winn
Treas: Tammie Crayne
Year Founded: 1974
Library: Y

◇Halton./Peel Chapter
Mailing: 1266 Monks Pass, Oakville ON L6M 1R4
905 825-3443
Executive:
Premier: Richard Olley
Editor: Marion Whate
Sec: Chuck Davey
Visiting Coord: Andrea Teixeira
Year Founded: 1983
Criteria: *none specific - however, most members wither have ostomy surgery or have a close friend or relative with ostomy surgery*
Budget: $1,000
Speakers Available
Membership: 80

◇United Ostomy Support Group Ottawa Inc
Mailing: PO Box 11134 Station H, Nepean ON K2H 7T8
613 447-0361
E: information@ostomyottawa.ca
W: www.ostomyottawa.ca
Executive:
Pres: Doug Graham

◈Quebec

◇l'estrie Chapter
Mailing: CP 661 Stn Pl de la Cite, Sherbrooke QC J1H 5K5
819 564-6052
E: apse@abacom.com
Executive:
Prés: Les Kehoe
VP: Janet Paquet
Sec: Ferne Oliver
Speakers Available
Membership: 200

PARKINSON'S DISEASE

Parkinson Society British Columbia
600-890 Pender St W, Vancouver BC V6C 1J9
604 662-3240; Fax: 604 687-1327
Toll-free: 800 668-3330
E: info@parkinson.bc.ca
W: www.parkinson.bc.ca

Executive:
Dir-Res Dev: Cecilia Tupper
Exec Dir: Diane Robinson
Info/Prog Mgr: Robbin Jeffereys
Res Dev Mgr: Betty Hum
Year Founded: 1969
Criteria: *Those living with PD & other interested parties.*
Budget: $950,000
No of Paid Staff: 6
Speakers Available
Library: Y *(Open to the public)*
Languages: English
Membership: 1,400
Membership Fee: $20

Parkinson Society Canada National Office
316-4211 Yonge St, Toronto ON M2P 2A9
416 227-9700; Fax: 416 227-9600
Toll-free: 800 565-3000
E: general.info@parkinson.ca
W: www.parkinson.ca
Executive:
Pres/CEO: Joyce Gordon
Year Founded: 1965
No of Paid Staff: 23
Speakers Available
Languages: English; French
Membership: 12 Regional organizations

◈Alberta:
Edmonton General Hospital
11111 Jasper Ave NW, Room 3Y18, Edmonton AB T5K 0L4
780 342-8993; Fax: 780 342-8969
E: info@parkinsonalberta.ca
W: www.parkinsonalberta.ca
Executive:
CEO: John Petryshen

◈Southern Alberta:
102-5636 Burbank Cres SE, Calgary AB T2H 1Z6
403 243-9901; Fax: 403 243-8283
Toll-free: 800 561-1911 Alberta
E: pssa@parkinsons-society.org
W: www.parkinsons-society.org
Executive:
CEO: John Petryshen
Exec Asst: Maria Iandolo
Year Founded: 1981
Criteria: *An interest in, or need for Parkinsons related information and or support.*
Budget: $500,000
No of Paid Staff: 5
Speakers Available
Library: Y *(Open to the public)*
Languages: French
Membership: 500

◈Manitoba:
7-414 Westmount Dr, Winnipeg MB R2J 1P2
204 786-2637; Fax: 204 786-2327
Toll-free: 866 999-5558
Executive:
Exec Dir: Howard Koks
Speakers Available
Library: Y *(Open to the public)*

◈Newfoundland & Labrador:
Viking Bldg
305-136 Crosbie Rd, St. John's NL A1B 3K3
709 754-4428; Fax: 709 754-5868
Toll-free: 800 567-7020
E: parkinson@nf.aibn.com
W: www.parkinson.ca
Year Founded: 1988
Criteria: *Person with Parkinson's or family or friend of*
No of Paid Staff: 1
Speakers Available
Library: Y *(Open to the public)*
Languages: English
Membership: 500 *(Lists available to the public)*

◈Maritime Region:
150-7071 Bayers Rd, Halifax NS B3L 2C2
902 422-3656; Fax: 902 422-3797
Toll-free: 800 663-2468 NS, NB & PEI
E: psmr@parkinsonmaritimes.ca
W: www.parkinsonmaritimes.ca
Executive:
Exec Dir: Mary Hatcher
Office Admin: Christopher Wirth Bulmer
Year Founded: 1983
Budget: $350,000
No of Paid Staff: 5
Speakers Available
Library: Y *(Open to the public)*
Languages: English
Membership: 24 *(Lists available to the public)*

◈Central & Northern Ontario Region:
321-4211 Yonge St, North York ON M2P 2A9
416 227-1200; Fax: 416 227-1520
Toll-free: 800 565-3000 3301
E: info.cno@parkinson.ca
W: www.parkinsoncno.ca
Speakers Available
Library: Y

◈Ontario:
Location: 300-381 Kent St, Ottawa ON K2P 2A8
Mailing: 1053 Carling Ave, Ottawa ON K1Y 4E9
613 722-9238; Fax: 613 722-3241
E: psoc@lri.ca
W: www.parkinsons.ca
Executive:
Dir-Resource Dev: Hilary Evans
Exec Dir: Dennise Taylor-Gilhen
Year Founded: 1978
No of Paid Staff: 4
Speakers Available
Library: Y *(Open to the public)*
Languages: English; French
Membership: 850
Membership Fee: $25 per year
Library:
PSOC Resource Library *(Open to the public)*

◈Southwestern Ontario Region:
117-4500 Blakie Rd, London ON N6L 1G5
519 652-9437; Fax: 519 652-9267
Toll-free: 888 851-7376
E: info@parkinsonsociety.ca
W: www.parkinsonsociety.ca
Executive:
CEO: Marilyn Matheson
Mgr-Admin: Joanne Bernard
Prog/Serv Mgr: Tracey Jones
Coord-Spec Events: Shelley Ralf
Year Founded: 1997
No of Paid Staff: 6
Speakers Available
Library: Y *(Open to the public)*
Languages: English

◈Société Parkinson du Québec:
Tour ouest
1080-550 rue Sherbrooke O, Montréal QC H3A 1B9
514 861-4422; Fax: 514 861-4510
Toll-free: 800 720-1307 Français
E: infos@parkinsonquebec.ca
W: www.parkinsonquebec.ca
Executive:
Coord commun/dév: Annie Turcot
Languages: French

◈Saskatchewan:
Mailing: 610 Duchess St, Saskatoon SK S7K 0R1
Toll-free: 888 685-0059
Toll-free Fax: 888 775-1402
E: pss@sasktel.net
W: www.parkinsonsaskatchewan.ca
Executive:
Exec Dir: Travis Low
Commun Outreach Coord: Jennifer Schoeck
Commun Coord: Sheena Miller
Year Founded: 1972
Criteria: *Open to all.*
No of Paid Staff: 3
Speakers Available
Library: Y *(Open to the public)*
Languages: English
Membership: 80 *(Lists available to the public)*
Membership Fee: $5

PRADER-WILLI SYNDROME

Ontario Prader - Willi Syndrome Association
Mailing: PO Box 73514 Rpo Wychwood, Toronto ON M6C 4A7
416 481-8657; Fax: 416 481-6706
E: opwsa@rogers.com
W: www.opwsa.com
Executive:
Admin: Debra Baptiste
Year Founded: 1982
No of Paid Staff: 1
Languages: English
Membership Fee: Agency/Professional: $30; Family: $25

PSORIASIS

Psoriasis Society of Canada
Location: 71 Noria Cres, Middle Sackville NS B4E 2L8
Mailing: PO Box 25015, RPO Clayton Park W, Halifax NS B3M 4H4
902 443-8680; Fax: 902 443-2073
Toll-free: 800 656-4494
W: www.psoriasissociety.org
Executive:
Pres: Judy Misner
Year Founded: 1983
Budget: $100,000
Speakers Available
Languages: English
Membership: 10,000
Membership Fee: $25

RHEUMATISM

Canadian Rheumatology Association (CRA)
244-16715 Yonge St, Newmarket ON L3X 1X4
905 952-0698; Fax: 905 952-0708
E: info@rheum.ca
W: www.rheum.ca
Executive:
Chair Mgmt Committee/Sec-Treas: Dr Jacob Karsh
Pres: Dr Carter Thorne
VP: Dr Cory Baillie
Criteria: *Open to any person involved in musculoskeletal care and nominated by two active members of the CRA.*
No of Paid Staff: 1
Languages: English; French
Membership: 400
Membership Fee: $100

SJOGREN'S SYNDROME

Association du Syndrome de Sjögren Inc.
001-3155 rue Hochelaga, Montréal QC H1W 1G4
514 934-3666; Fax: 514 934-1241
Toll-free: 877 934-3666
E: sjogren.montreal@qc.aira.com
W: www.sjogrens.ca
Executive:
Prés: Pierre Sébastien
VP: Ginette Texier
Trés: Raymond Groulx
Year Founded: 1994
Criteria: *Suffering from SS or friends of SS sufferers.*
Budget: $35,000
Speakers Available
Languages: English; French
Membership: 208

SPINA BIFIDA AND HYDROCEPHALUS

Spina Bifida and Hydrocephalus Association of Ontario
1006-555 Richmond St W, Box 103,
Toronto ON M5V 3B1
416 214-1056; Fax: 416 214-1446
Toll-free: 800 387-1575
E: provincial@sbhao.on.ca
W: www.sbhao.on.ca
Executive:
Chm: Marc Garson
Exec Dir: Joan Booth
Info/Serv Coord: Shauna Beaudoin
Year Founded: 1973
Criteria: *Open to all.*
No of Paid Staff: 9
Speakers Available
Library: Y *(Open to the public)*
Languages: English
Membership: 4,000
Membership Fee: Varies
Library:
SB & H Resource Centre *(Open to the public)*

◈***Toronto***
647-167 Lombard Ave, Winnipeg MB R3B 0V3
204 925-3650; Fax: 204 925-3654
Toll-free: 800 565-9488
E: info@sbhac.ca
W: www.sbhac.ca
Executive:
Pres: Colleen Talbot
Past Pres: Jody Sabroe
VP: Linda Randall
Natl Mgr: Bonnie Hidlebaugh
Treas: Pauline Dooley
Sec: Lorelei Fletcher
Year Founded: 1981
Criteria: *Open to all.*
Budget: $250,000
No of Paid Staff: 2
Speakers Available
Library: Y *(Open to the public)*
Languages: English; French
Membership: 2,500 *(Lists available to the public)*
Membership Fee: $20 Individual

SUDDEN ARRHYTHMIA DEATH SYNDROME

The Canadian Sudden Arrhythmia Death Syndromes (SADS) Foundation
9-6975 Meadowvale Town Centre Cir, Suite 314,
Mississauga ON L5N 2V7
905 826-6303; Fax: 905 826-9068
Toll-free: 877 525-5995
E: info@sads.ca
W: www.sads.ca
Executive:
Pres/Exec Dir: Pam Husband
Treas: Graham Davies
Year Founded: 1995
Speakers Available
Languages: English
Membership: 1,200

SYRINGOMYELIA

Canadian Syringomyelia Network
69 Penny Cres, Markham ON L3P 5X7
905 471-8278; Fax: 905 944-4844
E: barb@csn.ca
W: www.csn.ca
Executive:
Chair: Barbara Forrestall
Languages: English

TINNITUS

Canadian Tinnitus Foundation
202-15388 24 Ave, Surrey BC V4A 2J2
604 317-2952
E: info@findthecurenow.org
W: findthecurenow.org
Executive:
Exec Dir: Alexander Bridges

Tinnitus Association of Canada Inc.
23 Ellis Park Rd, Toronto ON M6S 2V4
416 762-1490
W: www.kadis.com/ta/tinnitus.htm
Executive:
Pres: Peter Austen
Board Member: Bryan Aubie
Board Member: Brian Cassidy
Board Member: Robin Fielding
Board Member: Ken Jones
Languages: English

TOURETTE SYNDROME

Tourette Syndrome Foundation of Canada
195-5945 Airport Rd, Mississauga ON L4V 1R9
905 673-2255; Fax: 905 673-2638
Toll-free: 800 361-3120
Toll-free Fax: 800 387-0120
E: tsfc@tourette.ca
W: www.tourette.ca
Executive:
Exec Dir: Lynn McLarnon
Year Founded: 1976
Criteria: *Open to those with an interest in Tourette syndrome. Consideration given to low income families.*
Budget: $500,000
No of Paid Staff: 3
Speakers Available
Library: Y *(Open to the public)*
Languages: English; French
Membership: 500 *(Lists available to the public)*
Membership Fee: Individual rates for low income families; Regular - $35
Library:
TSFC Library *(Open to the public)*

TUBEROUS SCLEROSIS

Tuberous Sclerosis Canada
125-92 Caplan Ave, Barrie ON L4N 0Z7
Toll-free: 866 558-7278 French
E: TSCanadaST@gmail.com
W: www.tscanada.ca
Executive:
Dir: Ray Marco
Dir: Karen Shulist
Criteria: *Open to all.*
Languages: English

TYROSINEMIA

Groupe d'Aide aux Enfants Tyrosinémiques du Québec
3162 rue Granville, Jonquière QC G7S 2B9
418 548-1580
E: gerard.tremblay@sympatico.ca
W: www.cegep-chicoutimi.qc.ca/gaetq
Executive:
Prés: Jean Harvey
Year Founded: 1989
Criteria: *Children affected by tyrosinemia.*
Languages: French
Membership: 120

MEDICAL & HEALTH (3) —Organ Donation

British Columbia Transplant
West Tower
555 12th Ave W, Floor 3, Vancouver BC V5Z 3X7
604 877-2240; Fax: 604 877-2111
Toll-free: 800 663-6189
W: www.transplant.bc.ca
Executive:
Prov Exec Dir: Dr Greg Grant
Languages: English

Canadian Society of Transplantation
774 Echo Dr, Ottawa ON K1S 5N8
905 415-3917; Fax: 613 730-1116
E: cst@royalcollege.ca
W: www.cst-transplant.ca
Executive:
Pres: Dr Tom Blydt-Hansen
Exec Dir: Hélène Samson
No of Paid Staff: 2
Languages: English; French
Membership: 425

The Canadian Transplant Association
11230 72 Ave NW, Edmonton AB T6G 0B5
780 430-5991
Toll-free: 877 779-5991
E: cta_national@hotmail.com
W: www.organ-donation-works.org

Executive:
Pres: David Smith
VP East: Aubrey Goldstein
Reg Dir AB/VP West: Jennifer Holman
Reg Dir ON: Sandra Holdsworth
Reg Dir Atlantic Prov: Mark Black
Reg Dir SK: Orest Saskiw
Reg Dir QC: Gaston Martin
Reg Dir BC: Margaret Benson
Dir-Membership Dev: Neil Felkins
Treas: Janice Locke
Sec: Kathy Tachynski
Year Founded: 1987
Languages: English; French

◈*British Columbia*
151 Osborne Rd E, North Vancouver BC V7N 1L8
604 985-6628
W: www.organ-donation-works.org
Executive:
VP-West: Margaret Benson
Languages: English

Eye Bank of Canada - Ontario Division
203-1929 Bayview Ave, Toronto ON M4G 3E8
416 978-7355; Fax: 416 978-1522
E: eye.bank@utoronto.ca
W: www.eyebank.utoronto.ca
Executive:
Mgr: Linda Sharpen
Exec Dir: William Dixon
Dir: Dr C Wedge
Languages: English

The Organ Donation & Transplant Association of Canada
444 Ontario St, Stratford ON N5A 3J2
Fax: 416 487-3908
Toll-free: 866 949-0003
Executive:
Chairman: Neil St. John
Vice Chair: John Balogh
CEO: Gabriel Etele
Dir: Francessa Hayes
Dir: Bobby Vincze
Dir: Ali Agat
Year Founded: 2004
Languages: English

Sarnia Organ Donors' Awareness Group
104-180 College Ave N, Sarnia ON N7T 7X2
519 344-7777; Fax: 519 344-7302
E: soda@ebtech.net
W: www.sarniaorgandonors.ca
Executive:
Dir: Connie Ellis
Office Admin: Susan Judas
Year Founded: 1994
Criteria: *Willingness to volunteer.*
Speakers Available
Library: Y *(Open to the public)*
Languages: English
Membership: 50

Southern Alberta Organ Tissue Donation Program - Lions Eye Bank
7007 14 St SW, Calgary AB T2V 1P9
403 943-3406; Fax: 403 943-3244
Executive:
Specialist: Roxanne Pennington
Asst Prog Mgr: Mijana Ridic
Year Founded: 1985
Criteria: *Open to all.*
Budget: $250,000
No of Paid Staff: 3
Speakers Available
Languages: English
Membership: 4,816

Trillium Gift of Life Network
900-522 University Ave, Toronto ON M5G 1W7
416 363-4001; Fax: 416 214-7807
Toll-free: 800 263-2833
E: info@giftoflife.on.ca
W: www.giftoflife.on.ca
Executive:
Pres/CEO: Dr Frank Markel
Languages: English

MEDICAL & HEALTH (4) —Professional & Administrative

Allergy, Asthma and Immunology Society of Ontario
2 Demaris Ave, Toronto ON M3N 1M1
416 633-2215; Fax: 416 633-3108
W: www.allergyasthma.on.ca
Executive:
Pres: Dr Howard Langer
Languages: English

Association canadienne des sages-femmes
59 rue Riverview, LaSalle QC H8R 3R9
514 807-3668; Fax: 514 738-0370
E: admin@canadianmidwives.org
W: www.canadianmidwives.org
Executive:
Dir gén: Tonia Occhionero
Year Founded: 2001
Languages: English
Membership: 850

◈*Alberta Association of Midwives*
63-4307 130 Ave SE, Suite 166, Calgary AB T2Z 3V8
403 214-1882
E: info@alberta-midwives.com
W: www.alberta-midwives.com
Executive:
Registrar: Theresa Barrett
Languages: English

◈*BC: Midwives Association of British Columbia*
2-175 15th Ave E, Vancouver BC V5T 2P6
604 736-5976; Fax: 604 736-5957
E: mabc.admin@telus.net
W: www.bcmidwives.com
Executive:
Exec Dir: Ganga Jolicoeur
Admv Asst: Ana Mirkovic
Year Founded: 1980
Languages: English; French

◈*Association of Midwives of Newfoundland & Labrador*
Location: Centre for Nursing Studies, 100 Forest Rd, Room 1017, St. John's NL A1A 1E5
Mailing: PO Box 78, North West River NL A0P 1M0
709 777-8140
E: pherbert@mun.ca
W: www.ucs.mun.ca/~pherbert/
Year Founded: 2001
Languages: English; French

◈*Association of Ontario Midwives*
301-365 Bloor St E, Toronto ON M4W 3L4
416 425-9974; Fax: 416 425-6905
Toll-free: 866 418-3773
E: admin@aom.on.ca
W: www.aom.on.ca
Executive:
Pres: Katrina Kilroy
Exec Dir: Kelly Stadelbauer
Year Founded: 1984
Criteria: *Registered midwives (voting members), student midwives (non-voting members), prior-learning and experience assessment candidates (non-voting members).*
No of Paid Staff: 13
Speakers Available
Library: Y *(Open to the public)*
Languages: English
Membership: 350

Association des radiologistes du Québec
Location: 3000-2 Complexe Desjardins, Montréal QC H5B 1G8
Mailing: CP 216 Succ Pl-Desjardins
514 350-5129; Fax: 514 350-5179
E: bureau@arq.qc.ca
W: www.arq.qc.ca
Executive:
Prés: Frédéric Desjardins
Adj admin: Lisette Pipon

Association d'Orthopédie du Québec
Location: 2 Complexe Desjardins, Montréal QC H5B 1G8
Mailing: CP 216 succ Pl-Desjardins
514 844-0803; Fax: 514 844-6786
E: aoq@fmsq.org
W: www.orthoquebec.ca
Executive:
Prés: Dr Louis Bellemare
Dir: Louise Leclaire
Languages: French

Association of Medical Microbiology and Infectious Disease Canada
192 Bank St, Ottawa ON K2P 1W8
613 260-3233; Fax: 613 260-3235
Toll-free: 866 467-1215 (Members Only)
E: info@ammi.ca
W: www.ammi.ca
Executive:
Exec Dir: Richard McCoy
Year Founded: 1977
Criteria: *Open to any ID & MED Micro Specialist holding a M.D. or Ph.D.*
Budget: $300,000
No of Paid Staff: 4
Speakers Available
Languages: English; French
Membership: 540

Association of Teaching Clinical Physicians of Montreal
Hôpital Sainte-Justine
4565 ch Queen-Mary, Montréal QC H3W 1W5
514 340-3515
Executive:
Prés: Dr Jean-Luc Senécal
Sec-trés: Dr Marie-Jeanne Kergoat
Year Founded: 1968
Criteria: *Professors of the Faculty of Medicine, University of Montreal.*
Speakers Available
Languages: French
Membership: 173

Athletic Therapists Association of British Columbia
Interuban Campus PISE306E,Camosun College
4371 Interurban Rd, Victoria BC V9E 2C5
250 508-6504
W: www.athletictherapybc.ca
Executive:
Pres/Registrar: Kelly Uniewski
Treas: Ashley Cornish

HEALTHCARE ASSOCIATIONS

British Columbia Podiatric Medical Association
220-445 Mountain Highway, North Vancouver BC V7J 2L1
604 985-3338; Fax: 604 682-2766
E: info@bcpodiatrists.ca
W: www.bcpodiatrists.ca
Executive:
Exec Dir: Susan Roberts
Year Founded: 1923
Criteria: *Open to any person with a DPM degree, and who has successfully completed the licensing examination.*
Budget: $125,000
No of Paid Staff: 1
Speakers Available
Languages: English
Membership: 89 *(Lists available to the public)*

Canadian Anesthesiologists' Society
208-1 Eglinton Ave E, Toronto ON M4P 3A1
416 480-0602; Fax: 416 480-0320
E: anesthesia@cas.ca
W: www.cas.ca
Year Founded: 1943
Criteria: *Open to any specialist anesthesiologist residing in Canada.*
Budget: $2,000,000
No of Paid Staff: 11
Speakers Available
Languages: English; French
Membership: 2,200
Membership Fee: $360/yr

Canadian Association of Emergency Physicians
104-1785 Alta Vista Dr, Ottawa ON K1G 3Y6
613 523-3343; Fax: 613 523-0190
Toll-free: 800 463-1158
E: admin@caep.ca
W: www.caep.ca
Executive:
Pres: Dr Bruce McLeod
Exec Dir: Vera Klein
Year Founded: 1978
Criteria: *Physicians*
No of Paid Staff: 8
Languages: English; French
Membership: 2,000
Membership Fee: $325

Canadian Association of Homeopathic Physicians
56-9703 41 Ave NW, Edmonton AB T6E 6M9
780 438-4465; Fax: 780 499-4203
Executive:
Exec Dir: Dr Sandhu Surinder
Languages: English

Canadian Association of Internes and Residents
412-151 Slater St, Ottawa ON K1P 5H3
613 234-6448; Fax: 613 234-5292
E: cair@cair.ca
W: www.cair.ca/
Executive:
Exec Dir: Cheryl Pellerin
Year Founded: 1973
No of Paid Staff: 5
Languages: English; French
Membership: 7,500

Canadian Association of Neuropathologists
Dept of Pathology,The Ottawa Hospital Civic Campus
Mack 738-5788 University Ave, Halifax NS B3H 1V8
902 473-3156; Fax: 902 473-1049
W: canp.medical.org
Executive:
Pres: Dr David Munoz
Sec-Treas: Dr Rob Macaulay
Year Founded: 1960
Criteria: *Medicine or Veterinary medicine, actively engaged in practice of neuropathology.*
Languages: English

Canadian Association of Optometrists
234 Argyle Ave, Ottawa ON K2P 1B9
613 235-7924; Fax: 613 235-2025
Toll-free: 888 263-4676
E: info@opto.ca
W: www.opto.ca
Executive:
Mgr Spec Prog/OA Course: Terry Theiss
Exec Dir: Glenn Campbell
Natl Dir /OA Course: Lise Loyer
Dir-Vision Care Plan: Doug Dean
Dir-Commun: Leslie Laskarin
Fin Off: Yuli Guo
Multimedia Dev: Tony Gibbs
Year Founded: 1941
No of Paid Staff: 7
Library: Y
Languages: English; French
Membership: 3,400

◈Alberta:
100-8407 Argyll Rd NW, Edmonton AB T6C 4B2
780 451-6824; Fax: 780 452-9918
Toll-free: 800 272-8843
E: alberta.association@optometrists.ab.ca
W: www.optometrists.ab.ca
Executive:
Exec Dir: Brian Wik
No of Paid Staff: 7
Languages: English
Membership: 520 *(Lists available to the public)*

◈British Columbia:
610-2525 Willow St, Vancouver BC V5Z 3N8
604 737-9907; Fax: 604 737-9967
Toll-free: 888 393-2226 BC only
E: info@optometrists.bc.ca
W: www.optometrists.bc.ca
Executive:
Pres: Dr Antoinette Dumala
CEO: Cheryl Williams
Year Founded: 1920
Criteria: *Licensed optometrist*
No of Paid Staff: 6
Speakers Available
Languages: English
Membership: 490 *(Lists available to the public)*

◈Manitoba:
200B-392 Academy Rd, Winnipeg MB R3N 0B8
204 943-9811; Fax: 204 943-1208
E: mao@optometrists.mb.ca
W: www.optometrists.mb.ca
Executive:
Exec Dir: Laureen Goodridge
Year Founded: 1909
Languages: English

◈New Brunswick:
1-490 Gibson St, Fredericton NB E3A 4E9
506 458-8759; Fax: 506 450-1271
E: nbao@nbnet.nb.ca
W: www.nbao.ca
Executive:
Pres: Dr Mark Inman
No of Paid Staff: 2
Speakers Available
Languages: English; French
Membership: 117

◈Newfoundland & Labrador
Mailing: PO Box 8042, St. John's NL A1B 3M7
709 739-8284; Fax: 709 739-8378
E: nlao@nl.rogers.com
W: www.nao.opto.ca
Executive:
Pres: Dr Mark Smith
VP: Dr Amy Oldford
Exec Dir: Ed Breen

◈Nova Scotia:
Location: 700-6009 Quinpool Rd, Halifax NS B3K 5J7
Mailing: PO Box 9410 Rpo Csc, Halifax NS B3K 5S3
902 435-2845; Fax: 902 425-2441
E: nsao@accesswave.ca
W: www.nsoptometrists.ca
Executive:
Exec Dir: John Sutherland
Year Founded: 1920
Languages: English
Membership: 89 *(Lists available to the public)*
Membership Fee: $2,075

◈Ontario:
Plaza 3
300-2000 Argentia Rd, Mississauga ON L5N 1V9
905 826-3522; Fax: 905 826-0625
Toll-free: 800 540-3837
W: www.eyecareoao.com
Executive:
CEO: Lesya Balych-Cooper
Year Founded: 1909
Criteria: *Open to any licensed optometrist in Ontario.*
No of Paid Staff: 7
Languages: English
Membership: 960
Membership Fee: $2,293

◈Quebec:
740-1265 rue Berri, Montréal QC H2L 4X4
514 288-6272; Fax: 514 288-7071
E: aoq@aoqnet.qc.ca
W: www.aoqnet.qc.ca
Executive:
Prés: Dr Steven Carrier
Dir gén: Erik de Pokomandy
Dir fin: Colette Elliott
Year Founded: 1966
No of Paid Staff: 6
Speakers Available
Languages: French
Membership: 1,300
Membership Fee: $800

◈Saskatchewan:
108-2366 Avenue C N, Saskatoon SK S7L 5X5
306 652-2069; Fax: 306 652-2642
Toll-free: 877 660-3937 Saskatchewan only
E: saskop@sasktel.net
W: www.optometrists.sk.ca
Executive:
Registrar: Dr Leland Kolbenson
Exec Dir: Sheila Spence
Occupational Vision Care Program Coord: Darren Mirau
Year Founded: 1909
Criteria: *Open to any person licensed to practise optometry in Saskatchewan.*
No of Paid Staff: 3
Languages: English
Membership: 140
Membership Fee: $2,200

Canadian Association of Pathologists
310-4 Cataraqui St, Kingston ON K7K 1Z7
613 507-8528; Fax: 866 531-0626
Toll-free: 800 668-3740
W: www.cap-acp.org
Executive:
Pres: Dr Ikakovina Alexopoulou
VP: Dr Martin Trotter
Sec-Treas: Dr Brian Cummings
Office of the Secretariat: Heather Dow
Year Founded: 1949
Criteria: *Ordinary Members: those persons who have graduated in medicine and who are licensed to practise in a Canadian province and who are: a) certified by or hold fellowship in The Royal College of Physicians and Surgeons of Canada in some recognized branch of laboratory medicine, or b) in possession of credentials which in the opinion of the Council are the equivalent of the paragraph above, or c) in possession of special skills and knowledge, by virtue of a minimum of four years' training in a medical laboratory science not recognized by The Royal College of Physicians and Surgeons of Canada and whom the Council consider as possessing qualifications equivalent to paragraphs (a) and (b) above.*
Associate Members: may include those persons who are: a) graduates in medicine, certified by or holding fellowship in The Royal College of Physicians and Surgeons of Canada in specialties other than laboratory sciences but who have an interest in certain phases of pathology, or
b) graduates in sciences other than medicine, who are recognized as authorities in their science and whose membership would further the aims and objectives of the Association; or c) in possession of credentials which in the opinion of the Council are the equivalent of paragraph (a) above and who may not necessarily be resident in Canada.
Junior Members: may include those persons who are graduates in medicine and who have expressed an interest to pursue a career in pathology, and are registered in a training program in pathology approved either by the Royal College of Physicians and Surgeons of Canada or by the Council, members in this category shall have their Junior membership terminated within two years after certification or fellowhsip in the Royal College of Physicians and Surgeons in Canada is obtained but, upon application to the Association, may be transferred to Ordinary membership on payment of the fee for Ordinary members. A year's free membership is available to residents who apply for Junior status.
No of Paid Staff: 2
Languages: English
Membership: 900

Canadian Association of Pediatric Surgeons
Children's Hospital of Winnipeg
AE403-840 Sherbrook St, Winnipeg MB R3A 1S1
204 787-1246; Fax: 204 787-4618
W: www.caps.ca
Executive:
Sec-Treas - CAPS: Dr B J Hancock
Criteria: *Qualified Pediatric General Sugeon*
Languages: English

Canadian Association of Physical Medicine and Rehabilitation
1937 Portobello Rd, PO Box 17059,
Ottawa ON K4A 4W0
613 707-0483; Fax: 613 707-0480
E: info@capmr.ca
W: www.capmr.ca
Executive:
Pres: Dr Rodney A Li Pi Shan
Exec Dir: Roberta Sulpher
Year Founded: 1952
Languages: English
Membership: 300

Canadian Association of Radiation Oncology
6-20 Crown Steel Dr, Markham ON L3R 9X9
905 415-3917; Fax: 905 415-0071
Toll-free: 855 415-3917
E: andrea@secretariatcentral.com
W: www.caro-acro.ca
Executive:
Pres/Dir ON: Dr Andrea Bezjak
Pres Elect/Dir BC: Dr Ross Halperin
Dir-ON/Sec-Treas: Dr Jacqueline Spayne
Dir Prairies: Dr Naseer Ahmed
Dir E Prov: Dr Teri Stuckless
Dir QC: Dr David Roberge
Dir QC: Dr Eric Vigneault
Association Coord: Andrea Smith
Year Founded: 1987
Criteria: *Limited to persons interested in furthering the objects of the society and shall consist of anyone whose application for admission as a member has been approved by the directors of the society. Categories: regular, resident, fellow, honorary, retired, and associate.*
Languages: English
Membership: 600
Membership Fee: $50 Associate; $200 Regular

Canadian College of Medical Geneticists
774 Echo Dr, Ottawa ON K1S 5N8
613 730-6250; Fax: 613 730-1116
E: ccmg@rcpsc.edu
W: www.ccmg-ccgm.org
Executive:
Mgr: Jessica E Séguin
Year Founded: 1975
Budget: $300
Languages: English
Membership: 200

Canadian Hematology Society
199-435 St. Laurent Blvd, Ottawa ON K1K 2Z8
613 748-9613; Fax: 613 748-6392
W: www.canadianhematologysociety.org
Executive:
Pres: Dr Stephen Couban
Languages: English; French
Membership Fee: $50

Canadian Laboratory Suppliers Association
131-525 Highland Rd W, Kitchener ON N2M 5P4
519 650-8028; Fax: 519 653-8749
E: jhowes@clsassoc.com
W: www.clsassoc.com
Executive:
Admin: Judy Howes

Canadian Medical Association
1867 Alta Vista Dr, Ottawa ON K1G 5W8
613 731-9331; Fax: 613 731-7314
Toll-free: 888 855-2555
E: pubs@cma.ca
W: www.cma.ca
Executive:
Pres: Dr Anna Reid
Year Founded: 1867
Criteria: *Open to any holder of a Canadian medical degree from a recognized Canadian medical school.*
No of Paid Staff: 125
Library: Y
Languages: English; French
Membership: 60,000
Library:
T. Clarence Routley Library

◈Alberta Medical Association
12230 106 Ave NW, Edmonton AB T5N 3Z1
780 482-2626; Fax: 780 482-5445
Toll-free: 800 272-9680
E: amamail@albertadoctors.org
W: www.albertadoctors.org
Executive:
Exec Dir: Michael A Gormley
Coord Corp Aff: Carol Hale
Asst Exec Dir-Corp Affrs: A Victor Taylor
Year Founded: 1905
Criteria: *Being a qualified medical doctor.*
Budget: $12,000,000
No of Paid Staff: 146
Languages: English
Membership: 10,000
Membership Fee: $1,513

◈British Columbia Medical Association
115-1665 Broadway W, Vancouver BC V6J 5A4
604 736-5551; Fax: 604 638-2911
Toll-free: 800 665-2262 BC only
E: communications@bcma.bc.ca
W: www.bcma.org
Executive:
CEO: Allan Seckel
Mgr-Exec Office: Susan Martin
Asst Dir-Sys: Peter Denny
Year Founded: 1900
Languages: English
Membership: 6,000

◈Manitoba Medical Association
20 Desjardins Dr, Winnipeg MB R3X 0E8
204 985-5888; Fax: 204 985-5844
Toll-free: 888 322-4242 MB only
E: general@docsmb.org
W: www.docsmb.org
Executive:
CEO: Robert Cram
Year Founded: 1908
No of Paid Staff: 17
Languages: English
Membership: 3000+

◈New Brunswick Medical Society
176 York St, Fredericton NB E3B 3N7
506 458-8860; Fax: 506 458-9853
E: nbms@nb.aibn.com
W: www.nbms.nb.ca
Executive:
CEO: Anthony Knight
Languages: English

◈Newfoundland and Labrador Medical Association
164 MacDonald Dr, St. John's NL A1A 4B3
709 726-7424; Fax: 709 726-7525
Toll-free: 800 563-2003 Within Province
E: nlma@nlma.nl.ca
W: www.nlma.nl.ca
Executive:
Dir-Ops/Membership: J David Mitchel
Exec Dir: Robert Ritter
Asst to Exec Dir: Donna Osmond
Year Founded: 1924
Criteria: *Open to any licensed physician.*
Budget: $1,500,000
No of Paid Staff: 11
Speakers Available
Languages: English
Membership: 1,600
Membership Fee: $1,094

◈Northwest Territories Medical Association
Mailing: PO Box 1732 Stn Main, Yellowknife NT X1A 2P3
867 920-4575; Fax: 867 920-4578
E: nwtmedassoc@ssimicro.com
W: www.nwtma.ca

Executive:
Exec Dir: Suzanne Burns Younge
Languages: English

◈Medical Society of Nova Scotia
25 Spectacle Lake Dr, Dartmouth NS B3B 1X7
902 468-1866; Fax: 902 468-6578
E: info@doctorsns.com
W: www.doctorsns.com
No of Paid Staff: 20
Speakers Available
Library: Y
Languages: English
Membership: 3,300

◈Ontario Medical Association
900-150 Bloor St W, Toronto ON M5S 3C1
416 599-2580; Fax: 416 340-2944
Toll-free: 800 268-7215
E: info@oma.org
W: www.oma.org
Executive:
Pres: Dr Stewart Kennedy
CEO: Ron Sapsford
Editor: Jeff Henry
Dir-Sys Tech: Patrick Song
Dir-Hum Res: Sandra Zidaric
Year Founded: 1881
Criteria: *For physicians only.*
No of Paid Staff: 6
Languages: English
Membership: 24,000 physicians

◈Medical Society of Prince Edward Island
2 Myrtle St, Stratford PE C1B 2W2
902 368-7303; Fax: 902 566-3934
Toll-free: 888 368-7303
W: www.mspei.pe.ca
Executive:
Exec Dir: Sandy Irwin
Dir-Commun: Kathy Maher
Accounting Tech: Marlene Guignion
Year Founded: 1855
Library: Y *(Open to the public)*
Languages: English
Membership: 275

◈Quebec Medical Association
3200-380 rue Saint-Antoine O, Montréal QC H2Y 3X7
514 866-0660; Fax: 514 866-0670
Toll-free: 800 363-3932
E: admin@amq.ca
W: www.amq.ca
Executive:
Dir admin: Monique Trottier
Year Founded: 1921
Criteria: *Membership open to physicians and medical students.*
No of Paid Staff: 10
Languages: English; French
Membership: 7,500

◈Saskatchewan Medical Association
402-321A 21st St E, Saskatoon SK S7K 0C1
306 244-2196; Fax: 306 653-1631
E: sma@sma.sk.ca
W: www.sma.sk.ca
Executive:
CEO: Dr Vino Padaychee
Dir-Commun: Scott Donaldson
No of Paid Staff: 15
Speakers Available
Library: Y
Languages: English
Membership: 1,800

Canadian Medical Protective Association
Location: 875 Carling Ave, Ottawa ON K1S 5P1
Mailing: PO Box 8225 Stn T CSC, Ottawa ON K1G 3H7
613 725-2000; Fax: 877 763-1300
Toll-free: 800 267-6522
E: mediainquiries@cmpa.org
W: www.cmpa-acpm.ca
Year Founded: 1901
Criteria: *Must be a physician.*
No of Paid Staff: 200
Languages: English; French
Membership: 62,000

Canadian Ophthalmological Society
610-1525 Carling Ave, Ottawa ON K1Z 8R9
613 729-6779; Fax: 613 729-7209
E: cos@eyesite.ca
W: www.eyesite.ca
Executive:
Exec Dir/CEO: Jennifer Brunet-Colvey
Mgr CPD: Inika Anderson
Man Editor CJO: Susan Gemmell
Coord CPD: Michael Peterson
Year Founded: 1937
Criteria: *Ophthalmological*
No of Paid Staff: 5
Languages: English
Membership: 1,013
Membership Fee: $500

Canadian Orthopaedic Association
450-4150 rue Sainte-Catherine O, Westmount QC H3Z 2Y5
514 874-9003; Fax: 514 874-0464
E: info@coa-aco.org
W: www.coa-aco.org
Executive:
Chef dir: Douglas C Thomson
Dir comm/d'adhes: Cynthia Vezina
Year Founded: 1945
Criteria: *Active membership: completed training in an approved program in orthopaedic surgery, obtained certification by the Royal College of Physicians and Surgeons of Canada or equivalent qualification as accepted by the association, obtained the endorsement of two active members as to the candidate's moral and ethical standing. Senior membership: at age 65, active members may become senior members. Under exceptional circumstances such as illness or retirement from practice, the board of directors may grant Senior membership to a member even though he/she may not be over 65 years of age. Associate membership: may be accorded to residents in an approved Canadian orthopaedic training program and to graduate fellows in orthopaedic training. Overseas membership: non-resident, practising in Canada or the U.S. Must hold an FRCSC in orthopaedics or equivalent, or must have received part or all of training in Canada and shown a continued interest in the affairs of the association and must be qualified orthopaedic consultant in his/her country and have fulfilled appropriate training and education standards. Must have letters of recommendation from two active members. Honourary membership: may be conferred upon members of the medical profession of acknowledged pre-eminence, and upon distinguished persons outside the medical profession, whom the association may wish to honour. Affiliate membership: open to fully trained orthopaedic surgeons who practise full-time orthopaedic surgery in Canada, but who do not possess an FRCSC (Orthopaedics), a Québec certification (Orthopaedics) or who are not diplomats of the American Board of Orthopaedic Surgery. Also open to basic scientists involved in orthopaedic research.*
Budget: $850,000
No of Paid Staff: 3
Speakers Available
Languages: English; French
Membership: 1,500
Membership Fee: $485

Canadian Psychiatric Association/Association des psychiatres du Canada
701-141 Laurier Ave W, Ottawa ON K1P 5J3
613 234-2815 230; Fax: 613 234-9857
E: cpa@cpa-apc.org
W: www.cpa-apc.org
Executive:
Admin Clerk/Pub: Christine Jenson
Man Editor Cdn Psychiatry Aujourd'hui: Jadranka Bacic
Exec Dir: Alex Saunders
Dir-Scientific Publications: Virginia Denis
Mgr-Pub Affairs: Kelly Masotti
Sr Commun Spec: Hélène Côté
Year Founded: 1951
No of Paid Staff: 24
Speakers Available
Languages: English; French
Membership: 3,200

Canadian Resident Matching Service
300-171 Nepean St, Ottawa ON K2P 0B4
613 237-0075; Fax: 613 563-2860
E: help@carms.ca
W: www.carms.ca
Executive:
Exec Dir: Sandra Banner
Year Founded: 1996
Criteria: *Open to any association concerned with medical education.*
No of Paid Staff: 7
Languages: English
Membership: 12 member organizations

Canadian Society for Aesthetic Plastic Surgery
2334 Heska Rd, Pickering ON L1V 2P9
905 831-7750; Fax: 905 831-7248
Toll-free: 800 263-4429
E: csacps@sympatico.ca
W: www.csaps.ca
Executive:
Pres/Pub Rel: Dr Brian Peterson
Pres: Wayne Carman
Past Pres: Dr Yvan Larocque
Exec Sec: Pat Hewitt
Year Founded: 1972
Criteria: *FRCSC or FACS Plastic Surgeon*
Languages: English
Membership: 165
Membership Fee: $500

Canadian Society of Internal Medicine
774 Echo Dr, Ottawa ON K1S 5N8
613 730-6244; Fax: 613 730-1116
E: csim@royalcollege.ca
W: www.csimonline.com
Executive:
Pres: Dr Finlay McAlister
Year Founded: 1984
Speakers Available
Languages: English
Membership: 700

Canadian Society Of Microbiologists
CSM Secretariat
305-1750 Courtwood Cres, Ottawa ON K2C 2B5
613 225-8889; Fax: 613 225-9621
E: info@csm-scm.org
W: www.csm-scm.org

Canadian Society of Nephrology
Mailing: CP 25255 Csp Riv-d-Prairies, Montréal QC H1E 7P9
514 643-4985
W: csnscn.ca
Executive:
Prés: Dr John Gill
Prés Elect: Dr Braden Manns
Sec-trés: Dr Sanjay Pandeya
Languages: English

Canadian Society of Otolaryngology - Head and Neck Surgery
221 Millford Cres, Elora ON N0B 1S0
519 846-0630; Fax: 519 846-9529
Toll-free: 800 655-9533
E: cso.hns@sympatico.ca
W: www.entcanada.org
Executive:
Pres: Dr Karen Kost
Sec/2nd VP Elect: Dr Peter Spafford
2nd VP: Dr Martin Corsten
1st VP: Dr Patrick Gullane
Exec Dir: Donna Humphrey
Treas: Dr Sam Daniel
Year Founded: 1947
Criteria: *Otolaryngologists or otolaryngologists-in-training.*
No of Paid Staff: 2
Languages: English; French
Membership: 700
Membership Fee: $335/yr

Canadian Society of Plastic Surgeons
4-1469 boul Saint-Joseph E, Montréal QC H2J 1M6
514 843-5415; Fax: 514 843-7005
E: csps_sccp@bellnet.ca
W: www.plasticsurgery.ca
Year Founded: 1947
Criteria: *Royal College certified plastic surgeons.*
No of Paid Staff: 1
Languages: English
Membership: 400 *(Lists available to the public)*
Membership Fee: $450

Collège des Médecins du Québec
2170 boul René-Lévesque O, Montréal QC H3H 2T8
514 933-4441; Fax: 514 933-1737
Toll-free: 888 633-3246
E: info@cmq.org
W: www.cmq.org
Executive:
PDG: Charles Bernard
Sec: Dr Yves Robert
Tech en doc: Hélène Landry
Year Founded: 1847
Budget: $20,000,000
No of Paid Staff: 110
Speakers Available
Languages: French
Membership: 18,748

The College of Family Physicians of Canada
2630 Skymark Ave, Mississauga ON L4W 5A4
905 629-0900
Toll-free: 800 387-6197
Toll-free Fax: 888 843-2372
E: info@cfpc.ca
W: www.cfpc.ca
Executive:
Exec Dir/CEO: Dr Francine Lemire
Dir-Commun/Publications/Pub: David Dehaas
Year Founded: 1954
Languages: French

◈Alberta:
Centre 170
370-10403 172 St NW, Edmonton AB T5S 1K9
780 488-2395; Fax: 780 488-2396
Toll-free: 800 361-0607
E: info@acfp.ca
W: www.acfp.ca
Executive:
Exec Dir: Peggy Maher
Languages: English

◈British Columbia:
350-1665 Broadway W, Vancouver BC V6J 1X1
604 736-1877; Fax: 604 736-4675
E: office@bccfp.bc.ca
W: www.bccfp.bc.ca
Executive:
Exec Dir: Dr Jim Thorsteinson
Project Dev/Membership Mgr: Ian Tang
Year Founded: 1987
Languages: English
Membership: 2,268

◈Manitoba:
240-1695 Henderson Hwy, Winnipeg MB R2G 1P1
204 668-3667; Fax: 204 668-3663
W: www.mcfp.mb.ca
Year Founded: 1954
Languages: English
Membership: 623

◈New Brunswick:
614 Dysart St, Dieppe NB E1A 4T9
506 852-1086; Fax: 506 855-7134
E: nbcfp@nb.sympatico.ca
W: www.cfpc.ca/local/nb/index.html
Executive:
Admin: Joanne Gallant
Year Founded: 1954
No of Paid Staff: 1
Languages: English; French
Membership: 501

◈Newfoundland & Labrador:
2422-300 Prince Philip Dr, St. John's NL A1B 3V6
709 782-4343; Fax: 709 782-4363
E: cfpcdebbie@hotmail.com
W: nl.cfpc.ca
Executive:
Pres: Dr Charlene Fitzgerald
Admin: Debbie Rideout
Languages: English

◈Nova Scotia:
Mill Cove Plaza
207-967 Bedford Hwy, Bedford NS B4A 1A9
902 499-0303; Fax: 902 457-2584
E: admin@nsfamdocs.com
W: www.cfpc.ca/nshome.htm
Executive:
Exec Dir: Cathie W Carroll
Year Founded: 1957
No of Paid Staff: 1
Languages: English
Membership: 650 *(Lists available to the public)*

◈Quebec:
202-3210 av Jacques-Bureau, Laval QC H7P 0A9
450 973-2228; Fax: 450 973-4329
Toll-free: 800 481-5962
E: cqmf@bellnet.ca
W: www.cqmf.qc.ca
Executive:
Prés: Dr Dominique Deschênes
Dir gén: Nicole Cloutier
Year Founded: 1954
Languages: English

◈Saskatchewan:
Mailing: PO Box 7111 Stn Main, Saskatoon SK S7K 4J1
306 665-7714; Fax: 306 665-7714
Executive:
Pres: Dr M Markentin
Admin: Lois Hislop
Languages: English

College of Physicians & Surgeons of Alberta
Telus Plaza South
2700-10020 100 St NW, Edmonton AB T5J 0N3
780 423-4764; Fax: 780 420-0651
Toll-free: 800 561-3899
E: info@cpsa.ab.ca
W: www.cpsa.ab.ca
Executive:
Registrar: Dr Trevor Theman
Commun Mgr: Kelly Eby
Year Founded: 1906
Criteria: *Available on website.*
Languages: English
Membership: 8,000 + *(Lists available to the public)*
Membership Fee: $950

College of Physicians and Surgeons of British Columbia
400-858 Beatty St, Vancouver BC V6B 1C1
604 733-7758; Fax: 604 733-3503
Toll-free: 800 461-3008
W: www.cpsbc.ca
Executive:
Registrar: Dr H M Oetter
Dept Registrar Legal: E Peaston
Dep Registrar Registrar Dept: Dr A J Burak
Dep Registrar: Dr S Kelleher
Dep Registrar: Dr W R Vroom
Year Founded: 1886
Library: Y
Languages: English
Membership: 9,600

College of Physicians and Surgeons of New Brunswick
300-1 Hampton Rd, Rothesay NB E2E 5K8
506 849-5050; Fax: 506 849-5069
Toll-free: 800 667-4641
E: info@cpsnb.org
W: www.cpsnb.org
No of Paid Staff: 3
Speakers Available
Languages: English; French
Membership list available to the public

The College of Physicians and Surgeons of Ontario
80 College St, Toronto ON M5G 2E2
416 967-2600; Fax: 416 961-3330
Toll-free: 800 268-7096
E: feedback@cpso.on.ca
W: www.cpso.on.ca
Executive:
Assoc Dir-Policy/Commun: Jill Hefley
Year Founded: 1866
No of Paid Staff: 320
Languages: English
Membership: 36,000
Membership Fee: $880

Fédération des Médecins Omnipraticiens du Québec

2 Place Alexis Nihon
2000-3500 boul de Maisonneuve O, étage 20,
Wesmount QC H3Z 3C1
514 878-1911; Fax: 514 878-4455
E: info@fmoq.org
W: www.fmoq.org
Executive:
PDG: Dr Louis Godin
Tech docum: Marie Paule Saint-Gelais
Dir de la planification/régionalisation: Dr Serge Dulude
Dir-affaires prof: Dr Michel Desrosiers
Dir-formation prof: Dr Claude Guimond
Year Founded: 1963
Criteria: *Médecin omnipracticien exerçant au Québec*
No of Paid Staff: 43
Speakers Available
Library: Y
Languages: English; French
Membership: 7,800

Fédération des Médecins Résidents du Québec

510-630 rue Sherbrooke O, Montréal QC H3A 1E4
514 282-0256; Fax: 514 282-0471
Toll-free: 800 465-0215
E: fmrq@fmrq.qc.ca
W: www.fmrq.qc.ca
Executive:
Prés: Charles Dussault
Adj à la direction: Laurence Auchère
Languages: English; French

Fédération des Médecins Spécialistes du Québec

Location: 3000-2 Complexe Desjardins,
Montréal QC H5B 1G8
Mailing: CP 216 succ Pl-Desjardins
514 350-5000; Fax: 514 350-5175
Toll-free: 800 561-0703
E: communications@fmsq.org
W: www.fmsq.org
Executive:
Prés: Dr Gaétan Barette
Dir aff pub/commun: Nicole Pelletier
Year Founded: 1965
Speakers Available
Languages: French
Membership: 9,000

Federation of Medical Regulatory Authorities of Canada

103-2283 St. Laurent Blvd, Ottawa ON K1G 5A2
613 738-0372; Fax: 613 738-9169
E: info@fmrac.com
W: www.fmrac.ca
Executive:
Pres: Dr Heidi Oetter
Exec Dir/CEO: Fleur-Ange Lefebvre
Year Founded: 1968
No of Paid Staff: 3
Languages: English; French
Membership list available to the public

Federation of Medical Women of Canada

780 Echo Dr, Ottawa ON K1S 5R7
613 569-5881; Fax: 613 569-4432
Toll-free: 877 771-3777
Toll-free Fax: 877 772-5777
E: fmwcmain@fmwc.ca
W: www.fmwc.ca
Executive:
Pres: Dr Nahid Azad

Limestone Dermatology

163 Brock St, Kingston ON K7L 1S2
613 549-6660; Fax: 613 547-2079
No of Paid Staff: 4
Languages: English

Médecins Francophones du Canada

8355 boul Saint-Laurent, Montréal QC H2P 2Z6
514 388-2228; Fax: 514 388-5335
Toll-free: 800 387-2228
E: info@medecinsfrancophones.ca
W: www.medecinsfrancophones.ca
Executive:
Prés: Dr Conrad Pelletier
Dir gén: Céline Monette
Year Founded: 1902
Languages: French
Membership: 5,000 +

Médecins Sans Frontières

402-720 Spadina Ave, Toronto ON M5S 2T9
416 964-0619; Fax: 416 963-8707
Toll-free: 800 982-7903
E: msfcan@msf.ca
W: www.msf.ca
Executive:
Exec Dir: Steve Cornish
Dir-Hum Res: Wang Ya
Dir-Fundraising: Rebecca Davies
Year Founded: 1991
No of Paid Staff: 44
Speakers Available
Languages: English; French

◈ Montréal

220-1470 rue Peel, Montréal QC H3A 1T1
514 845-5621; Fax: 514 845-3707
Toll-free: 866 878-5621
E: msfqc@msf.ca
W: www.msf.ca
Executive:
Coord: Jetske Duintjer
Year Founded: 1991
Criteria: *former aid MSF workers and Canadian office volunteers with more thqan one year's experience*
No of Paid Staff: 50
Speakers Available
Languages: English; French

Medical Council of Canada

Location: Business Bldg, 100-2283 St. Laurent Blvd, Ottawa ON K1G 5A2
Mailing: PO Box 8234 Stn T CSC, Ottawa ON K1G 3H7
613 521-6012; Fax: 613 521-9509
E: mcc_admin@mcc.ca
W: www.mcc.ca
Executive:
Exec Dir: Dr Ian Bowmer
Year Founded: 1912
No of Paid Staff: 102
Languages: English
Membership: 45

NONA Child Development Centre

2802 34 St, Vernon BC V1T 5X1
250 549-1281; Fax: 250 549-3771
E: administration@nona-cdc.com
W: www.nona-cdc.com
Executive:
Pres: Janice Foster
Dir: Tania Miliken-Heape
Dir: Peggy Graham
Dir: Jacquie Hansen
Dir: Marlene Sokol
Dir: Claire Abbott
Treas: Allen Dubeski
Sec: Nancy Hause
Year Founded: 1975
No of Paid Staff: 40
Speakers Available
Library: Y *(Open to the public)*
Languages: English
Membership: 20
Membership Fee: $2 per year

Occupational and Environmental Medical Association of Canada

503-386 Broadway, Winnipeg MB R3C 3R6
888 223-3808; Fax: 877 947-9767
E: info@oemac.org
W: www.oemac.org
Executive:
Exec Dir: Jonathan Strauss
Coord-Prog/Serv: Nikki Laurin
Year Founded: 1985
Criteria: *Open to any physician interested in occupational and environmental medicine.*
No of Paid Staff: 5
Speakers Available
Languages: English; French
Membership: 300 Membership Fees
Membership Fee: $250 + GST

Ontario College of Family Physicians (OCFP)

340 Richmond St W, Toronto ON M5V 1X2
416 867-9646; Fax: 416 867-9990
E: ocfp@cfpc.ca
W: www.ocfp.on.ca
Executive:
Pres/Reg Dir Region 4: Dr Frank Martino
Pres Elect/Reg Dir Region 7: Dr Jonathan Kerr
CEO: Jan Kasperski
Reg Dir Region 1: Dr Sarah-Lynn Newbery
Reg Dir/Sec-Treas Region 2: Dr Cathy Faulds
Reg Dir Region 3: Dr Michael Lee
Reg Dir Region 4: Dr Sanjeev Goel
Reg Dir Region 4: Dr Mary Manno
Reg Dir Region 5: Dr David White
Reg Dir Region 5: Dr Art Kushner
Reg Dir Region 5: Dr David Tannenbaum
Reg Dir Region 6: Dr Jennifer Young
Reg Dir Region 6: Dr Rosanna Pellizzari
Reg Dir Region 6: Dr Anne DuVal
Reg Dir Region 7: Dr Mark Fraser
Reg Dir Region 7: Dr John Brewer
Year Founded: 1954
No of Paid Staff: 10
Speakers Available
Library: Y
Languages: English
Membership: 7,300

Ontario Home Respiratory Services Association (OHRSA)

600-55 University Ave, Toronto ON M5J 2H7
416 961-8001 100; Fax: 416 961-9935
E: info@ohrsa.ca
W: www.ohrsa.ca
Executive:
Pres: Mattieu Giard
VP: Michael Pohanka
Sec-Treas: Al Benton
Consul: Paul Pellegrini

Year Founded: 1985
No of Paid Staff: 1
Languages: English
Membership: 19

Ontario Orthopaedic Association (OOA)
700-2 Bloor St W, Toronto ON M4W 3R1
416 498-4145; Fax: 416 972-5071
E: info@ooa.ca
W: www.ooa.ca
Executive:
Tariff Chair: Dr Dana Fleming
Pres: Dr Duncan MacKinlay
Treas: Dr Peter Kim
Sec: Dr Peter Schuringa
Exec Coord: Dafna Strauss
Year Founded: 1978
No of Paid Staff: 1
Library: Y *(Open to the public)*
Languages: English

Ontario Podiatric Medical Association
900-45 Sheppard Ave E, Toronto ON M2N 5W9
416 927-9111; Fax: 416 927-9111
Toll-free: 866 424-6762
E: contact@opma.ca
W: www.opma.ca
Executive:
Pres: Dr Bruce Ramsden
VP: Dr Kevan Orvitz
VP: Dr Stephen Haber
Treas: Dr Peter Higenell
Sec: Dr Martin Brain
Year Founded: 1943
Library: Y
Languages: English
Membership: 58 *(Lists available to the public)*

Ontario Society of Chiropodists
6519B Mississauga Rd, Mississauga ON L5N 1A6
905 567-3094; Fax: 905 567-7191
Toll-free: 877 823-1508
E: info@ontariochiropodist.com
W: www.ontariochiropodist.com
Executive:
Pres: Sarah Robinson
Languages: English

Ontario Society of Psychotherapists
1-189 Queen St E, Toronto ON M5A 1S2
416 923-4050; Fax: 416 968-6818
E: mail@psychotherapyontario.org
W: www.psychotherapyontario.org
Executive:
Pres: Pat Rayman
Treas: Rui Tian
Year Founded: 1992

Ontario Thoracic Society - A Div of Ontario Lung Association
401-18 Wynford Dr, Toronto ON M3C 0K8
416 864-9911 254; Fax: 416 864-9916
Toll-free: 888 344-5864
E: ots@on.lung.ca
W: www.on.lung.ca
Executive:
OTS Admin: Jeanne Castellanos
Med Dir: Dr Hedy Ginzberg
Year Founded: 1961
Criteria: *Doctors, scientists, residents, agencies, corporations with interest in respiratory health and who have demonstrated or expressed an interest in the objectives of the OTS.*
No of Paid Staff: 2
Languages: English
Membership: 310
Membership Fee: $60/year

Ordre des Optométristes du Québec
700-1265 rue Berri, Montréal QC H2L 4X4
514 499-0524; Fax: 514 499-1051
E: info@ooq.org
W: www.ooq.org
Executive:
Prés: Lise-Anne Chassé
Avocat/Dir gén: Marco Laverdière
Trés: Léo Breton
Year Founded: 1906
Budget: $1,087,000
No of Paid Staff: 5
Languages: French
Membership: 1,265

Ordre des Psychologues du Québec
Centre Médical René-Laénnec
510-1100 av Beaumont, Mont-Royal QC H3P 3H5
514 738-1881; Fax: 514 738-8838
E: info@ordrepsy.qc.ca
W: www.ordrepsy.qc.ca
Executive:
Prés: Rose-Marie Charest
Adj: Huguette Prosper
No of Paid Staff: 25
Languages: French

Pedorthic Association of Canada
503-386 Broadway, Winnipeg MB R3C 3R6
Fax: 204 947-9767
Toll-free: 888 268-4404
Toll-free Fax: 877 947-9767
E: info@pedorthic.ca
W: www.pedorthic.ca
Executive:
Sls/Serv Mgr: Chantal Champagne
Exec Dir: Jonathan N Strauss
Coord-Prog/Serv: Kirsten Parker
Year Founded: 1985
No of Paid Staff: 5
Speakers Available
Languages: English; French
Membership: 300

The Prince Edward Island College of Family Physicians
PEI College of Family Physicians
14 Royalty Rd, Charlottetown PE C1E 1T8
902 894-2605; Fax: 902 894-3975
E: pei.cfp@pei.aibn.com
W: pei.cfpc.ca
Executive:
Pres: Dr André Cellier
Treas: Dr Barbara Flanagan
Languages: English

Professional Association of Internes and Residents of Newfoundland (PAIRN)
Location: Health Sciences Complex, 300 Prince Philip Dr, Student Affairs Office Room 2713, St. John's NL A1B 3V6
Mailing: PO Box 4200 Stn C, St. John's NL A1C 5S7
709 737-7118; Fax: 709 737-6968
E: pairn@mun.ca
W: www.pairn.ca
Executive:
Pres: Angela Bussey
VP: Robert Mercer
Treas: Christopher Smith
Sec: Kathryn Sparrow
Languages: English
Membership: 200

Professional Association of Resident Physicians of Alberta
340-11044 82 Ave NW, Edmonton AB T6G 0T2
780 432-1749; Fax: 780 432-1778
E: para-ab@shawbiz.ca
W: www.para-ab.ca
Executive:
Exec Dir: Sarah Thomas
Year Founded: 1975
Criteria: *Physician completing further training.*
No of Paid Staff: 2
Speakers Available
Languages: English
Membership: 814

Professional Association of Residents and Interns of Manitoba
GF132-820 Sherbrook Ave, Winnipeg MB R3A 1R9
204 787-3673; Fax: 204 787-2692
E: parim.office@gmail.com
W: www.parim.org
Executive:
Co-Pres: Dr Elizabeth Berg
Co-Pres: Dr Markus Ziesmann
Year Founded: 1975
No of Paid Staff: 1
Languages: English
Membership: 482

Professional Association of Residents in the Maritime Provinces
Halifax Professional Ctr
460-5991 Spring Garden Rd, Halifax NS B3H 1Y6
902 404-3595; Fax: 902 404-3599
Toll-free: 877 972-7467
W: www.parimp.ca
Executive:
Exec Dir: Sandi Carew Flemming
Commun/MPRI Coord: Evie Sabean Croucher
Benefits/Events Coord: Leanne Bryan
Year Founded: 1969
Criteria: *Resident physicians with Dalhousie University.*
No of Paid Staff: 4
Languages: English
Membership: 480

Professional Association of Residents of British Columbia
2010-401 Georgia St W, Vancouver BC V6B 5A1
604 876-7636; Fax: 604 876-7690
E: par@par-bc.org
W: www.par-bc.org
Executive:
Exec Dir: Pria Sandhu
Languages: English

Quality Management Program - Laboratory Services
1500-393 University Ave, Toronto ON M5G 1E6
416 323-9540; Fax: 416 323-9324
E: mail@qmpls.org
W: www.qmpls.org
Executive:
Man Dir: Dr Greg Flynn
Proj Coord: Gertrude Welsh

Respiratory Therapy Society of Ontario
440-2 County Court Blvd, Brampton ON L6W 4V1
647 729-2717; Fax: 647 729-2715
Toll-free: 855 297-3089
E: office@rtso.ca
W: www.rtso.ca
Executive:
Bus Mgr: Stephen Laramee

Year Founded: 1972
Criteria: *Open to any practising or student respiratory therapist or corporate supplier to the respiratory therapy field.*
Speakers Available
Library: Y (Open to the public)
Languages: English
Membership: 1,300

The Royal College of Physicians and Surgeons of Canada
774 Echo Dr, Ottawa ON K1S 5N8
613 730-8177; Fax: 613 730-8830
Toll-free: 800 668-3740
E: feedback@royalcollege.ca
W: www.royalcollege.ca
Executive:
Pres: Cecil Rorabeck
Year Founded: 1929
Criteria: *Medical specialists who are Fellows of The Royal College of Physicians and Surgeons of Canada.*
Budget: $24,455,000
No of Paid Staff: 221
Speakers Available
Library: Y
Languages: English; French
Membership: 42,000
Membership Fee: $495 (residents excluded)

The Society of Obstetricians and Gynaecologists of Canada
780 Echo Dr, Ottawa ON K1S 5R7
613 730-4192; Fax: 613 730-4314
Toll-free: 800 561-2416
E: helpdesk@sogc.com
W: www.sogc.org
Executive:
Pres: Dr Douglas Black
Treas: Ian R Lange
Commun/Public Ed: Natalie Wright
Year Founded: 1944
Criteria: *Member Ob/Gyn: a person who is licensed to practise medicine in a province or territory of Canada and has a Specialist Certificate in Obstetrics and Gynaecology acceptable to Council, or whose specialty training in obstetrics and gynaecology is recognized by the Royal College of Physicians and Surgeons of Canada or the Collège des médecins du Québec.*
Life Member: a member Ob/Gyn who has reached the age of 65 years and is no longer in active practice or has been a Member Ob/Gyn for at least 35 years.
Honorary Member: any member of the Society may propose to the Council a distinguished individual for Honorary Membership. Upon approval by Council, and by a majority of members voting at the Annual Business Meeting, the distinguished individual shall become an Honorary Member. Honorary Members shall not be required to pay fees. They may not vote at meetings or hold office.
International member: a person who is licensed to practise medicine outside Canada and has a Specialist Certificate in obstetrics and gynaecology acceptable to the Council and recognized by the Royal College of Physicians and Surgeons of Canada or its equivalent organization in another country.
Junior member: a person who is enrolled in a post-graduate training program in Ob/Gyn acceptable to Council and is nominated by the Chairperson or Residency Director of the training program in which the person is enrolled.
Family practice resident member: a person who is enrolled in a family medicine residency program and is nominated by the Chairperson or Residency Program Director of the training program in which the applicant is enrolled.
Student member: a person who is enrolled in a canadian medical or nursing and midwifery school and is nominated by the Chairperson or Program Director of the training program in which the applicant is enrolled.
Associate member: a person who belongs to one of the following medical areas: basic or applied sciences; medicine (any branch of medicine other than those previously specified); nursing; midwifery; health care; allied health care (corporate).
No of Paid Staff: 55
Speakers Available
Library: Y
Languages: English; French
Membership: 3,200
Membership Fee: $20-$375/year

Society of Rural Physicians of Canada
Location: 269 rue Main, Shawville QC J0X 2Y0
Mailing: CP 893
819 647-7054; Fax: 819 647-2485
Toll-free: 877 276-1949
W: www.srpc.ca
Executive:
Ancien prés: Dr John Wootton
Prés: Dr Braam De Klerk
Agent admin: Lee Teperman
Year Founded: 1992
Library: Y
Languages: English; French
Membership Fee: $306 Active Member; $50 Retired; Free : Students & Residents, Honourary Members; $500 Affiliate Members; $100 Associate Members (non MDs)

University of Saskatchewan - Anatomy, & Cell Biology Department
Anatomy & Cell Biology,University of Saskatchewan
107 Wiggins Rd, Saskatoon SK S7N 5E5
306 966-4075; Fax: 306 966-4298
W: www.usask.ca/anatomy
Year Founded: 1956
Library: Y
Languages: English
Membership: Emeritus - 45; Paid - 100

Vancouver Medical Association
115-1665 Broadway W, Vancouver BC V6J 5A4
604 736-5551
Executive:
Coord: Diane Wong
Criteria: *Open to all qualified practitioners licensed to practise in BC.*
Languages: English
Membership: 500
Membership Fee: $75

MEDICAL & HEALTH (5) —Public Health & Health Promotion

Cardiac Fitness Association
1010 Hopewell Creek Rd, RR 2, Breslau ON N0B 1M0
519 648-2252; Fax: 519 648-3686
W: www.cfaheart.com
Executive:
Med Dir: Dr John Schaman
Year Founded: 1980
Criteria: *Rehabilitation program for cardiac patients.*
Languages: English

MEDICAL & HEALTH (6) —Specific Condition

MENTAL HEALTH

Anxiety Disorders Association of Manitoba
100-4 Fort St, Winnipeg MB R3C 1C4
204 925-0600; Fax: 204 925-0609
Toll-free: 800 805-8885
E: adam@adam.mb.ca
W: www.adam.mb.ca
Year Founded: 1986
Criteria: *Anyone who has an anxiety disorder or is concerned for people who have.*
Budget: $350,000
No of Paid Staff: 12
Speakers Available
Library: Y (Open to the public)
Languages: English

Association Ami du Déficient Mental Inc.
4960 7e Av, Montréal QC H1Y 2M9
514 527-7671; Fax: 514 527-7811
E: ldjadmi@hotmail.com
Executive:
Dir gén: Julie Archambault
Languages: French

Association des Groupes d'Intervention Défense de Droit Santé Mentale du Québec
210-4837 rue Boyer, Montréal QC H2J 3E6
514 523-3443; Fax: 514 523-0797
Toll-free: 866 523-3443
E: info@agidd.org
W: www.agidd.org
Executive:
Prés: Andrée Morneau
Dir gén: Doris Provencher

Association des Médecins Psychiatres du Québec
Tour est
2 Complexe Desjardins, étage 30, Montréal QC H5B 1G8
514 350-5128; Fax: 514 350-5198
E: ampq@fmsq.org
W: www.ampq.org
Executive:
Admin: Martine Dériger
Languages: French

Association of Psychologists of Nova Scotia
435-5991 Spring Garden Road, Halifax NS B3H 1Y6
902 422-9183; Fax: 902 462-9801
E: apns@apns.ca
W: www.apns.ca
Executive:
Exec Dir: Susan Marsh
Year Founded: 1965
No of Paid Staff: 1
Speakers Available
Languages: English
Membership: 360
Membership Fee: $150/yr

B.C. Association of Clinical Counsellors
14-2544 Dunlevy St, Victoria BC V8R 5Z2
250 595-4448; Fax: 250 595-2926
Toll-free: 800 909-6303 Cda
E: hoffice@bc-counsellors.org
W: www.bc-counsellors.org
Executive:
Exec Dir: Dr James A Browne
Year Founded: 1988

Criteria: *Master's Degree, Supervisory Experience, References, Criminal Record Check*
Budget: $1,000,000
No of Paid Staff: 8
Speakers Available
Library: Y
Languages: English
Membership: 2,400 *(Lists available to the public)*
Membership Fee: $435

Calgary Association of Self-Help

1019 7 Ave SW, Calgary AB T2P 1A8
403 266-8711; Fax: 403 266-2478
E: info@calgaryselfhelp.com
W: www.calgaryselfhelp.com
Executive:
CEO: Marion McGrath
Year Founded: 1973
Criteria: *Open to individuals interested in the Association's mandate.*
Budget: $2,081,500
No of Paid Staff: 24
Languages: English
Membership: 100
Membership Fee: $2

Canadian Association for Music Therapy

Mailing: 320-110 Cumberland St, Toronto ON M5R 3V5
416 944-0421; Fax: 416 944-0431
Toll-free Fax: 800 996-2268
E: camt@musictherapy.ca
W: www.musictherapy.ca
Executive:
Pres: Amy Clements-Cortes
Criteria: *The Canadian Association for Music Therapy (CAMT) is a federally incorporated, self-regulated non-profit professional association dedicated to fostering the practice of music therapy in clinical, educational, and community settings throughout Canada.*
CAMT serves as a forum for its members providing advice, guidance, information, and exchanges of professional experience concerning music therapy.
CAMT represents the interests of music therapists in matters related to standards of professional practice, salary scales, and government legislation.
No of Paid Staff: 1
Languages: English; French
Membership: 600
Membership Fee: $40 - Student; $75 - Associate; $150 - AV-1; $135 - AV-2; $40 - AV-R/1; $55 - Graduate Student; $300 - Corporate
Library:
CAMT Archives *(Open to the public)*

Canadian Counselling And Psychotherapy Association

114-223 Colonnade Rd, Nepean ON K2E 7K3
613 237-1099; Fax: 613 237-9786
Toll-free: 877 765-5565
E: info@ccpa-accp.ca
W: www.ccpa-accp.ca
Executive:
CEO: Barbara MacCallum
Office Mgr: Nicole Maurice
Year Founded: 1965
Criteria: *Full Category A: Individuals with a master's degree in counselling or related field from an institution recognized by the Association of Universities and Colleges of Canada (AUCC) or equivalent. Full Category B: Individuals with a university degree, college diploma in counselling or related field, or equivalent experience and training. Associate: Agencies or organizations not necessarily actively involved in counselling or related field but having an interest in the well being, role and function of CCA. Student: Individuals presently enrolled in a master's degree program in counselling or a related field at an institution recognized by the AUCC. Retired: Individuals who are members of CCA and are retired from the counselling profession.*
Budget: $500,000
No of Paid Staff: 4
Speakers Available
Languages: English; French
Membership: 3,100
Membership Fee: Full member - $120; Student/Retiree - $60; Assoc member - $100

Canadian Mental Health Association (National)

Phenix Professional Building
303-595 Montreal Rd, Ottawa ON K1K 4L2
613 745-7750; Fax: 613 745-5522
W: www.cmha.ca
Executive:
Chair: David Copus
CEO: Peter Coleridge
Year Founded: 1918
Budget: $750,000
Languages: English; French
Membership: 10,000
Membership Fee: $5-$20

◈ Alberta Division:

Capital Place
320-9707 110 St NW, Edmonton AB T5K 2L9
780 482-6576; Fax: 780 482-6348
E: alberta@cmha.ab.ca
W: www.cmha.ab.ca
Executive:
Mgr-Fin/Ops: Eveline Royer
Exec Dir: Tom Shand
Year Founded: 1955
Criteria: *Open to anyone interested in mental health issues.*
No of Paid Staff: 3
Library: Y *(Open to the public)*
Languages: English
Membership: 550 *(Lists available to the public)*
Membership Fee: Standard - $20; $50 Corporate; Special - $2.50; Basic - $5

◇ Alberta Central Region:

5017 50 Ave, Red Deer AB T4N 4B2
403 342-2266; Fax: 403 342-5684
E: education@reddeer.cmha.ab.ca
W: www.reddeer.cmha.ab.ca
Executive:
Exec Dir: Marion McGuigon
Office Mgr: Sherry Paterson
Speakers Available
Languages: English

◇ Alberta South Central Region:

Kahanoff Centre
400-105 12 Ave SE, Calgary AB T2G 1A1
403 297-1700; Fax: 403 270-3066
E: info@cmha.calgary.ab.ca
W: www.cmha.calgary.ab.ca
Executive:
Pres: Barbara Tate
Exec Dir: Judy Martin
IT Mgr: Hanif Hasham
Year Founded: 1955
No of Paid Staff: 75
Languages: English
Membership: 100

◇ East Central Region:

Location: 4870 51 St, Camrose AB T4V 1S1
Mailing: 4711 51 Ave, Camrose AB T4V 0V3
780 672-2570; Fax: 780 672-2574
E: cmhaecr@cable-lynx.net
W: www.camrose.cmha.ab.ca
Executive:
Exec Dir: Colleen Vennard
Emp Serv Prog Coord: Rhiannon Wegenast
Office Asst: Teri Sikstrom
Year Founded: 1918
Criteria: *People with mental illness that require support and assistance to live in the community and to prevent social isolation. Adults and seniors experiencing severe or persistent mental illness.*
No of Paid Staff: 20
Speakers Available
Languages: English
Membership: 47

◇ Edmonton Region:

Fifth Street Place
300-10010 105 St NW, Edmonton AB T5J 1C4
780 414-6300; Fax: 780 482-7498
E: main@cmha-edmonton.ab.ca
W: www.cmha-edmonton.ab.ca
Executive:
Exec Dir: Ione Challborn
Fin Admin: Barbara Baxter
Prog Mgr: Lyn Smedstad
Year Founded: 1986
Speakers Available
Languages: English
Membership list available to the public
Membership Fee: Corporate - $50; $2 Special; Basic - $5; Standard - $20

◇ North West Region:

10116 102 Ave, Grande Prairie AB T8V 1A1
780 814-5678; Fax: 780 513-4352
E: gpcmha@telus.net
W: www.grandeprairie.cmha.ca
Executive:
Exec Dir: Deborah Gregson
Exec Asst: Sheila Bird
Year Founded: 1985
No of Paid Staff: 10
Languages: English

◇ Pincher Creek:

Location: 696 Kettle St, Pincher Creek AB T0K 1W0
Mailing: PO Box 1052
403 627-2726; Fax: 403 627-1159
Executive:
Coord: Wayne Camber
Year Founded: 1984
No of Paid Staff: 1
Library: Y *(Open to the public)*
Languages: English

◇ South Region:

426 6 St S, Lethbridge AB T1J 2C9
403 329-4775; Fax: 403 320-7432
W: www.lethbridge.cmha.ab.ca

◇ South East Region:

204-1865 Dunmore Rd SE, Medicine Hat AB T1A 1Z8
403 504-1811; Fax: 403 504-2542
E: aser@cmha.ab.ca
W: www.ser.cmha.ab.ca
Executive:
Pres: Glen Allan
VP: Carol Drew
Exec Dir: Sharon Hayward
Treas: Derek Hirsch
Suicide Prevent Prog Coord: Micheline Payne
No of Paid Staff: 25
Speakers Available
Library: Y *(Open to the public)*
Languages: English
Membership Fee: $5
Library:
Resource Lending Library

◇ Wood Buffalo Region:

302-10011 Franklin Ave, Fort McMurray AB T9H 2K7
780 743-1053; Fax: 780 743-0959

E: admin@woodbuffalo.cmha.ab.ca
W: www.woodbuffalo.cmha.ca
Executive:
Exec Dir: Karen McMillan
No of Paid Staff: 4
Speakers Available
Library: Y *(Open to the public)*
Languages: English

◈ **British Columbia:**
1200-1111 Melville St, Vancouver BC V6E 3V6
604 688-3234; Fax: 604 688-3236
Toll-free: 800 555-8222
E: info@cmha.bc.ca
W: www.cmha.bc.ca
Executive:
Pres: Bill Wright
CEO: Beverley Gutray
Year Founded: 1953
Criteria: *Open to the general public.*
No of Paid Staff: 15
Speakers Available
Languages: English
Membership: 1,000
Membership Fee: $5 people on limited income; $20/year

◇ **100 Mile House:**
Location: 555B South Cedar Ave, 100 Mile House BC V0K 2E0
Mailing: PO Box 876
250 395-4883; Fax: 250 395-1183
E: southcariboo@cmha.bc.ca
Executive:
Exec Dir: Maggie Patterson-Dickey
Year Founded: 1993
Library: Y *(Open to the public)*
Languages: English

◇ **Cowichan Valley:**
371 Festubert St, Duncan BC V9L 3T1
250 746-5521; Fax: 250 748-2606
E: cmha-mi@shaw.ca
W: www.cowichanvalley.cmha.bc.ca
Executive:
Exec Dir: Anne Hodge
Admv Asst: Teri Vetter
Year Founded: 1992
Criteria: *Membership open to those who are interested in joining.*
Budget: $400,000
No of Paid Staff: 13
Library: Y
Languages: English
Membership: 65
Membership Fee: $20
Library:
Community Support, Education and Resources *(Open to the public)*

◇ **Delta Branch:**
4871 Delta St, Delta BC V4K 2T9
604 943-1878
E: cmha.delta@dccnet.com
W: www.delta.cmha.bc.ca
Executive:
Exec Dir: Judy Gray
Year Founded: 1996
Budget: $150,000
No of Paid Staff: 1
Speakers Available
Library: Y *(Open to the public)*
Languages: English
Membership: 60
Membership Fee: $20/year
Library:
CMHA Delta Resource Centre *(Open to the public)*

◇ **East Kootenay:**
39 13th Ave S, Cranbrook BC V1C 2V4
250 426-5222; Fax: 250 426-2134
E: jivan@cmhakootenays.org
W: www.kootenays.cmha.bc.ca
Executive:
Exec Dir: Janice Bradshaw
Housing Admin: Dana Hill
Dir-Women's/Childcare/Youth/Volunteer Serv: Jackie Donachie
Year Founded: 1994
Budget: $3,000,000
No of Paid Staff: 90
Speakers Available
Languages: English
Membership: 354 *(Lists available to the public)*

◇ **Kamloops:**
857 Seymour St, Kamloops BC V2C 2H6
250 374-0440; Fax: 250 374-8718
E: kamloops@cmha.bc.ca
W: www.kamloops.cmha.bc.ca
Executive:
Dir-Ops: Kimberly Wall
Exec Dir: Joan Mix
Languages: English

◇ **Kelowna:**
504 Sutherland Ave, Kelowna BC V1Y 5X1
250 861-3644; Fax: 250 763-4827
E: kelowna@cmha.bc.ca
W: www.kelowna.cmha.bc.ca
Languages: English

◇ **Nanaimo - Mid Island Branch:**
126 Haliburton St, Nanaimo BC V9R 4V8
250 244-4042; Fax: 250 244-4045
E: midisland@cmha.bc.ca
W: www.mid-island.cmha.bc.ca
Executive:
Fin Off: Suzie Tai
Languages: English

◇ **North & West Vancouver:**
Esplanade Centre
211-260 Esplanade W, North Vancouver BC V7M 3G7
604 987-6959; Fax: 604 980-0336
E: rebecca.bailey@cmha.bc.ca
W: www.northwestvancouver.cmha.bc.ca
Executive:
Exec Dir: Katie Hughes
Year Founded: 1958
Budget: $650,000
No of Paid Staff: 21
Speakers Available
Library: Y *(Open to the public)*
Languages: English
Membership: 70 *(Lists available to the public)*
Membership Fee: Family - $30; Individual - $20

◇ **Port Alberni:**
New Horizons Centre
3178 2nd Ave, Port Alberni BC V9Y 4C3
250 724-7199; Fax: 250 724-5635
E: b.hargreaves@cmhapa.ca
W: www.cmhapa.ca
Year Founded: 1992
Budget: $575,000
No of Paid Staff: 24
Speakers Available
Library: Y *(Open to the public)*
Languages: English
Membership: 200

◇ **Prince George:**
555 George St, Prince George BC V2L 1R8
250 564-8644; Fax: 250 564-6155
Toll-free: 866 564-8644
E: reception@cmhapg.ca
W: www.cmhapg.ca
Year Founded: 1962
No of Paid Staff: 30
Speakers Available
Library: Y *(Open to the public)*
Languages: English
Membership: 20
Membership Fee: $15/year

◇ **Richmond:**
7351 Elmbridge Way, Richmond BC V6X 1B8
604 276-8834; Fax: 604 276-0342
E: info@cmha-rmd.com
W: www.cmha-rmd.com
Executive:
Exec Dir: Dave MacDonald
Languages: English

◇ **Salmon Arm:**
Location: 433 Hudson Ave, Salmon Arm BC V1E 2S1
Mailing: PO Box 3275 Stn Main, Salmon Arm BC V1E 4S1
250 832-8477; Fax: 250 832-8410
E: info.sr@cmha.bc.ca
W: www.shuswap-revelstoke.cmha.bc.ca
Executive:
Exec Dir: Dawn Dunlop-Pugh
Prog Mgr: Dianna Churchill
Year Founded: 1990
Budget: $750,000
No of Paid Staff: 7
Speakers Available
Library: Y
Languages: English
Membership: 4,312
Membership Fee: $10
Library:
Shuswap Family Resource Centre *(Open to the public)*

◇ **Simon Fraser Branch:**
435 Sixth St, New Westminster BC V3L 3B1
604 516-8080; Fax: 604 524-2870
E: simonfraser@cmha.bc.ca
W: www.simonfraser.cmha.bc.ca/
Executive:
Exec Dir: Rodney Baker
Languages: English

◇ **South Fraser Branch:**
208-8334 128 St, Surrey BC V3W 4G2
604 543-1357; Fax: 604 543-1369
Languages: English

◇ **South Okanagan/Similkameen:**
2852 Skaha Lake Rd, Penticton BC V2A 6G1
250 493-8999; Fax: 250 493-5541
E: cmhasos@shaw.ca
W: www.sos.cmha.bc.ca
Executive:
Pres: Penny Nugent
Year Founded: 1988
Budget: $400,000
No of Paid Staff: 8
Library: Y
Languages: English
Membership: 240 *(Lists available to the public)*
Membership Fee: $2.50-$20.00

◇ **Trail & District:**
1939 Columbia Ave, Trail BC V1R 1K5
250 368-5223; Fax: 250 368-5230
E: sflagel@cmhakootenays.org
W: www.cmhakootenays.org
Languages: English

◇ **Vancouver/Burnaby:**
175 West Broadway, Vancouver BC V5Y 1P4
604 872-4902; Fax: 604 872-5934
E: info.vb@cmha.bc.ca
W: www.vb.cmha.bc.ca

Executive:
Employment Serv Mgr: Leigh Thomson
Volunteer Prog: Grace Kwok
No of Paid Staff: 25
Speakers Available
Library: Y *(Open to the public)*
Languages: English
Membership Fee: $20/year

◇ ***Vernon & District:***
3100 28 Ave, Vernon BC V1T 1W3
250 542-3114; Fax: 250 549-8446
E: vernon@cmha.bc.ca
W: www.vernon.cmha.bc.ca
Executive:
Exec Dir: Sandra Rysen
Year Founded: 1959
No of Paid Staff: 50
Speakers Available
Library: Y
Languages: English
Membership: 45
Membership Fee: Volunteer/Consumer - $5; General-$20

◇ ***Victoria:***
125 Skinner St, Victoria BC V9A 6X4
250 389-1211; Fax: 250 389-1263
E: info@miravictoria.ca
W: www.miravictoria.ca
Executive:
Exec Dir: Pam Edwards
IT Support: Sara Cawsey
Library: Y *(Open to the public)*
Languages: English

◇ ***Williams Lake:***
51 Fourth Ave S, Williams Lake BC V2G 1J6
250 398-8220; Fax: 250 392-4456
W: williamslake.cmha.bc.ca
Executive:
Exec Dir: Trevor Barnes
Year Founded: 1976
Criteria: *Interest in mental health issues.*
Budget: $1,500,000
No of Paid Staff: 20
Speakers Available
Languages: English
Membership: 40
Membership Fee: $20

◈ ***Manitoba:***
2633 Portage Ave, Winnipeg MB R3J 0P7
204 953-2350; Fax: 204 772-4969
E: info@cmhamanitoba.mb.ca
W: www.manitoba.cmha.ca
Executive:
Exec Dir: Tammy Watson
Coord-Admn/Fin Serv: Cheryl McClure
No of Paid Staff: 8
Speakers Available
Languages: English
Membership: 275
Membership Fee: $20/year

◇ ***Central Region:***
236 Saskatchewan Ave E, Portage la Prairie MB R1N 0K9
204 239-6590; Fax: 204 857-2869
E: cmhaplap@shawbiz.ca
W: www.cmhacentral.ca
Executive:
Reg Mgr: Leisa Miness
Year Founded: 1918
Budget: $400,000
No of Paid Staff: 7
Speakers Available
Languages: English
Membership: 20

◇ ***Eastman:***
Location: 689 Main St, Oakbank MB R0E 1J2
Mailing: PO Box 368, Oakbank MB R0E 1J0
204 444-4691; Fax: 204 444-7851
E: cmhaest@mts.net
Languages: English

◇ ***Interlake Region:***
217 Robinson Ave, Selkirk MB R1A 2M5
204 482-9723; Fax: 204 482-5684
E: cmhainlk@mts.net
W: www.interlake.cmha.ca
Executive:
Reg Dir: Brian Yuzdepski
No of Paid Staff: 9
Languages: English

◇ ***Norman Region:***
Location: 81 Edwards Ave, The Pas MB R9A 1M3
Mailing: PO Box 2605
204 623-7203; Fax: 204 623-6734
W: www.manitoba.cmha.ca
Languages: English

◇ ***Swan Valley Region:***
Location: 610 Main St, Swan River MB R0L 1Z0
Mailing: PO Box 1593
204 734-2734; Fax: 204 734-5727
E: cmha@mts.net
W: www.cmha.ca
Executive:
Reg Dir: Marvin Fried
Year Founded: 1988
Criteria: *Open to anyone who agress with CMHA principles and pays the membership fee.*
No of Paid Staff: 7
Speakers Available
Library: Y *(Open to the public)*
Languages: English
Membership: 178
Membership Fee: $20

◇ ***Thompson:***
Location: 43 Fox Bay, Thompson MB R8N 1E9
Mailing: PO Box 456, Thompson MB R8N 1N2
204 677-6050; Fax: 204 677-5534
Toll-free: 866 677-6057 Crisis Support
E: director@cmhathompson.ca
W: www.thompson.cmha.ca
Executive:
Exec Dir: Paullette Simkins
Admv/Fin Serv Coord: Lynda Kretchmann
Speakers Available
Library: Y *(Open to the public)*
Languages: English
Membership list available to the public
Library:
C.M.H.A. Library *(Open to the public)*

◇ ***Westman Region:***
23 12th St, Brandon MB R7A 4L6
204 727-5425; Fax: 204 571-6836
E: rcmha@mts.net
W: www.manitoba.cmha.ca
Executive:
Reg Mgr: Glen Kruck
Languages: English

◇ ***Winnipeg:***
930 Portage Ave, Winnipeg MB R3G 0P8
204 982-6100; Fax: 204 982-6128
E: office@cmhawpg.mb.ca
W: www.winnipeg.cmha.ca
Executive:
Chairperson: George Pasieka
Exec Dir: Nicole Chammartin
Year Founded: 1984
Library: Y *(Open to the public)*
Languages: English
Membership: 125
Membership Fee: $20/Year

◈ ***New Brunswick:***
202-403 Regent St, Fredericton NB E3B 3X6
506 455-5231; Fax: 506 459-3878
E: cmhanb@nb.aibn.com
W: www.nb.cmha.ca
Executive:
Dir-Ops: Kimberly Wall
Exec Dir: Joan Mix
No of Paid Staff: 15
Library: Y *(Open to the public)*
Languages: English; French
Membership Fee: $10-$15 per year

◇ ***Albert County:***
5295 Route 114, Hopewell Hill NB E4H 3M7
506 882-2604; Fax: 506 882-2884
E: avtc@nbnet.nb.ca
W: www.cmhanb.ca
Executive:
Pres: Rhonda McKinley
Admin: Paul Collins
Languages: English

◇ ***Charlotte County:***
5 Riverview Ave, St George NB E5C 3M1
506 755-4060; Fax: 506 755-4060
E: roz.allen@gnb.ca
W: www.novascotia.cmha.ca
Executive:
Reg Commun Worker: Rosslyn Allen
Languages: English; French

◇ ***Grand Falls:***
Location: 131 rue Pleasant, Grand Falls NB E3Z 1G1
Mailing: PO Box 5001 Stn Main
506 475-2415; Fax: 506 475-2452
E: danielle.d'amours@gnb.ca
W: www.nb.cmha.ca
Executive:
Reg Commun Worker: Bea Theriault
Languages: English; French

◇ ***Madawaska:***
Location: 331-121 Church St, Edmundston NB E3V 1L1
Mailing: CP 333 Stn Main, Edmundston NB E3V 3K9
506 739-9489; Fax: 506 737-4448
E: denyse.mazerolle2@gnb.ca
Executive:
Pres: Karine Levesque
Reg Commun Worker: Denyse Mazerolle
Languages: English; French

◇ ***Miramichi:***
Mental Health Clinic
506 773-7561; Fax: 506 778-5296
E: charline.mclean@gnb.ca
W: www.cmha.ca
Executive:
Reg'l Commun Worker: Charline McLean
Languages: English

◇ ***Moncton Region:***
104-30 Gordon St, Moncton NB E1C 1L8
506 859-8114; Fax: 506 859-9581
E: cmhamctn@nb.aibn.com
W: www.cmhamoncton.ca
Executive:
Exec Dir: Armand Savoie
Year Founded: 1951
No of Paid Staff: 6
Speakers Available
Languages: French; English
Membership: 250 *(Lists available to the public)*
Membership Fee: $20/Year

◇ ***Saint John:***
Saint John City Hall
1500-15 Market Sq, Saint John NB E2L 1E8
506 633-1705; Fax: 506 633-2892
E: cmha@nb.aibn.com
W: www.sj.cmha.ca

HEALTHCARE ASSOCIATIONS

Executive:
Exec Dir: Sherry LaPointe-Booy
Year Founded: 1960
No of Paid Staff: 2
Speakers Available
Languages: English

◇ ***Sussex***
30 Moffett Ave, Sussex NB E4E 1E8
506 432-2101; Fax: 506 432-7505
E: melissa.baxter@gnb.ca
W: www.nb.cmha.ca
Executive:
Reg Community Worker: Melissa Baxter
No of Paid Staff: 1
Speakers Available
Library: Y *(Open to the public)*
Languages: English; French
Membership list available to the public

◈ ***Sussex***
30 Moffett Ave, Sussex NB E4E 1E8
506 432-2101; Fax: 506 432-7505
E: melissa.baxter@gnb.ca
W: www.nb.cmha.ca
Executive:
Reg Community Worker: Melissa Baxter
No of Paid Staff: 1
Speakers Available
Library: Y *(Open to the public)*
Languages: English; French
Membership list available to the public

◈ ***Newfoundland/Labrador:***
70 The Boulevard, Floor 1, St. John's NL A1A 1K2
709 753-8550; Fax: 709 753-8537
Toll-free: 877 753-8550
E: office@cmhanl.ca
W: www.cmhanl.ca
Executive:
Exec Dir: George Skinner
Mgr-Corp Serv: Paul Fifield
Languages: English
Membership: 25 *(Lists available to the public)*

◈ ***Northwest Territories:***
Location: 5125 50 St, Yellowknife NT X1A 2P9
Mailing: PO Box 2580 Stn Main
867 873-3190; Fax: 867 873-4930
E: cmha@northwestel.net
W: www.nt-cmha.caha.ca
Executive:
Exec Dir: Sandra Beaton
Languages: English

◈ ***Nova Scotia:***
63 King St, Dartmouth NS B2Y 2R7
902 466-6600; Fax: 902 466-3300
Toll-free: 877 466-6606
W: www.novascotia.cmha.ca
Executive:
Exec Dir: Gail Gardiner
Speakers Available
Library: Y
Languages: English
Membership: 200
Membership Fee: $5
Library:
Resource Centre *(Open to the public)*

◇ ***Annapolis County Branch:***
Mailing: PO Box 249, Bridgetown NS B0S 1C0
902 665-4801; Fax: 902 655-5084
E: chapelcreekgallery@ns.sympatico.ca
Languages: English

◇ ***Annapolis County Branch:***
Location: 1043 Hwy 1, Cornwallis NS B0S 1H0
Mailing: PO Box 205
902 638-8164; Fax: 902 665-5084

◇ ***Cape Breton:***
1482 George St, Sydney NS B1P 1P3
902 567-7735; Fax: 902 567-7905
E: cmhacbrh@cbdha.nshealth.ca
Executive:
Exec Dir: Gail Gardiner
Languages: English

◇ ***Colchester/East Hants:***
Location: 25 Revere St, Truro NS B2N 5V2
Mailing: PO Box 1413 RPO Prince
902 895-4211; Fax: 902 895-4027
E: cmha@eastlink.ca
W: www.cmhaceh.ca
Executive:
Exec Dir: Susan Henderson
Year Founded: 1950
No of Paid Staff: 22
Speakers Available
Library: Y *(Open to the public)*
Languages: English
Membership Fee: $5

◇ ***Halifax-Dartmouth:***
Bloomfield Centre
2786 Agricola St, Room 216, Halifax NS B3K 4E1
902 455-5445; Fax: 902 455-7858
E: cmhahal@ns.aliantzinc.ca
W: www.cmhahaldart.ca
No of Paid Staff: 3
Speakers Available
Library: Y *(Open to the public)*
Languages: English
Membership: 200

◇ ***King's County:***
Location: 109-49 Cornwallis St, Kentville NS B4N 4H8
Mailing: PO Box 894 Stn Main
902 679-7464; Fax: 902 679-7470
E: programmanager@cmhakings.ns.ca
W: www.cmhakings.ns.ca
Executive:
Exec Dir: Michelle Ferdinand
Languages: English

◇ ***Lunenburg County:***
17-450 Lahave St, Bridgewater NS B4V 4A3
902 541-1153; Fax: 902 543-7082
E: cmha.lunenburg@gmail.com
W: www.cmhalq.com/
Year Founded: 1976
Languages: English

◇ ***Pictou:***
Location: 825 East River Rd, New Glasgow NS B2H 1S7
Mailing: PO Box 959 Stn Main, New Glasgow NS B2H 5K7
902 752-5578; Fax: 902 466-3300
Languages: English

◇ ***Yarmouth, Digby, Shelburne Branch:***
37 Brunswick St, Yarmouth NS B5A 2E7
902 742-0222; Fax: 902 742-9301
E: info@cmhayds.com
W: www.cmhayds.com/

◈ ***Durham Region***
60 Bond St W, Oshawa ON L1G 1A5
905 436-8760; Fax: 905 436-1569
E: cmha@cmhadurham.org
W: www.durham.cmha.ca
Executive:
CEO: Linda Gallacher
Year Founded: 1959
Criteria: *An interest in mental health issues and community support services.*
Budget: $2,900,000
No of Paid Staff: 58
Library: Y
Languages: English

Membership Fee: $20/Individual; $10/Student; $150/Corporation; $75/Organization; $35/Family
Library:
Resource Library *(Open to the public)*

◈ ***Ontario:***
2301-180 Dundas St W, Toronto ON M5G 1Z8
416 977-5580; Fax: 416 977-2813
Toll-free: 800 875-6213
E: info@ontario.cmha.ca
W: www.ontario.cmha.ca
Executive:
CEO: Camille Quenneville
Sr Dir-Fin: David Alge
No of Paid Staff: 23
Speakers Available
Library: Y
Languages: English
Library:
Mental Health Information Centre *(Open to the public)*

◇ ***Brant County:***
203-44 King St, Brantford ON N3T 3C7
519 752-2998; Fax: 519 752-2717
E: mail@cmhabrant.on.ca
W: www.cmhabrant.on.ca
Executive:
Exec Dir: Peg Purvis
Library: Y *(Open to the public)*
Languages: English

◇ ***Centre for Mental Health - Cambridge:***
3-9 Wellington St, Cambridge ON N1R 3Y4
519 740-7782; Fax: 519 740-0461
E: admin@cmhagrb.on.ca
W: www.cmhagrb.on.ca
Executive:
Exec Dir: Don Roth
Dir-Servs: Geoff Reekie
Team Leader: Tina Fish

◇ ***Centre for Mental Health - Guelph:***
147 Wyndham St N, Guelph ON N1H 4E9
519 836-6220; Fax: 519 836-6237
E: admin@cmhagrb.on.ca
W: www.cmhagrb.on.ca
Executive:
Exec Dir: Don Roth
Languages: English

◇ ***Centre for Mental Health - Orangeville:***
295A Broadway Ave, Orangeville ON L9W 1L2
519 938-8776; Fax: 519 938-9923
Toll-free: 866 938-8776
E: admin@cmhagrb.on.ca
W: www.cmhagrb.on.ca
Executive:
Resource Centre Coord: Rhonda Nalli
Languages: English

◇ ***Champlain East:***
329 Pitt St, Cornwall ON K6J 3R1
613 933-5845; Fax: 613 936-2323
Toll-free: 800 493-8271
E: office@cmha-east.on.ca
W: www.cmha-east.on.ca
Executive:
Ops Mgr: Bill Woodside
Exec Dir: Michael Lloyd
Languages: English

◇ ***Chatham-Kent:***
100-240 Grand Ave W, Chatham ON N7L 1C1
519 436-6100; Fax: 519 351-9203
E: dmeurkes@cmhakent.com
W: www.cmhakent.com
Executive:
CEO: Len Caro
Languages: English

HEALTHCARE ASSOCIATIONS

◇ ***Club Niagara/Mental Health Resource Centre/REAL Work***
2-6760 Morrison St, Niagara Falls ON L2E 6Z8
905 354-4576; Fax: 905 354-4577
E: info@cmhaniagara.ca
W: www.cmhaniagara.ca
Executive:
Pres: Laura Garner
VP: Rashmi Biswas
Br Mgr: Peggy Allen
Languages: English

◇ ***Cochrane Timiskaming:***
201-330 Second Ave, Timmins ON P4N 8A4
705 267-8100; Fax: 705 268-8742
E: cmhadm@cmhact.ca
W: www.cmhact.ca
Executive:
CEO: Liz Di Tullio
Exec Dir: Clark MacFarlane
Criteria: *Canadian citizen, 18 yrs. of age and over*
No of Paid Staff: 109
Languages: English
Membership: 352
Membership Fee: $5

◇ ***Cochrane Timiskmaming / Kirkland Lake:***
5 Kirkland St E, Kirkland Lake ON P2N 1N9
705 567-9596; Fax: 705 567-5211
E: cmhatmsk@cmhact.ca

◇ ***Cochrane Timiskmaming / New Liskeard:***
Location: 20 May St S, New Liskeard ON P0J 1P0
Mailing: PO Box 249
705 647-4444; Fax: 705 647-4434
E: cmhatmsk@cmhact.ca

◇ ***Consumer/Survivor Support Network & Eden Place Crop-In Centre***
101-2600 Edenhurst Dr, Mississauga ON L5A 3Z8
905 276-3302; Fax: 905 276-9646
W: www.cmhapeel.ca
Executive:
Mgr: Peter Mielke
Exec Dir: Sandy Milakovic
Languages: English

◇ ***Elgin County:***
110 Centre St, St Thomas ON N5R 2Z9
519 633-1781; Fax: 519 631-8273
E: cmhaelgin@execulink.com
W: www.cmhaelgin.ca
Executive:
Exec Dir: Heather DeBruyn
Languages: English

◇ ***Forest Outreach:***
59 King St W, Forest ON N0N 1J0
519 786-4545; Fax: 519 786-3023
Executive:
Clinical Case Mgr: Poonam Chhabra

◇ ***Fort Frances:***
Location: 612 Portage Ave, Fort Frances ON P9A 1A4
Mailing: PO Box 446 Stn Main, Fort Frances ON P9A 3M8
807 274-2347; Fax: 807 274-2473
E: cmha@cmhaff.ca
W: www.cmhaff.ca
Executive:
Pres/Chair: Trudy McCormick
Exec Dir: Shiela Shaw
Fin Mgr: Stacy Hahkala
Year Founded: 1980
Library: Y
Languages: English

◇ ***Grand River:***
Orchard Park
J100-5420 Hwy 6, RR 5, Guelph ON N1H 6J2
519 766-4450; Fax: 519 766-9211
E: admin@cmhagrb.on.ca
W: www.cmhagrb.on.ca
Executive:
Exec Dir: Don Roth

◇ ***Grey Bruce:***
1024 2nd Ave E, Owen Sound ON N4K 2H7
519 371-3642; Fax: 519 371-6485
E: admin@cmhagb.org
W: www.gb.cmha.ca
Executive:
Exec Dir: Claude Anderson
Br Admin: Brenda Hodgson
Speakers Available
Library: Y *(Open to the public)*
Languages: English

◇ ***Haldimand-Norfolk:***
204-150 West St, Simcoe ON N3Y 5C1
519 428-2380; Fax: 519 428-3424
Toll-free: 888 750-7778
E: info@cmha-hn.ca
W: www.cmha-hn.ca
Executive:
Exec Dir: Michael Benin
Asst Exec Dir: John Ranger
Year Founded: 1988
Budget: $2,500,000
No of Paid Staff: 25
Speakers Available
Library: Y
Languages: English; Spanish
Membership list available to the public

◇ ***Halton Region:***
388 Main St E, Milton ON L9T 1P8
905 693-4270; Fax: 905 693-9183
Toll-free: 877 693-4270
E: info.cmha@haltonhealthworks.ca
W: www.cmha-halton.ca
Executive:
CEO: Radhika Subramanyan
Dir-Fin/Admn: Marg O'Neill
Year Founded: 1918
No of Paid Staff: 53
Speakers Available
Library: Y *(Open to the public)*
Languages: English

◇ ***Hamilton:***
131 John St S, Hamilton ON L8N 2C3
905 521-0090; Fax: 905 521-0211
E: info@cmhahamilton.ca
W: www.cmhahamilton.ca/
Executive:
Case Mgr: Evelyn Krysinski
Exec Dir: Marilyn Jewell
Office Mgr: Louise Balcomb
Year Founded: 1966
Budget: $1,000,000
No of Paid Staff: 21
Languages: English

◇ ***Hastings & Prince Edward Counties:***
Century Place Building
530-199 Front St, Belleville ON K8N 5H5
613 969-8874; Fax: 613 969-8294
E: cmha.hastings@bellnet.ca
W: www.hastings-cmha.org
Executive:
Exec Dir: Shannan Mercer
No of Paid Staff: 8
Speakers Available
Languages: English

◇ ***Huron-Perth:***
540 Huron St, Stratford ON N5A 5T9
519 273-1391; Fax: 519 273-0505
E: geninfo@cmha-hp.on.ca
W: www.cmha-hp.on.ca
Executive:
Exec Dir: John Robertson
Languages: English

◇ ***Huron-Perth - Seaforth Office:***
Location: 92 Goderich St W, Seaforth ON N0K 1W0
Mailing: 540 Huron St, Stratford ON N5A 5T9
519 273-1391; Fax: 519 273-0505
Toll-free: 888 875-2944
E: geninfo@cmha-hp.on.ca
W: www.cmha-hp.on.ca
Executive:
Exec Dir: John Robertson
Languages: English

◇ ***Kawartha Lakes - Main Office:***
2 Kent St W, Floor 2, Lindsay ON K9V 2Y1
705 328-2704; Fax: 705 328-2456
Toll-free: 888 454-8875
E: info.cmha@cmhakawarthalakes.ca
W: www.cmhakawarthalakes.ca
Executive:
Pres: Doug Bothwell
VP: Judy Dickson
Exec Dir: Mark Graham
Languages: English

◇ ***Kawartha Lakes - Housing Office:***
51 Adelaide St N, Lindsay ON K9V 4L1
705 328-2798; Fax: 705 328-0711
E: info.cmha@cmhakawarthalakes.ca
W: www.cmhakawarthalakes.ca/

◇ ***Kingston:***
6 Ordnance St, Kingston ON K7K 5T9
613 549-7027; Fax: 613 549-7098
E: cmhstaff@kingston.net
W: www.kingston.org/cmha
Executive:
Br Mgr: Brenda Miller
Year Founded: 1978
Criteria: *Open to all.*
Budget: $150,000
No of Paid Staff: 3
Speakers Available
Library: Y *(Open to the public)*
Languages: English
Membership: 129 *(Lists available to the public)*
Membership Fee: $20

◇ ***Lambton County:***
210 Lochiel St, Sarnia ON N7T 4C7
519 337-5411; Fax: 519 337-2325
E: general@cmha.sarnia.net
W: www.cmhalambton.org
Executive:
CEO: Alan Stevenson
Dir-Client Serv: Penny Witcher
No of Paid Staff: 42
Speakers Available
Library: Y *(Open to the public)*
Languages: English

◇ ***Leeds-Grenville:***
3-25 Front Ave W, Brockville ON K6V 4J2
613 345-0950; Fax: 613 342-7937
E: info@cmha-lg.ca
W: www.cmha-lg.ca
Executive:
Exec Dir: Colin Slack
Year Founded: 1978
Languages: English

◇ ***London-Middlesex:***
648 Huron St, London ON N5Y 4J8
519 434-9191; Fax: 519 438-1167
E: aleena@london.cmha.ca
W: www.london.cmha.ca
Executive:
Chair: Elizabeth Abbott
Dir-Ops: Michele VanBeers

HEALTHCARE ASSOCIATIONS

Exec Dir: Mike Petrenko
Treas: Brian Soanes
Exec Coord: Aleena Needham
Year Founded: 1960
Criteria: *Anyone whose interest may be in the field of mental illness/health.*
Budget: $805,000
No of Paid Staff: 16
Speakers Available
Languages: English
Membership: 112
Membership Fee: $20
Library:
V. Spooner Resource Center *(Open to the public)*

◇ ***Mental Health Court Support - Brampton:***
102-2 County Court Blvd, Brampton ON L6W 3W8
905 451-7335; Fax: 905 456-7492
E: courtsupport@cmhapeel.ca
W: www.cmhapeel.ca
Executive:
Dir-Clinical Serv: Christine Devoy
Mgr-Justice Serv: Courtenay McGlashen
Speakers Available
Languages: English

◇ ***Mental Health Court Support - St. Catharines:***
1-59 Church St, St Catharines ON L2R 7N8
905 984-5423; Fax: 905 984-5019
W: www.cmhaniagara.ca
Executive:
Exec Dir: George Kurzawa
Languages: English

◇ ***Mississauga - Community Support Services***
601-7700 Hurontario St, Brampton ON L6Y 4M3
905 796-9030; Fax: 905 796-9035
E: partnershipplace@cmhapeel.ca
W: www.cmhapeel.ca
Executive:
Employment Developer: Ron Hesas
Employment Developer: Fran Kovacs
Year Founded: 1987
Criteria: *Adults over the age of 16, living in Mississauga, with a primary diagnosis of mental illness.*
No of Paid Staff: 4
Languages: English

◇ ***Niagara:***
15 Wellington St, St Catharines ON L2R 5P7
905 641-5222; Fax: 905 641-8821
E: info@cmhaniagara.ca
W: www.cmhaniagara.ca
Executive:
Exec Dir: George Kurzawa
Languages: English

◇ ***Niagara Falls - Counselling Project Share***
4129 Stanley Ave, Niagara Falls ON L2E 7H3
905 357-5121; Fax: 905 357-0143
W: www.projectshare.ca
Executive:
Chairperson: Brian Pellow
Vice Chairperson: Tom Snodgrass
Exec Dir: Elaine Pihach
Treas: Mick Wolfe
Sec: Paisley Janvary-Pool
Languages: English

◇ ***Nipissing:***
156 McIntyre St W, North Bay ON P1B 2Y6
705 474-1299; Fax: 705 474-5325
E: info@cmhanipissing.on.ca
W: www.cmhanipissing.on.ca
Executive:
Exec Dir: Georges Kristolaitis
Office Mgr: Jenny Leblond
Prog Mgr: Margi Clarke
Year Founded: 1977
Speakers Available
Languages: English

◇ ***Oxford County:***
522 Peel St, Woodstock ON N4S 1K3
519 539-8055; Fax: 519 539-8317
Toll-free: 800 859-7248
E: branch@cmhaoxford.on.ca
W: www.cmhaoxford.on.ca
Executive:
Exec Dir: Mike McMahon
Fin/Admn Mgr: Carrie Heron
Languages: English

◇ ***Oxford County***
29 Noxon St, Ingersoll ON N5C 1B8
519 485-1700 203; Fax: 519 485-9601
W: www.alexandrahospital.on.ca
Executive:
CEO: Crystal Houze
CFO: Frank Deutsch
Languages: English

◇ ***Ottawa:***
301-1355 Bank St, Ottawa ON K1H 8K7
613 737-7791; Fax: 613 737-7644
E: cmhaoc@magma.ca
W: www.cmhaottawa.ca
Executive:
Pres: Dr Andrew McCreary
Exec Dir: Tim Simboli
Treas: Dr Denis Trottier
Year Founded: 1953
Languages: English

◇ ***Peel Finance and Administration:***
28-241 Clarence St, Brampton ON L6W 4P2
905 451-1718; Fax: 905 451-1720
E: admin@cmhapeel.ca
W: www.cmhapeel.ca
Executive:
CEO: Sandy Milakovic
Mgr: Steve Farstad
Year Founded: 1962
Budget: $2,200,000
Speakers Available
Languages: English
Membership: 200 *(Lists available to the public)*
Membership Fee: Individual - $10; No charge to consumers; Business - $40; Family/Non-profit organization - $20

◇ ***Peterborough:***
466 George St N, Peterborough ON K9H 3R7
705 748-6711; Fax: 705 748-2577
E: info@peterborough.cmha.on.ca
W: www.peterborough.cmha.on.ca
Executive:
Exec Dir: Mark Graham
Dir-Hum Res: Linda Saunders

◇ ***Petrolia Outreach***
Location: 450 Blanche St, Floor 2, Petrolia ON N0N 1R0
Mailing: PO Box 1666
519 882-0013; Fax: 519 882-3058
W: www.cmhalambton.org
Executive:
CEO: Alan Steveson
Languages: English

◇ ***St. Catharines - Phoenix House/SafeBeds:***
15 Wellington St, St Catharines ON L2R 5P7
905 641-5222; Fax: 905 688-3316
E: info@cmhaniagara.ca
W: www.cmhaniagara.ca
Executive:
CEO: Camille Quenneville
Languages: English

◇ ***Sault Ste. Marie:***
386 Queen St E, Sault Ste. Marie ON P6A 1Z1
705 759-0458; Fax: 705 945-0261
E: annette@cmhassm.com
W: www.cmhassm.com
Executive:
Exec Dir: Annette Katajamaki
Year Founded: 1963
Budget: $1,500,000
No of Paid Staff: 21
Library: Y *(Open to the public)*
Languages: English

◇ ***Simcoe:***
15 Bradford St, Barrie ON L4N 1W2
705 726-5033; Fax: 705 726-8629
E: info@cmha-sos.on.ca
W: www.cmhasim.on.ca
Executive:
CEO: Nancy Roxborough
IT Specialist: Jason MacDonald
Languages: English

◇ ***Sudbury:***
100-111 Elm St, Sudbury ON P3C 1T3
705 675-7252; Fax: 705 675-7247
Toll-free: 866 285-2642
E: info@cmha-sm.on.ca
W: www.cmha-sm.on.ca
Executive:
CEO: Marion Quigley
Fin Admin: Sylvie Montpellier
Year Founded: 1984
Budget: $3,711,254
No of Paid Staff: 40
Speakers Available
Library: Y
Languages: Bilingual(English/French)
Membership: 56 *(Lists available to the public)*
Membership Fee: $20/year
Library:
Mental Health Resource Centre *(Open to the public)*

◇ ***Thunder Bay:***
200 Van Norman St, Thunder Bay ON P7A 4B8
807 345-5564; Fax: 807 345-4458
E: cmhatb@cmha-tb.on.ca
W: www.cmha-tb.on.ca
Executive:
Exec Dir: Maurice Fortin
Languages: English

◇ ***Tillsonburg Satellite Office:***
40 Brock St W, Tillsonburg ON N4G 2A2
519 842-8869; Fax: 519 842-9425
Toll-free: 800 859-7248
E: branch@cmhaoxford.on.ca
W: www.cmhaoxford.on.ca
Executive:
I-Exec Dir: Bob Fehir

◇ ***Toronto:***
480-700 Lawrence Ave W, Toronto ON M6A 3B4
416 789-7957; Fax: 416 789-9079
E: cmha.toronto@sympatico.ca
W: www.toronto.cmha.ca
Executive:
Exec Dir: Steve Lurie
Languages: English

◇ ***Toronto Markham Road Site:***
500-1200 Markham Rd, Scarborough ON M1H 3C3
416 289-6285; Fax: 416 289-6843
E: cmha.scar@bellnet.ca
W: www.toronto.cmha.ca
Executive:
Office Mgr: Diane Webber
Languages: English

◇ ***Windsor-Essex County:***
1400 Windsor Ave, Windsor ON N8X 3L9
519 255-7440; Fax: 519 255-7817
E: info@cmha-wecb.on.ca
W: www.cmha-wecb.on.ca

Executive:
CEO: Pamela Hines
Hum Res Mgr: Martha Young
IT Mgr: Mike Barlow
Languages: English

◇ ***York Region:***
300-1091 Gorham St, Newmarket ON L3Y 8X7
905 853-5700; Fax: 905 853-1051
E: yorkregion@cmha-yr.on.ca
W: www.cmha-yr.on.ca
Executive:
Exec Dir: Colleen Zakoor
Year Founded: 1984
No of Paid Staff: 62
Speakers Available
Library: Y *(Open to the public)*
Languages: Arabic; Bengali; Cantonese; Dari; Farsi; Finnish; Fookien; French; German; Hindi; Italian; Korean; Mandarin; Polish; Portuguese; Punjabi; Tagalog; Urdu; English

◇ ***Youth Net - Mississauga***
102-2 County Court Blvd, Brampton ON L6W 3W8
905 451-2123; Fax: 905 456-7492
E: info@cmhapeel.ca
W: www.youthnet.cmhapeel.ca
Executive:
Youth Net Coord: Tamara Farstad
Languages: English

◈ ***Oxford County***
29 Noxon St, Ingersoll ON N5C 1B8
519 485-1700 203; Fax: 519 485-9601
W: www.alexandrahospital.on.ca
Executive:
CEO: Crystal Houze
CFO: Frank Deutsch

◈ ***Petrolia Outreach***
Location: 450 Blanche St, Floor 2, Petrolia ON N0N 1R0
Mailing: PO Box 1666
519 882-0013; Fax: 519 882-3058
W: www.cmhalambton.org
Executive:
CEO: Alan Steveson
Languages: English

◈ ***Prince Eward Island:***
Location: 178 Fitzroy St, Charlottetown PE C1A 1S1
Mailing: PO Box 785 Stn Central, Charlottetown PE C1A 7L9
902 566-3034; Fax: 902 566-4643
E: division@cmha.pe.ca
W: www.cmha.pe.ca
Languages: English

◇ ***Prince County:***
11-67 Duke St, Summerside PE C1N 3R9
902 436-7399; Fax: 902 436-2209
E: assoc.executivedirector@cmha.pe.ca
W: www.cmha.pe.ca
Languages: English

◇ ***West Prince:***
Mailing: PO Box 537, Alberton PE C0B 1B0
902 853-3871; Fax: 902 853-3877
E: cmhawest@cmha.pe.ca
Languages: English

◈ ***Quebec:***
326-911 rue Jean-Talon E, Montréal QC H2R 1V5
514 849-3291
E: info@acsm.qc.ca
W: www.acsm.qc.ca
Executive:
Dir: Renée Ouimet
Year Founded: 1955
No of Paid Staff: 2
Library: Y *(Open to the public)*
Languages: English; French
Membership: 10 *(Lists available to the public)*
Membership Fee: $200

◇ ***Bas-du-Fleuve:***
315 av Rouleau, Rimouski QC G5L 5V5
418 723-6416 100; Fax: 418 721-5811
E: acsmbf@globetrotter.net
W: www.acsmbf.com
Year Founded: 1964
Budget: $200,000
No of Paid Staff: 6
Library: Y *(Open to the public)*
Languages: French
Membership: 175
Membership Fee: $10
Library:
Centre de documentation

◇ ***Chaudière-Appalaches:***
110-5935 rue Saint-Georges, Lévis QC G6V 4K8
418 835-5920; Fax: 418 835-1850
E: info@acsm-ca.qc.ca
W: www.acsm-ca.qc.ca
Executive:
Dir: Guylaine Gourgues
Year Founded: 1990
No of Paid Staff: 1
Languages: French; English

◇ ***Côte-Nord:***
Location: 10 av Boisvert, Port-Cartier QC G5B 1W7
Mailing: CP 323 succ Bureau-Chef, Port-Cartier QC G5B 2G9
418 766-4476; Fax: 418 766-4476
Toll-free: 800 364-4476
E: acsmcn@globetrotter.net
Executive:
Dir gén: Carole Chevarie
Year Founded: 1993
Budget: $70,000
No of Paid Staff: 2
Languages: French
Membership: 15

◇ ***Filiale de Montréal***
605-55 av du Mont-Royal O, Montréal QC H2T 2S6
514 521-4993; Fax: 514 521-3270
E: acsmmtl@cooptel.qc.ca
W: www.acsmmontreal.qc.ca
Executive:
Dir gén: Diane Vinet
Year Founded: 1979
Budget: $350,000
No of Paid Staff: 5
Languages: French
Membership: 400
Membership Fee: Ranges from $25-$30

◇ ***Haut-Richelieu:***
178B rue Mercier, St-Jean-sur-Richel QC J3B 6G9
450 346-5736; Fax: 450 346-2075
E: acsmhr@videotron.ca
W: www.acsmhr.com
Executive:
Dir gén: Cynthia Lambert
Languages: French; English

◇ ***Lac Saint-Jean:***
Location: 962 rue Paradis, Roberval QC G8H 2M1
Mailing: CP 214 succ Bureau-Chef, Roberval QC G8H 2N6
418 275-2405; Fax: 418 275-8746
E: acsmlsj@destination.ca
Executive:
Coord: Nancy Guillemetle
Year Founded: 1988
Languages: French; English
Membership: 15 *(Lists available to the public)*

◇ ***Québec:***
325 rue Raoul-Jobin, Québec QC G1K 1M9
418 529-1979; Fax: 418 529-1904
E: info@acsmquebec.org
W: www.acsmquebec.org
Executive:
Dir gén: Monique Boniewski
Languages: French; English

◇ ***Rive-Sud de Montréal:***
300-150 rue Grant, Longueuil QC J4H 3H6
450 616-1569
E: info@acsmrs.qc.ca
W: www.acsmrs.qc.ca
Executive:
Dir: Hélène Laramée
Languages: French; English

◇ ***Saguenay:***
371 rue Racine E, Chicoutimi QC G7H 1S8
418 549-0765; Fax: 418 549-7568
E: acsmsaguenay@videotron.ca
W: www.santementale.ca
Executive:
Dir gén: Christian Morin
Year Founded: 1966
Criteria: *Pour tout.*
No of Paid Staff: 49
Speakers Available
Languages: French
Membership: 32
Membership Fee: $5

◇ ***Sorel/Saint-Joseph/Tracy:***
Centre Sacré-Coeur
107-105 rue du Prince, Sorel-Tracy QC J3P 4J9
450 746-1497; Fax: 450 746-1073
Executive:
Dir gén: Francine Desjardins
Sec: Sylvette Pilon
Year Founded: 1965
Criteria: *Individuel, communautaire soutien, corporatif.*
Budget: $57,000
No of Paid Staff: 3
Speakers Available
Languages: French; English
Membership: 63

◈ ***Saskatchewan Division:***
2702 12th Ave, Regina SK S4T 1J2
306 525-5601; Fax: 306 569-3788
Toll-free: 800 461-5483
E: contactus@cmhask.com
W: www.cmhask.com
Executive:
Exec Dir: Dave Nelson
Year Founded: 1950
No of Paid Staff: 28
Speakers Available
Library: Y *(Open to the public)*
Languages: English
Membership: 700
Membership Fee: Professional - $50; Individual - $15
Library:
Friends for Life Resource Centre *(Open to the public)*

◇ ***Kindersley:***
Location: 113 2nd Ave E, Kindersley SK S0L 1S0
Mailing: PO Box 244
306 463-8052
E: a.w@sasktel.net
W: www.cmhask.ca
Executive:
Br Coord: Pam Welter
Criteria: *Open to all.*
Languages: English

HEALTHCARE ASSOCIATIONS

◇ ***Moose Jaw:***
650 Coteau St W, Room 324,
Moose Jaw SK S6H 5E6
306 692-4240
E: cmha.mj@sasktel.net
W: www.cmhamj.com/
Executive:
Br Dir: Donna Bowyer
Languages: English

◇ ***North Battleford:***
1011 103rd St, North Battleford SK S9A 1K3
306 446-7177; Fax: 306 445-7050
E: cmha.nb@sasktel.net
W: www.cmha.ca/branch_locations/north-battleford-branch/
Year Founded: 1953
No of Paid Staff: 3
Speakers Available
Library: Y
Languages: English
Membership: 120 *(Lists available to the public)*
Membership Fee: $2

◇ ***Prince Albert:***
1322 Central Ave, Prince Albert SK S6V 4W3
306 763-7747; Fax: 306 763-7717
E: pacmha@sasktel.net
W: www.citylightsnews.com/pacmha.htm
Executive:
Exec Dir: Douglas J Kinar
Year Founded: 1989
Criteria: *Open to all, but the majority of members suffer mental illness.*
Budget: $150,000
No of Paid Staff: 4
Speakers Available
Languages: English
Membership: 80 *(Lists available to the public)*

◇ ***Regina:***
1810 Albert St, Regina SK S4P 2S8
306 525-9543; Fax: 306 525-9579
E: info@cmharegina.com
Executive:
Admin: Kim Zazula
Languages: English

◇ ***Saskatoon***
1301 Avenue P N, Saskatoon SK S7L 2X1
306 384-9333; Fax: 306 978-5777
E: info@cmhasaskatoon.ca
W: www.saskatoon.cmha.ca
Executive:
Chair: Mike Petty
V-Chair: Bill Pringle
Year Founded: 1950
Budget: $350,000
No of Paid Staff: 7
Speakers Available
Languages: English
Membership: 200 *(Lists available to the public)*
Membership Fee: $15 Year

◇ ***Saskatoon***
2-804 Dufferin Ave, Saskatoon SK S7H 2B8
Executive:
Dir: Shauna Altroppe

◇ ***Swift Current:***
176 4th Ave NW, Swift Current SK S9H 0T6
306 778-2440; Fax: 306 773-0766
Executive:
Exec Dir: Ruth Smith
Year Founded: 1950

◇ ***Weyburn:***
404 Ashford St, Weyburn SK S4H 1K1
306 842-7959; Fax: 306 842-3096
E: cmhawey@sasktel.net
Executive:
Dir: Gladys Perepeluk
Languages: English

◇ ***Yorkton:***
Mailing: PO Box 1226 Stn Del.Centre,
Yorkton SK S3N 2X3
306 621-5925; Fax: 306 783-9662
E: ybranch@cmhask.com
W: www.cmhask.com
Executive:
Prog Dir: Dr Donia Alvarado-Okrainec
Languages: English

Canadian Mental Health Association - Oasis Centre
003-444 McGill St, Hawkesbury ON K6A 1R2
613 938-0435; Fax: 613 936-2323
W: www.cmha-east.on.ca
Executive:
Team Supv: Johanne Renaud
Languages: English

Canadian Mental Health Association - Shippagan
A-239 J D Gauthier Blvd, Shippagan NB E8S 1N2
506 336-4932; Fax: 506 336-3366
E: lucie.robichaud@gnb.ca
Executive:
Reg Commun Worker: Lucie Robichaud
Languages: English; French

Canadian Psychoanalytic Society Inc.
7000 ch de la Côte-des-Neiges, Montréal QC H3S 2C1
514 738-6105; Fax: 514 738-6393
E: psyanal@qc.aira.com
W: www.psychoanalysis.ca
Executive:
Prés: Dr Margaret-Ann Fitzpatrick-Hanly
Dir admin: Mena Iaciofano
Year Founded: 1966
Criteria: *Must be a psychoanalyst in good stantding with another Society, a candidate in good standing graduated from the Canadian Institute of Psychoanalysis*
No of Paid Staff: 5
Languages: English; French
Membership: 400
Library:
QC-SPM Library/Bibliothèque

◈ ***Toronto Psychoanalytic Society Inc.***
203-40 St Clair Ave E, Toronto ON M4T 1M9
416 922-7770; Fax: 416 922-9988
E: info@torontopsychoanalysis.com
W: www.torontopsychoanalysis.com
Executive:
Pres: Dr Rukhsana Bukhari
VP: Dr Christine Dunbar
Languages: English

◈ ***Société Psychanalytique de Québec***
1180 rue Charles-Albanel, Québec QC G1X 4T9
418 877-8445; Fax: 418 877-7056
Executive:
Psychanalyste didacticien: Dr François Sirois
Prés: Louise Mercier
Trés: André Renaud
Languages: French

Canadian Psychological Association
702-141 Laurier Ave W, Ottawa ON K1P 5J3
613 237-2144; Fax: 613 237-1674
Toll-free: 888 472-0657
E: cpa@cpa.ca
W: www.cpa.ca
Executive:
CEO: Dr Karen Cohen
CFO/Dir-Admn: Philippe Ramsay
Year Founded: 1939
Criteria: *Full Member: must possess at least a masters degree in psychology, or its academic equivalent, conferred by a graduate school of recognized standing,*
Student Affiliate: must be a graduate or undergraduate student enrolled full-time or part-time in a recognized university and engaged in the study (honours or equivalent) of psychology,
International Affiliate: must be a psychologist resident outside Canada who can provide evidence of membership in the psychological association of their country of residence,
Special Affiliate: must show an active interest in psychology, either as a profession or as a science, through work or study in psychology or a related field.
No of Paid Staff: 15
Speakers Available
Languages: English; French
Membership: 5,200
Membership Fee: $55.64-$222.56
Publications
Canadian Journal of Behavioural Science (English, Magazine, Quarterly, $70 - Individual; $110 - Institutional)
Canadian Journal of Experimental Psychology (English, Magazine, Quarterly, $70 - Individual; $110 - Institutional)

Capital Region Mental Health & Addictions Association, Inc.
292-65 Brunswick St, Fredericton NB E3B 1G5
506 458-1803; Fax: 506 443-9001
E: cmhafo@nb.aibn.com
W: www.crmhaa.ca
Executive:
Exec Dir: Dawn Maskill
Year Founded: 1957
No of Paid Staff: 11
Speakers Available
Languages: English

Centre for Addiction and Mental Health Foundation
1001 Queen St W, Toronto ON M6J 1H4
416 535-8501; Fax: 416 583-4316
Toll-free: 800 414-0471
E: foundation@camh.ca
W: www.supportcamh.net
Executive:
VP-Commun: Dean Hughes
Year Founded: 1998
No of Paid Staff: 14
Speakers Available
Languages: English

Children's Mental Health Ontario
309-40 St Clair Ave E, Toronto ON M4T 1M9
416 921-2109; Fax: 416 921-7600
Toll-free: 888 234-7054
E: info@cmho.org
W: www.kidsmentalhealth.ca
Executive:
Chair: Patricia Day
Pres/CEO: Gordon Floyd
Year Founded: 1972
No of Paid Staff: 12
Languages: English
Membership: 91

Coast Mental Health
293 11th Ave E, Vancouver BC V5T 2C4
604 872-3502; Fax: 604 879-2363
E: info@coastmentalhealth.com
W: www.coastmentalhealth.com
Executive:
Assoc Exec Dir: R Heather Edgar

College of Psychologists of New Brunswick
219-236 St. George St, Moncton NB E1C 1W1
506 382-1994; Fax: 506 857-9813
E: cpnb@nbnet.nb.ca
W: www.cpnb.ca
Executive:
Registrar: Cécile Mallais
Year Founded: 1967
No of Paid Staff: 3
Speakers Available
Languages: English; French
Membership: 400 *(Lists available to the public)*

Community Mental Health Centre
Location: 206-2741 Chamberland St, Rockland ON K4K 0B8
Mailing: PO Box 1240 Stn Main, Rockland ON K4K 1L8
613 446-5139; Fax: 613 446-5256
Executive:
Team Leader: Pascale Lavigne

Consumer/Survivor Association of Lambton
183 Christina St S, Sarnia ON N7T 2M9
519 344-5602; Fax: 519 344-6497
Executive:
Exec Dir: Mary Hopkins
Criteria: *Psychiatric survivors.*
No of Paid Staff: 5
Library: Y *(Open to the public)*
Languages: English
Membership: 500

CORE Association
412 3 St SE, Medicine Hat AB T1A 0H1
403 527-3302; Fax: 403 529-9022
E: core.main@coreassoc.net
W: www.coreassoc.net
Executive:
Exec Dir: Rita Bessant
No of Paid Staff: 150
Library: Y
Languages: English

Crest Support Services (Meadowcrest) Inc.
13570 Elginfield Rd, RR 1, Lucan ON N0M 2J0
519 227-6766; Fax: 519 227-6768
W: www.crestsupportservices.ca
Year Founded: 1971
Languages: English

East Metro Youth Services
200-1200 Markham Rd, Scarborough ON M1H 3C3
416 438-3697; Fax: 416 438-7424
E: emys@emys.on.ca
W: www.emys.on.ca
Executive:
Chair: Judy Marshall
Exec Dir: Claire Fainer

Echo Foundation
1050-1350 rue Sherbrooke O, Montréal QC H3G 1J1
514 843-5112; Fax: 514 843-4080
W: www.echofoundation.ca
Executive:
Dir gén: Kevin Leonard
Languages: English

Gateway Residential & Community Support Services of Niagara
CMHA ON Division
178 King St, Welland ON L3B 3J5
905 735-4445; Fax: 905 735-7570
Toll-free: 877 735-4445
W: www.gatewayofniagara.ca
Executive:
Exec Dir: John Osczypko
Resource/Commun Dev Mgr: Shelly Mousseau
Year Founded: 1993
No of Paid Staff: 25
Languages: English

General Practice Psychotherapy Association
312 Oakwood Crt, Newmarket ON L3Y 3C8
416 410-6644; Fax: 905 895-1630
E: info@gppaonline.ca
W: www.gppaonline.ca
Executive:
Assn Mgr: Carol Ford
Year Founded: 1984
Criteria: *MD or interest in Psychotherapy*
Budget: $115,000
Languages: English
Membership: 250
Membership Fee: $175

Healthy Minds Canada
2 Toronto St, Floor 5, Toronto ON M5C 2B6
416 351-7757; Fax: 416 351-7765
E: admin@healthymindscanada.ca
W: www.healthymindscanada.ca
Executive:
Exec Dir: Jean Milligan
Languages: English

Horizons Rennaissance Inc.
201-338 Montreal Rd, Vanier ON K1L 6B3
613 742-0988; Fax: 613 742-0986
E: aguillemette@horizons-renaissance.com
W: www.horizons-renaissance.com
Executive:
Dir Gen: Armel Guillemette

International Schizophrenia Foundation
16 Florence Ave, North York ON M2N 1E9
416 733-2117; Fax: 416 733-2352
E: centre@orthomed.org
W: www.orthomed.org
Executive:
Exec Dir: Steven Carter
Year Founded: 1968
No of Paid Staff: 4
Speakers Available
Library: Y *(Open to the public)*
Languages: English
Membership list available to the public
Membership Fee: $35/yr

Lambton County Developmental Services
Location: 339 Centre St, Petrolia ON N0N 1R0
Mailing: PO Box 1210
519 882-0933; Fax: 519 882-3386
E: administration@lcds.on.ca
W: www.lcds.on.ca
Executive:
Pres: Frank Huybers
Dir-Ops: Maureen MacSorley
Exec Dir: Candie Burchart-Etienne
Treas: Frank Backx
Sec: Corrine Nauta
Dir-Fin: Debbi Potter
Year Founded: 1985
Criteria: *Open to children and adults with developmental handicaps.*
Library: Y *(Open to the public)*
Languages: English

LivingWorks Education Inc.
4303D 11 St SE, Calgary AB T2G 4X1
403 209-0242; Fax: 403 209-0259
Toll-free Fax: 888 733-5484 222
E: info@livingworks.net
W: www.livingworks.net
Executive:
Pres: Richard F Ramsay
VP-Ops: Carole Thannhauser
VP-Bus Dev: Heather Stokes
Year Founded: 1991
No of Paid Staff: 19
Languages: English

MPA-Motivation, Power & Achievement Society
122 Powell St, Vancouver BC V6A 1G1
604 482-3700; Fax: 604 738-4132
E: info@mpa-society.org
W: www.mpa-society.org
Executive:
Exec Dir: David MacIntyre
Library: Y
Languages: English

Mental Health Rights Coalition
206A-20 Jackson St W, Hamilton ON L8P 1L2
905 545-2525; Fax: 905 545-0211
E: mhrced@bellnet.ca
W: www.mentalhealthrights.ca
Executive:
Exec Dir: Frances V Jewell
Criteria: *Consumer/Survivor (mental health) living, working or receiving services in Hamilton, and over 18 years of age.*
Budget: $131,000
No of Paid Staff: 11
Speakers Available
Library: Y *(Open to the public)*
Languages: English
Membership: 450

Mood Disorders Association of British Columbia - MDA
200-460 Nanaimo St, Vancouver BC V5L 4W3
604 873-0103; Fax: 604 873-3095
Toll-free: 855 282-7979
E: info@mdabc.net
W: www.mdabc.net
Executive:
Chair: Tom Dutta
Ops Mgr: Catherine St. Denis
Exec Dir: Sophia Van Norden
Treas: Spencer Dane
IT Coord: Jenny West
Year Founded: 1983
No of Paid Staff: 7
Speakers Available
Library: Y *(Open to the public)*
Languages: English; Chinese; Punjabi
Membership: 1,600
Membership Fee: Consumer - $15; Supporter - $50; Professional/Agency - $25

Mood Disorders Association of Ontario Inc.
602-36 Eglinton Ave W, Toronto ON M4R 1A1
416 486-8046; Fax: 416 486-8127
Toll-free: 888 486-8236
E: info@mooddisorders.on.ca
W: www.mooddisorders.on.ca

HEALTHCARE ASSOCIATIONS

Executive:
Pres/Chair: Anne Davis
Exec Dir: Ann Marie MacDonald
Treas: Peter Lane
Info Res Mgr: Eric Jonasson
Coord Family Youth Prog: Leeanne Needham
Support Mgr: Kim Umbach
Year Founded: 1985
Criteria: *Individuals, friends and family members of people dealing with depression or bipolar disorder.*
No of Paid Staff: 5
Speakers Available
Library: Y
Languages: English
Membership: 250

North Shore Connection Society
1070 Roosevelt Cres, North Vancouver BC V7P 1M3
604 984-9321; Fax: 604 984-9882
W: www.nsconnexions.org
Executive:
Exec Dir: Mary Mullen
IT Mgr: Kar-On Lee
Year Founded: 1959
Languages: English

North Shore Schizophrenia Society
205-1865 Marine Dr, West Vancouver BC V7V 1J7
604 926-0856; Fax: 604 926-0856
E: info@northshoreschizophrenia.org
W: www.northshoreschizophrenia.org
Executive:
Exec Dir: Cheryl Olney
Coord: Marguerite Hardin
Year Founded: 1983
No of Paid Staff: 2
Speakers Available
Languages: English; French
Membership: 150
Library:
Family Support Centre *(Open to the public)*

The Ontario Mental Health Foundation (OMHF)
441 Jarvis St, Floor 2, Toronto ON M4Y 2G8
416 920-7721; Fax: 416 920-0026
E: grants@omhf.on.ca
W: www.omhf.on.ca
Executive:
Exec Dir: Alexander Greer
Grant Officer: Emmanuelle Fontaine
No of Paid Staff: 4
Languages: English
Membership: 11

Ontario Psychological Association (OPA)
403-21 St Clair Ave E, Toronto ON M4T 1L9
416 961-5552; Fax: 416 961-5516
Toll-free: 800 268-0069
W: www.psych.on.ca
Executive:
Pres: Dr Margaret Weiser
Exec Dir: Dr Ruth Berman
Publications Mgr: Carla Mardonet
Year Founded: 1947
Budget: $500,000
No of Paid Staff: 5
Languages: English
Membership list available to the public

Open Door Group
100-112 3rd Ave E, Vancouver BC V5T 1C8
604 872-0770; Fax: 604 873-1758
W: www.opendoorgroup.org

Executive:
Prog Dir: Adele Kok
Exec Dir: Tom Burnell
Year Founded: 1976
Criteria: *Good working, mental health supporters.*
No of Paid Staff: 68
Library: Y *(Open to the public)*
Languages: English
Membership: 15 *(Lists available to the public)*
Membership Fee: $10

Partners in Psychiatry
Plaza 1
440-2000 Argentia Rd, Mississauga ON L5N 1P7
905 826-0067; Fax: 905 826-4267
Executive:
Owner: David Mackenzie

Le Phare Saint-Hyacinthe et régions Inc.
620 av Robert, Saint-Hyacinthe QC J2S 4L8
450 773-7202; Fax: 450 773-5117
Toll-free: 877 773-7202
E: reception@lephare-apamm.ca
W: www.lephare-apamm.ca
Executive:
Dir gén: Jocelyne Collard

Psychologists' Association of Alberta
103-1207 91 St SW, Edmonton AB T6X 1E9
780 424-0294; Fax: 780 423-4048
Toll-free: 888 424-0297
Toll-free Fax: 888 423-4048
E: paa@psychologistsassociation.ab.ca
W: www.psychologistsassociation.ab.ca
Executive:
Exec Dir: Pierre Bérubé
Exec Asst/Fin Mgr: Linda Forsythe
Year Founded: 1996
No of Paid Staff: 5
Speakers Available
Languages: English
Membership: 2,000

Reconnect Mental Health Services
400-56 Aberfoyle Cres, Etobicoke ON M8X 2W4
416 248-2050; Fax: 416 248-6557
E: contact@reconnect.on.ca
W: www.reconnect.on.ca

Schizophrenia Society of Canada - Head Office
4 Fort St, Winnipeg MB R3C 1C4
204 786-1616; Fax: 204 783-4898
Toll-free: 800 263-5545
E: info@schizophrenia.ca
W: www.schizophrenia.ca
Executive:
CEO: Chris Summerville
No of Paid Staff: 2
Speakers Available
Languages: English; French
Membership list available to the public

◈Alberta:
309-8989 MacLeod Trail SW, Calgary AB T2H 0M2
403 264-5161 33; Fax: 403 269-1727
Toll-free: 800 661-4644
Toll-free Fax: 866 273-1780
E: info@schizophrenia.ab.ca
W: www.schizophrenia.ab.ca
Executive:
Exec Dir: Rubyann Rice
Fund Dev/Data Base Coord: Sian Anderson
Year Founded: 1989
No of Paid Staff: 4
Speakers Available
Library: Y

Languages: English
Membership: 75 *(Lists available to the public)*
Membership Fee: $20 yearly
Library:
Lending Library *(Open to the public)*

◈British Columbia:
201-6011 Westminster Hwy, Richmond BC V7C 4V4
604 270-7841; Fax: 604 270-9861
Toll-free: 888 888-0029
E: bcss.prov@telus.net
W: www.bcss.org
Executive:
Exec Dir: Jane Duval
Office Admin: Sally Hull
Year Founded: 1982
Budget: $1,500,000
No of Paid Staff: 22
Speakers Available
Languages: English
Membership: 1,600
Membership Fee: $20 per year

◈Brandon & Assiniboine Region
Mailing: PO Box 817, Souris MB R0K 2C0
204 483-4054; Fax: 204 483-5065
E: da_beetle@hotmail.com
Executive:
Outreach Worker: Deanna Kowalchuk
Languages: English; French

◈Burntwood Region
43 Fox Bay, Thompson MB R8N 1E9
204 677-6051; Fax: 204 677-5534
E: selfhelp@cmhathompson.ca
Languages: English; French

◈Central Region
Location: 309 Main St, Winkler MB R6W 4A4
Mailing: PO Box 129 Stn Main
204 362-3027; Fax: 204 325-8742
E: msscentral@mts.net
Executive:
Outreach Worker: Diane Findlay
Library: Y *(Open to the public)*
Languages: English; French
Membership list available to the public

◈Interlake Region
Mailing: PO Box 101 Stn Main, Selkirk MB R1A 2B1
204 485-1253; Fax: 204 334-7880
E: bevking@mts.net
Executive:
Outreach Worker: Bev King
Languages: English; French

◈Manitoba:
100-4 Fort St, Winnipeg MB R3C 1C4
204 786-1616; Fax: 204 783-4898
Toll-free: 800 263-5545 (in Manitoba)
E: info@mss.mb.ca
W: www.mss.mb.ca
Executive:
Exec Dir: Chris Summerville
Year Founded: 1979
No of Paid Staff: 12
Speakers Available
Library: Y *(Open to the public)*
Languages: English
Membership list available to the public
Membership Fee: Family - $25/year; Single - $15/year

◇Brandon & Assiniboine Region
Mailing: PO Box 817, Souris MB R0K 2C0
204 483-4054; Fax: 204 483-5065
E: da_beetle@hotmail.com
Executive:
Outreach Worker: Deanna Kowalchuk
Languages: English; French

◇ ***Burntwood Region***
43 Fox Bay, Thompson MB R8N 1E9
204 677-6051; Fax: 204 677-5534
E: selfhelp@cmhathompson.ca
Languages: English; French

◇ ***Central Region***
Location: 309 Main St, Winkler MB R6W 4A4
Mailing: PO Box 129 Stn Main
204 362-3027; Fax: 204 325-8742
E: msscentral@mts.net
Executive:
Outreach Worker: Diane Findlay
Library: Y *(Open to the public)*
Languages: English; French
Membership list available to the public

◇ ***Interlake Region***
Mailing: PO Box 101 Stn Main, Selkirk MB R1A 2B1
204 485-1253; Fax: 204 334-7880
E: bevking@mts.net
Executive:
Outreach Worker: Bev King
Languages: English; French

◇ ***Norman Region***
Mailing: PO Box 3372 Stn Main, The Pas MB R9A 1R9
204 623-7346; Fax: 204 623-5528
E: mssnor@mts.net
Executive:
Outreach Worker: Nancy Shewchuck
Languages: English; French

◇ ***North Eastman Region***
21 Loewen Blvd, Steinbach MB R5G 0L4
204 371-0824; Fax: 204 346-0423
E: eastmanmss@mts.net
Executive:
Outreach Worker: Kim Heidinger

◇ ***Parkland Region***
112 6th Ave NE, Dauphin MB R7N 0W6
204 638-0433; Fax: 204 638-0433
E: parkmantim@hotmail.com
Executive:
Outreach Worker: Tim Shewchuk
Languages: English; French

◇ ***SMHC Region***
Mailing: PO Box 9600 Stn Main, Selkirk MB R1A 2B5
204 482-3810 416; Fax: 204 886-3821
Executive:
Outreach Worker: Kathy Sing
Languages: English; French

◈ ***North Eastman Region***
21 Loewen Blvd, Steinbach MB R5G 0L4
204 371-0824; Fax: 204 346-0423
E: eastmanmss@mts.net
Executive:
Outreach Worker: Kim Heidinger

◈ ***Parkland Region***
112 6th Ave NE, Dauphin MB R7N 0W6
204 638-0433; Fax: 204 638-0433
E: parkmantim@hotmail.com
Executive:
Outreach Worker: Tim Shewchuk
Languages: English; French

◈ ***SMHC Region***
Mailing: PO Box 9600 Stn Main, Selkirk MB R1A 2B5
204 482-3810 416; Fax: 204 886-3821
Executive:
Outreach Worker: Kathy Sing
Languages: English; French

◈ ***New Brunswick:***
Location: 130 Duke St, Miramichi NB E1V 3T7
Mailing: PO Box 562 Stn Main
506 622-1595; Fax: 506 622-8927
E: ssnbmiramichi@nb.aibn.com
W: www.schizophreniasociety.nb.ca
Executive:
Pres: Barbara Johnson
Admin: Natalie Thibeau-Rector
Year Founded: 1993
No of Paid Staff: 1
Speakers Available
Library: Y *(Open to the public)*
Languages: English
Membership list available to the public

◈ ***Newfoundland and Labrador:***
Location: 48 Kenmount Rd, St. John's NL A1B 1X0
Mailing: PO Box 28029
709 777-3335; Fax: 709 777-3524
E: info@ssnl.org
W: www.ssnl.org
Executive:
Exec Dir: Dave Banko
Year Founded: 1997
Criteria: *$15 per family, $10 per individual per year*
No of Paid Staff: 3
Speakers Available
Languages: English
Membership: 200
Membership Fee: Single - $10; Family - $15

◈ ***Nova Scotia:***
Location: E.C. Purdy Bldg, 300 Pleasant St, Room B23, Dartmouth NS B2Y 3S3
Mailing: PO Box 1004 Stn Main, Dartmouth NS B2Y 3Z9
902 465-2601; Fax: 902 465-5479
Toll-free: 800 465-2601 Within Nova Scotia
E: ssns@ns.sympatico.ca
W: www.ssns.ca
Executive:
Exec Dir: Dr Stephen Ayer
Year Founded: 1982
No of Paid Staff: 2
Speakers Available
Library: Y *(Open to the public)*
Languages: English
Membership: 180
Membership Fee: $10

◈ ***Ontario:***
302-130 Spadina Ave, Toronto ON M5V 2L4
800 449-6367; Fax: 416 449-8434
E: sso@schizophrenia.on.ca
W: www.schizophrenia.on.ca
Executive:
Pres: Norm Tasevski
Exec Dir: Mary Alberti
Year Founded: 1979
Criteria: *Family members, persons with schizophrenia, professionals.*
Budget: $2,500,000
No of Paid Staff: 30
Speakers Available
Languages: English
Membership: 1,500

◈ ***Prince Edward Island:***
Location: 92 Queen St, Floor 2, Charlottetown PE C1A 4B1
Mailing: PO Box 25020 Rpo Confederation, Charlottetown PE C1A 9N4
902 368-5850; Fax: 902 368-5467
E: schizophreniapei@pei.aibn.com
W: www.schizophrenia.ca
Year Founded: 1984
No of Paid Staff: 1
Speakers Available
Languages: English
Membership: 80
Membership Fee: $15 family; $10 single

◈ ***Quebec:***
Pavillon Bédard
7401 rue Hochelaga, Montréal QC H1N 3M5
514 251-4000 3400; Fax: 514 251-6347
Toll-free: 866 888-2323
E: info@schizophrenie.qc.ca
W: www.schizophrenie.qc.ca
Executive:
Dir gén: Francine Dubé
Year Founded: 1988
Criteria: *Famille et amis d'une personne atteinte de schizophrénie.*
No of Paid Staff: 5
Library: Y *(Open to the public)*
Languages: French
Membership: 820
Library:
Centre de documentation

◈ ***Saskatchewan:***
Location: 2123 Broad St, Regina SK S4P 1Y6
Mailing: PO Box 305 Stn Main, Regina SK S4P 3A1
306 584-2620; Fax: 306 584-0525
Toll-free: 877 584-2620
E: sssprov@sasktel.net
W: www.schizophrenia.sk.ca
Executive:
Exec Dir: Anita Hopfauf
Year Founded: 1982
Criteria: *none*
Budget: $300,000
No of Paid Staff: 5
Speakers Available
Library: Y *(Open to the public)*
Languages: English

◇ ***Saskatoon:***
219-230 Avenue R S, Saskatoon SK S7M 2Z1
306 374-2224; Fax: 306 477-5649
E: ssssaskatoon@sasktel.net
W: www.schizophrenia.sk.ca
Executive:
Coord: Ashlee Schmidt
Year Founded: 1982
Budget: $220,000
No of Paid Staff: 5
Speakers Available
Library: Y *(Open to the public)*
Languages: English
Membership: 264

STRIDE - Supported Training & Rehabilitation in Diverse Environments
388 Main St E, Milton ON L9T 1P8
905 693-4252; Fax: 905 693-9183
W: www.stride.on.ca
Executive:
Mgr South Halton: Mark Cox
Mgr North Halton: Jan McCabe
Exec Dir: Anita Lloyd
Year Founded: 1983
Languages: English

Tema Conter Memorial Trust
Location: 18 Doctors Lane, King City ON L7B 1G2
Mailing: PO Box 265 Stn Main, King City ON L7B 1A5
Fax: 905 893-1574
Toll-free: 888 288-8036
E: info@tema.ca
W: www.tema.ca
Executive:
Exec Dir: Vince Savoia
Languages: English

Winnserv Inc.
101-960 Portage Ave, Winnipeg MB R3G 0R4
204 783-8654; Fax: 204 786-8770
E: winnserv@shawcable.com
W: www.winnserv.ca
Executive:
Exec Dir: Karen Kowalchuk
Office Mgr: Toni Marks
Accnt: Joanne Minkus
Prog Coord: Leslie Udell
Prog Coord: Lorne Deviaene
Prog Coord: Lynn Woods

REHABILITATION

Ability Resource Centre - Div. of Rehabilitation Society of Southwestern Alberta
1610 29 St N, Lethbridge AB T1H 5L3
403 329-3911; Fax: 403 329-3581
E: staff@rehab.ab.ca
W: www.abilityresource.ca
Executive:
Ops Mgr: Irwin Wyrostok
Exec Dir: Ed Hinger
Year Founded: 1953
No of Paid Staff: 80
Languages: English

Alberta Athletic Therapists Association
Location: 402-1040 7 Ave SW, Calgary AB T2P 3G9
Mailing: PO Box 61115 RPO Kensington, Calgary AB T2N 4S6
403 440-6626; Fax: 403 440-6955
W: www.aata.ca
Executive:
Pres: Breda Lau
Treas: Kevin Wagner
Sec: Maggie Dunlop
Languages: English

Alberta College of Occupational Therapists
300-10436 81 Ave NW, Edmonton AB T6E 1X6
780 436-8381; Fax: 780 434-0658
Toll-free: 800 561-5429
E: info@acot.ca
W: www.acot.ca
Executive:
Registrar: Maggie Fulford
No of Paid Staff: 5
Speakers Available
Languages: English
Membership: 1,300
Membership Fee: $499 Year

Alberta Council of Disability Services
19-3220 5 Ave NE, Calgary AB T2A 5N1
403 250-9495; Fax: 403 291-9864
E: acds@acds.ca
W: www.acds.ca
Executive:
CEO: Ann Nicol
Year Founded: 1972
Criteria: *General Membership: Organizations in Alberta who primarily serve/support persons with disabilities.*
No of Paid Staff: 9
Languages: English
Membership: 115 *(Lists available to the public)*

Beit Halochem Canada, Aid to Disabled Veterans of Israel
219-1600 Steeles Ave W, Concord ON L4K 4M2
905 695-0611; Fax: 905 695-0612
Toll-free: 800 355-1648
E: info@beithalochem.ca
W: www.beithalochem.ca
Executive:
Pres: Toby Feldberg
Exec VP: Diane Shiffman
VP: Julia Sax
VP: Carolyn Lengyel
Exec Dir: Lisa Levy
Treas: Victor Peters
Sec: Rena Godfrey
Year Founded: 1978
No of Paid Staff: 3
Speakers Available
Library: Y *(Open to the public)*
Languages: English
Membership: 25 *(Lists available to the public)*

Canadian Association of Occupational Therapists
CTTC Bldg
3400-1125 Colonel By Dr, Ottawa ON K1S 5R1
613 523-2268; Fax: 613 523-2552
Toll-free: 800 434-2268
E: membership@caot.ca
W: www.caot.ca
Executive:
Exec Dir: Claudia von Zweck
Admn Mgr: Suzanne Kay
Year Founded: 1926
Criteria: *Graduation from an occupational therapy program accredited by CAOT or recognized by the World Federation of Occupational Therapists, successful completion of CAOT Certification Examination following completion of academic qualifications, payment of membership fee.*
Budget: $2,800,000
No of Paid Staff: 18
Languages: English
Membership: 7,600 *(Lists available to the public)*
Membership Fee: Varies

◊ Canadian Occupational Therapy Foundation
CTTC Bldg
3401-1125 Colonel By Dr, Ottawa ON K1S 5R1
613 523-2268; Fax: 613 523-2552
Toll-free: 800 434-2268
E: skamble@cotfcanada.org
W: www.cotfcanada.org
Executive:
Pres: Juliette Cooper
Exec Dir: Sangita Kamblé
Year Founded: 1983
Criteria: *All donors are members.*
Budget: $200,000
No of Paid Staff: 2
Speakers Available
Languages: English
Membership: 200

Canadian Athletic Therapists Association - National Office
402-1040 7 Ave SW, Calgary AB T2P 3G9
403 509-2282; Fax: 403 509-2280
E: info@athletictherapy.org
W: www.athletictherapy.org
Executive:
Exec Dir: Sandy Jespersen
Admv Asst: Helena De Fazio
Year Founded: 1963
Criteria: *Certified athletic therapist or certification Candidate with the CATA*
No of Paid Staff: 2
Speakers Available
Languages: English; French
Membership: 1,650
Membership Fee: $60/year

Canadian Council on Rehabilitation and Work
1202-1 Yonge St, Toronto ON M5E 1E5
416 260-3060; Fax: 416 260-3093
Toll-free: 800 664-0925
E: info@ccrw.org
W: www.ccrw.org
Executive:
Pres/CEO: Carole J Barron
Criteria: *Completion of membership application and payment of fees which covers a year's membership.*
Membership Fee Required: Y
Budget: $21,400,000
No of Paid Staff: 10
Speakers Available
Languages: English; French
Membership: 180
Library:
CCRW Reference Library

Canadian Physiotherapy Association
270-955 Green Valley Cres, Ottawa ON K2C 3V4
613 564-5454; Fax: 613 564-1577
Toll-free: 800 387-8679
E: information@physiotherapy.ca
W: www.physiotherapy.ca
Executive:
Pres: Rob Werstine
Year Founded: 1920
Criteria: *Different requirements based on type of member.*
Membership Fee Required: Y
No of Paid Staff: 30
Languages: English; French
Membership: 10,000

◊ British Columbia:
Business Bldg
402-1755 Broadway W, Vancouver BC V6J 4S5
604 736-5130; Fax: 604 736-5606
E: info@bcphysio.org
W: www.bcphysio.org
Executive:
CEO: Rebecca Tunnacliffe
Budget: $3,750,000
No of Paid Staff: 3
Languages: English
Membership: 2,000

◊ Newfoundland/Labrador:
Mailing: PO Box 28117 RPO Avalon Mall, St. John's NL A1B 4J8
Fax: 709 777-5920
Executive:
Pres: Sandra Gosse
Exec Dir: Lisa Pike
Speakers Available
Languages: English

◊ Saskatchewan:
118-1121 College Dr, Saskatoon SK S7N 0W3
306 955-7265; Fax: 306 955-7260
E: info@saskphysio.org
W: www.saskphysio.org
Executive:
Exec Dir: Lorna MacMillan
Criteria: *Must be a physiotherapist.*
No of Paid Staff: 1
Languages: English
Membership: 430
Membership Fee: $200

Centre Corps Âme et Esprit
595 côte de Beauvoir, Sherbrooke QC J1C 0B8
819 563-3323; Fax: 819 563-8260
E: ccae@abacom.com
W: www.corpsameesprit.ca

College of Occupational Therapists of Ontario
900-20 Bay St, Box 78, Toronto ON M5J 2N8
416 214-1177; Fax: 416 214-1173
Toll-free: 800 890-6570
E: info@coto.org
W: www.coto.org
Executive:
Registrar: Barb Worth
Year Founded: 1993
Budget: $1,400,000
No of Paid Staff: 12
Speakers Available
Languages: English; French
Membership list available to the public
Library:
Resource Room *(Open to the public)*

College of Physical Therapists of Alberta
Weber Centre
300-10357 109 St NW, Edmonton AB T5J 1N3
780 438-0338; Fax: 780 436-1908
E: info@physiotherapyalberta.ca
W: www.physiotherapyalberta.ca
Executive:
Registrar: Dianne Millette
Asst Registrar: Joyce Vogelgesang
Criteria: *Open to anyone with a degree in physical therapy.*
No of Paid Staff: 4
Languages: English
Membership: 1,800
Membership Fee: Inactive - $75; Active - $325

College of Physiotherapists of Manitoba
211-675 Pembina Hwy, Winnipeg MB R3M 2L6
204 287-8502; Fax: 204 474-2506
E: assocphysiomb@shaw.ca
W: www.manitobaphysio.com
Executive:
Registrar/Exec Dir: Brenda McKechnie
Office Mgr: Virginia Kaskiw
No of Paid Staff: 2
Languages: English
Membership: 700
Membership Fee: $300 per year

Golden Opportunity Vocational Rehabilitation Centre
Location: 32 Miner's Memorial Dr, Springhill NS B0M 1X0
Mailing: PO Box 887
902 597-3158; Fax: 902 597-2950
E: govrcworkshop10660@ns.aliantzinc.ca
Executive:
Exec Dir: Joanne Hunter
Year Founded: 1985
Budget: $500,000
No of Paid Staff: 3
Languages: English
Membership: 13 board members *(Lists available to the public)*

Manitoba Athletic Therapists Association
145 Pacific Ave, Winnipeg MB R3B 2Z6
204 925-5930
E: mail@mata.mb.ca
W: www.mata.mb.ca
Executive:
Pres: Dr Glen Bergeron
Prog Coord: Stephanie Somerville
Languages: English

Manitoba Physiotherapy Association
145 Pacific Ave, Winnipeg MB R3B 2Z6
204 925-5701; Fax: 204 925-5624
Toll-free: 877 925-5701 Manitoba only
E: ptassociation@mbphysio.org
W: www.mbphysio.org
Executive:
Pres: Lindo Catteeuw
Exec Dir: Merle MacAulay
Year Founded: 1954
Criteria: *Graduate physiotherapists.*
No of Paid Staff: 2
Speakers Available
Library: Y
Languages: English
Membership: 452 *(Lists available to the public)*
Membership Fee: $210

Manitoba Society of Occupational Therapists
7-120 Maryland St, Winnipeg MB R3G 1L1
204 957-1214; Fax: 204 775-2340
E: msot@msot.mb.ca
W: msot.mb.ca
Executive:
Contact: Sharon Eadie
Year Founded: 1963
Criteria: *Membership is open to occupational therapists.*
Budget: $30,000
Speakers Available
Languages: English
Membership: 305 *(Lists available to the public)*
Membership Fee: $60

Massage Therapist Association of Saskatchewan Inc
16-1724 Quebec Ave, Saskatoon SK S7K 1V9
306 384-7077; Fax: 306 384-7175
E: mtas@sasktel.net
W: www.saskmassagetherapy.com
Executive:
Pres: Julianne Heagy
VP: Christina Battyanie
Exec Dir: Lori Green
Treas: Kyla McDonald
Sec: Marles Kerns
Year Founded: 1966
No of Paid Staff: 2
Speakers Available
Languages: English
Membership: 813

Massage Therapists' Association of British Columbia
Airport Square
180-1200 73rd Ave W, Vancouver BC V6P 6G5
604 873-4467; Fax: 604 873-6211
Toll-free: 888 413-4467
E: mta@massagetherapy.bc.ca
W: www.massagetherapy.bc.ca
Executive:
Exec Dir: Brenda Locke
Mgr: Dee Willock
Year Founded: 1982
No of Paid Staff: 4
Speakers Available
Library: Y
Languages: English
Membership: 1,000

Massage Therapists' Association of Nova Scotia
Location: 700-6009 Quinpool Rd, Halifax NS B3K 5J7
Mailing: PO Box 9410 RPO CSC, Halifax NS B3K 5S3
902 429-2190; Fax: 902 425-2441
E: info@mtans.com
W: www.mtans.com
Executive:
Exec Dir: Donna Noddin
Languages: English

N.B. Massotherapy Association
Mailing: PO Box 353 Stn A, Fredericton NB E3B 4Z9
855 642-2662
Toll-free: 855 642-2662
E: info@nbma-amnb.ca
W: www.nbma-amnb.ca
Year Founded: 1988
Criteria: *Must be a registered massage therapist.*
No of Paid Staff: 2
Speakers Available
Languages: English; French
Membership: 224

New Brunswick Association of Occupational Therapists
Mailing: PO Box 184 Stn A, Fredericton NB E3B 4Y9
506 458-1001; Fax: 506 455-8846
E: info@nbaot.org
W: www.nbaot.org/
Executive:
Exec Asst: Suzanne Lateigne-Rioux
Languages: English

Newfoundland and Labrador Massage Therapists' Association
Mailing: PO Box 23212 RPO Churchill Sq, St. John's NL A1B 4J9
709 726-4006; Fax: 709 747-7767
E: nlmta@nlmta.ca
W: www.nlmta.ca
Executive:
Pres: Claudette Marie Warren
VP: Pamela Frampton
Treas: Pat Mennie
Year Founded: 1990
Languages: English
Membership: 128

Northern Association of Occupational Therapists (NAOT)
Location: Stanton Territorial Hospital, 550 Byrne Rd, Yellowknife NT X1A 2N1
Mailing: PO Box 10 Stn Main
867 669-4340; Fax: 867 669-4137
W: www.caot.ca
Executive:
Pres/Occup Ther: Amanda Johnson
Languages: English
Membership: 14
Membership Fee: $75

Nova Scotia Society of Occupational Therapists
2132B-6960 Mumford Rd, Halifax NS B3L 4P1
902 453-4537; Fax: 902 453-5899
Toll-free: 866 936-7768
E: nssot@nssot.ca
W: www.nssot.ca

Executive:
Pres Elect: Danielle Bissonnette
Pres: Jen Davis
Exec Dir: Anne Carswell
Treas: Meghan Bedun
Recording Sec: Vanessa McDermott
Corresponding Sec: Tania Angelucci
Office Mgr: Michelle Bregante
Rep East: Jennifer Keirstead
Rep West: Stephanie Anthony-Brown
Rep North: Sean Murphy
Languages: English

Ontario Athletic Therapists Association
498-283 Danforth Ave, Toronto ON M4K 1N2
905 845-4993
W: www.athletictherapist.on.ca
Executive:
Pres: Drew Laskoski
Exec VP: Paul Papoutsakis
VP-Fin: Andrea Prieur
VP-Mktg/Commun: Nelson Amaral
Languages: English
Membership: 550

Ontario Physiotherapy Association (OPA)
210-55 Eglinton Ave E, Toronto ON M4P 1G8
416 322-6866; Fax: 416 322-6705
E: physiomail@opa.on.ca
W: www.opa.on.ca
Executive:
Pres: Amanda Smart
CEO: Dorianne Sauvé
Corp Admin: Diane Unção
Sec: Christina Boyle
Board Member Kawartha/Quinte/St Lawrence: Mark Scheer
Board Member Hamilton/London/Niagara: Stephen Patton
Board Member Georgian Bay/Kitchener/Waterloo: Michael Major
Board Member Durham/York/Scarborough: Allan MacDonald
Board Member Eastern Ont: Liam Dessureault
Board Member Central Toronto/Grey Bruce: Joshua Williams
Prog/Mktg/Commun Mgr: Sara Pulins
Year Founded: 1920
Criteria: *Member of the Canadian Physiotherapy Association.*
No of Paid Staff: 5
Speakers Available
Library: Y *(Open to the public)*
Languages: English
Membership: 4,500
Membership Fee: $30
Library:
OPA

Ontario Society of Occupational Therapists
210-55 Eglinton Ave E, Toronto ON M4P 1G8
416 322-3011; Fax: 416 322-6705
Toll-free: 877 676-6768
E: osot@osot.on.ca
W: www.osot.on.ca
Executive:
Exec Dir: Christie Brenchley
Year Founded: 1921
Budget: $563,000
No of Paid Staff: 5
Library: Y
Languages: English
Membership: 3,100
Membership Fee: $176

Ordre professionnel de la physiothérapie du Québec
1000-7151 rue Jean-Talon E, Anjou QC H1M 3N8
514 351-2770; Fax: 514 351-2658
Toll-free: 800 361-2001
E: physio@oppq.qc.ca
W: www.oppq.qc.ca
Executive:
Prés: Lucie Forget
Dir gén/Sec de l'ordre: Claude Laurent
Dir serv admin: Dominique Serres
Dir commun: Thierry Vogler
Agente de commun: Sandra Chabannel
Asst à la dir gén: Caroline Forant
Year Founded: 1973
Budget: $4,000,000
No of Paid Staff: 26
Speakers Available
Languages: French
Membership list available to the public

Prince Edward Island Occupational Therapy Society
Mailing: PO Box 2248 Stn Central, Charlottetown PE C1A 8B9
902 892-1266
E: ycthompson@ihis.org
W: www.peiot.org
Executive:
Sec: Yvonne Thompson
Languages: English

Prison Fellowship Canada
5700-100 King St W, Toronto ON M5X 1C7
416 915-4102; Fax: 416 915-4103
Toll-free: 877 858-2891
E: info@prisonfellowship.ca
W: www.prisonfellowship.ca
Executive:
Co-Chair Board: Jennifer Jackson
Co-Chair Board: Michael Van Dusen
Exec Dir/CEO: Rev Eleanor Clitheroe
Dir Inmate Serv: Rick Arsenault
Man Dir: Judith Laus
Dir-Commun/Church Engagement: Stacey Campbell
Year Founded: 1980
Languages: English

Quebec Corporation of Athletic Therapists
165-7141 rue Sherbrooke O, Montréal QC H4B 1R6
514 848-2424 3311
E: admin@ctsq.qc.ca
W: www.ctsq.qc.ca
Executive:
Prés: Jaime Sochasky-Livingston
VP: Joan Seaman
Adj admin: Andrea Miller
Criteria: *Licensed athletic therapist or student in an undergraduate athletic therapy program.*
No of Paid Staff: 1
Speakers Available
Languages: English; French
Membership: 250

Registered Massage Therapists' Association of Ontario (RMTAO)
2943B Bloor St W, Toronto ON M8X 1B3
416 979-2010; Fax: 416 979-1144
Toll-free: 800 668-2022
E: info@rmtao.com
W: www.rmtao.com
Executive:
Exec Dir: Bryn Sumpton
Year Founded: 1936
Criteria: *Registered massage therapists in Ontario or students in recognized Ontario schools of massage therapy.*
Speakers Available
Languages: English
Membership: 1,400
Membership Fee: $350

Saskatchewan Association of Rehabilitation Centres/Sarcan
111 Cardinal Cres, Saskatoon SK S7L 6H5
306 933-0616; Fax: 306 653-3932
Toll-free: 800 667-3016 (Sask. only)
E: contact@sarcan.sk.ca
W: www.sarcsarcan.ca
Executive:
Exec Dir: Amy McNeil
Dir-Ops: Ken Homenick
Dir-Fin: Bob Hnetka
Year Founded: 1968
Criteria: *Facilities that provide support, training, activity or residential services to adults with disabilities.*
Budget: $12,000,000
No of Paid Staff: 365
Speakers Available
Languages: English
Membership: 73 *(Lists available to the public)*
Membership Fee: $200 per year

Saskatchewan Athletic Therapists Association
Mailing: PO Box 687 Stn Main, White City SK S4L 5B1
306 921-4881
E: dpitura@sasktel.net
W: www.saskathletictherapy.ca
Executive:
Pres: Dale Pitura
Registrar: Trevor Len
Treas: Chris Facca
Languages: English

Saskatchewan Society of Occupational Therapists (SSOT)
Mailing: PO Box 9089 Stn Main, Saskatoon SK S7K 7E7
306 956-7768
E: admin@ssot.sk.ca
W: www.ssot.sk.ca
Executive:
Pres: Sherry Just
Pres Elect: Jason Greville
Registrar: Jesse Dziad
Exec Dir/Sec-Treas: Coralie Lennea
Year Founded: 1971
Criteria: *Degree or equivalent in OT and completion of approved exams.*
Budget: $125,000
No of Paid Staff: 2
Speakers Available
Languages: English
Membership: 260 *(Lists available to the public)*
Membership Fee: $372 - Fulltime membership

SOCIAL ACTIVISM

Action Life Ottawa Inc.
1000 Brookfield Rd, Floor 2, Ottawa ON K1V 6J1
613 798-4494; Fax: 613 798-4496
E: info@actionlife.org
W: www.actionlife.org
Year Founded: 1971
Budget: $160,000
No of Paid Staff: 2
Speakers Available
Languages: English; French
Membership: 4,000
Membership Fee: $20

Alberni Valley Citizen Advocacy Society
5038 Argyle St, Port Alberni BC V9Y 1V4
250 723-8614; Fax: 250 723-8614
E: avcas@shaw.ca
Year Founded: 1967
Budget: $60,000
No of Paid Staff: 2
Speakers Available
Languages: English
Membership: 30 *(Lists available to the public)*
Membership Fee: $2/year

Alliance for Life Ontario
26 Norfolk St, Guelph ON N1H 4H8
519 824-7797; Fax: 519 836-2716
Toll-free: 800 665-0570 Pregnancy help-line
E: aflo@mgl.ca
W: www.allianceforlife.org
Executive:
Pres: Hetty Meijaard
Exec Dir: Jakki Jeffs
Treas: Michelle Knaap
Sec: Jennifer Snell
Criteria: *Open to all.*
Budget: $85,000
No of Paid Staff: 2
Speakers Available
Library: Y *(Open to the public)*
Languages: English
Membership list available to the public

Association d'Entraide le Chaînon Inc.
4373 av de l'Esplanade, Montréal QC H2W 1T2
514 845-0151; Fax: 514 844-4180
E: info@lechainon.org
W: www.lechainon.org
Executive:
Pres du conseil: René Goulet
Dir gén: Marcèle Lamarche
Trés: Monique Bérubé
Coord/Sec/Campagne de fin: Lynda Isabel
Adj: Marthe Menard
Year Founded: 1932
Budget: $2,000,000
No of Paid Staff: 85
Speakers Available
Languages: French
Membership: 40

Brant Right to Life Association
107 Wellington St, Brantford ON N3T 2M1
519 752-3041; Fax: 519 759-4863
Executive:
Pres: Linda Tensen
VP: Paul Vandervet
Budget: $1,200,000
Speakers Available
Library: Y *(Open to the public)*
Languages: English

CHF - Canadian Hunger Foundation
323 Chapel St, Ottawa ON K1N 7Z2
613 237-0180; Fax: 613 237-5969
Toll-free: 866 242-4243
E: info@chf.ca
W: www.chf.ca
Executive:
Pres/CEO: Garry Comber
Dir-Fin: M Forbes
Dir-Bus Dev: C Farrell
Commun Spec: Michael Jones
Year Founded: 1961
No of Paid Staff: 21
Languages: English

Canada Without Poverty
251 Bank St, Floor 2, Ottawa ON K2P 1X3
613 789-0096; Fax: 613 244-5777
Toll-free: 800 810-1076
E: info@cwp-csp.ca
W: www.cwp-csp.ca
Executive:
Exec Dir: Leilani Fartha
Dir-Partnerships/Dev: Rob Rainer
Year Founded: 1971
Criteria: *Regular members are those who are living in poverty. Associate members are those wo do not live in poverty wishing to support NAPO's work. Group membership - any group of low-income people and other non-profit organization with interest in poverty issues.*
No of Paid Staff: 3
Speakers Available
Languages: English; French
Membership: 3,600
Membership Fee: $2-$50
Library:
NAPO Resource Centre *(Open to the public)*

Canadians for Choice
Mailing: 251 Bank St, Floor 2, Ottawa ON K2P 1X3
613 789-9958; Fax: 613 566-3449
Toll-free: 888 642-2725
E: info@canadiansforchoice.ca
W: www.canadiansforchoice.ca
Executive:
A-Exec Dir: Agathe Gramet Kedzior
Year Founded: 2002
No of Paid Staff: 2
Speakers Available
Languages: English; French

Chisasibi Telecommunications Association
Location: 5 ch Center, étage 2, Chisasibi QC J0M 1E0
Mailing: CP 420
819 855-2527; Fax: 819 855-3186
Executive:
Four données: Raymond Menarick

Daily Bread Food Bank
191 New Toronto St, Toronto ON M8V 2E7
416 203-0050; Fax: 416 203-0049
E: info@dailybread.ca
W: www.dailybread.ca
Executive:
Mktg/Commun Mgr: Sarah Anderson
Exec Dir: Gail Nyberg
Year Founded: 1983
No of Paid Staff: 50
Speakers Available
Languages: English

Dying With Dignity Canada
802-55 Eglinton Ave E, Toronto ON M4P 1G8
416 486-3998; Fax: 416 486-5562
Toll-free: 800 495-6156
E: info@dyingwithdignity.ca
W: www.dyingwithdignity.ca
Executive:
Exec Dir: Wanda Morris
Client Support Prog Mgr: Margaret Johnston-Jones
Membership/Office Coord: Trudie Ross
Year Founded: 1980
No of Paid Staff: 2
Speakers Available
Languages: English
Membership: 4,000
Library:
DWD Library *(Open to the public)*

Environmentalists For Nuclear Energy (Canada) Inc.
1940 Hill 60, RR 5, Cobourg ON K9A 4J8
905 372-2410; Fax: 905 372-6274
E: nuc-ca@ecolo.org
W: www.ecolo.org/base/baseca.htm
Executive:
Founder: Rodney Anderson

Federation Of Northern Ontario Municipalities
Mailing: 88 Riverside Dr, Kapuskasing ON P5N 1B3
705 337-4252; Fax: 705 337-1741
E: fonom.info@gmail.com
W: www.fonom.org
Executive:
Sec: Barbara Major

Fighting Antisemitism Together
Location: 100 King St W, Floor 68, Toronto ON M5X 1A1
Mailing: PO Box 1 Stn 1st Can Place
416 867-7654; Fax: 416 867-5859
E: tony.comper@bmo.com
W: www.fightingantisemitism.com
Executive:
Co-Founder: Elizabeth Comper
Co-Founder: Tony Comper
Sr Admn Mgr: Nancy Greco
Year Founded: 2005
Languages: English

Fredericton Anti-Poverty Organization
242 Gibson St, Fredericton NB E3A 4E3
506 458-9102
E: fapo@antipoverty.com
W: www.antipoverty.com
Executive:
Chairman: Miriam McNeil
Treas: Peter Keith
Sec: Melynda Jarratt
Member-at-Large: Brenda Brawn
Member-at-Large: April Boone
Languages: English

Le Groupe Communautaire L'Itinéraire
2103 rue Sainte-Catherine E, Montréal QC H2K 2H9
514 597-0238; Fax: 514 597-1544
E: itineraire@itineraire.ca
W: www.itineraire.ca
Executive:
Dir: Serge Lareault
Adj: Sylvie Gamache

Hunger In Moose Jaw Inc.
269 Stadacona St W, Moose Jaw SK S6H 1Z4
306 692-1916; Fax: 306 694-0130
E: hunger.moosejaw@sasktel.net
Executive:
Admin: Carol Acton
Criteria: *Open to all.*
No of Paid Staff: 2
Speakers Available
Languages: English

International Centre for the Eradication of Poverty
83 Kingslake Rd, Toronto ON M2J 3E6
416 494-4763; Fax: 416 494-2185
E: bubale@pathcom.com
W: www.eradicatepoverty.org
Executive:
Pres: Dr Bhausaheb Ubale
Languages: English; French

La Montée

B-127 rue Galarneau, Saint-Pacôme QC G0L 3X0
418 852-2866; Fax: 418 852-2898
E: lamontee@videotron.ca
W: www.centrelamontee.com
Executive:
Chef dir: Réjeanne Hudon

Langley Pro-Life Society

Location: 20595 Fraser Hwy, Langley BC V3A 4G4
Mailing: PO Box 26012 RPO Langley Mall, Langley BC V3A 8J2
604 534-1195; Fax: 604 534-0028
E: langleyprolife@shaw.ca
W: www.langleyprolife.org
Executive:
Dir: Cathy Hetzler
Year Founded: 1979
Languages: English

Lethbridge and District Pro-Life Association

1801 9 Ave N, Lethbridge AB T1H 1H8
403 320-5433
Toll-free: 877 889-6626
E: lprolife@shaw.ca
W: www.lifelethbridge.org
Year Founded: 1977
No of Paid Staff: 3
Speakers Available
Library: Y *(Open to the public)*
Languages: English
Membership: 1,000
Membership Fee: $20 Year

MADD Canada - National Office

500-2010 Winston Park Dr, Oakville ON L6H 5R7
905 829-8805; Fax: 905 829-8860
Toll-free: 800 665-6233
E: info@madd.ca
W: www.madd.ca
Executive:
CEO: Andrew Murie
Victim Servs Mgr: Gloria Appleby
Year Founded: 1992
Criteria: *Open to all.*
Budget: $12,000,000
No of Paid Staff: 17
Speakers Available
Languages: English; French

◈ ***Edmonton & Area Chapter***
Strathcona Business Park
6-3908 97 St NW, Edmonton AB T6E 6N2
780 488-6233 221; Fax: 780 488-6040
E: maddedm@telus.net
W: www.madd.ca
Year Founded: 2001
No of Paid Staff: 1
Speakers Available
Library: Y *(Open to the public)*
Languages: English
Membership: 75-100 *(Lists available to the public)*
Membership Fee: $20

◈ ***MADD Alberta:***
Languages: English

◇ ***Calgary:***
Mailing: 6528 11 St NE, Calgary AB T2E 7J4
403 278-8081; Fax: 403 278-8891
E: info@maddcalgary.ca
W: www.maddcalgary.ca
Executive:
Pres: Terry Hughes
Year Founded: 2001
No of Paid Staff: 1
Speakers Available
Languages: English

◇ ***Cold Lake Region:***
Mailing: PO Box 8398 RPO Marine Lake, Cold Lake AB T9M 1N2
780 639-3202
E: maddcoldlake@gmail.com
W: www.madd.ca
Executive:
Pres: Germaine Gervais
VP: Beverly McKeown
Treas: Tammylin Gaudry
Sec: Heather-Lynn Rogers
Year Founded: 2001
Library: Y *(Open to the public)*
Languages: English
Membership: 18

◇ ***Medicine Hat & District:***
12-3307 Dunmore Rd SE, Medicine Hat AB T1B 3R2
403 504-4000; Fax: 403 548-3410
E: maddmh@telusplanet.net
W: www.maddmh.ca
Year Founded: 2004
Languages: English

◇ ***Red Deer & District:***
Location: CIRS Bldg, 4728 Ross St, Red Deer AB T4N 1S5
Mailing: PO Box 1115, Stn Postal Box Ctr, Red Deer AB T4N 6S5
403 347-9922; Fax: 403 347-9234
E: maddrd@telusplanet.net
Executive:
Pres: Aleta Neville
VP: Stacey Ferguson
Treas: Donna Meeder
Year Founded: 1993
No of Paid Staff: 1
Speakers Available
Languages: English

◇ ***Taber/Lethbridge & District:***
Location: Police Station, 5700 50 Ave, Taber AB T1G 2H7
Mailing: PO Box 4587 Stn Main, Taber AB T1G 2C9
403 223-0201; Fax: 403 223-5902
E: maddtaberlethbridge@telus.net
W: www.madd.ca
Executive:
Pres: Tracie Baceda
Year Founded: 1999
Languages: English

◈ ***MADD British Columbia:***
Languages: English

◇ ***Central Okanagan:***
Mailing: 9-3151 Lakeshore Rd, Suite 251, Kelowna BC V1W 3S9
250 317-9877
E: infomaddokanagan@gmail.com
W: www.madd.ca
Executive:
Pres: Carol Fazekas
Sec: Julie Johnson
Year Founded: 1997
Speakers Available
Languages: English

◇ ***Greater Vancouver:***
Mailing: PO Box 78043 RPO Northside, Port Coquitlam BC V3B 7H5
604 515-9212; Fax: 604 515-9213
E: maddvancouver@gmail.com
W: www.madd.ca/vancouver
Executive:
Pres: Manon Groulx
Year Founded: 1997
Speakers Available
Languages: English
Membership: 150
Membership Fee: $5

◇ ***North Island:***
Location: 7250 Market St, Port Hardy BC V0N 2P0
Mailing: PO Box 155
250 949-7789; Fax: 250 949-2617
Toll-free: 877 949-7789
E: MADD.NI.Chapter@gmail.com
W: www.madd.ca
Executive:
Pres: Norm Prince
Year Founded: 2001
Languages: English

◇ ***Upper Fraser Valley:***
8991 Young Rd, Chilliwack BC V2P 4R9
604 847-3784; Fax: 604 847-3785
E: info@madd-ufv.com
W: www.maddufv.com
Executive:
Pres: Angelina Bowen
Year Founded: 1999
Speakers Available
Library: Y *(Open to the public)*
Languages: English
Membership: 20

◈ ***MADD Manitoba:***
Languages: English

◇ ***Winnipeg:***
202-2621 Portage Ave, Winnipeg MB R3J 0P7
204 896-6233; Fax: 204 832-9235
E: maddwinnipeg@shaw.ca
W: www.madd.ca/winnipeg
Executive:
Pres: Melody Bodnarchuk
VP: Karen Magnusson
Past VP: Peter Oakes-Munro
Dir-Educ/Spokesperson/at Large: John Malyna
Treas: Wayne Bodnarchuk
Int Sec/Fundraising Chair: Connie Jaman
Year Founded: 1996
Speakers Available
Languages: English
Membership: 10 *(Lists available to the public)*

◇ ***Brandon:***
45 Garwood Dr, Brandon MB R7A 2K6
204 720-1254
E: brandonmaddchapter@gmail.com
W: www.madd.ca
Year Founded: 1999
Languages: English

◇ ***Eriksdale:***
Mailing: PO Box 246, Eriksdale MB R0C 0W0
204 739-2702
W: www.madd.ca
Executive:
Community Leader: Darcy Lamb

◈ ***MADD New Brunswick:***
Languages: English

◇ ***Saint John:***
Linden Place
199 Chesley Dr, Saint John NB E2K 4S9
506 672-6188; Fax: 506 672-6083
E: maddstj@nb.aibn.com
W: www.madd.ca/saintjohn
Executive:
Pres: Rick McNulty
Year Founded: 2001
No of Paid Staff: 1
Speakers Available
Languages: English

◇ ***Southeastern NB:***
205-236 St. George St, Moncton NB E1C 1W1
506 386-9815
E: maddsenb@nb.aibn.com
W: www.madd.ca/senb
Languages: English

◈ *MADD Newfoundland/Labrador:*
Languages: English

◇ *Avalon:*
121-120 Conception Bay Hwy, Conception Bay-S NL A1W 3A6
709 834-7663; Fax: 709 834-7663
E: maddavalon@nl.rogers.com
W: www.madd.ca
Year Founded: 1998
Languages: English

◇ *Bay St. George:*
PO Box 125 Stn Main, Stephenville NL A2N 2Y9
709 643-6996
Toll-free: 877 993-6996
E: maddbaystgeorge@nf.aibn.com
W: www.madd.ca
Year Founded: 2001
Languages: English

◇ *Corner Brook:*
Location: RR 1, Corner Brook NL A2H 6C9
Mailing: PO Box 725 Stn Main, Corner Brook NL A2H 6G7
709 634-6233; Fax: 709 637-4101
E: maddbayofislands@nf.aibn.com
W: www.madd.ca
Executive:
Pres: Karen Foley
Languages: English

◇ *Exploits Valley:*
Mailing: PO Box 420 Stn Main, Grnd-Falls-Windsor NL A2A 2J8
709 293-4965
E: exploitsmadd@gmail.com
W: www.madd.ca
Executive:
Pres: Lisa Lindahl
Languages: English

◇ *Gander:*
Location: RCMP Gander, 301 James Blvd, Gander NL A1V 1W7
Mailing: PO BOX 366 Stn Main
709 256-5843
E: donnabarrett.maddgander@hotmail.com
W: www.madd.ca
Executive:
Pres: Tracy Clarke
Languages: English

◇ *Labrador:*
Mailing: PO Box 7 Stn C, Happy-Valley-Goose NL A0P 1C0
709 896-8957; Fax: 709 896-8957
Toll-free: 800 963-6233
E: madd@hvgb.net
W: www.madd.ca
Executive:
Pres: Shawn Crann
Year Founded: 1993
Languages: English

◇ *Labrador West:*
708 Field St, Labrador City NL A2V 1H8
709 944-7471
Toll-free: 800 665-6233
E: jojo@crrstv.net
W: www.madd.ca
Executive:
Pres: Josephine Gaulton-Rowe
Languages: English

◇ *Mary's Harbour:*
Mailing: PO Box 62, Marys Harbour NL A0K 3P0
709 921-6939; Fax: 709 921-6345
E: jackierumbolt43@hotmail.com
W: www.madd.ca
Executive:
Commun Leader: Jackie Rumbolt
Year Founded: 2001
Languages: English

◈ *MADD Nova Scotia:*
Languages: English

◇ *Annapolis Valley:*
249 Redden Rd, RR 1, Windsor NS B0N 2T0
902 798-0912; Fax: 902 798-5013
Toll-free: 866 798-6233
E: atlantic@madd.ca
W: www.madd.ca/annapolisvalley/
Year Founded: 1995
Languages: English

◇ *Antigonish:*
Antigonish RCMP
4 Fairview St, Antigonish NS B2G 1R3
902 863-4344; Fax: 902 863-5770
E: kyla_neary@hotmail.com
W: www.madd.ca/antigonish
Executive:
Pres: Kyla Neary
Languages: English

◇ *Bordertown:*
11 Industrial Park Dr, Amherst NS B4H 4H7
902 661-0684; Fax: 902 667-3897
W: www.madd.ca
Executive:
Pres: Wendi Chase
Year Founded: 2004
Languages: English

◇ *Cape Breton:*
800 Grand Lake Rd, Sydney NS B1P 6S9
902 564-6790; Fax: 902 564-6759
E: maddcapebreton@seaside.ns.ca
W: www.madd.ca
Executive:
Pres: Steve Tortola
Year Founded: 2002
Languages: English

◇ *Cobequid:*
175 Victoria St, Truro NS B2N 1Z5
902 843-3111; Fax: 902 843-3314
E: maddcobequid@ns.aliantzinc.ca
W: www.maddcobequid.blogspot.com
Executive:
Pres: Margaret Miller
VP: Jeanne Atkinson
Languages: English

◇ *Halifax Regional:*
3115 Veith St, Halifax NS B3K 3G9
902 445-6233; Fax: 902 445-6233
E: maddhalifax@ns.aliantzinc.ca
W: www.maddhalifaxregional.com
Executive:
Pres: Anissa Aldridge
Treas: Patrick Daigle
Sec: Siobhan Shears
Year Founded: 1995
Speakers Available
Library: Y *(Open to the public)*
Languages: English

◇ *Lunenburg-Queens:*
Mailing: PO Box 561 Stn Main, Bridgewater NS B4V 2X6
902 354-5721
Toll-free: 866 798-6233
E: lqmadd@gmail.com
W: www.lqmadd.webs.com
Languages: English

◇ *Pictou County:*
Mailing: PO Box 502, Trenton NS B0K 1X0
902 752-3495
E: pcmadd@eastlink.ca
W: www.madd.ca/pictoucounty
Executive:
Pres: Terry Cornett
Year Founded: 2002
Languages: English

◇ *Yarmouth County*
Mailing: PO Box 103 Stn Main, Yarmouth NS B5A 4B1
902 748-0113
E: info@maddyarmouth.com
W: www.maddyarmouth.com
Executive:
Pres: Rick Allwright
VP: Donna Ouse
Year Founded: 2004
Languages: English
Membership: 25

◈ *Yarmouth County:*
Mailing: PO Box 103 Stn Main, Yarmouth NS B5A 4B1
902 748-0113
E: info@maddyarmouth.com
W: www.maddyarmouth.com
Executive:
Pres: Rick Allwright
VP: Donna Ouse
Year Founded: 2004
Languages: English
Membership: 25

◈ *Dufferin County:*
Mailing: PO Box 241 Stn A, Orangeville ON L9W 2Z6
519 939-7267
W: www.madd.ca
Executive:
Chapter Serv Coord: Samantha Stevenson
Year Founded: 1999
Criteria: *Anyone who is dedicated to the mission.*
No of Paid Staff: 1
Languages: English
Membership: 40

◈ *MADD Ontario:*
500-2010 Winston Park Dr, Oakville ON L6H 5R7
905 844-0096; Fax: 905 829-8860
Toll-free: 800 665-6233
E: info@maddhalton.org
W: www.maddhalton.org
Executive:
Pres: Ed Nicholson
Languages: English

◇ *Barrie/Simcoe:*
Mailing: PO Box 511 Stn Main, Barrie ON L4M 4T7
Toll-free: 866 466-5310
E: maddbarriesimcoe@rogers.com
W: www.madd.ca/barriesimcoe
Executive:
Pres: Jason Larkin
Year Founded: 2001
Languages: English

◇ *Chatham/Kent:*
369 Mercer St, Chatham ON N7M 6C8
519 359-7760
Toll-free: 800 665-6233
E: maddchathamkent@gmail.com
W: www.madd.ca/chathamkent
Year Founded: 2001
Languages: English

◇ *Dufferin County:*
Mailing: PO Box 241 Stn A, Orangeville ON L9W 2Z6
519 939-7267
W: www.madd.ca
Executive:
Chapter Serv Coord: Samantha Stevenson
Year Founded: 1999
Criteria: *Anyone who is dedicated to the mission.*
No of Paid Staff: 1
Languages: English
Membership: 40

◇ ***Durham Region:***
124-1288 Ritson Rd N, Oshawa ON L1G 8B2
905 576-7473; Fax: 905 576-4675
Toll-free: 877 876-7473
E: info@madd-durham.com
W: www.madd-durham.com
Executive:
Pres: Michelle Crabb
Year Founded: 2000
Languages: English

◇ ***Grey North Bruce:***
Location: 299 9th St E, Owen Sound ON N4K 1N8
Mailing: PO Box 2 Stn Main, Owen Sound ON N4K 5P1
519 371-5252
E: madd@bmts.com
W: www.madd.ca/greynorthbruce
Executive:
Pres: Drew Wilder
Dir Victim Serv: Sharon Lee Wideman
Year Founded: 1998
Languages: English

◇ ***Halton/Peel Chapter:***
500-2010 Winston Park Dr, Oakville ON L6H 5R7
905 844-0096; Fax: 905 829-8860
E: info@maddhalton.org
W: www.maddhalton.org
Executive:
Pres: Ed Nicholson
Year Founded: 1993
No of Paid Staff: 1
Languages: English

◇ ***Huron/Bruce County:***
Location: 153 John St W, Wingham ON N0G 2W0
Mailing: PO Box 388
519 357-4552; Fax: 519 357-4556
E: madd@hurontel.on.ca
W: www.hurontel.on.ca/~maddhb
Executive:
Pres: Barb Rintoul
Treas: Martina Aisenpreis
Year Founded: 1995
Languages: English

◇ ***Kawartha Lakes:***
6 Victoria Ave N, Lindsay ON K9V 4E5
705 328-9264
E: maddkawarthalakes@bellnet.ca
W: www.madd.ca/kawarthalakes/
Year Founded: 1995
Languages: English

◇ ***Kingston & District:***
National Office
500-2010 Winston Park Dr, Oakville ON L6H 5R7
800 665-6233 243
E: madd@kingston.net
W: www.madd.ca
Executive:
Mgr: Renata Cvitkovic
Year Founded: 1999
No of Paid Staff: 1
Speakers Available
Languages: English
Membership: 13 *(Lists available to the public)*

◇ ***London:***
Location: Ridgeview Community Church, 1470 Glenora Dr, London ON N5X 1V2
Mailing: PO Box 27066, London ON N5X 3X5
519 645-1350; Fax: 519 645-1380
E: admin@maddlondon.com
W: www.maddlondon.com
Year Founded: 1996
No of Paid Staff: 1
Speakers Available
Library: Y *(Open to the public)*
Languages: English
Membership Fee: $10 Per Year

◇ ***Nipissing:***
1133 Brookes St, North Bay ON P1B 2N9
705 474-6233; Fax: 705 474-6725
E: madd@efni.com
W: www.madd.ca
Executive:
Pres: Jackie McLeod
Year Founded: 1995
Library: Y *(Open to the public)*
Languages: English

◇ ***Ottawa***
Mailing: PO Box 24218 RPO Hazeldean, Kanata ON K2M 2C3
613 236-6233; Fax: 613 829-4660
E: madd.ottawa@bellnet.ca
W: www.maddottawa.ca
Executive:
Pres: Kathy Gagnier
Year Founded: 1995
Speakers Available
Library: Y *(Open to the public)*
Languages: English; French

◇ ***Quinte:***
Mailing: PO Box 662 Stn CSC, Belleville ON K8N 5B3
613 962-6233
E: info@maddquinte.ca
W: www.maddquinte.ca
Executive:
Pres: Kerri Jianopoulas
Year Founded: 1995
Speakers Available
Languages: English
Membership: 30

◇ ***Sarnia/Lambton:***
Royal LePage Bldg
404C-546 Christina St N, Sarnia ON N7T 5W6
519 339-9962; Fax: 519 336-6974
Toll-free: 800 665-6233
E: office@maddsarnialambton.com
W: www.madd.ca/sarnialambton.com
Executive:
Co-Pres: John Reurink
Year Founded: 1999
Languages: English

◇ ***St. Thomas:***
Location: 417 Wellington St, St Thomas ON N5R 6A3
Mailing: PO Box 23016 RPO Elgin Mall
519 637-3333
E: maddstthomas1@rogers.com
W: www.madd.ca
Executive:
Pres: Kathy Gilchrist

◇ ***Thunder Bay:***
Location: 18 Court St N, Thunder Bay ON P7A 4T3
Mailing: 166-1100 Memorial Ave, Thunder Bay ON P7B 4A3
807 344-1666; Fax: 807 344-1667
E: maddtbay@tbaytel.net
W: www.madd.ca
Year Founded: 1996
Languages: English

◇ ***Timiskaming & Area:***
Location: Dymond Fire Hall, 181 Drive-In-Theatre Rd, New Liskeard ON P0J 1P0
Mailing: PO Box 757, Haileybury ON P0J 1K0
705 672-5101
E: maddtemdongrosz@ntl.sympatico.ca
W: www.madd.ca
Executive:
Pres: Rob Clouston
VP: Sue Flaxey
Victim Serv Coord: Don Grosz
Year Founded: 2003
Languages: English

◇ ***Toronto:***
35 Lytton Blvd, Lower Level, Toronto ON M4R 1L2
416 924-2666; Fax: 416 924-3666
E: info@maddtoronto.ca
W: www.maddtoronto.ca
Executive:
Pres: Mary Sultana
No of Paid Staff: 1
Speakers Available

◇ ***York Region:***
York Region Police
16775 Yonge St, Newmarket ON L3Y 8J4
800 665-6233 243
E: maddyorkregion@live.ca
W: www.madd.ca/york
Executive:
Pres: Paulo Pecchia
Year Founded: 1992
Languages: English

◇ ***Waterloo Region:***
Mailing: PO Box 633 Stn Waterloo, Waterloo ON N2J 4B8
519 896-6233; Fax: 519 896-0291
E: maddwaterloo@hotmail.com
W: www.madd.ca
Executive:
Pres: Sandra Henderson
VP: Cat Spicer
Year Founded: 1992
Criteria: *No impaired driving charges/convictions.*
Languages: English
Membership list available to the public

◇ ***Windsor & Essex County:***
Extendicare Tecumseh Bldg
2475 St. Alphonse St, Tecumseh ON N8N 2X2
519 791-9623; Fax: 519 253-3657
E: maddwin@yahoo.ca
W: www.madd.ca/windsor
Executive:
Commun Leader: Chaouki Hamka
Languages: English

◈ ***MADD Prince Edward Island***

◇ ***Charlottetown Chapter***
46 Cardiff Lane, Stratford PE C1B 1P5
902 367-8988
E: gerardburke@eastlink.ca
W: www.madd.ca
Executive:
Pres: Amanda Burke
Languages: English

◈ ***Hautes Laurentides***
123 rue du Village, RR 1, Arundel QC J0T 1A0
819 429-3624
W: www.madd.ca
Executive:
Prés: Jason Dubeau

◈ ***Québec:***
Mailing: CP 41 Succ Saint-Canut, Mirabel QC J7N 1H7
Toll-free: 877 392-6233
E: mcmorin@madd.ca
W: www.madd.ca
Executive:
Dir serv aux sections: Marie Claude Morin
Year Founded: 1996
No of Paid Staff: 1
Speakers Available
Languages: French; English

◇ ***Beauceville***
Place Beauceville
494A rang Saint-Joseph, Beauceville QC G5X 2C6
418 774-1230
E: maddbeauce@live.fr
Executive:
Prés: Jean Poulin

◇ ***Hautes Laurentides***
123 rue du Village, RR 1, Arundel QC J0T 1A0
819 429-3624
W: www.madd.ca
Executive:
Prés: Jason Dubeau

◇ ***MADD - Montreal***
Mailing: A/S Pierro Hirsch
4575 rue Hutchison, Montréal QC H2V 4A1
514 729-6233
E: info@maddmontreal.ca
Executive:
Prés: Angeliki Souranis
VP: James Lawler

◈ ***MADD Saskatchewan:***
Languages: English

◇ ***Meadow Lake & Area:***
Location: 301 3rd St W, Meadow Lake SK S9X 1C8
Mailing: PO Box 1244 Stn Main,
Meadow Lake SK S9X 1Y9
306 240-9667; Fax: 306 236-4409
E: maddmeadowlake@gmail.com
W: www.madd.ca
Executive:
Pres: Darlene Quiring
Languages: English

◈ ***Yukon Territories:***

◇ ***Whitehorse:***
4-102 Gold Rd, Whitehorse YT Y1A 2W2
867 633-6230; Fax: 867 633-6230
E: maddwh@yahoo.ca
W: www.madd.ca
Executive:
Pres: Alvin Pederson
Year Founded: 2003
Languages: English

North Shore Pro-Life Society
Location: 1-1558 Lonsdale Ave, North Vancouver BC V7M 2J3
Mailing: PO Box 37521 RPO Lonsdale East, North Vancouver BC V7M 3L7
604 984-9094; Fax: 604 984-9094
Executive:
Dir: Elisa Bueno
Speakers Available
Library: Y *(Open to the public)*
Languages: English
Library:
NSPL Society Library *(Open to the public)*

Ontario Coalition for Abortion Clinics (OCAC)
Mailing: PO Box 495 Stn P, Toronto ON M5S 2T1
416 969-8463
E: ocac88@gmail.com
W: ocac-choice.com
Executive:
Organizer: Michelle Robidoux
Library: Y *(Open to the public)*
Languages: English

Right to Life Association of Newfoundland and Labrador
Location: 151 Lemarchant Rd, St. John's NL A1C 2H4
Mailing: PO Box 5427 Stn C, St. John's NL A1C 5W2
709 579-1500; Fax: 709 579-3818
E: nffriendsforlife@nl.rogers.com
W: www.nlrighttolife.com
Year Founded: 1974
Criteria: *To believe that: 1) human life begins at conception, 2) the right to life is a fundamental human right and all other rights depend on it. 3) All human beings share this right from conception to natural death. 4) Live in Newfoundland and Labrador.*
No of Paid Staff: 1
Speakers Available
Library: Y *(Open to the public)*
Languages: English

Right to Life Association of Toronto and Area (TRL)
302-120 Eglinton Ave E, Toronto ON M4P 1E2
416 483-7869
E: office@righttolife.to
W: www.rtl-toronto.org
Executive:
Pres: Katherine Ye
Exec Dir: Paul Klotz
Year Founded: 1971
No of Paid Staff: 2
Speakers Available
Languages: English
Library:
Right to Life Resource Library *(Open to the public)*

SWOVA Community Development and Research Society
344 Lower Ganges Rd, Salt Spring Island BC V8K 2V3
250 537-1336; Fax: 250 537-1336
E: info@swova.org
W: www.swova.org
Executive:
Board Chair: Lorna Cammaert
Exec Dir: Lynda Laushway
Office Admin: Megan Manning-Burton
Year Founded: 1996
Criteria: *Female, male, adult, youth, organizations: $25. per year per person org rates available.*
No of Paid Staff: 8
Library: Y *(Open to the public)*
Languages: English
Membership: 65 *(Lists available to the public)*
Membership Fee: $20 - sliding scale; $5 per year
Library:
SWOVA Resource Library *(Open to the public)*

Saskatchewan Pro-Life Association Inc.
Location: 493 Hoffer Dr, Regina SK S4N 6E2
Mailing: PO Box 27093 RPO Avonhurst, Regina SK S4R 8R8
306 352-3480; Fax: 306 352-3481
Toll-free: 888 842-7752
E: spla@sasktel.net
W: www.saskprolife.com
Executive:
Pres: Muriel Nielsen
Year Founded: 1974
Criteria: *Must believe in mandate.*
Budget: $212,000
No of Paid Staff: 2
Speakers Available
Library: Y *(Open to the public)*
Languages: English
Membership: 4,000
Membership Fee: $25

Servitor Foundation
295-704 Spadina Ave, Toronto ON M5S 2J2
Toll-free: 888 326-6886
E: info@servitorfoundation.org
W: www.servitorfoundation.org
Executive:
Pres: A J Butler

Society For Socialist Studies
Mailing: PO Box 3050 Stn CSC, Victoria BC V8W 3P5
250 807-8707; Fax: 403 342-7989
E: kanchan.sarker@ubc.ca
W: www.socialiststudies.ca
Executive:
Treas: David Huxtable
Sec: Mathew Brett

Syndicat des Débardeurs S C F P Section Local 375
7020 rue Notre-Dame E, Montréal QC H1N 3L6
514 255-8868; Fax: 514 255-8211
E: reception@syndicat375.org
W: www.syndicat375.org
Executive:
Sec-trés: Réjean Brunet

Together Against Poverty Society
302-895 Fort St, Victoria BC V8W 1H7
250 361-3521; Fax: 250 361-3541
E: tapsbc@shaw.ca
W: www.tapsbc.ca
Executive:
Pres: Joan McHardy
VP: Robin Bassett
Exec Dir: Kelly Newhook
Treas: Tony Pullman
Sec: Barb Amberstone
Year Founded: 1989
No of Paid Staff: 5
Speakers Available
Languages: English
Membership: 93 *(Lists available to the public)*
Membership Fee: $2 - Unemployed; $10 - Organization; $5 - Employed

Tourism Toronto
405-207 Queens Quay W, Toronto ON M5J 1A7
416 203-2600; Fax: 416 203-6753
E: toronto@torcvb.com
W: torontotourism.com/meetingplanners
Executive:
VP-Meeting/Convention Sls: Tara Gordon
Dir-Sls: Robert Kawamoto
Dir-Sls: Alice Au
Dir-Sls: Julie Holmen

Wilberforce Project
Mailing: PO Box 11479 Stn Main, Edmonton AB T5J 3K5
780 421-7747; Fax: 780 421-7749
E: director@albertaprolife.com
W: www.albertaprolife.com
Executive:
Exec Dir: Rosey Rosenke
Year Founded: 1985
No of Paid Staff: 2
Speakers Available
Languages: English

SPORTS (1) —Disabled

Alberta Amputee Sports and Recreation Association
Mailing: PO Box 708 Stn M, Calgary AB T2P 2J3
403 201-0507; Fax: 403 256-7611
Toll-free: 888 501-0507
E: info@aasra.ab.ca
W: www.aasra.ab.ca
Executive:
Pres: Hal Gibbens
VP: Rachael Pasay
Exec Dir: Gwendalyn Davies
Dir at Large: Shane Westin
Dir at Large: Donald Young
Treas: Chris Rodway
Sec: Elizabeth Starker
Year Founded: 1977

HEALTHCARE ASSOCIATIONS

Criteria: *Open to any amputee who has lost a limb(s) at a major joint and non-amputees as supporting members.*
No of Paid Staff: 1
Speakers Available
Languages: English
Membership: 200 +
Membership Fee: Full: $20 - $150 lifetime

Alberta Sports and Recreation Association for the Blind

007-15 Colonel Baker Pl NE, Calgary AB T2E 4Z3
403 262-5332; Fax: 403 265-7221
Toll-free: 888 882-7727
E: info@asrab.ab.ca
W: www.asrab.ab.ca
Executive:
Exec Dir: Linda MacPhail
Year Founded: 1975
No of Paid Staff: 2
Speakers Available
Languages: English
Membership: 300
Membership Fee: $25 Family; $10 Individual

Association Sportive des Aveugles du Québec Inc.

Location: 4545 av Pierre-de Coubertin, Montréal QC H1V 0B2
Mailing: 4545 av Pierre-De Coubertin
514 252-3178
E: infoasaq@sportsaveugles.qc.ca
W: www.sportsaveugles.qc.ca
Executive:
Dir gén: Nathalie Chartrand
Year Founded: 1979
Languages: French

British Columbia Blind Sports and Recreation Association

330-5055 Joyce St, Vancouver BC V5R 6B2
604 325-8638; Fax: 604 325-1638
Toll-free: 877 604-8638
E: info@bcblindsports.bc.ca
W: www.bcblindsports.bc.ca
Executive:
Pres: Brian Cowie
VP: Tami Grenon
Treas: Tom Ollis
Year Founded: 1978
No of Paid Staff: 5
Speakers Available
Languages: English
Membership: 775
Membership Fee: $5-$15/year
Library:
Members Resources Library *(Open to the public)*

British Columbia Deaf Sports Federation

3820 Cessna Dr, Room 225, Richmond BC V7B 0A2
604 333-3606; Fax: 604 333-3450
Toll-free: 800 855-0511 Through Telus Relay Service
E: bcdeafsports@telus.net
W: www.bcdeafsports.bc.ca
Executive:
VP: Jamie Finley
Treas: Douglas Hugill
Office Admin: Leonor Johnson
Year Founded: 1975
Budget: $100,000
No of Paid Staff: 1
Languages: English; American Sign Language
Membership: 200 *(Lists available to the public)*
Membership Fee: $25

Canadian Amputee Sports Association

104-3 Concorde Gate, Toronto ON M3C 3N7
416 426-7187; Fax: 416 426-7361
W: www.canadianamputeesports.ca
Executive:
Pres: James Reilly
VP: Alan Dean
Treas: Wayne Epp
Year Founded: 1977
Criteria: *Must be a member of a provincial amputee sport association.*
Speakers Available
Languages: English
Membership: 120
Membership Fee: Lifetime - $150; Individual - $20

◈Manitoba:
472 Speers Rd, Winnipeg MB R2J 1N2
204 926-7019; Fax: 204 945-5232
E: celands@shaw.ca
W: www.canadianamputeesports.ca
Executive:
Mgr: Christine Rickard
Criteria: *Open to all.*
Speakers Available
Languages: English
Membership: 5
Membership Fee: $10 per year

Canadian Association for Disabled Skiing

791 Strathcona Dr. SW, Calgary AB T3H 1N8
587 315-5870; Fax: 866 531-9644
E: executive.director@disabledskiing.ca
W: www.disabledskiing.ca
Executive:
Exec Dir: Maureen O'Hara-Leman
Year Founded: 1976
No of Paid Staff: 1
Speakers Available
Library: Y *(Open to the public)*
Languages: English

Canadian Cerebral Palsy Sports Association

Location: 1910 St. Laurent Blvd, Ottawa ON K1G 5K9
Mailing: PO Box 41009 RPO Elmvale
613 748-1430; Fax: 613 748-1355
E: info@ccpsa.ca
W: www.ccpsa.ca
Executive:
Pres: Sandy Hermiston
VP: Debra Bulmer
Exec Dir: Jennifer Larson
Year Founded: 2000
Budget: $1,500,000
No of Paid Staff: 3
Speakers Available
Library: Y
Languages: English; French

◈Alberta:
Percy Page Centre
11759 Groat Rd NW, Edmonton AB T5M 3K6
780 422-2904; Fax: 780 422-2663
E: contact@acpsa.ca
W: www.acpsa.ca
Executive:
Exec Dir: Brennan Nicoll
Year Founded: 1984
Criteria: *Have CP or related conditions*
Budget: $50,000
No of Paid Staff: 1
Speakers Available
Languages: English

◈British Columbia/SportAbility:
6235C 136 St, Surrey BC V3X 1H3
604 599-5240; Fax: 604 599-5241
Toll-free: 877 711-3111 in BC only
W: www.cpsports.com
Executive:
Pres: Megan Landels
Exec Dir: Terrie Moore
Treas: Carol Turnbull
Coord: Ross MacDonald
Year Founded: 1982
Criteria: *Athletes with a physical disability and volunteers.*
Budget: $250,000
No of Paid Staff: 4
Speakers Available
Languages: English
Membership: 1,200
Membership Fee: $20

◈Manitoba:
100-200 Main St, Winnipeg MB R3C 1A8
204 946-7600; Fax: 204 925-5703
E: mcpsa-swim@hotmail.com
W: www.ccpsa.ca
Languages: English

◈Quebec:
Location: 4545 boul Pierre-de Coubertin, Montréal QC H1V 3R2
Mailing: CP 1000, succ M
514 252-3143; Fax: 514 254-1069
E: secadmin@sportpc.qc.ca
W: www.sportpc.qc.ca
Executive:
Dir gén: Jo-ann Arvey
Year Founded: 1990
No of Paid Staff: 3
Languages: French
Membership: 1,500

Canadian Deaf Sports Association

202A-10217 boul Pie-IX, Montréal-Nord QC H1H 3Z5
514 321-8686; Fax: 514 252-3213
E: info@assc-cdsa.com
W: www.assc-cdsa.com
Executive:
Dir exéc: Craig Noonan
Languages: English

◈Nova Scotia:
Sport Nova Scotia
5516 Spring Garden Rd, Floor 4, Halifax NS B3J 1G6
902 425-5450; Fax: 902 425-5606
E: justin.debaie@ns.sympatico.ca
Executive:
NSDSA Pres: Justin DeBaie
Year Founded: 1984
Languages: English
Membership: 20

Canadian Wheelchair Sports Association

108-2255 St. Laurent Blvd, Ottawa ON K1G 4K3
613 523-0004; Fax: 613 523-0149
E: info@cwsa.ca
W: www.cwsa.ca
Executive:
Exec Dir: Cathy Cadieux
Dev Dir/Natl BTG Coord: Duncan Campbell
Prog Mgr: Don Lane
Commun Coord: Arley McNeney
Languages: English; French

◈Alberta:
11759 Groat Rd NW, Edmonton AB T5M 3K6
780 427-8699; Fax: 780 427-8723
Toll-free: 888 453-6770
E: wsa1@telus.net
W: www.abwheelchairsport.ca
Executive:
Exec Dir: Mike Sandomirsky
No of Paid Staff: 4

Speakers Available
Library: Y *(Open to the public)*
Languages: English; French

◈***British Columbia:***
210-3820 Cessna Dr, Richmond BC V7B 0A2
604 333-3520; Fax: 604 333-3450
Toll-free: 877 737-3090
E: info@bcwheelchairsports.com
W: www.bcwheelchairsports.com
Executive:
Exec Dir: Kathy Newman
Natl BTG Coord: Duncan Campbell
Year Founded: 1971
Budget: $700,000
No of Paid Staff: 4
Speakers Available
Library: Y *(Open to the public)*
Languages: English
Membership: 900
Membership Fee: $25 per year

◈***Manitoba:***
145 Pacific Ave, Winnipeg MB R3B 2Z6
204 925-5790; Fax: 204 925-5792
E: mwsa.proco@sportmanitoba.ca
W: www.mwsa.ca
Executive:
Exec Dir: Mandy Johnson
Year Founded: 1962
No of Paid Staff: 1
Speakers Available
Languages: English
Membership: 350
Membership Fee: $5

◈***New Brunswick***
1-209 Prince St, Saint John NB E2M 1P3
506 674-1205
W: www.cwsa.ca/resources/links
Executive:
Pres: Karen Ferguson

◈***Newfoundland/Labrador:***
48 Hollyberry Dr, Paradise NL A1L 0C1
709 782-0487; Fax: 709 747-4054
Executive:
Pres: Gary Power
No of Paid Staff: 1
Speakers Available
Languages: English

◈***Halifax NS***
13 Kincardine Dr, Dartmouth NS B2X 1H7
902 424-0096; Fax: 902 424-0627
W: www.nswheelchairsport.com/
Executive:
Pres: Ron Wheeler

◈***Ontario:***
Business Bldg
104-3 Concorde Gate, Toronto ON M3C 3N7
416 426-7189; Fax: 416 426-7361
E: info@ontwheelchairsports.org
W: www.ontwheelchairsports.org
Executive:
Exec Dir: Lynda Charters
Prog Coord: Carina Von Bredow
Languages: English

◈***Québec:***
Location: 4545 av Pierre-de Coubertin, Montréal QC H1V 3R2
Mailing: CP 1000 succ M
514 252-3108; Fax: 514 254-9793
E: info@parasportsquebec.com
W: www.parasportsquebec.com
Executive:
Dir adj: Isabelle Sinclair
Dir gén: Marc Antoine Ducharme
Year Founded: 1983
No of Paid Staff: 5
Speakers Available
Library: Y
Languages: French; Slovenian
Membership: 400

◈***Saskatchewan:***
510 Cynthia St, Saskatoon SK S7L 7K7
306 975-0824; Fax: 306 975-0825
E: swsa@shaw.ca
W: www.swsa.ca
Executive:
Exec Dir: Andrea Muir
Criteria: *Open to any person with with a mobility impairment and an interest in sport, recreation and leisure activities.*
No of Paid Staff: 3
Languages: English
Membership: 600
Membership Fee: $10/Active, $25/Family, $75/Club

Cochrane/Temiskaming Children's Treatment Centre
733 Ross Ave E, Timmins ON P4N 8S8
705 264-4700; Fax: 705 268-3585
Toll-free: 800 575-3210
E: children@ntl.sympatico.ca
W: www.nt.net/~children/index.html
Criteria: *Open to any child with a disability.*
Speakers Available
Languages: English; French

Manitoba Blind Sports Association
145 Pacific Ave, Winnipeg MB R3B 2Z6
204 925-5694; Fax: 204 925-5792
E: blindsport@shawbiz.ca
W: www.blindsport.mb.ca/
No of Paid Staff: 1
Speakers Available
Languages: English

Olympiques spéciaux Québec
2-5311 boul de Maisonneuve O, Montréal QC H4A 1Z5
514 843-8778; Fax: 514 843-8223
Toll-free: 877 743-8778
E: info@olympiquesspeciaux.qc.ca
W: www.olympiquesspeciaux.qc.ca
Executive:
Dir gén: Pierre Bélanger
Chef prog sportifs: Laurence Tétrault
Chef commun/événements: Marie-Josée Carroll
Coord commun: Joelle McGurrin

ParaSport & Recreation PEI
Location: Royalty Centre House of Sport, 40 Enman Cres, Room 115, Charlottetown PE C1E 1E6
Mailing: PO Box 841 Stn Central, Charlottetown PE C1A 7L9
902 368-4540; Fax: 902 368-4548
E: info@parasportpei.ca
W: www.parasportpei.ca/
Executive:
Pres: Richard Pettipas
VP: Don Spence
Exec Dir: Tracy Stevenson
Treas: Bob Kenny
Sec: Vicki Weldin
Bridging the Gap Coord: Cathleen MacKinnon
Year Founded: 1976
Budget: $110,000
No of Paid Staff: 1
Speakers Available
Languages: English
Membership: ~150
Membership Fee: $5

ParaSport Ontario
Business Bldg
104-3 Concorde Gate, Toronto ON M3C 3N7
416 426-7187; Fax: 416 426-7361
Toll-free: 800 265-1539
E: info@parasportontario.ca
W: www.parasportontario.ca
Executive:
Chair: Brian Skinner
VP-Sponsorship/Fundraising: Brian McLean
VP-Fin/Admn: Brian MacPherson
VP-Dev: Sheila Thomas
Exec Dir: Eric Cartlidge
Year Founded: 1981
No of Paid Staff: 6
Speakers Available
Languages: English
Membership: 1,800
Membership Fee: $20

Saskatchewan Blind Sports Association
510 Cynthia St, Saskatoon SK S7L 7K7
306 975-0888
E: sbsa.sk@shaw.ca
W: www.saskblindsports.ca
Executive:
Exec Dir: Tony Badger
Speakers Available
Languages: English
Membership: 299

Special Olympics Canada
600-21 St Clair Ave E, Toronto ON M4T 1L9
416 927-9050; Fax: 416 927-8475
Toll-free: 888 888-0608
E: info@specialolympics.ca
W: www.specialolympics.ca
Executive:
Pres/CEO: Lindsay Glassco
VP-Bus Dev/Mktg: Anthony Miceli
VP Sport: Sharon Bollenbach
Dir-Fin/Ops: Karen Forrest
Dir-Mktg/Pub Rel: Susana Petti
Dir-Sport/Competition: Marian Coulson
Dir-Bus Dev: Kevin Matchett
Year Founded: 1968
No of Paid Staff: 15
Speakers Available
Languages: English; French
Membership: 35,055 registered athletes

◈***Alberta:***
Percy Page Centre
11759 Groat Rd NW, Edmonton AB T5M 3K6
780 415-0719; Fax: 780 415-1306
Toll-free: 800 444-2883
E: info@specialolympics.ab.ca
W: www.specialolympics.ab.ca
Executive:
Pres/CEO: Kirk De Fazio
Dir-Mktg: Marvin Babiuk
Year Founded: 1980
Criteria: *Athletes with mental disabilities and volunteers.*
Budget: $1,000,000
No of Paid Staff: 10
Speakers Available
Languages: English
Membership: 4,000 *(Lists available to the public)*

◈***British Columbia:***
210-3701 Hastings St, Burnaby BC V5C 2H6
604 737-3078; Fax: 604 737-3080
Toll-free: 888 854-2276
E: info@specialolympics.bc.ca
W: www.specialolympics.bc.ca

Executive:
Pres/CEO: Dan Howe
Office Admin: Jennifer Cowell
Year Founded: 1980
No of Paid Staff: 10
Speakers Available
Languages: English
Membership: 3,000

◈***Manitoba:***
304-145 Pacific Ave, Winnipeg MB R3B 2Z6
204 925-5628; Fax: 204 925-5635
Toll-free: 888 333-9179
E: som@specialolympics.mb.ca
W: www.specialolympics.mb.ca
Executive:
Pres/CEO: Simon Mundey
Dir-Fin Serv: Carolyn Langtry
Year Founded: 1980
Budget: $1,800,000
No of Paid Staff: 14
Speakers Available
Languages: English
Membership: 1,300
Membership Fee: $25

◈***New Brunswick:***
13-900 Hanwell Rd, Fredericton NB E3B 6A2
506 455-0404; Fax: 506 455-0410
Toll-free: 888 362-5926
E: infosonb@specialolympics.ca
W: www.specialolympicsnb.ca
Executive:
Exec Dir: Josh Astle
Year Founded: 1979
Budget: $350,000
No of Paid Staff: 4
Speakers Available
Languages: English; French
Membership: 1,000

◈***Newfoundland and Labrador:***
16B-50 Pippy Place, St. John's NL A1B 4H7
709 738-1923; Fax: 709 738-0119
E: sonl@sonl.ca
W: www.sonl.ca
Executive:
Exec Dir: Trish Williams
No of Paid Staff: 7
Speakers Available
Library: Y
Languages: English

◈***Nova Scotia:***
Sovereign Bldg
201-5516 Spring Garden Rd, Halifax NS B3J 1G6
902 429-2266; Fax: 902 425-5606
Toll-free: 866 299-2019
W: www.sons.ca
Executive:
Pres/CEO: Michael Greek
No of Paid Staff: 3
Speakers Available
Languages: English
Membership: 1,500

◈***Ontario:***
200-65 Overlea Blvd, Toronto ON M4H 1P1
416 447-8326; Fax: 416 447-6336
Toll-free: 888 333-5515
W: www.specialolympicsontario.com
Executive:
Pres/CEO: Glenn MacDonell
VP: Linda Ashe
Mgr-Mktg Serv: Lynn Miller
Year Founded: 1979
Criteria: *Person must be diagnosed with a mental disability.*
Budget: $6,000,000
No of Paid Staff: 30
Speakers Available
Languages: English
Membership: 16,000 *(Lists available to the public)*

◈***Prince Edward Island:***
240-40 Enman Cres, Charlottetown PE C1E 1E6
902 368-8919; Fax: 902 892-4553
Toll-free: 800 287-1196
E: sopei@sopei.com
W: www.sopei.com
Executive:
Exec Dir: Valerie Downe
Year Founded: 1982
Criteria: *Open to any person with an intellectual disability.*
Budget: $250,000
No of Paid Staff: 3
Languages: English
Membership: 300 + *(Lists available to the public)*

◈***Saskatchewan:***
353 Broad St, Regina SK S4R 1X2
306 780-9247; Fax: 306 780-9441
Toll-free: 888 307-6226
E: sos@specialolympics.sk.ca
W: www.specialolympics.sk.ca
Executive:
CEO: Roger Dumont
Dir-Ops: Faye Matt
Admin/Ops Coord: Carrissa Trenton
Year Founded: 1975
No of Paid Staff: 5
Speakers Available
Library: Y *(Open to the public)*
Languages: English
Membership: 1,300
Membership Fee: $10/year

◈***Yukon:***
Location: 102-211 Hanson St, Whitehorse YT Y1A 1Y3
Mailing: 4061 4th Ave, Whitehorse YT Y1A 1H1
867 668-6511; Fax: 867 667-4237
E: info@specialolympicsyukon.ca
W: www.specialolympicsyukon.ca
Languages: English

Sunrise Therapeutic Riding & Learning Centre Inc.
6920 Concession 1, Puslinch ON N0B 2J0
519 837-0558; Fax: 519 837-1233
E: info@sunrise-therapeutic.ca
W: www.sunrise-therapeutic.ca
Executive:
Exec Dir: Ann Caine

SUPPORT GROUPS

Access Community Services Inc.
160 Walton St, Port Hope ON L1A 1N6
905 885-6358; Fax: 905 885-1753
E: info@accesscommunity.ca
W: www.accesscommunity.ca

Bay St. George Community Employment Corp.
35 Carolina Ave, Stephenville NL A2N 3P8
709 643-3470; Fax: 709 643-6398
Executive:
Contact: Ray McIsaac

Centre d'action bénévole Artisans de l'Aide
108-184 rue Saint-Eustache,
Saint-Eustache QC J7R 2L7
450 472-9540; Fax: 450 472-9586
E: info@cabartisans.org
Executive:
Dir gén: Ginette Bordeleau

Chilliwack Community Services
45938 Wellington Ave, Chilliwack BC V2P 2C7
604 792-4267; Fax: 604 792-6575
W: www.comserv.bc.ca
Executive:
Exec Dir: James Challman
Dir-Ops: Suzanne Cameron
Year Founded: 1928
No of Paid Staff: 102
Speakers Available

Circle of Care
4211 Yonge St, Floor 4, Toronto ON M2P 2A9
416 635-2860; Fax: 416 635-1692
E: info@circleofcare.com
W: www.circleofcare.com
Executive:
Pres/CEO: Michael Scheinert
Dir: Arnold Foss

Information Niagara
10-235 Martindale Rd, St Catharines ON L2W 1A5
905 682-6611; Fax: 905 682-4314
Toll-free: 800 223-3695
E: info@informationniagara.com
W: www.informationniagara.com
Executive:
Exec Dir: Rosanna Thoms

Life with a Baby
152 Hetherington Cres, Thornhill ON L4J 2M2
416 833-3860
E: info@lifewithababy.com
W: www.lifewithababy.com
Executive:
Founder: Claire Zoblin

Lions McInnes House
170 Henry St, Brantford ON N3S 5C7
519 752-6450; Fax: 519 752-9049
E: lionsmcinneshouse@rogers.com
Executive:
Chm: Margaret Small
Exec Dir: Joan Brintnell
Prog Dir: Laurie Marissen
Dir-Support Serv: Larry Noble

Parent Support Services Society of BC
204-5623 Imperial St, Burnaby BC V5J 1G1
604 669-1616; Fax: 604 669-1636
Toll-free: 877 345-9777
E: office@parentsupportbc.ca
W: www.parentsupportbc.ca
Executive:
Prog Dir: Bella Cenezero
Exec Dir: Carol Ross
Prov Office Admin: Viktor Panfilenok
Year Founded: 1974
Criteria: *Open to any person who supports the mission of child abuse prevention. Members will have voting privileges at annual general meetings and will receive a newsletter two times a year.*
Membership Fee Required: Y
Budget: $500,000
No of Paid Staff: 10
Speakers Available
Library: Y *(Open to the public)*
Languages: English; Cantonese; Mandarin; Russian; Spanish; Other language
Membership: 96
Membership Fee: Ranges from $5 to $50

Parents Together

7595 Victoria Dr, Vancouver BC V5P 3Z6
604 325-0556; Fax: 604 325-0596
E: parentstogether@bgc-gv.bc.ca
Executive:
Prog Coord: Wendy Smith
No of Paid Staff: 4
Speakers Available
Languages: English
Membership: 600 *(Lists available to the public)*
Membership Fee: $20/year

Rygiel Supports for Community Living

200-1550 Upper James St, Hamilton ON L9B 2L6
905 525-4311; Fax: 905 525-5933
E: info@rygiel.ca
W: www.rygiel.ca
Executive:
Chair: Dr Clint Davis
Exec Dir: Donna Marcaccio
Dir-Ops: John Baxter
Dir-Hum Res: Suzanne Gautreau
Dir-Serv: Chris Barone
Treas: Pat Mostacci

Saint Matthew's House

414 Barton St E, Hamilton ON L8L 2Y3
905 523-5546; Fax: 905 523-5553
E: admin@stmatthewshouse.ca
Executive:
Exec Dir: Steve Leighfield

Sleep-Wake Disorders Self-Help Group

434 Lower Malpeque Rd, Charlottetown PE C1E 1V1
902 628-2128; Fax: 902 367-6949
E: donfrizzell@bellaliant.net
Executive:
Facilitator: Don Frizzell
Languages: English

West Hillhurst Go-Getter's (S.C.) Association

1940 6 Ave NW, Calgary AB T2N 0W3
403 283-3720; Fax: 403 283-3744
E: hillhurs@telusplanet.net
Executive:
Pres: Sylvia Nelson
Admin: Tammy Cann
Year Founded: 1975
Criteria: *Any person 50 yrs. of age and older.*
No of Paid Staff: 4
Speakers Available
Library: Y *(Open to the public)*
Languages: English
Membership: 600
Membership Fee: $10 per year

SECTION 7 - 2012: THE YEAR IN REVIEW

2012: THE YEAR IN REVIEW

The material for this "Year in Review" was provided by the Canadian Medical Association and was based on articles from the *Canadian Medical Association Journal* (vol. 184). Full-text versions of *CMAJ* articles are available online in HTML and PDF formats at www.cmaj.ca. For more information on *CMAJ*, visit the CMA's website at www.cma.ca or contact CMA's Member Service Centre at 888 855-2555.

ABORIGINAL HEALTH

Double oppression

Aboriginal youths who are "two spirited" — i.e., gay, lesbian, bisexual or transgendered — are at higher risk of suicide because they face "double oppression: racism and heterosexism," the National Aboriginal Health Organization asserted. The organization unveiled a guide, *Suicide Prevention and Two-Spirited People*, that offered tips to mental health service providers on how to help such youths.
CMAJ 2012;184(9):E481-4
www.cmaj.ca/content/184/9/E481

Prescription drug abuse rising among Aboriginal youths

Indications of a staggering level of prescription drug abuse by Aboriginal youths left experts urging a more coordinated approach to the problem. *CMAJ* 2012;184(12):E647-8
www.cmaj.ca/content/184/12/E647

Aboriginal health programming under siege, critics charged

The federal government was deliberately undermining capacity to generate accurate Aboriginal health data and circulating discredited health data to downplay the severity of the Aboriginal health crisis in Canada, said critics. *CMAJ* 2012;184(14):E739-40
www.cmaj.ca/content/184/14/E739

ADDICTION MEDICINE

Changing attitudes about addiction

Stanbrook argued that society often thinks and behaves negatively toward addiction and the people who suffer from it. We must overcome these negative attitudes if we are to succeed in treating addiction as we do other chronic diseases, he said. *CMAJ* 2012;184(2):155
www.cmaj.ca/content/184/2/155

Chronic opioid dependence

Treating chronic opioid dependence with diacetylmorphine instead of methadone may result in lower societal costs and increased duration and quality of life. This cost-effectiveness analysis used a semi-Markov cohort model and data from a trial conducted in 2 Canadian cities. Cost savings were realized primarily because of reductions in crime, said Nosyk and colleagues. *CMAJ* 2012;184(6):E317-28
www.cmaj.ca/content/184/6/E317

Treatment gap

Drug use disorders were largely ignored and untreated globally, while just 82 of 147 countries included in a new World Health Organization information system offered some manner of special health services for drug dependent people. *CMAJ* 2012;184(11):E597-601
www.cmaj.ca/content/184/11/E597

ANESTHESIA AND ANALGESIA

Medically induced opioid addiction reaching alarming levels

Call it medically induced and law-abiding addiction. Experts were so astonished by the growing incidence of prescription opioid addiction that they were arguing for Canada to move immediately with a strategy to constrain its future effects on the health care system and the health of Canadians. *CMAJ* 2012;184(3):285-6
www.cmaj.ca/content/184/3/285

Minimizing anesthetic injection pain

Strazer and Lalonde outlined 5 practical tips for reducing the likelihood of pain for patients during injection of local anesthetic. These included choice of needle, temperature of the solution, use of a buffer and injection techniques. *CMAJ* 2012;184(18):2016
www.cmaj.ca/content/184/18/2016

CANCER

Second primary cancer

Five-year absolute risk per 100 of second primary cancer after first cancer in Danish population, 1980–2007

Type or site of first cancer	Type of second cancer: Cervix	Prostate	Breast	Colon	Lung	Skin
Cervix	0.34	–	0.61	0.28	0.34	0.31
Prostate	–	0.01	–	1.60	1.32	2.41
Breast	0.19	–	1.05	0.71	0.51	1.28
Colon	0.10	1.92	1.53	1.25	1.03	1.72
Lung	0.11	1.55	1.42	0.87	0.65	1.26
Skin	0.10	1.75	1.68	1.25	1.38	2.25

Cancer survivors have just over twice the risk of contracting another primary cancer of the same type but only a slightly increased risk of a primary cancer of another type. These findings came from a nationwide cohort study that followed close to 7.5 million people for more than 25 years using 3 linked administrative databases. Whether these associations were due to genetic factors or lifestyle risk could be the subject of future studies, said the authors. *CMAJ* 2012;184(1):E57-69
www.cmaj.ca/content/184/1/E57

Second primary cancer is a major concern for cancer survivors, their families and the health care professionals providing follow-up care. The absolute risk of each type of second primary cancer should influence clinical decisions about the frequency and type of follow-up care, said the authors. *CMAJ* 2012;184(1):19-20
www.cmaj.ca/content/184/1/19

Breast-screening guidelines fuelled firestorm

New guidelines for breast cancer screening that recommended women avoid routine mammography until age 50 were based on faulty methodology and would result in an "untold number of lives lost" if

implemented across Canada, the Canadian Association of Radiologists charged. *CMAJ* 2012;184(1):E17-8
www.cmaj.ca/content/184/1/E17

Advocacy groups continued to scorn screening guidelines

A national task force underestimated the benefits of early mammograms while overstating the harms when it recommended the scuttling of routine breast screening of women under the age of 50, breast cancer advocacy groups said. *CMAJ* 2012;184(6):E295-6
www.cmaj.ca/content/184/6/E295

Cervical screening in Aboriginal women

Recent data suggested that the rates of screening for cervical cancer among Aboriginal women were now similar to those among non-Aboriginal women in Canada. Whether this would translate to a reduced incidence of cervical cancer and associated mortality was unknown, said Demers and colleagues. *CMAJ* 2012;184(7):743-4
www.cmaj.ca/content/184/7/743

The impact of a cerebral glioma

Patients with glioma frequently feel acute psychological and existential distress during the diagnostic process and again as the tumour progresses. Cavers and colleagues repeated interviews with patients and caregivers over 2 years in this longitudinal qualitative study. Each patient is different, but understanding the typical patterns of social, psychological and existential distress alongside physical decline enables the provision of supportive care and appropriate communication, said the authors.
CMAJ 2012;184(7):E373-82
www.cmaj.ca/content/184/7/E373

Tumour lysis syndrome

A 76-year-old man presented to the emergency department with a 3-week history of nausea, vomiting and diarrhea. Despite extensive resuscitation efforts, he died within hours after admission. The diagnosis was spontaneous tumour lysis syndrome from an undiagnosed hepatocellular carcinoma. Kekra and colleagues emphasized that early recognition and treatment are essential to improving outcomes in this potentially fatal condition. *CMAJ* 2012;184(8):913-6
www.cmaj.ca/content/184/8/913

Family history and breast cancer

Obtaining a careful family history is central to identifying potential carriers of *BRCA* mutations who should be offered genetic counselling. Clinical interventions for carriers can substantially reduce the risk of breast or ovarian cancer, said Carroll and colleagues.
CMAJ 2012;184(12):1391
www.cmaj.ca/content/184/12/1391

Shingles does not increase cancer risk

Patients with a recent episode of herpes zoster are not at increased risk of cancer. A study used routine health insurance data to follow 35 871 people with newly diagnosed herpes zoster for a median follow-up of 3.68 years to count new cases of cancer. It is unnecessary to conduct extensive investigation for occult malignancy following an episode of herpes zoster, said the authors. *CMAJ* 2012;184(15):E804-9
www.cmaj.ca/content/184/15/E804

Tackling cancer in low-income countries

Five percent of global health spending on cancer occurred in low- and middle-income countries, which had almost 80% of the worldwide burden of cancer. According to Ginsburg and colleagues, Canadians could implement the innovative interventions and solutions that were urgently needed to reduce the growing burden of cancer in these countries. The authors called for the development of a Canadian global cancer network to help with planning, capacity building, research, and resources commitment. *CMAJ* 2012;184(15):1699-1704
www.cmaj.ca/content/184/15/1699

Breast cancer screening guidelines

In the 2011 update of its guidelines on screening for breast cancer, the Canadian Task Force on Preventive Health Care changed some of its previous recommendations. The authors of this primer reviewed these changes, the evidence supporting them and their implications for practice. *CMAJ* 2012;184(16):1803-7
www.cmaj.ca/content/184/16/1803

CARDIOVASCULAR MEDICINE

Diagnosed hypertension in Canada

The number of people with hypertension in Canada was increasing, while the number of new cases per year was decreasing. These findings came from an analysis of health administrative databases from each province and territory. Enhanced population programs were needed to prevent hypertension, said the authors. *CMAJ* 2012;184(1):E49-56
www.cmaj.ca/content/184/1/E49

Variations in coronary care

The mode of coronary revascularization was largely influenced by the recommendation of the physician performing the diagnostic angiography and factors related to the treating hospital. These findings came from an examination of routine hospital data and patient charts to identify factors associated with variations in revascularization practices in 17 cardiac centres. Opportunities existed to improve decision-making for revascularization, particularly for nonemergent multivessel disease, said the authors.
CMAJ 2012;184(2):179-86
www.cmaj.ca/content/184/2/179

The all-clear signal for rare heart arrhythmias

Clinicians argued that the advent of genetic testing had allowed for early identification of carriers of rare heart arrhythmias and the subsequent prescription of preventive therapeutics, thereby diminishing patient fears that they're at risk of keeling over.
CMAJ 2012;184(4):E213-4
www.cmaj.ca/content/184/4/E213

High-sensitivity troponin T assay

A high-sensitivity troponin T assay performed well at diagnosing myocardial infarction (MI) in patients with chest pain but without ST-segment elevation on electrocardiogram, especially those presenting 4 to 6 hours after onset of symptoms. This diagnostic cohort study involving 939 people with chest pain compared routine use of a troponin I assay with early measurement (at presentation and 2 hours later) with a high-sensitivity troponin T assay and examined prognosis over 1 year. The findings needed to be confirmed, but suggested that the new test could rule out MI for some patients as early as 2 hours after presentation, said Aldous and colleagues. *CMAJ* 2012;184(5):E260-8
www.cmaj.ca/content/184/5/E260

Ambulatory blood pressure monitoring

Hypertension was a major preventable cause of premature death and disability. Home and ambulatory blood pressure monitoring were useful in the diagnosis, but there was uncertainty about the exact therapeutic threshold, said Campbell and Hemmelgarn. *CMAJ* 2012;184(6):633-4
www.cmaj.ca/content/184/6/633

Atrial fibrillation and mental decline

Atrial fibrillation can cause cognitive and functional decline, even in the absence of overt stroke. A post-hoc analysis of 2 large randomized controlled trials involved more than 31 000 patients and measured cognitive decline during treatment with 2 blood pressure–lowering agents. Clinical trials involving patients with atrial fibrillation should include cognitive and functional measures, said Marzona and colleagues.
CMAJ 2012;184(6):E329-36
www.cmaj.ca/content/184/6/E329

Fever and multiorgan infarcts

A previously healthy 35-year-old man was brought to the emergency department by his family because he was confused. He also had experienced 5 days of fever, peripheral edema, orthopnea and blurred vision. He eventually underwent a surgical procedure, but the optimal timing required input from several specialties. *CMAJ* 2012;184(7):783-8
www.cmaj.ca/content/184/7/783

Q waves are important in prognosis

Patients with myocardial infarction who had Q waves at baseline fared worse than those without Q waves, even after adjustment for time from onset of symptoms and other prognostic features. This finding was based on an analysis of data from 4341 patients in the PLATO trial. This metric should prove useful in clinical decisions about patients with chest pain and ST-segment elevation, especially when time from symptom onset is unclear, said the authors. *CMAJ* 2012;184(10):1135-42
www.cmaj.ca/content/184/10/1135

We must ensure that Q waves are used in conjunction with, rather than as a replacement for, time to treatment for patients with ST-segment elevation myocardial infarction, said Mercuri and colleagues.
CMAJ 2012;184(10):1125-6
www.cmaj.ca/content/184/10/1125

Heart failure in Ontario

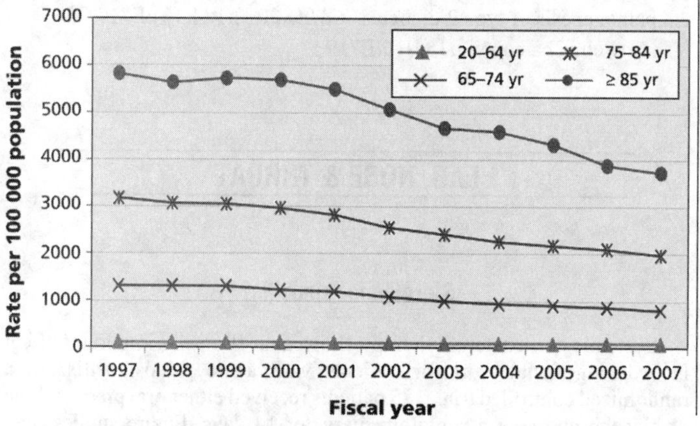

Sex-standardized trends in incidence of heart failure, by age group.

Failing organs, especially hearts, are hard to cure; best to avoid the failure in the first place. That appeared to be what was underway, at least in developed countries. In a population-based study using data from the publicly funded Ontario Health Insurance Plan, there was strong evidence of a declining incidence in heart failure. The disease itself, once established, had an undiminished ominous prognosis. The authors speculated that the decline was driven by a decrease in the incidence of ischemic heart disease. *CMAJ* 2012;184(14):E765-73
www.cmaj.ca/content/184/14/E765

Alcohol may cause atrial fibrillation

Moderate to high alcohol consumption was associated with an increased incidence of atrial fibrillation among people aged 55 years or older with cardiovascular disease or diabetes. This result was based on the combined data from 2 large antihypertensive drug treatment trials involving more than 30 000 participants. Recommendations about the protective effects of moderate alcohol consumption may need to be tempered with these findings, said the authors. *CMAJ* 2012;184(16):E857-66
www.cmaj.ca/content/184/16/E857

COMPLEMENTARY AND ALTERNATIVE MEDICINE

Homeopathic hubbub

It is "unethical for health practitioners to treat patients using homeopathy, for the reason that homeopathy (as a medicine or procedure) has been shown not to be efficacious," according to Australia's National Health and Medical Research Council. The Australian Association of Professional Homeopaths had been seeking the creation of a formal registration scheme for homeopaths, similar to that of physicians and nurses. *CMAJ* 2012;184(7):E354-6
www.cmaj.ca/content/184/7/E354

The new rules of naturopathy

Alberta became the fifth province in Canada to regulate naturopathic doctors, following a push by the profession to ensure consistent regulations and practice standards across the country.
CMAJ 2012;184(14):E743-4
www.cmaj.ca/content/184/14/E743

Needling toward essential health benefits

The era of acupuncture's existence as a practice on the margins of medicine appeared to be inexorably drawing to a close. An increasing number of Canadians were turning to this alternative therapy to treat chronic conditions, and an increasing number of physicians were willing to refer patients for such treatment. *CMAJ* 2012;184(16):1773
www.cmaj.ca/content/184/16/1773

CRITICAL CARE

Mother–infant ICU admissions

Mother–infant pairs in which both were admitted to intensive care units (ICUs) following delivery had the highest prevalence of separation due to interfacility transfer. In this study of routinely collected data, these mothers and babies also had the highest mortality compared with groups in which only the mother or the baby was admitted to an ICU. Coordination and communication of care plans could lessen the burden and frequency of separation of mother and newborn seen with concurrent ICU admissions, suggested the authors. *CMAJ* 2012;184(18):E956-62
www.cmaj.ca/content/184/18/E956

DERMATOLOGY

Chilblains

Most commonly idiopathic, these lesions may be associated with conditions such as systemic lupus erythematosus or antiphospholipid syndrome, cautioned Vano-Galvan and Martorell. *CMAJ* 2012;184(1):67
www.cmaj.ca/content/184/1/67

Unilateral laterothoracic exanthem

Unilateral laterothoracic exanthem, which is commonly mistaken for contact dermatitis, begins in the axilla and spreads centrifugally. It usually

occurs in children between 1 and 5 years of age in the winter and spring and resolves spontaneously within 4 to 6 weeks.
CMAJ 2012;184(3):322
www.cmaj.ca/content/184/3/322

Tattoo reactions and sarcoidosis

Reactions in cosmetic tattoos can be the only sign of cutaneous sarcoidosis. If a patient presents with inflammatory changes in tattoos, the possibility of cutaneous or systemic sarcoidosis should be considered. A tissue biopsy can help make the diagnosis. *CMAJ* 2012;184(4):432
www.cmaj.ca/content/184/4/432

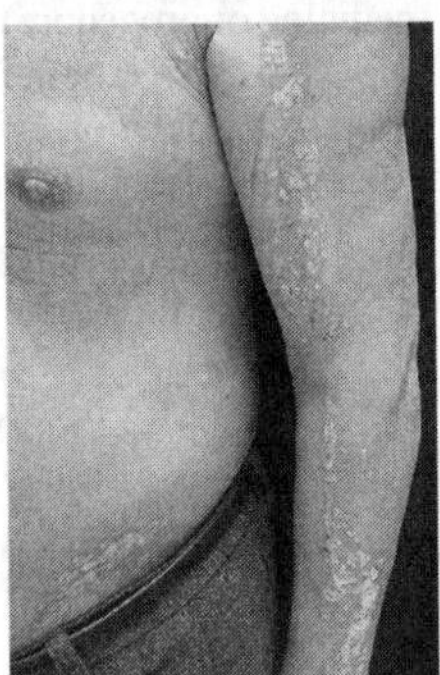

Linear psoriasis

A 69-year-old man presented with a 40-year history of recurrent scaly rashes in lines on the left side of his body. He was diagnosed with linear psoriasis, an unusual subtype of psoriasis characterized by a distribution of the rash along Blaschko lines. This condition is usually mild and responds well to topical treatment, said Li and Man. *CMAJ* 2012;184(7):789
www.cmaj.ca/content/184/7/789

Acne

Topical treatments for acne can be continued for years, whereas oral antibiotics can be gradually discontinued if the condition remains under control for 2 months, said Freiman and Barankin.
CMAJ 2012;184(13):1497
www.cmaj.ca/content/184/13/1497

DIABETES

Initiating insulin therapy

Although patients and physicians often have reservations about initiating insulin therapy in type 2 diabetes, insulin is a safe and effective agent in reducing glycated hemoglobin A_{1c}. Use of insulin is not associated with an increased risk of hypoglycemia in type 2 diabetes, said Lau and colleagues. Combination therapy that includes insulin and oral antihyperglycemic agents can reduce weight gain, insulin dose and the risk of hypoglycemia. *CMAJ* 2012;184(7):767-76
www.cmaj.ca/content/184/7/767

Macrosomia and maternal adiposity

Among pregnant women without gestational diabetes, mothers whose infants are large for gestational age are more likely to have a higher body mass index before pregnancy, greater weight gain during pregnancy and lower levels of leptin. Retnakaran and colleagues analyzed data for 472 pregnant women in their cohort study who underwent an oral glucose tolerance test late in pregnancy. Targeting healthy body weight in young women is a strategy to reduce the risk of infant macrosomia, said the authors. *CMAJ* 2012;184(12):1353-60
www.cmaj.ca/content/184/12/1353

New criteria had been proposed for the diagnosis of gestational diabetes that would increase the incidence to nearly 1 in 5 pregnancies. Because these changes in diagnostic criteria carried widespread implications for practice and health care funding, more general debate was needed before their acceptance. *CMAJ* 2012;184(12):1341-2
www.cmaj.ca/content/184/12/1341

Thiazolidinediones and bladder cancer

Adults with type 2 diabetes mellitus who use thiazolidinediones are at increased risk of bladder cancer. This finding came from a meta-analysis of 4 randomized controlled trials and 6 observational studies. The risk was observed specifically with pioglitazone, whereas the findings were inconclusive regarding rosiglitazone. These results may help inform clinical decision-making, because other treatment options exist that are not associated with cancer, said the authors.
CMAJ 2012;184(12):E675-83
www.cmaj.ca/content/184/12/E675

Charcot foot

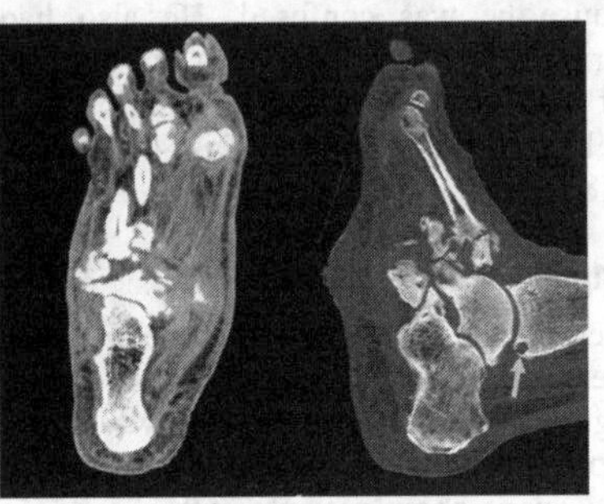

Lack of sensation can result in the development of Charcot foot or neuropathic arthropathy in up to 7.5% of those with diabetic neuropathy. Characterized by pathologic fractures, dislocations or subluxations that distort the foot's architecture, this condition requires prompt immobilization, absolute non–weight bearing and professional foot care. Some may require surgery.
CMAJ 2012;184(12):1392
www.cmaj.ca/content/184/12/1392

Bicarbonate and risk of diabetes

We still did not know why insulin receptors became less receptive as type 2 diabetes developed. In a cohort study of American nurses, chronically low plasma bicarbonate was shown to be associated with risk of diabetes; if confirmed, this finding could improve our understanding of the pathogenesis of type 2 diabetes. *CMAJ* 2012;184(13):E719-25
www.cmaj.ca/content/184/13/E719

EAR, NOSE & THROAT

Steroids for sinusitis?

Systemic corticosteroid therapy showed no clinically important effect in reducing facial pain for patients with acute rhinosinusitis. In a randomized controlled trial, 185 patients received either oral prednisolone or placebo and kept a symptom diary for 14 days. Future studies may reveal subgroups more likely to benefit, but in the meantime, there was no rationale for using corticosteroids in patients with acute rhinosinusitis, said the authors. *CMAJ* 2012;184(14):E751-7
www.cmaj.ca/content/184/14/E751

The "mother's kiss" technique

A foreign body stuck in a child's nostril may be safely removed by a trusted adult applying positive pressure through a short puff, using a technique similar to mouth-to-mouth resuscitation. A review of 8 case series and case reports described a high success rate for the technique. If promoted as a first-line approach, it could reduce the need for medical intervention and anesthesia in some cases, said the authors.
CMAJ 2012;184(17):E904-12
www.cmaj.ca/content/184/17/E904

EMERGENCY MEDICINE

Scombroid poisoning

People who have symptoms such as flushing, rash and urticaria after eating certain types of fish may be experiencing scombroid poisoning, a form of histamine poisoning. Despite elevated levels of histamine in the fish due to improper processing or storage, the fish may look, smell and taste normal, said Stratta and Badino. Most instances are self-limited and require no treatment. However, rapid-acting antihistamines and supportive care are commonly used for more severe symptoms.
CMAJ 2012;184(6):674
www.cmaj.ca/content/184/6/674

Turning to hospitals

More than 830 000 visits to hospital emergency departments in the United States in 2006 were for preventable dental conditions, an increase of 16% in just 3 years, according to the Pew Research Center. “A major driver of dental-related hospital visits is a failure by states to ensure that disadvantaged people have access to routine preventive care from dentists and other providers,” the study stated. *CMAJ* 2012;184(7):E354-6
www.cmaj.ca/content/184/7/E354

Pan-scanning for injury detection

Whole-body, contrast-enhanced computed tomography (pan-scanning) detected 1756 injuries in 982 patients with major trauma. Patients were scanned a median of 29 minutes after arrival in the trauma centre, and the results were compared to the final assessment. Pan-scanning showed promise for early detection of injuries, but 6.3% of injuries were missed by the initial pan-scanning. *CMAJ* 2012;184(8):869-76
www.cmaj.ca/content/184/8/869

ED wait times and mental illness

Patients visiting the emergency department for reasons related to mental illness waited less time to be seen by a physician than other patients when the emergency department was crowded and only slightly longer than other patients when it was not crowded. This observational study analyzed population-based health services data from Ontario for more than 8 million visits to 155 emergency departments between 2007 and 2009. The results allayed concerns that emergency departments had not been triaging patients with mental illness appropriately, said the authors. *CMAJ* 2012;184(18):E969-76
www.cmaj.ca/content/184/18/E969

ENDOCRINOLOGY

Hypothyroidism refractory to treatment

Serum thyroid-stimulating hormone (TSH) is the best marker for assessing appropriateness of thyroxine replacement in hypothyroidism, but what if the TSH does not respond to increasing doses of thyroxine? This article provided an algorithm and an approach to investigating the causes of treatment-refractory hypothyroidism.
CMAJ 2012;184(2):205-9
www.cmaj.ca/content/184/2/205

Levothyroxine dosing error

Inadequate replacement of levothyroxine can result in pituitary hyperplasia in severe primary hypothyroidism. Although poor adherence, malabsorption and drug interactions are more common causes of subtherapeutic responses to pharmacologic treatment, errors in dosing should be considered, said Clemens and Van Uum.
CMAJ 2012;184(2):210
www.cmaj.ca/content/184/2/210

Recurrent exercise-induced rhabdomyolysis

A previously healthy 29-year-old man presented with muscle aches and dark urine after a 4-hour hockey game. He had experienced similar episodes about once a year since he was 13 years old. A careful history revealed clues that led to the diagnosis, which was confirmed by some simple laboratory tests. The authors reviewed the diagnosis and management of single and recurrent episodes of rhabdomyolysis.
CMAJ 2012;184(4):426-30
www.cmaj.ca/content/184/4/426

ENVIRONMENTAL MEDICINE

Climate change posed health threats in the Arctic

As climate change and receding sea ice open new corridors into previously remote communities in the Arctic, residents can expect a wave of social ills and the introduction of diseases that may be as devastating as the Spanish flu was to those living in the north in the early 1990s, experts said. *CMAJ* 2012;184(1):E33-4
www.cmaj.ca/content/184/1/E33

Public health fallout from Japanese quake

A “culture of coverup” and inadequate cleanup efforts had combined to leave Japanese people exposed to “unconscionable” health risks 9 months after 2011’s meltdown of nuclear reactors at the Fukushima Daiichi power plant, health experts said. *CMAJ* 2012;184(2):E115-6
www.cmaj.ca/content/184/2/E115

EPIDEMIOLOGY

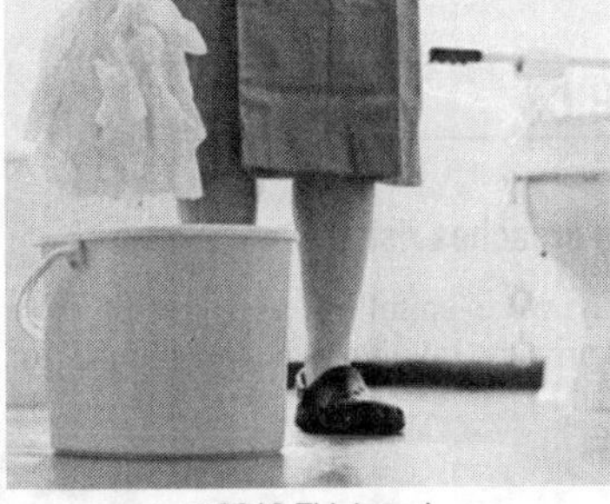

©2012 Thinkstock

Clostridium difficile in hospitals

Hospital-acquired infection with *C. difficile* significantly prolongs a patient’s stay in hospital, independent of baseline risk of death, and the estimated total cost of caring for patients who acquire this organism is substantial, said the authors.
CMAJ 2012;184(1):37-42
www.cmaj.ca/content/184/1/37

Infection with *C. difficile* is associated with high mortality and increases the length of a patient’s stay in hospital. Enoch and Aliyu suggested using a “care bundle” approach to rapidly reduce the transmission of this organism. *CMAJ* 2012;184(1):17-8
www.cmaj.ca/content/184/1/17

Research on drug use goes down the toilet

Sewers don’t lie. People may be less than forthright about what they put into their bodies, especially if that includes illicit drugs, but a chemical analysis of what comes out of their bodies removes all mystery. According to drug and addiction researchers, analyzing wastewater for remnants of illicit substances provides the only truly objective indicator of drug use patterns in a community. *CMAJ* 2012;184(2):165-7
www.cmaj.ca/content/184/2/165

Accuracy of depression screening

Suitable cut-off scores for the commonly used brief Patient Health Questionnaire (PHQ-9) depression screening tool include the range between 8 and 11. This meta-analysis of 18 diagnostic validation studies examined the variation in sensitivity and specificity with different cut-off scores. The optimal cut-off score may differ depending on the setting, said the authors. *CMAJ* 2012;184(3):E191-6
www.cmaj.ca/content/184/3/E191

Although the conventional score for diagnosing depression with the PHQ-9 has been 10, a wider range (8–12) may be more appropriate depending on the patient population, said Kroenke.
CMAJ 2012;184(3):281-2
www.cmaj.ca/content/184/3/281

Screening for depression

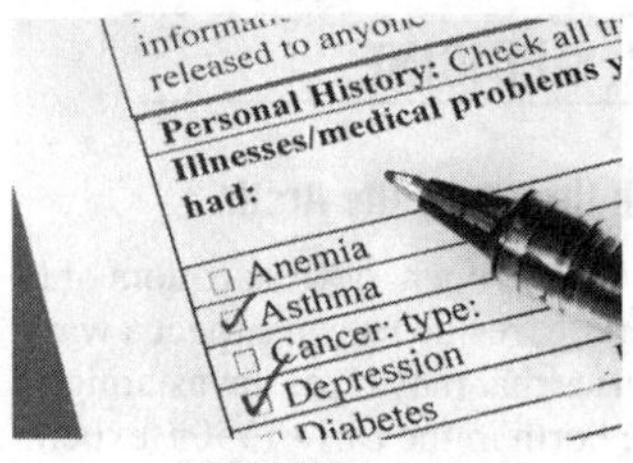

©2012 Thinkstock

The prevalence of depression and the availability of easy-to-use screening tools make it tempting to endorse widespread screening for the disease. However, according to Thombs and colleagues, screening in primary care is costly and does not yet show evidence of benefit. It may also have unintended negative effects for some patients. As Canada's guidelines were being updated, the authors wrote that recommendations to screen should require evidence of benefit that exceeds evidence of harm.
CMAJ 2012;184(4):413-8
www.cmaj.ca/content/184/4/413

Pass on PSA

The harms of regular screening with the prostate-specific antigen blood test, commonly called the PSA test, outweigh the benefits, according to the United States Preventive Services Task Force.
CMAJ 2012;184(10):E535-8
www.cmaj.ca/content/184/10/E535

ETHICS

Medical privacy breaches rising

Concerns about medical privacy were spiralling as a result of a whopping increase in breaches of privacy involving health records of patients. *CMAJ* 2012;184(4):E215-6
www.cmaj.ca/content/184/4/E215

Consent requirements for pelvic examinations performed for training purposes

According to Gibson and Downie, pelvic examinations performed for training purposes presumably constitute a battery in law, subject to defence of consent. They argued that the 2010 policy statement concerning pelvic examinations performed on women under anesthesia either needed to be revised to include residents or a new statement specific to residents needed to be drafted. *CMAJ* 2012;184(10):1159-61
www.cmaj.ca/content/184/10/1159

Choosing when and how to die

A report written for the Quebec National Assembly recommended the introduction of legislation to permit euthanasia. Flegel and Fletcher explored some of the implications of this report and asked if Canada was ready for such a change. *CMAJ* 2012;184(11):1227
www.cmaj.ca/content/184/11/1227

EVIDENCE-BASED MEDICINE

Prostate guidelines needed guidance

Guidelines for monitoring prostate cancer lacked a systematic approach because of inadequacies in the available evidence and its use. These findings came from a narrative review of guidelines from 9 organizations in North America, Europe and Australia. Guideline writers should take a more explicit and systematic approach to writing, said the authors. *CMAJ* 2012;184(2):169-77
www.cmaj.ca/content/184/2/169

Clinical experts should collaborate with methodologists in developing clinical guidelines to ensure that the recommendations made reflect high-quality scientific data. *CMAJ* 2012;184(2):159-60
www.cmaj.ca/content/184/2/159

Canadian task force guideline process

The Canadian Task Force on Preventive Health Care was re-established with a sustainable funding model. The authors outlined the process for guideline development by the task force and compared it with those from other major guideline development groups.
CMAJ 2012;184(14):1575-81
www.cmaj.ca/content/184/14/1575

FAMILY MEDICINE

Prognosis in back pain

Patients who presented with acute back pain improved markedly in the first 6 weeks, and by 1 year, the average levels of pain and disability were low. The initial pattern was similar for patients presenting with persistent back pain, but these patients had moderate levels of pain and disability after 1 year. These findings were based on a systematic review of 33 cohorts including 11 166 people. Summarizing prognostic factors is a challenge, said the authors, and could be a topic for future research.
CMAJ 2012;184(11):E613-24
www.cmaj.ca/content/184/11/E613

Most of the apparent benefits of treatment for back pain were likely unrelated to the effects of specific interventions, said Buchbinder and Underwood. *CMAJ* 2012;184(11):1229-30
www.cmaj.ca/content/184/11/1229

Iron to treat fatigue

Oral iron reduced the symptoms of fatigue compared to placebo in women with normal hemoglobin but reduced ferritin levels. This randomized controlled trial involving 198 women aged 18 to 53 years also showed effects on blood characteristics related to iron but did not detect a change in global measures of quality of life. Iron deficiency may be an underrecognized cause of fatigue in women of childbearing age, suggested Vaucher and colleagues. *CMAJ* 2012;184(11):1247-54
www.cmaj.ca/content/184/11/1247

GASTROENTEROLOGY

Suspected common bile duct stones

The management of patients suspected of having stones in the common bile duct depends on whether their probability of having such stones is high, intermediate or low. Recent advances in imaging and surgical techniques had led to substantial changes in the diagnosis and management of this condition, said Almadi and colleagues.
CMAJ 2012;184(8):884-92
www.cmaj.ca/content/184/8/884

Management of colonic diverticulitis

New insights into the pathogenesis of colonic diverticular disease were changing the management of acute and recurrent diverticulitis, said Tursi. Areas of particular interest included the use of mesalazine and probiotics in preventing recurrence. *CMAJ* 2012;184(13):1470-6
www.cmaj.ca/content/184/13/1470

Unusual presentation of typhoid fever

Typhoid fever is a well-characterized disease whose pathology had been known for 100 years. So, it was a surprise to report this case in which necrotizing granulomatous ileitis was associated and in which tuberculosis was excluded as a cause. *CMAJ* 2012;184(16):1808-10
www.cmaj.ca/content/184/16/1808

GENETICS

Testing the ethics of genetic testing in sports

Critics of direct-to-consumer genetic testing in sports questioned the ethics of assessing average athletes, particularly youth, for athletic potential. *CMAJ* 2012;184(1):E45-6
www.cmaj.ca/content/184/1/E45

Genetics privacy

Greater legal protection must be provided to Canadians to ensure that personal genetic data aren't used in an untoward manner by their employers or insurance companies, said a report by the British Columbia Civil Liberties Association. *CMAJ* 2012;184(4):E219-20
www.cmaj.ca/content/184/4/E219

Separating hype from reality in the era of the affordable genome

Despite lofty promises about personalized medicine, humans weren't getting healthier. *CMAJ* 2012;184(6):E287-8
www.cmaj.ca/content/184/6/E287

A race-based detour to personalized medicine

Some medical experts claimed race-based medicine was a step toward personalized medical care, but others believed it was unwise to push the field of medical genetics into the heated realm of racial politics. *CMAJ* 2012;184(7):E351-3
www.cmaj.ca/content/184/7/E351

Genetics of inflammatory bowel disease

There is genetic variation between white and First Nations people. Some genes associated with Crohn disease are more frequent in First Nations people, and some associated with ulcerative colitis are less frequent. Blood from 340 healthy First Nations people and 285 healthy white people was used to compare DNA for the presence of genes known to be associated with inflammatory bowel disease. These differences in the prevalence of genetic variants underline the complexity of inflammatory bowel disease, said Murdoch and colleagues. *CMAJ* 2012;184(8):E435-41
www.cmaj.ca/content/184/8/E435

Predisposed to risk but not change

Advocates for direct-to-consumer genetic testing had long argued that providing people with data about their predispositions toward health risks would motivate them to adopt healthier behaviours, but research provided little support for that proposition. *CMAJ* 2012;184(8):E407-8
www.cmaj.ca/content/184/8/E407

Unhealthy behaviours influenced by genes and environment

Neither genetics nor the environment, alone, can explain unhealthy behaviour. *CMAJ* 2012;184(8):E395-6
www.cmaj.ca/content/184/8/E395

Young women with breast cancer genes faced tough choices

As genetic testing increased, more young women were facing 3 choices: increased surveillance, chemoprevention or prophylactic surgery. *CMAJ* 2012;184(8):E401-2
www.cmaj.ca/content/184/8/E401

Screening embryos may lead to stigma

As advancing genetic screening technologies allowed for the detection of subtler mutations, including predisposition to late-onset diseases that could be treated, some ethicists were wondering if creating a list of "serious" conditions to be avoided may have unintended consequences. *CMAJ* 2012;184(9):E455-6
www.cmaj.ca/content/184/9/E455

Surge in Down syndrome prenatal testing anticipated

A new genetic test that could detect Down syndrome had some physicians concerned that the medical community was not prepared to educate and counsel a potentially huge number of pregnant women facing difficult family planning decisions. *CMAJ* 2012;184(9):E449-50
www.cmaj.ca/content/184/9/E449

GERIATRIC MEDICINE

Hospital-induced delirium hit hard

Hospital-acquired delirium was a common and dangerous condition that often went unnoticed and untreated, an oversight that experts in geriatric medicine said was costing the health care system untold millions of dollars. *CMAJ* 2012;184(1):23-4
www.cmaj.ca/content/184/1/23

Physicians open to ideas on how to assess and discuss fitness to drive

Physicians appeared eager to explore new ideas on how to broach the touchy subject of driving competency with older patients. *CMAJ* 2012;184(4):E207-8
www.cmaj.ca/content/184/4/E207

Graduated drivers' licences for seniors

A full driver's licence should default automatically to a restricted licence that allows seniors to drive only under favourable road conditions, argued Redelmeier and Stanbrook. However, graduated licensing must allow exemptions for healthy seniors. *CMAJ* 2012;184(10):1123
www.cmaj.ca/content/184/10/1123

Senior suicide

Suicide among senior citizens was an overlooked problem. *CMAJ* 2012;184(17):E885-6
www.cmaj.ca/content/184/17/E885

Aging successfully

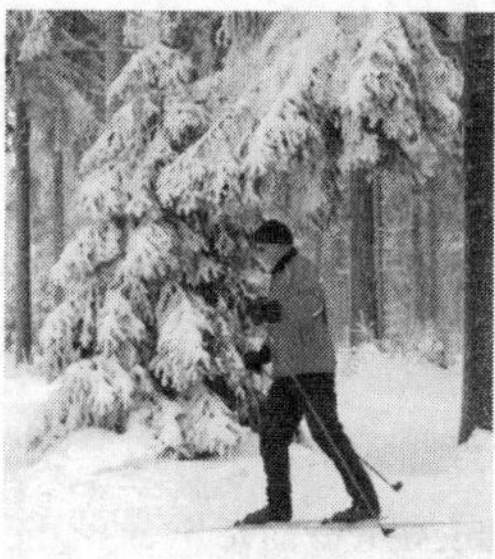

©2012 Thinkstock

We all know that living well leads to a better life, but the Whitehall II study revealed how good it can be. This high-quality cohort study showed that each of the following behaviours added in a measurable and independent way to survival free from major health problems: regular physical activity, daily fruit and vegetable consumption, not smoking and consuming alcohol moderately. Practitioners now had good evidence to counsel their patients on how to live longer. *CMAJ* 2012;184(18):1985-92
www.cmaj.ca/content/184/18/1985

Most of us would like to live longer if we can be healthy enough to enjoy the extra time. The 4 behaviours mentioned above may increase the odds of living in good health beyond 60 years of age. The future may yield

additional insights, as genomic, epigenomic, proteomic and metabolomic studies were just beginning to assess components of healthy aging. *CMAJ* 2012;184(18):1973-4
www.cmaj.ca/content/184/18/1973

Low vitamin D may not be so bad

Adults whose parents lived into very old age have lower blood levels of vitamin D than comparable adults. This analysis came from the Leiden Longevity Study, which compared the offspring of nonagenarians to their own partners. The authors suggested that this finding casted doubt on the possibility that the previously observed association between low blood levels of vitamin D and increased mortality was causal.
CMAJ 2012;184(18):E963-8
www.cmaj.ca/content/184/18/E963

GLOBAL HEALTH

Snakebite neglect rampant in Africa

Although it was estimated that as many as 1.5 million Africans were bit by snakes annually, leading to 32000 deaths, African health authorities largely ignored the snakebite problem, either because they were unaware of the incidence rates or did not think they could do anything about it.
CMAJ 2012;184(1):E27-8
www.cmaj.ca/content/184/1/E27

Food aid for children woefully substandard

Millions of malnourished children receive substandard food aid every year because of a lack of clear guidelines to hold donor nations accountable for the products they finance or distribute in the developing world, argued Médecins Sans Frontières. *CMAJ* 2012;184(1):E39-40
www.cmaj.ca/content/184/1/E39

The art of necessary compromise

Médecins Sans Frontières said it must often grapple with ethical conundrums, and make distasteful compromises, in order to provide relief in some environments. *CMAJ* 2012;184(5):E252-3
www.cmaj.ca/content/184/5/E252

Chan re-appointed

The World Health Assembly appointed Dr. Margaret Chan to serve a second term at the helm of the World Health Organization. In her acceptance speech, Chan urged that WHO continue to press for expanded health coverage for disadvantaged peoples. *CMAJ* 2012;184(10):E535-8
www.cmaj.ca/content/184/10/E535

Child survival

Pneumonia and diarrhea annually accounted for 29% of deaths among children under age 5 and about half of those were occurring in 5 nations: India, Nigeria, Democratic Republic of Congo, Pakistan and Ethiopia, according to a report by the United Nations Children's Fund.
CMAJ 2012;184(11):E597-601
www.cmaj.ca/content/184/11/E597

Micro-flush

Bill Gates hoped to spur innovation in toilet design to save lives in the developing world. The sanitary nightmare resulting from open defecation in many countries spread disease and caused millions of deaths, particularly among children under age 5. Western-style toilets, however, aren't the solution. They use too much water and require complex sewers. To address this problem, the Bill and Melinda Gates Foundation invested US$6.5 million in a "Reinvent the Toilet Challenge." The foundation awarded the California Institute of Technology US$100000 for its solar-powered design that recycles water and converts human waste into energy. *CMAJ* 2012;184(13):E691-2
www.cmaj.ca/content/184/13/E691

HEALTH POLICY & ECONOMICS

WHO signalled intent to trim sails

The year 2012 was poised to become a time of substantial change for the World Health Organization, which planned on initiating reforms but still faced major financing challenges. *CMAJ* 2012;184(1):E29-30
www.cmaj.ca/content/184/1/E29

Disclosing results of clinical trials

In the interest of protecting Canadians, Health Canada should publicly disclose the designs and results of clinical trials on the safety and efficacy of pharmaceuticals, biologics and medical devices. Matthew Herder argued that the law does not, in principle, preclude such disclosure. He stated that Canada should follow the lead of the US Food and Drug Administration and make the registration of clinical trials and disclosure of findings mandatory. *CMAJ* 2012;184(2):194-9
www.cmaj.ca/content/184/2/194

Crowdfunding for medical expenses

When a friend or relative needed help paying medical bills, many Americans were turning their social network into a safety net through a growing number of online fundraising platforms. But some observers said these websites were a symptom of the failing health care system in the United States – and hardly a solution. *CMAJ* 2012;184(2):E123-4
www.cmaj.ca/content/184/2/E123

Former Supreme Court justice blasted minimum sentences for marijuana offenders

Canada's new mandatory minimum sentences for drug offenders constituted a threat to public health and the concept of judicial proportionality, a former Supreme Court of Canada justice said.
CMAJ 2012;184(8):E391-2
www.cmaj.ca/content/184/8/E391

Everything in moderation, including vision

Call it a victory for incrementalism. The federal government's fiscal 2012/13 budget proved nowhere near as "transformative" as billed.
CMAJ 2012;184(8):E384-6
www.cmaj.ca/content/184/8/E384

Mental health strategy needed national buy-in

Canada's proposed mental health strategy would require a major grassroots advocacy campaign to ensure that it was adopted across all segments of society and that funds were generated to implement its recommended measures, proponents said. *CMAJ* 2012;184(9):E469-70
www.cmaj.ca/content/184/9/E469

Refugee health reforms assailed

A desire to dissuade "bogus" refugee claims, public envy over the level of health care that asylum seekers received, and cost savings were ample justification for limitations on hospital, physician and other medical services provided to refugee claimants and protected persons, Minister of Citizenship, Immigration and Multiculturalism Jason Kenney said. *CMAJ* 2012;184(10):E511-2
www.cmaj.ca/content/184/10/E511

Caring about the health of the poor

The poor, in general, have worse health than the rich. But there is, in fact, a social gradient of health such that everyone below the very top level of wealth has worse health than those above them. These socioeconomic inequalities in health arise from socioeconomic inequalities in society, including the conditions in which people are born, grow, live, work and age. According to Marmot, social inequality damages social cohesion, which may lead to violence (insecurity), and violates our sense of fairness. *CMAJ* 2012;184(11):1231-2
www.cmaj.ca/content/184/11/1231

Health disparities among income groups becoming more pronounced

Income levels were increasingly affecting the state of health of Canadians, as over the previous 4 years, the poor were more likely to be diagnosed with chronic conditions and were making greater use of health services. *CMAJ* 2012;184(13):E695-6
www.cmaj.ca/content/184/13/E695

Ontario fee cuts enraged nation's doctors

Canada's doctors voted to have their national association press for an amendment to the Canada Health Act to legally guarantee binding contracts and arbitration by a panel with an "independent chairman" in the event of contract disputes. *CMAJ* 2012;184(13):E697-8
www.cmaj.ca/content/184/13/E697

Recession repercussions

The downturn in the economy negatively affected the health of people in the United Kingdom, according to British doctors. More than three-quarters of 300 general practitioners surveyed claimed the recession made British residents unhealthier. *CMAJ* 2012;184(13):E691-2
www.cmaj.ca/content/184/13/E691

Billing protest

Members of the BC Health Coalition and Canadian Doctors for Medicare were protesting what they believed were illegal billing practices followed by private health clinics in Vancouver, British Columbia. The 2 clinics, the Cambie Surgery Centre and the Specialist Referral Clinic, were given a 30-day deadline in July 2012 by the Medical Services Commission to stop what it referred to as extra billing for publicly insured services. The clinics were founded by Dr. Brian Day (former president of the Canadian Medical Association), who filed a lawsuit against the Medical Services Commission and the province's minister of health and attorney-general. *CMAJ* 2012;184(13):E691-2
www.cmaj.ca/content/184/13/E691

Toward a patient charter with teeth

Many countries have adopted patient charters of rights, but to be meaningful, such charters must include an economical, accessible and independent complaints process. According to Flood and May, an ombudsman or commissioner can help reduce litigation and formal disciplinary proceedings against health care professionals.
CMAJ 2012;184(14):1583-7
www.cmaj.ca/content/184/14/1583

The costs of choice in senior care

Alberta's plan to move to a patient-based funding model for senior care was alarming some health care and advocacy groups, who feared the province was planning to increase privatization of elder care.
CMAJ 2012;184(14):E737-8
www.cmaj.ca/content/184/14/E737

Impact of Bill C-31 on refugees

The Canadian government was poised to adopt Bill C-31, which would allow the imprisonment of refugee claimants, including children aged 16–18 years, for at least 14 days and up to 6 months. According to Cleveland and Rousseau, numerous studies had shown high levels of psychiatric symptoms among detained refugee claimants, even after short periods. These symptoms tended to be aggravated over time and if family reunification was delayed after release. *CMAJ* 2012;184(15):1663-4
www.cmaj.ca/content/184/15/1663

Less health care for new refugees

People who arrived in Canada claiming refugee status would now be denied all health coverage, including coverage for emergencies. New federal government legislation also limited access to health insurance for preventive services, medications, emergency dental and vision care, and translation services for most refugees. According to Arya and colleagues, these changes shifted health care costs to vulnerable refugees and provincial health plans. *CMAJ* 2012;184(17):1875-6
www.cmaj.ca/content/184/17/1875

Reining in public spending on health care

The amount of public money devoted to health care in Canada was expected to grow by only 2.9% in 2012, a far cry from the 7% annual growth seen consistently for years until 2010.
CMAJ 2012;184(18):E927-8
www.cmaj.ca/content/184/18/E927

HEMATOLOGY

False-positive HTLV serology

After intravenous immunoglobulin transfusion for toxic myelopathy, a 29-year-old man with leukemia had positive tests for antibodies to several viruses. Savary Bélanger and colleagues traced the results of testing from before the transfusion to several months after and showed that the antibodies had been passively transferred during transfusion. The possibility of passive transfer of antibodies should be considered when interpreting a positive test result after transfusion.
CMAJ 2012;184(15):1709-12
www.cmaj.ca/content/184/15/1709

HIV / AIDS

The studies that launched a thousand snips

A series of influential clinical trials linking circumcision to reduced HIV transmission rates had given rise to mass circumcision campaigns in Africa, but anti-circumcision activists claimed the research was deeply flawed. *CMAJ* 2012;184(1):E37-8
www.cmaj.ca/content/184/1/E37

Global Fund cutback

The primary source of funding for AIDS treatment in the developing world announced that it would discontinue funding new grants for the next 2 years because of shortfalls in contributions from donor nations.
CMAJ 2012;184(1):E11-4
www.cmaj.ca/content/184/1/E11

Should hiding HIV status always be a crime?

Civil liberties advocates argued against compulsory disclosure of HIV status. *CMAJ* 2012;184(9):E479-80
www.cmaj.ca/content/184/9/E479

HIV laws

Governments should not have laws that criminalize HIV transmission or nondisclosure of HIV status, according to the Global Commission on HIV and the Law, an independent body established in 2010 to protect the human rights of people with HIV and help reduce spread of the virus. *CMAJ* 2012;184(12):E655-8
www.cmaj.ca/content/184/12/E655

HUMOUR

Holiday reading

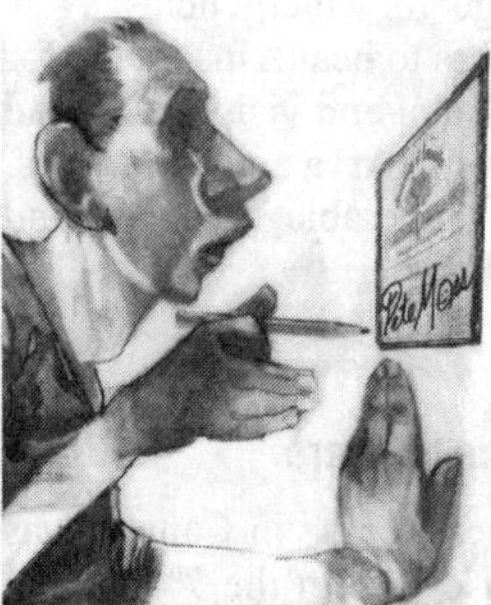
Image courtesy of Fred Sebastian

Humorous missives on the Mayan doomsday effect, an alarmingly green patient, how fake doctors use technology and the nebulous world of facts. *CMAJ* joyfully shared these treats for the holiday season.
CMAJ 2012;184(18):2021-2
www.cmaj.ca/content/184/18/2021
CMAJ 2012;184(18):2023
www.cmaj.ca/content/184/18/2023
CMAJ 2012;184(18):2024
www.cmaj.ca/content/184/18/2024
CMAJ 2012;184(18):2029
www.cmaj.ca/content/184/18/2029

IMMUNOLOGY

Systemic lupus erythematosus

A 60-year-old woman with systemic lupus erythematosus developed sudden bilateral loss of vision, along with a mild rash on her arms and legs. Although supporting test results were not back, emergency treatment was started after ophthalmologic examination.
CMAJ 2012;184(3):315-9
www.cmaj.ca/content/184/3/315

Bee pollen supplements

Bee pollen supplements consist of pollen granules collected by bees. Patients with pollen allergies may have allergic reactions, including anaphylaxis, from ingesting bee pollen, warned Jagdis and Sussman.
CMAJ 2012;184(10):1167-9
www.cmaj.ca/content/184/10/1167

INFECTIOUS DISEASES

Risk of infection in hospital

Elderly residents of long-term care facilities who visited the emergency department were more than 3 times as likely to have an acute infection in the following week. This finding came from a cohort study of 1269 residents of long-term care facilities that used chart review to assess infection and possible confounding factors. Additional precautions should be considered for residents following a visit to the emergency department, said Quach and colleagues. *CMAJ* 2012;184(4):E232-9
www.cmaj.ca/content/184/4/E232

Treating community-acquired pneumonia

Although community-acquired pneumonia is uncommon, it can be life-threatening. Leis and Gold emphasized that validated scoring systems can help triage patients into those who can receive treatment at home, those who require admission to hospital and those who should be referred promptly to intensive care. *CMAJ* 2012;184(5):559
www.cmaj.ca/content/184/5/559

Risk of infection after splenectomy

Patients who have undergone splenectomy are at risk of overwhelming infection. Petrescu and colleagues reviewed interventions that can be offered before and after splenectomy to substantially reduce this risk. *CMAJ* 2012;184(9):1053-4
www.cmaj.ca/content/184/9/1053

Acute bacterial meningitis in adults

If lumbar puncture is expected to be delayed, even for neuroimaging, antibiotic therapy for acute bacterial meningitis should not be postponed, said Moayedi and Gold. The authors added that select patients can undergo lumbar puncture without prior computed tomography of the brain. *CMAJ* 2012;184(9):1060
www.cmaj.ca/content/184/9/1060

Is zinc useful for the common cold?

Oral zinc treatment reduced the duration of cold symptoms in adults by 2.63 days. This systematic review of 17 trials involving 2121 people displayed considerable heterogeneity between trials, showed appreciable adverse events and did not detect an effect in children. There is only a weak rationale for physicians to recommend zinc for the treatment of the common cold, said the authors. *CMAJ* 2012;184(10):E551-61
www.cmaj.ca/content/184/10/E551

Clostridium difficile infection

A 66-year-old woman had diarrhea after receiving levofloxacin for pneumonia. Her stool tested positive for *Clostridium difficile* toxin. Kandel and colleagues reviewed the next steps in managing *C. difficile* infection, including treatment, monitoring and prevention of recurrence. *CMAJ* 2012;184(12):1383-5
www.cmaj.ca/content/184/12/1383

Herpes zoster

A 69-year-old man had a vesicular rash that was diagnosed as herpes zoster. Should he receive an oral antiviral agent? If postherpetic neuralgia develops, will anything decrease the pain? What about the herpes zoster vaccine? MacFadden and Gold addressed these and other common questions about herpes zoster. *CMAJ* 2012;184(13):1489-91
www.cmaj.ca/content/184/13/1489

Infectious disease experts monitored outbreaks of enterovirus 71 in Asia

Canadian infectious disease experts were monitoring a strain of enterovirus 71 that was killing children in Asia.
CMAJ 2012;184(15):E781-2
www.cmaj.ca/content/184/15/E781

Measles

Most cases of measles in Canada are caused by community transmission after international importation, said Desai and colleagues. Vaccination programs, early identification of cases and prompt containment are essential to maintaining the absence of endemic measles in Canada. *CMAJ* 2012;184(16):1811
www.cmaj.ca/content/184/16/1811

INFORMATICS

Nothing cutting edge about Canadian e-health strategy

New technologies such as tablets, smartphones and other mobile personal communications devices had long since outstripped Canada's e-health strategy, critics said. *CMAJ* 2012;184(1):E35-6
www.cmaj.ca/content/184/1/E35

Better literature searches

PubMed search filters can improve the efficiency of literature searches by physicians. This finding was based on a survey of nephrologists asking them to specify search terms to find medical literature to answer clinical questions. Improved searches may enhance the transfer of research into practice and improve patient care, said the authors.
CMAJ 2012;184(3):E184-E190
www.cmaj.ca/content/184/3/E184

UK unveiled patient-centred electronic health strategy

Completing a full retreat from an e-health strategy based on centralized national records, the government of the United Kingdom unveiled a 10-year blueprint that aimed to put the "power of information" in the hands of patients. *CMAJ* 2012;184(11):E579-80
www.cmaj.ca/content/184/11/E579

Use of electronic health records

Electronic health records afforded numerous potential benefits, but some clinicians were concerned that processing electronic information would reduce their productivity and increase their workload. Sittig and Singh tackled these concerns and others by presenting 10 "rights" and corresponding responsibilities to ensure that the quality of health care continued to improve. *CMAJ* 2012;184(13):1479-83
www.cmaj.ca/content/184/13/1479

Prescription drug monitoring databases

Implementing a centralized prescription network was associated with a dramatic reduction in the number of potentially inappropriate prescriptions filled for opioids and benzodiazepines. Dormuth and colleagues used 5 years of routine pharmacy data to evaluate the introduction of the network, comparing trends among patients over 65 years of age and among patients receiving social assistance, as well as patterns for commonly prescribed nonsteroidal anti-inflammatory drugs. Wider use of such networks could reduce the misuse of some prescription drugs, said the authors. *CMAJ* 2012;184(16):E852-6
www.cmaj.ca/content/184/16/E852

Prescription drug monitoring has the potential to prevent the misuse and abuse of controlled substances and fatal overdoses. However, to achieve optimal results, real-time access by health practitioners is essential, said Wilsey and Prasad. Real-time access allows clinicians to see when and from whom patients have received prescriptions for drugs, such as opioids, at the time the patient is being seen — information that can be helpful in making decisions about prescribing.
CMAJ 2012;184(16):1767-8
www.cmaj.ca/content/184/16/1767

INTERNATIONAL MEDICINE

Overhauling health care Down Under

Few developed nations in recent history had sought such systemic reform to their health care system as Australia, which over the course of the previous 4 years had squabbled over jurisdictional issues, funding, primary care reform and a host of other issues in a bid to implement its most substantial overhaul of health care since universality was introduced in 1975. *CMAJ* 2012;184(4):E205-6
www.cmaj.ca/content/184/4/E205

The Alzheimer front

United States President Barack Obama announced that his government would funnel US$156 million into Alzheimer disease research, treatment and awareness programs over the next 2 years in hopes of mitigating the effects of a disease that afflicted more than 5 million Americans.
CMAJ 2012;184(4):E219-20
www.cmaj.ca/content/184/4/E219

Taking the pulse of pulse oximetry in Africa

A potentially inexpensive means of providing pulse oximetry using mobile phones was being tested in sub-Saharan Africa in hopes of reducing the toll taken by deaths resulting from anesthesia complications in surgeries. *CMAJ* 2012;184(5):E244-5
www.cmaj.ca/content/184/5/E244

Mental health cuts

Mental health services in the United States were increasingly becoming a favoured target of legislators seeking to reduce budget deficits, according to the National Alliance on Mental Illness.
CMAJ 2012;184(5):E254-5
www.cmaj.ca/content/184/5/E254

Health in Colombia: a system in crisis

Colombia's health care provided dramatically inferior care to the less affluent. *CMAJ* 2012;184(6):E289-90
www.cmaj.ca/content/184/6/E289

Africa's road to blood ruin

Blood transfusion programs in African nations were rife with deficiencies. *CMAJ* 2012;184(7):E341-2
www.cmaj.ca/content/184/7/E341

India moved to contain organ donation havoc

Although nowhere near as endemic a problem as once was the case in India, payments for organ donations, which were made illegal in 1995, continued to blight the landscape and invited charges that the impoverished were being preyed upon. *CMAJ* 2012;184(8):E387-8
www.cmaj.ca/content/184/8/E387

Dementia leader

A doubling of funding for dementia research and the introduction of dementia screening as an element of the National Health Service program for people aged 40–74 were among measures introduced by the British government to address what Prime Minister David Cameron called "one of the great challenges of our time … the quiet crisis" of dementia.
CMAJ 2012;184(8):E413-6
www.cmaj.ca/content/184/8/E413

Bloom fading from e-health golden wattle

Australia's plan to create personally controlled electronic health records that would allow citizens to access and share medical records in a nationwide database was being assailed for its lack of functionality and its potential breaches of privacy. *CMAJ* 2012;184(9):E459-60
www.cmaj.ca/content/184/9/E459

Battle tolls

With tens of thousands of American soldiers scheduled to return home in the next few years as the United States withdrew from the war in Afghanistan, US Secretary of Veteran Affairs Eric K. Shinseki announced that his department would bolster its capacity to provide mental health services by increasing the mental health workforce by roughly 10%. *CMAJ* 2012;184(9):E481-4
www.cmaj.ca/content/184/9/E481

Deficient care

Only half of people with diabetes in England were receiving recommended care, and about 24 000 were dying from conditions that could have been prevented, according to the United Kingdom's National Audit Office. *CMAJ* 2012;184(10):E535-8
www.cmaj.ca/content/184/10/E535

India's "rural doctor" proposal stirred criticism

In a bid to resolve its severe shortage of medical professionals willing to toil in rural areas, the government of India proposed to create a new category of physician called the "rural doctor," whose training wouldn't be as intensive and thorough but who, theoretically, would be more willing to practise far from the beaten path. *CMAJ* 2012;184(12):E637-8
www.cmaj.ca/content/184/12/E637

Free medicine for all in India

India's proposed US$5.4-billion "free medicine for all" policy promised to be a game-changer for the lives of millions of poor and vulnerable people, many of whom could not afford their medications or were not being reached by public health facilities. *CMAJ* 2012;184(15):E783-4
www.cmaj.ca/content/184/15/E783

MEDIA

Baby basics

The *Canadian Medical Association Complete Book of Mother and Baby Care*, edited by Dr. Anne Biringer, is a practical, common-sense guide for parents on everything from planning for pregnancy to removing a splinter. *CMAJ* 2012;184(1):70
www.cmaj.ca/content/184/1/70

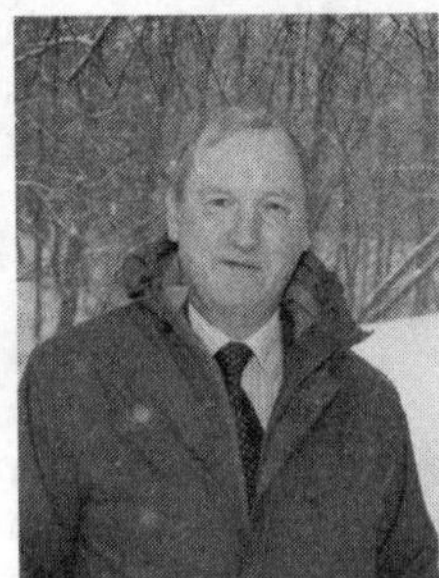
Dr. John Fletcher. Image courtesy of R. Collier

Utility, stability and a digital presence

Dr. John Fletcher took over the leadership of *CMAJ* from Dr. Rajendra Kale, interim editor-in-chief. Fletcher had 3 goals in mind for *CMAJ*: to see the journal improve its digital presence, attain financial stability and become more useful to practising physicians. *CMAJ* 2012;184(3):288-9
www.cmaj.ca/content/184/3/288

Squires Award

In selecting the study "CATCH: a clinical decision rule for the use of computed tomography in children with minor head injury" as the winner of the 2010 Bruce Squires Award, "we considered the study's potential to impact clinical practice, its originality, the quality of the methodology and its overall excellence. The CATCH study meets all of these criteria and certainly merits the Bruce Squires Award," said *CMAJ* Editor-in-Chief Dr. John Fletcher. *CMAJ* 2012;184(4):E219-20
www.cmaj.ca/content/184/4/E219

The view from the North

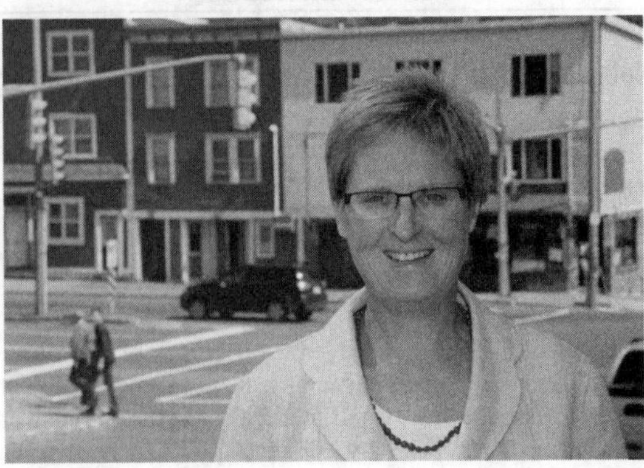
CMA President Dr. Anna Reid. Image courtesy of R. Collier

Incoming CMA President Dr. Anna Reid hoped Canada's doctors would come together to reduce health inequities among Aboriginal peoples and provide stressed physicians with the help they need to stay on the job. *CMAJ* 2012;184(13):E693-4
www.cmaj.ca/content/184/13/E693

Enough "unhelpful, over-the-top" rhetoric, Aglukkaq said

Critics who accuse the federal government of dodging its responsibilities to ensure national standards and equity are merely indulging in unhelpful rhetoric, said federal Health Minister Leona Aglukkaq at the Canadian Medical Association's 145th annual general meeting. *CMAJ* 2012;184(13):E707-8
www.cmaj.ca/content/184/13/E707

Master of re-invention elected to CMA helm

Dr. Louis Hugo Francescutti of Alberta — emergency physician, tenured professor, amateur stonemason, master storyteller — was to assume the CMA presidency in August 2013.
CMAJ 2012;184(13):E701-2
www.cmaj.ca/content/184/13/E701

MEDICAL CAREERS

More docs, better pay

The national physician pool grew by 2.3% to 69 700 doctors in 2010, the largest in history, according to the Canadian Institute for Health Information. Meanwhile, clinical payments for physicians reached nearly $19 billion in fiscal year 2009/10. *CMAJ* 2012;184(2):E106-8
www.cmaj.ca/content/184/2/E106

Are you kidding, doc?

Medical regulatory authorities who fail to conduct criminal records checks on physicians before issuing licences to practise are either "negligent" or "ridiculously naive," patient advocates said.
CMAJ 2012;184(4):E217-8
www.cmaj.ca/content/184/4/E217

Effects of assessing productivity

Strategies for assessing the productivity of faculty in academic medical centres appeared to improve productivity in research and clinical work, but not in teaching, and to lead to increases in compensation. A systematic review summarized findings from 8 studies of generally low methodologic quality, all conducted in the United States. Academic departments implementing strategies to assess the productivity of faculty

need to consider the associated challenges, uncertainties and intended consequences, said the authors. *CMAJ* 2012;184(11):E602-12
www.cmaj.ca/content/184/11/E602

Social media mishaps

It turned out that doctors who used Facebook, Twitter or other social media platforms were perfectly capable of embarrassing themselves — and the medical profession as a whole — by posting unprofessional material. *CMAJ* 2012;184(12):E627-8
www.cmaj.ca/content/184/12/E627

Logging on to tell your doctor off

Patients might not have been comfortable calling out their doctors for being unprofessional in person but appeared to have few qualms about expressing their frustrations online. Ratings websites for physicians were growing in number and popularity. *CMAJ* 2012;184(12):E629-30
www.cmaj.ca/content/184/12/E629

Attracting small-town docs a challenge

Loan forgiveness was one piece of the strategy to attract and retain rural doctors, according to educators, but Canada needed a systematic policy framework to tackle the problem. *CMAJ* 2012;184(14):E735-6
www.cmaj.ca/content/184/14/E735

MEDICAL EDUCATION

Residents called for duty hour reform

The fatigue from working long shifts was affecting the well-being and learning of medical residents, as well as putting patients at risk, and as a consequence, duty-hour reform was needed, according to the Canadian Association of Internes and Residents. *CMAJ* 2012;184(8):E411-2
www.cmaj.ca/content/184/8/E411

MCAT revisions finalized

Academic administrators were to reshape the Medical College Admission Test as part of a bid to produce more well-rounded physicians.
CMAJ 2012;184(9):E473-4
www.cmaj.ca/content/184/9/E473

Training Canadian hospitalists

In contrast to the United States, most Canadian hospitalists were family physicians. Although the issues of training and certification had begun to be addressed, this process was still in its infancy. A clear definition of the scope of practice of Canadian hospitalists and research on the impact these physicians had on the quality of care were needed.
CMAJ 2012;184(14):1557-8
www.cmaj.ca/content/184/14/1557

Promoting pride in practice

Advocates in the United Kingdom created a toolkit to educate and assess health providers on LGBT (lesbian, gay, bisexual, transsexual) issues such as using inclusive language and imagery, training staff on LGBT health problems and monitoring how people of various sexual orientations access health services. *CMAJ* 2012;184(15):E789-90
www.cmaj.ca/content/184/15/E789

The MD express lane

An Ontario university was proposing an accelerated path to a medical degree for select high school students. *CMAJ* 2012;184(16):E845-6
www.cmaj.ca/content/184/16/E845

MENTAL HEALTH

Outback blues

Mental illness in men aged 12–25 took an A$3.27-billion toll annually on the Australian economy and cost A$387 000 per hour "across a year in lost productivity," a report indicated. *CMAJ* 2012;184(10):E535-8
www.cmaj.ca/content/184/10/E535

Mental deficit

Though nearly half of all ill health among people under age 65 in the United Kingdom was due to mental illness, only a quarter of those with a mental illness were receiving treatment. This was true despite the low costs of psychological therapy and the potential savings through reduced disability benefits, according to a report by the Centre for Economic Performance's Mental Health Policy Group.
CMAJ 2012;184(11):E597-601
www.cmaj.ca/content/184/11/E597

Psychological distress and death

Psychological distress is associated with an increased risk of death from cerebrovascular disease. A study obtained data from a population-based cohort in the United Kingdom. Psychological distress was measured using the 12-item General Health Questionnaire. The results showed that the cardiovascular effects of psychological distress were not limited to coronary artery disease and may be useful for screening and preventive care. *CMAJ* 2012;184(13):1461-6
www.cmaj.ca/content/184/13/1461

Although the cardiovascular benefits of treating psychological stress remained unproven, clinicians should be mindful of traditional cardiovascular risk factors in people who are stressed and refer them for support and treatment, suggested Pan and Rexrode.
CMAJ 2012;184(13):1453-4
www.cmaj.ca/content/184/13/1453

NEPHROLOGY

Why patients might not want dialysis

Patients approaching end-stage kidney disease are willing to forgo considerable life expectancy to avoid dialysis. This result was based on a discrete choice experiment using questionnaire responses from 105 patients with renal disease that measured their preferences. Information about patients' preferences regarding the type and location of dialysis is important for the planning of future renal services, said Morton and colleagues. *CMAJ* 2012;184(5):E277-83
www.cmaj.ca/content/184/5/E277

Appropriate nephrology referrals

The number of appropriate referrals to nephrology increased in the year after routine reporting of the estimated glomerular filtration rate (eGFR) by laboratories was introduced. However, the proportion of referrals that was deemed appropriate did not change significantly because inappropriate referrals also increased. These findings came from a study involving 2672 patients referred to the nephrology service at a tertiary care hospital in the year before and the year after automatic reporting of the eGFR began. An increase in appropriate referrals would potentially improve patient care, said Akbari and colleagues.
CMAJ 2012;184(5):E269-76
www.cmaj.ca/content/184/5/E269

NEUROLOGY

Autonomic dysreflexia

Autonomic dysreflexia occurs in up to 90% of people with upper thoracic or cervical spine injury. Triggered by stimuli such as bladder distention or even a shoelace tied too tightly, this is a medical emergency and can be life-threatening. Awareness of the triggers is the key to prevention. *CMAJ* 2012;184(1):66
www.cmaj.ca/content/184/1/66

Physicians must be brought up to speed on concussion risks

Canadian physicians have often been uninformed about the long-term consequences of concussions sustained in sport, a specialist in athletic injuries argued. *CMAJ* 2012;184(2):E113-4
www.cmaj.ca/content/184/2/E113

Stop the fighting and play hockey

Kale argued that the brutal tradition of fighting in hockey should be given up now that research has shown that repeated head trauma can cause severe progressive brain damage. *CMAJ* 2012;184(3):275
www.cmaj.ca/content/184/3/275

Treating migraine

Four types of acupuncture, including a sham procedure, appeared to have similar effects in preventing migraine headache. A randomized controlled trial involving 480 people compared the number of days with migraine, as well as pain intensity, functional status and other secondary outcomes. The nonspecific effects of acupuncture may play a relevant role, said the authors. *CMAJ* 2012;184(4):401-10
www.cmaj.ca/content/184/4/401

Although there seems to be little difference between Chinese and non-Chinese acupuncture points, Chinese points might be marginally more effective, said Molsberger. *CMAJ* 2012;184(4):391-2
www.cmaj.ca/content/184/4/391

Giving more training to family physicians on how to treat migraine did not improve patients' symptoms. A pragmatic randomized controlled trial of 6 hours of training for doctors, and involving 490 patients, showed little difference in the frequency, severity or duration of attacks or number of days spent with headaches or away from work. Future interventions should target patients with frequent attacks who are not using preventive medication, said the authors. *CMAJ* 2012;184(4):E224-31
www.cmaj.ca/content/184/4/E224

Subarachnoid hemorrhage

About 1 in 14 patients presenting to an emergency department with a severe acute headache will have experienced a subarachnoid hemorrhage from an aneurysm. Do all patients with this presentation require computed tomography imaging and a lumbar puncture? Fine and colleagues discussed the latest literature that may change how clinicians assess these patients. *CMAJ* 2012;184(5):555-6
www.cmaj.ca/content/184/5/555

Stem cells for neurodegenerative disorders

Extravagant claims had been made of the potential for using stem cells to treat neurodegenerative disorders of the central nervous system. Barker argued that it is critical we understand the limitations of the technologies at our disposal, as well as the inherent difficulties in trying to take an *in vitro* cell culture system from the laboratory to the complexities of patients in the clinic. *CMAJ* 2012;184(6):631-2
www.cmaj.ca/content/184/6/631

Hockey concussion: Is it child abuse?

One critic said Hockey Canada's failure to implement more stringent anticoncussion measures constituted nothing short of "child abuse." *CMAJ* 2012;184(8):861-2
www.cmaj.ca/content/184/8/861

Dysphagia after stroke

Dysphagia after stroke was common, presenting in 55% of all patients admitted to hospital with acute disease, yet it was often underdiagnosed. Early detection of dysphagia with screening reduced comorbidity, such as pneumonia. *CMAJ* 2012;184(10):1127-8
www.cmaj.ca/content/184/10/1127

Smoked cannabis of some benefit in MS

People with multiple sclerosis who smoked cannabis had less pain and spasticity than patients smoking placebo. Thirty-seven people were included in this randomized crossover trial that also showed some impact on cognitive abilities. Larger studies were needed to determine optimum doses, said the authors. *CMAJ* 2012;184(10):1143-50
www.cmaj.ca/content/184/10/1143

Heavy hitting: concussions and safety law

Might occupational health and safety law be the foundation to compel Canadian sports associations and leagues to change their rules to ban actions that cause concussions, such as hitting in hockey, or heading the ball in soccer? *CMAJ* 2012;184(12):E641-2
www.cmaj.ca/content/184/12/E641

Melatonin

Although the use of melatonin for insomnia was controversial, melatonin had been shown to be effective against jet lag, particularly for people flying eastward and crossing many time zones. Short-term use appeared safe, but Carter and Juurlink reminded readers that melatonin was a synthetic hormone, not a herbal supplement.
CMAJ 2012;184(17):1923
www.cmaj.ca/content/184/17/1923

NUTRITION

Salt in fast food

The salt content of fast foods varied substantially by the country in which the food was produced. Data on salt content were collected for foods produced by 6 fast food chains in 6 countries. In the right regulatory environment, it is likely that fast food companies could substantially reduce salt in their products, said Dunford and colleagues.
CMAJ 2012;184(9):1023-8
www.cmaj.ca/content/184/9/1023

Inching toward universal nutrient disclosure

A proposed global standard for mandatory nutrition labelling would compel all food producers to articulate fat, protein, fibre, sodium, sugar and calorie content on the back of all processed food packages.
CMAJ 2012;184(10):E523-4
www.cmaj.ca/content/184/10/E523

The science of pesticide-free potato chips

There was no question that the organic food industry was booming. Even junk food makers were clambering aboard the organic train. The public perception appeared to be that organic foods were better, having been grown under strict conditions of purity that precluded the use of toxic

agricultural chemicals. Ergo, they must be "healthier" or more nutrient rich than conventionally produced fare, or, at a very minimum, free of traces of nasty compounds. But was there any concrete evidence in support of that proposition? *CMAJ* 2012;184(14):E741-2
www.cmaj.ca/content/184/14/E741

OBESITY

Managing obesity in adults

The 5A model can be useful in primary care for counselling patients who are obese or overweight. Measuring waist circumference can identify those with abdominal obesity who may have a normal body mass index. Adding psychological interventions to dietary or physical activity interventions improves their success, emphasized Plourde and Prud'Homme. *CMAJ* 2012;184(9):1039-44
www.cmaj.ca/content/184/9/1039

OBSTETRICS

Sex-selective abortions: no simple solution

While American legislators contemplated criminalizing sex-selective abortion, experts said the experience of other nations that had tried to impose such a prohibition indicated that it is difficult to enforce and easy to skirt. *CMAJ* 2012;184(3):286-8
www.cmaj.ca/content/184/3/286

Sex selection migrated to Canada

Easy access to abortion and advances in prenatal sex determination had combined to make Canada a haven for parents who would terminate female fetuses in favour of having sons, despite overwhelming censure of the practice, economists and bioethics experts said.
CMAJ 2012;184(3):E163-4
www.cmaj.ca/content/184/3/E163

Female feticide

Canada should prohibit disclosure of the sex of a fetus until after about 30 weeks of pregnancy to combat female feticide, an evil that was practised by some ethnic groups in North America.
CMAJ 2012;184(4):387-8
www.cmaj.ca/content/184/4/387

Screening for perinatal depression

Two simple case-finding questions showed acceptable accuracy at ruling out perinatal depression in women 2 months before or 1 to 3 months after delivery. Self-reported responses to these questions were compared against DSM-IV criteria for major depressive disorder among 152 women receiving perinatal care. These findings may assist the utility of clinical guidelines that advocate this brief case-finding approach, said the authors.
CMAJ 2012;184(8):E424-30
www.cmaj.ca/content/184/8/E424

Sex ratios in Canada

Multiparous women born in India were significantly more likely than multiparous women born in Canada to have a male infant. This finding was based on male:female ratios in Ontario calculated from registry data for 766 688 singleton live births between 2002 and 2007. Whether this difference was the result of prenatal sex selection should be determined by further studies, said Ray and colleagues. *CMAJ* 2012;184(9):E492-6
www.cmaj.ca/content/184/9/E492

Pregnancy complications among women born preterm

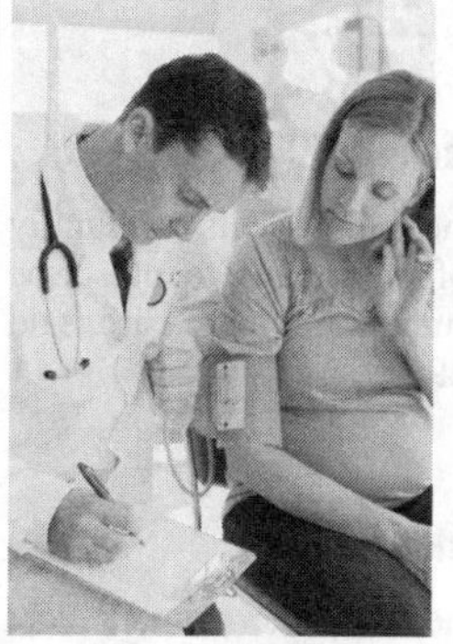

Women who were themselves born preterm are at increased risk of pregnancy complications later in life. Nuyt and colleagues compared pregnancy complications such as gestational diabetes, hypertension, preeclampsia and eclampsia in 7405 women who were born preterm and 16 714 women who were born at term between 1976 and 1995 and had later pregnancies between 1987 and 2008. The impact of preterm birth on obstetric care should be taken into account in the management of pregnant patients, said the authors. *CMAJ* 2012;184(16):1777-84
www.cmaj.ca/content/184/16/1777

Collaborative maternity care

Women attending a program of collaborative, interdisciplinary maternity care were more likely to have a physiologic birth than women receiving standard care. A retrospective study measured several outcomes among 1238 women attending an innovative birth program in Vancouver and observed favourable effects on rates of cesarean delivery, length of hospital stay and exclusive breast feeding at discharge. These results should encourage the implementation and evaluation of similar approaches elsewhere, said the authors. *CMAJ* 2012;184(17):1885-92
www.cmaj.ca/content/184/17/1885

OPHTHALMOLOGY

Acute-onset floaters and flashes

Usually caused by posterior vitreous detachment, acute-onset floaters and flashes are common in older adults and are usually benign. Because posterior vitreous detachment can progress to retinal detachment in a minority of cases, any patient with these symptoms and a defect in visual field or the presence of vitreous hemorrhage or pigment should be assessed by an ophthalmologist within 24 hours.
CMAJ 2012;184(4):431
www.cmaj.ca/content/184/4/431

Calculating risk in use of disposable contact lenses

Manufacturers suggested improper use of contact lenses could lead to serious problems, but many patients opted to ignore the risk.
CMAJ 2012;184(6):E297-8
www.cmaj.ca/content/184/6/E297

PALLIATIVE CARE

Line between acts and omissions blurred, euthanasia critics argued

Decriminalization of assisted suicide and voluntary euthanasia is an unethical alternative to redressing current deficiencies in palliative care in Canada, physicians, ethicists and patient advocates argued.
CMAJ 2012;184(1):E19-20
www.cmaj.ca/content/184/1/E19

Doctors offered different levels of palliative sedation

Physicians who used mild palliative sedation gave similar reasoning for choosing this approach as did physicians who used deep palliative sedation. During this qualitative study from the Netherlands, 54 physicians were interviewed about their most recent experience of providing palliative sedation. Proportionality of sedation should be seen

as a multidimensional notion that can result in different approaches, said the authors. *CMAJ* 2012;184(7):E360-6
www.cmaj.ca/content/184/7/E360

Opioids for dyspnea in advanced COPD

Discrepancies between the positive experiences of patients and family caregivers with opioids and the reluctance of physicians to prescribe opioids for refractory dyspnea constituted an important gap in care, said Rocker and colleagues. *CMAJ* 2012;184(9):E497-504
www.cmaj.ca/content/184/9/E497

Palliative care training substandard

Many experts in end-of-life care questioned whether primary care doctors had the skills necessary to ensure dying patients meet peaceful ends and were calling for more palliative experts and increased training for all physicians. *CMAJ* 2012;184(12):E643-4
www.cmaj.ca/content/184/12/E643

Palliative care subspecialty in the offing

The establishment of palliative medicine as a subspecialty, and certification of family physicians with added competence in palliative medicine, were logical steps in the provision of care to an aging population in Canada, experts contended. *CMAJ* 2012;184(12):E653-4
www.cmaj.ca/content/184/12/E653

PATHOLOGY

Cutaneous lymphoma or benign lesion?

A 66-year-old man presented with an erythematous nodule on his forearm, consistent with a pyogenic granuloma on inspection. The biopsy results, however, indicated a very different disorder.
CMAJ 2012;184(8):917
www.cmaj.ca/content/184/8/917

PATIENT CARE

Private rooms: the fiscal advantage

The architects of a new Canadian standard for hospitals said the justification for private rooms in Canadian hospitals was so overwhelming that they expected the new guidelines would be "widely utilized." *CMAJ* 2012;184(1):E47-8
www.cmaj.ca/content/184/1/E47

Networks delivered better primary care

Patients with diabetes managed in primary care networks received higher quality care and had slightly better clinical outcomes than those managed in other types of practice. These findings were based on routine health care data comparing processes of care, admissions to hospital and visits to emergency departments. Future studies should aim to determine how primary care networks can best implement equitable access, said the authors. *CMAJ* 2012;184(2):E144-52
www.cmaj.ca/content/184/2/E144

Who should be privy to your privates?

Uncertainty about who should chaperone intimate examinations may be undercutting the protections such attendants may afford patients and doctors, experts said. *CMAJ* 2012;184(6):E299-300
www.cmaj.ca/content/184/6/E299

Touch the screen now to see a doctor

Interactive self-registration kiosks were being touted as the next wave in efficiency in health facilities. *CMAJ* 2012;184(7):E339-40
www.cmaj.ca/content/184/7/E339

Chronic disparities

Sex and income level have an impact on the level of primary care that people with chronic diseases receive from their physicians, according to a Canadian Institute for Health Information study.
CMAJ 2012;184(7):E354-6
www.cmaj.ca/content/184/7/E354

Medical training and care under the rainbow umbrella

Surgical green joined the rainbow of colours at Toronto's 32nd Gay Pride Day, with 70 physicians joining the MD Pride March to promote better health care for lesbian, gay, bisexual, transgender and questioning (LGBTQ) people and improved working conditions for nonheterosexual physicians. *CMAJ* 2012;184(12):E633-4
www.cmaj.ca/content/184/12/E633

PATIENT SAFETY

Patients and families as safety experts

Families were keen to participate in a system to report adverse events during their children's hospital stay and frequently reported events that had not been noted by staff. These findings came from a questionnaire survey of 544 families following discharge of their children from a hospital ward. There was potential to recruit families to improve the safety of the health care system for children, said the authors.
CMAJ 2012;184(1):29-34
www.cmaj.ca/content/184/1/29

When questioned, patients report safety incidents that would otherwise go undetected. Furthermore, patients are highly motivated to report errors or problems with their care. Paying close attention to patients' and families' reports of safety issues may be our best early warning system for detecting deterioration of care, the authors argued.
CMAJ 2012;184(1):15-6
www.cmaj.ca/content/184/1/15

Medical ink

If your spouse's initials are "D.N.R.," you should probably think twice before tattooing them on your chest. Then again, if your end-of-life plans include a do-not-resuscitate order, maybe it's not such a bad idea after all.
CMAJ 2012;184(9):1018-20
www.cmaj.ca/content/184/9/1018

The lost sponge

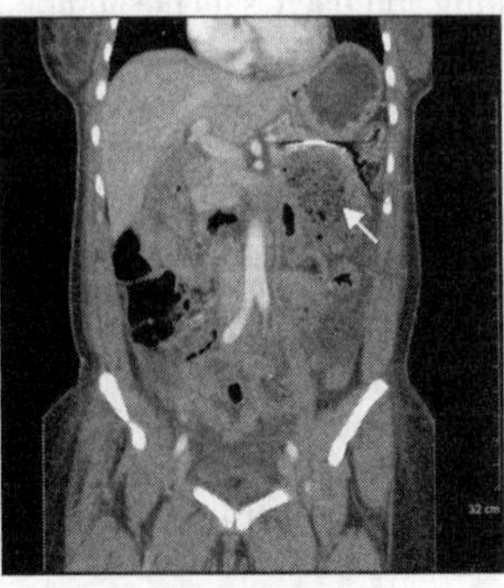

The sponge count was incorrect after a laparotomy for suspected small-bowel obstruction in a 43-year-old woman. Despite radiography and exploration of the abdomen, the sponge was not found until after computed tomography and a second laparotomy the next day. What went wrong? How can this type of event be prevented? Grant-Orser and colleagues shared the details of this case.
CMAJ 2012;184(11):1275-8
www.cmaj.ca/content/184/11/1275

Costly mistakes

Preventable mistakes in acute care settings were costing Canada nearly $400 million a year, according to the Canadian Patient Safety Institute. And that didn't include postdischarge costs and loss of occupational productivity. A greater focus on patient safety could lead to significant savings, the institute suggested. *CMAJ* 2012;184(12):E655-8
www.cmaj.ca/content/184/12/E655

PEDIATRICS

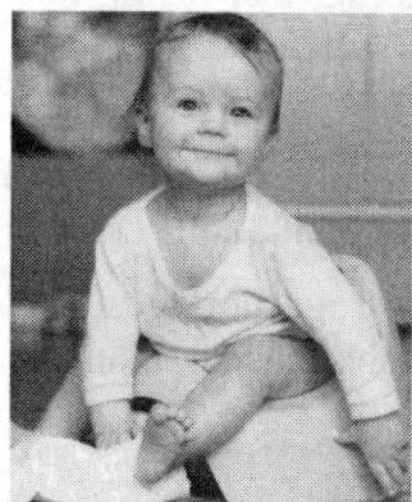
©2012 Thinkstock

Toilet training children

Toilet training should be started when both the child and parent are willing and able to participate. Moreover, a positive, consistent approach to toilet training is unlikely to cause long-term harm. *CMAJ* 2012;184(5):511-2
www.cmaj.ca/content/184/5/511

Is ADHD overdiagnosed in young boys?

Boys aged 6–12 years born in December, and hence the youngest in their grade, were 30% more likely to receive a diagnosis of attention-deficit/hyperactivity disorder than their older male classmates. Nearly 1 million children were included in this study, spanning 11 years, which identified relevant physician diagnoses and prescriptions. These findings raise concerns about the potential harms of overdiagnosis and overprescribing, said Morrow and colleagues. *CMAJ* 2012;184(7):755-62
www.cmaj.ca/content/184/7/755

Nocturnal enuresis

Very little advancement had been made recently in the treatment of nocturnal enuresis, said Kiddoo, but there was a greater understanding of the pathophysiology of this condition. Newer theories pointed to the role of the central nervous system, specifically the effects of sleep disruption. The bed alarm had the highest long-term success rate in managing this condition. *CMAJ* 2012;184(8):908-11
www.cmaj.ca/content/184/8/908

Jehovah's Witness teen with anemia

A 15-year-old girl refused transfusion for profound anemia because of her religious beliefs. Her symptoms worsened, and she ended up in the intensive care unit. What should the health care team do in this situation? *CMAJ* 2012;184(9):1055-9
www.cmaj.ca/content/184/9/1055

Impact of changing growth curves

Several organizations had recommended that physicians switch from using the Centers for Disease Control and Prevention (CDC) growth curves to the World Health Organization (WHO) growth curves to monitor growth for Canadian children aged 5–19 years. In their study, Kakinami and colleagues found that the WHO growth curves did not offer any discriminatory advantage over the CDC standards currently in practice for the detection of cardiometabolic abnormalities in children aged 9–16 years. *CMAJ* 2012;184(10):E539-50
www.cmaj.ca/content/184/10/E539

Outcome after childhood brain injury

After childhood brain injury, relatively good motor outcomes may obscure cognitive and behavioural problems. Widespread views that young brains make better recoveries are naive, said Forsyth and Kirkham. Outcomes after brain injury in children are highly variable. *CMAJ* 2012;184(11):1257-64
www.cmaj.ca/content/184/11/1257

Mental health crises in children

First Nations adolescents and adolescents from families receiving low-income subsidies made more visits to the emergency department for mental health crises than did children from families that did not receive subsidies. This study used routine health care data to count emergency visits and follow-up visits and to classify possible explanatory factors. Findings from this study could help improve discharge planning, said Newton and colleagues. *CMAJ* 2012;184(12):E665-74
www.cmaj.ca/content/184/12/E665

Physical punishment of children

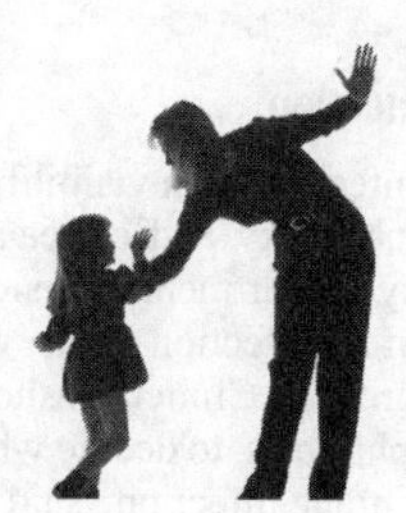
©2012 Thinkstock

With the growing body of research, physicians can confidently encourage parents to adopt constructive approaches to disciplining children. According to Durrant and Ensom, numerous studies have found that physical punishment increases the risk of broad and enduring negative developmental outcomes, including mental health disorders and slower cognitive development. Effective discipline depends on clear, age-appropriate expectations, effective communication and a safe environment. *CMAJ* 2012;184(12):1373-7
www.cmaj.ca/content/184/12/1373

Adolescent mental health

International development organizations needed to do more to address the mental health concerns of adolescents, according to the World Health Organization and the United Nations Children's Fund. About 20% of young people experienced a mental health problem each year, the most common being depression and anxiety. *CMAJ* 2012;184(12):E655-8
www.cmaj.ca/content/184/12/E655

Adverse events among children in hospital

Most responsible service for delivery of care at the time of each of the adverse events, by type of hospital

Most responsible service	Adverse events, no. (%) APC n = 210	CH n = 69	RR (95% CI)
Surgery	88 (41.9)	10 (14.5)	2.9 (1.6–5.7)
Medicine	60 (28.6)	23 (33.3)	0.9 (0.6–1.3)
Emergency	12 (5.7)	11 (15.9)	0.4 (0.2–0.8)
ICU	35 (16.7)	2 (2.9)	5.6 (1.4–34.4)
Maternity/obstetrics	7 (3.3)	8 (11.6)	0.3 (0.1–0.8)

Note: APC = academic pediatric centre, CH = community hospital, CI = confidence interval, ICU = intensive care unit, RR = relative risk.

About 1 in 9 children admitted to Canadian hospitals experienced an adverse event. Some of these were not preventable, but the authors of this study emphasized that there are many opportunities to reduce harm, particularly related to surgery, intensive care and diagnostic error. *CMAJ* 2012;184(13):E709-18
www.cmaj.ca/content/184/13/E709

Acetaminophen overdose in children

Acetaminophen overdose in children is a major cause of acute liver failure in children. A case reviewed developmental differences in drug metabolism between infants and older children, and highlighted controversies in the treatment of acute acetaminophen overdose. Ogilvie and coauthors emphasized that the widespread use and availability of

acetaminophen made the potential for overdose a population health concern. *CMAJ* 2012;184(13):1492-6
www.cmaj.ca/content/184/13/1492

Vitamin B_{12} deficiency in infants

Vitamin B_{12} deficiency in a breastfed infant usually results from a maternal deficiency in diet or through pernicious anemia. Symptoms can include poor feeding, weight loss and irritability, but neurologic manifestations (e.g., lethargy, gross motor developmental regression and slowing of brain growth) are most concerning, said Roumeliotis and colleagues. *CMAJ* 2012;184(14):1593-8
www.cmaj.ca/content/184/14/1593

Phimosis and urinary tract infection

There is no variation in risk of urinary tract infection with visibility of the urethral meatus in uncircumcised boys. Dubrovsky and colleagues screened 440 boys for whom the emergency department physician suspected urinary tract infection; they compared infection rates with respect to the presence or retractability of the foreskin. Clinicians should use circumcision status alone, not the degree of phimosis, to decide which boys should undergo investigation for urinary tract infection, said the authors. *CMAJ* 2012;184(15):E796-803
www.cmaj.ca/content/184/15/E796

Sleep in adolescents

Sleep disturbance was common among adolescents and was seen to be associated with an increased prevalence of cardiovascular risk factors, including higher levels of blood pressure, cholesterol and BMIs. However, duration of sleep did not show the same associations. A cross-sectional study used data from a prospective population-based study of 4104 high school students in Ontario. The findings called for intervention studies to evaluate the benefits of optimizing sleep in adolescents on cardiovascular risk, said the authors. *CMAJ* 2012;184(17):E913-20
www.cmaj.ca/content/184/17/E913

PHARMACEUTICALS

Illegal marketing

United States pharmaceutical giant Merck, Sharp & Dohne pleaded guilty to illegal promotion and marketing of the painkiller rofecoxib and agreed to pay a US$321 million criminal fine and US$628 million to resolve a civil claim regarding off-label marketing and false safety claims, the US Department of Justice announced. *CMAJ* 2012;184(1):E11-4
www.cmaj.ca/content/184/1/E11

Swallowing the pharmaceutical waters

A prescription drug may begin its life as a pretty little pill, but after a brief detour through a human digestive tract and miles of plumbing, some of it ends up in drinking water. Though the levels of pharmaceuticals in drinking water are minuscule, in the parts per trillion, some researchers were concerned that long-term exposure to this low-dose cocktail could prove harmful. *CMAJ* 2012;184(2):163-4
www.cmaj.ca/content/184/2/163

Prices gone wild: grey market "scalpers" scoring windfall in American drug market

Imagine a world where prices have gone completely haywire, spiking more than, say, 600%. A cup of coffee for $13? Gas at $7 a litre? Such was the plight of many hospitals and other health care providers in the United States as they grappled with extraordinary markups for vital drugs they couldn't get any other way. *CMAJ* 2012;184(2):E119-20
www.cmaj.ca/content/184/2/E119

Pfizer advertised smoking cessation drug despite health warnings

Pharmaceutical giant Pfizer Canada was using a national advertising campaign to persuade Canadians who wanted to quit smoking to use its smoking cessation drug varenicline (Champix), despite a study linking it to serious cardiovascular events. *CMAJ* 2012;184(2):E127-8
www.cmaj.ca/content/184/2/E127

Tracking opioid use vital to avoiding scourge

Vastly improved monitoring of addictive painkillers was needed to handle the scourge of inappropriate opioid prescribing, dispensing and use in Canada, experts said. *CMAJ* 2012;184(2):E129-30
www.cmaj.ca/content/184/2/E129

Online drug shortage registry "limited" in application

An online registry of current and impending drug shortages was launched as part of a bid to help physicians and pharmacists plan for pharmaceutical shortfalls. *CMAJ* 2012;184(3):E165-6
www.cmaj.ca/content/184/3/E165

Pharmaceutical intellectual property

Laws governing pharmaceutical intellectual property in Canada cost more than $100 million annually in litigation and kept consumer prices high. According to Grootendorst and colleagues, the problem stemmed from legal uncertainty created by the complex sets of regulations and rights over the period of market exclusivity. They proposed several options for reform, including offering fixed periods of market exclusivity for innovative drugs. *CMAJ* 2012;184(5):543-9
www.cmaj.ca/content/184/5/543

Bisphosphonate and ocular inflammation

People taking oral bisphosphonate for the first time may be at a higher risk of scleritis and uveitis. Using the British Columbia Linked Health Database, the authors studied more than 900 000 people, including 10 827 people who used bisphosphonates for the first time, between 2000 and 2007 to compare diagnoses of inflammatory eye diseases. Clinicians should inform their patients about the signs and symptoms of scleritis and uveitis so that they may seek help, said Etminan and colleagues. *CMAJ* 2012;184(8):E431-4
www.cmaj.ca/content/184/8/E431

Misuse in America

Roughly 63% of Americans fail to follow their clinician's instructions for taking prescription drugs, according to an analysis of 75 997 urine samples. Of the drug misusers, 60% tested positive for drugs that had not been prescribed by their physicians, putting them in danger of using lethal drug combinations, while in 40%, there was no evidence that they had taken the prescribed drug. *CMAJ* 2012;184(9):E481-4
www.cmaj.ca/content/184/9/E481

From outlier to trendsetter

India issued its first patent compulsory licensing order, for the kidney/liver cancer drug sorafenib, and started a deep ripple in the global pharmaceutical pond. *CMAJ* 2012;184(12):E635-6
www.cmaj.ca/content/184/12/E635

Generic savings

Generic prescription drugs saved US residents about US$1 trillion in the decade spanning 2003–2011, according to the Generic Pharmaceutical Association. Just in the last year of that period, 2011, generic drugs produced savings of US$192 billion, an increase of 22% over the prior year, stated the association's annual report. *CMAJ* 2012;184(12):E655-8
www.cmaj.ca/content/184/12/E655

Brand-name savings

Brand-name drug makers were offering coupons to customers in the United States in a bid to compete with generic versions of their products with expired patents. Pfizer Inc. offered copay coupons that allowed people with insurance low-cost access (as little as US$4 a month) to several of their products. Private insurers weren't happy about the coupons because they had to pay far more for brand-name drugs than for generic equivalents. *CMAJ* 2012;184(13):E691-2
www.cmaj.ca/content/184/13/E691

Should fluoroquinolones be avoided?

Moxifloxacin and levofloxacin were associated with almost twice the risk of admission to hospital for acute liver injury compared with clarithromycin. Juurlink and colleagues linked routine data from several databases to measure drug exposure in patients with liver injury and those without. If confirmed in other studies, these results suggest that both moxifloxacin and levofloxacin be considered for regulatory warnings, said the authors. *CMAJ* 2012;184(14):1565-70
www.cmaj.ca/content/184/14/1565

The relative risk of severe drug-induced liver injury is probably higher with moxifloxacin and levofloxacin compared with clarithromycin. However, because the absolute risk is very low, clinicians should choose the most efficacious antibiotic rather than try to avoid a very uncommon adverse reaction, said Hayashi and Chalasani.
CMAJ 2012;184(14):1555-6
www.cmaj.ca/content/184/14/1555

Feds must step up and restrict generic oxycodone, Ontario said

It would be a "complete abdication of responsibility" for the federal government to allow generic oxycodone onto the market, Ontario's health minister charged. *CMAJ* 2012;184(17):E893-4
www.cmaj.ca/content/184/17/E893

PREVENTIVE MEDICINE

Delivery of preventive care

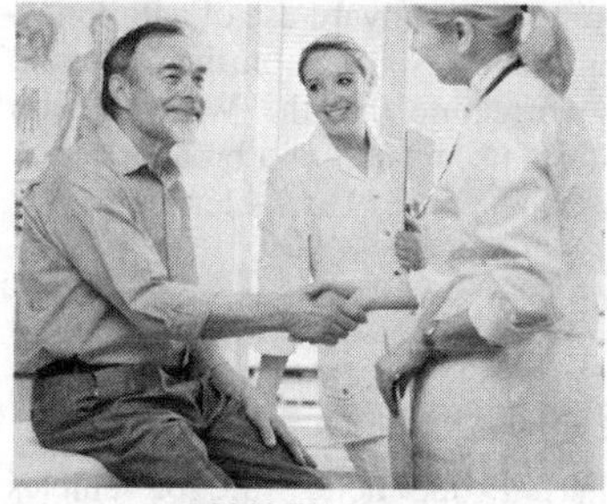
©2012 Thinkstock

Attempts to improve the delivery of preventive health care services will depend more on factors related to physician characteristics and practice structure than to how physicians are paid. A cross-sectional study of 137 primary care practices in 4 distinct funding models found little difference in the delivery of preventive care across the funding models. Practices with 1 or more female family physicians, a smaller patient load and an electronic reminder system provided superior preventive care. *CMAJ* 2012;184(2):E135-43
www.cmaj.ca/content/184/2/E135

PSYCHIATRY

Press that button again, please

Brain pacemakers had the potential to make obsolete the use of drugs and other therapies in the treatment of depression.
CMAJ 2012;184(5):E242-3
www.cmaj.ca/content/184/5/E242

Suicide among young people

Suicide rates were falling for boys but rising for girls, and suffocation was increasingly the method used. A descriptive study used data from Statistics Canada spanning the period from 1980 to 2008 showing different methods of suicide and trends over time. More research was needed to understand these trends and develop initiatives to prevent suicide. *CMAJ* 2012;184(9):1029-34
www.cmaj.ca/content/184/9/1029

Suicide rates among children and teens were higher in regions with social and economic deprivation, such as in some Aboriginal communities. Kirmayer commented that understanding the impact of social determinants on the identities, resilience and well-being of young people in these communities may hold the key to future reductions in suicide. *CMAJ* 2012;184(9):1015-6
www.cmaj.ca/content/184/9/1015

Diagnosing borderline personality disorder

Because individual symptoms of borderline personality disorder occur in other psychiatric disorders, patients with borderline personality disorder may receive treatment for other conditions for many years before a diagnosis is made. Aside from the ethical imperative of informing patients of their diagnosis, patients with borderline personality disorder benefit from an improved understanding of their condition, and this may help with avoiding improper treatments in the future, said Biskin and Paris. *CMAJ* 2012;184(16):1789-94
www.cmaj.ca/content/184/16/1789

Managing borderline personality disorder

Psychotherapy is the most important component in the treatment of borderline personality disorder, leading to large reductions in symptoms that persist over time, said Biskin and Paris. However, availability of these specialized psychotherapy techniques was limited. Pharmacotherapy may be beneficial as an adjunct to psychotherapy to reduce symptoms sufficiently for patients to stay in treatment.
CMAJ 2012;184(17):1897-902
www.cmaj.ca/content/184/17/1897

PUBLIC HEALTH

The redlining of harm reduction programs

Federal government opposition to Vancouver, British Columbia's safe injection site was but one indicator of a pattern of opposition to harm reduction programs, public health advocates charged.
CMAJ 2012;184(1):E21-2
www.cmaj.ca/content/184/1/E21

Crackdown on factory farm drug use urged

The federal government must crack down on the use of antibiotics such as cephalosporins and fluoroquinolones within the nation's meat industry because of the threat that antibiotic resistance poses to public health, said one of the government's leading veterinary drug safety officials.
CMAJ 2012;184(1):E23-4
www.cmaj.ca/content/184/1/E23

Europe clamped down on antibiotic misuse

In a bold plan to contain the deleterious effects of antimicrobial resistance, the European Commission called on all European Union countries to prohibit antibiotic use in animals and humans without veterinary or medical prescription. *CMAJ* 2012;184(1):E31-2
www.cmaj.ca/content/184/1/E31

The immunization stick

In a bid to increase immunization rates, the Australian government announced that it would commence withholding an annual A$726 tax benefit from parents whose children fail to receive primary vaccinations and subsequent booster shots. *CMAJ* 2012;184(1):E11-4
www.cmaj.ca/content/184/1/E11

Measles outbreak

Measles was on the rise in Europe as a consequence of declining vaccination rates, according to World Health Organization/Europe. *CMAJ* 2012;184(1):E11-4
www.cmaj.ca/content/184/1/E11

Prescribed but not taken

One in 10 Canadians did not take their prescription medications because of costs, said Law and colleagues. From their analysis of 5732 respondents to the Canadian Community Health Survey, the authors determined that insurance coverage was a major factor in explaining this finding. Reducing cost-related nonadherence would likely improve health, said the authors. *CMAJ* 2012;184(3):297-302
www.cmaj.ca/content/184/3/297

What coroners decide

When coroners have the freedom to decide, they are more likely to conduct an inquest into the death of a child than that of an elderly person and to investigate deaths following complications of medical care. They are least likely to investigate suicides. These findings came from an analysis of coroners' inquests in 5 Australian jurisdictions over 7.5 years. The processes of coroners' decisions are invisible but have an important influence on our understanding of death, said Walter and colleagues. *CMAJ* 2012;184(5):521-8
www.cmaj.ca/content/184/5/521

Provinces weighing HPV vaccination of boys

Provinces weighing the merits of offering human papillomavirus vaccine to boys and men aged 9–26 faced a tricky trade-off between benefits and costs. *CMAJ* 2012;184(5):E250-1
www.cmaj.ca/content/184/5/E250

Limiting WiFi in schools

The use of devices that emit non-ionizing electromagnetic radiation such as cellphones and WiFi networks in schools should be limited because they constitute a workplace hazard, according to the Ontario Catholic Teachers Association. *CMAJ* 2012;184(5):E254-5
www.cmaj.ca/content/184/5/E254

Helmets did not meet CSA requirements

Helmets were a no-brainer for skiers and snowboarders, but they did not meet the stringent requirements set by the Canadian Standards Association. *CMAJ* 2012;184(6):627
www.cmaj.ca/content/184/6/627

Flu vaccination good for pregnancy outcomes

Vaccinating pregnant women during the flu season reduced the number of babies who were small for gestational age. This finding came from a secondary analysis of a subgroup of women in a randomized controlled trial of seasonal flu vaccination in 340 pregnant women in Bangladesh. These data need confirmation, but they suggest that preventing influenza infection can influence intrauterine growth, said Steinhoff and colleagues. *CMAJ* 2012;184(6):645-53
www.cmaj.ca/content/184/6/645

End of modern medicine

Antimicrobial resistance was becoming so prevalent as a result of antibiotic overuse and, in the case of food production, "gross misuse," that the world may soon face "the end of modern medicine, as we know it," said the head of the World Health Organization.
CMAJ 2012;184(7):E354-6
www.cmaj.ca/content/184/7/E354

Waging war against rotavirus

Rotavirus was the most common cause of severe diarrhea in infants and young children worldwide. Canada supported the Global Alliance for Vaccines and Immunisation (GAVI) in its rollout of the rotavirus vaccination campaign for the world's poorest countries, but many Canadian provinces did not publicly fund this vaccine for Canadians. Policy-makers should ensure that all Canadian infants are offered this vaccination, said MacDonald and colleagues. *CMAJ* 2012;184(9):1011
www.cmaj.ca/content/184/9/1011

Better late than never

More than 7 months after the United States made the move, federal Health Minister Leona Aglukkaq indicated that the Canadian government planned to place methylenedioxypyrovalerone (MDPV), a key component of the street drug known as "bath salts," on schedule I of the Controlled Drugs and Substances Act. *CMAJ* 2012;184(10):E535-8
www.cmaj.ca/content/184/10/E535

Vaccinating children against anthrax

Should children be experimentally vaccinated against a threat that might never come? Or should a country hold off until an attack, in the meantime leaving children unprotected against life-threatening bacteria for which adults have a vaccine? *CMAJ* 2012;184(11):E577-8
www.cmaj.ca/content/184/11/E577

Farmyard drug use a US battlefield and a Canadian wasteland

The contrast was alarming. In the United States, judicial decisions and regulatory announcements were becoming daily fodder for news mills as the evidence mounted against subtherapeutic farmyard use of antibiotics. The consequences of growing antimicrobial resistance on the treatment of human diseases had become so worrisome that the World Health Organization urged a crackdown on farm use as part of a broader action plan to contain resistance. The Canadian response? Utter silence.
CMAJ 2012;184(11):E565
www.cmaj.ca/content/184/11/E565

Cycling safety

Mandatory helmets for adult cyclists, a "one-metre" rule for vehicles when passing cyclists, the removal of taxes from bicycle helmets to promote usage, and a community-based "complete streets" approach toward cycling were among measures recommended by a coroner's review of 129 deaths that occurred on Ontario's roads between 2006 and 2011. *CMAJ* 2012;184(11):E597-601
www.cmaj.ca/content/184/11/E597

Pathogen road map

A public database of the gene sequences of more than 100 000 food pathogens, such as *Salmonella*, *Campylobacter*, *E. coli* and *Listeria*, was to be established over the next 5 years by the United States Food and Drug Administration, the University of California/Davis and Agilent Technologies Inc. as part of a bid to improve scientific understanding of the organisms and develop new diagnostic tests to rapidly identify them.
CMAJ 2012;184(12):E655-8
www.cmaj.ca/content/184/12/E655

Plain victory

The World Health Organization (WHO) extended a hearty "Good on ya, mate!" to Australia for its victory against tobacco marketing. The country's high court dismissed a legal challenge from the tobacco industry to shoot down legislature requiring all tobacco products to be sold in plain packaging without branding. "With Australia's victory, public health enters a brave new world of tobacco control," WHO Director-General Dr. Margaret Chan said in a statement. "Plain packaging is a highly effective way to counter industry's ruthless marketing tactics." *CMAJ* 2012;184(13):E691-2
www.cmaj.ca/content/184/13/E691

Influenza vaccination coverage

All ethnic groups in Canada, with the exception of black Canadians, had higher uptake of influenza vaccination than white Canadians. These findings were based on 437 488 people's responses in several cycles of the Canadian Community Health Survey. Public health practitioners need to understand barriers affecting their communities to ensure optimal vaccine coverage, said the authors. *CMAJ* 2012;184(15):1673-81
www.cmaj.ca/content/184/15/1673

Although studies have consistently shown ethnic and racial disparities in vaccination coverage, the groups at risk will vary depending on the social and epidemiologic contexts at a particular time and place. Rather than focus on race and ethnicity, public health interventions to improve coverage should recognize the importance of such contexts to define appropriate risk groups, identify evidence-based interventions and measure effectiveness over time, said Gessner.
CMAJ 2012;184(15):1661-2
www.cmaj.ca/content/184/15/1661

"Bath salts"

The use of "bath salts," or synthetic cathinones, was increasing in Canada and elsewhere. Toxicity and dependence can occur with use. If a patient shows signs of a sympathomimetic toxidrome with negative urine toxicology results, cathinones toxicity should be considered.
CMAJ 2012;184(15):1713
www.cmaj.ca/content/184/15/1713

Bike helmets may save lives

Cyclists in a collision or accident who did not wear a helmet had 3.1 times the odds of dying compared with those who did wear a helmet. A case–control study included 129 fatalities and gathered information provided in coroners', police and accident reconstruction reports. The authors suggested that policies and campaigns that promote helmet use may decrease cycling mortality. *CMAJ* 2012;184(17):E921-3
www.cmaj.ca/content/184/17/E921

RADIOLOGY

Contrast-enhanced ultrasonography

Using microbubbles that do not infiltrate interstitial spaces makes the technique ideal for assessing vascular flow in renal, hepatic and other abdominal masses. *CMAJ* 2012;184(14):1599
www.cmaj.ca/content/184/14/1599

RESEARCH

CIHR/*CMAJ*: top achievements

CIHR and *CMAJ* celebrated top achievements in health research in Canada. *CMAJ* 2012;184(2):189-91
www.cmaj.ca/content/184/2/189

Ethical guidelines for research with humans

Canada and the United States had recently strengthened their guidelines and regulations for human research, but how they would be applied remained an issue. Canada's updated Tri-Council Policy Statement covered more current ethical issues than the US Advance Notice of Proposed Rulemaking, but both still applied to government-funded research only. According to Millum, the institution-based model of ethics review may lead to potential conflicts of interest in research ethics committees as well as underreview and overreview. Solutions put forward in these documents would require greater efforts for implementation by institutions and governments. *CMAJ* 2012;184(6):657-61
www.cmaj.ca/content/184/6/657

CIHR doubled support for clinical research

The Canadian government was to invest $150 million in a collaborative research program with drug companies. *CMAJ* 2012;184(7):E343-4
www.cmaj.ca/content/184/7/E343

Risk ratios in cohort studies and RCTs

Although odds ratios are often interpreted as risk ratios in cohort studies and clinical trials, odds ratios always overestimate the risk ratio. Knol and colleagues recommended that adjusted risk ratios should be presented in these types of studies and suggested several tools to estimate the correct risk ratio and confidence interval. *CMAJ* 2012;184(8):895-9
www.cmaj.ca/content/184/8/895

Missing-indicator method for analysis

Although the missing-indicator method is a popular and simple way to handle missing data in clinical research, it has been criticized for introducing bias. According to Groenwold and colleagues, in nonrandomized studies, the factor or test under study is often related to variables with missing values, in which case the missing-indicator method typically results in biased estimates. However, in randomized trials, the distribution of baseline covariates with missing values is likely balanced across treatment groups. This means the missing-indicator method will give unbiased estimates.
CMAJ 2012;184(11):1265-9
www.cmaj.ca/content/184/11/1265

Playing in the big leagues

Clinical medicine was among 6 research fields in which Canada punched above its international weight, according to the Council of Canadian Academies. *CMAJ* 2012;184(16):E833-4
www.cmaj.ca/content/184/16/E833

Boost RCTs in Canada

Randomized controlled trials (RCTs) in Canada received a disproportionately low level of funding compared with other forms of

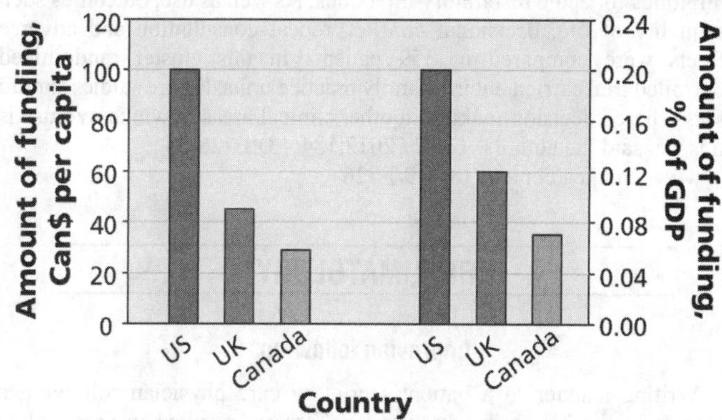

Federal funding for health research in 2010/11, by country.
GDP = gross domestic product, UK = United Kingdom, US = United States.

YEAR IN REVIEW / CMHF

research. According to Yusuf and Cairns, RCTs are important to the health of Canadians and the health care system. They argued that the Canadian Institutes of Health Research should increase funding for RCTs from 3.3% to 10% within 5 years. There also needed to be an appropriate infrastructure, an increase in partnerships, and strategies to overcome regulatory and institutional barriers to performing RCTs. *CMAJ* 2012;184(18):1997-2002
www.cmaj.ca/content/184/18/1997

RESPIROLOGY

Future concepts in pulmonary embolism

Can patients with acute pulmonary embolism receive treatment at home? When is it safe to stop anticoagulation? Geersing and colleagues showed how prognostic models could be used to answer these and other questions. *CMAJ* 2012;184(3):305-10
www.cmaj.ca/content/184/3/305

Statins may prevent pneumonia

Statin therapy modestly reduced the incidence of pneumonia among men over 50 years and women over 60 years of age. This finding came from a secondary analysis of 17 802 participants in the JUPITER trial of the effect of a statin on cardiovascular outcomes. This trial supported findings from observational studies, said Novack and colleagues. *CMAJ* 2012;184(7):E367-72
www.cmaj.ca/content/184/7/E367

Diffuse panbronchiolitis

Seen primarily in Asian populations, patients with diffuse panbronchiolitis may present with productive cough, shortness of breath and a history of sinusitis. Early recognition of this chronic sinobronchial inflammatory condition is important, as treatment with long-term and low-dose erythromycin improves prognosis. *CMAJ* 2012;184(10):1171
www.cmaj.ca/content/184/10/1171

Alpha-1 antitrypsin deficiency

About 5% of people with chronic obstructive pulmonary disease were thought to have alpha-1 antitrypsin deficiency, yet only 4%–5% of those had been identified. Why is it important to identify this deficiency? Brode and colleagues said that newer therapies may prevent further lung destruction and stabilize the disease. These patients are also at risk of liver disease and require monitoring. *CMAJ* 2012;184(12):1365-71
www.cmaj.ca/content/184/12/1365

Shared decisions reduced prescribing

A shared decision-making tool led to fewer patients deciding to use antibiotics for acute respiratory infections. As well as use, outcomes such as quality of life, decisional conflict, repeat consultation and adverse effects were compared in 359 patients in this cluster randomized controlled trial carried out in 9 family practice units. Future studies should assess shared decision-making in other clinical areas in which overuse is an issue, said the authors. *CMAJ* 2012;184(13):E726-34
www.cmaj.ca/content/184/13/E726

RHEUMATOLOGY

Improving follow-up

Writing a letter to a patient's primary care physician following a fracture of the hip, spine, humerus or forearm resulted in an absolute increase of 14.9% in people receiving testing and treatment for osteoporosis. More than 4000 patients were identified and followed up using routine data systems in this randomized controlled trial. This notification system is relatively simple to implement, said Leslie and colleagues. *CMAJ* 2012;184(3):290-6
www.cmaj.ca/content/184/3/290

Secondary prevention of osteoporosis among older patients who present with a fragility fracture should be associated with very high quality of care, but few patients receive bone mineral density testing or osteoporosis medications in the 6–12 months postfracture. Although the interventions reported by Leslie and colleagues show only modest improvements over usual care, they are worth pursuing. *CMAJ* 2012;184(3):279-80
www.cmaj.ca/content/184/3/279

Edema and elevated CA 125

A 56-year-old woman had an 18-month history of generalized edema with ascites. An elevated CA 125 level and an ovarian mass were suggestive of ovarian cancer, but the final diagnosis was something quite different. *CMAJ* 2012;184(6):671-3
www.cmaj.ca/content/184/6/671

SEXUAL MEDICINE

Age, sex, location ... sperm count?

A burgeoning online network of willing sperm donors and would-be mothers were bypassing licensed sperm banks.
CMAJ 2012;184(7):E347-8
www.cmaj.ca/content/184/7/E347

SURGERY

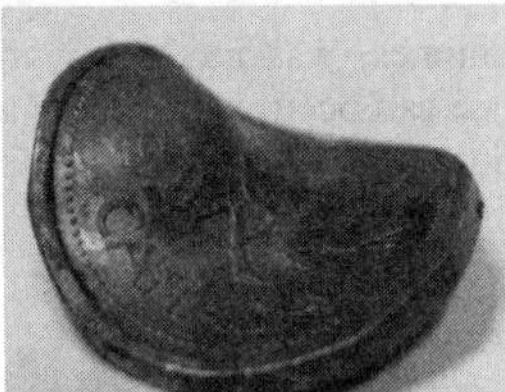

The lucky penny: the bullet rule

Identification of the trajectory of bullets in patients who sustain gunshot wounds is critical for determining the need for surgery and prognosis. The bullet rule can be helpful in ensuring that all bullets are accounted for, said Engels and Tien.
CMAJ 2012;184(1):63-5
www.cmaj.ca/content/184/1/63

The case for greening operating rooms

Canada's health care sector generated about 1.5% of our national greenhouse gas emissions and was a source of about 1% of solid waste. The operating room was one of the worst offenders. Kagoma and colleagues presented strategies and technologies to make operating rooms more ecologically sound without compromising patient care. These ranged from proper sorting of hazardous and nonhazardous materials, to innovative closed collection systems for fluid waste.
CMAJ 2012;184(17):1905-11
www.cmaj.ca/content/184/17/1905

TECHNOLOGY

All a twitter

The use of Twitter, Facebook and other social networking sites result in "negative" behavioural changes for over half of users, according to the registered British charity Anxiety UK. The charity said a set of studies, including a poll of 298 people, "revealed factors such as negatively comparing themselves to others, spending too much time in front of a computer, having trouble being able to disconnect and relax, as well as becoming confrontational online, thus causing problems in their relationships or job." *CMAJ* 2012;184(12):E655-8
www.cmaj.ca/content/184/12/E655

TRANSPLANTATION

Plan proposed to make organ donation less "ad hoc" in Canada

It appeared that a national agency or mechanism for allocating donated organs for transplantation wasn't in the cards. But after 4 years of wrangling with provincial governments and transplant programs, Canadian Blood Services proposed a strategic plan for an "integrated inter-provincial organ donation and transplantation system" to help reduce current inequities in access to organs and vastly improve Canada's current "mediocre" performance with respect to organ transplantation rates. *CMAJ* 2012;184(11):E575-6

www.cmaj.ca/content/184/11/E575

Organ donation's "silver bullet"?

Testing presumed consent for organ donation in a province or region where residents support the notion could help resolve the debate over whether a national "opt-out" system would improve Canada's chronic organ shortage, an expert said. *CMAJ* 2012;184(16):E835-6

www.cmaj.ca/content/184/16/E835

British docs urged elective ventilation

Some might call it harvesting organs. But the British Medical Association said the demand and need for transplantable organs was so acute that the time had come for Britain to consider keeping nearly brain-dead patients alive solely for the purpose of culling their hearts, livers and kidneys. *CMAJ* 2012;184(16):E837-8

www.cmaj.ca/content/184/16/E837

WOMEN'S HEALTH

Gender gap

Women in many parts of the world were less satisfied than men with their health. They also reported more instances of physical pain, health problems, worry and sadness, according to a Gallup survey. The largest gender gaps in satisfaction with health were reported in Pakistan (women: 63%; men: 83%), Belarus (women: 52%; men: 72%) and Ukraine (women: 44%; men: 63%). *CMAJ* 2012;184(12):E655-8

www.cmaj.ca/content/184/12/E655

CANADIAN MEDICAL HALL OF FAME

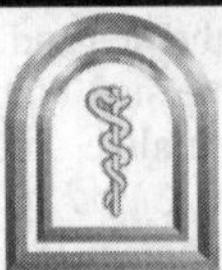

267 Dundas Street, London, ON N6A 1H2
Tel. (519) 488-2003 Fax (519) 488-2999
Email: cmhf@cdnmedhall.org
Website: http://www.cdnmedhall.org

Mission Statement

We create an enduring tribute to Canada's medical heroes who through discovery and innovation have contributed to improved health in Canada and around the world. Through the celebration of our laureates and the delivery of education programs, we inspire the pursuit of careers in health sciences fostering future innovators and leaders.

Vision Statement

A Canada that honours our medical heroes – those of the past, present and future

Nominations

The Canadian Medical Hall of Fame laureates must be Canadian citizens, or a major part of the achievement for which they are being nominated must have been developed during a period of residence in Canada. They are living or posthumous, whose outstanding contributions to medicine and the health sciences have led to extraordinary improvements in human health.

Their work may be a single meritorious contribution or a lifetime of superior accomplishments. Pioneers in their field, they are considered role models who inspire young Canadians to pursue careers in the health sciences.

Laureates may be recognized for their work in one or more of the following categories. Nominators are asked to indicate on the nomination form which of the categories most applies to their candidate.

The categories are:

1. Builder - Innovative leadership in health education and/or the creation of an institution or program that has endured to the benefit of human health services to humankind
2. Excellence in Health Care - Innovative leadership in health care exemplifying professionalism and services to humankind
3. Excellence in Health Research
   - Basic Research
   - Clinical Research
   - Health Services
   - Population and Public Health

Nomination and Selection Process

We accept nominations at any time. However, the deadline for each annual induction is the last Monday in June that precedes the induction ceremony.

Nominations remain active for three consecutive inductions and may be supplemented at any time during that period.

Nominations must be submitted according to the following guidelines:

- For nominations made by individuals, two individuals must serve as the nominators and they are required to submit a nomination letter. Each nominator may submit their own letter, or they may submit one letter that is co-signed
- For nominations made by an organization, one nomination letter signed on behalf of the organization is sufficient
- A nomination form must also be completed with particular attention given to the citation in which the contribution(s) justifying the nominee's induction into the Hall of Fame is clearly stated in a brief paragraph
- A curriculum vitae or biography is mandatory
- Supporting documents such as letters of support, news and journal articles are optional (max. 8 pages)

Visit http://www.cdnmedhall.org/process to submit your nomination electronically.

The selection process occurs in early September. All nominators will be notified of the outcome of their nomination after the successful candidates have been notified and before the public announcement in October.

Selection Committee 2013

Chair:
Dr. Alain Beaudet, President, Canadian Institutes of Health Research, Ottawa ON

Committee Members:
Professor Sir John Bell, President, Academy of Medical Sciences, London UK
Dr. Carol E. Cass, Associate Director (Research), Cross Cancer Institute, Edmonton AB
Dr. Colin McMillan, Parkdale Medical Centre, Charlottetown PE
Dr. David L. Sackett, Trout Research & Education Centre, Hamilton ON
Dr. Dominique Tessier, National Director, Medisys Health Group, Montréal QC
Dr. Aubrey J. Tingle, Associate Director, Maternal, Infant, Child and Youth Research Network, Richmond BC
Dr. Catharine Whiteside, Dean, Faculty of Medicine, University of Toronto, Toronto ON

Awards

Each inductee receives a gold Ivey Medallion engraved with his/her name and date of induction. A portrait of each inductee, created by renowned Canadian artist, Irma Coucil, is presented at the induction ceremony, and then hung in The Canadian Medical Hall of Fame. The induction ceremony took place on May 2, 2013 at the Cunard Centre in Halifax NS.

2013 INDUCTEES - CANADIAN MEDICAL HALL OF FAME

Dr. Antoine Hakim, OC

Category: Builder
Date of Birth: 1942
Education: PhD, Rensselaer Polytechnic Institute, 1971
MD, Albany Medical College, 1975

Major Contribution(s): Among the world's great neurologists, Dr. Hakim has changed the way neuroscience, especially strokes, have been understood and treated. Through his work at the University of Ottawa's Neuroscience Research Institute and his creation of the Canadian Stroke Network, Dr. Hakim has revolutionized the way strokes are being researched and treated in Canada and around the globe.

After obtaining his medical degree at the Albany Medical College in 1975, Dr. Hakim chose to focus his research on strokes, an unpopular area of study at the time. Completing his residency at the Montreal Neurological Institute and later becoming a professor at McGill University, he continued his stroke research using animal models that mimicked stroke conditions. He was amongst the first researchers ever to do so. Through his work and study at McGill, Dr. Hakim was better able to understand the process and damage caused by strokes which in turn led to a greater understanding of the types of treatments needed and their timing.

In 1992, Dr. Hakim moved to the nation's capital where he became chair of the University of Ottawa's Neurology Department and the director of the university's newly-established Neuroscience Research Institute. There he successfully recruited many talented young researchers and clinical investigators by offering an attractive balance of clinical application and research.

One of Dr. Hakim's crowning achievements is his leadership in the creation of the Canadian Stroke Network (CSN). Comprised of researchers, clinicians and healthcare workers in partnership with universities, governments and non-profit organizations, the CSN has been committed to the common goal of alleviating the burden of strokes on patients and their families, and providing the public with awareness on stroke prevention. As CEO and Scientific Director of the CSN, Dr. Hakim has been a pioneer in the fight against strokes, working with a team to champion the Canadian Stroke Strategy, a plan that most Canadian provinces have adopted. Dr. Hakim also helped develop the European Stroke Network in 2005.

In recognition of his hard work and dedication, Dr. Hakim has been honoured through various awards including the award for Excellence by the Canadian Stroke Consortium in 2000, the Ottawa Life Science Council Career Achievement Award in 2004, and was made an Officer of the Order of Canada in 2007.

ANTOINE HAKIM

Dr. David H. MacLennan, OC, OOnt

Category: Excellence in Health Research – Basic Research
Date of Birth: 1937
Education: PhD Purdue University

Major Contribution(s): Recognized nationally and internationally as one of Canada's foremost biomedical scientists, Dr. David MacLennan's studies provide a superb example of how basic research is developed to a point of clinical and veterinary application.

Born in Swan River, Manitoba in 1937 and raised on a farm, Dr. MacLennan obtained a BSA from the University of Manitoba in 1959, followed by MSc and PhD degrees in Biological Sciences from Purdue University. He was a postdoctoral fellow and then Assistant Professor in the Institute for Enzyme Research at the University of Wisconsin before returning to Canada in 1969 to become an Associate Professor in the Banting and Best Department of Medical Research at the University of Toronto. Subsequently, he was appointed as a University Professor, the University's highest academic rank, and was Chair of his Department for 12 years.

As a newly independent investigator in 1969, Dr MacLennan embarked on the isolation and characterization of a Ca^{2+} ATPase from a then obscure membrane system, the sarcoplasmic reticulum. His first paper describing this work in the Journal of Biological Chemistry was named a "classic JBC paper" on the 100th anniversary of that journal. In over 300 subsequent papers, he described the mechanism of action of the Ca^{2+} pump, the structure and function of many other muscle proteins involved in Ca^{2+} signalling in muscle, the genes encoding these proteins, and the genetic basis for muscle diseases caused by mutations in these genes.

Dr. MacLennan's studies of the genes encoding the Ca^{2+} release channels of both skeletal and cardiac muscle made it possible to identify patients who are susceptible to malignant hypothermia (MH) or to exercise-induced sudden cardiac death. MH Patients are at risk of fatal reactions to anaesthetics – if identified, they can be treated with safe anaesthetics. With millions of anaesthetics given each year, MH reactions are a worldwide health concern. An MH mutation in swine, also caused stress-induced death and lowered meat quality. By identifying the causal mutation and developing a diagnostic test for this disorder, Dr. MacLennan made it possible to eradicate the disease from herds, with substantial economic benefit to the swine industry.

Dr. MacLennan's research has been supported by the Canadian Institutes of Health Research, the Canadian Genetic Diseases Network of Centers of Excellence, the Heart and Stroke Foundation, the Muscular Dystrophy Association and the US National Institutes of Health. He is also recognized as an outstanding educator, overseeing the advanced research training of over 70 postdoctoral fellows, graduate students and visiting professors.

For his tireless efforts and dedication, Dr. MacLennan has received prestigious awards and honours such as the Gairdner Foundation International Award and election or appointment as a Fellow of both the Royal Society of Canada and the Royal Society of London UK, a Foreign Associate of the National Academy of Sciences USA, an Officer of the Order of Canada, and a Member of the Order of Ontario.

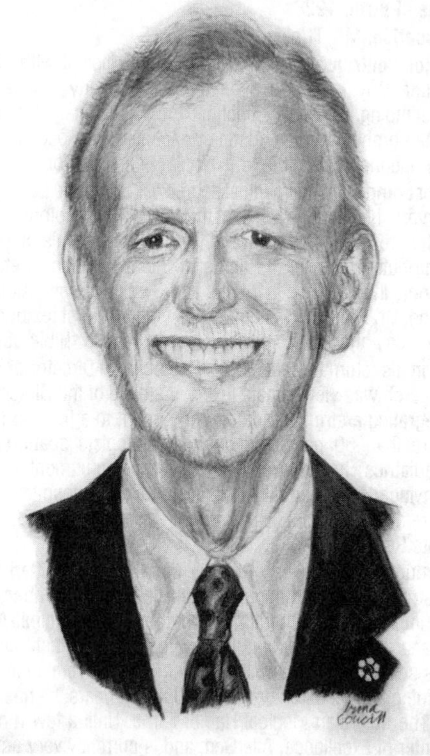

DAVID H. MACLENNAN

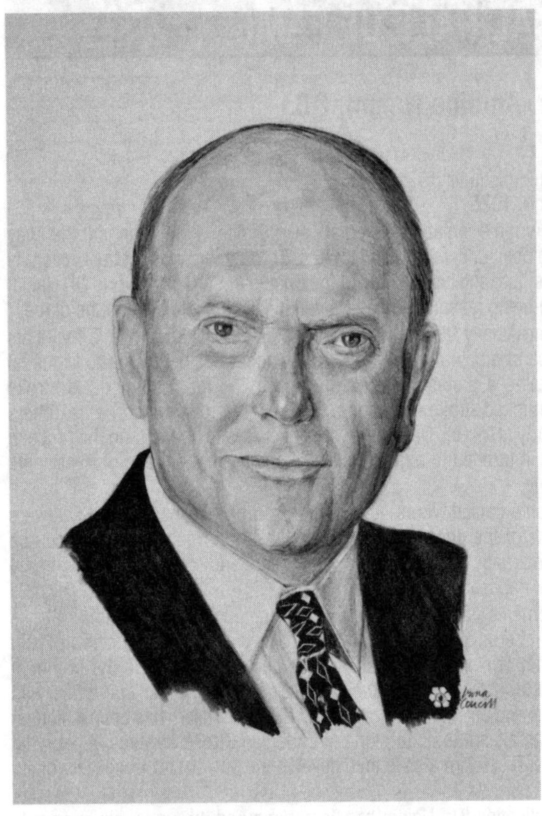

ARNOLD NAIMARK

Dr. Arnold Naimark, OC, OM

Category: Builder
Date of Birth: 1933
Education: MD, University of Manitoba, 1957
Major Contribution(s): A builder, a leader, a pioneer – these are some of the words used to describe the impact of Dr. Arnold Naimark. Dr. Naimark transformed the Faculty of Medicine at the University of Manitoba from a "clinically-focused prairie school" into one of Canada's major academic health sciences institutions. His leadership led to the development of a widely emulated model of integration of medical education and research with community needs.

Born and raised in Winnipeg, Dr. Naimark received his medical degree in 1957 from the University of Manitoba. He joined the faculty of medicine as an assistant professor in 1963 and in three short years he became the head of the medical department. By 1971, Dr. Naimark was serving as the faculty's dean.

In his role as dean, Dr. Naimark revolutionized the medical programs offered at the University of Manitoba. Some of his many accomplishments included the rejuvenation of the department of physiology and the department of social and preventive medicine (later the department of community health sciences). He championed the establishment of the department of family medicine and the growth of the department of medical microbiology and facilitated the creation of the Northern Medical Unit that provides healthcare to First Nations, Metis and Inuit people, which has become a model of excellence for health care delivery in northern and remote communities. Dr. Naimark played a seminal role in the establishment of the Manitoba Institute of Cell Biology, the St. Boniface Hospital Research Centre and the launch of the Manitoba Health Research Council. Through his innovative leadership as chair or president of several major national and international organizations concerned with medical education and research, Dr. Naimark introduced reforms that enhanced their effectiveness, influence and scope.

In 1981, Dr. Naimark was appointed ninth president and vice-chancellor of the University of Manitoba. As president, he set his sights on wider university issues but also continued working on the advancement of medicine and the health sciences generally. Latterly, he was the founding chair of the Canadian Health Services Research Foundation and of the Canadian Biotechnology Advisory Council and currently serves as chair of Genome Prairie and of CancerCare Manitoba. As one of the country's foremost educational administrators and champions of health research, he has been sought after for advice by prominent medical and educational institutions around the world and by federal and provincial agencies in Canada.

In recognition of his leadership and outstanding achievements, Dr. Naimark has been honoured with a series of awards. He was made a Fellow of the Royal Society of Canada in 1987 and an Officer of the Order of Canada in 1991. He was also awarded the Order of Manitoba in 2003 and was inducted into the Winnipeg's Citizen's Hall of Fame.

Dr. Claude Roy, OC

Categories: Excellence in Healthcare
Date of Birth: 1928
Education: MD, l'Université Laval, 1954
Major Contribution(s): Pairing scientific insight with compassion for his young patients, Dr. Claude Roy is regarded as one of the early pioneers in paediatric gastroenterology. An outstanding clinician, teacher and researcher, Dr. Roy has greatly contributed to the metamorphosis of Ste-Justine Hospital into the paediatric university hospital it is today with an international reputation for exemplary care and for superb training and research programs.

After completing his medical degree at l'Université Laval and his paediatric training at McGill and Harvard, he spent six years at the University of Colorado where he began an academic career in which research was always at the core of his academic activities. His major research contributions are in the areas of infant nutrition, metabolism of bile acids and fatty acids, chronic liver disease in infants and Cystic Fibrosis. Along with his Denver colleague and close friend, Dr. Arnie Silverman, he published the first textbook of the nascent subspecialty which is still today after its 4th edition regarded as the "Bible of the Subspecialty."

Upon his return to Canada, Dr. Roy became Director of Research at Ste-Justine at a time when research was viewed as a luxury. As head of the GI service, he emphasised the importance of integrating a strong research component to a training program which, over the years, trained more than 60 paediatric gastroenterologists scattered over three continents. As Chair of paediatrics, he led the charge for the recruitment of a number of clinician scientists and convinced the authorities that the future of the hospital would be played out in the research area. He remains very much involved with his institution and, until recently, he was Associate Director of its Research Centre.

Throughout his career, Dr. Roy has been committed to promoting recognition of paediatric gastroenterology through his activities with a number of professional organizations. He was Council member, Director of programs and principal Advisor to the President at the Medical Research Council of Canada, now the Canadian Institutes of Health Research. Over the years he has served as chair and board member of several disease-related foundations to support their training and research programs. Over the years, he has been a strong supporter of the mission of The Canadian Medical Hall of Fame. Until a few months ago, he was on the Board of the Center of Excellence, AllerGen, and is currently very active in the Canadian Nutrition Society.

Because of his dedication, hard work and contributions to science and medicine, Dr. Roy has been honoured with many national and international awards. He received an Honorary doctorate from the Université de Genève in 2003, and was made an Officer of the Order of Canada in 1990.

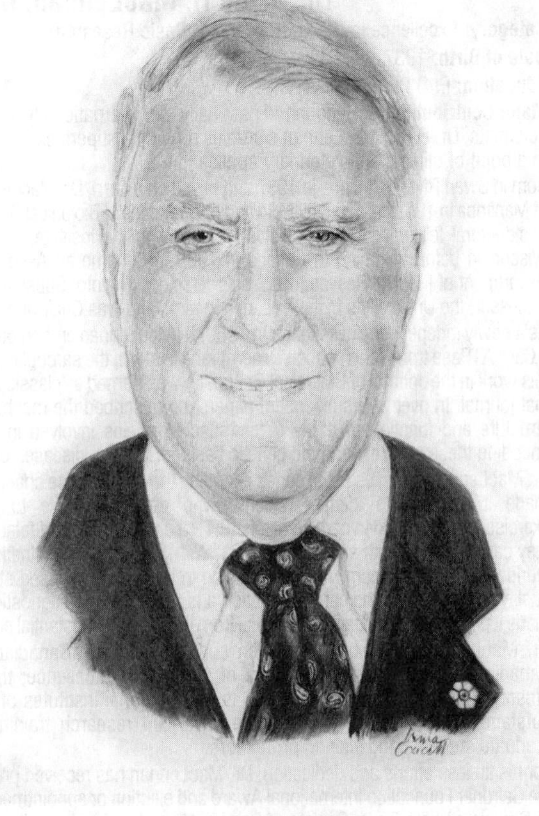

CLAUDE ROY

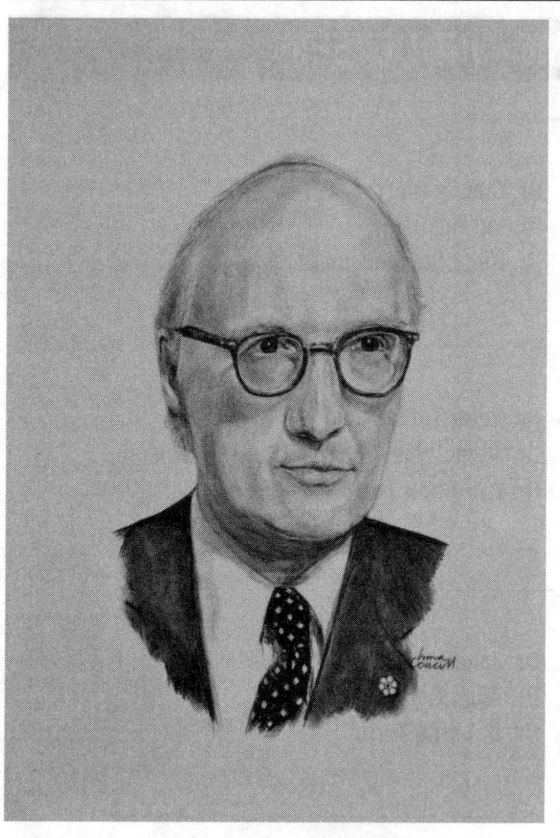

IAN RUSTED

Dr. Ian Rusted, OC

Category: Builder
Dates: 1921 – 2007
Education: MD, Dalhousie University, 1948

Major Contribution(s): Courage, dedication and perseverance. These are the qualities it took for Dr. Ian Rusted to fulfil his dream of establishing a medical school at Memorial University of Newfoundland. Prior to this, there was no medical school in the province of Newfoundland and Labrador and many questioned the feasibility of one in a poorer, underserved province. Undeterred by the naysayers, Dr. Rusted continued to pursue his vision and eventually founded Memorial's Faculty of Medicine, today a global leader in medical education.

Born in Upper Island Cove, Newfoundland in 1921, Dr. Rusted graduated from Memorial University College with a pre-medical diploma in 1940. From there he ventured to Trinity College, University of Toronto to complete his BA and following this, to Dalhousie University to earn his medical degree in 1948. Dr. Rusted continued his education at McGill University and at the Mayo Clinic in Minnesota. Although both institutions offered him positions, he chose to return to his home province.

Once back in Newfoundland, Dr. Rusted specialized in internal medicine and worked as a medical consultant for the provincial department of health. During this time he visited many cottage hospitals and worked with rural doctors. It was during this period that he began to see the need for a medical school in Newfoundland. After convincing the provincial and federal governments of his idea, he was appointed in 1966 director of post-graduate medical education and coordinator of planning for the proposed new medical school. In 1967, his vision materialized and he was appointed first dean and professor of medicine of the medical school at Memorial University of Newfoundland. He served as dean until 1979 and was then appointed vice-president (health sciences), a position he held until his retirement in 1988.

Today Memorial's Faculty of Medicine has over 2,000 medical graduates who have carried with them the legacy of Dr. Rusted. Through his belief in strong clinical skills and dedication to community-based learning, Dr. Rusted laid the foundation for superb medical education, training doctors working in both rural and urban areas around the world.

Dr. Rusted has been recognized with a series of awards and distinctions including three honorary degrees, the St. John's Citizen of the Year Award in 1979, Officer of the Order of Canada in 1985, an Honorary Life Membership Award from the Newfoundland Medical Association in 1989, and Master of the American College of Physicians in 1992.

Dr. Bette Stephenson, OC, OOnt

Categories: Builder
Date of Birth: 1921
Education: MD, University of Toronto, 1945

Major Contribution(s): A pioneer and role model for women, Dr. Bette Stephenson has had an outstanding career in the field of Canadian medicine, academics and politics. Dr. Stephenson is most notably recognized by her series of "firsts" as a woman in positions and offices traditionally held by men. She has successfully contributed to putting the practice of family medicine on the international medical map and, in turn, inspired countless women to pursue careers in medicine.

Born in Aurora, Ontario in 1921, Dr. Stephenson grew up with a deep admiration for the practice of medicine. Earning a medical degree from the University of Toronto in 1945, she was only one of ten girls to graduate out of a class of 142. After graduation, she and her husband opened a busy general practice that lasted for more than 40 years. Spurred on by the lack of medical professionals entering the field of family medicine, Dr. Stephenson helped create the College of Family Physicians in Canada which promoted the importance of family doctors. She became a member of the medical staff at the Women's College Hospital and later became the Outpatient Department and Chief of the Department of General Practice.

With a keen interest in political affairs, Dr. Stephenson became the first woman to serve on the Board of Directors of the Canadian Medical Association and the Ontario Medical Association. Subsequently, she became the first female president of both associations. In 1975 she was elected to the Legislative Assembly of Ontario and was the first female to hold various distinguished offices, such as the Minister of Education, Minister of Colleges and Universities, Minister of Finance/Treasurer, and to serve as Deputy Premier.

In addition to her medical and political careers, Dr. Stephenson helped promote medical research in Canada including the development of the Ontario Research Development Challenge Fund and the MaRS Discovery District. She is a founding member of the Canadian Institute of Advanced Research and a trustee of the Ontario Innovation Trust.

Dr. Stephenson has been honoured for her dedication to medicine in Canada through various awards. Among them she was appointed an Officer of the Order of Canada in 1992, awarded the Order of Ontario in 1999, and in 2009, an award was established in her name to honour her pivotal role and lifelong commitment to Ontario's publicly funded education system (The Dr. Bette M. Stephenson Recognition of Achievement).

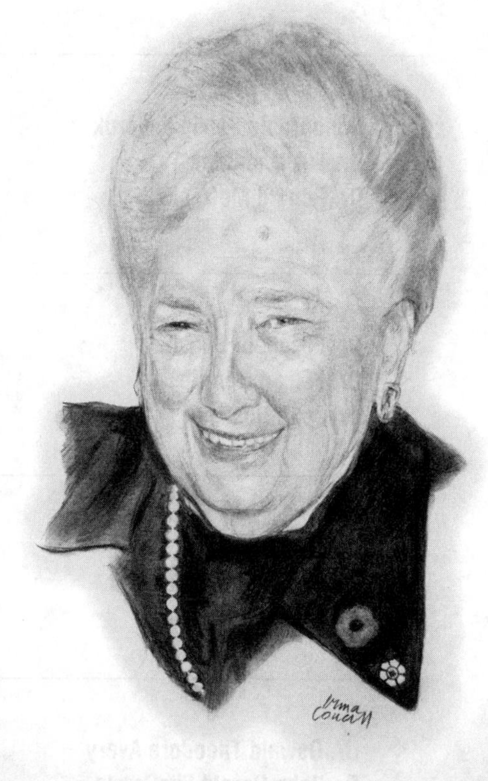

BETTE STEPHENSON

CANADIAN MEDICAL HALL OF FAME - INDUCTEES

2013

- Dr. Antoine Hakim
- Dr. David H. MacLennan
- Dr. Arnold Naimark
- Dr. Claude Roy
- Dr. Ian Rusted
- Dr. Bette Stephenson

2012

- Dr. John Dirks
- Terry Fox
- Dr. Armand Frappier
- Dr. F. Clarke Fraser
- Dr. Peter T. Macklem
- Dr. John James Rickard (J.J.R.) Macleod
- Dr. Lap-Chee Tsui

2011

- Dr. Albert Aguayo
- Dr. John Bienenstock
- Dr. Paul David
- Dr. Jonathan Campbell Meakins
- Dr. Allan Ronald
- Dr. D. Lorne Tyrrell

2010

- Dr. Alan Burton
- Dr. William Cochrane
- Dr. Phil Gold
- Dr. James Hogg
- Dr. Vera Peters
- Dr. Calvin Stiller

2009

- Honourable Sylvia Fedoruk
- Dr. Tak Wah Mak
- Dr. Ronald Melzack
- Dr. Charles H. Tator
- Dr. Mladen Vranic

2007

- Dr. Elizabeth Bagshaw
- Dr. Félix d'Hérelle
- Dr. Jean Dussault
- Senator Dr. Wilbert Keon
- Dr. Endel Tulving

2006

- Dr. David Hubel
- Dr. John S. McEachern
- Dr. Ian McWhinney
- Dr. Anthony Pawson
- Dr. Hans Selye

2004

- Dr. Oswald Theodore Avery
- Dr. John Gerald FitzGerald
- Honorable Marc Lalonde
- Dr. Maurice LeClair
- Dr. Ernest McCulloch
- Dr. James Edgar Till

2003

- Saint Marguerite d'Youville
- Dr. William Howard Feindel
- Dr. Donald O. Hebb
- Dr. Charles H. Hollenberg
- Dr. Charles B. Huggins
- Dr. J. Fraser Mustard

2001

- Dr. John E. Bradley
- Dr. Henry Friesen
- Dr. William E. Gallie
- Honorable Peter Lougheed
- Dr. Frederick Montizambert
- Dr. Charles Scriver
- Dr. Lucille Teasdale-Corti

2000

- Dr. Bernard Belleau
- Dr. G. Malcolm Brown
- Dr. John Evans
- Dr. Jack Hirsh
- Dr. Leonora King
- Dr. David Sackett

1998

- Dr. Murray Barr
- Dr. Norman Bethune
- Dr. Roberta Bondar
- Honorable Thomas C. Douglas
- Dr. Ray Farquharson
- Dr. C. Miller Fisher
- Dr. Claude Fortier
- Dr. Gustave Gingras
- Dr. Harold Johns
- Dr. Heinz Lehmann
- Dr. Maud Menten

1997

- Dr. Charles Thomas Beer
- Dr. Wilfred Gordon Bigelow
- Dr. Henri J. Breault
- Dr. Wilfred Thomason Grenfell
- Dr. Pierre Masson
- Dr. Brenda Milner
- Dr. Robert Laing Noble
- Dr. Louis Siminovitch

1995

- Dr. Henry J.M. Barnett
- Dr. Bruce Chown
- Dr. Herbert Jasper
- Dr. Charles P. Leblond
- Dr. William Thornton Mustard
- Dr. Robert Bruce Salter
- Dr. Michael Smith

1994

- Dr. Maude Elizabeth Seymour Abbott
- Dr. Frederick Grant Banting
- Dr. Charles Herbert Best
- Dr. John Symonds Lyon Browne
- Dr. James Bertram Collip
- Dr. Douglas Harold Copp
- Dr. Charles George Drake
- Dr. Jacques Genest
- Sir William Osler
- Dr. Wilder Graves Penfield